Clinical Anesthesia

Clinical Anesthesia

EIGHTH EDITION

EDITED BY

Paul G. Barash, MD
Emeritus Professor and Past Chair
Department of Anesthesiology
Yale University School of Medicine
Honorary Attending Anesthesiologist
Yale-New Haven Hospital
New Haven, Connecticut

Bruce F. Cullen, MD
Emeritus Professor
Department of Anesthesiology and Pain Medicine
University of Washington School of Medicine
Seattle, Washington

Robert K. Stoelting, MD
Emeritus Professor and Past Chair
Department of Anesthesia
School of Medicine
Indiana University
Indianapolis, Indiana

Michael K. Cahalan, MD
Professor and Chair
Department of Anesthesiology
School of Medicine
The University of Utah
Salt Lake City, Utah

M. Christine Stock, MD
Professor
Department of Anesthesiology
Feinberg School of Medicine
Northwestern University
Chicago, Illinois

Rafael Ortega, MD
Professor
Vice-Chairman of Academic Affairs
Department of Anesthesiology
Boston University School of Medicine
Boston, Massachusetts

Sam R. Sharar, MD
Professor
Vice-Chair for Faculty Affairs and Development
Department of Anesthesiology and Pain Medicine
University of Washington School of Medicine
Seattle, Washington

Natalie F. Holt, MD, MPH
Assistant Professor
Department of Anesthesiology
Yale University School of Medicine
Medical Director
Ambulatory Procedures Unit
VA Connecticut Healthcare System
West Haven, Connecticut

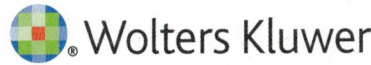

Philadelphia • Baltimore • New York • London
Buenos Aires • Hong Kong • Sydney • Tokyo

Acquisitions Editor: Keith Donnellan
Developmental Editor: Brendan Huffman
Production Project Manager: Priscilla Crater, Linda Van Pelt
Design Coordinator: Teresa Mallon
Senior Manufacturing Coordinator: Beth Welsh
Marketing Manager: Dan Dressler
Prepress Vendor: Aptara, Inc.

Eighth Edition

Copyright © 2017 Wolters Kluwer

Seventh Edition © 2013 by LIPPINCOTT WILLIAMS & WILKINS, a WOLTERS KLUWER business
Sixth Edition © 2009 by LIPPINCOTT WILLIAMS & WILKINS, a WOLTERS KLUWER business
Fifth Edition © 2005 by LIPPINCOTT WILLIAMS & WILKINS

All rights reserved. This book is protected by copyright. No part of this book may be reproduced or transmitted in any form or by any means, including as photocopies or scanned-in or other electronic copies, or utilized by any information storage and retrieval system without written permission from the copyright owner, except for brief quotations embodied in critical articles and reviews. Materials appearing in this book prepared by individuals as part of their official duties as U.S. government employees are not covered by the above-mentioned copyright. To request permission, please contact Wolters Kluwer at Two Commerce Square, 2001 Market Street, Philadelphia, PA 19103, via email at permissions@lww.com, or via our website at lww.com (products and services).

9 8 7 6 5 4 3 2 1

Library of Congress Cataloging-in-Publication Data

Names: Barash, Paul G., editor.
Title: Clinical anesthesia / edited by Paul G. Barash, Bruce F. Cullen,
   Robert K. Stoelting, Michael K. Cahalan, M. Christine Stock, Rafael
   Ortega, Sam R. Sharar, Natalie F. Holt.
Other titles: Clinical anesthesia (Barash)
Description: Eighth edition. | Philadelphia : Wolters Kluwer, [2017] |
   Includes bibliographical references and index.
Identifiers: LCCN 2016058322 | ISBN 9781496337009 (hardback)
Subjects: | MESH: Anesthesia | Anesthesiology | Anesthetics
Classification: LCC RD81 | NLM WO 200 | DDC 617.9/6–dc23
LC record available at https://lccn.loc.gov/2016058322

This work is provided "as is," and the publisher disclaims any and all warranties, express or implied, including any warranties as to accuracy, comprehensiveness, or currency of the content of this work.

This work is no substitute for individual patient assessment based upon healthcare professionals' examination of each patient and consideration of, among other things, age, weight, gender, current or prior medical conditions, medication history, laboratory data and other factors unique to the patient. The publisher does not provide medical advice or guidance and this work is merely a reference tool. Healthcare professionals, and not the publisher, are solely responsible for the use of this work including all medical judgments and for any resulting diagnosis and treatments.

Given continuous, rapid advances in medical science and health information, independent professional verification of medical diagnoses, indications, appropriate pharmaceutical selections and dosages, and treatment options should be made and healthcare professionals should consult a variety of sources. When prescribing medication, healthcare professionals are advised to consult the product information sheet (the manufacturer's package insert) accompanying each drug to verify, among other things, conditions of use, warnings and side effects and identify any changes in dosage schedule or contraindications, particularly if the medication to be administered is new, infrequently used or has a narrow therapeutic range. To the maximum extent permitted under applicable law, no responsibility is assumed by the publisher for any injury and/or damage to persons or property, as a matter of products liability, negligence law or otherwise, or from any reference to or use by any person of this work.

LWW.com

For All Students of Anesthesiology

Contributing Authors

Ramon Abola, MD
Assistant Professor
Department of Anesthesiology
Stony Brook Medicine
Stony Brook, New York

Ron O. Abrons, MD
Associate Professor
Department of Anesthesiology
The University of Iowa Hospitals and Clinics
Iowa City, Iowa

Shamsuddin Akhtar, MD
Associate Professor
Department of Anesthesiology and Pharmacology
Yale University School of Medicine
New Haven, Connecticut

Michael L. Ault, MD, FCCP, FCCM
Associate Professor of Anesthesiology, Medical Education, Neurological Surgery and Surgery
Chief and Fellowship Program Director, Section of Critical Care Medicine
Department of Anesthesiology
Northwestern University Feinberg School of Medicine
Chicago, Illinois

Douglas R. Bacon, MD, MA
Professor and Chair
Department of Anesthesiology
University of Mississippi Medical Center
Jackson, Mississippi

Gina C. Badescu, MD
Division of Cardiothoracic Anesthesiology
Maui Memorial Medical Center
Wailuku, Hawaii

Dalia Banks, MD, FASE
Clinical Professor
Division Chief of Cardiothoracic Anesthesiology
Director of Cardiothoracic Anesthesiology Fellowship
Clinical Director of Sulpizio CVC and PTU
University of California San Diego
San Diego, California

Paul G. Barash, MD
Professor Emeritus and Past Chair
Department of Anesthesiology
Yale University School of Medicine
Honorary Attending Anesthesiologist
Yale-New Haven Hospital
New Haven, Connecticut

John F. Bebawy, MD
Associate Professor of Anesthesiology & Neurological Surgery
Northwestern University
Feinberg School of Medicine
Chicago, Illinois

Itay Bentov, MD, PhD
Associate Professor
Anesthesiology and Pain Medicine
Adjunct Associate Professor
Department of Medicine
University of Washington School of Medicine
Harborview Medical Center
Seattle, Washington

Honorio T. Benzon, MD
Professor of Anesthesiology
Northwestern University Feinberg School of Medicine
Chicago, Illinois

Marcelle E. Blessing, MD
Assistant Professor of Anesthesiology
Yale University School of Medicine
New Haven, Connecticut

Michelle Y. Braunfeld, MD
Professor and Vice Chair
Department of Anesthesiology
David Geffen School of Medicine at UCLA
Chair, Department of Anesthesiology
Greater Los Angeles VA Hospital
Los Angeles, CA

Ferne R. Braveman, MD
Vice-Chair for Clinical Affairs
Director of Division of Obstetrical Anesthesiology
Professor of Anesthesiology and Obstetrics, Gynecology and Reproductive Medicine
Department of Anesthesiology
Yale School of Medicine
New Haven, Connecticut

Sorin J. Brull, MD, FCARCSI (Hon)
Professor of Anesthesiology
Department of Anesthesiology
Mayo Clinic College of Medicine
Mayo Clinic Florida
Jacksonville, Florida

Brenda A. Bucklin, MD
Professor of Anesthesiology
University of Colorado School of Medicine
Aurora, Colorado

Michael K. Cahalan, MD
Professor and Chair
Department of Anesthesiology
The University of Utah School of Medicine
Salt Lake City, Utah

Contributing Authors

Levon M. Capan, MD
Professor of Clinical Anesthesiology
New York University School of Medicine
Associate Director of Anesthesia Service
Bellevue Hospital Center
New York, New York

Louanne M. Carabini, MD
Assistant Professor
Department of Anesthesiology
Northwestern University Feinberg School of Medicine
Chicago, Illinois

Christopher G. Choukalas, MD, MS
Associate Clinical Professor
Department of Anesthesia and Perioperative Care
University of California, San Francisco
San Francisco VA Medical Center
San Francisco, California

Amalia Cochran, MD, MA
Associate Professor of Surgery
Vice-Chair of Education and Professionalism
University of Utah School of Medicine
Salt Lake City, Utah

Edmond Cohen, MD
Professor of Anesthesiology and Thoracic Surgery
Director of Thoracic Anesthesia
Icahn School of Medicine at Mount Sinai
New York, New York

Christopher M. Conley, MD
Clinical Assistant Professor of Anesthesiology
Boston University School of Medicine
Boston, Massachusetts

Christopher W. Connor, MD, PhD
Associate Professor of Anesthesiology and Biomedical Engineering
Department of Anesthesiology
Boston Medical Center
Boston, Massachusetts

C. Michael Crowder, MD, PhD
Allan J. Treuer Endowed Professor and Chair
Department of Anesthesiology and Pain Medicine
Adjunct Professor of Genome Sciences
University of Washington School of Medicine
Seattle, Washington

Marie Csete, MD, PhD
President and Chief Scientist
Huntington Medical Research Institutes
Pasadena, California
Professor of Anesthesiology
Keck USC School of Medicine
Los Angeles, California
Visiting Associate
Medical Engineering
California Institute of Technology
Pasadena, California

Bruce F. Cullen, MD
Emeritus Professor
Department of Anesthesiology and Pain Medicine
University of Washington School of Medicine
Seattle, Washington

Albert Dahan, MD, PhD
Department of Anesthesiology
Leiden University Medical Center
Leiden, The Netherlands

Rossemary De La Cruz, MD
Academic, Media, and Risk Management Associate
Department of Anesthesiology
Boston Medical Center
Boston, Massachusetts

Steven Deem, MD
Director, Neurocritical Care
Swedish Medical Center
Physicians Anesthesia Service
Clinical Professor of Anesthesiology
University of Washington
Seattle, Washington

Stephen F. Dierdorf, MD
Professor of Clinical Anesthesia
Department of Anesthesia and Perioperative Medicine
Medical University of South Carolina
Charleston, South Carolina

Karen B. Domino, MD, MPH
Professor and Vice-Chair for Clinical Research
Department of Anesthesiology and Pain Medicine
University of Washington School of Medicine
Seattle, Washington

Thomas J. Ebert, MD, PhD
Vice-Chair for Education
Professor of Anesthesiology
Medical College of Wisconsin and Zablocki VA Medical Center
Milwaukee, Wisconsin

Jan Ehrenwerth, MD
Professor Emeritus
Department of Anesthesiology
Yale University School of Medicine
New Haven, Connecticut

John H. Eichhorn, MD
Professor of Anesthesiology
College of Medicine
Provost's Distinguished Service Professor
Department of Anesthesiology
University of Kentucky Medical Center
Lexington, Kentucky

James B. Eisenkraft, MD
Professor
Department of Anesthesiology
Icahn School of Medicine at Mount Sinai
New York, New York

Alex S. Evers, MD
Henry S. Mallinckrodt Professor and Head
Department of Anesthesiology
Professor of Developmental Biology and Internal Medicine
Washington University School of Medicine
St. Louis, Missouri

Ana Fernandez-Bustamante, MD, PhD
Associate Professor
Department of Anesthesiology
University of Colorado School of Medicine
Aurora, Colorado

Lynne R. Ferrari, MD
Chief, Perioperative Anesthesia
Medical Director, Operating Rooms and Perioperative Programs
Department of Anesthesiology, Perioperative and Pain Medicine
Boston Children's Hospital
Boston, Massachusetts

Scott M. Fishman, MD
Professor, Department of Anesthesiology and Pain Medicine
Chief, Division of Pain Medicine
Vice-Chair, Department of Anesthesiology and Pain Medicine
Director, Center for Advancing Pain Relief
University of California Davis School of Medicine
Sacramento, California

Michael A. Fowler, MD, MBA
Assistant Professor
Residency Program Director
VCU Department of Anesthesiology
Richmond, Virginia

J. Sean Funston, MD
Professor
Department of Anesthesiology
The University of Texas Medical Branch
Galveston, Texas

Tong J. Gan, MD, MHS, FRCA
Professor and Chairman
Department of Anesthesiology
Stony Brook University
Stony Brook, New York

Steven I. Gayer, MD
Professor of Anesthesiology
University of Miami Health System
Miami, Florida

Sofia Geralemou, MD
Department of Anesthesiology
Stony Brook University Hospital
Stony Brook, New York

Loreta Grecu, MD
Clinical Associate Professor of Anesthesiology
Stony Brook University School of Medicine
Stony Brook, New York

Dhanesh K. Gupta, MD
Professor of Anesthesiology
Chief of Neuroanesthesiology
Department of Anesthesiology
Duke University Medical Center
Durham, North Carolina

Carin A. Hagberg, MD
Joseph C. Gabel Professor and Chair
Department of Anesthesiology
UTHealth Medical School
Houston, Texas

Matthew R. Hallman, MD
Assistant Professor
Department of Anesthesiology and Pain Medicine
University of Washington School of Medicine
Seattle, Washington

Kylene E. Halloran, MD
Assistant Professor of Anesthesiology
Dartmouth-Hitchcock Medical Center
Lebanon, New Hampshire

Stephen C. Haskins, MD
Assistant Anesthesiologist
Hospital for Special Surgery
Clinical Assistant Professor of Anesthesiology
Weill Cornell Medical College
New York, New York

J. Steven Hata, MD, MSc
Vice Chairman, Education Continuum
Center for Critical Care
Anesthesiology Institute
Cleveland Clinic
Cleveland, Ohio

Tara M. Hata, MD
Clinical Assistant Professor
Department of Pediatric Anesthesia
Cleveland Clinic
Cleveland, Ohio

Laurence M. Hausman, MD
Professor of Anesthesiology
Vice-Chair, Academic Affiliations
Director, Ambulatory Anesthesia
Department of Anesthesiology
Perioperative and Pain Medicine
Icahn School of Medicine at Mount Sinai
New York, New York

Salim M. Hayek, MD, PhD
Professor
Department of Anesthesiology
Case Western Reserve University
Chief, Division of Pain Medicine
University Hospitals Cleveland Medical Center
Cleveland, Ohio

Christopher L. Heine, MD
Assistant Professor
Department of Anesthesia and Perioperative Medicine
Medical University of South Carolina
Charleston, South Carolina

Thomas K. Henthorn, MD
Professor, Anesthesiology
Department of Anesthesiology
University of Colorado
Aurora, Colorado

Simon C. Hillier, MB, ChB
Professor
Departments of Anesthesiology and Pediatrics
Geisel School of Medicine
Dartmouth-Hitchcock Medical Center
Lebanon, New Hampshire

Natalie F. Holt, MD, MPH
Assistant Professor
Department of Anesthesiology
Yale University School of Medicine
Medical Director
Ambulatory Procedures Unit
VA Connecticut Healthcare System
West Haven, Connecticut

Robert S. Holzman, MD, MS (Hon), FAAP
Senior Associate in Perioperative Anesthesiology
Department of Anesthesiology, Perioperative and Pain Medicine
Boston Children's Hospital
Professor of Anesthesia
Harvard Medical School
Boston, Massachusetts

Harriet W. Hopf, MD
Professor and Vice-Chair
Department of Anesthesiology
University of Utah School of Medicine
Salt Lake City, Utah

Robert W. Hurley, MD, PhD
Professor and Vice-Chair
Department of Anesthesiology
Medical College of Wisconsin
Milwaukee, Wisconsin

Adam K. Jacob, MD
Associate Professor of Anesthesiology
Mayo Clinic College of Medicine
Rochester, Minnesota

Farid Jadbabaie, MD
Associate Professor of Medicine (Cardiology)
Director of Echocardiography Laboratory
VA Connecticut Healthcare System
Yale School of Medicine
New Haven, Connecticut

Rebecca L. Johnson, MD
Assistant Professor of Anesthesiology
Department of Anesthesiology
Mayo Clinic College of Medicine
Rochester, Minnesota

Sharma E. Joseph, MD
Instructor of Anesthesia
Boston University School of Medicine
Boston Medical Center
Boston, Massachusetts

Jonathan D. Katz, MD
Clinical Professor of Anesthesiology
Yale University School of Medicine
Professor of Anesthesiology
Frank H. Netter MD School of Medicine at Quinnipiac University
Attending Anesthesiologist
St. Vincent's Medical Center
Bridgeport, Connecticut

Christopher D. Kent, MD
Associate Professor
Department of Anesthesiology and Pain Medicine
University of Washington
Seattle, Washington

Meghan A. Kirksey, MD, PhD
Assistant Attending Anesthesiologist
Hospital for Special Surgery
Clinical Assistant Professor of Anesthesiology
Weill Cornell Medical College
New York, New York

Sandra L. Kopp, MD
Associate Professor of Anesthesiology
Department of Anesthesiology
Mayo Clinic College of Medicine
Rochester, Minnesota

Catherine Kuhn, MD
Director & Associate Dean, Graduate Medical Education
Designated Institutional Official
Professor of Anesthesiology
Department of Anesthesiology
Duke University
Durham, North Carolina

Jerrold Lerman, MD, FRCPC, FANZCA
Clinical Professor of Anesthesiology
Women and Children's Hospital of Buffalo
State University of New York
Buffalo, New York

Jerrold H. Levy, MD, FAHA, FCCM
Professor of Anesthesiology
Associate Professor of Surgery
Division of Cardiothoracic Anesthesiology and Critical Care
Duke University School of Medicine
Co-Director, Cardiothoracic ICU
Duke University Hospital
Durham, North Carolina

Adam D. Lichtman, MD, FASE
Associate Professor of Anesthesiology
Director of Vascular Anesthesia
Weill Cornell Medical College
New York Presbyterian Hospital
New York, New York

J. Lance Lichtor, MD
Department of Anesthesiology
Yale University School of Medicine
New Haven, Connecticut

Yi Lin, MD, PhD
Assistant Attending Anesthesiologist
Hospital for Special Surgery
New York, New York

Spencer S. Liu, MD
Clinical Professor of Anesthesiology
Weill College of Medicine at Cornell University
Department of Anesthesiology
Hospital for Special Surgery
New York, New York

Justin B. Long, MD, FAAP
Assistant Professor
Emory University School of Medicine
Department of Pediatric Anesthesiology
Children's Healthcare of Atlanta at Henrietta Egleston Hospital for Children
Atlanta, Georgia

Stephen M. Macres, MD, PharmD
Professor
Department of Anesthesiology and Pain Medicine
University of California Davis Medical Center
Sacramento, California

Peter Mancini, MD
Assistant Clinical Professor
Department of Anesthesiology
Yale University School of Medicine
New Haven, CT

Aaron J. Mancuso, MD
Assistant Professor of Anesthesiology
Geisel School of Medicine
Dartmouth-Hitchcock Medical Center
Lebanon, New Hampshire

Gerard Manecke, MD
Chair, Department of Anesthesiology
UCSD Medical Center
San Diego, California

Melissa M. Masaracchia, MD
Assistant Professor of Anesthesiology
Dartmouth-Hitchcock Medical Center
Geisel School of Medicine
Lebanon, New Hampshire

Joseph P. Mathew, MD, MHSC, MBA
Jerry Reves, MD, Professor and Chairman
Department of Anesthesiology
Duke University Medical Center
Durham, North Carolina

Kathryn E. McGoldrick, MD, FCAI (Hon)
Professor and Chair of Anesthesiology, Emeritus
Advisory Dean, Emeritus
New York Medical College
Valhalla, New York
Accreditation Council for Graduate Medical Education
Department of Institutional Accreditation
Chicago, Illinois

Joseph H. McIsaac III, MD, MS
Associate Clinical Professor of Anesthesiology
Associate Adjunct Professor of Biomedical Engineering
University of Connecticut
Avon, CT

Sanford M. Miller, MD
Clinical Professor (Emeritus) of Anesthesiology
NYU School of Medicine
Former Assistant Director of Anesthesiology
Bellevue Hospital Center
New York, New York

Shawn L. Mincer, MSW
Research Coordinator
Department of Anesthesiology and Pain Medicine
University of Washington
Seattle, Washington

Peter G. Moore, MBBS, PhD, FANZCA, FICM
Professor of Anesthesiology and Pain Medicine and Internal Medicine
University of California, Davis Health System
Sacramento, California

Candice Morrissey, MD, MSPH
Assistant Professor
Department of Anesthesiology
University of Utah
Salt Lake City, Utah

Michael J. Murray, MD, PhD
Department of Critical Care Medicine
Geisinger Medical Center
Danville, Pennsylvania

Sawyer A. Naze, MD
Resident
Department of Anesthesiology
Feinberg School of Medicine
Northwestern University
Chicago, Illinois

Steven M. Neustein, MD
Professor of Anesthesiology
Icahn School of Medicine at Mount Sinai
New York, New York

Marieke Niesters, MD, PhD
Department of Anesthesiology
Leiden University Medical Center
Leiden, The Netherlands

Mark C. Norris, MD
Director of Obstetric Anesthesia
Boston Medical Center
Clinical Professor of Anesthesiology
Boston University School of Medicine
Boston, Massachusetts

E. Andrew Ochroch, MD, MSCE
Professor of Anesthesiology, Critical Care, and Surgery
University of Pennsylvania
Philadelphia, Pennsylvania

Rafael Ortega, MD
Professor
Vice-Chairman of Academic Affairs
Department of Anesthesiology
Boston University School of Medicine
Boston, Massachusetts

Charles W. Otto, MD, FCCM
Professor of Anesthesiology
Associate Professor of Medicine
Department of Anesthesiology
University of Arizona College of Medicine
Tucson, Arizona

Frank Overdyk, MSEE, MD
Department of Anesthesiology
Roper St. Francis Health System
Charleston, South Carolina

Nathan Leon Pace, MD, MStat
Professor
Department of Anesthesiology
University of Utah
Salt Lake City, Utah

Paul S. Pagel, MD, PhD
Staff Physician
Anesthesiology Service
Clement J. Zablocki VA Medical Center
Milwaukee, Wisconsin

Ben Julian Palanca, MD, PhD, MSc
Assistant Professor
Department of Anesthesiology
Washington University School of Medicine
St. Louis, Missouri

Raymond S. Park, MD
Assistant in Perioperative Anesthesia
Department of Anesthesiology, Perioperative and Pain Medicine
Boston Children's Hospital
Instructor in Anaesthesia
Harvard Medical School
Boston, Massachusetts

Jeffrey J. Pasternak, MS, MD
Associate Professor of Anesthesiology
Mayo Clinic College of Medicine
Rochester, Minnesota

Albert C. Perrino Jr
Professor
Yale University School of Medicine
Chief, Anesthesiology
VA Connecticut Healthcare System
New Haven, Connecticut

Carly Peterson, MD, FRCPC
Division of Cardiothoracic Anesthesia
Department of Anesthesiology and Pain Medicine
University of Washington
Seattle, Washington

Andrew J. Pittaway, BM, BS FRCA
Associate Residency Program Director
Associate Professor
University of Washington
Attending Anesthesiologist
Department of Anesthesiology & Pain Medicine
Seattle Children's Hospital
Seattle, Washington

Mihai V. Podgoreanu, MD
Perioperative Genomics Program
Division of Cardiothoracic Anesthesia and Critical Care
Department of Anesthesiology
Duke University Medical Center
Durham, North Carolina

Wanda M. Popescu, MD
Associate Professor of Anesthesiology
Director, Thoracic and Vascular Anesthesia Division
Co-Director, Grand Rounds
Yale School of Medicine
New Haven, Connecticut

Karen L. Posner, PhD
Research Professor
Laura Cheney Professor in Anesthesia Patient Safety
Department of Anesthesia and Pain Medicine
University of Washington
Seattle, Washington

Jamie R. Privratsky, MD
Department of Anesthesiology
Duke University Medical Center
Durham, North Carolina

Donald S. Prough, MD
Rebecca Terry White Distinguished Professor
Chair of Anesthesiology
The University of Texas Medical Branch at Galveston
Galveston, Texas

Glenn Ramsey, MD
Professor
Department of Pathology
Feinberg School of Medicine
Northwestern University
Medical Director
Blood Bank
Northwestern Memorial Hospital
Chicago, Illinois

Kevin T. Riutort, MD, MS
USAP Colorado
Greenwood Village, Colorado

Gerardo Rodriguez, MD
Assistant Professor
Department of Anesthesiology
Boston University School of Medicine
Director, East Newton Surgical Intensive Care Unit
Boston Medical Center
Boston, Massachusetts

G. Alec Rooke, MD, PhD
Professor of Anesthesiology and Pain Medicine
University of Washington
Seattle, Washington

Stanley H. Rosenbaum, MA, MD
Professor of Anesthesiology, Internal Medicine and Surgery
Yale University School of Medicine
New Haven, Connecticut

Meg A. Rosenblatt, MD
Site Chair, Department of Anesthesiology, Mount Sinai West
Professor of Anesthesiology
Professor of Orthopaedics
Mount Sinai St. Luke's
New York, New York

William H. Rosenblatt, MD
Professor of Anesthesiology
Yale University School of Medicine
New Haven, Connecticut

Richard W. Rosenquist, MD
Chairman
Pain Management Department
Anesthesiology Institute
Cleveland Clinic
Cleveland, Ohio

Antonio F. Saad, MD, MFM/CCM
Fellow, Anesthesia and Obstetrics and Gynecology
University of Texas Medical Branch
Galveston, Texas

Aaron Sandler, MD
Assistant Professor of Anesthesiology
Department of Anesthesiology
Duke University
Durham, North Carolina

Barbara M. Scavone, MD
Professor of Anesthesia and Critical Care, and Obstetrics and Gynecology
University of Chicago
Chicago, Illinois

Corey Scher, MD
Clinical Professor of Anesthesiology
New York University School of Medicine-Bellevue Hospital Center
New York, New York

Jeffrey J. Schwartz, MD
Associate Professor
Department of Anesthesiology
Yale University School of Medicine
New Haven, Connecticut

Sam R. Sharar, MD
Professor
Vice-Chair for Faculty Affairs and Development
Department of Anesthesiology and Pain Medicine
University of Washington School of Medicine
Seattle, Washington

Aarti Sharma, MD
Associate Professor of Clinical Anesthesiology
Department of Anesthesiology
Weill Cornell Medical College
New York Presbyterian Hospital
New York, New York

Benjamin M. Sherman, MD
Cardiothoracic Anesthesiology
TeamHealth Anesthesia
Legacy Good Samaritan Hospital
Portland, Oregon

Nikolaos J. Skubas, MD, DSc, FASE, FACC
Professor of Anesthesiology and Cardiothoracic Surgery
Weill Cornell Medicine
Director, Cardiac Anesthesia
NewYork-Presbyterian Hospital
New York, New York

Hugh M. Smith, MD
Assistant Professor of Anesthesiology
Department of Anesthesiology and Perioperative Medicine
Mayo Clinic
Rochester, Minesota

Terry Smith, PhD
Associate Professor
Department of Anesthesiology
Leiden University Medical Center
Leiden, The Netherlands

Ellen M. Soffin, MD, PhD
Assistant Attending Anesthesiologist
Hospital for Special Surgery
New York, New York

Karen J. Souter, MB, BS, FRCA, MACM
Professor
Department of Anesthesiology and Pain Medicine
University of Washington
Seattle, Washington

Bruce D. Spiess, MD, FAHA
Professor and Associate Chair (Research)
Department of Anesthesiology
University of Florida
Gainesville, Florida

Mark Stafford-Smith, MD, CM, FRCP
Professor of Anesthesiology
Vice-Chair of Education
Fellowship Education Director
Adult Cardiothoracic Anesthesiology Fellowship
Department of Anesthesiology
Duke University Medical Center
Durham, North Carolina

Andrew F. Stasic, MD
Associate Professor of Clinical Anesthesia
Department of Anesthesia
Indiana University School of Medicine
Riley Hospital for Children
Indianapolis, Indiana

Randolph H. Steadman, MD, MS
Professor and Vice-Chair
Department of Anesthesiology and Perioperative Medicine
UCLA Health System
Los Angeles, California

Robert K. Stoelting, MD
Emeritus Professor and Past Chair
Department of Anesthesia
Indiana University School of Medicine
Indianapolis, Indiana

M. Christine Stock, MD
Professor
Department of Anesthesiology
Feinberg School of Medicine
Northwestern University
Chicago, Illinois

51 Anesthesia for Orthopedic Surgery   1441
MEGHAN A. KIRKSEY • STEPHEN C. HASKINS • ELLEN M. SOFFIN • SPENCER S. LIU

52 Transplant Anesthesia   1458
MARIE CSETE • GERARD MANECKE • DALIA BANKS

53 Trauma and Burns   1486
LEVON M. CAPAN • SANFORD M. MILLER • COREY SCHER

Section 9
POSTANESTHETIC MANAGEMENT, CRITICAL CARE, AND PAIN MANAGEMENT

54 Postanesthesia Recovery   1537
MICHAEL A. FOWLER • BRUCE D. SPIESS

55 Acute Pain Management   1562
STEPHEN M. MACRES • PETER G. MOORE • SCOTT M. FISHMAN

56 Chronic Pain Management   1607
HONORIO T. BENZON • ROBERT W. HURLEY • SALIM M. HAYEK

57 Critical Care Medicine   1632
MATTHEW R. HALLMAN • CHRISTOPHER G. CHOUKALAS • STEVEN DEEM

58 Cardiopulmonary Resuscitation   1661
CHARLES W. OTTO

59 Disaster Preparedness   1686
JOSEPH H. McISAAC III • CARIN A. HAGBERG • MICHAEL J. MURRAY

Section 10
APPENDICES

Appendix 1: Formulas   1708

Appendix 2: Atlas of Electrocardiography   1710
GINA C. BADESCU • BENJAMIN M. SHERMAN • JAMES R. ZAIDAN • PAUL G. BARASH

Appendix 3: Pacemaker and Implantable Cardiac Defibrillator Protocols   1724
GINA C. BADESCU • BENJAMIN M. SHERMAN • JAMES R. ZAIDAN • PAUL G. BARASH

Appendix 4: American Society of Anesthesiologists Standards, Guidelines, and Statements   1732

Appendix 5: The Airway Approach Algorithm and Difficult Airway Algorithm   1741

Appendix 6: Malignant Hyperthermia Protocol   1743

Appendix 7: Herbal Medications   1744

Appendix 8: Atlas of Ultrasound and Echocardiography (eBook only)
JOSHUA ZIMMERMAN • ROSSEMARY DE LA CRUZ • MICHAEL K. CAHALAN

Index   1749

Multimedia Contents

Narrated Interactive Clinical Vignettes

- 1.1 Historically Important Articles
- 2.1 Perioperative Surgical Home
- 3.1 Needlestick Injuries
- 5.1 Electrosurgical Unit
- 5.2 Convective Warming Blankets
- 5.3 Methylene Blue
- 5.4 Airway Fire
- 6.1 Genetic Variability and Pain Response
- 7.1 Statistical Methods
- 8.1 Methicillin-Resistant Staphylococcus Aureus
- 8.2 Surgical Site Infection
- 9.1 Transfusion Reaction
- 9.2 Anaphylaxis
- 9.3 Latex Allergy
- 10.1 Mechanism of Anesthesia
- 11.1 Serotonin Syndrome
- 12.1 Junctional Rhythm
- 12.2 Wolff-Parkinson White Syndrome
- 13.1 Catecholamines
- 13.2 Dopamine
- 13.3 Dexmedetomidine
- 13.4 Nitroprusside
- 14.1 Catecholamines
- 14.2 Postoperative Delirium
- 15.1 Venous Air Embolism
- 15.2 Postoperative Pulmonary Complications
- 16.1 Fluid Replacement
- 16.2 Hypertonic Saline
- 16.3 Syndrome of Inappropriate Antidiuretic Hormone Secretion (SIADH)
- 16.4 Hyperkalemia in ESRD
- 16.5 Hypercalcemia
- 16.6 Carcinoid Syndrome
- 17.1 Anti-thrombin III deficiency
- 17.2 Blood Type, Screening and Crossmatching
- 17.3 Amniotic Fluid Embolism
- 17.4 Jehovah's Witness
- 17.5 Von Willebrand Disease
- 17.6 Heparin-Induced Thrombocytopenia
- 17.7 Tranexamic Acid
- 18.1 Xenon
- 18.2 Postoperative Cognitive Dysfunction
- 18.3 CO_2 Elevation
- 19.1 Etomidate
- 19.2 Ketamine
- 19.3 Dexmedetomidine
- 20.1 Methadone
- 20.2 Naloxone
- 21.1 Sugammadex
- 22.1 Local Anesthestic Systemic Toxicity
- 23.1 Herbal Supplements
- 23.2 Bleomycin
- 23.3 Subacute Bacterial Endocarditis Prophylaxis
- 23.4 Implantable Cardiac Defibrillators (ICD)
- 23.5 Cigarette Smoking
- 23.6 Asthma
- 23.7 Obstructive Sleep Apnea
- 23.8 Preoperative Medication Management
- 23.9 Lithium
- 23.10 Prevention of Pulmonary Aspiration
- 24.1 Duchenne Muscular Dystrophy
- 24.2 Myasthenia Gravis
- 24.3 Multiple Sclerosis
- 24.4 Malignant Hyperthermia
- 24.5 Acute Intermittent Porphyria
- 24.6 Pseudocholinesterase Deficiency
- 24.7 G6PD Deficiency
- 24.8 Sickle Cell Disease
- 24.9 Rheumatoid Arthritis
- 25.1 Anesthesia Machine Checkout
- 25.2 Loss of Pipeline Oxygen
- 26.1 Central Venous Access
- 26.2 Pulmonary Artery Catheter Complications
- 26.3 Processed EEG Monitoring
- 27.1 Transesophageal Echocardiography (TEE)
- 27.2 Atrial Myxoma
- 27.3 Patent Foramen Ovale
- 28.1 Hereditary Hemorrhagic Telangiectasia (HHT)
- 28.2 Endobronchial Intubation
- 28.3 Aspiration Pneumonitis
- 28.4 Endotracheal Tube Cuff
- 28.5 Methemoglobinemia
- 29.1 Ulnar Nerve Neuropathy
- 29.2 Sitting Position
- 29.3 Venous Air Embolism
- 30.1 Failed Monitored Anesthesia Care
- 31.1 Ambulatory Anesthesia
- 31.2 Pediatric Upper Respiratory Infection
- 32.1 Office-Based Anesthesia
- 32.2 Tuberous Sclerosis
- 33.1 MRI Safety
- 33.2 Electroconvulsive Therapy
- 34.1 Elderly Changes
- 34.2 Elderly Changes 2
- 34.3 Geriatric Anesthesia
- 35.1 Loss of Resistance
- 35.2 Nausea after Spinal
- 35.3 Postdural Puncture Headache (PDPH)
- 35.4 Myomectomy
- 36.1 Trigeminal Neuralgia
- 36.2 Interscalene Block
- 36.3 Bier Block
- 37.1 Evoked Potentials
- 37.2 Mannitol
- 37.3 Postoperative Visual Loss
- 38.1 One Lung Ventilation

Multimedia Contents

38.2 Bronchial Blocker
38.3 Anterior Mediastinal Mass
38.4 Mediastinoscopy
39.1 Aortic Stenosis
39.2 Aortic Stenosis 2
39.3 Hypertrophic Obstructive Cardiomyopathy (HOCM)
39.4 Mitral Stenosis
39.5 Hypotension on Bypass
39.6 Intra-Aortic Balloon Pump (IABP)
39.7 Protamine Reaction
39.8 Cardiac Tamponade
39.9 Dextrocardia
40.1 Carotid Endarterectomy
40.2 Aortic Dissection
41.1 Nalbuphine
41.2 C-Section Difficult Airway
41.3 Preemclampsia
41.4 Placental Abruption
41.5 Uterine Atony
41.6 Electronic Fetal Monitoring
41.7 Neonatal Resuscitation
41.8 Pregnancy and Non-obstetrics Surgery
42.1 Caudal Block
42.2 TAP Block
42.3 Bronchopulmonary Dysplasia
42.4 Retinopathy of Prematurity
42.5 Tracheoesophageal Fistula
42.6 Neonatal anesthesia
42.7 Pyloric Stenosis
42.8 Patent Ductus Arteriosus (PDA)
43.1 Pediatric Airway
43.2 Superior Vena Cava Syndrome
43.3 Negative Pressure Pulmonary Edema
44.1 Carbon Dioxide
44.2 Nissen Fundoplication
45.1 Morbid Obesity
46.1 Cirrhosis
47.1 Thyroid Storm
47.2 Pheochromocytoma
48.1 Tympanoplasty
48.2 Epiglottitis
48.3 Vocal Cord Polyp
48.4 Laser Surgery
49.1 Ruptured Globe
49.2 Oculocardiac Reflex
49.3 Wrong Surgical Site
49.4 Corneal Abrasion
50.1 Robotic Prostatectomy
50.2 TUR Syndrome
50.3 Autonomic Hyperreflexia
50.4 Extracorporeal Shock Wave
50.5 Testicular Torsion
51.1 Spinal Anesthesia for Total Hip Replacement
51.2 Fat Embolism
51.3 Bone Cement Implantation Syndrome
51.4 Pulmonary Embolism
52.1 Brain Death
52.2 Organ Transplantation
52.3 Awareness
53.1 Massive Transfusion
53.2 Cardiac Arrest
53.3 Burns
53.4 Ruptured Globe
54.1 Obstructive Sleep Apnea
54.2 Corneal Abrasion
54.3 Hypothermia
54.4 Delayed Emergence
54.5 PACU Seizure
54.6 Post-operative Nausea and Vomiting
55.1 Surgical Stress Response
55.2 Opioid-Dependent Patient
55.3 Buprenorphine
56.1 Myofascial Pain Syndrome
56.2 Fibromyalgia
56.3 Postherpetic Neuralgia
56.4 Complex Regional Pain Syndrome (CRPS)
56.5 Cancer Pain
57.1 Septic Shock
57.2 Hemodynamic Changes
57.3 Weaning from Mechanical Ventilation
57.4 Acute Respiratory Distress Syndrome
58.1 Cardiac Arrest
58.2 Cardiac Arrest
59.1 Ebola Virus

Tutorial Videos

1.1 Ether Monument
1.2 Ether Controversy
1.3 ASA Seal
2.1 AIMS
3.1 Fixation Errors
3.2 ASA Seal
3.3 Needle Stick
3.4 Chain of Communication
4.1 Rates of Selected Anesthetic Complications
4.2 Accident Causation
5.1 Grounded Electrical Power
5.2 Electric Plugs
5.3 Line Isolation
5.4 Line Isolation Monitor
5.5 Return Plate
5.6 Fire in the Operating Room
6.1 Host Response to Injury
7.1 Graphing Data
8.1 Oxygen Tension in Wound Module
9.1 Type 3 Immune Complex Reaction
9.2 Anaphylaxis
10.1 Meyer-Overton Rule
11.1 Dose Response Relationships
11.2 Drug Concentration and Effect
12.1 Coronary Blood Flow
12.2 Laplace
12.3 Pressure-Volume Loop
14.1 Catecholamine Chemical Structures

14.2	Renin Angiotensin		26.14	CVP Waveforms
14.3	Antimuscarinics		26.15	Ultrasound Guided IJ Insertion
14.4	Reversible Anticholinesterases		26.16	Thermodilution Cardiac Output
15.1	Law of Laplace		26.17	Respiratory Variation
15.2	Lung Volumes		27.1	TEE Probe Movements
15.3	Lung Blood Flow Distribution		27.2	ME Four Chamber
15.4	Continuum of Ventilation and Perfusion		27.3	ME Two Chamber
15.5	Flow Volume		27.4	ME LAX
16.1	Renal Regulation of Water		27.5	ME Ascending Aortic LAX and SAX
16.2	Hyponatremia Rapid Correction		27.6	ME AV SAX
16.3	Hyperkalemia		27.7	ME RV Inflow-Outflow
17.1	Cerebral Aneurysm Coiling		27.8	ME Bicaval
17.2	Formation and Lysis of Fibrin		27.9	TG Mid SAX
18.1	Inhaled Anesthetic Formulas		27.10	TG Basal SAX
18.2	Inhaled Anesthetic Rate of Rise		27.11	Deep TG LAX
19.1	Drug Concentration and Effect		27.12	Desc Aortic SAX and LAX
20.1	Dose-Effect Curves		27.13	PLAX
20.2	Drug Concentration and Effect		27.14	PSAX
20.3	Vomiting Pharmacology		27.15	Apical 4-Chamber
21.1	Neuromuscular Blocking Agents		27.16	Subcostal 4-Chamber
21.2	Fasciculations		28.1	Indirect Laryngoscopy
21.3	Monitoring Nerve Block		28.2	Airway Evaluation
22.1	Peripheral Nerve Cross-Section		28.3	Vocal Chord Polyp
22.2	Ankle Block		28.4	Preoxygenation
23.1	Airway Exam		28.5	Preoxygenation Errors
24.1	Duchenne Muscular Dystrophy		28.6	ETT LMA Pressures
24.2	Dantrolene Mixing		28.7	LMA
24.3	Removing Anesthetics from the Breathing Circuit		28.8	Laryngoscopy Pitfalls
24.4	Raynauds		28.9	Laryngoscopy
24.5	Scleroderma		28.10	Right Endotracheal Intubation
24.6	Epidermolysis Bullosa		28.11	Colorimetric CO2 Detection
24.7	Pemphigus		28.12	Airway Trans-Illumination
25.1	Bourdon Tube		28.13	GlideScope
25.2	Circle System		28.14	Channel Scopes - Airtraq
25.3	Liquid Oxygen Storage Tank		28.15	Rapid-Sequence Intubation
25.4	E-Cylinder		28.16	Aspiration
25.5	Oxygen Proportioning Systems		28.17	Loose Teeth
25.6	Oxygen Flush Valve		28.18	Endotracheal Extubation Procedures
25.7	Vaporizer Interlocking Mechanism		28.19	Tracheostomy
25.8	Desflurane		28.20	O2 Dissociation Curve
25.9	CO2 Absorber		28.21	Nasal Intubation
25.10	Rebreathing CO2		28.22	FOB
25.11	Ventilator Bellows		28.23	Esophageal Intubation
25.12	Ascending Bellows Ventilator		28.24	Bougie
25.13	Wire Anenometers		28.25	Jet Ventilation
25.14	Scavenger System		29.1	Brachial Plexus Injury
26.1	Oximetry		29.2	Upper Extremity Neuropathy
26.2	Galvanic Oxygen Analyzers		29.3	Ulnar Nerve Compression
26.3	Capnogram		29.4	Ventilation and Perfusion in the Lateral Position
26.4	Cardiac Oscillation		29.5	Prone Position Facial
26.5	Arterial Line Tracing		29.6	Prone Position
26.6	Arterial Line Insertion		30.1	Continuous Infusion
26.7	Ultrasound Guided Radial Artery Cannulation		31.1	Vomiting Pharmacology
26.8	Transducer		32.1	Levels of Sedation
26.9	Arterial Line Infection		33.1	Anesthesia in Remote Locations
26.10	Arterial Line Complications		34.1	Age-Related Changes in Body Composition
26.11	NIBP Oscillations		34.2	Cardiovascular Response to Orthostasis
26.12	Swan Pressure Tracing		35.1	Dermatomes
26.13	Swan Real Life		35.2	Subarachnoid Block

35.3	Paresthesias	47.1	NIM Thyroid
35.4	Continuous Spinal	47.2	Vitamin D Metabolism
35.5	Hanging Drop	47.3	Catecholamines
36.1	Neck Anatomy	47.4	Metabolism of Endogenous Catecholamines
36.2	Brachial Plexus Block	48.1	Airway Abscess
36.3	Interscalene Block	48.2	Facial Nerve
36.4	Supraclavicular Block	48.3	Jet Ventilation
36.5	Sensory Innervation of the Hand	48.4	Epiglottis
36.6	TAP Block	48.5	Laser ENT
36.7	Penile Block	48.6	Tracheostomy
36.8	Femoral Nerve Block	49.1	Open Eye Injury
36.9	Ultrasound-Guided Saphenous Nerve Block	50.1	Laparoscopic
36.10	Ultrasound-Guided Popliteal Nerve Block	50.2	Robotic Prostatectomy
36.11	Ankle Block	51.1	Scoliosis
37.1	Intracranial Compliance	51.2	Brachial Plexus Injury
37.2	Mayfield Clamp	51.3	Prone Position
37.3		51.4	Prone Position Facial
38.1		51.5	Interscalene Block
38.2		51.6	Ankle Block
38.3		52.1	Left Liver Lobe Donation
38.4		53.1	Management of the Major Trauma Patient
38.5		53.2	Nail Trachea Case
38.6		53.3	Pneumothorax
38.7		54.1	Tracheostomy
38.8		54.2	Aspiration
38.9		55.1	Nociceptive Pathways
39.		55.2	Pain Sensitization
39.		55.3	Pain Processing
39.		55.4	Universal Pain Assessment Tool
39.		55.5	Brachial Plexus
39.		55.6	Interscalene Block
39.		55.7	Supraclavicular Block
39.		55.8	Femoral Nerve Block
39.		55.9	Ultrasound-Guided Saphenous Nerve Block
39.		55.10	Ultrasound-Guided Popliteal Nerve Block
40.		55.11	TAP Block
41.1	Lung Volumes	56.1	Nociceptive Pathways
41.2	Pudendal Nerve Block	56.2	Pain Sensitization
41.3	C-Section Spinal	57.1	Cerebral Blood Flow
41.4	Fetal Heart Rate	57.2	Swan Pressure Tracing
41.5	Surgery Recommendations in Pregnancy	57.3	Swan Real Life
42.1	Inhalation Induction	57.4	A-line Insertion
43.1	Single Breath Inhalational Induction	57.5	Mechanical Ventilation Pressure
44.1	Laparoscopic	57.6	A-line Infection
45.1	Sequelae of Obesity	58.1	Adult Bradycardia Algorithm
45.2	Sleep Apnea	58.2	Tachycardia Algorithm
46.1	Left Liver Lobe Donation	59.1	Disaster Preparedness

Appendix 2 Videos

1 Atrial Fibrillation
2 Atrial Flutter
3 Atrioventricular Block (First Degree)
4 Atrioventricular Block (Second Degree), Mobitz Type I/Wenckebach Block
5 Atrioventricular Block (Second Degree), Mobitz Type II
6 Atrioventricular Block (Third Degree), Complete Heart Block
7 Bundle Branch Block—Left (LBBB)
8 Bundle Branch Block—Right (RBBB)
9 Transmural Myocardial Infarction (TMI)
10 Subendocardial Myocardial Infarction (SEMI)
11 Myocardial Ischemia
12 Myocardial Ischemia
13 Digitalis Effect
14 Potassium
15 Paroxysmal Atrial Tachycardia (PAT)

16 Pericarditis
17 Premature Atrial Contraction (PAC)
18 Premature Ventricular Contraction (PVC)
19 Premature Ventricular Contraction (PVC)—Multifocal
20 Premature Ventricular Contraction (PVC)—Triplet
21 Premature Ventricular Contraction (PVC)—Bigeminy
22 Premature Ventricular Contraction (PVC)—Couplets
23 Sinus Bradycardia
24 Bradycardia Leading to Arrest
25 Agonal Rhythm
26 Sinus Arrhythmia
27 Sinus Tachycardia
28 Torsades de Pointes
29 Ventricular Fibrillation
30 Ventricular Tachycardia
31 Wolff-Parkinson-White Syndrome (WPW)
32 Atrial Pacing: Pacemaker Tracings
33 Ventricular Pacing
34 DDD Pacing

Section 1
INTRODUCTION AND OVERVIEW

1 The History of Anesthesia

ADAM K. JACOB • SANDRA L. KOPP • DOUGLAS R. BACON • HUGH M. SMITH

Anesthesia Before Ether
    Physical and Psychological Anesthesia
    Early Analgesics and Soporifics
    Inhaled Anesthetics
    Almost Discovery: Hickman, Clarke, Long, and Wells
    Public Demonstration of Ether Anesthesia
    Chloroform and Obstetrics
Anesthesia Principles, Equipment, and Standards
    Control of the Airway
    Tracheal Intubation
    Advanced Airway Devices
    Early Anesthesia Delivery Systems
    Alternative Circuits
    Ventilators
    Carbon Dioxide Absorption
    Flowmeters
    Vaporizers
    Patient Monitors
    Electrocardiography, Pulse Oximetry, and Capnography
    Safety Standards

The History of Anesthetic Agents and Adjuvants
    Inhaled Anesthetics
    Intravenous Anesthetics
    Local Anesthetics
    Opioids
    Muscle Relaxants
    Antiemetics
Anesthesia Subspecialties
    Regional Anesthesia
    Cardiovascular Anesthesia
    Neuroanesthesia
    Obstetric Anesthesia
    Transfusion Medicine
Professionalism and Anesthesia Practice
    Organized Anesthesiology
    Academic Anesthesia
    Establishing a Society
Conclusions

KEY POINTS

1. Anesthesiology is a young specialty historically, especially when compared with surgery or internal medicine.
2. Discoveries in anesthesiology have taken decades to build upon the observations and experiments of many people, and in some instances we are still searching. For example, the ideal volatile anesthetic has yet to be discovered.
3. Much of our current anesthesia equipment is the direct result of anesthesiologists being unhappy with existing tools and needing better ones to properly anesthetize patients.
4. Many safety standards have been established through the work of anesthesiologists who were frustrated by the status quo.
5. Regional anesthesia is the direct outgrowth of a chance observation by an intern who would go on to become a successful ophthalmologist.
6. Pain medicine began as an outgrowth of regional anesthesia.
7. Organizations of anesthesia professionals have been critical in establishing high standards in education and proficiency, which in turn has defined the specialty.
8. Respiratory critical care medicine started as the need by anesthesiologists to use positive-pressure ventilation to help polio victims.
9. Surgical anesthesia and physician specialization in its administration have allowed for increasingly complex operations to be performed on increasingly ill patients.

Surgery without adequate pain control may seem cruel to the modern reader, and in contemporary practice we are prone to forget the realities of preanesthesia surgery. Fanny Burney, a well-known literary artist from the early 19th century, described a mastectomy she endured after receiving a "wine cordial" as her sole anesthetic. As seven male assistants held her down, the surgery commenced: "When the dreadful steel was plunged into the breast-cutting through veins–arteries–flesh—nerves, I needed no injunction not to restrain my cries. I began a scream that lasted unintermittently during the whole time of the incision—and I almost marvel that it rings not in my Ears still! So excruciating was the agony. Oh Heaven!—I then felt the knife racking against the breast bone—scraping it! This performed while I yet remained in utterly speechless torture."[1] Burney's description illustrates the difficulty of overstating the impact of anesthesia on the human condition. An epitaph on a monument to William Thomas Green Morton, one of the founders of anesthesia, summarizes the contribution of anesthesia: "BEFORE WHOM in all time Surgery was Agony."[2] Although most human civilizations evolved some method for diminishing patient discomfort, *anesthesia*, in its modern and effective meaning, is a comparatively recent discovery with traceable origins in the mid-19th century. How we have changed perspectives, from one in which surgical pain was terrible and expected to one in which patients reasonably assume they will be safe, pain free, and unaware during extensive operations, is a fascinating story and the subject of this chapter.

Anesthesiologists are like no other physicians: We are experts at controlling the airway and at emergency resuscitation; we are real-time cardiopulmonologists achieving hemodynamic and respiratory stability for the anesthetized patient; we are pharmacologists and physiologists, calculating appropriate doses and desired responses; we are gurus of postoperative care and patient safety; we are internists performing perianesthetic medical evaluations; we are the pain experts across all medical disciplines and apply specialized techniques in pain clinics and labor wards; we manage the severely sick and injured in critical care units; we are neurologists, selectively blocking sympathetic, sensory, or motor functions with our regional techniques; and we are trained researchers exploring scientific mystery and clinical phenomenon.

Anesthesiology is an amalgam of specialized techniques, equipment, drugs, and knowledge that like the growth rings of a tree have built up over time. Current anesthesia practice is the summation of the individual efforts and fortuitous discoveries of centuries. Every component of modern anesthesia was at some point a new discovery and reflects the experience, knowledge, and inventiveness of our predecessors. Historical examination enables understanding of how these individual components of anesthesia evolved. Knowledge of the history of anesthesia enhances our appreciation of current practice and foretells where our specialty might be headed.

Anesthesia Before Ether

Physical and Psychological Anesthesia

The Edwin Smith Surgical Papyrus, the oldest known written surgical document, describes 48 cases performed by an Egyptian surgeon from 3000 to 2500 BC. Although this remarkable surgical treatise contains no direct mention of measures to lessen patient pain or suffering, Egyptian pictographs from the same era show a surgeon compressing a nerve in a patient's antecubital fossa while operating on the patient's hand. Another image displays a patient compressing his own brachial plexus while a procedure is performed on his palm.[3] In the 16th century, military surgeon Ambroise Paré became adept at nerve compression as a means of creating anesthesia.

Medical science has benefited from the natural refrigerating properties of ice and snow as well. For centuries anatomic dissections were performed only in winter because colder temperatures delayed deterioration of the cadaver. In the 17th century, Marco Aurelio Severino described the technique of "refrigeration anesthesia" in which snow was placed in parallel lines across the incisional plane such that the surgical site became insensate within minutes. The technique never became widely used, likely because of the challenge of maintaining stores of snow year-round.[4] Severino is also known to have saved numerous lives during an epidemic of diphtheria by performing tracheostomies and inserting trocars to maintain patency of the airway.[5]

Formal manipulation of the psyche to relieve surgical pain was undertaken by French physicians Charles Dupotet and Jules Cloquet in the late 1820s with hypnosis, then called *mesmerism*. Although the work of Anton Mesmer was discredited by the French Academy of Science after formal inquiry several decades earlier, proponents like Dupotet and Cloquet continued with mesmeric experiments and pleaded to the Academie de Medicine to reconsider its utility.[6] In a well-attended demonstration in 1828, Cloquet removed the breast of a 64-year-old patient while she reportedly remained in a calm, mesmeric sleep. This demonstration made a lasting impression on British physician John Elliotson, who became a leading figure of the mesmeric movement in England in the 1830s and 1840s. Innovative and quick to adopt new advances, Elliotson performed mesmeric demonstrations and in 1843 published *Numerous Cases of Surgical Operations Without Pain in the Mesmeric State*. Support for mesmerism faded when in 1846 renowned surgeon Robert Liston performed the first operation using ether anesthesia in England and remarked, "This Yankee dodge beats mesmerism all hollow."[7]

Early Analgesics and Soporifics

Dioscorides, a Greek physician from the first century AD, commented on the analgesia of mandragora, a drug prepared from the bark and leaves of the mandrake plant. He observed that the plant substance could be boiled in wine, strained, and used "in the case of persons...about to be cut or cauterized, when they wish to produce anesthesia."[8] Mandragora was still being used to benefit patients as late as the 17th century. From the ninth to the 13th centuries, the *soporific sponge* was a dominant mode of providing pain relief during surgery. Mandrake leaves, along with black nightshade, poppies, and other herbs, were boiled together and cooked onto a sponge. The sponge was then reconstituted in hot water and placed under the patient's nose before surgery. Prior to the hypodermic syringe and routine venous access, ingestion and inhalation were the only known routes for administering medicines to gain systemic effects. Prepared as indicated by published reports of the time, the sponge generally contained morphine and scopolamine—drugs used in modern anesthesia—in varying amounts.[9]

Alcohol was another element of the pre-ether armamentarium because it was thought to induce stupor and blunt the impact of pain. Although alcohol is a central nervous system depressant, in the amounts administered it produced little analgesia in the setting of true surgical pain. Fanny Burney's account underscores the ineffectiveness of alcohol as an anesthetic. Not only did alcohol provide minimal pain control, but it also did nothing to dull her recollection of events. Laudanum was an alcohol-based solution of opium first compounded by Paracelsus in the 16th century. It was wildly popular in the Victorian and Romantic periods and prescribed for a wide variety of ailments from the common cold to tuberculosis. Although appropriately used as an analgesic in some instances, it was frequently misused and abused. Laudanum was given by nursemaids to quiet wailing infants and abused by many upper-class women, poets, and artists who fell victim to its addictive potential.

In the first three decades of the 19th century, in Japan, Seisyu Hanaoka performed operations under what has been described as general anesthesia.[10] In the late 1900s, the manuscript "On the Use of Mafutsuto," the name given to the anesthetic method by Hanaoka, was translated into English. Written by Hajime Matsuoka, the manuscript details preanesthetic evaluation, the timing of anesthesia, and the proposed duration of surgery. The manuscript stated that care should be taken to ensure that lighting is appropriate; therefore it recommended that operations be performed at noon. Similarly, it stated that operations should not last more than 2 hours, because there was no way to replace intraoperative fluid or blood losses. The manuscript also contains a section on postoperative care.[11]

Inhaled Anesthetics

For many years nitrous oxide has been known for its ability to induce lightheadedness, and it was often inhaled by those seeking a thrill. It was made by heating ammonium nitrate in the presence of iron filings. The evolved gas was passed through water to eliminate toxic oxides of nitrogen before being stored. Nitrous oxide was first prepared in 1773 by Joseph Priestley, an English clergyman and scientist, who ranks among the great pioneers of chemistry. Without formal scientific training, Priestley prepared and examined several gases, including nitrous oxide, ammonia, sulfur dioxide, oxygen, carbon monoxide, and carbon dioxide.

At the end of the 18th century in England, there was a strong interest in the supposed wholesome effects of mineral water and gases, particularly with regard to treatment of scurvy, tuberculosis, and other diseases. Thomas Beddoes opened his Pneumatic Institute close to the small spa of Hotwells, in the city of Bristol, to study the beneficial effects of inhaled gases. He hired Humphry Davy in 1798 to conduct research projects for the institute. Davy performed brilliant investigations of several gases but focused much of his attention on nitrous oxide. His human experimental results, combined with research on the physical properties of the gas, were published in *Nitrous Oxide,* a 580-page book published in 1800. This impressive treatise is now best remembered for a few incidental observations. Davy commented that nitrous oxide transiently relieved a severe headache, obliterated a minor headache, and briefly quenched an aggravating toothache. The most frequently quoted passage was a casual entry: "As nitrous oxide in its extensive operation appears capable of destroying physical pain, it may probably be used with advantage during surgical operations in which no great effusion of blood takes place."[12] This is perhaps the most famous of the "missed opportunities" to discover surgical anesthesia. Davy's lasting nitrous oxide legacy was coining the phrase "laughing gas" to describe its unique property.

Almost Discovery: Hickman, Clarke, Long, and Wells

As the 19th century progressed, societal attitudes toward pain changed, perhaps best exemplified in the writings of the Romantic poets.[13] Thus, efforts to relieve pain were undertaken, and several more near-breakthroughs that occurred deserve mention. An English surgeon named Henry Hill Hickman searched intentionally for an inhaled anesthetic to relieve pain in his patients.[14] Hickman used high concentrations of carbon dioxide in his studies on mice and dogs. Carbon dioxide has some anesthetic properties, as shown by the absence of response to an incision in the animals of Hickman's study, but it was never determined whether the animals were insensate because of hypoxia rather than anesthesia. Hickman's concept was magnificent; his choice of agent was regrettable.

The discovery of surgical anesthetics in the modern era remains linked to inhaled anesthetics. The compound now known as *diethyl ether* had been known for centuries; it may have been synthesized first by eighth-century Arabian philosopher Jabir ibn Hayyan or possibly by Raymond Lully, a 13th-century European alchemist. But diethyl ether was certainly known in the 16th century, to both Valerius Cordus and Paracelsus, who prepared it by distilling sulfuric acid (oil of vitriol) with fortified wine to produce an *oleum vitrioli dulce* (sweet oil of vitriol). In one of the first "missed" observations on the effects of inhaled agents, Paracelsus observed that ether caused chickens to fall asleep and awaken unharmed. He must have been aware of its analgesic qualities because he reported that it could be recommended for use in painful illnesses.

For three centuries thereafter, this simple compound remained a therapeutic agent with only occasional use. Some of its properties were examined but without sustained interest by distinguished British scientists Robert Boyle, Isaac Newton, and Michael Faraday, none of whom made the conceptual link to surgical anesthesia. Its only routine application came as an inexpensive recreational drug among the poor of Britain and Ireland, who sometimes drank an ounce or two of ether when taxes made gin prohibitively expensive.[15] An American variation of this practice was conducted by groups of students who held ether-soaked towels to their faces at nocturnal "ether frolics."

William E. Clarke, a medical student from Rochester, New York, may have given the first ether anesthetic in January 1842. From techniques learned as a chemistry student in 1839, Clarke entertained his companions with nitrous oxide and ether. Emboldened by these experiences, he administered ether, from a towel, to a young woman named Hobbie. One of her teeth was then extracted without pain by a dentist named Elijah Pope.[16] However, it was suggested that the woman's unconsciousness was due to hysteria, and Clarke was advised to conduct no further anesthetic experiments.[17]

Two months later, on March 30, 1842, Crawford Williamson Long administered ether with a towel for surgical anesthesia in Jefferson, Georgia. His patient, James M. Venable, was a young man who was already familiar with ether's exhilarating effects, for he reported in a certificate that he had previously inhaled it and was fond of its use. Venable had two small tumors on his neck but refused to have them excised because he feared the pain that accompanied surgery. Knowing that Venable was familiar with ether's action, Dr. Long proposed that ether might alleviate pain and gained his patient's consent to proceed. After inhaling ether from the towel and having the procedure successfully completed, Venable reported that he was unaware of the removal of the tumors.[18] In determining the first fee for anesthesia and surgery, Long settled on a charge of $2.00.[19]

A common mid-19th century problem facing dentists was that patients refused beneficial treatment of their teeth for fear of the pain of the procedure. From a dentist's perspective, pain was not so much life-threatening as it was livelihood-threatening. One of the first dentists to engender a solution was Horace Wells of Hartford, Connecticut, whose great moment of discovery came on December 10, 1844. He observed a lecture-exhibition on nitrous oxide by an itinerant "scientist," Gardner Quincy Colton, who encouraged members of the audience to inhale a sample of the gas. Wells observed a young man injure his leg without pain while under the influence of nitrous oxide. Sensing that it might provide pain relief during dental procedures, Wells contacted Colton and boldly proposed an experiment in which Wells was to be the subject. The following day, Colton gave Wells nitrous oxide before a fellow dentist, William Riggs, extracted a tooth.[20] Afterward Wells declared that he had not felt any pain and deemed the experiment a success. Colton taught Wells to prepare nitrous oxide, which the dentist administered with success to patients in his practice. His apparatus probably resembled that used by Colton: a wooden tube placed in the mouth through which nitrous oxide was breathed from a small bag filled with the gas.

Public Demonstration of Ether Anesthesia

Another New Englander, William Thomas Green Morton, briefly shared a dental practice with Wells in Hartford. Wells' daybook shows that he gave Morton a course of instruction in anesthesia, but Morton apparently moved to Boston without paying for the lessons.[21] In Boston, Morton continued his interest in anesthesia and sought instruction from chemist and physician Charles T. Jackson. After learning that ether dropped on the skin provided analgesia, he began experiments with inhaled ether, an agent that proved to be much more versatile than nitrous oxide. Bottles of liquid ether were easily transported, and the volatility of the drug permitted effective inhalation. The concentrations required for surgical anesthesia were so low that patients did not become hypoxic when breathing ether vaporized in air. It also possessed what would later be recognized as a unique property among all inhaled anesthetics: the quality of providing surgical anesthesia without causing respiratory depression. These properties, combined with a slow rate of induction, gave the patient a significant safety margin even in the hands of relatively unskilled anesthetists.[22]

After anesthetizing a pet dog, Morton became confident of his skills and anesthetized patients with ether in his dental office. Encouraged by his success, Morton sought an invitation to give a public demonstration in the Bullfinch amphitheater of the Massachusetts General Hospital (the site where Wells' failed demonstration of the efficacy of nitrous oxide as a complete surgical anesthetic was incorrectly also thought to have occurred).[146] Many details of the October 16, 1846, demonstration are well known. Morton secured permission to provide an anesthetic to Edward Gilbert Abbott, a patient of surgeon John Collins Warren. Warren planned to excise a vascular lesion from the left side of Abbott's neck and was about to proceed when Morton arrived late. He had been delayed because he was obliged to wait for an instrument maker to complete a new inhaler (Fig. 1-1). It consisted of a large glass bulb containing a sponge soaked with oil of orange mixed with ether and a spout that was placed in the patient's mouth. An opening on the opposite side of the bulb allowed air to enter and be drawn over the ether-soaked sponge with each breath.[23]

The conversations of that morning were not accurately recorded; however, popular accounts state that the surgeon responded testily to Morton's apology for his tardy arrival by remarking, "Sir, your patient is ready." Morton directed his attention to his patient and first conducted a much abbreviated preoperative evaluation. He inquired, "Are you afraid?" Abbott responded that he was not and took the inhaler in his mouth. After a few minutes, Morton turned to the surgeon and said, "Sir, your patient is ready." Gilbert Abbott later reported that he was aware of the surgery but experienced no pain. It has been alleged that when the procedure ended, Warren immediately turned to his audience and uttered the statement, "Gentlemen, this is no humbug," but this has since been disputed.[24]

What would be recognized as America's greatest contribution to 19th century medicine had occurred. However, Morton, wishing to capitalize on his "discovery," refused to divulge what agent was in his inhaler. Some weeks passed before Morton admitted that the active component of the colored fluid, which he had called "Letheon," was simple diethyl ether. Morton, Wells, Jackson, and their supporters soon became drawn into a contentious, protracted, and fruitless debate over priority for the discovery. This debate has subsequently been termed *the ether controversy*. In short, Morton had applied for a patent for Letheon and, when it was granted, tried to receive royalties for the use of ether as an anesthetic.

When the details of Morton's anesthetic technique became public knowledge, the information was transmitted by train, stagecoach, and coastal vessels to other North American cities and by ship to the world. As ether was easy to prepare and administer, anesthetics were performed in Britain, France, Russia, South Africa, Australia, and other countries almost as soon as surgeons heard the welcome news of the extraordinary discovery. Even though surgery could now be performed with "pain put to sleep," the frequency of operations did not rise rapidly, and several years would pass before anesthesia was universally recommended.

Chloroform and Obstetrics

James Young Simpson was a successful obstetrician in Edinburgh, Scotland, and among the first to use ether for the relief of labor pain. Dissatisfied with ether, Simpson soon sought a more pleasant, rapid-acting anesthetic. He and his junior associates conducted a bold search by inhaling samples of several volatile chemicals collected for Simpson by British apothecaries. David Waldie suggested chloroform, which had first been prepared in 1831. Simpson and his friends inhaled it after dinner at a party in Simpson's home on the evening of November 4, 1847. They promptly fell unconscious and, when they awoke, were delighted with their success. Simpson quickly set about encouraging the use of chloroform. Within 2 weeks, he submitted his first account of its use for publication in *The Lancet*.

In the 19th century, the relief of obstetric pain had significant social ramifications and made anesthesia during childbirth a controversial subject. Simpson argued against the prevailing view, which held that relieving labor pain opposed God's will. The pain of the parturient was viewed as both a component of punishment and a means of atonement for Original Sin. Less than a year after administering the first anesthesia during childbirth, Simpson addressed these concerns in a pamphlet entitled *Answers to the Religious Objections Advanced Against the Employment of Anaesthetic Agents in Midwifery and Surgery and Obstetrics*. In it, Simpson recognized the Book of Genesis as being the root of this sentiment and noted that God promised to relieve the descendants of Adam and Eve of the curse. In addition, Simpson asserted that labor pain was a result of scientific and anatomic causes and not the result of religious condemnation. He stated that the upright position of humans necessitated strong pelvic muscles to support the abdominal contents. As a result, he argued that the uterus necessarily developed strong musculature to overcome the resistance of the pelvic floor and that great contractile power caused great pain. Simpson's pamphlet probably did not have a significant impact on the prevailing attitudes, but he did articulate many concepts that his contemporaries were debating at the time.[25]

Chloroform gained considerable notoriety after John Snow used it to deliver the last two children of Queen Victoria. The Queen's consort, Prince Albert, interviewed John Snow before he

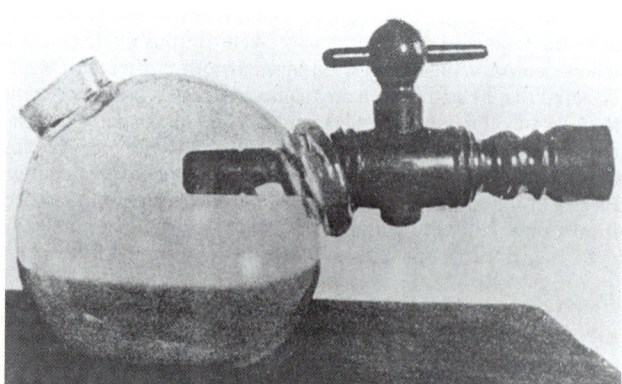

Figure 1-1 Morton's ether inhaler (1846).

was called to Buckingham Palace to administer chloroform at the request of the Queen's obstetrician. During the monarch's labor, Snow gave analgesic doses of chloroform on a folded handkerchief. This technique was soon termed *chloroform à la reine*. Victoria abhorred the pain of childbirth and enjoyed the relief that chloroform provided. She wrote in her journal, "Dr. Snow gave that blessed chloroform and the effect was soothing, quieting, and delightful beyond measure."[26] When the Queen, as head of the Church of England, endorsed obstetric anesthesia, religious debate over the management of labor pain terminated abruptly.

John Snow, already a respected physician, took an interest in anesthetic practice and was soon invited to work with many leading surgeons of the day. In 1848, Snow introduced a chloroform inhaler. He had recognized the versatility of the new agent and came to prefer it in his practice. At the same time, he initiated what was to become an extraordinary series of experiments that were remarkable in their scope and for anticipating sophisticated research performed a century later. Snow realized that successful anesthetics should abolish pain and unwanted movements. He anesthetized several species of animals with varying strengths of ether and chloroform to determine the concentration required to prevent reflex movement from sharp stimuli. This work approximated the modern concept of minimum alveolar concentration.[27] Snow assessed the anesthetic action of a large number of potential anesthetics but did not find any to rival chloroform or ether. His studies led him to recognize the relationship between solubility, vapor pressure, and anesthetic potency, which was not fully appreciated until after World War II. Snow published two remarkable books, *On the Inhalation of the Vapour of Ether* (1847) and *On Chloroform and Other Anaesthetics* (1858). The latter was almost completed when he died of a stroke at the age of 45, and it was published posthumously.

Anesthesia Principles, Equipment, and Standards

Control of the Airway

Definitive control of the airway, a skill anesthesiologists now consider paramount, developed only after many harrowing and apneic episodes spurred the development of safer airway management techniques. Preceding tracheal intubation, however, several important techniques were proposed toward the end of the 19th century that remain integral to anesthesiology education and practice. Joseph Clover was the first Englishman to urge the now-universal practice of thrusting the patient's jaw forward to overcome obstruction of the upper airway by the tongue. Clover also published a landmark case report in 1877 in which he created a surgical airway. Once his patient was asleep, Clover discovered that his patient had a tumor of the mouth that obstructed the airway completely, despite his trusted jaw-thrust maneuver. He averted disaster by inserting a small curved cannula of his design through the cricothyroid membrane. He continued anesthesia via the cannula until the tumor was excised. Clover, the model of the prepared anesthesiologist, remarked, "I have never used the cannula before although it has been my companion at some thousands of anaesthetic cases."[28]

Tracheal Intubation

The development of techniques and instruments for tracheal intubation ranks among the major advances in the history of anesthesiology. The first tracheal tubes were developed for the resuscitation of drowning victims but were not used in anesthesia until 1878. The first use of elective oral intubation for an anesthetic was undertaken by Scottish surgeon William Macewan. He had practiced passing flexible metal tubes through the larynx of a cadaver before attempting the maneuver on an awake patient with an oral tumor at the Glasgow Royal Infirmary on July 5, 1878.[29] Because topical anesthesia was not yet known, the experience must have demanded fortitude on the part of Macewan's patient. Once the tube was correctly positioned, an assistant began a chloroform–air anesthetic via the tube. Once anesthetized, the patient soon stopped coughing. Unfortunately, Macewan abandoned the practice following a fatality in which a patient had been successfully intubated while awake but the tube became dislodged once the patient was asleep. After the tube was removed, an attempt to provide chloroform by mask anesthesia was unsuccessful and the patient died.

An American surgeon named Joseph O'Dwyer is remembered for his extraordinary dedication to the advancement of tracheal intubation. In 1885, O'Dwyer designed a series of metal laryngeal tubes, which he inserted blindly between the vocal cords of children suffering a diphtheritic crisis. Three years later, O'Dwyer designed a second rigid tube with a conical tip that occluded the larynx so effectively that it could be used for artificial ventilation when applied with the bellows and T-piece tube designed by George Fell. The Fell–O'Dwyer apparatus, as it came to be known, was used during thoracic surgery by Rudolph Matas of New Orleans. Matas was so pleased with it that he predicted, "The procedure that promises the most benefit in preventing pulmonary collapse in operations on the chest is ... the rhythmical maintenance of artificial respiration by a tube in the glottis directly connected with a bellows."[147]

After O'Dwyer's death, the outstanding pioneer of tracheal intubation was Franz Kuhn, a surgeon of Kassel, Germany. From 1900 until 1912, Kuhn[148] published several articles and a classic monograph, "*Die perorale Intubation*," which were not well known in his lifetime but have since become widely appreciated. His work might have had a more profound impact if it had been translated into English. Kuhn described techniques of oral and nasal intubation that he performed with flexible metal tubes composed of coiled tubing similar to those now used for the spout of metal gasoline cans. After applying cocaine to the airway, Kuhn introduced his tube over a curved metal stylet that he directed toward the larynx with his left index finger. Although he was aware of the subglottic cuffs that had been used briefly by Victor Eisenmenger, Kuhn preferred to seal the larynx by positioning a supralaryngeal flange near the tube's tip before packing the pharynx with gauze. Kuhn even monitored the patient's breath sounds continuously through a monaural earpiece connected to an extension of the tracheal tube by a narrow tube.

Intubation of the trachea by palpation was an uncertain and sometimes traumatic act; surgeons even believed that it would be anatomically impossible to visualize the vocal cords directly. This misapprehension was overcome in 1895 by Alfred Kirstein in Berlin, who devised the first direct-vision laryngoscope.[30] Kirstein was motivated by a friend's report that a patient's trachea had been accidentally intubated during esophagoscopy. Kirstein promptly fabricated a handheld instrument that at first resembled a shortened cylindrical esophagoscope. He soon substituted a semicircular blade that opened inferiorly. Kirstein could now examine the larynx while standing behind his seated patient, whose head had been placed in an attitude approximating the currently termed "sniffing position." Although Alfred Kirstein's "autoscope" was not used by anesthesiologists, it was the forerunner of all modern laryngoscopes. Endoscopy was refined by Chevalier Jackson in Philadelphia, who designed a

U-shaped laryngoscope by adding a handgrip that was parallel to the blade. The Jackson blade has remained a standard instrument for endoscopists but was not favored by anesthesiologists. Two laryngoscopes that closely resembled modern L-shaped instruments were designed in 1910 and 1913 by two American surgeons, Henry Janeway and George Dorrance, but neither instrument achieved lasting use despite their excellent designs.[31]

Before the introduction of muscle relaxants in the 1940s, intubation of the trachea could be challenging. This challenge was made somewhat easier, however, with the advent of laryngoscope blades specifically designed to increase visualization of the vocal cords. Robert Miller of San Antonio, Texas, and Robert Macintosh of Oxford University created their respectively named blades within an interval of 2 years. In 1941, Miller brought forward the slender, straight blade with a slight curve near the tip to ease the passage of the tube through the larynx. Although Miller's blade was a refinement, the technique of its use was identical to that of earlier models as the epiglottis was lifted to expose the larynx.[32]

The Macintosh blade, which is placed in the vallecula rather than under the epiglottis, was invented as an incidental result of a tonsillectomy. Sir Robert Macintosh later described the circumstances of its discovery in an appreciation writing regarding the career of his technician, Mr. Richard Salt, who constructed the blade. As Sir Robert recalled, "A Boyle-Davis gag, a size larger than intended, was inserted for tonsillectomy, and when the mouth was fully opened the cords came into view. This was a surprise since conventional laryngoscopy, at that depth of anaesthesia, would have been impossible in those pre-relaxant days. Within a matter of hours, Salt had modified the blade of the Davis gag and attached a laryngoscope handle to it; and streamlined (after testing several models), the end result came into widespread use."[33] Macintosh underestimated the popularity of the blade, as more than 800,000 have been produced and many special-purpose versions have been marketed.

The most distinguished innovator in tracheal intubation was the self-trained British anesthetist Ivan (later, Sir Ivan) Magill.[34] In 1919, while serving in the Royal Army as a general medical officer, Magill was assigned to a military hospital near London. Although he had only rudimentary training in anesthesia, Magill was obliged to accept an assignment to the anesthesia service, where he worked with another neophyte, Stanley Rowbotham.[35] Together, Magill and Rowbotham attended casualties disfigured by severe facial injuries who underwent repeated restorative operations. These procedures required that the surgeon, Harold Gillies, have unrestricted access to the face and airway. These patients presented formidable challenges, but both Magill and Rowbotham became adept at tracheal intubation and quickly understood its current limitations. Because they learned from fortuitous observations, they soon extended the scope of tracheal anesthesia.

They gained expertise with blind nasal intubation after they learned to soften semirigid insufflation tubes for passage through the nostril. Even though their original intent was to position the tips of the nasal tubes in the posterior pharynx, the slender tubes frequently ended up in the trachea. Stimulated by this chance experience, they developed techniques of deliberate nasotracheal intubation. In 1920, Magill devised an aid to manipulating the catheter tip, the "Magill angulated forceps," which continues to be manufactured according to his original design over 90 years ago.

With the war over, Magill entered civilian practice and set out to develop a wide-bore tube that would resist kinking but be conformable to the contours of the upper airway. While in a hardware store, he found mineralized red rubber tubing that he cut, beveled, and smoothed to produce tubes that clinicians around the world would come to call "Magill tubes." His tubes remained the universal standard for more than 40 years until rubber products were supplanted by inert plastics. Magill also rediscovered the advantage of applying cocaine to the nasal mucosa, a technique that greatly facilitated awake blind nasal intubation.

In 1926, Arthur Guedel began a series of experiments that led to the introduction of the cuffed tube. Guedel transformed the basement of his Indianapolis home into a laboratory, where he subjected each step of the preparation and application of his cuffs to a vigorous review.[36] He fashioned cuffs from the rubber of dental dams, condoms, and surgical gloves that were glued onto the outer wall of tubes. Using animal tracheas donated by the family butcher as his model, he considered whether the cuff should be positioned above, below, or at the level of the vocal cords. He recommended that the cuff be positioned just below the vocal cords to seal the airway. Ralph Waters later recommended that cuffs be constructed of two layers of soft rubber cemented together. These detachable cuffs were first manufactured by Waters' children, who sold them to the Foregger Company.

Guedel sought ways to show the safety and utility of the cuffed tube. He first filled the mouth of an anesthetized and intubated patient with water and showed that the cuff sealed the airway. Even though this exhibition was successful, he searched for a more dramatic technique to capture the attention of those unfamiliar with the advantages of intubation. He reasoned that if the cuff prevented water from entering the trachea of an intubated patient, it should also prevent an animal from drowning, even if it were submerged under water. To encourage physicians attending a medical convention to use his tracheal techniques, Guedel prepared the first of several "dunked dog" demonstrations (Fig. 1-2). An anesthetized and intubated dog, Guedel's own pet, "Airway," was immersed in an aquarium. After the demonstration was completed, the anesthetic was discontinued before the animal was removed from the water. According to legend, Airway awoke promptly, shook water over the onlookers, saluted a post, then trotted from the hall to the applause of the audience.

After a patient experienced an accidental endobronchial intubation, Ralph Waters reasoned that a very long cuffed tube could be used to isolate the lungs. The dependent lung could be ventilated while the upper lung was being resected.[37] On learning of his friend's success with intentional one-lung anesthesia, Arthur Guedel proposed an important modification for chest surgery, the double-cuffed single-lumen tube, which was introduced by Emery Rovenstine. These tubes were easily

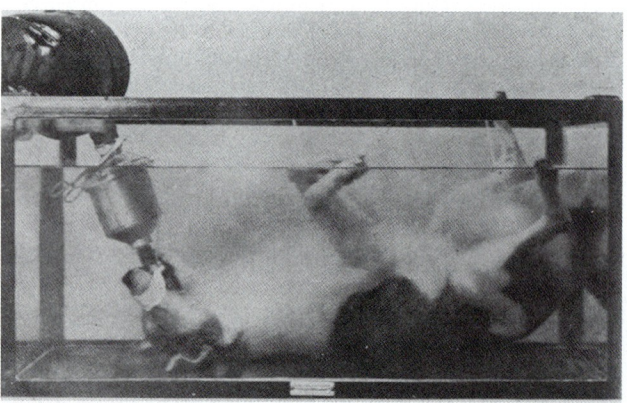

Figure 1-2 The "dunked dog."

positioned, an advantage over bronchial blockers that had to be inserted by a skilled bronchoscopist. In 1953, single-lumen tubes were supplanted by double-lumen endobronchial tubes. The double-lumen tube currently most popular was designed by Frank Robertshaw of Manchester, England, and is prepared in both right- and left-sided versions. Robertshaw tubes were first manufactured from mineralized red rubber but are now made of extruded plastic, a technique refined by David Sheridan. Sheridan was also the first person to embed centimeter markings along the side of tracheal tubes, a safety feature that reduced the risk of the tube's being incorrectly positioned.

Advanced Airway Devices

Conventional laryngoscopes proved inadequate for patients with "difficult airways." A few clinicians credit harrowing intubating experiences as the incentive for invention. In 1928, a rigid bronchoscope was specifically designed for examination of the large airways. Rigid bronchoscopes were refined and used by pulmonologists. Although it was known in 1870 that a thread of glass could transmit light along its length, technologic limitations were not overcome until 1964, when Shigeto Ikeda developed the first flexible fiberoptic bronchoscope. Fiberoptic-assisted tracheal intubation has become a common approach in the management of patients with difficult airways having surgery.

Roger Bullard desired a device to simultaneously examine the larynx and intubate the vocal cords. He had been frustrated by failed attempts to visualize the larynx of a patient with Pierre-Robin syndrome. In response, he developed the Bullard laryngoscope, whose fiberoptic bundles lie beside a curved blade. Similarly, the Wu-scope was designed by Tzu-Lang Wu in 1994 to combine and facilitate visualization and intubation of the trachea in patients with difficult airways.[38]

Dr. A. I. J. "Archie" Brain first recognized the principle of the laryngeal mask airway (LMA) in 1981 when, like many British clinicians, he provided dental anesthesia via a Goldman nasal mask. However, unlike any before him, he realized that just as the dental mask could be fitted closely about the nose, a comparable mask attached to a wide-bore tube might be positioned around the larynx. He not only conceived of this radical departure in airway management, which he first described in 1983,[39] but also spent years in single-handedly fabricating and testing several incremental modifications. Scores of Brain's prototypes are displayed in the Royal Berkshire Hospital, Reading, England, where they provide a detailed record of the evolution of the LMA. He fabricated his first models from Magill tubes and Goldman masks, then refined their shape by performing postmortem studies of the hypopharynx to determine the form of cuff that would be most functional. Before silicone rubber was selected, Brain had even mastered the technique of forming masks from liquid latex. Every detail of the LMA, the number and position of the aperture bars and the shape and the size of the masks, required repeated modification.[40]

Early Anesthesia Delivery Systems

The transition from ether inhalers and chloroform-soaked handkerchiefs to more sophisticated anesthesia delivery equipment occurred gradually, with incremental advances supplanting older methods. One of the earliest anesthesia apparatus designs was that of John Snow, who had realized the inadequacies of ether inhalers through which patients rebreathed via a mouthpiece. After practicing anesthesia for only 2 weeks, Snow created the first of his series of ingenious ether inhalers.[41] His best-known apparatus featured unidirectional valves within a malleable, well-fitting mask of his own design, which closely resembles the form of a modern face mask. The face piece was connected to the vaporizer by a breathing tube, which Snow deliberately designed to be wider than the human trachea so that even rapid respirations would not be impeded. A metal coil within the vaporizer ensured that the patient's inspired breath was drawn over a large surface area to promote the uptake of ether. The device also incorporated a warm water bath to maintain the volatility of the agent (Fig. 1-3). Snow did not attempt to capitalize on his creativity, in contrast to William Morton; he closed his account of its preparation with the generous observation, "There is no restriction respecting the making of it."[42]

Joseph Clover, another British physician, was the first anesthetist to administer chloroform in known concentrations through the "Clover bag." He obtained a 4.5% concentration of chloroform in air by pumping a measured volume of air with a bellows through a warmed evaporating vessel containing a known volume of liquid chloroform.[43] Although it was realized that nitrous oxide diluted in air often gave a hypoxic mixture and that the oxygen–nitrous oxide mixture was safer, Chicago surgeon Edmund Andrews complained about the physical limitations of delivering anesthesia to patients in their homes. The large bag was conspicuous and awkward to carry along busy streets. He observed that

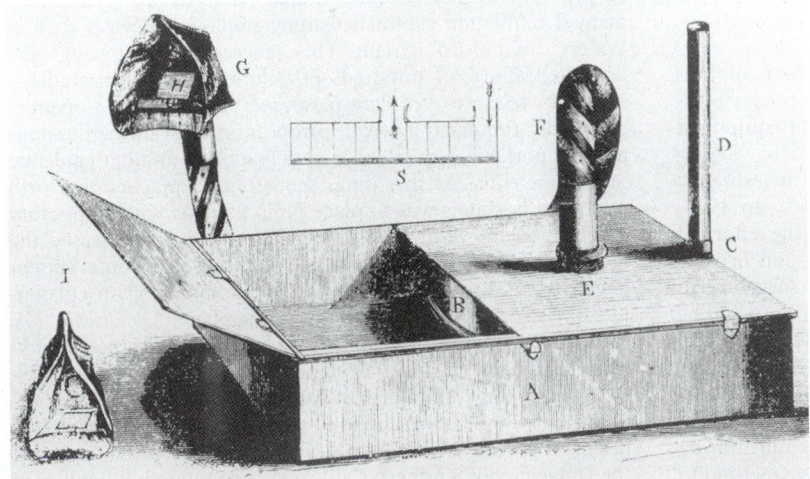

Figure 1-3 John Snow's inhaler (1847). The ether chamber (*B*) contained a spiral coil so that the air entering through the brass tube (*D*) was saturated by ether before ascending the flexible tube (*F*) to the face mask (*G*). The ether chamber rested in a bath of warm water (*A*).

"In city practice, among the higher classes, however, this is no obstacle as the bag can always be taken in a carriage, without attracting attention."[44] In 1872, Andrews was delighted to report the availability of liquefied nitrous oxide compressed under 750 pounds of pressure, which allowed a supply sufficient for three patients to be carried in a single cylinder.

Critical to increasing patient safety was the development of a machine capable of delivering a calibrated amount of gas and volatile anesthetic. In the late 19th century, demands in dentistry instigated development of the first freestanding anesthesia machines. Three American dentist-entrepreneurs, Samuel S. White, Charles Teter, and Jay Heidbrink, developed the original series of US instruments that used compressed cylinders of nitrous oxide and oxygen. Before 1900, the S. S. White Company modified Frederick Hewitt's apparatus and marketed its continuous-flow machine, which was refined by Teter in 1903. Heidbrink added reducing valves in 1912. In the same year, physicians initiated other important developments. Water–bubble flowmeters, introduced by Frederick Cotton and Walter Boothby of Harvard University, allowed the proportion of gases and their flow rate to be approximated. The Cotton and Boothby apparatus was transformed into a practical portable machine by James Tayloe Gwathmey of New York. The Gwathmey machine caught the attention of London anesthetist Henry E. G. "Cockie" Boyle, who acknowledged his debt to the American when he incorporated Gwathmey's concepts in the first of the series of "Boyle" machines that were marketed by Coxeter and British Oxygen Corporation. During the same period in Lubeck, Germany, Heinrich Draeger and his son, Bernhaard, adapted compressed gas technology, which they had originally developed for mine rescue equipment, to manufacture ether and chloroform–oxygen machines.

In the years after World War I, several US manufacturers continued to bring forward widely admired anesthesia machines. Richard von Foregger was an engineer who was exceptionally receptive to clinicians' suggestions for additional features for his machines. Elmer McKesson became one of the country's first specialists in anesthesiology in 1910 and developed a series of gas machines. In an era of flammable anesthetics, McKesson carried nitrous oxide anesthesia to its therapeutic limit by performing inductions with 100% nitrous oxide and thereafter adding small volumes of oxygen. If the resultant cyanosis became too profound, McKesson depressed a valve on his machine that flushed a small volume of oxygen into the circuit. Even though his techniques of primary and secondary saturation with nitrous oxide are no longer used, the oxygen flush valve is part of McKesson's legacy.

Alternative Circuits

A valveless device, the Ayre's T-piece, has found wide application in the management of intubated patients. Phillip Ayre practiced anesthesia in England when the limitations of equipment for pediatric patients produced what he described as "a protracted and sanguine battle between surgeon and anaesthetist, with the poor unfortunate baby as the battlefield."[45] In 1937, Ayre introduced his valveless T-piece to reduce the effort of breathing in neurosurgical patients. The T-piece soon became particularly popular for cleft palate repairs, as the surgeon had free access to the mouth. Positive-pressure ventilation could be achieved when the anesthetist obstructed the expiratory limb. In time, this ingenious, lightweight, nonrebreathing device evolved through more than 100 modifications for a variety of special situations. A significant alteration was Gordon Jackson Rees' circuit, which permitted improved control of ventilation by substituting a breathing bag on the outflow limb.[46] An alternative method to reduce the amount of equipment near the patient is provided by the coaxial circuit of the Bain–Spoerel apparatus.[47] This lightweight tube-within-a-tube has served very well in many circumstances since its Canadian innovators described it in 1972.

Ventilators

Mechanical ventilators are now an integral part of the anesthesia machine. Patients are ventilated during general anesthesia by electrical or gas-powered devices that are simple to control yet sophisticated in their function. The history of mechanical positive-pressure ventilation began with attempts to resuscitate victims of drowning by a bellows attached to a mask or tracheal tube. These experiments found little role in anesthetic care for many years. At the beginning of the 20th century, however, several modalities were explored before intermittent positive-pressure machines evolved.

A series of artificial environments were created in response to the frustration experienced by thoracic surgeons who found that the lung collapsed when they incised the pleura. Between 1900 and 1910, continuous positive- or negative-pressure devices were created to maintain inflation of the lungs of a spontaneously breathing patient once the chest was opened. Brauer (1904) and Murphy (1905) placed the patient's head and neck in a box in which positive pressure was continually maintained. Sauerbruch (1904) created a negative-pressure operating chamber encompassing both the surgical team and the patient's body and from which only the patient's head projected.[48]

In 1907, the first intermittent positive-pressure device, the Draeger "Pulmotor," was developed to rhythmically inflate the lungs. This instrument and later American models such as the E & J Resuscitator were used almost exclusively by firefighters and mine rescue workers. In 1934, a Swedish team developed the "Spiropulsator," which C. Crafoord later modified for use during cyclopropane anesthesia.[49] Its action was controlled by a magnetic control valve called *the flasher*, a type first used to provide intermittent gas flow for the lights of navigational buoys. When Trier Morch, a Danish anesthesiologist, could not obtain a Spiropulsator during World War II, he fabricated the Morch "Respirator," which used a piston pump to rhythmically deliver a fixed volume of gas to the patient.[48]

A major stimulus to the development of ventilators came as a consequence of a devastating epidemic of poliomyelitis that struck Copenhagen, Denmark, in 1952. As scores of patients were admitted, the only effective ventilatory support that could be provided to patients with bulbar paralysis was continuous manual ventilation via tracheostomy employing devices such as Waters' "to-and-fro" circuit. This succeeded only through the dedicated efforts of hundreds of volunteers. Medical students served in relays to ventilate paralyzed patients. The Copenhagen crisis stimulated a broad European interest in the development of portable ventilators in anticipation of another epidemic of poliomyelitis. At this time, the common practice in North American hospitals was to place polio patients with respiratory involvement in "iron lungs," metal cylinders that encased the body below the neck. Inspiration was caused by intermittent negative pressure created by an electric motor acting on a piston-like device occupying the foot of the chamber.

Some early American ventilators were adaptations of respiratory-assist machines originally designed for the delivery of aerosolized drugs for respiratory therapy. Two types employed the Bennett or Bird "flow-sensitive" valves. The Bennett valve was designed during World War II when a team of physiologists at the University of Southern California encountered difficulties in separating inspiration from expiration in an experimental apparatus designed to provide positive-pressure breathing for aviators at high altitude. An engineer, Ray Bennett, visited their laboratory, observed their problem, and resolved it with a mechanical flow-sensitive automatic valve. A second valving mechanism was later designed by an aeronautical engineer, Forrest Bird.

The use of the Bird and Bennett valves gained anesthetic application when the gas flow from the valve was directed into a rigid plastic jar containing a breathing bag or bellows as part of an anesthesia circuit. These "bag-in-bottle" devices mimicked the action of the clinician's hand as the gas flow compressed the bag, thereby providing positive-pressure inspiration. Passive exhalation was promoted by the descent of a weight on the bag or bellows.

Carbon Dioxide Absorption

Carbon dioxide (CO_2) absorption is a basic element of modern anesthetic machines. It was initially developed to allow rebreathing of gas and minimize loss of flammable gases into the room, thereby reducing the risk of explosion. In current practice, it permits decreased utilization of oxygen and anesthetic, thus reducing cost. The first CO_2 absorber in anesthesia came in 1906 from the work of Franz Kuhn, a German surgeon. His use of canisters developed for mine rescues by Draeger was innovative, but his circuit had unfortunate limitations. The exceptionally narrow breathing tubes and a large dead space explain its very limited use, and Kuhn's device was ignored.

A few years later, the first American machine with a CO_2 absorber was independently fabricated by a pharmacologist named Dennis Jackson. In 1915, Jackson developed an early technique of CO_2 absorption that permitted the use of a closed anesthesia circuit. He used solutions of sodium and calcium hydroxide to absorb CO_2. As his laboratory was located in an area of St. Louis, Missouri, heavily laden with coal smoke, Jackson reported that the apparatus allowed him the first breaths of absolutely fresh air he had ever enjoyed in that city. The complexity of Jackson's apparatus limited its use in hospital practice, but his pioneering work in this field encouraged Ralph Waters to introduce a simpler device using soda lime granules nine years later. Waters positioned a soda lime canister (Fig. 1-4) between a face mask and an adjacent breathing bag to which was attached the fresh gas flow. As long as the mask was held against the face, only small volumes of fresh gas flow were required and no valves were needed.[50]

Waters' device featured awkward positioning of the canister close to the patient's face. Brian Sword[51] overcame this limitation in 1930 with a freestanding machine with unidirectional valves to create a circle system and an inline CO_2 absorber. James Elam and his coworkers at the Roswell Park Cancer Institute in Buffalo, New York, further refined the CO_2 absorber, increasing the efficiency of CO_2 removal with a minimum of resistance for breathing.[52] Consequently, the circle system introduced by Sword in the 1930s, with a few refinements, became the standard anesthesia circuit in North America.

Flowmeters

As closed and semiclosed circuits became practical, gas flow could be measured with greater accuracy. Bubble flowmeters were replaced with dry bobbins or ball-bearing flowmeters, which, although they did not leak fluids, could cause inaccurate measurements if they adhered to the glass column. In 1910, M. Neu had been the first to apply rotameters in anesthesia for the administration of nitrous oxide and oxygen, but his machine

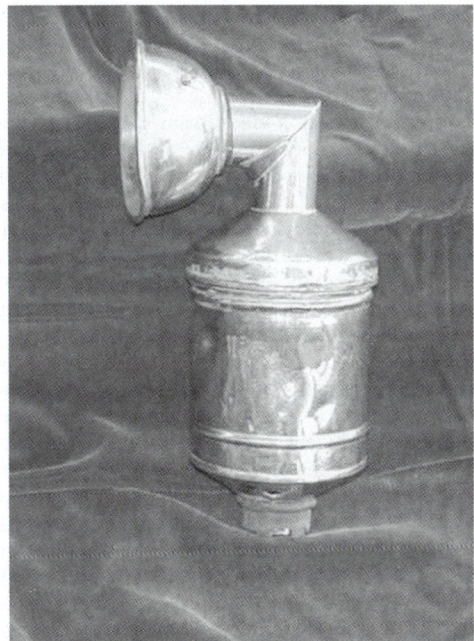

Figure 1-4 Waters' carbon dioxide absorbance canister.

was not a commercial success, perhaps because of the great cost of nitrous oxide in Germany at that time. Rotameters designed for use in German industry were first employed in Britain in 1937 by Richard Salt; but as World War II approached, the English were denied access to these sophisticated flowmeters. After World War II rotameters became regularly employed in British anesthesia machines, although most American equipment still featured nonrotating floats. The now-universal practice of displaying gas flow in liters per minute was not a customary part of all American machines until more than a decade after World War II.

Vaporizers

The art of a smooth induction with a potent anesthetic was a great challenge, particularly if the inspired concentration could not be determined with accuracy. Even the clinical introduction of halothane after 1956 might have been thwarted except for a fortunate coincidence: the prior development of calibrated vaporizers. Two types of calibrated vaporizers designed for other anesthetics had become available in the half decade before halothane was marketed. The prompt acceptance of halothane was in part because of an ability to provide it in carefully titrated concentrations.

The Copper Kettle was the first temperature-compensated, accurate vaporizer. It had been developed by Lucien Morris at the University of Wisconsin in response to Ralph Waters' plan to test chloroform by giving it in controlled concentrations.[53] Morris achieved this goal by passing a metered flow of oxygen through a vaporizer chamber that contained a sintered bronze disk to separate the oxygen into minute bubbles. The gas became fully saturated with anesthetic vapor as it percolated through the liquid. The concentration of the anesthetic inspired by the patient could be calculated by knowing the vapor pressure of the liquid anesthetic, the volume of oxygen flowing through the liquid, and the total volume of gases from all sources entering the anesthesia circuit. Although experimental models of Morris' vaporizer used a water bath to maintain vaporizer temperature stability, the excellent thermal conductivity of copper, especially when the device was attached to a metal anesthetic machine, was substituted in later models. When first marketed, the Copper Kettle did not feature a mechanism to indicate changes in the temperature (and vapor pressure) of the liquid. Shuh-Hsun Ngai proposed the incorporation of a thermometer, a suggestion that was later added to all vaporizers of that class.[54] The Copper Kettle (Foregger Company) and the Vernitrol (Ohio Medical Products) were universal vaporizers that could be charged with any anesthetic liquid, and, provided that its vapor pressure and temperature were known, the inspired concentration could be calculated quickly.

When halothane was first marketed in Britain, an effective temperature-compensated, agent-specific vaporizer had recently been placed in clinical use. The TECOTA (TEmperature COmpensated Trichloroethylene Air) vaporizer featured a bimetallic strip composed of brass and a nickel–steel alloy, two metals with different coefficients of expansion. As the anesthetic vapor cooled, the strip bent to move away from the orifice, thereby permitting more fresh gas to enter the vaporizing chamber. This maintained a constant inspired concentration despite changes in temperature and vapor pressure. After their TECOTA vaporizer was accepted into anesthetic practice, the technology was used to create the "Fluotec," the first of a series of agent-specific "tec" vaporizers for use in the operating room.

Patient Monitors

In many ways, the history of late-19th and early-20th century anesthesiology is the quest for the safest anesthetic. The discovery and widespread use of electrocardiography, pulse oximetry, blood gas analysis, capnography, and neuromuscular blockade monitoring have reduced patient morbidity and mortality and revolutionized anesthesia practice. Although safer machines assured clinicians that appropriate gas mixtures were delivered to the patient, monitors provided an early warning of acute physiologic deterioration before patients suffered irrevocable damage.

Joseph Clover was one of the first clinicians to routinely perform basic hemodynamic monitoring. Clover developed the habit of monitoring his patients' pulse, but, surprisingly, this was a contentious issue at the time. Prominent Scottish surgeons scorned Clover's emphasis on the action of chloroform on the heart. Baron Lister and others preferred that senior medical students give anesthetics and urged them to "strictly carry out certain simple instructions, among which is that of never touching the pulse, in order that their attention may not be distracted from the respiration."[55] Lister also counseled, "it appears that preliminary examination of the chest, often considered indispensable, is quite unnecessary, and more likely to induce the dreaded syncope, by alarming the patients, than to avert it."[56] Little progress in anesthesia could come from such reactionary statements. In contrast, Clover had observed the effect of chloroform on animals and urged other anesthetists to monitor the pulse at all times and to discontinue the anesthetic temporarily if any irregularity or weakness was observed in the strength of the pulse.

Two American surgeons, George W. Crile and Harvey Cushing, developed a strong interest in measuring blood pressure during anesthesia. Both men wrote thorough and detailed examinations of blood pressure monitoring; however, Cushing's contribution is better remembered because he was the first American to apply the Riva Rocci cuff, which he saw while visiting Italy. Cushing introduced the concept in 1902 and had blood pressure measurements recorded on anesthesia records.[57] In 1894, Cushing and a fellow student at Harvard Medical School, Charles Codman, initiated a system of recording patients' pulses to assess the course of the anesthetics they administered. In 1902, Cushing continued the practice of monitoring and recording patient blood pressures and pulses. The transition from manual to automated blood pressure devices, which first appeared in 1936 and operate on an oscillometric principle, has been gradual.

The first precordial stethoscope was believed to have been used by S. Griffith Davis at Johns Hopkins University.[41] He adapted a technique developed by Harvey Cushing in a laboratory in which dogs with surgically induced valvular lesions had stethoscopes attached to their chest wall so that medical students might listen to bruits characteristic of a specific malformation. Davis' technique was forgotten but was rehabilitated by Dr. Robert Smith, an energetic pioneer of pediatric anesthesiology in Boston in the 1940s. A Canadian contemporary, Albert Codesmith, of the Hospital for Sick Children, Toronto, became frustrated by the repeated dislodging of the chest piece under the surgical drapes and fabricated his first esophageal stethoscope from urethral catheters and Penrose drains. His brief report heralded its clinical role as a monitor of both normal and adventitious respiratory and cardiac sounds.[58]

Electrocardiography, Pulse Oximetry, and Capnography

Clinical electrocardiography began with Willem Einthoven's application of the string galvanometer in 1903. Within two decades, Thomas Lewis had described its role in the diagnosis of disturbances of cardiac rhythm, whereas James Herrick and Harold Pardee first drew attention to the changes produced by myocardial ischemia. After 1928, cathode ray oscilloscopes were available, but the risk of explosion owing to the presence of flammable anesthetics forestalled the introduction of the electrocardiogram into routine anesthetic practice until after World War II. At that time, the small screen of the heavily shielded "bullet" oscilloscope displayed only 3 seconds of data, but that information was highly prized.

Pulse oximetry, the optical measurement of oxygen saturation in tissues, is one of the more recent additions to the anesthesiologist's array of routine monitors. Although research in this area began in 1932, its first practical application came during World War II. An American physiologist, Glen Millikan, responded to a request from British colleagues in aviation research. Millikan set about preparing a series of devices to improve the supply of oxygen that was provided to pilots flying at high altitude in unpressurized aircraft. To monitor oxygen delivery and to prevent the pilot from succumbing to an unrecognized failure of his oxygen supply, Millikan created an oxygen-sensing monitor worn on the pilot's earlobe and coined the name *oximeter* to describe its action. Before his tragic death in a climbing accident in 1947, Millikan had begun to assess anesthetic applications of oximetry. Refinements of oximetry by a Japanese engineer, Takuo Aoyagi, led to the development of pulse oximetry. As John Severinghaus recounted the episode, Aoyagi had attempted to eliminate the changes in a signal caused by pulsatile variations when he realized that this fluctuation could be used to measure both the pulse and oxygen saturation.[56]

Anesthesiologists have recognized a need for breath-by-breath measurement of respiratory and anesthetic gases. After 1954, infrared absorption techniques gave immediate displays of the exhaled concentration of CO_2. The ability to confirm endotracheal intubation and monitor ventilation, as reflected by concentrations of

CO_2 in respired gas, began in 1943. At that time, Luft[59] described the principle of infrared absorption by CO_2 and developed an apparatus for measurement. Routine application of capnography in anesthesia practice was pioneered by Smalhout and Kalenda in the Netherlands. Breath-to-breath continuous monitoring and a waveform display of CO_2 levels help anesthesiologists recognize abnormalities in metabolism, ventilation, and circulation. More recently, infrared analysis has been perfected to enable breath-by-breath measurement of anesthetic gases as well. This technology has largely replaced mass spectrometry, which initially had only industrial applications before Albert Faulconer of the Mayo Clinic first used it to monitor the concentration of an exhaled anesthetic in 1954.

Safety Standards

The introduction of safety features was coordinated by the American National Standards Institute (ANSI) Committee Z79, which was sponsored from 1956 until 1983 by the American Society of Anesthesiologists. Since 1983, representatives from industry, government, and health-care professions have met on Committee Z79 of the American Society for Testing and Materials. They establish voluntary goals that may become accepted national standards for the safety of anesthesia equipment.

Ralph Tovell voiced the first call for standards during World War II while he was the US Army Consultant in Anesthesiology for Europe. Tovell found that because there were four different dimensions for connectors, tubes, masks, and breathing bags, supplies dispatched to field hospitals might not match their anesthesia machines. As Tovell[60] observed, "When a sudden need for accessory equipment arose, nurses and corpsmen were likely to respond to it by bringing parts that would not fit." Although Tovell's reports did not gain an immediate response, after the war Vincent Collins and Hamilton Davis took up his concern and formed ANSI Committee Z79. One of the committee's most active members, Leslie Rendell-Baker,[61] wrote an account of the committee's domestic and international achievements. He reported that Tovell encouraged all manufacturers to select the now-uniform orifice of 22 mm for all adult and pediatric face masks and to make every tracheal tube connector 15 mm in diameter. For the first time, a Z79-designed mask-tube elbow adapter would fit every mask and tracheal tube connector.

The Z79 Committee introduced other advances. Tracheal tubes of nontoxic plastic bear a Z79 or IT (implantation tested) mark. The committee also mandated touch identification of the oxygen flow control knob on the anesthesia machine at the suggestion of Roderick Calverley,[62] which reduced the risk that the wrong gas would be selected before internal mechanical controls prevented the selection of a hypoxic mixture. Pin indexing reduced the hazard of attaching a wrong cylinder in the place of oxygen. Diameter indexing of connectors prevented similar errors in high-pressure tubing. For many years, however, errors committed in reassembling hospital oxygen supply lines led to a series of tragedies before polarographic oxygen analyzers were added to the inspiratory limb of the anesthesia circuit.

The History of Anesthetic Agents and Adjuvants

Inhaled Anesthetics

Throughout the second half of the 19th century, other compounds were examined for their anesthetic potential. The pattern of fortuitous discovery that brought nitrous oxide, diethyl ether, and chloroform forward between 1844 and 1847 continued. The next inhaled anesthetics to be used routinely, ethyl chloride and ethylene, were also discovered as a result of unexpected observations. Ethyl chloride and ethylene were first formulated in the 18th century. Ethyl chloride was used as a topical anesthetic and counterirritant; it was so volatile that the skin transiently "froze" after ethyl chloride was sprayed on it. Its rediscovery as an anesthetic came in 1894, when a Swedish dentist named Carlson sprayed ethyl chloride into a patient's mouth to "freeze" a dental abscess. Carlson was surprised to discover that his patient suddenly lost consciousness.

As the mechanisms to deliver drugs were refined, entirely new classes of medications were also developed, with the intention of providing safer, more pleasant pain control. Ethylene gas was the first alternative to ether and chloroform, but it had some major disadvantages. The rediscovery of ethylene in 1923 also came from a serendipitous observation. After it was learned that ethylene gas had been used to inhibit the opening of carnation buds in Chicago greenhouses, it was speculated that a gas that put flowers to sleep might also have an anesthetic action on humans. Arno Luckhardt was the first to publish a clinical study in February 1923. Within a month, Isabella Herb in Chicago and W. Easson Brown in Toronto presented two other independent studies. Ethylene was not a successful anesthetic because high concentrations were required and it was explosive. An additional significant shortcoming was a particularly unpleasant smell, which could only be partially disguised by the use of oil of orange or a cheap perfume. When cyclopropane was introduced, ethylene was abandoned.

The anesthetic action of cyclopropane was inadvertently discovered in 1929.[63] Brown and Henderson had previously shown that propylene had desirable properties as an anesthetic when freshly prepared, but after storage in a steel cylinder, it deteriorated to create a toxic material that produced nausea and cardiac irregularities in humans. Velyien Henderson, a professor of pharmacology at the University of Toronto, suggested that the toxic product be identified. After a chemist, George Lucas, identified cyclopropane among the chemicals in the tank, he prepared a sample in low concentration with oxygen and administered it to two kittens. The animals fell asleep quietly but quickly recovered unharmed. Rather than being a toxic contaminant, Lucas saw that cyclopropane was a potent anesthetic. After its effects in other animals were studied and cyclopropane proved to be stable after storage, human experimentation began.

Henderson was the first volunteer; Lucas followed. They then arranged a public demonstration in which Frederick Banting, a Nobel Laureate for the discovery of insulin, was anesthetized before a group of physicians. Despite this promising beginning, further research was abruptly halted. Several anesthetic deaths in Toronto had been attributed to ethyl chloride, and concern about Canadian clinical trials of cyclopropane prevented human studies from proceeding. Rather than abandon the study, Henderson encouraged an American friend, Ralph Waters, to use cyclopropane at the University of Wisconsin. The Wisconsin group investigated the drug thoroughly and reported their clinical success in 1934.[64]

In 1930, Chauncey Leake and MeiYu Chen performed successful laboratory trials of Vinethene (divinyl ether) but were thwarted in its further development by a professor of surgery in San Francisco. Ironically, Canadians, who had lost cyclopropane to Wisconsin, learned of Vinethene from Leake and Chen in California and conducted the first human study in 1932 at the University of Alberta, Edmonton. International research collaboration enabled early anesthetic use of both cyclopropane and divinyl ether, advances that may not have occurred independently in either the United States or Canada.

All potent anesthetics of this period were explosive save for chloroform, whose hepatic and cardiac toxicity limited use in America. Anesthetic explosions remained a rare but devastating risk to both anesthesiologist and patient. To reduce the danger of explosion during the incendiary days of World War II, British anesthetists turned to trichloroethylene. This nonflammable anesthetic found limited application in America, as it decomposed to release phosgene when warmed in the presence of soda lime. By the end of World War II, however, another class of noninflammable anesthetics was prepared for laboratory trials. Ten years later, fluorinated hydrocarbons revolutionized inhalation anesthesia.

Fluorine, the lightest and most reactive halogen, forms exceptionally stable bonds. These bonds, although sometimes created with explosive force, resist separation by chemical or thermal means. For that reason, many early attempts to fluorinate hydrocarbons in a controlled manner were frustrated by the marked chemical activity of fluorine. In 1930, the first commercial application of fluorine chemistry came in the form of the refrigerant, Freon. This was followed by the first attempt to prepare a fluorinated anesthetic by Harold Booth and E. May Bixby in 1932. Although their drug, monochlorodifluoromethane, was devoid of anesthetic action, as were other drugs studied in that decade, their report predicted future developments. "A survey of the properties of 166 known gases suggested that the best possibility of finding a new noncombustible anesthetic gas lay in the field of organic fluoride compounds. Fluorine substitution for other halogens lowers the boiling point, increases stability, and generally decreases toxicity."[65]

After the war, a team at the University of Maryland under professor of pharmacology John C. Krantz, Jr., investigated the anesthetic properties of dozens of hydrocarbons over a period of several years, but only one, ethyl vinyl ether, entered clinical use in 1947. Because it was flammable, Krantz requested that it be fluorinated. In response, Julius Shukys prepared several fluorinated analogues. One of these, trifluoroethyl vinyl ether, or fluroxene, became the first fluorinated anesthetic. Fluroxene, which was nonflammable in concentrations needed for anesthesia, was marketed from 1954 until 1974. Despite its flammability at high concentrations, it was popular because, unlike halothane, it had favorable respiratory and circulatory depressant properties similar to its "cousin" diethyl ether.

In 1951, Charles Suckling, a British chemist at Imperial Chemical Industries, was asked to create a new anesthetic. Suckling, who already had an expert understanding of fluorination, began by asking clinicians to describe the properties of an ideal anesthetic. He learned from this inquiry that his search must consider several limiting factors, including the volatility, inflammability, stability, and potency of the compounds. After 2 years of research and testing, Charles Suckling created halothane. He first determined that halothane possessed anesthetic action by anesthetizing mealworms and houseflies before he forwarded it to pharmacologist James Raventos. Suckling also made accurate predictions as to the concentrations required for anesthesia in higher animals. After Raventos completed a favorable review, halothane was offered to Michael Johnstone, a respected anesthetist of Manchester, England, who recognized its great advantages over other anesthetics available in 1956. After Johnstone's endorsement, halothane use spread quickly and widely within the practice of anesthesia.[66]

Halothane was followed in 1960 by methoxyflurane, an anesthetic that remained popular for a decade. By 1970, however, it was learned that dose-related nephrotoxicity following protracted methoxyflurane anesthesia was caused by inorganic fluoride. Similarly, because of persisting concern that rare cases of hepatitis following anesthesia might be a result of a metabolite of halothane, the search for newer inhaled anesthetics focused on the resistance to metabolic degradation.

Two fluorinated liquid anesthetics, enflurane and its isomer isoflurane, were results of the search for increased stability. They were synthesized by Ross Terrell in 1963 and 1965, respectively. Because enflurane was easier to create, it preceded isoflurane. Its application was restricted after it was shown to be a marked cardiovascular depressant and to have some convulsant properties. Isoflurane was nearly abandoned because of difficulties in its purification, but after Louise Speers overcame this problem, several successful trials were published in 1971. The release of isoflurane for clinical use was delayed again for more than half a decade by calls for repeated testing in lower animals, owing to an unfounded concern that the drug might be carcinogenic. As a consequence, isoflurane received more thorough testing than any other drug heretofore used in anesthesia. The era when an anesthetic could be introduced following a single fortuitous observation had given way to a cautious program of assessment and reassessment. Remarkably, no anesthetics were introduced into clinical use for another 20 years. Finally, desflurane was released in 1992 and sevoflurane was released in 1994. Xenon, a gas having many properties of the ideal anesthetic, was administered to a few patients in the early 1950s but it never gained popularity because of the extreme costs associated with its removal from air. However, interest in xenon has been renewed now that gas concentrations can be accurately measured when administered at low flows, and devices are available to scavenge and reuse the gas.

Intravenous Anesthetics

Prior to William Harvey's description of a complete and continuous intravascular circuit in *De Motu Cordis* (1628), it was widely held that blood emanated from the heart and was propelled to the periphery where it was consumed. The idea that substances could be injected intravascularly and travel systemically probably originated with Christopher Wren. In 1657, Wren injected aqueous opium into a dog through a goose quill attached to a pig's bladder, rendering the animal "stupefied."[67] Wren similarly injected intravenous *crocus metallorum*, an impure preparation of antimony, and observed the animals to vomit and then die. Knowledge of a circulatory system and intravascular access spurred investigations in other areas, and Wren's contemporary, Richard Lower, performed the first blood transfusions of lamb's blood into dogs and other animals.

In the mid-19th century, equipment necessary for effective intravascular injections was conceived. Vaccination lancets were used in the 1830s to puncture the skin and force morphine paste subcutaneously for analgesia.[68] The hollow needle and hypodermic syringe were developed in the following decades but were not initially designed for intravenous use. In 1845, Dublin surgeon Francis Rynd created the hollow needle for injection of morphine into nerves in the treatment of "neuralgias." Similarly, Charles Gabriel Pravaz designed the first functional syringe in 1853 for perineural injections. Alexander Wood, however, is generally credited with perfecting the hypodermic glass syringe. In 1855, Wood published an article on the injection of opiates into painful spots by the use of hollow needle and his glass syringe.[69]

In 1872, Pierre Oré of Lyons performed what is perhaps the first successful intravenous surgical anesthesia by injecting chloral hydrate immediately prior to incision. His 1875 publication describes its use in 36 patients, but several postoperative deaths lent little to recommend this method to other practitioners.[70] In 1909, Ludwig Burkhardt produced surgical anesthesia by intravenous injections of chloroform and ether in Germany. Seven years later, Elisabeth Bredenfeld of Switzerland reported the use of intravenous morphine and scopolamine. The trials failed to show an improvement over inhaled techniques. Intravenous anesthesia found little application or popularity, primarily because of a lack of suitable drugs. In the following decades, this would change.

The first barbiturate, barbital, was synthesized in 1903 by Fischer and von Mering. Phenobarbital and all other successors of barbital had very protracted action and found little use in anesthesia. After 1929, oral pentobarbital was used as a sedative before surgery, but when it was given in anesthetic concentrations, long periods of unconsciousness followed. The first short-acting oxybarbiturate was hexobarbital (Evipal), available clinically in 1932. Hexobarbital was enthusiastically received by the anesthesia communities in Europe and North America because its abbreviated induction time was unrivaled by any other technique. A London anesthetist, Ronald Jarman, found that it had a dramatic advantage over inhalation inductions for minor procedures. Jarman instructed his patients to raise one arm while he injected hexobarbital into a vein of the opposite forearm. When the upraised arm fell, indicating the onset of hypnosis, the surgeon could begin. Patients were also amazed in that many awoke unable to believe they had been anesthetized.[71]

Even though the prompt action of hexobarbital had a dramatic effect on the conduct of anesthesia, it was soon replaced by two thiobarbiturates. In 1932, Donalee Tabern and Ernest H. Volwiler of the Abbott Company synthesized thiopental (Pentothal) and thiamylal (Surital). The sulfated barbiturates proved to be more satisfactory, potent, and rapid acting than were their oxybarbiturate analogues. Thiopental was first administered to a patient at the University of Wisconsin in March 1934, but the successful introduction of thiopental into clinical practice followed a thorough investigation conducted by John Lundy and his colleagues at the Mayo Clinic in June 1934.

When first introduced, thiopental was often given in repeated increments as the primary anesthetic for protracted procedures. Its hazards were soon appreciated. At first, depression of respiration was monitored by the simple method of observing the motion of a wisp of cotton placed over the nose. Only a few skilled practitioners were prepared to pass a tracheal tube if the patient stopped breathing. Such practitioners realized that thiopental without supplementation did not suppress airway reflexes, and they therefore encouraged the prophylactic provision of topical anesthesia of the airway beforehand. The vasodilatory effects of thiobarbiturates were widely appreciated only when thiopental caused cardiovascular collapse in hypovolemic burned civilian and military patients in World War II. In response, fluid replacement was used more aggressively and thiopental administered with greater caution.

In 1962, ketamine was synthesized by Dr. Calvin Stevens at the Parke Davis Laboratories in Ann Arbor, Michigan. One of the cyclohexylamine compounds that includes phencyclidine, ketamine was the only drug of this group that gained clinical utility. The other compounds produced undesirable postanesthetic delirium and psychotomimetic reactions. In 1966, the neologism "dissociative anesthesia" was created by Guenter Corrsen and Edward Domino to describe the trancelike state of profound analgesia produced by ketamine.[72] It was released for use in 1970, and although it remains primarily an agent for anesthetic induction, its analgesic properties are increasingly studied and used by pain specialists.

Etomidate was first described by Paul Janssen and his colleagues in 1964 and originally given the name hypnomidate. Its key advantages, minimal hemodynamic depression and lack of histamine release, account for its ongoing utility in clinical practice. It was released for use in 1974 and despite its drawbacks (pain on injection, myoclonus, postoperative nausea and vomiting [PONV], and inhibition of adrenal steroidogenesis), etomidate is often the drug of choice for anesthetizing hemodynamically unstable patients.

Propofol, or 2,6-diisopropylphenol, was first synthesized by Imperial Chemical Industries and tested clinically in 1977. Investigators found that it produced hypnosis quickly with minimal excitation and that patients awoke promptly once the drug was discontinued. In addition to its excellent induction characteristics, the antiemetic action of propofol made it an agent of choice in patient populations prone to nausea and emesis. Regrettably, Cremophor EL, the solvent with which it was formulated, produced several severe anaphylactic reactions, and it was withdrawn from use. Once propofol was reformulated with egg lecithin, glycerol, and soybean oil, the drug reentered clinical practice and gained great success. Its popularity in Britain coincided with the introduction of the LMA, and it was soon noted that propofol suppressed pharyngeal reflexes to a degree that permitted the insertion of an LMA without a need for either muscle relaxants or potent inhaled anesthetics.

Local Anesthetics

Centuries after the conquest of Peru, Europeans became aware of the stimulating properties of a local, indigenous plant that the Peruvians called *khoka*. *Khoka*, which meant *the plant*, quickly became known as *coca* in Europe. In 1860, shortly after the Austrian Carl von Scherzer imported enough coca leaves to allow for analysis, German chemists Albert Niemann and Wilhelm Lossen isolated the main alkaloid and named it *cocaine*. Twenty-five years later, at the recommendation of his friend Sigmund Freud, Carl Koller became interested in the effects of cocaine. After several animal experiments, Koller successfully demonstrated the analgesic properties of cocaine applied to the eye in a patient with glaucoma.[73] Unfortunately, nearly simultaneous with the first reports of cocaine use, there were reports of central nervous system and cardiovascular toxicity.[74,75] As the popularity of cocaine grew, so did the frequency of toxic reactions and cocaine addictions.[76] Skepticism about the use of cocaine quickly grew within the medical community, forcing the pharmacologic industry to develop alternative local anesthetics.

In 1898, Alfred Eihorn synthesized nivaquine the first amino amide local anesthetic.[77] Nirvaquine proved to be an irritant to tissues, and its use was immediately stopped. Returning his attention to the development of amino ester local anesthetics, Eihorn synthesized benzocaine in 1900 and procaine (Novocaine) shortly after in 1905. Amino esters were commonly used for local infiltration and spinal anesthesia despite their low potency and high likelihood to cause allergic reactions. Tetracaine, the last (and probably safest) amino ester local anesthetic developed, proved to be quite useful for many years.

In 1944, Nils Löfgren and Bengt Lundquist developed lidocaine, an amino amide local anesthetic.[76] Lidocaine gained immediate popularity because of its potency, rapid onset, decreased incidence of allergic reactions, and overall effectiveness for all types of regional anesthetic blocks. Since the introduction of lidocaine, all local anesthetics developed and marketed have been of the amino amide variety.

Because of the increase in lengthy and sophisticated surgical procedures, the development of a long-acting local anesthetic took precedence. From that demand, bupivacaine was introduced in 1965. Synthesized by B. Ekenstam[78] in 1957, bupivacaine was initially discarded after it was found to be highly toxic. By 1980, several years after being introduced to the United States, there were several reports of almost simultaneous seizures *and* cardiovascular collapse following unintended intravascular injection.[79] Shortly after this, as a result of the cardiovascular toxicity associated with bupivacaine and the profound motor block associated with etidocaine, the pharmaceutical industry began searching for a new long-acting alternative. Introduced in 1996, ropivacaine is structurally similar to mepivacaine and bupivacaine, although it is prepared as a single levorotatory isomer rather than a racemic mixture. The levorotatory isomer has less potential for toxicity than the dextrorotatory isomer.[80] The potential safety of ropivacaine is controversial because ropivacaine is approximately 25% less potent than bupivacaine. Therefore, at equal-potent doses the margin of safety between ropivacaine and bupivacaine becomes less apparent, although systemic toxicity with ropivacaine may respond more quickly to conventional resuscitation.[81]

Each local anesthetic developed has had its own positive and negative attributes, which is why some are still used today and others have fallen out of favor. The pharmaceutical industry is in the process of developing extended-release local anesthetics using liposomes and microspheres.[81-83]

Opioids

Opioids (historically referred to as *narcotics,* although semantically incorrect—see Chapter 19) remain the analgesic workhorse in anesthesia practice. They are used routinely in the perioperative period, in the management of acute pain, and in a variety of terminal and chronic pain states. The availability of short-, medium-, and long-acting opioids, as well as the many routes of administration, gives physicians considerable flexibility in the use of these agents. The analgesic and sedating properties of opium have been known for more than two millennia. Certainly the Greeks and Chinese civilizations harnessed these properties in medical and cultural practices. Opium is derived from the seeds of the poppy (*Papaver somniferum*) and is an amalgam of more than 25 pharmacologic alkaloids. The first alkaloid isolated, morphine, was extracted by Prussian chemist Freidrich A. W. Sertürner in 1803. He named this alkaloid after the Greek god of dreams, Morpheus. Morphine became commonly used as a supplement to inhaled anesthesia and for postoperative pain control during the latter half of the 19th century. Codeine, another alkaloid of opium, was isolated in 1832 by Robiquet, but its relatively weaker analgesic potency and nausea at higher doses limit its role in managing moderate-to-severe perioperative surgical pain.

Meperidine was the first synthetic opioid and was developed in 1939 by two German researchers at IG Farben, Otto Eisleb and O. Schaumann. Although many pharmacologists are remembered for the introduction of a single drug, one prolific researcher, Paul Janssen, has since 1953 brought forward more than 70 agents from among 70,000 chemicals created in his laboratory. His products have had profound effects on disciplines as disparate as parasitology and psychiatry. The pace of productive innovation in Janssen's research laboratory is astonishing. Chemical R4263 (fentanyl), synthesized in 1960, was followed only a year later by R4749 (droperidol), and then etomidate in 1964. Innovar, the fixed combination of fentanyl and droperidol, is less popular now but Janssen's phenylpiperidine derivatives, fentanyl, sufentanil, and alfentanil, are staples in the anesthesia pharmacopeia. Remifentanil, an ultra–short-acting opioid introduced by Glaxo–Wellcome in 1996, is a departure from other opioids in that it has very rapid onset and equally rapid offset owing to metabolism by nonspecific tissue esterases. Ketorolac, a nonsteroidal anti-inflammatory drug (NSAID) approved for use in 1990, was the first parenteral NSAID indicated for postoperative pain. With analgesic potency equivalent to 6 to 8 mg of morphine, Ketorolac provides significant postoperative pain control and has particular use when an opioid-sparing approach is essential. Ketorolac use is limited by side effects and may be inappropriate in patients with underlying renal dysfunction, bleeding problems, or compromised bone healing.

Muscle Relaxants

Muscle relaxants entered anesthesia practice nearly a century after inhalational anesthetics (Table 1-1). Curare, the first known neuromuscular blocking agent, was originally used in hunting and tribal warfare by native peoples of South America. The curares are alkaloids prepared from plants native to equatorial rain forests. The refinement of the harmless sap of several species of vines into toxins that were lethal (through creation of total muscular paralysis and apnea) only when injected was an extraordinary triumph introduced by paleopharmacologists in loincloths. Their discovery was more remarkable because it was independently repeated on three separate continents—South America, Africa, and Asia. These jungle tribes also developed nearly identical methods of delivering the toxin by darts, which, after being dipped in curare, maintained their potency indefinitely until they were propelled through blowpipes to strike the flesh of monkeys and other animals of the treetops. Moreover, the American Indians knew of the juice of a herb that would counteract the effects of the poison if administered in time.[84]

The earliest clinical use of curare in humans was to ameliorate the tortuous muscle spasms of infectious tetanus. In 1858, New York physician Louis Albert Sayres reported two cases in which he attempted to treat severe tetanus with curare at the Bellevue Hospital. Both his patients died. Similar efforts were undertaken to use muscle relaxants to treat epilepsy, rabies, and choreiform disorders. Treatment of Parkinson-like rigidity and the prevention of trauma from seizure therapy also preceded the use of curare in anesthesia.[85]

Interestingly, curare antagonists were developed well before muscle relaxants were ever used in surgery. In 1900, Jacob Pal, a Viennese physician, recognized that curare could be antagonized by physostigmine. This substance had been isolated from the Calabar bean some 36 years earlier by Scottish pharmacologist Sir T. R. Fraser. Neostigmine methylsulfate was synthesized in 1931 and was significantly more potent in antagonizing the effects of curare.[86]

In 1938, Richard and Ruth Gill returned to New York from South America, bringing with them 11.9 kg of crude curare collected near their Ecuadorian ranch. Their motivation was a mixture of personal and altruistic goals. Some months before, while on an earlier visit to the United States, Richard Gill learned that he had multiple sclerosis. His physician, Dr. Walter Freeman, mentioned the possibility that curare might have a therapeutic role in the management of spastic disorders. When the Gills returned to the United States with their supply of crude curare, they encouraged scientists at E. R. Squibb & Co. to take an interest in its unique properties. Squibb soon offered semirefined curare to two groups of American anesthesiologists, who assessed its action but quickly abandoned their studies when it

Table 1-1 Events in the Development of Muscle Relaxants

Year	Event
1516	Peter Martyr d'Anghera, *De orbe novo*, published account of South American Indian arrow poisons
1596	Sir Walter Raleigh provides detailed account of arrow poison effects and antidote
1745	Charles-Marie de la Condamine returns from Ecuador and conducts curare experiments with chickens and attempted to use sugar as an antidote
1780	Abbe Felix Fontana inserts curare directly into exposed sciatic nerve of rabbit without effect and concludes that mechanism is the destruction of the irritability of voluntary muscles. Publishes *On the American Poison Ticunas* (name of South American tribe)
1811	Benjamin Collins Brodie demonstrates that animals mechanically ventilated may survive significant doses of curare
1812	William Sewell suggests use of curare in "hydrophobia" (rabies) and tetanus
1844	Claude Bernard determines that death occurs by respiratory failure, motor nerves are unable to transmit stimuli from higher centers, differential effect on muscles with peripheral and thoracic muscles being affected before respiratory muscles. Bernard concludes that the site of action is the junction between muscles and nerves, neuromuscular junction
1858	Louis Albert Sayres, New York physician, uses curare to treat tetanus in two patients
1864	Physostigmine isolated from Calabar beans by Sir T. R. Fraser, a Scottish pharmacologist
1886–1897	R. Boehm, a German chemist, demonstrated three separate classes of alkaloids in each of three types of indigenous containers: tube-curares, pot-curares, and calabash-curares
1900	Jacob Pal recognizes that physostigmine can antagonize the effects of curare
1906	Succinylcholine, prepared by Reid Hunt and R. Taveau, experimented on rabbits pretreated with curare to learn of cardiac effects and so paralysis went unrecognized
1912	Arthur Lawen uses curare in surgery but report published in German so it goes largely unrecognized
1938	Richard and Ruth Gill bring large quantity of curare to New York for further study by pharmaceutical company
1939	Abram E. Bennett uses curare in children with spastic disorders and to prevent trauma from metrazol therapy (precursor to electroconvulsive therapy)
1942	Harold Griffith and Enid Johnson use curare for abdominal relaxation in surgery
1942	H. A. Halody develops rabbit head-drop assay for standardization and large-scale production of curare and d-tubocurarine
1948	Decamethonium, a depolarizing relaxant, is synthesized
1949	Succinylcholine prepared by Daniel Bovet and the following year by J. C. Castillo and Edwin de Beer
1956	Distinction between depolarizing and nondepolarizing neuromuscular blockade is made by William D. M. Paton
1964	Pancuronium released for use in humans, synthesized by Savage and Hewett
1979	Vecuronium introduced, specifically designed to be more hepatically metabolized than pancuronium
1993	Mivacurium released for clinical use
1994	Rocuronium introduced to clinical practice

caused total respiratory paralysis in two patients and the death of laboratory animals.

The earliest effective clinical application of curare in medicine occurred in physiatry. After A. R. McIntyre refined a portion of the raw curare in 1939, Abram E. Bennett of Omaha, Nebraska, injected it into children with spastic disorders. Although no persistent benefit could be observed in these patients, he next administered it to patients about to receive metrazol, a precursor to electroconvulsive therapy. Because it eliminated seizure-induced fractures, they termed it a "shock absorber." By 1941, other psychiatrists followed this practice and, when they found that the action of curare was protracted, occasionally used neostigmine as an antidote.

Curare was used initially in surgery by Arthur Lawen in 1912, but the published report was written in German and was ignored for decades. Lawen, a physiologist and physician from Leipzig, used curare in his laboratory before boldly producing abdominal relaxation at a light level of anesthesia in a surgical patient. Lawen's efforts were not appreciated for decades, and although his pioneering work anticipated later clinical application, safe use would have to await the introduction of regular intubation of the trachea and controlled ventilation of the lungs.[87]

Thirty years after Lawen, Harold Griffith, the chief anesthetist of the Montreal Homeopathic Hospital, learned of A. E. Bennett's successful use of curare and resolved to apply it in anesthesia. Because Griffith was already a master of tracheal intubation, he was much better prepared than were most of his contemporaries to attend to potential complications. On January 23, 1942, Griffith and his resident, Enid Johnson, anesthetized and intubated the trachea of a young man before injecting curare early in the course of his appendectomy. Satisfactory abdominal relaxation was obtained, and the surgery proceeded without incident. Griffith and Johnson's report of the successful use of curare in the 25 patients of their series launched a revolution in anesthetic care.[88]

Anesthesiologists who practiced before muscle relaxants recall the anxiety they felt when a premature attempt to intubate the trachea under cyclopropane caused persisting laryngospasm. Before 1942, abdominal relaxation was possible only if the patient tolerated high concentrations of an inhaled anesthetic, which might bring profound respiratory depression and protracted recovery. Curare and the drugs that followed transformed anesthesia profoundly. Because intubation of the trachea could now be taught in a deliberate manner, a neophyte could fail on a first attempt without compromising the safety of the patient. For the first time, abdominal relaxation could be attained when curare was supplemented by light planes of inhaled anesthetics or by a combination of intravenous agents providing "balanced anesthesia." New frontiers opened. Sedated and paralyzed patients could now successfully undergo the major physiologic trespasses of cardiopulmonary bypass, deliberate hypothermia, or long-term respiratory support after surgery.

Credit for successful and safe introduction of curare and d-tubocurarine into anesthesia must in part be given to a Squibb researcher named H. A. Holladay. Crude, unstandardized preparations of curare produced uncertain clinical effects and undesirable side effects related to various impurities. Isolation of d-tubocurarine in 1935 renewed clinical interest, but a method for standardizing "Intocostrin" and its purer derivative, d-tubocurarine, had yet to be devised. In the early 1940s, in part as a result of Griffith and Johnson's successful trials, Squibb embarked on wide-scale production. Holaday developed a reliable, easily reproducible method for standardizing curare doses that became known as the rabbit head-drop assay (Fig. 1-5). The assay consisted of aqueous curare solution injected intravenously in 0.1-mL doses every 15 seconds until the end point, when the rabbit became unable to raise its head, was reached.[89]

Successful clinical use of curare led to the introduction of other muscle relaxants. By 1948, gallamine and decamethonium had been synthesized. Metubine, a curare "rediscovered" in the 1970s, was used clinically in the same year. Succinylcholine was prepared by the Nobel Laureate Daniel Bovet in 1949 and was in wide international use before historians noted that the drug had been synthesized and tested long beforehand. In 1906, Reid Hunt and R. Taveaux prepared succinylcholine among a series of choline esters, which they had injected into rabbits to observe their cardiac effects. If their rabbits had not been previously paralyzed with curare, the depolarizing action of succinylcholine might have been recognized decades earlier.

The ability to monitor intraoperative neuromuscular blockade with nerve stimulators began in 1958. Working at St. Thomas' Hospital in London, T. H. Christie and H. Churchill-Davidson developed a method for monitoring peripheral neuromuscular blockade during anesthesia. It was not until 1970, however, that H. H. Ali et al.[90] devised the technique of delivering four supramaximal impulses delivered at 2 Hz (0.5 seconds apart), or a "train of four," as a method of quantifying the degree of residual neuromuscular blockade.

Research in relaxants was rekindled in 1960 when researchers became aware of the action of maloetine, a relaxant from the Congo basin. It was remarkable in that it had a steroidal nucleus. Investigations of maloetine led to pancuronium in 1968. In the 1970s and 1980s, research shifted toward identification of specific receptor biochemistry and development of receptor-specific drugs. From these isoquinolines, four related products emerged: vecuronium, pipecuronium, rocuronium, and rapacuronium. Rapacuronium, released in the early 1990s, was withdrawn from clinical use after several cases of intractable bronchospasm led to brain damage or death. Four clinical products based on the steroid parent drug d-tubocurarine (atracurium, mivacurium, doxacurium, and cis-atracurium) also made it to clinical use. Recognition that atracurium and cis-atracurium undergo spontaneous degradation by Hoffmann elimination has defined a role for these muscle relaxants in patients with liver and renal insufficiency.

Antiemetics

Effective treatment for PONV evolved relatively recently and has been driven by incentives to limit hospitalization expenses and improve patient satisfaction. But PONV is an old problem for which late-19th century practitioners recognized many causes including anxiety, severe pain, sudden changes in blood pressure, ileus, ingestion of blood, and the residual effects of opioids and inhalational anesthetics. Risk of pulmonary aspiration of gastric contents and subsequent death from asphyxia or aspiration pneumonia was a feared consequence of anesthesia, especially preceding use of cuffed endotracheal tubes. Vomiting and aspiration during anesthesia led to the practice of maintaining an empty stomach preoperatively, a policy that continues today despite evidence that clear fluids up to 3 hours before surgery do not increase gastric volumes, change gastric pH, or increase the risk of aspiration.

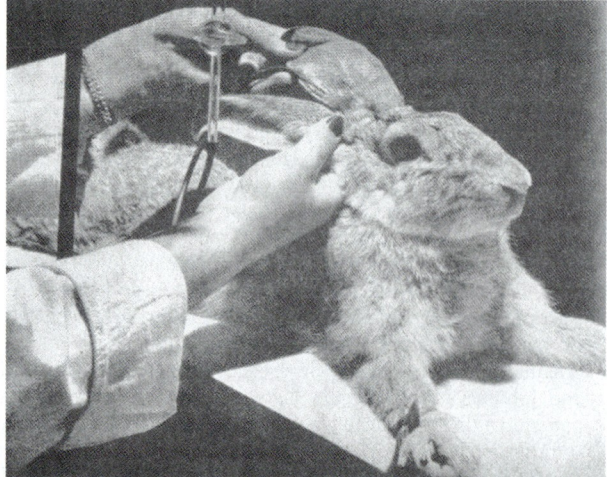 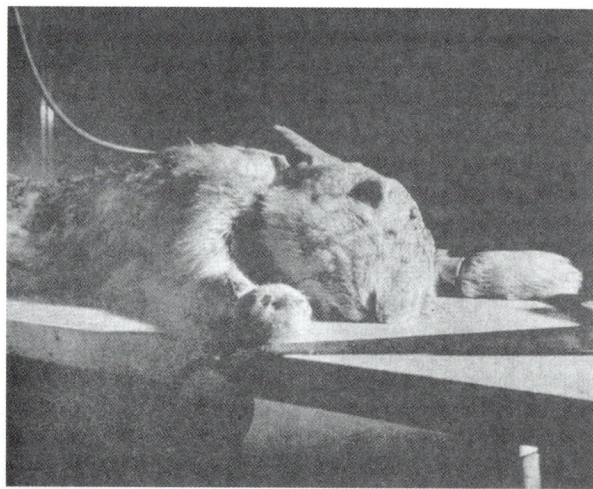

Figure 1-5 The rabbit head-drop assay. H. A. Halladay of Squibb pharmaceutical company developed a method of standardizing doses of curare and d-tubocurarine. A normal rabbit (**A**) had 0.1 mL of aqueous cecurane solution injected every 15 seconds until it could no longer raise its head (**B**).

A variety of treatments for nausea and vomiting were proposed by early anesthetists. James Gwathemy's 1914 publication, *Anesthesia*, commented that British surgeons customarily gave tincture of iodine in a teaspoonful of water every half hour for three or four doses. Inhalation of vinegar fumes and rectal injection of 30 to 40 drops of tincture of opium with 60 grains of sodium bromide were also thought to quiet the vomiting center.[91] Other practitioners attempted olfactory control by placing a piece of gauze moistened with essence of orange or an aromatic oil on the upper lip of the patient.[92] A 1937 anesthesia textbook encouraged treatment of PONV with lateral positioning, "iced soda water, strong black coffee, and chloretone.*" Counterirritation, such as mustard leaf on the epigastrium, was also believed useful in limiting emesis.[93] As late as 1951, anesthesia texts recommended oxygen administration, whiffs of ammonia spirits, and control of blood pressure and positioning.[94] The complex central mechanisms of nausea and vomiting were largely unaffected by most of these treatments. Newer drugs capable of intervening at specific pathways were needed to have an impact on PONV. As more short-acting anesthetics were developed, the problem received sharper focus in awake postoperative patients in the recovery room. The nausea accompanying use of newer chemotherapy agents provided additional impetus to the development of antiemetic medications.

In 1955, a nonrandomized study of patients demonstrated that the antihistamine cyclizine significantly reduced PONV. The following year, a more rigorous study by Knapp and Beecher reported a significant benefit from prophylaxis with the neuroleptic chlorpromazine. In 1957, promethazine (Phenergan) and chlorpromazine were both found to reduce PONV when used prophylactically. Thirteen years later, a double-blind study evaluating metoclopramide was published, and that drug became a first-line drug in the management of PONV. Droperidol, released in the early 1960s, became widely used until 2001, when concerns regarding prolongation of QT intervals prompted a warning from the Food and Drug Administration about its continued use.

The antiemetic effects of corticosteroids were first recognized by oncologists treating intracranial edema from tumors.[95] Subsequent studies have borne out the antiemetic properties of this class of drugs in treating PONV. Recognition of the serotonin 5-HT3 pathway in PONV has led to a unique class of drugs devoted only to addressing this particular problem. Ondansetron, the first representative of this drug class, was approved by the Food and Drug Administration in 1991. Additional serotonin 5-HT3 antagonists have been approved and are available today.

Anesthesia Subspecialties

Regional Anesthesia

Cocaine, an extract of the coca leaf, was the first effective local anesthetic. After Albert Niemann refined the active alkaloid and named it *cocaine*, it was used in experiments by a few investigators. It was noted that cocaine provided topical anesthesia and even produced local insensibility when injected, but Carl Koller, a Viennese surgical intern, first recognized the utility of cocaine in clinical practice.

In 1884, Carl Koller was completing his medical training at a time when many operations on the eye were performed without general anesthesia. Almost four decades after the discovery of ether, general anesthesia by mask still had limitations for ophthalmic surgery: lack of patient cooperation, interference of the anesthesia apparatus with surgical access, and a high incidence of PONV. At that time, because fine sutures were not available and surgical incisions of the eye were not closed, postoperative vomiting threatened the extrusion of the globe's contents, putting the patient at risk for irrevocable blindness.[96]

While a medical student, Koller had worked in a Viennese laboratory in a search of a topical ophthalmic anesthetic to overcome the limitations of general anesthesia. Unfortunately, the suspensions of morphine, chloral hydrate, and other drugs that he had used had been ineffectual. In 1884, Koller's friend, Sigmund Freud, became interested in the cerebral-stimulating effects of cocaine and gave him a small sample in an envelope, which he placed in his pocket. When the envelope leaked, a few grains of cocaine stuck to Koller's finger and he absentmindedly licked it with his tongue. When his tongue became numb, Koller instantly realized that he had found the object of his search. In his laboratory, he made a suspension of cocaine crystals that he and a laboratory associate tested in the eyes of a frog, a rabbit, and a dog. Satisfied with the anesthetic effects seen in the animal models, Koller dropped the solution onto his own cornea. To his amazement, his eyes were insensitive to the touch of a pin.[97] As an intern, Carl Koller could not afford to attend the Congress of German Ophthalmologists in Heidelberg on September 15, 1884. However, a friend presented his article at the meeting, and a revolution in ophthalmic surgery and other surgical disciplines began. Within the next year, more than 100 articles supporting the use of cocaine appeared in European and American medical journals. In 1888, Koller immigrated to New York, where he practiced ophthalmology for the remainder of his career.

American surgeons quickly developed new applications for cocaine. Its efficacy in anesthetizing the nose, mouth, larynx, trachea, rectum, and urethra was described in October 1884. The next month, the first reports of its subcutaneous injection were published. In December 1884, two young surgeons, William Halsted and Richard Hall, described blocks of the sensory nerves of the face and arm. Halsted[98] even performed a brachial plexus block but did so under direct vision while the patient received an inhaled anesthetic. Unfortunately, self-experimentation with cocaine was hazardous, as both surgeons became addicted.[99] Addiction was an ill-understood but frequent problem in the late 19th century, especially when cocaine and morphine were present in many patent medicines and folk remedies.

Other regional anesthetic techniques were attempted before the end of the 19th century. The term *spinal anesthesia* was coined in 1885 by Leonard Corning, a neurologist who had observed Hall and Halsted. Corning wanted to assess the action of cocaine as a specific therapy for neurologic problems. After first assessing its action in a dog, producing a blockade of rapid onset that was confined to the animal's rear legs, he performed a neuraxial block using cocaine on a man "addicted to masturbation." Corning administered one dose without effect, then after a second dose, the patient's legs "felt sleepy." The man had impaired sensibility in his lower extremity after about 20 minutes and left Corning's office "none the worse for the experience."[100] Although Corning did not describe escape of cerebrospinal fluid (CSF) in either case, it is likely that the dog had a spinal anesthetic and that the man had an epidural anesthetic. No therapeutic benefit was described, but Corning closed his account and his attention to the subject by suggesting that cocainization might in time be "a substitute for etherization in genitourinary or other branches of surgery."[101]

Two other authors, August Bier and Theodor Tuffier, described authentic spinal anesthesia, with mention of CSF,

---

*Chloretone (chlorobutanol) is prepared by mixing chloroform and acetone, and has a camphor-like odor that some find pleasant. Chloretone is now commonly used for euthanizing reptiles and amphibians.

injection of cocaine, and an appropriately short onset of action. In a comparative review of the original articles by Bier, Tuffier, and Corning, it was concluded that Corning's injection was extradural, and Bier merited the credit for introducing spinal anesthesia.[102]

Fourteen years passed before spinal anesthesia was performed for surgery. In the interval, Heinrich Quincke of Kiel, Germany, had described his technique of lumbar puncture. He offered the valuable observation that it was most safely performed at the level of the third or fourth lumbar interspace because entry at that level was below the termination of the spinal cord. Quincke's technique was used in Kiel for the first deliberate cocainization of the spinal cord in 1899 by his surgical colleague, August Bier. Six patients received small doses of cocaine intrathecally, but because some cried out during surgery and others vomited and experienced headaches, Bier considered it necessary to conduct further experiments before continuing this technique for surgery.

Professor Bier permitted his assistant, Dr. Hildebrandt, to perform a lumbar puncture, but after the needle penetrated the dura, Hildebrandt could not fit the syringe to the needle, and a large volume of the professor's spinal fluid escaped. They were at the point of abandoning the study when Hildebrandt volunteered to be the subject of a second attempt. Their persistence was rewarded with an astonishing success. Twenty-three minutes after the spinal injection, Bier noted: "A strong blow with an iron hammer against the tibia was not felt as pain. After 25 minutes: Strong pressure and pulling on a testicle were not painful."[92] They celebrated their success with wine and cigars. That night, both developed violent headaches, which they attributed at first to their celebration. Bier's headache was relieved after 9 days of bed rest. Hildebrandt, as a house officer, did not have the luxury of continued rest. Bier postulated that their headaches were a result of the loss of large volumes of CSF and urged that this be avoided if possible. The high incidence of complications following lumbar puncture with wide-bore needles and the toxic reactions attributed to cocaine explain his later loss of interest in spinal anesthesia.[103]

Surgeons in several other countries soon practiced spinal anesthesia, and progress occurred by many small contributions to the technique. Theodor Tuffier published the first series of 125 spinal anesthetics from France and later counseled that the solution should not be injected before CSF was seen. The first American report was by Rudolph Matas of New Orleans, whose first patient developed postanesthetic meningismus, a frequent complication that was overcome in part by the use of hermetically sealed sterile solutions recommended by E. W. Lee of Philadelphia and sterile gloves as advocated by Halsted. During 1899, Dudley Tait and Guidlo Caglieri of San Francisco performed experimental studies in animals and therapeutic spinals for orthopedic patients. They encouraged the use of fine needles to lessen the escape of CSF and urged that the skin and deeper tissues be infiltrated beforehand with local anesthesia.[104] This had been suggested earlier by William Halsted and the foremost advocate of infiltration anesthesia, Carl Ludwig Schleich of Berlin. An early American specialist in anesthesia, Ormond Goldan, published an anesthesia record appropriate for recording the course of "intraspinal cocainization" in 1900. In the same year, Heinrich Braun learned of a newly described extract of the adrenal gland, epinephrine, which he used to prolong the action of local anesthetics with great success. Braun developed several new nerve blocks, coined the term *conduction anesthesia*, and is remembered by European writers as the "father of conduction anesthesia." Braun was the first person to use procaine, which, along with stovaine, was one of the first synthetic local anesthetics produced to reduce the toxicity of cocaine.

Before 1907, anesthesiologists were sometimes disappointed to observe that their spinal anesthetics were incomplete. Most believed that the drug spread solely by local diffusion before the property of baricity was investigated by Arthur Barker, a London surgeon.[105] Barker constructed a glass tube shaped to follow the curves of the human spine and used it to demonstrate the limited spread of colored solutions that he had injected through a T-piece in the lumbar region. Barker applied this observation to use solutions of stovaine made hyperbaric by the addition of 5% glucose, which worked in a more predictable fashion. After the injection was complete, Barker placed his patient's head on pillows to contain the anesthetic below the nipple line. Lincoln Sise acknowledged Barker's work in 1935 when he introduced the use of hyperbaric solutions of tetracaine (Pontocaine). John Adriani advanced the concept further in 1946 when he used a hyperbaric solution to produce "saddle block," or perineal anesthesia. Adriani's patients remained seated after injection as the drug descended to the sacral nerves.

Tait, Jonnesco, and other early masters of spinal anesthesia used a cervical approach for thyroidectomy and thoracic procedures, but this radical approach was supplanted in 1928 by the lumbar injection of hypobaric solutions of "light" nupercaine by G. P. Pitkin. Although the use of hypobaric solutions is now limited primarily to patients positioned in the jackknife position, their former use for thoracic procedures demanded skill and precise timing. The enthusiasts of hypobaric anesthesia devised formulas to attempt to predict the time in seconds needed for a warmed solution of hypobaric nupercaine to spread in patients of varying size from its site of injection in the lumbar area to the level of the fourth thoracic dermatome.

The recurring problem of inadequate duration of single-injection spinal anesthesia led a Philadelphia surgeon, William Lemmon, to devise an apparatus for continuous spinal anesthesia in 1940.[106] Lemmon began with the patient in the lateral position. The spinal tap was performed with a malleable silver needle, which was left in position. As the patient was turned supine, the needle was positioned through a hole in the mattress and table. Additional injections of local anesthetic could be performed as required. Malleable silver needles also found a less cumbersome and more common application in 1942 when Waldo Edwards and Robert Hingson encouraged the use of Lemmon's needles for continuous caudal anesthesia in obstetrics. In 1944, Edward Tuohy of the Mayo Clinic introduced two important modifications of the continuous spinal techniques. He developed the now familiar Tuohy needle[107] as a means of improving the ease of passage of lacquered silk ureteral catheters through which he injected incremental doses of local anesthetic.[108]

In 1949, Martinez Curbelo of Havana, Cuba, used Tuohy's needle and a ureteral catheter to perform the first continuous epidural anesthetic. Silk and gum elastic catheters were difficult to sterilize and sometimes caused dural infections before being superseded by disposable plastics. Yet deliberate single-injection peridural anesthesia had been practiced occasionally for decades before continuous techniques brought it greater popularity. At the beginning of the 20th century, two French clinicians experimented independently with caudal anesthesia. Neurologist Jean Athanase Sicard applied the technique for a nonsurgical purpose, the relief of back pain. Fernand Cathelin used caudal anesthesia as a less dangerous alternative to spinal anesthesia for hernia repairs. He also demonstrated that the epidural space terminated in the neck by injecting a solution of India ink into the caudal canal of a dog. The lumbar approach was first used solely for multiple paravertebral nerve blocks before the Pagés–Dogliotti single-injection technique became accepted. Because they worked separately, the technique carries the names of both men. Captain Fidel Pagés prepared an elegant demonstration of segmental single-injection peridural anesthesia in 1921, but died soon after his article appeared in a Spanish military journal.[109] Ten years later, Achille M. Dogliotti of Turin, Italy, wrote a classic study that made the epidural technique well known.[72] Whereas Pagés used a tactile approach to identify the epidural space, Dogliotti identified it by the loss-of-resistance technique.

Surgery on the extremities lent itself to other regional anesthesia techniques. In 1902, Harvey Cushing coined the phrase *regional anesthesia* for his technique of blocking either the brachial or sciatic plexus under direct vision during general anesthesia to reduce anesthesia requirements and provide postoperative pain relief.[57] Fifteen years before his publication, George Crile advanced a similar approach to reduce the stress and shock of surgery. Crile, a dedicated advocate of regional and infiltration techniques during general anesthesia, coined the term *anoci-association*.[110]

An intravenous regional technique with procaine was reported in 1908 by August Bier, the surgeon who had pioneered spinal anesthesia. Bier injected procaine into a vein of the upper limb between two tourniquets. Even though the technique is termed the *Bier block*, it was not used for many decades until it was reintroduced 55 years later by Mackinnon Holmes, who modified the technique by introducing exsanguination before applying a single proximal cuff. Holmes used lidocaine, the very successful amide local anesthetic synthesized in 1943 by Lofgren and Lundquist of Sweden.

Several investigators achieved upper extremity anesthesia by percutaneous injections of the brachial plexus. In 1911, based on his intimate knowledge of the anatomy of the axillary area, Hirschel promoted a "blind" axillary injection. In the same year, Kulenkampff described a supraclavicular approach in which the operator sought out paresthesias of the plexus while keeping the needle at a point superficial to the first rib and the pleura. The risk of pneumothorax with Kulenkampff's approach led Mulley to attempt blocks more proximally by a lateral paravertebral approach, the precursor of what is now popularly known as the *Winnie block* (after Alon Winnie from Chicago).

Heinrich Braun wrote the earliest textbook of local anesthesia, which appeared in its first English translation in 1914. After 1922, Gaston Labat's *Regional Anesthesia* dominated the American market. Labat migrated from France to the Mayo Clinic in Minnesota, where he served briefly before taking a permanent position at the Bellevue Hospital in New York. He formed the first American Society for Regional Anesthesia.[112] After Labat's death, Emery A. Rovenstine was recruited to Bellevue to continue Labat's work, among other responsibilities. Rovenstein created the first American clinic for the treatment of chronic pain, where he and his associates refined techniques of lytic and therapeutic injections and used the American Society of Regional Anesthesia to further the knowledge of pain management across the United States.[112]

The development of the multidisciplinary pain clinic was one of the many contributions to anesthesiology made by John J. Bonica, a renowned teacher of regional techniques. During his periods of military, civilian, and university service at the University of Washington, Bonica formulated a series of improvements in the management of patients with chronic pain. His classic text *The Management of Pain* is regarded as a standard of the literature of anesthesia.

Cardiovascular Anesthesia

The earliest attempts to operate on the heart were limited to repairing cardiac wounds. These attempts generally failed until German surgeon Ludwig Rehn repaired a right ventricular stab wound in September 1896.[113] Despite this success, the field was not ready to advance. The taboo of cardiac surgery was summarized by Theodore Billroth when he supposedly said "any surgeon who would attempt an operation on the heart should lose the respect of his colleagues."[114] The resistance to such operations was partly because of fledgling anesthetic medications, lack of adequate monitors, and even a clear understanding of cardiovascular physiology that pervades modern anesthesia practice.

Fortunately, the turn of the 20th century saw many advances in anesthesia practice, blood typing and transfusion, anticoagulation, and antibiosis as well as surgical instrumentation and technique. Some continued to attempt procedures like closed mitral valvotomy in the midst of these technologic advancements, but outcomes were still very poor with mortality rates exceeding 80%. Many believe that the successful ligation of a 7-year-old girl's patent ductus arteriosus by Robert Gross in 1938 served as the landmark case for modern cardiac surgery. Soon after Gross' achievement, a host of new procedures were developed for repairing congenital cardiac lesions, including the first Blalock–Taussig shunt performed on a 15-month-old "blue baby" in 1944.[68] Although the shunt had been successfully demonstrated in animal models, Austin Lamont, Chief of Anesthesia at Johns Hopkins, was not supportive of the procedure. He emphatically stated "I will not put that child to death" and left the open drop ether–oxygen anesthetic to resident anesthesiologist Merel Harmel.[115] Lamont attended on the second Blalock–Taussig shunt 2 months later. Together, Harmel and Lamont[116] would publish the first article on anesthesia for cardiac surgery in 1946 based on 100 cases with Alfred Blalock and repair of congenital pulmonic stenosis.

Closed cardiac surgery ensued, and anesthesia pioneers like William McQuiston and Kenneth Keown worked side by side with surgeons during procedures like the first aortic–pulmonary anastomosis and the first transmyocardial mitral commissurotomy. Never before had anesthesia providers worked as intimately with surgeons for the patient's welfare. Anesthesiologist and World War II physician Max Samuel Sadove remarked, "the small-arms fire of the anesthesiologist joins the spy system of the lab to back up the surgeon's big artillery in a coordinated attack to conquer disease."[117]

Through the 1930s and 1940s, John Gibbon had been experimenting with several extracorporeal circuit designs and by 1947 was able to successfully place dogs on heart–lung bypass. The first successful use of Gibbon's cardiopulmonary bypass machine in humans in May 1953 was a monumental advance in the surgical treatment of complex cardiac pathology that stimulated international interest in open heart surgery and the specialty of cardiac anesthesia.

Over the next decade, rapid growth and expanded applications of cardiac surgery, including artificial valves and coronary artery bypass grafting, required many more anesthesiologists acquainted with these specialized techniques. In 1967, J. Earl Wynands published one of the first articles on anesthetic management of patients undergoing surgery for coronary artery disease.

As cardiac surgery evolved, so did the perioperative monitoring and care of patients undergoing cardiac surgery. Postoperative mechanical ventilation and surgical intensive care units appeared by the late 1960s. Devices like the left atrial pressure monitor and the intra-aortic balloon pump offered new methods of understanding cardiopulmonary physiology and treating postoperative ventricular failure. Cardiac anesthesiologists were quick to bring the pulmonary artery catheter (PAC) into the operating room, permitting more precise hemodynamic monitoring and intervention. Joel Kaplan, already known for using the V_5 lead to monitor for myocardial ischemia and nitroglycerin infusions to treat ischemia, popularized the use of the PAC to detect myocardial ischemia. At Texas Heart Institute, Stephen Slogoff and Arthur Keats demonstrated the negative impact of myocardial ischemia on clinical outcome. By the end of the 1980s, the same duo would reveal that the choice of anesthetic agent had little impact on outcome, challenging the earlier paradigm of "isoflurane steal" proposed by Sebastian Reiz.

Developments like cold potassium cardioplegia, monitoring and reversal of heparin, and reduction of blood loss with aprotinin would change the practice of cardiac anesthesia. Transesophageal echocardiography, introduced into cardiac surgery by Roizen, Cahalan, and Kremer in the 1980s, helped to further define the subspecialty of cardiac anesthesia.

Neuroanesthesia

Brain surgery is considered by some to be the oldest of the practiced medical arts. Evidence of trephination, a form of neurosurgery in which a hole is drilled or scraped into the skull to access the dura, was discovered in skulls dating back to 6500 BC at a French burial site. Prehistoric brain surgery was also practiced by civilizations in South America, Africa, and Asia.[118]

With the introduction of inhalational anesthesia in the mid-1800s, Scottish surgeon and neurosurgery pioneer Sir William Macewen used this novel practice while performing the first successful craniotomy for tumor removal in 1879. Macewen, well known for introducing the technique of orotracheal intubation, promoted the idea of teaching medical students at Glasgow Royal Infirmary the art of chloroform anesthesia.

Like Macewen, Sir Victor Horsely was a neurosurgeon with an interest in anesthesia. His experiments of how ether, chloroform, and morphine affected intracranial contents led him to conclude that "the agent of choice was chloroform and that morphine had some value because of its cerebral constriction effects."[119] He first published his anesthetic technique for brain surgery in the *British Medical Journal* in 1886.[120] Later, he omitted morphine from his regimen after discovering its tendency to produce respiratory depression.

Meanwhile, Harvard medical student and aspiring neurosurgeon Harvey Cushing developed the first charts to record heart rate, temperature, and respiration during anesthesia. Soon after, he would add blood pressure readings to the record. Cushing was one of the first surgeons to recognize the importance of dedicated, specially trained anesthesia personnel versed in neurosurgery. Charles Frazier,[121] a neurosurgical contemporary of Cushing, also recognized this need, stating that "no [cranial] operation be undertaken unless the services of a skilled anesthetizer are available."

Because ether and chloroform anesthesia had significant drawbacks, beginning in 1918 Cushing and his contemporaries explored the advantages of regional or local anesthesia for intracranial surgery. Part of the motivation driving this change was the increased duration in surgical time. Cushing and colleagues used a "slow" surgical technique for most surgical procedures, where the average duration for cranial operations was 5 hours.[122] In contrast, early neurosurgeons like Horseley and Sir Percy Sargeant could perform similar procedures in less than 90 minutes. Therefore, prolonged patient exposure to chloroform or ether anesthesia was likely to result in increased bleeding, postoperative headache, confusion, and/or vomiting. Cushing and his contemporaries thought the use of local or regional anesthesia lessened the risk of these complications.

After a decade, it was realized that the remote positioning of the anesthetist was troublesome when managing the airway of an awake or lightly sedated patient undergoing cranial surgery with regional anesthesia. Also, endotracheal tubes, although introduced at the beginning of the century, had become popular instruments for securing a patient's airway and providing inhalation anesthesia. Combined, these circumstances led to the rapid resurgence of popularity in general anesthesia for cranial surgery, a trend that would continue to the present day.

Although the introduction of agents like thiopental, curare, and halothane advanced the practice of anesthesiology in general, the development of methods to measure brain electrical activity, cerebral blood flow, and metabolic rate by Kety and Schmidt and intracranial pressure by Lundburg "put neuroanesthesia practice on a scientific foundation and opened doors to neuroanesthesia research."[123] Clinician-scientists like John D. (Jack) Michenfelder, later known as the father of neuroanesthesia, conducted basic science and clinical research on cerebral blood flow and brain function and protection in response to various anesthetic agents and techniques. Many lessons learned during this period of groundbreaking research are still commonly used in modern neuroanesthesia practice.

Obstetric Anesthesia

Social attitudes about pain associated with childbirth began to change in the 1860s, and women started demanding anesthesia for childbirth. Societal pressures were so great that physicians, although unconvinced of the benefits of analgesia, felt obligated to offer this service to their obstetric patients.[124] In 1907, an Austrian physician, Richard von Steinbüchel, used a combination of morphine and scopolamine to produce *Dämmerschlaff* or "Twilight Sleep."[125] Although these two drugs were well known, physicians remained skeptical that Twilight Sleep was essential to labor and delivery, which unfortunately contrasted with the opinion of most women. This method gained popularity after German obstetricians Carl Gauss and Bernhardt Krönig widely publicized the technique. Numerous advertisements touted the benefits of Twilight Sleep (analgesia, partial pain relief, and amnesia) as compared to ether and chloroform, which resulted in total unconsciousness.[126] Gauss recognized the narrow therapeutic margin of these medications and gave precise instructions on its use: The first injection (morphine 10 mg and scopolamine) was to be given shortly after active labor began—this was intended to blunt the pain of labor—and subsequent injections consisted of only scopolamine, which was dosed to obliterate the memory of labor. Because of the effects of scopolamine, many patients became disoriented and would scream and thrash about during labor and delivery. Gauss believed that he could minimize this reaction by decreasing the sensory input; therefore, he would put patients in a dark room, cover their eyes with gauze, and insert oil-soaked cotton into their ears. The patients were often confined to a padded bed and restrained with leather straps during the delivery.[127] Over time, the doses of morphine administered seemed to increase, although there were few, if any, reports of adverse neonatal effects. Virginia Apgar's landmark 1953 publication of a system for evaluating newborns (the Apgar Score) helped to demonstrate that there actually was a difference in the neonates of mothers who had general versus regional anesthesia.[128]

The bulk of the interest in Twilight Sleep appears to have been popular rather than medical and, for a brief period, was intensely followed in the United States.[129] Public enthusiasm for Twilight Sleep quickly subsided after a prominent advocate of the method died during childbirth. Her physicians claimed her death was not related to complications from the method of Twilight Sleep that was used.[130]

The first articles describing the obstetric application of spinal, epidural, caudal, paravertebral, parasacral, and pudendal nerve blocks appeared between 1900 and 1930. However, their benefits were underappreciated for many years because the obstetricians seldom used these techniques.[130] Continuous caudal anesthesia was introduced in 1944 by Hingson and Edwards,[131] and spinal anesthesia became popular shortly thereafter. Initially, spinal anesthesia could be administered by inexperienced personnel without monitoring. The combination of inexperienced providers and lack of patient monitoring led to higher rates of morbidity and mortality than those observed for general anesthesia.[132] Therefore, the use of spinal anesthesia was highly discouraged in the 1950s, leading to the "dark ages of obstetric anesthesia" when pain relief in obstetrics was essentially abandoned and women were forced to endure "natural childbirth" to avoid serious anesthesia-related complications.[133]

With an increased understanding of neuraxial anesthesia, involvement by well-trained anesthesiologists, and an appreciation for the physiologic changes during pregnancy, maternal and fetal safety greatly improved. At the onset of the 21st century, anesthesia-related deaths during cesarean sections under general anesthesia were reported as being more likely than neuraxial anesthesia-related deaths, making regional anesthesia the method of choice.[134,135] With the availability of safe and effective options for pain relief during labor and delivery, today's focus is on improving the quality of the birth experience for expectant parents.

Transfusion Medicine

Paleolithic cave drawings found in France depict a bear losing blood from multiple spear wounds, indicating that primitive man understood the simple relationship between blood and life.[136] More than 10,000 years later, modern anesthesiologists attempt to preserve this intimate relationship by replacing fluids and blood products when faced with intravascular volume depletion or diminished oxygen-carrying capacity from blood loss.

Blood transfusion was first attempted in 1667 by the physician to Louis XIV, Jean Baptiste Denis. Denis had learned of Richard Lower's transfusion of lamb's blood into a dog the previous year. Lamb's blood was most frequently used because the donating animal's essential qualities were thought to be transferred to the recipient. Despite this dangerous transspecies transfusion, Denis' first patient got better. His next two patients were not as fortunate, however, and Denis avoided further attempts. Given the poor outcomes of these early blood transfusions, and heated religious controversy regarding the implications of transferring animal-specific qualities across species, blood transfusion in humans was banned for more than a 100 years in both France and England beginning in 1670.[68]

In 1900, Karl Landsteiner and Samuel Shattock independently helped lay the scientific basis of all subsequent transfusions by recognizing that blood compatibility was based on different blood groups. Landsteiner, an Austrian physician, originally organized human blood into three groups based on substances present in the red blood cells. The fourth type, AB group, was identified in 1902 by two students, Decastrello and Sturli. On the basis of these findings, Reuben Ottenberg performed the first type-specific blood transfusion in 1907. Transfusion of physiologic solutions occurred in 1831, independently performed by O'Shaughnessy and Lewins in Great Britain. In his letter to *The Lancet*, Lewins described transfusing large volumes of saline solutions into patients with cholera. He reported that he would inject into adults 5 to 10 pounds of saline solution and repeat as needed.[137]

Despite its publication in a prominent journal, Lewins' technique was apparently overlooked for decades, and balanced physiologic solution availability would have to await the coming of analytical chemistry.

Professionalism and Anesthesia Practice

Organized Anesthesiology

Physician anesthetists sought to obtain respect among their surgical colleagues by organizing professional societies and improving the quality of training. The first American organization was founded by nine members on October 6, 1905, and called the Long Island Society of Anesthetists with annual dues of $1.00. In 1911, the annual assessment rose to $3.00 when the Long Island Society became the New York Society of Anesthetists. Although the new organization still carried a local title, it drew members from several states and had a membership of 70 physicians in 1915.[138]

One of the most noteworthy figures in the struggle to professionalize anesthesiology was Francis Hoffer McMechan. McMechan had been a practicing anesthesiologist in Cincinnati until 1911, when he suffered a severe first attack of rheumatoid arthritis, which eventually left him confined to a wheelchair and forced his retirement from the operating room in 1915. McMechan had been in practice for only 15 years, but he had written 18 clinical articles in this short time. A prolific researcher and writer, McMechan did not permit his crippling disease to sideline his career. Instead of pursuing goals in clinical medicine, he applied his talents to establishing anesthesiology societies.[139]

McMechan supported himself and his devoted wife through editing the *Quarterly Anesthesia Supplement* from 1914 until August 1926. He became editor of the first journal devoted to anesthesia, *Current Researches in Anesthesia and Analgesia*, the precursor of *Anesthesia and Analgesia*, the oldest journal of the specialty. As well as fostering the organization of the International Anesthesia Research Society (IARS) in 1925, McMechan and his wife, Laurette, became overseas ambassadors of American anesthesia. Because Laurette was French, it was understandable that McMechan combined his own ideas about anesthesiology with concepts from abroad.[123]

In 1926, McMechan held the Congress of Anesthetists in a joint conference with the Section on Anaesthetics of the British Medical Association. Subsequently, he traveled throughout Europe, giving lectures and networking with physicians in the field. On his final return to America, he was gravely ill and was confined to bed for 2 years. His hard work and constant travel paid dividends, however: In 1929, the IARS, which McMechan founded in 1922, had members not only from North America but also from several European countries, Japan, India, Argentina, and Brazil.[119] Most notable, McMechan influenced a young Australian anesthesiologist, Geoffry Kaye in a meeting in 1929 in Melbourne. Kaye become a devoted follower of McMechan, and in the following decades helped establish the Australian Society of Anesthesiologists, creating in the first floor of his home a meeting space, workshop, library, and museum.[140]

In the 1930s, McMechan expanded his mission from organizing anesthesiologists to promoting the academic aspects of the specialty. In 1931, work began on what would become the International College of Anesthetists. This body began to award fellowships in 1935. For the first time, physicians were recognized as specialists in anesthesiology. The certification qualifications were universal, and fellows were recognized as specialists in several countries. Although the criteria for certification were not strict, the college was a success in raising the standards of anesthesia practice in many nations.[141]

Academic Anesthesia

Many Americans promoted the growth of organized anesthesiology. Ralph Waters and John Lundy, among others, participated in evolving organized anesthesia. Waters' greatest contribution to the specialty was raising its academic standards. After completing his internship in 1913, he entered medical practice in Sioux City, Iowa, where he gradually limited his practice to anesthesia. His personal experience and extensive reading were supplemented by the only postgraduate training available, a 1-month course conducted in Ohio by E. I. McKesson. At that time, the custom of becoming a self-proclaimed specialist in medicine and surgery was not uncommon. Waters, who was frustrated by low standards and who would eventually have a great influence on establishing both anesthesia residency training and the formal examination process, recalled that before 1920, "The requirements for specialization in many Midwestern hospitals consisted of the possession of sufficient audacity to attempt a procedure and persuasive power adequate to gain the consent of the patient or his family."[142]

In an effort to improve anesthetic care, Waters regularly corresponded with Dennis Jackson and other scientists. In 1925, he relocated to Kansas City with a goal of gaining an academic post at the University of Kansas, but the professor of surgery failed to support his proposal. The larger city did allow him to initiate his freestanding outpatient surgical facility, "The Downtown Surgical Clinic," which featured one of the first postanesthetic recovery rooms.[130] In 1927, Erwin Schmidt, professor of surgery at the University of Wisconsin's medical school, encouraged Dean Charles Bardeen to recruit Waters.

In accepting the first American academic position in anesthesia, Waters described four objectives that have been since adopted by many other academic departments. His goals were as follows: "(1) to provide the best possible service to patients of the institution, (2) to teach what is known of the principles of Anesthesiology to all candidates for their medical degree, (3) to help long-term graduate students not only to gain a fundamental knowledge of the subject and to master the art of administration, but also to learn as much as possible of the effective methods of teaching, (4) to accompany these efforts with the encouragement of as much cooperative investigation as is consistent with achieving the first objectives."[129]

Waters' personal and professional qualities impressed talented young men and women who sought residency posts in his department. He encouraged residents to initiate research interests in which they collaborated with two pharmacologists whom Waters had known before arriving in Wisconsin, Arthur Loevenhart and Chauncey Leake, as well as others with whom he became associated in Madison. Clinical concerns were also investigated. As an example, anesthesia records were coded onto punch cards to form a database that was used to analyze departmental activities. Morbidity and mortality meetings, now a requirement of all training programs, also originated in Madison. Members of the department and distinguished visitors from other centers attended these meetings. As a consequence of their critical reviews of the conduct of anesthesia, responsibility for an operative tragedy gradually passed from the patient to the physician. In more casual times, a practitioner could complain, "The patient died because he did not take a good anesthetic."

Alternatively, the death might be attributed to a mysterious force such as "status lymphaticus," of which Arthur Guedel, a master of sardonic humor, observed, "Certainly status lymphaticus is at times a great help to the anesthetist. When he has a fatality under anesthesia with no other cleansing explanation he is glad to recognize the condition as an entity."[129]

In 1929, John Lundy at the Mayo Clinic organized the Anaesthetists' Travel Club, whose members were leading American or Canadian teachers of anesthesia. Each year one member was the host for a group of 20 to 40 anesthesiologists who gathered for a program of informal discussions. There were demonstrations of promising innovations for the operating room and laboratory, which were all subjected to what is remembered as a "high-spirited, energetic, critical review."[127] The Travel Club would be critical in the upcoming battle to form the American Board of Anesthesiology.

Even during the lean years of the Depression, international guests also visited Waters' department. For Geoffrey Kaye of Australia, Torsten Gordh of Sweden, Robert Macintosh and Michael Nosworthy of England, and scores of others, Waters' department was their "mecca of anesthesia." Ralph Waters trained 60 residents during the 22 years he was the "Chief." From 1937 onward, the alumni, who declared themselves the "Aqualumni" in his honor, returned annually for a professional and social reunion. Thirty-four Aqualumni took academic positions and, of these, 14 became chairpersons of departments of anesthesia. They maintained Waters' professional principles and encouraged teaching careers for many of their own graduates.[143] His enduring legacy was once recognized by the dean who had recruited him in 1927, Charles Bardeen, who observed, "Ralph Waters was the first person the University hired to put people to sleep, but, instead, he awakened a world-wide interest in anesthesia."[144]

Establishing a Society

Waters and Lundy, along with Paul Wood of New York City, had an important role in establishing organized anesthesia and the definition of the specialty. In the heart of the Great Depression, these three physicians realized that anesthesiology needed to have a process to determine who was an anesthetic specialist with American Medical Association (AMA) backing. Using the New York Society of Anesthetists, of which Paul Wood was secretary-treasurer, a new class of members, "Fellows," was created. The Fellows criteria followed established AMA guidelines for specialty certification. However, the AMA wanted a national organization to sponsor a specialty board. The New York Society of Anesthetists changed its name to the American Society of Anesthetists (ASA) in 1936. Combined with the American Society of Regional Anesthesia, whose president was Emery Rovenstein, the American Board of Anesthesiology (ABA) was organized as a subordinate board to the American Board of Surgery in 1938. With McMechan's death in 1939, the AMA favored independence for the ABA, and in 1940, independence was granted.[126,131]

A few years later, the officers of the American Society of Anesthetists were challenged by Dr. M. J. Seifert, who wrote, "An Anesthetist is a technician and an Anesthesiologist is the specific authority on anesthesia and anesthetics. I cannot understand why you do not term yourselves the American Society of Anesthesiologists."[133] Ralph Waters was declared the first president of the newly named ASA in 1945. In that year, when World War II ended, 739 (37%) of 1977 ASA members were in the armed forces. In the same year, the ASA's first Distinguished Service Award was presented to Paul M. Wood for his tireless service to the specialty, one element of which can be examined today in the extensive archives preserved in the Society's Wood Library-Museum at ASA headquarters, Park Ridge, Illinois.[144]

Conclusions

This overview of the development of anesthesiology is but a brief outline of the current roles in which anesthesiologists serve in hospitals, clinics, and laboratories. The operating room and obstetric delivery suite remain the central interest of most specialists. Aside from being the location where the techniques described in this chapter find regular application, service in these areas brings us into regular contact with new advances in pharmacology and bioengineering.

After surgery, patients are transported to the postanesthesia care unit or recovery room, an area that is now considered the anesthesiologist's "ward." Fifty years ago, patients were carried directly from the operating room to a surgical ward to be attended only by a junior nurse. That person lacked both the skills and the equipment to intervene when complications occurred. After the experiences of World War II taught the value of centralized care, physicians and nurses created recovery rooms, which were soon mandated for all major hospitals. By 1960, the evolution of critical care progressed through the use of mechanical ventilators. Patients who required many days of intensive medical and nursing management were cared for in a curtained corner of the recovery room. In time, curtains drawn about one or two beds gave way to fixed partitions and the relocation of those areas to form intensive care units. The principles of resuscitative and supportive care established by anesthesiologists transformed critical care medicine.

The future of anesthesiology is a bright one. The safer drugs that once revolutionized the care of patients undergoing surgery are constantly being improved. The role of the anesthesiologist continues to broaden as physicians with backgrounds in the specialty have developed clinics for chronic pain control and centers for outpatient surgery and assumed a role as administrative heads of perioperative units in major medical centers. Anesthesia practice continues to increase in scope, both inside and outside the operating suite, such that anesthesiologists have increasingly become an integral part of the entire perioperative experience.

REFERENCES

1. Joyce H. *The journals and letters of Fanny Burney.* Oxford: Clarendon; 1975. As quoted in: Papper EM. *Romance, Poetry, and Surgical Sleep.* Westport, CT: Greenwood Press; 1995:12.
2. Epitaph to W.T.G. Morton on a Memorial from the Mt. Auburn Cemetery. Cambridge, Massachusetts.
3. These Egyptian pictographs are dated approximately 2500 BC. See Ellis ES: *Ancient Anodynes: Primitive Anaesthesia and Allied Conditions.* London, UK: WM Heinemann Medical Books; 1946:80.
4. Bacon DR. Regional anesthesia and chronic pain therapy: a history. In: Brown DL, ed. *Regional Anesthesia and Analgesia.* Philadelphia, PA: WB Saunders; 1996:11.
5. Rutkow I. *Surgery, an Illustrated History.* St. Louis, MO: Mosby; 1993:215.
6. Winter A. *Mesmerized: Powers of Mind in Victorian Britain.* Chicago, IL: University of Chicago Press; 1998:42.
7. Marmer MJ. *Hypnosis in Anesthesiology.* Springfield, IL: Charles C Thomas; 1959:10.
8. Dioscorides. On mandragora. In: *Dioscorides Opera Libra.* Quoted in: Bergman N. *The Genesis of Surgical Anesthesia.* Park Ridge, IL: Wood Library-Museum of Anesthesiology; 1998:11.
9. Dote K. General anesthesia in Japan around 1830. *J Anesth Hist.* 2015;1:88
10. Dote K. *Mafutsutoron.* Japan: Ehime University School of Medicine; 2016.
11. Infusino M, O'Neill YV, Calmes S. Hog beans, poppies, and mandrake leaves: a test of the efficacy of the soporific sponge. In: Atkinson RS, Boulton TB, eds. *The History of Anaesthesia.* London, UK: Parthenon Publishing Group; 1989:31.
12. Davy H. *Researches Chemical and Philosophical Chiefly Concerning Nitrous Oxide or Dephlogisticated Nitrous Air, and Its Respiration.* London, UK: J Johnson; 1800:533.
13. Papper EM. *Romance, Poetry, and Surgical Sleep.* Westport, CT: Greenwood Press; 1995.
14. Hickman HH. A letter on suspended animation, containing experiments showing that it may be safely employed during operations on animals, with the view of ascertaining its probable utility in surgical operations on the human subject, addressed to T.A. Knight, Esq. Imprint Ironbridge, W. Smith, 1824.
15. Strickland RA. Ether drinking in Ireland. *Mayo Clin Proc.* 1996;71:1015.
16. Lyman HM. *Artificial Anaesthesia and Anaesthetics.* New York, NY: William Hood; 1881:6.
17. Stetson JB, William E. Clarke and the discovery of anesthesia. In: Fink BR, Morris L, Stephen ER, eds. *The History of Anesthesia: Third International Symposium Proceedings.* Park Ridge, IL: Wood Library-Museum of Anesthesiology; 1992:400.
18. Long CW. An account of the first use of sulphuric ether by inhalation as an anaesthetic in surgical operations. *South Med Surg J.* 1849;5:705.
19. Robinson V. *Victory Over Pain.* New York, NY: Henry Schuman; 1946:91.
20. Smith GB, Hirsch NP. Gardner Quincy Colton: pioneer of nitrous oxide anesthesia. *Anesth Analg.* 1991;72:382.
21. Menczer LF. Horace Wells's "day book A": a transcription and analysis. In: Wolfe RJ, Menczer LF, eds. *I Awaken to Glory.* Boston, MA: Boston Medical Library; 1994:112.
22. Greene NM. A consideration of factors in the discovery of anesthesia and their effects on its development. *Anesthesiology.* 1971;35:515–522.
23. Fenster J. *Ether Day.* New York, NY: Harper Collins; 2001:76.
24. Haridas RP. "Gentlemen! This Is no humbug!": Did John Collins Warren, M.D., proclaim these words on October 16, 1846, at Massachusetts General Hospital, Boston? *Anesthesiology.* 2016;124:553–560.
25. Caton D. *What a Blessing She Had Chloroform.* New Haven, CT: Yale University Press; 1999:103.
26. Journal of Queen Victoria. In: Strauss MB, ed. *Familiar Medical Quotations.* Boston, MA: Little Brown; 1968:17.
27. Eger EI, Saidman LJ, Brandstater B. Minimum alveolar anesthetic concentration: a standard of anesthetic potency. *Anesthesiology.* 1965;26:756–763.
28. Clover JT. Laryngotomy in chloroform anesthesia. *Br Med J.* 1877;1:132–133.
29. Macewan W. Clinical observations on the introduction of tracheal tubes by the mouth instead of performing tracheotomy or laryngotomy. *Br Med J.* 1880;2:122, 163–165.
30. Hirsch NP, Smith GB, Hirsch PO. Alfred Kirstein, pioneer of direct laryngoscopy. *Anaesthesia.* 1986;41:42–45.
31. Burkle CM, Zepeda FA, Bacon DR, et al. A historical perspective on use of the laryngoscope as a tool in anesthesiology. *Anesthesiology.* 2004;100:1003–1006.
32. Miller RA. A new laryngoscope. *Anesthesiology.* 1941;2:317.
33. Macintosh RR. Richard Salt of Oxford, anaesthetic technician extraordinary. *Anaesthesia.* 1976;31:855.
34. Thomas KB. Sir Ivan Whiteside Magill, KCVO, DSc, MB, BCh, BAO, FRCS, FFARCS (Hon), FFARCSI (Hon), DA: a review of his publications and other references to his life and work. *Anaesthesia.* 1978;33:628–634.
35. Condon HA, Gilchrist E. Stanley Rowbotham: twentieth century pioneer anaesthetist. *Anaesthesia.* 1986;41:46–52.
36. Calverley RK. Classical file. *Surv Anesth.* 1984;28:70.
37. Gale JW, Waters RM. Closed endobronchial anesthesia in thoracic surgery: preliminary report. *Curr Res Anesth Analg.* 1932;11:283.
38. Wu TL, Chou HC. A new laryngoscope: the combination intubating device (letter). *Anesthesiology.* 1994;81:1085–1087.
39. Brain AIJ. The laryngeal mask: a new concept in airway management. *Br J Anaesth.* 1983;55:801–805.
40. Van Zundert TC, Briacombe JR, Ferson DZ, et al. Archie Brain: celebrating 30 years of development in laryngeal mask airways. *Anaesthesia.* 2012;67(12):1375–1385.
41. Calverley RK. An early ether vaporizer designed by John Snow, a Treasure of the Wood Library-Museum of Anesthesiology. In: Fink BR, Morris LE, Stephen CR, eds. *The History of Anesthesiology.* Park Ridge, IL: Wood Library-Museum of Anesthesiology; 1992:91.
42. Snow J. *On the Inhalation of the Vapour of Ether.* London, UK: J Churchill; 1847:23. Reprinted by the Wood Library-Museum of Anesthesiology.
43. Calverley RK, Clover JT. A giant of Victorian anaesthesia. In: Rupreht J, van Lieburg MJ, Lee JA, Erdmann W, eds. *Anaesthesia: Essays on Its History.* Berlin: Springer-Verlag; 1985:21.
44. Andrews E. The oxygen mixture, a new anaesthetic combination. *Chicago Med Exam.* 1868;9:656.
45. Obituary of T. Philip Ayre. *Br Med J.* 1980;280:125.
46. Rees GJ. Anaesthesia in the newborn. *Br Med J.* 1950;2:1419–1422.
47. Bain JA, Spoerel WE. A stream-lined anaesthetic system. *Can Anaesth Soc J.* 1972;19:426–435.
48. Mushin WW, Rendell-Baker L. *Thoracic Anaesthesia Past and Present.* Springfield, IL: Charles C Thomas; 1953:44. Reprinted by the Wood Library-Museum of Anesthesiology, 1991.

49. Shephard DAE. Harvey Cushing and anaesthesia. *Can Anaesth Soc J.* 1965; 12:431–442.
50. Waters RM. Clinical scope and utility of carbon dioxide filtration in inhalation anesthesia. *Curr Res Anesth Analg.* 1923;3:20.
51. Sword BC. The closed circle method of administration of gas anesthesia. *Curr Res Anesth Analg.* 1930;9:198.
52. Sands RP, Bacon DR. An inventive mind: The career of James O. Elam, M.D. (1918–1995). *Anesthesiology.* 1998;88:1107–1112.
53. Morris LE. A new vaporizer for liquid anesthetic agents. *Anesthesiology.* 1952;13:587–593.
54. Sands R, Bacon DR. The copper kettle: a historical perspective. *J Clin Anesthesiol.* 1996;8:528–532.
55. Duncum BM. *The Development of Inhalation Anaesthesia.* London, UK: Oxford University Press; 1947:538.
56. Severinghaus JC, Honda Y. Pulse oximetry. *Int Anesthesiol Clin.* 1987;25: 205–214.
57. Cushing H. I. On the avoidance of shock in major amputations by cocainization of large nerve trunks preliminary to their division: with observations on blood-pressure changes in surgical cases. *Ann Surg.* 1902;36:321–345.
58. Codesmith A. An endo-esophageal stethoscope. *Anesthesiology.* 1954;15: 566.
59. Luft K. Methode der registrieren gas analyse mit hilfe der absorption ultraroten Strahlen ohne spectrale Zerlegung. *Z Tech Phys.* 1943;24:97.
60. Tovell RM. Problems in supply of anesthetic gases in the European theater of operations. *Anesthesiology.* 1947;8:303–311.
61. Rendell-Baker L. History of standards for anesthesia equipment. In: Rupreht J, van Lieburg MJ, Lee JA, et al., eds. *Anaesthesia: Essays on Its History.* Berlin, Germany: Springer-Verlag; 1985:161.
62. Calverley RK. A safety feature for anaesthesia machines: Touch identification of oxygen flow control. *Can Anaesth Soc J.* 1971;18:225–229.
63. Lucas GH. The discovery of cyclopropane. *Curr Res Anesth Analg.* 1961;40: 15–27.
64. Seevers MH, Meek WJ, Rovenstine EA, et al. Cyclopropane study with special reference to gas concentration, respiratory and electrocardiographic changes. *J Pharmacol Exp Ther.* 1934;51:1.
65. Calverley RK. Fluorinated anesthetics. I. The early years. *Surv Anesth.* 1986; 29:170.
66. Suckling CW. Some chemical and physical factors in the development of fluothane. *Br J Anaesth.* 1957;29:466–472.
67. Wren PC. *Philosophical Transactions.* Vol 1. London, UK: Anno; 1665 and 1666.
68. Keys TE. *The History of Surgical Anesthesia.* New York, NY: Dover Publications; 1945:38.
69. Dundee J, Wyant G. *Intravenous Anaesthesia.* Hong Kong: Churchill Livingstone; 1974:1.
70. Oré PC. Etudes, cliniques sur l'anesthésie chirurgicale par la methode des injection de choral dans les veines. Paris: JB Balliere et Fils; 1875. As quoted in: Hemelrijck JV, Kissin I. History of intravenous anesthesia. In: White PF, ed. *Textbook of Intravenous Anesthesia.* Baltimore: Williams & Wilkins; 1997:3.
71. Macintosh RR. Modern anaesthesia, with special reference to the chair of anaesthetics in Oxford. In: Rupreht J, van Lieburg MJ, Lee JA, et al., eds. *Anaesthesia: Essays on Its History.* Berlin: Springer-Verlag; 1985:352.
72. Hemelrijck JV, Kissin I. History of intravenous anesthesia. In: White PF, ed. *Textbook of Intravenous Anesthesia.* Baltimore: Williams & Wilkins; 1997:3.
73. Fink BR. Leaves and needles: the introduction of surgical local anesthesia. *Anesthesiology.* 1985;63:77–83.
74. Koller C. Über die Verwendung des Cocain zur Anästhesirung am Auge. *Wien Med Wochenschr.* 1884;34:1276.
75. Calatayud J, Gonzalez A. History of the development and evolution of local anesthesia since the coca leaf. *Anesthesiology.* 2003;98:1503–1508.
76. Fink BR. History of local anesthesia. In: Cousins MJ, Bridenbaugh PO, eds. *Neural Blockade.* Philadelphia, PA: JB Lippincott; 1980:12.
77. Ruetsch YA, Boni T, Borgeat A. From cocaine to ropivacaine: The history of local anesthetic drugs. *Curr Top Med Chem.* 2001;1:175.
78. Ekenstam B, Egnev B, Pettersson G. Local anaesthetics: I. N-alkyl pyrrolidine and N-alkyl piperidine carboxylic acid amides. *Acta Chem Scand.* 1957; 11:1183.
79. Albright GA. Cardiac arrest following regional anesthesia with etidocaine or bupivacaine. *Anesthesiology.* 1979;51:285.
80. Aberg G. Toxicological and local anaesthetic effects of optically active isomers of two local anaesthetic compounds. *Acta Pharmacol Toxicol (Copenh).* 1972;31:273–286.
81. Polley LS, Santos AC. Cardiac arrest following regional anesthesia with ropivacaine: here we go again! *Anesthesiology.* 2003;99:1253–1254.
82. Castillo J, Curley J, Hotz J, et al. Glucocorticoids prolong rat sciatic nerve blockade in vivo from bupivacaine microspheres. *Anesthesiology.* 1996;85:1157–1166.
83. Mowat JJ, Mok MJ, MacLeod BA, et al. Liposomal bupivacaine: extended duration nerve blockade using large unilamellar vesicles that exhibit a proton gradient. *Anesthesiology.* 1996;85:635–643.

84. McIntyre AR. *Curare, Its History, Nature, and Clinical Use.* Chicago: University of Chicago Press; 1947:6, 131.
85. Thomas BK. *Curare: Its History and Usage.* Philadelphia, PA: JB Lippincott Company; 1963:90.
86. Rushman GB, Davies NJH, Atkinson RS. *A Short History of Anaesthesia.* Oxford: Butterworth-Heinemann; 1996:78.
87. Knoefel PK. *Felice Fontana: Life and Works.* Trento: Societa de Studi Trentini; 1985:284.
88. Griffith HR, Johnson GE. The use of curare in general anesthesia. *Anesthesiology.* 1942;3:418.
89. McIntyre AR. Historical background, early use and development of muscle relaxants. *Anesthesiology.* 1959;20:409–415.
90. Ali HH, Utting JE, Gray C. Quantitative assessment of residual antidepolarizing block (part II). *Br J Anaesth.* 1971;43:478–485.
91. Gwathmey JT. *Anesthesia.* New York, NY: Appleton and Company; 1914:379.
92. Flagg PJ. *The Art of Anaesthesia.* Philadelphia, PA: JB Lippincott Company; 1918:80.
93. Hewer CL. *Recent Advances in Anaesthesia and Analgesia.* Philadelphia, PA: P Blakiston's Son & Co. Inc; 1937:237.
94. Collins VJ. *Principles and Practice of Anesthesiology.* Philadelphia, PA: Lea & Febiger; 1952:327.
95. Raeder J. History of postoperative nausea and vomiting. *Int Anesthesiol Clin.* 2003;41:1–12.
96. Koller C. Personal reminiscences of the first use of cocaine as local anesthetic in eye surgery. *Curr Res Anesth Analg.* 1928;7:9.
97. Becker HK. Carl Koller and cocaine. *Psychoanal Q.* 1963;32:309–373.
98. Halsted WS. Practical comments on the use and abuse of cocaine; suggested by its invariably successful employment in more than a thousand minor surgical operations. *N Y Med J.* 1885;42:294.
99. Olch PD, William S. Halstead and local anesthesia: Contributions and complications. *Anesthesiology.* 1975;42:479–486.
100. Marx G. The first spinal anesthesia: Who deserves the laurels? *Reg Anesth.* 1994;19:429–430.
101. Corning JL. Spinal anaesthesia and local medication of the cord. *N Y Med J.* 1885;42:483.
102. Bier AKG. Experiments in cocainization of the spinal cord, 1899. In: Faulconer A, Keys TE (trans), eds. *Foundations of Anesthesiology.* Springfield, IL: Charles C Thomas; 1965:854.
103. Goerig M, Agarwal K, Schulte am Esch J. The versatile August Bier (1861–1949), father of spinal anesthesia. *J Clin Anesth.* 2000;12:561–569.
104. Larson MD. Tait and Caglieri. The first spinal anesthetic in America. *Anesthesiology.* 1996;85:913–919.
105. Lee JA. Arthur Edward James Barker, 1850–1916: British pioneer of regional anaesthesia. *Anaesthesia.* 1979;34:885–891.
106. Lemmon WT. A method for continuous spinal anesthesia: a preliminary report. *Ann Surg.* 1940;111:141–144.
107. Martini JA, Bacon DR, Vasdev GM. Edward Tuohy: The man, his needle, and its place in obstetric anesthesia. *Reg Anesth Pain Med.* 2002;27:520–523.
108. Tuohy EB. Continuous spinal anesthesia: Its usefulness and technique involved. *Anesthesiology.* 1944;5:142.
109. Pagés F. Metameric anesthesia, 1921. In: Faulconer A, Keys TE (trans), eds. *Foundations of Anesthesiology.* Springfield, IL: Charles C Thomas; 1965:927.
110. Crile GW, Lower WE. *Anoci-Association.* Philadelphia, PA: WB Saunders Company; 1915.
111. Brown DL, Winnie AP. Biography of Louis Gaston Labat, M.D. *Reg Anesth.* 1992;17:249–262.
112. Bacon DR, Darwish H. Emery Rovenstine and regional anesthesia. *Reg Anesth.* 1997;22:273–279.
113. Rehn L. On penetrating cardiac injuries and cardiac suturing. *Arch Klin Chir.* 1897;55:315.
114. Naef AP. The mid-century revolution in thoracic and cardiovascular surgery: part 1. *Interact Cardiovasc Thorac Surg.* 2003;2:219–226.
115. Baum VC. Pediatric cardiac surgery: An historical appreciation. *Pediatr Anesth.* 2006;16:1213–1225.
116. Harmel M, Lamont A. Anesthesia in the treatment of congenital pulmonary stenosis. *Anesthesiology.* 1948;7:477–498.
117. With gas & needle. *Time.* Monday, October 19, 1953.
118. Tracy PT, Hanigan WC. The history of neuroanesthesia. In: Greenblatt SH, ed. *The History of Neurosurgery.* New York, NY: Thieme; 1997:213.
119. Samuels SI. The history of neuroanesthesia: a contemporary review. *Int Anesthesiol Clin.* 1996;34:1–20.
120. Horsley V. Brain surgery. *Br Med J.* 1886;2:670.
121. Frazier C. Problems and procedures in cranial surgery. *JAMA.* 1909;52: 1805.
122. Bacon DR. The World Federation of Societies of Anaesthesiologists: McMechan's final legacy? *Anesth Analg.* 1997;84:1130–1135.
123. Seldon TH. Francis Hoeffer McMechan. In: Volpitto PP, Vandam LD, eds. *Genesis of American Anesthesiology.* Springfield, IL: Charles C Thomas; 1982:5.
124. Canton D. The history of obstetric anesthesia. In: Chestnut DH, ed. *Obstetric Anesthesia: Principles and Practice.* Philadelphia, PA: Elsevier Mosby; 2004.

125. Barnett R. A horse named 'Twilight Sleep': the language of obstetric anaesthesia in 20th century Britain. *Int J Obstet Anesth.* 2005;14:310–315.
126. Canton D. *What a Blessing She Had Chloroform.* New Haven: Yale University Press; 1999.
127. MacKenzie RA, Bacon DR, Martin DP. Anaesthetists' Travel Club: a transformation of the Society of Clinical Surgery? *Bull Anesth Hist.* 2004;22:7–10.
128. Apgar V. A proposal for a new method of evaluation of the newborn infant. *Curr Res Anesth Analg.* 1953;32:260–267.
129. Guedel AE. *Inhalation Anesthesia: A Fundamental Guide.* New York, NY: Macmillan; 1937:129.
130. Waters RM. The down-town anesthesia clinic. *Am J Surg.* 1919;33:71.
131. Hingson RA. Continuous caudal analgesia in obstetrics, surgery, and therapeutics. *Br Med J.* 1949;2:777–781.
132. Gogarten W, Van Aken H. A century of regional analgesia in obstetrics. *Anesth Analg.* 2000;91:773–775.
133. Little DM Jr, Betcher AM. *The Diamond Jubilee 1905–1980.* Park Ridge, IL: American Society of Anesthesiologists; 1980:8.
134. Hawkins JL, Koonin LM, Palmer SK, et al. Anesthesia-related deaths during obstetric delivery in the United States, 1979–1990. *Anesthesiology.* 1997;86:277–284.
135. Hawkins JL. Anesthesia-related maternal mortality. *Clin Obstet Gynecol.* 2003;46:679–687.
136. Gottlieb AM. *A Pictorial History of Blood Practices and Transfusion.* Scottsdale, AZ: Arcane Publications; 1992:2.
137. Jenkins MT. *Epochs in Intravenous Fluid Therapy: From the Goose Quill and Pig Bladder to Balanced Salt Solutions.* Park Ridge, IL: The Lewis H. Wright Memorial Lecture, Wood Library-Museum Collection; 1993:4.
138. Betcher AM, Ciliberti BJ, Wood PM, et al. The jubilee year of organized anesthesia. *Anesthesiology.* 1956;17:226–264.
139. Bacon DR. The promise of one great anesthesia society. *Anesthesiology.* 1994;80:929–935.
140. Edwards ML, Waisel DB. 49 Mathoura Road: Geoffrey Kaye's letters to Paul M. Wood, 1939–1955. *Anesthesiology.* 2014;121:1150–1157.
141. Bacon DR, Lema MJ. To define a specialty: a brief history of the American Board of Anesthesiology's first written examination. *J Clin Anesth.* 1992;4:489–497.
142. Waters RM. Pioneering in anesthesiology. *Postgrad Med.* 1948;4:265–270.
143. Bacon DR, Ament R. Ralph waters and the beginnings of academic anesthesiology in the United States: the Wisconsin template. *J Clin Anesth.* 1995;7:534–543.
144. Bamforth BJ, Siebecker KL. Ralph M. Waters. In: Volpitto PP, Vandam LD, eds. *Genesis of American Anesthesiology.* Springfield, IL: Charles C Thomas; 1982.
145. Haridas RP: Horace wells' demonstration of nitrous oxide in Boston. *Anesthesiology.* 2013;119:1014–1022.
146. Duncum RM. The development of inhalation anaesthesia. London: Oxford University Press; 1947:86.
147. Kuhn F. Nasotracheal intubation (trans). In: Faulconer A, Keys AE, eds. *Foundations of Anesthesiology.* Springfield, IL: Charles C Thomas. 1965:677.

2 Scope of Practice

JOHN H. EICHHORN

Changing Anesthesiology Practice
  Bundled Payment Model
  Practice Model for Anesthesiologists: The Perioperative Surgical Home
  Practice Model Involving Anesthesiologists: The Service Line
  Large Group Practices: Anesthesia and Multispecialty
  Further Issues
Administrative Components of Anesthesiology Practice
  Operational and Information Resources
  The Credentialing Process and Clinical Privileges
  Maintenance of Certification in Anesthesiology
  Professional Staff Participation and Relationships
  Establishing Standards of Practice and Understanding the Standard of Care
  Policy and Procedure
  Meetings and Case Discussion
  Support Staff
  Anesthesia Equipment and Equipment Maintenance
  Malpractice Insurance
  Response to an Adverse Event
Practice Essentials
  The "Job Market" for Anesthesia Professionals
  Types of Practice
  Billing and Collecting
  Antitrust Considerations
  Exclusive Service Contracts
  Hospital Subsidies
  Evolving Practice Arrangements
  Accountable Care Organizations
  Management Intricacies
  Health Insurance Portability and Accountability Act
  Electronic Health ("Health") Records
  Expansion into Perioperative Medicine and Hospital Care
Operating Room Management
  Organization
  Scheduling Cases
  Anesthesiology Personnel Issues
Cost and Quality Issues
Conclusion

KEY POINTS

1. Anesthesia trainees, and many postgraduates, tend to lack sufficient knowledge (with sometimes unfortunate results) about modes of practice or employment, financial matters of all types, and the forces that shape them, but contracting in particular. They must educate themselves and also seek expert advice and counsel to survive (and hopefully flourish) in today's exceedingly intricate medical practice milieu.

2. Concerns about the unsustainable increases in the cost of health care in the United States have led to a major new emphasis on value (get more and better results for less cost) and quality (avoid expensive complications, both improving care and reducing costs). New models of surgical care that significantly impact the practice of clinical anesthesia and payment for it have been proposed and are progressing toward implementation. Anesthesia professionals must understand and appreciate these models and their potential changes to the practice and scope of anesthesia.

3. There are several very helpful detailed information resources concerning practice and operating room (OR) management available from the American Society of Anesthesiologists and other sources. Factors influencing anesthesiology practice conditions are changing rapidly, and today's anesthesia professionals must be armed with detailed information about concepts (such as "accountable care organizations," "quality reporting," and "pay for performance") that did not exist just a few years ago.

4. Securing hospital privileges is far more than a bureaucratic annoyance and must be taken seriously by anesthesiologists.

5. Anesthesiology is the leading medical specialty in establishing and promulgating standards of practice that have significantly influenced practice in a positive manner.

6. The immediate response to a major adverse anesthesia event is critical to the eventual result. An extremely valuable protocol is available at www.apsf.org, "Resource Center: Clinical Safety Tools."

7. Anesthesiologists must be involved, concerned, active participants and leaders in their institution and medical community in order to enhance their practice function and image.

8. Although the threatened impact of "managed care" largely failed to materialize regarding anesthesiology practice, other types of reorganization will matter. The impact of the "Great Recession" on the health-care system was substantial and will resonate into the future on budgets, availability of resources, and the economics of medical practice.

9. Anesthesiologists must participate in OR management in their facilities and should play a central leadership role. OR scheduling, staffing, utilization, and patient flow issues are complex, and anesthesiologists should work hard to both thoroughly understand and positively influence them.

10. Anesthesiology personnel issues involve an elaborate balancing act that is subject to complex conflicting forces. Anesthesiology groups/departments should give these issues, as well as their constituent personnel, more attention and energy than has been done traditionally in the past.

11. Attention to the many often-underemphasized details of infrastructure, organization, and administration can transform a merely endurable anesthesia practice into one that is safe, efficient, effective, productive, collegial, and even fun.

The structure and function of anesthesia practice are evolving rapidly in the United States in conjunction with the overhaul of the entire health-care system.

As the landscape shifts, many leaders of anesthesia professional organizations, along with some practitioners, have become engaged as activists attempting to influence the decisions that will ultimately affect the practice of anesthesiology.

This is in contrast to the past when anesthesia professionals as a group traditionally were little involved in the administration and management of many components of their practice beyond the strictly medical elements of applied physiology and pharmacology, pathophysiology, and therapeutics. This was perhaps somewhat understandable because anesthesia professionals traditionally spent most of their usually very long work hours in an OR. Business and regulatory matters were often left to the one or two members of the old-style traditional private practice group who were interested in or willing to deal with an outside-contractor billing agency, hospital administration, and so forth. In that era, very little formal teaching about factors affecting anesthesiology or practice management occurred. Today, the Anesthesiology Residency Review Committee of the Accreditation Council on Graduate Medical Education requires that the didactic curricula of anesthesiology residencies include material on "practice management." Training programs offer at least an introduction to such issues, but these may be insufficient to satisfactorily prepare professionals for the real infrastructure, administrative, business, and management challenges of the current practice of anesthesiology. All of the dramatic changes in anesthesiology practice further emphasize the need for insight and understanding.

This chapter presents a wide variety of topics that, a generation ago, were not included in anesthesiology textbooks or residency program curricula. Outlined are several basic components of the background and administrative, organizational (including both practice arrangements and daily functioning of the OR), and, especially, financial aspects of anesthesiology practice in the complex modern environment. Although many issues are undergoing almost constant and sometimes unpredictable change, it is important to understand the basic vocabulary and principles in this dynamic universe. Lack of understanding of these issues may well leave anesthesia professionals at a disadvantage when attempting to maximize the efficiency and impact of their daily activities, to make critical decisions about practice arrangements, and to secure fair compensation in an increasingly complex health-care system featuring greater and greater competition for scarcer and scarcer resources.

Changing Anesthesiology Practice

Pressure on the American health-care system to shift away from traditional models of organization and financing is significant. Concern about the fraction of the national gross domestic product devoted to health care has driven the dramatic emphasis on "value"[1] (get more and better results for less cost) in assessing and formulating the health-care "industry." There is widespread perception that inefficient, poorly coordinated, redundant efforts that are divided into "silos" that do not communicate well lead to suboptimal health-care outcomes at both the individual and population levels. Many American leaders from a wide diversity of perspectives have called for stopping the growth of health-care costs as a start and then actually reducing them to a much more manageable level. Accordingly, there are multiple initiatives focused on improving both the process and outcomes of health care, usually involving the concepts of "quality" (improved outcome and decreasing expensive complications) and also "value." This type of improvement is one of the main goals of the US Federal Government in promoting the creation of multidisciplinary integrated networked health-care delivery entities known as Accountable Care Organizations (ACOs), a central feature of the 2010 Patient Protection and Affordable Care Act (ACA).[2-4] The quality and value improvement initiatives in general often advocate standardization of care through adoption of evidence-based "best practices." This incorporates the desire to very sharply reduce individual variability in practice among practitioners, which is sometimes viewed negatively by health-care practitioners, including anesthesia professionals, who traditionally have evolved their own practice habits and preferences based on their personal education, training, and experience. It may yet be a long time before there are serious efforts to impose national protocols prescribing, for example, which muscle relaxant and which inhalation anesthetic will be used for all laparoscopic cholecystectomies. However, the current pervasive belief that the health-care system must be "smarter, better, safer, faster, and cheaper" with fixation on value cannot be ignored. Beyond going faster, reducing medication costs, placing fewer invasive monitors, and avoiding complications, value in clinical anesthesia practice can be difficult to define.[5] Overall, anesthesia professionals need to be aware of the involved forces and proposals regarding patterns of practice so they can participate constructively to further the interests of their patients, and their practices, rather than allowing themselves to become passive casualties of the inevitable changes that are coming.

Bundled Payment Model

One of the greatest changes affecting anesthesia practice is the concept that the organizations (and eventually individuals) who pay for health care are intending to alter radically the mechanism of rendering those payments. At its outset, this does not involve changing who pays (e.g., U.S. Federal Government, state government, private indemnity insurance companies, health plans, including health maintenance organizations, and cooperatives of many types), but rather how much is paid and to whom exactly. Whether this situation could be a harbinger of an attempt to totally revolutionize the U.S. health-care system by creating a universal-coverage single-payer (Federal Government administered) tax-supported system is unknown and impossible to predict.

A model program illustrates the concept of bundled payments for health care. The U.S. Federal Government agency, the Centers for Medicare and Medicaid Services (CMS), introduced in late 2015, with implementation in April 2016, their Comprehensive Care for Joint Replacement model. The stated aim is: "to support better and more efficient care for beneficiaries undergoing the most common inpatient surgeries for Medicare beneficiaries: hip and knee replacements.... This model tests bundled payment and quality measurement for an episode of care associated with hip and knee replacements to encourage hospitals, physicians, and postacute care providers to work together to improve the quality and coordination of care from the initial hospitalization through recovery."[6] The initial roll-out is complex, with all involved professional providers continuing to bill and collect from Medicare as always—until the end of the plan year, when CMS will compare a grand total of payments for the episode of care (defined as including 90 days after hospital discharge) for all covered patients at a given hospital within the test areas with calculated historic benchmarks. If the total cost is under the benchmark, CMS will pay the difference to the hospital to distribute as determined internally. If, on the other hand, the total paid by CMS exceeds the benchmark, the hospital will be required to refund (from what was already collected) the difference to CMS.[7] The source of the money refunded to CMS would be determined internally within the hospital, presumably involving collection (internal "clawback") of money from the various providers, including private practice anesthesia professionals, who already collected their professional fee reimbursement from CMS. Overall, the idea of this system is a blueprint for the future. CMS is a critical revenue source for most hospitals and many anesthesiology practices. Further, many health plans/health systems structure their payments for services parallel to the CMS system payment amounts, and more and more indemnity insurance companies are doing so also.

The fundamental concept introduced by the CMS Comprehensive Care for Joint Replacement model is straightforward. The ultimate goal is to transition to a prospective "bundled payment model" from all purchasers of health care for all defined "episodes of care," particularly including episodes involving surgical procedures. Thus, with implementation of such a system, when a patient has an operation, the involved physicians (primary care physician and/or internist, radiologist, surgeon, anesthesiologist, pathologist, consulting cardiologist, physical medicine/rehab physician, etc.) would not send any bills to the responsible payer for their professional services. Their traditional direct relationship with the payer will be ended. Rather, each of those physician specialists would be required to negotiate for a share of the bundled payment that comes directly to the hospital for the care episode for each patient the physician specialist cared for in any way. Obviously, this change would have a profound impact on what previously was the traditional fee-for-service private practice of anesthesiology, a model that still persists widely in the United States. Although the outcome of such a change is impossible to predict, popular speculation within organized anesthesiology in the United States is that income for involved anesthesia professionals would decrease, possibly significantly.

One important related consideration that is addressed in more detail below is the reference to traditional fee-for-service private practice of anesthesiology, usually involving organized groups of anesthesiologists (many employing Certified Registered Nurse Anesthetists [CRNAs]). These groups, in the past, included a large majority of the anesthesia professionals in the United States. The groups often had contracts to provide anesthesia care in private hospitals, but they were "independent practitioners," who were not employed by the hospital. The groups billed to and collected from third-party payers (and sometimes the patients directly) for anesthesia services. In those times, the small percentage of US anesthesia professionals who were employees of a health-care organization usually worked in university teaching hospitals or for integrated "clinics" or "systems" (e.g., Mayo, Cleveland, Kaiser, Inter-Mountain, Geisinger). Those employees received salaries, sometimes with additional variable (incentive) components. They authorized their employer to bill and collect for anesthesia professional services. Today, there has been a noteworthy trend of anesthesia professionals becoming full-time employees of private hospitals and health systems with prospectively negotiated salaries. They also authorize their employer to bill and collect for their services. These employees could reasonably expect that a transition to bundled payments directly to the hospital from third-party payers for episodes of surgical care would have less impact, if any, on their incomes—compared to anesthesia professionals still in independent traditional fee-for-service private practice situations.

Advancement of the concept of bundled payments for health care accelerated significantly in the United States after passage of the Patient Protection and Affordable Care Act in 2010, which stated "The Bundled Payments for Care Improvement (BPCI) initiative was developed by the Center for Medicare and Medicaid Innovation… [which]…was created by the Affordable Care Act to test innovative payment and service delivery models that have the potential to reduce…[CMS]…expenditures while preserving or enhancing the quality of care for beneficiaries."[8] The BPCI initiative seeks voluntary participants, and, as of January 1, 2016, had contracted with hundreds each of hospitals, skilled nursing facilities, and physician group practices. There is an evolution through four stages or "models" of payment in the transition from traditional fee-for-service to the final model, in which "CMS makes a single, prospectively determined bundled payment to the hospital that encompasses all services furnished by the hospital, physicians, and other practitioners during the episode of care," and the hospital divides and disburses the payment, as described above. This system can apply for any of 48 common "Medicare Service—Diagnosis Related Group" in-patient episodes, from "acute myocardial infarction" to "urinary tract infection," including many surgical episodes. Although this program is an initiative, it is expanding. The Comprehensive Care for Joint Replacement model described above, which directly impacts anesthesia professionals, is functionally a subset of a much larger testing ground for the eventual across-the-board elimination of traditional fee-for-service reimbursement by all payers for health care and the adoption of a universal bundled payment model. Anesthesia professionals in the United States must be aware of this likely impending/eventual dramatic restructuring of how they receive compensation for their professional services to patients and how this could impact their financial future.

Practice Model for Anesthesiologists: The Perioperative Surgical Home

Associated in some respects with the basic concept of bundling payments is a new practice model involving patient care provided by anesthesiologists and how it will be paid for. The Perioperative Surgical Home (PSH) model involves a controversial fundamental construct that is heavily promoted by the American Society of Anesthesiologists (ASA) and outlines a significantly expanded role for anesthesiologists in patient care.[9] In essence, the goal is a fully coordinated and integrated patient experience starting with the decision for a planned surgery and continuing through the preoperative, intraoperative, postoperative, and postdischarge phases of the surgical experience. The apparent intention as interpreted by many is that anesthesiologists will be the perioperative physicians who will essentially supervise the entire process and who will execute the coordination and integration of the care, for which they will be additionally compensated financially for this new role and responsibility by the applicable payer.

The ASA committee advancing this new approach states: "The PSH model is a patient-centered and physician-led multidisciplinary and team-based system of coordinated care that guides the patient throughout the entire surgical experience, from decision for the need for surgery to discharge from a medical facility and beyond. The goal is to create a better patient experience and make surgical care safer, efficient, and aligned in order to promote a better medical outcome at a lower cost."[10] An analysis of the PSH proposed concept[11] focused on a smooth continuum of care that reduces variability (imposes standardization) as a way to reduce errors and complications, thus improving care and decreasing cost. This report stated, "This can be achieved by having one team headed by anesthesiologists, to manage all aspects of this continuum from the time that the patient and the surgeon make the decision for surgery until 30 days after discharge…. [Throughout the process,] patients will be informed, educated, and involved in the decision making and treatment planning . . . By applying these concepts, anesthesiologists have a unique opportunity to improve outcomes, decrease length of stay and other metrics, and improve patient satisfaction." The potential for decreased costs for surgical care[12] has been promoted as a very positive feature that would increase the value of anesthesiologists and improve the stability and security of their position in the health-care arena into the future.

The elements of the PSH model involve new roles and responsibilities for anesthesiologists. Proponents maintain that anesthesiologists are in the best position to have an overview and maximum understanding of the entire perioperative interval and its process (Fig. 2-1). Coordination and direction by team-leading anesthesiologists of the patient's involved primary care physician, internist, surgeon, and specialist (cardiologist, endocrinologist, etc.) would decrease the number steps in the sequence, preventing duplication and waste of resources. Verification of nutrition status and optimization of chronic medications (for hypertension, diabetes, COPD, etc.) would increase the likelihood of smooth transit through surgery to a good outcome. Then, indicated preoperative consults would be ordered by the team leader to facilitate "prehabilitation" (e.g., pulmonary consultation and treatment, including smoking cessation) to optimize further the patient's condition prior to surgery, facilitating planned faster recovery and earlier discharge and also decreasing the risk of (expensive) complications. Prescription of standardized "best-practice" protocols for intraoperative anesthetic management, including limiting benzodiazepines, transfusions, excessive fluid administration, and unnecessary invasive monitors would not only enhance speedy recovery but also decrease OR anesthesia costs. Multimodal pain therapy postoperatively with minimal narcotics has the same goals. Aggressive intervention to promote rapid recovery and discharge would be directed by the team-leading anesthesiologists who would coordinate input and plans with the surgeon, hospitalist, primary care physician, involved specialists, and medical consultants, as well as rehab planners, social services, and the patient's family, thus preventing confusing and sometimes conflicting orders from the various potential sources. Discharge planning would specifically focus on medication reconciliation and assuring medication compliance, arranging needed follow-up appointments and treatments, and generally doing everything possible to prevent unplanned readmissions.

Predictably, beyond consideration of the substantial administrative, interprofessional, and financial challenges of actually

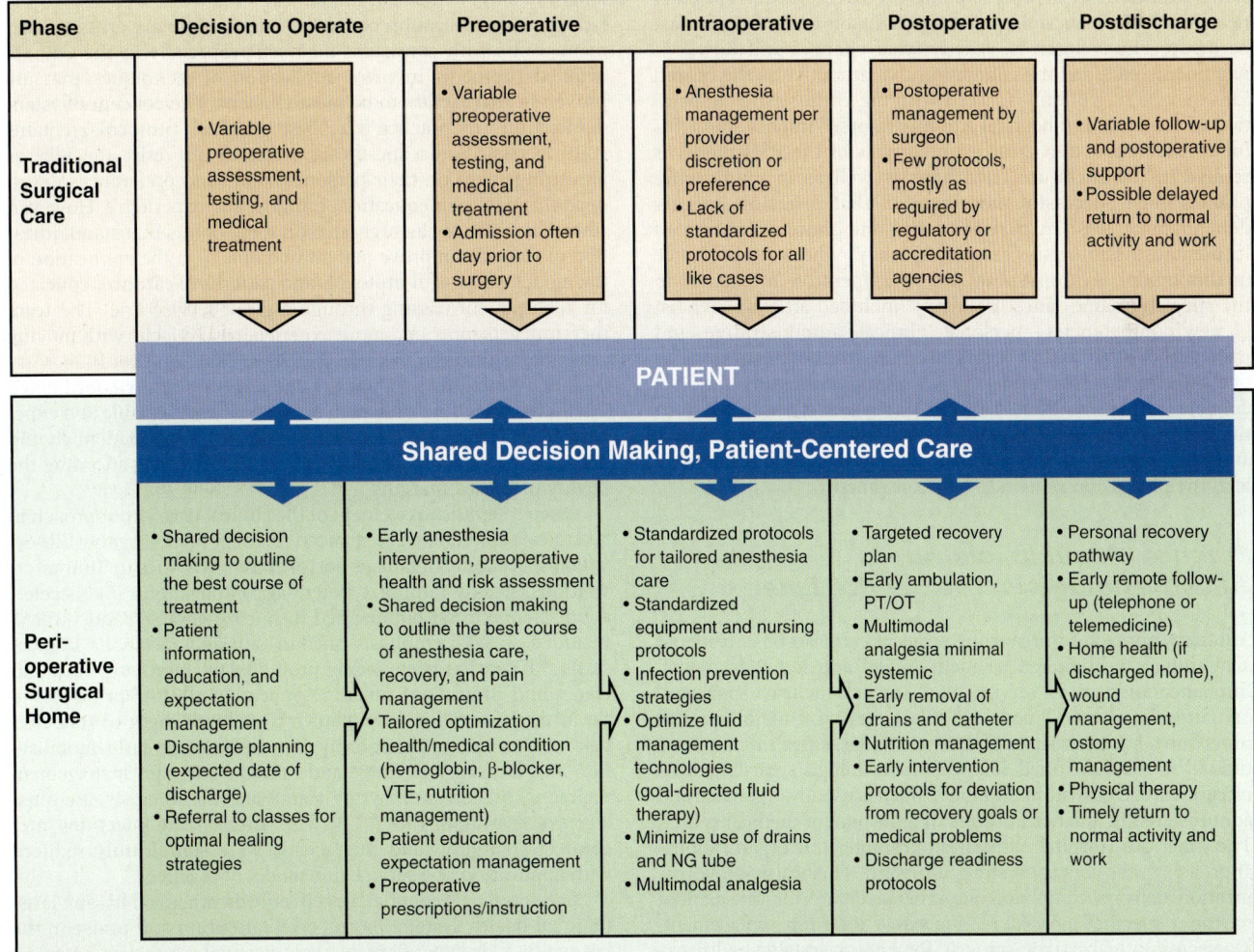

Figure 2-1 Elements of the perioperative surgical home model. PT, physical therapy; OT, occupational therapy; VTE, venous thromboembolism; NG, nasogastric. (Reproduced with permission from Kain ZN, Vakharia S, Garson L, et al. The perioperative surgical home as a future perioperative practice model. *Anesth Analg.* 2014;118:1126–1130. Copyright © 2014 International Anesthesia Research Society.)

implementing such a dramatically expanded practice model, some anesthesiologists apparently do not embrace the PSH concept. Reservations expressed include the concern that currently practicing anesthesiologists have not been trained and do not have the experience to assume some of the responsibilities and roles of primary care physicians, internists, hospitalists, or specialist consultants. Countering that point is the suggestion that larger anesthesiology groups would hire new members who are able and willing to perform those functions. Further, there is concern about strain in relationships between anesthesiologists and surgeons (and hospitalists), particularly if payments to them would be reduced, with the subtracted amounts going to the anesthesia physician or group supervising the perioperative process. Likewise, a reciprocal concern is that shifting of payments would not ultimately occur as planned/promised and that the supervising/coordinating anesthesiologists would be doing much more work for little or no increase in financial compensation. Finally, some anesthesiologists simply do not want to expand their scope of practice in this manner, stating that they are content to continue to practice as they envisioned when they became anesthesiologists: caring for patients at the time of their surgery or procedures. The proposals to implement PSH programs generated much scrutiny, analysis, and discussion that remain ongoing. There appears to be a consensus that essentially, although some evolution of the profession has occurred, the current practice model in anesthesiology is not sustainable and changes must be made. The concern is, exactly what changes and how?[13-15] Arguments included the contention that attractive as the overall idea may be, it will only succeed with the enthusiastic cooperation of surgeons and hospital administrators.[16] Intense, thoughtful consideration of a great many aspects of the PSH model is replete in the literature cited here as well as in many more publications. Successful movement in that direction appears dependent at least in part on wider and more education of future anesthesiologists (longer residency) who would practice in this model. A proposal to add "perioperative medicine" to the specialty name "anesthesiology" included an extensive list of new competencies—personal, clinical, administrative, and managerial—that will be required of anesthesiologists to practice fully in the PHS model.[17] All authors addressing the PSH concept emphasize how critically important the issues are to the future of anesthesia practice. The evolution will be complex and contentious. How it will have an impact and where it may lead the profession remain to be determined.

Practice Model Involving Anesthesiologists: The Service Line

Another approach to organizing surgical care can be considered a hybrid of the bundled payment model and the PSH model. Implementation of a "service line" (or "all-inclusive package" or "clinical pathway") model for selected elective major surgical procedures has been successful at several large health-care institutions across the United States. Anesthesiologists participate as integral caregivers within the model, but it is usually organized and administered by financial officers of a hospital or medical center. The American Hospital Association promotes this organizational approach.[18] The concept is straightforward. The health-care organization delivers complete comprehensive care for one patient having a specified procedure, such as a total hip replacement, a colectomy, or bariatric surgery, for one pre-established package price. This price is usually somewhat lower than the average cumulative total of the fee-for-service charges (facility, materials, and professional) customarily collected from third-party payers for that particular procedure. The established limited cost (which likely includes covering any necessary extended inpatient stay or complications within, e.g., 30 days postoperatively) is very attractive to third-party payers, who have an incentive to encourage or direct their patients to ward that health-care facility. There is no separate fee-for-service billing and no itemized bookkeeping by departments or practices. The facility collects the global fee and distributes a component of it to the various professional members of the integrated team, who would have, in the traditional model, submitted fee-for-service bills to the third-party payer.

Mutual benefits accrue with this model. The third-party payers benefit by possibly saving some money on each patient, but mostly by being able to predict their payments and budget accordingly. This gives them an advantage in pricing and marketing their insurance plans, which they hope will translate into more business. The health-care organization expects to be attractive to the payers and, thus, have more patients referred from the involved payers. Then, classically, the medical facility invests great effort into streamlining the care of patients in a given service line. This includes increased efficiency through coordination of efforts and services along with elimination of duplication and waste—in many of the same ways outlined earlier in the other models. Particular emphasis is on minimizing the risk of complications (and the associated expense) and reducing inpatient length of stay, which can dramatically reduce cost of care to the facility. Standardization of care by interdisciplinary cross-department teams with consistent members, especially in the OR, via detailed protocols involves application of techniques that are proven in that facility to be most efficient. The concept of "standardization" of practice via "best practice" protocols remains controversial. Some anesthesia professionals resist the idea as an infringement on their personal habits and preferences developed through their education, training, and experience. However, research evidence has suggested on some points that standardization of care can improve patient outcome.[19] In the application of the model, successful protocols and patterns of care are replicated for each patient passing through a given service line. The team therefore gets more and more experienced and facile with moving the patients through the line. Patient satisfaction should increase because, functionally, they are moving through a coordinated "well-oiled machine" in which everyone is very capable and experienced in their roles. Costs within the facility per patient should decrease, but revenue remains at the package price, affording the facility increased margins.

Often a significant element of the clinical pathway approach in a surgical service line is enhanced recovery after surgery (ERAS), which specifically organizes postoperative activities to limit interventions, strictly minimize potential complications, and accelerate discharge. First popularized in Europe and England,[20] ERAS included specific emphasis on nutrition and metabolic homeostasis.[21] ERAS has been widely promoted as improving both efficiency and clinical outcomes.[22] Application of ERAS principles in the United States has been shown to reduce length of stay after colorectal surgery, particularly by emphasizing early mobilization and feeding.[23] Creative and minimalistic pain management regimens, orchestrated by the team's anesthesiologists, are often a central feature of ERAS. Likewise, surgical site infections after colorectal surgery (and their costs) were significantly reduced with application of a service line model of practice.[24]

The service line model, specifically as practiced by one large regional health system, has received attention and praise in the lay media.[25] Independent of their particular practice settings, anesthesiologists can reasonably expect continued significant growth of the service line model in US surgical care now and in the near future. They should be prepared to contribute constructively, as should the involved surgeons. Resisting and holding out for exclusive preservation of the traditional itemized fee-for-service model may well lead to situations in which such uncooperative practitioners would be uncomfortable with attempting to continue practice in that facility.

Large Group Practices: Anesthesia and Multispecialty

A noteworthy trend in US anesthesia practice that interlocks with all the evolving practice models described previously is the dramatic proliferation of large (and in some cases, very large) group practices. This started initially as a burgeoning business model much as has been the case with other industries, such as the consolidation by merger of large US commercial airlines or pharmacy chains. In health care, there has been and is a widespread well-known movement in which health systems or large hospitals, usually in urban areas, purchase, merge with, or absorb smaller previously free-standing community hospitals in the surrounding area. Note that for actual anesthesia practice, however, and particularly "scope of practice" in its traditional sense, there are many spill-over implications for the day-to-day administration of individual anesthetics as well as for organizational, quality improvement, and research aspects of anesthesia care.

The business case for large urban hospitals taking over outlying community hospitals and enfolding their medical staffs into a centralized network is clear. The "core," "base," or "home" institution expands its "book of business" both by adding volume to its primary care role and by guaranteeing referrals for some secondary and most tertiary care to the core facility and its specialist medical staff. Economies of expanded scale (elimination of duplication, price bargaining advantage with suppliers, etc.) are similar to many other industries. Further, in the ACA, the significant financial incentives for implementation and use of electronic health records (EHRs) are perceived as functionally making these cross-platform integrated health information technology systems *mandatory*. Many smaller hospitals simply are unable to afford the cost of installing and maintaining their own EHR system, thus increasing the financial advantage of merging into a networked health system. Although details may vary from place to place, when a community hospital in which the hospital-based specialists (anesthesia, radiology, pathology, and emergency medicine) are private practitioners who are not hospital employees merges into a networked system, the practice arrangements for these specialists usually are re-evaluated. When such a community hospital has an exclusive contract with a private-practice anesthesia group, there are various potential eventualities. The group could attempt to maintain the same contract with the administration of the health system, or, alternatively, the group could dissolve and become direct employees of the health system. However, when the core facility has its contract with an anesthesia practice group, it is most likely that the community hospital anesthesia practice merges with the larger group based at the "home" hospital. This concept was one original impetus for the start of what evolved into some of the very large regional and national anesthesia practice groups.

As several of the consolidated anesthesia practice groups grew through merger after merger, administrative and financial support staffs evolved that accomplished significant economies of scale and organization. They became, in essence, successful startup businesses. It became clear to the physician and nonphysician leaders of these organizations that such a group could approach additional hospitals and ambulatory surgery centers that were not part of the original health system network and offer exclusive contracted anesthesia services to those facilities, wherever they might be located. The large group would seek to absorb or displace the anesthesia practice group that may have had an exclusive contract at a community hospital for many years. Because of the economies of scale (especially human resources and financial management), the large group frequently tries to offer a "better deal" to the community hospital than the local group, whether the terms involve more and more flexible staffing (more accommodation of surgeons' desires), decreased salary subsidy from the hospital, or other relevant considerations. Although the potential for conflict is clear, the large group can often offer to employ most or all of the existing members of the local group, whose work location and condition are then little affected, but they are relieved of all the administrative and overhead burdens of running a practice. Individual compensation arrangements change, and some anesthesiologists are willing to trade unpredictable income (albeit with upside potential for the partners) for a predictable guaranteed income that often comes with more predictable work hours. Likewise, the services (including educational), support, and benefits associated with being an employee along with hundreds or even thousands of other anesthesia professionals can be improvements over what existed with the small group. In the (relatively rare) cases in which the local small anesthesia group resists and refuses to cooperate, but the hospital awards an exclusive contract to the large regional or national group, that large organization moves in a new complement of employed anesthesia professionals, which may be mostly temporary personnel until permanent replacements from the large group's pool of employees relocate to the hospital's community.

Beyond the practice details described earlier, the large anesthesia groups can marshal special new resources. They can have dedicated directors devoted to quality improvement and patient safety efforts and projects. They can partner with an academic institution and then organize and offer their own internal continuing medical education (CME). Further, members can evolve or even be specifically hired to conduct clinical, epidemiologic, and organizational research using the sophisticated database that is a key component to the success of the large groups. Such research efforts can support the development of genuinely evidence-based best practice standardized protocols that are central to the PSH and service line practice models. Research results can be submitted for publication and presented at state, regional, or national anesthesia professional meetings, highlighting the thesis that the large anesthesia groups are not just business entities but also contributors to the development of the profession in general.

A variant on the concept of the large anesthesia group involves something of a similar construct, but as a component of a large multispecialty group that is part of a health system.[26] These may be regional networks (e.g., Kaiser Permanente or Inter-Mountain) or "clinics" (e.g., Mayo or Cleveland) with base locations and satellites. Anesthesia professionals, full-time employees like all other professional staff, are members of a department within those organizations. Some of the features and benefits of the large anesthesia groups exist, but the concept of growth by merger with or absorption of smaller entities applies to entire hospitals or health-care organizations. Integration of those anesthesiology departments into the whole of the multispecialty group and health system can have many of the features of the service-line approach to delivery of health care. Further, the resources accessible within these multispecialty-based health systems can be vast and can thus support major research, population health, and outreach initiatives, potentially affording anesthesia professionals new opportunities for engagement and impact not otherwise available.

As is the case with all aspects of change in anesthesiology practice, evolution continues regarding groups. The ASA[27] is making a concerted effort to engage and involve the large groups, even creating a standing Committee on Large Group Practice that emphasizes educational opportunities, advocacy, networking, participation in the Anesthesia Quality Institute and the Qualified Clinical Data Registry, practitioner surveys, and enhancing practice management. Overall, it seems unlikely, given the realities of health-care financing, organization, and politics now in the United States, that events would ever support dissolution of the large group practices and return to more locally based exclusive contract small anesthesia groups. Large groups, in all likelihood, will continue to proliferate and grow.

Further Issues

Payment Machinations

For the past several decades, great attention has been focused on payments from the US federal Medicare program for physician services in the current fee-for-service structure. Although fee-for-service appears to be slated for eventual phase-out, as outlined above, concern persists now because elements of fee-for-service payment from Medicare quite likely will persist at least through 2019. Interest is high because in some practices a substantial fraction of income is derived from Medicare. Moreover, a greater issue is that many private insurance companies consider Medicare payment rates when determining relative value of various services performed by practitioners. Accordingly, the vast majority of the US health-care establishment was pleased in 2015 when the US Congress repealed the so-called sustainable growth rate (SGR) formula component of Medicare payments that led to annual concerns that Medicare payments for professional services would be drastically reduced and annual drama with last-minute passage by Congress of an act to prevent that. However, the law that fixed the SGR problem known as the Medicare Access and CHIP Reauthorization Act of 2015 (MACRA) introduced new issues of concern. MACRA is cited by CMS as, "Making a new framework for rewarding health care providers for giving better care not just more care."[28] It is intended to be a bridge connecting quality to fee-for-service payment and employing a "value trajectory" into population health that eventually totally changes how practitioners are paid by Medicare. MACRA specifies modest annual automatic reductions in Medicare payments to practitioners until 2019 when a new Medicare payment model is scheduled to be implemented. The new system is very complex. It involves practitioners making a choice between two models that will determine their payment. First is the Merit Based Incentive Payment System, which retains some elements of fee-for-service but creates a functional zero-sum game. Practitioners who chose this method of determining their payment will be graded on four elements (Physician Quality Reporting System, Value Based Modifiers, Meaningful Use of EHRs, and Clinical Practice Improvement Activities). Practices whose scores exceed the median benchmark will receive payment bonuses, whereas, reciprocally, practices that underperform the benchmark will be penalized an equal amount. The other method of determining Medicare payments will be the "Alternative Payment Models,"[29] the details of which are being established, but that likely will significantly reward practice models configured along the lines of bundled payments, the PSH, and the service line model. The ASA leadership has expressed concern about how all these changes will impact the earnings of anesthesiologists, but at the same time is preparing its members for the transition to the new Medicare payment system mandated by CMS.[30]

APRN Consensus Model Implications

Because CRNAs in the United States are included in the large classification "advanced practice registered nurses" (APRN), evolving policies and regulations regarding scope of practice for APRNs are relevant to anesthesia professional practice. In 2008, the APRN Consensus Work Group and the National Council of State Boards of Nursing APRN Advisory Committee published an extensive document titled "Consensus Model for APRN Regulation: Licensure, Accreditation, Certification, and Education,"[31] that had been endorsed by 48 nursing professional organizations. It outlines a regulatory model that, in essence, eventually expands the scope of practice of APRNs to fully independent practice with full prescribing authority. One of the main themes is consistency throughout the United States because, often, regulations governing APRNs vary widely from state to state. Implementation of this model has been championed by the American Nurses Credentialing Center,[32,33] which is a subsidiary of the American Nurses Association that conducts the certifying process, including examinations, for APRNs (analogous in a sense to the American Board of Anesthesiology [ABA]). The main activities, which are ongoing and accelerating, are to promote and secure legislation in each state that adopts the model for APRN certification, accreditation, and licensure. The National Council of State Boards of Nursing maintains an online national map and scoring system that shows the implementation status for the APRN Consensus Model for each state, thus indicating "progress toward uniformity."[34] One of the stated main goals of this national effort is to increase access to primary care, particularly in less densely populated areas of the United States through allowing APRNs to practice to the "full extent of their education and training." Emphasis is in the areas of family practice, pediatrics, internal medicine, geriatrics, and women's health. In addition, subsumed within the same proposed policies and regulations are Certified Nurse Midwives and CRNAs. The American Association of Nurse Anesthetists (AANA) was one of the participating organizations in the creation and endorsement of the APRN Consensus Model. The relationship of CRNAs and physician anesthesiologists in the United States is long and complex—and beyond the scope of this chapter. The AANA advocates for increased independent practice for CRNAs and notes that as of the end of 2012, 17 states in the United States had adopted the so-called opt-out rule that removes the federal regulatory requirement for physician supervision of CNRAs. This "opt-out" has traditionally been opposed by the leadership of organized anesthesiologists, as was also consideration of a similar change within the Veterans' Administration health system. Although naturally concerned about the practice incomes and financial well-being of their members, both professional organizations, the AANA and the ASA, maintain that their positions regarding anesthesia practice characteristics in general and specifically of CRNAs are based on concerns about quality of care, patient safety, and patient outcomes. It seems virtually certain that extensive considerations of multiple aspects of these issues as they relate to anesthesia practice will continue into the foreseeable future.

Administrative Components of Anesthesiology Practice

Operational and Information Resources

Outlined in this chapter is an overview summary intended as an introduction to organization, administration, and practice management in anesthesiology. Further, the ASA, the professional association for physician anesthesiologists in the United States, for many years has made available to its members extensive resource material regarding practice in general and specific arrangements for its execution. Citation and availability of this material can be found on the ASA website, www.asahq.org. Elements are updated periodically by the ASA through its physician officers, committees, task forces, administrative and support staff, and its various offices. Although many of the documents and even the advice given in response to members' requests for help contain broad-brush generalities that must be interpreted in each individual practice situation, these nonetheless stand as a foundation on which many anesthesiology practices traditionally have been based. Prospective familiarity with the principles outlined in the ASA material likely could help avoid some of the problems leading to calls for help. Also, each spring, the ASA offers a Practice Management Conference at which both reviews and current updates of a wide variety of relevant administrative and financial topics are covered.

Background

The ASA[35] publishes the *Manual for Anesthesia Department Organization and Management,* an outline of a great many factors relevant to anesthesia practice and a large number of links to related ASA documents, such as information on physician responsibilities for medical care and on medical–administrative organization and responsibilities; the ASA *Guidelines for the Ethical Practice of Anesthesiology* (which incorporate sections on the principles of medical ethics); the definition of medical direction of nonphysician personnel (including the specific statement that an anesthesiologist engaged in medical direction should not personally be administering another anesthetic); the anesthesiologist's relationship to patients and other physicians; the anesthesiologist's duties, responsibilities, and relationship to the hospital; the anesthesiologist's relationship to nurse anesthetists and other nonphysician personnel; and quality improvement and data reporting resources. Further, beyond summaries such as this textbook chapter, reference to the great body of material created and presented by the ASA is an excellent starting point to help young anesthesia professionals during training prepare for the increasing rigors of starting and managing a career in practice. On the ASA website, within the "For Members" area, the "Practice Management" section is functionally a gold mine. It includes extensive information on the organization, administration, and business of anesthesia practice with reference to an extensive catalog of documents, webinars, and podcasts. Sections include the ASA Qualified Clinical Data Registry (QCDR), the National Anesthesia Clinical Outcomes Registry (NACOR), and the Physician Quality Reporting System (PQRS) regarding quality and data reporting. Also included are practice management educational resources; timely topics in payment and practice management; employment agreements; coding and billing; templates that satisfy the CMS "interpretative guidelines;" practice parameters; Quality Management and Departmental Administrative (QMDA) toolkit; Recovery Audit Contractor (RAC); and a bibliography of payment and practice management articles. Likewise, there is a great deal of other information on the ASA website concerning the most recent governmental regulations, rulings, and billing codes. Further, the *ASA Monitor* newsletter (mailed to members and on the ASA website) contains many articles on related current administrative, quality and regulatory, organizational, and financial developments.

In addition to the ASA and the AANA, the anesthesiology subspecialty societies and interest groups have web locations, as do most journals. Particularly, the website of the Anesthesia Patient Safety Foundation, www.apsf.org, has been cited as especially useful in promoting safe clinical practice. Electronic bulletin boards allow anesthesiology practitioners from around the world to exchange ideas in real time on diverse topics, both medical and administrative. One of the original sites that remains available is "GASNet" (http://anestit.unipa.it/homepage.html) and a web search ("anesthesiology + bulletin board") reveals a great number of sites that contain a variety of discussions about all manner of anesthesiology-related topics, including practice organization, administration, finance, and management. In addition, references to the entirety of the medical literature are readily accessible to any practitioner (such as by starting with www.nlm.nih.gov to access Medline). A modern anesthesiology practice cannot reasonably exist without readily available high-speed Internet connections.

The Credentialing Process and Clinical Privileges

The system of credentialing a health-care professional and granting clinical privileges in a health-care facility is motivated by a fundamental assumption that appropriate education, training, and experience, along with the absence of excessive numbers of bad patient outcomes, increase the chances that the individual will deliver acceptable-quality care. The process of credentialing health-care professionals has been the focus of considerable public attention (particularly in the mass media), in part the result of very rare incidents of untrained persons (impostors) infiltrating the health-care system and sometimes harming patients. The more common situation, however, involves health professionals who exaggerate past experience and credentials or fail to disclose adverse past experiences. In the past, there was justified publicity concerning physicians who lost their licenses sequentially in several states and simply moved on each time to start practice elsewhere (which should be much, much more difficult today).

Intense public and political pressure has been brought to bear on various lawmaking bodies, regulatory and licensing agencies, and health-care institution administrations to discover and purge both (1) fraudulent, criminal, and deviant health-care providers and (2) incompetent or simply poor-quality practitioners whose histories show sufficient poor patient outcomes to attract attention, usually through malpractice suits. Identifying and avoiding or correcting an incompetent practitioner is the goal. Verification of appropriate education, training, and experience on the part of a candidate for a clinical anesthesia position assumes special importance in light of the legal doctrine of *vicarious liability,* which can be described as follows: if an individual, group, or institution hires an anesthesia professional or even simply approves of that person (e.g., by granting clinical privileges through a hospital medical staff), those involved in the decision may later be held liable in the courts, along with the individual, for the individual's actions. This would be especially true if it were later discovered that the offending practitioner's past adverse outcomes had not been adequately investigated during the credentialing process.

Out of these various longstanding concerns has arisen the sometimes cumbersome process of obtaining state licenses to practice and obtaining hospital privileges. The stringent credentialing process for health-care practice is intended both to protect patients and to safeguard the integrity of the profession. Central credentialing systems have been developed, including those affiliated with the American Medical Association, American

Osteopathic Association, and, particularly, the Federation Credentials Verification Service of the Federation of State Medical Boards. These systems verify a physician's basic credentials (e.g., identity, citizenship or immigration status, medical education, postgraduate training, licensure examination history, prior licenses, and board actions) once, and then thereafter can certify the validity of these credentials to a state licensing board or medical facility. A few states do not yet accept this verification and most states seek specific supplemental information.

There are checklists of the requirements for the granting of medical staff privileges by hospitals (see the American Hospital Association Resource Center, www.aha.org/research/rc/index.shtml). In addition, the National Practitioner Data Bank and reporting system administered by the US government contains a great deal of information. This data bank is a central repository of licensing and credentials information about physicians. Virtually all adverse situations involving a physician—particularly, malpractice litigation and the revocation, suspension, or limitation of that physician's license to practice medicine or ability to hold hospital privileges—must be reported (via the particular state board of medical registration/licensure) to the National Practitioner Data Bank. It is a statutory requirement that all applications for hospital staff privileges be cross-checked against this national data bank. The potential medicolegal liability on the part of a facility's medical staff, and the anesthesiology group in particular, for failing to do so is significant. The data bank, however, is not a complete substitute for direct documentation and background checking. Often, practitioners reach private negotiated solutions following quality-driven medical staff problems, thereby avoiding the mandatory public reporting. In such cases, a practitioner in question may be given the option to resign medical staff privileges and avoid data bank reporting rather than undergo full involuntary privilege revocation (although most license and privilege applications contain a question specifically about this).

Documentation

The documentation for the credentialing process for each anesthesia practitioner must be complete. Privileges to administer anesthesia must be officially granted and delineated in writing. This can be straightforward or it can be more complex to accommodate institutional needs to identify practitioners specially qualified to practice in designated anesthesia subspecialty areas such as cardiac, infant/pediatric, obstetric, intensive care, or invasive pain management. Specific documentation of the process of granting or renewing clinical privileges is required and, unlike some other administrative records, the documentation likely is protected as confidential peer review information. Any questions about complex sensitive issues such as this should be referred to an experienced attorney familiar with applicable federal and state law. Verification of an applicant's credentials and experience is mandatory. Because of another type of legal case involving references, some examples of which have been highly publicized, medical practitioners may be hesitant to give an honest evaluation (or any evaluation at all) of individuals known to them who are seeking a professional position elsewhere. Obviously, someone writing a reference for a current or former coworker should be honest. Sticking to clearly documentable facts is advisable. Stating a fact that is in the public record (such as a malpractice case lost at trial) should not justify an objection from the subject of the reference. Whether such potentially "negative" facts can be omitted by a reference writer is complex. Including positive opinions and enthusiastic recommendations, of course, is no problem. Some fear that including facts that may be perceived as negative (e.g., the lost malpractice case or personal problems such as a history of treatment for substance abuse) and/or negative opinions will provoke a retaliatory lawsuit (such as for libel, defamation of character, or loss of livelihood) from the subject of the reference. Further, however, there have been cases of the facility doing the hiring suing reference writers for failing to mention (perceived as concealing) negative information about an applicant who later was charged with substandard practice. Because of the complexities and even apparent contradictions, many reference writers in these questionable situations confine their written material to brief, simple facts such as dates employed and position held. As always, questions about complex sensitive issues such as this should be referred to an experienced attorney familiar with applicable federal and state law. Further, one relevant strategy for investigating an anesthesia professional applying to a new institution traditionally has been seeking informal but important opinions from nurses in the OR where the applicant works or has worked. A call to the OR head nurse can often identify nurses who have worked with the applicant. Then, when speaking to them, simply asking whether they would be comfortable having the applicant care for a beloved member of his or her family can itself elicit valuable information and initiate a helpful conversation.

Because there should be no hesitation for a reference giver to include positive facts and opinions, receipt of a reference that includes nothing more than dates worked and position held can in some cases be a suggestion that there may be more to the story (although some entities have adopted such a policy in *all* cases simply to eliminate any value judgments as to what is positive or negative information). Receipt of such a "dates/position only" reference about a person applying for a position should usually provoke a telephone call to the writer. A telephone call to the writer is likely advisable in all cases, independent of whatever the written reference contains. Frequently, pertinent questions over the telephone can elicit more candid information. In rare instances, there may be dishonesty through omission by the reference giver even at this level. This may involve an applicant who an individual, a department or group, or an institution would like to see leave.

In all cases, new personnel in an anesthesia practice environment must be given a thorough and documented orientation and checkout. Policy, procedures, and equipment may be unfamiliar to even the most thoroughly trained, experienced, and safe practitioner. This may occasionally seem tedious, but it is a sound and critically important safety policy. Being in the midst of a crisis situation caused by unfamiliarity with a new setting is not the optimal orientation session.

After the initial granting of clinical privileges to practice anesthesia, anesthesia professionals must periodically renew their privileges within the institution or facility (e.g., annually or every other year). There are moral, ethical, and societal obligations on the part of the privilege-granting entity to take this process seriously. State licensing bodies often become aware of problems with health professionals very late in the evolution of any difficulties. An anesthesia professional's peers in the hospital or facility are much more likely to notice troublesome developments as they first appear. However, privilege renewals are often essentially automatic and receive little of the necessary attention. Judicious checking of renewal applications and awareness of relevant peer review information are absolutely essential. The anesthesia professionals or administrators responsible for evaluating staff members and reviewing their practices and privileges may be justifiably concerned about retaliatory legal action by a staff member who is censured or denied privilege renewal. Accordingly, such evaluating groups must be thoroughly objective (totally eliminating any hint of political or financial motives) and must have documentation that the staff person in question is in fact practicing below the standard of care. Court decisions have found liability by a hospital, its medical staff, or both, when the incompetence of a staff member was known, or should have been known, and was not acted upon. Again, questions about complex sensitive issues such as this should be referred to an experienced attorney familiar with applicable federal and state law.

A major issue in the granting of clinical privileges, especially in procedure-oriented specialties such as anesthesiology, is whether it is reasonable to continue the once common practice of "blanket" privileges. This process in effect authorizes the practitioner to attempt any treatment or procedure normally considered within the purview of the applicant's medical specialty. These considerations may have profound political and economic implications within medicine, such as which type of surgeon should be doing carotid endarterectomies or lumbar discectomies. More important, however, is whether the practitioner being evaluated is qualified to do everything traditionally associated with the specialty. Specifically, should the granting of privileges to practice anesthesia automatically approve the practitioner to handle pediatric cardiac cases, critically ill newborns (such as a day-old premature infant with a large diaphragmatic hernia), ablative pain therapy (such as an alcohol celiac plexus block under fluoroscopy), high-risk obstetric cases, and so forth? This question raises the issue of procedure-specific or limited privileges. The quality assurance (QA) and risk management considerations in this question are weighty if inexperienced or insufficiently qualified practitioners are allowed or even expected, because of peer or scheduling pressures, to undertake major challenges for which they are not prepared. The likelihood of complications and adverse outcomes will be higher, and the difficulty of defending the practitioner against a malpractice claim in the event of catastrophe will be significantly increased.

There is no clear answer to the question of procedure-specific credentialing and granting of privileges. Ignoring issues regarding qualifications to undertake complex and challenging procedures has clear negative potential. On the other hand, stringent procedure-specific credentialing is impractical in smaller groups, and in larger groups encourages many small "fiefdoms," with a consequent further atrophy of the clinical skills outside the practitioner's specific area(s). Each anesthesia department or group needs to address these issues. At the very least, the common practice of every applicant for privileges (new or renewal) checking off every line on the printed list of anesthesia procedures should be reviewed. In addition, board certification for physicians is now essentially a standard of QA of the minimum skills required for the consultant practice of anesthesiology. Subspecialty boards, such as those in pain management, critical care, and transesophageal echocardiography, further objectify the credentialing process. This is significant because initial board certification after the year 2000 by the ABA is time-limited and subject to periodic testing and recertification (see Maintenance of Certification below). Many states, some institutions, and even some regulatory bodies have requirements for a minimum number of hours of CME. Documentation of fulfilling such a standard again acts as one type of QA mechanism for the individual practitioner, while providing another objective credentialing measurement for those granting licenses or privileges.

Maintenance of Certification in Anesthesiology

American anesthesiologists certified as diplomates by the ABA after January 1, 2000, are issued a "time-limited" board certification valid for 10 years. A formal process culminating in the recertification of an anesthesiologist for an additional and then subsequent 10-year intervals has evolved and now appropriately is called "Maintenance of Certification in Anesthesiology" (MOCA). Because certification by a medical specialty board is now often expected or actually required by medical staff bylaws in order to obtain and maintain medical facility privileges, even anesthesiologists who were certified (without a time limit) prior to the year 2000 likely will be engaging in the MOCA process.

In 1999, the American Board of Medical Specialties (ABMS) initiated a process to better ensure continuing professional development of diplomates certified by the member boards. An enhancement of the traditional CME process, this initiative by the ABMS is designed to provide a transparent public system of accountability that the physician's skill and knowledge base do not wane after completion of formal training. Centered on the American Council for Graduate Medical Education core competencies of (1) patient-centered care, (2) medical knowledge, (3) interpersonal and communication skills, (4) professionalism, (5) system-based practice, and (6) practice-based learning improvement, each member board designs a curricular process to enhance and evaluate continued development of the competencies throughout the professional career of the certified clinician.

The MOCA program of the ABA has had significant evolution since its introduction (http://www.theaba.org/MOCA/MOCA-Timeline), much of which was prompted by input from participants in the program. As of the 2016 "MOCA 2.0" update, the elements of the program include Professionalism and Professional Standing; Lifelong Learning and Self-Assessment, based on CME; Assessment of Knowledge, Judgment, and Skills (based on the MOCA Minute concept that involves the anesthesiologist answering 30 questions per calendar quarter online—each of which includes an explanatory learning module—thus replacing the written examination component of the process); and Improvement in Medical Practice, for which participants complete activities (each with a point value counting toward the required total) during the 10-year cycle, demonstrating participation in practice improvement activities and evaluations of their clinical practice.

Clinicians with subspecialty training in Critical Care and Pain Medicine also have an MOCA process available. The updated version, also "MOCA 2.0," launches in 2017 and will have many of the same type of features as regular MOCA, but oriented to the specific subspecialty.

It is reasonable to project that the MOCA process will continue to evolve and likely will become more comprehensive over time as the overall emphasis on assuring both quality and efficiency of medical care in the United States increases further due to the expectations of accrediting bodies, government regulators, third-party payers, malpractice insurers, and, above all, the public.

Professional Staff Participation and Relationships

All medical care facilities and practice settings depend on their professional staffs, of course, for daily activities of the delivery of health care but, importantly, they also depend on those staffs to provide administrative structure and support. Medical staff activities are increasingly important in achieving favorable accreditation status from the "Joint Commission" (formerly known as the Joint Commission for the Accreditation of Healthcare Organizations or JCAHO) and in meeting a wide variety of governmental regulations and reviews. Principal medical staff activities involve sometimes time-consuming efforts, such as duties as a staff officer or committee member. Anesthesiologists should be participants in—in fact, should play a significant role in—credentialing, peer review, tissue review, transfusion review, OR management, and medical direction of same-day surgery units, postanesthesia care units (PACUs), intensive care units (ICUs), and pain management units. Also, it is very important that anesthesiology personnel be involved in fund-raising activities, benefits, community outreach projects sponsored by the facility, publicity, and social events of the facility staff.

Anesthesia professionals as a group have a reputation for lack of involvement in medical staff and facility issues, allegedly because of lack of time due to long hours in the OR or simply lack of interest. In fact, anesthesiology professionals are all-too-often perceived in a facility as the ones who slip in and out of the building essentially anonymously (often dressed very casually or even in the pajama-like comfort of scrub suits) and virtually unnoticed. This is an unfortunate state of affairs, and it has frequently come back in various painful ways to haunt those who have not been involved, or even noticed, within their own facility. Anesthesia professionals sometimes respond that the demands for anesthesiology service are so great that they simply never have the time or the opportunity to become involved in their facility and with their peers. If this is really true, it is clear that more anesthesia professionals must be added at that facility, even if doing so slightly reduces the income of those already there.

If anesthesia professionals are not involved and not perceived as interested, dedicated "team players," they will be shut out of critical negotiations and decisions relevant to their practice. Although one obvious instance in which others could make key decisions for uninvolved anesthesia professionals is the distribution of "bundled" professional payment income collected by a central "umbrella" medical practice organization or even the facility administration itself, there are many such situations, and the excluded uninvolved anesthesia professionals will be forced to comply with the resulting mandates.

Similarly, involvement with a facility, a professional staff, or a multispecialty group goes beyond formal organized governance and committee activity. Collegial relationships with professionals of other specialties and with administrators are central to maintenance of a recognized position and avoidance of the situation of exclusion just described. Being readily available for formal and informal consults, particularly regarding preoperative patient workup and the maximally efficient way to get surgeons' patients to the OR in a timely, expedient manner, is extremely important. No one individual can be everywhere all the time, but an anesthesiology group or department should strive to be always responsive to any request for help from physicians or administrators. It often appears that anesthesia professionals fail to appreciate just how great a positive impact a relatively simple involvement (starting an intravenous line for a pediatrician, helping an internist manage an ICU ventilator, or helping a facility administrator unclog a jammed recovery room) may have. Something as simple as having a departmental telephone extension within the facility that is always answered by a person, whoever it may be, who can direct the caller to the needed help is an extremely effective positive presentation for the facility's anesthesia professionals.

Establishing Standards of Practice and Understanding the Standard of Care

The increasing frequency and intensity of "production pressure,"[36] with the tacit (or even explicit) directive to anesthesia professionals to "go fast" no matter what, and to "do more with less," creates situations in which anesthesia professionals may conclude that they must cut corners and compromise safe patient care just to stay in business. This type of pressure has become even greater with the implementation of more and more protocols or parameters for practice, some from professional societies such as the ASA and some mandated by or developed in conjunction with purchasers of health care (government, insurance companies, heath plans, or managed care organizations [MCOs]). Many of these protocols are devised to fast-track patients through the medical care system, especially when an elective procedure is involved, in as absolutely little time as possible, thus minimizing costs. Do these fast-track protocols constitute or establish standards of care that health-care providers must implement? What are the implications of doing so? Of not doing so?

To better understand answers to such questions, it is important to have a basic background in the concept of the standard of care.

The *standard of care* is the conduct and skill of a prudent (or "reasonable") practitioner that can be expected by a reasonable patient. This is a very important medicolegal concept because a bad medical result due to failure to meet the standard of care is malpractice. Courts have traditionally relied on medical experts knowledgeable about the point in question to give opinions as to what is the standard of care and if it has been met in an individual case. This type of standard is somewhat different from the standards promulgated by various standard-setting bodies regarding, for example, the color of gas hoses connected to an anesthesia machine in the United States or the inability to open two vaporizers on that machine simultaneously. However, ignoring the equipment standards and tolerating an unsafe situation is a violation of the standard of care. Promulgated standards, such as the various safety codes and anesthesia machine specifications, rapidly become the standard of care because patients (through their attorneys, in the case of an untoward event) expect the published standards to be observed by the prudent practitioner.

Ultimately, the standard of care for an individual practitioner is what a jury says it is. However, it is possible to anticipate, at least in part, what knowledge and actions will be expected. There are two main sources of information as to exactly what is the expected standard of care. Traditionally, the beliefs offered by expert witnesses in medical liability lawsuits regarding what is actually being done in real life (de facto standards of care) were the main input juries had in deciding what was reasonable to expect from the defendant. The resulting problem is well known: except in the most egregious cases, it is usually possible for the lawyers to find experts who will support each of the two opposing sides, making the process more subjective than objective. (Because of this, there are even ASA *Guidelines for Expert Witness Qualifications and Testimony* and an equivalent document from the AANA). Of course, there can be legitimate differences of opinion among thoughtful, insightful experts, but even in these cases the jury still must decide who is more believable, looks better, or sounds better. The second, much more objective, source for defining certain component parts of the standard of care is the published standards of care, guidelines, practice parameters, and protocols that have become more and more common since the idea was originally introduced.[37] These serve as more objective evidence of what can be reasonably expected of practitioners and can make it easier for a jury evaluating whether a malpractice defendant failed to meet the applicable standard of care. Several types of documents exist and have differing implications.

Leading the Way

Anesthesiology likely is the medical specialty most involved with published standards of care. It has been suggested that the nature of anesthesia practice (having certain central critical functions relatively clearly defined and common to all situations and also having an emphasis on technology) makes it the most amenable of all the fields of medicine to the application of published standards. The original intraoperative monitoring standards[38] are a classic example. The ASA first adopted its own set of basic intraoperative monitoring standards in 1986 and has modified them many times. The text of all ASA standards, guidelines, statements, practice parameters, practice advisories, and other documents is readily available on the ASA website home page: select "Resources" and then "Standards, Guidelines, Statements, Practice Parameters" headings.

The Standards for Basic Anesthetic Monitoring document includes clear specifications for the presence of personnel during an anesthetic episode and for continual evaluation of oxygenation, ventilation, circulation, and temperature. These ASA monitoring standards very quickly became part of the accepted standard of care in anesthesia practice. This means they are important to practice management because they have profound medicolegal implications: a catastrophic accident occurring while the standards are being actively ignored is very difficult to defend in the consequent malpractice suit, whereas an accident that occurs during well-documented full compliance with the standards will automatically have a strong defense because the standard of care was being met. Several states in the United States have made compliance with these ASA standards mandatory under state regulations or even statutes. Various malpractice insurance companies offer discounts on malpractice insurance policy premiums for compliance with these standards, something quite natural to insurers because they are familiar with the idea of managing known risks to help minimize financial loss to the company. Note also that some malpractice insurance companies offer discounts to their insured anesthesia professionals for participating in simulation training, particularly for Crisis Resource Management of clinical emergencies during anesthesia care.

With many of the same elements of thinking, the ASA adopted "Basic Standards for Preanesthesia Care." This was supplemented significantly by another type of document, the ASA *Practice Advisory for Preanesthesia Evaluation*.[39] Also, the ASA adopted "Standards for Postanesthesia Care," in which there was consideration of and collaboration with the very detailed standards of practice for PACU care published by the American Society of Post Anesthesia Nurses (another good example of the sources of standards of care). This also was later supplemented by an extensive practice guideline.[40]

A slightly different situation exists with regard to the standards for conduct of anesthesia in obstetrics. These standards were originally passed by the ASA in 1988, in the same manner as the other ASA standards, but the ASA membership eventually questioned whether they reflected a realistic and desirable standard of care. Accordingly, the obstetric anesthesia standards were "downgraded" in 1990 to "guidelines," specifically to remove the mandatory nature of the document. Because there was no agreement as to what should be prescribed as the standard of care, the medicolegal imperative of published standards in this instance has been temporarily set aside. From a management perspective, this makes the guidelines no less valuable because the intent of optimizing care through the avoidance of complications is no less operative. However, in the event of the need to defend against a malpractice claim in this area, it is clear from this sequence of events that the exact standard of care is debatable and not yet finally established (an extremely important medicolegal consideration). A different ASA document has since been generated, *Practice Guidelines for Obstetrical Anesthesia*, with more detail and specificity as well as an emphasis on the meta-analytic approach.[41]

Practice Guidelines

Beyond formal standards that do prescribe the standard of care, an important type of related ASA document is the *Practice Guideline* (formerly "Practice Parameter"). This has some of the same elements as a standard of practice but is more intended to guide judgment, largely through algorithms with some element of guidelines, in addition to directing the details of specific procedures as would a formal standard. Beyond the details of the minimum standards for carrying out the procedure, these practice parameters set forth algorithms and guidelines for helping to determine under what circumstances and with what timing to perform it. Understandably, purchasers of health care (government, insurance companies, health plans, and MCOs) with a strong desire to limit the costs of medical care have great interest in practice parameters as potential vehicles for helping to eliminate "unnecessary" procedures and limit even the necessary ones.

The ASA has been very active in creating and publishing practice guidelines. The first published parameter (since revised) concerned the use of pulmonary artery (PA) catheters.[42] It considered the clinical effectiveness of PA catheters, public policy issues (costs and concerns of patients and providers), and recommendations (indications and practice settings). Also, the ASA *Difficult Airway Algorithm* has been updated periodically.[43] This thoughtful document synthesizes a strategy summarized in a decision tree diagram for dealing acutely with airway problems. The difficult airway algorithm has been discussed extensively in the literature, including suggestions regarding the role of supraglottic airways and, more recently, adding the various airway video imaging technologies. This illustrates that all the ASA practice guidelines involve fluid concepts that are subject to reconsideration, reinterpretation, and revision as experience and technology evolve. Undoubtedly, the difficult airway algorithm has great clinical value and helps many patients. However, there is concern that as with many modern things, it starts to outdate as soon as it is published. Such considerations are important, both clinically and because all these documents are readily noted by plaintiffs' lawyers as relevant to establishing the applicable standard of care.

An important question is whether guidelines and practice parameters from recognized entities such as the ASA *define* the standard of care. There is no simple answer. This will be decided over time by practitioners' actions, debates in the literature, mandates from malpractice insurers, and, of course, court decisions. Some guidelines, such as the concepts in the U.S. Food and Drug Administration (FDA) preanesthetic apparatus checkout, are accepted as the standard of care. There will be debate among experts, but the practitioner must make the decision as to how to apply practice parameters and guidelines such as those from the ASA. Practitioners have incorrectly assumed that they *must* do everything specified. This is clearly not true, yet there is a valid concern that these will someday be held up as defining the standard of care. Accordingly, prudent attention within the bounds of reason to the principles outlined in guidelines and parameters will put the practitioner in at least a reasonably defensible position, whereas radical deviation from them should be based only on obvious exigencies of the situation at that moment or clear, defensible alternative beliefs (with documentation).

The most recent type of document has been the "practice advisory," which can seem functionally similar to a guideline, but appears to have the implication of more consensus compromise than previous documents driven more by meta-analysis of the relevant literature. Examples of ASA Practice Advisories include "Intraoperative Awareness and Brain Function Monitoring," "Perioperative Management of Patients with Cardiac Rhythm Management Devices: Pacemakers and Implantable Cardioverter-Defibrillators," "Perioperative Visual Loss Associated with Spine Surgery," and "Practice Advisory on Anesthetic Care for Magnetic Resonance Imaging." At any given time, there are several additional topics under consideration and new advisories being prepared.

The potential QA and medicolegal implications of these documents are so important to anesthesia professionals and their practices that the ASA has what is essentially a guideline for the guidelines in its 2013 update of the "Policy Statement on Practice Parameters" in which the distinction is made between evidence-based documents and consensus-based documents with explanations of the background and formulation processes for each.

On the other hand, practice protocols, such as those for the fast-track management of coronary artery bypass graft patients, that are handed down by MCOs or health insurance companies are a different matter. Even though the desired implication is that practitioners must observe (or at least strongly consider) them, they do not have the same implications in defining the standard of care as the other documents. Practitioners must avoid getting trapped. It may well not be a valid legal defense to justify action or the lack of action because of a company or facility protocol. As difficult as it may be to reconcile with the payer, the practitioner still is subject to the classic definitions of standard of care.

The other types of standards associated with medical care are those of the Joint Commission, which is the best-known medical care quality regulatory agency. As noted, these standards were for many years concerned largely with structure (e.g., gas tanks chained down) and process (e.g., documentation complete), but in recent years they have been expanded to include reviews of the *outcome* of care and also review of the sequence of one individual inpatient's care through "tracer" sequences during an inspection. Joint Commission standards also focus on credentialing and privileges, verification that anesthesia services are of uniform quality throughout an institution, the qualifications of the director of the service, continuing education, and basic guidelines for anesthesia care (need for preoperative and postoperative evaluations, documentation, and so forth). Full Joint Commission accreditation of a health-care facility is usually for 3 years, although the process is considered "continuous." Even the best hospitals and facilities receive some citations of problems or deficiencies that are expected to be corrected, and an interim report of efforts to do so is required. If there are enough problems, accreditation can be conditional for 1 year, with a complete reinspection at that time. Being ready for a Joint Commission inspection (which is unannounced and can come at any time) starts with verification that an essential group/department structure is in place. The process of "constant preparation" ultimately involves a great deal of work, but because the standards usually do promote high-quality care, the majority of this work is highly constructive and of benefit to the institution and its medical staff.

Review Implications

"Peer review organizations"[44] were established in the 1980s and 1990s in every state, usually affiliated with state medical associations and/or state licensing agencies both to monitor quality of medical care and perform utilization reviews (URs), which were oriented to reducing health-care costs. These functions have migrated in recent years largely to the government insurers Medicare and Medicaid and have become fixated essentially exclusively on cost issues. Also, each private health insurance company has UR functions, whether internal or contracted out to a company that performs that function for the insurer.

The most likely interaction between a UR agency or office and anesthesia professionals will involve a request for perioperative admission of a patient whose care is mandated to be outpatient surgery (this could also occur in dealing with a health plan or MCO). If the anesthesiologist feels, for example, that either (1) preoperative admission for treatment to optimize cardiac, pulmonary, diabetic, or other medical status or (2) postoperative admission for monitoring of labile situations such as uncontrolled hypertension will reduce clear anesthetic risks for the patient, an application to UR for approval of admission must be made and vigorously supported. All too often, however, such issues surface a day or so before the scheduled procedure in a preanesthesia screening clinic or even in a preoperative holding area outside the OR on the day of surgery. This will continue to occur until anesthesia providers educate their constituent surgeon community as to what types of associated medical conditions may disqualify a proposed patient from the outpatient (ambulatory) surgical schedule. If adequate notice is given by the surgeon, the patient can be seen far enough in advance by an anesthesiologist to allow appropriate planning.

In the circumstance in which the first knowledge of a questionable patient comes 1 or 2 days before surgery, the anesthesiologist can try to have the procedure postponed, if possible, or can undertake the time-consuming task of multiple telephone calls to get the surgeon's agreement, get UR approval, and make the necessary arrangements. Because neither alternative is particularly attractive, especially from administrative and reimbursement perspectives, there may be a strong temptation to "let it slide" and try to deal with the patient as an outpatient even though this may be questionable. In almost all cases, it is likely that there would be no adverse result (the "get away with it" phenomenon). However, the patient might well be exposed to an avoidable risk. Both because of the workings of probability and because of the inevitable tendency to let sicker and sicker patients slip by as lax practitioners repeatedly "get away with it" and are lulled into a false sense of security, sooner or later there will be an unfortunate outcome or some preventable major morbidity or even mortality.

The situation is worsened when the first contact with a questionable ambulatory patient is preoperatively (or possibly even already in the OR) on the day of surgery. There may be intense pressure from the patient, the surgeon, or the OR administrator and staff to proceed with a case for which the anesthesia practitioner believes the patient is poorly prepared. The arguments made regarding patient inconvenience and anxiety are valid. However, they should not outweigh the best medical interests of the patient. Although this is a point in favor of screening all outpatients before the day of surgery, the anesthesia professional facing this situation on the day of operation should state clearly to all concerned the reasons for postponing the surgery, stressing the issue of avoidable risk and standards of care, and then help with alternative arrangements (including, if necessary, dealing with UR or an MCO).

Potential liability in this regard is the other side of the standard of care issue. Particularly concerning is the question of postoperative admission of ambulatory patients who have been unstable. It is an extremely poor defense against a malpractice claim to state that the patient was discharged home, only later to suffer a complication, because the UR process or a health plan or MCO deemed that operative procedure outpatient and not inpatient surgery. As bureaucratically annoying as it may be, it is a prudent management strategy to admit the patient if there is any legitimate question, thus minimizing the chance for complications, and later haggle with the UR bureaucracy.

Policy and Procedure

One important organizational point that is sometimes overlooked in anesthesia practice is the need for a complete policy and procedure manual. Such a compilation of documents is necessary for all practices, from the largest departments covering multiple hospitals to a single-room outpatient facility with one anesthesia provider. Such a manual can be extraordinarily valuable as, for example, when it provides crucial information during an emergency. Organizational and procedural elements should be included. A sample of a table of contents is in the ASA manual.[35] The organizational elements that should be present include a chart of organization and responsibilities that is not just a call schedule but a clear explanation of who is responsible for what functions of the department and when, with attendant details such as expectations for the practitioner's presence within the institution at designated hours, telephone availability, pager availability, the maximum permissible distance from the institution when on call, and so forth. Experience suggests it is especially important for there to be an absolutely clear specification of the availability of qualified anesthesiology personnel for emergency cesarean section, particularly in practice arrangements in which there are several people on call covering multiple locations. Sadly, these issues often are only considered after a disaster has occurred that involved miscommunication and the mistaken belief by one or more people that someone else would take care of an acute problem.

The organizational component of the policy and procedure manual should also include a clear explanation of the orientation and checkout procedure for new personnel, CME requirements and opportunities, the mechanisms for evaluating personnel and for communicating this evaluation to them, disaster plans (or reference to a separate disaster manual or protocol), QA activities of the department, and the format for statistical record keeping (number of procedures, types of anesthetics given, types of patients anesthetized, number and types of invasive monitoring procedures, number and type of responses to emergency calls, complications, or whatever the group/department decides).

The procedural component of the policy and procedure manual should give both handy practice tips and specific outlines of proposed courses of action for particular circumstances; it also should store little used but valuable information. Reference should be made to the statements, guidelines, practice parameters and advisories, and standards appearing on the ASA website. Also included should be references to or specific protocols for the areas mentioned in the Joint Commission standards: preanesthetic evaluation, immediate preinduction reevaluation, safety of the patient during the anesthetic period, release of the patient from any PACU, recording of all pertinent events during anesthesia, recording of postanesthesia visits, guidelines defining the role of anesthesia services in hospital infection control, and guidelines for safe use of general anesthetic agents. Other appropriate topics include the following:

1. Recommendations for preanesthesia apparatus checkout, such as from the ASA
2. Guidelines for admission to, minimal monitoring and duration of stay of an infant, child, or adult in, and then discharge from the PACU
3. Procedures for transporting patients to/from the OR, PACU, or ICU
4. Policy on ambulatory surgical patients—for example, screening, use of regional anesthesia, discharge home criteria
5. Policy on evaluation and processing of same-day admissions
6. Policy on ICU admission and discharge
7. Policy on physicians responsible for writing orders in recovery room and ICU
8. Policy on informed consent for anesthesia and its documentation
9. Policy on the use of patients in clinical research (if applicable)
10. Guidelines for the support of cadaveric organ donors and its termination (plus organ donation after cardiac death if applicable)
11. Guidelines on environmental safety, including pollution with trace gases and electrical equipment inspection, maintenance, and hazard prevention
12. Procedure for change of personnel during an anesthetic and documentation (particularly if a printed hand-off protocol is used)
13. Procedure for the introduction of new equipment, drugs, or clinical practices
14. Procedure for epidural and spinal narcotic administration and subsequent patient monitoring (e.g., type, minimum time, nursing units)
15. Procedure for initial treatment of cardiac or respiratory arrest (updated Advanced Cardiac Life Support guidelines)
16. Policy for handling patient's refusal of blood or blood products, including the mechanism to obtain a court order to transfuse
17. Procedure for the management of malignant hyperthermia
18. Procedure for the induction and maintenance of barbiturate coma
19. Procedure for the evaluation of suspected pseudocholinesterase deficiency
20. Protocol for responding to an adverse anesthetic event (such as a copy of the update of the "Adverse Event Protocol" [Eichhorn JH. Organized response to major anesthesia accident will help limit damage: Update of "Adverse Event Protocol" provides valuable plan. APSF Newsletter. 2006;21:11.])
21. Policy on resuscitation of do-not-resuscitate patients in the OR

Individual departments will add to and modify these suggestions as dictated by their specific needs. A thorough, carefully conceived policy and procedure manual is a valuable tool. The manual should be reviewed and updated as needed but at least annually. Each member of a group or department should review the manual at least annually and sign off in a log indicating familiarity with current policies and procedures.

Meetings and Case Discussion

There must be regularly scheduled departmental or group meetings. Although didactic lectures and continuing education meetings are valuable and necessary, there must also be regular opportunities for open clinical discussion about interesting cases and problem cases. Also, the Joint Commission requires that there be at least monthly meetings at which risk management and QA activities are documented and reported. Whether these meetings are called case conferences, morbidity and mortality conferences, or deaths and complications conferences, the entire department or group should gather for an interchange of ideas. More recently, these gatherings can be called *QA meetings*.

An open review of departmental statistics should be done, including all complications, even those that may appear trivial. Unusual patterns of small events may point toward a larger or systematic problem, especially if they are more frequently associated with one individual practitioner.

A problem case presented at the departmental meeting might be an overt accident, a near accident (critical incident), or an untoward outcome of unknown origin. Honest but constructive discussion, even of an anesthesia professional's technical deficiencies or lack of knowledge, should take place in the spirit of constructive peer review. The classic question, "What would you do differently next time?" is a good way to start the discussion. There may be situations in which inviting the surgeon or the internist involved in a specific case would be advantageous. The opportunity for each type of provider to hear the perspective of another discipline not only is inherently educational but also can promote communication and cooperation in future potential problem cases.

Records of these meetings must be kept for accreditation purposes, but the enshrining of overly detailed minutes (potentially subject to discovery by a plaintiff's attorney at a later date) may inhibit true educational and corrective interchanges about untoward events. In the circumstance of discussion of a case that seems likely to provoke litigation, it is appropriate to be certain that the meeting is classified as official "peer review" and possibly even invite the hospital attorney or legal counsel from the relevant malpractice insurance carrier (to guarantee the privacy of the discussion and minutes).

Support Staff

There is a fundamental need for support staff in every anesthesia practice. Even independent practitioners rely in some measure on facilities, equipment, and services provided by the organization maintaining the anesthetizing location. In large, well-organized departments, reliance on support staff is often very great. What is often overlooked, however, is a process analogous to that of credentialing and privileges for anesthesia professionals, although at a somewhat different level. The people expected to provide clinical anesthesia practice support must be qualified and must at all times understand what they are expected to do and how to do it. It is singularly unfortunate to realize only after an anesthesia catastrophe has occurred that basic details of simple work assignments, such as the changing of carbon dioxide absorbent, were routinely ignored. This indicates the need for supervision and monitoring of the support staff by the involved practitioners. Further, such support personnel are favorite targets of cost-cutting administrators who do not understand the function of anesthesia technicians or their equivalent. In the modern era, many administrators seem driven almost exclusively by the "bottom line" and cannot appreciate the connection between valuable workers such as these and the "revenue stream." Even though it is obvious to all who work in an OR that the anesthesia support personnel make it possible for there to be patients flowing through the OR, it is their responsibility to convince the facility's fiscal administrator that elimination of such positions is genuinely false economy because of the attendant loss in efficiency, particularly in turning over the room between surgeries. Further, it is also false economy to reduce the number of personnel below that genuinely needed to retrieve, clean, sort, disassemble, sterilize, reassemble, store, and distribute the tools of daily anesthesia practice. Vigorous defense (or initiation of new positions if the staff is inadequate) by the anesthesia professionals should be undertaken, even sometimes with the realization that it may be necessary in some circumstances for them to supplement the budget from the facility with some of their practice income to guarantee an adequate complement of competent workers.

Business and organizational issues in the management of an anesthesia practice are also critically dependent on the existence of a sufficient number of appropriately trained support staff. As noted, one frequently overlooked issue that contributes to the negative impression generated by some anesthesiology practices centers on being certain there is someone available to answer the telephone *at all times* during the hours surgeons, other physicians, and OR scheduling desks are likely to call. This seemingly trivial component of practice management is very important to the success of an anesthesiology practice as a business whose principal customers are the surgeons. Certainly there is a commercial server–client relationship both with the patient and the purchaser of health care; however, the uniquely symbiotic nature of the relationship between surgeons and anesthesiologists is such that availability even for simple "just wanted to let you know" telephone calls is genuinely important. The person who answers the telephone is the representative of the practice to the world and must take that responsibility seriously. From a management standpoint, significant impact on the success of the practice as a business often hinges on such details. Further, anesthesia professionals should always have reliable personal communication ability, whether electronic pagers (preferably with text, and even more preferably two-way) and/or mobile telephones (or the radio equivalent) to facilitate communications from other members of the department or group and from support or facility personnel. This may sound intrusive, but the unusual position of anesthesia professionals in the spectrum of health-care workers mandates this feature of managing an anesthesiology practice. Anesthesiology professionals should have no hesitation about spending their own practice income to do so. The symbolism alone is obvious.

Anesthesia Equipment and Equipment Maintenance

Problems with anesthesia equipment have been discussed extensively for many years.[45-47] However, compared with human error, overt equipment failure rarely causes intraoperative critical incidents[48] or deaths resulting from anesthesia care. Aside from the obvious human errors involving misuse of or unfamiliarity with the equipment, when the rare equipment failure does occur, it often appears that correct maintenance and servicing of the apparatus has not been done. These issues are part of anesthesia practice management efforts, which could have significant liability implications because there can often be confusion or even disputes about precisely who is responsible for arranging maintenance of the anesthesia equipment—the facility or the practitioners who use it and collect practice income from that activity. In many cases, the facility assumes the responsibility. In situations in which that is not true, however, it is necessary for the practitioners to recognize that responsibility and seek help securing a service arrangement, because this is likely an unfamiliar obligation for clinicians.

A distinction is made between failure resulting from progressive deterioration of equipment, which should be preventable because it is observable and should provoke appropriate remedial action, and catastrophic failure, which, realistically, often cannot be predicted. Preventive maintenance for mechanical parts is critical and involves periodic performance checks every 4 to 6 months. Also, an annual safety inspection of each anesthetizing location and the equipment itself is necessary. For equipment service, an excellent mechanism is a relatively elaborate cross-reference system (possibly kept handwritten in a notebook but ideal for maintenance on an electronic spreadsheet program) to identify both the device needing service and also the mechanism to secure the needed maintenance or repair. Most important, however, is the simple requirement that there is some type of reliable program for equipment maintenance and service for every anesthesia organization providing clinical care. Assuming that "someone must be taking care of it" without established certainty is an invitation to a potential medicolegal liability nightmare.

Equipment-handling principles are straightforward. Before purchase, it must be verified that a proposed piece of equipment meets all applicable standards, which will usually be true when dealing with new equipment from recognized major manufacturers. The renewed efforts of some facility administrators to save money by attempting to find "refurbished" anesthesia machines and monitoring systems (especially for "off-site," "satellite," or "office-based" locations) should provoke thorough review by the involved practitioners. On arrival, electrical equipment must be checked for absence of hazard (especially leakage of current) and compliance with applicable electrical standards. Complex equipment such as anesthesia machines, ventilators, and monitors should be assembled and checked out by a representative from the manufacturer or manufacturer's agent. There are potential adverse medicolegal implications when relatively untrained personnel certify a particular piece of new equipment as functioning within specification, even if they do it perfectly. On arrival, a sheet or section in the departmental master equipment log must be created with the make, model, serial number, and in-house identification for each piece of capital equipment (anything with a serial number). This not only allows immediate identification of any equipment involved in a future recall or product alert but also serves as the permanent repository of the record of every problem, problem resolution, maintenance, and servicing occurring until that particular equipment is scrapped. This log must be kept up-to-date at all times. There have been rare but frightening examples of potentially lethal problems with anesthesia machines leading to product alert notices requiring immediate identification of certain equipment and its service status. It is also very important to involve the manufacturer's representative in pre- and in-service training for those who will use the new equipment. Anesthesia systems with their ventilation and monitoring components have become significantly more integrated and more complex, particularly as they are increasingly electronic and less mechanical. Accordingly, it is critical that anesthesia professionals are properly trained to use their equipment safely. The perception that inadequate training is common and that this represents a threat to patient safety has led the Anesthesia Patient Safety Foundation to initiate a campaign urging anesthesia departments and groups to ensure organized verified complete training of all professionals who will use this new technology.[49]

Service

Beyond the administrative liability implications, precisely what type of support personnel should maintain and service major anesthesia equipment has been widely debated. Some groups or departments rely on factory service representatives from the equipment manufacturers for all attention to equipment, others engage independent service contractors, and still other (often larger) departments have access to personnel (either engineers and/or technicians) permanently within their facility. The single underlying principle is clear: The person(s) doing preventive maintenance and service on anesthesia equipment must be qualified. Anesthesia practitioners may wonder how they can assess these qualifications. The best way is to unhesitatingly ask pertinent questions about the education, training, and experience of those involved, including asking for references and speaking to supervisors and managers responsible for those doing the work. Whether an engineering technician who spent a week at a course at a factory can perform the most complex repairs depends on a variety of factors, which can be investigated by the practitioners ultimately using the equipment in the care of patients. Failure to be involved in this oversight function exposes the practice to increased liability in the event of an untoward outcome associated with improperly maintained or serviced equipment.

Replacement of obsolete anesthesia machines and monitoring equipment is a key element of a risk-modification program. Ten years is sometimes cited as an estimated useful life for an anesthesia machine, but although an ASA statement repeats that idea, it also notes that the ASA promulgated "Guidelines for Determining Anesthesia Machine Obsolescence" in 2004 does not subscribe to any specific time interval. Very old anesthesia machines likely do not meet certain safety standards now in force (such as vaporizer lockout, fresh gas ratio protection, and automatic enabling of the oxygen analyzer). Further, it appears likely that this technology will continue to advance, particularly because of the adoption of anesthesia workstation standards by the European Economic Union that are affecting anesthesia machine designs worldwide. Note that some anesthesia equipment manufacturers, anxious to minimize their own potential liability, have refused to support (with parts and service) some of the oldest of their pieces (particularly gas machines) still in use. This disowning of equipment by its own manufacturer is a very strong message to practitioners that such equipment must be replaced as soon as possible.

Should a piece of equipment fail, it must be removed from service and a replacement substituted. Groups, departments, and facilities are obligated to have sufficient backup equipment to cover any reasonable incidence of failure. The equipment removed from service must be clearly marked with a prominent label (so it is not returned into service by a well-meaning technician or practitioner) containing the date, time, person discovering, and the details of the problem. The responsible personnel must be notified so they can remove the equipment, make an entry in the log, and initiate the repair. As indicated in the protocol for response to an adverse event,[50] a piece of equipment involved or suspected in an injury-causing anesthesia accident must be immediately sequestered and not touched by anybody—particularly not by any equipment service personnel. If a severe accident occurred, it may be necessary for the equipment in question to be inspected at a later time by a group consisting of qualified representatives of the manufacturer, the service personnel, the plaintiff's attorney, the insurance companies involved, and the practitioner's defense attorney. The equipment should thus be impounded following a catastrophic adverse event and treated similarly to any object in a forensic "chain of evidence," with careful documentation of parties in contact with and responsible for securing the equipment in question following such an event. Also, major equipment problems may, in some circumstances, reflect a pattern of failure due to a design or manufacturing fault. These problems should be reported to the FDA's Medical Device Problem Reporting system via MedWatch on Form 3500 (found at www.fda.gov/medwatch/index.html, or telephone 800-FDA-1088). This system accepts voluntary reports from users and requires reports from manufacturers when there is knowledge of a medical device being involved in a serious incident. Whether or not filing such a report will have a positive impact in subsequent litigation is impossible to know, but it is a worthwhile practice management point that needs to be considered in the unlikely but important instance of a relevant event involving equipment failure.

Malpractice Insurance

All practitioners need liability insurance coverage specific for the specialty and role in which they are practicing. It is absolutely critical that applicants for medical liability insurance be completely honest in informing the insurer what duties and procedures they perform. Failure to do so, either from carelessness or from a foolishly misguided desire to reduce the resulting premium, may well result in retrospective denial of insurance coverage in the event of an untoward outcome from an activity the insurer did not know the insured engaged in.

Proof of adequate insurance coverage is usually required to secure or renew privileges to practice at a health-care facility. The facility may specify certain minimum policy limits in an attempt to limit its own liability exposure. It is difficult to suggest specific dollar amounts for policy limits because the details of practice vary so much among situations and locations. The malpractice crisis of the 1980s eased significantly in the early 1990s for anesthesia professionals, largely because of the decrease in number and severity of malpractice claims resulting from anesthesia catastrophes as anesthesia care in the United States became safer.[51–53] The exact analysis of this phenomenon can be debated,[54,55] but it is a simple fact that malpractice insurance risk ratings were decreased and premiums for anesthesia professionals have not been increased at the same rate as for other specialties over the same time and, in many cases, have actually decreased further. An ASA Committee on Professional Liability survey revealed: "In 2013, 72 percent of anesthesiologists had policy limits of $1 million/$3 million, 20 percent of anesthesiologists had higher limits, and greater than 8 percent had lower policy limits."[56] This policy specification usually means that the insurer will cover up to $1 million liability per claim and up to $3 million total per year, but this terminology is not necessarily universal. Therefore, anesthesia professionals must be absolutely certain what they are buying when they apply for malpractice insurance. There are specific parts of the United States known for a pattern of exorbitant settlements and jury verdicts, and liability insurance coverage limits of $2 to $5 million or even greater may be considered prudent in some circumstances. Note also that malpractice insurance premiums for anesthesiologists practicing chronic pain management are moderately higher due to the potential liabilities associated with pain procedures.[56] An additional feature in regard to choosing malpractice insurance policy limits is the potential to employ "umbrella" liability coverage above the limits of the base policy, as will be noted.

Background

The fundamental mechanism of medical malpractice insurance changed significantly some years ago because of the need for insurance companies to have better ways to predict their "losses" (amounts paid in settlements and judgments). Traditionally, medical liability insurance was sold on an "occurrence" basis, meaning that if the insurance policy was in force at the time of the occurrence of an incident resulting in a claim, whenever within the statute of limitations that claim might be filed, the practitioner would be covered. Occurrence insurance was somewhat more expensive than the alternative "claims-made" policies, but was seen as worth it by some (many) practitioners. These policies created some open-ended exposure for the insurer that sometimes led to unexpected large losses, even some large enough to threaten the existence of the insurance company. As a result, medical malpractice insurers over the years have converted almost exclusively to "claims-made" insurance, which covers only claims that are filed while the insurance is in force. Premium rates for the first year a physician is in practice are relatively low because there is less likelihood of a claim coming in (a majority of malpractice suits are filed 1 to 3 years after the event in question). The premiums usually increase yearly for the first 5 years and then the policy is considered "mature." The issue comes when the physician later, for whatever reason, must change insurance companies (e.g., because of relocation to another state). If the physician simply discontinues the policy and a claim is filed the next year, there will be no insurance coverage. Therefore, the physician must secure "tail coverage," sometimes for a minimum number of years (e.g., 5) or, more often, indefinitely to guarantee liability insurance protection for claims filed after the physician is no longer primarily covered by that insurance policy. It may be possible in some circumstances to purchase tail coverage from a different insurer than was involved with the primary policy, but by far the most common thing done is to simply extend the existing insurance coverage for the period of the tail. This very often yields a bill for the entire tail coverage premium, which can be quite sizable, potentially staggering a physician who simply wants to move to another state where his or her existing insurance company is not licensed to or refuses to do business. Individual situations will vary widely, but it is reasonable for anesthesiologists organized into a fiscal entity to consider this issue at the time of the inception of the group and record their policy decisions regarding providing tail coverage as a benefit in writing, rather than facing the potentially difficult question of how to treat one individual later. Other strategies have occasionally been employed when insuring the tail period, including converting the previous policy to part-time status for a period of years, or purchasing "nose" coverage from the new insurer—that is, paying an initial higher yearly premium with the new insurer, who then will cover claims that may occur during the tail period. Whatever strategy is adopted, it is critical that the individual practitioner is absolutely certain through personal verification that he or she is thoroughly covered at the time of any transition. The potential stakes are much too great to leave such important issues solely to an office clerk. Further, a practitioner arriving in a new location is often filling a need or void and is urged to begin clinical work as soon as possible by others who have been shouldering an increased load. It is essential that the new arrival verify with confirmation in writing (often called a "binder") that malpractice liability insurance coverage is in force before there is any patient contact.

Another component to the liability insurance situation is consideration of the advisability of purchasing yet another type of insurance called *umbrella coverage,* which is activated at the time of the need to pay a claim that exceeds the limits of coverage on the standard malpractice liability insurance policy. Because such an enormous claim is extremely unlikely, many practitioners are tempted to forgo the comparatively modest cost of such insurance coverage in the name of economy. As before, it is easy to see that this is potentially a very false economy—if there is a huge claim. Practitioners should consult with their financial managers and advisors, but it is likely that it would be considered wise management to purchase "umbrella" liability insurance coverage.

Medical malpractice insurers are becoming increasingly active in trying to prevent incidents that will lead to insurance claims. They often sponsor risk management seminars to teach practices and techniques to lessen the chances of liability claims and, in some cases, suggest (or even mandate) specific practices, such as strict documented compliance with the ASA "Standards for Basic Anesthetic Monitoring." In return for attendance at such events and/or the signing of contracts stating that the practitioner will follow certain guidelines or standards, the insurer often gives a discount on the liability insurance premium. Clearly, it is sound practice management strategy for practitioners to participate maximally in such programs. Likewise, some insurers make coverage conditional on the consistent implementation of certain strategies such as minimal monitoring, even stipulating that the practitioner will not be covered if it is found that the guidelines were being consciously ignored at the time of an untoward event. Again, it is obviously wise from a practice management standpoint to cooperate fully with such stipulations.

Response to an Adverse Event

Despite the decreased incidence of anesthesia catastrophes, even with the very best of practice, it is statistically likely that each anesthesiologist at least once in his or her professional life will be involved in a major anesthesia accident. Precisely because such an event is rare, very few are prepared for it. It is probable that the involved personnel will have no relevant past experience regarding what to do. Although an obvious resource is another anesthetist who has had some exposure or experience, one of these may not be available either. Suggestions have been published about what to do in that event.[57-59] Cooper et al.[60] thoughtfully presented the appropriate immediate response to an accident in a straightforward, logical, compact format (which has been updated[50]) that should periodically be reviewed by all anesthesiology practitioners and should be included in all anesthesia policy and procedure manuals. This "adverse events protocol" is also always immediately available at www.apsf.org ("Resource Center," then "Clinical Safety Tools"). Unfortunately, however, the principal personnel involved in a significant untoward event may react with such surprise or shock as to temporarily lose sight of logic. At the moment of recognition that a major anesthetic complication has occurred or is occurring, help must be called. A sufficient number of people to deal with the situation must be assembled on site as quickly as possible. For example, in the unlikely but still possible event that an esophageal intubation goes unrecognized long enough to cause a cardiac arrest, the immediate need is for enough skilled personnel to conduct the resuscitative efforts, including making the correct diagnosis and replacing the tube into the trachea. Whether the anesthesiologist apparently responsible for the complication should direct the immediate remedial efforts will depend on the person and the situation. In such a circumstance, it would seem wise for a senior or supervising anesthesiologist quickly to evaluate the scenario and make a decision. This person becomes the "incident supervisor" and has responsibility for helping prevent continuation or recurrence of the incident, for investigating the incident, and for ensuring documentation while the original and helping anesthesiologists focus on caring for the patient. As noted, involved equipment must be sequestered and not touched until such time as it is certain that it was not involved in the incident.

With the hope of preventing or mitigating catastrophic anesthesia accidents, the utilization of emergency manuals, usually including checklists, as "cognitive aids" within the application of "crisis resource management"[61] when an adverse threatening situation develops during an anesthetic has gained significant attention.[62,63] Although such documents containing suggested protocols can be stored and accessed electronically on a computer or smart phone at the time of a crisis in the OR, many anesthesia professionals who want these tools available prefer printed copies, often on thick laminated pages, actually attached to the anesthesia machine in each OR. Although the incident supervisor could seek guidance by reading a manual in real time during a crisis, having a "reader" who may or may not be another anesthesia professional whose sole activity during the crisis is to read out loud the relevant diagnostic and therapeutic suggestions in the protocol that applies to the crisis situation could be helpful. Overall, evidence from studies in simulated anesthesia crisis situations indicates on balance that the use of "emergency manual" type cognitive aids can improve patient outcome from an intraoperative anesthesia crisis.[64,65]

If the accident is not fatal, continuing care of the patient is critical. Measures may be instituted to help limit damage from brain hypoxia. Consultants may be helpful and should be called without hesitation. If not already involved, the chief of anesthesiology must be notified as well as the facility administrator, risk manager, and the anesthesiologist's insurance company. The latter are critical to allow consideration of immediate efforts to limit later financial loss. (Likewise, there are often provisions in medical malpractice insurance policies that might limit or even deny insurance coverage if the company is not notified of any reportable event immediately.) If there is an involved surgeon of record, he or she probably will first notify the family, but the anesthesiologist and others (risk manager, insurance loss control officer, or even legal counsel) might appropriately be included at the outset. Full disclosure of facts as they are best known—with no confessions, opinions, speculation, or placing of blame—is still believed by many to be the best presentation. Any attempt to conceal or shade the truth will later only confound an already difficult situation. Obviously, comfort and support should be offered, including, if appropriate, the services of facility personnel such as clergy, social workers, and counselors. Note that there is a strong movement in medical risk management and liability insurance advocating immediate full disclosure to the victim or survivors, including "confessions" of medical judgment and performance errors with attendant sincere apologies. If indicated, early offers of reasonable compensation may be included. There have been instances when this overall strategy has prevented the filing of a malpractice lawsuit and has been applauded by all involved as an example of a shift from the "culture of blame" with punishment to a "just culture" with restitution. A widespread movement to implement immediate disclosure and apology has received support.[66,67]

Certain states have enacted or proposed the so-called "I'm sorry!" legislation intended to prevent any explanation or apology by the involved practitioners from being used as plaintiff's evidence in a subsequent malpractice suit. The importance of the patient's perspective on a serious adverse anesthesia event was highlighted in a riveting account of the stories of both survivors of anesthesia catastrophes and the families of patients who died.[68] In each case, one main message was the enormous negative impact of the perceived failure of the involved anesthesia professionals and their institutions to share detailed information about what exactly happened. A general review summarized what patients want and expect following an adverse event.[69] Laudable as this policy of immediate full disclosure and apology may sound, it would be mandatory for an individual practitioner to check with the involved liability insurance carrier, the practice group, and the facility risk management officials and administration before attempting it.

The primary anesthesia provider and any others involved must document relevant information. Never, ever change any existing entries in the medical record. Write an amendment note if needed, with careful explanation of why amendment is necessary, particularly stressing explanations of professional judgments involved. State only facts as they are known. Make no judgments about causes or responsibility and do not "point fingers." The same guidelines hold true for the filing of the incident ("event") report in the facility, which should be done as soon as is practical. Further, all discussions with the patient or family should be carefully documented in the medical record. Because detailed memories of the events may fade in the 1 to 3 years that may pass before the practitioner faces deposition questions about exactly what happened, it is recommended that immediately after the incident, the involved clinical personnel sit down and write out their own personal notes, which will include opinions and impressions as well as maximally detailed accounts of the events as they unfolded. These personal notes are not part of the medical record or the facility files. These notes should be written in the physical presence of an involved attorney representing the practitioner, even if this is not yet the specific defense attorney secured by the malpractice insurance company, and then that attorney should take possession of and keep those notes as case material. This strategy is intended to make the personal notes "attorney–client work product," and thus not subject to forced "discovery" (revelation) by other parties to the case.

Follow-up after the immediate handling of the incident will involve the primary anesthesiologist but should again be directed by a senior supervisor, who may or may not be the same person as the incident supervisor. The "follow-up supervisor" verifies the adequacy and coordination of ongoing care of the patient and facilitates communication among all involved, especially with the risk manager. Lastly, it is necessary to verify that adequate postevent documentation is taking place.

Of course, it is expected that such an adverse event will be discussed in the applicable morbidity and mortality meeting. It is necessary, however, to coordinate this activity with the involved risk manager and attorney so as to be completely certain that the contents and conclusions of the discussion are clearly considered peer review activity, and thus are shielded (in most states) from discovery by the plaintiffs' attorney.

Unpleasant as this is to contemplate, it is better to have a clear plan and execute it in the event of an accident causing injury to a patient. Vigorous immediate intervention may improve the outcome for all concerned.

Practice Essentials

The "Job Market" for Anesthesia Professionals

Although there is and likely always will be debate about supply-and-demand considerations for anesthesia professionals in the United States, the aging of the Baby Boom population and the extension of health-care insurance coverage to a large number of underserved people by the ACA leads to the belief that there may be a shortage of all medical professionals in the United States, and this also includes anesthesia professionals. To this end, several new medical schools have opened in recent years in the United States. Also, the total number of anesthesia residents and fellows in training increased 13% from academic year 2007–2008 to 2014–2015.[70] Note also that the dramatic economic downturn ("Great Recession") late in the first decade of the twenty-first century complicated the issues of supply and demand. Some finishing residents (who would otherwise not have) sought fellowship training in order to be "more competitive" when seeking a practice position. Older practicing anesthesiologists who would have normally been expected to retire and thus open up practice spots were thought to be postponing retirement due to financial uncertainties. With the United States economic "recovery," in recent years, this may be less of a consideration. Also, state and federal budget support for medical schools and residency training positions were and continue to be threatened by economic uncertainties, and hospital budget pressures could influence subsidies for anesthesia practices. Another factor in the United States that may affect the decision of medical students to choose anesthesiology or of anesthesia residents projecting a career path is the complex issue noted above regarding independent practice by CRNAs and its potential impact. Although there will always be a need for anesthesia professionals, probably increasing now and in the immediate future, there likely will be more factors to consider in seeking a practice position than ever before. In an effort to assist anesthesiologists attempting to choose a practice mode, the ASA has created an online training course, Practice Management for Residents—Evaluating a Practice, the purpose of which is to "Provide the newly graduating anesthesiologist with basic knowledge and skills to make an informed choice regarding the type of anesthesiology practice that best fits their professional and personal goals and preferences." (http://www.asahq.org/shop-asa/detail?productId=133892)

Types of Practice

Anesthesiology professionals finishing their training still need to choose among three fundamental possibilities: academic practice in a teaching hospital environment, a practice of patient care in the private practice marketplace, or a practice of patient care as an employee of a health-care system, large group practice, organization, or facility.

Teaching hospitals with anesthesiology residency programs constitute only a very small fraction of the total number of facilities requiring anesthesia services. These academic departments tend to be among the larger groups of anesthesiologists, but the aggregate fraction of the entire anesthesiologist population is small. It is interesting, however, that by the nature of the system, most residents and fellows finishing their training have almost exclusively been exposed only to academic anesthesiology. Accordingly, finishing trainees in the past often were comparatively unprepared to evaluate and enter the anesthesiology job market.

Specialty certification by the ABA should be the goal of all anesthesia residency graduates. Some finishing trainees (residents or fellows) who know they are eventually headed for private practice have started their attending careers as full-time junior faculty in an academic department. This allows them to obtain some clinical practice and supervisory experience and offers them the opportunity to prepare for the ABA examinations in the nurturing, protected academic environment with which they are familiar. Most trainees, however, do not become junior faculty; they accept positions in practice immediately. But they should take into account the need to become ABA-certified and build into their new practice arrangements the stipulation that there will be time and consideration given toward this goal.

Academic Practice

For those who choose to stay in academic practice, a number of specific characteristics of academic anesthesia departments can be used as screening questions.

How big is the department? Junior faculty sometimes can get lost in very big departments and be treated as little better than glorified senior residents. On the other hand, the availability of subspecialty service opportunities and significant research and educational resources can make large departments extremely attractive. In smaller academic departments, there may be fewer resources, but the likelihood of being quickly accepted as a valued and contributing member of the teaching faculty (and research team, if appropriate) may be higher. In very small departments, the number of expectations, projects, and involvements could potentially be overwhelming. In addition, a small department may lack a dedicated research infrastructure, so it may be necessary for the faculty in this situation to collaborate with other, larger departments to accomplish meaningful academic work.

What exactly is expected of junior faculty? If teaching one resident class every other week is standard, the candidate must enthusiastically accept that assignment and the attendant preparation work and time up front. Likewise, if it is expected that junior faculty will, by definition, be actively involved in publishable research, specific plans for projects to which the candidate is amenable must be made. In such situations, clear stipulations about startup research funding and nonclinical time to carry out the projects should be obtained as much as possible (although clinical workload demands and revenue generation expectations may make this very difficult in some settings). Particularly important is determining what the expectation is concerning outside funding. For example, it can be a rude shock to realize that projects will suddenly halt after 2 years if extramural funding has not been secured.

What are the prospects for advancement? Many new junior faculty directly out of residency start with medical school appointments as instructors unless there is something else in their background that immediately qualifies them as assistant professors. It is wise to understand from the beginning what it takes in that department and medical school to facilitate academic advancement. There may be more than one academic "track"; the tenure track, for example, usually depends on published research whereas the clinical or teacher track relies more heavily on one's value in patient care and as a clinical educator. The criteria for promotion may be clearly spelled out by the institution—number of papers needed, involvement and recognition at various levels, grants submitted and funded, and so on—or the system may be less rigid and depend more heavily on the department chairman's and other faculty evaluations and recommendations. In either case, careful inquiry before accepting the position can avert later surprise and disappointment.

How much does it pay? Traditionally, academic anesthesiologists have not earned quite as much as those in private practice—in return for the advantage of more predictable schedules, continued intellectual stimulation, and the intangible rewards of academic success. There is now great activity and attention concerning reimbursement of anesthesiologists, and it is difficult to predict future income for any anesthesiology practice situation. However, all of the forces influencing payment for anesthesia care may significantly diminish the traditional income differential between academic and private practice. In many cases, a faculty member is exclusively an employee of the institution or a component financial entity, which bills and collects or negotiates group contracts for the patient care rendered by the faculty member, and then pays a negotiated amount (either an absolute dollar figure or a floating amount based on volume—or, especially, a combination of the two) that constitutes the faculty person's entire income. Under other much less and less common arrangements, faculty members themselves may be able to bill and collect or negotiate contracts for their clinical work. Some institutions have an (comparatively small) academic salary from the medical school for being on the faculty, but many do not; some channel variable amounts of money (from the so-called Part A clinical revenue) into the academic practice in recognition of teaching and administration or simply as a subsidy for needed service. Usually, the faculty will be members of some type of group or practice plan (either for the anesthesia department alone or for the entire faculty as a whole) that bills and collects or negotiates contracts and then distributes the practice income to the faculty under an arrangement that must be examined by the candidate. In most academic institutions, practice expenses such as all overhead and malpractice insurance as well as reasonable benefits, including discretionary funds for meetings, subscriptions, books, dues, and so forth, are automatically part of the compensation package, which often may not be true in private practice and must be counted in making any comparison. An important corollary issue is that of the source of the salaries of the department's primary anesthesia providers—residents and, in some cases, nurse anesthetists. Although the hospital usually pays for at least some and, often, most or all of these, arrangements vary, and it is important to ascertain whether the faculty practice income is also expected to cover the cost of the primary providers. Overall, it is appropriate for the candidate to ask probing questions about the commitment of the institution to the maintenance of reasonable compensation for faculty.

Private Practice in the Marketplace

Obviously, rotations to a private practice hospital in the final year of anesthesia residency could help greatly in regard to the realities of private practice, but not all residency programs offer such opportunities. In that case, the finishing trainee who is certain about going into traditional private practice must seek information on career development and mentors from the private sector.

In the past, independent individual practice was a viable option for some versus a position with a group (sole proprietorship, partnership, or corporation) that functions as a single financial entity. Independent practice became increasingly less viable in many locations because of the need to be able to bid for contracts with health systems, practice facilities, or managed care entities. However, where independent practice may still be possible, it usually first involves attempting to secure clinical privileges at a number of hospitals or facilities in the area in which one chooses to live. This may not always be easy, and this issue has been the subject of many (frequently unsuccessful) antitrust suits over recent years (see Antitrust Considerations). Then the anesthesiologist makes it known to the respective surgeon communities that he or she is available to render anesthesia services and waits until there is a request for his or her services. The anesthesiologist obtains the requisite financial information from the patient and then either individually bills and collects for services rendered or employs a service to do billing and collection for a percentage fee (which will vary depending on the circumstances, especially the volume of business; for billing [without scheduling services] it would be unlikely to be more than 7% or, at the most, 8% of actual collections).

How much of the needed equipment and supplies will be provided by the hospital or facility and how much by the independent anesthesiologist has varied widely. If an anesthesiologist spends considerable time in one operating suite, he or she may purchase an anesthesia machine exclusively for his or her own use and move it from room to room as needed. It is likely to be impractical to move a fully equipped anesthesia machine from hospital to hospital on a day-to-day basis. Among the features of this style of practice are the collegiality and relationships of a genuine private practice based on referrals and also the ability to decide independently how much time one wants to work.

The downside is the potential unpredictability of the demand for service and the time needed to establish referral patterns and obtain bookings sufficient to generate a livable income.

When seeking a position with a private group, the applicant should search for potential practice opportunities through word of mouth, recruiting letters received by the training program, journal and online announcements and advertisements, and placement services, either commercial or professional, such as that provided by the ASA Career Center (http://careers.asahq.org/). The growing availability and ease of access for online job searching has allowed prospective anesthesiologists and potential employers often to locate suitable candidates without the expense of commercial placement services. However, the most recent trend appears to be increasing reliance on placement services because these concerns vet an applicant for the practices, saving time and energy, and only present "qualified candidates" who look like a potential good fit for the practice. Traditional journal ads from private practices essentially disappeared by 2016. Some of the screening questions by the applicant are the same as for an academic position, but there must be even more emphasis on the exact details of clinical expectations and financial arrangements. Some trainees finish residency (or fellowship even more so) very highly skilled in complex, difficult anesthesia procedures. They can be surprised to find that in some private practice group situations, the junior-most anesthesiologist must wait some time, perhaps even years, before being eligible to do, for example, open heart anesthesia, and in the meantime will mostly be assigned more routine or less challenging anesthetics.

Financial arrangements in private group practices vary widely. A few groups may still be loose organizational alliances of independent practitioners who bill and collect separately and rotate clinical assignments and call for mutual convenience. Many groups act also as an umbrella fiscal entity, and there are many possible variations on this theme. In many circumstances in the past, new junior members started out as functional employees of the group for a probationary interval before being considered for full membership or partnership. This is not a classic employment situation because it is intended to be temporary as a prelude to full financial participation in the group. However, there have been enough instances of established groups abusing this arrangement that the ASA includes in its fundamental "Statement of Policy" the proviso: "Exploitation of anesthesiologists by other anesthesiologists is improper."[35] This goes on to say that after a reasonable trial period, income should reflect services rendered. These statements may have variable impact on groups in the marketplace. Some groups have a history of demanding excessively long trial periods during which the junior anesthesiologist's income is artificially low and then denying partnership and terminating the relationship to go on to employ a new probationer and start the cycle over again. Accordingly, new junior staff attempting to join groups should try to have such a "path to partnership" spelled out carefully in the agreement drafted by an expert representing the anesthesiologist. One key issue is the partnership "buy-in" once partnership is offered. This usually represents a percentage of the receivables (bills sent but not yet collected). As the cash outlay can be substantial, it is frequently "borrowed" from the group and paid back over time through a decrease in income, further delaying true equity participation in the group's profits. However, in times of great economic uncertainty and retrenchment, it could be theoretically possible that the equity partners in a group might take a cut in income while the employed junior associates continue to collect their full contracted compensation. At the very least, thorough investigation and understanding of the relationship is mandatory. Seeking assistance from an experienced medical practice contract attorney prior to any commitment is likely to be a very worthwhile investment.

Private Practice as an Employee

As noted in the opening section, there has been a major increasing trend toward anesthesiologists becoming permanent employees of any one of various fiscal entities. The key difference is that there is no intention or hope of achieving an equity position (share of ownership, usually of a partnership, thus becoming a full partner). Health systems, hospitals, outpatient surgery centers, multidisciplinary clinics, other facilities tied to a specific location where surgery is performed, physician groups that have umbrella fiscal entities specifically created to serve as the employer of physicians, and even surgeons may seek to hire anesthesiologists as permanent employees. The common thread in this idea is that these fiscal entities want guaranteed anesthesia services they can control. Also, they likely see the anesthesiologists as additional components for generating profits, or, worse yet, as a financial liability that must be mitigated. It has been argued occasionally that, in some cases, it may appear that employees are not paid compensation that is commensurate with their production of receivables, at least considering traditional collection for anesthesia services. That is, the fiscal entity will pay a salary plus appropriate overhead substantially below collections generated by the anesthesia professional's work. These arrangements seem particularly favored by some large MCOs in certain geographic areas that, uncharitably, view anesthesia professionals simply as expensive necessities that prevent facilities from realizing maximum profit (although sometimes there is a promise of a lighter or more manageable work schedule in these positions compared with marketplace private practice).

Negotiating for a position as a permanent full-time employee is somewhat simpler and more straightforward than it is in marketplace private practice. It parallels the usual understandings that apply to most regular employer–employee situations: job description, role expectations, working conditions, hours, pay, and benefits. Although some of the positions within large anesthesia groups may be quite similar to traditional marketplace private practice, the idea of anesthesiologists functionally becoming numbered shift workers disturbs many in the profession because it contradicts the traditional professional model. Again, the complex nature and multiple levels of such considerations make it a personal issue that must be carefully evaluated by each individual with full awareness and consideration of the issues outlined here and commensurate research of ASA resources and available data about common regional circumstances and details of any specific medical community (often involving efforts to seek out current and former employees of a given entity as sources of relevant information).

Practice as a Hospital Employee

Although CRNAs in some locations have traditionally practiced as hospital employees, until recently, it was less common outside full vertically integrated MCOs for physician anesthesiologists to be hospital (or facility) employees. One of the potential responses of hospitals to requests for subsidies from exclusive-contract private practice groups of anesthesiologists has been to offer the anesthesiologists full-time employment status rather than subsidize an independent practice group that has its own significant administrative and overhead costs. The hospital likely suggests that integrating the billing, collecting, and management functions as well as major overhead costs such as malpractice insurance into the existing larger hospital operation would be very cost-efficient, allowing more financial resources to go to physician salaries, and also with possibly a somewhat greater predictability in financially uncertain times. The hospital can also guarantee the availability of anesthesia care (a requirement to sustain the OR, one of the main hospital revenue sources) in an era when some anesthesiologist groups may simply walk away from a hospital in search of greater income elsewhere, leaving the hospital to seek a contract probably with one of the large and potentially expensive anesthesia management companies. Of course, in return for employee status, the anesthesiologists surrender some degree of independence and also, for the group's partners, their equity stake in sharing in any subsequent increased practice revenue. A hospital might counter that concern, particularly in the era of facilities subsidizing anesthesia practices, with the contention that traditional anesthesia fee-for-service private practice that has been so common for so long will *never again* yield enough revenue to maintain the compensation levels anesthesiologists have come to expect, so they will not be losing anything.

Practice for a Large Group Management Company

As noted in the opening section, in recent years there has been a proliferation of large state, regional, and national management companies that provide comprehensive anesthesia services on a contract basis with hospitals, surgery centers, and clinics. These companies, some started and/or managed by anesthesia professionals, promise the facility availability of anesthesia care during the specified hours in return for a contract to do so. This is intended to relieve the facility from any concern about recruiting, hiring/contracting, and retaining anesthesia professionals, virtually eliminating concern about disruption of OR schedules due to limited availability of anesthesia care. The only requirement of the facility is approval of the already prepared credentialing information for each anesthesia professional. Unlike many locum tenens companies in which anesthesia professionals are considered independent contractors and paid fixed contract amounts per hour, per day, or per job for a limited interval with no benefits, many of the large group management companies may employ anesthesia professionals full time on a salary with benefits (paid vacation, health insurance, retirement contribution, and so forth). The employment agreement would stipulate whether travel for temporary assignments in locations away from the employee's permanent home would be required as a condition of the full-time job or the position will always be in the practitioner's home community. When an existing company purchases an anesthesia practice and the former members of a group private practice agree to become employees of the company, usually the members remain in the community and practice at the same facility where they were previously located.

Practice in the Office-based Setting

Increasingly, anesthesia professionals are being recruited into the office-based practice of sedation and general anesthesia for a growing number of procedures. While the governance and oversight of this practice is evolving, there are several issues which are clear. A medical director must be appointed to determine the adequacy of facilities and to ensure that the procedures undertaken may be safely and effectively performed given the space, available equipment, and training of personnel involved. The anesthesia professional is a key component in determining patient selection. Practice situations should be avoided where the anesthesia professional does not have real input into the decision making about the patient and procedure. One danger in the office-based setting is that the hired anesthesia professional may feel intense production pressure if the owner/proceduralist (e.g., plastic surgeon, gastroenterologist, oral surgeon) is adamant about proceeding with a given patient despite a discussion about clinical concerns. Basic monitoring standards must be adhered to at all times and supervision of the patient until discharge from the facility must be factored into the time commitment on the part of the anesthesia professional. In addition, ensuring that all anesthesia equipment is up to date and in working order and that the protocols for cardiopulmonary emergencies and transfer of the patient to an outside facility are appropriate is required before accepting an office-based position or assignment. Some office-based centers allow the anesthesia professional to bill the patient and/or their third-party payer directly for services rendered in an application of the older and more independent fee-for-service model. Those considering office-based practice should review the information and guidelines published by the ASA.[71]

Billing and Collecting

In practices in which anesthesiologists are directly involved with the financial management, they need to understand as much as possible about the complex world of health-care reimbursement. This significant task is facilitated by the major section of the ASA website devoted to "Practice Management" (http://www.asahq.org/quality-and-practice-management/practice-management). One of its functions is helping ASA members understand and work with the sometimes confusing and convoluted issues of effective billing for anesthesiologists' services. There are several relevant sections of the ASA website regarding billing and coding, including a primer for residents (https://www.asahq.org/shop-asa/detail?productid=133891).

While dramatic plans and proposals for significant changes in payment for anesthesia care have been outlined (see above), the traditional basics have changed little in recent years. It is important to understand that many of the most contentious issues, such as the requirement for physician supervision of nurse anesthetists and the implications of that for reimbursement, apply in many circumstances mostly to Medicare and, in some states, Medicaid. Thus, the fraction of the patient population covered by these government payers is important in any consideration. Different practice situations have different arrangements regarding the financial relationships between anesthesiologists and nurse anesthetists, and this can affect the complex situation of who bills for what. The nurses may be employees of a hospital or surgery center, of the anesthesiologists who medically direct them, or of no one in that they are independent contractors billing separately (even in cases in which physician supervision—not medical direction—is required but where those physicians do not bill for that component). In 1998, Medicare mandated that an anesthesia care team of a nurse anesthetist medically directed by an anesthesiologist could bill as a team no more than 100% of the fee that would apply if the anesthesiologist did the case alone. The implications of this change were complex and variable among anesthesiology practices. However, the previously common practice of one anesthesiologist medically directing 2 to 4 CRNAs and billing a full professional fee for each case ended at that time. Also, complex related issues played out after that. In 2001, the federal government issued a new regulation allowing individual states to "opt out" of the requirement that nurse anesthetists be supervised by physicians and several states did so, as noted above. This was opposed by the ASA. Because perioperative patient care, one component of which is administering anesthesia, is traditionally considered the practice of medicine, the implications of this change as far as the role of surgeons (or no one) supervising nurse anesthetists and the malpractice liability status of nurse anesthetists practicing independently were believed to be unclear. Further, the implications of all this for billing insurers other than Medicare and Medicaid are exceedingly complex.

Classic Methodology

Because there is still application of the traditional method of billing for anesthesiology services, understanding can be important for anesthesia professionals entering or in practice. In this system, each anesthetic generates a value of so many "units," which represent effort and time. A conversion factor (dollars per unit) that can vary widely multiplied by the number of units generates a dollar amount to be billed. Each anesthetic has a base value number of units (which includes payment for standard preoperative evaluation and immediate postoperative care), for example, 8 for a cholecystectomy, and then the time taken for the anesthetic is divided into units, usually 15 minutes per unit. Thus, a cholecystectomy with anesthesia time of 1 hour and 10 minutes would have 8 base units and 4.66 time units for a total of 12.66 units. In some practice settings, it may be allowed to add modifiers, such as extra units for complex patients with multiple problems as reflected by an ASA physical status classification of 3 to 5 and/or E ("emergency") or for insertion of an arterial or PA catheter. The sum for all factors is the total billing unit value. Determining the base value for an anesthetic in units depends on full and correct understanding of what operation was done. Although this sounds easy, it is the most difficult component of traditional anesthesia billing. The process of determining the procedure done is known as *coding* because the procedure name listed on the anesthesia record is assigned an identifying code number from the universally used "current procedural terminology" (CPT)-4 coding book. This code is then translated through the ASA "Relative Value Guide," which assigns a base unit value to the type of procedure identified by the CPT-4 code. In the past, some anesthesiologists failed to understand the importance of correct coding to the success of the billing process. Placing this task in the hands of someone unfamiliar with the system and with surgical terminology can easily lead to incorrect coding. This can fail to capture charges and the resulting income to which the anesthesiologist is entitled or, worse, can systematically overcharge the payers, which will bring sanctions, penalties and, in certain cases, criminal prosecution. The international collection of diseases (ICD) terminology is the method by which providers and payers communicate concerning the type and classification of a given *diagnosis*. Usually, the diagnosis codes are entered by the facility billing for the time in the OR using the ICD-10 codes that went into effect in October 2015.

There has been a prevailing official governmental attitude that there are no simple, innocent coding errors. All upcoding (charging for more expensive services than were actually delivered) is considered to be prima facie evidence of fraud and is subject to severe disciplinary and legal action. All practices should have detailed compliance programs in place to ensure correct coding for services rendered. The ASA website has several relevant sections with information. Further, outside expert help (such as from a health-care law firm that specializes in compliance programs) can be highly desirable for the process of formulating and implementing a compliance plan regarding correct coding and billing.

Assembly and transfer of the information necessary to generate bills must be efficient and complete. Traditionally, this involved depositing in a secure central location an extra paper copy of the anesthesia record and often a "billing sheet" with it, on which was inscribed the names of all the involved personnel and any additional information about other potentially billable services, such as invasive monitors. Any practice involved with a comprehensive computerized electronic perioperative information management system in the facility should be using that to assemble this "front end" billing information. Short of that, some practices collect electronic information specifically generated by the anesthesia providers for that purpose. They have equipped each staff member with a handheld electronic device into which data are entered and then the device is synched with a departmental computer at the end of the day. If the OR suite has "Wi-Fi" (wireless electronic connection), the same function could be accomplished in real time with the providers entering the requisite information into a program on a computer or tablet affixed to each anesthesia machine (or carried by each staff member) or a smartphone with the appropriate application installed. Once the information has been secured, a mechanism must be employed to generate the actual bill and communicate it to the payer (on paper, on disk, or, usually, directly computer to computer: "Electronic claims submission"). The possible exact arrangements for doing this vary widely.

Whether an anesthesia practice that will be billing and collecting for anesthesia services should employ its own inhouse clerical and bookkeeping personnel to perform this function or should contract with an outside company whose sole function is medical billing and collecting (possibly, ideally, for anesthesiology only) can be debated endlessly. Whichever is chosen, knowledgeable oversight by the anesthesia professionals who ultimately will derive income from the revenue collected is required. Ultimately, the entity actually submitting the bill will verify that it has been paid (posting of receipts) and may or may not actually handle the incoming money. Very often, anesthesia practices or individuals who use a billing service (and even some who have inhouse billing staffs) will arrange that the actual payments go directly to a bank "lockbox," which is a post office box for paper checks (better individual than shared, even if more expensive) to which the payments come and then go directly into a bank account for the practice, which is also where electronic payments are received. This system avoids the situation of having the people who generate the bill actually handle the incoming receipts, a practice that has led to theft and fraud in a few cases. Eventual decisions about how hard to try to collect from payers who deny coverage and then from patients directly will depend on the circumstances, including local customs, and the associated expense balanced against expected returns.

Detailed summary statistics of the work done by an anesthesiology practice group are critical for logistic management of personnel, scheduling, and financial analysis. Spreadsheet and database computer programs customized for an individual practice's characteristics will be invaluable. A summary of the types of data an anesthesia practice should track is shown in Table 2-1. Once all the data are assembled and reviewed, at least monthly analysis by a business manager or equivalent, as well as officers/leaders of the practice group, can spot trends very early in their development and allow appropriate correction or planning. Often the responsible members of an anesthesiology group question how effective their financial services operation is, particularly regarding net collections. This is a complex issue[72] that, again, often requires outside help. Routine internal audits can be useful but could be self-serving. No billing office or company that is honest and completely above board should ever object to a client, in this case the anesthesiology practice group, engaging an independent outside auditor to come in and thoroughly examine both the efficiency of the operation and also "the books" concerning correctness and completeness of collections.

Anesthesia billing and collecting are among the most complex challenges in the medical reimbursement field. Traditional

Table 2-1 Types of Data an Anesthesiology Group Should Track and Maintain Concerning Its Own Practice

Types of Data the Anesthesiology Group's Computer System Should Track	Type of Information to Generate from These Data

• Transaction-based system (track each case and charge as separate record)
  ■ Track individual charges by CPT-4 code
  ■ Track individual payments by payer
• Track all data elements on an interrelated basis
  ■ By place of service
  ■ By charge, broken down
    ○ By number of units (time and base)
    ○ By ASA modifiers
    ○ By number of lines
  ■ By CPT-4 code
  ■ By payer
  ■ By payment code (full payment, discount, write-off, or refund)
  ■ By diagnosis (ICD-9 code)
  ■ By surgeon
  ■ By anesthesiologist
  ■ By anesthesia care team provider
  ■ By start and stop times
  ■ By age
  ■ By gender
  ■ By employer
  ■ By ZIP code
	• Aggregate number of cases per year for the group
	• Total number of cases per year for each provider within the group
	  ■ Number of cases performed by anesthesiologists
	  ■ Number of cases performed by the anesthesia care team
	• Average number of units per case (as one measure of intensity per case)
	• Average number of units per CPT-4 code
	• Average time units per case and per CPT-4 code
	  ■ Group should be able to calculate time units per individual surgeon
	• Average line charge per case
	• Charges per case by CPT-4 code
	• Payments per case by payer
	• Patient mix
	  ■ Percent traditional indemnity
	  ■ Percent managed care (broken down by each MCO for which services are provided)
	  ■ Percent self-pay
	  ■ Percent Medicare
	  ■ Percent Medicaid
	• Collection rate for each population served
	• Overall collection rate
	• Costs per unit (total costs, excluding compensation ÷ total units) (costs include liability insurance, rent, collection costs, and legal and accounting fees)
	• Compensation costs per unit (total compensation ÷ total units) for MCO populations, utilization patterns by age, gender, and diagnosis

CPT, current procedural terminology; ASA, American Society of Anesthesiologists; ICD-9, International Classification of Diseases, ninth revision; MCO, managed care organization.
Reprinted with permission, but without review for currency of the material, from *Managed Care Reimbursement Mechanisms: A Guide for Anesthesiologists.* Park Ridge, IL: American Society of Anesthesiologists; 1994, with permission.

anesthesia reimbursement is unique in all of medicine. The experience of many people over the years has suggested that it often is well advised to deal with an entity that is not only very experienced in anesthesia billing but also does anesthesia billing exclusively or as a large fraction of its efforts. It is very difficult for an anesthesiologist or a family member to do billing and collecting as a side activity to a normal life. This has led to inefficient and inadequate efforts in many cases, illustrating the value of paying a reasonable fee to a professional who will devote great time and energy to this challenging endeavor.

Antitrust Considerations

There can be antitrust implications of business arrangements involving anesthesiologists—particularly with all the realignments, consolidations, mergers, and contracts associated with the attempted implementation of managed care, expansion of health systems, the drive for cost efficiency and, more recently, the rise of ACOs. The applicable statutes and regulations are often poorly understood. Contrary to popular belief, the antitrust laws do not involve the rights of individuals to engage in business. Rather, the laws are concerned solely with the preservation of competition within a defined marketplace and the rights of the consumer, independent of whether any one vendor or provider of service is involved. When an anesthesiologist has been excluded from a particular hospital's staff or anesthesia group and then sues based on an alleged antitrust violation, the anesthesiologist loses virtually automatically. This is because there is still significant competition in the relevant medical care marketplace (community or region) and competition in that market is not threatened by the exclusion of one physician from one staff.

In essence, if there are *several* hospitals offering relatively similar services to an immediate community (the market), denial of privileges to one physician by one hospital is not anticompetitive. If, on the other hand, there is only *one* hospital in a smaller market, then the same act, the same set of circumstances, could be seen very differently. In that case, there would be a limitation of competition because the hospital dominates and, in fact, may control the market for hospital services. Exclusion of one physician, then, could limit access by the consumers to alternative competing services and hence would likely be judged an antitrust violation.

The Sherman Antitrust Act is a federal law more than 100 years old. Section 1 deals with contracts, combinations, conspiracy, and restraint of trade. By definition, two or more separate economic entities must be involved in an agreement that is challenged as illegal for this section to apply. Section 2 prohibits monopolies or conspiracy to create a monopoly, and it is possible that this could apply to a single economic entity that has illegally gained domination of a market. Consideration of possible monopolistic domination of a market involves a situation in which a single entity controls at least 50% of the business in that market. The stakes are high in that the antitrust legislation provides for triple damages if a lawsuit is successful. The US Department of Justice and the Federal Trade Commission are keenly interested in the current rapid evolution and consolidation in the health-care industry, and thus are actively involved in evaluating situations of possible antitrust violations. The potential for a "whistle-blower" to file a lawsuit and receive a fractional payment out of the eventual financial penalties against a guilty party has in some cases provoked employees or former employees of a health system or group practice to institute such lawsuits.

There are two ways to judge violations. Under the *per se rule*, which is applied relatively rarely, conduct that is obviously limiting competition in a market is automatically illegal. The other type of violation is based on the *rule of reason*, which involves a careful analysis of the market and the state of competition. The majority of complaints against physicians are judged by this rule. The more competitors there are in a market, the less likely that any one act is anticompetitive. In a community with two hospitals, one smaller than the other, with an anesthesiology group practice exclusively at each, if the larger anesthesiology practice group buys out and absorbs the smaller, leaving only one group for the only two hospitals in the community, that may be anticompetitive, particularly if a new anesthesiologist seeks to practice solo at those hospitals and is refused privileges.

Legal Implications

In the current era of rapidly evolving practice arrangements, the antitrust laws are important. If physicians (individuals or groups), who normally would be competitors because they are separate economic entities, meet and agree on the prices they will charge or the terms they will seek in a managed care, health system, or institutional contract, that can be anticompetitive, monopolistic, and hence possibly illegal. Note that sharing a common office and common billing service alone is not enough to constitute a true group. If, on the other hand, the same physicians join in a true economic partnership to form a new group (total integration), that is a single economic entity (and meets certain other criteria) that will set prices and negotiate contracts, that is perfectly legal. The other criteria are critical. There must be capital investment and also risk-sharing (if there is a profit or loss, it is distributed among the group members)—that is, total integration into a genuine partnership (that is usually incorporated, sometimes as a limited liability corporation). This issue is very important in considering the drive for new organizations to put together networks of physicians that then seek contracts with major employers to provide medical care. Sometimes, hospitals or clinics attempt to form a network comprising all the members of the medical staff so that the resulting entity can bid globally for total care contracts. Any network is a joint venture of independent practitioners. If the participating physicians of one specialty in a network are separate economic entities and the network advertises one price for their services, this would seem to suggest an antitrust violation (horizontal price fixing). In the past, if a network involved fewer than 20% of one type of medical specialist in a market, that was called a *safe harbor*, meaning that it was permissible for nonpartners to get together and negotiate prices. The federal government has tried to encourage formation of such networks to help reduce health-care costs, and as a result made some relevant exceptions to the application of these rules. As long as the network is nonexclusive (other non-network physicians of a given specialty are free to practice in the same facilities and compete for the same patients), the network can comprise up to 30% of the physicians of one specialty in a market. Note specifically that this does not allow a local specialty society in a big city to serve as a bargaining agent on fees for its members because it is very likely that more than 30% of the specialists in an area will be members of the society. The only real exception to this provision is in thinly populated rural areas where there may be just one physician network. In such cases (which are, so far, less common because the major managed care, health system, and network activity has occurred mainly in more heavily populated urban areas), there is no limit on how many of one specialty can become network members and have the network negotiate fees, as long as the network is nonexclusive.

Relevant legislation, regulations, and court actions all happen rapidly and often. Mergers among anesthesiology groups in a market area for the purposes of both efficiency and strength in negotiating fees have been very popular as a response to the rapidly changing marketplace. A list of questions must be answered to determine if such a merger would have anticompetitive implications. Some information may be available to ASA members, but it is important to consider independent expert advice and help. Obviously, anesthesiologists contemplating a merger or facing any one of a great number of other situations in the modern health-care arena must secure assistance from professional advisors, usually attorneys, whose job it is to be aware of the most recent developments, how they apply, and how best to forge agreements in formal contracts. Anesthesiologists hoping to find reputable advisors can start their search with word-of-mouth referrals from colleagues who have used such services. Local or state medical societies frequently know of attorneys who specialize in this area and it may be possible to get a referral through the ASA Washington, DC, office.

Exclusive Service Contracts

Often, one of the larger issues faced by anesthesiologists in the traditional fee-for-service private practice model seeking to define practice arrangements concerns the desirability of considering an exclusive contract with a health-care facility to provide anesthesia services. An exclusive contract states that anesthesiologists practicing at a given facility must be members of the group holding the exclusive contract and, sometimes, that members of the group will practice nowhere else. A hospital may want to give an exclusive contract in return for a guarantee of coverage as part of the contract. Also, the hospital may believe that such a contract can help ensure the quality of the anesthesia professionals because the contract can contain credentialing and performance criteria. It is important to understand that the hospital likely will exercise a degree of control over the anesthesiologists with such a contract in force, such as requiring them to participate as providers in any contracts the hospital makes with third-party payers and also tying hospital privileges to the existence of the contract (the so-called "clean-sweep provision" that bypasses any due process of the medical staff should the hospital terminate the contract). Certain of these types of provisions constitute *economic credentialing*, which is defined as the use of economic criteria unrelated to the quality of care or professional competency of physicians in granting or renewing hospital privileges (such as the acceptance of below-market fees associated with a hospital-negotiated care contract or even requiring financial contributions in some form to the hospital).

The ASA in the past has opposed economic credentialing. However, the anesthesiologists involved may accept such an exclusive services contract to guarantee that they alone will get the business from the surgeons on staff at that hospital, and hence the resulting income. There may be other considerations on both sides, and there is information on the ASA website (http://www.asahq.org/.../06/exclusive-contracts-and-closed-open-departments/en/1). However, it is critical that anesthesiologists faced with important practice management decisions, such as whether to enter into an exclusive contract, must seek outside advice and counsel. There are a great many nuances to these issues,[73–75] and anesthesiologists are at risk attempting to negotiate such complex matters alone, just as patients would be at risk if a contract attorney attempted to induce general anesthesia.

Denial of hospital privileges as a result of the existence of an exclusive contract with the anesthesiologists in place at the facility has been the source of many lawsuits, including the well-known Louisiana case of *Jefferson Parish Hospital District v Hyde*. In that case, the US Supreme Court found for the defendant anesthesiologists and the hospital, saying that there was no antitrust violation because there was no real adverse effect on competition as far as patients were concerned because there were several other hospitals within the market to which they could go, and therefore they could exercise their rights to take advantage of competition in the relevant market. Thus, existence of an exclusive contract only in the rare setting where anticompetitive effects on patients can be proved might lead to a legitimate antitrust claim by a physician denied privileges. This was proven true in the *Kessel v Monongahela County General Hospital* case in West Virginia in which an exclusive anesthesiology contract was held illegal. Therefore, again, these arrangements are by definition complex and fraught with hazard. Accordingly, outside advice and counsel are always necessary.

Hospital Subsidies

Modern economic realities have forced a great number of anesthesiology practice groups (in both private and academic settings) to recognize that their patient care revenue, after overhead is paid, does not provide sufficient compensation to attract and retain the number and quality of staff necessary to provide the expected clinical service (and fulfill any other group/department missions). Attempting to do the same (or more) work with fewer staff may temporarily provide increased financial compensation. Cutting benefits (discretionary personal professional expenses, retirement contributions, or even insurance coverage) may also be a component of a response to inadequate practice revenue. However, the resulting decrements in personal security, in convenience, and in quality of life as far as acute and chronic fatigue, decreased family and recreation time, and tension among colleagues fearful that someone else is getting a "better deal" will quickly overcome any brief advantage of a somewhat higher income. Therefore, many practice groups in such situations are requesting their hospital (or other health-care facility where they practice) pay them a direct cash subsidy that is used to augment practice revenue in order to maintain benefits and amenities while maintaining or even increasing the direct compensation to staff members, hopefully to a market-competitive level that will promote recruitment and retention of group members.

Obviously, requests by a practice group for a direct subsidy must be thoroughly justified to the facility administration receiving the petition. The group's business operation should already have been examined carefully for any possible defects or means to enhance revenue generation. Explanation of the general trend of declining reimbursements for anesthesia services should be carefully documented. Facts and figures on that and related topics can be obtained from journal articles and the ASA website and publications, including the *Monitor*. Demand for anesthesia coverage for the surgical schedule is a key component of this proposal. Scheduling and utilization, particularly if early-morning staffing is required for many ORs that are routinely unused later during the traditional work day, is a major issue to be understood and presented. Any other OR inefficiencies created by hospital support staff and previous efforts to deal with them should also be highlighted. Unfavorable payer mix, impact of contracts, and programs initiated by the hospital are also often major factors in situations of inadequate practice revenue. Always, the group's good will with the surgeons and the community in general should be emphasized, as well as of the indirect or "behind the scenes" services and benefits the anesthesiology group provides to the hospital. Note that the necessity for such a subsidy request is precisely the time when the anesthesia professionals will benefit from being perceived as "good citizens" of the health-care facility. An overly aggressive effort beyond the bounds of logic could provoke the facility to consider alternative arrangements, even up to the point of putting out a request for proposal from other anesthesiology practice groups. Therefore, thoughtful calculations are required and a careful balance must be sought, seeking enough financial support to supplement practice revenues so that members' compensation is competitive but not so much as to be excessive. Supporting statements and documents about offers and potential earnings elsewhere must be completely honest and not exaggerated or credibility and good faith will be lost. Further, part of any agreement will be the full sharing of the group's detailed financial information with the facility administration, both at the time of the request and on an ongoing basis if the payment is more than a one-time "bail out." Plans for review and renewal should be made once a subsidy is paid.

Any subsidy will likely require a formal contract. There may be concern about malpractice liability implications for the hospital even though the practice group stays an independent entity as before. There may be "inurement" or "private benefit" concerns that could be perceived as a threat to the tax-exempt status of a nonprofit hospital. Lack of understanding of the applicable laws may lead to fears that a subsidy could be an illegal "kickback" or a violation of the Stark II self-referral prohibition. As is almost always the case, expert outside professional consultant advice, usually from an attorney who specializes exclusively in health-care finance contracting, is mandatory in such circumstances. The ASA Washington, DC, office may be of help in identifying potential consultants, and the ASA has some basic information on subsidies to anesthesiology practice groups.[76–78]

Evolving Practice Arrangements

Even though managed care plans have not had the major impact anticipated, various iterations still exist and have ongoing implications for anesthesiology practice. Further, concern about disproportionate increases in health-care spending as a percentage of US gross domestic product noted above and the fear of the postulated bankruptcy of Medicare and Medicaid fuel the persistent specter of new efforts to impose managed care (nationalized or decentralized) or other arrangements designed to control costs.

In the initial stages of the evolution of a managed care marketplace, the MCO usually seeks contracts with providers based on discounted fee-for-service arrangements. This preserves the basic traditional idea of production-based physician reimbursement (do more, bill more) but the price of each act of services is lower (the providers are induced to give deep discounts with the promise of significant volumes of patients); also, the MCO gatekeeper primary care physicians and the MCO reviewers are strongly encouraged to limit complex and costly services as much as possible. There are other features intermittently along the way, such as the bundled payment models described above. In an application of the concept of risk-sharing (spend too much for patient care and lose income), this usually is initially manifest in the form of "withholds," the practice of the MCO holding back a fraction of the agreed-upon payment to the providers (e.g., 10% or 15%) and keeping this money until the end of the fiscal year. At that time, if there is any money left in the risk pool or withhold account after all the (partial) provider fees and MCO expenses are paid, it is distributed to the providers in proportion to their degree of participation during the year. This is a clever and powerful incentive to providers to reduce health-care expenses. However, it is not as powerful as the stage of full risk-sharing. At one point in time, experts predicted that managed care marketplaces would mature and MCOs would grow and succeed, with the existing organizations and, especially, any new ones, intending to shift to the model of prospective capitated payments for providers. Although it may be less likely today that this particular type of superstructure model will come to pass in the United States, the forces pushing cost control and fundamental reconfiguration of the US health-care establishment are powerful. It is valuable for anesthesiologists to understand one of the main models advocated by so-called reformers.

Prospective Payments

Prospective capitated payments constitute an entirely new world to health-care providers, involving prospective capitated payments for large populations of patients, in which each group of providers in the MCO receives a fixed amount per enrolled covered life (member) per month (PMPM) and agrees, except in the most unusual circumstances, to provide whatever care is needed by that population for that prospective payment. The most unusual circumstances involve "carve-out" arrangements in which specific very costly and unusual conditions or procedures (such as the birth of a child with disastrous multiple congenital anomalies) are covered separately on a discounted fee-for-service basis. If there were to ever be full capitation, the entire financial underpinning of American medical care would do a complete about-face from the traditional rewards for giving more care and doing more procedures to new rewards for giving and doing less. Some managed care contracts contain other features intended to protect the providers against unexpected overutilization by patients that would stretch the providers beyond the bounds of the original contract with the MCO. The provisions setting the boundaries are called *risk corridors,* and the "stop-loss clauses" add some discounted fee-for-service payment for the excess care beyond the risk corridor (capitated contract limit). Providers who were used to getting paid more for doing more can suddenly find themselves getting paid a fixed amount no matter how much or how little they do with regard to a specified population—hence, the perceived incentive to do, and consequently spend, less. If the providers render too much care within the defined boundary of the contract, they essentially will be working for free, the ultimate in risk-sharing.

There are clearly potential internal conflicts in such a system, and how patients reacted initially to this radical change in attitude on the part of physicians where it was actually implemented demonstrated that this overall mechanism is unlikely to be readily embraced by the general public. Health-care providers (physicians, other health-care professionals, and facilities), in turn, allied themselves in a wide variety of organizations to create strength and desirable resources to present to the MCOs in contract negotiations. "Management service organizations" are joint-venture network arrangements that do not involve true economic integration among the practitioners, but merely offer common services to physicians who may, as a loosely organized informal group, elect to seek MCO contracts. "Preferred provider organizations" are network arrangements of otherwise economically independent physicians who form a new corporate entity to seek managed care contracts in which there are significant financial incentives to patients to use the network providers and financial penalties for going to out-of-network providers. This has proved a relatively popular model and appeared to gain acceptance. Physician–hospital organizations are similar entities but involve understandings between groups of physicians and a hospital so that a large package or bundle of services can be constructed as essentially one-stop points of care. Independent practice associations are like preferred provider organizations but are specifically oriented toward capitated contracts for covered lives with significant risk-sharing by the providers. Groups (or clinics) "without walls" are collections of practitioners who fully integrate economically into a single fiscal entity (true partnership) and then compete for MCO contracts on the basis of risk-sharing incentives among the partners. Fully integrated groups or health maintenance organizations (such as Kaiser Permanente in California or Harvard Pilgrim Health in New England) house the group of partner provider physicians and associated support staff at a single location for the convenience of patients, a big selling point when they seek MCO or employer contracts.

Changing Paradigm

MCOs are unlikely to contract with just one solo independent anesthesiologist. Further, smaller private practice groups of anesthesiologists may find themselves at a competitive disadvantage[79] unless they become part of a vertically integrated (multispecialty) or horizontally integrated (with other anesthesiologists) organization. Negotiations with MCOs require expert advice, probably even more so than the traditional exclusive contracts with hospitals as previously noted. Before any negotiation can even be considered, the MCO must provide significant amounts of information about the covered patient population. The projected health-care utilization pattern of a large group of white-collar workers (and their families) from major upscale employers in an urban area will be quite different from that of a relatively rural Medicaid population. Specific demographics and past utilization histories are absolutely mandatory for each proposed population to be covered, and this information should go directly to the advising experts for evaluation, whether the proposed negotiation is for discounted fee-for-service, a fee schedule, global bundled fees, or full capitation.

Significant questions were pointedly raised about the reimbursement implications for anesthesiologists of the putative managed care/practice reorganization revolution. Much of that discussion has been rendered moot by the failure of the pure prospective capitated payment model to gain widespread adoption. However, if an anesthesia practice or its parent financial entity is ever asked to enter negotiation for a "per member per month" payment for anesthesia services, immediate consultation with independent experts should occur. Discounted fee-for-service arrangements are easier for anesthesiologists to understand because these are directly referable to existing traditional fee structures. Again, any negotiation requires outside help.

Another common feature of this discussion has been the tendency of private (nongovernmental) contracting organizations to attempt to tie their payments for professional services to the government's Medicare rate for specific CPT-4 codes. It is common for both commercial indemnity insurance entities (e.g., Blue

Shield, Aetna, Humana, United Health) and MCOs to offer primary care physicians, for example, 125% of the Medicare payment rate for specific services. Although groups of primary care physicians may view this as somewhat reasonable and, thus, they sign such contracts, anesthesiologists face unique challenges in this regard. Many leaders among anesthesia professionals believe that the Medicare reimbursement rate is unfairly low for the work involved in providing anesthesia care. The Medicare rate likely would remain less than half the per unit "conversion factor" that the large indemnity carriers traditionally have paid for anesthesia care in recent years. Therefore, 125% of what many anesthesia professionals consider woefully inadequate would still be inadequate. Thus, in spite of sometimes intense pressure, anesthesia professionals in many markets have been reluctant to accept indemnity insurance contract rates tied to Medicare rates. As always, anesthesia professionals faced with complex reimbursement situations and decisions should seek expert advice from the national offices of their professional practice organizations and from knowledgeable paid consultants and attorneys.

Pay for Performance

Commercial indemnity insurance entities, MCOs, and particularly, the US federal CMS all now emphasize the concept of "performance-based payments" as a significant way to limit the growth of (and even reduce) health-care costs,[80] especially by reducing expensive complications of medical care. This "pay-for-performance" movement began with the federal Tax Relief and Healthcare Act of 2006 and continued with the Physician Quality Reporting Initiative in 2008. The potential implications for anesthesia practice are many.[81]

In general, CMS made strenuous efforts to attempt to define and promulgate objective quality measures that could be documented as indicators of the "quality" of health care delivered. The main issue is the promotion of specific "best practices" care elements that help avoid expensive outcomes or complications that currently generate a disproportionate (preventable) fraction of health-care costs. The administration of aspirin and β-blockers within a fixed brief interval after the arrival of an acute myocardial infarction patient is a good example, as are various parameters in the care of patients with community-acquired pneumonia or congestive heart failure (all constituents of the CMS "core measures" on which quality is judged). Defining and validating objective and easily quantifiable so-called quality measures that will prevent expensive complications of anesthesia care has proved to be more difficult. The initial targeted parameter was somewhat indirect: the timing of the administration of prophylactic antibiotics prior to surgical incision. The anesthesia professional is judged to be in compliance when the antibiotic is administered within the prescribed limit prior to incision. This must be verifiably documented on the anesthesia record. Benchmark criteria such as 95% compliance for a specific financial entity billing Medicare and Medicaid must be met by members of the group or the reimbursement for anesthesia services by that financial entity will be reduced by a specific fraction (or a promised "bonus" will be withheld) as a compliance incentive, but also somewhat as an offset to the increased cost of the consequent complications associated with failure to comply. If performance is in compliance, CMS traditionally would pay the maximum allowable reimbursement (pay for performance).

The second target was catheter-related bloodstream infection, and the performance behavior expected of anesthesia professionals is observance of strict aseptic protocol during central vascular catheter placement (and avoiding the femoral route if at all possible). The third objective parameter of anesthesia care quality targeted temperature management of the surgical patient with the compliance behavior being met by achieving one of three possible goals: use of active warming intraoperatively or documented temperature 36°C or higher in either the last 30 minutes of anesthesia or the first 30 minutes in the PACU. Other potential objective performance criteria intended to encourage avoidance of costly complications of anesthesia care may include glucose control in major surgery, use of pencil-point spinal needles in obstetric anesthesia, ("meaningful") use of EHRs, preoperative screening for sleep apnea, preoperative fasting instructions, meperidine administration for postoperative shivering, and several others. In all cases when a parameter is adopted, benchmark criteria for degree of compliance will be established and reimbursement will be reduced one way or another for failure to comply, as documented on the relevant records and self-reported by the billing financial entity (subject to audit, of course).

Hospitals will have even more at stake in the sense that the pay-for-performance movement has created paradigms in which hospitals will not receive reimbursements for care associated with preventable complications such as catheter-related sepsis (blood or urinary), ventilator-acquired pneumonia, and decubitus ulcers. This concept has several implications. One is that smaller hospitals often populated by less acute patients will be more likely and quicker to transfer sicker patients to larger referral facilities in order to avoid losing reimbursement associated with the development of patient complications. Concomitantly, documentation of the timing of the development of complications has become critical. If a hospital or department has documented the pre-existing presence of a complication at the time of a patient's admission, it should not be penalized for the development of that condition. In this context, anesthesia professionals can have an important role documenting the existence of pneumonia, sacral decubitus ulcers, or sepsis in their records when they first see a newly admitted patient, usually for preoperative evaluation. This will be perceived as excellent institutional citizenship by the anesthesia professional because it may prevent significant reimbursement reduction to the hospital.

Accountable Care Organizations

The Patient Protection and ACA (nicknamed "ObamaCare") was signed into law in 2010. One area of significance to anesthesiology professionals concerned the creation of ACOs. After review of the 698-page final rule it became clear to ASA that there was little consideration to pre- and postoperative care. This was one of the original factors that led to the adaptation of the ACA-inspired "Patient-Centered Medical Home" (http://www.hhs.gov/about/news/2014/08/26/the-affordable-care-act-supports-patient-centered-medical-homes-in-health-centers.html) to a suggestion of the "Perioperative Surgical Home," discussed extensively in the opening section. As noted, in the PSH model, anesthesiologists are identified (and ultimately compensated) for their roles in preoperative evaluation of increasingly complex patient populations, intraoperative management of the anesthetic, and postoperative management of pain and critical care issues of the surgical patient. Included in this is the idea that even routine postoperative care of the patient is within the domain of the anesthesiologist, as is follow-up care for those patients suffering from subacute pain following surgical procedures. Clearly, in recent years, a growing number of institutions have come to rely on anesthesiologist-directed preoperative assessment clinics to ensure adequate preparation of the surgical patient for their procedure. Likewise most institutions have physicians (usually anesthesiologists) practicing pain medicine/management on staff. The PSH model merely seeks to bring these elements along with critical care together to provide a vertical integration of care during the perioperative period. Although most academic anesthesiology departments and some large community hospitals can assemble these teams into a "PHS" model, it remains to be seen how this concept could be executed in the medium to small community hospital setting or what partnerships would have to be developed to accomplish these goals. Although the current language of the ACA deals with the concept of primary care and does not comment on surgical care, the ACO format would in essence be similar to the prospective payment paradigm described above with payment distributed to members of the care team based upon participation in care of the patient and any savings rendered from the efficient delivery of care distributed to the stakeholders in a given ACO.

Management Intricacies

The complexities of modern medical practice are significant and increasing rapidly. Management consultants, both large national firms that cross all industries and also boutique firms that specialize in only medical practices, are advertising their services to anesthesiology group practices. A recent analysis (that might seem more fitting as an MBA school case study) of business strategies relevant to anesthesiology group practices suggested there are key elements that detrimentally go unrecognized.[82] Whether a specific anesthesiology practice should consider bringing in an outside management consultant to help bolster the function, efficiency, and profitability of the practice obviously must be an individual carefully considered decision. However, even such a suggestion is a recent phenomenon, reflecting the tensions of the modern medical marketplace. As in other related caveats, whenever considering engaging outside help, a rigorous vetting process is required, especially including reference checks and discussion with previous practices served by that consultant.

Health Insurance Portability and Accountability Act

The 2003 implementation of the Privacy Rule of the Health Insurance Portability and Accountability Act (HIPAA) of 1996 required significant changes in how medical records and patient information are handled in the day-to-day delivery of health care. An update on the implications for anesthesiologists titled "Payment and Practice Management Memo, October 2013: You Can't Be Too Careful When it Comes to HIPAA Privacy and Security" has been promulgated by the ASA (http://www.asahq.org/.../ttppm/Protected Health Information October 2013/en/1).

Attention is focused on "protected health information" (identifiable as from a specific patient by name). Patients must be notified of their privacy rights. Usually this will be covered by the health-care facility in which anesthesia professionals work, but if separate private records are maintained, separate notification may be necessary. Privacy policies must be created, adopted, and promulgated to all practitioners, all of whom then must be trained in application of those policies. Often, anesthesiology groups can combine with the facilities in which they practice as an "organized health-care arrangement" so that the anesthesia practitioners can be covered in part by the HIPAA compliance activities of the facility. A "privacy officer" must be appointed for the practice group. Finally, and most importantly, medical records containing protected health information must be secured so they are not readily available to those who do not need them to render care.

One of the most obvious applications for many anesthesiologists is concern about the assembled preoperative information and charts for tomorrow's cases that frequently were placed prominently in the OR holding area at the end of one work day in readiness for the next day's cases. HIPAA provisions require that all that patient information be locked away overnight. Another classic example is what many ORs refer to as "the board." Often, a large white dry-marker board occupies a prominent wall near the front desk of an OR suite, and the rooms, cases, and personnel assignments are inscribed thereon at the beginning of the day and modified or crossed off as the day progresses. Under HIPAA, patients' names may not be used on such a board if there is any chance that anyone not directly involved in their care could see them. Alternatively, some facilities tape a copy of the day's OR schedule (including patients' names, ages, and operations) on the wall, which would also be a violation. The same is true for similar boards or posted schedules in OR holding areas and PACUs. Another issue often overlooked that is very problematic and probably the one that concerns patients the most is the obtaining of history information in a location, such as a "bed slot" behind just a curtain in the OR holding area, where sensitive medical and personal information is spoken out loud within earshot of other patients, other patients' families, and noninvolved caregivers. This concern is difficult to address and there is no one universally applicable suggestion. However, anesthesia professionals who interact with patients in such environments should be as sensitive as physically possible to being overheard and also should bring such concerns to the attention of the facility administrators.

Further, many anesthesiology practices also must apply HIPAA provisions to their billing operations; the details will vary depending on the mechanisms used and a great deal will depend on which type of electronic claims submission software is being used by the billing entity actually submitting the claims. Telephone calls and faxes into offices must be handled specially if containing identifiable patient information. Presentation of patient information for QA or teaching purposes must be free of all identifiers unless specific individual permission has been obtained on prescribed printed forms. Requests for patient information from a wide variety of outside entities, including insurance companies and collection agencies, must be processed in HIPAA-compliant ways. HIPAA policy and actions, as well as enforcement activities, have been developed over time and as situations develop. This system depends in part on patient complaints for both enforcement and policy evolution. In many practices and practice locations, there have been few or even no formal complaints of violations of patient privacy, indicating that the initial implementation of HIPAA compliance may have largely had the desired effect.

Electronic Medical ("Health") Records

Databases, spreadsheets, and electronic transfer of information are nonspecific features that have been applied to health care. Replacing the classic medical record, on the other hand, has required the creation of entirely new software in an attempt to duplicate and also expand the function of the handwritten or dictated traditional "chart." This has afforded opportunities to multiple competing commercial entities to attempt to fill this need. Usually, competing proprietary systems are incompatible and do not "talk to each other." This fact severely limits one of the highly touted benefits of medical practices "going electronic." Cost is another great barrier, as is the formidable task of entering necessary information from the old paper records into the electronic system. There has been governmental and public pressure for health-care institutions, facilities, and practices to adopt electronic records because of the potential for increased legibility causing reduction in errors and confusion, greater speed of filing and retrieval, easy transmission of large amounts of information (such as from a surgeon's office to an anesthesia practice's booking office and also to a hospital's preoperative clinic or OR holding area), and QA monitoring or auditing of vast databases. Increased ease of transmission and filing of reimbursement claims and cost savings from clerical staff downsizing are claims intended to encourage physician practice groups to adopt EHRs. However, experience has suggested that the commercially available software systems (both for institutions and practice groups) are not as robust or reliable as advertised by their often aggressive manufacturers. Accordingly, the expected benefits did not materialize quite as predicted, particularly in that costs have been great, often far in excess of estimates, and cost savings have been minimal at best. Nonetheless, there was a federal mandate that health-care facilities and practices must implement "meaningful use" of EMR or face penalties in the form of reduced payments from Medicare and Medicaid. Practice groups of anesthesia professionals should consider all the noted points prior to investing in an EMR system (which can be called "AIMS" for "anesthesia information management system"). At minimum, careful study and evaluation of the same system already in place in another anesthesiology practice should be undertaken. ASA has attempted to answer members' questions (http://www.asahq.org/.../Advocacy/Electronic Health Records/ASAEHRFAQ/en/1) and there are multiple other resources on the ASA website, but the goal has seemed something of a moving target, so practitioners need to verify the most up-to-date information when they make decisions about EHRs.

If basic EHR implementation has been problematic for practices, true electronic AIMSs have been even more difficult. These include preoperative, intraoperative, postoperative, billing, and QA components. For the actual OR anesthesia record, several commercial versions are available. Various anesthesia professionals have various opinions about ease of implementation and subsequent use. Unless one massive bolus of fully integrated new technology from a single manufacturer is installed all at one time, integration of a new EHR with the existing anesthesia machines and monitors to ensure full accurate capture of all data parameters can often be difficult and frustrating. The function and value of electronic anesthesia records can be debated endlessly. All of them today will require computers on or in the anesthesia machine. These computers should be Internet-enabled so that demographic and billing information can be automatically uploaded to the facility's and the practice's database. Any such system must also integrate with the billing systems of the facility and the practice or the touted benefits will be largely negated. Likewise, such systems can be configured to report (upload) automatically case information (de-identified) to central repositories of clinical information, such as the QCDR and the NACOR, thus facilitating potential quality improvement projects and also satisfying requirements (EHR "meaningful use") that should prevent payment penalties and potentially even qualify for payment bonuses.

Again, the best, and in some senses, the only way to evaluate seriously and thoroughly a proposed major investment of money, effort, and time is to visit a fully functioning installation of a given electronic AIMS and talk directly in detail with the users. The costs, in all senses of the word, are so great that it remains a significant gamble to be the first to purchase and implement such a system.

Expansion into Perioperative Medicine and Hospital Care

The concept of the PSH is outlined in detail in the opening section and is being considered as a potential future model in some practices. Some anesthesiologists now practice for at least some of their time in preoperative screening clinics because of the great fraction of OR patients who do not spend the night before surgery in the hospital or who do not come to a hospital at all. In such settings, these anesthesiologists frequently assume a role analogous to that of a primary care physician, planning and executing a workup of one or more significant medical or surgical problems before the patient can reasonably be expected to undergo surgery. Likewise, this concept can apply in the postoperative period. An anesthesiologist, on site in the hospital, immediately available and completely free of OR or other duties, could not only make at least twice-daily rounds on patients after surgery and provide exceedingly comprehensive pain management service but also follow the surgical progress and make reports (likely via an EHR, instant messaging, or e-mail) to the surgeon's office or smartphone. A fundamental aspect of the practice of anesthesiology is the management of acute problems in the hospital setting. Though controversial, it is suggested by some that it is logical to maintain that anesthesiologists would be among the physicians best suited to provide primary care for hospitalized surgical patients. It is intended that the PSH would make the overall surgical episode more efficient. The involved anesthesiologists would need close working relationships with the participating surgeons so that the surgeons could remain involved in the technical and surgical details of the postoperative phase with which the anesthesiologists would be less familiar. As noted, the financial aspects of such arrangements could be complex in that third-party payers are unlikely to agree to new costs for a new class of providers, and the surgeons may be reluctant to have their compensation proportionately reduced, even if the new arrangement would free up time for them to see more new patients and do more cases. It could be argued that an anesthesia group with great insight may well be willing to provide such labor-intense service without expecting additional compensation because doing so will help insure the security of their existing positions and traditionally relatively high incomes. In the Rovenstine Lecture at the 2005 ASA Annual Meeting,[83] there was an emphatic plea for significantly expanding the scope of practice for anesthesiologists in perioperative care, patient care in general, and in health systems (facilitated by increasing the number trained and increasing use of nonphysicians supervised by anesthesiologists to care for healthy patients) as a way to secure a role for anesthesiologists among the leaders of the future of American health care. The concepts were reinforced in the 2014 Rovenstine Lecture, in which the imperative for anesthesiologists to change or be pushed aside by the reality of the unsustainable costs of the US health-care system was very strongly emphasized (https://education.asahq.org/drupal/2014/Rovenstine). Overall, to date, it appears that there has been comparatively little progress in this regard. The challenge persists for the young and upcoming generation of anesthesiologists.

An additional evolving opportunity within acute care hospitals is the creation and implementation of "rapid response teams." In essence, studies have revealed that patients on general care nursing floors sometimes begin to deteriorate and, for one reason or another (but often because of the responsible physician being unavailable or at a considerable distance at that moment), the patients are not evaluated or treated in a timely manner and often not until they have further deteriorated, sometimes to a critical status. Therefore, a national trend has developed in which hospitals create a team of knowledgeable professionals (who have other regular responsibilities) who usually have no prior knowledge of the deteriorating patient but who will respond within a very few minutes to the call from (usually) a floor nurse who detects a deteriorating patient (e.g., rapidly increasing fever, relative hypotension and tachycardia, absent urine output). Frequently, the rapid response team institutes immediate symptomatic treatment, arranges for a higher acuity level of care, and contacts the primary responsible physician. Importantly, in larger hospitals, it has been suggested that the in-house anesthesiologists are uniquely qualified to be key members of the rapid response team because the interventions almost always involve acute "bread-and-butter" resuscitative care. Although many anesthesiologists may believe they already have plenty of work in the OR, such participation when possible would be an outstanding and highly visible contribution to the hospital's mission of enhanced patient care. Also, such interventions theoretically could be separately billable encounters as consultations or, alternatively, excellent support in arguing for the maintenance or even increase of the hospital's financial subsidy to its anesthesia professional group.

Operating Room Management

The role of anesthesiologists in OR management has changed over time. Considering the potential shortage of anesthesia professionals, hospitals subsidizing many anesthesiology group practices, and an increasing workload, participation in OR management is essentially mandatory. The current emphasis on cost containment and efficiency is forcing anesthesiologists to take an active role in eliminating many dysfunctional aspects of OR practice that were previously ignored. First-case morning start times have changed from a hopeful suggestion to a genuine mandate. Delays of any sort are now often tracked electronically in real time and carefully scrutinized to eliminate waste and inefficiency. Together, anesthesiologists, surgeons, OR nurses and technicians, and increasingly, professional administrators/managers need to determine who is best qualified to be a leader in the day-to-day management of the OR.[84] Clearly, different groups have different perspectives. However, anesthesiologists are in the best position to see the "big picture," both overall and on any given day. Surgeons are commonly elsewhere before and after their individual cases (and sometimes for the beginning and the end of their cases); nurses and administrators may lack the medical knowledge to make appropriate, timely decisions, often "on the fly." It is the anesthesiologist with the insight, overview, and unique perspective who is best qualified to provide leadership in an OR community. The subsequent recognition and appreciation from the other groups (especially hospital administration) will clearly establish the anesthesiologists as concerned physicians genuinely interested in the welfare of the OR and the institution.

Organization

The symbiotic relationship between anesthesia professionals and surgeons remains unchanged. Both groups recognize this fact and also the common goal of having the OR function in a safe, expeditious manner. The age-old question, "Who is in charge of the OR?" still confronts many hospitals/institutions. Because some anesthesiology groups are subsidized by the hospital, the OR organization in such cases has changed accordingly. Many hospital administrators want to have input regarding who is in charge of the OR with an eye to increasing efficiency and throughput while reducing cost. Their wishes have an even added significance when more of their dollars are involved through the anesthesiology group subsidy. Sometimes there can be no real answer to, "Who's in charge?" because of the complexity of the interpersonal relationships in the OR. Some institutions have a professional manager (often a former OR registered nurse) whose sole job is to organize and run the OR. This individual may be vested with enough authority to be recognized by all as the person in charge. Other institutions ostensibly have a "medical director of the OR." However, the implications to the surgeons that an anesthesiologist is in charge, or vice versa, have caused many institutions to abandon the title or retain the position but assign no authority to it. In such instances, institutions usually resolve disputes through some authority with a physician's perspective. If there is no medical director with authority to make decisions stick, central authority usually resides with the OR committee, most often populated by physicians, senior nurses, and administrators. Every OR has this forum for major policy and fiscal decisions. As part of committee function, the standard practices of negotiation, diplomacy, and lobbying for votes are regularly carried out. The impact of such an OR committee varies widely among institutions.

Despite the constantly changing dynamics of the OR management and the attendant major frustrations, anesthesiologists should pursue a greater role in day-to-day management in every possible applicable practice setting. An anesthesiologist who is capable of facilitating the start of cases with minimal delays and solving problems "on the fly" as they arise will be in an excellent position to serve his or her department. Succeeding in this role will have a dramatic positive impact on all the OR constituents. The surgeons will be less concerned about who is in charge because their cases are getting done. The hospital administration will welcome the effort because they want something extra in return for any money they are now giving to the anesthesiology groups as a subsidy. Furthermore, the OR committee (or whatever system for dispute resolution is in place) is still functional and has not been circumvented (and will be thankful for the absence of disputes needing resolution).

Some institutions use the term *Clinical Director of the OR*. The person awarded this designation should be a senior-level individual with firsthand knowledge of the OR environment and function. Anesthesiologists have a better understanding of the perioperative process. They possess the medical knowledge to make appropriate decisions. Their intimate association with surgeons and their patients allows them to best allocate resources.

Contact and Communication

An important issue for the anesthesia professionals in any OR setting is who among the group will be the contact person to interact with the OR and its related administrative functions. In situations in which everyone is an independent contractor, there may be a titular chief who by design is the contact person. The anesthesiologist in this role commonly changes yearly to spread the duties among all the members. Larger groups or departments that function as the sole providing entity for that hospital/facility often identify an individual as the contact person to act as the voice for the department. Furthermore, these same groups delineate someone on a daily basis to be the operational clinical director, or the person "running the board." Frequently, this position is best filled by one from a small dedicated fraction of the group (e.g., three people) rather than rotating the responsibility among every member of the group. Experienced "board runners" have an instinctually derived better perspective on the nuances of managing the operating schedule in real time. Certain procedures may require specific training (e.g., transesophageal echocardiography skills) that not all members of the group possess. Clearly, changes sometimes have to be made in real time to match the ability of the anesthesia provider and the requirements of the procedure when urgent or emergent cases are posted.

Another benefit of a very small number of daily clinical directors is a relative consistency in the application of OR policies, particularly in relationship to the scheduling of cases, especially add-ons. One of the most frustrating aspects to both surgeons and OR personnel is unpredictability and inconsistency in the decisions made by the anesthesia group/department members. A patient deemed unacceptable for surgery by anesthesiologist X on Monday may be perfectly acceptable, in the same medical condition, for anesthesiologist Y on Tuesday. Differences of opinion are inevitable in any large group. However, day-to-day OR function may be hampered by a large number of these situations. Having one member of a very small group in charge will lead to more consistency in this process, especially if the board runner/clinical director has the authority to switch personnel to accommodate the situation. Without stifling individual practices, philosophies, and comfort levels, a certain amount of consistency applied to similar clinical scenarios will improve OR function immeasurably. These few dedicated directors should be able to accomplish both goals better than a large rotating number of people.

A newer potential component of intra-OR communications is the concept of checklists and team briefings. Analogous to the now-required "time-out" in each OR prior to surgical incision, when the correct identity of the patient, the intended procedure, and any laterality involved are verified, some ORs are attempting to have a similar interprofessional communication involving all relevant OR personnel (the team) prior to the patient's entering the OR. During this meeting the involved surgeon, anesthesia professional, circulating nurse, scrub person, and support persons each state a summary of what is projected to take place in this case, any anticipated need for extra or unusual resources or equipment, any anticipated difficulties or increased risks, and specific plans to deal with any feature of any of these points that would require intervention. In many models, a printed single-page checklist with routine prompts and fill-in boxes is used to facilitate the process. One study reported a two-third reduction in "communication failures" that have otherwise likely caused problems, risks, or inefficiencies.[85]

The World Health Organization's widely publicized "Surgery Safety Checklist" (http://www.who.int/patientsafety/safesurgery/checklist/en) is primarily an accident-prevention tool, but also promotes communication among everyone in the OR, particularly regarding planning—before, during, and after the actual operation—which is directly related to maximally efficient and safe conduct of the procedure.

Materials Management

Usually, the institutional component of the anesthesia service creates, maintains, and staffs a location ("the workroom") containing the specific supplies unique to the practice of anesthesia. Objectives necessary for efficient materials management include the standardization of equipment, drugs, and supplies. Volume purchasing, inventory reduction, and avoidance of duplication are also worthwhile. There needs to be coordination with the OR staff as to who is responsible for acquisition of routine hospital supplies such as syringes, needles, IV tubing, and IV fluids. Decisions as to which brands of which supplies to purchase ideally should be made as a group. Often, when several companies compete against each other in an open market, lower prices are negotiable. In many cases, however, hospitals belong to large buying groups that determine what brands and models of equipment and supplies will be available, with no exceptions possible except at greatly increased cost. Sometimes this is false economy if the provided items are inferior (cheap) or difficult to use—for example, if one must routinely open three or four intravenous cannulas to start a preoperative intravenous line as opposed to using a higher quality and reliable cannula that may cost more per unit but is less expensive overall because far fewer will be used. Dispassionate presentation of such logic by a respected team-player senior anesthesiologist to the OR committee or director of materials management may help resolve such conundrums.

Scheduling Cases

Anesthesiologists need to participate in the OR scheduling process at their facility or institution. In some facilities the scheduling office and the associated clerical personnel work under the anesthesia group. Commonly, scheduling falls under the OR staff's responsibility. Direct "control" of the schedule on a moment-to-moment basis often resides with the OR supervisor or charge person, frequently a nurse. Whatever the arrangements, the anesthesia group must have input and a direct line of communication to the scheduling system. The necessary number of anesthesia professionals that must be supplied often changes on a daily basis depending on the caseload and sometimes because of institutional policy decisions. After-hours calls must be arranged, policy changes factored in, and additions/subtractions to the surgical load (day to day, week to week, and long term as surgical practices come and go in that OR) dealt with as well. These issues are important even when all the anesthesia professionals are independently contracted and are not affiliated with each other. In such situations, the titular chief of anesthesia should be the one to act as the link to the scheduling system. When the anesthesia group/department functions as a single entity, the chairman/chief, clinical director, or appointed spokesperson will be the individual who represents his or her group at meetings in which scheduling decisions are made in conjunction with the OR supervisors, surgeons, and hospital administrators.

There are as many different ways to create scheduling policies as there are OR suites. Most hospitals/facilities follow proprietary patterns established over the years. Despite all the efforts directed toward its creation, the OR schedule (both weekly time allotments and day-to-day scheduling of specific cases) remains one of the most contentious subjects for the OR. Recognizing the fact that it is impossible to satisfy everyone, the anesthesia group should endeavor to facilitate the process as much as possible. Initially, anesthesiologists need to be sympathetic toward all the surgeons' desires/demands (stated or implied) and attempt to coordinate these requests with the institution's ability to provide rooms, equipment, and staff. Secondly, the anesthesia group should make every possible effort to provide enough anesthesia services and personnel to realistically meet the goals of the institution. In light of the potential shortage of anesthesia professionals in this country, these efforts need to be made with a great deal of open communication among all parties of the OR committee as well as every member of the anesthesia group.

Regarding scheduling, surgeons essentially fall into one of three groups. One group wants to operate any time they can get their cases scheduled. This group wants the OR open 24/7. Another larger group wants "first case of the day" as often as possible so they can then get to their offices. A smaller third group wants either the first time slot or an opening following that time slot, a several-hour hiatus, then to return to the OR after office hours to complete additional cases; usually starting after 5 PM. Clearly a compromise among these disparate constituencies must be reached. Anesthesiologists who approach the OR committee regarding this dilemma with a nonconfrontational attitude will greatly facilitate agreement on a compromise.

Types of Schedules

The majority of ORs use either block scheduling (preassigned guaranteed OR time for a surgeon or surgical service to schedule cases prior to an agreed-upon cut-off time; for example, 24 or 48 hours before) or, alternatively, open scheduling (first come, first serve). Most large institutions have a combination of both. Block scheduling inherently contains several advantages for creating a schedule. Block scheduling allows for more predictability in the daily OR function as well as an easy review of utilization of allotted time. Historic utilization data should be reviewed with surgeons, OR staff, and the OR committee to determine its validity. Many operating suites have found it useful to assemble rather comprehensive statistics about what occurs in each OR. Some computerized scheduling systems (see below) are part of a larger computerized perioperative information management system that automatically generates statistics. Graphic examples are 13-month "statistical control charts" or "run charts" that show the number of cases, number of OR minutes used for those cases (and when: such as in block, exceeding block, evenings, nights, weekends, and so forth), number of cancellations (and multiple other related parameters if desired) by service, by individual surgeon, and total for the current month and the 12 prior months, always with "control limits" (usually 2 standard deviations from the 13-month moving average) clearly indicated. All these data are valuable in that they generate a clear picture of what is actually going on in the OR. It is also extremely valuable in that block time allocation should be reviewed periodically and adjusted based on changes, degree of utilization, and projected needs. Inflexible block time scheduling can create a major point of contention if the assigned blocks are not regularly reevaluated. The surgeon or surgical service with the early starting block that habitually runs beyond his or her block time will create problems for the following cases. If this surgeon were made to schedule into the later block on a rotating basis, delays in his or her start caused by others may provoke improved accuracy of his or her subsequent early case postings. Adjustments in availability of block time can also be made in the setting of the "release time," the time prior to the operative date that a given block is declared not filled and becomes available for open scheduling. Surgeons prefer as late a release time as possible in order to maintain their access to their OR block time. However, unused reserved block time wastes resources and prevents another service from scheduling. A single release time rarely fits all circumstances, but negotiating service-specific release times may lead to improved satisfaction for all. In the *ideal* system, enough OR time and equipment should exist to provide for each surgical service's genuine needs while retaining the ability to add to the schedule (via open scheduling) as needed. Exactly such an environment does not exist. Invariably, in busy environments, surgical demand exceeds available block and open time, leading services to request additional block time. When this time is not granted, services may perversely then schedule procedures in open time before filling their block time. Surgeons who prefer open time would then be shut out of OR time. Open scheduling may reward those surgeons who run an efficient service, but it also may be a source of problems to those surgeons who have a significant portion of their service's cases arrive unscheduled, such as orthopedic surgeons. Some degree of flexibility will be necessary whichever system is used. The anesthesia group should adopt a neutral position in these discussions while being realistic about what can be accomplished given the number of ORs and the length of the normal operating day.

The handling of the urgent/emergent case posting precipitates a great deal of discussion in most OR environments. No studies allow determination of exactly what rate of OR utilization is the most cost-effective. However, some institutions reportedly subscribe to following parameters: adjusted utilization rates averaging below 70% are not associated with full use of available block time, wasting resources, whereas rates above 90% are frequently associated with the need for overtime hours. Different OR constituencies have different comfort zones for degrees of utilization. Most institutions cannot afford to have one or two ORs staffed, open, and waiting unless there is a reliable steady supply of late open-schedule additions, that is, urgent cases/emergencies, during the regular work day. A previously agreed-upon, clear algorithm for the acceptance and ordering of these cases will need to be adopted. In general, critical life-threatening emergencies and elective add-ons are fairly straightforward and at the two ends of the spectrum. The critical emergency goes in the next available room, whereas the elective case gets added to the end of the schedule. The so-called "urgent" patient requires the most judgment. Individual services should provide guidelines and limitations for their expected urgent cases. These "add-on case policy" guidelines should be common knowledge to everyone involved in running the OR. Consequently, these cases, such as ectopic pregnancies, open fractures, the patient with obstructed bowel, and eye injuries, can then be triaged and inserted into the elective schedule as needed with minimal discussion from the delayed surgeon. The surgeons whose urgent case is presented as one that must immediately bump another service's patient, yet conversely could wait several hours if it is their own patient that will be delayed, will have to face their own previously agreed-upon standards in a future OR committee meeting. A simple way to express one logical policy for urgent cases (e.g., acute appendicitis, unruptured ectopic pregnancy, intestinal obstruction) is: (1) bump the same surgeon's elective scheduled case; (2) if none, bump a scheduled case on the same service; (3) if none, bump a scheduled case from an open-schedule surgical service; and (4) if none, bump a scheduled case from a block schedule service. Some institutions require the attending surgeon of the posted urgent/emergent patient to speak personally with the surgeon of any bumped case.

Another area of burgeoning growth that must be accounted for in the daily work schedule is the non-OR "off-site" diagnostic test, or therapeutic intervention that requires anesthesia care. (In some locations, gastroenterologists expect anesthesia services for cases such as endoscopic retrograde cholangiopancreatography or other endoscopies on unusually sick patients, particularly after untoward emergencies beyond the capabilities of their sedation nurses have occurred and attracted attention in the facility.) In some instances the off-site procedures replace operations that, in the past, would have been posted on the OR schedule as urgent/emergency cases. For example, cerebral aneurysm coiling and computed tomography-guided abscess drainage, among other procedures, are done in imaging suites; some patients, adult as well as pediatric, require deep sedation or even general anesthesia for magnetic resonance imaging or computed tomography in radiology or for invasive procedures in catheterization laboratories. In addition, depending on distances involved and logistics, it may even be necessary to assign two people, a primary provider and an attending, exclusively to that one remote location when, had the case come to the OR, the attending may have been able to supervise one or more other cases also. Hospital administration or the OR committee may try to view these off-site cases as unrelated to OR function and, thus, purely a problem for the anesthesia group to solve. These cases must be treated the same as all the OR procedures.

In order to apportion hospital-based anesthesia resources reasonably, these off-site procedures should be subject to the same guidelines and processes for access and prioritization as any OR posting. Integration of the scheduling process with an institution-wide master program has been suggested as very helpful to maximize efficiency.[86] Most institutions have added at least one extra anesthetizing location ("line" on the printed schedule) to their formal operating schedule to designate these off-site procedures (occasionally with an imaginative classification such as "satellite," "road show," "outfield," or "safari"—which is an acronym for "safe anesthesia for all remote interventions"). For some of these off-site cases, there may be less or no reimbursement for anesthesia care. For example, government plans and also private insurance carriers may well not pay for the claustrophobic adult to receive monitored anesthesia care or even a general anesthetic for an obviously needed diagnostic magnetic resonance image, even though the patient, the surgeon, and the hospital benefit from the test results. The anesthesia group, the OR committee, and the hospital administration need to reach compromises for off-site procedures, regarding scheduling, allocation of anesthesia resources that would otherwise go to the OR, and even subsidization of the personnel costs in order to continue this obviously beneficial service that also does produce revenue for both the proceduralists and the facility.

Computerization

Computerized scheduling will likely benefit every OR regardless of size. Whether this scheduling function should be one component of a comprehensive EHR system is a complex question, as noted. In the OR, however, computerization allows for a faster, more efficient method of case posting than any handwritten system. Changes to the schedule can be made quickly without any loss of information. Rearranging the daily schedule is much simpler on a computer than erasing and rewriting on a ledger sheet. Furthermore, most hospitals have adopted a computer-determined average time for a given surgical procedure for a particular surgeon. Commonly, this time is the average of the last 10 (or 10 of the last 12, with the longest and shortest discarded) of the specific procedure (e.g., total knee replacement) with the potential to add a modifier (e.g., it is a repeat surgery) that shows a material difference in the projected time length (almost always longer) for one particular patient type. Suppose surgeon X has block time of 8 hours on a given day and wants to schedule four procedures in that allotted time. The computerized scheduling program looks at surgeon X's past performances and determines a projected length for each of the procedures that are identified to the computer, usually by CPT-4 codes or possibly some other code developed locally for frequent procedures done by surgeon X. (Note that the recorded time length includes the turnover time, thus making the case time definition from the time the patient enters the OR until the time any following patient enters that OR [unless an "exception" is entered specifically for an unusual circumstance].) The use of agreed-upon codes instead of just text descriptions helps ensure accuracy because it eliminates any need for the scheduling clerk to guess what the surgeon intends to do. Bookings in most circumstances should not be taken without the accompanying codes (surgeons' offices objections not withstanding). The computer then decides whether surgeon X will finish the four procedures in the allotted block time. If the computer concludes that the fourth case would finish significantly (the definition of which can be determined and entered into the program) beyond the available block time, it will not accept the fourth case into that room's schedule on that particular day. The surgeon will accept the computer's assigned times and adjust accordingly, planning only three cases, or appeal for an "exception" based on some factor not in the booking that is claimed will materially decrease the time needed for at least one of the four cases, which the surgeon must explain to the "exception czar" (anesthesiology clinical director or OR charge nurse) of the day. An alternative method has the computer simply add (to each case except the last) a projected turnover time that is agreed upon by all involved at an (often contentious) OR committee meeting. Computerizing the scheduling process significantly reduces any personal biases and should smooth out the entire operating day. The longstanding ritual of mid-to-late-afternoon disputes between the surgeons and the anesthesia group and/or OR staff about whether or not to start the last scheduled case may be eliminated or at least reduced by this more realistic prospective OR scheduling method.

There are many variables to consider in any OR scheduling system. The patient population served and the nature of the institution dictate the overall structure of the OR schedule. Inner-city level 1 trauma centers must accommodate emergencies on a regular basis, 24 hours a day. These centers are unlikely to create a workable schedule more than a day in advance. An ambulatory surgery center serving elective plastic surgery patients may see only the rare emergency bring-back bleeding patient. Their schedule may be accurate many days in advance, with a high degree of expectation that the patient will arrive on time properly prepared for surgery. The anesthesia group at this ambulatory center may rarely have to make changes to the schedule, allowing them to proceed with a fairly predictable daily workload. At the inner-city trauma hospital, a great deal of flexibility and constant communication with the surgeons will be required in an attempt to get the cases done in a reasonable time frame with the inherent constraints placed on the OR staff's resources and the time available. These two extreme examples from opposite ends of the scheduling process spectrum can provide guidelines for the majority of the institutions that fall somewhere in between. Beyond open communication, how best to work toward this mutual understanding depends on the particulars of the people involved and the environment, but some ORs report benefits from team-building exercises, leadership retreats, and even OR-wide social events. ORs with a particularly malignant history of finger-pointing and bad feelings among the personnel groups may constitute one of the few instances an outside consultant may really be valuable in that there are workplace psychologists who specialize in analyzing dysfunctional work environments and implementing changes to improve the situation for all involved.

Preoperative Clinic

An anesthesia preoperative evaluation clinic (APEC) that provides a comprehensive preoperative medical evaluation usually results in a more efficient running of the OR schedule.[87–89]

Unanticipated cancellations or delays are avoided when the anesthesia group evaluates complex patients prior to surgery. Even if the patient arrives to the OR on time the day of surgery, inadequate preoperative clearance mandating the ordering of additional tests will consume precious OR time during the delay waiting for results. Cancellations or delays adversely affect the efficiency of any OR. Subsequent cases in the delayed room, whether for the same or a different surgeon, may get significantly delayed or forced to be squeezed into an already busy schedule on another day. The financial impact of delays or cancellations on the institution is considerable. Revenue is lost with no offsetting absence of expenses. Worse, expenses may actually increase when overtime has to be paid, or the sterile equipment has to be discarded or repackaged after having been opened for the canceled procedure. Even worse, the inconvenienced patient and/or surgeon may go to another facility.

Optimal timing for preoperative evaluation should be related to the institution's scheduling preferences, patient convenience, and the overall health of the patient. Earlier completion of the preoperative evaluation may not reduce the overall cancellation rate when compared with a more proximate evaluation. However, an early evaluation and clearance may well provide a larger pool of patients available to place on the OR schedule (block or open) resulting in a more efficient use of OR time. Further, early evaluation creates an opportunity to "prehabilitate," as mentioned above. Diabetes, hypertension, asthma, and even COPD that appeared problematic upon evaluation can often be beneficially treated in even a few days—sometimes soon enough so the originally booked OR date need not be moved back. In addition, a protocol-driven evaluation process can anticipate possible or likely need for time-consuming investigations (such as a cardiology evaluation for the patient with likely previously undiagnosed angina). Early recognition of a failed preoperative test and need for postponement allows time for another patient to be moved into the now-vacant time slot. Also, early identification of certain problems requiring special care on the day of surgery (e.g., preoperative epidural, nerve block, or invasive monitoring placement) should lead to fewer unanticipated delays. Unfortunately, many issues precipitating delays are traditionally discovered on the day of surgery. Some of these preventable delays are unrelated to the patients' health status. Seemingly simple administrative issues such as verification of a ride home or incomplete financial information also contribute to unexpected delays. A properly functioning APEC may also be able to eliminate a majority of these annoying causes of preventable delays.

Regardless of the institutional specifics surrounding the service provided by the APEC, further cost savings can be obtained through its proper usage by the anesthesia group. The APEC frequently reduces dramatically the number of preoperative tests performed by focusing on which diagnostic tests and medical consults are really required for any specific patient (as opposed to the "shotgun approach" by some surgeons or the PCPs/internists consulted to give "medical clearance" who order excessive testing simply with the intent of trying to avoid some last-minute request, whatever it might be, for more data). In some circumstances, the APEC may also function as an additional source of revenue for the anesthesia group when a formal preoperative consult on a complicated patient is ordered well in advance by the surgeon, in the same manner as would have otherwise been directed to a primary care physician for the often nonreassuring "clearance for surgery." The ability to centralize pertinent information including admission precertification/clearance, financial data, diagnostic and laboratory results, consult reports, and preoperative recommendations improves OR function by decreasing the time spent searching for all these items after changes have been made to the schedule. Patient and family education performed by the APEC frequently leads to an increase in patients' overall satisfaction of the perioperative experience. In addition, patient anxiety may be reduced secondary to the more in-depth contact possibly inherent in the APEC process when compared with anesthesia practitioners meeting an ambulatory outpatient for the first time in an OR holding area immediately prior to surgery. The APEC model enables the anesthesia group to be more active and proactive in the perioperative process, improving their relations with the other OR constituents.

Anesthesiology Personnel Issues

In light of the putative shortage of anesthesia professionals, creating, managing, and maintaining an adequate supply of anesthesia practitioners is a top priority. Numbers of applicants for residency positions appeared robust in the first half of the second decade of the twenty-first century. The number of anesthesiology residency training programs remained fairly stable during this time. However, in 2016, there were approximately 100 fewer positions filled than in 2015 and a few programs did not fill all their slots. Anesthesiology training programs continue to be challenged in maintaining support of their educational missions.[90] Furthermore, the relative supply of nonphysician anesthesia professionals appears to be also decreasing. With the aging population of nurse anesthetists and the reportedly limited number of applications to schools in that profession, as well as the very limited number of training facilities for anesthesiology assistants, the overall supply of anesthesia professionals appeared potentially inadequate to meet current and, at least, short-term future demands. The need for anesthesia groups to create a flexible, attractive work environment in order to help retain professionals who might otherwise leave may increase. Note, however, that the "Great Recession" led to reduced turnover within practice groups for a few years because some anesthesia professionals, fearing economic uncertainty, chose to continue in practice positions that they likely would have vacated during normal economic conditions.

Another issue is consideration of what is a reasonable work load for an anesthesiologist and how best to measure, if possible, the clinical productivity of an anesthesia group/department. These questions have been the subject of considerable discussion.[91–93] Beyond the simple number of full-time equivalents, cases, and OR minutes, there must be consideration of factors such as the nature of the facility, types of surgical practice, patient acuity, and speed of the surgeons to allow fair comparisons. Thoughtful filtering of resulting data should take place before dissemination of the aggregate information to all members of a group because of the understandable extreme sensitivity among stressed and fatigued anesthesiologists to a suggestion that they are not working as hard as their group/department peers.

Except in highly unusual circumstances, flexible scheduling of anesthesia professionals and also fulfilling the demands placed on the group by the institution continues to be a constant balancing act. This demand assumes added significance because institutions subsidize many anesthesia groups. Even when a majority of providers in a facility are independent contractors where it is required that a specific surgeon request their services, there are time conflicts ranging from no one at all being available to unwanted down time. When the anesthesia group/department accepts the responsibility of providing anesthesia services for an institution, they must schedule enough providers for that OR suite on each given day. Ideally, a sufficient number of professionals would be hired so that there would always be enough personnel to staff the minimum number of rooms scheduled on any given day, as well as after-hours call duty. This situation rarely exists because it would be financially disadvantageous to have an excess number of providers with no or minimal clinical activity. Having exactly the right number of anesthesia professionals in a group for the clinical load works well until one (or more) of them is out with an unplanned absence such as an extended illness or a family emergency. Many academic departments have a natural buffer with some clinicians assigned intervals of nonclinical time for research, teaching, or administrative duties. However, repeated loss of these nonclinical days because of inadequate clinical staffing in the OR leads to undermining the academic/research mission of the department. Continued loss of this time will eventually lead to faculty resignations (and possible migration to private practice), thus eliminating the original buffer. Consequently, anesthesia groups/departments need to anticipate available clinical personnel and match them to the OR demands. Ideally, this information should be accurate for several months into the future. Meeting this specification has become more difficult. Hospital administrators must offer reasonable assurances to the anesthesia group providing service that a given OR utilization rate is likely, as well as accurate data regarding reimbursement (payer mix and any package contracts negotiated by the hospital). These data must be provided accurately and updated frequently if a health-care institution is to acquire and retain an anesthesia group staffed with the personnel to meet the expected demands.

Timing

Each operating environment has its own personnel scheduling system and expectations for the anesthesia group. Daily coordination between the anesthesia group's clinical director and the OR supervisor permits the construction of a reasonable schedule showing the number of ORs that day and when the schedule expects each of them to finish. Invariably, some cases take longer than anticipated or add-ons are posted, requiring the OR to run into the late afternoon or early evening. Many anesthesia professionals accept this occurrence as a matter of course. Few anesthesia professionals will tolerate this sequence of events as an essentially daily routine whether they are paid extra or not. These practitioners become exhausted and resent the burdens continuously placed on them. If the OR schedule is such that add-ons frequently occur and elective cases run well into the evening, many anesthesia professionals will opt to protect their personal and family time and cut back their working hours or resign. Neither would be welcome in a tight market. Under these circumstances, hiring additional personnel who are scheduled to arrive at a later time, for example, 11:00 AM, and then providing lunch relief and staying late (e.g., 7:30 PM or later if needed) to finish the schedule may well be a very worthwhile investment.

Another possible solution to the demands of an extended OR schedule on an anesthesia group's personnel may involve employing part-time anesthesia professionals. Part-time opportunities could enhance a group's ability to attract additional staff. Some anesthesia personnel will have personal or family situations or obligations that prevent them from committing to a full-time position, but who want to practice on schedules that work for them. Making accommodations (including pay, perks and benefits appropriate to the time worked) for this potential valuable source of help can prevent strain on the full-time people and smooth the overall function of the group/department.

Scheduling after-hours coverage also adds to the personnel difficulties facing the anesthesia group. The variations of call schemes are endless. The nature of the institution and the workload determine the degree of late-night/over-night coverage. Major referral centers and level 1 trauma centers require inhouse primary providers. If these providers include residents and/or nurse anesthetists, then the supervising attending staff likely will also be inhouse 24 hours a day. A common solution employed at many institutions is to staff the evening/night call shifts for an average workload based on historical statistics, recognizing that on some occasions there will be idle ORs, and, on other nights, the surgical demand will exceed the call team's numbers.

There are also medicolegal issues surrounding the call team's availability. Although this traditional model may be decreasing in numbers, it still exists: at a small community hospital with a limited number of independent anesthesiologists, these practitioners may agree to cover call on a rotating basis. The individuals not on call are usually not obligated to the OR and may well be truly unreachable. What happens then when the on-call anesthesiologist is administering an anesthetic and another true emergency case arrives in the OR suite and all the remaining staff anesthesiologists are legitimately unavailable? Does that anesthesiologist leave his or her current patient under the care of an OR nurse and go next door to tend to a more acutely (possibly critically) ill patient? Should the patient be transferred from the emergency department to another (hopefully nearby) hospital? These questions have no easy answers. Clearly, those practitioners on the scene have to assess in real time the relative risks and benefits and make the difficult decisions. Often in such settings, if at all possible, a second anesthesiologist will be on "back-up" call and available by pager or phone—with the understanding of being able to arrive within 30 minutes to help in a true emergency situation. In general, if the call duty requires the practitioner(s) frequently to work much or all of the night, leaving the individual(s) stressed and fatigued, they should not be required to work in the OR the next day during normal working hours.

A more complicated answer involves what to do when the call assignment rarely requires a long night's work and the on-call anesthesia professionals routinely have rooms assigned to them the next day, but at least one person has just finished a difficult 24-hour shift being awake and working all night. Anesthesia groups need to decide how to handle the possible call shift scenarios, with permutations and combinations, and clearly communicate prospectively their decisions to the OR committee before any difficult decision has to be made one morning. As always, the medicolegal aspects of any decision such as this need to be taken into consideration. Whether or not fatigue was a factor, the practitioner who worked throughout the night before and appeared to contribute to an anesthetic catastrophe the next morning would have a very difficult defense in court. Further, the anesthesiology group may also be held liable in that their practice/policy was in place, allegedly authorizing the supposedly dangerous situation.

Cost and Quality Issues

As noted at the outset, one of the more pervasive aspects of American medical care in today's environment is the drive to maintain and improve high-quality health care while simultaneously reducing the cost of that care. In 2015, health-care costs account for a remarkable 17.5% of the gross domestic product (CMS. National Health Expenditure Data: Historical. See: https://www.cms.gov/research-statistics-data-and-systems/statistics-trends-and-reports/nationalhealthexpenddata/nationalhealthaccountshistorical.html) nearly triple the fraction a generation ago. Even more alarming, if costs continue to increase at the current rate, by 2024, it will be 19.6% of the gross domestic product.[94] Consequently, all physicians, including anesthesiologists, are urged constantly to include cost-consciousness in decisions balancing the natural desire to provide the highest possible quality of care with the overall priorities of both the health-care system and the individual patient, all while facing increasingly limited resources. Complicated decisions are required regarding which patients are suitable for ambulatory surgery, what preoperative studies to order, what anesthetic drugs or technique is best for the patient, what monitors or equipment are reasonably required to run an OR, and the list goes on and on. With this as background, anesthesiologists legitimately can include economic considerations in their practice management decision processes. When presented with multiple options to provide for therapeutic intervention or patient assessment, one should not automatically choose the more expensive approach (just to "cover all the bases" or defend against later criticism or even a lawsuit) unless there is compelling evidence proving its value. Decisions that clearly materially increase cost should only be pursued when the benefit outweighs the risk. In anesthesia care as well as medicine in general, such decisions can be difficult regarding interventions that provide marginal benefit but contain significant cost increases. Because cost containment initially requires accurate cost awareness, anesthesiologists need to find out the actual costs and benefits of their anesthesia care techniques. Details will be unique to each practice setting. Because they will be excited that the anesthesiologists actually care, usually it is possible to get the cooperation of the facility administration's financial department members in researching and calculating the actual cost of anesthesia care so that thoughtful evaluations of potential reductions can be initiated.

Anesthesia drug expenses represent a small portion of the total perioperative costs (personnel costs being, by far, the greatest fraction). However, the great number of doses administered contributes significantly to aggregate total cost to the institution in actual dollars. Prudent drug selection combined with appropriate anesthetic technique can result in cost savings. Reducing fresh gas flow from 5 L/min to 2 L/min wherever possible has been estimated to potentially save approximately $150 million (inflation adjusted) annually in the United States.[95] A majority of anesthesia professionals usually attempt a practical approach to cost savings, but they are more frequently faced with difficult choices regarding methods of anesthesia that likely produce similar outcomes but at demonstrably different cost. When comparing the total costs of more expensive anesthetic drugs and techniques to lesser expensive ones, many variables need to be added to the formula. The cost of anesthetic drugs needs to include the costs of additional equipment such as extra infusion pumps and the associated maintenance, as well as the often-overlooked cost of anesthetic drug wastage in the OR.[96,97] There are other indirect costs that may be difficult to quantitate and are commonly overlooked. Some of these indirect costs include increased setup time, possibly increasing room turnover time, extended PACU recovery time, and additional expensive drugs required to treat side effects. Sometimes, more expensive techniques reduce indirect costs. A propofol infusion, although more expensive than inhaled vapor, commonly results in a decreased PACU stay after a short noninvasive procedure. If fewer PACU staff are needed or patient throughput is increased, the more expensive drug can possibly reduce overall cost. Conversely, using a comparatively expensive continuous propofol infusion for a long procedure definitely requiring postoperative admission to an ICU for which inhaled vapor would be just as good appears not to be cost justified. The impact of shorter-acting drugs and those with fewer side effects is context-specific. During long surgical procedures, such drugs may offer limited benefits over older, less expensive, longer-acting alternatives. Although newer, more expensive drugs may be easier to use, there is no objective evidence to support or refute the hypothesis that these drugs provide a "better" anesthetic experience when compared with carefully titrated older, less expensive, longer-acting drugs in the same class. This topic has been discussed for many years,[98] and likely will be for many to come.

Evaluation of outcomes and their subsequent application to cost analysis can be derived from two principle sources: data published in the literature and data collected from experience. As noted, computerized information management systems are useful tools to track outcomes and analyze the impact on the cost/benefit ledger, and large sophisticated databases with automatic input are in place and growing, with the intention of allowing "data mining" to reveal national trends. Using the collated data within a given institution in the same manner as for OR utilization and case load, practitioners can readily apply a statistical process to evaluate outcomes in their practice, possibly including correlation with cost. This information may take on added importance in that published incidence studies may not exist for the specific complication or outcome an anesthesia group is searching for. Cause-and-effect diagrams can track the parameters involved in the process and relate them to the various outcomes desired. An example could come from the extensive body of literature on the factors contributing to postoperative nausea and vomiting and the various possible preventions and treatments, many of which involve expensive medications. Information would be collected and stored in the database (locally and nationally). Ideally, the database would identify and track as many variables as needed/possible to delineate sources for possible improvement and its ultimate cost analysis. Once these sources for improvement and the ensuing cost impact are known, the anesthesia group can determine whether or not to pursue changing their practice. Various adverse outcomes can also be monitored. If analysis reveals a significant difference in the rate of an adverse outcome among practitioners, after all the other variables such as surgeon, patient mix, and so forth are eliminated, the outcome database can investigate the anesthetic techniques used by that practitioner (or group if comparing in the national database). If significant variations are identified, practitioner(s) would be able to learn of these variations in a nonthreatening manner because computer-derived data are used as opposed to a specific case analysis, which might lead that practitioner(s) to feel singled out for public criticism. The database can become a tool both for QA and professional education. These basic concepts are the underpinnings of both the US federal government's program within CMS, the Physician Quality Reporting System,[99] and the multiple programs within the ASA that start with reporting to the NACOR.[100] Both these programs have financial implications for payment to anesthesia professionals for their clinical care, but the idea of using such databases for their potential of genuine quality assessment and improvement (which, of course, should reduce costs also) is significant and should be embraced by everyone within the profession of clinical anesthesia.

Conclusion

Practice and OR "management" in anesthesiology today is more complex and more important than ever before. Attention to details that previously did not exist, were unknown, or were perceived as unimportant can likely make the difference between success and failure in anesthesiology practice.

Outlined here are basic descriptions and understandings of many different administrative, organizational, financial, and personnel components and factors in the practice of anesthesiology today. Ongoing significant changes in the health-care system will provide a continuing and expanding array of challenges.

Application of the knowledge and principles presented here will allow anesthesiologists to extrapolate creatively from these basics to their own individual circumstances and then forge ahead in anesthesiology practice that is safe, efficient, effective, productive, collegial, and even fun.

REFERENCES

1. Porter ME. What is value in health care? *N Engl J Med.* 2010;363:2477–2481.
2. CMS. Summary of final rule provisions for accountable care organizations under the Medicare shared savings program. https://www.cms.gov/medicare/medicare-fee-for-service-payment/sharedsavingsprogram/downloads/aco_summary_factsheet_icn907404.pdf. Accessed June 6, 2016.
3. Greaney TL. Accountable care organizations: the fork in the road. *N Engl J Med.* 2011;364:e1.
4. Inglehart JK. Assessing an ACO prototype: Medicare's physician group practice demonstration. *N Engl J Med.* 2011;364:198–200.
5. Meyer MJ, Hyder JA, Cole DJ, et al. The mandate to measure patient experience: how can patients "value" anesthesia care? *Anesth Analg.* 2016;122:1211–1215.
6. CMS. Comprehensive care for joint replacement model. https://innovation.cms.gov/initiatives/cjr. Accessed June 6, 2016.
7. American Health Care Association. Comprehensive care for joint replacement (CJR) final rule summary. https://www.ahcancal.org/facility_operations/medicare/Documents/AHCA%20Summary%20of%20CJR%20Final%20Rule.pdf. Accessed June 6, 2016.
8. CMS. Bundled payments for care improvement (BPCI) initiative: general information. See: https://innovation.cms.gov/initiatives/bundled-payments. Accessed June 6, 2016.
9. ASA. The need for the perioperative surgical home. http://www.asahq.org/~/media/sites/psh/files/psh-white-paper.pdf?la=en. Accessed June 6, 2016.
10. Schweitzer M, Fahy B, Leib M, et al. The perioperative surgical home model. *ASA Monit.* 2013;77:58–59.
11. Kain ZN, Vakharia S, Garson L, et al. The perioperative surgical home as a future perioperative practice model. *Anesth Analg.* 2014;118:1126–1130.
12. Dexter F, Wachtel R. Strategies for net cost reductions with the expanded role and expertise of anesthesiologists in the perioperative surgical home. *Anesth Analg.* 2014;118:1062–1071.
13. Prielipp RC, Morell RC, Coursin DB, et al. the future of anesthesiology: should the perioperative surgical home redefine us? *Anesth Analg.* 2015;120:1142–1148.
14. Warner MA, Apfelbaum JL. The perioperative surgical home: a response to a presumed burning platform or a thoughtful expansion of anesthesiology? *Anesth Analg.* 2015;120:1149–1151.
15. Vetter TR, Pittet J-F. The perioperative surgical home: a panacea or Pandora's box for the specialty of anesthesiology? *Anesth Analg.* 2015;120:968–973.
16. Butterworth JF, Green JA. The anesthesiologist-directed perioperative surgical home: a great idea that will succeed only if it is embraced by hospital administrators and surgeons. *Anesth Analg.* 2014;118:896–897.
17. Kain ZN, Fitch JCK, Kirsch JR, et al. Future of anesthesiology is perioperative medicine: a call for action. *Anesthesiology.* 2015;122:1192–1195.
18. Aston G. Service-line management: a behind the scenes road to value. Hospitals and Health Networks. http://www.hhnmag.com/articles/3757-service-line-management-a-behind-the-scenes-road-to-value. 2015. Accessed June 6, 2016.
19. Cook DJ, Pulido JN, Thompson JE, et al. Standardized practice design with electronic support mechanisms for surgical process improvement: reducing mechanical ventilation time. *Ann Surg.* 2014;260:1011–1015.
20. Knott A, Pathak S, McGrath JS, et al. Consensus views on implementation and measurement of enhanced recovery after surgery in England: Delphi study. *BMJ Open.* 2012;2(6):e001878.
21. Lassen K, Coolsen MM, Slim K, et al. Guidelines for perioperative care for pancreaticoduodenectomy: Enhanced Recovery After Surgery (ERAS®) Society recommendations. *World J Surg.* 2013;37:240–258.
22. Varadhan KK, Neal KR, Dejong CH, et al. The enhanced recovery after surgery (ERAS) pathway for patients undergoing major elective open colorectal surgery: a meta-analysis of randomized controlled trials. *Clin Nutr.* 2010;29:434–440.
23. Miller T, Thacker JK, White WD, et al. Reduced length of hospital stay in colorectal surgery after implementation of an enhanced recovery protocol. *Anesth Analg.* 2014;118:1052–1061.
24. Keenan JE, Speicher PJ, Thacker JK, et al. The preventive surgical site infection bundle in colorectal surgery: an effective approach to surgical site infection reduction and health care cost savings. *JAMA Surg.* 2014;149:1045–1052.
25. Abrams L. Where surgery comes with a 90-day guarantee. http://www.theatlantic.com/health/archive/2012/09/where-surgery-comes-with-a-90-day-guarantee/262841/. Accessed June 6, 2016.
26. Szokol JW, Stead S. The changing anesthesia economic landscape: emergence of large multispecialty practices and Accountable Care Organizations. *Curr Opin Anesthesiol.* 2014;27:183–189.
27. ASA. Large group practices and the ASA: our futures are intertwined. *ASA Monit.* 2016;80(1):42–44.
28. CMS. MACRA. https://www.cms.gov/Medicare/Quality-Initiatives-Patient-Assessment-Instruments/Value-Based-Programs/MACRA-MIPS-and-APMs/MACRA-MIPS-and-APMs.html. Accessed June 6, 2016.
29. American Medical Association. Medicare alternative payment models. http://www.ama-assn.org/ama/pub/advocacy/topics/medicare-alternative-payment-models.page. Accessed June 6, 2016.
30. ASA. SGR reform with MACRA: implications for anesthesiologists. http://www.asahq.org/…/aa2015bod/board-webinar-081015-macra/en/1. Accessed June 6, 2016.
31. National Council of State Boards of Nursing. https://www.ncsbn.org/Consensus_Model_for_APRN_Regulation_July_2008.pdf. Accessed June 6, 2016.
32. American Nurses Credentialing Center. About AANC. http://www.nursecredentialing.org/About-ANCC. Accessed June 6, 2016.
33. American Nurses Credentialing Center. Consensus model for APRN regulation: frequently asked questions. http://www.nursecredentialing.org/APRNRegulation-Consensus.pdf. Accessed June 6, 2016.
34. The National Council of State Boards of Nursing. Implementation status map. https://www.ncsbn.org/5397.htm. Accessed June 6, 2016.
35. ASA. Manual for anesthesia department and organization and management 2015. http://www.asahq.org/~/media/sites/asahq/files/public/resources/quality%20improvement/madom-summer-2015/2015-05-26_madom_summer-2015-full-version.pdf. Accessed June 6, 2016.
36. Gaba DM, Howard SK, Jump B. Production pressure in the work environment. *Anesthesiology.* 1994;81:488–500.
37. Eichhorn JH, Cooper JB, Cullen DJ, et al. Anesthesia practice standards at Harvard: a review. *J Clin Anesth.* 1988;1:55–65.
38. Eichhorn JH, Cooper JB, Cullen DJ, et al. Standards for patient monitoring during anesthesia at Harvard Medical School. *JAMA.* 1986;256:1017–1020.
39. ASA. Practice advisory for preanesthesia evaluation. *Anesthesiology.* 2012;116:522–538.
40. ASA. Practice guidelines for postanesthetic care. *Anesthesiology.* 2013;118:291–307.
41. ASA. Practice guidelines for obstetrical anesthesia. *Anesthesiology.* 2007;106:843–863.
42. ASA. Practice guidelines for pulmonary artery catheterization: An updated report by the American Society of Anesthesiologists Task Force on Pulmonary Artery Catheterization. *Anesthesiology.* 2003;99:988–1014.
43. ASA. Practice guidelines for management of the difficult airway. *Anesthesiology.* 2013;118:251–270.
44. Dans PE, Weiner JP, Otter SE. Peer review organizations: Promises and potential pitfalls. *N Engl J Med.* 1985;313:1131–1137.
45. Spooner RB, Kirby RR. Equipment-related anesthetic incidents. In: Pierce EC, Cooper JB, eds. *Analysis of Anesthetic Mishaps.* Boston, MA: International Anesthesiology Clinics; 1984;22:133.
46. Cooper JB, Newbower RS, Kitz RJ. An analysis of major errors and equipment failures in anesthesia management: considerations for prevention and detection. *Anesthesiology.* 1984;60:34–42.
47. Caplan RA, Vistica M, Posner KL, et al. Adverse anesthetic outcomes arising from gas delivery equipment: a closed claims analysis. *Anesthesiology.* 1997;87:741–748.
48. Cooper JB, Newbower RS, Long CD, et al. Preventable anesthesia mishaps: a study of human factors. *Anesthesiology.* 1978;49:399–406.
49. Olympio MA, Reinke B, Abramovich A. Challenges ahead in technology training: a report on the training initiative of the Committee on Technology. *APSF Newslett.* 2006;21:43.
50. Eichhorn JH. Organized response to major anesthesia accident will help limit damage: Update of "Adverse Event Protocol" provides valuable plan. *APSF Newslett.* 2006;21:11.
51. Eichhorn JH. Influence of practice standards on anesthesia outcome. *Baillieres Clin Anaesthesiol Int Pract Res.* 1992;6:663.
52. Eichhorn JH. Prevention of intraoperative anesthesia accidents and related severe injury through safety monitoring. *Anesthesiology.* 1989;70:572–577.
53. Keats AS. Anesthesia mortality in perspective. *Anesth Analg.* 1990;71:113–119.
54. Lagasse RS. Anesthesia safety: model or myth? *Anesthesiology.* 2002;97:1609.
55. Cooper JB, Gaba DM. No myth: anesthesia is a model for addressing patient safety. *Anesthesiology.* 2002;97:1335–1337.
56. Domino KB. Medical liability insurance: the calm before the storm? *ASA Newslett.* 2013;77:54–56.
57. Bacon AK. Death on the table: Some thoughts on how to handle an anaesthetic-related death. *Anaesthesia.* 1989;44:245–248.
58. Runciman WB, Webb RK, Klepper ID, et al. Crisis management: validation of an algorithm by analysis of 2000 incident reports. *Anaesth Intensive Care.* 1993;21:579–592.
59. Davies J, Webb RK. Adverse events in anaesthesia: the wrong drug. *Can J Anaesth.* 1994;41:83–86.
60. Cooper JB, Cullen DJ, Eichhorn JH, et al. Administrative guidelines for response to an adverse anesthesia event. *J Clin Anesth.* 1993;5:79–84.
61. Gaba DM, Fish KJ, Howard SK, Burden AR, eds. *Crisis Management in Anesthesiology.* 2nd ed. Philadelphia: Elsevier; 2014.
62. Harrison TK, Manser T, Howard SK, et al. Use of cognitive aids in a simulated anesthetic crisis. *Anesth Analg.* 2006;103:551–556.

63. Mulroy MF. For the Emergency Manual Implementation Collaborative. Emergency manuals: the time has come. *APSF Newslett.* 2013;28:9–10.
64. Goldhaber-Fiebert SN, Howard SK. Implementing emergency manuals: can cognitive aids help translate best practices for patient care during acute events? *Anesth Analg.* 2013;117:1149–1161.
65. Marshall S. The use of cognitive aids during emergencies in anesthesia: a review of the literature. *Anesth Analg.* 2013;117:1162–1171.
66. Kraman SS, Hamm G. Risk management: Extreme honesty may be the best policy. *Ann Intern Med.* 1999;131:963–967.
67. Lazare A. Apology in medical practice: an emerging clinical skill. *JAMA.* 2006;296:1401–1404.
68. Eichhorn JH. Patient perspective personalizes patient safety. *APSF Newslett.* 2005;20:61.
69. Cox W. The five A's: what do patients want after an adverse event? *J Healthcare Risk Manag.* 2007;27:25–29.
70. Accreditation Council for Graduate Medical Education. *Data Resource Book, Academic Year 2014–2015.* Chicago, IL: ACGME; 2015.
71. ASA. Guidelines for office-based anesthesia. http://www.asahq.org/~/media/Sites/ASAHQ/Files/Public/Resources/standards-guidelines/guidelines-for-office-based-anesthesia.pdf. October 15, 2014. Accessed June 6, 2016.
72. Locke J. The net collections fallacy and other performance metric myths. *Proceedings of the American Society of Anesthesiologists 2003 Conference on Practice Management.* Park Ridge, IL: American Society of Anesthesiologists; 2003:141.
73. Willett DE. Exclusive contracts: Update on legal issues. *Proceedings of the American Society of Anesthesiologists 2001 Conference on Practice Management.* Park Ridge, IL: American Society of Anesthesiologists; 2001:8.
74. Scott SJ, Blough GG. Exclusive contracts: Survey of hospital contracts. *Proceedings of the American Society of Anesthesiologists 2001 Conference on Practice Management.* Park Ridge, IL: American Society of Anesthesiologists; 2001:9.
75. Bierstein K. Pros and cons of exclusive contracts. *ASA Newsletter.* 2006;70(8):36.
76. Everett PC. Securing a hospital stipend: The business-like approach. *Proceedings of the American Society of Anesthesiologists 2003 Conference on Practice Management.* Park Ridge, IL: American Society of Anesthesiologists; 2003:189.
77. Semo JJ. Hospital stipend negotiations: Practical and legal issues. *Proceedings of the American Society of Anesthesiologists 2004 Conference on Practice Management.* Park Ridge, IL: American Society of Anesthesiologists; 2004:51.
78. Laden J, Monea M. Preparing the financial case for hospital support. *Proceedings of the American Society of Anesthesiologists 2008 Conference on Practice Management.* Park Ridge, IL: American Society of Anesthesiologists; 2008:258.
79. Adessa A. The vulnerability and potential extinction of independent, hospital-based practices. *Proceedings of the American Society of Anesthesiologists 2008 Conference on Practice Management.* Park Ridge, IL: American Society of Anesthesiologists; 2008:65.
80. Epstein AM, Lee TH, Hamel MB. Paying physicians for high-quality care. *N Engl J Med.* 2004;350:406–410.
81. Hannenberg AA. Progress report: Quality incentives in anesthesiology. *Proceedings of the American Society of Anesthesiologists 2008 Conference on Practice Management.* Park Ridge, IL: American Society of Anesthesiologists; 2008:57.
82. Scurlock C, Dexter F, Reich D, et al. Needs assessment for business strategies of anesthesiology groups' practices. *Anesth Analg.* 2011;113:170–174.
83. Warner M. Who better than anesthesiologists? The 44th Rovenstine lecture. *Anesthesiology.* 2006;104:1094–1101.
84. Sexton J, Makary MA, Tersigni AR, et al. Teamwork in the operating room. *Anesthesiology.* 2006;105:877.
85. Lingard L, Regehr G, Orser B, et al. Evaluation of a preoperative checklist and team briefing among surgeons, nurses, and anesthesiologists to reduce failures in communication. *Arch Surg.* 2008;143:12–17.
86. Dexter F, Xiao Y, Dow A, et al. Coordination of appointments for anesthesia care outside of operating rooms using an enterprise-wide scheduling system. *Anesth Analg.* 2007;105:1701–1710.
87. Pollard JB, Zboray AL, Mazze RI. Economic benefits attributed to opening a preoperative evaluation clinic for outpatients. *Anesth Analg.* 1996;83:407–410.
88. Fischer SP. Development and effectiveness of an anesthesia preoperative evaluation clinic in a teaching hospital. *Anesthesiology.* 1996;85:196–206
89. Yen C, Tsai M, Macario A. Preoperative evaluation clinics. *Curr Opin Anaesthesiol.* 2010;23:167–172.
90. Kheterpal S, Tremper K, Shanks A, et al. Workforce and finances of the United States anesthesiology training programs: 2009–2010. *Anesth Analg.* 2011;112:1480–1486.
91. Abouleish AE, Prough DS, Zornow MH, et al. Designing meaningful industry metrics for clinical productivity for anesthesiology departments. *Anesth Analg.* 2001;93:309–312.
92. Abouleish AE, Prough DS, Whitten CW, et al. Comparing clinical productivity of anesthesiology departments. *Anesthesiology.* 2002;97:608–615.
93. Abouleish AE, Prough DS, Barker SJ, et al. Organizational factors affect comparisons of clinical productivity of academic anesthesiology departments. *Anesth Analg.* 2003;96:802–812.
94. Keehan SP, Cuckler GA, Sisko AM, et al. National health expenditure projections, 2014–24: spending growth faster than recent trends. *Health Aff.* 2015;34:1407–1417.
95. Baum JA. Low flow anaesthesia: The sensible and judicious use of inhalation anaesthetics. *Acta Anaesthesiol Scand Suppl.* 1997;111:264–267.
96. Weinger MB. Drug wastage contributes significantly to the cost of routine anesthesia care. *J Clin Anesth.* 2001;13:491–497.
97. Rinehardt EK, Sivarajan M. Costs and wastes in anesthesia care. *Curr Opin Anaesthesiol.* 2012;25:221–225.
98. Johnstone R, Jozefczyk KG. Costs of anesthetic drugs: experiences with a cost education trial. *Anesth Analg.* 1994;78:766–771.
99. CMS. Physician quality reporting system. https://www.cms.gov/medicare/quality-initiatives-patient-assessment-instruments/pqrs/. Accessed June 6, 2016.
100. ASA. Quality reporting: NACOR. http://www.asahq.org/quality-and-practice-management/quality-reporting-nacor. Accessed June 6, 2016.

3 Occupational Health

JONATHAN D. KATZ • ROBERT S. HOLZMAN • AMY E. VINSON

Introduction
Physical Hazards
    Waste Anesthetic Gases
    Chemicals
    Allergic Reactions
    Radiation
    Noise Pollution
    Ergonomics/Human Factors
    Work Hours, Night Call, and Fatigue
Infectious Hazards
    OHSA Standards, Standard Precautions, and Transmission-based Precautions
    Respiratory Viruses
    Enteric Infections
    DNA Viruses
    Rubella
    Measles (Rubeola)
    Viral Hepatitis
    Pathogenic Human Retroviruses
    Prion Diseases
    Tuberculosis
    Viruses in Smoke Plumes
Emotional Considerations
    Stress
    Impact of Adverse Events
    Burnout
    Substance Use, Abuse, and Addiction
    Impairment and Disability
    The Aging Anesthesiologist
    Mortality Among Anesthesiologists
    Suicide
Wellness
    Nutrition, Diet, and Fitness
    Implementing Lifestyle Interventions for Lifestyle-related Diseases
    Mindfulness
Conclusion

KEY POINTS

1. Exposure to waste anesthetic gases can be reduced to levels below those recommended by the National Institute for Occupational Safety and Health by using waste gas scavenging equipment, routinely maintaining anesthesia machines, and following appropriate work practices.
2. Vigilance is one of the most critical tasks performed by anesthesiologists and may be adversely affected by several occupationally related issues including poor equipment engineering and design, excessive noise, interpersonal conflict, production pressures, and fatigue.
3. Sleep deprivation and fatigue are common among anesthesiologists and can adversely affect patient safety due to deleterious effects on the physician's cognition, mood, and health.
4. The risk of exposure to infectious pathogens can be reduced by the routine use of standard precautions, transmission-based precautions for infected patients, and safety devices designed to prevent needlestick injuries.
5. Hepatitis B vaccine is recommended for all anesthesia personnel because of the increased risk for occupational transmission of this blood-borne pathogen.
6. Substance use disorder, or chemical dependency, is a significant, often lethal, occupational hazard among anesthesiologists. An incidence of controlled substance abuse of 1% to 2% has been repeatedly reported within anesthesia training programs. Rates have not changed despite educational and systematic interventions.
7. Anesthesiologists have a disproportionately high rate of suicide. Factors include pre-existing personality traits, substance use disorder, and stress.
8. Physician wellness is integral to occupational health and patient safety. There is an evolving professional commitment to optimizing physician work style and lifestyle, as well as physical health (e.g., through better nutrition, fitness, and rest).
9. Mindfulness-based stress reduction techniques can improve physician wellness, physician performance, and patient safety.

Introduction

The health-care industry has the dubious distinction of being one of the most hazardous places to work in the United States. According to the U.S. Bureau of Labor, workers in the health-care and social assistance industry have the highest rate and greatest number of nonfatal occupational injuries among all workers in the private industry sector.[1] Unfortunately, in contrast to other well-known hazardous workplaces, such as agriculture and construction, the frequency of occupational injuries in the health-care sector continues to rise.

In addition to the occupational risks incurred by other members of the health-care team, commonly recognized workplace hazards for anesthesia personnel include exposure to waste anesthetic gases (WAG), ionizing radiation, fires, and infectious agents. In addition, anesthesia personnel are vulnerable to emotional and psychological disorders such as burnout and substance use disorder.

Despite heightened awareness and concerted efforts to minimize these occupational diseases, many continue to occur at disproportionate rates among anesthesiologists. This chapter will discuss these hazards and the work being done both to reduce occupational risks in the workplace and to improve patient safety through promotion of physician wellness.

Physical Hazards

Waste Anesthetic Gases

Levels of Waste Anesthetic Gases

In the absence of adequate air exchange and scavenging of WAG, high levels of anesthetic vapors can be detected in the ambient air surrounding anesthetizing locations. In 1969, prior to the routine use of scavenging devices, Linde and Bruce[2] observed an average concentration of halothane of 10 ppm and nitrous oxide of 130 ppm in the air surrounding an active anesthesia machine, with end-expired air samples from anesthesiologists as high as 12 ppm of halothane. Subsequent studies have reported even higher concentrations in poorly ventilated and/or unscavenged locations.[3]

Citing health concerns, the National Institute for Occupational Safety and Health (NIOSH) in 1977 recommended exposure limits of 2 ppm for halogenated anesthetic agents when used alone or 0.5 ppm for a halogenated agent and 25 ppm of nitrous oxide when used together (Time Weighted Average [TWA] during the period of anesthetic administration).[4] Scavenging equipment specifications and methods for monitoring WAG concentrations were also included in the report.

In a subsequent publication, NIOSH issued an alert to healthcare personnel that exposure to inhalation anesthetic agents, especially nitrous oxide, may produce "harmful effects" and included recommendations to monitor the air in operating rooms (ORs), implement appropriate engineering controls, enact certain work practices and equipment maintenance procedures, and institute a worker education program.[5] Other organizations, such as the American Conference of Governmental Industrial Hygienists, and some state departments of health, have established their own occupational exposure limits for WAG, in many cases higher than those recommended by NIOSH.

It has been well demonstrated that concentrations of WAG can usually be reduced to acceptable levels through strict compliance with the NIOSH recommendations.[6] However, there remain several potential sources for OR contamination and unavoidable situations, such as a mask induction (common in pediatric anesthesia), where levels of WAG can exceed these limits (Table 3-1).[3] Elevated levels of WAG have also been identified in the postanesthesia care unit (PACU),[7] typically occurring via exhaled gases from recovering patients.[8] Levels of WAG in the PACU can be reduced by ensuring adequate room ventilation and by discontinuing anesthetic gases in sufficient time before leaving the OR.

Health Consequences of WAG Exposure

The first published report of specific toxic effects from chronic occupational exposure to WAG appeared in a 1967 article that described a high incidence of fatigue, nausea, headaches, and miscarriage among female Russian anesthesiologists.[9] Although the study methodology has been subsequently questioned, it opened an ongoing dialogue about whether or not chronic exposure to WAG renders anesthesia providers more vulnerable to cellular injury, organ toxicity, adverse reproductive outcomes, impairment of psychomotor skills, substance use disorder, and premature death.

It is not surprising that chemicals with such widespread and profound physiologic effects as anesthetic agents would evidence toxic properties if applied in adequate concentrations to tissues. For example, there is ample evidence that cellular damage can be caused by chronic exposure of cultured cells and experimental animals to high concentrations of many anesthetic gases.[10–12] However, the clinical literature remains inconclusive regarding causality between adverse health effects and the level of occupational exposure to WAG experienced by most anesthesia personnel. Some limitations of the clinical studies include occupational exposure in the study population to other risk factors such as radiation, long work hours, stress, and unhealthy personal habits, as well as potential reporter bias that can occur in retrospective studies.

Most of the studies of possible health consequences to humans with occupational exposure to WAG have focused on cytotoxic changes, cancer, and reproductive outcomes. The reports on possible genotoxic effects of trace anesthetic exposure are conflicting. For example, in one study occupational exposure to sevoflurane (8.9 ± 5.6 ppm) and nitrous oxide (119 ± 39 ppm) was associated with increased levels of sister chromatid exchange (a marker of genotoxicity) with abnormal cytology returning to normal after 2 months of leave from the OR.[13] However, other studies have reported no findings of cellular damage among clinicians exposed to the levels of anesthetic gases that are encountered in an adequately ventilated and scavenged OR.[14] A conclusion that can be drawn from these conflicting reports is that the risk of genotoxicity is minimal under the low exposure to WAG usually experienced in a well-scavenged OR.[15,16]

The possibility of adverse reproductive outcomes has been the most intensively researched aspect of occupational WAG exposure. Early reports suggested an association between long-term occupational exposure to WAG and infertility, spontaneous abortions, and congenital abnormalities.[17] The American Society of Anesthesiologists (ASA) and NIOSH published a retrospective analysis in 1974 in which 49,585 OR personnel with occupational WAG exposure were compared with a nonexposed group of 23,911 health-care professionals.[18] Among the findings in this study was an increased risk of spontaneous abortion and congenital abnormalities in children of women who worked in the OR and an increased risk of congenital abnormalities in offspring of unexposed wives of male OR personnel.

In 1985, in response to criticism of the methodology and data analysis in this and other earlier reports, and in recognition of

---

Table 3-1 Sources of Operating Room Contamination

Anesthetic Techniques
- Filling of anesthesia vaporizers
- Flushing of the circuit
- Turning gas flow on before placing mask on patient
- Poorly fitting masks and laryngeal mask airways
- Uncuffed or leaking tracheal tubes
- Open pediatric circuits
- Failure to turn off gas flow control valves at the end of an anesthetic

Anesthesia Machine Delivery System and Scavenging System
- Open system
- Malfunction of hospital disposal system
- Leaks in high pressure hoses and connectors
- CO_2 absorbent canisters
- Mounting of gas tanks

Other Sources
- Cryosurgery units
- Cardiopulmonary bypass circuits

the fact that many of the studies were conducted prior to routine WAG scavenging, the ASA commissioned a meta-analysis of the existing data.[19] This study reported that the relative risks of spontaneous abortion for female physicians and female nurses working in the OR were 1.4 and 1.3, respectively. The increased relative risk for congenital abnormalities was of borderline statistical significance for exposed physicians only. The overall risk created by WAG exposure was small compared with other, better-documented, maternal risk factors, such as cigarette smoking and long working hours. The review also pointed out that duration and levels of anesthetic exposure were not measured in any of the studies and that other confounding factors were not adequately controlled.

The importance of adequate scavenging was highlighted in a subsequent meta-analysis of the risk of spontaneous abortion among hospital workers, dental assistants, veterinarians, and veterinary assistants.[20] The study identified a significant risk of spontaneous abortion in those studies conducted prior to the era of scavenging but no increased risk among personnel who worked in environments where WAG were scavenged.

Reports of elevated risks for adverse reproductive outcomes have continued to appear. Most of these reports concern personnel in locations where adequate scavenging of WAG is not universally practiced. Female dental assistants[21] and female veterinarians who work in large animal hospitals[22] have been specifically identified as at-risk for adverse reproductive outcomes.

It is likely that other job-associated conditions besides exposure to trace anesthetic gases, such as stress, infections, long work hours, shift work, and radiation exposure, may account for many of the adverse reproductive outcomes. A survey of 3,985 Swedish midwives demonstrated that night work was significantly associated with spontaneous abortions after the 12th week of pregnancy (odds ratio 3.33), whereas exposure to nitrous oxide appeared to have no effect.[23] Preterm birth in obstetric and neonatal nurses was associated with increased work hours, hours worked while standing, and occupational fatigue.[24] In addition, in a study of female veterinarians, the risks of birth defects were highest among those exposed to radiation and long working hours (>45 hr/wk) but not to those exposed to WAG.[22]

The literature on this subject remains inconclusive. Many of the epidemiologic studies continue to suffer from important design flaws. For example, the level of exposure to WAG is frequently unknown or not reported and the retrospective nature of the questionnaire lends itself to reporter bias. Still, the evidence taken as a whole suggests that there is a slight increase in the relative risk of spontaneous abortion and congenital abnormalities in offspring of females exposed to WAG. This risk is minimized when appropriate waste gas scavenging technology is applied.[25]

One of the principal reasons identified by NIOSH in their original publication on WAG was concern about "decrements in performance, cognition, audiovisual ability and dexterity."[26] The effect of WAG exposure on psychomotor performance among humans varies considerably depending upon the concentration of anesthetic gas to which the subjects are exposed. Temporary lethargy and fatigue are the most common symptoms described after brief exposures to subanesthetic concentrations of anesthetic gases. Longer exposures and higher concentrations have been associated with symptoms such as headache, depression, anxiety, loss of appetite, loss of memory, decreased reaction time, and decrements in cognitive function. Most of the measurable psychomotor and cognitive impairments produced by brief exposures are short-lived and disappear within 5 minutes of cessation of exposure.[27]

One other health consideration of WAG is the environmental impact and contribution to global warming. Among anesthetic gases, nitrous oxide is the greatest contributor to this effect because of the relatively large volumes that are used, the longer time period that it has been in use compared to other inhalation anesthetics, and the fact that nitrous oxide from a number of nonmedical sources is currently the dominant ozone-depleting gas.[28] Nitrous oxide from anesthetic use represents only a small fraction of that found in the stratosphere but nevertheless does contribute to the greenhouse effect.[29]

Chemicals

Methyl methacrylate is commonly used in many surgical procedures. Known cardiovascular complications of methyl methacrylate in surgical patients include hypotension, bradycardia, and cardiac arrest. Reported risks from repeated occupational exposure to methyl methacrylate include skin irritation and burns, systemic allergic reactions, eye irritation, headache, neurologic signs, adverse reproductive outcomes, and organ damage. In one report, a dental technician suffered significant lower limb neuropathy after repeated occupational exposure to methyl methacrylate.[30] Reported levels in modern ORs using scavenging devices are well below the U.S. Environmental Protection Agency recommended limit of an 8-hour TWA exposure of 100 ppm.

Allergic Reactions

Allergic reactions to volatile anesthetic agents and to some muscle relaxants have been associated with contact dermatitis, hepatitis, and anaphylaxis in individual anesthesiologists.[31,32] Analyses of sera from pediatric anesthesiologists exposed to halothane demonstrated an increased prevalence of autoantibodies to cytochrome P450 2E1 and hepatic endoplasmic reticulum protein (ERp58).[33] The pathophysiology appears more complex than antibody development and may be more of a halogenated hydrocarbon autoimmune reaction injuring the liver. These autoantibodies are also detectable in about one-third of patients with advanced alcoholic liver disease and chronic hepatitis C.[34] Despite the presence of these autoantibodies, only 1 of 105 anesthesiologists had findings of any hepatic injury. Therefore, although autoantibodies may occur in anesthesiologists frequently exposed to volatile anesthetics, they do not appear to commonly cause anesthetic-induced hepatitis.

Latex in surgical and examination gloves has become a common source of allergic reactions among OR personnel. In many cases, medical personnel who are allergic to latex experience their first adverse reactions while they are patients undergoing surgery. Although the majority of symptoms are mild, urticaria, bronchospasm, and rhinitis can occur. More severe symptoms are significantly related to a positive history of individual or family atopy. The prevalence of latex sensitivity among medical personnel can be as great as 16% to 20%.[35,36] For anesthesiologists the rate is approximately 12%.[37]

The latex found in medical products is actually a composite of proteins, polyisoprenes, lipids, and phospholipids combined with preservatives, accelerators, antioxidants, vulcanizing compounds, and lubricating agents (such as cornstarch or talc). The protein content is responsible for most of the generalized allergic reactions to latex-containing surgical gloves. These reactions are exacerbated by the presence of powder that enhances aerosolization.

Irritant or contact dermatitis accounts for the majority of reactions resulting from wearing latex-containing gloves (Table 3-2). True allergic reactions present as T-cell–mediated

Table 3-2 Types of Reactions to Latex Gloves

Category	Symptoms	Signs	Cause	Management
Contact dermatitis	Irritation, itching, pain	Scaling, drying, cracking of skin	Powders, soaps, gloves	Identify reaction, avoid irritant, use glove liner, use alternative product
Type IV—delayed hypersensitivity	Irritation, itching, pain (delayed 6–72 h)	Scaling, drying, cracking of skin; blistering	Chemical additives used in manufacturing (such as accelerators)	Identify offending chemical, possibly use alternative product without chemical additive, possibly use glove liner
Type I—immediate hypersensitivity			Proteins found in natural rubber latex-containing products	Identify reaction; avoid latex-containing products; use by coworkers of nonlatex or powder-free, low-protein gloves
Localized contact urticaria	Itchiness in localized area of contact (immediate)	Localized urticaria in a contact pattern; redness and swelling of skin resembling a "poison ivy" type of rash		Antihistamines, topical/systemic steroids
Generalized reaction	Itching, stuffy nose, shortness of breath, sense of foreboding, itching	Hives, runny nose, wheezing, hypoxemia, cardiovascular instability including hypotension and shock		Anaphylaxis protocol emphasizing epinephrine in appropriate doses

contact dermatitis (type IV) or as an immunoglobulin E–mediated anaphylactic reaction (type I).

Anesthesiologists who believe that they are allergic to latex must avoid all direct contact with latex-containing products. It is also important that coworkers wear nonlatex or powderless, low latex-allergen gloves to limit the levels of ambient allergens.

Radiation

Anesthesia personnel are at risk of radiation exposure from the primary x-ray beam and from scattered radiation reflected off surfaces such as tables, other equipment, and the patient. The biologic consequences of radiation exposure vary depending on age, gender, and the specific organ that is exposed. Well-documented consequences of radiation exposure include DNA damage, cell death, and organ injury. The development of cancer is an example of a radiation-induced injury with a long latency period and having no known threshold below which the risk entirely disappears.

The Occupational Safety and Health Administration (OSHA) has published occupational limits for workers exposed to ionizing radiation.[38] The annual limit is 5 rem with an allowable long-term limit of $(N - 18) \times 5$ rem, where N is the age in years. The recommended maximum occupational exposure to a pregnant or lactating worker should not exceed a monthly limit of 0.5 rem (excluding medical and natural background radiation).

Early studies reported that the exposure to radiation among anesthesia personnel is safely below the OSHA limits.[39] However, studies conducted subsequent to the increased utilization of ionizing radiation in ORs, cardiac catheterization, and interventional radiology suites, have revealed a trend toward increased exposure among anesthesia personnel (although still well below OSHA limits).[40,41] In one study, there was a doubling of the aggregate radiation exposure to members of a department of anesthesiology in the year following the introduction of an electrophysiology laboratory.[42] Preventative strategies for anesthesiologists to minimize their risk of radiation-induced injury include limiting the intensity and exposure time, distancing oneself from the source of the radiation, and using maximal shielding from both primary and scattered sources of radiation.

A second form of radiation with potential health consequence comes in the form of chronic exposure to low-frequency electromagnetic fields such as those emitted by magnetic resonance imaging (MRI) equipment.[43] Transient symptoms such as vertigo, nausea, dizziness, and visual phosphenes (light flashes) have all been reported. The severity of these symptoms is a function of the field strength of the scanner, the proximity to the scanner, and the rate of movement within the magnetic field. There are currently no published regulations in the United States that limit occupational exposure. Guidelines from the International Commission on Non-Ionizing Radiation Protection offer some suggestions regarding technique and worker practices to limit neurobehavioral effects.[44] No studies to date have identified any chronic adverse health effects from long-term exposure to high-intensity magnetic fields. However, until more information is available, it would seem prudent to conform to the general admonition regarding all forms of radiation exposure: keep it as low as reasonably achievable.

Noise Pollution

The magnitude of noise is determined by both the intensity of the sound (measured in decibels) and the duration of the exposure to that sound. A commonly accepted standard for the maximum level of safe noise exposure is 90 dB for 8 hours.[45] Each increase in noise of 5 dB halves the permissible exposure time, so that 100 dB is acceptable for just 2 hours per day. The maximum peak allowable exposure in an industrial setting is 115 dB.

Average noise levels in a modern OR usually far surpass recommended levels (Table 3-3). Ambient noise levels as great as 90 dB commonly result from high capacity heating and air conditioning systems, ventilators, suction equipment, forced-air patient warming devices, music, and conversations. Sporadic clatter from dropped instruments, surgical saws and drills, and anesthetic alarms adds to this background noise so that in some ORs noise levels of 100 dB or greater occur for 40% of the time, with peak levels exceeding 120 dB.[46]

Excessive noise can be distracting, especially to trainees and inexperienced clinicians.[47] Noise also interferes with the critical ability of clinicians in the OR to hear conversations and vital tones and alarms.[48,49] In order for voices and other auditory signals to be heard and accurately interpreted, these sounds must be elevated to 20 dB above background noise.[50] Anesthesia providers are especially vulnerable to noise pollution through its adverse effects on efficiency, short-term memory, and the ability to perform complex psychomotor tasks.[51] These hindrances can have their largest impact during induction and emergence, which are frequently the noisiest times in the OR.

Chronic exposure to excessive noise is a health hazard. The most direct complication of exposure to excessive noise is hearing loss.[52] The hearing loss occurs gradually, initially affecting higher frequencies (300 to 6,000 Hz), increases in severity with continued exposure, is frequently not realized until significant damage has occurred, and is irreversible. Although no direct causal relationship has been established with chronic exposure to excess noise in the OR, it is interesting that one study of hearing among anesthesiologists found that 66% had abnormal audiograms.[53] In 7% of those studied, the hearing impairment could potentially interfere with their ability to hear standard OR alarms. Other members of the surgical team, including surgeons and scrub nurses, have also been shown to suffer from accelerated hearing loss.[54]

One form of noise, music, deserves special consideration.[55] When properly selected, background music can help focus some members of the surgical staff and contribute toward work efficiency.[56,57] However, music also adds substantially to the already considerable ambient noise levels in the OR. Many members of the surgical team, particularly those in training or with limited experience, find music that is not self-selected distracting and a hindrance to their performance.[58] Anesthesiologists, in particular, frequently report that music can impair communication between team members and interfere with several of their tasks.[59] If music is to be played in the OR, the selection and the volume should be determined by mutual agreement of all of the parties present.

Table 3-3	Comparative Noise Levels
Source	**Noise Intensity**
EPA recommendation	45 dB
Continuous suction	75–85 dB
Clang of instruments	75–85 dB
Surgical saw	80–105 dB
Music	75–105 dB
Average OR noise	77 dB
OSHA limit (8 h)	90 dB
Subway	100 dB
OSHA limit (0 h)	115 dB

EPA, Environmental Protection Agency; OSHA, Occupational Safety and Health Administration.

Ergonomics/Human Factors

Human factor analysis, also called ergonomics, is the study of the interaction between humans and machines and the impact of equipment design on its use. It is a multidisciplinary science that applies diverse principles gleaned from anthropometry, ethnography, biomechanics, industrial and social psychology, architecture, education, and information technology. Human factor analysis has gained its widest acceptance in industries such as aviation and nuclear power where many well-publicized catastrophes have been linked to human error. The work performed by an anesthesiologist shares many of the characteristics found in these industries, including the intricacy of the tasks, a narrow margin of error, and the vulnerability to human error.

A number of human factor shortcomings exist in the anesthesiologist's workplace. For example, anesthesia equipment is often poorly designed or positioned. Anesthesia monitors and electronic medical records are frequently placed so that the anesthesiologist's attention is diverted away from the surgical field. Among those tasks most vulnerable to the distractions of poor workstation design is vigilance,[a] a duty so critical to the conduct of a safe anesthetic that the seal of the ASA bears as its only motto "Vigilance."

Other ergonomic factors can interfere with an anesthesiologist's ability to optimally perform his/her complex tasks. Any impediment that requires the expenditure of excessive mental or physical energy will eventually produce a decrement in performance. Poor engineering of the monitor displays, so that the manner of presentation is suboptimal, can increase the difficulty in extracting pertinent information and adversely influence the operator's performance.

Even alarms that were developed with the specific goal of augmenting the task of vigilance can have considerable shortcomings. In general, alarms are nonspecific (the same alarm signaling as many as 12 different deviations from "normal"), and are susceptible to artifacts and false positives that can cause "alarm fatigue," and distract the observer from more clinically significant information. It is not unusual for distractive alarms to be ignored or inactivated.[60] A positive trend that is emerging in alarm technology is the development of "knowledge-based alarms" that can integrate information from more than one monitor and suggest a list of diagnostic and therapeutic possibilities.

Organizational issues, such as failed communication with other team members, can adversely impact an anesthesiologist's performance. The potential for disaster as a result of poor communication has been well illustrated in a number of airline catastrophes. The possibility for miscommunication and resultant error is heightened in the OR as a result of the overlapping realms of professional responsibility, which may be at odds with established hierarchy. Poor communication can lead to conflict and compromised patient safety and has been identified as a root cause of many anesthesia-related sentinel events. Crisis resource management training, well established in the aerospace industry, has emerged to address this issue.[61,62]

Effective conflict resolution is an important element of the teamwork necessary for successful surgical outcomes. Some degree of conflict occurs during the management of as many as 78% of patients in high-intensity areas such as ORs or critical

---

[a]Vigilance is the ability to detect changes in a stimulus during prolonged monitoring tasks when the subject has no prior knowledge of whether or when any changes might occur.

care units.[63] Conflict and unpleasant interpersonal interactions among team members are among the most stressful aspects of the job of an anesthesiologist and can hinder safe anesthetic care.

Successful resolution of conflict is a skill that can be learned.[64] Mutual respect is required among team members along with a willingness to acknowledge differences of opinion. Intervention by a neutral third party is frequently helpful in finding an innovative solution. The airline industry has successfully implemented crew resource management programs to improve the performance of cockpit teams.[65] These can also be applied to OR personnel.

"Production pressure" has the potential to create an environment in which issues of productivity supersede those of safety, resulting in errors due directly to haste and/or deliberate deviations from safe practices.[66] The routine use of a preoperative checklist can help prevent multiple potential sources of error, including those directly related to production pressure.[67]

Work Hours, Night Call, and Fatigue

A circadian pattern of alertness and sleep is a fundamental element of healthy human physiology. Inadequate sleep caused by any number of factors, including obstructive sleep apnea or disruptive work schedules, can contribute to adverse health effects including cardiovascular disease and psychological illness.

Sleep-deprived workers are at greater risk of committing workplace errors and suffer more work-related accidents.[68] Accident susceptibility extends beyond work hours to other activities of daily living, such as driving. The changes resulting from sleep deprivation bear a striking similarity to those seen with alcohol intoxication.[69] Significant individual variations in impairment due to fatigue have been identified.[70] The contribution of sleep loss and fatigue to accidents has been documented in many well-publicized industrial catastrophes. Sleep deprivation was a contributing factor in catastrophic industrial accidents such as those at Chernobyl and Three Mile Island, and on the Exxon-Valdez oil tanker and the Challenger space shuttle.

A number of reports have also identified sleep deprivation as a causative factor in errors occurring in the health-care industry.[71] As early as 1971, Friedman et al.[72] reported that interns made almost twice as many errors reading electrocardiograms after an extended work shift than after a night of sleep. Intubation skills were reduced among emergency room physicians working night shifts when compared with other physicians working days, and physicians in both groups were more likely to commit errors during a simulated triage test toward the end of their work shifts.[73] In a study that examined the management by medical interns of medical admissions, 36% more medical errors occurred while on a "traditional" schedule (>24 hours work shifts) than when working a schedule that eliminated extended work shifts and reduced the number of hours worked per week.[74]

Anesthesiologists who take night call commonly suffer from each of the three well-defined classes of sleep deprivation: total, partial, and selective. Interruption of sleep during call frequently occurs between the hours of 2 AM and 4 AM when humans are most vulnerable to fatigue-induced errors.

The precise role of sleep deprivation on the specific end point of clinical outcomes remains unclear. A number of studies have identified consequences of sleep deprivation that could adversely impact the conduct of a safe anesthetic, including impaired cognition, short-term memory and clinical decision-making, prolonged reaction time, and reduced attention, vigilance, and performance. In a report by Howard et al.,[75] sleep-deprived residents managing a 4-hour simulated anesthetic demonstrated progressive impairment of alertness, mood, and performance and had longer response latency to vigilance probes. In a study of American anesthesia caregivers, more than 50% reported having committed an error in medical judgment that they attributed to fatigue.[76] And 58% of New Zealand anesthesiologists reported they had exceeded their self-defined limit for safe continuous administration of anesthesia, with 86% reporting that they had committed a fatigue-related error.[77] Similar reports of fatigue-related complications appear in the surgical literature with as many as 16% of preventable adverse surgical events attributed to surgeon fatigue.[78,79]

However, others have reported no evidence of suboptimal clinical management or poor outcomes from sleep-deprived clinicians. Chu et al.[80] found no increase in mortality or major morbidity in 4,000 consecutive cardiac surgical procedures performed by surgeons who had varying degrees of sleep (ranging from 0 to >6 hours) the night before surgery. Other studies of surgeons and critical care specialists corroborated these findings.[81,82]

Several factors help to explain the apparent disparity between reports of fatigue-related performance impairment and the failure to conclusively link these with medical errors or adverse outcomes. Sleep deprivation is often arbitrarily defined, with varying characterizations of the nonrested state. Also, there is great difficulty in eliminating confounding variables such as the impact of loss of continuity of care, errors occurring during "hand-offs" of patients, and the reallocation of many medical tasks from physicians to nonphysician providers. Finally, it can be difficult to extrapolate findings from simulation studies of volunteers in a laboratory to clinicians in real-life work conditions.

The health-care industry is slowly catching up with other industries, most notably the transport and airline industries, in identifying and regulating work practices that permit excessively long shifts. It was not until the well-publicized Libby Zion case in 1984 (which alleged that fatal, avoidable mistakes were made by exhausted, unsupervised residents) that medical organizations and state legislatures acted to limit excessive work hours among residents. In 2000, the Accreditation Council for Graduate Medical Education (ACGME) established the first set of standards to limit resident duty hours. These standards were revised by the ACGME in 2011 and updated in 2014.[83] The standards detail a list of work hours restrictions, including the well-known limit of 80 hours per week. Imposition of these standards has been controversial and a number of authors have commented on the failure of these changes to improve clinical outcomes. Somewhat ironically, at the end of a long list of duty hours restrictions, item VI.G.5.c states, "Residents in the final years of education must be prepared to enter the unsupervised practice of medicine and care for patients over irregular or extended periods." This statement recognizes that these restrictions on duty periods apply only to trainees and that work hours in medical practice remain unregulated.

Prolonged work hours and sleep deprivation are a ubiquitous component of many anesthesiologists' professional lives. Many academic faculty members now work longer hours than they did prior to house staff work hour limitations because of the shift of work from residents to faculty. A recent survey demonstrated an average work week of 57 hours among male and 51 hours among female American anesthesiologists.[84]

Several strategies have been devised to reduce fatigue and limit the adverse effects of sleep deprivation when long work periods are necessary. Recommendations include minimizing sleep debt by maximizing sleep before on-call shifts and utilizing maneuvers to overcome sleep inertia such as increasing ambient light levels, stretching, taking frequent breaks, and napping when possible. A number of pharmaceutical aids, such as caffeine and modafinil (a schedule IV drug), have been approved for military use and, if used under supervision and carefully monitored, may be helpful for clinicians with shift-work sleep disorder.[85]

Infectious Hazards

Anesthesia personnel are at risk for acquiring infections from patients, their families, and from numerous other personnel in the health-care workforce. This risk is likely to increase because as antimicrobial agents become more effective, the pathogens develop resistance and new survival strategies. Increasingly, immune-compromised patients become vectors for these resistant, opportunistic organisms. Furthermore, globalization brings increasing spread of organisms from less developed areas in the world, such as the 1999 outbreak in New York of West Nile Virus encephalitis and the 2003 epidemic of severe acute respiratory syndrome (SARS) in Hong Kong. Finally, diseases that were once thought to be noninfectious such as peptic ulcer disease (*Helicobacter pylori*), invasive cervical cancer (human papillomavirus), Kaposi's sarcoma (human herpesvirus type 8), and certain lymphomas such as Burkitt and non-Hodgkins (Epstein–Barr virus [EBV]) are now better understood as a long-term consequence of infection, making occupational health precautions even more important.

Viral infections are the most significant threat to medical personnel. Most commonly, these are spread through the respiratory route. Other infections are spread by hand-to-hand transmission and hand washing is the single most important protection strategy.[86] Immunity against some viral pathogens, such as hepatitis B, can be provided through vaccination.[87] Transmission of blood-borne pathogens such as hepatitis B virus (HBV), hepatitis C virus (HCV), and human immunodeficiency virus (HIV) can be prevented with mechanical barriers. Current recommendations from the Centers for Disease Control and Prevention (CDC) for pre-employment screening, infection control practices, vaccination, postexposure treatment, and work restrictions for infected personnel should be consulted for specific information related to each pathogen.[88,89]

OSHA Standards, Standard Precautions, and Transmission-based Precautions

In the late 1980s the CDC formulated recommendations ("universal precautions") for preventing transmission of blood-borne infections to medical personnel. The guidelines were based on the epidemiology of HBV as a worst-case model for transmission of blood-borne infections and available knowledge of the epidemiology of HIV and HCV. Since asymptomatic carriers of many blood-borne viruses cannot be identified, universal precautions were recommended for use during all patient contact. Although exposure to blood carries the greatest risk of occupationally related transmission of pathogens, it was recognized that universal precautions should also be applied to saliva, semen, vaginal secretions, human tissues, and cerebrospinal, synovial, pleural, peritoneal, pericardial, and amniotic fluids. Subsequently, the CDC aggregated the major features of universal precautions into "standard precautions" (Table 3-4) that should be applied to all patients,[90] now updated to include Ebola (Table 3-5).[91]

Table 3-4 Standard Precautions

Modes of Transmission

Direct contact transmission	Transmission of an infectious agent directly from one person to another; may occur via contact of blood or secretions with mucous membranes, open cuts, or mites.
Indirect contact transmission	Transmission of an infectious agent via an intermediate object (fomite) that has been previously contaminated. This may include (but is not limited to) patient-care devices, environmental surfaces, and clothing.

The particle size of emitted respiratory secretions is a continuum from aerosol size particles (≤5 μm) to droplets (>5 μm).

Droplet transmission	Droplets (>5 μm) remain suspended for short periods of time and tend to be deposited within 3 feet of where they are generated. The distance that a droplet travels may be affected by such things as temperature, humidity, and air currents. Droplets are preferentially deposited in the upper airways, whereas aerosols penetrate deeper into the lower respiratory tract.
Airborne transmission	Organisms that can remain infectious when disseminated over distance and time as the droplet nuclei (<5 μm particles) are dispersed on air currents.

Standard Precautions

Reduce the risk of transmission of infectious agents from patient to patient, patient to health-care worker (HCW), HCW to patient.

Apply to all patients, as anyone may be infected or colonized with a transmissible disease.

Wear gloves for all contact with blood, body fluids (except sweat), nonintact skin, and mucous membranes. Change gloves when they become soiled or when contact with a clean body part follows that with a contaminated part. Remove gloves after patient contact. Minimize environmental contamination.

Perform hand hygiene before patient contact and upon removal of gloves.

Gown, face, and eye protection should be worn if there is a risk of splash or spray.

Environmental cleaning after contamination by body substances.

Standard surgical mask when inserting a central line or performing neuraxial anesthesia.

Needle and sharp safety:
　Avoid recapping (when necessary, use one-handed technique).
　Avoid bending or breaking used sharps. Sharp disposal in puncture-resistant containers.

Practice and encourage respiratory hygiene/cough etiquette.

(continued)

Table 3-4 Standard Precautions (CONTINUED)

Contact Precautions (in addition to standard precautions)
- Signage outside room to indicate level of precautions.
- Gown and glove upon entering room and with any patient or environmental contact.
- Face and eye protection if there is a risk of splash or spray.
- Remove gloves and gown before exiting room. Avoid self-contamination when removing personal protective equipment (PPE).
- Perform hand hygiene after removal of PPE.
- Dedicated patient equipment whenever possible. Appropriately clean equipment prior to its use with other patients.
- Maintain contact precautions during transport and entire perioperative period.
- Communicate precaution level to those that will receive patient postoperatively.

Droplet Precautions (in addition to standard precautions)
- Single-patient room optimal. May cohort or keep patient with existing roommate when necessary.
- Spatial separation of patients of 3 feet. If curtain present, keep drawn.
- Signage outside room to indicate level of precautions.
- HCWs should wear standard surgical mask, gloves, gown, and eye protection as required under standard precautions.
- Patient should wear standard mask (if tolerated) when transport outside room required.
- Respiratory hygiene/cough etiquette.
- Maintain precautions throughout perioperative period.
- Communicate precaution level to those that will receive patient postoperatively.

Airborne Precautions (in addition to standard precautions)
- Place patient in an airborne infection isolation room (AIIR).
- Signage outside room to indicate level of precautions.
- N95 respirator or greater protection should be used when in the same room as the patient.
- Patient should remain in AIIR with door closed at all times, except for medically necessary procedures.
- Elective procedures should be postponed until patient no longer requires respiratory isolation.
- Patients should wear a standard surgical mask when transported outside the AIIR. The purpose of the mask is to prevent respiratory droplets from being expelled into the environment where they can become droplet nuclei.
- Operating rooms (ORs) are designed to have positive pressure in relation to the environment. Therefore, it is important to choose the most appropriate OR to minimize the risk of contaminating the OR suite. Options include the OR that is most remote from others, one with an antechamber, or installing a portable negative pressure isolation chamber at the OR door.
- The surgical procedure should be scheduled at a time when it will minimize exposure of other patients and medical staff to the airborne infectious disease.
- Postanesthesia recovery must take place with the same level of respiratory precautions.
- Communicate precaution level to receiving personnel.
- Room should remain vacant after the patient leaves until adequate time has elapsed to result in a 99.9% air turnover (duration dependent on number of air exchanges per hour in room).

Standard precautions include the appropriate application and use of hand washing, personal protective equipment (PPE), and respiratory hygiene/cough etiquette. The selection of specific barriers or PPE should be commensurate with the task being performed. Gloves may be sufficient during many procedures that involve contact with mucous membranes or oral fluids, such as routine endotracheal intubation or insertion of a peripheral intravenous catheter. However, additional personal protection, such as gown, mask, and face shield, may be required during endotracheal intubation when the patient has hematemesis or during bronchoscopy or endotracheal suctioning.

OSHA's Bloodborne Pathogens standard (29 CFR 1910.1030) prescribes safeguards to protect workers against the health hazards caused by blood-borne pathogens.[92] These standards require an exposure control plan specifically detailing the methods that the employer is providing to reduce employees' risk of exposure to blood-borne pathogens. The employer must encourage strategies to reduce blood exposures, furnish appropriate PPE (e.g., gloves, gowns), offer the HBV vaccine at no charge to personnel, and provide an annual education program to inform employees of their risk for blood-borne infection. Congressional testimony by OSHA reported an order of magnitude decrease in hepatitis B infection in a span of 8 years (1987–1995).[93]

The institution's employee health service is required to obtain and record a contagious disease history from new employees and provide immunizations and annual purified protein derivative (PPD) skin testing. In addition, the employee health service must have protocols for dealing with workers exposed to contagious diseases and those exposed to the blood of patients infected with HIV or HBV or HCV. Free consultation is available from the CDC Post-Exposure Prophylaxis Hotline (PEPline) at 1-888-448(HIV)-4911.

Table 3-5 Ebola Precautions

Ebola Hemorrhagic Fever

Site(s) of infection; transmission mode	As a rule infection develops after exposure of mucous membranes or RT, or through broken skin or percutaneous injury.
Incubation period	2–19 days, usually 5–10 days
Clinical features	Febrile illnesses with malaise, myalgias, headache, vomiting, and diarrhea that are rapidly complicated by hypotension, shock, and hemorrhagic features. Massive hemorrhage in <50% patients.
Diagnosis	Etiologic diagnosis can be made using RT-PCR, serologic detection of antibody and antigen, pathologic assessment with immunohistochemistry, and viral culture with EM confirmation of morphology.
Infectivity	Person-to-person transmission primarily occurs through unprotected contact with blood and body fluids; percutaneous injuries (e.g., needlestick) associated with a high rate of transmission; transmission in health-care settings has been reported but is prevented by use of barrier precautions.
Recommended precautions	Hemorrhagic fever-specific barrier precautions: If disease is believed to be related to intentional release of a bioweapon, epidemiology of transmission is unpredictable pending observation of disease transmission. Until the nature of the pathogen is understood and its transmission pattern confirmed, Standard, Contact, and Airborne Precautions should be used (see Table 3-4). Once the pathogen is characterized, if the epidemiology of transmission is consistent with natural disease, Droplet Precautions can be substituted for Airborne Precautions. Emphasize (1) use of sharps safety devices and safe work practices; (2) hand hygiene; (3) barrier protection against blood and body fluids upon entry into room (single gloves and fluid-resistant or impermeable gown, face/eye protection with masks, goggles or face shields); and (4) appropriate waste handling. Use N95 or higher respirators when performing aerosol-generating procedures. In settings where AIIRs are unavailable or the large numbers of patients cannot be accommodated by existing AIIRs, observe Droplet Precautions (plus Standard Precautions and Contact Precautions) and segregate patients from those not suspected of VHF infection. Limit blood draws to those essential to care.

Source: Infection Prevention and Control Recommendations for Hospitalized Patients Under Investigation (PUIs) for Ebola Virus Disease (EVD) in U.S. Hospitals (last reviewed January 24, 2016). http://www.cdc.gov/vhf/ebola/healthcare-us/hospitals/infection-control.html. RT, respiratory tract; PCR, polymerase chain reaction; EM, electron microscopy; AIIR, airborne infection isolation room; VHF, viral hemorrhagic fever.

Respiratory Viruses

Respiratory viruses account for half or more of all acute illnesses and are usually transmitted by one of two routes. Small-particle aerosols from viruses such as influenza and measles are produced by coughing, sneezing, or talking and can be propelled over large distances. Large droplets that have been produced by coughing or sneezing can contaminate the donor's hands or an inanimate surface. The virus is then transferred to the oral, nasal, or conjunctival mucous membranes of a susceptible person by self-inoculation. Rhinovirus and human respiratory syncytial virus (HRSV) are spread by this process.

Influenza Viruses

Influenza viruses (Orthomyxoviridae) are designated as type A, B, or C based on characteristics of the nucleoprotein (NP) and matrix (M) protein antigens. Influenza A viruses are subtyped on the basis of the surface hemagglutinin (H) and neuraminidase (N) antigens. Individual strains are designated according to the site of origin, isolate number, year of isolation, and subtype, for example, influenza A/California/07/2009 (the infamous H1N1 of 2009). Influenza A has 18 H subtypes and 11 N subtypes, of which only H1, H2, H3, N1, and N2 have been associated with epidemics of disease in humans. Influenza B viruses are not divided into subtypes but rather lineages and strains, whereas influenza C infections cause mild respiratory illness but are not associated with epidemics. Acutely ill patients shed virus for as long as 5 days after the onset of symptoms via small-particle aerosols. Because of their contact with nasopharyngeal secretions, anesthesiologists can easily become victims as well as vectors in the spread of influenza.

Influenza A (H1N1 or H3N2) and one or two influenza B viruses (depending on the vaccine) are included in each year's influenza vaccine. The CDC (Advisory Committee on Immunization Practices and the Healthcare Infection Control Practices Advisory Committee) recommends that all US health-care workers be immunized annually with the inactivated (killed virus) influenza virus vaccine. Through the efforts of the Society for Healthcare Epidemiology of America, there is evolving precedent to make this a condition of employment and medical staff credentialing.[94,95] Since the vaccine used in the United States and many other countries is produced in eggs, individuals with true hypersensitivity to egg products should be either desensitized or not vaccinated. A live attenuated influenza vaccine, approved for use in healthy nonpregnant persons 2 to 49 years of age and administered by intranasal spray, is now available. Inclusion and exclusion criteria are listed at http://www.cdc.gov/flu/about/qa/nasalspray.htm.

Influenza Pandemics

Influenza outbreaks occur almost every year, although their extent and severity vary widely. In the past century there have been three influenza pandemics (1918, 1957, and 1968) with the "Great Influenza" in 1918 killing between 40 and 50 million people worldwide. The most recent pandemic emerged in March 2009 and was caused by an influenza A/H1N1 virus that rapidly spread worldwide over several months. Containment requires early identification and isolation of infected individuals.

NIOSH-certified respirators (N95 or higher) should be used by personnel during activities or procedures likely to generate infectious respiratory aerosols.

Avian Influenza A

In 1997, human cases of influenza caused by avian influenza viruses (A/H5N1) were detected in Hong Kong during an extensive outbreak of influenza in poultry. Approximately 850 human cases have subsequently been reported worldwide with a mortality of more than 50%, nearly all associated with contact with infected poultry. Efficient person-to-person transmission has not been observed. Because of the absence of widespread immunity to the H5, H7, and H9 viruses, concern persists that avian-to-human transmission might contribute to the emergence of a pandemic strain.[96] A vaccine for prophylaxis against avian influenza H5N1 was approved for use in the United States in 2007.

Human Respiratory Syncytial Virus

HRSV is the most common cause of serious bronchiolitis and lower respiratory tract disease in infants and young children worldwide. During periods when HRSV is prevalent in the community (late November through May in the United States), many hospitalized infants and children may carry the virus. Large amounts of virus are present in respiratory secretions of infected children. Viable virus can be recovered for up to 6 hours on contaminated environmental surfaces. The virus is readily inactivated with soap and water and disinfectants. Infection of susceptible people occurs by self-inoculation when HRSV in secretions is transferred to the hands, which then contact the mucous membranes of the eyes or nose. Although most children have been exposed to HRSV early in life, immunity is not permanent and reinfection is common. HRSV may also be a significant cause of illness in healthy elderly patients and those with chronic cardiac or pulmonary disease.[96] HRSV is shed for approximately 7 days after infection. Careful hand washing and the use of standard precautions have been shown to reduce HRSV infection in hospital personnel.

Severe Acute Respiratory Syndrome

SARS is a respiratory tract infection produced by SARS-associated coronavirus (SARS-CoV). SARS typically presents with a fever greater than 38°C followed by symptoms of headache, generalized aches, and cough. Severe pneumonia may lead to acute respiratory distress syndrome and death. The mechanisms of transmission of SARS are incompletely understood. Spread may occur by both large and small aerosols and perhaps by the fecal–oral route, as well as close person-to-person contact. Aerosolization of respiratory secretions during coughing or endotracheal suctioning has been associated with transmission of the disease to medical personnel, including anesthesiologists and critical care nurses.[97] After the first cases were reported from Asia in late 2002, the disease quickly spread globally in 2003 before being controlled. Since 2004, global surveillance for SARS-CoV has detected no confirmed cases.

Enteric Infections

Diarrheal disease is second only to lower respiratory tract infections as the most common infectious cause of death worldwide. Infectious agents include viruses, bacteria, and parasites, acting via noninflammatory (enterotoxin), inflammatory (cytotoxin), or penetrating mechanisms. Traveler's diarrhea is the most common travel-related infectious illness (20% to 50%), with *Escherichia coli* the most common organism. Rotavirus is most common among children less than 2 years of age, especially children in day care. Rotavirus can spread rapidly in day care centers and pediatric wards. *Giardia lamblia* is more common in older children, as is norovirus, and there is a high rate of secondary cases among family members. *Clostridium difficile* is the main cause of nosocomial diarrhea among adult inpatients in the United States. One-third of elderly patients in nursing homes develop a significant diarrheal illness each year, and more than half of these are caused by *C. difficile,* especially following antibiotic therapy. Personal hygiene on the part of clinicians is directed to limiting secondary fecal–oral spread.

DNA Viruses

Herpes simplex viruses (HSV-1, HSV-2; *Herpesvirus hominis*) produce a variety of infections involving mucocutaneous surfaces, central nervous system (CNS), and visceral organs. Exposure to HSV at mucosal surfaces or abraded skin allows entry of the virus and initiation of viral replication. The primary infection with HSV type 1 is usually clinically inapparent but may involve severe oral lesions, fever, and adenopathy. After the primary infection subsides, the latent virus persists within the sensory nerve ganglion. Gingivostomatitis and pharyngitis are the most common clinical manifestations of first-episode HSV-1 infection, whereas recurrent herpes labialis is the most common clinical manifestation of reactivation HSV-2. Herpetic whitlow—HSV infection of the finger—may occur as a complication of primary oral or genital herpes by inoculation of virus through a break in the epidermal surface or by direct introduction of virus into the hand, a particularly important point for medical personnel. HSV infection of the eye is a common cause of corneal blindness in the United States. Of all HSV-infected populations, infants younger than 6 weeks have the highest frequency of visceral and/or CNS infection. Of note for obstetrical anesthesia practice, antibody to HSV-2 has been detected in 32% of pregnant women with no history of genital herpes. Asymptomatic HSV shedding was detected in 0.43% of women in late pregnancy and during delivery, and a first episode of clinical genital herpes was recognized by 16% of women during their pregnancy.[98] Medical personnel may be inoculated by direct contact with body fluids laden with either HSV type 1 or 2.

Varicella–zoster virus (VZV) causes two distinct clinical diseases: varicella (chickenpox) and zoster (shingles). Chickenpox, ubiquitous and highly contagious, is usually a benign illness of childhood with transmission by the respiratory route. Reactivation of latent VZV (herpes zoster), most common after the sixth decade of life, presents as a markedly painful dermatomal vesicular rash. Infection during pregnancy may result in fetal death or (rarely) congenital defects. Patients and medical personnel with active VZV infection can transmit the virus to others. Anesthesiologists working in pain clinics may be exposed to VZV when caring for patients who have discomfort from herpes zoster. Communicability begins 1 to 2 days before the onset of the rash and ends when all the lesions are crusted, usually 4 to 6 days after the rash appears.[99] Respiratory isolation should be used for patients with chickenpox or disseminated herpes zoster.[90] Use of gloves to avoid contact with vesicular fluid is adequate to prevent VZV spread from patients with localized herpes zoster.

Most adults in the United States have protective antibodies to VZV. Since there have been many reports of nosocomial transmission of VZV, it is recommended that all medical personnel have immunity to the virus. Anesthesia personnel with a negative or unknown history of infection should consider being serologically tested.[99] All medical personnel with negative titers should be restricted from caring for patients with active VZV infection and should be offered immunization with two doses of the live, attenuated varicella vaccine.

Susceptible personnel with a significant exposure to an individual with VZV infection are potentially infective from 10 to 21 days after exposure and should not contact patients during this period. The postexposure period during which a patient may receive varicella–zoster immune globulin (VariZIG) was recently increased from 4 to 10 days, although VariZIG should be administered as soon as possible after exposure.[100]

EBV, also a member of the family *Herpesviridae*, is the cause of heterophile-positive infectious mononucleosis, characterized by fever, sore throat, lymphadenopathy, and atypical lymphocytosis. About 15% of cases of Burkitt lymphoma in the United States and 90% of those in Africa are associated with EBV.[101] Anaplastic nasopharyngeal carcinoma is common in southern China and is uniformly associated with EBV. EBV has also been associated with Hodgkin disease, especially the mixed-cellularity type.

EBV is spread by contact with oral secretions. The virus is frequently transmitted from asymptomatic adults to infants and among young adults by transfer of saliva during kissing. Transmission by less intimate contact is rare. EBV has been transmitted by blood transfusion and bone marrow transplantation. More than 90% of asymptomatic seropositive individuals shed the virus in oropharyngeal secretions.

Cytomegalovirus (CMV) infects between 50% and 85% of individuals in the United States before age 40, with most infections producing minimal symptoms.[102] After the primary infection, the virus remains dormant, and recurrent disease only occurs with compromise of the individual's immune system. CMV is not readily spread by casual contact but rather by repeated or prolonged intimate exposure. It is unlikely that aerosols or small droplets play a role in CMV transmission.

Primary or recurrent CMV infection during pregnancy results in fetal infection in up to 2.5% of occurrences.[103] Congenital CMV syndrome may be found in up to 10% of infected infants. Thus, although CMV infection usually does not result in morbidity in healthy adults, it may have significant sequelae in pregnant women, and therefore becomes an occupational health concern for medical personnel.

The two major populations with CMV infection in the hospital include affected infants and immunocompromised patients. Routine infection control procedures (standard precautions) are sufficient to prevent CMV infection in health-care personnel.[104] Pregnant personnel should be made aware of the risks associated with CMV infection during pregnancy and of appropriate infection control precautions to be used when caring for high-risk patients.

Rubella

Although most adults in the United States are immune to rubella, up to 20% of women of childbearing age are still susceptible, allowing the potential for viral replication in the placenta and infection of fetal organs (congenital rubella syndrome [CRS]). The infection is persistent throughout fetal development and for up to 1 year after birth. Therefore, only individuals immune to rubella should have contact with infants who have CRS or who are congenitally infected with rubella virus but are not showing signs of CRS.[105]

Rubella is transmitted by contact with nasopharyngeal droplets spread by infected individuals through coughing or sneezing. Patients are most contagious while the rash is erupting but can transmit the virus from 1 week before to 5 to 7 days after the onset of the rash. Droplet precautions should be used to prevent transmission (Table 3-6).[90]

History is a poor indicator of immunity. Therefore, ensuring immunity at the time of employment (evidence of prior vaccination with live rubella vaccine or serologic confirmation) should prevent nosocomial transmission of rubella to personnel. A live, attenuated rubella virus vaccine (measles, mumps, rubella [MMR]) is available to produce immunity in susceptible personnel.[106] Many state or local health departments mandate rubella immunity for all medical personnel, and local regulations should be consulted.

Measles (Rubeola)

Measles virus is highly transmissible by large droplets and by the airborne route. The virus is found in the mucus of the nose and pharynx of the infected individual and is spread by coughing and sneezing. The disease can be transmitted from 4 days prior to the onset of the rash to 4 days after its onset. Airborne precautions should be used for infected patients (Table 3-6).[90,104] Secondary attack rates in susceptible household and institutional contacts generally exceed 90%.[107] In 2014, a record number of measles cases were reported in the United States, with 668 cases from 27 states reported to CDC's National Center for Immunization and Respiratory Diseases (NCIRD).[108] This is the greatest number of cases since measles elimination was prematurely reported in the United States in 2000. From January to August 2015, 188 people from 24 states and the District of Columbia were reported to have measles.[108] More than half of these cases were part of a large multistate outbreak linked to an amusement park in California.[108]

Medical settings are well-recognized sites of measles virus transmission. Highly infectious children may present to healthcare facilities during the prodrome when the diagnosis is not yet obvious. Medical personnel are at increased risk for acquiring measles and transmitting the virus to susceptible coworkers and patients. The CDC recommends that medical personnel have adequate immunity to measles, as documented by one of the following: evidence of two doses of live measles vaccine, a record of physician-diagnosed measles, or serologic evidence of measles immunity (Table 3-6).[106] Susceptible personnel born in or after 1957 should receive two doses of the live measles vaccine at the time of employment.[109]

Viral Hepatitis

Many viruses produce hepatitis. The most common are type A (infectious hepatitis), type B (HBV, serum hepatitis), and type C (HCV and non-A, non-B hepatitis [NANBH]), which is responsible for most cases of parenterally transmitted hepatitis in the United States. Delta hepatitis (HDV), caused by an incomplete virus, occurs only in people infected with HBV. Hepatitis E virus (HEV), previously labeled epidemic or enterically transmitted NANBH, is an enterically transmitted virus that occurs primarily in India, Asia, Africa, and Central America. In these locations, HEV is the most common cause of acute hepatitis. All types of viral hepatitis produce clinically similar illnesses. These range from asymptomatic and inapparent to fulminant and fatal infections, as well as subclinical to chronic persistent liver disease with cirrhosis and hepatocellular carcinoma, common to the blood-borne types (HBV, HCV, and HDV). The greatest risks of occupational transmission to anesthesia personnel are associated with HBV and HCV (Table 3-7).

(text continued on page 78)

Table 3-6 Prevention of Occupationally Acquired Infections

Infection/Condition	Precautions	Comments
Abscess		
Draining/major	Contact	
Draining/minor	Standard	
Acquired immune deficiency virus (HIV)	Standard	Postexposure prophylaxis (PEP) for some exposures
Avian influenza	Droplet	Enhanced precautions (i.e., airborne may be recommended)
Bronchiolitis	Contact	
Clostridium		
botulinum	Standard	Not transmitted person to person
difficile	Contact	
perfringens	Standard	Not transmitted person to person
Conjunctivitis		
Bacterial	Standard	
Viral	Contact	Most commonly: adenovirus, enterovirus, coxsackievirus A24
Creutzfeldt–Jakob disease	Standard	Single-use equipment preferred, special cleaning (NaOH, heat, and time requirements) for contaminated instruments and environment
Diphtheria, pharyngeal	Droplet	Until two cultures >24 h apart are negative
Escherichia coli	Standard	Contact precautions if patient incontinent
Haemophilus influenzae		
Seasonal	Droplet	Single-patient room or cohort, gown, and glove
Pandemic	Droplet	Enhanced precautions (airborne may be recommended)
Hepatitis, viral		
A	Standard	Contact precautions for incontinent patients
B	Standard	
C	Standard	
E	Standard	Contact precautions for incontinent patients
Herpes, zoster (varicella-zoster)		
Disseminated	Airborne, contact	Health-care workers (HCWs) without immunity should not care for patient if immune HCW available.
Localized	Standard	
Impetigo	Contact	
Legionnaires' disease	Standard	Not transmitted person to person
Lice		
Head	Contact	
Body	Standard	
Pubic	Standard	
Lyme disease	Standard	
Malaria	Standard	
Measles	Airborne	Susceptible HCW should not care for patient if immune HCW available. Maintain precautions for 4 days after onset of rash. Nonimmune exposed individuals may be infectious from days 5 to 21 after exposure. PEP available (vaccine, immune globulin).
Meningitis		
Bacterial	Standard	
Fungal	Standard	
Neisseria	Droplet	
Streptococcus	Standard	PEP available
Multidrug-resistant organisms (MDROs: MRSA, VRE, VISA/VRSA, ESBLs, resistant *Streptococcus pneumoniae*)	Standard/contact	

Table 3-6 Prevention of Occupationally Acquired Infections (CONTINUED)

Infection/Condition	Precautions	Comments
Mumps	Droplet	Susceptible HCWs should not care for patient if immune HCW available.
Mycoplasma	Droplet	
Mycobacterium tuberculosis	Airborne	
Parainfluenza	Contact	
Pertussis	Droplet	Single-patient room or cohort. PEP available. Tdap recommended
Poliomyelitis	Contact	
Rabies	Standard	
Respiratory syncytial virus	Contact	Standard mask should be worn.
Rhinovirus	Droplet	
Rubella	Droplet	Susceptible HCW should not care for patient if immune HCW available. Vaccine available. Nonimmune exposed individuals may be contagious from days 5–21 after exposure.
Salmonella	Standard	Contact precautions for incontinent patients
SARS-CoV	Airborne, droplet, contact	Maintain precautions until 10 days after resolution of fever.
Shigella	Standard	Contact precautions for incontinent patients
Smallpox	Airborne, contact	Maintain precautions until all scabs have crusted and separated (3–4 wks). Nonvaccinated HCW should not care for patient if immune HCW available
Staphylococcal		
Major, wound	Contact	
Streptococcal		
Major, wound	Contact, droplet	

MRSA, methicillin-resistant *Staphylococcus aureus;* VRE, vancomycin-resistant enterococci; VISA/VRSA, vancomycin-intermediate/resistant *Staphylococcus aureus;* ESBL, extended-spectrum beta-lactamase–producing organisms; SARS-CoV, severe acute respiratory syndrome-associated corona virus.
Adapted from CDC Guideline for Isolation Precautions: Preventing Transmission of Infectious Agents in Healthcare Settings, 2007. For a complete list of organisms, see Appendix A. Type and duration of precautions recommended for selected infections and conditions: http://www.cdc.gov/ncidod/dhqp/pdf/guidelines/Isolation2007.pdf.

Table 3-7 Risk of Occupational Infection with Blood-Borne Pathogens

1. The greatest risk of transmission of blood-borne infections with HIV, HBV, and HCV is from a blood-contaminated percutaneous injury.
2. The risk depends on the type of pathogen involved and increases when the source patient has higher viral titers (for HIV, HBV, HCV, respectively: acute or terminal HIV illness; hepatitis Be antigen–positive source; increased HCV RNA titers) and with increased quantity of inoculum volume transferred from the patient source.

Average risk after an accidental parenteral exposure (needlestick or cut):

	Clinical hepatitis risk	Seroconversion risk
Known HIV-infected patient	0.3%[a]	
Known hepatitis B surface antigen (HBsAg) positive/hepatitis Be antigen (HBeAg) negative	1–6%	23–37%
Known hepatitis B surface antigen (HBsAg) positive/hepatitis Be antigen (HBeAg) positive	22–31%	37–62%
Known hepatitis C positive		0.3–0.74%[b]

[a]Exceeds 0.3% for an exposure involving a greater infectious dose resulting from transfer of a larger blood volume, a higher HIV titer in the source patient's blood, or both. (Updated U.S. Public Health Service Guidelines for the Management of Occupational Exposures to HBV, HCV, and HIV and Recommendations for Postexposure Prophylaxis.)
[b]Jagger J, Puro V, De Carli G. Occupational transmission of hepatitis C virus. *JAMA.* 2002;288:1469.

Hepatitis A virus is the cause of about 20% to 40% of viral hepatitis in adults in the United States. Hepatitis A is usually a self-limited illness, and no chronic carrier state exists. Spread is predominantly by the fecal–oral route, either by person-to-person contact or by ingestion of contaminated food or water. Outbreaks are usually found in institutions or other closed groups where there has been a breakdown in normal sanitary conditions. Hospital personnel do not appear to be at increased risk for hepatitis A and nosocomial transmission is rare. Personnel exposed to patients with hepatitis A should receive immune globulin intramuscularly as soon as possible but not more than 2 weeks after the exposure to reduce the likelihood of infection.[110]

Hepatitis B is a significant occupational hazard for nonimmune anesthesiologists and other medical personnel who have frequent contact with blood and blood products. The prevalence of hepatitis B in the United States during 1999 to 2006 (anti-HBc = 4.7% and hepatitis B surface antigen [HBsAg] = 0.27%) was not statistically different from what it was during 1988 to 1994 (5.4% and 0.38%, respectively).[111] Following a decline since 1990 as a result primarily of effective vaccination, in 2013 the number of acute cases increased by 5.4% in the United States.[111] Although the increase may reflect the growing number of drug-related and health-care–related outbreaks associated with hepatitis B transmission, it is probably too early to interpret the causes.[111]

Acute HBV infection may be asymptomatic and usually resolves without significant hepatic damage. Less than 1% of acutely infected patients develop fulminant hepatitis.[112] Approximately 10% become chronic carriers of HBV (serologic evidence for >6 months). Within 2 years, half of the chronic carriers resolve their infection without significant hepatic impairment. Chronic active hepatitis, which may progress to cirrhosis and is linked to hepatocellular carcinoma, is found most commonly in individuals with chronic viral infection for more than 2 years.

The diagnosis and staging of HBV infection are made on the basis of serologic testing. The first marker is detectable in serum within 1 to 12 weeks (HBsAg). HBsAg becomes undetectable 1 to 2 months after the onset of jaundice and rarely persists beyond 6 months. After HBsAg disappears, antibody to HBsAg (anti-HBs) becomes detectable in serum and remains detectable indefinitely. Antibody to the surface antigen (anti-HBs) appears with resolution of the acute infection and confers lasting immunity against subsequent HBV infections (Fig. 3-1). Chronic HBV carriers are likely to have HBsAg and antibody to the core antigen (anti-HBc) present in serum samples. The presence of hepatitis B e antigen (HBeAg) in serum is indicative of active viral replication in hepatocytes.

Anesthesia personnel are at risk for occupationally acquired HBV infection as a result of accidental percutaneous or mucosal contact with blood or body fluids from infected patients. Patient groups with a high prevalence of HBV include immigrants from endemic areas, users of illicit parenteral drugs, homosexual men, and patients on hemodialysis.[112] Carriers are frequently not identified during hospitalization because the clinical history and routine preoperative laboratory tests may be insufficient for diagnosis. The risk for infection after an HBV-contaminated percutaneous exposure, such as an accidental needlestick, is 37% to 62% if the source patient is HBeAg-positive and 23% to 37% if HBeAg-negative (Table 3-7).[112] HBV can be found in saliva, but the rate of transmission is significantly less after mucosal contact with infected oral secretions than after percutaneous exposures to blood. HBV is a hardy virus that may be infectious for at least 1 week in dried blood on environmental surfaces.

Hepatitis B vaccine is the primary strategy to prevent occupational transmission of HBV to anesthesia personnel and other

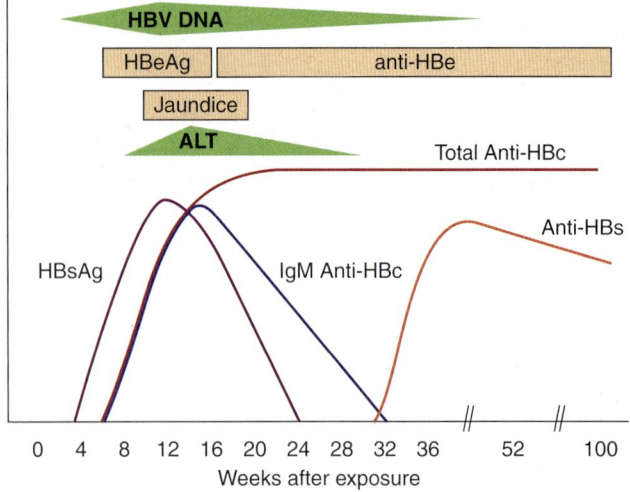

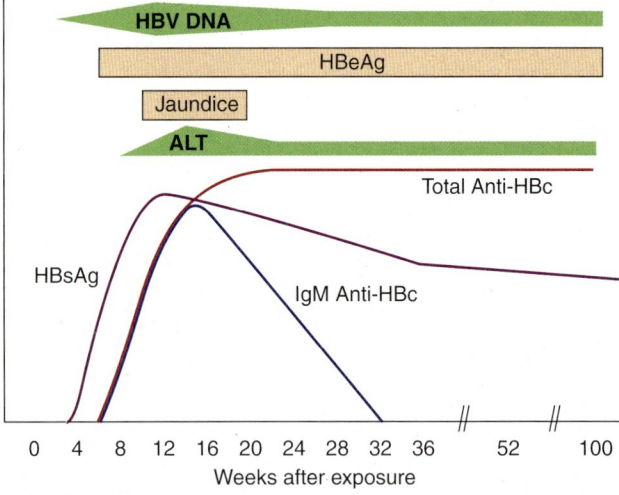

Figure 3-1 Clinical course and serologic profiles of acute and chronic hepatitis B. ALT, alanine aminotransferase. (Modified from Liang T. Hepatitis B: the virus and disease. *Hepatology*. 2009;49[5]:S13–S21.)

health personnel at increased risk. Administration of three doses of vaccine results in the production of protective antibodies (anti-HBs) in more than 90% of healthy personnel. Hospitals or anesthesia departments should have policies for educating, screening, and counseling personnel about their risk of acquiring HBV infection and should make vaccination available for susceptible personnel.[113] If adequate postvaccination immunity is not confirmed, a second three-dose vaccine series should be administered. Nonresponders to vaccination remain at risk for HBV infection and should be counseled on strategies to prevent infections and the need for postexposure prophylaxis (PEP). Vaccine-induced antibodies decline over time. The CDC states that for vaccinated adults with normal immune status, routine booster doses are not necessary and periodic monitoring of antibody concentration is not recommended.[113]

HCV causes most cases of parenterally transmitted NANBH and is a leading cause of chronic liver disease in the United States. Although antibody to HCV (anti-HCV) can be detected in most patients with hepatitis C, its presence does not correlate with resolution of the acute infection or progression of hepatitis, and it does not confer immunity against HCV infection.[114] Seropositivity for HCV RNA is a marker of chronic infection and continued viral presence. After HCV seroconversion, only 15% to 25% will clear the virus spontaneously.[115] Of those that develop chronic hepatitis, 20% will develop cirrhosis over the following 20 to 30 years and 1% to 2% of those will be diagnosed with hepatocellular carcinoma.[115]

Like HBV, HCV is transmitted through blood, but the rate of occupational HCV infection is less than for HBV. Although HCV transmission has been documented in health-care settings, the prevalence of anti-HCV in medical personnel in the United States is not greater than that found in the general population (1.6%).[113] The greatest risk of occupational HCV transmission is associated with exposure to blood from an HCV-positive source. HCV has been transmitted through blood splashes to the eye and with exposure via nonintact skin. HCV in dried blood on environmental surfaces may remain infectious for up to 16 hours, but environmental contamination does not appear to be a common route of transmission. HCV can be found in the saliva of infected individuals, but it is not believed to represent a great risk for occupational transmission.[113]

Prevention of exposure remains the primary strategy for protection against HCV infection. Personnel who have had a percutaneous or mucosal exposure to HCV-positive blood should have counseling and serologic testing in accordance with the guidelines in the section on Postexposure Treatment and Prophylactic Antiretroviral Therapy.[116]

Pathogenic Human Retroviruses

The family *Retroviridae* includes seven subfamilies, two of which produce disease in humans—human T lymphotropic viruses (HTLV)-I and HTLV-II, which are transforming retroviruses, and HIV-1 and HIV-2, which cause cytopathic effects either directly or indirectly. Tissue destruction may result directly from the viral infection or indirectly from malignant transformation of infected cells and an immune-deficient state in response to the virus, leading to neoplastic and infectious disease. HTLV-I infection is transmitted in at least three ways: from mother to child (especially via breast milk), through sexual activity, and parenterally via contaminated transfusions or contaminated needles. At the end of 2014, an estimated 36.9 million individuals were living with HIV infection according to the Joint United Nations Programme on HIV/AIDS (UNAIDS).[117] The global prevalence has increased approximately fourfold since 1990, reflecting the combined effects of continued high rates of new HIV infections and the beneficial (life-prolonging) impact of antiretroviral therapy. In 2014, there were an estimated 2 million new cases of HIV infection worldwide, including 220,000 in children under 15 years.[117] Approximately 1.1 million individuals in the United States are living with HIV infection; almost 20% are unaware of their infection.

The initial infection with HIV begins as a mononucleosis-like syndrome with lymphadenopathy and rash. Although the patient then enters an asymptomatic period, monocyte–macrophage cells serve as a viral reservoir and CD4+ T cells harbor the virus in the blood. Within a few weeks, an antibody may be detected by an enzyme immunoassay or rapid HIV antibody test, but a positive result must be confirmed using Western blot or immunofluorescent assay. After a variable length period of asymptomatic HIV infection, there is an increase in viral titer and impaired host immunity, resulting in opportunistic infections and malignancies characteristic of Acquired Immune Deficiency Syndrome (AIDS).

Risk of Occupational HIV Infection

There is a small but definite occupational risk of HIV transmission to medical personnel, laboratory personnel, and others who work with HIV-containing materials. An estimated 600,000 to 800,000 medical personnel are stuck with needles or other sharp medical instruments in the United States each year. Exposures that place personnel at potential risk of HIV infection are percutaneous injuries (a needlestick or cut with a sharp object) or contact of mucous membrane or nonintact skin with blood, tissue, or other potentially infectious body fluids. The risk of HIV transmission following skin puncture from a contaminated needle or a sharp object is 0.3% and after a mucous membrane exposure it is 0.09% if the injured and/or exposed person is not treated within 24 hours with antiretroviral drugs.[118] HIV transmission after nonintact skin exposure has been documented, but the average risk for transmission by this route has not been precisely determined. Transmission of HIV through intact skin has not been documented.

In the United States between 1985 and 2013, 58 medical personnel, for whom case investigations were completed, had confirmed seroconversions to HIV following occupational exposures; an additional 150 possible cases of occupationally acquired HIV infection were reported to CDC.[119] Since 1999, only one case has been reported. The routes of exposure were 49 percutaneous (puncture/cut injury); 5 mucocutaneous (mucous membrane and/or skin); 2 both percutaneous and mucocutaneous; and 2 of unknown route. The individuals with documented seroconversions included 20 laboratory workers (16 in clinical laboratories), 24 nurses, 6 physicians (nonsurgical), 2 surgical technicians, 1 dialysis technician, 1 respiratory therapist, 1 health aide, 1 embalmer/morgue technician, and 2 housekeeper/maintenance workers.[119]

Anesthesia personnel are frequently exposed to blood and body fluids during invasive procedures such as insertion of vascular catheters, arterial punctures, and endotracheal intubation.[120-122] Although many exposures are mucocutaneous and can be prevented by the use of PPE, these barriers do not prevent percutaneous exposures. Because of the tasks they perform, anesthesia personnel are likely to use and be injured by large-bore, hollow needles such as intravenous catheter stylets and needles on syringes. Needleless or protected needle safety devices can be used to replace standard devices to reduce the risk of needlestick injuries. Safety devices usually are more expensive than a comparable nonsafety item but may be more cost-effective when the financial cost of needlestick injury investigation and medical care for infected personnel is considered.

The occupational risk of HIV infection is a function of the annual number of blood exposures, the rate of HIV transmission with each exposure to infected blood, and the prevalence of HIV infection in the specific patient population. Greene et al.[120] prospectively collected data on 138 contaminated percutaneous injuries to anesthesia personnel. The rate of contaminated percutaneous injuries per year per full-time equivalent anesthesia worker was 0.42, and the average annual risk of HIV and HCV infection was estimated to be 0.0016% (0.16:10,000) and 0.015% (1.5:10,000), respectively.

Although HIV can be recovered in low titers from saliva in a small number of infected subjects, there is no convincing evidence that saliva can transmit HIV infection, either through kissing or through other exposures, such as those that occur occupationally. Saliva contains several antiviral factors including

HIV-specific immunoglobulins (IgA, IgG, and IgM isotypes). Moreover, there is no evidence that HIV transmission can occur as a result of exposure to tears, sweat, or urine. However, there have been isolated cases of transmission of HIV infection by body fluids that may or may not have been contaminated with blood.

Since the beginning of the HIV epidemic, there have been rare instances where transmission of infection from a medical personnel to patients seemed highly probable. An HIV-infected dentist in Florida may have infected as many as six of his patients, putatively through contaminated instruments.[123,124] Nevertheless, the risk of HIV transmission from medical personnel to patient is extremely low.

Postexposure Treatment and Prophylactic Antiretroviral Therapy

When personnel have been exposed to patients' blood or body fluids, the incident should immediately be reported to the employee health service or the designated individual within the institution. Based on the nature of the injury, the exposed worker and the source individual should be tested for serologic evidence of HIV, HBV, and HCV infection.[118] Current local laws must be consulted to determine policies for testing the source patient, and confidentiality must be maintained. U.S. Public Health Service recommendations include[118]:

1. PEP is recommended when occupational exposures to HIV occur.
2. The HIV status of the exposure source patient should be determined, if possible, to guide need for HIV PEP.
3. PEP medication regimens should be started as soon as possible after occupational exposure to HIV, and they should be continued for a 4-week duration.
4. PEP medication regimens should contain three (or more) antiretroviral drugs for all occupational exposures to HIV.
5. Expert consultation is recommended for any occupational exposures to HIV.
6. Close follow-up for exposed personnel should be provided that includes counseling, baseline and follow-up HIV testing, and monitoring for drug toxicity; follow-up appointments should begin within 72 hours of an HIV exposure.
7. If a newer fourth-generation combination HIV p24 antigen–HIV antibody test is utilized for follow-up HIV testing of the exposed medical personnel, HIV testing may be concluded 4 months after exposure; if a newer testing platform is not available, follow-up HIV testing is typically concluded 6 months after an HIV exposure.

The World Health Organization (WHO), in a push for early treatment and prevention, has revised its guidelines toward earlier treatment (as soon as possible after diagnosis) in substantially at-risk rather than high-risk individuals (pre-exposure prophylaxis [PrEP]) following the successful clinical trial of emtricitabine/tenofovir (Truvada).[125]

Failure of PEP has been attributed to a large viral inoculum, use of a single antiviral agent, drug resistance in the virus from the source patient, and delayed initiation or short duration of PEP therapy. For consultation on the treatment of occupational exposures to HIV and other blood-borne pathogens, the clinician managing the exposed patient can call the National Clinicians' Post-Exposure Prophylaxis Hotline (PEPline) at 1-888-448-4911.

Prion Diseases

Prions (from *pro*tein + infect*ion*) are composed of misfolded protein without nucleic acid. They are responsible for the transmissible spongiform encephalopathies: Bovine spongiform encephalopathy or "mad cow disease" in cattle and Creutzfeldt–Jakob disease (CJD) in humans. All are untreatable and fatal. When a prion enters a healthy organism, it provides a template to guide the misfolding of normal protein into the extremely stable prion form, highly resistant to denaturation by chemical and physical agents. This makes disinfection and sterilization of reusable medical instruments a unique challenge because effective prion decontamination relies upon protein hydrolysis or destruction of protein tertiary structure.

Prions cause neurodegenerative disease by aggregating extracellularly within the CNS to form amyloid plaques resulting in the histologically characteristic spongy architecture. CJD, caused by an infectious protein or prion, may be unsuspected in patients presenting with dementia.[126] There are specific guidelines for the disinfection and sterilization of prion-contaminated medical instruments.[127]

Tuberculosis

Tuberculosis (TB) is a major cause of death worldwide and, if properly treated, almost always curable. When untreated, TB can be fatal within 5 years in 50% to 65% of cases.[128] More than 5.8 million new cases of TB were reported to the WHO in 2009; 95% of cases were reported from developing countries. In 2014, 9,421 US cases of TB (0.3:10,000) were reported to the CDC,[129] 66% of which occurred among foreign-born persons.

Mycobacterium tuberculosis is most commonly transmitted from a person with infectious pulmonary TB to others by aerosolized droplet nuclei via coughing, sneezing, or speaking. As many as 3,000 infectious nuclei per cough can remain suspended in the air for several hours and can reach the terminal air passages when inhaled. The most infectious patients have cavitary pulmonary disease or, much less commonly, laryngeal TB and produce sputum containing as many as 10^5 to 10^7 acid-fast bacilli (AFB)/mL. Other routes of transmission are uncommon. Clinical illness directly following infection is classified as *primary TB* and is common among children in the first few years of life and among immune-compromised persons.

The best way to prevent TB is to diagnose and isolate infectious cases rapidly and to administer appropriate treatment until patients are noninfectious, usually 2 to 4 weeks after the start of proper treatment. In low-prevalence countries with adequate resources, screening of high-risk groups such as immigrants from high-prevalence countries, migratory workers, prisoners, homeless individuals, substance abusers, and HIV-seropositive persons is recommended.

Outbreaks of TB in health-care facilities have been attributed to delayed diagnosis of TB in the source patient, delayed initiation or inadequate deployment of airborne precautions, lapses in precautions during aerosol-generating procedures, and lack of adequate respiratory protection in health-care personnel.

Effective prevention of spread to medical personnel requires early identification of infected patients and immediate initiation of airborne infection isolation (Table 3-4). Patients must remain in isolation until adequate treatment is documented. Personnel should wear fit-tested respiratory protective devices when they enter an isolation room or when performing procedures that may induce coughing, such as endotracheal intubation or tracheal suctioning. The CDC recommends that respiratory protective devices worn to protect against TB should be able to filter 95% of particles 0.3 μm in size at flow rates of 50 L/min and should fit the face with a leak rate of less than 10% around the seal, documented by fit testing.[130] High-efficiency particulate air (HEPA) respirators (classified as N95) are NIOSH-approved devices that meet the CDC criteria for respiratory protective devices against TB.[131] It is reasonable to postpone elective surgery until infected patients have had an adequate course of chemotherapy. If surgery prior to the completion of treatment is required, bacterial filters (HEPA filters) should be used on the anesthetic breathing circuit for patients with TB. Patients must be recovered in a room that meets all the requirements for airborne precautions.

Routine periodic screening of employees for TB is frequently a part of a hospital's employee health policy with the frequency of screening dependent on the prevalence of infected patients in the hospitalized population. When a new conversion is detected by skin testing, a history of exposure should be sought to determine the source patient. Treatment or preventive therapy is based on the drug-susceptibility pattern of the TB in the source patient, if known.

Viruses in Smoke Plumes

The use of lasers and electrosurgical devices is associated with several hazards to patients and to OR personnel. Physical hazards include thermal burns, eye injuries, electrical hazards, fires, and explosions. Plume content consists of water and organic vapors, carbonized cell fragments, formaldehyde, acrolein, benzene, polyaromatic hydrocarbons, and carbon monoxide. Although airborne cancer cells have not been detected in laser plumes, potentially harmful particles varying from 0.5 to 5.0 μm have been detected (for comparison, a red blood cell = 7.5 μm). Intact and infectious viral DNA can be detected with laser treatment of verrucae. Viable viruses are carried on large particles that travel lower than 100 mm from the site being vaporized.[131,132]

Smoke-vacuuming systems as well as PPE are recommended when personnel are in proximity to surgical smoke.[133,134] The smoke-vacuuming systems should be held as close as 1 cm to within the target because at 2 cm there is a 50% loss of the evacuation ratio. HEPA or ultralow penetration air filters should be used, and charcoal filters should be used for odor and gas absorption. Venting should be to the outdoors, if possible, and venting systems should have the ability to detect filter overloading (i.e., pressure drop). These filtration guidelines do not address fluid aspiration, which must be carried out independently. In addition, OR personnel working in the vicinity of the laser plume should wear gloves, goggles, and high-efficiency filter masks (N95 respirators).[133]

Emotional Considerations

Stress

Anesthesia practice is mentally, emotionally, and physically stressful. The stress is continuous, and changes dynamically across life and career stages. Several aspects of practice are predictably stressful: a perioperative catastrophe, medical malpractice, and interpersonal conflict. How one responds to these challenges, whether in a constructive or maladaptive manner, will determine the effect on the individual.

Occupational stress is unavoidable and often motivating, but when it exceeds the capabilities of the worker, it can lead to poor mental and physical health, accidents, and burnout. Hans Selye described a three-component stress syndrome: the stressor, the psychological appraisal, and the coping mechanisms employed to address the challenge.[135] This is notably individualistic: one person's stress can be another's recreation. Stress has been linked to cardiovascular, musculoskeletal, and gastrointestinal disease; sleep and mood disturbances; and disruption of personal relationships. Stress is also costly, forecasting higher absenteeism, injuries, disability and decreased productivity.

In response to an awareness of the prevalence of depression, suicide, and substance use disorders among anesthesiologists, Jackson examined individual factors relating to the stress.[136] He defined stress as the "nonspecific adaptive response of the body to any change, demand, pressure, challenge, threat or trauma," and described the impact of personality type, gender, life cycle, and stress abatement programs on the personal response to stress. The perioperative environment supplies constant low-level stress, unpredictably punctuated by episodes of extreme stress, which are largely not controllable by anesthesiologists. Lack of an appropriate response can carry dire consequences, and anesthesiologists cite the following as particularly stressful: unpredictability of work, fear of an adverse event with a bad patient outcome, fear of litigation, need for sustained vigilance, production pressures, economic uncertainty, and strained relationships. Both resident and attending physicians have demonstrated objective evidence of stress at certain critical stages during anesthetic management.[137,138] There is evidence that acute stress can inhibit learning and working memory in the prefrontal cortex, making the appropriate management of stress critical for anesthesiologists.[139]

Personality traits like obsessive–compulsive behavior and dependence have been associated with maladaptive stress responses such as pessimism, self-doubt, internalization, and depression. These characteristics have correlated with future substance use disorder, psychiatric illness, and relational discord in undergraduate students.[140,141]

Impact of Adverse Events

An adverse event with a bad outcome is among the most significant stressors for an anesthesiologist. The description of a "second victim" being the involved medical provider and the "third victim" being subsequently cared-for patients, was proposed by Wu[142] in a 2000 editorial. This followed investigations in the United Kingdom of the impact of such events on surgeons and anesthesiologists after the 1998 sentinel loss of two elective orthopedic patients on the same day. Following an intraoperative death, 27% of surgeons and 26% of anesthesiologists felt they should cease working for the remainder of the day, and 53% of surgeons and 22% of anesthesiologists discontinued patient care for the remainder of the day.[143]

In a study of American Society of Anesthesiologists members, 84% had encountered a "perioperative catastrophe," with 88% requiring time to recover, 19% never fully recovering, 12% considering changing careers, 67% feeling care in the subsequent 4 hours was compromised and only 7% being given any time off.[144] An intense emotional response is normal following a medical error and conversations with peers was cited as the most helpful coping mechanism.[145] This was echoed in a study finding that peer support and individual meetings with department leadership were the most efficacious support modalities for residents following an adverse event.[146] Medical peer support systems have had varying degrees of participation and success.[146–148]

Burnout

Stress and burnout, although causally related, are distinct entities. Burnout is "exhaustion of physical or emotional strength or motivation usually as a result of prolonged stress or frustration,"[149] outlining its multidimensional nature and motivational outcome. The concept of burnout was originally studied in the 1970s[150] with quantitative investigation beginning in the 1980s with the Maslach Burnout Inventory (MBI),[151] which stratifies three major characteristics of burnout: emotional exhaustion, depersonalization/cynicism, and a low sense of personal accomplishment. Burnout typically arises in service industries where interpersonal dynamics and stressors are left unbalanced by job satisfaction and work–life balance. Freudenberger describes a cascade of events culminating in the "burnout syndrome."[150] Ironically, the initial steps are essentially requisite for successful medical school matriculation, starting with a compulsion to prove oneself, to work harder, and to neglect personal needs, and ending with withdrawal, behavior change, depersonalization, and depression. According to Maslach, engagement is the psychological converse to burnout.[152]

The effects of burnout on physicians are significant. Shanafelt published the first large study (7,288 respondents) of US physicians' burnout levels, finding that 45.8% of physicians expressed 1 or more major symptoms of burnout, a level much higher than the background rate of nonphysicians.[153] Amongst all physicians, anesthesiologists scored above the mean for burnout and near the mean for work–life balance. In subsequent reports, burnout has been shown in anesthesiologists (40% at risk for burnout),[154] academic anesthesiology chairs,[155] program directors,[156] nurse anesthetists,[157] and anesthesiologists globally.[158–160]

The health consequences of burnout (cardiovascular, musculoskeletal, and psychological maladies, substance use disorder and altered cortisol expression) have been well documented.[161–163] A correlation has also been shown between burnout and medical malpractice,[164] perceived medical errors and patient care in internal medicine residents,[165,166] empathy, suicidal ideation and professional conduct in medical students,[167,168] and career satisfaction and medical errors among surgeons.[169,170] Dyrbye[171] asserted that burnout is a threat to health-care reform and Wallace[172] proposes physician wellness as a quality indicator. A Canadian model revealed a greater than $200-million-dollar burnout impact, mostly in the form of reduced work hours and early retirement.[173] A population-based cohort study in Finland linked burnout to sickness absences and initiation of disability payments.[174,175]

Myriad solutions have been proposed to address the crisis of burnout in health care; the solution will likely involve an individualized "bundle" of interventions.

Substance Use, Abuse, and Addiction

Although drug proclivities have changed over time, society continues to struggle with the issue of substance use disorders. *Abuse* implies the use of a substance despite negative consequences and *addiction* is characterized by continued abuse despite attempts to curtail use, the need for increasing doses, physical dependence (withdrawal occurring in the absence of the substance), and increasing energy expended seeking the substance. Currently the skyrocketing use, misuse, and addiction to prescription opiate pain relievers (OPRs) has led to a quadrupling of deaths from OPR overdose between 1999 and 2011.[176] It is estimated that 10% to 12% of physicians will, at some point in their careers, develop a form of substance use disorder.[177] Although this prevalence is similar to the general US population, the drugs chosen are more often prescription and controlled medications,[178] with some studies suggesting higher rates than the general population.[179–181]

The medical community has held a longstanding concern for substance use disorder in physicians, and particularly among anesthesiologists.[182,183] Intriguingly, this issue does not spare the luminaries of medicine, with Sigmund Freud, Freeman Allen, and William Halsted being examples of high profile, yet addicted, physicians.[182,184] Data has even suggested that academic excellence (e.g., high test scores and Alpha Omega Alpha membership) is an independent predictor of admission for substance use disorder treatment.[185,186] Improved data collection began in the 1980s and the Medical Association of Georgia's Impaired Physician Program found that in their first 1,000 participants, anesthesiologists were disproportionately represented (12.1% of participants, but only 3.9% of US physicians; 33.7% of resident participants, but 4.6% of US residents). Further, anesthesiologists were much more likely to abuse narcotics, abuse multiple substances, and utilize the intravenous route than other physicians, who are more likely to abuse ethanol.[181] Recently, propofol has emerged as a drug of abuse, highlighting the more treacherous nature of the substances abused by anesthesiologists.[180,187–189] Unlike alcohol abuse, intravenous narcotic and hypnotic abuse has a short initiation to discovery phase and a high mortality and involves drug diversion.

When queried in a 2002 report, academic anesthesiology program chairs revealed a *known* incidence of drug abuse of 1% in faculty and 1.6% in residents.[190] More recent data substantiates this finding by following the outcomes of all physicians entering anesthesia residencies over a 40-year period. Substance use disorder occurred in 2.16 out of 1,000 resident-years, with the highest incidence occurring since 2003, despite educational, treatment, and drug accounting interventions. Of the 384 residents identified as having a substance use disorder (0.86% of the cohort), 28 died during their training period (all from drug-related causes). If one is to consider substance use disorder-related death an occupational hazard of anesthesia, the profession is more dangerous than being a firefighter.[191,192]

The disproportionate prevalence in anesthesiology residents is concerning and has been repeatedly shown.[181,190,193] In a retrospective study of 260 graduates of a single anesthesia program, 32% admitted to prior illicit drug use, 15.8% reported a history of problematic substance abuse, and 20% reported observing compromised teaching due to substance use by faculty.[194]

It is unclear why anesthesiologists appear particularly prone to substance use disorders, though a vulnerable host exposed to a "favorable" environment may account for a majority of the risk. Documented factors include a history of recreational drug use or other high-risk behaviors that are proven to make one susceptible to chemical dependency. Theorized factors include a stressful work environment, lack of external recognition, and low self-esteem, but there is no predictive tool that can identify all of those at risk for substance use disorders.[195] Additional explanations for the prevalence of substance use disorder among anesthesiologists include the availability of controlled substances as a motivator for pursuing an anesthetic career,[193,196] the ease of access and longstanding exposure to anesthetic agents,[197] and the actual personal administration of potent psychoactive medications. Drugs of choice among anesthesiologists have changed with availability. Initial reports indicated the popularity of meperidine, diazepam, and barbituates,[178] then synthetic opiates and inhalational agents,[190] and more recently propofol.[189]

Early recognition of addiction is critical to implementing life-saving interventions. It is important that anesthesiologists be able to recognize, not only in themselves but also in their colleagues, the constellation of physiologic, behavioral, and relational characteristics exhibited in substance use disorders (Table 3-8). Professional and personal withdrawal, while maintaining a façade of

Table 3-8 Signs of Substance Abuse and Dependence
Within the practice of anesthesia • Signing out increasing quantities of narcotics/hypnotics (often inappropriately high for the case) • Volunteering for cases requiring high-dose narcotics • Arriving early, staying late, taking extra call, and offering extra breaks to gain access to drugs (or calling in sick in the case of alcoholics) • Refusing lunch or breaks, personally administering medications in the recovery room, and preferring to work alone to mask drug diversion behavior • Asking for additional bathroom breaks, or staying in bathroom for long periods to use drugs • Being difficult to locate after breaks, as naps often follow drug use • Wearing long sleeves to hide needle marks • Illegible or sloppy charting • Frequent changes in job to maintain the secret
Behavioral changes • Mood swings and emotionally labile • Social withdrawal (from people and previously enjoyed activities) • Increased impulsivity • Leaving drug paraphernalia (bloody swabs, needles, etc.) in common areas • Decreased sexual drive • Increased domestic strife
Physical signs • Pinpoint pupils • Long sleeves worn due to cold sensitivity (associated with narcotics) • Alcohol odor on the breath or witnessing IV drug use • Weight loss and pallor • Narcotic withdrawal (sweating, tremors) • Coma and death—unfortunately a not uncommon presenting symptom

normality at work so as to preserve the access to drugs, is typical. By the time impairment is evident to most colleagues, the disease is in its end stages and often fatal.

Compared to internists, anesthesiologists have an increased relative rate (RR) of suicide from all causes (RR 1.45), drug-related suicide (RR 2), and drug-related death (RR 2.79).[198] Notably, drug-related deaths were far more prevalent in the 5 years subsequent to medical school graduation and account for 2,000 life-years lost for anesthesiologists younger than 65 years old. Warner found 28 drug-related deaths in residents who had been re-enrolled in anesthesia residencies following chemical dependency treatment,[191,192] echoing a study reporting 9 deaths in 100 residents returning to anesthesia residency after treatment.[193] Those re-entering and surviving residency training showed a significantly higher risk of death, with a hazard ratio of 7.9.[192]

There exist many state-specific legal ramifications to physician chemical impairment, which may be mitigated if the involved physician voluntarily seeks treatment. Failing to report impaired colleagues may even carry disciplinary and criminal penalties in certain states. By federal law, the National Practitioner Data Bank must be notified of disciplinary action taken against an impaired physician. There is a reluctance to seek help rooted deeply in physician culture, reinforced by years of self-denial required to complete training and practice medicine. A well-developed defense mechanism enables many physician-addicts to minimize evolving impairment and delay treatment, with often devastating consequences.[199]

One strategy aimed at prevention and early detection of substance use disorders is compulsory pre-employment and random drug screening of anesthesiologists, a practice standard in other high-profile industries (aviation, military, nuclear).[199] Although random drug screening is an element of re-entry contracts, few anesthesia departments randomly screen anesthesiologists.[200] Despite lingering questions regarding the legality and effectiveness of this approach, many academic anesthesiology chairs are in favor of testing.[194]

Controversy persists over the appropriate disposition of an anesthesiologist who has successfully completed substance use disorder treatment. Although the prognosis for sustained recovery is higher for physicians than the general public,[201] relapse is often fatal in those returning to practice in anesthesia. Death rates as high as 9% for anesthesia residents returning to training after substance use disorder treatment[193] are sobering and fuel the argument of a risk too great to take.[202] Countering that argument is that a risk stratification approach may be used, taking into account the three greatest factors linked to relapse[203]: family history of substance abuse, a major opioid as the abused drug, and a coexisting psychiatric disorder.[204] Return to practice can be achieved with relapse rates similar to other medical specialties for anesthesiologists following a rigorous treatment regimen.[205]

Re-entry into practice for a recovering physician must be collaborative, involving the recovering physician, the treating addiction counselor, occupational health, department leadership, organizational credentialing board, and others. Federal laws, such as the Americans with Disabilities Act, impose additional considerations. A carefully worded contract is essential and should include considerations for the following:

- Continued monitoring of sobriety (e.g., random drug screening, opiate antagonists)
- Continued treatment (addiction counseling, Alcoholics Anonymous [AA] or Narcotics Anonymous [NA])
- A period of supervised practice (e.g., not personally handling narcotics) or reduced call (e.g., no nights/weekends)

Despite precautions, relapse must be anticipated and the advice of a physician treatment center may be helpful. Those with the highest chance of successful re-entry into practice accept and understand their disease, have no concomitant psychiatric illness, have strong social support, are sponsored, are committed to their recovery, and have bonded with AA (http://www.aa.org/) or NA (http:/www.na.org/). In addition, their department and hospital must support their return. Those with active disease, severe psychiatric comorbidities, prolonged intravenous substance use, or with prior relapses or treatment failures should be redirected to another specialty.[206,207]

Substance use disorder prevention requires strict control of substances of abuse. Meticulous controlled substance regulation and accounting is essential, especially with the advent of conveniences like satellite pharmacies and automated drug dispensing machines. Systems are being developed to detect patterns and episodes of drug diversion.[208,209]

There is limited data linking substance abuse disorder and poor patient care.[210] However, the impact of the disease on the affected individual physician is great. The burden of substance use disorder is particularly great in anesthesiology and does not appear to be abating. Efforts must be made on multiple fronts to decrease this tragic occupational hazard, including education, controlled substance accounting, and systems of discovery, treatment, and recovery.

Impairment and Disability

Impairment[b] and disability[c] can arise from physical, mental, emotional, sensory, or developmental causes. The onset can be sudden, as occurs with injury or acute illness, or more gradual, as is the case with many chronic diseases.

Data regarding the number of impaired physicians[d] are difficult to obtain. Many cases of physician impairment are the result of substance-related disorders (see earlier). Other factors that can result in physician impairment include physical or mental illness. Unwillingness or inability to keep up with current literature and techniques can be considered a form of impairment.

Depression is a prominent finding among impaired physicians. Unfortunately, many of the personality traits that ensure success as a physician, such as self-sacrifice, competitiveness, achievement orientation, denial of feelings, and intellectualization of emotions, may also serve as risk factors for depression. Observations of alcoholic physicians have provided some insight into the association of achievement orientation and emotional disturbance. In one study, more than half of the alcoholic physicians graduated in the upper one-third of their medical school class, 23% were in the upper one-tenth of their class, and only 5% were in the lower one-third of their class.[211] Similarly, a report on alcohol use in medical school demonstrated better first-year grades and higher scores on Part I National Board of Medical Examiners tests among those students identified as alcohol abusers.[186]

It can be very challenging to appropriately respond to all of the problems imposed by the impaired or unsafe anesthesiologist.[212] Management protocols for dealing with the impaired physician are covered in a series of articles by Canavan and Baxter.[213]

The Aging Anesthesiologist

The natural and inevitable changes that accompany the aging process can impact the practice of anesthesiology.[214] Most notable are commonly observed anatomical and functional changes that appear in the CNS, such as decreases in short-term memory, creative thinking, and problem-solving abilities. Intellectual quickness, on-the-spot reasoning, learning, and reaction time all slow. These are frequently accompanied by other physiologic changes including impairments in hearing and vision that can exacerbate any cognitive impairment. The older anesthesiologist who is experiencing these neurologic changes is potentially more prone to difficulties in assimilation and application of new knowledge, rapid processing of information, complex decision making, and proper response initiation.[215] These potential deficiencies are especially exposed in the stressful environment of an OR.

There are also important changes in the cardiovascular and musculoskeletal systems that commonly occur and can affect the practice of an aging anesthesiologist. Older anesthesiologists may lack the strength to perform some of the more physically demanding aspects of practice, such as prolonged work shifts and night call, and may be more susceptible to late night errors. Failing eyesight, arthritic joints, and tremor may impair the anesthesiologist's ability to perform precision procedures such as vascular access or neural blockade.

These and other common physiologic changes associated with normal aging that might handicap an anesthesiologist are often accompanied by other changes that can provide an advantage. These include wisdom, judgment, and experience. There is a strong positive correlation between these attributes and certain elements of clinical performance.[215] It is less clear that this advantage extends to some of the more complex cognitive skills required to administer a safe anesthetic. As pointed out by Weinger,[216] experience is not synonymous with expertise.

Aging among all physicians, but particularly anesthesiologists, raises complex legal and ethical issues. Neither state licensure nor hospital privileges are specifically limited by the chronologic age of the practitioner. In many cases, the decision to limit or retire from practice remains at the discretion of the individual physician. A number of federal laws impact the aging physician's rights and responsibilities regarding continuation of work. These include the Age Discrimination Act, Title VII of the Civil Rights Act, the Medical and Family Leave Act, the Fair Labor Standards Act, and the Employee Retirement Income Security Act.

Age is an important factor in decisions about retirement. The median age of retirement for anesthesiologists as of 2012 was approximately 64 years.[217] Commonly cited reasons for retirement among older anesthesiologists include on-call responsibilities, financial considerations, lack of professional satisfaction, health concerns, and changes in governmental policies and the health-care operating environment. The decision to retire from anesthesiology is frequently precipitated by concerns about deteriorating clinical skills. In many cases, the retiring anesthesiologist just "felt it was time."[218] Older anesthesiologists who postpone retirement cite career satisfaction, unmet financial obligations, and the need to maintain health insurance for family members as the primary reason to remain in the workforce.

Mortality among Anesthesiologists

There have been a number of conflicting reports regarding how and at what age anesthesiologists most commonly die. Almost all of the studies report an increased rate of suicide.[198,219] Some earlier studies also reported an increased incidence of cancer, specifically leukemia and lymphoma, attributed at the time to chronic exposure to WAG, radiation, and stress.[18,19,220] Subsequent reports have failed to confirm an increased risk for cancer related mortality but continue to cite a disproportionate number of drug-related deaths and suicide.[198,221,222]

There are also contradictory reports about the average longevity of anesthesiologists. Using different databases, control populations, and methodologies, these studies have variously reported a shortened,[198,223] an average,[224,225] or a prolonged life expectancy.[219,222] A 2006 study reported a significant increase in longevity among anesthesiologists who had died throughout the 10-year study period 1992 to 2001, such that the average age at death in the last year of the study was 78 years, the same as the national average for all Americans.[226]

Suicide

There is a disproportionately high incidence of suicide among physicians.[227,228] Anesthesiologists have been singled out as being particularly vulnerable.[198] A partial explanation for this alarming observation lies with the high degree of stress that is an integral

---

[b]Impairment is any loss of use of any body part, organ system, or organ function.
[c]Disability is an impairment that substantially limits one or more major life activities.
[d]An impaired physician is one whose performance as a professional person and as a practitioner of the healing arts is impaired because of alcoholism, drug abuse, mental illness, senility, or disabling disease.

part of the job. There are a number of personality characteristics that may make an individual more susceptible to suicidal thoughts under extreme stress. These characteristics include high anxiety, insecurity, low self-esteem, impulsiveness, and poor self-control. In one study that examined personality traits among anesthesiologists, 20% manifested psychological profiles that reflected a predisposition to behavioral disintegration and attempted suicide when placed under extremes of stress.[229] This study raises the discomforting notion that "premorbid" personality characteristics exist before entering specialty training that could be identified during the admission process.

One specific type of stress for anesthesiologists, that resulting from a catastrophic adverse anesthetic outcome, and/or a malpractice lawsuit, may have a direct causative association with suicide.[144,230] Substance abuse among anesthesia personnel is another potential contributor to the increased suicide rate. Individuals with chemical dependence, who are not identified and are in the end stages of the disease, may die of drug overdose, a cause of death that can be difficult to distinguish from suicide. Drug abuse is among the highest causes of death and the most frequent method of suicide among anesthesiologists.[198] Drug overdose and death was the initial relapse symptom in 16% (13 of 79) of the parenteral opioid abusers who had reentered their residency in anesthesiology.[231] In a more recent survey that examined outcomes for residents who developed substance use disorder, 14.1% were dead within 12 years of onset of the disease.[192] Physicians who are impaired from substance abuse and whose privileges to practice medicine have been revoked are also at heightened risk for attempting suicide.[232]

Wellness

Sir William Osler said that "in no relationship is the physician more often derelict than in his duty to himself."[233] An emphasis on wellness has emerged as a codified component of anesthesia training internationally,[234] and in the United States with the adoption of the ACGME Milestones Project,[235] mandating that a trainee should demonstrate a "responsibility to maintain personal emotional, physical, and mental health." Despite the emphasis, little concrete guidance is offered regarding education and implementation, and varying wellness challenges encountered at different life-cycle stages further obfuscates the subject. External stressors, such as disease, disability, divorce, death, malpractice, and financial distress, may provoke maladaptive coping mechanisms with profound short- and long-term consequences.[136]

Half of the deaths in the United States are estimated to be premature and potentially "deferrable" with the modification of 10 behaviors: tobacco use, dietary pattern, physical activity level, alcohol consumption, exposure to microbial agents, exposure to toxic agents, use of firearms, sexual behavior, motor vehicle crashes, and illicit use of drugs.[236,237]

Nutrition, Diet, and Fitness

By the year 2025, it is predicted that the obesity pandemic will comprise 380 million cases.[238] More than a quarter (27.7%) of US workers fulfill BMI criteria for obesity, with working greater than 40 hours per week and in the health-care setting being independent risk factors for obesity.[239] Clearly anesthesiologists are not exempt from this health crisis.

At a cellular level, the beneficial effects of physical activity are evident. Nitric oxide (NO), one of the body's major bulwarks to oxidative stress, is increased in both sedentary and active men participating in both acute and chronic exercise. Those who exercise consistently have higher basal levels of NO.[240] In a rat model, physical activity led to modulation in hippocampal regenerative sprouting, implying improved learning capacity.[241]

A large (n = 17,549), longitudinal study of men entering Harvard College between 1916 and 1950 demonstrated a significant survival benefit to higher levels of physical activity with a 32% reduction in death rate between the lower and upper thirds.[242] A study of residents and fellows demonstrated 31% of participants adhered to U.S. Department of Health and Human Services levels of physical activity with 23% of invited trainees enrolling in an exercise program.[243] Those who participated in the exercise program had a higher objective quality of life and trended toward decreased burnout. A longitudinal study of Swedish healthcare workers utilizing objective measures of physical activity, burnout, depression, and anxiety showed that physical activity, particularly increases in physical activity, were associated with improved mental health.[244]

If the thought of becoming an elite athlete is daunting, there exists encouraging data that longer periods of moderate physical activity (e.g., walking) carry a similar overall survival benefit to shorter extremes of activity (e.g., running), with fewer injuries (Fig. 3-2).[245]

Implementing Lifestyle Interventions for Lifestyle-related Diseases

Given the number of premature preventable deaths due to tobacco use, sedentary lifestyle, and poor diet, lifestyle changes should focus on these factors.[236,237] A Cochrane review demonstrated that a multifaceted approach to weight loss involving counseling coupled with behavioral, dietary, and exercise components, yielded 3 to 4 kg of sustainable weight loss.[246] A meta-analysis of 33 trials revealed that dieting and exercise yielded greater weight loss than dieting alone and a greater likelihood of sustained weight loss.[247] Strategies to decrease and/or modify caloric intake (e.g., low-glycemic index foods, Mediterranean diet, reduced portions) can improve cardiovascular risk factors, prevent type 2 diabetes, improve hypertension, and lead to sustained weight loss.[248]

Smoking cessation is a difficult endeavor. A review and meta-analysis of 26 studies, showed that those who successfully quit smoking had improved mental health (less anxiety, depression, and stress), a more positive mood, and an overall improved quality of life.[249] There is currently controversy over the practice of not hiring smokers. Some argue discrimination, whereas others praise this as potentially lifesaving.[250,251] Regardless of the motivation, the practice of cessation is difficult, but can be successful by employing integrated pharmacologic and nonpharmacologic approaches.[252]

Mindfulness

Mindfulness, with its roots in Buddhist meditation practice, is an intentional, nonjudgmental practice of attention meant to cultivate awareness of the present moment.[253] The introduction of mindfulness-based stress reduction (MBSR) techniques to improve quality of life, decrease burnout, and supplement integrative approaches to medical therapy began appearing in the medical literature in the 1980s due largely to the work of Jon Kabat-Zinn.[254-256] Meditation techniques have been shown to change transcription profiles and the biochemical milieu

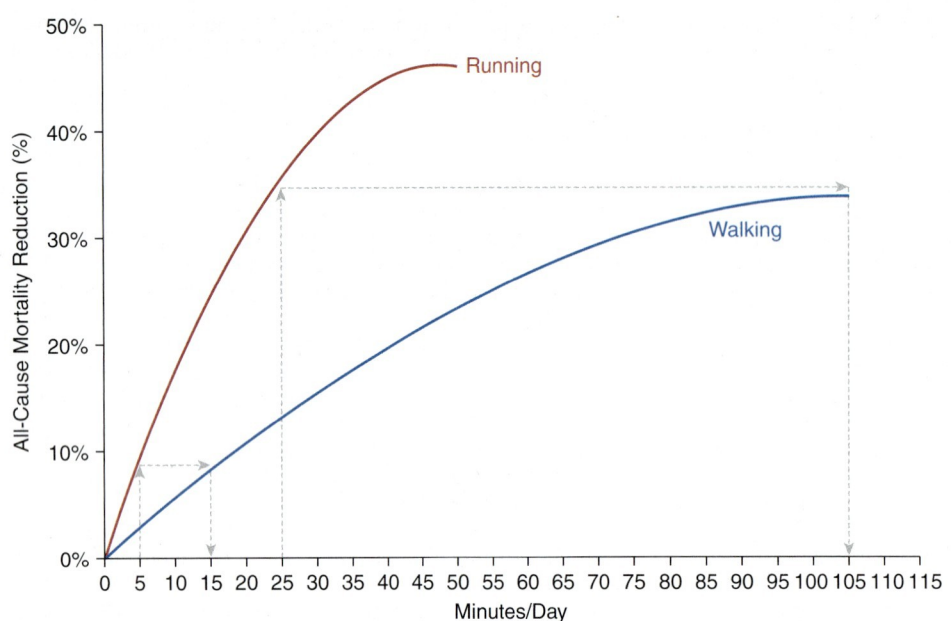

Figure 3-2 Demonstration of a similar reduction in all-cause mortality from longer periods of moderate physical activity when compared to shorter periods of vigorous activity. (Modified from Wen CP, Wai JPM, Tsai MK, et al. Minimal amount of exercise to prolong life: to walk, to run, or just mix it up? *J Am Coll Cardiol.* 2014;64[5]:482–484.)

(particularly in buffering oxidative stress and repairing cellular damage),[257–259] as well as affecting cortical structure and function (particularly relating to learning, memory, emotional stability, and positivity).[260–262] The use of MBSR with health-care providers has shown promise in decreasing burnout and improving physical and mental health.[263] A program designed to improve mindful communication in medical students led to decreased burnout, increased empathy, and overall enhancement of patient-centered care.[264]

Mindful practice requires mentoring and guidance through progressive phases from denial to generalizations, insight, new behaviors, compassion, and presence.[254] Many health-care organizations are rightfully pursuing the goal of becoming a "high reliability organization,"[265] which has been characterized as a consequence of "collective mindfulness."[266] The argument has been made that, in the name of patient safety, mindful practice is our ethical responsibility as anesthesiologists.[267]

Conclusion

The perioperative and critical care environments potentially expose anesthesiologists to physical hazards such as toxic chemicals, WAG, various forms of radiation and infectious agents. In addition, the sustained cognitive, emotional, and psychological demands can have significant bearing on performance and professional deportment. This chapter has reviewed some of the ongoing as well as emerging areas related to occupational illness and wellness of anesthesia personnel in these settings.

REFERENCES

1. Gomaa AE, Tapp LC, Luckhaupt SE, et al. Occupational traumatic injuries among workers in health care facilities - United States, 2012–2014. *MMWR Morb Mortal Wkly Rep.* 2015;64(15):405–410.
2. Linde HW, Bruce DL. Occupational exposure of anesthetists to halothane, nitrous oxide and radiation. *Anesthesiology.* 1969;30(4):363–368.
3. Hoerauf KH, Wallner T, Akça O, et al. Exposure to sevoflurane and nitrous oxide during four different methods of anesthetic induction. *Anesth Analg.* 1999;88(4):925–929.
4. National Institute for Occupational Safety and Health (NIOSH): Criteria for a Recommended Standard: Occupational Exposure to Waste Anesthetic Gases and Vapors. http://www.cdc.gov/niosh/docs/1970/77-140.html. Accessed November, 2015.
5. Centers for Disease Control and Prevention (CDC). NIOSH alert: request for assistance in controlling exposures to nitrous oxide during anesthetic administration. *MMWR Morb Mortal Wkly Rep.* 1994;43(28):522.
6. Panni MK, Corn SB. Scavenging in the operating room. *Curr Opin Anaesthesiol.* 2003;16(6):611–617.
7. McGlothlin JD, Moenning JE, Cole SS. Evaluation and control of waste anesthetic gases in the postanesthesia care unit. *J Perianesth Nurs.* 2014;29(4):298–312.
8. Sessler DI, Badgwell JM. Exposure of postoperative nurses to exhaled anesthetic gases. *Anesth Analg.* 1998;87(5):1083–1088.
9. Vaisman AI. [Working conditions in the operating room and their effect on the health of anesthetists]. *Eksp Khir Anesteziol.* 1967;12(3):44–49.
10. Matsuoka H, Kurosawa S, Horinouchi T, et al. Inhalation anesthetics induce apoptosis in normal peripheral lymphocytes in vitro. *Anesthesiology.* 2001;95(6):1467–1472.
11. Sanders RD, Weimann J, Maze M. Biologic effects of nitrous oxide: a mechanistic and toxicologic review. *Anesthesiology.* 2008;109(4):707–722.
12. Culley DJ, Raghavan SV, Waly M, et al. Nitrous oxide decreases cortical methionine synthase transiently but produces lasting memory impairment in aged rats. *Anesth Analg.* 2007;105(1):83–88.
13. Eroglu A, Celep F, Erciyes N. A comparison of sister chromatid exchanges in lymphocytes of anesthesiologists to nonanesthesiologists in the same hospital. *Anesth Analg.* 2006;102(5):1573–1577.
14. Wiesner G, Hoerauf K, Schroegendorfer K, et al. High-level, but not low-level, occupational exposure to inhaled anesthetics is associated with genotoxicity in the micronucleus assay. *Anesth Analg.* 2001;92(1):118–122.
15. Task Force on Trace Anesthetic Gases of the Committee on Occupational Health of Operating Room Personnel. *Waste Anesthetic Gases: Information for Management in Anesthetizing Areas and the Postanesthesia Care Unit (PACU)*. Park Ridge, IL: American Society of Anesthesiologists; 1999
16. Burm AGL. Occupational hazards of inhalational anaesthetics. *Best Pract Res Clin Anaesthesiol.* 2003;17(1):147–161.
17. Cohen EN, Bellville JW, Brown BW. Anesthesia, pregnancy, and miscarriage: a study of operating room nurses and anesthetists. *Anesthesiology.* 1971;35(4):343–347.
18. Occupational disease among operating room personnel: a national study. Report of an Ad Hoc Committee on the Effect of Trace Anesthetics on the Health of Operating Room Personnel, American Society of Anesthesiologists. *Anesthesiology.* 1974;41(4):321–340.
19. Buring JE, Hennekens CH, Mayrent SL, et al. Health experiences of operating room personnel. *Anesthesiology.* 1985;62(3):325–330.
20. Boivin JF. Risk of spontaneous abortion in women occupationally exposed to anaesthetic gases: a meta-analysis. *Occup Environ Med.* 1997;54(8):541–548.
21. Rowland AS, Baird DD, Shore DL, et al. Nitrous oxide and spontaneous abortion in female dental assistants. *Am J Epidemiol.* 1995;141(6):531–538.
22. Shirangi A, Fritschi L, Holman CDJ. Associations of unscavenged anesthetic gases and long working hours with preterm delivery in female veterinarians. *Obstet Gynecol.* 2009;113(5):1008–1017.

23. Axelsson G, Ahlborg G, Bodin L. Shift work, nitrous oxide exposure, and spontaneous abortion among Swedish midwives. *Occup Environ Med.* 1996;53(6):374–378.
24. Luke B, Mamelle N, Keith L, et al. The association between occupational factors and preterm birth: a United States nurses' study. Research Committee of the Association of Women's Health, Obstetric, and Neonatal Nurses. *Am J Obstet Gynecol.* 1995;173(3 Pt 1):849–862.
25. Lawson CC, Rocheleau CM, Whelan EA, et al. Occupational exposures among nurses and risk of spontaneous abortion. *Am J Obstet Gynecol.* 2012;206(4):327.e1–e8.
26. National Institute for Occupational Safety and Health (NIOSH): *Criteria for a Recommended Standard: Occupational Exposure to Waste Anesthetic Gases and Vapors.* Cincinnati, Ohio, Department of Health, Education, and Welfare (NIOSH), Publication No. 77–140. 1977. http://www.cdc.gov/niosh/docs/1970/77–140.html.
27. Zacny JP, Yajnik S, Lichtor JL, et al. The acute and residual effects of subanesthetic concentrations of isoflurane/nitrous oxide combinations on cognitive and psychomotor performance in healthy volunteers. *Anesth Analg.* 1996;82(1):153–157.
28. Ravishankara AR, Daniel JS, Portmann RW. Nitrous oxide (N_2O): the dominant ozone-depleting substance emitted in the 21st century. *Science.* 2009;326(5949):123–125.
29. Ryan SM, Nielsen CJ. Global warming potential of inhaled anesthetics: application to clinical use. *Anesth Analg.* 2010;111(1):92–98.
30. Sadoh DR, Sharief MK, Howard RS. Occupational exposure to methyl methacrylate monomer induces generalised neuropathy in a dental technician. *Br Dent J.* 1999;186(8):380–381.
31. Klatskin G, Kimberg DV. Recurrent hepatitis attributable to halothane sensitization in an anesthetist. *N Engl J Med.* 1969;280(10):515–522.
32. Vellore AD, Drought VJ, Sherwood-Jones D, et al. Occupational asthma and allergy to sevoflurane and isoflurane in anaesthetic staff. *Allergy.* 2006;61(12):1485–1486.
33. Njoku DB, Greenberg RS, Bourdi M, et al. Autoantibodies associated with volatile anesthetic hepatitis found in the sera of a large cohort of pediatric anesthesiologists. *Anesth Analg.* 2002;94(2):243–249.
34. Sutti S, Rigamonti C, Vidali M, et al. CYP2E1 autoantibodies in liver diseases. *Redox Biol.* 2014;3:72–78.
35. Amarasekera M, Rathnamalala N, Samaraweera S, et al. Prevalence of latex allergy among healthcare workers. *Int J Occup Med Environ Health.* 2010;23(4):391–396.
36. Filon FL, Radman G. Latex allergy: a follow up study of 1040 healthcare workers. *Occup Environ Med.* 2006;63(2):121–125.
37. Brown RH, Schauble JF, Hamilton RG. Prevalence of latex allergy among anesthesiologists. *Anesthesiology.* 1998;89(2):292–269.
38. Occupational Safety and Health Administration, United States Department of Labor. Maximum Permissible Dose Equivalent for Occupational Exposure. http://www.osha.gov/SLTC/radiationionizing/introtoionizing/ionizingattachmentsix.html. Accessed November, 2015.
39. McGowan C, Heaton B, Stephenson RN. Occupational x-ray exposure of anaesthetists. *Br J Anaesth.* 1996;76(6):868–869.
40. Anastasian ZH, Strozyk D, Meyers PM, et al. Radiation exposure of the anesthesiologist in the neurointerventional suite. *Anesthesiology.* 2011;114(3):512–520.
41. Ismail S, Khan F, Sultan N, et al. Radiation exposure to anaesthetists during interventional radiology. *Anaesthesia.* 2010;65(1):54–60.
42. Katz JD. Radiation exposure to anesthesia personnel: the impact of an electrophysiology laboratory. *Anesth Analg.* 2005;101(6):1725–1726.
43. Gorlin A, Hoxworth JM, Mueller J. Occupational hazards of exposure to magnetic resonance imaging. *Anesthesiology.* 2015;123(4):976–977.
44. International Commission on Non-Ionizing Radiation Protection. Guidelines on limits of exposure to static magnetic fields. *Health Phys.* 2009;96(4):504–514.
45. U.S. Department of Labor. Occupational Noise Exposure.29 CFR x1910.95. http://www.osha.gov/dts/osta/otm/noise/standards.html. Accessed November, 2015.
46. Kracht JM, Busch-Vishniac IJ, West JE. Noise in the operating rooms of Johns Hopkins Hospital. *J Acoust Soc Am.* 2007;121(5 Pt 1):2673–2680.
47. Gillie T, Broadbent D. What makes interruptions disruptive? A study of length, similarity, and complexity. *Psychol Res. American Medical Association;* 1989;50(4):243–250.
48. Way TJ, Long A, Weihing J, et al. Effect of noise on auditory processing in the operating room. *J Am Coll Surg.* 2013;216(5):933–938.
49. Stevenson RA, Schlesinger JJ, Wallace MT. Effects of divided attention and operating room noise on perception of pulse oximeter pitch changes: a laboratory study. *Anesthesiology.* 2013;118(2):376–381.
50. NIOSH Publication No. 98–126. Criteria for a Recommended Standard: Occupational Noise Exposure: Basis for the Exposure Standard. Chapter 3.3. http://www.cdc.gov/iosh/docs/98–126chap3.html. Accessed May 2, 2009.
51. Katz JD. Noise in the operating room. *Anesthesiology.* 2014;121(4):894–898.
52. Fritsch MH, Chacko CE, Patterson EB. Operating room sound level hazards for patients and physicians. *Otol Neurotol.* 2010;31(5):715–721.
53. Wallace MS, Ashman MN, Matjasko MJ. Hearing acuity of anesthesiologists and alarm detection. *Anesthesiology.* 1994;81(1):13–28.
54. Willett KM. Noise-induced hearing loss in orthopaedic staff. *J Bone Joint Surg Br.* 1991;73(1):113–115.
55. Moris DN, Linos D. Music meets surgery: two sides to the art of "healing". *Surg Endosc.* 2013;27(3):719–723.
56. Allen K, Blascovich J. Effects of music on cardiovascular reactivity among surgeons. *JAMA.* 1994;272(11):882–884.
57. George S, Ahmed S, Mammen KJ, et al. Influence of music on operation theatre staff. *J Anaesthesiol Clin Pharmacol.* 2011;27(3):354–357.
58. Miskovic D, Rosenthal R, Zingg U, et al. Randomized controlled trial investigating the effect of music on the virtual reality laparoscopic learning performance of novice surgeons. *Surg Endosc.* 2008;22(11):2416–2420.
59. Hawksworth C, Asbury AJ, Millar K. Music in theatre: not so harmonious. A survey of attitudes to music played in the operating theatre. *Anaesthesia.* 1997;52(1):79–83.
60. Edworthy J, Hellier E. Alarms and human behaviour: implications for medical alarms. *Br J Anaesth.* 2006;97(1):12–17.
61. Gaba DM. Crisis resource management and teamwork training in anaesthesia. *Br J Anaesth.* 2010;105(1):3–6.
62. Arriaga AF, Bader AM, Wong JM, et al. Simulation-based trial of surgical-crisis checklists. *N Engl J Med.* 2013;368(3):246–253.
63. Breen CM, Abernethy AP, Abbott KH, et al. Conflict associated with decisions to limit life-sustaining treatment in intensive care units. *J Gen Intern Med.* 2001;16(5):283–289.
64. Katz JD. Conflict and its resolution in the operating room. *J Clin Anesth.* 2007;19(2):152–258.
65. Helmreich RL, Merritt AC, Wilhelm JA. The evolution of Crew Resource Management training in commercial aviation. *Int J Aviat Psychol.* 1999;9(1):19–32.
66. Gaba DM, Howard SK, Jump B. Production pressure in the work environment. California anesthesiologists' attitudes and experiences. *Anesthesiology.* 1994;81(2):488–500.
67. Russ S, Rout S, Sevdalis N, et al. Do safety checklists improve teamwork and communication in the operating room? A systematic review. *Ann Surg.* 2013;258(6):856–871.
68. Fisman DN, Harris AD, Rubin M, et al. Fatigue increases the risk of injury from sharp devices in medical trainees: results from a case-crossover study. *Infect Control Hosp Epidemiol.* 2007;28(1):10–17.
69. Dawson D, Reid K. Fatigue, alcohol and performance impairment. *Nature.* 1997;388(6639):235.
70. King AC, Belenky G, Van Dongen HPA. Performance impairment consequent to sleep loss: determinants of resistance and susceptibility. *Curr Opin Pulm Med.* 2009;15(6):559–564.
71. Barger LK, Ayas NT, Cade BE, et al. Impact of extended-duration shifts on medical errors, adverse events, and attentional failures. *PLoS Med.* 2006;3(12):e487.
72. Friedman RC, Bigger JT, Kornfeld DS. The intern and sleep loss. *N Engl J Med.* 1971;285(4):201–203.
73. Smith-Coggins R, Rosekind MR, Hurd S, et al. Relationship of day versus night sleep to physician performance and mood. *Ann Emerg Med.* 1994;24(5):928–934.
74. Landrigan CP, Rothschild JM, Cronin JW, et al. Effect of reducing interns' work hours on serious medical errors in intensive care units. *N Engl J Med.* 2004;351(18):1838–1848.
75. Howard SK, Gaba DM, Smith BE, et al. Simulation study of rested versus sleep-deprived anesthesiologists. *Anesthesiology.* 2003;98(6):1345–1355.
76. Gravenstein JS, Cooper JB, Orkin FK. Work and rest cycles in anesthesia practice. *Anesthesiology.* 1990;72(4):737–742.
77. Gander PH, Merry A, Millar MM, et al. Hours of work and fatigue-related error: a survey of New Zealand anaesthetists. *Anaesth Intensive Care.* 2000;28(2):178–183.
78. Gawande AA, Zinner MJ, Studdert DM, et al. Analysis of errors reported by surgeons at three teaching hospitals. *Surgery.* 2003;133(6):614–621.
79. Haynes DF, Schwedler M, Dyslin DC, et al. Are postoperative complications related to resident sleep deprivation? *South Med J.* 1995;88(3):283–289.
80. Chu MWA, Stitt LW, Fox SA, et al. Prospective evaluation of consultant surgeon sleep deprivation and outcomes in more than 4000 consecutive cardiac surgical procedures. *Arch Surg.* 2011;146(9):1080–1085.
81. Ellman PI, Law MG, Tache-Leon C, et al. Sleep deprivation does not affect operative results in cardiac surgery. *Ann Thorac Surg.* 2004;78(3):906–911; discussion 906–911.
82. Schieman C, MacLean AR, Buie WD, et al. Does surgeon fatigue influence outcomes after anterior resection for rectal cancer? *Am J Surg.* 2008;195(5):684–687; discussion 687–688.
83. The Accreditation Council for Graduate Medical Education (ACGME). Common Duty Hour Requirements. Effective July 1, 2011. Updated June 18, 2014. https://www.acgme.org/acgmeweb/Portals/0/PDFs/dh-faqs2011.pdf. Accessed December, 2015.
84. Baird M, Daugherty L, Kumar KB, et al. Regional and gender differences and trends in the anesthesiologist workforce. *Anesthesiology.* 2015;123(5):997–1012.

85. Caldwell JA, Caldwell JL. Fatigue in military aviation: an overview of U.S. military-approved pharmacological countermeasures. *Aviat Space Environ Med.* 2005;76(7 Suppl):C39–C51.
86. Katz JD. Hand washing and hand disinfection: more than your mother taught you. *Anesthesiol Clin North America.* 2004;22(3):457–471; vi.
87. Prevention: Recommended Adult Immunization Schedule-United States-2015. U.S. Department of Health and Human Services; 2015. http://www.cdc.gov/vaccines/schedules/downloads/adult/adult-combined-schedule.pdf. Accessed November, 2015.
88. Centers for Disease Control and Prevention. Updated CDC recommendations for the management of Hepatitis B virus–infected health-care providers and students. *MMWR Recomm Rep.* 2012;61:1–10.
89. Centers for Disease Control and Prevention. Updated U.S. Public Health Service guidelines for the management of occupational exposures to HIV and recommendations for postexposure prophylaxis. *MMWR Morb Mortal Wkly Rep.* 2005;54:1–11.
90. Siegel JD, Rhinehart E, Jackson M. Health Care Infection Control Practices Advisory Committee. 2007 Guideline for Isolation Precautions: Preventing Transmission of Infectious Agents in Health Care Settings. *Am J Infect Control.* 2007;35(Suppl 2):S65–S164.
91. Centers for Disease Control and Prevention. *Infection Prevention and Control Recommendations for Hospitalized Patients Under Investigation (PUIs) for Ebola Virus Disease (EVD) in U.S. Hospitals.* Atlanta, GA, Centers for Disease Control and Prevention; 2015.
92. Occupational Safety and Health Administration. *Occupational Exposure to Bloodborne Pathogens; Needlestick and Other Sharps Injuries; Final Rule. 29 CFR Part 1910.* Washington, D.C: U.S. Government Printing Office; 2001.
93. Occupational Safety and Health Administration. Statement of Charles N. Jeffress, Assistant Secretary, Occupational Safety and Health Administration, U.S. Department of Labor, Subcommittee on Workforce Protections, House Education and the Workforce Committee, 2000.
94. Quach S, Pereira JA, Kwong JC, et al. Immunizing health care workers against influenza: a glimpse into the challenges with voluntary programs and considerations for mandatory policies. *Am J Infect Control.* 2013;41(11):1017–1023.
95. Talbot TR, Babcock H, Caplan AL, et al. Revised SHEA position paper: influenza vaccination of healthcare personnel. *Infect Control Hosp Epidemiol.* 2010;31(10):987–995.
96. Abdel-Ghafar A-N, Chotpitayasunondh T, Gao Z, et al. Writing Committee of the Second World Health Organization Consultation on Clinical Aspects of Human Infection with Avian Influenza A (H5N1) Virus. Update on avian influenza A (H5N1) virus infection in humans. *N Engl J Med.* 2008;358(3): 261–273.
97. Kamming D, Gardam M, Chung F. Anaesthesia and SARS. *Br J Anaesth.* 2003;90(6):715–718.
98. Frenkel LM. Clinical reactivation of Herpes simplex virus type 2 infection in seropositive pregnant women with no history of genital herpes. *Ann Intern Med.* 1993;118(6):414–418.
99. Marin M, Güris D, Chaves SS, et al. Advisory Committee on Immunization Practices, Centers for Disease Control and Prevention (CDC). Prevention of varicella: recommendations of the Advisory Committee on Immunization Practices (ACIP). *MMWR Recomm Rep.* 2007;1–40.
100. Centers for Disease Control and Prevention (CDC). FDA approval of an extended period for administering VariZIG for postexposure prophylaxis of varicella. *MMWR Morb Mortal Wkly Rep.* 2012;61(12):212.
101. Brady G, MacArthur GJ, Farrell PJ. Epstein-Barr virus and Burkitt lymphoma. *J Clin Pathol.* 2007;60(12):1397–1402.
102. National Center for Immunization and Respiratory Diseases, Division of Viral Diseases: Cytomegalovirus (CMV) and Congenital CMV Infection. Originally published July 28, 2010. http://www.cdc.gov/cmv/index.html. Accessed November, 29, 2015.
103. Cannon MJ, Schmid DS, Hyde TB. Review of cytomegalovirus seroprevalence and demographic characteristics associated with infection. *Rev Med Virol.* 2010;20(4):202–213.
104. Bolyard EA, Tablan OC, Williams WW, et al. Guideline for infection control in healthcare personnel, 1998. Hospital Infection Control Practices Advisory Committee. *Infect Control Hosp Epidemiol.* 1998;19(6):407–463.
105. Watson JC, Hadler SC, Dykewicz CA, et al. Measles, mumps, and rubella–vaccine use and strategies for elimination of measles, rubella, and congenital rubella syndrome and control of mumps: recommendations of the Advisory Committee on Immunization Practices (ACIP). *MMWR Recomm Rep.* 1998. 1–57.
106. Immunization of Health-Care Personnel. Recommendations of the Advisory Committee on Immunization Practices (ACIP), *MMWR Recomm Rep.* 2011.
107. Measles (Rubeola) Fact Sheet, CDC. http://www.cdc.gov/measles/. Accessed November, 29, 2015.
108. Clemmons NS, Gastanaduy PA, Fiebelkorn AP, et al. Centers for Disease Control and Prevention (CDC). Measles - United States, January 4–April 2, 2015. *MMWR Morb Mortal Wkly Rep.* 2015;64(14):373–376.
109. Advisory Committee on Immunization Practices. Centers for Disease Control and Prevention (CDC). Immunization of health-care personnel: recommendations of the Advisory Committee on Immunization Practices (ACIP). *MMWR Recomm Rep.* 2011. 1–45.
110. Advisory Committee on Immunization Practices (ACIP); Fiore AE, Wasley A, Bell BP. Prevention of hepatitis A through active or passive immunization: recommendations of the Advisory Committee on Immunization Practices (ACIP). *MMWR Recomm Rep.* 2006. 1–23.
111. Centers for Disease Control and Prevention. *Viral Hepatitis Surveillance: United States, 2013.* Atlanta, GA: U.S. Government Printing Office; 2013.
112. Updated U.S. Public Health Service Guidelines for the Management of Occupational Exposures to HBV. HCV, and HIV and Recommendations for Postexposure Prophylaxis. *MMWR Recomm Rep.* 2001;50:1–52.
113. U.S. Public Health Service. Updated U.S. Public Health Service Guidelines for the Management of Occupational Exposures to HBV, HCV, and HIV and Recommendations for Postexposure Prophylaxis. *MMWR Recomm Rep.* 2001. 1–52.
114. Scott JD, Gretch DR. Molecular diagnostics of hepatitis C virus infection: a systematic review. *JAMA.* 2007;297(7):724–732.
115. World Health Organization. Hepatitis C. Geneva, Switzerland: World Health Organization; 2002.
116. Diseases AAFTSOL. Recommendations for testing, managing, and treating hepatitis C. Revised March; 2014.
117. Joint United Nations Programme on HIV/AIDS (UNAIDS): *Global Aids Response Progress Reporting: 2014.* Geneva, Switzerland: World Health Organization; 2014.
118. Kuhar DT, Henderson DK, Struble KA, et al. Updated U.S. Public Health Service guidelines for the management of occupational exposures to human immunodeficiency virus and recommendations for postexposure prophylaxis. Infection control and hospital epidemiology. Cambridge University Press; 2013. pp. 875–892.
119. Joyce MP, Kuhar D, Brooks JT. Notes from the field: occupationally acquired HIV infection among health care workers - United States, 1985–2013. *MMWR Morb Mortal Wkly Rep.* 2015;63(53):1245–1246.
120. Greene ES, Berry AJ, Jagger J, et al. Multicenter study of contaminated percutaneous injuries in anesthesia personnel. *Anesthesiology.* 1998;89(6):1362–1372.
121. Greene ES, Berry AJ, Arnold WP, Jagger J. Percutaneous injuries in anesthesia personnel. *Anesth Analg.* 1996;83(2):273–278.
122. Task Force on Infection Control of the Committee on Occupational Health of Operating Room Personnel. *Recommendations for Infection Control for the Practice of Anesthesiology*, 3rd ed. Park Ridge, Ill: American Society of Anesthesiologists; 2011.
123. Barr S. The 1990 Florida Dental Investigation: is the case really closed? *Ann Intern Med.* 1996;124(2):250–254.
124. Ciesielski C, Marianos D, Ou CY, et al. Transmission of human immunodeficiency virus in a dental practice. *Ann Intern Med.* 1992;116(10):798–805.
125. *Guideline on When to Start Antiretroviral Therapy and on Pre-Exposure Prophylaxis for HIV.* Geneva: World Health Organization; 2015.
126. Johnson RT, Gibbs CJ. Creutzfeldt-Jakob disease and related transmissible spongiform encephalopathies. *N Engl J Med.* 1998;339(27):1994–2004.
127. Rutala WA, Weber DJ, Society for Healthcare Epidemiology of America. Guideline for disinfection and sterilization of prion-contaminated medical instruments. *Infection control and hospital epidemiology.* 2010. 107–117.
128. Blumberg HM, Burman WJ, Chaisson RE, et al. American Thoracic Society/Centers for Disease Control and Prevention/Infectious Diseases Society of America: treatment of tuberculosis. *Am J Respir Crit Care Med.* 2003;603–662.
129. CDC. *Reported Tuberculosis in the United States, 2014.* Atlanta, GA: U.S. Department of Health and Human Services, CDC, 2015.
130. Jensen PA, Lambert LA, Iademarco MF, et al. *Guidelines for preventing the transmission of Mycobacterium tuberculosis in health-care settings, 2005. MMWR.* 2005. 1–141.
131. Register F, U.S. Department of Health and Human Services. *Respiratory protective devices; final rule and notice.* Washington D.C, U.S. Government Printing Office; 1995:30336.
132. Hallmo P, Naess O. Laryngeal papillomatosis with human papillomavirus DNA contracted by a laser surgeon. *Eur Arch Otorhinolaryngol.* 1991;248(7): 425–427.
133. Sehulster L, Chinn R, Arduino MJ. Guidelines for environmental infection control in health-care facilities. *MMWR Recomm Rep.* 2003;52:1–48.
134. Control of smoke from laser/electric surgical procedures. *National Institute for Occupational Safety and Health. Applied occupational and environmental hygiene.* Taylor & Francis Group; 1999:71.
135. Selye H. *The Stress of Life.* New York: McGraw-Hill Book Co; 1984.
136. Jackson SH. The role of stress in anaesthetists' health and well-being. *Acta Anaesthesiol Scand.* 1999;43(6):583–602.
137. Kain ZN, Chan KM, Katz JD, et al. Anesthesiologists and acute perioperative stress: a cohort study. *Anesth Analg.* 2002;95(1):177–183.
138. Eisenach JH, Sprung J, Clark MM, et al. The psychological and physiological effects of acute occupational stress in New Anesthesiology Residents: A pilot trial. *Anesthesiology.* 2014:1.
139. Arnsten AF. Catecholamine modulation of prefrontal cortical cognitive function. *Trends Cogn Sci (Regul Ed).* 1998;2(11):436–447.
140. McDonald JS, Lingam RP, Gupta B, et al. Psychologic testing as an aid to selection of residents in anesthesiology. *Anesth Analg.* 1994;78(3):542–547.
141. Vaillant GE, Brighton JR, McArthur C. Physicians' use of mood-altering drugs. A 20-year follow-up report. *N Engl J Med.* 1970;282(7):365–370.

142. Wu AW. Medical error: the second victim. The doctor who makes the mistake needs help too. *BMJ*. 2000;320(7237):726–727.
143. Goldstone AR, Callaghan CJ, Mackay J, et al. Should surgeons take a break after an intraoperative death? Attitude survey and outcome evaluation. *BMJ*. 2004;328(7436):379.
144. Gazoni FM, Amato PE, Malik ZM, et al. The impact of perioperative catastrophes on anesthesiologists. *Anesth Analg*. 2012;114(3):596–603.
145. Schwappach DL, Boluarte TA. The emotional impact of medical error involvement on physicians: a call for leadership and organisational accountability. *Swiss Med Wkly*. 2009;139(1–2):9–15.
146. Vinson AE, Mitchell JD. Assessing levels of support for residents following adverse outcomes: a national survey of anesthesia residency programs in the United States. *Med Teach*. 2014;36(10):858–866.
147. van Pelt F. Peer support: healthcare professionals supporting each other after adverse medical events. *Qual Saf Health Care*. 2008;17(4):249–252.
148. Saadat H, Snow DL, Ottenheimer S, et al. Wellness program for anesthesiology residents: a randomized, controlled trial. *Acta Anaesthesiol Scand*. 2012;56(9):1130–1138.
149. burnout. 2015. In Merriam-Webster.com. Retrieved Dec 3, 2015, from http://www.merriam-webster.com/dictionary/burnout.
150. Freudenberger HJ. Staff Burn-Out. *J Soc Issues*. 1974;30(1):159–165.
151. Maslach C, Jackson SE, Leiter MP. Maslach burnout inventory. 1986.
152. Maslach C, Schaufeli WB, Leiter MP. Job burnout. *Annu Rev Psychol*. 2001;52:397–422.
153. Shanafelt TD, Boone S, Tan L, et al. Burnout and satisfaction with work-life balance among U.S. physicians relative to the general U.S. population. *Arch Intern Med*. 2012;172(18):1377–1385.
154. Nyssen AS, Hansez I, Baele P, et al. Occupational stress and burnout in anaesthesia. *Br J Anaesth*. 2003;90(3):333–337.
155. De Oliveira GSG, Ahmad SS, Stock MCM, et al. High incidence of burnout in academic chairpersons of anesthesiology: should we be taking better care of our leaders? *Anesthesiology*. 2011;114(1):181–193.
156. De Oliveira GS, Almeida MD, Ahmad S, et al. Anesthesiology residency program director burnout. *J Clin Anesth*. 2011;23(3):176–182.
157. Chipas A, McKenna D. Stress and burnout in nurse anesthesia. *AANA J*. 2011;79(2):122–128.
158. Chiron B, Michinov E, Olivier-Chiron E, et al. Job satisfaction, life satisfaction and burnout in French anaesthetists. *J Health Psychol*. 2010;15(6):948–958.
159. Kluger MT, Townend K, Laidlaw T. Job satisfaction, stress and burnout in Australian specialist anaesthetists. *Anaesthesia*. 2003;58(4):339–345.
160. Walsh AM, McCarthy D, Ghori K. Anesthesiology resident burnout-an Irish perspective. *Anesth Analg*. 2014;118(2):482–483.
161. Shirom A. Burnout and health: expanding our knowledge. *Stress and Health*. John Wiley & Sons, Ltd; 2009;25(4):281–285.
162. Honkonen T, Ahola K, Pertovaara M, et al. The association between burnout and physical illness in the general population—results from the Finnish Health 2000 Study. *J Psychosom Res*. 2006;61(1):59–66.
163. McCall SV. Chemically dependent health professionals. *West J Med*. 2001;174(1):50–54.
164. Jones JW, Barge BN, Steffy BD, et al. Stress and medical malpractice: Organizational risk assessment and intervention. *J Appl Psychol*. 1988;73(4):727–735.
165. West CP, Huschka MM, Novotny PJ, et al. Association of perceived medical errors with resident distress and empathy: a prospective longitudinal study. *JAMA*. 2006;296(9):1071–1078.
166. Shanafelt TD, Bradley KA, Wipf JE, et al. Burnout and self-reported patient care in an internal medicine residency program. *Ann Intern Med*. 2002;136(5):358–367.
167. Dyrbye LN, Thomas MR, Massie FS, et al. Burnout and suicidal ideation among U.S. medical students. *Ann Intern Med*. 2008;149(5):334–341.
168. Dyrbye LN, Massie FS, Eacker A, et al. Relationship between burnout and professional conduct and attitudes among U.S. medical students. *JAMA*. 2010;304(11):1173–1180.
169. Shanafelt TD, Balch CM, Bechamps GJ, et al. Burnout and career satisfaction among American surgeons. *Ann Surg*. 2009;250(3):463–471.
170. Shanafelt TD, Balch CM, Bechamps G, et al. Burnout and medical errors among American surgeons. *Ann Surg*. 2010;251(6):995–1000.
171. Dyrbye LN, Shanafelt TD. Physician burnout: a potential threat to successful health care reform. *JAMA*. 2011;305(19):2009–2010.
172. Wallace JE, Lemaire JB, Ghali WA. Physician wellness: a missing quality indicator. *The Lancet*. 2009;374(9702):1714–1721.
173. Dewa CS, Jacobs P, Thanh NX, et al. An estimate of the cost of burnout on early retirement and reduction in clinical hours of practicing physicians in Canada. *BMC Health Serv Res*. 2014;14(1):254.
174. Ahola K, Kivimäki M, Honkonen T, et al. Occupational burnout and medically certified sickness absence: a population-based study of Finnish employees. *J Psychosom Res*. 2008;64(2):185–193.
175. Ahola K, Gould R, Virtanen M, et al. Occupational burnout as a predictor of disability pension: a population-based cohort study. *Occup Environ Med*. 2009;66(5):284–290; discussion 282–283.

176. Kolodny A, Courtwright DT, Hwang CS, et al. The prescription opioid and heroin crisis: a public health approach to an epidemic of addiction. *Annu Rev Public Health*. 2015;36(1):559–574.
177. Hughes PH, Baldwin DC, Sheehan DV, et al. Resident physician substance use, by specialty. *Am J Psychiatry*. 1992;149(10):1348–1354.
178. Hughes PH, Brandenburg N, Baldwin DC, et al. Prevalence of substance use among U.S. physicians. *JAMA*. 1992;267(17):2333–2339.
179. Gold MS, Melker RJ, Dennis DM, et al. Fentanyl abuse and dependence: further evidence for second hand exposure hypothesis. *J Addict Dis*. 2006;25(1):15–21.
180. McLellan AT, Skipper GS, Campbell M, et al. Five year outcomes in a cohort study of physicians treated for substance use disorders in the United States. *BMJ*. 2008;337(nov04 1):a2038–8.
181. Talbott GD, Gallegos KV, Wilson PO, et al. The Medical Association of Georgia's Impaired Physicians Program. Review of the first 1000 physicians: analysis of specialty. *JAMA*. 1987;257(21):2927–2930.
182. Schonwald G, Skipper GE, Smith DE, et al. Anesthesiologists and substance use disorders. *Anesth Analg*. 2014;119(5):1007–1010.
183. Brewster JM. Prevalence of alcohol and other drug problems among physicians. *JAMA*. 1986;255(14):1913–1920.
184. Morris SD, Morris AJ, Rockoff MA. Freeman Allen: Boston's pioneering physician anesthetist. *Anesth Analg*. 2014;119:1186–1193.
185. Arnold WP. Substance abuse survey in anesthesiology training programs: A brief summary. *ASA Newsl*. 1995;59(10):12–13; 18.
186. Clark DC, Eckenfels EJ, Daugherty SR, et al. Alcohol-use patterns through medical school. *JAMA*. 1987;257(21):2921–2926.
187. Skipper GE, Campbell MD, Dupont RL. Anesthesiologists with substance use disorders: a 5-year outcome study from 16 state physician health programs. *Anesth Analg*. 2009;109(3):891–896.
188. Earley PH, Finver T. Addiction to propofol: a study of 22 treatment cases. *J Addict Med*. 2013;7(3):169–176.
189. Wischmeyer PE, Johnson BR, Wilson JE, et al. A survey of propofol abuse in academic anesthesia programs. *Anesth Analg*. 2007;105(4):1066–1071.
190. Booth JV, Grossman D, Moore J, et al. Substance abuse among physicians: a survey of academic anesthesiology programs. *Anesth Analg*. 2002;95(4):1024–1030.
191. Warner DO, Berge K, Sun H, et al. Substance use disorder among anesthesiology residents, 1975–2009. *JAMA*. 2013;310(21):2289–2296.
192. Warner DO, Berge K, Sun H, et al. Risk and outcomes of substance use disorder among anesthesiology residents: A matched cohort analysis. *Anesthesiology*. 2015;123(4):929–936.
193. Collins GB, McAllister MS, Jensen M, et al. Chemical dependency treatment outcomes of residents in anesthesiology: results of a survey. *Anesth Analg*. 2005;101(5):1457–1462.
194. Lutsky I, Abram SE, Jacobson GR, et al. Substance abuse by anesthesiology residents. *Acad Med*. 1991;66(3):164–166.
195. Moore RD, Mead L, Pearson TA. Youthful precursors of alcohol abuse in physicians. *Am J Med*. 1990;88(4):332–336.
196. Yarborough WH. Substance use disorders in physician training programs. *J Okla State Med Assoc*. 1999;92(10):504–507.
197. Hughes PH, Storr CL, Brandenburg NA, et al. Physician substance use by medical specialty. *J Addict Dis*. 1999;18(2):23–37.
198. Alexander BH, Checkoway H, Nagahama SI, et al. Cause-specific mortality risks of anesthesiologists. *Anesthesiology*. 2000;93(4):922.
199. Scott M, Fisher KS. The evolving legal context for drug testing programs. *Anesthesiology*. 1990 Nov;73(5):1022–1027.
200. Fitzsimons MG, Baker KH, Lowenstein E, et al. Random drug testing to reduce the incidence of addiction in anesthesia residents: preliminary results from one program. *Anesth Analg*. 2008;107(2):630–635.
201. Marshall EJ. Doctors' health and fitness to practise: treating addicted doctors. *Occup Med*. 2008;58(5):334–340.
202. Berge KH, Seppala MD, Lanier WL. The anesthesiology community's approach to opioid- and anesthetic-abusing personnel: time to change course. *Anesthesiology*. 2008;109(5):762–764.
203. Fitzsimons MG, Baker KH. Not all strikes are easy to call. *Anesth Analg*. 2009;109(3):693–694.
204. Domino KB, Hornbein TF, Polissar NL, et al. Risk factors for relapse in health care professionals with substance use disorders. *JAMA*. 2005;293(12):1453–1460.
205. Paris RT, Canavan DI. Physician substance abuse impairment: anesthesiologists vs. other specialties. *J Addict Dis*. 1999;18(1):1–7.
206. Angres DH, Talbott GD, Bettinardi-Angres K. *Anesthesiologist's Return to Practice, in Healing the Healer: The Addicted Physician*. Madison, CT: Psychosocial Press; 1998.
207. Task Force on Chemical Dependence of the Committee on Occupational Health of Operating Room Personnel. *Chemical Dependence in Anesthesiologists: What You Need to Know When You Need to Know It*. Park Ridge, IL: American Society of Anesthesiologists; 1998.
208. Epstein RH, Gratch DM, Grunwald Z. Development of a scheduled drug diversion surveillance system based on an analysis of atypical drug transactions. *Anesth Analg*. 2007;105(4):1053–1060.

209. Epstein RH, Gratch DM, McNulty S, et al. Validation of a system to detect scheduled drug diversion by anesthesia care providers. *Anesth Analg.* 2011;113(1):160–164.
210. Sivarajan M, Posner KL, Caplan RA, et al. Substance abuse among anesthesiologists. *Anesthesiology.* 1994;80(3):704.
211. Bissell L, Jones RW. The alcoholic physician: A survey. *Am J Psychiatry.* 1976.
212. Atkinson RS. The problem of the unsafe anaesthetist. *Br J Anaesth.* 1994;73(1):29–30.
213. Canavan DI, Baxter LE. The twentieth anniversary of the Physicians' Health Program of the Medical Society of New Jersey. *N J Med.* 2003;100(10):27–29.
214. Katz JD. Issues of concern for the aging anesthesiologist. *Anesth Analg.* 2001;92(6):1487–1492.
215. Eva KW. The aging physician: changes in cognitive processing and their impact on medical practice. *Acad Med.* 2002;77(10 Suppl):S1–S86.
216. Weinger MB. Experience not equal expertise: can simulation be used to tell the difference? *Anesthesiology.* 2007;107(5):691–694.
217. Orkin FK, McGinnis SL, Forte GJ, et al. United States anesthesiologists over 50: retirement decision making and workforce implications. *Anesthesiology.* 2012;117(5):953–963.
218. Travis KW, Mihevc NT, Orkin FK, et al. Age and anesthetic practice: a regional perspective. *J Clin Anesth.* 1999;11(3):175–186.
219. Carpenter LM, Swerdlow AJ, Fear NT. Mortality of doctors in different specialties: findings from a cohort of 20000 NHS hospital consultants. *Occup Environ Med.* 1997;54(6):388–395.
220. Bruce DL, Eide KA, Linde HW, et al. Causes of death among anesthesiologists: a 20-year survey. *Anesthesiology.* 1968;29(3):565–569.
221. Bruce DL, Eide KA, Smith NJ, et al. A prospective survey of anesthesiologist mortality, 1967–1971. *Anesthesiology.* 1974;41(1):71–74.
222. Lew EA. Mortality experience among anesthesiologists, 1954–1976. *Anesthesiology.* 1979;51(3):195–199.
223. Svärdsudd K, Wedel H, Gordh T. Mortality rates among Swedish physicians: a population-based nationwide study with special reference to anaesthesiologists. *Acta Anaesthesiol Scand.* 2002;46(10):1187–1195.
224. Katz JD. Do anesthesiologists die at a younger age than other physicians? Age-adjusted death rates. *Anesth Analg.* 2004;98(4):1111–1113.
225. Mostafa MS, Freeman RA. The specialty of physicians in relation to longevity and mortality, 1978–1979. *Ala Med.* 1985;54(11):13–18; 23.
226. Katz JD, Slade MD. Anesthesiologists are living longer: mortality experience 1992 to 2001. *J Clin Anesth.* 2006;18(6):405–408.
227. Center C, Davis M, Detre T, et al. Confronting depression and suicide in physicians: a consensus statement. *AMA.* 2003;3161–3166.
228. North CS, Ryall JE. Psychiatric illness in female physicians. Are high rates of depression an occupational hazard? *Postgrad Med.* 1997;101(5):233–236; 239–240; 242.
229. Reeve PE. Personality characteristics of a sample of anaesthetists. *Anaesthesia.* 1980;35(6):559–568.
230. Birmingham PK, Ward RJ. A high-risk suicide group: the anesthesiologist involved in litigation. *Am J Psychiatry.* 1985;142(10):1225–1226.
231. Menk EJ, Baumgarten RK, Kingsley CP, et al. Success of reentry into anesthesiology training programs by residents with a history of substance abuse. *JAMA.* 1990;263(22):3060–3062.
232. Crawshaw R, Bruce JA, Eraker PL, et al. An epidemic of suicide among physicians on probation. *JAMA.* 1980;243(19):1915–1917.
233. Osler W, Silverman ME, Murray TJ, et al., *2003 ACOP. The quotable Osler.* Philadelphia, PA: American College of Physicians; 2008.
234. Frank JR, Jabbour M, Frechette D. *Report of the CanMEDS Phase IV Working Groups.* Ottawa: The Royal College of Physicians and Surgeons of Canada; 2005. 2014.
235. The anesthesiology milestone project. *J Grad Med Educ.* 2014;6(1 Suppl 1):15–28.
236. McGinnis JM, Foege WH. Actual causes of death in the United States. *JAMA.* 1993;270(18):2207–2212.
237. Mokdad AH, Marks JS, Stroup DF, et al. Actual causes of death in the United States, 2000. *JAMA.* 2004;291(10):1238–1245.
238. Hossain P, Kawar B, Nahas El M. Obesity and diabetes in the developing world—a growing challenge. *N Engl J Med.* 2007;356(3):213–215.
239. Luckhaupt SE, Cohen MA, Li J, et al. Prevalence of obesity among U.S. workers and associations with occupational factors. *Am J Prev Med.* 2014;46(3):237–248.
240. Jenkins NT, Witkowski S, Spangenburg EE, et al. Effects of acute and chronic endurance exercise on intracellular nitric oxide in putative endothelial progenitor cells: role of NAPDH oxidase. *Am J Physiol Heart Circ Physiol.* 2009;297(5):H1798–H1805.
241. Ni H, Li C, Tao L-Y, et al. Physical exercise improves learning by modulating hippocampal mossy fiber sprouting and related gene expression in a developmental rat model of penicillin-induced recurrent epilepticus. *Toxicol Lett.* 2009;191(1):26–32.
242. Paffenbarger R. Physical exercise to reduce cardiovascular disease risk. *Proc Nutr Soc.* 2000;59(3):421–422.
243. Weight CJ, Sellon JL, Lessard-Anderson CR, et al. Physical activity, quality of life, and burnout among physician trainees: the effect of a team-based, incentivized exercise program. *Mayo Clin Proc.* 2013;88(12):1435–1442.
244. Lindwall M, Gerber M, Jonsdottir IH, et al. The relationships of change in physical activity with change in depression, anxiety, and burnout: a longitudinal study of Swedish healthcare workers. *Health Psychol.* 2014;33(11):1309–1318.
245. Wen CP, Wai JPM, Tsai MK, et al. Minimal amount of exercise to prolong life: to walk, to run, or just mix it up? *J Am Coll Cardiol.* 2014;64(5):482–484.
246. McTigue KM, Hess R, Ziouras J. Obesity in older adults: a systematic review of the evidence for diagnosis and treatment. *Obesity (Silver Spring).* 2006;14(9):1485–1497.
247. Curioni CC, Lourenço PM. Long-term weight loss after diet and exercise: a systematic review. *Int J Obes.* 2005;29(10):1168–1174.
248. Avenell A, Broom J, Brown TJ, et al. Systematic review of the long-term effects and economic consequences of treatments for obesity and implications for health improvement. *Health Technol Assess.* 2004;8(21):iii–iv; 1–182.
249. Taylor G, McNeill A, Girling A, et al. Change in mental health after smoking cessation: systematic review and meta-analysis. *BMJ.* 2014;348:g1151.
250. Asch DA, Muller RW, Volpp KG. Conflicts and compromises in not hiring smokers. *N Engl J Med.* 2013;368(15):1371–1373.
251. Schmidt H, Voigt K, Emanuel EJ. The ethics of not hiring smokers. *N Engl J Med.* 2013;368(15):1369–1371.
252. Rennard SI, Daughton DM. Smoking Cessation. *Clin Chest Med.* 2014;35(1):165–176.
253. Rapgay L, Bystrisky A. Classical mindfulness: an introduction to its theory and practice for clinical application. *Ann N Y Acad Sci.* 2009;1172:148–162.
254. Epstein RM. Mindful practice. *JAMA.* 1999;282(9):833–839.
255. Kabat-Zinn J, Massion AO, Kristeller J, et al. Effectiveness of a meditation-based stress reduction program in the treatment of anxiety disorders. *Am J Psychiatry.* 1992;149(7):936–943.
256. Kabat-Zinn J. An outpatient program in behavioral medicine for chronic pain patients based on the practice of mindfulness meditation: theoretical considerations and preliminary results. *Gen Hosp Psychiatry.* 1982;4(1):33–47.
257. Dusek JA, Otu HH, Wohlhueter AL, et al. Genomic counter-stress changes induced by the relaxation response. Awadalla P, ed. *PLoS ONE.* 2008;3(7):e2576.
258. Sharma H, Datta P, Singh A, et al. Gene expression profiling in practitioners of Sudarshan Kriya. *J Psychosom Res.* 2008;64(2):213–218.
259. Bhasin MK, Dusek JA, Chang B-H, et al. Relaxation response induces temporal transcriptome changes in energy metabolism, insulin secretion and inflammatory pathways. *PLoS ONE;* 2013;8(5):e62817.
260. Luders E, Kurth F, Toga AW, et al. Meditation effects within the hippocampal complex revealed by voxel-based morphometry and cytoarchitectonic probabilistic mapping. *Front Psychol.* 2013;4:398.
261. Hölzel BK, Carmody J, Vangel M, et al. Mindfulness practice leads to increases in regional brain gray matter density. *Psychiatry Res.* 2011;191(1):36–43.
262. Kilpatrick LA, Suyenobu BY, Smith SR, et al. Impact of mindfulness-based stress reduction training on intrinsic brain connectivity. *Neuroimage.* 2011;56(1):290–298.
263. Irving JA, Dobkin PL, Park J. Complementary Therapies in Clinical Practice. *Complement Ther Clin Pract.* 2009;15(2):61–66.
264. Krasner MS, Epstein RM, Beckman H, et al. Association of an educational program in mindful communication with burnout, empathy, and attitudes among primary care physicians. *JAMA.* 2009;302(12):1284–1293.
265. Christianson MK, Sutcliffe KM, Miller MA, et al. Becoming a high reliability organization. *Critical care.* 2011;15(6):314.
266. Weick KE, Sutcliffe KM, Obstfeld D. Organizing for high reliability: Processes of collective mindfulness. *Crisis management.* 2008:267.
267. Vinson AE, Wang J. Is Mindful Practice Our Ethical Responsibility as Anesthesiologists? *Int Anesthesiol Clin.* 2015;53(3):1–11.

4 Anesthetic Risk, Quality Improvement, and Liability

KAREN L. POSNER • CHRISTOPHER D. KENT • SHAWN L. MINCER • KAREN B. DOMINO

Anesthesia Risk
  Mortality and Major Morbidity Related to Anesthesia
  Risk Management
  National Practitioner Data Bank
Quality Improvement and Patient Safety in Anesthesia
  Structure, Process, and Outcome: The Building Blocks of Quality
  Difficulty of Outcome Measurement in Anesthesia
  Joint Commission Requirements for Quality Improvement
  Alternative Payment Models and Pay for Performance
Professional Liability
  The Tort System
  Causes of Anesthesia-related Lawsuits
  What to Do When Sued
Acknowledgments

KEY POINTS

1. Anesthetic mortality has decreased, but potentially preventable deaths and disabling complications still occur.
2. Risk management programs are broadly oriented toward reducing the liability exposure of the organization. Risk management programs complement quality improvement programs in minimizing liability exposure while maximizing quality of patient care.
3. Continuous quality improvement is a systems approach to identifying and improving quality of care. Quality improvement programs focus on improving the structure, process, and outcome of care.
4. Quality improvement programs are generally guided by the requirements of the Joint Commission that accredits health-care organizations and the reporting and performance requirements of the Centers for Medicare and Medicaid Services.
5. Medical malpractice refers to the legal concept of professional negligence. The patient-plaintiff must prove that the anesthesiologist owed the patient a duty and failed to fulfill this duty, that the anesthesiologist's actions caused an injury, and that the injury resulted from a breach in the standard of anesthesia care.
6. The most common lawsuits against anesthesiologists (excluding dental injuries) are for death, brain damage, nerve damage, and airway injury. Chronic pain management is the source of an increasing number of malpractice claims against anesthesiologists.

In anesthesia, as in other areas of life, everything does not always go as planned. Undesirable outcomes can occur regardless of the quality of care provided. Continuous quality improvement (CQI) programs are intended to maximize the collective learning from past near misses and undesirable outcomes to prevent their future occurrence. An anesthesia risk management program can work in conjunction with a program for quality improvement to minimize the liability risk of practice. Payers such as the Centers for Medicare and Medicaid Services (CMS) are increasingly depending on accreditation through bodies such as the Joint Commission to ensure that mechanisms are in place to deliver quality and safe care to all patients. In addition, there has been a move toward linking reimbursement to performance measurement and reporting. The legal aspects of American medical practice are important to the anesthesia community as the public turns to the courts for economic redress when their expectations of medical treatment are not met.

This chapter discusses anesthetic mortality and morbidity, risk management, CQI, performance measurement, and medical liability. The chapter provides background for the practitioner concerning the role of risk management activity in minimizing and managing liability exposure. Also described are the medical legal system, the most frequent causes of lawsuits for anesthesiologists, and appropriate actions for physicians to take in the event of a malpractice suit.

Anesthesia Risk

Mortality and Major Morbidity Related to Anesthesia

Estimates of anesthesia-related morbidity and mortality are difficult to quantify. Not only are there difficulties obtaining data on complications, but also different methods yield different estimates of anesthesia risk. Studies differ in their definitions of complications, in length of follow-up, and especially in approaches to evaluation of the contribution of anesthesia care to patient outcomes. A comprehensive review of anesthesia complications is beyond the scope of this chapter. A sampling of studies of anesthesia mortality and morbidity will be presented to provide historical perspective plus a limited overview of relatively recent findings.

Early studies estimated the anesthesia-related mortality rate as 1 per 1,560 anesthetics.[1] More recent studies use data from the 1990s, and later estimate the anesthesia-related death rate in the United States to be lower than 1 per 10,000 anesthetics.[2-7] Some examples of modern estimates of anesthesia-related death from throughout the world are provided in Table 4-1.[2-25] Differences in estimates may be influenced by different reporting methods, definitions, anesthesia practices, and patient populations, as well as actual differences in underlying complication rates.

Table 4-1 Estimates of Anesthesia-related Death

Reference	Country	Time	Data Sources/Methods	Rate of Death
Bainbridge et al.[8]	Global	1940s–2011 a. pre-1970s b. 1970s–1980s c. 1990s–2000s	Systematic review and meta-analysis of published studies in any language with a sample size over 3,000 of rates of anesthesia-related mortality of surgical patients who had undergone general anesthesia. (n = 87 studies including 21.4 million general anesthetics for patients undergoing surgery)	Anesthetic solely attributable mortality: a. 3.57/10,000 b. 0.52/10,000 c. 0.34/10,000 Anesthetic contributory mortality: a. 6.5/10,000 b. 3.23/10,000 c. 1.43/10,000
			Anesthetic mortality by national development status using the United Nations Human Development Index (HDI) over time to assess impact of country development on anesthetic mortality	Anesthetic solely attributable mortality: a. High HDI 3.57/10,000, Low HDI not reported b. High HDI 0.32/10,000, Low HDI 1.01/10,000 c. High HDI 0.25/10,000, Low HDI 1.41/10,000 Anesthetic contributory mortality: a. High HDI 6.84/10,000, Low HDI 3.26/10,000 b. High HDI 2.34/10,000, Low HDI 4.32/10,000 c. High HDI 0.85/10,000, Low HDI 4.67/10,000
Flick et al.[2]	USA	1988–2005	Perioperative cardiac arrest in pediatric patients at a tertiary referral hospital (n = 92,881 anesthetics)	Anesthesia-attributed deaths—0.22/10,000 anesthetics
Biboulet et al.[9]	France	1989–1995	ASA 1–4 patients undergoing anesthesia (n = 101,769 anesthetics); cardiac arrest within 12 h postanesthesia (n = 24)	Anesthesia-related death—0.6/10,000 anesthetics
Newland et al.[3]	USA	1989–1999	Cardiac arrests within 24 h of surgery (n = 72,959 anesthetics) in a teaching hospital	Death related to anesthesia-attributable perioperative cardiac arrest—0.55/10,000 anesthetics
Eagle and Davis[10]	Western Australia	1990–1995	Deaths within 48 h or deaths in which anesthesia was considered a contributing factor (n = 500 deaths)	Anesthesia-related death—0.025/10,000 anesthetics
Lagasse[4]	USA	a. 1992–1994 b. 1995–1999	a. Suburban teaching hospital (n = 115 deaths; n = 37,924 anesthetics) b. Urban teaching hospital (n = 232 deaths; n = 146,548 anesthetics)	Anesthesia-related death: a. 0.79/10,000 anesthetics b. 0.75/10,000 anesthetics
Khan and Khan[11]	Pakistan	1992–2003 a. 1992–1998 b. 1999–2003	University hospital. Deaths within 24 h of anesthesia (n = 111,289 anesthetics)	3.14/10,000 anesthetics; deaths totally attributable to anesthesia 0.35/10,000; anesthesia partially responsible for death 0.7/10,000 a. 0.68/10,000 anesthetics b. 0.18/10,000 anesthetics
Ahmed et al.[12]	Pakistan	1992–2006	Perioperative cardiac arrest in pediatric patients at a university hospital (n = 20,216 anesthetics)	Deaths primarily anesthesia-related 0.49/10,000 anesthetics
Davis[13]	Australia	1994–1996	Deaths reported to the committee (n = 8,500,000 anesthetics)	Anesthesia-related death—0.16/10,000 anesthetics
Morray et al.[5]	USA	1994–1997	Pediatric patients from 63 hospitals (n = 1,089,200 anesthetics)	Anesthesia-related death—0.36/10,000 anesthetics
Kawashima et al.[14]	Japan	1994–1998	Questionnaires to training hospitals (n = 2,363,038 anesthetics)	Death totally attributable to anesthesia—0.21/10,000 anesthetics

Table 4-1 Estimates of Anesthesia-related Death (CONTINUED)

Reference	Country	Time	Data Sources/Methods	Rate of Death
Arbous et al.[15]	Netherlands	1995–1997	All deaths within 24 h or patients who remained unintentionally comatose 24 h postanesthesia (n = 811 in 869,483 anesthetics)—64 hospitals	Anesthesia-related death—1.4/10,000 anesthetics
Braz et al.[16]	Brazil	1996–2005	Tertiary general teaching hospital (n = 53,718 anesthetics)	Anesthesia-related death—1.12/10,000 anesthetics Totally attributed—0.56/10,000 Partially attributed—0.56/10,000
Lienhart et al.[17]	France	1999	Nationwide survey of anesthesia-related deaths	Death totally related to anesthesia—0.069/10,000 Death partially related to anesthesia—0.47/10,000
Kawashima et al.[18]	Japan	1999	Questionnaires to training hospitals (n = 793,840 anesthetics)	Death totally attributable to anesthesia—0.13/10,000 anesthetics
Irita et al.[19]	Japan	1999–2002	Deaths as a result of life-threatening events in the operating room (n = 3,855,384 anesthetics) in training hospitals	Death totally attributable to anesthetic management—0.1/10,000 anesthetics
Li et al.[6]	USA	1999–2005	Deaths with anesthesia-related complication codes from death certificate data a. Population data from census records b. National hospital discharge survey data (inpatients)	Anesthesia-related deaths a. 1.1/million population/year b. 8.2/million hospital surgical discharges
Ellis et al.[7]	USA	1999–2009	Cardiac arrests within 24 h of surgery (n = 217,365 anesthetics) in a single hospital	Death due to anesthesia-attributable cardiac arrest—0.2/10,000 anesthetics Death due to anesthesia-contributable cardiac arrest—0.7/10,000 anesthetics
Charuluxananan et al.[20]	Thailand	2003–2004	Perioperative deaths within 24 h of surgery—20 hospitals (n = 163,403 anesthetics)	Death directly related to anesthesia—1.7/10,000 Death partially related to anesthesia—4.0/10,000
Gibbs[21]	Australia	2003–2005	Deaths reported to Anesthesia Mortality Committees (n = 5,983,704 anesthetics)	Anesthesia-related deaths 0.19/10,000
Rukewe et al.[22]	Nigeria	2005–2010	Cardiac arrest during surgery (n = 12,143) in a university hospital	Mortality related to anesthesia 11.5/10,000 anesthetics
Gonzalez et al.[23]	Brazil	2005–2010	Anesthesia related (totally or partially) pediatric cardiac arrest and mortality in a university hospital (n = 10,469)	Anesthesia-related mortality 0.0/10,000
van der Griend et al.[24]	Australia	2003–2008	Anesthesia related deaths in children ≤18 years from a single pediatric hospital (n = 101,885)	Anesthetic related death 0.98/10,000
De Bruin et al.[25]	Netherlands	2006–2012	Reported 30-day postoperative in-hospital mortality children <18 yrs from a single pediatric hospital (n = 45,182 anesthetics)	Partially anesthesia-related mortality within 24 h 0.7/10,000 Partially anesthesia-related mortality within 30 days 1.1/10,000

A systematic review and meta-analysis of mortality attributable to general anesthesia (GA) from before the 1970s through 2011 suggested a decrease worldwide, especially in developed countries.[8] This lends support to the generally accepted belief that anesthesia safety has improved over the past 50+ years.

Other complications related to anesthesia that have received relatively recent attention include postoperative nerve injury, awareness during GA, eye injuries and visual deficits, dental injury, postoperative cognitive dysfunction in elderly patients, and long-term cognitive impacts in pediatric patients (Table 4-2).[26–60]

(text continued on page 97)

Table 4-2 Rates of Selected Anesthesia Complications

Complication	Reference	Country	Time	Specific Complication	Results
Nerve injury	Brull et al.[26]	Various	1987–1999	Radiculopathy or peripheral neuropathy after spinal anesthesia	3.78/10,000 spinal anesthetics
				Radiculopathy or peripheral neuropathy after epidural anesthesia	2.19/10,000 epidural anesthetics
				Permanent neurologic injury after spinal anesthesia	0–4.2/10,000 spinal anesthetics
				Permanent neurologic injury after epidural anesthetic	0–7.6/10,000 epidural anesthetics
			Varies	Transient neurologic deficit after interscalene block	2.84/10,000 anesthetics
	Warner et al.[27]	USA	1995	Ulnar neuropathy in adults following noncardiac surgery (n = 1,502)	47/10,000
	Warner et al.[28]	USA	1997–1998	Lower extremity neuropathy in adult patients ≥18 under general anesthesia (GA) while in lithotomy position (n = 991)	151/10,000
	Welch et al.[29]	USA	1997–2007	Peripheral nerve injury within 48 h of sedation or anesthesia (n = 380,680)	2.9/10,000
	Auroy et al.[30]	France	1998–1999	Serious peripheral neuropathy related to regional anesthesia	Nonobstetric spinal blocks (SBs) (n = 35,439): 3.4/10,000 Obstetric SBs (n = 5,640): 3.5/10,000 Upper limb peripheral nerve blocks (PNBs) (n = 23,784): 1.7/10,000 Lower limb PNBs (n = 20,162): 4/10,000
	de Sèze et al.[31]	France	2000	Incapacitating neurologic complications lasting ≥3 months after central neuraxial blockade	Nonobstetric SBs (n = 67,884): 0.15/10,000; Nonobstetric epidural blocks (EBs) (n = 65,464): 0.015/10,000 Obstetric EBs (n = 116,639): 0.09/10,000
	Sites et al.[32]	USA	2003–2011	Postoperative sensory or motor dysfunction after ultrasound guided PNB with anatomic basis to support possible block contribution (n = 12,668)	Symptoms lasting >5 days 18/10,000 Symptoms lasting >6 months 9/10,000
	Barrington et al.[33]	USA	2006–2008	Late neurologic complications after PNB or plexus block (n = 7,156 blocks)	4.2/10,000 PNBs
Awareness	Errando et al.[34]	Spain	1995–1997 and 1998–2001	Awareness during GA (n = 3,921)	99.5/10,000
	Sandin et al.[35]	Sweden	1997–1998	Awareness associated with GA (n = 11,785)	15.3/10,000 procedures
	Sebel et al.[36]	USA	2001–2002	Awareness in patients ≥18 years old in seven academic medical centers (n = 19,575)	12.8/10,000

Table 4-2 Rates of Selected Anesthesia Complications (CONTINUED)

Complication	Reference	Country	Time	Specific Complication	Results
	Avidan et al.[37]	USA	2005–2006	Single-center prospective study in patients ≥18 years old (n = 1,941)	20.6/10,000
	Xu et al.[38]	China	NA	Multicenter cohort study of awareness after GA with muscle relaxants (n = 11,101)	41.4/10,000
	Mashour et al.[39]	United States	2008–2010	Randomized controlled trial of unselected surgical patients at three hospitals of a tertiary academic medical center assessing impact of interventions for awareness prevention. (n = 18,836)	Overall incidence of definite awareness in entire study group 10/10,000 Anesthetic concentration group 12/10,000 Bispectral index monitoring group 5/10,000 No intervention 15/10,000
	Pandit et al.[40]	United Kingdom	2011	Survey reports of accidental awareness under GA (n = 2,355,532)	Reported cases 0.65/10,000
	Pandit et al.[41]	United Kingdom	2012–2013	Patient reports of accidental awareness during GA (n = 2,766,600)	Certain/probable and possible cases 0.51/10,000
				Neuromuscular block (NMB) used (n = 1,272,700)	1.2/10,000
				During sedation (n = 308,800)	0.65/10,000
				No NMB (n = 1,494,000)	0.7/10,000
				Caesarean section (n = 8,000)	14.9/10,000
				Cardiothoracic surgery (n = 68,600)	1.16/10,000
				Pediatric surgery (n = 488,500)	0.16/10,000
Vision loss and eye injuries	Chang and Miller[42]	USA	1983–2002	Vision loss due to perioperative ischemic optic neuropathy (ION) associated with spine surgery (n = 14,102)	2.8/10,000
				Corneal abrasions	1.4/10,000
	Warner et al.[43]	USA	1986–1998	New-onset visual loss or visual changes lasting >30 days after noncardiac surgery (n = 125,234)	0.08/10,000 patients
	Roth et al.[44]	USA	1988–1992	Eye injury after nonocular surgery (n = 60,965)	5.6/10,000
				Corneal abrasions	3.4/10,000
				ION	0.16/10,000
	Patil et al.[45]	USA	1993–2002	Visual loss or disturbances after spine surgery (n = 4,728,815)	Any visual disturbance: 9.4/10,000 ION: 0.57/10,000 Central retinal artery occlusion: 0.10/10,000
	Holy et al.[46]	USA	1998–2004	Retrospective chart review for ION (n = 126,666)	ION: 1.3/10,000

(continued)

Table 4-2 Rates of Selected Anesthesia Complications (CONTINUED)

Complication	Reference	Country	Time	Specific Complication	Results
	Shen et al.[47]	USA	1996–2005	Vision loss in surgery	Overall: 2.35/10,000 Cardiac surgery: 8.64/10,000 Spinal fusion: 3.09/10,000 Cholecystectomy 0.66/10,000 Appendectomy: 0.12/10,000
	Warner et al.[48]	USA	1999	New-onset blurred vision lasting ≥3 days (n = 410,189 patients)	4.6/10,000
	Nandyala et al.[49]	USA	2002–2009	Postoperative visual loss after spinal fusion surgery from a national inpatient sample (n = 541,485)	1.9/10,000
	Martin et al.[50]	USA	2005	Postoperative corneal injury (n = 84,796) Baseline	15.1/10,000
			2006–2007	Performance initiative postoperative corneal injury	7.9/10,000
			2007–2008	Follow-up postoperative corneal injury	4.7/10,000
	Yu et al.[51]	Taiwan	2006–2008	Perioperative eye injuries during nonocular surgeries under GA at a university hospital (n = 75,120)	Corneal abrasion 1.3/10,000 Conjunctivitis 0.7/10,000 Prolonged blurred vision 0.1/10,000 Blindness 0.1/10,000
	Kara-Junior et al.[52]	Brazil	2007–2010	Ocular findings associated with nonocular surgeries under GA at a university hospital (n = 39,431)	Temporary ocular injury 2.3/10,000
Dental injury	Warner et al.[53]	USA	1987–1997	Dental injuries within 7 days of anesthesia that required intervention (n = 4,537)	2.2/10,000
				Dental injury under GA with tracheal intubation (n = 2,805)	3.6/10,000
	Newland et al.[54]	USA	1989–2003	Dental injury with anesthesia (n = 161,687 anesthetics)	4.8/10,000
	Adolphs et al.[55]	Germany	1990–2004	Dentoalveolar injury related to GA at a university hospital (n = 375,000)	2.2/10,000
	Vogel et al.[56]	Switzerland	1995–2005	Dental injuries during intubation in patients receiving GA at a university hospital (n = 115,151)	11/10,000
	Gaudio et al.[57]	Italy	2000–2009	Dental injuries in surgical procedures under GA with tracheal intubation (n = 62,898)	37.4/10,000

Table 4-2 Rates of Selected Anesthesia Complications (CONTINUED)

Complication	Reference	Country	Time	Specific Complication	Results
	Martin et al.[58]	USA	2001–2009	Dental injuries in adult non-operating room emergent intubations at a tertiary care hospital (n = 3,423)	17.5/10,000
	Vallejo et al.[59]	USA	2001–2008	Dental injuries in patients receiving anesthesia care at multiple locations of a large university hospital system (n = 816,690)	Overall incidence 4.4/10,000 GA 5.7/10,000 Monitored anesthesia care 0.8/10,000
	Mourao et al.[60]	Portugal	2011	Prospective study of dental damage diagnosed by a dentist after classic direct laryngoscopy at a university hospital (n = 536)	2,500/10,000

The incidence of ulnar neuropathy has been estimated to be 47 per 10,000 patients.[27] Lower-extremity neuropathy following surgery in the lithotomy position was observed in 151 per 10,000 patients.[28] Permanent neurologic injury following neuraxial anesthesia was estimated at 0 to 4.2 per 10,000 spinal anesthetics and 0 to 7.6 per 10,000 epidural anesthetics.[26,30,31] Peripheral nerve injury following peripheral nerve blocks (PNBs) was estimated to occur at a rate of 1.7 to 4.2 per 10,000 anesthetics.[29,30,33] Postoperative neurologic symptoms related to ultrasound-guided PNBs were estimated to occur at a rate 18/10,000 and 9/10,000 for symptoms lasting shorter than 5 days and greater than 6 months, respectively.[32] Awareness during GA has been estimated to occur in 15 to 100 per 10,000 patients.[34–41] The incidence of *patient reported* awareness during GA was 0.51 to 14.9 per 10,000 in the National Audit Project in Great Britain and Ireland.[41]

Eye injuries are a risk of anesthesia, including corneal abrasions as well as more rare complications such as blindness from ischemic optic neuropathy (ION) or central retinal artery occlusion.[42–52] Corneal abrasion has occurred at a rate of 1.4 to 15.1 per 10,000 procedures.[42,44,50] ION has been observed at 0.57 to 2.8 per 10,000 spine surgeries.[42,45] Risk factors for ION after spinal fusion have recently been identified and include a variety of patient, surgical, and anesthetic factors.[61] Among these include use of a Wilson surgical bed frame, obesity, and long anesthetic durations. All can contribute to increased venous congestion in the optic canal and potentially reduce optic nerve perfusion pressure. There was insufficient evidence to conclude that intraoperative anemia or transient periods of hypotension were causative factors. There is some evidence that the incidence of postoperative visual loss has been decreasing in the United States.[47]

Damage to teeth or dentures is the most common injury leading to anesthesia malpractice claims. Dental injury complaints are usually resolved by a hospital risk management department. Dental injuries after general endotracheal anesthesia were observed in approximately 1 per 2,000 to 3,000 patients in the United States.[53,54] A prospective study of dental damage diagnosed by a dentist after classic direct laryngoscopy in Portugal reported a high rate of 2,500/10,000.[60]

There has been increasing concern about the potential effect of anesthesia on cognitive function, especially among pediatric and elderly patients. It is difficult to sort out the potential contributions of surgery, anesthesia, and illness on neurocognitive function. Cognitive dysfunction, usually short term, has been observed in many adult patients after major surgery, and it has been hypothesized that the elderly may be at more significant risk for long-term cognitive problems.[62] While the role of anesthesia in postoperative cognitive dysfunction has not been definitively determined, recent evidence based on twin studies suggests that major surgery with anesthesia results in a negligible effect on cognitive function in middle-aged and elderly patients.[63] There is concern but limited data about the long-term cognitive impacts of pediatric anesthesia. One randomized controlled trial found no evidence for increased risk of neurodevelopment deficits at 2 years of age after 1 hour of GA in healthy infants undergoing inguinal herniorrhaphy. Follow-up at 5 years of age is pending.[64] For up-to-date research findings and a consensus statement from a diverse group of experts on the use of anesthetic drugs in infants and toddlers, see the web site for SmartTots at smarttots.org. SmartTots is a public/private partnership between the U.S. Food and Drug Administration and the International Anesthesia Research Society.

Risk Management

Conceptual Introduction

Risk management and quality improvement programs work hand in hand to minimize liability exposure while maximizing quality of patient care. Although the functions of these programs vary from one institution to another, they overlap in their focus on patient safety. They can generally be distinguished by their basic difference in orientation. A hospital risk management program is broadly oriented toward reducing the liability exposure of the organization. This includes not only professional liability (and therefore patient safety) but also contracts, employee safety, public safety, and any other liability exposure of the institution. Quality improvement programs have as their main goal the continuous maintenance and improvement of the quality of patient care. These programs may be broader in their patient safety focus than strictly risk management. Quality improvement (sometimes called *patient safety*) departments are responsible for providing the resources to provide safe, patient-centered, timely, efficient, effective, and equitable patient care.[65]

Risk Management in Anesthesia

Those aspects of risk management that are most directly relevant to the liability exposure of the anesthesiologist include prevention of patient injury, adherence to standards of care, documentation, and patient relations.

The key factors in the prevention of patient injury are vigilance, adequate monitoring, and up-to-date knowledge.[66] Physiologic monitoring of cardiopulmonary function, combined with monitoring of equipment function, might be expected to reduce anesthetic injury to a minimum. This was the rationale for the adoption by the American Society of Anesthesiologists (ASA) of *Standards for Basic Anesthetic Monitoring*.[67] Detailed information on anesthesia monitoring techniques can be found in Chapter 26, Commonly Used Monitoring Techniques.

The ASA website is an accessible resource that can be reviewed periodically for any changes in the published *Guidelines and Statements*. It should be noted that although membership in the ASA is not required for the practice of anesthesiology, expert witnesses will, with virtual certainty, hold any practitioner to the ASA standards. It is also possible that as a risk management strategy, a professional liability insurer or hospital may hold an individual anesthesiologist to standards higher than those promulgated by the ASA.

Another risk management tool is the use of checklists to prevent errors. Since the first checklists for pilots were developed for the military, checklists have been adopted by many industries wherein processes are too numerous and/or complex to rely on human memory. A checklist is a simple, yet powerful, tool that ensures no important detail is forgotten, and it removes variability, enhances consistency, and decreases likelihood of error. This patient safety tool helps to remind providers of key steps and thus works to facilitate safe and effective health-care delivery. Incorporation of checklists for routine anesthesia into regular anesthesia workflow processes has been advocated to improve patient safety.[68]

Historically, checklists have been used in anesthesia for anesthesia machine checkout procedures. Information pertaining to anesthesia workstation preuse procedures as well as safety considerations for workstations can be found in Chapter 25, The Anesthesia Workstation and Delivery Systems for Inhaled Anesthetics. Recently, checklists for clinical care have been promoted to improve patient safety and medical management in various clinical settings, for example, central venous catheterization, intraoperative emergencies, and perioperative care. Catheter-related bloodstream infections were reduced significantly with the implementation of a standardized process that included a checklist for catheter placement and management.[69] The ASA developed an algorithm for central venous catheter access.[70] During simulated emergency scenarios, checklists have improved performance in the management of local anesthesia systemic toxicity[71] and improved management of intraoperative crises such as malignant hyperthermia, massive hemorrhage, air embolism, and cardiac arrest.[72,73]

Perioperative use of the surgical safety checklist in a variety of global hospital settings reduced surgical complications and mortality.[74] In a staged fashion (prior to induction, prior to skin incision, prior to wound closure, and prior to patient leaving the OR), this checklist confirms patient information and presence of personnel, addresses potential case-specific concerns, and incorporates significant processes ranging from a surgical time-out to a postprocedural briefing (Table 4-3). The surgical safety checklist has been widely incorporated into practice in the

Table 4-3 World Health Organization Surgical Safety Checklist Elements

Preinduction
Patient confirms identity, site, procedure, and consent
Site marked
Anesthesia machine and medication check
Pulse oximeter on and functioning
Does the patient have:
   Known allergy?
   Risk for difficult airway or aspiration?

Before Incision
Team members introduce themselves by name and role
Confirm patient identity, procedure, and incision site
Antibiotics within last 60 min
Anticipated critical events:
   Critical or nonroutine steps in procedure
   Anticipated duration of surgery
   Anticipated blood loss
   Anesthesia concerns
   Sterility confirmed
   Equipment issues or concerns
Essential imaging displayed

Before Patient Leaves Operating Room
Confirm procedure
Complete instrument, sponge, and needle counts
Specimens labeled
Address equipment problems
What are the key concerns for recovery?

Adapted from the WHO Surgical Safety Checklist, http://whqlibdoc.who.int/publications/2009/9789241598590_eng_Checklist.pdf.

United States. Specific anesthesia preinduction checklists have also been developed and tested to improve information exchange and patient safety.[75]

Although it may seem obvious, qualified anesthesia personnel should be in continuous attendance during the conduct of all anesthetics. The only exceptions should be those that lay people (i.e., judge and jury) can understand, such as radiation hazards or an unexpected life-threatening emergency elsewhere. Even then, provisions should be made for monitoring the patient adequately. Adequate supervision of nurse anesthetists and residents is also important, as is good communication with surgeons when adverse anesthetic outcomes occur.

Informed Consent

Informed consent regarding anesthesia should be documented with a general surgical consent, which should include a statement to the effect that "I understand that all anesthetics involve risks of complications, serious injury, or, rarely, death from both known and unknown causes." In addition, there should be a note in the patient's record that the risks of anesthesia and alternatives were discussed and that the patient accepted the proposed anesthetic plan. A brief documentation in the record that the common complications and material risk of the proposed technique were discussed is helpful. In some institutions and states, a separate written anesthesia consent form must be used, which may include more detail about risks. If it is necessary to change the agreed-on anesthesia plan significantly after the patient is premedicated or anesthetized, the reasons for the change should be documented in the record.

Informed consent is problematic in that standard forms are often difficult for patients to understand, and patients often differ from physicians in their expectations and understanding of the risks and benefits associated with their treatments.[76–78] Patient complaints are commonly grounded in elements of informed consent, absorbing valuable health-care system resources even if they do not lead to a malpractice complaint.[79] Patient complaints can be leveraged to identify high-risk providers to target for interventions to improve communication skills.[80,81]

Shared decision-making is an enhanced form of informed consent applicable in elective situations when options for treatment are available to the patient. Shared decision-making is a strategy to empower the patient to actively make an evidence-based choice in his/her treatment.[82] In shared decision-making, evidence-based information is shared with the patient using educational materials ("decision-aids"), and patient preferences and values are elicited during the decision-making process. When all parties are satisfied that they understand the options and expectations, an informed decision can be made regarding treatment.[83,84]

There is an increasing body of evidence to suggest that sharing of information with patients, particularly when there may have been an adverse outcome, perhaps involving a medical error, can be beneficial. Effective disclosure can improve doctor–patient relations, facilitate better understanding of systems, and potentially decrease medical malpractice costs.[85]

Record Keeping

Good records can form a strong defense if they are adequate; however, records can be disastrous if inadequate. The anesthesia record itself should be as accurate, complete, and neat as possible. In addition to documenting vital signs at least every 5 minutes, special attention should be paid to ensure that the patient's ASA classification, monitors used, fluids administered, and doses and times of all administered drugs are accurately charted. Because the principal causes of hypoxic brain damage and death during anesthesia are related to ventilation and/or oxygenation, all respiratory variables that are monitored should be documented accurately. It is important to note when there is a change of anesthesia personnel during the conduct of a case. Sloppy, inaccurate anesthesia records, with gaps during critical events, can be extremely damaging to the defense when enlarged and placed before a jury.

The use of electronic health records (EHRs) has been mandated in health care, and currently in the United States anesthesia information management systems (AIMS) have supplanted the traditional anesthesia paper record in the majority of the operating rooms. CMS has implemented bonuses for practitioners who can demonstrate "meaningful use" of an EHR which may be followed by financial penalties for those who do not meet the standard. Some areas of anesthesia practice have received an exemption from the requirement to meaningfully use an EHR in their practices but it is unclear whether this will continue. Basic AIMS are connected to the patient monitors and the anesthesia machine and capture perioperative data specific to anesthesia (e.g., vital signs, times of induction, intubation and emergence, medications and fluids). There is improved patient care and cost savings at institutions where EHR are fully incorporated.[86] When properly configured, AIMS can increase provider efficiency,[87] improve quality of care,[88] improve coding and billing accuracy,[89,90] decrease paperwork, and be a legible, chronologic documentation of clinical care. Use of AIMS has substantial potential as a clinical-decision support mechanism.[91] AIMS can process information from multiple devices and the EHR, incorporate algorithms to remind physicians to perform critical clinical processes on time,[92,93] and alert physicians to changes in patient status.[94]

Some physicians are wary of EHRs and the possible increased risk of exposure to litigation. Concerns have been raised about the profuse amounts of data and the risk of electronic discovery being used in litigation.[95,96] Although there is a growing body of data and opinion, no definitive conclusions can yet be made regarding the impact of EHRs and the risk of malpractice.[97] EHRs were associated with fewer paid malpractice claims in one study.[98] The digital data reviewed in court may be detrimental to the physician-defendant case when shortcuts are taken and anomalies in time-stamped entries cast doubt on the integrity of the record; for example, engaging in the practice of documenting events before they actually occur.[99] Outside the operating room, in the documentation of preoperative assessments, pain management, and critical care consultation notes, the EHR presents a medicolegal and billing compliance risk if the practitioner engages in the use of copying and pasting, cloning, or carrying forward information from other notes without very careful review of those notes for accuracy and relevance to the care encounter they purport to document.

What to Do after an Adverse Outcome

If a critical incident occurs during the conduct of an anesthetic, the anesthesiologist should document, in narrative form, what happened, which drugs were used, the time sequence, and who was present. If there is no space or format appropriate to adequately summarize a complex catastrophic intra-anesthetic event in the usual anesthesia record, it should be documented in the patient's progress notes. The critical incident note should be written as soon as possible. For events where the etiology is unclear, speculation in the record regarding causation should be limited only to the generation of a differential diagnosis that might contribute to the ongoing care of the patient. The report should be as consistent as possible with concurrent records, such as the anesthesia, operating room, recovery room, and cardiac arrest records. If significant inconsistencies exist, they should be explained. Records should never be altered after the fact. If an error is made in record keeping, a line should be drawn through the error, leaving it legible, and the correction should be initialed and timed. Litigation is a lengthy process, and a court appearance to explain the incident to a jury may be years away, when memories have faded.

Whenever an anesthetic complication becomes apparent, appropriate consultation should be obtained quickly, and the departmental or institutional risk management group should be notified. If the complication is apt to lead to prolonged hospitalization or permanent injury, the liability insurance carrier should be notified. The patient should be followed closely while in the hospital, with telephone follow-up, if indicated, after discharge. The anesthesiologist(s), surgeon(s), consulting physicians, and the institution should coordinate and be consistent in their explanations to the patient or the patient's family as to the cause of any complication.

If anesthetic complications occur, the anesthesiologist should be honest with both the patient and the family about the cause. The providers should provide the facts about the event, express regret to the patient and family about the outcome, and give a formal apology if the unanticipated outcome is the result of an error or system failure.[85,100] Some states have laws mandating disclosure of serious adverse events to patients, and disclosure has been incorporated into quality reporting. Some states prohibit use of disclosure discussions as evidence in malpractice litigation.

Disclosure is considered the ethically right thing to do, and may reduce malpractice risk,[101] although malpractice risk reduction through disclosure is still subject to debate.[102] Some institutions, health systems, and insurers have adopted formal "communication and resolution" approaches to adverse events.[103,104] These approaches vary in their details but share the underlying premise that early disclosure and an offer of compensation may provide satisfactory resolution to the patient and avoid formal litigation proceedings.[105]

Special Circumstances: "Do Not Resuscitate" and Jehovah's Witnesses

It is important to recognize that patients have well-established rights, and that among these is the right to refuse specific treatments. Two situations most relevant to anesthesia care are "Do Not Resuscitate" (DNR) orders and the special circumstance of blood transfusion for Jehovah's Witnesses.

Patients with severe medical conditions may elect to forgo resuscitation attempts in the event of cardiac arrest. Such DNR orders may be specified at hospital admission or may be in place in the form of an advance directive prior to admission. DNR orders or advance directives may be general or specific, such as refusal of tracheal intubation or mechanical ventilation. When a patient with DNR status presents for anesthesia care, it is important to discuss this with the patient or patient's surrogate to clarify the patient's intentions. In many hospitals, the institutional policy is to suspend the DNR order during the immediate perioperative period since the cause for a cardiac arrest may be easily identified and treated. In other institutions, the patient may choose to suspend the DNR order during the entire perioperative period. It should be clarified when the DNR order should be reinstated (e.g., discharge from recovery or possibly later, when the patient has recovered from the procedure) and documented in the patient's chart. The perioperative status of DNR orders should also be clarified with the surgeon and other providers who will be involved in the patient's perioperative care. The ASA has published *Ethical Guidelines of the Anesthesia Care of Patients with Do-Not-Resuscitate Orders or Other Directives That Limit Treatment*.[106]

In the case of Jehovah's Witnesses, the treatment that may be refused is the administration of blood or blood products.[107] A central religious belief of many Jehovah's Witnesses is that the faithful will be forbidden salvation if they receive blood or blood products. Thus, for them to receive a transfusion is a mortal sin, and many Jehovah's Witnesses would rather die in grace than live with no possibility of salvation. Anesthesiologists must recognize and respect these beliefs, but also be cognizant that these convictions may conflict with their own personal, religious, or ethical codes.

As a general rule, physicians are not obligated to treat all patients who apply for treatment in elective situations. It is well within the rights of a physician to decline to care for any patient who wishes to place burdensome constraints on the physician or to unacceptably limit the physician's ability to provide optimal care. When presented with the opportunity to provide elective care for a Jehovah's Witness, the physician may decline to provide any care or may limit, by mutual consent with the patient, his or her obligation to adhere to the patient's religious beliefs. If such an agreement is reached, it must be documented clearly in the medical record, and it is desirable to have the patient co-sign the note. Not all Jehovah's Witnesses have identical beliefs regarding blood transfusions or which methods of blood preservation or sequestration will be allowed. Some patients will not allow any blood that has left the body to be reinfused, yet others will accept autotransfusion if their blood remains in constant contact with the body (via tubing).[107] Therefore, it is important to reach a clear understanding of which techniques for blood preservation are to be used and to document this plan in the record. Parents of a minor child may not legally prevent that child from receiving blood. It may be necessary to obtain a court order in this circumstance.

National Practitioner Data Bank

It is usually the obligation of the hospital risk management department to make reports and inquiries to the National Practitioner Data Bank (NPDB),[108] a nationwide information system that theoretically allows licensing boards and hospitals a means of detecting adverse information about physicians.[109] Simply moving into another state does not provide safe haven for incompetent physicians.

The NPDB requires notification of various adverse actions including medical malpractice payments, license actions by medical boards or states, negative actions or findings by a peer review organization or private accreditation entity, adverse clinical privilege actions, and adverse professional membership society actions.[110] There has been a great deal of effort to establish a minimum malpractice payment below which no report is necessary, but to date, any payment made on behalf of a physician in response to a written complaint or claim must be reported. Settlements made by cancellation of bills or settlements made on verbal complaints are not considered reportable payments.

Once a report has been submitted, the physician is notified and may dispute the accuracy of the report. At this time, the reporting entity may correct the form or void it. Failing that, the physician has the option of putting a brief statement in the file or appealing to the US Secretary of Health and Human Services, who may also either correct or void the form. A practitioner may make a query about his or her file at any time. A physician may also add a statement to a report at any time. Such statements will be included in any reports that are sent in response to inquiries. The existence of the NPDB reporting requirements has made physicians reluctant to allow settlement of nuisance suits because it will cause their names to be added to the data bank.

Quality Improvement and Patient Safety in Anesthesia

Quality is a concept that has continued to elude precise definition in medical practice. However, it is generally accepted that attention to quality will improve patient safety and satisfaction with anesthesia care. The field of quality improvement is continually evolving, as is the terminology used to describe such efforts. A more recent trend is emphasis on patient safety, the prevention of harm from medical care. At the time of this writing, patient safety initiatives are evolving and "pay for performance (P4P)" (direct linkage between care processes and outcomes and reimbursement) has been adopted by CMS. These will be discussed in a separate section.

Anesthesia quality improvement programs at the service level are generally guided by requirements of the Joint Commission that accredits hospitals and health-care organizations. Quality improvement programs are basically oriented toward improvement of the structure, process, and outcome of health-care delivery. An understanding of the fundamental principles of quality improvement may clarify the relationship between the continually evolving Joint Commission requirements and mandated quality improvement and other reporting initiatives.

Structure, Process, and Outcome: The Building Blocks of Quality

Although quality of care is difficult to define, it is generally accepted that it is composed of three components: structure, process, and outcome.[111] *Structure* refers to the setting in which care was provided, for example, personnel and facilities used to provide health-care services and the manner in which they are organized. This includes the qualifications and licensing of personnel, ratio of practitioners to patients, standards for the facilities and equipment used to provide care, and the organizational structure within which care is delivered. The *process* of care includes the sequence and coordination of patient care activities, that is, what was actually done. Was a preanesthetic evaluation performed and documented? Was the patient continuously attended and monitored throughout the anesthetic? *Outcome* of care refers to changes in health status of the patient following the delivery of medical care. A quality improvement program focuses on measuring and improving these basic components of care.

CQI takes a systems approach to identifying and improving quality of care.[112,113] The operator is just one part of a complex system. An important underlying premise is that poor results may be a result of either random or systematic error. Random errors are inherently difficult to prevent and programs focused in this direction are misguided. System errors, however, should be controllable and strategies to minimize them should be within reach. CQI is basically the process of continually evaluating anesthesia practice to identify systematic problems (opportunities for improvement) and implementing strategies to prevent their occurrence.

A CQI program may focus on undesirable outcomes as a way to identify opportunities for improvement in the structure and process of care. The focus is not on blame but rather on identification of the causes of undesirable outcomes. Instead of asking which practitioners have the highest patient mortality rates, a CQI program may focus on the relationship between the process of care and patient mortality. What proportion of deaths was related to the patient's disease process or debilitated condition? Are these patients being appropriately evaluated for anesthesia and surgery? Were there any controllable causes, such as lack of extra help during resuscitation? The latter may lead to a modification of personnel resources (structure) or assignments (process) to be sure that adequate personnel are available at all times.

Formally, the process of CQI involves the identification of opportunities for improvement through the continual assessment of important aspects of care. It is a process that is instituted from the bottom up, by those who are actually involved in the process to be improved, rather than from the top down by administrators. Identification of opportunities for improvement may be carried out by various means, from brainstorming sessions focusing on a systematic evaluation of care activities to the careful measurement of indicators of quality (such as morbidity and mortality). In any event, once areas are identified for improvement, their current status is measured and documented. This may involve measurement of outcomes, such as delayed recovery from anesthesia or peripheral nerve injury. The process of care leading to these problems is then analyzed. If a change is identified that should lead to improvement, it is implemented. After an appropriate time, the status is then measured again to determine whether improvement actually resulted. Attention may then be directed to continuing to improve this process or turning to a different process to target for improvement.

Difficulty of Outcome Measurement in Anesthesia

Improvement in quality of care is often measured by a reduction in the rate of adverse outcomes. However, adverse outcomes are relatively rare in anesthesia, making measurement of improvement difficult. For example, if an institution lowers its mortality rate of surgery patients from 1 in 1,000 to 0.5 in 1,000, this difference may not be statistically significant. In other words, it may be impossible to know if the change in outcome resulted from changes in care or is simply random fluctuation. Many adverse outcomes in anesthesia are sufficiently rare to render them problematic as quality improvement measures.

To complement outcome measurement, anesthesia CQI programs can focus on critical incidents, sentinel events, and human errors. *Critical incidents* are events that cause, or have the potential to cause, patient injury if not noticed and corrected in a timely manner. For example, a partial disconnect of the breathing circuit may be corrected before patient injury occurs, yet has the potential for causing hypoxic brain injury or death. Critical incidents are more common than adverse outcomes. Measurement of the occurrence rate of important critical incidents may serve as a proxy measure for rare outcomes in anesthesia in a CQI program designed to improve patient safety and prevent injury.

Sentinel events are single, isolated events that may indicate a systemic problem. The Joint Commission has a specific definition of sentinel events (any unexpected occurrences involving death or serious physical or psychological injury or risk thereof) that will be discussed later. In general, a sentinel event may be a significant or alarming critical incident that did not result in patient injury, such as a syringe swap and administration of a potentially lethal dose of medication that was noted and treated promptly, avoiding catastrophe. Or a sentinel event may be an unexpected significant patient injury such as intraoperative death. In either case, a CQI program may investigate sentinel events in an attempt to uncover systemic problems in the delivery of care that can be corrected. For example, a syringe swap may be analyzed for confusing or unclear labeling of medications or unnecessary medications routinely stocked on the anesthesia cart, setting the scene for unintended mix-up. In the case of death, all aspects of the patient's hospital course from selection for surgery to anesthetic management may be analyzed to determine if similar deaths can be prevented by a change in the care delivery system.

Human error has garnered much attention since a 1999 government report that 98,000 Americans may die annually from medical errors in hospitals.[114] Human errors are inevitable yet potentially preventable by appropriate system safeguards. Errors of planning involve use of a wrong plan to achieve an aim. Errors of execution are the failure of a planned action to be completed as intended. Modern anesthesia equipment is designed with safeguards such as alarm systems to detect errors that could lead to patient injury. Other anesthesia care processes are also amenable to human factors design principles, such as color coding of drug labels. A quality improvement program may identify human errors and institute safety systems to aid in error prevention.

Recently, many institutions have implemented "Communication and Resolution Programs" which have been shown to significantly reduce the incidence of medical errors.[115] In these institutions, when an error has occurred, the involved parties (including medical personnel, risk management, medical liability insurers, and the patient) immediately communicate with one another, the cause of the error is thoroughly investigated, the patient is rapidly remunerated financially (if necessary), and mechanisms are instituted to prevent recurrence of a similar error. Data from these institutions have shown a significant reduction in the incidence of error, dramatically reduced litigation, and improved patient satisfaction.

Joint Commission Requirements for Quality Improvement

The Joint Commission is a nonprofit organization that has its roots in an early twentieth century initiative of the American College of Surgeons. The organization became the Joint Commission on Accreditation of Hospitals in 1951 and then the Joint Commission on Accreditation of Healthcare Organizations in 1987 when it expanded its accreditation activities to facilities other than hospitals. The name of the organization was shortened to The Joint Commission in 2007.[116] Although Joint Commission accreditation of hospitals and surgery centers is officially voluntary, it is a requirement in order to participate in Medicaid billing in many states.

Joint Commission requirements for quality improvement activities are updated on an annual basis and are available online. In general, a hospital must adopt a method for systematically assessing and improving important functions and processes of care and their outcomes in a cyclical fashion. The general outline for this CQI cycle is the design of a process or function, measurement of performance, assessment of performance measures through statistical analysis or comparison with other data sources, and improvement of the process or function. Then the cycle repeats. The Joint Commission provides specific standards that must be met, with examples of appropriate measures of performance. The goal of this cycle of design, measurement, assessment, and improvement of performance of important functions and processes is to improve patient safety and quality of care.

Many of the specific Joint Commission requirements are outlined in its National Patient Safety Goals.[117] These include performance elements for all aspects of hospital care including processes for delivering perioperative care, such as medication labeling, the prevention of infections associated with urinary and central venous catheters, and the preprocedure "time-out."[117] The time-out is meant to ensure that the entire team (anesthesiologist, surgeon, nursing staff) agrees that the procedure, patient, and procedural details are correct. The surgical check list, described earlier in this chapter, is often used for this purpose. Since 2006 Joint Commission accreditation visits are unannounced or conducted on short notice and involve the inspection team watching patient care to see that safe and acceptable practices are routinely implemented. Surveyors may also talk to any staff member about organizational policies and procedures. Although the accreditation visits are by necessity episodic, the ORYX Performance Measurement Initiative[118] is a longstanding Joint Commission program that changed the focus of the accreditation process from simply taking a snapshot of institutional performance at the time of an inspection to a continuous process of reporting performance data using the ORYX tool. Unlike most programs in the quality arena that are primarily known by their acronyms, ORYX is named by the animal whose swiftness and graceful appearance was intended to be both memorable and evocative of positive attributes.[118]

The Joint Commission also requires all sentinel events (any unexpected occurrences involving death or serious physical or psychological injury or risk thereof) to undergo root cause analysis.[119] A root cause analysis is typically facilitated by the hospital and includes everyone involved in the care of the affected patient in reconstructing the events to identify system process flaws that facilitated medical error. Any surgery on the wrong patient or wrong body part is included in this policy. The Joint Commission publishes sentinel event alerts so health-care organizations can learn from the experiences of others and prevent future medical errors.

Alternative Payment Models and Pay for Performance

Alternative Payment Models (APMs) are part of the move away from traditional volume driven fee-for-service systems to other payment formulas that are intended to promote quality, patient value, and efficiency in health care. The models attempt to do this by shifting some of the down-side risk of excess costs due to complications and inefficient care to the providers through capitation and/or bundled payments. Some models also share the upside risk of cost savings gained through improved efficiency with the providers. A full exploration of this trend in reimbursement and health-care organization and its potential impact on the manner in which anesthesiologists will practice in the future is beyond the scope of this chapter and is mentioned here due to its importance as part of the forces shaping quality improvement programs.

Pay for Performance (P4P) is a broad term that encompasses programs and initiatives aimed at improving the quality and efficiency of health care by providing financial incentives to hospitals and health-care professionals to measure and report health-care outcomes and to meet specific goals and standards for outcomes and processes. There are a large number of initiatives in the private sector but historically the best known P4P programs have been those of the CMS; the Value-Based Purchasing program for hospitals and institutions and the Physician Quality Reporting System (PQRS) for individual health professionals and group practices. Within these programs performance parameters were divided into the domains of: clinical process of care, structure, outcome, efficiency, and patient experience. The programs were initially introduced with a formula that paid a percentage bonus to institutions and providers for having reported and met applicable performance goals. As the programs have evolved negative payment adjustments or penalties were introduced for participants that failed to report data or did not meet performance goals. Performance parameters directly applicable to the delivery of perioperative care are only a small subset of all the parameters in these programs. An item-specific, comprehensive outline of the parameters and goals relevant to perioperative care will not be included here as these have changed and will continue to change, such that they may not be relevant over the longer term. For example, one of the previously perennial performance parameters, which had also been aligned with the Joint Commission's Surgical Care Improvement Project (SCIP) was the delivery of antibiotic prophylaxis for surgical infection prevention within 60 minutes prior to incision. This parameter was dropped by CMS because adherence was close to 100%, so it was no longer providing information that could discriminate between the practices of participating providers.[120,121]

The next CMS P4P program on the horizon in 2018 will combine and streamline the PQRS program and the Value-Based Purchasing program into one system created under the Medicare Access and CHIP Reauthorization Act (MACRA). Over a 10-year timeline this system will incentivize practitioners through Merit-Based Incentive Payments (MIPS) or through participation in APMs to replace traditional fee-for-service payments. The MIPS system will assess individual physician performance in four categories: quality, resource use, meaningful use of certified EHR technology, and clinical practice improvement activities to generate a composite score on a 0- to 100-point scale. After full implementation of the program in 2019 physicians participating in the MIPS will have their Medicare payments adjusted positively or negatively according to their ranking above or below the mean composite score. Because APMs have already ostensibly been created to move practitioners from volume to quality-based practice, those practitioners who receive a "significant portion" of their Medicare payments through an eligible APM entity, will be exempt from the MIPS requirements and will be considered "qualifying APM participants."

The concept of P4P has been around for a sufficient length of time that there is evidence accumulating on how well the idea has performed in meeting the intended goals. This evidence primarily pertains to general initiatives, rather than the parameters that apply specifically to the delivery of perioperative care. The evidence is mixed as to whether processes and practitioner behavior are changed by P4P initiatives and there are very limited data to support the idea that patient outcomes are improved. A study of hospitals in the United Kingdom[122] found that the mortality due to pneumonia was improved after the introduction of P4P initiatives. However, a major study in the United States[123] did not demonstrate any similar improvements and a Cochrane Review[124] did not find any evidence for the effectiveness of P4P programs. Some investigators have suggested that there are major gaps between the documentation of care and the delivery of care,[125] and that P4P incentivizes providers to focus more on the documentation of certain elements of care but may divert resources and efforts from the actual delivery of care.[121] Regardless of any present lack of evidence for the effectiveness of these measures, MACRA and MIPS will ensure that they will remain part of the health-care landscape and anesthesiologists should adopt a proactive approach to shaping and improving any future P4P programs.

The Anesthesia Quality Institute (AQI) has developed a National Anesthesia Clinical Outcomes Registry (NACOR) that can serve as a benchmarking resource for anesthesiologists. The AQI is a resource chartered by ASA in 2009.[126] The AQI was developed to assist members in maintaining certification and meeting emerging standards and to collect digital case information. NACOR is the registry of accumulated digital data acquired through periodic transfer of case-specific data directly from one electronic system (electronic billing and health records, EHR, AIMS, etc.) to another. NACOR data can be used to meet current CMS P4P measures. The NACOR registry is a rich bank of data for future outcomes analysis that may be used for personal benchmarking, comparing quality of care, maintaining licensure and certification, and research. Through NACOR, acquired data (practice demographics, case-specific data, outcome data, and risk adjustment data) can be analyzed, changes can be implemented, and health care can be improved.

Professional Liability

This section addresses the basic concepts of medical liability. A more detailed discussion of liability issues and the steps of the lawsuit process and appropriate actions for physicians to take when sued is available in the ASA Manual on Professional Liability.[127]

The Tort System

Although physicians may become involved in the criminal law system in a professional capacity, they more commonly become involved in the legal system of civil laws. Civil law is broadly divided into *contract law* and *tort law*. A tort may be loosely defined as a civil wrongdoing; negligence is one type of tort. *Malpractice* actually refers to any professional misconduct, but its use in legal terms typically refers to professional negligence.

To be successful in a malpractice suit, the patient-plaintiff must prove four things:
1. Duty: That the anesthesiologist owed the patient a duty
2. Breach of duty: That the anesthesiologist failed to fulfill his or her duty
3. Causation: That a reasonably close causal relation exists between the anesthesiologist's acts and the resultant injury
4. Damages: That actual damage resulted because of a breach of the standard of care.

Failure to prove any one of these four elements will result in a decision for the defendant-anesthesiologist.

Duty

As a physician, the anesthesiologist establishes a duty to the patient when a doctor–patient relationship exists. When the patient is seen preoperatively and the anesthesiologist agrees to provide anesthesia care for the patient, a duty to the patient has been established. In the most general terms, the duty the anesthesiologist owes to the patient is to adhere to the *standard of care* for the treatment of the patient. Because it is virtually impossible to delineate specific standards for all aspects of medical practice and all eventualities, the courts have created the concept of the *reasonable and prudent* physician. For all specialties, there is a national standard that has displaced the local standard.

Breach of Duty

In a malpractice action, expert witnesses will review the medical records of the case and determine whether the anesthesiologist acted in a reasonable and prudent manner in the specific situation and fulfilled his or her duty to the patient. If they find that the anesthesiologist either did something that should not have been done or failed to do something that should have been done, then the duty to adhere to the standard of care has been breached. Therefore, the second requirement for a successful suit will have been met.

Causation

Judges and juries are interested in determining whether the breach of duty was the *proximate cause* of the injury. If the odds are better than even that the breach of duty led, however circuitously, to the injury, this requirement is met.

There are two common tests employed to establish causation. The first is the *but for* test and the second is the *substantial factor* test. If the injury would not have occurred but for the action of the defendant-anesthesiologist, or if the act of the anesthesiologist was a substantial factor in the injury despite other causes, then proximate cause is established.

Although the burden of proof of causation ordinarily falls on the patient-plaintiff, it may, under special circumstances, be shifted to the physician-defendant under the doctrine of *res ipsa loquitur* (literally, "the thing speaks for itself"). Applying this doctrine requires proving the following:
1. The injury is of a kind that typically would not occur in the absence of negligence.
2. The injury must be caused by something under the exclusive control of the anesthesiologist.

3. The injury must not be attributable to any contribution on the part of the patient.
4. The evidence for the explanation of events must be more accessible to the anesthesiologist than to the patient.

Because anesthesiologists render patients insensible to their surroundings and unable to protect themselves from injury, the doctrine of *res ipsa loquitur* may be invoked in anesthesia malpractice cases. If the plaintiff can successfully argue that the injury would not have occurred in the absence of negligence, then the defendant-anesthesiologist must prove that he/she was not negligent in the case under consideration.

Damages

The law allows for three different types of damages. *General damages* are those such as pain and suffering that directly result from the injury. *Special damages* are those actual damages that are a consequence of the injury, such as medical expenses, lost income, and funeral expenses. *Punitive damages* are intended to punish the physician for negligence that was reckless, wanton, fraudulent, or willful. Punitive damages are exceedingly rare in medical malpractice cases. More likely in the case of gross negligence is a loss of the license to practice anesthesia. In extreme cases, criminal charges may be brought against the physician, although this is rare. Determination of the dollar amount is usually based on some assessment of the plaintiff's condition versus the condition he or she would have been in had there been no negligence. Plaintiffs' attorneys generally charge a percentage of the damages and will, therefore, seek to maximize the award given. Some states have legislated caps on damages. Such caps are more common for general damages, although some states cap total compensation for malpractice awards.

Standard of Care

Because medical malpractice usually involves issues beyond the comprehension of lay jurors and judges, the court establishes the standard of care in a particular case by the testimony of *expert witnesses*. These witnesses differ from factual witnesses mainly in that they may give opinions. The trial court judge has sole discretion in determining whether a witness may be qualified as an expert. Although any licensed physician may be an expert, information will be sought regarding the witness's education and training, the nature and scope of the person's practice, memberships and affiliations, and publications. The purpose in gathering this information is not only to establish the qualifications of the witness to provide expert testimony but also to determine the weight to be given to that testimony by the jury. In many cases the success of a lawsuit depends primarily on the stature and believability of the expert witnesses.

Unfortunately, there is a tendency for experts to link severe injury with inappropriate care (i.e., a bias that "bad outcomes mean bad care"). To investigate the influence of the severity of the injury on the assessment of standard of care, a group of 112 practicing anesthesiologists judged appropriateness of care in 21 cases involving adverse anesthetic outcomes.[128] The original outcome in each case was either temporary or permanent. For each original case, a matching alternate case was created that was identical to the original in every respect, except that a plausible outcome of the opposite severity was substituted. Reviewers judged the standard of care in each case. Knowledge of the severity of injury produced a significant inverse effect on the judgment of appropriateness of care.[128] The proportion of ratings for appropriate care decreased when the outcome was changed from temporary to permanent and increased when the outcome was changed from permanent to temporary. These results suggest that outcome bias in the assessment of standard of care may contribute to the frequency and size of payments.

In certain circumstances, the standard of care may also be determined from published societal guidelines, written policies of a hospital or department, or textbooks and monographs. Some medical specialty societies have carefully avoided applying the term *standards* to their guidelines in the hope that no binding behavior or mandatory practices have been created. The essential difference between standards and guidelines is that guidelines *should* be adhered to and standards *must* be adhered to. The ASA has a searchable database of all standards, guidelines, and practice parameters on their website.[67] The ASA also has extensive material on quality improvement and practice management on their website.[129]

Causes of Anesthesia-related Lawsuits

Relatively few adverse outcomes end up in a malpractice suit. It has been estimated that less than 1 of 25 patient injuries result in malpractice litigation.[130] The ASA Committee on Professional Liability has conducted a nationwide analysis of malpractice claims against anesthesiologists, excluding dental damage, since 1985 (i.e., the *Closed Claims Project*).[131-133] While most malpractice claims continue to be associated with surgical anesthesia care, obstetric anesthesia, acute pain management, and chronic pain management together represent one-third of anesthesia malpractice claims (Fig. 4-1).

The leading injuries in anesthesia-related malpractice claims in the 2000s were death (30%), nerve damage (22%), permanent brain damage (10%), and airway injury (6%) (Fig. 4-2). Burns from cautery fires, especially during monitored anesthesia care, increased over previous decades.[134,135] The causes of death and permanent brain damage were predominantly problems in airway management (e.g., inadequate ventilation, difficult intubation, premature extubation) and other complications such as pulmonary embolism, inadequate fluid therapy, stroke, hemorrhage, and myocardial infarction.[136] Nerve damage, especially to the ulnar nerve, often occurs despite apparently adequate positioning.[137,138] Nerve injury was also the most common complication leading to claims after PNBs.[139] Spinal cord injury was the most common cause of nerve damage claims against anesthesiologists in the 1990s.[137]

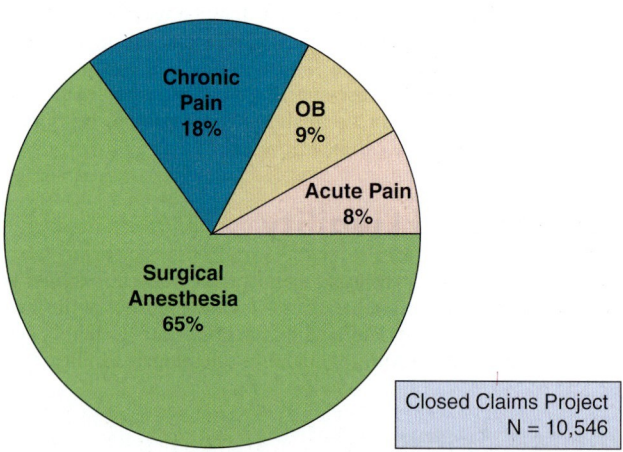

Figure 4-1 Types of anesthesia care in malpractice claims in the year 2000 or later. Most claims are associated with surgical anesthesia care. Anesthesia Closed Claims Project (*n* = 10,546). OB, obstetric.

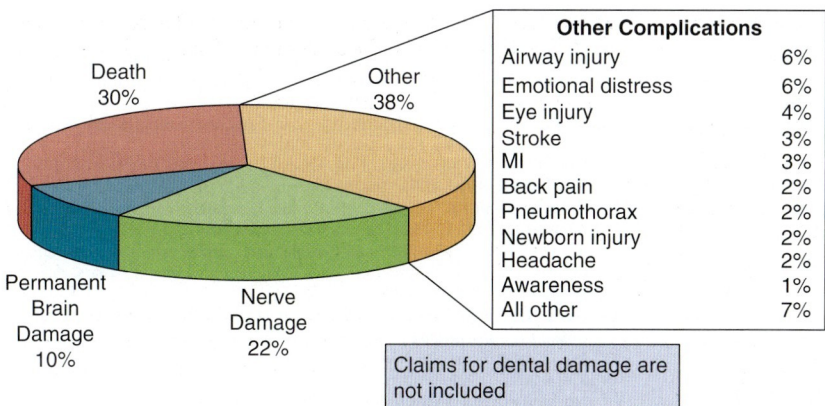

Figure 4-2 The most common injuries leading to anesthesia malpractice claims in the year 2000 or later. Damage to teeth and dentures excluded. Anesthesia Closed Claims Project (n = 10,546). MI, myocardial infarction.

Chronic pain management is an increasing source of malpractice claims against anesthesiologists.[133,140,141] Cervical spine interventions for chronic pain management were the most common nonneurolytic injections in the 2000s, representing 27% of recent pain medicine malpractice claims. Permanent nerve injury, generally to the spinal cord, was the outcome in 54% of these claims.[141,142] Medication management represented 17% of recent chronic pain management claims, with death as the most common outcome.[141,143] Lumbar injections decreased over time, representing 17% of pain medicine claims in the 2000s, with permanent disabling nerve injury the outcome in 26% of lumbar injection claims.[141] Claims associated with implanted devices increased over time, representing 16% of pain medicine claims in the 2000s.[141]

The anesthesiologist is likely to be the target of a lawsuit if an untoward outcome occurs because the physician–patient relationship is usually tenuous at best. The patient rarely chooses the anesthesiologist, the preoperative visit is brief, and the anesthesiologist who sees the patient preoperatively may not actually anesthetize the patient. Communication between anesthesiologists and surgeons about complications is often lacking, and the tendency is for the surgeon to "blame anesthesia." In addition, anesthesiologists are often sued along with the surgeon in the case of an adverse outcome. This may occur even if the outcome was in no way related to the anesthetic care. However, as mentioned earlier, there is an increasing body of evidence that early full disclosure of adverse events to patients, probably best done by individuals properly trained in the process of disclosure, may significantly reduce the incidence of malpractice claims.[85,100,115]

What to Do When Sued

A lawsuit begins when the patient-plaintiff's attorney files a *complaint* and demands for jury trial with the court. The anesthesiologist is then served with the complaint and a summons requiring an answer to the complaint. Until this happens, no lawsuit has been filed. Insurance carriers must be notified immediately after the receipt of the complaint. The anesthesiologist will need assistance in answering the complaint, and there is a time limit placed on the response.

Specific actions at this point include the following:
1. Do not discuss the case with anyone, including colleagues who may have been involved, operating room personnel, or friends. (Although in many jurisdictions the courts will look favorably upon a physician who speaks to the patient soon after an adverse outcome occurs, and offers sympathy and an apology without necessarily admitting guilt.)[115]
2. Never alter any records.
3. Gather together all pertinent records, including a copy of the anesthetic record, billing statements, and correspondence concerning the case.
4. Make notes recording all events recalled about the case.
5. Cooperate fully with the attorney provided by the insurer.

The first task the anesthesiologist must perform with an attorney is to prepare an answer to the complaint. The complaint contains certain facts and allegations with which the defense may either agree or disagree. Defense attorneys rely on the frank and totally candid observations of the physician in preparing an answer to the complaint. Physicians should be willing to educate their attorneys about the medical facts of the case, although most medical malpractice attorneys will be knowledgeable and medically sophisticated.

The next phase of the malpractice suit is called *discovery*. The purpose of discovery is the gathering of facts and clarification of issues in advance of the trial. In all likelihood the anesthesiologist will initially receive a written interrogatory, which will request factual information. In consultation with the defense attorney, the interrogatory should be answered in writing because carelessly or inadvertently misstated facts can become troublesome later.

Depositions are a second mechanism of discovery. The defendant-anesthesiologist will be deposed as a fact witness, and depositions will be obtained from other anesthesiologists who will act as expert witnesses. A nationally recognized expert in the area in question, recommended by the defendant but who is not a personal friend, and who agrees with the defense position, may be very valuable.

The plaintiff's attorney, not the defense attorney, will depose the anesthesiologist. Despite the apparent informality of the deposition, the anesthesiologist must be constantly aware that what is said during the deposition carries as much weight as what would be said in court. It is important to be factually prepared for the deposition by review of personal notes, the anesthetic record, and the medical record. The physician should dress conservatively and professionally because appearance and image are very important. The opposition is assessing the physician to see how he or she will appear to a jury. Answer only the question asked, and do not volunteer information. Rely on one's attorney for assistance when preparing for a deposition.

There will be depositions from expert witnesses, both for the plaintiff and for the defense. The anesthesiologist should work with his or her attorney to suggest questions and rebuttals. The better educated the attorney is about the medical facts, the reasons the anesthesiologist did what was done, and the alternative approaches, the better able the attorney will be to conduct these expert depositions.

If there is some merit in the case but the damages are minimal, or if proof of innocence will be difficult, there will probably be a settlement offer. There is a high cost incurred by both plaintiffs and defendants in pursuing a malpractice claim up through a jury trial. Unless there is a strong probability of a large dollar award, reputable plaintiffs' attorneys are not likely to pursue the claim. Thus, even if physicians believe that they are totally innocent of any wrongdoing, they should not be offended or angered about settling of the case: This is solely a matter of money, not medicine.

If a settlement is not reached during the discovery phase, a trial will occur. Only about 1 in 20 malpractice cases ever reach the point of a jury trial. Only those cases in which both sides think they can win, and which are likely to have significant financial impact, will proceed to trial.

The discussion of deposition testimony also applies to testimony in court, but there are a few additional points to consider during the trial. The members of the jury will not be as sophisticated medically as the attorneys who deposed the anesthesiologist during discovery. However, do not underestimate the intelligence of the jury. Talking down to them will create an unfavorable impression. If the answer to a question is not known, avoid guessing. If specific facts cannot be remembered, say so. Nobody expects total recall of events that may have occurred years before.

The defendant-physician should be present during the entire trial, even when not testifying, and should dress professionally. Displays of anger, remorse, relief, or hostility will hurt the physician in court. The physician should be able to give his or her testimony without using notes or documents. When it is necessary to refer to the medical record, it will be admitted into evidence. The anesthesiologist's goal is to convince the jury that he or she behaved in this case as any other competent and prudent anesthesiologist would have behaved.

It is important to keep in mind that *proof* in a malpractice case means only "more likely than not." The patient-plaintiff must "prove" the four elements of negligence, not to absolute certainty, but only to a probability greater than 50%. On the positive side, this means that the defendant-anesthesiologist must only show that his or her actions were, more likely than not, within an acceptable standard of care.

Acknowledgments

The authors wish to thank F. W. Cheney, MD, and D. A. Kroll, MD, whose material from previous editions of this chapter has been retained in the current edition.

REFERENCES

1. Beecher HK, Todd DP. A study of the deaths associated with anesthesia and surgery: based on a study of 599,548 anesthesias in 10 institutions 1948–1952, inclusive. *Ann Surg.* 1954;140:2–35.
2. Flick RP, Sprung J, Harrison TE, et al. Perioperative cardiac arrests in children between 1988 and 2005 at a tertiary referral center: a study of 92,881 patients. *Anesthesiology.* 2007;106:226–237.
3. Newland MC, Ellis SJ, Lydiatt CA, et al. Anesthetic-related cardiac arrest and its mortality: a report covering 72,959 anesthetics over 10 years from a US teaching hospital. *Anesthesiology.* 2002;97:108–115.
4. Lagasse RS. Anesthesia safety: Model or myth? A review of the published literature and analysis of current original data. *Anesthesiology.* 2002;97:1609–1617.
5. Morray JP, Geiduschek JM, Ramamoorthy C, et al. Anesthesia-related cardiac arrest in children: initial findings of the Pediatric Perioperative Cardiac Arrest (POCA) Registry. *Anesthesiology.* 2000;93:6–14.
6. Li G, Warner M, Lang BH, et al. Epidemiology of anesthesia-related mortality in the United States, 1999–2005. *Anesthesiology.* 2009;110(4):759–765.
7. Ellis SJ, Newland MC, Simonsen JA, et al. Anesthesia-related cardiac arrest. *Anesthesiology.* 2014;120;829–838.
8. Bainbridge D, Martin J, Arango M, et al. Perioperative and anesthesia-related mortality in developed and developing countries: a systematic review and meta-analysis. *Lancet.* 2012;380:1075–1081.
9. Biboulet P, Aubas P, Dubourdieu J, et al. Fatal and non fatal cardiac arrests related to anesthesia. *Can J Anaesth.* 2001;48:326–328.
10. Eagle CC, Davis NJ. Report of the Anaesthetic Mortality Committee of Western Australia 1990–1995. *Anaesth Intensive Care.* 1997;25:51–59.
11. Khan M, Khan FA. Anesthetic deaths in a developing country. *Middle East J Anesthesiol.* 2007;19:159–172.
12. Ahmed A, Ali M, Khan M, et al. Perioperative cardiac arrests in children at a university teaching hospital of a developing country over 15 years. *Paediatr Anaesth.* 2009;19:581–586.
13. Davis NJ, ed. *Anaesthesia Related Mortality in Australia 1994. Report of the Committee convened under the auspices of the Australian and New Zealand College of Anaesthetists.* Melbourne: Capitol Press; 1999.
14. Kawashima Y, Takahashi S, Suzuki M, et al. Anesthesia-related mortality and morbidity over a 5-year period in 2,363,038 patients in Japan. *Acta Anaesthesiol Scand.* 2003;47:809–817.
15. Arbous MS, Grobbee DE, van Kleef JW, et al. Mortality associated with anaesthesia: a qualitative analysis to identify risk factors. *Anaesthesia.* 2001;56:1141–1153.
16. Braz LG, Modolo NSP, do Nascimento P, et al. Perioperative cardiac arrest: a study of 53,718 anaesthetics over 9 yr from a Brazilian teaching hospital. *Br J Anaesth.* 2006;96:569–575.
17. Lienhart A, Auroy Y, Pequignot F, et al. Survey of anesthesia-related mortality in France. *Anesthesiology.* 2006;105:1087–1097.
18. Kawashima Y, Seo N, Morita K, et al. Annual study of perioperative mortality and morbidity for the year of 1999 in Japan: THE outlines report of the Japan Society of Anesthesiologists Committee on Operating Room Safety (in Japanese). *Masui.* 2001;50:1260–1274.
19. Irita K, Kawashima Y, Iwao Y, et al. Annual mortality and morbidity in operating rooms during 2002 and summary of morbidity and mortality between 1999 and 2002 in Japan: a brief review (in Japanese). *Masui.* 2004;53:320–335.
20. Charuluxananan S, Chinachoti T, Pulnitiporn A, et al. The Thai Anesthesia Incidents Study (THAI Study) of perioperative death: ANALYSIS of risk factors. *J Med Assoc Thai.* 2005;88(7):S30–S40.
21. Gibbs N, ed. *Safety of Anaesthesia: A Review of Anaesthesia-Related Mortality Reporting in Australia and New Zealand 2003–2005. Report of the mortality working group convened under the auspices of the Australian and New Zealand College of Anaesthetists.* Melbourne: Australian and New Zealand College of Anaesthetists; 2009.
22. Rukewe A, Fatiregun A, Osunlaja TO. Cardiac arrest during anesthesia at a university hospital in Nigeria. *Niger J Clin Pract.* 214;17:28–31.
23. Gonzalez LP, Braz JR, Modolo MP, et al. Pediatric perioperative cardiac arrest and mortality: a study from a tertiary teaching hospital. *Pediatr Crit Care Med.* 2014;18:878–884.
24. van der Griend BF, Lister NA, McKenzie IM, et al. Postoperative mortality in children after 101,885 anesthetics at a tertiary pediatric hospital. *Anesth Analg.* 2011;112:1440–1447.
25. de Bruin L, Pasma W, van der Werff DBM, et al. Perioperative hospital mortality at a tertiary paediatric institution. *Br J Anaesth.* 2015;115:608–615.
26. Brull R, McCartney CJ, Chan VW, et al. Neurological complications after regional anesthesia: contemporary estimates of risk. *Anesth Analg.* 2007;104:965–974.
27. Warner MA, Warner DO, Matsumoto JY, et al. Ulnar neuropathy in surgical patients. *Anesthesiology.* 1999;90:54–59.
28. Warner MA, Warner DO, Harper CM, et al. Lower extremity neuropathies associated with lithotomy positions. *Anesthesiology.* 2000;93:938–942.
29. Welch MB, Brummett CM, Welch TD, et al. Perioperative peripheral nerve injuries: a retrospective study of 380,680 cases during a 10-year period at a single institution. *Anesthesiology.* 2009;111:490–497.
30. Auroy Y, Benhamou D, Bargues L, et al. Major complications of regional anesthesia in France: the SOS Regional Anesthesia Hotline Service. *Anesthesiology.* 2002;97:1274–1280.
31. de Sèze MP, Sztark F, Janvier G, et al. Severe and long-lasting complications of the nerve root and spinal cord after central neuraxial blockade. *Anesth Analg.* 2007;104:975–979.
32. Sites BD, Taenzer AH, Herrick MD, et al. Incidence of local anesthetic systemic toxicity and postoperative neurologic symptoms associated with 12,668 ultrasound-guided nerve blocks: an analysis from a prospective clinical registry. *Reg Anesth Pain Med.* 2012;37:478–482.
33. Barrington MJ, Watts SA, Gledhill SR, et al. Preliminary results of the Australasian Regional Anaesthesia Collaboration: a prospective audit of more than 7000 peripheral nerve and plexus blocks for neurologic and other complications. *Reg Anesth Pain Med.* 2009;34:534–541.
34. Errando CL, Sigl JC, Robles M, et al. Awareness with recall during general anesthesia: a prospective observational evaluation of 4001 patients. *Br J Anaesth.* 2008;101:178–185.

35. Sandin RH, Enlund G, Samuelsson P, et al. Awareness during anaesthesia: a prospective case study. Lancet. 2000;355:707–711.
36. Sebel PS, Bowdle TA, Ghoneim MM, et al. The incidence of awareness during anesthesia: a multicenter United States study. Anesth Analg. 2004;99:833–839.
37. Avidan MS, Zhang L, Burnside BA, et al. Anesthesia awareness and the bispectral index. N Engl J Med. 2008;358:1097–1108.
38. Xu L, Wu AS, Yue Y. The incidence of intra-operative awareness during general anesthesia in China: a multi-center observational study. Acta Anaesthesiol Scand. 2009;53:873–882.
39. Mashour GA, Shanks A, Tremper KK, et al. Prevention of intraoperative awareness with explicit recall in an unselected surgical population: a randomized comparative effectiveness trial. Anesthesiology. 2012;117:717–725.
40. Pandit JJ, Cook TM, Jonker WR, et al. A national survey of anaesthetists (NAP5 Baseline) to estimate an annual incidence of accidental awareness during general anaesthesia in the UK. Br J Anaesth. 2013;110:501–509.
41. Pandit JJ, Andrade J, Bogod DG, et al. 5th National Audit Project (NAP5) on accidental awareness during general anaesthesia: summary of main findings and risk factors. Br J Anaesth. 2014;113:549–559.
42. Chang SH, Miller NR. The incidence of vision loss due to perioperative ischemic optic neuropathy associated with spine surgery: the Johns Hopkins experience. Spine. 2005;30:1299–1302.
43. Warner ME, Warner MA, Garrity JA, et al. The frequency of perioperative vision loss. Anesth Analg. 2001;93:1417–1421.
44. Roth S, Thisted RA, Erickson JP, et al. Eye injuries after nonocular surgery: a study of 60,965 anesthetics from 1988 to 1992. Anesthesiology. 1996;85:1020–1027.
45. Patil CG, Lad EM, Lad SP, et al. Visual loss after spine surgery: a population-based study. Spine. 2008;33:1491–1496.
46. Holy SE, Tsai JH, McAllister RK, et al. Perioperative ischemic optic neuropathy: a case control analysis of 126,666 surgical procedures at a single institution. Anesthesiology. 2009;110:246–253.
47. Shen Y, Drum M, Roth S. The prevalence of perioperative visual loss in the United States: a 10-year study from 1996 to 2005 of spinal, orthopedic, cardiac, and general surgery. Anesth Analg. 2009;109:1534–1545.
48. Warner ME, Fronapfel PJ, Hebl JR, et al. Perioperative visual changes. Anesthesiology. 2002;96:855–859.
49. Nandyala SV, Marquez-Lara A, Fineberg SJ, et al. Incidence and risk factors for perioperative visual loss after spine fusion. Spine J. 2014;14:1866–1872.
50. Martin DP, Weingarten TN, Gunn PW, et al. Performance improvement system and postoperative corneal injuries: incidence and risk factors. Anesthesiology. 2009;111:320–326.
51. Yu HD, Chou AH, Yang MW, et al. An analysis of perioperative eye injuries after nonocular surgery. Acta Anaesthesiol Taiwan. 2010;48:122–129.
52. Kara-Junior N, Espindola RF, Valverde Filho J, et al. Ocular risk management in patients undergoing general anesthesia: an analysis of 39,431 surgeries. Clinics (Sao Paulo). 2015;70:541–543.
53. Warner ME, Benenfeld SM, Warner MA, et al. Perianesthetic dental injuries: frequency, outcomes, and risk factors. Anesthesiology. 1999;90:1302–1305.
54. Newland MC, Ellis SJ, Peters KR, et al. Dental injury associated with anesthesia: a report of 161,687 anesthetics given over 14 years. J Clin Anesth. 2007;19:339–345.
55. Adolphs N, Kessler B, von Heyman C, et al. Dentoalveolar injury related to general anaesthesia: a 14 years review and a statement from the surgical point of view based on a retrospective analysis of the documentation of a university hospital. Dent Traumatol. 2011;27:10–14.
56. Vogel J, Stubinger S, Kaufmann M, et al. Dental injuries resulting from tracheal intubation—a retrospective study. Dent Traumatol. 2009;25:73–77.
57. Gaudio RM, Barbieri S, Feltracco P, et al. Traumatic dental injuries during anaesthesia. Part II: medico-legal evaluation and liability. Dent Traumatol. 2011;27:40–45.
58. Martin LD, Mhyre JM, Shanks AM, et al. 3,423 emergency tracheal intubations at a university hospital: airway outcomes and complications. Anesthesiology. 2011;114:42–48.
59. Vallejo MC, Best MW, Phelps AL, et al. Perioperative dental injury at a tertiary care health system: an eight-year audit of 816,690 anesthetics. J Healthcare Risk Manag. 2012;31:25–32.
60. Mourao J, Neto J, Luis C, et al. Dental injury after conventional direct laryngoscopy: a prospective observational study. Anaesthesia. 2013;68:1059–1065.
61. The Postoperative Visual Loss Study Group. Risk factors associated with ischemic optic neuropathy after spinal fusion surgery. Anesthesiology. 2012;116:15–24.
62. Avidan MS, Evers AS. The fallacy of persistent postoperative cognitive decline. Anesthesiology. 2016;124:255–258.
63. Dokkedal U, Hansen TG, Rasmussen LS, et al. Cognitive functioning after surgery in middle-aged and elderly Danish twins. Anesthesiology. 2016;124:312–321.
64. Davidson AJ, Disma N, de Graff JC, et al. Neurodevelopmental outcome at 2 years of age after general anaesthesia and awake-regional anaesthesia in infancy (GAS): an international multicentre, randomized controlled trial. Lancet. 2016;387:239–250.
65. Committee on Quality of Health Care in America, Institute of Medicine. Crossing the Quality Chasm, A New Health System for the 21st Century. Washington, DC: National Academy Press; 2001.
66. Gaba DM, Maxwell M, DeAnda A. Anesthetic mishaps: breaking the chain of accident evolution. Anesthesiology. 1987;66:670–676.
67. Standards & Guidelines. American Society of Anesthesiologists website http://asahq.org/quality-and-practice-management/standards-and-guidelines. Accessed February 19, 2016.
68. Krombach JW, Marks JD, Dubowitz G, et al. Development and implementation of checklists for routine anesthesia care: a proposal for improving patient safety. Anesth Analg. 2015;121:1097–1103.
69. Provonost P, Needham D, Berenholtz S, et al. An intervention to decrease catheter-related bloodstream infections in the ICU. N Engl J Med. 2006;355:2725–2732.
70. American Society of Anesthesiologists (ASA). Task Force on Central Venous Access: practice guidelines for central venous access. Anesthesiology. 2012;116:539–573.
71. Neal JM, Hsiung RL, Mulroy MF, et al. ASRA checklist improves trainee performance during a simulated episode of local anesthetic systemic toxicity. Reg Anesth Pain Med. 2012;37:8–15.
72. Ziewacz JE, Arriaga AF, Bader AM, et al. Crisis checklists for the operating room: development and pilot testing. J Am Coll Surg. 2011;213:212–219.
73. Arriga AF, Bader AM, Wong JM, et al. Simulation-based trial of surgical trial checklists. N Engl J Med. 2013;368:246–253.
74. Haynes AB, Weiser TG, Berry WR, et al. A surgical safety checklist to reduce morbidity and mortality in a global population. N Engl J Med. 2009;360:491–499.
75. Tscholl DW, Weiss M, Kolbe M, et al. An anesthesia preinduction checklist to improve information exchange, knowledge of critical information, perception of safety, and possibly perception of teamwork in anesthesia teams. Anesth Analg. 2015;121:948–956.
76. Etchells E, Ferrari M, Kiss A, et al. Informed decision-making in elective major vascular surgery: analysis of 145 surgeon-patient consultations. Can J Surg. 2011;54:173–178.
77. Ankuda CK, Block SD, Copper Z, et al. Measuring critical deficits in shared decision making before elective surgery. Patient Educ Couns. 2014;94:328–333.
78. Whittle J, Conigliaro J, Good CB, et al. Understanding of the benefits of coronary revascularization procedures among patients who are offered such procedures. Am Heart J. 2007;154:662–668.
79. Posner KL, Severson JR, Domino KB. The role of informed consent in patient complaints: Reducing hidden health system costs and improving patient engagement through shared decision-making. J Healthcare Risk Manag. 2015;35:38–45.
80. Hickson GB, Jenkins DA. Identifying and addressing communication failures as a means of reducing unnecessary malpractice claims. NC Med J. 2007;68:362–364.
81. Pichert JW, Moore IN, Karrass J, et al. An intervention model that promotes accountability: peer messengers and patient/family complaints. Jt Comm J Qual Patient Saf. 2013;39:435–446.
82. Charles C, Gafni A, Whelan T. Shared decision-making in the medical encounter: what does it mean? (Or it takes at least two to tango). Soc Sci Med. 1997;44:681–692.
83. Cooper Z, Sayal P, Abbett SK, et al. A conceptual framework for appropriateness in surgical care: reviewing past approaches and looking ahead to patient-centered shared decision making. Anesthesiology. 2015;123:1450–1454.
84. Fowler FJ Jr, Levin CA, Sepucha KR. Informing and involving patients to improve the quality of medical decisions. Health Aff. 2011;30:699–706.
85. Souter KJ, Gallagher TH. The disclosure of unanticipated outcomes of care and medical errors: what does this mean for anesthesiologists? Anesth Analg. 2012;114:615–621.
86. Hillestad R, Bigelow J, Bower A, et al. Can electronic medical record systems transform health care? Potential health benefits, savings and costs. Health Aff (Millwood). 2005;24:1103–1117.
87. McLellan S, Galvin M, McMaugh D. Benefits measurement from the use of an automated anaesthetic record keeping system (AARK). Electron J Health Inform. 2011;6(1):e6.
88. Chaudhry B, Wang J, Wu S, et al. Systematic review: impact of health information technology on quality, efficiency, and costs of medical care. Ann Intern Med. 2006;144:742–752.
89. Reich DL, Kahn RA, Wax D, et al. Development of a module for point-of-care charge capture and submission using an anesthesia information management system. Anesthesiology. 2006;105:179–186.
90. Spring SF, Sandberg WS, Anupama S, et al. Automated documentation error detection and notification improves anesthesia billing performance. Anesthesiology. 2007;106:157–163.
91. Wanderer JP, Sandberg WS, Ehrenfeld JM. Real-time alerts and reminders using information systems. Anesthesiol Clin. 2011;29:389–396.
92. Nair BG, Grunzweig K, Peterson GN, et al. Intraoperative blood glucose management: impact of a real-time decision support system on adherence to institutional protocol. J Clin Monit Comput. 2015.
93. Nair BG, Newman SF, Peterson GN, et al. Feedback mechanisms including real-time electronic alerts to achieve near 100% timely prophylactic antibiotic administration in surgical cases. Anesth Analg. 2010;111:1293–1300.

94. Nair BG, Horibe M, Newman SF, et al. Anesthesia information management system-based near real-time decision support to manage intraoperative hypotension and hypertension. *Anesth Analg*. 2014;118:206–214.
95. Vigoda MM, Lubarsky DA. Failure to recognize loss of incoming data in an anesthesia record-keeping system may have increased medical liability. *Anesth Analg*. 2006;102:1798–1802.
96. Miller AR, Tucker CE. Electronic discovery and the adoption of information technology. *J Law Econ Organ*. 2014;30:217–243.
97. Mangalmurti SS, Murtagh L, Mello MM. Medical malpractice liability in the age of electronic health records. *N Engl J Med*. 2010;363:2060–2067.
98. Virapongse A, Bates DW, Shi P, et al. Electronic health records and malpractice claims in office practice. *Arch Intern Med*. 2008;168:2362–2367.
99. Vigoda MM, Lubarsky DA. The medicolegal importance of enhancing timeliness of documentation when using an anesthesia information system and the response to automated feedback in an academic practice. *Anesth Analg*. 2006;103:131–136.
100. Gallagher TH, Studdert D, Levinson W. Disclosing harmful medical errors to patients. *N Engl J Med*. 2007;356:2713–2719.
101. Kachalia A, Bates DW. Disclosing medical errors: the view from the USA. *Surgeon*. 2014;12:64–67.
102. Studdert DM, Mello M, Gawande AA, et al. Disclosure of medical injury to patients: an improbable risk management strategy. *Health Aff*. 2007;26:215–226.
103. Mello MM, Gallagher TH. Malpractice reform: opportunities for leadership by health care institutions and liability insurers. *N Engl J Med*. 2010;362:1353–1356.
104. Boothman RC, Blackwell AC, Campbell DA, et al. A better approach to medical malpractice claims? The University of Michigan experience. *J Health Life Sci Law*. 2009;2:125–159.
105. Quinn RE, Iechler MC. The 3Rs Program: the Colorado experience. *Clin Obstet Gynecol*. 2008;51:709–718.
106. Ethical Guidelines of the Anesthesia Care of Patients with Do-Not-Resuscitate Orders or Other Directives That Limit Treatment. American Society of Anesthesiologists website. http://www.asahq.org/~/media/sites/asahq/files/public/resources/standards-guidelines/ethical-guidelines-for-the-anesthesia-care-of-patients.pdf. Updated October 16, 2013. Accessed February 19, 2016.
107. Lawson T, Ralph C. Perioperative Jehovah's Witnesses: a review. *Br J Anaesthesia*. 2015;115(5):676–687.
108. National Practitioner Data Bank for Adverse Information on Physicians and Other Health Care Practitioners. Code of Federal Regulations. Title 45, Subtitle A, Subchapter A, Part 60 (2002). http://www.ecfr.gov/cgi-bin/text-idx?tpl=/ecfrbrowse/Title45/45cfr60_main_02.tpl. Accessed February 19, 2016.
109. Baldwin LM, Hart LG, Oshel RE, et al. Hospital peer review and the National Practitioner Data Bank: clinical privileges action reports. *JAMA*. 1999;282:349–355.
110. Health Resources and Services Administration (HRSA), HHS. National Practitioner Data Bank for adverse information on physicians and other health care practitioners: reporting on adverse and negative actions. Final rule. *Fed Regist*. 2010;75(18):4655–4682.
111. Donabedian A. The quality of care: how can it be assessed? *JAMA*. 1988;260:1743–1748.
112. Deming WE. *Out of the Crisis*. Cambridge: Massachusetts Institute of Technology; 1986.
113. Juran JM. *Juran on Planning for Quality*. New York: Free Press; 1988.
114. Kohn LT, Corrigan JM, Donaldson MS, eds. Committee on Quality of Health Care in America, Institute of Medicine. *To Err Is Human: Building a Safer Health System*. Washington, DC: National Academy Press; 1999.
115. Mello MM, Boothman RC, McDonald T, et al. Communication and resolution programs: the challenges and lessons learned from six early adopters. *Health Aff*. 2014;1;11–19.
116. Roberts JS, Coale JG, Redman RR. A history of the Joint Commission on Accreditation of Hospitals. *JAMA*. 1987;258:936–940.
117. National patient safety goals. The Joint Commission website. http://www.jointcommission.org/standards_information/npsgs.aspx. Accessed February 19, 2016.
118. What does "ORYX" stand for? The Joint Commission website. March 29, 2013. https://manual.jointcommission.org/Manual/Questions/UserQuestion100049. Accessed February 19, 2016.
119. Sentinel event policy and procedures. The Joint Commission website. http://www.jointcommission.org/Sentinel_Event_Policy_and_Procedures./ Updated January 6, 2016. Accessed February 19, 2016.
120. Hospital value-based purchasing. The Centers for Medicare & Medicaid Services website. https://www.cms.gov/Medicare/Quality-Initiatives-Patient-Assessment-Instruments/hospital-value-based-purchasing/index.html?redirect = /Hospital-Value-Based-Purchasing. Updated October 30, 2015. Accessed February 19, 2016.
121. Schonberger RB, Barash PG, Lagasse RS. The Surgical Care Improvement Project antibiotic guidelines: should we expect anything more than good intentions? *Anesth Analg*. 2015;121:397–403.
122. Sutton M, Nikolova S, Boaden P, et al. Reduced mortality with hospital pay for performance in England. *N Engl J Med*. 2012;367:1821–1828.
123. Jha AK, Joynt KE, Orav EJ, et al. The long-term effect of Premier pay for performance on patient outcomes. *N Engl J Med*. 2012;366:1606–1615.
124. Flodgren G, Eccles MP, Shepperd S, et al. An overview of reviews evaluating the effectiveness of financial incentives in changing healthcare professional behaviours and patient outcomes. *Cochrane Database Syst Rev*. 2011;7:CD009255.
125. Hawkins RB, Levy SM, Senter CE, et al. Beyond surgical care improvement program compliance: antibiotic prophylaxis implementation gaps. *Am J Surg*. 2013;206:451–456.
126. Dutton RP, DuKatz A. Quality improvement using automated data sources: the Anesthesia Quality Institute. *Anesthesiol Clin*. 2011;29:439–454.
127. Committee on Professional Liability, American Society of Anesthesiologists. *Manual on Professional Liability*. Schaumburg, IL: American Society of Anesthesiologists, 2010.
128. Caplan RA, Posner KL, Cheney FW. Effect of outcome on physician judgments of appropriateness of care. *JAMA*. 1991;265:1957–1960.
129. Quality and practice management. American Society of Anesthesiologists website. http://www.asahq.org/quality-and-practice-management. Accessed on February 19, 2016.
130. Localio AR, Lawthers AG, Brennan TA, et al. Relation between malpractice claims and adverse events due to negligence: results of the Harvard Medical Practice Study III. *N Engl J Med*. 1991;325:245–251.
131. Cheney FW, Posner K, Caplan RA, et al. Standard of care and anesthesia liability. *JAMA*. 1989;261:1599–1603.
132. Cheney FW. The American Society of Anesthesiologists Closed Claims Project: what have we learned, how has it affected practice, and how will it affect practice in the future? *Anesthesiology*. 1999;91:552–556.
133. Metzner J, Posner KL, Lam MS, et al. Closed claims' analysis. *Best Pract Res Clin Anaesthesiol*. 2011;25:263–276.
134. Bhananker SM, Posner KL, Cheney FW, et al. Injury and liability associated with monitored anesthesia care: a closed claims analysis. *Anesthesiology*. 2006;104:228–234.
135. Mehta SP, Bhananker SM, Posner KL, et al. Operating room fires: a closed claims analysis. *Anesthesiology*. 2013;118:1133–1139.
136. Cheney FW, Posner KL, Lee LA, et al. Trends in anesthesia-related death and brain damage: a closed claims analysis. *Anesthesiology*. 2006;105:1081–1086.
137. Cheney FW, Domino KB, Caplan RA, et al. Nerve injury associated with anesthesia: a closed claims analysis. *Anesthesiology*. 1999;90:1062–1069.
138. Warner MA, Warner ME, Martin JT. Ulnar neuropathy: incidence, outcome, and risk factors in sedated or anesthetized patients. *Anesthesiology*. 1994;81:1332–1340.
139. Lee LA, Posner KL, Kent CD, et al. Complications associated with peripheral nerve blocks: Lessons from the ASA closed claims project. *Int Anesthesiol Clin*. 2011;49:56–67.
140. Fitzgibbon DR, Posner KL, Domino KB, et al. Chronic pain management: American Society of Anesthesiologists Closed Claims Project. *Anesthesiology*. 2004;100:98–105.
141. Pollak KA, Stephens LS, Posner KL, et al. Trends in pain medicine liability. *Anesthesiology*. 2015;123:1133–1141.
142. Rathmell JP, Michna E, Fitzgibbon DR, et al. Injury and liability associated with cervical procedures for chronic pain. *Anesthesiology*. 2011;114:918–926.
143. Fitzgibbon DR, Rathmell JP, Michna E, et al. Malpractice claims associated with medication management for chronic pain. *Anesthesiology*. 2010;112:948–956.

5 Electrical and Fire Safety*

JAN EHRENWERTH

Principles of Electricity
  Direct and Alternating Currents
  Impedance
  Capacitance
  Inductance
Electrical Shock Hazards
  Alternating and Direct Currents
  Source of Shocks
  Grounding
Electrical Power: Grounded
Electrical Power: Ungrounded
The Line Isolation Monitor
Ground Fault Circuit Interrupter
Double Insulation
Microshock
Electrosurgery
  Conductive Flooring
Environmental Hazards
Electromagnetic Interference
Construction of New Operating Rooms
Fire Safety

KEY POINTS

1. A basic principle of electricity is known as *Ohm's law* (Voltage = current × resistance).
2. To have the completed circuit necessary for current flow, a closed loop must exist and a voltage source must drive the current through the impedance.
3. To receive a shock, one must contact the electrical circuit at two points, and there must be a voltage source that causes the current to flow through an individual.
4. In electrical terminology, *grounding* is applied to two separate concepts: the grounding of electrical power and the grounding of electrical equipment.
5. To provide an extra measure of safety from gross electrical shock (macroshock), the power supplied to most operating rooms (ORs) is ungrounded.
6. The line isolation monitor is a device that continuously monitors the integrity of an isolated power system.
7. The ground fault circuit interrupter is a popular device used to prevent individuals from receiving an electrical shock in a grounded power system.
8. An electrically susceptible patient (i.e., one who has a direct, external connection to the heart) may be at risk from very small currents; this is called *microshock*.
9. Problems can arise if the electrosurgical return plate is improperly applied to the patient or if the cord connecting the return plate to the electrosurgical unit is damaged or broken.
10. Fires in the OR are just as much a danger today as they were 100 years ago when patients were anesthetized with flammable anesthetic agents.
11. The necessary components for a fire consist of the triad of heat or an ignition source, a fuel, and an oxidizer.
12. The two major ignition sources for OR fires are the electrosurgical unit and the laser.
13. It is known that desiccated carbon dioxide absorbent can, in rare circumstances, react with sevoflurane to produce a fire.
14. All OR personnel should be familiar with the location and operation of fire extinguishers.

The myriad of electrical and electronic devices in the modern operating room (OR) greatly improve patient care and safety. However, these devices also subject both the patient and OR personnel to increased risks. To reduce the risk of electrical shock, most ORs have electrical systems that incorporate special safety features. It is incumbent upon the anesthesiologist to have a thorough understanding of the basic principles of electricity and an appreciation of the concepts of electrical safety applicable to the OR environment.

---

*This chapter and images were developed in whole for both Barash PG, Cullen BF, Stoelting RK, et al., eds. *Clinical Anesthesia*, 8th ed. Philadelphia, PA: Wolters Kluwer Health/Lippincott Williams & Wilkins, and Ehrenwerth J, Eisenkraft JB, Berry JM, eds. *Anesthesia Equipment: Principles and Applications*. 2nd ed. Philadelphia, PA: Elsevier, with permission of the editors and publishers.

Principles of Electricity

A basic principle of electricity is known as *Ohm's law*, which is represented by the equation:

$$E = I \times R$$

where E is electromotive force (in volts), I is current (in amperes), and R is resistance (in ohms). Ohm's law forms the basis for the physiologic equation BP = CO × SVR; that is, blood pressure (BP) is equal to the cardiac output (CO) times the systemic vascular resistance (SVR). In this case, the BP of the vascular system is analogous to voltage, the CO to current, and the SVR to the forces opposing the flow of electrons. Electrical power (P) is measured in watts (W). Power is the product of the voltage (E) and the current (I), as defined by the formula:

$$P = E \times I$$

The amount of electrical work done is measured in watts multiplied by a unit of time. The watt-second (a joule, J) is a common designation for electrical energy expended in doing work. The energy produced by a defibrillator is measured in watt-seconds (or joules). The kilowatt-hour is used by electrical utility companies to measure larger quantities of electrical energy.

Power can be thought of as a measure not only of work done but also of heat produced in any electrical circuit. Substituting Ohm's law in the formula:

$$P = E \times I$$
$$P = (I \times R) \times I$$
$$P = I^2 \times R$$

Thus, power is equal to the square of the current I^2 (amperage) times the resistance R. Using these formulas, it is possible to calculate the number of amperes and the resistance of a given device if the wattage and the voltage are known. For example, a 60-W light bulb operating on a household 120-V circuit would require 0.5 A of current for operation. Rearranging the formula so that:

$$I = P/E$$

We have:

$$I = (60 \text{ watts})/120 \text{ volts}$$
$$I = 0.5 \text{ ampere}$$

Using this in Ohm's law:

$$R = E/I$$

The resistance can be calculated to be 240 ohms:

$$R = (120 \text{ volts})/(0.5 \text{ ampere})$$
$$R = 240 \text{ ohms}$$

It is obvious from the previous discussion that 1 V of electromotive force (EMF) flowing through a 1-ohm resistance will generate 1 A of current. Similarly, 1 A of current induced by 1 V of EMF will generate 1 W of power.

Direct and Alternating Currents

Any substance that permits the flow of electrons is called a *conductor*. Current is characterized by electrons flowing through a conductor. If the electron flow is always in the same direction, it is referred to as *direct current* (DC). However, if the electron flow reverses direction at a regular interval, it is termed *alternating current* (AC). Either of these types of current can be pulsed or continuous in nature.

The previous discussion of Ohm's law is accurate when applied to DC circuits. However, when dealing with AC circuits, the situation is more complex because the flow of the current is opposed by a more complicated form of resistance, known as *impedance*.

Impedance

Impedance, designated by the letter Z, is defined as the sum of the forces that oppose electron movement in an AC circuit. Impedance consists of resistance (ohms) but also takes capacitance and inductance into account. In actuality, when referring to AC circuits, Ohm's law is defined as:

$$E = I \times Z$$

An *insulator* is a substance that opposes the flow of electrons. Therefore, an insulator has a high impedance to electron flow, whereas a conductor has a low impedance to electron flow.

In AC circuits, the capacitance and inductance can be important factors in determining the total impedance. Both capacitance and inductance are influenced by the frequency (cycles per second or hertz, Hz) at which the AC current reverses direction. The impedance is directly proportional to the frequency (f) times the inductance (IND):

$$Z \propto (f \times IND)$$

and the impedance is inversely proportional to the product of the frequency (f) and the capacitance (CAP):

$$Z \propto 1/(f \times CAP)$$

As the AC current increases in frequency, the net effect of both capacitance and inductance increases. However, because impedance and capacitance are inversely related, total impedance decreases as the product of the frequency and the capacitance increases. Thus, as frequency increases, impedance falls and more current is allowed to pass.

Capacitance

A *capacitor* consists of any two parallel conductors that are separated by an insulator (Fig. 5-1). A capacitor has the ability to store charge. *Capacitance* is the measure of that substance's ability to store charge. In a DC circuit the capacitor plates are charged by a voltage source (i.e., a battery) and there is only a momentary current flow. The circuit is not completed and no further current can flow unless a resistance is connected between the two plates and the capacitor is discharged.

In contrast to DC circuits, a capacitor in an AC circuit permits current flow even when the circuit is not completed by a resistance. This is because of the nature of AC circuits, in which the current flow is constantly being reversed. Because current flow results from the movement of electrons, the capacitor plates are alternately charged—first positive and then negative with every reversal of the AC current direction—resulting in an effective current flow as far as the remainder of the circuit is concerned, even though the circuit is not completed.

Since the effect of capacitance on impedance varies directly with the AC frequency in hertz, the greater the AC frequency, the lower the impedance. Therefore, high-frequency currents (0.5 to 2 million Hz), such as those used by electrosurgical units (ESUs), will cause a marked decrease in impedance.

Electrical devices use capacitors for various beneficial purposes. There is, however, a phenomenon known as *stray capacitance*—capacitance that was not designed into the system but is incidental to the construction of the equipment. All AC-operated equipment produces stray capacitance. An ordinary power cord, for example, consisting of two insulated wires running next to each other will generate significant capacitance simply by being plugged into a 120-V circuit, even though the piece of equipment is not turned on. Another example of stray capacitance is found in electric motors. The circuit wiring in

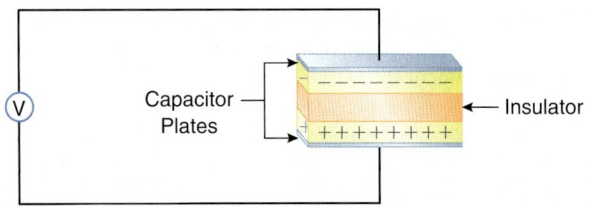

Figure 5-1 A capacitor consists of two parallel conductors separated by an insulator. The capacitor is capable of storing charge supplied by a voltage source.

electric motors generates stray capacitance to the metal housing of the motor. The clinical importance of capacitance will be emphasized later in the chapter.

Inductance

Whenever electrons flow in a wire, a magnetic field is induced around the wire. If the wire is coiled repeatedly around an iron core, as in a transformer, the magnetic field can be very strong. *Inductance* is a property of AC circuits in which an opposing EMF can be electromagnetically generated in the circuit. The net effect of inductance is to increase impedance. Since the effect of inductance on impedance also depends on AC frequency, increases in frequency will increase the total impedance. Therefore, the total impedance of a coil will be much greater than its simple resistance.

Electrical Shock Hazards

Alternating and Direct Currents

Whenever an individual contacts an external source of electricity, an electrical shock is possible. An electrical current can stimulate skeletal muscle cells to contract, and thus can be used therapeutically in devices such as pacemakers or defibrillators. However, casual contact with an electrical current, whether AC or DC, can lead to injury or death. Although it takes approximately three times as much DC as AC to cause ventricular fibrillation, this by no means renders DC harmless. Devices such as an automobile battery or a DC defibrillator can be sources of DC shocks.

In the United States, utility companies supply electrical energy in the form of ACs of 120 V at a frequency of 60 Hz. The 120 V of EMF and 1 A of current are the effective voltage and amperage in an AC circuit. This is also referred to as *RMS* (root-mean-square). It takes 1.414 A of peak amperage in the sinusoidal curve to give an effective amperage of 1 A. Similarly, it takes 170 V (120 × 1.414) at the peak of the AC curve to get an effective voltage of 120 V. The 60 Hz refers to the number of times in 1 second that the current reverses its direction of flow. Both the voltage and current waveforms form a sinusoidal pattern (Fig. 5-2).

To have the completed circuit necessary for current flow, a closed loop must exist and a voltage source must drive the current through the impedance. If current is to flow in the electrical circuit, there has to be a *voltage differential*, or a drop in the driving pressure across the impedance. According to Ohm's law, if the resistance is held constant, then the greater the current flow, the larger the voltage drop must be.

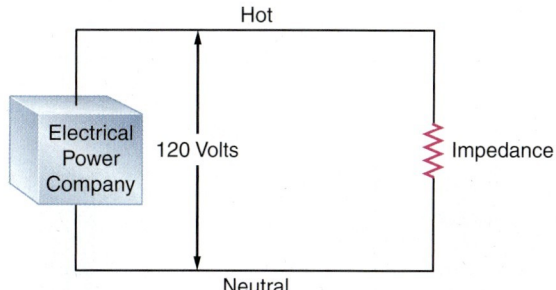

Figure 5-3 A typical AC circuit where there is a potential difference of 120 V between the hot and neutral sides of the circuit. The current flows through a resistance, which in AC circuits is more accurately referred to as *impedance,* and then returns to the electrical power company.

The power company attempts to maintain the line voltage constant at 120 V. Therefore, by Ohm's law, the current flow is inversely proportional to the impedance. A typical power cord consists of two conductors. One, designated as *hot* carries the current to the impedance; the other is *neutral,* and it returns the current to the source. The potential difference between the two is effectively 120 V (Fig. 5-3). The amount of current flowing through a given device is frequently referred to as the *load.* The load of the circuit depends on the impedance. A very high impedance circuit allows only a small current to flow and thus has a small load. A very low impedance circuit will draw a large current and is said to be a large load. A *short circuit* occurs when there is a zero impedance load with a very high current flow.[1]

Source of Shocks

Electrical accidents or shocks occur when a person becomes part of, or completes, an electrical circuit. To receive a shock, one must contact the electrical circuit at two points, and there must be a voltage source that causes the current to flow through an individual (Fig. 5-4).

When an individual contacts a source of electricity, damage occurs in one of two ways. First, the electrical current can disrupt the normal electrical function of cells. Depending on its magnitude, the current can contract muscles, alter brain function, paralyze respiration, or disrupt normal heart function, leading to ventricular fibrillation. The second mechanism involves the dissipation of electrical energy throughout the body's tissues. An electrical current passing through any resistance raises the temperature of that substance. If enough thermal energy is released, the temperature will rise sufficiently to produce a burn. Accidents involving household currents usually do not result in severe burns. However, in accidents involving very high voltages (i.e., power transmission lines), severe burns are common.

The severity of an electrical shock is determined by the amount of current (number of amperes) and the duration of the current flow. For the purpose of this discussion, electrical shocks are divided into two categories. *Macroshock* refers to large amounts of current flowing through a person, which can cause harm or death. *Microshock* refers to very small amounts of current and applies only to the electrically susceptible patient. This is an individual who has an external conduit that is in direct

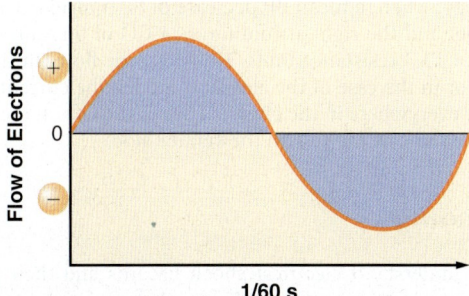

Figure 5-2 Sine wave flow of electrons in a 60-Hz AC.

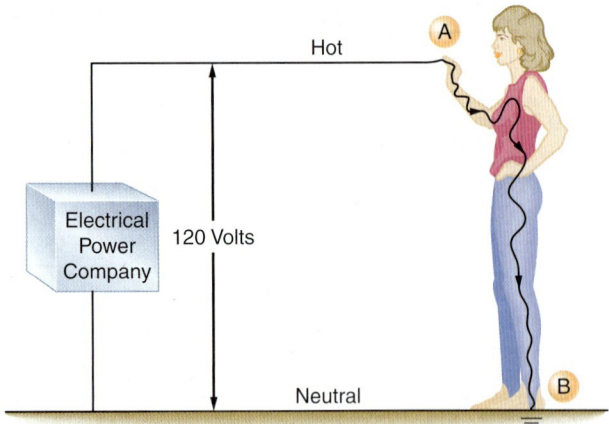

Figure 5-4 An individual can complete an electric circuit and receive a shock by coming in contact with the hot side of the circuit (point A). This is because he or she is standing on the ground (point B) and the contact point A and the ground point B provide the two contact points necessary for a completed circuit. The severity of the shock that the individual receives depends on his or her skin resistance.

contact with the heart. This can be a pacing wire or a saline-filled catheter such as a central venous or pulmonary artery catheter. In the case of the electrically susceptible patient, even minute amounts of current (microshock) may cause ventricular fibrillation.

Table 5-1 shows the effects typically produced by various currents following a 1-second contact with a 60-Hz current. When an individual contacts a 120-V household current, the severity of the shock will depend on his or her skin resistance, the duration of the contact, and the current density. Skin resistance can vary from a few thousand to 1 million ohms. If a person with a skin resistance of 1,000 ohms contacts a 120-V circuit, he or she would receive 120 mA of current, which would probably be lethal. However, if that same person's skin resistance is 100,000 ohms, the current flow would be 1.2 mA, which would barely be perceptible.

$$I = E/R = (120 \text{ volts})/(1,000 \text{ ohms}) = 120 \text{ mA}$$
$$I = E/R = (120 \text{ volts})/(100,000 \text{ ohms}) = 1.2 \text{ mA}$$

The longer an individual is in contact with the electrical source, the more dire the consequences, because more energy will be released and more tissue damaged. Also, there will be a greater chance of ventricular fibrillation from excitation of the heart during the vulnerable period of the electrocardiogram (ECG) cycle.

Current density is a way of expressing the amount of current that is applied per unit area of tissue. The diffusion of current in the body tends to be in all directions. The greater the current or the smaller the area to which it is applied, the higher the current density. In relation to the heart, a current of 100 mA (100,000 µA) is generally required to produce ventricular fibrillation when applied to the surface of the body. However, only 100 µA (0.1 mA) is required to produce ventricular fibrillation when that minute current is applied directly to the myocardium through an instrument having a very small contact area, such as a pacing wire electrode. In this case, the current density is 1,000-fold greater when applied directly to the heart; therefore, only 1/1,000 of the energy is required to cause ventricular fibrillation. In this case, the electrically susceptible patient can be electrocuted with currents well below 1 mA, which is the threshold of perception for humans. The frequency at which the current reverses is also an important factor in determining the amount of current an individual can safely contact. Utility companies in the United States produce electricity at a frequency of 60 Hz. They use 60 Hz because higher frequencies cause greater power loss through transmission lines and lower frequencies cause a detectable flicker from light sources.[2] The "let-go" current is defined as that current above which sustained muscular contraction occurs and at which an individual would be unable to let go of an energized wire. The let-go current for a 60-Hz AC power is 10 to 20 mA,[1,3,4] whereas at a frequency of 1 million Hz, up to 3 A (3,000 mA) is generally considered safe. It should be noted that very high frequency currents do not excite contractile tissue; consequently, they do not cause cardiac dysrhythmias.

It can be seen that Ohm's law governs the flow of electricity. For a completed circuit to exist, there must be a closed loop with a driving pressure to force a current through a resistance, just as in the cardiovascular system there must be a BP to drive the CO through the peripheral resistance. Figure 5-5 illustrates that a hot wire carrying a 120-V pressure through the resistance of a 60-W light bulb produces a current flow of 0.5 A. The voltage in the neutral wire is approximately 0 V, whereas the current in the neutral wire remains at 0.5 A. This correlates with our cardiovascular analogy, where a mean BP decrease of 80 mmHg between the aortic root and the right atrium forces a CO of 6 L/min through an SVR of 13.3 resistance units. However, the flow (in this case, the CO, or in the case of the electrical model, the current) is still the same everywhere in the circuit. That is, the CO on the arterial side is the same as the CO on the venous side.

Grounding

To fully understand electrical shock hazards and their prevention, one must have a thorough knowledge of the concepts of grounding. These concepts of grounding probably constitute the

Table 5-1 Effects of 60-Hz Current on an Average Human for a 1-Second Contact

Current	Effect
Macroshock	
1 mA (0.001 A)	Threshold of perception
5 mA (0.005 A)	Accepted as maximum harmless current intensity
10–20 mA (0.01–0.02 A)	"Let-go" current before sustained muscle contraction
50 mA (0.05 A)	Pain, possible fainting, mechanical injury; heart and respiratory functions continue
100–300 mA (0.1–0.3 A)	Ventricular fibrillation will start, but respiratory center remains intact
6,000 mA (6 A)	Sustained myocardial contraction, followed by normal heart rhythm; temporary respiratory paralysis; burns if current density is high
Microshock	
100 µA (0.1 mA)	Ventricular fibrillation
10 µA (0.01 mA)	Recommended maximum 60-Hz leakage current

A, amperes; mA, milliamperes; µA, microamperes.

5 Electrical and Fire Safety

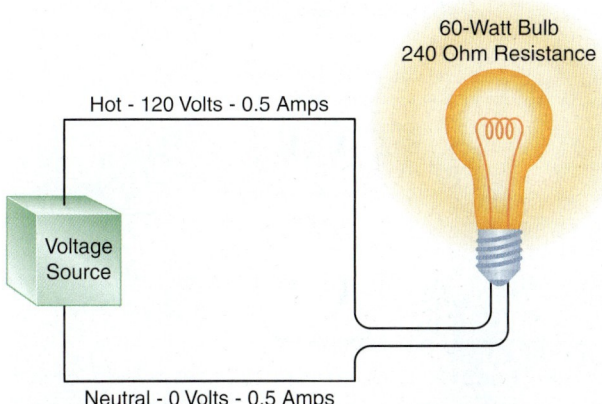

Figure 5-5 A 60-W light bulb has an internal resistance of 240 ohms and draws 0.5 A of current. The voltage drop in the circuit is from 120 in the hot wire to 0 in the neutral wire, but the current is 0.5 A in both the hot and neutral wires.

Table 5-2 Differences Between Power and Equipment Grounding in the Home and the Operating Room

	Power	Equipment
Home	+	±
Operating room	−	+

+, grounded; −, ungrounded; ±, may or may not be grounded.

most confusing aspects of electrical safety because the same term is used to describe several different principles. In electrical terminology, grounding is applied to two separate concepts. The first is the grounding of electrical *power,* and the second is the grounding of electrical *equipment.* Thus, the concepts that (1) power can be grounded or ungrounded and that (2) power can supply electrical devices that are themselves grounded or ungrounded are not mutually exclusive. It is vital to understand this point as the basis of electrical safety (Table 5-2). Whereas electrical *power* is grounded in the home, it is usually ungrounded in the OR. In the home, electrical *equipment* may be grounded or ungrounded, but it should always be grounded in the OR.

Electrical Power: Grounded

Electrical utilities universally provide power that is grounded (by convention, the earth-ground potential is zero, and all voltages represent a difference between potentials). That is, one of the wires supplying the power to a home is intentionally connected to the earth. The utility companies do this as a safety measure to prevent electrical charges from building up in their wiring during electrical storms. This also prevents the very high voltages used in transmitting power by the utility from entering the home in the event of an equipment failure in their high-voltage system.

The power enters the typical home via two wires. These two wires are attached to the main fuse or the circuit breaker box at the service entrance. The "hot" wire supplies power to the "hot" distribution strip. The neutral wire is connected to the neutral distribution strip and to a service entrance ground (i.e., a pipe buried in the earth; Fig. 5-6). From the fuse box, three wires leave to supply the electrical outlets in the house. In the United States, the hot wire is color-coded black and carries a voltage 120 V above ground potential. The second wire is the neutral wire color-coded white; the third wire is the ground wire, which is either color-coded green or uninsulated (bare wire). The ground and the neutral wires are attached at the same point in the circuit breaker box and then further connected to a cold-water pipe (Figs. 5-7 and 5-8). Thus, this grounded power system is also referred to as a *neutral grounded power system.* The black wire is not connected to the ground, as this would create a short circuit. The black wire is attached to the hot (i.e., 120 V above ground) distribution strip on which the circuit breakers or fuses are located. From here, numerous branch circuits supply electrical power to the outlets in the house. Each branch circuit is protected by a circuit breaker or fuse that limits current to a specific maximum amperage. Most electrical circuits in the house are 15- or 20-A circuits. These typically supply power to the electrical outlets and lights in the house. Several higher amperage circuits are also provided for devices such as an electric stove or an electric clothes dryer. These devices are powered

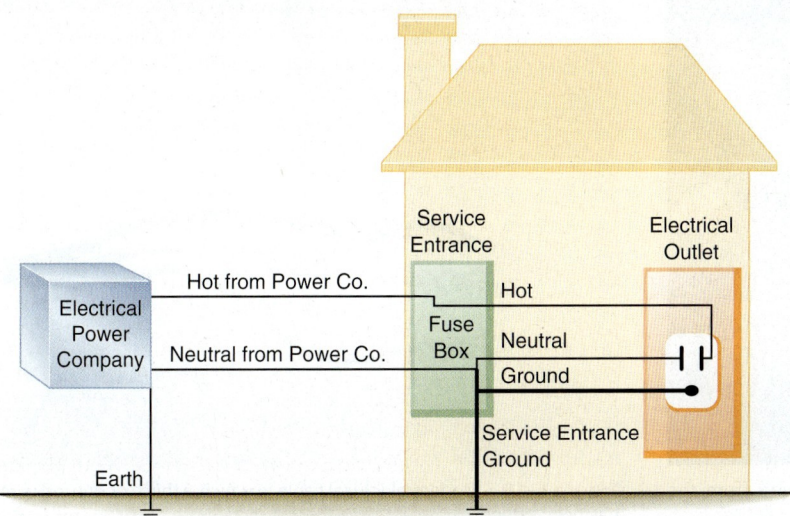

Figure 5-6 In a neutral grounded power system, the electric company supplies two lines to the typical home. The neutral wire is connected to ground by the power company and again connected to a service entrance ground when it enters the fuse box. Both the neutral and ground wires are connected together in the fuse box at the neutral bus bar, which is also attached to the service entrance ground.

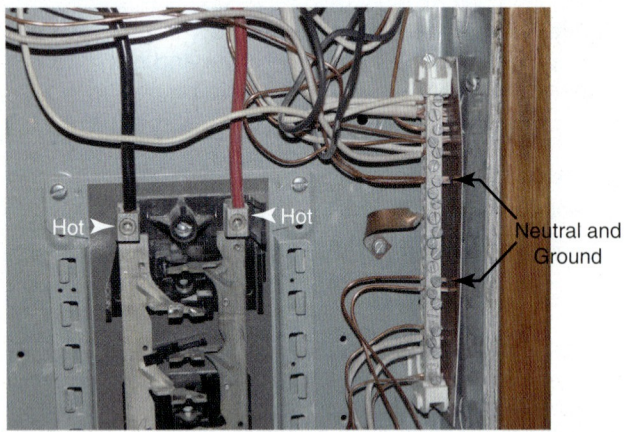

Figure 5-7 Inside a fuse box with the circuit breakers removed. The *arrowheads* indicate the hot wires energizing the strips where the circuit breakers are located. The *arrows* point to the neutral bus bar where the neutral and ground wires are connected.

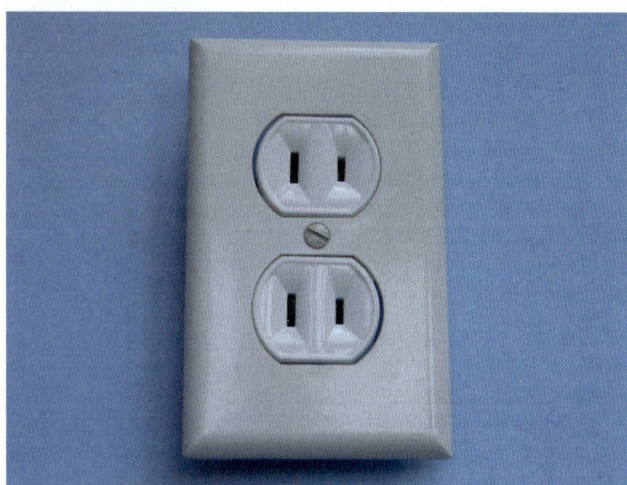

Figure 5-9 An older style electrical outlet consisting of just two wires (a hot and a neutral). There is no ground wire.

by 240-V circuits, which can draw from 30 to 50 A of current. The circuit breaker or fuse will interrupt the flow of current on the hot side of the line in the event of a short circuit or if the demand placed on that circuit is too high. For example, a 15-A branch circuit will be capable of supporting 1,800 W of power.

$$P = E \times I$$
$$P = 120 \text{ volts} \times 15 \text{ amperes}$$
$$P = 1,800 \text{ watts}$$

Therefore, if two 1,500-W hair dryers were simultaneously plugged into one outlet, the load would be too great for a 15-A circuit, and the circuit breaker would open (trip) or the fuse would melt. This is done to prevent the supply wires in the circuit from melting and starting a fire. The amperage of the circuit breaker on the branch circuit is determined by the thickness of the wire that it supplies. If a 20-A breaker is used with wire rated for only 15 A, the wire could melt and start a fire before the circuit breaker would trip. It is important to note that a 15-A circuit breaker does not protect an individual from lethal shocks. The 15 A of current that would trip the circuit breaker far exceeds the 100 to 200 mA that will produce ventricular fibrillation.

The wires that leave the circuit breaker supply the electrical outlets and lighting for the rest of the house. In older homes, the electrical cable consists of two wires, a hot and a neutral, which supply power to the electrical outlets (Fig. 5-9). In newer homes, a third wire has been added to the electrical cable (Fig. 5-10). This third wire is either green or uninsulated (bare) and serves as a ground wire for the power receptacle (Fig. 5-11). On one end, the ground wire is attached to the electrical outlet (Fig. 5-12); on the other, it is connected to the neutral distribution strip in the circuit breaker box along with the neutral (white) wires (Fig. 5-13).

It should be realized that in both the old and new situations, the power is grounded. That is, a 120-V potential exists between the hot (black) and the neutral (white) wire and between the hot wire and ground. In this case, the ground is the earth (Fig. 5-14). In modern home construction, there is still a 120-V potential difference between the hot (black) and the neutral (white) wire as well as a 120-V difference between the equipment ground wire

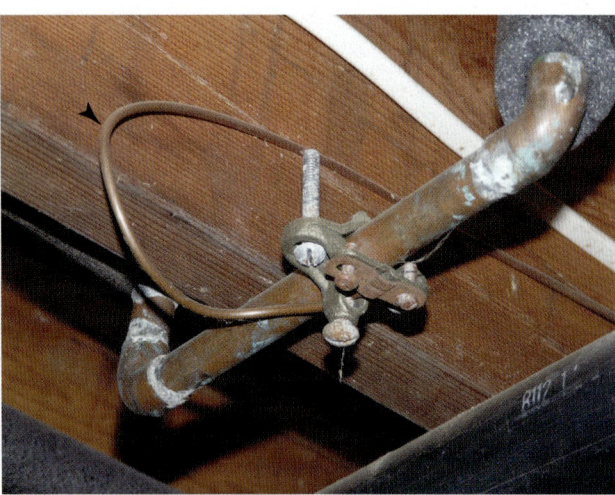

Figure 5-8 The *arrowhead* indicates the ground wire from the circuit breaker box attached to a cold-water pipe.

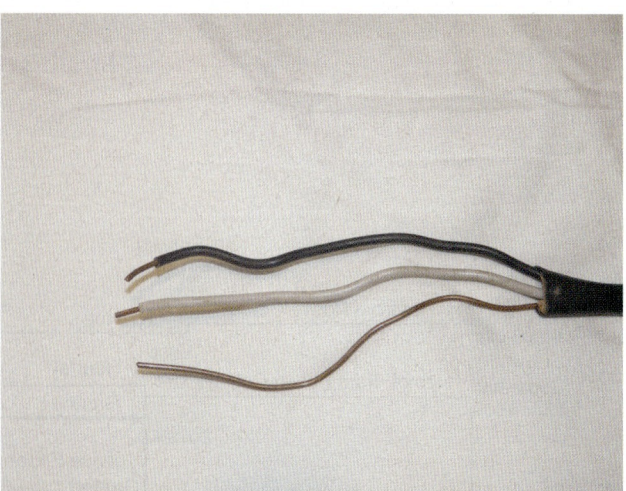

Figure 5-10 Modern electrical cable in which a third, or ground wire has been added.

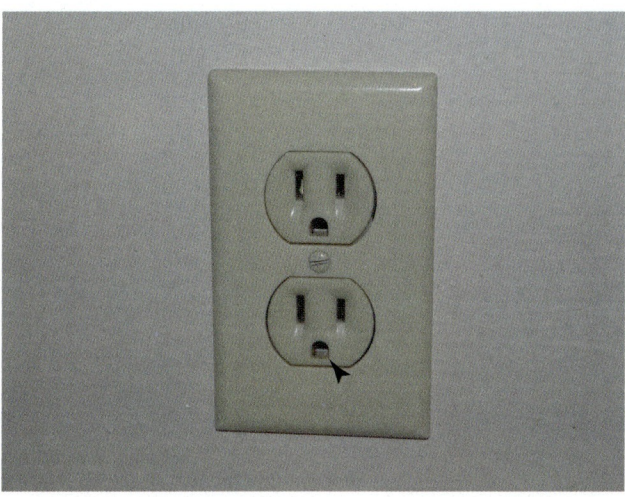

Figure 5-11 Modern electrical outlet in which the ground wire is present. The *arrowhead* points to the part of the receptacle where the ground wire connects.

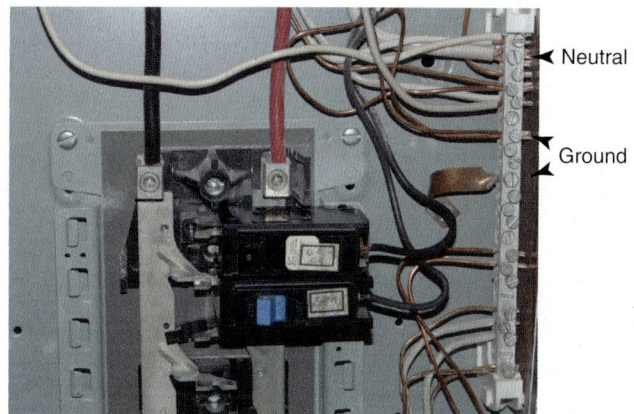

Figure 5-13 The ground wires (bare wires) from the power outlet are run to the neutral bus bar, where they are connected with the neutral wires (white wires) (*arrowheads*).

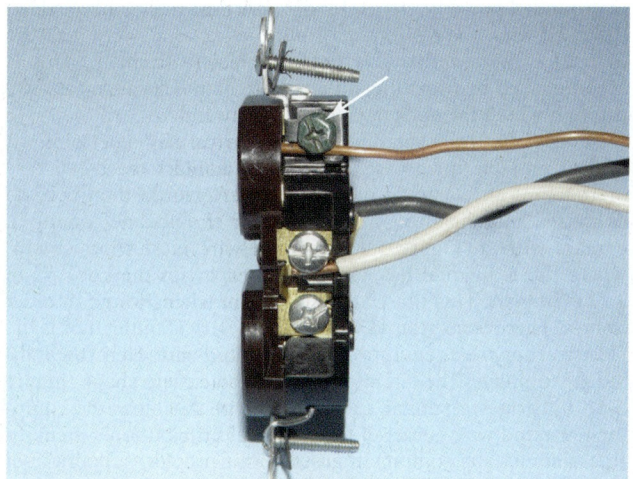

Figure 5-12 Detail of modern electrical power receptacle. The *arrow* points to the ground wire (bare wire), which is attached to the green grounding screw on the power receptacle.

(which is the third wire), and between the hot wire and earth (Fig. 5-15).

A 60-W light bulb can be used as an example to further illustrate this point. Normally, the hot and neutral wires are connected to the two wires of the light bulb socket, and throwing the switch will illuminate the bulb (Fig. 5-16). Similarly, if the hot wire is connected to one side of the bulb socket and the other wire from the light bulb is connected to the equipment ground wire, the bulb will still illuminate. If there is no equipment ground wire, the bulb will still light if the second wire is connected to any grounded metallic object such as a water pipe or a faucet. This illustrates the fact that the 120-V potential difference exists not only between the hot and the neutral wires but also between the hot wire and any grounded object. Thus, in a grounded power system, the current will flow between the hot wire and any conductor with an earth ground.

As previously stated, current flow requires a closed loop with a source of voltage. For an individual to receive an electric shock, he or she must contact the loop at two points. Because we may be standing on the ground or be in contact with an object that is referenced to ground, only one additional contact point is necessary to complete the circuit and thus receive an electrical shock. This is an unfortunate and inherently dangerous consequence

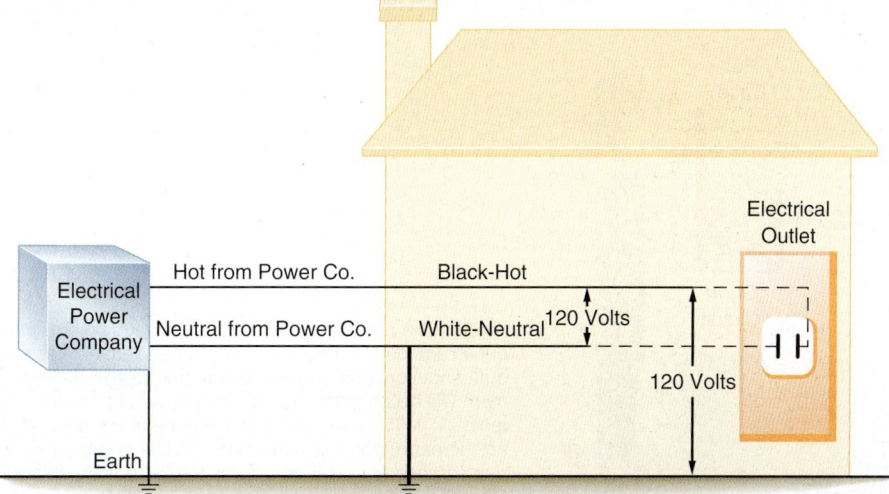

Figure 5-14 Diagram of a house with older style wiring that does not contain a ground wire. A 120-V potential difference exists between the hot and the neutral wires, as well as between the hot wire and the earth.

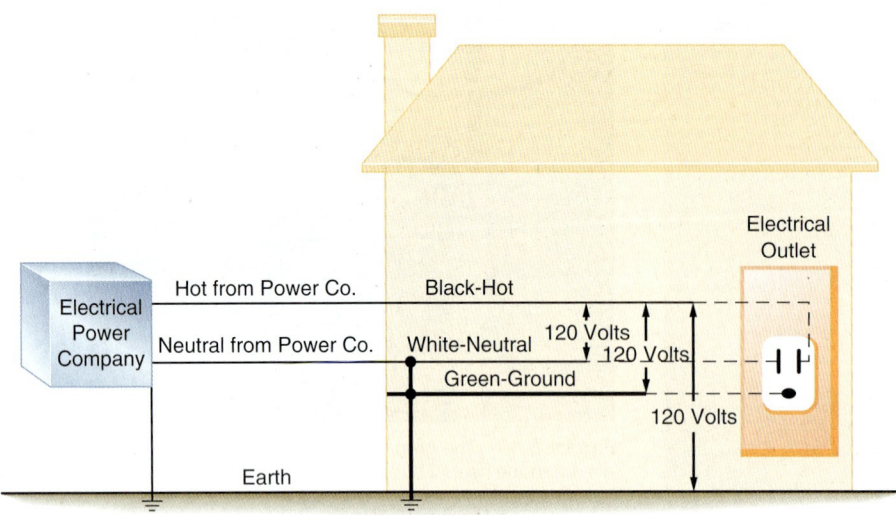

Figure 5-15 Diagram of a house with modern wiring in which the third, or ground, wire has been added. The 120-V potential difference exists between the hot and neutral wires, the hot and the ground wires, and the hot wire and the earth.

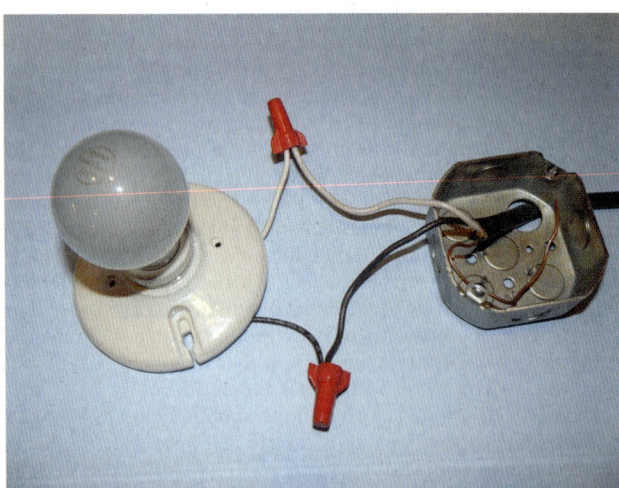

Figure 5-16 A simple light bulb circuit in which the hot (*black*) and neutral (*white*) wires are connected with the corresponding wires from the light bulb fixture.

of grounded power systems. Modern wiring systems have added the third wire, the equipment ground wire, as a safety measure to reduce the severity of a potential electrical shock. This is accomplished by providing an alternate, low-resistance pathway through which the current can flow to ground.

Over time, the insulation covering wires may deteriorate. It is then possible for a bare, hot wire to contact the metal case or frame of an electrical device. The case would then become energized and constitute a shock hazard to someone coming in contact with it. Figure 5-17 illustrates a typical short circuit, where the individual has come in contact with the hot case of an instrument. This illustrates the type of wiring found in older homes. There is no ground wire in the electrical outlet, nor is the electrical apparatus equipped with a ground wire. Here, the individual completes the circuit and receives a severe shock. Figure 5-18 illustrates a similar example, except that now the equipment ground wire is part of the electrical distribution system. In this example, the equipment ground wire provides a pathway of low impedance through which the current can travel; therefore, most of the current would travel through the ground wire. In this case, the person may get a shock, but it is unlikely to be fatal.

The electrical power supplied to homes is always grounded. A 120-V potential always exists between the hot conductor and the ground or earth. The third or equipment ground wire used in

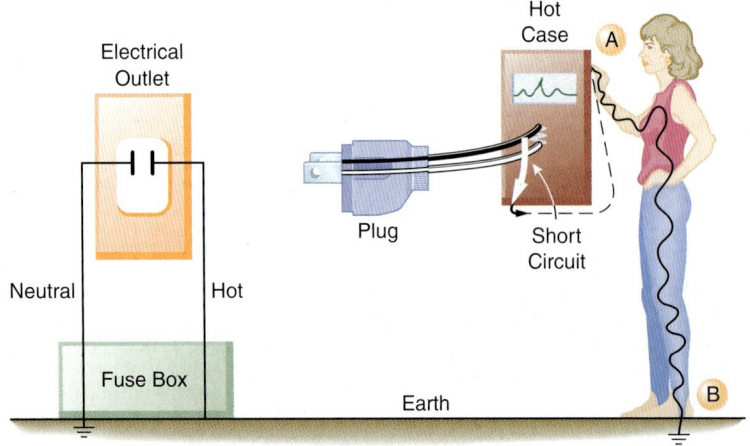

Figure 5-17 When a faulty piece of equipment without an equipment ground wire is plugged into an electrical outlet not containing a ground wire, the case of the instrument will become hot. An individual touching the hot case (point *A*) will receive a shock because he or she is standing on the earth (point *B*) and completes the circuit. The current (*dashed line*) will flow from the instrument through the individual touching the hot case.

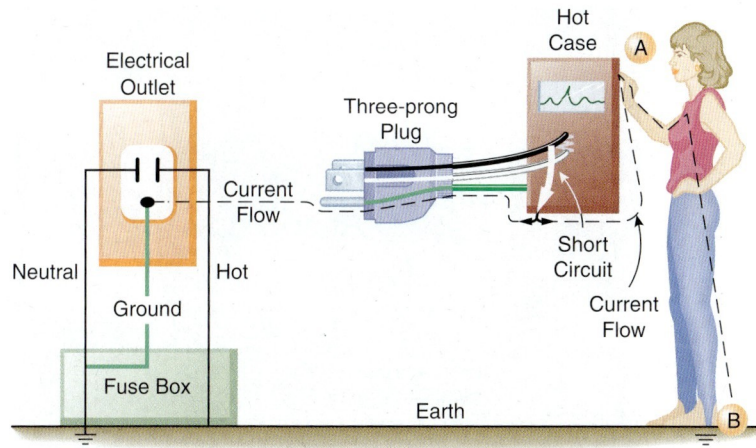

Figure 5-18 When a faulty piece of equipment containing an equipment ground wire is properly connected to an electrical outlet with a grounding connection, the current (*dashed line*) will preferentially flow down the low-resistance ground wire. An individual touching the case (point *A*) while standing on the ground (point *B*) will still complete the circuit; however, only a small part of the current will go through the individual.

modern electrical wiring systems does not normally have current flowing through it. In the event of a short circuit, an electrical device with a three-prong plug (i.e., a ground wire connected to its case) will conduct the majority of the short-circuited or "fault" current through the ground wire and away from the individual. This provides a significant safety benefit to someone accidentally contacting the defective device. If a large enough fault current exists, the ground wire also will provide a means to complete the short circuit back to the circuit breaker or fuse, and this will either melt the fuse or trip the circuit breaker. Thus, in a grounded power system, it is possible to have either grounded or ungrounded equipment, depending on when the wiring was installed and whether the electrical device is equipped with a three-prong plug containing a ground wire. Obviously, attempts to bypass the safety system of the equipment ground should be avoided. Devices such as a "cheater plug" (Fig. 5-19) should never be used because they defeat the safety feature of the equipment ground wire.

Electrical Power: Ungrounded

Numerous electronic devices, together with power cords and puddles of saline solutions on the floor, make the OR an electrically hazardous environment for both patients and personnel.

Bruner et al.[5] found that 40% of electrical accidents in hospitals occurred in the OR. The complexity of electrical equipment in the modern OR demands that electrical safety be a factor of paramount importance. To provide an extra measure of safety from macroshock, the power supplied to most ORs is ungrounded. In this ungrounded power system, the current is isolated from the ground potential. The 120-V potential difference exists only between the two wires of the isolated power system (IPS), but no circuit exists between the ground and either of the isolated power lines.

Supplying ungrounded power to the OR requires the use of an *isolation transformer* (Fig. 5-20). This device uses electromagnetic induction to induce a current in the ungrounded or secondary winding of the transformer from energy supplied to the primary winding. There is no direct electrical connection between the power supplied by the utility company on the primary side and the power induced by the transformer on the ungrounded or secondary side. Thus, the power supplied to the OR is isolated from the ground (Fig. 5-21). Since the 120-V potential exists only between the two wires of the isolated circuit, neither wire is hot nor neutral with reference to ground. In this case, they are simply referred to as line 1 and line 2 (Fig. 5-22). Using the example of the light bulb, if one connects the two wires of the bulb socket to the two wires of the IPS, the light will illuminate. However, if one connects one

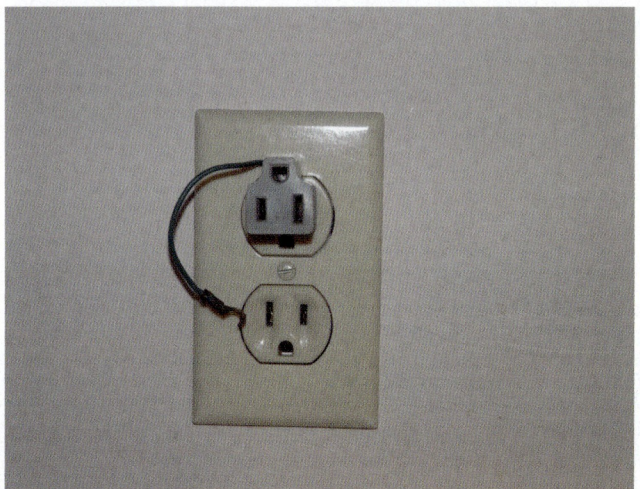
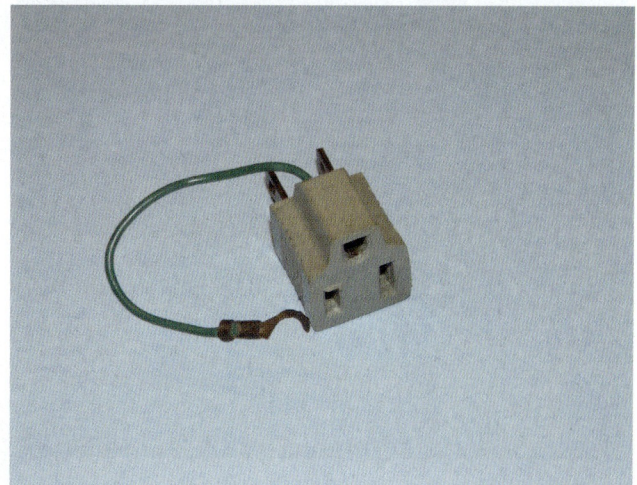

Figure 5-19 Right: a "cheater plug" that converts a three-prong power cord to a two-prong cord. **Left:** The wire attached to the cheater plug is rarely connected to the screw in the middle of the outlet. This totally defeats the purpose of the equipment ground wire.

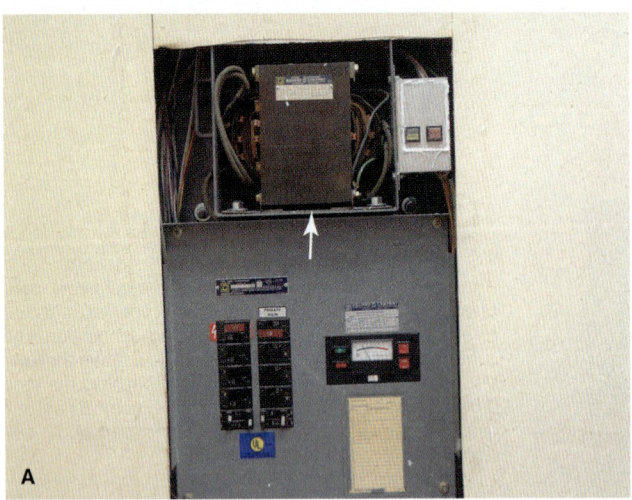
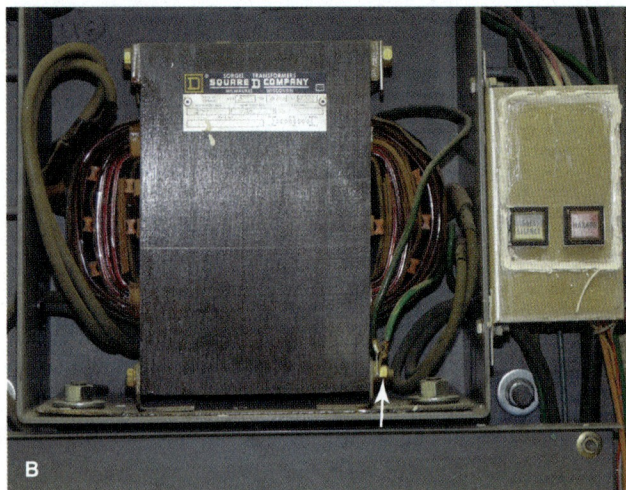

Figure 5-20 **A:** Isolated power panel showing circuit breakers, LIM, and isolation transformer (*arrow*). **B:** Detail of an isolation transformer with the attached warning lights. The *arrow* points to ground wire connection on the primary side of the transformer. Note that no similar connection exists on the secondary side of the transformer.

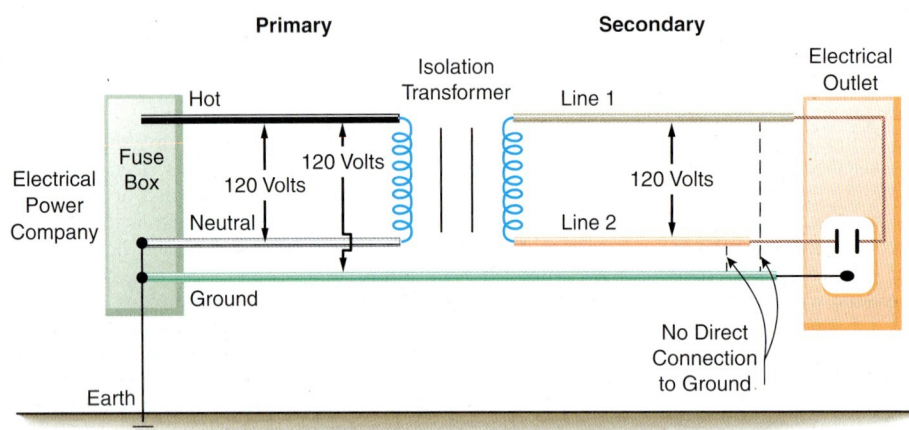

Figure 5-21 In the OR, the isolation transformer converts the grounded power on the primary side to an ungrounded power system on the secondary side of the transformer. A 120-V potential difference exists between line 1 and line 2. There is no direct connection from the power on the secondary side to ground. The equipment ground wire, however, is still present.

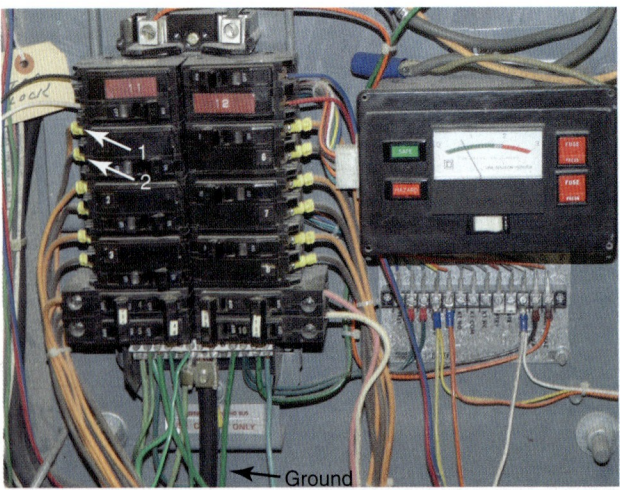

Figure 5-22 Detail of the inside of a circuit breaker box in an isolated power system. The *bottom arrow* points to ground (*green*) wires meeting at the common ground terminal. *Arrows 1* and *2* indicate lines 1 and 2 (*orange* and *brown*) from the isolated power circuit breaker. Neither line 1 nor line 2 is connected to the same terminals as the ground wires. This is in marked contrast to Figure 5-13, where the neutral and ground wires are attached at the same point.

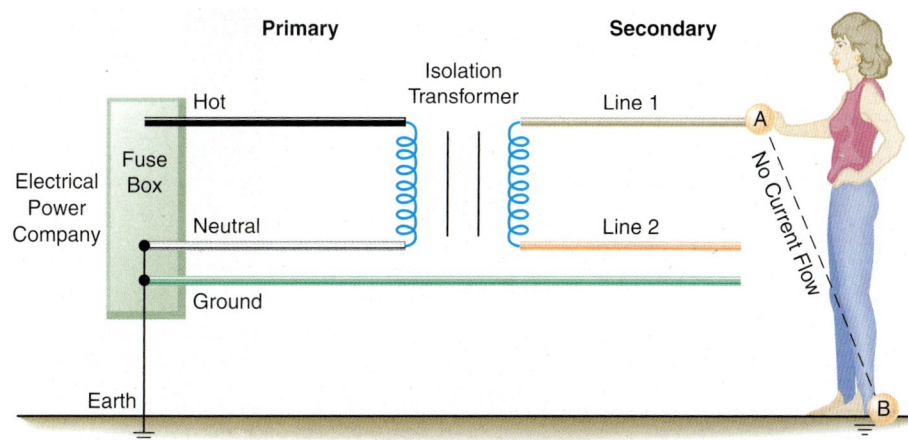

Figure 5-23 A safety feature of the isolated power system is illustrated. An individual contacting one side of the isolated power system (point A) and standing on the ground (point B) will not receive a shock. In this instance, the individual is not contacting the circuit at two points and thus is not completing the circuit. Point A is part of the isolated power system, and point B is part of the primary or grounded side of the circuit.

of the wires to one side of the isolated power and the other wire to the ground, the light will not illuminate. If the wires of the IPS are connected, the short circuit will trip the circuit breaker. In comparing the two systems, the standard grounded power has a direct connection to ground, whereas the isolated system imposes a very high impedance to any current flow to ground. The added safety of this system can be seen in Figure 5-23. In this case, a person has come in contact with one side of the IPS (point A). Since standing on the ground (point B) does not constitute a part of the isolated circuit, the individual does not complete the loop and will not receive a shock. This is because the ground is part of the primary circuit (*solid lines*), and the person is contacting only one side of the isolated secondary circuit (*cross-hatched lines*). The person does not complete either circuit (i.e., have two contact points); therefore, this situation does not pose an electric shock hazard. Of course, if the person contacts both lines of the IPS (an unlikely event), he or she would receive a shock.

If a faulty electrical appliance with an intact equipment ground wire is plugged into a standard household outlet, and the home wiring has a properly connected ground wire, then the amount of electrical current that will flow through the individual is considerably less than what will flow through the low-resistance ground wire. Here, an individual would be fairly well protected from a serious shock. However, if that ground wire were broken, the individual might receive a lethal shock. No shock would occur if the same faulty piece of equipment were plugged into the IPS, even if the equipment ground wire were broken. Thus, the IPS provides a significant amount of protection from macroshock. Another feature of the IPS is that the faulty piece of equipment, even though it may be partially short-circuited, will not usually trip the circuit breaker. This is an important feature because the faulty piece of equipment may be part of a life-support system for a patient. It is important to note that even though the power is isolated from ground, the case or frame of all electrical equipment is still connected to an equipment ground. The third wire (equipment ground wire) is necessary for a total electrical safety program.

Figure 5-24 illustrates a scenario involving a faulty piece of equipment connected to the IPS. This does not represent a hazard; it merely converts the isolated power back to a grounded power system as exists outside the OR. In fact, a *second* fault is necessary to create a hazard.

The previous discussion assumes that the IPS is perfectly isolated from ground. Actually, perfect isolation is impossible to achieve. All AC-operated power systems and electrical devices manifest some degree of capacitance. As previously discussed, electrical power cords, wires, and electrical motors exhibit capacitive coupling to the ground wire and metal conduits and "leak"

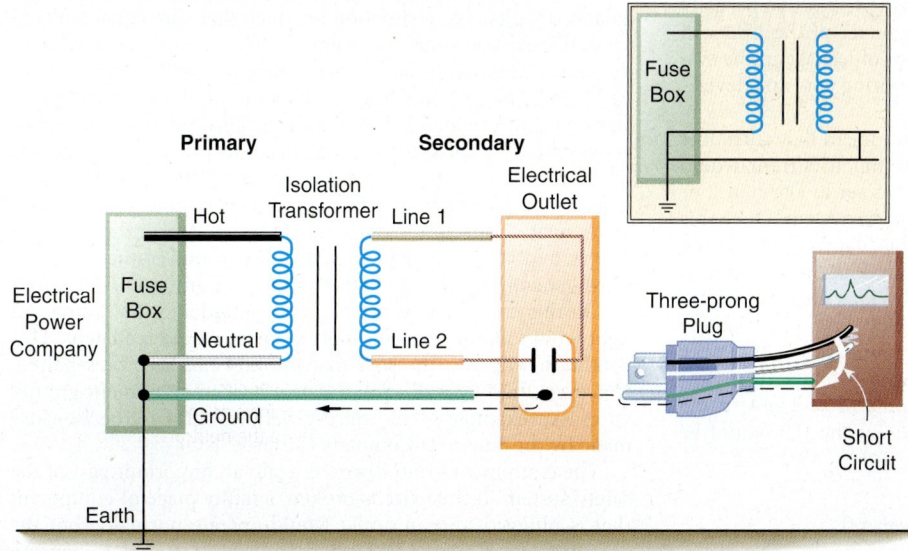

Figure 5-24 A faulty piece of equipment plugged into the isolated power system does not present a shock hazard. It merely converts the isolated power system into a grounded power system. The figure inset illustrates that the isolated power system is now identical to the grounded power system. The *dashed line* indicates current flow in the ground wire.

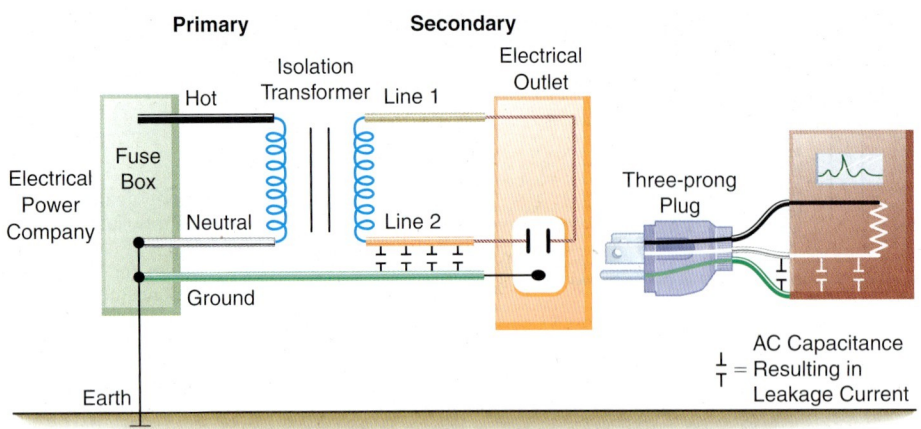

Figure 5-25 The capacitance that exists in alternating current (AC) power lines and AC-operated equipment results in small "leakage currents" that partially degrade the isolated power system.

small amounts of current to the ground (Fig. 5-25). This so-called *leakage current* partially ungrounds the IPS. This does not usually amount to more than a few milliamperes in an OR. So an individual coming in contact with one side of the IPS would receive only a very small shock (1 to 2 mA). Although this amount of current would be perceptible, it would not be dangerous.

The Line Isolation Monitor

The *line isolation monitor* (LIM) is a device that continuously monitors the integrity of an IPS. If a faulty piece of equipment is connected to the IPS, this will, in effect, change the system back to a conventional grounded system. Also, the faulty piece of equipment will continue to function normally. Therefore, it is essential that a warning system be in place to alert the personnel that the power is no longer ungrounded. The LIM continuously monitors the isolated power to ensure that it is indeed isolated from ground, and the device has a meter that displays a continuous indication of the integrity of the system (Fig. 5-26). The LIM is actually measuring the impedance to the ground of each side of the IPS. As previously discussed, with perfect isolation, impedance would be infinitely high and there would be no current flow in the event of a first fault situation ($Z = E/I$; if $I = 0$, then $Z = \infty$). Because all AC wiring and all AC-operated electrical devices have some capacitance, small leakage currents are present that partially degrade the isolation of the system. The meter of the LIM will indicate (in milliamperes) the total amount of leakage in the system resulting from capacitance, electrical wiring, and any devices plugged into the IPS.

The reading on the LIM meter does not mean that current is actually flowing; rather, it indicates how much current would flow in the event of a first fault. The LIM is set to alarm at 2 or 5 mA, depending on the age and brand of the system. Once this preset limit is exceeded, visual and audible alarms are triggered to indicate that the isolation from the ground has been degraded beyond a predetermined limit (Fig. 5-27). This does not necessarily mean that there is a hazardous situation, but rather that the system is no longer totally isolated from ground. It would require a second fault to create a dangerous situation.

For example, if the LIM were set to alarm at 2 mA, using Ohm's law, the impedance for either side of the IPS would be 60,000 ohms:

$$Z = E/I$$
$$Z = (120 \text{ volts})/(0.002 \text{ ampere})$$
$$Z = 60,000 \text{ ohms}$$

Therefore, if either side of the IPS had less than 60,000 ohms impedance to the ground, the LIM would trigger an alarm. This might occur in two situations. In the first situation, a faulty piece of equipment is plugged into the IPS. In this case, a true fault to ground exists from one line to ground. Now the system would be converted to the equivalent of a grounded power system. This faulty piece of equipment should be removed and serviced as soon as possible. However, this piece of equipment could still be used safely if it were essential for the care of the patient. It should be remembered, however, that continuing to use this faulty piece of equipment would create the potential for a serious electrical shock. This would occur if a second faulty piece of equipment were simultaneously connected to the IPS.

The second situation involves connecting many perfectly normal pieces of equipment to the IPS. Although each piece of equipment has only a small amount of leakage current, if the total leakage exceeds 2 mA, the LIM will trigger an alarm. Assume that in the same OR there are 30 electrical devices, each having 100 µA of leakage current. The total leakage current (30 × 100 µA) would be 3 mA. The impedance to ground would still be 40,000 ohms (120/0.003). The LIM alarm would sound because the 2 mA set point was violated. However, the system is still safe and represents a state significantly different from that in the first situation. For this reason, the newer LIMs are set to alarm at 5 mA instead of 2 mA.

The newest LIMs are referred to as *third-generation monitors*. The first-generation monitor, or static LIM, was unable to detect balanced faults (i.e., a situation in which there are equal faults to ground from both line 1 and line 2). The second-generation, or dynamic, LIM did not have this problem but could interfere with physiologic monitoring. Both of these monitors would trigger an alarm at 2 mA, which led to annoying "false" alarms. The third-generation LIM corrects the problems of its predecessors and has the alarm threshold set at 5 mA.[6] Proper functioning of the LIM depends on having both intact equipment ground wires as well as its own connection to ground. First- and second-generation LIMs could not detect the loss of the LIM ground connection. The third-generation LIM can detect this loss of ground to the monitor. In this case the LIM alarm would sound and the red hazard light would illuminate, but the LIM meter would read zero. This condition will alert the staff that the LIM needs to be repaired. However, the LIM still cannot detect broken equipment ground wires. An example of the third-generation LIM is the *Iso-Gard* made by the Square D Company (Monroe, NC).

The equipment ground wire is again an important part of the safety system. If this wire is broken, a faulty piece of equipment that is plugged into an outlet would operate normally, but the LIM would not alarm. A second fault could therefore cause a

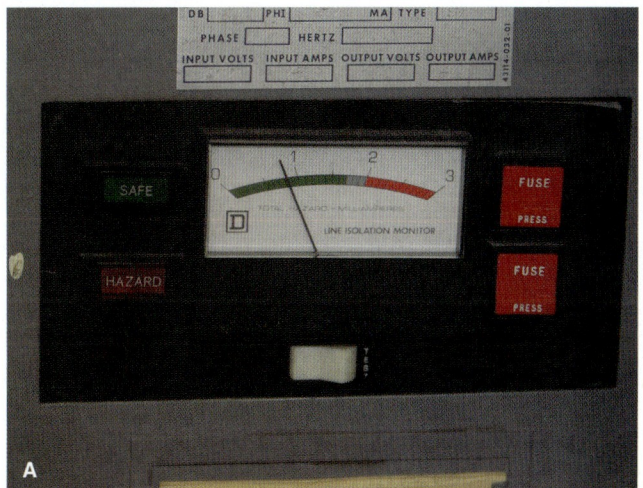
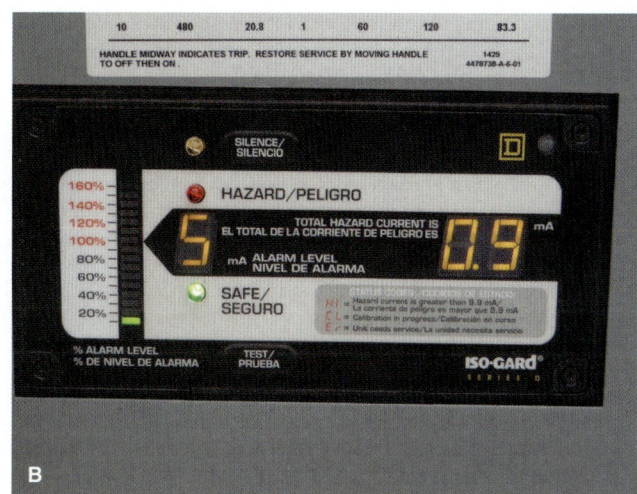
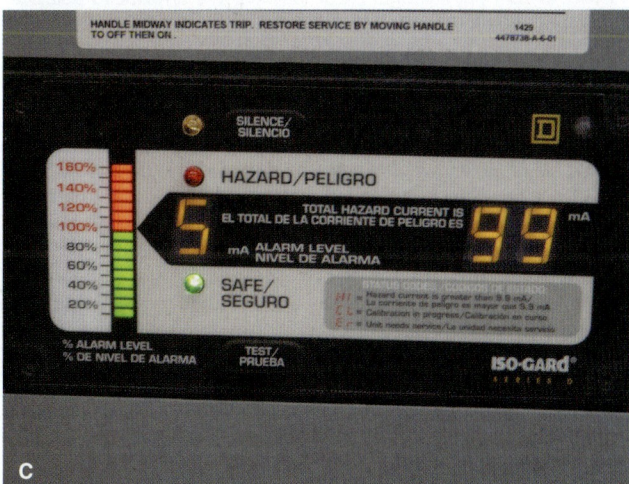

Figure 5-26 The meter of the LIM is calibrated in milliamperes. If the isolation of the power system is degraded such that more than 2 mA (5 mA in newer systems) of current could flow, the hazard light will illuminate and a warning buzzer will sound. Note the button for testing the hazard warning system. **A:** Older LIM that will trigger an alarm at 2 mA. **B:** Newer LIM that will trigger an alarm at 5 mA. **C:** The LIM alarm is triggered, and the red hazard stripe is illuminated, and the number on the right shows 9.9 mA of potential current flow.

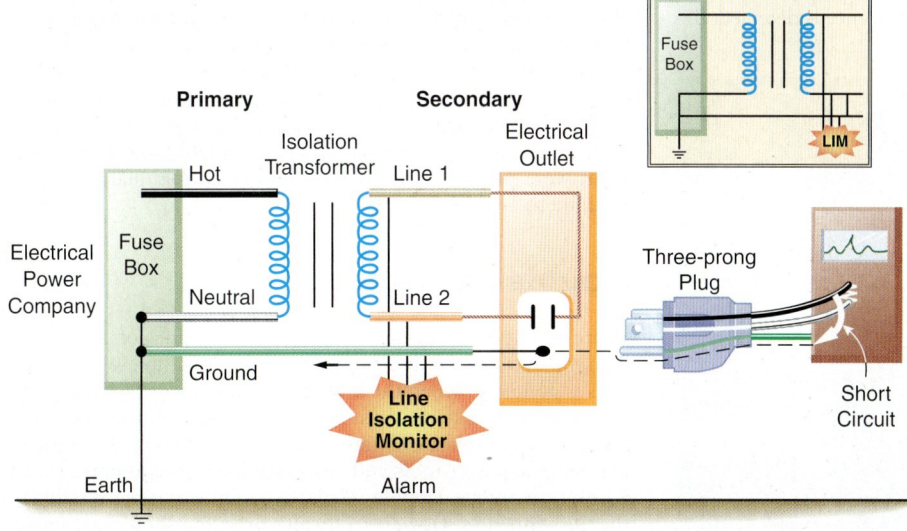

Figure 5-27 When a faulty piece of equipment is plugged into the isolated power system, it will markedly decrease the impedance from line 1 or line 2 to ground. This will be detected by the line isolation monitor (LIM), which will sound an alarm.

shock, without any alarm from the LIM. Also, in the event of a second fault, the equipment ground wire provides a low-resistance path to ground for most of the fault current (Fig. 5-24). The LIM will only be able to register leakage currents from pieces of equipment that are connected to the IPS and have intact ground wires.

If the LIM alarm is triggered, the first thing to do is to check the gauge to determine if it is a true fault. The other possibility is that too many pieces of electrical equipment have been plugged in and the 2 mA limit has been exceeded. If the gauge is between 2 and 5 mA, it is probable that too much electrical equipment has been plugged in. If the gauge reads greater than 5 mA, most likely there is a faulty piece of equipment present in the OR. The next step is to identify the faulty equipment, which is done by unplugging each piece of equipment until the alarm ceases. If the faulty piece of equipment is not of a life-support nature, it should be removed from the OR. If it is a vital piece of life-support equipment, it can be safely used. (Note: If a critical piece of life support equipment—like the cardio-pulmonary bypass machine—is suspected as causing the alarm, do not disconnect it until it is no longer needed.) However, it must be remembered that the protection of the IPS and the LIM is no longer operative. Therefore, if possible, no other electrical equipment should be connected during the remainder of the case, or until the faulty piece of equipment can be safely removed.

Ground Fault Circuit Interrupter

The ground fault circuit interrupter (GFCI, or occasionally abbreviated as GFI) is another popular device used to prevent individuals from receiving an electrical shock in a grounded power system. Electrical codes for most new construction require that a GFCI circuit be present in potentially hazardous (e.g., wet) areas such as bathrooms, kitchens, or outdoor electrical outlets. The GFCI may be installed as an individual power outlet (Fig. 5-28) or may be a special circuit breaker to which all the individual protected outlets are connected at a single point. The special GFCI circuit breaker is located in the main fuse/circuit breaker box and can be distinguished by its red test button (Fig. 5-29). As Figure 5-5 demonstrates, the current flowing in both the hot and neutral wires is usually equal. The GFCI monitors both sides of the circuit for the equality of current flow; if a difference is detected, the

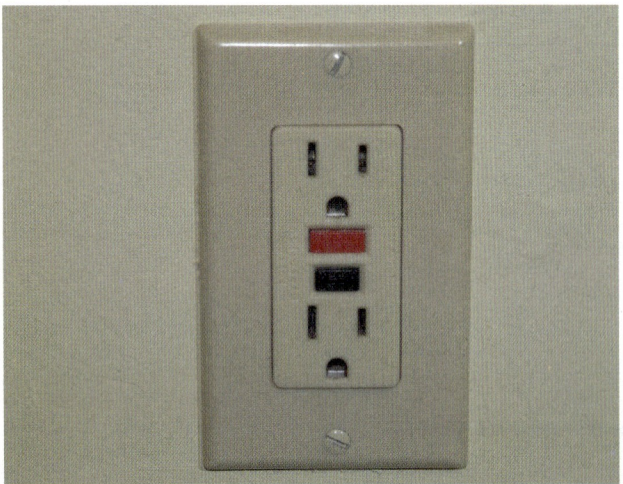

Figure 5-28 A GFCI electrical outlet with integrated test (*black*) and reset (*red*) buttons.

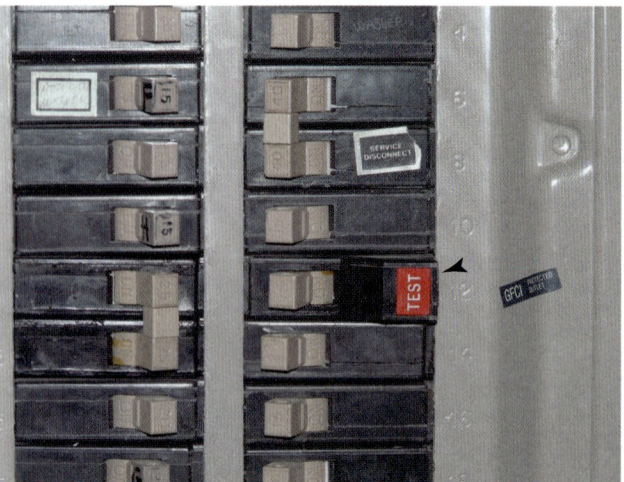

Figure 5-29 Special GFCI circuit breaker. The *arrowhead* points to the distinguishing red test button.

power is immediately interrupted. If an individual should contact a faulty piece of equipment such that current flowed through the individual, an imbalance between the two sides of the circuit would be created, which would be detected by the GFCI. Since the GFCI can detect very small current differences (in the range of 5 mA), the GFCI will open the circuit in a few milliseconds, thereby interrupting the current flow before a significant shock occurs. Thus, the GFCI provides a high level of protection at a very modest cost. If the OR has a GFCI that tripped, then one should first attempt to reset it by pushing the reset button. This is because a surge may have caused the GFCI to trip. If it cannot be reset, then the equipment must be removed from service and checked by the biomedical engineering staff. It is essential that when GFCIs are used in an OR, only one outlet be protected by each GFCI. They should never be "daisy-chained," so that one GFCI protects multiple outlets. This was illustrated in a report by Courtney et al.[7] when they lost all power to their monitors and the anesthesia machine. The cause was a power cord to a warming blanket that got pinched in the OR table causing a short circuit. The GFCI tripped and shut off the power to the warming blanket. However, that GFCI also controlled the outlets where the anesthesia machine and monitors were connected.

The disadvantage of using a GFCI in the OR is that it interrupts the power without warning. A defective piece of equipment could no longer be used, which might be a problem if it were of a life-support nature, whereas if the same faulty piece of equipment were plugged into an IPS, the LIM would alarm but the equipment could still be used.

Double Insulation

There is one instance in which it is acceptable for a piece of equipment to have only a two-prong and not a three-prong plug. This is permitted when the instrument has what is termed *double insulation*. These instruments have two layers of insulation and usually have a plastic exterior. Double insulation is found in many home power tools and is seen in hospital equipment such as infusion pumps. Double-insulated equipment is permissible in the OR with IPSs. However, if water or saline should get inside the unit, there could be a hazard because the double insulation is bypassed. This is even more serious if the OR has no isolated power or GFCIs.[8]

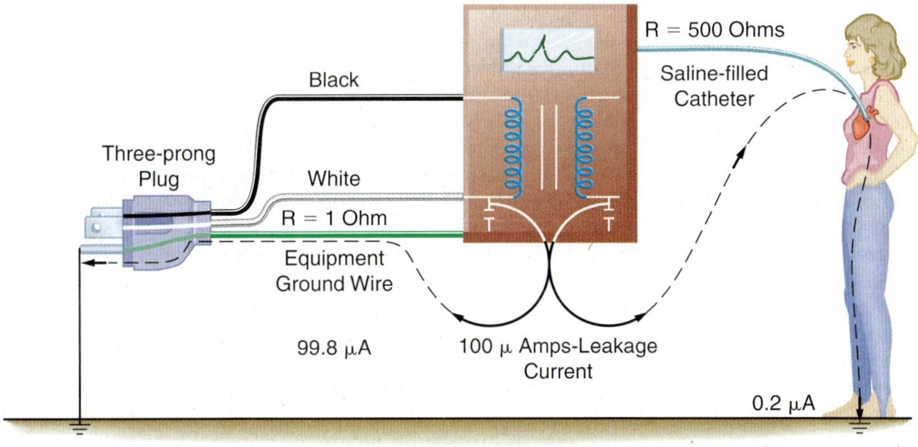

Figure 5-30 The electrically susceptible patient is protected from microshock by the presence of an intact equipment ground wire. The equipment ground wire provides a low-impedance path in which the majority of the leakage current (*dashed lines*) can flow. R, resistance.

Microshock

As previously discussed, macroshock involves relatively large amounts of current applied to the surface of the body. The current is conducted through all the tissues in proportion to their conductivity and area in a plane perpendicular to the current. Consequently, the "density" of the current (amperes per meter squared) that reaches the heart is considerably less than what is applied to the body surface. However, an electrically susceptible patient (i.e., one who has a direct, external connection to the heart, such as through a central venous pressure catheter or transvenous cardiac pacing wires) may be at risk from very small currents; this is called *microshock*.[9] The catheter orifice or electrical wire with a very small surface area in contact with the heart produces a relatively large current density at the heart.[10] Stated another way, even very small amounts of current applied directly to the myocardium will cause ventricular fibrillation. Microshock is a particularly difficult problem because of the insidious nature of the hazard.

In the electrically susceptible patient, ventricular fibrillation can be produced by a current that is below the threshold of human perception. The exact amount of current necessary to cause ventricular fibrillation in this type of patient is unknown. Whalen et al.[11] were able to produce fibrillation with 20 µA of current applied directly to the myocardium of dogs. Raftery et al.[12] produced fibrillation with 80 µA of current in some patients. Hull[13] used data obtained by Watson et al.[14] to show that 50% of patients would fibrillate at currents of 200 µA. Since 1,000 µA (1 mA) is generally regarded as the threshold of human perception with 60-Hz AC, the electrically susceptible patient can be electrocuted with one-tenth the normally perceptible currents. This is not only of academic interest but also of practical concern because many cases of ventricular fibrillation from microshock have been reported.[15-19]

The stray capacitance that is part of any AC-powered electrical instrument may result in significant amounts of charge buildup on the case of the instrument. If an individual simultaneously touches the case of an instrument where this has occurred and the electrically susceptible patient, he or she may unknowingly cause a discharge to the patient that results in ventricular fibrillation. Once again, the equipment ground wire constitutes the major source of protection against microshock for the electrically susceptible patient. In this case, the equipment ground wire provides a low-resistance path by which most of the leakage current is dissipated instead of stored as a charge.

Figure 5-30 illustrates a situation involving a patient with a saline-filled catheter in the heart with a resistance of approximately 500 ohms. The ground wire with a resistance of 1 ohm is connected to the instrument case. A leakage current of 100 µA will divide according to the relative resistances of the two paths. In this case, 99.8 µA will flow through the equipment ground wire and only 0.2 µA will flow through the fluid-filled catheter. This extremely small current does not endanger the patient. However, if the equipment ground wire were broken, the electrically susceptible patient would be at great risk because all 100 µA of leakage current could flow through the catheter and cause ventricular fibrillation (Fig. 5-31). Currently, electronic equipment is permitted 100 µA of leakage current.

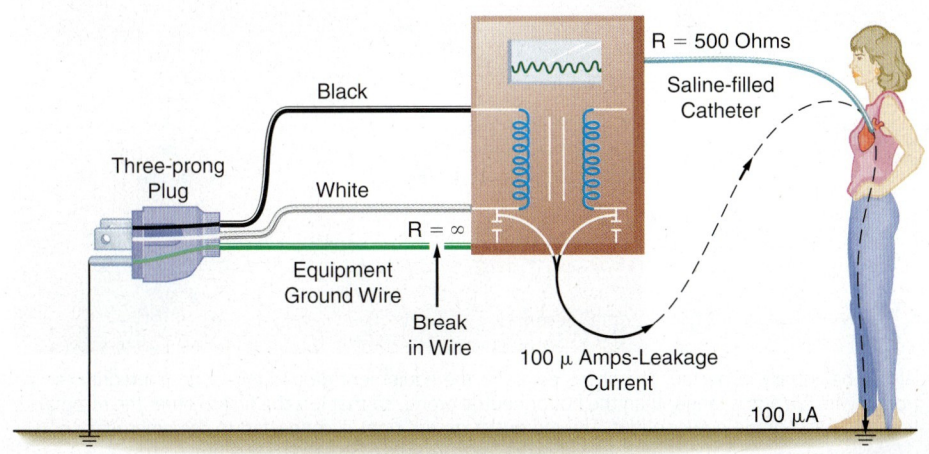

Figure 5-31 A broken equipment ground wire results in a significant hazard to the electrically susceptible patient. In this case, the entire leakage current can be conducted to the heart and may result in ventricular fibrillation. R, resistance.

Modern patient monitors incorporate another mechanism to reduce the risk of microshock for electrically susceptible patients.[20] This mechanism involves electrically isolating all direct patient connections from the power supply of the monitor by placing a very high impedance between the patient and any device. This limits the amount of internal leakage through the patient connection to a very small value. The standard currently is less than 10 μA. For instance, the output of an ECG monitor's power supply is electrically isolated from the patient by placing a very high impedance between the monitor and the patient's ECG leads.[21] Isolation techniques are designed to inhibit hazardous electrical pathways between the patient and the monitor while allowing the passage of the physiologic signal.

An intact equipment ground wire is probably the most important factor in preventing microshock. There are, however, other things that the anesthesiologist can do to reduce the incidence of microshock. One should never simultaneously touch an electrical device and a saline-filled central catheter or external pacing wires. Whenever one is handling a central catheter or pacing wires, it is best to insulate oneself by wearing rubber gloves. Also, one should never let any external current source, such as a nerve stimulator, come into contact with the catheter or wires. Finally, one should be alert to potential sources of energy that can be transmitted to the patient. Even stray radiofrequency current from the ESU (cautery) can, with the right conditions, be a source of microshock.[22] It must be remembered that the LIM is not designed to provide protection from microshock. The microampere currents involved in microshock are far below the LIM threshold of protection. In addition, the LIM does not register the leakage of individual monitors, but rather indicates the status of the total system. The LIM reading indicates the total amount of leakage current resulting from the entire capacitance of the system. This is the amount of current that would flow to ground in the event of a first-fault situation.

The essence of electrical safety is a thorough understanding of all the principles of grounding. The objective of electrical safety is to make it difficult for electrical current to pass through people. For this reason, both the patient and the anesthesiologist should be isolated from ground as much as possible. That is, their resistance to current flow should be as high as is technologically feasible. In the inherently unsafe electrical environment of an OR, several measures can be taken to help protect against contacting hazardous current flows. First, the grounded power provided by the utility company can be converted to ungrounded power by means of an isolation transformer. The LIM will continuously monitor the status of this isolation from ground and warn that the isolation of the power (from ground) has been lost in the event that a defective piece of equipment is plugged into one of the isolated circuit outlets. In addition, the shock that an individual could receive from a faulty piece of equipment is determined by the capacitance of the system and is limited to a few milliamperes. Second, all equipment plugged into the IPS has an equipment ground wire that is attached to the case of the instrument. This equipment ground wire provides an alternative low-resistance pathway enabling potentially dangerous currents to flow to ground. Thus, the patient and the anesthesiologist should be as insulated from ground as possible and all electrical equipment should be grounded.

The equipment ground wire serves three functions. First, it provides a low-resistance path for fault currents to reduce the risk of macroshock. Second, it dissipates leakage currents that are potentially harmful to the electrically susceptible patient. Third, it provides information to the LIM on the status of the ungrounded power system. If the equipment ground wire is broken, a significant factor in the prevention of electrical shock is lost. In addition, the IPS will appear safer than it actually is because the LIM is unable to detect broken equipment ground wires.

Because power cord plugs and receptacles are subjected to greater abuse in the hospital than in the home, the Underwriters Laboratories (Melville, NY) has issued a strict specification for special "hospital-grade" plugs and receptacles (Fig. 5-32). The plugs and receptacles that conform to this specification are marked by a green dot.[23] The hospital-grade plug is one that can be visually inspected or easily disassembled to ensure the integrity of the ground wire connection. Molded opaque plugs are not acceptable. Edwards[24] reported that of 3,000 non–hospital-grade receptacles installed in a new hospital building, 1,800 (60%) were defective after 3 years. When 2,000 of the non–hospital-grade receptacles were replaced with ones of hospital grade, no failures occurred after 18 months of use.

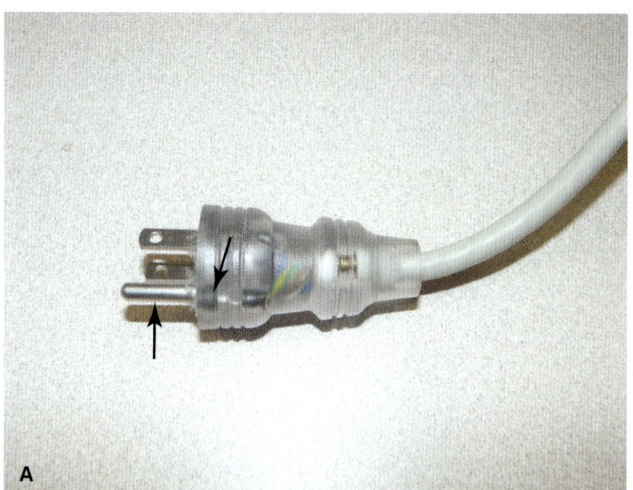 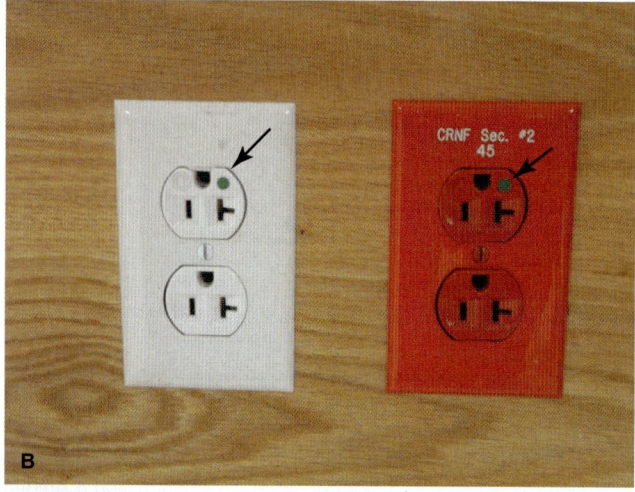

Figure 5-32 **A:** A hospital-grade plug that can be visually inspected. The *arrow* points to the equipment ground wire whose integrity can be readily verified Note that the prong for the ground wire (*arrow*) is longer than the hot or neutral prong, so that it is the first to enter the receptacle. **B:** The *arrows* point to the green dot denoting a hospital-grade power outlet. The red outlet on the right is connected to the emergency power (generator) system.

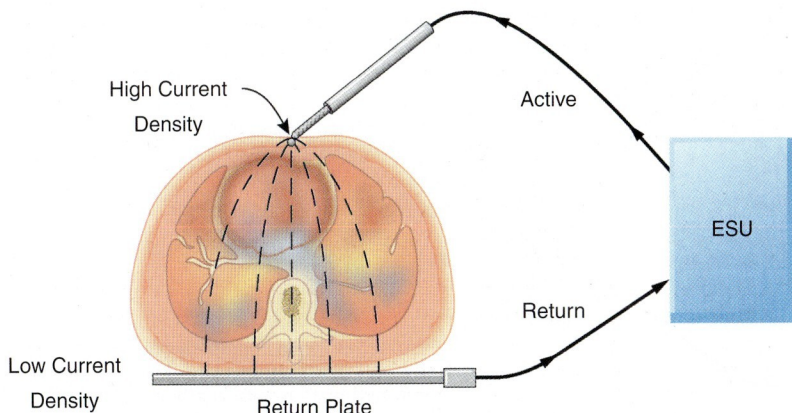

Figure 5-33 A properly applied electrosurgical unit (ESU) return plate. The current density at the return plate is low, resulting in no danger to the patient.

Electrosurgery

On that fateful October day in 1926 when Dr. Harvey W. Cushing first used an ESU machine invented by Professor William T. Bovie to resect a brain tumor, the course of modern surgery and anesthesia was forever altered.[25] The ubiquitous use of electrosurgery attests to the success of Professor Bovie's invention. However, this technology was not adopted without a cost. The widespread use of electrocautery has, at the very least, hastened the elimination of explosive anesthetic agents from the OR. In addition, as every anesthesiologist is aware, few things in the OR are immune to interference from the "Bovie." The high-frequency electrical energy generated by the ESU interferes with everything from the ECG signal to CO computers, pulse oximeters, and even implanted cardiac pacemakers.[26]

The ESU operates by generating very-high-frequency currents (radiofrequency range) of anywhere from 500,000 to 1 million Hz. These currents pass through tissue, and heat is created by the resistance of the tissues to current flow. The amount of heat (H) produced is proportional to the square of the current and inversely proportional to the area through which the current passes ($H = I^2/A$).[27] By concentrating the energy at the tip of the "Bovie pencil," the surgeon can produce either a cut or a coagulation at any given spot. This very-high-frequency current behaves differently from the standard 60-Hz AC current and can pass directly across the precordium without causing ventricular fibrillation.[27] This is because high-frequency currents have a low tissue penetration and do not excite contractile cells.

The term electrocautery is often mistakenly used interchangeably with electrosurgery. Electrocautery is usually a small, hand held, battery operated device that uses an electrical current to heat a metal wire. The heated wire is then applied directly to the tissue to achieve a desired effect.

Although the ESU is used safely hundreds of thousands of times each year, there is evidence that under certain circumstances it has been the cause of ventricular fibrillation.[28–31] The mechanism is thought to be low frequency (50 to 60 Hz) "stray current" that is generated when the ESU is activated. Current in the 50- to 60-Hz range can cause ventricular fibrillation. These cases have been associated with the use of the coagulation mode, when the surgeon is using the device near the heart, and when the patient has a conductor in the heart such as a CVP or pulmonary artery catheter. However, the exact mechanism has not been elucidated.

The large amount of energy generated by the ESU can pose other problems to the operator and the patient. Dr. Cushing became aware of one such problem. He wrote, "Once the operator received a shock which passed through a metal retractor to his arm and out by a wire from his headlight, which was unpleasant to say the least."[32] The ESU cannot be safely operated unless the energy is properly routed from the ESU through the patient and back to the unit. Ideally, the current generated by the active electrode is concentrated at the ESU tip, constituting a very small surface area. This energy has a high current density and is able to generate enough heat to produce a therapeutic cut or coagulation. The energy then passes through the patient to a dispersive electrode of large surface area that returns the energy safely to the ESU (Fig. 5-33).

One unfortunate quirk in terminology concerns the return (dispersive) plate of the ESU. This plate, often incorrectly referred to as a *ground plate*, is actually a dispersive electrode of large surface area that safely returns the generated energy to the ESU via a low current density pathway. When inquiring whether the dispersive electrode has been attached to the patient, OR personnel frequently ask, "Is the patient grounded?" As the aim of electrical safety is to isolate the patient from the ground, this expression is worse than erroneous; it can lead to confusion. Because the area of the return plate is large, the current density is low; therefore, no harmful heat is generated and no tissue destruction occurs. In a properly functioning system, the only tissue effect is at the site of the active electrode that is held by the surgeon.

Problems can arise if the electrosurgical return plate is improperly applied to the patient or if the cord connecting the return plate to the ESU is damaged or broken. In these instances, the high-frequency current generated by the ESU will seek an alternate return pathway. Anything attached to the patient, such as ECG leads or a temperature probe, can provide this alternate return pathway. The current density at the ECG pad will be considerably higher than normal because its surface area is much less than that of the ESU return plate. This may result in a serious burn at this alternate return site. Similarly, a burn may occur at the site of the ESU return plate if it is not properly applied to the patient or if it becomes partially dislodged during the operation (Fig. 5-34). This is not merely a theoretical possibility but is evidenced by the numerous case reports involving patients who have received ESU burns.[33–39]

The original ESUs were manufactured with the power supply connected directly to the ground by the equipment ground wire. These devices made it extremely easy for ESU current to return by alternate pathways. The ESU would continue to operate normally even without the return plate connected to the patient. In most modern ESUs, the power supply is isolated from ground to protect the patient from burns.[40] It was hoped that by isolating the return pathway from ground, the only route for current flow would be via the return electrode. Theoretically, this

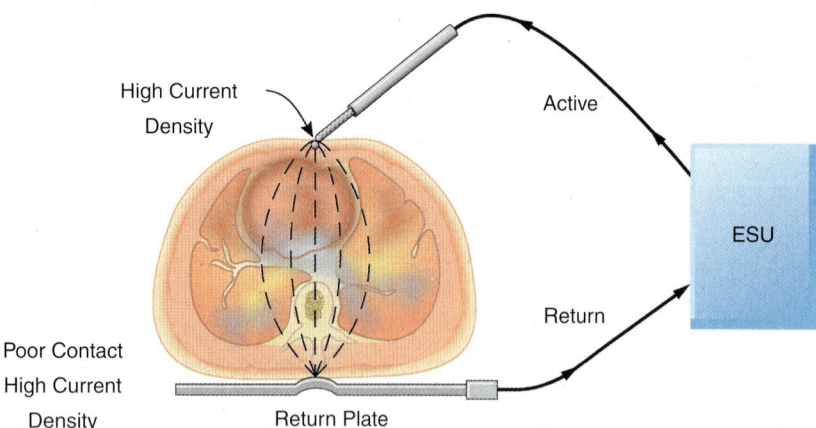

Figure 5-34 An improperly applied electrosurgical unit (ESU) return plate. Poor contact with the return plate results in a high current density and a possible burn to the patient.

would eliminate alternate return pathways and greatly reduce the incidence of burns. However, Mitchell[41] found two situations in which the current could return via alternate pathways, even with the isolated ESU circuit. If the return plate were left either on top of an uninsulated ESU cabinet or in contact with the bottom of the OR table, then the ESU could operate fairly normally and the current would return via alternate pathways. It will be recalled that the impedance is inversely proportional to the capacitance times the current frequency. The ESU operates at 500,000 to more than 1,000,000 Hz, which greatly enhances the effect of capacitive coupling and causes a marked reduction in impedance. Therefore, even with isolated ESUs, the decrease in impedance allows the current to return to the ESU by alternate pathways. In addition, the isolated ESU does not protect the patient from burns if the return electrode does not make proper contact with the patient. Although the isolated ESU does provide additional patient safety, it is by no means foolproof protection against the patient receiving a burn.

Preventing patient burns from the ESU is the responsibility of all professional staff in the OR. Not only the circulating nurse, but also the surgeon and the anesthesiologist must be aware of proper techniques and be vigilant to potential problems. The most important factor is the proper application of the return plate. It is essential that the return plate has the appropriate amount of electrolyte gel and an intact return wire. Reusable return plates must be properly cleaned after each use, and disposable plates must be checked to ensure that the electrolyte has not dried out during storage. In addition, it is prudent to place the return plate as close as possible to the site of the operation. ECG pads should be placed as far from the site of the operation as is feasible. OR personnel must be alert to the possibility that pools of flammable "prep" solutions such as alcohol and acetone can ignite when the ESU is used. If the ESU must be used on a patient with a demand pacemaker, the return electrode should be located below the thorax, and preparations for treating potential dysrhythmias should be available, including a magnet to convert the pacemaker to a fixed rate, a defibrillator, and an external pacemaker. It is best to keep the pacemaker out of the path between the surgical site and the dispersal plate.

The ESU has also caused other problems in patients with pacemakers, including reprogramming and microshock.[42,43] If the surgeon requests higher than normal power settings on the ESU, this should alert both the circulating nurse and the anesthesiologist to a potential problem. The return plate and cable must be immediately inspected to ensure that it is functioning and properly positioned. If this does not correct the problem, the return plate should be replaced.[44,45] If the problem remains, the entire ESU should be taken out of service. Finally, an ESU that is dropped or damaged must be removed immediately from the OR and thoroughly tested by a qualified biomedical engineer. Following these simple safety steps will prevent most patient burns from the ESU.

The previous discussion concerned only *unipolar* ESUs. There is a second type of ESU, in which the current passes only between the two blades of a pair of forceps. This type of device is referred to as a *bipolar* ESU. Because the active and return electrodes are the two blades of the forceps, it is not necessary to attach another dispersive electrode to the patient, unless a unipolar ESU is also being used. The bipolar ESU generates considerably less power than the unipolar and is mainly used for ophthalmic and neurologic surgery.

In 1980, Mirowski et al.[46] reported the first human implantation of a device to treat intractable ventricular tachydysrhythmias. This device, known as the *automatic implantable cardioverter-defibrillator* (AICD), is capable of sensing ventricular tachycardia and ventricular fibrillation and then automatically defibrillating the patient. Since 1980, thousands of patients have received AICD implants.[47,48] Because some of these patients may present for noncardiac surgery, it is important that the anesthesiologist be aware of potential problems.[47] The use of a unipolar ESU may cause electrical interference that could be interpreted by the AICD as a ventricular tachydysrhythmia. This would trigger a defibrillation pulse to be delivered to the patient and would likely cause an actual episode of ventricular tachycardia or ventricular fibrillation. The patient with an AICD is also at risk for ventricular fibrillation during electroconvulsive therapy.[49] In both cases, the AICD should be disabled by placing a magnet over the device or by use of a specific protocol to shut it off. Therefore, it is best to consult with someone experienced with the device before starting surgery. The device can be reactivated by reversing the process. Also, an external defibrillator and a noninvasive pacemaker should be in the OR whenever a patient with an AICD is anesthetized.

Electrical safety in the OR is a matter of combining common sense with some basic principles of electricity. Once OR personnel understand the importance of safe electrical practice, they are able to develop a heightened awareness to potential problems. All electrical equipment must undergo routine maintenance, service, and inspection to ensure that it conforms to designated electrical safety standards. Records of these test results must be kept for future inspection because human error can easily compound electrical hazards. Starmer et al.[50] cited one case concerning a newly constructed laboratory where the ground wire was not attached to a receptacle. In another study, Albisser et al.[51] found a 14% (198/1,424) incidence of improperly or incorrectly wired outlets. Furthermore, potentially hazardous situations should be recognized and corrected before they become a problem. For instance, electrical power cords are frequently placed on the floor where they can be crushed by various carts or the anesthesia machine. These cords could be located overhead or placed in an area of low traffic flow. Multiple-plug extension boxes should not be left on the floor where they can come in contact with electrolyte solutions. These could easily be mounted on a cart or the anesthesia machine. Pieces of equipment that have been damaged or have obvious defects in the power cord must not be used until they have been properly repaired. If everyone is aware of what constitutes a potential hazard, dangerous situations can be prevented with minimal effort.

Sparks generated by the ESU may provide the ignition source for a fire with resulting burns to the patient and OR personnel. This is a particular risk when the ESU is used in an oxygen-enriched environment as may be present in the patient's airway or in close proximity to the patient's face. The administration of high-flow nasal oxygen to a sedated patient during procedures on the face and eye is particularly hazardous. Most plastics such as tracheal tubes and components of the anesthetic breathing system that would not burn in room air will ignite in the presence of oxygen and/or nitrous oxide. Tenting of the drapes to allow dispersion of any accumulated oxygen and/or its dilution by room air will decrease the risk of ignition from a spark generated by a nearby ESU. The risk of fire can also be reduced by use of a circle anesthesia breathing system with minimal to no leak of gases around the anesthesia mask.

Conductive Flooring

In past years, conductive flooring was mandated for ORs where flammable anesthetic agents were being administered. This would minimize the buildup of static charges that could cause a flammable anesthetic agent to ignite. The standards have now been changed to eliminate the necessity for conductive flooring in anesthetizing areas where flammable agents are no longer used.

Environmental Hazards

There are a number of potential electrically related hazards in the OR that are of concern to the anesthesiologist. There is the potential for electrical shock not only to the patient but also to OR personnel. In addition, cables and power cords to electrical equipment and monitoring devices can become hazardous. Finally, all OR personnel should have a plan of what to do in the event of a power failure.

In today's OR, there are literally dozens of pieces of electrical equipment. It is not uncommon to have numerous power cords lying on the floor, where they are vulnerable to damage. If the insulation on the power cable becomes damaged, it is fairly easy for the hot wire to come in contact with a piece of metal equipment. If the OR does not have isolated power, that piece of equipment would become energized and be a potential electrical shock hazard.[52] Having isolated power minimizes the risk to the patient and OR personnel. Clearly, getting electrical power cords off the floor is desirable. This can be accomplished by having electrical outlets in the ceiling or by having ceiling-mounted articulated arms that contain electrical outlets. Also, the use of multioutlet extension boxes that sit on the floor can be hazardous and should be avoided. These can be contaminated with fluids, which could easily trip the circuit breaker. In one case, it apparently tripped the main circuit breaker for the entire OR, resulting in a loss of all electrical power except for the overhead lights.[53]

Modern monitoring devices have many safety features incorporated into them. Virtually all of them have isolated the patient input from the power supply of the device. This is frequently done with optocoupler isolation circuits, which transfer electrical signals by utilizing light waves. This was an important feature that was lacking from the original ECG monitors. In the early days, patients could actually become part of the electrical circuit of the monitor. There have been relatively few problems with patients and monitoring devices since the advent of isolated inputs. However, between 1985 and 1994, the Food and Drug Administration (FDA) received approximately 24 reports in which infants and children had received an electrical shock (including five children who died by electrocution).[54,55] These electrical accidents occurred because the electrode lead wires from either an ECG monitor or an apnea monitor were plugged directly into a 120-V electrical outlet instead of the appropriate patient cable. In 1997, the FDA issued a new performance standard for electrode lead wires and patient cables that requires that the exposed male connector pins from the electrode lead wires be eliminated. Therefore, the lead wires must have female connections and the connector pins must be housed in a protected patient cable (Fig. 5-35). This effectively eliminates the possibility of the patient being connected directly to an AC source since there are no exposed connector pins on the lead wires.

All health-care facilities are required to have a source of emergency power. This generally consists of one or more electrical generators. These generators are configured to start up automatically and provide power to the facility within 10 seconds after detecting the loss of power from the utility company. The facility is required to test these generators on a regular basis. However, in the past, not all health-care facilities tested them under actual load. There are numerous anecdotal reports of generators not functioning properly during an actual power failure. If the generators are not tested under actual load, it is possible that many years will pass before a real power outage puts a severe demand on the generator. If the facility has several generators and one of them fails, the increased demand on the others may be enough to cause them to fail in rapid succession.[56] Hospitals (under the current National Fire Protection Association [NFPA] 99 standards) must test their emergency power supply systems (generators) under connected load once a month for at least 30 minutes. If the generator is oversized for the application and cannot be loaded to at least 30% of its rating, it must be load-banked and run for a total of 2 hours every year. A fairly recent requirement

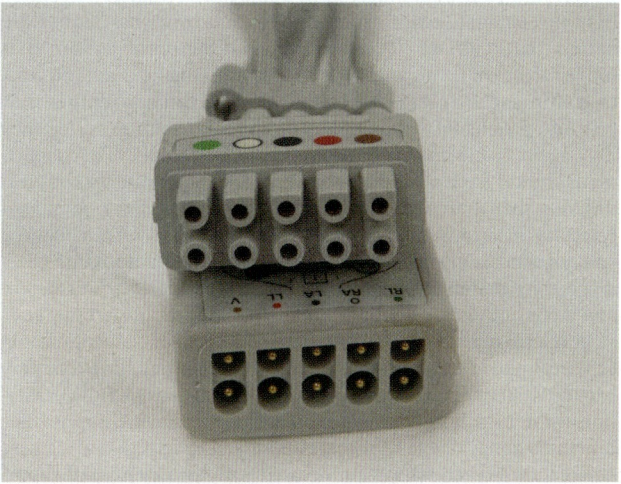

Figure 5-35 The current standard for patient lead wires (**top**) requires a female connector. The patient cable (**bottom**) has shielded connector pins that the lead wires plug into.

is for emergency power supply systems to be tested once every 3 years for 4 continuous hours, with a recommendation that this be performed during peak usage of the system.[57,58]

Although all hospitals are required to have emergency generators to power essential equipment in the event of a power failure, these generators do not function in every circumstance. If there is a loss of power from the electrical utility, then this is detected by a relay switch, which in turn causes a series of events to activate the transfer of the power generation to the backup system. This usually happens seamlessly. However, if the transfer switch or the generator fails, then there will be no backup electricity.

Another cause of partial or total power failure has to do with construction mishaps.[56] As hospitals frequently remodel, add new wings, or upgrade existing facilities, there is always a chance that the power will be accidentally interrupted. This may be due to a worker tripping a GFI, a relay failure that caused a power transfer to a nonworking generator, or a fire in the electrical vault of the hospital.[59–61] Since the electrical utility is still supplying power, the generators may not be activated.

The causes of a power failure are numerous. Local events can usually be corrected in a few hours. However, the effects of a natural disaster can be devastating. A hospital may have to operate on emergency power for days or even several weeks. If the power cannot be restored in a reasonable time frame, some or all of the patients may have to be evacuated.

Some disasters, like a hurricane will allow the hospital several days to prepare. However, a tornado or an earthquake will strike without warning. OR managers need to know what equipment will operate on emergency power. While the ventilation system will usually be powered by the generators, the air conditioning systems may not operate. This can be devastating on hot humid summer days. How long will the generators operate? Two days is a minimum, but is there fuel for them to run longer?[62] During a major hurricane and the flood that followed, a major New York City hospital had its generators safely located on an upper level. However, the fuel pumps for the generators were located in the basement which flooded, and left the hospital with no emergency power.

It is vitally important that each OR has a contingency plan for a power failure. There should be a supply of battery-operated light sources available in each OR. A laryngoscope can serve as a readily available source of light that allows one to find flashlights and other pieces of equipment. The overhead lights in the OR should also be connected to some sort of battery-operated lighting system. Traditional anesthesia machines have a backup battery that will last 30 to 60 minutes. If the power failure lasts longer than that, the anesthesiologist must make plans on how to continue the anesthetic. The newer electronic machines may be more problematic than older traditional machines, since they may have electronic gas or vaporization systems. The department should have a supply of battery-powered monitors, but it is unlikely that there will be enough for every OR. Syringe pumps typically have a battery, and BPs can be taken with a manual sphygmomanometer. Since many ORs employ automated drug dispensing systems, these devices will not work without power and a communication link to the hospital information system.

Modern anesthesia workstations are heavily dependent on electrical power to function properly. Therefore, all have a battery backup system. Typically, these batteries can power the workstation for 1 to 2 hours. Once the battery is exhausted, only basic functions are available to the anesthesiologist. This would include emergency oxygen which can be used with a conventional vaporizer to provide inhalational anesthesia. However, the Desflurane Tec 6 vaporizer and many of the newer electronic vaporizers cannot deliver anesthetic agent without electrical power. The Arkon Workstation (Spacelabs Healthcare, Snoqualmie, WA) has a unique feature. The workstation has the capability to hold up to 4 batteries which extend the usable function up to 4 hours. These batteries can be easily added or changed by the user during a power failure.

In reality, the backup generators will usually supply power in the event of an emergency. However, there are many circumstances where the hospital can experience partial or total power loss. The cost of these contingencies is relatively small but the benefits can be incomparable in an emergency.

Electromagnetic Interference

Rapid advances in technology have led to an explosion in the number of wireless communication devices in the marketplace. These devices include cellular telephones, cordless telephones, walkie-talkies, and wireless Internet access devices. All of these devices have something in common: They emit electromagnetic interference (EMI). This most commonly manifests itself when traveling on airplanes. Most airlines require that these devices be turned off when the plane is taking off or landing or, in some cases, during the entire flight. There is concern that the EMI emitted by these devices may interfere with the plane's navigation and communication equipment.

In recent years, the number of people who own these devices has increased exponentially. Indeed, in some hospitals, they form a vital link in the regular or emergency communication system. It is not uncommon for physicians, nurses, paramedics, and other personnel to have their own cellular telephones. In addition, patients and visitors may also have cellular telephones and other types of communication devices. Hospital maintenance and security personnel frequently have walkie-talkie–type radios and some hospitals have even instituted an in-house cellular telephone network that augments or replaces the paging system. There has been concern that the EMI emitted by these devices may interfere with implanted pacemakers or various types of monitoring devices and ventilators in critical care areas.[63] One case of a patient death has been reported when a ventilator malfunctioned secondary to EMI.[64]

Several studies have been done to find out if cellular telephones cause problems with cardiac pacemakers. One report by Hayes et al.[65] studied 980 patients with five different types of cellular telephones. They conducted more than 5,000 tests and found that in more than 20% of the cases they could detect some interference from the cellular telephone. Patients were symptomatic in 7.2% of the cases, and clinically significant interference occurred in 6.6% of the cases. When the telephone was held in the normal position over the ear, clinically significant interference was not detected. In fact, the interference that caused clinical symptoms occurred only if the telephone was directly over the pacemaker. Other studies have demonstrated changes such as erroneous sensing and pacer inhibition.[66,67] Again, these occurred only when the telephone was close to the pacemaker. The changes were temporary, and the pacemaker reverted to normal when the cellular telephone was moved to a safe distance. Currently, the FDA guidelines are that the cellular telephones be kept at least 6 inches from the pacemaker. Therefore, a patient with a pacemaker should not carry a cellular telephone in the shirt pocket, which is adjacent to the pacemaker. There appears to be little risk if hospital personnel carry a cellular telephone and if they ensure that it is kept at a reasonable distance from patients with a pacemaker.

AICDs comprise another group of devices of concern to biomedical engineers. Fetter et al.[68] conducted a study of 41 patients who had AICDs. They concluded that the cellular telephones did not interfere with the AICDs. They did, however, recommend keeping the cellular telephone at least 6 inches from the device.

EMI extends well beyond that of cellular telephones. Walkie-talkies, which are frequently used by hospital maintenance and security personnel, paging systems, police radios, and even televisions all emit EMI, which could potentially interfere with medical devices of any nature. Although there are many anecdotal reports, the amount of available scientific information on this problem is scant. Reports of interference include ventilator and infusion pumps that have been shut down or reprogrammed, interference with ECG monitors, and even an electronic wheelchair that was accidentally started because of EMI. It is a difficult problem to study because there are many different types of devices that emit EMI and a vast array of medical equipment that has the potential to interact with these devices. Even though a device may seem "safe" in the medical environment, if two or three cellular telephones or walkie-talkies are brought together in the same area at the same time, there may be unanticipated problems or interference.

Any time a cellular telephone is turned on, it is actually communicating with the cellular network, even though a call is not in progress. Therefore, the potential to interfere with devices exists. The ECRI Institute reported in October 1999 that walkie-talkies were far more likely to cause problems with medical devices than cellular telephones.[69] This is because they operate on a lower frequency than cellular telephones and have a higher power output. The ECRI recommends that cellular telephones be maintained at a distance of 1 m from medical devices, while walkie-talkies be kept at a distance of 6 to 8 m.

Some hospitals have made restrictive policies on the use of cellular telephones, particularly in critical care areas.[70] These policies are supported by little scientific documentation and are nearly impossible to enforce. The ubiquitous presence of cellular telephones carried by hospital personnel and visitors makes enforcing a ban virtually impossible. Even when people try to comply with the ban, failure is nearly inevitable because the general public is usually unaware that a cellular telephone in the standby mode is still communicating with the tower and generating EMI.

The real solution is to "harden" devices against EMI. This is difficult to do because of the many different frequencies on which these devices operate. Education of medical personnel is essential. When working in an OR or critical care area, all personnel must be alert to the fact that electronic devices and pacemakers can be interfered with by EMI. Creating a restrictive policy would certainly irritate personnel and visitors, and in some cases, may actually compromise emergency communications.[71]

Construction of New Operating Rooms

Frequently, an anesthesiologist is asked to consult with hospital administrators and architects in designing new, or remodeling older, ORs. In the past, a strict electrical code was enforced because of the use of flammable anesthetic agents. This code included a requirement for IPSs and LIMs. The NFPA revised its standard for health-care facilities in 1984 (NFPA 99–1984). These standards did not require IPS or LIMs in areas designated for use of nonflammable anesthetic agents only.[72,73] Although not mandatory, NFPA standards are usually adopted by local authorities when revising their electrical codes.

This change in the standard created a dilemma. The NFPA 99–2012 and NFPA 99–2015—*Health Care Facilities Code,* mandates that "wet procedure locations shall be provided with special protection against electrical shock." Section 6.3.2.2.8.2 further states that "this special protection shall be provided as follows: (1) Power distribution system that inherently limits the possible ground-fault current due to a first fault to a low value, without interrupting the power supply, (2) power distribution system in which the power supply is interrupted if the ground-fault current does, in fact, exceed the trip value of a Class A GFCI."[74]

The decision of whether to install isolated power hinged on two factors. The first was whether or not the OR was considered a wet location, and, if so, whether an interruptible power supply was tolerable. When power interruption was tolerable, a GFCI was permitted as the protective means. However, the standard also stated that "the use of an isolated power system (IPS) shall be permitted as a protective means capable of limiting ground fault current without power interruption."

Most people who have worked in an OR would attest to its being a wet procedure location. The presence of blood, body fluids, and saline solutions spilled on the floor all contribute to making this a wet environment. The cystoscopy suite serves as a good example.

Once the premise that the OR is a wet location is accepted, it must be determined whether a GFCI can provide the means of protection. The argument against using GFCIs in the OR is illustrated by the following example. Assume that during an open heart procedure, the cardiopulmonary bypass pump and the patient monitors are plugged into outlets on the same branch circuit. Also assume that during bypass, the circulating nurse plugs in a faulty headlight. If there is a GFCI protecting the circuit, the fault will be detected and the GFCI will interrupt all power to the pump and the monitors. This undoubtedly would cause a great deal of confusion and consternation among the OR personnel and may place the patient at risk for injury. The pump would have to be manually operated while the problem was being resolved. In addition, the GFCI could not be reset (and power restored) until the headlight is identified as the cause of the fault and unplugged from the outlet. However, if the OR were protected with an IPS and LIM, the same scenario would cause the LIM to alarm, but the pump and patient monitors would continue to operate normally. There would be no interruption of power and the problem could be resolved without risk to the patient.

It should be realized that a GFCI is an active system. That is, a potentially hazardous current is already flowing and must be actively interrupted, whereas the IPS (with LIM) is designed to be safe during a first-fault situation. Thus, it is a passive system because no mechanical action is required to activate the protection.[75]

Many hospital administrators and engineers wanted to eliminate IPSs in new OR construction by advocating that it was unnecessary and costly. They also grossly inflated the maintenance costs of the IPS. In fact, the maintenance costs of modern systems are minimal, and the installation costs are approximately 1% to 2% of the cost of constructing a new OR. The American Society of Anesthesiologists (ASA) and others, however, had advocated for the retention of IPSs.[75–78] In 2006, the ASA, through its representatives to NFPA 99 and its technical committee on Electrical Systems, launched a major campaign to have ORs default to being a wet procedure location. This was vigorously opposed by the American Hospital Association and the American Society of Healthcare engineers. The final version of the NFPA 99–2012 and NFPA 99–2015 edition, contains the following language: "Section 6.3.2.2.8.4 ORs shall be considered to be a wet procedure location, unless a risk assessment conducted by the health care governing body determines otherwise." In addition section 6.3.2.2.8.7 states: "Operating rooms defined as wet procedure locations shall be protected by either isolated power or ground fault circuit interrupters." Although, this code applies only to new or remodeled ORs, it is nonetheless a major victory for ASA, our patients, and OR personnel. In the event that the health-care facility wants to classify an OR as a "dry" location, then they have to do a risk assessment, and the NFPA 99 annex (A.6.3.2.2.8.4) states that among others this should include clinicians.[74]

Although not perfect,[79] the IPS and LIM do provide both the patient and OR personnel with a significant amount of protection in an electrically hazardous environment. IPSs provide clean stable voltages, which is important for sensitive diagnostic equipment.[80] Also, modern LIMs, which are microprocessor-based, require only yearly instead of monthly testing.

The value of the IPS is illustrated in a report by Day[81] in 1994. He reported four instances of electrical shock to OR personnel in a 1-year period. The operating suite had been renovated and the IPS removed, and it was not until the OR personnel received a shock that a problem was discovered. Also, in 2010, Wills et al.[82] reported an incident where an OR nurse received a severe electrical shock while plugging in a piece of equipment. This case further illustrates the consequences of having a wet floor in an OR with no IPS or GFCIs.

Anesthesiologists need to be aware of these new regulations and strongly encourage that new ORs be constructed with IPSs. The relatively small cost savings that the alternative would represent do not justify the elimination of such a useful safety system. The use of GFCIs in the OR environment can be acceptable if carefully planned and engineered. In order to avoid the loss of power to multiple instruments and monitors at one time, each outlet must be an individual GFCI. If that is done, then a fault will result in only one piece of equipment losing power. Using GFCIs also precludes the use of multiple plug strips in the OR.

Finally, in 2011, August reported on the opening of 24 new ORs in his facility. To their dismay, they found that the electrical service panels outside each OR were locked, and that the ORs had been reclassified as "dry" locations, without the knowledge of the anesthesia department.[83] Barker also reported an incident where a PACU monitor overheated and was billowing smoke. An attempt to shut off the power, was met with a locked circuit breaker box.[84] He too, commented on the need to have ORs designated as wet procedure locations.

Hopefully, with the new NFPA 99 code, there will be far fewer incidents of new ORs being designated as "dry" locations, especially without the knowledge of the anesthesia department. Electrical safety should be the concern of everyone in the OR. Accidents can be prevented only if proper installation and maintenance of the appropriate safety equipment in the OR have occurred and the OR personnel understand the concepts of electrical safety and are vigilant in their efforts to detect new hazards.[85]

Fire Safety

Fires in the OR are just as much a danger today as they were 100 years ago when patients were anesthetized with flammable anesthetic agents.[86,87] Because the potential consequences of a fire or explosion with ether or cyclopropane were well known and potentially devastating, OR fire safety practices were routinely followed.[88,89]

Today, the risk of an OR fire is probably as great or greater than the days when ether and cyclopropane were used, in part because of the routine use of potential sources of ignition (including electrosurgical cauteries) in an environment rich in fuel sources (i.e., flammable materials) and oxidizers (e.g., oxygen and nitrous oxide). Although the number of OR fires that occur annually in the United States is unknown, some estimates suggest that there are 550 to 650 fires each year, with as many as 5% to 10% associated with serious injury or death.[90] In contrast to the era of flammable anesthetics, there currently appears to be a lack of awareness of the potential for an OR fire. In response to the risks presented by this situation, in 2008 and updated in 2013, the ASA released a Practice Advisory on the Prevention and Management of Operating Room Fires (Table 5-3).[91]

Table 5-3 Recommendations for The Prevention and Management of Operating Room Fires

Preparation
- Train personnel in operating room fire management
- Practice responses to fires (fire drills)
- Assure that fire-management equipment is readily available
- Determine if a high-risk situation exists
- Team decides how to prevent/manage a fire
- Each person assigned a task (e.g., remove endotracheal tube or disconnect circuit)

Prevention
- Allow flammable skin preparations to dry before draping
- Configure surgical drapes to avoid buildup of oxidizer
- Anesthesiologist collaborates with team throughout the procedure to minimize oxidizer-enriched environment near ignition source
- Keep O_2 concentration as low as clinically possible
- Avoid N_2O
- Notify surgeon if oxidizer ↔ ignition source are in proximity to each other
- Moisten gauze and sponges that are near an ignition source

Management
- Look for early warning sign of a fire (e.g., pop, flash, or smoke)
- Stop procedure and each team member immediately carries out assigned task

Airway Fire
- *Simultaneously* remove the endotracheal tube and stop gases/disconnect circuit
- Pour saline into airway
- Remove burning materials
- Mask ventilate patient, assess injury, consider bronchoscopy, reintubate

Fire on the Patient
- Turn off gases
- Remove drapes and burning materials
- Extinguish flames with water, saline, or fire extinguisher
- Assess patient's status, devise care plan, assess for smoke inhalation

Failure to Extinguish
- Use CO_2 fire extinguisher
- Activate fire alarm
- Consider evacuation of room: Close door and do not reopen
- Turn off medical gas supply to room

Risk Management
- Preserve scene
- Notify hospital risk manager
- Follow local regulatory reporting requirements
- Treat fire as an adverse event
- FIRE DRILLS

Adapted from: Practice Advisory for the Prevention and Management of Operating Room Fires: An updated report by the American Society of Anesthesiologists Task Force on Operating Room Fires: American Society of Anesthesiologists: Schaumburg, IL. Approved by the ASA House of Delegates in October 2012; published in Anesthesiology, February 2013.

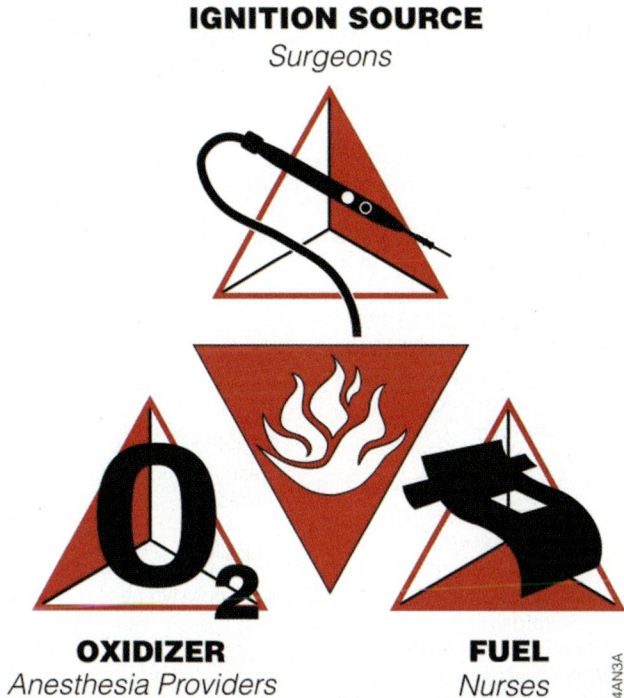

Figure 5-36 The fire triangle. (Copyright © ECRI Institute. Used with permission.)

For a fire to start, three components are necessary. The limbs of the "fire triad" are a heat or ignition source, fuel, and an oxidizer (Fig. 5-36).[92] A fire occurs when there is a chemical reaction of a fuel rapidly combining with an oxidizer to release energy in the form of heat and light. In the OR, there are many heat or ignition sources, such as the ESU, lasers, and the ends of fiberoptic light cords. The main oxidizers in the OR are air, oxygen, and nitrous oxide. Oxygen and nitrous oxide function equally well as oxidizers, so a combination of 50% oxygen and 50% nitrous oxide would avidly support combustion, as would 100% oxygen. Fuel for a fire can be found everywhere in the OR. Paper drapes, which have largely replaced cloth drapes, are much easier to ignite and can burn with greater intensity.[93,94] Other sources of fuel include gauze dressings, endotracheal tubes, gel mattress pads, and even facial or body hair (Table 5-4).[95]

Fire prevention is accomplished by not allowing all three of the elements of the fire triad to come together at the same time.[96] The challenge in the OR is that frequently each of the limbs of the fire triad is controlled by a different individual. For instance, the surgeon is frequently in charge of the ignition source, the anesthesiologist is usually administering the oxidizer, and the OR nurse frequently controls the fuel sources. It is not always evident to any one individual that all of these elements may be coming together at the same time. This is especially true in any case in which there is the possibility of oxygen or an oxygen–nitrous oxide mixture being delivered around the surgical site. In these circumstances, the risk of an OR fire is markedly increased and the need for communication among the surgeon, the anesthesiologist, and the OR nurses throughout the procedure is essential.

There are several dangers that may result from an OR fire. The most obvious is that the patient and OR personnel can suffer severe burns. However, a less obvious but potentially more deadly risk can be posed by the products of combustion (called *toxicants*). When materials, such as plastics, burn a variety of injurious compounds can be produced. These include carbon monoxide, ammonia, hydrogen chloride, and even cyanide. Toxicants can produce injury by damaging airways and lung tissue, and can cause asphyxia. OR fires can often produce significant amounts of smoke and toxicants, but may not cause enough heat to activate overhead sprinkler systems. If enough smoke is produced, the OR personnel may have to evacuate the area. Therefore, it is essential to have an evacuation plan for both the OR personnel and the patient, which was planned and carefully considered before a fire could occur.

OR fires can be divided into two different types. The more common type of fire occurs *in* or *on* the patient, especially during high-risk procedures in which an ignition source is used in an oxidizer-rich environment. These would include airway fires (including endotracheal tube fires, fires in the oropharynx, which may occur during a tonsillectomy, fires in the breathing circuit), and fires during laparoscopy. In 2005, Katz and Campbell[97] reported on a fire during a thoracotomy. A dry gauze lap pad was set on fire, because 100% oxygen was present in the thoracic cavity while the surgeon was using the electrocautery. Cases that involve stripping of the pleura or resection of pulmonary blebs, tracheobronchopleural fistula, can easily result in high concentrations of oxygen in the thoracic cavity when the lung is reinflated due to gas leakage.[98,99] Solutions to this problem include making sure that the lap pads are always wet, and if the surgeon needs the lung inflated, then doing CPAP with air instead of oxygen will greatly reduce the risk of a fire.

Fires occurring on the patient mainly involve head and neck surgery done under regional anesthesia (RA) or monitored anesthesia care (MAC) when the patient is receiving high flows of supplemental oxygen. Because these fires occur in an oxygen-enriched environment, items such as surgical towels, drapes, or even the body hair can be readily ignited and produce a severe burn. The ECRI Institute warns that "oxygen enriched atmospheres lower the temperature at which a fuel will ignite."[90] In addition, these fires will burn more vigorously, and spread faster. The other type of OR fire is one that is remote from the patient. This would include an electrical fire in a piece of equipment, or a carbon dioxide (CO_2) absorber fire. A report by Lepiane describes a case where the power cord to the OR table was trapped beneath the base of the table. When the bed control was activated, a shower of sparks arose and ignited the sheets on the bed.[100]

All materials burn in the presence of an oxygen-enriched environment. Wolf et al.[101] tested a number of surgical drape materials in 21%, 50%, and 95% oxygen. They found that the higher the concentration of oxygen, the more readily the material could be set on fire. In 50% and 95% O_2, all the materials burned. In the case of the cotton huck towel, the time to ignition in 21% O_2 was a mean of 12 seconds. The same material ignited in 0.1 seconds in 95% O_2. Recent studies by Goldberg[102] and Culp et al.[103] showed similar results with a variety of common OR materials. Namely, that all materials ignited in an oxygen-enriched environment, and there was a dramatic increase in flammability especially with 100% oxygen.

In an editorial accompanying the Culp article, Eichhorn urged the elimination of open oxygen delivery in MAC cases involving the head and neck or upper body. He stressed that anesthesiologists must stop the routine administration of oxygen in these cases simply because "it's the way we always do it."[104]

The two major ignition sources for OR fires are the ESU and the laser. However, the ends of some fiberoptic light cords can also become hot enough to start a fire if they are placed on paper drapes. Although the ESU is responsible for igniting the majority

Table 5-4 Fuel Sources Commonly Found in the Operating Room

"Prep" agents
  Alcohol
  Degreasers (acetone, ether)
  Adhesives (tincture of benzoin, Aeroplast)
  Chlorhexidine digluconate (Hibitane)
  Iodophor (Dura-Prep)
Drapes and covers
  Patient drapes (paper, plastic, cloth)
  Equipment drapes (paper, plastic, cloth)
  Blankets and sheets
  Pillows, mattresses, and padding
  Gowns
  Masks
  Shoe covers
  Gloves (latex, nonlatex)
  Clothing
  Compression (antiembolism) stockings
Patient
  Hair
  Alimentary tract gases (methane, hydrogen)
  Desiccated tissue
Dressings
  Gauze and sponges
  Petrolatum-impregnated dressings
  Xeroform
  Adhesive tape (cloth, plastic, paper)
  Elastic bandages
  Stockinettes
  Sutures
  Steri-strips
  Collodion
Ointments
  Petrolatum
  Antibiotics (bacitracin, neomycin, polymyxin B)
  Nitropaste (Nitro-Bid)
  EMLA
  Lip balms
Anesthesia equipment
  Breathing circuit hoses
  Masks
  Endotracheal tubes
  Oral and nasal airways
  Laryngeal mask airways
  Nasogastric tubes
  Suction catheters and tubing
  Scavenger hoses
  Volatile anesthetics
  CO_2 absorbers
  Intravenous tubing
  Pressure monitor tubing and plastic transducers
Other equipment
  Charts and records
  Cardboard, wooden, and particleboard boxes and cabinets
  Packing materials (cardboard, expanded polystyrene [Styrofoam])
  Fiberoptic cable covers
  Wire covers and insulation
  Fiberoptic endoscope coverings
  Sphygmomanometer cuffs and tubing
  Pneumatic tourniquet cuffs and tubing
  Stethoscope tubing
  Vascular shunts (Gore-Tex, Dacron)
  Dialysis and extracorporeal circulation circuits
  Wound drains and collection systems
  Mops and brooms
  Textbooks and instruction manuals

of the fires,[105] it is the laser that has generated the most attention and research. Laser is the acronym for *light amplification by stimulated emission of radiation*. A laser consists of an energy source and material that the energy excites to emit light.[106–108] The material that the energy excites is called the *lasing medium* and provides the name of the particular type of laser. Laser light has several important properties. It is coherent radiation (meaning all the waves have the same frequency and phase), it is monochromatic (of a single color or wavelength), and it is collimated (the beam does not disperse as the distance from the source increases). This coherent light can be focused into very small spots that have very high power density.

There are many different types of medical lasers, and each has a specific application. The argon laser is used in eye and dermatologic procedures because it is absorbed by hemoglobin and has a modest tissue penetration of between 0.05 and 2.0 mm. The potassium titanyl phosphate (KTP) or frequency-doubled yttrium aluminum garnet (YAG) lasers are also absorbed by hemoglobin and have tissue penetrations similar to that of the argon laser. The tunable dye laser has a wavelength that is easily changed and can be used in different applications, particularly in dermatologic procedures. The neodymium-doped yttrium aluminum garnet (Nd:YAG) laser is the most powerful of the medical lasers. Since the tissue penetration is between 2 and 6 mm, it can be used for tumor debulking, particularly in the trachea and main stem bronchi, or in the upper airway. The energy can be transmitted through a fiberoptic cable that is placed down the suction port of a fiberoptic bronchoscope (FOB). The laser can then be used in a contact mode to treat a tumor mass. The CO_2 laser has very little tissue penetration and can be used where great precision is needed. It is also absorbed by water, so that minimal heat is dispersed to surrounding tissues. The CO_2 laser is used primarily for procedures in the oropharynx and in and around the vocal cords. The helium–neon (He–Ne) laser produces an intense red light and thus can be used for aiming the CO_2 and the Nd:YAG lasers. It has very low power and thus will present no significant danger to OR personnel.

One of the most devastating types of OR fires occurs when an endotracheal tube is ignited *in* the patient.[109–114] If the patient is being ventilated with oxygen and/or nitrous oxide, the endotracheal tube will essentially emit a blowtorch type of flame that can result in severe injury to the trachea, lungs, and surrounding tissues (Fig. 5-37). Red rubber, polyvinyl chloride, and silicone endotracheal tubes all have oxygen-flammability indices (defined as the minimum O_2 fraction in N_2 that will just support a candle-like flame for a given fuel source using a standard ignition source)[115] of less than 26%.[116] Historically, anesthesiologists attempted to improve the safety of these tubes by wrapping red rubber or polyvinyl chloride tubes with some sort of reflective tape. However, taped–wrapped tubes often became kinked, gaps

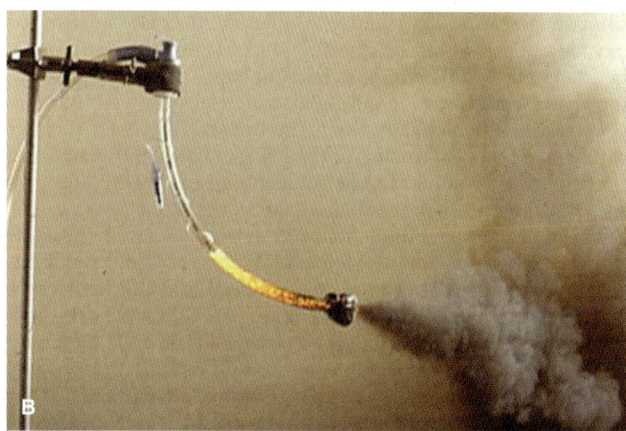

Figure 5-37 **A:** A burning ET tube with a high concentration of O_2 or O_2/N_2O will exhibit a "blowtorch" effect. (Copyright © ECRI Institute. Used with permission.) **B:** A burning ET tube will produce a large amount of debris. (Copyright © ECRI Institute. Used with permission.)

in the tape exposed areas of the tube to the laser, and non–laser-resistant tape was sometimes unintentionally used. To prevent these problems during high-risk procedures, "laser-resistant" endotracheal tubes have been developed.[117–119] Anesthesiologists can now use an endotracheal tube that is designed to be resistant to ignition by the specific type of laser that will be used during surgery. For instance, when using the CO_2 laser, the LaserFlex (Mallinckrodt, Pleasanton, CA) (Fig. 5-38) is an excellent choice. This is a flexible metal tube that has two cuffs that can be inflated with saline colored with methylene blue. The methylene blue enables the surgeon to easily recognize if he or she has accidentally penetrated one of the cuffs. The LaserFlex tube is highly resistant to being struck by the laser. If the Nd:YAG laser is being used, then the Lasertubus (Rüsch Inc., Duluth, GA) can be used (Fig. 5-39). The Lasertubus has a soft rubber shaft that is covered by a corrugated silver foil that is in turn covered in a Merocel sponge jacket. In order to provide maximum protection, the Merocel must be kept moist with saline. It should be noted that only the portion of the tube covered with the Merocel is laser resistant.

Another potential source of ignition for an OR fire is the ESU.[120,121] A typical example of how an ESU could cause ignition would be during a tonsillectomy in a child in whom the anesthesiologist was using an uncuffed, flammable endotracheal tube. In this case, the oxygen or oxygen–nitrous oxide mixture could leak around the endotracheal tube and pool at the operative site, providing an oxidizer-enriched environment. When the surgeon uses the ESU (or laser) to cauterize the tonsil bed, the combination of a high concentration of oxidizer (oxygen or oxygen–nitrous oxide mixture), fuel (endotracheal tube), and ignition source (the ESU or laser) could easily start a fire.[122–124]

The best way to prevent this type of fire is to take steps to prevent the three legs of the fire triad from coming together. For example, mixing the oxygen with air will keep the inspired oxygen concentration as low as possible, thus reducing the available oxidizer. Another possibility would be to place wet pledgets around the endotracheal tube, which would prevent the escape of oxygen or oxygen–nitrous oxide mixture from the trachea into the operative field. This reduces the available oxidizer and would keep the endotracheal tube and tissues from becoming desiccated, thus reducing their suitability as fuel sources. However, the pledgets must be kept moist, lest they dry out and become an additional source of fuel for a fire.

A related situation that requires a different solution can arise when a critically ill patient requires a tracheostomy.[125–128] These patients may require very high concentrations of inspired oxygen

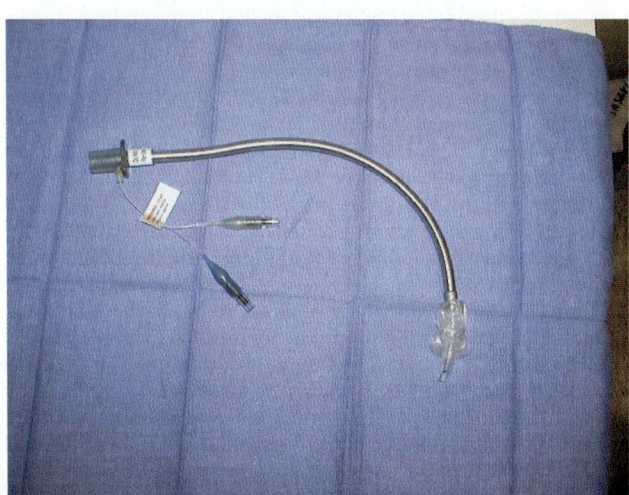

Figure 5-38 LaserFlex laser resistant ET tube.

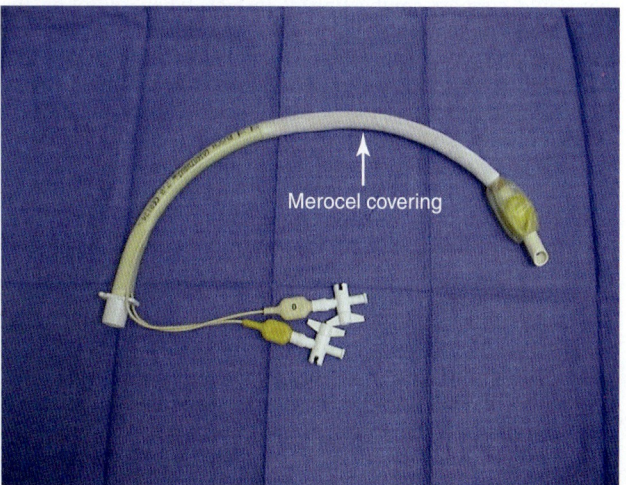

Figure 5-39 Lasertubus laser resistant ET tube.

to maintain tissue oxygenation so that any decrease in inspired oxygen concentration or interruption of ventilation would not be tolerated. In this circumstance, the best option for preventing a fire would be to avoid the use of electrocautery (ignition source) when the surgeon enters the trachea. The Nd:YAG laser can be used to treat tumors of the lower trachea and main stem bronchi. Most commonly, the surgeon will use a FOB and pass the laser fiber through the suction port of the bronchoscope. The FOB can be used in conjunction with a rigid metal bronchoscope or passed through an 8.5 or 9.0 mm polyvinyl chloride endotracheal tube. A special laser-resistant tube would not be used in this circumstance because the FOB and laser fiber pass through the endotracheal tube and focus on tissue distal to the tube. Fire safety precautions available in this setting include titrating the concentration of inspired oxygen to as low a concentration as the patient can tolerate while maintaining a saturation of between 90% and 95% (ideally keeping the inspired oxygen below 30%), keeping the tip of the endotracheal tube and FOB away from the site of surgery and out of the "line of fire" of the laser, and removing charred and desiccated tissue from the surgical field.

The use of a rigid metal bronchoscope instead of an endotracheal tube will eliminate the possibility of setting the tube on fire but does not eliminate the possibility of setting the FOB on fire. This would also necessitate the use of a jet Venturi system to ventilate the patient, which would, in turn, deliver an inspired oxygen concentration of between 40% and 60%.

There are a number of basic safety precautions that should be taken whenever a laser is used in surgery. Since laser light can be reflected off any metal surface, it is important that all OR personnel wear protective goggles that are specific to the type of laser being used. The anesthesiologist needs to be aware that the laser goggles may make it difficult to read certain monitor displays. In addition, it is important that the patient's eyes be covered with wet gauze or eye packs. OR personnel should also wear high filtration masks because the laser "plume" may contain vaporized virus particles or chemical toxins. Finally, all doors to the OR should have warning signs that a laser is in use, and all windows should be covered with black window shades.

Laparoscopic surgery in the abdomen is another potential risk for a surgically related fire. Ordinarily, the abdomen is inflated with CO_2, which does not support combustion. It is important to verify that, indeed, only CO_2 is being used, as erroneous inclusion of oxygen can be disastrous.[129,130] Also, nitrous oxide administered to the patient as part of the anesthetic can, over 30 minutes, diffuse into the abdominal cavity and attain a concentration that could support combustion.[131] In fact, when sampling the abdominal gas contents after 30 minutes, the mean nitrous oxide concentration was 36%; however, in certain patients it reached a concentration of 47%. Both methane and hydrogen are flammable gases that are frequently present in bowel gas in significant concentrations. Methane concentration in bowel gas can be up to 56% and hydrogen has been reported as high as 69%. With the maximum abdominal concentration of 47% nitrous oxide mixed with CO_2, it would require the maximum of 56% of methane to be flammable. Therefore, this represents a relatively small hazard. In contrast, a concentration of 69% hydrogen is flammable if the nitrous oxide concentration is above 29%. Therefore, a fire is possible if the surgeon, while using the ESU, enters the bowel with a high concentration of hydrogen and the intra-abdominal nitrous oxide content is more than 29%. The risk is greater during emergent colon surgery, when an unprepped or ruptured colon can release hydrogen or methane that can be ignited by the ESU.[132] In recent years, fires *on* the patient have become the most frequent type of OR fire. These cases occur most often during surgery in and around the head and neck, where the patient is receiving MAC and supplemental oxygen is being administered by either a face mask or nasal cannulae.[133–137] The higher the oxygen flow rate, the higher the oxygen concentration will be under the drapes, and the longer it will take to dissipate.[138,139] In these cases, the oxygen can collect under the drapes if not properly vented, and when the surgeon uses the ESU or the laser, a fire can easily start. Placing a modified nasal cannula into a nasopharyngeal airway, has been shown to reduce the oxygen concentration under the drapes.[140,141]

There are many things that can act as fuel, such as the surgical towels, paper drapes, disinfecting preparation solutions, sponges, plastic tubing from the oxygen face mask, and even the body hair. These fires start very quickly and can turn into an intense blaze in only a few seconds. Even if the fire is quickly extinguished, the patient will usually sustain a significant burn.

Currently, the majority of OR fires occur with MAC during head and neck surgery. Invariably, this involves an oxygen-enriched atmosphere since the majority of surgical fires are oxygen enriched. Currently, the Anesthesia Patient Safety Foundation (APSF), and ECRI Institute recommend that there be no open delivery of oxygen during these cases.[90,142] If the patient needs increased levels of sedation during a time when the surgeon is using the ESU or laser, then the airway needs to be secured with an LMA or an endotracheal tube. Occasionally, there are cases during which the patient and the anesthesiologist need to communicate. An example of this might be an awake craniotomy or a carotid endarterectomy under RA. In these cases it is prudent to use an FiO_2 of less than 30%. Preferably, the patient should receive only room air during these cases.

The ASA Closed Claims Study provides some further insights into the problem.[143] They have maintained a database of closed malpractice claims since 1985. Analysis of the database showed there were 103 claims for OR fires between 1985 and 2009. This amounted to 1.9% of the total claims (n = 5,297). Of those, 78 (76%) occurred during MAC or RA. Twenty-five (24%) of the cases happened when the patient was receiving general anesthesia.

The ESU was found to be the ignition source in 90% of the fire cases. There has been an increase in the incidence of the ESU being the ignition source in recent years. From 1985 to 1994, these totaled 1% of all surgical claims, but increased to 4.4% of claims from 2000 to 2009. Eighty-five percent (85%) of the ESU fires involved the head, neck, or upper chest, and 97% of the MAC/RA fires occurred in the head, neck, or upper chest region. Oxygen was the oxidizer in 95% of the ESU-induced fires, and in 84% there was open delivery of oxygen.

The most important principle that the anesthesiologist has to keep in mind to minimize the risk of fire is to titrate the inspired oxygen to the lowest concentration necessary to keep patient's oxygenation within safe levels. If the anesthesia machine has the ability to deliver air, then the nasal cannula or face mask can be attached to the anesthesia circuit by using a small no. 3 or no. 4, 15-mm endotracheal tube adapter.[144] This is attached to the right-angle elbow of the circuit. If the anesthesia machine is equipped with an auxiliary oxygen flowmeter that has a removable nipple adapter, then a humidifier can be installed in place of the nipple adapter. The humidifier has a Venturi mechanism through which room air is entrained and thus the oxygen concentration that is delivered to the face mask can be varied from 28% to 100%. Finally, if this machine has a common gas outlet that is easily accessible, a nasal cannula or face mask can be attached at this point using the same small 3- or 4-mm endotracheal tube adaptor (Fig. 5-40). If it is necessary to deliver more than 30% oxygen to the patient, then delivering 5 to 15 L/min of

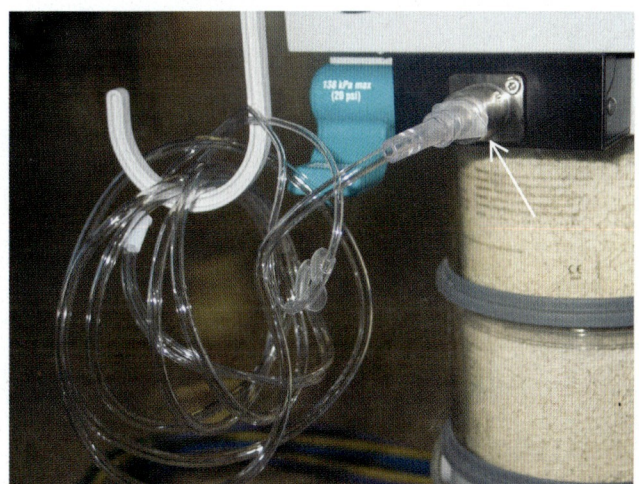

Figure 5-40 A nasal cannula connected to the alternate fresh gas outlet (*arrow*) on a GE-Datex-Ohmeda Aestiva anesthesia machine.

air under the drapes will dilute the oxygen.[145] The oxygen should always be discontinued at least 1 minute before the surgeon uses the ESU. Also the bipolar ESU is preferable to the monopolar ESU. It is important that the drapes be arranged in such a manner that there is no oxygen buildup beneath them. Venting the drapes and having the surgeon use an adhesive sticky drape that seals the operative site from the oxygen flow are steps that will help reduce the risk of a fire.[146] However, the seal of the adhesive drape may break down during the case and allow oxygen into the operative field. Therefore, this technique cannot be counted on to reliably protect the patient.

It is potentially possible to discontinue the use of oxygen before the surgeon plans to use the electrocautery or laser. This would have to be done several minutes beforehand in order to allow any oxygen that has built up to dissipate. If the surgeon is planning to use the electrosurgery or laser during the entire case, this may not be practical. Also the bipolar ESU is preferable to the monopolar ESU.

Some newer surgical preparation solutions can contribute to surgically related fires.[147-150] These solutions typically come prepackaged in a "paint stick" applicator with a sponge on the end (e.g., DuraPrep, 3M, St. Paul, MN; ChloraPrep or Prevail, Becton Dickinson, Franklin Lakes, NJ). They consist of an Iodophor or CHG mixed with at least 70% isopropyl alcohol. This is highly flammable and can easily be the fuel for an OR fire. In 2001, Barker and Polson[133] reported such a case. In a laboratory recreation, they found that if the DuraPrep had been allowed to dry completely (4 to 5 minutes), the fire did not occur (Fig. 5-41). The other problem with these types of preparation solutions is that small pools of the solution can accumulate if the person doing the preparation is not careful. The alcohol in these small puddles will continue to evaporate for a period of time, and the alcohol vapors are also extremely flammable. Flammable skin preparation solutions should be allowed to dry at least 3 minutes, and puddles removed before the site is draped (Fig. 5-42). If the preparation solution gets into the patient's hair, then drying can take up to 60 minutes.

It is important to bear in mind that halogenation of hydrocarbon anesthetics confers relative, but not absolute, resistance to combustion. Even the newer, "nonflammable" volatile anesthetics can, under certain circumstances, present fire hazards. For example, sevoflurane is nonflammable in air, but can serve as a fuel at concentrations as low as 11% in oxygen and 10% in nitrous oxide.[151] In addition, sevoflurane and desiccated CO_2 absorbent (either soda lime or Baralyme) can undergo exothermic chemical reactions that have been implicated in several fires that involved the anesthesia breathing circuit.[152-155] In 2003, the manufacturer of sevoflurane published a "Dear Health Care Provider" letter and advisory alert.[156] To prevent future fires, the manufacturer of sevoflurane has recommended that anesthesiologists employ several measures, including avoiding the use of desiccated CO_2 absorbent and monitoring the temperature of the absorbers and the inspired concentration of sevoflurane; if elevated temperature or an inspired sevoflurane concentration that differed unexpectedly from the vaporizer setting is detected, it is recommended that the patient be disconnected from the anesthesia circuit and monitored for signs of thermal or chemical injury, and that the CO_2 absorbent be removed from the circuit and/or replaced.

Another way to prevent this type of fire is to use a CO_2 absorbent that does not contain a strong alkali, as do soda lime and Baralyme (Chemetron Medical Division, Allied Healthcare Products, St. Louis, Missouri). Amsorb (Armstrong Medical Limited, Coleraine, Northern Ireland) is a CO_2 absorbent that contains calcium hydroxide and calcium chloride, but no strong alkali.[157] In experimental studies, it was found that Amsorb is unreactive with currently used volatile anesthetics and does not produce carbon monoxide or Compound A with desiccated absorbent. Therefore, it would not interact with sevoflurane and undergo an exothermic chemical reaction.[155]

If a fire does occur, it is important to extinguish it as soon as possible. The first step is to interrupt the fire triad by removing one component. This is usually best accomplished by removing the oxidizer from the fire. Therefore, if a tracheal tube is on fire, disconnecting the circuit from the tube or disconnecting the inspiratory limb of the circuit will usually result in the fire immediately going out. Simultaneously the surgeon should remove the burning endotracheal tube. Once the fire is extinguished, the airway is inspected via bronchoscopy, and the patient reintubated.

If the fire is on the patient, then extinguishing it with a basin of saline may be the most rapid and effective method to deal with this type of fire. There is also a method to use a sheet or towel to extinguish the fire. If the drapes are burning, particularly if they are paper drapes, then they must be removed and placed on the floor. Paper drapes are impervious to water; thus, throwing water or saline on them will do little to extinguish the fire. Once the burning drapes are removed from the patient, the fire can then be extinguished with a fire extinguisher. In most OR fires, the sprinkler system is not activated. This is because the sprinklers are not located directly over the OR table and because OR fires seldom get hot enough to activate the sprinklers.

All OR personnel should receive OR fire safety education, which should include training in institutional fire safety protocols and learning the location and operation of the fire extinguishers. Fire safety education, including fire drills, allows each member of the OR team to learn and practice what his or her responsibilities and actions should be if a fire were to occur.[158] Fire drills are an important part of the plan and can help personnel become familiar with the exits, evacuation routes, location of fire extinguishers, and how to shut off medical gas and electrical supplies. Although institutional fire safety protocols vary, the general principles of responding to an OR fire can be summarized by the mnemonic ERASE: Extinguish, rescue, activate, shut, and evaluate. In sequence: First, the team should generally attempt to extinguish a fire on, in, or near the patient. Depending on the situation, this may include the use of saline or a CO_2 fire extinguisher (see later discussion). If the initial attempts at

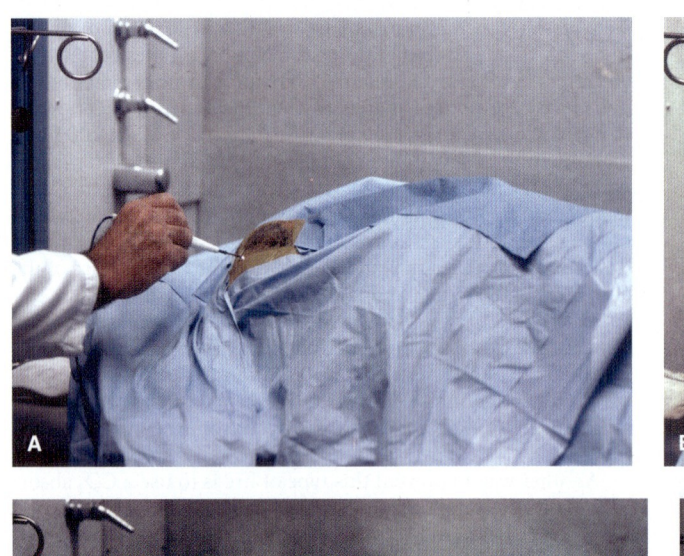
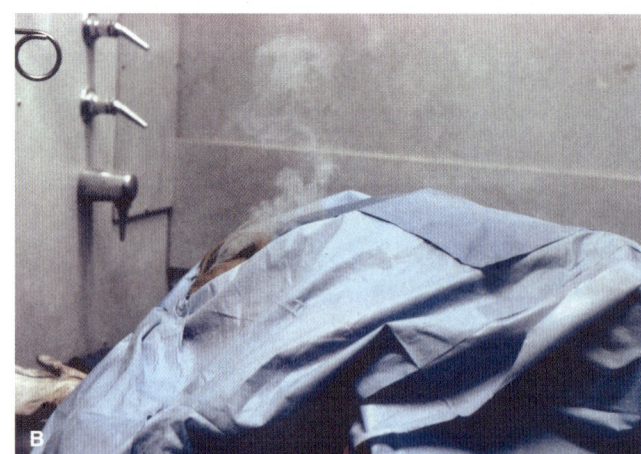
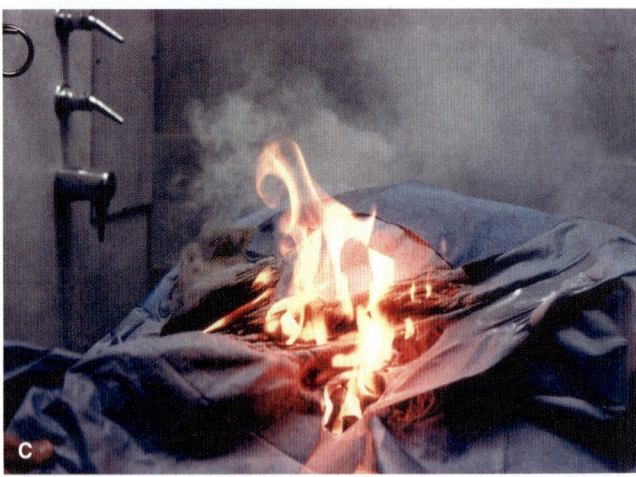
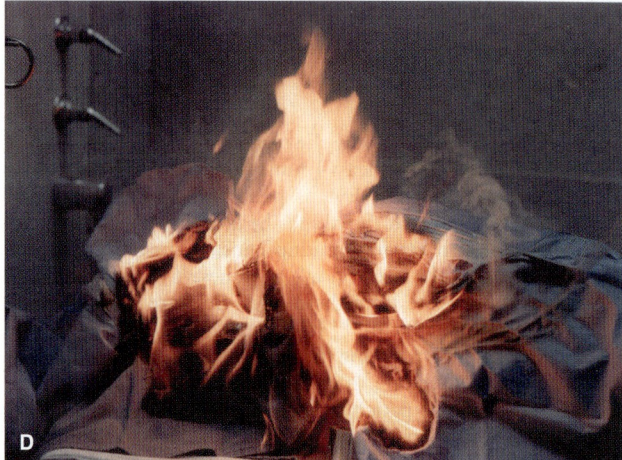

Figure 5-41 Simulation of fire caused by ESU electrode during surgery. **A:** Mannequin prepared and draped for surgery. Electrosurgical unit monopolar pencil electrode applied to operative site at start of surgery. **B:** Six seconds after electrosurgical unit application. Smoke appears from under the drapes. **C:** Fourteen seconds after electrosurgical unit application. Flames burst through the drapes. **D:** Twenty-four seconds after electrosurgical unit application. Entire patient head and drapes in flames. (Reprinted with permission from Barker SJ, Polson JS. Fire in the operating room: A case report and laboratory study. *Anesth Analg.* 2001;93:960. Copyright © 2001, International Anesthesia Research Society.)

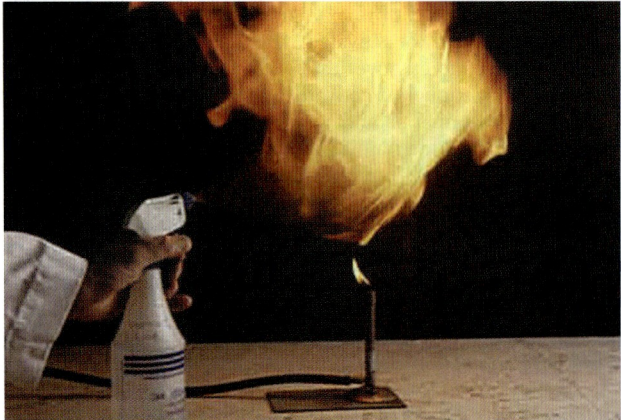

Figure 5-42 A demonstration of the intense heat and flame that is present in an alcohol fire. (Photograph courtesy of Mark Bruley of Emergency Care Research Institute. Reprinted with permission, Copyright 2009, ECRI Institute. www.ecri.org.)

extinguishing the fire are unsuccessful, the patient and all other persons at risk should be rescued and the OR evacuated, if possible, and the fire alarm should be activated. Once the OR is emptied of personnel, the doors should be shut and the medical gas supply to the room should be shut off. The patient should then be evaluated and any injuries should be appropriately managed.

Preventing an OR fire should be the hallmark of all fire safety programs and training. The first step is to determine whether a high risk situation exists. This can be accomplished by doing a "fire time out" prior to starting the case. The risk factors include: (1) open delivery of oxygen/oxygen-enriched environment; (2) an ignition/heat source, such as ESU, laser, or electrocautery; (3) surgery in the head, neck, or upper chest area; (4) an alcohol prep solution. If three or more of these factors are present, then a high fire risk situation exists, and the team should take necessary steps to prevent a fire.

Other safety measures to prevent a fire include keeping the oxygen concentration as low as clinically possible. Notify the surgeon if an oxygen-enriched environment is in proximity to an ignition source. Allow sufficient time for the

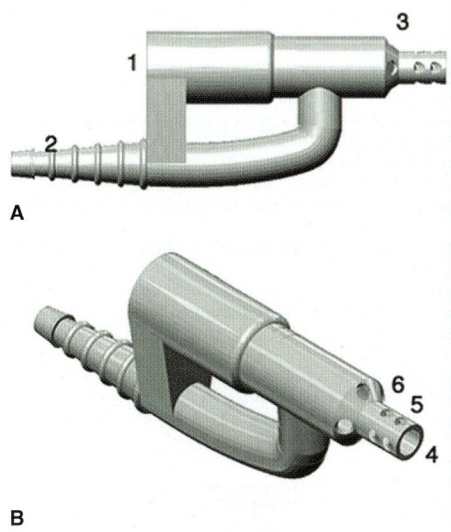
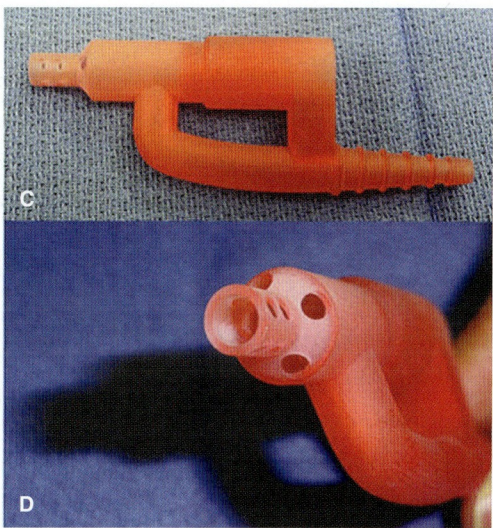

Figure 5-43 The figure shows the CO_2 fire protection device. Panels **A** and **B** illustrate a 3-dimensional model, and Panels **C** and **D** show the polymer prototype. Number 1, is the barrel for the ESU; Number 2 is the inlet for the CO_2; Numbers 3 to 6 are the sleeve and exit ports for the CO_2. (Reprinted with permission from Culp WC Jr, Kimbrough BA, Luna S, et al. Operating room fire prevention: creating an electrosurgical unit fire safety device. *Annals of Surgery*. 2014;260:214–217.)

oxygen-enriched environment to dissipate before activating the ESU or laser. Ensure that alcohol preps are dry before draping the patient, and moisten all sponges that are in proximity to an ignition source.[159–161]

The ESU has been implicated as the ignition source in as many as 90% of OR fires.[143] This is exacerbated when there is an oxygen-enriched environment, as fuel sources will ignite more rapidly, and burn faster and hotter. If there was an engineering solution to mitigate this problem, then fire safety would be greatly enhanced.[162] Culp et al.[163,164] might have developed just such a device. Their device consists of a polymer sleeve that fits over an ESU pencil. They then connected a continuous flow of carbon dioxide to the sleeve which flowed around the ESU pencil tip. The CO_2 acted as a fire suppressant and in laboratory tests none of the tested materials was ignited even in the presence of 100% oxygen (Fig. 5-43 and Fig. 5-44.).

Fire extinguishers are divided into three classes, termed *A, B,* and *C,* based on the types of fires for which they are best suited. Class A extinguishers are used on paper, cloth, and plastic materials; Class B extinguishers are used for fires when liquids or grease are involved; Class C extinguishers are used for energized electrical equipment. A single fire extinguisher may be useful for any one, two, or all three types of fires. Probably the best fire extinguisher for the OR is the CO_2 extinguisher. This can be used on Class B and C fires and some Class A fires. Other extinguishers are water mist and new environmentally friendly fluorocarbons that replaced the Halon fire extinguisher. Finally, many ORs are equipped with a fire hose that supplies pressurized water at a rate of 50 gallons per minute. Such equipment is best left to the fire department to use, unless there is a need to rescue someone from a fire. In order to effectively use a fire extinguisher, the acronym "PASS" can be used. This stands for *p*ull the pin to activate the fire extinguisher, *a*im at the base of the fire, *s*queeze the trigger, and *s*weep the extinguisher back and forth across the base of the fire. When responding to a fire, the acronym RACE is useful. This stands for *r*escue; *a*larm; *c*onfine; *e*xtinguish. Clearly, having a plan that everyone is familiar with will greatly facilitate extinguishing the fire and minimizing the harm to the patient and equipment.

However, neither fire drills nor the presence and use of fire extinguishers should be relied on to provide a fire-safe operating environment. Only through heightened awareness, continuing education, and ongoing communication can the legs of the fire triad be kept apart and the risk of an OR fire minimized.

Figure 5-44 The CO_2 fire protection device with white smoke exiting the device (simulating carbon dioxide flow) and surrounding the ESU pencil tip. (Reprinted with permission from Culp WC Jr, Kimbrough BA, Luna S, et al. Operating room fire prevention: creating an electrosurgical unit fire safety device. *Annals of Surgery*. 2014;260:214–217.)

REFERENCES

1. Harpell TR. Electrical shock hazards in the hospital environment. Their causes and cures. *Can Hosp.* 1970;47:48–53.
2. Buczko GB, McKay WP. Electrical safety in the operating room. *Can J Anaesth.* 1987;34:315–322.
3. Wald A. Electrical safety in medicine. In: Skalak R, Chien S, ed. *Handbook of Bioengineering.* New York, NY: McGraw-Hill; 1987.
4. Dalziel CF, Massaglia FP. Let-Go Currents and Voltages. *IEEE Transactions on Education.* 1956;75.
5. Bruner JM, Aronow S, Cavicchi RV. Electrical incidents in a large hospital: a 42 month register. *J Assoc Adv Med Instrum.* 1972;6:222–230.
6. Bernstein MS. Isolated power and line isolation monitors. *Biomed Instrum Technol.* 1990;24:221–223.
7. Courtney NM, McCoy EP, Scolaro RJ, et al. A serious and repeatable electrical hazard–compressed electrical cord and an operating table. *Anaesth Intensive Care.* 2006;34:392–396.
8. Gibby GL. Shock and electrocution. In: Lobato EB GN, Kirby Robert R, eds. *Complications in Anesthesiology.* Philadelphia, PA: Wolters Kluwer/Lippincott Williams & Wilkins; 2008.
9. Weinberg DI, Artley JL, Whalen RE, et al. Electric shock hazards in cardiac catheterization. *Circ Res.* 1962;11:1004–1009.

10. Starmer CF, Whalen RE. Current density and electrically induced ventricular fibrillation. *Med Instrum.* 1973;7:158–161.
11. Whalen RE, Starmer CF, McIntosh HD. Electrical hazards associated with cardiac pacemaking. *Ann N Y Acad Sci.* 1964;111:922–931.
12. Raftery EB, Green HL, Yacoub MH. Disturbances of heart rhythm produced by 50 Hz leakage currents in human subjects. *Cardiovasc Res.* 1975;9:263–265.
13. Hull CJ. Electrocution hazards in the operating theatre. *Br J Anaesth.* 1978;50:647–657.
14. Watson AB, Wright JS, Loughman J. Electrical thresholds for ventricular fibrillation in man. *Med J Aust.* 1973;1:1179–1182.
15. Furman S, Schwedel JB, Robinson G, et al. Use of an intracardiac pacemaker in the control of heart block. *Surgery.* 1961;49:98–108.
16. Noordijk JA, Oey FT, Tebra W. Myocardial electrodes and the danger of ventricular fibrillation. *Lancet.* 1961;1:975–977.
17. Pengelly LD, Klassen GA. Myocardial electrodes and the danger of ventricular fibrillation. *Lancet.* 1961;277:1234.
18. Rowe GG, Zarnstorff WC. Ventricular fibrillation during selective angiocardiography. *JAMA.* 1965;192:947–950.
19. Hopps JA, Roy OZ. Electrical hazards in cardiac diagnosis and treatment. *Med Electron Biol Eng.* 1:133–134.
20. Baas LS, Beery TA, Hickey CS. Care and safety of pacemaker electrodes in intensive care and telemetry nursing units. *Am J Crit Care.* 1997;6:302–311.
21. Leeming MN. Protection of the "electrically susceptible patient": a discussion of systems and methods. *Anesthesiology.* 1973;38:370–383.
22. McNulty SE, Cooper M, Staudt S. Transmitted radiofrequency current through a flow directed pulmonary artery catheter. *Anesth Analg.* 1994;78:587–589.
23. Cromwell L, Weibell FJ, Pfeiffer EA. *Biomedical Instrumentation and Measurements.* Englewood Cliffs, NJ: Prentice-Hall; 1973.
24. Edwards NK. Specialized electrical grounding needs. *Clin Perinatol.* 1976;3:367–374.
25. Goldwyn RM. Bovie: the man and the machine. *Ann Plast Surg.* 1979;2:135–153.
26. Lichter I, Borrie J, Miller WM. Radio-frequency hazards with cardiac pacemakers. *Br Med J.* 1965;1:1513–1518.
27. Dornette WHL. An electrically safe surgical environment. *Arch Surg.* 1973;107:567–573.
28. Klop WM, Lohuis PJ, Strating RP, et al. Ventricular fibrillation caused by electrocoagulation during laparoscopic surgery. *Surg Endosc.* 2002;16:362.
29. Fu Q, Cao P, Mi WD, et al. Ventricular fibrillation caused by electrocoagulation during thoracic surgery. *Acta Anaesthesiol Scand.* 2010;54:256.
30. Yan CY, Cai XJ, Wang YF, et al. Ventricular fibrillation caused by electrocoagulation in monopolar mode during laparoscopic subphrenic mass resection. *Surg Endosc.* 2011;25:309–311.
31. Dalibon N, Pelle-Lancien E, Puyo P, et al. Recurrent asystole during electrocauterization: an uncommon hazard in common situations. *Eur J Anaesthesiol.* 2005;22:476–478.
32. Cushing H, Bovie W. Electro-surgery as an aid to the removal of intracranial tumors: With a preliminary note on a new surgical-current generator. *Surg Gyn Obs.* 1928;47:751.
33. Meathe EA. Electrical safety for patients and anesthetists. In: Saidman LJ, Smith NT, eds. *Monitoring in Anesthesia.* 2nd ed. Boston: Butterworth-Heinemann; 1984.
34. Rolly G. Two cases of burns caused by misuse of coagulation unit and monitoring. *Acta Anaesthesiol Belg.* 1978;29:313–316.
35. Parker EO 3rd. Electrosurgical burn at the site of an esophageal temperature probe. *Anesthesiology.* 1984;61:93–95.
36. Schneider AJ, Apple HP, Braun RT. Electrosurgical burns at skin temperature probes. *Anesthesiology.* 1977;47:72–74.
37. Bloch EC, Burton LW. Electrosurgical burn while using a battery-operated Doppler monitor. *Anesth Analg.* 1979;58:339–342.
38. Becker CM, Malhotra IV, Hedley-Whyte J. The distribution of radiofrequency current and burns. *Anesthesiology.* 1973;38:106–122.
39. Russell MJ, Gaetz M. Intraoperative electrode burns. *J Clin Monitor Comp.* 2004;18:25–32.
40. Jones CM, Pierre KB, Nicoud IB, et al. Electrosurgery. *Curr Surg.* 2006;63:458–463.
41. Mitchell JP. The isolated circuit diathermy. *Ann R Coll Surg Engl.* 1979;61:287–290.
42. Titel JH, el-Etr AA. Fibrillation resulting from pacemaker electrodes and electrocautery during surgery. *Anesthesiology.* 1968;29:845–846.
43. Domino KB, Smith TC. Electrocautery-induced reprogramming of a pacemaker using a precordial magnet. *Anesth Analg.* 1983;62:609–612.
44. ECRI Institute. Damaged reusable ESU return electrode cables. *Health Devices.* 1985;14:214.
45. ECRI Institute. Sparking from and ignition of damaged electrosurgical electrode cables. *Health Devices.* 1998;27:301–303.
46. Mirowski M, Reid PR, Mower MM, et al. Termination of malignant ventricular arrhythmias with an implanted automatic defibrillator in human beings. *N Engl J Med.* 1980;303:322–324.
47. Crozier IG, Ward DE. Automatic implantable defibrillators. *Br J Hosp Med.* 1988;40:136–139.
48. Elefteriades JA, Biblo LA, Batsford WP, et al. Evolving patterns in the surgical treatment of malignant ventricular tachyarrhythmias. *Ann Thorac Surg.* 1990;49:94–100.
49. Carr CM, Whiteley SM. The automatic implantable cardioverter-defibrillator. Implications for anaesthetists. *Anaesthesia.* 1991;46:737–740.
50. Starmer CF, McIntosh HD, Whalen RE. Electrical hazards and cardiovascular function. *N Engl J Med.* 1971;284:181–186.
51. Albisser AM, Parson ID, Pask BA. A survey of the grounding systems in several large hospitals. *Med Instrum.* 1973;7:297–302.
52. McLaughlin AJ, Campkin NT. Electrical safety—a reminder. *Anaesthesia.* 1998;53:608–609.
53. Nixon MC, Ghurye M. Electrical failure in theatre—a consequence of complacency? *Anaesthesia.* 1997;52:88–89.
54. ECRI Institute. Medical devices; establishment of a performance standard for electrode lead wires and patient cables. *Federal Register.* 1997;62:25477.
55. ECRI Institute. FDA establishes performance standards for electrode lead wires. *Health Devices.* 1998;27:34.
56. Tye JC, Chamley D. Complete power failure. *Anaesthesia.* 2000;55:1133–1134.
57. National Fire Protection Association. *NFPA-99, Health Care Facilities Code, 2015 Edition, Article 6.4.4.1.1. Maintenance and Testing of Alternate Power Source and Transfer Switches.* Quincy, MA.
58. National Fire Protection Association. *NFPA-110, Standard for Emergency and Standby Power Systems.* Chapter 8, 2016 Edition. Quincy, MA.
59. Pagan A, Curty R, Rodriguez MI, et al. Emergency—total power outage in the OR. *AORN Journal.* 2001;74:514–516.
60. Carpenter T, Robinson ST. Case reports: response to a partial power failure in the operating room. *Anesth Analg.* 2010;110:1644–1646.
61. Eichhorn JH, Hessel EA 2nd. Electrical power failure in the operating room: a neglected topic in anesthesia safety. *Anesth Analg.* 2010;110:1519–1521.
62. Mathias JM. Blackout, Isabel offer lessons in preparing for emergencies. *Or Manager.* 2003;19:1, 7–8.
63. Jones RP, Conway DH. The effect of electromagnetic interference from mobile communication on the performance of intensive care ventilators. *Eur J Anaesthesiol.* 2005;22:578–583.
64. Lawrentschuk N, Bolton DM. Mobile phone interference with medical equipment and its clinical relevance: a systematic review. *Med J Aust.* 2004;181:145–149.
65. Hayes DL, Wang PJ, Reynolds DW, et al. Interference with cardiac pacemakers by cellular telephones. *N Engl J Med.* 1997;336:1473–1479.
66. Schlegel RE, Grant FH, Raman S, et al. Electromagnetic compatibility study of the in-vitro interaction of wireless phones with cardiac pacemakers. *Biomed Instrum Technol.* 1998;32:645–655.
67. Chen WH, Lau CP, Leung SK, et al. Interference of cellular phones with implanted permanent pacemakers. *Clin Cardiol.* 1996;19:881–886.
68. Fetter JG, Ivans V, Benditt DG, et al. Digital cellular telephone interaction with implantable cardioverter-defibrillators. *J Am Coll Cardiol.* 1998;31:623–628.
69. ECRI Institute. Cell phones and walkie-talkies. Is it time to relax your restrictive policies? *Health Devices.* 1999;28:409–413.
70. Adler D, Margulies L, Mahler Y, et al. Measurements of electromagnetic fields radiated from communication equipment and of environmental electromagnetic noise: impact on the use of communication equipment within the hospital. *Biomed Instrum Technol.* 1998;32:581–590.
71. Schwartz J, Ehrenwerth J. Electrical safety. In: Lake C, Hines R, Blitt C, eds. *Clinical Monitoring: Practical Applications for Anesthesia and Critical Care.* Philadelphia, PA: WB Saunders; 2000.
72. Kermit E, Staewen WS. Isolated power systems: Historical perspective and update on regulations. *Biomed Tech Today.* 1986;1:86.
73. National Fire Protection Association. *NFPA-70:National Electric Code (NEC). 2014 Edition, Article 6.4.4.1.1. Maintenance and Testing of Alternate Power Source and Transfer Switches.* Quincy, MA.
74. National Fire Protection Association. *NFPA-99:Health Care Facilities Code. 2015 Edition.* Quincy, MA.
75. Bruner JMR, Leonard PF. *Electricity, Safety and the Patient.* Chicago, IL: Year Book Medical Publishers; 1989.
76. Matjasko MJ, Ashman MN. All you need to know about electrical safety in the operating room. In: Barash PG, Deutsch S, Tinker J, eds. *ASA Refresher Courses in Anesthesiology.* Philadelphia, PA: JB Lippincott; 1990:251.
77. Lennon RL, Leonard PF. A hitherto unreported virtue of the isolated power system. *Anesth Analg.* 1987;66:1056–1057.
78. Barker SJ, Doyle DJ. Editorial: electrical safety in the operating room: Dry versus wet. *Anesth Analg.* 2010;110:1517–1518.
79. Gilbert TB, Shaffer M, Matthews M. Electrical shock by dislodged spark gap in bipolar electrosurgical device. *Anesth Analg.* 1991;73:355–357.
80. Van Kerckhove K. Re-evaluating the isolated power equation. *Electrical Products and Solutions.* 2008;25–27.
81. Day FJ. Electrical safety revisited: a new wrinkle. *Anesthesiology.* 1994;80:220–221.
82. Wills JH, Ehrenwerth J, Rogers D. Electrical injury to a nurse due to conductive fluid in an operating room designated as a dry location. *Anesth Analg.* 2010;110:1647–1649.
83. August DA. Locked out of a box and a process. *Anesth Analg.* 2011;112:1248–1249.

84. Barker SJ. In response to August DA. *Anesth Analg.* 2011;112:1249.
85. Litt L, Ehrenwerth J. Electrical safety in the operating room: important old wine, disguised new bottles. *Anesth Analg.* 1994;78:417–419.
86. Seifert HA. Fire safety in the operating room. In: Eisenkraft J, ed. *Progress in Anesthesiology*. Philadelphia, PA: WB Saunders; 1994.
87. Neufeld GR. Fires and explosions. In: Orkin FK, Cooperman LH, eds. *Complications in Anesthesiology*. Philadelphia: Lippincott; 1983:671.
88. Moxon MA, Ward ME. Fire in the operating theatre. Evacuation pre-planning may save lives. *Anaesthesia.* 1986;41:543–546.
89. Vickers MD. Fire and explosion hazards in operating theatres. *Br J Anaesth.* 1978;50:659–664.
90. ECRI Institute. New clinical guide to surgical fire prevention. Patients can catch fire—here's how to keep them safer. *Health Devices.* 2009;38:314–332.
91. Apfelbaum JL, Caplan RA, Barker SJ, et al. Practice advisory for the prevention and management of operating room fires: an updated report by the American Society of Anesthesiologists Task Force on Operating Room Fires. *Anesthesiology.* 2013;118:271–290.
92. de Richemond AL. The patient is on fire! *Health Devices.* 1992;21:19.
93. Cameron BG, Ingram GS. Flammability of drape materials in nitrous oxide and oxygen. *Anaesthesia.* 1971;26:281–288.
94. Johnson RM, Smith CV, Leggett K. Flammability of disposable surgical drapes. *Arch Ophthalmol.* 1976;94:1327–1329.
95. Simpson JI, Wolf GL. Flammability of esophageal stethoscopes, nasogastric tubes, feeding tubes, and nasopharyngeal airways in oxygen- and nitrous oxide-enriched atmospheres. *Anesth Analg.* 1988;67:1093–1095.
96. Ponath RE. Preventing surgical fires. *JAMA.* 1984;252:1762.
97. Katz JA, Campbell L. Fire during thoracotomy: a need to control the inspired oxygen concentration. *Anesth Analg.* 2005;101:612.
98. Errando CL, Garcia-Covisa N, Del-Rosario E, et al. An infrequent case of fire in the operating room during open surgery of a tracheobronchopleural fistula. *J Cardiothorac Vasc Anesth.* 2005;19:556–557.
99. Hudson DW, Guidry OF, Abernathy JH 3rd, et al. Case 4–2012. Intrathoracic fire during coronary artery bypass graft surgery. *J Cardiothorac Vasc Anesth.* 2012;26:520–521.
100. Lepiane SE. Fire in the OR: this can't be happening to me. *ORL - Head & Neck Nursing.* 2001;19:18–19.
101. Wolf GL, Sidebotham GW, Lazard JL, et al. Laser ignition of surgical drape materials in air, 50% oxygen, and 95% oxygen. *Anesthesiology.* 2004;100:1167–1171.
102. Goldberg J. Brief laboratory report: surgical drape flammability. *AANA Journal.* 2006;74:352–354.
103. Culp WC Jr, Kimbrough BA, Luna S. Flammability of surgical drapes and materials in varying concentrations of oxygen. *Anesthesiology.* 2013;119:770–776.
104. Eichhorn JH. A burning issue: preventing patient fires in the operating room. *Anesthesiology.* 2013;119:749–751.
105. Food and Drug Administration. Surgical Fires Reported January 1995-June 1998. FDA Databases MDR/MAUDE. 1999.
106. Rampil IJ. Anesthetic considerations for laser surgery. *Anesth Analg.* 1992; 74:424–435.
107. Pashayan AG, Ehrenwerth J. Lasers and electrical safety in the operating room. In: Ehrenwerth J, Eisenkraft, JB, eds. *Anesthesia Equipment: Principles and Applications*. St. Louis, MO: Mosby; 1993.
108. ECRI Institute. Lasers in medicine—An introduction. *Health Devices.* 1984; 13:151.
109. Casey KR, Fairfax WR, Smith SJ, et al. Intratracheal fire ignited by the Nd-YAG laser during treatment of tracheal stenosis. *Chest.* 1983;84:295–296.
110. Burgess GE 3rd, LeJeune FE Jr. Endotracheal tube ignition during laser surgery of the larynx. *Arch Otolaryngol.* 1979;105:561–562.
111. Cozine K, Rosenbaum LM, Askanazi J, et al. Laser-induced endotracheal tube fire. *Anesthesiology.* 1981;55:583–585.
112. Geffin B, Shapshay SM, Bellack GS, et al. Flammability of endotracheal tubes during Nd-YAG laser application in the airway. *Anesthesiology.* 1986;65:511–515.
113. Hirshman CA, Smith J. Indirect ignition of the endotracheal tube during carbon dioxide laser surgery. *Arch Otolaryngol.* 1980;106:639–641.
114. Krawtz S, Mehta AC, Wiedemann HP, et al. Nd-YAG laser-induced endobronchial burn. Management and long-term follow-up. *Chest.* 1989;95: 916–918.
115. Goldblum K. Oxygen index: Key to precise flammability ratings. *Soc Plast Eng J.* 1969;25:50–52.
116. Wolf GL, Simpson JI. Flammability of endotracheal tubes in oxygen and nitrous oxide enriched atmosphere. *Anesthesiology.* 1987;67:236–239.
117. de Richemond AL. Laser resistant endotracheal tubes—Protection against oxygen enriched airway fires during surgery? In: Stoltzfus JM, McIlroy K, eds. *Flammability and Sensitivity of Material in Oxygen-Enriched Atmospheres*, vol 5 (ASTM STP 1111). Philadelphia, PA: American Society for Testing and Materials; 1991:157.
118. ECRI Institute. Airway fires: reducing the risk during laser surgery. *Health Devices.* 1990;19:109–139.
119. ECRI Institute. Laser-resistant tracheal tubes. *Health Devices.* 1992;21: 4–14.
120. Aly A, McIlwain M, Duncavage JA. Electrosurgery-induced endotracheal tube ignition during tracheotomy. *Ann Otol Rhinol Laryngol.* 1991;100:31–33.
121. Simpson JI, Wolf GL. Endotracheal tube fire ignited by pharyngeal electrocautery. *Anesthesiology.* 1986;65:76–77.
122. Gupte SR. Gauze fire in the oral cavity: a case report. *Anesth Analg.* 1972;51: 645–646.
123. Snow JC, Norton ML, Saluja TS, et al. Fire hazard during CO2 laser microsurgery on the larynx and trachea. *Anesth Analg.* 1976;55:146–147.
124. Kaddoum RN, Chidiac EJ, Zestos MM, et al. Electrocautery-induced fire during adenotonsillectomy: report of two cases. *J Clin Anesth.* 2006;18:129–131.
125. Lew EO, Mittleman RE, Murray D. Endotracheal tube ignition by electrocautery during tracheostomy: case report with autopsy findings. *J Forensic Sci.* 1991;36:1586–1591.
126. Marsh B, Riley RH. Double-lumen tube fire during tracheostomy. *Anesthesiology.* 1992;76:480–481.
127. Thompson JW, Colin W, Snowden T, et al. Fire in the operating room during tracheostomy. *Southern Med J.* 1998;91:243–247.
128. Paugh DH, White KW. Fire in the operating room during tracheotomy: a case report. *AANA Journal.* 2005;73:97–100.
129. Neuman GG, Sidebotham G, Negoianu E, et al. Laparoscopy explosion hazards with nitrous oxide. *Anesthesiology.* 1993;78:875–879.
130. Di Pierro GB, Besmer I, Hefermehl LJ, et al. Intra-abdominal fire due to insufflating oxygen instead of carbon dioxide during robot-assisted radical prostatectomy: case report and literature review. *Eur Urol.* 2010;58:626–628.
131. Greilich PE, Greilich NB, Froelich EG. Intraabdominal fire during laparoscopic cholecystectomy. *Anesthesiology.* 1995;83:871–874.
132. Raghavan K, Lagisetty KH, Butler KL, et al. Intraoperative fires during emergent colon surgery. *American Surgeon.* 2015;81:E82–E83.
133. Barker SJ, Polson JS. Fire in the operating room: a case report and laboratory study. *Anesth Analg.* 2001;93:960–965.
134. Bruley ME, Lavanchy C. *Oxygen-Enriched Fires During Surgery of the Head and Neck. Symposium on Flammability and Sensitivity of Material in Oxygen-Enriched Atmospheres(ASTM STP 1040)*. Philadelphia, PA: American Society for Testing and Materials; 1989:392.
135. de Richemond AL, Bruley ME. Head and neck surgical fires. In: Eisele DW, ed. *Complications in Head and Neck Surgery*. St. Louis, MO: Mosby; 1993.
136. ECRI Institute. Fires during surgery of the head and neck area (hazard). *Health Devices.* 1979;9:50.
137. Ramanathan S, Capan L, Chalon J, et al. Minienvironmental control under the drapes during operations on the eyes of conscious patients. *Anesthesiology.* 1978;48:286–288.
138. Greco RJ, Gonzalez R, Johnson P, et al. Potential dangers of oxygen supplementation during facial surgery. *Plast Reconstr Surg.* 1995;95:978–984.
139. Barnes AM, Frantz RA. Do oxygen-enriched atmospheres exist beneath surgical drapes and contribute to fire hazard potential in the operating room? *AANA Journal.* 2000;68:153–161.
140. Engel SJ, Patel NK, Morrison CM, et al. Operating room fires: part II. Optimizing safety. *Plastic & Reconstructive Surgery.* 2012;130:681–689.
141. Meneghetti SC, Morgan MM, Fritz J, et al. Operating room fires: optimizing safety. *Plastic & Reconstructive Surgery.* 2007;120:1701–1708.
142. Anesthesia Patient Safety Foundation. Prevention and management of operating room fires (Video). apsf.org; 2010.
143. Mehta SP, Bhananker SM, Posner KL, et al. Operating room fires: a closed claims analysis. *Anesthesiology.* 2013;118:1133–1139.
144. Lampotang S, Gravenstein N, Paulus DA, et al. Reducing the incidence of surgical fires: supplying nasal cannulae with sub-100% O_2 gas mixtures from anesthesia machines. *Anesth Analg.* 2005;101:1407–1412.
145. Rinder CS. Fire safety in the operating room. *Curr Opin Anaesthesiol.* 2008; 21:790–795.
146. Tao JP, Hirabayashi KE, Kim BT, et al. The efficacy of a midfacial seal drape in reducing oculofacial surgical field fire risk. *Ophthal Plast Reconstr Surg.* 2013; 29:109–112.
147. Patel R, Chavda KD, Hukkeri S. Surgical field fire and skin burns caused by alcohol-based skin preparation. *J Emerg Trauma Shock.* 2010;3:305.
148. Prasad R, Quezado Z, St Andre A, et al. Fires in the operating room and intensive care unit: awareness is the key to prevention. *Anesth Analg.* 2006; 102:172–174.
149. ECRI Institute. Improper use of alcohol-based skin preps can cause surgical fires. *Health Devices.* 2003;32:441–443.
150. Rocos B, Donaldson LJ. Alcohol skin preparation causes surgical fires. *Ann R Coll Surg Engl.* 2012;94:87–89.
151. Wallin RF, Regan BM, Napoli MD, et al. Sevoflurane: a new inhalational anesthetic agent. *Anesth Analg.* 1975;54:758–766.
152. Fatheree RS, Leighton BL. Acute respiratory distress syndrome after an exothermic Baralyme-sevoflurane reaction. *Anesthesiology.* 2004;101:531–533.
153. Castro BA, Freedman LA, Craig WL, et al. Explosion within an anesthesia machine: Baralyme, high fresh gas flows and sevoflurane concentration. *Anesthesiology.* 2004;101:537–539.
154. Wu J, Previte JP, Adler E, et al. Spontaneous ignition, explosion, and fire with sevoflurane and barium hydroxide lime. *Anesthesiology.* 2004;101: 534–537.
155. Laster M, Roth P, Eger EI 2nd. Fires from the interaction of anesthetics with desiccated absorbent. *Anesth Analg.* 2004;99:769–774.

156. Abbott A. Dear healthcare provider (letter). November 17, 2003. [http://www.fda.gov/downloads/Safety/MedWatch/SafetyInformation/SafetyAlertsforHumanMedicalProducts/UCM169499.pdf].
157. Murray JM, Renfrew CW, Bedi A, et al. Amsorb: a new carbon dioxide absorbent for use in anesthetic breathing systems. *Anesthesiology*. 1999;91:1342–1348.
158. Flowers J. Code red in the OR—implementing an OR fire drill. *AORN Journal*. 2004;79:797–805.
159. ECRI Institute. ECRI's latest audio conference targets surgical fires. Training and communication are key, say speakers. *Health Devices*. 2003;32:396–398.
160. ECRI Institute. A clinician's guide to surgical fires. How they occur, how to prevent them, how to put them out. *Health Devices*. 2003;32:5–24.
161. Guglielmi CL, Flowers J, Dagi TF, et al. Empowering providers to eliminate surgical fires. *AORN Journal*. 2014;100:412–428.
162. Feldman JM, Ehrenwerth J, Dutton RP. Thinking outside the triangle: a new approach to preventing surgical fires. *Anesth Analg*. 2014;118:704–705.
163. Culp WC Jr, Kimbrough BA, Luna S, et al. Operating room fire prevention: creating an electrosurgical unit fire safety device. *Annals of Surgery*. 2014;260:214–217.
164. Culp WC Jr, Kimbrough BA, Luna S, et al. Mitigating operating room fires: development of a carbon dioxide fire prevention device. *Anesth Analg*. 2014;118:772–775.

Section 2
BASIC SCIENCE AND FUNDAMENTALS

6 Genomic Basis of Perioperative Medicine

MIHAI V. PODGOREANU • JOSEPH P. MATHEW

Scientific Rationale for Perioperative Precision Medicine
   Human Genomic Variation
   Profiling the Regulatory Genome to Understand Perioperative Biology and Discover Biomarkers of Adverse Outcomes
   Epigenetics: The Link between Environment and Genes
   Overview of Genetic Epidemiology and Functional Genomic Methodology
Genomics and Perioperative Risk Profiling
   Predictive Biomarkers for Perioperative Adverse Cardiac Events
   Genetic Variants and Postoperative Event-free Survival
   Genetic Susceptibility to Adverse Perioperative Neurologic Outcomes
   Genetic Susceptibility to Adverse Perioperative Kidney Outcomes
   Genetic Variants and Risk for Postoperative Lung Injury
Pharmacogenomics and Anesthesia
   Genetic Variability in Response to Anesthetic Agents
   Genetic Variability in Pain Response
   Genetic Variability in Response to Other Drugs Used Perioperatively
Conclusions and Future Directions
Acknowledgments

KEY POINTS

1. Candidate gene studies and recent genome-wide association studies suggest that susceptibility to a range of common adverse perioperative events including cardiac (myocardial infarction, ventricular dysfunction, atrial fibrillation), neurologic, and renal, among others, is genetically and epigenetically determined. Ongoing emphasis is placed on prioritizing genetic variants that warrant clinical action.
2. Potential applications of biomarkers in perioperative medicine include prognosis, diagnosis and monitoring of adverse events, as well as informing therapeutic decisions. Very few have been rigorously evaluated to demonstrate incremental discriminatory accuracy when added to existing risk stratification models (clinical validity), or change therapy (clinical utility). Among the most promising are natriuretic peptides and C-reactive protein (CRP) for cardiovascular risk prediction, postoperative troponin surveillance to diagnose myocardial injury, and procalcitonin to assess infection in the critically ill.
3. Interindividual variability in response to anesthetic agents is as high as 24%, and has underlying genetic mechanisms.
4. Individual variability in analgesic responsiveness is attributed to genetic control of peripheral nociceptive pathways and descending central pain modulatory pathways.
5. Pharmacogenomic variation in genes modulating drug actions explains part of the variability in drug response, and has shown promising clinical utility for several classes of drugs used perioperatively.
6. To facilitate translation to medical practice, systematic evaluation of existing genomic evidence for clinical decisions in the perioperative continuum, updating the practice guidelines, as well as identifying the revenue sources to reimburse the generation and use of genomic information are still required.

Scientific Rationale for Perioperative Precision Medicine

Intrinsic variability exists across the human population in morphology, behavior, physiology, development, and disease susceptibility. Of particular relevance to our specialty, responses to stressful stimuli and drug therapy are also variable. As we appreciate in our daily practices in the operating rooms and intensive care units, one hallmark of perioperative physiology is the wide range of patient responses to the acute and sometimes repeated exposures to a collection of robust perturbations to homeostasis induced by surgical injury, hemodynamic challenges, vascular cannulations, mechanical circulatory support, intra-aortic balloon counterpulsation, mechanical ventilation, partial/total organ resection, transient limb/organ ischemia-reperfusion, transfusions, anesthetic agents, and the pharmacopoeia used in the perioperative period (the *perioperative exposome*). This translates into substantial interindividual variability in immediate adverse perioperative events (mortality or incidence/severity of organ dysfunction), as well as long-term outcomes (i.e., phenotypes; Table 6-1). For decades we have attributed this variability only

Table 6-1 Categories of Perioperative Phenotypes

Immediate perioperative outcomes	• Inhospital mortality • Perioperative myocardial infarction • Perioperative low cardiac output syndrome/acute decompensated heart failure/ventricular dysfunction • Perioperative vasoplegic syndrome • Perioperative arrhythmias (atrial fibrillation, QTc prolongation) • Postoperative bleeding • Perioperative venous thrombosis • Acute postoperative stroke • Postoperative delirium • Perioperative acute kidney injury • Acute perioperative lung injury/prolonged postoperative mechanical ventilation • Acute allograft dysfunction/rejection • Postoperative sepsis • Multiple organ dysfunction syndrome • Postoperative nausea and vomiting • Acute postoperative pain • Variability in response to anesthetics, analgesics and other perioperative drugs • Intermediate phenotypes (plasma biomarker levels)
Long-term postoperative outcomes	• Event-free survival/major adverse cardiac events • Progression of vein graft disease • Chronic allograft dysfunction/rejection • Postoperative cognitive dysfunction • Postoperative depression • Transition from acute to chronic pain • Cancer progression • Quality of life

to factors that increase an individual's biologic susceptibility or reduce resilience to surgical trauma (such as age, gender, frailty, cardiopulmonary fitness, nutritional state, comorbidities)—what we colloquially call "protoplasm"—or to heterogeneity in the intensity of exposure to perioperative stressors. Now we are beginning to appreciate that genomic and epigenomic variation is also partially responsible for this observed variability in patient vulnerability and outcomes. An individual's susceptibility to adverse perioperative events stems not only from genomic contributions to the development of co-morbid risk factors (such as coronary artery disease or reduced preoperative cardiopulmonary reserve) during his or her lifetime, but also from genomic variability in specific biologic pathways participating in the host response to surgical injury (Fig. 6-1). With increasing evidence suggesting that genomic and epigenomic regulation can significantly modulate risk of adverse perioperative events,[1–7] the emerging field of *perioperative genomics* aims to apply functional genomic approaches to uncover biologic mechanisms that explain why similar patients have such dramatically different outcomes after surgery, and is justified by a unique combination of exposures to environmental insults and postoperative phenotypes that characterize surgical and critically ill patient populations.

Traditional epidemiologic approaches have been limiting our ability to examine factors contributing to such differential individual susceptibility to adverse perioperative events, often having to generalize from otherwise limited homogenous cohorts to the effects on the overall population. However, it has become apparent that heterogeneity in response at the individual level tends to "stretch out" the population-level response distribution curve (Fig. 6-1).[9] *Precision medicine* is an emerging approach for disease prevention and treatment that takes into account individual variability in genes, environment, and lifestyle for each patient. Although not new, this concept has been recently brought within our reach by three converging opportunities: a rapid and significant expansion of large-scale biologic databases (such as the reference human genome, catalogs of human genetic variation, RNA and protein databases, and curated biologic pathway databases); powerful methods to characterize and monitor patients (including the ability to conduct molecular profiles at the genome, proteome, metabolome and microbiome levels, cellular assays, multiparameter data streaming, mobile health technologies, patient-activated social networks); and refinement of computational tools for managing and analyzing large datasets ("Big Data" analytics).[10] The presidential Precision Medicine Initiative, launched in 2015, seeks to extend precision medicine to all diseases by building a national research cohort of more than 1 million participants reflecting the diversity of the US population, with commitment to protecting participant privacy, regulatory modernization, and public–private partnerships.

Several unique characteristics of the perioperative continuum suggest it may represent an ideal acute care paradigm to implement precision medicine strategies. First, as a planned event (for the most part), surgery allows for preemptive molecular or genetic profiling that can inform preoperative optimization strategies. Second, the perioperative environment involves intense perturbations and stressors that can unmask underlying genetic susceptibilities. A third unique feature of the perioperative setting is the dynamic decision-making process, which involves multiple decision points over a relatively short period of time, several medications amenable to pharmacogenomics-driven decision support in order to improve their efficacy and safety, and a clinical need for such guidance regarding patient-specific drug choices and dosing (Fig. 6-2). Fourth, the acuity of the initial surgical episode is similarly followed by a rapid convalescence period or a short time to developing adverse events, thus allowing for rapid assessment of clinical outcomes and interventions.[1] Perioperative physicians are generally familiar with risk prediction tools, their implementation in clinical practice including incorporating interindividual variability into risk decisions, communicating risks, and the intricacies of managing longitudinal care transitions throughout the perioperative continuum. Finally, perioperative health-care delivery systems have been early adopters of electronic medical records (EMRs), with several large multi-institutional data integration efforts like the Multicenter Perioperative Group (www.mpogresearch.org) and the Anesthesiology Performance Improvement and Reporting Exchange (www.aspirecqi.org) well underway to enable perioperative medicine research, improve adherence to evidence-based standards of care, and reduce variability in both clinical practice and in common adverse postoperative outcomes, hospital length of stay, and cost.

Perioperative precision medicine aims to classify individuals into subpopulations that differ in their susceptibility to develop certain adverse perioperative events, in the biology or prognosis of these adverse outcomes, or in their responses to specific treatments and interventions throughout the perioperative period. Decisions regarding preventive or therapeutic interventions, informed by precision medicine molecular and analytical approaches, would then be concentrated on patients likely to benefit, sparing expense

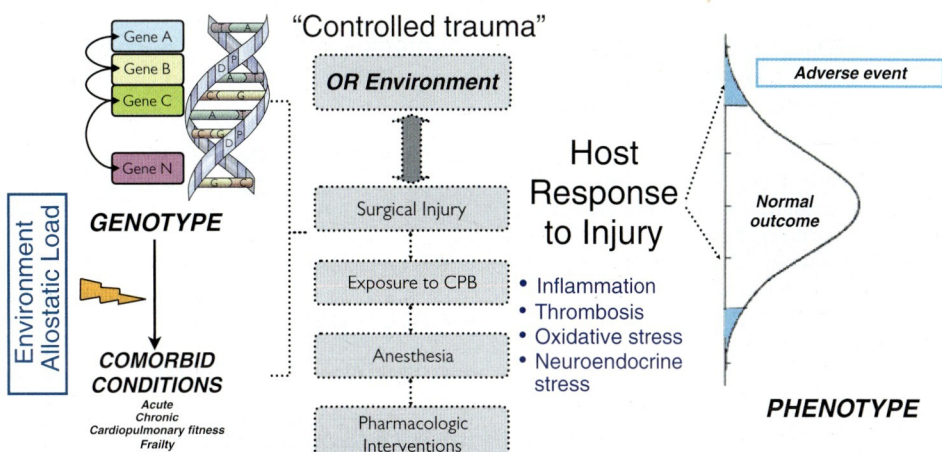

Figure 6-1 The perioperative period represents a unique and extreme example of gene–environment interactions. Perioperative adverse events are complex traits, characteristically involving an interaction between acute exposures to robust operative environmental perturbations (surgical trauma, hemodynamic challenges, exposure to extracorporeal circulation, drug administration—the *perioperative exposome*) occurring on a landscape of susceptibility determined by an individual's clinical and genetic characteristics (constitutive factors). The observed variability in perioperative outcomes can be in part attributed to genetic and epigenetic variability modulating the host response to surgical injury. Adverse outcomes will develop only in patients whose combined burden of genetic and environmental risk factors exceeds a certain threshold, which may vary with age. In fact, physiologic stress associated with life-threatening injury exposes genetic anomalies that might otherwise go unnoticed. Identification of such genetic contributions not only to disease causation and susceptibility but also to the individual patient's *responses* to disease and drug therapy, and incorporation of genetic risk information in clinical decision-making, may lead to improved health outcomes and reduced costs. However, some individuals are more sensitive than others to any given exposure to perioperative stressors, making them more susceptible to develop adverse events. Heterogeneity in response at the individual level tends to "stretch out" the population-level dose–response curve for any perioperative stress exposure.[8] The occurrence of perioperative adverse events is further determined by the effectiveness of adaptive (hormetic) responses to perioperative stressors, which can mitigate injurious systemic host responses. OR, operating room; CPB, cardiopulmonary bypass.

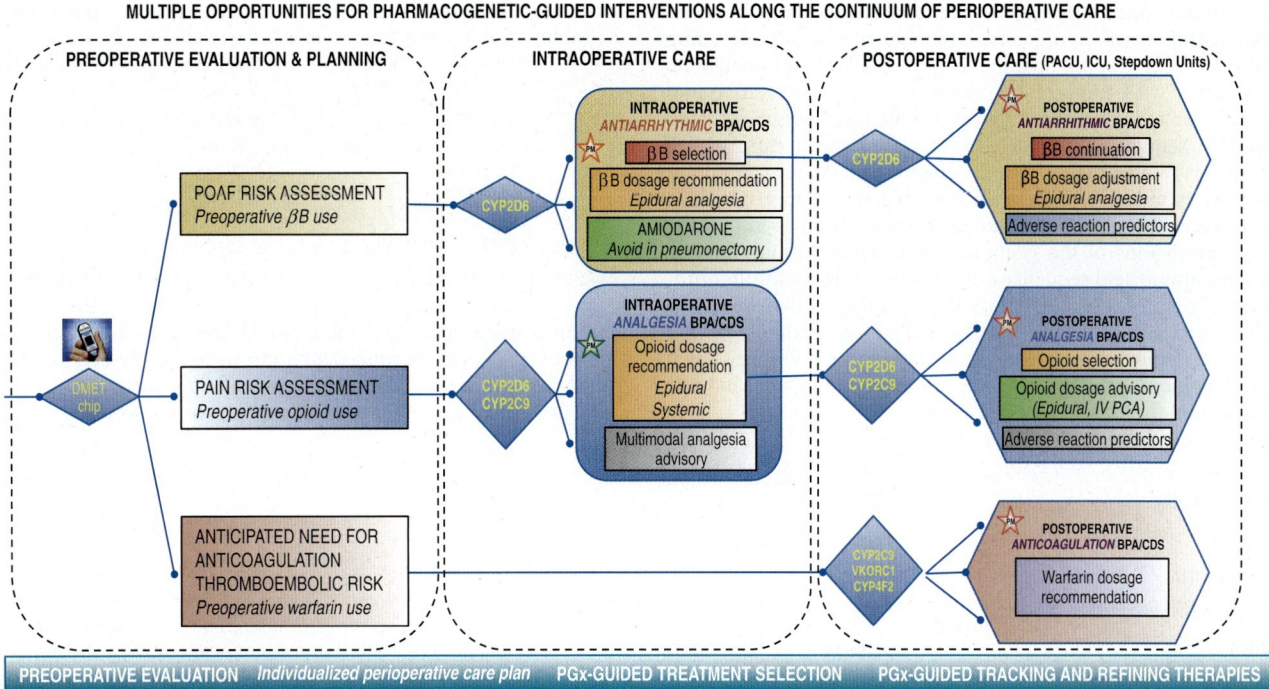

Figure 6-2 Multiple opportunities exist for implementation of a set of actionable, accessible, and sustainable clinical decision support tools to provide pharmacogenomics (PGx)-guided drug prescription along the continuum of perioperative care, under a new clinical paradigm to reduce hospital length of stay and cost. POAF, postoperative atrial fibrillation; βB, beta blocker; PACU, postanesthesia care unit; ICU, intensive care unit; PCA, patient-controlled analgesia.

and side effects for those who will not. Adoption of this new generation of molecular tests into clinical practice is predicated, however, on perioperative physicians becoming increasingly familiar with several key concepts, including patterns of human genome variation, gene regulation, basic population genetic methodology, gene and protein expression analysis, and most importantly the general principles for evaluating biomarker performance. This chapter serves as a primer in genomic and precision medicine by highlighting the evolving applications of genomic technologies to refine perioperative risk stratification, outcome prediction, understanding the complex biologic mechanisms underlying surgical stress responses, as well as identification and validation of novel targets for perioperative organ protection.

Human Genomic Variation

In elucidating the genetic basis of disease, much of what has been investigated in the pre-Human Genome Project era focused on identifying rare genetic variants (*mutations*) responsible for more than 1,500 monogenic disorders such as hypertrophic cardiomyopathy, long-QT syndrome, sickle cell anemia, cystic fibrosis, or familial hypercholesterolemia. However, most of the genetic diversity in the population is attributable to more widespread DNA sequence variations (*polymorphisms*), typically single nucleotide base substitutions (*single nucleotide polymorphisms*, SNPs), or to a broader category of *structural genetic variants* which include short sequence repeats (*microsatellites*), insertion/deletion (I/D) of one or more nucleotides (*indels*), inversions, and copy number variants (*CNVs*, large segments of DNA that vary in number of copies),[11] all of which may or may not be associated with a specific phenotype (Fig. 6-3). In addition to the nuclear genome, the mitochondrial genome encodes for 37 genes essential to mitochondrial function. Variability in the mitochondrial DNA is implicated in a growing number of diseases including neurodegenerative, myopathic, cardiovascular, and metabolic conditions, with important implications for perioperative and critical care management.[12] To be classified as a polymorphism, the DNA sequence alternatives (i.e., *alleles*) must exist with a frequency greater than 1% in the population. About 15 million SNPs are estimated to exist in the human genome, approximately once every 300 base pairs, located in genes as well as in the surrounding regions of the genome. Polymorphisms may directly alter the amino acid sequence and therefore potentially alter protein function, or alter regulatory DNA sequences that modulate protein expression. Sets of nearby SNPs on a chromosome are inherited in blocks, referred to as *haplotypes*. As it will be shown later, haplotype analysis is a useful way of applying genotype information in disease gene discovery.

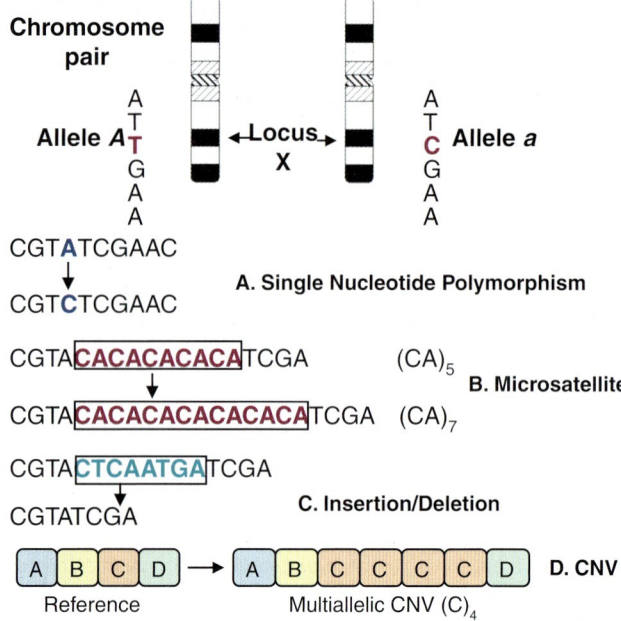

Figure 6-3 Categories of common human genetic variation. **A:** *Single nucleotide polymorphisms* (SNP) can be silent or have functional consequences: changes in amino acid sequence or premature termination of protein synthesis (if they occur in the coding regions of the gene) or alterations in the expression of the gene, resulting in more or less protein (if they occur in regulatory regions of the gene such as the promoter region or the intron/exon boundaries). Structural genetic variants include: **B:** *Microsatellites* with varying number of dinucleotide $(CA)_n$ repeats; **C:** *Insertions–deletions;* **D:** *Copy number variation* (CNV), A-D are long DNA segments, segment D shows variation in copy number. Glossary: *locus*, the location of a gene/genetic marker in the genome; *alleles*, alternative forms of a gene/genetic marker; *genotype*, the observed alleles for an individual at a genetic locus; *heterozygous*, two different alleles are present at a locus; *homozygous*, two identical alleles are present at a locus. An SNP at position 1691 of a gene, with alleles G and A would be written as 1691G>A.

Profiling the Regulatory Genome to Understand Perioperative Biology and Discover Biomarkers of Adverse Outcomes

Genomic approaches are anchored in the "central dogma" of molecular biology, the concept of transcription of messenger RNA (mRNA) from a DNA template, followed by translation of RNA into protein (Fig. 6-4). Since transcription is a key regulatory

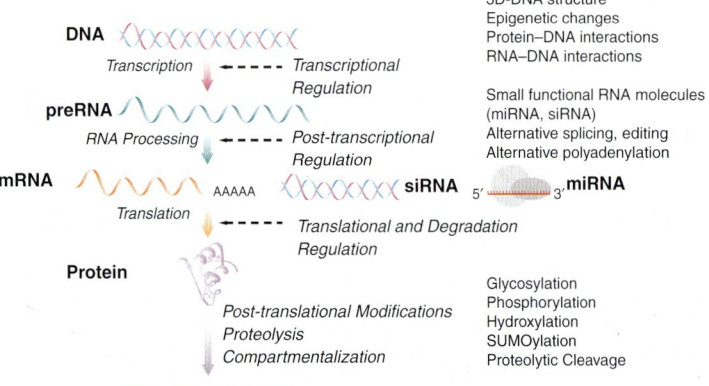

Figure 6-4 Increasing complexity of the central dogma of molecular biology. Protein expression involves two main processes: RNA synthesis (*transcription*) and protein synthesis (*translation*), with many intermediate regulatory steps. A single gene can give rise to multiple protein products (isoforms) via processing of preRNA molecules yielding multiple RNA products, including microRNA (miRNA) and small interfering RNA (siRNA) molecules, as well as alternative splicing and RNA editing. Thus functional variability at the protein level, ultimately responsible for biologic effects, is the cumulative result of genetic variability as well as extensive transcriptional, posttranscriptional, translational, and posttranslational modifications.

step that may eventually signal many other cascades of events, the study of RNA abundance in a cell or organ (i.e., quantifying gene expression) can improve the understanding of a wide variety of biologic systems. Furthermore, although the human genome contains only about 26,000 genes, functional variability at the protein level is far more diverse, resulting from extensive posttranscriptional and posttranslational modifications. It is believed that there are approximately 200,000 distinct proteins in humans, further subjected to a wide array of dynamic posttranslational modifications (such as phosphorylation, glycosylation, acetylation, S-nitrosylation, carbonylation, SUMOylation, and disulfide structures, among others), which are implicated in protein stability, coordinate protein–protein interactions, and serve key regulatory functions. Increasing evidence suggests that variability in gene expression levels underlies complex disease and is determined by regulatory DNA polymorphisms affecting transcription, splicing, and translation efficiency in a tissue- and stimulus-specific manner.[13] Thus, in addition to the assessment of genetic variability at the DNA sequence level (*static genomics*), analysis of large-scale variability in the pattern of RNA and protein expression both at baseline and in response to exposure to the multidimensional perioperative stimuli (*dynamic genomics*) using microarray, next-generation sequencing, and proteomic approaches provides a much needed understanding of the overall regulatory networks involved in the pathophysiology of adverse postoperative outcomes (Table 6-2). Such dynamic genomic markers can be incorporated in genomic classifiers and used clinically to improve perioperative risk stratification or monitor

Table 6-2 Summary of Gene Expression Studies with Implications for Perioperative Cardiovascular Outcomes

Tissue (Species)	Stimulus/Method	Genomic Signature: Number/Types of Genes	Reference
Myocardium (rat)	Ischemia/μA	14 (wound-healing, Ca-handling)	17
Myocardium (human)	CPB/circulatory arrest/μA	58 (inflammation, transcription activators, apoptosis, stress response)-adults 50 (cardioprotective, antiproliferative, antihypertrophic)-neonates	18 19
Myocardium (human)	CPB/cold cardioplegia-induced ischemia/RNA-seq	Downregulation of 3,724 transcripts (90%), including humoral immune response and complement pathway genes; upregulation of 374 transcripts (9.1%), including hemoglobin genes	20
Myocardium (rat)	IPC vs. APC/μA	566 differentially regulated/56 jointly regulated (cell defense)	21
Myocardium (rat)	APC vs. ApostC/μA	Opposing genomic profiles, 8 gene clusters, <2% jointly regulated genes	22
Myocardium (human)	APC, OPCAB, postoperative LV function/μA	319 upregulated and 281 downregulated gene sets in response to OPCAB; deregulation of fatty acid oxidation, DNA-damage signaling and G-CSF survival (perioperative) and PGC-1α (constitutive) pathways predict improved LV function in sevoflurane treated patients	23
PBMC (human)	APC, sevoflurane/μA	Deregulation of late preconditioning, PGC-1α, fatty acid oxidation, and L-selectin pathways	24
Atrial myocardium (pig)	Pacing-induced AF/μA+P	81 (MCL-2 ventricular/atrial isoform shift)	25
Atrial myocardium (human)	AF/μA	1,434 (ventricular-like genomic signature)	26
PBMC (human)	Cardiac surgery, PoAF/μA	1,302 genes uniquely deregulated in PoAF/401 upregulated (oxidative stress), 902 downregulated	27
PBMC (human)	Cardiac surgery, POCD/μA	1,201 genes uniquely deregulated in POCD/531 upregulated, 670 downregulated (inflammation, antigen presentation, cell adhesion, and apoptosis)	28
PBMC (human)	Heart transplant/μA	30 (profile correlated with biopsy-proven rejection; persistent immune activation in response to treatment)	29
PBMC (human)	Heart transplant/RT-PCR	11 (AlloMap, AlloMap score)	30
Myocardium (human)	Heart transplant/P	2 (increased αB-crystallin and tropomyosin serum levels)	31
PBMC, plasma (human)	TAAA/μA+P	138 genes and 7 plasma proteins predicted MODS	16
PBMC (human)	Obstructive CAD in non-diabetic patients/RT-PCR	23-gene expression signature	32
Ventricular myocardium (human)	End-stage cardiomyopathy on LVAD/μA	Combined signature of 28 microRNAs and 29 mRNAs had superior performance to classify status and predict recovery	33

AF, atrial fibrillation; APC, anesthetic preconditioning, APostC, anesthetic postconditioning; CPB, cardiopulmonary bypass; CAD, coronary artery disease; G-CSF, granulocyte colony stimulating factor; IPC, ischemic preconditioning; LV, left ventricle; μA, microarray; MCL-2, myosin light chain 2; MODS, multiple organ dysfunction syndrome; OPCAB, off-pump coronary artery bypass; P, proteomics; PBMC, peripheral blood mononuclear cells; PGC-1α, peroxisome proliferators-activated receptor γ cofactor-1α; PoAF, postoperative atrial fibrillation; POCD, postoperative cognitive decline; RT-PCR, real time polymerase chain reaction; TAAA, thoracoabdominal aortic aneurysm repair; LVAD, left ventricular assist device.

postoperative recovery.[14] An example of using the interplay between static genomic and dynamic genomic information for perioperative risk prediction in the case of thoracic aortic disease follows. Although surgical repair of thoracic aortic aneurysms is typically recommended when the aortic diameter reaches 5.0 to 5.5 cm, studies indicate that 60% of aortic dissections occur at aortic diameters smaller than 5.5 cm. However, DNA variants in specific genes (static genomics) can not only distinguish patients at risk for thoracic aortic disease but also predict the risk of early dissection at diameters smaller than 5.0 cm, thus potentially personalizing the timing of aortic surgery.[15] Moreover, combined genomic and proteomic analysis (dynamic genomics) using expression patterns of 138 genes from peripheral blood leukocytes and levels of seven circulating plasma proteins accurately discriminated patients who developed multiple organ dysfunction syndrome (MODS) after thoracoabdominal aortic aneurysm repair from those who did not. Importantly, these genome-wide gene expression and plasma protein concentration patterns were observed *before* surgical trauma and visceral ischemia-reperfusion injury, suggesting that patients who developed MODS differed preoperatively in either their genetic predisposition or pre-existing inflammatory state.[16]

In addition to their applications for risk prediction, dynamic genomic markers can improve mechanistic understanding of perioperative stress, by evaluating and cataloguing organ-specific responses to surgical injury and severe systemic stimuli such as cardiopulmonary bypass (CPB), ischemia-reperfusion, and endotoxemia, which can be subsequently used to identify and validate novel targets for organ protective strategies. We illustrate such applications with several examples from the perioperative period. Using an integrated approach of transcriptomic and proteomic analyses of peripheral blood, the molecular response signatures to cardiac surgery with and without CPB have been characterized,[34] offering novel insights into the concepts of contact activation and compartmentalization of inflammatory responses to major surgery. Although CPB has been traditionally thought to be a robust trigger of systemic inflammation, similar systemic levels of key inflammatory mediators were in fact seen following off-pump cardiac surgery, but with a delayed onset. Rather than being the primary source of serum cytokines as previously believed, peripheral blood leukocytes only assume a primed phenotype upon contact with the extracorporeal circuit which facilitate their trapping and subsequent tissue-associated inflammatory response. Similar whole blood transcriptomic analyses in cardiac surgical patients have identified convergent regulatory mechanisms triggered by ischemia-reperfusion (e.g., HIF-1α), priming of leukocytes by exposure to CPB (e.g., TLR4, TLR6), and downstream signaling of pro- and anti-inflammatory genes (pentraxin 3, resistin), which were previously thought to be distinct.[35] Yet other studies have identified genomic differences in circulating blood leukocytes between patients developing postoperative neurocognitive decline[28] or new-onset postoperative atrial fibrillation (AF).[27] Using circulating blood cells as a sentinel or reporter tissue is complemented by a large number of reports describing gene expression changes directly in myocardial tissue in response to acute ischemia, such as alterations in immediate-early genes (c-*fos*, *jun*B), genes coding for calcium-handling proteins (calsequestrin, phospholamban), extracellular matrix, and cytoskeletal proteins in ischemic myocardium,[17] as well as upregulation of transcripts involved in cytoprotection (heat shock proteins), resistance to apoptosis, and cell growth in areas of stunned myocardium.[36] Moreover, cardiac gene expression profiling after CPB and cardioplegic arrest has identified age-related upregulation of inflammatory and transcription activators, apoptosis, and stress genes.[18,19]

Conversely, next-generation RNA sequencing of human ventricular myocardium during cold cardioplegia-induced ischemia identified significant downregulation of immune inflammatory and complement genes, and interesting targets in transcription factors regulating reactive oxygen species production, apoptosis, and inflammatory response.[20] Whole-genome expression analysis has also been utilized to study molecular changes associated with myocardial preconditioning. The main functional categories of genes identified as potentially involved in cardioprotective pathways include a host of transcription factors, heat shock proteins, antioxidant genes (heme-oxygenase, glutathione peroxidase), and growth factors, but different gene programs were found to be activated in ischemic versus anesthetic preconditioning, resulting in two distinct molecular cardioprotective phenotypes.[21] More recently, a transcriptional response pattern consistent with late preconditioning has been reported in peripheral blood leukocytes following sevoflurane administration in healthy volunteers, characterized by reduced expression of L-selectin as well as downregulation of genes involved in fatty acid oxidation and the PCG1α (peroxisome activated receptor gamma coactivator 1α) pathway,[24] which mirrors changes observed in the myocardium from patients undergoing off-pump coronary artery bypass grafting (CABG) (Table 6-2).[23] Deregulation of these conserved survival pathways thus appears to generalize across tissues, making them important targets for cardioprotection, but further studies are needed to correlate perioperative gene expression response patterns in end organs such as the myocardium to those in readily available surrogate tissues such as peripheral blood leukocytes.

A limitation of gene expression studies evaluating RNA abundance like those described earlier is that changes in the *transcriptome* (the complete collection of transcribed elements of the genome) is not fully representative of the *proteome* (the complement of proteins encoded by the genome), since many transcripts are not targeted for translation, as evidenced by the concept of gene silencing by RNA interference. Alternative splicing, a wide variety of posttranslational modifications, and protein–protein interactions responsible for biologic function, would therefore remain undetected by gene expression profiling (Fig. 6-4). This has led to the emergence of *proteomics,* a field seeking to study the sequence, abundance, modification, localization, and function of proteins in a biologic system at a given time and in response to a disease state, trauma, stress, or therapeutic intervention.[37] Thus, proteomics offers a more global and integrated view of biology, complementing other functional genomic approaches. Several preclinical proteomic studies relevant to perioperative medicine have characterized the temporal changes in brain protein expression in response to various inhaled anesthetics,[38,39] or following cardiac surgery with hypothermic circulatory arrest.[40] This may focus further studies aimed to identify new anesthetic binding sites, and the development of neuroprotective strategies. The natural cardioprotective adaptations invoked by mammalian hibernators to cope with ischemia-reperfusion injury have been recently characterized using comparative proteomic approaches, and involve extensive metabolic remodeling with increased expression of fatty acid metabolic proteins and reduced levels of toxic lipid metabolites, offering insights into novel strategies for metabolic optimization as a transformative approach for perioperative organ protection.[41] Furthermore, detailed knowledge of the plasma proteome has profound implications in perioperative transfusion medicine,[42] in particular, related to peptide and protein changes that occur during storage of blood products.

Innate and adaptive immune host responses to surgery play key roles in the pathogenesis of perioperative organ injury and dysfunction, prompting the use of comprehensive immune monitoring via *flow cytometry* (exact quantification of surface marker expression on blood immune cells) and cytokine determination for outcome prediction. Monocytic HLA-DR surface expression and plasma IL-10 were the best predictors of infection risk after cardiac surgery,[43] whereas surface expression of CD99 and CD47 (markers of neutrophil migratory responses) predict acute kidney injury and, when combined with the EuroSCORE, improve prediction of postoperative intensive care unit (ICU) length of stay after cardiac surgery.[44]

Emerging *metabolomic* tools have created the opportunity to establish metabolic signatures of tissue injury. In a population of patients undergoing alcohol septal ablation for hypertrophic obstructive cardiomyopathy, a human model of planned myocardial infarction, targeted mass spectrometry-based metabolite profiling identified changes in circulating levels of metabolites participating in pyrimidine metabolism, the TCA cycle, and the pentose phosphate pathway as early as 10 minutes after myocardial infarction (MI) in an initial derivation group and were validated in a second, independent group. Coronary sinus sampling distinguished cardiac-derived from peripheral metabolic changes. To assess generalizability, the planned MI-derived metabolic signature (consisting of aconitic acid, hypoxanthine, trimethylamine N-oxide, and threonine) differentiated with high accuracy patients with spontaneous MI.[45] We applied a similar approach to cardiac surgical patients undergoing planned global myocardial ischemia/reperfusion, and identified clear differences in metabolic fuel uptake based on the pre-existing ventricular state (left ventricular dysfunction, coronary artery disease, or neither) as well as altered metabolic signatures predictive of postoperative hemodynamic course and perioperative myocardial infarction.[46] Although simultaneous assessment of coronary sinus effluent in addition to the peripheral blood improves cardiac specificity of the observed signatures, direct measurements of metabolites in myocardial tissue allows marked enrichment and easier detection of potential biomarkers compared to plasma, as well as an assessment of how metabolic substrates are utilized in the tissue of interest. Such studies are possible in cardiac surgical patients where atrial tissues are routinely removed; for example, one study using high-resolution ¹H-NMR spectroscopy identified alterations in myocardial ketone metabolism associated with persistent atrial fibrillation (AF), and the ratio of glycolytic to lipid metabolism end-products correlated positively with time of onset of postoperative AF.[47]

Epigenetics: The Link between Environment and Genes

In response to outside stimuli, the genome can undergo potentially heritable alterations that can substantially affect gene expression and regulation without altering the DNA sequence—hence termed epigenetic. Whereas DNA is the blueprint, epigenetic information provides the instruction for using that blueprint. The epigenetic code—consisting of DNA-based modifications (e.g., DNA methylation), posttranslational modifications of histone proteins (e.g., acetylation), and a growing array of noncoding RNAs (e.g., micro RNA)—is responsive to the environment, differs between cell types, and is susceptible to change, thus representing an excellent target to impact health outcomes. Evidence from animal and human studies suggests that epigenetic mechanisms can explain susceptibility to acute and chronic pain, making them potential therapeutic targets. Specific epigenetic mechanisms relevant to perioperative analgesia involve the developmental expression of opioid receptors and opioid-induced hyperalgesia. In general, opiates tend to increase global DNA methylation levels, whereas local anesthetics conversely have a demethylating effect. This local anesthetic effect may have potential in the development of chronic pain and perioperative cancer medicine.[7] Furthermore, important pathophysiologic processes relevant to the perioperative period like stress-induced proinflammatory responses are regulated by epigenetic factors such as histone acetylation. Again, lidocaine has been shown to both demethylate DNA and have strong anti-inflammatory properties, but a direct epigenetic link has not yet been investigated. Finally, the ability of noncoding RNAs to mediate important organ protective phenomena like anesthetic preconditioning, have recently been reported.[6,48]

Next we review the common genomic strategies used to study disease and drug responses.

Overview of Genetic Epidemiology and Functional Genomic Methodology

Most ongoing research on complex disorders focuses on identifying genetic variants that modify susceptibility to given conditions or drug responses. Often the design of such studies is complicated by the presence of multiple risk factors, gene–environment interactions and a lack of even rough estimates of the number of genes underlying such complex traits. Genetic association studies examine the frequency of specific genetic or epigenetic variants in a population-based sample of unrelated diseased individuals and appropriately matched unaffected controls. The nature of most complex diseases in general, and perioperative adverse outcomes in particular (surgical patients are typically elderly), makes the study of extended multigenerational family pedigrees impractical (with few exceptions, e.g., malignant hyperthermia), due to the lack of availability of pedigree information and/or DNA samples. Even a detailed family history, the first tool in the genomic toolbox, is seldom available for most categories of adverse perioperative events. Feasibility without requiring family-based sample collections, and the increased statistical power to uncover small clinical effects of multiple genes constitute the main advantages of the genetic association approach over traditional linkage analysis methodology.

Two broad strategies have been employed to identify complex trait loci through association analysis. The *candidate gene* approach is motivated by what is known about the trait biologically, with genes selected because of *a priori* hypotheses about their potential etiologic role in disease based on current understanding of the disease pathophysiology,[49] and can be characterized as a hypothesis-testing approach, but is intrinsically biased. Until recently however, most significant results were gathered from candidate gene association studies. As it will be presented in more detail later, this includes most published reports on specific genotypes associated with a variety of organ-specific perioperative adverse outcomes, including myocardial infarction,[50,51] neurocognitive dysfunction,[52-54] renal compromise,[55-57] vein graft restenosis,[58,59] postoperative thrombosis,[60] vascular reactivity,[61] severe sepsis,[62,63] transplant rejection,[64] and death (for reviews, see references 1 and 4).

The second strategy is the *genome-wide scan*, in which thousands of markers uniformly distributed throughout the genome or epigenome are used to locate regions that may harbor genes or regulatory regions influencing phenotypic variability. Examples include genome-wide association studies (GWAS) or epigenome-wide association studies (EWAS), as well as next-generation sequencing (NGS) technologies involving whole-exome sequencing (all the protein-coding genes in a genome) or whole-genome sequencing. These are unbiased approaches, in the sense that no prior assumptions are being made about the biologic processes involved and no weight is given to known genes, thus allowing the detection of previously unknown trait loci. Within the past decade, an explosion of adequately powered and successfully replicated GWAS have identified very significant genetic contributors to risk for common polygenic diseases like CAD,[65-67] MI,[68] diabetes (type I and II),[69,70] AF,[71] obesity, blood pressure,[72] asthma, common cancers, rheumatoid arthritis, Crohn disease, and others. More recently, the GWAS methodology has also been extended to study key perioperative adverse outcomes like MI,[73] AF,[74] ventricular dysfunction,[75] and acute kidney injury.[76] Although the ability to predict disease remains limited, the newly discovered genetic associations have provided insight into unsuspected mechanisms for disease, many of them located in known drug targets.[77] These studies were facilitated by the completion of several key extensions of the Human Genome Project—the International HapMap Project (a high-resolution map of human genetic variation and haplotypes),[78] the 1,000 Genomes Project (an initial catalog of human genetic variation across ethnically diverse populations),[79] and the Encyclopedia of DNA Elements (ENCODE, a map of functional elements in the human genome, their tissue distribution, and their roles in affecting gene function and regulation),[80]—coupled with advances in high-throughput genotyping technologies. At the time of this publication, the NHGRI-EBI GWAS Catalog (www.ebi.ac.uk/gwas) included 2,193 publications and 16,976 associations, with the list growing every day.[81] Several important themes have emerged from GWAS. First, most SNPs associated with common diseases collectively explain only a small proportion of the observed contribution of heredity to the risk of disease (e.g., 6% for type-2 diabetes), or other complex traits (e.g., 2% for body mass index and 5% for height). This *"missing heritability"* problem is in part explained by the underlying rationale for GWAS—the "Common Disease-Common Variant" hypothesis—postulating that common diseases may arise secondary to cumulative effects of common variants. Most genes however lack a common functional coding variant with a detectable functional effect, yet they typically contain several rare variants. A counter-hypothesis has emerged stating that there are additional novel genes harboring such low frequency variants (possibly with larger effects) that may be the primary drivers of common disease. Currently these variants are poorly detected by genotyping microarrays, but with the advent of next-generation sequencing technologies the potential exists to revolutionize complex traits genetics by identifying and typing rare variants and thus rendering virtually every gene susceptible for genetic analysis. Nevertheless, GWAS results also underscored that small genetic effect sizes do not necessarily translate into limited therapeutic effectiveness of intervening in the respective biologic pathways. Case in point, although the risk variant in HMG CoA reductase was associated in GWAS with only 2.3 mg/dL variability in LDL cholesterol,[82] up to 60% reductions in LDL levels can be achieved by intervening in the LDL metabolic pathway. Secondly, more than two-thirds of the variants identified so far are located either in intergenic regions or in genes of unknown function. This, among other findings, has challenged the very concept of "gene" as the traditional unit of heredity. Discovery of the diverse and ubiquitous roles of new classes of RNA (including *microRNAs* and *short interfering RNAs*) led to an emerging picture of gene regulation as interdependent layers of control consisting of interactions of DNA with regulatory proteins and RNA (Fig. 6-4).[83] Furthermore, as discussed earlier, on top of the DNA sequence lays another (*epigenetic*) code, that influences when and what genes should be transcribed or silenced. The epigenome is laid down during prenatal and postnatal development, and is heritable through cell divisions.

One of the main weaknesses of the genetic association approach is that, unless the marker of interest "travels" (i.e., is in *linkage disequilibrium*) with a functional variant, or the marker allele *is* the actual functional (causal) variant, the power to detect and map complex trait loci will be reduced. Newer ("next-generation") approaches based on direct *whole-genome sequencing* depart from the concept of linkage by attempting to directly identify causal alleles.[84] One particular application of genome-scale sequencing is *whole-exome sequencing*. The *exome*, defined as the protein coding portion of the genome, is comprised in humans of approximately 30 megabases (1%) split amongst approximately 200,000 exons. Aside from the ability to identify rare variants and the obvious substantial cost reduction (~20-fold), this approach has the advantage of focusing on nonsynonymous variants in coding genes for which there are well-established methods of functional validation and interpretation of biologic effects, thus enabling their implication as causal variants. However, it completely misses noncoding and structural variation in the genome. Early results suggest that whole-exome sequencing is an effective approach to identify causal mutations for monogenic disorders but also to distinguish signal (causal rare variants) from noise (background rate of rare mutations) for complex traits. Successful studies so far (e.g., early-onset MI) sequenced individuals informed by the following key observations: the younger the age when developing MI, the greater the heritability; selecting extremes of the phenotype distribution (e.g., young with MI versus old without MI as a "hyper-normal" control group) is likely to improve power; and that genetic discovery may be enhanced by studying multiple ethnicities. These studies have demanded the development of novel statistical methods to associate rare variants with the phenotype. One such promising solution for overcoming the statistical challenges revolving around sequencing low frequency variants is to combine all nonsynonymous SNPs (by gene or biologic pathway) into a single statistical test. The first integrated analysis of a complete human genome in a clinical context, in a patient with a family history of vascular disease and early sudden death has been reported in the *Lancet* in 2010.[85] The analysis revealed increased genetic risk for CAD, MI, type 2 diabetes, and some cancers, as well as rare variants in three genes clinically associated with sudden cardiac death. Furthermore, the patient had variants associated with clopidogrel resistance, a positive response to lipid-lowering therapies, and a low initial dosing requirement for warfarin, suggesting that routine whole-genome sequencing can yield clinically relevant information for individual patients. Several additional advantages of next-generation technologies involve sequencing of multiple genomes per person, such as matched tumor and blood DNA samples from 20 common types of cancer in the Cancer Genome Atlas, which enable development of targeted therapeutics based on a detailed molecular understanding of pathogenesis. Equally important for medical progress is the sequencing of genomes of the billions of microorganisms that dwell within us as part of the Human Microbiome Project.

Other known limitations of genetic association studies include potential false positive findings resulting from population stratification (i.e., admixture of different ethnic or genetic backgrounds in the case and control groups), and multiple comparison issues when large numbers of genes or variants are being assessed.[86] Replication of findings across different populations or related phenotypes remains the most reliable method of validating a true relationship between genetic polymorphisms and disease, but poor reproducibility in subsequent studies has been one of the main criticisms of the candidate gene association approach.[87] Therefore, it is particularly important to follow initial association analysis results with functional analyses using in silico, in vitro, and in vivo experiments aimed at identifying the causal genetic variants, causal epigenetics, and affected biologic pathways.

Translation of genomic findings to the clinic ultimately revolves around either new disease mechanisms (better disease definition or disease stratification) or new therapeutic strategies (new targets, drug repurposing, or drug response stratification). A particular focus of recent efforts to translate genome sequence information into clinical-decision making revolves around the "actionability" of specific genetic variants, and the level of evidence required to establish whether a variant is actionable. In the context of incidental findings or in an asymptomatic individual, *clinical actionability* represents the degree to which an intervention exists that can mitigate harm before a clinical diagnosis is made. Related terms are *clinical validity*, the accuracy and reliability of a variant in identifying or predicting an event with biologic or medical significance in an asymptomatic individual, and *clinical utility*, the usefulness of information in clinical-decision making and improving health outcomes.[88] The National Institutes of Health has created the Clinical Genome Resource (ClinGen) to serve as an authoritative public portal defining the clinical relevance of genomic variants for use in precision medicine (www.clinicalgenome.org).[89] Several applications to perioperative medicine are presented in the following sections.

Genomics and Perioperative Risk Profiling

More than 40 million patients undergo surgery annually in the United States at a cost of $450 billion. Each year approximately 1 million patients sustain medical complications after surgery, resulting in costs of $25 billion annually. The proportion of the US population above 65 years of age is estimated to double in the next two decades, leading to a 25% increase in the number of surgeries, a 50% increase in surgery-related costs, and a 100% increase in complications from surgery. Although many preoperative predictors have been identified and are constantly being refined, risk stratification based on clinical, procedural, and biologic markers explains only a small part of the variability in the incidence of perioperative complications. As mentioned earlier, it is becoming increasingly recognized that perioperative morbidity arises as a direct result of the environmental stress of surgery occurring on a landscape of susceptibility that is determined by an individual's clinical and genetic characteristics, and may even occur in otherwise healthy individuals. Such adverse outcomes will develop only in patients whose combined burden of genetic and environmental risk factors exceeds a certain threshold, which may vary with age. Identification of such genetic contributions not only to disease causation and susceptibility but also to the *response* to disease and drug therapy, and incorporation of genetic risk information in clinical decision-making, may lead to improved health outcomes and reduced costs. For instance, understanding the role of genetic variation in proinflammatory and prothrombotic pathways, the main pathophysiologic mechanisms responsible for perioperative complications, may contribute to the development of target-specific therapies, thereby limiting the incidence of adverse events in high-risk patients. To increase clinical relevance for the practicing perioperative physician, we summarize next existing evidence by specific outcome while highlighting candidate genes in relevant mechanistic pathways (Tables 6-3 through 6-5).

Table 6-3 Representative Genetic Polymorphisms Associated with Altered Susceptibility to Adverse Perioperative Cardiovascular Events

Gene	Polymorphism	Type of Surgery	Effect Size	Reference
Perioperative Myocardial Infarction, Ventricular Dysfunction, Early Vein Graft Failure				
IL6	−572G>C	Cardiac/CPB	2.47	50
	−174G>C	Thoracic	1.8	90
ICAM-1	E469 L	Cardiac/CPB	1.88	50
SELE	98G>T		0.16	50
MBL2	LYQA secretor haplotype	CABG/CPB	3.97	51
ITGB3	L33P	CABG/CPB	2.5[a]	91
	(Pl^{A1}/Pl^{A2})	Major vascular	2.4	92
GP1 BA	T145M	Major vascular	3.4	92
TNFA	−308G>A	Thoracic	2.5	90
TNFB (LTA)	TNFB2	Cardiac/CPB	3.84	93
IL10	−1082G>A		n.r.	94
F5	R506Q(FVL)	CABG/CPB	3.29	95
CMA1	−1905 A>G		n.r.	58
ANRIL	rs10116277 G>T (9p21)		1.7	96
NPR3	rs700923 A>G		4.28	97
	rs16890196 A>G		4.09	
	rs765199 C>T		4.27	
	rs700926 A>C		3.89	
NPPA_NPPB	rs632793 T>C		0.52	97
	rs6668352 G>A		0.44	
	rs549596 T>C		0.48	
	rs198388 C>T		0.51	
	rs198389 A>G		0.54	

(continued)

Table 6-3 Representative Genetic Polymorphisms Associated with Altered Susceptibility to Adverse Perioperative Cardiovascular Events (CONTINUED)

Gene	Polymorphism	Type of Surgery	Effect Size	Reference
PAI-1	4G/5G		n.r.	98
PAR4	rs773857		2.4	99
PAPPA2[g]	rs10454444		0.46[b]	73
	rs10913237		0.46[b]	
HDAC4[g]	rs10200850		2.23[b]	
SEC24D[g]	rs4834703		1.98[b]	
	rs6822035		1.65[b]	
3p22.3[g]	rs17691914		2.01[b]	75
Perioperative Vasoplegia, Vascular Reactivity, Coronary Tone				
DDAH II	−449G>C	Cardiac/CPB	0.4	100
NOS3	E298D		n.r.	101,102
ACE	In/del		n.r.	61,103
AGTRAP	rs11121816	CABG/CPB, septic shock	1.42[d]	104
ADRB2	Q27E	Tracheal intubation	11.7[c]	105
GNB3	825 C>T	Response to α-AR agonists	n.r.	102
PON1	Q192R	Resting coronary tone	n.r.	102
TNFβ+250	−1082G>A	Hyperdynamic state		106
Postoperative Arrhythmias: Atrial Fibrillation, QTc Prolongation				
IL6	−174G>C	CABG/CPB	3.25	107,108
		β-blocker failure	n.r.	109
		Thoracic	1.8	90
RANTES	−403G>A	β-blocker failure	n.r.	109
TNFA	−308G>A	Thoracic	2.5	90
ATFB5 (4q25)	rs2200733 C>T	Cardiac/CPB	1.97[b]	110,111
	rs2220427 T>G		1.76[b]	
	rs10033464		1.28[d]	
IL1B	−511 T>C		1.44	
	5810G>A		0.66	112
ADRB1	rs1801253 (Arg389Gly)		2.63[b]	113
GRK5	rs3740563	CABG/CPB	2.6[b]	114
LY96[g]	rs10504554	CABG/CPB	0.48[b]	74
Postoperative MACE, Late Vein Graft Failure				
ADRB1	R389G	Noncardiac with spinal block	1.87[d]	115
ACE	In/del	CABG/CPB	3.1[e]	116
ITGB3	L33P		4.7	117
MTHFR	A222 V	PTCA and CABG/CBP	2.8	118
ADRB2	R16G	Cardiac surgery/CPB	1.96	119
	Q27E		2.82	
HP	Hp1/Hp2	CABG	n.r.	120
CR1,KDR		CABG/CPB	n.r.	59
MICA				
HLA-DPB1				
VTN				
LPL	HindIII		n.r.	121
THBD	A455 V		2.78	122
ATFB5 (4q25)	rs2200733		1.57[d]	111
IL6	−174G>C	Noncardiac vascular surgery	2.14	123
	nt565 G>A		1.84	123

Table 6-3 Representative Genetic Polymorphisms Associated with Altered Susceptibility to Adverse Perioperative Cardiovascular Events (CONTINUED)

Gene	Polymorphism	Type of Surgery	Effect Size	Reference
IL10	−1082 G>A			
	−819 C>T			
	−592 C>A			
	ATA haplotype		2.16	
Cardiac Allograft Rejection				
TNFA	−308G>A	Cardiac transplant	n.r.	124
IL10	−1082G>A		n.r.	124
ICAM1	K469E		n.r.	125
IL1RN	86-bp VNTR	Thoracic transplant	2.02	126
IL1B	3953 C>T		20.5[f]	126
TGF-β	915G>C	Cardiac transplant	n.r.	127

ACE, angiotensin converting enzyme; ADRB1, β₁ adrenergic receptor; ADRB2, β₂ adrenergic receptor; AGTRAP, angiotensin II type 1 receptor-associated protein; ANRIL, antisense noncoding RNA in the INK4 locus; ATFB5, Atrial fibrillation, familial 5; CABG, coronary artery bypass grafting; CMA1, heart chymase; CPB, cardiopulmonary bypass; CR1, complement component 3b/4b; DDAH II, dimethylarginine dimethylaminohydrolase II; F5, factor V; GNB3, G-protein β₃ subunit; GP1 BA, glycoprotein Ibα; HLA-DPB1, β chain of class II major histocompatibility complex; HP, haptoglobin; ICAM1, intercellular adhesion molecule 1; IL1B, interleukin 1β; IL1RN, interleukin 1 receptor antagonist; IL6, interleukin 6; IL10, interleukin 10; ITGB3, glycoprotein IIIa; KDR, kinase inert domain receptor; LPL, lipoprotein lipase; MACE, major adverse cardiac event; MBL2, mannose binding lectin 2; MICA, MHC I polypeptide; MTHFR, methylenetetrahydrofolate reductase; n.r., not reported; NOS3, endothelial nitric oxide synthase; NPPA/NPPB, natriuretic peptide precursor A/B; NPR3, natriuretic peptide receptor 3 precursor; OR, odds ratio; PAI-1, plasminogen activator inhibitor 1; PON1, paraoxonase 1; RANTES, regulated upon activation normally T-expressed and secreted; SELE, E-selectin; SELP, P-selectin; TGF-β, transforming growth factor-beta; TNFA, tumor necrosis factor α; VNTR, variable number tandem repeat; VTN, vitronectin.
[a]relative risk; [b]odds ratio; [c]F-value; [d]hazard ratio; [e]β-coefficient; [f]in haplotype with IL1RN VNTR; [g]locus identified in perioperative GWAS.

Predictive Biomarkers for Perioperative Adverse Cardiac Events

Perioperative Myocardial Infarction and Ventricular Dysfunction

Patients with underlying cardiovascular disease can be at increased risk for perioperative cardiac complications. Over the last few decades several multifactorial risk indices have been developed and validated for both noncardiac (e.g., Lee's Revised Cardiac Risk Index) and cardiac surgical patients (e.g., Hannan scores), with the specific aim of stratifying risk for perioperative adverse events. However, these multifactorial risk indices have only limited predictive value for identifying patients at the highest risk of postoperative MI (PMI).[143] In this context, it has been proposed that genomic approaches could aid in refining an individual's risk profile. The incidence of PMI following cardiovascular surgery remains between 7% and 19%,[144,145] despite advances in

Table 6-4 Representative Genetic Polymorphisms Associated with Altered Susceptibility to Adverse Perioperative Neurologic Events

Gene	Polymorphism	Type of Surgery	OR	Reference
Perioperative Stroke				
IL6	−174G>C	Cardiac/CPB	3.3	128
CRP	1846 C>T			
Perioperative Cognitive Dysfunction, Neurodevelopmental Dysfunction				
SELP	E298D	Cardiac/CPB	0.51	52
CRP	1059G>C	Cardiac/CPB	0.37	52
ITGB3	L33P (Pl[A1]/Pl[A2])	Cardiac/CPB	n.r.	53
APOE	ε4	CABG/CPB (adults)	n.r.	129
	ε2	Cardiac/CPB (children)	7; 11	130,131
APOE	ε4	CABG/CPB	1.26	132
Postoperative Delirium				
APOE	ε4	Major noncardiac	3.64	133
		Critically ill	7.32	134
SLC6A3	rs393795	Cardiac and noncardiac, elderly	0.4	135

IL6, interleukin 6; CPB, cardiopulmonary bypass; CRP, C-reactive protein; SELP, P-selectin; ITGB3, platelet glycoprotein IIIa; APOE, apolipoprotein E; SLC6A3, solute carrier family 6, member 3; OR, odds ratio; n.r., not reported.

Table 6-5 Representative Genetic Polymorphisms Associated with Other Adverse Perioperative Outcomes

Gene	Polymorphism	Type of Surgery	Effect Size	Reference
Perioperative Thrombotic Events				
F5	FVL	Noncardiac, Cardiac	n.r.	60
Perioperative Bleeding				
F5	R506Q(FVL)	Cardiac/CPB	−1.25[a]	136
PAI-1	4G/5G		10[b]	137
ITGA2	−52 C>T, 807 C>T		−0.15[a]	138,139
GP1 BA	T145M		−0.22[a]	138
TF	−603 A>G		−0.03[a]	138
TFPI	−399 C>T		−0.05[a]	138
F2	20210G>A		0.38[a]	138
ACE	In/del		0.15[a]	138
ITGB3	L33P (Pl^A1/Pl^A2)		n.r.	140
PAI-1	4G/5G		10[b]	137
ELAM-1	98 G>T, 561 A>C	CABG/CPB	n.r.	141
PROC	rs1799809	Cardiac/CPB	1.97[b]	139
ABO	rs630014		1.83[b]	139
F9	rs6048		1.72[b]	139
TNFA	−238G>A	Brain AVM treatment	3.5[c]	142
APOE	ε2		10.9[c]	142
Perioperative Acute Kidney Injury				
IL6	−572G>C	CABG/CPB	20.04[d]	55
AGT	M235 T		32.19[d]	55
NOS3	E298D		4.29[d]	55
APOE	ε4		−0.13[a]	55,57
3p21.6[f]	rs13317787	Cardiac/CPB	21.7[a]	76
BBS9[f]	rs10262995		12.8[a]	
Perioperative Severe Sepsis				
APOE	ε3		0.28[e]	63

ABO, ABO blood group; ACE, angiotensin converting enzyme; AGT, angiotensinogen; APOE, apolipoprotein E; AVM, arteriovenous malformation; BBS9, Bardet–Biedl Syndrome 9; CPB, cardiopulmonary bypass; CRP, C-reactive protein; ELAM-1, endothelial-leukocyte adhesion molecule-1; F2, prothrombin; F5, factor V; FVL, factor V Leiden; F9, factor IX; GP1 BA, glycoprotein Ibα; IL6, interleukin 6; ITGA2, glycoprotein Ialla; ITGB3, glycoprotein IIIa; NOS3, endothelial nitric oxide synthase; n.r., not reported; OR, odds ratio; PROC, protein C; TF, tissue factor; TFPI, tissue factor pathway inhibitor.
[a]β-coefficient; [b]odds ratio; [c]hazard ratio; [d]F-value; [e]relative risk; [f]locus identified in perioperative GWAS.

surgical, cardioprotective, and anesthetic techniques, and is consistently associated with reduced short- and long-term survival in these patients. The pathophysiology of PMI after cardiac surgery involves systemic and local inflammation, "vulnerable" blood, and neuroendocrine stress.[1] In noncardiac surgery, PMI occurs as a result of two distinct mechanisms: (1) coronary plaque rupture and subsequent thrombosis triggered by a number of perioperative stressors including catecholamine surges, proinflammatory, and prothrombotic states; and (2) myocardial oxygen supply–demand imbalance.[146] Interindividual genetic variability in these mechanistic pathways is extensive, which may combine in any given patient to modulate overall susceptibility to perioperative stress and ultimately the magnitude of myocardial injury. Nevertheless, until recently, only a few studies have explored the role of genetic factors in the development of PMI,[58,116,120] mainly conducted in patients undergoing CABG surgery (Table 6-3).

Inflammation biomarkers and perioperative adverse cardiac events. Although the role of inflammation in cardiovascular disease biology has long been established, we are just beginning to understand the relationship between genetically controlled variability in inflammatory responses to surgery and PMI pathogenesis. Several studies reported independent predictive value for incident PMI after cardiac surgery with CPB of polymorphisms in proinflammatory genes interleukin-6 (*IL6*), intercellular adhesion molecule-1 (*ICAM1*), and E-selectin (*SELE*),[50] or a combined haplotype in the mannose-binding lectin gene (*MBL2* LYQA secretor haplotype), an important recognition molecule in the complement pathway.[51] Similarly, genetic variants in *IL6* and *TNFA* have also been described in association with increased incidence of postoperative cardiovascular complications including PMI after lung surgery for cancer.[90] Several polymorphisms in key proinflammatory genes have been associated with robust increases in perioperative inflammatory responses in patients undergoing cardiac surgery with CPB. These include the promoter SNPs in *IL6* (-572G>C and -174G>C),[147] also shown to prolong the hospital length of stay[148]; the apolipoprotein E genotype (the ε4 allele)[149]; SNPs in the tumor necrosis factor genes (*TNFA*-308G>A and -863 C>A, *LTA*+250G>A),[150,151] further associated with postoperative left ventricular dysfunction[93]; and a functional SNP in the macrophage migration inhibitory factor (MIF).[152] Conversely, a genetic variant is modulating the release of the anti-inflammatory cytokine interleukin-10 (*IL10*–1082G>A) in response to CPB, with high levels of IL10 surprisingly being associated with postoperative cardiovascular dysfunction.[94] In patients undergoing elective surgical revascularization for peripheral vascular disease, several SNPs in *IL6* (-174 G>C, nt565 G>A) and *IL10* (-1082 G>A, -819 C>T, -592 C>A, and the ATA haplotype) were associated with endothelial dysfunction and an increased risk of a composite endpoint of acute postoperative cardiovascular events.[123]

CRP is the prototypical acute-phase reactant and the most extensively studied inflammatory marker in clinical studies, and high sensitivity CRP (hs-CRP) has emerged as a robust predictor of cardiovascular risk at all stages, from healthy subjects to patients with acute coronary syndromes and acute decompensated heart failure.[153] Whether CRP is merely a marker or also a mediator of inflammatory processes is yet unclear, but several lines of evidence support the latter theory. In perioperative medicine, elevated preoperative CRP levels have been associated with increased short- and long-term morbidity and mortality in patients undergoing primary elective CABG (cutoff >3 mg/L)[154] as well as in higher-acuity CABG patients (cutoff >10 mg/L).[155] Interestingly, in a retrospective analysis of patients with elevated baseline hs-CRP levels undergoing off-pump CABG surgery, preoperative statin therapy was associated with reduced postoperative myocardial injury and need for dialysis.[156] In elective major noncardiac surgery patients, preoperative CRP levels (cutoff >3.4 mg/L) independently predicted perioperative major cardiovascular events (composite of MI, pulmonary edema, cardiovascular death) and significantly improved the predictive power of RCRI in receiver operating characteristic analysis.[157] In addition to the already established heritability of elevated baseline plasma CRP levels, recent reports indicate that the acute-phase rise in postoperative plasma CRP levels is also genetically determined. The *CRP*1059G>C polymorphism was associated with lower peak postoperative serum CRP following both elective CABG with CPB,[158] as well as esophagectomy for thoracic esophageal cancer.[159] Furthermore, *CRP*-717 C>T polymorphism was associated with stress hyperglycemia in patients undergoing esophagectomy for cancer, leading to increased postoperative infectious complications and ICU length of stay.[160]

Hemostatic biomarkers and perioperative adverse cardiac events. The host response to surgery is also characterized by alterations in the coagulation system, manifested as increased fibrinogen concentration, platelet adhesiveness, and plasminogen activator inhibitor-1 (PAI-1) production. These changes can be more pronounced after cardiac surgery, where the complex and multifactorial effects of hypothermia, hemodilution, and CPB-induced activation of coagulation, fibrinolytic, and inflammatory pathways are combined. Dysfunction of the coagulation system following cardiac surgery may manifest on a continuum ranging from increased thrombotic complications such as coronary graft thrombosis, PMI, stroke, pulmonary embolism at one end of the spectrum, to excessive bleeding as the other extreme. The balance between normal hemostasis, bleeding, and thrombosis is markedly influenced by the rate of thrombin formation and platelet activation, with genetic variability known to modulate each of these mechanistic pathways,[161] suggesting significant heritability of the prothrombotic state (see Table 6-5 for an overview of genetic variants associated with postoperative bleeding). Several genotypes in hemostatic genes have been associated with increased risk of coronary graft thrombosis and myocardial injury following CABG. A genetic variant in the promoter of the *PAI-1* gene, consisting of an insertion (5G)/deletion (4G) polymorphism, has been associated with changes in the plasma levels of PAI-1. Since PAI-1 is an important negative regulator of fibrinolytic activity, its polymorphism has been associated with increased risk of early graft thrombosis after CABG,[98] and in a meta-analysis, with increased incidence of MI.[162] Functional genetic variants regulating platelet activation have also been associated with adverse postoperative outcomes. These include a polymorphism in the platelet glycoprotein IIIa gene (*ITGB3*), resulting in increased platelet aggregation (Pl[A2] polymorphism), associated with increased perioperative myocardial injury,[91] risk of thrombotic coronary graft occlusion, MI, and 1-year mortality,[117] as well as a variant in the protease-activated receptor-4 (*PAR4*) gene associated with PMI after CABG.[99] Advanced heart failure patients requiring ventricular mechanical support represent a unique population that might benefit from a thorough preoperative risk profiling, given that implantation of ventricular assist devices can unmask previously undiagnosed thrombophilia. In the setting of noncardiac surgery, two polymorphisms in platelet glycoprotein receptors (*ITGB3* and *GP1 BA*) have been shown to be independent risk predictors of PMI in patients undergoing major vascular surgery, and resulted in improved discrimination of an ischemia risk assessment tool when added to historic and procedural risk factors.[92] Finally, a point mutation in coagulation factor V (1691G>A) resulting in resistance to activated protein C (factor V Leiden), was also associated with various postoperative thrombotic complications following noncardiac surgery.[60] Conversely, in patients undergoing cardiac surgery, factor V Leiden was associated with significant reductions in postoperative blood loss and overall risk of transfusion.[136] Nevertheless, in a prospective study of CABG patients with routine 3-month postoperative angiographic follow-up, carriers of factor V Leiden had a higher incidence of graft occlusion.[95]

Natriuretic peptides and perioperative adverse cardiac events. Circulating B-type natriuretic peptide (BNP) is a powerful biomarker of cardiovascular outcomes in many circumstances. Produced mainly in the ventricular myocardium, BNP is formed by cleavage of its prohormone by the enzyme corin into the biologically active C-terminal fragment (BNP), and an inactive N-terminal fragment (NT-proBNP). Known stimuli of BNP activation are myocardial mechanical stretch (from volume or pressure overload), acute ischemic injury, and a variety of other proinflammatory and neurohormonal stimuli inducing myocardial stress. Although secreted in 1:1 ratio, circulating levels of BNP and NT-proBNP differ considerably due to different clearance characteristics. A large number of studies have reported consistent associations of baseline plasma BNP or NT-proBNP levels with a variety of postoperative short- and long-term morbidity and mortality end points, independent of the traditional risk factors. For noncardiac surgery, these have been summarized in two meta-analyses that overall indicate an approximately 20-fold increase in risk of adverse perioperative cardiovascular outcomes.[163,164] Similarly, for cardiac surgery patients, preoperative BNP was a strong independent predictor of inhospital postoperative ventricular dysfunction, hospital length of stay, and 5-year mortality following primary CABG,[165] performing better than peak postoperative BNP.[166] Perioperative plasma corin concentrations decrease in patients undergoing CABG surgery, and larger relative decreases are associated with risk of long-term heart failure hospitalization and death.[167] The current guidelines for preoperative cardiac risk assessment in noncardiac surgery list BNP and NT-proBNP measurements as class IIa/level B indications.[168] However, despite the large number of studies conducted in both cardiac and noncardiac surgery, precise cut-off levels for BNP still need to be determined and adjusted for age, gender, and renal function. Similarly, no BNP-based goal-directed therapies have been reported in the perioperative period, although a role for BNP assays in monitoring aortic valve disease for optimal timing of surgery has been proposed.[169] Furthermore, a recent study by Fox et al.[97] identified genetic variation in natriuretic peptide precursor genes (*NPPA/NPPB*) to be independently associated with decreased risk of postoperative ventricular dysfunction following primary CABG, whereas variants in natriuretic peptide receptor *NPR3* were associated with an increased risk (Table 6-3), offering additional clues into the molecular mechanisms underlying postoperative ventricular dysfunction.

Genetic variation in vascular reactivity and perioperative adverse cardiac events. The perioperative period is characterized by robust activation of the sympathetic nervous system, which plays an important role in the pathophysiology of PMI. Thus, patients with CAD who carry specific polymorphisms in adrenergic receptor (AR) genes can be at high risk for catecholamine toxicity and cardiovascular complications. Several functionally important SNPs modulating the AR pathways have been described.[170] One of them is the Arg389Gly polymorphism in β_1-AR gene (*ADRB1*), an SNP associated with increased risk of composite cardiovascular morbidity at 1 year after noncardiac surgery under spinal anesthesia.[115] Of note, perioperative β-blockade had no effect. These findings prompted the investigators to suggest that stratification on AR genotype in future trials may help identify patients likely to benefit from perioperative β-blocker (BB) therapy. Significantly increased vascular responsiveness to α-adrenergic stimulation (phenylephrine) has been observed in carriers of the endothelial nitric oxide synthase (*NOS3*) 894>T polymorphism,[101] and angiotensin-converting enzyme (*ACE*) I/D polymorphism[61,103] undergoing cardiac surgery with CPB. Conversely, certain patients, especially those undergoing CPB for cardiac surgery, exhibit a form of vasodilatory shock known as vasoplegic syndrome, with a reported incidence of 8% to 20%. Although the precise mechanisms remain unclear, vasoplegic syndrome and vasopressor requirements have been associated with a common polymorphism in the dimethylarginine dimethylaminohydrolase II (*DDAH II*) gene, an important regulator of nitric oxide synthase activity,[100] whereas a functional SNP in angiotensin II type 1 receptor-associated protein (*AGTRAP*), the negative regulator of angiotensin II receptor type 1, is associated with decreased postoperative blood pressure following CABG as well as increased mortality in septic shock.[104] Regulation of pulmonary vascular tone is also subject to genetic regulation, and pediatric patients carrying the Glu298Asp polymorphism in *NOS3* are more likely to develop acute postoperative pulmonary hypertension following intracardiac repair of congenital cardiac disease with CPB.[171] Significant alterations in postoperative endothelial function are observed following on-pump cardiac surgery, and are associated with pronounced changes in biomarkers of endothelial origin like soluble P- and E-selectin, tetranectin, von Willebrand factor, and ACE activity.[172] Moreover, plasma concentrations of IL1β, soluble TREM-1, endocan, and cell-free DNA are early predictive biomarkers of sterile-SIRS after cardiovascular surgery.[173] In addition to variability in perioperative vascular tone, a genetic susceptibility to disturbed fluid handling following cardiac surgery has also been identified, with a common polymorphism in uromodulin (*UMOD*) gene as well as a genetic risk score comprising 14 SNPs related to inflammatory and hemodynamic pathways associated with risk of postoperative fluid overload.[174] Differences in perioperative vascular reactivity in relation to genetic variants of the β_2-AR (*ADRB2*) have similarly been noted in patients undergoing noncardiac surgery. A common functional *ADRB2* SNP (Glu27) was associated with increased blood pressure responses to endotracheal intubation,[105] whereas the incidence and severity of maternal hypotension and response to treatment in obstetric patients following spinal anesthesia for cesarean delivery was affected by *ADRB2* genotype (Gly16 and/or Glu27 led to lower vasopressor use for the treatment of hypotension).[175]

Genome-wide association studies and perioperative myocardial adverse events. A common SNP at the 9p21 locus has been identified in several replicated GWAS analyses to be associated with a wide array of vascular phenotypes in ambulatory populations, including CAD, MI, carotid atherosclerosis, abdominal aortic aneurysms, and intracranial aneurysms. Two studies have validated the association of polymorphisms at the 9p21 locus with both perioperative myocardial injury[176] and all-cause mortality after primary CABG.[96] The mechanism of action of this SNP in the development of PMI and mortality is not completely understood, but involves altered regulation of cell proliferation, senescence, and apoptosis. It seems that cardiac surgery with CPB may trigger the effects of the 9p21 gene variant leading to accumulation of senescent cells or cells that show evidence of necrotic death with cellular edema and lysis.

More recently, polymorphisms in the pregnancy-associated plasma protein A2 (*PAPPA2*), histone deacetylase-4 (*HDAC4*), and SEC24 family, member D (*SEC24D*, a member of the cytoplasmatic coat protein complex II) and two intergenic regions were identified as part of a GWAS in patients undergoing CABG to be associated with postoperative MI.[73] These novel findings implicate regulation of insulin-like growth factor bioavailability and repair processes (*PAPPA2*), myocardial cell cycle progression, differentiation and apoptosis, with potential use in predicting individual patient responsiveness to HDAC inhibition (*HDAC4*), and endoplasmic reticulum trapping of misfolded proteins under conditions of endoplasmic reticulum stress such as ischemia and oxidative injury (*SEC24D*). Although these observations are intriguing, future follow-up studies will be needed to translate these initial findings into biologic insights that could lead to predictive and therapeutic advances in perioperative care.

Perioperative Atrial Fibrillation

Perioperative atrial fibrillation (PoAF) remains a significant clinical problem after cardiac and noncardiac thoracic procedures. With an incidence of 27% to 40%, PoAF is associated with increased morbidity, hospital length of stay, rehospitalization, health-care costs, and reduced survival. This has prompted several investigators to develop comprehensive indices for PoAF risk prediction based on demographic, clinical, electrocardiographic, and procedural risk factors. Nevertheless, the predictive accuracy of these risk indices remains limited,[177] suggesting that genetic variation may play a significant role in the occurrence of PoAF. Heritable forms of AF have been described in the ambulatory nonsurgical population, and it appears both monogenic forms like "lone" AF as well as polygenic predisposition to more common acquired forms like PoAF do exist. A GWAS found two polymorphisms on chromosome 4q25 to be significantly associated with AF,[71] findings replicated in other patient groups from Sweden, the United States, and Hong Kong. Subsequently, this locus was also associated with new onset PoAF after cardiac surgery with CPB (CABG with or without concurrent valve surgery).[110] The mechanism of action of this genetic locus is unknown, but it lies close to several genes involved in the development of pulmonary myocardium, or the sleeve of cardiomyocytes extending from the left atrium into the initial portion of the pulmonary veins. Clinical studies have demonstrated that ectopic foci of electric activity arising from within the pulmonary veins and posterior left atrium play a substantial role in initiating and maintaining AF.

Other candidate susceptibility genes for PoAF include those determining the duration of action potential (voltage-gated ion channels, ion transporters), responses to extracellular factors (adrenergic and other hormone receptors, heat shock proteins), remodeling processes, and magnitude of inflammatory and oxidative stress. It has been described that inflammation, reflected by elevated baseline CRP or IL6 levels and exaggerated postoperative leukocytosis, predicts the occurrence of PoAF. A link between inflammation and the development of PoAF is also supported by evidence that postoperative administration of nonsteroidal anti-inflammatory drugs may reduce the incidence of PoAF. Several studies implicated a functional SNP in the *IL6* promoter (-174G>C) to be associated with higher perioperative plasma IL-6 levels and adverse outcomes after CABG, including PoAF.[107,108,178] Activation of innate immune responses has also recently been suggested by results from the first GWAS of PoAF following CABG, which identified a variant in lymphocyte antigen 96 (*LY96*) to be associated with decreased incidence of new-onset PoAF after adjustment for clinical and procedural risk factors.[74] In noncardiac surgery, polymorphisms in *IL6* and *TNFA* genes have been shown to be associated with an increased risk of postoperative morbidity, including new-onset arrhythmias.[90] There is however a contradictory lack of association between CRP levels (strongly regulated by IL-6) and PoAF in women undergoing cardiac surgery,[179] which may reflect gender-related differences. On the other hand, both pre- and postoperative PAI-1 levels were independently associated with development of PoAF following cardiac surgery.[180]

Polymorphisms in adrenergic pathway genes have also been implicated in susceptibility to develop new-onset PoAF after CABG. A functional variant in the β_1-AR gene (*ADRB1* Arg389Gly) was associated with PoAF, with effects modulated by BB therapy, being stronger among patients without BB prophylaxis compared to those receiving BBs.[113] Furthermore, in patients undergoing CABG, polymorphisms in G protein-coupled kinase 5 (*GRK5*) were associated with PoAF despite perioperative BB therapy.[114] GRK5 is expressed in the normal human heart, and regulates cardiac inotropic and chronotropic actions of catecholamines by physiologically modulating β-AR activity through receptor phosphorylation, β-arrestin recruitment, uncoupling from G proteins, and β-AR desensitization. Although the mechanism of action is incompletely understood, functional variants in *GRK5* modify the β_1-adreneregic receptor signaling pathway similar to partial receptor antagonism by BBs, thus altering their effectiveness. In summary, these polymorphisms may provide new insights into new-onset PoAF pathogenesis and differential responses to BB therapy, which can inform development of personalized perioperative treatment strategies for this common complication.

Investigations in the transcriptional responses to AF in human atrial appendage myocardium collected at the time of cardiac surgery or in preclinical models (Table 6-2) have identified a ventricular-like genomic signature in fibrillating atria, with increased ratios of ventricular to atrial isoforms, suggesting dedifferentiation.[26] It remains unclear whether this "ventricularization" of atrial gene expression reflects cause or effect of AF, but likely represents an adaptive energy-saving process to the high metabolic demand of fibrillating atrial myocardium, akin to chronic hibernation. Because atrial tissue gene expression profiling may help to determine how differentially expressed genes in the human atrium before CPB are related to subsequent biologic pathway activation patterns, and whether specific expression profiles are associated with an increased risk for PoAF or altered response to BB therapy after CABG surgery, we recently reported an expression quantitative trait locus (eQTL) analysis of PoAF.[181] We found significant upregulation of *VOPP1* gene (vesicular overexpressed in cancer-prosurvival protein 1) in patients with PoAF, which was associated with transactivating variants in G-protein coupled kinase 5 (*GRK5*), suggesting potential pathophysiologic roles of VOPP1 in PoAF despite perioperative BB therapy. Patients who exhibit PoAF after cardiac surgery also display a differential genomic response to CPB in their peripheral blood leukocytes, characterized by upregulation of oxidative stress genes correlated with a significant increase in oxidant stress both systemically (as measured by total peroxide levels) as well as at the myocardial level (as measured in the right atrium).[27] Finally, one study used high-resolution ^{1}H-NMR spectroscopy to conduct combined metabolomic and proteomic analyses of atrial tissue samples obtained at the time of cardiac surgery identified alterations in myocardial ketone metabolism associated with persistent AF, and the ratio of glycolytic end products to end products of lipid metabolism correlated positively with time of onset of PoAF.[47]

Genetic Variants and Postoperative Event-free Survival

Large randomized clinical trials examining the benefits of CABG surgery and percutaneous coronary interventions relative to medical therapy and/or to one another have refined our knowledge of early and long-term survival after CABG. Although these studies have helped define subgroups of patients who benefit from surgical revascularization, they also revealed substantial variability in long-term survival after CABG, altered by important demographic and environmental risk factors. Increasing evidence suggests that the *ACE* gene indel polymorphism may influence post-CABG complications, with carriers of the *D* allele having higher mortality and restenosis rates after CABG surgery compared with the *I* allele.[116] As discussed earlier, a prothrombotic amino acid alteration in the β_3-integrin chain of the glycoprotein IIb/IIIa platelet receptor (the Pl^{A2} polymorphism) is associated with an increased risk for major adverse cardiac events (composite of MI, coronary bypass graft occlusion, or death) following CABG surgery (Table 6-3).[117] And variation at the chromosome 9p21 locus described earlier was associated with 5-year all-cause mortality following CABG, and improved the predictive ability of the EuroSCORE.[96] We found preliminary evidence for association of two functional SNPs modulating β_2-AR activity (Arg16Gly and Gln27Glu) with incidence of death or major adverse cardiac events following cardiac surgery,[119] and further identified a functional polymorphism in thrombomodulin gene (*THBD* Ala455Val) associated with increased 5-year mortality after CABG independent of EuroSCORE.[122]

Genetic Susceptibility to Adverse Perioperative Neurologic Outcomes

Despite advances in surgical and anesthetic techniques, significant neurologic morbidity continues to occur following cardiac surgery, ranging in severity from coma and focal stroke (incidence 1% to 3%) to more subtle cognitive deficits (incidence up to 69%), with a substantial impact on the risk of perioperative death, quality of life, and resource utilization. Variability in the reported incidence of both early and late neurologic deficits remains poorly explained by procedural risk factors, suggesting that environmental (operative) and genetic factors may interact to determine disease onset, progression, and recovery. The pathophysiology of perioperative neurologic injury is thought to involve complex interactions between primary pathways associated with atherosclerosis and thrombosis, and secondary response pathways like inflammation, vascular reactivity, and direct cellular injury. Many functional genetic variants have been reported in each of these mechanistic pathways involved in modulating the magnitude and the response to neurologic injury, which may have implications in chronic as well as acute perioperative neurocognitive outcomes. For example, the interaction of minor alleles of the CRP (1846 C>T) and IL-6 promoter SNP -174G>C significantly increases the risk of acute stroke after cardiac surgery.[128] Similarly, P-selectin and CRP genes both modulate the susceptibility to postoperative cognitive decline (POCD) following cardiac surgery.[52] Specifically, the loss-of-function minor alleles of CRP 1059G>C and SELP 1087G>A are independently associated with a *reduction* in the observed incidence of POCD after adjustment for known clinical and demographic covariates (Table 6-4).

Our group has demonstrated a significant association between the apolipoprotein E (*APOE*) E4 genotype and adverse cerebral outcomes in cardiac surgery patients.[129,182] This is consistent with the role of the *APOE* genotype in recovery from acute brain injury, such as intracranial hemorrhage,[183] closed head injury,[184] and stroke,[185] as well as experimental models of cerebral ischemia-reperfusion injury[186]; two subsequent studies in CABG patients, however, have not replicated these initial findings. Furthermore, the incidence of postoperative delirium following major noncardiac surgery in the elderly[133] and in critically ill patients[134] is increased in carriers of the *APOE* ε4 allele. Unlike adult cardiac surgery patients, infants possessing the *APOE* ε2 allele are at increased risk for developing adverse neurodevelopmental sequelae following cardiac surgery.[130,131] The mechanisms by which the *APOE* genotypes might influence neurologic outcomes have yet to be determined, but do not seem to be related to alterations in global cerebral blood flow or oxygen metabolism during CPB[187]; however, genotypic effects in modulating the inflammatory response,[149] extent of aortic atheroma burden,[188] and risk for premature coronary atherosclerosis[189] may play a role.

Consistent with the observed role of platelet activation in the pathophysiology of adverse neurologic sequelae, genetic variants in surface platelet membrane glycoproteins, important mediators of platelet adhesion and platelet–platelet interactions, increase the susceptibility to prothrombotic events. Among these, the Pl^{A2} polymorphism in glycoprotein IIb/IIIa has been related to various adverse thrombotic outcomes, including acute coronary thrombosis[190] and atherothrombotic stroke.[191] We found the Pl^{A2} allele to be associated with more severe neurocognitive decline after CPB,[53] which could represent exacerbation of platelet-dependent thrombotic processes associated with plaque embolism.

Cardiac surgical patients who develop POCD demonstrate inherently different genetic responses to CPB from those without POCD, as evidenced by acute deregulation of gene expression pathways involving inflammation, antigen presentation, and cellular adhesion in peripheral blood leukocytes.[28] These findings corroborate with proteomic changes, in which patients with POCD similarly have significantly higher serologic inflammatory indices compared with those patients without POCD,[192,193] and adds to the increasing level of evidence that CPB does not cause an indiscriminate variation in gene expression, but rather distinct patterns in specific pathways that are highly associated with the development of postoperative complications such as POCD. The implications for perioperative medicine include identifying populations at risk who might benefit not only from an improved informed consent, stratification, and resource allocation, but also from targeted anti-inflammatory strategies.

In noncardiac surgery, a study conducted in patients undergoing carotid endarterectomy concluded that preoperative plasma levels of fibrinogen and high-sensitivity CRP (hsCRP) were independently associated with new periprocedural cerebral ischemic lesions caused by microembolic events, as determined by MRI diffusion-weighted imaging.[194]

Genetic Susceptibility to Adverse Perioperative Kidney Outcomes

Acute kidney injury (AKI) is a common, serious complication of cardiac surgery; about 8% to 15% of patients develop moderate renal injury (>1.0 mg/dL peak creatinine rise), and up to 5% of them develop renal failure requiring dialysis.[195] AKI is independently associated with inhospital mortality rates, exceeding 60% in patients requiring dialysis.[195] Several studies have demonstrated that inheritance of genetic polymorphisms in the APOE gene (ε4 allele)[57] and in the promoter region of the IL6 gene (-174 C allele)[178] are associated with AKI following CABG surgery (Table 6-5). We have reported that major differences in peak postoperative serum creatinine rise after CABG are predicted by carrying combinations of polymorphisms that interestingly differ by race: the angiotensinogen (*AGT*) 842 T>C and IL6 -572G>C variants in Caucasians, and the endothelial nitric oxide synthase (*NOS3*) 894G>T and *ACE* I/D in African Americans are associated with more than 50% reduction in postoperative glomerular filtration rate.[55] A recent GWAS of cardiac surgery–associated AKI identified two novel susceptibility loci, one located in the Bardet–Biedl syndrome 9 (*BBS9*) gene, potentially implicating abnormalities in the primary renal cilia function in the pathogenesis of AKI.[76] Further identification of genotypes predictive of adverse perioperative renal outcomes may facilitate individually tailored therapy, risk stratify the patients for interventional trials targeting the gene product itself, and aid in medical-decision making (e.g., selecting medical over surgical management).

Genetic Variants and Risk for Postoperative Lung Injury

Prolonged mechanical ventilation (inability to extubate patient by 24 hours postoperatively) is a significant complication following cardiac surgery, occurring in 5.6% and 10.5% of patients undergoing first and repeat CABG surgery, respectively.[196] Several pulmonary and nonpulmonary causes have been identified, and scoring systems based on preoperative and procedural risk factors have been proposed and validated. Recently, genetic variants in the renin–angiotensin pathway and in proinflammatory cytokine genes have been associated with respiratory complications post-CPB. The D allele of a common functional I/D polymorphism in the *ACE* gene, accounting for 47% of variance in circulating ACE levels,[197] is associated with prolonged mechanical ventilation following CABG,[198] and with susceptibility to and prognosis of acute respiratory distress syndrome (ARDS).[199] Furthermore, a hyposecretor haplotype in the neighboring genes tumor necrosis factor alpha (*TNFA*) and lymphotoxin alpha (*LTA*) on chromosome 6 (*TNFA*-308G/*LTA*+250G haplotype)[200] and a functional polymorphism modulating postoperative interleukin 6 levels (*IL6*–174G>C)[178] are independently associated with higher risk of prolonged mechanical ventilation post-CABG. The association is more dramatic in patients undergoing conventional CABG than in those undergoing off-pump CABG (OPCAB), suggesting that in high-risk patients identified by preoperative genetic screening OPCAB may be the optimal surgical procedure. In children, plasma gelsolin and sRAGE have been reported to improve prediction of CPB-induced acute lung injury.[201,202]

A next crucial step in understanding the complexity of adverse perioperative outcomes is to assess the contribution of variations in many genes simultaneously and their interaction with traditional risk factors to the longitudinal prediction of outcomes in individual patients. The use of such outcome predictive models incorporating genetic information may help stratify mortality and morbidity in surgical patients, improve prognostication, direct medical decision-making both intraoperatively and during postoperative follow-up, and even suggest novel targets for therapeutic intervention in the perioperative period.

Pharmacogenomics and Anesthesia

Interindividual variability in response to drug therapy, both in terms of efficacy and safety, is a rule by which anesthesiologists live. In fact, much of the art of anesthesiology is the astute clinician being prepared to deal with outliers. The term *pharmacogenomics* is used to describe how inherited variations in genes modulating drug actions are related to interindividual variability in drug response. Such variability in drug action may be *pharmacokinetic* or *pharmacodynamic* (Fig. 6-5). Pharmacokinetic variability refers to variability in a drug's absorption, distribution, metabolism, and excretion that mediates its efficacy and/or toxicity. The molecules involved in these processes include drug-metabolizing enzymes (such as members of the cytochrome P450, or CYP, superfamily), and drug transport molecules that mediate drug uptake into, and efflux from, intracellular sites. Pharmacodynamic variability refers to variable drug effects despite equivalent drug delivery to molecular sites of action. This may reflect variability in the function of the molecular target of the drug, or in the pathophysiologic context in which the drug interacts with its receptor-target (e.g., affinity, coupling, expression).[203] Thus, pharmacogenomics investigates complex, polygenically determined phenotypes of drug efficacy or toxicity, with the goal of identifying novel therapeutic targets and customizing drug therapy.

Historically, characterization of the genetic basis for plasma pseudocholinesterase deficiency in 1956 was of fundamental importance to anesthesia and the further development and understanding of genetically determined differences in drug response.[204] Pharmacogenetic testing is currently not recommended in the population at large, but only as an explanation for an adverse event.[205] Moreover, research to refine the genetic underpinnings of malignant hyperthermia, a rare autosomal dominant genetic disease of skeletal muscle calcium metabolism triggered by administration of general anesthesia with volatile anesthetic agents or succinylcholine in susceptible individuals, revealed that MH susceptibility results from a complex interaction between multiple genes and environment.[206] Although direct DNA testing in the general population for susceptibility to MH is currently not recommended, testing individuals with a positive family history has the potential to greatly reduce mortality and morbidity.[205]

Genetic Variability in Response to Anesthetic Agents

Anesthetic potency, defined by the minimum alveolar concentration (MAC) of an inhaled anesthetic that abolishes purposeful movement in response to a noxious stimulus, varies among individuals, with a coefficient of variation (the ratio of standard deviation to the mean) of approximately 10%.[207] This observed variability may be explained by interindividual differences in multiple genes that underlie responsiveness to anesthetics, by environmental or physiologic factors (brain temperature,

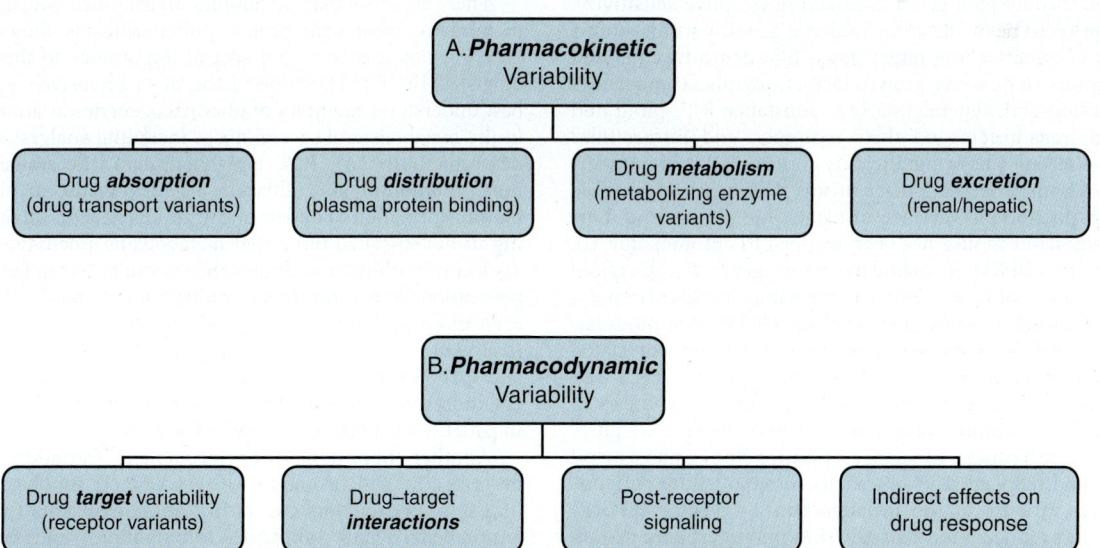

Figure 6-5 Pharmacogenomic determinants of individual drug response operate by pharmacokinetic and pharmacodynamic mechanisms. **A:** Genetic variants in *drug transporters* (e.g., ATP-binding cassette sub-family B member 1 or *ABCB1* gene) and *drug metabolizing enzymes* (e.g., cytochrome P450 2D6 or *CYP2D6* gene, *CYP2C9* gene, N-acetyltransferase or *NAT2* gene, plasma cholinesterase or *BCHE* gene) are responsible for *pharmacokinetic* variability in drug response. **B:** Polymorphisms in *drug targets* (e.g., β_1 and β_2-adrenergic receptor *ADRB1*, *ADRB2* genes; angiotensin-I converting enzyme *ACE* gene), *postreceptor signaling molecules* (e.g., guanine nucleotide binding protein β_3 or *GNB3* gene), or *molecules indirectly affecting drug response* (e.g., various ion channel genes involved in drug-induced arrhythmias) are sources of *pharmacodynamic* variability.

age), or by measurement errors. With growing public concern over intraoperative awareness, understanding the mechanisms responsible for this variability may facilitate implementation of patient-specific preventative strategies. Evidence of a genetic basis for increased anesthetic requirements is beginning to emerge, suggested for instance by variability in the immobilizing dose of sevoflurane (as much as 24%) in populations with different ethnic (and thus genetic) backgrounds.[208]

Based on combined pharmacologic and genetic in vivo studies to date, several receptors are unlikely to be direct mediators of MAC, including the $GABA_A$ (despite their compelling role in IV anesthetic-induced immobility), 5-HT_3, AMPA, kainate, acetylcholine and α_2-ARs, and potassium channels.[209] Glycine, NMDA receptors, and sodium channels remain likely candidates.[210] These conclusions, however, do not apply to other anesthetic end points, such as hypnosis, amnesia, and analgesia. Several preclinical proteomic analyses have identified in a more unbiased way a group of potential anesthetic targets for halothane,[37] desflurane,[38] and sevoflurane,[39] which should provide the basis for more focused studies of anesthetic binding sites. Such "omic" approaches have the potential to evolve into preoperative screening profiles useful in guiding individualized therapeutic decisions, such as prevention of anesthetic awareness in patients with a genetic predisposition to increased anesthetic requirements.

Genetic Variability in Pain Response

Similar to the observed variability in anesthetic potency, the response to painful stimuli and analgesic manipulations varies among individuals. Increasing evidence suggests that pain behavior in response to noxious stimuli and its modulation by the central nervous system in response to drug administration or environmental stress, as well as the development of persistent pain conditions through pain amplification, are strongly influenced by genetic factors.[211–213] Results from studies in twins[214] and inbred mouse strains[215] indicate a moderate heritability for chronic pain syndromes and nociceptive sensitivity, which appears to be mediated by multiple genes. Various strains of knockout mice lacking target genes like neurotrophins and their receptors (e.g., nerve growth factor), peripheral mediators of nociception and hyperalgesia (e.g. substance P), opioid and nonopioid transmitters and their receptors, and intracellular signaling molecules have significantly contributed to the understanding of pain processing mechanisms.[216] A locus responsible for 28% of phenotypic variance in magnitude of systemic morphine analgesia in mouse has been mapped to chromosome 10, in or near the OPRM (μ-opioid receptor) gene. The μ-opioid receptor is also subject to pharmacodynamic variability; polymorphisms in the promoter region of the OPRM gene modulating interleukin4-mediated gene expression have been correlated with morphine antinociception. The much quoted OPRM 188 A>G polymorphism is associated with decreased responses to morphine-6-glucuronide, resulting in altered analgesic requirements, but also reduced incidence of postoperative nausea and vomiting, and reduced risks of toxicity in renal failure patients. Conversely, variants of the melanocortin 1 receptor (MC1R) gene, which produce a red hair-fair skin phenotype, are associated with increased analgesic responses to κ-opioid agonists in women but not men, providing evidence for a gene-by-gender interaction in regulating analgesic response (for a review, see Somogyi et al.[217]). Very recent reports suggest that peripherally located β_2-ARs (ADRB2) also contribute to basal pain sensitivity and the development of chronic pain states, as well as opioid-induced hyperalgesia.[213] Functionally important haplotypes in the ADRB2[212] and catechol-O-methyltransferase (COMT)[218] genes are associated with enhanced pain sensitivity in humans.

In addition to the genetic control of peripheral nociceptive pathways, considerable evidence exists for genetic variability in the descending central pain modulatory pathways, further explaining the interindividual variability in analgesic responsiveness. One good example relevant to analgesic efficacy is cytochrome P450D6 (CYP2D6), a member of the superfamily of microsomal enzymes that catalyze phase I drug metabolism, and responsible for the metabolism of a large number of therapeutic compounds. The relationship between the CYP2D6 genotype and the enzyme metabolic rate has been extensively characterized, with at least twelve known mutations leading to a tetramodal distribution of CYP2D6 activity: ultrarapid metabolizers (5% to 7% of the population), extensive metabolizers (60%), intermediate metabolizers (25%), and poor metabolizers (10%). Currently, pharmacogenomic screening tests predict CYP2D6 phenotype with more than 95% reliability. The consequences of inheriting an allele that compromises CYP2D6 function include the inability to metabolize codeine (a prodrug) to morphine by O-demethylation, leading to lack of analgesia but increased side effects from the parent drug (e.g., fatigue) in poor metabolizers.[205,211]

Genetic Variability in Response to Other Drugs Used Perioperatively

A wide variety of drugs used in the perioperative period display significant pharmacokinetic or pharmacodynamic variability that is genetically modulated (Table 6-6). Although such genetic variation in drug metabolizing enzymes or drug targets usually result in unusually variable drug response, genetic markers associated with rare but life-threatening side effects have also been described. Of note, the most commonly cited categories of drugs involved in adverse drug reactions include cardiovascular, antibiotic, psychiatric, and analgesic medications, and interestingly, each category has a known genetic basis for increased risk of adverse reactions.

There are more than 30 families of drug-metabolizing enzymes in humans, most with genetic polymorphisms shown to influence enzymatic activity. Of special importance to the anesthesiologist is the CYP2D6, one of the most intensively studied and best understood examples of pharmacogenetic variation, involved in the metabolism of several drugs including analgesics (codeine, dextromethorphan), BBs, antiarrhythmics (flecainide, propafenone, quinidine), and diltiazem. CYP2D6 is also involved in the biotransformation of ondansetron, and its genetic variation resulting in the so-called ultrarapid metabolizing phenotype has been associated with increased incidence of ondansetron failure for the prevention of postoperative vomiting but not nausea,[219] which was even more pronounced if tropisetron was used as an antiemetic treatment.[220] Joint assessment of genotype-dependent CYP2D6 and CYP3A4 activities revealed that ondansetron metabolism is enantioselective, and doubling the ondansetron dose is ineffective in patients with high CYP2D6/3A4 activity.[221]

Another important pharmacogenetic variation has been described in cytochrome P450C9 (CYP2C9), involved in metabolizing anticoagulants (warfarin), anticonvulsants (phenytoin), antidiabetic agents (glipizide, tolbutamide), and nonsteroidal anti-inflammatory drugs (celecoxib, ibuprofen), among others. Three known CYP2C9 variant alleles result in different enzyme activities (extensive, intermediate, and slow metabolizer phenotypes), and have clinical implications in the increased risk of life-threatening bleeding complications in slow metabolizers during standard warfarin therapy. This illustrates the concept of "high-risk pharmacokinetics," which applies to drugs with low

Table 6-6 Examples of Genetic Polymorphisms Involved In Variable Responses to Drugs Used in the Perioperative Period

Drug Class	Gene Name (Gene Symbol)	Effect of Polymorphism
Pharmacokinetic Variability		
β-blockers	Cytochrome P450 2D6 (CYP2D6)	Enhanced drug effect
Codeine, dextromethorphan	CYP2D6	Decreased drug effect
Ca-channel blockers	Cytochrome P450 3A4 (CYP3A4)	Uncertain
Alfentanil	CYP3A4	Enhanced drug response
Angiotensin-II receptor type 1 blockers	Cytochrome P450 2C9 (CYP2C9)	Enhanced blood pressure response
Warfarin	CYP2C9	Enhanced anticoagulant effect, risk of bleeding
Phenytoin	CYP2C9	Enhanced drug effect
ACE-inhibitors	Angiotensin-I converting enzyme (ACE)	Blood pressure response
Procainamide	N-acetyltransferase 2 (NAT2)	Enhanced drug effect
Succinylcholine	Butyrylcholinesterase (BCHE)	Enhanced drug effect
Digoxin	P-glycoprotein (ABCB1, MDR1)	Increased bioavailability
Pharmacodynamic Variability		
β-blockers	$β_1$ and $β_2$ adrenergic receptors (ADRB1, ADRB2)	Blood pressure and heart rate response, airway responsiveness to $β_2$-agonists
QT-prolonging drugs (antiarrhythmics, cisapride, erythromycin, etc.)	Sodium and potassium ion channels (SCN5 A, KCNH2, KCNE2, KCNQ1)	Long QT-syndrome, risk of torsade de pointes
Aspirin, glycoprotein IIb/IIIa inhibitors	Glycoprotein IIIa subunit of platelet glycoprotein IIb/IIIa (ITGB3)	Variability in antiplatelet effects
Phenylephrine	Endothelial nitric oxide synthase (NOS3)	Blood pressure response

therapeutic ratios eliminated by a single pathway (in this case CYP2C9-mediated oxidation); genetic variation in that pathway may lead to large changes in drug clearance, concentrations, and effects.[203] Dose adjustments based on the pharmacogenetic phenotype have been proposed for drugs metabolized via both CYP2D6 and CYP2C9 pathways,[205] and a commercially available, FDA-approved test (CYP450 AmpliChip, Roche Molecular Diagnostics) allows clinicians for the first time to test patients for a wide spectrum of genetic variation in drug metabolizing enzymes. The strongest evidence to date for use of pharmacogenomic testing is to aid in the determination of warfarin dosage by using genotypes in the CYP2C9 and vitamin K epoxide reductase complex 1 (VKORC1) genes, with four FDA-approved tests now commercially available. Furthermore, CYP2C9 genotypes and age could be used in patients on chronic warfarin therapy awaiting elective surgery to inform the time required to discontinue the drug preoperatively (rather than uniformly applying the 5-day recommended guidelines) and thus potentially avoiding the costs associated with surgical delays.[222]

Genetic variation in drug targets (receptors) can have profound effect on drug efficacy, and over 25 examples have already been identified. For example, functional polymorphisms in the $β_2$-AR (Arg16Gly, Gln27Glu) influence the bronchodilator and vascular responses to β-agonists, and $β_1$-AR variants (Arg-389Gly) modulate responses to BBs and may impact postoperative cardiovascular adverse events.[115,170] An excellent recent review by Nagele[223] provides a strong rationale for using pharmacogenomic variation in BB metabolism (CYP2D6) and receptor signaling pathways (both ADRB1, ADRB2, and downstream genes) to determine the effectiveness and safety of perioperative β-blockade for prevention of perioperative MI, particularly given the conflicting results raised by the POISE trial.[224] Finally, clinically important genetic polymorphisms with indirect effects on drug response have been described. These include variants in candidate genes like sodium (SCN5 A) and potassium ion channels (KCNH2, KCNE2, KCNQ1), which alter susceptibility to drug-induced long-QT syndrome and ventricular arrhythmias (torsade de pointes) associated with the use of drugs like erythromycin, terfenadine, disopyramide, sotalol, cisapride, or quinidine. Carriers of such susceptibility alleles have no manifest QT-interval prolongation or family history of sudden death until QT-prolonging drug challenge is superimposed.[203] Predisposition to QT-interval prolongation (considered a surrogate for risk of life-threatening ventricular arrhythmias) has been responsible for more drug withdrawals from the market than any other category of adverse event in recent times, so understanding genetic predisposing factors constitutes one of the highest priorities of current pharmacogenomic efforts.

Pharmacogenomics is emerging as an additional modifying component to anesthesia along with age, gender, co-morbidities, and medication usage. Specific testing and treatment guidelines allowing clinicians to appropriately modify drug utilization (e.g., adjust dose or change drug) already exist for a few compounds,[205] and will likely be expanded to all relevant therapeutic compounds (Fig. 6-2), together with identification of novel therapeutic targets.

Conclusions and Future Directions

The Human Genome Project has revolutionized all aspects of medicine, allowing us to assess the impact of genetic variability on disease taxonomy, characterization, and outcome, and individual responses to various drugs and injuries. Mechanistically, information gleaned through genomic approaches is already unraveling longstanding mysteries behind general anesthetic action and adverse responses to drugs used perioperatively. To take full advantage of the unique opportunities offered by the genomic revolution and begin implementing precision medicine concepts, the cycle of innovation in perioperative medicine must shift to a new framework which includes comprehensive and standardized definitions of the phenotypes of interest (including short- and long-term adverse outcomes such as organ injury/dysfunction, adverse drug responses, transition to chronic pain) by developing and refining EMR-driven phenotyping algorithms,[225] followed by identification of the underlying genes, characterization of the mechanism from DNA to phenotype, and rigorous development and validation of actionable companion diagnostics implemented at the point-of-care using EMR-integrated clinical decision support tools (Fig. 6-2).[226] For the anesthesiologist, this may soon translate into prospective risk assessment incorporating genetic profiling of markers important in thrombotic, inflammatory, vascular, and neurologic responses to perioperative stress, with implications ranging from individualized additional preoperative testing and physiologic optimization, to choice of perioperative monitoring strategies and critical care resource utilization. Furthermore, genetic profiling of drug metabolizing enzymes, carrier proteins, and receptors, using currently available high-throughput molecular technologies, will enable personalized choice of drugs and dosage regimens tailored to suit a patient's pharmacogenetic profile. At that point, perioperative physicians will have far more robust information to use in designing the most appropriate and safest anesthetic plan for a given patient.

Although one of the aims of the Human Genome Project is to improve therapy through genome-based prediction, the birth of personal genomics opens up a Pandora's box of ethical issues, including privacy and the risk for discrimination against individuals who are genetically predisposed for a medical disorder. Such discrimination may include barriers to obtaining health, life, or long-term care insurance, or obtaining employment. Thus, extensive efforts are made to protect patients participating in genetic research from prejudice, discrimination, or uses of genetic information that will adversely affect them. To address the concerns of both biomedical research and health communities, the U.S. Senate has approved in 2003 the Genetic Information and Nondiscrimination Act, which provides the strong safeguards required to protect the public participating in human genome research. Another ethical concern is the transferability of genetic tests across ethnic groups, particularly in the prediction of adverse drug responses. It is known that most polymorphisms associated with variability in drug response show significant differences in allele frequencies among populations and racial groups. Furthermore, the patterns of linkage disequilibrium are markedly different between ethnic groups, which may lead to spurious findings when markers, instead of causal variants, are used in diagnostic tests extrapolated across populations. In exploring racial disparities in health and disease outcomes, considerable debate has focused on whether race and ethnic identity are primarily social or biologic constructs, and the contribution of genetic variability in explaining observed differences in the rates of disease between racial groups. With the goal of personalized medicine being the prediction of risk and treatment of disease on the basis of an individual's genetic profile, some have argued that biologic consideration of race will become obsolete. However, in this discovery phase of the postgenome era, continuing to incorporate racial information in genetic studies should improve our understanding of the architecture of the human genome, and its implications for novel strategies aiming at identifying variants protecting against, or conferring susceptibility to, common diseases and modulating drug effects.[227]

Acknowledgments

Supported in part by NIH grants HL075273 and HL092071 (to MVP).

REFERENCES

1. Podgoreanu MV, Schwinn DA. New paradigms in cardiovascular medicine: emerging technologies and practices: perioperative genomics. *J Am Coll Cardiol.* 2005;46:1965–1977.
2. Fox AA, Shernan SK, Body SC. Predictive genomics of adverse events after cardiac surgery. *Semin Cardiothorac Vasc Anesth.* 2004;8:297–315.
3. Stuber F, Hoeft A. The influence of genomics on outcome after cardiovascular surgery. *Curr Opin Anaesthesiol.* 2002;15:3–8.
4. Ziegeler S, Tsusaki BE, Collard CD. Influence of genotype on perioperative risk and outcome. *Anesthesiology.* 2003;99:212–219.
5. Neudecker V, Brodsky KS, Kreth S, et al. Emerging roles for MicroRNAs in perioperative medicine. *Anesthesiology.* 2016;124:489–506.
6. Stary CM, Patel HH, Roth DM. Epigenetics: the epicenter for future anesthesia research? *Anesthesiology.* 2015;123(4):743–744.
7. Lirk P, Fiegl H, Weber NC, et al. Epigenetics in the perioperative period. *Br J Pharmacol.* 2015;172:2748–2755.
8. National Research Council. *Science and Decisions: Advancing Risk Assessment.* Washington, DC: The National Academies Press; 2009.
9. Betts K, Shelton-Davenport M, Rapporteurs, et al. *Interindividual Variability: New Ways to Study and Implications for Decision Making: Workshop in Brief. Interindividual Variability: New Ways to Study and Implications for Decision Making: Workshop in Brief.* Washington, DC: National Academies Press; 2016.
10. Collins FS, Varmus H. A new initiative on precision medicine. *N Engl J Med.* 2015;372:793–795.
11. Redon R, Ishikawa S, Fitch KR, et al. Global variation in copy number in the human genome. *Nature.* 2006;444:444–454.
12. Niezgoda J, Morgan PG. Anesthetic considerations in patients with mitochondrial defects. *Paediatr Anaesth.* 2013;23:785–793.
13. Stranger BE, Nica AC, Forrest MS, et al. Population genomics of human gene expression. *Nat Genet.* 2007;39:1217–1224.
14. Hopf HW. Molecular diagnostics of injury and repair responses in critical illness: what is the future of "monitoring" in the intensive care unit? *Crit Care Med.* 2003;31:S518–S523.
15. Milewicz DM, Regalado ES. Use of genetics for personalized management of heritable thoracic aortic disease: how do we get there? *J Thorac Cardiovasc Surg.* 2015;149:S3–S5.
16. Feezor RJ, Baker HV, Xiao W, et al. Genomic and proteomic determinants of outcome in patients undergoing thoracoabdominal aortic aneurysm repair. *J Immunol.* 2004;172:7103–7109.
17. Sehl PD, Tai JT, Hillan KJ, et al. Application of cDNA microarrays in determining molecular phenotype in cardiac growth, development, and response to injury. *Circulation.* 2000;101:1990–1999.
18. Ruel M, Bianchi C, Khan TA, et al. Gene expression profile after cardiopulmonary bypass and cardioplegic arrest. *J Thorac Cardiovasc Surg.* 2003;126:1521–1530.
19. Konstantinov IE, Coles JG, Boscarino C, et al. Gene expression profiles in children undergoing cardiac surgery for right heart obstructive lesions. *J Thorac Cardiovasc Surg.* 2004;127:746–754.
20. Muehlschlegel JD, Christodoulou DC, McKean D, et al. Using next-generation RNA sequencing to examine ischemic changes induced by cold blood cardioplegia on the human left ventricular myocardium transcriptome. *Anesthesiology.* 2015;122:537–550.
21. Sergeev P, da Silva R, Lucchinetti E, et al. Trigger-dependent gene expression profiles in cardiac preconditioning: evidence for distinct genetic programs in ischemic and anesthetic preconditioning. *Anesthesiology.* 2004;100:474–488.
22. Lucchinetti E, da Silva R, Pasch T, et al. Anaesthetic preconditioning but not postconditioning prevents early activation of the deleterious cardiac remodelling programme: evidence of opposing genomic responses in cardioprotection by pre- and postconditioning. *Br J Anaesth.* 2005;95:140–152.
23. Lucchinetti E, Hofer C, Bestmann L, et al. Gene regulatory control of myocardial energy metabolism predicts postoperative cardiac function in patients undergoing off-pump coronary artery bypass graft surgery: inhalational versus intravenous anesthetics. *Anesthesiology.* 2007;106:444–457.
24. Lucchinetti E, Aguirre J, Feng J, et al. Molecular evidence of late preconditioning after sevoflurane inhalation in healthy volunteers. *Anesth Analg.* 2007;105:629–640.
25. Lai LP, Lin JL, Lin CS, et al. Functional genomic study on atrial fibrillation using cDNA microarray and two-dimensional protein electrophoresis techniques and identification of the myosin regulatory light chain isoform reprogramming in atrial fibrillation. *J Cardiovasc Electrophysiol.* 2004;15:214–223.
26. Barth AS, Merk S, Arnoldi E, et al. Reprogramming of the human atrial transcriptome in permanent atrial fibrillation: expression of a ventricular-like genomic signature. *Circ Res.* 2005;96:1022–1029.

27. Ramlawi B, Otu H, Mieno S, et al. Oxidative stress and atrial fibrillation after cardiac surgery: a case-control study. *Ann Thorac Surg.* 2007;84:1166–1172.
28. Ramlawi B, Otu H, Rudolph JL, et al. Genomic expression pathways associated with brain injury after cardiopulmonary bypass. *J Thorac Cardiovasc Surg.* 2007;134:996–1005.
29. Horwitz PA, Tsai EJ, Putt ME, et al. Detection of cardiac allograft rejection and response to immunosuppressive therapy with peripheral blood gene expression. *Circulation.* 2004;110:3815–3821.
30. Pham MX, Teuteberg JJ, Kfoury AG, et al. Gene-expression profiling for rejection surveillance after cardiac transplantation. *N Engl J Med.* 2010;362:1890–1900.
31. Borozdenkova S, Westbrook JA, Patel V, et al. Use of proteomics to discover novel markers of cardiac allograft rejection. *J Proteome Res.* 2004;3:282–288.
32. Rosenberg S, Elashoff MR, Beineke P, et al. Multicenter validation of the diagnostic accuracy of a blood-based gene expression test for assessing obstructive coronary artery disease in nondiabetic patients. *Ann Intern Med.* 2010;153:425–434.
33. Matkovich SJ, Van Booven DJ, Youker KA, et al. Reciprocal regulation of myocardial microRNAs and messenger RNA in human cardiomyopathy and reversal of the microRNA signature by biomechanical support. *Circulation.* 2009;119:1263–1271.
34. Tomic V, Russwurm S, Moller E, et al. Transcriptomic and proteomic patterns of systemic inflammation in on-pump and off-pump coronary artery bypass grafting. *Circulation.* 2005;112:2912–2920.
35. Liangos O, Domhan S, Schwager C, et al. Whole blood transcriptomics in cardiac surgery identifies a gene regulatory network connecting ischemia reperfusion with systemic inflammation. *PLoS One.* 2010;5:e13658.
36. Depre C, Tomlinson JE, Kudej RK, et al. Gene program for cardiac cell survival induced by transient ischemia in conscious pigs. *Proc Natl Acad Sci U S A.* 2001;98:9336–9341.
37. Atkins JH, Johansson JS. Technologies to shape the future: proteomics applications in anesthesiology and critical care medicine. *Anesth Analg.* 2006;102:1207–1216.
38. Futterer CD, Maurer MH, Schmitt A, et al. Alterations in rat brain proteins after desflurane anesthesia. *Anesthesiology.* 2004;100:302–308.
39. Kalenka A, Hinkelbein J, Feldmann RE Jr, et al. The effects of sevoflurane anesthesia on rat brain proteins: a proteomic time-course analysis. *Anesth Analg.* 2007;104:1129–1135.
40. Sheikh AM, Barrett C, Villamizar N, et al. Proteomics of cerebral injury in a neonatal model of cardiopulmonary bypass with deep hypothermic circulatory arrest. *J Thorac Cardiovasc Surg.* 2006;132:820–828.
41. Quinones QJ, Zhang Z, Ma Q, et al. Proteomic profiling reveals adaptive responses to surgical myocardial ischemia-reperfusion in hibernating arctic ground squirrels compared to rats. *Anesthesiology.* 2016;124:1296–1310.
42. Queloz PA, Thadikkaran L, Crettaz D, et al. Proteomics and transfusion medicine: future perspectives. *Proteomics.* 2006;6:5605–5614.
43. Strohmeyer JC, Blume C, Meisel C, et al. Standardized immune monitoring for the prediction of infections after cardiopulmonary bypass surgery in risk patients. *Cytometry B Clin Cytom.* 2003;53:54–62.
44. Kennedy SA, McEllistrem B, Kinsella A, et al. EuroSCORE and neutrophil adhesion molecules predict outcome post-cardiac surgery. *Eur J Clin Invest.* 2012;42:881–890.
45. Lewis GD, Wei R, Liu E, et al. Metabolite profiling of blood from individuals undergoing planned myocardial infarction reveals early markers of myocardial injury. *J Clin Invest.* 2008;118:3503–3512.
46. Turer AT, Stevens RD, Bain JR, et al. Metabolomic profiling reveals distinct patterns of myocardial substrate use in humans with coronary artery disease or left ventricular dysfunction during surgical ischemia/reperfusion. *Circulation.* 2009;119:1736–1746.
47. Mayr M, Yusuf S, Weir G, et al. Combined metabolomic and proteomic analysis of human atrial fibrillation. *J Am Coll Cardiol.* 2008;51:585–594.
48. Qiao S, Olson JM, Paterson M, et al. MicroRNA-21 Mediates isoflurane-induced cardioprotection against ischemia-reperfusion injury via Akt/nitric oxide synthase/mitochondrial permeability transition pore pathway. *Anesthesiology.* 2015;123:786–798.
49. Tabor HK, Risch NJ, Myers RM. Opinion: candidate-gene approaches for studying complex genetic traits: practical considerations. *Nat Rev Genet.* 2002;3:391–397.
50. Podgoreanu MV, White WD, Morris RW, et al. Inflammatory gene polymorphisms and risk of postoperative myocardial infarction after cardiac surgery. *Circulation.* 2006;114:I275–I281.
51. Collard CD, Shernan SK, Fox AA, et al. The MBL2 'LYQA secretor' haplotype is an independent predictor of postoperative myocardial infarction in whites undergoing coronary artery bypass graft surgery. *Circulation.* 2007;116:I106–I112.
52. Mathew JP, Podgoreanu MV, Grocott HP, et al. Genetic variants in P-selectin and C-reactive protein influence susceptibility to cognitive decline after cardiac surgery. *J Am Coll Cardiol.* 2007;49:1934–1942.
53. Mathew JP, Rinder CS, Howe JG, et al. Platelet PlA2 polymorphism enhances risk of neurocognitive decline after cardiopulmonary bypass. Multicenter Study of Perioperative Ischemia (McSPI) Research Group. *Ann Thorac Surg.* 2001;71:663–666.
54. Bartels K, Li YJ, Li YW, et al. Apolipoprotein epsilon 4 genotype is associated with less improvement in cognitive function five years after cardiac surgery: a retrospective cohort study. *Can J Anaesth.* 2015;62:618–626.
55. Stafford-Smith M, Podgoreanu M, Swaminathan M, et al. Association of genetic polymorphisms with risk of renal injury after coronary bypass graft surgery. *Am J Kidney Dis.* 2005;45:519–530.
56. Chew ST, Newman MF, White WD, et al. Preliminary report on the association of apolipoprotein E polymorphisms, with postoperative peak serum creatinine concentrations in cardiac surgical patients. *Anesthesiology.* 2000;93:325–331.
57. MacKensen GB, Swaminathan M, Ti LK, et al. Preliminary report on the interaction of apolipoprotein E polymorphism with aortic atherosclerosis and acute nephropathy after CABG. *Ann Thorac Surg.* 2004;78:520–526.
58. Ortlepp JR, Janssens U, Bleckmann F, et al. A chymase gene variant is associated with atherosclerosis in venous coronary artery bypass grafts. *Coron Artery Dis.* 2001;12:493–497.
59. Ellis SG, Chen MS, Jia G, et al. Relation of polymorphisms in five genes to long-term aortocoronary saphenous vein graft patency. *Am J Cardiol.* 2007;99:1087–1089.
60. Donahue BS. Factor V Leiden and perioperative risk. *Anesth Analg.* 2004;98:1623–1634.
61. Lasocki S, Iglarz M, Seince PF, et al. Involvement of renin-angiotensin system in pressure-flow relationship: role of angiotensin-converting enzyme gene polymorphism. *Anesthesiology.* 2002;96:271–275.
62. Stuber F, Petersen M, Bokelmann F, et al. A genomic polymorphism within the tumor necrosis factor locus influences plasma tumor necrosis factor-alpha concentrations and outcome of patients with severe sepsis. *Crit Care Med.* 1996;24:381–384.
63. Moretti EW, Morris RW, Podgoreanu M, et al. APOE polymorphism is associated with risk of severe sepsis in surgical patients. *Crit Care Med.* 2005;33:2521–2526.
64. Slavcheva E, Albanis E, Jiao Q, et al. Cytotoxic T-lymphocyte antigen 4 gene polymorphisms and susceptibility to acute allograft rejection. *Transplantation.* 2001;72:935–940.
65. The Wellcome Trust Case-Control Consortium. Genome-wide association study of 14000 cases of seven common diseases and 3000 shared controls. *Nature.* 2007;447:661–678.
66. Samani NJ, Erdmann J, Hall AS, et al. Genomewide association analysis of coronary artery disease. *N Engl J Med.* 2007;357:443–453.
67. McPherson R, Pertsemlidis A, Kavaslar N, et al. A common allele on chromosome 9 associated with coronary heart disease. *Science.* 2007;316:1488–1491.
68. Helgadottir A, Thorleifsson G, Manolescu A, et al. A common variant on chromosome 9p21 affects the risk of myocardial infarction. *Science.* 2007;316:1491–1493.
69. Todd JA, Walker NM, Cooper JD, et al. Robust associations of four new chromosome regions from genome-wide analyses of type 1 diabetes. *Nat Genet.* 2007;39:857–864.
70. Saxena R, Voight BF, Lyssenko V, et al. Genome-wide association analysis identifies loci for type 2 diabetes and triglyceride levels. *Science.* 2007;316:1331–1336.
71. Gudbjartsson DF, Arnar DO, Helgadottir A, et al. Variants conferring risk of atrial fibrillation on chromosome 4q25. *Nature.* 2007;448:353–357.
72. International Consortium for Blood Pressure Genome-Wide Association Studies, Ehret GB, Munroe PB, et al. Genetic variants in novel pathways influence blood pressure and cardiovascular disease risk. *Nature.* 2011;478:103–109.
73. Kertai MD, Li YJ, Li YW, et al.; Duke Perioperative Genetics and Safety Outcomes Investigative Team. Genome-wide association study of perioperative myocardial infarction after coronary artery bypass surgery. *BMJ Open.* 2015;5:e006920.
74. Kertai MD, Li YJ, Ji Y, et al; Duke Perioperative Genetics and Safety Outcomes Investigative Team. Genome-wide association study of new-onset atrial fibrillation after coronary artery bypass grafting surgery. *Am Heart J.* 2015;170:580–590.
75. Fox AA, Pretorius M, Liu KY, et al. Genome-wide assessment for genetic variants associated with ventricular dysfunction after primary coronary artery bypass graft surgery. *PLoS One.* 2011;6:e24593.
76. Stafford-Smith M, Li YJ, Mathew JP, et al. Genome-wide association study of acute kidney injury after coronary bypass graft surgery identifies susceptibility loci. *Kidney Int.* 2015;88:823–832.
77. Collins FS. Reengineering translational science: the time is right. *Sci Transl Med.* 2011;3:90cm17.
78. Frazer KA, Ballinger DG, Cox DR, et al. A second generation human haplotype map of over 3.1 million SNPs. *Nature.* 2007;449:851–861.
79. 1000 Genomes Project Consortium, Abecasis GR, Auton A, Brooks LD, et al. An integrated map of genetic variation from 1092 human genomes. *Nature.* 2012;491:56–65.
80. Kellis M, Wold B, Snyder MP, et al. Defining functional DNA elements in the human genome. *Proc Natl Acad Sci U S A.* 2014;111:6131–6138.
81. Welter D, MacArthur J, Morales J, et al. The NHGRI GWAS Catalog, a curated resource of SNP-trait associations. *Nucleic Acids Res.* 2014;42:D1001–D1006.
82. Kathiresan S, Willer CJ, Peloso GM, et al. Common variants at 30 loci contribute to polygenic dyslipidemia. *Nat Genet.* 2009;41:56–65.

83. Feero WG, Guttmacher AE, Collins FS. Genomic medicine: an updated primer. *N Engl J Med.* 2010;362:2001–2011.
84. Wheeler DA, Srinivasan M, Egholm M, et al. The complete genome of an individual by massively parallel DNA sequencing. *Nature.* 2008;452:872–876.
85. Ashley EA, Butte AJ, Wheeler MT, et al. Clinical assessment incorporating a personal genome. *Lancet.* 2010;375:1525–1535.
86. Cardon L, Bell JI. Association study designs for complex diseases. *Nat Rev Genet.* 2001;2:91–99.
87. Hirschhorn JN, Lohmueller K, Byrne E, et al. A comprehensive review of genetic association studies. *Genet Med.* 2002;4:45–61.
88. Beachy SH, Johnson SG, Olson S, et al.; Institute of Medicine (U.S.). *Roundtable on Translating Genomic-Based Research for Health. Assessing Genomic Sequencing Information for Health Care Decision Making: Workshop Summary.* Washington, DC: The National Academies Press; 2014.
89. Rehm HL, Berg JS, Brooks LD, et al. ClinGen: the clinical genome resource. *N Engl J Med.* 2015;372:2235–2242.
90. Shaw AD, Vaporciyan AA, Wu X, et al. Inflammatory gene polymorphisms influence risk of postoperative morbidity after lung resection. *Ann Thorac Surg.* 2005;79:1704–1710.
91. Rinder CS, Mathew JP, Rinder HM, et al. Platelet PlA2 polymorphism and platelet activation are associated with increased troponin I release after cardiopulmonary bypass. *Anesthesiology.* 2002;97:1118–1122.
92. Faraday N, Martinez EA, Scharpf RB, et al. Platelet gene polymorphisms and cardiac risk assessment in vascular surgical patients. *Anesthesiology.* 2004;101:1291–1297.
93. Tomasdottir H, Hjartarson H, Ricksten A, et al. Tumor necrosis factor gene polymorphism is associated with enhanced systemic inflammatory response and increased cardiopulmonary morbidity after cardiac surgery. *Anesth Analg.* 2003;97:944–949.
94. Galley HF, Lowe PR, Carmichael RL, et al. Genotype and interleukin-10 responses after cardiopulmonary bypass. *Br J Anaesth.* 2003;91:424–426.
95. Moor E, Silveira A, van't Hooft F, et al. Coagulation factor V (Arg506–>Gln) mutation and early saphenous vein graft occlusion after coronary artery bypass grafting. *Thromb Haemost.* 1998;80:220–224.
96. Muehlschlegel JD, Liu KY, Perry TE, et al. Chromosome 9p21 variant predicts mortality after coronary artery bypass graft surgery. *Circulation.* 2010;122: S60–S65.
97. Fox AA, Collard CD, Shernan SK, et al. Natriuretic peptide system gene variants are associated with ventricular dysfunction after coronary artery bypass grafting. *Anesthesiology.* 2009;110:738–747.
98. Rifon J, Paramo JA, Panizo C, et al. The increase of plasminogen activator inhibitor activity is associated with graft occlusion in patients undergoing aorto-coronary bypass surgery. *Br J Haematol.* 1997;99:262–267.
99. Muehlschlegel JD, Perry TE, Liu KY, et al. Polymorphism in the protease-activated receptor-4 gene region associates with platelet activation and perioperative myocardial injury. *Am J Hematol.* 2012;87:161–166.
100. Ryan R, Thornton J, Duggan E, et al. Gene polymorphism and requirement for vasopressor infusion after cardiac surgery. *Ann Thorac Surg.* 2006;82: 895–901.
101. Philip I, Plantefeve G, Vuillaumier-Barrot S, et al. G894 T polymorphism in the endothelial nitric oxide synthase gene is associated with an enhanced vascular responsiveness to phenylephrine. *Circulation.* 1999;99:3096–3098.
102. Heusch G, Erbel R, Siffert W. Genetic determinants of coronary vasomotor tone in humans. *Am J Physiol Heart Circ Physiol.* 2001;281:H1465–H1468.
103. Henrion D, Benessiano J, Philip I, et al. The deletion genotype of the angiotensin I-converting enzyme is associated with an increased vascular reactivity in vivo and in vitro. *J Am Coll Cardiol.* 1999;34:830–836.
104. Nakada TA, Russell JA, Boyd JH, et al. Association of angiotensin II type 1 receptor-associated protein gene polymorphism with increased mortality in septic shock. *Crit Care Med.* 2011;39:1641–1648.
105. Kim NS, Lee IO, Lee MK, et al. The effects of beta2 adrenoceptor gene polymorphisms on pressor response during laryngoscopy and tracheal intubation. *Anaesthesia.* 2002;57:227–232.
106. Iribarren JL, Sagasti FM, Jimenez JJ, et al. TNFbeta+250 polymorphism and hyperdynamic state in cardiac surgery with extracorporeal circulation. *Interact Cardiovasc Thorac Surg.* 2008;7:1071–1074.
107. Gaudino M, Andreotti F, Zamparelli R, et al. The -174G/C interleukin-6 polymorphism influences postoperative interleukin-6 levels and postoperative atrial fibrillation: is atrial fibrillation an inflammatory complication? *Circulation.* 2003;108(Suppl 1):II195–II199.
108. Motsinger AA, Donahue BS, Brown NJ, et al. Risk factor interactions and genetic effects associated with post-operative atrial fibrillation. *Pac Symp Biocomput.* 2006:584–595.
109. Donahue BS, Roden D. Inflammatory cytokine polymorphisms are associated with beta-blocker failure in preventing postoperative atrial fibrillation. *Anesth Analg.* 2005;100:SCA30 (abstract).
110. Body SC, Collard CD, Shernan SK, et al. Variation in the 4q25 chromosomal locus predicts atrial fibrillation after coronary artery bypass graft surgery. *Circ Cardiovasc Genet.* 2009;2:499–506.
111. Virani SS, Brautbar A, Lee VV, et al. Usefulness of single nucleotide polymorphism in chromosome 4q25 to predict in-hospital and long-term development of atrial fibrillation and survival in patients undergoing coronary artery bypass grafting. *Am J Cardiol.* 2011;107:1504–1509.
112. Kertai MD, Ji Y, Li YJ, et al. Interleukin 1-beta gene variants are associated with QTc interval prolongation following cardiac surgery. *Can J Anaesth.* 2016; 63(4):397–410.
113. Jeff JM, Donahue BS, Brown-Gentry K, et al. Genetic variation in the beta1-adrenergic receptor is associated with the risk of atrial fibrillation after cardiac surgery. *Am Heart J.* 2014;167:101–108.
114. Kertai MD, Li YW, Li YJ, et al.; Duke Perioperative G and Safety Outcomes Investigative Team. G protein-coupled receptor kinase 5 gene polymorphisms are associated with postoperative atrial fibrillation after coronary artery bypass grafting in patients receiving beta-blockers. *Circ Cardiovasc Genet.* 2014;7:625–633.
115. Zaugg M, Bestmann L, Wacker J, et al. Adrenergic receptor genotype but not perioperative bisoprolol therapy may determine cardiovascular outcome in at-risk patients undergoing surgery with spinal block. The Swiss Beta Blocker in Spinal Anesthesia (BBSA) study: a double-blinded, placebo-controlled, multi-center trial with 1-year follow-up. *Anesthesiology.* 2007;107:33–44.
116. Volzke H, Engel J, Kleine V, et al. Angiotensin I-converting enzyme insertion/deletion polymorphism and cardiac mortality and morbidity after coronary artery bypass graft surgery. *Chest.* 2002;122:31–36.
117. Zotz RB, Klein M, Dauben HP, et al. Prospective analysis after coronary-artery bypass grafting: platelet GP IIIa polymorphism (HPA-1b/PIA2) is a risk factor for bypass occlusion, myocardial infarction, and death. *Thromb Haemost.* 2000;83:404–407.
118. Botto N, Andreassi MG, Rizza A, et al. C677 T polymorphism of the methylenetetrahydrofolate reductase gene is a risk factor of adverse events after coronary revascularization. *Int J Cardiol.* 2004;96:341–345.
119. Podgoreanu MV, Booth JV, White WD, et al. Beta adrenergic receptor polymorphisms and risk of adverse events following cardiac surgery. *Circulation.* 2003;108:IV-434.
120. Delanghe J, Cambier B, Langlois M, et al. Haptoglobin polymorphism, a genetic risk factor in coronary artery bypass surgery. *Atherosclerosis.* 1997; 132:215–219.
121. Taylor KD, Scheuner MT, Yang H, et al. Lipoprotein lipase locus and progression of atherosclerosis in coronary-artery bypass grafts. *Genet Med.* 2004;6: 481–486.
122. Lobato RL, White WD, Mathew JP, et al. Thrombomodulin variants are associated with increased mortality following CABG surgery in replicated analyses. *Circulation.* 2010;122:A13651 (abstract).
123. Stoica AL, Stoica E, Constantinescu I, et al. Interleukin-6 and interleukin-10 gene polymorphism, endothelial dysfunction, and postoperative prognosis in patients with peripheral arterial disease. *J Vasc Surg.* 2010;52:103–109.
124. Holweg CT, Weimar W, Uitterlinden AG, et al. Clinical impact of cytokine gene polymorphisms in heart and lung transplantation. *J Heart Lung Transplant.* 2004;23:1017–1026.
125. Borozdenkova S, Smith J, Marshall S, et al. Identification of ICAM-1 polymorphism that is associated with protection from transplant associated vasculopathy after cardiac transplantation. *Hum Immunol.* 2001;62:247–255.
126. Vamvakopoulos JE, Taylor CJ, Green C, et al. Interleukin 1 and chronic rejection: possible genetic links in human heart allografts. *Am J Transplant.* 2002;2:76–83.
127. Benza RL, Coffey CS, Pekarek DM, et al. Transforming growth factor-beta polymorphisms and cardiac allograft rejection. *J Heart Lung Transplant.* 2009;28: 1057–1062.
128. Grocott HP, White WD, Morris RW, et al. Genetic polymorphisms and the risk of stroke after cardiac surgery. *Stroke.* 2005;36:1854–1858.
129. Tardiff BE, Newman MF, Saunders AM, et al. Preliminary report of a genetic basis for cognitive decline after cardiac operations. The Neurologic Outcome Research Group of the Duke Heart Center. *Ann Thorac Surg.* 1997;64:715–720.
130. Gaynor JW, Gerdes M, Zackai EH, et al. Apolipoprotein E genotype and neurodevelopmental sequelae of infant cardiac surgery. *J Thorac Cardiovasc Surg.* 2003;126:1736–1745.
131. Zeltser I, Jarvik GP, Bernbaum J, et al. Genetic factors are important determinants of neurodevelopmental outcome after repair of tetralogy of Fallot. *J Thorac Cardiovasc Surg.* 2008;135:91–97.
132. McDonagh DL, Mathew JP, White WD, et al. Cognitive function after major noncardiac surgery, apolipoprotein E4 genotype, and biomarkers of brain injury. *Anesthesiology.* 2010;112:852–859.
133. Leung JM, Sands LP, Wang Y, et al. Apolipoprotein E e4 allele increases the risk of early postoperative delirium in older patients undergoing noncardiac surgery. *Anesthesiology.* 2007;107:406–411.
134. Ely EW, Girard TD, Shintani AK, et al. Apolipoprotein E4 polymorphism as a genetic predisposition to delirium in critically ill patients. *Crit Care Med.* 2007;35:112–117.
135. van Munster BC, de Rooij SE, Yazdanpanah M, et al. The association of the dopamine transporter gene and the dopamine receptor 2 gene with delirium, a meta-analysis. *Am J Med Genet B Neuropsychiatr Genet.* 2010;153B:648–655.
136. Donahue BS, Gailani D, Higgins MS, et al. Factor V Leiden protects against blood loss and transfusion after cardiac surgery. *Circulation.* 2003;107: 1003–1008.

137. Duggan E, O'Dwyer MJ, Caraher E, et al. Coagulopathy after cardiac surgery may be influenced by a functional plasminogen activator inhibitor polymorphism. *Anesth Analg.* 2007;104:1343–1347.
138. Welsby IJ, Podgoreanu MV, Phillips-Bute B, et al. Genetic factors contribute to bleeding after cardiac surgery. *J Thromb Haemost.* 2005;3:1206–1212.
139. Greiff G, Pleym H, Stenseth R, et al. Genetic variation influences the risk of bleeding after cardiac surgery: novel associations and validation of previous findings. *Acta Anaesthesiol Scand.* 2015;59:796–806.
140. Morawski W, Sanak M, Cisowski M, et al. Prediction of the excessive perioperative bleeding in patients undergoing coronary artery bypass grafting: role of aspirin and platelet glycoprotein IIIa polymorphism. *J Thorac Cardiovasc Surg.* 2005;130:791–796.
141. Welsby IJ, Podgoreanu MV, Phillips-Bute B, et al. Association of the 98 T ELAM-1 polymorphism with increased bleeding after cardiac surgery. *J Cardiothorac Vasc Anesth.* 2010;24:427–433.
142. Achrol AS, Kim H, Pawlikowska L, et al. Association of tumor necrosis factor-alpha-238G>A and apolipoprotein E2 polymorphisms with intracranial hemorrhage after brain arteriovenous malformation treatment. *Neurosurgery.* 2007;61:731–739.
143. Howell SJ, Sear JW. Perioperative myocardial injury: individual and population implications. *Br J Anaesth.* 2004;93:3–8.
144. Mangano DT. Effects of acadesine on myocardial infarction, stroke, and death following surgery. A meta-analysis of the 5 international randomized trials. The Multicenter Study of Perioperative Ischemia (McSPI) Research Group. *JAMA.* 1997;277:325–332.
145. Mahaffey KW, Roe MT, Kilaru R, et al. Creatine kinase-MB elevation after coronary artery bypass grafting surgery in patients with non-ST-segment elevation acute coronary syndromes predict worse outcomes: results from four large clinical trials. *Eur Heart J.* 2007;28:425–432.
146. Landesberg G, Beattie WS, Mosseri M, et al. Perioperative myocardial infarction. *Circulation.* 2009;119:2936–2944.
147. Brull DJ, Montgomery HE, Sanders J, et al. Interleukin-6 gene -174 g>c and -572 g>c promoter polymorphisms are strong predictors of plasma interleukin-6 levels after coronary artery bypass surgery. *Arterioscler Thromb Vasc Biol.* 2001;21:1458–1463.
148. Burzotta F, Iacoviello L, Di Castelnuovo A, et al. Relation of the -174 G/C polymorphism of interleukin-6 to interleukin-6 plasma levels and to length of hospitalization after surgical coronary revascularization. *Am J Cardiol.* 2001;88:1125–1128.
149. Grocott HP, Newman MF, El-Moalem H, et al. Apolipoprotein E genotype differentially influences the proinflammatory and anti-inflammatory response to cardiopulmonary bypass. *J Thorac Cardiovasc Surg.* 2001;122:622–623.
150. Roth-Isigkeit A, Hasselbach L, Ocklitz E, et al. Inter-individual differences in cytokine release in patients undergoing cardiac surgery with cardiopulmonary bypass. *Clin Exp Immunol.* 2001;125:80–88.
151. Boehm J, Hauner K, Grammer J, et al. Tumor necrosis factor-alpha -863 C/A promoter polymorphism affects the inflammatory response after cardiac surgery. *Eur J Cardiothorac Surg.* 2011;40:e50–e54.
152. Lehmann LE, Schroeder S, Hartmann W, et al. A single nucleotide polymorphism of macrophage migration inhibitory factor is related to inflammatory response in coronary bypass surgery using cardiopulmonary bypass. *Eur J Cardiothorac Surg.* 2006;30:59–63.
153. Willerson JT, Ridker PM. Inflammation as a cardiovascular risk factor. *Circulation.* 2004;109:II2–II10.
154. Perry TE, Muehlschlegel JD, Liu KY, et al. Preoperative C-reactive protein predicts long-term mortality and hospital length of stay after primary, nonemergent coronary artery bypass grafting. *Anesthesiology.* 2010;112:607–613.
155. Kangasniemi OP, Biancari F, Luukkonen J, et al. Preoperative C-reactive protein is predictive of long-term outcome after coronary artery bypass surgery. *Eur J Cardiothorac Surg.* 2006;29:983–985.
156. Song Y, Kwak YL, Choi YS, et al. Effect of preoperative statin therapy on myocardial protection and morbidity endpoints following off-pump coronary bypass surgery in patients with elevated C-reactive protein level. *Korean J Anesthesiol.* 2010;58:136–141.
157. Choi JH, Cho DK, Song YB, et al. Preoperative NT-proBNP and CRP predict perioperative major cardiovascular events in non-cardiac surgery. *Heart.* 2010;96:56–62.
158. Perry TE, Muehlschlegel JD, Liu KY, et al. C-Reactive protein gene variants are associated with postoperative C-reactive protein levels after coronary artery bypass surgery. *BMC Med Genet.* 2009;10:38.
159. Motoyama S, Miura M, Hinai Y, et al. C-reactive protein 1059G>C genetic polymorphism influences serum C-reactive protein levels after esophagectomy in patients with thoracic esophageal cancer. *J Am Coll Surg.* 2009;209:477–483.
160. Motoyama S, Miura M, Hinai Y, et al. C-reactive protein -717 C>T genetic polymorphism associates with esophagectomy-induced stress hyperglycemia. *World J Surg.* 2010;34:1001–1007.
161. Voetsch B, Loscalzo J. Genetic determinants of arterial thrombosis. *Arterioscler Thromb Vasc Biol.* 2004;24:216–229.
162. Iacoviello L, Burzotta F, Di Castelnuovo A, et al. The 4G/5G polymorphism of PAI-1 promoter gene and the risk of myocardial infarction: a meta-analysis. *Thromb Haemost.* 1998;80:1029–1030.
163. Karthikeyan G, Moncur RA, Levine O, et al. Is a pre-operative brain natriuretic peptide or N-terminal pro-B-type natriuretic peptide measurement an independent predictor of adverse cardiovascular outcomes within 30 days of noncardiac surgery? A systematic review and meta-analysis of observational studies. *J Am Coll Cardiol.* 2009;54:1599–1606.
164. Ryding AD, Kumar S, Worthington AM, et al. Prognostic value of brain natriuretic peptide in noncardiac surgery: a meta-analysis. *Anesthesiology.* 2009;111:311–319.
165. Fox AA, Shernan SK, Collard CD, et al. Preoperative B-type natriuretic peptide is as independent predictor of ventricular dysfunction and mortality after primary coronary artery bypass grafting. *J Thorac Cardiovasc Surg.* 2008;136:452–461.
166. Fox AA, Muehlschlegel JD, Body SC, et al. Comparison of the utility of preoperative versus postoperative B-type natriuretic peptide for predicting hospital length of stay and mortality after primary coronary artery bypass grafting. *Anesthesiology.* 2010;112:842–851.
167. Barnet CS, Liu X, Body SC, et al. Plasma corin decreases after coronary artery bypass graft surgery and is associated with postoperative heart failure: a pilot study. *J Cardiothorac Vasc Anesth.* 2015;29:374–381.
168. Poldermans D, Bax JJ, Boersma E, et al. Guidelines for pre-operative cardiac risk assessment and perioperative cardiac management in non-cardiac surgery. *Eur Heart J.* 2009;30:2769–2812.
169. Shaw SM, Lewis NT, Williams SG, et al. A role for BNP assays in monitoring aortic valve disease for optimal timing of surgery. *Int J Cardiol.* 2008;127:328–330.
170. Zaugg M, Schaub MC. Genetic modulation of adrenergic activity in the heart and vasculature: implications for perioperative medicine. *Anesthesiology.* 2005;102:429–446.
171. Loukanov T, Hoss K, Tonchev P, et al. Endothelial nitric oxide synthase gene polymorphism (Glu298Asp) and acute pulmonary hypertension post cardiopulmonary bypass in children with congenital cardiac diseases. *Cardiol Young.* 2011;21:161–169.
172. Panagiotopoulos I, Palatianos G, Michalopoulos A, et al. Alterations in biomarkers of endothelial function following on-pump coronary artery revascularization. *J Clin Lab Anal.* 2010;24:389–398.
173. Stoppelkamp S, Veseli K, Stang K, et al. Identification of predictive early biomarkers for sterile-SIRS after cardiovascular surgery. *PLoS One.* 2015;10:e0135527.
174. Enger TB, Pleym H, Stenseth R, et al. Genetic and clinical risk factors for fluid overload following open-heart surgery. *Acta Anaesthesiol Scand.* 2014;58:539–548.
175. Smiley RM, Blouin JL, Negron M, et al. Beta2-adrenoceptor genotype affects vasopressor requirements during spinal anesthesia for cesarean delivery. *Anesthesiology.* 2006;104:644–650.
176. Liu KY, Muehlschlegel JD, Perry TE, et al. Common genetic variants on chromosome 9p21 predict perioperative myocardial injury after coronary artery bypass graft surgery. *J Thorac Cardiovasc Surg.* 2010;139:483–488.
177. Mathew JP, Fontes ML, Tudor IC, et al. A multicenter risk index for atrial fibrillation after cardiac surgery. *JAMA.* 2004;291:1720–1729.
178. Gaudino M, Di Castelnuovo A, Zamparelli R, et al. Genetic control of postoperative systemic inflammatory reaction and pulmonary and renal complications after coronary artery surgery. *J Thorac Cardiovasc Surg.* 2003;126:1107–1112.
179. Hogue CW Jr, Palin CA, Kailasam R, et al. C-reactive protein levels and atrial fibrillation after cardiac surgery in women. *Ann Thorac Surg.* 2006;82:97–102.
180. Pretorius M, Donahue BS, Yu C, et al. Plasminogen activator inhibitor-1 as a predictor of postoperative atrial fibrillation after cardiopulmonary bypass. *Circulation.* 2007;116:I1–I7.
181. Kertai MD, Qi W, Li YJ, et al.; Duke Perioperative G and Safety Outcomes Investigative Team. Gene signatures of postoperative atrial fibrillation in atrial tissue after coronary artery bypass grafting surgery in patients receiving beta-blockers. *J Mol Cell Cardiol.* 2016;92:109–115.
182. Newman MF, Booth JV, Laskowitz DT, et al. Genetic predictors of perioperative neurological and cognitive injury and recovery. *Best Pract Res Clin Anesthesiol.* 2001;15:247–276.
183. Alberts MJ, Graffagnino C, McClenny C, et al. ApoE genotype and survival from intracerebral haemorrhage. *Lancet.* 1995;346:575.
184. Teasdale GM, Nicoll JA, Murray G, et al. Association of apolipoprotein E polymorphism with outcome after head injury. *Lancet.* 1997;350:1069–1071.
185. Slooter AJ, Tang MX, van Duijn CM, et al. Apolipoprotein E epsilon4 and the risk of dementia with stroke. A population-based investigation. *JAMA.* 1997;277:818–821.
186. Sheng H, Laskowitz DT, Bennett E, et al. Apolipoprotein E isoform-specific differences in outcome from focal ischemia in transgenic mice. *J Cereb Blood Flow Metab.* 1998;18:361–366.
187. Ti LK, Mathew JP, Mackensen GB, et al. Effect of apolipoprotein E genotype on cerebral autoregulation during cardiopulmonary bypass. *Stroke.* 2001;32:1514–1519.
188. Ti LK, Mackensen GB, Grocott HP, et al. Apolipoprotein E4 increases aortic atheroma burden in cardiac surgical patients. *J Thorac Cardiovasc Surg.* 2003;125:211–213.

189. Newman MF, Laskowitz DT, White WD, et al. Apolipoprotein E polymorphisms and age at first coronary artery bypass graft. *Anesth Analg.* 2001;92:824–829.
190. Weiss EJ, Bray PF, Tayback M, et al. A polymorphism of a platelet glycoprotein receptor as an inherited risk factor for coronary thrombosis. *N Engl J Med.* 1996;334:1090–1094.
191. Carter AM, Catto AJ, Bamford JM, et al. Platelet GP IIIa PlA and GP Ib variable number tandem repeat polymorphisms and markers of platelet activation in acute stroke. *Arterioscler Thromb Vasc Biol.* 1998;18:1124–1131.
192. Ramlawi B, Rudolph JL, Mieno S, et al. Serologic markers of brain injury and cognitive function after cardiopulmonary bypass. *Ann Surg.* 2006;244:593–601.
193. Ramlawi B, Rudolph JL, Mieno S, et al. C-Reactive protein and inflammatory response associated to neurocognitive decline following cardiac surgery. *Surgery.* 2006;140:221–226.
194. Heider P, Poppert H, Wolf O, et al. Fibrinogen and high-sensitive C-reactive protein as serologic predictors for perioperative cerebral microembolic lesions after carotid endarterectomy. *J Vasc Surg.* 2007;46:449–454.
195. Mangano CM, Diamondstone LS, Ramsay JG, et al. Renal dysfunction after myocardial revascularization: risk factors, adverse outcomes, and hospital resource utilization. The Multicenter Study of Perioperative Ischemia Research Group. *Ann Intern Med.* 1998;128:194–203.
196. Yende S, Wunderink R. Causes of prolonged mechanical ventilation after coronary artery bypass surgery. *Chest.* 2002;122:245–252.
197. Rigat B, Hubert C, Alhenc-Gelas F, et al. An insertion/deletion polymorphism in the angiotensin I-converting enzyme gene accounting for half the variance of serum enzyme levels. *J Clin Invest.* 1990;86:1343–1346.
198. Yende S, Quasney MW, Tolley EA, et al. Clinical relevance of angiotensin-converting enzyme gene polymorphisms to predict risk of mechanical ventilation after coronary artery bypass graft surgery. *Crit Care Med.* 2004;32:922–927.
199. Marshall RP, Webb S, Bellingan GJ, et al. Angiotensin converting enzyme insertion/deletion polymorphism is associated with susceptibility and outcome in acute respiratory distress syndrome. *Am J Respir Crit Care Med.* 2002;166:646–650.
200. Yende S, Quasney MW, Tolley E, et al. Association of tumor necrosis factor gene polymorphisms and prolonged mechanical ventilation after coronary artery bypass surgery. *Crit Care Med.* 2003;31:133–140.
201. Shi S, Chen C, Zhao D, et al. The role of plasma gelsolin in cardiopulmonary bypass induced acute lung injury in infants and young children: a pilot study. *BMC Anesthesiol.* 2014;14:67.
202. Liu X, Chen Q, Shi S, et al. Plasma sRAGE enables prediction of acute lung injury after cardiac surgery in children. *Crit Care.* 2012;16:R91.
203. Roden DM. Cardiovascular pharmacogenomics. *Circulation.* 2003;108:3071–3074.
204. Lehmann H, Ryan E. The familial incidence of low pseudocholinesterase level. *Lancet.* 1956;271:124.
205. Bukaveckas BL, Valdes R Jr, Linder MW. Pharmacogenetics as related to the practice of cardiothoracic and vascular anesthesia. *J Cardiothorac Vasc Anesth.* 2004;18:353–365.
206. Pessah IN, Allen PD. Malignant hyperthermia. *Best Pract Res Clin Anaesthesiol.* 2001;15:277–288.
207. Eger EI II. *Anesthetic uptake and action.* Baltimore: Williams & Wilkins; 1974.
208. Ezri T, Sessler D, Weisenberg M, et al. Association of ethnicity with the minimum alveolar concentration of sevoflurane. *Anesthesiology.* 2007;107:9–14.
209. Gerstin KM, Gong DH, Abdallah M, et al. Mutation of KCNK5 or Kir3.2 potassium channels in mice does not change minimum alveolar anesthetic concentration. *Anesth Analg.* 2003;96:1345–1349.
210. Sonner JM, Antognini JF, Dutton RC, et al. Inhaled anesthetics and immobility: mechanisms, mysteries, and minimum alveolar anesthetic concentration. *Anesth Analg.* 2003;97:718–740.
211. Sternberg WF, Mogil JF. Genetic and hormonal basis of pain states. *Best Pract Res Clin Anaesthesiol.* 2001;15:229–245.
212. Diatchenko L, Anderson AD, Slade GD, et al. Three major haplotypes of the beta2 adrenergic receptor define psychological profile, blood pressure, and the risk for development of a common musculoskeletal pain disorder. *Am J Med Genet B Neuropsychiatr Genet.* 2006;141:449–462.
213. Diatchenko L, Nackley AG, Tchivileva IE, et al. Genetic architecture of human pain perception. *Trends Genet.* 2007;23:605–613.
214. Bengtsson B, Thorson J. Back pain: a study of twins. *Acta Genet Med Gemellol (Roma).* 1991;40:83–90.
215. Mogil JS, Wilson SG, Bon K, et al. Heritability of nociception I: responses of 11 inbred mouse strains on 12 measures of nociception. *Pain.* 1999;80:67–82.
216. Lacroix-Fralish ML, Ledoux JB, Mogil JS. The Pain Genes Database: An interactive web browser of pain-related transgenic knockout studies. *Pain.* 2007;131:3–4.
217. Somogyi AA, Barratt DT, Coller JK. Pharmacogenetics of opioids. *Clin Pharmacol Ther.* 2007;81:429–444.
218. Diatchenko L, Nackley AG, Slade GD, et al. Catechol-O-methyltransferase gene polymorphisms are associated with multiple pain-evoking stimuli. *Pain.* 2006;125:216–224.
219. Candiotti KA, Birnbach DJ, Lubarsky DA, et al. The impact of pharmacogenomics on postoperative nausea and vomiting: do CYP2D6 allele copy number and polymorphisms affect the success or failure of ondansetron prophylaxis? *Anesthesiology.* 2005;102:543–549.
220. Kaiser R, Sezer O, Papies A, et al. Patient-tailored antiemetic treatment with 5-hydroxytryptamine type 3 receptor antagonists according to cytochrome P-450 2D6 genotypes. *J Clin Oncol.* 2002;20:2805–2811.
221. Stamer UM, Lee EH, Rauers NI, et al. CYP2D6- and CYP3 A-dependent enantioselective plasma concentrations of ondansetron in postanesthesia care. *Anesth Analg.* 2011;113:48–54.
222. Abohelaika S, Wynne H, Cope L, et al. The impact of genetics on the management of patients on warfarin awaiting surgery. *Age Ageing.* 2015;44:721–722.
223. Nagele P, Liggett SB. Genetic variation, beta-blockers, and perioperative myocardial infarction. *Anesthesiology.* 2011;115:1316–1327.
224. Devereaux PJ, Yang H, Yusuf S, et al. Effects of extended-release metoprolol succinate in patients undergoing non-cardiac surgery (POISE trial): a randomised controlled trial. *Lancet.* 2008;371:1839–1847.
225. Liao KP, Cai T, Savova GK, et al. Development of phenotype algorithms using electronic medical records and incorporating natural language processing. *BMJ.* 2015;350:h1885.
226. Castaneda C, Nalley K, Mannion C, et al. Clinical decision support systems for improving diagnostic accuracy and achieving precision medicine. *J Clin Bioinforma.* 2015;5:4.
227. Phimister EG. Medicine and the racial divide. *N Engl J Med.* 2003;348:1081–1082.

7 Experimental Design and Statistics

NATHAN LEON PACE

Introduction
Foundations
    Data Structure
    Descriptive Statistics
    Central Location
    Spread or Variability
    Types of Research Design
Experimental Medicine: Management of Bias
    Sampling
    Experimental Constraints
    Control Groups
    Random Allocation of Treatment Groups
    Blinding
Experimental Medicine: Statistical Analysis
    Hypothesis Formulation
    Logic of Proof
    Sample Size Calculations

Inferential Statistics
    The Fickle P Value
    The Bayesian Alternative
Experimental Medicine: Statistical Tests
    Interval Data
    Binary Variables
    Linear Regression
    Epidemiology
    Multivariable Linear Regression
    Univariable and Multivariable Logistic Regression
    Propensity Score Matching and Analysis
    Systematic Reviews and Meta-analyses
    Big Data
Conclusions
    Interpretation of Results
    Statistical Resources
    Statistics and Anesthesia

KEY POINTS

1. Statistics and mathematics are the language of scientific medicine.
2. Good research planning includes a clear biologic hypothesis, the specification of outcome variables, the choice of anticipated statistical methods, and sample size planning.
3. To minimize the risk of bias in clinical research of interventions, the crucial elements of good research design include concurrent control groups; random allocation of subjects to treatment groups; concealment of random allocation; blinding of treatment assignment to patients, caregivers, and outcome assessors; and full reporting of outcomes for all study patients.
4. Visual presentation of data by graphs, descriptive statistics (e.g., mean, standard deviation), and inferential statistics (e.g., t test, confidence interval) are all essential methods for the presentation of research results.
5. Bayesian statistical methods report research results as a function of both observed data and historical (prior) knowledge; the more common Frequentist statistical methods report research results only as a function of observed data.
6. Multivariable logistic regression and propensity score matching are statistical techniques for identifying associations between risk factors and outcomes in nonrandomized studies.
7. Systematic review and meta-analysis summarize the results of individual studies and permit more powerful inferences for the comparison of interventions.
8. Anesthesia data does not yet have the Volume, Velocity, and Variety characteristics of Big Data.
9. Resources and guidance for experimental design and statistical methods include policy statements, textbooks, journal articles, and public domain software.

Introduction

If a physician is to be a practitioner of scientific medicine, he or she must read the language of science to be able to independently assess and interpret the scientific report. Without exception, the language of the medical report is increasingly statistical. Readers of the anesthesia literature, whether in a community hospital or a university environment, cannot and should not totally depend on the editors of journals to banish all errors of statistical analysis and interpretation. In addition, there are regularly questions about simple statistics in examinations required for anesthesiologists. Finally, certain statistical methods have everyday applications in clinical medicine. This chapter briefly scans some elements of experimental design and statistical analysis.

Foundations

Statistics is a method for working with *sets* of numbers. Statistics involves the description of number sets, the comparison of number sets with theoretical models, comparison between number sets, and comparison of recently acquired number sets with those from the past. A typical scientific hypothesis asks which of two methods (treatments), X and Y, is better. Statistical methods are necessary because there are sources of variation in any data set, including random biologic variation and measurement error. These errors in the data cause difficulties in avoiding bias and in being precise. Bias keeps the true value from being known and fosters incorrect decisions; precision deals with the problem of the data scatter and with quantifying the uncertainty about the value in the population from which a sample is drawn. These statistical methods are relatively independent of the particular field of study.

Data Structure

Data collected in an experiment include the defining characteristics of the experiment and the values of events or attributes that vary over time or conditions. The former are called *explanatory variables* and the latter are called *response variables*. Variables such as gender, age, and doses of accompanying drugs reflect the variability of the experimental subjects. Explanatory variables, it is hoped, explain the systematic variations in the response variables. In a sense, the response variables depend on the explanatory variables.

Response variables are also called *dependent variables*. Response variables reflect the primary properties of experimental interest in the subjects. Research in anesthesiology is particularly likely to have repeated measurement variables; that is, a particular measurement recorded more than once for each individual. Some variables can be both explanatory and response; these are called *intermediate response variables*. Suppose an experiment is conducted comparing electrocardiography and myocardial responses between five doses of an opioid. One might analyze how ST segments depended on the dose of opioids; here, maximum ST segment depression is a response variable. Maximum ST segment depression might also be used as an explanatory variable to address the subtler question of the extent to which the effect of an opioid dose on postoperative myocardial infarction can be accounted for by ST segment changes.

The mathematical characteristics of the possible values of a variable fit into five classifications (Table 7-1). Properly assigning a variable to the correct data type is essential for choosing the correct statistical technique. For *interval variables*, there is equal distance between successive intervals; the difference between 15 and 10 is the same as the difference between 25 and 20. *Discrete interval data* can have only integer values; for example, number of living children. *Continuous interval data* are measured on a continuum and can be a decimal fraction; for example, blood pressure can be described as accurately as desired (e.g., 136, 136.1, or 136.14 mmHg). The same statistical techniques are used for discrete and continuous data.

Putting observations into two or more discrete categories derives *categorical variables*; for statistical analysis, numeric values are assigned as labels to the categories. *Dichotomous data* allow only two possible values; for example, male versus female. *Ordinal data* have three or more categories that can logically be ranked or ordered; however, the ranking or ordering of the variable indicates only relative and not absolute differences between values; there is not necessarily the same difference between American Society of Anesthesiologists Physical Status score I and II as there is between III and IV. Although ordinal data are often treated as interval data in choosing a statistical technique, such analysis may be suspect; alternative techniques for ordinal data are available. *Nominal variables* are placed into categories that have no logical ordering. The eye colors blue, hazel, and brown might be assigned the numbers 1, 2, and 3, but it is nonsense to say that blue is lower than hazel is lower than brown.

Descriptive Statistics

Although the results of a particular experiment might be presented by repeatedly showing the entire set of numbers, there are concise ways of summarizing the information content of the data set into a few numbers. These numbers are called *sample* or *summary statistics*; summary statistics are calculated using the numbers of the sample. By convention, the symbols of summary statistics are roman letters. The two summary statistics most frequently used for interval variables are the *central location* and the *variability*, but there are other summary statistics. Other data types have analogous summary statistics. Although the first purpose of descriptive statistics is to describe the sample of numbers obtained, there is also the desire to use the summary statistics from the sample to characterize the population from which the sample was obtained. The population also has measures of central location and variability called the *parameters* of the population; Greek letters denote population parameters. Usually, the population parameters cannot be directly calculated because data from all population members cannot be obtained. The beauty of properly chosen summary statistics is that they are the best possible estimators of the population parameters.

These sampling statistics can be used in conjunction with a probability density function to provide additional descriptions of the sample and its population. Also commonly described as a probability distribution, a probability density function is an algebraic equation, $f(x)$, which gives a theoretical percentage distribution of x. Each value of x has a probability of occurrence given by $f(x)$. The most important probability distribution is the *normal* or *Gaussian function* $f(x) = \frac{1}{\sqrt{2\pi\sigma^2}} \exp\left[-\frac{1}{2}\left(\frac{x-\mu}{\sigma}\right)^2\right]$. There are two parameters (population mean and population variance) in the equation of the normal function that are denoted μ and σ^2. Often called the *normal equation*, it can be plotted and produces the familiar bell-shaped curve. Why are the mathematical properties of this curve so important to biostatistics? First, it has been empirically noted that when a biologic variable is sampled repeatedly, the pattern of the numbers plotted as a histogram resembles the normal curve; thus, most biologic data are said to follow or to obey a normal distribution. Second, if it is reasonable to assume that a sample is from a normal population, the mathematical properties of the normal equation can be used with the sampling statistic estimators of the population parameters

Table 7-1 Data Types

Data Type	Definition	Examples
Interval		
Discrete	Data measured with an integer only scale	Parity, number of teeth
Continuous	Data measured with a constant scale interval	Blood pressure, temperature
Categorical		
Dichotomous	Binary data	Mortality, gender
Nominal	Qualitative data that cannot be ordered or ranked	Eye color, drug category
Ordinal	Data ordered, ranked, or measured without a constant scale interval	ASA physical status score, pain score

to describe the sample and the population. Third, a mathematical theorem (the central limit theorem) allows the use of the assumption of normality for certain purposes, even if the population is not normally distributed.

Central Location

The three most common summary statistics of central location for interval variables are the arithmetic *mean*, the *median*, and the *mode*. The mean is merely the average of the numbers in the data set. Being a summary statistic of the sample, the arithmetic mean is denoted by the Roman letter x under a bar or $\bar{x} = \frac{1}{n}\sum_{i=1}^{n} x_i$ where i is the index of summation and n is the count of objects in the sample. If all values in the population could be obtained, then the population mean μ could be calculated similarly. Because all values of the population cannot be obtained, the sample mean is used. (Statisticians describe the sample mean as the unbiased, consistent, minimum variance, sufficient estimator of the population mean. Thus, the sample mean $\bar{x}$ is the estimator of the population mean μ.)

The median is the middlemost number or the number that divides the sample into two equal parts—first, ranking the sample values from lowest to highest and then counting up halfway to obtain the median. The concept of ranking is used in nonparametric statistics. A virtue of the median is that it is hardly affected by a few extremely high or low values. The mode is the most popular number of a sample; that is, the number that occurs most frequently. A sample may have ties for the most common value and be bi- or polymodal; these modes may be widely separated or adjacent. The raw data should be inspected for this unusual appearance. The mode is always mentioned in discussions of descriptive statistics, but it is rarely used in statistical practice.

Spread or Variability

Any set of interval data has variability unless all the numbers are identical. The range of ages from lowest to highest expresses the largest difference. This spread, diversity, and variability can also be expressed in a concise manner. Variability is specified by calculating the *deviation* or *deviate* of each individual x_i from the center (mean) of all the x_i's. The *sum of the squared deviates* is always positive unless all set values are identical. This sum is then divided by the number of individual measurements. The result is the *average squared deviation*; the average squared deviation is ubiquitous in statistics.

The concept of describing the spread of a set of numbers by calculating the average distance from each number to the center of the numbers applies to both a sample and a population; this average squared distance is called the *variance*. The population variance is a parameter and is represented by σ^2. As with the population mean, the population variance is not usually known and cannot be calculated. Just as the sample mean is used in place of the population mean, the sample variance is used in place of the population variance. The sample variance is $VAR = SD^2 = \frac{\sum_{i=1}^{n}(x_i - \bar{x})^2}{(n-1)}$.

Statistical theory demonstrates that if the divisor in the formula for SD^2 is $(n-1)$ rather than n, the sample variance is an unbiased estimator of the population variance. Although the variance is used extensively in statistical calculations, the units of variance are squared units of the original observations. The square root of the variance has the same units as the original observations; the square roots of the sample and population variances are called the *sample (SD)* and *population (σ) standard deviations*.

It was previously mentioned that most biologic observations appear to come from populations with normal distributions. By accepting this assumption of a normal distribution, further meaning can be given to the sample summary statistics (mean and SD) that have been calculated. This involves the use of the expression $\bar{x} \pm k \times SD$ where $k = 1, 2, 3$, and so forth. If the population from which the sample is taken is unimodal and roughly symmetric, then the bounds for 1, 2, and 3 encompasses roughly 68%, 95%, and 99% of the sample and population members.

Types of Research Design

Ultimately, research design consists of choosing what subjects to study, what experimental conditions and constraints to enforce, and which observations to collect at what intervals. A few key features in this research design largely determine the strength of scientific inference on the collected data. These key features allow the classification of research reports (Table 7-2). This classification reveals the variety of experimental approaches and indicates strengths and weaknesses of the same design applied to many research problems.

The first distinction is between *longitudinal* and *cross-sectional* studies. The former is the study of changes over time, whereas the latter describes a phenomenon at a certain point in time. For example, reporting the frequency with which certain drugs are used during anesthesia is a cross-sectional study, whereas investigating the hemodynamic effects of different drugs during anesthesia is a longitudinal one.

Longitudinal studies are next classified by the method with which the research subjects are selected. These methods for choosing research subjects can be either *prospective* or *retrospective*; these two approaches are also known as *cohort* (prospective) or *case-control* (retrospective). A prospective study assembles groups of subjects by some input characteristic that is thought to change an output characteristic; a typical input characteristic would be the opioid drug administered during anesthesia; for example, remifentanil or fentanyl. A retrospective study gathers subjects by an output characteristic; an output characteristic is the status of the subject after an event; for example, the occurrence of a myocardial infarction. A prospective (cohort) study would be one in which a group of patients undergoing neurologic surgery was divided in two groups, given two different opioids (remifentanil or fentanyl), and followed for the development of a perioperative myocardial infarction. In a retrospective (case-control) study, patients who suffered a perioperative myocardial infarction would be identified from hospital records; a group of subjects of similar age, gender, and disease who did not suffer a

Table 7-2 Classification of Clinical Research Reports

I. Longitudinal studies
   A. Prospective (cohort) studies
      1. Studies of deliberate intervention
         a. Concurrent controls
         b. Historical controls
      2. Observational studies
   B. Retrospective (case-control) studies
II. Cross-sectional studies

perioperative myocardial infarction also would be chosen, and the two groups would then be compared for the relative use of the two opioids (remifentanil or fentanyl). Retrospective studies are a primary tool of epidemiology. A case-control study can often identify an association between an input and output characteristic, but the causal link or relationship between the two is more difficult to specify.

Prospective studies are further divided into those in which the investigator performs a deliberate intervention and those in which the investigator merely observes. In a study of *deliberate intervention,* the investigator would choose several anesthetic maintenance techniques and compare the incidence of postoperative nausea and vomiting. If it were performed as an *observational study,* the investigator would observe a group of patients receiving anesthetics chosen at the discretion of each patient's anesthesiologist and compare the risk of postoperative nausea and vomiting among the anesthetics used. Obviously, in this example of an observational study, there has been an intervention; an anesthetic has been given. The crucial distinction is whether the investigator controlled the intervention. An observational study may reveal differences among treatment groups, but whether such differences are the consequence of the treatments or of other differences among the patients receiving the treatments will remain obscure. The comparison of cohorts with interventions not assigned under experimental control is a prominent technique of epidemiology.

Studies of deliberate intervention are further subdivided into those with concurrent controls and those with historical controls. Concurrent controls are either a simultaneous parallel control group or a self-control study; historical controls include previous studies and literature reports. A *randomized controlled trial* (RCT) is thus a longitudinal, prospective study of deliberate intervention with concurrent controls.

Although most of this discussion about experimental design has focused on human experimentation, the same principles apply and should be followed in animal experimentation. The randomized, controlled clinical trial is the most potent scientific tool for evaluating medical treatment; randomization into treatment groups is relied on to equally weigh the subjects of the treatment groups for baseline attributes that might predispose or protect the subjects from the outcome of interest.

Experimental Medicine: Management of Bias

Case reports engender interest, suspicion, doubt, wonder, and perhaps the desire to experiment; however, the case report is not sufficient evidence to advance scientific medicine. The experimenter attempts to constrain and control, as much as possible, the environment in which he or she collects numbers to test a hypothesis. The elements of experimental design are intended to prevent and minimize the possibility of bias, that is, a deviation of results or inferences from the truth.

Sampling

Two words of great importance to statisticians are *population* and *sample.* In statistical language, each has a specialized meaning. Instead of referring only to the count of individuals in a geographic or political region, population refers to any target group of things (animate or inanimate) in which there is interest. For anesthesia researchers, a typical target population might be mothers in the first stage of labor or head-trauma victims undergoing craniotomy. A target population could also be cell cultures or hospital bills. A sample is a subset of the target population. Samples are taken because of the impossibility of observing the entire population; it is generally not affordable, convenient, or practical to examine more than a relatively small fraction of the population. Nevertheless, the researcher wishes to generalize from the results of the small sample group to the entire population.

Although the subjects of a population are alike in at least one way, these population members are generally quite diverse in other ways. Because the researcher can work only with a subset of the population, he or she hopes that the sample of subjects in the experiment is representative of the population's diversity. Head-injury patients can have open or closed wounds, a variety of coexisting diseases, and normal or increased intracranial pressure. These subgroups within a population are called *strata.* Often the researcher wishes to increase the sameness or homogeneity of the target population by further restricting it to just a few strata; perhaps only closed and not open head injuries will be included. Restricting the target population to eliminate too much diversity must be balanced against the desire to have the results be applicable to the broadest possible population of patients.

The best hope for a representative sample of the population would be realized if every subject in the population had the same chance of being observed; this is called *random sampling.* If there were several strata of importance, random sampling from each stratum would be appropriate. Unfortunately, in most clinical anesthesia studies researchers are limited to using those patients who happen to show up at their hospitals; this is called *convenience sampling.* Convenience sampling is also subject to the nuances of the surgical schedule, the goodwill of the referring physician and attending surgeon, and the willingness of the patient to cooperate. At best, the convenience sample is representative of patients at that institution, with no assurance that these patients are similar to those elsewhere. Convenience sampling is also the rule in studying new anesthetic drugs; such studies are typically performed on healthy, young volunteers.

Experimental Constraints

The researcher must define the conditions to which the sample members will be exposed. Particularly in clinical research, one must decide whether these conditions should be rigidly standardized or whether the experimental circumstances should be adjusted or individualized to the patient. In anesthetic drug research, should a fixed dose be given to all members of the sample or should the dose be adjusted to produce an effect or to achieve a specific end point? Standardizing the treatment groups by fixed doses simplifies the research work. There are risks to this standardization, however: (1) a fixed dose may produce excessive numbers of side effects in some patients, (2) a fixed dose may be therapeutically insufficient in others, and (3) a treatment standardized for an experimental protocol may be so artificial that it has no broad clinical relevance, even if demonstrated to be superior. The researcher should carefully choose and report the adjustment/individualization of experimental treatments.

Control Groups

Even if a researcher is studying just one experimental group, the results of the experiment are usually not interpreted solely in terms of that one group but are also contrasted and compared with other experimental groups. Examining the effects of a new drug on blood pressure during anesthetic induction is important, but what is more important is comparing those results with the effects of one or more standard drugs commonly used in the same situation. Where can the researcher obtain these comparative data? There are several possibilities: (1) each patient could receive the standard drug under identical experimental circumstances at another time, (2) another group of patients receiving the standard drug could be studied simultaneously, (3) a group of patients could have been studied previously with the standard drug under similar circumstances, and (4) literature reports of the effects of the drug under related but not necessarily identical circumstances could be used. Under the first two possibilities, the control group is contemporaneous—either a *self-control* (crossover) or *parallel control* group. The second two possibilities are examples of the use of *historical controls*.

Because historical controls already exist, they are convenient and seemingly cheap to use. Unfortunately, the history of medicine is littered with the "debris" of therapies enthusiastically accepted on the basis of comparison with past experience. A classic example is operative ligation of the internal mammary artery for the treatment of angina pectoris—a procedure now known to be of no value. Proposed as a method to improve coronary artery blood flow, the lack of benefit was demonstrated in a trial where some patients had the procedure and some had a sham procedure; both groups showed benefit.[1] There is now firm empirical evidence that studies using historical controls usually show a favorable outcome for a new therapy, whereas studies with concurrent controls, that is, parallel control group or self-control, less often reveal a benefit.[2] Nothing seems to increase the enthusiasm for a new treatment as much as the omission of a concurrent control group. If the outcome with an old treatment is not studied simultaneously with the outcome of a new treatment, one cannot know if any differences in results are a consequence of the two treatments, or of unsuspected and unknowable differences between the patients, or of other changes over time in the general medical environment. One possible exception would be in studying a disease that is uniformly fatal (100% mortality) over a very short time.

Random Allocation of Treatment Groups

Having accepted the necessity of an experiment with a control group, the question arises as to the method by which each subject should be assigned to the predetermined experimental groups. Should it depend on the whim of the investigator, the day of the week, the preference of a referring physician, the wish of the patient, the assignment of the previous subject, the availability of a study drug, a hospital chart number, or some other arbitrary criterion? All such methods have been used and are still used, but all can ruin the purity and usefulness of the experiment. It is important to remember the purpose of sampling: By exposing a small number of subjects from the target population to the various experimental conditions, one hopes to make conclusions about the entire population. Thus, the experimental groups should be as similar as possible to each other in reflecting the target population; if the groups are different, selection bias is introduced into the experiment. Although randomly allocating subjects of a sample to one or another of the experimental groups requires additional work, this principle prevents selection bias by the researcher, minimizes (but cannot always prevent) the possibility that important differences exist among the experimental groups, and disarms the critics' complaints about research methods. Random allocation is most commonly accomplished by the use of computer-generated random numbers. Even with a random allocation process, selection bias can occur if research personnel are allowed knowledge of the group assignment of the next patient to be recruited for a study. Failure to conceal random allocation leads to biases in the results of clinical studies.[3,4]

Blinding

Blinding refers to the masking from the view of patient and experimenters the experimental group to which the subject has been or will be assigned. In clinical trials, the necessity for blinding starts even before a patient is enrolled in the research study; this is called the *concealment of random allocation*. There is good evidence that, if the process of random allocation is accessible to view, the referring physicians, the research team members, or both are tempted to manipulate the entrance of specific patients into the study to influence their assignment to a specific treatment group[5]; they do so having formed a personal opinion about the relative merits of the treatment groups and desiring to get the "best" for someone they favor. This creates bias in the experimental groups.

Each subject should remain, if possible, ignorant of the assigned treatment group after entrance into the research protocol. The patient's expectation of improvement, a placebo effect, is a real and useful part of clinical care. But when studying a new treatment, one must ensure that the fame or infamy of the treatments does not induce a bias in outcome by changing patient expectations. A researcher's knowledge of the treatment assignment can bias his or her ability to administer the research protocol and to observe and record data faithfully; this is true for clinical, animal, and in vitro research. If the treatment group is known, those who observe data cannot trust themselves to record the data impartially and dispassionately. The appellations *single-blind* and *double-blind* to describe blinding are commonly used in research reports, but often applied inconsistently; the researcher should carefully plan and report exactly who is blinded.

Experimental Medicine: Statistical Analysis

Hypothesis Formulation

The researcher starts work with some intuitive feel for the phenomenon to be studied. Whether stated explicitly or not, this is the *biologic hypothesis*; it is a statement of experimental expectations to be accomplished by the use of experimental tools, instruments, or methods accessible to the research team. An example would be the hope that isoflurane would produce less myocardial ischemia than fentanyl; the experimental method might be the electrocardiography determination of ST segment changes. The biologic hypothesis of the researcher becomes a *statistical hypothesis* during research planning. The researcher measures quantities that can vary—variables such as heart rate or temperature or ST segment change—in samples from populations of interest. In a statistical hypothesis, statements are made about the relationship among parameters of one or more populations. (To restate, a *parameter* is a number describing a variable of a population; Greek letters are used to denote parameters.) The typical statistical hypothesis can be established in a somewhat rote fashion for every research project, regardless of the methods, materials, or goals. The most frequently used method of setting up the algebraic formulation of the statistical hypothesis is to create two mutually exclusive statements about some parameters of the study population (Table 7-3); estimates for the values for these parameters are acquired by sampling data. In

Table 7-3 Algebraic Statement of Statistical Hypotheses

H_0: $\phi_1 = \phi_2$ (null hypothesis)
H_a: $\phi_1 \neq \phi_2$ (alternative hypothesis)
ϕ_1 = Parameter estimated from sample of first population
ϕ_2 = Parameter estimated from sample of second population

the hypothetical example comparing isoflurane and fentanyl, ϕ_1 and ϕ_2 would represent the ST segment changes with isoflurane and with fentanyl. The *null hypothesis* is the hypothesis of no difference of ST segment changes between isoflurane and fentanyl. The *alternative hypothesis* is usually nondirectional, that is, either ϕ_1 is less than ϕ_2 or ϕ_1 is more than ϕ_2; this is known as a *two-tail alternative hypothesis*. This is a more conservative alternative hypothesis than assuming that the inequality can only be either less than or greater than.

Logic of Proof

One particular decision strategy is used most commonly to choose between the null and alternative hypothesis. The approach is to assume that the null hypothesis is true even though the goal of the experiment is to show that there is a difference. One examines the consequences of this assumption by examining the actual sample values obtained for the variable(s) of interest. This is done by calculating what is called a *sample test statistic*; sample test statistics are calculated from the sample numbers. Associated with a sample test statistic is a *probability*. One also chooses the *level of significance*; the level of significance is the probability level considered too low to warrant support of the null hypothesis being tested. If sample values are sufficiently unlikely to have occurred by chance (i.e., the probability of the sample test statistic is less than the chosen level of significance), the null hypothesis is rejected; otherwise, the null hypothesis is not rejected.

Because the statistics deal with probabilities, not certainties, there is a chance that the decision concerning the null hypothesis is erroneous. These errors are best displayed in table form (Table 7-4); condition 1 and condition 2 could be different drugs, two doses of the same drug, or different patient groups. Of the four possible outcomes, two decisions are clearly undesirable. The error of wrongly rejecting the null hypothesis (false-positive) is called the *type I* or α-*error*. The experimenter should choose a probability value for α before collecting data; the experimenter decides how cautious to be against falsely claiming a difference. The most common choice for the value of α is 0.05. What are the consequences of choosing an α of 0.05? Assuming that there is, in fact, no difference between the two conditions and that the experiment is to be repeated 20 times, then during one of these experimental replications (5% of 20), a mistaken conclusion that there is a difference would be made. The probability of a type I error depends on the chosen level of significance and the existence or nonexistence of a difference between the two experimental conditions. The smaller the chosen α, the smaller will be the risk of a type I error.

The error of failing to reject a false null hypothesis (false-negative) is called a *type II* or β-*error*. (The power of a test is $1-\beta$.) The probability of a type II error depends on four factors. Unfortunately, the smaller the α, the greater the chance of a false-negative conclusion; this fact keeps the experimenter from automatically choosing a very small α. Second, the more variability there is in the populations being compared, the greater the chance of a type II error. This is analogous to listening to a noisy radio broadcast; the more static there is, the harder it will be to discriminate between words. Next, increasing the number of subjects will lower the probability of a type II error. The fourth and most important factor is the magnitude of the difference between the two experimental conditions. The probability of a type II error goes from very high, when there is only a small difference, to extremely low, when the two conditions produce large differences in population parameters.

Sample Size Calculations

Formerly, researchers typically ignored the latter error in experimental design. The practical importance of worrying about type II errors reached the consciousness of the medical research community several decades ago. Some controlled clinical trials that claimed to find no advantage of new therapies compared with standard therapies lacked sufficient statistical power to discriminate between the experimental groups and would have missed an important therapeutic improvement. As an example, the formula for calculating the size of each sample in a study comparing the means of two populations is: $n = 2\left[\dfrac{(z_\alpha - z_\beta)\sigma}{\mu_1 - \mu_2}\right]^2$. The z values are taken from the normal probability distribution and represent assumptions about the prespecified α and β; the sigma (σ) is the assumed common SD; the mu's (μ) are the assumed population values. There are four options for decreasing type II error (increasing statistical power): (1) raise α, (2) reduce population variability, (3) make the sample bigger, and (4) make the difference between the conditions greater. Under most circumstances, only the sample size can be varied. Sample size planning has become an important part of research design for controlled clinical trials. Some published research still fails the test of adequate sample size planning.

Table 7-4 Errors in Hypothesis Testing: The Two-Way Truth Table

		Reality (population parameters)	
		Conditions 1 and 2 Equivalent	**Conditions 1 and 2 Not Equivalent**
Conclusion from sample (sample statistics)	Conditions 1 and 2 equivalent[a]	Correct conclusion	False-negative type II error (β-error)
	Conditions 1 and 2 not equivalent[b]	False-positive type I error (α-error)	Correct conclusion

[a]Do not reject the null hypothesis: condition 1 = condition 2.
[b]Reject the null hypothesis: condition 1 ≠ condition 2.

Inferential Statistics

The testing of hypotheses or *significance testing* has been the main focus of inferential statistics. Hypothesis testing allows the experimenter to use data from the sample to make inferences about the population. Statisticians have created formulas that use the values of the samples to calculate test statistics. Statisticians have also explored the properties of various theoretical probability distributions. Depending on the assumptions about how data are collected, the appropriate probability distribution is chosen as the source of critical values to accept or reject the null hypothesis. If the value of the test statistic calculated from the sample(s) is greater than the critical value, the null hypothesis is rejected. The critical value is chosen from the appropriate probability distribution after the magnitude of the type I error is specified.

There are parameters within the equation that generate any particular probability distribution; for the normal probability distribution, the parameters are μ and σ^2. For the normal distribution, each set of values for μ and σ^2 will generate a different shape for the bell-like normal curve. All probability distributions contain one or more parameters and can be plotted as curves; these parameters may be discrete (integer only) or continuous. Each value or combination of values for these parameters will create a different curve for the probability distribution being used. Thus, each probability distribution is actually a family of probability curves. Some additional parameters of theoretical probability distributions have been given the special name *degrees of freedom* and are represented by Latin letters such as m, n, and s.

Associated with the formula for computing a test statistic is a rule for assigning integer values to the one or more parameters called degrees of freedom. The number of degrees of freedom and the value for each degree of freedom depend on (1) the number of subjects, (2) the number of experimental groups, (3) the specifics of the statistical hypothesis, and (4) the type of statistical test. The correct curve of the probability distribution from which to obtain a critical value for comparison with the value of the test statistic is obtained with the values of one or more degrees of freedom.

To accept or reject the null hypothesis, the following steps are performed: (1) confirm that experimental data conform to the assumptions of the intended statistical test; (2) choose a significance level (α); (3) calculate the test statistic; (4) determine the degree(s) of freedom; (5) find the critical value for the chosen α and the degree(s) of freedom from the appropriate probability distribution; (6) if the test statistic exceeds the critical value, reject the null hypothesis; (7) if the test statistic does not exceed the critical value, do not reject the null hypothesis.

The Fickle P Value

There is an extremely common misapprehension about the meaning of the *P* value in the typical null hypothesis/alternative hypothesis testing.[6,7] If a statistical test is declared to be significant at $P = 0.05$, most physicians will state that there is 95% certainty that the null hypothesis is incorrect.[6] As Goodman[6] stated: "This is an understandable but categorically wrong interpretation because the P value is calculated on the assumption that the null hypothesis is true. It cannot, therefore, be a direct measure of the probability that the null hypothesis is false." The odds that the desired outcome, the alternative hypothesis, is true will depend not just on the data of the experiment, but also on how plausible was that hypothesis before conducting the research. This interaction of hypothesis plausibility and statistical results can be displayed graphically (Fig. 7-1).[8,9] A long shot, implausible

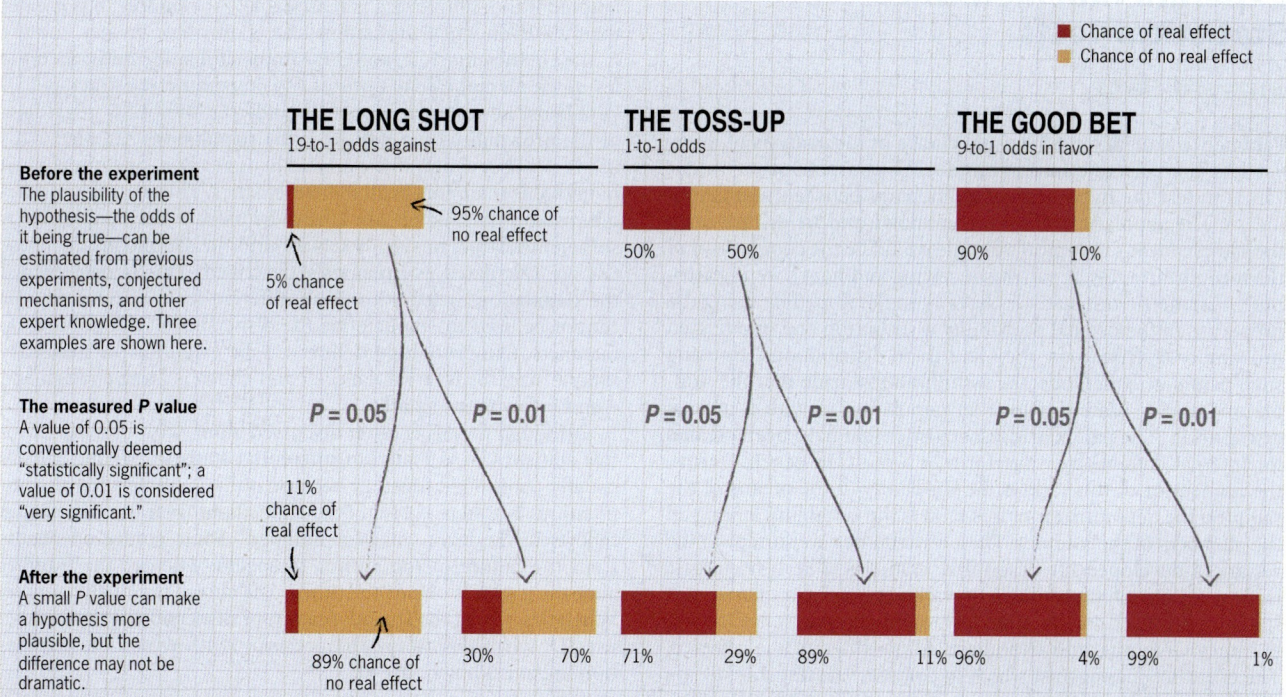

Figure 7-1 Probable cause. A *P* value measures whether an observed result can be attributed to chance. But it cannot answer a researcher's real question: What are the odds that a hypothesis is correct? Those odds depend on how strong the result was and, most importantly, on how plausible the hypothesis is in the first place. (Reprinted with permission from Nuzzo R. Statistical errors. P values, the 'gold standard' of statistical validity, are not as reliable as many scientists assume. *Nature*. 2014;506:150–152. Copyright © 2014 *Nature*, with permission of Macmillan Publishers Ltd.)[9]

hypothesis (19-to-1 odds against) stills remains implausible (11% chance of a real effect) if the P value of the experiment is 0.05.

The Bayesian Alternative

Be it an RCT or an observational study report, the results and claims of medical research are not and should not be considered in isolation from prior knowledge. Yet the most commonly used methods of statistical inference used in medical research (see supra) explicitly uses only the newly obtained data. This is the Frequentist approach or inference, so called because the precise definition of probability values depends on assumptions about hypothetical repeated replication of data collection. The new information of a study is a function only of the data.

A competing approach is called Bayesian inference that explicitly reports the new information of a study as a function of both observed data and historical (prior) knowledge. Both Frequentist and Bayesian inferences make statements about parameters. But Bayesian methods involve the multiplication of the prior knowledge represented as a probability distribution of the parameter(s) times the likelihood of the observed data; the product is the new (posterior) probability distribution of the parameter.[10,11] Bayesian methods have been proposed to resolve the conundrum that some highly cited clinical research whose evidence is interpreted by a Frequentist P value is later contradicted or found to be excessively optimistic in the magnitude of effect.[12–15] Among reasons for the slower adoption of Bayesian methods are concerns about the subjectivity in defining the prior probability distribution and the considerably greater computational difficulty in performing an analysis.

Experimental Medicine: Statistical Tests

Interval Data

Parametric statistics are the usual choice in the analysis of interval data, both discrete and continuous. The purpose of such analysis is to test the hypothesis of a difference between population means. The population means are unknown and are estimated by the sample means. A typical example would be the comparison of the mean heart rates of patients receiving and not receiving atropine. Parametric test statistics have been developed by using the properties of the normal probability distribution and two related probability distributions, the t and the F distributions. In using such parametric methods, the assumption is made that the sample or samples is/are drawn from population(s) with a normal distribution. The parametric test statistics that have been created for interval data all have the form of a ratio. In general terms, the numerator of this ratio is the variability of the means of the samples; the denominator of this ratio is the variability among all the members of the samples. These variabilities are similar to the variances developed for descriptive statistics. The test statistic is thus a ratio of variabilities or variances. All parametric test statistics are used in the same fashion; if the test statistic ratio becomes large, the null hypothesis of no difference is rejected. The critical values against which to compare the test statistic are taken from tables of the three relevant probability distributions (normal, t, or F). In hypothesis testing at least one of the population means is unknown, but the population variance(s) may or may not be known. Parametric statistics can be divided into two groups according to whether or not the population variances are known. If the population variance is known, the test statistic used is called the z score; critical values are obtained from the normal distribution. In most biomedical applications, the population variance is rarely known and the z score is little used.

Confidence Intervals

The other major areas of statistical inference are the estimation of parameters with associated *confidence intervals* (CIs). In statistics, a CI is an interval estimate of a population parameter. A CI describes how likely it is that the population parameter is estimated by any particular sample statistic such as the mean. (The technical definition of the CI of the mean is more rigorous. A 95% CI implies that if the experiment were done over and over again, 95 of each 100 CIs would be expected to contain the true value of the mean.) CIs are a range of the following form: summary statistic ± (confidence factor) × (precision factor).

The *precision factor* is derived from the sample itself, whereas the *confidence factor* is taken from a probability distribution and also depends on the specified confidence level chosen. For a sample of interval data taken from a normally distributed population for which CIs are to be chosen for $\bar{x}$ the precision factor is called the *standard error of the mean* and is obtained by dividing SD by the square root of the sample size or $SE = \dfrac{SD}{\sqrt{n}} = \sqrt{\sum_{i=1}^{n}(x_i - \bar{x})^2 / n(n-1)}$.

The confidence factors are the same as those used for the dispersion or spread of the sample and are obtained from the normal distribution. The CIs for confidence factors 1, 2, and 3 have roughly a 68%, 95%, and 99% chance of containing the population mean. Strictly speaking, when the SD must be estimated from sample values, the confidence factors should be taken from the t *distribution*, another probability distribution. These coefficients will be larger than those used previously. This is usually ignored if the sample size is reasonable; for example, n is greater than 25. Even when the sample size is only 5 or greater, the use of the coefficients 1, 2, and 3 is simple and sufficiently accurate for quick mental calculations of CIs on parameter estimates.

Almost all research reports include the use of SE, regardless of the probability distribution of the populations sampled. This use is a consequence of the *central limit theorem*, one of the most remarkable theorems in all of mathematics. The central limit theorem states that the SE can always be used, if the sample size is sufficiently large, to specify CIs around the sample mean. These CIs are calculated as previously described. This is true even if the population distribution is so different from normal that SD cannot be used to characterize the dispersion of the population members. Only rough guidelines can be given for the necessary sample size; for interval data, 25 and above is large enough and 4 and below is too small.

Although the SE is often discussed along with other descriptive statistics, it is really an inferential statistic. SE and SD are usually mentioned together because of their similarities of computation, but there is often confusion about their use in research reports in the form "mean ± number." Some confusion results from the failure of the author to specify whether the number after the ± sign is one or the other. The choice is actually simple. When describing the spread, scatter, or dispersion of the sample, use SD; when describing the precision with which the population mean is known, use SE.

t Test

An important advance in statistical inference came early in the twentieth century with the creation of *Student's t test statistic* and the *t distribution*, which allowed the testing of hypotheses when the population variance is not known. The most common use of Student's *t* test is to compare the mean values of two populations. There are two types of *t* test. If each subject has two measurements taken, for example, one before (x_i) and one after (y_i) a drug, then a one sample or *paired t test* procedure is used; each control measurement taken before drug administration is paired with a measurement in the same patient after drug administration. Of course, this is a self-control experiment. This pairing of measurements in the same patient reduces variability and increases statistical power. The difference $d_i = x_i - y_i$ of each pair of values is calculated and the average $\bar{d}$ is calculated. In the formula for Student's *t* statistic, the numerator is $\bar{d}$ whereas the denominator is the SE of $\bar{d}$ denoted $(SE_{\bar{d}})$ so the test statistic is $t = \frac{\bar{d}}{SE_{\bar{d}}}$.

All *t* statistics are created in this way; the numerator is the difference of two means, whereas the denominator is the SE of the two means. If the difference between the two means is large compared with their variability, then the null hypothesis of no difference is rejected. The critical values for the *t* statistic are taken from the *t* probability distribution. The *t* distribution is symmetric and bell-shaped but more spread out than the normal distribution. The *t* distribution has a single integer parameter; for a paired *t* test, the value of this single degree of freedom is the sample size minus one. There can be some confusion about the use of the letter *t*. It refers both to the value of the test statistic calculated by the formula and to the critical value from the theoretical probability distribution. The critical *t* value is determined by looking in a *t* table after a significance level is chosen and the degree of freedom is computed.

More commonly, measurements are taken on two separate groups of subjects. For example, one group receives blood pressure treatment with sample values x_i, whereas no treatment is given to a control group with sample values y_i. The number of subjects in each group might or might not be identical; regardless of this, in no sense is an individual measurement in the first group matched or paired with a specific measurement in the second group. An *unpaired* or *two-sample t test* is used to compare the means of the two groups. The numerator of the *t* statistic is $\bar{x} - \bar{y}$. The denominator is a weighted average of the SDs of each sample so that the test statistic *t* is $t = \frac{\bar{x} - \bar{y}}{\sqrt{\left(\frac{1}{n_x} + \frac{1}{n_y}\right)\left(\frac{(n_x - 1)s_x^2 + (n_y - 1)s_y^2}{n_x + n_y - 2}\right)}}$.

The degree of freedom for an unpaired *t* test is calculated as the sum of the subjects of the two groups minus two. As with the paired *t* test, if the *t* ratio becomes large, the null hypothesis is rejected.

The results of a comparison of samples from two populations should be complete. In addition to displaying the individual mean values of $\bar{x}$ and $\bar{y}$ with their CIs and the results of the *t* test, the mean difference, $\bar{x} - \bar{y}$, is also included with its associated CI. This difference of means is the effect size, a quantitative measure of the magnitude of effect. The reporting of the effect size facilitates the interpretation of the clinical importance, as opposed to the statistical significance of a research result.

Analysis of Variance

Experiments in anesthesia, whether they are with humans or with animals, may not be limited to one or two groups of data for each variable. It is very common to follow a variable longitudinally; heart rate, for example, might be measured five times before and during anesthetic induction. These are also called *repeated measurement experiments*; the experimenter will wish to compare changes between the initial heart rate measurement and those obtained during induction. The experimental design might also include several groups receiving different induction drugs; for example, comparing heart rate across groups immediately after laryngoscopy. Researchers have mistakenly handled these analysis problems with just the *t* test. If heart rate is collected five times, these collection times could be labeled A, B, C, D, and E. Then A could be compared with B, C, D, and E; B could be compared with C, D, and E; and so forth. The total of possible pairings is ten; thus, ten paired *t* tests could be calculated for all the possible pairings of A, B, C, D, and E. A similar approach can be used for comparing more than two groups for unpaired data.

The use of *t* tests in this fashion is inappropriate. In testing a statistical hypothesis, the experimenter sets the level of type I error; this is usually chosen to be 0.05. When using many *t* tests, as in the example given earlier, the chosen error rate for performing all these *t* tests is much higher than 0.05, even though the type I error is set at 0.05 for each individual comparison. In fact, the type I error rate for all *t* tests simultaneously; that is, the chance of finding at least one of the multiple *t* test statistics significant merely by chance is given by the formula $\alpha = 1 - 0.95^\kappa$. If 13 *t* tests are performed ($\kappa = 13$), the real error rate is 49%. Applying *t* tests over and over again to all the possible pairings of a variable will misleadingly identify statistical significance when in fact there is none.

The most versatile approach for handling comparisons of means between more than two groups or between several measurements in the same group is called *analysis of variance* and is frequently cited by the acronym ANOVA. Analysis of variance consists of rules for creating test statistics on means when there are more than two groups. These test statistics are called *F ratios*, after Ronald Fisher; the critical values for the *F* test statistic are taken from the *F* probability distribution that Fisher derived.

Suppose that data for three groups are obtained. What can be said about the mean values of the three target populations? The *F* test is actually asking several questions simultaneously: Is group 1 different from group 2; is group 2 different from group 3; and is group 1 different from group 3? As with the *t* test, the *F* test statistic is a ratio; in general terms, the numerator expresses the variability of the mean values of the three groups, whereas the denominator expresses the average variability or difference of each sample value from the mean of all sample values. The formulas to create the test statistic are computationally elegant but are rather hard to appreciate intuitively. The *F* statistic has two degrees of freedom, denoted *m* and *n*; the value of *m* is a function of the number of experimental groups; the value for *n* is a function of the number of subjects in all experimental groups. The analysis of multigroup data is not necessarily finished after the ANOVAs are calculated. If the null hypothesis is rejected and it is accepted that there are differences among the groups tested, how can it be decided where the differences are? A variety of techniques are available to make what are called *multiple comparisons* after the ANOVA test is performed.

Robustness and Nonparametric Tests

Most statistical tests depend on certain assumptions about the nature of the distribution of values in the underlying populations from which experimental samples are taken. For the parametric statistics, that is, *t* tests and analysis of variance, it is assumed that the populations follow the normal distribution. However, for some data, experience or historical reasons suggests that these assumptions of a normal distribution do not hold; some examples include proportions, percentages, and response times. What should the experimenter do if he or she fears that the data are not normally distributed?

The experimenter might choose to ignore the problem of non-normal data and inhomogeneity of variance, hoping that everything will work out. Such insouciance is actually a very practical and reasonable approach to the problem. Parametric statistics are called *robust* statistics; they stand up to much adversity. To a statistician, robustness implies that the magnitude of type I errors is not seriously affected by ill-conditioned data. Parametric statistics are sufficiently robust that the accuracy of decisions reached by means of t tests and analysis of variance remains very credible, even for moderately severe departures from the assumptions.

Another possibility would be to use statistics that do not require any assumptions about probability distributions of the populations. Such statistics are known as *nonparametric tests;* they can be used whenever there is very serious concern about the shape of the data. Nonparametric statistics are also the tests of choice for ordinal data. The basic concept behind nonparametric statistics is the ability to rank or order the observations; nonparametric tests are also called *order statistics.*

Most nonparametric statistics still require the use of theoretical probability distributions; the critical values that must be exceeded by the test statistic are taken from the binomial, normal, and chi-square distributions, depending on the nonparametric test being used. The *nonparametric sign test, Mann–Whitney rank sum test,* and *Kruskal–Wallis one-way analysis of variance* are analogous to the paired t test, unpaired t test, and one-way analysis of variance, respectively. The currently available nonparametric tests are not used more commonly because they do not adapt well to complex statistical models and because they are less able than parametric tests to distinguish between the null and alternative hypotheses if the data are, in fact, normally distributed. There are general guidelines that relate the variable type and the experimental design to the choice of statistical test (Table 7-5).

Binary Variables

Confidence Intervals on Proportions

Categorical binary data, also called *enumeration data,* provide counts of subject responses. Given a sample of subjects of whom some have a certain characteristic (e.g., death, female sex), a ratio of responders to the number of subjects can be easily calculated as $p = x/n$; this ratio or rate can be expressed as a decimal fraction or as a percentage. It should be clear that this is a measure of central location of binary data. In the population from which the sample is taken, the ratio of responders to total subjects is a population parameter, denoted π. (This is not related to the geometry constant $\pi = 3.14159....$) The sample proportion p is the estimator $(\hat{\pi})$ of the population proportion π. As with other data types, π is usually not known, but must be estimated from the sample. The sample ratio p is the best estimate of π.

Because the population is not generally known, the experimenter usually wishes to estimate π by the sample ratio p and to specify with what precision π is known. If the sample is sufficiently large ($n \times p \geq 5; n \times (1 - p) \geq 5$), advantage is taken of the central limit theorem to derive an SE analogous to that derived for interval data: $SE = \sqrt{\dfrac{p \times (1 - p)}{n}}$. This sample SE is exactly analogous to the sample SE of the mean for interval data, except that it is an SE of the proportion. Just as a 95% CI of the mean was calculated, so may a CI on the proportion may be obtained. Larger samples will make the CI more precise.

If nothing goes wrong, is everything all right? This question was proposed by Henley and Lippman-Hand[16] to discuss the interpretations of zero numerators using the 3 over n rule. Consider an observational study that reports no morbidity in 167 patients receiving a new intravenous anesthetic. Is there really no risk? Although the best estimate of the population parameter π is 0/167 or 0%, an upper bound on the 95% CI is relevant to consider how high the rate of adverse events might be. As the probability of binary data is provided by the *binomial probability distribution function,* this upper bound may be derived from $1 - (0.05)^{1/n}$ where n is the denominator; for n is greater than 30, this is well approximated by $3/n = 3/167 \approx 1.8\%$.

The zero numerator example can be used to illustrate a difference between a Bayesian and Frequentist approach. If there is no prior information (Bayes–Laplace β-*probability distribution function*), the upper bound is $3/(n + 1) = 3/168 \approx 1.8\%$; the Bayesian equivalent of a CI is called a Credible Interval (CI).[17] As the sample size increases, $3/n$ and $3/(n + 1)$ becomes closer and closer. By contrast, when there is prior information Bayesian inference will provide a more informative CI than a Frequentist approach. Suppose a prior study with the same new anesthetic had found 15 morbid events in 10,000 (0.15%) patients. Then with the new data the estimate of the population rate of morbidity is 0.12% (upper bound 95% CI = 0.36%).[17] Using prior information and the new data of 0 events in 167 patients, the population rate estimate has been reduced from 0.15% to 0.12% and the upper bound of the 95% CI is much lower (0.36% vs. 1.8%) than by Frequentist estimation.

Hypothesis Testing

In the experiment negating the value of mammary artery ligation, five of eight patients (62.5%) having ligation showed benefit, and five of nine patients (55.6%) having sham surgery also had benefit.[1] Is this difference real? This experiment sampled patients from two populations—those having the real procedure and those having the sham procedure. A variety of statistical techniques allow a comparison of the success rate. These include *Fisher's exact test* and (*Pearson's*) *chi-square test.* The chi-square test offers the advantage of being computationally simpler; it can also analyze contingency tables with more than two rows and

Table 7-5 When to Use What

Variable Type	One-sample Tests	Two-sample Tests	Multiple-sample Tests
Dichotomous or nominal	Binomial distribution	Chi-square test, Fisher's exact test	Chi-square test
Ordinal	Chi-square test	Chi-square test, nonparametric tests	Chi-square test, nonparametric tests
Continuous or discrete	z distribution or t distribution	Unpaired t test, paired t test, nonparametric tests	Analysis of variance, nonparametric analysis of variance

two columns; however, certain assumptions of sample size and response rate are not achieved by this experiment. Fisher's exact test fails to reject the null hypothesis for this data.

The results of such experiments are often presented as a rate/risk ratio (RR), an effect size. (Other effect sizes for comparison of two populations with binary outcomes are the odds ratio [OR], the risk difference, and the number needed to treat.) The rate of improvement for the experimental group (5/8 = 62.5%) is divided by the rate of improvement for the control group (5/9 = 55.6%). An RR of 1.00 (100%) fails to show a difference of benefit or harm between the two groups. In this example the RR is 1.125. Thus, the experimental group had a 12.5% greater chance of improvement compared with the control group. A CI can be calculated for the RR; in this example it is (0.40, 3.13), thus widely spread to either side of the RR of no difference. (If such an experiment were performed now, the sample size would be much larger to have adequate statistical power.)

Linear Regression

Often a goal of an experiment is to find relationships between two variables so that in new patients the prediction of the value of one characteristic may be made by knowledge of another characteristic. The most commonly used technique for this purpose is linear regression analysis. Experiments for this purpose collect data pairs (x_i, y_i); these data pairs may be captured in either clinical trials or observational studies. The y variable is called the dependent or response variable, and the x variable is denoted the independent or explanatory variable. These data should be displayed in a scatter plot; in the simplest type, a straight line (linear relationship) is assumed between two variables; the y variable is considered a function of the x variable. This is expressed as the linear regression equation $y = a + bx$; the parameters of the regression equation are a and b. (Strictly defined, a and b are estimators of the population parameters alpha [α] and beta [β].) The parameter b is the slope of the straight line relating x and y; for each 1 unit change in x, there are b unit changes in y. The parameter a is the intercept (value of y when x equals 0). Estimates of the parameters are obtained from a least squares method that sets the slope b value to minimize the sum of the vertical distances from the data pairs to the regression

line: $b = \dfrac{\sum_{i=1}^{n}(x_i - \bar{x})(y_i - \bar{y})}{\sum_{i=1}^{n}(x_i - \bar{x})^2}$; $a = \bar{y} + b\bar{x}$. The parameter of

greatest interest in regression is usually the slope, especially whether the slope is nonzero; a zero valued slope implies that x and y are not linearly related. With the additional assumption of bivariate normality (both x and y normally distributed), a t test statistic is used to check the statistical significance of the slope.

The same (x_i, y_i) data pairs are usually subjected to correlation analysis. The correlation coefficient r is a measure of the linear covariation of x and y; r ranges from -1 to 1. There is no linear correlation between x and y if r is zero valued. It is estimated by

$r = \dfrac{\sum_{i=1}^{n}(x_i - \bar{x})(y_i - \bar{y})}{\sqrt{\sum_{i=1}^{n}(x_i - \bar{x})^2}\sqrt{\sum_{i=1}^{n}(y_i - \bar{y})^2}}$. The test of the statistical

significance of r is equivalent to the test for the significance of the regression slope b. The squared value of r, known as the coefficient of determination (r^2) varies between 0 and 1 and is sometime expressed as a percentage. The coefficient of determination has a very useful interpretation: the fraction of the variation of y explained by the variation of x.

As a hypothetical example, suppose that age and a plasma biomarker of physical maturity are collected in 11 children. The (x_i, y_i) values recorded are (10, 8.04), (8, 6.95), (13, 7.58), (9, 8.81), (11, 8.33), (14, 9.96), (6, 7.24), (4, 4.26), (12, 10.84), (7, 4.82), and (5, 5.68). Neither an inspection of these values nor of the summary statistics ($\bar{x} = 9.00$, $\bar{y} = 7.50$) permit the reader to detect any relationship. The calculation of the coefficient of determination ($r^2 = 0.67$) does allow the inference that 67% of the variation in the biomarker is explained by the variation in age.

A researcher or reader should not be satisfied to see only the statistical results of regression and correlation. The statistician Anscombe[18] created four hypothetical data sets to illustrate the importance of visual inspection of data. Each data set has 11 paired (x_i, y_i) observations (Fig. 7-2). The hypothetical example (listed earlier) is displayed in the upper left quadrant; a linear relationship is displayed. For the data in the upper right quadrant, the relationship between x and y is curvilinear (quadratic). For the lower right quadrant, there is no relationship between x and y; with one exception all data pairs have the same x value. For the lower left quadrant, there is a near perfect correlation between x and y except for one data pair with a much higher y value. Nevertheless, all summary statistics, regression, and correlation values of the four data sets including means, SDs, slopes, intercepts, standard errors of regression parameters, statistical significance of regression parameters, and correlation coefficients are equal. There are clearly four different patterns that can only be detected by visual inspection. Even this simplest form of regression and correlation analysis is based on the strong assumption of an underlying linear relationship between x and y; failure of that assumption leads to erroneous statistical inference. Using just the summary, regression, and correlation statistics, the four data sets would have been thought to have very similar/identical underlying relationships.

Epidemiology

Epidemiology is the study of the patterns, causes, and effects of health and disease conditions. Epidemiology is based on observations collected systematically, but without the interventions (anesthetic drugs and techniques) being allocated to patients under experimental control. Major areas of epidemiologic study relevant to anesthesia care are nonrandomized studies (NRSs) of the effectiveness of anesthetic drugs and techniques on outcomes following anesthesia and surgery, the properties of diagnostic tests for the identification of perioperative complications, the determination of risk factors for outcomes, and the estimation of risk prognosis models for individual predication. Systematic reviews (SRs) and meta-analysis (MA) also come under the banner of epidemiology as does the advent of "Big Data."

A fundamental axiom of epidemiology is "Association does not necessarily imply causation." In 1965, the epidemiologist Bradford Hill suggested guidelines for assessing evidence of causation when presented with an observed association between the environment and disease. Fifty years later Ioannidis[19] revisited these criteria, assessed which of these had worked, and identified two: Consistency and Experiment. Of the former, Hill[20] offered this question: "Has it (an association) been repeatedly observed by different persons, in different places, circumstances, and times?" But nothing can replace Experiment. Ioannidis[13]

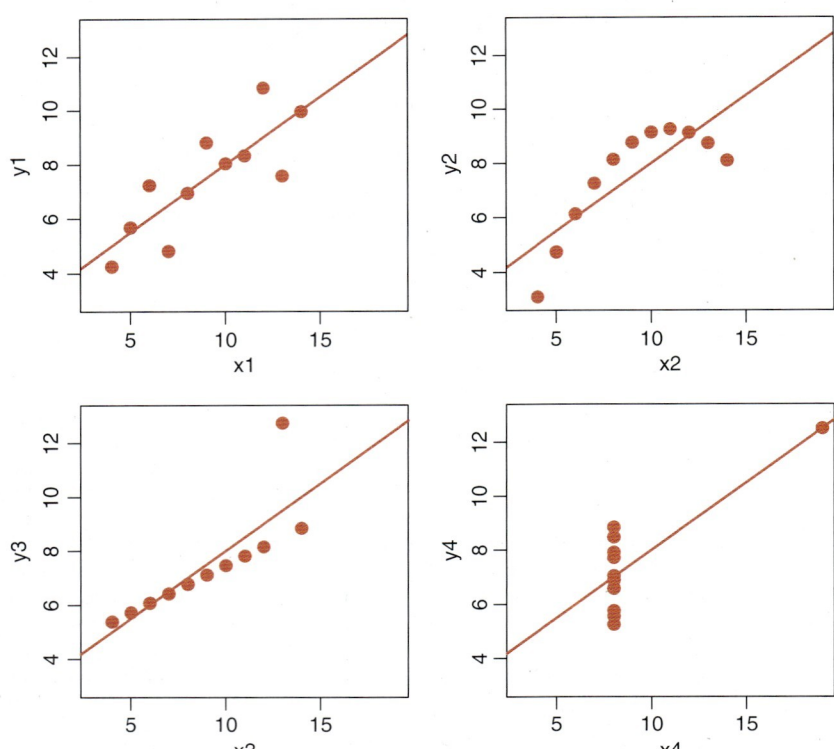

Figure 7-2 Four scatter plots from the Anscombe data sets. For each data set, $n = 11$, $\bar{x} = 9.00$, $SD_x = 3.31$, $\bar{y} = 7.50$, $SD_y = 2.03$, $y = 3.00 + 0.50x$, $SE_a = 1.12$, $SE_b = 0.12$, $r^2 = 0.67$, and so forth. All statistics are equal up to the fourth decimal place.

reported: "Among the most highly cited papers in the biomedical literature, five out of six observational studies have been 'refuted' by subsequent randomized trials…" Be it an RCT or an observational study report, the results and claims of medical research are not and should not be considered in isolation from prior knowledge. The precision with which the *P* value is calculated by statistical software by itself should not replace a consideration of all evidence.

Multivariable Linear Regression

Regression methods can be extended to data sets in which one response variable is linearly related to many explanatory variables. This regression includes methods for choosing which of the explanatory variables have a statistically significant (i.e., nonzero) regression slope. Multivariable linear regression is the creation of a model relating some continuous response such as heart rate to *k* explanatory variables; these are also called covariates. This regression starts with data from *n* patients of the form $(y_i, x_{i,1}, x_{i,2}, \ldots, x_{i,k})$, where the subscript *i* denotes the *i*th patient, y_i is the response in the *i*th patient, x_i is the value of a covariate in the *i*th patient, and the second subscript of x_i denotes the *1* to *k* covariates. The linear model equation for the *i*th individual is:

$$\mu_i = \beta_0 + \beta_1 x_{i,1} + \beta_2 x_{i,2} + \ldots + \beta_k x_{i,k} = \sum_{j=1}^{k} \beta_j x_{i,j}.$$ The β_js are the

unknown coefficients (parameters) of the model that will be estimated from the observed data. For the *i*th individual, the expected value of the model, μ_i, is the linear sum of each covariate value multiplied by its coefficient. The difference between the observed (y_i) and expected value (μ_i) reflects biologic variability, measurement error, and so forth.

Univariable and Multivariable Logistic Regression

If the response variable is binary (alive/dead, complication/no complication), linear regression has been extended. Thus, the typical sigmoidally shaped regression of a binary outcome (e.g., movement) versus anesthetic dose. There are multiple methods for regression of binary outcomes, the most common being logistic regression. The most commonly used format of the logistic method is the multivariable logistic regression model. The response variable y_i denotes the value of the binary outcome in the *i*th individual and is generally coded as 0 or 1, representing the absence or presence of an event (e.g., day-of-surgery mortality). Letting π represent the probability that the response variable has value 1, then the logit transformation, log *of the odds ratio* $= \ln\left(\dfrac{\pi}{1-\pi}\right)$,

allows π to be expressed as the linear combination of the covariates: $\ln\left(\dfrac{\pi_i}{1-\pi_i}\right) = \beta_0 + \beta_1 x_{i,1} + \beta_2 x_{i,2} + \ldots + \beta_k x_{i,k} = \sum_{j=1}^{k} \beta_j x_{i,j}.$

The logit transformation is the link function relating the sum of the covariates to the probability of the binary outcome.

Multivariable regression is used to control for confounding. Confounding occurs when the apparent association between a covariate and an outcome is affected by the relationship of a third variable to the covariate and to the outcome; the third variable is a confounder. As contrasted to sequentially regressing each covariate against the response variable, this is done by simultaneously fitting all explanatory variables simultaneously.[21] For example, in exploring the relationship between tobacco and myocardial infarction, male sex, poverty, and sedentary lifestyle could be confounders because they are associated with both smoking and coronary heart disease.

Each year thousands of reports are published in the medical literature using stepwise, multivariable logistic regression on observational data to identify "independent" predictors for various clinical outcomes.[22] In the anesthesia literature PONV has been a very common topic for such statistical modeling.[23–26] Stepwise, multivariable logistic regression is an automatic procedure where there are a large number of potential explanatory variables and no underlying theory on which to base the selection of prediction model risk factors.[27] Once these prediction models have been created, there is a framework for assessing their performance.[28–30] Great skepticism should be shown for most of these prognostic models, especially those concerning mortality, as they usually have not been validated, have modest accuracy, and do not have documented clinical utility.[31,32]

Propensity Score Matching and Analysis

Another approach for providing estimation of treatment-effect in NRSs is the methodology of propensity score matching.[33] This use of NRS data is intended to investigate the effect of treatment X on a specified dichotomous outcome Y; the good outcome can be denoted Y^+, for example, survival, with Y^- being the opposite. It is usually the case that one or more baseline prognostic covariates (confounders $C_1, C_2, ..., C_k$) may be imbalanced between the patients that did (X^+) and did not (X^-) receive the treatment of interest. The favorable outcome, conditional on receiving treatment X^+, is denoted $Y^+|X^+$ with $Y^+|X^-$ being a favorable outcome in those not receiving the treatment. Any difference between interventions on the outcome Y may be a consequence of the confounders influencing both the treatment and the outcome; a failure to observe a difference in outcome may also be a consequence of confounding. As an example, pulmonary artery catheterization (PAC) in the care of the critically ill was adopted about 40 years ago and widely disseminated without rigorous evaluation. The enthusiasm of intensivists for such monitoring even forced the cessation of an RCT comparing care with and without PACs because of the unwillingness of physicians to allow patient participation in the study.[34] Using data of 5,735 critically ill patients, Connors et al.[35] reported lower 6-month survival in the 2,184 patients with PACs ($Y^+|X^+$ = 46.3% vs. $Y^+|X^-$ = 53.7%), but far more X^+ patients had multiorgan system failure (MOSF: 57% vs. 35%) at the time of PAC placement; there were other imbalances of initial covariates. Was the higher mortality attributable to the use of PACs or to a greater severity of illness? Using propensity matching, Connors created a pair of subsets (1,008 patients vs. 1,008 patients) with similar proportions of prognostic factors in both groups (e.g., MOSF: 34%); 6-month survival was still lower ($Y^+|X^+$ = 46.0% vs. $Y^+|X^-$ = 51.2%).

Propensity score matching is a statistical technique within the general concept of matching. If only one prognostic factor was important, for example, sex, then a pair of matched subsets could be created easily by repeatedly and randomly placing one man and one woman into each subset—matching the groups just by sex. However, there is usually a great deal of baseline information about patients observed in an NRS; Connors et al.[35] had details for about 40+ baseline covariates. In addition, it is often not evident which baseline characteristics are predictive of outcome. Creating matched groups by simple matching is not generally possible using more than a very few covariates.

The propensity score is defined as a subject's probability of receiving a specific treatment conditional on the many baseline covariates. The propensity score is usually estimated by multivariable logistic regression. In contrast to the attempt to create a parsimonious model with a few independent predictors of outcome by logistic regression modeling of NRS data, all available covariates are left in the model for a propensity score whether or not they are statistically significant. These covariates must be restricted to those that are known prior to the intervention. In the study by Connors, the presence/absence of MOSF on hospital admission should be included in propensity score; MOSF developing a week later should not.

For each patient in the data set, the z score obtained from the sum of each covariate times its regression coefficient is calculated: $z = \beta_0 + \beta_1 C_{i,1} + \beta_2 C_{i,2} + \ldots + \beta_k C_{i,k} = \sum_{j=1}^{k} \beta_j C_{i,j}$. Taking the antilogit of the z score ($p = \frac{1}{1+e^{-z}}$) yields the probability that a patient with those covariate values received the intervention. Of course, it is in fact known whether or not a patient received the intervention. Propensity matched subsets of patients are created by randomly choosing and matching one patient receiving the intervention to one patient not receiving the intervention with the same probability from the z score; usually the propensity probabilities (scores) are matched to the third or greater decimal place. The success of propensity score matching in balancing many covariates was well displayed in an observational comparison of epidural anesthesia for intermediate-to-high risk noncardiac surgery by Wijeysundera et al.[36] As graphed by Gayat et al.[37] (Fig. 7-3), 45 baseline characteristics of two matched subsets of about 44,000 patients each became extremely well balanced. In the original data set, an arterial line was used in 59% versus 33%; after balancing, an arterial line was used in 48% for both. The total of patients in the two matched subsets will always be less than the total count of patients in the NRS data set; some patients cannot be matched. Simple paired statistics are used to compare the outcomes of the two subsets.

Propensity score methods are being used in NRSs to reduce the effect of selection bias in estimating causal treatment effects. Besides propensity score matching, the effect of selection bias can also be reduced by using propensity scores for stratification, regression adjustment, and weighting. It is now routine to see NRS using propensity analysis in the intensive care and anesthesia literature—most commonly using matching.[37] A propensity score matching analysis should include: (1) details of propensity score building; (2) matching method; and (3) demonstration of covariate balancing by tabular or graphical display.[37] The propensity score can reduce bias due to observed covariates.

But propensity score methods cannot replace the RCT because randomization minimizes covariate imbalance between treatment groups for observed, unobserved, and unobservable covariates. In 2007, Murphy et al.[38] reported outcomes following cardiac surgery using a database of operations on about 8,700 patients; propensity scores estimated from preoperative risk factors and intraoperative events were used to adjust all statistical comparisons for this potential confounding. Mortality, morbidity, and cost of care was increased in patients receiving blood. In 2015 Murphy et al.[39] reported the 2,000-patient TITRe2 trial with the hypothesis that a restrictive threshold for red-cell transfusion would reduce

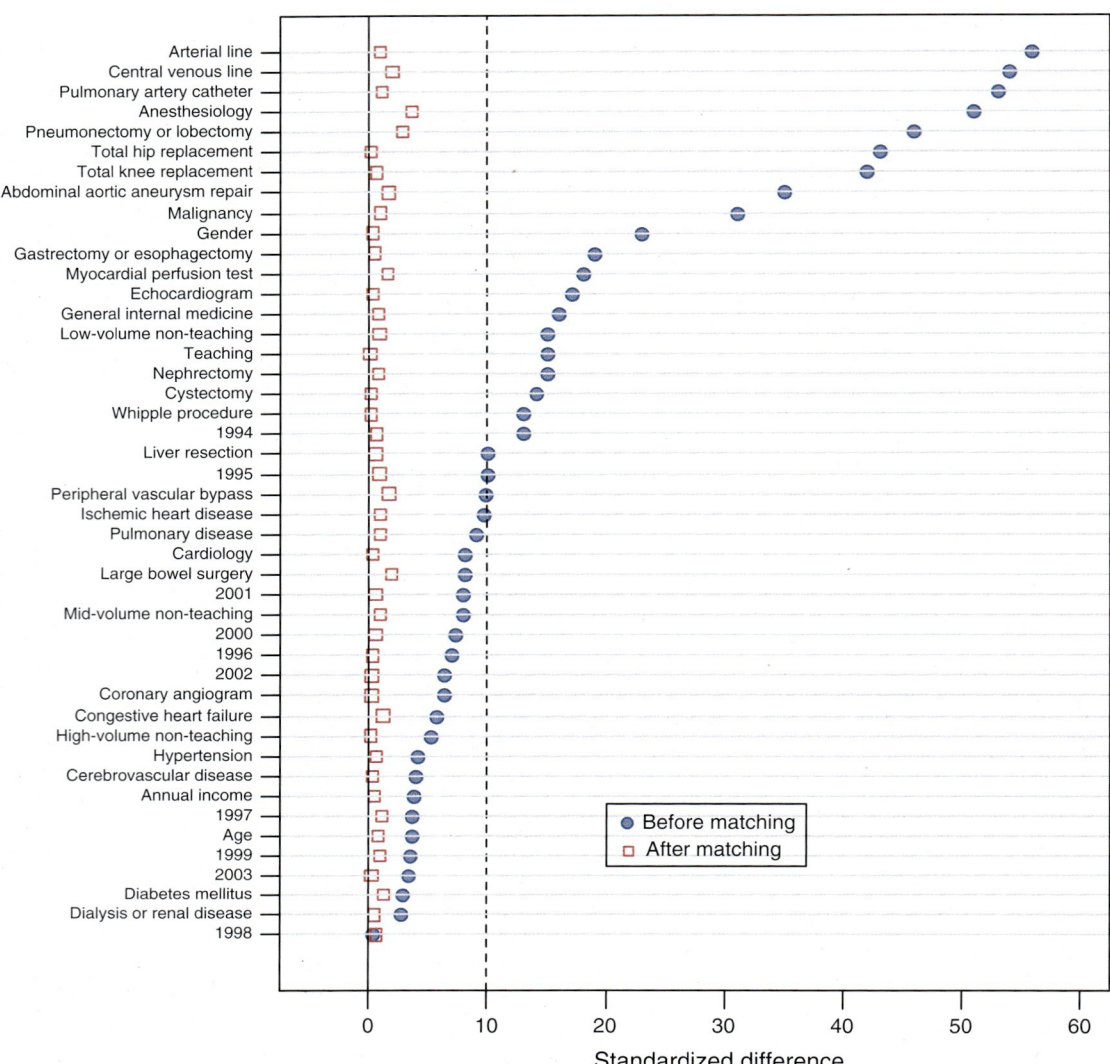

Figure 7-3 Graphical representation of 45 baseline covariates before and after propensity score matching using data from Wijeysundera et al.[36] The standardized difference for each covariate is the average difference between groups divided by the average standard deviation of the two groups. The standardized difference increases directly with increasing imbalance between groups. With propensity score matching, the standardized difference is close to zero for all covariates. (Reprinted from Gayat E, Pirracchio R, Resche-Rigon M, et al. Propensity scores in intensive care and anaesthesiology literature: a systematic review. *Intensive Care Med.* 36;2010;1997.[37] With kind permission from Springer Science+Business Media.)

postoperative morbidity. There was no difference by transfusion strategy in the primary, composite outcome (serious infections or ischemic events); indeed, mortality was higher (4.2% vs. 2.6%) at 3 months in the restrictive-threshold group. Contrasting RCTs and NRS, the authors concluded: "The difference is probably due to the fact that observational analyses are confounded by prognostic factors that influence the decision to transfuse red cells." Even a well-conducted propensity adjusted analysis cannot remove confounding for unobserved or unobservable covariates.

Systematic Reviews and Meta-analyses

7 It is over 25 years since the first systematic review (SR) with an accompanying meta-analysis (MA) was published in an anesthesia journal[40] and reports using these research methods are now commonplace in anesthesia journals.[41–44] The focused question of an SR of interventions can be subsumed by the acronym PICO: P, Population; I, Intervention; C, Comparison; and O, Outcome. The structured title of an SR usually contains most of the PICO elements.

Data are obtained from controlled trials (usually randomized) already in the medical literature rather than from newly conducted clinical trials; the basic unit of analysis of this observational research is the published study. A structured protocol is followed that includes in part: (1) choice of study inclusion/exclusion criteria; (2) explicitly defined literature searching; (3) abstraction of data from included studies; (4) appraisal of risk bias within each study; (5) systematic pooling of data; and (6) discussion of inferences. This structured protocol is intended to minimize bias. Even RCTs may have sources of bias such as

(1) selection bias: systematic differences between the patients receiving each intervention; (2) performance bias: systematic differences in care being given to study patients other than the preplanned interventions being evaluated; (3) attrition bias: systematic differences in the withdrawal of patients from each of the two intervention groups; and (4) detection bias: systematic differences in the ascertainment and recording of outcomes. The main focus of bias detection in the trials incorporated into an SR is (1) the randomization process, (2) the concealment of random allocation, (3) the use of blinding, and (4) the reporting/analysis of dropouts.

Binary outcomes (yes/no, alive/dead, presence/absence) within a study are usually compared by the RR or OR effect size; for continuous variables, the effect size is the mean difference. If there is sufficient clinical similarity among the included studies, a summary value of the overall effect size of the intervention versus comparison treatments is estimated by MA. MA is a set of statistical techniques for combining results from different studies. The results of an MA are usually present in a figure called a *Forest plot* (Fig. 7-4). The far left column identifies the included studies; the center left columns display the observed data. The center right columns lists the RRs with 95% CIs for the individual studies and the summary statistics. The horizontal lines and diamond shapes in the figures of the far right column are graphical representations of individual study relative risk and summary relative risk, respectively. There are also descriptive and inferential statistics concerning the statistical heterogeneity of the MA and the significance of the summary statistics. Methods for MA continue to be refined. For example, the assessment of statistical power of MAs has prompted new statistical approaches to maintain the Type I error rate with MA updating.[45] Also, it has been noted that the initial estimates of benefit in an SR are generally inflated when compared to the effect size estimated when the SR is later updated.[46]

An examination of Figure 7-4 shows that 11 of 15 individual comparisons had wide, nonsignificant CIs that touch or cross the RR of identity (RR = 1). However, the overall consistency of effect is easily seen with lidocaine being "favored" in only one study. The RR calculated from all studies was 7.31 with a 95% CI [4.16, 12.86]. The power of summary statistics to combine evidence is clear. About every seventh patient (92/637) who had a lidocaine spinal block had Transient Neurologic Syndrome (TNS); this risk of TNS was about seven times higher compared to other local anesthetics.[47]

The production of SRs comes from several sources. Many come from the individual initiative of researchers who publish their results as stand-alone reports in the journals of medicine and anesthesia. The American Society of Anesthesiologists has developed a process for the creation of practice parameters that includes among other things a variant form of SRs. A prominent proponent of SRs is the Cochrane Collaboration: an international network of more than 30,000 volunteers from over 100 countries that have published over 6,500 SRs online in The Cochrane Library.[a] An important distinction between Cochrane and non-Cochrane SRs is an obligation by the authors to maintain and update Cochrane SRs periodically as new research reports become available; an SR is provisional, an update with new evidence always being possible. The Cochrane Collaboration has extensive documentation, tutorials, and software available electronically explaining the techniques of SRs and MA.[48] There are more than 50 collaborative review groups within the Cochrane Collaboration that provide the editorial control and supervision of SRs; one of these is responsible for reviews of interventions in anesthesia, and critical and emergency care.[49]

Big Data

Big data has the attributes of the three "V"s (Volume, Velocity, and Variety). How big is Big Data? The volume usually cited is billions of records produced at a velocity of millions each day encompassing many variable types. The computer storage of Big Data requires a new nomenclature beyond gigabyte (GB) and terabyte: petabyte = 10^6 GBs; exabyte = 10^9 GBs; and even higher. Big Data is now a formal activity at the National Institutes of Health, the Big Data to Knowledge (BD2 K) Initiative.[50] The mission statement of BD2 K includes: "To conduct research and develop the methods, software, and tools needed to analyze biomedical Big Data."[b]

Big Data can be also defined to include studies that required new approaches to the collection, management, and analysis of data beyond those commonly used or available; historically, two epidemiology reports in anesthesia published 50 or more years ago can claim inclusion within Big Data. The first was a 5-year (1948–1952) study of all postoperative deaths following about 600,000 anesthetics at 10 academic medical centers distributed across the United States.[51] The other was the National Halothane Study, which reported the rate of deaths and fatal hepatic necrosis during four years (1959–1962) following about 850,000 anesthetics at 34 hospitals.[52] Both studies required a scaling up of resources for data collection and management and both included new statistical methods.

Besides the Big Data of genomics and medical images, what else does Big Data promise? Messages posted to social media and inquiries on web search engines tally in the millions each day. The logs of this activity have been called the digital exhaust of our age. Is there usable health content therein? Authors from the search engine company Google reported that by tallying search topics, for example, "Cold/flu remedy" or "Influenza complication," this social media data predicted accurately flu trends across several years of flu epidemics; these predictions mirrored official health statistics of the rise and fall of infections.[53] It was proposed that by harnessing the collective intelligence of millions of users, even faster surveillance of disease activity was possible. A more skeptical reexamination of these social media models found them not sufficient to replace timely local and national surveillance of health trends.[54]

Whither Big Data in anesthesia?[55-57] There is much use of institutional and governmental administrative and billing databases in epidemiology reports of anesthesia. And there are now several national repositories of perioperative data including the National Clinical Outcomes Registry (NACOR), the Multicenter Perioperative Outcomes Group (MPOG), the National Surgery Quality Program (NSQIP), and the Society of Thoracic Surgeons National Database.[56] Although all have millions of patient records, only MPOG routinely captures all physiologic monitoring data at 5-minute or more frequent intervals. Even with this perioperative data, no repository or administrative database meets the definition of Big Data. The routine digitation of waveforms (e.g., electrocardiogram) at high resolution with storage in a national repository would quickly create Big Data.[58] The use of prospective genotyping of patients prior to anesthesia and surgery would also create Big Data.[56,59] Until then, anesthesia does not fit under Big Data.

---

[a]See http://www.cochrane.org.

[b]See https://datascience.nih.gov/bd2 k/about.

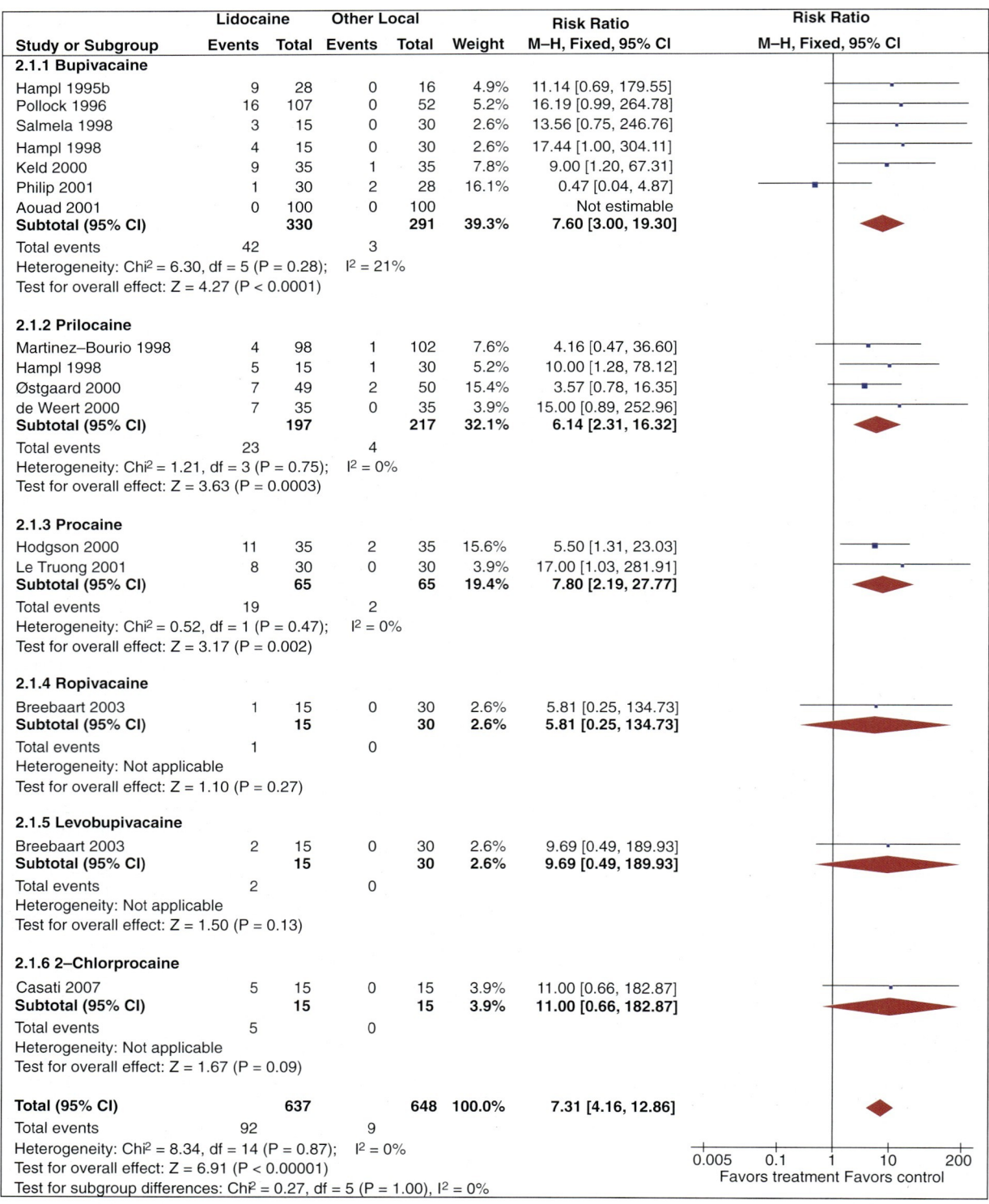

Figure 7-4 A Forest plot illustrates the relative strength of treatment effect across multiple studies. The point estimate for each study is represented by a square with 95% CIs represented by horizontal lines. In a Forest plot of RRs or ORs, the x-axis of the graph is on a logarithmic scale so that CIs are symmetrical about the point estimate. The vertical line of no effect is at 1. The area of each square is proportional to the weight of that study in the summary RR. The summary RRs are diamonds whose lateral points indicate the 95% CI of the summary value. Reprinted by permission and is published within a Cochrane Review in the Cochrane Database of Systematic Reviews 2009, Issue 2. Cochrane Reviews are regularly updated as new evidence emerges and in response to comments and criticisms, and the Cochrane Database of Systematic Reviews should be consulted for the most recent version of the Review. (Reprinted with permission from Zaric D, Pace NL. Transient neurologic symptoms [TNS] following spinal anaesthesia with lidocaine versus other local anaesthetics. Cochrane Database of Systematic Reviews 2009, Issue 2. Art. No.: CD003006. DOI: http://dx.doi.org/10.1002/14651858.CD003006.pub3. Copyright John Wiley & Sons.)[47]

Conclusions

Interpretation of Results

Scientific studies do not end with the statistical test.[60] The experimenter must submit an opinion as to the generalizability of his or her work to the rest of the world. Even if there is a statistically significant difference, the experimenter must decide if this difference is medically or physiologically important. Statistical significance does not always equate with biologic relevance. The questions an experimenter should ask about the interpretation of results are highly dependent on the specifics of the experiment. First, even small, clinically unimportant differences between groups can be detected if the sample size is sufficiently large. On the other hand, if the sample size is small, one must always worry that identified or unidentified confounding variables may explain any difference; as the sample size decreases, randomization is less successful in assuring homogenous groups. Second, if the experimental groups are given three or more doses of a drug, do the results suggest a steadily increasing or decreasing dose–response relationship? Suppose the observed effect for an intermediate dose is either much higher or much lower than that for both the highest and lowest dose; a dose–response relationship may exist, but some skepticism about the experimental methods is warranted. Third, for clinical studies comparing different drugs, devices, and operations on patient outcome, are the patients, clinical care, and studied therapies sufficiently similar to those provided at other locations to be of interest to a wide group of practitioners? This is the distinction between *efficacy*—does it work under the best (research) circumstances—and *effectiveness*—does it work under the typical circumstances of routine clinical care?

Finally, in comparing alternative therapies, the confidence that a claim for a superior therapy is true depends on the study design. The strength of the evidence concerning efficacy will be least for an anecdotal case report; next in importance will be a retrospective study, then a prospective series of patients compared with historical controls, and finally a randomized, controlled clinical trial. The greatest strength for a therapeutic claim is a series of randomized, controlled clinical trials confirming the same hypothesis.

Statistical Resources

Accompanying the exponential growth of medical information has been the creation of a wealth of biostatistical knowledge. The increased emphasis on evidence-based medicine creates a great need for educating future and current physicians in quantitative reasoning, probability, and statistics. Detailed expositions of specific and recommended topics within these domains are available.[61] Textbooks oriented toward medical statistics and with expositions of basic, intermediate, and advanced statistics abound.[62–67] There are journals of biomedical statistics, including *Epidemiology, Research Synthesis Methods, Systematic Reviews, Statistics in Medicine*, and *Statistical Methods in Medical Research*, whose audiences are both statisticians and biomedical researchers. Some medical journals, for example, the *British Medical Journal*, regularly publish expositions of both basic and newer advanced statistical methods. Extensive Internet resources including free online courses of data analysis methods, electronic textbooks of basic statistical methods, online statistical calculators, standard data sets, and reviews of statistical software can be easily found. High performance statistical software is freely available from the R Foundation for Statistical Computing, Vienna, Austria.[c]

There is a continuing expansion in the resources giving guidance in methodology. Much of the improvement has been driven by epidemiologists and statisticians associated with the Cochrane Collaboration. Standards for the reporting of the clinical trials and observational studies and for the SR and MA techniques include: (1) the 2010 CONSORT (Consolidated Standards of Reporting Trials) statement[68,69]; (2) the STROBE (Strengthening the Reporting of Observational Studies in Epidemiology) statement[70,71]; (3) the PRISMA (Preferred Reporting Items for Systematic reviews and Meta-Analyses) statement[72,73]; and (4) the MOOSE (Meta-analysis of Observational Studies in Epidemiology) statement.[74] There is a centralized resource for obtaining these and other guidelines at the Equator-Network.[d]

Statistics and Anesthesia

Reports in journals of anesthesia now include many newer methods that have not been mentioned in this chapter. To mention just three: (1) studies of the pharmacokinetics and pharmacokinetics of a drug or a combination of drugs typically use linear mixed effects or generalized linear mixed effects models, (2) techniques of survival analysis are applied to hospital discharge times or postoperative morbidity/mortality outcomes, and (3) methods of interim analysis or sequential trial design are used in RCTs to stop futile or dangerous treatments.

Academic anesthesia needs more workers to immerse themselves in these statistical fundamentals. Having done so, these statistically knowledgeable academic anesthesiologists will be prepared to improve their own research projects, to assist their colleagues in research, to efficiently seek consultation from the professional statistician, to strengthen the editorial review of journal articles, and to expound to the clinical reader the whys and wherefores of statistics. The clinical reader also needs to expend his or her own effort to acquire some basic statistical skills. Journals are increasingly difficult to understand without some basic statistical understanding. Finally, understanding principles of experimental design and statistical inference can prevent premature acceptances of new therapies from faulty studies.

REFERENCES

1. Cobb LA, Thomas GI, Dillard DH, et al. An evaluation of internal-mammary-artery ligation by a double-blind technic. *N Engl J Med*. 1959;260:1115–1118.
2. Sacks H, Chalmers TC, Smith HJ. Randomized versus historical controls for clinical trials. *Am J Med*. 1982;72:233–240.
3. Kunz R, Oxman AD. The unpredictability paradox: review of empirical comparisons of randomised and non-randomised clinical trials. *BMJ*. 1998;317:1185–1190.
4. Herbison P, Hay-Smith J, Gillespie WJ. Different methods of allocation to groups in randomized trials are associated with different levels of bias: a meta-epidemiological study. *J Clin Epidemiol*. 2011;64:1070–1075.
5. Schulz KF, Chalmers I, Hayes RJ, et al. Empirical evidence of bias: dimensions of methodological quality associated with estimates of treatment effects in controlled trials. *JAMA*. 1995;273:408–412.
6. Goodman SN. Toward evidence-based medical statistics: 1. The P value fallacy. *Ann Intern Med*. 1999;130:995–1004.
7. Goodman SN. Toward evidence-based medical statistics: 2. The Bayes factor. *Ann Intern Med*. 1999;130:1005–1013.
8. Goodman SN. Of P-values and Bayes: a modest proposal. *Epidemiology*. 2001;12:295–297.
9. Nuzzo R. Scientific method: statistical errors. *Nature*. 2014;506:150–152.
10. Little RJ. Calibrated Bayes: A Bayes/Frequentist roadmap. *Am Stat*. 2006;60:213–223.
11. Sterne JA, Davey Smith G. Sifting the evidence-what's wrong with significance tests? *BMJ*. 2001;322:226–231.
12. Ioannidis JP. Why most published research findings are false. *PLoS Med*. 2005;2:e124.

---

[c]See http://www.R-project.org.

[d]See http://www.equator-network.org.

13. Ioannidis JP. Contradicted and initially stronger effects in highly cited clinical research. *JAMA*. 2005;294:218–228.
14. Ioannidis JP. Effect of formal statistical significance on the credibility of observational associations. *Am J Epidemiol*. 2008;168:374–383.
15. Katki HA. Invited commentary: evidence-based evaluation of p values and Bayes factors. *Am J Epidemiol*. 2008;168:384–388.
16. Hanley JA, Lippman-Hand A. If nothing goes wrong, is everything all right? Interpreting zero numerators. *JAMA*. 1983;249:1743–1745.
17. Tuyl F, Gerlach R, Mengersen K. A comparison of Bayes-Laplace, Jeffreys, and other priors: the case of zero events. *Am Stat*. 2008;62:40–44.
18. Anscombe FJ. Graphs in statistical analysis. *Am Stat*. 1973;27:17–21.
19. Ioannidis JP. Exposure-wide epidemiology: revisiting Bradford Hill. *Stat Med*. 2016;35:1749–1762.
20. Hill AB. The environment and disease: association or causation? *Proc R Soc Med*. 1965;58:295–300.
21. Katz MH. Multivariable analysis: a primer for readers of medical research. *Ann Intern Med*. 2003;138:644–650.
22. Brotman DJ, Walker E, Lauer MS, et al. In search of fewer independent risk factors. *Arch Intern Med*. 2005;165:138–145.
23. Eberhart LH, Morin AM. Risk scores for predicting postoperative nausea and vomiting are clinically useful tools and should be used in every patient. Con: 'life is really simple, but we insist on making it complicated.' *Eur J Anaesthesiol*. 2011;28:155–159.
24. Kranke P. Effective management of postoperative nausea and vomiting: let us practise what we preach! *Eur J Anaesthesiol*. 2011;28:152–154.
25. Pierre S. Risk scores for predicting post-operative nausea and vomiting are clinically useful tools and should be used in every patient: 'Don't throw the baby out with the bathwater.' *Eur J Anaesthesiol*. 2011;28:160–163.
26. Pace NL, Eberhart LH, Kranke PR. Quantifying prognosis with risk predictions. *Eur J Anaesthesiol*. 2012;29:7–16.
27. Pace NL. Independent predictors from stepwise logistic regression may be nothing more than publishable p values. *Anesth Analg*. 2008;107:1775–1778.
28. Cook NR. Statistical evaluation of prognostic versus diagnostic models: beyond the ROC curve. *Clin Chem*. 2008;54:17–23.
29. Cook NR, Ridker PM. Advances in measuring the effect of individual predictors of cardiovascular risk: the role of reclassification measures. *Ann Intern Med*. 2009;150:795–802.
30. Steyerberg EW, Vickers AJ, Cook NR, et al. Assessing the performance of prediction models: a framework for traditional and novel measures. *Epidemiology*. 2010;21:128–138.
31. Siontis GC, Tzoulaki I, Ioannidis JP. Predicting death: an empirical evaluation of predictive tools for mortality. *Arch Intern Med*. 2011;171:1721–1726.
32. Wyatt JC, Altman DG. Prognostic models: clinically useful or quickly forgotten? *BMJ*. 1995;311:1539–1541.
33. Haukoos JS, Lewis RJ. The propensity score. *JAMA*. 2015;314:1637–1638.
34. Guyatt G. A randomized control trial of right-heart catheterization in critically ill patients. Ontario Intensive Care Study Group. *J Intensive Care Med*. 1991;6:91–95.
35. Connors AF, Jr., Speroff T, Dawson NV, et al. The effectiveness of right heart catheterization in the initial care of critically ill patients. SUPPORT Investigators. *JAMA*. 1996;276:889–897.
36. Wijeysundera DN, Beattie WS, Austin PC, et al. Epidural anaesthesia and survival after intermediate-to-high risk non-cardiac surgery: a population-based cohort study. *Lancet*. 2008;372:562–569.
37. Gayat E, Pirracchio R, Resche-Rigon M, et al. Propensity scores in intensive care and anaesthesiology literature: a systematic review. *Intensive Care Med*. 2010;36:1993–2003.
38. Murphy GJ, Reeves BC, Rogers CA, et al. Increased mortality, postoperative morbidity, and cost after red blood cell transfusion in patients having cardiac surgery. *Circulation*. 2007;116:2544–2552.
39. Murphy GJ, Pike K, Rogers CA, et al. Liberal or restrictive transfusion after cardiac surgery. *N Engl J Med*. 2015;372:997–1008.
40. Pace NL. Prevention of succinylcholine myalgias: a meta-analysis. *Anesth Analg*. 1990;70:477–483.
41. Biondi-Zoccai G, Lotrionte M, Landoni G, et al. The rough guide to systematic reviews and meta-analyses. *HSR Proc Intensive Care Cardiovasc Anesth*. 2011;3:161–173.
42. Carlisle JB. Systematic reviews: how they work and how to use them. *Anaesthesia*. 2007;62:702–707.
43. Kranke P. Evidence-based practice: how to perform and use systematic reviews for clinical decision-making. *Eur J Anaesthesiol*. 2010;27:763–772.
44. Pace NL. Research methods for meta-analyses. *Best Pract Res Clin Anaesthesiol*. 2011;25:523–533.
45. Imberger G, Gluud C, Boylan J, et al. Systematic reviews of anesthesiologic interventions reported as statistically significant: problems with power, precision, and type 1 error protection. *Anesth Analg*. 2015;121:1611–1622.
46. Pereira TV, Ioannidis JP. Statistically significant meta-analyses of clinical trials have modest credibility and inflated effects. *J Clin Epidemiol*. 2011;64:1060–1069.
47. Zaric D, Pace NL. Transient neurologic symptoms (TNS) following spinal anaesthesia with lidocaine versus other local anaesthetics. *Cochrane Database Syst Rev*. 2009;(2):CD003006.
48. Cochrane Handbook for Systematic Reviews of Interventions. Version 5.1.0: The Cochrane Collaboration; 2011. Available from: http://www.cochrane-handbook.org.
49. Pedersen T, Møller A. The Cochrane Collaboration and the Cochrane Anaesthesia Review Group. In: Møller A, Pedersen T, Cracknell J, eds. *Evidence-Based Anaesthesia and Intensive Care*. New York, NY: Cambridge University Press; 2006:77–87.
50. Margolis R, Derr L, Dunn M, et al. The National Institutes of Health's Big Data to Knowledge (BD2 K) initiative: capitalizing on biomedical big data. *J Am Med Inform Assoc*. 2014;21:957–958.
51. Beecher HK, Todd DP. A study of the deaths associated with anesthesia and surgery: based on a study of 599548 anesthesias in ten institutions 1948–1952, inclusive. *Ann Surg*. 1954;140:2–35.
52. Summary of the national Halothane Study. Possible association between halothane anesthesia and postoperative hepatic necrosis. *JAMA*. 1966;197:775–788.
53. Ginsberg J, Mohebbi MH, Patel RS, et al. Detecting influenza epidemics using search engine query data. *Nature*. 2009;457:1012–1014.
54. Olson DR, Konty KJ, Paladini M, et al. Reassessing Google Flu Trends data for detection of seasonal and pandemic influenza: a comparative epidemiological study at three geographic scales. *PLoS Comput Biol*. 2013;9:e1003256.
55. Giambrone GP, Hemmings HC, Sturm M, et al. Information technology innovation: the power and perils of big data. *Br J Anaesth*. 2015;115:339–342.
56. Levin MA, Wanderer JP, Ehrenfeld JM. Data, big data, and metadata in anesthesiology. *Anesth Analg*. 2015;121:1661–1667.
57. Simpao AF, Ahumada LM, Rehman MA. Big data and visual analytics in anaesthesia and health care. *Br J Anaesth*. 2015;115:350–356.
58. Liu D, Gorges M, Jenkins SA. University of Queensland vital signs dataset: development of an accessible repository of anesthesia patient monitoring data for research. *Anesth Analg*. 2012;114:584–589.
59. Pulley JM, Denny JC, Peterson JF, et al. Operational implementation of prospective genotyping for personalized medicine: the design of the Vanderbilt PREDICT project. *Clin Pharmacol Ther*. 2012;92:87–95.
60. Sutherland WJ, Spiegelhalter D, Burgman MA. Policy: Twenty tips for interpreting scientific claims. *Nature*. 2013;503:335–337.
61. Baldi B, Utts J. What your future doctor should know about statistics: must-include topics for introductory undergraduate biostatistics. *Am Stat*. 2015;69:231–240.
62. Campbell MJ, Machin D, Walters SJ. *Medical Statistics: A Textbook for the Health Sciences*. 4th ed. Chichester, England: John Wiley & Sons; 2007.
63. Dalgaard P. *Introductory Statistics with R*. 2nd ed. New York, NY: Springer; 2008.
64. Dawson B, Trapp R. *Basic & Clinical Biostatistics*. 4th ed. New York, NY: McGraw-Hill; 2004.
65. Glantz SA. *Primer of Biostatistics*. 7th ed. New York, NY: McGraw-Hill; 2012.
66. Guyatt G, Rennie D, Meade MO, et al. *Users Guides' Manual for Evidence-Based Clinical Practice*. 3rd ed. New York, NY: McGraw-Hill Education; 2014.
67. Riffenburgh RH. *Statistics in Medicine*. 3rd ed. San Diego, CA: Academic Press; 2012.
68. Moher D, Hopewell S, Schulz KF, et al. CONSORT 2010 explanation and elaboration: updated guidelines for reporting parallel group randomised trials. *BMJ*. 2010;340:c869.
69. Schulz KF, Altman DG, Moher D. CONSORT 2010 statement: updated guidelines for reporting parallel group randomised trials. *BMJ*. 2010;340:c332.
70. Vandenbroucke JP, von Elm E, Altman DG, et al. Strengthening the Reporting of Observational Studies in Epidemiology (STROBE): explanation and elaboration. *PLoS Med*. 2007;4:e297.
71. von Elm E, Altman DG, Egger M, et al. Strengthening the Reporting of Observational Studies in Epidemiology (STROBE) statement: guidelines for reporting observational studies. *BMJ*. 2007;335:806–808.
72. Liberati A, Altman DG, Tetzlaff J, et al. The PRISMA statement for reporting systematic reviews and meta-analyses of studies that evaluate healthcare interventions: explanation and elaboration. *BMJ*. 2009;339:b2700.
73. Moher D, Liberati A, Tetzlaff J, et al. Preferred reporting items for systematic reviews and meta-analyses: the PRISMA statement. *BMJ*. 2009;339:b2535.
74. Stroup DF, Berlin JA, Morton SC, et al. Meta-analysis of observational studies in epidemiology: a proposal for reporting: Meta-analysis of Observational Studies in Epidemiology (MOOSE) group. *JAMA*. 2000;283:2008–2012.

8 Inflammation, Wound Healing, and Infection

HARRIET W. HOPF • AMALIA COCHRAN • CRISTIANE M. UENO • CANDICE MORRISSEY

Infection Control
  Hand Hygiene
  Antisepsis
  Antibiotic Prophylaxis
Mechanisms of Wound Repair
  The Initial Response to Injury
  Resistance to Infection
  Proliferation
  Maturation and Remodeling

Wound Perfusion and Oxygenation
Patient Management
  Preoperative Preparation
  Intraoperative Management
  Postoperative Management
Summary
  Areas for Future Research

KEY POINTS

1. The most crucial component of infection prevention is frequent and effective hand hygiene. Wearing gloves does not reduce the need for hand hygiene.

2. The ideal hand hygiene agent kills a broad spectrum of microbes, has antimicrobial activity that persists for at least 6 hours after application, is simple to use, and has few side effects. Antibiotic prophylaxis has become standard for surgeries in which there is more than a minimum risk of infection. The most commonly used antibiotic for surgical prophylaxis is cefazolin, a first-generation cephalosporin, as the potential pathogens for most surgeries are gram-positive cocci from the skin.

3. The exact timing for the administration of the antibiotic depends on the pharmacology and half-life of the drug, but should generally be 0 to 60 minutes before incision. Anesthesiologists should work in consultation with surgeons to use guidelines determined by the local infection control committee to take initiative for administering prophylactic antibiotics because they have access to the patient during the 60 minutes prior to incision and can optimize timing of administration. The standard teaching that oxygen delivery depends more on hemoglobin-bound oxygen (oxygen content) than on arterial PO_2 may be true of working muscle, but it is not true of wound healing.

4. Although oxygen consumption is relatively low in wounds, it is consumed by processes that require oxygen at a high concentration. Delivery of oxygen to wounds depends on arterial PO_2 rather than hemoglobin-bound oxygen (oxygen content). High oxygen tensions (>100 mmHg) can be reached in wounds but only if perfusion is normal and arterial PO_2 is high. Peripheral vasoconstriction, which results from central sympathetic control of subcutaneous vascular tone, is probably the most frequent and clinically the most important impediment to wound oxygenation and wound healing. All vasoconstrictive stimuli must be corrected simultaneously to allow optimal healing. Modifiable risks for wound infections include smoking, malnutrition, obesity, hyperglycemia, hypercholesterolemia, and hypertension. These should be assessed and corrected when possible prior to surgery.

5. Prevention or correction of hypothermia has been shown to decrease wound infections and increase collagen deposition in patients undergoing major abdominal surgery. Maintenance of a high room temperature or active warming before, during, and after the operation is significantly more effective than other methods of warming, such as application of warmed blankets, circulating water blankets placed on the surface of the operating table, and humidification of the breathing circuit.

6. Optimizing the volume of perioperative fluid administration to minimize morbidity and mortality remains a significant and controversial challenge. Current best recommendations for volume management include replacing fluid losses based on standard recommendations for the type of surgery, replacement of blood loss, and replacement of other ongoing fluid losses (e.g., high urine output due to diuretic or dye administration, hyperglycemia, or thermoregulatory vasoconstriction).

7. Administration of supplemental oxygen via face mask or nasal cannulae increases safety in patients receiving systemic opioids. As a side benefit, it may also improve wound healing. Pain control also appears important since it favorably influences both pulmonary function and vascular tone.

8. In patients with moderate to high risk of surgical site infection, anesthesiologists have the opportunity to enhance wound healing and reduce the incidence of wound infections by simple, inexpensive, and readily available means.

Introduction

Despite major advances in the management of patients undergoing surgery—including aseptic technique, prophylactic antibiotics, and advances in surgical approaches such as laparoscopic surgery—surgical wound infection and wound failure remain common complications of surgery (Fig. 8-1).[1] The Centers for Disease Control and Prevention (CDC) estimates that 18 million operative procedures were performed in acute care hospitals in the United States in 2010 and there were approximately 157,500

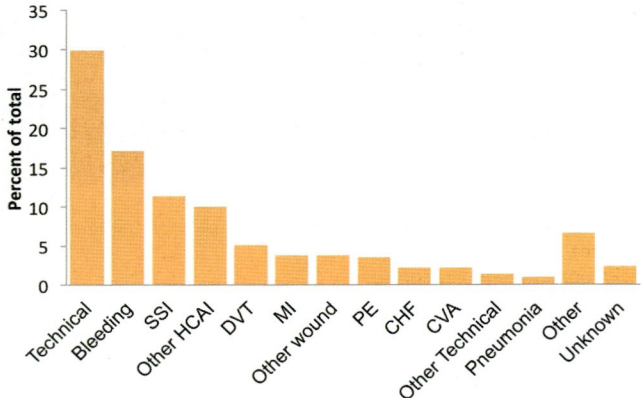

Figure 8-1 Thomas et al. reviewed the records of 15,000 nonpsychiatric patients discharged from a representative sample of Utah and Colorado hospitals in 1992 for adverse events. There were 17,912 adverse events identified, or 2.9 ± 0.2% of hospitalizations. Of these, almost half (45%) were related to operative care. The graph shows the distribution of adverse events within the subcategory of operative care (7,716 operative adverse events). About 20% were infection related and about 15% were wound related. SSI, surgical site infection; HCAI, health-care–associated infection; DVT, deep venous thrombosis; MI, myocardial infarction; PE, pulmonary embolus; CHF, congestive heart failure; CVA, cerebrovascular accident. (Data from Thomas EJ, Studdert DM, Burstin HR, et al. Incidence and types of adverse events and negligent care in Utah and Colorado. *Med Care.* 2000;38:261–271.)

surgical site infections (SSIs) in 2011 (Table 8-1).[2] Wound complications are associated with prolonged hospitalization, increased resource consumption, and even increased mortality. A growing body of literature supports the concept that patient factors are a major determinant of wound outcome following surgery. Comorbidities such as diabetes and cardiac disease clearly contribute, and a patient's genetic make-up may also contribute.[3] Environmental stressors and the individual response to stress are also important. In particular, wounds are exquisitely sensitive to hypoxia, which is both common and preventable. Perioperative management can be adapted to promote postoperative wound healing and resistance to infection. Along with aseptic technique and prophylactic antibiotics, maintaining perfusion and oxygenation of the wound is paramount. This chapter discusses how knowledge of the principles of infection control and the biology and physiology of wound repair and resistance to infection can improve outcomes.

Infection Control

1 Hand Hygiene

Perhaps the most crucial component of infection prevention is frequent and effective hand hygiene. In 1847, Ignaz Semmelweis made the observation that women who delivered their babies in the First Clinic at the General Hospital of Vienna, staffed by medical students and physicians, had a mortality rate of 5% to 15%, largely the result of puerperal infections; this was substantially higher than the 2% rate of women who delivered at Clinic 2, which was staffed by midwife students and midwives.[4] Students and physicians at Clinic 1 usually started the day performing autopsies (including on patients who died of puerperal fever) and then moved on to the clinic, where they performed examinations on women in labor. Semmelweis made the connection, and although germ theory was some years off, he insisted that physicians and medical students wash their hands in a chlorinated solution when leaving the pathology laboratory. This reduced the rate of puerperal fever to the same rate as at Clinic 2. Soon, Semmelweis identified cases of transmission from an infected to an uninfected patient, and instituted the use of chlorinated solution hand washing between cases as well. He also demonstrated that the chlorinated solution was more effective than soap and water. Unfortunately, his innovation was not widely adopted, resulting from a combination of his delay in publishing his results, the reluctance of his colleagues to accept that they might be responsible for transmitting disease, and his lack of tact in trying to convince health-care workers to adopt his measures. Despite our current knowledge of germ theory, hand hygiene remains an inexplicably neglected component of infection control: Studies consistently demonstrate about a 40% rate of adherence (range, 5% to 81%) to hand hygiene guidelines,[4] and compliance by anesthesiologists in the operating room (OR) is notably lower.[5]

Bacteria are resident in the skin and can never be completely eliminated.[6] Resident flora are embedded in the deeper folds of the skin and are more resistant to removal, but are also infrequently pathogenic. Coagulase-negative Staphylococci and diphtheroids are the most common. Transient flora colonize the superficial layers of the skin and thus are easier to remove with hand hygiene. Transient flora are also the source of most health-care–associated infections, as health-care worker skin can become contaminated from patient contact or contact with contaminated surfaces. Contamination from surfaces is most commonly with organisms such as Staphylococci and Enterococci, which are resistant to drying. Even "clean" activities such as taking a patient's pulse or applying monitors can lead to hand contamination: 100 to 1,000 colony-forming units of *Klebsiella* species were measured on nurses' hands following such activities in one study.[7] No studies have related hand contamination to actual transmission of infection to patients; however, numerous studies, starting with those of Semmelweis, have demonstrated a reduction in health-care–associated infections following institution of hand hygiene or improved adherence to hand hygiene.[6]

2

A number of products are available for hand hygiene. The ideal agent kills a broad spectrum of microbes, has antimicrobial activity that persists for at least 6 hours after application, is simple to use, and has few side effects. The most commonly used and efficacious agents are reviewed here.

Plain (not antiseptic) soap and water are generally the least effective at reducing hand contamination.[8] Although obvious dirt is removed by the detergent effect of soap and the mechanical action of washing, bacterial load is not greatly reduced. Further, soap and water hand hygiene is associated with high rates of skin irritation and drying, both of which are risk factors for an increased bacterial load. Soap and water are, however, the most effective at removing spores, and therefore should be used when contamination with *Clostridium difficile* or *Bacillus anthracis* is a concern.[6]

Alcohol-based rinses, gels, and foams denature proteins, and this confers their antimicrobial activity.[6] Ethanol is most commonly used because it has more antiviral activity than isopropanol. Antiseptics containing 60% to 95% ethanol with a water base are germicidal and effective against gram-positive and gram-negative bacteria, lipophilic viruses such as herpes simplex, human immunodeficiency, influenza, respiratory syncytial, and vaccinia viruses, and hepatitis B and C viruses. They have little persistent activity, although regrowth of bacteria does occur slowly after use of alcohol-based products. Combination with low doses of other agents such as chlorhexidine, quaternary ammonium compounds, or triclosan can confer persistent

Table 8-1 Criteria for Defining a Surgical Site Infection (SSI)

Superficial Incisional SSI
- Infection occurs within 30 days after the operation
  and
- Infection involves only skin or subcutaneous tissue of the incision
  and
- At least *one* of the following:
  1. Purulent drainage, with or without laboratory confirmation, from the superficial incision
  2. Organisms isolated from an aseptically obtained culture of fluid or tissue from the superficial incision
  3. At least one of the following signs or symptoms of infection: Pain or tenderness, localized swelling, redness, or heat *and* superficial incision is deliberately opened by the surgeon, *unless* the incision is culture-negative
  4. Diagnosis of superficial incisional SSI by the surgeon or attending physician
- Do *not* report the following conditions as superficial incisional SSI:
  1. Stitch abscess (minimal inflammation and discharge confined to the points of suture penetration)
  2. Infection of an episiotomy or newborn circumcision site
  3. Infected burn wound
  4. Incisional SSI that extends into the facial and muscle layers (see "Deep Incisional SSI")

Note: Specific criteria are used for identifying infected episiotomy and circumcision sites and burn wounds

Deep Incisional SSI
- Infection occurs within 30 days after the operation if no implant is left in place or within 1 year if implant is in place and the infection appears to be related to the operation
  and
- Infection involves deep soft tissues (e.g., fascial and muscle layers) of the incision
  and
- At least *one* of the following:
  1. Purulent drainage from the deep incision but not from the organ/space component of the surgical site
  2. A deep incision spontaneously dehisces or is deliberately opened by a surgeon when the patient has at least one of the following signs or symptoms: Fever (>38°C), localized pain, or tenderness, unless site is culture-negative
  3. An abscess or other evidence of infection involving the deep incision is found on direct examination, during reoperation, or by histopathologic or radiologic examination
  4. Diagnosis of a deep incisional SSI by a surgeon or attending physician

Notes:
  1. Report infection that involves both superficial and deep incision sites as deep incisional SSI
  2. Report an organ/space SSI that drains through the incision as a deep incisional SSI

Organ/Space SSI
- Infection occurs within 30 days after the operation if no implant is left in place or within 1 year if implant is in place and the infection appears to be related to the operation
  and
- Infection involves any part of the anatomy (e.g., organs or spaces), other than the incision, which was opened or manipulated during an operation
  and
- At least *one* of the following:
  1. Purulent drainage from a drain that is placed through a stab wound into the organ/space
  2. Organisms isolated from an aseptically obtained culture of fluid or tissue in the organ/space
  3. An abscess or other evidence of infection involving the organ/space that is found on direct examination, during reoperation, or by histopathologic or radiologic examination
  4. Diagnosis of an organ/space SSI by a surgeon or attending physician

From Mangram AJ, Horan TC, Pearson ML, et al. Guideline for Prevention of Surgical Site Infection, 1999. Centers for Disease Control and Prevention (CDC) Hospital Infection Control Practices Advisory Committee. *Am J Infect Control.* 1999;27:97–132, with permission.

---

activity. Efficacy depends on volume applied (3 mL is superior to 1 mL) and duration of contact (ideally, 30 seconds).

Chlorhexidine is a cationic bisbiguanide that disrupts cytoplasmic membranes, resulting in precipitation of cellular contents.[6] It is germicidal against gram-positive bacteria and lipophilic viruses, with somewhat less activity against gram-negative bacteria and fungi, and minimal against tubercle bacilli. It has substantial persistence on the skin. The CDC has identified chlorhexidine as the topical agent of choice. It may cause severe corneal damage after direct contact with the eye, ototoxicity after direct contact with the inner or middle ear, and neurotoxicity after direct contact with the brain or meninges. There are reports of bacteria that have acquired reduced susceptibility to chlorhexidine, but these are of questionable clinical pertinence since the concentrations at which resistance was found were substantially lower than that of commercially available products. Recent reports have identified immunoglobulin E–mediated allergic reactions to chlorhexidine.[9] Cases are likely underreported because of the difficulty identifying the source of anaphylactic reactions perioperatively. Chlorhexidine is present in a wide range of medical and community-based products,

Table 8-2 Indications for Hand Hygiene

When hands are visibly dirty or contaminated with proteinaceous material or are visibly soiled with blood or other body fluids, wash hands with either a nonantimicrobial soap and water or an antimicrobial soap and water.
If hands are not visibly soiled, use an alcohol-based hand rub for routinely decontaminating hands. Alternatively, wash hands with an antimicrobial soap and water.
Decontaminate hands before having direct contact with patients.
Decontaminate hands before donning sterile gloves when inserting a central intravascular catheter.
Decontaminate hands before inserting indwelling urinary catheters, peripheral vascular catheters, or other invasive devices that do not require a surgical procedure.
Decontaminate hands after contact with a patient's intact skin (e.g., applying monitors, moving patient).
Decontaminate hands after contact with body fluids or excretions, mucous membranes, nonintact skin, and wound dressings if hands are not visibly soiled.
Decontaminate hands if moving from a contaminated-body site (e.g., mouth during tracheal intubation) to a clean-body site (e.g., adjusting gas flow, turning on ventilator, starting IV) during patient care.
Decontaminate hands after contact with inanimate objects (including medical equipment) in the immediate vicinity of the patient. Take care to reduce contamination of the anesthesia machine (e.g., after tracheal intubation) as well!
Decontaminate hands after removing gloves.
Before eating and after using a restroom, wash hands with a nonantimicrobial soap and water or with an antimicrobial soap and water.
Antimicrobial-impregnated wipes (i.e., towelettes) may be considered as an alternative to washing hands with nonantimicrobial soap and water. Because they are not as effective as alcohol-based hand rubs or washing hands with an antimicrobial soap and water for reducing bacterial counts on the hands of HCWs, they are not a substitute for using an alcohol-based hand rub or antimicrobial soap.

IV, intravenous (tube); HCW, health-care worker.
Modified from Boyce JM, Pittet D. Guideline for hand hygiene in health-care settings. Recommendations of the Healthcare Infection Control Practices Advisory Committee and the HIPAC/SHEA/APIC/IDSA Hand Hygiene Task Force. *Am J Infect Control*. 2002;30(8):S1.

---

including wipes, impregnated central venous catheters, toothpaste, mouthwash, contact lens cleanser, and food preservatives. Therefore, potentially sensitizing exposures are common.

Iodine and iodophors (iodine with a polymer carrier) penetrate the cell wall and impair protein synthesis and cell membrane function.[6] They are bactericidal against gram-positive, gram-negative, and some spore-forming bacteria including clostridia and *Bacillus* species, although inactive against spores. They also have activity against mycobacteria, viruses, and fungi. Their persistence is generally fairly poor. They cause more contact dermatitis than other commonly used agents, and allergies to this class of topical agent are common. Iodophors generally cause fewer side effects than iodine agents.

The choice of an antiseptic depends on the expected pathogens, acceptability by health-care workers, and cost. In general, antiseptics cost about $1 per patient day, far less than the cost of health-care–associated infections. In nine studies that examined the effect of improved hand hygiene adherence on health-care–associated infections, the majority demonstrated that as hand hygiene practices improved, infection rates decreased.[6]

Barriers to hand hygiene include skin irritation and fear of skin irritation, inaccessibility, time, and health-care worker acceptance (largely related to the other factors mentioned). Although alcohol-based agents have long been believed to cause more skin irritation, several recent trials have demonstrated less skin irritation and better acceptance with emollient-containing, alcohol-based hand rubs compared with either antimicrobial or nonantimicrobial soaps. The use of appropriate (glove-compatible) lotions twice a day also reduces skin irritation—as well as leading to a 50% increase in hand hygiene frequency in one study.[6] Alcohol-based gels and foams are also generally more accessible than antiseptic soap and water, as the dispenser may be pocket-sized or placed conveniently near sites of patient care. It has been estimated that alcohol-based gels and foams require only about 25% of the time of going to a sink to wash one's hands. However, soap and water should be used to remove particulate matter including blood and other body fluids or after five to ten applications of alcohol-based agent.

Adherence to hand hygiene guidelines (Tables 8-2 to 8-4) generally decreases as the frequency of indicated hand washing increases, as the workload increases, and as staffing decreases. CDC guidelines for health-care providers traditionally focused on hand hygiene prior to entering and after leaving a patient room. More recently, the World Health Organization has developed a campaign highlighting the "5 Moments" of hand hygiene

Table 8-3 Hand Hygiene Technique

When decontaminating hands with an alcohol-based hand rub, apply the recommended volume of product to the palm of one hand and rub hands together, covering all surfaces of hands and fingers, until hands are dry.
When washing hands with soap and water, wet hands first with water, apply an amount of the product recommended by the manufacturer to hands, and rub hands together vigorously for at least 15 seconds, covering all surfaces of the hands and fingers. Rinse hands with water and dry thoroughly with a disposable towel. Use towel to turn off the faucet. Avoid using hot water because repeated exposure to hot water may increase the risk of dermatitis.
Liquid, bar, leaflet, or powdered forms of plain soap are acceptable when washing hands with a nonantimicrobial soap and water. When bar soap is used, soap racks that facilitate drainage and small bars of soap should be used.

Modified from Boyce JM, Pittet D. Guideline for hand hygiene in health-care settings. Recommendations of the Healthcare Infection Control Practices Advisory Committee and the HIPAC/SHEA/APIC/IDSA Hand Hygiene Task Force. *Am J Infect Control*. 2002;30(8):S1.

Table 8-4 Skin Care
Provide health-care workers with hand lotions or creams to minimize the occurrence of irritant contact dermatitis associated with hand antisepsis or hand washing. Solicit information from manufacturers regarding any effects that hand lotions, creams, or alcohol-based hand antiseptics may have on the persistent effects of antimicrobial soaps being used in the institution, as well as on glove integrity. Select a combination of products that minimizes these effects.

Modified from Boyce JM, Pittet D. Guideline for hand hygiene in health-care settings. Recommendations of the Healthcare Infection Control Practices Advisory Committee and the HIPAC/SHEA/APIC/IDSA Hand Hygiene Task Force. *Am J Infect Control.* 2002;30(8):S1.

(Fig. 8-2). The campaign emphasizes the need to perform hand hygiene after each contact with a patient or their immediate environment.[10]

In an intensive care unit (ICU), hand hygiene for nurses is generally indicated about 20 times per hour, as compared with lower acuity units, where this number decreases to eight times per hour.[6] In the operating room (OR), frequent patient contact by the anesthesiologist requires frequent hand hygiene, probably at about the level of nurses in the ICU, while accessibility is often quite limited. Sinks are available only outside the OR. Therefore, alcohol-based agents should be available within hand's reach of the anesthesia machine. Loftus et al.[11] studied bacterial contamination of the anesthesia work area (adjustable pressure limiting valve complex and agent flowmeter) and cross-contamination of the sterile anesthesia stopcock during 61 first cases in their OR. They found an average increase in bacterial contamination of the work area of 115 colonies per surface area sampled during cases (95% confidence interval: 62–169; $p < 0.001$). Transmission of bacteria from the work area to the sterile stopcock in the patients' intravenous tubing occurred in 32% of cases, including transmission of methicillin-resistant *Staphylococcus aureus* (MRSA) in two cases and vancomycin-resistant *Enterococcus* in one case. A high level of contamination of the work area (>100 colonies per surface area sampled) increased the risk of stopcock contamination 4.7-fold (95% confidence interval: 1.42–15.42; $p = 0.011$).

In a follow-up study, Koff et al.[5] demonstrated that increased hand hygiene episodes (7 to 9 per hour compared to <0.5 per hour during the control period) triggered by an alarm and encouraged by education decreased work area contamination, decreased stopcock contamination from 32% to 8%, and decreased health-care–associated infections significantly. Opportunities were not measured and hand hygiene episodes were not necessarily coordinated with one of the 5 Moments. Thus, transmission of bacterial contamination by the anesthesia provider appears to be common, a potential source of nosocomial infections, and largely preventable.[11] More recent studies by the same group demonstrate anesthesia provider hands as a source of cross-contamination between patients.[12] Frequent hand hygiene by anesthesia providers has a direct and positive impact on patient outcomes.

Wearing gloves does not reduce the need for hand hygiene. Although gloves provide protection, bacterial flora from patients may be cultured from up to 30% of health-care workers who wear gloves during patient contact.[6] Therefore, hand hygiene should be practiced both before putting on gloves and immediately after removal. Moreover, gloves should be removed or changed immediately after each procedure, including vascular access, intubation, and neuraxial anesthesia, because gloves become contaminated by patient contact just as hands do. Balancing hand hygiene with close attention to the patient during critical portions of the case (e.g., securing the airway) can be challenging. Double gloving and providing a convenient location for contaminated equipment have been suggested as effective approaches.[13,14]

Artificial and long fingernails, as well as chipped fingernail polish, are associated with higher concentrations of bacteria on the hands of health-care workers. Artificial nails have been identified as a source in several hospital-associated outbreaks of infection with gram-negative bacilli and yeast, and CDC guidelines discourage wearing of artificial nails by health-care workers in high-risk settings; many hospitals have banned wearing of artificial nails by any employee who has direct patient contact.[6] It may also be appropriate to counsel patients scheduled for surgery that artificial nails may increase their risk of infection, although this has not been investigated. Large quantities of bacteria are typically trapped under the fingernails, and 2002 CDC guidelines recommend that health-care workers keep their nail tips trimmed to less than ¼ inch.[6]

Bacteria may be cultured at higher concentrations from the skin beneath a ring. On the other hand, wearing a ring does not increase overall bacterial levels measured on the hands of health-care workers. Therefore, it remains unclear whether transmission of infection could be reduced by prohibiting health-care workers from wearing rings.[6]

Antisepsis

Masks have long been advocated as preventing SSI and are used almost universally in ORs in the US. Tunevall[15] studied the rate of wound infections in 3,088 patients over 115 weeks. In alternating weeks, OR personnel either wore masks or did not (personnel with active respiratory infections continued to wear masks). There was no difference in the rate of surgical wound infections (4.7% vs. 3.5%, respectively) in the two groups, nor in bacterial species cultured from the wounds. Friberg et al.[16] demonstrated comparable air and surface contamination during sham surgery in a horizontal laminar airflow unit whether OR personnel wore a nonsterile hood and mask or a sterilized helmet aspirator system. However, when the head cover but not the mask was omitted, contamination increased three- to fivefold. These data suggest that wearing a head cover is useful for preventing SSI, while wearing a mask is not. Nonetheless, the study by Tunevall is a small one, and most hospitals continue to require a mask in the OR while surgical instruments are open. Moreover, the mask does serve the purpose of protecting the health-care provider, particularly when combined with eye protection, and thus should most likely be used during tracheal intubation, emergence from anesthesia, and at other times when exposure to body fluids is likely.

Although the preponderance of postoperative surgical infections is caused by flora that are endogenous to the patient, environmental and airborne contaminants may also play a causative role. An important, but frequently overlooked, consideration is the role that traffic patterns into an OR can play in patient exposure to airborne organisms. A recent Israeli study of risk factors for surgical infection after total knee replacement demonstrated a trend toward increased infection rates with increased number of orthopedic surgeons or anesthetists present in the OR.[17] This study reconfirmed a prior study showing a trend toward increased incidence of SSI as the number of people in the operating suite increases.[18] However, it has been noted in one audit that physicians and nurses did little to limit the number of people through ORs during procedures.[19] Current recommended practices are that traffic patterns should limit the flow of people through an

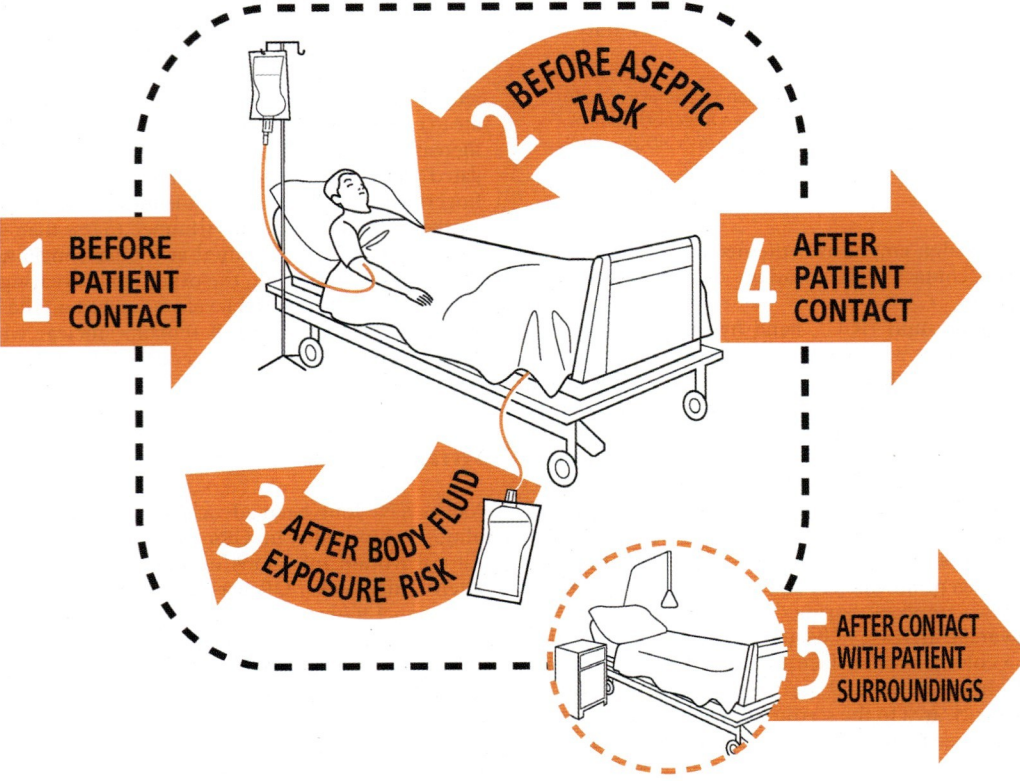

Figure 8-2 World Health Organization schematic of the 5 Moments for Hand Hygiene.

OR that is in use, and that no more people than necessary should be in an OR during a procedure.[20] The anesthesiologist is clearly in a position to play a leadership role in controlling human traffic through the OR.

Mermel et al.[21] demonstrated in 1991 that central venous lines placed by the anesthesiologist in the OR became infected more often (relative risk [RR], 2.1; $p = 0.03$) than those placed by surgeons or other providers, whether in or out of the OR. Contributing factors appeared to be site of placement and the stringency of aseptic technique. Infection risk is significantly higher with femoral (HR 3.5) or jugular (HR 2.1) site selection as compared to subclavian placement; however, subclavian placement does have a higher associated rate of pneumothorax.[22] Chlorhexidine–alcohol skin preparation results in a lower rate of central venous catheter–associated bloodstream infection than povidone-iodine with alcohol and should be used preferentially.[23] Raad et al.[24] demonstrated that use of a maximal sterile barrier technique versus sterile gloves and small sterile drapes led to a significant reduction in central venous catheter-related infection from 7.2% to 2.2% ($p = 0.03$). Therefore, gowning and gloving, careful aseptic technique, and use of a wide sterile field should be routine.[25] Use of ultrasound guidance for placement is not associated with an increased infection rate, and therefore is recommended since it decreases mechanical complications during placement.[26] In anesthetized patients, the central line is ideally placed before the surgical site is draped in order to avoid contamination of the wire on the underside of the surgical drape.

Epidural abscess formation is an extremely rare but potentially catastrophic complication of neuraxial anesthesia and epidural catheter placement. Therefore, careful attention to aseptic technique and infection control is required. The most important consideration is to prevent contamination of the needle and catheter. Thus, hand washing, skin preparation, draping, and maintenance of a sterile field should be carefully observed. Gowning and wearing a mask likely play a smaller role, but are reasonable given the devastating consequences of infection. Finally, epidurals should probably be avoided in patients known or suspected to have bacteremia or deferred until after appropriate antibiotics are administered.

Antibiotic Prophylaxis

After antibiotics came into widespread use in the 1940s and 1950s, there was much debate over the possibility that antibiotic prophylaxis might prevent SSI. In 1957, Miles et al.[27] used a guinea pig model for proof of the principle that administration of an antibiotic prior to contamination (incision) could reduce the risk of SSI. When appropriate antibiotics were given within 2 hours before or after intradermal injection of bacteria, they were effective in preventing invasive infection and necrosis. When given outside this window, they were not effective. This gave rise to the concept of a "decisive period" in which antibiotics will be effective, which remains a guiding principle of antibiotic prophylaxis. Miles et al. also demonstrated that injection of epinephrine intradermally prior to administration of antibiotics led to antibiotic failure, as demonstrated by an increased wound infection rate. This demonstrated the crucial role of local perfusion in delivering antibiotics to the site. Knighton et al.[28] using the same model, demonstrated that increased inspired oxygen was equally as effective as antibiotics in preventing infection, and that the two effects were additive (Fig. 8-3). Knighton et al.[29] also delayed the administration of oxygen for up to 6 hours after inoculation and demonstrated no reduction in effect. Thus, the decisive period for oxygen is considerably longer than that for antibiotics.

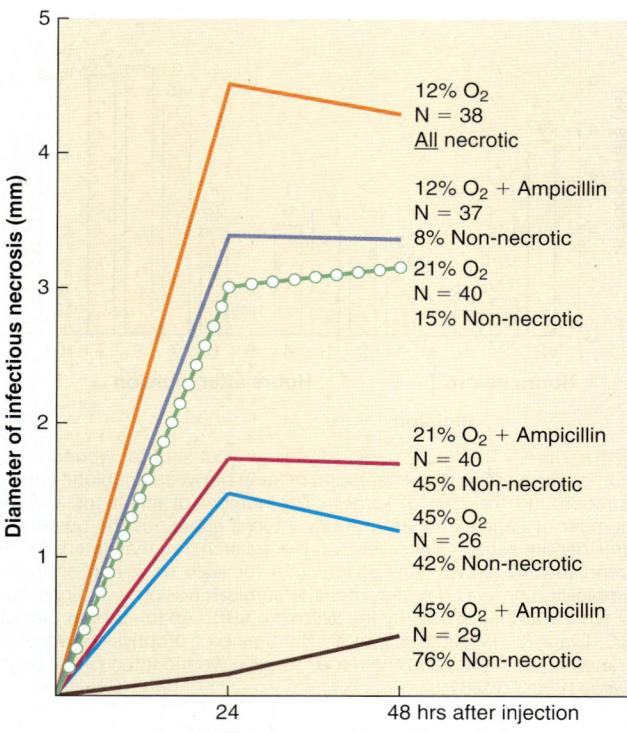

Figure 8-3 The effect of oxygen and/or antibiotics on lesion diameter after intradermal injection of bacteria into guinea pigs. Note that at every level, oxygen adds to the effect of antibiotics and that increasing oxygen in the breathing mixture from 12% to 20% or from 20% to 45% exerts an effect comparable to that of appropriately timed antibiotics. (Reprinted with permission from Rabkin J, Hunt TK. Infection and oxygen. In: Davis J, Hunt TK, eds. *Problem Wounds: The Role of Oxygen*. New York: Elsevier; 1988:1.)

Two surgeons at Washington University in St. Louis, Harvey Bernard and William Cole,[30] reported on the first controlled clinical trial of the efficacy of antibiotic prophylaxis in 1964 and demonstrated a benefit in abdominal operations. Thereafter, numerous clinical trials were performed with somewhat variable results. Eventually these served to define the timing and population in which prophylactic antibiotics work. By the 1970s, antibiotic prophylaxis for high-risk surgery—meaning clean-contaminated and contaminated cases—was becoming well accepted and widely used, although some skeptics remained. In 1992, Classen et al.[31] published their prospective series including 2,847 patients undergoing clean or clean-contaminated surgical procedures at LDS Hospital in Salt Lake City, UT (Fig. 8-4). They demonstrated that the decisive period for SSI in humans undergoing surgery was essentially the same as for experimental infections in guinea pigs. That is, they found the lowest infection rate when antibiotics were given within 2 hours before or after incision, and a rapid increase in SSI rate when they were given outside that range. The best results, though only by a small margin and not statistically significant, were within 0 and 60 minutes of surgery, and this subsequently became the clinical standard.

Antibiotic prophylaxis has now become standard for surgeries in which there is more than a minimum risk of infection. Although not every surgery and situation has been studied, a strong rationale for the approach to prophylactic antibiotics has

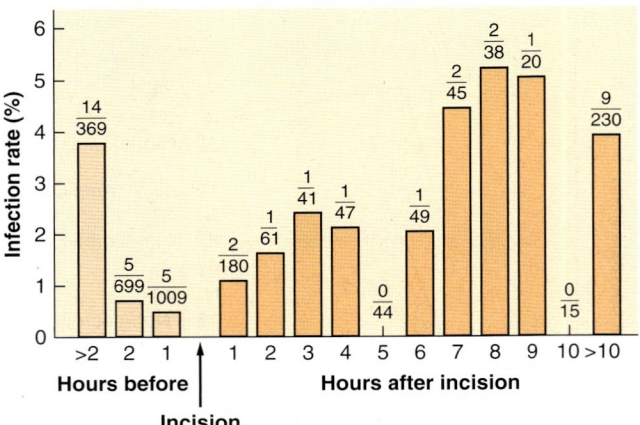

Figure 8-4 The figure demonstrates rates of surgical wound infection corresponding to the temporal relation between antibiotic administration and the start of surgery. The number of infections and the number of patients for each hourly interval appear as the numerator and denominator, respectively, of the fraction for that interval. The trend toward higher rates of infection for each hour that antibiotic administration was delayed after the surgical incision was significant (z score = 2.00; $p < 0.05$ by the Wilcoxon test). (Adapted from Classen DC, Evans RS, Pestotnik KS, et al. The timing of prophylactic administration of antibiotics and the risk of surgical-wound infection. *N Engl J Med*. 1992:326;281.)

including *Staphylococcus aureus* and coagulase-negative staphylococci (e.g., *Staphylococcus epidermidis*). In clean-contaminated procedures, the most common pathogens include gram-negative rods, and enterococci in addition to skin flora. Data from the National Nosocomial Infections Surveillance (NNIS) system for 2006 to 2007 indicate that the proportion of SSI caused by *S. aureus* has increased to 30%, with about half caused by MRSA. Infections caused by MRSA are associated with higher mortality rates, prolonged hospital stays, and higher hospital costs than infections caused by other agents. Nevertheless, it is not recommended that vancomycin be used as a routine agent for surgical antimicrobial prophylaxis.[32]

Several groups separately developed guidelines for use of surgical prophylactic antibiotics, culminating in recommendations published in 2004 by the National Surgical Infection Prevention Project and updated in 2013.[32] These guidelines emphasize timing and choice of appropriate agents; a number of agents are recommended as appropriate for each procedure, allowing for choices to be guided by local sensitivity patterns and providing for alternate agents in the case of drug sensitivity or allergy. (See Table 8-5 for general recommendations.) The most commonly used antibiotic for surgical prophylaxis is cefazolin, a first-generation cephalosporin, because it is the most widely studied agent, with proven efficacy, safety, and desirable duration of action, and its spectrum of activity covers the organisms commonly encountered in surgery.[32,33]

By definition, prophylactic antibiotics are given pre- or intraoperatively. The exact timing for the administration of the antibiotic depends on the pharmacology and half-life of the drug. It has been suggested that administration of prophylactic antibiotics is ideal within 30 minutes to 1 hour of incision.[33,34] Drugs given by bolus administration (e.g., cefazolin) achieve adequate tissue concentration rapidly, so that giving these drugs within 0 and 30 minutes of incisions appears equally efficacious. Giving the antibiotics too early (so that the incision is more than 60 minutes after the dose) is a recurrent issue at many hospitals, especially

emerged. Ideally, the antimicrobial of choice for prophylaxis should prevent SSI, prevent SSI-related morbidity and mortality, be cost-effective, avoid adverse effects, and have no adverse consequences on the microbial flora of the patient or of the hospital.[32] The agent for antibiotic prophylaxis must cover the most likely spectrum of bacteria presented in the surgical field. The most common surgical-site pathogens in clean procedures are skin flora,

Table 8-5 General Recommendations for Antibiotic Prophylaxis

- Antibiotic prophylaxis choice, dose, and timing should be determined by a hospital committee based on national guidelines,[32] local patterns of antibiotic sensitivity, and other considerations.
- Always confirm the antibiotic selection with surgeons at the time-out or earlier.
  - The surgeon may wish to delay antibiotics until after culture.
  - Antibiotics may not be indicated (e.g., low-risk, elective procedures such as laparoscopic cholecystectomy or breast biopsy where implants will not be used).
  - Make sure to record the reason for not giving antibiotics on the record.
- β-Lactam allergies.
  - Penicillin allergy is almost never a contraindication to cefazolin or other cephalosporin administration. A *documented* history of anaphylaxis or other serious reaction (angioedema, hives, bronchospasm, Stevens–Johnson syndrome or toxic epidermal necrolysis) is the exception. Determine the severity of a patient's β-lactam allergy prior to choosing an alternative antimicrobial.
  - Lack of understanding of a true allergic reaction can lead to choosing an antimicrobial with reduced efficacy, increased cost, and greater risk of side effects.
- Ideally an antibiotic infusion should be completed before incision, but CMS guidelines consider starting the infusion before incision adequate. When possible, for drugs requiring slow (>30 min) infusion, the infusion should be initiated preoperatively.
- When a tourniquet is used, the dose should be completed at least 5 minutes before the tourniquet is inflated.
- Dosing schedules are more frequent than for therapeutic use to maintain wound tissue levels throughout surgery and ongoing contamination. Renal insufficiency may delay redosing, although initial dose is usually not affected.
- Additional intraoperative doses should be given when there is significant blood loss (~ half to one blood volume). Use the recommended second dose for this purpose.
- When *therapeutic* antibiotics are given preoperatively for an infection or presumed infection (e.g., acute appendicitis), prophylactic antibiotics are not required. Each situation should be examined individually: In some cases, coverage of skin flora may be appropriate prior to skin incision, but often continuation of the therapeutic antibiotics is all that is required.

Used with permission from University of Utah Health Care.

in cases that require complex patient positioning. Giving the antibiotics closer to the incision time prevents this problem. Providing timely prophylactic antibiotics is relatively uncomplicated for antibiotics that can be given as a bolus dose (e.g., cephalosporins) or as an infusion over a few minutes (e.g., clindamycin) and thus provide tissue levels within minutes. For drugs like vancomycin that require infusion over an hour or more, coordination of administration is more complex. In general, it is considered acceptable if the infusion is started within 120 minutes before incision. Vancomycin is usually given in the context of known or suspected MRSA colonization; giving a dose of cefazolin in addition within an hour of incision is a way to ensure adequate antibiotic levels at the time of incision while providing coverage for MRSA with the vancomycin. When a tourniquet is used, the infusion must be complete prior to inflation of the tourniquet. An appropriate dose based on body weight and volume of distribution should be given. Depending on the half-life, antibiotics should be repeated during long operations or operations with large blood loss.[32] For example, cefazolin is normally dosed every 8 hours but the dose should be repeated every 4 hours intraoperatively.[32] Finally, prophylactic antibiotics should be discontinued by 24 hours following surgery if postoperative dosing is selected at all. Prolonging the course of prophylactic antibiotics does not reduce the risk of infection but does increase the risk of adverse consequences of antibiotic administration,[32] including resistance, C. difficile infection, and sensitization.

Because they have access to the patient during the 60 minutes prior to incision and can optimize timing of administration, anesthesiologists should work in consultation with the surgeon to use guidelines determined by the local infection control committee to take initiative for administering prophylactic antibiotics. In this way, anesthesiologists can make a major contribution to preventing SSI. The Centers for Medicare and Medicaid Services has identified timely and appropriate antibiotic prophylaxis administration as a cornerstone of SSI prevention. Physician and hospital reimbursements are increasingly tied to such performance measures, meaning anesthesiologists also have an economic interest in ensuring adherence to guidelines.

Mechanisms of Wound Repair

Wound healing is a complex process, requiring a coordinated repair response including inflammation, matrix production, angiogenesis, epithelialization, and remodeling (Fig. 8-5). Many factors may impair wound healing. Systemic factors such as medical comorbidities, nutrition,[35] sympathetic nervous system activation,[36] and age[37-39] have a substantial effect on the repair process.

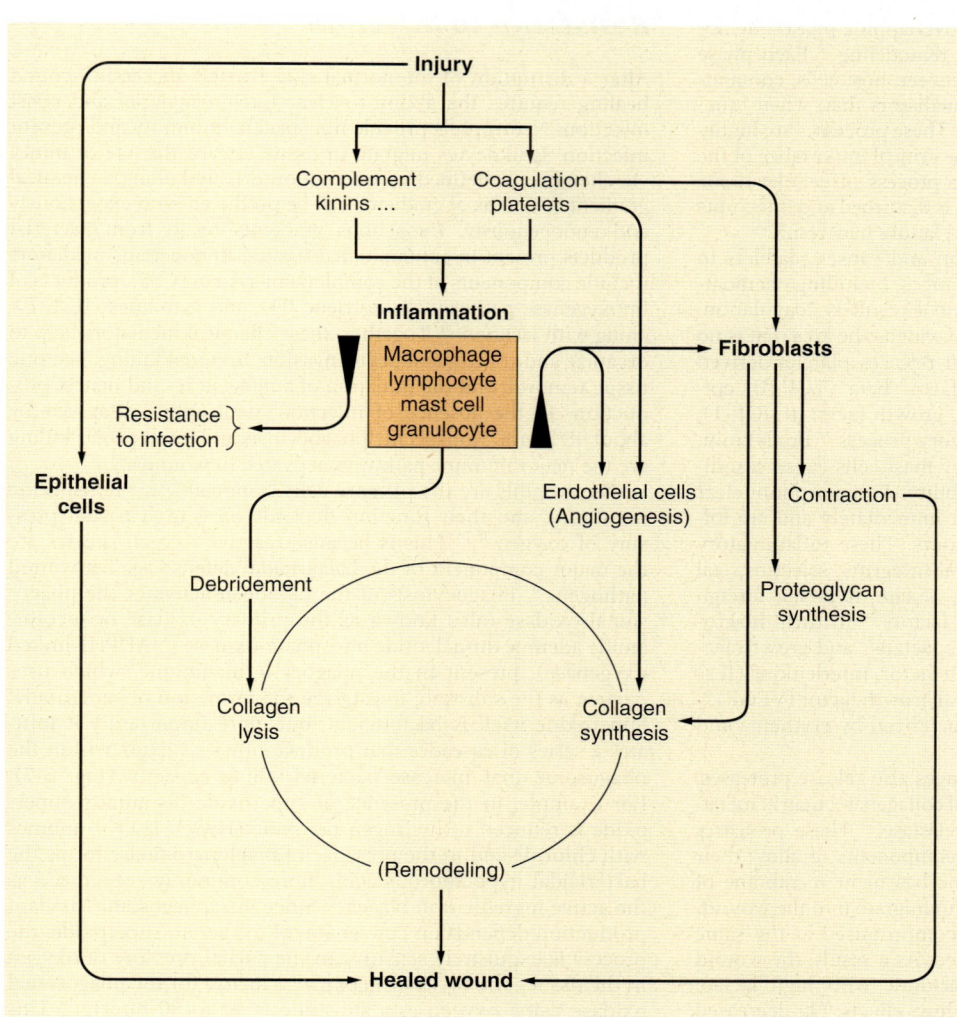

Figure 8-5 Schematic of the processes of wound healing. (Reprinted with permission from Hunt T. *Fundamentals of Wound Management in Surgery, Wound Healing: Disorders of Repair.* South Plainfield, NJ: Chirugecom, Inc., 1976.)

Local environmental factors in and around the wound including bacterial load,[40] degree of inflammation, moisture content,[41] oxygen tension,[42] and vascular perfusion[43] also have a profound effect on healing. Although all of these factors are important, perhaps the most critical element is oxygen supply to the wound. Wound hypoxia impairs each of the components of healing.[44]

Although the role of oxygen is usually thought of in terms of aerobic respiration and energy production via oxidative phosphorylation, in wound healing oxygen is required as a cofactor for enzymatic processes and for cell-signaling mechanisms. Oxygen is a rate-limiting component in leukocyte-mediated bacterial killing and collagen formation because specific enzymes require oxygen at a partial pressure of at least 40 mmHg.[45,46] The mechanisms by which the other processes are oxygen-dependent are less clear, but these processes also require oxygen at a concentration much above that required for cellular respiration.[47–49]

The Initial Response to Injury

A surgical incision disrupts the skin barrier, creating an acute wound, and an effective initial response to injury depends on the ability to clean out foreign material and to resist infection. This response initiates a sequence of events that starts with any source of injury that disrupts homeostasis in the local environment and eventually leads to healing.

Wound healing is described in four overlapping phases: hemostasis, inflammation, proliferation, and remodeling.[50] Each phase is composed of complex interactions between host cells, contaminants, cytokines, and other chemical mediators that, when functioning properly, lead to repair of injury. These processes are highly conserved across species,[51] indicating the critical importance of the inflammatory response that directs the process of cellular/tissue repair. When any component of healing is disturbed and interrupts the orderly progression of repair, wound failure may result.[50]

Injury damages the local circulation and causes platelets to aggregate and release a variety of substances, including chemoattractants and growth factors.[50] The initial result is coagulation, which prevents exsanguination but also widens the area that is no longer perfused. Platelet degranulation releases platelet-derived growth factor, transforming growth factor beta (TGF-β), epidermal growth factor, and insulin-like growth factor-1 (IGF-1), which conjointly initiate the inflammatory process.[50] Bradykinin, complement, and histamine released by mast cells cause vasodilation and increased vascular permeability. Polymorphonuclear leukocytes arrive at the wound almost immediately and are followed by macrophages at 24 to 48 hours. These inflammatory cells activate in response to endothelial integrins, selectins, cell adhesion molecules, cadherins, fibrin, lactate, hypoxia, foreign bodies, infectious agents, and growth factors.[50] In turn, macrophages and lymphocytes produce more lactate[52] and growth factors, including IGF-1, leukocyte growth factor, interleukins (ILs) 1 and 2, TGF-β, and vascular endothelial growth factor (VEGF).[53] This early inflammatory phase is characterized by erythema and edema of the wound edges.

Activated neutrophils and macrophages also release proteases, including neutrophil elastase, neutrophil collagenase, matrix metalloproteinase, and macrophage metalloelastase.[50] These proteases degrade damaged extracellular matrix components to allow their replacement. Proteases also degrade the basement membrane of capillaries to enable inflammatory cells to migrate into the wound.

In wounds, local blood supply is compromised at the same time that metabolic demand is increased. As a result, the wound environment becomes hypoxic and acidotic with high lactate levels.[54,55] This represents the sum of three effects: (1) decreased oxygen supply due to vascular damage and coagulation, (2) increased metabolic demand due to the heightened cellular response (anaerobic glycolysis), and (3) aerobic glycolysis by inflammatory cells.[56,57] Leukocytes contain few mitochondria and therefore acquire energy from glucose, primarily by production of lactate and even in the presence of adequate oxygen supply.[56] In activated neutrophils, the respiratory burst, in which oxygen and glucose are converted to superoxide, hydrogen ion, and lactate, accounts for up to 98% of oxygen consumption; in the setting of injury, this activity increases by up to 50-fold over baseline.[58]

Local hypoxia is a normal and inevitable result of tissue injury.[59,60] Hypoxia acts as a stimulus to repair,[61] but also leads to poor healing[42] and increased susceptibility to infection.[62,63] Numerous experimental models[27,62,64,65] as well as human clinical experience[63,66] have led to the conclusion that wound healing is delayed in hypoxic wounds. The partial pressure of oxygen in dermal wounds is heterogeneous, ranging from 0 to 10 mmHg in the central ("dead space") portion of the wound, to 80 to 100 mmHg (near arterial) adjacent to perfused arterioles and capillaries (Fig. 8-6).[60] The PO_2 of a given area depends on diffusion of oxygen from perfused capillaries, and thus wound PO_2 depends on capillary density, arterial PO_2, and the metabolic activity of the cells, with some contribution from shifts in the oxyhemoglobin dissociation curve associated with wound pH and temperature.

Resistance to Infection

After a disruption of the normal skin barrier, successful wound healing requires the ability to clear foreign material and resist infection. Neutrophils provide nonspecific immunity and prevent infection. Leukocytes migrate in tissue toward the site of injury via chemotaxis, defined as locomotion oriented along a chemical gradient.[50] Chemical gradients can be produced both exogenously and endogenously. Exogenous gradients result from bacterial products present in contaminated tissues. Endogenous mediators include components of the complement system (C5a), products of lipoxygenase pathway (leukotriene B4), and cytokines (IL-1, 8), along with lactate.[67,68] Together, these chemical mediators help to organize and control leukocyte invasion, bacterial killing, necrotic tissue removal, and the initiation of angiogenesis and matrix production. In the absence of infection, neutrophils disappear by about 48 hours. Nonspecific phagocytosis and intracellular killing are the major immune pathways activated in wounds.[69]

Neutrophils are the primary cells responsible for nonspecific immunity, and their function depends on a high partial pressure of oxygen.[46,70] This is because reactive oxygen species are the major component of the bactericidal defense against wound pathogens.[69] Phagocytosis of the pathogen activates the phagosomal oxidase (also known as the primary oxidase or nicotinamide adenine dinucleotide phosphate-oxidase [NADPH]-linked oxygenase), present in the phagocytic membrane, which uses oxygen as the substrate to catalyze the formation of superoxide. Superoxide itself is bactericidal, but more importantly it initiates a series of cascades that produce other oxidants within the phagosome that increase bacterial-killing capacity (Fig. 8-7). For example, in the presence of superoxide dismutase, superoxide is reduced to hydrogen peroxide (H_2O_2). H_2O_2 combines with chloride and in the presence of myeloperoxidase forms the bactericidal hypochlorous acid, more commonly recognized as the active ingredient in bleach.[71] Since intraphagosomal oxidant production depends on conversion of oxygen to superoxide, the process is exquisitely sensitive to the partial pressure of oxygen in the tissue. The K_m (half-maximal velocity) for the phagosomal oxidase using oxygen as a substrate is 40 to 80 mmHg.[46] This

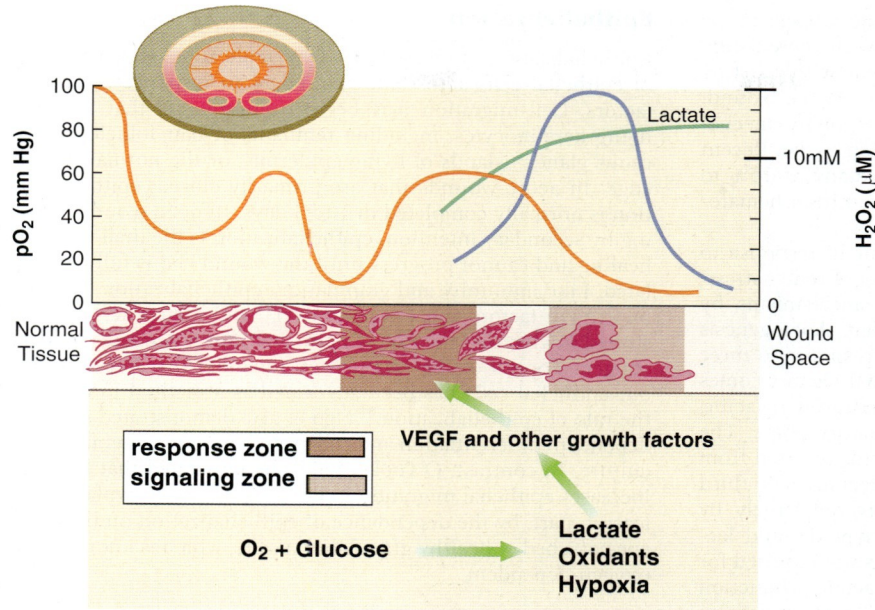

Figure 8-6 The varying oxygen tension in the wound module. Cross-section of the wound module in a rabbit ear chamber is in left upper corner of figure. PO$_2$, depicted graphically above the cross-section (*orange line*), is highest next to the vessels, with a gradient down to zero at the wound edge. Note also the lactate gradient (*green line*), high in the dead space and lower (but still above plasma) toward the vasculature. Hydrogen peroxide (H$_2$O$_2$) is present at fairly high concentrations (*blue line*) and is also a major stimulus to wound repair.[67] Growth factors such as VEGF are produced by inflammatory cells in the hypoxic, high lactate, high hydrogen peroxide "signaling zone" and then diffuse to the "response zone" where they act on fibroblasts and endothelial cells to promote healing. VEGF, vascular endothelial growth factor. (Modified from Silver IE. The physiology of wound healing. In: Hunt TK, Dunphy JE, eds. *Fundamentals of Wound Management*. New York: Appleton-Century-Crofts, 1980:30.)

means that resistance to infection is critically impaired by wound hypoxia and becomes more efficient as PO$_2$ increases even to very high levels (500 to 1,000 mmHg).[46] Such levels do not occur naturally in tissue, but can be achieved by the administration of hyperbaric oxygen.[72-74] This is one mechanism for the proposed benefit of hyperbaric oxygen therapy as an adjunctive treatment for necrotizing infections and chronic refractory osteomyelitis.[75]

Oxidants produced by inflammatory cells have a dual role in wound repair. Not only are they central to resistance to infection, but they also play a major role in initiating and directing the healing process. Oxidants, and in particular hydrogen peroxide produced via the respiratory burst, increase neovascularization and collagen deposition in vitro and in vivo.[67]

Proliferation

The proliferative phase normally begins approximately 4 days after injury, concurrent with a waning of the inflammatory phase. It consists of granulation tissue formation and epithelialization. Granulation involves neovascularization and synthesis of collagen and connective tissue proteins.

Neovascularization

New blood vessels must replace the injured microcirculation. Neovascularization in wounds proceeds both by angiogenesis and vasculogenesis. Angiogenesis is the phenomenon of new vessel growth via budding from existing vessels. In the setting of wounds, new vessels grow from mature vessels, usually intact postcapillary venules in the undamaged tissue immediately adjacent to the site of injury. Normally, the oxygen tension in adjacent tissue is sufficient to support this process. The new vessel growth extends and enters into the damaged areas that are typically high in lactate and have a low partial pressure of oxygen. Mature extracellular matrix is required for ingrowth of mature vessels.[76]

In vasculogenesis, bone marrow–derived endothelial precursor cells (EPCs) populate the tissue and differentiate and grow

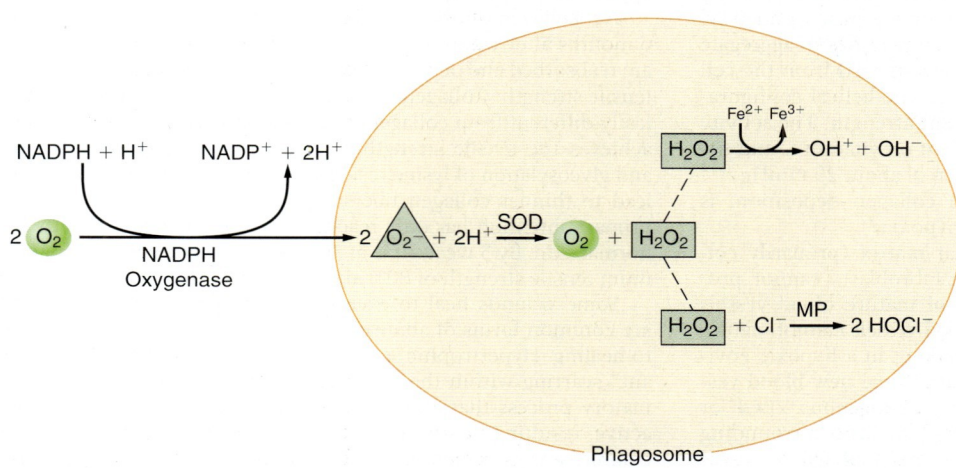

Figure 8-7 Schematic of superoxide and other oxidant production within the phagosome. NADPH, nicotinamide adenine dinucleotide phosphate-oxidase; NADP, nicotinamide adenine dinucleotide phosphate; SOD, superoxide dismutase; MP, myeloperoxidase. (Reprinted with permission from Hunt TK, Hopf HW. Wound healing and wound infection. What surgeons and anesthesiologists can do. *Surg Clin North Am*. 1997;77[3]:587–606.)

into new vessel tubules. In wounds, these tubules appear in the damaged area before any direct anastomosis with pre-existing vessels are made. These tubules must connect with existing vasculature to establish an intact blood supply in the wound. Angiogenesis has long been held to be the primary mechanism for new blood vessel growth in granulation tissue. Recent research, however, has demonstrated that as many as 15% to 20% of new blood vessels in wounds are derived from hematopoietic stem cells.[76–78]

Angiogenesis and vasculogenesis both occur in response to similar stimuli, consisting of some combination of redox stress, hypoxia, and lactate. However, the specific mechanisms by which they proceed appear to differ somewhat. Angiogenesis involves the movement of endothelial cells in response to three waves of growth factors. The first wave of growth factors comes with the release by platelets of platelet-derived growth factor, TGF-β, IGF-1, and others during the inflammatory phase. The second wave comes from fibroblast growth factor released from normal binding sites on connective tissue molecules. The third and dominant wave comes from VEGF, delivered largely by macrophages stimulated by fibrinopeptides, hypoxia, and lactate.[79] Although it is usually present, hypoxia is not required for granulation because of constitutive (aerobic) lactate production by inflammatory cells and fibroblasts. Too little lactate leads to inadequate granulation, while levels in excess of about 15 mM—usually associated with inflammation or infection—delay granulation.[80] The capillary endothelial response to angiogenic agents requires oxygen so that angiogenesis progresses in proportion to blood perfusion and arterial PO_2.[81]

Vasculogenesis occurs in response to similar stressors as angiogenesis. EPCs are mobilized from the bone marrow into the circulation via a nitric oxide–mediated mechanism. Tissue hypoxia induces release of VEGF-A, which activates bone marrow stromal nitric oxide synthase. Increased bone marrow nitric oxide leads to release of EPCs into the circulation. These circulating EPCs home to the wound via tissue-hypoxia–induced upregulation of stromal cell-derived factor 1α. Within the wound, EPCs undergo differentiation and participate in the formation of new blood vessels.[77]

Collagen and Extracellular Matrix Deposition

New blood vessels grow into the matrix that is produced by fibroblasts. Although fibroblasts replicate and migrate mainly in response to growth factors and chemoattractants, production of mature collagen requires oxygen.[45] Lactate, hypoxia, and some growth factors induce collagen mRNA synthesis and procollagen production. Posttranslational modification by prolyl and lysyl hydroxylases is required to allow collagen peptides to aggregate into triple helices. Collagen can only be exported from the cell when it is in this triple helical structure. The helical configuration is also primarily responsible for tissue strength. The activity of the hydroxylases is critically dependent on vitamin C and tissue oxygen tension, with a K_m for oxygen of about 25 mmHg.[45,82] Wound strength, which results from collagen deposition, is therefore highly vulnerable to wound hypoxia.[42]

Neovascularization and extracellular matrix (primarily collagen) production are closely linked. Fibroblasts cannot produce mature collagen in the absence of mature blood vessels that deliver oxygen to the site. New blood vessels cannot mature without a strong collagen matrix. Mice kept in a hypoxic environment of 13% inspired oxygen develop some new blood vessels in a test wound with the addition of exogenous VEGF or lactate, but these vessels are immature with little surrounding matrix and demonstrate frequent areas of hemorrhage.[47]

Epithelialization

Epithelialization is characterized by replication and migration of epithelial cells across the skin edges in response to growth factors. Cell migration may begin from any site that contains living keratinocytes, including remnants of hair follicles, sebaceous glands, islands of living epidermis, or the normal wound edge. In acute wounds that are primarily closed, epithelialization is normally completed in 1 to 3 days. In open wounds healing by secondary intention, epithelialization is the final phase of healing and cannot progress until the wound bed is fully granulated. Like immunity and granulation, epithelialization depends on growth factors and oxygen. Silver[83] and Medawar[49] demonstrated in vivo that the rate of epithelialization depends on local oxygen. Topical oxygen applied in a manner that does not dry out epithelial cells has been advocated as a method to increase the rate of epithelialization.[84] Ngo et al.[85] demonstrated oxygen-dependent differentiation and cell growth in human keratinocyte culture. In contrast, O'Toole et al.[86] demonstrated that hypoxia increases epithelial migration in vitro. This may be explained, at least in part, by the dependence of epithelialization on the presence of a bed of healthy granulation tissue, which is known to be oxygen-dependent.

Maturation and Remodeling

The final phase of wound repair is maturation, which involves ongoing remodeling of the granulation tissue and increasing wound tensile strength. As the matrix becomes denser with thicker, stronger collagen fibrils, it becomes stiffer and less compliant. Fibroblasts are capable of adapting to changing mechanical stress and loading. Fibroblasts migrate throughout the matrix to help mold the wound to new stresses. Matrix metalloproteinases and other proteases help with fibroblast migration and continued matrix remodeling in response to mechanical stress. Some fibroblasts differentiate into myofibroblasts under the influence of TGF-β, resulting in contractile cells. As the myofibroblasts contract, the collagenous matrix cross-links in the shortened position. This helps to strengthen the matrix and minimize scar size. Contraction is inhibited by the use of high doses of corticosteroids.[87] Even steroids given several days after injury have this effect. In those wounds where contraction is detrimental, this effect can be used for benefit. Although there is little definitive evidence, one dose of dexamethasone intraoperatively to prevent postoperative nausea and vomiting does not appear to impair healing.

Net collagen synthesis continues for at least 6 weeks and up to 6 months after wounding. Over time, the initial collagen threads are reabsorbed and deposited along stress lines, conferring greater tensile strength. Collagen found in granulation tissue is biochemically different from collagen of uninjured skin, and a scar never achieves the tensile strength of uninjured skin. Hydroxylation and glycosylation of lysine residues in granulation tissue collagen lead to thinner collagen fibers. At 1 week, a wound closed by primary intention has only reached 3% of the tensile strength of normal skin. By 3 weeks it is at 30%, and it only reaches its maximum tensile strength of 80% after 3 to 6 months.

Some wounds heal to excess. Hypertrophic scar and keloid are common forms of abnormal scar due to abnormal responses to healing. Hypertrophic scarring may be thought of as "exuberant" scarring within the boundaries of the wound. The inflammatory process that allows wound healing remains excessively active, resulting in stiff, rubbery, nonmobile scar tissue. Hypertrophic scars are most commonly seen following burns and in incisions over areas of tension and are thought to correlate with the length of time required to close the wound and opposing tension forces present in the wound, although other factors are also believed to play a role and are being actively explored. Keloids are scars that outgrow the boundaries of the initial scar, and are most typically seen following skin incisions. Keloid formation is most likely due to a genetic predisposition, although exogenous inflammatory factors may also play a role.

Wound Perfusion and Oxygenation

Complications of wounds include failure to heal, infection, and excessive scarring or contracture. Rapid repair has the least potential for infection and excess scarring. The perioperative physician's goals, therefore, are to avoid contamination, ensure rapid tissue synthesis, and optimize the immune response. All surgical procedures lead to some degree of contamination that must be controlled by local host defenses. The initial hours after contamination represent a decisive period during which inadequate local defenses may allow an infection to become established.

Normally, wounds on the extremities and trunk heal more slowly than those on the face. The major difference in these wounds is the degree of tissue perfusion and thus the wound tissue oxygen tension. As a rule, repair proceeds most rapidly and immunity is strongest when wound oxygen levels are high, and this is only achieved by maintaining perfusion of injured tissue.[88] Ischemic or hypoxic tissue, on the other hand, is highly susceptible to infection and heals poorly, if at all.[66] Wound tissue oxygenation is complex and depends on the interaction of blood perfusion, arterial oxygen tension, hemoglobin dissociation conditions, carrying capacity, mass transfer resistances, and local oxygen consumption. Wound oxygen delivery depends on vascular anatomy, the degree of vasoconstriction, and arterial PO_2.

The standard teaching that oxygen delivery depends more on hemoglobin-bound oxygen (oxygen content) than on arterial PO_2 may be true of working muscle, but it is not true of wound healing. In muscle, intercapillary distances are small and oxygen consumption is high. In contrast, intercapillary distances are large and oxygen consumption is relatively low in subcutaneous tissue.[48] In wounds, where the microvasculature is damaged, diffusion distances are substantially increased. Peripheral vasoconstriction further increases diffusion distance.[60] The driving force of diffusion is partial pressure. Hence, a high PO_2 is needed to force oxygen into injured and healing tissues, particularly in subcutaneous tissue, fascia, tendon, and bone, the tissues most at risk for poor healing.

Although oxygen consumption is relatively low in wounds, it is consumed by processes that require oxygen at a high concentration. Inflammatory cells use little oxygen for respiration, producing energy largely via the hexose monophosphate shunt.[46] Most of the oxygen consumed in wounds is used for oxidant production (bacterial killing), with a significant contribution as well for collagen synthesis, angiogenesis, and epithelialization. The rate constants (K_m) for oxygen for these components of repair all fall within the physiologic range of 25 to 100 mmHg.[45,46,49,70,89]

Because of the high rate constants for oxygen substrate for the components of repair, the rate at which repair proceeds varies according to tissue PO_2 from zero to at least 250 mmHg. In vitro fibroblast replication is optimal at a PO_2 of about 40 to 60 mmHg. Neutrophils lose their ability to kill bacteria in vitro below a PO_2 of about 40 mmHg.[90,91] These in vitro observations are clinically relevant. "Normal" subcutaneous PO_2, measured in test wounds in uninjured, euthermic, euvolemic volunteers breathing room air, is 65 ± 7 mmHg.[92] Thus, any reduction in wound PO_2 may impair immunity and repair. In surgical patients, the rate of wound infections is inversely proportional[63] and collagen deposition is directly proportional[42] to postoperative subcutaneous wound tissue oxygen tension.

High oxygen tensions (>100 mmHg) can be reached in wounds but only if perfusion is rapid and arterial PO_2 is high.[42,88] This is because subcutaneous tissue serves a reservoir function, so there is normally flow in excess of nutritional needs and wound cells consume relatively little oxygen, about 0.7/100 mL of blood flow at a normal perfusion rate.[48,93] When arterial oxygen tension (PaO_2) is high, this small volume can be carried by plasma alone. Contrary to popular belief, therefore, oxygen-carrying capacity, that is, hemoglobin concentration, is not particularly important to wound healing, provided that perfusion is normal.[94,95] Wound PO_2 and collagen synthesis remain normal in individuals who have hematocrit levels as low as 15% to 18% provided they can appropriately increase cardiac output, and vasoconstriction is prevented.[95,96]

Peripheral vasoconstriction, which results from central sympathetic control of subcutaneous vascular tone, is probably the most frequent and clinically the most important impediment to wound oxygenation. Subcutaneous tissue is both a reservoir to maintain central volume and a major site of thermoregulation. There is little local regulation of blood flow, except by local heating.[97] Therefore, subcutaneous tissue is particularly vulnerable to vasoconstriction. Sympathetically induced peripheral vasoconstriction is stimulated by cold, pain, fear, and blood volume deficit,[98,99] and by various pharmacologic agents including nicotine,[92] β-adrenergic antagonists, and $α_1$-agonists, all commonly present in the perioperative environment. Use of low doses of vasopressor agents to correct anesthesia (vasodilation)-induced hypotension, however, does not generally impair wound perfusion or free-flap survival.[100] Perioperative hypothermia is common and results from anesthetic drugs, exposure to cold, and redistribution of body heat from the core to the periphery.[101] Blood loss and increases in insensible losses increase fluid requirements in the perioperative period, thereby leaving the patient vulnerable to inadequate fluid replacement. Thus, vasomotor tone is, to a large degree, under the perioperative physician's control.[98,99]

Prevention or correction of hypothermia[102] and blood volume deficits[103] have been shown to decrease wound infections and increase collagen deposition in patients undergoing major abdominal surgery. Preoperative systemic (forced air warmer) or local (warming bandage) warming have also been shown to decrease wound infections, even in clean, low-risk surgeries such as breast surgery and inguinal hernia repair.[104] Subcutaneous tissue oxygen tension is significantly higher in patients with good pain control than in those with poor pain control after arthroscopic knee surgery.[105] Stress also causes wound hypoxia and significantly impairs wound healing and resistance to infection.[106,107] These effects are clearly mediated, in large part, by changes in the partial pressure of oxygen in the injured tissue.

A number of groups have evaluated whether increasing inspired oxygen during surgery can reduce SSI by increasing wound oxygen levels. Most found benefit. Greif et al.[108] demonstrated in a randomized, controlled, double-blind trial including 500 patients that in warm, volume-replete patients with good pain control undergoing major colon surgery, administration of 80% versus 30% oxygen intraoperatively and for the first 2 hours after surgery significantly reduced the wound infection rate by 50%. Wound oxygen levels were significantly higher (almost double) intraoperatively and in the postanesthesia care unit (PACU) in the 80% oxygen group. Belda et al.[109] replicated these results (significant 40% reduction in SSI) in a randomized, controlled, double-blind trial in 300 colon surgery patients randomized to 80% versus 30% oxygen intraoperatively and during the first 6 hours after surgery. Surgical and anesthetic management were standardized and intended to support optimal perfusion. Myles et al.[110] demonstrated a significant reduction in major postoperative complications, as well as specifically wound infections in 2,050 major surgery patients randomized to 80% oxygen in 20% nitrogen versus 30% oxygen in 70% nitrous oxide intraoperatively. Bickel et al.[111] demonstrated a significant reduction in SSI (5.6% vs. 13.5%; $p = 0.04$) in patients undergoing open appendectomy ($n = 210$) who received 80% oxygen intraoperatively and high flow oxygen for 2 hours after surgery versus those who received 30% oxygen intraoperatively. Schietroma et al.[112] demonstrated in patients undergoing major rectal cancer surgery ($n = 72$) that the risk of anastomotic leak was 46% lower in the 80% inspired oxygen group (RR, 0.63; 95% confidence interval, 0.42–0.98) versus the 30% group. In a retrospective case–control study of patients undergoing spine surgery,[113] intraoperative administered fraction of inspired oxygen of less than 50% was the strongest predictor of SSI (OR, 12; 94% CI, 4.5–33; $P < 0.001$).

Pryor et al.[114] demonstrated a doubling of SSI in patients randomized to 80% versus 35% oxygen intraoperatively ($n = 165$). There were a number of methodologic flaws in the study, but, more importantly, the two groups of patients were not equivalent, which likely explained the increase in infections seen in the 80% oxygen group. Meyhoff et al.[115] found no difference in SSI rate (20.1% vs. 19.1%, $p = NS$) as a function of oxygen administration in 1,400 patients undergoing colon and gynecologic surgery. A major difference in design from the studies that demonstrated benefit was the use of a highly restricted volume replacement regimen. The stated aim was that patients were to gain no more than 1 kg by the second day after operation. Without data on wound oxygen (which was not measured), it is difficult to determine the reason for the difference in outcome compared to the Greif, Belda, and Myles studies, but wound vasoconstriction and a resulting lack of increase in wound oxygen tension is a strong possibility.

Although the preponderance of evidence indicates that use of high-inspired oxygen intraoperatively and providing supplemental oxygen postoperatively in *well-perfused* patients undergoing major abdominal surgery will reduce the risk of wound infection, there remains controversy about the benefits of high-inspired oxygen. One factor in the hesitation to adopt high-inspired oxygen is concern about potential side effects or toxicity of 80% oxygen. Two of the above studies examined this question in detail and found no difference in pulmonary complications or atelectasis.[115,116] A randomized controlled trial in patients at low risk for SSI ($n = 100$) found no difference in postoperative oxygen requirement in patients randomized to 30% oxygen intraoperatively versus those randomized to more than 90%.[117] A recent Cochrane analysis of studies of high perioperative inspired oxygen[118] found no significant effect on mortality, although the authors point out that the sample size is not sufficient to rule out the possibility of harm. Thus, high-inspired oxygen appears to be a low-risk approach to enhancing host defenses and reducing SSI.

Perfusion and oxygen also play a key role in the effectiveness of antibiotic prophylaxis. Delivery of antibiotics depends on perfusion. Parenteral antibiotics given so that high levels are present in the blood at the time of wounding clearly diminish but do not eliminate wound infections.[31] In about one-third of all wound infections, the bacteria cultured from the wound are sensitive to the prophylactic antibiotic given to the patient, even when the antibiotics were given according to standard procedure.[31] The vulnerable third of patients appear to be the hypoxic and vasoconstricted group. When antibiotics are present in the wound at the time of injury, they are trapped in the fibrin clot at the wound site where they may have efficacy against contaminating organisms. Antibiotics diffuse poorly into the fibrin clot; however, so that later administration, whether more than 2 hours after injury or in response to wound infection, will have little effect. On the other hand, oxygen diffuses easily through the fibrin clots and is effective even 6 hours after contamination.[29]

Bactericidal antibodies currently in use employ oxygen to kill organisms in much the same way as phagocytes. Kohanski[119] has demonstrated that quinolones, β-lactams, and aminoglycosides kill *S. aureus* and *Escherichia coli* by stimulating hydroxyl radical production from oxygen, even though all have different mechanisms for entering bacteria. Suller and Lloyd[120] observed a logarithmic reduction in bacterial cell counts in 10 to 15 hours in aerobic conditions compared with more than 60 hours to achieve the same result in an anaerobic environment for four facultative anaerobic staphylococcal strains exposed to vancomycin in air-equilibrated versus hypoxic conditions. Thus, maintaining conditions that optimize wound oxygen will also optimize the effectiveness of many commonly used antibiotics.

Patient Management

A recent meta-analysis of 16 randomized controlled trials, quasiexperimental studies, and cohort studies[121] demonstrated that the use of "bundles" of evidence-based care in patients undergoing colorectal surgery significantly reduced the risk of SSI. Unfortunately, as the authors note, there is currently "no consensus as to what comprises the optimal colorectal surgical care bundle." Standardization of care is likely responsible for some of the benefit. Further study is required to identify individual best practices. In the meantime, the following are approaches that anesthesiologists can take with the aim of improving wound healing and resistance to infection in their patients.

Preoperative Preparation

Given knowledge of the physiology of wound healing, what are the best strategies for an anesthesiologist to pursue to ensure optimal healing? SSI result from a multitude of factors that include the health of the patient, the type of surgery, the number and type of organisms contaminating the surgical site, and surgical technique. To the degree they are predictable, interventions can be targeted at those patients most at risk (Table 8-6).

The CDC, in the Study of the Effect of Nosocomial Infection Control (SENIC),[122] developed a remarkably useful and simple predictive tool based on a score of 0 or 1 for each of the following four patient factors: an abdominal operation, an operation that lasts 2 hours or more, a surgical site that is contaminated or infected, and a patient who will have three or more diagnoses at discharge, exclusive of wound infection. The risk of infection with a score of 0 is 1%, with a score of 1 is 3.6%, with a score of 2 is 9%, with a score of 3 is 17%, and with a score of 4 is 27%. These percentages may seem high, but this index was constructed on 3% of the American surgical patients from 1975–1976 and 1983, and the overall results are consistent with numerous other studies. More recent risk analyses by the same group, based on simpler predictors (e.g., American Society of Anesthesiologists Physical Status Classification) have yielded less sensitivity, but about the same overall infection rate.[123]

Modifiable or potentially modifiable risks include smoking, malnutrition, obesity, diabetes and hyperglycemia, steroid use,

Table 8-6	Preoperative Checklist

Assess and optimize cardiopulmonary function. Correct hypertension.
Treat vasoconstriction: Attend to blood volume, thermoregulatory vasoconstriction, pain, and anxiety.
Assess recent nutrition and treat as appropriate.
Treat existing infection. Among other actions, clean and treat skin infections.
Assess wound risk by SENIC score in order to decide on the extent to which prophylactic measures should be taken.
Start vitamin A or anabolic steroids in patients taking prednisone.
Improve or maintain blood sugar control.

From Hunt TK, Hopf HW. Wound healing and wound infection. What surgeons and anesthesiologists can do. *Surg Clin North Am.* 1997;77:587, with permission.

Table 8-7	Intraoperative Management

Appropriate prophylactic antibiotics should be given at the start of any procedure in which infection is highly probable and/or has potentially disastrous consequences. Maintain antibiotic levels during long operations.
Keep patients warm.
Observe gentle surgical technique with minimal use of ties and cautery.
Keep wounds moist.
Antibiotic irrigation in contaminated cases.
Elevate PaO_2.
Delayed closure for heavily contaminated wounds.
Use appropriate sutures (and skin tapes).
Use appropriate dressings.

From Hunt TK, Hopf HW. Wound healing and wound infection. What surgeons and anesthesiologists can do. *Surg Clin North Am.* 1997;77:587, with permission.

anemia, hypercholesterolemia, and hypertension. These should be assessed and corrected when possible prior to surgery. The decision to delay surgery must take into account both the urgency of the surgery and the severity of the risk.

Stress also predisposes to poor wound healing. Adverse psychosocial circumstances at the time of surgery may put patients at risk for poor wound healing. Kiecolt-Glaser et al.[124] studied the impact of hostile marital interactions on the healing of experimental blister wounds. High-hostile couples produced more proinflammatory cytokines and healed more slowly than low-hostile couples. Using a tape-stripping model, Muizzuddin et al.[125] investigated the effect of marital dissolution on skin barrier recovery and found that high stress was associated with slower recovery. Bosch et al.[126] studied the healing of a circular wound on the oral hard palate in subjects who varied in depression and/or dysphoria. High-dysphoric individuals had higher wound sizes from day 2 onward and depressive symptoms predicted slower wound healing. Collectively, these studies point to links between psychosocial distress, dysregulation at the system level, and impaired capacity for wound healing. It seems likely that stress-reduction techniques will reduce wound complications, and well-designed clinical trials are needed in this area.

Intraoperative Management

Careful surgical technique is fundamental to optimal wound healing (Table 8-7). Delicate handling of the tissue, adequate hemostasis, and surgeon experience lead to healthier wounds. Incisions should be planned with regard to blood supply, particularly when operating near or in old incisions. Mechanical retractors should be released from time to time to allow perfusion to the wound edges. Judicious antibiotic irrigation of contaminated areas may be effective. Because dried wounds lose perfusion, wounds should be kept moist, especially during long operations. Not all wounds can be anatomically closed. Edema, obesity, the possibility of unacceptable respiratory compromise, or the need to debride grossly contaminated or necrotic soft tissues can all interfere with closure of the wound.

As the operation proceeds, new wounds are made and contamination continues. All anesthetic agents tend to cause hypothermia—first, by causing vasodilation, which redistributes heat from core to periphery in previously vasoconstricted patients, and second, by increasing heat loss and decreasing heat production.[101] Vasoconstriction is uncommon intraoperatively, as the threshold for thermoregulatory vasoconstriction is decreased, but is often severe in the immediate postoperative period when anesthesia is discontinued and the thermoregulatory threshold returns to normal in the face of core hypothermia. The onset of pain with emergence from anesthesia adds to this vasoconstriction because of the associated catecholamine release.[105] Rapid rewarming using a forced air warmer for hypothermic patients in the post-anesthesia care unit (PACU) does appear to be effective,[127] although prevention of hypothermia is clearly the goal.[102] Maintenance of a high room temperature or active warming before, during, and after the operation is significantly more effective than other methods of warming such as application of warm blankets, circulating water blankets placed on the operating table surface, and humidification of the breathing circuit.[128]

Forced air warming was the first practical means of keeping patients warm intraoperatively. More recently, a number of other effective approaches have been introduced, including resistive warming, negative pressure warming, and thin, adhesive circulating water pads that are applied directly to the skin.[129]

Volume Management

Intravascular volume management during surgery has implications for tissue perfusion and, therefore, wound healing. Numerous factors, including patient comorbidities, medications such as diuretics, fever, preoperative volume state, surgical procedure, blood and insensible losses, and surgical stress all influence fluid requirements during surgery. It is widely agreed that the goal of intraoperative fluid management is to ensure sufficient intravascular volume to maintain perfusion and maximize oxygen delivery to the tissues, while avoiding the ill effects of hypervolemia, namely interstitial edema; what is difficult to determine is how to achieve that goal. Patient monitoring, fluid choice, and fluid administration strategy are topics of much debate, with a poorly standardized and often contradictory literature. For a comprehensive review of fluid management, see Chapter 16: Fluids, Electrolytes and Acid-Base Physiology.

Estimating preoperative volume status can be challenging, as there are many factors to consider. Preoperative fluid state may be reduced by fasting, mechanical bowel preparation, or medication use. Pre-existing medical conditions such as systolic and diastolic heart failure may cause hypervolemia and physiology that is exquisitely sensitive to fluid overload. While hemodialysis reliably induces hypovolemia, patients with end-stage renal disease are also susceptible to fluid overload, and intraoperative fluid replacement is complex. Patient history and physical examination, for more straightforward patients, and other tools such as preoperative echocardiography, for complex patients, can give the anesthesiologist an idea of presurgical patient's general volume status.

There are known serious complications of both hyper- and hypovolemia, particularly in the perioperative period. The major complications of hypovolemia, aside from hemodynamic instability, include decreased oxygenation of surgical wounds (which predisposes to wound infection),[42,63,88,130–132] decreased collagen formation,[42,103] impaired wound healing, and increased wound breakdown. The major complications associated with hypervolemia include pulmonary edema, congestive heart failure, edema of gut with prolonged ileus, and possibly an increase in cardiac arrhythmias.[133] Inappropriately high fluid administration may result in elevated atrial natriuretic peptide, inducing endothelial glycocalyx dysfunction, with resultant vascular permeability and extravascular fluid shifts.[134]

Recent studies suggest patients benefit from ingestion of high-carbohydrate, clear liquids 2 to 3 hours prior to surgery in order to achieve a euvolemic state at the start of surgery. In addition to providing hydration, there is evidence that this is a safe practice with the additional benefits of increased patient satisfaction[135] and decreased postoperative insulin resistance.[136]

Intraoperative assessment of fluid status is necessary for optimization of intravascular volume. Estimates of blood loss, third-space fluid losses, and maintenance requirements are notoriously inaccurate and may lead to either over- or underreplacement if used as guides. Surgical stress can result in increased intravenous fluid requirements. The increased fluid requirement may be partly due to substances like IL-6, TNF, substance-P, and bradykinin, which are released in response to, and in proportion to, surgical stress.[137] These inflammatory mediators cause both vasodilation and an increase in vascular permeability.[138] However, the concept of third spacing as a cause of functional intravascular fluid depletion has been challenged.[139]

6 Optimizing the volume of perioperative fluid administration to minimize morbidity and mortality remains a significant and controversial challenge. Currently, most practitioners rely on clinical acumen, vital signs such as heart rate and blood pressure, and urine output to manage perioperative fluids. Surgical patients can be markedly hypovolemic without a change in any one of these variables because of the compensatory action of peripheral vasoconstriction.[42,88,132] Unfortunately, this shunts blood away from skin, increases wound hypoxemia, and increases the risk of surgical wound infection. Static monitors such as heart rate, blood pressure, urine output, central venous pressure,[42,63,103,140] and pulmonary artery catheters have been shown to be limited. More dynamic monitors such as stroke volume assessment, pulse pressure variation, and systolic pressure variation can be predictive of fluid responsiveness[141]; however, these have limitations, including the requirements of a regular R to R interval, closed chest, and adequate tidal volumes. Echocardiography, including assessment of stroke volume and other indices for preload, afterload, and contractility, can be a helpful intraoperative guide,[142] but large-scale clinical trials are needed to validate its use as a dynamic modality for monitoring. Additional limitations include lack of available hardware and expertise.

Intraoperative fluid optimization strategies have ranged from liberal, to restrictive (also known as zero-balance), to goal-directed (SV optimization). There is evidence that increased volume may be beneficial for skin perfusion. Arkilic et al.[130] randomized 56 patients to liberal (16 to 18 mL/kg/hr) or conservative (8 mL/kg/hr) intraoperative fluid therapy and measured tissue perfusion and oxygen tension as a surrogate for wound healing. The liberal fluid regimen was associated with significantly greater intraoperative subcutaneous oxygen tension as measured by a tissue oxygen sensor. The study was too small to evaluate the effect on wound complications. Kabon et al.[143] performed a randomized, controlled trial to compare standard (8 mL/kg/hr) versus high (16 to 18 mL/kg/hr) volume administration in 253 patients undergoing elective colon resection. They found a trend toward reduced wound infections in the group that received high volume (8.5% vs. 11.3%), which would be a clinically significant reduction. Unfortunately, the study was terminated early, so it had inadequate power. Patients at high risk for heart failure or with end-stage renal disease were excluded, so the study also has limited generalizability. On the other side, there is concern that liberal fluid administration may be excessive and may be detrimental to patients. In a systematic review, Holte et al.[138] found benefit in avoiding excessive fluid administration in major surgery.

The discussion of "liberal" and "restricted" fluids requires consideration of whether colloids or crystalloids are preferable for intraoperative fluid administration. Synthetic colloids have been associated with coagulopathy when large volumes are delivered, which appears to be in large part mediated by dilution of coagulation factors.[144] Crystalloids, on the other hand, may cause a hypercoagulable state.[143] The intravascular half-life of colloids, either albumin or synthetic colloids, is much longer than that of crystalloids, allowing the total volume of fluid administered to be reduced by including colloids in surgical fluid resuscitation.[144] Edema formation may also be decreased. A number of studies[133,144–147] purport to evaluate intraoperative or postoperative fluid administration in terms of restrictive versus traditional fluid management. Virtually all have compared colloid ("restrictive" group) with crystalloid ("traditional" group) administration. Thus, the "restricted" volume group likely received a larger amount of effective intravascular volume than the traditional or "liberal" group. In general, these studies have demonstrated improved outcomes (reduction in SSI, earlier return of bowel function) for the colloid group. The mechanism for the benefit is unclear, however, as on the basis of effective intravascular volume delivered, the crystalloid groups might actually have been less well volume replaced than the colloid groups.

What is clear is that fluid overload to the point of interstitial edema is not beneficial for most organ function, including kidneys, liver, lungs, and heart. Interstitial edema can result in poor wound healing and infection due to decreased oxygen diffusion distance. Finding the balance between appropriate volume supplementation for adequate perfusion and avoiding tissue edema is the challenge. One of the difficulties in interpreting the literature on volume management is the lack of standardization of definitions such as "liberal" and "restricted," the amount and combinations of fluid used for replacement, and the lack of standardization of targets and outcomes. At this time, an individualized plan based on preoperative and intraoperative volume assessment, and appropriate monitoring, depending on the complexity of comorbidities and the surgical procedure, is required to attempt to find this balance for every patient. Goal-directed therapy, using stroke volume variation or echocardiography, holds promise, but much work remains to be done to define and implement reliable standards.

Current best recommendations include replacing fluid losses based on standard recommendations (Table 8-8) for the type of surgery, replacement of blood loss, and replacement of other ongoing fluid losses (e.g., high urine output due to diuretic or dye administration, hyperglycemia, or thermoregulatory vasoconstriction). Maintenance of normothermia is also critical to

Table 8-8 Standard Volume Management Guidelines for Surgical Patients

Fluid requirement = deficit + maintenance (baseline plus replacement) + estimated blood loss and other sensible fluid losses
Deficit = maintenance (1.5 mL/kg/hr) × hours NPO
Adjust for fever, high NG output, bowel preparation, and other sources of ongoing preoperative increased fluid loss
Use goal-directed therapy as available
Replace EBL 3:1 with crystalloid, 1:1 with colloid

Maintenance requirements for different surgeries:
Superficial surgical trauma: 1–2 mL/kg/hr
  Peripheral surgery
Minimal surgical trauma: 3–4 mL/kg/hr
  Head and neck, hernia, knee surgery
Moderate surgical trauma: 5–6 mL/kg/hr
  Major surgery without exposed abdominal contents
Severe surgical trauma: 8–10 mL/kg/hr
  Major abdominal, especially with exposed abdominal contents

NPO, nothing by mouth; NG, nasogastric; EBL, estimated blood loss.

Table 8-9 Postoperative Management

Keep patient warm.
Provide analgesia to keep patient comfortable, if not pain free. Patient report and the ability to move freely are the best signs of adequate pain relief.
Only one more dose of antibiotic unless an infection is present or contamination continues.
Keep up with third-space losses. Remember that fever increases fluid losses.
Assess perfusion and react to abnormalities.
Avoid diuresis until pain is gone and patient is warm.
Assess losses (including thermal losses) if wound is open.
Assess need for parenteral or enteral nutrition and respond.
Continue to control hypertension and hyperglycemia.

From Hunt TK, Hopf HW. Wound healing and wound infection. What surgeons and anesthesiologists can do. *Surg Clin North Am.* 1997;77:587, with permission.

---

optimal volume management. Warm patients are unlikely to develop pulmonary edema with a high rate of fluid administration because they have excess capacitance due to vasodilation. Cold patients, on the other hand, are highly susceptible to pulmonary edema even after relatively small fluid boluses. Thermoregulatory vasoconstriction increases afterload, causing increased cardiac work. Moreover, administered fluid cannot open up constricted vessels until the hypothermic stimulus is removed; thus, there is virtually no excess capacitance in the system.

Pain control should be addressed intraoperatively so that patients do not have severe pain on emergence. Achieving the goal is more important than the technique used to do so. Although regional anesthesia and analgesia may provide superior pain relief, the effects of specific analgesic regimens on wound outcome have not yet adequately been studied.

Postoperative Management

Wounds are most vulnerable in the first few hours after surgery (Table 8-9). Although antibiotics lose their effectiveness after the first hours, oxygen-mediated natural wound immunity lasts longer.[29] Even a short period of vasoconstriction during the first day is sufficient to reduce oxygen supply and increase infection risk.[63] Correction and prevention of vasoconstriction in the first 24 to 48 hours after surgery will have significant beneficial effects.[63] Given the large number of diabetic patients who undergo surgery, along with the fact that the stress response frequently induces hyperglycemia intraoperatively even in nondiabetic patients, guidelines for controlling blood sugar in perioperative patients are critical to prevention of SSI. Unfortunately, balancing a narrow therapeutic window between hypoglycemia and hyperglycemia is a complex issue in blood sugar control. Clinical trials have provided conflicting results. A 2001 randomized controlled trial demonstrated a 25% reduction in risk of septicemia in critically ill surgical patients whose blood glucose levels were more tightly controlled than a comparison group.[148] On the other hand, in 2007 Gandhi et al.[149] found no difference in SSI in 400 cardiac surgery patients comparing a target blood sugar of 80 to 100 versus less than 200 mg/dL. The NICE-SUGAR study in 6,104 ICU patients demonstrated excess mortality in the tight control (81 to 108 mg/dL) versus standard (<180 mg/dL) group.[150] The current recommendation is to keep glucose close to normal (e.g., 100 to 180 or 200 mg/dL).[151]

All vasoconstrictive stimuli must be corrected simultaneously to allow optimal healing. Volume is the last to be corrected because vasoconstriction for other reasons induces diuresis and renders the patient relatively hypovolemic (peripherally, not centrally). These measures are particularly important in any patients at high risk for wound complications for other reasons (e.g., malnutrition, steroid use, diabetes), or when vasoconstrictive drugs such as β-blockers and α-agonists are required for other reasons.

Local perfusion is not assured until patients have a normal blood volume, are warm and pain free, and are receiving no vasoconstrictive drugs; that is, until the sympathetic nervous system is inactivated. Warming should continue until patients are thoroughly awake and active and can maintain their own thermal balance. After major operations, warming may be useful for many hours or even days. The goal is to achieve warmth at the skin; wound vasoconstriction due to cold surroundings often coexists with core hyperthermia. Moderate hyperthermia is not, itself, a problem. When extensive wounds are left open, warmth should be continued, and heat losses due to evaporation should be prevented to avoid vasoconstriction and to minimize caloric losses.

Assessing perfusion, especially in the PACU, is critical. Unfortunately, urine output is a poor, often misleading guide to peripheral perfusion.[131] Markedly low output may indicate decreased renal perfusion, but normal or even high urine output has little correlation to wound or tissue PO_2. Many factors commonly present in the perioperative period, including hyperglycemia, dye administration, thermoregulatory vasoconstriction, adrenal insufficiency, and various drugs, may cause inappropriate diuresis in the face of mild hypovolemia.

Physical examination of the patient is a better guide to hypovolemia and vasoconstriction. Assess vasoconstriction by a capillary return time of more than 2 to 3 seconds at the forehead and more than 5 seconds over the patella. Eye turgor is another good measure of volume status. Finally, patients can usually distinguish thirst from a dry mouth. Skin should be warm and dry.

After major abdominal surgery, third-space losses continue for about 12 to 24 hours, so that increased fluid requirements continue. In general, for large abdominal cases, 2 to 3 mL/kg/hr of IV fluids is sufficient for the first 12 to 24 postoperative hours. After that period, the IV rate should be decreased below calculated maintenance levels because edema fluid begins to be mobilized, thus increasing circulating intravascular volume.

When excessive tissue fluids have accumulated, diuresis should be undertaken gently so that transcapillary refill can maintain blood volume. This applies to patients who need renal dialysis as well. The average dialysis patient vasoconstricts sufficiently to lower tissue PO_2 by 30% or more during dialysis and needs about 24 hours to return vasomotor tone and wound and tissue PO_2 to normal.[152] Fluid losses from the vascular system are not necessarily replaced from the tissues as rapidly as they are sustained. Tissue edema may be the price paid for adequate intravascular volume. Edema increases intracapillary distance, so that there may be a delicate balance between excessive edema and peripheral vasoconstriction (which worsens the hypoxia caused by edema).

Vasoconstrictive drugs should be avoided. The most common and most avoidable is nicotine in the form of cigarettes. β-Blockers should be used only when clearly medically indicated. Both are known to reduce wound and tissue PO_2. Clonidine is an alternative drug for heart rate control[153,154] that also induces vasodilation and may increase wound PO_2.[155] High-dose α-adrenergic agonists or other vasopressors may cause harm by decreasing tissue PO_2, but lower doses have little or no effect on wound/tissue PO_2.[100] It is important to remember that decreasing cardiac output may also reduce wound perfusion. Thus, a balance must be maintained between minimizing use of vasopressors and maintaining adequate cardiac output.

Maintenance of tissue PO_2 requires attention to pulmonary function postoperatively. Administration of supplemental oxygen via face mask or nasal cannulae increases safety in patients receiving systemic opioids[156] and one study demonstrated a reduction in SSI after lower extremity revascularization.[157] Pain control also appears important since it favorably influences both pulmonary function and vascular tone. This is particularly true in patients at high risk for pulmonary complications postoperatively, such as morbidly obese patients and those with pulmonary disease.[158] Epidural analgesia may be the route of choice in these patients. It has several advantages over parenterally administered opioids in that it generally achieves lower pain scores with less sedation. Nonetheless, opioid-induced pruritus is more common with epidural administration, and in some patients may be severe enough to counteract the benefits of pain control.

Patient-controlled analgesia is also quite effective at achieving low pain scores. It also has the benefit of giving control to the patient, leading to patient satisfaction as high as with epidural analgesia in many cases.[159] Nurse-administered, as-needed doses of IV or intramuscular opioids should be avoided as inadequate pain control often exceeds 50% using this approach.[160] The key to pain control is recognition of the need for analgesia and attention to the patient's complaints of pain. Opioid requirements vary enormously and are not always predictable, but even tolerant patients (IV drug abusers or those with cancer pain) can be given adequate pain relief with sufficient attention. Multimodal analgesia appears to be a valuable approach, reducing pain while minimizing respiratory depression.

Summary

In patients with moderate to high risk of SSI, anesthesiologists have the opportunity to enhance wound healing and reduce the incidence of wound infections by simple, inexpensive, and readily available means. Intraoperatively, appropriate antibiotic use, prevention of vasoconstriction through volume and warming, and maintenance of a high PaO_2 (300 to 500 mmHg) are key. Postoperatively, the focus should remain on prevention of vasoconstriction through pain relief, warming, and adequate volume administration in the PACU. The addition of measures to reduce and prevent the stress response is likely to be effective as well, although further study is required.

Areas for Future Research

- Does universal adherence to the "5 Moments for Hand Hygiene" improve outcomes?
- Is delay of antibiotics for culture justified?
- Psychological preparation and intervention can modulate the stress response. Will this reduce wound complications?
- Do nonsteroidal anti-inflammatory agents increase risk of wound complications?
- Does dexamethasone for postoperative nausea and vomiting prophylaxis increase the risk of wound complications?
- Do epidurals reduce the risk of SSI? Are they cost-effective (vs. time and risk)?
- How much fluid is required? Does goal-directed fluid therapy improve outcomes?
- Who should get a high FiO_2? Is there potential toxicity?
- Does postoperative oxygen reduce wound complications? How long should patients receive supplemental oxygen postoperatively?

REFERENCES

1. Brennan TA, Leape LL, Laird NM, et al. Incidence of adverse events and negligence in hospitalized patients: results of the Harvard Medical Practice Study I. *N Engl J Med.* 1991;324:370–376.
2. Magill SS, Edwards JR, Bamberg W, et al. Multistate point-prevalence survey of health care–associated infections. *N Engl J Med.* 2014;370:1198–1208.
3. Lee JP, Hopf HW, Cannon-Albright L. Empiric evidence for a genetic contribution to predisposition to surgical site infection. *Wound Rep Regen.* 2013;21:211–215.
4. Noakes TD, Borresen J, Hew-Butler T, et al. Semmelweis and the aetiology of puerperal sepsis 160 years on: an historical review. *Epidemiol Infect.* 2007;136(1):1–9.
5. Koff MD, Loftus RW, Burchman CC, et al. Reduction in intraoperative bacterial contamination of peripheral intravenous tubing through the use of a novel device. *Anesthesiology.* 2009;110:978–985.
6. Boyce JM, Pittet D. Healthcare Infection Control Practices Advisory Committee; HICPAC/SHEA/APIC/IDSA Hand Hygiene Task Force. Guideline for Hand Hygiene in Health-Care Settings. Recommendations of the Healthcare Infection Control Practices Advisory Committee and the HIPAC/SHEA/APIC/IDSA Hand Hygiene Task Force. *Am J Infect Control.* 2002;30:S1–S46.
7. Casewell M, Phillips I. Hands as route of transmission for *Klebsiella* species. *Br Med J.* 1977;2:1315–1317.
8. Ehrenkranz NJ, Alfonso BC. Failure of bland soap handwash to prevent hand transfer of patient bacteria to urethral catheters. *Infect Control Hosp Epidemiol.* 1991;12:654–662.
9. Sivathasan N, Goodfellow PB. Skin cleansers: the risks of chlorhexidine. *J Clin Pharmacol.* 2011;51:785–786.
10. Sax H, Allegranzi B, Uçkay I, et al. 'My five moments for hand hygiene': a user-centered design approach to understand, train, monitor and report hand hygiene. *J Hosp Infect.* 2007;67:9–21.
11. Loftus RW, Koff MD, Burchman CC, et al. Transmission of pathogenic bacterial organisms in the anesthesia work area. *Anesthesiology.* 2008;109:399–407.
12. Loftus RW, Koff MD, Birnbach DJ. The dynamics and implications of bacterial transmission events arising from the anesthesia work area. *Anesth Analg.* 2015;120:853–860.
13. Mecham E, Hopf HW. A proposal to minimize work area contamination during induction. *Anesthesiology.* 2011;116:712.
14. Birnbach DJ1, Rosen LF, Fitzpatrick M, et al. Double gloves: a randomized trial to evaluate a simple strategy to reduce contamination in the operating room. *Anesth Analg.* 2015;120:848–852.
15. Tunevall TG. Postoperative wound infections and surgical face masks: a controlled study. *World J Surg.* 1991;15:383–387.
16. Friberg B, Friberg S, Ostensson R, et al. Surgical area contamination—comparable bacterial counts using disposable head and mask and helmet aspirator system, but dramatic increase upon omission of head-gear: an experimental study in horizontal laminar air-flow. *J Hosp Infect.* 2001;47:110–115.

17. Babkin Y, Raveh D, Lifschitz M, et al. Incidence and risk factors for surgical infection after total knee replacement. *Scand J Infect Dis.* 2007;39:890–895.
18. Pryor F, Messmer PR. The effect of traffic patterns in the OR on surgical site infections. *AORN J.* 1998;68:649–660.
19. Moro ML. Health care-associated infections. *Surg Infect (Larchmt).* 2006;7:S21–S23.
20. Allo MD, Tedesco M. Operating room management: operative suite considerations, infection control. *Surg Clin North Am.* 2005;85:1291–1297.
21. Mermel LA, McCormick RD, Springman SR, et al. The pathogenesis and epidemiology of catheter-related infection with pulmonary artery Swan-Ganz catheters: a prospective study utilizing molecular subtyping. *Am J Med.* 1991;91:197S–205S.
22. Parienti JJ, Mongardon N, Megarbane B, et al. Intravascular complications of central venous catheterization by site. *N Engl J Med.* 2015;373:1220–1229.
23. Mimoz O, LocetJC, Kerforne T, et al. Skin antisepsis with chlorhexidine-alcohol versus povidone iodine-alcohol, with and without skin scrubbing, for prevention of intravascular-catheter-related infection (CLEAN): an open-label, multicentre, randomised, controlled, two-by-two factorial trial. *Lancet.* 2015;386:2069–2077.
24. Raad II, Hohn DC, Gilbreath BJ, et al. Prevention of central venous catheter-related infections by using maximal sterile barrier precautions during insertion. *Infect Control Hosp Epidemiol.* 1994;15:231–238.
25. O'Grady NP, Alexander M, Dellinger EP, et al. Guidelines for the prevention of intravascular catheter-related infections. *Infect Control Hosp Epidemiol.* 2002;23:759–769.
26. Carier V, Haenny A, Inan C, et al. No association between ultrasound-guided insertion of central venous catheters and bloodstream infection: a prospective observational study. *J Hosp Infect.* 2014;87:103–108.
27. Miles AA, Miles EM, Burke J. The value and duration of defence reactions of the skin to the primary lodgement of bacteria. *Br J Exp Pathol.* 1957;38:79–96.
28. Knighton DR, Halliday B, Hunt TK. Oxygen as an antibiotic: the effect of inspired oxygen on infection. *Arch Surg.* 1984;119:199–204.
29. Knighton DR, Halliday B, Hunt TK. Oxygen as an antibiotic: a comparison of the effects of inspired oxygen concentration and antibiotic administration on in vivo bacterial clearance. *Arch Surg.* 1986;121:191–195.
30. Bernard HR, Cole WR. The prophylaxis of surgical infection: the effect of prophylactic antimicrobial drugs on the incidence of infection following potentially contaminated operations. *Surgery.* 1964;56:151–157.
31. Classen D, Evans R, Pestotnik S, et al. The timing of prophylactic administration of antibiotics and the risk of surgical-wound infection. *N Engl J Med.* 1992;326:281–286.
32. Bratzler DW, Dellinger EP, Olsen KM Clinical practice guidelines for antimicrobial prophylaxis in surgery. *Am J Health Syst Pharm.* 2013;70:195–283.
33. Nichols RL, Condon RE, Barie PS. Antibiotic prophylaxis in surgery: 2005 and beyond. *Surg Infect (Larchmt).* 2005;6 349–361.
34. Burke JP. Maximizing appropriate antibiotic prophylaxis for surgical patients: an update from LDS Hospital, Salt Lake City. *Clin Infect Dis.* 2001;33(Suppl 2):S78–S83.
35. Arnold M, Barbul A. Nutrition and wound healing. *Plast Reconstr Surg.* 2006;117:42S–58S.
36. Jensen JA, Jonsson K, Goodson WH III, et al. Epinephrine lowers subcutaneous wound oxygen tension. *Curr Surg* 1985;42:472–474.
37. Mogford JE, Tawil N, Chen A, et al. Effect of age and hypoxia on TGFbeta1 receptor expression and signal transduction in human dermal fibroblasts: Impact on cell migration. *J Cell Physiol.* 2002;190:259–265.
38. Mogford JE, Sisco M, Bonomo SR, et al. Impact of aging on gene expression in a rat model of ischemic cutaneous wound healing. *J Surg Res.* 2004;118:190–196.
39. Lenhardt R, Hopf HW, Marker E, et al. Perioperative collagen deposition in elderly and young men and women. *Arch Surg.* 2000;135:71–74.
40. Robson MC, Mannari RJ, Smith PD, et al. Maintenance of wound bacterial balance. *Am J Surg.* 1999;178:399–402.
41. Winter GD. Formation of the scab and the rate of epithelisation of superficial wounds in the skin of the young domestic pig. 1962. *J Wound Care.* 1995;4:366–367.
42. Jonsson K, Jensen J, Goodson W, et al. Tissue oxygenation, anemia, and perfusion in relation to wound healing in surgical patients. *Ann Surg.* 1991;214:605–613.
43. Hopf HW, Ueno C, Aslam R, et al. Guidelines for the treatment of arterial insufficiency ulcers. *Wound Repair Regen.* 2006;14:693–710.
44. Ueno C, Hunt TK, Hopf HW. Using physiology to improve surgical wound outcomes. *Plast Reconstr Surg.* 2006;117:59S–71S.
45. De Jong L, Kemp A. Stoichiometry and kinetics of the prolyl 4-hydroxylase partial reaction. *Biochim Biophys Acta.* 1984;787:105–111.
46. Allen DB, Maguire JJ, Mahdavian M, et al. Wound hypoxia and acidosis limit neutrophil bacterial killing mechanisms. *Arch Surg.* 1997;132:991–996.
47. Hopf HW, Gibson JJ, Angeles AP, et al. Hyperoxia and angiogenesis. *Wound Repair Regen.* 2005;13:558–564.
48. Evans NTS, Naylor PFD. Steady states of oxygen tension in human dermis. *Respir Physiol.* 1966;2:46–60.
49. Medawar PS. The behavior of mammalian skin epithelium under strictly anaerobic conditions. *Q J Microsc Sci.* 1947;88:27.
50. Schultz G. Molecular regulation of wound healing. In: Bryant R, Nix D, eds. *Acute and Chronic Wounds: Current Management Concepts.* 3rd ed. St. Louis, MO: Mosby Elsevier; 2006:82–99.
51. Adams JC. Functions of the conserved thrombospondin carboxy-terminal cassette in cell-extracellular matrix interactions and signaling. *Int J Biochem Cell Biol.* 2004;36:1102–1114.
52. Constant J, Suh D, Hussain M, et al. Wound healing angiogenesis: the metabolic basis of repair. In: *Molecular, Cellular, and Clinical Aspects of Angiogenesis.* New York: Plenum Press; 1996:151–159.
53. Dvonch VM, Murphey RJ, Matsuoka J, et al. Changes in growth factor levels in human wound fluid. *Surgery.* 1992;112:18–23.
54. Zabel DD, Feng JJ, Scheuenstuhl H, et al. Lactate stimulation of macrophage-derived angiogenic activity is associated with inhibition of poly(ADP-ribose) synthesis. *Lab Invest.* 1996;74:644–649.
55. Heppenstall RB, Littooy FN, Fuchs R, et al. Gas tensions in healing tissues of traumatized patients. *Surgery.* 1974;75:874–880.
56. Trabold O, Wagner S, Wicke C, et al. Lactate and oxygen constitute a fundamental regulatory mechanism in wound healing. *Wound Repair Regen.* 2003;11:504–509.
57. Caldwell MD, Shearer J, Morris A, et al. Evidence for aerobic glycolysis in lambda-carrageenan-wounded skeletal muscle. *J Surg Res.* 1984;37:63–68.
58. Klebanoff SJ. Oxygen metabolism and the toxic properties of phagocytes. *Ann Intern Med.* 1980;93:480–489.
59. Niinikoski J, Hunt TK, Dunphy JE. Oxygen supply in healing tissue. *Am J Surg.* 1972;123:247–252.
60. Silver IA. Cellular microenvironment in healing and non-healing wounds. In: Hunt TK, Heppenstall RB, Pines E, eds. *Soft and Hard Tissue Repair.* New York: Praeger; 1984:50–66.
61. Falcone PA, Caldwell MD. Wound metabolism. *Clin Plast Surg.* 1990;17:443–456.
62. Chang N, Mathes SJ. Comparison of the effect of bacterial inoculation in musculocutaneous and random-pattern flaps. *Plast Reconstr Surg.* 1982;70(1):1–10.
63. Hopf HW, Hunt TK, West JM, et al. Wound tissue oxygen tension predicts the risk of wound infection in surgical patients. *Arch Surg.* 1997;132:997–1004.
64. Schwentker A, Evans SM, Partington M, et al. A model of wound healing in chronically radiation-damaged rat skin. *Cancer Lett.* 1998;128:71–78.
65. Bauer SM, Goldstein LJ, Bauer RJ, et al. The bone marrow-derived endothelial progenitor cell response is impaired in delayed wound healing from ischemia. *J Vasc Surg.* 2006;43:134–141.
66. Wütscher R, Bounameaux H. Determination of amputation level in ischemic limbs: reappraisal of the measurement of TcPo2. *Diab Care.* 1997;20:1315–1318.
67. Sen CK, Khanna S, Babior BM, et al. Oxidant-induced vascular endothelial growth factor expression in human keratinocytes and cutaneous wound healing. *J Biol Chem.* 2002;277:33284–33290.
68. Beckert S, Farrahi F, Aslam RS, et al. Lactate stimulates endothelial cell migration. *Wound Repair Regen.* 2006;14:321–324.
69. Babior BM. Oxygen-dependent microbial killing by phagocytes (first of two parts). *N Engl J Med.* 1978;298:659–668.
70. Edwards S, Hallett MB, Campbell AK. Oxygen-radical production during inflammation may be limited by oxygen concentration. *Biochem J.* 1984;217:851–854.
71. Lam GY, Huang J, Brumell JH. The many roles of NOX2 NADPH oxidase-derived ROS in immunity. *Semin Immunopathol.* 2010;32:415–430.
72. Smith BM, Desvigne LD, Slade JB, et al. Transcutaneous oxygen measurements predict healing of leg wounds with hyperbaric therapy. *Wound Repair Regen.* 1996;4:224–229.
73. Fife CE, Buyukcakir C, Otto GH, et al. The predictive value of transcutaneous oxygen tension measurement in diabetic lower extremity ulcers treated with hyperbaric oxygen therapy: a retrospective analysis of 1,144 patients. *Wound Repair Regen.* 2002;10:198–207.
74. Rollins MD, Gibson JJ, Hunt TK, et al. Wound oxygen levels during hyperbaric oxygen treatment in healing wounds. *Undersea Hyperb Med.* 2006;33:17–25.
75. Thom SR. Hyperbaric oxygen: its mechanisms and efficacy. *Plast Reconstr Surg.* 2011;127(Suppl 1):131S–141S.
76. Hunt TK, Aslam RS, Beckert S, et al. Aerobically derived lactate stimulates revascularization and tissue repair via redox mechanisms. *Antioxid Redox Signal.* 2007;9:1115–1124.
77. Velazquez OC. Angiogenesis and vasculogenesis: inducing the growth of new blood vessels and wound healing by stimulation of bone marrow–derived progenitor cell mobilization and homing. *J Vasc Surg.* 2007;45(Suppl A):A39–A47.
78. Capla JM, Ceradini DJ, Tepper OM, et al. Skin graft vascularization involves precisely regulated regression and replacement of endothelial cells through both angiogenesis and vasculogenesis. *Plast Reconstr Surg.* 2006;117:836–844.
79. Schultz GS, Grant MB. Neovascular growth factors. *Eye (Lond).* 1991;5:170–180.

80. Beckert S, Hierlemann H, Muschenborn N, et al. Experimental ischemic wounds: correlation of cell proliferation and insulin-like growth factor I expression and its modification by different local IGF-I release systems. *Wound Repair Regen.* 2005;13:278–283.
81. Knighton DR, Silver IA, Hunt TK. Regulation of wound-healing angiogenesis-effect of oxygen gradients and inspired oxygen concentration. *Surgery.* 1981;90: 262–270.
82. Uitto J, Prockop DJ. Synthesis and secretion of under-hydroxylated procollagen at various temperatures by cells subject to temporary anoxia. *Biochem Biophys Res Commun.* 1974;60:414.
83. Silver IA. Oxygen tension and epithelialization. In: Maibach HI, Rovee DT, eds. *Epidermal Wound Healing.* Chicago: Year Book Medical Publishers; 1972:291.
84. Feldmeier JJ, Hopf HW, Warriner RA III, et al. UHMS position statement: Topical oxygen for chronic wounds. *Undersea Hyperb Med.* 2005;32:157–168.
85. Ngo MA, Sinitsyna NN, Qin Q, et al. Oxygen-dependent differentiation of human keratinocytes. *J Invest Dermatol.* 2007;127:354–361.
86. O'Toole EA, Marinkovich MP, Peavey CL, et al. Hypoxia increases human keratinocyte motility on connective tissue. *J Clin Invest.* 1997;100:2881–2891.
87. Doughty DB. Preventing and managing surgical wound dehiscence. *Adv Skin Wound Care.* 2005;18:319–322.
88. Gottrup F, Firmin R, Rabkin J, et al. Directly measured tissue oxygen tension and arterial oxygen tension assess tissue perfusion. *Crit Care Med.* 1987; 15:1030–1036.
89. Hutton JJ, Tappel AL, Udenfriend S. Cofactor and substrate requirements of collagen proline hydroxylase. *Arch Biochem Biophys.* 1967;118:231–240.
90. Jönsson K, Hunt TK, Mathes SJ. Oxygen as an isolated variable influences resistance to infection. *Ann Surg.* 1988;208:783–787.
91. Hohn DC, MacKay RD, Halliday B, et al. Effect of O_2 tension on microbicidal function of leukocytes in wounds and in vitro. *Surg Forum.* 1976;27:18–20.
92. Jensen JA, Goodson WH, Hopf HW, et al. Cigarette smoking decreases tissue oxygen. *Arch Surg.* 1991;126:1131–1134.
93. Hopf H, Hunt T, Jensen J. Calculation of subcutaneous tissue blood flow. *Surg Forum.* 1988;39:33–36.
94. Hopf HW, Viele M, Watson JJ, et al. Subcutaneous perfusion and oxygen during acute severe isovolemic hemodilution in healthy volunteers. *Arch Surg.* 2000;135:1443–1449.
95. Hopf H, Hunt T. Does—and if so, to what extent—normovolemic dilutional anemia influence post-operative wound healing? *Chir Gastroenterol.* 1992;8:148–150.
96. Jensen JA, Goodson WH III, Vasconez LO, et al. Wound healing in anemia. *West J Med.* 1986;144:465–467.
97. Sheffield CW, Sessler DI, Hopf HW, et al. Centrally and locally mediated thermoregulatory responses alter subcutaneous oxygen tension. *Wound Repair Regen.* 1996;4:339–345.
98. Derbyshire DR, Smith G. Sympathoadrenal responses to anaesthesia and surgery. *Br J Anaesth.* 1984;56:725–739.
99. Halter JB, Pflug AE, Porte D Jr. Mechanism of plasma catecholamine increases during surgical stress in man. *J Clin Endocrinol Metab.* 1977;45:936–944.
100. Motakef S, Mountziaris PM, Ismail IK, et al. Emerging paradigms in perioperative management for microsurgical free tissue transfer: review of the literature and evidence-based guidelines. *Plast Reconstr Surg.* 2015;135(1): 290–299.
101. Matsukawa T, Sessler DI, Sessler AM, et al. Heat flow and distribution during induction of general anesthesia. *Anesthesiology.* 1995;82:662–673.
102. Kurz A, Sessler DI, Lenhardt R. Perioperative normothermia to reduce the incidence of surgical-wound infection and shorten hospitalization: study of wound infection and temperature group. *N Engl J Med.* 1996;334: 1209–1215.
103. Hartmann M, Jönsson K, Zederfeldt B. Effect of tissue perfusion and oxygenation on accumulation of collagen in healing wounds: randomized study in patients after major abdominal operations. *Eur J Surg.* 1992;158:521–526.
104. Melling AC, Ali B, Scott EM, et al. Effects of preoperative warming on the incidence of wound infection after clean surgery: a randomised controlled trial. *Lancet.* 2001;358:876–880.
105. Akça O, Melischek M, Scheck T, et al. Postoperative pain and subcutaneous oxygen tension [letter]. *Lancet.* 1999;354:41–42.
106. Rojas IG, Padgett DA, Sheridan JF, et al. Stress-induced susceptibility to bacterial infection during cutaneous wound healing. *Brain Behav Immun.* 2002;16:74–84.
107. Horan MP, Quan N, Subramanian SV, et al. Impaired wound contraction and delayed myofibroblast differentiation in restraint-stressed mice. *Brain Behav Immun.* 2005;19:207–216.
108. Greif R, Akça O, Horn EP, et al. Supplemental perioperative oxygen to reduce the incidence of surgical-wound infection. Outcomes Research Group. *N Engl J Med.* 2000;342:161–167.
109. Belda FJ, Aguilera L, Garcia de la Asuncion J, et al. Supplemental perioperative oxygen and the risk of surgical wound infection: a randomized controlled trial. *JAMA.* 2005;294:2035–2042.
110. Myles PS, Leslie K, Chan MT, et al. Avoidance of nitrous oxide for patients undergoing major surgery: a randomized controlled trial. *Anesthesiology.* 2007; 107:221–231.
111. Bickel A, Gurevits M, Vamos R, et al. Perioperative hyperoxygenation and wound site infection following surgery for acute appendicitis: a randomized, prospective, controlled trial. *Arch Surg.* 2011;146:464–470.
112. Schietroma M, Carlei F, Cecilia E, et al. Colorectal infraperitoneal anastomosis: The effects of perioperative supplemental oxygen administration on the anastomotic dehiscence. *J Gastrointest Surg.* 2012;16:427–434.
113. Maragakis LL, Cosgrove SE, Martinez EA, et al. Intraoperative fraction of inspired oxygen is a modifiable risk factor for surgical site infection after spinal surgery. *Anesthesiology.* 2009;110:556–562.
114. Pryor KO, Fahey TJ 3rd, Lien CA, et al. Surgical site infection and the routine use of perioperative hyperoxia in a general surgical population: a randomized controlled trial. *JAMA.* 2004;291:79–87.
115. Meyhoff C, Wetterslev J, Jorgensen LN, et al. Effect of high perioperative oxygen fraction on surgical site infection and pulmonary complications after abdominal surgery: the PROXI randomized clinical trial. *JAMA.* 2009;302:1543–1550.
116. Akça O, Podolsky A, Eisenhuber E, et al. Comparable postoperative pulmonary atelectasis in patients given 30% or 80% oxygen during and 2 hours after colon resection. *Anesthesiology.* 1999;91:991–998.
117. Mackintosh N, Gertsch MC, Hopf HW, et al. High intraoperative inspired oxygen does not increase postoperative supplemental oxygen requirements. *Anesthesiology.* 2012;117:271–279.
118. Wetterslev J, Meyhoff CS, Jørgensen LN, et al. The effects of high perioperative inspiratory oxygen fraction for adult surgical patients. *Cochrane Database Syst Rev.* 2015;6:CD008884
119. Kohanski MA, Dwyer DJ, Hayete B, et al. A common mechanism of cellular death induced by bactericidal antibiotics. *Cell.* 2007;130:797–810.
120. Suller MT, Lloyd D. The antibacterial activity of vancomycin towards *Staphylococcus aureus* under aerobic and anaerobic conditions. *J Appl Microbiol.* 2002;92:866–872.
121. Tanner J, Padley W, Assadian O. Do surgical care bundles reduce the risk of surgical site infections in patients undergoing colorectal surgery? A systematic review and cohort meta-analysis of 8,515 patients. *Surgery.* 2015;158:66–77.
122. Haley RW, Culver DH, Morgan WM, et al. Identifying patients at high risk of surgical wound infection: a simple multivariate index of patient susceptibility and wound contamination. *Am J Epidemiol.* 1985;121:206–215.
123. Culver DH, Horan TC, Gaynes RP, et al. Surgical wound infection rates by wound class, operative procedure, and patient risk index. National Nosocomial Infections Surveillance System. *Am J Med.* 1991;91:152S–157S.
124. Kiecolt-Glaser JK, Loving TJ, Stowell JR, et al. Hostile marital interactions, proinflammatory cytokine production, and wound healing. *Arch Gen Psychiatry.* 2005;62:1377–1384.
125. Muizzuddin N, Matsui MS, Marenus KD, et al. Impact of stress of marital dissolution on skin barrier recovery: tape stripping and measurement of transepidermal water loss (TEWL). *Skin Res Technol.* 2003;9:34–38.
126. Bosch JA, Engeland CG, Cacioppo JT, et al. Depressive symptoms predict mucosal wound healing. *Psychosom Med.* 2007;69:597–605.
127. West J, Hopf H, Sessler D, et al. The effect of rapid postoperative rewarming on tissue oxygen. *Wound Repair Regen.* 1993;1:93.
128. Kurz A, Kurz M, Poeschl G, et al. Forced-air warming maintains intraoperative normothermia better than circulating water mattresses. *Anesth Analg.* 1993;77:89–95.
129. Galvão CM, Marck PB, Sawada NO, et al. A systematic review of the effectiveness of cutaneous warming systems to prevent hypothermia. *J Clin Nurs.* 2010;18:627–636.
130. Arkiliç CF, Taguchi A, Sharma N, et al. Supplemental perioperative fluid administration increases tissue oxygen pressure. *Surgery.* 2003;133:49–55.
131. Jonsson K, Jensen JA, Goodson WH III, et al. Assessment of perfusion in postoperative patients using tissue oxygen measurements. *Br J Surg.* 1987;74: 263–267.
132. Gosain A, Rabkin J, Reymond JP, et al. Tissue oxygen tension and other indicators of blood loss or organ perfusion during graded hemorrhage. *Surgery.* 1991;109:523–532.
133. Nisanevich V, Felsenstein I, Almogy G, et al. Effect of intraoperative fluid management on outcome after intraabdominal surgery. *Anesthesiology.* 2005;103: 25–32.
134. Alphonsus CS, Rodseth RN. The endothelial glycocalyx: a review of the vascular barrier. *Anaesthesia.* 2014;69:777–784.
135. Hausel J, Nygren J, Lagerkranser M, et al. A carbohydrate-rich drink reduces preoperative discomfort in elective surgery patients. *Anesth Analg.* 2001;93: 1344–1350.
136. Nygren J, Soop M, Thorell A, et al. Preoperative oral carbohydrate administration reduces postoperative insulin resistance. *Clin Nutr.* 1998;17:65–71.
137. Kehlet H. Surgical stress response: does endoscopic surgery confer an advantage? *World J Surg.* 1999;23:801–807
138. Holte K, Sharrock NE, Kehlet H. Pathophysiology and clinical implications of perioperative fluid excess. *Br J Anaesth.* 2002;89:622–632.
139. Chappell D, Jacob M, Hofmann-Kiefer K, et al. A rational approach to perioperative fluid management. *Anesthesiology.* 2008;109:723–740.
140. Marik PE, Baram M, Vahid B. Does central venous pressure predict fluid responsiveness? A systematic review of the literature and the tale of seven mares. *Chest.* 2008;134:172–178.

141. Marik PE, Cavallazzi R, Vasu T, et al. Dynamic changes in arterial waveform derived variables and fluid responsiveness in mechanically ventilated patients: a systematic review of the literature. *Crit Care Med*. 2009;37:2642–2647.
142. Porter TR, Shillcutt SK, Adams MS, et al. Guidelines for the use of echocardiography as a monitor for therapeutic intervention in adults. *J Am Soc Echocardiogr*. 2015;28:40–56.
143. Kabon B, Akca O, Taguchi A, et al. Supplemental intravenous crystalloid administration does not reduce the risk of surgical wound infection. *Anesth Analg*. 2005;101:1546–1553.
144. Grocott MP, Mythen MG, Gan TJ. Perioperative fluid management and clinical outcomes in adults. *Anesth Analg*. 2005;100:1093–1106.
145. Ruttmann TG, James MF, Aronson I. In vivo investigation into the effects of haemodilution with hydroxyethyl starch (200/0.5) and normal saline on coagulation. *Br J Anaesth*. 1998;80:612–616.
146. Lobo DN, Bostock KA, Neal KR, et al. Effect of salt and water balance on recovery of gastrointestinal function after elective colonic resection: a randomised controlled trial. *Lancet*. 2002;359:1812–1818.
147. Brandstrup B, Tønnesen H, Beier-Holgersen R. Effects of intravenous fluid restriction on postoperative complications: comparison of two perioperative fluid regimens: a randomized assessor-blinded multicenter trial. *Ann Surg*. 2003;238:641–648.
148. van den Berghe G, Wouters P, Weekers F, et al. Intensive insulin therapy in the critically ill patients. *N Engl J Med*. 2001;345:1359–1367.
149. Gandhi GY, Nuttall GA, Abel MD, et al. Intensive intraoperative insulin therapy versus conventional glucose management during cardiac surgery: a randomized trial. *Ann Intern Med*. 2007;146:233–243.
150. Finfer S, Chittock DR, Su SY, et al. Intensive versus conventional glucose control in critically ill patients. *N Engl J Med*. 2009;360:1283–1297.
151. Griesdale DE, de Souza RJ, van Dam RM, et al. Intensive insulin therapy and mortality among critically ill patients: a meta-analysis including NICE-SUGAR study data. *CMAJ*. 2009;180:821–827.
152. Jensen JA, Goodson WH III, Omachi RS, et al. Subcutaneous tissue oxygen tension falls during hemodialysis. *Surgery*. 1987;101:416–421.
153. Stühmeier K, Mainzer B, Cierpka J, et al. Small, oral dose of clonidine reduces the incidence of intraoperative myocardial ischemia in patients having vascular surgery. *Anesthesiology*. 1996;85:706–712.
154. Wallace AW, Galindez D, Salahieh A, et al. Effect of clonidine on cardiovascular morbidity and mortality after noncardiac surgery. *Anesthesiology*. 2004;101:284–293.
155. Hopf H, West J, Hunt T. Clonidine increases tissue oxygen in patients with local tissue hypoxia in non-healing wounds. *Wound Repair Regen*. 1996;4:A129.
156. Stone JG, Cozine KA, Wald A. Nocturnal oxygenation during patient-controlled analgesia. *Anesth Analg*. 1999;89:104–110.
157. Turtiainen J, Saimanen E, Partio T, et al. Supplemental postoperative oxygen in the prevention of surgical wound infection after lower limb vascular surgery: a randomized controlled trial. *World J Surg*. 2011;35:1387–1395.
158. Wisner D. A stepwise logistic regression analysis of factors affecting morbidity and mortality after thoracic trauma: effect of epidural analgesia. *J Trauma*. 1990;30:799–804.
159. Owen H, McMillan V, Rogowski D. Postoperative pain therapy: a survey of patients' expectations and their experiences. *Pain*. 1990;41:303–307.
160. Donovan M, Dillon P, McGuire L. Incidence and characteristics of pain in a sample of medical-surgical inpatients. *Pain*. 1987;30:69–78.

9 The Allergic Response

JERROLD H. LEVY

Introduction
Basic Immunologic Principles
  Antigens
  Thymus-derived (T-cell) and Bursa-derived (B-cell)
    Lymphocytes
  Antibodies
  Effector Cells and Proteins of the Immune Response
  Effects of Anesthesia on Immune Function
Hypersensitivity Responses (Allergy)
  Type I Reactions
  Type II Reactions
  Type III Reactions (Immune Complex Reactions)

Type IV Reactions (Delayed Hypersensitivity Reactions)
Intraoperative Allergic Reactions
Anaphylactic Reactions
  IgE-mediated Pathophysiology
  Non–IgE-mediated Reactions
  Treatment Plan
Perioperative Management of the Patient with Allergies
  Immunologic Mechanisms of Drug Allergy
  Evaluation of Patients with Allergic Reactions
  Agents Implicated in Allergic Reactions
Summary

KEY POINTS

1. Anesthesiologists routinely administer multiple agents in the perioperative period including drugs (antibiotics, anesthetic agents, neuromuscular blocking agents [NMBAs]), polypeptides (i.e., protamine), and blood products, or patients are exposed to environmental antigens (i.e., latex) all of which can produce an allergic reaction.
2. Cytokines are inflammatory cell activators that are synthesized to act as secondary messengers and activate endothelial cells and white cells.
3. Antibodies are specific proteins called immunoglobulins that can recognize and bind to a specific antigens, and usually IgE or IgG is implicated.
4. Immune competence during surgery can be affected by direct and hormonal effects of anesthetic drugs, by immunologic effects of other drugs used, by the surgery, by coincident infection, and by transfused blood products.
5. Most of the allergic reactions evoked by intravenous drugs occur within 5 minutes of administration. In the anesthetized patient, the most common life-threatening manifestation of an allergic reaction is circulatory collapse, reflecting vasodilation with resulting decreased venous return.
6. Many diverse molecules administered during the perioperative period release histamine in a dose-dependent, nonimmunologic fashion.
7. A plan for treating anaphylactic reactions must be established before the event. Airway maintenance, 100% oxygen administration, intravascular volume expansion, and epinephrine are essential to treat the hypotension and hypoxia that result from vasodilation, increased capillary permeability, and bronchospasm. Vasopressin and additional diagnostic monitoring should be considered for refractory shock.
8. After an anaphylactic reaction, it is important to attempt to identify the causative agent to prevent readministration.
9. Health-care workers and children with spina bifida, urogenital abnormalities, or certain food allergies have been recognized as people at increased risk for anaphylaxis to latex.
10. NMBAs have several unique molecular features that make them potential antigens.

Introduction

Allergic reactions represent an important cause of perioperative complications. Anesthesiologists routinely administer multiple drugs and blood products and manage patients during their perioperative medical care where they are exposed to multiple agents including drugs (i.e., antibiotics, anesthetic agents, neuromuscular blocking agents [NMBAs]), polypeptides (protamine), blood products, and environmental antigens (i.e., latex). Anesthesiologists must be able to rapidly recognize and treat anaphylaxis, the most life-threatening form of an allergic reaction.[1]

The allergic response represents just one aspect of the pathologic response that the immune system evolved to recognize foreign substances. As part of normal host surveillance mechanisms, a series of cellular and humoral elements oversees foreign surfaces of cell surfaces and molecular structures called *antigens* to provide host defense. These foreign substances (antigens) consist of molecular arrangements found on cells, bacteria, viruses, proteins, or complex macromolecules.[2,3] Immunologic mechanisms (1) involve antigen interaction with antibodies or specific effector cells; (2) are reproducible; and (3) are specific and adaptive, distinguishing foreign substances and amplifying reactivity through a series of inflammatory cells and proteins. The immune system serves to protect the body against external microorganisms and toxins, as well as internal threats from neoplastic cells; however, it can respond inappropriately to cause hypersensitive (allergic) reactions. Life-threatening allergic reactions to drugs and other foreign substances observed perioperatively may represent different expressions of the immune response.[2,3]

Basic Immunologic Principles

The immune system protects the body from invasion by organisms by recognizing and removing foreign substances called *antigens* that are molecular structures, usually proteins and/or carbohydrates. The body also has mechanisms to tolerate similar molecular configurations of the host (self-tolerance); however, problems arise when the immune system is dysfunctional as in cases of autoimmunity that can give rise to serious diseases including rheumatoid arthritis and lupus. The immune response includes both cell-mediated immunity and humoral immunity. Cell-mediated immunity involves immune cells directed at elimination or destruction of pathogens or cells. Humoral immunity comprises different antibodies and proteins, such as complement, that can directly or in concert with cellular immunity orchestrate cell injury and destruction. The purpose is to provide host defense mechanisms.

As part of humoral immune responses, protein mediators called cytokines and chemokines are released initially by inflammatory responses to bring other immune cells to the site of the injury or infection, cause further inflammatory responses and fever, and increase capillary permeability to allow other immune cells to migrate and translocate to the site of injury. This inflammatory response also causes hemostatic activation and produces pain, erythema, and edema locally and potentially systemically depending on the extent of the injury. Cytokines have an extensive spectrum of inflammatory effects, an issue studied extensively in sepsis.[4] The immune response can be variable in onset from immediate in anaphylaxis to days, and can remember antigens for many years, especially following immunization.

Although this is a simplified review of the immune system, it is important to consider individual aspects of the immune response and their importance.

Antigens

As mentioned, molecules stimulating an immune response (antibody production or lymphocyte stimulation) are called *antigens*.[5,6] Only a few drugs used by anesthesiologists, such as polypeptides (protamine) and other large macromolecules (dextrans), are complete antigens (Table 9-1). Most commonly used drugs are simple organic compounds of low molecular weight (around 1,000 Da). For most drugs that are small molecules, to become immunogenic they must bind two circulating proteins or tissues to result in an antigen (hapten–macromolecular complex). Small molecular weight substances such as drugs or drug metabolites that bind to host proteins or cell membranes to sensitize patients are called *haptens*. Haptens are not antigenic by themselves. Often, a reactive drug metabolite (i.e., penicilloyl derivative of penicillin) is believed to bind with macromolecules to become antigens. Certain molecular structures in bacteria or fungi are immediately recognized as foreign by multiple aspects of the immune system.

Thymus-derived (T-cell) and Bursa-derived (B-cell) Lymphocytes

The thymus of the fetus differentiates immature lymphocytes into thymus-derived cells (T cells). T cells have receptors that are activated by binding with foreign antigens and secrete mediators that regulate the immune response. The subpopulations of T cells that exist in humans include helper, suppressor, cytotoxic, and killer cells.[5,6] The two types of regulatory T cells are helper cells (OKT4) and suppressor cells (OKT8). Helper cells are important for key effector cell responses, whereas suppressor cells inhibit immune function. Infection of helper T cells with a retrovirus, the human immunodeficiency virus, produces a specific increase in the number of suppressor cells. Cytotoxic T cells destroy mycobacteria, fungi, and viruses. Other lymphocytes, called natural killer cells, do not need specific antigen stimulation to set up their role. Both the cytotoxic T cells and natural killer cells take part in defense against tumor cells and in transplant rejection. T cells produce mediators that influence the response of other cell types involved in the recognition and destruction of foreign substances.[5,6]

B cells represent a specific lymphocyte cell line that can differentiate into specific plasma cells that synthesize antibodies, a step controlled by both helper and suppressor T-cell lymphocytes. B cells are also called bursa-derived cells because in birds, the bursa of Fabricius is important in producing cells responsible for antibody synthesis.

Antibodies

Antibodies are specific proteins called *immunoglobulins* (Igs) that can recognize and bind to a specific antigen. The basic structure of the antibody molecule is illustrated in Figure 9-1. Each antibody

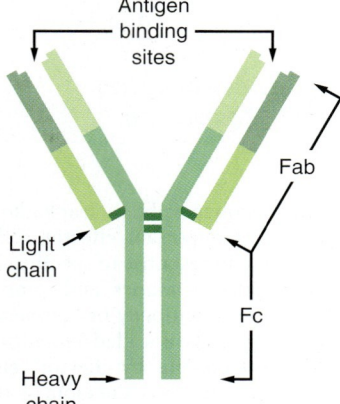

Figure 9-1 Basic structural configuration of the antibody molecule representing human immunoglobulin G (IgG). Immunoglobulins are composed of two heavy chains and two light chains bound by disulfide linkages (represented by *crossbars*). Papain cleaves the molecule into two Fab fragments and one Fc fragment. Antigen binding occurs on the Fab fragments, whereas the Fc segment is responsible for membrane binding or complement activation. (Reprinted with permission from: Levy JH. *Anaphylactic Reactions in Anesthesia and Intensive Care.* 2nd ed. Boston, MA: Butterworth-Heinemann; 1992.)

Table 9-1 Agents Administered during Anesthesia That Act as Antigens

Haptens	Macromolecules
Penicillin and its derivatives	Aprotinin
Anesthetic drugs	Blood products
	Chymopapain
	Colloid volume expanders
	Neuromuscular blocking agents
	Protamine
	Latex

Table 9-2 Biologic Characteristics of Immunoglobulins

	IgG	IgM	IgA	IgE	IgD
Heavy chain	γ	μ	α	ε	δ
Molecular weight	160,000	900,000	170,000	188,000	184,000
Subclasses	1, 2, 3, 4	1, 2	1, 2		
Serum concentration (mg/dL)	6–14	0.5–1.5	1–3	$<0.5 \times 10^3$	<0.1
Complement activation	All but IgG$_4$	+	–	–	–
Placental transfer	+	–	–	–	–
Serum half-life (days)	23	5	6	1–5	2–8
Cell binding	Mast cells (IgG$_4$) Neutrophils Lymphocytes Mononuclear cells Platelets	Lymphocytes		Mast cells Basophils	Neutrophils Lymphocytes

Modified with permission from: Levy JH. *Anaphylactic Reactions in Anesthesia and Intensive Care.* 2nd ed. Boston, MA: Butterworth-Heinemann; 1992.

has at least two heavy chains and two light chains that are bound together by disulfide bonds. The Fab fragment has the ability to bind antigen, and the Fc, or crystallizable, fragment is responsible for the unique biologic properties of the different classes of Igs (cell binding and complement activation). Antibodies function as specific receptor molecules for immune cells and proteins. When antigen binds covalently to the Fab fragments, the antibody undergoes conformational changes to activate the Fc receptor. The results of antigen–antibody binding depend on the cell type, which causes a specific type of activation (i.e., lymphocyte proliferation and differentiation into antibody-secreting cells, mast cell degranulation, and complement activation). Multiple therapeutic agents are based on Fab fragments that bind irreversibly to a specific molecular configuration or drug and include such agents as abciximab (a platelet inhibitor that binds the IIb/IIIa receptor) and idarucizumab (that binds to dabigatran to reverse its anticoagulant effect).

Five major classes of antibodies occur in humans: IgG, IgA, IgM, IgD, and IgE. The heavy chain determines the structure and function of each molecule. The basic properties of each antibody are listed in Table 9-2.

Effector Cells and Proteins of the Immune Response

Cells

Monocytes, neutrophils (polymorphonuclear leukocytes [PMNs]), and eosinophils represent important effector cells that migrate into areas of inflammation in response to specific chemotactic factors, including lymphokines, cytokines, and complement-derived mediators. The deposition of antibody or complement fragments on the surface of foreign cells is called *opsonization*, a process that promotes killing foreign cells by effector cells. In addition, lymphokines and cytokines produce chemotaxis of other inflammatory cells in a manner described in the following sections.[5,6] Activation of this cellular process is orchestrated by multiple mechanisms, as best recently reviewed.[7]

Monocytes and Macrophages

Macrophages regulate immune responses by processing and presenting antigens to effect inflammatory, tumoricidal, and microbicidal functions. Macrophages arise from circulating monocytes or may be confined to specific organs such as the lung. They are recruited and activated in response to microorganisms or tissue injury. Macrophages ingest antigens before they interact with receptors on the lymphocyte surface to regulate their action. Macrophages synthesize mediators to facilitate both B-lymphocyte and T-lymphocyte responses.

Polymorphonuclear Leukocytes (Neutrophils)

The first cells to appear in acute inflammatory reaction are neutrophils that contain acid hydrolases, neutral proteases, and lysosomes. Once activated, they produce hydroxyl radicals, superoxide, and hydrogen peroxide, which aid in microbial killing.

Eosinophils

The exact function of the eosinophil in host defense is unclear; however, inflammatory cells recruit eosinophils to collect at sites of parasitic infections, tumors, and allergic reactions.

Basophils

Basophils comprise 0.5% to 1% of circulating granulocytes in the blood. On the surface of basophils are IgE receptors, which function similarly to those on mast cells.

Mast Cells

Mast cells are important cells for immediate hypersensitivity responses. They are tissue fixed and located in the perivascular spaces of the skin, lung, and intestine. On the surface of mast cells are IgE receptors, which bind to specific antigens. Once activated, these cells release physiologically active mediators important to immediate hypersensitivity responses (see IgE-mediated Pathophysiology section under Anaphylactic Reactions). Mast cells can be activated by a series of both immune and nonimmune stimuli.

Proteins

Cytokines/Interleukins

Cytokines are inflammatory cell activators that are synthesized by macrophages to act as secondary messengers and activate endothelial cells and white cells.[8] Interleukin-1 and tumor necrosis factor are examples of cytokines considered to be important mediators of the biologic responses to infection and other inflammatory reactions. Liberation of interleukin-1 and tumor necrosis factor produces fever, neuropeptide release, endothelial cell activation, increased adhesion molecule expression, neutrophil priming, hypotension, myocardial suppression, and a catabolic state.[8] The term *interleukin* was coined for a group of cytokines that promotes communication between and among ("inter") leukocytes ("leukin"). Interleukins are a group of different regulatory proteins that act to control many aspects of the immune and inflammatory responses. The interleukins are polypeptides synthesized in response to cellular activation; they produce their inflammatory effects by activating specific receptors on inflammatory cells and vasculature. T-cell lymphocytes influence the activity of other immunologic and nonimmunologic cells by producing an array of interleukins that they secrete. Different interleukins of this class have been isolated and characterized; they function as short-range or intracellular soluble mediators of the immune and inflammatory responses. The interleukin family of cytokines has been rapidly growing in number because of advances in gene cloning.

Complement

The primary humoral response to antigen and antibody binding is activation of the complement system.[9,10] The complement system consists of around 20 different proteins that bind to activated antibodies, other complement proteins, and cell membranes. The complement system is an important effector system of inflammation. Complement activation can be initiated by IgG or IgM binding to antigen, by plasmin through the classic pathway, by endotoxin, or by drugs through the alternate (properdin) pathway (Fig. 9-2). Specific fragments released during complement activation include C3a, C4a, and C5a, which have important humoral and chemotactic properties (see Non–IgE-mediated Reactions section). The major function of the complement system is to recognize bacteria both directly and indirectly by attracting phagocytes (chemotaxis), as well as the increased adhesion of phagocytes to antigens (opsonization), and cell lysis by activation of the complete cascade.[9,10]

A series of inhibitors regulates activation to ensure regulation of the complement system. Hereditary (autosomal dominant) or acquired (associated with lymphoma, lymphosarcoma, chronic lymphatic leukemia, and macroglobulinemia) angioedema is an example of a deficiency in an inhibitor of the C1 complement system (C1 esterase deficiency). This syndrome is characterized by recurrent increased vascular permeability of specific subcutaneous and serosal tissues (angioedema), which produces laryngeal obstruction and respiratory and cardiovascular abnormalities after tissue trauma and surgery, or even without any obvious precipitating factor.[11] One of the important pathologic manifestations of complement activation is acute pulmonary vasoconstriction associated with protamine administration.[1]

Effects of Anesthesia on Immune Function

Anesthesia and surgery depress nonspecific host resistance mechanisms, including lymphocyte activation and phagocytosis.[12] Immune competence during surgery can be affected by direct and hormonal effects of anesthetic drugs, by immunologic effects of other drugs used, by the surgery, by coincident infections, and by transfused blood products. Blood represents a complex of humoral and cellular elements that may alter immunomodulation to various antigens. Although multiple studies demonstrate in vitro changes of immune function, no studies have ever proved their importance.[12] Besides, such changes are likely of minor importance compared with the hormonal aspects of stress responses.

Hypersensitivity Responses (Allergy)

Gell and Coombs first described a scheme for classifying immune responses to understand specific diseases mediated by immunologic processes. The immune pathway functions as a protective mechanism, but can also react inappropriately to produce a hypersensitivity or allergic response. They defined four basic types of hypersensitivity, types I to IV. It is useful first to review all four mechanisms to understand the different immune reactions that occur in humans.

Type I Reactions

Type I reactions are anaphylactic or immediate-type hypersensitivity reactions (Fig. 9-3). Physiologically active mediators are released from mast cells and basophils after antigen binding to IgE antibodies on the membranes of these cells. Type I hypersensitivity reactions include anaphylaxis, extrinsic asthma, and allergic rhinitis.

Type II Reactions

Type II reactions are also known as antibody-dependent cell-mediated cytotoxic hypersensitivity or cytotoxic reactions

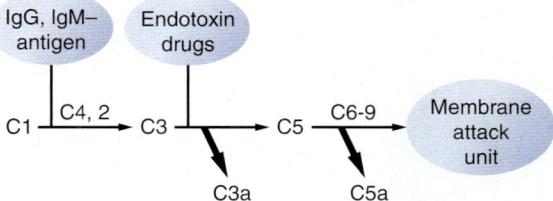

Figure 9-2 Diagram of complement activation. Complement system can be activated by either the classic pathway (IgG, IgM–antigen interaction) or the alternate pathway (endotoxin, drug interaction). Small peptide fragments of C3 and C5 called anaphylatoxins (C3a, C5a) that are released during activation are potent vasoactive mediators. Formation of the complete complement cascade produces a membrane attack unit that lyses cell walls and membranes. An inhibitor of the complement cascade, the C1 esterase inhibitor, ensures the complement system is turned off most of the time.

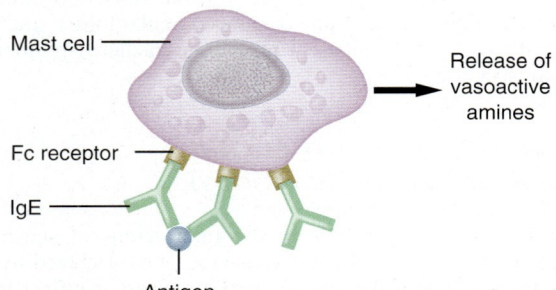

Figure 9-3 Type I immediate hypersensitivity reactions (anaphylaxis) involve IgE antibodies binding to mast cells or basophils by way of their Fc receptors. On encountering immunospecific antigens, the IgE becomes cross-linked, inducing degranulation, intracellular activation, and release of mediators. This reaction is independent of complement.

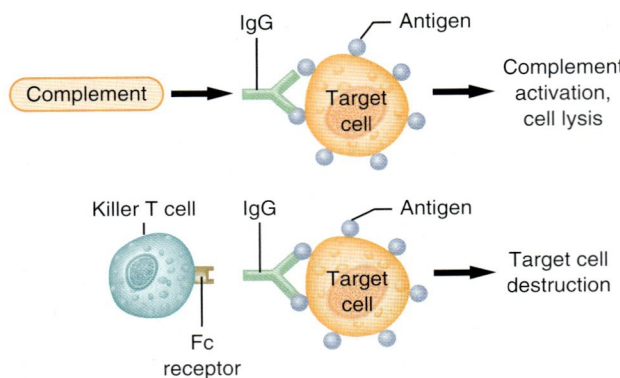

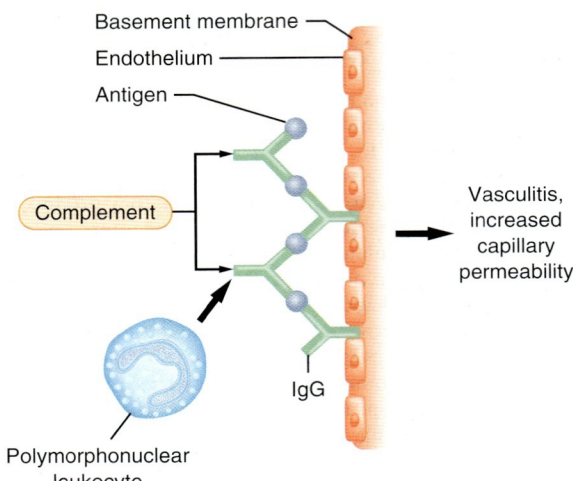

Figure 9-4 Type II or cytotoxic reactions. Antibody of an IgG or IgM class is directed against antigens on an individual's own cells (target cells). The antigens may be integral membrane components or foreign molecules that have been absorbed. This may lead to complement activation, including cell lysis (*upper figure*) or cytotoxic action by killer T-cell lymphocytes (*lower figure*).

Figure 9-5 Type III immune complex reactions. Antibodies of an IgG or IgM type bind to the antigen in the soluble base and are subsequently deposited in the microvasculature. Complement is activated, resulting in chemotaxis and activation of polymorphonuclear leukocytes at the site of antigen–antibody complexes and subsequent tissue injury.

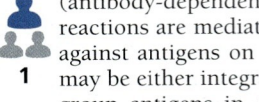

(antibody-dependent cell-mediated cytotoxic) (Fig. 9-4). These reactions are mediated by either IgG or IgM antibodies directed against antigens on the surface of foreign cells. These antigens may be either integral cell membrane components (A or B blood group antigens in ABO incompatibility reactions) or haptens that absorb to the surface of a cell, stimulating the production of antihapten antibodies (autoimmune hemolytic anemia). The cell damage in type II reactions is produced by (1) direct cell lysis after complete complement cascade activation, (2) increased phagocytosis by macrophages, or (3) killer T-cell lymphocytes producing antibody-dependent cell-mediated cytotoxic effects. Examples of type II reactions in humans are ABO-incompatible transfusion reactions, drug-induced immune hemolytic anemia, and heparin-induced thrombocytopenia.

Type III Reactions (Immune Complex Reactions)

Type III reactions result from circulating soluble antigens and antibodies that bind to form insoluble complexes that deposit in the microvasculature (Fig. 9-5). Complement is activated, and neutrophils are localized to the site of complement deposition to produce tissue damage. Type III reactions include classic serum sickness observed after snake antisera or antithymocyte globulin, and immune complex vascular injury, and may occur through mechanisms of protamine-mediated pulmonary vasoconstriction.[1]

Type IV Reactions (Delayed Hypersensitivity Reactions)

Type IV reactions result from the interactions of sensitized lymphocytes with specific antigens (Fig. 9-6). Delayed hypersensitivity reactions are mainly mononuclear, manifest in 18 to 24 hours, peak at 40 to 80 hours, and disappear in 72 to 96 hours. Antigen–lymphocyte binding produces lymphokine synthesis, lymphocyte proliferation, and generation of cytotoxic T cells, attracting macrophages and other inflammatory cells. Cytotoxic T cells are produced specifically to kill target cells that bear antigens identical with those that triggered the reaction. This form of immunity is important in tissue rejection, graft-versus-host reactions, contact dermatitis (e.g., poison ivy), and tuberculin immunity.

Intraoperative Allergic Reactions

Understanding perioperative anaphylaxis is important because of the potential for morbidity and mortality.[13] However, most estimates of the incidence are based on retrospective data, which may account for variability in the incidence. The risk of perioperative anaphylaxis is reported as between 1:3,500 and 1:20,000, with a mortality rate of 4% and an additional 2% surviving with severe brain damage.[13,14] More than 90% of the allergic reactions evoked by intravenous drugs occur within 5 minutes of administration. In the anesthetized patient, the most common life-threatening manifestation of an allergic reaction is circulatory collapse, reflecting vasodilation with resulting decreased venous return (Table 9-3). The only manifestation of an allergic reaction may be refractory hypotension. Portier and Richet first used the word *anaphylaxis* (from *ana*, "against," and *prophylaxis*, "protection") to describe the profound shock and resulting death that sometimes occurred in dogs immediately after a

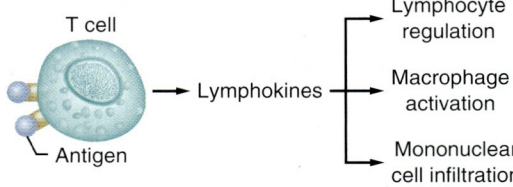

Figure 9-6 Type IV immune complex reactions (delayed hypersensitivity or cell-mediated immunity). Antigen binds to sensitized T-cell lymphocytes to release lymphokines after a second contact with the same antigen. This reaction is independent of circulating antibody or complement activation. Lymphokines induce inflammatory reactions and activate, as well as attract, macrophages and other mononuclear cells to produce delayed tissue injury.

Table 9-3 Recognition of Anaphylaxis during Regional and General Anesthesia		
Systems	**Symptoms**	**Signs**
Respiratory	Dyspnea Chest discomfort	Coughing Wheezing Sneezing Laryngeal edema Decreased pulmonary compliance Fulminant pulmonary edema Acute respiratory failure
Cardiovascular	Dizziness Malaise Retrosternal oppression	Disorientation Diaphoresis Loss of consciousness Hypotension Tachycardia Dysrhythmias Decreased systemic vascular resistance Cardiac arrest Pulmonary hypertension
Cutaneous	Itching Burning Tingling	Urticaria (hives) Flushing Periorbital edema Perioral edema

Reprinted with permission from: Levy JH. *Anaphylactic Reactions in Anesthesia and Intensive Care*. 2nd ed. Boston, MA: Butterworth-Heinemann; 1992.

Anaphylactic Reactions

IgE-mediated Pathophysiology

Antigen binding to IgE antibodies initiates anaphylaxis (Fig. 9-7). Prior exposure to the antigen or to a substance of similar structure is needed to produce sensitization, although an allergic history may be unknown to the patient. On reexposure, binding of the antigen to bridge two immunospecific IgE antibodies found on the surfaces of mast cells and basophils releases stored mediators, including histamine, tryptase, and chemotactic factors.[13,16,17] Arachidonic acid metabolites (leukotrienes and prostaglandins), kinins, and cytokines are subsequently synthesized and released in response to cellular activation.[18] The released mediators produce a symptom complex of bronchospasm and upper airway edema in the respiratory system, vasodilation and increased capillary permeability in the cardiovascular system, and urticaria in the cutaneous system. Different mediators are released from mast cells and basophils after activation.

Chemical Mediators of Anaphylaxis

Histamine stimulates H_1, H_2, and H_3 receptors. H_1 receptor activation releases endothelium-derived relaxing factor (nitric oxide) from vascular endothelium, increases capillary permeability, and contracts airway and vascular smooth muscle.[16,19] H_2 receptor activation causes gastric secretion, inhibits mast cell activation, and contributes to vasodilation. When injected into skin, histamine produces the classic wheal (increased capillary permeability producing tissue edema) and flare (cutaneous vasodilation) response in humans.[20,21] Histamine undergoes rapid metabolism in humans by the enzymes histamine N-methyltransferase and diamine oxidase found in endothelial cells.

Peptide Mediators of Anaphylaxis

Factors are released from mast cells and basophils that cause granulocyte migration (chemotaxis) and collection at the site of the inflammatory stimulus.[17,18] Eosinophilic chemotactic factor

second challenge with a foreign antigen.[15] When life-threatening allergic reactions mediated by antibodies occur, they are defined as anaphylactic. Although the term *anaphylactoid* has been used in the past to describe nonimmunologic reactions, this term is now rarely used.

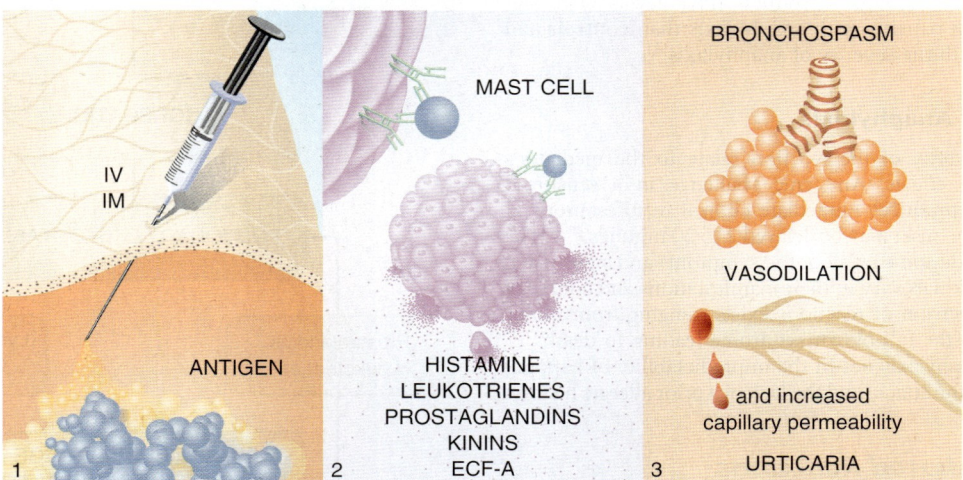

Figure 9-7 During anaphylaxis (type I immediate hypersensitivity reaction), (1) antigen enters a patient during anesthesia through a parenteral route. (2) It bridges two IgE antibodies on the surface of mast cells or basophils. In a calcium-dependent and energy-dependent process, cells release various substances—histamine, eosinophilic chemotactic factor of anaphylaxis, leukotrienes, prostaglandins, and kinins. (3) These released mediators produce the characteristic effects in the pulmonary, cardiovascular, and cutaneous systems. The most severe and life-threatening effects of the vasoactive mediators occur in the respiratory and cardiovascular systems. (Reprinted with permission from: Levy JH. *Identification and Treatment of Anaphylaxis: Mechanisms of Action and Strategies for Treatment Under General Anesthesia*. Chicago, IL: Smith Laboratories; 1983.)

of anaphylaxis (ECF-A) is a small molecular weight peptide chemotactic for eosinophils.[22] Although the exact role of ECF-A or the eosinophil in acute allergic response is unclear, eosinophils release enzymes that can inactivate histamine and leukotrienes.[18] In addition, a neutrophilic chemotactic factor is released that causes chemotaxis and activation.[18,23] Neutrophil activation may be responsible for recurrent manifestations of anaphylaxis.

Arachidonic Acid Metabolites

Leukotrienes and prostaglandins are both synthesized after mast cell activation from arachidonic acid metabolism of phospholipid cell membranes through either lipoxygenase or cyclooxygenase pathways.[22] The classic slow-reacting substance of anaphylaxis is a combination of leukotrienes C_4, D_4, and E_4. Leukotrienes produce bronchoconstriction (more intense than that produced by histamine), increased capillary permeability, vasodilation, coronary vasoconstriction, and myocardial depression.[24] Prostaglandins are potent mast cell mediators that produce vasodilation, bronchospasm, pulmonary hypertension, and increased capillary permeability. Prostaglandin D_2, the major metabolite of mast cells, produces bronchospasm and vasodilation. Elevated plasma levels of thromboxane B_2 (the metabolite of thromboxane A_2), also a prostaglandin synthesized by mast cells as well as by PMNs, have been demonstrated after protamine reactions associated with pulmonary hypertension.

Kinins

Small peptides called *kinins* are synthesized in mast cells and basophils to produce vasodilation, increased capillary permeability, and bronchoconstriction. Kinins can stimulate vascular endothelium to release vasoactive factors, including prostacyclin, and endothelial-derived relaxing factors such as nitric oxide.

Platelet-Activating Factor

Platelet-activating factor (PAF), an unstored lipid synthesized in activated human mast cells, is a potent biologic material. PAF aggregates and activates human platelets, and perhaps leukocytes, to release inflammatory products. PAF levels were significantly higher in patients with anaphylaxis than controls and were correlated with the severity of anaphylaxis.[23]

Recognition of Anaphylaxis

The onset and severity of the reaction relate to the mediator's specific end-organ effects. Antigenic challenge in a sensitized individual usually produces immediate clinical manifestations of anaphylaxis, but the onset may be delayed 2 to 20 minutes.[24–27] The reaction may include some or all of the symptoms and signs listed in Table 9-3. Individuals vary in their manifestations and course of anaphylaxis. A spectrum of reactions exists, ranging from minor clinical changes to the full-blown syndrome leading to death.[24,28] The enigma of anaphylaxis lies in the unpredictability of happening, the severity of the attack, and the lack of a prior allergic history.

Non–IgE-mediated Reactions

Other immunologic and nonimmunologic mechanisms release many of the mediators previously discussed independent of IgE, creating a clinical syndrome identical with anaphylaxis. Specific pathways important in producing the same clinical manifestations are considered later.

Table 9-4 Biologic Effects of Anaphylatoxins

Biologic Effects	C3a	C5a
Histamine release	+	+
Smooth muscle contraction	+	+
Increased vascular permeability	+	+
Chemotaxis		+
Leukocyte and platelet aggregation		+
Interleukin release	+	+

Complement Activation

Complement activation follows both immunologic (antibody mediated; i.e., classic pathway) or nonimmunologic (alternative) pathways to include a series of multimolecular, self-assembling proteins that release biologically active complement fragments of C3 and C5.[9,10] C3a and C5a are called *anaphylatoxins* because they release histamine from mast cells and basophils, contract smooth muscle, increase capillary permeability, and cause interleukin synthesis (Table 9-4). C5a interacts with specific high-affinity receptors on PMNs and platelets, causing leukocyte chemotaxis, aggregation, and activation.[9,10] Aggregated leukocytes embolize to various organs, producing microvascular occlusion and liberation of inflammatory products such as arachidonic acid metabolites, oxygen free radicals, and lysosomal enzymes (Fig. 9-8). Antibodies of the IgG class directed against antigenic determinants or granulocyte surfaces can also produce leukocyte aggregation.[29] These antibodies are called *leukoagglutinins*.

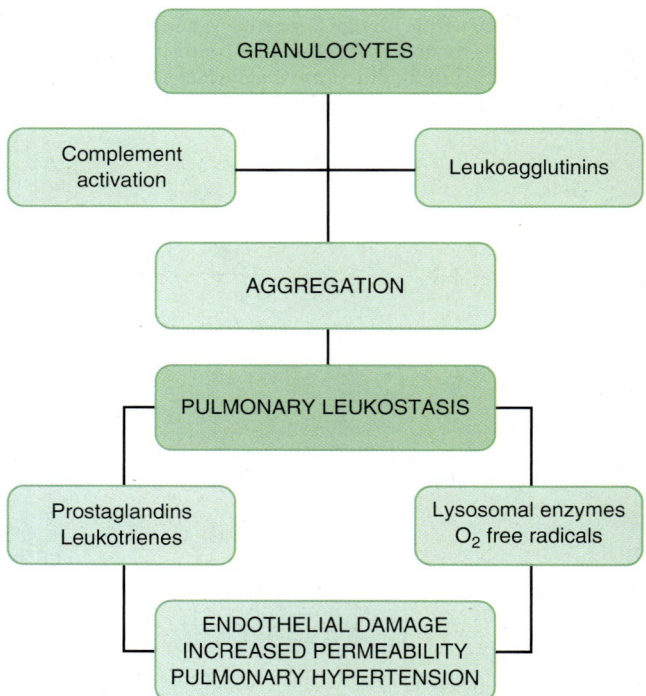

Figure 9-8 Sequence of events producing granulocyte aggregation, pulmonary leukostasis, and cardiopulmonary dysfunction. (Reprinted with permission from: Levy JH. *Anaphylactic Reactions in Anesthesia and Intensive Care.* 2nd ed. Boston, MA: Butterworth-Heinemann; 1992.)

Table 9-5 Drugs Capable of Nonimmunologic Histamine Release

Antibiotics (vancomycin, pentamidine)
Basic compounds
Hyperosmotic agents
Muscle relaxants (d-tubocurarine, metocurine, atracurium, mivacurium, doxacurium)
Opioids (morphine, meperidine, codeine)
Thiobarbiturates

Investigators have associated complement activation and PMN aggregation in producing the clinical expression of transfusion reactions, pulmonary vasoconstriction after protamine reactions, adult respiratory distress syndrome, and septic shock.[1]

Angioedema can also occur from allergic reactions but also from complement deficiency states.[11] Hereditary angioedema (HAE) is an example of the complement deficiency state that can present with life-threatening episodes of airway edema and gastrointestinal edema/diarrhea requiring emergency or urgent interventions. Several variants of HAE exist that occur due to unopposed activation of multiple kinins and mediators including kallikrein and bradykinin causing increased vascular permeability and edema.[11] Older treatment was anabolic steroids and antifibrinolytics. C1 esterase inhibitor (C1-INH) concentrates are licensed in the United States for use in HAE patients, one for prophylaxis (Cinryze, ViroPharma, administered every 3 or 4 days for routine prophylaxis against angioedema attacks in HAE patients) and the other for treating acute abdominal and facial HAE attacks (Berinert P, CSL Behring).[11] The first kinin pathway modulator, ecallantide (Kalbitor, Dyax), is also licensed in the United States for treating HAE attacks.[11]

Nonimmunologic Release of Histamine

Many diverse molecules administered during the perioperative period release histamine in a dose-dependent, nonimmunologic fashion (Table 9-5 and Fig. 9-9).[1] The mechanisms involved in nonimmunologic histamine release are not well understood, but represent selective mast cell and not basophil activation (Fig. 9-10).[30,31] Human cutaneous mast cells are the only cell population that releases histamine in response to both drugs and endogenous stimuli (neuropeptides). Nonimmunologic histamine release may involve mast cell activation through specific cell-signaling activation (Fig. 9-11). Different molecular structures release histamine in humans, which suggests that different mechanisms are involved. Histamine release is not dependent on the μ-receptor because fentanyl and sufentanil, the most potent μ-receptor agonists clinically available, do not release histamine in human skin.[32] Although the newer muscle relaxants may be more potent at the neuromuscular junction, drugs that are mast cell degranulators are equally capable of releasing histamine.[33] On an equimolar basis, atracurium is as potent as d-tubocurarine or metocurine in its ability to degranulate mast cells.[33] Newer aminosteroidal agents such as rocuronium and rapacuronium at clinically recommended doses have minimal effects on histamine release.[34,35]

Antihistamine pretreatment before administration of drugs that are known to release histamine in humans does not inhibit histamine release; rather, the antihistamines compete with histamine at the receptor and may attenuate decreases in systemic vascular resistance.[1] However, the effect of any drug on systemic vascular resistance may depend on other factors in addition to histamine release.

Treatment Plan

A plan for treating anaphylactic reactions must be established before the event. Airway maintenance, 100% oxygen administration, intravascular volume expansion, and epinephrine are essential to treat the hypotension and hypoxemia that result from vasodilation, increased capillary permeability, and bronchospasm.[1] Table 9-6 lists a protocol for managing anaphylaxis during general anesthesia, with representative doses for a 70-kg adult. Therapy must be titrated to cardiopulmonary stability with monitoring.[1] Severe reactions need aggressive therapy and may be protracted, with persistent hypotension, pulmonary hypertension, lower respiratory obstruction, or laryngeal obstruction that

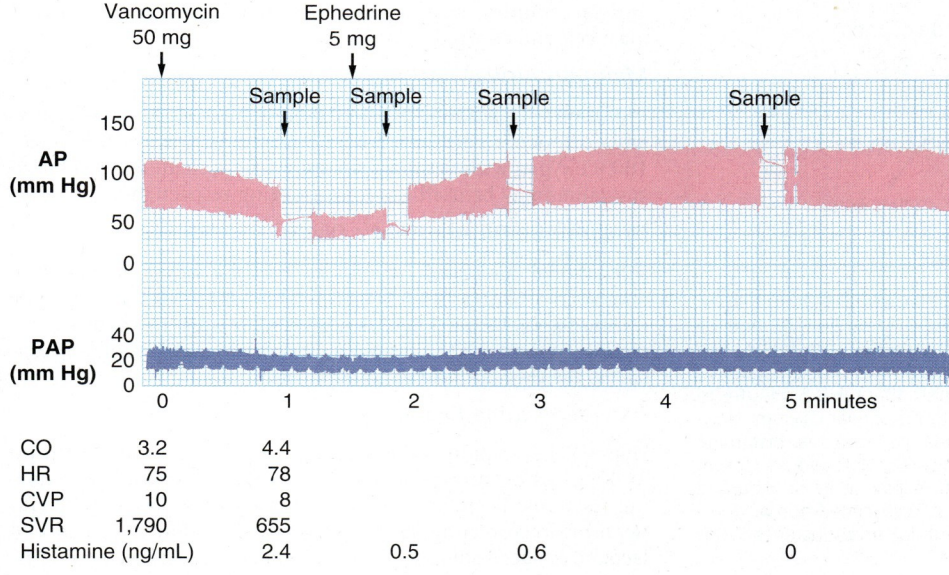

Figure 9-9 Example of an anaphylactic reaction after rapid vancomycin administration in a patient. Hypotension is associated with an increased cardiac output and decreased calculated systemic vascular resistance. Plasma histamine levels 1 minute after vancomycin administration were 2.4 ng/mL and subsequently decreased to zero. The patient was given ephedrine 5 mg, and blood pressure returned to baseline values. AP, arterial pressure; PAP, pulmonary artery pressure; CO, cardiac output; HR, heart rate; CVP, central venous pressure; SVR, systemic vascular resistance. (Reprinted with permission from: Levy JH, Kettlekamp N, Goertz P, et al. Histamine release by vancomycin: A mechanism for hypotension in man. Anesthesiology. 1987;67:122.)

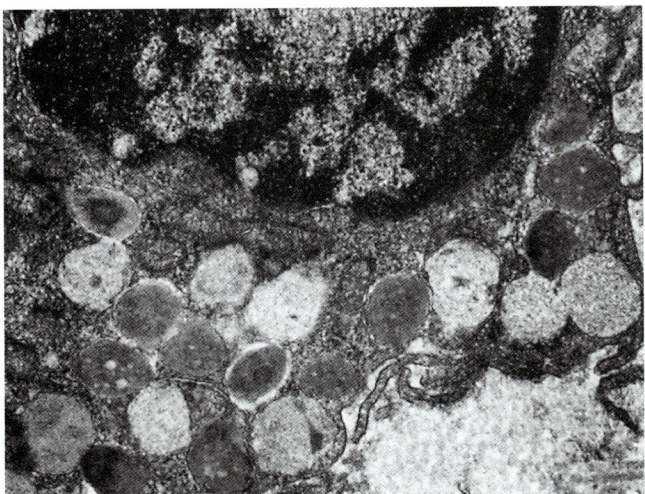

Figure 9-10 Electron micrograph of human cutaneous mast cell after injection of dynorphin, a κ-opioid agonist. The cell outline is rounded and most of the cytoplasmic granules are swollen, exhibiting varying degrees of decreased electron density and flocculence consistent with ongoing degranulation. The perigranular membranes of the adjacent granules at the periphery of the cell are fused to each other and to the plasma membrane. Original magnification ×72,000. (Reprinted with permission from: Casale TB, Bowman S, Kaliner M. Induction of human cutaneous mast cell degranulation by opiates and endogenous opioid peptides: Evidence for opiate and nonopiate receptor participation. *J Allergy Clin Immunol.* 1984;73:778.)

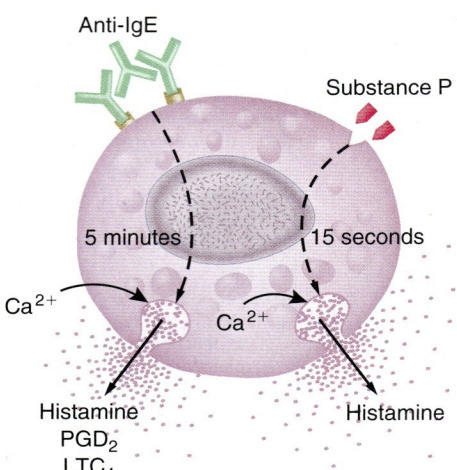

Figure 9-11 Different mechanisms of mediator release from human cutaneous mast cells stimulated immunologically by anti-IgE and by nonimmunologic stimuli with substance P. Anti-IgE stimulation, like antigen stimulation, initiates the release of histamine, prostaglandin D_2 (PGD_2), or leukotriene C_4 (LTC_4) by a mechanism that takes 5 minutes to reach completion and requires the influx of intracellular calcium. Nonimmunologic activation with drugs or substance P releases histamine but not PGD_2 or LTC_4 by a mechanism that is complete within 15 seconds and uses calcium mobilized from intracellular sources. (Adapted from: Caulfield JP, El-Lati S, Thomas G, et al. Dissociated human foreskin mast cells degranulate in response to anti-IgE and substance P. *Lab Invest.* 1990;63:502.)

Table 9-6 Management of Anaphylaxis during General Anesthesia

Initial Therapy

1. Stop administration of antigen
2. Maintain airway and administer 100% O_2
3. Discontinue all anesthetic agents
4. Start intravascular volume expansion (2–4 L of crystalloid/colloid with hypotension)
5. Give epinephrine (5–10 μg IV bolus with hypotension, titrate as needed; 0.1–1.0 mg IV with cardiovascular collapse)

Secondary Treatment

1. Antihistamines (0.5–1 mg/kg diphenhydramine)
2. Catecholamine infusions (starting doses: Epinephrine 4–8 μg/min; norepinephrine 4–8 μg/min; or isoproterenol 0.5–1 μg/min as an infusion; titrated to desired effects)
3. Bronchodilators: Inhaled albuterol, terbutaline, and/or anticholinergic agents with persistent bronchospasm)
4. Corticosteroids (0.25–1 g hydrocortisone; alternatively, 1–2 g methylprednisolone)[a]
5. Sodium bicarbonate (0.5–1 mEq/kg with persistent hypotension or acidosis)
6. Airway evaluation (before extubation)
7. Refractory shock: vasopressin and additional monitoring/echocardiography

[a]Methylprednisolone may be the drug of choice if the reaction is suspected to be mediated by complement.
IV, intravenous administration.
Reprinted with permission from: Levy JH. *Anaphylactic Reactions in Anesthesia and Intensive Care*. 2nd ed. Boston, MA: Butterworth-Heinemann; 1992:162.

---

may persist 5 to 32 hours despite vigorous therapy. All patients who have experienced an anaphylactic reaction should be admitted to an intensive care unit for 24 hours of monitoring because manifestations may recur after successful treatment.

Initial Therapy

Although it may not be possible to stop the administration of antigen, limiting antigen administration may prevent further mast cell and basophil activation.

Maintain Airway and Administer 100% Oxygen

Profound ventilation–perfusion abnormalities producing hypoxemia can occur with anaphylactic reactions. Always administer 100% oxygen with ventilatory support as needed. Arterial blood gas values may be useful to follow during resuscitation.

Discontinue All Anesthetic Drugs

Inhalational anesthetic drugs are not the bronchodilators of choice in treating bronchospasm after anaphylaxis, especially during hypotension. These drugs interfere with the body's compensatory response to cardiovascular collapse, and halothane sensitizes the myocardium to epinephrine.

Provide Volume Expansion

Hypovolemia rapidly follows during anaphylactic shock with up to 40% loss of intravascular fluid into the interstitial space during reactions. Therefore, volume expansion is important with epinephrine in correcting the acute hypotension. Initially, 2 to 4 L of lactated Ringer's solution, or colloid or normal saline, should be administered, keeping in mind that an additional 25 to 50 mL/kg may be necessary if hypotension persists. Refractory hypotension after volume and epinephrine administration requires additional hemodynamic monitoring. The use of transesophageal echocardiography for rapid assessment of intraventricular volume and ventricular function, and to determine other occult causes of acute cardiovascular dysfunction, can be important for accurate assessment of intravascular volume and guidance of rational therapeutic interventions.[1] Fulminant noncardiogenic pulmonary edema with loss of intravascular volume can occur after anaphylaxis. This condition requires intravascular volume repletion with careful hemodynamic monitoring until the capillary defect improves. Colloid volume expansion has not proved to be more effective than crystalloid volume expansion for treating anaphylactic shock.

Administer Epinephrine

Epinephrine is the drug of choice when resuscitating patients during anaphylactic shock. α-Adrenergic effects vasoconstrict to reverse hypotension; β_2-receptor stimulation bronchodilates and inhibits mediator release by increasing cyclic adenosine monophosphate (cAMP) in mast cells and basophils. The route of epinephrine administration and the dose depend on the patient's condition. Rapid and timely intervention is important when treating anaphylaxis. Furthermore, patients under general anesthesia may have altered sympathoadrenergic responses to acute anaphylactic shock, whereas the patient under spinal or epidural anesthesia may be partially sympathectomized and may need even larger doses of catecholamines.

In hypotensive patients, 5 to 10 μg boluses of epinephrine should be administered intravenously and incrementally titrated to restore blood pressure. (This dose of epinephrine can be obtained with 0.05 to 0.1 mL of a 1:10,000 dilution [100 μg/mL] or by mixing 2 mg epinephrine with 250 mL of fluid to yield an 8 μg/mL solution.) Additional volume and incrementally increased doses of epinephrine should be administered until hypotension is corrected. Although infusion is an ideal method of administering epinephrine, it is usually impossible to infuse the drug through peripheral intravenous access lines during acute volume resuscitation. With cardiovascular collapse, full intravenous cardiopulmonary resuscitative doses of epinephrine, 0.1 to 1.0 mg, should be administered and repeated until hemodynamic stability resumes. Patients with laryngeal edema without hypotension should receive subcutaneous epinephrine. Epinephrine should not be administered IV to patients with normal blood pressures.

Secondary Treatment

Antihistamines

Because H_1 receptors mediate many of the adverse effects of histamine, the intravenous administration of 0.5 to 1 mg/kg of an H_1 antagonist such as diphenhydramine may be useful in treating acute anaphylaxis. Antihistamines do not inhibit anaphylactic reactions or histamine release, but compete with histamine at receptor sites. H_1 antagonists are indicated in all forms of anaphylaxis. The H_1 antagonists available for parenteral administration may have antidopaminergic effects and should be given slowly to prevent precipitous hypotension in potentially hypovolemic patients.[1] The indications for administering an H_2 antagonist once anaphylaxis has occurred remain unclear.

Catecholamines

Epinephrine infusions may be useful in patients with persistent hypotension or bronchospasm after initial resuscitation.[1] Epinephrine infusions should be started at 0.05 to 0.1 μg/kg/min (5 to 10 μg/min) and titrated to correct hypotension. Norepinephrine infusions may be needed in patients with refractory hypotension due to decreased systemic vascular resistance. It may be started at 0.05 to 0.1 μg/kg/min (5 to 10 μg/min) and adjusted to correct hypotension.[1]

Bronchodilators

Inhaled β-adrenergic agents include inhaled albuterol or terbutaline if bronchospasm is a major feature.[36] Inhaled ipratropium may be especially useful for treatment of bronchospasm in patients receiving β-adrenergic blockers.[36] Special adaptors allow administration of bronchodilators through the endotracheal tube.

Corticosteroids

Corticosteroids have anti-inflammatory effects that are mediated by multiple mechanisms, including altering the activation and migration of other inflammatory cells (i.e., PMNs) after an acute reaction. Consider infusing high-dose corticosteroids early in the course of therapy although beneficial effects are delayed at least 4 to 6 hours.[36] Despite their unproven usefulness in treating acute reactions, they are often administered as adjuncts to therapy when refractory bronchospasm or refractory shock occurs after resuscitative therapy. Although the exact corticosteroid dose and preparation are unclear, investigators have recommended 0.25 to 1 g intravenously of hydrocortisone in IgE-mediated reactions. Alternatively, 1 to 2 g of methylprednisolone (30 to 35 mg/kg) intravenously may be useful in reactions believed to be complement mediated, such as catastrophic pulmonary vasoconstriction after protamine transfusion reactions. Administering corticosteroids after an anaphylactic reaction may also be important in attenuating the late-phase reactions reported to occur 12 to 24 hours after anaphylaxis.

Bicarbonate

Acidosis develops rapidly in patients with persistent hypotension. This acidosis reduces the effect of epinephrine on the heart and systemic vasculature. Therefore, with refractory hypotension or acidemia, sodium bicarbonate, 0.5 to 1 mEq/kg, may be given and repeated every 5 minutes or as dictated by arterial blood gas values.

Airway Evaluation

Because profound laryngeal edema can occur, the airway should be evaluated before extubation of the trachea. Persistent facial edema suggests airway edema. The tracheas of these patients should remain intubated until the edema subsides. Developing a significant air leak after endotracheal tube cuff deflation and before extubation of the trachea is useful in assessing airway patency. If there is any question of airway edema, direct laryngoscopy should be performed before the trachea is extubated.

Refractory Hypotension

Vasopressin is an important drug for refractory shock, including vasodilatory shock associated with anaphylaxis. Vasodilatory shock is characterized by hypotension association with a high cardiac output and is thought to be due to the multiple activation of vasodilator mechanisms and the inability of α-adrenergic mechanisms to compensate. Starting doses to consider are 0.01 units/min as an infusion, although bolus administration is part of Advanced Cardiopulmonary Life Support (ACLS) guidelines.[36] Vasopressin may attenuate pathologic-induced vasodilation. Further, additional monitoring, including echocardiography should be considered in patients with refractory hypotension to better evaluate cardiac function or hypovolemia.

Perioperative Management of the Patient with Allergies

Allergic drug reactions account for 6% to 10% of all adverse reactions, and the risk of an allergic drug reaction occurring is approximately 1% to 3% for most drugs, and around 5% of adults in the United States may be allergic to one or more drugs.[37–39] Unfortunately, patients often refer to adverse drug effects as being allergic in nature. For example, opioid administration can produce nausea, vomiting, or even local release of histamine along the vein of administration. Patients will say they are "allergic" to a specific drug when in fact their adverse reaction is independent of allergy. Nearly 15% of adults in the United States believe they are allergic to specific medication(s) and therefore may be denied treatment with an indicated drug. To understand allergic reactions, the spectrum of adverse reactions to drugs needs to be considered.

Predictable adverse drug reactions account for about 80% of adverse drug effects. They are often dose dependent, related to known pharmacologic actions of the drug, and typically occur in normal patients. Most serious, predictable adverse drug reactions are toxic and are directly related to the drug in the body (overdosage) or to an unintentional route of administration (e.g., lidocaine-induced seizures or cardiovascular collapse). Side effects are the most common adverse drug reactions and are undesirable pharmacologic actions of the drugs occurring at usual prescribed dosages. Most anesthetic drugs present multiple side effects that can produce precipitous hypotension. For example, morphine dilates the venous capacitance bed, thereby decreasing preload; releases histamine from cutaneous mast cells, thereby producing arterial and venous dilation; slows the heart rate; and decreases sympathetic tone. However, the net effects of morphine on blood pressure and myocardial function depend on the patient's blood volume, sympathetic tone, and ventricular function. Hypotension rapidly develops in a volume-depleted trauma patient in pain who is given morphine. Drug interactions also represent important predictable adverse drug reactions. Intravenous fentanyl administration to a patient who has just received intravenous benzodiazepines or other sedative-hypnotic drugs may produce precipitous hypotension that results from decreased sympathetic tone or direct vasodilation from propofol administration.[40] This represents a dose-dependent, predictable adverse drug reaction that is independent of allergy.

Unpredictable adverse drug reactions are usually dose independent and usually not related to the drug's pharmacologic actions, but are often related to the immunologic response (allergy) of the individual. On occasion, adverse reactions can be related to genetic differences (i.e., idiosyncratic) in a susceptible individual who has an isolated genetic enzyme deficiency. In most allergic drug reactions, an immunologic mechanism is present or, more often, presumed. Determining whether the causing event involves a reaction between the drug or drug metabolites with drug-specific antibodies or sensitized T lymphocytes is often impractical. Without direct immunologic evidence, which may be helpful in distinguishing an allergic reaction from other adverse reactions, including allergic reactions that occur in only a small percentage of patients receiving the drug, the clinical manifestations do not resemble known pharmacologic actions. In the absence of prior drug exposure, allergic symptoms rarely appear after less than 1 week of continuous treatment. After sensitization, the reaction develops rapidly on re-exposure to the drug. In general, drugs that have been administered without complications for several months or longer are rarely responsible for producing drug allergy. The time span between exposure to the drug and noticed manifestations is often the most vital information in deciding which drugs administered were the cause of a suspected allergic reaction.

Although the reaction may produce a life-threatening response in the cardiopulmonary system (anaphylaxis), various cutaneous manifestations, fever, and pulmonary reactions have been attributed to drug hypersensitivity. Usually, the reaction may be reproduced by small doses of the suspected drug or other agents having similar or cross-reacting chemical structures. On occasion, drug-specific antibodies or lymphocytes have been identified that react with the suspected drug, although the relationship is seldom diagnostically useful in practice. Even when an immune response to a drug is demonstrated, it may not be associated with a clinical allergic reaction. As with adverse drug reactions in general, the reaction usually subsides within several days of discontinuation of the drug.

Immunologic Mechanisms of Drug Allergy

Different immunologic responses to any antigen can occur. Drugs have been associated with all the immunologic mechanisms proposed by Gell and Coombs. Although more than one mechanism may contribute to a particular reaction, any one can occur. Penicillin may produce different reactions in different patients or a spectrum of reactions in the same patient. In one patient, penicillin can produce anaphylaxis (type I reaction), hemolytic anemia (type II reaction), serum sickness (type III reaction), and contact dermatitis (type IV reaction).[5,6] Therefore, any one antigen has the ability to produce a diffuse spectrum of allergic responses in humans. Why some patients have localized rashes or angioedema in response to penicillin whereas others suffer complete cardiopulmonary collapse is unknown. Most anesthetic drugs and agents administered perioperatively have been reported to produce anaphylactic reactions (Table 9-7).[31,39] Muscle relaxants are the most common drugs responsible for evoking intraoperative allergic reactions. In this regard, there is cross-sensitivity between succinylcholine and the nondepolarizing muscle relaxants. Unexplained intraoperative cardiovascular collapse has been attributed to anaphylaxis triggered by latex (natural rubber).

Life-threatening allergic reactions are potentially thought to occur more likely in patients with a history of allergy, atopy, or asthma, although this concept is also controversial and in part based on older data.[41] Nevertheless, because the incidence is low, the history is not a reliable predictor that an allergic reaction will occur and does not mandate that such patients should be investigated or pretreated or that specific drugs should be selected or avoided. Although different mechanisms have been proposed, no one theory has been proved. The drugs and foreign substances listed in Table 9-7 may have both immunologic and nonimmunologic mechanisms for adverse drug reactions in humans.

Evaluation of Patients with Allergic Reactions

Identifying the drug responsible for a suspected allergic reaction still depends on circumstantial evidence suggesting the temporal sequence of drug administration. Conventional in vivo and in vitro methods of diagnosing allergic reactions to most anesthetic drugs are unavailable or not applicable. The most important factor in diagnosis is the awareness of the physician that an untoward event may be related to a drug the patient received. The physician must always be aware of the capacity of any drug to produce an allergic reaction. The history is important when

Table 9-7 Agents Implicated in Allergic Reactions during Anesthesia

Anesthetic Agents
Induction agents (cremophor-solubilized drugs, barbiturates, etomidate, propofol)
Local anesthetics (para-aminobenzoic ester agents)
Muscle relaxants (succinylcholine, gallamine, pancuronium, d-tubocurarine, metocurine, atracurium, vecuronium, mivacurium, doxacurium)
Opioids (meperidine, morphine, fentanyl)

Other Agents
Antibiotics (cephalosporins, penicillin, sulfonamides, vancomycin)
Aprotinin
Blood products (whole blood, packed cells, plasma/fresh frozen plasma, platelets, cryoprecipitate, fibrin glue, immunoglobulins)
Bone cement
Chymopapain
Corticosteroids
Cyclosporine
Drug additives (preservatives)
Furosemide
Insulin
Mannitol
Methyl methacrylate
Nonsteroidal anti-inflammatory drugs
Protamine
Radiocontrast dye
Latex (natural rubber)
Streptokinase
Vascular graft material
Vitamin K
Colloid volume expanders (dextrans, protein fractions, albumin, hydroxyethyl starch)

Reprinted with permission from: Levy JH. *Anaphylactic Reactions in Anesthesia and Intensive Care.* 2nd ed. Boston, MA: Butterworth-Heinemann; 1992.

evaluating whether an adverse drug reaction is allergic and whether the drug can be readministered. Although a prior allergic reaction to the drug in question is important, this is rarely the case. Direct challenge of a patient with a test dose of drug is the only way to prove a reaction, but this is potentially dangerous and not recommended. Although the anesthesiologist commonly gives small test doses of anesthetic drugs, these are pharmacologic test doses and have nothing to do with immunologic dosages. The demonstration of drug-specific IgE antibodies is accepted as evidence that the patient may be at risk for anaphylaxis if the drug is administered. Different clinical tests are of historical interest, and few of them are actually available to confirm or diagnose drug allergy, but these are considered in the following section.

Testing for Allergy

After an anaphylactic reaction, it is important to identify the causative agent to prevent readministration. When one particular drug has been administered and there is a clear correlation between the time of administration and the occurrence of a reaction, testing may be unnecessary, and general avoidance of the drug should be instituted. However, when patients have simultaneously received multiple drugs (e.g., an opioid, muscle relaxant, hypnotic, and antibiotic), it is often difficult to prove which particular drug caused the reaction. Further, the reaction might have been caused by the vehicle or by one of the preservatives. For patients who want to know which drug was responsible and for patients scheduled for subsequent procedures, some degree of allergy evaluation should be undertaken to evaluate the drug at risk. Unfortunately, few *laboratory* tests exist for anesthetic drugs; therefore, the available allergy tests are discussed.

Leukocyte Histamine Release

Leukocyte histamine is performed by incubating the patient's leukocytes with the offending drug and measuring histamine release as a marker for basophil activation, although false-positive results can occur. This test is not easy to perform, although variations allow the use of whole blood instead of isolated PMNs, and is generally not available nor used.

In Vitro Immunologic Testing

The enzyme-linked immunosorbent assay (ELISA) measures antigen-specific antibodies. The ELISA evaluates immunospecific IgE directed against the antigen in question by adding an anti-IgE coupled to an enzyme such as peroxidase that acts as a chromogen. A colorless substrate is acted on by peroxidase to produce a colored byproduct. The ELISA has been used to prove IgE antibodies to proteins such as protamine, has been developed to screen for other antibodies to diverse agents, and has become the mainstay of immunologic testing. Although antibodies can occur, patients may be asymptomatic. An older test previously used was the radioallergosorbent test (RAST), which used radiolabeled antibodies directed against human IgE and was counted in a scintillation counter, and has been largely replaced by ELISA assays. Major limitations to in vitro immunologic testing too many anesthetic drugs include the commercial availability of the drug prepared as an antigen.

Intradermal Testing (Skin Testing)

Skin testing is the method most often used in patients after anaphylactic reaction to anesthetic drugs after the history has suggested the relevant antigens for testing.[42] Within minutes after antigen introduction, histamine released from cutaneous mast cells causes vasodilation (flare) and localized edema from increased vascular permeability (wheal). Fisher suggested that this is a simple, safe, and useful method of establishing a diagnosis in most cases of anaphylactic reactions occurring in the perioperative period. If the strict protocols established by Fisher are used, intradermal reactions are helpful.[42] Intradermal testing is of no value in reactions to contrast media or colloid volume expanders. Cross-sensitivity between drugs of similar structures can often be evaluated based on skin testing.

Agents Implicated in Allergic Reactions

Any drug or biologic agent can cause anaphylaxis in a patient. However, the agents most often implicated in the perioperative period include antibiotics, blood products, chlorhexidine, neuromuscular blocking drugs (NMBDs), polypeptides (aprotinin, latex, and protamine), and intravascular volume expanders. Most of the information about perioperative anaphylaxis is from Australia, Europe, the United Kingdom, and New Zealand, where centers have existed for many years to investigate perioperative anaphylaxis when it occurs.[43–48] In one of the largest reports, perioperative anaphylaxis was evaluated over an 8-year period from 1997 to 2004 in France. Among the 2,516 patients with anaphylaxis, IgE-mediated reactions occurred in 1,816 cases (72.2%). The most common causes for the IgE-mediated events were NMBDs in 58% (n = 1067), latex in 19.6% (n = 316), and antibiotics in 12.8% (n = 236).[49] One of the concerns regarding NMBA allergy is that if patients are allergic to a muscle relaxant, there is a potential for cross-reactivity because of the similarity of the active site, a quaternary ammonium molecule, among the different types of relaxants, and alternatives cannot be chosen without some degree of immunologic testing.

From the United States/North American perspective, only a few reports note either the incidence or agents implicated for perioperative anaphylaxis. Older reports from 1990 noted barbiturates were the most likely causative agent for 38% of IgE-mediated anaphylaxis, an agent that has disappeared from clinical practice in the United States.[50] However, European reports suggest the most frequent agent reported for perioperative IgE-mediated anaphylaxis is NMBAs.[51] A recent report from 2011 in the United States examined a skin test database of 38 patients with perioperative anaphylaxis who were tested to medications implicated in the reactions.[52] The history obtained by an allergist, skin test results, and tryptase measurements were reported.[52] Of note, 40% of the surgical procedures were aborted, and 58% of events resulted in intensive care unit admissions, suggesting the severity of the responses.[52] Of the 38 patients, 18 were considered IgE-mediated reactions by skin testing, 6 were non–IgE-mediated anaphylactic reactions as determined by elevated tryptase levels and negative skin testing, and 14 were probable non–IgE-mediated anaphylactic reactions because tryptase levels were normal or not obtained and skin testing was negative. Of the IgE-mediated anaphylactic reactions, antibiotics were the causative agents in half of the patients while NMBAs were implicated solely as a likely causative agent in only one reaction. The authors noted causative agents could not be determined in the other half of the patients.[52] The authors identified only one true IgE-mediated reaction to an NMBA; however, another patient had positive skin tests to three agents including vecuronium, propofol, and cefazolin, making the diagnosis uncertain. A previous Danish study reported 68 patients, of which 36 underwent complete investigations with in vitro testing and skin testing, and found that only one patient tested positive for NMBAs (4.8%: 1/21), while chlorhexidine accounted for 19.1% of reactions and antibiotics, 14.3%.[53] In the current study chlorhexidine was tested in only 4% of cases and may account for some of the undiagnosed reactions with elevated tryptase.[52] Because of this information, antibiotics, latex, and NMBAs will be considered in more detail, along with local anesthetic (LA) agents.

Antibiotics

Most surgical patients receive an antibiotic that includes a cephalosporin or vancomycin for prophylaxis. Despite their widespread use, the incidence of antibiotic allergy and its reported prevalence vary widely, as cutaneous manifestations are often the presenting reaction.[39] As reviewed in a recent article,[1] anaphylaxis to penicillins is low, occurring in an estimated 0.004% to 0.015%, but this widely quoted reference is old and penicillin is rarely used.[54] Further, data on anaphylaxis to cephalosporins is also uncommon, occurring from 0.0001% to 0.1%; however, this number is not zero.[55] Anaphylactic reactions to vancomycin are rare, but as we have demonstrated, it is a potent histamine-releasing agent that can cause severe hypotension and flushing on administration especially with rapid infusion.[30,31]

As reviewed previously, managing the patient with a history of penicillin allergy when the surgeon requests cephalosporin administration is still not clear based on reported data.[1]

Older data suggest cross-reactivity to cephalosporins among penicillin-allergic patients is high and suggest choosing another agent, a practice that developed from case reports[56] of anaphylaxis following first-generation cephalosporins together with in vitro and skin testing, which showed extensive cross-reactivity between penicillins and first-generation cephalosporins.[1] The clinical relevance of this in vitro cross-reactivity was never demonstrated.[56] However, the risk of acute cephalosporin reactions among patients with positive penicillin skin tests is reported to be ~4.4%, compared with 0.6% among patients with negative penicillin skin tests.[56,57] Anaphylactic reactors were selectively omitted from these open studies. Further, an allergic reaction to a cephalosporin may occur independently of prior penicillin sensitization. One authority has concluded that most patients who have a history of penicillin allergy will tolerate cephalosporins, but that indiscriminate administration cannot be recommended, especially for patients who have had serious acute reactions to any β-lactam antibiotic.[39] Penicillin skin testing when available can be useful in identifying the 85% of patients with histories of penicillin allergy who no longer have (or never had) IgE antibodies to major and minor determinants and are therefore at negligible risk of cephalosporin reactions. For the remaining patients who are skin test positive, gradual escalation of the first dose of a cephalosporin under careful observation will further mitigate against uncommon but potentially serious acute reactions.

If a patient has a penicillin allergy history that is consistent with anaphylaxis and penicillin skin testing is unavailable, then cephalosporins should be used with caution, with graded dose escalation of the first dose. A patient who has experienced an allergic reaction to a specific cephalosporin should probably not receive that cephalosporin again. However, the risk of an acute reaction when a different cephalosporin is administered appears to be low, but systemic evaluations of reaction risks when administering other cephalosporins or β-lactam antibiotics to patients with IgE antibodies to a particular cephalosporin are not available. Unfortunately, patient histories are often unreliable in this circumstance.

Latex Allergy

For the anesthesiologist, latex represents an environmental agent often implicated as an important cause of perioperative anaphylaxis. Latex is the milky sap derived from the tree *Hevea brasiliensis*, to which multiple agents, including preservatives, accelerators, and antioxidants are added to make the final rubber product. Latex is present in a variety of different products. Latex allergy is an IgE-dependent immediate hypersensitivity reaction to latex proteins. The first case of an allergic reaction because of latex was reported in 1979 and was manifested by contact urticaria. In 1989, the first reports of intraoperative anaphylaxis because of latex were reported.

Health-care workers and children with spina bifida, urogenital abnormalities, or certain food allergies have also been recognized as people at increased risk for anaphylaxis to latex. Brown and colleagues reported a 24% incidence of irritant or contact dermatitis and a 12.5% incidence of latex-specific IgE positivity in anesthesiologists. Of this group, 10% were clinically asymptomatic, although IgE positive.[58] A history of atopy was also a significant risk factor for latex sensitization. Brown and colleagues suggested that these people are in their early stages of sensitization and perhaps, by avoiding latex exposure, their progression to symptomatic disease can be prevented.[58] Patients allergic to bananas, avocados, and kiwis have also been reported to have antibodies that cross-react with latex.[59,60] Multiple attempts are being made to reduce latex exposure to both health-care workers and patients. If latex allergy occurs, then strict avoidance of latex from gloves and other sources needs to be considered, following recommendations as reported by Holzman.[61,62] Although latex was previously a common environmental antigen, ongoing effort by suppliers of hospital equipment has significantly reduced latex exposure in recent years.

More importantly, anesthesiologists must be prepared to treat the life-threatening cardiopulmonary collapse that occurs after anaphylaxis, as previously discussed. The most important preventive therapy is to avoid antigen exposure; although clinicians have used pretreatment with antihistamine (diphenhydramine and cimetidine) and corticosteroids, there are no data in the literature to suggest that pretreatment prevents anaphylaxis or decreases its severity.[1] Patients in whom latex allergy is suspected should be referred to an allergist for proper evaluation and potential testing for definitive diagnosis. When this is not possible, patients should be treated as if they were latex allergic, and the antigen avoided. Patients with a documented history of latex allergy should wear Medic Alert bracelets.

Local Anesthetics

Skin testing to local anesthetics (LAs) is considered a direct challenge or provocative dose testing. LA drugs are injected in increasing quantities under controlled circumstances. This testing decides if the person can safely receive amide derivatives (e.g., lidocaine) and can also be used to decide if the person is sensitive to *para*-aminobenzoic ester agents (e.g., procaine, tetracaine). Because the immediate hypersensitivity reactions to LAs are unknown, they are commonly regarded as "pseudo-allergic" or "nonimmune type" anaphylaxis, as immunologically mediated reactions have rarely been observed with positive skin-prick tests.[63] Other ingredients in LA preparations have to be considered as elicitors; for example, preservatives like benzoates or sulfites or latex contaminants in injection bottles. Practical management of patients with a history of LA reaction includes a careful allergy history and skin-prick and intradermal tests. Undiluted LA solutions may elicit false-positive intradermal test reactions. If prick and intradermal tests are negative, the procedure of subcutaneous provocation testing is applied in a placebo-controlled manner. When patients are constantly reacting to placebo, a regimen of "reverse placebo provocation" with injection of an LA (verum) is applied while the patient is informed about receiving placebo in order to "rule out psychosomatic involvement." With this regimen it is possible to eliminate anxiousness and fear, and the patient has proof that he has tolerated the respective LA substance.[63]

However, the diagnostic evaluation of patients with suspected allergy to LAs who have experienced a reaction remains controversial. One of the largest reports of skin testing for LA allergy evaluation is a retrospective chart review of patients following LA skin testing who underwent prick and intradermal skin testing followed by incremental subcutaneous and open subcutaneous challenge.[64] A total of 178 patients underwent 227 LA skin tests of which 220 (97%) were negative, and 214 (97%) had negative challenge or probable non–IgE-mediated events during challenge while three patients with six negative skin tests had a local reaction during the challenge. Only seven skin tests per five patients met the criteria for a positive skin test, and one patient had a skin reaction without systemic effects, three patients had a negative subcutaneous challenge, and one patient did not undergo a challenge. Overall, 98% of patients receiving LAs after open subcutaneous challenge tolerated the medications. The negative predictive value of the LA skin test was 97% with few positive skin tests. Positive LA skin tests are uncommon and the LA skin tests have an excellent negative predictive value.[64]

Neuromuscular Blocking Agents

NMBAs have several unique molecular features that make them potential antigens. All NMBAs are functionally divalent and are thus capable of cross-linking cell-surface IgE and causing mediator release from mast cells and basophils without binding or haptenating to larger carrier molecules. NMBAs have also been implicated in epidemiologic studies of anesthetic drug-induced anaphylaxis. Epidemiologic data from France suggest that NMBAs are responsible for 62% to 81% of reactions, depending on the time period evaluated.

In more recent years, NMBAs, especially steroid-derived agents, have been reported as potential causative agents of anaphylactic reactions during anesthesia. The data associating NMBAs in the most recent reports from France are mainly based on skin testing; however, studies have previously reported that steroidal-derived NMBAs and other molecules produce false-positive skin tests (i.e., weal and flare). One of the major problems is that anaphylaxis to NMBAs is rare in the United States but has been reported more often in Europe. Although suggestions have been made that this is because of underreporting, the severity of anaphylaxis and its sequelae to produce adverse outcomes clearly make this unlikely based on the current medicolegal climate that exists in the United States. One of the only ways to explain this widely divergent perspective is to understand how the diagnosis is made, because the recommended threshold test concentrations have not been defined, resulting in unreliable results.

We have previously reported that steroid-derived agents can induce positive weal and flare responses independent of mast cell degranulation, even at low concentrations, following intradermal injection. This effect is likely because of a direct effect on the cutaneous vasculature that occurs for most NMBAs at concentrations as low as 10^{-5} M, using intradermal skin tests in 30 volunteers. A positive cutaneous reaction without evidence of mast cell degranulation was noted at low concentrations (100 μg/mL) of rocuronium in almost all the volunteers. We have used intradermal injections to compare cutaneous effects of anesthetic and other agents.

Other investigators have also reported similar results. Because prick tests are often used for authenticating NMBAs as causative drugs, Dhonneur and colleagues evaluated 30 volunteers, using prick testing. Each subject received 10 prick tests (50 μL) on both forearms.[65] The investigators studied the weal and flare responses to prick tests with rocuronium and vecuronium, using four dilutions (1/1,000, 1/100, 1/10, and 1) and two controls, and measured weal and flare immediately after and at 15 minutes. They noted 50% and 40% of the subjects had a positive skin reaction to undiluted rocuronium and vecuronium, respectively. To avoid false-positive results, they suggested that prick testing with rocuronium and vecuronium should be performed in subjects who have experienced a hypersensitivity reaction during anesthesia, with concentrations below that commonly inducing positive reactions in anesthesia-naive, healthy subjects (i.e., for men in a dilution of 1/10 and for women in a dilution of 1/100).[65] Guidelines for prick testing that are internationally agreed on need to be established. Many of these differences may explain the various incidences of allergy to NMBAs among countries. Concentration–skin response curves to rocuronium and vecuronium have showed that prick tests should be performed with dilution of the commercially available preparation. Female volunteers significantly ($P < 0.01$) reacted to lower vecuronium and rocuronium concentrations more frequently than did males. In female subjects, positive skin reactions were reported with dilutions of 1/100 of both relaxants. In male subjects, positive skin reactions were noted with the undiluted concentration, except for one volunteer who reacted to rocuronium (1/10 dilution).[65]

Summary

Although the immune system functions to provide host defense, it can respond inappropriately to produce hypersensitivity or allergic reactions. A spectrum of life-threatening allergic reactions to any drug or agent can occur in the perioperative period. The enigma of these reactions lies in their unpredictable nature. Certain patients undergoing high-risk procedures with multiple blood product exposures are also at higher risk. However, a high index of suspicion, prompt recognition, and appropriate and aggressive therapy can help avoid a disastrous outcome.

REFERENCES

1. Levy JH, Adkinson NF Jr. Anaphylaxis during cardiac surgery: Implications for clinicians. *Anesth Analg.* 2008;106:392–403.
2. Kay AB. Allergy and allergic diseases. First of two parts. *N Engl J Med.* 2001;344:30–37.
3. Kay AB. Allergy and allergic diseases. Second of two parts. *N Engl J Med.* 2001;344:109–113.
4. Hotchkiss RS, Karl IE. The pathophysiology and treatment of sepsis. *N Engl J Med.* 2003;348:138–150.
5. Delves PJ, Roitt IM. The immune system. Second of two parts. *N Engl J Med.* 2000;343:108–117.
6. Delves PJ, Roitt IM. The immune system. First of two parts. *N Engl J Med.* 2000;343:37–49.
7. Skrupky LP, Kerby PW, Hotchkiss RS. Advances in the management of sepsis and the understanding of key immunologic defects. *Anesthesiology.* 2011;115:1349–1362.
8. Pober JS, Cotran RS. Cytokines and endothelial cell biology. *Physiol Rev.* 1990;70:427–451.
9. Walport MJ. Complement. Second of two parts. *N Engl J Med.* 2001;344:1140–1144.
10. Walport MJ. Complement. First of two parts. *N Engl J Med.* 2001;344:1058–1066.
11. Levy JH, Freiberger DJ, Roback J. Hereditary angioedema: current and emerging treatment options. *Anesth Analg.* 2010;110:1271–1280.
12. Stevenson GW, Hall SC, Rudnick S, et al. The effect of anesthetic agents on the human immune response. *Anesthesiology.* 1990;72:542–552.
13. Sampson HA, Munoz-Furlong A, Bock SA, et al. Symposium on the definition and management of anaphylaxis: summary report. *J Allergy Clin Immunol.* 2005;115:584–591.
14. Mertes PM, Laxenaire MC, Alla F. Anaphylactic and anaphylactoid reactions occurring during anesthesia in France in 1999–2000. *Anesthesiology.* 2003;99:536–545.
15. Portier P, Richet CR. De l'action anaphylactique de certains venins. *C R Soc Biol.* 1902;54:170–172.
16. MacGlashan D Jr. Histamine: a mediator of inflammation. *J Allergy Clin Immunol.* 2003;112:S53–S59.
17. Kalesnikoff J, Galli SJ. Anaphylaxis: mechanisms of mast cell activation. *Chem Immunol Allergy.* 2011;95:45–66.
18. Wedemeyer J, Tsai M, Galli SJ. Roles of mast cells and basophils in innate and acquired immunity. *Curr Opin Immunol.* 2000;12:624–631.
19. Marone G, Bova M, Detoraki A, et al. The human heart as a shock organ in anaphylaxis. *Novartis Found Symp.* 2004;257:133–149.
20. Majno G, Palade GE. Studies on inflammation. 1. The effect of histamine and serotonin on vascular permeability: an electron microscopic study. *J Biophys Biochem Cytol.* 1961;11:571–605.
21. Majno G, Palade GE, Schoefl GI. Studies on inflammation. II. The site of action of histamine and serotonin along the vascular tree: a topographic study. *J Biophys Biochem Cytol.* 1961;11:607–626.
22. Holgate ST, Peters-Golden M, Panettieri RA, et al. Roles of cysteinyl leukotrienes in airway inflammation, smooth muscle function, and remodeling. *J Allergy Clin Immunol.* 2003;111:S18–S34, discussion S34–S36.
23. Vadas P, Gold M, Perelman B, et al. Platelet-activating factor, PAF acetylhydrolase, and severe anaphylaxis. *N Engl J Med.* 2008;358:28–35.
24. Pumphrey RS. Lessons for management of anaphylaxis from a study of fatal reactions. *Clin Exp Allergy.* 2000;30:1144–1150.
25. Pumphrey R. Anaphylaxis: can we tell who is at risk of a fatal reaction? *Curr Opin Allergy Clin Immunol.* 2004;4:285–290.
26. Pumphrey RS. Fatal anaphylaxis in the UK, 1992–2001. *Novartis Found Symp.* 2004;257:116–128.
27. Delage C, Irey NS. Anaphylactic deaths: a clinicopathologic study of 43 cases. *J Forensic Sci.* 1972;17:525–540.
28. Pumphrey RS, Roberts IS. Postmortem findings after fatal anaphylactic reactions. *J Clin Pathol.* 2000;53:273–276.
29. Sheppard CA, Logdberg LE, Zimring JC, et al. Transfusion-related acute lung injury. *Hematol Oncol Clin North Am.* 2007;21:163–176.
30. Veien M, Szlam F, Holden JT, et al. Mechanisms of nonimmunological histamine and tryptase release from human cutaneous mast cells. *Anesthesiology.* 2000;92:1074–1081.
31. Levy JH, Kettlekamp N, Goertz P, et al. Histamine release by vancomycin: a mechanism for hypotension in man. *Anesthesiology.* 1987;67:122–125.
32. Levy JH, Brister NW, Shearin A, et al. Wheal and flare responses to opioids in humans. *Anesthesiology.* 1989;70:756–760.
33. Levy JH, Adelson D, Walker B. Wheal and flare responses to muscle relaxants in humans. *Agents Actions.* 1991;34:302–308.
34. Levy JH, Davis GK, Duggan J, et al. Determination of the hemodynamics and histamine release of rocuronium (Org 9426) when administered in increased doses under $N_2 O/O_2$-sufentanil anesthesia. *Anesth Analg.* 1994;78:318–321.
35. Levy JH, Pitts M, Thanopoulos A, et al. The effects of rapacuronium on histamine release and hemodynamics in adult patients undergoing general anesthesia. *Anesth Analg.* 1999;89:290–295.
36. 2005 CARE AHAGFCRAEC. Part 10.6: anaphylaxis. *Circulation.* 2005;112:IV143–IV145.
37. DeSwarte RD. Drug allergy: problems and strategies. *J Allergy Clin Immunol.* 1984;74:209–224.
38. Gruchalla RS. Drug allergy. *J Allergy Clin Immunol.* 2003;111:S548–S559.
39. Gruchalla RS, Pirmohamed M. Clinical practice: antibiotic allergy. *N Engl J Med.* 2006;354:601–609.
40. Reich DL, Hossain S, Krol M, et al. Predictors of hypotension after induction of general anesthesia. *Anesth Analg.* 2005;101:622–628.
41. Laforest M, More D, Fisher M. Predisposing factors in anaphylactoid reactions to anaesthetic drugs in an Australian population: the role of allergy, atopy and previous anaesthesia. *Anaesth Intensive Care.* 1980;8:454–459.
42. Fisher MM, Bowey CJ. Intradermal compared with prick testing in the diagnosis of anaesthetic allergy. *Br J Anaesth.* 1997;79:59–63.
43. Galletly DC, Treuren BC. Anaphylactoid reactions during anaesthesia: seven years' experience of intradermal testing. *Anaesthesia.* 1985;40:329–333.
44. Laxenaire MC. Drugs and other agents involved in anaphylactic shock occurring during anaesthesia: a French multicenter epidemiological inquiry. *Ann Fr Anesth Reanim.* 1993;12:91–96.
45. Laxenaire MC, Mertes PM. Anaphylaxis during anaesthesia: RESULTS of a two-year survey in France. *Br J Anaesth.* 2001;87:549–558.
46. Harboe T, Guttormsen AB, Irgens A, et al. Anaphylaxis during anesthesia in Norway: a 6-year single-center follow-up study. *Anesthesiology.* 2005;102:897–903.
47. Mertes PM. Anaphylactic reactions during anaesthesia: let us treat the problem rather than debating its existence. *Acta Anaesthesiol Scand.* 2005;49:431–433.
48. Fisher M, Baldo BA. Anaphylaxis during anaesthesia: current aspects of diagnosis and prevention. *Eur J Anaesthesiol.* 1994;11:263–284.
49. Mertes PM, Alla F, Trechot P, et al. Anaphylaxis during anesthesia in France: an 8-year national survey. *J Allergy Clin Immunol.* 2011;128(2):366–367.
50. Moscicki RA, Sockin SM, Corsello BF, et al. Anaphylaxis during induction of general anesthesia: subsequent evaluation and management. *J Allergy Clin Immunol.* 1990;86:325–332.
51. Levy JH. Anaphylactic reactions to neuromuscular blocking drugs: are we making the correct diagnosis? *Anesth Analg.* 2004;98:881–882.
52. Gurrieri C, Weingarten TN, Martin DP, et al. Allergic reactions during anesthesia at a large United States referral center. *Anesth Analg.* 2011;113(5):1202–1212.
53. Garvey LH, Roed-Petersen J, Menne T, et al. Danish anaesthesia allergy centre: preliminary results. *Acta Anaesthesiol Scand.* 2001;45:1204–1209.
54. Idsoe O, Guthe T, Willcox RR, et al. Nature and extent of penicillin side-reactions, with particular reference to fatalities from anaphylactic shock. *Bull World Health Organ.* 1968;38:159–188.
55. Kelkar PS, Li JT. Cephalosporin allergy. *N Engl J Med.* 2001;345:804–809.
56. Pichichero ME. A review of evidence supporting the American Academy of Pediatrics recommendation for prescribing cephalosporin antibiotics for penicillin-allergic patients. *Pediatrics.* 2005;115:1048–1057.
57. Pichichero ME. Cephalosporins can be prescribed safely for penicillin-allergic patients. *J Fam Pract.* 2006;55:106–112.
58. Brown RH, Schauble JF, Hamilton RG. Prevalence of latex allergy among anesthesiologists: Identification of sensitized but asymptomatic individuals. *Anesthesiology.* 1998;89:292–299.
59. Lavaud F, Prevost A, Cossart C, et al. Allergy to latex, avocado pear, and banana: Evidence for a 30 kd antigen in immunoblotting. *J Allergy Clin Immunol.* 1995;95:557–564.
60. Blanco C, Carrillo T, Castillo R, et al. Latex allergy: Clinical features and cross-reactivity with fruits. *Ann Allergy.* 1994;73:309–314.
61. Holzman RS. Clinical management of latex-allergic children. *Anesth Analg.* 1997;85:529–533.
62. Holzman RS, Katz JD. Occupational latex allergy: the end of the innocence. *Anesthesiology.* 1998;89:287–289.
63. Ring J, Franz R, Brockow K. Anaphylactic reactions to local anesthetics. *Chem Immunol Allergy.* 2011;95:190–200.
64. McClimon B, Rank M, Li J. The predictive value of skin testing in the diagnosis of local anesthetic allergy. *Allergy Asthma Proc.* 2011;32:95–98.
65. Dhonneur G, Combes X, Chassard D, et al. Skin sensitivity to rocuronium and vecuronium: a randomized controlled prick-testing study in healthy volunteers. *Anesth Analg.* 2004;98:986–989.

10 Mechanisms of Anesthesia and Consciousness

C. MICHAEL CROWDER • BEN JULIAN PALANCA • ALEX S. EVERS

What Is Anesthesia?
How Is Anesthesia Measured?
What Is the Chemical Nature of Anesthetic Target Sites?
  The Meyer–Overton Rule
  Exceptions to the Meyer–Overton Rule
  Lipid versus Protein Targets
  Lipid Theories of Anesthesia
  Protein Theories of Anesthesia
  Evidence for Anesthetic Binding to Proteins
  Summary
How Do Anesthetics Interfere with the Electrophysiologic Function of the Nervous System?
  Neuronal Excitability
  Synaptic Transmission
  Summary

Anesthetic Actions on Ion Channels
  Anesthetic Effects on Voltage-dependent Ion Channels
  Anesthetic Effects on Ligand-gated Ion Channels
  Summary
How Are the Molecular Effects of Anesthetics Linked to Anesthesia in the Intact Organism?
  Pharmacologic Approaches
  Genetic Approaches
  Summary
Where in the Central Nervous System Do Anesthetics Work?
  Immobility
  Autonomic Control
  Amnesia
  Unconsciousness
  Summary
Conclusions
Acknowledgments

KEY POINTS

1. The components of the anesthetic state include unconsciousness, amnesia, analgesia, immobility, and attenuation of autonomic responses to noxious stimulation.
2. Minimum alveolar concentration (MAC) remains the most robust measurement and the standard for determining the potency of volatile anesthetics.
3. Direct interactions of anesthetic molecules with proteins would not only satisfy the Meyer–Overton rule, but would also provide the simplest explanation for compounds that deviate from this rule.
4. Current evidence strongly indicates protein rather than lipid as the molecular target for anesthetic action.
5. While current data still support the prevailing view that neuronal excitability is only slightly affected by general anesthetics, this small effect may nevertheless contribute significantly to the clinical actions of volatile anesthetics.
6. The synapse is generally thought to be the most likely relevant site of anesthetic action. Existing evidence indicates that even at this one site, anesthetics produce various effects, including presynaptic inhibition of neurotransmitter release, inhibition of excitatory neurotransmission, and enhancement of inhibitory neurotransmission. Furthermore, the effects of anesthetics on synaptic function differ among various anesthetic agents, neurotransmitters, and neuronal preparations.
7. Existing evidence suggests that most voltage-dependent calcium channels (VDCCs) are modestly sensitive or insensitive to anesthetics. However, some sodium channel subtypes are inhibited by volatile anesthetics and this effect may be responsible in part for a reduction in neurotransmitter release at some synapses.
8. Activation of background K^+ channels could be an important and general mechanism through which volatile and gaseous anesthetics regulate neuronal resting membrane potential and thereby excitability.
9. Hyperpolarization-activated cyclic nucleotide-gated channels are a relatively recently discovered channel type inhibited by volatile anesthetics and some intravenous anesthetics at clinical concentrations.
10. A large body of evidence shows that clinical concentrations of many anesthetics potentiate GABA-activated currents in the central nervous system. Other members of the ligand-activated ion channel family, including glycine receptors, neuronal nicotinic receptors, and $5-HT_3$ receptors, are also affected by clinical concentrations of anesthetics and remain plausible anesthetic targets.
11. Genetic experiments in mice provide definitive evidence for roles of specific $GABA_A$ receptor channels, two-pore potassium channels, and HCN channels in particular anesthetic behavioral effects. Genetically engineered mice also show that distinct anesthetic targets mediate different anesthetic endpoints and that not all anesthetics have the same targets.
12. While anesthetic action to produce immobility occurs largely at the spinal cord, specific molecular targets for amnesia lie in the hippocampus.

13 Anesthetic-induced unconsciousness can be viewed as impairment of both arousal and awareness. These actions are mediated by targets distributed across the brainstem, hypothalamus, thalamus, and cerebral cortex.
14 Anesthetic ablation of arousal relies on disruption of redundant subcortical systems that regulate sleep and patterns of cortical activity.
15 Anesthetics alter the interaction of cortical networks responsible for cognitive functions and may thereby alter awareness by limiting the capacity to both represent and integrate information.

The introduction of general anesthetics into clinical practice over 150 years ago stands as one of the seminal innovations of medicine. This single discovery facilitated the development of modern surgery and spawned the specialty of anesthesiology. Despite the importance of general anesthetics, and despite more than 100 years of active research, the molecular mechanisms responsible for anesthetic action are only partially understood.

Why have mechanisms of anesthesia been so difficult to elucidate? Anesthetics, as a class of drugs, are challenging to study for three major reasons:

1. Anesthesia, by definition, is a change in the responses of an *intact animal* to external stimuli. Making a definitive link between anesthetic effects observed in vitro and the anesthetic state observed and defined in vivo has proven difficult.
2. No structure–activity relationships are apparent among anesthetics; a wide variety of structurally unrelated compounds, ranging from steroids to elemental xenon, are capable of producing clinical anesthesia. This suggests that there are multiple molecular mechanisms that can produce clinical anesthesia.
3. Anesthetics work at very high concentrations in comparison to drugs, neurotransmitters, and hormones that act at specific receptors. This implies that if anesthetics do act by binding to specific receptor sites, they must bind with very low affinity and probably stay bound to the receptor for very short periods of time. Low-affinity binding is much more difficult to observe and characterize than is high-affinity binding.

Despite these difficulties, molecular and genetic tools are now available that should allow for major insights into anesthetic mechanisms in the next decade. The aim of this chapter is to provide a conceptual framework for the reader to catalog current knowledge and integrate future developments about mechanisms of anesthesia. Five specific questions will be addressed in this chapter:

1. What is anesthesia and how do we measure it?
2. What are the molecular targets of anesthetics?
3. What are the cellular neurophysiologic mechanisms of anesthesia (e.g., effects on synaptic function vs. effects on action potential generation) and what anesthetic effects on ion channels and other neuronal proteins underlie these mechanisms?
4. How are the molecular and cellular effects of anesthetics linked to the behavioral effects of anesthetics observed in vivo?
5. What are the major anatomic sites of anesthetic action in the central nervous system (CNS), and how do anesthetics interfere with their interactions?

What Is Anesthesia?

General anesthesia can be broadly defined as a drug-induced reversible depression of the CNS resulting in the loss of response to and perception of all external stimuli. Unfortunately, such a broad definition is inadequate for two reasons. First, the definition is not actually broad enough. Anesthesia is not simply a deafferented state; amnesia and unconsciousness are important aspects of the anesthetic state. Second, the definition is too broad, as all general anesthetics do not produce equal depression of all sensory modalities. For example, barbiturates are considered to be anesthetics but produce minimal analgesia. A more practical description of the anesthetic state is a collection of five "component" changes in behavior or perception–unconsciousness, amnesia, analgesia, immobility, and attenuation of autonomic responses to noxious stimulation.

Regardless of which definition of anesthesia is used, rapid and reversible drug-induced changes in behavior or perception are essential to anesthesia. As such, anesthesia can only be defined and measured in the intact organism. Changes in behavior such as unconsciousness or amnesia can be intuitively understood in higher organisms such as mammals, but become increasingly difficult to define as one descends the phylogenetic tree. Thus, while anesthetics have effects on organisms ranging from worms to man, it is difficult to map with certainty the effects of anesthetics observed in lower organisms to any of our behavioral definitions of anesthesia. This contributes to the difficulty of using simple organisms as models in which to study the molecular mechanisms of anesthesia. Similarly, any cellular or molecular effects of anesthetics observed in higher organisms can be extremely difficult to link with the constellation of behaviors that constitute the anesthetic state. The absence of a simple and concise definition of anesthesia has clearly been one of the stumbling blocks to elucidating the mechanisms of anesthesia at a molecular and cellular level. Precise definitions for each of the component behaviors of the anesthetic state will be an important tool in dissecting the molecular and cellular mechanisms of each of the clinically important effects of anesthetic agents.

An additional difficulty in defining anesthesia is that our understanding of the mechanisms of consciousness is rather amorphous at present. One cannot easily define anesthesia when the neurobiologic phenomena ablated by anesthesia are not well understood. As discussed later in this chapter, the neural substrates for consciousness are beginning to be unraveled[1,2] and new theories[3,4] have incorporated this new anatomic knowledge leading to identification of surrogate physiologic markers of consciousness.[5] These new insights into mechanisms of consciousness are discussed in the section *Where in the Central Nervous System Do Anesthetics Work?*

Finally, it has long been assumed that anesthesia is a state that is achieved when an anesthetic agent reaches a specific concentration at its effect site in the brain and that if tolerance to the anesthetic develops, increasing concentrations of anesthetic might be required to maintain a constant level of anesthesia during prolonged anesthetic administration. The finding that it takes a higher anesthetic brain concentration to induce anesthesia than to maintain anesthesia (i.e., emergence occurs at a significantly lower concentration than induction) contradicts these assumptions.[6] This phenomenon, referred to as neural inertia, adds a wrinkle to the definition of anesthesia, suggesting that the mechanisms of anesthetic induction and emergence may be different. This suggestion is supported by the recent finding that the sedative component of anesthesia can be reversed by stimulation of specific arousal pathways in the brain, even in the presence of "anesthetic" concentrations of inhalational agents.[7,8]

How Is Anesthesia Measured?

In order to study the pharmacology of anesthetic action, quantitative measurements of anesthetic potency are absolutely essential. To this end, Quasha et al.[9] have defined the concept of minimum alveolar concentration (MAC). MAC is defined as the alveolar partial pressure of a gas at which 50% of humans do not respond to a surgical incision. In animals, MAC is defined as the alveolar partial pressure of a gas at which 50% of animals do not respond to a noxious stimulus, such as tail clamp,[10] or at which they lose their righting reflex. The use of MAC as a measure of anesthetic potency has two major advantages. First, it is an extremely reproducible measurement that is remarkably constant over a wide range of species.[9] Second, the use of end-tidal gas concentration provides an index of the "free" concentration of drug required to produce anesthesia since the end-tidal gas concentration is in equilibrium with the free concentration in plasma.

The MAC concept has several important limitations, particularly when trying to relate MAC values to anesthetic potency observed in vitro. First, the endpoint in a MAC determination is quantal: A subject is either anesthetized or unanesthetized; it cannot be partially anesthetized. Furthermore, MAC represents the average response of a whole population of subjects rather than the response of a single subject. The quantal nature of the MAC measurement makes it very difficult to compare MAC measurements to concentration–response curves obtained in vitro, where the graded response of a single preparation is measured as a function of anesthetic concentration. The second limitation of MAC measurements is that they can only be directly applied to anesthetic gases. Parenteral anesthetics (barbiturates, neurosteroids, propofol) cannot be assigned a MAC value, making it difficult to compare the potency of parenteral and volatile anesthetics. A MAC equivalent for parental anesthetics is the free concentration of the drug in plasma required to prevent response to a noxious stimulus in 50% of subjects; this value has been estimated for several parenteral anesthetics.[11] A third limitation of MAC is that it is highly dependent on the anesthetic endpoint used to define it. For example, if loss of response to a verbal command is used as an anesthetic endpoint, the MAC values obtained (MAC_{awake}) will be much lower than classic MAC values based on response to a noxious stimulus. Indeed, each behavioral component of the anesthetic state will likely have a different MAC value. Despite its limitations, MAC remains the most robust measurement and the standard for determining the potency of volatile anesthetics.

Because of the limitations of MAC, monitors that measure some correlate of anesthetic depth have been introduced into clinical practice.[12] The most popular of these monitors converts spontaneous electroencephalogram (EEG) waveforms into a single value that correlates with anesthetic depth for some general anesthetics. To date, these monitors have not been shown to be more effective at preventing awareness during anesthesia than simply maintaining an adequate end-tidal anesthetic concentration[13,14] or giving a standard dose of intravenous anesthetic. Nonetheless it is logical to think that different individuals may have different sensitivities to anesthetics and that measuring a surrogate endpoint such as a processed EEG value,[15] an evoked potential,[16] or a functional neuroimaging signal indicative of integrated cortical activity[1] might be a better indicator of anesthetic depth than merely measuring delivered concentration.

What Is the Chemical Nature of Anesthetic Target Sites?

The Meyer–Overton Rule

More than 100 years ago, Meyer[17] and Overton[18] independently observed that the potency of gases as anesthetics was strongly correlated with their solubility in olive oil (Fig. 10-1). Since a wide variety of structurally unrelated compounds obey the Meyer–Overton rule, it has been reasoned that all anesthetics are likely to act at the same molecular site. This idea is referred to as the *unitary theory of anesthesia*. It has also been argued that since solubility in a specific solvent strongly correlates with anesthetic potency, the solvent showing the strongest correlation between anesthetic solubility and potency is likely to most closely mimic the chemical and physical properties of the anesthetic target site in the CNS. On the basis of this reasoning, the anesthetic target site was assumed to be hydrophobic in nature. Since olive oil/gas partition coefficients can be determined for gases and volatile liquids, but not for liquid anesthetics, attempts have been made to correlate anesthetic potency with solvent/water partition coefficients. To date, the octanol/water partition coefficient best correlates with anesthetic potency. This correlation holds for a variety of classes of anesthetics and spans a 10,000-fold range of anesthetic potencies.[19] The properties of the solvent octanol suggest that the anesthetic site is likely to be amphipathic, having both polar and nonpolar characteristics.

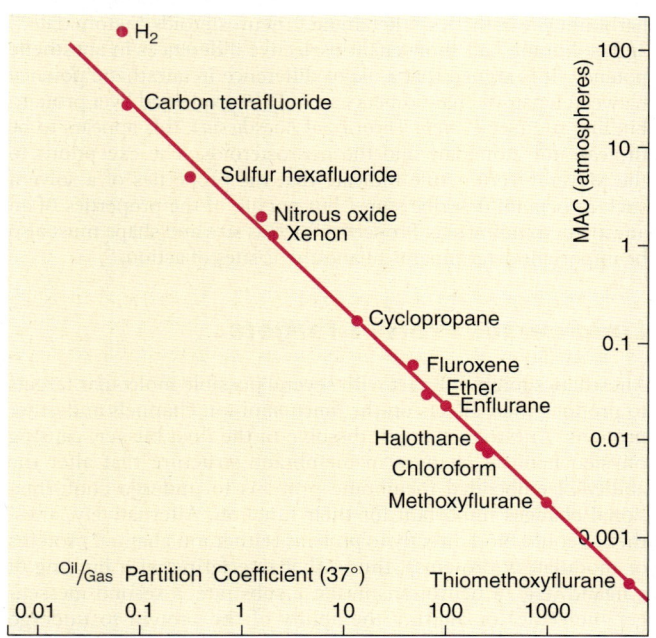

Figure 10-1 The Meyer–Overton rule. There is a linear relationship (on a log–log scale) between the oil/gas partition coefficient and the anesthetic potency (minimum alveolar concentration, MAC) of a number of gases. The correlation between lipid solubility and MAC extends over a 70,000-fold difference in anesthetic potency. (Reproduced with permission from Tanfiuji Y, Eger EI, Terrell RC. Some characteristics of an exceptionally potent inhaled anesthetic: thiomethoxyflurane. *Anesth Analg*. 1977;56:387.)

Exceptions to the Meyer–Overton Rule

Compounds exist that are structurally similar to halogenated anesthetics,[20] barbiturates,[21] and neurosteroids,[22] yet are convulsants rather than anesthetics. On the basis of olive oil/gas partition coefficients of the halogenated convulsant compounds, anesthesia should have been achieved within the range of concentrations studied.[23] Halogenated compounds have also been identified that are neither anesthetic nor convulsant, despite oil/gas partition coefficients that would predict they should be anesthetics.[23] Interestingly, some of these polyhalogenated compounds do produce amnesia in animals[24] and are thus referred to as *nonimmobilizers* rather than as nonanesthetics.

In several homologous series of anesthetics, anesthetic potency increases with increasing chain length until a certain critical chain length is reached. Beyond this critical chain length, compounds are unable to produce anesthesia, even at the highest attainable concentrations. In the series of n-alkanols, for example, anesthetic potency increases from methanol through dodecanol; all longer alkanols are unable to produce anesthesia.[25] This phenomenon is referred to as the *cutoff effect*. Cutoff effects have been described for several homologous series of anesthetics including n-alkanes, n-alkanols, cycloalkanemethanols,[26] and perfluoroalkanes.[27] While the anesthetic potency in each of these homologous series of anesthetics shows a cutoff, a corresponding cutoff in octanol/water or oil/gas partition coefficients has not been demonstrated. Therefore, compounds above the cutoff represent a deviation from the Meyer–Overton rule.

A final deviation from the Meyer–Overton rule is the observation that enantiomers of anesthetics differ in their potency as anesthetics. Enantiomers (mirror-image compounds) are a class of stereoisomers that have identical physical properties, including identical solubility in solvents such as octanol or olive oil. Animal studies of barbiturate anesthetics,[28] ketamine,[29] neurosteroids,[30] etomidate,[31] and isoflurane[32] all show enantioselective differences in anesthetic potency. It is argued that a *major* difference in anesthetic potency between a pair of enantiomers can only be explained by a protein-binding site (see *Protein Theories of Anesthesia*); this appears to be the case for etomidate and the neurosteroids. The exceptions to the Meyer–Overton rule indicate that the properties of a solvent such as octanol describe some, but not all, of the properties of an anesthetic-binding site. Properties such as size and shape must also be important determinants of anesthetic sites of action.

Lipid versus Protein Targets

Anesthetics might interact with several possible molecular targets to produce their effects on the *function* of ion channels and other proteins. Anesthetics might dissolve in the *lipid* bilayer, causing physicochemical changes in membrane structure that alter the ability of embedded membrane proteins to undergo conformational changes important for their function. Alternatively, anesthetics could bind directly to *proteins* (either ion channel proteins or modulatory proteins), thus either interfering with binding of a ligand (e.g., a neurotransmitter, a substrate, a second messenger molecule) or altering the ability of the protein to undergo conformational changes important for its function. The following section summarizes the arguments for and against lipid theories and protein theories of anesthesia.

Lipid Theories of Anesthesia

In its simplest incarnation, the lipid theory of anesthesia postulates that anesthetics dissolve in the lipid bilayers of biologic membranes and produce anesthesia when they reach a critical concentration in the membrane. Consistent with this hypothesis, the membrane/gas partition coefficients of anesthetic gases in pure lipid bilayers correlate strongly with anesthetic potency.[33] Also, consistent with the lipid theories, various membrane perturbations are produced by general anesthetics; however, the magnitude of these changes produced by clinical concentrations of anesthetics are quite small and are thought to be very unlikely to disrupt nervous system function.[34] While some of the more sophisticated lipid theories can account for the cutoff effect and for the ineffectiveness of nonimmobilizers, no lipid theory can plausibly explain all anesthetic pharmacology. Thus, most investigators do not consider lipids as the most likely target of general anesthetics.

Protein Theories of Anesthesia

The Meyer–Overton rule could also be explained by the direct interaction of anesthetics with hydrophobic sites on proteins. Three types of hydrophobic sites on proteins might interact with anesthetics:

1. Hydrophobic amino acids comprise the core of water-soluble proteins. Anesthetics could bind in hydrophobic pockets that are fortuitously present in the protein core.
2. Hydrophobic amino acids also form the lining of binding sites for hydrophobic ligands. For example, there are hydrophobic pockets in which fatty acids tightly bind on proteins such as albumin and the low–molecular-weight fatty acid–binding proteins. Anesthetics could compete with endogenous ligands for binding to such sites on either water-soluble or membrane proteins.
3. Hydrophobic amino acids are major constituents of the α-helices, which form the membrane-spanning regions of membrane proteins; hydrophobic amino acid side chains form the protein surface that faces the membrane lipid. Anesthetic molecules could interact with pockets formed between the α-helices or with the hydrophobic surface of these membrane proteins, disrupting normal lipid–protein interactions and possibly directly affecting protein conformation.

Direct interaction of anesthetic molecules with proteins not only satisfies the Meyer–Overton rule, but would also provide the simplest explanation for compounds that deviate from this rule. Any protein-binding site is likely to be defined by properties such as size and shape in addition to its solvent properties. Limitations in size and shape could reduce the binding affinity of compounds beyond the cutoff, thus explaining their lack of anesthetic effect. Enantioselectivity is also most easily explained by a direct binding of anesthetic molecules to defined sites on proteins; a protein-binding site of defined dimensions could readily distinguish between enantiomers on the basis of their different shapes. Protein-binding sites for anesthetics could also explain the convulsant effects of some polyhalogenated alkanes. Different compounds binding (in slightly different ways) to the same binding pocket can produce different effects on protein conformation and hence on protein function. For example, polyhalogenated alkanes (*nonimmobilizers*) could be inverse agonists, binding at the same protein sites at which halogenated alkane anesthetics are agonists. The evidence for direct interactions between anesthetics and proteins is briefly reviewed in the following section.

Evidence for Anesthetic Binding to Proteins

A breakthrough in protein theories of anesthesia was the demonstration that a purified water-soluble protein, firefly luciferase, could be inhibited by general anesthetics. This provided the important proof of principle that anesthetics could bind to proteins in the absence of membranes. Numerous studies have extensively characterized the anesthetic inhibition of firefly luciferase activity and have shown that inhibition occurs at concentrations very similar to those required to produce clinical anesthesia, is consistent with the Meyer–Overton rule, is competitive with respect to the substrate D-luciferin, and exhibits a cutoff in anesthetic potency for both n-alkanes and n-alkanols.[35,36] These data suggest that the luciferin-binding pocket may have physical and chemical characteristics similar to those of a putative anesthetic-binding site in the CNS. To address proteins more relevant to anesthetic effects on the nervous system, numerous studies have employed site-directed mutagenesis of anesthetic-sensitive ion channels to identify amino acid residues that are crucial to anesthetic action. While the residues identified in these studies may contribute to anesthetic-binding sites, they may alternatively be sites that are essential for anesthetic-induced conformational changes in the protein. The literature on site-directed mutagenesis studies to identify putative anesthetic-binding sites on ion channels is extensively reviewed in the section *Anesthetic Actions on Ion Channels*.

More direct approaches to study anesthetic binding to proteins have included NMR spectroscopy and photoaffinity labeling. Early studies using ^{19}F-NMR spectroscopy demonstrated that isoflurane binds to the fatty acid–binding sites on bovine serum albumin (BSA), and that binding is competitively inhibited by halothane, methoxyflurane, sevoflurane, and octanol.[37,38] Using this BSA model, it was subsequently shown that anesthetic-binding sites could be identified and characterized using photoaffinity labeling with ^{14}C-labeled halothane.[39,40] Photoaffinity-labeling reagents have subsequently been developed for a variety of anesthetics, including etomidate,[41] propofol,[42,43] barbiturates,[44] and neurosteroids.[45] These photoaffinity-labeling reagents can be used to identify putative anesthetic-binding sites, the functional significance of which can be validated using site-directed mutagenesis.

The most extensive photolabeling studies have used etomidate analogue photolabeling reagents to identify etomidate-binding sites on purified $GABA_A$ receptors. An initial study used azi-etomidate, a photolabeling reagent that preferentially labels nucleophilic amino acids, to photolabel-purified $GABA_A$ receptors from bovine brain.[46] This study identified two methionine residues that were sites of attachment for azi-etomidate: One site on the TM1 helix (Met-236) of the α_1 subunit and the other (Met-286) on the TM3 helix of the β_3 subunit. These data suggest an etomidate-binding pocket in the transmembrane domain at the interface between the α_1 and β_3 subunits. A subsequent study using TDBzl-etomidate, a photolabeling reagent with broader amino acid side chain reactivity, identified additional amino acids that confirmed and further defined this intersubunit–binding site.[44] The combined results of site-directed mutagenesis studies and photoaffinity-labeling studies identified a specific, functionally relevant binding site for etomidate on $GABA_A$ receptors, definitively refuting lipid theories of anesthetic action. Photoaffinity-labeling studies with other anesthetic agents including propofol[43,47] and barbiturates[48] have identified binding pockets for anesthetics, which are currently being tested and validated using site-directed mutagenesis.

Although photoaffinity-labeling techniques can provide extensive information about anesthetic-binding sites on proteins, they cannot reveal the details of the three-dimensional structure of these sites. X-ray diffraction crystallography can provide this kind of three-dimensional detail and has been used to study anesthetic interactions with a small number of proteins. Firefly luciferase has been crystallized in the presence and absence of the anesthetic bromoform, confirming that anesthetics bind in the D-luciferin–binding pocket.[49] Human serum albumin has also been crystallized in the presence of either propofol or halothane, demonstrating binding of both anesthetics to preformed fatty acid–binding pockets. While these data provide insight into the structure of anesthetic-binding sites, x-ray crystallographic studies of anesthetic-binding sites on biologically relevant targets such as ion channels have been hampered by difficulties with crystallizing membrane proteins. Recently, a bacterial homolog of the ligand-gated ion channels, GLIC, has been crystallized and its crystal structure has been solved.[50] GLIC has been shown to be sensitive to clinical concentrations of anesthetics, and furthermore the crystal structure of GLIC complexed with either desflurane or propofol has been solved.[51] These data reveal a preformed binding cavity in the interface between the transmembrane domains of each subunit of the ion channel. The recent description of the high-resolution crystal structure of a $GABA_A$ receptor[52] should soon make it possible to define the precise dimensions and location of anesthetic-binding pockets on a relevant anesthetic target protein. It is important to recognize that even the x-ray crystal structures of anesthetics bound to target ion channels may not fully elucidate how and where anesthetics act. Ion channels are allosteric proteins that fluctuate between multiple conformations, whereas x-ray structures are static "snapshots" of just one conformation. Anesthetics bind to and stabilize specific conformations of proteins, which may or may not be the same conformation in which the protein is crystallized.

Summary

Evidence from studies using water-soluble proteins demonstrates that anesthetics can bind to hydrophobic pockets on proteins and that anesthetic–protein interactions can account for the Meyer–Overton rule and deviations from it. Photoaffinity-labeling studies demonstrate that etomidate binds to a pocket in the interface between the α_1 and β_3 subunits of the $GABA_A$ receptor. Mutagenesis of amino acids within this etomidate-binding pocket eliminates the anesthetic effect of etomidate, providing unequivocal evidence that anesthetic action can be mediated by binding to a specific protein site. Studies with propofol and barbiturate analogue photoaffinity-labeling reagents have also demonstrated putative binding sites on the $GABA_A$ receptor. Finally, recent x-ray crystallographic studies using the bacterial ion channel GLIC provide the first glimpse of the three-dimensional structure of an anesthetic-binding site on a relevant protein model. While the long-standing controversy between lipid and protein theories of anesthesia may be behind us, numerous unanswered questions remain about the details of anesthetic–protein interactions, including:

1. What is the stoichiometry of anesthetic binding to a protein (i.e., do many anesthetic molecules interact with a single protein molecule or only a few)?
2. Do anesthetics compete with endogenous ligands for binding to hydrophobic pockets on protein targets or do they bind to fortuitous cavities in the protein?
3. Do all anesthetics bind to the same pocket on a protein or are there multiple hydrophobic pockets for different anesthetics?
4. How many proteins have hydrophobic pockets in which anesthetics can bind at clinically relevant concentrations?

How Do Anesthetics Interfere with the Electrophysiologic Function of the Nervous System?

The functional unit of the CNS is the neuron, and ultimately general anesthetics must disrupt the function of neurons mediating behavior, consciousness, and memory. In the simplest terms, anesthetics could accomplish this by altering the intrinsic firing rate of individual neurons, termed neuronal excitability, and/or by altering communication between neurons, generally occurring via synaptic transmission.

Neuronal Excitability

Neurons transmit information down their axons through action potentials. The propensity of a neuron to generate and propagate action potentials from the cell body to their nerve terminals is called its excitability. Intrinsic neuronal excitability is chiefly determined by three parameters: resting membrane potential, the threshold potential for action-potential generation, and the size/propagation of the action potential. Anesthetics can hyperpolarize (create a more negative resting membrane potential) both spinal motor neurons and cortical neurons,[53,54] and this ability to hyperpolarize neurons correlates with anesthetic potency. In general, the hyperpolarization produced by anesthetics is small in magnitude and is unlikely to alter *propagation* of an action potential down an axon. Small changes in resting potential may, however, inhibit the *initiation* of an action potential generated in response to synaptic excitation or in a spontaneously firing neuron. Indeed, isoflurane has been shown to hyperpolarize thalamic neurons, leading to an inhibition of tonic firing of action potentials.[55] Anesthetics have not been shown to reliably alter the threshold potential of a neuron for action-potential generation. However, the data are conflicting on whether the size of the action potential, once initiated, is diminished by general anesthetics. A classic article by Larrabee and Posternak[56] demonstrated that concentrations of ether and chloroform that completely block synaptic transmission in mammalian sympathetic ganglia have no effect on presynaptic action-potential amplitude. Similar results have been obtained with fluorinated volatile anesthetics in mammalian brain preparations.[57,58] This dogma that the action potential is relatively resistant to general anesthetics has been challenged by more recent reports that volatile anesthetics at clinical concentrations produce a small but significant reduction in the size of the action potential in mammalian neurons.[59-61] At a large synapse, amenable to direct measurement of the action potential and transmitter release in the same neuron, the slightly smaller action potential was shown to produce a substantial reduction in transmitter release due to the exponential relationship between the two.[60] Thus, while current data still support the prevailing view that neuronal excitability is only slightly affected by general anesthetics, this small effect may nevertheless contribute significantly to the clinical actions of volatile anesthetics.

Synaptic Transmission

Synaptic transmission is widely considered to be the most likely subcellular site of general anesthetic action. Neurotransmission across both excitatory and inhibitory synapses is markedly altered by general anesthetics. General anesthetics inhibit excitatory synaptic transmission in a variety of preparations, including sympathetic ganglia,[56] olfactory cortex,[57] hippocampus,[58] and spinal cord.[62] However, not all excitatory synapses appear to be equally sensitive to anesthetics; indeed, transmission across some hippocampal excitatory synapses is enhanced by inhalational anesthetics.[63] In a similar fashion, general anesthetics both enhance and depress inhibitory synaptic transmission in various preparations. In a classic article in 1975, Nicoll et al.[64] showed that barbiturates enhanced inhibitory synaptic transmission by prolonging the decay of the GABAergic inhibitory postsynaptic current. Enhancement of inhibitory transmission has also been observed with many other general anesthetics including etomidate,[65] propofol,[66] inhalational anesthetics,[67] and neurosteroids.[68] As discussed below, a growing body of genetic experiments in mice demonstrate that the potentiation of GABAergic inhibitory postsynaptic currents is necessary for a significant portion of the behavioral effects of each of these classes of anesthetics.

Presynaptic Effects

Neurotransmitter release at glutamatergic synapses has consistently been found to be inhibited by clinical concentrations of volatile anesthetics. For example, a study by Perouansky et al.[69] conducted in mouse hippocampal slices showed that halothane inhibited excitatory postsynaptic potentials elicited by presynaptic electrical stimulation, but not those elicited by direct application of glutamate. This indicates that halothane must be acting to prevent the release of glutamate. MacIver and Roth[63] extended these observations by finding that the inhibition of glutamate release from hippocampal neurons is not due to effects at GABAergic synapses that could indirectly decrease transmitter release from glutamatergic neurons. Reduction of glutamate release by intravenous anesthetics has also been demonstrated, but the evidence is more limited and the effects potentially indirect.[70,71]

The data for anesthetic effects on inhibitory neurotransmitter release are mixed. Inhibition,[72] stimulation,[73,74] and no effect[75] on GABA release have been reported for both volatile and intravenous anesthetics. In a brain synaptosomal preparation where both GABA and glutamate release could be studied simultaneously, Westphalen and Hemmings[76] found that glutamate and, to a lesser degree, GABA release were inhibited by clinical concentrations of isoflurane. More recently the same group has shown that release from norepinephrine, dopamine, and acetylcholine-containing synaptosomes is also inhibited by isoflurane, although again less potently compared to glutamatergic synaptosomes.[77] The mechanism underlying anesthetic effects on transmitter release has not been established. The mechanism does not appear to involve reduced neurotransmitter synthesis or storage, but rather is a direct effect on neurosecretion. A variety of evidence argues that at some synapses a substantial portion of the anesthetic effect is upstream of the transmitter release machinery,[78] perhaps on presynaptic sodium channels or potassium leak channels (see later discussion). However, genetic data in *Caenorhabditis elegans* show that mutations in the transmitter release machinery strongly influence volatile anesthetic sensitivity.[79,80] Recent evidence in rodent preparations suggests that this mechanism may be conserved in mammals.[81]

Postsynaptic Effects

At a variety of synapses, anesthetics alter the postsynaptic response to released neurotransmitter. Anesthetic modulation of excitatory neurotransmitter receptor function varies depending on the receptor type, anesthetic agent, and preparation. In a classic study, Richards and Smaje[82] examined the effects of several anesthetic agents on the response of olfactory cortical neurons to application of glutamate, the major excitatory neurotransmitter in the CNS. They found that while pentobarbital, diethyl ether, methoxyflurane, and alphaxalone depressed the electrical response to glutamate, halothane did not. In contrast, when acetylcholine was applied to the same olfactory cortical preparation, halothane and methoxyflurane stimulated the electrical response, whereas pentobarbital had no effect; only alphaxalone depressed the electrical response to acetylcholine.[82,83]

Anesthetic modulation of neuronal responses to inhibitory neurotransmitters is more consistent. A wide variety of

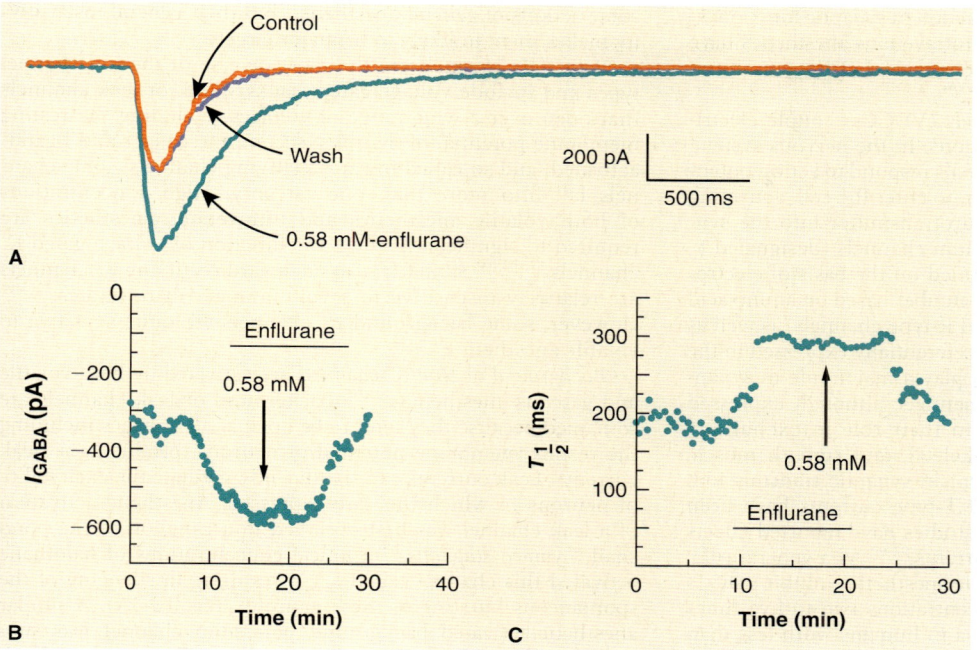

Figure 10-2 Enflurane potentiates the ability of GABA (γ-aminobutyric acid) to activate a chloride current in cultured rat hippocampal cells. This potentiation is rapidly reversed by removal of enflurane (wash; **A**). Enflurane increases both the amplitude of the current (**B**) and the time ($\tau_{1/2}$) it takes for the current to decay (**C**). (Reproduced with permission from Jones MV, Brooks PA, Harrison L. Enhancement of γ-aminobutyric acid-activated Cl⁻ currents in cultured rat hippocampal neurones by three volatile anaesthetics. *J Physiol.* 1992;449:289.)

anesthetics, including barbiturates, etomidate, neurosteroids, propofol, and the fluorinated volatile anesthetics, have been shown to potentiate the electrical response to exogenously applied GABA (for reviews, see Refs.[84,85]). For example, Figure 10-2 illustrates the ability of enflurane to increase both the amplitude and the duration of the current elicited by application of GABA to hippocampal neurons.[86]

Summary

Anesthetics alter the two fundamental determinants of neuronal communication, neuronal excitability and synaptic transmission. Anesthetics have powerful and widespread effects on synaptic transmission that would logically contribute to general anesthesia. Thus, the synapse is generally thought to be the more relevant site of anesthetic action. Existing evidence indicates that even at the synapse, anesthetics have diverse actions, including presynaptic inhibition of neurotransmitter release, inhibition of excitatory neurotransmitter effect, and enhancement of inhibitory neurotransmitter effect. Furthermore, the synaptic effects of anesthetics differ among various anesthetic agents, neurotransmitters, and neuronal preparations.

Anesthetic Actions on Ion Channels

Ion channels are a likely target of anesthetic action. The advent of patch clamp techniques in the early 1980s made it possible to measure directly the currents from single ion channel proteins. Accordingly, during the 1980s and 1990s a major effort was directed at describing the effects of anesthetics on the various kinds of ion channels. The following section summarizes and distills this effort. For the purposes of this discussion, ion channels are cataloged according to the stimuli to which they respond by opening or closing (i.e., their mechanism of gating).

Anesthetic Effects on Voltage-dependent Ion Channels

A variety of ion channels can sense a change in membrane potential and respond by either opening or closing their pores. These channels include voltage-dependent sodium, potassium, and calcium channels, all of which share significant structural homologies. Voltage-dependent sodium and potassium channels are largely involved in generating and shaping action potentials. The effects of anesthetics on these channels have been extensively studied by Haydon and Urban[87] in the squid giant axon. These studies show that these invertebrate sodium and potassium channels are remarkably insensitive to volatile anesthetics. For example, the halothane concentration required to inhibit 50% of the peak sodium channel current is eight times the halothane concentration required to produce anesthesia. The delayed rectifier potassium channel was even less sensitive, requiring halothane concentrations more than 20 times those required to produce anesthesia. Similar results have been obtained in a mammalian cell line (GH₃ pituitary cells) where both sodium and potassium currents were inhibited by halothane only at concentrations greater than five times those required to produce anesthesia.[88] However, more recent studies with volatile anesthetics have challenged the notion that voltage-dependent sodium channels are insensitive to anesthetics.[89] Rehberg et al.[90] expressed rat brain IIA sodium channels in a mammalian cell line, and showed that clinically relevant concentrations of a variety of inhalational anesthetics suppressed voltage-elicited sodium currents. Ratnakumari and Hemmings[91] showed that sodium flux mediated by rat brain sodium channels was significantly inhibited by clinical concentrations of halothane. Shiraishi and Harris[92] documented the effects of isoflurane on a variety of sodium channel subtypes and found that several but not all subtypes are sensitive to clinical concentrations. Finally, as previously described, in a rat brainstem neuron, Wu et al.[60] found that a small inhibition of sodium currents by isoflurane resulted in a large inhibition of synaptic activity. Thus, sodium channel activity not only appears to be inhibited by volatile anesthetics, but this inhibition results in a significant reduction in synaptic function, at least at some mammalian synapses. Intravenous anesthetics have also been shown to inhibit sodium channels, but the concentrations for this effect are supraclinical.[93,94]

Voltage-dependent calcium channels (VDCCs) couple electrical activity to specific cellular functions. In the nervous system, VDCCs located at presynaptic terminals respond to action potentials by opening. This allows calcium to enter the cell, activating calcium-dependent secretion of neurotransmitter into the synaptic cleft. At least six types of calcium channels (designated L, N, P, Q, R, and T) have been identified on the basis of electrophysiologic properties, and a larger number based on amino acid sequence similarities. N-, P-, Q-, and R-type channels, as well as some of the untitled channels, are preferentially expressed in the nervous system and are thought to play a major role in synaptic transmission. L-type calcium channels, although expressed in brain, have been best studied in their role in excitation–contraction coupling in cardiac, skeletal, and smooth muscle and are thought to be less important in synaptic transmission. The anesthetics' actions on L- and T-type currents have been well characterized,[88,95,96] and some studies have reported effects of anesthetics on N- and P-type currents.[97–99] As a general rule, these studies have shown that volatile anesthetics inhibit VDCCs (50% reduction in current) at concentrations two to five times those required to produce anesthesia in humans, with less than a 20% inhibition of calcium current at clinical concentrations of anesthetics. However, some studies have found VDCCs that are extremely sensitive to anesthetics. Takenoshita and Steinbach[100] reported a T-type calcium current in dorsal root ganglion neurons that was inhibited by subanesthetic concentrations of halothane. Additionally, Ffrench-Mullen et al.[101] have reported a VDCC of unspecified type in guinea pig hippocampus that is inhibited by pentobarbital at concentrations identical to those required to produce anesthesia. Thus, VDCCs could well mediate

some actions of general anesthetics, but their general insensitivity makes them unlikely to be major targets.

Potassium channels are the most diverse of the ion channel types and include voltage-gated, background, or leak channels that open over a wide range of voltages, including the resting membrane potential of neurons, second messenger and ligand-activated, and so-called inward rectifying channels; some channels fall into more than one category. High concentrations of both volatile anesthetics and intravenous anesthetics are required to significantly affect the function of voltage-gated K^+ channels.[87,102,103] Similarly, classic inward rectifying K^+ channels are relatively insensitive to sevoflurane and barbiturates.[104–106] However, some background K^+ channels are quite sensitive to volatile anesthetics.

Background or *leak K^+ channels* are activated by both volatile and gaseous anesthetics.[107,108] Background or leak channels are so named because they tend to be open at all voltages including the resting membrane potential of neurons, producing a "leak current." Leak currents can significantly regulate the excitability of neurons in which they are expressed. Anesthetic activation of a leak channel was first observed in a ganglion of the pond snail, *Lymnea stagnalis*.[109] Clinical concentrations of halothane activated this channel called $I_{K(AN)}$, resulting in silencing of the spontaneous bursting of these neurons (Fig. 10-3A). A similar anesthetic-activated background potassium channel was subsequently found by Winegar and Yost[110] in the marine mollusk *Aplysia*. The importance of volatile anesthetic activation of these invertebrate potassium channels has now become apparent with the discovery of a large family of background potassium channels in mammals. These mammalian potassium channels share a unique structure with two pore-forming domains in tandem, plus four transmembrane segments (2P/4TM; Fig. 10-3C,D).[111] Patel et al.[112] have studied the effects of volatile anesthetics on several members of the mammalian 2P/4TM family. They have shown that

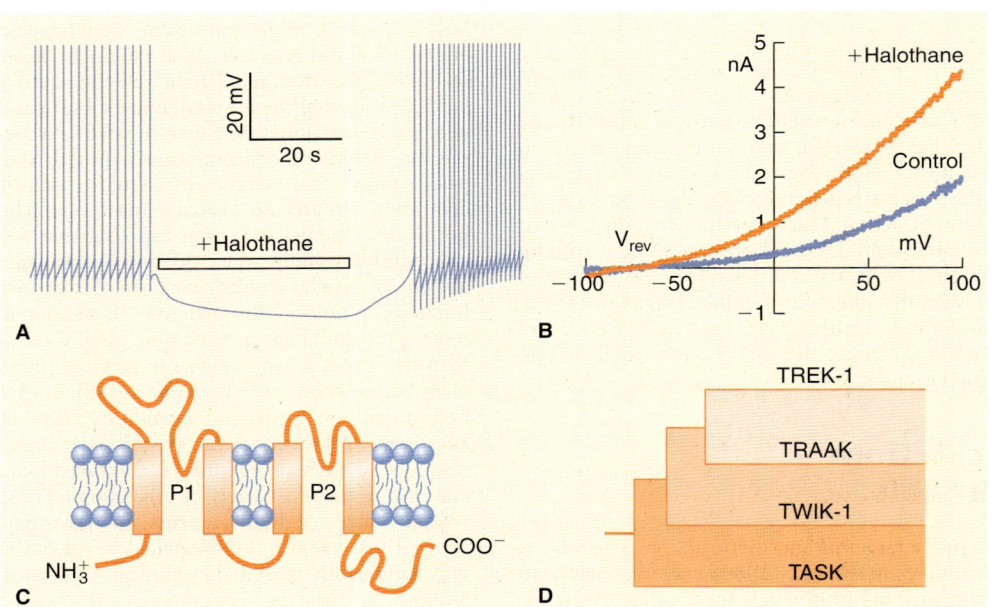

Figure 10-3 Volatile anesthetics activate background K^+ channels. **A:** Halothane reversibly hyperpolarizes a pacemaker neuron from *Lymnaea stagnalis* (the pond snail) by activating I_{Kan}. **B:** Halothane (300 μM) activates human recombinant TREK-1 channels expressed in COS cells. The figure shows current–voltage relationships with reversal potential (V_{rev}) of –88 mV, indicative of a K^+ channel. **C:** Predicted structure of a typical subunit of the mammalian background K^+ channels. Note the four transmembrane spanning segments (*orange rectangles*) and the two pore-forming domains (P1 and P2). Some, but not all of these 2P/4TM K^+ channels are activated by volatile anesthetics. **D:** Phylogenetic tree for the 2P/4TM family. (Reproduced with permission from Franks NP, Lieb WR. Background K^+ channels: an important target for anesthetics? *Nat Neurosci.* 1999;2:395.)

TREK-1 channels are activated by clinical concentrations of chloroform, diethyl ether, halothane, and isoflurane (Fig. 10-3B). In contrast, closely related TRAAK channels are insensitive to all the volatile anesthetics, and TASK channels are activated by halothane and isoflurane, inhibited by diethyl ether, and unaffected by chloroform. These authors further showed that the C-terminal regions of TASK and TREK-1 contain amino acids essential for anesthetic action. TREK-1 but not TASK was found to be activated by clinical concentrations of the gaseous anesthetics xenon, nitrous oxide, and cyclopropane.[113] Thus, activation of background K$^+$ channels in mammalian vertebrates could be an important and general mechanism through which inhalational and gaseous anesthetics regulate neuronal resting membrane potential and thereby excitability. Indeed, genetic evidence argues for a role of these channels in producing anesthesia (see later discussion).

Hyperpolarization-activated cyclic nucleotide-gated channels (HCN channels) are a relatively recently discovered channel type that is modulated by clinical concentrations of both volatile and some intravenous anesthetics. HCN channels pass a depolarizing current (termed I_h in the CNS) consisting of a mix of sodium and potassium ions and are activated by membrane hyperpolarization, the voltage dependence of which is shifted to a more depolarized range with the second messenger cyclic AMP.[114] Therefore, cAMP activates HCN channels under most physiologic conditions. HCN channels are composed of homomeric and heteromeric combinations of four subunits—HCN1, 2, 3, 4, all of which are expressed in both brain and heart. HCN channels have been shown to regulate resting membrane potential and rhythmic firing of both the sinoatrial node and spontaneously spiking neurons. Thus, they are important for synchronous oscillations of neuronal networks.[114]

Volatile anesthetics, propofol, and ketamine have been shown to inhibit HCN-mediated currents in both cell culture and native mouse neurons. The Bayliss group has shown that halothane shifted to more negative membrane potentials the voltage-dependent activation of the I_h current, and also inhibited its maximal amplitude.[115] Expression of HCN1 and HCN2 homomeric channels in cultured cells showed that halothane altered voltage-dependence of activation of HCN1 channels while reducing the maximal amplitude of HCN2 currents. In isolated spinal motor neurons, halothane reduced the I_h current, consistent with inhibition of HCN channels. Similar inhibition of HCN1 channels was subsequently observed with clinical concentrations of propofol and ketamine.[116,117] The inhibition of HCN1 by ketamine was stereoselective in the same manner as its stereoselectivity for general anesthesia.[116] Notably in this same study, etomidate was not found to inhibit HCN1 channel activation. Thus, HCN1 channels may be important for the actions of both volatile anesthetics and a subset of intravenous anesthetics. Genetic experiments described below argue that anesthetic inhibition of HCN1 and HCN2 channels may contribute to anesthesia.

Summary

Existing evidence suggests that most VDCCs are modestly sensitive or insensitive to anesthetics. However, some sodium channel subtypes are inhibited by volatile anesthetics, and this effect may be responsible in part for a reduction in neurotransmitter release at some synapses. Recent evidence suggests that members of the 2P/4TM family of background potassium channels may be important in producing some components of the anesthetic state. Additionally, the HCN family of channels has emerged as a potentially relevant anesthetic target for both volatile and intravenous anesthetics.

Anesthetic Effects on Ligand-gated Ion Channels

Fast excitatory and inhibitory neurotransmission is mediated by the actions of ligand-gated ion channels. Synaptically released glutamate or GABA diffuse across the synaptic cleft and bind to channel proteins that open as a consequence of neurotransmitter release. The channel proteins that bind GABA (GABA$_A$ receptors) are members of a superfamily of structurally related ligand-gated ion channel proteins that include nicotinic acetylcholine receptors, glycine receptors, and 5-HT$_3$ receptors. Based on the structure of the nicotinic acetylcholine receptor, each ligand-gated channel is thought to be composed of five subunits. The glutamate receptors comprise another family, with each receptor thought to be a tetrameric protein composed of structurally related subunits. These ligand-gated ion channels provide a logical target for anesthetic action because selective effects on these channels could inhibit fast excitatory synaptic transmission and/or facilitate fast inhibitory synaptic transmission. The effects of anesthetic agents on ligand-gated ion channels have been thoroughly cataloged in several reviews.[34,84,118,119] The following section provides a brief summary of this large body of work.

Glutamate-activated Ion Channels

Glutamate-activated ion channels have been classified, based on selective agonists, into three categories: AMPA receptors, kainate receptors, and NMDA receptors. AMPA and kainate receptors are relatively nonselective monovalent cation channels involved in fast excitatory synaptic transmission, whereas NMDA channels conduct not only Na$^+$ and K$^+$, but also Ca^{++}. They are involved in long-term modulation of synaptic responses (long-term potentiation). Studies from the early 1980s in mouse and rat brain preparations showed that AMPA- and kainate-activated currents are insensitive to clinical concentrations of halothane,[120] enflurane,[121] and the neurosteroid allopregnanolone.[122] In contrast, kainate- and AMPA-activated currents were shown to be sensitive to barbiturates. In rat hippocampal neurons, 50 μM pentobarbital (pentobarbital produces anesthesia at approximately 50 μM) inhibited kainate and AMPA responses by 50%.[122] Studies using cloned and expressed glutamate receptor subunits show that submaximal agonist responses of GluR3 (AMPA-type) receptors are inhibited by fluorinated volatile anesthetics, whereas agonist responses of GluR6 (kainate-type) receptors are enhanced.[123] In contrast, both GluR3 and GluR6 receptors are inhibited by pentobarbital. The directionally opposite effects of the volatile anesthetics on different glutamate receptor subtypes may explain the earlier inconclusive effects observed in tissue, where multiple subunit types are expressed. These opposite effects have also been used as a strategy to identify critical sites on the molecules involved in anesthetic effect. By producing GluR3/GluR6 receptor chimeras (receptors made up of various combinations of sections of the GluR3 and GluR6 receptors) and screening for volatile anesthetic effect, specific areas of the protein required for volatile anesthetic potentiation of GluR6 have been identified. Subsequent site-directed mutagenesis studies have identified a specific glycine residue (Gly-819) as critical for volatile anesthetic action on GluR6-containing receptors.[124]

NMDA-activated currents are also sensitive to a subset of anesthetics. Electrophysiologic studies show virtually no effects of clinical concentrations of volatile anesthetics,[120,121] neurosteroids, or barbiturates[122] on NMDA-activated currents. On the other hand, biochemical flux studies have shown that volatile anesthetics may inhibit NMDA-activated channels. A study in rat brain

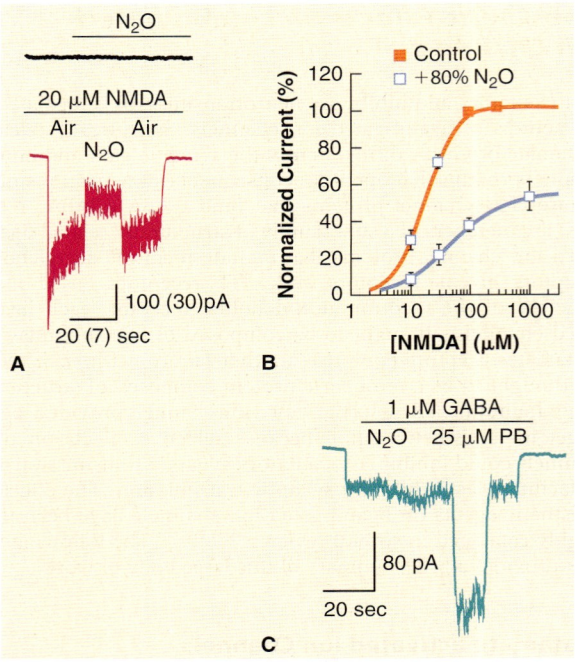

ketamine in intact animals show the same stereoselectivity as that observed in vitro,[29] consistent with the hypothesis that the NMDA receptor is a relevant molecular target for the anesthetic actions of ketamine. Two other recent findings suggest that NMDA receptors may also be an important target for nitrous oxide and xenon. These studies show that N_2O[129,130] and xenon[131] are potent and selective inhibitors of NMDA-activated currents. This is illustrated in Figure 10-4, showing that N_2O inhibits NMDA-elicited, but not GABA-elicited, currents in hippocampal neurons.

GABA-activated Ion Channels

GABA is the most important inhibitory neurotransmitter in the mammalian CNS. GABA-activated ion channels ($GABA_A$ receptors) mediate the postsynaptic response to synaptically released GABA by selectively allowing chloride ions to enter, and thereby hyperpolarize neurons. $GABA_A$ receptors are pentameric multisubunit proteins consisting of various combinations of α, β, δ, and ε subunits, and there are many subtypes of each of these subunits. The function of $GABA_A$ receptors is modulated by a wide variety of pharmacologic agents including convulsants, anticonvulsants, sedatives, anxiolytics, and anesthetics.[84] The effects of these various drugs on $GABA_A$ receptor function varies across brain regions and cell types. The following section briefly reviews the effects of anesthetics on $GABA_A$ receptor function.

Barbiturates, anesthetic steroids, benzodiazepines, propofol, etomidate, and the volatile anesthetics all modulate $GABA_A$ receptor function.[86,132–135] These drugs produce three kinds of effects on the electrophysiologic behavior of the $GABA_A$ receptor channels: potentiation, direct gating, and inhibition. *Potentiation* refers to the ability of anesthetics to increase markedly the current elicited by low concentrations of GABA. Potentiation is illustrated in Figure 10-5, showing the effects of halothane on currents elicited by a range of GABA concentrations in dissociated cortical neurons. Anesthetic potentiation of $GABA_A$ currents generally occurs at concentrations of anesthetics within the clinical range. *Direct gating* refers to the ability of anesthetics to activate $GABA_A$ channels in the absence of GABA. Generally, direct gating of $GABA_A$ currents occurs at anesthetic concentrations higher than those used clinically, but the concentration–response curves for potentiation and for direct gating can overlap. It is not known whether direct gating of $GABA_A$ channels is either required for or contributes to the effects of

Figure 10-4 Nitrous oxide inhibits NMDA-elicited, but not GABA-elicited currents in rat hippocampal neurons. **A:** Eighty percent N_2O has no effect on holding current (upper trace), but inhibits the current elicited by NMDA. **B:** N_2O causes a rightward and downward shift of the NMDA concentration–response curve, indicating a mixed competitive/noncompetitive antagonism. **C:** Eighty percent N_2O has little effect on GABA-elicited currents. In contrast, an equipotent anesthetic concentration of pentobarbital markedly enhances the GABA-elicited current. (Reproduced with permission from Jevtovic-Todorovic V, Todorovic SM, Mennerick S, et al. Nitrous oxide (laughing gas) is an NMDA antagonist, neuroprotectant, and neurotoxin. *Nat Med*. 1998;4:460.)

microvesicles showed that anesthetic concentrations (0.2 to 0.3 mM) of halothane and enflurane inhibited NMDA-activated calcium flux by 50%.[125] Ketamine is a potent and selective inhibitor of NMDA-activated currents. Ketamine stereoselectively inhibits NMDA currents by binding to the phencyclidine site on the NMDA receptor protein.[126–128] The anesthetic effects of

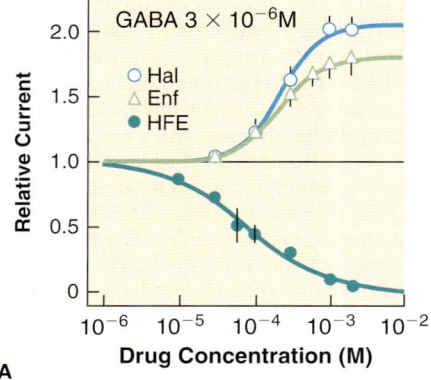
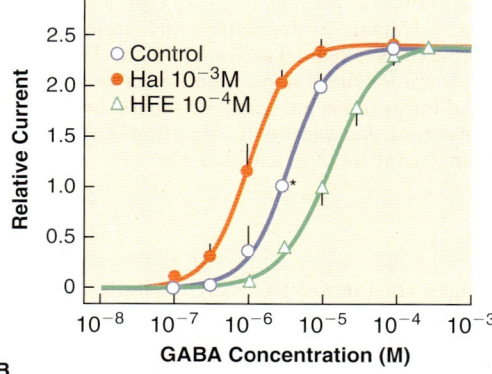

Figure 10-5 The effects of halothane (Hal), enflurane (Enf), and fluorothyl (HFE) on GABA-activated chloride currents in dissociated rat CNS neurons. **A:** Clinical concentrations of halothane and enflurane potentiate the ability of GABA to elicit a chloride current. The convulsant fluorothyl antagonizes the effects of GABA (γ-aminobutyric acid). **B:** GABA causes a concentration-dependent activation of a chloride current. Halothane shifts the GABA concentration–response curve to the left (increases the apparent affinity of the channel for GABA), whereas fluorothyl shifts the curve to the right (decreases the apparent affinity of the channel for GABA). (Reproduced with permission from Wakamori M, Ikemoto Y, Akaike N. Effects of two volatile anesthetics and a volatile convulsant on the excitatory and inhibitory amino acid responses in dissociated CNS neurons of the rat. *J Neurophysiol*. 1991;66:2014.)

anesthetics on GABA-mediated inhibitory synaptic transmission in vivo. In the case of anesthetic steroids, strong evidence indicates that potentiation, rather than direct gating of GABA$_A$ currents, is required for producing anesthesia.[30] Anesthetics can also inhibit GABA-activated currents. *Inhibition* refers to the ability of anesthetics to prevent GABA from initiating current flow through GABA$_A$ channels, and has generally been observed at high concentrations of both GABA and anesthetics.[136,137] Inhibition of GABA$_A$ channels may help to explain why volatile anesthetics have, in some cases, been observed to inhibit rather than facilitate inhibitory synaptic transmission.[138]

Effects of anesthetics have also been observed on the function of single GABA$_A$ channels. These studies show that barbiturates,[135] propofol,[133] and volatile anesthetics[139] do not alter the conductance (rate at which ions traverse the open channel) of the channel; instead, they increase the frequency with which the channel opens and/or the average length of time that the channel remains open. Collectively, the whole cell and single channel data are most consistent with the idea that clinical concentrations of anesthetics produce a change in the conformation of GABA$_A$ receptors that increases the affinity of the receptor for GABA. This is consistent with the ability of anesthetics to increase the duration of inhibitory postsynaptic potentials, since higher affinity binding of GABA would slow the dissociation of GABA from postsynaptic GABA$_A$ channels. Anesthetics would not be expected to increase the peak amplitude of a GABAergic inhibitory postsynaptic potential, since synaptically released GABA probably reaches very high concentrations in the synapse. Higher concentrations of anesthetics can produce additional effects, either directly activating or inhibiting GABA$_A$ channels. For example, a study by Banks and Pearce[140] showed that isoflurane and enflurane simultaneously increased the duration and decreased the amplitude of GABAergic inhibitory postsynaptic currents in hippocampal slices.

Despite the similar effects of many anesthetics on GABA$_A$ receptor function, different anesthetics act on distinct subtypes of GABA$_A$ receptors. This is well illustrated for benzodiazepine sensitivity, which requires the presence of the γ_2 subunit subtype.[141] Sensitivity to etomidate has been shown to require the presence of a β_2 or β_3 subunit.[142] The presence of a δ or ϵ subunit in a GABA$_A$ receptor has been shown to confer insensitivity to the potentiating effects of some anesthetics.[143,144] Interestingly, GABA$_A$ receptors composed of ρ-type subunits (referred to as *GABA$_C$ receptors*) have been shown to be inhibited rather than potentiated by volatile anesthetics.[145] This property has been exploited to construct chimeric receptors composed of part of the ρ-receptor coupled to part of an α, β, or glycine receptor subunit. By screening these chimeras for anesthetic sensitivity, regions of the α, β, and glycine subunits responsible for anesthetic sensitivity have been identified. Based on the results of these chimeric studies, site-directed mutagenesis studies were performed to identify the specific amino acids responsible for conferring anesthetic sensitivity. These studies revealed two critical amino acids, near the extracellular regions of transmembrane domains 2 and 3 (TM2, TM3) of the glycine and GABA$_A$ receptors, that are required for volatile anesthetic potentiation of agonist effect.[146] It is not yet clear if these amino acids represent a volatile anesthetic binding site, or whether they are sites critical to transducing anesthetic-induced conformational changes in the receptor molecule. Interestingly, one of the amino acids shown to be critical to volatile anesthetic effect (TM3 site) has also been shown to be required (in the β_2/β_3 subunit) for the potentiating effects of etomidate.[147] In contrast, the TM2 and TM3 sites do not appear to be required for potentiation by propofol, barbiturates, or neurosteroids.[148] A distinct amino acid in the TM3 region of the β_1 subunit of the GABA$_A$ receptor has been shown to selectively modulate the ability of propofol to potentiate GABA agonist effects. Neurosteroid effects on GABA$_A$ receptors occur via interactions with specific sites within the transmembrane spanning regions of the α_1 and β_2 subunits, distinct from those in which benzodiazepines and pentobarbital act.[149] Collectively, these data provide strong evidence that anesthetics act at multiple unique sites on the GABA$_A$ receptor protein.

Other Ligand-activated Ion Channels

Ligand-gated receptors structurally similar to the GABA$_A$ receptor, including the nicotinic acetylcholine receptors (muscle and neuronal types), glycine receptors, and 5-HT$_3$ receptors, have been shown to be modulated by general anesthetics.[150] The muscle nicotinic receptor has served as a useful model because of its abundance and the wealth of knowledge about its structure. This nicotinic receptor subtype has been shown to be inhibited by anesthetic concentrations in the clinical range[151] and to be desensitized by higher concentrations of anesthetics.[152] Neuronal nicotinic receptors are structurally similar to the muscle type and are widely expressed in the mammalian CNS. Neuronal nicotinic receptors in molluscan neurons[153] and in bovine chromaffin cells[154] were found to be inhibited by clinical concentrations of volatile anesthetics. Studies using cloned and expressed neuronal nicotinic receptor subunits have shown a high degree of subunit and anesthetic selectivity. In receptors composed of various combinations of α_2, α_4, β_2, and β_4 subunits, acetylcholine-elicited currents are inhibited by *subanesthetic* concentrations of halothane[155] or isoflurane.[156] In contrast, these receptors are relatively insensitive to propofol, and receptors composed of only α_7 subunits are insensitive to both isoflurane and propofol.[156,157] Subsequent pharmacologic experiments using selective inhibitors of neuronal nicotinic receptors led to the conclusion that these receptors are unlikely to have a major role in immobilization by volatile anesthetics.[158,159] However, they might play a role in the amnestic or hypnotic effects of volatile anesthetics.[160]

Glycine is an important inhibitory neurotransmitter, particularly in the spinal cord and brainstem. The glycine receptor is a member of the ligand-activated channel superfamily that, like the GABA$_A$ receptor, is chloride-selective. A large number of studies have shown that clinical concentrations of volatile anesthetics potentiate glycine-activated currents in intact neurons[120] and in cloned glycine receptors expressed in oocytes.[161,162] Volatile anesthetics appear to produce their potentiating effect by increasing the affinity of the receptor for glycine, much like for GABA$_A$ receptors.[161] Propofol,[133] alphaxalone, and pentobarbital also potentiate glycine-activated currents, whereas etomidate and ketamine do not.[162] Potentiation of glycine receptor function may contribute to the anesthetic action of volatile anesthetics and some parenteral anesthetics.

The 5-HT$_3$ receptors are also members of the genetically related superfamily of ligand-gated receptor channels. Clinical concentrations of volatile anesthetics potentiate currents activated by 5-hydroxytryptamine in intact cells[163] and in cloned receptors expressed in oocytes.[164] In contrast, thiopental inhibits 5-HT$_3$ receptor currents[163] and propofol is without effect on these receptor channels.[164] The 5-HT$_3$ receptors may play some role in the anesthetic state produced by volatile anesthetics and may also contribute to some unpleasant anesthetic side effects such as nausea and vomiting.

Summary

Several ligand-gated ion channels are modulated by clinical concentrations of anesthetics. Ketamine, N$_2$O, and xenon inhibit NMDA-type glutamate receptors, and this effect may play a major role in their mechanism of action. A large body of evidence shows that many anesthetics potentiate GABA-activated currents in the CNS. This suggests that GABA$_A$ receptors are a probable molecular target of anesthetics. Other members of the ligand-activated ion channel family, including glycine receptors, neuronal nicotinic receptors, and 5-HT$_3$ receptors, are also affected by anesthetics and remain plausible anesthetic targets.

How Are the Molecular Effects of Anesthetics Linked to Anesthesia in the Intact Organism?

The previous sections have described how anesthetics affect the function of a number of ion channels and signaling proteins, probably via direct anesthetic–protein interactions. However, these *in vitro* experiments do not allow for determining which, if any, of these effects of anesthetics on protein function are necessary and/or sufficient to produce anesthesia in an intact organism. A number of approaches have been employed to try to link anesthetic effects observed at a molecular level to anesthesia in intact animals. These approaches and their pitfalls are briefly explored in the following section.

Pharmacologic Approaches

An experimental paradigm frequently used to study anesthetic mechanisms is to administer a drug thought to act specifically at a putative anesthetic target (e.g., a receptor agonist or antagonist, an ion channel activator or antagonist), then determine whether the drug has either increased or decreased the animal's sensitivity to a given anesthetic. The underlying assumption is that if a change in anesthetic sensitivity is observed, then the anesthetic is likely to act via an action on the specific target of the administered drug. However, conclusions from this approach must be tempered by a number of considerations. The drugs used to modulate anesthetic sensitivity usually have their own direct effects on CNS excitability and thus may *indirectly* affect anesthetic requirements. For example, while α$_2$-adrenergic agonists decrease halothane MAC,[165] they are profound CNS depressants in their own right and produce anesthesia by mechanisms distinct from those used by volatile anesthetics. Thus, the "MAC-sparing" effects of α$_2$-agonists provide little insight into how halothane works. A more useful pharmacologic strategy would be to identify drugs that have no effect on CNS excitability but prevent the effects of given anesthetics. Currently, however, there are no such anesthetic antagonists. Development of specific antagonists for anesthetic agents would provide a major tool for linking anesthetic effects at the molecular level to anesthesia in the intact organism, and might also be of significant clinical utility.

An alternative pharmacologic approach is to develop "litmus tests" for the relevance of anesthetic effects observed in vitro. One such test takes advantage of compounds that are nonanesthetic despite the predictions of the Meyer–Overton rule.[23] Another test uses anesthetic stereoselectivity as the discriminator, with the assumption that a target not affected with the same stereoselectivity as that observed for whole animal anesthesia is unlikely to be relevant to the production of anesthesia.[166] Although these tests may increase the plausibility of a particular target, they cannot be used definitively to rule out a potential target. For example, a nonanesthetic might depress CNS excitability via its actions on an important anesthetic target site while simultaneously producing counterbalancing excitatory effects at a second site. In this case the "litmus test" would incorrectly eliminate the anesthetic site as irrelevant to whole-animal anesthesia. This example is quite plausible given the convulsant effects of many of the nonanesthetic polyhalogenated hydrocarbons. Likewise, anesthetics may act stereoselectively on some relevant targets and nonstereoselectively on others. Another sort of litmus test is to antagonize the putative anesthetic target. If anesthetic effects are mediated through this target, inactivation of the target by the antagonist should result in anesthetic resistance. Using this logic, the modest MAC-sparing effects of GABA$_A$ and glycine receptor antagonists were used to argue that both GABA$_A$ and glycine receptors mediate some but not all of the immobilizing effects of volatile anesthetics in rodents.[167–169] This same group used the lack of effect of neuronal nicotinic antagonists on isoflurane MAC to conclude that these receptors had no role in volatile anesthetic immobilization.[158] Issues of specificity and efficacy of the antagonists prevent these experiments from being definitive. Nevertheless, these results are important and consistent with the conclusions that volatile anesthetics affect the function of a large number of important neuronal proteins, and no one target is likely to mediate all of the effects of these drugs.

Genetic Approaches

An alternative approach to study the relationship between anesthetic effects observed in vitro and whole-animal anesthesia is to alter the structure or abundance of putative anesthetic targets and determine how this affects whole-animal anesthetic sensitivity. While they also have potential flaws, genetic techniques provide the most specific and versatile methods for changing the structure or abundance of putative anesthetic targets. The first true genetic screen for mutants with altered general anesthetic sensitivity was performed in the nematode *C. elegans* by Phil Morgan and Margaret Sedensky.[170] They screened for altered sensitivity to immobilization of *C. elegans* by halothane, which occurs at supraclinical concentrations. The first mutant isolated had a threefold reduction in its EC$_{50}$ for halothane and had an interesting locomotion defect in the absence of halothane called *fainting*. Normal *C. elegans* worms crawl almost continuously whereas "fainter" mutants spontaneously stop moving for extended periods of time. In testing other previously isolated fainter mutants, Morgan and Sedensky found that, in general, fainters were hypersensitive to halothane.[171] Subsequent genetic screens and mapping of fainting mutants have led to a focus on a novel presumptive cation channel, NCA-1/NCA-2, that controls halothane sensitivity in both *C. elegans* and in the fruit fly *Drosophila*.[172] This remarkable conservation of the anesthetic hypersensitivity phenotype across such divergent species argues for a fundamental role of NCA-1/NCA-2 in the action of halothane.

Clinical concentrations of volatile anesthetics do not immobilize *C. elegans*, but they do produce behavioral effects including loss of coordinated movement.[173] Crowder et al. have screened for mutants that are resistant to anesthetic-induced uncoordination and found that mutations in a set of genes encoding proteins regulating neurotransmitter release control anesthetic sensitivity.[79,80] The gene with the largest effect encoded syntaxin 1A, a neuronal protein highly conserved from *C. elegans* to humans and essential for fusion of neurotransmitter vesicles with the presynaptic membrane.[80] Importantly, some syntaxin mutations produced hypersensitivity to volatile anesthetics while others conferred resistance. These allelic differences in anesthetic sensitivity could not be accounted for by effects on the process of transmitter release itself; rather, the genetic data argued that syntaxin interacts with a protein critical for volatile anesthetic action, perhaps an anesthetic target. Subsequent experiments by others in rats have shown that expression of the same mutant syntaxin in cultured rat neurons reduces the potency of isoflurane at inhibiting neurotransmitter release in mammals.[81] A highly evolutionarily conserved presynaptic protein called UNC-13 in *C. elegans* has been implicated in this syntaxin-regulated volatile anesthetic mechanism.[174] *C. elegans unc-13* mutants are fully resistant to the effects of clinical concentrations of isoflurane, and isoflurane prevents the normal synaptic localization of UNC-13 in *C. elegans*. Whether UNC-13 is a direct target of volatile anesthetics is unknown. This same laboratory has also shown by mutant analysis that an NMDA glutamate receptor subunit is essential for nitrous oxide sensitivity in *C. elegans*[175] and that another glutamate receptor subunit is required for the effects of xenon.[176]

In *Drosophila*, clinical concentrations of volatile anesthetics disrupt negative geotaxis behavior and response to a noxious light or heat stimulus.[177–179] Using one or more of these anesthetics effects, Krishnan and Nash[179] performed a forward genetic screen for halothane resistance. The results of this screen have led to a focus on the *Drosophila* homolog of NCA-1/NCA-2. As previously discussed, mutants in the *Drosophila* homolog of NCA-1/NCA-2 are hypersensitive to halothane like the *C. elegans* mutants.[172] The synergy of both *Drosophila* and *C. elegans* genetics should lead to an understanding of how this channel controls volatile anesthetic sensitivity.

In mammals, the most powerful genetic model organism is the mouse, where techniques have been developed to alter or delete any gene of interest. The GABA$_A$ receptor has been extensively studied using mouse genetic techniques.[180] Mice carrying mutations in α, β, and δ GABA$_A$ receptor subunits have been tested for their effects on anesthetic endpoints (Table 10-1). For α subunits,

Table 10-1 Mouse Genetics of Anesthesia

Gene Product	Mutation	Anesthetic Behavioral Effect				References
		Hypnosis	Immobility	Sedation	Amnesia	
GABA$_A$ α$_1$	Global and forebrain KO	**Hal**; Iso, Pentobarb	Iso, Hal, Des		**Iso**	Sonner (2005), Blednov (2003)
GABA$_A$ α$_1$	S270H/L277A	**Iso, Enf, Etom**; Hal	Iso, Hal, Des		**Etom**; Pentobarb	Borghese (2006), Sonner (2007), Werner (2006)
GABA$_A$ α$_4$	Global KO	**Hal**; Iso	Iso, Hal		**Iso**	Rau (2009)
GABA$_A$ α$_5$	Global KO	Etom		Etom	**Etom**; Ket	Cheng (2006), Martin (2009)
GABA$_A$ α$_6$	Global KO	Hal, Enf, Pentobarb	Enf			Homanics (1997)
GABA$_A$ β$_2$	Global KO	Etom, Pentobarb	Etom	**Etom**		Blednov (2003), O'Meara (2004)
GABA$_A$ β$_2$	N265S	**Etom**; Prop, Pentobarb	**Etom**; Prop	**Etom**; Prop		Reynolds (2003), Cirone (2004)
GABA$_A$ β$_3$	Global and forebrain KO	**Etom**; Hal, Enf, Pentobarb	**Hal, Enf**; Iso		**Iso**; Etom	Quinlan (1998), Rau (2011)
GABA$_A$ β$_3$	N265M	**Etom, Prop, Pentobarb**; Neurosteroids, Hal, Enf	*Etom, Prop, Pentobarb*; **Hal, Iso, Enf, Cyclo**; Neurosteroids	Etom	Prop, Iso	Zeller (2007), Zeller (2007), Jurd (2003), Lambert (2005), Liao (2005)
GABA$_A$ δ	Global KO	**Neurosteroids**; Etom, Prop, Ketam, Pentobarb, Hal, Enf	Hal, Enf	Neurosteroids		Mihalek (1999)
TREK-1	Global KO	**Chloro, Des, Iso, Hal, Sevo**; Pentobarb	**Chloro, Des, Hal, Iso, Sevo**			Herteaux (2004)
TASK-1	Global KO	**Iso**; Hal	**Hal**; Iso			Linden (2006), Linden (2008)
TASK-2	Global KO		Hal, Iso, Des			Gerstin (2003)
TASK-3	Global KO	**Hal**; Cyclo, Prop	**Hal**; Iso			Linden (2007), Pang (2009)
HCN1	Global and forebrain KO	**Ket, Prop, Iso, Sevo**; Etom			**Iso**, **Sevo**	Chen (2009), Zhou (2015)
HCN2	Global KO			Xenon		Mattusch (2015)

Bold indicates decreased sensitivity to that anesthetic; italics indicates lack of sensitivity.

four knockout mutations (where the gene is fully inactivated), and one knockin mutation (where a functional but altered gene product is produced), have been examined. Knockout of the α_1 and α_4 subunits produced similar phenotypes, with a large reduction of the efficacy of isoflurane at blocking learning and memory tasks in the mutant mice compared to wild type controls.[181-183] Similarly, an α_5 knockout mouse was strongly resistant to the amnestic effects of etomidate.[184] The α_1 and α_4 knockouts also had small differences for halothane potency in assays of hypnosis. An α_6 knockout strain had normal sensitivities to halothane, enflurane, and pentobarbital in hypnosis and immobility assays.[185] A knockin α_1 mouse strain expressing a double mutated α_1(S270H, L277A) subunit, has also been tested for its anesthetic sensitivity.[186-188] The α_1(S270H) mutation had been shown to block GABA potentiation by volatile anesthetics,[189] but the mutation also increased native sensitivity to GABA, confounding interpretation of the data. Moreover, α_1(S270H) single-mutant mice are quite abnormal behaviorally and are prone to anesthetic-induced seizure activity.[190] Thus, a second mutation, L277A, was introduced into the α_1 subunit that compensated for the change in native gating properties.[186] The α_1(S270H, L277A) mice are viable and demonstrate grossly normal behavior. These mice are mildly resistant to the hypnotic effects of isoflurane, enflurane, and etomidate, as well as to the ataxic effects of etomidate; however, the potency of the drugs in MAC and fear-conditioning assays (a measure of learning) are not altered by the double-mutant α_1 subunit.

While the anesthetic behavioral phenotypes of the α-subunit mutant mice were only incrementally different from wild type mice, β subunit mutants have profound differences for the intravenous anesthetics etomidate and propofol. The electrophysiologic experiments that formed the foundation for generation of the mutant mice showed that etomidate potently inhibited β_2- and β_3-containing GABA$_A$ receptors and was much less potent against β_1-containing receptors.[142,147] Mouse β_2 and β_3 both differ from β_1 at amino residue 265 in the second transmembrane domain with an asparagine (N) in β_2 and β_3, but a serine (S) in β_1 and a methionine (M) in an etomidate-insensitive insect GABA receptor. Electrophysiologic testing of recombinant β_3(N265M) receptors revealed that these mutations blocked potentiation of the receptor by etomidate and propofol.[147,191] An important confirmation of the relevance of these in vitro studies came from Rudolph et al., who showed that a mouse β_3(N265M) knockin strain was fully resistant to the immobilizing effects of etomidate, propofol, and pentobarbital (Fig. 10-6).[192,193] These results provided the first definitive link between an anesthetic in vitro action and a mammalian behavioral endpoint. However, the β_3(N265M) mice were not completely resistant to the hypnotic action of these anesthetics, indicating that other targets mediate this behavioral effect (Table 10-1). Interestingly, the respiratory depressant effects of etomidate and propofol are also blocked by the β_3(N265M) mutation, but the cardiovascular and hypothermic actions of the drugs are not.[194,195] The β_3(N265M) mice also have a modest reduction in sensitivity to the immobilizing actions of volatile anesthetics, suggesting that the β_3 subunit may play a minor role in immobilization, but the mutant has unaltered sensitivity to the amnestic effects of isoflurane and propofol.[194,196] Additional evidence for the importance of the β_3 subunit comes from selective knockout of β_3 in mouse forebrain. In context fear conditioning assays (a measure of hippocampal-dependent memory formation), this strain was found to have an EC_{50} for isoflurane of about threefold higher than that of the wild type strain.[197] The β_2 subunit has also been shown to be important for anesthetic sensitivity. A β_2(N265S) mutant mouse has reduced sensitivity to etomidate, although no anesthetic endpoint is fully blocked by this mutation (Fig. 10-6).[198,199] Finally, strains carrying a knockout mutation of the δ subunit of the GABA$_A$ receptor have a shorter duration of neurosteroid-induced loss-of-righting reflex, whereas their sensitivity to other intravenous and volatile anesthetics is unchanged.[200] Thus, the δ subunit may play a relatively specific role in neurosteroid action.

The roles in anesthetic sensitivity of several background potassium channels have been tested in limited mouse genetic studies. A TREK-1 knockout mouse was found to be significantly, but not fully resistant to multiple volatile anesthetics for hypnotic and immobility endpoints.[201] The volatile anesthetic resistance of the TREK-1 knockout is substantial, particularly for halothane, where MAC was increased by 48%. Importantly, the TREK-1 knockout mice have a normal sensitivity to pentobarbital, indicating specificity for volatile anesthetics consistent with previous electrophysiologic data. Recently, Westphalen et al.[202] has used the TREK-1 knockout strain to test the hypothesis that TREK-1 mediates some of the presynaptic inhibitory effects of volatile anesthetics. Indeed, glutamate release from synaptosomes prepared from the TREK-1 knockout strain is significantly resistant to inhibition by halothane compared to release from wild type control synaptosomes. The role of TASK-2, another two-pore background potassium channel, has been similarly tested by measuring the MAC of a TASK-2 knockout mouse. However, unlike for TREK-1, the TASK-2 knockout has MAC values similar to wild type controls for desflurane, halothane, and isoflurane.[104] This result is somewhat surprising given that TASK-2 is strongly activated by halothane and isoflurane and may be explained by an overall reduced expression in the nervous system compared to TREK-1.[107] Knockout strains for TASK-1 and TASK-3 have modest, but significant volatile anesthetic resistance to hypnosis and immobility (Table 10-1),[203-205] consistent with a role for these channels in anesthesia.

Finally, both global and forebrain-specific knockout mouse strains of the HCN1 subunit and a global knockout of the HCN2 subunit have been generated and tested for their anesthetic sensitivity.[48,116,206-208] The HCN1 global knockout strain is strongly resistant to ketamine (85% increased ED_{50}) and propofol (47% increased ED_{50}) and normally sensitive to etomidate.[116] The lack of effect of etomidate indicates that the increase is not due to some nonspecific increase in sensitivities to all hypnotics. Both global and forebrain-specific HCN1 knockout strains were also mildly but significantly resistant to isoflurane and sevoflurane in assays of hypnosis and amnesia.[206] An HCN2 global knockout strain had reduced sensitivity to the effects of xenon on thalamic neuron currents, thalamocortical signaling, and sedation.[207]

Summary

Results from both invertebrate and vertebrate genetics indicate that multiple proteins control volatile anesthetic sensitivity. Some of these may be anesthetic targets and some not. The evidence for β_3-containing GABA$_A$ receptors as relevant targets for etomidate and propofol, however, is quite strong. Both drugs potentiate β_3-containing receptors expressed heterologously; however, a missense mutation blocks this potentiation. Mice expressing this mutant receptor are fully resistant to immobilization by etomidate and propofol, but are normally sensitive to the neurosteroid anesthetic alphaxalone. Other anesthetic endpoints are not fully dependent on the β_3 subunit, therefore other targets must be involved. For propofol and ketamine, but not etomidate, electrophysiologic and genetic data implicate the HCN1 channel as one such target. Volatile anesthetics appear to have multiple relevant targets, including GABA$_A$ receptors, some two-pore

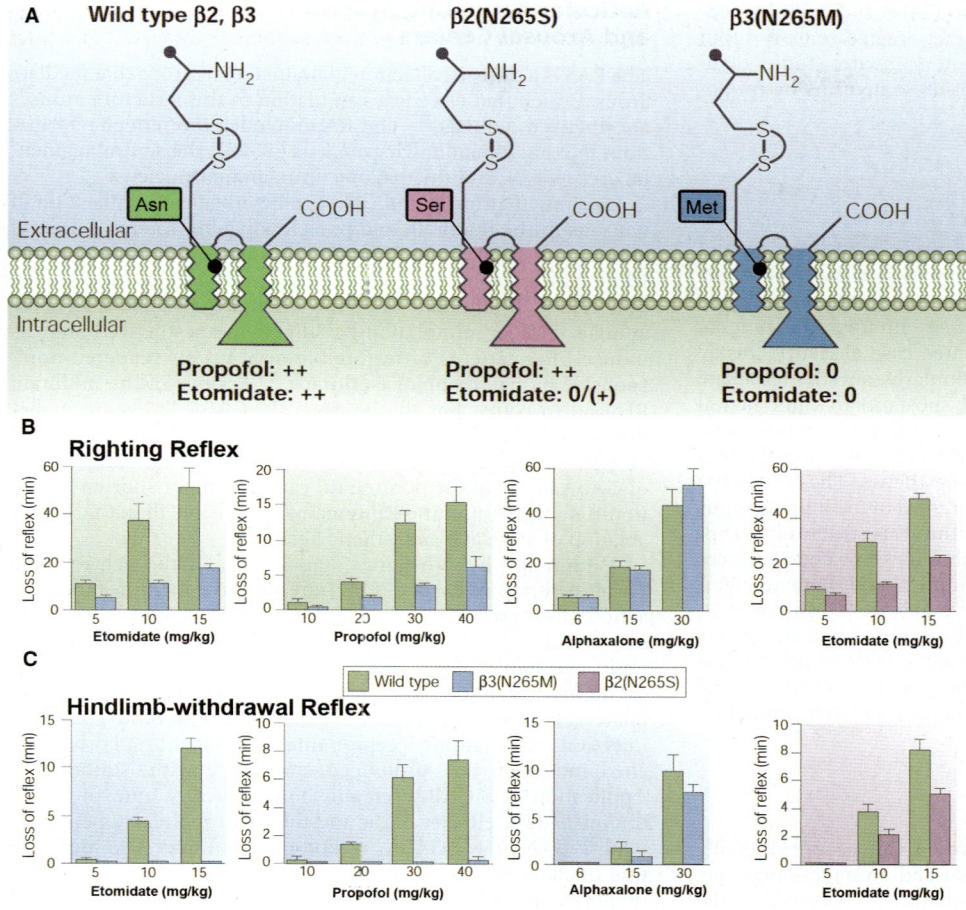

Figure 10-6 Mutations in the β_2 and β_3 subunits of the $GABA_A$ receptor reduce sensitivity to etomidate and propofol. **A:** Knockin transgenic mice were generated with mutation of a conserved asparagine (Asn) in the second transmembrane domain to a serine (Ser) in the β_2 subunit or a methionine (Met) in the β_3 subunit. **B:** The sensitivities of the wild type and the two knockin mice strains were measured in a loss of righting reflex assay, which is thought to model hypnosis. Mutant sensitivities to etomidate and propofol are highly significantly different compared to wild type. The neurosteroid alphaxalone is equally potent in wild type and in the β_3(N265M) strain. **C:** The sensitivities of the wild type and the two knockin mice strains were measured in a hindlimb withdrawal reflex to a painful stimulus assay, which is thought to model immobility. Note the lack of significant sensitivities to either etomidate or propofol in the β_3(N265M) strain. (Adapted from Rudolph U, Antkowiak B. Molecular and neuronal substrates for general anaesthetics. *Nat Rev Neurosci.* 2004;5:709.)

potassium channels, and HCN1 channels. Genetic evidence points to glutamate receptors and HCN2 channels as relevant to xenon's action. Other plausible anesthetic targets such as certain sodium channels, presynaptic proteins, and glycine receptors remain to be tested genetically in mice.

Where in the Central Nervous System Do Anesthetics Work?

Immobility

Several lines of evidence indicate that the spinal cord is the main site at which anesthetics inhibit motor responses to noxious stimulation. This is, of course, the endpoint used in most measurements of anesthetic potency. Rampil et al.[209,210] have shown that MAC values for fluorinated volatile anesthetics are unaffected in the rat by either decerebration[209] or cervical spinal cord transection.[210] Antognini and Schwartz[211] have used the strategy of isolating the cerebral circulation of goats to explore the contribution of brain and spinal cord to the determination of MAC. They found that when isoflurane is administered only to the brain, MAC is 2.9%, whereas when it is administered to the body and brain, MAC is 1.2%. Surprisingly, when isoflurane was preferentially administered to the body and not to the brain, isoflurane MAC was reduced to 0.8%,[212] suggesting that anesthetic action on the brain may actually sensitize the cord to noxious stimuli, through

neurons in the mesencephalic locomotor region.[213] Anesthetic action at the spinal cord underlies MAC through multiple targets. Volatile anesthetics directly reduce excitatory synaptic transmission of spinal neurons.[62,214–216] Propofol depresses activity in ventral horn neurons via a GABAergic mechanism that can be blocked by the antagonist picrotoxin.[217] In contrast, while isoflurane inhibits both dorsal horn neurons and motoneurons, the mechanism appears to be independent of GABA receptors.[217] Isoflurane also suppresses interneurons of central pattern generators involved in coordinated movements.[218] Thus, anesthetics can alter descending, afferent, efferent, and modulatory limbs of reflex arcs for reacting to noxious stimulation.

Autonomic Control

Anesthetics exert profound effects on cardiopulmonary and thermoregulatory homeostatic circuitry within autonomic centers in the brainstem and hypothalamus. Inspiratory neurons in the medulla drive phrenic motor neurons to activate diaphragmatic contraction. Halothane suppresses the spontaneous activity of these neurons in dogs by reducing glutamatergic input.[219] Anesthetics also perturb cardiovascular reflexes mediated by nuclei in the brainstem. For example, the nucleus ambiguus contains cardiac vagal neurons whose efferents are critical in the regulation of heart rate by the parasympathetic nervous system. In rats, both propofol and isoflurane augment the inhibitory potentials of cardiac vagal neurons in response to GABA.[220] Similarly, neurons in the nucleus of the solitary tract receive sensory input from carotid and aortic body baroreceptors; in vitro studies demonstrate GABA-mediated inhibition of these neurons by propofol[221] and isoflurane.[222]

Amnesia

While the neurobiologic mechanisms underlying learning and memory remain unclear, the hippocampus is a plausible anesthetic target for the suppression of memory formation. Bilateral resection of these structures induces anterograde amnesia, as demonstrated by the well-documented case of Henry Gustav Molaison, known as "Patient H.M." Similarly, anesthetics ablate the formation of new memories and substantially alter neural activity, while leaving prior memories seemingly intact. Genetic and pharmacologic experiments support a crucial role of the hippocampus in the amnestic actions of anesthetics. The α_5 subtype of the $GABA_A$ receptor is primarily expressed in the hippocampus and controls synaptic transmission within this structure.[223] Hippocampal GABA receptors with α_5 subunits show conductances that are exquisitely sensitive to isoflurane[224] and mediate memory deficits that persist after anesthetic exposure.[225] Moreover, α_5 $GABA_A$ receptor knockout mice are resistant to amnestic effects of etomidate.[184] Thus, α_5 $GABA_A$ receptors in the hippocampus are targets of different anesthetic agents, with potential clinical significance for both intraoperative and postoperative amnesia.

Unconsciousness

Consciousness is a complex state, which can be operationally divided into the components of arousal and awareness that may have differential susceptibility to anesthetics.[226] *Awareness* is the ability to process and store information in order to interact with internal or external environment. In contrast, *arousal* or *wakefulness* is the state of receptivity to the external environment and is likely mediated through subcortical structures such as the reticular activating system (RAS) and other arousal centers (Fig. 10-7).

Reticular Activating System and Arousal Centers

The RAS is a diffuse collection of brainstem neurons that mediate arousal, such that electrical stimulation in this structure arouses anesthetized animals.[227] The RAS includes the reticular formation, the tuberomammillary nucleus (TMN), the ventral tegmental area (VTA), and the thalamic intralaminar nucleus.

The reticular formation (RF) is a heterogeneous collection of neurons in the midbrain and pons involved in the regulation of arousal and sleep. Lesions of the midbrain RF can induce coma, while classic experiments by Moruzzi and Magoun have shown that electrical stimulation of the midbrain awakened sleeping animals. Similar stimulation paradigms in anesthetized animals induce EEG patterns of restored arousal in rats rendered unresponsive by halothane or isoflurane.[228] Lesions of the midbrain RF lead to coma. For the pontine RF, GABA levels are higher during wakefulness than in rapid eye movement (REM) sleep[229] or isoflurane-induced unconsciousness.[230] As the manipulation of GABA levels in the pontine RF can prolong or shorten induction time,[230] the pontine RF remains a plausible direct target for ablation of arousal by anesthetic agents.

Within the hypothalamus, the TMN and the ventrolateral posterior optic nucleus (VLPO) are putative loci for anesthetic action in suppressing arousal (Fig. 10-7). These mutually inhibitory structures form a bistable control of wakefulness and non-rapid eye movement sleep.[231] The TMN is the sole source of excitatory histaminergic efferents in the CNS. Rats that have had bilateral lesions of the TMN or been treated with intraventricular injections of histamine receptor antagonists manifest both shortened induction and prolonged emergence with isoflurane.[232] Application of a GABAergic antagonist directly onto the TMN diminished the efficacy of the anesthetics propofol and pentobarbital.[233] β_3(N265M) $GABA_A$ receptor mutant mice also implicate this nucleus as a target of propofol; the inhibitory postsynaptic potentials of their TMN neurons and the hypnotic effects of propofol are reduced.[234] In addition to direct antagonism of the TMN, inhibitory afferents of the VLPO suppress the locus coeruleus (LC) and the perifornical area (PF) (Fig. 10-7). Although anesthetics have been shown to activate VLPO neurons, ablation of this structure does not chronically impair induction of general

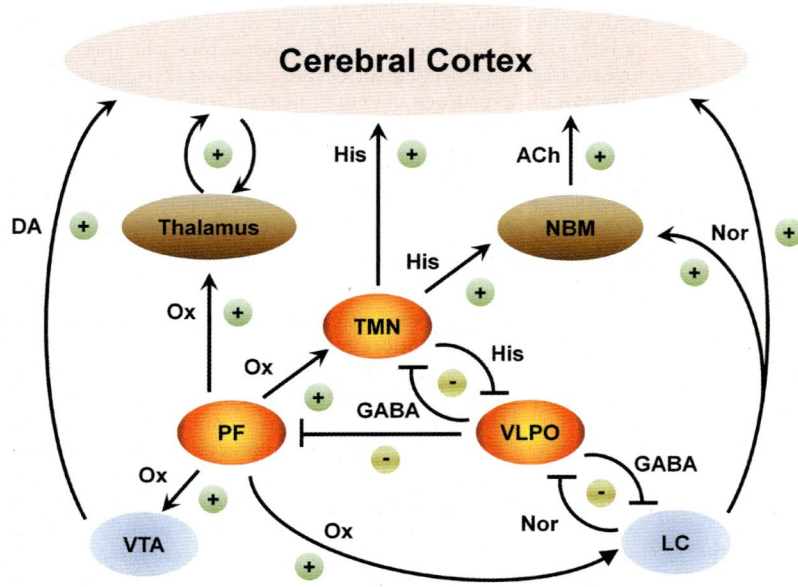

Figure 10-7 Diagram of subcortical arousal circuitry implicated in anesthetic-induced unconsciousness. The tuberomammillary nucleus (TMN) and ventrolateral preoptic nucleus (VLPO) form a bistable sleep/wake switch. The TMN also provides histaminergic output to the cerebral cortex and enhances excitatory cholinergic release from the nucleus basalis of Meynert (NBM). Orexin release from perifornical area (PF) stabilizes the VLPO/TMN sleep switch and plays a key role in modulating outputs of the dopaminergic ventral tegmental area (VTA), the noradrenergic locus coeruleus (LC), and thalamic outputs involved in maintaining recurrent thalamocortical excitability and the integrity of networks linking distributed cortical areas. Ox, orexin; Nor, norepinephrine; His, histamine; GABA, γ-aminobutyric acid; ACh, acetylcholine; DA, dopamine.

anesthesia.[235] Thus, the VLPO may contribute only indirectly to anesthetic-induced unconsciousness, whereas experimental support for the TMN as a site of anesthetic action is stronger.

The PF in the lateral hypothalamus appears to be critical in anesthetic emergence, rather than induction of unconsciousness. It is the sole source of orexin, a neurotransmitter that stabilizes the flip-flopping of the VLPO/TMN sleep switch to favor activation of the arousal-promoting TMN (Fig. 10-7). Orexin knockout animals show frequent sleep/wake transitions akin to narcolepsy. In rodents anesthetized by isoflurane, intraventricular injections of orexin A shift the EEG from burst-suppression to arousal-like patterns.[236] Shortened emergence from propofol[234,237] or dexmedetomidine[234] can also be induced by orexin-A injections into CSF. While ablation of arousal by either isoflurane or sevoflurane is not affected in orexin knockout animals, recovery from anesthesia is delayed,[238] suggesting asymmetry in the neural mechanisms underlying induction and emergence.

Suppression of the nucleus basalis of Meynert (NBM) is likely important in mediating anesthetic suppression of arousal and awareness. The NBM receives input from arousal centers (Fig. 10-7) and is the major source of excitatory cholinergic input to the thalamus, RAS, and the cerebral cortex. Norepinephrine infused into the NBM induces arousal in rats with righting reflexes ablated by desflurane.[239] Activation of the NBM by histamine reverses EEG slowing[232] and accelerates emergence from isoflurane, but not intravenous anesthetics.[240] Whether the NBM represents a target specific for volatile agents remains an open question.

The VTA provides dopaminergic inputs to the prefrontal cortical areas, the hippocampus, and amygdala. In contrast, the LC within the pons is the primary adrenergic source to the cortex, thalamus, and hypothalamus (Fig. 10-7). Dual inhibitors of these two pathways restore righting reflex in isoflurane-anesthetized rats.[7] Recent data highlight the importance of the VTA and the dopamine D1 receptor in isoflurane,[241] sevoflurane,[242] and propofol anesthesia. LC activation prolongs induction, antagonizes cortical suppression during anesthetic maintenance, and facilitates emergence through α_1 adrenergic receptor mechanisms.[243] These studies suggest that both the VTA and LC play important roles in anesthetic unconsciousness.

Thalamus

The thalamus regulates widespread cortical excitability and relays information to specialized cortical regions, and is a likely target for anesthetic ablation of arousal and awareness.[244] Anesthetic agents do not appear to induce thalamic deafferentiation in relay nuclei for vision (lateral geniculate nucleus) or other sensory modalities; peripheral sensory stimulation leads to activation of corresponding cortical areas during general anesthesia[245] and even burst suppression.[246] In contrast, neurons in the thalamic reticular nuclei (TRN) and medial thalamic nuclei remain plausible potential anesthetic targets. TRN neurons process excitatory input from the cerebral cortex, dorsal thalamic nuclei, and the RAS. They are in a key position to dampen recurrent loops between thalamic and cortical neurons.[244] While TRN neurons are inhibited by etomidate[247] and isoflurane,[248] demonstration of their role in vivo has not been reported. Elsewhere in the thalamus, stimulation or ablation of the centromedian nuclei alter attention and arousal. Microinfusions targeting Kv1.2 potassium channels[249] or nicotinic cholinergic receptors[250] in these regions reverse volatile anesthetic hypnosis. Correlated neural activity between midline thalamic regions and cortical regions involved in attention and introspection are weakened in humans rendered unconscious by propofol[251] or sevoflurane.[252] Future study will elucidate whether anesthetics induce unconsciousness primarily at these thalamic nuclei, in their recurrent interactions with specific cortical regions, or within the cerebral cortical regions mediating awareness of space and time.

Cerebral Cortex

The cerebral cortex is the major site for generating awareness of the external environment. Primary sensory areas provide focused, feed-forward activity to association and "higher" cortical areas that provide reciprocal diffuse feedback.

The disruption of feedback connections by anesthetics may contribute to impaired consciousness by attenuating the integration of information distributed among cortical regions. The late components of rat visual neuron responses to flashed stimuli are attenuated by desflurane.[253] These high latency responses are associated with feedback activity and mediate contextual modulation from higher cortical areas. Electrode recordings in rats have also compared the directional bias of activity between frontal and parietal cortical areas in both awake and anesthetized states. While interactions are balanced during wakefulness, feedback interactions were preferentially diminished when rats were anesthetized by isoflurane.[254] Human fMRI[255–257] and EEG studies have yielded similar findings of reduced feedback from frontal to posterior areas, with propofol,[258–261] sevoflurane,[262] or ketamine.[261] Direct evidence to substantiate this mechanism is pending.

The effects of anesthetics on both cortical firing rates and timing of action potentials may contribute to the ablation of awareness by limiting both the diversity of information that can be represented and the integration of neural information.[1] Anesthetics alter the topology of distinct networks of distributed cortical areas subserving attention and higher cognitive processes through patterns of correlated activity. With induction of propofol- or sevoflurane-induced unconsciousness, two such networks have shown weaker correlations among constituent cortical areas: the default mode network,[252,255] associated with memory and consciousness,[263,264] and the ventral attention network,[252,256,265] linked with externally directed attention.[266,267] These networks represent potential cortical targets of anesthetic action. The weakening of correlated brain activity between regions of different networks[255,256] suggests that the blurring of boundaries between specialized groups of cortical areas may also contribute to impaired consciousness.

Anesthetics weaken high-frequency synchronized oscillatory cortical activity involved in integrating information into coherent representations.[268] In rats, isoflurane reduces high gamma range (70 to 140 Hz) synchrony in the frontal cortex, visual cortex, and hippocampus.[269] Recordings from humans implanted with subdural electrocorticographic electrodes revealed a reduction in high gamma band power (>75 Hz) on induction with propofol and recovery during emergence from propofol.[270] Analysis of EEG from humans rendered unresponsive by propofol revealed a reduction in information integration in the gamma band,[258] and multiple anesthetic agents cause widespread reduction in gamma band power.[271]

Summary

Anesthetics suppress circuits in the spinal cord and brainstem to induce immobility and disrupt autonomic homeostasis. The hippocampus is a major site of anesthetic action for anterograde amnesia. As the neurobiologic underpinnings of arousal and awareness are distributed across brainstem, subcortical, and cortical structures, no single anatomic site is responsible for anesthetic-induced unconsciousness. Recent work has revealed that networks of subcortical and thalamic nuclei are altered in the ablation of arousal. Cortical networks critical for cognitive processing of awareness are the tentative substrates for extinction of subjective percepts, noxious and otherwise. Network perturbations in both frequency and temporal coding of information are putative mechanisms for altered integration and neural representation.

Conclusions

In this chapter, evidence has been reviewed concerning the anatomic, physiologic, and molecular loci of anesthetic action. It is clear that all anesthetic effects cannot be localized to a specific anatomic site in the CNS. Indeed, considerable evidence supports the conclusion that different components of the anesthetic state are mediated by actions at disparate anatomic sites. Likewise, the actions of anesthetics cannot be localized to a single physiologic process. While there is consensus that anesthetics ultimately affect synaptic function, as opposed to intrinsic neuronal excitability, their particular effects on presynaptic and postsynaptic function vary by agent and synapse. At a molecular level, volatile anesthetics show some selectivity, but still affect the function of multiple ion channels and synaptic proteins. The intravenous anesthetics, etomidate, propofol, and barbiturates, are more specific with the $GABA_A$ receptor as their major target. Although these effects are likely mediated via direct protein–anesthetic interactions, numerous proteins can directly interact with anesthetics. Genetic data plainly demonstrate that the unitary theory of anesthesia is not correct. No single mechanism is responsible for the effects of all general anesthetics, nor does a single mechanism account for all effects of a single anesthetic. Figure 10-8 provides a simple model of how the known molecular and cellular effects of general anesthetics might summate to produce anesthesia. This cartoon is not meant to include all potential molecular targets of general anesthetics; rather, only those molecules with strong support from multiple distinct investigational approaches are shown.

Although the precise set of molecular interactions responsible for producing anesthesia have not been fully elucidated, anesthetics do act via selective effects on specific molecular targets. The technological revolutions in molecular biology, genetics, neurophysiology, and neuroimaging make it likely that the next decade will provide additional answers to the anesthetic mechanism puzzle.

Acknowledgments

The authors acknowledge generous ongoing funding support from National Institute of General Medical Sciences, National Institute of Neurological Disorders and Stroke, National Center for Research Resources, the National Center for Advancing Translational Sciences, and the Taylor Institute for Innovative Psychiatry (ASE), for ASE-R01 GM108799, CMC-RO1 NS045905, R21 NS084360 and BJP- UL1TR000448, subaward KL2 TR000450.

REFERENCES

1. Alkire MT, Hudetz AG, Tononi G. Consciousness and anesthesia. *Science*. 2008;322:876–880.
2. Mashour GA. Top-down mechanisms of anesthetic-induced unconsciousness. *Front Syst Neurosci*. 2014;8:115.
3. Tononi G. Consciousness as integrated information: a provisional manifesto. *Biol Bull*. 2008;215:216–242.
4. Tononi G, Koch C. Consciousness: here, there and everywhere? *Phil Trans Royal Soc Lond Series B Biol Sci*. 2015;370(1668). pii: 20140167.
5. Akeju O, Loggia ML, Catana C, et al. Disruption of thalamic functional connectivity is a neural correlate of dexmedetomidine-induced unconsciousness. *eLife*. 2014;3:e04499.
6. Friedman EB, Sun Y, Moore JT, et al. A conserved behavioral state barrier impedes transitions between anesthetic-induced unconsciousness and wakefulness: evidence for neural inertia. *PLoS ONE*. 2010;5:e11903.
7. Solt K, Cotten JF, Cimenser A, et al. Methylphenidate actively induces emergence from general anesthesia. *Anesthesiology*. 2011;115:791–803.
8. Solt K, Van Dort CJ, Chemali JJ, et al. Electrical stimulation of the ventral tegmental area induces reanimation from general anesthesia. *Anesthesiology*. 2014;121:311–319.
9. Quasha AL, Eger EI II, Tinker JH. Determination and applications of MAC. *Anesthesiology*. 1980;53:315–334.
10. White PF, Johnston RR, Eger EI 2nd. Determination of anesthetic requirement in rats. *Anesthesiology*. 1974;40:52–57.
11. Franks NP, Lieb WR. Molecular and cellular mechanisms of general anaesthesia. *Nature*. 1994;367:607–614.
12. Bowdle TA. Depth of anesthesia monitoring. *Anesthesiol Clin*. 2006;24: 793–822.
13. Avidan MS, Jacobsohn E, Glick D, et al. Prevention of intraoperative awareness in a high-risk surgical population. *N Engl Jo Med*. 2011;365:591–600.
14. Avidan MS, Zhang L, Burnside BA, et al. Anesthesia awareness and the bispectral index. *N Engl J Med*. 2008;358:1097–1108.
15. Palanca BJ, Mashour GA, Avidan MS. Processed electroencephalogram in depth of anesthesia monitoring. *Curr Opin Anaesthesiol*. 2009;22:553–559.
16. Bruhn J, Myles PS, Sneyd R, et al. Depth of anaesthesia monitoring: what's available, what's validated and what's next? *Br J Anaesth*. 2006;97:85–94.
17. Meyer H. Theorie der alkoholnarkose. *Arch Exp Pathol Pharmacol*. 1899;42: 109–118.
18. Overton CE. *Studies of Narcosis*. London, UK: Chapman and Hall; 1891.
19. Franks NP, Lieb WR. Where do general anaesthetics act? *Nature*. 1978;274: 3393–3342.
20. Larson ER. Fluorine compounds in anesthesiology. In: Trarrant P, ed. *Fluorine Chemistry Reviews*. 3rd ed. New York, NY: Dekker; 1969.
21. Andrews PR, Jones GP, Poulton DB. Convulsant, anticonvulsant and anaesthetic barbiturates: in vivo activities of oxo- and thiobarbiturates related to pentobarbitone. *Eur J Pharmacol*. 1982;79:61–65.
22. Paul SM, Purdy RH. Neuroactive steroids. *FASEB J*. 1992;6:2311–2322.
23. Koblin DD, Chortkoff BS, Laster MJ, et al. Polyhalogenated and perfluorinated compounds that disobey the Meyer–Overton hypothesis. *Anesth Analg*. 1994;79:1043–1048.
24. Kandel L, Chortkoff BS, Sonner J, et al. Nonanesthetics can suppress learning. *Anesth Analg*. 1996;82:321–326.
25. Alifimoff JK, Firestone LL, Miller KW. Anaesthetic potencies of primary alkanols: implications for the molecular dimensions of the anaesthetic site. *Br J Pharmacol*. 1989;96:9–16.

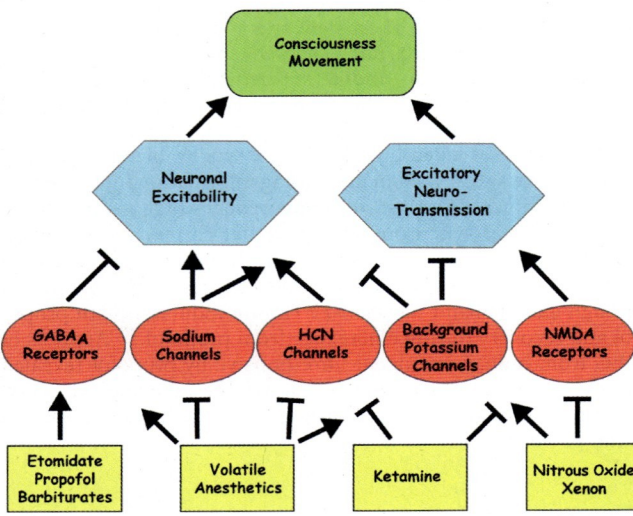

Figure 10-8 A multisite model for anesthesia. Anesthetics are grouped according to similarity of mechanism. Arrows indicate activation or potentiation, and Ts indicate inhibition or antagonism. The neurophysiologic effects of general anesthetics are lumped into neuronal excitability (the probability of a neuron firing and propagating an axon potential) and excitatory neurotransmission (synaptic activity at excitatory synapses such as glutamatergic). Neuronal excitability in this context is the sum of both intrinsic and extrinsic factors (e.g., GABAergic inhibition).

26. Raines DE, Korten SE, Hill AG, et al. Anesthetic cutoff in cycloalkanemethanols: a test of current theories. *Anesthesiology*. 1993;78:918–927.
27. Liu J, Laster MJ, Koblin DD, et al. A cutoff in potency exists in the perfluoroalkanes. *Anesth Analg*. 1994;79:238–244.
28. Andrews PR, Mark LC. Structural specificity of barbiturates and related drugs. *Anesthesiology*. 1982;57:314–320.
29. Ryder S, Way WL, Trevor AJ. Comparative pharmacology of the optical isomers of ketamine in mice. *Eur J Pharmacol*. 1978;49:15–23.
30. Wittmer LL, Hu Y, Kalkbrenner M, et al. Enantioselectivity of steroid-induced gamma-aminobutyric acid A receptor modulation and anesthesia. *Mol Pharmacol*. 1996;50:1581–1586.
31. Tomlin SL, Jenkins A, Lieb WR, et al. Stereoselective effects of etomidate optical isomers on gamma-aminobutyric acid type A receptors and animals. *Anesthesiology*. 1998;88:708–717.
32. Lysko GS, Robinson JL, Casto R, et al. The stereospecific effects of isoflurane isomers in vivo. *Eur J Pharmacol*. 1994;263:25–29.
33. Smith RA, Porter EG, Miller KW. The solubility of anesthetic gases in lipid bilayers. *Biochim Biophys Acta*. 1981;645:327–338.
34. Franks NP. Molecular targets underlying general anaesthesia. *Br J Pharmacol*. 2006;147(Suppl 1):S72–S81.
35. Franks NP, Lieb WR. Do general anaesthetics act by competitive binding to specific receptors? *Nature*. 1984;310:599–601.
36. Franks NP, Lieb WR. Mapping of general anaesthetic target sites provides a molecular basis for cutoff effects. *Nature*. 1985;316:349–351.
37. Dubois BW, Cherian SF, Evers AS. Volatile anesthetics compete for common binding sites on bovine serum albumin: a 19F-NMR study. *Proc Natl Acad Sci U S A*. 1993;90:6478–6482.
38. Dubois BW, Evers AS. 19F-NMR spin-spin relaxation (T2) method for characterizing volatile anesthetic binding to proteins: analysis of isoflurane binding to serum albumin. *Biochemistry*. 1992;31:7069–7076.
39. Eckenhoff RG, Shuman H. Halothane binding to soluble proteins determined by photoaffinity labeling. *Anesthesiology*. 1993;79:96–106.
40. Eckenhoff RG. Amino acid resolution of halothane binding sites in serum albumin. *J Biol Chem*. 1996;271:15521–15526.
41. Husain SS, Ziebell MR, Ruesch D, et al. 2-(3-Methyl-3H-diaziren-3-yl)ethyl 1-(1-phenylethyl)-1H-imidazole-5-carboxylate: a derivative of the stereoselective general anesthetic etomidate for photolabeling ligand-gated ion channels. *J Med Chem*. 2003;46:1257–1265.
42. Hall MA, Xi J, Lor C, et al. m-Azipropofol (AziPm) a photoactive analogue of the intravenous general anesthetic propofol. *J Med Chem*. 2010;53:5667–5675.
43. Yip GM, Chen ZW, Edge CJ, et al. A propofol binding site on mammalian $GABA_A$ receptors identified by photolabeling. *Nat Chem Biol*. 2013;9:715–720.
44. Chiara DC, Dostalova Z, Jayakar SS, et al. Mapping general anesthetic binding site(s) in human α1β3 γ-aminobutyric acid type A receptors with [3H]TDBzl-etomidate, a photoreactive etomidate analog. *Biochemistry*. 2012;51:836–847.
45. Chen ZW, Wang C, Krishnan K, et al. 11-Trifluoromethyl-phenyldiazirinyl neurosteroid analogues: potent general anesthetics and photolabeling reagents for $GABA_A$ receptors. *Psychopharmacology*. 2014;231:3479–3491.
46. Li GD, Chiara DC, Sawyer GW, et al. Identification of a $GABA_A$ receptor anesthetic binding site at subunit interfaces by photolabeling with an etomidate analog. *J Neurosci*. 2006;26:11599–11605.
47. Jayakar SS, Zhou X, Chiara DC, et al. Multiple propofol-binding sites in a γ-aminobutyric acid type A receptor ($GABA_AR$) identified using a photoreactive propofol analog. *J Biol Chem*. 2014;289:27456–2768.
48. Chiara DC, Jayakar SS, Zhou X, et al. Specificity of intersubunit general anesthetic-binding sites in the transmembrane domain of the human α1β3γ2 gamma-aminobutyric acid type A ($GABA_A$) receptor. *J Biol Chem*. 2013;288:19343–19357.
49. Franks NP, Jenkins A, Conti E, et al. Structural basis for the inhibition of firefly luciferase by a general anesthetic. *Biophysical Journal*. 1998;75:2205–2211.
50. Bocquet N, Nury H, Baaden M, et al. X-ray structure of a pentameric ligand-gated ion channel in an apparently open conformation. *Nature*. 2009;457:111–114.
51. Nury H, Bocquet N, Le Poupon C, et al. Crystal structure of the extracellular domain of a bacterial ligand-gated ion channel. *J Mol Biol*. 2010;395:1114–1127.
52. Miller PS, Aricescu AR. Crystal structure of a human $GABA_A$ receptor. *Nature*. 2014;512:270–275.
53. MacIver MB, Kendig JJ. Anesthetic effects on resting membrane potential are voltage-dependent and agent-specific. *Anesthesiology*. 1991;74:83–88.
54. Madison DV, Nicoll RA. General anaesthetics hyperpolarize neurons in the vertebrate central nervous system. *Science*. 1982;217:1055–1057.
55. Ries CR, Puil E. Mechanism of anesthesia revealed by shunting actions of isoflurane on thalamocortical neurons. *J Neurophysiol*. 1999;81:1795–1801.
56. Larrabee MG, Posternak JM. Selective action of anesthetics on synapses and axons in mammalian sympathetic ganglia. *J Neurophysiol*. 1952;15:91–114.
57. Richards CD, Russell WJ, Smaje JC. The action of ether and methoxyflurane on synaptic transmission in isolated preparations of the mammalian cortex. *J Physiol*. 1975;248:121–142.
58. Richards CD, White AE. The actions of volatile anaesthetics on synaptic transmission in the dentate gyrus. *J Physiol*. 1975;252:241–257.
59. Langmoen IA, Larsen M, Berg-Johnsen J. Volatile anaesthetics: cellular mechanisms of action. *Eur J Anaesthesiol*. 1995;12:51–58.
60. Wu XS, Sun JY, Evers AS, et al. Isoflurane inhibits transmitter release and the presynaptic action potential. *Anesthesiology*. 2004;100:663–670.
61. Purtell K, Gingrich KJ, Ouyang W, et al. Activity-dependent depression of neuronal sodium channels by the general anaesthetic isoflurane. *Br J Anaesth*. 2015;115:112–121.
62. Kullmann DM, Martin RL, Redman SJ. Reduction by general anaesthetics of group Ia excitatory postsynaptic potentials and currents in the cat spinal cord. *J Physiol*. 1989;412:277–296.
63. MacIver MB, Roth SH. Inhalational anaesthetics exhibit pathway-specific and differential actions on hippocampal synaptic responses in vitro. *Br J Anaesth*. 1988;60:680–691.
64. Nicoll RA, Eccles JC, Oshima T, et al. Prolongation of hippocampal inhibitory postsynaptic potentials by barbiturates. *Nature*. 1975;258:625–627.
65. Proctor WR, Mynlieff M, Dunwiddie TV. Facilitatory action of etomidate and pentobarbital on recurrent inhibition in rat hippocampal pyramidal neurons. *J Neurosci*. 1986;6:3161–3168.
66. Collins GG. Effects of the anaesthetic 2,6-diisopropylphenol on synaptic transmission in the rat olfactory cortex slice. *Br J Pharmacol*. 1988;95:939–949.
67. Nicoll RA. The effects of anaesthetics on synaptic excitation and inhibition in the olfactory bulb. *J Physiol*. 1972;223:803–814.
68. Harrison NL, Vicini S, Barker JL. A steroid anesthetic prolongs inhibitory postsynaptic currents in cultured rat hippocampal neurons. *J Neurosci*. 1987;7:604–609.
69. Perouansky M, Baranov D, Salman M, et al. Effects of halothane on glutamate receptor-mediated excitatory post-synaptic currents: a patch-clamp study in adult mouse hippocampal slices. *Anesthesiology*. 1995;83:109–119.
70. Buggy DJ, Nicol B, Rowbotham DJ, et al. Effects of intravenous anesthetic agents on glutamate release: a role for GABAA receptor-mediated inhibition. *Br J Pharmacol*. 1988;95:939–949.
71. Kendall TJ, Minchin MC. The effects of anaesthetics on the uptake and release of amino acid neurotransmitters in thalamic slices. *Br J Pharmacol*. 1982;75:219–227.
72. Larsen M, Haugstad TS, Berg-Johnsen J, et al. Effect of isoflurane on release and uptake of gamma-aminobutyric acid from rat cortical synaptosomes. *Br J Anaesth*. 1998;80:634–638.
73. Collins GG. Release of endogenous amino acid neurotransmitter candidates from rat olfactory cortex slices: possible regulatory mechanisms and the effects of pentobarbitone. *Brain Research*. 1980;190:517–528.
74. Murugaiah KD, Hemmings HC Jr. Effects of intravenous general anesthetics on [3H]GABA release from rat cortical synaptosomes. *Anesthesiology*. 1998;89:919–928.
75. Mantz J, Lecharny JB, Laudenbach V, et al. Anesthetics affect the uptake but not the depolarization-evoked release of GABA in rat striatal synaptosomes. *Anesthesiology*. 1995;82:502–511.
76. Westphalen RI, Hemmings HC Jr. Selective depression by general anesthetics of glutamate versus GABA release from isolated cortical nerve terminals. *J Pharmacol Exp Ther*. 2003;304:1188–1196.
77. Westphalen RI, Desai KM, Hemmings HC Jr. Presynaptic inhibition of the release of multiple major central nervous system neurotransmitter types by the inhaled anaesthetic isoflurane. *Br J Anaesth*. 2013;110:592–599.
78. Baumgart JP, Zhou ZY, Hara M, et al. Isoflurane inhibits synaptic vesicle exocytosis through reduced Ca^{2+} influx, not Ca^{2+}-exocytosis coupling. *Proc Natl Acad Sci U S A*. 2015;112:11959–11964.
79. Hawasli AH, Saifee O, Liu C, et al. Resistance to volatile anesthetics by mutations enhancing excitatory neurotransmitter release in Caenorhabditis elegans. *Genetics*. 2004;168:831–843.
80. van Swinderen B, Saifee O, Shebester L, et al. A neomorphic syntaxin mutation blocks volatile-anesthetic action in Caenorhabditis elegans. *Proc Natl Acad Sci U S A*. 1999;96:2479–2484.
81. Herring BE, Xie Z, Marks J, et al. Isoflurane inhibits the neurotransmitter release machinery. *J Neurophysiol*. 2009;102:1265–1273.
82. Richards CD, Smaje JC. Anaesthetics depress the sensitivity of cortical neurones to L-glutamate. *Br J Pharmacol*. 1976;58:347–357.
83. Smaje JC. General anaesthetics and the acetylcholine-sensitivity of cortical neurones. *Br J Pharmacol*. 1976;58:359–366.
84. Olsen RW, Li GD. $GABA_A$ receptors as molecular targets of general anesthetics: identification of binding sites provides clues to allosteric modulation. *Can J Anaesth*. 2011;58:206–215.
85. Akk G, Steinbach JH. Structural studies of the actions of anesthetic drugs on the gamma-aminobutyric acid type A receptor. *Anesthesiology*. 2011;115:1338–1348.
86. Jones MV, Brooks PA, Harrison NL. Enhancements of gamma-aminobutyric acid-activated Cl- currents in cultured rat hippocampal neurones by three volatile anaesthetics. *J Physiol*. 1992;449:279–293.
87. Haydon DA, Urban BW. The actions of some general anaesthetics on the potassium current of the squid giant axon. *J Physiol*. 1986;373:311–327.
88. Herrington J, Stern RC, Evers AS, et al. Halothane inhibits two components of calcium current in clonal (GH_3) pituitary cells. *J Neurosci*. 1991;11:2226–2240.
89. Herold KF, Hemmings HC Jr. Sodium channels as targets for volatile anesthetics. *Front Pharmacol*. 2012;3:50.
90. Rehberg B, Xiao YH, Duch DS. Central nervous system sodium channels are significantly suppressed at clinical concentrations of volatile anesthetics. *Anesthesiology*. 1996;84:1223–1233.

91. Ratnakumari L, Hemmings HC Jr. Inhibition of presynaptic sodium channels by halothane. *Anesthesiology.* 1998;88:1043–1054.
92. Shiraishi M, Harris RA. Effects of alcohols and anesthetics on recombinant voltage-gated Na+ channels. *J Pharmacol Exp Ther.* 2004;309:987–994.
93. Frenkel C, Weckbecker K, Wartenberg HC, et al. Blocking effects of the anaesthetic etomidate on human brain sodium channels. *Neurosc Lett.* 1998;249:131–134.
94. Rehberg B, Duch DS. Suppression of central nervous system sodium channels by propofol. *Anesthesiology.* 1999;91:512–520.
95. Eskinder H, Rusch NJ, Supan FD, et al. The effects of volatile anesthetics on L- and T-type calcium channel currents in canine cardiac Purkinje cells. *Anesthesiology.* 1991;74:919–926.
96. Terrar DA. Structure and function of calcium channels and the actions of anaesthetics. *Br J Anaesth.* 1993;71:39–46.
97. Gundersen CB, Umbach JA, Swartz BE. Barbiturates depress currents through human-brain calcium channels studied in xenopus oocytes. *J Pharmacol Exp Ther.* 1988;247:824–829.
98. Hall AC, Lieb WR, Franks NP. Insensitivity of P-type calcium channels to inhalational and intravenous general anesthetics. *Anesthesiology.* 1994;81:117–1123.
99. Study RE. Isoflurane inhibits multiple voltage-gated calcium currents in hippocampal pyramidal neurons. *Anesthesiology.* 1994;81:104–116.
100. Takenoshita M, Steinbach JH. Halothane blocks low-voltage-activated calcium current in rat sensory neurons. *J Neurosci.* 1991;11:1404–1412.
101. Ffrench-Mullen JM, Barker JL, Rogawski MA. Calcium current block by (-)-pentobarbital, phenobarbital, and CHEB but not (+)-pentobarbital in acutely isolated hippocampal CA1 neurons: comparison with effects on GABA-activated Cl- current. *J Neurosci.* 1993;13:3211–3221.
102. Correa AM. Gating kinetics of Shaker K+ channels are differentially modified by general anesthetics. *Am J Physiol.* 1998;275:C1009–C1021.
103. Friederich P, Urban BW. Interaction of intravenous anesthetics with human neuronal potassium currents in relation to clinical concentrations. *Anesthesiology.* 1999;91:1853–1860.
104. Gerstin KM, Gong DH, Abdallah M, et al. Mutation of KCNK5 or Kir3.2 potassium channels in mice does not change minimum alveolar anesthetic concentration. *Anesth Analg.* 2003;96:1345–1349.
105. Gibbons SJ, Nunez-Hernandez R, Maze G, et al. Inhibition of a fast inwardly rectifying potassium conductance by barbiturates. *Anesth Analg.* 1996;82:1242–1246.
106. Stadnicka A, Bosnjak ZJ, Kampine JP, et al. Effects of sevoflurane on inward rectifier K+ current in guinea pig ventricular cardiomyocytes. *Am J Physiol.* 1997;273:H324–H332.
107. Patel AJ, Honore E. Anesthetic-sensitive 2P domain K+ channels. *Anesthesiology.* 2001;95:1013–1021.
108. Steinberg EA, Wafford KA, Brickley SG, et al. The role of K_2p channels in anaesthesia and sleep. *Pflugers Arch.* 2015;467:907–916.
109. Franks NP, Lieb WR. Volatile general anaesthetics activate a novel neuronal K+ current. *Nature.* 1988;333:662–664.
110. Winegar BD, Yost CS. Volatile anesthetics directly activate baseline S K+ channels in aplysia neurons. *Brain Res.* 1998;807:255–262.
111. Honore E. The neuronal background K2P channels: focus on TREK1. *Nat Rev Neurosci.* 2007;8:251–261.
112. Patel AJ, Honore E, Lesage F, et al. Inhalational anesthetics activate two-pore-domain background K+ channels. *Nat Neurosci.* 1999;2:422–426.
113. Gruss M, Bushell TJ, Bright DP, et al. Two-pore-domain K+ channels are a novel target for the anesthetic gases xenon, nitrous oxide, and cyclopropane. *Mol Pharmacol.* 2004;65:443–452.
114. Postea O, Biel M. Exploring HCN channels as novel drug targets. *Nat Rev Drug Discov.* 2011;10:903–914.
115. Chen X, Sirois JE, Lei Q, et al. HCN subunit-specific and cAMP-modulated effects of anesthetics on neuronal pacemaker currents. *J Neurosci.* 2005;25:5803–5814.
116. Chen X, Shu S, Bayliss DA. HCN1 channel subunits are a molecular substrate for hypnotic actions of ketamine. *J Neurosci.* 2009;29:600–609.
117. Cacheaux LP, Topf N, Tibbs GR, et al. Impairment of hyperpolarization-activated, cyclic nucleotide-gated channel function by the intravenous general anesthetic propofol. *J Pharmacol Exp Ther.* 2005;315:517–525.
118. Akk G, Mennerick S, Steinbach JH. Actions of anesthetics on excitatory transmitter-gated channels. *Handb Exp Pharmacol.* 2008:53–84.
119. Krasowski MD, Harrison NL. General anaesthetic actions on ligand-gated ion channels. *Cell Mol Life Sci.* 1999;55:1278–1303.
120. Wakamori M, Ikemoto Y, Akaike N. Effects of two volatile anesthetics and a volatile convulsant on the excitatory and inhibitory amino acid responses in dissociated CNS neurons of the rat. *J Neurophysiol.* 1991;66:2014–2021.
121. Lin L, Chen LL, Harris RA. Enflurane inhibits NMDA, AMPA and kainate-induced currents in *Xenopus* oocytes expressing mouse and human brain mRNA. *FASEB J.* 1992;7:479–485.
122. Weight FF, Lovinger DM, White G, et al. Alcohol and anesthetic actions on excitatory amino acid-activated ion channels. *Ann NY Acad Sci.* 1991;625:97–107.
123. Dildy-Mayfield JE, Eger EI II, Harris RA. Anesthetics produce subunit-selective actions on glutamate receptors. *J Pharmacol Exp Ther.* 1996;276:1058–1065.
124. Minami K, Wick MJ, Stern-Bach Y, et al. Sites of volatile anesthetic action on kainate (glutamate receptor 6) receptors. *J Biol Chem.* 1998;273:8248–8255.
125. Aronstam RS, Martin DC, Dennison RL. Volatile anesthetics inhibit NMDA-stimulated ^{45}Ca uptake by rat brain microvesicles. *Neurochem Res.* 1994;19:1515–1520.
126. Anis NA, Berry SC, Burton NR, et al. The dissociative anaesthetics, ketamine and phencyclidine, selectively reduce excitation of central mammalian neurones by N-methyl-aspartate. *Br J Pharmacol.* 1983;79:565–575.
127. Lodge D, Anis NA, Burton NR. Effects of optical isomers of ketamine on excitation of cat and rat spinal neurons by amino-acids and acetylcholine. *Neurosci Lett.* 1982;29:281–286.
128. Zeilhofer HU, Swandulla D, Geisslinger G, et al. Differential effects of ketamine enantiomers on NMDA receptor currents in cultured neurons. *Eur J Pharmacol.* 1992;213:155–158.
129. Jevtovic-Todorovic V, Todorovic SM, Mennerick S, et al. Nitrous oxide (laughing gas) is an NMDA antagonist, neuroprotectant and neurotoxin. *Nat Med.* 1998;4:460–463.
130. Mennerick S, Jevtovic-Todorovic V, Todorovic SM, et al. Effect of nitrous oxide on excitatory and inhibitory synaptic transmission in hippocampal cultures. *J Neurosci.* 1998;18:9716–9726.
131. Franks NP, Dickinson R, de Sousa SL, et al. How does xenon produce anaesthesia?. *Nature.* 1998;396:324.
132. Barker JL, Harrison NL, Lange GD, et al. Potentiation of gamma-aminobutyric-acid-activated chloride conductance by a steroid anesthetic in cultured rat spinal neurons. *J Physiol Lond.* 1987;386:485–501.
133. Hales TH, Lambert JJ. Modulation of the $GABA_A$ receptor by propofol. *Br J Pharmacol.* 1988;93:84P.
134. Macdonald RL, Olsen RW. GABAA receptor channels. *Annu Rev Neurosci.* 1994;17:569–602.
135. Macdonald RL, Rogers CJ, Twyman RE. Barbiturate regulation of kinetic properties of the GABAA receptor channels of mouse spinal neurones in culture. *J Physiol.* 1989;417:483–500.
136. Hall AC, Lieb WR, Franks NP. Stereoselective and non-stereoselective actions of isoflurane on the $GABA_A$ receptor. *Br J Pharmacol.* 1994;112:906–910.
137. Nakahiro M, Yeh JZ, Brunner E, et al. General anesthetics modulate GABA receptor channel complex in rat dorsal root ganglion neurons. *FASEB J.* 1989;3:1850–1854.
138. Fujiwara N, Higashi H, Nishi S, et al. Changes in spontaneous firing patterns of rat hippocampal neurones induced by volatile anaesthetics. *J Physiol.* 1988;402:155–175.
139. Yeh JZ, Quandt FN, Tanguy J, et al. General anesthetic action on gamma-aminobutyric acid-activated channels. *Ann NY Acad Sci.* 1991;625:155–173.
140. Banks MI, Pearce RA. Dual actions of volatile anesthetics on GABA(A) IPSCs: dissociation of blocking and prolonging effects. *Anesthesiology.* 1999;90:120–134.
141. Pritchett DB, Sontheimer H, Shivers BD, et al. Importance of a novel $GABA_A$ receptor subunit for benzodiazepine pharmacology. *Nature.* 1989;338:582–585.
142. Hill-Venning C, Belelli D, Peters JA, et al. Subunit-dependent interaction of the general anaesthetic etomidate with the gamma-aminobutyric acid type A receptor. *Br J Pharmacol.* 1997;120:749–756.
143. Davies PA, Hanna MC, Hales TG, et al. Insensitivity to anaesthetic agents conferred by a class of $GABA_A$ receptor subunit. *Nature.* 1997;385:820–823.
144. Zhu WJ, Wang JF, Krueger KE, et al. Delta subunit inhibits neurosteroid modulation of GABAA receptors. *J Neurosci.* 1996;16:6648–6656.
145. Mihic SJ, Harris RA. Inhibition of rho1 receptor GABAergic currents by alcohols and volatile anesthetics. *J Pharmacol Exp Ther.* 1996;277:411–416.
146. Mihic SJ, Ye Q, Wick MJ, et al. Sites of alcohol and volatile anaesthetic action on GABA(A) and glycine receptors. *Nature.* 1997;389:385–389.
147. Belelli D, Lambert JJ, Peters JA, et al. The interaction of the general anesthetic etomidate with the gamma-aminobutyric acid type A receptor is influenced by a single amino acid. *Proc Natl Acad Sci U S A.* 1997;94:11031–11036.
148. Krasowski MD, Koltchine VV, Rick CE, et al. Propofol and other intravenous anesthetics have sites of action on the gamma-aminobutyric acid type A receptor distinct from that for isoflurane. *Molec Pharmacol.* 1998;53:530–538.
149. Hosie AM, Wilkins ME, da Silva HM, et al. Endogenous neurosteroids regulate GABAA receptors through two discrete transmembrane sites. *Nature.* 2006;444:486–489.
150. Forman SA, Miller KW. Anesthetic sites and allosteric mechanisms of action on Cys-loop ligand-gated ion channels. *Can J Anaesth.* 2011;58:191–205.
151. Dilger JP, Vidal AM, Mody HI, et al. Evidence for direct actions of general anesthetics on an ion channel protein: an new look at a unified mode of action. *Anesthesiology.* 1994;81:431–442.
152. Firestone LL, Sauter JF, Braswell LM, et al. Actions of general anesthetics on acetylcholine receptor-rich membranes from Torpedo californica. *Anesthesiology.* 1986;64:694–702.
153. Franks NP, Lieb WR. Stereospecific effects of inhalational general anesthetic optical isomers on nerve ion channels. *Science.* 1991;254:427–430.
154. Charlesworth P, Richards CD. Anaesthetic modulation of nicotinic ion channel kinetics in bovine chromaffin cells. *Br J Pharmacol.* 1995;114:909–917.
155. Violet JM, Downie DL, Nakisa RC, et al. Differential sensitivities of mammalian neuronal and muscle nicotinic acetylcholine receptors to general anesthetics. *Anesthesiology.* 1997;86:866–874.
156. Flood P, Ramirez-Latorre J, Role L. Alpha 4 beta 2 neuronal nicotinic acetylcholine receptors in the central nervous system are inhibited by isoflurane

157. Evers AS, Steinbach JH. Supersensitive sites in the central nervous system. Anesthetics block brain nicotinic receptors. *Anesthesiology*. 1997;86:760–762.
158. Eger EI 2nd, Zhang Y, Laster M, et al. Acetylcholine receptors do not mediate the immobilization produced by inhaled anesthetics. *Anesth Analg*. 2002;94:1500–1504.
159. Wong SM, Sonner JM, Kendig JJ. Acetylcholine receptors do not mediate isoflurane's actions on spinal cord in vitro. *Anesth Analg*. 2002;94:1495–1499.
160. Raines DE, Claycomb RJ. The role of electrostatic interactions in governing anesthetic action on the torpedo nicotinic acetylcholine receptor. *Anesth Analg*. 2002;95:356–361.
161. Downie DL, Hall AC, Lieb WR, et al. Effects of inhalational general anaesthetics on native glycine receptors in rat medullary neurons and recombinant glycine receptors in *Xenopus* oocytes. *Br J Pharmacol*. 1996;118:493–502.
162. Mascia MP, Machu TK, Harris RA. Enhancement of homomeric glycine receptor function by long-chain alcohols and anaesthetics. *Br J Pharmacol*. 1996;119:1331–1336.
163. Jenkins A, Franks NP, Lieb WR. Actions of general anaesthetics on 5-HT3 receptors in N1E-115 neuroblastoma cells. *Br J Pharmacol*. 1996;117:1507–1515.
164. Machu TK, Harris RA. Alcohols and anesthetics enhance the function of 5-hydroxytryptamine3 receptors expressed in *Xenopus laevis* oocytes. *J Pharmacol Exp Ther*. 1994;271:898–905.
165. Segal IS, Vickery RG, Walton JK, et al. Dexmedetomidine diminishes halothane anesthetic requirements in rats through a postsynaptic alpha-2 adrenergic-receptor. *Anesthesiology*. 1988;69:818–823.
166. Moody EJ, Harris BD, Skolnick P. The potential for safer anesthesia using stereoselective anesthetics. *Trends Pharmacol Sci*. 1994;15:387–391.
167. Zhang Y, Laster MJ, Hara K, et al. Glycine receptors mediate part of the immobility produced by inhaled anesthetics. *Anesth Analg*. 2003;96:97–101.
168. Zhang Y, Sonner JM, Eger EI II, et al. Gamma-aminobutyric acid$_A$ receptors do not mediate the immobility produced by isoflurane. *Anesth Analg*. 2004;99:85–90.
169. Zhang Y, Wu S, Eger EI, et al. Neither GABA(A) nor strychnine-sensitive glycine receptors are the sole mediators of MAC for isoflurane. *Anesth Analg*. 2001;92:123–127.
170. Morgan PG, Cascorbi HF. Effect of anesthetics and a convulsant on normal and mutant Caenorhabditis elegans. *Anesthesiology*. 1985;62:738–744.
171. Sedensky MM, Meneely PM. Genetic analysis of halothane sensitivity in Caenorhabditis elegans. *Science*. 1987;236:952–954.
172. Humphrey JA, Hamming KS, Thacker CM, et al. A putative cation channel and its novel regulator: cross-species conservation of effects on general anesthesia. *Curr Biol*. 2007;17:624–629.
173. Crowder CM, Shebester LD, Schedl T. Behavioral effects of volatile anesthetics in Caenorhabditis elegans. *Anesthesiology*. 1996;85:901–912.
174. Metz LB, Dasgupta N, Liu C, et al. An evolutionarily conserved presynaptic protein is required for isoflurane sensitivity in Caenorhabditis elegans. *Anesthesiology*. 2007;107:971–982.
175. Nagele P, Metz LB, Crowder CM. Nitrous oxide (N(2)O) requires the N-methyl-D-aspartate receptor for its action in Caenorhabditis elegans. *Proc Natl Acad Sci U S A*. 2004;101:8791–8796.
176. Nagele P, Metz LB, Crowder CM. Xenon acts by inhibition of non-N-methyl-D-aspartate receptor-mediated glutamatergic neurotransmission in Caenorhabditis elegans. *Anesthesiology*. 2005;103:508–513.
177. Campbell DB, Nash HA. Use of drosophila mutants to distinguish among volatile general-anesthetics. *Proc Natl Acad Sci U S A*. 1994;91:2135–2139.
178. Campbell JL, Nash HA. The visually-induced jump response of Drosophila melanogaster is sensitive to volatile anesthetics. *J Neurogenet*. 1998;12:241–251.
179. Krishnan KS, Nash HA. A genetic study of the anesthetic response: mutants of *Drosophila melanogaster* altered in sensitivity to halothane. *Proc Natl Acad Sci U S A*. 1990;87:8632–8636.
180. Drexler B, Antkowiak B, Engin E, et al. Identification and characterization of anesthetic targets by mouse molecular genetics approaches. *Can J Anaesth*. 2011;58:178–190.
181. Bledno YA, Jung S, Alva H, et al. Deletion of the alpha1 or beta2 subunit of GABAA receptors reduces actions of alcohol and other drugs. *J Pharmacol Exp Ther*. 2003;304:30–36.
182. Rau V, Iyer SV, Oh I, et al. Gamma-aminobutyric acid type A receptor alpha 4 subunit knockout mice are resistant to the amnestic effect of isoflurane. *Anesth Analg*. 2009;109:1816–1822.
183. Sonner JM, Cascio M, Xing Y, et al. Alpha 1 subunit-containing GABA type A receptors in forebrain contribute to the effect of inhaled anesthetics on conditioned fear. *Mol Pharmacol*. 2005;68:61–68.
184. Cheng VY, Martin LJ, Elliott EM, et al. Alpha$_5$GABA$_A$ receptors mediate the amnestic but not sedative-hypnotic effects of the general anesthetic etomidate. *J Neurosci*. 2006;26:3713–3720.
185. Homanics GE, Ferguson C, Quinlan JJ, et al. Gene knockout of the alpha6 subunit of the gamma-aminobutyric acid type A receptor: lack of effect on responses to ethanol, pentobarbital, and general anesthetics. *Mol Pharmacol*. 1997;51:588–596.
186. Borghese CM, Werner DF, Topf N, et al. An isoflurane- and alcohol-insensitive mutant GABA$_A$ receptor α1 subunit with near-normal apparent affinity for GABA: characterization in heterologous systems and production of knockin mice. *J Pharmacol Exp Ther*. 2006;319:208–218.
187. Sonner JM, Werner DF, Elsen FP, et al. Effect of isoflurane and other potent inhaled anesthetics on minimum alveolar concentration, learning, and the righting reflex in mice engineered to express alpha1 gamma-aminobutyric acid type A receptors unresponsive to isoflurane. *Anesthesiology*. 2007;106:107–213.
188. Werner DF, Bledno YA, Ariwodola OJ, et al. Knockin mice with ethanol-insensitive alpha1-containing gamma-aminobutyric acid type A receptors display selective alterations in behavioral responses to ethanol. *J Pharmacol Exp Ther*. 2006;319:219–227.
189. Nishikawa K, Jenkins A, Paraskevakis I, et al. Volatile anesthetic actions on the GABAA receptors: contrasting effects of alpha 1(S270) and beta 2(N265) point mutations. *Neuropharmacology*. 2002;42:337–345.
190. Homanics GE, Elsen FP, Ying SW, et al. A gain-of-function mutation in the GABA receptor produces synaptic and behavioral abnormalities in the mouse. *Genes Brain Behav*. 2005;4:10–19.
191. Siegwart R, Jurd R, Rudolph U. Molecular determinants for the action of general anesthetics at recombinant α2β3γ2γ-aminobutyric acid$_A$ receptors. *J Neurochem*. 2002;80:140–148.
192. Jurd R, Arras M, Lambert S, et al. General anesthetic actions in vivo strongly attenuated by a point mutation in the GABA(A) receptor beta3 subunit. *Faseb J*. 2003;17:250–252.
193. Zeller A, Arras M, Jurd R, et al. Identification of a molecular target mediating the general anesthetic actions of pentobarbital. *Mol Pharmacol*. 2007;71:852–859.
194. Zeller A, Arras M, Jurd R, et al. Mapping the contribution of beta3-containing GABAA receptors to volatile and intravenous general anesthetic actions. *BMC Pharmacol*. 2007;7:2.
195. Zeller A, Arras M, Lazaris A, et al. Distinct molecular targets for the central respiratory and cardiac actions of the general anesthetics etomidate and propofol. *FASEB J*. 2005;19:1677–1679.
196. Liao M, Sonner JM, Jurd R, et al. Beta3-containing gamma-aminobutyric acidA receptors are not major targets for the amnesic and immobilizing actions of isoflurane. *Anesth Analg*. 2005;101:412–418.
197. Rau V, Oh I, Liao M, et al. Gamma-aminobutyric acid type A receptor beta3 subunit forebrain-specific knockout mice are resistant to the amnestic effect of isoflurane. *Anesth Analg*. 2011;113:500–504.
198. Cirone J, Rosahl TW, Reynolds DS, et al. Gamma-aminobutyric acid type A receptor beta 2 subunit mediates the hypothermic effect of etomidate in mice. *Anesthesiology*. 2004;100:1438–1445.
199. Reynolds DS, Rosahl TW, Cirone J, et al. Sedation and anesthesia mediated by distinct GABA(A) receptor isoforms. *J Neurosci*. 2003;23:8608–8617.
200. Mihalek RM, Banerjee PK, Korpi ER, et al. Attenuated sensitivity to neuroactive steroids in gamma-aminobutyrate type A receptor delta subunit knockout mice. *Proc Natl Acad Sci U S A*. 1999;96:12905–12910.
201. Heurteaux C, Guy N, Laigle C, et al. TREK-1, a K+ channel involved in neuroprotection and general anesthesia. *EMBO J*. 2004;23:2684–2695.
202. Westphalen RI, Krivitski M, Amarosa A, et al. Reduced inhibition of cortical glutamate and GABA release by halothane in mice lacking the K+ channel, TREK-1. *Br J Pharmacol*. 2007;152:939–945.
203. Linden AM, Aller MI, Leppa E, et al. The in vivo contributions of TASK-1-containing channels to the actions of inhalation anesthetics, the alpha(2) adrenergic sedative dexmedetomidine, and cannabinoid agonists. *J Pharmacol Exp Ther*. 2006;317:615–626.
204. Linden AM, Sandu C, Aller MI, et al. TASK-3 knockout mice exhibit exaggerated nocturnal activity, impairments in cognitive functions, and reduced sensitivity to inhalation anesthetics. *J Pharmacol Exp Ther*. 2007;323:924–934.
205. Pang DS, Robledo CJ, Carr DR, et al. An unexpected role for TASK-3 potassium channels in network oscillations with implications for sleep mechanisms and anesthetic action. *Proc Natl Acad Sci U S A*. 2009;106:17546–17551.
206. Zhou C, Liang P, Liu J, et al. HCN1 channels contribute to the effects of amnesia and hypnosis but not immobility of volatile anesthetics. *Anesth Analg*. 2015;121:661–666.
207. Mattusch C, Kratzer S, Buerge M, et al. Impact of hyperpolarization-activated, cyclic nucleotide-gated cation channel type 2 for the xenon-mediated anesthetic effect: evidence from in vitro and in vivo experiments. *Anesthesiology*. 2015;122:1047–1059.
208. Zhou C, Douglas JE, Kumar NN, et al. Forebrain HCN1 channels contribute to hypnotic actions of ketamine. *Anesthesiology*. 2013;118:785–795.
209. Rampil IJ, Mason P, Singh H. Anesthetic potency (MAC) is independent of forebrain structures in the rat. *Anesthesiology*. 1993;78:707–712.
210. Rampil IJ. Anesthetic potency is not altered after hypothermic spinal cord transection in rats. *Anesthesiology*. 1994;80:606–610.
211. Antognini JF, Schwartz K. Exaggerated anesthetic requirements in the preferentially anesthetized brain. *Anesthesiology*. 1993;79:1244–1249.
212. Borges M, Antognini JF. Does the brain influence somatic responses to noxious stimuli during isoflurane anesthesia? *Anesthesiology*. 1994;81:1511–1515.
213. Jinks SL, Bravo M, Satter O, et al. Brainstem regions affecting minimum alveolar concentration and movement pattern during isoflurane anesthesia. *Anesthesiology*. 2010;112:316–324.

214. Takenoshita M, Takahashi T. Mechanisms of halothane action on synaptic transmission in motoneurons of the newborn rat spinal cord in vitro. *Brain Res*. 1987;402:303–310.
215. Zorychta E, Esplin DW, Capek R. Action of halothane on transmitter release in the spinal monosynaptic pathway. *Fed Proc Am Soc Exp Biol*. 1975;34.
216. Fujiwara N, Higashi H, Fujita S. Mechanism of halothane action on synaptic transmission in motoneurons of the newborn rat spinal cord in vitro. *J Physiol*. 1988;412.
217. Kungys G, Kim J, Jinks SL, et al. Propofol produces immobility via action in the ventral horn of the spinal cord by a GABAergic mechanism. *Anesth Analg*. 2009;108:1531–1537.
218. Jinks SL, Atherley RJ, Dominguez CL, et al. Isoflurane disrupts central pattern generator activity and coordination in the lamprey isolated spinal cord. *Anesthesiology*. 2005;103:567–575.
219. Stucke AG, Zuperku EJ, Tonkovic-Capin V, et al. Halothane depresses glutamatergic neurotransmission to brain stem inspiratory premotor neurons in a decerebrate dog model. *Anesthesiology*. 2003;98:897–905.
220. Wang X. Propofol and isoflurane enhancement of tonic gamma-aminobutyric acid type a current in cardiac vagal neurons in the nucleus ambiguus. *Anesth Analg*. 2009;108:142–148.
221. McDougall SJ, Bailey TW, Mendelowitz D, et al. Propofol enhances both tonic and phasic inhibitory currents in second-order neurons of the solitary tract nucleus (NTS). *Neuropharmacology*. 2008;54:552–563.
222. Peters JH, McDougall SJ, Mendelowitz D, et al. Isoflurane differentially modulates inhibitory and excitatory synaptic transmission to the solitary tract nucleus. *Anesthesiology*. 2008;108:675–683.
223. Collinson N, Kuenzi FM, Jarolimek W, et al. Enhanced learning and memory and altered GABAergic synaptic transmission in mice lacking the alpha 5 subunit of the GABAA receptor. *J Neurosci*. 2002;22:5572–5580.
224. Caraiscos VB, Newell JG, You-Ten KE, et al. Selective enhancement of tonic GABAergic inhibition in murine hippocampal neurons by low concentrations of the volatile anesthetic isoflurane. *J Neurosci*. 2004;24:8454–8458.
225. Zurek AA, Bridgwater EM, Orser BA. Inhibition of alpha5 gamma-aminobutyric acid type A receptors restores recognition memory after general anesthesia. *Anesth Analg*. 2012;114:845–855.
226. Laureys S. The neural correlate of (un)awareness: lessons from the vegetative state. *Trends Cogn Sci*. 2005;9:556–555.
227. French JD, Verzeano M, Magoun HW. A neural basis of the anesthetic state. *AMA Arch Neurol Psychiatry*. 1953;69:519–529.
228. Orth M, Bravo E, Barter L, et al. The differential effects of halothane and isoflurane on electroencephalographic responses to electrical microstimulation of the reticular formation. *Anesth Analg*. 2006;102:1709–1714.
229. Vanini G, Wathen BL, Lydic R, et al. Endogenous GABA levels in the pontine reticular formation are greater during wakefulness than during rapid eye movement sleep. *J Neurosci*. 2011;31:2649–2656.
230. Vanini G, Watson CJ, Lydic R, et al. Gamma-aminobutyric acid-mediated neurotransmission in the pontine reticular formation modulates hypnosis, immobility, and breathing during isoflurane anesthesia. *Anesthesiology*. 2008;109:978–988.
231. Saper CB, Chou TC, Scammell TE. The sleep switch: hypothalamic control of sleep and wakefulness. *Trends Neurosci*. 2001;24:726–731.
232. Luo T, Leung LS. Involvement of tuberomamillary histaminergic neurons in isoflurane anesthesia. *Anesthesiology*. 2011;115:36–43.
233. Nelson LE, Guo TZ, Lu J, et al. The sedative component of anesthesia is mediated by GABA(A) receptors in an endogenous sleep pathway. *Nat Neurosci*. 2002;5:979–984.
234. Zecharia AY, Nelson LE, Gent TC, et al. The involvement of hypothalamic sleep pathways in general anesthesia: testing the hypothesis using the GABAA receptor beta3N265M knock-in mouse. *J Neurosci*. 2009;29:2177–2187.
235. Eikermann M, Vetrivelan R, Grosse-Sundrup M, et al. The ventrolateral preoptic nucleus is not required for isoflurane general anesthesia. *Brain Res*. 2011;1426:30–37.
236. Yasuda Y, Takeda A, Fukuda S, et al. Orexin a elicits arousal electroencephalography without sympathetic cardiovascular activation in isoflurane-anesthetized rats. *Anesth Analg*. 2003;97:1663–1666.
237. Zhang LN, Li ZJ, Tong L, et al. Orexin-A facilitates emergence from propofol anesthesia in the rat. *Anesth Analg*. 2012;115:789–796.
238. Kelz MB, Sun Y, Chen J, et al. An essential role for orexins in emergence from general anesthesia. *Proc Natl Acad Sci U S A*. 2008;105:1309–1314.
239. Pillay S, Vizuete JA, McCallum JB, et al. Norepinephrine infusion into nucleus basalis elicits microarousal in desflurane-anesthetized rats. *Anesthesiology*. 2011;115:733–742.
240. Luo T, Leung LS. Basal forebrain histaminergic transmission modulates electroencephalographic activity and emergence from isoflurane anesthesia. *Anesthesiology*. 2009;111:725–733.
241. Taylor NE, Chemali JJ, Brown EN, et al. Activation of D1 dopamine receptors induces emergence from isoflurane general anesthesia. *Anesthesiology*. 2013;118:30–39.
242. Kenny JD, Taylor NE, Brown EN, et al. Dextroamphetamine (but not atomoxetine) induces reanimation from general anesthesia: implications for the roles of dopamine and norepinephrine in active emergence. *PLoS One*. 2015;10:e0131914.
243. Vazey EM, Aston-Jones G. Designer receptor manipulations reveal a role of the locus coeruleus noradrenergic system in isoflurane general anesthesia. *Proc Natl Acad Sci U S A*. 2014;111:3859–3864.
244. Alkire MT, Haier RJ, Fallon JH. Toward a unified theory of narcosis: brain imaging evidence for a thalamocortical switch as the neurophysiologic basis of anesthetic-induced unconsciousness. *Conscious Cogn*. 2000;9:370–386.
245. Imas OA, Ropella KM, Wood JD, et al. Halothane augments event-related gamma oscillations in rat visual cortex. *Neuroscience*. 2004;123:269–278.
246. Hudetz AG, Imas OA. Burst activation of the cerebral cortex by flash stimuli during isoflurane anesthesia in rats. *Anesthesiology*. 2007;107:983–991.
247. Herd MB, Lambert JJ, Belelli D. The general anaesthetic etomidate inhibits the excitability of mouse thalamocortical relay neurons by modulating multiple modes of GABAA receptor-mediated inhibition. *Eur J Neurosci*. 2014;40:2487–2501.
248. Yen CT, Shaw FZ. Reticular thalamic responses to nociceptive inputs in anesthetized rats. *Brain Res*. 2003;968:179–191.
249. Alkire MT, Asher CD, Franciscus AM, et al. Thalamic microinfusion of antibody to a voltage-gated potassium channel restores consciousness during anesthesia. *Anesthesiology*. 2009;110:766–773.
250. Alkire MT, McReynolds JR, Hahn EL, et al. Thalamic microinjection of nicotine reverses sevoflurane-induced loss of righting reflex in the rat. *Anesthesiology*. 2007;107:264–272.
251. Liu X, Lauer KK, Ward BD, et al. Differential effects of deep sedation with propofol on the specific and nonspecific thalamocortical systems: a functional magnetic resonance imaging study. *Anesthesiology*. 2013;118:59–69.
252. Palanca BJ, Mitra A, Larson-Prior L, et al. Resting-state functional magnetic resonance imaging correlates of sevoflurane-induced unconsciousness. *Anesthesiology*. 2015;123:346–356.
253. Hudetz AG, Vizuete JA, Imas OA. Desflurane selectively suppresses long-latency cortical neuronal response to flash in the rat. *Anesthesiology*. 2009;111:231–239.
254. Imas OA, Ropella KM, Ward BD, et al. Volatile anesthetics disrupt frontal-posterior recurrent information transfer at gamma frequencies in rat. *Neurosci Lett*. 2005;387:145–150.
255. Boveroux P, Vanhaudenhuyse A, Bruno MA, et al. Breakdown of within- and between-network resting state functional magnetic resonance imaging connectivity during propofol-induced loss of consciousness. *Anesthesiology*. 2010;113:1038–1053.
256. Schrouff J, Perlbarg V, Boly M, et al. Brain functional integration decreases during propofol-induced loss of consciousness. *Neuroimage*. 2011;57:198–205.
257. Jordan D, Ilg R, Riedl V, et al. Simultaneous electroencephalographic and functional magnetic resonance imaging indicate impaired cortical top-down processing in association with anesthetic-induced unconsciousness. *Anesthesiology*. 2013;119:1031–1042.
258. Lee U, Mashour GA, Kim S, et al. Propofol induction reduces the capacity for neural information integration: implications for the mechanism of consciousness and general anesthesia. *Conscious Cogn*. 2009;18:56–64.
259. Ku SW, Lee U, Noh GJ, et al. Preferential inhibition of frontal-to-parietal feedback connectivity is a neurophysiologic correlate of general anesthesia in surgical patients. *PLoS One*. 2011;6:e25155.
260. Lee U, Kim S, Noh GJ, et al. The directionality and functional organization of frontoparietal connectivity during consciousness and anesthesia in humans. *Conscious Cogn*. 2009;18:1069–1078.
261. Lee U, Ku S, Noh G, et al. Disruption of frontal-parietal communication by ketamine, propofol, and sevoflurane. *Anesthesiology*. 2013;118:1264–1275.
262. Blain-Moraes S, Tarnal V, Vanini G, et al. Neurophysiological correlates of sevoflurane-induced unconsciousness. *Anesthesiology*. 2015;122:307–316.
263. Raichle ME, MacLeod AM, Snyder AZ, et al. A default mode of brain function. *Proc Natl Acad Sci U S A*. 2001;98:676–682.
264. Greicius MD, Krasnow B, Reiss AL, et al. Functional connectivity in the resting brain: a network analysis of the default mode hypothesis. *Proc Natl Acad Sci U S A*. 2003;100:253–258.
265. Guldenmund P, Demertzi A, Boveroux P, et al. Thalamus, brainstem and salience network connectivity changes during propofol-induced sedation and unconsciousness. *Brain Connect*. 2013;3:273–285.
266. Corbetta M, Shulman GL. Control of goal-directed and stimulus-driven attention in the brain. *Nat Rev Neurosci*. 2002;3:201–215.
267. Seeley WW, Menon V, Schatzberg AF, et al. Dissociable intrinsic connectivity networks for salience processing and executive control. *J Neurosci*. 2007;27:2349–2356.
268. Mashour GA. Consciousness unbound: toward a paradigm of general anesthesia. *Anesthesiology*. 2004;100:428–433.
269. Hudetz AG, Vizuete JA, Pillay S. Differential effects of isoflurane on high-frequency and low-frequency gamma oscillations in the cerebral cortex and hippocampus in freely moving rats. *Anesthesiology*. 2011;114:588–595.
270. Breshears JD, Roland JL, Sharma M, et al. Stable and dynamic cortical electrophysiology of induction and emergence with propofol anesthesia. *Proc Natl Acad Sci U S A*. 2010;107:21170–21175.
271. John ER, Prichep LS, Kox W, et al. Invariant reversible QEEG effects of anesthetics. *Conscious Cogn*. 2001;10:165–183.

11 Basic Principles of Clinical Pharmacology

DHANESH K. GUPTA • THOMAS K. HENTHORN

Pharmacokinetic Principles
  Drug Absorption and Routes of Administration
  Drug Distribution
  Drug Elimination
Pharmacokinetic Models
  Physiologic versus Compartmental Models
  Pharmacokinetic Concepts
  Compartmental Pharmacokinetic Models
  Noncompartmental (Stochastic) Pharmacokinetic Models
Pharmacodynamic Principles
  Drug–Receptor Interactions
  Dose–Response Relationships
  Concentration–Response Relationships
Drug Interactions
  Pharmaceutical (Physicchemical) Interactions
  Pharmacokinetic Interactions
  Pharmacodynamic Interactions

Clinical Applications of Pharmacokinetics and Pharmacodynamics to the Administration of Intravenous Anesthetics
  Rise to Steady-state Concentration
  Manual Bolus and Infusion Dosing Schemes
  Isoconcentration Nomogram
  Context-sensitive Decrement Times
  Soft Pharmacology and Anesthesiology
  Target-controlled Infusions
  Time to Maximum Effect Compartment Concentration (T_{max})
  Volume of Distribution at Peak Effect (V_{DPE})
  Front-end Pharmacokinetics
  Closed-loop Infusions
  Response Surface Models of Drug–Drug Interactions
Conclusion

KEY POINTS

1. Most drugs must pass through cell membranes to reach their sites of action. Consequently, drugs tend to be relatively lipophilic, rather than hydrophilic.
2. The highly lipophilic anesthetic drugs have a rapid onset of action because they rapidly diffuse into the highly perfused brain tissue. They have a very short duration of action because of redistribution of drug from the CNS to the blood.
3. The cytochrome P450 (CYP) superfamily is the most important group of enzymes involved in drug metabolism. It and other drug-metabolizing enzymes exhibit genetic polymorphism.
4. The kidneys eliminate hydrophilic drugs and relatively hydrophilic metabolites of lipophilic drugs. Renal elimination of lipophilic compounds is negligible.
5. The liver is the most important organ for metabolism of drugs. Hepatic drug clearance depends on three factors: the intrinsic ability of the liver to metabolize a drug, hepatic blood flow, and the extent of binding of the drug to blood components.
6. The volume of distribution quantifies the extent of drug distribution. The greater the affinity of tissues for a drug relative to blood, the greater its volume of distribution (i.e., lipophilic drugs have greater volumes of distribution).
7. Elimination clearance is the parameter that characterizes the ability of drug-eliminating tissues to irreversibly remove drugs from the body. The efficiency of the body in removing drug from the body is proportional to the elimination clearance.
8. All else being equal, an increase in the volume of distribution of a drug will increase its elimination half-life; an increase in elimination clearance will decrease elimination half-life.
9. Most drugs bring about a pharmacologic effect by binding to a specific receptor that results in a change in cellular function to produce the pharmacologic effect.
10. Although most pharmacologic effects can be characterized by both dose–response curves and concentration–response curves, dose–response curves cannot be used to determine whether variations in pharmacologic response are caused by differences in pharmacokinetics, pharmacodynamics, or both.
11. Integrated pharmacokinetic–pharmacodynamic models allow temporal characterization of the relationship between dose, plasma concentration, and pharmacologic effect.
12. In vitro drug–drug interactions due to pharmaceutical (physicochemical) properties of drugs can significantly alter drug bioavailability and produce unintended toxic byproducts.
13. Novel approaches to antagonizing neuromuscular blockade have been developed that take advantage of in vivo physiochemical drug–drug interactions, thereby avoiding some of the systemic side effects associated with inhibition of plasma acetylcholinesterase.
14. Distribution clearance is influenced by changes in cardiac output and regional blood flow.

15. Inhibition of CYP isozyme activity can make it difficult to achieve adequate analgesia when using opioids such as codeine and Tramadol that require CYP 2D6 activity for conversion to the biologically active opioid.
16. Serotonin syndrome can be precipitated by a wide array of drugs that are associated with serotonergic activity, including SSRIs, NSRIs, and phenylpiperidine opioids.
17. Simulations of multicompartmental pharmacokinetic models that describe intravenous anesthetics demonstrate that for most anesthetic dosing regimens, the distribution of drug from the plasma to the inert peripheral tissues has a greater influence on the plasma concentration profile of the drug than the elimination of drug from the body.
18. Target-controlled infusions are achieved with computer-controlled infusion pumps worldwide (not yet FDA-approved in the United States), and permit clinicians to make use of the drug concentration–effect relationship, optimally accounting for pharmacokinetics, and predicting the offset of drug effect.
19. Classic pharmacokinetic models inaccurately describe the initial several minutes of drug distribution that occur during the time of drug onset, and, therefore, overestimate the interindividual pharmacodynamic variability.
20. By understanding the interactions between the opioids and the sedative-hypnotics (e.g., response surface models), it is possible to select target concentration pairs of the two drugs that produce the desired clinical effect while minimizing unwanted side effects associated with high concentrations of a single drug.

In 1943, Halford[1] labeled thiopental as "an ideal method of euthanasia" for war surgical patients and pronounced that "open drop ether still retains primacy!" Based on this recount of the experience with thiopental at Pearl Harbor, it is impressive that cooler heads prevailed—Adams and Gray[2] detailed a case of a civilian gunshot wound where they carefully titrated incremental doses of thiopental without any adverse respiratory or cardiovascular events. To highlight the importance of the quiet case report versus the animated condemnation of intravenous (IV) anesthesia for patients with hemorrhagic shock, an anonymous editorial appeared in the same issue of *Anesthesiology* that attempted to give some scientific justification for the discrepancy in opinions.[3] As the editorial detailed, thiopental has a small therapeutic index, and the tolerance to normal doses is decreased in extreme physical conditions (e.g., blood loss, sepsis). Therefore, just like with open drop ether, small doses of thiopental should be titrated to achieve the desired effects and avoid side effects associated with overdose. Fortuitously, the anesthesia community did not simply abandon the use of thiopental, and in 1960, Price[4] utilized mathematical models in order to describe the effects of hypovolemia on thiopental distribution.

Anesthetic drugs are administered with the goal of rapidly establishing and maintaining a therapeutic effect while minimizing undesired side effects. Although open-drop ether and chloroform were administered using knowledge of a dose–effect relationship, the more potent volatile agents, along with the IV hypnotics, neuromuscular junction blocking agents, and IV opioids, all require a sound knowledge of pharmacokinetics and pharmacodynamics in order to accurately achieve the desired pharmacologic effect for the desired period of time without any drug toxicity.

This chapter attempts to guide the reader through the fundamental knowledge of what the body does to a drug (i.e., pharmacokinetics) and what a drug does to the body (i.e., pharmacodynamics). The initial section of this chapter discusses the biologic and pharmacologic factors that influence the absorption, distribution, and elimination of a drug from the body. Where necessary, quantitative analyses of these processes are discussed to give readers insight into the intricacies of pharmacokinetics that cannot be easily described by text alone. The second section concentrates on the factors that determine the relationship between drug concentration and pharmacologic effect. Once again, mathematical models are presented as needed in order to clarify pharmacodynamic concepts. The third section applies concepts from the first two sections in order to describe the clinically important drug–drug interactions that are encountered in the perioperative period. The final section builds on the reader's knowledge gained from the first two sections to apply the principles of pharmacokinetics and pharmacodynamics to determine the target concentration of IV anesthetics required and the dosing strategies necessary to produce an adequate anesthetic state. Understanding these concepts should allow the reader to integrate the anesthetic drugs of the future into a rational anesthetic regimen. Although specific drugs are utilized to illustrate pharmacokinetic and pharmacodynamic principles throughout this chapter, the principles discussed are universal. Detailed pharmacologic information of anesthetic pharmacopeia are presented in subsequent chapters of this book.

Pharmacokinetic Principles

Drug Absorption and Routes of Administration

Transfer of Drugs across Membranes

For even the simplest drug that is directly administered into the blood to exert its action, it must move across at least one cell membrane to its site of action. Because biologic membranes are lipid bilayers composed of a lipophilic core sandwiched between two hydrophilic layers, only small lipophilic drugs can passively diffuse across the membrane down their concentration gradients. In order for water-soluble drugs to passively diffuse across the membrane down its concentration gradient, transmembrane proteins that form a hydrophilic channel are required. Because of the abundance of these nonspecific hydrophilic channels in the capillary endothelium of all organs except for the central nervous system (CNS), where the blood–brain barrier capillary endothelial cells have very limited numbers of transmembrane hydrophilic channels, *passive transport* of drugs from the intravascular space into the interstitium of various organs is limited by blood flow, not by the lipid solubility of the drug.[5]

Hydrophilic drugs can only enter the CNS after binding to drug-specific transmembrane proteins that actively transport the hydrophilic drug across the capillary endothelium into the CNS interstitium. When these transmembrane carrier proteins require energy to transport the drug across the membrane, they are able to shuttle compounds against their concentration gradients, a process called *active transport*. In contrast, when these carrier proteins do not require energy to shuttle drugs, they cannot overcome concentration gradients, a process called *facilitated diffusion*. Active transport is not limited to the CNS, but is also found in the organs related to drug elimination (e.g., hepatocytes, renal tubular cells, pulmonary capillary endothelium), where the ability to transport drugs against the concentration gradient has specific biologic advantages. Both active transport and facilitated diffusion of drugs are saturable processes that are primarily limited by the number of carrier proteins available to shuttle a specific drug.[5]

For lipophilic compounds transporters are not needed for the drug to diffuse across the capillary wall into tissues, but the presence of transporters does affect the concentration gradients that exist. For instance, some lipophilic drugs are transported out of tissues by ATP-dependent transporters such as p-glycoprotein (P-gp). The lipophilic potent μ-opioid agonist, loperamide, used for the treatment of diarrhea, has limited bioavailability because of P-gp transporters at the intestine-portal capillary interface and then what does reach the circulation has its CNS penetrance limited by P-gp at the blood–brain barrier.[6] Conversely, lipophilic compounds can be transported into tissues, increasing the tissue concentration of the drug beyond what would be accomplished by passive diffusion. The class of transporters called organic anion polypeptide transporters (OATPs) are located in the microvascular endothelium of the brain and transports endogenous opioids into the brain.[7,8] These OATPs also transport drugs. The degree to which transporter proteins may account for intra- and interindividual responses to anesthetic drugs has not been well studied to date.[9]

Intravenous Administration

In order for a drug to be delivered to the site of drug action, it must be absorbed into the systemic circulation. Therefore, IV administration results in immediate delivery of a drug with 100% bioavailability. Although this can lead to rapid overshoot of the desired plasma concentration which can potentially result in immediate and severe side effects for drugs that have a low *therapeutic index* (the ratio of the blood concentration that produces a toxic effect in 50% of the population to the blood concentration that produces a therapeutic effect in 50% of the population). Except for IV administration, the absorption of a drug into the systemic circulation is an important determinant of the time course of drug action and the maximum drug effect produced. As the absorption of drug is slowed, the maximum plasma concentration achieved, and therefore the maximum drug effect achieved, is limited. However, as long as the plasma concentration is maintained at a level above the minimum effective plasma concentration, the drug will produce a drug effect.[10] Therefore, non-IV methods of drug administration can produce a sustained and significant drug effect that may be more advantageous than administering drugs by the IV route.[11]

Bioavailability is the *relative amount* of a drug dose that reaches the systemic circulation unchanged and the *rate* at which this occurs. For most intravenously administered drugs, the absolute bioavailability of drug available is close to unity and the rate is nearly instantaneous. However, the pulmonary endothelium can slow the rate at which intravenously administered drugs reach the systemic circulation if distribution into the alveolar endothelium is extensive, such as occurs with the pulmonary uptake of fentanyl. The pulmonary endothelium also contains enzymes that may metabolize intravenously administered drugs (e.g., propofol) on first pass and reduce their absolute bioavailability.[12]

Oral Administration

For almost all therapeutic agents in all fields of medicine, oral administration is the safest and most convenient method of administration. However, this route is not utilized significantly in anesthetic practice because of the limited and variable rate of bioavailability. The absorption rate in the gastrointestinal tract is highly variable because the main determinant of the timing of absorption is gastric emptying into the small intestines, where the surface area for absorption is several orders of magnitude greater than that of the stomach or large intestines. In addition, the active metabolism of drug by the small intestine mucosal epithelium, and the obligatory path through the portal circulation before entering the systemic circulation, contribute to decreased bioavailability of orally administered drugs.[13] In fact, the metabolic capacity of the liver for drugs is so high that only a small fraction of most lipophilic drugs actually reach the systemic circulation. Because of this extensive *first-pass metabolism*, the oral dose of most drugs must be significantly higher than IV to generate a therapeutic plasma concentration. The prolonged and variable time until peak concentrations are usually achieved from oral administration (between tens of minutes to hours), makes it impractical to utilize this mode to administer perioperative anesthetic agents.

Highly lipophilic drugs that can maintain a high contact time with nasal or oral (sublingual) mucosa can be absorbed without needing to traverse the gastrointestinal tract. Sublingual administration of drug has the additional advantage over gastrointestinal absorption in that absorbed drug directly enters the systemic venous circulation and therefore is able to bypass the metabolically active intestinal mucosa and the hepatic first-pass metabolism. Therefore, small doses of drug can rapidly produce significant increases in drug plasma concentration and therapeutic effect.[14] However, because of formulation limitations and the small surface area available for absorption, there are a limited number of drugs that are appropriate for sublingual administration (e.g., nitroglycerin, fentanyl).

Transcutaneous Administration

A few lipophilic drugs have been manufactured in formulations that are sufficient to allow penetration of intact skin. Although scopolamine, nitroglycerin, opioids, and clonidine all produce therapeutic systemic plasma concentrations when administered as "drug patches," the extended amount of time that it takes to achieve an effective therapeutic concentration limits practical application except for maintenance therapy. Attempts to speed the passive diffusion of these drugs utilizing an electric current has been described for fentanyl,[15] but it is still limited in its practicality.

Intramuscular and Subcutaneous Administration

Absorption of drugs from the depots in the subcutaneous tissue or in muscle tissue is directly dependent on the drug formulation and the blood flow to the depot. Because of the high blood flow to muscles in most physiologic states, intramuscular absorption of drugs in solution is relatively rapid and complete. Therefore, some aqueous drugs can be administered as intramuscular injection with rapid and predictable effects (e.g., neuromuscular junction blocking agents). The subcutaneous route of drug absorption is more variable in its onset because of the variability of subcutaneous blood flow during varying physiologic states—this is the primary reason that subcutaneous heparin and regular insulin administered perioperatively have variable times of onset and maximum effect.

Intrathecal, Epidural, and Perineural Injection

Because the spinal cord is the primary site of action of many anesthetic agents, direct injection of local anesthetics and opioids into the intrathecal space bypasses the limitations of drug absorption and drug distribution of any other route of administration. This is not the case for epidural and perineural administration of local anesthetics, because not delivering the drug directly into the cerebrospinal fluid necessitates that the drug be absorbed through the dura or nerve sheath in order to reach the site of drug action. The major downside to all of these techniques is the relative expertise required to perform regional anesthetics to oral, IV, and inhalational administration of drug.

Inhalational Administration

The large surface area of the pulmonary alveoli available for exchange with the large volumetric flow of blood found in the pulmonary capillaries makes inhalational administration an extremely attractive method by which to administer drugs.[16] New technologies have been developed which can rapidly and predictably aerosolize a wide range of drugs and thus approximate IV administration.[17] These devices are currently in Phase II FDA trials.

Drug Distribution

Once drug has entered the systemic circulation, it is transported through bulk flow of blood to all of the organs throughout the body. The relative distribution of cardiac output among organ vascular beds determines the speed at which organs are exposed to drug. The highly perfused core circulatory components—the brain, lungs, heart, and kidneys—receive the highest relative distribution of cardiac output and therefore are the initial organs to reach equilibrium with plasma drug concentrations.[4] Drug concentrations then equilibrate with the less well-perfused muscles and liver and then, finally, with the relatively poorly perfused splanchnic vasculature, adipose tissue, and bone.

Whether by passive diffusion or transporter-mediation, drug transport at the capillaries is not usually saturable, so the amount of drug uptake by tissues and organs is limited by the blood flow they receive (i.e., flow-limited drug uptake).

Although the rate to initial drug delivery may be dependent on the relative blood flow to the organ, the rate of drug equilibration by the tissue is dependent on the ratio of blood flow to tissue content. Therefore, drug uptake rapidly approaches equilibrium in the highly perfused, but low volume, brain, kidneys, and lungs in a matter of minutes, whereas drug transfer to the less well-perfused, intermediate volume muscle tissue may take hours to approach equilibrium, and drug transfer to the poorly perfused, large cellular volumes of adipose tissue does not equilibrate for days.[11]

Redistribution

Highly lipophilic drugs such as thiopental and propofol rapidly begin to diffuse into the highly perfused brain tissue usually less than a minute after IV injection. Because of the low tissue volume but high perfusion of the brain, the drug concentration in the cerebral arterial blood rapidly equilibrates, usually within 3 minutes, with the concentration in the brain tissue. As drug continues to be taken up by other tissues with lower blood flows and higher tissue mass, the plasma concentration of the drug continues to rapidly decrease. Once the concentration of drug in the brain tissue is higher than the plasma concentration of drug, there is a reversal of the drug concentration gradient so that the lipophilic drug readily diffuses back into the blood and is *redistributed* to the other tissues that are still taking up drug.[4,18,19] This process continues for each of the organ beds, until ultimately the adipose tissue will contain the majority of the lipophilic drug that has not been removed from the body by metabolism or excretion. However, after a single bolus of a highly lipophilic drug, the brain's tissue concentration rapidly decreases below therapeutic levels due to redistribution of drug to muscle tissue, which has a larger perfusion than adipose tissue.[4,19] Although single, moderate doses of highly lipophilic drugs have a very short CNS duration of action because of redistribution of drug from the CNS to the blood and other, less well-perfused tissues, repeated injections of a drug allow the rapid establishment of significant peripheral tissue concentrations. When the tissue concentrations of a drug are high enough, the decrease in plasma drug concentration below therapeutic threshold becomes solely dependent on drug elimination from the body.[20]

Drug Elimination

Besides being excreted unchanged from the body, a drug can be biotransformed (metabolized) into one or more new compounds that are then eliminated from the body. Either mechanism of elimination will decrease the drug concentration in the body such that the concentration will eventually be negligible and therefore unable to produce drug effect. Elimination is the pharmacokinetic term that describes all the processes that remove a drug from the body. Although the liver and the kidneys are considered the major organs of drug elimination, drug metabolism can occur at many other locations that contain active drug metabolizing enzymes (e.g., pulmonary vasculature, red blood cells) and drug can be excreted unchanged from other organs (e.g., lungs).

Elimination clearance (drug clearance) is the theoretical volume of blood from which drug is completely and irreversibly removed in a unit of time.[21] *Total* drug clearance can be calculated with pharmacokinetic models of blood concentration versus time data.

Biotransformation Reactions

Most drugs that are excreted unchanged from the body are hydrophilic and therefore readily pass into urine or stool. Drugs that are not sufficiently hydrophilic to be able to be excreted unchanged require modification into more hydrophilic, excretable compounds. Enzymatic reactions that metabolize drugs can be classified into Phase I and Phase II biotransformation reactions. Phase I reactions tend to transform a drug into one or more polar, and hence potentially excretable compounds. Phase II reactions transform the original drug by conjugating a variety of endogenous compounds to a polar functional group of the drug, making the metabolite even more hydrophilic. Often drugs will undergo a Phase I reaction to produce a new compound with a polar functional group that will then undergo a Phase II reaction. However, it is possible for a drug to undergo either a Phase I reaction alone or a Phase II reaction alone.

Phase I Reactions

Phase I reactions may hydrolyze, oxidize, or reduce the parent compound. *Hydrolysis* is the insertion of a molecule of water into another molecule, which forms an unstable intermediate compound that subsequently splits apart. Thus, hydrolysis cleaves the original substance into two separate molecules. Hydrolytic reactions are the primary way amides, such as lidocaine and other amide local anesthetics, and esters, such as succinylcholine, are metabolized.

Many drugs are biotransformed by oxidative reactions. *Oxidations* are defined as reactions that remove electrons from a molecule. The common element of most, if not all, oxidations is an enzymatically mediated reaction that inserts a hydroxyl group (OH) into the drug molecule. In some instances, this produces a chemically stable, more polar hydroxylated metabolite. However, hydroxylation usually creates unstable compounds that spontaneously split into separate molecules. Many different biotransformations are effected by this basic mechanism. Dealkylation (removal of a carbon-containing group), deamination (removal of nitrogen-containing groups), oxidation of nitrogen-containing groups, desulfuration, dehalogenation, and dehydrogenation all follow an initial hydroxylation. Hydrolysis and hydroxylation are comparable processes. Both have an initial, enzymatically mediated step that produces an unstable compound that rapidly dissociates into separate molecules.

Some drugs are metabolized by *reductive reactions,* that is, reactions that add electrons to a molecule. In contrast to oxidations, where electrons are transferred from NADPH to an oxygen atom, the electrons are transferred to the drug molecule. Oxidation of xenobiotics requires oxygen, but reductive biotransformation is inhibited by oxygen, so it is facilitated when the intracellular oxygen tension is low.

Cytochrome P450 Enzymes

The cytochrome P450 (CYP) are the superfamily of constitutive and inducible enzymes that catalyze most Phase I biotransformations. CYP3A4 is the single most important enzyme, accounting for 40% to 45% of all CYP-mediated drug metabolism. CYPs are incorporated into the smooth endoplasmic reticulum of hepatocytes and the membranes of the upper intestinal enterocytes in high concentrations. CYPs are also found in the lungs, kidneys, and skin, but in much smaller numbers. CYP isoenzymes oxidize their substrates primarily by the insertion of an atom of oxygen in the form of a hydroxyl group, while another oxygen atom is reduced to water.

Several constitutive CYPs are involved in the production of various endogenous compounds, such as cholesterol, steroid hormones, prostaglandins, and eicosanoids. In addition to the constitutive forms, production of various CYPs can be induced by a wide variety of xenobiotics. CYP drug-metabolizing activity increases after exposure to various exogenous chemicals, including many drugs. The number and type of CYPs present at any time depends on exposure to different xenobiotics. The CYP system is able to protect the organism from the deleterious effects of accumulation of exogenous compounds because of its two fundamental characteristics—broad substrate specificity and the capability to adapt to exposure to different substances by induction of different CYP isoenzymes. Table 11-1 groups drugs encountered in anesthetic practice according to the CYP isoenzymes responsible for their biotransformation.

Biotransformations can be inhibited if different substrates compete for the drug-binding site on the same CYP member. The effect of two competing substrates on each other's metabolism depends on their relative affinities for the enzyme. Biotransformation of the compound with the lower affinity is inhibited to a greater degree. This is the mechanism by which the H_2 receptor antagonist cimetidine inhibits the metabolism of many drugs, including meperidine, propranolol, and diazepam. The newer H_2 antagonist ranitidine has a different structure and causes fewer clinically significant drug interactions. Other drugs, notably calcium channel blockers and antidepressants, also inhibit oxidative drug metabolism in humans. This information allows clinicians to predict which combinations of drugs are more likely to lead to clinically significant interactions because of altered drug metabolism by the cytochrome P450 system.

Table 11-1   Substrates for CYP Isoenzymes Encountered in Anesthesiology

CYP3A4	CYP2D6
Acetaminophen	Captopril
Alfentanil	Codeine
Alprazolam	Hydrocodone
Bupivacaine	Metoprolol
Cisapride	Ondansetron
Codeine	Oxycodone
Diazepam	Propranolol
Digitoxin	Timolol
Diltiazem	**CYP2B6**
Fentanyl	Methadone
Lidocaine	Propofol
Midazolam	**CYP2C9**
Nicardipine	Diclofenac
Nifedipine	Ibuprofen
Omeprazole	Indomethacin
Ropivacaine	**CYP2C19**
Statins	Diazepam
Sufentanil	Omeprazole
Verapamil	Propranolol
Warfarin	Warfarin

Phase II Reactions

Phase II reactions are also known as *conjugation* or *synthetic reactions.* Many drugs do not have a polar chemical group suitable for conjugation, so conjugation occurs only after a Phase I reaction. Other drugs, such as morphine, already have a polar group that serves as a "handle" for conjugation, and they undergo these reactions directly. Various endogenous compounds can be attached to parent drugs or their Phase I metabolites to form different conjugation products. These endogenous substrates include glucuronic acid, acetate, and amino acids. Mercapturic acid conjugates result from the binding of exogenous compounds to glutathione. Other conjugation reactions produce sulfated or methylated derivatives of drugs or their metabolites. Like the cytochrome P450 system, the enzymes that catalyze Phase II reactions are inducible. Phase II reactions produce conjugates that are polar, water-soluble compounds. This facilitates the ultimate excretion of the drug via the kidneys or hepatobiliary secretion. Like CYP, there are different families and superfamilies of the enzymes that catalyze Phase II biotransformations.

Genetic Variations in Drug Metabolism

For most enzymes involved in Phase I and Phase II reactions, there are several biologically available isoforms. Drug metabolism varies substantially among individuals because of variability in the genes controlling the numerous enzymes responsible for biotransformation. For most drugs, the distribution of the rates of metabolism of the population is a unimodal distribution. If there are genetic variants (polymorphisms) that affect the rate of drug metabolism, the distribution of the rates of metabolism of the population will be a multimodal distribution. More detailed analysis of this multimodal distribution will reveal subpopulations with different rates of drug elimination, and each of the rates of drug metabolism of each of these subpopulations will be described by a unimodal distribution. For example, different genotypes result in either normal, low, or (rarely) absent plasma pseudocholinesterase activity, accounting for the well-known differences in individuals' responses to succinylcholine, which is hydrolyzed by this enzyme.

Many drug-metabolizing enzymes exhibit genetic polymorphism, including CYP and various transferases that catalyze phase II reactions. However, none of these has a sex-related difference.

Chronologic Variations in Drug Metabolism

The activity and capacity of the CYP enzymes increases from subnormal levels in the fetal and neonatal periods to reach normal levels at about 1 year of age. Although age is a covariate in mathematical models of drug elimination, it is not clear if these changes are related to chronologic changes in organ function (age related organ dysfunction) or to a decrease in CYP levels with increasing age. In contrast, it is clear that the neonate has a limited ability to perform phase II conjugation reactions, but after normalizing phase II activity over the initial year of life, advanced age does not affect the capacity to perform phase II reactions.

Renal Drug Clearance

4 The primary role of the kidneys in drug elimination is to excrete into urine the unchanged, hydrophilic drugs, and the hepatic derived metabolites from Phase I and Phase II reactions of lipophilic drugs. The passive elimination of drugs by passive glomerular filtration is a very inefficient process—any significant degree of binding of the drug to plasma proteins or erythrocytes will decrease the renal drug clearance below the glomerular filtration rate. In order to make renal elimination more efficient, discrete active transporters of organic acids and bases exist in the proximal renal tubular cells. Although these transporters are saturable, they allow for the renal clearance of drugs to approach the entire renal blood flow.

In reality, renal drug clearance of actively secreted drugs can be inhibited by both passive tubular reabsorption of lipophilic drugs and active, carrier-mediated tubular reabsorption of hydrophilic drugs. Therefore, the small amount of filtered and secreted lipophilic drug is easily reabsorbed in the distal tubules, making the net renal clearance negligible. In contrast, the large amount of filtered and secreted hydrophilic drug can be passively reabsorbed if renal tubular flow decreases substantially (e.g., oliguria) and/or the urine pH favors the un-ionized form of the hydrophilic drug. Renal drug clearance, even for drugs eliminated primarily by tubular secretion, is dependent on renal function. Therefore, in patients with acute and chronic causes of decreased renal function (usually indicated by reduced creatinine clearance), including age, low cardiac output states, and hepatorenal syndrome, drug dosing must be altered in order to avoid accumulation of parent compounds and potentially toxic metabolites (e.g., lidocaine, meperidine) (Table 11-2).

Hepatic Drug Clearance

5 Drug elimination by the liver depends on the intrinsic ability of the liver to metabolize the drug (intrinsic clearance, Cl_i), and the amount of drug available to diffuse into the liver. Many types of mathematical models have been developed to attempt to accurately describe the relationship between hepatic artery blood flow, portal artery blood flow, intrinsic clearance, and drug binding to plasma proteins.[22,23] According to these models, the unbound concentration of drug in the hepatic venous blood (C_v) is in equilibrium with the drug within the liver that is available for elimination. These models also make the assumption that all of the drug delivered to the liver is available for elimination and that the elimination is a first-order process—a constant *fraction* of the available drug is eliminated per unit time. The fraction of the drug removed from the blood passing through the liver is the hepatic extraction ratio, E:

$$E = \frac{C_a - C_v}{C_a} \quad (11\text{-}1)$$

where C_a is the mixed hepatic arterial–portal venous drug concentration and C_v is the mixed hepatic venous drug concentration. The total hepatic drug clearance, Cl_H, is:

$$Cl_H = Q \cdot E \quad (11\text{-}2)$$

where Q is hepatic blood flow. Therefore, hepatic clearance is a function of hepatic blood flow and the ability of the liver to extract drug from the blood.

The ability to extract drug depends on the activity of drug-metabolizing enzymes and the capacity for hepatobiliary excretion—the intrinsic clearance of the liver (Cl_i).

Intrinsic clearance represents the ability of the liver to remove drug from the blood in the absence of any limitations imposed by blood flow or drug binding. The relationship of total hepatic drug clearance to the extraction ratio and intrinsic clearance, Cl_i, is:

$$Cl_H = Q \cdot E = Q\left(\frac{Cl_i}{Q + Cl_i}\right) \quad (11\text{-}3)$$

The right-hand side of Equation 11-3 indicates that if intrinsic clearance is very high (many times larger than hepatic blood flow, $Cl_i \gg Q$), total hepatic clearance approaches hepatic blood flow. On the other hand, if intrinsic clearance is very small ($Q + Cl_i \approx Q$), hepatic clearance will be similar to intrinsic clearance. These relationships are shown in Figure 11-1.

Thus, hepatic drug clearance and extraction are determined by two independent variables, intrinsic clearance and hepatic blood flow. Changes in either will change hepatic clearance. However, the extent of the change depends on the initial relationship between intrinsic clearance and hepatic blood flow, according to the nonlinear relationship:

$$E = \frac{Cl_i}{Q + Cl_i} \quad (11\text{-}4)$$

If the initial intrinsic clearance is small relative to hepatic blood flow, then the extraction ratio is also small, and Equation 11-4 reduces to the following relationship:

$$E = \frac{Cl_i}{Q} \ll 1 \quad (11\text{-}4a)$$

Equation 11-4a indicates that doubling intrinsic clearance will produce an almost proportional increment in the extraction ratio, and, consequently, hepatic elimination clearance (Fig. 11-1, inset). However, if intrinsic clearance is much greater

Table 11-2 Drugs with Significant Renal Excretion Encountered in Anesthesiology

Aminoglycosides	Pancuronium
Atenolol	Penicillins
Cephalosporins	Procainamide
Digoxin	Pyridostigmine
Edrophonium	Quinolones
Nadolol	Rocuronium
Neostigmine	Sugammadex

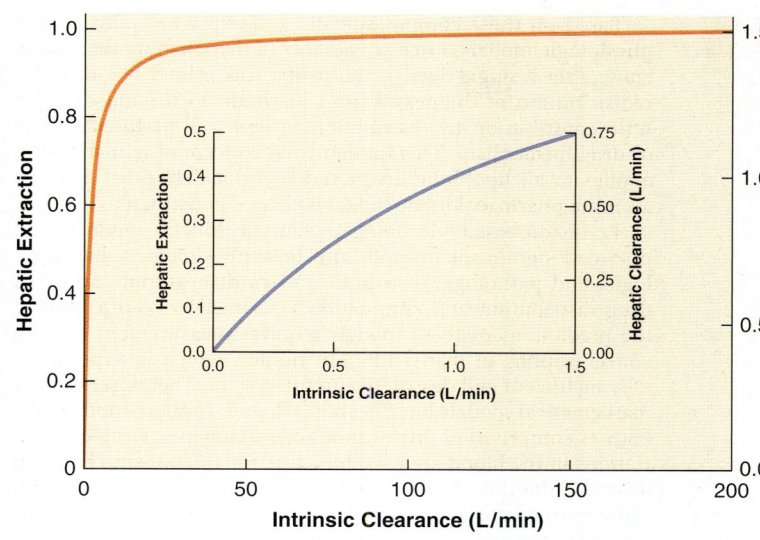

Figure 11-1 The relationship between hepatic extraction ratio (E, right y-axis), intrinsic clearance (Cl_i, x-axis), and hepatic clearance (Cl_H, left y-axis) at the normal hepatic blood flow (Q) of 1.5 L/min. For drugs with a high intrinsic clearance ($Cl_i \gg Q$), increasing intrinsic clearance has little effect on hepatic extraction, and total hepatic clearance approaches hepatic blood flow. In contrast, if the intrinsic clearance is small ($Cl_i \leq Q$), the extraction ratio is similar to the intrinsic clearance (inset). (Adapted from Wilkinson GR, Shand DG. A physiologic approach to hepatic drug clearance. *Clin Pharmacol Ther*. 1975;18:377.)

than hepatic blood flow, Equation 11-4 reduces to the following relationship:

$$E = \frac{Cl_i}{Cl_i} \approx 1 \quad (11\text{-}4b)$$

Equation 11-4b demonstrates that the extraction ratio is independent of intrinsic clearance and therefore a change in intrinsic clearance has a negligible effect on the extraction ratio and hepatic drug clearance (Fig. 11-1). In nonmathematical terms, high intrinsic clearance indicates efficient hepatic elimination. It is hard to enhance an already efficient process, whereas it is relatively easy to improve on inefficient drug clearance because of low intrinsic clearance.

For drugs with a high extraction ratio and a high intrinsic clearance, hepatic elimination clearance is directly proportional to hepatic blood flow. Therefore, any manipulation of hepatic blood flow will be directly reflected by a proportional change in hepatic elimination clearance (Fig. 11-2). In contrast, when the intrinsic clearance is low, changes in hepatic blood flow produce inversely proportional changes in extraction ratio (Fig. 11-3), and therefore the hepatic elimination clearance is essentially independent of hepatic blood flow and exquisitely related to intrinsic clearance. Therefore, classifying drugs as having either low, intermediate, or high extraction ratios (Table 11-3), allows predictions to be made on how intrinsic hepatic clearance and hepatic blood flow affect hepatic elimination clearance. This allows gross adjustments to be made in hepatically metabolized drug dosing to avoid excess accumulation of drugs (decreased hepatic elimination without dose adjustment) or subtherapeutic dosing strategies (increased hepatic elimination without dose adjustment).

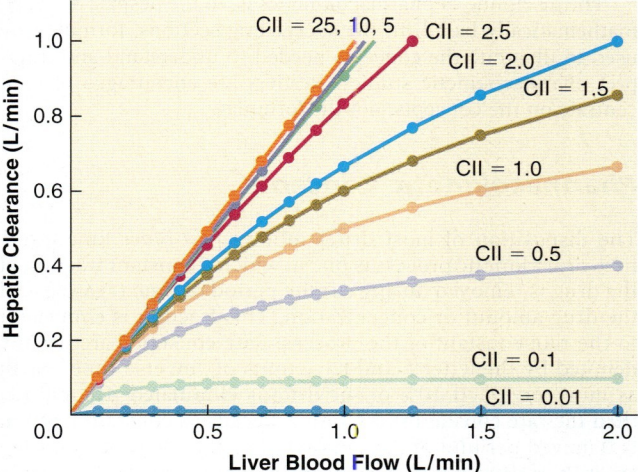

Figure 11-2 The relationship between liver blood flow (Q, x-axis) and hepatic clearance (Cl_H, y-axis) for different values of intrinsic clearance (Cl_i). When the intrinsic clearance is low, hepatic elimination clearance is independent of liver blood flow—the drug elimination is limited by the capacity of the liver to metabolize the drug (i.e., the intrinsic clearance). In contrast, as intrinsic clearance increases, the hepatic elimination becomes more dependent on hepatic blood flow—the liver is able to metabolize all of the drug that it is exposed to and therefore only limited by the amount of drug that is delivered to the liver (i.e., flow limited metabolism).

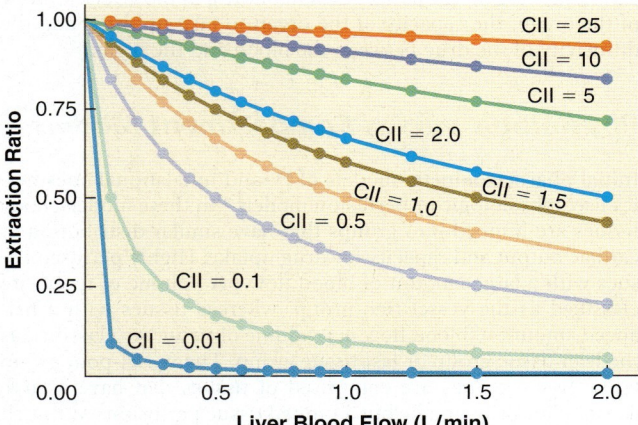

Figure 11-3 The relationship between liver blood flow (Q, x-axis) and hepatic extraction ratio (E, y-axis) for different values of intrinsic clearance (Cl_i). When the intrinsic clearance is low, increases in blood flows cause a decrease in the extraction ratio because the liver has limited metabolic capabilities. In contrast, when the intrinsic clearance is high, the extraction ratio is essentially independent of hepatic blood flow because the liver's ability to eliminate drug is well above the amount of drug provided by normal hepatic blood flow.

Table 11-3 Classification of Drugs Encountered in Anesthesiology According to Hepatic Extraction Ratios	
Low	**High**
Diazepam	Alprenolol
Lorazepam	Bupivacaine
Methadone	Diltiazem
Phenytoin	Fentanyl
Rocuronium	Ketamine
Theophylline	Lidocaine
Thiopental	Meperidine
	Metoprolol
Intermediate	Morphine
Alfentanil	Naloxone
Methohexital	Nifedipine
Midazolam	Propofol
Vecuronium	Propranolol

Pharmacologic and pathologic manipulations of cardiac output, with its consequences on hepatic/splanchnic blood flow and renal blood flow, are important covariates when designing drug dosing strategies.[24] As detailed above, in states where cardiac output is decreased (e.g., heart failure, shock, spinal anesthesia), high extraction ratio drugs will have a decrease in hepatic elimination, whereas low extraction rate drugs will have minimal change in clearance.[25,26] In contrast, autoregulation of renal blood flow maintains a relatively constant renal elimination clearance until low urine output states eventually allow increased reabsorption of drugs from the distal tubules.[27]

Pharmacokinetic Models

The concentration of drug at its site or sites of action is the fundamental determinant of a drug's pharmacologic effects. Although the blood is rarely the site of action of drug effect, the tissue drug concentration of an individual organ is a function of the blood flow to the organ, the concentration of drug in the arterial inflow of the organ, the capacity of the organ to take up drug, and the diffusivity of the drug between the blood and the organ.

Physiologic versus Compartment Models

Initial pharmacokinetic models of IV and inhalational anesthetics used physiologic or perfusion models.[4] In these models, body tissues are lumped into groups that have similar distribution of cardiac output and capacity for drug uptake. Highly perfused tissues with a large amount of blood flow per volume of tissue are classified as the vessel rich group, whereas tissues with a balanced amount of blood flow per volume of tissue are classified as the lean tissue group or fast tissue group. The vessel-poor group (slow tissue group) are comprised of tissues that have a large capacity for drug uptake but a limited tissue perfusion. Although identification of the exact organs that make up each tissue group is not possible from the mathematical model, it is apparent that the highly perfused tissues are composed of the brain, lungs, kidneys, and a subset of muscle; the fast equilibrating tissue would be consistent with the majority of muscle and some of the splanchnic bed (e.g., liver), and the slowly equilibrating tissues contain the majority of the adipose tissue and the remainder of the splanchnic organs.

Based on these computationally and experimentally intense physiologic models, Price[4,18] was able to demonstrate that awakening after a single dose of thiopental was primarily a result of redistribution of thiopental from the brain to the muscle with little contribution by distribution to less well-perfused tissues or drug metabolism. This fundamental concept of redistribution applies to all lipophilic drugs and was not delineated until an accurate pharmacokinetic model had been constructed.

Perfusion-based physiologic pharmacokinetic models have provided significant insights into how physiologic, pharmacologic, and pathologic distribution of cardiac output can effect drug distribution and elimination.[28,29] However, verification of the predictions of these models requires measurement of drug concentrations in many different tissues, which is experimentally inefficient and destructive to the system. Therefore, simpler mathematical models have been developed. In these models, the body is comprised of one or more compartments. Drug concentrations in the blood are used to define the relationship between dose and the time course of changes in the drug concentration. The compartments of the compartmental pharmacokinetic models cannot be equated with the tissue groups that make up physiologic pharmacokinetic models because the compartments are theoretical entities that are used to mathematically characterize the blood concentration profile of a drug. These models allow the derivation of pharmacokinetic parameters that can be used to quantify drug distribution and elimination—volume of distribution, clearance, and half-lives.

Although the simplicity of compartmental models, compared to physiologic pharmacokinetic models, has its advantages, it also has some disadvantages. For example, cardiac output is not a parameter of compartmental models, and compartmental models therefore cannot be used to predict directly the effect of cardiac failure on drug disposition.[30] However, compartmental pharmacokinetic models can still quantify the effects of reduced cardiac output on the disposition of a drug if a group of patients with cardiac failure is compared to a group of otherwise healthy subjects.

The discipline of pharmacokinetics is, to the despair of many, mathematically based. In the succeeding sections, formulas are used to illustrate the concepts needed to understand and interpret pharmacokinetic studies. Readers are encouraged to concentrate on the concepts, not the formulas.

Pharmacokinetic Concepts

The disposition of most drugs follows *first-order* kinetics. A first-order kinetic process is one in which a constant fraction of the drug is removed during a finite period of time regardless of the drug amount or concentration. This fraction is equivalent to the rate constant of the process. Rate constants are usually denoted by the letter k and have units of "inverse time," such as min^{-1} or h^{-1}. If 10% of the drug is eliminated per minute, then the rate constant is $0.1\ \text{min}^{-1}$. Because a constant fraction is removed per unit of time in first-order kinetics, the absolute amount of drug removed is proportional to the concentration of the drug. It follows that, in first-order kinetics, the rate of change of the amount of drug at any given time is proportional to the concentration present at that time. When the concentration is high, more drug will be removed than when it is low. First-order kinetics apply not only to elimination, but also to absorption and distribution.

Rather than using rate constants, the rapidity of pharmacokinetic processes is often described with half-lives—the time required for the concentration to change by a factor of 2. Half-lives are calculated directly from the corresponding rate constants with this simple equation:

$$t_{1/2} = \frac{\ln 2}{k} = \frac{0.693}{k} \quad (11\text{-}5)$$

Thus, a rate constant of 0.1 min^{-1} translates into a half-life of 6.93 minutes. The half-life of any first-order kinetic process, including drug absorption, distribution, and elimination, can be calculated. First-order processes asymptotically approach completion, because a constant fraction of the drug, not an absolute amount, is removed per unit of time. However, after five half-lives, the process will be almost 97% complete (Table 11-4). For practical purposes, this is essentially 100%, and therefore there is a negligible amount of drug remaining in the body.

Volume of Distribution

The volume of distribution quantifies the extent of drug distribution. The physiologic factor that governs the extent of drug distribution is the overall capacity of tissues versus the capacity of blood for that drug. Overall tissue capacity for uptake of a drug is in turn a function of the total mass of the tissues into which a drug distributes and their average affinity for the drug. In compartmental pharmacokinetic models, drugs are envisaged as distributing into one or more "boxes," or compartments. These compartments cannot be equated directly with specific tissues. Rather, they are hypothetical entities that permit analysis of drug distribution and elimination and description of the drug concentration versus time profile.

The volume of distribution is an "apparent" volume because it represents the size of these hypothetical boxes, or compartments, that are necessary to explain the concentration of drug in a reference compartment, usually called the *central* or *plasma compartment*. The volume of distribution, V_d, relates the total amount of drug present to the concentration observed in the central compartment:

$$V_d = \frac{amount\ of\ drug\ administered}{initial\ drug\ plasma\ concentration} \quad (11\text{-}6)$$

If a drug is extensively distributed, then the concentration will be lower relative to the amount of drug present, which equates to a larger volume of distribution. For example, if a total of 10 mg of drug is present and the concentration is 2 mg/L, then the apparent volume of distribution is 5 L. On the other hand, if the concentration was 4 mg/L, then the volume of distribution would be 2.5 L.

Simply stated, the apparent volume of distribution is a numeric index of the extent of drug distribution that does not have any relationship to the actual volume of any tissue or group of tissues. It may be as small as plasma volume, or, if overall tissue uptake is extensive, the apparent volume of distribution may greatly exceed the actual total volume of the body. In general, lipophilic drugs have larger volumes of distribution than hydrophilic drugs. Because the volume of distribution is a mathematical construct to model the distribution of a drug in the body, the volume of distribution cannot provide any information regarding the actual tissue concentration in any specific real organ in the body. However, this simple mathematical construct provides a useful summary description of the behavior of the drug in the body. In fact, the loading dose of drug required to achieve a target plasma concentration can be easily calculated by rearranging Equation 11-6 as follows:

$$Loading\ Dose = V_d \times Target\ Concentration \quad (11\text{-}7)$$

Based on this equation, it is clear that an increase in the volume of distribution means that a larger loading dose will be required to "fill up the box" and achieve the same concentration. Therefore, any change in state because of changes in physiologic and pathologic conditions can alter the volume of distribution, necessitating therapeutic adjustments.

Total Drug (Elimination) Clearance

Elimination clearance (drug clearance) is the theoretical volume of blood from which drug is completely and irreversibly removed in a unit of time. Elimination clearance has the units of flow—[volume per time]. *Total* drug clearance can be calculated with pharmacokinetic models of blood concentration versus time data. Drug clearance is often corrected for weight or body surface area, in which case the units are mL/min/kg or mL/min/m^2, respectively.

Elimination clearance, Cl, can be calculated from the declining blood levels observed after an IV injection, as follows:

$$Cl = \frac{dose\ of\ drug\ administered}{area\ under\ the\ concentration\ versus\ time\ curve} \quad (11\text{-}8)$$

If a drug is rapidly removed from the plasma, its concentration will fall more quickly than the concentration of a drug that is less readily eliminated. This results in a smaller area under the concentration versus time curve, which equates to greater clearance (Fig. 11-4).

Without additional organ-specific data (e.g., urine drug concentration measurements, drug arterial inflow concentration) calculating elimination clearance from compartmental pharmacokinetic models usually does not specify the relative contribution of different organs to drug elimination. Nonetheless, estimation of drug clearance with these models has made important contributions to clinical pharmacology. In particular, these models have provided a great deal of clinically useful information regarding altered drug elimination in various pathologic conditions.

Elimination Half-Life

Although the elimination clearance is the pharmacokinetic parameter that best describes the physiologic process of drug elimination (i.e., drug delivery to organs of elimination coupled with the capacity of the organ to eliminate the drug), the pharmacokinetic variable most often reported in textbooks and literature is the *elimination half-life* of a drug ($t_{1/2}\beta$). The elimination half-life is the time during which the amount of drug in the body decreases by 50%. Although this parameter appears to be a simple summary of the physiology of drug elimination, it is

Table 11-4 Half-lives and Corresponding Percentage of Drug Removed

Number of Half-lives	Percentage of Drug Remaining	Percentage of Drug Removed
0	100	0
1	50	50
2	25	75
3	12.5	87.5
4	6.25	93.75
5	3.125	96.875

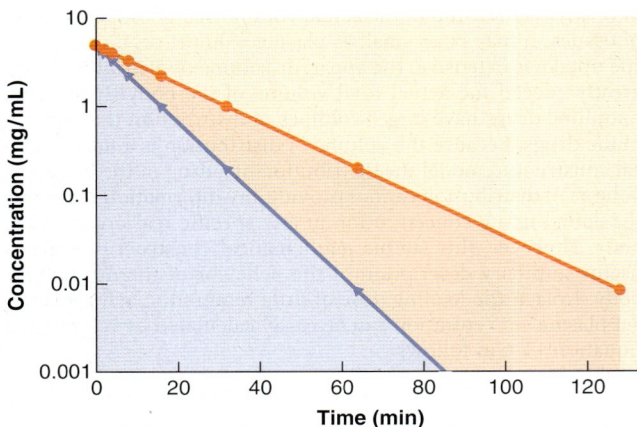

Figure 11-4 The plasma concentration (*y*-axis) versus time (*x*-axis) curve for two drugs which only differ in their elimination clearance. Notice that the areas under the curves are different, signifying that the drug that has the smaller area under the curve is more rapidly eliminated from the body than the drug that has the slower elimination clearance.

actually a complex parameter, influenced by the distribution and the elimination of the drug, as follows:

$$t_{1/2_\beta} = \frac{\ln 2}{k_\beta} = 0.693 \times \frac{V_d}{Cl_E} \qquad (11\text{-}9)$$

Therefore, when a physiologic or pathologic perturbation changes the elimination half-life of a drug, it is not a simple reflection of the change in the body's ability to metabolize or eliminate the drug. For example, the elimination half-life of thiopental is prolonged in the elderly; however, the elimination clearance is unchanged and the volume of distribution is increased.[31] Therefore, elderly patients need dosing strategies that accommodate for the change in the distribution of the drug rather than a decreased metabolism of the drug. In contrast, in patients with renal insufficiency, the increase in the elimination half-life of pancuronium is due to a simple decrease in renal elimination of the drug, and the volume of distribution is unchanged.[32]

Aside from its inability to give insight into the mechanism by which a drug is retained in the body, the elimination half-life is unable to give insight into the time that it takes for a single dose or a series of repeated drug doses to terminate its effect. Although elimination of drug from the body begins the moment the drug is delivered to the organs of elimination, the rapid termination of effect of a bolus of an IV agent is due to redistribution of drug from the brain to the blood and subsequently other tissues (e.g., muscle). Therefore, the effects of most anesthetics have waned long before even one elimination half-life has been completed, making this measure of drug kinetics incapable of providing useful information regarding the duration of action following the administration of IV agents. Thus the elimination half-life has limited utility in anesthetic practice.[10]

Effect of Hepatic or Renal Disease on Pharmacokinetic Parameters

Diverse pathophysiologic changes preclude precise prediction of the pharmacokinetics of a given drug in individual patients with hepatic or renal disease. In addition, liver function tests (e.g., transaminases) are unreliable predictors of the degree of liver function and the remaining metabolic capacity for drug elimination. However, some generalizations can be made. In patients with hepatic disease, the elimination half-life of drugs metabolized or excreted by the liver is often increased because of decreased clearance, and, possibly, increased volume of distribution caused by ascites and altered protein binding.[10,33] Drug concentration at steady-state is inversely proportional to elimination clearance. Therefore, when hepatic drug clearance is reduced, repeated bolus dosing or continuous infusion of such drugs as benzodiazepines, opioids, and barbiturates may result in excessive accumulation of drug as well as excessive and prolonged pharmacologic effects. Since recovery from small doses of drugs such as thiopental and fentanyl is largely the result of redistribution, recovery from conservative doses will be minimally affected by reductions in elimination clearance. In patients with renal failure, similar concerns apply to the administration of drugs excreted by the kidneys. It is almost always better to underestimate a patient's dose requirement, observe the response, and give additional drug if necessary.

Nonlinear Pharmacokinetics

The physiologic and compartmental models thus far discussed are based on the assumption that drug distribution and elimination are first-order processes. Therefore, their parameters, such as clearance and elimination half-life, are independent of the dose or concentration of the drug. However, the rate of elimination of a few drugs is dose dependent, or *nonlinear*.

Elimination of drugs involves interactions with either enzymes catalyzing biotransformation reactions or carrier proteins for transmembrane transport. If sufficient drug is present, the capacity of the drug-eliminating systems can be exceeded. When this occurs, it is no longer possible to excrete a constant fraction of the drug present, and a constant amount of drug is excreted per unit time. Phenytoin is a well-known example of a drug that exhibits nonlinear elimination at therapeutic concentrations,[34] whereas in anesthetic practice, the extremely high doses of thiopental utilized for cerebral protection can demonstrate zero-order elimination.[35] In theory, all drugs are cleared in a nonlinear fashion. In practice, the capacity to eliminate most drugs is so great that this is usually not evident, even with toxic concentrations.

Compartmental Pharmacokinetic Models

One-Compartment Model

Although for most drugs the one-compartment model is an oversimplification, it does serve to illustrate the basic relationships among clearance, volume of distribution, and the elimination half-life. In this model, the body is envisaged as a single homogeneous compartment. Drug distribution after injection is assumed to be instantaneous, so there are no concentration gradients within the compartment. The concentration can decrease only by elimination of drug from the system. The plasma concentration versus time curve for a hypothetical drug with one-compartment kinetics is shown in Figure 11-5. The decrease in plasma concentration (*C*) with time from the initial concentration (C_0) can be characterized by the simple monoexponential function:

$$C(t) = C_0 \times e^{-k_e \times t} \qquad (11\text{-}10)$$

With the concentration plotted on a logarithmic scale, the concentration versus time curve becomes a straight line. The slope of the logarithm of concentration versus time is equal to the first-order elimination rate constant (k_e).

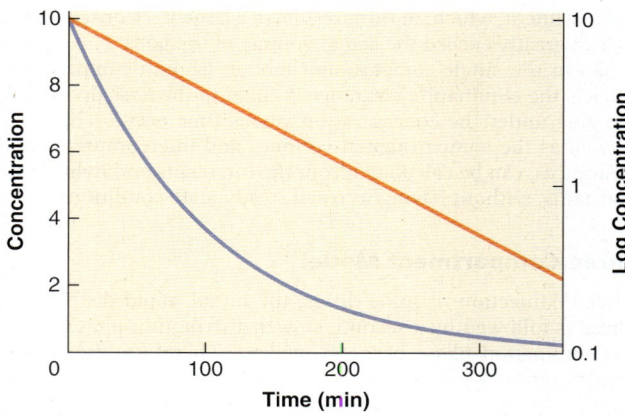

Figure 11-5 The plasma concentration versus time profile plotted on both linear (*blue line*, left y-axis) and logarithmic (*red line*, right y-axis) scales for a hypothetical drug exhibiting one-compartment, first-order pharmacokinetics. Note that the slope of the logarithmic concentration profile is equal to the elimination rate constant (k_e) and related to the elimination half-life ($t_{1/2}\beta$) as described in Equation 11-9.

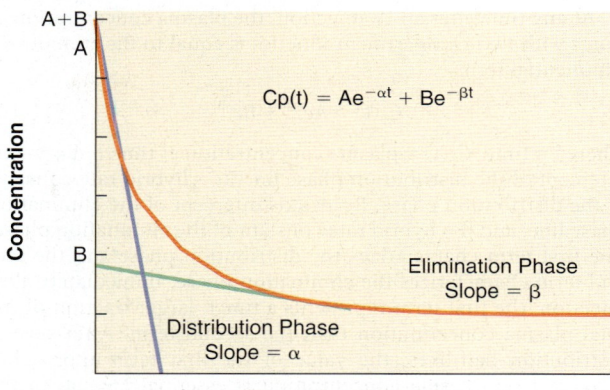

Figure 11-6 The logarithmic plasma concentration versus time profile for a hypothetical drug exhibiting two-compartment, first-order pharmacokinetics. Note that the distribution phase has a slope that is significantly larger than that of the elimination phase, indicating that the process of distribution is not only more rapid than elimination of the drug from the body, but also responsible for most of the decline in plasma concentration in the several minutes after drug administration.

In the one-compartment model, drug clearance, Cl, is equal to the product of the elimination rate constant, k_e, and the volume of distribution:

$$Cl = k_e \cdot V_d \qquad (11\text{-}11)$$

Combining Equations 11-5 and 11-10 yields Equation 11-9 (where $k_e = k_\beta$):

$$t_{1/2\beta} = \frac{\ln 2}{k_e} = 0.693 \times \frac{V_d}{Cl_E} \qquad (11\text{-}9)$$

Therefore, when it is appropriate to make the simplifying assumption of instantaneous mixing of drug into a single compartment, the elimination half-life is inversely proportional to the slope of the concentration time curve. For drugs which require consideration of their multicompartmental pharmacokinetics, the relationship among clearance, volume of distribution, and the elimination half-life is not a simple linear one such as Equation 11-9. However, the same principles apply. All else being equal, the greater the clearance, the shorter the elimination half-life; the larger the volume of distribution, the longer the elimination half-life. Thus, the elimination half-life depends on two other variables, clearance and volume of distribution, that characterize, respectively, the extent of drug distribution and efficiency of drug elimination.

Two-Compartment Model

For many drugs, a graph of the logarithm of the plasma concentration versus time after an IV injection is similar to the schematic graph shown in Figure 11-6. There are two discrete phases in the decline of the plasma concentration. The first phase after injection is characterized by a very rapid decrease in concentration. The rapid decrease in concentration during this "distribution phase" is largely caused by passage of drug from the plasma into tissues. The distribution phase is followed by a slower decline of the concentration owing to drug elimination. Elimination also begins immediately after injection, but its contribution to the drop in plasma concentration is initially much smaller than the fall in concentration because of drug distribution.

To account for this biphasic behavior, one must consider the body to be made up of two compartments: a central compartment, which includes the plasma, and a peripheral compartment (Fig. 11-7). This two-compartment model assumes that it is the central compartment into which the drug is injected and from which the blood samples for measurement of concentration are obtained, and that drug is eliminated only from the central compartment. Drug distribution within the central compartment is considered to be instantaneous. In reality, this last assumption cannot be true. However, drug uptake into some of the highly perfused tissues is so rapid that it cannot be detected as a discrete phase on the plasma concentration versus time curve.

The distribution and elimination phases can be characterized by graphic analysis of the plasma concentration versus time curve, as shown in Figure 11-6. The elimination phase line is extrapolated back to time zero (the time of injection). In Figure 11-6, the zero time intercepts of the distribution and elimination lines are points A and B, respectively. The *hybrid rate constants*, α and β, are equal to the slopes of the two lines, and are used to calculate the distribution and elimination half-lives; α and β are called hybrid rate constants because they depend on both distribution and elimination processes.

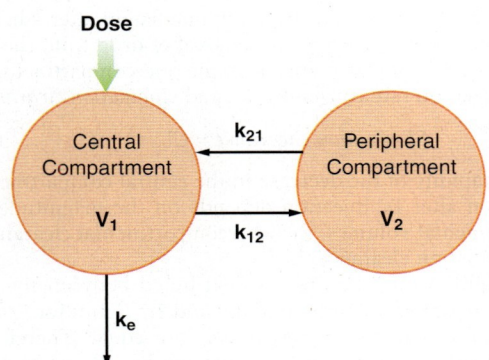

Figure 11-7 A schematic of a two-compartment pharmacokinetic model. See text for explanation.

At any time after an IV injection, the plasma concentration of drugs with two-compartment kinetics is equal to the sum of two exponential terms:

$$C_p(t) = Ae^{-\alpha t} + Be^{-\beta t} \quad (11\text{-}12)$$

where t = time, $C_p(t)$ = plasma concentration at time t, A = y-axis intercept of the distribution phase line, α = hybrid rate constant of the distribution phase, B = y-axis intercept of the elimination phase line, and β = hybrid rate constant of the elimination phase. The first term characterizes the distribution phase and the second term characterizes the elimination phase. Immediately after injection, the first term represents a much larger fraction of the total plasma concentration than the second term. After several distribution half-lives, the value of the first term approaches zero, and the plasma concentration is essentially equal to the value of the second term (Fig. 11-6).

In multicompartmental models, the drug is initially distributed only within the central compartment. Therefore, the initial apparent volume of distribution is the volume of the central compartment. Immediately after injection, the amount of drug present is the dose, and the concentration is the extrapolated concentration at time $t = 0$, which is equal to the sum of the intercepts of the distribution and elimination lines. The volume of the central compartment, V_1, is calculated by modifying Equation 11-6:

$$V_1 = \frac{dose}{initial\ plasma\ concentration} = \frac{dose}{A+B} \quad (11\text{-}13)$$

The volume of the central compartment is important in clinical anesthesiology because it is the pharmacokinetic parameter that determines the peak plasma concentration after an IV bolus injection. Hypovolemia, for example, reduces the volume of the central compartment. If doses are not correspondingly reduced, the higher plasma concentrations will increase the incidence of adverse pharmacologic effects.

Immediately after IV injection, all of the drug is in the central compartment. Simultaneously, three processes begin. Drug moves from the central to the peripheral compartment, which also has a volume, V_2. This intercompartmental transfer is a first-order process, and its magnitude is quantified by the rate constant k_{12}. As soon as drug appears in the peripheral compartment, some passes back to the central compartment, a process characterized by the rate constant k_{21}. The transfer of drug between the central and peripheral compartments is quantified by the *distributional* or *intercompartmental clearance*:

$$Intercompartmental\ Clearance = Cl_{12} = Cl_{21} = V_1 \times k_{12} = V_2 \times k_{21} \quad (11\text{-}14)$$

The third process that begins immediately after administration of the drug is irreversible removal of drug from the system via the central compartment. As in the one-compartment model, the elimination rate constant is k_e, and *elimination clearance* is:

$$Elimination\ Clearance = Cl_E = V_1 \times k_e \quad (11\text{-}15)$$

The rapidity of the decrease in the central compartment concentration after IV injection depends on the magnitude of the compartmental volumes, the intercompartmental clearance, and the elimination clearance.

At equilibrium, the drug is distributed between the central and the peripheral compartments, and by definition, the drug concentrations in the compartments are equal. Therefore, the ultimate volume of distribution, termed the volume of distribution at steady-state (V_{ss}), is the sum of V_1 and V_2. Extensive tissue uptake of a drug is reflected by a large volume of the peripheral compartment, which, in turn, results in a large V_{ss}. Consequently, V_{ss} can greatly exceed the actual volume of the body.

As in the single-compartment model, in multicompartment models the elimination clearance is equal to the dose divided by the area under the concentration versus time curve. This area, as well as the compartmental volumes and intercompartmental clearances, can be calculated from the intercepts and hybrid rate constants, without having to reach steady-state conditions.

Three-Compartment Model

After IV injection of some drugs, the initial, rapid distribution phase is followed by a second, slower distribution phase before the elimination phase becomes evident. Therefore, the plasma concentration is the sum of three exponential terms:

$$C_p(t) = Ae^{-\alpha t} + Be^{-\beta t} + Ge^{-\gamma t} \quad (11\text{-}16)$$

where t = time, $C_p(t)$ = plasma concentration at time t, A = intercept of the rapid distribution phase line, α = hybrid rate constant of the rapid distribution phase, B = intercept of the slower distribution phase line, β = hybrid rate constant of the slower distribution phase, G = intercept of the elimination phase line, and γ = hybrid rate constant of the elimination phase. This triphasic behavior is explained by a three-compartment pharmacokinetic model (Fig. 11-8). As in the two-compartment model, the drug is injected into and eliminated from the central compartment. Drug is reversibly transferred between the central compartment and two peripheral compartments, which accounts for two distribution phases. Drug transfer between the central compartment and the more rapidly equilibrating, or "shallow," peripheral compartment is characterized by the first-order rate constants k_{12} and k_{21}. Transfer in and out of the more slowly equilibrating, "deep" compartment is characterized by the rate constants k_{13} and k_{31}. In this model, there are three compartmental volumes: V_1, V_2, and V_3, whose sum equals V_{ss}; and three clearances: the rapid intercompartmental clearance, the slow intercompartmental clearance, and elimination clearance.

The pharmacokinetic parameters of interest to clinicians, such as clearance, volumes of distribution, and distribution and elimination half-lives, are determined by calculations analogous to those used in the two-compartment model. Accurate estimates of these parameters depend on accurate characterization of the measured plasma concentration versus time data. A frequently encountered problem is that the duration of sampling is not long enough to define accurately the elimination phase. Similar problems arise if the assay cannot detect low concentrations of the drug. Conversely, samples are sometimes obtained too infrequently following drug administration to be able to characterize the distribution phases accurately.[36,37] Whether a drug

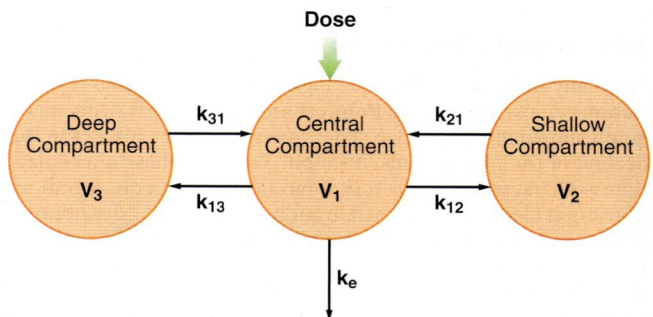

Figure 11-8 A schematic of a three-compartment pharmacokinetic model. See text for details.

exhibits two- or three-compartment kinetics is of no clinical consequence.[10] In fact, some drugs have two-compartment kinetics in some patients and three-compartment kinetics in others. In selecting a pharmacokinetic model, the most important factor is that it accurately characterizes the measured concentrations.

In general, the model with the smallest number of compartments or exponents that accurately reflects the data is used. However, it is good to consider that the data collected in a particular study may not be reflective of the clinical pharmacologic issues of concern in another situation, making published pharmacokinetic model parameters potentially irrelevant. For instance, new data indicate that hypotension following IV administration of drug X is related to peak arterial plasma drug X concentrations 1 minute after injection, but previous pharmacokinetic models are based on venous plasma drug X concentrations beginning 5 minutes after the dose. In this case, the pharmacokinetic models will not be of use in designing dosing regimens for drug X that avoid toxic drug concentrations at 1 minute.[10,38,39]

Almost all earlier pharmacokinetic studies used *two-stage modeling*. With this technique, pharmacokinetic parameters were estimated independently for each subject and then averaged to provide estimates of the typical parameters for the population. One problem with this approach is that if outliers are present, averaging parameters could result in a model that does not accurately predict typical drug concentrations. Currently, most pharmacokinetic models are developed using *population pharmacokinetic modeling*, which has been made feasible because of advances in modeling software and increased computing power. With these techniques, the pharmacokinetic parameters are estimated using all the concentration versus time data from the entire group of subjects in a single stage, using sophisticated nonlinear regression methods. This modeling technique provides single estimates of the typical parameter values for the population.

Noncompartmental (Stochastic) Pharmacokinetic Models

Often investigators performing pharmacokinetic analyses of drugs want to avoid the experimental requirements of a physiologic model—data or empirical estimations of individual organ inflow and outflow concentration profiles and organ tissue drug concentrations are required in order to identify the components of the model.[40] Although compartmental models do not assume any physiologic or anatomic basis for the model structure, investigators often attribute anatomic and physiologic function to these empiric models.[41] Even if the disciplined clinical pharmacologist avoids overinterpretation of the meaning of compartment models, the simple fact that several competing models can provide equally good descriptions of the mathematical data, or that some subjects in a data set may better fit with a three-compartment model rather than the two-compartment model that provides the best fit for the other data set subjects, leads many to question whether there is a true best model architecture for any given drug. Therefore, some investigators choose to employ mathematical techniques to characterize a pharmacokinetic data set that attempt to avoid any preconceived notion of structure, and yet yield the pharmacokinetic parameters that summarize drug distribution and elimination. These techniques are classified as noncompartmental techniques or stochastic techniques and are similar to the methods based on moment analysis utilized in process analysis of chemical engineering systems. Although these techniques are often called model-independent, like any mathematical construct, assumptions must be made to simplify

the mathematics. The basic assumptions of noncompartmental analysis are that all of the elimination clearance occurs directly from the plasma, the distribution and elimination of drug is a linear and first-order process, and the pharmacokinetics of the system does not vary over the time of the data collection (time-invariant). All of these assumptions are also made in the basic compartmental, and most physiologic, models. Therefore, the main advantage of the noncompartmental pharmacokinetic methods is that a general description of drug absorption, distribution, and elimination can be made without resorting to more complex mathematical modeling techniques.[40]

Another appealing facet of noncompartmental analysis is that the parameters that describe drug distribution (volume of distribution at steady-state, Vd_{ss}) and drug elimination (elimination clearance, Cl_E) are analogous to parameters found in other pharmacokinetic techniques. In fact, when properly defined, the estimates of these parameters from the noncompartmental approach and a well-defined compartmental model yield similar values. The main unique parameter of noncompartmental analysis is the Mean Residence Time (MRT), which is the average time a drug molecule spends in the body before being eliminated.[42] The MRT unfortunately suffers from the main failings of the elimination half-life derived from compartmental models—not only does it fail to capture the contribution of extensive distribution versus limited elimination to allow a drug to linger in the body, but both parameters also fail to describe the situation where the drug effect can dissipate by redistribution of drug from the site of action back into blood and then into other, less well-perfused tissues.[43]

Pharmacodynamic Principles

Much of the clinical pharmacology efforts of the late eighties through nineties were devoted to applying new computational power of desktop personal computers to deciphering the pharmacokinetics of IV anesthetics. However, the premise behind developing models to better characterize and understand the effects of various physiologic and pathologic states on drug distribution and elimination was that the relationship between a dose of drug and its effect(s) had already been characterized. As computational power and drug assay technology grew, it became possible to characterize the relationship between a drug concentration and the associated pharmacologic effect. As a result, pharmacodynamic studies since the nineties have focused on the quantitative analysis of the relationship between the drug concentration in the blood and the resultant effects of the drug on physiologic processes.

Drug–Receptor Interactions

Most pharmacologic agents produce their physiologic effects by binding to a drug specific receptor, which brings about a change in cellular function. The majority of pharmacologic receptors are cell membrane bound proteins, although some receptors are located in the cytoplasm or the nucleoplasm of the cell.

Binding of drugs to receptors, like the binding of drugs to plasma proteins, is usually reversible, and follows the Law of Mass Action:

$$[drug] + [receptor] \leftrightarrow [drug - receptor\ complex] \quad (11\text{-}17)$$

This relationship demonstrates that the higher the concentration of free drug or unoccupied receptor, the greater the tendency to form the drug–receptor complex. Plotting the percentage of receptors occupied by a drug against the logarithm

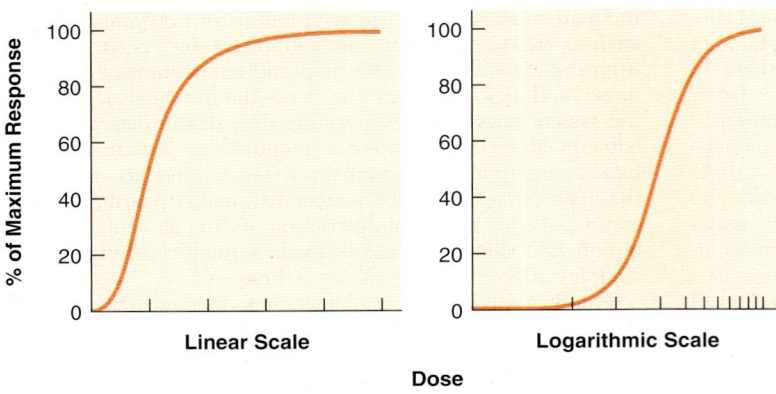

Figure 11-9 A schematic curve of the effect of a drug plotted against dose. In the left panel, the response data is plotted against the dose data on a linear scale. In the right panel, the same response data are plotted against the dose data on a logarithmic scale yielding a sigmoid dose–response curve that is linear between 20% and 80% of the maximal effect.

of the concentration of the drug yields a sigmoid curve, as shown in Figure 11-9.[44]

The percentage of receptors occupied by a drug is not equivalent to the percentage of maximal effect produced by the drug. In fact, most receptor systems have more receptors than required to obtain the maximum drug effect.[45] The presence of "extra" unoccupied receptors will promote the formation of the drug–receptor complex (Law of Mass Action, Equation 11-17); therefore, near-maximal drug effects can occur at very low drug concentrations. This not only allows extremely efficient responses to drugs, but it provides a large margin of safety—an extremely large number of a drug's receptors must be bound to an antagonist before the drug is unable to produce its pharmacologic effect. For example, at the neuromuscular junction, only 20% to 25% of the postjunctional nicotinic cholinergic receptors need to bind acetylcholine to produce contraction of all the fibers in the muscle, while 75% of the receptors must be blocked by a nondepolarizing neuromuscular antagonist to produce a significant drop in muscle strength. This accounts for the "margin of safety" of neuromuscular transmission.[45]

The binding of drugs to receptors and the resulting changes in cellular function are the last two steps in the complex series of events between administration of the drug and production of its pharmacologic effects. There are two primary schemes by which the binding of an agonist to a receptor changes cellular function: receptor-linked membrane ion channels called *ionophores*, and guanine nucleotide binding proteins, referred to as *G-proteins*. The nicotinic cholinergic receptor in the neuromuscular postsynaptic membrane is one example of a receptor–ionophore complex. Binding of acetylcholine opens the cation ionophore, leading to an influx of Na^+ ions, propagation of an action potential, and, ultimately, muscle contraction. The β-amino butyric acid (GABA) receptor–chloride ionophore complex is another example of this type of effector mechanism. Binding of either endogenous neurotransmitters (GABA) or exogenous agonists (benzodiazepines and IV anesthetics) increases Cl^- conductance, which hyperpolarizes the neuron and decreases its excitability. Adrenergic receptors are the prototypical G-protein coupled receptors. G-proteins change the intracellular concentrations of various so-called second messengers, such as Ca^{2+} and cyclic AMP, in order to transduce their signal and produce modified cellular behavior.

Desensitization and Downregulation of Receptors

Receptors are not static entities. Rather, they are dynamic cellular components that adapt to their environment. Prolonged exposure of a receptor to its agonist leads to desensitization—subsequent doses of the agonist will produce lower maximal effects. With sustained elevation of the cytosolic second messengers downstream of the G-proteins, pathways to prevent further G-protein signaling are activated. Phosphorylation by G-protein receptor kinases and arrestin-mediated blockage of the coupling site needed to form the active heterotrimeric G protein complex prevents G protein coupled receptors from becoming active. Arrestins and other cell membrane proteins can tag receptors that have sustained activity, so that these non–G-protein receptors are internalized and sequestered so they are no longer accessible to agonists. Similar mechanisms will prevent the trafficking of stored receptors to the cell membrane. The combined increased rate of internalization and decreased rate of replenishing of receptor results in *downregulation*—a decrease in the total number of receptors. Signals that produce downregulation with sustained receptor activation are essentially reversed in the face of constant receptor inactivity. Therefore, chronically denervated neuromuscular junctions, just like cardiac tissue constantly bathed with adrenergic antagonists, will upregulate the specific receptors in an attempt to produce a signal in the face of lower concentrations of agonists.

Agonists, Partial Agonists, and Antagonists

Drugs that bind to receptors and produce an effect are called *agonists*. Different drugs that act on the same receptor may be capable of producing the same maximal effect (E_{max}), although they may differ in the concentration that produces the effect (i.e., potency). Agonists that differ in potency but bind to the same receptors will have parallel concentration–response curves (Fig. 11-10, curves *A* and *B*). Differences in potency of agonists reflect differences in affinity for the receptor. *Partial agonists* are drugs that are not capable of producing the maximal effect, even at very high concentrations (Fig. 11-10, curve *C*).

Compounds that bind to receptors without producing any changes in cellular function are referred to as *antagonists*—antagonists make it impossible for agonists to bind their receptors. *Competitive antagonists* bind reversibly to receptors, and their blocking effect can be overcome by high concentrations of an agonist (i.e., competition). Therefore, competitive antagonists produce a parallel shift in the dose–response curve, but the maximum effect is not altered (Fig. 11-10, curves *A* and *B*). *Noncompetitive antagonists* bind irreversibly to receptors. This has the same effect as reducing the number of receptors and shifts the dose–response curve downward and to the right, decreasing both the slope and the maximum effect (Fig. 11-10, curves *A* and *C*). The effect of noncompetitive antagonists is reversed only by synthesis of new receptor molecules.

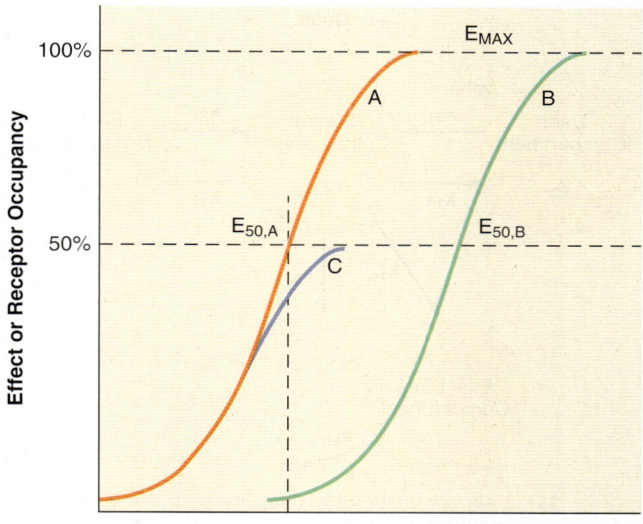

Figure 11-10 Schematic pharmacodynamic curves, with dose or concentration on the x-axis and effect or receptor occupancy on the y-axis, that illustrate agonism, partial agonism, and antagonism. Drug A produces a maximum effect, E_{max}, and a 50% of maximal effect at dose or concentration $E_{50,A}$. Drug B, a full agonist, can produce the maximum effect, E_{max}; however, it is less potent ($E_{50,B} > E_{50,A}$). Drug C, a partial agonist, can only produce a maximum effect of approximately 50% E_{max}. If a competitive antagonist is given to a patient, the dose response for the agonist would shift from curve A to curve B—although the receptors would have the same affinity for the agonist, the presence of the competitor would necessitate an increase in agonist in order to produce an effect. In fact, the agonist would still be able to produce a maximal effect, if a sufficient overdose was given to displace the competitive antagonist. However, the competitive antagonist would not change the binding characteristics of the receptor for the agonist and so curve B is simply shifted to the right but remains parallel to curve A. In contrast, if a noncompetitive antagonist binds to the receptor, the agonist would no longer be able to produce a maximal effect, no matter how much of an overdose is administered (curve C).

Agonists produce a structural change in the receptor molecule that initiates changes in cellular function. Partial agonists may produce a qualitatively different change in the receptor, whereas antagonists bind without producing a change in the receptor that results in altered cellular function. The underlying mechanisms by which different compounds that bind to the same receptor act as agonists, partial agonists, or antagonists are not fully understood.

Dose–Response Relationships

Dose–response studies determine the relationship between increasing doses of a drug and the ensuing changes in pharmacologic effects. Schematic dose–response curves are shown in Figure 11-9, with the dose plotted on both linear and logarithmic scales. There is a curvilinear relationship between dose and the intensity of response. Low doses produce little pharmacologic effect. Once effects become evident, a small increase in dose produces a relatively large change in effect. At near-maximal response, large increases in dose produce little change in effect. Usually the dose is plotted on a logarithmic scale (Fig. 11-9, right panel), which demonstrates the linear relationship between the logarithm of the dose and the intensity of the response between 20% and 80% of the maximum effect.

Acquiring the pharmacologic effect data from a population of subjects exposed to a variety of doses of a drug provides four key characteristics of the drug dose–response relationship—potency, drug-receptor affinity, efficacy, and population pharmacodynamic variability. The *potency* of the drug—the dose required to produce a given effect—is usually expressed as the dose required to produce a given effect in 50% of subjects, the *ED50*. The *slope* of the curve between 20% and 80% of the maximal effect indicates the rate of increase in effect as the dose is increased and is a reflection of the affinity of the receptor for the drug. The maximum effect is referred to as the *efficacy* of the drug. Finally, if curves from multiple subjects are generated, the *variability* in potency, efficacy, and the slope of the dose–response curve can be estimated.

The dose needed to produce a given pharmacologic effect varies considerably, even in "normal" patients. The patient most resistant to the drug usually requires a dose two- to threefold greater than the patient with the lowest dose requirements. This variability is caused by differences among individuals in the relationship between drug concentration and pharmacologic effect, superimposed on differences in pharmacokinetics. Dose–response studies have the disadvantage of not being able to determine whether variations in pharmacologic response are caused by differences in pharmacokinetics, pharmacodynamics, or both.

Concentration–Response Relationships

The onset and duration of pharmacologic effects depend not only on pharmacokinetic factors but also on the pharmacodynamic factors governing the degree of temporal disequilibrium between changes in concentration and changes in effect. The magnitude of the pharmacologic effect is a function of the amount of drug present at the site of action, so increasing the dose increases the peak effect. Larger doses have a more rapid onset of action because pharmacologically active concentrations at the site of action occur sooner. Increasing the dose also increases the duration of action because pharmacologically effective concentrations are maintained for a longer time.

Ideally, the concentration of drug at its site of action should be used to define the concentration–response relationship. Unfortunately, these data are rarely available, so the relationship between the concentration of drug in the blood and pharmacologic effect is studied instead. This relationship is easiest to understand if the changes in pharmacologic effect that occur during and after an IV infusion of a hypothetical drug are considered. If a drug is infused at a constant rate, the plasma concentration initially increases rapidly and asymptotically approaches a steady-state level after approximately five elimination half-lives have elapsed (Fig. 11-11). The effect of the drug initially increases very slowly, then more rapidly, and eventually also reaches a steady state. When the infusion is discontinued, indicated by point C in Figure 11-11, the plasma concentration immediately decreases because of drug distribution and elimination. However, the effect stays the same for a short period, and then also begins to decrease—there is always a time lag between changes in plasma concentration and changes in pharmacologic response. Figure 11-11 also demonstrates that the same plasma concentration is associated with different responses if the concentration is changing. At points A and B in Figure 11-11, the plasma concentrations are the same, but the effects at each time differ. When the concentration is increasing, there is a concentration gradient from blood to the site of action. When the infusion is discontinued, the concentration gradient is reversed. Therefore, at the same plasma concentration, the concentration at the site

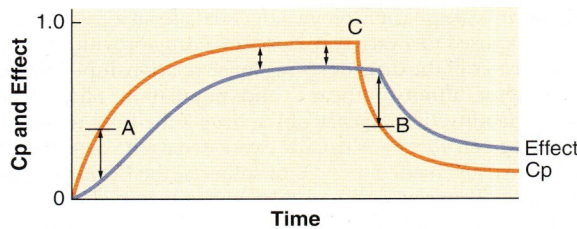

Figure 11-11 The changes in plasma drug concentration and pharmacologic effect during and after an intravenous infusion. See text for explanation. (Adapted from Stanski DR, Sheiner LB. Pharmacokinetics and pharmacodynamics of muscle relaxants. *Anesthesiology*. 1979;51:103.)

of action is higher after, compared to during, the infusion. This is associated with a correspondingly greater effect.

In theory, there must be some degree of temporal disequilibrium between plasma concentration and drug effect for all drugs with extravascular sites of action. However, for some drugs, the time lag may be so short that it cannot be demonstrated. The magnitude of this temporal disequilibrium depends on several factors:

- The perfusion of the organ on which the drug acts
- The tissue:blood partition coefficient of the drug
- The rate of diffusion or transport of the drug from the blood to the cellular site of action
- The rate and affinity of drug–receptor binding
- The time required for processes initiated by the drug–receptor interaction to produce changes in cellular function

The consequence of this time lag between changes in concentration and changes in effects is that the plasma concentration will have an unvarying relationship with pharmacologic effect only under steady-state conditions. At steady state, the plasma concentration is in equilibrium with the concentrations throughout the body, and is thus directly proportional to the steady-state concentration at the site of action. Plotting the logarithm of the steady-state plasma concentration versus response generates a curve identical in appearance to the dose–response curve shown in the right panel of Figure 11-9. The $Cp_{ss}50$, the steady-state plasma concentration producing 50% of the maximal response, is determined from the concentration–response curve. Like the ED50, the $Cp_{ss}50$ is a measure of sensitivity to a drug, but the $Cp_{ss}50$ has the advantage of being unaffected by pharmacokinetic variability. Because it takes five elimination half-lives to approach steady-state conditions, it is not practical to determine the $Cp_{ss}50$ directly. For drugs with long elimination half-lives, the pseudoequilibrium during the elimination phase can be used to approximate steady-state conditions, because the concentrations in plasma and at the site of action are changing very slowly.

Combined Pharmacokinetic–Pharmacodynamic Models

Integrated pharmacokinetic–pharmacodynamic models fully characterize the relationships among time, dose, plasma concentration, and pharmacologic effect. This is accomplished by adding a hypothetical "effect compartment" (biophase) to a standard compartmental pharmacokinetic model (Fig. 11-12).[46–48] Transfer of drug between central compartment and the effect compartment is assumed to be a first-order process, and the pharmacologic effect is assumed to be directly related to the concentration in the biophase. The biophase is a "virtual" compartment, although linked to the pharmacokinetic model, and does not actually receive or return drug to the model and, therefore, ensures that the effect site processes do not influence the pharmacokinetics of

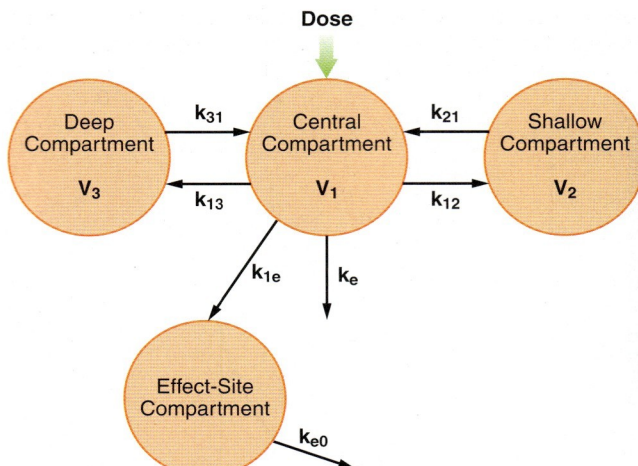

Figure 11-12 A schematic of a three-compartment pharmacokinetic model with the effect site linked to the central compartment. The rate constant for transfer between the plasma (central compartment) and the effect site, k_{1e}, and the volume of the effect site are both presumed to be negligible to ensure that the effect site does not influence the pharmacokinetic model. The rate constant for drug removal from the effect site, which relates the concentration in the central compartment to the pharmacologic effect is k_{e0}.

the rest of the body. By simultaneously characterizing the pharmacokinetics of the drug and the time course of drug effect, the combined pharmacokinetic–pharmacodynamic model is able to quantify the temporal dissociation between the plasma (central compartment) concentration and effect with the rate constant for equilibration between the plasma and the biophase, k_{e0}. By quantifying the time lag between changes in plasma concentration and changes in pharmacologic effect, these models can also define the $Cp_{ss}50$, even without steady-state conditions. These models have contributed greatly to our understanding of factors influencing the response to IV anesthetics, opioids, and nondepolarizing muscle relaxants in humans.

The rate of equilibration between the plasma and the biophase, k_{e0}, can also be characterized by the half-life of effect site equilibration ($T_{1/2ke0}$) using the formula:

$$T_{1/2k_{e_0}} = \frac{\ln 2}{k_{e0}} = \frac{0.693}{k_{e0}} \quad (11\text{-}18)$$

$T_{1/2ke0}$ is the time for the effect site concentration to reach 50% of the plasma concentration when the plasma concentration is held constant. For anesthetics with a short $T_{1/2ke0}$ (high k_{e0}), equilibration between the plasma and the biophase is rapid and therefore there is little delay before an effect is reached when a bolus of drug is administered or an infusion of drug is initiated. However, because the decline in the effect site concentration will also depend on the concentration gradient between the effect site and the plasma, drugs that rapidly equilibrate with the biophase may take longer to redistribute away.[49] Therefore, the offset of drug effect is more dependent on the pharmacokinetics of the body than on the rapidity of biophase-plasma equilibration.[20,49]

Population Pharmacokinetic–Pharmacodynamic Models

Population pharmacokinetic–pharmacodynamic (PKPD) modeling has emerged as a nearly essential part of study design and data analysis in the clinical pharmacology of anesthetic drugs.[50] Despite the term "population," these techniques are designed to bring an individual's specific physiologic characteristics into dose regimen selection. These analyses were made possible through the combined efforts of a theoretical statistician, Stuart Beal, and a leading clinical pharmacologist, Lewis Sheiner, and found early adoption in anesthesiology.[51,52] Sheiner and Beal termed their technique nonlinear mixed effects (meaning both fixed and random effects) modeling and wrote a computer program (NONMEM) to fit PKPD data from multiple individuals, and even from multiple studies, while building an overarching statistical description.[53] In this way a typical (or median) value for each parameter (e.g., clearance, volume, EC_{50}) of the PKPD model (called fixed effects, or thetas, θ, in NONMEM terminology) could be combined with a random effect variable (eta, η, in NONMEM) that described where on the distribution (e.g., Gaussian) of all ηs each individual η lies for each parameter, θ.[50]

With nonlinear mixed effects modeling it is possible to include the interindividual variability of each parameter into a PKPD model for the population(s) studied; an important concept when trying to predict the next dose administered to the next patient. Furthermore, the spread of the random effects (ηs) can be reduced by including each individual's demographic data, for example, genomic and physiologic factors, into the model in the form of covariates to refine the model and enhance its ability to predict the next patient's response to a drug by inclusion of demographic data in the dose calculation.

Allometric scaling has developed as a corollary to population PKPD modeling. Allometry derives from an observation that interspecies metabolism varies by an animal's weight raised to the 0.75 power (instead of 1.0).[54] It has been widely applied to scale pharmacokinetic models across species. More recently, allometry has been applied to intraspecies (human) scaling when developing population mixed effects PKPD models at the extremes of age (i.e., pediatric and geriatric) or size (i.e., morbid obesity).[55-57]

Population PKPD models were developed to facilitate individualized medicine in drug therapy. However, dosing regimens are rapidly becoming calculation-intensive, with the inclusion of increasing numbers of important covariates, especially with additional nonlinear allometric considerations. Thus, to allow precision dosing in the practice of anesthesiology, these complex calculations should ideally be incorporated into drug-specific infusion pumps (e.g., TCI pumps) or into apps the clinician can have on a PDA at the bedside.

Therapeutic Thresholds and Therapeutic Window

The timing of the onset and the offset of drug action is not only dependent on the effect site's concentration profile (i.e., the drug's pharmacokinetics and pharmacodynamics), but it also depends on the minimum concentration that produces a discernible level of drug effect—the therapeutic threshold of the drug. The therapeutic threshold of a drug depends on the magnitude of the desired effect or the intensity of the stimulus being treated. For example, superficial procedures (i.e., mastectomy, melanoma excision, etc) are not as painful (Fig. 11-13, dashed green line) as orthopedic procedures (i.e., long bone instrumentation, spine fusion, etc., dotted green line). Therefore, the dose of fentanyl that produces analgesia for superficial procedures (black solid concentration profile) does not produce clinically discernible analgesia for the orthopedic procedures (i.e., below the therapeutic threshold). In contrast, the dose of fentanyl that produces analgesia for the orthopedic procedures (blue solid concentration profile) will not only provide analgesia for the superficial

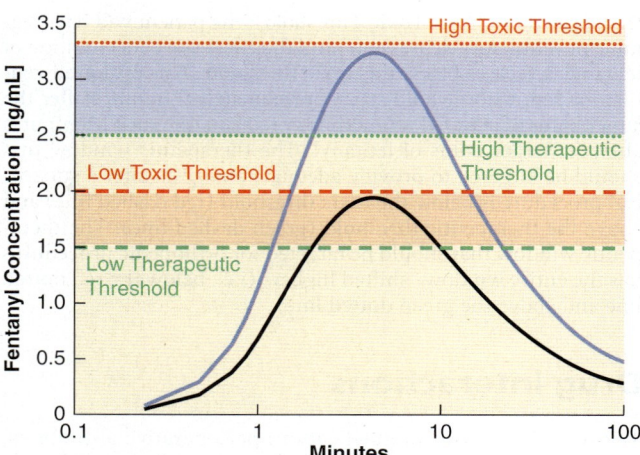

Figure 11-13 The effect site concentration versus time profiles after a small intravenous bolus (*solid black line*) and a larger intravenous bolus (*solid blue line*) of fentanyl. Representative therapeutic thresholds (the minimum concentration required to produce clinically discernible analgesia), and toxic threshold (the concentration above which profound opioid induced ventilatory depression occurs) are demonstrated superficial procedures, such as mastectomy (*green dashed line*, low therapeutic threshold), and for orthopedic procedures, such as long bone instrumentation (*dotted green line*, high therapeutic threshold). A given bolus of fentanyl only produces clinically discernible analgesia from the time it produces an effect site concentration above the therapeutic threshold concentration for a patient until the time when the effect site concentration decreases below the therapeutic threshold concentration. If the effect site concentration does not exceed the toxic threshold for a patient, then it does not produce profound opioid induced ventilatory depression. In contrast, if the bolus does produce an effect site concentration above the toxic threshold concentration, it will produce profound ventilatory depression that is sustained until the effect site concentration decreases below the toxic threshold concentration. For example, after superficial surgery, a small dose of fentanyl (*solid black line*) will initially produce detectable analgesia approximately 2 minutes after administration (when it crosses the low therapeutic threshold, *dashed green line*) which will last until approximately 10 minutes after administration (when the concentration decreases below the low therapeutic threshold, *green dashed line*). Since the dose does not produce a concentration above the low toxic threshold (*dashed red line*), hypoventilation will not occur after this single bolus. In contrast, for the same superficial procedure, a larger bolus of fentanyl (*solid blue line*) will initially produce analgesia less than 1 minute after administration (when it crosses the low therapeutic threshold, *dashed green line*), which will last until approximately 30 minutes after administration (when the concentration decreases below the low therapeutic threshold, *green dashed line*). Since the dose produces an effect site concentration above the toxic threshold (*dashed red line*), it will produce profound hypoventilation from approximately 2 minutes until the effect site concentration decreases below the same toxic threshold at approximately 18 minutes. So, although the larger bolus produces a quicker onset of action and a longer duration of action, it produces toxicity for a portion of this time. After orthopedic procedures (*dotted green line* for high therapeutic threshold and *dotted red line* for high toxic threshold), a small bolus of fentanyl will be subtherapeutic and ineffective (*black solid line*) because it does not produce a concentration above the high therapeutic threshold (*dotted green line*). In contrast, a larger bolus of fentanyl produces clinically discernible analgesia from approximately 2 through 10 minutes after administration (time that *blue line* is above *green dotted line*).

procedures, but it will also have a faster onset of effect because it reaches the therapeutic threshold quicker. In addition, since the larger bolus of fentanyl results in concentrations of drug that are above the toxic threshold for the superficial procedures (red dashed line, Low Toxic Threshold), the patient will have significant ventilatory depression until the effect site concentration of fentanyl decreases below this toxic threshold. This profound ventilatory depression would start approximately 2 minutes after the larger bolus of fentanyl was administered and last until 18 minutes after the larger bolus of fentanyl. The therapeutic window that should be targeted to provide adequate analgesia after a superficial procedure is below the toxic threshold (red dashed line) and above the therapeutic threshold (green dashed line). The therapeutic window that should be targeted for orthopedic procedures has the entire window "shifted higher" (i.e., below the red dotted line and above the green dotted line).

Drug Interactions

Taking into account premedication, perioperative antibiotics, IV agents used for induction or maintenance, inhalational anesthetics, opioids, muscle relaxants, the drugs used to restore neuromuscular transmission, and postoperative analgesics, 10 or more drugs may be given as relatively "routine" anesthetics. Consequently, thorough understanding of the mechanisms of drug interactions and knowledge of specific interactions with drugs used in anesthesia are essential to the safe practice of anesthesiology. Indeed, anesthesiologists often deliberately take advantage of drug interactions. For example, moderate to high doses of opioid are often utilized to decrease the amount of volatile anesthetic required to provide immobility and hemodynamic stability to surgical incision (e.g., MAC* and MAC_{BAR}), thereby avoiding the side effects of higher concentrations of inhaled anesthetics (e.g., vasodilation, prolonged awakening). In this section, we will examine the major classes of drug–drug interactions by detailing common examples encountered in the perioperative period.

Pharmaceutical (Physiochemical) Interactions

In Vitro Interactions

Anesthesiologists often overlook the drug interactions produced by pharmaceutical (physicochemical) properties because most perioperative drugs are administered intravenously or via inhalation, and therefore have a high bioavailability. However, in vitro drug–drug interactions due to physiochemical properties of drugs can significantly alter drug bioavailability and produce unintended toxic byproducts. Basic acid–base chemistry can predict many of the observed in vitro interactions. One classic example of a physiochemical drug–drug interaction that alters drug bioavailability is the formation of insoluble salts that precipitate when acidic drugs, such as thiopental, and basic drugs, such as opioids or muscle relaxants, are "mixed" when the two drugs are administered into IV tubing with an insufficient fluid flow rate.[58] Another example is the observation that commercial preparations of local anesthetic solutions that contain epinephrine would have a lower pH than plain local anesthetic solutions to which epinephrine is added shortly prior to administration,

---

*MAC: Minimum alveolar concentration is the pseudo-steady state end-tidal alveolar concentration at which 50% of patients do not move in response to surgical incision or do not have an increase in heart rate or blood pressure in response to surgical incision (BAR: blocks autonomic responses).

because of the high acidity of the antioxidant stabilizers used in commercial preparations (i.e., sodium bisulfite or sodium pyrosulfite).[59] The unintended consequence of this commercial formulation is that the local anesthetic appears less effective owing to the increased concentration of the less permeable ionized form of local anesthetic that exists in acidic environments.

Although physiochemical drug interactions that affect the bioavailability of drugs are relatively easy to avoid or, at least, overcome by increasing the drug dose, some physiochemical interactions can result in unintended toxic compounds. One chemical agent often overlooked by anesthesiologists is the soda lime or Baralyme that is used in modern anesthesia machines to remove carbon dioxide from the exhaled gases. Although patients are not directly administered this agent, the gas that they inhale from the anesthesia machine often contains the byproducts of the interaction between the constituents of the exhaled gas and the carbon dioxide absorbent. While this allows the patient to receive a "heated and humidified" inhaled gas mixture, if conditions are correct, the halogenated volatile anesthetics can undergo degradation by the strong base (i.e., sodium and/or potassium hydroxide) contained in the carbon dioxide absorber.[60] This chemical reaction led the FDA to recommend that sevoflurane exposure should not exceed 2 MAC-hours at using fresh gas flow rates of 1 to less than 2 L/min, in order to minimize exposure to the potentially nephrotoxic haloalkene ("compound A") formed by dehydrofluorination of sevoflurane by soda lime or Barolyme.[61] Although the effects of compound A on human renal function are not of great clinical concern, the strong bases in the carbon dioxide can also degrade the difluorom-ethyl containing halogenated volatile anesthetics (i.e., desflurane and isoflurane) to carbon monoxide.[62] These patient safety concerns led to the development and the increased use of Amsorb, a carbon dioxide adsorbent that contains calcium hydroxide lime in place of sodium and/or potassium hydroxide, and therefore causes minimal to no carbon monoxide or compound A formation.[63]

In Vivo Interactions

Whereas many of the in vitro physiochemical interactions can result in unintended toxicity due to exposure to either subtherapeutic drug concentrations or toxic degradation products, physiochemical interactions have been exploited to develop two novel approaches to antagonize neuromuscular junction blocking agents. The first approach, which was approved for use in the European Union in 2008 and in the United States in 2016, is the selective relaxant binding agent, sugammadex. Sugammadex is a synthetic cyclodextrin that encapsulates and electrostatically binds rocuronium. By essentially irreversibly binding plasma rocuronium, sugammadex acts as a chelator that not only rapidly decreases the free plasma rocuronium concentration but also promotes redistribution of rocuronium from the neuromuscular junction (extracellular space) to the intravascular space.[64] Therefore, if there is an excess of sugammadex molecules relative to rocuronium molecules, the neuromuscular blockade is antagonized. Although sugammadex was developed to antagonize neuromuscular blockade produced by rocuronium, it is also able to antagonize profound neuromuscular blockade produced by the other commonly used steroidal neuromuscular blocking agents, vecuronium and pipecuronium.[65,66] However, sugammadex is unable to antagonize neuromuscular blockade produced by the benzylisoquinoline neuromuscular blocking agent, cisatracurium. However, molecules from the cucurbit[n]uril family can encapsulate both the steroidal and benzylisoquinoline family of neuromuscular blocking agents in preclinical models and may be a more comprehensive solution for antagonism of neuromuscular blockade via molecular encapsulation.[67–69] An alternative approach to neuromuscular blockade antagonism is to design a molecule that can be inactivated via nonbiologic routes. This approach has led to Phase 1 studies of a new class of nondepolarizing neuromuscular blocking drugs called the fumarates (olefinic diester isoquinolinium compounds). These molecules are rapidly inactivated by the nonenzymatic formation of cysteine adducts when combined with plasma cysteine.[70] Therefore, cysteine administration antagonizes the neuromuscular blockade. These two novel approaches to drug development could be used to develop designer drugs that can be readily antagonized via nonbiologic routes, if the important receptor targets for sedation and amnesia components of general anesthesia are identified.

Pharmacokinetic Interactions

Drugs can alter each other's absorption, distribution, and elimination. Understanding the basis for alterations in the pharmacokinetics allows anesthesiologists to not only avoid unintentional supratherapeutic or subtherapeutic concentrations of the perioperative medications, but also to strategically employ alterations in pharmacokinetics to achieve the desired concentration profile.

Absorption (Uptake)

Some drugs can alter the absorption of other drugs, by either altering the delivery of drug to site of drug absorption (uptake) or by altering the local blood flow to the site of drug administration. Although this type of drug–drug interaction will alter bioavailability, it should not alter any other pharmacokinetic parameter. Drugs like ranitidine, which alters gastric pH, and metoclopramide, which speeds gastric emptying, alter absorption from the GI tract. Vasoconstrictors that decrease local blood flow and decrease systemic uptake of drug can be beneficial when added to local anesthetic solutions because they prolong the duration of action of the local anesthetic at the site of injection and can decrease the risk of systemic toxicity from rapid absorption. However, when systemically administered, vasoactive drugs can decrease blood flow to skin and muscle, and decrease the systemic uptake of drugs given by subcutaneous or intramuscular injection. In a similar manner, vasoactive agents can alter the ventilation–perfusion ratio, thereby altering pulmonary uptake of volatile anesthetics, despite a constant inspired concentration. Because of the variability produced by vasoactive agents in drug uptake, careful thought must be given when choosing to administer drugs via non-IV route in perioperative patients.

Distribution

Some drugs can alter the systemic distribution of other drugs. Alterations in drug distribution will change some or all of a pharmacokinetic model's volume parameters. It can also alter one or all of the *intercompartmental* clearance parameters of a multicompartmental pharmacokinetic model. There are two main mechanisms purported in textbooks and the clinical pharmacology literature by which drug–drug interactions alter drug distribution—(a) changing the volume of tissue available for drug uptake and (b) changing the amount of drug available for tissue uptake. Since the drug dose required to achieve a desired drug concentration is intimately linked to systemic drug distribution, understanding what common drug–drug interactions produce real alterations in drug distribution can avoid unintentional exposure to subtherapeutic and supratherapeutic drug concentrations.

Although a drug cannot alter the actual volume of tissue available for drug uptake, changing the exposure of blood to different tissue beds changes a drug's apparent tissue volume of distribution. Therefore, drug-induced alterations of cardiac output and the distribution of cardiac output to tissues can change the distribution clearance of other drugs. Once again, vasoactive agents can alter tissue distribution by altering regional blood flow even if the total cardiac output is unchanged. Because the change in the plasma drug concentration produced by a prescribed dosing regimen is inversely related to the distribution clearance, the drug dose must be decreased when vasoactive drugs decrease cardiac output or the distribution of cardiac output; otherwise the patient will be exposed to supratherapeutic drug concentrations.[71–73] In addition, the unintended cardiovascular effects of anesthetic drugs, such as the decrease in cardiac output with increasing doses of the direct myocardial depressant, halothane, or the direct arterial dilator, isoflurane, can lead to similar increases in the plasma drug concentration.[74,75]

There is an overabundance of clinical pharmacology literature that examines the ability of one drug to displace another drug from its protein-binding site(s), thereby increasing the concentration of unbound drug in the blood that could cause supratherapeutic concentrations and potential toxicity. When examining specific pharmacokinetic parameters, an increase in the fraction of unbound drug in the plasma could theoretically increase the total apparent volume of distribution (V_{ss}), as more molecules of drug are available for distribution into the tissue. Although most changes in protein binding will not influence clinical drug exposure, analysis of the equations governing the steady-state pharmacokinetics suggests that drugs that are extensively protein bound, have a high hepatic extraction ratio, and have a low therapeutic index may be the exception that require dose adjustment.[76] However, the clinical importance of protein binding in anesthetic drugs is based on several common misconceptions regarding drug distribution. First, the number of unoccupied binding sites is several orders of magnitude higher than the number of molecules of anesthetic drug administered in clinical practice. Therefore, it is hard to envision a scenario where a significant amount of displacement could occur. Even if a drug could displace a significant amount of another drug from its protein-binding site, the liver has the capacity available to metabolize this sudden influx of free drug, thereby returning the free drug concentration to the predisplacement concentrations (i.e., flow limited metabolism). Finally, the theoretical argument supporting the importance of protein binding on highly lipophilic drugs ignores the fact that lipophilic drugs not only have flow-limited elimination clearance, but also flow-limited tissue distribution. Therefore, the equations supporting the negligible role of protein binding on flow-limited elimination clearance also generalize to include flow-limited tissue distribution.[76] Indirect proof of this is provided by the fact that there are no examples in the literature of drug–drug interactions that produce changes in protein binding of opioids and hypnotics that are clinically relevant.[77]

Metabolism

Drugs that alter hepatic blood flow (i.e., vasoactive drugs, volatile anesthetics) can proportionally alter hepatic metabolism of drugs with flow-limited clearance.[71–75] In addition, drugs that inhibit or induce the enzymes that catalyze biotransformation

Table 11-5   Inducers and Inhibitors of Hepatic Drug Metabolism

Inducers
Carbamazepine
Ethanol
Glucocorticoids
Phenobarbital
Phenytoin
Rifampin
St John's wort
Tamoxifen

Inhibitors
Azole antifungal drugs (i.e., ketoconazole, itraconazole)
Cimetidine
Disulfiram
Grapefruit juice
Macrolide antibiotics (i.e., clarithromycin and erythromycin)
Protease inhibitors (i.e., ritonavir, indinavir, saquinavir)
Quinidine
Selective serotonin reuptake inhibitors (i.e., fluoxetine and sertraline)
CYP3A4 and CYP2D6

---

reactions can affect clearance of other concomitantly administered drugs (Table 11-5). The concomitant use of CYP isozyme inducers can usually be overcome by increasing the administered dose, especially if an easy measure of biologic activity is available or the therapeutic concentration range is known. For example, the anticonvulsant phenytoin shortens the duration of action of the nondepolarizing neuromuscular junction blocking agents by inducing CYP3A4 and therefore increasing elimination clearance of the drug.[78] In contrast, when CYP isozyme inhibition is present, it is more difficult to adjust the drug dose without achieving supratherapeutic, and possibly toxic drug concentrations, unless a suitable rapidly responsive measure of biologic activity is available. While it may be possible to safely administer opioids in the presence of protease inhibitors such as ritonavir, because opioids can be titrated in small doses to clinical effect, it is more difficult to titrate warfarin or glyburide when instituting short-term antifungal therapy. Furthermore, prodrugs that require CYP isozyme activity for conversion to active moieties may be difficult to titrate to adequate clinical effect if there are other sources of interindividual variability in drug dose–response. The opioid prodrugs codeine, oxycodone, hydrocodone, and tramadol all require CYP2D6 for conversion to the biologically active opioid.[77] Because of the high polymorphic character of the CYP2D6 enzyme, it is difficult to determine which patients who are taking selective serotonin reuptake inhibitors, that also inhibit CYP2D6 activity, would receive adequate analgesia from these opioids. Therefore, other opioids may have less variability in opioid dose–response and be better choices than these prodrugs.

Pharmacodynamic Interactions

Pharmacodynamic interactions fall into two broad classifications. Drugs can interact, either directly or indirectly, at the same receptors. Opioid antagonists directly displace opioids from opiate receptors. Cholinesterase inhibitors indirectly antagonize the effects of neuromuscular blockers by increasing the amount of acetylcholine, which displaces the blocking drug from nicotinic receptors. Pharmacodynamic interactions can also occur if two drugs affect a physiologic system at different sites.[79,80] For example, μ-opioid receptor-mediated ventilatory depression can be selectively antagonized by ampakines that potentiate AMPA receptor-mediated glutamatergic excitation without mitigating opioid-induced analgesia.[81]

The most common example of pharmacodynamic interactions that are used to the advantage of anesthesiologists (and their patients) is the interaction between hypnotics and opioids. Hypnotics and opioids, each acting on their own specific receptors, appear to interact synergistically.[82] The pharmacodynamic interaction between two drugs can be characterized by utilizing response surface models.[83–88] The three-dimensional models are useful in delineating the concentration pairs of a hypnotic (e.g., volatile anesthetic, propofol, midazolam) and an opioid (e.g., remifentanil, alfentanil, fentanyl) that produce adequate anesthesia while minimizing undesired side effects.[89] (See Response Surface Models, below.)

Serotonin Syndrome

One pharmacodynamic interaction that has become more common with the widespread use of medications that modulate the serotonergic pathway is the potentially fatal serotonin syndrome (syndrome toxicity).[90,91] High CNS concentrations of serotonin, can produce mental status changes (confusion, hyperactivity, memory problems), muscle twitching, excessive sweating, shivering, and fever. Classically, excessive CNS serotonin levels are associated with inhibition of monoamine oxidase, an enzyme responsible for breaking down serotonin in the brain. However, excessive intrasynaptic serotonin levels from decreased reuptake of serotonin have been associated with other antidepressant medications, including serotonin reuptake inhibitors and serotonin norepinephrine reuptake inhibitors (Table 11-6). The interaction of meperidine with MAOIs is the most classic drug–drug interaction associated with serotonin syndrome. It is important to know that other common perioperative medications, such as methylene blue, which is a potent reversible MAOI, and the phenylpiperidine series of opioids (i.e., fentanyl and its congeners, methadone, meperidine, tramadol), which act as weak serotonin reuptake inhibitors, have been reported to be associated with serotonin toxicity in small case reports.[91–94] Ideally, the serotonergic drug would be held until sufficient CNS drug washout can occur to mitigate any interaction. Because the SSRIs with long elimination half-lives require greater than 4 weeks for adequate CNS washout, withholding these drugs can result in worsening depression or neuropathic pain, depending on the indication for the initial serotonergic medication. Therefore, when adequate washout cannot be obtained and methylene blue must be administered, the serotonergic drug should be stopped and not reinstated for 24 hours after the last dose of methylene blue.[93] When methylene blue or phenylpiperidine opioids must be administered to patients taking serotonergic psychiatric medications, clinicians should have a high clinical suspicion for the development of serotonin toxicity. This is especially important in the perioperative period when other more common clinical states, such as postoperative delirium or perioperative fever, can be associated with the common symptoms of serotonin toxicity, thereby delaying diagnosis. Although cyproheptadine, a serotonin receptor antagonist, is the most common treatment for moderate to severe serotonin toxicity, it is only available as an oral formulation, thereby limiting its bioavailability in critically ill perioperative patients. Intravenous chlorpromazine is an alternative serotonin receptor antagonist that has been used successfully with concomitant supportive care.

Table 11-6 Serotonergic Psychiatric Drugs Implicated in the Cases of Serotonin Syndrome with Methylene Blue[a]

Class	Generic	Brand Name(s)
Selective serotonin reuptake inhibitors (SSRIs)	Paroxetine	Paxil, Paxil CR, Pexeva
	Fluvoxamine	Luvox, Luvox CR
	Fluoxetine	Prozac, Sarafem, Symbyax
	Sertraline	Zoloft
	Citalopram	Celexa
	Escitalopram	Lexapro
	Vilazodone	Viibryd
Serotonin–norepinephrine reuptake inhibitors (SNRIs)	Venlafaxine	Effexor, Effexor XR
	Desvenlafaxine	Pristiq
	Duloxetine	Cymbalta
Tricyclic antidepressants (TCAs)	Amitriptyline	Amitid, Amitril, Elavil, Endep, Etrafon, Limbitrol, Triavil
	Desipramine	Norpramin, Pertofrane
	Clomipramine	Anafranil
	Imipramine	Tofranil, Tofranil PM, Janimine, Pramine, Presamine
	Nortriptyline	Pamelor, Aventyl hydrochloride
	Protriptyline	Vivactil
	Doxepin	Sinequan, Zonalon, Silenor
	Trimipramine	Surmontil
Monoamine oxidase inhibitors (MAOIs)	Isocarboxazid	Marplan
	Phenelzine	Nardil
	Selegiline	Emsam, Eldepryl, Zelapar
	Tranylcypromine	Parnate
Others	Amoxapine	Asendin
	Maprotiline	Ludiomil
	Nefazodone	Serzone
	Trazodone	Desyrel, Oleptro, Trialodine
	Bupropion	Wellbutrin, Wellbutrin SR, Wellbutrin XL, Zyban, Aplenzin
	Buspirone	Buspar
	Mirtazapine	Remeron, Remeron Soltab

[a] Adapted from U.S. Food & Drug Administration website, updated 11/08/2011 (http://www.fda.gov/Drugs/DrugSafety/ucm276119.htm)

Clinical Applications of Pharmacokinetics and Pharmacodynamics to the Administration of Intravenous Anesthetics

While no new inhaled anesthetics have been synthesized since the 1960s, IV drugs that act on the CNS continue to be developed. Anesthesiologists have become accustomed to the exquisite control of anesthetic blood (and effect site) concentrations afforded by modern volatile anesthetic agents and their vaporizers, coupled to end-tidal anesthetic gas monitoring. Although pharmacokinetic and pharmacodynamic principles and data have contributed greatly to our understanding of the behavior of IV anesthetics, their primary utility and ultimate purpose are to determine optimal dosing with as much mathematical precision and clinical accuracy as possible. In most pharmacotherapeutic scenarios outside of anesthesia care, the time scales for onset of drug effect, its maintenance, and its offset are measured in days, weeks, or even years. In such cases, global pharmacokinetic variables (and one-compartment models) such as total volume of distribution (V_{SS}), elimination clearance (Cl_e), and half-life ($t_{1/2}$) are sufficient and utilitarian parameters for calculating dose regimens. However, in the OR and ICU, the temporal tolerances for onset and offset of desired drug effects are measured in minutes.[38,39] Consequently, these global variables are insufficient to describe the details of kinetic behavior of drugs in the minutes following IV administration. This is particularly true of lipid-soluble hypnotics and opioids that rapidly and extensively distribute throughout the various tissues of the body, because distribution processes dominate pharmacokinetic behavior during the time frame of most anesthetics. In addition, the therapeutic indices of many IV anesthetic drugs are small and two-tailed (e.g., an underdose, resulting in awareness, which is a "toxic" effect). Optimal dosing in these situations requires use of all the variables of a multicompartmental pharmacokinetic model to account for drug distribution in blood and other tissues.

It is not easy to intuit the pharmacokinetic behavior of a multicompartmental system by simple examination of the kinetic variables.[10] Computer simulation is required to meaningfully interpret dosing or to accurately devise new dosing regimens. In addition, there are several pharmacokinetic concepts that are uniquely applicable to IV administration of drugs with multicompartmental kinetics and must be taken into account when administering IV infusions.

To achieve similar degrees of control of intravenously administered anesthetic drug concentrations in blood and in the CNS, new technologies aimed at improving IV infusion devices, as well as new software to manage the daunting pharmacokinetic principles involved, are needed. This section examines the current state of infusion devices and the pharmacokinetic and pharmacodynamic principles specifically required for precise delivery of anesthetic agents.

Rise to Steady-state Concentration

The drug concentration versus time profile for the rise to steady state is the mirror image of its elimination profile. In a one-compartment model with a decline in concentration versus time that is monoexponential following a single dose, the rise of drug concentration to the steady-state concentration (C_{ss}) is likewise monoexponential during a continuous infusion. That is, in one elimination half-life an infusion is halfway to its eventual steady-state concentration, in another half-life it reaches half of what remains between halfway and steady state (i.e., 75% of the eventual steady state is reached in two elimination half-lives), and so on for each half-life increment. The equation describing this behavior is:

$$C_p(t) = C_{ss}[1 - e^{-kt}] \quad (11\text{-}19)$$

where $C_p(t)$ = the concentration at time t, k is the rate constant related to the elimination half-life, and t is the time from the start of the infusion. This relationship can also be described by:

$$C_p(n) = C_{ss}[1 - (1/2)^n] \quad (11\text{-}20)$$

in which $C_p(n)$ is the concentration at n half-lives. Equation 11-20 indicates that during a constant infusion, the concentration reaches 90% of C_{ss} after 3.3 half-lives, which is usually deemed close enough for clinical purposes.

However, for a drug such as propofol, which partitions extensively to pharmacologically inert body tissues (e.g., muscle, gut), a monoexponential equation, or single-compartment model, is insufficient to describe the time course of propofol concentrations in the first minutes and hours after beginning drug administration. Instead, a multicompartmental or multiexponential model must be used. With such a model, the picture changes drastically for the plasma drug concentration rise toward steady state. The rate of rise toward steady state is determined by the distribution rate constants to the degree that their respective exponential terms contribute to the total area under the concentration versus time curve. Thus, for the three-compartment model describing the pharmacokinetics of propofol, Equation 11-19 becomes:

$$C_p(t) = C_{SS}\left[\frac{A}{A+B+G}(1-e^{-\alpha t}) + \frac{B}{A+B+G}(1-e^{-\beta t}) + \frac{G}{A+B+G}(1-e^{-\gamma t})\right] \quad (11\text{-}21)$$

in which t = time; $C_p(t)$ = plasma concentration at time; A = coefficient of the rapid distribution phase and α = hybrid rate constant of the rapid distribution phase; B = coefficient of the slower distribution phase and β = hybrid rate constant of the slower distribution; and G = coefficient of elimination phase and γ = hybrid rate constant of the elimination phase. $A + B + G$s is the sum of the coefficients of all the exponential terms. For most lipophilic anesthetics and opioids, A is typically one order of magnitude greater than B, and B is in turn an order of magnitude greater than G. Therefore, distribution-phase kinetics for IV anesthetics have a much greater influence on the time to reach C_{ss} than do elimination-phase kinetics.[49]

For example, with propofol having an elimination half-life of approximately 6 hours, the simple one-compartment rule in Equation 11-20 tells us that it would take 6 hours from the start of a constant rate infusion to reach even 50% of the eventual steady-state propofol plasma concentration and 12 hours to reach 75%. In contrast, with a full three-compartment propofol kinetic model, Equation 11-21 accurately predicts that 50% of steady state is reached in less than 30 minutes and 75% will be reached in less than 4 hours. This example emphasizes the necessity of using multicompartment models to describe the clinical pharmacokinetics of IV anesthetics.

Manual Bolus and Infusion Dosing Schemes

Based on a one compartment pharmacokinetic model, a stable steady-state plasma concentration ($C_{p,ss}$) can be maintained by administering an infusion at a rate (I) that is proportional to the elimination of drug from the body (Cl_E):

$$I = C_{p,SS} \times Cl_E \quad (11\text{-}22)$$

However, if the drug was only administered by initiating and maintaining this infusion, it would take one-elimination half-time to reach 50% of the target plasma concentration and three times that long to reach 90% of the target plasma concentration. In order to decrease the time until the target plasma concentration is achieved, an initial bolus (loading dose) of drug can be administered that would produce the target plasma concentration—

$$Bolus = C_{p,SS} \times V_{d,SS} \quad (11\text{-}23)$$

Although this method is very efficient in achieving and maintaining the target plasma concentration of a drug that instantaneously mixes and equilibrates throughout the tissues of the body (e.g., drugs modeled with a one-compartment pharmacokinetic model), utilizing the steady-state elimination clearance and volume of distribution to calculate the loading dose and maintenance infusion rate will result in plasma drug concentrations that are higher throughout the initial distribution phase (Fig. 11-14).

Using Equations 11-22 and 11-23 and $V_{d,SS}$ = 262 L and Cl_E = 1.7 L/min (for a 50-year-old man who is 178 cm tall and weighs 70 kg, from Schnider et al.), the loading dose and infusion rate of propofol that is needed to achieve a steady-state plasma concentration of 5 μg/mL is 1,300 mg (18 mg/kg) and 120 μg/kg/min. Obviously, the loading dose of propofol is too high, compared to clinically utilized doses (1 to 2 mg/kg) while the infusion rate appears to be a clinically acceptable dose. The erroneous estimate of the loading dose is due to the fact that the initial bolus of drug is not instantaneously mixed and equilibrated with the entire volume of tissue that will eventually take up drug. Therefore, manual dosing strategies for IV anesthetics need to be modified to account for the fact that when a bolus of drug is administered, it rapidly mixes and equilibrates with the blood and only a small volume of tissue (e.g., the central compartment), and then will distribute over time into other tissues.

To design a manual bolus that more precisely achieves the desired target plasma concentration, it is necessary to choose a bolus that is based on the small, initial volume of distribution (V_c). To maintain the target plasma concentration, a series of infusions of decreasing rate can be used that match the elimination clearance and compensate for drug loss from the central to the peripheral compartments during the initial period of extensive drug distribution and the second period of moderate drug

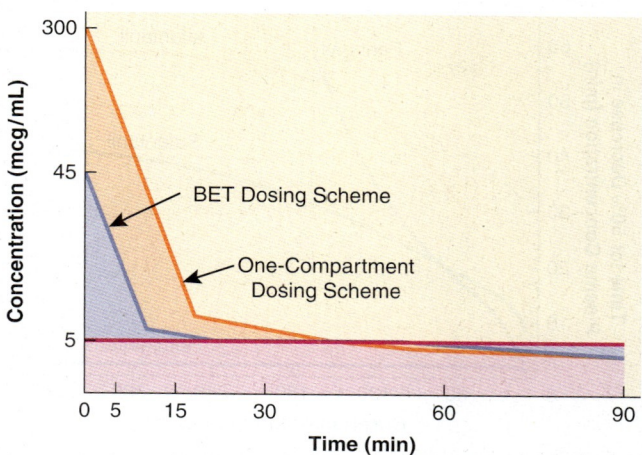

Figure 11-14 A computer simulation of the plasma propofol concentration profile during and after the administration of a single bolus and infusion scheme calculated using the steady-state, one-compartment pharmacokinetic parameters (*red line*) and the BET scheme from Table 11-7 (*blue line*) to achieve a plasma concentration of 5 μg/mL. $V_{d,ss}$ = 262 L and Cl_E = 1.7 L/min for a 50-year old male who is 178 cm tall and weighs 70 kg.

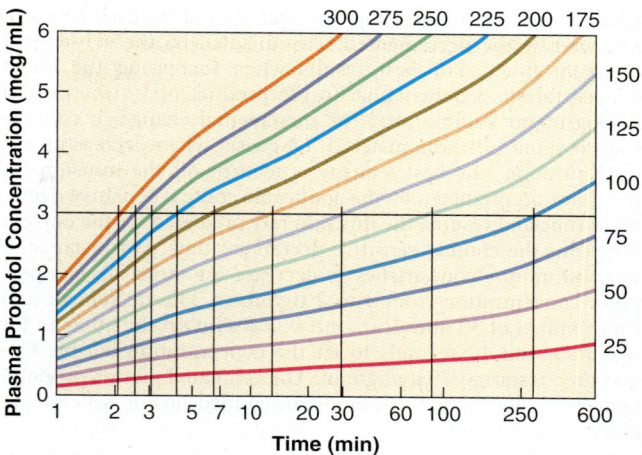

Figure 11-15 Isoconcentration nomogram for determining propofol infusion rates designed to maintain a desired plasma propofol concentration. This nomogram is based on the pharmacokinetics of Schnider et al. and is plotted on a log–log scale to better delineate the early time points. Curved lines represent the plasma propofol concentration versus time plots, resulting from the various continuous infusion rates indicated along the right and upper borders (units in μg/kg/min). A horizontal line is placed at the desired target plasma propofol concentration (3 μg/mL in this case) and vertical lines are placed at each intersection of a curved concentration–time plot. The vertical lines indicate the times that the infusion rate should be set to the one represented by the next intersected curve as one moves from left to right along the horizontal line drawn at 3 μg/mL. In this example, the infusion rate would be reduced from 300 μg/kg/min to 275 μg/kg/min at 2.5 minutes, to 250 μg/kg/min at 3 minutes, to 225 μg/kg/min at 4.5 minutes, and so on until it is turned to 100 μg/kg/min at 260 minutes.

distribution. This manual dosing scheme has been termed the BET scheme, where B is the loading bolus dose, E is the infusion to replace drug removed by elimination clearance, and T is a continuously decreasing infusion that compensates for transfer of drug to the peripheral tissues (i.e., distribution).[95] An example of a BET scheme for propofol to achieve a target plasma concentration of 5 μg/mL is shown in Table 11-7.

Isoconcentration Nomogram

To make the calculations of the various infusion rates required to maintain a target plasma concentration for a drug that follows multicompartment pharmacokinetics, a clinician would need access to a basic computer and the software to perform the appropriate simulations. With the appropriate formulas, this is quite feasible to do on any basic computer with any basic spreadsheet. However, even with more sophisticated pharmacokinetic software (e.g., SAAM II, WinNonLin, RugLoop, Stanpump), this is a time-consuming process that diverts the clinician's attention from the patient. In 1994, Shafer[96] introduced an isoconcentration nomogram for propofol that used the rise toward steady state described by a multicompartmental system (Fig. 11-15). This graphic tool allows users to employ concentration–effect, rather than dose–effect, relationships when determining optimal dosing of IV anesthetic agents. The nomogram is constructed by calculating the plasma drug concentration versus time curve for a constant-rate infusion from a set of pharmacokinetic variables for a particular drug. From this single simulation, one can readily visualize (and estimate) the rise toward steady-state plasma drug concentration described by the drug's pharmacokinetic model. By simulating a range of potential infusion rates, a series of curves of identical shape are then plotted on a single graph, with drug concentrations at any time that are directly proportional to the infusion rate.

By placing a horizontal line at the desired plasma drug concentration (*y*-axis), the times (*x*-axis) at which the horizontal intersects the line for a particular infusion rate will represent the times at which the infusion rate should be set to the rate on the intercepting line. In the example shown (Fig. 11-15) with 25-μg/kg/min increments, the predicted plasma propofol concentrations remain within 10% of the target from 2 minutes onward with a bias of underestimation. If it is desired that the estimated concentration never falls below the target, then the time to decrease to the next lower infusion should be at the midpoint of the subsequent interval. Extending the infusions to the subsequent midpoint times will introduce a maximum overestimation bias of approximately 17% with the illustrated infusion increments. Biases will be increased or decreased by constructing nomograms with larger or smaller infusion increments, respectively.

The nomogram can also be used to increase or reduce the targeted plasma propofol concentration. To target a new plasma drug concentration, a new horizontal line can be drawn at the desired concentration. The infusion rate that is closest to the

Table 11-7 The Bolus–Elimination–Infusion (BET) Scheme to Achieve a Propofol Plasma Concentration of 5 μg/mL for 120 Minutes

Bolus	2.8 mg/kg	
Infusion	238 μg/kg/min	0–10 min
	187 μg/kg/min	10–20 min
	136 μg/kg/min	20–60 min
	112 μg/kg/min	60–120 min

current time intersect is the one that should be used initially, followed by the decremented rates dictated by the subsequent intercept times. For best results when increasing the target concentration, a bolus equal to the product of V_c (the central compartment volume) and the incremental change in concentration should be administered. Likewise, when decreasing the concentration, the best strategy is to turn off the infusion for the duration predicted by the applicable context-sensitive decrement time and resume the infusion rate predicted for the current time plus the context-sensitive decrement time. For instance, if after 30 minutes one wishes to decrease the target plasma propofol concentration from 3 to 2 μg/mL (a 33% decrement at a time context of 30 minutes), one would shut off the infusion for 1 minute and 10 seconds to let the concentration fall by 33% and then restart at 75 μg/kg/min. The estimated plasma propofol concentrations from this nomogram-guided dosing scheme are shown in Figure 11-16.

Context-sensitive Decrement Times

During an infusion, drug is taken up by the inert, peripheral tissues.[18] Once drug delivery is terminated, recovery occurs when the effect site concentration decreases below a threshold concentration for producing a pharmacologic effect (e.g., MAC$_{AWAKE}$—the concentration where 50% of patients follow commands).[49,88] Although the rate of elimination of the drug from the body can give some indication for the time required to reach a subtherapeutic effect, site, drug concentration, and distribution to and from the peripheral tissues also contribute to the time course of decreasing drug concentrations of the central and the effect site. For drugs with multicompartmental kinetics, the elimination half-life will always overestimate the time to recovery from anesthetic drugs. The *context-sensitive half-time* is defined as the time required for the drug concentration of the plasma to decrease by 50%, where the context is the duration of the infusion.[97] The context-sensitive half-time for the common synthetic opioids fentanyl, alfentanil, sufentanil, and remifentanil are illustrated in Figure 11-17.

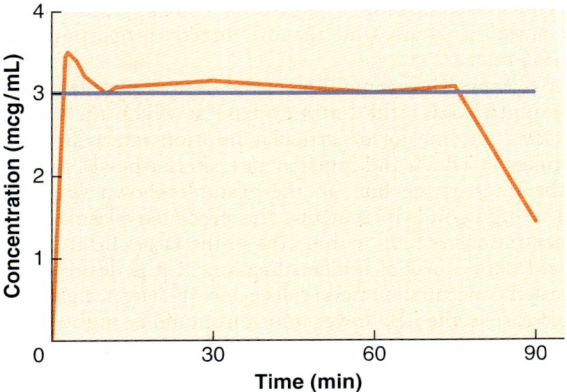

Figure 11-16 Simulated plasma propofol concentration history resulting from the information in the isoconcentration nomogram in Figure 11-15 and extending the times to switch the infusion to the next lower increment to the midpoint of the subsequent time segment (i.e., the switch from 250 to 225 μg/kg/min was at 5 minutes, rather than at 4.5 minutes). Note that for the first 30 minutes, this sequence predicts plasma propofol concentrations that are always slightly above 3 μg/mL (see text). The infusion is stopped at 90 minutes in this case.

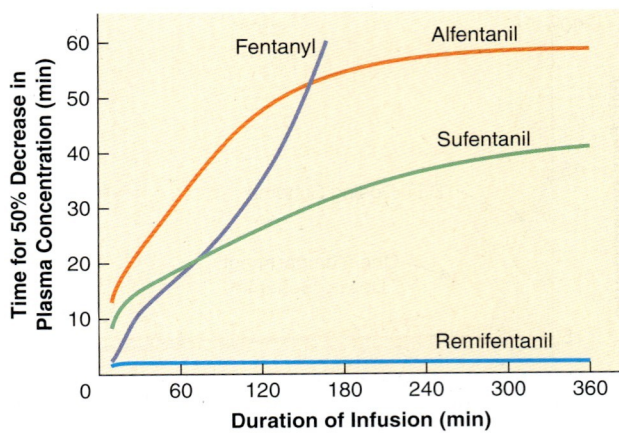

Figure 11-17 The context-sensitive plasma half-time for fentanyl, alfentanil, sufentanil, and remifentanil.

The context-sensitive half-time is not a pharmacokinetic parameter per se. It is calculated by simulating a target-controlled infusion (TCI) of a particular length (the length is the context) and then observing the time required for the plasma concentration to reach one-half of the target concentration from the time the infusion is terminated. As the length of the infusion increases, the value of the half-time increases and will eventually asymptotically approach a maximum half-time at steady state. Generally, for multicompartmental pharmacokinetic models, the half-time will always be less than the elimination half-life.

When an infusion is terminated at steady state, input into the system's central compartment is lost and net transfer of drug is no longer zero. Instead, net drug distribution immediately begins moving toward the central compartment from the peripheral compartments rather than away, as was the case during infusion, and elimination from the central compartment continues unabated by the infusion's input. Plasma or central compartment concentrations will fall relatively rapidly, compared to the elimination half-life, until set concentration ratios of central:fast and central:slow are achieved. These ratios with higher peripheral compartment drug concentrations will achieve the net drug distribution flux into the central compartment that will balance the elimination flux to create a constant elimination rate.

During the elimination phase, the multicompartmental system behaves, kinetically, as a single compartment, but only does so because there are (fixed) drug concentration ratios among the compartments. With a short infusion, the peripheral compartment drug concentrations will have only achieved low drug concentrations, and the plasma drug concentration will have to fall quite far to reach the central:peripheral drug concentration ratios needed to enter the constant elimination phase. Thus, the half-time is less with shorter infusion contexts. After a very long infusion with peripheral compartment drug concentrations reaching higher drug concentrations as they approach their steady state, plasma drug concentrations will not need to fall as much to reach the concentration ratios required for the elimination phase, and the rate of plasma drug decline will begin approaching the elimination half-life sooner, resulting in longer half-times.

One must be aware of the limitations of the context-sensitive half-time concept.[10,20] First, it is not a kinetic parameter; it only describes a specific simulation event. This means it cannot be extrapolated backward or, more importantly, forward to lesser or greater drug concentration decrements, as is possible with true kinetic parameters. Secondly, it cannot be directly calculated

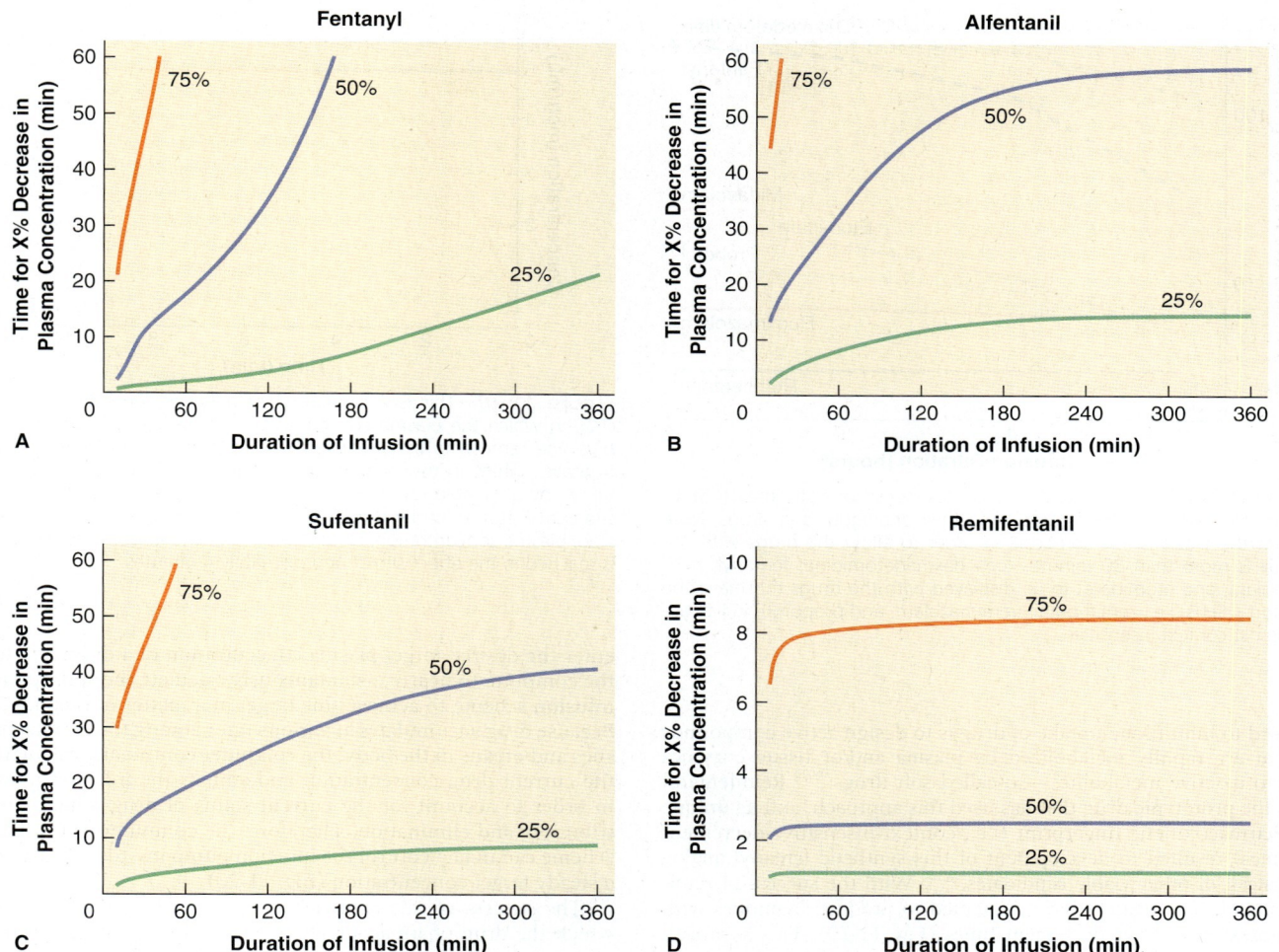

Figure 11-18 The context-sensitive 25%, 50%, and 75% plasma decrement times for fentanyl, alfentanil, sufentanil, and remifentanil.

from other kinetic parameters. Rather, a model of the specific drug pharmacokinetics is programmed into a simulation with a set drug infusion regimen; tedious for pencil and paper or handheld calculator, but a simple matter for even a modest computing device (e.g., tricyclic antidepressant [TCA] pumps and applications for smartphones). Third, the most relevant concentration decrease may not be one-half. It could be less than one-half or, as is likelier in practice, more than one-half. Therefore, simulating both the specific infusion context as well as the required percentage decrease from the target concentration should be done to get the best estimate of when a drug's effect will reach the clinically desired end point.

Although a 50% decrease in plasma concentration is an appealing and comprehensible parameter, larger or smaller decreases in plasma concentrations may be required for recovery from the drug. Simulations show that the times for different percent decreases in plasma concentration are not linear.[10,20] Therefore, if a 25% or 75% decrease in plasma concentration is required, simulations must be performed to calculate the context-sensitive 25% decrement time or context-sensitive 75% decrement time (Fig. 11-18). In addition, if the concentration of interest is the effect site concentration rather than the plasma concentration, simulations can be performed to calculate the context-sensitive effect site decrement time. Finally, if a constant plasma or effect site concentration is not maintained throughout the delivery of the drug (which is typically the case with manual bolus and infusion schemes and also with varying drug requirements depending on surgical stimulation, etc.), the context-sensitive decrement times are guidelines of recovery rather than an absolute prediction of the decay in drug concentration. If precise drug administration data are known, it is possible to compute the context-sensitive decrement time for the individual situation or context. Even though the context-sensitive decrement times are limited, this concept has changed the way that IV anesthetics are described and has helped foster an increase in accurately and safely administering IV anesthetics.

Soft Pharmacology and Anesthesiology

Accumulation of drug in well perfused but inactive tissue beds (i.e., skeletal muscle) results in tissue depots of drug. When the arterial concentration of drug is less than the tissue concentration of drug in any of these tissue depots, the drug redistributes from the tissue back into the plasma, thereby slowing the rate of decline of the plasma concentration. One strategy that has been

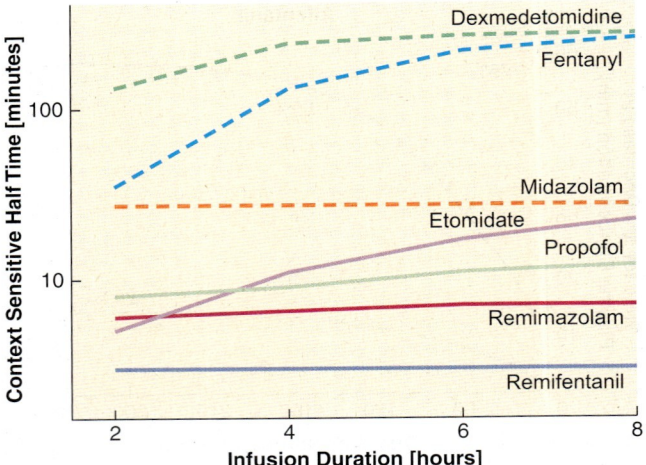

Figure 11-19 The effect site context-sensitive half-times (CSHTs) for the classic anesthetic drugs and their analogous soft drugs. Note that the y-axis is in a log scale in order to allow the drugs with the CSHTs more than 30 minutes (i.e., dexmedetomidine, fentanyl, midazolam, and etomidate) to be displayed with the drugs that have the short CSHTs (i.e., remifentanil, remimazolam, and propofol), which are almost context insensitive.

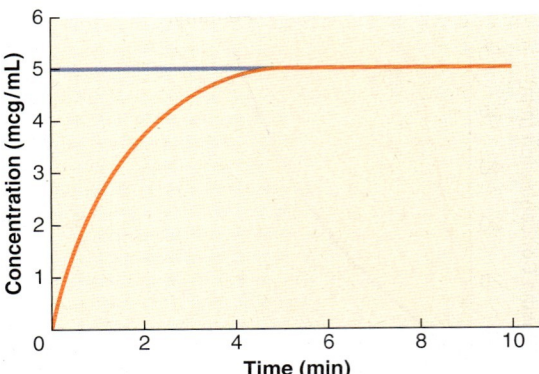

Figure 11-20 This is a simulation of a target-controlled infusion (TCI) in which the plasma concentration is targeted at 5 μg/mL. The *blue line* represents the predicted plasma propofol concentration of 5 μg/mL, which in theory is attained at time t = 0 and is then maintained by a variable rate infusion. The *red line* is the predicted effect site concentration under the conditions of a constant pseudo–steady-state plasma concentration. Note that 95% of the target concentration is reached in the effect site at approximately 4 minutes.

used to limit tissue uptake of drug is to design active compounds that are rapidly metabolized by plasma and/or tissue enzymes into inactive metabolites—so-called soft drugs.[98,99] Remifentanil is the prototypic drug that has used this approach, and its unique pharmacokinetic fingerprint (i.e., context-insensitive decrement times) resulted in development of this synthetic fentanyl analog instead of other viable candidates.[48,100] With the success of remifentanil, investigators have attempted to produce hypnotics with context-insensitive decrement times (Fig. 11-19). This approach has resulted in a new benzodiazepine, several etomidate analogues, and a novel hypnotic that inhibits $GABA_A$ receptors.[101–104] Remimazolam, a plasma and tissue esterase metabolized benzodiazepine, is currently in Phase II studies investigating its applications to procedural sedation as well as to general anesthesia.[105–107] The etomidate analogues are not yet in Phase I studies. However, the preclinical data have resulted in selection of an etomidate analog that has context insensitive decrement times as well as limited adrenal suppression.[108–114] Further studies will determine if the etomidate analogues have a safer profile in the setting of cerebral ischemia than does etomidate.[115–117] Phase I studies of AZD-3043 have shown rapid onset, rapidly titratable hypnosis with a context-insensitive recovery profile.[104,118–120]

Target-controlled Infusions

Prior to performing an anesthetic, it is possible to perform the calculations above and derive a BET scheme targeted to a pre-determined plasma or effect site concentration. However, in the operating room, once the anesthetic has commenced, without the help of a computer, software, and possibly an assistant, it is laborious and difficult to make any calculations to determine how to adjust the infusion or how to bolus (or stop the infusion) to increase or decrease the target plasma concentration.[121] By linking a computer with the appropriate pharmacokinetic model to an infusion pump, it is possible for the physician to enter the desired target plasma concentration of a drug, and for the computer to nearly instantaneously calculate the appropriate infusion scheme to achieve this target in a matter of seconds.[122] Because drug accumulates at various rates among the various tissues and organs in the body, the computer continually calculates the current drug concentration and adjusts the infusion pump in order to account for the current status of drug uptake, distribution, and elimination. Therefore, the computer driven BET scheme can in fact control the infusion pump in order to achieve a steady target concentration (Fig. 11-20).

The success of this approach is influenced by the extent to which the drug pharmacokinetic and pharmacodynamic parameters programmed into the computer match those of the particular patient at hand. While this same limitation applies to the more rudimentary (non-TCI) dosing done routinely in every clinical setting, we must examine the special ramifications of pharmacokinetic–pharmacodynamic model misspecification with TCI in any discussion of its future importance in the clinical setting.

The mathematical principles governing TCI are actually quite simple. For a computer-control pump to produce and maintain a plasma drug concentration it must first administer a dose equal to the product of the central compartment, V_1, and the target concentration (Fig. 11-21). Then for each moment after that, the amount of drug to be administered into the central compartment to maintain the target concentration is equal to drug eliminated from the central compartment *plus* drug distributed from the central compartment to peripheral compartments *minus* drug returning to the central compartment from peripheral compartments. The software keeps track of the estimated drug in each compartment over time and applies the rate constants for intercompartmental drug transfer from the pharmacokinetic model to these amounts to determine drug movement at any given time. It then matches the estimated concentrations to the target concentration at any time to determine the amount of drug that should be infused. The software can also predict future concentrations, usually with the assumption that the infusion will be stopped so that emergence from anesthesia or the dissipation of drug effect will occur optimally according to the context-sensitive decrement time.

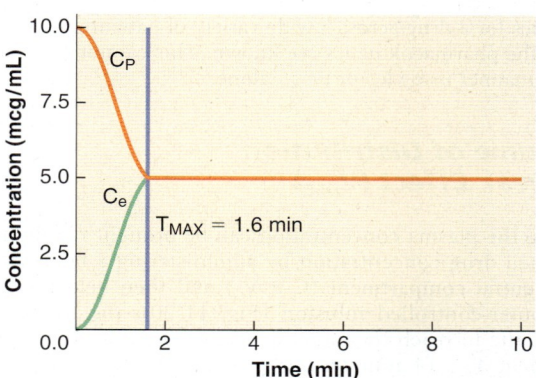

Figure 11-21 This is a simulation of a target-controlled infusion (TCI) in which the effect site concentration (C_e) is targeted at 5 µg/mL. The *orange line* represents the predicted plasma propofol concentration (C_p) that results from a bolus dose, given at time t = 0, that is predicted to purposely overshoot the plasma propofol concentration target until time t = T_{max} (1.6 minutes). At T_{max} pseudo-equilibration between the effect site and the plasma occurs and both concentrations are then predicted to be the same until the target is changed. Note that the effect site attains the target in less than half the time with effect site targeting compared to the plasma concentration targeting seen in Figure 11-20.

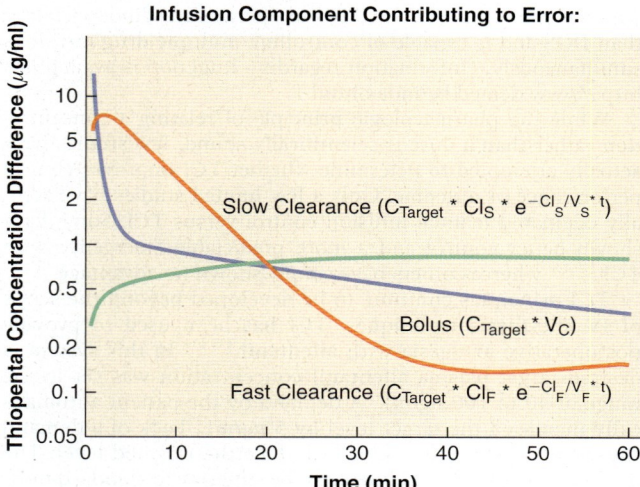

Figure 11-22 The influence of the misspecification of each of the components of the traditional three compartment pharmacokinetic models on the prolonged discrepancy (overshoot) between predicted and targeted concentrations with target-controlled infusions. The error resulting from elimination clearance was negligible and therefore not illustrated. Notice that the loading dose (based on V_c) produces a large amount of error in the initial minutes; however, from 1 to 20 minutes, the deviation from the target concentration is largely due to the overestimation of Cl_F. The equations listed are for the respective BET infusions of the TCI system. (Reprinted with permission from Avram MJ, Krejcie TC. Using front-end kinetics to optimize target-controlled drug infusions. *Anesthesiology*. 2003; 99:1078–1086.)

Because there is a delay or hysteresis between the attainment of a drug concentration in the plasma and the production of a drug effect, it is advantageous to have the mathematics of this delay incorporated into TCI. By adding the kinetics of the effect site it is possible to target effect site concentrations as would be in keeping with the principle of working as closely to the relevant concentration–effect relationship as possible. A dose scheme that targets concentrations in a compartment remote from the central compartment (i.e., the effect site) has no closed form solution for calculating the infusion rate(s) needed. Instead, the solution is solved numerically and involves some additional concepts that must be considered, namely the time to peak effect, T_{max}, and the volume of distribution at peak effect, V_{DPE}. These are discussed later. In principle, targeting the effect site necessitates producing an overshoot in plasma drug concentrations during induction and for subsequent target increases. This is similar in concept to overpressurizing inhaled anesthetic concentrations to achieve a targeted end-tidal concentration. However, unlike the inspiratory limb of an anesthesia circuit, the plasma compartment seems to be closely linked to cardiovascular effects, and large overshoots in plasma drug concentration may produce unwanted side effects.

The performance of TCI is influenced by the pharmacokinetic model chosen. Although most modern TCI models, whether they target the plasma or the effect site, seem to be similar in performance, they all produce overshoot for 10–20 minutes when increasing the target concentration.[36] This is because the dose adjustments made are based on calculations that utilize a central compartment that ignores the complexity of intravascular mixing, thereby overestimating the central compartment's true volume (V_C) and overestimating the rate of transfer to the fast peripheral tissue (Cl_F) and the size of the peripheral tissue compartment (V_F) (Fig. 11-22). The performance of TCI is also influenced by the variance between pharmacokinetic parameters determined from group or population studies and the individual patient. Median absolute performance errors for fentanyl,[123] alfentanil,[124] sufentanil,[125] midazolam,[126,127] and propofol[127,128] are in the range of ±30% when literature values for pharmacokinetic parameters are used to drive the TCI device and fall to approximately ±7% when the average kinetics of the test subjects themselves are used.[124] Divergence (the percentage change of the absolute performance error) is generally quite low (approximately 1%) when target concentrations remain relatively stable, but increase to nearly 20% when the frequency of concentration steps is as frequent as every 12 minutes.[36,128] These data suggest that while a considerable error may exist (±30%) between the targeted drug concentration and the one actually achieved in a patient, the concentration attained will not vary much over time. Thus, incremental adjustments in the target should result in incremental and stable new concentrations in the patient as long as the incremental adjustments are not too frequent.

The introduction of the concept of TCI, was first described by Schwilden et al. in early 1980s. Other software systems were developed in North America by groups at Stanford University and Duke University. By the late 1990s a commercially available TCI system for propofol (Diprifusor) was introduced. This greatly increased both anesthesiologists' interest in this mode of delivery and their understanding of the concentration–effect relationships for hypnotics and opioids. In most of the world, devices for delivering propofol by TCI are commercially available from at least three companies (Graseby, Alaris, and Fresenius) with similar performance parameters.[129] In the United States, there are still no FDA-approved devices. For investigational purposes, Stanpump (developed by Steve Shafer at Stanford University) can be interfaced via an RS232 port to an infusion pump. Stanpump currently provides pharmacokinetic parameters for 19 different drugs, but has the ability to accept any kinetic model for any drug provided by the user. RugLoop is TCI software (developed by Michel Struys of Ghent University), which is similar to STANPUMP but operates in Windows rather than DOS and is capable of controlling multiple drug infusions simultaneously. (Information regarding RugLoop is available at http://www.demed.be/index.html.)

While the pharmacologic principle of relating a concentration rather than a dose is scientifically sound, few studies have actually attempted to determine whether TCI improves clinical performance or outcome. Only a few limited studies have actually compared manual infusion control versus TCI. Some have shown better control and a more predictable emergence with TCI,[129,130] whereas others have simply shown no advantage.[131,132]

TCI principles continue to be developed beyond the scope of IV anesthesia techniques. TCI has been used to provide postoperative analgesia with alfentanil.[133,134] In this system, a desired target plasma alfentanil concentration was set in the range of 40 to 100 ng/mL. A demand by the patient automatically increased the target level by 5 ng/mL. Lack of a demand caused the system to gradually reduce the targeted level. The quality of analgesia was judged to be superior to standard morphine PCA.

Similarly, TCI has been used to provide patient-controlled sedation with propofol.[135,136] The TCI was set to 1 µg/mL and a demand by the patient increased the level by 0.2 µg/mL. As with the TCI analgesia system, the lack of a demand caused the system to gradually reduce the targeted plasma propofol concentration. The timing and increment of the decrease were adjusted by the clinician. Over 90% of patients were satisfied with this method of sedation.

Time to Maximum Effect Compartment Concentration (T_{max})

Earlier in this chapter, the delay between attaining a plasma concentration and an effect site concentration was described (Fig. 11-11). This delay, or hysteresis, is presumed to be a result of transfer of drug between the plasma compartment, V_C, and an effect compartment, V_e, as well as the time required for a cellular response. By simultaneously modeling the plasma drug concentration versus time data (pharmacokinetics) and the measured drug effect (pharmacodynamics), an estimate of the drug transfer rate constant, k_{e0}, between plasma and the putative effect site can be estimated.[47] However, estimates of k_{e0}, like all rate constants, are model specific.[137,138] That is, k_{e0} cannot be transported from one set of kinetic parameters determined in one specific pharmacokinetic–pharmacodynamic study to any other set of pharmacokinetic parameters. Likewise, it is not valid to compare estimates of k_{e0} among studies of the same drug or across different drugs and, therefore, one should not be surprised that reported values for k_{e0} for the same drug vary markedly among studies. The model-independent parameter that characterizes the delay between the plasma and effect site is the time to maximal effect, or T_{max}.[138] Accordingly, if the T_{max} and the pharmacokinetics for a drug are known from independent studies, a k_{e0} can be estimated by numeric techniques for the independent kinetic set that would produce the known effect site T_{max}.

The concept of a transportable, model-independent parameter that characterizes the kinetics of the effect site is important for robust effect site–targeted, computer-controlled infusions. This is because there are many more pharmacokinetic studies characterizing a wider variety of patient types and groups in the literature than there are complete pharmacokinetic–pharmacodynamic studies. By making the generally valid assumption that interindividual differences are small in a drug's rate of effect site equilibration, it is possible with a known T_{max} to estimate effect site kinetics for a drug across a wide variety of patient groups where only the pharmacokinetics are known. This cannot be done in a valid manner using k_{E0} or $t\frac{1}{2}\ _{Ke0}$ alone.[137,138]

Volume of Distribution at Peak Effect (V_{DPE})

While the plasma concentration can be brought rapidly to the targeted drug concentration by administering a bolus dose to the central compartment ($C \times V_C$) and then held there by a computer-controlled infusion (Fig. 11-20), the time for the effect site to reach the target concentration will be much longer than T_{max} (4 minutes for propofol effect site concentration to reach 95% of that targeted). It is possible to calculate a bolus dose that will attain the estimated effect site concentration at T_{max} without overshoot in the effect site. However, plasma drug concentration will be overshot (Fig. 11-19). This is done by combining the concept of describing drug distribution as an expanding volume of distribution that starts at V_C and approaches V_β (the apparent volume of distribution during the elimination phase) over time with the concept of T_{max}.[139,140]

Volume of distribution over time is calculated by dividing the total amount of drug remaining in the body by the plasma drug concentration at each time, t. The time-dependent volume at the time of peak effect (or T_{max}) is V_{DPE}. The product of the targeted effect site concentration and V_{DPE} plus the amount lost to elimination in the time to T_{max} becomes the proper bolus dose that will attain the target concentration at the effect site as rapidly as possible without overshoot. In practical terms this bolus is given at time $t = 0$, after which the infusion stops until time $t = T_{max}$. It then resumes infusing drug in its normal "stop loss" manner.

Some software programs for controlling TCIs include this concept in their algorithms. In the case of the propofol kinetics used to construct the isoconcentration nomogram in Figure 11-15, the pharmacokinetic–pharmacodynamic parameter set of Schnider et al.[141] predicts a T_{max} of 1.6 minutes, a V_{DPE} of 16.62 L, and an elimination loss of 23.8% of the dose over 1.6 minutes in a 70-kg man. Thus the proper propofol bolus for a targeted effect site propofol concentration of 5 µg/mL is 109 mg. The computer-controlled infusion pump will deliver this dose as rapidly as possible and then begin a targeted infusion for 5 µg/mL at $t = 1.6$ minutes (Fig. 11-21).

Front-end Pharmacokinetics

Classic PK-PD models make the simplifying assumptions that there is instantaneous and complete mixing of drug in the intravascular space—a mathematical construct without regard for the physiology that drives drug disposition.[142-144] Therefore, the classic PK models inaccurately describe the initial/central distribution volume (V_C), as a result of which they misestimate intercompartmental clearances and are unable to characterize cardiac output and its distribution.[36,39,71,142,144-147] Misspecification of V_C also results in misspecification of the effect site kinetics and compensates by overestimating interindividual PD variability.[36,144,147] Physiologically based PK-PD models that can accurately estimate distribution volumes and clearances result in more realistic estimates of PD variability (Fig. 11-23).[147] Another source of PK and PD variability is cardiac output and its distribution.[71,144,145,147,148] Cardiac output and its distribution influences PK by modifying the distribution of drug to tissue compartments. In addition, cardiac output influences PD by changing the blood-effect site equilibration rate (Fig. 11-24).[147] Because they cannot characterize

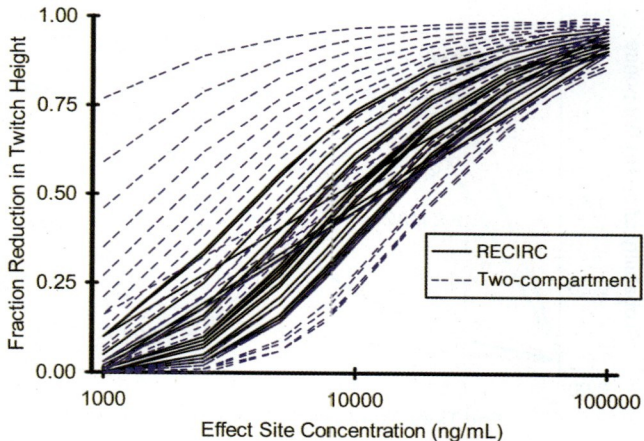

Figure 11-23 The misestimation of the central distribution volume (Vc) by a traditional compartmental PK-PD model results in more interindividual variability in pharmacodynamic estimates than pharmacodynamic estimates from a high-resolution, recirculatory PK-PD model. This figure uses Monte-Carlo simulation of the effect site concentration–pharmacologic effect relationships to demonstrate the interindividual variability from a traditional compartmental PK-PD model (2 COMP, blue dashed lines) and a high-resolution recirculatory PK-PD model (RECIRC, black solid lines). (Adapted from the rocuronium data of Kuipers JA, Boer F, Olofsen E, et al. Recirculatory pharmacokinetics and pharmacodynamics of rocuronium in patients: the influence of cardiac output. Anesthesiology. 2001;94:47–55.)

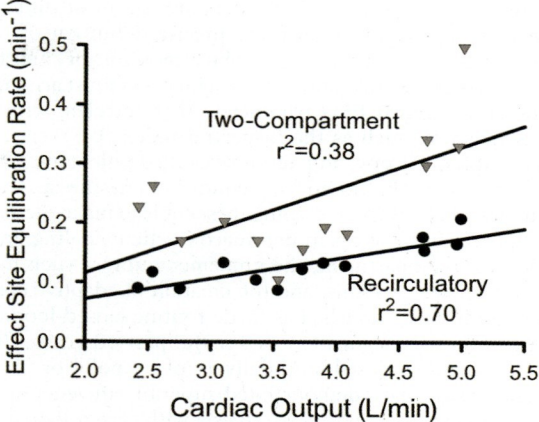

Figure 11-24 The effects of cardiac output on the blood–effect site equilibration rate (k_{e0}) when the PK-PD model is a high-resolution "recirculatory" model (black circles) versus a traditional compartmental model (triangles). While the traditional model has a moderate correlation between measured cardiac output and k_{e0} and significant systematic error (grey line), the high-resolution recirculatory model has a very strong correlation between measured cardiac output and k_{e0} (black line). Therefore, for lipophilic drugs with flow limited tissue-distribution (i.e., opioids, hypnotics, etc.), a high-resolution PK-PD model provides a physiologic basis for transfer of drug from the blood to the effect site. In addition, these high-resolution PK-PD models can quantitate the effects of physiologic perturbations on the PK and PD of these drugs more accurately than the traditional compartmental models. (Adapted from the rocuronium data of Kuipers JA, Boer F, Olofsen E, et al. Recirculatory pharmacokinetics and pharmacodynamics of rocuronium in patients: the influence of cardiac output. Anesthesiology. 2001;94:47–55.)

cardiac output and its distribution, classic PK-PD models will be unable to identify the changes in cardiac output and its distribution that are the result of alterations in physiology related to sex, age, body composition, or pathologic processes.[149,150] Therefore, classic PK-PD models will not identify factors that solely alter cardiac output and its distribution as a source of PK variability and will overestimate the true PD.[36,147,151,152]

The term *front-end pharmacokinetics* refers to the intravascular mixing, pulmonary uptake, and recirculation events that occur in the first few minutes during and after IV drug administration.[39] These kinetic events and the drug concentration versus time profile that results are important because the peak effect of rapidly acting drugs occurs during this temporal window.[38,147,153,154] Although it has been suggested that front-end pharmacokinetics be used to guide drug dosing,[36] current TCI does not incorporate front-end kinetics into the models from which drug infusion rates are calculated. As described above, not doing so introduces further error.

TCI relies on pharmacokinetic models that are based on the simplifying assumption of instantaneous and complete mixing within V_C. However, the determination of V_C is routinely overestimated in most pharmacokinetic studies. Overestimation of V_C, when used to calculate TCI infusion rates, results in plasma drug concentrations that overshoot the desired target concentration, especially in the first few minutes after beginning TCI. Furthermore, correct description of drug distribution to tissues is dependent on an accurate V_C estimate, so inaccuracies caused by not taking front-end pharmacokinetics into account may be persistent and result in undershoot as well as overshoot. Simulation indicates that pharmacokinetic parameters derived from studies in which the drug is administered by a short (approximately 2 minutes) infusion better estimate V_C and tissue-distribution kinetics than those from a rapid IV bolus infusion.[36,37] When the latter drug administration method is used, full characterization of the front-end recirculatory pharmacokinetics is required to obtain valid estimates of V for use in TCI.[36,37]

Closed-loop Infusions

When a valid, and nearly continuous, measure of drug effect is available, drug delivery can be automatically titrated by feedback control. Such systems have been used experimentally for control of blood pressure,[155] oxygen delivery,[156] blood glucose,[157] neuromuscular blockade,[158] and depth of anesthesia.[159–165] A target value for the desired effect measure (the output of the system) is selected and the rate of drug delivery (the input into the system) is dependent on whether the effect measure is above, below, or at the target value. Thus the output feeds back and controls the input. Standard controllers (referred to as *proportional-integral-derivative* [*PID*] *controllers*) adjust drug delivery based on both the integral, or magnitude, of the deviation from target and the rate of deviation, or the derivative.

Under a range of responses, standard PID controllers work quite well. However, they have been shown to develop unstable characteristics in situations where the output may vary rapidly and widely. Schwilden et al.[161] proposed a controller in which the output (measured response) controls not only the input (drug infusion rate), but also the pharmacokinetic model driving the infusion rate. This is known as a *model-driven* or *adaptive* closed-loop system. Such a system has performed well in clinical trials,[160] and in a simulation of extreme conditions it was demonstrated to outperform a standard PID controller.[163]

Closed-loop systems for anesthesia are the most difficult to design and implement because the precise definition of "anesthesia" remains elusive, as does a robust monitor for "anesthetic depth."[88] Because modification of consciousness must accompany anesthesia, processed EEG parameters that correlate with level of consciousness, such as the Bispectral Index (BIS), electroencephalographic entropy, and auditory evoked potentials, make it possible to undertake closed-loop control of anesthesia. There is keen interest in further developing these tools to make them more reliable, because advances in pharmacokinetic modeling, including the effect compartment, the implementation of such models into drug delivery systems, and the creation of adaptive controllers based on these models, has made routine closed-loop delivery of anesthesia imaginable.[159] Over the past 10 years, clinical trials investigating closed-loop delivery of propofol or propofol and remifentanil have demonstrated superior efficiency in drug delivery and emergence from anesthesia with closed-loop devices compared to manual titration by experienced anesthesia providers.[167-172] So far it has been difficult to bring a true closed-loop system to market in medical applications, because of the regulatory agency hurdles. From a regulatory point of view, an open-loop TCI system is much easier to attain and offers many of the benefits of actual closed-loop systems. Unless there is a regulatory or a design "breakthrough," closed-loop systems for anesthesia will likely remain in the theoretical and experimental realms.[173,174]

Response Surface Models of Drug–Drug Interactions

During the course of an operation, the level of anesthetic drug administered is adjusted to ensure amnesia to ongoing events, provide immobility to noxious stimulation, and blunt the sympathetic response to noxious stimulation. Although it is possible to achieve an adequate anesthetic state with a high dose of a sedative-hypnotic alone (i.e., a volatile anesthetic or propofol), the effect site drug concentration necessary is often associated with excessive hemodynamic depression[80] and excessively deep plane of hypnosis that may be associated with longstanding morbidity or mortality.[175,176] Therefore, to limit side-effects, an opioid and a sedative-hypnotic are administered together. Although the administration of two volatile anesthetics or a volatile anesthetic and propofol produce a net-additive effect, the combination of an opioid and a sedative-hypnotic are synergistic for most pharmacologic effects. By understanding the interactions between the opioids and the sedative-hypnotics, it is possible to select target concentration pairs of the two drugs that produce the desired clinical effect while minimizing unwanted side-effects associated with high concentrations of a single drug (e.g., hemodynamic instability, prolonged respiratory depression).

Studies designed to evaluate the pharmacodynamic interactions between an opioid and a sedative-hypnotic have traditionally focused on the effects of adding one or two fixed doses or concentrations of the opioid to several defined concentrations or doses of the sedative-hypnotic.[79,80,177-184] Graphic demonstrations of these interaction data are most commonly performed by demonstrating a shift of parallel dose–response curves (Fig. 11-25). An alternative mathematical model is the isobologram—iso-effect curves that show dose combinations that result in equal effect (Fig. 11-26). Isobolographic analysis has the additional benefit of characterizing the interaction between the two drugs as additive, antagonistic, or synergistic (Fig. 11-27), whereas shifts of dose–response curves require more complex concentrations to determine if the interaction demonstrated by a leftward shift in the curve is more than additive.

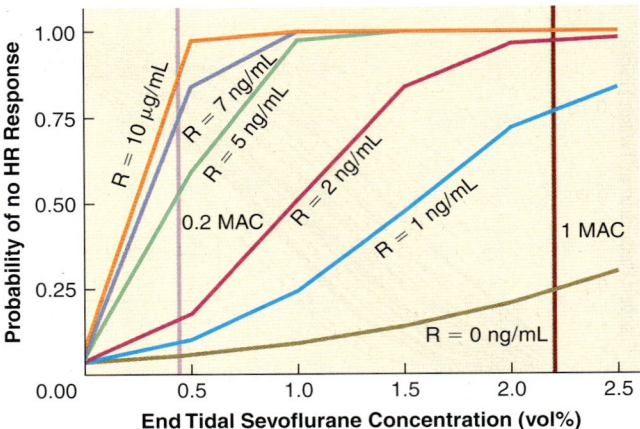

Figure 11-25 The effect of adding remifentanil on the concentration–effect curve for sevoflurane induced analgesia (no hemodynamic response to a 5 second, 50 mA tetanic stimulation in volunteers). Each curve represents the concentration–effect relation for sevoflurane with a fixed effect site concentration of remifentanil. The leftward shift in the curves indicates that remifentanil decreases the amount of sevoflurane needed to produce adequate analgesia. The changes in the slopes of the concentration–response curves indicate that there is significant pharmacodynamic synergy between sevoflurane–remifentanil. Also note that there is a ceiling effect to this pharmacodynamic interaction—the magnitude of the leftward shift decreases as the remifentanil concentration increases. (Adapted from Manyam SC, Gupta DK, Johnson KB, et al. Opioid-volatile anesthetic synergy: a response surface model with remifentanil and sevoflurane as prototypes. *Anesthesiology*. 2006;105:267–278.)

An alternative mathematical model that can fully characterize the complete spectrum of interaction between two drugs for all possible concentrations and effects is the response surface model.[84,87] The surface morphology of a response surface not only demonstrates whether the interaction is additive, synergistic, or antagonistic, but the model itself can quantitatively

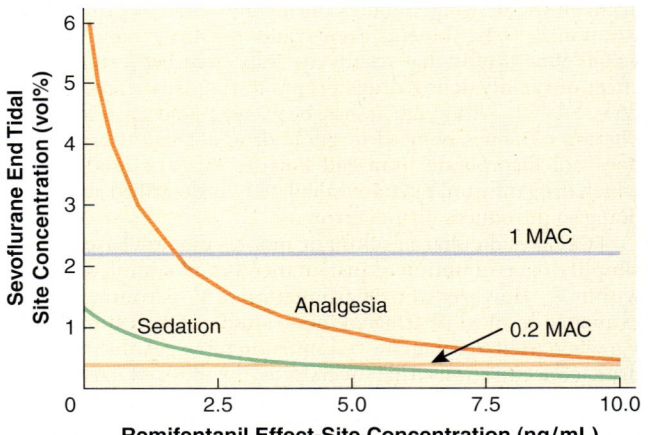

Figure 11-26 Remifentanil–sevoflurane interaction for sedation (*green line*) and analgesia to electrical tetanic stimulation (*red line*) for volunteers. The respective 95% isoboles demonstrate the myriad target concentration pairs of remifentanil and sevoflurane that have a 95% probability of producing the desired pharmacodynamic end point. (Adapted from Manyam SC, Gupta DK, Johnson KB, et al. Opioid-volatile anesthetic synergy: a response surface model with remifentanil and sevoflurane as prototypes. *Anesthesiology*. 2006;105:267–278.)

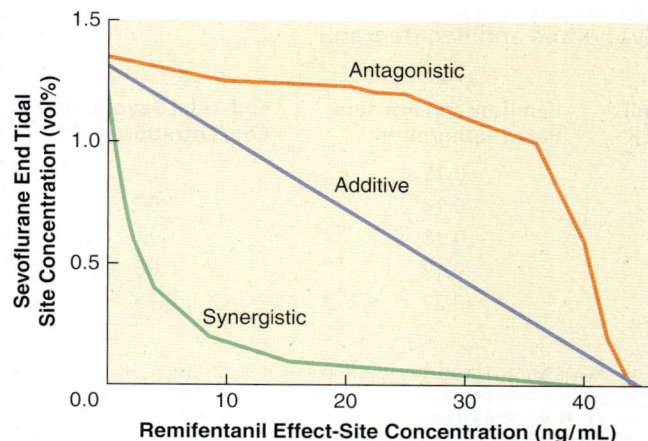

Figure 11-27 Isoboles to demonstrate additive (*blue line*), synergistic (*green line*), and antagonistic (*red line*) interactions between Drug A and Drug B.

describe the degree of interaction between the two drugs. Furthermore, isobolograms can be derived from the projection of the response surface onto the appropriate horizontal effect plane (Fig. 11-28), and concentration–response curves can be derived from taking a vertical slice through a response surface in the plane perpendicular to the fixed-opioid concentration of interest (Fig. 11-28).[84,87,88] Therefore, response surface models can be viewed as generalizations of the traditional pharmacodynamic methods of analysis. The major limitation of response surface models is that they require a large number of pharmacodynamic measurements across all possible concentration pairing to accurately characterize the entire surface.[185] This is most efficiently done in the laboratory setting utilizing volunteers who can be exposed to subtherapeutic (e.g., below the level that guarantees amnesia) and supratherapeutic drug concentration pairs. However, because response surface models characterize the drug concentration pairs that provide adequate anesthesia and also adequate recovery from anesthesia, these models provide information that are not normally available from studies that generate an isobologram from surgical patients.

Isobolograms and response surface models clearly demonstrate that there are multiple target concentration pairs of an opioid and a sedative-hypnotic that can provide adequate anesthesia—a 95% probability of no hemodynamic response to a noxious stimulus and 95% probability of clinically adequate sedation.[85,86,89] Combining the response surface pharmacodynamic models with pharmacokinetic models allows computer simulations to be performed to identify the target concentration pair of the opioid and the sedative-hypnotic that produces an adequate anesthetic and yet optimizes one or more pharmacodynamic end points, such as the speed of awakening from anesthesia, drug-induced respiratory depression, or drug acquisition costs.[82,86] For sevoflurane–remifentanil anesthetics, these types of pharmacokinetic–pharmacodynamic simulations demonstrate the benefit of minimizing the administered dose of even the low solubility volatile anesthetic sevoflurane to near 0.5 MAC to take advantage of the pharmacokinetic efficiency of remifentanil, especially as the duration of anesthesia increases (Fig. 11-29 and Table 11-8).[86] These response surface models can accurately predict loss of responsiveness and loss of response to painful stimuli as well as emergence from anesthesia and the time at which a patient will require analgesia in the recovery room.[186–189] In addition, these pharmacodynamic targets can be incorporated into closed-loop controllers to deliver closed-loop anesthesia.[172]

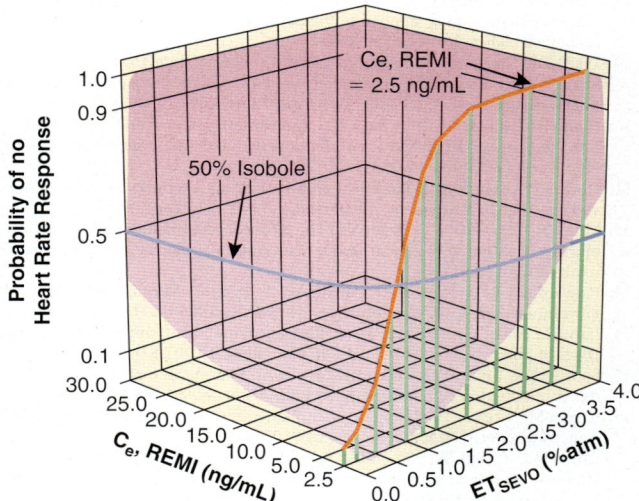

Figure 11-28 A response surface model characterizing the remifentanil–sevoflurane interaction for analgesia to electrical tetanic stimulation. The projection of the response surface onto the 50% probability horizontal plane results in the 50% effect isobole while the projection of the response surface onto the 2.5 ng/mL remifentanil effect site concentration vertical plane results in the sevoflurane concentration–response curve under 2.5 ng/mL of remifentanil. (Adapted from Manyam SC, Gupta DK, Johnson KB, et al. Opioid-volatile anesthetic synergy: a response surface model with remifentanil and sevoflurane as prototypes. *Anesthesiology*. 2006;105:267–278.)

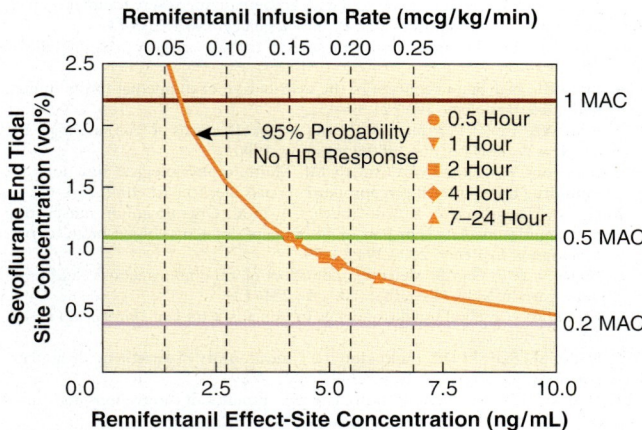

Figure 11-29 The optimal target concentration pairs of remifentanil and sevoflurane to maintain adequate analgesia (95% isobole for analgesia to electrical tetanic stimulation) and result in the most rapid emergence for anesthetics of various durations. For example, for a 2-hour anesthetic, target concentrations of 0.93 vol% sevoflurane, and 4.9 ng/mL remifentanil would result in a 5.8-minute time to awakening. As the duration of anesthesia increases, a minimum sevoflurane target concentration of 0.75 vol% is reached. (Adapted from Manyam SC, Gupta DK, Johnson KB, et al. Opioid-volatile anesthetic synergy: a response surface model with remifentanil and sevoflurane as prototypes. *Anesthesiology*. 2006;105:267–278.)

Table 11-8 The Optimal Target Concentration Pairs of Sevoflurane and Remifentanil for Anesthetics 30 to 900 Minutes in Duration

Duration of Anesthetic (h)	Shortest Recovery Time (min)	Effect Site Remifentanil Concentration (ng/mL)	Remifentanil Infusion Rate (µg/kg/min)	End-Tidal Sevoflurane Concentration (vol%)
0.5	4.5	4.1	0.15	1.1
1	5.0	4.3	0.16	1.05
2	5.8	4.9	0.18	093
4	6.7	5.2	0.19	0.88
7–24	7.2–7.7	6.1	0.22	0.75

Conclusion

Since World War II, we have moved from characterizing all anesthetics by a dose–response relationship to developing sophisticated models to characterize the synergistic interaction between sedative-hypnotics and opioids and having the physical devices and the computer support to accurately administer drugs to achieve the desired concentrations at the effect site of drug action. The rational selection of drug target concentrations required to achieve adequate anesthesia and minimize side effects (e.g., prolonged awakening, hemodynamic depression) and the methods by which to efficiently achieve those concentration targets with minimal overshoot requires a solid understanding of the clinical pharmacology of anesthetics. As new drugs enter the anesthetic armamentarium, careful characterization of their pharmacokinetic and pharmacodynamic properties will allow them to be safely and appropriately utilized as part of a balanced anesthetic.[88]

REFERENCES

1. Halford FJ. A critique of intravenous anesthesia in war surgery. *Anesthesiology*. 1943;4:67–96.
2. Adams RC, Gray HK. Intravenous anesthesia with pentothal sodium in the case of gunshot wound associated with accompanying severe traumatic shock and loss of blood: report of a case. *Anesthesiology*. 1943;4:70–73.
3. The question of intravenous anesthesia in war surgery. *Anesthesiology*. 1943;4:74–77.
4. Price HL. A dynamic concept of the distribution of thiopental in the human body. *Anesthesiology*. 1960;21:40–45.
5. Pratt WB, Taylor P. *Principles of Drug Action: The Basis of Pharmacology*. 3rd ed. New York, NY: Churchill Livingstone; 1990.
6. Johnstone RW, Ruefli AA, Smyth MJ. Multiple physiological functions for multidrug transporter P-glycoprotein?. *Trends Biochem Sci*. 2000;25:1–6.
7. Gao B, Hagenbuch B, Kullak-Ublick GA, et al. Organic anion-transporting polypeptides mediate transport of opioid peptides across blood-brain barrier. *J Pharmacol Exp Ther*. 2000;294:73–79.
8. Hagenbuch B, Gao B, Meier PJ. Transport of xenobiotics across the blood-brain barrier. *News Physiol Sci*. 2002;17:231–234.
9. Upton RN. Cerebral uptake of drugs in humans. *Clin Exp Pharmacol Physiol*. 2007;34:695–701.
10. Shafer SL, Stanski DR. Improving the clinical utility of anesthetic drug pharmacokinetics. *Anesthesiology*. 1992;76:327–330.
11. Stanski DR, Greenblatt DJ, Lowenstein E. Kinetics of intravenous and intramuscular morphine. *Clin Pharmacol Ther*. 1978;24:52–59.
12. Kuipers JA, Boer F, Olieman W, et al. First-pass lung uptake and pulmonary clearance of propofol: assessment with a recirculatory indocyanine green pharmacokinetic model. *Anesthesiology*. 1999;91:1780–1787.
13. Ding X, Kaminsky LS. Human extrahepatic cytochromes P450: function in xenobiotic metabolism and tissue-selective chemical toxicity in the respiratory and gastrointestinal tracts. *Annu Rev Pharmacol Toxicol*. 2003;43:149–173.
14. Stanley TH, Hague B, Mock DL, et al. Oral transmucosal fentanyl citrate (lollipop) premedication in human volunteers. *Anesth Analg*. 1989;69:21–27.
15. Ashburn MA, Streisand J, Zhang J, et al. The iontophoresis of fentanyl citrate in humans. *Anesthesiology*. 1995;82:1146–1153.
16. Eger EI 2nd, Severinghaus JW. Effect of uneven pulmonary distribution of blood and gas on induction with inhalation anesthetics. *Anesthesiology*. 1964;25:620–626.
17. Avram MJ, Henthorn TK, Spyker DA, et al. Recirculatory pharmacokinetic model of the uptake, distribution, and bioavailability of prochlorperazine administered as a thermally generated aerosol in a single breath to dogs. *Drug Metab Dispos*. 2007;35:262–267.
18. Price HL, Kovnat PJ, Safer JN, et al. The uptake of thiopental by body tissues and its relationship to the duration of narcosis. *Clin Pharmacol Ther*. 1960;1:16.
19. Saidman LJ, Eger EI II. The effect of thiopental metabolism on duration of anesthesia. *Anesthesiology*. 1966;27:118–126.
20. Shafer SL, Varvel JR. Pharmacokinetics, pharmacodynamics, and rational opioid selection. *Anesthesiology*. 1991;74:53–63.
21. Wilkinson GR. Clearance approaches in pharmacology. *Pharmacol Rev*. 1987;39:1–47.
22. Ahmad AB, Bennett PN, Rowland M. Models of hepatic drug clearance: discrimination between the 'well stirred' and 'parallel-tube' models. *J Pharm Pharmacol*. 1983;35:219–224.
23. Wilkinson GR, Shand DG. Commentary: a physiological approach to hepatic drug clearance. *Clin Pharmacol Ther*. 1975;18:377–390.
24. Weiss M, Krejcie TC, Avram MJ. Transit time dispersion in pulmonary and systemic circulation: effects of cardiac output and solute diffusivity. *Am J Physiol Heart Circ Physiol*. 2006;291:H861–H870.
25. Nies AS, Shand DG, Wilkinson GR. Altered hepatic blood flow and drug disposition. *Clin Pharmacokinet*. 1976;1:1351–1355.
26. Wilkinson GR. Pharmacokinetics of drug disposition: hemodynamic considerations. *Annu Rev Pharmacol*. 1975;15:11–27.
27. Rane A, Villeneuve JP, Stone WJ, et al. Plasma binding and disposition of furosemide in the nephrotic syndrome and in uremia. *Clin Pharmacol Ther*. 1978;24:199–207.
28. Ebling WF, Wada DR, Stanski DR. From piecewise to full physiologic pharmacokinetic modeling: applied to thiopental disposition in the rat. *J Pharmacokinet Biopharm*. 1994;22:259–292.
29. Wada DR, Bjorkman S, Ebling WF, et al. Computer simulation of the effects of alterations in blood flows and body composition on thiopental pharmacokinetics in humans. *Anesthesiology*. 1997;87:884–899.
30. Henthorn TK, Avram MJ, Krejcie TC. Intravascular mixing and drug distribution: the concurrent disposition of thiopental and indocyanine green. *Clin Pharmacol Ther*. 1989;45:56–65.
31. Homer TD, Stanski DR. The effect of increasing age on thiopental disposition and anesthetic requirement. *Anesthesiology*. 1985;62:714–724.
32. Miller RD, Stevens WC, Way WL. The effect of renal failure and hyperkalemia on the duration of pancuronium neuromuscular blockade in man. *Anesth Analg*. 1973;52:661–666.
33. Patwardhan RV, Johnson RF, Hoyumpa A Jr, et al. Normal metabolism of morphine in cirrhosis. *Gastroenterology*. 1981;81:1006–1011.
34. Lund L, Alvan G, Berlin A, et al. Pharmacokinetics of single and multiple doses of phenytoin in man. *Eur J Clin Pharmacol*. 1974;7:81–86.
35. Stanski DR, Mihm FG, Rosenthal MH, et al. Pharmacokinetics of high-dose thiopental used in cerebral resuscitation. *Anesthesiology*. 1980;53:169–171.
36. Avram MJ, Krejcie TC. Using front-end kinetics to optimize target-controlled drug infusions. *Anesthesiology*. 2003;99:1078–1086.
37. Chiou WL, Peng GW, Nation RL. Rapid estimation of volume of distribution after a short intravenous infusion and its application to dosing adjustments. *J Clin Pharmacol*. 1978;18:266–271.
38. Fisher DM. (Almost) everything you learned about pharmacokinetics was (somewhat) wrong! *Anesth Analg*. 1996;83:901–903.
39. Krejcie TC, Avram MJ. What determines anesthetic induction dose? It's the front-end kinetics, doctor! *Anesth Analg*. 1999;89:541–544.
40. Weiss M, Krejcie TC, Avram MJ. A minimal physiological model of thiopental distribution kinetics based on a multiple indicator approach. *Drug Metab Dispos*. 2007;35:1525–1532.
41. Hull CJ. How far can we go with compartmental models? *Anesthesiology*. 1990;72:399–402.
42. Kong AN, Jusko WJ. Definitions and applications of mean transit and residence times in reference to the two-compartment mammillary plasma clearance model. *J Pharm Sci*. 1988;77:157–165.

43. Jacobs JR, Shafer SL, Larsen JL, et al. Two equally valid interpretations of the linear multicompartment mammillary pharmacokinetic model. *J Pharm Sci.* 1990;79:331–333.
44. Norman J. Drug-receptor reactions. *Br J Anaesth.* 1979;51:595–601.
45. Waud BE, Waud DR. The margin of safety of neuromuscular transmission in the muscle of the diaphragm. *Anesthesiology.* 1972;37:417–422.
46. Segre G. Kinetics of interaction between drugs and biological systems. *Farmaco [Sci].* 1968;23:907–918.
47. Sheiner LB, Stanski DR, Vozeh S, et al. Simultaneous modeling of pharmacokinetics and pharmacodynamics: application to d-tubocurarine. *Clin Pharmacol Ther.* 1979;25:358–371.
48. Kern SE, Stanski DR. Pharmacokinetics and pharmacodynamics of intravenously administered anesthetic drugs: concepts and lessons for drug development. *Clin Pharmacol Ther.* 2008;84:153–157.
49. Jacobs JR, Reves JG. Effect site equilibration time is a determinant of induction dose requirement. *Anesth Analg.* 1993;76:1–6.
50. Olofsen E, Dahan A. Population pharmacokinetics/pharmacodynamics of anesthetics. *AAPS J.* 2005;7:E383–E389.
51. Sheiner LB, Beal SL. Evaluation of methods for estimating population pharmacokinetics parameters. I. Michaelis-Menten model: routine clinical pharmacokinetic data. *J Pharmacokinet Biopharm.* 1980;8:553–571.
52. Maitre PO, Vozeh S, Heykants J, et al. Population pharmacokinetics of alfentanil: the average dose-plasma concentration relationship and interindividual variability in patients. *Anesthesiology.* 1987;66:3–12.
53. Group NP. *NONMEN User's Guide.* San Francisco, CA: University of California; 1999.
54. West GB, Brown JH, Enquist BJ. A general model for the origin of allometric scaling laws in biology. *Science.* 1997;276:122–126.
55. Mahmood I. Dosing in children: a critical review of the pharmacokinetic allometric scaling and modelling approaches in paediatric drug development and clinical settings. *Clin Pharmacokinet.* 2014;53:327–346.
56. Cortinez LI, De la Fuente N, Eleveld DJ, et al. Performance of propofol target-controlled infusion models in the obese: pharmacokinetic and pharmacodynamic analysis. *Anesth Analg.* 2014;119:302–310.
57. Mahmood I. Prediction of drug clearance in premature and mature neonates, infants and children ≤2 years of age: a comparison of the predictive. *J Clin Pharmacol.* 2016;56(6):733–739.
58. Morton WD, Lerman J. The effect of pancuronium on the solubility of aqueous thiopentone. *Can J Anaesth.* 1987;34:87–89.
59. Dejong RH, Cullen SC. Buffer-demand and Ph of local anesthetic solutions containing epinephrine. *Anesthesiology.* 1963;24:801–807.
60. Anders MW. Formation and toxicity of anesthetic degradation products. *Annu Rev Pharmacol Toxicol.* 2005;45:147–176.
61. Kharasch ED. Adverse drug reactions with halogenated anesthetics. *Clin Pharmacol Ther.* 2008;84:158–162.
62. Baxter PJ, Garton K, Kharasch ED. Mechanistic aspects of carbon monoxide formation from volatile anesthetics. *Anesthesiology.* 1998;89:929–941.
63. Kharasch ED, Powers KM, Artru AA. Comparison of Amsorb, sodalime, and Baralyme degradation of volatile anesthetics and formation of carbon monoxide and compound a in swine in vivo. *Anesthesiology.* 2002;96:173–812.
64. Bom A, Bradley M, Cameron K, et al. A novel concept of reversing neuromuscular block: chemical encapsulation of rocuronium bromide by a cyclodextrin-based synthetic host. *Angew Chem Int Ed Engl.* 2002;41:266–270.
65. Suy K, Morias K, Cammu G, et al. Effective reversal of moderate rocuronium- or vecuronium-induced neuromuscular block with sugammadex, a selective relaxant binding agent. *Anesthesiology.* 2007;106:283–288.
66. Tassonyi E, Pongracz A, Nemes R, et al. Reversal of pipecuronium-induced moderate neuromuscular block with sugammadex in the presence of a sevoflurane anesthetic: a randomized trial. *Anesth Analg.* 2015;121:373–380.
67. Haerter F, Eikermann M. Reversing neuromuscular blockade: inhibitors of the acetylcholinesterase versus the encapsulating agents sugammadex and calabadion. *Exp Opin Pharmacother.* 2016;17:819–833.
68. Haerter F, Simons JC, Foerster U, et al. Comparative effectiveness of calabadion and sugammadex to reverse non-depolarizing neuromuscular-blocking agents. *Anesthesiology.* 2015;123:1337–1349.
69. Hoffmann U, Grosse-Sundrup M, Eikermann-Haerter K, et al. Calabadion: a new agent to reverse the effects of benzylisoquinoline and steroidal neuromuscular-blocking agents. *Anesthesiology.* 2013;119:317–325.
70. Heerdt PM, Malhotra JK, Pan BY, et al. Pharmacodynamics and cardiopulmonary side effects of CW002, a cysteine-reversible neuromuscular blocking drug in dogs. *Anesthesiology.* 2010;112:910–916.
71. Avram MJ, Krejcie TC, Henthorn TK, et al. Beta-adrenergic blockade affects initial drug distribution due to decreased cardiac output and altered blood flow distribution. *J Pharmacol Exp Ther.* 2004;311:617–624.
72. Niemann CU, Henthorn TK, Krejcie TC, et al. Indocyanine green kinetics characterize blood volume and flow distribution and their alteration by propranolol. *Clin Pharmacol Ther.* 2000;67:342–350.
73. Krejcie TC, Wang Z, Avram MJ. Drug-induced hemodynamic perturbations alter the disposition of markers of blood volume, extracellular fluid, and total body water. *J Pharmacol Exp Ther.* 2001;296:922–930.
74. Avram MJ, Krejcie TC, Niemann CU, et al. Isoflurane alters the recirculatory pharmacokinetics of physiologic markers. *Anesthesiology.* 2000;92:1757–1768.
75. Avram MJ, Krejcie TC, Niemann CU, et al. The effect of halothane on the recirculatory pharmacokinetics of physiologic markers. *Anesthesiology.* 1997;87:1381–1393.
76. Benet LZ, Hoener BA. Changes in plasma protein binding have little clinical relevance. *Clin Pharmacol Ther.* 2002;71:115–121.
77. Gupta DK, Krejcie TC, Avram MJ. Pharmacokinetics of opioids. In: Evers A, Maze M, Kharasch ED, eds. *Anesthetic Pharmacology: Physiologic Principles and Clinical Practice.* 2nd ed. Cambridge, UK: Cambridge University Press; 2011:509–530.
78. Wright PM, McCarthy G, Szenohradszky J, et al. Influence of chronic phenytoin administration on the pharmacokinetics and pharmacodynamics of vecuronium. *Anesthesiology.* 2004;100:626–633.
79. Zbinden AM, Maggiorini M, Petersen-Felix S, et al. Anesthetic depth defined using multiple noxious stimuli during isoflurane/oxygen anesthesia. I. Motor reactions. *Anesthesiology.* 1994;80:253–260.
80. Zbinden AM, Petersen-Felix S, Thomson DA. Anesthetic depth defined using multiple noxious stimuli during isoflurane/oxygen anesthesia. II. Hemodynamic responses. *Anesthesiology.* 1994;80:261–267.
81. Oertel BG, Felden L, Tran PV, et al. Selective antagonism of opioid-induced ventilatory depression by an ampakine molecule in humans without loss of opioid analgesia. *Clin Pharmacol Ther.* 2010;87:204–211.
82. Vuyk J, Mertens MJ, Olofsen E, et al. Propofol anesthesia and rational opioid selection: determination of optimal EC50-EC95 propofol-opioid concentrations that assure adequate anesthesia and a rapid return of consciousness. *Anesthesiology.* 1997;87:1549–1562.
83. Bouillon TW, Bruhn J, Radulescu L, et al. Pharmacodynamic interaction between propofol and remifentanil regarding hypnosis, tolerance of laryngoscopy, bispectral index, and electroencephalographic approximate entropy. *Anesthesiology.* 2004;100:1353–1372.
84. Greco WR, Bravo G, Parsons JC. The search for synergy: a critical review from a response surface perspective. *Pharmacol Rev.* 1995;47:331–385.
85. Kern SE, Xie G, White JL, et al. A response surface analysis of propofol-remifentanil pharmacodynamic interaction in volunteers. *Anesthesiology.* 2004;100:1373–1381.
86. Manyam SC, Gupta DK, Johnson KB, et al. Opioid-volatile anesthetic synergy: a response surface model with remifentanil and sevoflurane as prototypes. *Anesthesiology.* 2006;105:267–278.
87. Minto CF, Schnider TW, Short TG, et al. Response surface model for anesthetic drug interactions. *Anesthesiology.* 2000;92:1603–1616.
88. Shafer SL, Stanski DR. Defining depth of anesthesia. *Handb Exp Pharmacol.* 2008:409–423.
89. Manyam SC, Gupta DK, Johnson KB, et al. When is a bispectral index of 60 too low? Rational processed electroencephalographic targets are dependent on the sedative-opioid ratio. *Anesthesiology.* 2007;106:472–483.
90. Boyer EW, Shannon M. The serotonin syndrome. *N Engl J Med.* 2005;352:1112–1120.
91. Rastogi R, Swarm RA, Patel TA. Case scenario: opioid association with serotonin syndrome: implications to the practitioners. *Anesthesiology.* 2011;115:1291–1298.
92. Gillman PK. Monoamine oxidase inhibitors, opioid analgesics and serotonin toxicity. *Br J Anaesth.* 2005;95:434–441.
93. Gillman PK. CNS toxicity involving methylene blue: the exemplar for understanding and predicting drug interactions that precipitate serotonin toxicity. *J Psychopharmacol.* 2011;25:429–436.
94. Schwiebert C, Irving C, Gillman PK. Small doses of methylene blue, previously considered safe, can precipitate serotonin toxicity. *Anaesthesia.* 2009;64:924.
95. Schuttler J, Schwilden H, Stoekel H. Pharmacokinetics as applied to total intravenous anaesthesia: practical implications. *Anaesthesia.* 1983;38(Suppl):53–56.
96. Shafer SL. Towards optimal intravenous dosing strategies. *Semin Anesth.* 1994;12:222.
97. Hughes MA, Glass PS, Jacobs JR. Context-sensitive half-time in multicompartment pharmacokinetic models for intravenous anesthetic drugs. *Anesthesiology.* 1992;76:334–341.
98. Egan TD. Is anesthesiology going soft? Trends in fragile pharmacology. *Anesthesiology.* 2009;111:229–230.
99. Johnson KB. New horizons in sedative hypnotic drug development: fast, clean, and soft. *Anesth Analg.* 2012;115:220–222.
100. Egan TD, Muir KT, Hermann DJ, et al. The electroencephalogram (EEG) and clinical measures of opioid potency: defining the EEG-clinical potency relationship ('fingerprint') with application to remifentanil. *Int J Pharmaceutical Med.* 2001;15:11–19.
101. Kilpatrick GJ, McIntyre MS, Cox RF, et al. CNS 7056: a novel ultra-short-acting benzodiazepine. *Anesthesiology.* 2007;107:60–66.
102. Cotten JF, Husain SS, Forman SA, et al. Methoxycarbonyl-etomidate: a novel rapidly metabolized and ultra-short-acting etomidate analogue that does not produce prolonged adrenocortical suppression. *Anesthesiology.* 2009;111:240–249.

103. Jonsson Fagerlund M, Sjodin J, Dabrowski MA, et al. Reduced efficacy of the intravenous anesthetic agent AZD3043 at GABA(A) receptors with beta2 (N289M) and beta3 (N290M) point-mutations. *Eur J Pharmacol.* 2012;694:13–19.
104. Egan TD, Obara S, Jenkins TE, et al. AZD-3043: a novel, metabolically labile sedative-hypnotic agent with rapid and predictable emergence from hypnosis. *Anesthesiology.* 2012;116:1267–1277.
105. Antonik LJ, Goldwater DR, Kilpatrick GJ, et al. A placebo- and midazolam-controlled phase I single ascending-dose study evaluating the safety, pharmacokinetics, and pharmacodynamics of remimazolam (CNS 7056). Part I. Safety, efficacy, and basic pharmacokinetics. *Anesth Analg.* 2012;115:274–283.
106. Wiltshire HR, Kilpatrick GJ, Tilbrook GS, et al. A placebo- and midazolam-controlled phase I single ascending-dose study evaluating the safety, pharmacokinetics, and pharmacodynamics of remimazolam (CNS 7056). Part II. Population pharmacokinetic and pharmacodynamic modeling and simulation. *Anesth Analg.* 2012;115:2842–2896.
107. Pambianco DJ, Borkett KM, Riff DS, et al. A phase IIb study comparing the safety and efficacy of remimazolam and midazolam in patients undergoing colonoscopy. *Gastrointest Endosc.* 2016;83:984–992.
108. Cotten JF, Forman SA, Laha JK, et al. Carboetomidate: a pyrrole analog of etomidate designed not to suppress adrenocortical function. *Anesthesiology.* 2010;112:637–644.
109. Cotten JF, Le Ge R, Banacos N, et al. Closed-loop continuous infusions of etomidate and etomidate analogs in rats: a comparative study of dosing and the impact on adrenocortical function. *Anesthesiology.* 2011;115:764–773.
110. Ge R, Pejo E, Husain SS, et al. Electroencephalographic and hypnotic recoveries after brief and prolonged infusions of etomidate and optimized soft etomidate analogs. *Anesthesiology.* 2012;117:1037–1043.
111. Husain SS, Pejo E, Ge R, et al. Modifying methoxycarbonyl etomidate interester spacer optimizes in vitro metabolic stability and in vivo hypnotic potency and duration of action. *Anesthesiology.* 2012;117:1027–1036.
112. Ge R, Pejo E, Cotten JF, et al. Adrenocortical suppression and recovery after continuous hypnotic infusion: etomidate versus its soft analogue cyclopropyl-methoxycarbonyl metomidate. *Crit Care.* 2013;17:R20.
113. Pejo E, Santer P, Jeffrey S, et al. Analogues of etomidate: modifications around etomidate's chiral carbon and the impact on in vitro and in vivo pharmacology. *Anesthesiology.* 2014;121:290–301.
114. Pejo E, Liu J, Lin X, et al. Distinct hypnotic recoveries after infusions of methoxycarbonyl etomidate and cyclopropyl methoxycarbonyl metomidate: the role of the metabolite. *Anesth Analg.* 2016;122:1008–1014.
115. Edelman GJ, Hoffman WE, Charbel FT. Cerebral hypoxia after etomidate administration and temporary cerebral artery occlusion. *Anesth Analg.* 1997;85:821–825.
116. Hoffman WE, Charbel FT, Edelman G, et al. Comparison of the effect of etomidate and desflurane on brain tissue gases and pH during prolonged middle cerebral artery occlusion. *Anesthesiology.* 1998;88:1188–1194.
117. Drummond JC, McKay LD, Cole DJ, et al. The role of nitric oxide synthase inhibition in the adverse effects of etomidate in the setting of focal cerebral ischemia in rats. *Anesth Analg.* 2005;100:841–846.
118. Kalman S, Koch P, Ahlen K, et al. First human study of the investigational sedative and anesthetic drug AZD3043: a dose-escalation trial to assess the safety, pharmacokinetics, and efficacy of a 30-minute infusion in healthy male volunteers. *Anesth Analg.* 2015;121:885–893.
119. Norberg A, Koch P, Kanes SJ, et al. A bolus and bolus followed by infusion study of AZD3043, an investigational intravenous drug for sedation and anesthesia: safety and pharmacodynamics in healthy male and female volunteers. *Anesth Analg.* 2015;121:894–903.
120. Bjornsson MA, Norberg A, Kalman S, et al. A recirculatory model for pharmacokinetics and the effects on bispectral index after intravenous infusion of the sedative and anesthetic AZD3043 in healthy volunteers. *Anesth Analg.* 2015;121:904–913.
121. Maitre PO, Shafer SL. A simple pocket calculator approach to predict anesthetic drug concentrations from pharmacokinetic data. *Anesthesiology.* 1990;73:332–336.
122. Egan TD. Target-controlled drug delivery: progress toward an intravenous "vaporizer" and automated anesthetic administration. *Anesthesiology.* 2003;99:1214–1219.
123. Shafer SL, Varvel JR, Aziz N, et al. Pharmacokinetics of fentanyl administered by computer-controlled infusion pump. *Anesthesiology.* 1990;73:1091–1102.
124. Barvais L, Cantraine F, D'Hollander A, et al. Predictive accuracy of continuous alfentanil infusion in volunteers: variability of different pharmacokinetic sets. *Anesth Analg.* 1993;77:801–810.
125. Barvais L, Heitz D, Schmartz D, et al. Pharmacokinetic model-driven infusion of sufentanil and midazolam during cardiac surgery: assessment of the prospective predictive accuracy and the quality of anesthesia. *J Cardiothorac Vasc Anesth.* 2000;14:402–408.
126. Barvais L, D'Hollander AA, Cantraine F, et al. Predictive accuracy of midazolam in adult patients scheduled for coronary surgery. *J Clin Anesth.* 1994;6:297–302.
127. Veselis RA, Glass P, Dnistrian A, et al. Performance of computer-assisted continuous infusion at low concentrations of intravenous sedatives. *Anesth Analg.* 1997;84:1049–1057.
128. Vuyk J, Engbers FH, Burm AG, et al. Performance of computer-controlled infusion of propofol: an evaluation of five pharmacokinetic parameter sets. *Anesth Analg.* 1995;81:1275–1282.
129. Schraag S, Flaschar J. Delivery performance of commercial target-controlled infusion devices with Diprifusor module. *Eur J Anaesthesiol.* 2002;19:357–360.
130. Passot S, Servin F, Allary R, et al. Target-controlled versus manually-controlled infusion of propofol for direct laryngoscopy and bronchoscopy. *Anesth Analg.* 2002;94:1212–1216.
131. Gale T, Leslie K, Kluger M. Propofol anaesthesia via target controlled infusion or manually controlled infusion: effects on the bispectral index as a measure of anaesthetic depth. *Anaesth Intensive Care.* 2001;29:579–584.
132. Suttner S, Boldt J, Schmidt C, et al. Cost analysis of target-controlled infusion-based anesthesia compared with standard anesthesia regimens. *Anesth Analg.* 1999;88:77–82.
133. Checketts MR, Gilhooly CJ, Kenny GN. Patient-maintained analgesia with target-controlled alfentanil infusion after cardiac surgery: a comparison with morphine PCA. *Br J Anaesth.* 1998;80:748–751.
134. van den Nieuwenhuyzen MC, Engbers FH, Burm AG, et al. Target-controlled infusion of alfentanil for postoperative analgesia: contribution of plasma protein binding to intra-patient and inter-patient variability. *Br J Anaesth.* 1999;82:580–585.
135. Campbell L, Imrie G, Doherty P, et al. Patient maintained sedation for colonoscopy using a target controlled infusion of propofol. *Anaesthesia.* 2004;59:127–132.
136. Irwin MG, Thompson N, Kenny GN. Patient-maintained propofol sedation: assessment of a target-controlled infusion system. *Anaesthesia.* 1997;52:525–530.
137. Gentry WB, Krejcie TC, Henthorn TK, et al. Effect of infusion rate on thiopental dose–response relationships: assessment of a pharmacokinetic-pharmacodynamic model. *Anesthesiology.* 1994;81:316–324.
138. Minto CF, Schnider TW, Gregg KM, et al. Using the time of maximum effect site concentration to combine pharmacokinetics and pharmacodynamics. *Anesthesiology.* 2003;99:324–333.
139. Henthorn TK, Krejcie TC, Shanks CA, et al. Time-dependent distribution volume and kinetics of the pharmacodynamic effector site. *J Pharm Sci.* 1992;81:1136–1138.
140. Shafer SL, Gregg KM. Algorithms to rapidly achieve and maintain stable drug concentrations at the site of drug effect with a computer-controlled infusion pump. *J Pharmacokinet Biopharm.* 1992;20:147–169.
141. Schnider TW, Minto CF, Gambus PL, et al. The influence of method of administration and covariates on the pharmacokinetics of propofol in adult volunteers. *Anesthesiology.* 1998;88:1170–1182.
142. Chiou WL. Potential pitfalls in the conventional pharmacokinetic studies: effects of the initial mixing of drug in blood and the pulmonary first-pass elimination. *J Pharmacokinet Biopharm.* 1979;7:527–536.
143. Henthorn TK. The effect of altered physiological states on intravenous anesthetics. *Handb Exp Pharmacol.* 2008:363–377.
144. Henthorn TK, Krejcie TC, Avram MJ. Early drug distribution: a generally neglected aspect of pharmacokinetics of particular relevance to intravenously administered anesthetic agents. *Clin Pharmacol Ther.* 2008;84:18–22.
145. Krejcie TC, Henthorn TK, Gentry WB, et al. Modifications of blood volume alter the disposition of markers of blood volume, extracellular fluid, and total body water. *J Pharmacol Exp Ther.* 1999;291:1308–1316.
146. Krejcie TC, Henthorn TK, Niemann CU, et al. Recirculatory pharmacokinetic models of markers of blood, extracellular fluid and total body water administered concomitantly. *J Pharmacol Exp Ther.* 1996;278:1050–1057.
147. Kuipers JA, Boer F, Olofsen E, et al. Recirculatory pharmacokinetics and pharmacodynamics of rocuronium in patients: the influence of cardiac output. *Anesthesiology.* 2001;94:47–55.
148. Avram MJ, Sanghvi R, Henthorn TK, et al. Determinants of thiopental induction dose requirements. *Anesth Analg.* 1993;76:10–17.
149. Forbes GB, Hursh JB. Age and sex trends in lean body mass calculated from K40 measurements: with a note on the theoretical basis for the procedure. *Ann N Y Acad Sci.* 1963;110:255–263.
150. Sathyaprabha TN, Pradhan C, Rashmi G, et al. Noninvasive cardiac output measurement by transthoracic electrical bioimpedance: influence of age and gender. *J Clin Monit Comput.* 2008;22:401–408.
151. Avram MJ, Henthorn TK, Spyker DA, et al. Recirculatory kinetic model of fentanyl administered as a thermally generated aerosol to volunteers. *Anesthesiology.* 2008;109:A815.
152. Avram MJ, Henthorn TK, Spyker DA, et al. Recirculatory pharmacokinetic model of fentanyl aerosol in volunteers. *Clin Pharmacol Ther.* 2008;83:PI-76.
153. Avram MJ, Krejcie TC, Henthorn TK. The concordance of early antipyrine and thiopental distribution kinetics. *J Pharmacol Exp Ther.* 2002;302:594–600.
154. Kuipers JA, Boer F, Olofsen E, et al. Recirculatory and compartmental pharmacokinetic modeling of alfentanil in pigs: the influence of cardiac output. *Anesthesiology.* 1999;90:1146–1157.
155. Woodruff EA, Martin JF, Omens M. A model for the design and evaluation of algorithms for closed-loop cardiovascular therapy. *IEEE Trans Biomed Eng.* 1997;44:694–705.
156. Tehrani F, Rogers M, Lo T, et al. Closed-loop control if the inspired fraction of oxygen in mechanical ventilation. *J Clin Monit Comput.* 2002;17:367–376.

157. Renard E. Implantable closed-loop glucose-sensing and insulin delivery: the future for insulin pump therapy. *Curr Opin Pharmacol*. 2002;2:708–716.
158. O'Hara DA, Hexem JG, Derbyshire GJ, et al. The use of a PID controller to model vecuronium pharmacokinetics and pharmacodynamics during liver transplantation: proportional-integral-derivative. *IEEE Trans Biomed Eng*. 1997;44:610–619.
159. De Smet T, Struys MM, Greenwald S, et al. Estimation of optimal modeling weights for a Bayesian-based closed-loop system for propofol administration using the bispectral index as a controlled variable: a simulation study. *Anesth Analg*. 2007;105:1629–1638.
160. Mortier E, Struys M, De Smet T, et al. Closed-loop controlled administration of propofol using bispectral analysis. *Anaesthesia*. 1998;53:749–754.
161. Schwilden H, Schuttler J, Stoeckel H. Closed-loop feedback control of methohexital anesthesia by quantitative EEG analysis in humans. *Anesthesiology*. 1987;67:341–347.
162. Schwilden H, Stoeckel H. Effective therapeutic infusions produced by closed-loop feedback control of methohexital administration during total intravenous anesthesia with fentanyl. *Anesthesiology*. 1990;73:225–229.
163. Struys MM, De Smet T, Greenwald S, et al. Performance evaluation of two published closed-loop control systems using bispectral index monitoring: a simulation study. *Anesthesiology*. 2004;100:640–647.
164. Struys MM, De Smet T, Mortier EP. Closed-loop control of anaesthesia. *Curr Opin Anaesthesiol*. 2002;15:421–425.
165. Struys MM, De Smet T, Versichelen LF, et al. Comparison of closed-loop controlled administration of propofol using Bispectral Index as the controlled variable versus "standard practice" controlled administration. *Anesthesiology*. 2001;95:6–17.
166. Tzabazis A, Ihmsen H, Schywalsky M, et al. EEG-controlled closed-loop dosing of propofol in rats. *Br J Anaesth*. 2004;92:564–569.
167. Liu N, Chazot T, Genty A, et al. Titration of propofol for anesthetic induction and maintenance guided by the bispectral index: closed-loop versus manual control: a prospective, randomized, multicenter study. *Anesthesiology*. 2006;104:686–695.
168. Liu N, Chazot T, Hamada S, et al. Closed-loop coadministration of propofol and remifentanil guided by bispectral index: a randomized multicenter study. *Anesth Analg*. 2011;112:546–557.
169. Liu N, Lory C, Assenzo V, et al. Feasibility of closed-loop co-administration of propofol and remifentanil guided by the bispectral index in obese patients: a prospective cohort comparison. *Br J Anaesth*. 2015;114:605–614.
170. Orliaguet GA, Benabbes Lambert F, Chazot T, et al. Feasibility of closed-loop titration of propofol and remifentanil guided by the bispectral monitor in pediatric and adolescent patients: a prospective randomized study. *Anesthesiology*. 2015;122:759–767.
171. Puri GD, Mathew PJ, Biswas I, et al. A multicenter evaluation of a closed-loop anesthesia delivery system: a randomized controlled trial. *Anesth Analg*. 2016;122:106–114.
172. Short TG, Hannam JA, Laurent S, et al. Refining target-controlled infusion: an assessment of pharmacodynamic target-controlled infusion of propofol and remifentanil using a response surface model of their combined effects on bispectral index. *Anesth Analg*. 2016;122:90–97.
173. Manberg PJ, Vozella CM, Kelley SD. Regulatory challenges facing closed-loop anesthetic drug infusion devices. *Clin Pharmacol Ther*. 2008;84:166–169.
174. Liu N, Rinehart J. Closed-loop propofol administration: routine care or a research tool? What impact in the future? *Anesth Analg*. 2016;122:4–6.
175. Monk TG, Saini V, Weldon BC, et al. Anesthetic management and one-year mortality after noncardiac surgery. *Anesth Analg*. 2005;100:4–10.
176. Monk TG, Weldon BC, Garvan CW, et al. Predictors of cognitive dysfunction after major noncardiac surgery. *Anesthesiology*. 2008;108:18–30.
177. Katoh T, Ikeda K. The effects of fentanyl on sevoflurane requirements for loss of consciousness and skin incision. *Anesthesiology*. 1998;88:18–24.
178. Katoh T, Kobayashi S, Suzuki A, et al. The effect of fentanyl on sevoflurane requirements for somatic and sympathetic responses to surgical incision. *Anesthesiology*. 1999;90:398–405.
179. Katoh T, Nakajima Y, Moriwaki G, et al. Sevoflurane requirements for tracheal intubation with and without fentanyl. *Br J Anaesth*. 1999;82:561–565.
180. Katoh T, Uchiyama T, Ikeda K. Effect of fentanyl on awakening concentration of sevoflurane. *Br J Anaesth*. 1994;73:322–325.
181. McEwan AI, Smith C, Dyar O, et al. Isoflurane minimum alveolar concentration reduction by fentanyl. *Anesthesiology*. 1993;78:864–869.
182. Sebel PS, Glass PS, Fletcher JE, et al. Reduction of the MAC of desflurane with fentanyl. *Anesthesiology*. 1992;76:52–59.
183. Vuyk J, Lim T, Engbers FH, et al. Pharmacodynamics of alfentanil as a supplement to propofol or nitrous oxide for lower abdominal surgery in female patients. *Anesthesiology*. 1993;78:1036–1045.
184. Vuyk J, Lim T, Engbers FH, et al. The pharmacodynamic interaction of propofol and alfentanil during lower abdominal surgery in women. *Anesthesiology*. 1995;83:8–22.
185. Short TG, Ho TY, Minto CF, et al. Efficient trial design for eliciting a pharmacokinetic-pharmacodynamic model-based response surface describing the interaction between two intravenous anesthetic drugs. *Anesthesiology*. 2002;96:400–408.
186. Johnson KB, Syroid ND, Gupta DK, et al. An evaluation of remifentanil propofol response surfaces for loss of responsiveness, loss of response to surrogates of painful stimuli and laryngoscopy in patients undergoing elective surgery. *Anesth Analg*. 2008;106:471–479.
187. Johnson KB, Syroid ND, Gupta DK, et al. An evaluation of remifentanil-sevoflurane response surface models in patients emerging from anesthesia: model improvement using effect-site sevoflurane concentrations. *Anesth Analg*. 2010;111:387–394.
188. Syroid ND, Johnson KB, Pace NL, et al. Response surface model predictions of emergence and response to pain in the recovery room: an evaluation of patients emerging from an isoflurane and fentanyl anesthetic. *Anesth Analg*. 2010;111:380–386.
189. Ting CK, Johnson KB, Teng WN, et al. Response surface model predictions of wake-up time during scoliosis surgery. *Anesth Analg*. 2014;118:546–553.

Section 3
CORE CARE PRINCIPLES

12 Cardiac Anatomy and Physiology*

PAUL S. PAGEL • DAVID F. STOWE

Introduction
Gross Anatomy
   Architecture
   Valve Structure
   Coronary Blood Supply
   Impulse Conduction
Coronary Physiology
Cardiac Myocyte Anatomy and Function
   Ultrastructure
   Contractile Apparatus
   Calcium–Myofilament Interaction
   Myosin–Actin Interaction
Law of Laplace

The Cardiac Cycle
The Pressure–Volume Diagram
Determinants of Systolic Function
   Heart Rate
   Preload
   Afterload
   Myocardial Contractility
Determinants of Diastolic Function
   Invasive Assessment of LV Relaxation
   Invasive Assessment of LV Filling and Compliance
   Noninvasive Evaluation of Diastolic Function
   Pericardium
   Atrial Function

KEY POINTS

1. The heart's cartilaginous skeleton, myocardial fiber orientation, valves, coronary blood supply, and conduction system determine its mechanical capabilities.
2. The cardiac myocyte is engineered for contraction and relaxation.
3. Changes in sarcomere muscle tension and length observed in isolated cardiac muscle are translated into alterations in pressure and volume in the intact heart.
4. The pressure–volume diagram provides a useful framework for the analysis of atrial and ventricular systolic and diastolic function.
5. The end-systolic and end-diastolic pressure–volume relations determine the operating range of each cardiac chamber.
6. Heart rate, preload, afterload, and myocardial contractility determine pump performance.
7. Preload is the quantity of blood that a chamber contains immediately before contraction.
8. Afterload is the external resistance to chamber emptying after contraction begins and the aortic valve opens.
9. Myocardial contractility is the force of contraction under controlled heart rate and loading conditions; contractility may be quantified using pressure–volume relation, isovolumic contraction, or ejection phase analysis.
10. The ability of a cardiac chamber to effectively collect blood at a normal filling pressure defines its diastolic function.
11. Diastole is a complex sequence of temporally related, heterogeneous events; no single index comprehensively describes diastolic function.
12. Left ventricular diastolic dysfunction is responsible for heart failure in as many as 50% of patients.
13. Invasive analysis of diastolic function may be conducted using the pressure–volume model.
14. Transmitral and pulmonary venous blood flow velocities derived using pulse wave Doppler echocardiography are commonly used to noninvasively measure diastolic function.
15. The restraining forces of the pericardium are important determinants of chamber filling and ventricular interdependence.
16. The atria are reservoirs, conduits, and contractile chambers.

---

*From the Anesthesia Service, the Clement J. Zablocki Veterans Affairs Medical Center, Milwaukee, Wisconsin (PSP and DFS) and the Departments of Anesthesiology and Physiology, the Medical College of Wisconsin, Milwaukee, Wisconsin (DFS). This work was supported entirely by departmental funds. The authors have no conflicts of interest pursuant to this work. The authors thank our mentor and former Chairman John P. Kampine, MD, PhD, for his contributions to previous versions of this chapter.

Introduction

The heart is a phasic, variable speed, electrically self-activating muscular pump that provides its own blood supply. The two pair of atria and ventricles are elastic chambers arranged in series that supply equal amounts of blood to the pulmonary and systemic vasculature. Myocardium in the atria and ventricles responds to stimulation rate and muscle stretch before (preload) and after (afterload) contraction begins. Coronary arterial blood vessels supply oxygen and metabolic substrates to the heart. The mechanical characteristics of the myocardium and its response to changes in autonomic nervous system activity allow the heart to adapt to rapidly changing physiologic conditions. The inherent contractile properties of the atria and ventricles and the ability of these chambers to adequately fill without excessive pressure are the major determinants of overall cardiac performance. As a result, abnormalities in either systolic or diastolic function may cause heart failure. Comprehensive knowledge of cardiac anatomy and physiology is essential for the practice of anesthesiology. This chapter describes the fundamentals of cardiac anatomy and physiology in adults. The authors will focus on the left atrium and ventricle (LA and LV, respectively) for the vast majority of the subsequent discussion unless otherwise noted.

Gross Anatomy

Architecture

A flexible, cartilaginous structure forms the heart's skeleton composed of the annuli of the cardiac valves, the aortic and pulmonary arterial (PA) roots, the central fibrous body, and the left and right fibrous trigones. This foundation creates support for the valves and maintains the heart's structural integrity as internal pressures vary. A small quantity of superficial subepicardial muscle also inserts into the cartilaginous skeleton, but most atrial and ventricular muscle directly arises from and inserts within adjacent surrounding myocardium. Myocardial fibers are continuously interwoven and cannot be separated into distinct "layers." The atria contain two relatively thin orthogonal bands of myocardium, whereas the LV and, to a lesser extent the right ventricle (RV), consist of the interdigitating deep sinospiral, the superficial sinospiral, and the superficial bulbospiral muscles (Fig. 12-1). The angle of the myocardial fibers changes within the ventricular wall's thickness from the subendocardium to the subepicardium. Myocardial fibers of the LV are oriented in perpendicular, oblique, and helical planes from the cardiac base (superior in the mediastinum) to its apex. This arrangement reverses direction at approximately the LV's midpoint, creating an overall fiber architecture that mimics a flattened "figure of eight." This fiber orientation facilitates LV chamber shortening along the heart's longitudinal axis and produces a distinctive torsional twisting (analogous to "wringing" of a wash cloth) motion during contraction. The twisting effect substantially enhances the LV's ability to eject blood, as loss of this helical–rotational action reduces ejection fraction in patients with heart failure.[1] Elastic recoil of the systolic twist during LV relaxation is also an important determinant of early diastolic filling, especially during hypovolemia and exercise.[2] In contrast to the subepicardial and subendocardial layers, midmyocardial fibers are arranged in a circumferential orientation and act almost exclusively to decrease chamber diameter during contraction.

The LV free walls taper in thickness from base to apex because the relative amount of midmyocardium gradually declines. LV and RV subendocardium and LV midmyocardium extending from the LV anterior wall contribute to the interventricular septum, which thickens toward the LV chamber during contraction under normal conditions because the majority of the septum is composed of LV myocardium. However, RV hypertrophy resulting from an increase in afterload (e.g., pulmonary arterial [PA] hypertension) may cause paradoxical motion of the interventricular septum. Regional differences in LV wall thickness and fiber orientation also contribute to load-dependent alterations in LV mechanics.[3] Irregular ridges of subendocardium ("trabeculae carnae" [Latin for "meaty ridges"]) are present within the RV chamber, and to a lesser extent, in the LV apex. The precise physiologic significance of the trabeculae carnae is unknown.

The LV apex and interventricular septum are relatively fixed in space within the mediastinum during contraction and relaxation. In contrast, the LV's lateral and posterior walls shift position to the anterior and to the right during systole. This motion changes the orientation of the LV longitudinal axis from a position that favors LV filling (perpendicular to the mitral valve) to one that facilitates ejection (orthogonal to the LV outflow tract and aortic valve). The movement of the lateral and posterior LV walls during contraction is also responsible for the point of maximal impulse palpable on the left chest wall. The combined effects of subendocardial and subepicardial contraction, papillary muscle shortening, and elastic recoil produced by ejection of blood into the aortic root causes the LV base to descend toward the apex during contraction. Thus, normal electrical activation of the LV causes its long axis to shorten, reduces its chamber diameter, and produces torsional rotation of its apex in an anterior-right direction (Fig. 12-2). Differential changes in wall tension also create an apex-to-base intraventricular pressure gradient during LV ejection. This action enhances the transfer of stroke volume from the LV to the ascending aorta and proximal great vessels.

The crescent-shaped RV is located anterior and to the right of the LV. The RV propels venous blood into the compliant, low-pressure PA vasculature. The RV's walls are thinner and contain fewer cardiac myocytes than the LV. The RV is exposed to only 15% to 20% of the LV's peak systolic wall stress. Embryologically distinct inflow and outflow tracts exist in the RV. As a result, RV contraction is less temporally uniform than the LV and is more peristaltic in nature. The RV free wall uses the interventricular septum for structural support during contraction. The contracting LV also provides additional external assistance to RV during the latter chamber's contraction. These two factors combine to improve the RV's

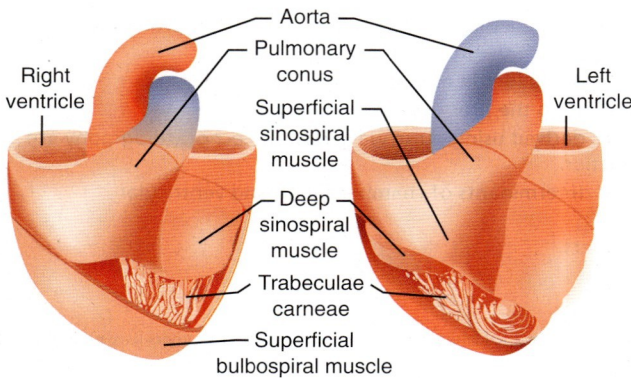

Figure 12-1 Illustration depicting the components of the myocardium. The outer muscle layers pull the base of the heart toward the apex. The inner circumferential layers constrict the lumen, particularly of the LV.

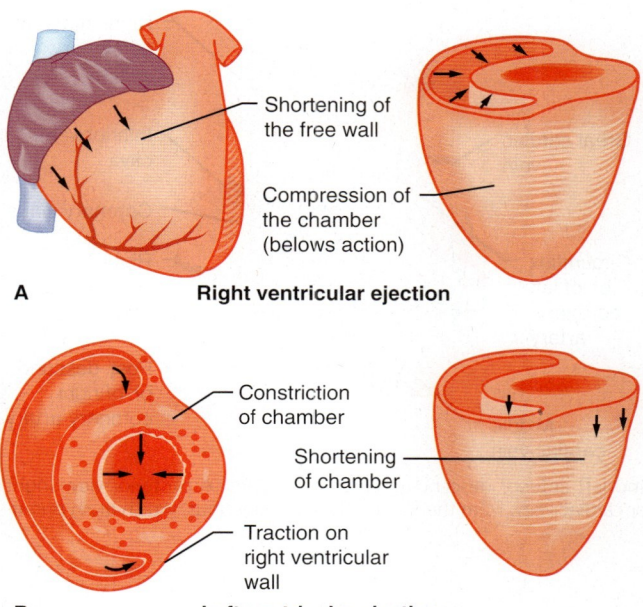

Figure 12-2 Illustration depicting the contraction characteristics and modes of emptying of the RV and LV. The volumes ejected by each ventricle are equal, but the LV requires a more circumferential muscular wall to eject its volume at a pressure that is approximately four to five times greater than that in the right ventricle.

mechanical advantage above its contractile ability alone, and in so doing, partially compensate for the chamber's thinner walls. This allows the RV to eject an identical stroke volume to the LV during each cardiac cycle. Nevertheless, the RV more easily decompensates when afterload increases because the RV is able to produce less than 20% of the total stroke work than the thicker, more muscular LV generates. However, the RV's greater compliance allows the chamber to more easily accommodate acute increases in preload than the stiffer LV.

Valve Structure

Two pairs of translucent, macroscopically avascular valves ensure unidirectional movement of blood through the normal heart. The pulmonic and aortic valves separate the RV and LV from the PA and aorta, respectively. The valves open and close passively in response to pressure gradients produced during contraction and relaxation, respectively. The pulmonic valve leaflets are named for their anatomic locations (right, left, and anterior), whereas the aortic valve leaflets correspond to the adjacent coronary artery ostium if present (right, left, and non). The orifice areas of the pulmonic and aortic valves are nearly equal to the corresponding cross-sectional areas of their annuli during ejection. The sinuses of Valsalva are dilated segments of aortic root immediately superior to each aortic leaflet. Hydraulic flow vortices occur within the sinuses that prevent adherence of the valve leaflets to the aortic wall during ejection and facilitate valve closure by preserving leaflet mobility during diastole.[4] These actions prevent the valve leaflets from inadvertently occluding the right and left coronary ostia. The proximal PA does not contain sinuses of Valsalva.

Located between the LA and the LV, the mitral valve has two leaflets (the oval-shaped anterior and the crescent-shaped posterior) and a prolate ellipsoid (saddle-shaped) three-dimensional structure.[5,6] Coaptation of the leaflets occurs along a central curve with the anterior leaflet creating a convex border. Despite the differences in their shapes, the anterior and posterior leaflets have similar cross-sectional areas because the posterior leaflet occupies a greater percentage of the annular circumference. Anterior-lateral and posterior-medial commissures connect the leaflets in these annular locations and are located above each corresponding papillary muscle. A positive pressure gradient between the LA and LV develops during late LV relaxation as LV pressure falls below LA pressure, driving open the mitral valve and allowing blood to flow from the LA into the LV (early ventricular filling). LV untwisting and elastic recoil of the chamber further contribute to this process. The mitral valve closes as rapidly increasing LV hydraulic pressure during early systole forces the leaflets in a superior direction. The chordae tendinae act as restricting cables to limit this superior motion of the mitral leaflets, facilitating their coaptation. When functioning properly, the chordae tendinae prevent the mitral leaflets from prolapsing or inverting into the LA. Conversely, chordal rupture is a common cause of mitral regurgitation because excessive leaflet motion beyond the coaptation zone occurs, allowing unobstructed retrograde blood flow from the pressurized LV into the low-pressure LA outlet. Primary and secondary chordae tendinae attach to the leaflet edges and bodies, respectively, whereas tertiary chordae insert into the distal posterior leaflet or the myocardium immediately adjacent to the annulus. The papillary muscles are composed of subendocardial myocardium that contract with the LV. Each papillary muscle normally has chordal attachments to both mitral leaflets. Papillary muscle contraction tensions the chordae, providing another mechanism by which the chordae prevent excessive leaflet motion. Tightening of the mitral annulus through a sphincter-like contraction of the surrounding subepicardium also aids in mitral valve closure. The mitral valve apparatus is very important for normal LV function for two major reasons. First, the valve apparatus assures unidirectional blood flow from the LA to the LV by preventing reflux of blood into the LA and pulmonary veins during LV contraction. In addition to chordal rupture previously mentioned, papillary muscle ischemia or infarction may cause the mitral apparatus to fail, resulting in acute mitral regurgitation. Second, the mitral apparatus also contributes to LV systolic function because papillary muscle shortening assists LV apical contraction. This latter effect often becomes apparent during mitral valve replacement because many chordal attachments to the papillary muscles are intentionally severed. This compromise of mitral apparatus structure reduces LV ejection fraction and may contribute to difficult weaning from cardiopulmonary bypass in some patients undergoing mitral valve replacement, especially those with pre-existing LV systolic dysfunction.

The tricuspid valve is normally composed of anterior, posterior, and septal leaflets.[7] The posterior leaflet is usually smaller than the anterior and septal leaflets. The tricuspid valve assures unidirectional movement of blood from the RA and RV. Identification of a septal papillary muscle can be used to distinguish the morphologic RV from the LV in patients with some forms of congenital heart disease (e.g., transposition of the great vessels). A lateral segment of myocardium stretching between the apical aspects of anterior and septal papillary muscles, known as the moderator band, separates the embryologic RV inflow and outflow tracts. Unlike the mitral valve, the tricuspid valve does not have a collagenous annulus. Instead, the tricuspid leaflets originate from the atrioventricular groove that separates the RA from the RV. Notably, the proximal right coronary artery lies within this groove, and the vessel must be carefully avoided during tricuspid valve repair or replacement.

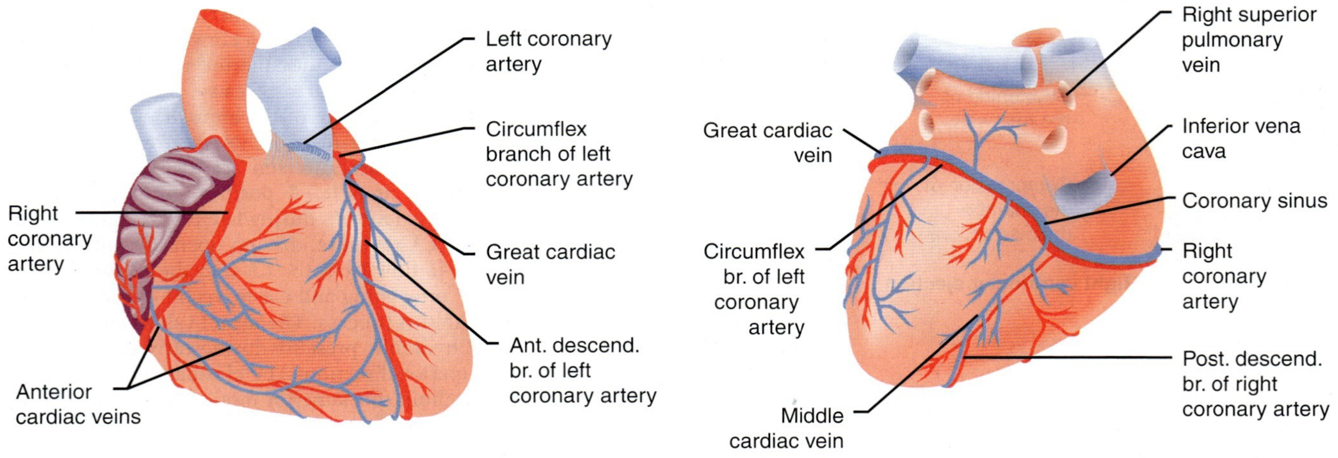

Figure 12-3 An anterior view of the heart (left) shows right coronary and left anterior descending coronary arteries. A posterior view (right) shows left circumflex and posterior descending coronary arteries. The anterior cardiac veins from the RV and the coronary sinus, which drain primarily the LV, empty into the RA.

Coronary Blood Supply

The left anterior descending, left circumflex, and right coronary arteries (LAD, LCCA, and RCA, respectively) supply blood to the LV (Fig. 12-3). Most coronary blood flow to the LV myocardium occurs during diastole because aortic pressure exceeds LV pressure. A critical stenosis or acute occlusion of the LAD, LCCA, or RCA almost invariably produces myocardial ischemia or infarction accompanied by regional contractile dysfunction that is easily predicted based on the known distribution of each coronary artery's blood supply. The LAD and its diagonal branches supply the medial LV anterior wall, the anterior two-thirds of the interventricular septum, and the LV apex. The LCCA and its marginal branches perfuse the anterior and posterior aspects of the lateral wall. The RCA provides blood flow to the medial portions of the posterior wall and the posterior one-third of the interventricular septum. The major epicardial coronary vessel that feeds the posterior descending coronary artery (PDA) determines the "dominance" of the coronary circulation. A "right dominant" circulation (RCA supplies blood to the PDA) is observed in approximately 80% of patients, whereas a "left dominant" circulation (LCCA perfuses the PDA) occurs in the remaining 20%. Distal connections or collateral vessels between the major coronary arteries may also provide an alternative route of blood flow to regions of myocardium that lie distal to a severe stenosis or occlusion. Notably, the development of coronary collaterals in response to chronic myocardial ischemia is highly variable and quite unpredictable in patients with coronary artery disease. A single coronary artery (2:1 ratio of RCA to LCCA) provides blood flow to the posterior-medial papillary muscle in two-thirds of patients. Thus, RCA or LCCA occlusion may produce acute posterior-medial papillary muscle ischemia or infarction and, as a result, new mitral regurgitation. However, this is not always the case, as both vessels perfuse the posterior-medial papillary muscle in the remaining patients.[8] In contrast to the variable blood supply to the posterior-medial papillary muscle, the anterior-lateral papillary muscle has a robust dual supply (LAD and LCCA), rendering this papillary muscle less susceptible to ischemic dysfunction than its counterpart.

Coronary blood flow to the RA, LA, and RV occurs during both systole and diastole because aortic pressure most often exceeds the pressure within each of these chambers unless profound hypotension is present (Fig. 12-4). The RCA and its branches supply blood flow to most of the RV, although distal diagonal and septal branches of the LAD also perfuse the RV anterior wall. Thus, either RCA or LAD occlusion may cause RV ischemia or infarction with resulting contractile dysfunction. Branches of the LCCA are the major sources of blood supply to the LA. As a result, LCCA occlusion often causes acute decompensation of LA contractility, whereas a compensatory increase in LA contractility

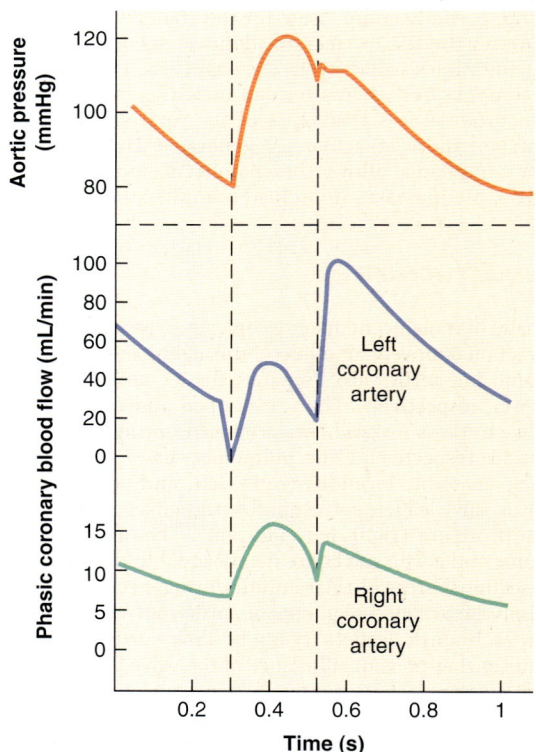

Figure 12-4 Schematic representation of blood flow in the left and right coronary arteries during phases of the cardiac cycle. Note that most left coronary flow occurs during diastole while right coronary flow (and coronary sinus flow) occurs mostly during late systole and early diastole.

(based on a Frank–Starling mechanism) is most often observed if the LAD is acutely occluded.[9] Branches of both the RCA and the LCCA supply the RA. For example, either the RCA (55% of patients) or the LCCA perfuses the sinoatrial (SA) node. The RCA usually supplies blood to the atrioventricular (AV) node, but the LCCA may also perfuse the AV node depending on the coronary circulation's right or left dominance. The clinical implications of these relationships are clear: Critical stenosis or acute occlusion of either the RCA or LCCA may interrupt normal atrial or AV node conduction and cause bradyarrhythmias.

The proximal branches of the RCA, LCCA, and LAD are located on the epicardial surface of the heart and give rise to intramural vessels that penetrate perpendicularly or obliquely deep into the myocardium. Except for the thin tissue layer on the endocardial surface of each chamber, the heart's blood supply is derived almost entirely from perforating branches of the three major epicardial coronary arteries. The penetrating branches divide into dense capillary networks located parallel to the myocardial bundles. Arterial branches with diameters between 50 and 500 μm form interconnecting anastomoses (Fig. 12-5), whereas vessels between 100 and 200 μm in diameter form a plexus within the subendocardium. Coronary collaterals between different branches of the same coronary artery or between branches of two different coronary arteries are also variably present. Coronary collateral blood flow is usually minimal in the absence of a hemodynamically significant stenosis because the driving pressure across the collateral vessel is equal. However, if a main artery supplying one branch of a collateral vessel is severely stenotic or occluded, a pressure gradient develops that diverts blood flow from the patent artery into the myocardial distribution of the occluded artery through the collateral vessel. It stands to reason that the degree of coronary collateral formation often determines whether patients with coronary artery disease will develop anginal symptoms in response to increases in myocardial oxygen consumption.

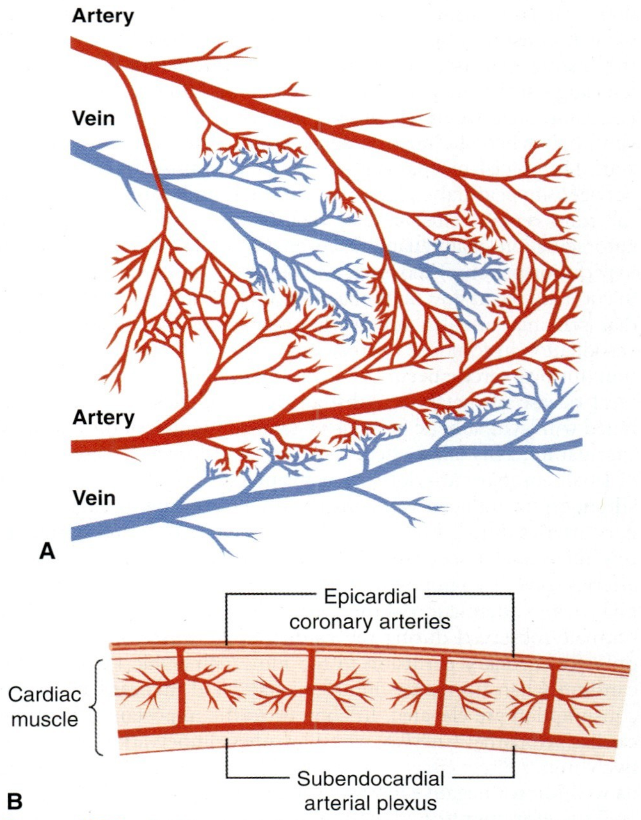

The main coronary venous drainage of the heart retraces the course of the major coronary arteries along the AV and interventricular grooves. There are three major coronary veins: the great cardiac vein courses along the AV groove and the LAD; the anterior cardiac vein is located adjacent to the RCA; and the middle cardiac vein is associated with PDA. Most often, there are two coronary veins located along either side of each major coronary arterial branch. The main coronary veins converge into the coronary sinus that empties into the posterior aspect of the right atrium immediately above the tricuspid valve.[10] Approximately 85% of total coronary blood flow returning from the LV empties into the coronary sinus, whereas the remaining flow drains directly into the atrial and ventricular cavities through the Thebesian veins. The RV veins drain into the anterior cardiac veins that empty individually into the RA.

The coronary capillary network is similar in structure to that observed in other tissue beds. The capillary to myofibril density in myocardium is approximately 1:1 because of the heart's exceptionally high metabolic demand. Adjacent capillaries are usually separated by the diameter of single myocyte. The capillary distribution is quite uniform throughout the atria and ventricles (3,000 and 4,000/mm^2) except in the AV node and interventricular septum, where it is substantially reduced. This observation provides an anatomic rationale explaining why the proximal portion of the RV and LV conduction system may be more vulnerable to ischemia. As in other capillary beds, coronary capillaries are the sites for oxygen and carbon dioxide exchange and for the movement of larger molecules (e.g., glucose) across the endothelium without the impediment of vascular smooth muscle.

Impulse Conduction

The mechanism by which the heart is electrically activated is critical for its performance. The SA node is the primary cardiac pacemaker. Decreases in firing rate, delays or blockade of normal conduction, or the presence of secondary pacemakers (e.g., AV node, bundle of His) may supersede the dominance of SA automaticity. The anterior, middle (Wenckebach), and posterior (Thorel) internodal pathways rapidly transmit the initial SA node depolarization across the RA to the AV node. Bachmann's bundle (a branch of the anterior internodal pathway) transmits the SA node depolarization across the LA through the atrial septum. Histologic examination of atrial myocytes rarely allows differentiation of cells that are specifically involved in the internodal pathway, but the unique conducting characteristics of these specialized myocytes may be clearly identified in the electrophysiology laboratory. The heart's cartilaginous skeleton electrically isolates the atria from the ventricles. As a result, atrial depolarization is directed solely to the RV and LV through the AV node, which pierces this cartilaginous framework. Because AV node conduction velocity is quite slow compared with the pathways proximal and distal to it, the AV node is responsible for the sequential contraction pattern of the atria and the ventricles. Accessory pathways that bypass the AV node and establish abnormal conduction between the atria and ventricles may precipitate supraventricular tachyarrhythmias. This is the putative mechanism

Figure 12-5 **A:** Diagram of the arterial-to-arterial and venous-to-venous anastomoses of the coronary arterial system, which allow diversion of flow if one distribution becomes blocked. **B:** Diagram of the epicardial coronary vessels lying on the cardiac muscle surface, the penetrating deep vessels, and the subendocardial arterial plexus connecting the deep vessels.

by which the bundle of Kent produces Wolff–Parkinson–White syndrome. The AV node transmits its depolarization to the His bundle, which further transmits the signal to the RV and LV via the right and left bundle branches, respectively, through Purkinje fibers within the endocardium. The conduction velocity through the His bundle, the bundle branches, and the Purkinje network is very rapid, assuring coordinated RV and LV depolarization and contraction. The relatively homogeneous distribution of Purkinje fibers throughout the LV myocardium produces temporally uniform contractile activation of the chamber (functional syncytium). Notably, artificial RV epicardial pacing (as is sometimes used during cardiac surgery) does not rely on this normal conduction sequence and, as a result, causes dyssynchronous LV activation that may be erroneously interpreted as a new ischemia-induced regional wall motion abnormality. Chronic RV apical pacing may also contribute to LV dysfunction and subsequent heart failure because of long-term imposition of contractile dyssynchrony.[11] Indeed, restoration of the normal electrical activation sequence is the basis upon which cardiac resynchronization therapy improves LV contractile function in patients with heart failure.[12]

Coronary Physiology

Blood supply to the LV is directly dependent on the difference between the aortic diastolic pressure and LV end-diastolic pressure (coronary perfusion pressure) and inversely related to the vascular resistance to flow, which varies to the fourth power of the vessel radius (Poiseuille law). Two other determinants of coronary flow are vessel length and blood viscosity, but these factors are relatively constant. Resting coronary blood flow in the adult is approximately 250 mL/min (1 mL/min/g; 5% of normal adult cardiac output). Cyclical changes in aortic pressure and the resistance to flow resulting from physical compression of the intramural coronary arteries govern the pulsatile pattern of LV coronary flow. The LV subendocardium is exposed to a higher pressure than the subepicardium during systole, and the intraventricular tissue pressure actually exceeds peak developed LV pressure. As a result, the subendocardial layer is much more susceptible to ischemia when a flow-limiting coronary stenosis, pressure-overload hypertrophy, or pronounced tachycardia is present. Coronary blood flow is also reduced when aortic diastolic pressure is low, such as occurs in severe aortic valvular insufficiency. Elevated LV end-diastolic pressure, as typically observed in heart failure, also reduces coronary perfusion pressure and blood flow. Venous blood flow in the coronary sinus peaks during late systole because the contracting LV compresses major venous drainage channels.

Another important determinant of coronary blood flow is coronary vascular resistance (estimated using the ratio of coronary blood flow to perfusion pressure), which also varies substantially during the cardiac cycle. While coronary perfusion certainly changes in response to aortic, intramyocardial, and coronary venous pressures, the primary regulator of coronary blood flow is the variable resistance imparted by coronary vascular smooth muscle. For example, activation of the sympathetic nervous system increases coronary vascular smooth muscle tone, thereby making coronary vascular resistance greater. The degree of smooth muscle stretch (myogenic factor) also influences coronary vascular tone and resistance. However, metabolic factors are the primary physiologic determinants of coronary vascular tone and myocardial perfusion. The ratio of subepicardial to subendocardial blood flow remains near unity throughout the cardiac cycle despite the differentially greater systolic compressive forces exerted on the subendocardium. β adrenoceptor-mediated vasodilation and local release of metabolic autocrine substances (e.g., adenosine) produced by the myocardium itself act to offset this greater resistance to flow in the subendocardium. The relative maintenance of subendocardial blood flow despite compression is also related to the redundancy of arteriolar and capillary anastomoses within the subendocardium.

The heart normally extracts between 75% and 80% of arterial oxygen content, by far the greatest oxygen extraction of all the body's organs. The majority of myocardial oxygen consumption results from the magnitude of LV pressure during isovolumic contraction and the rate at which this pressure develops. The LV's diameter and wall thickness also have profound effects on myocardial oxygen consumption as dictated by the Law of Laplace (see below). Heart rate is the primary determinant of myocardial oxygen consumption in the intact heart. Increases in myocardial contractility, preload, and afterload are also associated with greater myocardial oxygen consumption. Cardiac oxygen extraction is near maximal under resting conditions and cannot substantially increase during exercise. As a result, the primary mechanism by which myocardium is able to meets its oxygen requirements during exercise is through enhanced oxygen delivery, which is proportional to coronary blood flow when hemoglobin concentration is constant. Thus, it is not surprising that myocardial oxygen consumption is the most important determinant of coronary blood flow. For example, myocardial oxygen consumption and corresponding coronary blood flow increase by a magnitude of four- to fivefold during strenuous physical exercise. The difference between maximal and resting coronary blood flow (coronary reserve) determines the magnitude with which coronary blood flow can rise during exercise-induced increases in myocardial oxygen consumption. Coronary vascular resistance is greater in the resting, perfused heart than in the contracting heart. These data suggest that increases in coronary blood flow exceed those of perfusion pressure in response to greater myocardial oxygen consumption when the heart is contracting versus when it is quiescent. The precise mechanisms responsible for this close correlation between myocardial oxygen consumption and coronary vasomotor tone remain elusive. The factors responsible for coronary autoregulation (maintenance of coronary blood flow despite changes in perfusion pressure) and reactive hyperemia (the several-fold increase in coronary blood flow above baseline after a brief period of myocardial ischemia) are also not clearly understood. Metabolic coronary vasodilation in response to enhanced myocardial oxygen consumption during exercise occurs, at least in part, as a result of enhanced local release of metabolic substrates (e.g., adenosine, ADP) combined with sympathetic nervous system stimulation of the coronary vasculature. This latter effect causes a "feed-forward" vasodilation of small coronary arterioles by activating β adrenoceptors.[13] An α adrenoceptor-induced vasoconstriction also occurs in larger coronary arteries during exercise. Although seemingly counterintuitive, this differential vasoconstriction of larger caliber upstream coronary arteries serves two important functions: reduction of vascular compliance and attenuation of the wide swings in coronary blood flow normally observed during the cardiac cycle. These actions act to preserve coronary perfusion to the more vulnerable LV subendocardium when heart rate, inotropic state, and myocardial oxygen consumption are elevated. In contrast to the important role of the cardiac sympathetic nerves, parasympathetic innervation has a relatively minor direct effect on coronary blood flow regulation despite its well-known negative inotropic and chronotropic actions.

The aforementioned conclusions about sympathetic nervous system control of the coronary circulation are based on alterations in the slope of the myocardial oxygen consumption–coronary venous oxygen tension relation during graded exercise in the presence of exogenous α or β adrenoceptor blockade. The β adrenoceptor appears to account for only one-fourth of the total coronary vasodilation observed during exercise-induced hyperemia, but most of this vasodilation is most likely related to local or autocrine metabolic factors that act on coronary vascular smooth muscle with or without the additional modulation by vascular endothelium. Adenine nucleotides from red blood cells or the myocardium itself may activate endothelial purinergic receptors to produce coronary vasodilation during exercise.[14] Many factors have been proposed to individually or collectively modulate coronary blood flow at the arteriolar or capillary level, including adenosine, bradykinin, nitric oxide, arterial oxygen or carbon dioxide tension, acid–base status, osmolarity, plasma electrolyte (e.g., K^+, Ca^{2+}) concentrations, and various products of arachidonic acid metabolism. Many of these factors exert predictable direct effects. For example, hypoxia or ischemia decreases arterial oxygen tension and pH concomitant with increases in carbon dioxide tension, adenosine release, and the plasma concentrations of K^+ and Ca^{2+}. These changes collectively augment coronary blood flow during exercise, but none individually is solely responsible for this vasodilation. Adenosine receptor blockade does not alter coronary blood flow under resting conditions or during exercise. Similarly, inhibition of nitric oxide (NO) production or antagonism of adenosine triphosphate-sensitive potassium (K_{ATP}) channels does not affect the myocardial oxygen consumption–coronary venous oxygen content relationship during graded exercise. Nevertheless, it is quite clear that NO and K_{ATP} channels are important regulators of myocardial oxygen supply–demand relations under resting conditions. Adenosine released during hypoxia or ischemia also causes coronary vasodilation, and K_{ATP} channel activation mediates this effect. Adenosine and K_{ATP} channels also play a central role in reactive hyperemia after brief myocardial ischemia, but neither mediator appears to be required for coronary autoregulation. Indeed, the K_{ATP} channel may act to reduce coronary vascular smooth muscle tone and maintain a higher basal level of coronary blood flow during resting conditions. While not acting as a local metabolic vasodilator of small coronary arteries and arterioles per se, NO may dilate larger epicardial coronary vessels in response to downstream vasodilation and prevent excessive sheer stress on coronary vascular endothelium. Endothelin and thromboxane A_2 produce direct coronary vasoconstriction in vitro, but the precise role of these substances on the regulation of coronary blood flow in vivo has not been defined.

Cardiac Myocyte Anatomy and Function

Ultrastructure

The heart contracts and relaxes nearly three billion times during an average lifetime, based on an average heart rate of 70 beats per minute and a life expectancy of 75 years. A review of cardiac myocyte ultrastructure provides important insights into how this remarkable feat is possible. The sarcolemma is the external membrane of the cardiac muscle cell. The sarcolemma contains ion channels (e.g., Na^+, K^+, Ca^{2+}), ion pumps and exchangers (e.g., Na^+–K^+ ATPase, Ca^{2+}-ATPase, Na^+–Ca^{2+} or Na^+–H^+ exchangers), G protein-coupled and other receptors (e.g., β_1 adrenergic, muscarinic, adenosine, opioid), and transporter enzymes that regulate intracellular ion concentrations, facilitate signal transduction, and provide metabolic substrates required for energy production. Deep invaginations of the sarcolemma, known as transverse (T) tubules, penetrate the internal structure of the myocyte at regular intervals. The T-tubules assure rapid, simultaneous transmission of the depolarizing impulses that initiate myocyte contraction. The cardiac myocyte is densely packed with mitochondria that are responsible for production of large quantities of high-energy phosphates (e.g., ATP) needed for contraction and relaxation. The sarcomere is the fundamental contractile unit of cardiac muscle. The myofilaments within each sarcomere are arranged in parallel cross-striated bundles of thin (containing actin, tropomyosin, and the troponin complex) and thick (primarily composed of myosin and its supporting proteins) fibers. Sarcomeres are connected in series and produce characteristic shortening and thickening of the long and short axes of each myocyte, respectively, during contraction.

Observations from light and electron microscopy led to the definition of the sarcomere's distinctive structural features. The area of overlap of thick and thin fibers characterizes the "A" band. This band lengthens as the sarcomere shortens during contraction. The "I" band represents the region of the sarcomere that contains thin filaments alone, and this band is reduced in width as the cell contracts. Each "I" band is bisected by a "Z" (from the German *zuckung* [twitch]) line, which delineates the border between two adjacent sarcomeres. As a result, the length of each sarcomere contains a complete "A" band and two symmetric one-half "I" bands located between "Z" lines. A central "M" band is also present within the "A" band. This "M" band is composed of thick filaments spatially constrained in a cross-sectional hexagonal matrix by myosin-binding protein C. A densely intertwined network of sarcoplasmic reticulum (SR) invests each bundle of contractile proteins and functions as a Ca^{2+} reservoir. This SR network assures homogeneous distribution and reuptake of activator Ca^{2+} throughout the myofilaments during contraction and relaxation, respectively. The SR subsarcolemmal cisternae are specialized structures located immediately adjacent to, but not continuous with, the sarcolemmal and transverse tubular membranes. The cisternae are packed with ryanodine receptors that function as the primary Ca^{2+} release channel for the SR. The contractile machinery and the mitochondria that power it occupy more than 80% of the total volume of the cardiac myocyte. This observation emphasizes that mechanical function, and not new protein synthesis, is the predominant activity of the cardiac myocyte. Intercalated discs connect adjacent myocytes through the fascia adherens and desmosomes that link actin and other proteins between cells, respectively. The intercalated discs also provide a seamless electrical connection between myocytes via large, nonspecific ion channels (known as "gap junctions") that facilitate intercellular cytosolic diffusion of ions and small molecules.

Contractile Apparatus

Myosin, actin, tropomyosin, and the three-protein troponin complex compose the six major components of the contractile apparatus. Myosin (molecular weight of approximately 500 kDa; length, 0.17 μm) contains two interwoven chain helices with two globular heads that bind to actin and two additional pairs of light chains. Enzymatic digestion of myosin divides the structure into light (containing the tail section of the complex) and heavy (composed of the globular heads and the light chains) meromyosin. The elongated tail section of the myosin complex (light meromyosin) functions as the main structural support of the molecule (Fig. 12-6). The globular heads of the myosin dimer contain two "hinges," located at the junction of the distal light chains and the tail helix, that play an essential role in myofilament shortening during contraction. These globular structures bind to actin, thereby activating an ATPase that is involved in hinge rotation and release of actin during contraction and relaxation, respectively. The activity of this actin-activated myosin ATPase is a

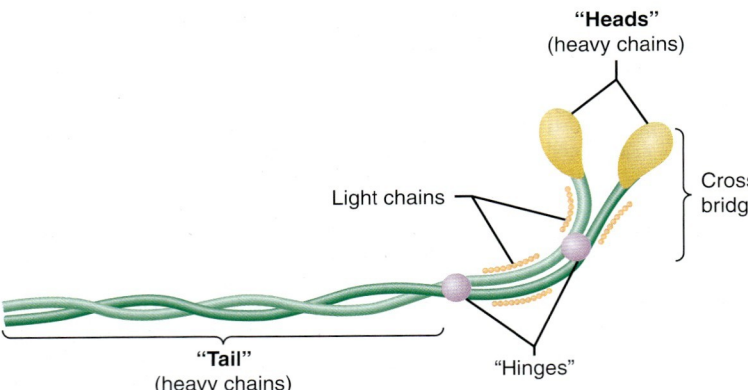

Figure 12-6 Schematic illustration of the myosin molecule demonstrating double helix tail, globular heads that form cross bridges with actin during contraction, two pairs of light chains, and "hinges" (cleavage sites of proteolytic enzymes) that divide the molecule into meromyosin fragments (see text).

major determinant of the maximum velocity of sarcomere shortening. Notably, adult and neonatal atrial and ventricular myocardium contain several different myosin ATPase isoforms that are distinguished by their relative ATPase activity. The myosin molecules are primarily arranged in series along the length of the thick filament, but are abutted "tail-to-tail" in the center of the thick filament. This orientation facilitates shortening of the distance between "Z" lines during contraction as the thin filaments are drawn symmetrically toward the sarcomere's center.

The light chains contained within the myosin complex serve "regulatory" or "essential" roles. Regulatory myosin light chains may favorably modulate myosin–actin interaction through Ca^{2+}-dependent protein kinase phosphorylation, whereas essential light chains serve an as yet undefined obligate function in myosin activity because their removal denatures the myosin molecule. Discussion of myosin light chain isoforms is beyond the scope of this chapter, but it is important to note that isoform switches from ventricular to atrial forms have been observed in left ventricular hypertrophy that may contribute to contractile dysfunction.[15] In addition to myosin and its binding protein, thick filaments contain titin, a long elastic protein that attaches myosin to the "Z" lines. Titin is thought to be a "length sensor" that establishes progressively greater passive restoring forces as sarcomere length approaches its maximum or minimum (similar to a bidirectional spring).[16] Compression and stretching of titin occur during decreases and increases in muscle load, thereby resisting further sarcomere shortening and lengthening, respectively. Thus, titin is a third important elastic element (in addition to actin and myosin) that contributes to the stress-strain mechanical properties of cardiac muscle.[17]

Actin is the major component of the thin filament. Actin is a 42-kDa, ovoid-shaped, globular protein ("G" form; 5.5 nm in diameter) that exists as a filamentous (F) polymer in cardiac muscle. F-actin binds ADP and a divalent cation (Ca^{2+} or Mg^{2+}), but unlike myosin, the molecule does not directly hydrolyze high-energy nucleotides (e.g., ATP). F-actin is wound in double-stranded helical chains of G-actin monomers that resemble two intertwined strands of pearls. A single complete helical revolution of filamentous actin is approximately 77 nm in length and contains 14 G-actin monomers. Actin derives its name from its function as the "activator of myosin" ATPase through its reversible binding with myosin. The hydrolysis of ATP by this actin–myosin complex provides the chemical energy required to produce the conformational changes in the myosin heads that drive the contraction–relaxation cycle within the sarcomere. Tropomyosin is one of two major inhibitors of actin–myosin interaction. Tropomyosin (length of 40 nm; weight between 68 and 72 kDa) is a rigid double-stranded α-helix protein. A single disulfide bond links the two helices of tropomyosin. Human tropomyosin contains both α and β isoforms (34 and 36 kDa, respectively) and may be present as a homo- or heterodimer.[18] Tropomyosin serves to stiffen the thin filament through its position within the longitudinal cleft between intertwined F-actin polymers (Fig. 12-7). However, the primary function of tropomyosin is its Ca^{2+}-dependent interaction with troponin complex proteins. This tropomyosin–troponin interaction provides the microscopic link between sarcolemmal membrane depolarization to actin–myosin binding (excitation–contraction coupling). Cytoskeletal proteins, including actinin and nebulette, anchor the thin filaments to the "Z" lines.[19]

The troponin proteins serve complementary yet distinct roles as regulators of the contractile apparatus.[20] The troponin complexes are arranged at 40-nm intervals along the length of the thin filament. Troponin C (so named because this molecule binds Ca^{2+}) exists in a highly conserved, single isoform in cardiac muscle. Troponin C is composed of a central nine-turn α helix separating two globular regions that contain four discrete amino acid sequences capable of binding divalent cations. Two (termed sites I and II) of the four amino acid–cation binding sequences are Ca^{2+}-specific. This feature allows the troponin C molecule to respond to the acute changes in intracellular Ca^{2+} concentration that accompany contraction and relaxation. Cardiac troponin I (inhibitor) is a 23-kDa protein that exists in a single isoform. Troponin I alone weakly prevents the interaction between actin and myosin, but when combined with tropomyosin, the troponin I–tropomyosin complex becomes the primary inhibitor of actin–myosin binding. Troponin I contains a serine residue that may be phosphorylated by protein kinase A via cAMP, reducing troponin C–Ca^{2+} binding and enhancing relaxation during administration

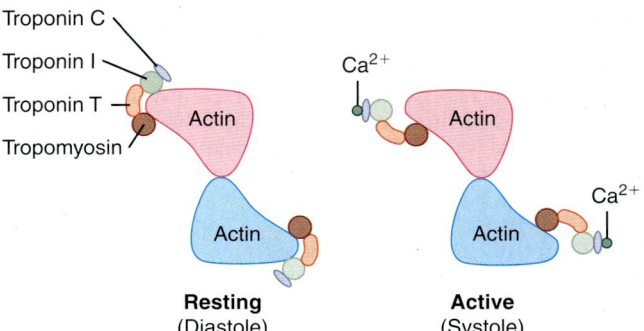

Figure 12-7 Cross-sectional schematic illustration demonstrating the structural relationship between the troponin–tropomyosin complex and actin under resting conditions (left panel) and after Ca^{2+} binding to troponin C (right panel, see text).

of β_1 adrenoceptor agonists (e.g., dobutamine) or phosphodiesterase fraction III inhibitors (e.g., milrinone). Troponin T (so named because it binds other troponin molecules and tropomyosin) is the largest of the troponin proteins and exists in four major isoforms. Troponin T anchors the other troponin molecules and influences the relative Ca^{2+} sensitivity of the complex.[21]

Calcium–Myofilament Interaction

A series of conformational changes in the troponin–tropomyosin complex occur as a result of Ca^{2+}–troponin C binding that culminate in exposure of the myosin-binding site on the actin molecule. During conditions in which intracellular Ca^{2+} concentration is low (10^{-7} M; diastole), very little Ca^{2+} is bound to troponin C, and a troponin complex constrains each tropomyosin molecule to the outer region of the groove between F-actin filaments. This configuration blocks cross-bridge formation and prevents myosin–actin interaction. Thus, the troponin–tropomyosin complex creates a basal inhibitory state under resting conditions. A 100-fold increase in intracellular Ca^{2+} concentration (10^{-5} M) occurs as a result of sarcolemmal depolarization (systole). Opening of L- and T-type sarcolemmal Ca^{2+} channels allows Ca^{2+} influx into the myocyte from the extracellular compartment and stimulates Ca^{2+}-dependent Ca^{2+} release from the SR through its ryanodine receptors. When Ca^{2+} is bound to troponin C, troponin C elongates and its interactions with troponin I and T are enhanced. This allosteric rearrangement and the altered binding characteristics that it produces weaken the interaction between troponin I and actin, allow repositioning of the tropomyosin molecule along the F-actin filaments, and reverse the baseline inhibition of actin–myosin binding by tropomyosin.[22] As a result, Ca^{2+} binding to troponin C is directly linked to a series of changes in regulatory protein structure, negating inhibition of the binding site for myosin on the actin molecule and allowing cross-bridge formation to occur. This antagonism of inhibition is fully reversible: Ca^{2+} dissociation from troponin C restores the original troponin–tropomyosin conformation on F-actin and facilitates relaxation.

A Ca^{2+}-ATPase located in the SR membrane (sarcoendoplasmic reticulum Ca^{2+}-ATPase, SERCA) removes most of the Ca^{2+} ions from the myofilaments and the cytosol after membrane repolarization. This Ca^{2+} is stored (approximately 10^{-3} M) in the SR bound to calsequestrin and calreticulin until the next sarcolemmal depolarization. The Na^+–Ca^{2+} exchanger and a Ca^{2+}-ATPase located within the sarcolemmal membrane also remove a small quantity of Ca^{2+} from the sarcoplasm. Phospholamban is a small protein (6 kDa) located in the SR membrane that partially inhibits the activity of the dominant form (type 2a) of cardiac SERCA under baseline conditions. However, phosphorylation of this protein by protein kinase A blocks this inhibition and enhances the rate of SERCA uptake of Ca^{2+} into the SR.[23] This action increases the rate and extent of relaxation (positive lusitropic effect) and augments the amount of Ca^{2+} available for the next contraction (positive inotropic effect). Thus, a cAMP-dependent protein kinase that is responsive to β_1 adrenoceptor stimulation or phosphodiesterase fraction III inhibition regulates SERCA activity. This observation explains why positive inotropic drugs such as dobutamine and milrinone also augment relaxation.

Myosin–Actin Interaction

The biochemistry of sarcomere contraction is most often described using a simplified four-component model (Fig. 12-8).[24] High-affinity binding of ATP to the catalytic domain of myosin initiates the series of events that cause sarcomere contraction. Myosin ATPase hydrolyzes the ATP molecule into ADP and inorganic phosphate, but the reaction products do not immediately dissociate from myosin. Instead, an "active" complex is

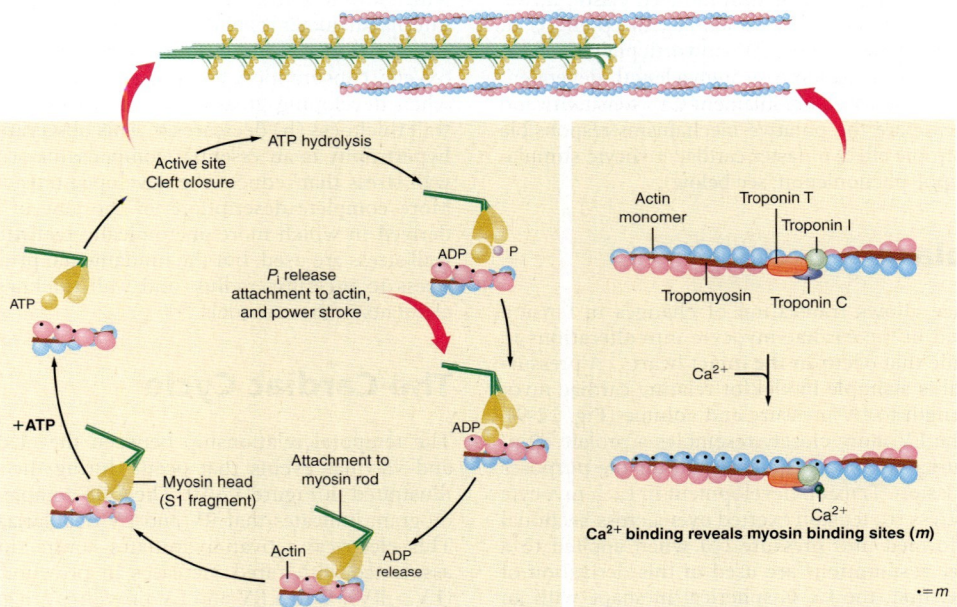

Figure 12-8 Schematic illustration of the actin filaments and its individual monomers and active myosin-binding sites (*m*; left panel). The myosin head is dissociated from actin by binding with adenosine triphosphate (ATP). Subsequent ATP hydrolysis and release of inorganic phosphate (P_i) "cocks" the head group into a tension-generating configuration. Attachment of the myosin head to actin allows the head to apply tension to the myosin rod and the actin filament. The right panel illustrates Ca^{2+} binding to troponin C, which causes troponin I to decrease its affinity for actin. As a result in a conformational shift in tropomyosin position (see text), seven sites on actin monomers are revealed.

formed that retains the reaction's chemical energy as potential energy. In the absence of actin, subsequent dissociation of ADP and phosphate from myosin is the rate-limiting step of myosin ATPase. The muscle remains relaxed under these conditions. However, the activity of myosin ATPase is markedly increased when the myosin–ADP–phosphate complex is bound to actin, and the chemical energy obtained from ATP hydrolysis is transferred into mechanical work. Attachment of myosin to its binding site on the actin molecule releases the phosphate anion from the myosin head, producing a unique molecular conformation within the cross-bridge structure that generates tension in both myofilaments.[25] Release of ADP and the stored potential energy from this activated conformation produce rotation of the cross-bridge (power stroke) at the hinge point separating the myosin helical tail region from the globular myosin head and its associated light chain proteins. Each cross-bridge rotation generates 3 to 4×10^{-12} N of force and moves myosin 11 nm along the actin molecule.[26] Completion of myosin head rotation and ADP release does not immediately dissociate the myosin-active complex, but leaves it in a low-energy bound (rigor) state. Separation of myosin and actin requires binding of a new ATP molecule to myosin. The process is then repeated, provided that there is an adequate ATP supply and troponin–tropomyosin inhibition does not block the myosin-binding site on actin.

Several factors may affect the efficiency of cross-bridge biochemistry and myocardial contractility independent of autonomic nervous system activity or administration of vasoactive drugs. A direct relationship between myosin ATPase activity and the maximal velocity of unloaded muscle shortening (V_{max}) exists. The normal increase in intracellular Ca^{2+} concentration that occurs after sarcolemmal depolarization (from 10^{-7} to 10^{-5} M) enhances baseline myosin ATPase activity fivefold before it interacts with actin, increasing V_{max}. Contractile force also depends on sarcomere length immediately before sarcolemmal depolarization. This length-dependent activation (Frank–Starling effect) may be related to an increase in myofilament Ca^{2+} sensitivity, favorable alterations in spacing between myofilaments, or titin-induced elastic recoil. An abrupt increase in load during contraction (Anrep effect) or after a prolonged pause between beats (Woodworth phenomenon) transiently enhances contractile force through a length-dependent activation mechanism. Increased myofilament Ca^{2+} sensitivity and greater SR Ca^{2+} release are the putative mechanisms responsible for the positive inotropic effect of faster cardiac myocyte stimulation frequency (Treppe phenomenon; see below).

Law of Laplace

The Law of Laplace allows translation of changes in tension and length observed in the cardiac myocyte into alterations in pressure and volume that occur in the intact heart.[27] A pressurized, spherical shell is a simple model for relating cardiac myocyte tension and length to LV pressure and volume (Fig. 12-9). The geometry of the LV more closely resembles a prolate ellipsoid,[28] but a pressurized sphere is quite useful for the purposes of the current discussion. Tension development in each myocyte increases LV wall stress (σ; tension exerted over a cross-sectional area) that is transformed into pressure (p) when applied to a fluid (blood). Three assumptions are used in this derivation of the Law of Laplace: first, the LV is spherical in shape with an internal radius (r) and uniform wall thickness (h); second, σ is presumed to be constant throughout the thickness of the LV wall; and third, the LV exists in static equilibrium (i.e., is not actively contracting). In this model, "p" is the force acting to distend the LV, whereas "σ" represents the force resisting this distension. It

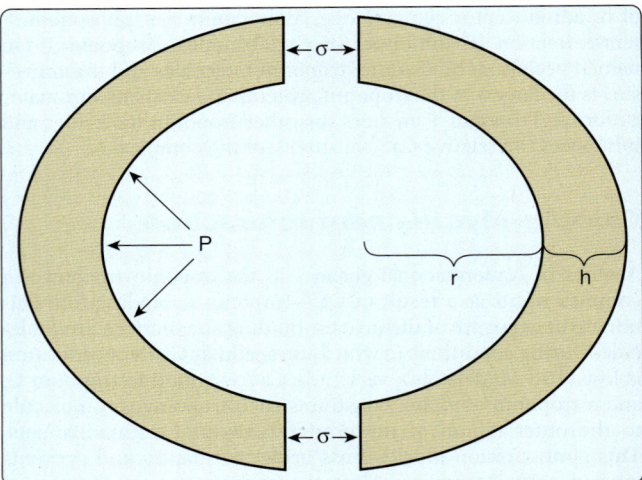

Figure 12-9 This schematic diagram depicts the opposing forces within a theoretical LV sphere that determine the Law of Laplace. LV pressure (P) pushes the sphere apart, whereas wall stress (σ) holds the sphere together. r, LV radius; h, LV thickness. (Reproduced with permission from Kaplan JA, Reich DL, Savino JS. *Kaplan's Cardiac Anesthesia: The Echo Era*. 6th ed. St. Louis, MO: Elsevier Saunders; 2011:105.)

can be easily shown that σ = pr/2h, indicating that wall stress varies directly with pressure and chamber radius and inversely with wall thickness. Despite the model's assumptions and simplicity, this version of the Law of Laplace allows appreciation of the factors that alter LV wall stress and how cardiac pathology influences them. For example, the chronically elevated LV pressure (p) that occurs in the presence of severe aortic valve stenosis or uncontrolled essential hypertension increases σ because these variables are directly related. Similarly, LV dilation associated with chronic mitral regurgitation also increases σ because the internal diameter (r) of the LV is larger. Notably, increases in wall stress in either of these circumstances causes greater myocardial oxygen consumption because each myocyte uses more energy when developing greater tension.[29] Conversely, an increase in wall thickness (h) decreases σ. This observation emphasizes that hypertrophy is an essential compensatory response to elevated wall stress that reduces the developed tension in each myocyte. More complete descriptions of the Law of Laplace have been derived in which more anatomically realistic LV geometry and wall stress are used, but the fundamental principles relating wall stress to pressure, radius, and wall thickness remain essential elements in these models.[30,31]

The Cardiac Cycle

The temporal relationship between the electrical, mechanical, and valvular events that occur during the cardiac cycle[32] are illustrated in Figure 12-10. The QRS complex of the electrocardiogram indicates that RV and LV depolarization has occurred. This electrical activation initiates contraction (systole) and is associated with rapid increases in pressure in both chambers (LV > RV). When RV and LV pressures are greater than RA and LA pressures, the tricuspid and mitral valves close, respectively, and produce first heart sound (S_1). Isovolumic contraction, rapid ejection, and slower ejection phases are the three major phases of LV systole. During LV isovolumic contraction, LV volume is constant because both the aortic and mitral valves are closed.

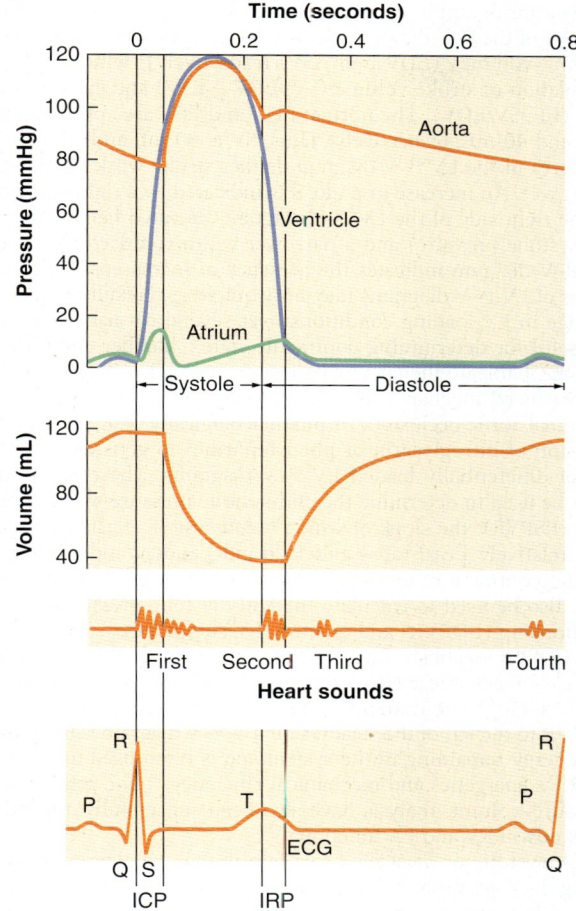

Figure 12-10 Mechanical and electrical events of the cardiac cycle showing also the LV volume curve and the heart sounds. Note the LV isovolumic contraction (ICP) and the relaxation period (IRP), during which there is no change in LV volume because aortic and mitral valves are closed. The LV decreases in volume as it ejects its contents into the aorta. During the first third of systolic ejection (the rapid ejection period), the curve of emptying is steep. ECG, electrocardiogram.

However, LV shape becomes more spherical because of decreases in longitudinal dimension. The maximal rate of increase in LV pressure (+dP/dt), a commonly used index of myocardial contractility, also occurs during LV isovolumic contraction. In contrast to the synchronous LV, the peristaltic-like contraction of the RV inflow and outflow tracts precludes true isovolumic contraction in the RV.[33,34] The pressures in the aortic and pulmonic roots reach their minima before the corresponding valves open. When LV and RV pressures are greater than aortic and PA pressures, respectively, rapid ejection of approximately two-thirds of the end-diastolic volume of each chamber occurs. The kinetic energy of LV and RV contraction is stored as potential energy in the elastic aorta and PA, respectively, which is then released to the corresponding distal vascular beds during diastole. The relative compliance of the proximal systemic and PA vasculature determines the magnitude of this stored potential energy. As aortic and PA pressures reach their maximum values, ejection falls dramatically and stops entirely when the ventricles begin to repolarize. Aortic and PA pressures briefly exceed LV and RV pressures as this slower ejection phase comes to an end,

and the corresponding valves close in response to these reversed pressure gradients. Valve closure causes the second heart sound (S_2); this event denotes end-systole. S_2 is normally split because the pulmonic valve closes slightly after the aortic valve.

Isovolumic relaxation, early ventricular filling, diastasis, and atrial systole are the four phases of LV diastole. LV volume is constant during isovolumic relaxation because both the aortic and mitral valves are closed. LV pressure very rapidly declines as the myofilaments uncouple. The mitral valve opens when LA pressure exceeds LV pressure, and the pressure gradient between the chambers drives blood stored in the LA into the LV. LV pressure continues to fall after the mitral valve opens[35] because sarcomere relaxation is incomplete and recoil of compressed elastic components occurs. This process establishes a time-dependent pressure gradient between the LA and LV.[36] The instantaneous LA pressure immediately before mitral valve opening combined with the rate and extent with which LV pressure declines are the primary determinants of the pressure gradient between the two chambers.[37] Early LV filling is quite rapid: the peak velocities of mitral blood flow during early filling and aortic blood flow during ejection are similar (approximately 1 m/s).[38] Transmitral blood flow causes a vortex ring to form within the LV, which facilitates selective filling of the LV outflow tract because of the LV's structural asymmetry.[39] Age and cardiac disease (e.g., myocardial ischemia, pressure-overload hypertrophy) often delay LV relaxation, an important cause of diastolic dysfunction because the LA-to-LV pressure gradient is reduced, early LV filling is attenuated, and vortex ring formation is partially inhibited.[40,41] LV pressure will continue to fall to subatmospheric values if blood flow across the mitral valve is experimentally prevented.[42] This "diastolic suction" effect assures that the LV continues to fill even if LA pressure is zero (e.g., during profound hypovolemia or intense exercise).[43] The early filling phase of diastole normally provides 70% to 75% of final stroke volume. During the third phase of diastole, the LA acts as a conduit for pulmonary venous blood flow to flow freely through the open mitral valve into the LV. Less than 5% of total stroke volume enters the LV during diastasis, which may be shortened or eliminated by tachycardia.[44] The final phase of diastole is atrial systole. LA contraction again creates a positive pressure LA to LV gradient and stimulates active blood flow. The sphincter-like anatomy of the pulmonary venous–LA junction largely prevents retrograde blood flow into the pulmonary veins unless LA pressure is markedly elevated (e.g., heart failure, severe mitral regurgitation). Atrial systole normally generates 15% to 25% of final stroke volume, but this percentage increases when delayed LV relaxation or reduced LV compliance is present. Thus, it is common for patients with such abnormalities to develop acute hemodynamic instability when LA contraction suddenly becomes timed improperly (e.g., AV conduction block) or disappears entirely (e.g., atrial fibrillation).

Three major deflections are observed in the LA pressure waveform during sinus rhythm. LA contraction follows the P wave of atrial depolarization and produces the "a" wave of atrial systole. An increase in LA preload or contractility augments the magnitude of the "a" wave. The rate of deceleration of the "a" wave is an index of LA relaxation.[45] A second small increase in LA pressure occurs with the onset of LV contraction because the mitral valve closes. This deflection is known as the "c" wave. The final "v" wave results from LA filling during LV systole and early relaxation as pulmonary venous return enters the LA while the mitral valve is closed. Mitral regurgitation or reduction in LA compliance enhances the magnitude of this "v" wave.[46] Similar changes in the RA pressure waveform deflections also occur. Indeed, the RA "a-c-v" morphology is easily observed in the external jugular veins when examining most patients in supine position.

The Pressure–Volume Diagram

A simultaneous temporal plot of continuous LV pressure and volume creates a phase–space diagram that is useful for analysis of LV systolic and diastolic function (Fig. 12-11). The LV pressure–volume (P–V) diagram proceeds in a counterclockwise direction. End-diastole initiates the cardiac cycle (point A, Fig. 12-11). This is followed by isovolumic contraction, in which a rapid increase in LV pressure occurs without change in LV volume. When LV pressure is greater than aorta pressure, the aortic valve opens (point B, Fig. 12-11). Ejection of blood from the LV volume into the aorta and the proximal great vessels causes a precipitous decline in LV volume. The aortic valve closes when LV pressure drops below aortic pressure (point C, Fig. 12-11). When LV pressure falls below LA pressure during isovolumic relaxation, the mitral valve opens (point D, Fig. 12-11) and LV filling then occurs, causing a large increase in LV volume concomitant with a small increase in LV pressure during the remainder of diastole. This final stage completes a single circuit (cardiac cycle) around the P–V diagram.

The LV P–V diagram allows recognition of major cardiac events (e.g., aortic and mitral valve opening and closing) without formal electrocardiographic correlation. The lower right and upper left corners of the P–V diagram identify the LV end-diastolic and end-systolic volumes (EDV and ESV, respectively), which facilitate calculation of stroke volume (SV; EDV − ESV) and ejection fraction (EF; SV/EDV). The normal EDV and ESV are approximately 120 and 40 mL, respectively. Thus, SV is 80 mL and EF is 67%. The area of the LV P–V diagram defines stroke work for the cardiac cycle. An increase in preload is indicated by a rightward shift of the right side of the LV P–V diagram. Elevated height (greater LV systolic pressure) and a narrower width (reduced SV) of the LV P–V diagram indicates the presence of increased afterload. A series of LV P–V diagrams may be acquired as a result of an acute change in LV loading conditions over several cardiac cycles and is useful for determining contractile state, chamber compliance, and mechanical efficiency. Changes in preload or afterload may be produced mechanically (e.g., transient inferior vena caval or proximal aortic occlusion) or pharmacologically (e.g., intravenous infusion of nitroglycerin or phenylephrine) to generate a nested set of differentially loaded LV P–V diagrams. These loops may then be used to determine the end-systolic pressure–volume relation (ESPVR), the slope of which ("end-systolic elastance" [E_{es}]) is a relatively heart-rate– and load-independent index of myocardial contractility in vivo.[47] The same set of LV P–V diagrams may also be used to calculate the end-diastolic pressure–volume relationship (EDPVR) and quantify LV compliance.[27] The ESPVR and EDPVR establish the operational range of the LV and define the LV's mechanical characteristics during systole and diastole, respectively.[48] The triangular space that lies between ESPVR and EDPVR to the left of the steady-state LV P–V diagram is the potential energy remaining in the system and is often used to quantify the LV's energetics and mechanical efficiency.[49] The principles of pressure–volume analysis have also been successfully applied to the study of RV and LA function.[50,51]

LV systolic or diastolic heart failure may be clearly depicted using P–V analysis.[52] Pure LV systolic dysfunction is represented by a reduction in the ESPVR slope and often occurs in conjunction with LV dilation, as illustrated by a right shift of the P–V diagram without a substantial change in the position of EDPVR (Fig. 12-12). The increase in preload (right shift) is a compensatory response to depression of myocardial contractility that serves to maintain stroke volume, but occurs at a cost of elevated LV filling pressure, greater LV volume, and increased myocardial oxygen consumption. An increase in EDPVR defines a reduction in LV compliance consistent with LV diastolic dysfunction because LV pressure is greater for a given LV volume. In pure diastolic heart failure, myocardial contractility is preserved (ESPVR is unchanged), but clinical symptoms are present because LV filling pressures are elevated. Simultaneously depressed ESPVR and elevated EDPVR are observed in the presence of combined LV systolic and diastolic dysfunction. Under these circumstances, the LV operates in a restricted range of preload and afterload conditions. Stroke volume and cardiac output are often substantially compromised as a result, leading to global tissue malperfusion.

Determinants of Systolic Function

The LV's ability to collect and eject blood determines its overall performance. The amount of blood that the LV contains before the onset of contraction (preload), the arterial resistance to emptying that the LV must overcome during ejection (afterload), and the contractile properties of the LV myocardium (inotropic state) determine the stroke volume for each cardiac cycle (Fig. 12-13). These three factors combine with the heart rate and rhythm to

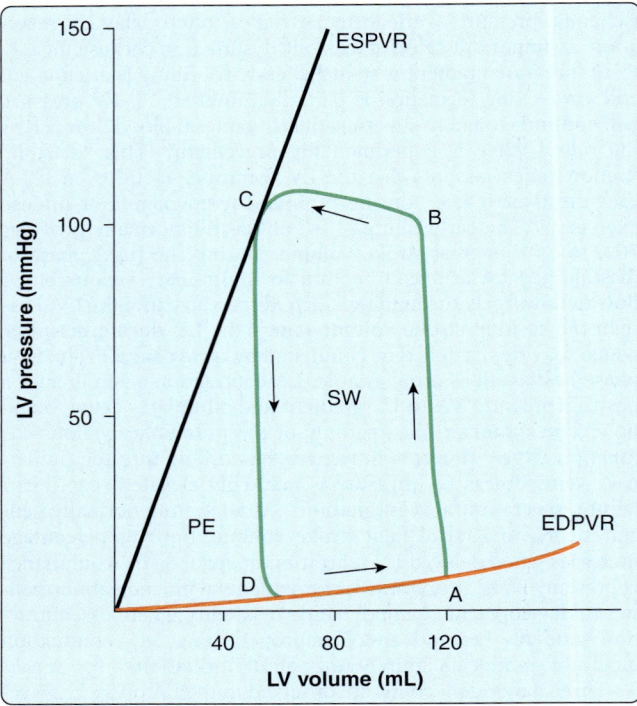

Figure 12-11 This illustration depicts the steady-state LV pressure–volume diagram. The cardiac cycle proceeds in a time-dependent counterclockwise direction (*arrows*). Points A, B, C, and D correspond to LV end-diastole (closure of the mitral valve), opening of the aortic valve, LV end-systole (closure of the aortic valve), and opening of the mitral valve, respectively. Segments AB, BC, CD, and DA represent isovolumic contraction, ejection, isovolumic relaxation, and filling, respectively. The LV is constrained to operate within the boundaries of the end-systolic and end-diastolic pressure–volume relations (ESPVR and EDPVR, respectively). The area inscribed by the LV pressure–volume diagram is stroke work (SW) performed during the cardiac cycle. The area to the left of the LV pressure–volume diagram between ESPVR and EDPVR is the remaining potential energy (PE) of the system. (Reproduced with permission from Kaplan JA, Reich DL, Savino JS. *Kaplan's Cardiac Anesthesia: The Echo Era.* 6th ed. St. Louis, MO: Elsevier Saunders; 2011:107.)

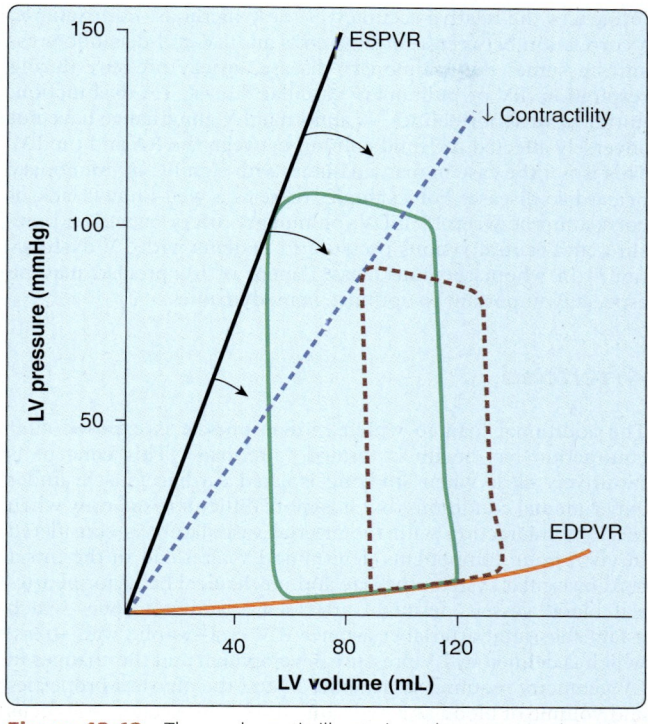 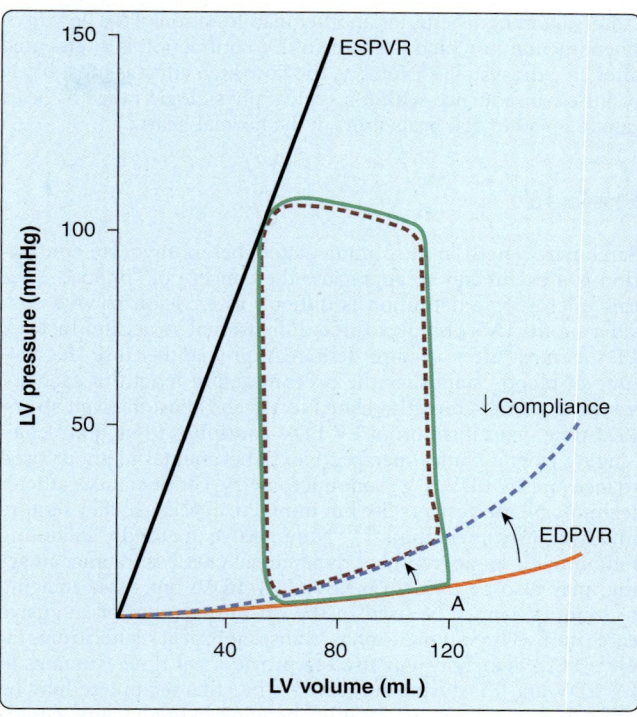

Figure 12-12 These schematic illustrations demonstrate alterations in the steady-state LV pressure–volume diagram produced by a reduction in myocardial contractility as indicated by a decrease in the slope of the end-systolic pressure–volume relation (ESPVR; left panel) and a decrease in LV compliance as indicated by an increase in the position of the end-diastolic pressure–volume relation (EDPVR; right panel). These diagrams emphasize that heart failure may result from LV systolic or diastolic dysfunction independently. Reproduced with permission from Kaplan JA, Reich DL, Savino JS. *Kaplan's Cardiac Anesthesia: The Echo Era*. 6th ed. St. Louis, MO: Elsevier Saunders; 2011:109.)

determine cardiac output. The LV's structural integrity is essential to its efficiency as a pump. For example, an anomalous route of blood flow from the chamber (e.g., a ventricular septal defect with left to right shunt) or valvular dysfunction (e.g., severe mitral regurgitation) may reduce forward flow because blood is diverted into lower pressure outlets (the RV or the LA in these examples, respectively) and is not ejected directly into the aorta. Pulmonary venous blood flow, LA and mitral valve function, pericardial forces, and the active (relaxation) and passive (compliance) diastolic properties of the LV determine the LV's ability to fill properly at normal pressure (approximately 10 mmHg).[53] Perturbations in any of these variables attenuates optimal LV filling and may contribute to the development of heart failure independent of LV systolic dysfunction per se.

Heart Rate

The contractile state of isolated cardiac muscle is directly related to its stimulation frequency. This phenomenon is known as the Bowditch, "staircase," or "Treppe" effect, or the "force-frequency" relationship. Improved Ca^{2+} cycling efficiency and increased myofilament Ca^{2+} sensitivity are most likely responsible for the Bowditch effect. Maximal contractile force is generated at 150 to 180 stimulations/min in isolated cardiac muscle. These experimental data support the clinical observation of ideal matching of cardiac output to venous return at heart rates of approximately 175 beats/min during intense aerobic exercise in trained endurance athletes. Contractility begins to decrease at heart rates exceeding 175 beats/min because LV relaxation abnormalities begin to develop. Insufficient Ca^{2+} uptake from the contractile apparatus, attenuated LV diastolic filling time, and reduced coronary perfusion resulting from an inadequate duration of diastole combine to contribute to the reduction in inotropic state and cardiac output during profound tachycardia. Thus, tachyarrhythmias or rapid pacing may cause profound hemodynamic compromise, even in otherwise healthy individuals. The Bowditch effect is a particularly important mechanism by which contractility is enhanced and adequate arterial blood pressure is maintained in disease states characterized by profound impairments in LV filling (e.g., pericardial tamponade, constrictive pericarditis). The

Figure 12-13 This illustration depicts the major factors that determine LV diastolic (left) and systolic (right) function. Note that pulmonary venous (PV) blood flow, LA function, mitral valve integrity, LA relaxation, and LV compliance combine to determine LV preload. (Reproduced with permission from Kaplan JA, Reich DL, Savino JS. *Kaplan's Cardiac Anesthesia: The Echo Era*. 6th ed. St. Louis, MO: Elsevier Saunders; 2011:111.)

"interval-strength" effect is another manifestation of the Bowditch phenomenon in which the force of LV contraction is augmented after an extrasystole.[54] Notably, the Bowditch effect is most likely of little consequence within a typical physiologic range of heart rate (e.g., 50 to 150 beats/min) in the normal heart.[55]

Preload

Sarcomere length in vitro immediately before myocyte contraction is a useful way to appreciate the concept of "preload," but this microscopic definition is difficult to envision in vivo considering the LV's complex three-dimensional structure. Instead, EDV is most often used to define LV preload because this volume of blood establishes the precontraction length of each LV sarcomere and is directly related to LV end-diastolic wall stress. Real-time quantification of LV EDV continues to be quite challenging from a clinical perspective. Experimental methods used to measure LV EDV (e.g., sonomicrometry, conductance catheter technology) are very precise but impractical because they require invasive instrumentation.[56,57] Noninvasive methods, including radionuclide angiography or dynamic magnetic resonance imaging, may also be used to measure LV EDV, but these imaging techniques cannot be used in the operating room or intensive care unit. Three-dimensional transesophageal echocardiography (TEE) is increasingly used to provide real-time estimates of LV EDV and EF during surgery,[58-60] but this technique may be difficult to apply during rapidly changing hemodynamic conditions. Cardiac anesthesiologists often estimate LV EDV using two-dimensional TEE in the transgastric LV midpapillary short axis view to measure or visually estimate LV end-diastolic area or diameter. A decrease in LV preload is usually inferred when there is a reduction in end-diastolic area and diameter, although marked arterial vasodilation may also produce similar findings.

Other clinically used indices of LV preload have inherent limitations (Fig. 12-14). Advancing a fluid-filled catheter into the LV allows measurement of LV end-diastolic pressure, which is related to EDV through the exponential EDPVR curve. This invasive technique is possible only in the cardiac catheterization laboratory or the operating room. In lieu of this method, other pressures "upstream" from the LV are more commonly used to estimate LV EDV, including mean LA, pulmonary capillary occlusion (wedge), pulmonary arterial diastolic, RV end-diastolic, and RA (central venous) pressures. The integrity of the structures that separate each site of measurement from the LV influences the relative accuracy of these methods. For example, a correlation between central venous and LV end-diastolic pressures assumes that pulmonary disease, airway pressure during respiration, RV or pulmonary vascular disease, LA dysfunction, mitral valve abnormalities, or abnormal LV compliance have not adversely affected the fluid column between the RA and the LV. This is not the case in many patients with significant pulmonary or cardiac disease. For example, there is a well-known lack of correlation between LV EDV, pulmonary artery occlusion pressure, and central venous pressure in patients with LV dysfunction,[61] in whom accurate measurement of LV preload may be especially important to optimize hemodynamics.

Afterload

The additional load to which cardiac muscle is exposed after contraction has begun is termed "afterload." This concept is intuitively clear when studying isolated cardiac muscle under experimental conditions, but it is more difficult to quantify when the LV's interaction with the arterial vasculature is considered in vivo. Four components determine LV afterload in the intact cardiovascular system: the size and mechanical behavior of arterial blood vessels; terminal arteriolar vasomotor tone, which establishes total arterial resistance; LV end-systolic wall stress, which is defined by LV pressure development and the changes in LV geometry required to generate it; and the physical properties and volume of blood as a hydraulic fluid. This section will focus on LV afterload, but the methods used to estimate RV afterload are virtually identical to those used to quantify LV afterload.[62] Nevertheless, the reader should appreciate that two major differences exist between the LV and the RV afterload systems: the systemic circulation is substantially less compliant that pulmonary arterial vasculature and, as mentioned previously, the LV is less sensitive to changes in afterload than is the RV.

The most comprehensive description of LV afterload is aortic input impedance $[Z_{in}(\omega)]$, defined as the ratio of continuous aortic pressure (the forces acting on the blood) to blood flow (the motion that those forces creates). Power spectral or Fourier series analysis is used to calculate $Z_{in}(\omega)$ from high-fidelity measurements of pressure and blood flow. $Z_{in}(\omega)$ includes the frequency-dependent characteristics of the arterial vasculature, including its viscoelastic effects and wave reflection properties. This methodology is quite useful from a biomechanical engineering perspective, but has limited practical applicability. Another definition of LV afterload

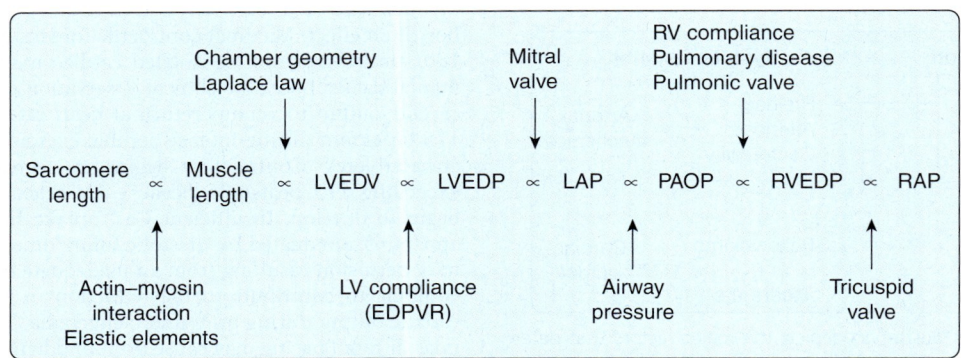

Figure 12-14 This schematic diagram depicts factors that influence experimental and clinical estimates of sarcomere length as a pure index of the preload of the contracting LV myocyte. LVEDV and LVEDP, LV end-diastolic volume and end-diastolic pressure, respectively; EDPVR, end-diastolic pressure–volume relation; LAP, left atrial pressure; PAOP, pulmonary artery occlusion pressure; RV, right ventricle; RVEDP, RV end-diastolic pressure; RAP, right atrial pressure. (Reproduced with permission from Kaplan JA, Reich DL, Savino JS. *Kaplan's Cardiac Anesthesia: The Echo Era*. 6th ed. St. Louis, MO: Elsevier Saunders; 2011:112.)

quantifies the mechanical forces to which the LV is exposed at the end of ejection as LV end-systolic wall stress. As previously mentioned, a large decline in LV volume occurs after the aortic valve opens, concomitant with elevated LV pressure and increased wall thickness. The Law of Laplace indicates that changes in these variables cause a pronounced increase in LV end-systolic wall stress, which reaches its maximum value during early LV ejection and subsequently falls.[28] These alterations in LV systolic wall stress during ejection are important. Maximal LV systolic wall stress is a potent stimulus for myocyte hypertrophy in the presence of chronic increases in afterload, such as may be observed in patients with severe aortic valve stenosis or uncontrolled essential hypertension.[63] The area under the LV systolic wall stress curve is directly related to myocardial oxygen consumption.[64] At end-systole, the forces driving further ejection and those resisting it are equal. Thus, LV end-systolic wall stress is also a determinant of stroke volume.

Afterload may also be approached from a mechanical systems perspective, because the LV and the arterial vasculature must be appropriately matched to assure optimal energy transfer between them. In this "coupling" model, the LV and arterial circulation are considered elastic chambers in series. LV-arterial coupling is described using the ratio of LV elastance (E_{es}) and effective arterial elastance (E_a), each of which is determined in the P–V plane (Fig. 12-15).[65] E_a may also be estimated as the ratio of end-systolic arterial pressure to stroke volume, and has been clinically applied to approximate LV afterload using this definition. Arteriolar resistance and the compliance of the proximal great vessels influence E_a, but E_a does not include arterial frequency dependence or wave reflection properties and cannot be used as a quantitative index of LV afterload as a result.

The most commonly used clinical estimate of LV afterload is systemic vascular resistance calculated as ([MAP − RAP] • 80)/CO, where MAP and RAP are mean arterial and right atrial pressures, respectively, CO is cardiac output, and 80 is a constant that converts $mmHg \cdot min^{-1} \cdot L^{-1}$ to $dynes \cdot sec \cdot cm^{-5}$. Systemic vascular resistance primarily reflects the resistance of terminal arterioles, which is a major component of afterload. However, similar to LV end-systolic wall stress and E_a, systemic vascular resistance does not consider the mechanical properties of the blood and arterial walls, ignores the frequency-dependence of arterial pressure and blood flow, and does not account for arterial wave reflection. Notably, these components of LV afterload are of greater importance in elderly patients or in the presence of atherosclerosis,[66] clinical circumstances in which quantitative evaluation of afterload may be especially relevant. In general, systemic vascular resistance is best used as a nonparametric estimate, but not as a quantitative index, of LV afterload produced by vasoactive medications or cardiovascular disease.[67]

The failing LV is especially sensitive to increases in afterload.[68] Activation of the sympathetic nervous system serves to improve contractility in the presence of LV systolic dysfunction, but this response also causes unintentional but equally important increases in LV afterload that often negates the expected increase in cardiac output. LV hypertrophy is also an important adaptation response to chronic increases in LV afterload that reduces LV wall stress by increasing wall thickness (Fig. 12-16). However, this

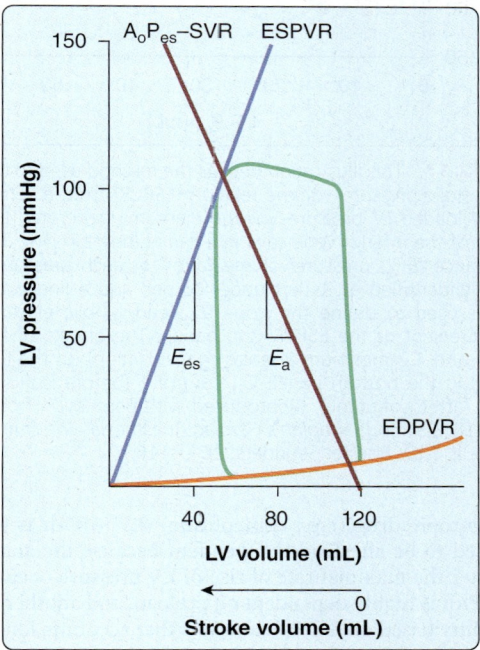

Figure 12-15 This schematic diagram illustrates the LV end-systolic pressure–volume and aortic end-systolic pressure-stroke volume relations (ESPVR and A_oP_{es}-SVR, respectively) used to determine LV-arterial coupling as the ratio of end-systolic elastance (E_{es}; the slope of ESPVR) and effective arterial elastance (E_a; the slope of A_oP_{es}-SVR). EDPVR = end-diastolic pressure–volume relation. (Reproduced with permission from Kaplan JA, Reich DL, Savino JS. *Kaplan's Cardiac Anesthesia: The Echo Era.* 6th ed. St. Louis, MO: Elsevier Saunders; 2011:114.)

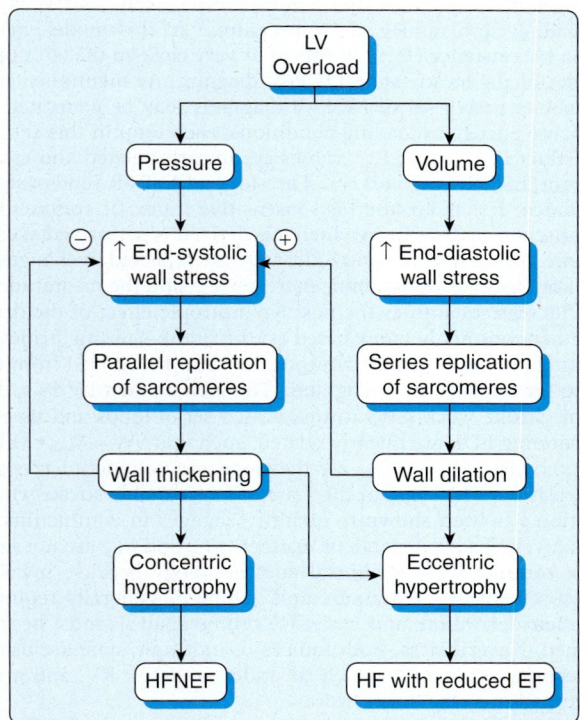

Figure 12-16 LV pressure- and volume-overload produce compensatory responses based on the nature of the inciting stress. Wall thickening reduces (−) whereas chamber dilation increases (+) end-systolic wall stress as predicted by the Law of Laplace. LV pressure-overload hypertrophy has been linked to heart failure with normal ejection fraction (HFNEF), but LV volume-overload most often causes heart failure (HF) with reduced ejection fraction (EF). (Reproduced with permission from Kaplan JA, Reich DL, Savino JS. *Kaplan's Cardiac Anesthesia: The Echo Era.* 6th ed. St. Louis, MO: Elsevier Saunders; 2011:114.)

compensatory response also inadvertently increases myocardial oxygen consumption and reduces LV compliance. These effects make the hypertrophied LV more susceptible to myocardial ischemia and diastolic dysfunction, respectively. Thus, decreasing LV afterload by reducing the inciting stress is the most important objective in the clinical management of heart failure.

Myocardial Contractility

Myocardial contractility is the force that cardiac muscle is capable of producing during contraction under controlled loading conditions and stimulation rate. Determining myocardial contractility is relatively easy in isolated cardiac muscle, but this measurement is remarkably difficult in the intact heart. The ability to quantify inotropic state has important implications during the clinical management of patients with LV or RV contractile dysfunction, but a "gold standard" of myocardial contractility independent of heart rate and loading conditions remains elusive. Inotropic state and loading conditions are inextricably connected in the sarcomere[69] and thus, it most likely not feasible to measure contractility as an independent variable. To date, indices derived from LV P–V analysis, isovolumic contraction, and ejection are the major approaches to the measurement of contractility in vivo, all of which have limitations.

The ratio of continuous LV pressure-to-volume during the cardiac cycle is termed "time-varying elastance" $[E(t)]$, such that $E(t) = P(t)/[V(t)-V_0]$, where $P(t)$ and $V(t)$ are the time-dependent changes in LV pressure and volume, respectively, and V_0 is LV volume at zero mmHg of LV pressure.[70] In this model, maximum LV elastance (E_{max}) occurs at or very close to the left upper corner of the steady-state LV P–V diagram. As mentioned previously, a nested set of LV P–V diagrams may be generated by an acute change in loading conditions; each loop in this set has a distinct E_{max}. These E_{max} values are linearly related and establish the ESPVR (Fig. 12-17). The slope of ESPVR (end-systolic elastance; E_{es}) is an afterload-insensitive index of contractility because the analysis from which it is derived is performed at end-systole. Alterations in contractile state are reflected in changes in E_{es}. For example, dobutamine increases E_{es}, and the magnitude of this increase quantifies the positive inotropic effect of the drug. Another contractile index based on the Frank–Starling principle relating preload to cardiac output may also be derived from the same series of LV P–V diagrams. The area of each LV P–V diagram (stroke work; SW) in this nested set of loops and its corresponding EDV are linearly related, such that SW = M_{sw} • (EDV − V_{sw}), where M_{sw} and V_{sw} are the slope and volume intercept of the relation. The slope of this "preload recruitable stroke work" relation has been shown to quantify changes in contractility in a relatively load-independent manner.[71] E_{es} and M_{sw} are not used on a routine basis in clinical anesthesiology because invasive measurement of LV pressure and volume is generally required for their derivation, and extensive offline analysis must be performed. Nevertheless, both indices of inotropic state are useful conceptual tools with which to understand LV, RV, and atrial contractility in the intact heart.

Indices of global myocardial contractility may also be derived during isovolumic contraction using the LV pressure waveform. The most commonly used isovolumic index of contractility is dP/dt. This index requires invasive measurement of continuous LV pressure and is most often recorded in the cardiac catheterization laboratory, but may also be estimated noninvasively using TEE.[72] LV +dP/dt sensitively indicates changes in contractile state, but its absolute value is less important than the magnitude of its change in response to an intervention such as administration

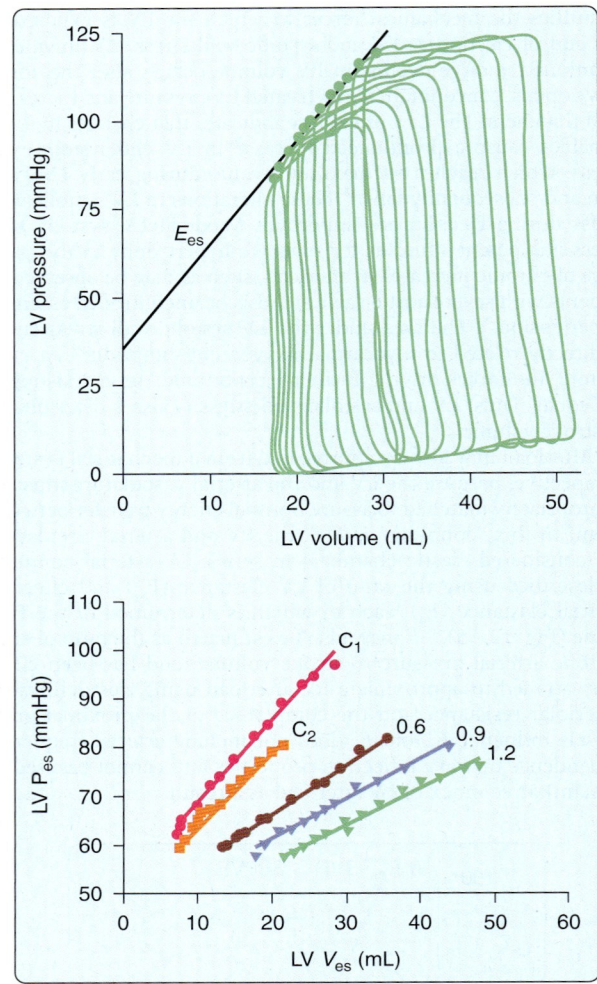

Figure 12-17 This illustration depicts the method used to derive the LV end-systolic pressure–volume relation (ESPVR) from a series of differentially loaded LV pressure–volume diagrams generated by abrupt occlusion of the inferior vena cava in a canine heart *in vivo*. The maximal elastance (E_{max}; pressure/volume ratio) for each pressure–volume diagram is identified as its left upper corner, and a linear regression analysis is used to define the slope (E_{es}; end-systolic elastance) and volume intercept of the ESPVR (top panel). The effects of isoflurane (0.6, 0.9, and 1.2 minimum alveolar concentration) on the ESPVR are illustrated in the bottom panel. C_1, control 1 (before isoflurane); C_2, control 2 (after isoflurane). (Reproduced with permission from Kaplan JA, Reich DL, Savino JS. *Kaplan's Cardiac Anesthesia: The Echo Era*. 6th ed. St. Louis, MO: Elsevier Saunders; 2011:116.)

of an inotropic drug (e.g., epinephrine). LV +dP/dt is generally considered to be afterload-independent because the aortic valve opens after the maximal rate of rise of LV pressure occurs. However, +dP/dt is highly dependent on preload, and another index of contractility based on LV P–V analysis that accounts for this preload dependence has been developed and applied in laboratory and clinical settings.[73] LV mass, chamber geometry, and valve disease also influence +dP/dt. Decreases in global LV inotropic state caused by regional myocardial ischemia may also not be accurately quantified with +dP/dt, because compensatory increases in contractility occur in the surrounding nonischemic myocardium, thereby effectively normalizing overall function. Other isovolumic indices of contractility based on +dP/dt, including the rate of rise of LV pressure at a predetermined LV pressure (e.g., dP/dt measured at 40 mmHg) or the ratio of dP/dt to maximum LV pressure (dP/dt/P) have also been used, but these measures do not provide unique information compared with +dP/dt.

Ejection fraction is the most commonly used clinical index of LV contractility. Ejection fraction is usually measured with two- or three-dimensional echocardiography, but other methods, including radionuclide angiography and magnetic resonance imaging (MRI), also provide reliable estimates of this ejection phase index of inotropic state. In the operating room, two-dimensional TEE midesophageal four- or two-chamber windows can obtained at end-systole and end-diastole and analyzed using Simpson rule of discs to determine EF. However, this technique is rather time-consuming and is impractical when hemodynamics are unstable. Instead, regional approximations of EF, such as fractional shortening and fractional area change (FAC), are often used by examining midpapillary short axis diameter and area, respectively, at end-systole and end-diastole. For example, FAC is determined as EDA − ESA/EDA, where EDA and ESA are end-diastolic and end-systolic areas, respectively, measured by tracing the LV's endocardial borders (Fig. 12-18). All ejection phase indices of contractility are dependent on loading conditions and inotropic state. Thus, interpretation of EF, FAC, or fractional shortening must be considered within the clinical context under which the data were obtained. For example, profoundly depressed EF in a patient with severe hypertension may occur because afterload is markedly increased, and not because myocardial contractility is grossly impaired. Ejection phase indices may also be inaccurate in the presence of mitral or aortic valve disease or a ventricular septal defect. Indeed, EF may be greater than normal during acute mitral regurgitation because a substantial portion of blood flow from the LV is diverted into the LA during systole and not because the LV is inherently "hyperdynamic."

Determinants of Diastolic Function

Each chamber of the heart must fill adequately under normal pressures to facilitate optimal function during the subsequent contraction. We will emphasize LV diastolic function in the current section of this chapter, but the readers should be aware that the diastolic properties of the RV and atria are also important for the heart's overall performance. Because diastole is an inherently complex sequence of temporally related events (Table 12-1), no single index of LV diastolic function completely characterizes this phase of the cardiac cycle or selectively predicts those patients who may be at greatest risk of developing heart failure related to abnormal diastolic function.[74] Notably, nearly one-half of patients with heart failure do not have overt evidence of LV systolic dysfunction (e.g., a reduction in LV EF).[75] Hypertensive elderly women who are obese and have renal insufficiency, anemia, or atrial fibrillation appear to be at greatest risk of developing this "heart failure with normal ejection fraction" (HFNEF; also known as "diastolic heart failure").[76] Delayed LV relaxation, reduced compliance, and abnormal LV-arterial coupling have been implicated in the pathophysiology of HFNEF

Table 12-1 Determinants of Left Ventricular Diastolic Function

Heart rate and rhythm
LV systolic function
Wall thickness
Chamber geometry
Duration, rate, and extent of myocyte relaxation
LV untwisting and elastic recoil
Magnitude of diastolic suction
LA–LV pressure gradient
Passive elastic properties of LV myocardium
Viscoelastic effects (rapid LV filling and atrial systole)
LA structure and function
Mitral valve structure and function
Pulmonary venous blood flow
Pericardial restraint
RV loading conditions and function
Ventricular interdependence
Coronary blood flow and vascular engorgement
Compression by mediastinal masses

LV, left ventricle; LA, left atrium; RV, right ventricle.
Reprinted with permission from Kaplan JA, Reich DL, Savino JS. *Kaplan's Cardiac Anesthesia: The Echo Era*. 6th ed. St. Louis, MO: Elsevier Saunders; 2011:121.

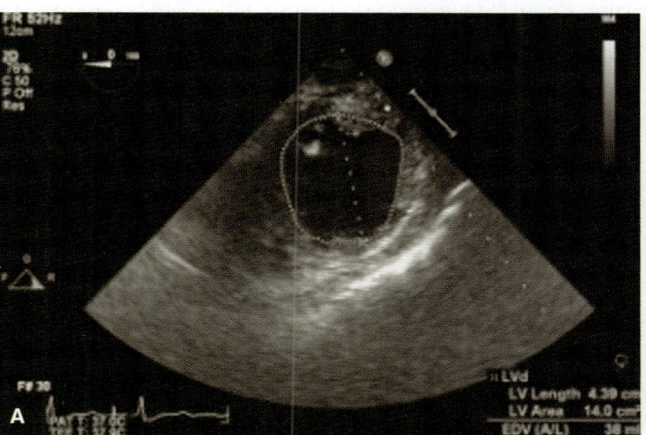 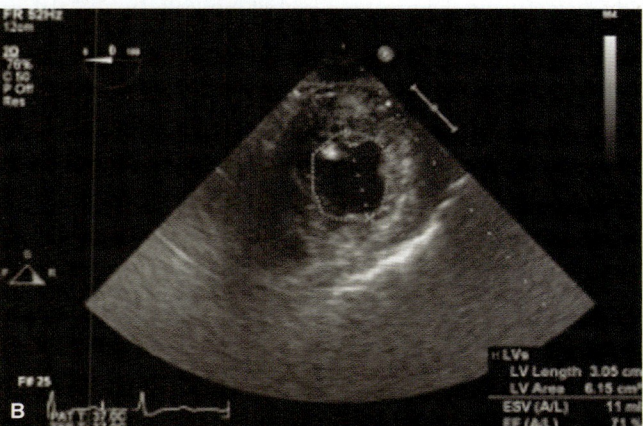

Figure 12-18 Calculation of fractional area change from LV midpapillary short axis images obtained at end-diastole (left panel) and end-systole (right panel). The LV endocardial border is manually traced (excluding the papillary muscles). The software integrates the area inscribed in the LV chamber. (Reproduced with permission from Kaplan JA, Reich DL, Savino JS. *Kaplan's Cardiac Anesthesia: The Echo Era*. 6th ed. St. Louis, MO: Elsevier Saunders; 2011:119.)

> **Table 12-2** Common Causes of Left Ventricular Diastolic Dysfunction
>
> Age > 60 years
> Acute myocardial ischemia (supply or demand)
> Myocardial stunning, hibernation, or infarction
> Ventricular remodeling after infarction
> Pressure-overload hypertrophy (e.g., aortic stenosis, hypertension)
> Volume-overload hypertrophy (e.g., aortic or mitral regurgitation)
> Hypertrophic obstructive cardiomyopathy
> Dilated cardiomyopathy
> Restrictive cardiomyopathy (e.g., amyloidosis, hemochromatosis)
> Pericardial diseases (e.g., tamponade, constrictive pericarditis)
>
> Reprinted with permission from Kaplan JA, Reich DL, Savino JS. *Kaplan's Cardiac Anesthesia: The Echo Era*. 6th ed. St. Louis, MO: Elsevier Saunders; 2011:121.

(Table 12-1).[77,78] Thus, LV diastolic dysfunction is a major cause of HFNEF. The severity of and response to medical therapy in HFNEF are key factors that establish exercise tolerance[79] and predict prognosis.[80] From the anesthesiologist's perspective, LV diastolic function is a major determinant of the LV's response to changes in loading conditions. Many volatile and intravenous anesthetics affect LV relaxation and filling in the normal and failing heart.[81] As a result, preoperative determination of the presence, severity, and underlying etiology of LV diastolic dysfunction (Table 12-2) is important when caring for patients undergoing surgery in which large shifts in intravascular volume are anticipated. Isolated LV diastolic dysfunction is also an independent risk factor for adverse cardiovascular events, including mortality, in patients undergoing major surgery.[82]

Invasive Assessment of LV Relaxation

Removal of Ca^{2+} from the contractile apparatus and the sarcoplasm is an active, energy-dependent process that results in rapid dissociation of contractile proteins and recoil of compressed elastic elements. Failure of actin–myosin cross bridges to properly dissociate or abnormal removal of intracellular Ca^{2+} delays relaxation in the intact LV.[83] As mentioned previously, early LV filling is dependent on the rate and extent of LV relaxation and thus, is attenuated when relaxation is delayed. Under these circumstances, final EDV becomes more dependent on the contribution of atrial systole. As a result, acute onset of atrial fibrillation often causes heart failure in patients with disease states in which pronounced delays in LV relaxation occur (e.g., hypertrophic cardiomyopathy). Myocardial ischemia caused by acute occlusion of a major coronary artery is also a frequent cause of delayed LV relaxation and may be accompanied by reductions in LV compliance that further limit LV filling, cause LA and pulmonary venous hypertension, and contribute to the development of pulmonary edema.[84]

Measuring the rate with which LV pressure declines during isovolumic relaxation is the most common technique for quantifying LV relaxation. This type of analysis generally requires invasive measurement of continuous LV pressure and is usually reserved for the cardiac catheterization laboratory. Several indices of LV relaxation may be derived using this method, among which the maximum rate of LV pressure decline (−dP/dt; analogous to +dP/dt during isovolumic contraction) and a time constant (τ) of LV relaxation are the most common. LV −dP/dt is not an ideal as an index of LV relaxation because this parameter is essentially a "snapshot" of relaxation that is affected by the value of LV end-systolic pressure. LV pressure decay during relaxation is exponential between aortic valve closure and mitral valve opening. A time constant (τ) derived using the equation: $P(t) = P_0 e^{-t/\tau}$, where $P(t)$ is time-dependent LV pressure, P_0 is LV pressure at end-systole, e is the natural exponent, and t is time after LV end-systole, is used to quantify relaxation. Despite the limitations of this simple model,[85,86] an increase in τ indicates that a delay in LV relaxation has occurred. This technique has been used to quantify delays in LV relaxation during cardiac disease (e.g., myocardial ischemia,[87] pressure-overload hypertrophy[88]) or as a result of administration of negative inotropic medications including volatile anesthetics.[89] In contrast, reductions in τ (indicative of more rapid relaxation) are observed during tachycardia, sympathetic nervous system activation, or administration of positive inotropic drugs. From a clinical standpoint, LV relaxation and its pharmacologic modulation are very important in heart failure. LV relaxation is modestly dependent on afterload under normal conditions,[27] but this afterload-sensitivity of LV relaxation is especially pronounced in the failing heart.[90] Thus, medications that reduce afterload not only augment LV systolic function but also simultaneously enhance LV relaxation (decrease τ) in patients with heart failure.[68] This latter effect improves early LV filling dynamics and reduces congestive signs and symptoms.

Invasive Assessment of LV Filling and Compliance

Indices of LV filling may be calculated using invasive or noninvasive (e.g., two-or three-dimensional echocardiography, radionuclide angiography, cardiac MRI) measurement of continuous LV volume. The first derivative of LV volume waveform with respect to time (dV/dt) creates a biphasic waveform with peaks occurring during early LV filling (E) and atrial systole (A). The transmitral blood flow velocity signal acquired during LV filling using pulse wave Doppler echocardiography (see below) closely resembles this dV/dt waveform. Development of heart failure causes characteristic changes in dV/dt morphology that are identical to the "delayed relaxation," "pseudonormal," and "restrictive" filling patterns measured using pulse wave Doppler (Fig. 12-19).[91] Invasive analysis of LV filling with continuous LV volume and its first derivative is limited almost exclusively to the laboratory and is of little practical value in clinical anesthesiology except as a teaching tool.

As mentioned earlier in the discussion, EDPVR is an index of LV compliance derived from a nested set of LV P–V diagrams. The relationship between end-diastolic pressure (EDP) and EDV is exponential such that $EDP = Ae^{K(EDV)} + B$, where K is the modulus of chamber stiffness and A and B are curve-fitting constants. An increase in K indicates that the LV is less compliant, that is, higher LV pressure is required to distend the LV to a given volume. Parallel upward shifts in the EDPVR, such as seen in pericardial tamponade, represent an exception, because the value of K remains constant under these circumstances even though LV pressure is greater at each LV volume.[52] Thus, the relative position of the EDPVR in P–V phase space may be more important than the actual value of K itself because a shift in EDPVR up or to the left indicates that a higher LV pressure is required to achieve a similar LV volume.[92]

The diastolic stress–strain relation is another model frequently used to experimentally describe LV compliance. Myocardium is

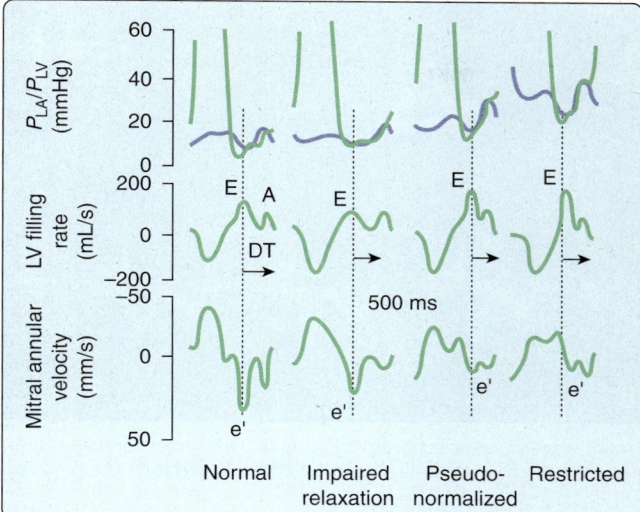

Figure 12-19 This illustration depicts the simultaneous relationships between LA and LV pressures (P_{LA} and P_{LV}, respectively; top panels), LV filling rate during early filling (E) and atrial systole (A; middle panels), and early mitral annular velocity (e; bottom panels) under normal conditions and during evolving diastolic dysfunction (impaired relaxation, pseudonormal, and restrictive). Note the initial lengthening of E wave deceleration time (DT) during impaired relaxation and the subsequent shortening of DT as diastolic function worsens. (Reproduced with permission from Kaplan JA, Reich DL, Savino JS. *Kaplan's Cardiac Anesthesia: The Echo Era*. 6th ed. St. Louis, MO: Elsevier Saunders; 2011:122.)

an elastic material that follows Hooke law, developing resisting forces (stress; σ) as muscle length (strain; ε) increases during LV filling. The relationship is also exponential such that $\sigma = \alpha(e^{\beta\varepsilon} - 1)$, where α is the coefficient of gain and β is the modulus of myocardial stiffness.[93] Similar to the EDPVR, an increase in β occurs when the stress–strain relationship shifts up or to the left and may be observed in pathologic conditions characterized by fundamental structural abnormalities that adversely influence myocardial stiffness (e.g., hypertrophic cardiomyopathy, amyloidosis). EDPVR and myocardial stress–strain relations are generally not used clinically because analysis required to examine these relationships is complicated, time-consuming, and limited to steady-state hemodynamic conditions.

Noninvasive Evaluation of Diastolic Function

The duration between aortic valve closure (end-systole) and mitral valve opening (onset of transmitral blood flow) defines isovolumic relaxation time (IVRT), a commonly used noninvasive index of LV relaxation that is usually measured using M-mode or pulse wave Doppler echocardiography. The rate of LV relaxation and the difference between LV end-systolic pressure and LA pressure when the mitral valve opens determines IVRT in the absence of aortic or mitral valve disease.[94] It should be readily apparent that IVRT is dependent on both LV relaxation and loading conditions. Indeed, IVRT is seldom used alone to quantify LV relaxation, but is most often combined with the transmitral blood flow velocity pattern to more comprehensively define the rate and extent of LV relaxation.

Noninvasive analysis of LV diastolic function is based on Doppler echocardiographic evaluation of transmitral blood flow velocity.[95] A pulse wave Doppler echocardiography sample volume is placed between the tips of the mitral leaflets to obtain a high-resolution transmitral blood flow velocity envelope. The normal pattern of transmitral blood flow velocity has two peaks: an early "E" peak associated with early LV filling and a late "A" peak corresponding to LA systole.[96] The ratio of the peak E and A wave velocities is commonly used to quantify the relative contributions of early LV filling and atrial systole to EDV. The time elapsed as the E wave velocity declines from its peak value to zero is known as the deceleration time; this parameter is often used with IVRT to quantify LV relaxation. For example, an increase in E wave deceleration time indicates that early LV filling is prolonged because LV relaxation is delayed. Age affects LV diastolic function because a progressive slowing of LV relaxation occurs. As a result, IVRT, deceleration time, and A wave velocity increase with age, whereas E wave velocity and E/A ratio decrease.[97] The aging heart becomes less compliant, especially in the presence of coexisting essential hypertension and LV hypertrophy. This change predisposes the elderly to develop heart failure.[98]

The reversal of E/A with advancing age is an example of a "delayed relaxation" pattern of LV diastolic dysfunction. This transmitral blood flow velocity pattern is the least severe of three abnormal LV filling patterns that describe the continuum of abnormal LV diastolic function. Clinical symptoms, exercise tolerance, New York Heart Association (NYHA) functional class, and mortality are closely correlated with the relative severity of LV diastolic dysfunction quantified using this method.[99] E/A < 1 characterizes "delayed relaxation" and indicates that early LV filling is attenuated and the LA's contribution to filling is enhanced (atrial kick).[91] The "delayed relaxation" pattern is often observed in patients with essential hypertension, pressure-overload LV hypertrophy, and myocardial ischemia (Fig. 12-20).

As diastolic dysfunction worsens, a "pseudonormal" pattern replaces the "delayed relaxation" profile. This pseudonormal pattern occurs because E/A becomes > 1 (similar to the normal profile, thus the term "pseudonormal") as LA pressures increase to compensate for the further reduction in LV compliance. Thus, E wave velocity "normalizes" because the LA–LV pressure gradient increases when the mitral valve opens. Other indices of diastolic function (e.g., pulmonary venous blood flow velocity, tissue Doppler imaging) are required to distinguish the "pseudonormal" from a normal transmitral blood flow velocity profile. Alternatively, administration of a small bolus of a vasodilator (e.g., nitroglycerin) may convert a "pseudonormal" profile into a "delayed relaxation" pattern by transiently reducing LA pressure.[100] A "restrictive pattern" of transmitral blood flow velocity is the most severe form of LV diastolic dysfunction in which LA hypertension is present and LV compliance is further reduced. The E/A becomes > 2 as the LA–LV pressure gradient is further augmented by increased LA pressure (causing a larger peak E wave velocity), concomitant with progressive LA contractile dysfunction (decline in peak A wave velocity). Failure of a "restrictive" filling pattern to respond to administration of a vasodilator and revert to a "pseudonormal" or "delayed relaxation" pattern carries a grim prognosis in patients with heart failure, unless a mechanical circulatory support device is implanted or cardiac transplantation is performed.[95]

Abnormal LV diastolic function may also be determined using analysis of the pulmonary venous blood flow velocity pattern obtained with pulse wave Doppler echocardiography.[101] Most often, the pulmonary venous blood flow velocity is used in combination with transmitral blood flow velocity when quantifying the severity of LV diastolic dysfunction.[102] Two large positive deflections (forward flow from the pulmonary veins into the LA) and a single, small negative deflection

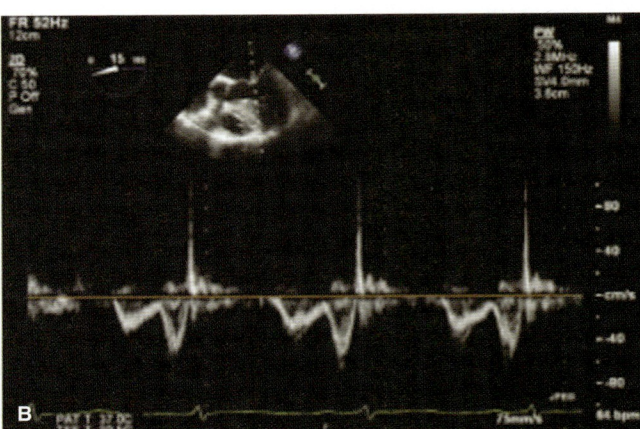

Figure 12-20 Transmitral blood flow velocity waveforms obtained using pulse wave Doppler echocardiography under normal conditions (left) and during delayed relaxation (right). (Reproduced with permission from Kaplan JA, Reich DL, Savino JS. *Kaplan's Cardiac Anesthesia: The Echo Era*. 6th ed. St. Louis, MO: Elsevier Saunders; 2011:123.)

(retrograde flow from the LA to the pulmonary veins, termed "atrial reversal") establish the normal pulmonary venous blood flow velocity pattern. The first positive deflection is known as the "S" (systolic) wave, and occurs while the mitral valve is closed (LV systole and early diastole).[103] This "S" wave results from LA relaxation, which stimulates forward movement of blood from the pulmonary veins into the LA. The mitral valve annulus also descends toward the LV apex during systole, drawing additional blood from the pulmonary veins into the LA (similar to an engine piston).[104] This latter action is attenuated when LV contractility is depressed, emphasizing that the LV systolic function has a direct impact on LA filling. Transmission of the RV systolic pressure pulse through the pulmonary circulation further contributes to LA filling. After the mitral valve opens, blood stored in the LA during LV systole enters the LV, an event which allows additional blood to flow from the pulmonary veins into the LA. This causes the second positive deflection ("D" [diastolic] wave) of the pulmonary venous blood flow velocity pattern. The "D" wave is dependent on the extent of early LV filling and LV compliance.[105] LA preload, LA contractility, and LV pressure during late diastole determine the magnitude of the "atrial reversal" (Ar) wave.[106]

The ratio of "S" to "D" waves and the peak velocity of the "Ar" wave increase with age.[96] These findings emphasize that LA function is more important to LV filling in the elderly. As LV diastolic function worsens, LA pressures increase and the "S" wave is attenuated (Fig. 12-21). The presence of this blunted "S" wave allows the echocardiographer to distinguish between normal and "pseudonormal" transmitral blood flow velocity patterns because S/D < 1 in the latter condition.[101] Such alterations in S/D become even more exaggerated in the presence of a "restrictive" filling pattern because LV diastolic and LA pressures are further elevated. Indeed, the "S" wave may be entirely abolished or even reversed (blood flow refluxing from the LA into the pulmonary veins) concomitant with an enhanced "D" wave in the presence of "restrictive" pathophysiology. Thus, pulmonary venous blood flow velocity patterns provide very useful information about LV diastolic dysfunction. Pulmonary venous blood flow patterns are also important when grading the severity of mitral regurgitation because LA pressure rises rapidly during the "S" phase as a result of regurgitant blood flow from the LV to the LA. Profound blunting or reversal of the "S" wave under these circumstances indicates that moderate or severe mitral regurgitation is present, respectively. Other indices of diastolic function, including tissue Doppler imaging[107] and color M-mode propagation velocity,[108] may also be used to define the progression of LV diastolic dysfunction. The reader is referred to Chapter 27 for a detailed discussion of the echocardiographic assessment of diastolic function.

Pericardium

The pericardium contains the heart, proximal great vessels, vena cavae, and pulmonary veins. The pericardium acts to separate the heart from other structures in the mediastinum and limits the heart's movement through its diaphragmatic and great vessel attachments. The fluid in the pericardium acts as a lubricant and consists of a combination of plasma ultrafiltrate, lymph, and myocardial interstitial fluid (total volume of 15 to 35 mL). The pericardium is much less compliant than myocardium, and has very limited volume reserve (Fig. 12-22).[109] As a result, an acute increase in pericardial volume (e.g., tamponade) causes a

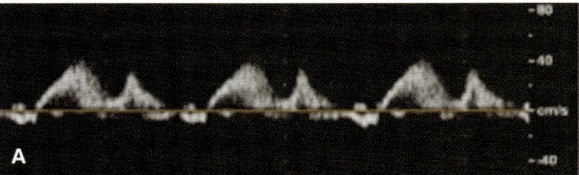
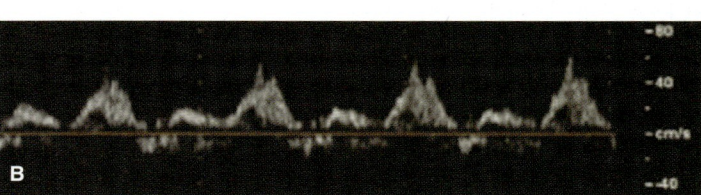

Figure 12-21 Pulmonary venous blood flow velocity waveforms obtained using pulse wave Doppler echocardiography under normal conditions (left panel) and in the presence of increased LA pressure (right panel). (Reproduced with permission from Kaplan JA, Reich DL, Savino JS. *Kaplan's Cardiac Anesthesia: The Echo Era*. 6th ed. St. Louis, MO: Elsevier Saunders; 2011:125.)

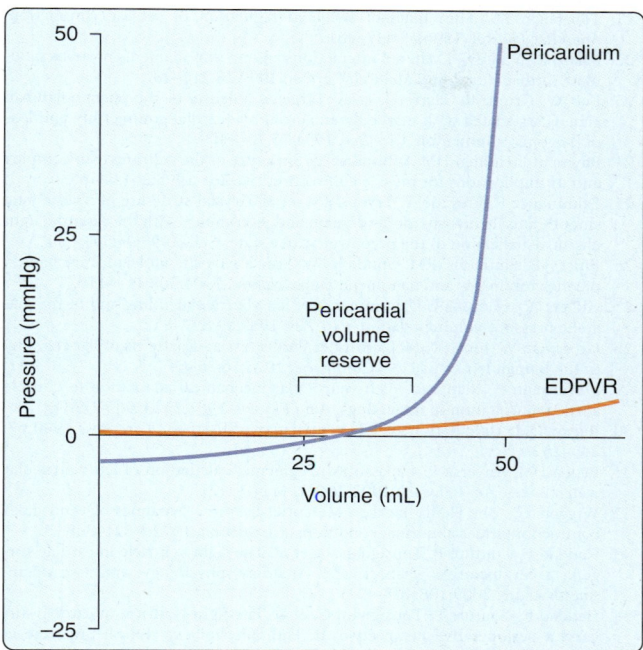

Figure 12-22 Pressure–volume relation of the pericardium (*blue line*) compared with the LV end-diastolic pressure–volume relation (EDPVR; *red line*). Note that large increases in pericardial volume occur after reserve volume is exceeded. (Reproduced with permission from Kaplan JA, Reich DL, Savino JS. *Kaplan's Cardiac Anesthesia: The Echo Era*. 6th ed. St. Louis, MO: Elsevier Saunders; 2011:127.)

during spontaneous ventilation.[115] Because intrathoracic pressure declines during inspiration, venous return to the right side of the heart increases and produces modest dilation of the RV. The result of this RV distention is a corresponding increase in pericardial restraint of the LV, which limits LV filling and causes a small decrease in stroke volume and mean arterial pressure. This ventricular interaction effect between the RV and LV is reversed during expiration. Directly opposite effects on RV and LV filling occur during inspiration and expiration in the presence of positive-pressure ventilation. The hemodynamic consequences of ventricular interdependence form the basis of respiratory cycle-induced pulse pressure and stroke volume variation, which have been shown to the useful dynamic indices of preload in conscious and anesthetized patients.[116] Notably, pericardial tamponade[117] or constrictive pericarditis[118] exaggerates the normal respiratory changes in RV and LV filling and produces pulsus paradoxus. It is especially important to appreciate that spontaneous ventilation is crucial in these conditions because negative intrathoracic pressure assists venous return, whereas cardiovascular collapse may occur with the initiation of positive pressure ventilation because venous return becomes profoundly limited.

Atrial Function

The mechanical properties of the LA are often overlooked in discussions of cardiac physiology. This is unfortunate because the LA acts as a contractile chamber, a reservoir (storage of blood before mitral valve opening), and a conduit (an extension of the pulmonary veins). The LA's function is critical to LV performance. The maximum velocity of shortening of LA myocardium is equal to or greater than LV myocardium under similar loading conditions.[119] LA emptying fraction (similar to LV EF) is dependent on LA contractility, preload, and LV compliance, unless the LA becomes so dilated that its myofilaments are stretched far beyond their normal operating length.[120] This magnitude of LA dilation may occur when LA pressures are chronically elevated because of severe LV diastolic dysfunction or mitral regurgitation. Under these conditions, the LA may no longer be capable of contributing to EDV as a contractile chamber. The LA's response to changes in autonomic nervous system activity, inotropic medications, and anesthetics is very similar to that of the LV.[121,122] LV compliance and pressure during late diastole determine the afterload with which the LA is confronted during its contraction. Thus, the LA must perform greater work in the presence of LV diastolic dysfunction because its afterload is increased. Like the RV, the LA is more susceptible to acute increases in afterload than is the LV, because the LA has less muscle mass and thinner walls. As a result, the LA emptying fraction may initially increase early during developing LV failure,[123] but subsequently decline as LA contractile dysfunction occurs concomitant with chamber dilatation.[124] LV diastolic dysfunction also causes remodeling and reduced compliance of the LA, which also further limit pulmonary venous return.

The LA also serves reservoir and conduit functions. LA relaxation, LV base descent during systole, transmission of RV stroke volume, and LA compliance determine LA reservoir function. LA ischemia, hypertrophy, or dilation attenuate reservoir function, as do LV or RV contractile dysfunction.[104,106] Disease states in which LA compliance is selectively reduced are associated with impaired LA filling and contribute to pulmonary venous congestion.[46,125] The LA appendage plays an important role in LA filling, as exclusion or excision of the LA appendage reduces the compliance of the LA chamber as a whole.[126,127] LA appendage exclusion procedures are often performed during cryoablation

pronounced elevation in pericardial pressure that substantially restricts filling of the cardiac chambers.[110] The pericardium normally restrains expansion of the low-pressure atria and RV because these chambers have thinner walls than the LV. Indeed, pericardial restraint is the primary determinant of the diastolic pressure–volume relations of the RA, LA, and RV, whereas the compliance of these chambers alone is less important. The pericardium also profoundly affects LV filling.[111] As mentioned earlier, a parallel upward shift of the EDPVR occurs in response to an acute increase in pericardial pressure.[112] This shift in the EDPVR indicates that LV pressure must be greater for each LV volume and explains why LV filling is impaired during tamponade physiology. While the pericardium is acutely noncompliant, a slow increase in pericardial pressure (e.g., chronic pericardial effusion or biventricular dilatation) causes the pericardium to gradually expand in size. This compensatory response increases the pericardium's compliance and reduces its restraining forces, thereby allowing the heart to continue functioning without imminent hemodynamic collapse.

Ventricular interdependence is the influence of the pressure and volume of one ventricle on the function of the other. The pericardium plays a central role in ventricular interdependence because it provides equal restraint of the RV and the LV. As a result, a rapid increase in RV pressure and volume (e.g., volume overload, acute increase in pulmonary arterial pressure) causes the pressure within the pericardium to increase as well. This action compresses the LV, reducing its effective compliance and impairing its filling.[113] Not surprisingly, LV distention has a similar effect on the RV and limits RV filling through an identical mechanism.[114] Ventricular interdependence may be readily appreciated by examining changes in RV and LV filling for treatment of chronic atrial fibrillation, and reduced LA compliance concomitant with elevated pulmonary venous pressures may be anticipated despite restoration of sinus rhythm.

Exercise enhances both LA contractility and reservoir function.[128] The latter effect is important because greater reservoir capacity causes a larger LA–LV pressure gradient during early LV filling, thereby facilitating additional blood flow to the LV during conditions requiring greater LV stroke volume and cardiac output. Conduit function is also augmented in endurance athletes.[129] As the LA begins to dilate in healthy elderly subjects, compensatory increases in LA emptying fraction and declines in passive LA emptying occur.[130] LA dilation initially augments the ratio of LA reservoir to LV stroke volume (termed "storage fraction"),[131] but this beneficial effect comes at a cost: the dilation increases in LA wall stress, which may contribute to eventual LA contractile dysfunction and the development of atrial arrhythmias.[132]

REFERENCES

1. Buckberg GD, Coghlan HC, Torrent-Guasp F. The structure and function of the helical heart and its buttress wrapping. VI. Geometric concepts of heart failure and use for structural correction. *Semin Thorac Cardiovasc Surg.* 2001;13:386–401.
2. Cheng C-P, Noda T, Nozawa T, et al. Effect of heart failure on the mechanism of exercise-induced augmentation of mitral valve flow. *Circ Res.* 1993;72:795–806.
3. Takayama Y, Costa KD, Covell JW. Contribution of laminar myofiber architecture to load-dependent changes in mechanics of LV myocardium. *Am J Physiol Heart Circ Physiol.* 2002;282:H1510–H1520.
4. Gharib M, Rambod E, Kheradvar A, et al. Optimal vortex formation as an index of cardiac health. *Proc Natl Acad Sci U S A.* 2006;103:6305–6308.
5. Sidebotham DA, Allen SJ, Gerber IL, et al. Intraoperative transesophageal echocardiography for surgical repair of mitral regurgitation. *J Am Soc Echocardiogr.* 2014;27:345–366.
6. Pagel PS, Diciaula G, Schroeder AR. Edible model of mitral valve leaflet surface geometry. *J Cardiothorac Vasc Anesth.* 2015;29:e4–e5.
7. Montealegre-Gallegos M, Bergman R, Jiang L, et al. Tricuspid valve: an intraoperative echocardiographic perspective. *J Cardiothorac Vasc Anesth.* 2014;28:761–770.
8. Voci P, Bilotta F, Caretta Q, et al. Papillary muscle perfusion pattern. A hypothesis for ischemic papillary muscle dysfunction. *Circulation.* 1995;91:1714–1718.
9. Stefanadis C, Dernellis J, Tsiamis E, et al. Effects of pacing-induced and balloon coronary occlusion ischemia on left atrial function in patients with coronary artery disease. *J Am Coll Cardiol.* 1999;33:687–696.
10. Katti K, Patil NP. The Thebesian valve: gatekeeper to the coronary sinus. *Clin Anat.* 2012;25:379–385.
11. Tops LF, Schalij MJ, Bax JJ. The effects of right ventricular apical pacing on ventricular function and dyssynchrony implications for therapy. *J Am Coll Cardiol.* 2009;54:764–776.
12. Epstein AE, DiMarco JP, Ellenbogen KA, et al. ACC/AHA/HRS 2008 Guidelines for Device-Based Therapy of Cardiac Rhythm Abnormalities: a report of the American College of Cardiology/American Heart Association Task Force on Practice Guidelines (Writing Committee to Revise the ACC/AHA/NASPE 2002 Guideline Update for Implantation of Cardiac Pacemakers and Antiarrhythmia Devices): developed in collaboration with the American Association for Thoracic Surgery and Society of Thoracic Surgeons. *Circulation.* 2008;117:e350–e408.
13. Gorman MW, Tune JD, Richmond KN, et al. Feedforward sympathetic coronary vasodilation in exercising dogs. *J Appl Physiol.* 2000;89:1892–1902.
14. Gorman MW, Rooke GA, Savage MV, et al. Adenine nucleotide control of coronary blood flow during exercise. *Am J Physiol Heart Circ Physiol.* 2010;299:H1981–H1989.
15. Schaub MC, Hefti MA, Zuellig RA, et al. Modulation of contractility in human cardiac hypertrophy by myosin essential light chain isoforms. *Cardiovasc Res.* 1998;37:381–404.
16. Cazorla O, Vassort G, Garnier D, et al. Length modulation of active force in rat cardiac myocytes: is titin the sensor? *J Mol Cell Cardiol.* 1999;31:1215–1227.
17. Helmes M, Trombitas K, Granzier H. Titin develops restoring force in rat cardiac myocytes. *Circ Res.* 1996;79:619–626.
18. Schiaffino S, Reggiani C. Molecular diversity of myofibrillar proteins: gene regulation and functional significance. *Physiol Rev.* 1996;76:371–423.
19. Moncman CL, Wang K. Nebulette: a 107 kD nebulin-like protein in cardiac muscle. *Cell Motil Cytoskel.* 1995;32:205–225.
20. Solaro RJ, Rarick HM. Troponin and tropomyosin. Proteins that switch on and tune in the activity of cardiac myofilaments. *Circ Res.* 1998;83:471–480.
21. Tobacman LS. Thin filament-mediated regulation of cardiac contraction. *Annu Rev Physiol.* 1996;58:447–481.
22. Solaro RJ, Van Eyk J. Altered interactions among thin filaments proteins modulate cardiac function. *J Mol Cell Cardiol.* 1999;28:217–230.
23. Luo W, Grupp IL, Harrer J, et al. Targeted ablation of the phospholamban gene is associated with markedly enhanced myocardial contractility and loss of β-agonist stimulation. *Circ Res.* 1994;75:401–409.
24. Rayment I, Holden HM, Whittaker M. Structure of the actin-myosin complex and its implications for muscle contraction. *Science.* 1993;261:58–65.
25. Dominguez R, Freyzon Y, Trybus KM, et al. Crystal structure of a vertebrate smooth muscle myosin motor domain and its complex with the essential light chain: visualization of the prepower stroke state. *Cell.* 1998;94:559–571.
26. Finer JT, Simmons RM, Spudich JA. Single myosin molecule mechanics: piconewton forces and nanometer steps. *Nature.* 1994;368:113–119.
27. Gilbert JC, Glantz SA. Determinants of left ventricular filling and of the diastolic pressure-volume relation. *Circ Res.* 1989;64:827–852.
28. Grossman W, Jones D, McLaurin LP. Wall stress and patterns of hypertrophy in the human left ventricle. *J Clin Invest.* 1975;56:56–64.
29. Florenzano F, Glantz SA. Left-ventricular mechanical adaptation to chronic aortic regurgitation in intact dogs. *Am J Physiol.* 1987;252:H969–H984.
30. Regen DM. Calculation of left ventricular wall stress. *Circ Res.* 1990;67:245–252.
31. Regen DM, Anversa P, Capasso JM. Segmental calculation of left ventricular wall stresses. *Am J Physiol.* 1993;264:H1411–H1421.
32. Wiggers CJ. The Henry Jackson Memorial Lecture. Dynamics of ventricular contraction under abnormal conditions. *Circulation.* 1952;5:321–348.
33. Haddad F, Couture P, Tousignant C, et al. The right ventricle in cardiac surgery, a perioperative perspective: I. Anatomy, physiology, and assessment. *Anesth Analg.* 2009;108:407–421.
34. Haddad F, Couture P, Tousignant C, et al. The right ventricle in cardiac surgery, a perioperative perspective: II. Pathophysiology, clinical importance, and management. *Anesth Analg.* 2009;108:422–433.
35. Cheng C-P, Freeman GL, Santamore WP, et al. Effect of loading conditions, contractile state, and heart rate on early diastolic left ventricular filling in conscious dogs. *Circ Res.* 1990;66:814–823.
36. Courtois M, Kovacs SJ Jr, Ludbrook PA. Transmitral pressure-flow velocity relation. Importance of regional pressure gradients in the left ventricle during diastole. *Circulation.* 1988;78:661–671.
37. Ishida Y, Meisner JS, Tsujioka K, et al. Left ventricular filling dynamics: influence of left ventricular relaxation and left atrial pressure. *Circulation.* 1986;74:187–196.
38. Little WC, Oh JK. Echocardiographic evaluation of diastolic function can be used to guide clinical care. *Circulation.* 2009;120:802–809.
39. Kheradvar A, Gharib M. On mitral valve dynamics and its connection to early diastolic flow. *Ann Biomed Eng.* 2009;37:1–13.
40. Pagel PS, Gandhi SD, Iqbal Z, et al. Cardiopulmonary bypass transiently inhibits intraventricular vortex ring formation in patients undergoing coronary artery bypass graft surgery. *J Cardiothorac Vasc Anesth.* 2012;26:376–380.
41. Pagel PS, Hudetz JA. Chronic pressure-overload hypertrophy attenuates vortex formation time in patients with severe aortic stenosis and preserved left ventricular systolic function undergoing aortic valve replacement. *J Cardiothorac Vasc Anesth.* 2013;27:660–664.
42. Yellin EL, Nikolic S, Frater RWM. Left ventricular filling dynamics and diastolic function. *Prog Cardiovasc Dis.* 1990;32:247–271.
43. Suga H, Yasumura Y, Nozawa T, et al. Pressure-volume relation around zero transmural pressure in excised cross-circulated dog left ventricle. *Circ Res.* 1988;63:361–372.
44. Keren G, Meisner JS, Sherez J, et al. Interrelationship of mid-diastolic mitral valve motion, pulmonary venous flow, and transmitral flow. *Circulation.* 1986;74:36–44.
45. Barbier P, Solomon SB, Schiller NB, et al. Left atrial relaxation and left ventricular systolic function determine left atrial reservoir function. *Circulation.* 1999;100:427–436.
46. Mehta S, Charbonneau F, Fitchett DH, et al. The clinical consequences of a stiff left atrium. *Am Heart J.* 1991;122:1184–1191.
47. Sagawa K. The end-systolic pressure-volume relation of the ventricle: definition, modifications and clinical use. *Circulation.* 1981;63:1223–1227.
48. Kass DA, Maughan WL, Guo ZM, et al. Comparative influence of load versus inotropic states on indexes of ventricular contractility: experimental and theoretical analysis based on pressure-volume relationships. *Circulation.* 1987;76:1422–1436.
49. Suga H. Ventricular energetics. *Physiol Rev.* 1990;70:247–277.
50. Brown KA, Ditchey RV. Human right ventricular end-systolic pressure-volume relation defined by maximal elastance. *Circulation.* 1988;78:81–91.
51. Pagel PS, Kehl F, Gare M, et al. Mechanical function of the left atrium: new insights based on analysis of pressure-volume relations and Doppler echocardiography. *Anesthesiology.* 2003;98:975–994.
52. Grossman W. Diastolic dysfunction and congestive heart failure. *Circulation.* 1990;81(2 suppl):III1–7.
53. Little WC, Downes TR. Clinical evaluation of left ventricular diastolic performance. *Prog Cardiovasc Dis.* 1990;32:273–290.

54. Wier W, Yue DT. Intracellular [Ca^{++}] transients underlying the short-term force-interval relationship in ferret ventricular myocardium. *J Physiol (Lond)*. 1986;376:507–530.
55. Vatner SF. Sympathetic mechanisms regulating myocardial contractility in conscious animals. In: Fozzard HA, Haber E, Jennings RB, et al., eds. *The Heart and Cardiovascular System: Scientific Foundations*. 2nd ed. New York: Raven Press; 1991:1709–1728.
56. Little WC, Freeman GL, O'Rourke RA. Simultaneous determination of left ventricular end-systolic pressure-volume and pressure-dimension relationships in closed-chest dogs. *Circulation*. 1985;71:1301–1308.
57. Burkhoff D. The conductance method of left ventricular volume estimation. Methodologic limitations put into perspective. *Circulation*. 1990;81:703–706.
58. Dorosz JL, Lezotte DC, Weitzenkamp DA, et al. Performance of 3-dimensional echocardiography in measuring left ventricular volumes and ejection fraction: a systematic review and meta-analysis. *J Am Coll Cardiol*. 2012;59:1799–1808.
59. Cowie B, Kluger R, Kalpokas M. Left ventricular volume and ejection fraction assessment with transoesophageal echocardiography: 2D vs 3D imaging. *Br J Anesth*. 2013;110:201–206.
60. Meris A, Santambrogio L, Casso G, et al. Intraoperative three-dimensional versus two-dimensional echocardiography for left ventricular assessment. *Anesth Analg*. 2014;118:711–720.
61. Hansen RM, Viquerat CE, Matthay MA, et al. Poor correlation between pulmonary arterial wedge pressure and left ventricular end-diastolic volume after coronary artery bypass graft surgery. *Anesthesiology*. 1986;64:764–770.
62. Tousignant C, Van Orman JR. Pulmonary impedance and pulmonary Doppler trace in the perioperative period. *Anesth Analg*. 2015;121:601–609.
63. Borow KM, Colan SD, Neumann A. Altered left ventricular mechanics in patients with valvular aortic stenosis and coarctation of the aorta: effects on systolic performance and late outcome. *Circulation*. 1985;72:515–522.
64. Weber KT, Janicki JS. Myocardial oxygen consumption: the role of wall force and shortening. *Am J Physiol*. 1977;233:H421–H430.
65. Little WC, Cheng CP. Left ventricular-arterial coupling in conscious dogs. *Am J Physiol*. 1991;261:H70–H76.
66. Nichols WW, Nicolini FA, Pepine CJ. Determinants of isolated systolic hypertension in the elderly. *J Hypertens*. 1992;10:S73–S77.
67. Lang RM, Borow KM, Neumann A, et al. Systemic vascular resistance: an unreliable index of left ventricular afterload. *Circulation*. 1986;74:1114–1123.
68. Little WC. Enhanced load dependence of relaxation in heart failure. Clinical implications. *Circulation*. 1992;85:2326–2328.
69. de Tombe PP, Little WC. Inotropic effects of ejection are myocardial properties. *Am J Physiol*. 1994;266:H1202–H1213.
70. Suga H, Sagawa K, Shoukas AA. Load-independence of the instantaneous pressure-volume ratio of the canine left ventricle and effects of epinephrine and heart rate on the ratio. *Circ Res*. 1973;32:314–322.
71. Glower DD, Spratt JA, Snow ND, et al. Linearity of the Frank-Starling relationship in the intact heart: the concept of preload recruitable stroke work. *Circulation*. 1985;71:994–1009.
72. Chen C, Rodriguez L, Guerrero JL, et al. Noninvasive estimation of the instantaneous first derivative of left ventricular pressure using continuous-wave Doppler echocardiography. *Circulation*. 1991;83:2101–2110.
73. Little WC. The left ventricular dP/dt$_{max}$-end-diastolic volume relation in closed-chest dogs. *Circ Res*. 1985;56:808–815.
74. Yew WYW. Evaluation of left ventricular diastolic function. *Circulation*. 1989;79:1393–1397.
75. Gaasch WH, Zile MR. Left ventricular diastolic dysfunction and diastolic heart failure. *Annu Rev Med*. 2004;55:373–394.
76. Maeder MT, Kaye DM. Heart failure with normal left ventricular ejection fraction. *J Am Coll Cardiol*. 2009;53:905–918.
77. Zile MR, Baicu CF, Gaasch WH. Diastolic heart failure – abnormalities in active relaxation and passive stiffness of the left ventricle. *N Engl J Med*. 2004;350:1953–1959.
78. Bench T, Burkhoff D, O'Connell JB, et al. Heart failure with normal ejection fraction: consideration of mechanisms other than diastolic dysfunction. *Curr Heart Fail Rep*. 2009;6:57–64.
79. Grewal J, McCully RB, Kane GC, et al. Left ventricular function and exercise capacity. *JAMA*. 2009;301:286–294.
80. Traversi E, Pozzoli M, Cioffi G, et al. Mitral flow velocity changes after 6 months of optimized therapy provides important hemodynamic and prognostic information in patients with heart failure. *Am Heart J*. 1996;132:809–819.
81. Pagel PS, Farber NE. Inhaled anesthetics: cardiovascular pharmacology. In: Miller R D, Cohen N, Eriksson LI, et al. *Miller's Anesthesia*, 8th ed. Philadelphia, PA: Elsevier Churchill Livingstone; 2014:706–751.
82. Flu WJ, van Kuijk JP, Hoeks SE, et al. Prognostic implications of asymptomatic left ventricular dysfunction in patients undergoing vascular surgery. *Anesthesiology*. 2010;112:1316–1324.
83. Morgan JP, Erny RE, Allen PD, et al. Abnormal intracellular calcium handling, a major cause of systolic and diastolic dysfunction in ventricular myocardium from patients with heart failure. *Circulation*. 1990;81(Suppl III):21–32.
84. Carroll JD, Hess OM, Hirzel HO, et al. Left ventricular systolic and diastolic function in coronary artery disease: effects of revascularization on exercise-induced ischemia. *Circulation*. 1985;72:119–129.
85. Weiss JL, Frederiksen JW, Weisfeldt ML. Hemodynamic determinants of the time course of fall in canine left ventricular pressure. *J Clin Invest*. 1976;58:751–760.
86. Raff GL, Glantz SA. Volume loading slows left ventricular isovolumic relaxation rate: evidence of load-dependent relaxation in the intact dog heart. *Circ Res*. 1981;48:813–824.
87. Serizawa T, Vogel WM, Apstein CS, et al. Comparison of acute alterations in left ventricular relaxation and diastolic chamber stiffness induced by hypoxia and ischemia. Role of myocardial oxygen supply-demand imbalance. *J Clin Invest*. 1981;68:91–102.
88. Eichhorn P, Grimm J, Koch R, et al. Left ventricular relaxation in patients with left ventricular hypertrophy secondary to aortic valve disease. *Circulation*. 1982;65:1395–1404.
89. Pagel PS, Kampine JP, Schmeling WT, et al. Alteration of left ventricular diastolic function by desflurane, isoflurane, and halothane in the chronically instrumented dog with autonomic nervous system blockade. *Anesthesiology*. 1991;74:1103–1114.
90. Eichhorn EJ, Willard JE, Alvarez L, et al. Are contraction and relaxation coupled in patients with and without congestive heart failure? *Circulation*. 1992;85:2132–2139.
91. Ohno M, Cheng C-P, Little WC. Mechanism of altered patterns of left ventricular filling during the development of congestive heart failure. *Circulation*. 1994;89:2241–2250.
92. Glantz SA. Computing indices of diastolic stiffness has been counterproductive. *Fed Proc*. 1980;39:162–168.
93. Mirsky I. Assessment of diastolic function: suggested methods and future considerations. *Circulation*. 1984;69:836–841.
94. Myreng Y, Smiseth OA. Assessment of left ventricular relaxation by Doppler echocardiography. Comparison of isovolumic relaxation time and transmitral flow velocities with time constant of isovolumic relaxation. *Circulation*. 1990;81:260–266.
95. Nishimura RA, Tajik AJ. Evaluation of diastolic filling of left ventricle in health and disease: Doppler echocardiography is the clinician's Rosetta stone. *J Am Coll Cardiol*. 1997;30:8–18.
96. Nagueh SF, Appleton CP, Gillebert TC, et al. Recommendations for the evaluation of left ventricular diastolic function by echocardiography. *J Am Soc Echocardiogr*. 2009;22:107–133.
97. Klein AL, Burstow DJ, Tajik AJ, et al. Effects of age on left ventricular dimensions and filling dynamics in 117 normal persons. *Mayo Clin Proc*. 1994;69:212–224.
98. Genovesi-Ebert A, Marabotti C, Palombo C, et al. Left ventricular filling: relationship with arterial blood pressure, left ventricular mass, age, heart rate, and body build. *J Hypertens*. 1991;9:345–353.
99. Cohen GI, Petrolungo JF, Thomas JD, et al. A practical guide to assessment of ventricular diastolic function using Doppler echocardiography. *J Am Coll Cardiol*. 1996;27:1753–1760.
100. Hurrell DG, Nishimura RA, Ilstrup DM, et al. Utility of preload alteration in assessment of left ventricular filling pressure by Doppler echocardiography: a simultaneous catheterization and Doppler echocardiographic study. *J Am Coll Cardiol*. 1997;30:459–467.
101. Rakowski H, Appleton C, Chan KL, et al. Canadian consensus recommendations for the measurement and reporting of diastolic dysfunction by echocardiography: from the Investigators of Consensus on Diastolic Dysfunction by Echocardiography. *J Am Soc Echocardiogr*. 1996;9:736–760.
102. Dini FL, Dell'Anna R, Micheli A, et al. Impact of blunted pulmonary venous flow on the outcome of patients with left ventricular systolic dysfunction secondary to either ischemic or idiopathic dilated cardiomyopathy. *Am J Cardiol*. 2000;85:1455–1460.
103. Smiseth OA, Thompson CR, Lohavanichbutr K, et al. The pulmonary venous systolic flow pulse. Its origin and relationship to left atrial pressure. *J Am Coll Cardiol*. 1999;34:802–809.
104. Fujii K, Ozaki M, Yamagishi T, et al. Effect of left ventricular contractile performance on passive left atrial filling: clinical study using radionuclide angiography. *Clin Cardiol*. 1994;17:258–262.
105. Appleton CP, Gonzalez MS, Basnight MA. Relationship of left atrial pressure and pulmonary venous flow velocities: importance of baseline mitral and pulmonary venous flow velocity patterns in lightly sedated dogs. *J Am Soc Echocardiogr*. 1994;7:264–275.
106. Keren G, Bier A, Sherez J, et al. Atrial contraction is an important determinant of pulmonary venous flow. *J Am Coll Cardiol*. 1986;7:693–695.
107. Garcia MJ, Thomas JD, Klein AL. New Doppler echocardiographic applications for the study of diastolic function. *J Am Coll Cardiol*. 1998;32:865–875.
108. Takatsuji H, Mikami T, Urasawa K, et al. A new approach for evaluation of left ventricular diastolic function: spatial and temporal analysis of left ventricular filling flow propagation by color M-mode Doppler echocardiography. *J Am Coll Cardiol*. 1996;27:365–371.
109. Watkins MW, LeWinter MM. Physiologic role of the normal pericardium. *Annu Rev Med*. 1993;44:171–180.
110. Maruyama Y, Ashikawa K, Isoyama S, et al. Mechanical interactions between four heart chambers with and without the pericardium in canine hearts. *Circ Res*. 1982;50:86–100.

111. Refsum H, Junemann M, Lipton MJ, Skioldebrand C, Carlsson E, Tyberg JV. Ventricular diastolic pressure-volume relations and the pericardium. Effects of changes in blood volume and pericardial effusion in dogs. *Circulation.* 1981;64:997–1004.
112. Junemann M, Smiseth OA, Refsum H, et al. Quantification of effect of pericardium on LV diastolic PV relation in dogs. *Am J Physiol.* 1987;252:H963–H968.
113. Santamore WP, Dell'Italia LJ. Ventricular interdependence: significant left ventricular contributions to right ventricular systolic function. *Prog Cardiovasc Dis.* 1998;40:289–308.
114. Weber KT, Janicki JS, Shroff S, et al. Contractile mechanics and interaction of the right and left ventricles. *Am J Cardiol.* 1981;47:686–695.
115. Gonzalez MS, Basnight MA, Appleton CP. Experimental cardiac tamponade: a hemodynamic and Doppler echocardiographic reexamination of the relation of right and left heart ejection dynamics to the phase of respiration. *J Am Coll Cardiol.* 1991;18:243–252.
116. Pinsky MR. Functional hemodynamic monitoring. *Crit Care Clin.* 2015;31:89–111.
117. Santamore WP, Heckman JL, Bove AA. Right and left ventricular pressure-volume response to elevated pericardial pressure. *Am Rev Respir Dis.* 1986;134:101–107.
118. Santamore WP, Bartlett R, Van Buren SJ, et al. Ventricular coupling in constrictive pericarditis. *Circulation.* 1986;74:597–602.
119. Goldman S, Olajos M, Morkin E. Comparison of left atrial and left ventricular performance in conscious dogs. *Cardiovasc Res.* 1984;18:604–612.
120. Payne RM, Stone HL, Engelken EJ. Atrial function during volume loading. *J Appl Physiol.* 1971;31:326–331.
121. Dernellis J, Tsiamis E, Stefanadis C, et al. Effects of postural changes on left atrial function in patients with hypertrophic cardiomyopathy. *Am Heart J.* 1998;136:982–987.
122. Gare M, Schwabe DA, Hettrick DA, et al. Desflurane, sevoflurane, and isoflurane affect left atrial active and passive mechanical properties and impair left atrial-left ventricular coupling in vivo. Analysis using pressure-volume relations. *Anesthesiology.* 2001;95:689–698.
123. Prioli A, Marino P, Lanzoni L, et al. Increasing degrees of left ventricular filling impairment modulate left atrial function in humans. *Am J Cardiol.* 1998;82:756–761.
124. Ito T, Suwa M, Kobashi A, et al. Reversible left atrial dysfunction possibly due to afterload mismatch in patients with left ventricular dysfunction. *J Am Soc Echocardiogr.* 1998;11:274–279.
125. Plehn JF, Southworth J, Cornwell GG III. Brief report: atrial systolic failure in primary amyloidosis. *N Engl J Med.* 1992;327:1570–1573.
126. Tabata T, Oki T, Yamada H, et al. Role of left atrial appendage in left atrial reservoir function as evaluated by left atrial appendage clamping during cardiac surgery. *Am J Cardiol.* 1998;81:327–332.
127. Hoit BD, Shao Y, Tsai LM, et al. Altered left atrial compliance after atrial appendectomy. Influence on left atrial and ventricular filling. *Circ Res.* 1993;72:167–175.
128. Nishikawa Y, Roberts JP, Tan P, et al. Effect of dynamic exercise on left atrial function in conscious dogs. *J Physiol.* 1994;481:457–468.
129. Toutouzas K, Trikas A, Pitsavos C, et al. Echocardiographic features of left atrium in elite male athletes. *Am J Cardiol.* 1996;78:1314–1317.
130. Triposkiadis F, Tentolouris K, Androulakis A, et al. Left atrial mechanical function in the healthy elderly: new insights from a combined assessment of changes in atrial volume and transmitral flow velocity. *J Am Soc Echocardiogr.* 1995;8:801–809.
131. Nishigaki K, Arakawa M, Miwa H, et al. A study of left atrial transport function. Effect of age or left ventricular ejection fraction on left atrial storage function. *Angiology.* 1994;45:953–962.
132. Zuccala G, Cocchi A, Lattanzio F, et al. Effect of age on left atrial function in patients with coronary artery disease. *Cardiology.* 1994;85:8–13.

13 Cardiovascular Pharmacology

PAUL S. PAGEL • LORETA GRECU

Introduction
Cholinergic Drugs
Cholinergic Agonists
Cholinesterase Inhibitors
Muscarinic Antagonists
Muscarinic Antagonist Toxicity
Fundamentals of Catecholamine Pharmacology
Epinephrine
Norepinephrine
Dopamine
Dobutamine
Isoproterenol
Selective β_2-Adrenoceptor Agonists
Fenoldopam
Sympathomimetics
    Ephedrine
    Phenylephrine
α_1-Adrenoceptor Antagonists
α_2-Adrenoceptor Agonists: Clonidine and Dexmedetomidine
β-Adrenoceptor Antagonists (β-Blockers)
    Propranolol
    Metoprolol
    Atenolol
    Esmolol
    Labetalol
    Carvedilol
Phosphodiesterase Inhibitors
Levosimendan
Digitalis Glycosides
Vasopressin
Nitrovasodilators
    Nitroglycerin
    Sodium Nitroprusside
Hydralazine
Calcium Channel Blockers
    Nifedipine
    Nicardipine
    Clevidipine
    Nimodipine
    Diltiazem
    Verapamil
Angiotensin-converting Enzyme Inhibitors
Angiotensin Receptor Blockers

KEY POINTS

1. Drugs that mimic the effects of acetylcholine are most commonly used in ophthalmology.
2. Anticholinesterases prolong the actions of acetylcholine by preventing its metabolism; these drugs are used clinically for reversal of neuromuscular blockade and treatment of central anticholinergic syndrome.
3. Muscarinic antagonists inhibit the effects of acetylcholine mediated through the parasympathetic nervous system.
4. The cardiovascular effects of endogenous and synthetic catecholamines are dependent on their specificity for α- and β-adrenoceptor subtypes.
5. Catecholamines have well-documented utility in the treatment of acute left ventricular dysfunction, but may cause arrhythmias, hypertension, and myocardial ischemia.
6. α_1-Adrenoceptor antagonists not only reduce arterial pressure but also produce reflex tachycardia and orthostatic hypotension, especially in patients with hypovolemia.
7. The α_2-adrenoceptor agonists clonidine and dexmedetomidine are used extensively for sedation, anxiolysis, and analgesia.
8. β-Blockers play major roles in the treatment of hypertension, coronary artery disease, myocardial infarction, and heart failure.
9. Milrinone and levosimendan are important medications for the management of acute left ventricular dysfunction and cause synergistic positive inotropic effects when administered with catecholamines by enhancing intracellular cAMP-mediated signaling.
10. Vasopressin is the most potent arterial vasoconstrictor currently available and is useful for treatment of vasoplegia associated with sepsis or cardiac surgery.
11. Calcium channel blockers reduce arterial pressure and dilate coronary arteries, but some of these drugs also affect sinoatrial node automaticity and atrioventricular node conduction. These latter actions may be beneficial in the presence of supraventricular tachyarrhythmias.
12. Angiotensin-converting enzyme inhibitors and angiotensin receptor blockers are useful for the treatment of hypertension and heart failure.

From the Anesthesia Service, the Clement J. Zablocki Veterans Affairs Medical Center, Milwaukee, Wisconsin (PSP) and the Department of Anesthesiology, Yale University, New Haven, Connecticut (LG). This work was supported entirely by departmental funds. The authors have no conflicts of interest pursuant to this work.

Introduction

This chapter discusses the pharmacology of medications that affect the autonomic nervous and cardiovascular systems. A thorough understanding of the pharmacology of cholinergic and anticholinergic drugs, endogenous and synthetic catecholamines, sympathomimetics, α_1-antagonists, α_2-agonists, β-blockers, phosphodiesterase inhibitors, digitalis glycosides, vasopressin, and antihypertensive medications including nitrovasodilators, calcium (Ca^{2+}) channel blockers, and angiotensin-converting enzyme (ACE) inhibitors is essential for the practice of anesthesiology. Each of these drug classifications will be reviewed in detail, with primary emphasis on their cardiovascular actions.

Cholinergic Drugs

Cholinergic drugs mimic (e.g., agonists such as methacholine), enhance (e.g., anticholinesterase inhibitors including neostigmine), or block (e.g., antagonists such as atropine) the actions of acetylcholine (ACh) in autonomic ganglia and skeletal muscle at nicotinic receptors or in parasympathetic postganglionic neurons through muscarinic receptors. In general, cholinergic drugs have greater site-specificity and exert more prolonged effects than the primary neurotransmitter. Compared with the plethora of medications that affect the sympathetic nervous system (see below), there are relatively few drugs in current clinical use that influence the function of parasympathetic nervous system by modulating ACh's actions or metabolism. ACh itself has virtually no therapeutic applications because of its diffuse action, extensive side effect profile, and rapid hydrolysis by acetylcholinesterase and butyrylcholinesterase (pseudocholinesterase). Topical ACh eye drops are occasionally used when acute miosis is required during ophthalmologic surgery (e.g., cataract extraction) or for the treatment of glaucoma. Under these circumstances, systemic cholinergic effects are usually not observed because little ACh uptake occurs and ACh is quickly metabolized.

Cholinergic Agonists

Synthetic cholinergic agonists are not used in anesthesia practice, but understanding of their pharmacology remains important because anesthesiologists often encounter patients who are treated with them (Fig. 13-1; Table 13-1). ACh is a quaternary ammonium compound that causes changes in membrane conformation when it interacts with postsynaptic receptors, increasing the permeability to Na^+, K^+, and Cl^- ions down their respective electrochemical gradients and causing membrane depolarization. Structure–activity relationships identified two important binding sites on the postsynaptic ACh receptor that are crucial for this process: the "ester" site that binds this moiety of the molecule and an "ion" site through which the quaternary amine is bound. Subtle differences in the chemical structure of cholinergic drugs

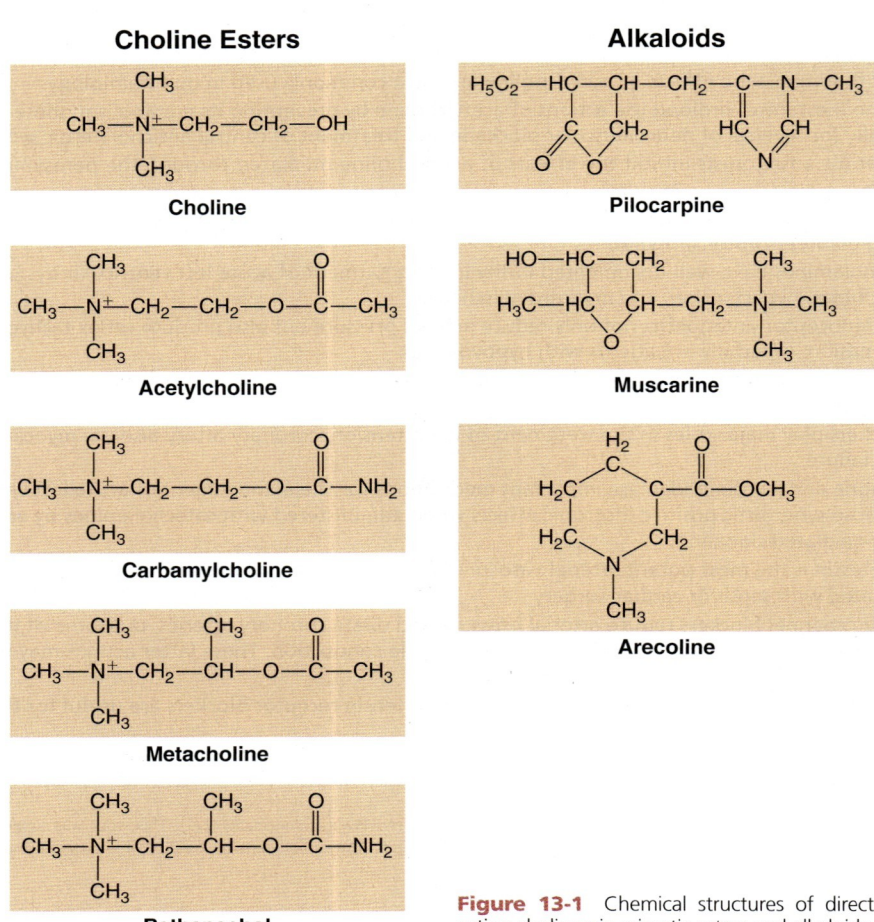

Figure 13-1 Chemical structures of direct acting cholinergic-mimetic esters and alkaloids.

Table 13-1 Comparative Muscarinic Actions of Direct Cholinomimetic Agents

	Systemic				
	Acetylcholine	Methacholine	Carbamylcholine	Bethanechol	Pilocarpine
Esterase Hydrolysis	+++	+	0	0	0
Eye (Topical)					
Iris	++	++	+++	+++	+++
Ciliary	++	++	+++	+++	++
Heart					
Rate	−	−	−	−	
Contractility	−	−	−	−	
Conduction	−	−	−	−	
Smooth Muscle					
Vascular	−	−	−	−	− −
Bronchial	++	++	+	+	++
Gastrointestinal motility	++	++	+++	+++	++
Gastrointestinal sphincters	−	−	−	−	++
Biliary	++	++	+++	+++	++
Bladder					
Detrusor	++	++	+++	+++	++
Sphincter	−	−	−	−	−
Exocrine Glands					
Respiratory	+++	++	+++	++	++++
Salivary	++	++	++	++	+++++
Pharyngeal	++	++	++	++	++++
Lacrimal	++	++	++	++	++++
Sweat	++	++	++	++	+++++
Gastrointestinal acid and secretions	++	++	++	++	++++
Nicotinic Actions	+++	+	+++	−	+++

+, stimulation; −, inhibition.

are capable of producing more muscarinic and less nicotinic specificity while simultaneously reducing the rate of the drug's metabolism. Two major classes of cholinergic agonists have been developed based on modification of these structural components: choline esters and alkaloids. For example, β-methylation of the choline moiety produces methacholine, a synthetic cholinergic drug that is a muscarinic agonist and is almost entirely resistant to cholinesterase hydrolysis. Methacholine is used almost exclusively as a provocative agent for identifying the presence of reactive airway disease in subjects who do not have clinically apparent signs or symptoms of asthma. Methacholine causes bronchoconstriction, increases airway secretions, and reduces peak expiratory flow rate via activation of bronchial muscarinic M_3 receptors.[1] Not surprisingly, methacholine may also produce bradycardia and hypotension as a result of M_3 receptor activation in myocardium and vascular endothelium, respectively. Methacholine-induced stimulation of M_3 receptors activates the pertussis toxin-insensitive $G_{q/11}$ protein coupled-phospholipase C-inositol triphosphate (IP_3)-mediated signaling cascade, culminating in endothelial nitric oxide synthase activation, nitric oxide production, and dilation of vascular smooth muscle.[2] Use of methacholine is relatively contraindicated in patients with known asthma or chronic obstructive pulmonary disease, essential hypertension, recent cerebrovascular accident, or myocardial infarction because marked bronchospasm or profound hypotension may occur. Indeed, emergency airway equipment, oxygen, inhaled $β_2$-adrenoceptor agonists, and resuscitative medications should be readily available during methacholine provocative testing.

Bethanechol is a choline ester (a carbamate derivative of methacholine) that is relatively selective for the M_3 receptors in the urinary and gastrointestinal tracts with relative sparing of the cardiovascular and respiratory systems. Bethanechol is useful for treatment of nonobstructive urinary retention during the postoperative period or in some cases of neurogenic bladder as an alternative to chronic catheterization.[3] Bethanechol also increases gastrointestinal motility and stimulates peristalsis. The drug was previously used for treatment of postoperative abdominal distention, gastric atony, and gastroesophageal reflux disease, but more efficacious medications are now available for these conditions. Carbamylcholine is another choline ester derivative that is used topically to produce miosis in patients with wide-angle glaucoma. Pilocarpine is an alkaloid cholinergic agonist used as a topical miotic agent to reduce intraocular pressure in patients with glaucoma. Oral pilocarpine may also be used to increase salivary and lacrimal gland production in patients with xerostomia after head and neck irradiation or in those with Sjögren syndrome.[4] Finally, muscarinic agonists may also be useful for treatment of cognitive impairment in patients with Alzheimer disease.

Cholinesterase Inhibitors

2 Cholinesterase inhibitors (anticholinesterases) are essential to anesthesiologists because these medications are used to produce the sustained cholinergic effect necessary to overcome nondepolarizing neuromuscular blockade. These drugs are also used for treatment of myasthenia gravis, glaucoma, and, less commonly, intestinal or urinary bladder atony and have important anesthetic implications. The pharmacology of anticholinesterases as neuromuscular blockade reversal medications is described in detail in Chapter 21; the current discussion will focus solely on the actions of these drugs as cholinergic-mimetics. In contrast to organophosphate compounds (e.g., pesticides such as malathion and parathion; nerve toxins including sarin, soman, and VX) that irreversibly inhibit acetylcholinesterase and butyrylcholinesterase, clinically used cholinesterase inhibitors (e.g., neostigmine, edrophonium) reversibly inhibit these enzymes, which very rapidly hydrolyze ACh (half-life of microseconds) into acetate and choline molecules under normal conditions, thereby inactivating the neurotransmitter. This inhibition of acetylcholinesterase and butyrylcholinesterase allows the actions of ACh at postganglionic muscarinic receptors to be markedly amplified, resulting in intense parasympathetic nervous system activity similar to that produced by direct cholinergic agonists. The unimpeded accumulation of ACh also causes dual actions on autonomic nervous system ganglia and skeletal muscle, initially stimulating but subsequently depressing neurotransmission through their nicotinic receptors. Similar initial stimulation followed by depression of central nervous system cholinergic receptors also occurs with exposure to a lethal dose of an anticholinesterase, for example, when an organophosphate overdose occurs during its use as a pesticide or when the agent is used as a chemical weapon during warfare or a terrorist attack.[5]

Clinically used cholinesterase inhibitors are either carbamoyl esters (including neostigmine, physostigmine, and pyridostigmine) or quaternary ammonium alcohols (edrophonium; Fig. 13-2). Three areas on the acetylcholinesterase molecule are capable of binding inhibitory ligands: two are located in the active center of the enzyme (the acyl pocket and a choline subsite, referred to collectively as the "esteratic" site), whereas the third is a peripheral "anionic" site.[6] The specificity and duration of action of cholinesterase inhibitors depend on their binding site, affinity, and rate of hydrolysis. For example, edrophonium reversibly binds to the choline subsite, but the cholinesterase inhibitor's chemical structure facilitates its rapid renal excretion and contributes to the drug's relatively short duration of action (approximately 1 hour). The carbamate cholinesterase inhibitors also bind to acetylcholinesterase's "esteratic" site, but these drugs are more slowly metabolized because their carbamoyl ester linkage is less susceptible to hydrolysis, thereby extending their clinical duration of action to approximately 4 hours. In contrast, organophosphates bind irreversibly to the active center of anticholinesterase and require stimulated hydrolysis of the phosphate–enzyme complex to restore the enzyme's activity with drugs such as pralidoxime (2-PAM). Organophosphates are particular insidious toxins because they may be odorless, are rapidly absorbed through the skin, are very lipid-soluble, and move freely into the central nervous system.[7]

The most prominent pharmacologic effects of the cholinesterase inhibitors are their actions on muscarinic receptors, but when used to reverse nondepolarizing neuromuscular blockade, the intended target of these drugs is the nicotinic receptors at the motor endplate of skeletal muscle. Notably, higher concentrations of ACh are required to activate nicotinic than muscarinic receptors. Thus, the relative excess of ACh needed to overcome nondepolarizing neuromuscular blockade of nicotinic receptors predictably causes profound stimulation of muscarinic receptors and cholinergic side effects. As a result, administration of a muscarinic antagonist (e.g., atropine, glycopyrrolate) is most often required to block the side effects of cholinesterase inhibitors (e.g., bradycardia, hypotension, bronchospasm, sialorrhea, miosis, increased intestinal motility, sphincter relaxation) while sparing the actions of these drugs at the nicotinic receptors. Unlike neostigmine, pyridostigmine, and edrophonium, physostigmine is a tertiary amine that readily crosses the blood–brain barrier and inhibits acetylcholinesterase in the central nervous system. As a result, physostigmine is effective for the treatment of atropine or scopolamine overdose (these muscarinic antagonists also penetrate the blood–brain barrier) and central anticholinergic syndrome (see below).[8]

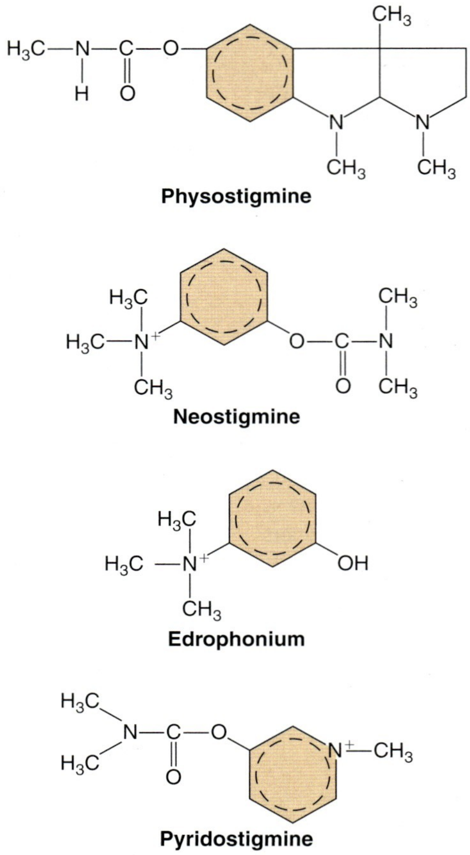

Figure 13-2 Chemical structures of clinical anticholinesterases.

Echothiophate iodide is the only clinically used organophosphate cholinesterase inhibitor, which is applied topically for the treatment of glaucoma because of its miotic effect. The drug's primary advantage over other topical glaucoma medications is its prolonged duration of action. Indeed, echothiophate may remain clinically effective for several weeks after cessation of therapy. Topical absorption of echothiophate is highly variable but can be considerable. As a result, succinylcholine may have a prolonged duration of action in patients treated with echothiophate. Despite this theoretical concern, the use of succinylcholine should not be expressly avoided when the depolarizing neuromuscular blocker is clinically indicated.

Muscarinic Antagonists

3 The muscarinic antagonists atropine, scopolamine, and glycopyrrolate are commonly used in anesthesia practice (Table 13-2).

Table 13-2 Comparative Effects of Muscarinic Antagonists

Name	Chemical Structure	Duration IV (hrs)	Duration IM (hrs)	CNS	Heart Rate	Antisialagogue Effect	Mydriasis Cycloplegia
Atropine		0.25–0.5	2–4	Stimulation	+++	+	+
Scopolamine		0.5–1	4–6	Sedation	0	++	+
Glycopyrrolate		2–4	6–8	0	+	++	0

Atropine and scopolamine are belladonna alkaloids that are derived from a variety of plant species (including deadly nightshade shrub, jimson weed, and henbane) and have been used for millennia as toxins and therapeutic agents. Muscarinic antagonists are competitive inhibitors of ACh at parasympathetic muscarinic receptors and act to increase heart rate; inhibit salivary, bronchial, and gastrointestinal secretions; attenuate gastric acid production; reduce gastrointestinal motility; cause bronchodilation; and antagonize the muscarinic side effects of anticholinesterases during reversal of neuromuscular blockade. Notably, the drugs also bind to presynaptic muscarinic receptors on norepinephrine-secreting postganglionic neurons. This action may enhance sympathetic nervous system activity because ACh-induced stimulation of these presynaptic receptors normally inhibits norepinephrine release, whereas muscarinic blockade abolishes this inhibition.[9] Anesthesiologists first used atropine to mitigate excessive salivation and attenuate vagal-mediated bradycardia during open-drop ether or chloroform anesthesia. These antiquated indications are no longer of relevance in modern practice, but anesthesiologists continue to exploit the antisialagogue effect of muscarinic antagonists (particularly glycopyrrolate) in preparation for fiberoptic intubation or during some otolaryngology or dental procedures in adults and children. Although the potencies of atropine, scopolamine, and glycopyrrolate are quite different, the drugs have little or no muscarinic receptor subtype specificity, and as a result, exert similar anticholinergic effects in most target organs except for the heart and central nervous system. In contrast, selective muscarinic subtype receptor antagonists have also been synthesized and are now used extensively for treatment of overactive bladder conditions[10] without causing pronounced adverse systemic anticholinergic effects.

Atropine and scopolamine are tertiary amines that easily penetrate the blood–brain barrier and produce central nervous system effects. For example, scopolamine is primarily a central nervous system depressant that causes sedation, amnesia, and euphoria. When combined with an intravenous long-acting opioid (e.g., morphine, meperidine), these properties made scopolamine particularly useful as intramuscular premedication for patients undergoing cardiac or major noncardiac surgery before midazolam was introduced into clinical practice in the 1980s. Transdermal scopolamine is currently used for prophylaxis against kinetosis (motion sickness) and is also effective for the treatment of postoperative nausea and vomiting, but the drug may be associated with anticholinergic side effects despite this route of administration. Lower doses of atropine are relatively devoid of central nervous system effects, but higher doses (≥2 mg; used most often in combination with an anticholinesterase inhibitor to reverse neuromuscular blockade or for the treatment of symptomatic bradyarrhythmias) often produce restlessness, disorientation, hallucinations, and delirium. In contrast to atropine and scopolamine, the synthetic muscarinic antagonist glycopyrrolate is a quaternary amine that does not cross the blood–brain barrier and is devoid of central nervous system effects. When combined with glycopyrrolate's more prolonged duration of action, this latter property makes the muscarinic antagonist more attractive for routine clinical use in anesthesiology than atropine.

Atropine, and to a lesser extent glycopyrrolate, increase heart rate when sinus bradycardia occurs as a result of vagal stimulation (e.g., peritoneal traction during abdominal surgery) or inhibition of cardiac sympathetic nerve traffic during spinal or epidural anesthesia. Atropine is also a treatment of choice for symptomatic bradyarrhythmias (e.g., second- or third-degree heart block). Conversely, atropine must be used with extreme caution when tachycardia is deleterious (e.g., coronary artery stenosis, aortic valve stenosis, hypertrophic obstructive cardiomyopathy, pheochromocytoma, thyroid storm). Paradoxically, very low doses of atropine (<0.1 mg) may decrease heart rate[11] through blockade of presynaptic parasympathetic neuron M_1 receptors.[12] Scopolamine most often produces little or no change in heart rate when administered through an intramuscular route for premedication. Notably, both clinically used belladonna alkaloids are capable of producing a paradoxical bradycardia when lower doses of these drugs are administered (scopolamine to a greater extent than atropine). Atropine and scopolamine cause mydriasis and cycloplegia because they exert muscarinic antagonist effects on ACh-mediated cranial nerve II (afferent) and III (efferent) control of pupillary reactivity and ocular accommodation. Indeed, atropine-mimetics are widely used in ophthalmology because

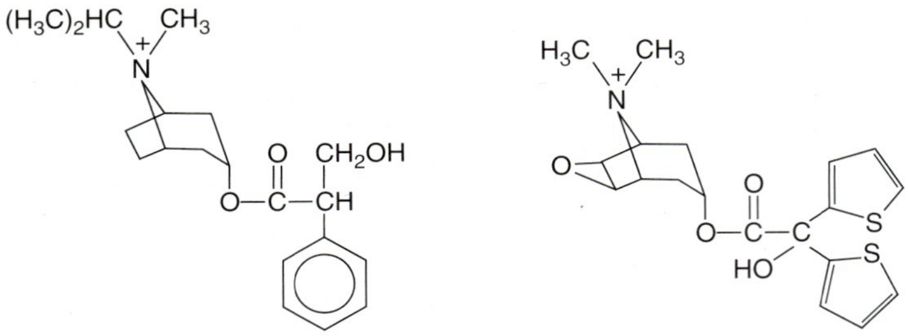

Figure 13-3 Chemical structures of inhaled muscarinic antagonists.

pupillary dilation facilitates visual inspection of the posterior chamber and retina. Not surprisingly, muscarinic antagonists are relatively contraindicated in patients with narrow-angle glaucoma because pupillary dilation thickens the peripheral iris and narrows the iridocorneal angle, thereby mechanically impairing aqueous humor drainage and increasing intraocular pressure. Muscarinic antagonists inhibit sympathetic nervous system innervation of sweat glands because ACh is the neurotransmitter in these postganglionic neurons. Pediatric patients are particularly susceptible to develop hyperthermia when treated with these drugs because children are more reliant on sweating to maintain normal body temperature than adults. Muscarinic antagonists may also be relatively contraindicated in febrile patients for similar reasons.

Ipratropium and tiotropium are muscarinic antagonists that resemble atropine and are used for the treatment of reactive airway disease (Fig. 13-3).[13,14] The drugs are bronchial smooth muscle dilators that are administered using metered-dose inhalers. Bronchodilation produced by ipratropium and tiotropium is less pronounced than that observed with β_2-adrenoceptor agonists. Nevertheless, ipratropium and tiotropium effectively inhibit airway reactivity induced by a variety of provocative substances (methacholine, histamine, prostaglandin $F_{2-\alpha}$), but they are ineffective against leukotriene-induced bronchoconstriction. Neither drug substantially affects mucociliary clearance. Because of their quaternary ammonium structures, ipratropium and tiotropium are poorly absorbed into the systemic circulation and do not produce adverse anticholinergic side effects with the exception of xerostomia. The inhaled muscarinic antagonists may be more efficacious in patients with chronic obstructive pulmonary disease than in those suffering from asthma.[15]

Muscarinic Antagonist Toxicity

Atropine and other muscarinic antagonists cause symptoms associated with blockade of Ach at parasympathetic and sympathetic (sweat glands) postganglionic neurons (Table 13-3). The familiar medical school mnemonic "dry as a bone; red as a beet; blind as a bat; hot as a hare; mad as a hatter" summarizes these effects. The central nervous system effects of muscarinic antagonists are particularly noteworthy because muscarinic ACh receptors are abundant in the brain, blockade of which may result in psychoactive effects including excitation, restlessness, sedation, confusion, hallucinations, stupor, delirium, psychosis, seizures, or coma. These alterations in sensorium associated with centrally acting muscarinic antagonists are characteristic features of central anticholinergic syndrome (known as "postoperative delirium" when it occurs after emergence from general anesthesia) and may persist well beyond the expected duration of the offending drug's metabolism. Antihistamines, tricyclic antidepressants, phenothiazines, benzodiazepines, and a variety of other medications are also associated with central anticholinergic syndrome (Table 13-4). As mentioned previously, the treatment of choice for central anticholinergic syndrome is the tertiary amine anticholinesterase physostigmine, which crosses the blood–brain barrier and increases ACh concentrations in the central nervous system. Physostigmine is most often administered in 1 or 2 mg doses to avoid producing peripheral cholinergic activity. Importantly, the duration of action of physostigmine may be shorter than that of the muscarinic antagonist. As a result, repeated treatment with physostigmine may be required if symptoms recur. Nevertheless, the drug must be used with caution because of unopposed cholinergic agonist effects in the absence of a muscarinic antagonist.

Fundamentals of Catecholamine Pharmacology

α-, β-, and dopamine-adrenergic receptor subtypes mediate the cardiovascular effects of endogenous (epinephrine, norepinephrine, dopamine) and synthetic (dobutamine, isoproterenol) catecholamines (Table 13-5). These substances stimulate β_1-adrenoceptors located on the sarcolemmal membrane of atrial and ventricular myocytes to varying degrees. Activation of β_1-adrenoceptors causes positive chronotropic (increase in heart rate), dromotropic (faster conduction velocity), inotropic (greater contractility), and lusitropic (shorter relaxation) effects. A stimulatory guanine nucleotide-binding (G_s) protein couples the β_1-adrenoceptor to the intracellular enzyme adenylyl cyclase (Fig. 13-4). Agonist occupation of the β_1-adrenoceptor accelerates

Table 13-3	Atropine Toxicity
Dose Range (mg)	**Muscarinic Antagonist Effects**
0.5–1.0	Increased heart rate; xerostomia (dry mouth); thirst; lack of sweating; mild pupillary dilation
2–5	Tachycardia; palpitations; mydriasis; cycloplegia; restlessness or confusion; inability to swallow, urinate, defecate, or sweat; hot skin
10 or greater	Profound tachycardia, mydriasis, and cycloplegia; hot, red skin; fever; hallucinations; delirium; coma; death

Adapted with permission from Brown JA, Laiken N. Muscarinic receptor agonists and antagonists. In: Brunton LL, Chabner BA, Knollmann BC, eds. *Goodman & Gilman's The Pharmacological Basis of Therapeutics*. 12th ed. New York, NY: McGraw-Hill Medical; 2011:226.

Table 13-4 Antimuscarinic Compounds Associated with Central Anticholinergic Syndrome

Belladonna Alkaloids
Atropine sulfate
Scopolamine hydrobromide

Synthetic and Natural Tertiary Amine Compounds
Dicyclomine antispasmodic with local anesthetic activity
Thiphenamil antispasmodic with local anesthetic activity
Procaine
Cocaine
Cyclopentolate mydriatic

Quaternary Derivatives of Belladonna Alkaloids
Methscopolamine bromide—antispasmodic
Homatropine methylbromide—sedative, antispasmodic
Homatropine hydrobromide—ophthalmic solution—mydriatic

Synthetic Quaternary Compounds
Methantheline bromide
Propantheline bromide

Antihistamines
Chlorpheniramine
Diphenhydramine

Plants
Deadly nightshade (atropine)
Bittersweet
Potato leaves and sprouts
Jimson or loco weed
Coca plant (cocaine)

Over-the-counter
Asthmador—atropine-like
Compoz—scopolamine sedation
Sleep Eze—scopolamine sedation
Sominex—scopolamine sedation

Antiparkinson Drugs
Benztropine
Trihexyphenidyl
Biperiden
Ethopropazine
Procyclidine

Antipsychotic Drugs
Chlorpromazine
Thioridazine
Haloperidol
Droperidol
Promethazine

Tricyclic Antidepressants
Amitriptyline
Imipramine
Desipramine

Synthetic Opioids
Meperidine
Methadone

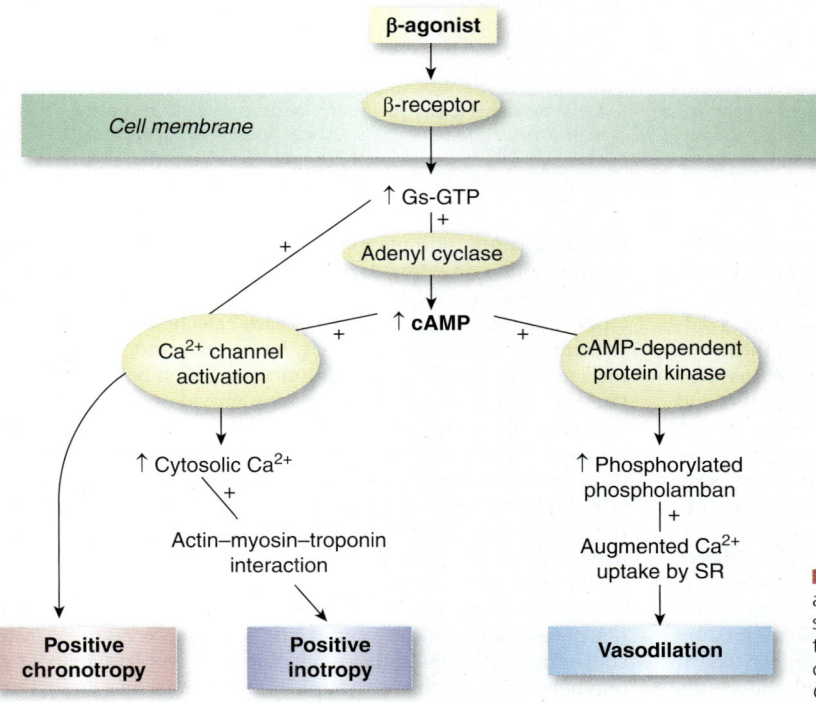

Figure 13-4 Schematic illustration of β-adrenoceptor agonist mechanism of action. (Adapted with permission from Gillies M, Bellomo R, Doolan L, et al. Bench-to-bedside review: Inotropic drug therapy after adult cardiac surgery: a systematic literature review. *Crit Care.* 2005;9:266–279.)

Table 13-5 Comparative Effects of Endogenous and Synthetic Catecholamines

Name	Chemical Structure	β_1	β_2
Epinephrine		++++	+++
Norepinephrine		+++	+
Dopamine		++++	++
Dobutamine		+++++	+++
Isoproterenol		+++++	+++++
Phenylephrine		0	0

Abbreviations: IV, intravenous; IM, intramuscular; CHF, congestive heart failure; AS, aortic stenosis; HCM, hypertrophic obstructive cardiomyopathy. Modified from Linn KA, Pagel PS. Cardiovascular pharmacology. In: Barash PG, Cullen BF, Stoelting RK, et al., eds. *Clinical Anesthesia Fundamentals*. Philadelphia, PA: Wolters Kluwer; 2015:234–235.

the formation of the second messenger cyclic adenosine monophosphate (cAMP) from adenosine triphosphate (ATP). Activation of this signaling cascade has three major consequences in myocardial calcium (Ca^{2+}) homeostasis: first, greater Ca^{2+} availability for contractile activation; second, increased efficacy of activator Ca^{2+} at troponin C of the contractile apparatus; and third, faster removal of Ca^{2+} from the contractile apparatus and the sarcoplasm after contraction. The first two of these actions directly increase contractility (inotropic effect), whereas the third facilitates more rapid myocardial relaxation during early diastole (lusitropic effect). Not surprisingly, treatment of left ventricular (LV) dysfunction is the major reason why catecholamines are used during the perioperative period. The relative density and functional integrity of the β_1-adrenoceptor and its downstream signaling cascade substantially influence the clinical efficacy of catecholamines because receptor downregulation and abnormal intracellular Ca^{2+} homeostasis commonly occur in the presence of LV dysfunction.[16,17] Notably, β_2-adrenoceptors are also present in myocardium (atrial > ventricular).[18] These β_2-adrenoceptors are also linked to adenylyl cyclase through G_s proteins and act to partially preserve myocardial responsiveness to catecholamine stimulation in the presence of β_1-adrenoceptor dysfunction or downregulation.[19,20]

The tissue-specific distribution of α- and β-adrenoceptor subtypes combines with differences in each catecholamine's chemical structure and its relative selectivity for adrenoceptors to determine the actions of catecholamines in other perfusion beds. This selectivity is often dose-related. Dopamine provides a particular useful (although not strictly accurate) pedagogical illustration of this principle. Lower doses of this catecholamine ($<3\ \mu g \cdot kg^{-1} \cdot min^{-1}$) predominantly stimulate dopamine subtype 1 and 2 receptors (DA_1 and DA_2, respectively) and cause splanchnic and renal arterial vasodilation. Progressively larger doses of dopamine sequentially activate β_1- (5 to 10 $\mu g \cdot kg^{-1} \cdot min^{-1}$) and α_1-adrenoceptors (>10 $\mu g \cdot kg^{-1} \cdot min^{-1}$), enhancing contractility and causing arterial vasoconstriction, respectively. α_1-Adrenoceptors are major regulators of vasomotor tone in arteries, arterioles, and veins. Thus, catecholamines with substantial α_1-adrenoceptor agonist activity (e.g., norepinephrine) increase systemic vascular resistance and reduce venous capacitance through arterial and venous vasoconstriction, respectively. Phospholipase-inositol 1,4,5-triphosphate signaling through an inhibitory guanine nucleotide-binding (G_i) protein

α_1	Dopamine$_1$	Dose Range	Clinical Indications	Major Side Effects
+++++	0	IV: 0.01–0.2 µg/kg/min Bolus: 1 mg IV q 3–5 min IM(1:1,000): 0.1–0.5 mg	Shock (cardiogenic, vasodilatory) Bronchospasm Anaphylaxis Symptomatic bradycardia unresponsive to atropine/pacing	Arrhythmias Myocardial Ischemia Sudden cardiac death Hypertension Stroke
+++++	0	IV: 0.01–0.2 µg/kg/min	Shock (cardiogenic, vasodilatory)	Arrhythmias Bradycardia Peripheral ischemia Hypertension Tissue necrosis with extravasation
+++	+++++	IV: 2–20 µg/kg/min	Shock (cardiogenic, vasodilatory) Symptomatic bradycardia unresponsive to atropine/pacing	Hypertension Arrhythmias Myocardial ischemia Peripheral ischemia (high doses)
+	0	IV: 2–20 µg/kg/min	Low cardiac output (CHF, cardiogenic shock, sepsis-induced myocardial dysfunction) Symptomatic bradycardia unresponsive to atropine/pacing	Tachycardia Arrhythmias Myocardial ischemia Hypertension Hypotension
0	0	IV: 2–10 µg/kg/min	Bradyarrhythmias Denervated heart	Arrhythmias Myocardial ischemia Hypertension Hypotension
+++++	0	IV: 0.15–0.75 µg/kg/min Bolus: 0.1–0.5 mg	Hypotension with tachycardia Hypotension in AS or HCM	Reflex bradycardia Hypertension Peripheral and visceral vasoconstriction Tissue necrosis with extravasation

mediates this α_1-adrenoceptor vasoconstriction (Fig. 13-5). This cascade opens Ca^{2+} channels, releases Ca^{2+} from intracellular stores (sarcoplasmic reticulum and calmodulin), and activates several Ca^{2+}-dependent protein kinases. These actions act in concert to increase intracellular Ca^{2+} concentration and cause contraction of vascular smooth muscle. α_1-Adrenoceptors predominate in many vascular beds, but β_2-adrenoceptors are the most common adrenoceptor subtype in skeletal muscle. Catecholamine-induced activation of β_2-adrenoceptors produces arteriolar vasodilation through adenylyl cyclase-mediated signaling. The result of this vasodilation is increased blood flow to skeletal muscle, which facilitates the "fight or flight" response to a perceived threat.

The actions of each specific catecholamine on heart rate, myocardial contractility, and LV preload and afterload combine to determine its overall effect on arterial pressure. For example, if a catecholamine acts primarily through the α_1-adrenoceptor, an increase in arterial pressure may be predicted because enhanced arterial and venous vasomotor tone increases systemic vascular resistance (greater afterload) and facilitates venous return to the heart (increased preload), respectively. In contrast, a catecholamine with primarily β-adrenoceptor activity and little or no effect on the α_1-adrenoceptor should modestly decrease arterial pressure because reductions in systemic vascular resistance (through β_2-adrenoceptor activation) offset increases in cardiac output caused by tachycardia and enhanced myocardial contractility (β_1-adrenoceptor effects). All catecholamines have the potential to cause detrimental increases in myocardial oxygen consumption in patients with flow-limiting coronary artery stenoses and may produce acute myocardial ischemia as a result. Thus, the use of a catecholamine to support LV function in a patient with heart failure and coronary artery disease should be approached with caution. For this reason, afterload reduction is usually a more prudent approach to improve cardiac output and reduce congestive symptoms in a patient with coronary artery disease complicated by heart failure.

Epinephrine

Methylation of norepinephrine by phenylethanolamine N-methyltransferase converts the norepinephrine into epinephrine in adrenal medullary chromaffin cells. Epinephrine is stored in

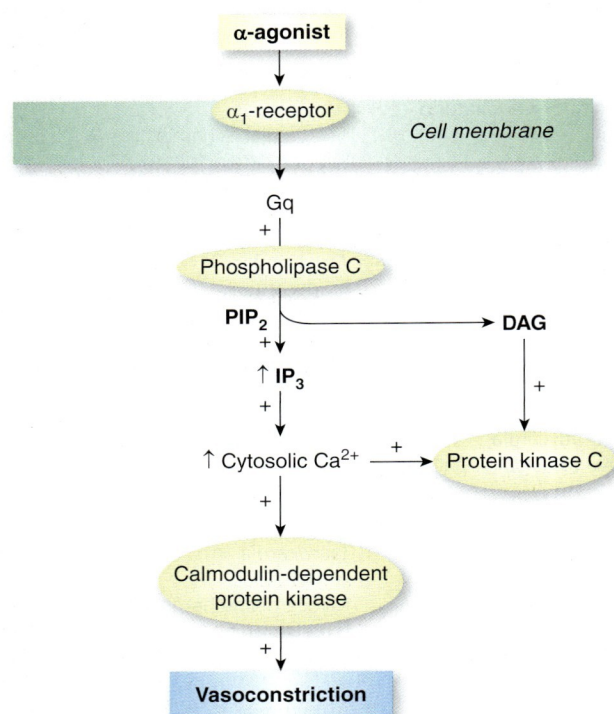

Figure 13-5 Schematic illustration of α-adrenoceptor agonist mechanism of action. (Adapted with permission from Gillies M, Bellomo R, Doolan L, et al. Bench-to-bedside review: Inotropic drug therapy after adult cardiac surgery: a systematic literature review. *Crit Care.* 2005;9:266–279.)

and released from specific chromaffin cells that differ from those that store norepinephrine. These epinephrine- and norepinephrine-containing chromaffin cell types appear to release their respective catecholamines somewhat selectively to differing stimuli. For example, chromaffin cells storing epinephrine are especially sensitive and release this catecholamine in response to histamine exposure, whereas nicotinic agonists cause release of norepinephrine.[21] Epinephrine exerts its major cardiovascular effects through activation of α_1-, β_1-, and β_2-adrenoceptors. Epinephrine is the quintessential positive inotropic molecule. Epinephrine stimulates β_1-adrenoceptors located on the cell membranes of sinoatrial (SA) node cells and cardiac myocytes to increase heart rate and myocardial contractility, respectively. Epinephrine-induced activation of β_1-adrenoceptors also enhances the rate and extent of myocardial relaxation. This action improves ventricular filling during early diastole. The combination of these actions on heart rate and LV systolic and diastolic function markedly increases cardiac output. For example, increases in cardiac index of 0.1, 0.7, and 1.2 L min^{-1}·m^2 were observed during intravenous infusion of epinephrine (0.01, 0.02, and 0.04 µg·kg^{-1}·min^{-1}) in humans.[22] The initial tachycardia that occurs during administration of an intravenous infusion of epinephrine is often partially attenuated over time as baroreceptor-mediated reflexes are activated. Epinephrine is particularly useful for the treatment of acute biventricular failure during cardiac surgery because it predictably increases cardiac output. Epinephrine (0.01 to 0.03 µg·kg^{-1}·min^{-1}) caused similar hemodynamic effects with less pronounced tachycardia compared with dobutamine (2.5 to 5.0 µg·kg^{-1}·min^{-1}) in patients after coronary artery bypass graft surgery.[23] The authors recommend the use of epinephrine as the primary inotropic drug for the treatment of acute LV dysfunction after cardiopulmonary bypass because it produces very predictable increases in cardiac output compared with its synthetic derivatives. Data indicating that routine use of dobutamine in cardiac surgery adversely affects outcome support this recommendation.[24] Epinephrine also enhances cardiac output and oxygen delivery without producing deleterious tachycardia in patients with sepsis. However, epinephrine's efficacy as an inotropic drug is often limited because of the catecholamine's propensity to cause atrial or ventricular arrhythmias. Epinephrine increases conduction velocity and reduces refractory period in the AV node, His bundle, Purkinje fibers, and ventricular muscle. The positive dromotropic effect of epinephrine on AV nodal conduction may produce supraventricular tachyarrhythmias or cause pronounced increases in ventricular rate in the presence of atrial flutter or fibrillation. Either of these clinical conditions may inadvertently cause hypotension because profound tachycardia compromises coronary perfusion and LV filling time. Epinephrine may also increase the automaticity of latent pacemakers because spontaneous diastolic depolarization is enhanced. Irritability in other parts of the conduction system may also precipitate ventricular arrhythmias including premature ventricular contractions, ventricular tachycardia, and ventricular fibrillation, especially in the presence of a pre-existing arrhythmogenic substrate (e.g., regional myocardial ischemia or infarction, cardiomyopathy).

Epinephrine causes vasoconstriction in cutaneous, mesenteric, splenic, and renal perfusion territories because it is an α_1-adrenoceptor agonist, but the catecholamine also simultaneously vasodilates arterial blood vessels supplying skeletal muscle as a result of β_2-adrenoceptor activation.[25] Thus, epinephrine's overall effects on blood flow are dependent on the organ-specific distribution of α_1- and β_2-adrenoceptors. These actions are also dose-dependent: lower doses (<0.02 µg·kg^{-1}·min^{-1}) of epinephrine stimulate β_2-adrenoceptors, causing vasodilation and modest declines in arterial pressure. In contrast, higher doses (>0.1 µg·kg^{-1}·min^{-1}) of the catecholamine activate α_1-adrenoceptors, increasing systemic vascular resistance and arterial pressure. Higher doses of epinephrine also cause intense renal arterial vasoconstriction resulting from the combination of direct α_1-adrenoceptor agonist effects and indirect facilitation of renin release. The increase in arterial pressure associated with a large bolus dose (e.g., 1 mg in adults) of epinephrine improves coronary blood flow and survival during cardiopulmonary resuscitation.[26] As a result, epinephrine is the drug of choice in the American Heart Association Adult Advanced Cardiac Life Support protocols for malignant ventricular arrhythmias, pulseless electrical activity, and asystole.[27]

The venous circulation also contains a high density of α_1-adrenoceptors. As a result, epinephrine produces venoconstriction and enhances venous return to the heart (preload). Epinephrine causes vasoconstriction of the pulmonary arterial vascular smooth muscle and increases pulmonary arterial pressures through α_1-adrenoceptor activation. These actions may be especially pronounced in patients with pulmonary arterial hypertension (e.g., cor pulmonale, congenital heart diseases with left-to-right shunt). α_1- and β_2-adrenoceptors exist in the coronary circulation, but selective activation of either of these receptor subtypes does not represent the major mechanism by which epinephrine affects coronary blood flow. Instead, increases in coronary blood flow observed during administration of epinephrine occur principally because of metabolic autoregulation. Indeed, increases in myocardial oxygen consumption resulting from increases in heart rate, contractility, preload, and afterload are responsible for coronary vasodilation. Nevertheless, epinephrine may directly constrict epicardial coronary arteries and reduce coronary blood flow in the presence of pre-existing maximal coronary vasodilation (e.g., acute myocardial ischemia distal to a severe coronary stenosis) through direct α_1-adrenoceptor stimulation.

The vasoconstrictor properties of epinephrine make it useful for several other clinical applications. Subcutaneous infiltration of epinephrine is used to substantially reduce or nearly eliminate bleeding during dental, otolaryngology, plastic surgery, and orthopedic surgery procedures. The mixture of a local anesthetic (e.g., lidocaine) with a dilute concentration of epinephrine reduces blood loss associated with tumescent anesthesia for liposuction. The vasoconstriction produced by epinephrine also substantially decreases the risk of adverse cardiovascular side effects (e.g., hypertension, arrhythmias) because the catecholamine is slowly absorbed under these circumstances. Anesthesiologists routinely use epinephrine as a vasoconstrictor to delay the absorption of local anesthetics and thereby prolong the duration of neuraxial anesthesia or peripheral nerve blocks. This effect also decreases serum anesthetic concentration and reduces the risk of systemic toxicity. Mucosal vasoconstriction resulting from inhalation of aerosolized racemic epinephrine (containing a mixture of the levo- and dextrorotary optical isomers) is frequently used to treat airway edema associated with prolonged endotracheal intubation, airway trauma, or croup. Intramuscular injection of epinephrine may be preferred to inhalation of the catecholamine in pediatric patients with severe croup because rebound edema may occur when using the latter technique as a result of the relatively short half-life of inhaled epinephrine.[28] Finally, epinephrine-induced activation of β_2-adrenoceptors in airway smooth muscle causes bronchodilation in patients with reactive airway disease. Epinephrine also decreases antigen-mediated release of histamine and leukotrienes from mast cells, which makes the catecholamine useful for the treatment of bronchospasm associated with anaphylaxis.[29]

Prior administration of α- or β-adrenoceptor antagonists profoundly influences the epinephrine's cardiovascular effects. For example, epinephrine causes more pronounced increases in systemic vascular resistance and arterial pressure when administered in the presence of the nonselective β-blocker propranolol because β_2-adrenoceptor–mediated arterial vasodilation no longer opposes α_1-adrenoceptor-induced vasoconstriction. β-Blockade also competitively inhibits epinephrine-induced β_1-adrenoceptor activation. This competitive inhibition attenuates the positive chronotropic and inotropic effects of the catecholamine. Indeed, the hemodynamic effects of epinephrine may be quite similar to those of the synthetic pure α_1-adrenoceptor agonist phenylephrine (see below) in the presence of complete β_1- and β_2-adrenoceptor blockade. Conversely, epinephrine's β_2-adrenoceptor–mediated vasodilation is unmasked in the presence of α_1-adrenoceptor blockade, and the catecholamine may produce hypotension under these conditions. α_2-Adrenoceptor antagonists (e.g., cocaine) enhance the intensity and duration of action of the epinephrine's cardiovascular effects by inhibiting its reuptake.

Norepinephrine

Norepinephrine is the endogenous neurotransmitter released from postganglionic sympathetic nervous system nerve terminals. Norepinephrine activates α_1-, α_2-, and β_1-adrenoceptors, but this catecholamine has little effect on β_2-adrenoceptors, unlike its methylated derivative epinephrine. As a result of this adrenoceptor selectivity, norepinephrine predictably enhances myocardial contractility and causes intense arterial vasoconstriction. These actions dramatically increase arterial pressure while cardiac output remains relatively unchanged. In contrast, administration of a pure α_1-adrenoceptor agonist (e.g., phenylephrine) produces dose-related declines in cardiac output in normal and failing myocardium by increasing LV afterload because β_1-adrenoceptors are not stimulated and resulting increases in contractility do not occur. Unlike epinephrine, norepinephrine usually does not cause tachycardia because elevated arterial pressure activates baroreceptor-mediated reflexes, effectively balancing the direct positive chronotropic effects of β_1-adrenoceptor stimulation. In general, greater increases in diastolic arterial pressure and systemic vascular resistance occur during administration of norepinephrine compared with similar doses of epinephrine. Norepinephrine constricts venous capacitance vessels through α_1-adrenoceptor stimulation. This action increases venous return (preload), and combined with a β_1-adrenoceptor–mediated positive inotropic effect, modestly augments stroke volume despite concomitant increases in LV afterload.

Norepinephrine is most often used for treatment of refractory hypotension resulting from pronounced vasodilation. Norepinephrine is an established treatment in patients with septic shock[30] that is unresponsive to volume administration or other vasoactive medications because the catecholamine increases arterial pressure, cardiac index, and urine output. Norepinephrine, most often in combination with nitric oxide scavenger methylene blue, is also useful for the management of vasoplegic syndrome.[31] This hypotensive state is associated with low systemic vascular resistance and frequently occurs during or after prolonged cardiopulmonary bypass in patients undergoing cardiac surgery. The potent vasoconstrictor vasopressin has largely supplanted norepinephrine in this clinical setting. Norepinephrine increases coronary perfusion pressure in patients with severe coronary artery disease, but the catecholamine also dramatically increases myocardial oxygen consumption and may produce acute myocardial ischemia in the presence of flow-limiting coronary stenoses despite the improvement in diastolic arterial pressure. Norepinephrine may also cause spasm of internal mammary or radial artery grafts used during coronary artery surgery as a result of activation of α_1-adrenoceptors. Ventricular and supraventricular arrhythmias are sometimes observed during administration of norepinephrine, but the arrhythmogenic potential of norepinephrine is less than that of epinephrine. As a result, substitution of norepinephrine for epinephrine may be appropriate when hemodynamically significant atrial or ventricular arrhythmias are present.

Norepinephrine stimulates pulmonary arterial α_1-adrenoceptors and causes dose-related increases in pulmonary arterial pressures that may precipitate right ventricular (RV) dysfunction or failure because the RV is relatively intolerant to acute increases in afterload compared with the more muscular, thicker walled LV. An inhaled selective pulmonary vasodilator (e.g., nitric oxide, prostacyclin) may help to attenuate norepinephrine's direct pulmonary vasoconstrictor effects when the catecholamine is used in patients with pulmonary hypertension and depressed myocardial contractility. Alternatively, lower doses of norepinephrine may be administered directly through a left atrial catheter in patients with LV failure and pulmonary hypertension because metabolism in peripheral tissues reduces the quantity of norepinephrine that is returned to the pulmonary vasculature through the venous circulation. This selective left atrial route of norepinephrine administration enhances coronary perfusion pressure while simultaneously increasing LV contractility. These actions may decrease biventricular filling pressures and increase cardiac output. When arterial pressure is normal or modestly reduced, norepinephrine causes dose-dependent decreases in hepatic, skeletal muscle, splanchnic, and renal blood flow through α_1-adrenoceptor–induced vasoconstriction. However, norepinephrine increases perfusion pressure and blood flow to these vascular beds when arterial pressure is profoundly reduced. Nevertheless, sustained reductions in renal, mesenteric, and peripheral vascular blood flow represent a major limitation of prolonged use of norepinephrine. Activation of renal dopamine receptors with low-dose dopamine or the selective DA_1 agonist fenoldopam to partially counteract the deleterious actions of norepinephrine on renal blood flow may preserve renal perfusion and urine output but most likely does not reduce the incidence or severity of acute kidney injury in patients with hypotension. Norepinephrine should be administered through a central venous catheter to avoid the possibility of tissue necrosis from extravasation.

Dopamine

Dopamine is the biochemical precursor of norepinephrine. The catecholamine activates several adrenergic and dopaminergic receptor subtypes in a dose-related fashion. Lower doses (below 3 $\mu g \cdot kg^{-1} \cdot min^{-1}$) selectively activate DA_1 receptors to dilate renal, mesenteric, and splenic arterial blood vessels and increase renal and splanchnic blood flow. Lower doses of dopamine also reduce norepinephrine release from pre- and postganglionic sympathetic neurons through a DA_2-receptor–mediated mechanism. As a result of these actions, lower doses of dopamine modestly decrease arterial pressure. Moderate doses (3 to 8 $\mu g \cdot kg^{-1} \cdot min^{-1}$) of dopamine activate both α_1- and β_1-adrenoceptors, resulting in elevated arterial pressure and positive inotropic effects. In contrast, high doses (in excess of 10 $\mu g \cdot kg^{-1} \cdot min^{-1}$) of dopamine act primarily on α_1-adrenoceptors to increase arterial pressure through arteriolar vasoconstriction. Unfortunately, this dose–response description of dopamine pharmacodynamics is overly simplistic because differences in receptor density and regulation, drug interactions, and patient variability cause a wide, often unpredictable range of clinical responses[32] even in healthy individuals.[33] For example, it was once presumed that low doses of dopamine provided renal protective effects through DA_1-receptor–mediated increases in renal blood flow. However, this hypothesis was subsequently not supported because even low doses of dopamine are capable of producing simultaneous α_1- and β_1-adrenoceptor activation that may attenuate or abolish the catecholamine's intended renal dopaminergic effect. Conversely, renal blood flow and urine output may be preserved (and are certainly not reduced) during administration of higher doses of dopamine because DA_1 receptors continue to be activated despite a predominant α_1-adrenoceptor agonist effect. Varied responses such as these may explain why the results of several clinical trials indicated that dopamine does not consistently provide renal protective effects despite improvements in renal perfusion and urine output. A meta-analysis of 61 clinical trials involving 3,359 patients demonstrated that low-dose dopamine transiently increased urine output, but the catecholamine did not reduce the incidence or severity of renal dysfunction or prevent mortality.[34] Thus, the use of low-dose dopamine to maintain or enhance renal function and prevent acute kidney injury is no longer recommended.[35]

Dopamine is still occasionally used as a positive inotropic medication in patients with acute LV dysfunction, although the authors prefer to use more potent catecholamines that have more predictable pharmacodynamic profiles (e.g., epinephrine, norepinephrine) with or without a cardiac phosphodiesterase fraction III inhibitor (e.g., milrinone) for this purpose in their practices. Dopamine increases myocardial contractility through activation of β_1-adrenoceptors. Dopamine also stimulates arterial and venous α_1-adrenoceptors, increasing LV afterload and enhancing venous return, respectively. As a result of these combined actions on α_1- and β_1-adrenoceptors, dopamine increases arterial pressure and cardiac output. The use of dopamine for the treatment of hypotension in the presence of depressed contractility is limited to some degree in patients with pre-existing pulmonary arterial hypertension or heart failure with elevated LV filling pressures. For example, right atrial, mean pulmonary arterial, and pulmonary capillary occlusion pressures were greater in patients undergoing cardiac surgery receiving dopamine compared with dobutamine despite producing similar increases in cardiac output. Dopamine may also cause more pronounced tachycardia than epinephrine in cardiac surgery patients. An arterial vasodilator (e.g., sodium nitroprusside) may be used to blunt dopamine-induced increases in LV afterload and thereby further enhance cardiac output. However, inotrope-vasodilators (e.g., milrinone, levosimendan) are more commonly used for this purpose in modern anesthesia practice than this older "dopamine plus nitroprusside ('dopride')" strategy. Like epinephrine and norepinephrine, dopamine directly increases myocardial oxygen consumption and may cause or worsen myocardial ischemia in the presence of hemodynamically significant coronary stenoses.

Dobutamine

Commercial preparations of the synthetic catecholamine dobutamine contain two stereoisomers (− and +), both of which stimulate β-adrenoceptors, but these (−) and (+) stereoisomers cause opposing agonist and antagonist effects on α_1-adrenoceptors, respectively.[36] As a result, dobutamine is a potent stimulator of β-adrenoceptors, but the drug has little effect on α_1-adrenoceptors when it is administered at infusion rates less than 5 $\mu g \cdot kg^{-1} \cdot min^{-1}$. This unique pharmacology allows dobutamine to enhance myocardial contractility and simultaneously reduce arterial vasomotor tone through β_1- and β_2-adrenoceptor activation, respectively. These actions combine to markedly improve LV-arterial coupling, enhance myocardial efficiency, and increase cardiac output in the presence or absence of LV dysfunction.[37] The favorable effects of dobutamine on mechanical matching between the LV and the arterial vasculature also partially explain the declines in mitral regurgitation observed when dobutamine is administered to patients with dilated cardiomyopathy and increased LV filling pressures.[38] The dobutamine (−) isomer progressively stimulates the α_1-adrenoceptor as infusion rates increase above 5 $\mu g \cdot kg^{-1} \cdot min^{-1}$. This action mitigates the magnitude of vasodilation resulting from β_2-adrenoceptor activation and effectively preserves LV preload, afterload, and arterial pressure. The α_1-adrenoceptor agonist effect of higher doses of dobutamine also serves to blunt the baroreceptor reflex-mediated tachycardia that might otherwise occur. Nevertheless, dobutamine often increases heart rate by direct β_1-adrenoceptor-mediated positive chronotropic and dromotropic effects. In fact, dobutamine produced significantly higher heart rates than epinephrine at equivalent values of cardiac index in patients after coronary artery surgery.[23] Dobutamine directly increases myocardial oxygen consumption and may cause acute myocardial ischemia in patients with flow-limiting coronary stenoses. This is the underlying principle behind dobutamine stress echocardiography as a diagnostic tool for the detection of coronary artery disease because regional wall motion abnormalities in the affected coronary perfusion territories occur in response to the myocardial oxygen supply–demand mismatch during transient infusion of the drug.[39] Conversely, dobutamine often reduces heart rate in patients with heart failure because increases in cardiac output and oxygen delivery improve tissue perfusion and reduce chronically elevated sympathetic nervous system tone. Dobutamine may also favorably decrease myocardial oxygen consumption in the failing heart because stimulation of β_2-adrenoceptors decreases LV preload and afterload and, consequently, LV end-diastolic and end-systolic wall stress, respectively.

Dobutamine modestly decreases pulmonary arterial pressures and pulmonary vascular resistance through β_2-adrenoceptor stimulation. Thus, dobutamine may be a useful positive inotropic drug in intensive care unit patients with pulmonary arterial hypertension.[40] As previously mentioned, dopamine, in contrast to dobutamine, activates α_1-adrenoceptors in the pulmonary arterial and venous capacitance vessels, and these effects increase pulmonary arterial pressures and LV preload, respectively. As a result, dobutamine may be preferred over dopamine in heart failure patients with elevated pulmonary vascular resistance and LV filling pressures. However, this dobutamine-induced pulmonary vasodilation has the potential to exacerbate ventilation–perfusion mismatch, increase transpulmonary shunt, and contribute to relative hypoxemia. Dobutamine may also improve renal perfusion by increasing cardiac output, but unlike dopamine, the drug does not directly activate DA_1 receptors to cause renal arterial vasodilation. Unfortunately, several clinical trials demonstrated that use of dobutamine was linked to an increased incidence of major adverse cardiac events including mortality in patients with decompensated heart failure despite the theoretical beneficial cardiovascular effects of the drug.[41,42] Dobutamine also produced adverse events in patients undergoing cardiac surgery.[24] As a result of these and other compelling data, the authors have personally eliminated the use of dobutamine for positive inotropic support in patients with LV dysfunction undergoing cardiac surgery. Nevertheless, dobutamine remains a useful drug for the treatment of depressed myocardial contractility in patients with sepsis.[43]

Isoproterenol

Isoproterenol is a nonselective β-adrenoceptor agonist synthetic catecholamine derived from dopamine. Isoproterenol has a low affinity for and does not exert activity at the α-adrenoceptor. As a result, isoproterenol increases heart rate and myocardial contractility and decreases arterial pressure through β_1- and β_2-adrenoceptor agonist effects, respectively. Historically, isoproterenol was used for "pharmacologic pacing" in patients with symptomatic bradyarrhythmias or AV conduction block (e.g., Mobitz type II second-degree block, third-degree block) because of the drug's positive chronotropic effects. Isoproterenol was also used during cardiac transplantation to increase heart rate and enhance myocardial contractility in the denervated donor organ. However, transcutaneous or transvenous pacing has largely replaced the catecholamine for heart rate control in modern practice, especially in view of the drug's propensity to precipitate adverse supraventricular and ventricular tachyarrhythmias.[44] Isoproterenol was previously used to treat RV dysfunction resulting from severe pulmonary arterial hypertension because the drug reduces pulmonary vascular resistance by stimulating β_2-adrenoceptors in pulmonary arterial vascular smooth muscle, but selective inhaled pulmonary vasodilators (e.g., nitric oxide, prostaglandin I_2) are more effective and are associated with fewer adverse side effects. Thus, although the clinical applicability of isoproterenol is quite limited at present, the comparison of the pharmacology of isoproterenol with other catecholamines merits continued discussion.

Isoproterenol causes β_2-adrenoceptor–mediated arteriolar vasodilation in renal, mesenteric, splenic, and skeletal muscle circulations. These actions reduce systemic vascular resistance and decrease arterial pressure. Isoproterenol causes direct positive chronotropic and dromotropic effects and increases heart rate because of β_1-adrenoceptor activation. Tachycardia also occurs because hypotension stimulates baroreceptor reflex-mediated increases in heart rate. Isoproterenol is a positive inotropic drug, but cardiac output may not increase because tachycardia interferes with LV filling dynamics and β_2-adrenoceptor–mediated venodilation decreases LV preload. For example, isoproterenol, unlike dobutamine, did not increase cardiac output in patients undergoing coronary artery or valve replacement surgery. Predictably, the hemodynamic effects of isoproterenol cause dose-related increases in myocardial oxygen consumption. The synthetic catecholamine also reduces coronary perfusion pressure and decreases diastolic filling time. These alterations in myocardial oxygen supply–demand relations may contribute to the development of acute myocardial ischemia or cause subendocardial necrosis, even in the absence of coronary artery disease. Thus, isoproterenol may be especially deleterious in patients with flow-limiting coronary stenoses.

Selective β_2-Adrenoceptor Agonists

A number of short- and long-acting selective β_2-adrenoceptor agonists, including metaproterenol, albuterol, salmeterol, and fenoterol, are currently in clinical use for treatment of asthma and chronic obstructive pulmonary disease. A hydroxyl substitution on the phenyl ring or a large moiety attached to the amino group of a catecholamine's basic chemical structure increases the molecule's relative β_2-adrenoceptor affinity. These drugs stimulate β_2-adrenoceptors in bronchial smooth muscle to produce bronchodilation, reduce airway resistance, and improve obstructive symptoms. Reductions in histamine and leukotriene release from pulmonary mast cells, and improvements in mucociliary function may also contribute to beneficial effects of selective β_2-adrenoceptor agonists in patients with reactive airway disease.[45] To minimize the systemic side effects of β_2-adrenoceptor activation (e.g., tremor, anxiety, restlessness), the drugs are usually aerosolized and administered using a metered-dose inhaler. However, the β_2-adrenoceptor selectivity of these drugs progressively decreases and β_1-adrenoceptor–mediated adverse effects (e.g., tachycardia, arrhythmias) become more apparent as larger doses are used. Terbutaline is another β_2-adrenoceptor agonist that is administered subcutaneously or intramuscularly and may be useful in the management of status asthmaticus.

Fenoldopam

Fenoldopam mesylate is an intravenous selective DA_1-receptor agonist that does not exert activity at α- or β-adrenoceptors.[35] The drug dilates mesenteric, splenic, and renal arterioles, increases renal blood flow, decreases renal vascular resistance, reduces systemic vascular resistance, improves creatinine clearance, and promotes both natriuretic and diuretic effects. Fenoldopam was initially developed as an antihypertensive medication because of its actions as a vasodilator,[46] but the drug may also be capable of protecting the kidney against radiographic contrast-induced nephropathy, presumably by virtue of enhanced renal blood flow.[47,48] This potential to block renal injury, particularly in the presence of hypotension or pre-existing kidney damage, prompted intense investigation of fenoldopam as a possible renal protective agent. For example, a large meta-analysis based primarily on small single center studies suggested that fenoldopam may reduce the risk of acute tubular necrosis, the need for renal replacement therapy, and overall mortality in patients with or at risk for acute kidney injury.[49] Unfortunately, large randomized controlled clinical trials have failed to support these promising early results. Fenoldopam did not provide renal protection against contrast-induced nephropathy.[50] Similarly, fenoldopam did not decrease the need for dialysis in intensive care unit patients with early acute tubular necrosis,[51] nor did the DA_1-receptor agonist reduce the requirement for renal replacement therapy or 30-day mortality in patients with acute kidney injury undergoing cardiac surgery.[52] Thus, despite the fact that fenoldopam is a potent direct renal vasodilator and promotes increased urine output, the drug does not appear to exert clinically meaningful protection against renal injury. Intravenous fenoldopam has a rapid onset of action as an antihypertensive medication. The drug undergoes hepatic metabolism and is excreted in the urine. The elimination half-life of fenoldopam is approximately 5 minutes. Unlike the findings with intravenous nitrovasodilators (see below), tolerance to fenoldopam's antihypertensive effects does not appear to occur. Rebound hypertension has also not been observed with abrupt discontinuation of the drug. The most common adverse effects of fenoldopam are related to its effects as a vasodilator and include hypotension, tachycardia, flushing, dizziness, headache, tachycardia, and nausea.

Sympathomimetics

Ephedrine

The sympathomimetic drug ephedrine exerts both direct and indirect actions on adrenoceptors. Endocytosis of ephedrine into α_1- and β_1-adrenoceptor presynaptic postganglionic nerve terminals displaces norepinephrine from the synaptic vesicles. The displaced norepinephrine is then released to activate the corresponding postsynaptic receptors to cause arterial and venous vasoconstriction and increased myocardial contractility, respectively. This indirect action is the ephedrine's predominant pharmacologic effect. Indeed, ephedrine's initial cardiovascular effects resemble those of epinephrine because dose-related increases in heart rate, cardiac output, and systemic vascular resistance are observed. However, ephedrine is less potent than epinephrine, and the indirect acting sympathomimetic's duration of action is longer than that of the endogenous catecholamine. Ephedrine also directly stimulates β_2-adrenoceptors, which limits the increases in arterial pressure that occur as a result of α_1-adrenoceptor activation. Tachyphylaxis to ephedrine's hemodynamic effects occurs with repetitive administration of the drug because presynaptic norepinephrine stores are quickly depleted and ephedrine is released from synaptic vesicles as a false neurotransmitter instead. In contrast, tachyphylaxis does not occur with epinephrine because the endogenous catecholamine directly stimulates α- and β-adrenoceptors independent of norepinephrine displacement and release. Notably, drugs that block the ephedrine uptake into adrenergic nerves (e.g., cocaine) and those that deplete norepinephrine reserves (e.g., reserpine) predictably attenuate the cardiovascular effects of ephedrine. The most common clinical use of ephedrine during anesthesia is treatment of acute decreases in arterial pressure concomitant with bradycardia. Ephedrine was previously used for the treatment of hypotension in laboring parturients because the drug increases uterine blood flow, but phenylephrine may be preferred in this setting because ephedrine crosses the placenta and may cause fetal acidosis.[53]

Phenylephrine

The chemical structure of phenylephrine is similar to epinephrine: unlike the endogenous catecholamine, the sympathomimetic drug does not contain a hydroxyl group on the phenyl ring. As a result of this minor structural difference, phenylephrine almost exclusively stimulates α_1-adrenoceptors to increase venous and arterial vasomotor tone while exerting little or no effect on β-adrenoceptors. In contrast to ephedrine, phenylephrine acts directly on the α_1-adrenoceptor and is not dependent on presynaptic norepinephrine displacement to produce its cardiovascular effects. Phenylephrine constricts venous capacitance vessels and causes cutaneous, skeletal muscle, mesenteric, splenic, and renal vasoconstriction. These actions increase LV preload and afterload and cause dose-related increases in arterial pressure. Predictably, baroreceptor reflex-mediated decreases in heart rate also occur. Cardiac output usually remains relatively constant when LV function is normal, but cardiac output may decline when LV function is impaired[54] because failing myocardium is more sensitive to acute increases in afterload.[55] Phenylephrine also increases pulmonary artery pressures through pulmonary arterial vasoconstriction and greater venous return. Unlike endogenous or synthetic catecholamines, phenylephrine is not arrhythmogenic. Intravenous boluses or infusions of phenylephrine are most often used for treatment of hypotension in the presence of normal or elevated heart rate.

α_1-Adrenoceptor Antagonists

On the basis of the previous discussion, it should be readily apparent that blockade of the α_1-adrenoceptor in arterial and venous vascular smooth muscle causes vasodilation by inhibiting the actions of endogenous catecholamines and other sympathomimetic amines at this receptor subtype. For this reason, α_1-adrenoceptor blockers were previously used for the treatment of essential hypertension, but β-blockers, ACE inhibitors, angiotensin II receptor blockers (ARBs), Ca^{2+} channel blockers, diuretics, and nitrates have largely replaced these drugs for this clinical indication in modern practice. α_1-Adrenoceptor antagonists (e.g., prazosin) are certainly very effective antihypertensive medications, but many patients complained that the side effect profile, including debilitating orthostatic hypotension, baroreceptor reflex-mediated tachycardia[56] with or without palpitations, nasal congestion, and fluid retention, was intolerable during chronic use of these drugs. The presence of α_1-adrenoceptor blockade also has the potential to cause unopposed β_1- and β_2-adrenoceptor activity. For example, epinephrine will activate only β_1- and β_2-adrenoceptors because the α_1-adrenoceptor agonist effects of the catecholamine are inhibited. As a result, epinephrine produces pronounced tachycardia (a β_1 effect) and severe hypotension (activation of β_2 receptors causing arterial and venous vasodilation) when administered in the presence of an α_1-adrenoceptor blocker. Similarly, norepinephrine and ephedrine only activate β_1-adrenoceptors because their α_1-adrenoceptor agonist actions are inhibited. The pure α_1-agonist phenylephrine also exerts little or no effect as a vasoconstrictor under these conditions. The response of a given vascular bed to an α_1-adrenoceptor antagonist is dependent on its intrinsic level of vasoconstriction, as blood vessels with higher vascular smooth muscle tone will generally be more responsive to α_1-adrenoceptor blockade.

Phenoxybenzamine is an orally administered, relatively nonselective α-adrenoceptor antagonist that binds irreversibly to α_1- and α_2-adrenoceptors (the ratio of selectivity for these receptor subtypes is approximately 100:1). Because phenoxybenzamine's actions at α-adrenoceptors are irreversible, synthesis of new receptors is required to reverse the drug's effects as a vasodilator. Phenoxybenzamine's prolonged half-life after oral administration also contributes to its sustained actions at the α-adrenoceptor. Phenoxybenzamine is used almost exclusively to normalize arterial pressure before surgery in patients with pheochromocytoma.[57] The slow onset of α-adrenoceptor blockade produced by phenoxybenzamine occurs because the molecule requires structural modification to become pharmacologically active. As a result, several weeks of treatment may be required to obtain adequate control of arterial pressure. Restoration of normal intravascular volume status is also an important goal of phenoxybenzamine therapy because hypovolemia resulting from elevated serum norepinephrine and epinephrine concentrations contributes to hemodynamic instability during pheochromocytoma resection. Subsequent addition of a β-adrenoceptor antagonist also helps in achieving these goals and also serves to protect the myocardium from the adverse effects of chronic catecholamine stimulation. These combined interventions facilitate greater cardiovascular stability during pheochromocytoma resection, which is usually associated with additional release of norepinephrine and epinephrine into the circulation during tumor manipulation. The most prominent side effect of phenoxybenzamine therapy is orthostatic hypotension, which may be especially severe in the presence of pre-existing hypertension or hypovolemia. Vasopressin may be required to treat refractory hypotension associated with phenoxybenzamine overdose.

The competitive α_1- and α_2-adrenoceptor antagonist phentolamine is also used in patients with pheochromocytoma. In contrast to phenoxybenzamine, the effects of phentolamine are reversible (half-life less than 10 minutes) and new receptor synthesis is not required to restore α-adrenoceptor activity and vascular smooth muscle tone. Phentolamine is a potent intravenous vasodilator that rapidly decreases arterial pressure, but in doing so, also causes baroreceptor reflex-mediated tachycardia. Blockade of cardiac α_2-adrenoceptors by phentolamine may contribute to the development of arrhythmias. Phentolamine also exerts antihistamine and cholinergic activity, the latter of which may produce abdominal cramping and diarrhea. Because the drug causes hypotension and tachycardia, phentolamine is relatively contraindicated and should only be used with extreme caution in patients with flow-limiting coronary artery stenoses. Phentolamine is occasionally used as a local vasodilator to prevent tissue necrosis when iatrogenic extravasation of a vasoconstrictor (e.g., norepinephrine, phenylephrine) has occurred. The α-adrenoceptor antagonist may also be effective when treating refractory hypertension associated with clonidine withdrawal or tyramine exposure in patients receiving a monoamine oxidase inhibitor.

Unlike phenoxybenzamine and phentolamine, prazosin is a relatively selective antagonist of α_1-adrenoceptors (α_1 to α_2 ratio of approximately 1,000:1) that causes arterial and venous vasodilation. α_2-Adrenoceptor modulation of norepinephrine release from postganglionic sympathetic neurons remains intact. As a result, baroreceptor reflex-mediated tachycardia is substantially attenuated after administration of prazosin. Nevertheless, orthostatic hypotension is an important clinical side effect of prazosin when the drug is used for the treatment of hypertension. Prazosin undergoes hepatic metabolism. The drug also increases the ratio of high- to low-density lipoproteins. In contrast with ACE inhibitors, prazosin does not improve survival in patients with heart failure and the drug is no longer recommended for this clinical indication as a result. Other α_1-adrenoceptor antagonists (e.g., terazosin, doxazosin, tamsulosin) are used for the treatment of benign prostatic hyperplasia because the prostate contains a large number of α_{1A}-adrenoceptors.[58] Patients who are treated with these medications occasionally present for surgery, and anesthesiologists should be aware that anesthetic-induced vasodilation might be exacerbated in the presence of these urologic α_1-adrenoceptor antagonists.

α_2-Adrenoceptor Agonists: Clonidine and Dexmedetomidine

The α_2-adrenoceptor agonists clonidine and dexmedetomidine are commonly used by anesthesiologists and pain medicine specialists for sedation, anxiolysis, and analgesia.[59,60] Clonidine binds to α_2-adrenoceptors and inhibits norepinephrine release from presynaptic postganglionic sympathetic neurons. α_2-Adrenoceptor agonists block sympathetic nerve traffic through pre- and postsynaptic mechanisms in the central nervous system and also inhibit spinal presynaptic sympathetic nerve transmission. Clonidine is a partial α_2-adrenoceptor agonist with relative selectivity for α_2- versus α_1-receptors of approximately 200:1. Because of its sympatholytic effects, clonidine was originally used for the treatment of hypertension. Activation of α_2-adrenoceptors in the vasomotor center, attenuation of peripheral norepinephrine release from postganglionic sympathetic neurons, and stimulation of central nervous system imidazoline receptors are postulated mechanisms for the antihypertensive effect of clonidine.[61,62] Clonidine blunts centrally mediated sympathetic nervous system tone, decreases serum norepinephrine and norepinephrine concentrations, and reduces activation of the renin–angiotensin–aldosterone axis. In addition, clonidine stimulates parasympathetic nervous system activity, which, when combined with withdrawal of sympathetic tone, produces bradycardia. Unlike other antihypertensive medications, clonidine does not affect baroreceptor-mediated reflex control of heart rate.[63] The α_2-adrenoceptor agonist is generally not associated with orthostatic hypotension when used in patients with hypertension, unlike α_1-antagonists or ACE inhibitors. Nevertheless, hypotension and bradycardia may occur when large doses of the drug are administered. These effects are easily reversed with conventional vasoactive medications.

Clonidine continues to be used as an antihypertensive medication, but the drug also reduces volatile and intravenous anesthetic requirements, blunts the hemodynamic responses to laryngoscopy and endotracheal intubation, promotes intraoperative cardiovascular stability, partially attenuates the sympathetic stress response associated with surgery, and decreases postoperative tissue oxygen requirements.[64–66] Clonidine and other α_2-adrenoceptor agonists including dexmedetomidine were shown to reduce the risk of myocardial ischemia and infarction and decrease perioperative mortality in patients undergoing major vascular or cardiac surgery, in a meta-analysis of 23 controlled trials in which more than 3,395 patients were enrolled.[67] These anti-ischemic actions were presumably related to the drug's sympatholytic effects, which reduce myocardial oxygen consumption. Clonidine augments the effects of local anesthetics and opioids and increases their duration of action when used for neuraxial and regional anesthesia.[68] As a result, clonidine decreases the incidence and severity of side effects associated with local anesthetics and opioids because the quantities of these latter drugs required for anesthesia and analgesia are reduced. Clonidine is effective as a postoperative analgesic and also has well-documented utility in the treatment of chronic regional pain syndrome and neuropathic pain. The sedative and anxiolytic effects of clonidine are attributed to activation of α_2-adrenoceptors in the locus coeruleus. Notably, clonidine does not substantially inhibit respiratory drive in the presence or absence of opioids despite the α_2-adrenoceptor agonist's sedative effect.[69] Thus, clonidine's sedative–analgesic effects may be exploited without undo concern about the potential for respiratory depression. Hyperglycemia may occur in patients treated with clonidine because the α_2-adrenoceptor agonist inhibits insulin release. This side effect may be especially important in patients with poorly controlled diabetes mellitus. Finally, anesthesiologists may occasionally encounter patients who are receiving clonidine to mitigate withdrawal symptoms associated with treatment of a substance abuse disorder.[70]

Discontinuation of clonidine may be necessary during the perioperative period if a patient is unable to ingest oral medications, but abrupt withdrawal of the α_2-adrenoceptor agonist often results in severe hypertension associated with tachycardia, headache, anxiety, tremor, and diaphoresis. Under these circumstances, invasive monitoring of arterial pressure in an intensive care unit setting and treatment of hypertension with other intravenous medications may be necessary until oral clonidine therapy can be resumed. β-Blockers should not be used alone under such circumstances because unopposed α_1-adrenoceptor stimulation causes profound vasoconstriction, thereby worsening the hypertensive emergency. Alternatively, transdermal clonidine may be used to mitigate or prevent drug withdrawal–induced hypertensive emergency in those patients who are unable to consume the medication. It is important to note that transdermal clonidine requires approximately 48 hours after initial application to achieve therapeutic serum concentrations.

Dexmedetomidine is approximately sevenfold more selective for the α_2-adrenoceptor (α_2 to α_1 ratio of 1,600:1) and has a substantially shorter context-sensitive half-life than clonidine. These characteristics make an intravenous infusion of dexmedetomidine useful for sedation, amnesia, and analgesia in the operating room and intensive care unit.[71,72] Like clonidine, dexmedetomidine reduces anesthetic requirements during general, neuraxial, and regional anesthesia; decreases heart rate, arterial pressure, and plasma catecholamine concentrations; attenuates intraoperative cardiovascular lability; and does not cause clinically significant respiratory depression. This latter feature is especially beneficial in the setting of elective fiberoptic intubation or weaning from mechanical ventilation. Dexmedetomidine's relative preservation of respiratory drive and its lack of effects on electrophysiologic monitoring make the α_2-adrenoceptor agonist useful for functional neurosurgery.[73] Dexmedetomidine exerts neuroprotective effects against cerebral ischemia and hypoxia; this neuroprotection appears to be related to a direct cytoprotective effect.[74] Dexmedetomidine also facilitates perioperative care of obese patients with obstructive sleep apnea and those undergoing bariatric surgery because the drug provides analgesia, reduces opioid requirements, and does not substantially depress respiration.[75] When used as a sedative in the intensive care patients, dexmedetomidine reduced the incidence of delirium, the duration of mechanical ventilation, the length of intensive care unit stay, and mortality compared with midazolam.[76] Dexmedetomidine may be associated with hypothermia because the drug lowers the threshold body temperature at which compensatory thermoregulation mechanisms are activated.

β-Adrenoceptor Antagonists (β-Blockers)

Many of the cardiovascular effects of β-adrenoceptor antagonists (more commonly called "β-blockers") may be anticipated based on the previous discussion of catecholamines. The peer-reviewed literature describing the actions, uses, and potential limitations of β-blockers is exhaustive. It is not the authors' intention to review this literature in detail; instead, we wish to highlight the major effects and clinical applications of the most ubiquitous drugs in cardiovascular pharmacology. β-Blockers produce important anti-ischemic effects and are a first-line therapy for patients with ST- and non–ST-segment elevation, myocardial infarction in the absence of cardiogenic shock, hemodynamically significant bradyarrhythmias, or reactive airway disease. These medications have been repeatedly shown to reduce morbidity and mortality associated with myocardial infarction in a large number of clinical trials. β-Blockers bind to β_1-adrenoceptors and inhibit the actions of circulating catecholamines and norepinephrine released from postganglionic sympathetic neurons. As a result, heart rate and myocardial contractility are reduced. The decrease in heart rate produced by β-blockers prolongs diastole, increases coronary blood flow to the LV, enhances coronary collateral perfusion to ischemic myocardium, and improves oxygen delivery to the coronary microcirculation. These combined effects serve to reduce myocardial oxygen demand while simultaneously increasing supply. β-Blockers have also been shown to inhibit platelet aggregation. This latter action is particularly important during acute myocardial ischemia or evolving myocardial infarction because platelet aggregation at the site of an atherosclerotic plaque may worsen a coronary stenosis or produce acute occlusion of the vessel. β-Blockers are very effective for the treatment of essential hypertension, produce antiarrhythmic effects through negative chronotropic actions, and have well-established roles in the treatment of heart failure, hypertrophic obstructive cardiomyopathy, aortic dissection, thyrotoxicosis, pheochromocytoma, and migraine headache prophylaxis. Topical β-blockers are also used for treatment of open-angle glaucoma. Perhaps, of most relevance to anesthesiologists, perioperative administration of β-blockers has been shown to reduce the incidence of nonfatal myocardial infarction in patients undergoing noncardiac surgery.[77,78] These drugs are specifically recommended for patients with documented or multiple risk factors for myocardial ischemia,[79] but not those without convincing evidence of coronary artery disease.[80,81]

Propranolol is the prototypical β-blocker against which all other medications in this pharmacologic class are compared (Table 13-6). Propranolol and other β-blockers are chemically related to isoproterenol and contain an aromatic moiety linked to the ethanolamine group, the latter of which allows interaction with the β-adrenoceptor. Additions to the molecule's aromatic group determine the degree of β_1-adrenoceptor specificity. All β-blockers have a chiral center; the negative enantiomer of each drug is biologically active. The relative selectivity of β-blockers for β_1- and β_2-adrenoceptors, their lipid solubility, and the presence or absence of intrinsic sympathomimetic ability (e.g., partial stimulation of the β_1-adrenoceptor), myocardial membrane stabilizing activity, and additional cardiovascular actions combine with each drug's pharmacokinetic effects to distinguish

Table 13-6 Comparative Effects of β-blockers

Name	Chemical Structure	Selectivity β1	Selectivity β2	α1	Plasma Half-life (hrs)	Intrinsic Sympathomimetic Activity	Membrane Stabilizing Activity	Lipid Solubility	Metabolism
Propranolol		+	+	0	3–4	0	+	+++	Liver
Metoprolol		+	0	0	3–4	0	0	++	Liver
Atenolol		+	0	0	6–9	0	0	+	Renal
Esmolol		+	0	0	0.15	0	0	+	RBC esterase
Labetalol		+	+	+	6	+	0	+	Liver
Carvedilol		+	+	+	2–8	0	0	+++	Liver

RBC, red blood cell.

individual β-blockers from one another. The ability to prevent isoproterenol-induced increases in heart rate defines each β-blocker's potency (propranolol is considered the standard in these determinations). Propranolol is a "first-generation" (nonselective) β-blocker that competitively inhibits both $β_1$- and $β_2$-adrenoceptors, whereas metoprolol, atenolol, and esmolol are classified as "second-generation" β-blockers because these drugs are selective for the $β_1$-adrenoceptor. Notably, this $β_1$-adrenoceptor selectivity is relative because larger doses of second-generation β-blockers inhibit both $β_1$- and $β_2$-adrenceptors. "Third-generation" β-blockers exert other cardiovascular effects in addition to their actions at β-adrenoceptors. For example, labetalol blocks $α_1$-adrenoceptors; carvedilol exerts antioxidant and anti-inflammatory actions; bucindolol has intrinsic sympathomimetic effects because it is a partial agonist of $β_1$-adrenoceptors; and nebivolol produces nitric oxide–mediated vasodilation through its actions on vascular endothelium.

The reductions in heart rate and myocardial contractility produced by β-blockers are more pronounced in the presence of increased sympathetic nervous system tone (e.g., surgical stress, exercise, heart failure) because vagal activity is usually the predominant factor regulating cardiovascular homeostasis during basal conditions. Nonselective β-blockers initially reduce cardiac output as a result of negative chronotropic and inotropic effects concomitant with arterial vasoconstriction mediated through blockade of vascular smooth muscle $β_2$-adrenoceptors and compensatory sympathetic stimulation of $α_1$-adrenoceptors. The initial increase in systemic vascular resistance that occurs with a nonselective β-blocker gradually declines during long-term administration.[82] Selective $β_1$-blockers with or without $α_1$-adrenoceptor antagonist activity, and those with direct vasodilator effects, generally reduce systemic vascular resistance and preserve cardiac output to varying degrees despite simultaneous depression of myocardial contractility. β-Blockers are used extensively for the treatment of hypertension, but the precise mechanisms by which β-blockers that do not have specific additional vasodilating properties are able to reduce arterial blood pressure remain to be clearly defined (Fig. 13-6). Stimulation of $β_1$-adrenoceptors in renal juxtaglomerular cells by the sympathetic postganglionic neurons causes renin secretion and activates the renin–angiotensin–aldosterone axis (see below). Many β-blockers inhibit this renin release, but their antihypertensive effects usually occur before plasma renin concentrations decline.[83] Similarly, some β-blockers also do not substantially affect renin metabolism and yet are quite effective at reducing arterial pressure in hypertensive patients. It is also unlikely that β-blockers cause antihypertensive effects through a decrease in centrally mediated sympathetic nervous system tone because drugs with markedly different lipid solubility are equally effective at decreasing arterial pressure. β-Blockers most likely do not favorably modulate postganglionic sympathetic neuron norepinephrine release despite the presence of presynaptic β-adrenoceptors that are known to stimulate release of the neurotransmitter. Clearly, selective β-blockers that do not affect $β_2$-adrenoceptor viability ("second-generation") and those that inhibit $α_1$-adrenoceptors or produce vasodilation through other mechanisms also decrease arterial pressure (Fig. 13-6).[84] Nevertheless, nonselective β-blockers such as propranolol are valuable antihypertensive medications independent of these alternative vasodilating characteristics.

β-Blockers have been a mainstay in the pharmacologic treatment of acute myocardial ischemia and infarction since their introduction into clinical practice in the 1960s. As mentioned previously, β-blockers directly reduce myocardial oxygen consumption and improve coronary perfusion, thereby enhancing myocardial oxygen supply–demand relations and decreasing ischemic burden. These actions reduce the magnitude of myocardial necrosis, preserve LV systolic function, attenuate the development of malignant ventricular arrhythmias, decrease mortality, and improve long-term functional capacity. The results supporting the use of β-blockers in acute myocardial infarction are among the most convincing data ever published in the medical literature. Many placebo-controlled randomized double-blind clinical trials demonstrated unequivocally that β-blockers are not only effective for treatment of acute myocardial infarction but also substantially decrease the risk of developing a subsequent infarction in patients with coronary artery disease.[85,86] Indeed, the estimated overall reduction in mortality associated with use of β-blockers in myocardial infarction is approximately 25%.[87] β-Blockers also have well-established efficacy for the chronic treatment of heart failure. The use of β-blockers in heart failure was initially viewed with skepticism because administration of a drug that further depresses myocardial contractility would appear to be counterintuitive. However, sympathetic nervous system tone is chronically elevated in heart failure, and this excessive sympathetic activity produces a series of alterations in

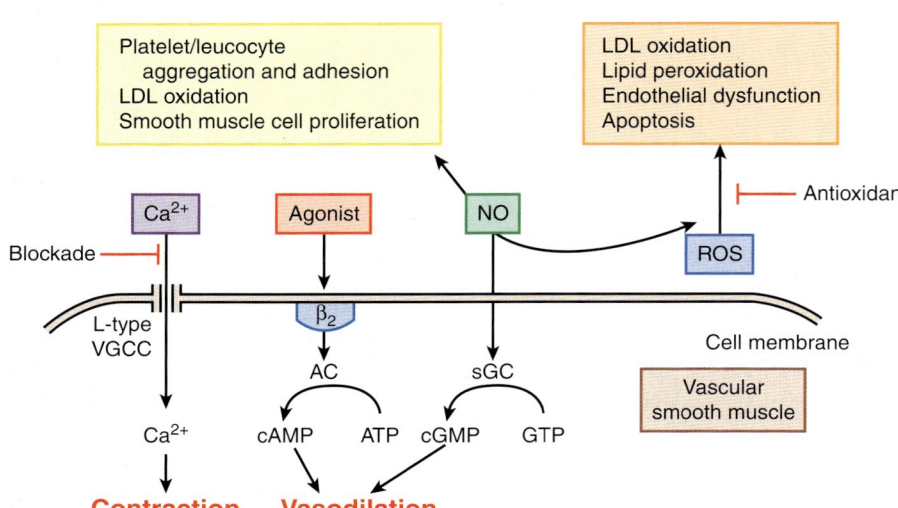

Figure 13-6 Schematic illustration of potential mechanism by which β-blockers produce vasodilation; abbreviations: VGCC, voltage-gated Ca^{2+} channel; AC, adenylyl cyclase; NO, nitric oxide; sGC, soluble guanylyl cyclase; ROS, reactive oxygen species; LDL, low-density lipoprotein. (Modified with permission from Toda N. Vasodilating β-adrenoceptor blockers as cardiovascular therapeutics. Pharmacol Ther, 2003, 100:215–234. Copyright 2003 Elsevier Inc. All rights reserved.)

β_1-adrenoceptor density and function, intracellular signal transduction, contractile protein expression, and Ca^{2+} homeostasis that promote mitochondrial dysfunction, stimulate myocyte apoptosis (programmed cell death), cause pathologic ventricular remodeling, and accelerate disease progression.[88,89] Clinical trials demonstrated that β-blockers significantly decrease mortality in patients with heart failure independent of disease severity.[90] In fact, some large randomized studies were halted before completion because patients with moderate to severe heart failure receiving β-blockers had markedly improved mortality compared with those treated with placebo.[91] β-Blockers mitigate clinical symptoms, improve exercise tolerance, reduce the need for and duration of subsequent hospitalization, and decrease the risk of sudden cardiac death in patients with heart failure.[92]

The electrophysiologic effects of β-blockers make these drugs quite useful for the treatment of tachyarrhythmias. β-Blockers reduce SA node automaticity, inhibit the activity of subsidiary ectopic pacemakers, decrease impulse conduction velocity through atrial conduction pathways, prolong conduction time through the AV node, and increase the AV node's refractory period. Both β_1- and β_2-adrenoceptors mediate these negative chronotropic and dromotropic effects.[20] Some β-blockers also exert membrane-stabilizing activity that may theoretically contribute to their antiarrhythmic efficacy, but these "quinidine-like" actions are most likely only of clinical relevance when a β-blocker overdose has occurred. β-Blockers are used to reduce ventricular rate in patients with sinus tachycardia, atrial fibrillation or flutter, supraventricular tachycardia, and re-entrant tachyarrhythmias (e.g., Wolff–Parkinson–White, Lown–Ganong–Levine). β-Blockers inhibit tachycardia in response to laryngoscopy and endotracheal intubation. β-Blockers also attenuate baroreceptor-mediated reflex sinus tachycardia in response to vasodilator therapy. For example, administration of a β-blocker mitigates the reflex tachycardia associated with an α_1-adrenoceptor antagonist used to reduce arterial pressure in pheochromocytoma. β-Blockers also attenuate the development of cardiomyopathy resulting from elevated catecholamine concentrations in this disease. When combined with intravenous vasodilator therapy (e.g., sodium nitroprusside, clevidipine), the negative chronotropic and inotropic effects of β-blockers reduce heart rate and proximal ascending aortic shear stress in acute Stanford type A (Debakey type I or II) aortic dissection. Analogously, β-blockers reduce the risk of aortic dissection and the rate of ascending aortic dilatation in patients with Marfan's syndrome by decreasing pulsatile hydraulic forces on the proximal aortic root.[93] β-Blockers decrease heart rate and inhibit the development of tachyarrhythmias in hyperthyroidism and thyroid storm, in part by preventing the peripheral conversion of thyroxine to its more active triiodothyronine form. As a result, β-blockers are useful adjuncts to propylthiouracil in the treatment of hyperthyroidism. β-Blocker–induced declines in heart rate concomitant with depression of myocardial contractility substantially reduce dynamic LV outflow tract pressure gradient and the magnitude-associated mitral regurgitation while improving symptoms in patients with hypertrophic obstructive cardiomyopathy.[94]

Topical β-blockers (e.g., timolol, betaxolol) are used for the treatment of open-angle glaucoma. These drugs reduce aqueous humor production but do not affect pupil size or accommodation, unlike topical anticholinergic medications. It is important to recognize that these topical β-blockers may be systemically absorbed and thus, may exert adverse cardiovascular or pulmonary side effects. As a result, topical β-blockers may be relatively contraindicated in patients with symptomatic bradyarrhythmias or bronchospastic lung disease. A role for β-blockers in prophylaxis against migraine headache is well established, but the mechanism for this beneficial effect remains unclear.[95] β-Blockers may also be useful for reducing sympathetically mediated symptoms, including palpitations, tachycardia, and tremor, associated with performance situations that provoke anxiety (e.g., public speaking, oral examinations). Similarly, β-blockers may also be helpful in controlling sympathetic nervous system activation that occurs with drug withdrawal in patients with substance use disorders.

β-Blockers are associated with a number of important adverse effects. Despite the well-established beneficial effects of β-blockers in patients with heart failure, the negative inotropic effects of these drugs may worsen heart failure symptoms and lead to further decompensation in some patients with severe LV dysfunction. Abrupt withdrawal of a β-blocker after long-term treatment may produce myocardial ischemia and infarction or cause sudden cardiac death in susceptible patients with critical coronary artery stenoses. Because of the electrophysiologic effects of β-blockers, second- or third-degree heart block may occur in patients with pre-existing AV conduction abnormalities or those treated with other negative dromotropic drugs (e.g., diltiazem, verapamil).[96] Nonselective β-blockers inhibit β_2-adrenoceptors in arterial vascular smooth muscle. The resulting vasoconstriction may occasionally worsen vascular insufficiency in patients with peripheral vascular disease or precipitate Raynaud's phenomenon in susceptible individuals. Nevertheless, β-blockers remain a mainstay in the treatment of patients with peripheral vascular disease because the vast majority of these patients also have clinically significant coronary artery disease that substantially increases their risk of myocardial ischemia, arrhythmias, and mortality. Propranolol and other first-generation β-blockers inhibit bronchial β_2-adrenoceptors and may cause potentially fatal bronchoconstriction in patients with asthma or chronic obstructive pulmonary disease. Long-term use of β_1-blockers (e.g., atenolol) for the treatment of hypertension, myocardial ischemia and infarction, or heart failure must be approached with caution in patients with reactive airway disease because the β_1-selectivity of these drugs is not absolute and suitable alternative medications are available (e.g., Ca^{2+} channel blockers, nitrates, ACE inhibitors) to manage these conditions. Nevertheless, a selective β_1-adrenoceptor antagonist may be advantageous in some patients with coronary artery disease who also suffer from chronic obstructive pulmonary disease.[97] β-Blockers also interfere with carbohydrate and lipid metabolism. Endogenous catecholamines stimulate glycogenolysis, lipolysis, and gluconeogenesis, promoting the release of glucose into the circulation when hypoglycemia is present. Nonselective β-blockers may inhibit this physiologic response to and recovery from hypoglycemia, especially in patients with type I diabetes mellitus. Nonselective β-blockers also attenuate the sympathetically mediated tremor, tachycardia, and anxiety associated with hypoglycemia. Thus, nonselective β-blockers may be relatively contraindicated in patients with poorly controlled diabetes who often develop hypoglycemic episodes, and drugs with β_1-selectivity may be preferred in this setting.[98]

Propranolol

As mentioned previously, propranolol is the prototypical nonselective β-blocker. Available in oral and intravenous forms, propranolol inhibits β_1- and β_2- but not α_1-adrenoceptors and possesses some degree of membrane stabilization activity at higher doses, but does not exert intrinsic sympathetic activity. The medication is highly lipophilic, easily absorbed from the stomach, and undergoes extensive first-pass hepatic metabolism. A high degree of variability between patients is observed in propranolol metabolism between patients. Liver disease and reductions in hepatic blood flow, but not renal impairment, delay the drug's metabolism and require dose adjustment. Propranolol is used for treatment of hypertension and symptomatic coronary artery disease. Despite a relatively short half-life (approximately 4 hours), propranolol can most often be administered using a twice-per-day dosing regimen because of a persistent antihypertensive effect. Several weeks of propranolol treatment are often required to achieve optimal reduction in arterial pressure. Inhibition of tachycardia during exercise indicates adequate β-blockade. Intravenous propranolol was used for treatment of tachyarrhythmias, but esmolol is preferred for this indication in current clinical practice because of its short half-life. The landmark Beta-Blocker Heart Attack Trial demonstrated that propranolol therapy substantially decreases mortality (7.2% compared with 9.8%) in patients with acute myocardial infarction.[99] Use of propranolol has gradually decreased with the widespread application of other $β_1$-selective blockers and third-generation drugs with other cardiovascular actions.

Metoprolol

Metoprolol is relatively selective for $β_1$-adrenoceptors but has no intrinsic sympathetic or membrane stabilization activity. The drug is available in oral and intravenous forms. Like propranolol, oral metoprolol is rapidly absorbed, but the drug does undergo first-pass hepatic metabolism by cytochrome P450 2D6 that limits its initial availability. The kidney excretes less than 10% of the drug in its original form. Metoprolol's half-life of 3 to 4 hours allows twice-per-day dosing in patients with normal metabolism, but an extended release form is also available that allows once-daily administration. The half-life of metoprolol is doubled in patients who are poor cytochrome P450 2D6 metabolizers; these individuals are approximately fivefold more likely to develop adverse side effects after oral metoprolol administration.[100] Metoprolol is commonly used for treatment of hypertension, angina pectoris, acute myocardial infarction, and chronic heart failure.[101]

Atenolol

Like metoprolol, atenolol is a selective inhibitor of $β_1$-adrenoceptors and does not possess intrinsic sympathetic or membrane stabilization activity. The drug has a longer half-life (6 to 9 hours) than metoprolol that facilitates a daily dosing regimen. The liver does not metabolize atenolol, most of which is excreted in its original form by the kidney. As a result, the dose of atenolol must be reduced in patients with moderate to severe renal insufficiency. The lack of first-pass hepatic metabolism reduces variability in plasma atenolol concentrations between patients after oral administration.[102] Similar to other β-blockers, atenolol is used for the treatment of hypertension, coronary artery disease, acute myocardial infarction, and heart failure.

Esmolol

Esmolol is a relatively selective $β_1$-blocker. The chemical structure of esmolol is very similar to that of propranolol and metoprolol, but esmolol contains an additional methylester group that facilitates the drug's rapid metabolism via hydrolysis by red blood cell esterases, resulting in an elimination half-life of approximately 9 minutes. The quick onset and rapid metabolism of esmolol makes the drug very useful for the treatment of acute tachycardia and hypertension during surgery. Esmolol is most often administered as an intravenous bolus, which causes almost immediate dose-related decreases in heart rate and myocardial contractility; arterial pressure most often falls as a result of these direct negative chronotropic and inotropic effects. Esmolol is often used to attenuate the sympathetic nervous system response to laryngoscopy, endotracheal intubation, or surgical stimulation, particularly in patients with known or suspected coronary artery disease who may be at risk for acute myocardial ischemia. Esmolol is also useful for rapid control of heart rate in patients with supraventricular tachyarrhythmias (e.g., atrial fibrillation, atrial flutter). Finally, esmolol effectively blunts the sympathetically mediated tachycardia and hypertension that occur shortly after the onset of seizure activity during electroconvulsive therapy. Because esmolol does not appreciably block $β_2$-adrenoceptors due to its relative $β_1$-selectivity, hypotension is more commonly observed after administration of this drug compared with other nonselective β-blockers.

Labetalol

Labetalol is composed of four stereoisomers that inhibit α- and β-adrenoceptors to varying degrees.[103] One of the four stereoisomers is an $α_1$-adrenoceptor antagonist, another is a nonselective β-blocker, and the remaining two do not appreciably affect adrenergic receptors. The net effect of this mixture is a drug that selectively inhibits $α_1$-adrenoceptors while simultaneously blocking $β_1$- and $β_2$-adrenoceptors in a nonselective manner. The intravenous formulation of labetalol contains a ratio of $α_1$- to β-blockade of approximately 1:7. Blockade of the $α_1$-adrenoceptor causes arteriolar vasodilation and decreases arterial pressure through a reduction in systemic vascular resistance. This property makes the drug very useful for the treatment of perioperative hypertension. Despite its nonselective β-blocking properties, labetalol is also a partial $β_2$-adrenoceptor agonist; this latter characteristic also contributes to vasodilation. Labetalol-induced inhibition of $β_1$-adrenoceptors decreases heart rate and myocardial contractility. Stroke volume and cardiac output are essentially unchanged as a result of the combined actions of labetalol on $α_1$- and $β_2$-adrenoceptors. Unlike other vasodilators, labetalol produces vasodilation without triggering baroreceptor reflex tachycardia because the drug blocks anticipated increases in heart rate mediated through $β_1$-adrenoceptors. This latter action is beneficial for the treatment of hypertension in the setting of acute myocardial ischemia. Labetalol is also useful for controlling arterial pressure without producing tachycardia in patients with hypertensive emergencies and those with acute aortic dissection. Labetalol has been shown to attenuate the sympathetic nervous system response to laryngoscopy and endotracheal intubation, although the drug's relatively long elimination half-life (approximately 6 hours) limits its utility in this setting.

Carvedilol

Carvedilol is another third-generation β-blocker that inhibits $β_1$-, $β_2$-, and $α_1$-adrenoceptors.[104] Like labetalol, the drug causes arterial vasodilation because it is an $α_1$-adrenoceptor antagonist. The drug is a membrane stabilizer but lacks intrinsic sympathomimetic activity. Carvedilol exerts important antioxidant and anti-inflammatory effects: the drug not only suppresses production of reactive oxygen species, but it also is a scavenger of these free radical intermediates. The antioxidant and anti-inflammatory actions of carvedilol inhibit the uptake of deleterious reduced low-density lipoproteins into coronary vascular endothelium and protect myocardium against ischemia-reperfusion injury, in part by attenuating recruitment, chemotaxis, and activation of cytotoxic neutrophils.[105] Carvedilol is commonly used in the treatment of hypertension, stable angina pectoris, and acute myocardial infarction, but the drug has been shown to be particularly efficacious in patients with heart failure. Several large clinical trials provided convincing evidence that carvedilol improves LV function, reverses or slows the progression of pathologic LV remodeling, decreases the need for and the duration of subsequent hospitalization, and substantially reduces mortality in chronic heart failure resulting from a variety of underlying causes including coronary artery disease.[106] In fact, the beneficial effects of carvedilol appear to be greater than those of metoprolol in heart failure, and several experts have opined that carvedilol should be the preferred therapeutic option in this clinical setting.[107] Carvedilol is very lipophilic, is nearly entirely absorbed after oral administration, and, similar to propranolol and metoprolol, undergoes extensive first-pass hepatic oxidative metabolism via cytochrome P450 2D6 with little or no dependence on the kidney for elimination.

Phosphodiesterase Inhibitors

The phosphodiesterases are structurally related enzymes that hydrolyze the second messengers cAMP and cGMP and terminate their physiologic effects in a variety of tissues. At least seven different phosphodiesterase isoform subtypes have been identified. Inhibitors of these enzymes enhance the intracellular effects of cAMP and cGMP by preventing their metabolism. The phosphodiesterase inhibitors currently in clinical use are somewhat isoenzyme-selective at lower doses, but this selectivity is lost when higher doses of these medications are used. Myocardium and vascular smooth muscle contain the type III phosphodiesterase isoenzyme (PDE III), which is bound to the sarcoplasmic reticulum and cleaves cAMP to adenosine monophosphate (AMP).[108] Selective inhibition of cardiac PDE III by bipyridine compounds such as milrinone and inamrinone alters intracellular Ca^{2+} regulation to enhance myocardial contractility without affecting catecholamine release or activation of $beta_1$-adrenoceptors. PDE III inhibitors increase cAMP concentration, enhance protein kinase A activity, and phosphorylate voltage-dependent Ca^{2+} channels[109] and phospholamban, the major sarcoplasmic reticulum regulatory protein.[110] These actions combine to increase transsarcolemmal Ca^{2+} influx into the cardiac myocyte and promote Ca^{2+}-induced Ca^{2+} release from its sarcoplasmic reticulum, thereby exerting a positive inotropic effect because larger quantities of Ca^{2+} are available for contractile activation. Inhibition of cAMP metabolism also stimulates greater Ca^{2+} uptake into the sarcoplasmic reticulum. As a result, PDE III inhibitors enhance the rate and extent of myocardial relaxation. This positive lusitropic effect serves to improve diastolic function in many patients with heart failure.

PDE III inhibitors cause pronounced arterial and venous vasodilation by blocking cGMP-metabolism and facilitating the actions of this second messenger in vascular smooth muscle. The proclivity of PDE III inhibitors to simultaneously enhance contractility and cause vasodilation defines these medications as "inodilators." PDE III inhibitors cause relatively greater vasodilation than drugs with $β_2$-adrenoceptor agonist activity, including dobutamine and isoproterenol. This reduction in LV afterload increases cardiac output, improves LV-arterial coupling, and enhances mechanical efficiency. Intravenous or inhalational administration of PDE III inhibitors also reduces pulmonary vascular resistance, an action that may be particularly helpful in patients with pulmonary arterial hypertension who are undergoing cardiac surgery or transplantation.[111,112] However, this pulmonary vasodilation is capable of increasing intrapulmonary shunt and contributing to the development of hypoxemia. PDE III inhibitors also dilate venous capacitance vessels and reduce preload. Notably, decreases in preload and afterload resulting from administration of a PDE III inhibitor often lead to reductions in myocardial oxygen consumption in patients with heart failure despite simultaneous positive inotropic, lusitropic, and chronotropic effects.[113] In general, mean arterial pressure is either maintained or may be modestly reduced during administration of PDE III inhibitors provided that intravascular volume is adequately supplemented because increases in cardiac output are capable of compensating for reductions in afterload.

PDE III inhibitors cause increases in heart rate that are less pronounced than those observed during administration of catecholamines. Indeed, a selective $β_1$ adrenoceptor antagonist may abolish the positive chronotropic effects of a PDE III inhibitor without depressing the latter drug's positive inotropic effect. PDE III inhibitors may precipitate the development of malignant ventricular arrhythmias because these drugs increase intracellular cAMP and Ca^{2+} concentrations.[114] PDE III inhibitors block platelet aggregation, suppress neointimal hyperplasia associated with endothelial injury, and attenuate the proinflammatory effects of cardiopulmonary bypass.[115] In addition, these drugs dilate native epicardial coronary arteries and arterial bypass conduits.[116] As a result, PDE III inhibitors have the potential to exert important anti-ischemic effects in patients with coronary artery disease undergoing CABG surgery. The efficacy of PDE III inhibitors is reduced in the failing heart, but not to the extent observed with $β_1$ adrenoceptor agonists. Thus, PDE III inhibitors will continue to enhance myocardial contractility despite concomitant β adrenoceptor downregulation and dysfunction.[113] This pharmacologic property stimulated the conduct of a number of large clinical trials designed to evaluate the utility of orally administered PDE III inhibitors for the treatment of chronic severe heart failure. Although PDE III inhibitors did enhance cardiac performance and improve apparent quality of life in these studies, the drugs also significantly increased mortality resulting from ventricular arrhythmias and sudden cardiac death.[117] Hence, while the use of PDE III inhibitors is contraindicated for the treatment of chronic heart failure, these drugs continue to be of central importance for the treatment of acute LV dysfunction during cardiac surgery and in the intensive care unit. The authors often use the combination of a PDE III inhibitor and a $β_1$-adrenoceptor agonist when weaning patients with pre-existing LV systolic dysfunction from cardiopulmonary bypass because these drugs produce synergistic effects on cAMP-mediated intracellular signaling.

Milrinone (Table 13-7) and inamrinone are PDE III inhibitors that have been used extensively for inotropic support during and after cardiac surgery. Milrinone is 15- to 20-fold more potent than the chemically similar compound inamrinone. Milrinone enhances myocardial contractility and causes arterial and venous vasodilation, thereby improving the likelihood of successful weaning of patients with poor LV function from cardiopulmonary bypass.[118] The pharmacokinetics and pharmacodynamics of milrinone were extensively studied in patients undergoing cardiac surgery[119] and those in the intensive care unit.[120] Milrinone loading doses of 25 or 50 $µg·kg^{-1}$ and infusion rates ranging between 0.375 and 0.75 $µg·kg^{-1}·min^{-1}$ are useful for increasing cardiac output and oxygen delivery in these clinical settings. Inamrinone was the first clinically used phosphodiesterase III inhibitor and exerted cardiovascular effects that were almost identical to those

Table 13-7 Comparative Effects of Milrinone, Levosimendan, and Vasopressin

Name	Chemical Structure	Mechanism of Action	Dose Range	Clinical Indications	Major Side Effects
Milrinone		PDE III inhibition	Load: 25–50 µg/kg IV: 0.375–0.75 µg/kg/min	Acute LV dysfunction	Arrhythmias Myocardial ischemia Sudden cardiac death Hypertension Stroke
Levosimendan		Myofilament Ca^{2+} sensitization PDE III Inhibition K_{ATP} channel opener	Load: 12–24 µg/kg IV: 0.05–0.2 µg/kg/min	Acute LV dysfunction Heart failure	Tachycardia Hypotension
Vasopressin		V_1 (vascular smooth muscle) and V_2 (renal collecting tubules) agonist	IV: 0.01–0.1 U/min	Shock (vasodilatory, cardiogenic) Cardiac arrest	Arrhythmias Hypertension Myocardial ischemia Reduced cardiac output Peripheral ischemia Splanchnic vasoconstriction

Abbreviations: IV, intravenous; LV, left ventricular; Ca^{2+}, calcium; PDE, phosphodiesterase; K_{ATP}, adenosine triphosphate-sensitive potassium channel.
Modified from Linn KA, Pagel PS. Cardiovascular pharmacology. In: Barash PG, Cullen BF, Stoelting RK, et al., eds. *Clinical Anesthesia Fundamentals*. Philadelphia, PA: Wolters Kluwer; 2015:234–235.

of milrinone, but use of the drug for the treatment of LV dysfunction was abandoned because of its propensity to cause profound thrombocytopenia during prolonged use.[121]

Levosimendan

Myofilament Ca^{2+} sensitizers are positive inotropic, vasodilating drugs that enhance myocardial contractility by increasing the Ca^{2+} sensitivity of the contractile apparatus.[122] Levosimendan (Table 13-7) is the only drug in this class that is currently available, although a number of other myofilament Ca^{2+} sensitizers were previously studied in clinical trials. Levosimendan is used extensively in Europe for short-term treatment of heart failure[123] and for inotropic support in patients undergoing cardiac surgery.[124] However, use of the drug in the United States is relatively limited because it remains unclear whether levosimendan provides any clinically meaningful unique advantages over conventional therapy.[125] Levosimendan was initially touted as a treatment for acute decompensation of chronic heart failure that would decrease morbidity and mortality, but the myofilament Ca^{2+} sensitizer did not reduce the incidence of death or major adverse cardiac events compared with dobutamine.[126] Intermittent ambulatory treatment with levosimendan also did not improve functional capacity or quality of life in patients with advanced heart failure.[127] Levosimendan produced rapid improvement of symptoms in patients with acute decompensated heart failure, but the drug also increased the risk of cardiovascular-related complications.[128] As a result of these and other recent clinical trials, the future of levosimendan as a treatment for heart failure is uncertain.

Levosimendan exerts its positive inotropic and vasodilator actions through three major mechanisms.[128] First, levosimendan binds to troponin C (TnC) and stabilizes the Ca^{2+}-bound conformation of the regulatory protein in a Ca^{2+}-dependent manner. This action prolongs the interaction between actin and myosin filaments and enhances the rate and extent of myocyte contraction to increase myocardial contractility. The Ca^{2+}-dependence of levosimendan–TnC binding prevents relaxation abnormalities that would otherwise be expected to occur. Second, levosimendan is a potent PDE III inhibitor that produces positive inotropic and lusitropic effects and causes systemic, pulmonary, and coronary vasodilation. Finally, levosimendan opens ATP-dependent K^+ (K_{ATP}) channels, which contribute to the drug's vasodilator properties and may also produce the additional benefit of myocardial protection against reversible[129] and irreversible[130] ischemic injury. Levosimendan decreases LV filling pressures, mean arterial pressure, and pulmonary and systemic vascular resistances and increases cardiac output in patients with heart failure. The modest reductions in arterial pressure observed with levosimendan are similar to those produced by milrinone and usually respond to volume administration. Levosimendan also improves LV-arterial coupling and mechanical efficiency, while causing only minimal increases in heart rate and myocardial oxygen consumption. Similar to the findings in the setting of heart failure, levosimendan also improves cardiac performance concomitant with reductions in pulmonary capillary occlusion pressure and systemic vascular resistance in patients with normal and depressed LV systolic function undergoing cardiac surgery.[131] Levosimendan has a biologically active metabolite (OR-1896) that most likely contributes to the parent drug's more prolonged hemodynamic effects compared with catecholamines or PDE III inhibitors.[132]

Digitalis Glycosides

The search for new drugs that chronically enhance myocardial contractility in failing heart has been astonishingly disappointing despite decades of intense cardiovascular pharmacology research.[133] Digitalis glycosides continue to be the only currently available class of positive inotropic drugs for oral treatment of mild to moderate heart failure, and these medications have been used for centuries. Digitalis glycosides are naturally occurring substances found in several plant species including "foxglove" (*Digitalis purpurea*). The most commonly prescribed digitalis glycosides are digoxin and digitoxin, but a number of related compounds are also used clinically. Digitalis glycosides enhance contractile function, but this positive inotropic effect is relatively minor when compared with other drugs used for the treatment of acute LV dysfunction. Digitalis glycosides selectively bind to the α-subunit of the sarcolemmal Na^+-K^+ ATPase on its extracellular surface and reversibly inhibit the enzyme.[134] An increase in extracellular K^+ concentration partially inhibits this digitalis-Na^+-K^+ ATPase binding. As a result, administration of K^+ is capable of reversing digitalis toxicity resulting from hypokalemia. Inhibition of sarcolemmal Na^+-K^+ ATPase indirectly increases Ca^{2+} availability, thereby enhancing myocardial contractility. The Na^+-K^+ ATPase enzyme normally trades three Na^+ ions (intracellular to extracellular) for two K^+ ions (extracellular to intracellular) against their corresponding cation concentration gradients. Inhibition of this energy-dependent ion exchange produces modestly increases intracellular Na^+ concentration, which reduces Ca^{2+} extrusion from the myoplasm by the sarcolemmal Na^+-Ca^{2+} exchanger. The additional Ca^{2+} is stored in the sarcoplasmic reticulum and then released during the next contraction. In contrast to other drugs that increase myocardial contractility, tachyphylaxis to the positive inotropic effects of digitalis glycosides does not occur. The mechanism of action of digitalis glycosides is similar to that implicated for the Treppe ("staircase") phenomenon (see Chapter 12), in which a rapid increase in heart rate causes a delay in Na^+-K^+ ATPase activity, leading to a transient increase in intracellular Na^+ concentration and enhanced contractile force mediated by favorable Na^+-Ca^{2+} exchange.

The increase in myocardial contractility produced by digitalis glycosides is associated with declines in LV preload and afterload, LV wall tension, and myocardial oxygen consumption in the failing heart. Heart rate remains unchanged. Because digitalis glycosides augment contractility and improve cardiac output, these drugs reduce the chronically elevated sympathetic nervous system activity that is a characteristic feature of heart failure. Reductions in norepinephrine concentrations and consequently, declines in LV afterload, also occur in response to this withdrawal of sympathetic tone. The decrease in sympathetic nervous system activity observed with digitalis glycosides is also related to the direct actions of these drugs on cardiac baroreceptors. These combined actions play important roles in reducing morbidity and mortality in patients with heart failure.[135] However, digitalis-induced inhibition of Na^+-K^+ ATPase also causes profound alterations in electrophysiology (e.g., SA and AV nodes, conduction pathways, His–Purkinje fibers) because the enzyme maintains normal resting membrane potential. Withdrawal of sympathetic and increases in parasympathetic nervous system activity further modulate the direct electrophysiologic effects of digitalis glycosides. Thus, it is not surprising that digitalis glycosides often cause a wide variety of arrhythmias including sinus bradycardia or arrest, AV conduction delays, and second- or third-degree heart block. Notably, toxic levels of digitalis glycosides may paradoxically increase sympathetic nervous system tone and precipitate the development of ventricular tachyarrhythmias. Digitalis glycosides have a low therapeutic ratio and narrow margin of safety. As a result, mortality resulting from arrhythmias is directly related to a digitalis drug's plasma concentration. Digitalis glycosides are most often used for management of supraventricular tachyarrhythmias with rapid ventricular response during the perioperative period because the drugs prolong conduction time in the AV node.

Vasopressin

Vasopressin (antidiuretic hormone; Table 13-7) is a peptide hormone released from the posterior pituitary that regulates water reabsorption in the kidney and exerts potent hemodynamic effects independent of adrenoceptors. Vasopressin receptors consist of three subtypes (V_1, V_2, and V_3), all of which are five-subunit helical membrane proteins coupled to G proteins. Vasopressin's cardiovascular effects are predominately mediated through V_1 receptors, which are located in the cell membrane of vascular smooth muscle.[136] Activation of the V_1 receptor subtype stimulates phospholipase C and triggers hydrolysis of inositol 4,5-bisphosphate (PIP_2) to inositol 1,4,5-triphosphate (IP_3) and diacyl glycerol (DAG). These second messengers increase intracellular Ca^{2+} concentration and produce contraction of the vascular smooth muscle cell. V_2 receptors are present on renal collecting duct cells and, when activated, increase reabsorption of free water, whereas V_3 receptors are located in the pituitary gland itself and act as autacoid modulators.

Along with the sympathetic nervous system and renin–angiotensin–aldosterone axis, endogenous vasopressin plays an essential role in the maintenance of arterial pressure. Exogenous administration of vasopressin does not substantially affect arterial pressure in conscious, healthy patients because activation of central V_1 receptors in the area postrema enhances baroreceptor reflex-mediated inhibition of efferent sympathetic nervous outflow that counterbalances the elevated system vascular resistance resulting from V_1-induced arterial vasoconstriction. In contrast, vasopressinergic mechanisms are essential for maintaining arterial pressure under conditions in which sympathetic nervous system or renin–angiotensin–aldosterone axis dysfunction is present. Indeed, exogenous administration of vasopressin has been shown to effectively support arterial pressure when a relative vasopressin deficiency exists (e.g., catecholamine-refractory hypotension, vasodilatory shock, sepsis, cardiac arrest). ACE inhibitors and ARBs used to treat hypertension also affect autonomic nervous system and renin–angiotensin–aldosterone axis function. Intraoperative hypotension that is relatively refractory to administration of catecholamines or sympathomimetics has been repeatedly described in patients who are treated with these medications. General or neuraxial anesthesia also reduces sympathetic nervous system tone, resulting in decreased plasma stress hormone concentrations including vasopressin. Under these circumstances, administration of vasopressin activates V_1 vascular smooth muscle receptors and rapidly increases arterial pressure during anesthesia by causing arterial vasoconstriction. Vasopressin therapy has been shown to reduce mortality associated with acute vasodilatory states such as anaphylaxis. In addition, infusion of vasopressin is indicated for the treatment of severe hypotension after prolonged cardiopulmonary bypass in patients who are otherwise unresponsive to phenylephrine or norepinephrine (vasoplegia).

Vasopressin is a useful drug for the treatment of sepsis and cardiac arrest. Vasodilation that is refractory to fluid resuscitation combined with a relative deficiency of endogenous vasopressin is a characteristic feature of sepsis. Inadequate sympathetic nervous system and renin–angiotensin–aldosterone axis responses to hypotension are also present in sepsis. Administration of vasopressin in the absence or presence of other vasoactive medications often stabilizes hemodynamics and improves survival in patients with sepsis. The combined use of vasopressin with other vasoactive medications reduces the overall dose of vasopressin required to maintain arterial pressure, thereby limiting the adverse effects of vasopressin on organ perfusion. In fact, sustained administration of higher doses of vasopressin may produce mesenteric ischemia, peripheral vascular insufficiency, and cardiac arrest because the drug causes pronounced vasoconstriction of cutaneous, skeletal muscle, splanchnic, and coronary vascular beds, concomitant with reduced perfusion of and oxygen delivery to these tissues. Bolus intravenous administration of vasopressin is also used as part of the American Heart Association Adult Advanced Cardiac Life Support algorithm for cardiac arrest resulting from ventricular fibrillation, pulseless electrical activity, or asystole.

Nitrovasodilators

Organic nitrates (e.g., nitroglycerin) and nitric oxide (NO) donors (e.g., sodium nitroprusside) are nitrovasodilators that release NO through enzymatic sulfhydryl group reduction or through a spontaneous mechanism that occurs independent of metabolism, respectively. Like endogenous NO produced by vascular endothelium, exogenous NO stimulates guanylate cyclase within the vascular smooth muscle cell to convert guanosine triphosphate to cGMP. The second messenger activates a cGMP-dependent protein kinase (protein kinase G) that dephosphorylates myosin light chains and contributes to relaxation of vascular smooth muscle. NO stimulates Ca^{2+} reuptake into the sarcoplasmic reticulum by activating the sarcoplasmic reticulum Ca^{2+} ATPase through a cGMP-independent mechanism. This action decreases intracellular Ca^{2+} concentration and causes relaxation. NO also stimulates K^+ efflux from the cell by activating the K^+ channel. This shift in K^+ balance produces cellular hyperpolarization, which, in turn, closes the voltage-gated Ca^{2+} channel and facilitates relaxation.

Nitrovasodilators are often used to improve hemodynamics and myocardial oxygen supply–demand relations in patients with heart failure. Venodilation reduces venous return, contributing to declines in LV and RV end-diastolic volume, pressure, and wall stress. Arterial vasodilation also reduces systemic and pulmonary arterial pressures, which decreases LV and RV end-systolic wall stress, respectively. These actions combine to decrease myocardial oxygen consumption. Simultaneously, nitrovasodilators increase myocardial oxygen supply through direct dilation of epicardial coronary arteries in the absence of flow-limiting stenoses. The reduction in LV end-diastolic pressure observed during administration of nitrovasodilators coupled with coronary vasodilation substantially enhances subendocardial perfusion. The clinical efficacy of nitrovasodilators may display some initial variability between patients, but the cardiovascular effects of these drugs inevitably diminish with prolonged use. Some patients may be relatively resistant to the effects of organic nitrates in the presence of oxidative stress because superoxide anions scavenge NO, cause reversible oxidation of guanylate cyclase, and inhibit aldehyde dehydrogenase. The latter action prevents the release of NO from organic nitrates. A progressive attenuation of hemodynamic responses to nitrovasodilators may develop in other patients as a result of sympathetic nervous system and renin–angiotensin–aldosterone axis activation. This phenomenon, termed "pseudotolerance," accounts for the rebound hypertension that may be observed after abrupt discontinuation of nitrovasodilator therapy. Inhibition of guanylate cyclase activity is most likely responsible for true tolerance to organic nitrates. A daily "drug holiday" is a useful strategy for reversing this effect in patients requiring prolonged treatment. Administration of N-acetylcysteine, a sulfhydryl donor, may also be effective for reversing true tolerance. Notably, prolonged use of organic nitrates may also cause methemoglobinemia, interfere with platelet aggregation, and produce heparin resistance. It is important to recognize that organic nitrates should also be used with caution in patients receiving phosphodiesterase type V inhibitors (e.g., sildenafil) because NO-induced vasodilation is enhanced, and profound hypotension, myocardial ischemia or infarction, and death may result.

Nitroglycerin

Nitroglycerin dilates venules to a greater degree than arterioles. At lower doses, the organic nitrate produces venodilation without causing a significant decrease in systemic vascular resistance. Arterial pressure and cardiac output fall in response to the reduction in preload despite a modest baroreceptor reflex-mediated increase in heart rate. Nitroglycerin also decreases pulmonary arterial pressures and vascular resistance. At higher doses, nitroglycerin dilates arterioles and reduces LV afterload. These effects cause more pronounced decreases in arterial pressure and stimulate greater reflex tachycardia. Overshoot hypotension and tachycardia is particularly common in the setting of hypovolemia, such as is often observed in patients with poorly controlled essential hypertension and parturients with pregnancy-induced hypertension.

Nitroglycerin improves the balance of myocardial oxygen supply to demand through its actions as a direct coronary vasodilator (which increase supply) and its systemic hemodynamic effects (which reduce demand). Nitroglycerin dilates both normal and poststenotic epicardial coronary arteries, enhances blood flow through coronary collateral vessels, and preferentially improves subendocardial perfusion. The drug also inhibits coronary vasospasm and dilates arterial conduits (e.g., internal mammary artery, radial artery) used during CABG surgery. Nitroglycerin decreases myocardial oxygen demand by reducing LV preload, and to a lesser extent afterload, thereby producing corresponding reductions in LV end-diastolic and end-systolic wall stress. These effects are particularly important in patients with acutely decompensated heart failure resulting from myocardial ischemia. Thus, nitroglycerin is a very effective first-line drug for the treatment of myocardial ischemia. Nevertheless, caution should be exercised when using nitroglycerin in patients with ischemia who are also hypovolemic because the drug may precipitate life-threatening hypotension by further compromising coronary perfusion pressure and reducing coronary blood flow despite epicardial vasodilation. These actions may inadvertently worsen myocardial ischemia.

Sodium Nitroprusside

Sodium nitroprusside is an ultra–short-acting direct NO donor. It is a potent venous and arterial vasodilator that rapidly reduces arterial pressure by decreasing LV preload and afterload, respectively. Not surprisingly, sodium nitroprusside is a first-line drug for the treatment of hypertensive emergencies. Sodium nitroprusside is also useful for the treatment of cardiogenic shock because arterial vasodilation improves forward flow by reducing impedance to LV ejection while venodilation decreases LV filling pressures. Unlike nitroglycerin, sodium nitroprusside is relatively contraindicated in patients with acute myocardial ischemia because the drug causes abnormal redistribution of coronary blood flow away from ischemic myocardium ("coronary steal"). This effect occurs because sodium nitroprusside produces greater coronary vasodilation in vessels that perfuse normal myocardium compared with those that supply the ischemic territory, the latter of which are already maximally vasodilated. Baroreceptor reflex-mediated tachycardia is also more pronounced during administration of sodium nitroprusside compared with nitroglycerin because the direct NO donor is a more potent arteriolar vasodilator than the organic nitrate. This reflex tachycardia dramatically increases heart rate and myocardial oxygen consumption, thereby exacerbating acute myocardial ischemia. Sodium nitroprusside is often combined with a β_1-adrenoceptor antagonist such as esmolol to decrease arterial pressure, depress myocardial contractility, and reduce ascending aortic wall stress in patients with acute aortic dissection until direct surgical control of the injury can be achieved. Clinical use of sodium nitroprusside is limited by its toxic metabolites, which predictably accumulate when administration is prolonged or relatively high doses are used. Metabolism of sodium nitroprusside produces cyanide, which binds with cytochrome C to inhibit aerobic metabolism and cause lactic acidosis. Cyanide derived from sodium nitroprusside metabolism also binds with hemoglobin to form methemoglobin and with sulfur to form thiocyanate. The latter metabolite may accumulate in patients with renal insufficiency and produce neurologic complications including delirium and seizures.

Hydralazine

Hydralazine is a direct vasodilator that reduces intracellular Ca^{2+} concentration in vascular smooth muscle. Activation of K_{ATP} channels is partially responsible for this effect, which results in direct relaxation of small arteries and arterioles in coronary, cerebral, splanchnic, and renal vascular beds, declines in systemic vascular resistance, and decreases in arterial pressure. LV preload is relatively preserved because hydralazine does not dilate venous capacitance vessels. The primary reduction in afterload stimulates baroreceptor reflex-mediated tachycardia and increases cardiac output. The magnitude of tachycardia observed with administration of hydralazine is often greater than expected based solely on baroreceptor reflexes alone and may reflect a direct effect of the drug on cardiovascular regulation in the central nervous system. This pronounced tachycardia might produce acute myocardial ischemia in patients with critical coronary stenoses based on increases in myocardial oxygen demand. Hydralazine-induced tachycardia responds appropriately to β_1-adrenoceptor antagonists, but caution should be exercised because further declines in arterial pressure may also occur. Hydralazine is commonly used for management of sustained postoperative hypertension in the absence of tachycardia.

Calcium Channel Blockers

Ca^{2+} channels are asymmetric biochemical pores consisting of at least four subunits (α_1, α_2/δ, and β with or without gamma) that traverse many biologic membranes.[137] Ca^{2+} channels are closed under quiescent conditions, but they may open through a voltage-dependent or receptor-operated mechanism to allow Ca^{2+} entry into the cell or an organelle (e.g., mitochondria, sarcoplasmic reticulum). Myocardial and vascular smooth muscle cell membranes contain two types of voltage-dependent Ca^{2+} channels that are defined on the basis of the duration of opening: T (transient) and L (long). The L-type Ca^{2+} channel is the predominant target of Ca^{2+} channel blockers in current clinical use. These drugs do not block the T-type Ca^{2+} channel. Ca^{2+} channel blockers may be divided into four chemical groups including 1,4-dihydropyridines (e.g., nifedipine, nicardipine, nimodipine, clevidipine), benzothiazepines (diltiazem), phenylalkylamines (verapamil), and diarylaminopropylamine ethers (bepridil), the first three of which are used clinically (Table 13-8).

In general, Ca^{2+} channel blockers produce varying degrees of vasodilation; direct negative chronotropic, dromotropic, and inotropic effects; and baroreceptor reflex-mediated increases in heart rate, depending on each drug's selectivity for myocardial and vascular smooth muscle L-type Ca^{2+} channels. All Ca^{2+} channel blockers produce greater relaxation of arterial, compared with venous, vascular smooth muscle. As a result, LV afterload is reduced while preload is relatively preserved. Ca^{2+} channel blockers cause coronary arterial vasodilation and inhibit coronary artery vasospasm. These actions may enhance coronary blood flow assuming that coronary perfusion pressure is not substantially reduced as a result of arterial vasodilation. In addition to causing declines in LV afterload, some Ca^{2+} channel blockers (e.g., diltiazem, verapamil) also reduce myocardial oxygen consumption by decreasing heart rate and myocardial contractility. However, other Ca^{2+} channel blockers (e.g., dihydropyridines) may increase myocardial oxygen consumption because of baroreceptor reflex-induced tachycardia. As a result, these Ca^{2+} channel blockers may not exert anti-ischemic effects in patients with hemodynamically significant coronary artery stenoses.

Nifedipine

Nifedipine and other related dihydropyridine Ca^{2+} channel blockers (e.g., amlodipine, felodipine, isradipine) are most often used for chronic treatment of essential hypertension. Like other Ca^{2+} channel blockers, nifedipine is a relatively selective arterial vasodilator that does not substantially affect venous vasomotor tone. This effect decreases arterial pressure, but in so doing, activates the sympathetic nervous system and elicits baroreceptor reflex-mediated increases in heart rate. Nifedipine produces direct myocardial depression in vitro, but this negative inotropic effect is not evident when the drug is used clinically because arterial vasodilation occurs at plasma concentrations that are substantially less than those required for reductions in myocardial contractility. Similarly, typical doses of nifedipine only minimally alter SA node automaticity and AV conduction. Maintenance of venous return and contractility state combined with modest tachycardia and a decline in LV afterload result in small increases in cardiac output. Nifedipine is frequently used in patients with coronary artery disease, most often in combination with a β_1-adrenoceptor antagonist to abolish baroreceptor reflex-mediated tachycardia,[138] because the Ca^{2+} channel blocker decreases myocardial oxygen consumption via a reduction in LV afterload and is a direct epicardial coronary vasodilator. Another more specific indication for this Ca^{2+} channel blocker is variant angina, a disease process in which reductions in coronary blood flow occur as a result of regional coronary vasoconstriction independent of coronary artery stenoses.[138] Nifedipine is probably more effective than nitrates for the treatment of variant

Table 13-8 Comparative Effects of Ca²⁺ Channel Blockers

Name	Chemical Structure	Myocardial Depression	Coronary Blood Flow	Suppression of SA Node (Automaticity)	Suppression of AV Node (Conduction)
Nifedipine		+	+++++	+	0
Nicardipine		0	+++++	+	0
Clevidipine		+	+++++	+	0
Nimodipine		+	++++	+	0
Diltiazem		++	+++	+++++	++++
Verapamil		++++	++++	+++++	++++

SA, sinoatrial; AV, atrioventricular.
Adapted with permission from Michel T, Hoffman BB. Treatment of myocardial ischemia and hypertension. In: Brunton LL, Chabner BA, Knollman BC, eds. *Goodman and Gilman's The Pharmacological Basis of Therapeutics*. 12th ed. New York, NY: McGraw-Hill Medical; 2011:756.

angina because the Ca^{2+} channel blocker causes more profound, consistent coronary vasodilation. Vasospasm may also occur in patients with unstable angina resulting from atherosclerosis, and nifedipine may also be beneficial in this setting.[139] Despite these salutary effects, nifedipine does not improve and may worsen mortality when used in patients with acute myocardial infarction, in contrast to other Ca^{2+} channel blockers such as diltiazem and verapamil.[140] Nifedipine is also used to provide arterial vasodilation in patients with Raynaud's phenomenon.[141]

Nicardipine

Nicardipine is another dihydropyridine Ca^{2+} channel antagonist that is highly selective for vascular smooth muscle. Nicardipine produces cardiovascular effects that are similar to nifedipine, but has a longer half-life than the latter drug. Nicardipine is a profound vasodilator because of its pronounced inhibition of Ca^{2+} influx in vascular smooth muscle. Like other dihydropyridine Ca^{2+} channel antagonists, nicardipine preferentially dilates arteriolar vessels; this effect decreases arterial pressure. In contrast to diltiazem and verapamil, nicardipine does not substantially depress myocardial contractility nor does the drug affect the rate of SA node firing. As a result, stroke volume and cardiac output are relatively preserved or may increase. Nicardipine-induced decreases in arterial pressure trigger increases in heart rate through activation of baroreceptor reflexes, but the tachycardia observed during administration of nicardipine is less pronounced than typically occurs with sodium nitroprusside at comparable levels of arterial pressure. Nicardipine is also a highly potent coronary vasodilator and is often used to dilate arterial conduits during coronary artery bypass graft surgery. Because of its relatively long half-life, nicardipine is primarily used for treatment of sustained perioperative hypertension and not for acute, often transient hypertensive episodes that are commonly observed during surgery.

Clevidipine

Clevidipine is an ultra–short-acting dihydropyridine Ca^{2+} channel antagonist with a plasma half-life of approximately 2 minutes after intravenous administration.[142,143] Like nicardipine and nifedipine, clevidipine exerts pronounced effects at the less negative resting membrane potentials typically observed in vascular smooth muscle cells, but demonstrates lower potency in cardiac myocytes in which resting membrane potentials are substantially more negative. As a result of these differences in cellular electrophysiology, clevidipine is highly selective for arterial vascular smooth muscle and is nearly devoid of negative chronotropic or inotropic effects. This hemodynamic profile may be especially useful for the treatment of hypertension in patients with compromised LV function in the absence or presence of acute heart failure.[144] Clevidipine causes dose-related arteriolar vasodilation while sparing venous vasomotor tone, thereby reducing systemic vascular resistance and arterial pressure without affecting LV preload. These actions may combine to augment cardiac output. Modest increases in heart rate may also occur during administration of clevidipine as a result of baroreceptor reflex activation. Unlike other short-acting antihypertensive drugs, clevidipine is not associated with the development of tachyphylaxis, and abrupt discontinuation of the drug does not appear to cause rebound hypertension. Because tissue and plasma esterases are responsible for clevidipine metabolism, little to no accumulation of the drug occurs even in the setting of hepatic or kidney dysfunction. Clevidipine compares favorably with nitroglycerin, sodium nitroprusside, and nicardipine for the treatment of acute hypertension in cardiac surgery patients.[145] Clevidipine has also demonstrated efficacy for treatment of hypertension associated with pheochromocytoma[146] and acute intracerebral hemorrhage.[147] The short-acting Ca^{2+} channel blocker is also useful for producing controlled hypotension during spinal surgery.[148]

Nimodipine

The dihydropyridine nimodipine is more lipophilic and more easily crosses the blood–brain barrier than other drugs in this class of Ca^{2+} channel blockers. As a result, nimodipine exerts more cerebral arterial vasodilation than other dihydropyridines. Nimodipine is currently the only medication approved by the U.S. Food and Drug Administration for treatment of cerebral vasospasm after aneurysmal subarachnoid hemorrhage.[149,150] Several clinical trials demonstrated that nimodipine significantly reduces the severity of symptoms resulting from cerebral vasospasm, the incidence of cerebral infarction, the occurrence of delayed neurologic deficits, and the risk of mortality while improving long-term neurologic functional status after the initial hemorrhage.[151,152] Nimodipine does not affect the incidence of recurrent hemorrhage or prevent other adverse reactions.[152] Nimodipine also does not reverse angiographic evidence of vasospasm, indicating that the mechanism by which the Ca^{2+} channel blocker improves outcome in this setting is most likely not related to dilation of large cerebral arteries. Instead, nimodipine appears to reduce cerebral arteriolar resistance and enhance blood flow through pia mater collateral vessels. In addition, nimodipine may attenuate Ca^{2+}-mediated neurotoxicity and thereby exert clinically beneficial neuroprotective effects.[153]

Diltiazem

Diltiazem is the only benzothiazepine Ca^{2+} channel blocker in current clinical use.[154] The cardiovascular effects of diltiazem are somewhat different from those produced by the dihydropyridines. Intravenous administration of diltiazem produces arterial vasodilation and decreases arterial pressure. These actions initially stimulate baroreceptor reflex-mediated tachycardia and increase cardiac output, but heart rate subsequently falls because, in contrast to dihydropyridine Ca^{2+} channel blockers, diltiazem exerts potent negative chronotropic and dromotropic effects on SA node automaticity and AV node conduction, respectively. Oral administration of diltiazem reduces heart rate, arterial pressure, and myocardial oxygen consumption. Both routes of administration cause coronary vasodilation and moderate negative inotropic effects. These combined properties make diltiazem a useful alternative medication for the treatment of patients with hypertension and symptomatic coronary artery disease[155] in clinical situations in which β-adrenoceptor antagonists may be relatively contraindicated (e.g., asthma, chronic obstructive pulmonary disease). Similarly, diltiazem may also prevent subsequent myocardial infarction in patients who have already suffered an infarction but cannot receive a β-adrenoceptor antagonist.[138] Because diltiazem prolongs AV node conduction, the drug may be effective for ventricular rate control in patients with chronic atrial fibrillation, atrial flutter, or supraventricular tachycardia.[156,157] However, adenosine or cardioversion (depending on the magnitude of accompanying hypotension) remains the recommended treatment for symptomatic supraventricular tachycardia in the 2015

American Heart Association Advanced Adult Cardiovascular Life Support guidelines.[158]

Verapamil

The phenylalkylamine Ca^{2+} channel blocker verapamil produces less arterial vasodilation, but exerts more potent effects on automaticity, conduction, and myocardial contractility than the dihydropyridines. As a result, baroreceptor reflex-mediated increases in heart rate that may be expected because of reductions in arterial vasomotor tone and systemic vascular resistance do not occur. The sympathetic nervous system activation resulting from arterial vasodilation generally compensates for the direct negative inotropic effect of verapamil, and cardiac output is maintained or modestly increased because of the decline in LV afterload in patients with normal LV function. However, verapamil has the potential to markedly worsen pre-existing LV systolic dysfunction in patients with heart failure because of the Ca^{2+} channel blocker's myocardial depressant effects. Like diltiazem, verapamil is a coronary vasodilator and decreases myocardial oxygen consumption as a result of its hemodynamic effects. Thus, verapamil may be effective for the treatment of angina pectoris and myocardial infarction in patients who may be unable to tolerate β_1-adrenoceptor antagonists.[159]

The actions of verapamil on cardiac electrophysiology make the Ca^{2+} channel antagonist a useful alternative to adenosine for the treatment of supraventricular tachyarrhythmias.[158] Re-entry through the SA node or AV node is responsible for the vast majority of supraventricular tachyarrhythmias except when an aberrant conduction ("pre-excitation") pathway is present (e.g., the bundle of Kent in Wolff–Parkinson–White syndrome).[160] Similar to but to a greater extent than diltiazem, verapamil reduces the rate of SA node discharge, markedly decreases AV node conduction velocity, and increases the refractory period of the AV node consistent with a class IV antiarrhythmic. These actions predictably prolong PR interval and increase AV conduction time. For example, verapamil has been shown to significantly reduce the risk of supraventricular tachyarrhythmias in patients undergoing cardiac and noncardiac surgery because of these actions on the proximal cardiac conduction system.[161,162] Verapamil may also be useful for the treatment of atrial fibrillation or flutter with rapid ventricular response because the drug substantially reduces ventricular rate and may occasionally facilitate conversion of the atrial arrhythmia to sinus rhythm. Verapamil is contraindicated in the presence of an aberrant re-entry supraventricular tachyarrhythmia because blockade of AV conduction leaves direct transmission from the atrium to the ventricle through the aberrant pathway unopposed, thereby exposing the patient to the risk of malignant ventricular arrhythmias and sudden cardiac death.[163] Administration of verapamil in the presence of a β_1-adrenoceptor antagonist may cause complete heart block or profound myocardial depression. Verapamil is also contraindicated in patients with sick sinus syndrome or atrioventricular node dysfunction.[164]

Angiotensin-converting Enzyme Inhibitors

The renin–angiotensin–aldosterone system is another major regulator of cardiovascular homeostasis. Renal cortical juxtaglomerular cells secrete renin in response to decreases in Na^+ reabsorption by the macula densa, reduced perfusion pressure to preglomerular arterioles, and β_1-adrenoceptor stimulation resulting from

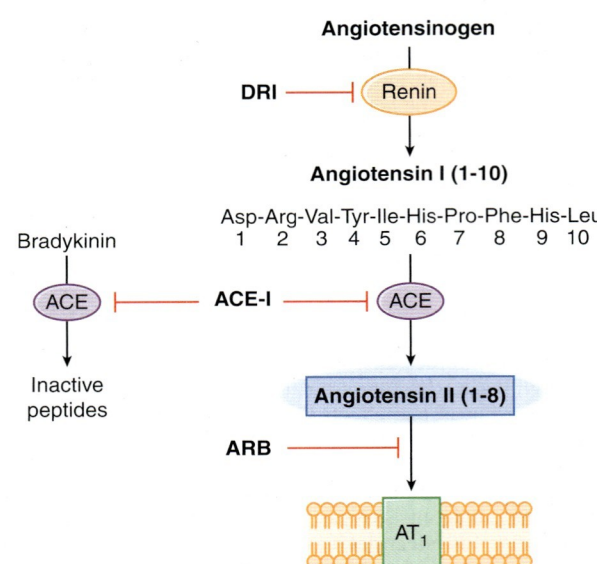

Figure 13-7 Schematic illustration of inhibitors of the renin–angiotensin system; abbreviations: DRI, direct renin inhibitor; ACE, angiotensin-converting enzyme; ACE I, angiotensin-converting enzyme inhibitor; ARB, angiotensin receptor blocker; AT_1, angiotensin subtype 1 receptor. (Adapted with permission from Hilal-Dandan R. Renin and angiotensin. In: Brunton LL, Chabner BA, Knollman BC, eds. *Goodman and Gilman's The Pharmacological Basis of Therapeutics*. 12th ed. New York, NY: McGraw-Hill Medical; 2011:731.)

sympathetic nervous system activation. Renin cleaves angiotensinogen into the 10 amino acid peptide angiotensin I (Fig. 13-7). Angiotensin-converting enzyme (synthesized in pulmonary vascular endothelium) then excises the C-terminal histidine and leucine residues from the angiotensin I molecule to form the biologically active octapeptide angiotensin II. A potent vasoconstrictor of renal and mesenteric arterioles through its actions at the angiotensin subtype I (AT_1) receptor mediated through G_q protein-phospholipase C-inositol triphosphate-Ca^{2+} signaling,[165] angiotensin II also facilitates the release of norepinephrine from sympathetic postganglionic neurons and augments the actions of the endogenous catecholamine in vascular smooth muscle. In addition, angiotensin II enhances release of norepinephrine and epinephrine from the adrenal medulla and attenuates baroreceptor-mediated reductions in sympathetic nervous system tone that occur in response to compensatory elevations in arterial pressure. Angiotensin II inhibits renal tubular reabsorption of Na^+, thereby reducing Na^+ and water excretion and enhancing K^+ excretion. Angiotensin II further stimulates the synthesis and release of aldosterone from the zona glomerulosa of the adrenal cortex. Aldosterone augments the actions of angiotensin II on renal tubular Na^+ retention and K^+ excretion. The net result of these collective effects is elevated arterial pressure and increased intravascular volume.

ACE inhibitors block the conversion of angiotensin I to angiotensin II. As may be predicted based on the aforementioned effects of angiotensin II, ACE inhibitors are potent antihypertensive medications. There are currently eleven ACE inhibitors in clinical use in the United States, which differ in potency, duration of action, metabolism and clearance, and whether hepatic esterase conversion of a prodrug form to a metabolite is required for activity (e.g., enalapril, quinapril, ramipril). Captopril was the first ACE inhibitor, but its use has diminished to some extent because the drug is associated with a greater number of adverse side effects and possible drug interactions than other ACE inhibitors. Enalapril is the only ACE inhibitor available in an intravenous form (enalaprilat), whereas lisinopril is the only orally administered drug in this class with a prolonged half-life that does not require multiple daily dosing. ACE inhibitors reduce LV afterload and decrease arterial pressure through a reduction in arterial vasomotor tone in patients with essential or renal vascular hypertension, but not in those with primary aldosteronism. Cardiac output remains unchanged or modestly increases while LV preload is unaffected. Sympathetic nervous system tone does not change despite the decrease in arterial pressure, and baroreceptor-mediated reflexes remain intact. As a result, patients do not develop orthostatic hypotension or limited exercise capacity when treated with an ACE inhibitor unless relative hypovolemia is present because of concomitant diuretic therapy; the ACE inhibitor is administered with another arterial vasodilator (e.g., Ca^{2+} channel blocker); or elevated plasma renin concentrations are present.

ACE inhibitors have been shown to be very effective in the treatment of LV systolic dysfunction with or without heart failure. Several large-scale, randomized, controlled double blind clinical trials provided convincing evidence that ACE inhibitors halt or delay the progression of heart failure and improve quality of life in patients resulting from LV systolic or diastolic dysfunction. ACE inhibitors also cause declines in the need for hospitalization, the incidence of myocardial infarction, and the risk of sudden cardiac death. In the presence of LV dysfunction, ACE inhibitors decrease LV afterload, improve arterial compliance, reduce arterial pressure, enhance cardiac output, increase renal blood flow, and facilitate natriuresis. The hemodynamic effects serve to reduce chronically elevated sympathetic nervous system tone because tissue perfusion improves, whereas the renal actions result in beneficial reductions in intravascular volume. ACE inhibitors have well-documented salutary effects in patients with acute myocardial infarction, especially those with diabetes mellitus and hypertension.[166] ACE inhibitors also substantially reduced the incidence of myocardial infarction, cerebrovascular accident, and mortality in patients at high risk for major adverse cardiovascular events.[167] Finally, ACE inhibitors exert renal protective effects in diabetic patients and mitigate the progression of renal dysfunction in other forms of nephropathy as well.[168]

ACE inhibitors produce several side effects, the most common of which is a dry cough that affects as many as 20% of patients treated with these medications. Blockade of ACE-induced degradation of bradykinin exacerbates the pulmonary effects of the inflammatory mediator and contributes to this clinical problem. Nonsteroidal anti-inflammatory drugs attenuate the ability of ACE inhibitors to reduce arterial pressure in patients with hypertension. ACE inhibitors may also cause hyperkalemia in patients with chronic kidney injury and in those with normal renal function who are treated with K^+-sparing diuretics (e.g., spironolactone, triamterene) or K^+ supplements. Conversely, ACE inhibitors blunt the hypokalemic effects of thiazide and loop diuretics. Acute renal failure, reversible neutropenia, fetal teratogenicity, and dermatitis are other adverse effects of ACE inhibitors. Angioedema is a potentially life-threatening, although rare (0.1% to 0.5% of patients), complication of ACE inhibitors in which rapidly developing edema of the lips, nose, tongue, mouth, hypopharynx, and glottis occurs that may quickly jeopardize airway integrity.[169] Angioedema resulting from an ACE inhibitor usually occurs with the initial dose of the drug and may require emergent endotracheal intubation or a surgical airway to prevent death from asphyxia. Notably, African-Americans are approximately 4.5-fold more likely to develop this complication than are their Caucasian counterparts.[170] Perhaps of most relevance to the anesthesiologist, chronic treatment with an ACE inhibitor may precipitate profound hypotension in the presence of vasodilating general anesthetics that is refractory to treatment with phenylephrine, ephedrine, or norepinephrine.[171,172] Vasopressinergic V_1 agonists (e.g., terlipressin) are more effective than norepinephrine in treating this form of intraoperative hypotension.[173,174] Discontinuation of ACE inhibitor therapy before elective surgery is recommended to avoid this complication.

Angiotensin Receptor Blockers

Angiotensin receptor blockers inhibit the AT_1 receptor with high affinity and thereby markedly attenuate the cardiovascular, endocrine, and renal effects of angiotensin II.[175] All ARBs are potent antihypertensive medications that more effectively inhibit the actions of angiotensin II at AT_1 receptors than do ACE inhibitors. In contrast to ACE inhibitors, ARBs do not affect angiotensin II-induced activation of angiotensin subtype 2 (AT_2) receptors. The clinical implications of these differences in pharmacodynamics between ARBs and ACE inhibitors remain unclear. ARBs and ACE inhibitors reduce arterial pressure to equivalent degrees, but angiotensin receptor blockers produce fewer side effects. Similar to ACE inhibitors, ARBs (e.g., losartan, candesartan, valsartan) improved functional capacity and reduced morbidity and mortality in patients with heart failure[176] and acute myocardial infarction complicated by LV dysfunction.[177] Whether the combination of an ARB and an ACE inhibitor provides any added clinical benefits in these settings has not been resolved.[178] ARBs are most often used in patients with heart failure who are unable to tolerate the side effects of ACE inhibitors, the latter of which continue to be used as first-line medications in heart failure pharmacotherapy. Like ACE inhibitors, ARBs provide renal protection in patients with diabetes mellitus independent of the effects of these drugs on arterial pressure.[179] ARBs also reduce the risk of stroke in patients with hypertension, maintain sinus rhythm after cardioversion in patients with long-term atrial fibrillation, and improve symptoms in patients with hepatic cirrhosis-induced portal hypertension. As predicted by their pharmacologic mechanism of action, ARBs are less likely to cause cough, dermatitis, or angioedema than ACE inhibitors. However, angiotensin receptor blockers exert fetal toxicity and may cause hyperkalemia in patients treated with K^+-sparing diuretics or those with renal insufficiency similar to ACE inhibitors.

REFERENCES

1. Crapo RO, Casaburi R, Coates AL, et al. Guidelines for methacholine and exercise challenge testing—1999. This official statement of the American Thoracic Society was adopted by the ATS Board of Directors, July 1999. *Am J Respir Crit Care Med*. 2000;161:309–329.
2. Ignarro LJ, Cirino G, Casini A, et al. Nitric oxide as a signaling molecule in the vascular system. *J Cardiovasc Pharmacol*. 1999;34:879–886.
3. Wein AJ: Practical uropharmacology. *Urol Clin North Am*. 1991;18:269–281.
4. Porter SR, Scully C, Hegarty AM. An update of the etiology and management of xerostomia. *Oral Srug Oral Med Oral Pathol Oral Radiol Endod*. 2004;97:28–46.
5. Nozaki H, Aikawa N. Sarin poisoning in Tokyo subway. *Lancet*. 1995;346:1446–1447.
6. Taylor P, Radic Z. The cholinesterases: from genes to proteins. *Annu Rev Pharmacol Toxicol*. 1994;34:281–320.
7. Storm JE, Rozman KK, Doull J. Occupational exposure limits for 30 organophosphate pesticides based on inhibition of red blood cell acetylcholinesterase. *Toxicology*. 2000;150:1–29.
8. Nilsson E. Physostigmine treatment in various drug-induced intoxications. *Ann Clin Res*. 1982;14:165–172.
9. Dampney RA, Coleman MJ, Fontes MA, et al. Central mechanisms underlying short- and long-term regulation of the cardiovascular system. *Clin Exp Pharmacol Physiol*. 2002;29:261–268.

10. Chapple C, Khullar V, Gabriel Z, et al. The effects of antimuscarinic treatments on overactive bladder: a systematic review and meta-analysis. *Eur Urol.* 2005;48:5–26.
11. Alcalay M, Izraeli S, Wallach-Kapon R, et al. Paradoxical pharmacodynamic effect of atropine on parasympathetic control: a study of spectral analysis of heart rate fluctuations. *Clin Pharmacol Ther.* 1992;52:518–527.
12. Wellstein A, Pitschner HF. Complex dose-response curves of atropine in man explained by different functions of M1- and M2-cholinoreceptors. *Naunyn Schmiedbergs Arch Pharmacol.* 1988;338:19–27.
13. Gross NJ. Ipratropium bromide. *N Engl J Med.* 1988;319:486–494.
14. Gross NJ. Tiotropium bromide. *Chest.* 2004;126:1946–1953.
15. Barnes PJ, Hansel TT. Prospect for new drugs for chronic obstructive pulmonary disease. *Lancet.* 2004;364:985–996.
16. Morgan JP, Erny RE, Allen PD, et al. Abnormal intracellular calcium handling, a major cause of systolic and diastolic dysfunction in ventricular myocardium from patients with heart failure. *Circulation.* 1990;81(Suppl III):21–32.
17. Post SR, Hammond HK, Insel PA. Beta-adrenergic receptors and receptor signaling in heart failure. *Annu Rev Pharmacol Toxicol.* 1999;39:343–360.
18. Vanhees L, Aubert A, Fagard R, et al. Influence of beta1- versus beta2-adrenoceptor blockade on left ventricular function in humans. *J Cardiovasc Pharmacol.* 1986;8:1086–1091.
19. Brodde O. The functional importance of beta 1 and beta 2 adrenoceptors in the human heart. *Am J Cardiol.* 1988;62:24C–29C.
20. Brodde OE, Michel MC. Adrenergic and muscarinic receptors in the human heart. *Pharmacol Rev.* 1999;51:651–690.
21. Marley PD, Livett BG. Differences between the mechanisms of adrenaline and noradrenaline secretion from isolated, bovine, adrenal chromaffin cells. *Neurosci Lett.* 1987;77:81–86.
22. Leenen FH, Chan YK, Smith DL, et al. Epinephrine and left ventricular function in humans: effects of beta-1 vs nonselective beta blockade. *Clin Pharmacol Ther.* 1988;43:519–528.
23. Butterworth JF IV, Prielipp RC, Royster RL, et al. Dobutamine increases heart rate more than epinephrine in patients recovering from aortocoronary bypass surgery. *J Cardiothorac Vasc Anesth.* 1992;6:535–541.
24. Fellehi JL, Parienti JJ, Hanouz JL, et al. Perioperative use of dobutamine in cardiac surgery and adverse cardiac outcome: propensity-adjusted analyses. *Anesthesiology.* 2008;108:979–987.
25. Allwood MJ, Cobbold AF, Ginsberg J. Peripheral vascular effects of noradrenaline, isopropylnoradrenaline, and dopamine. *Br Med Bull.* 1963;19:132–136.
26. Paradis NA, Martin GB, Rivers EP, et al. Coronary perfusion pressure and the return of spontaneous circulation in human cardiopulmonary resuscitation. *JAMA.* 1990;263:1106–1113.
27. Link MS, Berkow LC, Kudenchuck PJ, et al. Part 7: Adultadvanced cardiovascular life support: 2015 American Heart Association Guidelines for Cardiopulmonary Resuscitation and Emergency Cardiovascular Care. *Circulation.* 2015;132:S444–S464.
28. Walker DM: Update on epinephrine (adrenaline) for pediatric emergencies. *Curr Opin Pediatr.* 2009;21:313–319.
29. Bochner BS, Lichtenstein LM: Anaphylaxis. *N Engl J Med.* 1991;324:1785–1790.
30. Russell JA, Walley KR, Singer J, et al. Vasopressin versus norepinephrine in patients with septic shock. *N Engl J Med.* 2008;358:877–887.
31. Leyh RG, Kofidis T, Struber M, et al. Methylene blue: the drug of choice for catecholamine-refractory vasoplegia after cardiopulmonary bypass? *J Thorac Cardiovasc Surg.* 2003;125:1426–1431.
32. Griffin MJ, Hines RL. Management of perioperative ventricular dysfunction. *J Cardiothorac Vasc Anesth.* 2001;15:90–106.
33. MacGregor DA, Smith TE, Prielipp RC, et al. Pharmacokinetics of dopamine in healthy male subjects. *Anesthesiology.* 2000;92:338–346.
34. Friedrich JO, Adhikari N, Herridge MS, et al. Meta-analysis: low-dose dopamine increases urine output but does not prevent renal dysfunction or death. *Ann Intern Med.* 2005;142:510–524.
35. Venkataraman R. Can we prevent acute kidney injury? *Crit Care Med.* 2008;36:S166–S171.
36. Ruffalo RR. The pharmacology of dobutamine. *Am J Med Sci.* 1987;294:244–248.
37. Binkley PF, Van Fossen DB, Nunziata E, et al. Influence of positive inotropic therapy on pulsatile hydraulic load and ventricular-vascular coupling in congestive heart failure. *J Am Coll Cardiol.* 1990;15:1127–1135.
38. Keren G, Laniado S, Sonnenblick EH, et al. Dynamics of functional mitral regurgitation during dobutamine therapy in patients with severe congestive heart failure: A Doppler echocardiograhic study. *Am Heart J.* 1989;118:748–754.
39. Aronson S, Dupont F, Savage R, et al. Changes in regional myocardial function after coronary artery bypass are predicted by intraoperative low-dose dobutamine echocardiography. *Anesthesiology.* 2000;93:685–692.
40. Zamanian RT, Haddad F, Doyle RL, et al. Management strategies for patients with pulmonary hypertension in the intensive care unit. *Crit Care Med.* 2007;35:2037–2050.
41. Abraham WT, Adams KF, Fonarow GC, et al. In-hospital mortality in patients with acute decompensated heart failure requiring intravenous vasoactive medications: an analysis from the Acute Decompensated Heart Failure National Registry (ADHERE). *J Am Coll Cardiol.* 2005;46:57–64.
42. Follath F, Cleland JG, Just H, et al. Efficacy and safety of intravenous levosimendan compared with dobutamine in severe low-output heart failure (the LIDO study): a randomised double-blind trial. *Lancet.* 2002;360:196–202.
43. Dellinger RP, Levy MM, Carlet JM, et al. Surviving Sepsis Campaign: international guidelines for management of severe sepsis and septic shock: 2008. *Crit Care Med.* 2008;36:296–327.
44. Altschuld RA, Billman GE. Beta2-adrenoceptors and ventricular fibrillation. *Pharmacol Ther.* 2000;88:1–14.
45. Seale JP. Whither beta-adrenoceptor agonists in the treatment of asthma? *Prog Clin Biol Res.* 1988;263:367–377.
46. Feneck R. Drugs for the perioperative control of hypertension: current issues and future directions. *Drugs.* 2007;67:2023–2044.
47. Kini AS, Mitre CA, Kim M, et al. A protocol for prevention of radiographic contrast nephropathy during percutaneous coronary intervention: effect of select dopamine receptor agonist fenoldopam. *Catheter Cardiovasc Interv.* 2002;55:169–173.
48. Tumlin JA, Wang A, Murray PT, et al. Fenoldopam mesylate blocks reductions in renal plasma flow after radiocontrast dye infusion: a pilot trial in the prevention of contrast nephropathy. *Am Heart J.* 2002;143:894–903.
49. Landoni G, Biondi-Zoccai GG, Tumlin JA, et al. Beneficial impact of fenoldopam in critically ill patients with or at risk for acute renal failure: a meta-analysis of randomized clinical trials. *Am J Kidney Dis.* 2007;49:56–68, 2007.
50. Stone GW, McCullough PA, Tumlin JA, et al. Fenoldopam mesylate for the prevention of contrast-induced nephropathy: a randomized controlled trial. *JAMA.* 2003;290:2284–2291.
51. Tumlin JA, Finkel KW, Murray PT, et al. Fenoldopam mesylate in early acute tubular necrosis: a randomized, double-blind, placebo-controlled clinical trial. *Am J Kidney Dis.* 2005;46:26–34.
52. Bove T, Zangrillo A, Guarracino F, et al. Effect of fenoldopam on use of renal replacement therapy among patients with acute kidney injury after cardiac surgery: a randomized clinical trial. *JAMA.* 2014;312:2244–2253.
53. Ngan Kee WD. Prevention of maternal hypotension after regional anaesthesia for caesarean section. *Curr Opin Anaesthesiol.* 2010;23:304–309.
54. Rooke GA, Freund PR, Jacobson AF. Hemodynamic response and change in organ blood volume during spinal anesthesia in elderly men with cardiac disease. *Anesth Analg.* 1997;85:99–105.
55. Little WC: Enhanced load dependence of relaxation in heart failure. Clinical implications. *Circulation.* 1992;85:2326–2328.
56. Starke K, Gothert M, Kilbinger H. Modulation of neurotransmitter release by presynaptic autoreceptors. *Physiol Rev.* 1989;69:864–989.
57. Pacak K. Preoperative management of the pheochromocytoma patient. *J Clin Endocrinol Metab.* 2007;92:4069–4079.
58. Michel MD, Vrydag W. Alpha1-, alpha2-, and beta-adrenoceptors in the urinary bladder urethra and prostate. *Br J Pharmacol.* 2006;147:S88–S119.
59. Hayashi Y, Maze M. Alpha$_2$-adrenoceptor agonists and anaesthesia. *Br J Anaesth.* 1993;71:108–118.
60. Sanders RD, Maze M. Alpha2-adrenoceptor agonists. *Curr Opin Investig Drugs.* 2007;8:25–33.
61. van Zwieten PA. Centrally acting antihypertensives: a renaissance of interest. Mechanisms and haemodynamics. *J Hypertens.* 1997;15(Suppl):S3–S8.
62. Zhu QM, Lesnick JD, Jasper JR, et al. Cardiovascular effects of rilmenidine, moxonidine and clonidine in conscious wild-type and D79N alpha2A-adrenoceptor transgenic mice. *Br J Pharmacol.* 1999;126:1522–1530.
63. Muzi M, Goff DR, Kampine JP, et al. Clonidine reduces sympathetic activity but maintains baroreflex responses in normotensive humans. *Anesthesiology.* 1992;77:864–871.
64. Flacke JW, Bloor BC, Flacke WE, et al. Reduced narcotic requirement by clonidine with improved hemodynamic and adrenergic stability in patients undergoing coronary bypass surgery. *Anesthesiology.* 1987;67:11–19.
65. Quintin L, Viale JP, Annat G, et al. Oxygen uptake after major abdominal surgery: effect of clonidine. *Anesthesiology.* 1991;74:236–241.
66. Quintin L, Roudot F, Roux C, et al. Effect of clonidine on the circulation and vasoactive hormones after aortic surgery. *Br J Anaesth.* 1991;66:108–115.
67. Wijeysundera DN, Naik JS, Beattie WS. Alpha-2 adrenergic agonists to prevent perioperative cardiovascular complications: a meta-analysis. *Am J Med.* 2003;114:742–752.
68. Eisenach JC, De Kock M, Klimscha W. Alpha2-adrenergic agonists for regional anesthesia. A clinical review of clonidine (1984–1995). *Anesthesiology.* 1996;85:655–674.
69. Bailey PL, Sperry RJ, Johnson GK, et al. Respiratory effects of clonidine alone and combined with morphine, in humans. *Anesthesiology.* 1991;74:43–48.
70. Gold MS, Pottash AC, Sweeney DR, et al. Opiate withdrawal using clonidine. A safe, effective, and rapid nonopiate treatment. *JAMA.* 1980;243:343–346.
71. Arain SR, Ebert TJ. The efficacy, side effects, and recovery characteristics of dexmedetomidine versus propofol when used for intraoperative sedation. *Anesth Analg.* 2002;95:461–466.
72. Hoy SM, Keating GM. Dexmedetomidine: a review of its use for sedation in mechanically ventilated patients in an intensive care setting and for procedural sedation. *Drugs.* 2011;71:1481–1501.
73. Rozet I. Anesthesia for functional neurosurgery: the role of dexmedetomidine. *Curr Opin Anaesthesiol.* 2008;21:537–543.

74. Ma D, Hossain M, Rajakumaraswamy N, et al. Dexmedetomidine produces its neuroprotective effect via the alpha 2A-adrenoceptor subtype. *Eur J Pharmacol.* 2004;502:87–97.
75. Carollo DS, Nossaman BD, Ramadhyani U. Dexmedetomidine: a review of clinical applications. *Curr Opin Anaesthesiol.* 2008;21:457–461.
76. Shehabi Y, Riker RR, Bokesch PM, et al. Delirium duration and mortality in lightly sedated mechanically ventilated intensive care patients. *Crit Care Med.* 2010;38:2311–2318.
77. Wijeysundera DN, Duncan D, Nkonde-Price C, et al. Perioperative beta blockade in noncardiac surgery: a systematic review for the 2014 ACC/AHA guideline on perioperative cardiovascular evaluation and management of patients undergoing noncardiac surgery: a report of the American College of Cardiology/American Heart Association Task Force on practice guidelines. *J Am Coll Cardiol.* 2014;64:2406–2425.
78. Fleisher LA, Fleischmann KE, Auerbach AD, et al. 2014 ACC/AHA guideline on perioperative cardiovascular evaluation and management of patients undergoing noncardiac surgery: a report of the American College of Cardiology/American Heart Association Task Force on practice guidelines. *J Am Coll Cardiol.* 2014;64:e77–e137.
79. Fleischmann KE, Beckman JA, Buller CE, et al. 2009 ACCF/AHA focused update on perioperative beta blockade: a report of the American College of Cardiology Foundation/American Heart Association Task Force on Practice Guidelines. *Circulation.* 2009;120:2123–2151.
80. Lindenauer PK, Pekow P, Wang K, et al. Perioperative beta-blocker therapy and mortality after major noncardiac surgery. *N Engl J Med.* 2005;353:349–361.
81. Devereaux PJ, Yang H, Yusuf S, et al. Effects of extended-release metoprolol succinate in patients undergoing non-cardiac surgery (POISE trial): a randomised controlled trial. *Lancet.* 2008;371:1839–1847.
82. Man in't Veld AJ, Van den Meiracker AH, Schalekamp MA. Do beta blockers really increase peripheral vascular resistance? Review of the literature and new observations under basal conditions. *Am J Hypertens.* 1988;1:91–96.
83. van den Meiracker AH, Man in't Veld AJ, van Eck HJ, et al. Hemodynamic and hormonal adaptations to beta-adrenoceptor blockade. A 24-hour study of acebutolol, atenolol, pindolol, and propranolol in hypertensive patients. *Circulation.* 1988;11:413–423.
84. Toda N. Vasodilating beta-adrenoceptor blockers as cardiovascular therapeutics. *Pharmacol Ther.* 2003;100:215–234.
85. Antman EM, Hand M, Armstrong PW, et al. 2007 Focused Update of the ACC/AHA 2004 Guidelines for the Management of Patients with ST-Elevation Myocardial Infarction: a report of the American College of Cardiology/American Heart Association Task Force on Practice Guidelines: developed in collaboration with the Canadian Cardiovascular Society endorsed by the American Academy of Family Physicians: 2007 Writing Group to Review New Evidence and Update the ACC/AHA 2004 Guidelines for the Management of Patients with ST-Elevation Myocardial Infarction, Writing on Behalf of the 2004 Writing Committee. *Circulation.* 2008;117:296–329.
86. Amsterdam EA, Wenger NK, Brindis RG, et al. 2014 AHA/ACC Guideline for the Management of Patients with Non-ST-Elevation Acute Coronary Syndromes: a report of the American College of Cardiology/American Heart Association Task Force on Practice Guidelines. *J Am Coll Cardiol.* 2014;64:e139–e228.
87. Freemantle N, Cleland J, Young P, et al. Beta blockade after myocardial infarction: systematic review and meta regression analysis. *BMJ.* 1999;318:1730–1737.
88. Lefkowitz RJ, Rockman HA, Koch WJ. Catecholamines, beta-adrenergic receptors, and heart failure. *Circulation.* 2000;101:1634–1637.
89. Ding B, Abe J, Wei H, et al. A positive feedback loop of phosphodiestersase 3 (PDE3) and inducible cAMP early repressor (ICER) leads to cardiomyocyte apoptosis. *Proc Natl Acad Sci USA.* 2005;102:14771–14776.
90. Cleland JG: Beta-blockers for heart failure: Why, which, when, and where. *Med Clin North Am.* 2003;87:339–371.
91. Packer M, Colucci WS, Sackner-Bernstein JD, et al. Double-blind, placebo-controlled study of the effects of carvedilol in patients with moderate to severe heart failure. The PRECISE Trial. Prospective Randomized Evaluation of Carvedilol on Symptoms and Exercise. *Circulation.* 1996;94:2793–2799.
92. Bolger AP, Al-Nasser F. Beta-blockers for chronic heart failure: surviving longer but feeling better? *Int J Cardiol.* 2003;92:1–8.
93. Lacro RV, Dietz HC, Sleeper LA, et al. Atenolol versus losartan in children and young adults with Marfan's syndrome. *N Engl J Med.* 2014;371:2061–2071.
94. Nishimura RA, Holmes DR Jr. Clinical practice. Hypertrophic obstructive cardiomyopathy. *N Engl J Med.* 2004;350:1320–1327.
95. Tfelt-Hansen P. Efficacy of beta-blockers in migraine. A critical review. *Cephalalgia.* 1986;6(Suppl 2):15–24.
96. Strauss WE, Parisi AF. Combined use of calcium-channel and beta-adrenergic blockers for the treatment of chronic stable angina. Rationale, efficacy, and adverse effects. *Ann Intern Med.* 1988;109:570–581.
97. Salpeter SR, Ormiston TM, Sapleter EE. Cardioselective beta-blockers for chronic obstructive pulmonary disease. *Cochrane Database Sys Rev.* 2005;CD003566.
98. DiBari M, Marchionni N, Pahor M. Beta-blockers after acute myocardial infarction in elderly patients with diabetes mellitus: Time to reassess. *Drugs Aging.* 2003;20:13–22.
99. National Heart Lung and Blood Institute. A randomized trial of propranolol in patients with acute myocardial infarction. I. Mortality results. *JAMA.* 1982;247:1707–1714.
100. Wuttke H, Rau T, Heide R, et al. Increased frequency of cytochrome P450 2D6 poor metabolizers among patients with metoprolol-associated adverse effects. *Clin Pharmacol Ther.* 2002;72:429–437.
101. Prakash A, Markham A. Metoprolol: a review of its use in chronic heart failure. *Drugs.* 2000;60:647–678.
102. Feldman RD, Hussain Y, Kuyper LM, et al. Intraclass differences among antihypertensive drugs. *Annu Rev Pharmacol Toxicol.* 2015;55:333–352.
103. Donnelly R, Macphee GJ. Clinical pharmacokinetics and kinetic-dynamic relationships of dilevalol and labetalol. *Clin Pharmacokinet.* 1991;21:95–109.
104. DiNicolantonio JJ, Hackam DG. Carvedilol: a third-generation beta-blocker should be a first-choice beta-blocker. *Expert Rev Cardiovasc Ther.* 2012;10:13–25.
105. Vinten-Johansen J. Involvement of neutrophils in the pathogenesis of lethal myocardial reperfusion injury. *Cardiovasc Res.* 2004;61:481–497.
106. Keating GM, Jarvis B. Carvedilol: a review of its use in chronic heart failure. *Drugs.* 2003;63:1697–1741.
107. Doughty RN, White HD. Carvedilol: use in chronic heart failure. *Expert Rev Cardiovasc Ther.* 2007;5:21–31.
108. Movsesian MA, Smith CJ, Krall J, et al. Sarcoplasmic reticulum-associated cyclic adenosine 5′-monophosphate phosphodiesterase activity in normal and failing human hearts. *J Clin Invest.* 1991;88:15–19.
109. Kajimoto K, Hagiwara N, Kasanuki H, et al. Contribution of phosphodiesterase isozymes to the regulation of L-type calcium current in human cardiac myocytes. *Br J Pharmacol.* 1997;121:1549–1556.
110. Koss KL, Kranias EG: Phospholamban: a prominent regulator of myocardial contractility. *Circ Res.* 1996;79:1059–1063.
111. Doolan LA, Jones EF, Kalman J, et al. A placebo-controlled trial verifying the efficacy of milrinone in weaning high-risk patients from cardiopulmonary bypass. *J Cardiothorac Vasc Anesth.* 1997;11:37–41.
112. Chen EP, Bittner HB, Davis RD, et al. Hemodynamic and inotropic effects of milrinone after heart transplantation in the setting of recipient pulmonary hypertension. *J Heart Lung Transplant.* 1998;17:669–678.
113. Konstam MA, Cody RJ. Short-term use of intravenous milrinone for heart failure. *Am J Cardiol.* 1995;75:822–826.
114. Tisdale JE, Patel R, Webb CR, et al. Electrophysiologic and proarrhythmic effects of intravenous inotropic agents. *Prog Cardiovasc Dis.* 1995;38:167–180.
115. Hayashida N, Tomoeda H, Oda T, et al. Inhibitory effect of milrinone on cytokine production after cardiopulmonary bypass. *Ann Thorac Surg.* 1999;68:1661–1667.
116. Cracowski JL, Stanke-Labesque F, Chavanon O, et al. Vasorelaxant actions of enoximone, dobutamine, and the combination on human arterial coronary bypass grafts. *J Cardiovasc Pharmacol.* 1999;34:741–748.
117. Packer M, Carver JR, Rodeheffer RJ, et al. Effect of oral milrinone on mortality in severe chronic heart failure. THE PROMISE Study Research Group. *N Engl J Med.* 1991;325:1468–1475.
118. Rathmell JP, Prielipp RC, Butterworth JF IV, et al. A multicenter, randomized, blind comparison of amrinone and milrinone after elective cardiac surgery. *Anesth Analg.* 1998;86:683–690.
119. Butterworth IV JF, Hines RL, Royster RL, et al. A pharmacokinetic and pharmacodynamic evaluation of milrinone in adults undergoing cardiac surgery. *Anesth Analg.* 1995;81:783–792.
120. Prielipp RC, MacGregor DA, Butterworth JF IV, et al. Pharmacodynamics and pharmacokinetics of milrinone administration to increase oxygen delivery in critically ill patients. *Chest.* 1996;109:1291–1301.
121. Kikura M, Lee MK, Safon RA, et al. The effects of milrinone on platelets in patients undergoing cardiac surgery. *Anesth Analg.* 1995;81:44–48.
122. Toller WG, Stranz C. Levosimendan: a new inotropic and vasodilator agent. *Anesthesiology.* 2006;104:556–569.
123. Packer M, Colucci W, Fisher L, et al. Effect of levosimendan on the short-term clinical course of patients with acutely decompensated heart failure. *JACC Heart Fail.* 2013;1:103–111.
124. Toller W, Heringlake M, Guarracino F, et al. Preoperative and perioperative use of levosimendan in cardiac surgery: European expert opinion. *Int J Cardiol.* 2015;184:323–336.
125. Pagel PS. Levosimendan in cardiac surgery: a unique drug for the treatment of perioperative left ventricular dysfunction or just another inodilator searching for a clinical application? *Anesth Analg.* 2007;104:759–761.
126. Mebazaa A, Nieminen MS, Packer M, et al. Levosimendan vs dobutamine for patients with acute decompensated heart failure: the SURVIVE Randomized Trial. *JAMA.* 2007;297:1883–1891.
127. Altenberger J, Parissis JT, Costard-Jaeckle A, et al. Efficacy and safety of pulsed infusions of levosimendan in outpatients with advanced heart failure (LevoReP) study: a multicentre randomized trial. *Eur J Heart Fail.* 2014;16:898–906.
128. Papp Z, Edes I, Fruhwald S, et al. Levosimendan: molecular mechanisms and clinical implications: consensus of experts on the mechanisms of action of levosimendan. *Int J Cardiol.* 2012;159:82–87.
129. Sonntag S, Sundberg S, Lehtonen LA, et al. The calcium sensitizer levosimendan improves the function of stunned myocardium after percutaneous transluminal coronary angioplasty in acute myocardial ischemia. *J Am Coll Cardiol.* 2004;43:2177–2182.

130. Kersten JR, Montgomery MW, Pagel PS, et al. Levosimendan, a positive inotropic agent, decreases myocardial infarct size via activation of K_{ATP} channels. *Anesth Analg*. 2000;90:5–11.
131. De Hert SG, Lorsomradee S, Cromheecke S, et al. The effects of levosimendan in cardiac surgery patients with poor left ventricular function. *Anesth Analg*. 2007;104:766–773.
132. Kivikko M, Lehtonen L, Colucci WS. Sustained hemodynamic effects of intravenous levosimendan. *Circulation*. 2003;107:81–86.
133. Armstrong PW, Moe GW. Medical advances in the treatment of congestive heart failure. *Circulation*. 1993;88:2941–2952.
134. Hauptman PJ, Kelly RA. Digitalis. *Circulation*. 1999;99:1265–1270.
135. The Digitalis Investigation Group. The effect of digoxin on mortality and morbidity in patients with heart failure. *N Engl J Med*. 1997;336:525–533.
136. Treschan TA, Peters J. The vasopressin system: physiology and clinical strategies. *Anesthesiology*. 2006;105:599–612.
137. Schwartz A. Molecular and cellular aspects of calcium channel antagonism. *Am J Cardiol*. 1992;70:6F–8F.
138. Gibbons RJ, Abrams J, Chatterjee K, et al. ACC/AHA guideline update for the management of patients with chronic stable angina–summary article: a report of the American College of Cardiology/American Heart Association Task Force on Practice Guidelines (Committee on the Management of Patients With Chronic Stable Angina). *Circulation*. 2003;107:149–158.
139. Yeghiazarians Y, Braunstein JB, Askari A, et al. Unstable angina pectoris. *N Engl J Med*. 2000;342:101–114.
140. Opie LH, Yusuf S, Kubler W. Current status of safety and efficacy of calcium channel blockers in cardiovascular diseases: A critical analysis based on 100 studies. *Prog Cardiovasc Dis*. 2000;43:171–196.
141. Thompson AE, Pope JE. Calcium channel blockers for primary Raynaud's phenomenon: a meta-analysis. *Rheumatology*. 2005;44:145–150.
142. Kenyon KW. Clevidipine: an ultra short-acting calcium channel antagonist for acute hypertension. *Ann Pharmacother*. 2009;43:1258–1265.
143. Keating GM. Clevidipine: a review of its use for managing blood pressure in perioperative and intensive care settings. *Drugs*. 2014;74:1947–1960.
144. Peacock WF, Chandra A, Char D, et al. Clevidipine in acute heart failure: Results of the A Study of Blood Pressure Control in Acute Heart Failure-A Pilot Study (PRONTO). *Am Heart J*. 2014;167:529–536.
145. Aronson S, Dyke CM, Stierer KA, et al. The ECLIPSE trial: comparative studies of clevidipine to nitroglycerin, sodium nitroprusside, and nicardipine for acute hypertension treatment in cardiac surgery patients. *Anesth Analg*. 2008;107:1110–1121.
146. Lord MS, Augoustides JG. Perioperative management of pheochromocytoma: focus on magnesium, clevidipine, and vasopressin. *J Cardiothorac Vasc Anesth*. 2012;26:526–531.
147. Graffagnino C, Bergese S, Love J, et al. Clevidipine rapidly and safely reduces blood pressure in acute intracerebral hemorrhage: the ACCELERATE trial. *Cerebrovasc Dis*. 2013;36:173–180.
148. Tobias JD, Hoernschemeyer DG. Clevidipine for controlled hypotension during spinal surgery in adolescents. *J Neurosurg Anesthesiol*. 2011;23:347–351.
149. Mocco J, Zacharia BE, Komotar RJ, et al. A review of current and future medical therapies for cerebral vasospasm following aneurysmal subarachnoid hemorrhage. *Neurosurg Focus*. 2006;21:E9.
150. Adamcyzk P, He S, Amar AP, et al. Medical management of cerebral vasospasm following aneurysmal subarachnoid hemorrhage: a review of current and emerging therapeutic interventions. *Neurol Res Int*. 2013;2013:462–491.
151. Pickard JD, Murray GD, Illingworth R, et al. Effect of oral nimodipine on cerebral infarction and outcome after subarachnoid haemorrhage: British aneurysm nimodipine trial. *BMJ*. 1989;298:636–642.
152. Liu GJ, Luo J, Zhang LP, et al. Meta-analysis of the effectiveness and safety of prophylactic use of nimodipine in patients with aneurysmal subarachnoid hemorrhage. *CNS Neurol Disord Drug Targets*. 2011;10:834–844.
153. Feigin VL, Rinkel GJ, Algra A, et al. Calcium antagonists in patients with aneurysmal subarachnoid hemorrhage: a systematic review. *Neurology*. 1998;50:876–883.
154. Grossman E, Messerli FH. Calcium antagonists. *Prog Cardiovasc Dis*. 2004;47:34–57.
155. Claas SA, Glasser SP. Long-acting diltiazem HCl for chronotherapeutic treatment of hypertension and chronic stable angina pectoris. *Expert Opin Pharmacother*. 2005;6:765–776.
156. Wattanasuwan N, Khan IA, Mehta NJ, et al. Acute ventricular rate control in atrial fibrillation: IV combination of diltiazem and digoxin vs. IV diltiazem alone. *Chest*. 2001;119:502–506.
157. Lim SH, Anantharaman V, Teo WS, et al. Slow infusion of calcium channel blockers compared with intravenous adenosine in the emergency treatment of supraventricular tachycardia. *Resuscitation*. 2009;80:523–528.
158. Link MS, Berkow LC, Kudenchuk PJ, et al. Part 7: Adult Advanced Cardiovascular Life Support. 2015 American Heart Association Guidelines Update for Cardiopulmonary Resuscitation and Emergency Cardiovascular Care. *Circulation*. 2015;132(18 Suppl 2):S444–S464.
159. Eisenberg MJ, Brox A, Bestawros AN. Calcium channel blockers: an update. *Am J Med*. 2004;116:35–43.
160. Cohen MI, Triedman JK, Cannon BC, et al. PACES/HRS expert consensus statement on the management of the asymptomatic young patient with Wolff-Parkinson-White (WPW, ventricular preexcitation) electrocardiographic pattern: developed in partnership between the Pediatric and Congenital Electrophysiology Society (PACES) and the Heart Rhythm Society (HRS). Endorsed by the governing bodies of PACES, HRS, the American College of Cardiology Foundation (ACCF), the American Heart Association (AHA), the American Academy of Pediatrics (AAP), and the Canadian Heart Rhythm Society (CHRS). *Heart Rhythm*. 2012;9:1006–1024.
161. Wijeysundera DN, Beattie WS. Calcium channel blockers for reducing cardiac morbidity after noncardiac surgery: a meta-analysis. *Anesth Analg*. 2003;97:634–641.
162. Wijeysundera DN, Beattie WS, Rao V, et al. Calcium antagonists reduce cardiovascular complications after cardiac surgery: a meta-analysis. *J Am Coll Cardiol*. 2003;41:1496–1505.
163. Redfearn DP, Krahn AD, Skanes AC, et al. Use of medications in Wolff-Parkinson-White syndrome. *Expert Opin Pharmacother*. 2005;6:955–963.
164. Arroyo AM, Kao LW. Calcium channel blocker toxicity. *Pediatr Emerg Care*. 2009;25:532–538.
165. Mehta PK, Griendling KK. Angiotensin II cell signaling: Physiological and pathological effects in the cardiovascular system. *Am J Physiol Cell Physiol*. 2007;292:C82–C97.
166. ACE Inhibitor Myocardial Infarction Collaborative Group. Indications for ACE inhibitors in the early treatment of acute myocardial infarction: systematic review of individual data from 100,000 patients in randomized trials. *Circulation*. 1998;97:2202–2212.
167. Heart Outcomes Prevention Study Investigators. Effects of an angiotensin-converting enzyme inhibitor ramipril on cardiovascular events in high-risk patients. The Heart Outcomes Prevention Evaluation Study Investigators. *N Engl J Med*. 2000;342:145–153.
168. Ruggenenti P, Cravedi P, Remuzzi G. The RAAS in the pathogenesis and treatment of diabetic nephropathy. *Nat Rev Nephrol*. 2010;6:319–330.
169. Warner NJ, Rush JE. Safety profiles of angiotensin-converting enzyme inhibitors. *Drugs*. 1988;35(Suppl 5):89–97.
170. Brown NJ, Ray WA, Snowden M, et al. Black Americans have an increased rate of angiotensin converting enzyme inhibitor-associated angioedema. *Clin Pharmacol Ther*. 1996;60:8–13.
171. Kheterpal S, Khodaparast O, et al. Chronic angiotensin-converting enzyme inhibitor or angiotensin receptor blocker therapy combined with diuretic therapy is associated with increased episodes of hypotension during noncardiac surgery. *J Cardiothorac Vasc Anesth*. 2008;22:180–186.
172. Lange M, Van Aken H, Westphal M, et al. Role of vasopressinergic V1 receptor agonists in the treatment of perioperative catecholamine-refractory arterial hypotension. *Best Pract Res Clin Anaesthesiol*. 2008;22:369–381.
173. Boccara G, Ouwattara A, Godet G, et al. Terlipressin versus norepinephrine to correct refractory arterial hypotension after general anesthesia in patients chronically treated with renin-angiotensin system inhibitors. *Anesthesiology*. 2003;98:1338–1344.
174. Morelli A, Tritapepe L, Rocco M, et al. Terlipressin versus norepinephrine to counteract anesthesia-induced hypotension in patients treated with renin-angiotensin system inhibitors: effects on systemic and regional hemodynamics. *Anesthesiology*. 2005;102:12–19.
175. Csajka C, Buslin T, Brunner HR, et al. Pharmacokinetic-pharmacodynamic profile of angiotensin II receptor antagonists. *Clin Pharmacokinet*. 1997;32:1–29.
176. Maggioni AP, Anand I, Gottlieb SO, et al. Effect of valsartan on morbidity and mortality in patients with heart failure not receiving angiotensin-converting enzyme inhibitors. *J Am Coll Cardiol*. 2002;40:1414–1421.
177. Pfeffer MA, McMurray JJ, Velazquez EJ, et al. Valsartan, captopril, or both in myocardial infarction complicated by heart failure, left ventricular dysfunction, or both. *N Engl J Med*. 2003;349:1893–1906.
178. McMurray JJ, Ostergren J, Swedberg K, et al. Effects of candesartan in patients with chronic heart failure and reduced left ventricular systolic function taking angiotensin-converting-enzyme inhibitors: the CHARM-Added Trial. *Lancet*. 2003;362:767–771.
179. Viberti G, Wheeldon NM, MicroAlbuminuria Reduction with VALsartan (MARVAL) Study Investigators. Microalbuminuria reduction with valsartan in patients with type 2 diabetes mellitus: a blood pressure-independent effect. *Circulation*. 2002;106:672–678.

14 Autonomic Nervous System Anatomy and Physiology

LORETA GRECU

Anesthesia and the Autonomic Nervous System
Functional Anatomy
    Central Autonomic Organization
    Peripheral Autonomic Nervous System Organization
Receptors
    Cholinergic Receptors
    Adrenergic Receptors
Autonomic Nervous System Reflexes and Interactions
    Baroreceptors
    Denervated Heart
    Interaction of Autonomic Nervous System Receptors
    Interaction with Other Regulatory Systems

Clinical Autonomic Nervous System Pharmacology*
    Mode of Action
    Ganglionic Drugs
    Cholinergic Drugs
Autonomic Syndromes and Autonomic Regulation
    Horner Syndrome
    Diabetic Neuropathy
    Orthostatic Hypotension
    Monoamine Oxidase Inhibitors
    Tricyclic Antidepressants
    Selective Serotonin Reuptake Inhibitors

KEY POINTS

1. The autonomic nervous system (ANS) includes that part of the central and peripheral nervous system concerned with involuntary regulation of cardiac muscle, smooth muscle, glandular and visceral functions.
2. The sympathetic and parasympathetic nervous systems (SNS, PNS) affect cardiac pump function in three ways: (1) by changing the rate (chronotropism), (2) by changing the strength of contraction (inotropism), and (3) by modulating coronary blood flow.
3. SNS nerves are by far the most important regulators of the peripheral circulation.
4. The ANS can be pharmacologically subdivided by the neurotransmitter secreted at the effector cell: Acetylcholine (ACh) released by the PNS, and the catecholamines epinephrine (EPI) and norepinephrine (NE), which are the mediators of peripheral SNS activity.
5. An agonist is a substance that interacts with a receptor to evoke a biologic response. An antagonist is a substance that interferes with the triggering of the response at a receptor site by an agonist.
6. The adrenergic receptors are termed adrenergic or noradrenergic, depending on their responsiveness to EPI and NE.
7. The numbers and sensitivity of adrenergic receptors can be influenced by normal, genetic, and developmental factors.
8. The ANS reflex comprises (1) sensors, (2) afferent pathways, (3) CNS integration, and (4) efferent pathways to the receptors and efferent organs.
9. The clinical application of ANS pharmacology is based on the knowledge of ANS anatomy, physiology, and molecular pharmacology.
10. Clinically, anticholinesterase drugs may be divided into two types: the reversible and nonreversible cholinesterase inhibitors.

Anesthesia and the Autonomic Nervous System

Anesthesiology is the practice of autonomic medicine. Drugs that produce anesthesia may also have potent autonomic side effects. The greater part of our training and practice is spent acquiring skills in utilizing or averting the autonomic nervous system (ANS) side effects of anesthetic drugs under a variety of pathophysiologic conditions. The success of any anesthetic depends upon how well homeostasis is maintained. The anesthetic record reflects ANS function.

The ANS includes that part of the central and peripheral nervous system concerned with involuntary regulation of cardiac muscle, smooth muscle, and glandular and visceral functions. ANS activity refers to visceral reflexes that function below the conscious level. The ANS is also responsive to changes in somatic motor and sensory activities of the body. The physiologic evidence of visceral reflexes as a result of somatic events is abundantly clear. The ANS is therefore not as distinct an entity as the term suggests. Neither somatic nor ANS activity occurs in isolation.[1] The ANS organizes visceral support for somatic behavior and adjusts body states in anticipation of emotional behavior or responses to the stress of disease. In brief, it organizes fight or flight responses.

Afferent fibers from visceral structures are the first link in the reflex arcs of the ANS, and may relay visceral pain or changes in vessel stretch. Most ANS efferent fibers are accompanied by sensory fibers that are now commonly recognized as components of the ANS. However, the afferent components of the ANS cannot be as distinctively divided as can the efferent nerves. ANS visceral sensory nerves are anatomically indistinguishable from somatic sensory nerves. The clinical importance

---

*See Chapter 59 for additional information regarding the sympathomimetic, adrenergic antagonists and sympatholytic drugs.

of visceral afferent fibers is closely implicated in the management of chronic pain states.

Functional Anatomy

The ANS is organized into two divisions based on anatomy, physiology, and pharmacology. Langley divided this nervous system into two parts in 1921. He retained the term *sympathetic* (sympathetic nervous system [SNS]) introduced by Willis in 1665 for the first part, and introduced the term "parasympathetic" (parasympathetic nervous system [PNS]) for the second. The term ANS was adopted as a comprehensive name for both. Table 14-1 lists the complementary effects of SNS (adrenergic, sympathetic) and PNS (cholinergic, parasympathetic) activity of organ systems.

Central Autonomic Organization

Pure central ANS versus somatic centers are not known. Integration of ANS activity occurs at all levels of the cerebrospinal axis. Efferent ANS activity can be initiated locally and by centers located in the spinal cord, brainstem, and hypothalamus. The cerebral cortex is the highest level of ANS integration. Fainting at the sight of blood is an example of this higher level of somatic and ANS integration. ANS function has also been successfully modulated through conscious, intentional efforts demonstrating that somatic responses are always accompanied by visceral responses and vice versa.

The principal site of ANS organization is the *hypothalamus*. SNS functions are controlled by nuclei in the posterolateral hypothalamus. Stimulation of these nuclei results in a massive discharge of the sympathoadrenal system. PNS functions are

Table 14-1 Homeostatic Balance between Adrenergic and Cholinergic Effects

Organ System	Response	
	Adrenergic	*Cholinergic*
Heart		
Sinoatrial node	Tachycardia	Bradycardia
Atrioventricular node	Increased conduction	Decreased conduction
His-Purkinje	Increased automaticity and conduction velocity	Minimal
Myocardium	Increased contractility, conduction velocity, automaticity	Minimal decrease in contractility
Coronary vessels	Constriction (α_1) and dilation (β_1)	Dilation and constriction[a]
Blood Vessels		
Skin and mucosa	Constriction	Dilation
Skeletal muscle	Constriction (α_1) > dilation (β_2)	Dilation
Pulmonary	Constriction	Dilation
Bronchial Smooth Muscle	Relaxation	Contraction
Gastrointestinal Tract		
Gallbladder and ducts	Relaxation	Contraction
Gut motility	Decreased	Increased
Secretions	Decreased	Increased
Sphincters	Constriction	Relaxation
Bladder		
Detrusor	Relaxation	Contraction
Trigone	Constriction	Relaxation
Glands		
Nasal	Vasoconstriction and reduced secretion	Stimulation of secretions
Lacrimal		
Parotid		
Submandibular		
Gastric		
Pancreatic		
Sweat Glands	Diaphoresis (cholinergic)	None
Apocrine Glands	Thick, odiferous secretion	None
Eye		
Pupil	Mydriasis	Miosis
Ciliary muscle	Relaxation for far vision	Contraction for near vision

[a]See "Interaction of Autonomic Nervous System Receptors."

governed by nuclei in the midline and some anterior nuclei of the hypothalamus. The anterior hypothalamus is involved with regulation of temperature. The supraoptic hypothalamic nuclei regulate water metabolism and are anatomically and functionally associated with the posterior lobe of the pituitary (see Interaction of Autonomic Nervous System Receptors). This hypothalamic–neurohypophyseal connection represents a central ANS mechanism that affects the kidney by means of antidiuretic hormone (ADH). Long-term blood pressure control, reactions to physical and emotional stress, sleep, and sexual reflexes are regulated by the hypothalamus.

The *medulla oblongata* and *pons* are vital centers of acute ANS organization. Together, they integrate momentary hemodynamic adjustments and maintain the sequence and automaticity of ventilation. Integration of afferent and efferent ANS impulses at this central nervous system (CNS) level is responsible for the tonic activity exhibited by the ANS. Tonicity holds visceral organs in a state of intermediate activity that can be either diminished or augmented by altering the rate of nerve firing. The nucleus tractus solitarius, located within the medulla, is the primary area for relay of afferent chemoreceptor and baroreceptor information from the glossopharyngeal and vagus nerves. Increased afferent impulses from these two nerves inhibit peripheral SNS vascular tone, producing vasodilation; it also increases vagal tone, producing bradycardia. Studies of patients with high spinal cord lesions show that a number of reflex changes are mediated at the spinal or segmental level. ANS hyperreflexia is an example of spinal cord mediation of ANS reflexes without integration of function from higher inhibitory centers.[1]

Peripheral Autonomic Nervous System Organization

The peripheral ANS is the efferent (motor) component of the ANS and consists of the same two complementary parts: The SNS and the PNS. Most organs receive fibers from both divisions (Fig. 14-1). In general, activities of the two systems produce opposite but complementary effects (Table 14-1). A few tissues, such as sweat glands and spleen, are innervated by only SNS fibers. Although the anatomy of the somatic and ANS sensory pathways is identical, the motor pathways are characteristically different. The efferent somatic motor system, like somatic afferents, is composed of a single (unipolar) neuron with its cell body in the ventral gray matter of the spinal cord. Its myelinated axon extends directly to the voluntary striated muscle unit. In contrast, the efferent (motor) ANS is a two-neuron (bipolar) chain

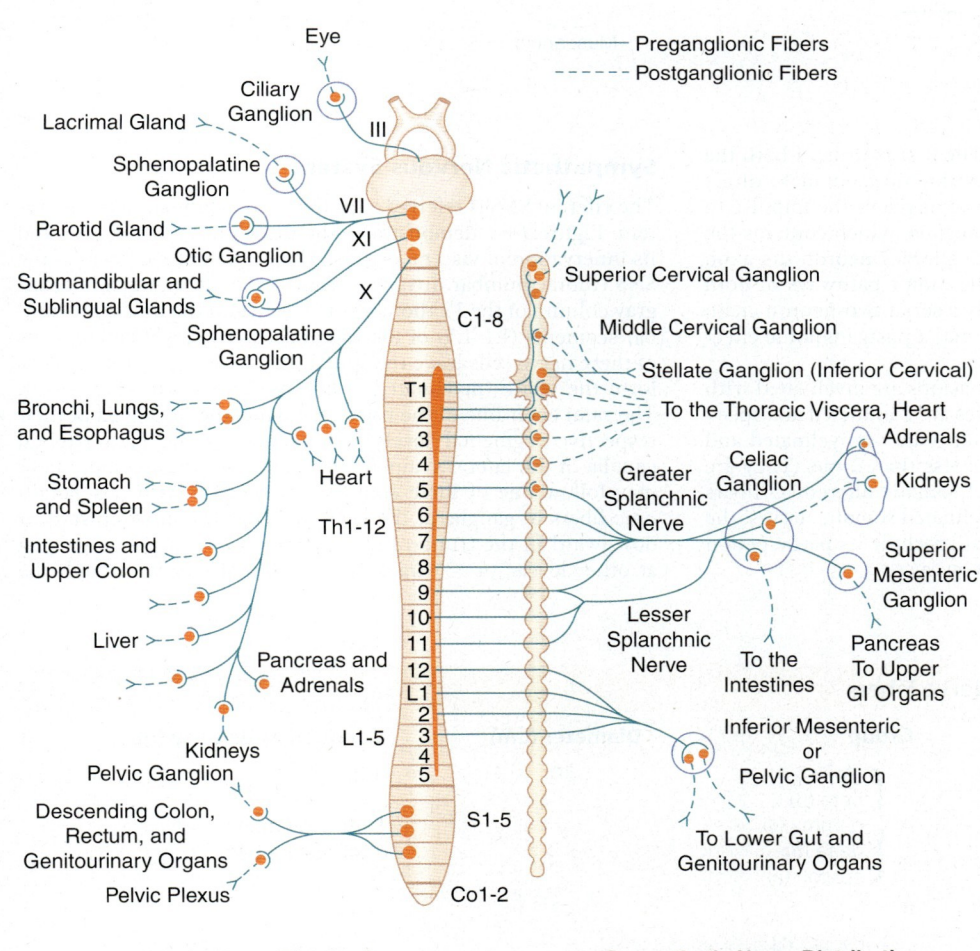

Figure 14-1 Schematic distribution of the craniosacral (parasympathetic) and thoracolumbar (sympathetic) nervous systems. Parasympathetic preganglionic fibers pass directly to the organ that is innervated. Their postganglionic cell bodies are situated near or within the innervated viscera. This limited distribution of parasympathetic postganglionic fibers is consistent with the discrete and limited effect of parasympathetic function. The postganglionic sympathetic neurons originate in either the paired sympathetic ganglia or one of the unpaired collateral plexuses. One preganglionic fiber influences many postganglionic neurons. Activation of the SNS produces a more diffuse physiologic response rather than a discrete, localized effect. GI, gastrointestinal.

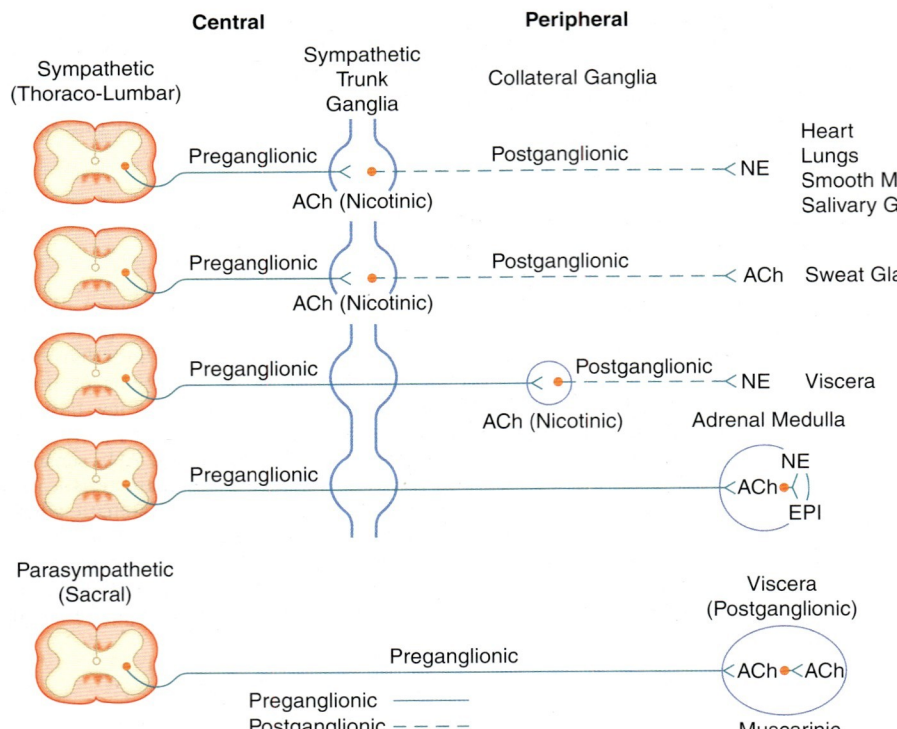

Figure 14-2 Schematic diagram of the efferent ANS. Efferent impulses are integrated centrally and sent reflexly to the adrenergic and cholinergic receptors. Sympathetic fibers ending in the adrenal medulla are preganglionic, and acetylcholine (ACh) is the neurotransmitter. Stimulation of the chromaffin cells, acting as postganglionic neurons, releases epinephrine (EPI) and norepinephrine (NE).

from the CNS to the effector organ. The first neuron of both the SNS and PNS originates within the CNS but does not make direct contact with the effector organ. Instead, it relays the impulse to a second station known as an *ANS ganglion*, which contains the cell body of the second ANS (postganglionic) neuron. Its axon contacts the effector organ. Thus, the motor pathways of both divisions of the ANS are schematically a serial two-neuron chain consisting of a preganglionic neuron and a postganglionic effector neuron (Fig. 14-2).

Preganglionic fibers of both subdivisions are myelinated with diameters of less than 3 mm.[1] Impulses are conducted at a speed of 3 to 15 m/s. The postganglionic fibers are unmyelinated and conduct impulses at slower speeds of less than 2 m/s. They are similar to unmyelinated visceral and somatic afferent C fibers (Table 14-2). Compared with the myelinated somatic nerves, the ANS conducts impulses at speeds that preclude its participation in the immediate phase of a somatic response.

Sympathetic Nervous System

The efferent SNS is referred to as the thoracolumbar nervous system. Figure 14-1 demonstrates the distribution of the SNS and its innervation of visceral organs. The preganglionic fibers of the SNS (thoracolumbar division) originate in the intermediolateral gray column of the 12 thoracic (T1–T12) and the first three lumbar segments (L1–L3) of the spinal cord. The myelinated axons of these nerve cells leave the spinal cord with the motor fibers to form the white (myelinated) communicating rami (Fig. 14-3). The rami enter one of the paired 22 sympathetic ganglia at their respective segmental levels. Upon entering the paravertebral ganglia of the lateral sympathetic chain, the preganglionic fiber may follow one of three courses: (1) synapse with postganglionic fibers in ganglia at the level of exit, (2) course upward or downward in the trunk of the SNS chain to synapse in ganglia at other levels, or (3) track for variable distances through the

Table 14-2 Classification of Nerve Fibers

Description of Nerve Fibers	Group		Diameter (μm)	Conduction Velocity (m/s)
Myelinated somatic	A	alpha (α)	20	120
		beta (β)		
		gamma (γ)		5–40 (pain fibers)
		delta (δ)	3–4	5–40 (pain fibers)
		epsilon (ε)	2	5
Myelinated visceral (preganglionic autonomic)	B		<3	3–15
Unmyelinated somatic	C		<2	0.5–2.0 (pain fibers)

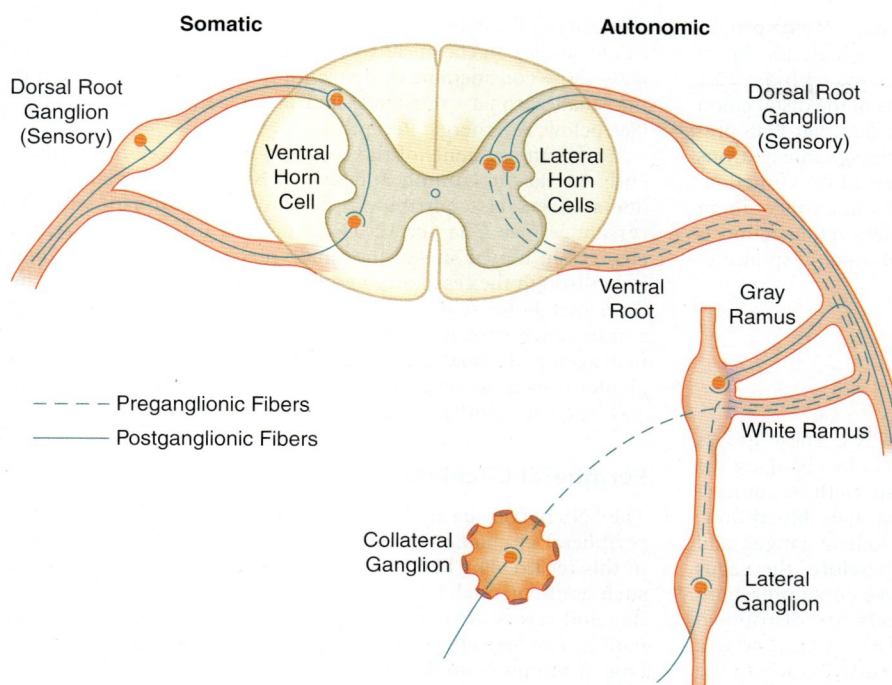

Figure 14-3 The spinal reflex arc of the somatic nerves is shown on the left. The different arrangements of neurons in the sympathetic system are shown on the right. Preganglionic fibers coming out through white rami may make synaptic connections following one of three courses: (1) synapse in ganglia at the level of exit, (2) course up or down the sympathetic chain to synapse at another level, or (3) exit the chain without synapsing to an outlying collateral ganglion.

sympathetic chain and exit without synapsing to terminate in an outlying, unpaired, SNS collateral ganglion. The adrenal gland is an exception to the rule. Preganglionic fibers pass directly into the adrenal medulla without synapsing in a ganglion (Fig. 14-2). The cells of the medulla are derived from neuronal tissue and are analogous to postganglionic neurons.

The sympathetic postganglionic neuronal cell bodies are located in ganglia of the paired lateral SNS chain or unpaired collateral ganglia in more peripheral plexuses. Collateral ganglia, such as the celiac and inferior mesenteric ganglia (plexus), are formed by the convergence of preganglionic fibers with many postganglionic neuronal bodies. SNS ganglia are almost always located closer to the spinal cord than to the organs they innervate. The sympathetic postganglionic neurons can therefore originate in either the paired lateral paravertebral SNS ganglia or one of the unpaired collateral plexuses. The unmyelinated postganglionic fibers then proceed from the ganglia to terminate within the organs they innervate. Many of the postganglionic fibers pass from the lateral SNS chain back into the spinal nerves, forming the gray (unmyelinated) communicating rami at all levels of the spinal cord (Fig. 14-2). They are distributed distally to sweat glands, pilomotor muscle, and blood vessels of the skin and muscle. These nerves are unmyelinated C type fibers (Table 14-2) and are carried within the somatic nerves. Approximately 8% of the fibers in the average somatic nerve are sympathetic.

The first four or five thoracic spinal segments generate preganglionic fibers that ascend in the neck to form three special paired ganglia. These are the superior cervical, middle cervical, and cervicothoracic ganglia. The last is known as the stellate ganglion and is actually formed by the fusion of the inferior cervical and first thoracic SNS ganglia. These ganglia provide sympathetic innervation of the head, neck, upper extremities, heart, and lungs. Afferent pain fibers also travel with these nerves, accounting for chest, neck, or upper extremity pain with myocardial ischemia.

Activation of the SNS produces a diffuse physiologic response (mass reflex) rather than discrete effects. SNS postganglionic neurons outnumber the preganglionic neurons in an average ratio of 20:1 to 30:1.[2] One preganglionic fiber influences a larger number of postganglionic neurons, which are dispersed to many organs.

Parasympathetic Nervous System

The PNS, like the SNS, has both preganglionic and postganglionic neurons. The preganglionic cell bodies originate in the brainstem and sacral segments of the spinal cord. PNS preganglionic fibers are found in cranial nerves III (oculomotor), VII (facial), IX (glossopharyngeal), and X (vagus). The sacral outflow originates in the intermediolateral gray horns of the second, third, and fourth sacral nerves. Figure 14-1 shows the distribution of the PNS division and its innervation of visceral organs.

The vagus (cranial nerve X) nerve has the most extensive distribution of all the PNS, accounting for more than 75% of PNS activity. The paired vagus nerves supply PNS innervation to the heart, lungs, esophagus, stomach, small intestine, proximal half of the colon, liver, gallbladder, pancreas, and upper portions of the ureters. The sacral fibers form the pelvic visceral nerves, or nervi erigentes. These nerves supply the remainder of the viscera that are not innervated by the vagus. They supply the descending colon, rectum, uterus, bladder, and lower portions of the ureters and are primarily concerned with emptying. Various sexual reactions are also governed by the sacral PNS. The PNS is responsible for penile erection, but SNS stimulation governs ejaculation.

In contrast to the SNS division, PNS preganglionic fibers pass directly to the organ that is innervated. The postganglionic cell bodies are situated near or within the innervated viscera and generally are not visible. The proximity of PNS ganglia to or within the viscera provides a limited distribution of postganglionic fibers. The ratio of postganglionic to preganglionic fibers in many organs appears to be 1:1 to 3:1 compared with the 20:1 found in the SNS system. The Auerbach plexus in the distal colon is the exception, with a ratio of 8,000:1. The fact that PNS preganglionic fibers synapse with only a few postganglionic neurons is consistent with the discrete and limited effect of PNS function. For example, vagal bradycardia can occur without a concomitant change in intestinal motility or salivation. Mass reflex action is not a characteristic of the PNS. The effects of organ response to PNS stimulation are outlined in Table 14-1.

Autonomic Innervation

Heart

The heart is well supplied by the SNS and PNS. These nerves affect cardiac pump function in three ways: (1) by changing the rate (chronotropism), (2) by changing the strength of contraction (inotropism), and (3) by modulating coronary blood flow. The PNS cardiac vagal fibers approach the stellate ganglia and then join the efferent cardiac SNS fibers; therefore, the vagus nerve to the heart and lungs is a mixed nerve containing both PNS and SNS efferent fibers. The PNS fibers are distributed mainly to the sinoatrial and atrioventricular (AV) nodes and to a lesser extent to the atria. There is little or no distribution to the ventricles. Therefore, the main effect of vagal cardiac stimulation to the heart is chronotropic. Vagal stimulation decreases the rate of sinoatrial node discharge and decreases excitability of the AV junctional fibers, slowing impulse conduction to the ventricles. A strong vagal discharge can completely arrest sinoatrial node firing and block impulse conduction to the ventricles.[3]

The physiologic importance of the PNS on myocardial contractility is not as well understood as that of the SNS. Cholinergic blockade can double the heart rate (HR) without altering contractility of the left ventricle. Vagal stimulation of the heart can reduce left ventricular maximum rate of tension development (dP/dT) and decrease contractile force by as much as 10% to 20%. However, PNS stimulation is relatively unimportant in this regard compared with its predominant effect on HR. The SNS has the same supraventricular distribution as the PNS, but with stronger representation to the ventricles. SNS efferents to the myocardium funnel through the paired stellate ganglia. The right stellate ganglion distributes primarily to the anterior epicardial surface and the interventricular septum. Right stellate stimulation decreases systolic duration and increases HR. The left stellate ganglion supplies the posterior and lateral surfaces of both ventricles. Left stellate stimulation increases mean arterial pressure and left ventricular contractility without causing a substantial change in HR. Normal SNS tone maintains contractility approximately 20% above that in the absence of any SNS stimulation.[4] Therefore, the dominant effect of the ANS on myocardial contractility is mediated primarily through the SNS. Intrinsic mechanisms of the myocardium, however, can maintain circulation quite well without the ANS, as evidenced by the success of cardiac transplants (see Chapter 51). The heart and ANS are in perfect symbiosis. ANS via its components imprints the cardiac electrophysiology by potentially inducing significant dysrhythmias or electrocardiographic abnormalities, which in the end may lead to global cardiac dysfunction. The precise role of the ANS is unknown, specifically if it is an active component or just an accompaniment. Future research interests concern the modification of the autonomic cardiac innervation through pharmacology or using alternative approaches.[5] Early investigations, performed in anesthetized, open-chest animals, demonstrated that cardiac ANS nerves exert only slight effects on the coronary vascular bed; however, more recent studies on chronically instrumented, intact, conscious animals show considerable evidence for a strong SNS regulation of the small coronary resistance and larger conductance vessels[6,7] (see below, Adrenergic Receptors).

Different segments of the coronary arterial tree react differently to various stimuli and drugs. Normally, the large conductance vessels contribute little to overall coronary vascular resistance (see Chapter 12). Fluctuations in resistance reflect changes in lumen size of the small, precapillary vessels. Blood flow through the resistance vessels is regulated primarily by the local metabolic requirements of the myocardium. The larger conductance vessels, however, can constrict markedly due to neurogenic stimulation. Neurogenic influence also assumes a greater role in the resistance vessels when they become hypoxic and lose autoregulation.

Peripheral Circulation

The SNS nerves are by far the most important regulators of the peripheral circulation. The PNS nerves play only a minor role in this regard. The PNS dilates vessels, but only in limited areas such as the genitalia. SNS stimulation produces both vasodilation and vasoconstriction, with vasoconstrictor effects predominating. The SNS effect on the vascular bed is determined by the type of receptors on which the SNS fiber terminates (see below, Adrenergic Receptors). SNS constrictor receptors are distributed to all segments of the circulation. Blood vessels in the skin, kidneys, spleen, and mesentery have an extensive SNS distribution, whereas those in the heart, brain, and muscle have less SNS innervation.

Basal vasomotor tone is maintained by impulses from the lateral portion of the vasomotor center in the medulla oblongata that continually transmits impulses through the SNS, maintaining partial arteriolar and venular constriction. Circulating epinephrine (EPI) from the adrenal medulla has additive effects. This basal ANS tone maintains arteriolar constriction at an intermediate diameter. The arteriole, therefore, has the potential for either further constriction or dilation. If the basal tones were not present, the SNS could only affect vasoconstriction and not vasodilation.[8] The SNS tone in the venules produces little resistance to flow compared with the arterioles and the arteries. The importance of SNS stimulation of veins is to reduce or increase their capacity. By functioning as a reservoir for approximately 80% of the total blood volume, small changes in venous capacitance produce large changes in venous return and, thus, cardiac preload.

Lungs

The lungs are innervated by both the SNS and PNS. Postganglionic SNS fibers from the upper thoracic ganglia (stellate) pass to the lungs to innervate the smooth muscles of the bronchi and pulmonary blood vessels. PNS innervation of these structures is via the vagus nerve. SNS stimulation produces bronchodilation and pulmonary vasoconstriction.[9] Little else has been proven conclusively about the vasomotor control of the pulmonary vessels other than that they adjust to accommodate the output of the right ventricle. The effect of stimulation of the pulmonary SNS nerves on pulmonary vascular resistance is not ideal but may be important in maintaining hemodynamic stability during stress and exercise by balancing right and left ventricular output. Stimulation of the vagus nerve produces almost no vasodilation of the pulmonary circulation. Hypoxic pulmonary vasoconstriction is a local phenomenon capable of providing a faster adjustment to the requirements of the organism.

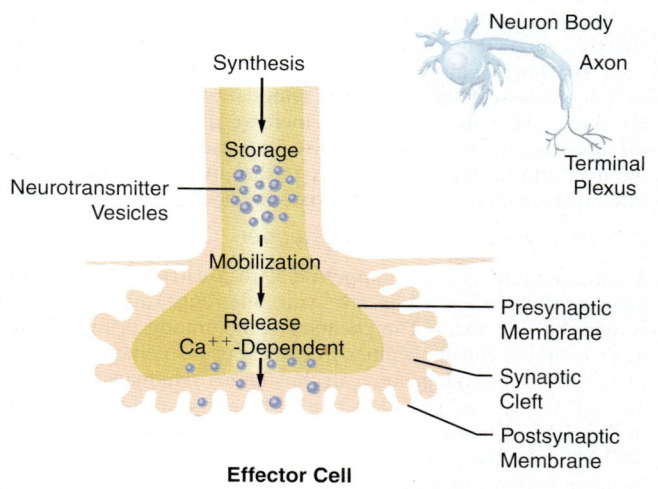

Figure 14-4 The anatomy and physiology of the terminal postganglionic sympathetic and parasympathetic fibers are similar.

the sympathetic postganglionic fibers (see Fig. 14-2). Cotransmission of adenosine triphosphate (ATP), neuropeptide Y (NPY), and NE has been demonstrated at vascular sympathetic nerve terminals in a number of different tissues including muscle, intestine, kidney, and skin. The preganglionic neurons of both systems secrete ACh.

The terminations of the postganglionic fibers of both ANS subdivisions are anatomically and physiologically similar. The terminations are characterized by multiple branching called *terminal effector plexuses* or *reticulae*. These filaments surround the elements of the effector unit "like a mesh stocking."[8] Thus, one SNS postganglionic neuron, for example, can innervate approximately 25,000 effector cells, for example, vascular smooth muscle. The terminal filaments end in presynaptic enlargements called varicosities. Each varicosity contains vesicles, approximately 500 Å in diameter, in which the neurotransmitters are stored (Fig. 14-4). The rate of synthesis depends on the level of ANS activity and is regulated by local feedback. The distance between the varicosity and the effector cell (synaptic or junctional cleft) varies from 100 Å in ganglia and arterioles to as much as 20,000 Å in large arteries. The time for diffusion is directly proportional to the width of the synaptic gap. Depolarization on the nerve releases the vesicular contents into the synaptic cleft by exocytosis.

Both the SNS and the vagus nerve provide active bronchomotor control. SNS stimulation causes bronchodilation, whereas vagal stimulation produces constriction. PNS stimulation may also increase secretions of the bronchial glands. Vagal receptor endings in the alveolar ducts also play an important role in the reflex regulation of the ventilation cycle. The lung has important nonventilatory activity as well. It serves as a metabolic organ that removes local mediators such as norepinephrine (NE) from the circulation and converts others, such as angiotensin 1, to active compounds[10] (see below, Interaction with Other Regulatory Systems).

Autonomic Nervous System Transmission

Transmission of excitation across the terminal junctional sites (synaptic clefts) of the peripheral ANS occurs through the mediation of released chemicals (Fig. 14-4). Transmitters interact with receptors on the end organ to evoke a biologic response.

The ANS can be pharmacologically subdivided by the neurotransmitter secreted at the effector cell. Pharmacologic parlance designates the SNS and PNS as adrenergic and cholinergic, respectively. The terminals of the PNS postganglionic fibers release acetylcholine (ACh). With the exception of sweat glands, NE is the principal neurotransmitter released at the terminals of

Parasympathetic Nervous System Transmission

Synthesis

ACh is considered the primary neurotransmitter of the PNS. ACh is formed in the presynaptic terminal by acetylation of choline with acetyl coenzyme A. This step is catalyzed by choline acetyl transferase (Fig. 14-5). ACh is then stored in a concentrated form in presynaptic vesicles. A continual release of small amounts of ACh, called quanta, occurs during the resting state. Each quantum results in small changes in the electrical potential of the synaptic end plate without producing depolarization. These are known as miniature end-plate potentials. Arrival of an action potential causes a synchronous release of hundreds of quanta, resulting in depolarization of the end plate. Release of ACh from the vesicles is dependent on influx of calcium (Ca^{2+}) from the interstitial space. ACh is not reused like NE; therefore, it must be synthesized constantly.

Metabolism

The ability of a receptor to modulate function of an effector organ is dependent upon rapid recovery to its baseline state after stimulation. For this to occur, the neurotransmitter must be quickly removed from the vicinity of the receptor. ACh removal

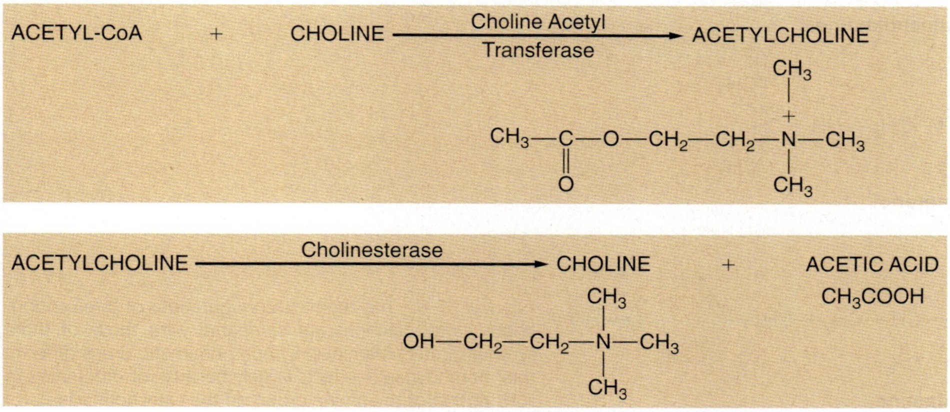

$$ACETYL\text{-}CoA + CHOLINE \xrightarrow{\text{Choline Acetyl Transferase}} ACETYLCHOLINE$$

$$CH_3-\underset{O}{\underset{\|}{C}}-O-CH_2-CH_2-\overset{+}{\underset{CH_3}{\underset{|}{N}}}-CH_3$$

$$ACETYLCHOLINE \xrightarrow{\text{Cholinesterase}} CHOLINE + ACETIC\ ACID\ (CH_3COOH)$$

$$OH-CH_2-CH_2-\underset{CH_3}{\underset{|}{N}}-CH_3$$

Figure 14-5 Synthesis and metabolism of acetylcholine.

occurs by rapid hydrolysis by acetylcholinesterase (Fig. 14-5). This enzyme is found in neurons, at the neuromuscular junction, and in various other tissues of the body. A similar enzyme, pseudocholinesterase or plasma cholinesterase is also found throughout the body but only to a limited extent in neural tissue. It does not appear to be physiologically important in termination of the action of ACh. Both acetylcholinesterase and pseudocholinesterase hydrolyze ACh as well as other esters (such as the ester-type local anesthetics), and they may be distinguished by specific biochemical tests.[3]

Sympathetic Nervous System Transmission

Traditionally, the catecholamines EPI and NE are considered the main mediators of peripheral SNS activity. NE is released from localized presynaptic vesicles of nearly all postganglionic sympathetic nerves. Vascular SNS nerve terminals, however, also release ATP. Thus, ATP and NE are co-neurotransmitters. They are released directly to their site of action. Their postjunctional effects appear to be synergistic in tissues.

The SNS fibers ending in the adrenal medulla are preganglionic, and ACh is the neurotransmitter (Fig. 14-2). It interacts with the chromaffin cells in the adrenal medulla, causing release of EPI and NE. The chromaffin cells take the place of the postganglionic neurons. Stimulation of the sympathetic nerves innervating the adrenal medulla, however, causes the release of large quantities of a mixture of EPI and NE into the circulation. The greater portion of this hormonal surge is normally EPI. EPI and NE, when released into the circulation, are classified as hormones in that they are synthesized, stored, and released from the adrenal medulla to act at distant sites.

Hormonal EPI and NE have essentially the same effects on effector cells as those caused by local direct sympathetic stimulation. The hormonal effects, although brief, last about 10 times as long as those caused by direct stimulation. EPI has a greater metabolic effect than NE. It can increase the metabolic rate of the body as much as 100%. It also increases glycogenolysis in the liver and muscle with glucose release into the blood. These functions are all necessary to prepare the body for fight or flight.

Catecholamines: The First Messenger

A catecholamine is any compound with a catechol nucleus (a benzene ring with two adjacent hydroxyl groups) and an amine-containing side chain. The chemical configuration of five of the more common catecholamines in clinical use is demonstrated in Figure 14-6. The endogenous catecholamines in humans are dopamine (DA), NE, and EPI. Dopamine is a neurotransmitter present in the CNS, primarily involved in coordinating motor activity in the brain. It is the precursor of NE. NE is synthesized and stored in nerve endings of postganglionic SNS neurons. It is also synthesized in the adrenal medulla and is the chemical precursor of EPI. Stored EPI is located chiefly in chromaffin cells of the adrenal medulla. About 80% to 85% of the catecholamine content of the adrenal medulla is EPI and 15% to 20% is NE. The brain contains both noradrenergic and dopaminergic receptors, but circulating catecholamines do not cross the blood–brain barrier. The catecholamines present in the brain are synthesized there.

Catecholamines are often referred to as adrenergic drugs because their effector actions are mediated through receptors specific for the SNS. Sympathomimetics can activate these same receptors because of their structural similarity. For example, clonidine is an α_2-receptor agonist that does not possess a

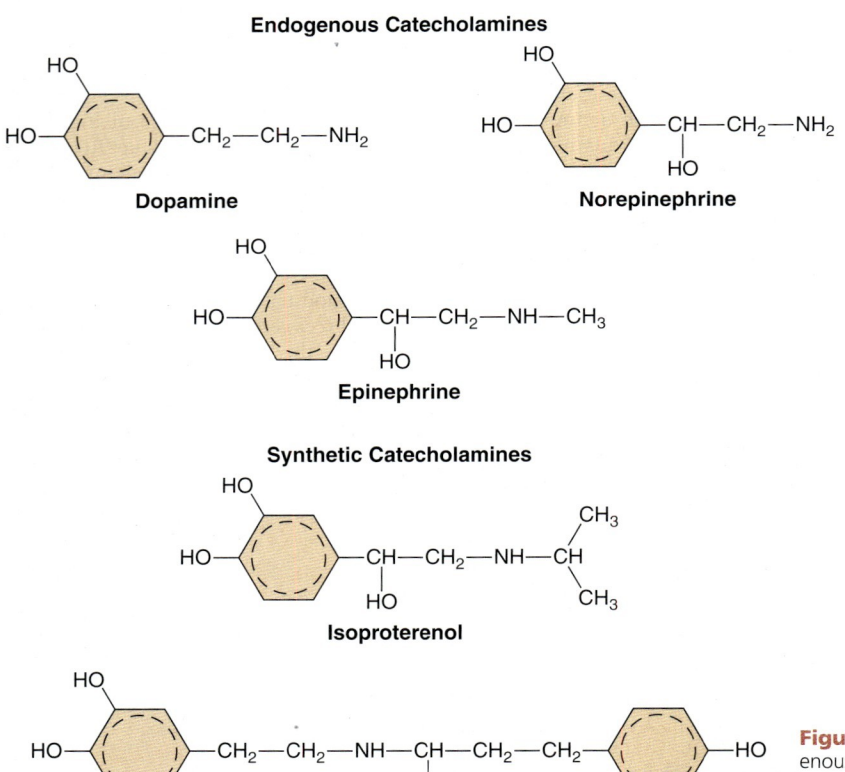

Figure 14-6 The chemical configurations of three endogenous catecholamines are compared with those of three synthetic catecholamines. Sympathomimetic drugs differ in their hemodynamic effects largely because of differences in substitution of the amine group on the catechol nucleus.

catechol nucleus and even has two ring systems that are aplanar to each other. However, clonidine enjoys a remarkable spatial similarity to NE that allows it to activate the α receptor. Drugs that produce sympathetic-like effects but lack basic catecholamine structure are defined as sympathomimetics. All clinically useful catecholamines are sympathomimetics, but not all sympathomimetics are catecholamines. The effects of endogenous or synthetic catecholamines on adrenergic receptors can be direct or indirect. Indirect-acting catecholamines (i.e., ephedrine) have little intrinsic effect on adrenergic receptors but produce their effects by stimulating release of the stored neurotransmitter from SNS nerve terminals. Some synthetic and endogenous catecholamines stimulate adrenergic receptor sites directly (e.g., phenylephrine), whereas others have a mixed mode of action. The actions of direct-acting catecholamines are independent of endogenous NE stores; however, the indirect-acting catecholamines are entirely dependent on adequate neuronal stores of endogenous NE.

Synthesis

The main site of NE synthesis is in or near the postganglionic nerve endings. Some synthesis does occur in vesicles near the cell body that pass to the nerve endings. Phenylalanine or tyrosine is taken up into the axoplasm of the nerve terminal and modified into either NE or EPI. Figure 14-7 demonstrates this synthesis cascade. Tyrosine hydroxylase catalyzes the conversion of tyrosine to dihydroxyphenylalanine. This is the rate-limiting step at which NE synthesis is controlled through feedback inhibition. Dopamine

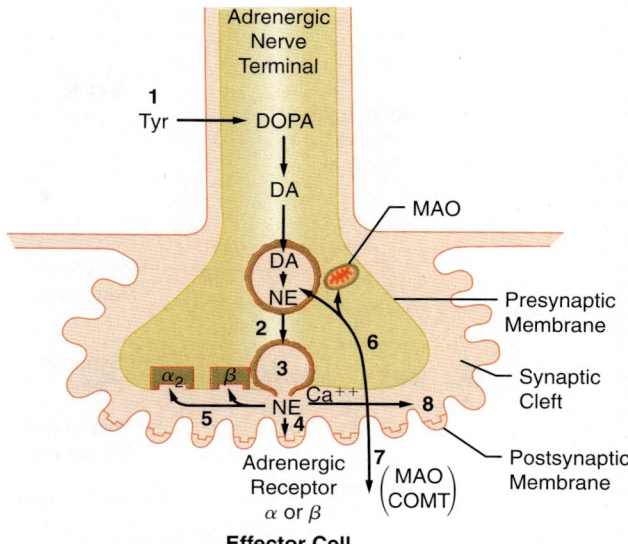

Figure 14-8 Schematic of the synthesis and disposition of NE in adrenergic neurotransmission. (1) Synthesis and storage in neuronal vesicles; (2) Action potential permits calcium entry with (3) exocytosis of NE into synaptic gap. (4) Released NE reacts with receptors on effector cell. NE (5) may react with presynaptic α_2 receptor to inhibit further NE release or with presynaptic β-receptor to enhance reuptake of NE (6) (uptake 1). Extraneuronal uptake (uptake 2) absorbs NE into effector cell (7) with overflow occurring systemically (8). MAO, monoamine oxidase; COMT, catechol-O-methyltransferase; Tyr, tyrosine; DOPA, dihydroxyphenylalanine; NE, norepinephrine.

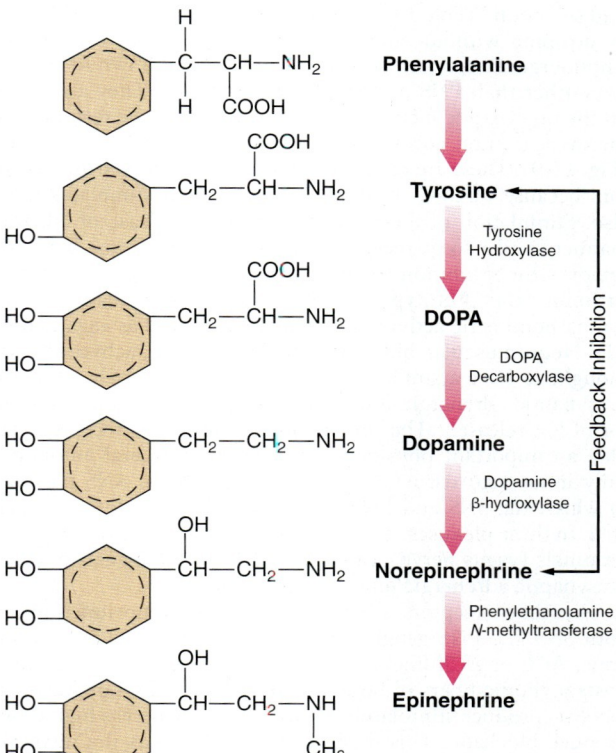

Figure 14-7 Schematic of the synthesis of catecholamines. The conversion of tyrosine to DOPA by tyrosine hydroxylase is inhibited by increased NE synthesis. Epinephrine is shown in these steps but is primarily synthesized in the adrenal medulla. DOPA, dihydroxyphenylalanine.

(DA) synthesis occurs in the cytoplasm of the neuron. The vesicles of peripheral postganglionic neurons contain the enzyme dopamine-β-hydroxylase, which converts dopamine to NE. The adrenal medulla additionally contains phenylethanolamine-N-methyltransferase, which converts NE to EPI. This reaction takes place outside the medullary vesicles, and the newly formed EPI then enters the vesicle for storage (Fig. 14-8). All the endogenous catecholamines are stored in presynaptic vesicles and released on arrival of an action potential. Excitation–secretion coupling in sympathetic neurons is Ca^{2+}-dependent.

Regulation

Increased SNS nervous activity, as in congestive heart failure or chronic stress, stimulates the synthesis of catecholamines. Glucocorticoids from the adrenal cortex stimulate an increase in phenylethanolamine-N-methyltransferase that methylates NE to EPI.

The release of NE is dependent upon depolarization of the nerve and an increase in calcium ion permeability. This release is inhibited by colchicine and prostaglandin E_2, suggesting a contractile mechanism. NE inhibits its own release by stimulating presynaptic (prejunctional) α_2 receptors. Phenoxybenzamine and phentolamine, α-receptor antagonists, increase the release of NE by blocking inhibitory presynaptic α_2 receptors (Fig. 14-9). Other receptors are also important in NE regulation (see below, Other Receptors).

Inactivation

The catecholamines are removed from the synaptic cleft by three mechanisms (Fig. 14-8). These are reuptake into the presynaptic terminals, extraneuronal uptake, and diffusion. Termination of NE action at the effector site is almost entirely by reuptake

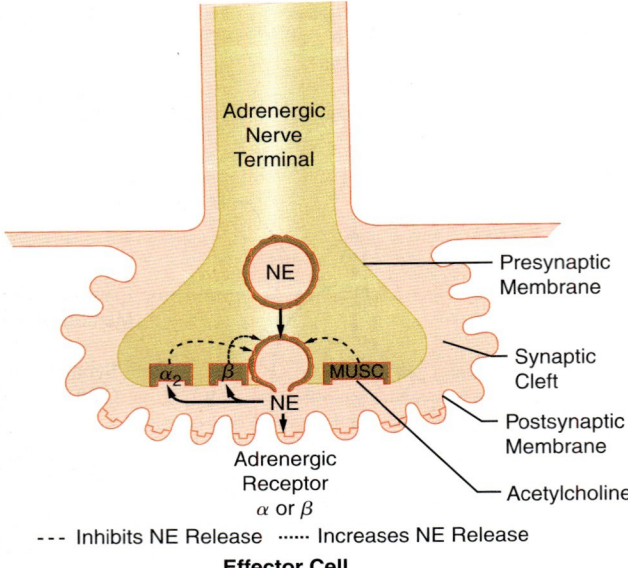

Figure 14-9 This schematic demonstrates just a few of the presynaptic adrenergic receptors thought to exist. Agonist and antagonist drugs are clinically available for these receptors (Table 14-5). The α_2 receptors serve as a negative feedback mechanism whereby NE stimulation inhibits its own release. Presynaptic β-stimulation increases NE uptake, augmenting its availability. Presynaptic muscarinic (MUSC) receptors respond to ACh diffusing from nearby cholinergic terminals. They inhibit NE release and can be blocked by atropine. NE, norepinephrine.

of NE into the terminals of the presynaptic neuron. This is an active, energy-requiring, and temperature-dependent process. The reuptake of NE in the presynaptic terminals is also a stereospecific process. Structurally similar compounds (guanethidine, metaraminol) may enter the vesicles and displace the neurotransmitter. Tricyclic antidepressants and cocaine inhibit the reuptake of NE, resulting in high synaptic NE concentrations and accentuated receptor response. In addition, evidence suggests that NE reuptake is mediated by a presynaptic β-adrenergic mechanism because β-blockade causes marked elevations of EPI and NE (Figs. 14-8 and 14-9).[11] Extraneuronal uptake is a minor pathway for inactivating NE. Effector cells and other extraneuronal tissues take up NE. The NE that is taken up by the extraneuronal tissue is metabolized by monoamine oxidase (MAO) and by catechol-O-methyltransferase (COMT) to form vanillylmandelic acid. The minute amount of catecholamine that escapes these two mechanisms diffuses into the circulation, where it is metabolized by the liver and kidney. The same enzymes inactivate EPI. Reuptake is the predominant pathway for inactivation of the endogenous catecholamines, while metabolism by the liver and kidney is the predominant pathway for catecholamines given exogenously. This accounts for the longer duration of action of the exogenous catecholamines than that noted at the local synapse.

The final metabolic product of the catecholamines is vanillylmandelic acid. Vanillylmandelic acid constitutes the major metabolite (80% to 90%) of NE found in the urine. Less than 5% of released NE appears unchanged in the urine. The metabolic products excreted in the urine provide a gross estimate of SNS activity and can facilitate the clinical diagnosis of pheochromocytoma (see Chapter 46).

Receptors

An agonist is a substance that interacts with a receptor to evoke a biologic response. ACh, NE, EPI, DA, and ATP are the major agonists of the ANS. An antagonist is a substance that interferes with the evocation of a response at a receptor site by an agonist. Receptors are therefore target sites that lead to a response by the effector cell when activated by an agonist. Receptors are protein macromolecules and are located in the plasma membrane. Several thousand receptors have been demonstrated in a single cell. The enormity of this network becomes apparent when one considers that ~25,000 single cells can be innervated by a single neuron.

Cholinergic Receptors

ACh is the neurotransmitter for three distinct classes of receptors. These receptors can be differentiated by their anatomic location and their affinity for various agonists and antagonists. ACh mediates the "first messenger" function of transmitting impulses within the PNS, the ganglia of the SNS, and the neuroeffector junction of striated, voluntary muscle (Fig. 14-2). Cholinergic receptors are further subdivided into muscarinic and nicotinic receptors because muscarine and nicotine stimulate them selectively. However, both muscarinic and nicotinic receptors respond to ACh (see below, Cholinergic Drugs). Muscarine activates cholinergic receptors at the postganglionic PNS junctions of cardiac and smooth muscle. Muscarinic stimulation is characterized by bradycardia, decreased inotropism, bronchoconstriction, miosis, salivation, gastrointestinal hypermotility, and increased gastric acid secretion (Table 14-1). Muscarinic receptors can be blocked by atropine without effect on nicotinic receptors (see below, Cholinergic Drugs). Muscarinic receptors are known to exist in sites other than PNS postganglionic junctions. They are found on the presynaptic membrane of sympathetic nerve terminals in the myocardium, coronary vessels, and peripheral vasculature (Fig. 14-9). These are referred to as adrenergic muscarinic receptors because of their location; however, ACh stimulates them also. Stimulation of these receptors inhibits release of NE in a manner similar to α_2-receptor stimulation. Muscarinic blockade removes the inhibition of NE release, augmenting SNS activity. Atropine, the prototypical muscarinic blocker, may produce sympathomimetic activity in this manner as well as vagal blockade. Neuromuscular blocking drugs that cause tachycardia are thought to have a similar mechanism of action. ACh acting on presynaptic adrenergic muscarinic receptors is a potent inhibitor of NE release.[11] The prejunctional muscarinic receptor may play an important physiologic role because several autonomically innervated tissues (e.g., the heart) possess ANS plexuses in which the SNS and PNS nerve terminals are closely associated. In these plexuses, ACh, released from the nearby PNS nerve terminals (vagus nerve), can inhibit NE release by activation of presynaptic adrenergic muscarinic receptors.

Nicotinic receptors are found at the synaptic junctions of both SNS and PNS ganglia. Because both junctions are cholinergic, ACh or ACh-like substances such as nicotine will excite postganglionic fibers of both systems (Fig. 14-2). Low doses of nicotine produce stimulation of ANS ganglia whereas high doses produce blockade. This dualism is referred to as the nicotinic effect (see below, Ganglionic Drugs). Nicotinic stimulation of the SNS ganglia produces hypertension and tachycardia by causing the release of EPI and NE from the adrenal medulla. Adrenal hormone release is mediated by ACh in the chromaffin cells, which are analogous to postganglionic neurons. A further increase in nicotine concentration produces hypotension and neuromuscular weakness, as it becomes a ganglionic blocker. The cholinergic neuroeffector junction of skeletal muscle also contains nicotinic receptors, although they are not identical to the nicotinic receptors in ANS ganglia.

Adrenergic Receptors

The adrenergic receptors are termed adrenergic or noradrenergic, depending on their responsiveness to EPI or NE. The dissimilarities of these two drugs led Ahlquist in 1948 to propose two types of opposing adrenergic receptors, termed alpha (α) and beta (β). The development of new agonists and antagonists with relatively selective activity allowed subdivision of the β-receptors into β_1 and β_2; α-receptors were subsequently divided into α_1 and α_2. These were later further subdivided using molecular cloning. The sympathomimetic adrenergic drugs in current use differ from one another in their effects, largely because of differences in substitution on the amine group, which influences the relative α or β effect (Fig. 14-6).

Another major peripheral adrenergic receptor specific for dopamine is termed the dopaminergic (DA) receptor. Further studies have revealed not only subsets of the α and β receptors but also the DA receptor. These DA receptors have been identified in the CNS and in renal, mesenteric, and coronary vessels. The physiologic importance of these receptors is a matter of controversy because there are no identifiable peripheral DA neurons. Dopamine measured in the circulation is assumed to result from spillover from the brain.

The function of dopamine in the CNS has long been known, but the peripheral dopamine receptor has been elucidated only within the past 25 years. The presence of the peripheral DA receptor was obscured because dopamine does not affect the DA receptor exclusively. It also stimulates α and β receptors in a dose-related manner. However, DA receptors function independently of α or β blockade and are modified by DA antagonists such as haloperidol, droperidol, and phenothiazines. Thus, there is a necessity for the addition of the DA receptor and its subsets (DA_1 and DA_2).

The distribution of adrenergic receptors in organs and tissues is not uniform and their function differs not only by their location but also in their numbers and/or distribution. Adrenergic receptors are found in two loci in the sympathetic neuroeffector junction. They are found in both the presynaptic (prejunctional) and postsynaptic (postjunctional) sites as well as extrasynaptic sites (Fig. 14-10). Table 14-3 is a review of the function and synaptic location of some of the clinically important receptors and their subtypes.

α-Adrenergic Receptors

The α-adrenergic (α) receptors have been further subdivided into two clinically important classes, α_1 and α_2. This classification is based on their response to the α-antagonists yohimbine and prazosin. Prazosin is a more potent antagonist of α_1 receptors, whereas α_2 receptors are more sensitive to yohimbine. Recently, pharmacologic experiments have demonstrated the existence of two subtypes within the α_1 group, namely α_{1A} and α_{1B}, and at least two subtypes within the α_2 group, respectively, α_{2A} and α_{2B}. The importance of these subsets is still emerging, with evidence that the spleen and liver contain mainly α_{1B} receptors, and the heart, neocortex, kidney, vas deferens, and hippocampus contain equal amounts of α_{1A} and α_{1B} receptors. The α_1-adrenergic receptors are found in the smooth muscle cells of the peripheral

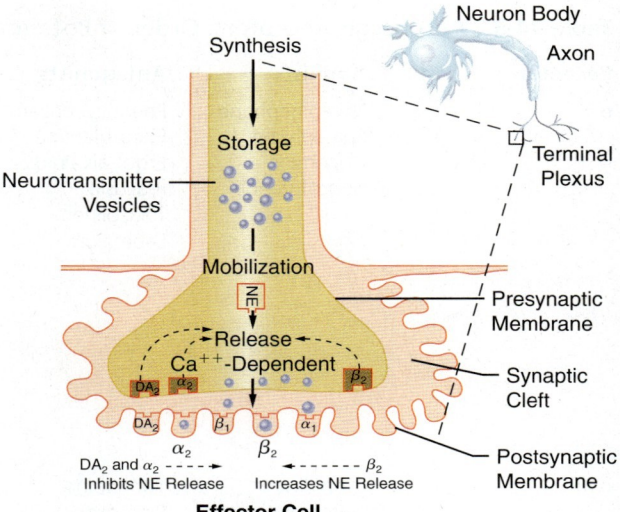

Figure 14-10 Location of several known adrenergic receptors. The presynaptic α_2 and DA receptors serve as a negative feedback mechanism, whereby stimulation of NE inhibits its own release. Presynaptic β_2 stimulation increases NE uptake, augmenting its availability. Postsynaptic α_2 and β_2 receptors are extrasynaptic and are considered noninnervated hormonal receptors. DA, dopamine; NE, norepinephrine.

vasculature, coronary arteries, skin, uterus, intestinal mucosa, and splanchnic beds (Table 14-4).[12] The α_1 receptors serve as postsynaptic activators of vascular and intestinal smooth muscle as well as of endocrine glands. Their activation results in either decreased or increased tone, depending upon the effector organ. The response in resistance and capacitance vessels is constriction, whereas in the intestinal tract it is relaxation. There is now a large body of evidence documenting the presence of postjunctional α_1 adrenoceptors in the mammalian heart. α_1-Adrenergic receptors have been shown to have a positive inotropic effect on cardiac tissues in most mammals studied, including humans. Experimental work strongly supports the concept that enhanced myocardial α_1 responsiveness plays a primary role in the genesis of malignant arrhythmias induced by catecholamines during myocardial ischemia and reperfusion. Drugs possessing potent α_1-antagonist activity such as prazosin and phentolamine provide significant antiarrhythmic activity. The clinical mechanism and significance of these findings are not yet clear. However, there is no doubt that α_1-adrenergic antagonists prevent catecholamine-induced ventricular arrhythmias.[13] In contrast, studies of the effects of β-antagonists in experimental and clinical myocardial infarction have provided conflicting results.

The discovery of presynaptic α-adrenoceptors and their role in the modulation of NE transmission provided the stimulus for the subclassification of α receptors into α_1 and α_2 subtypes. Presynaptic α_1 receptors have not been identified; receptors appear confined only to the postsynaptic membrane. On the other hand, α_2 receptors are found on both presynaptic and postsynaptic membranes of the adrenergic neuroeffector junction. Table 14-4 reviews these sites. Postsynaptic membranes contain a near equal mix of α_1 and α_2 receptors.

The α_2 adrenoceptors may be subdivided even further into as many as four possible subtypes. The postsynaptic α_2 receptors have many actions, which include arterial and venous vasoconstriction, platelet aggregation, inhibition of insulin release, inhibition of bowel motility, stimulation of growth hormone release, and inhibition of ADH release.

Table 14-3 Adrenergic Receptors: Order of Potency of Agonists and Antagonists

Receptor	Agonists[a]		Antagonists	Location	Action
α_1	++++	Norepinephrine	Phenoxybenzamine[b]	Smooth muscle (vascular, iris, radial, ureter, pilomotor, uterus, trigone, gastrointestinal, and bladder sphincters)	Contraction Vasoconstriction
	+++	Epinephrine	Phentolamine[b]		
	++	Dopamine	Ergot alkaloids[b]		
	+	Isoproterenol	Prazosin		
			Tolazoline[b]	Brain	Neurotransmission
			Labetalol[b]	Smooth muscle (gastrointestinal)	Relaxation
				Heart	Glycogenolysis
				Salivary glands	Increased force,[c] glycolysis
				Adipose tissue	Secretion (K$^+$, H$_2$O)
				Sweat glands (localized)	Glycogenesis
				Kidney (proximal tubule)	Secretion
					Gluconeogenesis Na$^+$ reabsorption
α_2	++++	Clonidine	Yohimbine	Adrenergic nerve endings Presynaptic—CNS	Inhibition norepinephrine release
	+++	Norepinephrine	Piperoxan		
	++	Epinephrine	Phentolamine[b]		
	++	Norepinephrine	Phenoxybenzamine[b]	Platelets	Aggregation, granule release
	+	Phenylephrine	Tolazoline[b]		
			Labetalol[b]	Adipose tissue	Inhibition lipolysis
				Endocrine pancreas	Inhibition insulin release
				Vascular smooth muscle—?	Contraction
				Kidney	Inhibition renin disease
				Brain	Neurotransmission
β_1	++++	Isoproterenol[b]	Acebutolol	Heart	Increased rate, contractility, conduction velocity
	+++	Epinephrine	Practolol		
	++	Norepinephrine	Propranolol[b]		Coronary vasodilation
	+	Dopamine	Alprenolol[b]	Adipose tissue	Lipolysis
			Metoprolol		
			Esmolol		
β_2	++++	Isoproterenol[a]	Propranolol[b]	Liver	Glycogenolysis, gluconeogenesis
	+++	Epinephrine	Butoxamine		
	++	Norepinephrine	Alprenolol		
	+	Dopamine	Esmolol	Skeletal muscle	Glycogenolysis, lactate release
			Nadolol		
			Timolol	Smooth muscle (bronchi, uterus, vascular, gastrointestinal, detrusor, spleen capsule)	Relaxation
			Labetalol		
				Endocrine pancreas	Insulin secretion
				Salivary glands	Amylase secretion
DA$_1$	++++	Fenoldopam		Vascular smooth muscle Renal and mesentery	Vasodilation
	++	Dopamine	Haloperidol		
	+	Epinephrine	Droperidol		
	+	Metoclopramide	Phenothiazines		
DA$_2$	++	Dopamine	Domperidone	Presynaptic—adrenergic nerve endings	Inhibits norepinephrine release
	+	Bromocriptine			

DA, dopamine.
[a]Listed in decreasing order of potency.
[b]Nonselective.
[c]β_1-Adrenergic responses are greater.
Pluses indicate strength of potency.

Table 14-4 Adrenergic Receptors

Receptor	Synaptic Site	Anatomic Site	Action	LV Function and Stroke Volume
α_1	Postsynaptic	Peripheral vascular smooth muscle	Constriction	Decreased
		Renal vascular smooth muscle	Constriction	
		Coronary arteries, epicardial	Constriction	
		Myocardium 30%–40% of resting tone	Positive inotropism	Improved
		Renal tubules	Antidiuresis	
α_2	Presynaptic	Peripheral vascular smooth muscle release	Inhibit NE	
			Secondary vasodilation	Improved
		Coronaries		
		CNS	Inhibition of CNS activity	
			Sedation	
			Decrease MAC	
	Postsynaptic	Coronaries, endocardial	Constriction	Decreased
		CNS	Inhibition of insulin release	
			Decreased bowel motility	
			Inhibition of antidiuretic hormone	
			Analgesia	
		Renal tubule	Promotes Na^{2+} and H_2O excretion	
β_1	Postsynaptic NE sensitive	Myocardium	Positive inotropism and chronotropism	Improved
		Sinoatrial (SA) node		
		Ventricular conduction		
		Kidney	Renin release	
		Coronaries	Relaxation	
β_2	Presynaptic NE sensitive	Myocardium	Accelerates NE release	Improved
		SA node ventricular conduction vessels	Opposite action to presynaptic α_2 agonism	
			Constriction	
	Postsynaptic (extrasynaptic) (EPI sensitive)	Myocardium	Positive inotropism and chronotropism	Improved
		Vascular smooth muscle	Relaxation	Improved
		Bronchial smooth muscle	Relaxation	Improved
		Renal vessels	Relaxation	
DA_1	Postsynaptic	Blood vessels (renal, mesentery, coronary)	Vasodilation	Improved
		Renal tubules	Natriuresis	
			Diuresis	
		Juxtaglomerular cells	Renin release (modulates diuresis)	
		Sympathetic ganglia	Minor inhibition	
DA_2	Presynaptic	Postganglionic sympathetic nerves	Inhibit NE release	Improved
			Secondary vasodilation	
	Postsynaptic	Renal and mesenteric vasculature	? Vasoconstriction	

LV, left ventricular; NE, norepinephrine; MAC, minimum alveolar concentration; EPI, epinephrine; DA, dopamine.

α_2 Receptors can be found in cholinergic pathways as well as in adrenergic pathways. They can significantly modulate parasympathetic activity as well. Current research implies that α_2 stimulation of the parasympathetic pathways plays a role in the modulation of the baroreceptor reflex (increased sensitivity), vagal mediation of heart rate (bradycardia), bronchoconstriction, and salivation (dry mouth). However, cholinergic receptors can also be found in adrenergic pathways; thus, muscarinic and nicotinic receptors have been found in presynaptic and postsynaptic locations, where in turn they modulate sympathetic activity (Fig. 14-9). There is speculation that the features that are desirable to the anesthesiologist, such as sedation, anxiolysis, analgesia, and hypnosis, are mediated through this site.

Stimulation of presynaptic α_2 receptors mediates inhibition of NE release into the synaptic cleft, serving as a negative feedback mechanism. The central effects are primarily related to a reduction in sympathetic outflow with a concomitantly enhanced parasympathetic outflow (e.g., enhanced baroreceptor activity). This results in a decreased systemic vascular resistance, decreased cardiac output (CO), decreased inotropic state in the myocardium, and decreased HR. The peripheral presynaptic α_2 effects are similar, and NE release is inhibited in postganglionic neurons. However, stimulation of postsynaptic α_2 receptors, like the α_1 postsynaptic receptor, affects vasoconstriction. NE acts on both α_1 and α_2 receptors. Thus, NE not only activates smooth muscle vasoconstriction (postsynaptic α_1 and α_2 receptors) but also stimulates presynaptic α_2 receptors and inhibits its own release. Selective stimulation of the presynaptic α_2 receptor could produce a beneficial reduction of peripheral vascular resistance. Unfortunately, most known presynaptic α_2 agonists also stimulate the postsynaptic α_2 receptors, causing vasoconstriction. Blockade of α_2 presynaptic receptors, however, ablates normal inhibition of NE, causing vasoconstriction. Vasodilation occurs with the blockade of postsynaptic α_1 and α_2 receptors.

α-Adrenergic Receptors in the Cardiovascular System

Postsynaptic α_1 and α_2 receptors in the mammalian myocardium and coronary arteries mediate a number of responses.

Coronary Arteries

The presence of postsynaptic α_1 and α_2 receptors in mammalian models has been demonstrated. Sympathetic nerves cause coronary vasoconstriction, which is mediated predominately by postsynaptic α_2, more so than α_1 receptors. The larger epicardial arteries possess mainly α_1 receptors, whereas α_2 receptors and some α_1 receptors are present in the small coronary artery resistance vessels.[14] Epicardial vessels contribute only 5% to the total resistance of the coronary circulation; therefore, α_1 agonists such as phenylephrine have little influence on coronary resistance.[15,16] Myocardial ischemia has been shown to increase α_2 receptor density in the coronary arteries. Ischemia has also been shown to cause a reflex increase in sympathetic activity mediated by α mechanisms. This cascade may further increase coronary constriction. Postsynaptic α_1 receptors do not rely upon extracellular Ca^{2+} to constrict the vessel, whereas the α_2-constrictor response is highly dependent upon extracellular influx and exquisitely sensitive to calcium channel inhibitors.[17]

Myocardium

The role of β receptors in mediating catecholamine-induced inotropism and arrhythmogenesis is well known (see below, β-Adrenergic Receptors). Studies have shown the presence of postsynaptic myocardial α_1 receptors, which also exert a major, facilatory, positive inotropic effect on the myocardium of several species of mammals including humans. Their contribution to malignant reperfusion arrhythmogenesis has also been recognized.

Phenylephrine, an α_1 agonist, can increase myocardial contractility two- to threefold compared with a six- to sevenfold increase produced by isoproterenol, a pure β agonist. Myocardial postsynaptic α_1 receptors mediate perhaps as much as 30% to 50% of the basal inotropic tone of the normal heart.

Postsynaptic myocardial α_1 receptors play a more prominent inotropic role in the failing heart by serving as a reserve to the normally predominant β_1 receptors. Although the response to both α_1 and β_1 agonists is reduced in the failing myocardium, the interaction between the two receptors is more apparent. Chronic heart failure is known to produce a reduced density (downregulation) of myocardial β_1 receptors as a result of high levels of circulating catecholamines. However, there is no evidence of downregulation of either α_1 or β_2 receptors in cardiac failure. The increase in density of myocardial α_1 adrenoreceptors is more pronounced with failure and myocardial ischemia.[18] Thus, enhanced myocardial α_1-receptor numbers and sensitivity may contribute to the positive inotropism seen during ischemia as well as to the malignant arrhythmias that occur with reperfusion.

Intracellular mobilization of cytosolic Ca^{2+} by the activated α_1-myocardial receptors during ischemia appears to contribute to these arrhythmias. The α_1 receptor also increases the sensitivity of the contractile elements to Ca^{2+}. Drugs possessing potent α_1 antagonism such as prazosin and phentolamine have been shown to possess significant antiarrhythmic activity, but are of limited usefulness because of hypotension. Enhanced α_1 activity with myocardial ischemia may explain why the antiarrhythmic benefits of β antagonists in patients with acute myocardial infarction are far from certain. The contribution of β receptors to positive inotropism and arrhythmogenesis during ischemia and reperfusion may be overshadowed by the α receptors during acute failure and ischemia.

Peripheral Vessels

Activation of the presynaptic α_2-vascular receptors produces vasodilation, whereas the postsynaptic α_1- and α_2-vascular receptors subserve vasoconstriction. Presynaptic vascular α_2 receptors inhibit NE release. This represents a negative feedback mechanism by which NE inhibits its own release via the prejunctional receptor. Presynaptic α_2 agonists, such as clonidine, inhibit NE release at the neurosympathetic junction, producing vasodilatation. The effect of selective presynaptic α_2-receptor agonists to ameliorate coronary vasoconstriction in humans is unclear. Excitation of the inhibitory presynaptic α_2 receptors by endogenous or synthetic catecholamines also inhibits NE release. However, most sympathomimetics are nonselective α agonists that will excite equally presynaptic α_2 vasodilating receptors and vasoconstrictive postsynaptic α_1 and α_2 receptors. Postsynaptic α_1 and α_2 receptors coexist in both the arterial and venous sides of the circulation with the relative distribution of α_2 receptors being greater on the venous side.[12] This may explain why pure α_1 agonists, such as methoxamine, produce little venoconstriction, whereas many nonselective agonists such as phenylephrine produce significant venoconstriction. NE is the most potent venoconstrictor of all the catecholamines. Clinically, venoconstriction would have the effect of preloading by shifting venous capacitance centrally, whereas stimulation of arterial postsynaptic α_1 and α_2 receptors would affect afterloading by increasing arterial resistance.

α-Adrenergic Receptors in the Central Nervous System

All subtypes of the α, β, and DA receptors have been found in various regions of the brain and spinal cord. The functional role of the cerebral α and β receptors suggests a close association with blood pressure and HR control. Cerebral and spinal cord presynaptic α_2 receptors are also involved in inhibition of presynaptic NE release. Although the brain contains adrenergic and dopaminergic receptors, circulating catecholamines do not cross the blood–brain barrier. The catecholamines in the brain are synthesized there. Many actions have been attributed to the cerebral postsynaptic α_2 receptor. This includes inhibition of insulin release, inhibition of bowel motility, stimulation of growth hormone release, and inhibition of ADH release. Central neuraxial injections of α_2 agonists, such as clonidine, induce analgesia, sedation, and cardiovascular depression. The increased duration of epidural or intrathecal anesthesia by the addition of nonselective α agonists to the local anesthetic may produce additional analgesia through this mechanism.

α Receptors in the Kidney

The kidney has an extensive and exclusive adrenergic innervation of the afferent and efferent glomerular arterioles, proximal and distal renal tubules, ascending loop of Henle, and juxtaglomerular apparatus. The greatest density of innervation is in the thick ascending loop of Henle, followed by the distal convoluted tubules and proximal tube. Both α_1 and α_2 subtypes are found in the kidney with the α_2 receptor dominating. The α_1 receptor is predominant in the renal vasculature and elicits vasoconstriction, which modulates renal blood flow. Tubular α_1 receptors enhance sodium and water reabsorption, leading to antinatriuresis, whereas tubular α_2 receptors promote sodium and water excretion.

β-Adrenergic Receptors

The β-adrenergic receptors, like the α receptor, have been divided into subtypes. They are designated as the β_1 and β_2 subtypes. Recently, molecular cloning has demonstrated the existence of a third subtype, namely β_3 receptor. Activation of all these receptor subtypes induces the activation of adenylyl cyclase and increased conversion of ATP to cyclic adenosine-3′,5′-monophosphate (cAMP). β_1 Receptors predominate in the myocardium, the sinoatrial node, and the ventricular conduction system. The β_1 receptors also mediate the effects of the catecholamines on the myocardium. These receptors are equally sensitive to EPI and NE, which distinguishes them from the β_2 receptors. Effects of β_1 stimulation are outlined in Table 14-4, which include their effects specifically on the cardiovascular system.

The β_2 receptors are located in the smooth muscles of the blood vessels in the skin, muscle, mesentery, and in bronchial smooth muscle. Stimulation produces vasodilation and bronchial relaxation. The β_2 receptors are more sensitive to EPI than NE. β Receptors are found in both presynaptic and postsynaptic membranes of the adrenergic neuroeffector junction. β_1 Receptors are distributed to postsynaptic sites and have not been identified on the presynaptic membrane. Presynaptic β receptors are of the β_2 subtype. The effects of activation of the presynaptic β_2 receptor are diametrically opposed to those of the presynaptic α_2 receptor. The presynaptic β_2 receptor accelerates endogenous NE release, whereas blockade of this receptor will inhibit NE release. Antagonism of the presynaptic β_2 receptors produces a physiologic result similar to activation of the presynaptic α_2 receptor. The postsynaptic β_1 receptors are located on the synaptic membrane and respond primarily to neuronal NE. The postsynaptic β_2 receptors, like the postsynaptic α_2 receptor, respond primarily to circulating EPI.

β Receptors in the Cardiovascular System

Myocardium

Myocardial β receptors were originally classified as β_1 receptors. Those in the vascular and bronchial smooth muscle were called the β_2 subtype. However, studies have confirmed the coexistence of β_1 and β_2 receptors in the myocardium.[19] Both β_1 and β_2 receptors are functionally coupled to adenylate cyclase, suggesting a similar involvement in the regulation of inotropism and chronotropism. Postsynaptic β_1 receptors are distributed predominantly to the myocardium, the sinoatrial node, and the ventricular conduction system. The β_2 receptors have the same distribution but are presynaptic. Activation of the presynaptic β_2 receptor accelerates the release of NE into the synaptic cleft. The β_2 receptor comprises 20% to 30% of the β receptors in the ventricular myocardium and up to 40% of the β receptors in the atrium.

The effect of NE on inotropism in the normal heart is mediated entirely through the postsynaptic β_1 receptor, whereas the inotropic effects of EPI are mediated through both the β_1- and β_2-myocardial receptors. The β_2 receptors may also mediate the chronotropic responses to EPI which explains why selective β_1 antagonists are less effective in suppressing induced tachycardia than the nonselective β_1 antagonist propranolol.

Peripheral Vessels

The postsynaptic vascular β receptors are virtually all of the β_2 subtype. The β_2 receptors are located in the smooth muscle of the blood vessels of the skin, muscle, mesentery, and bronchi. Stimulation of the postsynaptic β_2 receptor produces vasodilation and bronchial relaxation. Modest vasoconstriction occurs when subjected to blockade because the actions of the vascular postsynaptic β_2 receptors no longer oppose the actions of the α_1- and α_2-postsynaptic receptors.

β Receptors in the Kidney

The kidney contains both β_1 and β_2 receptors, with the β_1 being predominant. Renin release from the juxtaglomerular apparatus is enhanced by β stimulation. The β_1 receptor evokes renin release in humans. Renal β_2 receptors also appear to regulate renal blood flow at the vascular level. They have been identified pharmacologically and mediate a vasodilatory response.

Dopaminergic Receptors

Dopamine, synthesized in 1910, was recognized in 1959 not only as a vasopressor and the precursor of NE and EPI, but also as an important central and peripheral neurotransmitter. Dopamine receptors (DA) are localized in the CNS, on blood vessels and postganglionic sympathetic nerves (Table 14-4). Two clinically important types of DA receptors have been recognized: DA_1 and DA_2, while other subtypes such as DA_4 and DA_5 are still being investigated. The DA_1 receptors are postsynaptic, whereas the DA_2 receptors are both presynaptic and postsynaptic. The presynaptic DA_2 receptors, like the presynaptic α_2 receptor, inhibit NE release and can produce vasodilatation. The postsynaptic DA_2 receptor may subserve vasoconstriction similar to that of the postsynaptic α_2 receptor. This effect is opposite to that of the postsynaptic DA_1 renal vascular receptor. The zona glomerulosa of the adrenal cortex also contains DA_2 receptors, which inhibit the release of aldosterone.

Myocardium

Defining specific dopaminergic receptors has been difficult because dopamine also exerts effects on the α and β receptors. DA receptors have not been described in the myocardium. Effects of dopamine are those related to activation of β_1 receptors, which promote positive inotropism and chronotropism. β_2 Activation may produce some systemic vasodilatation.

Peripheral Vessels

The greatest numbers of DA_1-postsynaptic receptors are found on vascular smooth muscle cells of the kidney and mesentery, but are also found in the other systemic arteries including coronary, cerebral, and cutaneous arteries. The vascular receptors are, like the β_2 receptors, linked to adenylate cyclase and mediate smooth muscle relaxation. Activation of these receptors produces vasodilatation, increasing blood flow to these organs. Concurrent activation of vascular presynaptic DA_2 receptors also inhibits NE release at presynaptic α_2 receptors, which may also contribute to peripheral vasodilatation. Higher doses of dopamine can mediate vasoconstriction via the postsynaptic α_1 and α_2 receptors. The constrictive effect is relatively weak in the cardiovascular system, where the action of dopamine on adrenergic receptors is 1/35 and 1/50 as potent as that of EPI and NE, respectively.[20]

Central Nervous System

DA receptors have been identified in the hypothalamus where they are involved in prolactin release. They are also found in the basal ganglia where they coordinate motor function. Degeneration of dopaminergic neurons in the substantia nigra is the cause of Parkinson disease. Another central action of dopamine is to stimulate the chemoreceptor trigger zone of the medulla, producing nausea and vomiting. Dopamine antagonists such as haloperidol and droperidol are clinically effective in countering this action.

Kidney and Mesentery

Apart from their effect on the vessels of the kidney and mesentery, DA receptors on the smooth muscle of the esophagus, stomach, and small intestine enhance secretion production and reduce intestinal motility.[20,21] Metoclopramide, a dopamine antagonist, is useful for aspiration prophylaxis by promoting gastric emptying. The distribution of DA receptors in the renal vasculature is well known, but DA receptors have other functions within the kidney. DA_1 receptors are located on renal tubules, which inhibit sodium reabsorption with subsequent natriuresis and diuresis. The natriuresis may be the result of a combined renal vasodilatation, improved CO, and tubular action of the DA_1 receptors. Juxtaglomerular cells also contain DA_1 receptors, which increase renin release when activated. This action modulates the diuresis produced by DA_1 activation of the tubules.

Dopamine has unique autonomic effects by activating specific peripheral dopaminergic receptors, which promote natriuresis and reduce afterload via dilatation of the renal and mesenteric arterial beds. Peripheral dopaminergic activity serves as a natural antihypertensive mechanism. Its actions are overshadowed by the opposite effect of its main biologic partner, NE. Plasma NE levels are known to increase with aging, likely the result of reduced clearance, while peripheral dopaminergic activity is known to diminish. Subtle changes in the DA–NE balance with aging may account for the diminished ability of the aged kidney to excrete a salt load.

Other Receptors

Adenosine Receptors

Adenosine produces inhibition of NE release. The effect of adenosine is blocked by caffeine and other methylxanthines. The physiologic function of these receptors may be the reduction of sympathetic tone under hypoxic conditions when adenosine production is enhanced. As a consequence of reduced NE release, cardiac work would be decreased and oxygen demand reduced. Adenosine has been effectively used to produce controlled hypotension.[22]

Serotonin

Serotonin (5-hydroxytryptamine) depresses the response of isolated blood vessels to SNS stimulation and decreases release of labeled NE in these preparations. Raising the external calcium ion concentration antagonizes this inhibitory action of serotonin. Thus, serotonin may inhibit neuronal NE release by a mechanism that limits the availability of calcium ions at the nerve terminal.

Prostaglandin E2, Histamine, and Opioids

Prostaglandin E2, histamine, and several opioids have been reported to act on prejunctional receptor sites to inhibit NE release in certain sympathetically innervated tissue. However, these inhibitory receptors are unlikely to play a physiologic role in limiting NE release since their direct antagonists, compounds such as inhibitors of cyclooxygenase, histamine antagonists, and naloxone do not increase an NE release.

Histamine acts in a manner similar to the neurotransmitters of the SNS. The cell membrane has specific receptors for histamine, with the individual response being determined by the type of cell being stimulated (see Chapter 9). Two receptors for histamine have been determined. These have been designated H_1 and H_2, for which it has been possible to develop specific agonists and antagonists. Stimulation of the H_1 receptors produces bronchoconstriction and intestinal contraction. The major role of the H_2 receptors is related to acid production by the parietal cells of the stomach; however, histamine is also present in relatively high concentrations in the myocardium and cardiac conducting tissue, where it exerts positive inotropic and chronotropic effects while depressing dromotropism. The positive inotropic and chronotropic effects of histamine are H_2 receptor effects that are not blocked by β antagonism. These effects are blocked by H_2 antagonists, such as cimetidine, which accounts for the occasional report of cardiovascular collapse following the use of cimetidine. The negative dromotropic effect and that of coronary spasm caused by histamine are H_1 receptor effects.

Adrenergic Receptor Numbers and Sensitivity

Receptors, once thought to be static entities, are now thought to be dynamically regulated by a variety of conditions and to be in a constant state of flux. Receptors are synthesized in the sarcoplasmic reticulum (SR) of the parent cell, where they may remain extrasynaptic or externalize to the synaptic membranes where they may cluster. Membrane receptors may be removed or internalized to intracellular sites for either dehydration or recycling.

The numbers and sensitivity of adrenergic receptors can be influenced by normal, genetic, and developmental factors. Changes in the number of receptors alter the response to catecholamines. Alteration in the number or density of receptors is referred to as either upregulation or downregulation. As a rule, the number of receptors is inversely proportional to the ambient concentration of the catecholamines. Extended exposure of receptors to their agonists markedly reduces, but does not ablate, the biologic response to catecholamines. For example, increased adrenergic activity occurs in response to reduced perfusion as a result of acute or chronic myocardial dysfunction. Plasma catecholamines are increased. Subsequently, the myocardial postsynaptic $β_1$ receptors are "downregulated" (see Chapter 11). This is thought to explain the diminished inotropic and chronotropic response to $β_1$ agonists and exercise in patients with chronic heart failure. However, calcium-induced inotropism is not impaired because extrasynaptic $β_2$-receptor numbers remain relatively intact. The $β_2$ receptors may account for up to 40% of the inotropism of the failing heart compared with 20% in the normal heart.[18,23] Tachyphylaxis to infused catecholamines is also thought to be the result of acute "downregulation" of receptors. There appears to be a reduction in numbers or sensitivity of β receptors in hypertensive patients who also have elevated plasma catecholamines. Downregulation is the presumptive explanation for the lack of correlation between plasma catecholamine levels and the blood pressure elevation in patients with pheochromocytoma. Chronic use of β agonists such as terbutaline, isoproterenol, or EPI for the treatment of asthma can result in tachyphylaxis because of downregulation. Even short-term use (1 to 6 hours) of β agonists may cause downregulation of receptor numbers. Downregulation is reversible on termination of the agonist. Chronic treatment of animals with nonselective β blockade causes a 100% increase in the number of β receptors. This accounts for the propranolol withdrawal syndrome in which the acute discontinuation of the β antagonist leaves the α receptors unopposed, in addition to an increased number of β receptors. Clonidine withdrawal can be explained by the same mechanism. Up- or downregulation of receptor numbers may not alter sensitivity of the receptor. Likewise, sensitivity may be increased or decreased in the presence of normal numbers of receptors. The pharmacologic factors affecting up- or downregulation of the α and β receptors are similar.

Autonomic Nervous System Reflexes and Interactions

8 The ANS reflex has been compared to a computer circuit. This control system, as in all reflex systems, has (1) sensors, (2) afferent pathways, (3) CNS integration, and (4) efferent pathways to the receptors and efferent organs. Fine adjustments are made at the local level through positive and negative feedback mechanisms. The baroreceptor is an example. The variable to be controlled (blood pressure) is sensed (carotid sinus), integrated (medullary vasomotor center), and adjusted through specific effector–receptor sites. Drugs or disease can interrupt this circuit at any point. β Blockers may attenuate the effector response, whereas an α agonist such as clonidine may alter both the effector and the integrator functions of blood pressure control.

Baroreceptors

Several reflexes in the cardiovascular system help govern arterial blood pressure, and control cardiac output (CO) and heart rate (HR). The aim of the circulation is to provide blood flow to all the body organs (see Chapter 12). Yet, the most important controlled variable to which the sensors are attuned is blood pressure, a product of the blood flow and vascular resistance. Étienne Marey noted in 1859 that the pulse rate is inversely proportional to the blood pressure, and this is known as Marey law. Subsequently, Hering, Koch, and others demonstrated that the alterations in HR evoked by changes in blood pressure are dependent on baroreceptors located in the aortic arch and the carotid sinuses. These pressure sensors react to alterations in stretch caused by blood pressure. Impulses from the carotid sinus and aortic arch reach the medullary vasomotor center by the glossopharyngeal and vagus nerves, respectively. Increased sensory traffic from the baroreceptors, caused by increased blood pressure, inhibits SNS effector traffic. The relative increase in vagal tone produces vasodilation, slowing of the HR, and a lowering of blood pressure. Real increases in vagal tone occur when blood pressure exceeds normal limits. The Valsalva maneuver can best demonstrate the arterial baroreceptor reflex (Fig. 14-11). The Valsalva maneuver raises the intrathoracic pressure by forced expiration against a closed glottis. The arterial blood pressure rises momentarily as the intrathoracic blood is forced into the heart (increased preload). Sustained intrathoracic pressure diminishes venous return, reduces the CO, and drops the blood pressure. Reflex vasoconstriction and tachycardia ensue. Blood pressure returns to normal with release of the forced expiration, but then briefly "overshoots" because of the vasoconstriction and increased venous return. A slowing of the HR accompanies the overshoot in pressure. The cardiovascular responses to the Valsalva maneuver require an intact ANS circuit from peripheral sensor to peripheral adrenergic receptors. The

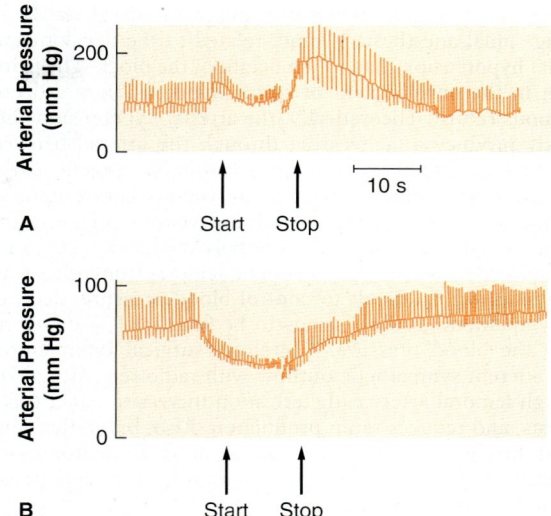

Figure 14-11 A: The normal blood pressure response to the Valsalva maneuver is demonstrated. Pulse rate moves in a reciprocal direction according to Marey law of the heart. **B:** An abnormal Valsalva response is shown in a patient with C5 quadriplegia.

Valsalva maneuver has been used to identify patients at risk for anesthesia due to ANS instability. This was once a major concern in patients receiving drugs that depleted catecholamines, such as reserpine. Dysfunction of the SNS is implicated if exaggerated and prolonged hypotension develops during the forced expiration phase (50% from resting mean arterial pressure). In addition, the overshoot at the end of the Valsalva maneuver is absent. Dysfunction of the PNS can be assumed if the HR does not respond appropriately to the blood pressure changes.

Venous baroreceptors may be more dominant in the moment-to-moment regulation of CO. Baroreceptors in the right atrium and great veins produce an increase in HR when stretched by increased right atrial pressure. Reduced venous pressure decreases HR. Unlike the arterial baroreceptors, venous sensors are not thought to alter vascular tone; however, venoconstriction is postulated to occur when atrial pressures decline. Stretch of the venous receptors produces changes in HR opposite to those produced when the arterial pressure sensors are stimulated. The arterial and venous pressure receptors separately monitor two of the four major determinants of CO: afterload and preload, respectively. Venous baroreceptors sample preload by stretch of the atrium. Arterial baroreceptors survey resistance, or afterload, as reflected in the mean arterial pressure. Afterload and preload produce opposite effects on CO; thus, one should not be surprised that the venous and arterial baroreceptors produce opposing effects after a similar stretch stimulus—pressure.

Bainbridge described the venous baroreceptor reflex and demonstrated that it can be abolished by vagal resection. Numerous investigators have confirmed the acceleration of the HR in response to volume. However, the magnitude and direction of the HR response are dependent on the prevailing HR at the time of stimulation. The denervated, transplanted mammalian heart also accelerates in response to volume loading. HR, like CO, can apparently be adjusted to the quantity of blood entering the heart. The Bainbridge reflex relates to the characteristic but paradoxical slowing of the heart seen with spinal anesthesia. Blockade of the SNS levels of T1–T4 ablates the efferent limb of the cardiac accelerator nerves. This source of cardiac deceleration is obvious, as the vagus nerve is unopposed. However, bradycardia during spinal anesthesia is more related to the development of arterial hypotension than to the height of the block. The primary defect in the development of spinal hypotension is a decrease in venous return. Theoretically, the arterial hypotension should reflexly produce a tachycardia through the arterial baroreceptors. Instead, bradycardia is more common. Greene suggests that in the unmedicated person, the venous baroreceptors are dominant over the arterial. A reduced venous pressure, therefore, slows HR.[24] In contrast, humorally mediated tachycardia is the usual response to hypotension or acidosis from other causes. In patients with difficult to control blood pressure, decreasing the sympathetic outflow seems to be beneficial in better regulating the blood pressure. Therefore, surgical interruption of renal efferent sympathetic outflow with radiofrequency ablation through femoral artery catheterization increases natriuresis and diuresis, and reduces renin production. Also, baroreflex sensitization through an implantable carotid sinus stimulator seems to be extremely promising in patients with refractory hypertension, with more research underway.[25]

Denervated Heart

Reflex modulation of the adrenergic agonists is best seen in the denervated transplant heart, which retains the recipient's innervated sinoatrial node and the donor's denervated sinoatrial node[26] (see Chapter 51). NE infusion in the transplanted heart produces a slowing of the recipient's atrial rate through vagal feedback as the blood pressure rises. In the unmodulated donor heart, atrial rate increases. The baroreceptors are therefore not operant in the transplanted heart. Isoproterenol, a pure β agonist, increases the discharge rate of both the recipient and donor node by direct action, with the donor rate near doubling that of the recipient node. Atropine accelerates the recipient's atrial rate, whereas no effect is seen on the donor rate, which now controls HR.

β blockade produces comparable slowing of the sinoatrial node of both recipient and donor. The exercise capability of the denervated heart is conspicuously reduced by β blockade, presumably because of its reliance on circulating catecholamines. Propranolol has also been demonstrated to reduce the β response to chronotropic effects of NE and isoproterenol in the transplanted heart. The CO of the transplanted heart varies appropriately with changes in preload and afterload.

Interaction of Autonomic Nervous System Receptors

Strong interactions have been noted between SNS and PNS nerves in organs that receive dual, antagonistic innervation. Release of NE at the presynaptic terminal is modified by the PNS. For example, vagal inhibition of left ventricular contractility is accentuated as the level of SNS activity is raised. This interaction is termed "accentuated antagonism" and is mediated by a combination of presynaptic and postsynaptic mechanisms. The coronary arteries present an example of this phenomenon and deserve special attention.

The myocardium and coronary vessels are abundantly supplied with adrenergic and cholinergic fibers. Strong activity of both α and β receptors has been demonstrated in the coronary vascular bed. Selective stimulation of both the α_1 and postsynaptic α_2 receptors increases coronary vascular resistance, whereas selective α blockade eliminates this effect. Therefore, both β_1 and α_1 adrenoreceptors are present on coronary arteries and accessible to NE released by sympathetic nerves.[6,15]

The presynaptic adrenergic terminals of the myocardium and coronary vessels, like all blood vessels studied, contain muscarinic receptors.[11] Recent observations confirm that muscarinic agents and vagal stimulation, acting on the presynaptic, SNS muscarinic receptor, inhibit the release of NE in a manner similar to that of the presynaptic α_2 and DA_2 receptors (Fig. 14-9). Conversely, blockade of the muscarinic receptors with atropine markedly augments the positive inotropic responses to catecholamines.[6] Suppression of NE release explains, in part, vagal-induced attenuation of the inotropic response to strong SNS stimulation (accentuated antagonism) and only a weak negative inotropic effect of vagal stimulation when there is low background SNS activity. This may also explain why vagal activity reduces the vulnerability of the myocardium to fibrillation during infusions of NE.

ACh may cause coronary spasm during periods of high SNS tone.[6] Inhibition of NE release by presynaptic adrenergic muscarinic receptors of the smooth muscle of coronary vessels would lessen the coronary relaxation normally produced by NE on the β_1 receptor (Fig. 14-9). In anesthetized dogs, the rate of NE outflow into the coronary sinus blood, evoked by cardiac SNS stimulation, is markedly diminished by simultaneous vagal efferent stimulation.[27] This action is known to be prevented by atropine, which also causes coronary vasodilation.

Interaction with Other Regulatory Systems

The ANS is integrally related to several endocrine systems that ultimately summate to control blood pressure and regulate homeostasis. These include the renin–angiotensin system, ADH, glucocorticoids, and insulin (see Chapter 46). Both α and β receptors have been found in the endocrine pancreas and modulate insulin release (Table 14-4). β Stimulation increases insulin release, whereas α stimulation decreases it. The overall importance of this interaction is not entirely clear, but decreased tolerance to glucose and potassium has been noted in subjects taking β-blocking drugs. The renin–angiotensin system 2 is a complex endocrine system that modulates both blood pressure and water–electrolyte homeostasis (Fig. 14-12). Renin is a proteolytic enzyme released by the cells of the juxtaglomerular apparatus of the renal cortex. Renin acts on plasma angiotensinogen to form angiotensin I. Angiotensin I is then converted to angiotensin II by a converting enzyme in the lung. Angiotensin II is a powerful angiotensin direct arterial vasoconstrictor. It also acts on the adrenal cortex to release aldosterone and on the adrenal medulla to release EPI. In addition to its direct effects on vascular smooth muscle, angiotensin II augments NE release via presynaptic receptors, thus enhancing peripheral SNS tone. Captopril, enalapril, and lisinopril inhibit the action of angiotensin-converting enzyme, thus preventing the conversion of angiotensin I to angiotensin II. Renin is released in response to hyponatremia, decreased renal perfusion pressure, and ANS stimulation via β receptors on juxtaglomerular cells. Changes in sympathetic tone may thus alter renin release and affect homeostasis in a variety of ways. The ANS is also intimately related to adrenocortical function. As outlined above, glucocorticoid release modulates phenylethanolamine-N-methyltransferase formation and thus synthesis of EPI. Glucocorticoids are also important in regulating the response of peripheral tissues to changes in SNS tone. Thus, the ANS is intimately related to other homeostatic mechanisms.

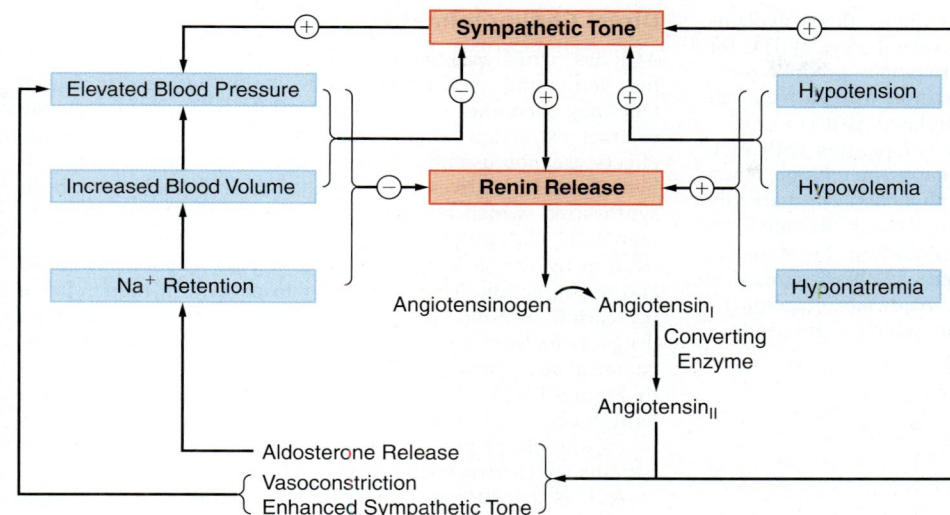

Figure 14-12 The interactions of the renin–angiotensin and SNS in regulating homeostasis are shown schematically along with the physiologic variables that modulate their function. Arrows with a plus sign (+) represent stimulation, and those with a minus sign (–) represent inhibition.

Clinical Autonomic Nervous System Pharmacology

[9] The clinical application of ANS pharmacology is based on the knowledge of ANS anatomy, physiology, and molecular pharmacology. Drugs that modify ANS activity can be classified by their site of action, mechanism of action, or the pathology for which they are most commonly used. Antihypertensive drugs are an example of the third category. This classification is a matter of degree because considerable functional overlap occurs. An example of classification by site relates to the ganglionic agonists or blocking agents. ANS drugs can be further categorized as those that act at the prejunctional membrane and those acting postjunctionally. They can then be more specifically classified by the predominant receptor or receptors on which they act.

Mode of Action

ANS drugs may be broadly classified by mode of action according to their mimetic or lytic actions. This may also be termed agonist or antagonist. A sympathomimetic, such as ephedrine, mimics SNS sympathetic activity by stimulation of adrenergic receptor sites both directly and indirectly. Sympatholytic drugs cause dissolution of SNS activity at these same receptor sites. β Receptor blockers are examples of sympatholytic drugs. Several modes of ANS drug action become evident when one follows the cascade of neurotransmission. Drugs that act on prejunctional membranes may therefore (1) interfere with transmitter synthesis (α-methyl paratyrosine), (2) interfere with transmitter storage (reserpine), (3) interfere with transmitter release (clonidine), (4) stimulate transmitter release (ephedrine), or (5) interfere with reuptake of transmitter (cocaine). Drugs may also (6) modify metabolism of the neurotransmitter in the synaptic cleft (anticholinesterase). Drugs acting at postjunctional sites may (7) directly stimulate postjunctional receptors and (8) interfere with the transmitter agonist at the postjunctional receptor.

The ultimate response of an effector organ to an agonist or antagonist depends on (1) the drug, (2) its plasma concentration, (3) the number of receptors in the effector organ, (4) binding by the receptor, (5) the concurrent activities of other drugs and hormones, (6) the cellular metabolic status, and (7) reflex adjustments by the organism.

Ganglionic Drugs

SNS and PNS ganglia are pharmacologically similar in that the transmission through these ANS ganglia is effected by ACh (Fig. 14-2). Most ganglionic agonists and antagonists are not selective and affect SNS and PNS ganglia equally. This nonselective property creates many undesirable and unpredictable side effects, which have limited the clinical usefulness of this category of drug.

Agonists

There are essentially no clinically useful ganglionic agonists. Nicotine is the prototypical ganglionic agonist. In low doses, it stimulates ANS ganglia and the neuromuscular junction of striated muscle. High doses produce ganglionic and neuromuscular blockade. The protean side effects of nicotinic stimulation render it useful only as an investigative tool.

Antagonists

Drugs that interfere with neurotransmission at ANS ganglia are known as ganglionic blocking agents. Nicotine, in high doses, is the prototypical ganglionic blocking agent also; however, early stimulatory nicotinic activity can be blocked both at the ganglia and at the muscle end plates with other ganglionic blockers and muscle relaxants, respectively, without blocking muscarinic effects. Ganglionic blockers produce their nicotinic effects by competing, mimicking, or interfering with ACh metabolism. Hexamethonium, trimethaphan, and pentolinium produce a selective nondepolarizing blockade of neurotransmission at ANS ganglia without producing nicotinic neuromuscular blockade. They compete with ACh in the ganglia without stimulating the receptors. The introduction of drugs that produce vasodilation directly or by action on the SNS vasomotor center has made the ganglionic blockers obsolete. D-Tubocurare (dTC) produces a competitive nondepolarizing block of both motor end plates and ANS ganglia. The action of motor paralysis predominates, but the concomitant ganglionic blockade at higher doses explains part of the hypotensive effect often seen with the use of dTC for muscle relaxation. Anticholinesterase drugs may produce nicotinic type ganglionic blockade by competition with ACh as well as by persistent depolarization via accumulated ACh.

Trimethaphan produces blockade by competition with ACh for receptors, thus stabilizing the postsynaptic membrane. However, side effects and rapid onset tachyphylaxis have markedly reduced its use in anesthesia.[28] The patient's pupils become fixed and dilated during administration, which obscures eye signs, an important consideration for neurosurgery. In this regard, it is distinctly inferior to nitroprusside. The major advantage of trimethaphan is its short duration of action, which is the result of pseudocholinesterase hydrolysis.

Cholinergic Drugs

Muscarinic Agonists

The cholinomimetic muscarinic drugs act at sites in the body where ACh is the neurotransmitter of the nerve impulse. These drugs may be divided into three groups, the first two of which are direct muscarinic agonists. The third group acts indirectly. These groups are choline esters (ACh, methacholine, carbamylcholine, bethanechol), alkaloids (pilocarpine, muscarine), and anticholinesterases (physostigmine, neostigmine, pyridostigmine, edrophonium, echothiophate).

Direct Cholinomimetics

ACh has virtually no therapeutic applications because of its diffuse action and rapid hydrolysis by cholinesterase (Fig. 14-5). One may encounter the use of topical ACh (1%) drops during cataract extraction when a rapid miosis is desired. Systemic effects are not usually seen because of the rapidity of ACh hydrolysis. Derivatives of ACh, other choline esters, have been synthesized, which possess more selective muscarinic activity than ACh. They differ from ACh in being more resistant to inactivation by cholinesterase and thus having a more prolonged and useful action. They also differ from ACh in their relative muscarinic and nicotinic activities. The best studied of these drugs are methacholine, bethanechol, and carbamylcholine. The chemical structures of ACh and these choline esters are shown in Figure 14-13. Their pharmacologic actions are compared with those of ACh in Table 14-5. These are not important drugs in anesthesiology practice but anesthesiologists may encounter patients who are receiving them. (See Chapter 23.)

ACh is a quaternary ammonium compound that interacts with postsynaptic receptors, causing conformational membrane changes. This results in increased permeability to small ions and, thus, depolarization. All the receptors translate the reversible binding of ACh into openings of discrete channels in excitable membranes, allowing Na^+ and K^+ ions to flow along their electrochemical gradients. Structure–activity relationships point to the presence of two important binding sites on the receptor, an esteratic site that binds the ester end of the molecule and an ionic

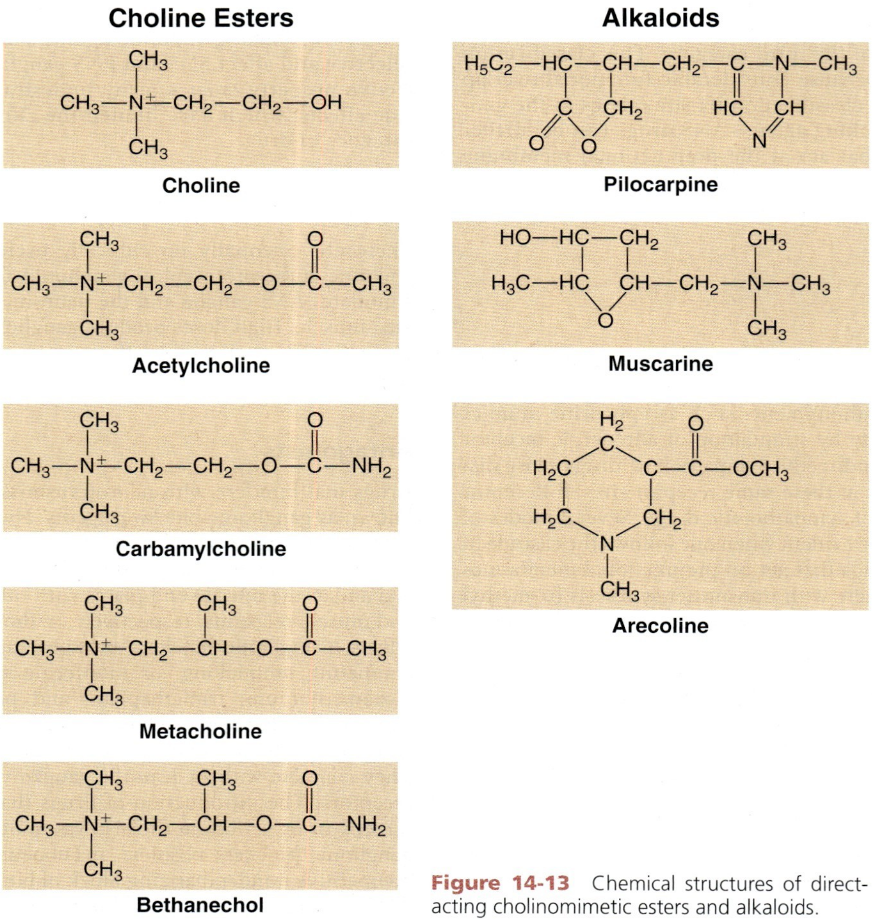

Figure 14-13 Chemical structures of direct-acting cholinomimetic esters and alkaloids.

Table 14-5 Comparative Muscarinic Actions of Direct Cholinomimetic Agents

	Systemic				
	Acetylcholine	Methacholine	Carbamylcholine	Bethanechol	Pilocarpine
Esterase Hydrolysis	+++	+	0	0	0
Eye (Topical)					
Iris	++	++	+++	+++	+++
Ciliary	++	++	+++	+++	++
Heart					
Rate	−	−		−	
Contractility	−	−		−	
Conduction	−	−		−	
Smooth Muscle					
Vascular	−	−		−	−
Bronchial	++	++	+	+	++
Gastrointestinal motility	++	++	+++	+++	++
Gastrointestinal sphincters	−	−	−	−	++
Biliary	++	++	+++	+++	++
Bladder					
Detrusor	++	++	+++	+++	++
Sphincter	−	−	−	−	−
Exocrine Glands					
Respiratory	+++	++	+++	++	++++
Salivary	++	++	++	++	+++++
Pharyngeal	++	++	++	++	++++
Lacrimal	++	++	++	++	++++
Sweat	++	++	++	++	+++++
Gastrointestinal acid and secretions	++	++	++	++	++++
Nicotinic Actions	+++	+	+++	−	+++

+, stimulation; −, inhibition.

site that binds the quaternary amine portion (Fig. 14-5). Subtle changes in the structure of the compound can markedly alter the responses among different tissue groups. The degree of muscarinic activity falls if the acetyl group is replaced, but this confers a resistance to enzymatic hydrolysis. Bethanechol is resistant to hydrolysis but possesses mainly muscarinic activity. β-Methyl substitution produces methacholine, which is less resistant to hydrolysis and is primarily a muscarinic agonist. Methacholine slows the heart and dilates peripheral blood vessels. It is used to terminate supraventricular tachydysrhythmias, especially paroxysmal tachycardia, when other measures have failed. It also increases intestinal tone. Methacholine should not be given to patients with asthma. Hypertensive patients may also develop marked hypotension. Side effects are those of PNS stimulation such as nausea, vomiting, and flushed sweating. Overdose is treated with atropine. Bethanechol is relatively selective for the gastrointestinal and urinary tracts. In usual doses it does not slow the heart or lower the blood pressure. Bethanechol is of value in treating postoperative abdominal distention (nonobstructive paralytic ileus), gastric atony following bilateral vagotomy, congenital megacolon, nonobstructive urinary retention, and some cases of neurogenic bladder.

Direct-acting cholinomimetic alkaloids include muscarine and pilocarpine. They act at the same sites as ACh, and their effects are similar to those of ACh as described in Table 14-5. There are no uses for these drugs in anesthesiology. Pilocarpine is the only drug of this group used therapeutically in the United States. Its sole use is for the treatment of glaucoma, for which it is the standard. It is used as a topical miotic drug in ophthalmologic practice to reduce intraocular pressure in glaucoma.

Muscarinic agonists are particularly dangerous in patients with myasthenia gravis (who are receiving anticholinesterases), bulbar palsy, cardiac disease, asthma, peptic ulcer, progressive muscular atrophy, or mechanical intestinal obstruction or urinary retention because they intensify these conditions.

Indirect Cholinomimetics

The indirect-acting cholinomimetic drugs are of greater importance to the anesthesiologist than are the direct-acting drugs. These drugs produce cholinomimetic effects indirectly as a result of inhibition or inactivation of the enzyme acetylcholinesterase, which normally destroys ACh by hydrolysis. They are referred to as cholinesterase inhibitors or anticholinesterases. Most of these drugs inhibit both acetylcholinesterase and pseudocholinesterase. Inhibition of acetylcholinesterase permits the accumulation of ACh transmitter in the synapse, resulting in intense PNS activity similar to that of the direct cholinomimetic agents.

The accumulation of ACh by the anticholinesterases potentially can produce all of the following: (1) stimulation of muscarinic receptors at ANS-effect organs, (2) stimulation followed by depression of all ANS ganglia and skeletal muscle (nicotinic), and (3) stimulation with later depression of cholinergic receptor sites in the CNS. All of these effects may be seen with lethal doses of anticholinesterase drugs, but therapeutic doses only produce the first two.

Actions of therapeutic significance of the anticholinesterase drugs to the anesthesiologist concern the eye, the intestine, and the neuromuscular junction. The effects of anticholinesterases are useful in the treatment of myasthenia gravis, glaucoma, and atony of the gastrointestinal and urinary tracts. Anticholinesterase drugs are used routinely in anesthesia to reverse nondepolarizing neuromuscular block. The most prominent pharmacologic effects of the anticholinesterase drugs are muscarinic. Their most useful actions are their nicotinic effects. Muscarinic activity is evoked by lower concentrations of ACh than are necessary to produce the desired nicotinic effect. For example, the anticholinesterase neostigmine reverses neuromuscular blockade by increasing ACh concentration at the muscle end plate, a nicotinic receptor. Nicotinic reversal of neuromuscular blockade can usually be produced safely only when the patient has been protected by atropine or other muscarinic blockers. This prevents the untoward muscarinic effects of bradycardia, hypotension, bronchospasm, or intestinal spasm. Reversal of neuromuscular blockade in patients who have had bowel anastomosis was at one time a major controversy. (See Chapter 21.) Some thought that the muscarinic effects of anticholinesterase drugs (hypermotility) increased the risk of anastomotic leakage whereas others found no association between their use and subsequent breakdown. National experience has favored the latter opinion.

Clinically, anticholinesterase drugs may be divided into two types: the reversible and nonreversible cholinesterase inhibitors.[28] Reversible cholinesterase inhibitors delay the hydrolysis of ACh from 1 to 8 hours. Nonreversible drugs are so named because their inhibitory effects may last from days to weeks. The differences in duration of various anticholinesterases likely depend on whether they inhibit the anionic or esteratic site of acetylcholinesterase. Therefore, the anticholinesterase drugs have also been pharmacologically subdivided. Drugs that inhibit the anionic site are called competitive inhibitors. Their action is due to competition between the anticholinesterase and ACh for the anionic site. These drugs tend to be short-acting. Edrophonium is an example of this type. Drugs that inhibit the esteratic site are called acid-transferring inhibitors. These drugs include the longer-acting neostigmine, pyridostigmine, and physostigmine.

Most of the reversible cholinesterase inhibitors are quaternary ammonium compounds and do not cross the blood–brain barrier. Physostigmine is a tertiary amine that readily passes into the CNS (Fig. 14-14). It produces central muscarinic stimulation and, thus, is not used to reverse neuromuscular blockade but can be used to treat atropine poisoning. Conversely, atropine is used to treat physostigmine poisoning. Physostigmine has also been found to be a specific antidote in the treatment of postoperative delirium (see below, Central Anticholinergic Syndrome).[3]

The irreversible cholinesterase inhibitors are mostly organophosphate compounds. The organophosphate compounds are highly lipid-soluble, readily pass into the CNS, and are rapidly absorbed through the skin. They are used as the active ingredient in potent insecticides and chemical warfare agents known as nerve gases (see Chapter 53). The only therapeutic drug of this group is echothiophate, which is available in the form of topical drops for the treatment of glaucoma. Its primary advantage is its prolonged duration of action. Topical absorption is variable but considerable. Echothiophate can remain effective for 2 or 3 weeks following cessation of therapy. A history of use of echothiophate is important in avoiding prolonged action of succinylcholine, which requires pseudocholinesterase for its hydrolysis. Organophosphate poisoning manifests all the signs and symptoms of excess ACh. The antidote cartridges dispensed to troops to counter the effects of anticholinesterase nerve gases contain only atropine, which would effectively counter the muscarinic effects of the gas; however, atropine does little to counter the high-dose nicotinic muscle paralysis or the central ventilation depression that contributes to death from nerve gases. Treatment requires high doses of atropine, 35 to 70 mcg/kg IV every 3 to 10 minutes until muscarinic symptoms abate. Lower doses at less frequent intervals may be required for several days. Central ventilatory depression and weakness require respiratory support and specific therapy of the cholinesterase lesion. Pralidoxime has been reported to reactivate cholinesterase activity by hydrolysis of the phosphate enzyme complex. It is particularly effective with parathion poisoning and is the only cholinesterase reactivator available in the United States.[28]

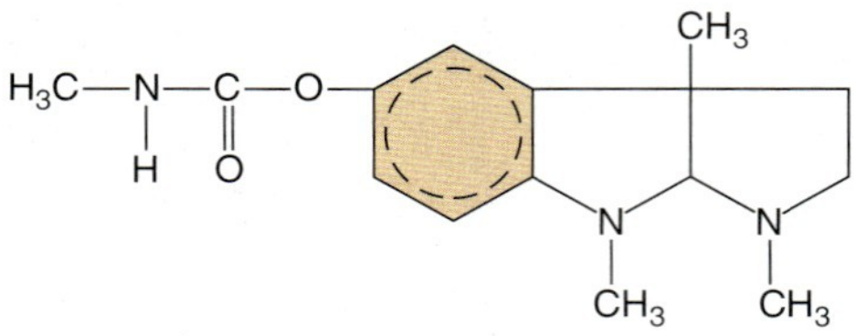

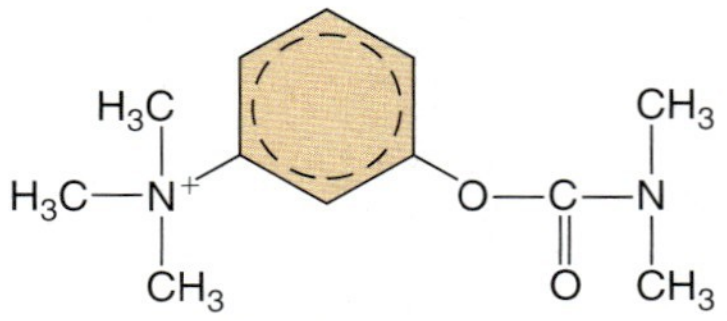

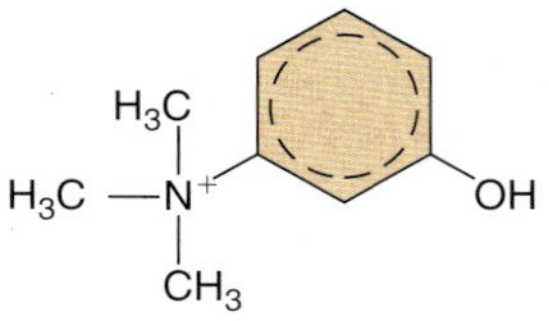

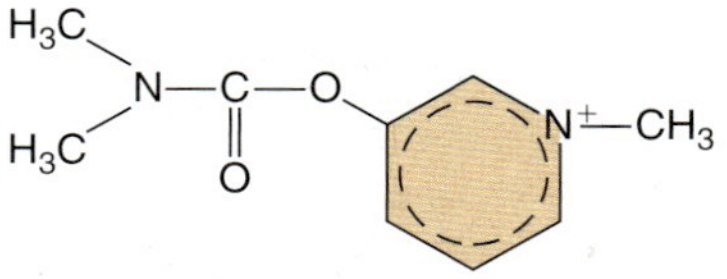

Figure 14-14 Structural formulas of clinically useful reversible anticholinesterase drugs. Physostigmine is a tertiary amine and crosses the blood–brain barrier. It is useful in treating the central anticholinergic syndrome.

Muscarinic Antagonists

Muscarinic antagonist refers to a specific drug action for which the term anticholinergic is widely used. Any drug that interferes with the action of ACh as a transmitter can be considered

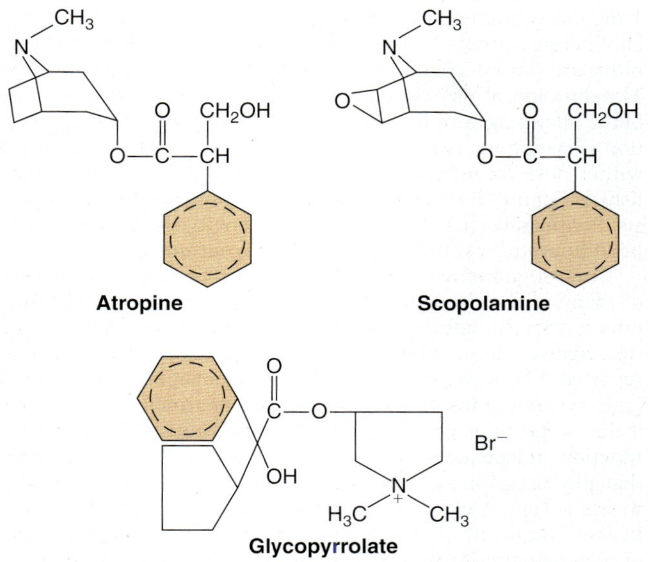

Figure 14-15 Structural formulas of the clinically useful antimuscarinic drugs.

Atropine-like Drugs

Atropine, scopolamine, and glycopyrrolate are the most commonly used muscarinic antagonists used in anesthesia (Fig. 14-15). The actions of these drugs include inhibition of salivary, bronchial, pancreatic, and gastrointestinal secretions, and they antagonize the muscarinic side effects of anticholinesterases during reversal of muscle relaxants. Historically, atropine was introduced to anesthesia practice to prevent excessive secretions during ether anesthesia and to prevent vagal bradycardia during the administration of chloroform.[28] Antimuscarinic agents do not inhibit transmission equally, and there are marked variations in sensitivity at different muscarinic sites owing to differences in penetration and affinities of the various receptors. Differences in relative potency between the different antimuscarinics are outlined in Table 14-6. Atropine and scopolamine are tertiary amines (Fig. 14-15) and easily penetrate the blood–brain barrier and placenta. Glycopyrrolate is a quaternary amine that, like the reversible anticholinesterase drugs, does not easily penetrate these barriers. Glycopyrrolate, a synthetic antimuscarinic, has gained popularity because it avoids the central effects of the other two

an anticholinergic agent. The term anticholinergic refers to a broader classification that also includes the nicotinic antagonists.

drugs. Clinical observations suggested that bradycardia associated with spinal anesthesia is refractory to the administration of glycopyrrolate, and that atropine and ephedrine are the drugs of choice in order to prevent a possible cardiac arrest. Nevertheless, recent data (69 parturients) demonstrated that prophylactic administration of glycopyrrolate does prevent bradycardia associated with spinal anesthesia for cesarean delivery.[29] Atropine and scopolamine have notable CNS effects that are dissimilar. Scopolamine differs from atropine mainly in its central depressant effects, which produce sedation, amnesia, and euphoria. Such properties are widely used for premedication for cardiac patients in combination with morphine and a major tranquilizer. Scopolamine also has been used to induce amnesia in patients who have a high risk for intraoperative awareness, such as trauma victims who are hemodynamically unstable and cannot receive adequate anesthesia. Atropine, as a premedication, has slight effects on the CNS, including mild stimulation. Higher doses such as those given for reversal of muscle relaxants (1 to 2 mg) may produce restlessness, disorientation, hallucinations, and delirium (see below, Central Anticholinergic Syndrome).

Atropine is useful in increasing CO when sinus bradycardia due to vagal stimulation is present. Atropine and scopolamine are noted to produce a paradoxical bradycardia when given in low doses. Scopolamine (0.1 to 0.2 mg) usually causes more slowing than atropine but also produces less cardiac acceleration at higher doses. The usual intramuscular premedicant doses of scopolamine cause either a decrease or no change in HR. Atropine may also produce sympathomimetic effects by blocking presynaptic muscarinic receptors found on adrenergic nerve terminals.[30] ACh stimulation of these receptors inhibits NE release, and blockade by atropine releases this inhibition (see Cholinergic Receptors: Muscarinic). Atropine-like drugs that cross the blood–brain barrier also produce dilation of the pupil (mydriasis) and paralysis of accommodation (cycloplegia). Atropine-like drugs are widely used in ophthalmology as mydriatics and cycloplegics. Atropine is contraindicated in patients with narrow-angle glaucoma (see Chapter 48). Pupillary dilation thickens the peripheral part of the iris, which narrows the iridocorneal angle. This leads to impaired drainage of aqueous humor, and increase of the intraocular pressure. Doses of atropine used for premedication have little effect in this regard, whereas equal doses of scopolamine cause mydriasis. Prudence would dictate avoidance of either agent in patients with narrow-angle glaucoma. The need for antimuscarinic premedication is questionable in this situation.

Atropine and scopolamine also possess antiemetic action. Atropine, however, reduces the opening pressure of the lower esophageal sphincter, which theoretically increases the risk of passive regurgitation. The belladonna alkaloids (atropine and scopolamine) also block ACh transmission to sweat glands, which, although they are cholinergic, are innervated by the SNS.

Table 14-6 Comparison of Antimuscarinic Drugs

	Duration		CNS	GI Tone	Gastric Acid	Airway Secretions[a]	Heart Rate
	IV	IM (hr)					
Atropine	15–30 min	2–4	++	–	–	–	+++[c]
Scopolamine	30–60 min	4–6	+++[b]	–	–	–	–0[c]
Glycopyrrolate	2–4 hr	6–8	0	–	–	–	+0

IV, intravenous; IM, intramuscular; GI, gastrointestinal.
[a]Secretions may be reduced by inspissations.
[b]CNS effect often manifest as sedation before stimulation.
[c]May decelerate initially.

Antimuscarinic agents produce antinicotinic actions at higher doses and result in important actions on CNS transmission that are pharmacologically similar to the postganglionic cholinergic function. Atropine is best avoided where tachycardia would be harmful, as may occur in thyrotoxicosis, pheochromocytoma, or obstructive coronary artery disease. Atropine should be avoided in hyperpyrexial patients because it inhibits sweating.

Central Anticholinergic Syndrome

The belladonna alkaloids have long been known to produce undesirable side effects ranging from stupor (scopolamine) to delirium (atropine). This syndrome has been called postoperative delirium, atropine toxicity, and central anticholinergic syndrome. Biochemical studies have demonstrated abundant muscarinic ACh receptors in the brain that can be affected by any drug possessing antimuscarinic activity and capable of crossing the blood–brain barrier. Hundreds of drugs exist that meet these criteria and with which this syndrome has been associated. Table 14-7 lists some of those drugs.[3] High doses of atropinic alkaloids rapidly produce dryness of the mouth, blurred vision with photophobia (mydriasis), hot and dry skin (flushed), and fever. Mental symptoms range from sedation, stupor, and coma to anxiety, restlessness, disorientation, hallucinations, and delirium. Convulsions may occur if lethal poisoning has occurred. Although an alarming reaction may occur, fatalities are rare. Intoxication is usually short-lived and followed by amnesia. These reactions can be controlled by the intravenous injection of physostigmine. Physostigmine is an anticholinesterase that, by virtue of being a tertiary amine, readily passes into the CNS to counter antimuscarinic activity. It should be given slowly in 1 mg doses, not exceeding 3 mg, to avoid producing peripheral cholinergic activity. Neostigmine, pyridostigmine, and edrophonium are not effective because they cannot pass into the CNS. The duration of physostigmine action may be shorter than that of the offending antimuscarinic agent and require repeated injection if symptoms recur. Physostigmine appears safe when used within dose recommendations and when indications are established. Central disorientation alone does not establish a diagnosis. Peripheral signs of antimuscarinic activity should be present in addition to a central anticholinergic syndrome.

Physostigmine has been reported to reverse the CNS effects of many of the drugs listed in Table 14-7, including antihistamines, tricyclic antidepressants, and tranquilizers. Reversal of the sedative effects of opioids and benzodiazepines has also been reported.[31] However, anticholinesterase agents potentiate cholinergic synaptic transmission and increase neuronal activity, even if no receptor antagonist is present. Thus, arousal may not be a function independent of its cholinesterase activity, and claims that physostigmine is a nonspecific CNS stimulant may not be warranted and could, in fact, be dangerous. These considerations, in association with possible significant bradycardia, made the use of physostigmine fairly scarce in the postanesthesia care units.

Autonomic Syndromes and Autonomic Regulation

Recent research in different clinical fields seems to connect the autonomic system and its regulation with the course of various diseases, which can prove its importance beyond the classical role of fight or flight.

Table 14-7 Antimuscarinic Compounds Associated with Central Anticholinergic Syndrome

Belladonna Alkaloids
Atropine sulfate
Scopolamine hydrobromide

Synthetic and Natural Tertiary Amine Compounds
Dicyclomine antispasmodic with local anesthetic activity
Thiphenamil antispasmodic with local anesthetic activity
Procaine
Cocaine
Cyclopentolate mydriatic

Quaternary Derivatives of Belladonna Alkaloids
Methscopolamine bromide—antispasmodic
Homatropine methylbromide—sedative, antispasmodic
Homatropine hydrobromide—ophthalmic solution—mydriatic

Synthetic Quaternary Compounds
Methantheline bromide
Propantheline bromide

Antihistamines
Chlorpheniramine
Diphenhydramine

Plants
Deadly nightshade (atropine)
Bittersweet
Potato leaves and sprouts
Jimson or loco weed
Coca plant (cocaine)

Over-the-Counter
Asthmador—atropine-like
Sleep-Eze (diphenhydramine)—scopolamine sedation
Sominex (diphenhydramine)—scopolamine sedation

Antiparkinson Drugs
Benztropine
Trihexphenidyl
Biperiden
Ethopropazine
Procyclidine

Antipsychotic Drugs
Chlorpromazine
Thioridazine
Haloperidol
Droperidol
Promethazine

Tricyclic Antidepressants
Amitriptyline
Imipramine
Desipramine

Synthetic Opioids
Meperidine
Methadone

This type of association between the afferent-pathway-sensing proinflammatory cytokines, which is informing the brain with subsequent vagal feedback from the nucleus tractus solitarius to the periphery and release of ACh, may be a mechanism by which an anti-inflammatory action occurs, with possible vagal regulation of the oncologic processes; it may ultimately lead to extended survival of these patients, which is a promising avenue, especially since vagal activity may be manipulated by behavioral, surgical, and pharmacologic interventions, including the use of β-blockers.[33]

At the onset of temporal seizures, there appears to be a decrease in parasympathetic tone, which returns slowly to normal at the end of the seizure episode. This phenomenon is inversely correlated with patient's age and duration of the seizure episode, and also with postictal hypoxemia, which in extreme cases may increase the risk for patient death.[34]

Even more importantly, cardiac autonomic dysregulation plays a central role in the evolution of several cardiovascular syndromes such as hypertension, arrhythmias, heart failure, and even myocardial infarction.[35] Therefore, addressing the ANS and specifically the upregulation of sympathetic nerve abnormalities in heart failure may have a great impact upon treatment of these conditions.

Explicitly, higher sympathetic tone may precipitate malignant arrhythmias. Therefore, some forms of autonomic testing may be useful to predict which patients are at risk, and subsequently decide on how to proceed with the management. Thus, cardiac autonomic testing includes heart rate variability, baroreflex sensitivity, heart rate turbulence, heart rate deceleration capacity, and T-wave alternans. Of the possible occurring pathology, one can name a few, such as atrial fibrillation, ventricular tachyarrhythmias due to ischemia, cardiomyopathy, heart failure, prolonged QT syndrome, Brugada syndrome, and idiopathic ventricular fibrillation.[35] Implicitly, vagal nerve stimulation is a possible avenue for the management of these arrhythmias as well as heart failure.[36]

Some authors suggest that atrial fibrillation may be due to simultaneous and thus imbalanced discharge of both sympathetic and parasympathetic discharges, with the stellate ganglion and vagus nerve playing an essential part in this process. Renal denervation has been proposed as an adjunct therapy for hypertension, atrial fibrillation, and ventricular arrhythmias, since it appears to lead to a reduction in heart rate, as well as atrioventricular conduction, and therefore it decreases the secretion of NE. Acupuncture has been proposed as a useful, albeit less traditional, tool for atrial fibrillation management. Other possible avenues for further research as well as therapeutic interventions include low-level vagus nerve stimulation, spinal cord stimulation, left cardiac sympathetic denervation, ganglionated plexus ablation, and cutaneous stimulation, which may prove to be a better alternative in patients who cannot tolerate pharmacologic treatment; some of these techniques can be utilized as well for patients with chronic heart failure.[37–40] Explicitly, patients with resistant hypertension may benefit from bilateral renal nerve ablation by catheters delivering high-frequency ultrasound, as well as bilateral, and more recently unilateral carotid baroreceptor stimulation via an implanted stimulator. However, some negative results have been found as well, with no significant difference between tested subjects, which leads to the need for more randomized studies to elucidate this important clinical issue.[41] There are still some unanswered questions regarding the use of β blockers in patients with heart failure, especially since central inhibition of SNS seems to be associated with increase in mortality; therefore it appears that a better approach remains with receptor inhibition, and that the β blockers' beneficial effects reside in counteracting the effects of tachycardia.[42]

Even beyond our ability to manipulate the ANS, it appears that just by observing a cohort of patients admitted to the Emergency Department, one can predict their short-term mortality by determining their deceleration capacity, a factor assessed using heart rate and R-R interval, which ultimately appear to be significantly lower in nonsurvivors rather than in survivors.[43] In addition, autonomic impairment in patients with traumatic brain injury, which is measured by heart rate variability and baroreflex sensitivity, appears to worsen the risk of death in these patients.[44] The ANS seems to be implicated as a cause of sudden cardiac death in epilepsy by several possible mechanisms, such as long or short QT interval, Brugada syndrome, Dravet syndrome, decreased heart rate variability, chronic autonomic changes, ventricular arrhythmias, bradycardia, asystole, and antiepileptic medications.[45] Also, obese patients with insulin resistance may benefit from sympathetic blockade, either with pharmacologic methods or through renal denervation, but more studies are needed in the future for complete elucidation of these mechanisms.[46]

Horner Syndrome

Horner syndrome, also known as oculosympathetic paresis, classically manifests as miosis, ptosis, and anhidrosis (Fig. 14-16). Its occurrence is the result of a lesion alongside a three-neuron adrenergic pathway from the hypothalamus, through the brachial plexus to the superior cervical ganglion, and then through the cavernous sinus within the adventitia of the internal carotid artery toward the eye. There it converges with the ophthalmic division of the trigeminal nerve, and it ends up innervating the iris dilator muscle, Muller's muscle, which induces a lower lid retraction as well as minor portion of upper lid elevation.

The causes of Horner syndrome are stroke, tumor, trauma, demyelinating diseases, dissections, or aneurysms of the internal carotid artery, as well as idiopathic events.

It is essential to differentiate more precisely the location of the injury along the sympathetic tract, such as first-, second-, or third-order neuron in order to facilitate more specific testing, which will lead to a more accurate diagnosis. For example, injuries along the first-order neuron include commonly lateral medullary infarction, as well as strokes, tumors, and demyelinating afflictions, and usually are associated with other neurologic signs such as weakness, sensory deficits, hoarseness, and possible vertigo. Second-order neuron injuries include apical pulmonary tumors and thyroid malignancies. Several regional anesthesia procedures such as epidural nerve blocks may produce Horner

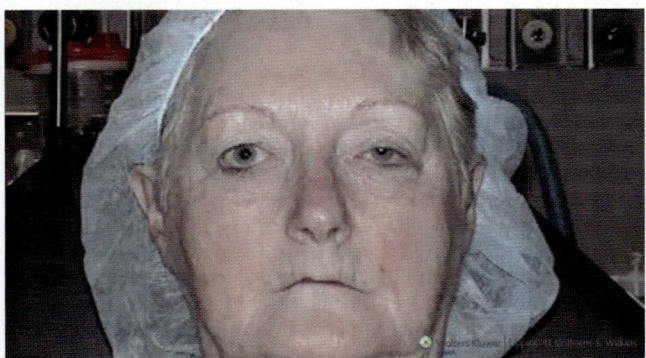

Figure 14-16 Horner Syndrome (left eye). Note miosis and ptosis. Loss of sweating not shown.

syndrome symptoms due to the effect of local anesthetics on the preganglionic neuron. Finally, third-order syndrome includes disease of the carotid artery, such as aneurysm, dissection, thrombosis, and even carotid endarterectomy. In these cases, common symptoms are face and neck pain.[47]

If the diagnosis can be done clinically, the next step is localizing the culprit; otherwise confirmation is performed by utilizing either a few drops of cocaine, which block the reuptake of NE and induce pupillary dilatation more in the normal eye than in the affected pupil, or apraclonidine, a direct α-adrenergic receptor agonist that reverses the anisocoria.

In order to determine the location of the lesion along the sympathetic tract, one can utilize a few drops of hydroxyl amphetamine, or its derivative pholedrine, which release NE, and in cases of first- or second-order Horner's the pupils will dilate, while in third-order Horner's the pupils will not dilate. Clearly, neuroimaging with CT scanning, and even MRI, are required for a more precise diagnosis.

Treatment is mainly supportive, and based on the cause, that is why clear identification of the location of the lesion is of utmost importance.[48,49]

Diabetic Neuropathy

Diabetic neuropathy is probably the best-known affliction associated with ANS dysfunctions. There is a progression of the symptoms with sensory loss initially and, as the disease progresses, with motor weakness as well. The first symptoms relate to a deficiency in vibratory sensation, as well as impairment of sensation to pain, light touch, and temperature, classically characterized as stocking-glove sensorial deficit. These symptoms are associated with depressed ankle reflexes, with a gradual evolution toward a more generalized motor weakness and loss of reflexes. This is not an uncommon occurrence in adult-onset diabetes, with a prevalence of approximately 41.9% to 26.4%, in a more recent study.[50,51] The most significant reason why it is important to follow this particular development is due to the fact that it can lead to foot ulcers, either acute and chronic, as well as muscle and joint pathology, with muscle atrophy, arthropathies, and stress fractures.

There are several methods of assessing the severity of the neuropathy, which can be normal, mild, moderate, or severe, by evaluating both symptoms and clinical signs.

Electrodiagnostic testing is necessary for atypical presentations, as well as for classification in clinical and epidemiologic studies.[52,53]

Monitoring of patients should be done at diagnosis and at regular intervals, to prevent development of complications associated with the diabetic foot.

Orthostatic Hypotension

Orthostatic hypotension is characterized by a decrease in blood pressure after standing or eating, and can be manifested by dizziness and syncope, which may progress to angina and, in rare cases, even to death.

In normal circumstances, upon standing, a certain volume of blood is pooled by gravity toward the splanchnic vessels and lower extremities, which leads to a decrease in venous return and subsequently a drop in blood pressure. The normal response is a compensatory mechanism that involves the central and peripheral nervous system, and consists of an increase in sympathetic outflow that instead raises the peripheral vascular resistance, venous return, and cardiac output and maintains blood pressure within normal limits, ultimately allowing standing upright.

The main conditions that lead to orthostatic hypotension are autonomic dysfunction and significant hypovolemia, and they appear to be more common in the elderly population.

These conditions are different from short-lived reflex syncope, which includes vasovagal, situational, and carotid sinus syncope; reflex syncope manifests with vasodilation and bradycardia instead of expected tachycardia, which subsequently determines hypotension followed by cerebral hypoperfusion, and thus causes the main symptom of temporary loss of consciousness.[54]

This condition may be due to neurodegenerative diseases whose common denominator is inappropriately low release of NE from the postganglionic sympathetic neurons, followed by inadequate vasoconstriction, reduced intravascular volume, and orthostatic hypotension. These disease include Parkinson disease, dementia with Lewy bodies, multiple system atrophy, and pure autonomic failure. In addition, there are peripheral neuropathies, as well as autoimmune blockade of ganglionic transmission, that produce the same manifestations, and here we can include diabetes mellitus, Guillain–Barré, paraneoplastic autonomic neuropathy, and familial dysautonomia. Orthostatic hypotension is among the side effects of several medications including alcohol, α-blockers, antidepressants, sympathetic nervous system blockers, antiparkinsonism drugs, β-blockers, diuretics, muscle relaxants, morphine, phosphodiesterase inhibitors, sedatives, and vasodilators. Aging contributes to a decrease in baroreceptor sensitivity, and it may be related to milder forms of orthostatic hypotension.

Symptoms, which vary in intensity, consist of dizziness, lightheadedness, weakness, blurred vision, and in severe cases syncope, angina, or even stroke. Less specific symptoms may include generalized weakness, fatigue, cognitive slowing, neck pain, and localized headache in the posterior cervical and shoulder region, also called coat hanger headache.

Diagnosis is made when there is at least a 20 mmHg drop in systolic blood pressure and/or 10 mmHg decrease in diastolic blood pressure, associated commonly with increase in heart rate within 2 to 5 minutes after changing posture from supine to standing.[55–57]

Treatment is symptomatic, starting with removal of medications that may possibly induce this pathology, lifestyle modification, avoiding dehydration, exercise, physical maneuvers such as crossing legs when standing, increasing the salt and water intake, avoiding large meals, and drinking water with meals. Medications that can be used to alleviate symptoms include fludrocortisone, sympathetic agents such as ephedrine, phenylephrine, midodrine, other supplements such as pyridostigmine, nonsteroidal agents, caffeine, and erythropoietin. Other experimental agents including vasopressin analogues, yohimbine, somatostatin, dihydroergotamine, dihydroxyphenylserine, dopamine antagonists such as metoclopramide, atomoxetine, and even ambulatory NE infusion have been attempted with some positive results.[58]

Monoamine Oxidase Inhibitors

Monoamine oxidase inhibitors (MAOIs) and tricyclic antidepressants are used to treat psychotic depression.[61–63] These drugs are not used in the practice of anesthesia but are a source of potentially serious anesthetic interactions in patients who take them chronically (see Chapter 22). Their use is rapidly declining, as the nontricyclic antidepressants such as fluoxetine (Prozac) are more efficacious and produce fewer side effects. Few of the MAOIs or tricyclic antidepressants will be encountered in an anesthesia practice today, with the exceptions of phenelzine (Nardil) and amitriptyline (Amitril, Elavil). Their pharmacologic actions and side effects are the direct result of their effect on the cascade of catecholamine metabolism. MAOIs block the oxidative deamination of endogenous catecholamines into inactive vanillylmandelic acid. They do not inhibit synthesis. Thus, blockade of MAO would produce an accumulation of NE, EPI, dopamine, and 5-hydroxytryptamine in adrenergically active tissues, including the brain. The action of sympathomimetic amines is potentiated in patients taking MAOIs. Indirect acting sympathomimetics (ephedrine, tyramine) produce an exaggerated response as they trigger the release of accumulated catecholamines. Foods containing a high tyramine content such as cheese, red Italian wine, and pickled herring can also precipitate hypertensive crises.[28] Meperidine has been reported to produce hypertensive crisis, convulsions, and coma with MAO inhibitors. Hepatotoxicity has been reported that does not seem to be related to dosage or duration of treatment. Its incidence is low but remains a factor in selecting anesthesia.

The anesthetic management of patients taking MAOIs remains controversial. Currently, recommendations for management include discontinuation of the drugs for at least 2 weeks before surgery; however, this recommendation is not based on controlled studies but rather is the result of limited case reports that suggest potent drug interactions.

Tricyclic Antidepressants

On the basis of their chemical structure, this group of antidepressant drugs is referred to as tricyclic antidepressants. These drugs have almost replaced MAOIs, since they have fewer side effects.[62,63] All of these agents block uptake of NE into adrenergic nerve endings. Just as with MAOIs, high doses of tricyclic antidepressants can induce seizure activity that is responsive to diazepam. Neuroleptic drugs may potentiate the effects of tricyclic antidepressants by competition with metabolism in the liver. Chronic barbiturate use increases metabolism of tricyclic antidepressants by microsomal enzyme induction. Other sedatives, however, potentiate the tricyclic antidepressants in a manner similar to that occurring with MAOIs. Atropine also has an exaggerated effect because of the anticholinergic effect of tricyclic antidepressants. Prolonged sedation from thiopental has been reported. Ketamine may also be dangerous in patients taking tricyclic antidepressants by producing acute hypertension and cardiac dysrhythmia. Despite these serious interactions, discontinuation of these drugs before surgery is probably not necessary. The latency of onset of these drugs is from 2 to 5 weeks; however, the excretion of tricyclic antidepressants is rapid, with approximately 70% of a dose appearing in the urine during the first 72 hours. The long latency period for resumption of treatment militates against interrupted treatment. A thorough knowledge of the possible drug interactions and autonomic countermeasures now available obviates postponement.

Selective Serotonin Reuptake Inhibitors

Mechanism of action of SSRIs appears to be the selective inhibition of neuronal uptake of serotonin. This potentiates the behavioral changes induced by the serotonin precursor 5-hydroxytryptophan.[62,63] The availability of sympathetic antagonists for treatment of possible side effects during anesthesia weighs in favor of continuation of therapy versus the risk of exacerbation of a severe depression. Prozac (fluoxetine) is a popular oral nontricyclic antidepressant. The elimination half-life of Prozac is 1 to 3 days and can lead to significant accumulation of the drug. Prozac's metabolism, like that of other compounds, including tricyclic antidepressants, phenobarbital, ethanol, and pentothal, involves the P450 II D6 system; concomitant therapy with drugs also metabolized by this enzyme system may lead to drug interactions and prolongation of effect of the benzodiazepines. Bupropion hydrochloride is available in a both a regular (Wellbutrin) and sustained-release (Zyban) form. Wellbutrin is used as an antidepressant, whereas Zyban is marketed as a nonnicotine aid to smoking cessation. The neurochemical mechanism of the antidepressant effect of bupropion is not known. It does not inhibit MAO and is a weak blocker of the neuronal uptake of serotonin and NE. It also inhibits the neuronal uptake of dopamine to some extent. No systematic data have been collected on the interactions of bupropion and other drugs. Patients with heart disease have emerged as a special category due to the finding that depression significantly affects cardiovascular health. Several studies support the safety of SSRIs in these patients due to their association with a decrease in morbidity and mortality, and the need for continuous treatment, especially in the elderly. Nevertheless, there is some evidence, although small, that these drugs may increase the risk of bleeding. Since these patients may use concomitantly other antiplatelet/anticoagulation therapies, increased vigilance is mandatory.[61-63]

REFERENCES

1. Guyton AC, Hall JE. The autonomic nervous system and the adrenal medulla. In: Guyton AC, Hall JE, eds. *Textbook of Medical Physiology*. 13th ed. Philadelphia, PA: Saunders/Elsevier; 2015:773–786.
2. Eisenhofer G. Sympathetic nerve function: assessment by radioisotope dilution analysis. *Clin Auton Res*. 2005;15:264–283.
3. Flacke WE, Flacke JW. Cholinergic and anticholinergic agents. In: Smith NT, Corbascio AN, eds. *Drug Interactions in Anesthesia*. 2nd ed. Philadelphia, PA: Lea & Febiger; 1986:160–175.
4. Guyton AC, Hall JE. Cardiac output, venous return, and their regulation. In: Guyton AC, Hall JE, eds. *Textbook of Medical Physiology*. 13th ed. Philadelphia, PA: Saunders/Elsevier; 2015:245–258.
5. Kapa S, Venkatachalam KL, Asirvatham SJ. The autonomic nervous system in cardiac electrophysiology: An elegant interaction and emerging concepts. *Cardiol Rev*. 2010;18:275–284.
6. Ajani AE, Yan BP. The mystery of coronary artery spasm. *Heart Lung Circ*. 2007;16:10–15.
7. Kawano H, Ogawa H. Endothelial dysfunction and coronary artery spasm. *Curr Drug Targets Cardiovasc Haematol Disord*. 2004;4:23–33.
8. Bevan JA. Some bases of differences in vascular response to sympathetic activity. *Circ Res*. 1979;45:161–171.
9. O'Rourke ST, Vanhoutte PM. Adrenergic and cholinergic regulation of bronchial vascular tone. *Am Rev Respir Dis*. 1992;146:S11–S14.
10. Pearl RG, Maze M, Rosenthal MH. Pulmonary and systemic hemodynamic effects of central venous and left atrial sympathomimetic drug administration in the dog. *J Cardiothorac Anesth*. 1987;1:29–35.
11. Sinski M, Lewandowski J, Abramczyk P, et al. Why study sympathetic nervous system? *J Physiol Pharmacol*. 2006;57(Suppl 11):79–92.
12. Civantos Calzada B, Aleixandre de Artiñano A. Alpha-adrenoceptor subtypes. *Pharmacol Res*. 2001;44:195–208.
13. Aubry ML, Davey MJ, Petch B. Cardioprotective and antidysrhythmic effects of alpha 1-adrenoceptor blockade during myocardial ischaemia and reperfusion in the dog. *J Cardiovasc Pharmacol*. 1985;7(Suppl 6):S93–102.
14. Cohen RA, Shepherd JT, Vanhoutte PM. Effects of the adrenergic transmitter on epicardial coronary arteries. *Fed Proc*. 1984;43:2862–2866.
15. Baumgart D, Haude M, Görge G, et al. Augmented alpha-adrenergic constriction of atherosclerotic human coronary arteries. *Circulation*. 1999;99:2090–2097.
16. Griggs DM Jr, Chilian WM, Boatwright RB, et al. Evidence against significant resting alpha-adrenergic coronary vasoconstrictor tone. *Fed Proc*. 1984;43:2873–2877.
17. Heusch G, Baumgart D, Camici P, et al. Alpha-adrenergic coronary vasoconstriction and myocardial ischemia in humans. *Circulation*. 2000;101:689–694.
18. Lymperopoulos A, Rengo G, Koch WJ. Adrenal adrenoceptors in heart failure: Fine-tuning cardiac stimulation. *Trends Mol Med*. 2007;13:503–511.
19. Vanhoutte PM. Endothelial adrenoceptors. *J Cardiovasc Pharmacol*. 2001;38:796–808.
20. Tobata D, Takao K, Mochizuki M, et al. Effects of dopamine, dobutamine, amrinone and milrinone on regional blood flow in isoflurane anesthetized dogs. *J Vet Med Sci*. 2004;66:1097–1105.
21. Hilberman JM, Maseda J, Stinson EB, et al. The diuretic properties of dopamine in patients after open-heart operation. *Anesthesiology*. 1984;61:489–494.

22. Owall A, Gordon E, Lagerkranser M, et al. Clinical experience with adenosine for controlled hypotension during cerebral aneurysm surgery. *Anesth Analg.* 1987;66:229–234.
23. Brodde OE. Beta-adrenoceptors in cardiac disease. *Pharmacol Ther.* 1993;60:405–430.
24. Pitkänen M. Spinal (subarahnoid) neural blockade. In: Cousins MJ, Carr DB, Horlocker TT, et al., eds. *Cousins & Bridenbaugh's Neural Blockade in Clinical Anesthesia and Pain Medicine*. 4th ed. Philadelphia, PA: Lippincott Williams & Wilkins; 2009:213–240.
25. Krum H, Sobotka P, Mahfoud F, et al. Device-based antihypertensive therapy: therapeutic modulation of the autonomic nervous system. *Circulation.* 2011;123:209–215.
26. Valantine H. Cardiac allograft vasculopathy after heart transplantation: risk factors and management. *J Heart Lung Transpl.* 2004;23:S187–S193.
27. Levy MN, Blattberg B. Effect of vagal stimulation on the overflow of norepinephrine into the coronary sinus during cardiac sympathetic nerve stimulation in the dog. *Circ Res.* 1976;38:81–84.
28. Flood P, Rathmell JP, Shafer S. *Pharmacology & Physiology in Anesthetic Practice.* 5th ed. Philadelphia, PA: Lippincott Williams & Wilkins; 2014:960.
29. Chamchad D, Horrow JC, Nakhamchik L, et al. Prophylactic glycopyrrolate prevents bradycardia after spinal anesthesia for cesarean section: a randomized, double-blinded, placebo-controlled prospective trial with heart rate variability correlation. *J Clin Anesth.* 2011;23:361–366.
30. Dampney RA, Coleman MJ, Fontes MA, et al. Central mechanisms underlying short- and long-term regulation of the cardiovascular system. *Clin Exp Pharmacol Physiol.* 2002;29:261–268.
31. Spaulding BC, Choi SD, Gross JB, et al. The effect of physostigmine on diazepam-induced ventilatory depression: a double-blind study. *Anesthesiology.* 1984;61:551–554.
32. Miano TA, Crouch MA. Evolving role of vasopressin in the treatment of cardiac arrest. *Pharmacotherapy.* 2006;26:828–839.
33. Giese-Davis J, Wilhelm FH, Tamagawa R, et al. Higher vagal activity as related to survival in patients with advanced breast cancer: An analysis of autonomic dysregulation. *Psychosom Med.* 2015;77(4):346–355.
34. Szurhaj W, Troussière AC, Logier R, et al. Ictal changes in parasympathetic tone: Prediction of postictal oxygen desaturation. *Neurology.* 2015;85(14):1233–1239.
35. Fukuda K, Kanazawa H, Aizawa Y, et al. Cardiac innervation and sudden cardiac death. *Circ Res.* 2015;116(12):2005–2019.
36. Tomaselli GF. Introduction to a compendium on sudden cardiac death: epidemiology, mechanisms, and management. *Circ. Res.* 2015;116:1883–1886.
37. Shen MJ, Zipes DP. Role of autonomic nervous system in modulating cardiac arrhythmias. *Circ Res.* 2014;114:1004–1021.
38. Schwartz PJ, La Rovere MT, De Ferrari GT, et al. Autonomic modulation for the management of patients with chronic heart failure. *Circ Heart Fail.* 2015;8:619–628.
39. Chen PS, Chen LS, Fishbein MC, et al. Role of the autonomic nervous system in atrial fibrillation: pathophysiology and therapy. *Circ Res.* 2014;114;1500–1515.
40. Zannad F, Stough WG, Mahfoud F, et al. Design considerations for clinical trials of autonomic modulation therapies targeting hypertension and heart failure. *Hypertension.* 2015;65:5–15.
41. Mancia G, Grassi G. The autonomic nervous system and hypertension. 2014;114:1804–1814.
42. Florea VG, Cohn JN. The autonomic nervous system and heart failure. *Circ Res.* 2014;114:1816–1826.
43. Eick C, Rizas KD, Meyer-Zurn CS, et al. Autonomic nervous system activity as risk predictor in the medical emergency department: a prospective cohort study. *Crit Care Med.* 2015;43:1079–1086.
44. Bermeo-Ovalle AC, Kennedy JD, Schuele SU. Cardiac and autonomic mechanisms contributing to SUDEP. *J Clin Neurophysiol.* 2015;32:21–29.
45. Sykora M, Czosnyka M, Liu X, et al. Autonomic impairment in severe traumatic brain injury: a multimodal neuromonitoring study. *Crit Care Med.* Epub 2016.
46. Gamboa A, Okamoto LE, Arnold AC, et al. Autonomic blockade improves insulin sensitivity in obese patients. *Hypertension.* 2014;64;867–874.
47. Lyrer PA, Brandt T, Metso TM, et al. Clinical import of Horner syndrome in internal carotid and vertebral artery dissection. *Neurology.* 2014;82:1653–1659.
48. Chen PL, Chen JT, Lu DW, et al. Comparing efficacies of 0.5% alpraclonidine with 4% cocaine in the diagnosis of Horner syndrome in pediatric patients. *J Ocul Pharmacol Ther.* 2006;22:182–187.
49. Wilhelm H, Ochsner H, Kopycziok E, et al. Horner's syndrome: a retrospective analysis of 90 cases and recommendations for clinical handling. *Ger J Ophthalmol.* 1992;1:96–102.
50. Partanen J, Niskanen L, Lehtinen J, et al. Natural history of peripheral neuropathy in patients with non-insulin-dependent diabetes mellitus. *N Engl J Med.* 1995;333:89–94.
51. Davies M, Brophy S, Williams R, et al. The prevalence, severity, and impact of painful diabetic peripheral neuropathy in typ2 diabetes. *Diabetic Care.* 2006;29:1518–1522.
52. Young MJ, Boulton AJ, Macleod AF, et al. A multicenter study of the prevalence of diabetic peripheral neuropathy in the United Kingdom hospital clinic population. *Diabetologia.* 1993;36:150–154.
53. Feldman EL, Stevens MJ, Thomas PK, et al. A practical two-step quantitative clinical and electrophysiological assessment for the diagnosis ad staging of diabetic neuropathy. *Diabetes Care.* 1994;17:1281–1289.
54. Task Force for the Diagnosis and Management of Syncope, European Society of Cardiology (ESC), European Heart Rhythm Association (EHRA), et al. Guidelines for the diagnosis and management of syncope (version 2009). *Eur Heart J.* 2009; 30:2631–2671.
55. Freeman R, Wieling W, Axelrod FB, et al. Consensus statement on the definition of orthostatic hypotension, neutrally mediated syncope and the postural tachycardia syndrome. *Clic Auton Res.* 2011;21:69–72.
56. Feldstein C, Weder AB. Orthostatic hypotension: a common, serious and underrecognized problem in hospitalized patients. *J Am Soc Hypertens.* 2012;6:27–39.
57. Metzler M, Duerr S, Granata R, et al. neurogenic orthostatic hypotension: pathophysiology, evaluation, and management. *J Neurol.* 2013;260:2212–2219.
58. Mills PB, Fung CK, Travlos A, et al. Nonpharmacologic management of orthostatic hypotension: a systematic review. *Arch Phys Med Rehabil.* 2015;96:366–375.
59. Lanier JB, Mote MB, Clay EC. Evaluation and management of orthostatic hypotension. *Am Fam Physician.* 2011;84:527–536.
60. Izcovich A, Gonzalez Malla C, Manzotti M, et al. Midorine for orthostatic hypotension and recurrent reflex syncope: a systematic review. *Neurology.* 2014;83;1170–1177.
61. Krings-Ernst I, Ulrich S, Adl M. Antidepressant treatment with MAO-inhibitors during general and regional anesthesia: a review and case report of spinal anesthesia without discontinuation of tranylcypromine. *Int J Clin Pharmacol Ther.* 2013;51:763.
62. Peck TP, Wong A, Norman E. Anaesthetic implications of psychoactive drugs. *Cont Educ Anaes Crit Care Pain.* 2010;10:177.
63. Bromhead H, Feeney A. Antidepressant and psychiatric drugs. Part 1. Antidepressants. *Anaesthesia Tutorial of the Week.* 2009;14:1.

15 Respiratory Function in Anesthesia

PAUL C. TAMUL • MICHAEL L. AULT

Functional Anatomy of the Lungs
   Thorax
   Muscles of Ventilation
   Lung Structures
   Pulmonary Vascular Systems
Lung Mechanics
   Elastic Work
   Resistance to Gas Flow
Control of Ventilation
   Terminology
   Generation of Ventilatory Pattern
   Medullary Centers
   Pontine Centers
   Higher Respiratory Centers
   Reflex Control of Ventilation
   Chemical Control of Ventilation
Oxygen and Carbon Dioxide Transport
   Bulk Flow of Gas (Convection)
   Gas Diffusion
   Distribution of Ventilation and Perfusion
   Physiologic Dead Space
   Assessment of Physiologic Dead Space
   Physiologic Shunt
   Assessment of Arterial Oxygenation and Physiologic Shunt
   Physiologic Shunt Calculation
Pulmonary Function Testing
   Lung Volumes and Capacities
   Pulmonary Function Tests
   Practical Application of Pulmonary Function Tests
Anesthesia and Obstructive Pulmonary Disease
Anesthesia and Restrictive Pulmonary Disease
Effects of Cigarette Smoking on Pulmonary Function
Postoperative Pulmonary Function
   Postoperative Pulmonary Complications

KEY POINTS

1. In a person with normal lungs, breathing can be performed exclusively by the diaphragm.
2. In the adult, the tip of an orotracheal tube moves an average of 3.8 cm with flexion/extension of the neck, but can travel as much as 6.4 cm. In infants and children, displacement of even 1 cm can move the tube above the vocal cords or below the carina.
3. The following anatomy should be considered when contemplating use of a double-lumen tube. The adult right main stem bronchus is about 2.5 cm long before it branches into lobar bronchi. In 10% of adults, the right upper lobe bronchus departs from the right main stem bronchus less than 2.5 cm below the carina. In 2% to 3% of adults, the right upper lobe bronchus opens directly into the trachea, above the carina.
4. When lung compliance is reduced, larger changes in pleural pressure are needed to create the same tidal volume (Vt). Patients with low lung compliance breathe with smaller Vt and more rapidly, making spontaneous respiratory rate the most sensitive clinical index of lung compliance.
5. Carotid and aortic bodies are stimulated by PaO_2 values less than 60 to 65 mmHg. Thus, patients who depend on hypoxic ventilatory drive must have PaO_2 values below 65 mmHg. The response of the peripheral receptors will not reliably increase ventilatory rate or minute ventilation to herald the onset of hypoxemia during general anesthesia or recovery.
6. There are three etiologies of hyperventilation: arterial hypoxemia, metabolic acidemia, and central etiologies (e.g., intracranial hypertension, hepatic cirrhosis, anxiety, pharmacologic agents).
7. Increases in dead space ventilation primarily affect CO_2 elimination (with minimal influence on arterial oxygenation), whereas increases in physiologic shunt primarily affect arterial oxygenation (with minimal influence on CO_2 elimination).
8. During spontaneous ventilation, the ratio of alveolar ventilation to dead space ventilation is 2:1. The alveolar-to–dead space ventilation ratio during positive-pressure ventilation is 1:1. Thus, minute ventilation during mechanical ventilatory support must be greater than that during spontaneous ventilation to achieve the same $PaCO_2$.
9. $PaCO_2 \geq PETCO_2$ unless the patient inspires or receives exogenous CO_2. The difference between $PaCO_2$ and $PETCO_2$ is due to dead space ventilation. The most common reason for an acute increase in dead space ventilation is decreased cardiac output.
10. Calculation of the shunt fraction is the best tool for evaluating the lungs' efficiency in oxygenating the arterial blood. It is the only index of oxygenation that takes into account the contribution of mixed venous blood to arterial oxygenation.
11. When functional residual capacity (FRC) is reduced, lung compliance falls (causing tachypnea) and venous admixture increases, creating arterial hypoxemia.
12. There is no compelling evidence that defines rules for ordering preoperative pulmonary function tests. Rather, they should only be obtained to ascertain the presence of reversible pulmonary dysfunction (bronchospasm) or to define the severity of advanced pulmonary disease.

13 Patients who smoke should be advised to *stop* smoking at least 2 months prior to an elective operation to decrease the risk of postoperative pulmonary complications (PPCs).

14 The operative site is one of the most important determinants of the risk of PPC. The highest risk for PPC is associated with nonlaparoscopic upper abdominal operations, followed by lower abdominal and intrathoracic operations.

15 The single most important aspect of postoperative pulmonary care and prevention of PPC is early ambulation. Patients should be encouraged to get out of bed and walk.

Anesthesiologists directly manipulate pulmonary function. Thus, a sound and thorough working knowledge of applied pulmonary physiology is essential to the safe conduct of anesthesia. This chapter discusses pulmonary anatomy, the control of ventilation, oxygen and carbon dioxide transport, ventilation–perfusion relationships, lung volumes and pulmonary function testing, abnormal physiology and anesthesia, the effect of smoking on pulmonary function, and risk assessment for postoperative pulmonary complications (PPCs).

Functional Anatomy of the Lungs

This section emphasizes functional lung anatomy, with structure described as it applies to the mechanical and physiologic function of the lungs.

Thorax

The thoracic cage is shaped like a truncated cone, with a small superior aperture and a larger inferior opening to which the diaphragm is attached. The sternal angle is located in the horizontal plane that passes through the vertebral column at the T4 or T5 level. This plane separates the superior from the inferior mediastinum. During ventilation, the predominant changes in thoracic diameter occur in the anteroposterior direction in the upper thoracic region and in the lateral or transverse direction in the lower thorax.

Muscles of Ventilation

Work of breathing is the energy expenditure of ventilatory muscles. Similar to other skeletal muscles, the ventilatory muscles are endurance muscles subject to fatigue from inadequate oxygen delivery, poor nutrition, and increased work secondary to chronic obstructive pulmonary disease (COPD) with gas trapping or increased airway resistance. The ventilatory muscles include the diaphragm, intercostal muscles, abdominal muscles, cervical strap muscles, sternocleidomastoid muscles, and the large back and intervertebral muscles of the shoulder girdle. During nonstrenuous breathing, the diaphragm performs most of the muscle work. Work contribution from the intercostal muscles in nonstrenuous breathing is minor. Normally, at rest, inspiration requires work while exhalation is passive. As work of breathing increases, abdominal muscles assist with rib depression and increase intra-abdominal pressure to facilitate forced exhalation causing the "stitch," or rib pain athletes experience when they actively exhale. When a further increase in work is required, the cervical strap muscles are recruited to help elevate the sternum and upper portions of the chest to optimize the dimensions of the thoracic cavity. Finally, during periods of maximal work, recruitment of large back and paravertebral muscles of the shoulder girdle contribute to ventilatory effort. The muscles of the abdominal wall, the most powerful muscles of expiration, are important for expulsive efforts such as coughing.[1] However, with normal lungs, breathing can be performed solely by the diaphragm.

Breathing is an endurance phenomenon involving fatigue-resistant muscle fibers, characterized by a slow-twitch response to electrical stimulation that must create sufficient force to lift the ribs and generate subatmospheric pressure in the intrapleural space. These fatigue-resistant fibers comprise approximately 50% of the total diaphragmatic muscle fibers. The high oxidative capacity of these fibers creates endurance units.[2] Fast-twitch muscle fibers, more susceptible to fatigue, have rapid responses to electrical stimulation, imparting strength and allowing greater force over less time. The combination of fast-twitch fibers useful during brief periods of maximal ventilatory effort (coughing, sneezing) and slow-twitch fibers providing endurance (breathing without rest) underscores the unique dual function of the diaphragm as a muscle.[3]

A working muscle like the diaphragm must be firmly anchored at both its origin and insertion. However, its unique insertion is mobile—a central tendon originates from fibers attached to the vertebral bodies, as well as the lower ribs and sternum. Diaphragmatic contraction results in descent of the diaphragmatic dome and expansion of the thoracic base, creating decreases in intrathoracic and intrapleural pressure and an increase in intra-abdominal pressure.

The cervical strap muscles, active even during restful breathing, are the most important inspiratory accessory muscles. When diaphragm function is impaired, as in patients with cervical spinal cord transection, they can become the primary inspiratory muscles.

Lung Structures

In an intact respiratory system, the expandable lung tissue fills the pleural cavity. The visceral and parietal pleurae oppose each other, creating a potential intrapleural space where pressure decreases when the diaphragm descends and the rib cage expands. At the end of inspiration, the resultant subatmospheric intrapleural pressure is a reflection of the opposing and equal forces between the natural tendency of the lungs to collapse and the chest wall musculature to remain expanded. These equal and opposing forces at end-inspiration result in the functional residual capacity (FRC), the volume of gas remaining in the lungs at passive end-expiration. At FRC, the intrapleural space normally has a slightly subambient pressure (−2 to −3 mmHg). Major divisions of the right and left lung are listed in Table 15-1. Knowledge of the bronchopulmonary segments is important for localizing lung pathology, interpreting lung radiographs, identifying lung regions during bronchoscopy, and operating on the lung. Each bronchopulmonary segment is separated from its adjacent segments by well-defined connective tissue planes that often anatomically confine initial lung pathologies.

Table 15-1	Major Divisions of the Lung
Lung Side/Lobe	Bronchopulmonary Segment
Right	
Upper	Apical
	Anterior
	Posterior
Middle	Medial
	Lateral
Lower	Superior
	Medial basal
	Lateral basal
	Anterior basal
	Posterior basal
Left	
Upper	Apical posterior
	Anterior
Lingula	Superior
	Inferior
Lower	Superior
	Posterior basal
	Anteromedial basal
	Lateral basal

The lung parenchyma can be subdivided into three airway categories based on functional lung anatomy (Table 15-2). The conductive airways allow basic gas transport without gas exchange. The next group of airways, which have smaller diameters, are transitional airways. Transitional airways are not only conduits for gas movement, but also allow limited gas diffusion and exchange. Finally, the primary function of the smallest respiratory airways is gas exchange.

Conventionally, large airways with diameters more than 2 mm create 90% of total airway resistance. The number of alveoli increases progressively with age, from approximately 24 million at birth, and reaches its final adult count of 300 million by the age of 8 or 9 years. These alveoli are associated with about 250 million precapillaries and 280 billion capillary segments, resulting in a surface area of approximately 70 m^2 for gas exchange.

Conductive Airways

In the adult, the trachea is a fibromuscular tube about 10 to 12 cm long with an outer diameter of approximately 20 mm. Structural support is provided by 20 U-shaped structures composed of hyaline cartilage, with the opening of the U facing posteriorly. The cricoid membrane tethers the trachea to the cricoid cartilage at the level of the sixth cervical vertebral body. The trachea enters the superior mediastinum and bifurcates at the sternal angle (the lower border of the fourth thoracic vertebral body). Normally, half of the trachea is intrathoracic and half is extrathoracic. Because both ends of the trachea are attached to mobile structures, the adult carina can move superiorly as much as 5 cm from its normal resting position. Awareness of airway "motion" is essential to proper care of the intubated patient. In the adult, the tip of an orotracheal tube moves an average of 3.8 cm with flexion and extension of the neck, but can travel as far as 6.4 cm.[4] In infants and children, tracheal tube movement with respect to the trachea is even more critical: displacement of even 1 cm can result in unintentional extubation or bronchial intubation.

The next airway generation below the carina is composed of the right and left main stem bronchi. The diameter of the right bronchus is generally greater than that of the left. In the adult, the right bronchus leaves the trachea at approximately 25 degrees from the vertical tracheal axis, whereas the angle of the left bronchus is about 45 degrees. Thus, unintentional endobronchial intubation or aspiration of foreign material is more likely to occur on the right than the left. Furthermore, the right upper lobe bronchus dives almost directly posterior at approximately 90 degrees from the right main bronchus, facilitating aspiration of foreign bodies and fluid into the right upper lobe in the supine patient. In children younger than 3 years of age, the angles created by the right and left main stem bronchi are approximately equal, with takeoff angles of about 55 degrees.

The adult right main bronchus is about 2.5 cm long before it initially branches into lobar bronchi. However, in 10% of adults, the right upper lobe bronchus departs from the right main stem bronchus less than 2.5 cm from the carina. Furthermore, in 2% to 3% of adults, the right upper lobe bronchus opens into the trachea, superior to the carina. Patients with these anomalies require special consideration when placing double-lumen tracheal tubes, especially if one contemplates inserting a right-sided endobronchial tube. After the right upper and middle lobe bronchi divide from the right main bronchus, the main channel becomes the right lower lobe bronchus.

The left main bronchus is about 5 cm long before its initial branching point to the left upper lobe and the lingula; it then continues as the left lower lobe bronchus.

The bronchioles, typically 1 mm in diameter, are devoid of cartilaginous support and have the highest proportion of smooth muscle in their walls. Of the three to four bronchiolar generations, the final generation is the terminal bronchiole, which is the last airway component incapable of gas exchange.

Transitional Airways

The respiratory bronchiole, which follows the terminal bronchiole, is the first site in the tracheobronchial tree where gas exchange occurs. In adults, two or three generations of respiratory bronchioles lead to alveolar ducts, of which there are four to five generations, each with multiple openings into alveolar sacs. The final divisions of alveolar ducts terminate in alveolar sacs that open into alveolar clusters.

Respiratory Airways and the Alveolar–capillary Membrane

The alveolar-capillary membrane has two primary functions: transport of respiratory gases (oxygen and carbon dioxide), and the production of a wide variety of local and humoral substances. Gas transport is facilitated by the pulmonary capillary beds that are the densest capillary networks in the body. This extensive

Table 15-2	Functional Airway Divisions	
Type	Function	Structure
Conductive	Bulk gas movement	Trachea to terminal bronchioles
Transitional	Bulk gas movement	Respiratory bronchioles
	Limited gas exchange	Alveolar ducts
Respiratory	Gas exchange	Alveoli
		Alveolar sacs

vascular branching system starts with pulmonary arterioles in the region of the respiratory bronchioles. Each alveolus is closely associated with some 1,000 short capillary segments.

The alveolar–capillary interface is complicated, but well designed to facilitate gas exchange. Viewed with electron microscopy, the alveolar wall consists of a thin capillary epithelial cell, a basement membrane, a pulmonary capillary endothelial cell, and a surfactant lining layer. The flattened, squamous type I alveolar cells cover about 80% of the alveolar surface. Type I cells contain flattened nuclei and extremely thin cytoplasmic extensions that provide the surface suitable for gas exchange. Type I cells are highly differentiated and metabolically limited, which makes them highly susceptible to injury. When type I cells are damaged severely (during acute lung injury or adult respiratory distress syndrome), type II cells replicate and modify to form new type I cells.[5]

Type II alveolar cells are interspersed among type I cells, primarily at alveolar–septal junctions. These polygonal cells have vast metabolic and enzymatic activity, and manufacture surfactant. The enzymatic activity required to produce surfactant is only 50% of the total enzymatic activity present in type II alveolar cells.[6] The remaining enzymatic activity modulates local electrolyte balance, as well as endothelial and lymphatic cell functions. Both type I and type II alveolar cells have tight intracellular junctions, providing a relatively impermeable barrier to fluids.

Type III alveolar cells, alveolar macrophages, are an important element of immunologic lung defense. Their migratory and phagocytic activities permit ingestion of foreign materials within alveolar spaces.[7] Although functional pulmonary macrophages reduce the incidence of lung infection,[8] they also play an integral role in the organ-wide pulmonary inflammatory response. Thus, it is highly controversial whether the presence of these cells is beneficial (reducing the sequelae of infection) or harmful (contributing to the inflammatory response).[9]

Pulmonary Vascular Systems

Two major circulatory systems supply blood to the lungs: the pulmonary and bronchial vascular networks. The pulmonary vascular system delivers mixed-venous blood from the right ventricle to the pulmonary capillary bed via two pulmonary arteries. After gas exchange occurs in the pulmonary capillary bed, blood is returned to the left atrium via four pulmonary veins. The pulmonary veins run independently along the intralobar connective tissue planes. The pulmonary capillary system adequately provides the metabolic and oxygen needs of the alveolar parenchyma. The bronchial arterial system provides oxygen to the conductive airways and pulmonary vessels. Anatomic connections between the bronchial and pulmonary venous circulations create an absolute shunt of about 2% to 5% of the total cardiac output, and represent "normal" shunt.

Lung Mechanics

Lung movement occurs secondary to forces external to the lungs. During spontaneous ventilation, the external forces are produced by ventilatory muscles. The response of the lungs to these external forces is governed by two main characteristics: ease of elastic recoil of the chest wall and resistance to gas flow within airways.

Elastic Work

The natural tendency of the lungs is to collapse because of elastic recoil; thus, expiration at rest is normally passive as gas flows out of the lungs. The thoracic cage exerts an outward-directed force, and the lungs exert an inward-directed force. Because the outward force of the thoracic cage exceeds the inward force of the lung, the overall tendency of the lung within the thoracic cage is to remain inflated. FRC represents the gas volume in the lungs when the outward and inward forces on the lung are equal. Gravitational forces create a more subatmospheric pressure in nondependent areas of the lung than in dependent areas. In the upright adult, the difference in intrapleural pressure from the top to the bottom of the lung is about 7 cm H_2O.

Surface tension at an air–fluid interface produces forces that tend to further reduce the area of interface. For a bubble to remain inflated, the gas pressure within the bubble is contained by surface tension and must be higher than the surrounding gas pressure. Alveoli resemble bubbles in this respect, but unlike a bubble, alveolar gas communicates with the atmosphere via the airways. The Laplace equation describes this phenomenon: $P = 2T/R$, where P is the pressure within the bubble (dyn $\times$ cm^{-2}), T is the surface tension of the liquid (dyn $\times$ cm^{-1}), and R is the radius of the bubble (cm).

During inspiration, the surface tension of the liquid in the lung increases to 40 mN/m, a value close to that of plasma. During expiration, this surface tension falls to 19 mN/m, a value lower than that of most other fluids. This change in surface tension creates hysteresis of the alveoli, the phenomenon of different pressure–volume relationships of the alveoli during inspiration versus expiration. Unlike a bubble, the pressure within an alveolus decreases as the radius of curvature decreases, creating gas flow from larger to smaller alveoli that maintains structural stability and prevents lung collapse.

The alveolar transmural pressure gradient, or transpulmonary pressure, is the difference between intrapleural and alveolar pressure, and is directly proportional to lung volume. Intrapleural pressure can be safely measured with a percutaneously inserted catheter[10]; however, clinicians rarely perform this technique. When measured with an esophageal balloon in the midesophagus, esophageal pressure can be used as a reflection of intrapleural pressure.[11] Commercially available esophageal pressure monitors increase the ease and accuracy of measuring esophageal pressure as a reflection of intrapleural pressure.[12] These monitors are useful for estimating the elastic work performed by the patient during spontaneous ventilation, mechanical ventilation, or a combination of spontaneous and mechanical ventilation. By estimating intrapleural pressure on a real-time basis, it is possible to quantitate the patient's work of breathing. For example, low levels of inspiratory pressure support can compensate for the work of breathing imposed by the endotracheal tube.[13]

Physiologic work of breathing includes elastic work (inspiratory work required to overcome the elastic recoil of the pulmonary system) and resistive work (work to overcome resistance to gas flow in the airway). For a patient in whom breathing apparatus is employed—such as an endotracheal tube or a ventilator demand valve—the concept of total work of breathing encompasses physiologic work plus equipment-imposed ventilatory work to overcome the resistance imposed by the breathing apparatus.

If the lungs are slowly inflated and deflated, the pressure–volume curve during inflation differs from that obtained during deflation. The two curves form a hysteresis loop that becomes progressively broader as the tidal volume is increased (Fig. 15-1). To inflate the lungs, pressure greater than the recoil pressure of deflation is needed. This means that the lung accepts deformation poorly and, once deformed, reforms to its original shape slowly. Elastic hysteresis is important for the maintenance of normal lung compliance, but is not clinically significant.

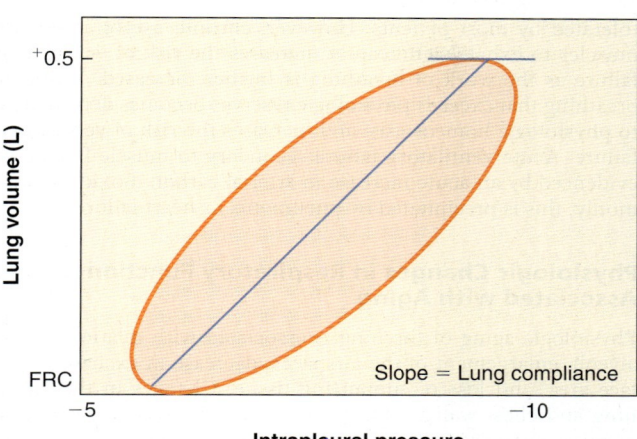

Figure 15-1 Dynamic pressure–volume loop of resting tidal volume. Quiet, normal breathing is characterized by hysteresis of the pressure–volume loop. The lung is more resistant to deformation than expected and returns to its original configuration less easily than expected. The slope of the line connecting the zenith and nadir lung volumes is lung compliance, about 500 mL/3 cm H_2O = 167 mL/cm H_2O.

The sum of the pressure–volume relationships of the thorax and lung results in a sigmoidal curve (Fig. 15-2). The vertical line drawn at end-expiration coincides with FRC. Normally, humans breathe on the steepest part of the sigmoidal curve, where compliance ($\Delta V/\Delta P$) or slope is highest. In restrictive pulmonary diseases, the compliance curve shifts to the right, has decreased slope ($\Delta V/\Delta P$), or both. This decreased lung compliance results in smaller FRCs. When lung compliance is reduced, larger changes in intrapleural pressure are required to create the same tidal volume; that is, the thorax has to work harder to move the same

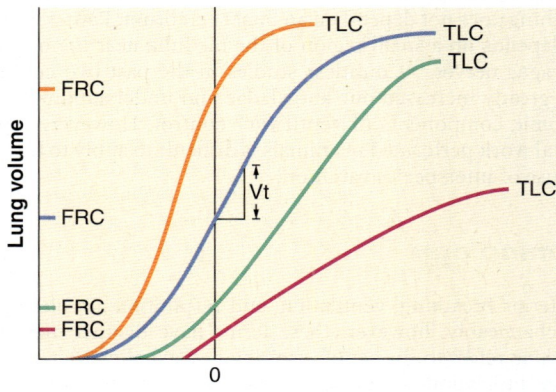

Figure 15-2 Pulmonary pressure–volume relationships at different values of total lung capacity (TLC), ignoring hysteresis. The *blue* depicts the normal pulmonary pressure–volume relationships. Humans normally breathe on the linear, steep part of this sigmoidal curve, where the slope (equal to compliance) is greatest. The *black vertical line* at zero defines functional residual capacity (FRC), regardless of the position of the curve on the graph. Mild restrictive lung disease, indicated by the *green line*, shifts the curve to the right with little change in slope. However, with restrictive disease, the patient breathes on a lower FRC, at a point on the curve where the slope is less. Severe restrictive pulmonary disease profoundly depresses the FRC and diminishes the slope of the entire curve (*red line*). Obstructive disease (*orange line*) elevates both FRC and compliance.

volume of gas into the lungs. The body, being an energy conserving organism, prefers to move less gas with each breath rather than working harder to achieve the same tidal volume. Thus, patients with restrictive lung disease typically breathe with smaller tidal volumes at more rapid rates, making spontaneous ventilatory rate one of the most sensitive indices of lung compliance. When lung compliance is decreased, the benefit of therapeutic continuous positive airway pressure (CPAP) is its ability to shift the vertical FRC line to the right, allowing the patient to breathe on a steeper, more efficient portion of the volume–pressure curve. In other words, CPAP can increase the FRC, which allows for a slower ventilatory rate with a larger tidal volume.

At the other end of the spectrum, patients with diseases that increase lung compliance expend less elastic work to inspire, but have decreased elastic recoil, resulting in larger than normal FRC (gas trapping). In such cases, their volume–pressure curves shift to the left and steepen. Chronic obstructive lung disease and acute asthma are the most common examples of diseases with high lung compliance. If lung compliance and FRC are sufficiently high that elastic recoil is minimal, the patient must use ventilatory muscles to actively exhale. The difficulty these patients experience in emptying the lungs is compounded by increased airway resistance.

Both compliance and inspiratory elastic work can be measured for a single breath by measuring airway pressure (Paw), intrapleural (Ppl) pressure, and tidal volume. If esophageal pressure is measured correctly, the esophageal pressure values can be substituted for Ppl values. Lung compliance (C_L) is the slope of the volume–pressure curve, and calculated by the equation

$$C_L = \frac{\Delta V}{\Delta P_L} + \frac{Vt}{P_{L_i} - P_{L_e}} = \frac{Vt}{(Paw_i - Ppl_i) - (Paw_e - Ppl_e)} \quad (15\text{-}1)$$

where P_L is transpulmonary pressure, P_{L_i} and P_{L_e} are transpulmonary pressures at end-inspiration and end-expiration, Vt is tidal volume, Paw_e and Paw_i are expiratory and inspiratory airway pressures, and Ppl_e and Ppl_i are expiratory and inspiratory intrapleural pressures.

Elastic work (W_{el}) is performed during inspiration only because expiration is passive during normal breathing. The area within the triangle in Figure 15-2 describes the work required to inspire. The equation that yields elastic work (and the area of the triangle) is

$$\begin{aligned} W_{el} &= \frac{1}{2}(Vt)(P_{L_i} - P_{L_e}) \\ &= \frac{1}{2}(Vt)[(Paw_i - Ppl_i) - (Paw_e - Ppl_e)] \end{aligned} \quad (15\text{-}2)$$

Resistance to Gas Flow

Both laminar and turbulent flows exist within the respiratory tract, usually in mixed patterns. The physics of each, however, is significantly different.

Laminar Flow

Below critical flow rates that create turbulent flow, gas proceeds through a straight tube as a series of concentric cylinders that slide over one another. Fully developed flow has a parabolic profile with a velocity of zero at the cylinder wall and a maximum velocity at the center of the advancing "cone." This type of streamlined flow is usually inaudible. The advancing conical front means that some fresh gas reaches the end of the tube before the tube has been completely filled with fresh gas. Thus, laminar flow in the airways results in alveolar ventilation that can occur even when the tidal volume (Vt) is less than anatomic dead space. This phenomenon has significant clinical implications. As noted by Rohrer[14] in 1915, it allows high-frequency ventilation to achieve adequate alveolar ventilation.

Resistance (R) to laminar gas flows in a straight, unbranched cylinder can be calculated by the following equation of Poiseuille:

$$R = \frac{8 \times length \times viscosity}{\pi \times (radius)^4} = \frac{P_B - P_A}{flow} \quad (15\text{-}3)$$

where P_B and P_A are barometric and alveolar pressures. It is essential to note that as radius decreases in narrowed airways, resistance will increase by a power of four. Viscosity is the only physical gas property that is relevant under conditions of laminar flow. Helium has a low density, but its viscosity is close to that of air. Therefore, helium will not improve gas flow if the flow is laminar. However, if flow is turbulent due to critical airway narrowing or abnormally high airway resistance, low-density helium is potentially useful therapy (see next section).

Turbulent Flow

High flow rates, particularly through branched or irregularly shaped tubes, disrupt the orderly flow of laminar gas. When resistance to gas flow is significant, turbulent flow occurs and is usually audible. Turbulent flow usually presents with a square front; fresh gas will not reach the end of the tube until the amount of gas entering the tube is almost equal to the volume of the tube. Thus, turbulent flow effectively purges the contents of a tube. Four conditions that will change laminar flow to turbulent flow are high gas flows, sharp angles within the tube, branching in the tube, and a decrease in the diameter of the tube. During laminar flow, resistance is inversely proportional to gas flow rate. Conversely, during turbulent flow, resistance increases significantly in proportion to the flow rate. A detailed description of these phenomena is beyond the scope of this chapter, but the reader is referred to descriptions by Nunn.[15]

Increased Airway Resistance

Bronchiolar smooth muscle hyperreactivity (true bronchospasm), mucosal edema, mucous plugging, epithelial desquamation, tumors, and foreign bodies all increase airway resistance. The conscious subject can detect small increases in inspiratory resistance.[16] The normal response to increased inspiratory resistance is increased inspiratory muscle effort, with little change in FRC.[17] Emphysematous patients retain remarkable ability to preserve an adequate alveolar ventilation, even with gross airway obstruction. In patients with preoperative FEV_1 values lower than 1 L, $PaCO_2$ is normal in most patients. Furthermore, asthmatic patients compensate well for increased airway resistance and also keep the mean $PaCO_2$ in the lower end of normal range.[18] Thus, an increased $PaCO_2$ in the setting of increased airway resistance warrants serious attention as it suggests that the patient's compensatory mechanisms are nearly exhausted. Mild expiratory resistance does not result in muscle use for active exhalation in conscious or anesthetized subjects. Instead, the initial work to overcome expiratory resistance is performed by augmenting inspiratory force until a sufficiently high lung volume is achieved that allows elastic recoil to overcome expiratory resistance.[19] Only when expiratory resistance becomes excessive are accessory muscles recruited to expel gas from the lungs. During acute increases in expiratory resistance, this response is well tolerated by most patients. However, chronic use of accessory muscles to exhale significantly increases the risk of ventilatory failure as the work of breathing is further increased. Work of breathing that exceeds physiologic reserves becomes detrimental to physiologic homeostasis, and increases the risk of ventilatory failure. Acute ventilatory failure secondary to muscle fatigue is evidenced by an acute increase in arterial carbon dioxide. Commonly, this is precipitated by pneumonia or heart failure.

Physiologic Changes in Respiratory Function Associated with Aging

Physiologic aging of the lung is associated with dilation of the alveoli, enlargement of the airspaces, decrease in exchange surface area, and loss of supporting tissue. Changes in the aging lung and chest wall result in decreased lung recoil (elastance) creating an increased residual volume and FRC. In addition, compliance of the chest wall diminishes, thereby increasing the work of breathing compared with younger subjects. Respiratory muscle strength decreases with aging and is strongly correlated with nutritional status and cardiac index. Expiratory flow rates decrease with a flow–volume curve suggestive of small airway resistance. Despite these changes, the respiratory system is normally able to maintain adequate gas exchange at rest and during exertion throughout life, with only modest decrements in PaO_2 and no change in $PaCO_2$. With aging, respiratory centers in the nervous system demonstrate decreased sensitivity to hypoxemia and hypercapnia resulting in a blunted ventilatory response when challenged by heart failure, airway obstruction, or pneumonia.[20]

Control of Ventilation

Mechanisms that control ventilation are extremely complex, requiring integration with many parts of the central and peripheral nervous systems (Fig. 15-3). LeGallois, who localized the respiratory centers in the brainstem in 1812, demonstrated that breathing does not depend on an intact cerebrum. Rather, breathing depends on a small region of the medulla near the origin of the vagus nerves.[21] Countless studies in the past two centuries have greatly increased our knowledge and understanding of the anatomic components of ventilatory control. However, experimental work performed in animals is difficult to apply to humans because of interspecies variation.

Terminology

The terms breathing, ventilation, and respiration are often used interchangeably; however, these terms have distinct meanings. *Breathing* refers to the act of inspiring and exhaling that requires energy utilization for muscle work; therefore, it is limited by energy reserves. *Ventilation,* on the other hand, is the movement of gas in and out of the lungs. When spontaneous, ventilation requires energy for muscle work and is thus, breathing. *Respiration* occurs when energy is released from organic molecules. Such energy release is dependent on the movement of gas molecules such as carbon dioxide and oxygen across membranes, whether alveolar or mitochondrial. Thus, humans breathe to ventilate and ventilate to respire. Despite what appears to be clear distinctions in terminology, vernacular use of these terms is often confused in daily dialogue. For example: *respirators* are used to treat those who have succumbed to *respiratory* arrest and do not have a *respiratory* rate, and residents are sometimes advised to *breathe* down a patient using a potent anesthetic agent.

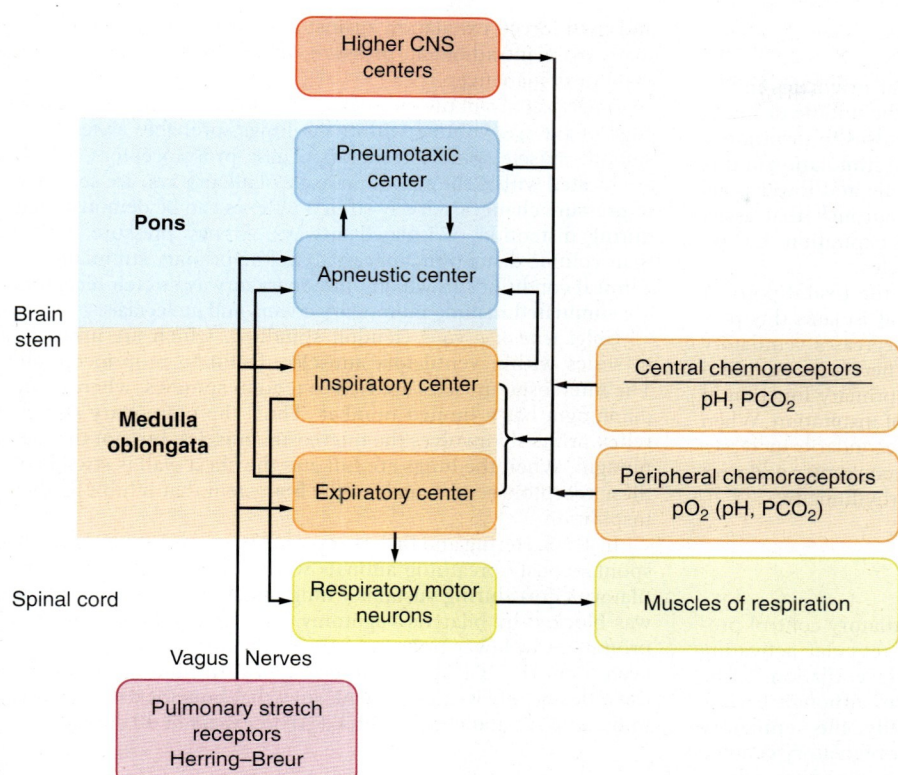

Figure 15-3 Classic central nervous system (CNS) respiratory centers. Diagram illustrates major respiratory centers, neurofeedback circuits, primary neurohumoral sensory inputs, and mechanical outputs.

Generation of Ventilatory Pattern

Refer to Table 15-3 for definitions of terms used in this section. A *respiratory center* is a specific area in the brain that integrates neural traffic to produce spontaneous ventilation. Within the pontine and medullary reticular formations, there are several discrete respiratory centers that function as the control system (Fig. 15-3).

Initial descriptions of brainstem respiratory functions are based on classic ablation and electrical stimulation studies.

Table 15-3 Definition of Respiratory Pattern Terminology

Word	Definition
Eupnea	"Good breathing": continuous inspiratory and expiratory movement without interruption
Apnea	"No breathing": cessation of ventilatory effort at passive end-expiration (lung volume = FRC)
Apneusis	Cessation of ventilatory effort with lungs filled at TLC
Apneustic ventilation	Apneusis with periodic expiratory spasms
Biot	Ventilatory gasps interposed between periods of ventilation apnea; *also* "agonal ventilation"

FRC, functional residual capacity; TLC, total lung capacity.

Another method for localizing respiratory centers entails the recording of action potentials from different areas of the brainstem with microelectrodes. This method is based on the assumption that local brain activity that occurs in phase with respiratory activity identifies "respiratory neurons."[22] These techniques are imperfect for precisely localizing discrete respiratory centers.

Medullary Centers

The medulla oblongata contains the most basic ventilatory control centers in the brain. Specific medullary areas are primarily active during inspiration or during expiration, with many neural inspiratory or expiratory interconnections. The inspiratory centers that reside in the dorsal respiratory group (DRG) are located in the dorsal medullary reticular formation. The DRG is the source of elementary ventilatory rhythmicity[23,24] and serves as the "pacemaker" for the respiratory system.[25] Whereas resting lung volume occurs at end-expiration, the electrical activity of the ventilatory centers is at rest at end-inspiration. The rhythmic activity of the DRG persists even when all incoming peripheral and interconnecting nerves are sectioned or blocked completely. Isolating the DRG in this manner results in ataxic, gasping ventilation with frequent maximum inspiratory efforts (apneustic breathing).

The ventral respiratory group (VRG) is located in the ventral medullary reticular formation and serves as the expiratory coordinating center. The inspiratory and expiratory neurons function by a system of reciprocal innervation, or negative feedback.[22] When the DRG creates an impulse to inspire, inspiration occurs and the DRG impulse is quenched by a reciprocating VRG impulse. This VRG transmission prohibits further use of the inspiratory muscles, thus allowing passive expiration to occur.

Pontine Centers

The pontine centers process information that originates in the medulla. The apneustic center is located in the middle or lower pons. With activation, this center sends impulses to inspiratory DRG neurons to sustain inspiration. Electrical stimulation of this area results in inspiratory spasm.[26] The middle and lower pons contain specific areas for phase-spanning neurons[27] that assist with the transition between inspiration and expiration, but do not exert direct control over ventilatory muscles.

The pneumotaxic respiratory center is in the rostral pons. A simple transection through the brainstem that isolates this portion of the pons from the upper brainstem decreases ventilatory rate and increases tidal volume. If both vagus nerves are additionally transected, apneusis results.[28] Thus, the primary function of the pneumotaxic center is to limit the depth of inspiration. When maximally activated, the pneumotaxic center secondarily increases ventilatory frequency. However, the pneumotaxic center performs no pacemaking function and has no intrinsic rhythmicity.

Higher Respiratory Centers

Many higher brain structures can affect ventilatory control processes. In the midbrain, stimulation of the reticular activating system increases the rate and amplitude of ventilation.[29] The cerebral cortex also affects breathing pattern, although precise neural pathways are not known. Occasionally, the ventilatory control process becomes subservient to other regulatory centers. For example, the respiratory system plays an important role in the control of body temperature because it supplies a large surface area for heat exchange. This is especially important in animals in which panting is a primary means of dissipating heat. Thus, the ventilatory pattern is influenced by neural input from descending pathways from the anterior and posterior hypothalamus to the pneumotaxic center of the upper pons.

Vasomotor control and certain respiratory responses are closely linked. Stimulation of the carotid sinus not only decreases vasomotor tone, but also inhibits ventilation. Alternatively, stimulation of the carotid body chemoreceptors (see Chemical Control of Ventilation section) results in an increase in both ventilatory activity and vasomotor tone.

Reflex Control of Ventilation

Reflexes that directly influence ventilatory pattern usually do so to prevent airway obstruction. *Deglutition*, or swallowing, involves the glossopharyngeal and vagus nerves. Stimulation of the anterior and posterior pharyngeal pillars of the posterior pharynx induces swallowing. During swallowing, inspiration ceases momentarily, is usually followed by a single large breath, and briefly increases ventilation.

Vomiting significantly modifies normal ventilatory activity.[30] Swallowing, salivation, gastrointestinal reflexes, rhythmic spasmodic ventilatory movements, and significant diaphragmatic and abdominal muscular activity must be coordinated over a very brief interval. Because of the obvious risk of aspirating gastric contents, it is advantageous to inhibit inspiration during vomiting. Input into the respiratory centers occurs from both cranial and spinal cord nerves.

Coughing results from stimulation of the tracheal subepithelium, especially along the posterior tracheal wall and carina.[31] Coughing also requires coordination of both airway and ventilatory muscle activity. An effective cough requires deep inspiration and then forced exhalation against a momentarily closed glottis to increase intrathoracic pressure, thus allowing an expulsive expiratory maneuver.

Proprioception in the pulmonary system, the qualitative knowledge of the gas volume within the lungs, probably arises from smooth muscle spindle receptors. These proprioceptors, which are located within the smooth muscle of all airways, are sensitive to pressure changes. Airway stretch reflexes can be demonstrated during distention of isolated airways. Airway pressure, rather than volume distention, appears to be the primary stimulation.[32] Clinical conditions in which pulmonary airway stretch receptors are stimulated include pulmonary edema and atelectasis.

Golgi tendon organs (tendon spindles), which are arranged in series within ventilatory muscles, facilitate proprioception. The intercostal muscles are rich in tendon spindles, whereas the diaphragm has a limited number. Thus, the pulmonary stretch reflex primarily involves the intercostal muscles, but not the diaphragm. When the lungs are full and the chest wall is stretched, these receptors send signals to the brainstem that inhibit further inspiration.

In 1868, Hering and Breuer reported that lightly anesthetized, spontaneously breathing animals would cease or decrease ventilatory effort during sustained lung distention.[33] This response was blocked by bilateral vagotomy. The *Hering–Breuer reflex* is prominent in lower-order mammals and sufficiently active that even 5 cm H_2O CPAP will induce apnea. In humans, however, the reflex is only weakly present, such that humans will continue to breathe spontaneously with CPAP in excess of 40 cm H_2O.

Chemical Control of Ventilation

Peripheral Chemoreceptors

In a simplistic view of chemical ventilatory control, the peripheral chemoreceptors respond primarily to lack of oxygen, and the central nervous system (CNS) receptors respond primarily to changes in PCO_2, pH, and acid–base disturbances.

The peripheral chemoreceptors are composed of the carotid and aortic bodies. The carotid bodies, located at the bifurcation of the common carotid artery, have predominantly ventilatory effects. The aortic bodies are scattered about the aortic arch and its branches, and have predominantly circulatory effects. The neural output from the carotid body reaches the central respiratory centers via the afferent glossopharyngeal nerves. Output from the aortic bodies travels to the medullary centers via the vagus nerve. Both carotid and aortic bodies are stimulated by decreased PaO_2, but not by decreased SaO_2 or CaO_2. When PaO_2 falls to less than 100 mmHg, neural activity from these receptors begins to increase. However, it is not until the PaO_2 reaches 60 to 65 mmHg that neural activity increases sufficiently to substantially augment minute ventilation. Thus, patients who depend on hypoxic ventilatory drive have PaO_2 values in the mid-60s. Once these patients' PaO_2 values exceed 60 to 65 mmHg, ventilatory drive diminishes and PaO_2 falls until ventilation is again stimulated by arterial hypoxemia. Thus, during withdrawal of mechanical ventilatory support in the patient who depends on hypoxic ventilatory drive, the PaO_2 must fall to less than 65 mmHg for spontaneous ventilation to resume.

The carotid bodies are also sensitive to decreased pH_a, but this response is minor. Similarly, changes in $PaCO_2$ do not stimulate these receptors sufficiently to alter minute ventilation. Increases in blood temperature, hypoperfusion of the carotid bodies themselves, and some chemicals will stimulate these receptors. Sympathetic ganglion stimulation by nicotine or acetylcholine will stimulate the carotid and aortic bodies; this effect is blocked by hexamethonium. Blockade of the cytochrome electron transport system by cyanide will prevent oxidative metabolism and will also stimulate these receptors.

Increased ventilatory rate and tidal volume result from stimulation of these receptors. Hemodynamic changes resulting from stimulation of these receptors include bradycardia, hypertension, increases in bronchiolar tone, and increases in adrenal secretion. The carotid body chemical receptors have been termed *ultimum moriens* ("last to die"). Although the response of peripheral receptors to hypoxemia was formerly believed to be resistant to the influences of anesthesia, potent inhaled anesthetics appear to depress hypoxic ventilatory response by depressing carotid body response to hypoxemia.[34] The response of the peripheral receptors during general anesthesia or recovery from anesthesia is not sufficiently robust to reliably increase ventilatory rate or minute ventilation to herald the onset of arterial hypoxemia. Furthermore, flumazenil only partially reversed the diazepam-induced depression of hypoxic ventilatory drive,[35] and suggests that humans may develop tolerance to respiratory depressant effects of diazepam.

Central Chemoreceptors

Approximately 80% of the ventilatory response to inhaled carbon dioxide originates in the central medullary centers. Acid–base regulation involving carbon dioxide, H$^+$, and bicarbonate is related primarily to chemosensitive receptors located in the medulla close to or in contact with the cerebrospinal fluid (CSF). The chemosensitive areas of the brainstem are in the inferolateral aspects of the medulla near the origin of the glossopharyngeal and vagus nerves. The area just beneath the surface of the ventral medulla is exquisitely sensitive to the extracellular fluid H$^+$ concentration.[36] Although this central response is the major regulator of breathing, carbon dioxide has little direct stimulating effect on these chemosensitive areas. These receptors are primarily sensitive to changes in H$^+$ concentration. Carbon dioxide has a potent but indirect effect by reacting with water to form carbonic acid, which dissociates into hydrogen and bicarbonate ions.[37]

An acute increase in PaCO$_2$ is a more potent ventilatory stimulus than an acute increase in arterial H$^+$ concentration from a metabolic source. Carbon dioxide, but not H$^+$, passes readily through the blood–brain and blood–CSF barriers. Although local buffering systems in arterial blood and body fluids immediately neutralize H$^+$, the CSF has minimal buffering capacity. Thus, once carbon dioxide crosses into the CSF, H$^+$ are created and trapped in the CSF, resulting in a CSF H$^+$ concentration considerably greater than that found in the blood. Because carbon dioxide crosses the blood–brain barrier readily, the PCO$_2$ values in the CSF, cerebral tissue, and jugular venous blood rise quickly and to the same degree as the PaCO$_2$, although the central values are about 10 mmHg higher than those measured in arterial blood.

The ventilatory response to changes in PaCO$_2$ (increased Vt, increased respiratory rate) is rapid and peaks within 1 to 2 minutes after an acute change in PaCO$_2$. With persistent levels of carbon dioxide stimulation, however, the resultant increase in ventilation declines over a period of several hours. This is probably the result of bicarbonate ions that are actively transported from the blood into the CSF through the arachnoid villi that increase CSF pH toward the normal range.[38]

With chronic carbon dioxide retention, CSF pH is renormalized, which then determines ventilatory response to subsequent changes in arterial carbon dioxide tension. This phenomenon explains the differing effects of acute versus chronic hypercapnia on the CNS-mediated ventilatory response. Because of this difference, the goals of mechanical ventilatory support in a patient with chronic CO$_2$ retention are different from a normal patient. Providing mechanical support that allows a PaCO$_2$ range to generate a pH that is normal for a specific patient is referred to as "eucapnic ventilation." Attempting to achieve a normal PaCO$_2$ (normocarbia) in a patient with chronic carbon dioxide retention will iatrogenically result in alkalemia, further increasing CSF pH and raising the apneic threshold.[39] Finally, central medullary chemoreceptors also respond to temperature change. Cold CSF (with normal pH) or local anesthetic applied to the medullary surface will depress ventilation.

Ventilatory Response to Altitude

Ventilatory response and adaptation to high altitude are good examples of how peripheral and central chemoreceptors integrate in the control of ventilation. The following mechanism of acclimatization was proposed by Severinghaus et al.[40] in 1963 and has since been confirmed.

Following ascent from sea level to 4,000 m, acute exposure to high altitude and low PIO$_2$ results in arterial hypoxemia. This decrease in PaO$_2$ activates the peripheral hypoxemic ventilatory drive by stimulating the carotid and aortic bodies, and causes increased minute ventilation. As minute ventilation increases, PaCO$_2$ and CSF PCO$_2$ decrease, causing concomitant increases in pH$_a$ and CSF pH. The alkaline shift of the CSF decreases ventilatory drive via medullary chemoreceptors, partially offsetting hypoxemic drive. A temporary equilibrium is attained within minutes, with PaCO$_2$ only 2 to 5 mmHg less than normal and PaO$_2$ approximately 45 mmHg. This initially profound hypoxemia probably causes the acute respiratory distress and other associated symptoms (headache, diarrhea) associated with rapid ascent. However, the CNS is able to restore CSF pH to normal (7.326) by pumping bicarbonate ions out of the CSF over 2 to 3 days. In 2 to 3 days, CSF bicarbonate concentration decreases approximately 5 mEq/L and restores CSF pH to within 0.01 pH unit of values at sea level. Then, centrally mediated ventilatory drive returns to normal, and hypoxic drive and stimulation of peripheral receptors can proceed unopposed. Thus, after 3 days' exposure to 4,000 m altitude, ventilatory adaptation would result in a new equilibrium, with PaCO$_2$ approximately 30 mmHg and PaO$_2$ approximately 55 mmHg. Following descent to sea level, the low CSF bicarbonate concentration persists for several days, and the climber "overbreathes" until CSF bicarbonate and pH values return to normal.

Breath-holding

Most adults with normal lungs and gas exchange can hold their breath for about 1 minute when breathing room air without previously hyperventilating. After 1 minute of breath-holding under these circumstances, PaO$_2$ decreases to approximately 65 to 70 mmHg and PaCO$_2$ increases by about 12 mmHg. In the absence of supplemental oxygen and hyperventilation, the "breakpoint" at which normal people are compelled to breathe is remarkably constant at a PaCO$_2$ of 50 mmHg.[41,42] However, if the individual breathes 100% oxygen prior to breath-holding, he or she should be able to hold his or her breath for 2 to 3 minutes, or until PaCO$_2$ rises to 60 mmHg. Hyperventilation prior to breath-holding reducing PaCO$_2$ to 20 mmHg can lengthen the period of breath-holding to 3 to 4 minutes.[43] Hyperventilation with 100% oxygen prior to breath-holding should extend the apneic period to 6 to 10 minutes. The rate of PaCO$_2$ rise in awake, preoxygenated adults with normal lungs who hold their breath without previous hyperventilation is 7 mmHg/min in the first 10 seconds, 2 mmHg/min in the next 10 seconds, and 6 mmHg/min thereafter.[42]

The duration of voluntary breath-holding is directly proportional to lung volume at onset, and is probably related both to oxygen stores in the alveoli and to the rate at which $PaCO_2$ rises. With smaller lung volumes, the same amount of carbon dioxide is emptied into a smaller volume during the apneic period, thus increasing the carbon dioxide concentration more rapidly than occurs with larger lung volumes. Of note, apneic patients during general anesthesia actually "breath-hold" at FRC rather than at vital capacity, which tends to accelerate the rate of $PaCO_2$ rise. Despite this difference in lung volume, the rate of rise of $PaCO_2$ in apneic anesthetized patients is 12 mmHg during the first minute and 3.5 mmHg/min thereafter, significantly lower than in the awake state.[43,44] During anesthesia, metabolic rate and carbon dioxide production are significantly less than during ambulatory wakefulness, which likely accounts for the lower rate of $PaCO_2$ rise under anesthesia.

Hyperventilation with room air prior to prolonged breath-holding during exercise is inadvisable. During underwater swimming after poolside hyperventilation, the urge to breathe is first stimulated by a rising $PaCO_2$. Swimmers who hyperventilate with room air prior to swimming long distances frequently lose consciousness from arterial hypoxemia before the $PaCO_2$ is sufficiently increased to stimulate the "need" to breathe.

Hyperventilation is rarely followed by an apneic period in awake humans, despite a markedly depressed $PaCO_2$. However, minute ventilation may decrease significantly. Aggressive intermittent positive-pressure breathing treatments for patients with COPD who continue to have a carbon dioxide–based ventilatory drive can depress minute ventilation sufficiently to create arterial hypoxemia if they breathe room air after cessation of therapy.[45] In contrast, even mild hyperventilation during general anesthesia will produce prolonged apneic periods.[46]

Quantitative Aspects of Chemical Control of Breathing

The ventilatory responses to oxygen and carbon dioxide can be assessed quantitatively. Unfortunately, the quantitative indices of hypoxemic sensitivity are not clinically useful because the normal range is wide and confounded by many environmental factors. The reader is referred to a classical discussion of the quantitative indices of hypoxemic sensitivity.[47]

Ventilatory responses to $PaCO_2$ changes are measured in several ways, provided that carbon dioxide production remains constant. When subjects voluntarily increase minute ventilation to a prescribed level, the $PaCO_2$ decreases nonlinearly. The plot of minute ventilation (independent variable) and $PaCO_2$ (dependent variable) is the metabolic hyperbola (Fig. 15-4). This curve is cumbersome to evaluate and difficult to use clinically.

The curve more commonly used is the $PaCO_2$ ventilatory response curve (Fig. 15-4) that describes the effect of changing $PaCO_2$ on minute ventilation. Usually, subjects inspire carbon dioxide to raise $PaCO_2$, and the effect on minute ventilation is measured. The carbon dioxide response curve can be generated more rapidly by increasing the fraction of inspired carbon dioxide (F_{ICO_2}) and requiring the subject to rebreathe exhaled gas. However, the results obtained with this technique are less pure because the F_{ICO_2} is not controlled.

Creating these curves and observing how they change in various circumstances allows quantitative study of factors that affect carbon dioxide control of ventilation. The carbon dioxide response curve approaches linearity in the range most often encountered in life: at $PaCO_2$ values between 20 and 80 mmHg. Once the $PaCO_2$ exceeds 80 mmHg, the curve becomes parabolic, with its peak ventilatory response at a $PaCO_2$ between 100 and 120 mmHg. Increasing the

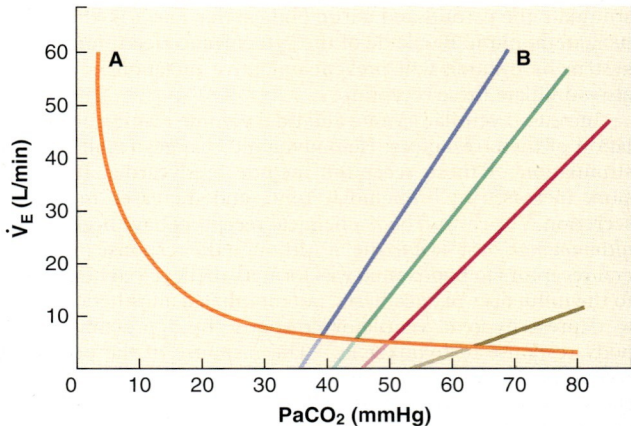

Figure 15-4 Carbon dioxide–ventilatory response curve. The metabolic hyperbola, curve A, is generated by varying minute ventilation (V_E) and measuring changes in carbon dioxide concentration. The hyperbolic configuration makes it cumbersome for clinical use. The carbon dioxide–ventilatory response curve, B, is linear between approximately 20 and 80 mmHg. It is generated by varying $PaCO_2$ (usually by controlling inspired carbon dioxide concentration) and measuring the resultant V_E. This is the most commonly used test of ventilatory response. The slope defines "sensitivity"; the setpoint, or resting $PaCO_2$, occurs at the intersection of the metabolic hyperbola and the carbon dioxide–ventilatory response curve; and the apneic threshold can be obtained by extrapolating the carbon dioxide–ventilatory response curve to the x-intercept. In the absence of surgical stimulation, increasing doses of potent inhaled anesthesia or opioids will shift the curve to the right and eventually depress the slope (*green, red, and brown lines*). Painful stimulation will reverse these changes to varying and unpredictable degrees.

$PaCO_2$ to higher than 100 mmHg allows carbon dioxide to act as a ventilatory and CNS depressant, the origin of the term "carbon dioxide narcosis," with 1 minimum alveolar concentration (MAC) being approximately 200 mmHg.

The slope of the carbon dioxide response curve represents carbon dioxide sensitivity. When $PaCO_2$ reaches 100 mmHg, carbon dioxide sensitivity is at its peak. The *setpoint*—the intersection of the carbon dioxide response curve and the metabolic hyperbola—defines normal resting $PaCO_2$. Extrapolation of the carbon dioxide response curve to the x-intercept (where minute ventilation is 0) defines the apneic threshold. In awake, normal adults, the apneic threshold normally occurs at a $PaCO_2$ of around 32 mmHg, although awake adults usually continue to breathe when they achieve the apneic threshold because the sensation of apnea is disturbing. The slope of the curve is a measure of the response of the entire ventilatory mechanism to carbon dioxide stimulation.

Once PaO_2 exceeds 100 mmHg, it no longer influences the carbon dioxide response curve. When the PaO_2 is between 65 and 100 mmHg, its effect on the carbon dioxide response curve is small. However, when PaO_2 falls to less than 65 mmHg, the carbon dioxide response curve shifts to the left and its slope increases, probably as a result of increased ventilatory drive stimulated by the peripheral chemoreceptors. Thus, during measurements of carbon dioxide ventilatory response, the subject should breathe supplemental oxygen to prevent hypoxic ventilatory drive interference. Three clinical states result in a left shift and/or a steepened slope of the carbon dioxide response curve, and are the only causes of true hyperventilation, that is, an increase in minute ventilation such that the decreased $PaCO_2$ creates either primary or compensatory respiratory alkalosis. These three causes of hyperventilation are arterial hypoxemia, metabolic acidemia, and CNS etiologies. Examples of central etiologies include drug administration, intracranial hypertension, hepatic cirrhosis, and nonspecific arousal states such as anxiety and fear. Aminophylline, doxapram, salicylates, and norepinephrine stimulate ventilation independent of peripheral chemoreceptors. Opioid antagonists given in the absence of opioids do not stimulate ventilation. However, when given after opiate administration, they do reverse the effects of opioids on the carbon dioxide response curve.

Conversely, ventilatory depressants either shift the carbon dioxide response curve to the right, decrease its slope, or both. Changes in physiology that depress ventilation include metabolic alkalemia, denervation of peripheral chemoreceptors, normal sleep, and drugs. During normal sleep, the carbon dioxide response curve is displaced to the right, with the degree of displacement depending on the depth of sleep. Usually, $PaCO_2$ increases up to 10 mmHg during deep sleep. Hypoxemic responses are not impaired by sleep, which is convenient for continued survival at high altitude while sleeping.

Opioids displace the carbon dioxide response curve to the right with little change in slope at sedative doses. With higher, "anesthetic" doses, the curve shifts farther to the right and its slope is depressed, simulating the effect of potent inhalation agents on the carbon dioxide response curve (Fig. 15-4). In the absence of other ventilatory depressant drugs, opioids induce pathognomonic changes in ventilatory patterns: a decreased ventilatory rate with an increased tidal volume. Not until opioids nearly induce apnea is tidal volume decreased. Large narcotic doses usually result in apnea responsive to verbal encouragement before consciousness is lost.

Barbiturates in sedative or light hypnotic doses have little effect on the carbon dioxide response curve. However, in doses adequate to allow skin incision, barbiturates shift the carbon dioxide response curve to the right. The ventilatory pattern resulting from barbiturate administration is characterized by decreased tidal volume and increased ventilatory rate. Potent inhaled anesthetics displace the carbon dioxide response curve to the right and decrease the slope to a degree dependent on both the anesthetic dose and the level of surgical stimulation. Like barbiturates, the ventilatory pattern following administration of potent inhaled anesthetics is initially represented by a decreased tidal volume and increased ventilatory rate. As more potent anesthetic agent is administered, however, ventilatory rate decreases toward an apneic end point. This clinical response occurs when the carbon dioxide response curve eventually becomes horizontal (slope = 0), resulting in essentially no ventilatory response to $PaCO_2$ changes.

Potent inhaled anesthetics and opioids displace the setpoint to the right, implying that the resting, steady-state $PaCO_2$ is higher and minute ventilation lower. Furthermore, when the carbon dioxide response curve shifts to the right, the apneic threshold also increases (Fig. 15-4). Surgical stimulation reverses the ventilatory response changes induced by inhaled anesthetics and opioids, but the degree of reversal is not predictable.

Oxygen and Carbon Dioxide Transport

This chapter discusses only external respiration, in which oxygen moves from the ambient environment into the pulmonary capillaries, and carbon dioxide leaves the pulmonary capillaries to enter the atmosphere. The movement of gas across the alveolar–capillary membrane depends on the integrity of the pulmonary and cardiac systems. Unless otherwise stated, the reader should assume the ventilation and perfusion of alveolar–capillary units are normal. Abnormal distribution of ventilation or perfusion of the lungs is discussed later (see Ventilation–Perfusion Relationships section).

Bulk Flow of Gas (Convection)

Convection, in which all gas molecules move in the same direction, is the primary mechanism responsible for gas flow in large and most small airways, from the bronchi down to the bronchiolar airways of the fourteenth or fifteenth generation. Resistance can be defined with Poiseuille law (Equation 15-2), and increases rapidly as the radius or cross-sectional area of a tube decreases. Although a single isolated fourteenth-generation bronchiolar airway may have greater resistance to air flow compared to a bronchus, the overall total resistance in a system is also dependent on the number of parallel pathways present. The overall total resistance of the system will be less than any individual tube's resistance, as illustrated by the equation:

$$1/R_{total} = 1/R_1 + 1/R_2 + 1/R_3 + \text{etc.} \qquad (15\text{-}4)$$

The anatomy of the tracheobronchial tree is organized in such a way that there is an increase in total parallel pathways and total cross-sectional area with each generation toward the periphery. Therefore, total airway resistance to gas flow is lower at the periphery compared to the large bronchi.

The exponential increase in total cross-sectional area of parallel airways toward the lung periphery also affects airflow velocity. Similar to airflow resistance, velocity is inversely proportional to a system's overall total cross-sectional area. Therefore, airflow velocity at the lower generations of the tracheobronchial tree is lower than that of the bronchi. In other words, the velocity of airflow decreases from the trachea down to the peripheral distal airways. During normal quiet ventilation, gas flow within convective airways is mainly laminar.

Gas Diffusion

Diffusion within a gas-filled space is random molecular motion that results in complete mixing of all gases. In the distal airways of the lung beginning with the terminal bronchioles (sixteenth airway generation), diffusion becomes the predominant mode of gas transport. Once gas reaches the small alveolar ducts, alveolar sacs, and alveoli, both diffusion and regional $\dot{V}/\dot{Q}$ relationships influence gas transport. Historically, clinicians assumed defects in gas diffusion were responsible for arterial hypoxemia. However, the most frequent cause of arterial hypoxemia is shunt effect (see Ventilation–Perfusion Relationships section).[48]

The other usage of "diffusion" refers to the passive movement of molecules across a membrane that is governed primarily by concentration gradient. In this sense, carbon dioxide is 20 times more diffusible across human membranes than is oxygen; therefore, carbon dioxide crosses alveoli easily. As a result, hypercapnia is *never* the result of defective diffusion; rather, it is the result of inadequate alveolar ventilation relative to carbon dioxide production.

True diffusion defects that create arterial hypoxemia are rare. The most common reason for a measured decrease in diffusing capacity (see Pulmonary Function Testing section) is mismatched ventilation and perfusion, which functionally results in a decreased surface area available for diffusion.

Distribution of Ventilation and Perfusion

The efficiency with which oxygen and carbon dioxide exchange at the alveolar–capillary level highly depends on the matching of capillary perfusion and alveolar ventilation. At this level, the marriage between the lung and the circulatory system must be well matched and intimate.

Distribution of Blood Flow

Blood flow within the lung is mainly gravity dependent. Because the alveolar–capillary beds are not composed of rigid vessels, the pressure of the surrounding tissues can influence the resistance to flow through the individual capillaries. Thus, blood flow depends on the relationship between pulmonary artery pressure (P_{pa}), alveolar pressure (P_A), and pulmonary venous pressure (P_{pv}) (Fig. 15-5). West created a lung model that divides the lung into three zones.[48,49] Zone 1 conditions occur in the most gravity-independent part of the lung (lung apex). In this region, alveolar pressure is approximately equal to atmospheric pressure. Pulmonary artery pressure always exceeds pulmonary venous pressure, which is subatmospheric in Zone 1. Therefore, Zone 1 can be described by the following relationship: $P_A > P_{pa} > P_{pv}$. In Zone 1, alveolar pressure transmitted to the pulmonary capillaries promotes their collapse, with a consequent theoretical blood flow of zero to this lung region. Thus, Zone 1 receives ventilation in the absence of perfusion. This relationship is referred to as alveolar dead space ventilation. Normally, Zone 1 areas exist only to a limited extent. However, in conditions of decreased pulmonary artery pressure, such as hypovolemic shock, Zone 1 enlarges, thus increasing alveolar dead space ventilation.

Zone 2 occurs from the lower limit of Zone 1 to the upper limit of Zone 3, where $P_{pa} > P_A > P_{pv}$. The pressure difference between pulmonary artery and alveolar pressure determines blood flow in Zone 2. Pulmonary venous pressure has little influence. Well-matched ventilation and perfusion occur in Zone 2, which contains the majority of alveoli.

Finally, Zone 3 occurs in the most gravity-dependent areas of the lung where $P_{pa} > P_{pv} > P_A$ and blood flow is primarily governed by the pulmonary arterial to venous pressure difference. Because gravity also increases pulmonary venous pressure, the pulmonary capillaries become distended. Thus, perfusion in Zone 3 is lush, resulting in capillary perfusion in excess of ventilation, or physiologic shunt.

Distribution of Ventilation

Alveolar pressure is the same throughout the lung; therefore, the more negative intrapleural pressure at the apex (or the least gravity-dependent area) results in larger, more distended apical alveoli than in other areas of the lung. The transpulmonary pressure ($P_{aw} - P_{pl}$), or distending pressure of the lung, is greater at the top and lower at the bottom, where intrapleural pressure is less negative. Despite the smaller alveolar size, more ventilation is delivered to dependent pulmonary areas. The decrease in intrapleural pressure at the base of the lungs during inspiration is greater than at the apex because of diaphragmatic proximity. Thus, because the dependent area of the lung generates the greatest change in transpulmonary pressure, more gas is sucked into dependent areas of the lung.

Ventilation–Perfusion Relationships

As discussed previously, the majority of blood flow is distributed to the gravity-dependent part of the lung. During a spontaneous breath, the largest portion of the tidal volume also reaches the gravity-dependent part of the lung. Thus, the nondependent area of the lung receives a lower proportion of both ventilation (V_A) and perfusion (Q), and dependent lung receives greater proportions of ventilation and perfusion. Nevertheless, ventilation and perfusion are not matched perfectly, and various $\dot{V}/\dot{Q}$ ratios result throughout the lung. The ideal $\dot{V}/\dot{Q}$ ratio of 1 is believed to occur at approximately the level of the third rib. Above this level, ventilation occurs slightly in excess of perfusion, whereas below the third rib the $\dot{V}/\dot{Q}$ ratio becomes less than 1 (Fig. 15-6).

In a simplified model, gas exchange units can be divided into normal ($\dot{V}/\dot{Q}$ 1:1), dead space ($\dot{V}/\dot{Q} = 1:0$), shunt ($\dot{V}/\dot{Q} = 0:1$), or a silent unit ($\dot{V}/\dot{Q} = 0:0$) (Fig. 15-7). Although this model is helpful in understanding $\dot{V}/\dot{Q}$ relationships and their influences on gas exchange, $\dot{V}/\dot{Q}$ really occurs as a continuum. In the lungs of a healthy, upright, spontaneously breathing individual, the majority

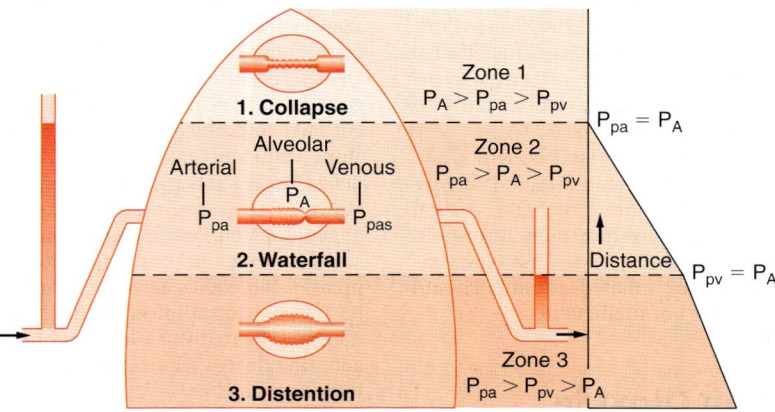

Figure 15-5 Distribution of blood flow in the isolated lung. In Zone 1, alveolar pressure (P_A) exceeds pulmonary artery pressure (P_{pa}), and no flow occurs because the vessels are collapsed. In Zone 2, arterial pressure exceeds alveolar pressure, but alveolar pressure exceeds pulmonary venous pressure (P_{pv}). Flow in Zone 2 is determined by the arterial–alveolar pressure difference ($P_{pa} - P_A$), which steadily increases down the zone. In Zone 3, pulmonary venous pressure exceeds alveolar pressure, and flow is determined by the arterial–venous pressure difference ($P_{pa} - P_{pv}$), which is constant down this pulmonary zone. However, the pressure across the vessel walls increases down the zone so their caliber increases, as does flow. (Adapted from West JB, Dollery CT, Naimark A. Distribution of blood flow in isolated lung: Relation to vascular and alveolar pressures. *J Appl Physiol.* 1964;19:713–724.)

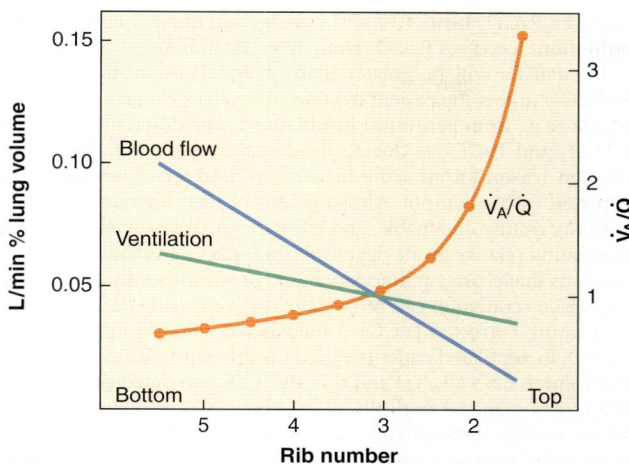

Figure 15-6 Distribution of ventilation, blood flow, and ventilation–perfusion ratio in the normal, upright lung. Straight lines have been drawn through the ventilation and blood flow data. Because blood flow falls more rapidly than ventilation with distance up the lung, ventilation–perfusion ratio rises, slowly at first, then rapidly. (Reprinted with permission from West JB. Ventilation/Blood Flow and Gas Exchange, 4th ed. Oxford, England, Blackwell Scientific, 1985.)

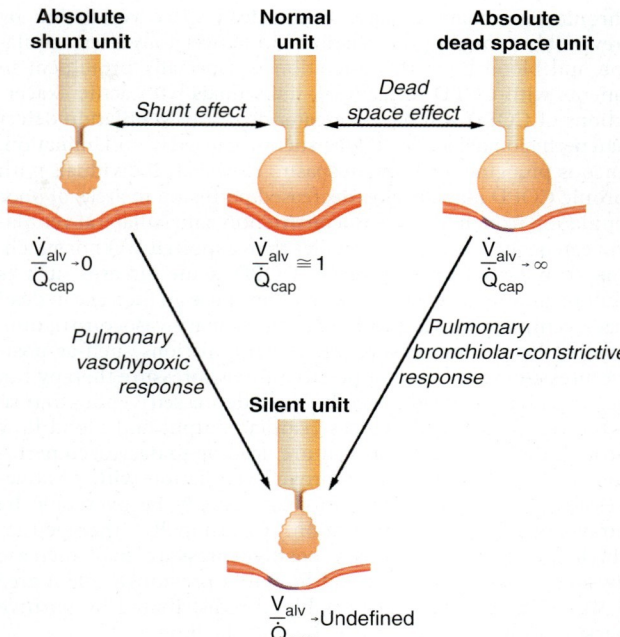

Figure 15-7 Continuum of ventilation–perfusion relationships. Gas exchange is maximally effective in normal lung units and only partially effective in shunt and dead space effect units. It is totally absent in silent units, absolute shunt, and dead space units.

of alveolar–capillary units are normal gas exchange units. The $\dot{V}/\dot{Q}$ ratio varies between absolute shunt (in which $\dot{V}/\dot{Q} = 0$) to absolute dead space (in which $\dot{V}/\dot{Q} = \infty$). Rather than absolute shunt, most units with low $\dot{V}/\dot{Q}$ mismatch receive a small amount of ventilation relative to blood flow. Similarly, most dead space units are not absolute, but rather are characterized by low blood flow relative to ventilation. During acute lung injury and adult respiratory distress syndrome, areas of low $\dot{V}/\dot{Q}$ matching commonly lie adjacent to areas of high $\dot{V}/\dot{Q}$ matching.[50] Thus, the West lung zone model should be used to aid the understanding of pulmonary physiology and not be regarded as an incontrovertible anatomic truism.

Hypoxic pulmonary vasoconstriction and bronchoconstriction allow the lungs to maintain optimal $\dot{V}/\dot{Q}$ matching. Hypoxic pulmonary vasoconstriction, stimulated by alveolar hypoxia, severely decreases blood flow. Thus, poorly ventilated alveoli also receive minuscule blood flow. Furthermore, decreased regional pulmonary blood flow results in bronchiolar constriction and diminishes the degree of dead space ventilation.[51,52] When either phenomenon occurs, the shunt or dead space units effectively become silent units in which little ventilation or perfusion occurs.

Many pulmonary diseases result in both physiologic shunt and dead space abnormalities. However, most disease processes can be characterized as producing either primarily shunt or dead space in their early stages. Increases in dead space ventilation primarily affect carbon dioxide elimination and have little influence on arterial oxygenation until dead space ventilation exceeds 80% to 90% of minute ventilation ($\dot{V}_E$). Similarly, physiologic shunt primarily affects arterial oxygenation with little effect on carbon dioxide elimination until the physiologic shunt fraction exceeds 75% to 80% of the cardiac output. Defective to absent gas exchange can be the net effect of either abnormality in the extreme.

Physiologic Dead Space

Each inspired breath is composed of gas that contributes to alveolar ventilation (V_A) and gas that becomes dead space ventilation (V_D). Thus, tidal volume (Vt) = $V_A + V_D$. In the normal, spontaneously breathing person, the ratio of alveolar-to-dead space ventilation (V_A/V_D) for each breath is 2:1. Conveniently, the rule of "1, 2, 3" applies to normal, spontaneously breathing persons. For each breath, 1 mL/lb (lean body weight) becomes V_D, 2 mL × lb^{-1} becomes V_L, and 3 mL × lb^{-1} constitutes the Vt.

Physiologic dead space consists of anatomic and alveolar dead space. Anatomic dead space ventilation, approximately 2 mL/kg ideal body weight, accounts for the majority of physiologic dead space. It arises from ventilation of structures that do not exchange respiratory gases: the oronasopharynx to the terminal and respiratory bronchioles. Clinical conditions that modify anatomic dead space include tracheal intubation, tracheostomy, and large lengths of ventilator tubing between the tracheal tube and the ventilator Y-piece. It is important to note that ventilation occurs because gas flows into and out of the alveoli. In contrast, the inspiratory or expiratory limb of the anesthesia circle system has unidirectional flow, and therefore, is not a component of anatomic dead space ventilation.

Alveolar dead space ventilation arises from ventilation of alveoli with inadequate or no perfusion. Since disease produces little change in anatomic dead space, physiologic dead space is primarily influenced by changes in alveolar dead space. Rapid changes in physiologic dead space ventilation most often arise from changes in pulmonary blood flow, resulting in decreased perfusion to ventilated alveoli. The most common etiology of acutely increased physiologic dead space is an abrupt decrease in cardiac output. Another pathologic condition that interferes with pulmonary blood flow, and thereby creates dead space, is pulmonary embolism, whether due to thrombus, fat, air, or amniotic fluid. Although there may be obstruction to blood flow with some types of pulmonary emboli, the greatest decrease in pulmonary blood flow is due to vasoconstriction induced by locally released vasoactive substances such as leukotrienes.

Chronic pulmonary diseases create dead space ventilation by irreversibly changing the relationship between alveolar ventilation and blood flow; this alteration is especially prominent in patients with COPD. In general, individuals with acute exacerbations of COPD will have a greater degree of ventilation defect than perfusion defect due to obstruction caused by inflammation, mucous plugging, or bronchospasm. However, individuals with chronic COPD may develop decreased perfusion in areas of poor ventilation from hypoxic vasoconstriction, and collateral ventilation can occur, leading to a smaller than expected $\dot{V}/\dot{Q}$ mismatch. Similar to acute exacerbations of COPD, acute diseases such as adult respiratory distress syndrome can cause an increase in dead space ventilation owing to intense pulmonary vasoconstriction. Finally, therapeutic or supportive manipulations such as positive-pressure ventilation or positive airway pressure therapy can increase alveolar dead space because depressed venous return to the right heart will decrease cardiac output and blood flow through the pulmonary vasculature, leading to decreased perfusion of the alveoli despite improved ventilation with positive-pressure therapy. However, this can usually be overcome by intravenous fluid administration. Occasionally, therapeutics which create intrapulmonary positive pressure may increase physiologic shunt, when blood flow to a previously silent area of $\dot{V}/\dot{Q}$ matching now receives blood redistributed by positive pressure from more compliant areas of the lung.

Assessment of Physiologic Dead Space

As the lung receives nearly 100% of the cardiac output, assessment of physiologic dead space ventilation in the acute setting yields valuable information about pulmonary blood flow and, ultimately, about cardiac output. If pulmonary blood flow decreases, the most likely cause is a decreased cardiac output. Thus, it is clinically useful to be able to readily assess the degree of physiologic dead space ventilation.

There are two easy and several difficult ways to assess dead space ventilation. A comparison of minute ventilation and $PaCO_2$ allows a gross qualitative assessment of physiologic dead space ventilation. The $PaCO_2$ is determined only by alveolar ventilation and carbon dioxide production ($\dot{V}CO_2$). If $\dot{V}CO_2$ remains constant, $PaCO_2$ will also remain constant as long as minute ventilation supplies the same degree of alveolar ventilation. If the spontaneously breathing individual must increase minute ventilation to maintain the same $PaCO_2$, he or she will experience an increase in dead space ventilation because less of the minute ventilation is contributing to alveolar ventilation. Alternatively, a mechanically ventilated patient with a fixed minute ventilation and no increases in $\dot{V}CO_2$ also experiences an increased dead space ventilation if the $PaCO_2$ rises. Hence, when $PaCO_2$ in a mechanically ventilated patient increases, it is necessary to determine if the cause is increased dead space ventilation or an increased $\dot{V}CO_2$.

Because positive-pressure ventilation increases alveolar pressure, the mechanically ventilated patient with normal lungs has a dead space to alveolar ventilation ratio (V_D/V_A) of 1:1 (more West Zone 1) rather than 1:2, as during spontaneous ventilation. If mechanical Vt is 1,000 mL, 500 mL contributes to V_A, and 500 mL contributes to V_D. At rest, the required $\dot{V}_A$ with normal $\dot{V}CO_2$ is approximately 60 mL/kg/min. A 70-kg man would then require a $\dot{V}_A$ of 4,200 mL/min. During spontaneous breathing, the required $\dot{V}_E$ would be 6,300 mL/min, but during mechanical ventilation $\dot{V}_E$ would have to be 8,400 mL/min. Using this calculation, if a 70-kg resting patient requires $\dot{V}_E$ much in excess of 8,400 mL/min, either $\dot{V}_D$ or $\dot{V}CO_2$ is increased. A rule of thumb for mechanically ventilated patients is that doubling baseline minute ventilation decreases $PaCO_2$ from 40 to 30 mmHg, and quadrupling minute ventilation decreases $PaCO_2$ from 40 to 20 mmHg.

The $PaCO_2$ will be greater than or equal to end-tidal $PaCO_2$ ($PETCO_2$) unless the patient inspires or receives exogenous carbon dioxide (e.g., from peritoneal insufflation). The difference between $PETCO_2$ and $PaCO_2$ is due to dead space ventilation. The most common reason for an acute increase in dead space ventilation is decreased cardiac output. Measurement of this difference—which is simple, readily obtainable, and fairly inexpensive—yields reliable information relative to the degree of dead space ventilation. Clinical situations that change pulmonary blood flow sufficiently to increase dead space ventilation can be detected by comparing $PETCO_2$ with temperature-corrected $PaCO_2$. Yamanaka and Sue[53] found that the $PETCO_2$ in ventilated patients varied linearly with the dead space to tidal volume ratio (V_D/Vt) and that $PETCO_2$ correlated poorly with $PaCO_2$. Thus, in the critically ill, mechanically ventilated patient, and in anesthetized patients, monitoring $PETCO_2$ gives far more information about ventilatory efficiency or dead space ventilation than it does about the absolute value of $PaCO_2$.

Anesthesiologists commonly measure $PETCO_2$ to detect venous air embolism during anesthesia. A lowered cardiac output alone, in the absence of venous air embolism, may sufficiently decrease pulmonary perfusion, so dead space ventilation increases and $PETCO_2$ falls. Thus, a depressed $PETCO_2$ is sensitive for decreased cardiac output but not specific for pulmonary embolism. Air in the pulmonary arteries mechanically interferes with blood flow and also causes pulmonary arterial constriction, further decreasing pulmonary blood flow. A decreased $PETCO_2$ suggests that a physiologically significant air embolism has occurred. The same physiologic considerations apply to detecting pulmonary thromboembolism.

Some clinicians use the divergence of $PETCO_2$ from $PaCO_2$ as a reflection of pulmonary blood flow for other applications. During intentional pharmacologic or surgical manipulation of pulmonary blood flow, the difference between $PaCO_2$ and $PETCO_2$ serves as a useful physiologic monitor for the effectiveness of these interventions. Furthermore, $PETCO_2$ reflects pulmonary perfusion, is a useful tool for studying and monitoring the effectiveness of resuscitation efforts, and may provide a marker for survival after resuscitation.[54]

The most quantitative technique used to measure physiologic dead space uses a modification of the Bohr equation:

$$\frac{V_D}{Vt} = \frac{PaCO_2 - P\bar{E}CO_2}{PaCO_2} \qquad (15\text{-}5)$$

where $P\bar{E}CO_2$ is the PCO_2 from the mixture of all expired gases over the period of time during which measurements are made. This calculation estimates the fraction of each breath that does not contribute to gas exchange. In spontaneously breathing patients, normal V_D/Vt is between 0.2 and 0.4, or approximately 0.33. In patients receiving positive-pressure ventilation, V_D/Vt becomes about 0.5. The major limitation of performing this calculation is the difficulty in collecting exhaled gas for $P\bar{E}CO_2$ measurement. Exhaled gases, collected in cumbersome Douglas bags, can be easily contaminated with inspired air or supplemental oxygen. The measurement will also be inaccurate if the patient does not maintain a steady ventilatory pattern. Therefore, extreme care must be taken to ensure all measurements are performed accurately. In practice, this measurement is rarely performed.

Physiologic Shunt

Whereas physiologic dead space ventilation applies to areas of the lung that are ventilated but poorly perfused, physiologic shunt occurs in lung that is perfused but poorly ventilated. The physiologic shunt ($\dot{Q}_{SP}$) is that portion of the total cardiac output ($\dot{Q}_T$) that returns to the left heart and systemic circulation without receiving oxygen in the lung. When pulmonary blood is not exposed to alveoli or when those alveoli are devoid of ventilation, the result is *absolute or true shunt*, in which $\dot{V}_A/\dot{Q} = 0$. *Shunt effect*, or *venous admixture*, is the more common clinical phenomenon and occurs in areas where alveolar ventilation is deficient compared with the degree of perfusion: $0 < \dot{V}_A/\dot{Q} < 1$.

Because blood passing through areas of absolute shunt receives no oxygen, arterial hypoxemia resulting from absolute shunt is minimally reversed with supplemental oxygen. Alternatively, supplemental oxygen supplied to patients with arterial hypoxemia due to venous admixture will increase the PaO_2. Although ventilation to these alveoli is deficient, they do carry a small amount of oxygen to the capillary bed. Thus, assessment of arterial oxygen responsiveness to supplemental oxygen administration is a helpful diagnostic tool.

A small percentage of venous blood normally bypasses the right ventricle and empties directly into the left atrium. This anatomic, absolute, or true shunt arises from the venous return of the pleural, bronchiolar, and thebesian veins. This venous admixture accounts for 2% to 5% of total cardiac output and represents the small shunt that normally occurs. Anatomic shunts of greatest magnitude are usually associated with congenital heart diseases that cause right-to-left shunt. Intrapulmonary anatomic shunts can also cause anatomic shunt. For example, the arterial hypoxemia associated with advanced hepatic failure (hepatopulmonary syndrome) is due, in part, to arteriovenous malformations.[55,56] Diseases that may cause absolute or true shunt include acute lobar atelectasis, extensive acute lung injury, advanced pulmonary edema, and consolidated pneumonia. Disease entities that tend to produce venous admixture include mild pulmonary edema, postoperative atelectasis, and COPD.

Assessment of Arterial Oxygenation and Physiologic Shunt

The simplest assessment of oxygenation is qualitative comparison of the patient's F_{IO_2} and PaO_2. The highest possible PaO_2 for any given F_{IO_2} (and $PaCO_2$) can be calculated from the alveolar gas equation:

$$PaO_2 = F_{IO_2}(P_b - P_{H_2O}) - \frac{PaCO_2}{R} \quad (15\text{-}6)$$

where PaO_2 and $PaCO_2$ are alveolar PO_2 and PCO_2, P_{H_2O} is water vapor pressure at 100% saturation and 37°C, P_b is barometric pressure, and R is respiratory quotient. Assuming one makes the calculation for a well-perfused alveolus, the alveolar and arterial PCO_2 are equal. Therefore, $PaCO_2$ can be substituted for $PaCO_2$. Respiratory quotient (R) is the ratio of O_2 consumed ($\dot{V}O_2$) to CO_2 produced ($\dot{V}CO_2$):

$$\frac{\dot{V}_{CO_2}}{\dot{V}_{O_2}} = \frac{200 \text{ mL/min}}{250 \text{ mL/min}} = 0.8 \quad (15\text{-}7)$$

Oxygen tension–based indices do not reflect mixed venous contribution to arterial oxygenation and can be misleading.[57] Even if venous admixture is small, mixed venous blood with very low oxygen content will magnify the effect of a small shunt. Oxygen tension–based indices, for example, PaO_2/F_{IO_2}, alveolar to arterial PO_2 difference ($P[A\text{-}a]O_2$), and ratio PaO_2/PAO_2, do not take into account the influence of mixed venous oxygen content ($C\bar{v}O_2$) on arterial oxygenation. Therefore, in critically ill patients who are hypoxemic, the insertion of a pulmonary artery catheter to assess shunt and to measure cardiac output may be essential to understanding the influence of cardiac function on arterial oxygenation.

The alveolar gas equation has important clinical utility in recognizing alveolar hypoventilation due to its effect on arterial oxygenation. Dalton's law refers to the fact that each gas in a mixture will exert its own partial pressure, and in sum will equal the total pressure of the mixture.[58] The first term in the equation describes the partial pressure of oxygen in the alveolus, while the second represents carbon dioxide. In the event of significant alveolar hypoventilation, carbon dioxide accumulates in arterial blood and subsequently the alveolus. While inspiring room air the concentration of oxygen is reduced and arterial hypoxemia will occur. Using a $PaCO_2$ value of 80 mmHg, the alveolar gas equation will calculate the PaO_2 as approximately 50 mmHg. Assuming a normal P_{50} for hemoglobin and normal A-a gradient, this arterial oxygen tension will correspond to an arterial saturation value in the 80% range, modestly above the value for mixed venous saturation.[39] In response to hypoxemia, alveolar hyperventilation produces a decrease in $PaCO_2$ and $PaCO_2$. While inspiring room air, if the $PaCO_2$ were to decrease, a concomitant increase in the partial pressure of oxygen must occur to preserve the total pressure in the alveolus. For example, if the $PaCO_2$ were to decrease to 20 mmHg, the resulting PaO_2 would increase by approximately 25 mmHg, thereby increasing arterial oxygen saturation, oxygen content, and oxygen delivery.

The assessment of arterial oxygenation requires, at least, knowledge of F_{IO_2} and either PaO_2 or SaO_2. Oxygen tension–based indices of oxygenation are useful, but they do not take into account the contribution of mixed venous blood to arterial oxygenation. Mixed venous blood can become extremely desaturated in the critically ill patient owing to inadequate cardiac output, anemia, arterial hypoxemia, increased $\dot{V}O_2$, or abnormal hemoglobin moieties. The best knowledge of the efficiency with which the lungs oxygenate the arterial blood can be obtained only by calculating shunt fraction.

Physiologic Shunt Calculation

The clinical reference standard for the calculation of physiologic shunt fraction is derived from a two-compartment pulmonary blood flow model. One compartment performs ideal gas exchange and contains perfectly married alveolar–capillary units while the other is the shunt compartment and contains pulmonary capillaries that have no exposure to ventilated alveoli. Using the Fick relationship, the following equation can be derived:

$$\frac{\dot{Q}_{SP}}{\dot{Q}_T} = \frac{Cc'O_2 - CaO_2}{Cc'O_2 - C\bar{v}O_2} \quad (15\text{-}8)$$

where $\dot{Q}_{SP}/\dot{Q}_T$ is the shunt fraction ($\dot{Q}_{SP}$ is blood flow through the physiologic shunt compartment, $\dot{Q}_T$ is total cardiac output), and $Cc'O_2$, CaO_2, and $C\bar{v}O_2$ are end-capillary, arterial, and mixed-venous oxygen contents, respectively. Normal intrapulmonary shunt is approximately 5%. Because this equation is based on an artificial two-compartment model, the absolute value is physically meaningless. A calculated $\dot{Q}_{SP}/\dot{Q}_T$ of 25% means that if the lung existed in two compartments, 25% of the cardiac output would travel through the shunt compartment. Since the lung does not truly exist in two compartments, this equation grossly estimates pulmonary oxygen exchange defects. Nevertheless, it remains our best tool for clinically evaluating the lungs' efficiency in oxygenating arterial blood. Observing changes in shunt fraction corresponding to therapeutic intervention or disease progression is more valuable than knowing the absolute value per se.

Since hemoglobin concentration is uniform throughout the vascular system, the oxygen contents in the shunt equation are determined primarily by oxyhemoglobin saturation. Thus, the shunt equation can be approximated by substituting saturation values for each term; the new value, called *ventilation–perfusion ratio* (VQI),[56] is determined as follows:

$$VQI = \frac{Sc'O_2 - SaO_2}{Sc'O_2 - S\bar{v}O_2} \cong \frac{1 - SaO_2}{1 - S\bar{v}O_2} \quad (15\text{-}9)$$

If the patient is neither breathing a hypoxic gas mixture nor has a methemoglobin or carboxyhemoglobin value in excess of 5% to 6%, $Sc'O_2$ must equal 1 because the model requires a perfect alveolar–capillary interface. This substitution results in the final expression in the previous equation. The absolute values of VQI are meaningless, although "normal" should be 0% to 4%. Like $\dot{Q}_{SP}/\dot{Q}_T$, the importance of these values lies in their trend as disease and treatment progress.

SaO_2 and $S\bar{v}O_2$ can be estimated continuously with pulse oximetry and by using a pulmonary artery catheter with oximetry capability. By interfacing the outputs of these two devices with a computer, VQI can be calculated continuously. The greatest advantage of calculating $\dot{Q}_{SP}/\dot{Q}_T$ or VQI to assess arterial oxygenation efficiency is that these values include the contribution of mixed venous blood.

Pulmonary Function Testing

Because anesthesiologists frequently care for patients with significant pulmonary dysfunction, they must be able to interpret tests of pulmonary function (and dysfunction) intelligently. This section discusses lung volumes, tests of pulmonary mechanics, and diffusing capacity.

Lung Volumes and Capacities

Known, reproducible pulmonary gas volumes and capacities provide a reliable basis for comparison between normal and abnormal measurements.[59] Because normal measurements vary with size, height is most frequently used to define "normal." Lung capacities are composed of two or more lung volumes. Lung volumes and capacities are schematically illustrated in Figure 15-8.

Tidal volume is the volume of gas that moves in and out of the lungs during quiet breathing and is about 6 to 8 mL/kg. Tidal volume falls with decreased lung compliance or when the patient has reduced ventilatory muscle strength.

Vital capacity is usually around 60 mL/kg but may vary as much as 20% from normal in healthy individuals. Vital capacity correlates well with deep breathing and effective coughing. It is decreased by restrictive pulmonary disease such as pulmonary edema or atelectasis. Vital capacity may also be reduced by mechanically induced, extrapulmonary restriction seen in pleural effusion, pneumothorax, pregnancy, large ascites, or ventilatory muscle weakness.

The *inspiratory capacity* is the largest volume of gas that can be inspired from the resting expiratory level and is frequently decreased in the presence of significant extrathoracic airway obstruction. This measurement is one of the few simple tests that can detect extrathoracic airway obstruction. Most routine pulmonary function tests measure only exhaled flows and volumes, which may be relatively unaffected by extrathoracic obstruction until it is severe. Changes in the absolute volume of inspiratory capacity usually parallel changes in vital capacity. *Expiratory reserve volume* is not of great diagnostic value.

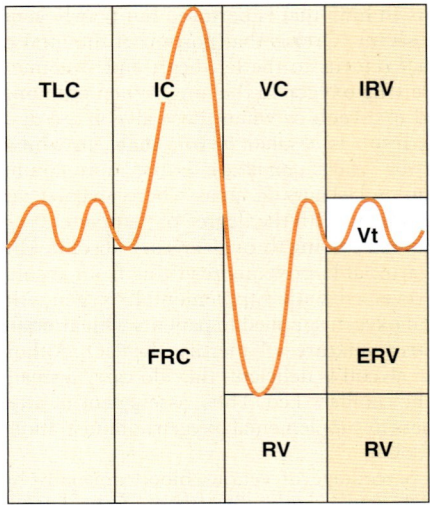

Figure 15-8 Lung volumes and capacities. The *darkest shaded bar* on the far right depicts the four basic lung volumes that sum to create TLC. Other lung capacities are composed of two or more lung volumes. The overlying spirographic tracing orients the reader to the relationship between the lung volumes and capacities and the spirogram. ERV, expiratory reserve volume; FRC, functional residual capacity; IC, inspiratory capacity; IRV, inspiratory reserve volume; RV, residual volume; TLC, total lung capacity; VC, vital capacity; Vt, tidal volume.

FRC is the volume of gas remaining in the lungs at passive end-expiration. *Residual volume* is the gas remaining within the lungs at the end of forced maximal expiration. The FRC serves two primary physiologic functions. First, it determines the point on the pulmonary volume–pressure curve for resting ventilation (Fig. 15-2). The tangent defined by the midportion pulmonary volume–pressure curve at FRC defines lung compliance. Thus, FRC determines the elastic pressure–volume relationships within the lung. Furthermore, FRC is the resting expiratory volume of the lung and is the primary determinant of oxygen reserve in humans when apnea occurs. As such, it greatly influences ventilation–perfusion relationships within the lung. When FRC is reduced, venous admixture (low $\dot{V}_A/\dot{Q}$) increases and results in arterial hypoxemia (see Oxygen and Carbon Dioxide Transport and Lung Mechanics sections).

Further, the FRC may be used to quantify the degree of pulmonary restriction. Disease processes that reduce FRC and lung compliance include acute lung injury, pulmonary edema, pulmonary fibrotic processes, and atelectasis. Mechanical factors also reduce FRC, for example, pregnancy, obesity, pleural effusion, and posture. The FRC decreases 10% when a healthy subject lies supine. Ventilatory muscle weakness or paralysis will also decrease FRC. In contrast, patients with COPD have excessively compliant lungs that recoil less forcibly. Their lungs retain an abnormally large volume at the end of passive expiration, a phenomenon called *gas trapping*.

FRC Measurement

The FRC and residual volume must be measured indirectly because residual volume cannot be removed from the lung.

The multiple-breath nitrogen washout test is performed by having the subject breathe 100% oxygen for several minutes to enable alveolar nitrogen to gradually "wash out." With each breath, the volume of gas and the concentration of nitrogen in the exhaled gas are measured. A rapid nitrogen analyzer coupled to a spirometer or pneumotachometer provides a breath-by-breath analysis of nitrogen washout. Electronic signals proportional to nitrogen concentrations and exhaled volumes (or flow, if a pneumotachometer is used) are integrated to derive the exhaled volume of nitrogen for each breath. Then, the values for all breaths are summed to provide a total volume of nitrogen washed out of the lungs. The test proceeds until the alveolar nitrogen concentration is reduced to less than 7%, usually requiring 7 to 10 minutes. FRC is calculated using the equation:

$$FRC = N_2 \text{ volume} \times \frac{[N_2]_f}{[N_2]_i} \quad (15\text{-}10)$$

where $[N_2]_i$ and $[N_2]_f$ are the fractional concentrations of alveolar nitrogen at the beginning and end of the test, respectively.

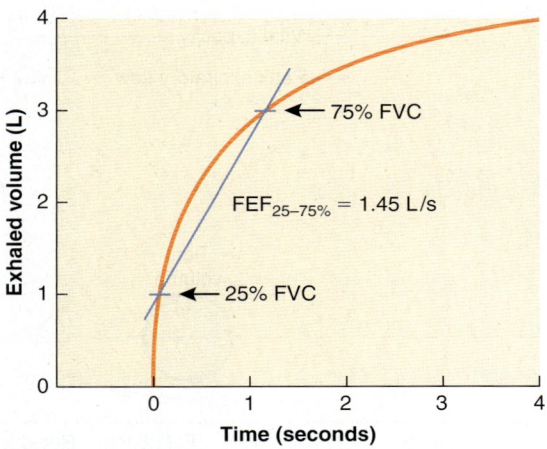

Figure 15-9 $FEF_{25\%-75\%}$. The spirogram depicts a 4 L FVC on which the points representing 25% and 75% FVC are marked. The slope of the line connecting these points is the $FEF_{25\%-75\%}$.

Pulmonary Function Tests

Forced Vital Capacity

The forced vital capacity (FVC) is the volume of gas that can be expired as forcefully and rapidly as possible after maximal inspiration. Normally, FVC is equal to vital capacity. Although forced expiration significantly increases intrapleural pressures yet changes airway pressure minimally, bronchiolar collapse, obstructive lesions, and gas trapping are exaggerated. Thus, FVC may be reduced in chronic obstructive diseases even when the vital capacity appears near normal. FVC is nearly always decreased by restrictive diseases. FVC values lower than 15 mL/kg are associated with an increased incidence of PPCs, probably because these patients cough ineffectively.[60] FVC reduced to this level represents a profound defect, most commonly seen in quadriplegics or severe neuromuscular disease. Finally, FVC is largely dependent on patient effort and cooperation.

Forced Expiratory Volume

FEV_T is the forced expiratory volume of gas over a given time interval during the FVC maneuver. The interval, described by the subscript T, is the time elapsed in seconds from the onset of expiration. Because FEV_T records a volume of gas expired over time, it is actually a measure of flow. By measuring expiratory flow at specific intervals, the severity of airway obstruction can be ascertained. Decreased FEV_T values are common in both obstructive and restrictive disease patterns. The most important application of FEV_T is its comparison with the patient's FVC. Normal subjects can expire at least three-fourths of FVC within the first second of the forced expiratory maneuver. The FEV_1, the most frequently employed value, is normally greater than or equal to 75% of the FVC, or $FEV_1/FVC \geq 0.75$.

Normally, an individual can expire 50% to 60% of FVC in 0.5 second, 75% to 85% in 1 second, 94% in 2 seconds, and 97% in 3 seconds. Cooperative patients with obstructive disease will exhibit a reduced FEV_1/FVC in most cases. However, patients with restrictive disease usually have normal FEV_1/FVC ratios. The validity of the evaluation of the FEV_1/FVC is highly dependent on patient cooperation and effort. It is possible to deliberately produce an artificially low FEV_1/FVC.

Forced Expiratory Flow

$FEF_{25\%-75\%}$ is the average forced expiratory flow during the middle half of the FEV maneuver. This test is also called maximum mid-expiratory flow rate. The length of time required for a subject to expire the middle half of the FVC is divided into 50% of the FVC. The spirogram in Figure 15-9 marks the place from 25% to 75% of FVC, constituting the middle 50% of FVC. The straight line connecting the 25% and 75% volumes has a slope approximately equal to average flow. A normal value for a healthy 70-kg man is approximately 4.7 L/sec (or 280 L/min). Normally, both the absolute value and the percentage of predicted value for the individual being studied are recorded. A normal value is 100 ± 25% of predicted. Decreased flow rates from this middle 50% of FVC are indicative of obstructive disease of medium size airways. This value is typically normal in restrictive diseases. This test is fairly sensitive in the early stages of obstructive airway disease. Decreased $FEV_{25\%-75\%}$ frequently will be observed before other obstructive manifestations occur. Although somewhat effort dependent, the test is much more reliable and reproducible than FEV_1/FVC.

Maximum Voluntary Ventilation

Maximum voluntary ventilation (MVV) is the largest volume of gas that can be breathed in 1 minute by voluntary effort. The MVV is measured by having the subject breathe as deeply and as rapidly as possible for 10, 12, or 15 seconds. The results are extrapolated to 1 minute. The subject is instructed to set his or her own ventilatory rate and move more than tidal volume but less than vital capacity in each breath.

MVV measures the endurance of the ventilatory muscles and indirectly reflects lung–thorax compliance and airway resistance. MVV is the best ventilatory endurance test that can be performed in the laboratory. Values that vary by as much as 30% from predicted values may be normal, so only large reductions in MVV are significant. Healthy, young adults average about 170 L/min. Values are lower in women and decrease with age in both sexes. Because this maneuver exaggerates air trapping and exerts the ventilatory muscles, MVV is decreased greatly in patients with moderate to severe obstructive disease. MVV is usually normal in patients with restrictive disease.

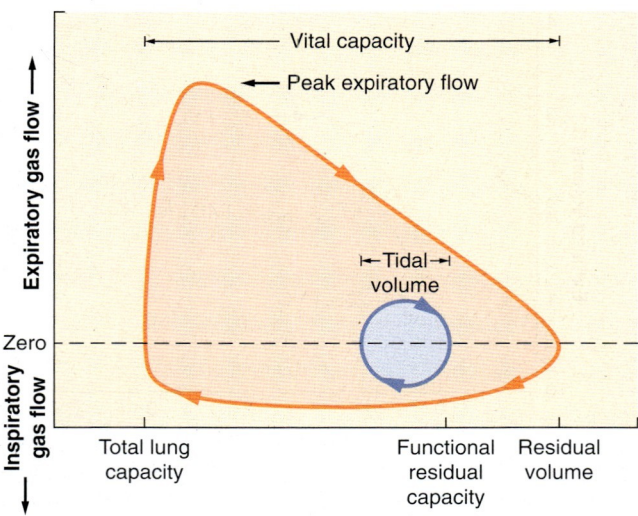

Figure 15-10 Flow–volume loop. The figure depicts a normally configured adult flow–volume loop. The slope of the loop after the subject reaches peak expiratory flow is nearly linear.

Flow–Volume Loops

The flow–volume loop graphically demonstrates the flow generated during a forced expiratory maneuver followed by a forced inspiratory maneuver, plotted against the volume of gas expired (Fig. 15-10). The subject forcefully exhales completely, then immediately forcefully inhales to vital capacity. The expired and inspired volumes are plotted on the abscissa and flow is plotted on the ordinate. Although various numbers can be generated from the flow–volume loop, the configuration of the loop itself is probably the most informative part of the test.

Flow–volume loops were formerly useful in the diagnosis of large airway and extrathoracic airway obstruction prior to the availability of precise imaging techniques. Imaging techniques such as MRI give more precise and useful information in the diagnosis of upper airway and extrathoracic obstruction and superseded the use of flow–volume loops for diagnosis of these conditions. Therefore, it is rare that flow–volume loops are useful for preoperative pulmonary evaluation in the modern era of imaging.

Carbon Monoxide Diffusing Capacity

Since PO_2 in the pulmonary capillary blood varies with time as it moves through the pulmonary microvasculature, oxygen cannot be used to assess diffusing capacity. Instead, a gas mixture containing carbon monoxide is traditionally used to measure diffusing capacity. The partial pressure of carbon monoxide in the blood is nearly zero, and its affinity for hemoglobin is 200 times that of oxygen.[61] Carbon monoxide diffusing capacity (D_{LCO}) collectively measures all the factors that affect diffusion across the alveolar–capillary membrane. The D_{LCO} is recorded in mL CO/min/mmHg at STPD. In persons with normal hemoglobin concentrations and normal V/Q matching, the main factor limiting diffusion is the alveolar–capillary membrane. There are several methods for determining D_{LCO}, but all measure diffusing capacity according to the equation

$$D_{LCO} = V_A \times (60/t) \times [1/(P_B-47)] \times \ln(F_{ACOo}/F_{ACOt}) \quad (15\text{-}11)$$

The average value for resting subjects when the single-breath method is used is 25 mL CO/min/mmHg. D_{LCO} values can increase to two or three times normal during exercise.

The D_{LO_2} may be estimated from the D_{LCO} by multiplying D_{LCO} by 1.23, although the D_{LCO} is usually the reported value. D_{LCO} can be divided by the lung volume at which the measurement was made to obtain an expression of diffusing capacity per unit lung volume.

Some of the other factors that can influence D_{LCO} are as follows:

1. Hemoglobin concentration: decreased hemoglobin concentration decreases the D_{LCO}
2. Alveolar PCO_2: an increased $PaCO_2$ raises D_{LCO}
3. Body position: the supine position increases D_{LCO}
4. Pulmonary capillary blood volume

Diffusing capacity is decreased in alveolar fibrosis associated with sarcoidosis, asbestosis, berylliosis, oxygen toxicity, and pulmonary edema. These states are frequently categorized as diffusion defects, but low D_{LCO} is probably more closely related to loss of lung volume or capillary bed perfusion. D_{LCO} is decreased in obstructive disease because of the decreased alveolar surface area, loss of capillary bed, the increased distance from the terminal bronchiole to the alveolar–capillary membrane, and V/Q mismatching. In short, few disease states truly inhibit oxygen diffusion across the alveolar–capillary membrane.

Practical Application of Pulmonary Function Tests

Of the many pulmonary function tests, spirometry is the most useful, cost-effective, and commonly used test.[62] Screening spirometry yields VC, FVC, and FEV_1. From these values, two basic types of pulmonary dysfunction can be identified and quantitated: obstructive defects and restrictive defects. The primary criterion for airflow obstruction is decreased FEV_1/FVC ratio. Other measurements, such as $FEF_{25\%-75\%}$, can be used to support the diagnosis of an obstructive defect or to assist in management (e.g., use of bronchodilators). A restrictive defect is a proportional decrease in all lung volumes (VC, FVC, and FEV_1), but FEV_1/FVC remains normal. When there is a question about whether a decreased VC is due to restriction, TLC should be measured. Reduced TLC defines a restrictive defect, but is not necessary unless VC on screening spirometry is reduced. The American Thoracic Society published an experts' consensus concerning interpretation of lung function tests.[63] Table 15-4 summarizes the distinctions between results from those with restrictive versus obstructive defects.

Preoperative Pulmonary Assessment

Markedly impaired pulmonary function is likely in patients who have the following:

1. Any chronic disease that involves the lung
2. Smoking history, persistent cough, and/or wheezing
3. Chest wall and spinal deformities
4. Morbid obesity
5. Surgical need for single-lung anesthesia or lung resection
6. Severe neuromuscular disease

Preoperative pulmonary evaluation must include history and physical examination, and may include chest radiograph, arterial blood gas analysis, and screening spirometry, depending on the patient's history. A history of sputum production, wheezing or dyspnea, exercise intolerance, or limited daily activities may yield more practical information than does formal testing.

Table 15-4 Pulmonary Function Tests in Restrictive and Obstructive Lung Disease

Value	Restrictive Disease	Obstructive Disease
Definition	Proportional decreases in all lung volumes	Small airway obstruction to expiratory flow
FVC	↓↓↓	Normal or slightly ↑
FEV_1	↓↓↓	Normal or slightly ↓
FEV_1/FVC	Normal	↓↓↓
$FEF_{25–75\%}$	Normal	↓↓↓
FRC	↓↓↓	Normal or ↑ if gas trapping
TLC	↓↓↓	Normal or ↑ if gas trapping

FEV, forced expiratory volume; FRC, functional residual capacity; FVC, forced vital capacity; TLC, total lung capacity; ↓↓↓, ↑↑↑ = large decrease or increase, respectively; ↓, ↑ = small/moderate decrease or increase, respectively.

Arterial blood analysis while the patient breathes room air adds information regarding gas exchange and acid–base balance. It is most useful if the patient's history suggests chronic hypoxemia or carbon dioxide retention, and can guide perioperative ventilatory management. Blood gas results should be interpreted in the context of measured bicarbonate levels, which are frequently elevated in those with chronic acidemia.

The goals of preoperative pulmonary function testing are to predict the likelihood of pulmonary complications, obtain quantitative baseline information to guide perioperative management, and identify patients who may benefit from preoperative therapy to improve pulmonary function. For patients undergoing lung resections, pulmonary function testing provides some predictive benefit.[64] For all other patients, however, evidence suggests that preoperative pulmonary function testing does not predict or assign risk for PPCs.[65,66]

In 2012, the American Society of Anesthesiologists' Taskforce on Preanesthetic Evaluation published an updated practice advisory[67] stating that "there is insufficient evidence to identify explicit decision parameters or rules for ordering preoperative tests on the basis of specific clinical characteristics." The literature[68] also reveals that specific measurements of lung function do not predict PPCs. Rather, testing should be performed to identify reversible pulmonary disease (bronchospasm) or to define the severity of advanced pulmonary disease, because the clinician obtains valuable information from the patient's history. In a series of 272 adults undergoing nonthoracic surgery, McAlister et al.[69] reported the following historical factors to independently increase the risk of PPC: age above 65 years, smoking more than 40 pack-years, COPD, asthma, productive cough, and exercise tolerance of less than one flight of stairs.

The need to obtain baseline pulmonary function data should be reserved for those patients with severely impaired preoperative pulmonary function, such as quadriplegics or myasthenics, so that liberation from mechanical ventilation and/or tracheal extubation can be based on objective baseline pulmonary function.

Arterial blood gases are not indicated unless the patient's history suggests arterial hypoxemia or severe COPD. Then, the arterial blood gas should be used in a similar manner as preoperative pulmonary function testing—to identify reversible disease or to define the severity of the disease at baseline. Defining baseline PaO_2 and $PaCO_2$ is particularly important if one anticipates postoperative ventilation of a patient with severe COPD.

Anesthesia and Obstructive Pulmonary Disease

Patients with marked obstructive pulmonary disease are at increased risk for both intraoperative and postoperative pulmonary complications. For example, patients with reduced FEV_1/FVC or reduced mid-expiratory flow exhibit both small airway obstruction and increased airway reactivity. Because of the hazard of provoking reflex bronchoconstriction during laryngoscopy and tracheal intubation, patients with COPD or asthma should receive aggressive bronchodilator therapy prior to instrumentation of the airway. Adjunctive intravenous administration of opioids and lidocaine prior to airway instrumentation will decrease airway reactivity by deepening anesthesia. High alveolar concentrations of most potent inhalational anesthetics will blunt reflex bronchoconstriction. Furthermore, a single dose of corticosteroids may help prevent postoperative increases in airway resistance.

In patients with severe obstructive disease, spontaneous ventilation during general anesthesia is more likely to result in hypercapnia than in patients with normal pulmonary function.[70] Preoperative FEV_1 reduction correlates with the $PaCO_2$ increase during anesthesia. Slower rates of mechanical ventilation (8 to 10 breaths min^{-1}) should be used to allow sufficient time for exhalation. Low ventilatory rates necessitate a larger Vt to maintain a normal $PaCO_2$; however, the larger Vt may predispose the patient to pulmonary barotrauma due to higher peak airway pressure. Tidal volume and inspiratory flows should be adjusted to keep peak airway pressure less than 40 cm H_2O,[71,72] if possible. Higher inspiratory flows produce a shorter inspiratory time and, usually a higher peak airway pressure. Thus, a balance that avoids high peak airway pressure and excessively large Vt, yet allows a long expiratory time should be sought.

In most cases, one would extubate the patient's trachea at the end of surgery because the endotracheal tube increases both airway resistance and reflex bronchoconstriction, limits the ability of the patient to clear secretions effectively, and increases the risk of iatrogenic infection. Because endotracheal tubes can trigger reflex bronchospasm during emergence from general anesthesia, in some patients with obstructive disease (e.g., the young asthmatic), tracheal extubation is performed during deep levels of anesthesia at the conclusion of the operation.

Anesthesia and Restrictive Pulmonary Disease

Restrictive disease is characterized by proportional decreases in all lung volumes. The decreased FRC produces low lung compliance and also results in arterial hypoxemia because of low V̇/Q̇ conditions. These patients typically breathe rapidly and shallowly.

Positive-pressure ventilation of patients with restrictive disease is fraught with high peak airway pressures because more pressure is required to expand stiff lungs. Use of a lower Vt at more rapid rates can reduce the risk of barotrauma, but may increase the chances of developing atelectasis. Large Vt should be avoided because of the increased risks of both barotrauma[73] and volutrauma.[50] Various lung protective strategies have been developed to ventilate patients with profound restrictive lung disease (see Chapters 36 and 56).

Patients with severe restrictive diseases tolerate apnea poorly because the FRC is reduced, and a lower oxygen store is available during apneic periods. Even preoxygenation with an F_{IO_2} of 1.0 can result in arterial hypoxemia within seconds after the cessation of breathing or disconnection from a ventilator circuit. Because arterial hypoxemia develops so rapidly, transportation of these patients within the hospital should be performed with a pulse oximeter.

Even healthy individuals develop mild restrictive defects during anesthesia. FRC decreases 10% to 15% when healthy, spontaneously breathing individuals lie supine. Tracheal intubation also minimally reduces FRC. General anesthesia decreases FRC by an additional 5% to 10%,[74] which usually results in decreased lung compliance.[75] The FRC reaches its nadir within the first 10 minutes of anesthesia,[74,76,77] independent of whether ventilation is spontaneous or controlled. The diminished FRC persists into the postoperative period, but is improved with positive end-expiratory pressure or CPAP.[74,78,79] However, once positive airway pressure is removed, FRC falls to previously diminished levels, and reaches a postoperative nadir 12 hours after operation.[80]

Effects of Cigarette Smoking on Pulmonary Function

Smoking affects pulmonary function in many ways. The irritant smoke decreases ciliary motility and increases sputum production. Thus, these patients have a high volume of sputum and decreased ability to clear it effectively. In addition, airway reactivity and the development of obstructive disease become problematic. Studies of the pathogenesis of COPD suggest that smoking results in an excess of pulmonary proteolytic enzymes that directly damage the lung parenchyma.[81] Exposure to smoke increases synthesis and release of elastolytic enzymes from alveolar macrophages—cells instrumental in the genesis of COPD due to smoking. Further damage to the lung tissue is likely caused by reactive metabolites of oxygen (hydroxyl radicals and hydrogen peroxide) that macrophages use to kill microorganisms. The immunoregulatory function of the macrophages is also changed by cigarette smoking, including presentation of antigens and interaction with T lymphocytes.[82] Other adverse effects of smoking on lung tissue include increased epithelial permeability[83] and changed pulmonary surfactant.[84] The airway irritation or small airway reactivity evoked by inhaling cigarette smoke results from nicotine-mediated activation of sensory endings located in the central airways.[85]

Early in the disease, mild V/Q mismatch, bronchitis, and airway hyperreactivity are present, and with time progress to the hallmarks of COPD: gas trapping, flattened diaphragmatic configuration (decreasing the diaphragm's efficiency), and barrel chest deformity. Lung compliance increases significantly and limited elastic recoil prevents complete passive exhalation. As a result, many COPD patients exhale forcibly to reduce gas trapping.

With gas trapping, V/Q mismatch increases, resulting in large areas of dead space ventilation and venous admixture. Carbon dioxide elimination is inefficient because of increased dead space ventilation. The typical minute ventilation for patients with advanced obstructive lung disease can be up to twice normal. In addition, venous admixture produces arterial hypoxemia that is exquisitely sensitive to low concentrations of supplemental oxygen. Gas exchange is further impaired by the increased carboxyhemoglobin concentration from inspired smoke. Normal carboxyhemoglobin concentration in nonsmokers is approximately 1%; in smokers, however, it can be as high as 8% to 10%. Cessation of smoking, even for 12 to 24 hours preoperatively, can decrease carbon monoxide concentration to near normal.

Smoking is one of the main and most prevalent risk factors associated with postoperative morbidity.[86] COPD patients who smoke have a two-fold to six-fold[87] risk of developing postoperative pneumonia compared with nonsmokers. Furthermore, smokers' relative risk of PPCs is doubled, even if they do not have evidence of clinical pulmonary disease or abnormal pulmonary function.[88] The incidence of PPCs in smokers can be reduced by abstinence from smoking, although there is no consensus on the minimal or optimal duration of preoperative smoking abstinence.[89–91] Warner et al.[86] studied 200 patients undergoing coronary artery bypass grafting and found that patients who continued to smoke or stopped less than 8 weeks before the operation had a complication rate nearly four times that of patients who had quit smoking more than 8 weeks preoperatively. Normalization of mucociliary function requires 2 to 3 weeks of abstinence from smoking, during which time sputum production increases. Several months of smoking abstinence is required to return sputum clearance to normal.[92] In a study of bupropion-assisted smoking cessation, Hurt et al.[93] demonstrated a decreased risk of postoperative complications even after 4 weeks of abstinence from smoking.

Nonetheless, Public Health Service guidelines published in 2000 emphasize the responsibility of health-care facilities to coordinate interventions aimed at tobacco dependence treatment. The guidelines note that tobacco dependence often necessitates repeated interventions, although "every patient who uses tobacco should be offered at least brief treatment" as brief tobacco dependence therapy has been shown to be effective. These guidelines recognize five first-line pharmacologic adjuncts that increase smoking cessation success: bupropion SR, nicotine gum, nicotine inhaler, nicotine nasal spray, and nicotine patch. In addition, clonidine and nortriptyline were identified as second-line pharmacologic adjuncts.[94]

Following publication of these 2000 guidelines, a randomized controlled trial utilizing the partial nicotinic acetylcholine agonist, varenicline, showed improved smoking abstinence rates compared to bupropion SR treatment.[95] Based on this information, the utilization of varenicline in a smoking cessation program should be considered.

Smokers who decrease, but do not stop cigarette consumption without the aid of nicotine replacement therapy, continue to acquire equal amounts of nicotine from fewer cigarettes by changing their technique of smoking to maximize nicotine intake.[96] Levels of serum nicotine and cotinine and urinary mutagenesis levels remain unchanged. Thus, *reduction* in the number of cigarettes smoked will likely have little effect on the risk of developing PPCs.[87] Smoking patients should be advised to *stop* smoking 2 months prior to elective operations to maximize their benefit,[86] or for at least 4 weeks to benefit from improved mucociliary function and some reduction in PPC rate. If patients cannot stop smoking for 4 to 8 weeks preoperatively, it is controversial whether they should be advised to stop smoking 24 hours preoperatively. A 24-hour smoking abstinence would allow carboxyhemoglobin levels to fall to normal, but may increase the risk of PPC.

Postoperative Pulmonary Function

The changes in pulmonary function that occur postoperatively are primarily restrictive, with proportional decreases in all lung volumes and no change in airway resistance. The decrease in

FRC, however, is the yardstick by which the severity of the restrictive defect is gauged. This defect is generated by abdominal contents that impinge on and prevent normal movement of the diaphragm, and by an abnormal respiratory pattern devoid of sighs and characterized by shallow, rapid respirations. The normal resting respiratory rate for adults is 12 breaths per minute, whereas the postoperative patient usually breathes approximately 20 breaths per minute. Furthermore, most (but not all) factors that tend to make the restrictive defect worse are also associated with a higher risk of PPCs.

The operative site is the single most important determinant of postoperative pulmonary dysfunction and the risk of PPCs. Nonlaparoscopic upper abdominal operations cause the most profound restrictive defect, precipitating a 40% to 50% decrease in FRC compared with preoperative levels, when conventional postoperative analgesia is employed. Lower abdominal and thoracic operations cause the next most severe change in pulmonary function, with decreases in FRC to 30% of preoperative levels. Most other operative sites—intracranial, peripheral vascular, otolaryngologic—have approximately the same effect on FRC, with reductions of 15% to 20% of preoperative levels.

Postoperative Pulmonary Complications

Two problems confound interpretation of the literature examining PPCs. First, there is no clear definition of what constitutes a PPC. For example, some clinical studies include only pneumonia, whereas others add atelectasis and/or ventilatory failure. Thus it is important to discern what complications are specifically being addressed. Second, the criteria by which diagnoses of postoperative pneumonia or atelectasis is made varies from study to study. For this discussion, PPCs include atelectasis and pneumonia only. Reasonable, well-accepted diagnostic criteria for pneumonia include change in the color and quantity of sputum, oral temperature exceeding 38.5°C, and a new infiltrate on chest radiograph.

The operative site is an important risk factor for the development of PPCs. Nonlaparoscopic upper abdominal operations increase PPC risk at least two-fold,[90] with rates of occurrence varying from 20% to 70%.[96] Lower abdominal and intrathoracic operations are associated with slightly less risk, but still higher risk than extremity, intracranial, and head/neck operations.

Patients with COPD are at high risk for PPC. This risk can be minimized by ensuring they do not have an active pulmonary infection, and that any increased airway resistance is minimized by the use of bronchodilator therapy. Interestingly, those with asthma are not at increased risk for atelectasis or pneumonia. However, exacerbation of asthma in the postoperative period can be problematic. Careful attention must be given to ensuring the bronchodilating regimens and steroid administration (either inhaled or systemic) are continued throughout the perioperative period.

There are several strategies to reduce risk of PPC: the use of postoperative lung-expanding therapies, choice of analgesia,[97] and cessation of smoking. After upper abdominal operations, FRC typically recovers over 3 to 7 days. However, with the use of intermittent CPAP by mask, FRC will recover within 72 hours.[97] Patients correctly use incentive spirometers only 10% of the time unless therapy is supervised.[98] Combinations of deep breathing cough, mobilization, and pain management are as effective as incentive spirometry at preventing PPCs,[99] and they are less expensive than supervised incentive spirometry; thus, they are preferred over incentive spirometry therapy.

After median sternotomy for cardiac operations, FRC does not return to normal for several weeks, regardless of postoperative pulmonary therapy.[100] The persistently low FRC in this population is probably due to mechanical factors such as a widened mediastinum, intrapleural fluid, and altered chest wall compliance. The single most important aspect of postoperative pulmonary care is getting the patient out of bed, preferably walking.

The choice of anesthetic technique for intraoperative anesthesia does not change the risk for PPCs independent of the operative site or duration of the operation. Operations exceeding 3 hours are associated with a higher rate of PPCs. Choice of postoperative analgesia strongly influences the risk of PPCs.[90] The use of postoperative epidural analgesia, particularly for abdominal and thoracic operations, markedly decreases the risk of PPCs, and may decrease length of hospital stay.

Although obesity is associated with marked restrictive defects, it is controversial whether obesity independently increases the risk of PPCs.[101] However, data support[101] advanced age as an independent risk factor for PPCs.

Several authors have attempted to assess the influence of overall health on PPC risk. Indices that weigh and score various aspects of physiology and health demonstrate that patients who are in a poor state of health preoperatively tend to be at higher risk of PPCs.[91]

Patients with obstructive airway disease and decreased expiratory flows may benefit from preoperative bronchodilator therapy and formal pulmonary toilet.[102] High-risk patients with COPD who receive bronchodilation, chest physical therapy, deep breathing, forced oral fluids (>3 L/day), and preoperative instruction in postoperative respiratory techniques, as well as those who stop smoking for more than 2 months preoperatively, experience a PPC rate approximately equal to that observed in normal patients.[103] Interestingly, although such a regimen significantly reduces the incidence of PPCs,[104] airway obstruction and arterial hypoxemia are not measurably reversed during the 48 to 72 hours of preoperative therapy.[105] It is possible that the reduced PPC rate results from the additional attention that these patients receive, rather than from the specific regimen employed.

REFERENCES

1. Lieberma.DA, Faulkner JA, Craig AB Jr, et al. Performance and histochemical composition of guinea-pig and human diaphragm. J Appl Physiol. 1973;34(2):233–237.
2. Roussos CS, Macklem PT. Diaphragmatic fatigue in man. J Appl Physiol. 1977;43(2):189–197.
3. Campbell EJ, Green JH. The behavior of the abdominal muscles and intra-abdominal pressure during quiet breathing and increases pulmonary ventilation: A study in man. J Physiol (Lond). 1955;127:423–426.
4. Conrady PA, Goodman LR, Lainge F, et al. Alteration of endotracheal tube position: Flexion and extension of the neck. Crit Care Med. 1976;4:8–12.
5. Bachofen M, Weibel ER. Basic pattern of tissue repair in human lungs following unspecific injury. Chest. 1974;65(4):14S–19S.
6. Fishman A. Non-respiratory function of lung. Chest. 1977;72.
7. Hocking WG, Golde DW. The pulmonary-alveolar macrophage (first of two parts). N Engl J Med. 1979;301(11):580–587.
8. Whitehead TC, Zhang H, Mullen B, et al. Effect of mechanical ventilation on cytokine response to intratracheal hypopolysaccharide. Anesthesiology. 2004;101(1):52–58.
9. Dreyfuss D, Rouby JJ. Mechanical ventilation-induced lung release of cytokines: a key for the future or pandora's box? Anesthesiology. 2004;101(1):1–3.
10. Downs JB. A technique for direct measurement of intrapleural pressure. Crit Care Med. 1976;4(4):207–210.
11. Baydur A, Behrakis PK, Zin WA, et al. A simple method for assessing the validity of the esophageal balloon technique. Am Rev Respir Dis. 1982;126(5):788–791.
12. Banner MJ, Kirby RR, Gabrielli A, et al. Partially and totally unloading respiratory muscles based on real-time measurements of work of breathing. A clinical approach. Chest. 1994;106(6):1835–1842.
13. Brochard L, Rua F, Lorino H, et al. Inspiratory pressure support compensates for the additional work of breathing caused by the endotracheal-tube. Anesthesiology. 1991;75(5):739–745.
14. Rohrer F. Der Strömungswiderstand in den menschlichen Atemwegen. Pflugers Arch. 1915;162:225.
15. Nunn J. Resistance to gas flow and airway closure. 1987.

16. Campbell EJ, Freedman S, Smith PS, et al. The ability of man to detect added elastic loads to breathing. *Clin Sci*. 1961;20:223–231.
17. Fink BR, Ngai SH, Holaday DA. Effect of air flow resistance on ventilation and respiratory muscle activity. *J Am Med Assoc*. 1958;168(17):2245–2249.
18. Palmer KN, Diament ML. Effect of aerosol isoprenaline on blood-gas tensions in severe bronchial asthma. *Lancet*. 1967;2(7528):1232–1233.
19. Campbell EJ. The effects of increased resistance to expiration on the respiratory behavior of the abdominal muscles and intraabdominal pressure. *J Physiol*. 1957;136:556–562.
20. Janssens JP, Pache JC, Nicod LP. Physiologic changes in respiratory function associated with aging. *Eur Respir J*. 1999;13:197–205.
21. LeGallois C. Expériences sur le Principe de la Vie. 1812.
22. Salmoiraghi GC, Burns BD. Localization and patterns of discharge of respiratory neurons in the brainstem of a cat. *J Neurophysiol*. 1960;23:2–13.
23. Cohen MI. Neurogenesis of respiratory rhythm in the mammal. *Physiol Rev*. 1979;59(4):1105–1173.
24. Guz A. Regulation of respiration in man. *Annu Rev Physiol*. 1975;37:303–323.
25. Pitts RF, Magoun HW, Ranson SW. The origin of respiratory rhythmicity. *Am J Physiol*. 1939;127(4):654–670.
26. Lumsden T. Observations on the respiratory centers in the cat. *J Physiol*. 1923;57(3–4):153–160.
27. Cohen MI, Wang SC. Respiratory neuronal activity in pons of the cat. *Am J Physiol*. 1956;187(3):592.
28. Stella G. On the mechanism of production and the physiologic significance of "apneusis." *J Physiol (Lond)*. 1938;93(1):10–23.
29. Kabat H. Electrical stimulation of points in the forebrain and mid-brain: The resultant alterations in respiration. *J Comp Neurol*. 1936;64(187).
30. Wang SC, Borison HL. The vomiting center—a critical experimental analysis. *Arch Neurol Psych*. 1950;63(6):928–941.
31. Gaylor J. The intrinsic nervous mechanisms of the human lung. *Brain*. 1934;57(143).
32. Davis HL, Fowler WS, Lambert EH. Effect of volume and rate of inflation and deflation on transpulmonary pressure and response of pulmonary stretch receptors. *Am J Physiol*. 1956;187(3):558–566.
33. Hering EB, J. Die Sebsteuerung der Atmung durch den Nervus vagus. *Stizber Akad Wiss Wien*. 1868;57(682).
34. Ide T, Sakurai Y, Aono M, et al. Contribution of peripheral chemoreception to the depression of the hypoxic ventilatory response during halothane anesthesia in cats. *Anesthesiology*. 1999;90(4):1084–1091.
35. Mora CT, Torjman M, White PF. Effects of diazepam and flumazenil on sedation and hypoxic ventilatory response. *Anesth Analg*. 1989;68(4):473–478.
36. Leusen I. Regulation of cerebrospinal fluid composition with reference to breathing. *Physiol Rev*. 1972;52(1):1–56.
37. Cohen M. Discharge patterns of brainstem respiratory neurons in relation to carbon dioxide tension. *J Neurophysiol*. 1968;31(2):142–165.
38. Heinemann HO, Goldring RM. Bicarbonate and the regulation of ventilation. *Am J Med*. 1974;57(3):361–370.
39. Shapiro BA PW, Kozlowski-Templin R, eds. *Clinical Application of Blood Gases*. 5 ed. Elsevier Health Sciences; 1993.
40. Severinghaus JW, Mitchell RA, Richardson BW, et al. Respiratory control at high altitude suggesting active transport regulation of CSF pH. *J Appl Physiol*. 1963;18:1155–1156.
41. Ferris EB, Engel GL, Stevens CD, et al. Voluntary breath holding. *J Clin Invest*. 1946;25:734–743.
42. Stock MC, Downs JB, McDonald JS, et al. The carbon dioxide rate of rise in awake apneic man. *J Clin Anesth*. 1988;1:96–103.
43. Eger EI, Severinghaus JW. The rate of rise of $PaCO_2$ in the apneic anesthetized patient. *Anesthesiology*. 1961;22:419–425.
44. Stock MC, Schisler JQ, McSweeney TD. The $PaCO_2$ rate of rise in anesthetized patients with airway obstruction. *J Clin Anesth*. 1989;1(5):328–332.
45. Wright FG, Jr., Foley MF, Downs JB, et al. Hypoxemia and hypocarbia following intermittent positive-pressure breathing. *Anesth Analg*. 1976;55(4):555–559.
46. Fink BR. The stimulant effect of wakefulness on respiration: clinical aspects. *Br J Anaesth*. 1961;33:97–101.
47. Berger AJ, Mitchell RA, Severinghaus JW. Regulation of respiration (third of three parts). *N Engl J Med*. 1977;297(4):194–201.
48. West JB, Dollery CT, Naimark A. Distribution of blood flow in isolated lung; relation to vascular and alveolar pressures. *J Appl Physiol*. 1964;19:713–724.
49. West JD, Dollery CT. Distribution of blood flow and the pressure-flow relations of the whole lung. *J Appl Physiol*. 1965;20:175–183.
50. Gattinoni L, Pesenti A, Avalli L, et al. Pressure-volume curve of total respiratory system in acute respiratory-failure—computed tomographic scan study. *Am Rev Respirat Dis*. 1987;136(3):730–736.
51. Benumof JP, Pirlo AF, Johanson I, et al. Interaction of PvO_2 with PaO_2 on hypoxic pulmonary vasoconstriction. *J Appl Physiol*. 1981;51:871–874.
52. Swenson EW, Finley TN, Guzman SV. Unilateral hypoventilation in man during temporary occlusion of one pulmonary artery. *J Clin Invest*. 1961;40(5):828–835.
53. Yamanaka MS, Sue DY. Comparison of arterial-end-tidal PCO_2 difference and deadspace/tidal volume ratio in respiratory failure. *Chest*. 1987;92:832–835.
54. Tyburski JG, Collinge JD, Wilson RF, et al. End-tidal CO2-derived values during emergency trauma surgery correlated with outcome: A prospective study. *J Trauma*. 2002;53(4):738–743.
55. Huffmyer JL, Nemergut EC. Respiratory dysfunction and pulmonary disease in cirrhosis and other hepatic disorders. *Respir Care*. 2007;41:1030–1036.
56. Gaines DI, Fallon MB. Hepatopulmonary syndrome. *Liver Int*. 2004;24(5):397–401.
57. Räsänen J, Downs JB, Malec DJ, et al. Oxygen tensions and oxyhemoglobin saturations in the assessment of pulmonary gas exchange. *Crit Care Med*. 1987;15:1058–1061.
58. Cruickshank S HN. The alveolar gas equation. *Contin Educ Anaesth Crit Care Pain*. 2004;4(1):24–27.
59. Christi RV. The lung volume and its subdivisions: I. Methods of measurement. *J Clin Invest*. 1932;11:1099–1118.
60. Tisi GM. Preoperative evaluation of pulmonary-function—validity, indications, and benefits. *Am Rev Respirat Dis*. 1979;119(2):293–310.
61. Apthorp GM, Marshall R. Pulmonary diffusing capacity: A comparison of breath-holding and steady-state methods using carbon monoxide. *J Clin Invest*. 1961;40:1775–1784.
62. Crapo RO. Pulmonary-function testing—reply. *N Eng J Med*. 1994;331(19):1313–1314.
63. American Thoracic Society. Lung function testing: Selection of reference values and interpretive strategies. *Am Rev Respir Dis*. 1991;144:1202–1218.
64. Kearney DJ, Lee TH, Reilly JJ, et al. Assessment of operative risk in patients undergoing lung resection—importance of predicted pulmonary-function. *Chest*. 1994;105(3):753–759.
65. Ferguson MK. Preoperative assessment of pulmonary risk. *Chest*. 1999;115(5):58s–63s.
66. Bapoje SR, Whitaker JF, Schulz T, et al. Preoperative evaluation of the patient with pulmonary disease. *Chest*. 2007;132:1637–1645.
67. American Society of Anesthesiologists Task Force on Preanesthesia Evaluation. Practice advisory for preanesthetic evaluation: A report by the American Society of Anesthesiologists. *Anesthesiology*. 2002;96:485–496.
68. Zollinger AH, C Pasch T. Preoperative pulmonary evaluation: Fact and myth. *Curr Opin Anaesth*. 2002;14:59.
69. McAlister FA, Khan NA, Strauss SE, et al. Accuracy of the preoperative assessment in predicting pulmonary risk after non-thoracic surgery. *Am J Respir Crit Care Med*. 2003;167:741–744.
70. Pietak S, Weenig CS, Hickey R, et al. Anesthetic effects on ventilation in patients with chronic obstructive pulmonary disease. *Anesthesiology*. 1975;42(2):160–166.
71. Connors AF, Jr., McCaffree DR, Gray BA. Effect of inspiratory flow rate on gas exchange during mechanical ventilation. *Am Rev Respir Dis*. 1981;124(5):537–543.
72. Tuxen DL, Lane S. The effects of ventilatory pattern on hyperinflation, airway pressures, and circulation in mechanical ventilation of patients with severe airflow obstruction. *Am Rev Respir Dis*. 1987;136:872–879.
73. Petersen GW, Baier H. Incidence of pulmonary barotrauma in a medical ICU. *Crit Care Med*. 1983;11(2):67–69.
74. Brisner B, Hedenstierna G, Lundquist H, et al. Pulmonary densities during anesthesia with muscular relaxation: A proposal of atelectasis. *Anesthesiology*. 1985;62:422–428.
75. Don HF, Robson JG. The mechanics of the respiratory system during anesthesia. *Anesthesiology*. 1965;26:168–178.
76. Don HF, Wahba M, Cuadrado L, et al. The effects of anesthesia and 100 percent oxygen on the functional residual capacity of the lungs. *Anesthesiology*. 1970;32:521–529.
77. Westbrook PR, Stubbs SE, Sessler AD, et al. Effects of anesthesia and muscle paralysis on respiratory mechanics in normal man. *J Appl Physiol*. 1973;34(1):81–86.
78. Wyche MQ, Teichner RL, Kallos T, et al. Effects of continuous positive-pressure breathing on functional residual capacity and arterial oxygenation during intra-abdominal operation. *Anesthesiology*. 1973;38:68–74.
79. Rose DM, Downs JB, Heenan TJ. Temporal responses of functional residual capacity and oxygen tension to changes in positive end-expiratory pressure. *Crit Care Med*. 1981;9(2):79–82.
80. Craig DB. Postoperative recovery of pulmonary function. *Anesth Analg*. [Review]. 1981;60(1):46–52.
81. Diamond L, Lai YL. Augmentation of elastase-induced emphysema by cigarette smoke: effects of reducing tar and nicotine content. *J Toxicol Environ Health*. [Research Support, Non-U.S. Gov't]. 1987;20(3):287–301.
82. DeShazo RD, Banks BD, Diem JE, et al. Bronchoalveolar lavage cell-lymphocyte interactions in normal non-smokers and smokers. *Am Rev Respir Dis*. 1983;127:545–548.
83. Hogg JC. The effect of smoking on airway permeability. *Chest*. [Editorial]. 1983;83(1):1–2.
84. Clements JA. Smoking and pulmonary surfactant. *N Engl J Med*. 1972;286(5):261–262.
85. Lee LY, Gerhardstein DC, Wang AL, et al. Nicotine is responsible for airway irritation evoked by cigarette smoke inhalation in men. *J Appl Physiol*. 1993;75:1955–1961.

86. Warner MA, Divertie MB, Tinker JH. Preoperative cessation of smoking and pulmonary complications in coronary artery bypass patients. *Anesthesiology*. [Comparative Study]. 1984;60(4):380–383.
87. Bluman LG, Mosca L, Newman N, et al. Preoperative smoking habits and postoperative pulmonary complications. *Chest*. 1998;113(4):883–889.
88. Chalon J, Tayyab MA, Ramanathan S. Cytology of respiratory epithelium as a predictor of respiratory complications after operation. *Chest*. 1975;67(1):32–35.
89. Theadom A, Cropley M. Effects of preoperative smoking cessation on the incidence and risk of intraoperative and postoperative complications in adult smokers: a systematic review. *Tob Control*. 2006;15:352–358.
90. Quraishi SA, Orkin FK, Roizen MF. The anesthesia preoperative assessment: an opportunity for smoking cessation intervention. *J Clin Anesth*. 2006;18:635–640.
91. Warner MA, Offord KP, Warner ME, et al. Role of preoperative cessation of smoking and other factors in postoperative pulmonary complications: a blinded prospective study of coronary artery bypass patients. *Mayo Clin Proc*. 1989;64(6):609–616.
92. Beckers S, Camu F. The anesthetic risk of tobacco smoking. *Acta Anaesthesiol Belg*. [Review]. 1991;42(1):45–56.
93. Hurt RD, Sachs DP, Glover ED, et al. A comparison of sustained-release bupropion and placebo for smoking cessation. *N Engl J Med*. 1997;337(17):1195–1202.
94. Fiore MB. US public health service clinical practice guideline: treating tobacco use and dependence. *Respir Care*. 2000;45(10):1200–1262.
95. Gonzales D, Rennard SI, Nides M, et al. Varenicline, an alpha4beta2 nicotinic acetylcholine receptor partial agonist, vs sustained-release bupropion and placebo for smoking cessation: a randomized controlled trial. *JAMA*. 2006;296(1):47–55.
96. Benowitz NL, Jacob P, 3rd, Kozlowski LT, et al. Influence of smoking fewer cigarettes on exposure to tar, nicotine, and carbon monoxide. *N Engl J Med*. 1986;315(21):1310–1313.
97. Gust R, Pecher S, Gust A, et al. Effect of patient-controlled analgesia on pulmonary complications after coronary artery bypass grafting. *Crit Care Med*. 1999;27:2218–2223.
98. Stock MC, Downs JB, Gauer PK, et al. Prevention of postoperative pulmonary complications with CPAP, incentive spirometry, and conservative therapy. *Chest*. 1985;87(2):151–157.
99. Lyager S, Wernberg M, Rajani N, et al. Can postoperative pulmonary complications be improved by treatment with Bartlett Edwards incentive spirometer after upper abdominal surgery? *Acta Anaesthesiol Scand*. 1979;23:312–319.
100. Stock MC, Downs JB, Cooper RB, et al. Comparison of continuous positive airway pressure, incentive spirometry, and conservative therapy after cardiac operations. *Crit Care Med*. [Clinical Trial Comparative Study Randomized Controlled Trial]. 1984;12(11):969–972.
101. Smetana GW, Lawrence VA, Cornell JE. Preoperative pulmonary risk stratification for non-cardiothoracic surgery: a systematic review for the American College of Physicians. *Ann Intern Med*. 2006;144:581–595.
102. Chumillas S, Ponce JL, Delgado F, et al. Prevention of postoperative pulmonary complications through respiratory rehabilitation: A controlled clinical study. *Arch Phys Med Rehabilit*. 1998;79(1):5–9.
103. Brooks-Brunn JA. Validation of a predictive model for postoperative pulmonary complications. *Heart Lung*. 1998;27(3):151–158.
104. Gracey DR, Divertie MB, Didier EP. Preoperative pulmonary preparation of patients with chronic obstructive pulmonary-disease—prospective-study. *Chest*. 1979;76(2):123–129.
105. Petty TL, Brink GA, Miller MW, et al. Objective functional improvement in chronic airway obstruction. *Chest*. 1970;57(3):216–223.

16 Fluids, Electrolytes, and Acid–Base Physiology

DONALD S. PROUGH • J. SEAN FUNSTON • ANTONIO F. SAAD • CHRISTER H. SVENSÉN

Acid–Base Interpretation and Treatment
  Overview of Acid–Base Equilibrium
  Metabolic Alkalosis
  Metabolic Acidosis
  Respiratory Alkalosis
  Respiratory Acidosis
Practical Approach to Acid–Base Interpretation
  Examples
Fluid Management
  Physiology
  Fluid Replacement Therapy

Surgical Fluid Requirements
Colloids, Crystalloids, and Hypertonic Solutions
Fluid Status: Assessment and Monitoring
Electrolytes
  Sodium
  Potassium
  Calcium
  Phosphate
  Magnesium

KEY POINTS

1. The Henderson–Hasselbalch equation describes the relationship between pH, $PaCO_2$, and serum bicarbonate. The Henderson equation defines the previous relationship but substitutes calculated hydrogen ion concentration for pH.

2. The pathophysiology of metabolic alkalosis is divided into generating and maintenance factors. A particularly important maintenance factor is the renal response to hypovolemia.

3. The addition of iatrogenic respiratory alkalosis to metabolic alkalosis can produce severe alkalemia.

4. Metabolic acidosis occurs as a consequence of the use of bicarbonate to buffer endogenous organic acids or as a consequence of external bicarbonate loss. The former causes an increase in the anion gap, calculated as $[Na^+] - ([Cl^-] + [HCO_3^-])$.

5. When substituting mechanical ventilation for spontaneous ventilation in a patient with severe metabolic acidosis, appropriate ventilatory compensation should be maintained, pending effective treatment of the primary cause for the metabolic acidosis.

6. Sodium bicarbonate, never proved to alter outcome in acidemic patients, should be reserved for those patients with severe acidemia.

7. Control of blood glucose in critically ill surgical patients has been associated with improvements in clinical outcomes. However, a blood glucose target of 180 mg/dL or less is associated with a lower mortality than a target of 81 to 108 mg/dL.

8. In patients undergoing moderate surgical procedures, generous administration of fluids is associated with fewer minor complications, such as nausea, vomiting, and drowsiness.

9. In patients undergoing colon surgery, careful perioperative fluid restriction has been associated with lower mortality and better wound healing.

10. Homeostatic mechanisms are usually adequate for the maintenance of electrolyte balance. However, critical illnesses and their treatment strategies can cause significant perturbations in electrolyte status, possibly leading to worsened patient outcome.

11. Disorders of the concentration of sodium, the principal extracellular cation, depend on the total body water (TBW) concentration and can lead to neurologic dysfunction. Disorders of potassium, the principal intracellular cation, are influenced primarily by insults that result in increased total body losses of potassium or changes in the distribution between extracellular and intracellular compartments.

12. Calcium, phosphorus, and magnesium are all essential for maintenance and function of the cardiovascular system. In addition, they also provide the milieu that ensures neuromuscular transmission. Disorders affecting any one of these electrolytes may lead to significant dysfunction and possibly result in cardiopulmonary arrest.

As a consequence of underlying diseases and of therapeutic manipulations, surgical patients develop potentially harmful disorders of acid–base equilibrium, intravascular and extravascular volume, and serum electrolytes. Precise perioperative management of acid–base status, fluids, and electrolytes may limit perioperative morbidity and mortality.

Acid–Base Interpretation and Treatment

Management of perioperative acid–base disturbances requires an understanding of the four simple acid–base disorders—metabolic alkalosis, metabolic acidosis, respiratory alkalosis, and respiratory acidosis—as well as more complex combinations of disturbances. This section will review the pathogenesis, major complications, physiologic compensatory mechanisms, and treatment of common perioperative acid–base abnormalities.

Overview of Acid–Base Equilibrium

Conventionally, acid–base equilibrium is described using the Henderson–Hasselbalch equation:

$$pH = 6.1 + \log \frac{[HCO_3^-]}{0.03 \times PaCO_2} \quad (16\text{-}1)$$

where 6.1 = the pK_a of carbonic acid and 0.03 is the solubility coefficient in blood of carbon dioxide (CO_2).[1] Within this context, pH is the dependent variable, while the bicarbonate concentration ($[HCO_3^-]$) and $PaCO_2$ are independent variables; therefore, metabolic alkalosis and acidosis are defined as disturbances in which $[HCO_3^-]$ is primarily increased or decreased, and respiratory alkalosis and acidosis are defined as disturbances in which $PaCO_2$ is primarily decreased or increased. pH, the negative logarithm of the hydrogen ion concentration ($[H^+]$), defines the acidity or alkalinity of solutions or blood. The simpler Henderson equation, after calculation of $[H^+]$ from pH, also describes the relationship between the three major variables measured or calculated in blood gas samples:

$$[H^+] = \frac{24 \times PaCO_2}{[HCO_3^-]} \quad (16\text{-}2)$$

To approximate the logarithmic relationship of pH to $[H^+]$, assume that $[H^+]$ is 40 mmol/L at a pH of 7.4; that an increase in pH of 0.10 pH units reduces $[H^+]$ to $0.8 \times$ the starting $[H^+]$ concentration; that a decrease in pH of 0.10 pH units increases the $[H^+]$ by a factor of 1.25; and that small changes (i.e., <0.05 pH units) produce reciprocal increases or decreases of 1 mmol/L in $[H^+]$ for each 0.01 decrease or increase in pH units.

The alternative "Stewart" approach to acid–base interpretation distinguishes between the independent variables and dependent variables that determine pH.[2,3] The independent variables are $PaCO_2$, the strong (i.e., highly dissociated) ion difference, and the concentration of proteins, which usually are not strong ions. The strong ions include sodium (Na^+), potassium (K^+), chloride (Cl^-), and lactate. The strong ion difference, calculated as ($Na^+ + K^+ - Cl^-$), is approximately 42 mEq/L. Although the Stewart approach provides more insight into the mechanisms underlying acid–base disturbances than does the more descriptive Henderson–Hasselbalch approach, the clinical interpretation or treatment of common acid–base disturbances is rarely handicapped by the simpler constructs of the conventional Henderson–Hasselbalch or Henderson equations.[4]

Metabolic Alkalosis

Metabolic alkalosis, characterized by hyperbicarbonatemia (>27 mEq/L) and usually by an alkalemic pH (>7.45), occurs frequently in postoperative and critically ill patients. Factors that generate metabolic alkalosis include vomiting and diuretic administration (Table 16-1).[5] Maintenance of metabolic alkalosis depends on a continued stimulus, such as renal hypoperfusion, hypokalemia, hypochloremia, or hypovolemia, for distal tubular reabsorption of $[HCO_3^-]$ (Table 16-2).[5]

Metabolic alkalosis is associated with hypokalemia, ionized hypocalcemia, secondary ventricular arrhythmias, increased digoxin toxicity, and compensatory hypoventilation (hypercarbia), although compensation rarely results in $PaCO_2$ above 55 mmHg (Table 16-3). Alkalemia may reduce tissue oxygen availability by shifting the oxyhemoglobin dissociation curve to the left and by decreasing cardiac output.[5] During anesthetic management, inadvertent addition of iatrogenic respiratory alkalosis to pre-existing metabolic alkalosis may produce severe alkalemia and precipitate cardiovascular depression, dysrhythmias, and hypokalemia.

In patients in whom arterial blood gases have not yet been obtained, serum electrolytes and a history of major risk factors, such as vomiting, nasogastric suction, or chronic diuretic use, can suggest metabolic alkalosis. Estimates of $[HCO_3^-]$ on serum electrolyte results (often abbreviated as total CO_2) should be about 1 mEq/L greater than $[HCO_3^-]$ on simultaneously obtained arterial blood gases. If either calculated $[HCO_3^-]$ on the arterial blood gases or "CO_2" on the serum electrolytes exceeds normal (24 and 25 mEq/L, respectively) by more than 4 mEq/L, the patient either has a primary metabolic alkalosis or has conserved bicarbonate in response to chronic hypercarbia. Recognition of hyperbicarbonatemia on the preoperative serum electrolytes justifies arterial blood gas analysis and should alert the anesthesiologist to the likelihood of factors that generate or maintain metabolic alkalosis (Tables 16-1 and 16-2).

Table 16-1 Generation of Metabolic Alkalosis

Generation	Examples
I. Loss of acid from extracellular space	Vomiting
A. Loss of gastric fluid (HCl)	Primary aldosteronism plus diuretic
B. Acid loss in the urine: Increased distal Na delivery in presence of hyperaldosteronism	Potassium deficiency
C. Acid shifts into cells	Congenital chloride-losing diarrhea
D. Loss of acid into stool	Milk–alkali syndrome
II. Excessive HCO_3^- loads	Lactate, acetate, or citrate administration
A. Absolute	$NaHCO_3$ dialysis
1. Oral or parenteral HCO_3^-	Correction (e.g., by mechanical ventilatory support) of chronic hypercapnia
2. Metabolic conversion of the salts of organic acids to HCO_3^-	
B. Relative	
III. Posthypercapnic states	

Modified from Khanna A, Kurtzman NA. Metabolic alkalosis. *J Nephrol.* 2006;19(Suppl 9):S86–S96.

Table 16-2 Factors That Maintain Metabolic Alkalosis

Factor	Proposed Mechanism
Decreased GFR	Increases fractional HCO_3^- reabsorption and prevents the elevated plasma $[HCO_3^-]$ from exceeding Tm
Volume contraction	Stimulates proximal tubular HCO_3 reabsorption
Hypokalemia	Decreases GFR and increases proximal tubular HCO_3^- reabsorption; stimulates Na-independent/K-dependent (low) secretion in CCT
Hypochloremia[a]	Increases renin, decreases GFR, and decreases distal chloride delivery (↑ proton secretion in MCT)
Passive backflux of HCO_3^-	Creates a favorable concentration gradient for passive HCO_3^- movement from proximal tubular lumen to blood
Aldosterone	Increases Na-dependent proton secretion in CCT and Na-independent proton secretion in CCT and MCT

All factors decrease urinary HCO_3 excretion in vivo.
[a]Animal models are associated with hypokalemia; thus, the precise role of chloride in humans is not clearly understood.
GFR, glomerular filtration rate; CCT, cortical collecting tubule; MCT, medullary collecting tubule. TM, transport maximum for HCO_3^-.
Modified from Khanna A, Kurtzman NA. Metabolic alkalosis. *J Nephrol.* 2006;19(Suppl 9):S86–S96.

Treatment of metabolic alkalosis consists of etiologic and nonetiologic therapies. Etiologic therapy consists of measures such as expansion of intravascular volume or the administration of potassium. Infusion of 0.9% saline will dose-dependently increase serum $[Cl^-]$ and decrease serum $[HCO_3^-]$.[6] Nonetiologic therapy includes administration of acetazolamide (a carbonic anhydrase inhibitor that causes renal bicarbonate wasting), dialysis against a high-chloride/low bicarbonate dialysate or infusion of $[H^+]$ in the form of ammonium chloride, arginine hydrochloride, or 0.1 N hydrochloric acid (100 mmol/L).[5] Of the previously mentioned factors, 0.1 N hydrochloric acid most rapidly corrects life-threatening metabolic alkalosis but must be infused into a central vein; peripheral infusion will cause severe tissue damage.

Table 16-3 Respiratory Compensation in Response to Metabolic Alkalosis and Metabolic Acidosis

Metabolic Alkalosis
1. $PaCO_2$ increases ~0.5–0.6 mmHg per 1 mEq/L increase in $[HCO_3^-]$
2. The last two digits of the pH should approximate the $[HCO_3^-]$ + 15

Metabolic Acidosis
1. $PaCO_2 = [HCO_3^-] \times 1.5 + 8$
2. $PaCO_2$ decreases 1.2 mmHg per 1 mEq/L in $[HCO_3^-]$ to a minimum of 10–15 mmHg
3. The last two digits of the pH – $[HCO_3^-]$ + 15

Metabolic Acidosis

Metabolic acidosis, characterized by hypobicarbonatemia (<21 mEq/L) and usually by an acidemic pH (<7.35), can be innocuous or reflect a life-threatening emergency. Metabolic acidosis occurs as a consequence of buffering by bicarbonate of endogenous or exogenous acid loads or as a consequence of abnormal external loss of bicarbonate.[7–9] Approximately 70 mmol of acid metabolites are produced, buffered, and excreted daily; these include about 25 mmol of sulfuric acid from amino acid metabolism, 40 mmol of organic acids, and phosphoric and other acids. Extracellular volume (ECV) in a 70-kg adult contains 336 mmol of bicarbonate buffer (24 mEq/L × 14 L of ECV). Glomerular filtration of plasma volume (PV) necessitates reabsorption of 4,500 mmol of bicarbonate daily, of which 85% is reabsorbed in the proximal tubule and 10% in the thick ascending limb, and the remainder is titrated by proton secretion in the collecting duct.

Calculation of the anion gap [AG; $[Na^+] - ([Cl^-] + [HCO_3^-])$] distinguishes between two types of metabolic acidosis (Table 16-4).[10] The AG is normal (<13 mEq/L) in situations such as diarrhea, biliary drainage, and renal tubular acidosis, in which bicarbonate is lost externally, and is also normal or reduced in hyperchloremic acidosis associated with perioperative infusion of substantial quantities of 0.9% saline.[6,11] Metabolic acidosis associated with a high AG (>13 mEq/L) occurs because of excess production or decreased excretion of organic acids or ingestion of one of several toxic compounds (Table 16-4). In metabolic acidosis associated with a high AG, bicarbonate ions are consumed in buffering hydrogen ions, while the associated anion replaces bicarbonate in serum. Three quarters of the normal AG consists of albumin; to correct the calculated AG for hypoalbuminemia, add to the calculated AG the difference between measured serum albumin and normal albumin concentration (4 g/dL) multiplied by 2 to 2.5.[12] The albumin-corrected

Table 16-4 Differential Diagnosis of Metabolic Acidosis

Elevated Anion Gap[a]

Three diseases
- Uremia
- Ketoacidosis
- Lactic acidosis

Toxins
- Methanol
- Ethylene glycol
- Salicylates
- Paraldehyde

Normal Anion Gap[b]
- Renal tubular acidosis
- Diarrhea
- Carbonic anhydrase inhibition
- Ureteral diversions
- Early renal failure
- Hydronephrosis
- HCl administration
- Saline administration

[a]Correction of the anion gap for hypoalbuminemia is essential for effective perioperative use.
[b]To correct the anion gap for hypoalbuminemia, add to the calculated anion gap twice the difference between normal serum albumin (4 g/L) and actual serum albumin.

Table 16-5 Failure to Maintain Appropriate Ventilatory Compensation for Metabolic Acidosis[a]

		Spontaneous Ventilation		Mechanical Hypoventilation
Arterial blood gases	pH	7.29		7.13
	$PaCO_2$ (mmHg)	29	→→→→→→→	49
	$[HCO_3^-]$ (mEq/L)	14		16

[a]In the presence of metabolic acidosis, an otherwise modest increase in $PaCO_2$ may create a life-threatening decrease in pH.

AG should exceed the normal anion gap by an amount (ΔAG) approximately equal to the decrease below normal of serum $[HCO_3^-]$ (ΔHCO_3^-).[13] A ratio of $\Delta AG:\Delta HCO_3^-$ that is below 0.8 or above 1.2 should prompt consideration of a mixed acid–base disturbance.

Sufficient reductions in pH may reduce myocardial contractility, increase pulmonary vascular resistance, and decrease systemic vascular resistance. It is particularly important to note that failure of a patient to appropriately hyperventilate in response to metabolic acidosis is physiologically equivalent to respiratory acidosis[7] and suggests clinical deterioration. If a patient with metabolic acidosis requires mechanical ventilation, for example, during general anesthesia, every attempt should be made to maintain an appropriate level of ventilatory compensation (Table 16-3) until the primary process can be corrected. Table 16-5 illustrates failure to maintain compensatory hyperventilation.

The anesthetic risk associated with metabolic acidosis is proportional to the severity of the underlying process that produces the metabolic acidosis. Although a patient with hyperchloremic metabolic acidosis may be relatively healthy, those with lactic acidosis, ketoacidosis, uremia, or toxic ingestions will be chronically or acutely ill. Preoperative assessment should emphasize volume status and renal function. If shock has caused metabolic acidosis, direct arterial pressure monitoring may be necessary, and preload may require assessment via echocardiography or pulmonary arterial catheterization. Intraoperatively, one should be concerned about the possibility of exaggerated hypotensive responses to drugs and positive pressure ventilation. In planning intravenous fluid therapy, consider that balanced salt solutions tend to increase pH and $[HCO_3^-]$ (i.e., by metabolism of lactate to bicarbonate) and 0.9% saline tends to decrease pH and $[HCO_3^-]$.

The treatment of metabolic acidosis consists of treatment of the primary pathophysiologic process, for example, hypoperfusion or hypoxia, and if pH is severely decreased, administration of $NaHCO_3$. Hyperventilation, although an important compensatory response to metabolic acidosis, is not a definitive therapy for metabolic acidosis. The initial dose of $NaHCO_3$ can be calculated as:

$$NaHCO_3 (mEq/L) = \frac{Wt(kg) \times 0.3(24\ mEq/L - Actual\ HCO_3^-)}{2}$$

(16-3)

where 0.3 = the assumed distribution space for bicarbonate and 24 mEq/L is the normal value for $[HCO_3^-]$ on arterial blood gas determination. The calculation markedly underestimates dosage in severe metabolic acidosis. In infants and children, a customary initial dose is 1 to 2 mEq/kg of body weight.

Both evidence and opinion suggest that $NaHCO_3$ should rarely be used to treat acidemia induced by metabolic acidosis.[7,8,14] In critically ill patients with lactic acidosis, there were no important differences between the physiologic effects (other than changes in pH) of 0.9 M $NaHCO_3$ and 0.9 M sodium chloride.[15] Importantly, $NaHCO_3$ did not improve the cardiovascular response to catecholamines and actually reduced plasma ionized calcium.[15] Although many clinicians choose to administer $NaHCO_3$ to patients with persistent lactic acidosis and ongoing deterioration, there are no clinical trials that demonstrate improved outcome. In contrast to $NaHCO_3$, the buffer tris-hydroxymethyl aminomethane (THAM) effectively reduces $[H^+]$, does not increase plasma $[Na^+]$, does not generate CO_2 as a byproduct of buffering, and does not decrease plasma $[K^+]$[16]; however, there is no generally accepted indication for THAM.

Respiratory Alkalosis

Respiratory alkalosis, always characterized by hypocarbia ($PaCO_2 \leq 35$ mmHg) and usually characterized by an alkalemic pH (>7.45), results from an increase in minute alveolar ventilation (V_A) that is greater than that required to excrete metabolic CO_2 production. Because respiratory alkalosis may be a sign of pain, anxiety, hypoxemia, central nervous system disease, or systemic sepsis, the development of spontaneous respiratory alkalosis in a previously normocarbic patient requires prompt evaluation. The hyperventilation syndrome, a diagnosis of exclusion, is most often encountered in the emergency department.[17]

Respiratory alkalosis may produce hypokalemia, hypocalcemia, cardiac dysrhythmias, bronchoconstriction, and hypotension, and may potentiate the toxicity of digoxin. In addition, both brain pH and cerebral blood flow are tightly regulated and respond rapidly to changes in $PaCO_2$.[18] Doubling V_A reduces $PaCO_2$ to 20 mmHg and halves cerebral blood flow; conversely, halving minute ventilation doubles $PaCO_2$ and doubles cerebral blood flow. Therefore, acute hyperventilation may be useful in neurosurgical procedures to reduce brain bulk and to control intracranial pressure (ICP) during emergent surgery for noncranial injuries associated with acute closed head trauma. In those situations, intraoperative monitoring of arterial blood gases, correlated with capnography, will document adequate reduction of $PaCO_2$. Acute profound hypocapnia (<20 mmHg) may produce electroencephalographic evidence of cerebral ischemia. If $PaCO_2$ is maintained at abnormally high or low levels for 8 to 24 hours, cerebral blood flow will return toward previous levels, associated with a return of cerebrospinal fluid $[HCO_3^-]$ toward normal.

Treatment of respiratory alkalosis per se is often not required. The most important steps are recognition and treatment of the underlying cause.[17] For instance, correction of hypoxemia or effective management of sepsis should result in resolution of the associated increases in respiratory drive. Preoperative recognition of chronic hyperventilation necessitates intraoperative maintenance of a similar $PaCO_2$.

Respiratory Acidosis

Respiratory acidosis, always characterized by hypercarbia ($PaCO_2$ >45 mmHg) and usually characterized by a low pH (<7.35), occurs because of a decrease in V_A, an increase in production of carbon dioxide (VCO_2) or both, from the equation:

$$Pa_{CO_2} = K \frac{V_{CO_2}}{V_A} \quad (16\text{-}4)$$

where K = constant (rebreathing of exhaled, carbon dioxide–containing gas may also increase $PaCO_2$). Respiratory acidosis may be either acute, without compensation by renal [HCO_3^-] retention, or chronic, with [HCO_3^-] retention, offsetting the decrease in pH (Table 16-6). A reduction in V_A may be due to an overall decrease in total minute ventilation (V_E) or to an increase in the amount of wasted ventilation (V_D), according to the equation:

$$V_A = V_E - V_D \quad (16\text{-}5)$$

Decreases in V_E may occur because of central ventilatory depression by drugs or central nervous system injury, because of increased work of breathing, or because of airway obstruction or neuromuscular dysfunction. Increases in V_D occur with chronic obstructive pulmonary disease, pulmonary embolism, decreased cardiac output, and most forms of respiratory failure. VCO_2 may be increased by sepsis, high-glucose parenteral feeding, or fever.

Patients with chronic hypercarbia due to intrinsic pulmonary disease require careful preoperative evaluation. The ventilatory restriction imposed by upper abdominal or thoracic surgery may aggravate ventilatory insufficiency after surgery. Administration of narcotics and sedatives, even in small doses, may cause hazardous ventilatory depression. Preoperative evaluation should consider direct arterial pressure monitoring and frequent intraoperative blood gas determinations, as well as strategies to manage postoperative pain with minimal doses of systemic opioids. Intraoperatively, a patient with chronically compensated hypercarbia should be ventilated to maintain a normal pH. Inadvertent restoration of normal V_A may result in profound alkalemia. Postoperatively, prophylactic ventilatory support may be required for selected patients with chronic hypercarbia.

The treatment of respiratory acidosis depends on whether the process is acute or chronic. Acute respiratory acidosis may require mechanical ventilation unless a simple etiologic factor (i.e., narcotic overdosage or residual muscular blockade) can be treated quickly. Bicarbonate administration is never indicated unless severe metabolic acidosis is also present or unless mechanical ventilation is ineffective in reducing acute hypercarbia. In contrast, chronic respiratory acidosis is rarely managed with ventilation but rather with efforts to improve pulmonary function. In patients requiring mechanical ventilation for acute respiratory failure, ventilation with a lung-protective strategy may result in hypercapnia, which occasionally may require administration of buffers to avoid excessive acidemia.[19]

Practical Approach to Acid–Base Interpretation

Rapid interpretation of a patient's acid–base status involves the integration of three sets of data: arterial blood gases, electrolytes, and history. A systematic approach facilitates interpretation (Table 16-7). Acid–base assessment usually can be completed before initiating therapy; however, the first step should be to determine whether there are life-threatening pH disturbances (e.g., respiratory acidosis or metabolic acidosis with pH < 7.1) that require immediate attention.

The second step is to determine whether a patient is acidemic (pH < 7.35) or alkalemic (pH > 7.45). The pH status will usually indicate the predominant primary process, that is, acidosis produces acidemia and alkalosis produces alkalemia. Note that the suffix "-osis" indicates a primary process that, if unopposed, will produce the corresponding pH change. The suffix "-emia" refers to the pH. A compensatory process is not considered an "-osis." Of course, a patient may have mixed "-oses," that is, more than one primary process.

The third step is to determine whether the entire arterial blood gas picture is consistent with a simple acute respiratory alkalosis or acidosis (Table 16-6). For example, a patient with acute hypocarbia ($PaCO_2$ 30 mmHg) would have a pH increase of 0.10 units to a pH of 7.50 and a decrease of calculated [HCO_3^-] to 22 mEq/L.

As the fourth step, recognition that changes in $PaCO_2$, pH, and [HCO_3] which are not consistent with a simple acute respiratory disturbance should prompt consideration of chronic respiratory acidosis (≥24 hours) or metabolic acidosis or alkalosis. In chronic respiratory acidosis, pH returns to nearly normal as bicarbonate is retained by the kidneys (Table 16-6), usually at a ratio of 4 to 5 mEq/L per 10 mmHg chronic increase in $PaCO_2$.[20] For example, chronic hypoventilation at a $PaCO_2$ of 60 mmHg would be

---

Table 16-6 Changes of [HCO_3^-] and pH in Response to Acute and Chronic Changes in $PaCO_2$

Decreased $PaCO_2$
- pH increases 0.10 per 10-mmHg decrease in $PaCO_2$
- [HCO_3^-] decreases 2 mEq/L per 10-mmHg decrease in $PaCO_2$
- pH will nearly normalize if hypocarbia is sustained
- [HCO_3^-] will decrease 5–6 mEq/L per 10-mmHg chronic decrease in $PaCO_2$[a]

Increased $PaCO_2$
- pH will decrease 0.05 per acute 10 mmHg increase $PaCO_2$
- [HCO_3^-] will increase 1 mEq/L per 10 mmHg increase $PaCO_2$
- pH will return toward normal if hypercarbia is sustained
- [HCO_3^-] will increase 4–5 mEq/L per chronic 10 mmHg increase in $PaCO_2$

[a]Hospitalized patients rarely develop chronic compensation for hypocarbia because of stimuli that enhance distal tubular reabsorption of sodium.

Table 16-7 Sequential Approach to Acid–Base Interpretation

1. Is the pH life-threatening, requiring immediate intervention?
2. Is the pH acidemic or alkalemic?
3. Could the entire arterial blood gas picture represent only an acute increase or decrease in $PaCO_2$?
4. If the answer to question 3 is "No," is there evidence of a chronic respiratory disturbance or of an acute metabolic disturbance?
5. If an acute metabolic disturbance is present, is it accompanied by appropriate respiratory compensatory changes?
6. Is an anion gap present?
7. Are the clinical data consistent with the proposed interpretation?

associated with an increase in [HCO_3^-] of 8 to 10 mEq/L so that [HCO_3^-] would be expected to range from 32 to 34 mEq/L and pH would be expected to be within the low normal range (7.35 to 7.38). If neither an acute nor chronic respiratory change appears to explain the arterial blood gas data, then a metabolic disturbance must also be present.

The fifth question addresses respiratory compensation for metabolic disturbances, which occurs more rapidly than renal compensation for respiratory disturbances (Table 16-3). Several general rules describe compensation. First, overcompensation is rare. Second, inadequate or excessive compensation suggests an additional primary disturbance. Third, hypobicarbonatemia associated with an increased anion gap is never compensatory.

The sixth question, whether an anion gap is present, should be assessed even if the arterial blood gases appear straightforward. The simultaneous occurrence of metabolic alkalosis and metabolic acidosis may result in an unremarkable pH and [HCO_3^-]; therefore, the combined abnormality may only be appreciated by examining the anion gap (if the cause of the metabolic acidosis is associated with a high anion gap). As noted previously, correct assessment of the anion gap requires correction for hypoalbuminemia.[12] Metabolic acidoses associated with increased anion gaps require specific treatments, thus necessitating a correct diagnosis and differentiation from hyperchloremic metabolic acidosis. For instance, if metabolic acidosis results from administration of large volumes of 0.9% saline, no specific treatment of metabolic acidosis would usually be necessary.

The seventh and final question is whether the clinical data are consistent with the proposed acid–base interpretation. Failure to integrate clinical findings with arterial blood gas and plasma electrolyte data may lead to serious errors in interpretation and management.

Examples

The following two hypothetical cases illustrate the use of the algorithm and rules of thumb previously discussed.

Example 1

A 65-year-old woman has undergone 12 hours of an expected 16-hour radical neck dissection and flap construction. Estimated blood loss is 1,000 mL. She has received three units of packed red blood cells and 6 L of 0.9% saline. Her blood pressure and heart rate have remained stable while anesthetized with 0.5% to 1% isoflurane in 70:30 nitrous oxide and oxygen. Urinary output is adequate. Arterial blood gas levels are shown in Table 16-8.

The step-by-step interpretation is as follows:
1. The pH requires no immediate treatment.
2. The pH is normal.
3. The arterial blood gases cannot be adequately explained by acute hypocarbia. The predicted pH would be 7.48 and the predicted [HCO_3^-] would be 22 mEq/L (Table 16-6).
4. A metabolic acidosis appears to be present.
5. Patients under general anesthesia with controlled mechanical ventilation cannot compensate for metabolic acidosis. However, spontaneous hypocarbia of this magnitude would represent slight overcompensation for metabolic acidosis (Table 16-3) and would suggest the presence of a primary respiratory alkalosis.
6. Metabolic acidosis occurring during prolonged anesthesia and surgery could suggest lactic acidosis and prompt additional fluid therapy or other attempts to improve perfusion. However, serum electrolytes reveal an AG that is slightly less than normal (Table 16-8), suggesting that the metabolic acidosis is probably the result of dilution of the ECV with a high-chloride fluid. Correction of the AG for the serum albumin of 3 g/dL only increases the anion gap to 10 to 11 mEq/L, again consistent with hyperchloremic metabolic acidosis. After differentiation from high-AG metabolic acidoses, hyperchloremic acidosis secondary to infusion of high-chloride fluid usually requires no treatment. The arterial blood gases and serum electrolytes are compatible with the clinical picture.

Table 16-8 Hyperchloremic Metabolic Acidosis during Prolonged Surgery

Parameter	Value
Arterial blood gases	
pH	7.40
$PaCO_2$	32 mmHg
[HCO_3^-]	19 mEq/L
Electrolytes	
[Na^+]	140 mEq/L
[Cl^-]	114 mEq/L
CO_2	20 mEq/L
Anion gap	8 mEq/L
Serum albumin	3 g/dL

Example 2

A 35-year-old man, 3 days after appendectomy, develops nausea with recurrent emesis persisting for 48 hours. An arterial blood gas reveals the results shown in the third column of Table 16-9.
1. The pH of 7.50 requires no immediate intervention.
2. The pH is alkalemic, suggesting a primary alkalosis.
3. An acute $PaCO_2$ of 46 mmHg would yield a pH of approximately 7.37; therefore, this is not simply an acute ventilatory disturbance.
4. The patient has a primary metabolic alkalosis as suggested by the [HCO_3^-] of 35 mEq/L.
5. The limits of respiratory compensation for metabolic alkalosis are wide and difficult to predict for individual patients.

Table 16-9 Metabolic Alkalosis Secondary to Nausea and Vomiting with Subsequent Lactic Acidosis Secondary to Hypovolemia

Parameter	Normal	Metabolic Alkalosis	Metabolic Acidosis
Blood Gases			
pH	7.40	7.50	7.40
$PaCO_2$ (mmHg)	40	46	40
[HCO_3^-] (mEq/L)	24	35	24
Serum Electrolytes			
[Na^+] (mEq/L)	140	140	140
[Cl^-] (mEq/L)	105	94	94
CO_2 (mEq/L)	25	36	25
Anion gap (mEq/L)	10	10	21

The rules of thumb, summarized in Table 16-3, suggest that [HCO_3^-] + 15 should equal the last two digits of the pH and that the $PaCO_2$ should increase 5 to 6 mmHg for every 10 mEq/L change in serum [HCO_3^-]; that is, a pH of 7.50 and a $PaCO_2$ of 46 mmHg are within the expected range.
6. The anion gap is 10 mEq/L.
7. The diagnosis of a primary metabolic alkalosis with compensatory hypoventilation is consistent with the history of recurrent vomiting. Consider how the arterial blood gases could change if vomiting were sufficiently severe to produce hypovolemic shock and lactic acidosis (fourth column of Table 16-9).

This sequence illustrates the important concept that the final pH, $PaCO_2$, and [HCO_3^-] represent the result of all of the vectors operating on acid–base status. Complex or "triple disturbances" can only be interpreted using a thorough, stepwise approach.

Fluid Management

Physiology

Body Fluid Compartments

Accurate replacement of fluid deficits necessitates an understanding of the expected volumes of distribution spaces for water, sodium, and colloid. The sum of intracellular volume (ICV; 40% of total body weight), ECV (20% of body weight), equals total body water (TBW), which therefore approximates 60% of total body weight. Plasma volume equals about 3 L, one-fifth of ECV, the remainder of which is interstitial fluid volume (IFV). Red cell volume, approximately 2 L, is part of ICV.

The volume of distribution of sodium-free water is TBW while the distribution volume of infused sodium is ECV. The sodium concentrations ([Na^+]) in PV and IFV, the two components of the ECV, are approximately 140 mEq/L. The predominant intracellular cation, potassium, has an intracellular concentration ([K^+]) approximating 150 mEq/L. The volume of distribution for colloid solutions is the ECV. Albumin, the most important oncotically active colloid in the ECV, is unequally distributed in PV (~4 g/dL) and IFV (~1 g/dL). However, the IFV concentration of albumin varies greatly among tissues.

Distribution of Infused Fluids

Conventionally, clinical prediction of PV expansion after fluid infusion assumes that body fluid spaces are static. Kinetic analysis of PV expansion replaces the static assumption with a dynamic description. As an example of the static approach, assume that a 70-kg patient has suffered an acute blood loss of 2,000 mL, approximately 40% of the predicted 5 L blood volume. The formula describing the effects of replacement with 5% dextrose in water (D_5W), lactated Ringer solution, or 5% or 25% human serum albumin is as follows:

$$\text{Expected PV increment} = \text{volume infused} \times \text{normal PV/distribution volume} \quad (16\text{-}6)$$

Calculating the volume of a given fluid required to produce a certain PV increment requires the following rearrangement of the equation:

$$\text{Volume infused} = \text{expected PV increment} \times \text{distribution volume/normal PV} \quad (16\text{-}7)$$

To restore blood volume using D_5W, assuming a distribution volume for sodium-free water of TBW, requires 28 L:

$$28\ L = 2\ L \times 42\ L/3\ L \quad (16\text{-}8)$$

where 2 L is the desired PV increment, 42 L = TBW in a 70-kg person, and 3 L is the normal estimated PV.

To restore blood volume using lactated Ringer solution requires 9.1 L:

$$9.1\ L = 2\ L \times 14\ L/3\ L \quad (16\text{-}9)$$

where 14 L = ECV in a 70-kg person.

If 5% albumin, which exerts colloid osmotic pressure similar to plasma, were infused, the infused volume initially would remain in the PV, perhaps attracting additional interstitial fluid intravascularly. Twenty-five percent human serum albumin, a concentrated colloid, expands PV by approximately 400 mL for each 100 mL infused.

However, these static analyses are simplistic. Infused fluid does not simply equilibrate throughout an assumed distribution volume but is added to a complex system that regulates intravascular, interstitial, and ICV. A more comprehensive kinetic model was proposed by Svensén and Hahn.[21] Kinetic models of intravenous fluid therapy allow clinicians to predict more accurately the time course of volume changes produced by infusions of fluids of various compositions. Kinetic analysis permits estimation of peak volume expansion and rates of clearance of infused fluid and complements analysis of "pharmacodynamic" effects, such as changes in cardiac output or cardiac filling pressures.[22]

Using a kinetic approach to fluid therapy permits analysis of the effects of common physiologic and pharmacologic influences on fluid distribution in experimental animals or humans. For example, in chronically instrumented sheep, fluid infusion during isoflurane anesthesia was associated with greater expansion of extravascular volume than in the conscious state.[23] The kinetics of PV expansion after fluid infusion were similar in conscious and anesthetized sheep, but reduced urinary output under anesthesia was associated with greater expansion of extravascular volume; this effect was attributable to isoflurane and not to mechanical ventilation.[23] Similar studies in volunteers suggested that the influence of anesthesia on fluid kinetics could be related to lower mean arterial pressures and activation of the renin/angiotensin/aldosterone system.[24] In subsequent studies in sheep, administration of catecholamine infusions before and during fluid infusions profoundly altered intravascular fluid retention, with phenylephrine diminishing and isoproterenol enhancing intravascular fluid retention (Fig. 16-1).[25]

The influence of rapid fluid infusion on the integrity of the endothelial glycocalyx potentially confounds volume kinetic assessment of PV. Rapid infusion of crystalloid fluids can potentially release noncirculating fluid volume that is trapped within the endothelial glycocalyx,[26] resulting in apparent rather than actual plasma dilution.

Regulation of Osmolarity and Effective Circulating Volume

TBW content is the net result of intake and output of water. Water intake includes ingested liquids plus an average of 750 mL ingested in solid food and 350 mL that is generated metabolically. Water output consists of insensible losses (~1,000 mL/day), gastrointestinal losses (100 to 150 mL/day), and urinary output, the volume of which is regulated to maintain TBW. Thirst, the primary mechanism of controlling water intake, is triggered by an increase in body fluid tonicity or by a decrease in effective circulating volume.

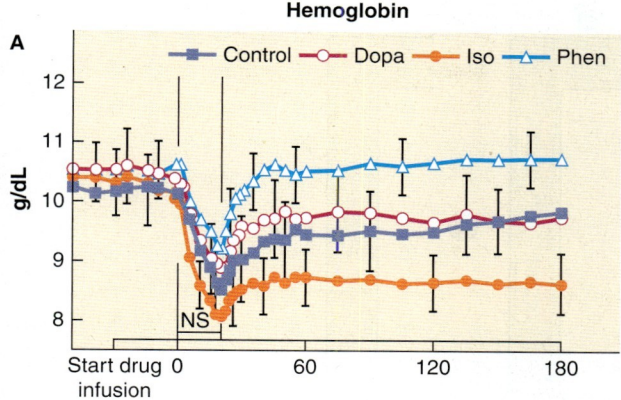

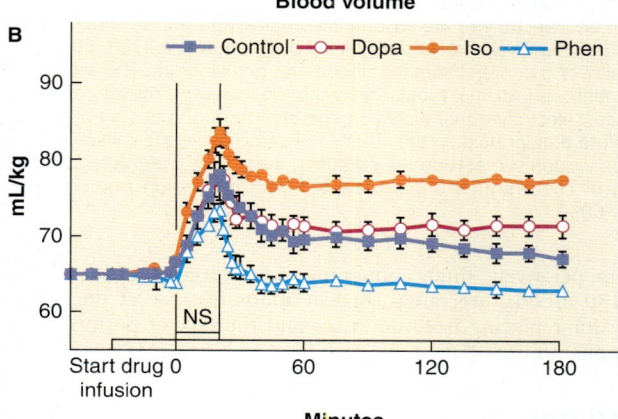

Figure 16-1 **A:** Blood hemoglobin (mean ± SEM) sampled at three baseline periods during a 30-minute catecholamine infusion and for 3 hours after starting a 20-minute 0.9% NaCl bolus of 24 mL/kg. Catecholamine protocols are dopamine (Dopa, *open diamonds*), isoproterenol (Iso, closed circles), phenylephrine (Phen, open triangles), and no-drug control (Control, closed squares). The 0.9% NaCl bolus decreased hemoglobin in all protocols at the end of the 20-minute 0.9% NaCl infusion and in all protocols except the Phen protocol thereafter. Postinfusion protocol differences were Phen > Dopa = Control > Iso. **B:** Calculated blood volume (mean ± SEM) at three baseline periods during a catecholamine infusion and for 3 hours after starting a 20-minute 0.9% NaCl bolus of 24 mL/kg. The 0.9% NaCl bolus increased blood volume in all protocols at T_{20} and in all protocols except the Phen protocol thereafter. Postinfusion protocol differences were Iso > Dopa = Control > Phen. NS, normal saline bolus. (Adapted with permission from Vane LA, Prough DS, Kinsky MA, et al. Effects of different catecholamines on the dynamics of volume expansion of crystalloid infusion. *Anesthesiology.* 2004;101:1136–1144.)

Renal reabsorption of filtered water and sodium is regulated by the renin/angiotensin/aldosterone system, antidiuretic hormone (ADH), and natriuretic peptides.[27] Renal water handling has three important components: (1) delivery of tubular fluid to the diluting segments of the nephron, (2) separation of solute and water in the diluting segment, and (3) variable reabsorption of water in the collecting ducts. In the descending loop of Henle, water is reabsorbed while solute is retained to achieve a final osmolality of tubular fluid of approximately 1,200 mOsm/kg (Fig. 16-2). This concentrated fluid is then diluted by the active reabsorption of sodium via the $NaKCl_2$ transporter in the ascending limb of the loop of Henle[28] and via the Na/Cl transporter in the distal tubule, both of which are relatively impermeable to water. Within the collecting duct, water reabsorption is modulated by ADH (also called *vasopressin*).[29] Vasopressin binds to V_2 receptors (G-protein coupled receptors) along the basolateral membrane of the collecting duct cells; the resulting increased cAMP levels then stimulate the synthesis and insertion of the aquaporin-2 water channel into the apical membrane of collecting duct cells.[30,31]

Plasma hypotonicity suppresses ADH release, resulting in excretion of dilute urine. Hypertonicity stimulates ADH secretion, which increases the permeability of the collecting duct to water and enhances water reabsorption. In response to changing plasma [Na^+], changing secretion of ADH can vary urinary osmolality from 50 to 1,200 mOsm/kg and urinary volume from 0.4 to 20 L/day (Fig. 16-3).[32] Nonosmotic modulators of ADH secretion include hemodynamic (hypotension, hypovolemia, congestive heart failure, cirrhosis, nephrotic syndrome, and adrenal insufficiency) and nonhemodynamic stimuli (nausea, pain, and medications, including opiates).[33]

Two powerful hormonal systems regulate total body sodium. The natriuretic peptides, ANP, brain natriuretic peptide, and C-type natriuretic peptide, defend against sodium overload[34,35] and the renin–angiotensin–aldosterone axis defends against sodium depletion and hypovolemia. ANP, released from the cardiac atria in response to increased atrial stretch, exerts vasodilatory effects and increases the renal excretion of sodium and water. ANP secretion is decreased during hypovolemia. Even in patients with chronic (nonoliguric) renal insufficiency, infusion of ANP in low, nonhypotensive doses increased sodium excretion and augmented urinary losses of retained solutes.[34]

Aldosterone is the final common pathway in a complex response to decreased effective arterial volume, whether decreased effective arterial volume is absolute or relative, as in edematous states or hypoalbuminemia. In this pathway, decreased stretch in the baroreceptors of the aortic arch and carotid body and stretch receptors in the great veins, pulmonary vasculature, and atria result in increased sympathetic tone. Increased sympathetic tone, in combination with decreased renal perfusion, leads to renin release and formation of angiotensin I from angiotensinogen. Subsequently, in the lungs, angiotensin-converting enzyme (ACE) converts angiotensin I to angiotensin II, which stimulates the adrenal cortex to synthesize and release aldosterone.[36] Acting primarily in the distal tubules, high concentrations of aldosterone cause sodium reabsorption and may reduce urinary excretion of sodium nearly to zero. Intrarenal physical factors are also important in regulating sodium balance. Sodium loading decreases colloid osmotic pressure, thereby increasing the glomerular filtration rate (GFR), decreasing net sodium reabsorption, and increasing distal sodium delivery, which, in turn, suppresses renin secretion.

Fluid Replacement Therapy

Maintenance Requirements for Water, Sodium, and Potassium

Calculation of maintenance fluid requirements is of limited value in determining intraoperative fluid requirements. However, calculation of maintenance fluid requirements (Table 16-10) is useful for estimating water and electrolyte deficits that result from preoperative restriction of oral food and fluids and for estimating the ongoing requirements for patients with prolonged postoperative bowel dysfunction. In healthy adults, sufficient water is required to balance gastrointestinal losses (100 to 200 mL/day), insensible losses (500 to 1,000 mL/day), and urinary losses of

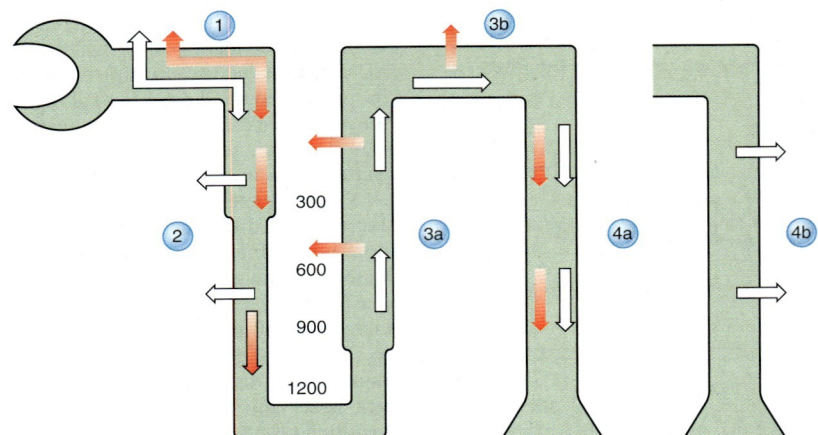

Figure 16-2 Renal filtration, reabsorption, and excretion of water. *Open arrows* represent water and *solid arrows* represent electrolytes. Water and electrolytes are filtered by the glomerulus. In the proximal tubule *(1)*, water and electrolytes are absorbed isotonically. In the descending loop of Henle *(2)*, water is absorbed to achieve osmotic equilibrium with the interstitium while electrolytes are retained. The numbers (300, 600, 900, and 1,200) between the descending and ascending limbs represent the osmolality of the interstitium in milliosmoles per kilogram. The delivery of solute and fluid to the distal nephron is a function of proximal tubular reabsorption; as proximal tubular reabsorption increases, delivery of solute to the medullary *(3a)* and cortical *(3b)* diluting sites decreases. In the diluting sites, electrolyte-free water is generated through selective reabsorption of electrolytes while water is retained in the tubular lumen, generating a dilute tubular fluid. In the absence of vasopressin, the collecting duct *(4a)* remains relatively impermeable to water and diluted urine is excreted. When vasopressin acts on the collecting ducts *(4b)*, water is reabsorbed from these vasopressin-responsive nephron segments, allowing the excretion of concentrated urine. (Adapted with permission from Fried LF, Palevsky PM. Hyponatremia and hypernatremia. *Med Clin North Am.* 1997:585–609.)

1,000 mL/day. Urinary losses exceeding 1,000 mL/day may represent an appropriate physiologic response to ECV expansion or pathophysiologic inability to conserve salt or water.

Daily adult requirements for sodium and potassium are approximately 75 and 40 mEq respectively, although wider ranges of sodium intake than potassium intake are physiologically tolerated because renal sodium conservation and excretion are more efficient than potassium conservation and excretion. Therefore, healthy, 70-kg adults require 2,500 mL/day of water containing [Na$^+$] of 30 mEq/L and [K$^+$] of 15 to 20 mEq/L.

Intraoperatively, fluids containing sodium-free water (i.e., [Na$^+$] < 130 mEq/L) are rarely used in adults because of the necessity for replacing isotonic losses and the risk of postoperative hyponatremia.[37–40]

Dextrose

Traditionally, glucose-containing intravenous fluids have been given in an effort to prevent hypoglycemia and limit protein catabolism. However, because of the hyperglycemic response

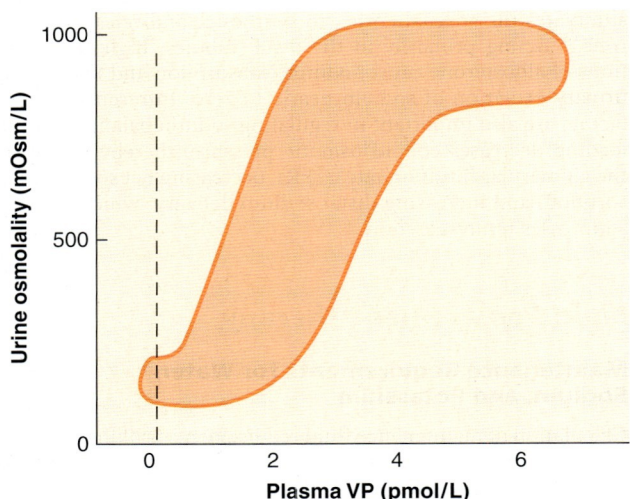
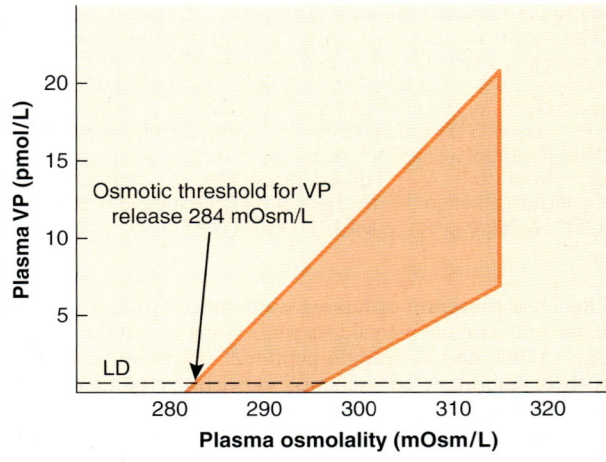

Figure 16-3 Left: The sigmoid relationship between plasma vasopressin (VP) and urinary osmolality. Data were obtained during water loading and fluid restriction in a group of healthy adults. Maximum urinary concentration is achieved by plasma VP values of 3 to 4 pmol/L. **Right:** The linear relationship between plasma osmolality and plasma VP. Increases in VP in response to hypertonicity induced by infusion of 855 mmol/L saline in a group of healthy adults. The *shaded area* represents the reference range response. LD represents the limit of detection of the VP assay, 0.3 pmol/L. (Adapted with permission from Ball SG. Vasopressin and disorders of water balance: the physiology and pathophysiology of vasopressin. *Ann Clin Biochem.* 2007;44:417–431.)

Table 16-10	Hourly and Daily Maintenance Water Requirements	
Weight (kg)	Water (mL/kg/hr)	Water (mL/kg/day)
1–10	4	100
11–20	2	50
21–n+	1	20

associated with surgical stress, only infants and patients receiving insulin or drugs that interfere with glucose synthesis are at risk for hypoglycemia. Iatrogenic hyperglycemia can limit the effectiveness of fluid resuscitation by inducing an osmotic diuresis and, in animals, may aggravate ischemic neurologic injury.[41] Although associated with worsened clinical outcome after subarachnoid hemorrhage[42] and traumatic brain injury,[43] hyperglycemia may also constitute a hormonally mediated response to more severe injury. In a meta-analysis of studies performed in critically ill patients, targeted blood glucose management, at a target of 180 mg/dL or less, was associated with reduced mortality and morbidity in comparison with a tighter control target of 81 to 108 mg/dL.[44]

Surgical Fluid Requirements

Water and Electrolyte Composition of Fluid Losses

Surgical patients require replacement of PV and ECV losses secondary to wound or burn edema, ascites, and gastrointestinal secretions. The fluid composition of wound and burn edema and ascitic fluid is protein-rich, with electrolyte concentrations similar to those of plasma. Although gastrointestinal secretions vary greatly in composition, the composition of replacement fluid need not be closely matched if ECV is adequate and renal and cardiovascular functions are normal. Substantial loss of gastrointestinal fluids requires more accurate replacement of electrolytes (i.e., potassium, magnesium, phosphate). Chronic gastric losses may produce hypochloremic metabolic alkalosis that can be corrected with 0.9% saline; chronic diarrhea may produce hyperchloremic metabolic acidosis that may be prevented or corrected by infusion of fluid containing bicarbonate or bicarbonate substrate (e.g., lactate). If cardiovascular or renal function is impaired, more precise replacement may require frequent assessment of serum electrolytes.

Influence of Perioperative Fluid Infusion Rates on Clinical Outcomes

Conventionally, intraoperative fluid management included replacement of fluid ("third space fluid") that was assumed to accumulate extravascularly in surgically manipulated tissue.[45] Until recently, perioperative clinical practice included, in addition to replacement of estimated blood loss, 4 to 6 mL/kg/hr for procedures involving minimal tissue trauma, 6 to 8 mL/kg/hr for those involving moderate trauma, and 8 to 12 mL/kg/hr for those involving severe trauma.

However, clinical trials strongly link perioperative fluid management to both minor and major morbidities. Moreover, the influence of fluid volume and composition appear to be specific to the type of surgery used. Maharaj et al.[46] randomized 80 ASA I–II patients scheduled for gynecologic laparoscopy to either large volume, defined as 2 mL/kg/hr of fasting over 20 minutes preoperatively (e.g., 1,440 mL/60 kg in a patient who had been fasting for 12 hours) or small volume, defined as total fluid of 3 mL/kg over 20 minutes preoperatively. In patients receiving the higher dose, postoperative nausea and vomiting and pain were significantly reduced (Fig. 16-4).[46] Holte et al.[47] randomized 48 ASA I–II patients undergoing laparoscopic cholecystectomy to receive either 15 or 40 mL/kg of lactated Ringer solution intraoperatively; the higher dose of fluid was associated with improved postoperative pulmonary function and exercise capacity, reduced neurohumoral stress response, and improvements in nausea, general sense of well-being, thirst, dizziness, drowsiness, fatigue, and balance function. Holte et al.[48] randomized 48 ASA I–III patients undergoing fast-track elective knee arthroplasty under intraoperative epidural/spinal anesthesia and

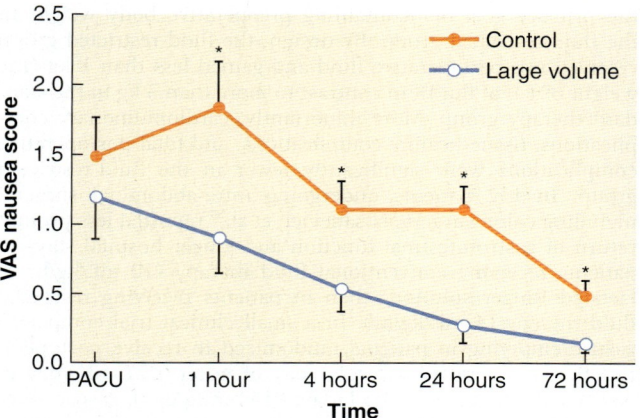
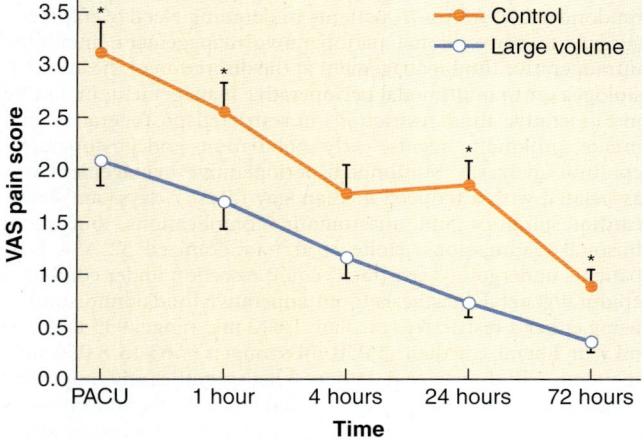

Figure 16-4 Top: Mean postoperative verbal analogue scale (VAS) nausea scores in each group over the first 72 postoperative hours. Mean VAS nausea scores were significantly lower in the group that received the large-volume intravenous fluid infusion compared with the control group at 1, 4, 24, and 72 hours postoperatively. **Bottom:** Mean postoperative VAS pain scores in each group over the first 72 postoperative hours. Mean VAS pain scores were significantly lower in the group that received the large-volume intravenous fluid infusion compared with the control group at 0, 1, 24, and 72 hours postoperatively. *Significantly higher ($p < 0.05$, t-test postanalysis of variance) VAS score compared with the large volume group. PACU, postanesthesia care unit. (Adapted with permission from Maharaj CH, Kallam SR, Malik A, et al. Preoperative intravenous fluid therapy decreases postoperative nausea and pain in high risk patients. *Anesth Analg.* 2005;100:675–682.)

postoperative epidural analgesia to either liberal or restricted fluids. Median intravenous fluid administered intraoperatively and in the postanesthesia care unit in the restrictive group was 1,740 mL (range, 1,100–2,165 mL) of lactated Ringer solution and in the liberal group was 3,275 mL (range, 2,400–4,000 mL). Restrictive fluid administration was associated with a higher incidence of vomiting but less hypercoagulability and no difference in short-term postoperative mobility or ileus. Therefore, in patients undergoing surgery of limited scope, fluid restriction appears to be less well tolerated than more liberal fluid therapy, but perhaps at the expense of hypercoagulability.

In patients undergoing major intra-abdominal surgery, recent randomized controlled trials also suggest that restrictive fluid administration is associated with a combination of positive and negative effects. Brandstrup et al.[49] randomized 172 elective colon surgery patients to either restrictive perioperative fluid management or standard perioperative fluid management, with the primary goal of maintaining preoperative body weight in the fluid-restricted group. By design, the fluid-restricted group received less perioperative fluid and gained less than 1 kg (the weight of 1 L of fluid), in contrast to more than 3 kg in the standard therapy group. More importantly, cardiopulmonary complications, tissue-healing complications, and total postoperative complications were significantly fewer in the fluid-restricted group. In 152 patients undergoing intra-abdominal surgery, including colon surgery, Nisanevich et al.[50] reported less prompt return of gastrointestinal function and longer hospital stays in patients receiving conventional fluid therapy (10 mL/kg/hr of lactated Ringer solution) than in patients receiving restricted fluid therapy (4 mL/kg/hr). In a small clinical trial comparing gastric emptying in patients randomized to receive postoperative fluids at a restricted (≤2 L/day of water; ≤77 mEq/day of Na$^+$) or liberal regimen (≥3 L/day; ≥154 mEq/day), gastric emptying time for both liquids and solids was significantly reduced in patients receiving restricted fluids (Fig. 16-5).[51] Khoo et al.[52] randomized 70 ASA I–III patients undergoing elective colorectal surgery to conventional perioperative management, including intraoperative fluid management at the discretion of the anesthesiologist, or to multimodal perioperative management, including intraoperative fluid restriction, unrestricted postoperative oral intake, prokinetic agents, early ambulation, and postoperative epidural analgesia. Multimodal perioperative management was associated with a reduced median stay (5 vs. 7 days) and fewer cardiorespiratory and anastomotic complications, but more hospital readmissions. Holte et al.[53] randomized 32 ASA I–III patients undergoing "fast-track" colon resection under combined epidural/general anesthesia to intraoperative fluid administration using either a restrictive (median: 1,640 mL; range: 935 to 2,250 mL) or liberal (median: 5,050 mL; range: 3,563 to 8,050 mL) regimen. Fluid-restricted patients had significantly improved postoperative forced vital capacity and fewer, less severe episodes of oxygen desaturation, but at the expense of increased stress responses (aldosterone, ADH, and angiotensin II measurements), and a statistically insignificantly increased number of complications. In a recent meta-analysis, Corcoran et al.[54] reviewed 23 randomized trials involving 3,861 patients assigned to liberal or goal-directed therapy during major surgery. Patients in both the liberal and goal-directed therapy groups received more fluid during surgery than their respective comparative groups (restrictive fluid administration). However, the patients in the liberal groups had a higher risk of pneumonia (risk ratio 2.2), pulmonary edema (risk ratio 3.8), and longer hospital stay (mean difference 2 days) than their comparative groups. The patients in the goal-directed therapy groups had a lower risk of pneumonia and renal complications (risk ratio 0.7), and shorter hospital

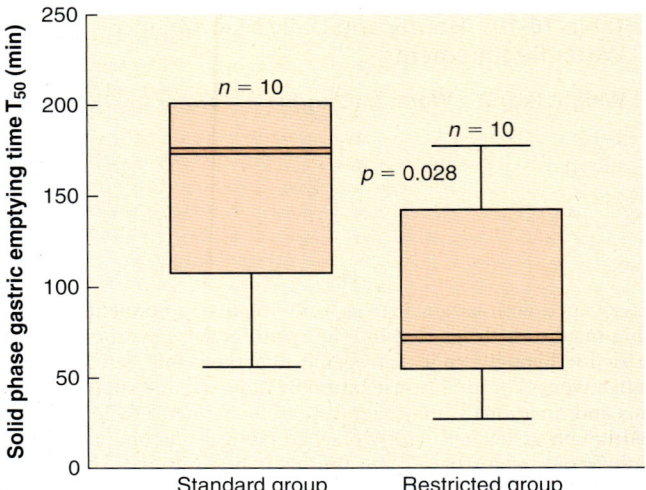

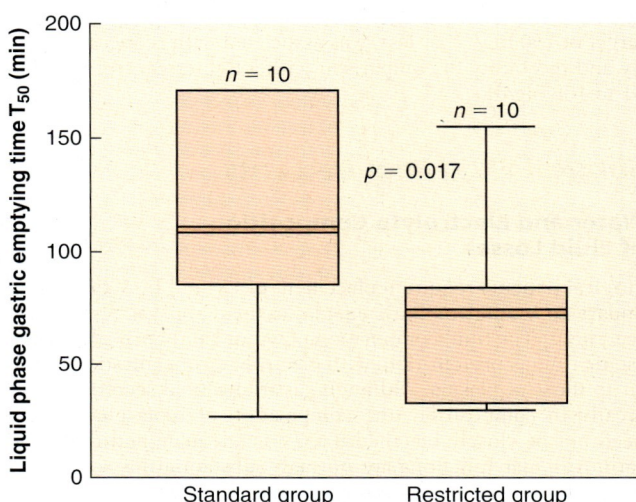

Figure 16-5 Solid and liquid phase gastric emptying times (T_{50}) after 4 days of standard or restricted intravenous postoperative fluid therapy. *Solid lines* are medians, *shaded areas* interquartile ranges, and *whiskers* represent extreme values. Differences between medians for solid and liquid phase T_{50} were 56 minutes (95% confidence interval: 12 to 132 minutes) and 52 minutes (9 to 95 minutes), respectively. (Adapted with permission from Lobo DN, Bostock KA, Neal KR, et al. Effect of salt and water balance on recovery of gastrointestinal function after elective colonic resection: a randomised controlled trial. *Lancet*. 2002;359:1812.)

stay (mean difference 2 days) compared to the patients in the non–goal-directed therapy group. These authors concluded that goal-directed fluid therapy was associated with fewer adverse outcomes than non–goal-directed, liberal fluid administration. However, they also concluded that the data do not establish whether goal-directed fluid therapy is superior to non–goal-directed restrictive fluid therapy.

Critically ill patients with acute lung injury represent an important group that may benefit from careful regulation of fluid intake. The ARDS Clinical Trials Network[55] randomized 1,000 patients with acute lung injury to a 7-day trial comparing a conservative fluid strategy with a liberal fluid strategy. Over the course of the trial the conservative strategy group had a cumulative net fluid balance that was slightly negative in comparison to a mean net cumulative fluid balance in the liberal group of nearly 7 L. Although overall mortality was no different in the two groups, the conservative fluid group had improved oxygenation and required fewer days of mechanical ventilation and intensive care. Despite achieving a negative fluid balance, the conservative strategy group had no greater incidence of acute renal failure.

Colloids, Crystalloids, and Hypertonic Solutions

Physiology and Pharmacology

Osmotically active particles attract water across semipermeable membranes until equilibrium is attained. *Osmolarity* is defined as the number of osmotically active particles per *liter* of solvent; *osmolality*, defined as the number of osmotically active particles per *kilogram*, can be estimated as follows:

$$\text{Osmolality} = ([Na^+] \times 2) + (\text{Glucose}/18) + (\text{BUN}/2.8) \quad (16\text{-}10)$$

where osmolality is expressed in mmol/kg, $[Na^+]$ is expressed in mEq/L, serum glucose is expressed in mg/dL, and BUN is blood urea nitrogen expressed in mg/dL. Sugars, alcohols, and radiographic dyes increase measured osmolality, generating an increased "osmolal gap" between the measured and calculated values.

High concentrations of osmotically active particles lead to hyperosmolar states. Both uremia (increased BUN) and hypernatremia (increased serum sodium) increase serum osmolality. However, because urea distributes throughout TBW, an increase in BUN does not cause *hypertonicity*. Sodium, largely restricted to the ECV, causes hypertonicity, that is, osmotically mediated redistribution of water from ICV to ECV. The term *tonicity* is also used colloquially to compare the osmotic pressure of a parenteral solution to that of plasma.

Although only a small proportion of the osmotically active particles in blood consist of plasma proteins, those particles are essential in determining the equilibrium of fluid between the interstitial and plasma compartments of ECV. The reflection coefficient (σ) describes the permeability of capillary membranes to individual solutes, with 0 representing free permeability and 1 representing complete impermeability. The reflection coefficient for albumin ranges from 0.6 to 0.9 in various capillary beds. Because capillary protein concentrations exceed interstitial concentrations, the osmotic pressure exerted by plasma proteins (termed *colloid osmotic pressure* or *oncotic pressure*) is higher than interstitial oncotic pressure and tends to preserve PV. The filtration rate of fluid from the capillaries into the interstitial space is the net result of a combination of forces, including the gradient from intravascular to interstitial colloid osmotic pressures and the hydrostatic gradient between intravascular and interstitial pressures. The net fluid filtration at any point within a systemic or pulmonary capillary is approximated by Starling law of capillary filtration, as expressed in the equation:

$$Q = \underline{kA} \left[(P_c - P_i) + \sigma(\pi_i - \pi_c) \right] \quad (16\text{-}11)$$

where Q = fluid filtration, k = capillary filtration coefficient (conductivity of water), A = area of the capillary membrane, P_c = capillary hydrostatic pressure, P_i = interstitial hydrostatic pressure, σ = the reflection coefficient for albumin, π_i = interstitial colloid osmotic pressure, and π_c = capillary colloid osmotic pressure. However, it is important to note that the Starling law does not account for the influence on fluid filtration of the capillary glycocalyx, which is strongly influenced by disease processes and fluid administration.[56] Attachment of albumin to the endothelial glycocalyx results in the colloid osmotic pressure gradient actually being the difference between π_c and the colloid osmotic pressure in the space between the endothelial glycocalyx and the capillary wall.[57]

The IFV is determined by the relative rates of capillary filtration and lymphatic drainage. P_c, the most powerful factor promoting fluid filtration, is determined by capillary flow, arterial resistance, venous resistance, and venous pressure. If capillary filtration increases, the rates of water and sodium filtration usually exceed protein filtration, resulting in preservation of π_c, dilution of π_i, and preservation of the oncotic pressure gradient, the most powerful factor opposing fluid filtration. When coupled with increased lymphatic drainage, preservation of the oncotic pressure gradient limits the accumulation of IF. If P_c increases at a time when lymphatic drainage is maximal, then IFV accumulates, forming edema. However, because of the influence of the glycocalyx, theoretical rates of fluid filtration usually substantially exceed actual filtration rates, a phenomenon termed the "low lymph flow paradox."[57]

Clinical Implications of Choices between Alternative Fluids

If membrane permeability is intact, colloids such as albumin or hydroxyethyl starch (HES) preferentially expand PV rather than IFV. Concentrated colloid-containing solutions (e.g., 25% albumin) exert sufficient oncotic pressure to translocate substantial volumes of IFV into the PV, thereby increasing PV by a volume that exceeds the original infused volume. PV expansion unaccompanied by IFV expansion offers apparent advantages: Lower fluid requirements, less peripheral and pulmonary edema accumulation, and reduced concern about the cardiopulmonary consequences of later fluid mobilization (Table 16-11). However, exhaustive research has failed to establish the superiority of either colloid-containing or crystalloid-containing fluids for either intraoperative or postoperative use.

Despite the lack of conclusive evidence of efficacy, albumin has been used in critically ill patients for decades.[58] In patients with sepsis or septic shock, the Early Albumin Resuscitation during Septic Shock (EARSS) study[59] and the Albumin Italian Outcome Sepsis (ALBIOS) trial[60] failed to find any overall difference in mortality. However, in the ALBIOS trial, time to discontinue vasoactive agents was shorter in the albumin group and, in a post hoc analysis, the subgroup of patients presenting with septic shock had a significantly reduced 90-day mortality if they received albumin. This benefit remained after adjustment of confounding variables.[61]

Meta-analyses have generated conflicting information regarding the influence of albumin administration on outcome. In burn patients who received albumin, mortality and the incidence of abdominal compartment syndrome were reduced.[62] In hypoalbuminemic patients who were resistant to diuretics, coadministration of albumin and furosemide transiently improved urinary output and sodium excretion.[63] In a meta-analysis of clinical trials in patients with acute respiratory distress syndrome (ARDS), albumin administration was associated with improved oxygenation but no increase in survival.[64] Overall, the findings of these reviews are confounded by heterogeneity and by the paucity of available clinical data, thus making it more difficult to elucidate the benefit of albumin resuscitation in critically ill patients.

HES, once a commonly used synthetic colloid, has been linked in critically ill patients to increased mortality and morbidity such

Table 16-11 Claimed Advantages and Disadvantages of Colloid Versus Crystalloid Intravenous Fluids

Solution	Advantages	Disadvantages
Colloid	Smaller infused volume Prolonged increase in plasma volume Less peripheral edema	Greater cost Coagulopathy (dextran > HES) Pulmonary edema (capillary leak states) Decreased GFR Osmotic diuresis (low-molecular-weight dextran) Greater duration of excessive volume expansion
Crystalloid	Lower cost Greater urinary flow Interstitial fluid replacement	Transient increase in intravascular volume Transient hemodynamic improvement Peripheral edema (protein dilution) Pulmonary edema (protein dilution plus high PAOP)

HES, hydroxyethyl starch; GFR, glomerular filtration rate; PAOP, pulmonary arterial occlusion pressure.

as coagulopathy, pruritus, nephrotoxicity, and acute renal failure.[65] In the "6S Trial," HES was associated with an increased risk of death and end-stage renal failure in comparison to Ringer acetate.[66] As a consequence, the Surviving Sepsis Campaign recommended that HES be eliminated from treatment of septic patients.[67] Subsequently, the US Food and Drug Administration banned all marketing of HES due to lack of evidence of clinical benefit in any patient population, with abundant evidence of harm, especially kidney failure. Eventually, HES was recalled from the US market.

Colloids and Traumatic Brain Injury

Two-year follow-up of a subset of 460 patients with traumatic brain injury (Glasgow Coma Scale score ≤ 13) demonstrated a nearly twofold increased risk of death in patients receiving colloid fluid management.[68] A subsequent secondary analysis suggested that patients receiving 4% albumin had a higher incidence of refractory intracranial hypertension.[69] Van Aken et al.[70] offered a plausible explanation, in that the 4% albumin solution used in the SAFE trial was suspended in a hypo-osmolar carrier solution, so that the adverse effects of the infusion could have been due to reduced osmolality, independent of the colloid content.

Cirrhotic patients may represent a specific subset of patients in whom albumin infusion could be beneficial. In patients with decompensated cirrhosis, infusion of albumin reduced prostaglandin E_2 and improved macrophage function.[71] In rodents with cirrhosis and ascites, albumin improved cardiac function, apparently by reducing production of TNFα and nitric oxide.[72] Clinical trials will be needed to confirm the therapeutic value of albumin in cirrhosis.

Implications of Crystalloid and Colloid Infusions on Intracranial Pressure

Because the cerebral capillary membrane, the blood–brain barrier, is highly impermeable to sodium, abrupt changes in serum osmolality produced by changes in serum sodium produce reciprocal changes in brain water. The effects of acute changes in colloid osmotic pressure are less clear. In anesthetized rabbits, reducing plasma osmolality from 295 to 282 mOsm/kg (which decreases plasma osmotic pressure by ~250 mmHg) increased cortical water content and ICP; in contrast, reducing colloid osmotic pressure from 20 to 7 mmHg produced no significant change in either variable.[73] In anesthetized rats subjected to fluid percussion TBI followed by hemorrhage of 20 mL/kg, resuscitation with 90 mL/kg of isotonic lactated Ringer solution was associated with equivalent blood volume expansion to 20 mL/kg of 5% albumin, but at the expense of higher brain water. Resuscitation with only 50 mL/kg of isotonic lactated Ringer solution did not increase brain water, but also failed to restore blood volume.[74] In this experimental study, the 5% albumin was suspended in a slightly hyperosmolar solution in contrast to the hypo-osmolar 4% solution used in the SAFE clinical trial.[70] Although the role of colloid in resuscitation of brain-injured patients remains unclear, it is appropriate to avoid large volumes of hypo-oncotic fluids such as lactated Ringer solution.[75]

Clinical Implications of Hypertonic Fluid Administration

An ideal alternative to conventional crystalloid and colloid fluids would be inexpensive, would produce minimal peripheral or pulmonary edema, would generate sustained hemodynamic effects, and would be effective even if administered in small volumes. Hypertonic, hypernatremic solutions, with or without added colloid, appear to fulfill some of these criteria (Table 16-12).

Hypertonic solutions exert favorable effects on cerebral hemodynamics, in part because of the reciprocal relationship between plasma osmolality and brain water.[73] ICP increased during resuscitation from hemorrhagic shock with lactated Ringer solution but remained unchanged if 7.5% saline was infused in a sufficient volume to comparably improve systemic hemodynamics.[76] However, a delayed increase in ICP was reported after hypertonic resuscitation from hypovolemic shock accompanied by an intracranial mass lesion.[77]

Despite concerns about central nervous system dysfunction due to hypertonicity and hypernatremia associated with hypertonic saline, acute increases in serum sodium to 155 to 160 mEq/L produced no apparent harm in hypovolemic trauma patients resuscitated with hypertonic saline.[78] Central pontine myelinolysis, which follows rapid correction of severe, chronic hyponatremia, has not been observed in clinical trials of hypertonic resuscitation. Despite theoretical considerations favoring the use of hypertonic saline in resuscitation of patients with traumatic brain injury, a subsequent randomized trial failed to demonstrate an improvement in outcome.[79]

Will clinicians routinely use hypertonic, or a combination of hypertonic/hyperoncotic, fluids for resuscitation in the future? Pending further preclinical work, the theoretical advantages of such fluids appear most attractive in the acute resuscitation of hypovolemic patients who have decreased intracranial compliance.[80]

Table 16-12 Hypertonic Resuscitation Fluids: Advantages and Disadvantages

Solution	Advantages	Disadvantages
Hypertonic crystalloid	Inexpensive Promotes urinary flow Small initial volume Arteriolar dilation Reduced peripheral edema Lower intracranial pressure	Hypertonicity Subdural hemorrhage Transient effect Potential rebound intracranial hypertension
Hypertonic crystalloid plus colloid (in comparison to hypertonic crystalloid alone)	Sustained hemodynamic response Reduced subsequent volume requirements	Added expense Osmotic diuresis Hypertonicity

Reprinted with permission from Prough DS, Johnston WE. Fluid resuscitation in septic shock: no solution yet. *Anesth Analg.* 1989;69:699–704.

Hypertonic solutions are also used to reduce brain water and intracranial volume during neurosurgery and in critical care. Although this goal is conventionally accomplished with mannitol, some clinicians prefer hypertonic saline solutions.[81,82] Hypertonic saline solutions and mannitol solutions of similar osmolality have similar effects on brain water, intracranial volume, and ICP. However, infusion of hypertonic saline increases intravascular volume, while diuresis secondary to mannitol decreases intravascular volume.[83] While few complications relate specifically to osmotic therapy, acute severe hyperosmolality could, theoretically, precipitate BBB opening. Clinical use of hypertonic saline is associated, as is 0.9% saline, with hyperchloremic acidosis, which usually requires no treatment, but must be differentiated from other causes of metabolic acidosis.

Fluid Status: Assessment and Monitoring

For most surgical patients, conventional clinical assessment of the adequacy of intravascular volume is appropriate. For high-risk patients, goal-directed hemodynamic management may be superior.

Conventional Clinical Assessment

Assessment of blood volume and ECV begins with identification of predisposing factors such as bowel obstruction, preoperative bowel preparation, chronic diuretic use, sepsis, burns, and trauma. Assessment of hypovolemia is mainly based on physical signs that include oliguria, supine hypotension, and a positive tilt test. In general, oliguria implies hypovolemia, keeping in mind that hypovolemic patients can have adequate urinary output and that urinary output can be misleadingly high. Supine hypotension suggests a blood volume deficit greater than 30%, although in elderly or chronic hypertensive patients, an arterial blood pressure within the normal range could represent relative hypotension.

A positive tilt test, defined as an increase in heart rate of at least 20 beats per minute and a decrease in systolic blood pressure of 20 mmHg or more when the subject assumes the upright position, can be falsely negative. Young, healthy subjects can withstand acute loss of 20% of blood volume while exhibiting only postural tachycardia and variable postural hypotension. In contrast, orthostasis may occur in 20% to 30% of elderly patients despite normal blood volume. In volunteers, withdrawal of 500 mL of blood[84] was associated with a greater increase in heart rate on standing than before blood withdrawal, but with no significant difference in the response of blood pressure or cardiac index.

Laboratory markers of hypovolemia or ECV depletion include azotemia, low urinary sodium, metabolic alkalosis (if hypovolemia is mild), and metabolic acidosis (if hypovolemia is severe). In acute hemorrhage, hematocrit decreases slowly as fluid shifts from the interstitial to the intravascular space and more rapidly during administration of fluids. The sensitivities and specificities of measurements of blood and urinary variables to hypovolemia are poor. Conditions other than hypovolemia that increase BUN include high-protein intake, gastrointestinal bleeding, or accelerated catabolism. Severe liver dysfunction is associated with a low BUN. Serum creatinine (SCr), a product of muscle catabolism, may be misleadingly low in elderly adults, females, and debilitated or malnourished patients. In contrast, in muscular or acutely catabolic patients, SCr may exceed the normal range (0.5 to 1.5 mg/dL) because of greater muscle protein metabolism. SCr is a late marker of acute kidney injury and an insensitive indicator of chronic kidney dysfunction, because 40% to 50% of nephrons must become dysfunctional before SCr exceeds the normal range. A ratio of BUN to SCr exceeding normal (10 to 20) suggests dehydration. In prerenal oliguria, enhanced sodium reabsorption should reduce urinary [Na$^+$] to 20 mEq/L or less and enhanced water reabsorption should increase urinary concentration (i.e., urinary osmolality >400 mOsm/kg, urine/plasma creatinine ratio >40:1). Although hypovolemia does not generate metabolic alkalosis, ECV depletion is a potent stimulus for the maintenance of metabolic alkalosis. Severe hypovolemia may result in systemic hypoperfusion and lactic acidosis.

Intraoperative Clinical Assessment

Both surgeons and anesthesiologists tend to underestimate blood loss, based on assessment of blood on surgical gauze pads, pooled on the floor, and accumulated in the surgical field and suction containers. Assessment of the adequacy of intraoperative fluid resuscitation integrates multiple clinical variables, including heart rate, blood pressure, urinary output, arterial oxygenation, and pH. In patients receiving potent inhalational agents, maintenance of blood pressure within the normal range implies adequate intravascular volume. When measured, a central venous pressure of 6 to 12 mmHg suggests adequate blood volume. Tachycardia is an insensitive and nonspecific indicator of hypovolemia that is also altered by anesthetic drugs. In severe hypovolemia, the accuracy of indirect measurements of blood pressure diminishes. Under those circumstances, direct arterial pressure measurements are more accurate than indirect techniques. Arterial cannulation also provides convenient access for obtaining blood samples and assessing pulse pressure variation (PPV) accompanying positive pressure ventilation in the presence of hypovolemia.[85,86]

Urinary output usually declines precipitously during moderate to severe hypovolemia. Therefore, in the absence of glycosuria or diuretic administration, a urinary output of 0.5 to 1.0 mL/kg/hr during anesthesia suggests adequate renal perfusion. Lactic acidosis and acidemia occur only when tissue hypoperfusion becomes severe. Cardiac output can be normal despite severely reduced regional blood flow. Mixed venous hemoglobin desaturation, a specific indicator of poor systemic perfusion, reflects average perfusion in multiple organs and cannot supplant regional monitors such as urinary output.

Assessing the adequacy of intravascular volume and targeting a goal related to intravascular volume are common components of Enhanced Recovery After Surgery (ERAS).[87] Assessing physiologic responses to fluid administration can indicate the adequacy of cardiac preload and facilitate management of hemodynamics. Assessment increasingly depends on dynamic physiologic variables rather than static variables such as central venous pressure. Common physiologic variables that have been developed include PPV, passive leg raising (PLR), the 250-L bolus challenge test,[88] and assessment of corrected flow time (FTc) and descending aortic stroke volume using the esophageal Doppler.[87]

Several clinical studies have shown that goal-directed hemodynamic therapy during high-risk surgery, including cardiac, hip, and major bowel surgery, is associated with improved postoperative outcome.[87,89–91] In general, monitoring techniques are used to estimate whether additional fluid administration will improve cardiac output, hopefully while avoiding excessive fluid administration. If, after PLR or a bolus challenge (250 mL), cardiac output increases over 15%, or a PPV of over 13% decreases below that threshold, an increase in cardiac preload will be associated with an increase in cardiac output. PLR cannot be used in patients with abdominal hypertension or in patients with traumatic brain injury because PLR may increase ICP. PPV requires direct arterial pressure monitoring, full mechanical ventilation with tidal volumes above 8 mL/kg without dyssynchrony, and absence of cardiac arrhythmias.

Esophageal Doppler assessment of blood flow in the descending aorta is another promising technique in measuring adequacy of cardiac preload during high-risk surgical procedures.[92,93] In general, a corrected flow time less than 0.35 second suggests that volume expansion should improve cardiac output, while a corrected flow time greater than 0.4 second suggests that further volume expansion will be ineffective. Using the esophageal Doppler to guide administration of colloid boluses, Venn et al.[94] and Gan et al.[91] have reported shortened length of hospital stay after hip surgery and major surgery, respectively. Of note, Horowitz and Kumar[95] speculated that the infusion of colloid rather than the monitor-driven algorithm was responsible for the improved results. Large multicenter trials are needed in order to ascertain the benefits of the described novel techniques in perioperative outcomes of patients undergoing high-risk surgery.

Oxygen Delivery as a Goal of Management

Because of the assumption that tissue hypoperfusion could be subclinical, the concept arose that maintenance of systemic oxygen delivery (DO_2) above a somewhat arbitrary threshold could limit the frequency and severity of clinically inapparent tissue hypoperfusion. In high-risk surgical patients, a DO_2 index (DO_2I) of at least 600 mL O_2/m^2/min (equivalent to a cardiac index of 3 L/m^2/min, a [Hgb] of 14 g/dL, and 98% oxyhemoglobin saturation) has been associated with improved outcome.[96] However, there is no apparent benefit for patients other than surgical patients and patients undergoing initial resuscitation from septic shock in the emergency department.[97] In addition, outcome may be strongly influenced by the choice of methods to increase DO_2, that is, the choice of fluid administration or various inotropic agents. Lobo et al.[98] randomized 50 high-risk patients, defined as elderly patients with coexistent pathologies who were undergoing major elective surgery, to goal-directed hemodynamic therapy ($DO_2I > 600$ mL O_2/m^2/min) intraoperatively and for the first 24 hours postoperatively either with fluids alone or with fluids plus dobutamine. Postoperative cardiovascular complications occurred significantly more frequently in the group receiving fluids alone (13/25, 52%, vs. 4/25, 16%; relative risk, 3.25; 95% CI, 1.22–8.60; $p < 0.05$); in addition, mortality was greater, but not statistically significantly greater in the group receiving fluids alone. Another specific risk associated with use of fluids to achieve goal-oriented resuscitation is an increased incidence of abdominal compartment syndrome in trauma patients.[99]

Electrolytes

Sodium

Physiologic Role

Sodium, the principal extracellular cation and solute, is essential for generation of action potentials in neurologic and cardiac tissues. Disorders (pathologic increases or decreases) of *total body sodium* are associated with corresponding increases or decreases of ECV and PV. Disorders of sodium *concentration*, that is, hyponatremia and hypernatremia, usually result from relative excesses or deficits, respectively, of water. Regulation of total body sodium and [Na^+] is accomplished primarily by the endocrine and renal systems (Table 16-13). Secretion of aldosterone and ANP control *total body sodium*. ADH, which is secreted in response to increased osmolality or decreased blood pressure, primarily regulates [Na^+]. Therefore, primary

Table 16-13	Regulation of Total Body Electrolyte Mass and Plasma Concentrations
Electrolyte	**Regulated by**
Sodium	Total body sodium regulated by aldosterone, ANP, [Na^+] altered by ADH
Potassium	Total body potassium regulated by aldosterone, intrinsic renal mechanisms; [K^+] regulated by epinephrine, insulin
Calcium	Both total body calcium and [Ca^{++}] regulated by PTH, vitamin D
Phosphate	Both total body phosphate and [HPO_4^-] regulated primarily by renal mechanisms with a minor contribution from PTH
Magnesium	Both total body magnesium and [Mg^{++}] regulated primarily by renal mechanisms with a minor contribution from PTH and vitamin D

ANP, atrial natriuretic peptide; [Na^+], sodium concentration; ADH, antidiuretic hormone; PTH, parathyroid hormone.

hyperaldosteronism is associated with hypervolemia and with hypertension, but not with abnormal [Na$^+$].[100,101]

Hyponatremia

Hyponatremia, defined as [Na$^+$] below 130 mEq/L, is the most common electrolyte disturbance in hospitalized patients.[102] In the majority of hyponatremic patients, total body sodium is normal or increased. The most common clinical scenarios associated with hyponatremia include the postoperative state, acute intracranial disease, malignant disease, medications, and acute pulmonary disease. Recently, hyponatremia, as well as hypokalemia and hypophosphatemia, have been recognized as complications of immunologic treatment of cancers such as hepatocellular carcinoma and melanoma.[103,104] Hyponatremia is associated with increased mortality, both as a direct effect of hyponatremia and because of the association between hyponatremia and severe systemic disease, and with prolonged hospital stay, increased frequency of readmission and increased costs of care.[102]

The signs and symptoms of hyponatremia depend on both the rate and severity of the decrease in plasma [Na$^+$]. Symptoms that can accompany severe hyponatremia ([Na$^+$] < 120 mEq/L) include loss of appetite, nausea, vomiting, cramps, weakness, altered level of consciousness, coma, and seizures.[105]

Acute central nervous system manifestations of hyponatremia result from brain overhydration. Because the blood–brain barrier is poorly permeable to sodium but freely permeable to water, a rapid decrease in plasma [Na$^+$] promptly increases both extracellular and intracellular brain water. Because the brain does not rapidly compensate for changes in osmolality,[106] acute hyponatremia produces more severe symptoms than chronic hyponatremia. The symptoms of chronic hyponatremia probably relate to depletion of brain electrolytes. Once brain volume has compensated for hyponatremia, rapid increases in [Na$^+$] may lead to abrupt brain dehydration.

In hyponatremic patients, serum osmolality may be normal, high, or low (Fig. 16-6). Hyponatremia with a normal or high serum osmolality results from the presence of a nonsodium solute,

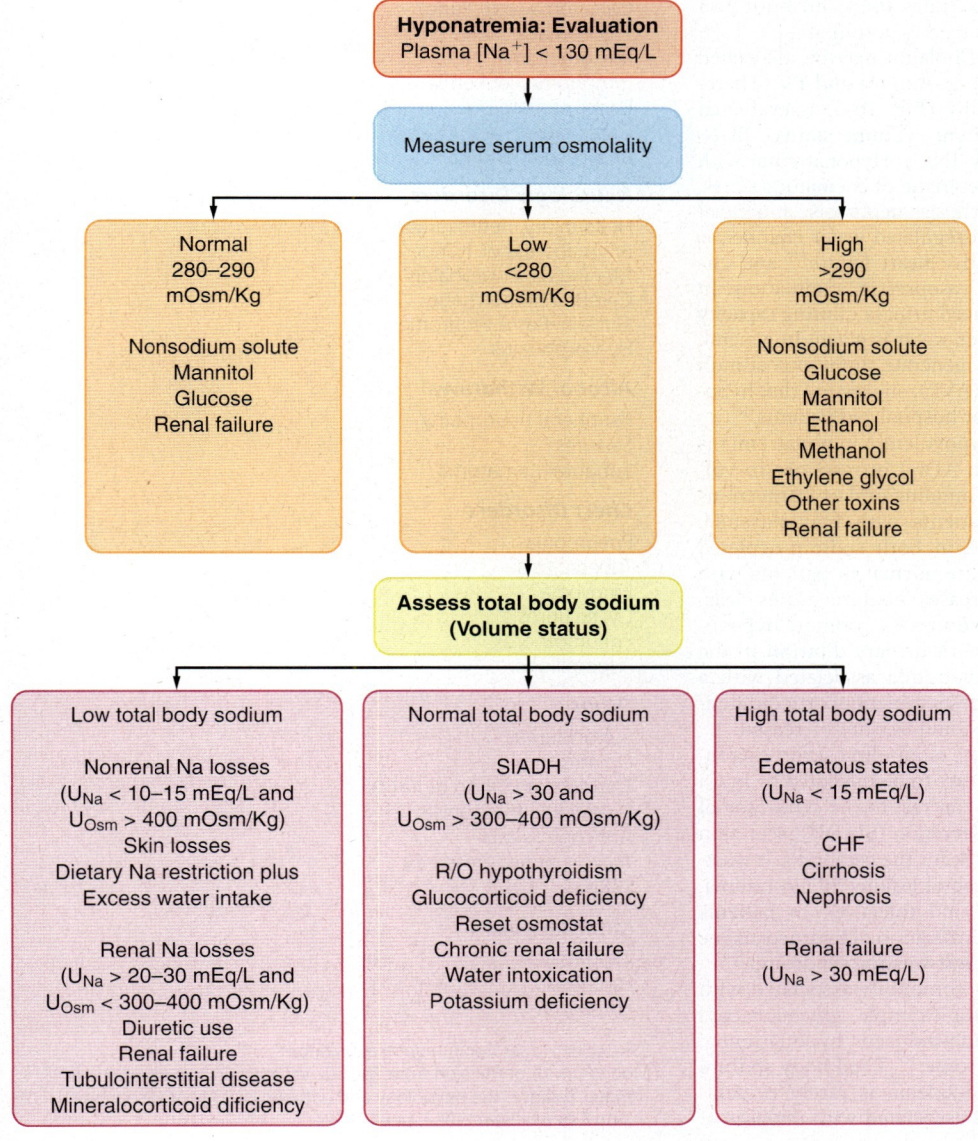

Figure 16-6 Algorithm by which hyponatremia can be evaluated. SIADH, syndrome of inappropriate antidiuretic hormone secretion; R/O, rule out; CHF, congestive heart failure.

such as glucose or mannitol, which holds water within the extracellular space and results in dilutional hyponatremia. The presence of a nonsodium solute may be inferred if measured osmolality exceeds calculated osmolality by over 10 mOsm/kg. For example, plasma [Na$^+$] decreases approximately 2.4 mEq/L for each 100 mg/dL rise in glucose concentration, with perhaps even greater decreases at glucose concentration above 400 mg/dL.[107] In anesthesia practice, a common cause of hyponatremia associated with a normal osmolality is the absorption of large volumes of sodium-free irrigating solutions (containing mannitol, glycerin, or sorbitol as the solute) during transurethral resection of the prostate.[108]

Hyposmolality is more important in generating symptoms than is hyponatremia per se.[108] Neurologic symptoms are minimal if mannitol is the unmeasured osmole because mannitol does not cross the blood–brain barrier and is excreted with water in the urine. In contrast, as glycine or sorbitol is metabolized, hyposmolality will gradually develop, and cerebral edema may appear as a late complication. Hyponatremia with a normal or elevated serum osmolality also may accompany renal insufficiency. BUN, included in the calculation of total osmolality, distributes throughout both ECV and ICV. Calculation of *effective* osmolality (2[Na$^+$] + glucose/18) excludes the contribution of urea to osmolality and demonstrates true hypotonicity.

Hyponatremia with low serum osmolality may be associated with a high, low, or normal total body sodium and PV. Therefore, hyponatremia with hyposmolality (Fig. 16-6) is evaluated by assessing total body sodium content (volume status), BUN, SCr, urinary osmolality, and urinary [Na$^+$]. Hyponatremia with increased total body sodium is characteristic of edematous states, that is, congestive heart failure, cirrhosis, nephrosis, and renal failure. Aquaporin 2, the vasopressin-regulated water channel, is upregulated in experimental congestive heart failure[109] and cirrhosis[110] and decreased by chronic vasopressin stimulation. In patients with renal insufficiency, reduced urinary diluting capacity can lead to hyponatremia if excess free water is given. In general, diseases that prompt hospitalization generate numerous stimuli for secretion of arginine vasopressin (AVP), suggesting that hyponatremic fluids are rarely indicated for hospitalized patients.[37]

The underlying mechanism of hypovolemic hyponatremia is secretion of AVP (synonymous with ADH) in response to volume contraction in association with ongoing oral or intravenous intake of hypotonic fluid.[111] In patients with hyponatremia, plasma copeptin levels are elevated in both sodium-depleted and sodium-expanded patients but are normal in patients with SIADH.[112,113] Angiotensin II also decreases renal free water clearance. Thiazide diuretics, unlike loop diuretics, promote hypovolemic hyponatremia by interfering with urinary dilution in the distal tubule.[111] Hypovolemic hyponatremia associated with a urinary [Na$^+$] above 20 mmol/L suggests mineralocorticoid deficiency, especially if serum [K$^+$], BUN, and SCr are increased.[111]

The cerebral salt-wasting syndrome is an often severe, symptomatic salt-losing diathesis that appears to be mediated by brain natriuretic peptide and in which, in contrast to the syndrome of inappropriate antidiuretic hormone secretion (SIADH), secretion of AVP is *appropriate*[111]; patients at risk for the cerebral salt-wasting syndrome include those with cerebral lesions due to trauma, subarachnoid hemorrhage, tumors, and infection. In patients after subarachnoid hemorrhage, administration of hydrocortisone 1,200 mg/day prevented the cerebral salt-wasting syndrome.[114]

Euvolemic hyponatremia is most commonly associated with nonosmotic vasopressin secretion, for example, glucocorticoid deficiency, hypothyroidism, thiazide-induced hyponatremia, SIADH, and the reset osmostat syndrome.[111] Total body sodium and ECV are relatively normal and edema is rarely evident. SIADH may be idiopathic but also is associated with diseases of the central nervous system and with pulmonary disease (Table 16-14). Euvolemic hyponatremia is usually associated with exogenous AVP administration, pharmacologic potentiation of AVP action, drugs that mimic the action of AVP in the renal tubules, or excessive ectopic AVP secretion. Tissues from some small cell lung cancers, duodenal cancers, and pancreatic cancers increase AVP production in response to osmotic stimulation.[111]

At least 4% of postoperative patients experience plasma [Na$^+$] below 130 mEq/L. Although neurologic manifestations usually do not accompany mild postoperative hyponatremia, signs of hypervolemia are occasionally present. Much less frequently, postoperative hyponatremia is accompanied by mental status changes, seizures, and transtentorial herniation,[115] attributable in part to intravenous administration of hypotonic fluids, secretion

Table 16-14 Common Associations with the Syndrome of Inappropriate Antidiuretic Hormone Secretion

Neoplastic Disease
Carcinoma (e.g., lung)
Thymoma
Mesothelioma
Lymphoma, leukemia
Ewing sarcoma
Carcinoid
Bronchial adenoma

Neurologic Disorders
Head injury, neurosurgery
Brain abscess or tumor
Meningitis, encephalitis
Cerebral hemorrhage
Guillain–Barré syndrome
Hydrocephalus

Alcohol Withdrawal
Peripheral neuropathy
Seizures
Subdural hematoma

Chest Disorders
Pneumonia
Tuberculosis
Empyema
Cystic fibrosis
Pneumothorax
Aspergillosis

Drugs
Sulfonylureas
Opiates
Thiazides and loop diuretics
Dopamine antagonists
Anticonvulsants
Tricyclic antidepressants
SSRIs

Miscellaneous
Idiopathic
Psychosis
Porphyria

SSRI, selective serotonin reuptake inhibitor.
Modified with permission from Ball SG. Vasopressin and disorders of water balance: the physiology and pathophysiology of vasopressin. *Ann Clin Biochem.* 2007;44:417–431.

of AVP, and other factors, including drugs and altered renal function that influence perioperative water balance. Women appear to be more vulnerable than men, and premenopausal women appear to be more vulnerable than postmenopausal women to brain damage secondary to postoperative hyponatremia.[105] If AVP is persistently increased, postoperative hyponatremia can develop even with infusion of isotonic fluids.

If both [Na^+] and measured osmolality are below the normal range, hyponatremia is further evaluated by first assessing volume status using physical findings and laboratory data. In hypovolemic patients or edematous patients, the ratio of BUN to SCr should be above 20:1. Urinary [Na^+] is generally below 15 mEq/L in edematous states and volume depletion and above 20 mEq/L in hyponatremia secondary to renal salt wasting or renal failure with water retention.

The criteria for the diagnosis of SIADH are listed in Table 16-15. Urinary [Na^+] should be above 20 mEq/L unless fluids have been restricted. Arieff[116] has argued that the diagnosis of SIADH may be inaccurately applied to functionally hypovolemic postoperative patients, in whom, by definition, AVP secretion would be "appropriate." In addition, the definition of SIADH is changing due to identification of distinctive molecular characteristics that differentiate among patients with SIADH.[117,118]

Treatment of hyponatremia associated with a normal or high serum osmolality requires reduction of the elevated concentrations of the responsible solute, for example, urea or mannitol. Uremic patients are treated by free water restriction or dialysis. Treatment of edematous (hypervolemic) patients necessitates restriction of both sodium and water, usually accompanied by efforts to improve cardiac output and renal perfusion and to use diuretics to inhibit sodium reabsorption (Fig. 16-7). In hypovolemic, hyponatremic patients, blood volume must be restored, usually by infusion of 0.9% saline, and excessive sodium losses must be curtailed. Correction of hypovolemia usually results in removal of the stimulus for AVP release, accompanied by a rapid water diuresis.

The cornerstone of SIADH management is free water restriction and elimination of precipitating causes. Water restriction, sufficient to decrease TBW by 0.5 to 1 L/day, decreases ECV even if excessive AVP secretion continues. The resultant reduction in GFR enhances proximal tubular reabsorption of salt and water, thereby decreasing free water generation, and stimulates aldosterone secretion. As long as free water losses (i.e., renal, skin, gastrointestinal) exceed free water intake, plasma [Na^+] will increase. During treatment of hyponatremia, increases in plasma [Na^+] are determined both by the composition of the infused fluid and by the rate of renal free water excretion. Free water excretion can be increased by administering furosemide.

Table 16-15 Diagnostic Criteria for Syndrome of Inappropriate Antidiuretic Hormone Secretion

Hyponatremia with appropriately low plasma osmolality
Urinary osmolality greater than plasma osmolality
Renal sodium excretion >20 mmol/L
Absence of hypotension, hypovolemia, and edematous states
Normal renal and adrenal functions
Absence of drugs that directly influence renal water and sodium handling

Modified from Ball SG. Vasopressin and disorders of water balance: the physiology and pathophysiology of vasopressin. *Ann Clin Biochem*. 2007;44:417–431.

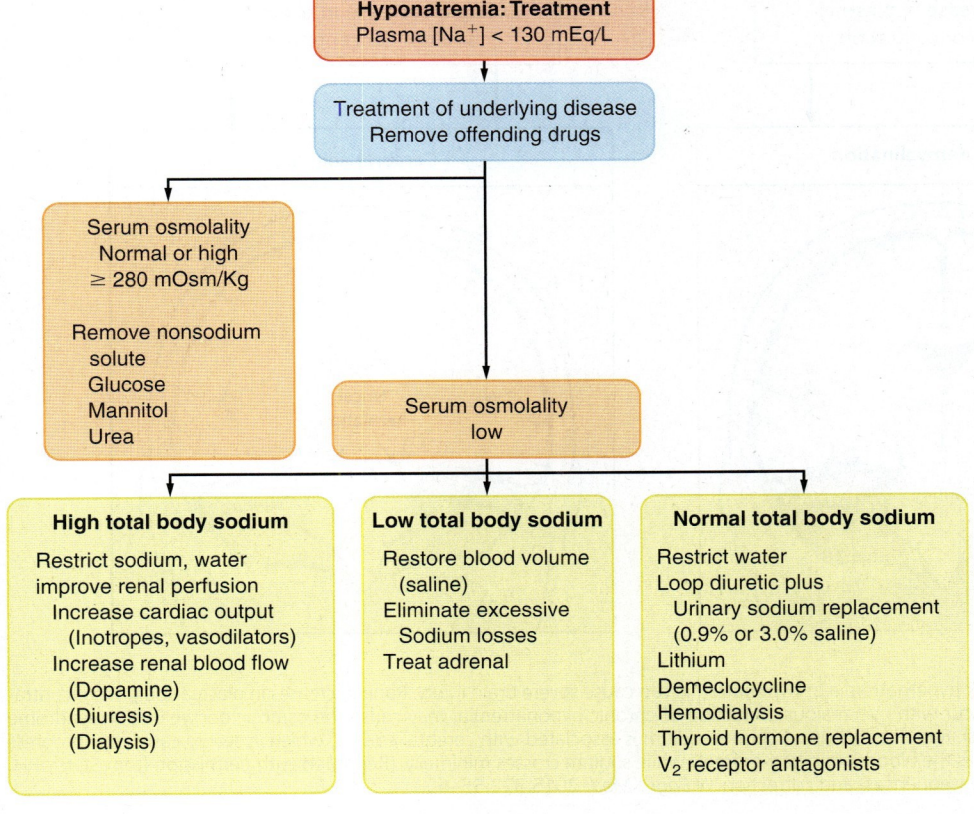

Figure 16-7 Hyponatremia is treated according to the etiology of the disturbance, the level of serum osmolality, and a clinical estimation of total body sodium.

Vasopressin receptor blocking agents inhibit the action of AVP on the renal collecting ducts.[119–122] These agents have proven to be safe and efficacious in hyponatremic patients, appearing to have particular value in patients with hypervolemic hyponatremia secondary to congestive heart failure.[119] Conivaptan, which inhibits both V_{1a} and V_2 receptors, has been approved for the treatment of normovolemic and hypervolemic, hyponatremic patients.[121] However, potential decreases in blood pressure associated with V_{1a} receptor blockade necessitate caution in patients with borderline low blood pressure.[122] Tolvaptan, a selective V_2 receptor antagonist, also has proven effective in clinical trials.[123] Vaptans are rapidly becoming a mainstay of therapy for normovolemic and hypervolemic hypernatremia.[122,124]

Neurologic symptoms or profound hyponatremia ([Na+] < 115 to 120 mEq/L) require more aggressive therapy. Hypertonic (3%) saline is most clearly indicated in patients who have seizures or who acutely develop symptoms of water intoxication secondary to intravenous fluid administration. In such patients, acute hyponatremia is associated with severe brain swelling that can lead to herniation.[125] In patients with severe neurologic symptoms, 3% saline may be administered at a rate of 1 to 2 mL/kg/hr, to increase plasma [Na+] by 1 to 2 mEq/L/hr; however, this treatment should not continue for more than a few hours with the goal being to increase [Na+] by no more than 4 to 8 mEq/L/day.[125] An increase in [Na+] of 4 mEq/L is usually sufficient to markedly reduce acute symptoms.[118] Three percent saline may only transiently increase plasma [Na+] because ECV expansion results in increased urinary sodium excretion. Intravenous furosemide, combined with quantitative replacement of urinary sodium losses with 0.9% or 3% saline, can rapidly increase plasma [Na+], in part by increasing free water clearance.

The rate of treatment of hyponatremia continues to generate controversy, extending from "too fast, too soon" to "too slow, too late." Although delayed correction may result in neurologic injury, inappropriately rapid correction may result in abrupt brain dehydration (Fig. 16-8) or permanent neurologic sequelae (i.e., osmotic demyelination syndrome),[126] cerebral hemorrhage, or congestive heart failure. The symptoms of the osmotic demyelination syndrome vary from mild (transient behavioral disturbances or seizures) to severe (including pseudobulbar palsy and quadriparesis). The principal determinants of neurologic injury appear to be the severity and chronicity of hyponatremia and the rate of correction. The osmotic demyelination syndrome is more likely when hyponatremia has persisted for longer than 48 hours. Most patients in whom the osmotic demyelination syndrome is fatal have undergone correction of plasma [Na+] of more than 20 mEq/L/day. Other risk factors for the development of osmotic demyelination syndrome include alcoholism, poor nutritional status, liver disease, burns, and hypokalemia.[127]

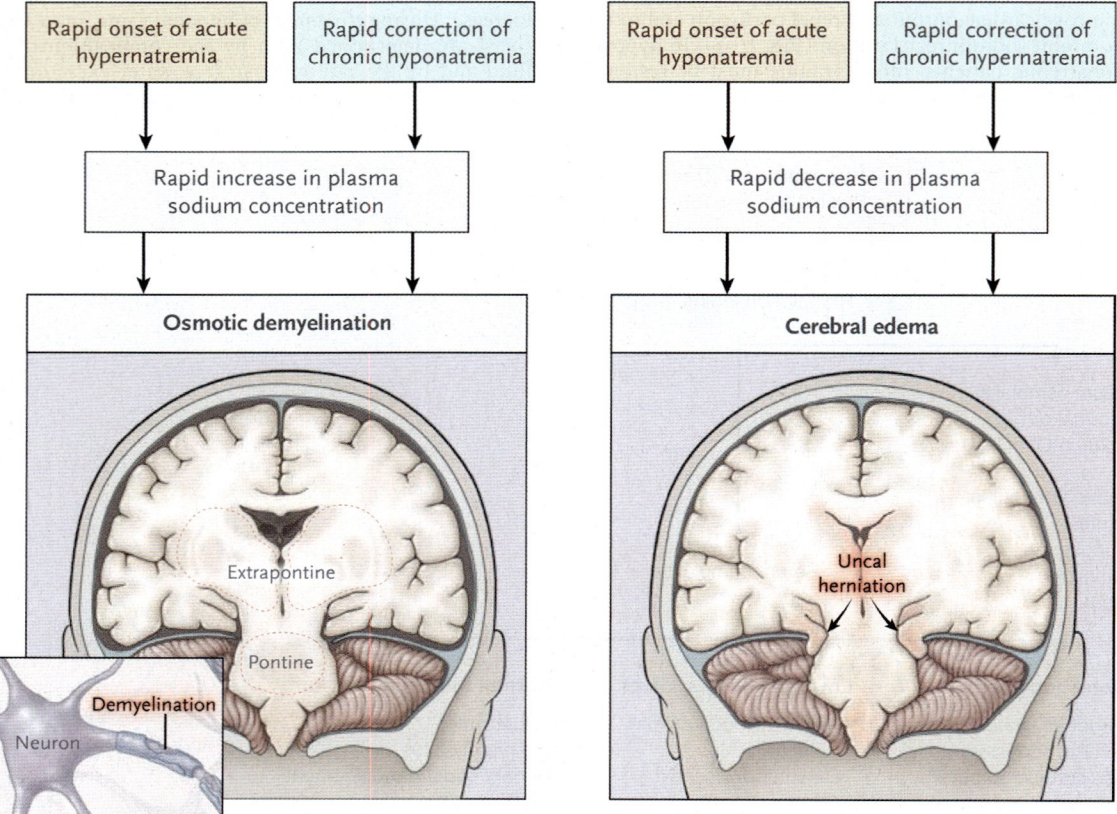

Figure 16-8 Rapid correction of either hypernatremia or hyponatremia can cause severe brain injury. Rapid increases in plasma sodium concentration, especially when those increases occur with overzealous correction of chronic hyponatremia, may cause the osmotic demyelination syndrome (also termed central pontine myelinolysis). Rapid reduction of plasma sodium is associated with cerebral edema, which in severe cases may progress to brain herniation, because water crosses the blood–brain barrier freely while sodium crosses minimally. (Reprinted with permission from Sterns RH. Disorders of plasma sodium—causes, consequences, and correction. *N Engl J Med.* 2015;372:55–65.)

The clinician faces formidable difficulties in predicting the rate at which plasma [Na⁺] will increase because increases in plasma [Na⁺] are determined both by the composition of the infused fluid and by the rate of renal free water excretion. The expected change in plasma [Na⁺] resulting from 1 L of selected infusate can be estimated using the following equation[128]:

$$\Delta [Na^+]_s = \frac{[Na^+]_{inf} - [Na^+]_s}{TBW + 1} \quad (16\text{-}12)$$

where $\Delta[Na^+]_s$ = the change in the patient's serum [Na⁺], $[Na^+]_{inf}$ = the [Na⁺] of the infusate, $[Na^+]_s$ = serum [Na⁺], TBW = estimated total body water in liters, and 1 is a factor added to take into account the volume of infusate.

Treatment should be interrupted or slowed when symptoms improve. Frequent determinations of [Na⁺] are important to prevent correction at a rate above 1 to 2 mEq/L in any 1 hour and above 8 mEq/L in 24 hours.[127] Initially, plasma [Na⁺] may be increased by 1 to 2 mEq/L/hr; however, the rate of correction should then be slowed to avoid excessively rapid correction. Hypernatremia should be avoided. Once plasma [Na⁺] exceeds 120 to 125 mEq/L, water restriction alone is usually sufficient to normalize [Na⁺]. As acute hyponatremia is corrected, central nervous system signs and symptoms usually improve within 24 hours, although 96 hours may be necessary for maximal recovery.

For patients who require long-term pharmacologic therapy of hyponatremia, vasopressin receptor antagonists are the current most promising therapies.[129] Hemodialysis is occasionally necessary in severely hyponatremic patients who cannot be adequately managed with drugs or hypertonic saline. Once hyponatremia has improved, careful fluid restriction is necessary to avoid recurrence of hyponatremia.

Hypernatremia

Hypernatremia ([Na⁺] > 150 mEq/L) indicates an absolute or relative water deficit.[126] Normally, slight increases in tonicity or [Na⁺] stimulate thirst and AVP secretion. Therefore, severe, persistent hypernatremia occurs only in patients who cannot respond to thirst by voluntary ingestion of fluid, that is, obtunded patients, anesthetized patients, and infants.

Hypernatremia produces neurologic symptoms (including stupor, coma, and seizures), hypovolemia, renal insufficiency (occasionally progressing to renal failure), and decreased urinary concentrating ability. Because hypernatremia frequently results from diabetes insipidus (DI) or osmotically induced losses of sodium and water, many patients are hypovolemic or bear the stigmata of renal disease. Postoperative neurosurgical patients who have undergone pituitary surgery are at particular risk of developing transient or prolonged DI. Polyuria may be present for only a few days within the first week of surgery, may be permanent, or may demonstrate a triphasic sequence: early DI, return of urinary concentrating ability, then recurrent DI.[130]

The clinical consequences of hypernatremia are most serious at the extremes of age and when hypernatremia develops abruptly. Geriatric patients are at increased risk of hypernatremia because of decreased renal concentrating ability and decreased thirst. Brain shrinkage secondary to rapidly developing hypernatremia may damage delicate cerebral vessels, leading to subdural hematoma, subcortical parenchymal hemorrhage, subarachnoid hemorrhage, and venous thrombosis. Polyuria may cause bladder distention, hydronephrosis, and permanent renal damage. Although the mortality of patients with hypernatremia is 40% to 55%, it is unclear whether hypernatremia contributes to mortality or is simply a marker of severe associated disease.

Surprisingly, if plasma [Na⁺] is initially normal, moderate acute increases in plasma [Na⁺] do not appear to precipitate central pontine myelinolysis. However, larger accidental increases in plasma [Na⁺] have produced severe consequences in children. In experimental animals, acute severe hypernatremia (acute increase from 146 mEq/L to 170 mEq/L) caused neuronal damage at 24 hours, suggestive of early central pontine myelinolysis.[131]

By definition, hypernatremia indicates an absolute or relative water deficit and is always associated with hypertonicity. Hypernatremia can be generated by hypotonic fluid loss, as in burns, gastrointestinal losses, diuretic therapy, osmotic diuresis, renal disease, mineralocorticoid excess or deficiency, and iatrogenic causes or can be generated by isolated water loss, as in central or nephrogenic DI. The acquired form of nephrogenic DI is more common and usually less severe than the congenital form. As chronic renal failure advances, most patients have defective concentrating ability, resulting in resistance to AVP associated with hypotonic urine. Because hypovolemia accompanies most pathologic water loss, signs of hypoperfusion also may be present. In many patients, before the development of hypernatremia, an increased volume of hypotonic urine suggests an abnormality in water balance. Although uncommon as a cause of hypernatremia, isolated sodium gain occasionally occurs in patients who receive large quantities of sodium, such as treatment of metabolic acidosis with 8.4% sodium bicarbonate, in which [Na⁺] is approximately 1,000 mEq/L, or perioperative or prehospital treatment with hypertonic saline resuscitation solutions.

Hypernatremic patients can be separated into three groups—hypovolemic, normovolemic, and hypervolemic—based on clinical assessment of ECV (Fig. 16-9). Note that plasma [Na⁺] does not reflect total body sodium, which must be estimated separately based on signs of the adequacy of ECV. Polyuric, hypernatremic patients may be undergoing solute diuresis or may have DI. Measurement of urinary sodium and osmolality can help to differentiate the various causes. Hypotonic urine (osmolality < 150 mOsm/kg) in the setting of hypertonicity and polyuria is diagnostic of DI.

Treatment of hypernatremia produced by water loss requires repletion of water as well of associated deficits in total body sodium and other electrolytes (Table 16-16). Common errors in treating hypernatremia include excessively rapid correction as well as failing to appreciate the magnitude of the water deficit and failing to account for ongoing maintenance requirements and continued fluid losses in planning therapy.[132–134]

Table 16-16 Hypernatremia: Acute Treatment

Sodium Depletion (Hypovolemia)
Hypovolemia correction (0.9% saline)
Hypernatremia correction (hypotonic fluids)

Sodium Overload (Hypervolemia)
Enhance sodium removal (loop diuretics, dialysis)
Replace water deficit (hypotonic fluids)

Normal Total Body Sodium (Euvolemia)
Replace water deficit (hypotonic fluids)
Control diabetes insipidus
   Central diabetes insipidus:
     DDAVP, 10–20 μg intranasally; 2–4 μg SC
     Aqueous vasopressin, 5 U q2–4h IM or SC
   Nephrogenic diabetes insipidus:
     Restrict sodium, water intake
     Thiazide diuretics

DDAVP, desmopressin.

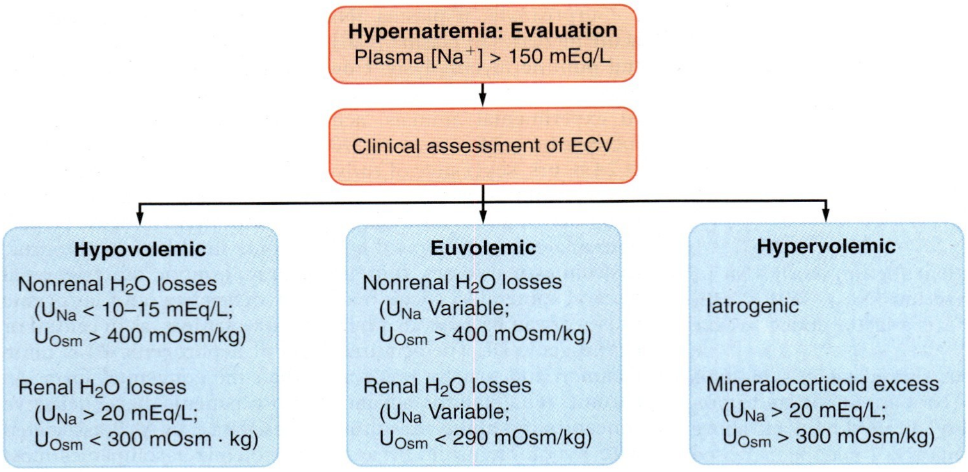

Hypernatremia: Evaluation
Plasma [Na⁺] > 150 mEq/L

Clinical assessment of ECV

Hypovolemic
Nonrenal H₂O losses
(U_{Na} < 10–15 mEq/L;
U_{Osm} > 400 mOsm/kg)

Renal H₂O losses
(U_{Na} > 20 mEq/L;
U_{Osm} < 300 mOsm · kg)

Euvolemic
Nonrenal H₂O losses
(U_{Na} Variable;
U_{Osm} > 400 mOsm/kg)

Renal H₂O losses
(U_{Na} Variable;
U_{Osm} < 290 mOsm/kg)

Hypervolemic
Iatrogenic

Mineralocorticoid excess
(U_{Na} > 20 mEq/L;
U_{Osm} > 300 mOsm/kg)

Figure 16-9 Severe hypernatremia is evaluated by first separating patients into hypovolemic, euvolemic, and hypervolemic groups based on assessment of extracellular volume (ECV). Next, potential etiologic factors are diagnostically assessed. [Na⁺], serum sodium concentration; U_{Na}, urinary sodium concentration; U_{Osm}, urinary osmolality.

The first step in treating hypernatremia is to estimate the TBW deficit, which can be accomplished by inserting the measured plasma [Na⁺] into the equation:

$$\text{TBW deficit} = 0.6 \times \text{body weight (kg)} \times [([Na^+] - 140)/140] \quad (16\text{-}13)$$

where 140 is the middle of the normal range for [Na⁺]. Adrogué and Madias[132] proposed a useful equation (Eq. 16-12) to predict the expected change in serum [Na⁺] produced by infusion of 1 L of infusate.

Hypernatremia must be corrected slowly because of the risk of neurologic sequelae such as seizures or cerebral edema (Fig. 16-8). At the cellular level, restoration of cell volume occurs quickly after tonicity is altered; as a consequence, acute treatment of hypertonicity may result in overshooting the original, normotonic cell volume. The water deficit should be replaced over 24 to 48 hours, and the plasma [Na⁺] should not be reduced by more than 1 to 2 mEq/L/hr for the first few hours and, if the hypernatremia has been present for more than 2 days, no more than 10 mEq/L/day.[126,132] Reversible underlying causes should be treated. Hypovolemia should be corrected promptly with 0.9% saline. Although the [Na⁺] of 0.9% saline is 154 mEq/L, the solution is effective in treating volume deficits and will reduce [Na⁺] that exceeds 154 mEq/L in hypovolemic, hypernatremic patients. Once hypovolemia is corrected, water can be replaced orally or with intravenous hypotonic fluids, depending on the ability of the patient to tolerate oral hydration. In the occasional sodium-overloaded patient, sodium excretion can be accelerated using loop diuretics or dialysis. In acute, severe hypernatremia, treatment with venovenous hemofiltration was associated with lower mortality than was calculation of water deficit and infusion of hypotonic fluids.[134,135]

The management of hypernatremia secondary to DI varies according to whether the cause is central or nephrogenic (Table 16-16). The two most suitable agents for correcting central DI (an AVP deficiency syndrome) are desmopressin (DDAVP) and aqueous vasopressin. DDAVP, given subcutaneously in a dose of 1 to 4 μg or intranasally in a dose of 5 to 20 μg every 12 to 24 hours, is effective in most patients. DDAVP is preferred because it has a longer duration of action than AVP and lacks vasoconstrictor effects.[135] Incomplete AVP deficits (partial DI) often are effectively managed with pharmacologic agents that stimulate AVP release or enhance the renal response to AVP.

Chlorpropamide, which potentiates the renal effects of vasopressin, and carbamazepine, which enhances vasopressin secretion, have been used to treat partial central DI, but are associated with clinically important side effects. In nephrogenic DI, salt and water restriction or thiazide diuretics induce contraction of ECV, thereby enhancing fluid reabsorption in the proximal tubules. If less filtrate passes through into the collecting ducts, less water will be excreted. However, thiazide diuretics exert limited therapeutic effects.[134]

Potassium

Physiologic Role

Potassium plays an important role in cell membrane physiology, especially in maintaining resting membrane potentials and in generating action potentials in the central nervous system and heart. Potassium is actively transported into cells by a Na/K adenosine triphosphatase (ATPase) pump, which maintains an intracellular [K⁺] that is at least 30-fold greater than extracellular [K⁺]. Intracellular potassium concentration ([K⁺]) is normally 150 mEq/L, while the extracellular concentration is only 3.5 to 5 mEq/L. Serum [K⁺] measures about 0.5 mEq/L higher than plasma [K⁺] because of cell lysis during clotting. Total body potassium in a 70-kg adult is approximately 4,256 mEq, of which 4,200 mEq is intracellular; of the 56 mEq in the ECV, only 12 mEq is located in the PV. The ratio of intracellular to extracellular potassium contributes to the resting potential difference across cell membranes and therefore to the integrity of cardiac and neuromuscular transmissions. The primary mechanism that maintains potassium inside cells is the negative voltage created by the transport of three sodium ions out of the cell for every two potassium ions transported in. Both insulin and β-agonists promote potassium entry into cells.[136,137] Metabolic and respiratory acidoses tend to shift potassium out of cells, while metabolic and respiratory alkaloses favor movement into cells.

Usual potassium intake varies between 50 and 150 mEq/day. Freely filtered at the glomerulus, most potassium excretion is urinary, with some fecal elimination. Most filtered potassium is reabsorbed; usually, excretion is approximately equal to daily intake. As long as GFR is above 8 mL/min, dietary potassium intake, unless greater than normal, can be excreted. Assuming a plasma [K⁺] of 4 mEq/L and a normal GFR of 180 L/day, 720 mEq of potassium are filtered daily, of which 85% to 90% is reabsorbed in the proximal convoluted tubule and loop of Henle. The remaining 10% to 15% reaches the distal convoluted tubule, which is the major site at which potassium excretion is regulated. Excretion of potassium ions is a function of open potassium channels and the electrical driving force in the cortical collecting duct.

The two most important regulators of potassium excretion are plasma [K^+] and aldosterone. Potassium secretion into the distal convoluted tubules and cortical collecting ducts is increased by hyperkalemia, aldosterone, alkalemia, increased delivery of Na^+ to the distal tubule and collecting duct, high urinary flow rates, and the presence in luminal fluid of nonreabsorbable anions such as carbenicillin, phosphates, and sulfates. As sodium reabsorption increases, the electrical driving force opposing reabsorption of potassium is increased. Aldosterone increases sodium reabsorption by inducing a more open configuration of the epithelial sodium channel; potassium-sparing diuretics (amiloride and triamterene) and trimethoprim block the epithelial sodium channel, thereby increasing potassium reabsorption. Magnesium depletion contributes to renal potassium wasting.

Hypokalemia

Uncommon among healthy persons, hypokalemia ([K^+] < 3.5 mEq/L) is a frequent complication of treatment with diuretic drugs and occasionally complicates other diseases and treatment regimens (Table 16-17). Plasma [K^+] poorly reflects total body potassium; hypokalemia may occur with normal, low, or high total body potassium. However, as a general rule, a chronic decrement of 1 mEq/L in the plasma [K^+] corresponds to a total body deficit of approximately 200 to 300 mEq. In uncomplicated hypokalemia, the total body potassium deficit exceeds 300 mEq if plasma [K^+] is below 3 mEq/L and 700 mEq if plasma [K^+] is below 2 mEq/L.

The symptoms and signs of hypokalemia primarily relate to neuromuscular and cardiovascular functions. Hypokalemia causes muscle weakness and, when severe, may even cause paralysis. With chronic potassium loss, the ratio of intracellular to extracellular [K^+] remains relatively stable; in contrast, acute redistribution of potassium from the extracellular to the intracellular space substantially changes resting membrane potentials. Cardiac rhythm disturbances are among the most dangerous complications of potassium deficiency. Acute hypokalemia causes hyperpolarization of the cardiac cell and may lead to ventricular escape activity, re-entrant phenomena, ectopic tachycardias, and delayed conduction. In patients treated with digoxin, hypokalemia increases toxicity by increasing myocardial digoxin binding and pharmacologic effectiveness. Hypokalemia contributes to systemic hypertension, especially when combined with a high-sodium diet. In diabetic patients, hypokalemia impairs insulin secretion and end-organ sensitivity to insulin. Although no clear threshold has been defined for a level of hypokalemia below which safe conduct of anesthesia is compromised, [K^+] below 3.5 mEq/L in cardiac surgical patients has been associated with an increased incidence of perioperative dysrhythmias, especially atrial fibrillation/flutter.[138]

Potassium depletion also induces defects in renal concentrating ability, resulting in polyuria and a reduction in GFR. Potassium replacement improves GFR, although the concentrating deficit may not improve for several months after treatment. If hypokalemia is sufficiently prolonged, chronic renal interstitial damage may occur. In experimental animals, hypokalemia was associated with intrarenal vasoconstriction and a pattern of renal injury similar to that produced by ischemia.[139]

Hypokalemia may result from chronic depletion of total body potassium or from acute redistribution of potassium from the ECV to the ICV. Redistribution of potassium into cells occurs when the activity of the sodium–potassium ATPase pump is acutely increased by extracellular hyperkalemia or increased intracellular concentrations of sodium, as well as by insulin, carbohydrate loading (which stimulates release of endogenous insulin), $β_2$-agonists, and aldosterone. Both metabolic and respiratory alkaloses lead to decreases in plasma [K^+].

Causes of chronic hypokalemia include those etiologies associated with renal potassium conservation (extrarenal potassium losses; low urinary [K^+]) and those with renal potassium wasting (Fig. 16-10).[140] A low urinary [K^+] suggests inadequate dietary intake or extrarenal depletion (in the absence of recent diuretic use). Diuretic-induced urinary potassium losses are frequently associated with hypokalemia, secondary to increased aldosterone secretion, alkalemia, and increased renal tubular flow. Aldosterone does not cause renal potassium wasting unless sodium ions are present; that is, aldosterone primarily controls sodium reabsorption, not potassium excretion. Renal tubular damage due to nephrotoxins such as aminoglycosides or amphotericin B may also cause renal potassium wasting.

Initial evaluation of hypokalemia includes a medical history (e.g., diarrhea, vomiting, diuretic, or laxative use), physical examination (e.g., hypertension, cushingoid features, edema), measurement of serum electrolytes (e.g., magnesium), arterial pH assessment, and evaluation of the electrocardiogram (ECG). Measurement of 24-hour urinary excretion of sodium and potassium may distinguish extrarenal from renal causes. Magnesium deficiency, associated with aminoglycoside and cisplatin therapy, can generate hypokalemia that is resistant to potassium replacement therapy. Plasma renin and aldosterone levels

Table 16-17 Causes of Renal Potassium Loss

Drugs
  Diuretics
    Thiazide diuretics
    Loop diuretics
    Osmotic diuretics
  Antibiotics
    Penicillin and penicillin analogs
    Amphotericin B
    Aminoglycosides

Hormones
  Aldosterone
  Glucocorticoids

Bicarbonaturia
  Distal renal tubular acidosis
  Treatment of proximal renal tubular acidosis
  Correction phase of metabolic alkalosis

Magnesium Deficiency

Other Less Common Causes
  Cisplatin
  Carbonic anhydrase inhibitors
  Leukemia
  Diuretic phase of acute tubular necrosis

Intrinsic Renal Transport Defects
  Bartter syndrome
  Gitelman syndrome

Modified from Weiner ID, Wingo CS. Hypokalemia: consequences, causes, and correction. *J Am Soc Nephrol*. 1997;8:1179–1188.

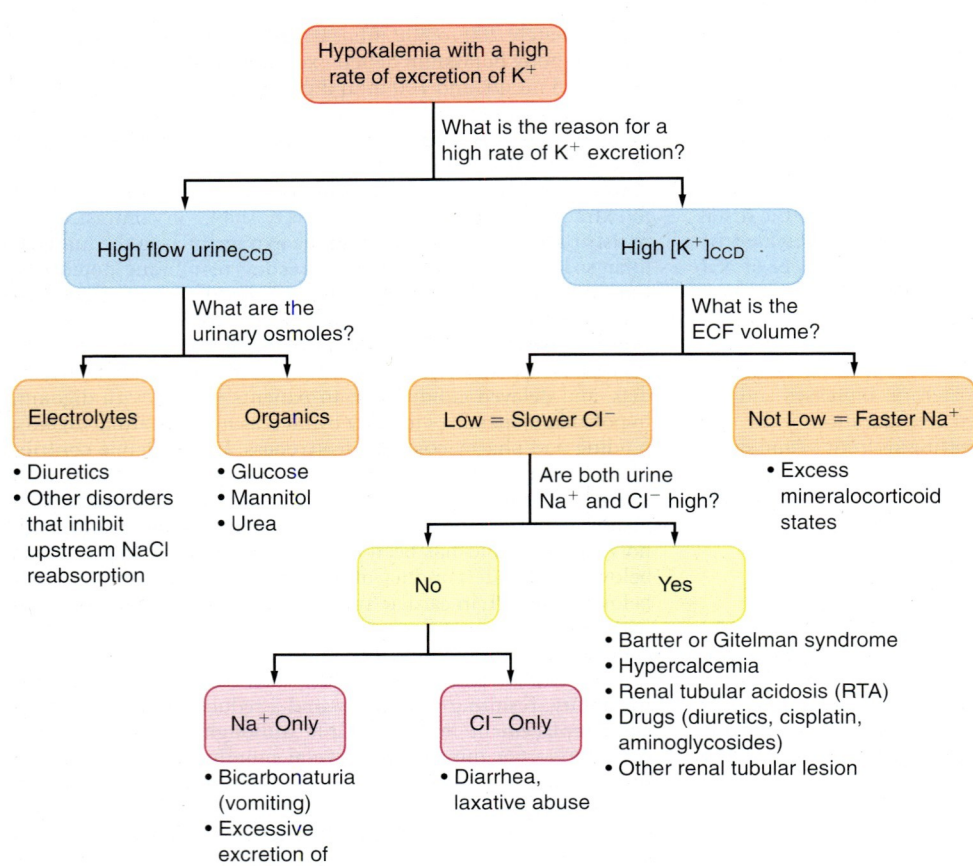

Figure 16-10 A diagnostic flow chart for hypokalemia with a high rate of K^+ excretion. ECF, extracellular fluid; CCD, cortical collecting duct. (Adapted from Lin SH, Halperin ML. Hypokalemia: a practical approach to diagnosis and its genetic basis. *Curr Med Chem.* 2007;14:1551–1565.)

may be helpful in the differential diagnosis of hypokalemia of unclear origin, especially if primary hyperaldosteronism is suspected.[141] Characteristic electrocardiographic changes associated with hypokalemia include flat or inverted T waves, prominent U waves, and ST segment depression.

The treatment of hypokalemia consists of potassium repletion, correction of alkalemia, and removal of offending drugs (Table 16-18). Hypokalemia secondary only to acute redistribution (e.g., secondary to acute alkalemia) may not require treatment. There is no urgent need for potassium replacement therapy in mild-to-moderate hypokalemia (3 to 3.5 mEq/L) in patients who have no symptoms or signs. If total body potassium is decreased, oral potassium supplementation is preferable to intravenous replacement. Potassium is usually replaced as the chloride salt because coexisting chloride deficiency may limit the ability of the kidney to conserve potassium.

Intravenous potassium repletion, when necessary, must be performed cautiously (i.e., usually at a rate of 10 to 20 mEq/hr) of the risk of excessively rapid increases in plasma $[K^+]$. The plasma $[K^+]$ and the ECG must be monitored during rapid repletion (10 to 20 mEq/hr) to avoid hyperkalemic complications. Particular care should be taken in patients who have concurrent acidemia, type IV renal tubular acidosis, or diabetes mellitus, or in those patients receiving nonsteroidal anti-inflammatory agents, ACE inhibitors, or β_2-blockers, all of which delay movement of extracellular potassium into cells. β_1-Blockers do not delay movement of extracellular potassium into cells or predispose patients to hyperkalemia.[142]

However, in patients with life-threatening dysrhythmias secondary to hypokalemia, serum $[K^+]$ must be rapidly increased. Assuming that PV in a 70-kg adult is 3 L, administration of 6 mEq/L of potassium in 1 minute will acutely increase plasma $[K^+]$ by no more than 2 mEq/L; subsequent redistribution into interstitial fluid and ICV will rapidly decrease plasma $[K^+]$.

Hypokalemia associated with hyperaldosteronemia (e.g., primary aldosteronism, Cushing syndrome) usually responds favorably to reduced sodium intake and increased potassium intake. Hypomagnesemia, if present, aggravates the effects of hypokalemia, impairs potassium conservation, and should be treated. Potassium supplements or potassium-sparing diuretics should be given cautiously to patients who have diabetes

Table 16-18 Hypokalemia: Treatment

Correct Precipitating Factors
Increased pH
Decreased $[Mg^{2+}]$
Drugs

Mild Hypokalemia ($[K^+] > 2$ mEq/L)
Intravenous KCl infusion ≤10 mEq/hr

Severe Hypokalemia ($[K^+] \leq 2$ mEq/L, paralysis or ECG changes)
Intravenous KCl infusion ≤40 mEq/hr
Continuous electrocardiographic monitoring
If life-threatening, 5–6 mEq bolus

mellitus or renal insufficiency, which limit compensation for acute hyperkalemia. In patients such as those who have diabetic ketoacidosis, who are both hypokalemic and acidemic, potassium administration should precede correction of acidosis to avoid a precipitous decrease in plasma [K$^+$] as pH increases.

In patients with normal serum potassium accompanied by symptoms of potassium depletion (e.g., muscle fatigue) or history of potassium loss or insufficient intake, or in patients in whom potassium depletion may be of special threat (e.g., patients on diuretics, digitalis, or β$_2$-agonists), muscle biopsy with measurement of muscle potassium concentration may be a useful procedure to detect and quantify potassium depletion.

Hyperkalemia

The most lethal manifestations of hyperkalemia ([K$^+$] > 5 mEq/L) involve the cardiac conducting system and include dysrhythmias, conduction abnormalities, and cardiac arrest. In anesthesia practice, the classic example of hyperkalemic cardiac toxicity is associated with the administration of succinylcholine to paraplegic, quadriplegic, or severely burned patients.[143] If plasma [K$^+$] is below 6 mEq/L, cardiac effects are negligible. As the concentration increases further, the ECG shows tall, peaked T waves, especially in the precordial leads. With further increases, the PR interval becomes prolonged, followed by a decrease in the amplitude of the P wave. Finally, the QRS complex widens into a pattern resembling a sine wave, as a prelude to cardiac standstill (Fig. 16-11).[136] Hyperkalemic cardiotoxicity is enhanced by hyponatremia, hypocalcemia, or acidosis. Because progression to fatal cardiotoxicity is unpredictable and often swift, the presence of hyperkalemic ECG changes mandates immediate therapy. The life-threatening cardiac effects usually require more urgent treatment than other manifestations of hyperkalemia. However, ascending muscle weakness appears when plasma [K$^+$] approaches 7 mEq/L, and may progress to flaccid paralysis, inability to phonate, and respiratory arrest.

The most important diagnostic issues are medical history, emphasizing recent drug therapy, and assessment of renal function. Although the ECG may provide the first suggestion of hyperkalemia in some patients, and despite the well-described effects of hyperkalemia on cardiac conduction and rhythm, the ECG is an insensitive and nonspecific method of detecting hyperkalemia. If hyponatremia is also present, adrenal function should be evaluated.

Hyperkalemia may occur with normal, high, or low total body potassium stores. A deficiency of aldosterone, a major regulator of potassium excretion, leads to hyperkalemia in adrenal insufficiency, renal insufficiency, advanced age, and hyporeninemic hypoaldosteronism, a state associated with diabetes mellitus.[144] Because the kidneys excrete potassium, severe renal insufficiency commonly causes hyperkalemia. Patients with chronic renal insufficiency can maintain normal plasma [K$^+$] despite markedly decreased GFR because urinary potassium excretion depends on tubular secretion rather than glomerular filtration if GFR exceeds 8 mL/min.

Drugs are now the most common cause of hyperkalemia, especially in elderly patients. Drugs that may limit potassium excretion include nonsteroidal anti-inflammatory drugs, ACE inhibitors, cyclosporine, and potassium-sparing diuretics such as triamterene. Drug-induced hyperkalemia most commonly occurs in patients with other predisposing factors, such as diabetes mellitus, renal insufficiency, advanced age, or hyporeninemic hypoaldosteronism. ACE inhibitors are particularly likely to produce hyperkalemia in patients who have congestive heart failure.[145,146] Up to 38% of patients receiving ACE inhibitors develop hyperkalemia.[147] Two promising newer potassium binders, patiromer and sodium zirconium cyclosilicate, may be useful for chronic prevention of hyperkalemia in patients receiving ACE inhibitors.[148–150]

In patients who have normal total body potassium, hyperkalemia may accompany a sudden shift of potassium from the ICV to the ECV because of acidemia, increased catabolism, or rhabdomyolysis. Metabolic acidosis and respiratory acidosis tend to cause an increase in plasma [K$^+$]. However, organic acidoses (i.e., lactic acidosis, ketoacidosis) have little effect on [K$^+$], whereas mineral acids cause significant cellular shifts. In response to increased hydrogen ion activity because of addition

Serum potassium	Typical ECG appearance	Possible ECG abnormalities
Mild (5.5–6.5 mEq/L)	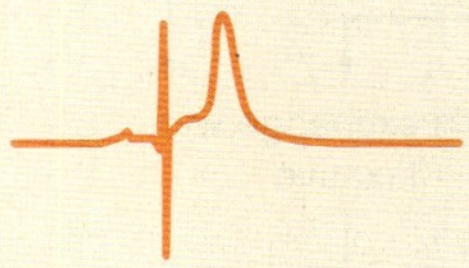	Peaked T waves Prolonged PR segment
Moderate (6.5–8.0 mEq/L)	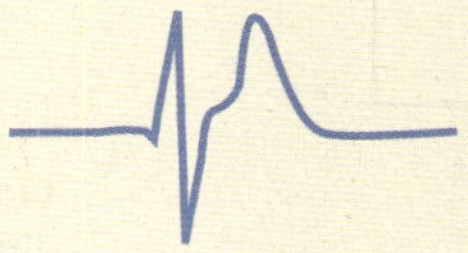	Loss of P wave Prolonged QRS complex ST-segment elevation Ectopic beats and escape rhythms
Severe (>8.0 mEq/L)	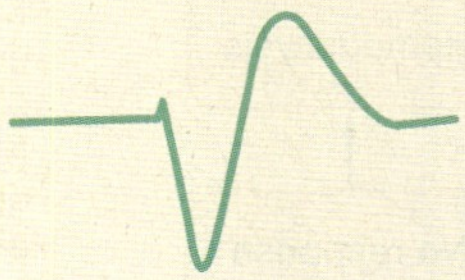	Progressive widening of QRS complex Sine wave Ventricular fibrillation Asystole Axis deviations Bundle branch blocks Fascicular blocks

Figure 16-11 Electrocardiographic (ECG) manifestations of hyperkalemia. (Adapted with permission from Sood MM, Sood AR, Richardson R. Emergency management and commonly encountered outpatient scenarios in patients with hyperkalemia. *Mayo Clin Proc.* 2007;82:1553–1561.)

of acids, potassium will increase if the anion remains in the ECV. Neither lactate nor ketoacids remain in the extracellular fluid. Therefore, hyperkalemia in these circumstances reflects tissue injury or lack of insulin. Pseudohyperkalemia, which occurs when potassium is released from cells in blood collection tubes, can be diagnosed by comparing serum and plasma K^+ levels from the same blood sample. Hyperkalemia usually accompanies malignant hyperthermia.

The treatment of hyperkalemia is aimed at eliminating the cause, reversing membrane hyperexcitability, and removing potassium from the body (Fig. 16-12).[136,137,146,151] Mineralocorticoid deficiency can be treated with 9-α-fludrocortisone (0.025 to 0.10 mg/day). Hyperkalemia secondary to digitalis intoxication may be resistant to therapy because attempts to shift potassium from the ECV to the ICV are often ineffective. In this situation, use of digoxin-specific antibodies has been successful.

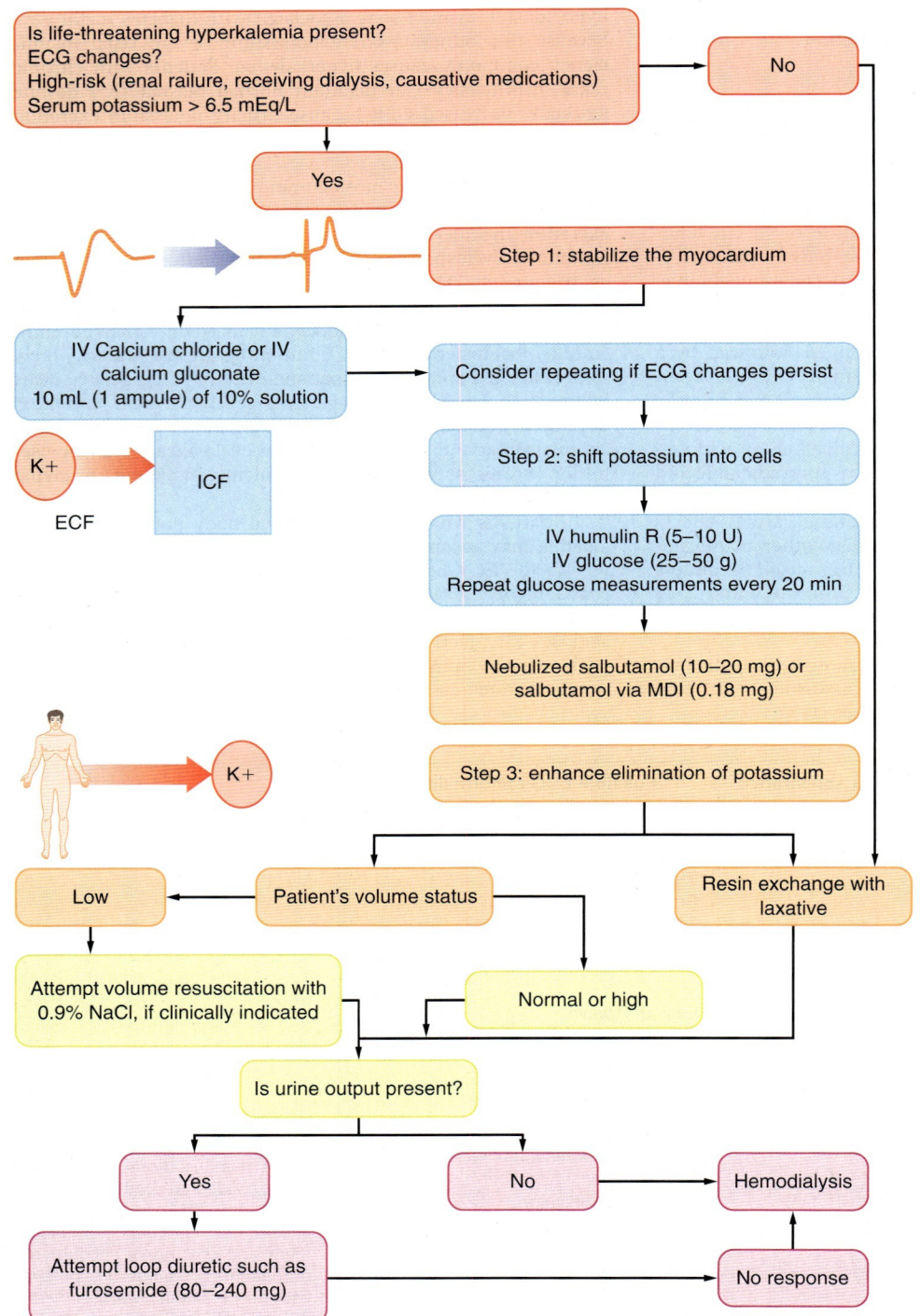

Figure 16-12 Algorithmic management of hyperkalemia. ECG, electrocardiographic; IV, intravenous; K, potassium; ECF, extracellular fluid; ICF, intracellular fluid; MDI, metered-dose inhaler; NaCl, sodium chloride. (Adapted with permission from Sood MM, Sood AR, Richardson R. Emergency management and commonly encountered outpatient scenarios in patients with hyperkalemia. *Mayo Clin Proc.* 2007;82:1553–1561.)

Table 16-19 Severe Hyperkalemia[a] Treatment
Reverse Membrane Effects
Calcium (10 mL of 10% calcium chloride IV over 10 min)
Transfer Extracellular [K+] into Cells
Glucose and insulin ($D_{10}W$ + 5–10 U regular insulin per 25–50 g glucose)
Sodium bicarbonate (50–100 mEq over 5–10 min)
β_2-agonists
Remove Potassium from Body
Diuretics, proximal or loop
Potassium-exchange resins (sodium polystyrene sulfonate)
Hemodialysis
Monitor Electrocardiogram and Serum [K+] Level

[a]Potassium concentration ([K+]) > 6.5 mEq/L or electrocardiographic changes. IV, intravenous; $D_{10}W$, 10% dextrose in water.

Emergent management of severe hyperkalemia is described in detail in Table 16-19. Membrane hyperexcitability can be antagonized by translocating potassium from the ECV to the ICV, removing excess potassium, or (transiently) by infusing calcium chloride to depress the membrane threshold potential.[152] Pending definitive treatment, rapid infusion of calcium chloride (1 g of $CaCl_2$ over 3 minutes, or two or three ampules of 10% calcium gluconate over 5 minutes) may stabilize cardiac rhythm (Table 16-19). Calcium should be given cautiously if digitalis intoxication is likely. Insulin, in a dose-dependent fashion, causes cellular uptake of potassium by increasing the activity of the sodium/potassium ATPase pump. Insulin increases cellular uptake of potassium best when high insulin levels are achieved by intravenous injection of 5 to 10 units of regular insulin, accompanied by 50 mL of 50% glucose.[136,145] Larger doses of insulin are no more effective and risk hypoglycemia.[153] β_2-Adrenergic drugs such as salbutamol and albuterol also increase potassium uptake by skeletal muscle and reduce plasma [K+], an action that may explain hypokalemia with severe, acute illness. Salbutamol, a selective β_2-agonist, decreases serum potassium acutely by 1 mEq/L or more when given by inhalation or intravenously, although cardiac dysrhythmias may occasionally complicate treatment with selective β_2-agonists.[136] Although administration of sodium bicarbonate has long been considered a part of the treatment of hyperkalemia, bicarbonate, when used alone, is relatively ineffective and is no longer favored, except for patients with metabolic acidosis.[150]

Potassium may be removed from the body by the renal or gastrointestinal routes. Furosemide promotes kaliuresis in a dose-dependent fashion. Sodium polystyrene sulfonate resin (Kayexalate), which exchanges sodium for potassium, can be given orally (30 to 60 g)[154] or as a retention enema (50 g in 200 mL of 20% sorbitol). However, sodium overload and hypervolemia are potential risks. Hemodialysis and continuous renal replacement therapy may be necessary for patients with acute kidney injury or chronic renal failure.[151]

Calcium

Physiologic Role

Calcium is a divalent cation found primarily in the extracellular fluid. The free calcium concentration [Ca^{2+}] in ECV is approximately 1 mM, whereas the free [Ca^{2+}] in the ICV approximates 100 nM, an intracellular:extracellular gradient of 10,000 to 1. Circulating calcium consists of a protein-bound fraction (40% to 50%), a fraction bound to inorganic anions (10% to 15%), and an ionized fraction (45% to 50%), which is the physiologically active and homeostatically regulated component. Acute acidemia increases and acute alkalemia decreases ionized calcium.[155] Because mathematical formulae that "correct" total calcium measurements for albumin concentration are inaccurate in critically ill patients,[156] ionized calcium should be directly measured.

In general, calcium is essential for all movement that occurs in mammalian systems. Essential for normal excitation–contraction coupling, calcium is also necessary for proper function of muscle tissue, ciliary movement, mitosis, neurotransmitter release, enzyme secretion, and hormonal secretion. Cyclic adenosine monophosphate (cAMP) and phosphoinositides, which are major second messengers regulating cellular metabolism, function primarily through the regulation of calcium movement. Activation of numerous intracellular enzyme systems requires calcium. Calcium is important both for generation of the cardiac pacemaker activity and for generation of the cardiac action potential and therefore is the primary ion responsible for the plateau phase of the action potential. Calcium also serves vital functions in membrane and bone structure.

Serum [Ca^{2+}] is regulated by multiple factors (Fig. 16-13),[157] including a calcium receptor[157,158] and several hormones. Parathyroid hormone (PTH) and calcitriol, the most important neurohumoral mediators of serum [Ca^{2+}],[159] mobilize calcium from bone, increase renal tubular reabsorption of calcium, and enhance intestinal absorption of calcium. Vitamin D, after ingestion or cutaneous manufacture under the stimulus of ultraviolet light, is 25-hydroxylated to calcidiol in the liver and then is 1-hydroxylated to calcitriol, the active metabolite, in the kidney. Even in the absence of dietary calcium intake, PTH and vitamin D can maintain a normal circulating [Ca^{2+}] by mobilizing calcium from bone. In addition to the key roles played by PTH and calcitriol in regulating serum [Ca^{2+}], other recently described pathways play key molecular roles in bone resorption. The receptor activator of nuclear factor κB (RANK), RANK ligand (RANKL), and osteoprotegerin play key molecular roles; binding of RANKL to RANK stimulates osteoclast activity, whereas binding of RANKL to osteoprotegerin, a soluble decoy receptor, disrupts binding to RANK.[160]

Hypocalcemia

Hypocalcemia (ionized [Ca^{2+}] <4 mg/dL or <1 mmol/L) occurs as a result of failure of PTH or calcitriol action or because of calcium chelation or precipitation, not because of calcium deficiency alone. PTH deficiency can result from suppression of the parathyroid glands by severe hypo- or hypermagnesemia or from surgical damage or removal of the parathyroid glands. Permanent hypocalcemia occurs in about 5% of patients who undergo thyroidectomy, with the incidence somewhat higher in patients who undergo central neck dissection.[161] Burns, sepsis, and pancreatitis may suppress parathyroid function and interfere with vitamin D action. Vitamin D deficiency may result from lack of dietary vitamin D or from vitamin D malabsorption in patients who lack sunlight exposure. Hyperphosphatemia-induced hypocalcemia may occur as a consequence of overzealous phosphate therapy, from cell lysis secondary to chemotherapy, or as a result of cellular destruction from rhabdomyolysis. Precipitation of $CaHPO_4$ complexes occurs with hyperphosphatemia. However, ionized [Ca^{2+}] only decreases approximately 0.019 mM

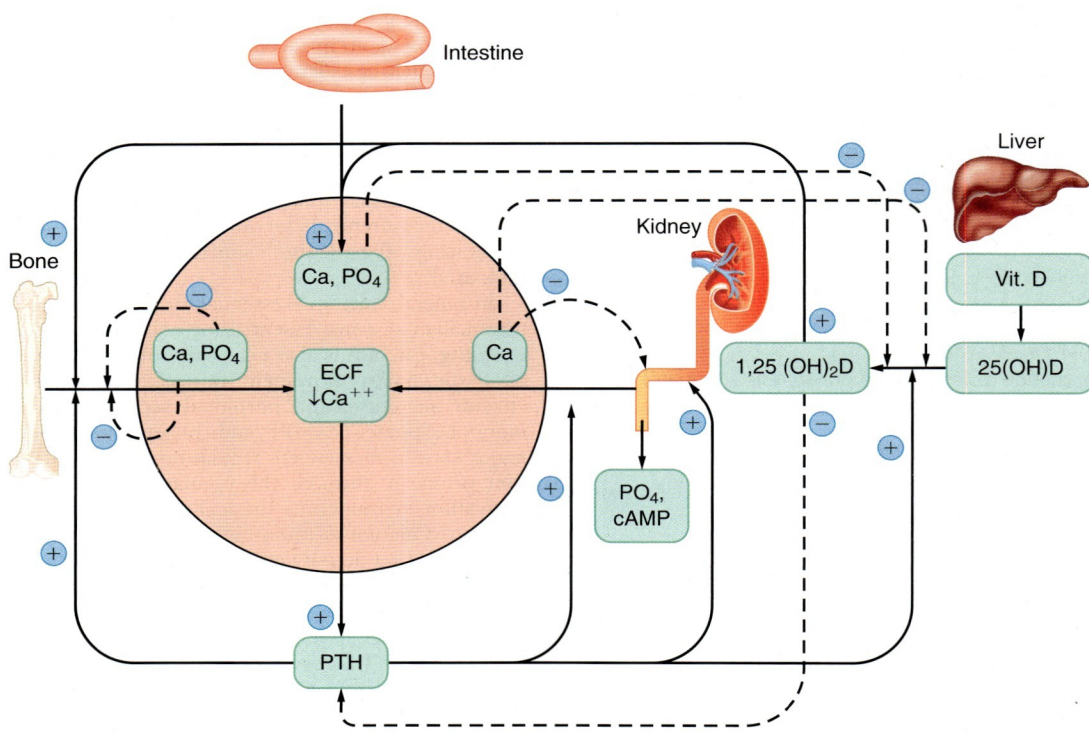

Figure 16-13 Schematic representation of the regulatory system maintaining Ca²⁺ homeostasis. The *solid arrows* and *lines* delineate effects of parathyroid hormone (PTH) and 1,25 (OH)$_2$D$_3$ (dihydroxyvitamin D) on their target tissues; *dashed arrows* and *lines* show examples of how extracellular Ca²⁺ or phosphate ions act directly on tissues regulating mineral ion metabolism. Ca, calcium; PO$_4$, phosphate; ECF, extracellular fluid; cAMP, cyclic adenosine monophosphate; 25(OH)D, 25-hydroxyvitamin D; minus signs indicate inhibitory actions and plus signs indicate stimulatory effects. (Adapted with permission from Brown EM, Pollak M, Hebert SC. The extracellular calcium-sensing receptor: Its role in health and disease. *Annu Rev Med.* 1998;49:15–29.)

for each 1 mM increase in phosphate concentration. Alkalemia resulting from hyperventilation or sodium bicarbonate injection can acutely decrease [Ca²⁺]. In massive transfusion, citrate may produce hypocalcemia by chelating calcium; however, decreases are usually transient and produce negligible cardiovascular effects, unless citrate clearance is decreased (e.g., by hepatic or renal disease or hypothermia). In massive transfusion, a high proportion of patients develop moderate or severe hypocalcemia.[162]

The hallmark of hypocalcemia is increased neuronal membrane irritability and tetany (Table 16-20). Early symptoms include sensations of numbness and tingling involving fingers, toes, and the circumoral region. In frank tetany, tonic contraction of respiratory muscles may lead to laryngospasm, bronchospasm, or respiratory arrest. Smooth muscle spasm can result in abdominal cramping and urinary frequency. Mental status alterations include irritability, depression, psychosis, and dementia. Hypocalcemia also may cause acute symptomatic seizures.[163] Hypocalcemia may impair cardiovascular function and has been associated with heart failure, hypotension, dysrhythmias, insensitivity to digitalis, and impaired β-adrenergic action.

Reduced *ionized* serum calcium occurs in as many as 88% of critically ill patients, 66% of less severely ill intensive care unit patients, and 26% of hospitalized non–intensive care unit patients.[164] Patients at particular risk include patients after multiple trauma and cardiopulmonary bypass. In most such patients, ionized hypocalcemia is clinically mild ([Ca²⁺] 0.8 to 1 mmol/L).

Table 16-20 Hypocalcemia: Clinical Manifestations

Cardiovascular
Dysrhythmias
Digitalis insensitivity
Electrocardiographic changes
Heart failure
Hypotension

Neuromuscular
Tetany
Muscle spasm
Papilledema
Seizures
Weakness

Respiratory
Apnea
Laryngeal spasm
Bronchospasm

Psychiatric
Anxiety
Dementia
Depression
Psychosis

Fatigue

Initial diagnostic evaluation should concentrate on history and physical examination, laboratory evaluation of renal function, and measurement of serum phosphate concentration. Latent hypocalcemia can be diagnosed by tapping on the facial nerve to elicit *Chvostek sign* or by inflating a sphygmomanometer to 20 mmHg above systolic pressure, which produces radial and ulnar nerve ischemia and causes carpal spasm known as *Trousseau sign*. The differential diagnosis of hypocalcemia can be approached by addressing four issues: age of the patient, serum phosphate concentration, general clinical status, and duration of hypocalcemia. Low or normal phosphate concentrations imply vitamin D or magnesium deficiency. An otherwise healthy patient with chronic hypocalcemia probably is hypoparathyroid. High phosphate concentrations suggest renal failure or hypoparathyroidism. In renal insufficiency, reduced phosphorus excretion results in hyperphosphatemia, which downregulates the 1α-hydroxylase responsible for the renal conversion of calcidiol to calcitriol. This, in combination with decreased production of calcitriol secondary to reduced renal mass, causes reduced intestinal absorption of calcium and hypocalcemia.[164] Chronically ill adults with hypocalcemia often have disorders such as malabsorption, osteomalacia, or osteoblastic metastases.

The definitive treatment of hypocalcemia necessitates identification and treatment of the underlying cause (Table 16-21). Symptomatic hypocalcemia usually occurs when serum ionized [Ca^{2+}] is less than 0.7 mM.

Unnecessary offending drugs should be discontinued. Hypocalcemia resulting from hypomagnesemia or hyperphosphatemia is treated by repletion of magnesium or removal of phosphate. Treatment of a patient who has tetany and hyperphosphatemia requires coordination of therapy to avoid the consequences of metastatic soft-tissue calcification. Potassium and other electrolytes should be measured and abnormalities should be corrected. Hyperkalemia and hypomagnesemia potentiate hypocalcemia-induced cardiac and neuromuscular irritability. In contrast, hypokalemia protects against hypocalcemic tetany; therefore, correction of hypokalemia without correction of hypocalcemia may provoke tetany.

Mild, ionized hypocalcemia should not be overtreated. For instance, in most patients after cardiac surgery, administration of calcium only increases blood pressure and actually attenuates the β-adrenergic effects of epinephrine. Therefore, calcium infusions should be of limited value in surgical patients unless there is demonstrable evidence of ionized hypocalcemia. Calcium salts appear to confer no benefit to patients already receiving inotropic or vasoactive agents.

The cornerstone of therapy for confirmed, symptomatic, ionized hypocalcemia ([Ca^{2+}] < 0.7 mM) is calcium administration. In patients who have severe hypocalcemia or hypocalcemic symptoms, calcium should be administered intravenously. In emergency situations, in an averaged-sized adult, the "rule of 10s" advises infusion of 10 mL of 10% calcium gluconate (93 mg elemental calcium) over 10 minutes, followed by a continuous infusion of elemental calcium, 0.3 to 2 mg/kg/hr (i.e., 3 to 16 mL/hr of 10% calcium gluconate for a 70-kg adult). Calcium salts should be diluted in 50 to 100 mL D_5W (to limit venous irritation and thrombosis), should not be mixed with bicarbonate (to prevent precipitation), and must be given cautiously to digitalized patients because calcium increases the toxicity of digoxin. Continuous ECG monitoring during initial therapy will detect cardiotoxicity (e.g., heart block, ventricular fibrillation). During calcium replacement, clinicians should monitor serum calcium, magnesium, phosphate, potassium, and creatinine. Once the ionized [Ca^{2+}] is stable in the range of 4 to 5 mg/dL (1 to 1.25 mM), oral calcium supplements can substitute for parenteral therapy. Urinary calcium should be monitored in an attempt to avoid hypercalciuria (>5 mg/kg/24 hr) and urinary tract stone formation.

When supplementation fails to maintain serum calcium within the normal range, or if hypercalciuria develops, vitamin D or vitamin D analogs may be added. Although the principal effect of vitamin D is to increase enteric calcium absorption, osseous calcium resorption is also enhanced. When rapid changes in dosage are anticipated or an immediate effect is required (e.g., postoperative hypoparathyroidism), shorter-acting calciferols such as dihydrotachysterol may be preferable. Because the effect of vitamin D is not regulated, the dosages of calcium and vitamin D should be adjusted to raise the serum calcium into the low normal range.

Adverse reactions to calcium and vitamin D include hypercalcemia and hypercalciuria. If hypercalcemia develops, calcium and vitamin D should be discontinued and appropriate therapy given. The toxic effects of vitamin D metabolites persist in proportion to their biologic half-lives (ergocalciferol, 20 to 60 days; dihydrotachysterol, 5 to 15 days; calcitriol, 2 to 10 days). Glucocorticoids antagonize the toxic effects of vitamin D metabolites.

Another therapeutic option for patients with persistent hypoparathyroidism is recombinant human PTH, although the expense of the recombinant hormone is a barrier to wider use.[165]

Hypercalcemia

Although ionized [Ca^{2+}] most accurately defines hypercalcemia (ionized [Ca^{2+}] > 1.5 mmol/L), hypercalcemia customarily is discussed in terms of total serum calcium (total serum calcium > 10.5 mg/dL). In hypoalbuminemic patients, total serum calcium can be estimated (albeit inaccurately) by assuming an increase of 0.8 mg/dL for every 1 g/dL of albumin concentration below 4 g/dL. Patients in whom total serum calcium is below 11.5 mg/dL are usually asymptomatic. Patients with moderate hypercalcemia (total serum calcium 11.5 to 13 mg/dL) may show symptoms of lethargy, anorexia, nausea, and polyuria. Severe hypercalcemia (total serum calcium > 13 mg/dL) is associated with more severe neuromyopathic symptoms, including muscle weakness, depression, impaired memory, emotional lability, lethargy, stupor, and coma. The cardiovascular effects of hypercalcemia include hypertension, arrhythmias, heart block, cardiac arrest, and digitalis sensitivity. Skeletal disease may occur secondary to direct osteolysis or humoral bone resorption.

Hypercalcemia impairs urinary concentrating ability and renal excretory capacity for calcium by irreversibly precipitating calcium salts within the renal parenchyma and by reducing renal blood flow and GFR. In response to hypovolemia, renal tubular reabsorption of sodium enhances renal calcium reabsorption.

Table 16-21 Hypocalcemia: Acute Treatment

Administer Calcium
  IV: 10 mL 10% calcium gluconate[a] over 10 min, followed by elemental calcium 0.3–2 mg/kg/hr
  Oral: 500–100 mg elemental calcium q6h

Administer Vitamin D
  Ergocalciferol, 1,200 μg/day ($T_{1/2}$ = 30 days)
  Dihydrotachysterol, 200–400 μg/day ($T_{1/2}$ = 7 days)
  1,25-dihydroxycholecalciferol, 0.25–1 μg/day ($T_{1/2}$ = 1 day)

Monitor Electrocardiogram

[a]Calcium gluconate contains 93 mg elemental calcium per 10-mL vial.
IV, intravenous; $T_{1/2}$, half-life.

Effective treatment of severe hypercalcemia is necessary to prevent progressive dehydration and renal failure leading to further increases in total serum calcium, because volume depletion exacerbates hypercalcemia.

Hypercalcemia occurs when calcium enters the ECV more rapidly than the kidneys can excrete the excess. Clinically, hypercalcemia most commonly results from an excess of bone resorption over bone formation, usually secondary to malignant disease, hyperparathyroidism, hypocalciuric hypercalcemia, thyrotoxicosis, immobilization, and granulomatous diseases. Granulomatous diseases produce hypercalciuria and hypercalcemia because of conversion by granulomatous tissue of calcidiol to calcitriol.

Malignancy may produce hypercalcemia through either bone destruction or secretion by malignant tissue of hormones that promote hypercalcemia. Examples of malignancy-associated hormonal effects include secretion by solid tumors of parathormone-like peptides and derangement of the RANKL/osteoprotegerin system in multiple myeloma.[166] Primary hyperparathyroidism is associated with weakness, weight loss, and anemia, symptoms that suggest malignancy but may result simply from hyperparathyroidism.[167] To compensate for increased gut absorption or bone resorption of calcium, renal excretion can readily increase from 100 to more than 400 mg/day. Factors that promote hypercalcemia may be offset by coexisting disorders, such as pancreatitis, sepsis, or hyperphosphatemia, that cause hypocalcemia.

Although definitive treatment of hypercalcemia requires correction of underlying causes, temporizing therapy may be necessary to avoid complications and to relieve symptoms. Total serum calcium exceeding 14 mg/dL represents a medical emergency. General supportive treatment includes hydration, correction of associated electrolyte abnormalities, removal of offending drugs, dietary calcium restriction, and increased physical activity. Because anorexia and antagonism by calcium of ADH action result in sodium and water depletion, infusion of 0.9% saline will dilute serum calcium, promote renal excretion, and can reduce total serum calcium by 1.5 to 3 mg/dL. Urinary output should be maintained at 200 to 300 mL/hr. As GFR increases, sodium ions increase calcium excretion by competing with calcium ions for reabsorption in the proximal renal tubules and the loop of Henle.

Furosemide further enhances calcium excretion by increasing tubular sodium. Patients who have renal impairment may require higher doses of furosemide. During saline infusion and forced diuresis, careful monitoring of cardiopulmonary status and electrolytes, especially magnesium and potassium, is required. Intensive diuresis and saline administration can achieve net calcium excretion rates of 2,000 to 4,000 mg/24 hr, a rate eight times greater than saline alone, but still less than the 6,000 mg every 8 hours that can be removed by hemodialysis.[166] Patients treated with phosphates for hypercalcemia should be well hydrated.

Bone resorption, the primary cause of hypercalcemia, can be minimized by increasing physical activity and initiating drug therapy with bisphosphonates, calcitonin, glucocorticoids, or calcimetrics.[166] Bisphosphonates, currently the first-line therapy for acute hypercalcemia, inhibit osteoclast function and viability. Bisphosphonates are the principal drugs for the management of hypercalcemia mediated by osteoclastic bone resorption.[166] Pamidronate, unlike earlier bisphosphonates, does not appear to worsen renal insufficiency. Risedronate has been associated with less gastrointestinal morbidity than alendronate.[168,169] Zoledronate has the most rapid onset of action among the bisphosphonates and prolongs the duration before relapse of hypercalcemia; however, zoledronate has been associated with compromised renal function.[170] Bisphosphonates also are used to control osteoporosis in both men and women.[171]

Calcitonin, usually reserved as a secondary treatment for life-threatening hypercalcemia, lowers serum calcium within 24 to 48 hours and is more effective when combined with glucocorticoids.[166] Usually calcitonin reduces total serum calcium by only 1 to 2 mg/dL. Although calcitonin is relatively nontoxic, more than 25% of patients may not respond. Thus, calcitonin is unsuitable as a first-line drug during life-threatening hypercalcemia. Hydrocortisone is effective in treating hypercalcemic patients with lymphatic malignancies, vitamin D or A intoxication, and diseases associated with production by tumor or granulomas of $1,25(OH)_2D$ or osteoclast-activating factor. Glucocorticoids rarely improve hypercalcemia secondary to malignancy or hyperparathyroidism. Control of hypercalcemia associated with malignancy usually requires control of the underlying cancer.[172]

Primary hyperparathyroidism most commonly occurs secondary to parathyroid adenomas (80% to 85%) with hyperplasia (10% to 15%) and carcinoma (1% to 5%) accounting for the remainder.[167] Although either minimally invasive parathyroidectomy or bilateral neck dissection effectively manages hyperparathyroidism, minimally invasive parathyroidectomy appears to be associated with less frequent postoperative hypocalcemia and less frequent recurrent laryngeal nerve injury.[173] Calcimimetics have become an attractive treatment option for suppressing primary, secondary, and tertiary hyperparathyroidism, especially in poor surgical candidates. With the first agent, cinacalcet, recently released for clinical use in the United States and others undergoing clinical trials, calcimimetic agents also reduce inorganic phosphate concentration (Pi) and the calcium × phosphate product.[174-176] Although parathyroidectomy remains the treatment of choice for primary hyperparathyroidism, calcimimetics represent an alternative for patients who are not acceptable candidates for surgery.[176] In hyperparathyroidism secondary to chronic renal failure, conventional treatment with calcium supplements, phosphate binders, and vitamin D analogues reduces the associated secondary hyperparathyroidism but also generates undesirable side effects, including hypercalcemia.[176] In effect, such patients develop a variation of the milk–alkali syndrome.[177] In chronic renal failure patients, calcimimetics reduce serum calcium, Pi and the calcium × phosphate product by sensitizing the parathyroid calcium receptor to calcium.[175] In addition, calcimimetics appear to be effective in tertiary hyperparathyroidism, which develops after renal transplantation in 25% to 50% of renal allograft recipients.[175]

Phosphates lower serum calcium by causing deposition of calcium in bone and soft tissue. Because the risk of extraskeletal calcification of organs such as the kidneys and myocardium is less if phosphates are given orally, the intravenous route should be reserved for patients with life-threatening hypercalcemia and those in whom other measures have failed.

Phosphate

Physiologic Role

Phosphorus, in the form of inorganic phosphate (Pi), is distributed in similar concentrations throughout the intracellular and the extracellular fluids. Of total body phosphorus, 90% exists in bone, 10% is intracellular, and the remainder, less than 1%, is found in the extracellular fluid. Phosphate circulates as the free ion (55%), complexed ion (33%), and in a protein-bound form (12%). Blood levels vary widely: The normal total Pi ranges from 2.7 to 4.5 mg/dL in adults.

Control of Pi is achieved by altered renal excretion and redistribution within the body compartments.[178] Absorption occurs in the duodenum and jejunum and is largely unregulated. Phosphate reabsorption in the kidney is primarily regulated by PTH, dietary intake, and insulin-like growth factor. Phosphate is freely filtered at the glomerulus, and its concentration in the glomerular ultrafiltrate is similar to that of plasma. The filtered phosphate is then reabsorbed in the proximal tubule, where it is cotransported with sodium. Cotransport is regulated by phosphorus intake and PTH. Phosphate excretion is increased by volume expansion and decreased by respiratory alkalosis.

Phosphates provide the primary energy bond in ATP and creatine phosphate. Therefore, severe phosphate depletion results in cellular energy depletion. Phosphorus is an essential element of second-messenger systems, including cAMP and phosphoinositides, and is a major component of nucleic acids, phospholipids, and cell membranes. As part of 2,3-diphosphoglycerate, phosphate promotes release of oxygen from the hemoglobin molecule. Phosphorus also functions in protein phosphorylation and acts as a urinary buffer.[178]

Hypophosphatemia

Hypophosphatemia is characterized by low levels of phosphate-containing cellular components, including ATP, 2,3-diphosphoglycerate, and membrane phospholipids. Serious life-threatening organ dysfunction may occur when the serum Pi falls below 1 mg/dL. Neurologic manifestations of hypophosphatemia include paresthesias, myopathy, encephalopathy, delirium, seizures, and coma.[179] Hematologic abnormalities include dysfunction of erythrocytes, platelets, and leukocytes. Because hypophosphatemia limits the chemotactic, phagocytic, and bactericidal activity of granulocytes, associated immune dysfunction may contribute to the susceptibility of hypophosphatemic patients to sepsis.[180] Muscle weakness and malaise are common. Respiratory muscle failure and myocardial dysfunction are potential problems of particular concern to anesthesiologists. Rhabdomyolysis is a complication of severe hypophosphatemia.

Common in postoperative and traumatized patients, hypophosphatemia (Pi < 2.5 mg/dL) is caused by three primary abnormalities in Pi homeostasis: An intracellular shift of Pi, an increase in renal Pi loss, and a decrease in gastrointestinal Pi absorption. Carbohydrate-induced hypophosphatemia (the "refeeding syndrome"),[181] by insulin-induced cellular Pi uptake, may occur as catabolic patients become anabolic and during medical management of diabetic ketoacidosis.[182] Acute alkalemia, which may reduce serum Pi to 1 to 2 mg/dL, increases intracellular consumption of Pi by increasing the rate of glycolysis. Hyperventilation significantly reduces Pi and, importantly, the effect is progressive after cessation of hyperventilation.[183] Acute correction of respiratory acidemia may also result in severe hypophosphatemia. Respiratory alkalosis probably explains the hypophosphatemia associated with gram-negative bacteremia and salicylate poisoning. Excessive renal loss of Pi explains the hypophosphatemia associated with hyperparathyroidism, hypomagnesemia, hypothermia, diuretic therapy, and renal tubular defects in Pi absorption. Excess gastrointestinal loss of Pi is most commonly secondary to the use of Pi-binding antacids or to malabsorption syndromes. Hypophosphatemia is associated with anticancer drugs, especially alkylating agents, monoclonal antibodies, and estrogens.[184]

Measurement of urinary Pi aids in differentiation of hypophosphatemia due to renal losses from that due to excessive gastrointestinal losses or redistribution of Pi into cells. Extrarenal causes of hypophosphatemia cause avid renal tubular Pi reabsorption, reducing urinary excretion to below 100 mg/day.

Table 16-22 Hypophosphatemia: Acute Treatment
Parenteral phosphate, 0.2 mM–0.68 mM/kg (5–16 mg/kg) over 12 hr
Potassium phosphate (93 mg/mL of phosphate)
Sodium phosphate (93 mg/mL of phosphate)

Patients who have severe (<1 mg/dL) or symptomatic hypophosphatemia require intravenous phosphate administration (Table 16-22).[179] In chronically hypophosphatemic patients, 7 to 15 mmol of phosphate can be infused per hour, with the magnitude of the dose proportional to the severity of symptoms.[178] The dosage must be adjusted as indicated by the serum Pi level because the cumulative deficit cannot be predicted accurately. Oral therapy can be substituted for parenteral Pi once the serum Pi level exceeds 2 mg/dL. Continued therapy with Pi supplements is required for 5 to 10 days in order to replenish body stores.

Phosphate should be administered cautiously to hypocalcemic patients because of the risk of precipitating more severe hypocalcemia. In hypercalcemic patients, Pi may cause soft-tissue calcification. Phosphorus must be given cautiously to patients with renal insufficiency because of impaired excretory ability. During treatment, close monitoring of serum Pi, calcium, magnesium, and potassium is essential to avoid complications.

Hyperphosphatemia

Renal failure is the most common cause of hyperphosphatemia. Renal excretion of Pi remains adequate until the GFR falls below 20 to 25 mL/min. Accumulation of Pi in patients with chronic renal failure merits the inclusion of Pi as a uremic toxin.[185] The clinical features of hyperphosphatemia (Pi > 5 mg/dL) relate primarily to the development of hypocalcemia and ectopic calcification. Hyperphosphatemia is caused by three basic mechanisms: inadequate renal excretion, increased movement of Pi out of cells, and increased Pi or vitamin D intake. Rapid cell lysis from rhabdomyolysis, sepsis, and the tumor lysis syndrome,[184] can cause hyperphosphatemia, especially when renal function is impaired.

Measurements of BUN, creatinine, GFR, and urinary Pi are helpful in the differential diagnosis of hyperphosphatemia. Normal renal function accompanied by high Pi excretion (>1,500 mg/day) indicates an oversupply of Pi. An elevated BUN, elevated creatinine, and low GFR suggest impaired renal excretion of Pi. Normal renal function and Pi excretion less than 1,500 mg/day suggest increased Pi reabsorption (i.e., hypoparathyroidism).

Hyperphosphatemia is corrected by eliminating the cause of the Pi elevation and correcting the associated hypocalcemia. Calcium supplementation of hyperphosphatemic, hypocalcemic patients should be delayed until serum phosphate has fallen below 2 mmol/L (6 mg/dL).[164] The serum concentration of Pi is reduced by restricting intake, increasing urinary excretion with saline and acetazolamide (500 mg every 6 hours), and increasing gastrointestinal losses by enteric administration of aluminum hydroxide (30 to 45 mL every 6 hours).

Although calcimimetics may replace Pi-binders for managing hyperphosphatemia in patients with chronic renal failure, several Pi-binders remain in common use. Calcium-based binders may contribute to hypercalcemia, sevelamer hydrochloride binds bile acids, and lanthanum carbonate offers the advantage of requiring patients to ingest fewer pills. Hemodialysis and peritoneal dialysis are effective in removing Pi in patients who have renal failure.[179]

Magnesium

Physiologic Role

Magnesium is an important, multifunctional, divalent cation located primarily in the intracellular space. Approximately 50% of the typical adult's 24 g of magnesium is located in bone, 12 g is located intracellularly (approximately half in muscle), and less than 1% (<240 mg) of total body magnesium circulates in the serum.[186] Of the normal circulating total magnesium concentration (1.5 to 1.9 mEq/L or 0.75 to 0.95 mmol/L or 1.8 to 2.3 mg/dL), there are three components: protein-bound (30%), anion-bound (15%), and ionized (55%), of which only ionized magnesium is active.

Magnesium is necessary for enzymatic reactions involving DNA and protein synthesis, energy metabolism, glucose utilization, and fatty acid synthesis and breakdown.[187] As a primary regulator or cofactor in many enzyme systems, magnesium is important for the regulation of the sodium–potassium pump, Ca-ATPase enzymes, adenylyl cyclase, proton pumps, and slow calcium channels. Magnesium has been called an *endogenous calcium antagonist* because regulation of slow calcium channels contributes to maintenance of normal vascular tone, prevention of vasospasm, and perhaps the prevention of calcium overload in many tissues. Because magnesium partially regulates PTH secretion and is important for the maintenance of end-organ sensitivity to both PTH and vitamin D, abnormalities in ionized magnesium concentration ($[Mg^{2+}]$) may result in abnormal calcium metabolism. Magnesium functions in potassium metabolism primarily through regulating sodium–potassium ATPase, an enzyme that controls potassium entry into cells, especially in potassium-depleted states, and controls reabsorption of potassium by the renal tubules. In addition, magnesium functions as a regulator of membrane excitability and serves as a structural component in both cell membranes and the skeleton.

Because magnesium stabilizes axonal membranes, hypomagnesemia decreases the threshold of axonal stimulation and increases nerve conduction velocity. Magnesium also influences the release of neurotransmitters at the neuromuscular junction by competitively inhibiting the entry of calcium into the presynaptic nerve terminals. The concentration of calcium required to trigger calcium release and the rate at which calcium is released from the sarcoplasmic reticulum are inversely related to the ambient magnesium concentration. Thus, the net effect of hypomagnesemia is muscle that contracts more in response to stimuli and is tetany-prone.

Magnesium is widely available in foods and is absorbed through the gastrointestinal tract, although dietary consumption appears to have decreased over several decades.[187] Seventy percent of plasma magnesium is filtered through the glomerular membrane; of the filtered magnesium, 30% is absorbed in the proximal tubule, 60% in the thick ascending loop of Henle, and 10% to 15% in the distal tubule.[186] While both magnesium and Pi are primarily regulated by intrinsic renal mechanisms, PTH exerts a greater effect on renal loss of Pi.

Magnesium has been used to help manage an impressive array of clinical problems in patients who are not hypomagnesemic. Therapeutic hypermagnesemia is used to treat patients with premature labor, preeclampsia, and eclampsia. Because magnesium blocks the release of catecholamines from adrenergic nerve terminals and the adrenal glands, magnesium has been used to reduce the effects of catecholamine excess in patients with tetanus and pheochromocytoma.[187] In patients awaiting liver transplantation, administration of magnesium significantly improved hypocoagulability.[188] Although clinical data are inconsistent, magnesium also may exert an analgesic effect on postoperative pain,[189] perhaps in part due to magnesium's antagonism of the N-methyl-D-aspartate glutamate receptor.[189] Magnesium has been proposed as part of an antivasospasm regimen after subarachnoid hemorrhage, but its efficacy may be limited by induction of hypocalcemia, which in turn could aggravate cerebral vasospasm.[190] Surprisingly, redistribution of magnesium after subarachnoid hemorrhage has been correlated with ECG changes.[191]

Magnesium administration may influence dysrhythmias by direct effects on myocardial membranes, by altering cellular potassium and sodium concentrations, by inhibiting cellular calcium entry, by improving myocardial oxygen supply and demand, by prolonging the effective refractory period, by depressing conduction, by antagonizing catecholamine action on the conducting system, and by preventing vasospasm. Administration of magnesium reduces the incidence of dysrhythmias after myocardial infarction and in patients with congestive heart failure.[192] In addition, magnesium often reverses torsades de pointes, even in normomagnesemic patients.[193] Treatment of hypomagnesemia during cardiopulmonary bypass decreased the incidence of postoperative ventricular tachycardia from 30% to 7% and increased the frequency of continuous sinus rhythm from 5% to 34%.[194]

Hypomagnesemia

The clinical features of hypomagnesemia ($[Mg^{2+}] < 1.8$ mg/dL), like those of hypocalcemia, are characterized by increased neuronal irritability and tetany (Table 16-23).[195] Symptoms are rare when the serum $[Mg^{2+}]$ is 1.5 to 1.7 mg/dL; in most symptomatic patients serum $[Mg^{2+}]$ is below 1.2 mg/dL. Patients frequently complain of weakness, lethargy, muscle spasms, paresthesias, and depression. When severe, hypomagnesemia may induce seizures, confusion, and coma. Cardiovascular abnormalities include coronary artery spasm, cardiac failure, dysrhythmias, and hypotension. Hypomagnesemia can aggravate digoxin toxicity and congestive heart failure.

Rarely resulting from inadequate dietary intake, hypomagnesemia most commonly is caused by inadequate gastrointestinal absorption, excessive magnesium losses, or failure of renal magnesium conservation. Recently reports demonstrate that hypomagnesemia is associated with administration with proton pump inhibitors, a complication that is resolved if an H_2 antagonist is substituted.[195,196] Hypomagnesemia is particularly frequent in alcoholic patients and in patients in intensive care.[195] Excessive loss of magnesium is associated with prolonged nasogastric suctioning, gastrointestinal or biliary fistulas, and intestinal drains. Inability of the renal tubules to conserve magnesium complicates a variety of systemic and renal diseases, although advanced renal disease with a decreased GFR may lead to magnesium retention. Polyuria, whether secondary to ECV expansion or to pharmacologic or pathologic diuresis, may result in excessive urinary magnesium excretion. Various drugs, including aminoglycosides, *cis*-platinum, cardiac glycosides, and diuretics, enhance urinary magnesium excretion. Intracellular shifts of magnesium as a result of thyroid hormone or insulin administration may also decrease serum $[Mg^{2+}]$.

Because the sodium–potassium pump is magnesium-dependent, hypomagnesemia increases myocardial sensitivity to digitalis preparations and may cause hypokalemia as a result of renal potassium wasting. Attempts to correct potassium deficits with

Table 16-23 Manifestations of Altered Serum Magnesium Concentrations			
Magnesium Level			
mg/dL	mEq/L	mmol/L	**Manifestation**
<1.2	<1	<0.5	Tetany Seizures Arrhythmias
1.2–1.8	1–1.5	0.5–0.75	Neuromuscular irritability Hypocalcemia Hypokalemia
1.8–2.5	1.5–2.1	0.75–1.05	Normal magnesium level
2.5–5	2.1–4.2	1.05–2.1	Typically asymptomatic
5–7	4.2–5.8	2.1–2.9	Lethargy Drowsiness Flushing Nausea and vomiting Diminished deep tendon reflex
7–12	5.8–10	2.9–5	Somnolence Loss of deep tendon reflexes Hypotension ECG changes
>12	>10	>5	Complete heart block Cardiac arrest Apnea Paralysis Coma

ECG, electrocardiogram.
Reprinted with permission from Topf JM, Murray PT. Hypomagnesemia and hypermagnesemia. *Rev Endocr Metab Disord.* 2003;4:195–206.

Table 16-24 Hypomagnesemia: Acute Treatment
Intravenous Mg[a]: 8–16 mEq (1–2 g MgSO$_4$) bolus over 1 hr, followed by 2–4 mEq/hr (250–500 mg/hr MgSO$_4$) as continuous infusion
Intramuscular Mg[a]: 10 mEq q4–6h

[a]MgSO$_4$: 1 g = 8 mEq/mg; MgCl$_2$: 1 g = 10 mEq/mg.

potassium-replacement therapy alone may not be successful without simultaneous magnesium therapy. Magnesium is important in the regulation of potassium channels. The interrelationships of magnesium and potassium in cardiac tissue have probably the greatest clinical relevance in terms of dysrhythmias, digoxin toxicity, and myocardial infarction. Both severe hypomagnesemia and hypermagnesemia suppress PTH secretion and can cause hypocalcemia. Severe hypomagnesemia may also impair end-organ response to PTH.

Hypomagnesemia is associated with hypokalemia, hyponatremia, hypophosphatemia, and hypocalcemia. The reported prevalence of hypomagnesemia in hospitalized and critically ill patients varies from 12 to 65%.[195] Patients who develop hypomagnesemia while in intensive care have an increased mortality.[192] Serum [Mg^{2+}] may not reflect intracellular magnesium content. Peripheral lymphocyte magnesium concentration correlates well with skeletal and cardiac magnesium content.

Measurement of 24-hour urinary magnesium excretion is useful in separating renal from nonrenal causes of hypomagnesemia. Normal kidneys can reduce magnesium excretion to below 1 to 2 mEq/day in response to magnesium depletion. Hypomagnesemia accompanied by high urinary excretion of magnesium (>3 to 4 mEq/day) suggests a renal etiology. In the magnesium-loading test, urinary [Mg^{2+}] excretion is measured for 24 hours after an intravenous magnesium load.

Magnesium deficiency is treated by the administration of magnesium supplements (Table 16-24). One gram of magnesium sulfate provides approximately 4 mmol (8 mEq or 98 mg) of elemental magnesium. Mild deficiencies can be treated with diet alone. Replacement must be added to daily magnesium requirements (0.3 to 0.4 mEq/kg/day). Symptomatic or severe hypomagnesemia ([Mg^{2+}] <1 mg/dL) should be treated with parenteral magnesium: 1 to 2 g (8 to 16 mEq) of magnesium sulfate as an intravenous bolus over the first hour, followed by a continuous infusion of 2 to 4 mEq/hr. Therapy should be guided subsequently by the serum magnesium level. The rate of infusion should not exceed 1 mEq/min, even in emergency situations, and the patient should receive continuous cardiac monitoring to detect cardiotoxicity. Because magnesium antagonizes calcium, blood pressure and cardiac function should be monitored, although blood pressure and cardiac output usually change little during magnesium infusion.

During repletion, patellar reflexes should be monitored frequently and magnesium withheld if they become suppressed. Patients who have renal insufficiency have a diminished ability to excrete magnesium and require careful monitoring during therapy. Repletion of systemic magnesium stores usually requires 5 to 7 days of therapy, after which daily maintenance doses of magnesium should be provided. Magnesium can be given orally, usually in a dose of 60 to 90 mEq/day of magnesium oxide. Hypocalcemic, hypomagnesemic patients should receive magnesium as the chloride salt because the sulfate ion can chelate calcium and further reduce the serum [Ca^{2+}].

Hypermagnesemia

Most cases of hypermagnesemia ([Mg^{2+}] > 2.5 mg/dL) are iatrogenic, resulting from the administration of magnesium in antacids, enemas, or parenteral nutrition, especially to patients with impaired renal function. Other rarer causes of mild hypermagnesemia are hypothyroidism, Addison disease, lithium intoxication, and familial hypocalciuric hypercalcemia. Hypermagnesemia is rarely detected in routine electrolyte determinations. Hypermagnesemia antagonizes the release and effect of acetylcholine at the neuromuscular junction. The result is depressed skeletal muscle function and neuromuscular blockade. Magnesium potentiates the action of nondepolarizing muscle relaxants and decreases potassium release in response to succinylcholine. The clinical features of progressive hypermagnesemia are listed in Table 16-23.

The neuromuscular and cardiac toxicity of hypermagnesemia can be acutely, but transiently, antagonized by giving intravenous calcium (5 to 10 mEq) to buy time while more definitive therapy is instituted.[179] All magnesium-containing preparations must be stopped. Urinary excretion of magnesium can be increased by expanding ECV and inducing diuresis with a combination of saline and furosemide. In emergency situations and in patients with renal failure, magnesium may be removed by dialysis.

REFERENCES

1. Corey HE. Stewart and beyond: new models of acid–base balance. *Kidney Int.* 2004;64(3):777–787.
2. Gomez H, Kellum JA. Understanding acid–base disorders. *Crit Care Clin.* 2015;31(4):849–860.
3. Magder S, Emami A. Practical approach to physical-chemical acid–base management. Stewart at the bedside. *Ann Am Thorac Soc.* 2015;12(1):111–117.
4. Rastegar A. Clinical utility of Stewart's method in diagnosis and management of acid–base disorders. *Clin J Am Soc Nephrol.* 2009;4(7):1267–1274.
5. Khanna A, Kurtzman NA. Metabolic alkalosis. *Respir Care.* 2001;46(4):354–365.
6. Prough DS, Bidani A. Hyperchloremic metabolic acidosis is a predictable consequence of intraoperative infusion of 0.9% saline. *Anesthesiology* 1999;90:1247–1249.
7. Adrogue HJ. Metabolic acidosis: pathophysiology, diagnosis and management. *J Nephrol.* 2006;19 Suppl 9:S62–S69.
8. Morris CG, Low J. Metabolic acidosis in the critically ill. Part 2. Causes and treatment. *Anaesthesia.* 2008;63(4):396–411.
9. Morris CG, Low J. Metabolic acidosis in the critically ill. Part 1. Classification and pathophysiology. *Anaesthesia.* 2008;63(3):294–301.
10. Kraut JA, Madias NE. Serum anion gap: its uses and limitations in clinical medicine. *Clin J Am Soc Nephrol.* 2007;2(1):162–174.
11. Scheingraber S, Rehm M, Sehmisch C, et al. Rapid saline infusion produces hyperchloremic acidosis in patients undergoing gynecologic surgery. *Anesthesiology.* 1999;90(5):1265–1270.
12. Carvounis CP, Feinfeld DA. A simple estimate of the effect of the serum albumin level on the anion Gap. *Am J Nephrol.* 2000;20(5):369–372.
13. Carmody JB, Norwood VF. Paediatric acid–base disorders: a case-based review of procedures and pitfalls. *Paediatr Child Health.* 2013;18(1):29–32.
14. Gehlbach BK, Schmidt GA. Bench-to-bedside review: treating acid–base abnormalities in the intensive care unit - the role of buffers. *Crit Care.* 2004;8(4):259–265.
15. Cooper DJ, Walley KR, Wiggs BR, et al. Bicarbonate does not improve hemodynamics in critically ill patients who have lactic acidosis. A prospective, controlled clinical study. *Ann Intern Med.* 1990;112:492–498.
16. Hoste EA, Colpaert K, Vanholder RC, et al. Sodium bicarbonate versus THAM in ICU patients with mild metabolic acidosis. *J Nephrol.* 2005;18(3):303–307.
17. Foster GT, Vaziri ND, Sassoon CSH. Respiratory alkalosis. *Respir Care.* 2001;46(4):384–391.
18. Chesler M. Regulation and modulation of pH in the brain. *Physiol Rev.* 2003;83(4):1183–1221.
19. Kallet RH, Liu K, Tang J. Management of acidosis during lung-protective ventilation in acute respiratory distress syndrome. *Respir Care Clin North Am.* 2003;9(4):437–456.
20. Martinu T, Menzies D, Dial S. Re-evaluation of acid–base prediction rules in patients with chronic respiratory acidosis. *Can Respir J.* 2003;10(6):311–315.
21. Svensén C, Hahn RG. Volume kinetics of Ringer solution, dextran 70, and hypertonic saline in male volunteers. *Anesthesiology.* 1997;87:204–212.
22. Svensen CH, Rodhe PM, Prough DS. Pharmacokinetic aspects of fluid therapy. *Best Pract Res Clin Anaesthesiol.* 2009;23(2):213–224.
23. Connolly CM, Kramer GC, Hahn RG, et al. Isoflurane but not mechanical ventilation promotes extravascular fluid accumulation during crystalloid volume loading. *Anesthesiology.* 2003;98(3):670–681.
24. Norberg A, Hahn RG, Li H, et al. Population volume kinetics predicts retention of 0.9% saline infused in awake and isoflurane-anesthetized volunteers. *Anesthesiology.* 2007;107(1):24–32.
25. Vane LA, Prough DS, Kinsky MA, et al. Effects of different catecholamines on the dynamics of volume expansion of crystalloid infusion. *Anesthesiology.* 2004;101(5):1136–1144.
26. Chappell D, Dorfler N, Jacob M, et al. Glycocalyx protection reduces leukocyte adhesion after ischemia/reperfusion. *Shock.* 2010;34(2):133–139.
27. Danziger J, Zeidel ML. Osmotic homeostasis. *Clin J Am Soc Nephrol.* 2015;10(5):852–862.
28. Pallone TL, Edwards A, Mattson DL. Renal medullary circulation. *Compr Physiol.* 2012;2(1):97–140.
29. Knepper MA, Kwon TH, Nielsen S. Molecular physiology of water balance. *N Engl J Med.* 2015;373(2):196.
30. Schrier RW. The sea within us: disorders of body water homeostasis. *Curr Opin Investig Drugs.* 2007;8(4):304–311.
31. Nielsen S, Chou CL, Marples D, et al. Vasopressin increases water permeability of kidney collecting duct by inducing translocation of aquaporin-CD water channels to plasma membrane. *Proc Natl Acad Sci U S A.* 1995 Feb 14;92(4):1013–1017.
32. Ball SG. Vasopressin and disorders of water balance: the physiology and pathophysiology of vasopressin. *Ann Clin Biochem.* 2007;44(Pt 5):417–431.
33. Schrier RW. Body water homeostasis: clinical disorders of urinary dilution and concentration. *J Am Soc Nephrol.* 2006;17(7):1820–1832.
34. Potter LR, Yoder AR, Flora DR, et al. Natriuretic peptides: their structures, receptors, physiologic functions and therapeutic applications. *Handb Exp Pharmacol.* 2009;(191):341–366.
35. Volpe M. Natriuretic peptides and cardio-renal disease. *Int J Cardiol.* 2014 Oct 20;176(3):630–639.
36. von Lueder TG, Sangaralingham SJ, Wang BH, et al. Renin-angiotensin blockade combined with natriuretic peptide system augmentation: novel therapeutic concepts to combat heart failure. *Circ Heart Fail.* 2013;6(3):594–605.
37. Moritz ML, Ayus JC. Hospital-acquired hyponatremia: why are hypotonic parenteral fluids still being used? *Nat Clin Pract Nephrol.* 2007;3(7):374–382.
38. Carandang F, Anglemyer A, Longhurst CA, et al. Association between maintenance fluid tonicity and hospital-acquired hyponatremia. *J Pediatr.* 2013;163(6):1646–1651.
39. Anderson RJ, Chung HM, Kluge R, et al. Hyponatremia: a prospective analysis of its epidemiology and the pathogenetic role of vasopressin. *Ann Intern Med.* 1985;102:164–168.
40. Chung H, Kluge R, Schrier RW, et al. Postoperative hyponatremia: a prospective study. *Arch Intern Med.* 1986;146:333–336.
41. Baughman VL. Brain protection during neurosurgery. *Anesthesiol Clin North Am.* 2002;20(2):315–327.
42. Lanzino G, Kassell NF, Germanson T, et al. Plasma glucose levels and outcome after aneurysmal subarachnoid hemorrhage. *J Neurosurg.* 1993;79:885–891.
43. Rovlias A, Kotsou S. The influence of hyperglycemia on neurological outcome in patients with severe head injury. *Neurosurgery.* 2000;46:335–343.
44. Griesdale DE, de Souza RJ, van Dam RM, et al. Intensive insulin therapy and mortality among critically ill patients: a meta-analysis including NICE-SUGAR study data. *CMAJ.* 2009;180(8):821–827.
45. Jacob M, Chappell D, Rehm M. The 'third space': fact or fiction? *Best Pract Res Clin Anaesthesiol.* 2009;23(2):145–157.
46. Maharaj CH, Kallam SR, Malik A, et al. Preoperative intravenous fluid therapy decreases postoperative nausea and pain in high risk patients. *Anesth Analg.* 2005;100(3):675–682.
47. Holte K, Klarskov B, Christensen DS, et al. Liberal versus restrictive fluid administration to improve recovery after laparoscopic cholecystectomy: a randomized, double-blind study. *Ann Surg.* 2004;240(5):892–899.
48. Holte K, Kristensen BB, Valentiner L, et al. Liberal versus restrictive fluid management in knee arthroplasty: a randomized, double-blind study. *Anesth Analg.* 2007;105(2):465–474.
49. Brandstrup B, Tonnesen H, Beier-Holgersen R, et al. Effects of intravenous fluid restriction on postoperative complications: Comparison of two perioperative fluid regimens: a randomized assessor-blinded multicenter trial. *Ann Surg.* 2003;238(5):641–648.
50. Nisanevich V, Felsenstein I, Almogy G, et al. Effect of intraoperative fluid management on outcome after intraabdominal surgery. *Anesthesiology.* 2005;103(1):25–32.
51. Lobo DN, Bostock KA, Neal KR, et al. Effect of salt and water balance on recovery of gastrointestinal function after elective colonic resection: a randomised controlled trial. *Lancet.* 2002;359(9320):1812–1818.
52. Khoo CK, Vickery CJ, Forsyth N, et al. A prospective randomized controlled trial of multimodal perioperative management protocol in patients undergoing elective colorectal resection for cancer. *Ann Surg.* 2007;245(6):867–872.
53. Holte K, Foss NB, Andersen J, et al. Liberal or restrictive fluid administration in fast-track colonic surgery: a randomized, double-blind study. *Br J Anaesth.* 2007;99(4):500–508.
54. Corcoran T, Rhodes JE, Clarke S, et al. Perioperative fluid management in major surgery: a stratified meta-analysis. *Anesth Analg.* 2012;114(3):640–651.
55. Wiedemann HP, Wheeler AP, Bernard GR, et al. Comparison of two fluid-management strategies in acute lung injury. *N Engl J Med.* 2006;354(24):2564–2575.
56. Collins SR, Blank RS, Deatherage LS, et al. Special article: the endothelial glycocalyx: emerging concepts in pulmonary edema and acute lung injury. *Anesth Analg.* 2013;117(3):664–674.
57. Alphonsus CS, Rodseth RN. The endothelial glycocalyx: a review of the vascular barrier. *Anaesthesia.* 2014;69(7):777–784.
58. Vincent JL, Russell JA, Jacob M, et al. Albumin administration in the acutely ill: what is new and where next? *Crit Care.* 2014;18(4):231.
59. Charpentier J, Mira JP; EARSS Study Group. Efficacy and tolerance of hyperoncotic albumin administration in septic shock patients: the EARSS study. *Intensive Care Med.* 2011;37(Suppl 1):315.
60. Caironi P, Tognoni G, Masson S, et al. Albumin replacement in patients with severe sepsis or septic shock. *N Engl J Med.* 2014;370(15):1412–1421.
61. Caironi P, Gattinoni L. Proposed benefits of albumin from the ALBIOS trial: a dose of insane belief. *Crit Care.* 2014;18(5):510.
62. Navickis RJ, Greenhalgh DG, Wilkes MM. Albumin in burn shock resuscitation: a meta-analysis of controlled clinical studies. *J Burn Care Res.* 2016;37(3):e268–e278.
63. Kitsios GD, Mascari P, Ettunsi R, et al. Co-administration of furosemide with albumin for overcoming diuretic resistance in patients with hypoalbuminemia: a meta-analysis. *J Crit Care.* 2014;29(2):253–259.
64. Uhlig C, Silva PL, Deckert S, et al. Albumin versus crystalloid solutions in patients with the acute respiratory distress syndrome: a systematic review and meta-analysis. *Crit Care.* 2014;18(1):R10.
65. Hartog C, Reinhart K. CONTRA: Hydroxyethyl starch solutions are unsafe in critically ill patients. *Intensive Care Med.* 2009;35(8):1337–1342.
66. Perner A, Haase N, Guttormsen AB, et al. Hydroxyethyl starch 130/0.42 versus Ringer's acetate in severe sepsis. *N Engl J Med.* 2012;367(2):124–134.

67. Dellinger RP, Levy MM, Rhodes A, et al. Surviving sepsis campaign: international guidelines for management of severe sepsis and septic shock: 2012. *Crit Care Med.* 2013;41(2):580–637.
68. Myburgh J, Cooper DJ, Finfer S, et al. Saline or albumin for fluid resuscitation in patients with traumatic brain injury. *N Engl J Med.* 2007;357(9):874–884.
69. Cooper DJ, Myburgh J, Heritier C, et al. Albumin resuscitation for traumatic brain injury: is intracranial hypertension the cause of increased mortality? *J Neurotrauma.* 2013;30(7):512–518.
70. Van Aken HK, Kampmeier TG, Ertmer C, et al. Fluid resuscitation in patients with traumatic brain injury: what is a SAFE approach? *Curr Opin Anaesthesiol.* 2012;25(5):563–565.
71. O'Brien AJ, Fullerton JN, Massey KA, et al. Immunosuppression in acutely decompensated cirrhosis is mediated by prostaglandin E2. *Nat Med.* 2014;20(5):518–523.
72. Bortoluzzi A, Ceolotto G, Gola E, et al. Positive cardiac inotropic effect of albumin infusion in rodents with cirrhosis and ascites: molecular mechanisms. *Hepatology.* 2013;57(1):266–276.
73. Zornow MH, Todd MM, Moore SS. The acute cerebral effects of changes in plasma osmolality and oncotic pressure. *Anesthesiology.* 1987;67:936–941.
74. Jungner M, Grande PO, Mattiasson G, et al. Effects on brain edema of crystalloid and albumin fluid resuscitation after brain trauma and hemorrhage in the rat. *Anesthesiology.* 2010;112(5):1194–1203.
75. Lira A, Pinsky MR. Choices in fluid type and volume during resuscitation: impact on patient outcomes. *Ann Intensive Care.* 2014;4:38.
76. Prough DS, Whitley JM, Taylor CL, et al. Regional cerebral blood flow following resuscitation from hemorrhagic shock with hypertonic saline: Influence of a subdural mass. *Anesthesiology.* 1991;75:319–327.
77. Prough DS, Whitley JM, Taylor CL, et al. Rebound intracranial hypertension in dogs after resuscitation with hypertonic solutions from hemorrhagic shock accompanied by an intracranial mass lesion. *J Neurosurg Anesth.* 1999;11:102–111.
78. Vassar MJ, Fischer RP, O'Brien PE, et al. A multicenter trial for resuscitation of injured patients with 7.5% sodium chloride: the effect of added dextran 70. *Arch Surg.* 1993;128:1003–1013.
79. Cooper DJ, Myles PS, McDermott FT, et al. Prehospital hypertonic saline resuscitation of patients with hypotension and severe traumatic brain injury: a randomized controlled trial. *JAMA.* 2004;291(11):1350–1357.
80. Chesnut RM. Avoidance of hypotension: condition sine qua non of successful severe head-injury management. *J Trauma.* 1997;42:S4–S9.
81. Bentsen G, Breivik H, Lundar T, et al. Predictable reduction of intracranial hypertension with hypertonic saline hydroxyethyl starch: a prospective clinical trial in critically ill patients with subarachnoid haemorrhage. *Acta Anaesthesiol Scand.* 2004;48(9):1089–1095.
82. Thongrong C, Kong N, Govindarajan B, et al. Current purpose and practice of hypertonic saline in neurosurgery: a review of the literature. *World Neurosurg.* 2014;82(6):1307–1318.
83. Forsyth LL, Liu-Deryke X, Parker D Jr, et al. Role of hypertonic saline for the management of intracranial hypertension after stroke and traumatic brain injury. *Pharmacotherapy.* 2008;28(4):469–484.
84. Wong DH, O'Connor D, Tremper KK, et al. Changes in cardiac output after acute blood loss and position change in man. *Crit Care Med.* 1989;17:979–983.
85. Marik PE, Cavallazzi R, Vasu T, et al. Dynamic changes in arterial waveform derived variables and fluid responsiveness in mechanically ventilated patients: a systematic review of the literature. *Crit Care Med.* 2009;379:2642–2647.
86. Renner J, Scholz J, Bein B. Monitoring fluid therapy. *Best Pract Res Clin Anaesthesiol.* 2009;23(2):159–171.
87. Thiele RH, Bartels K, Gan TJ. Inter-device differences in monitoring for goal-directed fluid therapy. *Can J Anaesth.* 2015;622:169–181.
88. Carsetti A, Cecconi M, Rhodes A. Fluid bolus therapy: monitoring and predicting fluid responsiveness. *Curr Opin Crit Care.* 2015;21(5):388–394.
89. Mythen MG, Webb AR. Perioperative plasma volume expansion reduces the incidence of gut mucosal hypoperfusion during cardiac surgery. *Arch Surg.* 1995;130:423–429.
90. Sinclair S, James S, Singer M. Intraoperative intravascular volume optimisation and length of hospital stay after repair of proximal femoral fracture: randomised controlled trial. *BMJ.* 1997;315(7113):909–912.
91. Gan TJ, Soppitt A, Maroof M, et al. Goal-directed intraoperative fluid administration reduces length of hospital stay after major surgery. *Anesthesiology.* 2002;97(4):820–826.
92. Madan AK, UyBarreta VV, Aliabadi-Wahle S, et al. Esophageal Doppler ultrasound monitor versus pulmonary artery catheter in the hemodynamic management of critically ill surgical patients. *J Trauma.* 1999;46:607–612.
93. DiCorte CJ, Latham P, Greilich PE, et al. Esophageal Doppler monitor determinations of cardiac output and preload during cardiac operations. *Ann Thorac Surg.* 2000;696.:1782–1786.
94. Venn R, Steele A, Richardson P, et al. Randomized controlled trial to investigate influence of the fluid challenge on duration of hospital stay and perioperative morbidity in patients with hip fractures. *Br J Anaesth.* 2002;88(1):65–71.
95. Horowitz P, Kumar A. It's the colloid, not the esophageal Doppler monitor. *Anesthesiology.* 2003;99:238–239.
96. Kern JW, Shoemaker WC. Meta-analysis of hemodynamic optimization in high-risk patients. *Crit Care Med.* 2002;30(8):1686–1692.
97. Otero RM, Nguyen HB, Huang DT, et al. Early goal-directed therapy in severe sepsis and septic shock revisited: concepts, controversies, and contemporary findings. *Chest.* 2006;130(5):1579–1595.
98. Lobo SM, Lobo FR, Polachini CA, et al. Prospective, randomized trial comparing fluids and dobutamine optimization of oxygen delivery in high-risk surgical patients. *Crit Care.* 2006;10(3):R72.
99. Balogh Z, McKinley BA, Cocanour CS, et al. Supranormal trauma resuscitation causes more cases of abdominal compartment syndrome. *Arch Surg.* 2003;138(6):637–642.
100. Young WF. Primary aldosteronism: renaissance of a syndrome. *Clin Endocrinol (Oxf).* 2007;66(5):607–618.
101. Karagiannis A, Tziomalos K, Papageorgiou A, et al. Spironolactone versus eplerenone for the treatment of idiopathic hyperaldosteronism. *Expert Opin Pharmacother.* 2008;9(4):509–515.
102. Corona G, Giuliani C, Parenti G, et al. The economic burden of hyponatremia: systematic review and meta-analysis. *Am J Med.* 2016.
103. Berardi R, Santoni M, Rinaldi S, et al. Risk of hyponatraemia in cancer patients treated with targeted therapies: a systematic review and meta-analysis of clinical trials. *PLoS One.* 2016;11(5):e0152079.
104. Wanchoo R, Jhaveri KD, Deray G, et al. Renal effects of BRAF inhibitors: a systematic review by the Cancer and the Kidney International Network. *Clin Kidney J.* 2016;9(2):245–251.
105. Lien YH, Shapiro JI. Hyponatremia: clinical diagnosis and management. *Am J Med.* 2007;120(8):653–658.
106. Pham PM, Pham PA, Pham SV, et al. Correction of hyponatremia and osmotic demyelinating syndrome: have we neglected to think intracellularly? *Clin Exp Nephrol.* 2015;19(3):489–495.
107. Kashyap AS. Hyperglycemia-induced hyponatremia: is it time to correct the correction factor? *Arch Intern Med.* 1999;159(22):2745–2746.
108. Gravenstein D. Transurethral resection of the prostate (TURP) syndrome: a review of the pathophysiology and management. *Anesth Analg.* 1997;84(2):438–446.
109. Xu DL, Martin PY, Ohara M, et al. Upregulation of aquaporin-2 water channel expression in chronic heart failure rat. *J Clin Invest.* 1997;99(7):1500–1505.
110. Fujita N, Ishikawa SE, Sasaki S, et al. Role of water channel AQP-CD in water retention in SIADH and cirrhotic rats. *Am J Physiol.* 1995;269(6Pt 2):F926–F931.
111. Verbalis JG, Goldsmith SR, Greenberg A, et al. Hyponatremia treatment guidelines 2007: expert panel recommendations. *Am J Med.* 2007;120(11 Suppl 1):S1–S21.
112. Christ-Crain M, Fenske W. Copeptin in the diagnosis of vasopressin-dependent disorders of fluid homeostasis. *Nat Rev Endocrinol.* 2016;12(3):168–176.
113. Christ-Crain M, Morgenthaler NG, Fenske W. Copeptin as a biomarker and a diagnostic tool in the evaluation of patients with polyuria-polydipsia and hyponatremia. *Best Pract Res Clin Endocrinol Metab.* 2016;30(2):235–247.
114. Katayama Y, Haraoka J, Hirabayashi H, et al. A randomized controlled trial of hydrocortisone against hyponatremia in patients with aneurysmal subarachnoid hemorrhage. *Stroke.* 2007;38(8):2373–2375.
115. Fraser CL, Arieff AI. Fatal central diabetes mellitus and insipidus resulting from untreated hyponatremia: a new syndrome. *Ann Intern Med.* 1990;112:113–119.
116. Arieff AI. Postoperative hyponatraemic encephalopathy following elective surgery in children. *Paediatr Anesth.* 1998;8:1–4.
117. Fenske W, Sandner B, Christ-Crain M. A copeptin-based classification of the osmoregulatory defects in the syndrome of inappropriate antidiuresis. *Best Pract Res Clin Endocrinol Metab.* 2016;30(2):219–233.
118. Cuesta M, Thompson CJ. The syndrome of inappropriate antidiuresis (SIAD). *Best Pract Res Clin Endocrinol Metab.* 2016;30(2):175–187.
119. Kumar S, Rubin S, Mather PJ, et al. Hyponatremia and vasopressin antagonism in congestive heart failure. *Clin Cardiol.* 2007;30(11):546–551.
120. Decaux G. V2-antagonists for the treatment of hyponatraemia. *Nephrol Dial Transplant.* 2007;22(7):1853–1855.
121. Cawley MJ. Hyponatremia: current treatment strategies and the role of vasopressin antagonists. *Ann Pharmacother.* 2007;41(5):840–850.
122. Madias NE. Effects of tolvaptan, an oral vasopressin V2 receptor antagonist, in hyponatremia. *Am J Kidney Dis.* 2007;50(2):184–187.
123. Schrier RW, Gross P, Gheorghiade M, et al. Tolvaptan, a selective oral vasopressin V2-receptor antagonist, for hyponatremia. *N Engl J Med.* 2006;355(20):2099–2112.
124. Rondon-Berrios H, Berl T. Vasopressin receptor antagonists: characteristics and clinical role. *Best Pract Res Clin Endocrinol Metab.* 2016;30(2):289–303.
125. Sterns RH, Silver SM. Complications and management of hyponatremia. *Curr Opin Nephrol Hypertens.* 2016;25(2):114–119.
126. Sterns RH. Disorders of plasma sodium: causes, consequences, and correction. *N Engl J Med.* 2015;372(1):55–65.
127. Biswas M, Davies JS. Hyponatraemia in clinical practice. *Postgrad Med J.* 2007;83(980):373–378.
128. Adrogué HJ, Madias NE. Aiding fluid prescription for the dysnatremias. *Intensive Care Med.* 1997;23:309–316.
129. Esposito P, Piotti G, Bianzina S, et al. The syndrome of inappropriate antidiuresis: pathophysiology, clinical management and new therapeutic options. *Nephron Clin Pract.* 2011;119(1):c62–c73.
130. Loh JA, Verbalis JG. Disorders of water and salt metabolism associated with pituitary disease. *Endocrinol Metab Clin North Am.* 2008;37(1):213–234, x.

131. Ayus JC, Armstrong DL, Arieff AI. Effects of hypernatraemia in the central nervous system and its therapy in rats and rabbits. *J Physiol*. 1996;492:243–255.
132. Adrogué HJ, Madias NE. Hypernatremia. *N Engl J Med*. 2000;342:1493–1499.
133. Liamis G, Kalogirou M, Saugos V, et al. Therapeutic approach in patients with dysnatraemias. *Nephrol Dial Transplant*. 2006;21(6):1564–1569.
134. Muhsin SA, Mount DB. Diagnosis and treatment of hypernatremia. *Best Pract Res Clin Endocrinol Metab*. 2016;30(2):189–203.
135. Adler SM, Verbalis JG. Disorders of body water homeostasis in critical illness. *Endocrinol Metab Clin North Am*. 2006;35(4):873–894, xi.
136. Sood MM, Sood AR, Richardson R. Emergency management and commonly encountered outpatient scenarios in patients with hyperkalemia. *Mayo Clin Proc*. 2007;82(12):1553–1561.
137. Gilligan P, Pountney A, Wilson B, et al. SOCRATES Episode II synopsis of Cochrane reviews applicable to emergency services Episode II): the return of series III. *Emerg Med J*. 2007;24(7):489–491.
138. Wahr JA, Parks R, Boisvert R, et al. Preoperative serum potassium levels and perioperative outcomes in cardiac surgery patients. *JAMA*. 1999;281:2203–2210.
139. Suga SI, Phillips MI, Ray PE, et al. Hypokalemia induces renal injury and alterations in vasoactive mediators that favor salt sensitivity. *Am J Physiol Renal Physiol*. 2001;281(4):F620–F629.
140. Lin SH, Halperin ML. Hypokalemia: a practical approach to diagnosis and its genetic basis. *Curr Med Chem*. 2007;14(14):1551–1565.
141. Khosla N, Hogan D. Mineralocorticoid hypertension and hypokalemia. *Semin Nephrol*. 2006;26(6):434–440.
142. Furgeson SB, Chonchol M. Beta-blockade in chronic dialysis patients. *Semin Dial*. 2008;21(1):43–48.
143. Gronert GA. Succinylcholine hyperkalemia after burns. *Anesthesiology*. 1999;91(1):320–322.
144. Sousa AG, Cabral JV, El-Feghaly WB, et al. Hyporeninemic hypoaldosteronism and diabetes mellitus: pathophysiology assumptions, clinical aspects and implications for management. *World J Diabetes*. 2016;7(5):101–111.
145. Kim HJ, Han SW. Therapeutic approach to hyperkalemia. *Nephron*. 2002;92 Suppl 1:33–40.
146. Putcha N, Allon M. Management of hyperkalemia in dialysis patients. *Semin Dial*. 2007;20(5):431–439.
147. Aggarwal S, Topaloglu H, Kumar S. Systematic review of hyperkalemia due to angiotensin enzyme converting inhibitors. *Value Health*. 2015;18(7):A396.
148. Zannad F, Rossignol P, Stough WG, et al. New approaches to hyperkalemia in patients with indications for renin angiotensin aldosterone inhibitors: considerations for trial design and regulatory approval. *Int J Cardiol*. 2016;216:46–51.
149. Rastogi A, Arman F, Alipourfetrati S. New agents in treatment of hyperkalemia: an opportunity to optimize use of RAAS inhibitors for blood pressure control and organ protection in patients with chronic kidney disease. *Curr Hypertens Rep*. 2016;18(7):55.
150. Sterns RH, Grieff M, Bernstein PL. Treatment of hyperkalemia: something old, something new. *Kidney Int*. 2016;89(3):546–554.
151. Yessayan L, Yee J, Frinak S, et al. continuous renal replacement therapy for the management of acid-base and electrolyte imbalances in acute kidney Injury. *Adv Chronic Kidney Dis*. 2016;23(3):203–210.
152. McDonald TJ, Oram RA, Vaidya B. Investigating hyperkalaemia in adults. *BMJ*. 2015;351:h4762.
153. Harel Z, Kamel KS. Optimal dose and method of administration of intravenous insulin in the management of emergency hyperkalemia: a systematic review. *PLoS One*. 2016;11(5):e0154963.
154. Mistry M, Shea A, Giguere P, et al. Evaluation of sodium polystyrene sulfonate dosing strategies in the inpatient management of hyperkalemia. *Ann Pharmacother*. 2016;50(6):455–462.
155. Shepard MM, Smith JW, III. Hypercalcemia. *Am J Med Sci*. 2007;334(5):381–385.
156. Slomp J, van der Voort PHJ, Gerritsen RT, et al. Albumin-adjusted calcium is not suitable for diagnosis of hyper-and hypocalcemia in the critically ill. *Crit Care Med*. 2003;31(5):1389–1393.
157. Brown EM, Pollak M, Hebert SC. The extracellular calcium-sensing receptor: its role in health and disease. *Annu Rev Med*. 1998;49:15–29.
158. Brown EM, Pollak M, Seidman CE, et al. Calcium-ion-sensing cell-surface receptors. *N Engl J Med*. 1995;333(4):234–240.
159. Bushinsky DA, Monk RD. Calcium. *Lancet*. 1998;352:306–311.
160. Blair JM, Zheng Y, Dunstan CR. RANK ligand. *Int J Biochem Cell Biol*. 2007;39(6):1077–1081.
161. Seo GH, Chai YJ, Choi HJ, et al. Incidence of permanent hypocalcaemia after total thyroidectomy with or without central neck dissection for thyroid carcinoma: a nationwide claim study. *Clin Endocrinol (Oxf)*. 2016;85(3):483–487.
162. Giancarelli A, Birrer KL, Alban RF, et al. Hypocalcemia in trauma patients receiving massive transfusion. *J Surg Res*. 2016;202(1):182–187.
163. Nardone R, Brigo F, Trinka E. Acute symptomatic seizures caused by electrolyte disturbances. *J Clin Neurol*. 2016;12(1):21–33.
164. Dickerson RN. Treatment of hypocalcemia in critical illness. Part 1. *Nutrition*. 2007;23(4):358–361.
165. Hod T, Riella LV, Chandraker A. Recombinant PTH therapy for severe hypoparathyroidism after kidney transplantation in pre-transplant parathyroidectomized patients: review of the literature and a case report. *Clin Transplant*. 2015;29(11):951–957.
166. Zojer N, Ludwig H. Hematological emergencies. *Ann Oncol*. 2007;18(Suppl 1):i45–i48.
167. Duan K, Gomez HK, Mete O. Clinicopathological correlates of hyperparathyroidism. *J Clin Pathol*. 2015;68(10):771–787.
168. Kane S, Borisov NN, Brixner D. Pharmacoeconomic evaluation of gastrointestinal tract events during treatment with risedronate or alendronate: a retrospective cohort study. *Am J Manag Care*. 2004;10(7):S216–S223.
169. Miller RG, Bolognese M, Worley K, et al. Incidence of gastrointestinal events among bisphosphonate patients in an observational setting. *Am J Manag Care*. 2004;10(7):S207–S215.
170. Valverde P. Pharmacotherapies to manage bone loss-associated diseases: a quest for the perfect benefit-to-risk ratio. *Curr Med Chem*. 2008;15(3):284–304.
171. Olszynski WP, Davison KS. Alendronate for the treatment of osteoporosis in men. *Expert Opin Pharmacother*. 2008;9(3):491–498.
172. Galindo RJ, Romao I, Valsamis A, et al. Hypercalcemia of malignancy and colorectal cancer. *World J Oncol*. 2016;7(1):5–12.
173. Singh Ospina NM, Rodriguez-Gutierrez R, Maraka S, et al. Outcomes of parathyroidectomy in patients with primary hyperparathyroidism: a systematic review and meta-analysis. *World J Surg*. 2016;40(10):2359–2377.
174. Ogata H, Koiwa F, Ito H, et al. Therapeutic strategies for secondary hyperparathyroidism in dialysis patients. *Ther Apher Dial*. 2006;10(4):355–363.
175. Shahapuni I, Monge M, Oprisiu R, et al. Drug Insight: renal indications of calcimimetics. *Nat Clin Pract Nephrol*. 2006;2(6):316–325.
176. Wuthrich RP, Martin D, Bilezikian JP. The role of calcimimetics in the treatment of hyperparathyroidism. *Eur J Clin Invest*. 2007;37(12):915–922.
177. Felsenfeld AJ, Levine BS. Milk alkali syndrome and the dynamics of calcium homeostasis. *Clin J Am Soc Nephrol*. 2006;1(4):641–654.
178. Kraft MD. Phosphorus and calcium: a review for the adult nutrition support clinician. *Nutr Clin Pract*. 2015;30(1):21–33.
179. Chang WT, Radin B, McCurdy MT. Calcium, magnesium, and phosphate abnormalities in the emergency department. *Emerg Med Clin North Am*. 2014;32(2):349–366.
180. Giovannini I, Chiarla C, Nuzzo G. Pathophysiologic and clinical correlates of hypophosphatemia and the relationship with sepsis and outcome in postoperative patients after hepatectomy. *Shock*. 2002;18(2):111–115.
181. Brooks MJ, Melnik G. The refeeding syndrome: an approach to understanding its complications and preventing its occurrence. *Pharmacology*. 1995;15:713–726.
182. Konstantinov NK, Rohrscheib M, Agaba EI, et al. Respiratory failure in diabetic ketoacidosis. *World J Diabetes*. 2015;6(8):1009–1023.
183. Paleologos M, Stone E, Braude S. Persistent, progressive hypophosphataemia after voluntary hyperventilation. *Clin Sci (Lond)*. 2000;98(5):619–625.
184. Liamis G, Filippatos TD, Elisaf MS. Electrolyte disorders associated with the use of anticancer drugs. *Eur J Pharmacol*. 2016;777:78–87.
185. Burke SK. Phosphate is a uremic toxin. *J Ren Nutr*. 2008;18(1):27–32.
186. Gums JG. Magnesium in cardiovascular and other disorders. *Am J Health Syst Pharm*. 2004;61(15):1569–1576.
187. Dube L, Granry JC. The therapeutic use of magnesium in anesthesiology, intensive care and emergency medicine: a review. *Can J Anaesth*. 2003;50(7):732–746.
188. Choi JH, Lee J, Park CM. Magnesium therapy improves thromboelastographic findings before liver transplantation: a preliminary study. *Can J Anaesth*. 2005;52(2):156–159.
189. Lysakowski C, Dumont L, Czarnetzki C, et al. Magnesium as an adjuvant to postoperative analgesia: a systematic review of randomized trials. *Anesth Analg*. 2007;104(6):1532–1539, table.
190. Van De Water JM, van den Bergh WM, Hoff RG, et al. Hypocalcaemia may reduce the beneficial effect of magnesium treatment in aneurysmal subarachnoid haemorrhage. *Magnes Res*. 2007;20(2):130–135.
191. van den Bergh WM, Algra A, Rinkel GJ. Electrocardiographic abnormalities and serum magnesium in patients with subarachnoid hemorrhage. *Stroke*. 2004;35(3):644–648.
192. Soliman HM, Mercan D, Lobo SS, et al. Development of ionized hypomagnesemia is associated with higher mortality rates. *Crit Care Med*. 2003;31(4):1082–1087.
193. Tzivoni D, Banai S, Schuger C, et al. Treatment of torsade de pointes with magnesium sulfate. *Circulation*. 1988;77:392–397.
194. Wilkes NJ, Mallett SV, Peachey T, et al. Correction of ionized plasma magnesium during cardiopulmonary bypass reduces the risk of postoperative cardiac arrhythmia. *Anesth Analg*. 2002;95(4):828–834.
195. Agus ZS. Mechanisms and causes of hypomagnesemia. *Curr Opin Nephrol Hypertens*. 2016;25(4):301–307.
196. Janett S, Camozzi P, Peeters GG, et al. Hypomagnesemia induced by long-term treatment with proton-pump inhibitors. *Gastroenterol Res Pract*. 2015;2015:951768.

17 Hemostasis and Transfusion Medicine

LOUANNE M. CARABINI • GLENN RAMSEY

Introduction
Hemostasis and Coagulation
   Primary Hemostasis
   Secondary Hemostasis
   Fibrinolysis
Laboratory Evaluation of Hemostasis
   Laboratory Evaluation of Primary Hemostasis
   Laboratory Evaluation of Secondary Hemostasis and Coagulation
   Viscoelastic Testing
   Diagnosis of Thromboembolic Disorders
   Monitoring Anticoagulation Therapeutic Agents
Blood Component Production
   Blood Collection
   Component Processing and Storage
   Plasma Derivatives
   Pathogen Inactivation
   RBC and Platelet Substitutes
Blood Products and Transfusion Thresholds
   Compatibility Testing
   Red Blood Cells
   Platelets
   Plasma Products
   Cryoprecipitate
   Fibrinogen Concentrate
The Risks of Blood Product Administration
   Infectious Risks of Blood Product Administration
   Noninfectious Risks of Blood Product Administration
Blood Conservation Strategies
   Autologous Blood Transfusion
Disorders of Hemostasis: Diagnosis and Treatment
   Disorders of Primary Hemostasis
   Disorders of Secondary Hemostasis
   Hereditary Hypercoagulability
   Acquired Disorders of Hemostasis
Anticoagulation and Pharmacologic Therapy
   Anticoagulation Regimens and Associated Anesthetic Concerns
   Recombinant Activated Factor VII
   Prothrombin Complex Concentrates
   Desmopressin
   Antifibrinolytic Therapy
Conclusions

KEY POINTS

1. Modern transfusion medicine focuses on patient-centered blood component therapy.
2. Blood must not only be maintained as a fluid in normal circulation, but also be capable of forming a solid clot to stanch leaks in the vascular wall, and then dismantling the clot when the need has passed.
3. Clotting factors in the plasma are activated at sites of endothelial injury and assemble in enzymatic complexes to activate thrombin.
4. Fibrin clots must be broken down after their job is done, and fibrinolysis is a complex process with checks and balances.
5. The first screening test for hemostatic problems should always be the patient's medical history.
6. Platelet aggregation is the most detailed overall platelet function test (PFT).
7. A general oversight of plasma clotting factor activity is obtained by the prothrombin time (PT) for the extrinsic (tissue) pathway and the activated partial thromboplastin time (aPTT) for the intrinsic (contact) pathway.
8. Disseminated intravascular coagulopathy (DIC) describes unchecked coagulation initiated by pathologic systemic activation of the intrinsic clotting pathway.
9. The risk for venous thromboembolism is increased by intercurrent factors such as physical inactivity or immobilization, malignancy, oral contraceptives, estrogen therapy, and pregnancy.
10. Most anticoagulant therapies need ongoing or selective testing for assessment of therapeutic effect.
11. Leukoreduction (LR) to remove WBCs from red blood cells (RBCs) and platelets reduces the risk of HLA alloimmunization, febrile nonhemolytic transfusion reactions (FNHTRs), and CMV transmission in patients who require these precautions.
12. Plasma derivatives are proteins processed from plasma for therapeutic infusions.
13. Techniques have been developed to kill microbial pathogens in blood components.
14. Many years of effort have gone into the search for an oxygen-carrying substitute for RBCs.
15. Routine RBC compatibility testing includes ABO and RhD typing, an antibody screen for IgG non-ABO RBC antibodies, and an RBC cross-match.
16. Over the past decade, transfusion practices for medical and surgical patients shifted from a liberal strategy to more restrictive management with lower thresholds and careful consideration of the balance between transfusion risks and the physiologic consequences of anemia.
17. Oxygen delivery to the tissues (DO_2) is dependent on cardiac output (CO), regional blood flow, and oxygen-carrying capacity, also known as the oxygen content (CaO_2) of blood.
18. Numerous recommendations provide guidance for the transfusion management of thrombocytopenia and acquired or inherited platelet disorders.

19. Cryoprecipitate is created by a controlled thaw of frozen plasma, which allows for precipitation of large molecules, most notably fibrinogen and vWF.
20. Over the past few decades, the risk–benefit ratio of blood product transfusion has been the subject of several studies and review articles.
21. Given the extensive use of more sensitive methods for screening and controlling the infectious risks of blood product transfusion, noninfectious complications have emerged as the major source of transfusion-related morbidity and mortality.
22. Transfusion-related acute lung injury (TRALI) is a clinical diagnosis that can be clouded by confounding comorbidities or patient acuity; therefore, TRALI tends to be underreported in the literature and is extremely difficult, if not impossible, to study with randomized prospective clinical trials.
23. Preoperative autologous donation programs are most effective when double units are donated with ample time for erythrogenesis prior to the date of surgery.
24. Over the past decade, RBC salvage techniques have improved drastically and now offer an efficient, cost-effective, and safe method for perioperative blood conservation.
25. Disorders of hemostasis can be classified as those that cause a propensity for hemorrhage and those that facilitate inappropriate thrombosis.
26. Symptomatically, disorders of primary hemostasis often present with superficial signs of bleeding on the skin or mucosa.
27. Von Willebrand disease (vWD) is the most common hereditary bleeding disorder, with a prevalence of approximately 1% in the general population.
28. Hemophilia is a genetic disease that results from deficiencies or dysfunction of specific clotting factors.
29. Antiplatelet therapy is indicated for patients at risk for cerebral vascular accident, myocardial infarction, or other vascular thrombosis complications.
30. Heparin-induced thrombocytopenia (HIT) is a clinical disorder that develops after extended use of heparin therapy. It occurs in approximately 1% to 5% of patients receiving heparin and is associated with morbidity from thromboembolic complications.
31. Recombinant activated factor VII (rFVIIa) is only indicated for the treatment of hemophiliacs with inhibitors/antibodies and factor VII deficiency.
32. Prothrombin complex concentrates are now the drug of choice for emergent reversal of warfarin in place of rFVIIa and fresh frozen plasma (FFP).
33. Antifibrinolytic agents have been used to prevent and treat surgical blood loss for several decades.

Introduction

Recent focus on quality, safety, and cost effectiveness in health care extends into the practice of transfusion medicine. Patient-centered blood management emphasizes the use of evidence-based decisions and blood conservation strategies. There continues to be significant variability in blood product transfusion practices despite consistent guidelines from experts and task forces from the American Society of Anesthesiologists (ASA), the American Association of Blood Banks (AABB), the Society of Cardiac Anesthesiologists (SCA), and the Society of Critical Care Medicine (SCCM).[1,2] Restrictive transfusion practices continue to demonstrate improved outcomes with noninferior or reduced morbidity and mortality; however, it remains unclear which patient characteristics determine the appropriate transfusion goal for a given health-care situation. Therefore, it is imperative for the anesthesia provider to understand the treatment benefits, the rare and common adverse effects, and the specific therapeutic details of blood product preparation, conservation, and delivery in order to best manage their patients.

This chapter begins with a review of primary and secondary hemostasis, fibrinolysis, and regulation of the coagulation pathway. We continue with a description of the most common coagulation profile tests, followed by the method for blood product collection and storage. The therapeutic indications and risks associated with blood component therapy are discussed at length. The chapter also includes extensive clinical sections discussing congenital and acquired deficiencies in hemostasis and coagulation, as well as an up-to-date presentation of available pharmacologic treatment medications to maintain a balanced hemostatic mechanism.

Hemostasis and Coagulation

Primary Hemostasis

Blood must not only be maintained as a fluid in normal circulation, but also be capable of forming a solid clot to stanch leaks in the vascular wall, and then dismantling the clot when the need has passed. This delicate equilibrium between anticoagulation and coagulation is maintained by a complex system of counterbalanced blood proteins and cells (platelets). Many congenital and acquired disorders can push the system toward either bleeding or thrombosis. The patient care team has a number of tests to evaluate the system, and many therapeutic modalities to correct these imbalances.

Platelets adhere to sites of endothelial disruption, undergo activation to recruit more platelets and amplify the platelet response, and then cross-link with fibrin, the end product of the plasma clotting factor cascade, to form a platelet plug. *Primary hemostasis* (Fig. 17-1) describes the initiation of the platelet plug and clotting mechanism.

Adherence

When the endothelial lining is disrupted to expose the underlying matrix, platelets attach to collagen via surface integrin

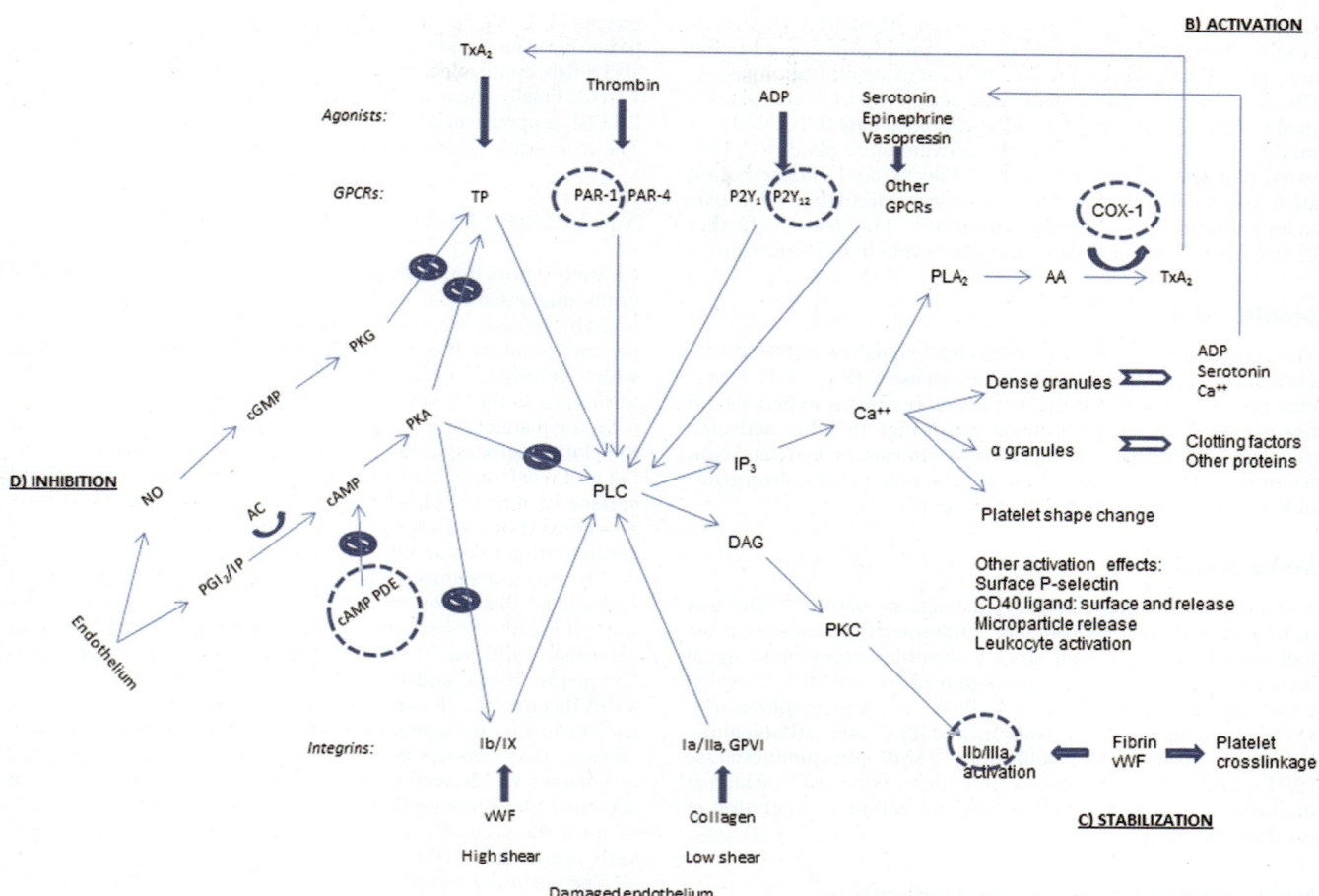

Figure 17-1 Overview of platelet pathways for adherence, activation, stabilization, and physiologic inhibition. Many pathway intermediaries and other elements are not shown, but are reviewed elsewhere.[3,5] *Thin arrows:* signaling pathways. *Thick arrows:* ligand binding. *Curved arrows:* catalysis. *Clear arrows:* secretion. *Slashed circles:* inhibitory signaling pathways. *Round circles:* antiplatelet drug targets. (**A**) Adherence. vWF, von Willebrand factor. Glycoproteins Ib/IX, Ia/IIa, and VI. (**B**) Activation. Agonists: TxA_2, thromboxane A_2; ADP, adenosine diphosphate. Receptors: GPCR, G-protein–coupled receptor; TP, thromboxane prostanoid; PAR, protease-activated receptor. Intermediaries: PLC, phospholipase C; IP_3, inositol-1,4,5-triphosphate; DAG, diacylglycerol; PKC, protein kinase C; Ca^{2+}, calcium; PLA_2, phospholipase A_2; AA, arachidonic acid; COX, cyclooxygenase. (**C**) Stabilization. Glycoprotein IIb/IIIa. (**D**) Inhibition. NO, nitric oxide; PGI_2, prostaglandin I_2 (prostacyclin); IP, PGI_2 receptor; AC, adenylate cyclase; cAMP, cyclic adenosine monophosphate; PDE, phosphodiesterase; cGMP, cyclic guanosine monophosphate; PKA, protein kinase A; PKG, protein kinase G. Targets of antiplatelet drugs. COX-1: aspirin, triflusal. $P2Y_{12}$: clopidogrel, prasugrel, ticlopidine, cangrelor, ticagrelor. cAMP PDE: dipyridamole, cilostazol. IIb/IIIa: abciximab, eptifibatide, tirofiban.

receptors—glycoproteins (GP) Ia/IIa and GP VI (Fig. 17-1A). Collagen adherence is favored in low-shear conditions such as venous circulation.[3] In high-shear arterial blood flow, von Willebrand factor (vWF) from endothelial cells and from pre-existing clot binds to integrin Ib/IX, the other major adherence anchor.[4] In capillary blood flow, platelets are pushed to the periphery by red blood cells (RBCs), so anemia lessens platelet contact and reduces platelet function.[3]

Activation

Platelet activation can be mediated by numerous signaling pathways from the platelet surface (Fig. 17-1B). In "outside-in" signaling, a central target is phospholipase C (PLC). The above adherence integrins trigger pathways to activate PLC.[3] Another set of surface receptors, G-protein–coupled receptors (GPCRs), are activated by an array of corresponding agonists, including thrombin from the factor clotting cascade, adenosine diphosphate (ADP), thromboxane A_2 (TxA_2), serotonin, epinephrine, and vasopressin. Each of these agonist–GPCR pairings set off activation pathways for PLC as well.[5]

Activated PLC leads to several structural changes in the platelets. Via inositol-1,4,5-triphosphate (IP_3), calcium (Ca^{2+}) is released from storage tubules. Calcium ions catalyze release of dense granules and α-granules at the platelet surface. These granules contain ADP, serotonin, and more Ca^{2+}, all of which can activate more platelets.[3] The α-granules contain numerous proteins, including factor V, fibrinogen, and platelet factor 4 (PF4), which promotes clotting by binding and neutralizing heparin-like compounds and heparin.[3] (This heparin–PF4 complex is the target antigen for the antibodies causing heparin-induced thrombocytopenia [HIT], discussed in depth later in this chapter.)

Calcium also facilitates rearrangement of the platelet microskeleton to change the platelet shape from round and discoid to flat and spiky. Furthermore, the Ca^{2+} helps activate phospholipase A_2 (PLA_2), which releases arachidonic acid (AA) from the platelet membrane. AA, as catalyzed by cyclooxygenase-1 (COX-1), is modified to TxA_2, which can then activate more platelets.[4] Activated platelets also have surface P-selectin and surface-bound and released CD40 ligand. They also release circulating microparticles and attract and activate leukocytes; these features further contribute to hemostasis and also play a role in inflammation.[3]

Stabilization

The activated PLC initiates "inside-out" signaling of GP IIb/IIIa via diacylglycerol (DAG) and protein kinase C (Fig. 17-1C). This changes the shape of GP IIb/IIIa, which permits it to better bind fibrin and vWF. These proteins can bridge to other activated platelets.[4] The fibrin binding can also enmesh the platelets, contributing to the formation of the platelet plug in the convergence of the platelet and clotting factor systems.

Inhibition

To maintain hemostatic balance, platelets are naturally inhibited in their endothelial environment. Endothelial cells secrete prostaglandin I_2 (PGI_2), which binds to a surface receptor to signal increased cyclic adenosine monophosphate (cAMP). Elevated cAMP activates protein kinase A (PKA), a multisite inhibitor of vWF adherence, TxA_2 activation, and PLC internal signaling. However, cAMP is metabolized by cAMP phosphodiesterase (PDE). Endothelial cells also secrete nitric oxide (NO), which at high levels initiates a signaling pathway leading to inhibition of the TxA_2 receptor.[5]

Mechanisms of Antiplatelet Medications

Figure 17-1 shows the sites of action for current antiplatelet medications.[6] No drugs are available to counteract the first step, platelet adherence (Fig. 17-1A). Aspirin and triflusal dampen the secretion of TxA_2 by inhibiting COX-1, the enzyme which converts AA into TxA_2 (Fig. 17-1B). Another agonist, ADP, has its $P2Y_{12}$ receptor blocked by clopidogrel and several other drugs. The protease-activated receptor-1 (PAR-1) for thrombin activation is blocked by vorapaxar. Formation and stabilization of the platelet plug is blocked by abciximab, eptifibatide, and tirofiban, which act at GP IIb/IIIa (Fig. 17-1C). Finally, the major inhibitory pathway mediated by endothelial PGI_2 is upregulated by dipyridamole and cilostazol (Fig. 17-1D).[6] These medications are discussed later in this chapter.

Secondary Hemostasis

Clotting factors in the plasma are activated at sites of endothelial injury and assemble in enzymatic complexes to activate thrombin. This *initiates* secondary hemostasis. Thrombin then *amplifies* production of itself by activating other more efficient enzymes, which *propagate* a thrombin burst. Thrombin also converts fibrinogen to fibrin, which cross-links with activated platelets to form the platelet plug. Each of the three enzymatic complexes in the clotting process consists of four parts: an enzyme in the serine protease family, a cofactor, a plasma membrane phospholipid surface such as the platelet, and calcium ion (Ca^{2+}). The proteases convert other clotting factors from their inactive circulating configuration to an active form (termed [factor number] a).[7]

The extrinsic pathway (Fig. 17-2). The process begins when endothelial disruption exposes tissue factor (TF) on underlying cell membranes extrinsic to the circulation—hence the term "extrinsic pathway." TF binds both VII and VIIa, which circulate at low levels, and is a cofactor for the activation of factor VII. VIIa enzyme, TF cofactor, cell membrane phospholipid, and Ca^{2+} form the first complex, a low-efficiency extrinsic-pathway "tenase" that activates factor X and factor IX. Then Xa enzyme, its cofactor Va (derived in large part from factor V released from activated platelet α-granules), phospholipid, and Ca^{2+} assemble to form the second complex, a "prothrombinase," which converts prothrombin (II) to thrombin (IIa).[7]

The intrinsic pathway (Fig. 17-2). Thrombin has several central functions. It activates platelets via surface receptors PAR-1 and PAR-4 (see Primary Hemostasis), cleaves more V to Va, and initiates the "intrinsic" (intravascular) coagulation pathway by cleaving factor XI to XIa. XIa cleaves more IX to IXa. Thrombin also activates VIII to VIIIa. (VIII is carried and stabilized in the plasma by vWF until needed, so vWF deficiency also results in low plasma VIII levels.) The third complex is then formed: IXa

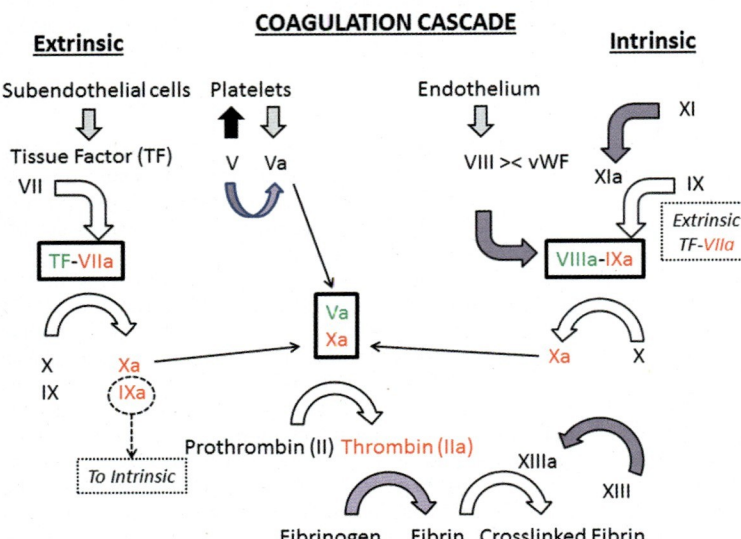

Figure 17-2 Schematic diagram of the coagulation cascade of clotting factors, with extrinsic, intrinsic, and common pathways. Von Willebrand factor (vWF) and factor VIII circulate together (><). *Gray arrows:* secretion. *Red:* vitamin K–dependent factors. *Green:* cofactors. *Purple arrows:* thrombin activation. *Black arrow:* uptake. *Dotted lines:* intrinsic–extrinsic crossover. *Solid boxes:* also Ca++ and platelet phospholipid.

enzyme, VIIIa cofactor, phospholipid, and Ca^{2+}. This is a high-efficiency intrinsic-pathway "tenase," which provides many times more Xa for more prothrombinase complex. Ultimately, thrombin cleaves fibrinogen to fibrin monomers, which then polymerize extensively. Fibrin polymers are cross-linked by factor XIIIa (also activated by thrombin) to form the stable fibrin clot. Fibrin also cross-links activated platelets by their GP IIb/IIIa receptors to enmesh platelets and fibrin in the platelet plug (see Primary Hemostasis).[7]

All of these clotting factors are primarily produced in the liver, except for VIII, which is also released by endothelial cells and is well maintained in liver disease. The plasma half-life of most clotting factors is around 1.5 to 3 days, except for the initiating factor VII (6 hours) and the cofactors V and VIII (8 to 12 hours), which are much shorter. Four critical enzyme factors—VII in the extrinsic tenase, IX in the intrinsic tenase, X in the prothrombinase, and prothrombin (II)—must be carboxylated at multiple glutamic acid residues after translation, in order to interact with phospholipid and Ca^{2+}. Vitamin K in its reduced form is the cofactor for the glutamyl-carboxylase enzyme, and thus these four factors (II, VII, IX, X) are vitamin K–dependent.[7]

Inhibition of Clotting Factors

The clotting pathways have three main regulatory inhibitors (Fig. 17-3)[3-5,7,8]:

1. TF pathway inhibitor (TFPI) inhibits the external tenase complex by binding to the VIIa protease and to its Xa product. TFPI is produced in endothelial cells, and its release is stimulated by heparin. Heparin in turn binds to and raises the inhibitory efficiency of TFPI.
2. Antithrombin-III (AT-III) is a serine protease inhibitor or serpin. Serpins disrupt the active sites and increase the clearance of their target proteases. AT-III inhibits proteases in all clotting pathways: VIIa in extrinsic tenase, Xa in prothrombinase, XIa and IXa in the intrinsic tenase pathway, and thrombin. AT-III's inhibitory function is greatly increased when bound to heparin.
3. Protein C-ase is an enzymatic complex with the same four-part structure as the coagulation complexes above:

an enzyme, thrombin, its cofactor thrombomodulin, phospholipid, and Ca^{2+}. Thrombomodulin is expressed on endothelial cell membranes. In the protein C-ase complex, thrombin cleaves and activates protein C. Activated protein C (APC) brakes clotting by cleaving VIIIa and Va, the cofactors for the external tenase and the prothrombinase complexes. Protein C has a short half-life of 6 hours. Protein S is thought to be a cofactor for protein C; both are vitamin K–dependent.[7]

Fibrinolysis

Fibrin clots must be broken down after their job is done (fibrinolysis), and is a complex process with checks and balances. Plasminogen is activated to plasmin, which breaks down fibrin polymers (Fig. 17-4).[9] The major activator of plasminogen in the blood is tissue plasminogen activator (tPA), which is secreted from endothelial cells and platelets. Both plasminogen and tPA bind to lysine sites on fibrin. When associated with cross-linked fibrin, tPA becomes much more efficient. Once some plasmin is formed, it cleaves tPA to a more active form. tPA also directly cleaves fibrin polymers.

In tissues, urokinase is the main plasminogen activator. Urokinase is secreted from the endothelium, monocytes, macrophages, and urinary epithelium. These cells also bind plasminogen with two receptors, the annexin A2 complex and the urokinase receptor, which facilitate its conversion to plasmin. Plasmin also activates urokinase to a more active form. Urokinase and tPA can be administered as medications to lyse thrombi.

Inhibition of Fibrinolysis

Plasminogen activation inhibitor-1 (PAI-1) is a serpin which binds to tPA and urokinase and accelerates their clearance from plasma (Fig. 17-4). Activated platelets release PAI-1 from α-granules. PAI-2, which acts similarly to PAI-1, is secreted by the placenta and is prominent in pregnancy. Thrombin-activated fibrinolysis inhibitor (TAFI) is secreted from endothelial cells and is activated by the thrombin–thrombomodulin

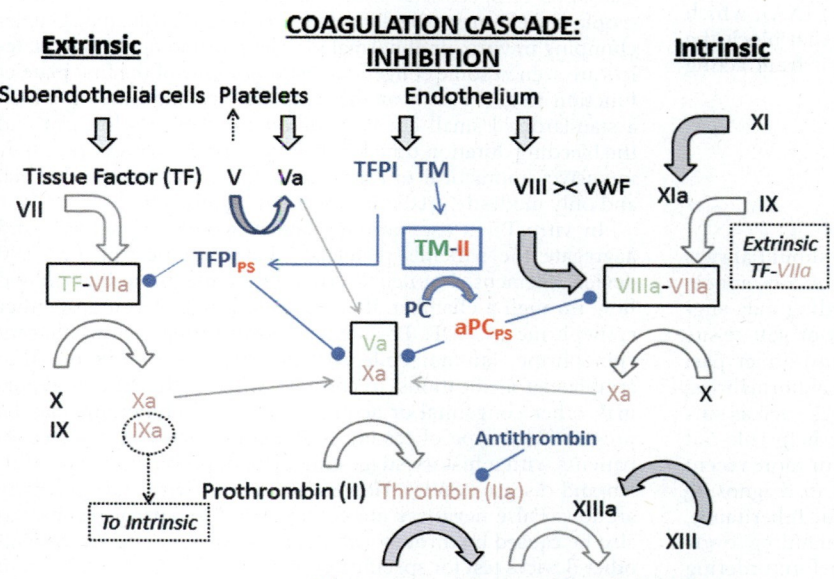

Figure 17-3 Schematic diagram of inhibitory control of the coagulation cascade. *Purple arrows:* thrombin activation. *Blue circle-head arrows:* inhibition. TM, thrombomodulin; TFPI, tissue factor pathway inhibitor. *Red:* vitamin K–dependent factors. *Green:* cofactor.

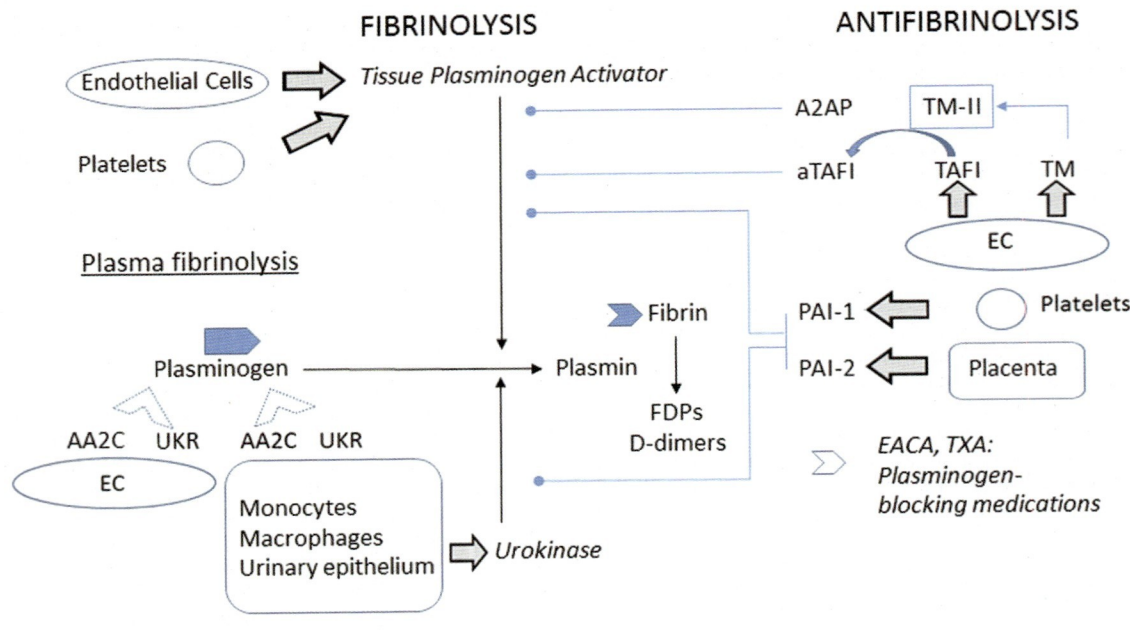

Figure 17-4 Fibrinolysis and antifibrinolysis pathways. AA2C, annexin A2 complex; A2AP, α-2-antiplasmin; EACA, epsilon-aminocaproic acid; EC, endothelial cells; FDPs, fibrin degradation products; PAI, plasminogen activator inhibitor; (a)TAFI, (activated) thrombin-activated fibrinolysis inhibitor; TM, thrombomodulin; II, factor II (thrombin); TXA, tranexamic acid; UKR, urokinase receptor. *Gray arrows*: secretion. *Black arrows*: enzyme activation. *Curved arrow*: thrombin activation. *Round-headed lines*: inhibition. *Dotted angles*: AA2C and UKR cell-membrane receptors binding to plasminogen. *Solid pentagon* on plasminogen: lysine-binding sites attaching to fibrin. *Solid chevron* on fibrin: lysines to which plasminogen binds. *Clear chevron*: antifibrinolytic medications blocking the lysine-binding sites on plasminogen. *Italics*: pharmacologic therapies promoting (tPA, urokinase) or inhibiting (EACA, TXA) fibrinolysis.

complex. TAFI cleaves fibrin and fibrin polymers in a fashion that inhibits the action of tPA, and TAFI also inhibits the action of plasmin on fibrin. α_2-Antiplasmin binds to plasmin and blocks its action, although this also slows the metabolism of plasmin.

Fibrinolysis is inhibited pharmacologically by epsilon-aminocaproic acid (EACA) and tranexamic acid (TXA), which stabilize clots. These drugs are lysine analogues that block the lysine-binding sites of plasminogen, preventing it from acting on fibrin.

Laboratory Evaluation of Hemostasis

[5] The first screening test for hemostatic problems should always be the patient's medical history.[10] The nature of any abnormal bleeding is helpful; dermal or mucosal bleeding may suggest platelet dysfunction, whereas hemarthroses or soft tissue bleeding suggests factor deficiencies. Besides any direct past history of bleeding, thrombosis, or laboratory abnormalities, the patient's experience with hemostatic challenges such as surgery, dental procedures, and menstruation may help rule-out clinical problems or suggest a lifelong congenital or more recent acquired disorder. The family history is helpful in diagnosing a congenital problem and the possible pattern of inheritance. Anticoagulants and antiplatelet medications, including over-the-counter drugs, should always be reviewed before ordering laboratory analysis.

Laboratory Evaluation of Primary Hemostasis

The normal automated platelet count in adults is approximately 150,000 to 400,000/µL. The peripheral blood smear should be examined in specimens with abnormal platelet counts. Microscopic review may reveal clotted specimens, artifactual platelet clumping in vitro, or abnormal platelet morphology. Large platelets are seen in some congenital disorders. One of the first platelet function tests (PFTs) was the template bleeding time, in which a standardized small cut is made on the subject's forearm and the bleeding duration timed. However, this test is invasive, labor-intensive, impractical to repeat frequently, poorly reproducible, and only modestly predictive for bleeding problems.

In vitro PFTs use various platelet agonists to activate and aggregate the patient's platelets.[11] For example, the PFA-100 device (Siemens, Munich, Germany) simulates capillary blood flow through a chamber after activation by collagen and either epinephrine or ADP. Prolonged "closure time" with collagen/epinephrine, but not collagen/ADP, suggests aspirin or other antiplatelet medications. In contrast, when both pairs are abnormal, other congenital or acquired platelet dysfunctions may be present. This type of testing is sometimes used as a screen in patients with a history suggesting platelet problems or von Willebrand disease (vWD). However, the sensitivity and specificity are low. False negatives are common and abnormal results can also be caused by thrombocytopenia, uremia, or anemia. Several other devices test for specific antiplatelet medication effects from aspirin or $P2Y_{12}$ inhibitors.[11]

6   Platelet aggregation is the most detailed overall PFT. Platelets are tested with multiple isolated agonists to assess their patterns of physical aggregation and, in turn, the platelets' own agonist release. Some uncommon congenital disorders lack responses to specific agonists in a characteristic fashion. More detailed testing may be needed for a specific diagnosis, such as electron microscopy for granule defects, flow cytometry for surface receptors and granule markers, or genetic testing.[12]

vWD is a factor deficiency with clinical features of platelet dysfunction, due to the central role of vWF in cross-linking activated platelets to form the platelet plug.[13] Up to 1% of all patients have vWD, with a wide range of severity due to either quantitative or functional defects of vWF. Diagnostic testing is integral to deciphering the specific defect and type of vWD to ensure the appropriate treatment. Since vWF is the carrier for factor VIII (FVIII) in plasma, vWF protein levels usually correlate with FVIII levels. Initial testing for vWD should include the vWF antigen level, vWF activity level, and FVIII activity level for comparison with vWF. Blood group O persons have shorter plasma half-life and lower normal levels of vWF, so ABO blood typing is needed to interpret a borderline vWF level. Type 1 vWD is a quantitative deficiency, with decreased antigen and activity. Type 2 vWD may have normal antigen levels, but decreased activity from a defective protein. Within type 2, there are several subtypes with different molecular defects, and specialized identification is needed in order to determine the best therapy. Type 3 vWD is a rare, very severe autosomal recessive deficiency.[13] Acquired vWD occurs through removal of vWF from the plasma by adsorption to paraproteins or high number of platelets (hematologic disorders), autoantibodies to vWF, or depletion by turbulent blood flow in congenital heart disease, dysfunctional heart valves, and left ventricular assist devices.[14] The clinical features and management of vWD are discussed later in this chapter.

Laboratory Evaluation of Secondary Hemostasis and Coagulation

7   A general oversight of plasma clotting factor activity is obtained by the *prothrombin time (PT)* for the extrinsic (tissue) pathway and the *aPTT* for the intrinsic (contact) pathway (Fig. 17-2), with both tests relevant to the common pathway.[10] These clotting tests are performed in blood specimens collected in a chelator (3.2% citrate), which binds Ca^{2+} to prevent clotting in the tube. The in vitro clotting test is activated by TF in the PT, or by negatively charged surfaces in the aPTT, using phospholipid as a platform (substituting for platelets). Ca^{2+} is then added to overcome the specimen chelation, and the time until complete fibrin clotting is measured. Representative normal ranges are around 12 to 15 seconds for the PT and 25 to 35 seconds for the aPTT, but are defined by each laboratory using its own equipment, reagents, and normal specimens. Testing is routinely performed at 37°C, but hypothermia in the patient impairs the enzymatic reactions of clot formation.

Clotting physiology is more complicated than the traditional diagrams of separate cascade pathways for these two tests. For example, thrombin from the extrinsic pathway can activate the intrinsic pathway. In vitro, the aPTT clotting test is activated by synthetic contact materials that initiate via factor XII, so deficiencies of XII and other related contact factors cause a prolonged aPTT. However, deficiencies of these contact factors do not cause bleeding and may be associated with impaired fibrinolysis and thrombosis. Fibrinogen activity is also a critical parameter. Most assays measure the functional conversion of fibrinogen to fibrin, although the fibrinogen protein level can also be measured for comparison to assess fibrinogen dysfunction. Normal fibrinogen levels are around 150 to 400 mg/dL.

Mixing Studies

To investigate elevated PT or aPTT values, the test should be repeated after mixing the patient's plasma with equal volumes of normal plasma. Even in severe factor deficiencies, the PT or aPTT shows substantial correction toward normal in a mixing study. However, if the patient's plasma contains an inhibitor or an anticoagulant, the normal plasma will also be affected and the PT or aPTT will not be corrected.

Individual factor level activities are determined by the degree of correction observed when patient plasma is mixed with factor-deficient plasma. The classic congenital factor deficiencies are FVIII deficiency (hemophilia A) and factor IX deficiency (hemophilia B). Both are X-linked and thus nearly always in males. Factor XI deficiency is most often seen in persons of Ashkenazi Jewish descent. Acquired factor deficiencies usually involve multiple factors.[15] The vitamin K–dependent factors are II (thrombin), VII, IX, and X. In liver disease, all-factor synthesis is deficient except FVIII, which also comes from endothelium. However, FVIII and other factors can be low in disseminated intravascular coagulation (DIC). As noted, FVIII may be low as part of vWD. Isolated factor X deficiency occurs in some patients with amyloidosis because the abnormal protein absorbs this factor. Assessing factors V (liver disease), VII (liver disease or vitamin K deficiency), and VIII (consumption) may suggest a pattern to aid in the diagnosis of specific clinical syndromes.

Coagulation inhibitors are substances, usually antibodies, that block one or more clotting factors. Most do not cause bleeding; the most common examples are lupus anticoagulants (LAs), a type of antiphospholipid antibodies (APLA). However, factor-specific inhibitor antibodies can block clotting in vivo and cause bleeding.[15] They are identified by their effect on the plasma factor's activity and semiquantified by assessing how much interference the patient's plasma gives to factor level measurements in normal plasma. Some severe hemophiliacs and other factor-deficient patients develop alloantibodies to therapeutic clotting factors, interfering with treatment and necessitating alternative factor therapies or immunosuppression. Bovine thrombin used for topical hemostasis can induce cross-reacting antibodies to the patient's own factor V. Autoantibodies to specific clotting factors, most commonly FVIII, can cause serious coagulopathy.

8   DIC describes unchecked coagulation initiated by pathologic systemic activation of the intrinsic clotting pathway. The specific pathophysiology of DIC is discussed later in this chapter, but diagnostic criteria require an inciting condition such as extensive tissue injury or a systemic inflammatory response secondary to infection, obstetrical complication, or malignancy. Intravascular platelet activation and fibrin formation lead to thrombocytopenia, hypofibrinogenemia, and RBCs sheared by fibrin strands (schistocytes). The results of coagulation testing vary, but often show prolonged PT and aPTT. In some patients, thrombosis is the most prominent clinical finding, but in most patients, the depletion of platelets and clotting factors with accompanying activation of fibrinolysis leads to diffuse consumptive coagulopathy. Fibrin formation followed by fibrinolysis generates the fibrin fragments called D-dimers, which when quantified in immunologic testing are a useful indicator of DIC.

Three other tests are commonly performed during surgery with whole-blood specimens: the *activated clotting time (ACT)*, *ecarin clotting time (ECT)*, and viscoelastic whole-blood clotting. The ACT, a point of care test, assesses the intrinsic clotting pathway and is used mainly to monitor heparin anticoagulation and its protamine reversal during cardiopulmonary bypass or vascular surgery. The ECT also describes the intrinsic clotting function, but it is primarily used for measuring the clinical effects of direct thrombin inhibitors (DTIs) such as bivalirudin and dabigatran. The ACT and aPTT also reflect the clinical efficacy of DTIs, but at high doses required for cardiopulmonary bypass, ECT is more accurate.[16] However, the ECT is not widely available.

Viscoelastic Testing

Whole-blood clotting and fibrinolysis can be assessed by viscoelastic testing in thromboelastography (TEG, Haemoscope Corp., Niles, IL, USA) or rotation thromboelastometry (ROTEM, Pentapharm GmBH, Munich, Germany).[17] These tests measure the rate, strength, and lysis, if any, of clot formation. Numerous parameters can be measured with these tests; accordingly, the TEG–ROTEM working group attempted to standardize the parameters obtained from both testing modalities in order to make them more clinically relevant. There are minor differences in the mechanisms for TEG versus ROTEM; however, both involve the use of whole blood in a heated cup with the addition of a sensor pin. The cup or the pin oscillates while the blood clots. The increasing resistance to oscillation is transmitted through the sensor pin, resulting in a graphic depiction of clot formation. The patterns obtained can implicate defects in factor levels, platelet function, fibrinogen concentration, and/or the presence of abnormal fibrinolysis, the last of which is difficult to measure rapidly otherwise. Testing can be performed in the presence of inhibitors of heparin or fibrinolysis to help judge whether these drugs would be effective therapies. This test format has also been adapted to assess antiplatelet therapy in patients with ventricular assist devices.[18] Viscoelastic testing is helpful in determining the appropriate therapy, including platelets, plasma, fibrinogen replacement, or antifibrinolytics, particularly complex bleeding syndromes such as massive hemorrhage with consumptive or dilutional coagulopathy progress.

Diagnosis of Thromboembolic Disorders

9 The risk for deep venous thrombosis (DVT), pulmonary embolism (PE), venous thromboembolism (VTE), and other thromboses is increased by intercurrent factors such as physical inactivity or immobilization, malignancy, oral contraceptives, estrogen therapy, and pregnancy. However, in addition to or especially in the absence of such factors, laboratory testing often identifies an underlying congenital or acquired predisposing abnormality that tips the hemostatic systems toward thrombosis. Discovery of one or more risk factors may influence the course of therapy and suggest benefit from family studies.

Congenital Risk Factors for Thrombosis

The most commonly tested congenital problems discussed below increase the risk of VTE.[19] Although arterial thrombosis may involve a few of these factors, platelets are more directly involved on the arterial side, and congenital contributions are less well defined. Some investigators have described a "sticky platelet syndrome," with hyperactive platelet aggregometry. Although severe congenital problems may present in childhood, they are rare; most thrombotic presentations are in adulthood over a lifetime of potential risk. Congenital problems are mostly categorized as deficiencies in antithrombotic pathways or hypercoagulable clotting factors.

Several congenital factors involve the protein C-ase complex and its function. The most common hypercoagulable mutation is factor V Leiden (FVL), in about 5% of Caucasians.[20] FV is the cofactor for FX when the latter activates prothrombin to thrombin. APC is the natural brake on FV, by cleaving it at Arg506. FVL carries the autosomal dominant mutation Arg506Gln, rendering FV fairly resistant to APC. Thus, FV is overactive and thrombin formation is favored. The FVL polymorphism is readily identified genetically. However, a small percentage of persons with resistance to APC have other mutations in FV or other conditions. Therefore, slightly more inclusive is the functional clotting test for APC resistance, which assesses plasma clotting time with and without reagent APC.

Protein C itself is functionally deficient in up to 0.5% of the population, with autosomal dominant inheritance. This leads to overactive FVIII and FV cofactors in their respective intrinsic tenase and prothrombinase complexes. Most have low activity and antigen (type I), but some have low activity with normal antigen levels (type II). Homozygous protein C deficiency is a very severe thrombotic disorder beginning in infancy. Protein S deficiency can lead to thrombosis because of its cofactor role to protein C. Around 1 in 700 persons has autosomal dominant deficiency. Protein S circulates partly bound to the complement C4 binding protein and partly as the unbound (free) active form. Nearly all cases of protein S deficiency can be identified by assaying the free antigen and then categorized as to whether the total antigen is low (type I) or normal (type II). Type II is rare, and has low function but normal antigen levels. Both protein C and protein S are vitamin K–dependent, and therefore vitamin K deficiency or warfarin interferes with laboratory assessment of their activities. Warfarin-induced skin necrosis in protein C or S deficiencies is discussed in antithrombotic therapy testing below. In AT-III deficiency, the relative lack of its normal blocking function on the key enzymes VIIa, IXa, Xa, and XIa leads to thrombosis risk. Testing for AT-III activity will detect both quantitative and qualitative defects.

The best characterized congenital gain in thrombotic function is the prothrombin mutation G20210A (guanine to adenine). This autosomal dominant condition is found in about 1 in 50 Caucasians, but is much less prevalent in African and Asian backgrounds. Persons with this variant have high circulating prothrombin levels as the reason for thrombosis risk. Genetic testing for the mutation is more definitive than prothrombin levels. Elevated FVIII levels may be a modest risk factor for thrombosis, but FVIII is an acute-phase reactant and rises in many intercurrent conditions. Whether there is an inherited element to persistently elevated FVIII levels is unclear.

Acquired Risk Factors for Thrombosis

Several factors increase the risk of thrombosis.[21] APLA are associated with both arterial and venous thrombosis risk. These antibodies bind to phospholipid–protein complexes. Several possible mechanisms for their in vivo effects have been proposed. They may bind to and activate endothelial cells, which in turn could directly initiate coagulation and/or cause vascular injury. They may interfere with phospholipids in the protein C-ase enzyme complex, leading to diminution of protein C's regulatory function. The various antigenic targets and mechanisms of APLA require multiple tests for their detection. Studies should include tests of clotting function, most notably LA tests, and tests of solid-phase binding to antigen targets, such as anticardiolipin antibodies (ACLA) and anti-β_2-glycoprotein-1 (AβGP). AβGP is a protein often present in the phospholipid–protein complex targeted by these antibodies.

LA antibodies are a common cause of prolonged aPTT that does not correct by mixing with normal plasma. It should be emphasized that the prolonged aPTT is a phenomenon of the in vitro test and is NOT associated with bleeding. However, not all LAs prolong the aPTT. Laboratories testing for LA should use at least two different tests to improve detection. One is usually a test based on the aPTT, but modified with phospholipid reagent selected to be sensitive to LA interference. A second clotting-based test is also recommended, such as the dilute Russell viper venom time (DRVVT), in which the snake venom activates FX in the common pathway, leading to thrombin formation. This test's reagent phospholipid is adjusted by dilution to be LA sensitive, but because the venom bypasses the usual initiating factors, the DRVVT is not affected by autoantibody inhibitors of FVIII or other upstream factors, a potential cause of confusion in the PTT-based assays.

ACLA and AβGP antibody tests usually employ enzyme immunoassays (EIAs). AβGP may be more specific for physiologic thrombotic effect, by presenting an actual target of in vivo antibodies, whereas ACLA may develop in other conditions such as infections. For example, false-positive nontreponemal syphilis serology is sometimes seen with ACLA.

Hyperhomocysteinemia is a risk factor for venous and possibly arterial thrombosis. This amino acid is made from methionine and is then either converted back or processed to cysteine. The mechanism for thrombosis risk is unclear, but endothelial cell injury has been proposed. Fasting total homocysteine is the initial screening test. Hyperhomocysteinemia can be due to various congenital mutations in homocysteine's metabolic pathways, or can be acquired via vitamin deficiencies affecting its metabolism (folate, B_{12}, B_6) or in many other medical conditions.

Monitoring Anticoagulation Therapeutic Agents

Most anticoagulant therapies need ongoing or selective testing for assessment of therapeutic effect. Appropriate monitoring ensures that these agents are maintained within the therapeutic range; otherwise patients are at risk for thromboembolism and bleeding complications, which can have devastating consequences.

Warfarin Anticoagulation

Warfarin therapy must be monitored by the PT and its analogue for this purpose, the international normalized ratio (INR), in order to avoid under- or overcoagulation. PT methods and reagents can widely differ between laboratories, yielding varying PT values for the same degree of factor deficiency. However, each PT test vendor supplies a conversion parameter to express the PT as the INR for patients on warfarin. The INR is a normalized value which is intended to compare results across laboratories for evaluating combined deficiencies of factors II, VII, IX, and X, the warfarin-dependent factors. The INR's therapeutic range for warfarin anticoagulation is generally 2.0 to 3.0, except for mechanical heart valves and prevention of myocardial infarction (INR 2.5 to 3.5).[22]

When warfarin is started or stopped, the factors with the fastest plasma turnover (i.e., the shortest half-lives) decline or rise the fastest, respectively. Thus, the inhibitor protein C, with a 6-hour half-life, declines faster than most clotting factors as warfarin takes effect. This can cause an imbalance toward clotting during the initiation of warfarin therapy. Warfarin-induced skin necrosis is a thrombotic complication often occurring when previously unrecognized congenital protein C deficiency accentuates this imbalance.

Warfarin's pharmacology is affected by genetic variations in the metabolism of the drug (cytochrome P450, CYP2C9) or its counterbalancing vitamin K (vitamin K epoxide reductase complex subunit 1, VKORC1). Genetic polymorphism testing has been advocated for achieving more rapid therapeutic effect when initiating therapy or in assessing difficulty achieving the target INR, but clinical trials are divided on its benefit.[23] The INR is not calibrated to evaluate nonwarfarin deficiencies such as liver disease, which affects most other clotting factors. Thus, the INR is not intended to be used in other conditions, including liver disease.

Heparin Anticoagulation Testing

The aPTT is used to assess heparin anticoagulation. Each laboratory determines its own therapeutic target range for heparin anticoagulation, typically of the order of 1.5 to 2.5 times the normal mean. The laboratory determines the exact range for their test system based on a functional enzymatic test for heparin action, the antifactor Xa activity (aFXa). (This is a different test than the clotting factor X activity level). Using the aFXa assay, therapeutic target heparin levels of 0.3 to 0.7 aFXa units/mL are correlated with aPTT results for that range. aFXa testing can be helpful in assessing heparin resistance.

Low–molecular-weight heparin (LMWH) drugs and their analogue, synthetic pentasaccharide (e.g., fondaparinux), do not affect the aPTT assay, and coagulation testing is usually not needed. However, if necessary, the drugs' plasma activity levels can be assessed by aFXa assays calibrated for each drug.[24] This may be helpful in renal failure affecting drug excretion, or in pregnant women, obese patients, and neonates for whom drug levels are less certain after subcutaneous injection. Like heparin, these agents inhibit factor Xa indirectly via their enhancing effect on AT.

Heparin (and to a lesser degree LMWH) can stimulate the production of antibodies against the heparin–PF4 complex. These antibodies can in turn cause HIT and/or activation of platelets to induce thrombosis.[25] If thrombocytopenia or thrombosis develops in a patient on these drugs, tests for HIT antibodies are available by EIA or by functional measures such as serotonin release. Patients with HIT must avoid heparin and LMWH.

Several newer anticoagulants have become widely used alternatives to warfarin for some indications. These are direct anticoagulants that are not mediated by AT. The oral "xaban" class of drugs, including rivaroxaban and apixaban, directly inhibit factor Xa.[26] Monitoring is not routinely needed. If drug activity must be assessed, the PTT is prolonged but is unreliable; aFXa assays calibrated for each specific drug are used.[27]

DTIs also pose challenges for coagulation testing. These include hirudin from leeches, its recombinant "-rudin" mimicking molecules (intravenous bivalirudin, desirudin), and small synthetic molecules acting at the same site as hirudin on thrombin (intravenous argatroban, oral dabigatran). They all prolong the PT and aPTT and interfere with clot-based fibrinogen assays. There is no consensus on how to quantify the effect of these drugs. The ECT has been promulgated.[27] In the ECT, ecarin, an enzyme in snake venom, cleaves prothrombin to a metabolic intermediate, which is inhibited by hirudin and its analogues. The dilute thrombin time has also been used. However, neither of these tests are widely available.

Emergency reversal of these anticoagulants is becoming available.[28] Idarucizumab, a monoclonal antibody fragment that functionally neutralizes dabigatran, was recently approved by the FDA. Clotting tests are usually corrected by the drug, but additional drug can be given if clotting tests become reelevated and bleeding recurs. Two drugs that block the action of anti-Xa inhibitors are in clinical trials.

Blood Component Production

Blood Collection

The production of blood components is highly controlled by regulations and accreditation requirements in the interests of donor and recipient safety, as well as therapeutic efficacy. Blood donors are carefully screened and tested, and blood products are made in specialized laboratories and other facilities. Regional blood centers collect and provide most blood components for transfusion, although some hospitals collect blood or platelets to augment their supply. Virtually all blood components come from volunteer unpaid donors. Pharmaceutical companies process plasma into various derivatives or synthesize some desired proteins for infusion.

Blood donors undergo a confidential interview to screen for medical problems for their own donation safety, as well as for risks of disease transmission to their recipients.[29] They are questioned about risk factors, exposure, or signs of human immunodeficiency virus (HIV), hepatitis, and other infections. There are geographically based deferral criteria for tropical exposure to malaria and (in US donors) European exposure to variant Creutzfeldt–Jakob disease (vCJD). The donor's pulse, blood pressure, and hemoglobin/hematocrit level (US minimum 12.5 g/dL or 38%) are checked. Phlebotomy is performed with validated antiseptic measures to reduce the risk of bacterial contamination in the blood bags. In the United States, donors are deferred for 8 weeks after a whole-blood donation to avoid iron deficiency.

Table 17-1 shows the contents and storage parameters for blood components. In whole-blood donations, 450 to 500 mL of blood is collected into citrate anticoagulant and then separated by centrifugation into RBCs, platelets, and/or plasma. The RBC units usually have most plasma removed and replaced with preservative. In the United States, the plasma must be frozen within 6 hours of collection to be labeled fresh frozen plasma (FFP). A large proportion of plasma is now made as plasma frozen within 24 hours, with minimal effect on clotting factor content compared to FFP. Cryoprecipitate is made from barely thawed FFP, which yields a precipitate rich in fibrinogen; the precipitate is isolated by centrifugation and refrozen.[30] Five bags of "cryo" comprise a typical adult dose. Whole-blood–derived platelets (sometimes called "random-donor platelets") are derived from platelet-rich plasma in the United States and from the buffy-coat centrifugation layer in other countries.[31] Four to six units are pooled to yield one adult-sized dose of platelets. Traditionally, pooling was done at the hospital just before transfusion, but blood centers can now provide pre-pooled platelets to hospitals.

Blood components are also collected by apheresis, in which the donor's blood is processed by ex vivo centrifugation, the desired component(s) are siphoned off into citrate anticoagulant, and the remainder returned to the donor. Most platelets are produced by apheresis (sometimes called single-donor platelets). Plasma and RBCs can also be collected by apheresis, and if the donor's blood volume and cell counts permit, two doses of the desired component can be obtained in one collection session.

All donors are checked against files of deferred donors, and all donations are tested for blood-borne infectious agents. Tests for HIV, hepatitis B virus (HBV), and hepatitis C virus (HCV) are universally required.[32] The addition of sensitive nucleic acid testing (NAT; e.g., polymerase chain reaction) to routine serology shortens the window period in a recently infected donor down to 7 to 10 days for HIV and HCV and 1 month for HBV. The US FDA also requires testing for syphilis, human T-cell lymphotropic virus (HTLV), and West Nile virus (WNV). Also available for donors at risk is a test for *Trypanosoma cruzi* (Chagas disease). Cytomegalovirus (CMV) is found mainly in leukocytes (WBCs). Selected patients at risk for complications of infection from cellular components can receive either CMV-negative units or leukoreduced units.

At some centers, directed donations can be made by family or friends for a specific patient. These donations augment the overall supply of blood and donors, and potentially reduce the number of donor exposures by using the same donor(s) more than once. However, the infectious risk from these units is not considered any less than from community volunteer donors. Cellular components from blood relatives must be irradiated to prevent the risk of transfusion graft-versus-host disease (GVHD) from closely matched donor lymphocytes that are not rejected by the recipient.

Autologous donations by the patient can be made in advance of scheduled surgery, with physician approval. The usual minimum hemoglobin or hematocrit is 11 g/dL or 33%, respectively, which is lower than the minimum allowed for regular donors. Patients should be on erythropoietin or iron supplementation to support RBC replenishment. In order to achieve a net gain in RBC mass, donations should be scheduled with some lead time within the 6-week storage period to permit erythropoiesis before surgery. Erythropoietin assists with multiple donations. Autologous units are only used for the patient and cannot be given to anyone else, since they often have a lower RBC content than normal requirements, and surgical patients frequently have conditions disqualifying them for regular donation. Autologous donations often create iatrogenic anemia with limited efficacy; they are best reserved for patients with difficult cross-match problems.

Component Processing and Storage

Leukoreduction (LR) to remove WBCs from RBCs and platelets reduces the risk of human leukocyte antigen (HLA)

Table 17-1 Blood Components

Component	Average Volume	Storage Parameters
Packed red blood cells	300 mL	1°–6°C for 21–35 d or 42 d with additive solution
Red blood cells, frozen	300 mL	<−65°C for 10 yr
Platelets, whole-blood derived	50 mL per bag, usual dose 4–6 bags	20°–24°C for 5 d
Platelets, apheresis	300 mL	20°–24°C for 5 d
Plasma, fresh frozen	250 mL	<−18°C for 1 yr or <−65°C for 7 yr
Plasma, frozen within 24 h	250 mL	<−18°C for 1 yr
Cryoprecipitate	15 mL per bag, usual dose 4–6 bags	<−18°C for 1 yr

alloimmunization, febrile nonhemolytic transfusion reactions (FNHTRs), and CMV transmission in patients who require these precautions. LR is usually performed by filtration, although some apheresis collections have sufficiently precise cell separation to minimize WBC content. The WBC content is typically reduced from around 10^9 WBCs/unit to less than 10^6 WBCs/unit.

In addition to the routine indications above, LR has been studied for the prevention of transfusion-related acute lung injury (TRALI) and so-called transfusion-related immunomodulation (TRIM)—possible immunosuppressive and proinflammatory effects mediated by donor WBCs. "Universal" LR of all cellular components is done in many countries; however, randomized controlled trials have been mostly inconclusive for benefit. Meta-analysis of available data has highlighted cardiac surgery as a setting in which there may be postoperative survival benefit associated with leukoreduced blood components.[33]

Washing cellular components with saline is mostly done to remove plasma in patients with allergic transfusion reactions such as those who are IgA deficient. It does not affect the antigens on the cells and does not remove enough WBCs to prevent GVHD or HLA alloimmunization.

Irradiation of cellular components is performed to prevent transfusion GVHD from directed-donor units from blood relatives, or in highly immunosuppressed patients at risk for this complication because of leukemia, lymphoma, hematopoietic stem cell transplants, congenital cellular immunodeficiencies, and purine analogues such as fludarabine.[34] The units are exposed to gamma irradiation (2,500 cGy) to damage donor WBC DNA and prevent a cellular immune proliferative response to the recipient's tissues. Irradiation is often performed in cesium-137 blood irradiators. The blood units do not come in contact with the radioisotope and are not radioactive, but laboratory personnel must comply with radiation safety regulations. In recent years, x-ray generators that do not contain radioisotopes have been approved for blood components.

Platelets are stored at room temperature to preserve clotting function, but this increases the risk of bacterial growth in contaminated units, compared to other blood components. Accordingly, bacterial detection has become routine in many countries. Platelet testing must be done after a short period of storage in order to detect growing bacteria. Blood centers can take culture samples from platelet pheresis units and prepooled whole-blood–derived platelets before product release. However, culturing is not feasible from the small volumes of individual whole-blood–derived platelets when the transfusion service is pooling the units just before use. In this situation, bacterial antigen testing is available to transfusion services and is required by accrediting agencies in the United States.

RBC preservation solutions use CPDA—Citrate for anticoagulation, Phosphate as a buffer, 1 to 2 g of Dextrose (D-glucose), and Adenine—to maintain adenosine triphosphate (ATP) levels and RBC membrane integrity. However, despite preservatives, several metabolic changes occur during RBC storage. 2,3-Diphosphoglycerate (2,3-DPG) is depleted in the first 2 weeks, and shifts the oxygen dissociation curve to the left, increasing hemoglobin binding of oxygen (although this reverses after transfusion). Furthermore, by the end of the 42-day shelf life of additive-solution RBCs, the pH is 6.5, the plasma K^+ is 50 mmol/L from RBC leakage and hemolysis, and 15% to 20% of the RBCs are nonviable.[35] RBC storage lesions may be related to observations linking older units to adverse outcomes such as short-term mortality and multiple organ failure.[36] However, randomized trials comparing outcomes with fresher RBCs versus routinely stored RBCs have thus far not shown overall benefit for fresher units.[37]

Plasma Derivatives

Plasma derivatives are proteins processed from plasma for therapeutic infusions. They include albumin, immunoglobulins (IGs), clotting factors, and other proteins. Derivatives are purified from plasma using physicochemical fractionation methods initially developed by Edwin J. Cohn in the 1930s. Donors for plasma derivatives are screened and tested similarly to blood component donors, and the separation techniques provide a degree of purification from microbial pathogens. However, the large number of donor units that must be pooled together for production of plasma derivatives introduces the possibility of contamination of an entire lot by a small number of infected donors. Such was the case in the early years of HIV when factor concentrates infected a large proportion of hemophiliacs before the risk was known. Because intact cells are not required, many derivatives can undergo purification and pathogen inactivation methods which are impractical for blood components.

Albumin is produced in large quantities for intravascular volume support and is pasteurized at 60°C for sterility. IGs are given for immune support or for immunomodulation to suppress native antibody production. IGs can also withstand robust pathogen inactivation processes, and in some cases are nanofiltered to remove viruses. To be given intravenously, IGs need extra processing to avoid reaction-provoking protein aggregates. Hyperimmune globulins are fractionated from the plasma of donors with high levels of antibody to specific antigens of interest, such as viruses (HBV, CMV, varicella zoster) or the Rh blood group D antigen (RhIG to prevent anti-D formation in RhD-negative women).

Factor concentrates for patients with congenital deficiencies are made with special techniques to ultrapurify factors VIII, IX, X, XIII, vWF, fibrinogen, and in some countries, factor XI, while also applying pathogen inactivation methods and viral filtration to remove microbes. However, recombinant factors VIII, IX, and vWF are also available to further allay concern about disease transmission, and recombinant activated factor VII (rFVIIa) is approved for rare VII-deficient patients. Some hemophiliacs develop inhibitory antibodies to the FVIII or factor IX they are missing. These inhibitor patients often need products that "bypass" their missing clotting step. The therapeutic potential of prothrombin complex concentrates (PCCs) containing multiple factors or rFVIIa to bypass secondary hemostasis and generate a thrombin burst is discussed later in this chapter. On the antithrombotic side of hemostasis, AT concentrate is available.

Other plasma proteins that are purified for selected deficiencies include complement C1 esterase inhibitor (for hereditary angioedema) and α_1-antitrypsin.

Pathogen Inactivation

Techniques have been developed to inactivate microbial pathogens in blood components.[38] The major advantage of this approach is protection against unrecognized infectious agents. The methods vary by blood component. Solvent–detergent treatment is approved for plasma, and psoralen treatment for plasma and platelets, although these products are not yet widely available in the United States. In Europe and other countries, these types of products are broadly used, along with methylene blue treatment for plasma and riboflavin treatment for plasma and platelets.

Cell-free plasma, either in pools or as individual units, can be treated with membrane-disrupting solvent–detergent treatments for enveloped viruses. Nonenveloped viruses, most prominently hepatitis A and parvovirus, are less susceptible to this process, but NAT can be added to detect these agents.

More robust methods involve agents that damage nucleic acids. When methylene blue, psoralen, or riboflavin is added to the blood bag, they bind to nucleic acids. Then photoinactivation is performed with agent-specific wavelengths of light, cross-linking DNA, and RNA to prevent microbial function. Not yet approved (but under investigation) is ultraviolet light treatment of platelets alone, without a photosensitizer chemical. RBC units are less amenable to photoinactivation because of the hemoglobin, but nucleic acid alkylation technology is under development.

The nucleic acid damage agents also inactivate donor WBCs and thus prevent transfusion GVHD. Adverse effects of these techniques include somewhat reduced platelet counts and plasma clotting factor levels, and potential toxicity from some of the added agents if they are not sufficiently removed after treatment.[39]

RBC and Platelet Substitutes

Many years of effort have gone into the search for an oxygen-carrying substitute for RBCs. Oxygen-avid perfluorocarbon chemicals underwent international trials, but 100% O_2 administration was needed and clinical trials were unsuccessful.[40] Several hemoglobin solutions have been made from pools of human or bovine hemoglobin, or from recombinant hemoglobin, all of which were chemically modified to facilitate extracellular O_2 offloading.[41] However, the potentially toxic effects of free hemoglobin, including intravascular binding of the vasodilator nitrous oxide (NO), are not sufficiently understood for regulatory approval. US clinical trials were unsuccessful in demonstrating clinical advantage in prehospital trauma management. None of these agents appear to hold much promise for clinical application in the near future. A more recent avenue of exploration is the possibility of "growing" RBCs in cell culture systems. They would be biocompatible and low in pathogen risk, and their RBC antigens could be engineered to some extent to maximize compatibility. The biology of cultivating mature normal RBCs in large scale is under investigation.

Platelets are so complex that it would be difficult to replace their functions fully. However, some early work has emerged on preserved platelets (e.g., freeze dried or fixed) and on biocompatible platforms bearing hemostatic proteins, such as fibrinogen-coated albumin beads, which could supply some degree of platelet-like clotting function. Culturing platelets in vitro for therapeutic uses is also being pursued.[42]

Blood Products and Transfusion Thresholds

Compatibility Testing

Routine RBC compatibility testing includes ABO and RhD typing, an antibody screen for IgG non-ABO RBC antibodies, and an RBC cross-match.[43] RBCs must be ABO compatible to avoid intravascular hemolysis, and RhD-negative patients should receive D-negative RBCs to avoid anti-D alloimmunization. Rh, Kell, Kidd, Duffy, and some other non-ABO antibodies can also hemolyze transfused RBCs; 1% of all patients and 5% to 20% of heavily transfused patients have such antibodies. If no antibodies are present, the cross-match can be electronic; that is, RBC units are selected by the laboratory computer to be ABO and RhD compatible. But if hemolytic antibodies are detected or are on record, RBC units negative for the incompatible antigen(s) must be found, and a serologic cross-match of patient plasma versus donor RBCs is performed to confirm compatibility. Most hospitals have blood order schedules for their most common surgical procedures, which set forth a recommended number of RBC units to cover 80% to 90% of patients undergoing each procedure.

RBC compatibility testing takes 45 to 60 minutes, and much longer if antibodies are found. Hence, testing in advance of scheduled surgery is desirable. In emergencies, uncross-matched group O RBCs can be given, albeit with the risk of non-ABO antibody incompatibility. Group AB is the universal donor plasma and avoids transfusing anti-A or anti-B versus the patient's RBCs.

Red Blood Cells

Over the past decade, transfusion practices for medical and surgical patients shifted from a liberal to a more restrictive strategy, with lower thresholds for transfusion and careful consideration of the balance between transfusion risks and the physiologic consequences of anemia. The ASA's most recent update to the *Practice Guidelines for Perioperative Blood Management* defines restrictive practices as "hemoglobin criteria for transfusion less than 8 g/dL and hematocrit values less than 25%." The ASA recommendations for RBC transfusion thresholds are consistent with the guidelines published by other international societies in perioperative management and critical care medicine, whose goals for hemoglobin range between 7 and 10 g/dL (Table 17-2).[44]

There are countless studies comparing liberal versus restrictive transfusion practices for acute anemia, but the most critical large randomized controlled trials include the Transfusion Requirements in Critical Care (TRICC), the Transfusion Requirements After Cardiac Surgery (TRACS) trial, the Functional Outcomes in Cardiovascular Patients Undergoing Surgical hip fracture repair (FOCUS) study, and a recent randomized controlled trial with patients suffering from acute upper gastrointestinal bleeding.[45-48] Unfortunately, there is still little evidence to support a clear recommendation for hemoglobin thresholds in patients at high risk of tissue hypoxia and end-organ dysfunction in the setting of acute coronary syndrome, sepsis, and acute neurologic injury as often these patients are excluded from studies with restrictive transfusion practices.

The TRICC trial included critically ill, but euvolemic patients in a large multicenter randomized controlled trial. The investigators compared the survival of patients transfused to hemoglobin levels greater than 10 g/dL in the liberal group, with patients treated under a restrictive strategy with a goal hemoglobin greater than 7 g/dL. Overall survival for more than 800 patients did not differ between the groups.[47] Subsequent subgroup analysis and several meta-analyses and systematic reviews confirmed these results, and also established the risks associated with liberal transfusion management for various patient populations, including those less than 55 years old, trauma patients, and those with stable cardiovascular disease.[46,49]

Traditionally, patients with cardiovascular disease and anemia were considered to be at significant risk of tissue ischemia and thought to benefit from higher hemoglobin goals in the perioperative and critical care settings. These recommendations were based on two studies that showed an association between anemia and mortality that improved with transfusion.[50] Several retrospective studies and systematic reviews have since contradicted these findings by documenting the safety of hematocrits less than 24% during cardiac surgery with cardiopulmonary

Table 17-2 International Society Transfusion Guidelines

Guideline Sponsoring Society	Asymptomatic ICU Patients	ACS	Neurologic Injury	Other
American Society of Anesthesiologists (ASA), *Anesthesiology 2015*				Restrictive goal: 6–10 g/dL
British Committee for Standards in Haemotology (BCSH), *BJH 2013*	>7 g/dL	8–9 g/dL	TBI: 7–9 g/dL Ischemia: >9 g/dL	Early sepsis: >9 g/dL Late sepsis: 7–9 g/dL
European Society of Anaesthesiology (ESA), *Eur J Anaesthesia 2013*			TBI: 7–9 g/dL	7–9 g/dL for active bleeding
AABB (Former American Association of Blood Banks), *JAMA 2016*	>7 g/dL	>8 g/dL	No supportive evidence	Postoperative: >8 g/dL
Society of Cardiovascular Anesthesiologists and Society of Thoracic Surgeons (SCA/STS), *Ann Thor Surg 2011*	>6–7 g/dL			Higher goal >7 g/dL for at-risk patients
Society of Critical Care Medicine (SCCM), *CCM 2009*	>7 g/dL	>8 g/dL	No supportive evidence	

ICU, intensive care unit; ACS, acute coronary syndrome; TBI, traumatic brain injury.

bypass.[46] The TRACS trial randomized postcardiac surgery patients to restrictive (hematocrit >24%) versus liberal (hematocrit >30%) transfusion strategies and found no difference in 30-day mortality or severe morbidity. Furthermore, transfusion was found to be an independent risk factor for morbidity and mortality.[46] Accordingly, the most recent Society of Thoracic Surgeons (STS) and the SCA's *Blood Conservation Clinical Practice Guidelines* recognizes that all cardiac surgery patients are at risk for tissue hypoxia and transfusion. These guidelines report that tissue oxygenation does not improve with transfusion for hemoglobin levels greater than 10 g/dL, stating that "Transfusion is reasonable in most postoperative patients whose hemoglobin is less than 7 g/dL." For patients with hemoglobin levels between 7 and 10 g/dL the two societies recommend transfusion in patients with "critical noncardiac end-organ ischemia," active blood loss, or clinical indication of tissue hypoxia (low mixed venous oxygen saturation or electrocardiographic or echocardiographic evidence of myocardial ischemia).[51]

The noninferiority of restrictive transfusion practice for at-risk patients was again confirmed with the FOCUS trial, which enrolled 2016 patients over 50 years old undergoing hip fracture repair with a history of cardiovascular disease, diabetes, peripheral vascular disease, or smoking. This trial is most influential for reporting functional outcomes in the form of a walking test, in addition to 30- and 60-day mortality and morbidity. The investigators found no difference in outcomes, despite the restrictive group receiving a third of the transfusions, compared to the liberal group, with 59% of patients receiving no RBCs compared to only 3% in the liberal group.[45] Villanueva et al. demonstrated improved mortality and morbidity in the restrictive arm of a study involving patients with active upper gastrointestinal hemorrhage. These authors also showed an association in the liberal group between receiving more RBC transfusions and demonstrating progressive bleeding and poor hemostasis.[48] These large trials in acute care or perioperative patients confirm the recommendations of the ASA and SCA/STS as well as the AABB, the European Society of Anaesthesiology (ESA), and the British Committee for Standards in Haematology (BCSH) guidelines for patient blood management outlined in Table 17-2.[44,51–54]

Patients with acute neurologic illness such as ischemic stroke, subarachnoid hemorrhage, and traumatic brain injury are at significant risk for secondary injury from tissue hypoxia. Acute and chronic anemia both initiate physiologic compensatory mechanisms discussed below, as well as neuroprotective strategies for tolerating decreases in cerebral oxygen delivery at critically low hemoglobin levels between 4 and 5 g/dL, as demonstrated by studies in Jehovah's Witness patients. However, the hemoglobin level at which anemia induces detrimental patient outcomes for those with acute neurologic injury remains unclear.[55] Evidence indicates that a hemoglobin level less than 9 g/dL is independently predictive of poor outcome, especially in patients with cerebrovascular injury. However, transfused RBCs do not function as well as endogenous erythrocytes. Therefore, it remains controversial whether RBC transfusion significantly improves tissue oxygenation and overall patient outcomes.[56] This leaves the clinician with little guidance to decide when and who should be transfused.

Physiologic Compensation for Anemia

There is ample evidence for the human tolerance of both acute and chronic anemia. Oxygen delivery to the tissues (DO_2) is dependent on cardiac output (CO), regional blood flow, and the blood's oxygen-carrying capacity (i.e., oxygen content [CaO_2]). The relationship between these variables and oxygen consumption (VO_2) is shown in Table 17-3.[57,58] Hemoglobin plays an integral role in oxygen transport and delivery to the tissues. The clinical justification for RBC transfusion assumes that increasing the hemoglobin will improve oxygen-carrying capacity and therefore avoid tissue hypoxia. However, given the ability of the body to compensate for anemia, it is unclear whether increasing hemoglobin in a stable anemic patient actually improves tissue oxygenation. There are several compensatory mechanisms for anemia, most notably increased CO, altered microcirculatory blood flow, and improved tissue oxygen extraction from hemoglobin. These physiologic changes, together with the detrimental impact of RBC storage limit the therapeutic effects of transfusion.[59]

1. *Increased CO.* There are several mechanisms that increase CO as compensation for isovolemic hemodilution. First, the heart rate increases secondary to a sympathetic surge initiated by anemia and hypoxia.[57,58,60] Second, higher stroke volume results from increased preload secondary

Table 17-3	Equations for Tissue Oxygenation	
Parameter	Unit	Equation
Oxygen delivery (DO_2)	mL O_2/min	$DO_2 = CO$ (L/min) $\times C_aO_2$ (mL/dL)
Arterial oxygen content (C_aO_2)	mL O_2/dL	$C_aO_2 = 1.36 \times Hgb$ (g/dL) $\times S_aO_2$ (%) $+ [P_aO_2 \times 0.003]$
Venous oxygen content (C_vO_2)	mL O_2/dL	$C_vO_2 = 1.36 \times Hgb$ (g/dL) $\times S_vO_2$ (%) $+ [P_vO_2 \times 0.003]$
Blood flow, cardiac output (CO)	L/min	Flow $= \pi r^4 \Delta P/8\eta L$ (r = radius, ΔP = change in pressure, η = viscosity, and L = length of the vessel)
Oxygen consumption (VO_2)	mL O_2/min	$VO_2 = CO$ (L/min) $\times [C_aO_2 - C_vO_2]$
Oxygen extraction ratio (O_2EF)	%	$O_2EF = [C_aO_2 - C_vO_2]/C_aO_2 \times 100\%$ or $= VO_2/DO_2 \times 100\%$

Hgb, hemoglobin; P_aO_2, partial pressure of oxygen in arterial blood; P_vO_2, partial pressure of oxygen in venous blood.

to decreases in both systemic vascular resistance and afterload. Isovolemic hemodilution occurs when acute blood loss is resuscitated with crystalloid or colloid fluids, thereby maintaining blood volume with a lower hemoglobin. The resultant decrease in blood viscosity reduces shear stress in the microvasculature, which significantly increases flow and venous return. Furthermore, tissue acidosis induces arteriolar vasodilation, thereby decreasing overall afterload.[57,58,60]

2. *Altered microcirculatory blood flow.* The decrease in blood viscosity associated with isovolemic hemodilution and chronic anemia improves blood flow through the microcirculation secondary to lower shear force in capillary beds.[57,60] Furthermore, microcirculatory blood flow increases with dilation of arterioles secondary to the release of NO from endothelial cells in response to tissue hypoxia. NO also induces arteriovenous shunting and recruitment of new circulatory beds, thereby increasing blood flow to ischemic tissue. Patients with chronic anemia also increase angiogenesis and overall microcirculatory blood volume to compensate for the decreased oxygen-carrying capacity.[60] These mechanisms are extremely efficient. In fact, studies in anemic critically ill patients fail to show additional improvements in tissue oxygenation measures after transfusion.[59]

3. *Increased tissue oxygen extraction.* Anemia causes the oxyhemoglobin disassociation curve to shift to the right secondary to increased levels of 2,3-DPG in RBCs. This adaptive process is particularly influential for the physiologic compensation of chronic anemia, and often is the only mechanism necessary to maintain oxygen delivery. Isovolemic hemodilution to hematocrit levels less than 25% generates an increase in 2,3-DPG levels. Furthermore, acidemia associated with acute hemorrhage also shifts the oxygen dissociation curve to the right, thereby decreasing the affinity of oxygen for hemoglobin and improving the tissue oxygen extraction ratio.[57,60]

There continues to be controversy about RBC transfusion given the lack of evidence to support a universal transfusion threshold. Despite the wealth of literature documenting its potential harm, transfusion continues to be the mainstay of treatment for acute and chronic anemia. Healthy patients are most often able to compensate for anemia and tolerate critically low hemoglobin levels; however, the risk of tissue hypoxia in acute situations or in patients who are unable to compensate remains unclear. As CO increases to compensate for anemia with increased heart rates and a disproportionate increase in coronary blood flow, the critical hemoglobin level for each patient varies with their amount of cardiovascular reserve.[57]

Further studies of restrictive versus liberal transfusion strategies for patients with acute coronary syndrome, including ST-elevation and non–ST-elevation myocardial infarction or unstable angina, are needed to answer the question of transfusion thresholds for these patients. Pilot studies are inconclusive—the CRIT Randomized Pilot Study by Cooper et al. reported noninferiority of restrictive transfusion, but Carson et al. demonstrated that liberal management improved mortality in nonbleeding patients with acute coronary syndrome.[61,62]

Overall, each clinician must take into account the patient's comorbidities, the acuity of anemia, and their ability to compensate adequately without signs or symptoms of tissue hypoxia (Table 17-4). Furthermore, it is important to measure the response to transfusion with follow-up hemoglobin levels in order to identify consumptive anemia, hemolysis, or ongoing bleeding as well as to guide further transfusions. In stable patients without ongoing bleeding, the hemoglobin should rise 1 g/dL (approximately 3% rise in hematocrit) for each unit of packed RBCs given.[49,52,54]

The above discussion focuses on isovolemic hemodilution secondary to chronic anemia or acute hemorrhage and fluid resuscitation, when compensatory mechanisms allow adaptation to the detrimental effects of decreased hemoglobin levels. It is important to recognize that further transfusion may be necessary prior to the availability of measured hemoglobin and hematocrit levels during acute hemorrhage, intraoperative bleeding, or trauma resuscitation. In the case of uncompensated blood

Table 17-4 Clinical Indications of Tissue Hypoxia

• Unstable vital signs
  ▪ Tachycardia
  ▪ Hypotension
  ▪ Tachypnea or dyspnea
• Laboratory and invasive monitor indices
  ▪ Mixed venous O_2 saturation (SV_mO_2) <50%
  ▪ Central venous O_2 saturation (SV_cO_2) <60%
  ▪ Increased O_2 extraction ratio (O_2ER) >50%
  ▪ Lactic acidosis (metabolic acidemia with lactate >2 mmol/L)
• Signs of end-organ dysfunction
  ▪ Electrocardiographic (ST changes, onset of arrhythmias) or echocardiographic indications of myocardial ischemia
  ▪ Electroencephalographic indications of cerebral hypoperfusion
  ▪ New onset oliguria (less than 0.5 mL/kg/h for >6 h)

loss, hemoglobin levels may be normal or misleadingly high. In these situations, the clinician must estimate blood loss from the patient's hemodynamic picture and assessment of the operative field, in order to guide transfusion management. The BCSH and AABB guidelines recommend a goal of hemoglobin over 8 g/dL, and the ESA recommends a target hemoglobin between 7 and 9 g/dL for the patients with acute hemorrhage.[52,54]

Platelets

Numerous recommendations provide guidance for the transfusion management of thrombocytopenia and acquired or inherited platelet disorders.[51,63–65] The indications for platelet transfusion depend on both quantitative and qualitative measures of platelet activity and the clinical setting. Table 17-5 outlines typical platelet thresholds for transfusion based on the clinical situation and patient history. For stable patients with severe thrombocytopenia, transfusion can be held until counts fall below 10,000 μL, in the absence of signs or symptoms of bleeding.[66] Prophylactic platelet transfusion is necessary for patients with severe thrombocytopenia (below 50,000/μL) who are about to undergo major surgery or invasive procedures such as lumbar puncture, liver biopsy, neuraxial anesthesia, or endoscopy with biopsy.[44,63] The most recent guidelines from the AABB recommend a threshold of less than 20,000/μL for prophylaxis prior to placement of a central venous catheter.[67] In preparation for surgery on the eye or the central nervous system, the platelet count should be raised to above 100,000/μL. Any patient with critical blood loss or hemorrhagic shock should be transfused to a platelet target of 75,000 to 100,000/μL.[65]

Transfusion is not necessary for platelet counts over 100,000/μL in clinically stable patients without suspicion of platelet dysfunction, whereas most patients with counts below 50,000/μL and clinical bleeding require therapeutic transfusion.[44,63,67] There are several relative indications for transfusion of platelet counts between 50,000 and 100,000/μL. In particular, patients having surgery on the eye or central nervous system, or patients with multiple traumatic injuries benefit from higher transfusion goals.[63,65,67] Furthermore, patients undergoing massive transfusion or hemorrhage with estimated blood loss of more than two blood volumes and ongoing bleeding should have a transfusion threshold of at least 75,000/μL to ensure the level does not fall below 50,000/μL.[65]

Platelet transfusion should not be guided by platelet counts alone, but also by the clinical suspicion of platelet dysfunction that can be inherited or acquired. Qualitative dysfunction is often associated with systemic diseases such as uremia, liver failure, and disseminated intravascular coagulopathy (DIC). It also occurs after cardiopulmonary bypass, extracorporeal circulation such as dialysis or plasmapheresis, and as a result of medication side effects (Table 17-6).[44,67] Regardless of the platelet count, if bleeding is out of proportion to the level of thrombocytopenia, qualitative deficiency should be suspected and treated.

The average dose of platelets is one concentrate from apheresis donation, or pools of five to eight concentrates from whole-blood or buffy-coat collections. These "units" generally contain about 3×10^{11} to 4×10^{11} platelets each.[63] Once platelets are given, a posttransfusion response should be followed to guide further therapy and to rule-out ongoing consumptive pathophysiology. Refractoriness at 20 to 24 hours is generally associated with older platelets or increased consumption secondary to fever, infection, bleeding, or medications. Adjunctive therapy for platelet dysfunction can be established with antifibrinolytics, DDAVP (1-deamino-8-D-arginine vasopressin, desmopressin), or PCCs as discussed later in this chapter.[44,51,63]

Plasma Products

Plasma contains all the factors involved in hemostasis. Modern preparations of plasma now include fresh frozen within 8 hours of phlebotomy (FFP), plasma frozen within 24 hours of collection (PF24), or "thawed plasma," which includes units of frozen plasma that have been thawed for more than 24 hours yet remain usable for up to 4 additional days. The preparation and storage method for each formulation involves either

Table 17-5 Indications for Platelet Transfusion

Stable patients without evidence of bleeding or coagulopathy	<10,000/μL
Prophylaxis for central venous catheterization	<20,000/μL
Prophylaxis for invasive procedures such as lumbar puncture, neuraxial anesthesia, endoscopy with biopsy, liver biopsy, or major nonneuraxial surgery	<50,000/μL
Stable patients with clinical evidence of bleeding or coagulopathy including DIC	<50,000/μL
Patients undergoing massive transfusion	<75,000–100,000/μL
Patients having surgery at critical sites such as the eye or central nervous system	<80,000–100,000/μL
Microvascular bleeding attributed to platelet dysfunction such as uremia, liver disease, postcardiopulmonary bypass	Clinician judgment

DIC, disseminated intravascular coagulation.

Table 17-6 Causes of Acquired Platelet Dysfunction

Uremia
Liver disease
Paraproteinemia (multiple myeloma, Waldenström macroglobulinemia, monoclonal gammopathy, or polyclonal hypergammaglobulinemia)
Myeloproliferative disease
Myelodysplastic syndrome
Disseminated intravascular coagulopathy
Extracorporeal circulation (dialysis, cardiopulmonary bypass, plasmapheresis)
Medications (aspirin, NSAIDs, thienopyridines, GPIIb/IIIa antagonists, β-lactam antibiotics, antidepressants, phenothiazines)
Herbal remedies (fish oil, flaxseed oil, ginger, Ginkgo biloba, garlic, grape seed extract, saw palmetto, feverfew, bilberry, bromelain)

NSAIDs, nonsteroidal anti-inflammatory drugs; GP, glycoprotein.

Table 17-7 Indications for the Use of Plasma Products

- Correction of inherited factor deficiencies when there is no specific factor concentrate (e.g., factor V) and when the PT or aPTT is >1.5 times the mean control or INR >2.0.
- Replacement of multifactor deficiencies with clinical bleeding after transfusion of more than one blood volume (>70 mL/kg) when PT, INR, or aPTT cannot be obtained immediately.
- Correction of acquired multifactor deficiencies with clinical evidence of bleeding or in anticipation of major surgery or an invasive procedure with PT or aPTT >1.5 times the control, or INR >2.0.
  - Liver dysfunction with clinical signs of bleeding.
  - DIC with clinical signs of bleeding.
  - Reversal of vitamin K antagonists (warfarin) *when PCCs are not available*.
  - Heparin resistance secondary to AT deficiency when AT concentrate is not available.
  - Treatment of thrombotic microangiopathies (thrombotic thrombocytopenic purpura, HELLP syndrome, or hemolytic uremic syndrome).
- Treatment of hereditary angioedema when C1-esterase inhibitor is not available.

DIC, disseminated intravascular coagulation; PT, prothrombin time; aPTT, activated partial thromboplastin time; PCCs, prothrombin complex concentrates; AT, antithrombin; HELLP, hemolytic anemia elevated liver enzymes and low platelet count.

separation from whole blood or apheresis; both maintain normal levels of stable factors and at least 70% normal levels of labile factors such as FVIII and FV. Prior to use, each unit must be thawed at 30° to 37°C, but can be stored at 4° ± 2°C for up to 24 hours as thawed FFP or 5 days as thawed plasma.[68–70] Throughout this chapter, the inclusive term, "plasma" will be used for FFP, PF24, and thawed plasma unless otherwise specified. During preparation and distribution, care must be taken to ensure ABO compatibility for plasma transfusion to avoid transfusion of donor anti-A and anti-B antibodies that may lead to hemolysis.[71]

Plasma is indicated for the treatment of coagulopathy secondary to congenital or acquired factor deficiencies. The specific indications for plasma products outlined in Table 17-7 are based on one of the most recent guidelines from the ASA, BCSH, SCA/STS, and AABB.[44,51,69,71] The initial therapeutic dose of plasma averages 10 to 15 mL/kg in an attempt to obtain at least 30% factor activity. Repeat dosing is guided by serial diagnostic coagulation tests such as the PT, INR, and aPTT.[44,51,71] Recent updates to these guidelines are guarded in their recommendations for prophylactic use of plasma for patients at risk for hemorrhage but without clinical evidence of bleeding. Systematic reviews fail to demonstrate the efficacy of prophylactic plasma to reduce RBC transfusion, morbidity, or mortality, especially when given to patients with mild derangements in PT, INR, or aPTT and no clinical signs of bleeding.[69,72,73] The administration of plasma carries risks of several transfusion reactions, most notably TRALI, allergic reactions, and transfusion-associated circulatory overload (TACO). Together with limited prophylactic benefits and high frequency of inappropriate use, these risks arguably make plasma the riskiest blood component currently in use.[69,72,73]

Over the past decade there has been growing debate over "damage control" resuscitation protocols for trauma patients with major bleeding. Traditionally, trauma patients were resuscitated first with fluid and RBCs, and only received plasma based on the results of coagulation tests.[65] However, it has been argued that this method perpetuates dilutional coagulopathy and prolonged microvascular bleeding, especially when long turn-around-time coagulation assays are used to assess hemostasis.[74,75] Numerous observational studies originally showed improved outcomes with higher ratios of plasma to RBC units (more than 2:3) and with transfusion protocols that provide a balanced ratio of platelets, plasma coagulation factors, and RBCs.[76] However, these retrospective findings are likely confounded by injury severity and potential "survivor bias" that occurs when patients die of massive hemorrhage before plasma can be thawed and transfused.[76,77]

Two large prospective multicenter trials—the Prospective, Observational, Multicenter Major Trauma Transfusion (PROMMTT) trial and the Pragmatic, Randomized Optimal Platelets, and Plasma Ratios (PROPPR) trial—were both designed to definitively answer the question of whether fixed ratio transfusion protocols for trauma resuscitation can improve patient outcomes. Both trials demonstrated the feasibility of providing patients with thawed plasma in a timely manner, although this practice significantly increases the wastage rate.[74,78,79] When plasma resuscitation is delayed, patients are at increased risk of hemorrhagic shock and death, supporting one trauma society's recommendations that Level I trauma centers have thawed universal donor plasma available. However, neither trial demonstrated a survival benefit at either 24 hours or 30 days for patients receiving a higher ratio of platelets to plasma to RBCs (1:1:1 vs. 1:1:2).[74,78] Those with the higher ratio of plasma were less likely to expire secondary to exsanguination at 6 hours; however, overall mortality at 24 hours and 30 days did not differ between groups and most commonly resulted from traumatic brain injury, sepsis, and multiorgan system failure.[78] The influence of plasma use in traumatic brain injury raises additional questions, as many studies demonstrate increased mortality with the use of plasma products over normal saline.[73] Accordingly, guidelines from the AABB, ASA, and SCA/STS continue to recommend using fixed ratios of plasma only for resuscitation of massive hemorrhage, until coagulation profile assay results become available to further guide blood product transfusion.[44,51,69]

Cryoprecipitate

Cryoprecipitate is created by a controlled thaw of FFP, which allows for precipitation of large molecules. It is then centrifuged, the supernatant removed, and the final product resuspended in 10 to 15 mL of plasma, containing fibrinogen (about 15 g/L), fibronectin, vWF, FVIII, and FXIII.[30,68] These small concentrates are typically combined for a single adult dose from five pools and frozen at −18°C for up to 12 months. This dose should increase fibrinogen levels by approximately 50 g/dL.[30,68] Current use of cryoprecipitate is limited to a few countries (United States and Canada) and generally only indicated for hypofibrinogenemia (Table 17-8). Compared to plasma, cryoprecipitate contains more fibrinogen per volume (15 vs. 2.5 g/L in plasma)[71] and therefore functions as a low-volume alternative for fibrinogen replacement, especially during acquired hypofibrinogenemia states such as DIC and massive hemorrhage. It carries similar transfusion risks as plasma, and consequently has been replaced in several countries, including in Europe, with fibrinogen concentrates that can be virally inactivated.[30,68]

> **Table 17-8** Indications for Fibrinogen Replacement
>
> - Microvascular bleeding with hypofibrinogenemia
>   - DIC with fibrinogen <150 mg/dL
>   - Hemorrhage or massive transfusion with fibrinogen <180–200 mg/dL
> - Prophylaxis in patients with hemophilia A and vWD (if specific factor concentrates are unavailable or ineffective due to inhibitors)
> - Prophylaxis for patients with congenital dysfibrinogenemias
>
> DIC, disseminated intravascular coagulation; vWD, von Willebrand disease.

Fibrinogen Concentrate

Fibrinogen concentrates are derived from plasma after several steps of viral inactivation that also minimize antibodies and antigens to produce a lyophilized powder formulation that can be stored at room temperature and reconstituted for administration in less than 10 minutes. They are used frequently around the world as a safe, low-volume alternative to cryoprecipitate, but are only are available in the United States for treatment of congenital hypofibrinogenemias. Several studies demonstrate the efficacy of fibrinogen concentrates in settings of acute hemorrhage, cardiac surgery, and obstetrical hemorrhage; however large randomized controlled trials have not been reported.[30,68]

Fibrinogen is primarily responsible for clot stabilization, but it also assists with platelet activation and aggregation and, at adequate concentrations, may compensate for low thrombin states.[80,81] Traditionally, the threshold for fibrinogen replacement has been at levels less than 80 to 100 mg/dL. This continues to be included in many blood management guidelines, despite little evidence to support its validity.[30,44,68,82] Several studies and subspecialty societies have suggested more conservative goals (fibrinogen concentrations of 180 to 200 g/dL) to optimize clot stability.[30,68,82,83]

The Risks of Blood Product Administration

According to the 2011 update from the National Blood Collection and Utilization Survey, over 20 million blood products are transfused annually throughout the United States. The Center for Disease Control and Prevention (CDC)-supported Hemovigilance Module of the National Healthcare Safety Network (NHSN) has small, but growing participation from transfusion centers and hospitals (4.5%). Data from this module suggest that the overall risk of a transfusion reaction is approximately 239.5 per 100,000 components with 8% of reactions, infectious and noninfectious, being severe or life-threatening.[8,84,85]

National hemovigilance networks worldwide suspect both underreporting of transfusion reactions and avoidable morbidity and mortality secondary to clerical errors or inadequate clinical evaluation of patients undergoing blood product transfusion. Patients receiving blood component therapy should be continuously monitored for fever, hypotension, and cardiopulmonary complications. Mild fever with or without pruritus or rash is still the most common reaction, and can be treated symptomatically with antihistamines or antipyretics. In the event of a more severe fever (≥39°C, or ≥2°C rise in temperature) with constitutional symptoms (e.g., rigors, myalgia, nausea, vomiting, or diaphoresis), transfusion should be halted and the product returned to the blood bank for retesting of compatibility and antibodies. Sepsis should be ruled out if fever is persistent. Pulmonary symptoms should be investigated for TRALI, TACO, or anaphylaxis. Typically, acute hemolytic reactions will involve hypotension, shock, and cardiopulmonary collapse. Transfusion should not be discontinued if shock symptoms are likely secondary to hemorrhage.[86]

Infectious Risks of Blood Product Administration

In the mid-1980s, the realization of transfusion-transmissible infections such as HIV and hepatitis raised concerns about the infectious risks of blood product administration. Since the introduction of Nucleic Acid Amplification Testing (NAT) for major transfusion-transmittable viral infections (HCV in 2000, HIV in 2003, and HBV in 2006), the risk of infection from blood product transfusion has decreased substantially.[87,88] Prior to the institution of NAT, the blood supply was simply tested for the presence of viral antibodies. This left a long window period when the blood was potentially infectious, but with insufficient time for the donor to mount an antibody response detectable by conventional testing. NAT increased the sensitivity of donor screening by testing for the presence of specific viral DNA or RNA. This significantly shortened the window period between when a donor gets infected and when the viral load is detectable. The residual risk of transfusion-transmitted infections now depends mostly on the length of this window period, relative to the reproductive rate of each virus and the prevalence of the disease. There are additional risks of false negatives NATs or the mistaken release of quarantined blood products; however, these events account for less than 0.5% of the residual risk of transfusion-transmitted viral infection.[89,90]

The true risk of transfusion-transmittable infections is difficult to accurately quantify given the variability of donor response to inoculation and the immune state of the recipient. However, the residual risk can be mathematically modeled from the prevalence of infection in donors and the known window period of each viral illness. The estimated residual risk of major viral infection and the viral-specific window periods are shown in Table 17-9, based on the reported incidence of infection in donors for the American Red Cross Blood Services.[89,90] These residual risks are likely overestimates, since not all transfusions of known infected blood products result in recipient infection.[91,92] The mathematical modeling of residual risk assumes 100% infectivity with even one infectious unit of viral particles per blood bag. It also presumes that the collection and storage process is harmless to viral reproduction. Furthermore, viral infectivity will vary depending on the acute phase of infection when an immunocompetent recipient could resist transmission or the chronic phase of infection when antibodies are present and reduce infectivity.[92]

Transfusion-transmitted viral infections traditionally receive the most attention from patients due to their associated morbidity and mortality. Despite increased awareness and public health initiatives, the prevalence of HIV and HCV in the donor population continues to increase secondary to prolonged survival of patients, making the prevalence of HIV and HCV in the general population higher. Contrary to HIV and HCV, the prevalence of HBV has decreased since 1999 presumably due to high vaccination rates. Overall, the prevalence of disease in the general population is now the largest determinant of transfusion-transmittable infection risk.[90]

Table 17-9 Residual Risk of Transfusion-transmitted Infections

Infection	Residual Risk	Window Period and Comments
Viral infections		
Human immunodeficiency virus (HIV)	1/2,300,000	7–10-d window
Hepatitis C (HCV)	1/1,800,000	7–10-d window
Hepatitis B (HBV)	1/280,000–1/352,000	38-d window
Human T-cell lymphotropic virus (HTLV)	1/2,993,000	51-d window, cell associated
West Nile virus (WNV)	Rare	11 cases reported from 2003–2010
Cytomegalovirus (CMV)—all donors	1–3%	
Leukoreduced products	0.023%	
Emerging infections	Rare	Incidence is too small to estimate
Chagas and malaria		Donor screening limits risk in the United States
Creutzfeldt–Jakob (vCJD)		Incubation for years
Dengue virus and *Babesia* species		Transient epidemics increase risks
Parvovirus (B19v)		May cause aplastic anemia in immunosuppressed patients
Bacterial contamination—all types	1/3,000	
Packed red blood cells	1/35,000	Lower risk than platelet concentrates
Platelets, apheresis	1/15,000	Apheresis decreases risk

Data derived from: Allain JP, Stramer SL, Carneiro-Proietti AB, et al. Transfusion-transmitted infectious diseases. *Biologicals.* 2009;37(2):71–77; Lindholm PF, Annen K, Ramsey G. Approaches to minimize infection risk in blood banking and transfusion practice. *Infect Disord Drug Targets.* 2011;11(1):45–56; Zou S, Stramer SL, Dodd RY. Donor testing and risk: current prevalence, incidence, and residual risk of transfusion-transmissible agents in US allogeneic donations. *Transfus Med Rev.* 2012;26(2):119–128; Dwyre DM, Fernando LP, Holland PV. Hepatitis B, hepatitis C and HIV transfusion-transmitted infections in the 21st century. *Vox sanguinis.* 2011;100(1):92–98.

Many patients inquire about directed donations from family and friends. They should be made aware of the stringent processes for random donor screening for infectious risk factors, as well as the significantly increased prevalence of viral infections—especially HCV and HBV—in directed donations.[93]

Human Immunodeficiency Virus

As a retrovirus, HIV is transmitted as RNA and requires translation into DNA prior to replication. This virus was highly transmittable in the US blood supply until sensitive NAT and donor screening became available. The incidence of transfusion transmission of HIV was as high as 1 in every 100 donations in the early 1980s, but only 1 in every 400,000 donations in 1997.[94] The residual risk of HIV has fallen to lower than 1 per 2.3 million blood product transfusions.[89] However, despite a short window period of 7 to 10 days, the residual risk of HIV transmission via blood supply is expected to increase slightly or remain stagnant secondary to increased prevalence of HIV in the general population due to improved treatments and prolonged survival.[90]

Hepatitis C Virus

Although HCV is rarer than the other types of transmittable hepatitis and has a relatively benign acute phase, it progresses to chronic carrier state in up to 80% to 85% of infections and is associated with significant risk of fulminant hepatic failure, cirrhosis, hepatocellular carcinoma, and death.[89,91] Similar to HIV, the transfusion risk of HCV decreased drastically with the increased sensitivity of NAT testing and donor screening. However, the prevalence of donor HCV increased over the past 5 to 7 years due to increases in both incidence and prevalence in the general population. Recent reports have implicated higher infectivity rates in non–hospital-based health-care facilities and endoscopic procedures.[90,91] Furthermore, HCV infections become more aggressive and transmittable in patients coinfected with HIV due to the increased viral load that results from immunosuppression.[87]

Hepatitis B Virus

HBV is a common blood-borne pathogen with fairly high incidence of infection in the general population and over 300 million carriers worldwide.[91] The United States has a low prevalence rate of 2%, compared with 8% to 15% in the Middle East, Africa, and parts of South America and Asia.[87,91] The acute infection associated with HBV is asymptomatic in most patients, or limited to mild constitutional signs and jaundice. Rarely, however, it can progress to fulminant hepatic failure. The residual risk of transfusion-transmitted HBV remains high, given the common prevalence of the disease and a long window period. This risk is now decreasing with substantial prevalence reductions in the general population that are likely secondary due to the increased availability of and compliance with HBV vaccine.[89–91]

Human T-Cell Lymphotropic Virus-1 and Virus-2

HTLV-1 causes T-cell leukemia and lymphoma, or HTLV-associated myelopathy in a small percentage of infected persons. HTLV-2 does not have any significant consequences for immunocompetent or even HIV coinfected patients.[89] Regardless of the relatively infrequent disease association with HTLV, the US blood supply is routinely tested for anti-HTLV antibodies indicative of previous infection.[89,90] Given that HTLV is cell associated, the transmission via transfusion may be eradicated with LR.

Cytomegalovirus

CMV is ubiquitous in the general population with a prevalence of about 40% to 80%.[89] Consequently, it is the most common transfusion-transmitted infection with an incidence of 1% to 3%.[90] In immunocompetent recipients the infection is often asymptomatic or mild and self-limited. However, in immunocompromised patients—in particular, neonates, patients with HIV, and transplant recipients—the disease can be associated with severe multiorgan system failure involving the liver, lungs, kidneys, hematologic system, gastrointestinal tract, and the central nervous system.[90,95] The CMV virus is carried by white blood cells and transmitted via CMV-seropositive cellular components. LR decreases the infectivity of CMV-positive donor products, but has not completely eradicated the transfusion transmission of CMV.[89,95] Therefore, it is recommended that patients at highest risk for CMV infection, such as neonates and pregnant women, receive LR blood products from CMV-seronegative–only donors.[89,90,96]

Emerging Infections

HIV remains the most noteworthy microbe to recently infect the blood. Several pathogens have also emerged through changes in ecologic and geographic factors such as travel, climate change, or new insect and animal vectors. The most recent example of a significant new transfusion-transmissible infection is the West Nile Virus (WNV), a mosquito-borne flavivirus that emerged in 1999. WNV causes only a mild febrile illness in healthy patients, but may progress to encephalitis or meningitis in up to 40% of immunosuppressed patients.[89] The peak of the WNV epidemic occurred in 2002 to 2003, with 23 transfusion-transmitted illnesses that year. However, since the institution of donor screening with NAT testing in 2003, the incidence of transfusion-transmitted WNV has dropped to only 11 reported cases from 2003 to 2010.[89,90] Surveillance studies continue to investigate the virulence of various strains of WNV worldwide and the ability of the current NAT test to recognize seroconversion in donors.[97]

A few other pathogens have been red flagged by the AABB Transfusion-Transmitted Disease Committee as potential threats to the safety of the US blood supply. Most concerning are human vCJD, *Babesia* species, Chagas, dengue virus, and the *Plasmodium* species, which causes malaria.[89] vCJD is the human form of bovine spongiform encephalitis. It results in fatal degenerative neurologic disease secondary to prion proteins that precipitate an abnormal formation and structure of other proteins. It gained attention after an epidemic of cases in the 1980s to 1990s throughout the United Kingdom. Thus far, there have been three cases of confirmed transfusion-transmitted vCJD.[89] There are no known effective treatments, and the incubation period is reported in years. Currently no testing regimens exist for diagnosis of prion disease in donors or collected blood, but donor deferral for those who resided in the United Kingdom during the epidemic has avoided any known transfusion transmissions within the United States.[89] The incidence and infectivity of other viral and parasitic pathogens is so rare that they do not warrant a careful discussion here. However, it is important to remember that there may be emerging infections that are yet unrecognized, leaving the blood supply at constant risk. Western countries continue to evaluate the risk–benefit ratios and ethical cost considerations for screening tests and donor deferrals, with the knowledge that testing to ensure 100% sensitivity is highly unlikely and adds significant costs.[88]

Bacterial Contamination

Despite significant public concern for transfusion-transmitted viral disease, bacterial contamination of blood components poses the largest risk of transfusion-related infection by two or three orders of magnitude. Bacteremia may progress to sepsis and continues to be one of the major causes of transfusion-associated fatality, according to the FDA.[98] Frequent pathogens implicated in bacterial contamination of blood products stem from skin flora, including *Staphylococcus* and *Bacillus* species, but gram-negative species such as *Escherichia coli* and *Enterobacter cloacae* more frequently lead to sepsis.[89] Platelet concentrates carry the highest risk of bacterial contamination, since they are stored at 20° to 24°C, which provides a more suitable environment for bacterial replication, as opposed to RBCs, which are stored at 4°C, or plasma, which is frozen.[89]

Several methods aimed at reducing the risk of transfusion-transmitted bacterial infections have proven beneficial. Single-donor collections are associated with less contamination than platelet concentrates from pooled units, likely due to fewer venipunctures and exposures to skin flora, and to collection processes. It is now standard practice to divert the first 20 to 40 mL of collected blood into a separate collection chamber to avoid contaminating the whole donation with blood and epidermal tissue from the initial venipuncture. Standards for skin preparation prior to blood donation and sterile techniques for collection and processing procedures have also decreased contaminants. Furthermore, all apheresis platelets are culture tested prior to storage.[89,99] Bacterial sepsis continues to be a significant cause of transfusion morbidity and mortality, with increasing interest in development of efficient product testing to minimize the risks.[100] Traditional testing of platelet products in the United States relied on indirect testing of pH, glucose, and platelet morphology. As new methodologies such as automated cultures and rapid immunoassays become available, sensitivity for detecting infection increases; however, a residual risk of bacterial transmission remains. New techniques for pathogen reduction (e.g., photoactivity) are currently in use in Europe, but not approved for use in the United States at this time.[31]

Noninfectious Risks of Blood Product Administration

Given the extensive use of more sensitive methods for screening and controlling the infectious risks of blood product transfusion, noninfectious complications have emerged as the major source of transfusion-related morbidity and mortality.[98] Table 17-10 summarizes the relative incidences and main features of the most common noninfectious risks of blood product administration.

Immune-Mediated Transfusion Reactions

Febrile Nonhemolytic Transfusion Reactions

Allergic and febrile reactions are the most common complications of transfused blood products, although the incidence of both has decreased with increased use of LR and single-donor apheresis platelet units.[85] FNHTRs classically present within 4 hours of transfusion with an increase in temperature of 1° to

Table 17-10 Noninfectious Transfusion Reactions

Adverse Reaction	Incidence	Notes
Immune-mediated Reactions		
Febrile nonhemolytic transfusion reaction	0.03–2%	
Minor allergic reactions (urticaria, flushing)	1–3%	
Anaphylactic/toid reactions		IgA deficiency increases risk
Packed red blood cells	0.5/100,000	Washing may avoid reaction
Fresh frozen plasma and platelets	2–3/100,000	More prevalent with plasma-containing products
Acute hemolytic transfusion reaction (AHTR)	1/80,000	
Delayed hemolytic transfusion reaction (DHTR)	1/1,500	Associated with alloantibodies to minor RBC antigens, Kidd, or Rh; One-third have clinical reaction
Transfusion-related immunomodulation (TRIM)	100%	
Alloimmunization	2%	For all patients, risk increases with number of units transfused
Transfusion-related acute lung injury (TRALI)	1/1,300–5,000	Varies with blood product component and patient population
Graft-versus-host disease (TA-GVHD)	1/5,000	Related to immunosuppression; reduced risk with irradiation
Posttransfusion purpura (PTP)	Rare	Attributed to antihuman platelet antigen-1a
Reactions Related to Patient Comorbidities or Transfusion Practice		
Transfusion-associated cardiovascular overload (TACO)	1–8%	Higher in patients with CHF and CRI
Metabolic derangements		
Hyperkalemia		
Citrate toxicity		
Iron overload		
Hypothermia		

Frequencies are presented as percentages when >0.1% and otherwise as ratios.
IgA, immunoglobulin A; CHF, congestive heart failure; CRI, chronic renal insufficiency.

2°C, and may be associated with chills, rigors, anxiety, and headache.[86] They are typically self-limited, but can be prevented or treated with anti-inflammatory or antipyretic medications. The pathophysiology of FNHTRs involves recipient alloimmunization to HLAs from donor WBCs and the release of leukocyte-derived cytokines during product storage.[101] As a result, the risk of febrile reactions increases with repetitive transfusions. Prior to the widespread institution of LR, the incidence of FNHTR was as high as 30%, but currently it is between 0.03% and 2.18%.[101] Although these reactions are common, more serious adverse effects of transfusion, such as sepsis, anaphylaxis, and hemolysis may also present with fever, and should be ruled out prior to diagnosing an FNHTR.

Allergic Reactions

Minor allergic reactions, a relatively common type of transfusion reaction, occur in about 1% to 3% of transfusions. Symptoms are most commonly described as urticaria, hives with or without pruritus, and angioedema.[86,102] The specific cause of allergic reactions is unclear, but likely involves an immune response to recipient WBC antigens or transfused plasma proteins.[86,102] Prophylaxis with antihistamines is common practice for patients with a history of allergic reactions to blood products, but several studies have demonstrated no symptom reduction with pretreatment. Best practice should be to reduce the rate of transfusion and treat supportively when symptoms arise.[86] If symptoms become severe with recurrent or frequent transfusion needs, cellular products can be washed.

Major allergic reactions present as anaphylactoid or anaphylactic reactions with hemodynamic instability, bronchospasm, rash, flushing, and/or angioedema.[86,103] These reactions are rare—only 1 in 50,000 transfusions for absolute IgA-deficient individuals when premedication and product preparation are ensured (Table 17-10)—but the reaction can be fatal if unrecognized.[103] Pathophysiologically, the recipient—typically patients who are IgA deficient with anti-IgA antibodies—mounts an immediate immune response to transfused plasma proteins or cellular antigens. Classically, anaphylaxis requires an immediate type I hypersensitivity IgE-mediated reaction; however, most major allergic responses to blood transfusions do not show laboratory evidence of IgE antibodies, and are therefore anaphylactoid reactions.[102] These transfusion complications can be prevented in patients with known IgA deficiency by washing blood products prior to transfusion or by using products obtained from IgA-deficient donors.[103]

Acute hemolytic transfusion reactions (AHTRs) remain one of the leading causes of transfusion-related fatalities. They occur with the transfusion of incompatible blood products when pre-existing IgM or IgG antibodies in recipients form complexes with donor RBC antigens, causing complement activation and immediate intravascular hemolysis. Classically, AHTRs result from ABO incompatibility secondary to native anti-A or anti-B IgM. Careful adherence to protocols for specimen phlebotomy and blood component administration is vital for prevention. However, growing evidence exists for the implication of other RBC antigens such as Kidd, Kell, and Duffy, causing acute hemolytic reactions in patients with a history of transfusion exposure and alloimmunization.[104] Rarely, the transfusion of incompatible plasma (type O plasma or whole blood to a patient with type A, B, or AB blood) has resulted in AHTRs as well.[104,105] These reactions are rare and have become less frequent with the institution of safety measures to reduce clerical error and improve the availability of cross-matched blood products. Data from national surveillance databases in the United States and the United Kingdom report AHTR as the third leading cause of transfusion-related mortalities. Fortunately, less than half of patients transfused with incompatible blood products become symptomatic. The overall fatality rate from incompatible transfusion is 10%, but is significantly dependent on the volume transfused with fatality risk more than 20% with the infusion of more than 50 mL.[85,98,104]

AHTRs occur secondary to IgM-mediated antibody–antigen complexes that activate complement and result in intravascular and extravascular hemolysis in the spleen and liver. The release of bradykinin causes fever, hypotension, and hemodynamic instability, while histamine release from mast cells leads to bronchospasm and urticaria, as well as symptoms of dyspnea, flushing, and severe anxiety. Hemolysis results in the release of free hemoglobin that is bound by haptoglobin and plasma proteins, but will also be eliminated by the kidney when these proteins are unavailable.[104] Severe hemolysis may lead to renal failure, DIC, and death. General anesthesia can mask several of the presenting symptoms of AHTRs; therefore, vigilance during transfusion of an anesthetized patient must remain high, as survival depends on discontinuing the transfusion.

The diagnosis of hemolytic reactions is confirmed with laboratory findings of free hemoglobin, low haptoglobin, bilirubin increases, a positive direct antiglobulin (Coombs) test, and hematuria. Suspicion of a transfusion reaction should prompt immediate discontinuation of the transfusion, and investigation into the donor and recipient blood types and antigen–antibody components. Treatment of AHTR involves supportive care for hemodynamic instability and microvascular bleeding, as well as maintenance of adequate urine output to avoid renal failure associated with hemaglobinuria. Anemia can be profound, as the immediate hemolysis can destroy over 200 mL of blood per hour.[104]

Delayed hemolytic transfusion reactions (DHTRs) result from passive transfusion of RBC antibodies to native antigens in the recipient, or more commonly, alloantibodies in the recipient to minor RBC antigens in the Rh, Kell, Kidd, Duffy, MNSs, and other blood groups. There are at least 35 recognized blood groups at this time.[104,105] DHTRs generally present 3 to 10 days after transfusion of an apparently "compatible" blood component. Typically, the recipient has IgG alloantibodies to a particular RBC antigen, and will mount an amnestic immune response; however, the pretransfusion antibody levels are too low for serologic detection. Symptoms of DHTRs are much milder than AHTRs and rarely result in major morbidity or mortality because the hemolysis occurs extravascularly in the reticuloendothelial system, liver, and spleen. Patients experience mild fever and possible rash, with laboratory and clinical signs of hemolysis such as jaundice, hemaglobinuria, low haptoglobin, positive direct Coombs test, and decreasing hemoglobin levels. The incidence of DHTRs is likely underreported as symptoms are subtle and may be attributed to the patient's underlying systemic illness. Studies estimate the risk of alloimmunization is up to 30% of transfusions. Symptoms are generally self-limited and treated supportively with hydration to protect the renal tubules during hemolysis, with further compatible transfusions to support anemia as indicated. Anemia is typically not severe, with less than 400 mL of RBCs destroyed over a 24-hour period.[104]

Transfusion-related Immunomodulation

In the 1970s, transfusion-related immunomodulation (TRIM) was discovered from improved survival of renal allografts in patients who had received a transfusion pretransplant. This highlighted the potential immunosuppressant effects of stored allogeneic blood products. However, these beneficial effects are patient-specific. Immunosuppression also proved to increase the recurrence of malignancies and the incidence of serious health-care–associated infections, as well as long-term mortality after cardiac surgery.[106–108] Given multiple studies demonstrating the detrimental effects of just one transfused unit (including TRALI, multiorgan system failure, and increased rates of infection), efforts to define its immunomodulation mechanisms are in progress.[106,109,110]

Results point to a multifactorial pathophysiology that implicates transfused WBCs, donor plasma HLA class 1 peptides, cytokines, and immune mediators released during blood product storage, as well as the immune function of transfused RBCs within the microvasculature of the recipient.[109,110] Several experts propose a "two-insult" model for TRIM similar to the pathophysiologic mechanism for TRALI and acute respiratory distress syndrome.[109] Presumably, most patients requiring blood products are suffering from a precondition that "primes" both the immune system and vascular endothelium (e.g., trauma, surgery, or acute illness). This constitutes the first insult and causes active neutrophils to adhere to vascular endothelial cells and become hypersensitive to blood-borne immune mediators. The second insult occurs with the infusion of transfused blood products that contain WBCs with HLA class I antigens, as well as soluble immune response modifiers in the form of cytokines, complement factors, and the breakdown products of lipid membranes.[106,109,110] Several studies demonstrate a decrease in T-cell responsiveness and the inhibition of monocyte function after transfusion of RBCs.

The degree of TRIM-induced injury has been attributed to progressive storage lesions thought to be related to the age of RBC products at the time of transfusion. However, several recent trials, including the ARIPI trial in premature infants, the ABLE trial in critically ill patients, the RECESS trial in cardiac surgery, and the TOTAL trial in children with hemorrhagic shock, consistently report no significant association between RBC storage duration and mortality or other adverse transfusion outcomes.[37,111–113] Also, prestorage LR and poststorage WBC filtration have been investigated as a means of limiting the deleterious effects of TRIM; however, results thus far are variable and inconclusive.[100,106] Nevertheless, evidence collected over the past 30 years from clinical trials and animal studies supports the hypothesis that TRIM involves both proinflammatory mechanisms and systemic immunosuppression.

Alloimmunization

Alloimmunization refers to the induction of an immune response to allogenic antigen exposure. This process occurs occasionally through pregnancy, but the majority of alloimmunization results from transfusion of blood products containing immunogenic antigens on the surface of RBCs. Unlike classic ABO antigens, which consist of carbohydrate chains, most of the non-ABO alloantigens (Kell, Kidd, Duffy, etc.) result from single amino acid polymorphisms between the recipient and donor.[114] Healthy donor populations are expected to have an incidence of approximately 1% for blood group antibodies other than ABO.[104] AHTRs result in an immediate IgM-mediated immune response to ABO incompatibility with naturally occurring anti-A or anti-B antibodies. In contrast, alloimmunization prompts an amnestic IgG-mediated humoral immunity to foreign proteins and does not result in RBC destruction until the second antigen exposure, which may cause complement activation and delayed extravascular hemolysis.[104,114] Thus, the clinical consequences of alloimmunization are rarely immediate or fatal, but the generation of antibodies may cause DHTRs and adds difficulty to subsequent cross-matching.

The incidence of alloimmunization is estimated between 4.4% and 10.5% from multiple longitudinal studies, but up to 40% to 58% in chronically transfused patients such as those with sickle cell disease, hematologic malignancy, or thalassemia.[115,116] This is especially evident for patients who require frequent platelet transfusions. Platelets carry significant levels of multiple human platelet antigens (HPA 1 to 15) and other polymorphisms that can result in the destruction of transfused platelets and refractory thrombocytopenia.[114] The use of single-donor apheresis units may limit the exposure to HPA and HLA. Furthermore, early studies demonstrate that preemptive matching of RBC units beyond just ABO blood groups reduces the risk of alloimmunization by up to 64%.[116] This practice could significantly alter the long-term prognosis for chronic transfusion patients.

Transfusion-Related Acute Lung Injury

For at least the past decade, TRALI has been internationally recognized as the leading cause of transfusion-associated mortality, according to the United Kingdom's SHOT database. In recent data from the FDA, TRALI accounts for over 40% of US transfusion-related fatalities.[85,98,117] The incidence of TRALI is estimated to range from 0.04% to 8.0%, depending on patient risk factors and blood products used. A recent study of noncardiac surgery patients reported an incidence of 1.3% for all blood components.[118] Other estimates predict an incidence of 1 in 5,000 products (highest with plasma-containing products), and mortality rates of 5% to 25%.[119] Over the past decade, more consistent criteria have been used to diagnose TRALI—acute onset hypoxemia occurring within 6 hours of transfusion ($PaO_2/FiO_2 \leq 300$ mmHg or oxygen saturation ≤90% on room air) and no evidence of left atrial hypertension. Possible TRALI can be diagnosed when alternative risk factors for acute lung injury are present, such as trauma or sepsis.[118,120,121] TRALI remains a clinical diagnosis that can be confounded by comorbidities or patient acuity. Consequently, TRALI tends to be underreported in the literature and difficult to study with randomized prospective clinical trials.

The pathophysiology of TRALI is complex and not yet fully understood. The clinical picture involves low-pressure pulmonary edema secondary to neutrophil activation and sequestration in the lungs. This results in endothelial injury and capillary leakage of proteinaceous fluid into the interstitium and intraalveolar spaces. There are two leading theories on the mechanism of lung injury, both with sound experimental and clinical evidence. The antibody-mediated model stems from evidence of antibody–antigen complexes in the plasma of transfusion recipients who suffered from TRALI.[119,120] These antibodies are mostly against HLAs (class I and II) and human neutrophil antigens (HNAs).[119,120] Antibodies form in the donor plasma after alloimmunization from pregnancy, prior transfusion, or prior transplantation. Accordingly, plasma donation from multiparous women has been implicated as one of the highest risks associated with TRALI.[119] Once the antibodies are transfused into the recipient, they complex with native WBC antigens on the surface of monocytes (HLA class II), endothelial cells (HLA class I), and neutrophils (HNAs and HLA class I), thereby activating the neutrophils to facilitate aggregation and release of cytotoxic mediators. Subsequently, the endothelial lining of capillaries in the lung is damaged, resulting in extravasation of WBCs and leakage of edema fluid.[119]

The second proposed mechanism of TRALI was termed the "Two-Hit Model" in the late 1990s by Silliman et al., when they discovered the role of biologic response modifiers in its pathophysiology. Stored blood components accumulate lipid degradation products (mostly phosphatidylcholine derivatives) that function to activate neutrophils primed and sequestered on the endothelial vascular lining of lung tissue.[122] Patients with the highest incidence of TRALI often suffer from a pre-existing proinflammatory state such as active infection, trauma, surgery, or multiple transfusions.[118,120] Acute illness causes the immune system to be hyperreactive, with neutrophils poised on the microvasculature endothelium and "primed" to be activated by various biologic response modifiers, including cytokines, complement, and leukotrienes.[122] The transfusion of stored blood products and associated reactive lipid particles marks the second "hit," which activates primed neutrophils and results in the destruction of the capillary lining of lung microvasculature.[120,122] The overall pathophysiology of TRALI likely involves both of these mechanisms.

The management of TRALI focuses on supportive measures to limit lung injury and optimize oxygenation. This includes maximizing positive end-expiratory pressures, avoiding volume overload, and using low tidal volume strategies. Several studies have demonstrated decreased incidence of TRALI with deferral of high risk alloimmunization donors such as those with history of pregnancy, transfusion, or high antibody titers. Laboratory testing for antibody titers is time-consuming and inefficient; however, forcing many blood management services to use male-only donors for platelet and plasma products.[120] LR is also used to minimize the incidence and severity of TRALI, and likely has a significant clinical benefit for patients at high risk with critical illness or immunosuppression.[96] However, a recent systematic review demonstrated no definitive evidence to support universal leukoreduction for all patients.[96] Overall, prevention is the best treatment for TRALI, and is currently a major focus of clinical and experimental study, with emphasis on blood conservation strategies and restrictive transfusion practices.

Transfusion-Associated Graft-versus-Host Disease

Transfusion-associated GVHD (TA-GVHD) is a rare but fulminant and fatal complication of blood products containing cellular components (platelets and RBCs). Although its incidence is decreasing secondary to preventative γ irradiation and LR, mortality is more than 90%. It occurs when donor lymphocytes engraft in the recipient and attack host cells they recognize as foreign. Patients at risk for TA-GVHD include those immunocompromised from stem cell transplants, B-cell malignancies (e.g., multiple myeloma, non-Hodgkin lymphoma) or acute lymphocytic leukemia, or with Hodgkin's disease or congenital immunodeficiency syndromes.[123] Immunocompetent patients may also be at risk when transfused with directed donations from blood relations with similar HLA types because transfused donor lymphocytes are not recognized as foreign, yet still reject the recipient's tissue.[119] TA-GVHD classically presents 4 to 21 days after transfusion, but clinical suspicion should exist for up to 6 weeks. Symptoms progress rapidly and generally affect the skin, hepatic, digestive, and hematopoietic organ systems causing fever, rash, liver dysfunction, diarrhea, and pancytopenia.[119,123]

Posttransfusion Purpura

Defined as severe thrombocytopenia with purpura occurring 5 to 10 days posttransfusion, posttransfusion purpura (PTP) is a very rare complication of transfusion, but associated with high morbidity and mortality. Most patients are female and have platelet-specific alloantibodies such as anti-HPA-1a.[124] These antibodies are almost exclusively found in previously pregnant women and cause platelet destruction of both transfused and autologous platelets. Intravenous IG is the first line of treatment, but plasmapheresis may be necessary to remove antibody and avoid bleeding complications.[124]

Nonimmune-Mediated Transfusion Reactions

Transfusion-Associated Cardiovascular Overload

Transfusion-associated cardiovascular overload (TACO) describes the occurrence of hydrostatic pulmonary edema after transfusion of blood component therapy. It differs from TRALI in that it is not immune mediated or associated with increased capillary permeability, and it responds rapidly to diuretic therapy and afterload reduction. The recent CDC definition requires evidence of acute respiratory distress within 6 hours of transfusion with features of left heart failure including increased central venous pressure or increased brain natriuretic peptide.[125] Similar to TRALI, TACO can be difficult to diagnose and is likely underreported in the literature. The overall incidence of TACO ranges from 1% to 8% of transfused patients, and is more prevalent in critically ill and postoperative patients with a history of congestive heart failure, chronic diuretic dependence, and underlining renal insufficiency.[126,127] Other risk factors for TACO include the volume and rate of transfusion, plasma products, and positive fluid balance.[125,127]

Recent reports from the FDA and the United Kingdom's SHOT database describe significant morbidity and mortality risks associated with TACO, the second leading cause of transfusion-related fatality over the past 5 years.[98,117] Furthermore, TACO increases the length of both ICU and hospital stay.[127] Preventative measures include slowing the rate of transfusion when appropriate, administering one blood product at a time, frequent assessment of vital signs, symptoms, and pulmonary status, and rapid treatment of volume overload with diuretics.

Metabolic Derangements

The metabolic derangements from transfusion are usually not evident unless patients received a large volume transfusion or rapid infusion rates, but often include hyperkalemia, citrate toxicity, and hypothermia.[128] As storage time for blood products increases, the cellular components leak potassium and metabolize glucose into lactate, resulting in hyperkalemia and/or acidemia in the transfused product. The acidosis is quickly cleared by physiologic buffers, as citrate preservative in blood products is metabolized to bicarbonate; therefore, ongoing acidosis in patients undergoing massive transfusion is likely secondary to tissue hypoxia and not to transfusion of acidemic blood products. However, hyperkalemia results from high-volume transfusion, especially when infusion rates exceed 100 to 150 mL/hr. Packed RBCs can contain over 7 mEq/dL of potassium depending on the storage age and can produce consequences of hyperkalemia, such as ventricular arrhythmia or sudden cardiac arrest, particularly in neonates and patients with renal insufficiency.[128]

Citrate is a common anticoagulant used in stored blood products and is readily metabolized by the liver and quickly eliminated. However, with rapid infusion rates, massive transfusion, or in patients with liver dysfunction, citrate accumulates in the plasma and chelates calcium, resulting in hypocalcemia. Severe hypocalcemia leads to muscle weakness, tetany, arrhythmias, myocardial dysfunction, and acquired coagulopathy.[128]

Blood product transfusion can also lead to hypothermia, especially during rapid infusion of previously cold or recently thawed blood products. Coagulation factor activity decreases by 10% for every 1°C decrease in core body temperature. Fluid warmers are standard of care for rapid transfusion; nevertheless, hypothermia is commonly associated with massive transfusion and can result in platelet and coagulation factor dysfunction, arrhythmias, hepatic dysfunction, decreased citrate and drug metabolism, and myocardial depression. Additional preventative measures include warming the surrounding environment, surface warming, heated and humidified inspired gases, and fluid warmers for all infusion lines.[128]

Iron Overload

Packed RBCs carry increasing concentrations of iron as a result of hemolysis during storage and transfusion. Iron stores accumulate in patients who require frequent transfusions for chronic anemia or hemoglobinopathies, with increased mortality demonstrated for patients who receive more than 20 units of PRBCs. Iron overload occurs when deposits in the liver, heart, and endocrine systems result in organ dysfunction. Stored iron is not directly detrimental to organ systems; however, iron metabolism produces harmful intracellular free radicals, which in turn cause cellular dysfunction and organ failure. Patients often suffer from cardiomyopathy and cirrhosis.[129] Furthermore, iron availability for microorganisms increases the risk of recurrent infections to patients with chronic transfusion requirements. Chelation therapy is the first line of treatment, but difficult to administer secondary to the bioavailability and side effect profile of chelating agents. Exchange transfusion therapy decreases the iron load better than traditional transfusion, but it is expensive and associated with complications from central venous access and a larger amount of blood products.[129]

Blood Conservation Strategies

Most healthy patients undergoing routine surgery will not require allogenic blood transfusion. However, there are some elective procedures such as liver resection, orthopedic surgery, cardiac surgery, and scoliosis correction where the risk of blood transfusion exceeds 30%.[130] As discussed in detail earlier, blood component therapy is associated with significant morbidity and mortality for all patient populations. It is also scarce and costly. Several methodologies have been suggested to conserve perioperative transfusion (Table 17-11), with the most recent guidelines from the ASA emphasizing many of these adjunctive techniques.[44]

Autologous Blood Transfusion

Autologous blood conservation (ABC) first gained popularity because of the rising risk of transfusion-transmitted viral infections. All forms of ABC reduce the need for allogenic blood components; however, now that the incidence of infectious risks with allogenic blood has declined substantially, the utility and cost-effectiveness of ABC is not as certain, especially when the process involves blood storage. ABC encompasses three separate processes: (1) preoperative autologous blood donation (PAD); (2) acute normovolemic hemodilution (ANH); and (3) perioperative blood cell salvage.

Table 17-11 Perioperative Blood Conservation Strategies

Technique	Comments
Preoperative autologous donation (PAD)	Increased overall transfusion requirement; lower preoperative hemoglobin
Acute normovolemic hemodilution (ANH)	Limited benefit; contains clotting factors and platelets
Intraoperative blood salvage (IOBS)	Cost-effective, low risk, and highly efficacious
Postoperative blood salvage (POBS)	Efficacious for high-risk orthopedic surgery
Pharmacologic agents	
Stimulants of erythropoiesis	Erythropoietin, vitamin B_{12}, folate
Prohemostatic agents	Vitamin K, DDAVP, antifibrinolytics, factor concentrates

DDAVP, 1-deamino-8-D-arginine vasopressin.

PAD summarizes the process of patients donating their own whole blood in the weeks preceding a planned surgical procedure to ensure that they receive autologous blood, should red cell replacement be necessary. PAD was initially popular in the 1980s, when concern for transfusion-transmitted HIV was high; however, it has since become less frequently used given the reduced risk of viral infections and new concerns about the risks and adverse effects of stored blood. PAD eliminates the risk of transfusion-transmitted infection and alloimmunization, and it may also decrease the risk of TRALI. However, recipients of stored autologous blood remain at risk for clerical error, TACO, bacterial infection, metabolic derangements, and TRIM. PAD reduces the need for allogenic blood transfusion when performed with appropriate protocols that include early donation and erythrocyte-stimulating agents (ESA) to allow for sufficient erythrogenesis. However, intraoperative blood salvage (IOBS) techniques have improved their efficiency. Given the increased tolerance for lower perioperative hemoglobin levels, the increased wastage of PAD units (up to 45%), diminishes the efficacy and cost effectiveness of its routine use.[130,131]

PAD is currently indicated for use in patients in whom it would be difficult to find compatible blood products due to multiple antibodies or rare blood types, those who refuse to receive allogenic transfusion, and those undergoing elective surgery where more than 4 units of RBC transfusion is anticipated.[130,131] Typically, each donation session collects a single or double unit of whole blood and can technically be repeated weekly until 72 hours prior to the scheduled procedure.[131] Patients are rarely able to donate more than 4 units because of the limited storage time, and hemoglobin must remain above 11 g/dL before donation.[130] However, the earlier the donation, the more time a patient has to recover from iatrogenic anemia. Despite the ability to donate up until 72 hours before surgery, it is not recommended to undergo donation within 28 days of planned surgery as PAD rapidly loses its effectiveness when donation occurs in proximity to surgery and patients present with preoperative anemia.[130,131] PAD is most effective when used in conjunction with erythropoietin, which increases the tolerance for repeat donations. Iron supplementation is not indicated and generally not helpful in patients who are already iron replete; however, oral iron should be administered to patients known to be iron deficient prior to autologous donation and surgery.[130,131]

PAD should be avoided if the scheduled procedure is at risk of postponement because autologous donated units may become outdated if surgery does not proceed on time. Furthermore, directed donations are not subjected to the same testing or deferral procedures as allogenic blood collection, and therefore cannot be used by the general population if they are not transfused into the patient. Transfusion of autologous blood should still be guided by the same indications for transfusion of allogenic RBCs— avoiding wastage is not an appropriate reason to transfuse autologous units. In other words, patients should not be overtransfused simply because they have stored autologous blood. In large retrospective studies comparing PAD to IOBS techniques, PAD is less effective at reducing allogenic transfusion rates and presents several risks such as symptomatic donation, preoperative anemia (average preoperative hemoglobin level 1.1g/dL below controls), increased rates of overall transfusion, and higher costs.[130,131] As with any perioperative management plan, the advantages and disadvantages should be individually considered in the context of the patient's history, planned procedure, and physical state before implementing a PAD program.

ANH is the process of extracting multiple units of blood immediately before surgical incision while maintaining euvolemia with crystalloid or colloid supplementation. The withdrawn blood is high in hematocrit and contains clotting factors and functional platelets. After ANH, the patient loses blood with lower hemoglobin and fewer red cells. This process reduces the oxygen-carrying capacity of blood, but healthy patients maintain oxygen delivery with intact compensatory mechanisms such as increased CO and oxygen extraction. At the end of surgery, the autologous units are reinfused, thereby replacing RBCs, platelets, and plasma proteins active in hemostasis. This process eliminates the infectious and alloimmunization risks of allogenic transfusion, as well as the immunomodulatory risks of blood storage. ANH was first introduced in the 1970s and gained popularity in the 1990s, when transfusion-transmitted infectious risks were high. In the last 20 years, however, three large meta-analyses documented only modest decreases in the risk of allogenic transfusion rates, and highlighted limitations and controversy associated with publication bias for ANH trials.[132,133] Furthermore, a recent mathematical modeling study demonstrated ANH to be inferior to high-efficiency IOBS and protocolized PAD.[131]

Procedurally, ANH involves the removal of a predetermined volume of blood after the induction of anesthesia, but prior to surgical incision. Target hematocrit nadirs will vary based on individual patient history and baseline physiologic state; however, these usually range from 25% to 30%.[133] The simple formula for allowable blood loss is used to calculate the volume to be removed. Volume to be removed = $EBV \times [(Hct_i - Hct_t)/Hct_{ave}]$ where EBV is the estimated blood volume; Hct_i, the starting hematocrit; Hct_t, the target low hematocrit; Hct_{ave}, the average of Hct. Euvolemia should be maintained with either crystalloids at a ratio of 3:1 with colloids at a ratio of 1:1 relative to the volume of blood removed.[131]

Given the limited evidence of benefit, ANH is not recommended for routine use. However, it may be considered for patients with multiple antibodies or a rare blood type that creates difficulty with finding compatible products, or for patients who refuse allogenic transfusion or stored blood component therapy such as Jehovah's Witnesses. ANH is most effective in patients with high preoperative hemoglobin levels, minimal cardiovascular comorbidities that allow intraoperative anemia, and a surgical risk for large volume blood loss. This technique of autologous transfusion is favorable compared to PAD in selected patient populations.[132]

Perioperative Erythropoietin

Erythropoietin is the primary regulator of erythropoiesis. Its endogenous release is stimulated by anemia or physiologic hypoxia. It is currently FDA-approved for treatment of anemia in oncology patients with chemotherapy-induced anemia and patients with chronic renal failure. It has also been used to optimize patients with preoperative anemia undergoing surgery with significant risk of transfusion and patients undergoing PAD[134] (because conventional PAD programs maintain hematocrit levels well above the threshold for endogenous erythropoietin release, causing insufficient native stimulation of erythropoiesis). Several studies have shown a clear decrease in the requirements for allogenic blood transfusion, when erythropoietin is used in conjunction with a PAD program for adolescent spine, orthopedic, or cardiac surgery that maintains preoperative hemoglobin concentrations between 10 and 13 g/dL.[134,135] However, there is ongoing concern for increased risk of thromboembolic events and overall safety issues when erythropoietin is used routinely. For these reasons, its generalized use is not recommended at this time.

Perioperative Blood Salvage

RBC salvage was first attempted in the early nineteenth century for patients with postpartum hemorrhage. Not surprisingly, it was fraught with complications throughout its early development. It was not until the 1970s that commercial cell salvage devices became available for clinical use, yet there were still frequent complications such as hemolysis, air embolism, and coagulopathy.[136] Over the past decade RBC salvage techniques have improved significantly and now offer an efficient, cost-effective, and safe method for perioperative blood conservation. In general, cell salvage involves the collection of shed surgical blood, which is filtered and/or washed prior to reinfusion. This process can be carried out intraoperatively with direct suction of the surgical field, or postoperatively in the case of orthopedic, cardiac, and thoracic surgery with the use of blood from wound drainage.

IOBS requires the use of a double-lumen suction catheter with one port for aspiration from the surgical field and the other for the addition of an anticoagulant solution, usually heparin or citrate. Suctioned blood is then collected in a reservoir, filtered to remove large debris, and centrifuged to produce RBC concentrates. The final step of washing clears the product of residual contaminants such as plasma, platelets, free hemoglobin, cellular fragments, WBCs, and the remaining heparin or citrate. The resultant red cells are resuspended in saline and ready for reinfusion. This is usually reinfused to the patient immediately through standard blood filters, but may be stored at 4°C for up to 6 hours with careful patient and product identification. On average, IOBS yields a hematocrit ranging from 50% to 80%.[131,136] The efficiency depends on several factors including the volume of blood processed at a time, the length of time that blood remains in the wound, and the rate and precision of suctioning, since increased turbulence from the surgical field adds shear stress, which damages RBCs. Most modern-day cell savers, when used appropriately, provide RBC concentrates with a hematocrit of 60% to 70%.[131,136]

IOBS has proven benefits for reducing allogenic blood transfusion in major surgery, particularly multilevel spine fusions and cardiac surgery.[136–139] However, recent studies and a meta-analysis on the use of cell salvage in routine knee and hip arthroplasty demonstrate reduced efficacy and cost effectiveness for IOBS. This is likely secondary to more restrictive transfusion practices, better preoperative optimization of hemoglobin levels, and the use of antifibrinolytics.[135,140,141] However, IOBS continues to be indicated for patients with low preoperative hemoglobin who cannot tolerate PAD or ANH, those unwilling to consent to allogenic transfusion, and patients with pre-existing bleeding risks or multiple alloantibodies.[131,142,143] Evidence shows that salvaged blood has better oxygen-carrying capacity and tissue oxygenation than stored blood, secondary to retention of red cell's biconcave disc shape and increased levels of 2,3-DPG and ATP.[136,144] There are very few studies directly comparing IOBS to ANH and PAD. One mathematical modeling study demonstrated the superiority of IOBS to PAD and ANH when high-efficiency systems are able to recover more than 70% of blood loss.[131] Overall, IOBS is cost-effective, convenient, and advantageous for emergency procedures and surgeries with high risk of significant perioperative blood loss.

The complications of IOBS are rare and are mostly associated with either the method of suctioning or contamination from the surgical field. Risks include nonimmunogenic hemolysis, fever, and contamination with various substances such as topical anticoagulants, urine, amniotic fluid, or bacteria. Washing the salvaged blood clears most contaminants, and variable suction devices limit the sheer stress that causes hemolysis. Reinfusion of salvaged blood in volumes greater than 50% of the estimated blood volume can result in dilutional coagulopathy similar to massive transfusion of allogenic RBCs, since neither contains clotting factors or platelets. Lastly, IOBS can cause gas embolism if the reinfusion bag is connected in a continuous circuit with the patient.[136,145] Careful adherence to the recommended application of modern cell-saver devices effectively eliminates many of these concerns.

Traditionally, cell salvage was contraindicated in cancer surgery and operations where blood loss is contaminated by urine, anticoagulants, or amniotic fluid. However, several studies now demonstrate the safety of cell salvage when blood is processed, washed, and administered through a leukodepletion filter.[136,145] Use in surgery for prostate cancer and gynecologic oncology, which often involves urine and malignant cells contaminating the field, has not shown significant increases in morbidity, mortality, or cancer recurrence. However, it is recommended that IOBS be filtered and irradiated when there is concern for malignancy, and avoided completely when the tumor is ruptured causing an overwhelming concentration of cancer cells in shed blood.[136] The use of IOBS for obstetric cases raises concerns about inducing alloimmunization or amniotic fluid embolism, recently termed "anaphylactoid syndrome of pregnancy." Because this syndrome is very rare, it is difficult to establish the safety of a new technique. However, Goucher et al.[145] reviewed the results of seven IOBS trials for almost 300 obstetric patients and found no increased incidence of amniotic fluid emboli. Leukodepletion filters remove most of the amniotic fluid, immune mediators, and debris. Although fetal RBCs cannot be differentiated from maternal red cells and may potentiate alloimmunization, this risk is already present during delivery and not exacerbated by the use of IOBS. Cell salvage should be considered for high-risk obstetric patients such as those undergoing planned cesarean hysterectomy or those with placenta accreta.[145] The only absolute contraindications to IOBS are microbial contamination of the surgical field, and cancer surgery where tumor rupture or direct manipulation is likely.[136]

Postoperative blood salvage (POBS) involves the collection and reinfusion of blood shed into surgical wound drains in the immediate postoperative period. The recovered blood product can be processed in one of the two ways: "washed" POBS is centrifuged, washed, and resuspended as RBC concentrates, whereas "unwashed" POBS is simply filtered before reinfusion. The resultant hematocrit of unwashed POBS ranges from 20% to 30% and should not be expected to increase the patient's hemoglobin level. Rather, it will aid in avoidance of dilutional anemia associated with the fluid resuscitation for postoperative bleeding. There are advantages and disadvantages to both techniques, resulting in continued controversies over the safety and efficacy of POBS.

POBS studies are limited, but meta-analyses demonstrate efficacy in orthopedic procedures such as knee and hip arthroplasty. Unwashed POBS is most commonly used in orthopedics, as it is highly efficacious, cost-effective, and requires little additional training in comparison to use of washed POBS.[146,147] POBS has also been studied in postcardiac surgery patients and shown to be efficacious at reducing the need for allogenic blood transfusion.[146] However, shed blood from surgical wounds, involving the thorax and mediastinum, contains inflammatory mediators, activated clotting factors, fibrin and fibrin split products, and the products of hemolysis such as free hemoglobin. These substances can precipitate renal damage, lung injury, or coagulopathy. POBS for cardiac surgery should be washed prior to reinfusion in accordance with the most recent guidelines from the SCA.[51,148]

POBS continues to be part of the multimodal approach to perioperative patient blood management. Complications include concern for hemolysis and immunomodulation, and its overall efficacy and cost effectiveness remain unclear. However, POBS continues to be used in routine orthopedic and cardiac surgery.[146-148] It is contraindicated for patients with pre-existing hemoglobinopathies such as sickle cell disease and thalassemia.[146] Furthermore, similar to IOBS, blood should not be reinfused if it has been contaminated with microbials or drugs used topically in the surgical field that are not indicated for systemic use (e.g., betadine, chlorhexidine, and topical antibiotics).[146]

Jehovah's Witnesses belong to an international and well-established religious society with over 7.8 million followers who believe in a literal translation of the Bible. Passages such as Genesis 9, verse 4 ("But you shall not eat flesh with its life, that is, its blood") and Leviticus 17, verse 10 ("If any one of the house of Israel…eats any blood, I will … cut him off from among his people") lead to a proscription against receiving blood product transfusions. Followers believe that once blood has left the body it should not be consumed in any way. Receipt of a blood transfusion is believed to cause irreversible death to a member's soul without hope of eternal life.[142,143] Most Jehovah's Witnesses understand and accept the threat of death as a possible result of refusing therapeutic transfusion. Clearly this is challenging for treating physicians, especially in the case of emergent hemorrhage. The best management for Jehovah's Witnesses is to have a well-prescribed perioperative management plan to maximize blood conservation strategies and a clear conversation about the patient's individual concerns and beliefs. Some patients consent to blood component therapy, factor concentrates derived from blood (e.g., albumin or PCCs), or extracorporeal circulation, which may include cardiopulmonary bypass, ANH, and IOBS if left in continuous circulation with the body. These decisions can be made based on a patient's review of their conscience and their own interpretation of religious scripture.[143]

Jehovah's Witnesses are fully aware of how their belief system affects medical management with routine life-sustaining treatments. Accordingly, there are over 1,700 Hospital Liaison Committees worldwide designed to assist with personal healthcare management plans that provide both patient autonomy and the best medical care available.[143] Some of the most challenging questions arise with minors, emergencies, and unconscious patients, when the physician is unable to have a clear conversation about the patient's specific beliefs. There is a great deal of individual variability within the religion that can lead to drastically different management plans for bleeding and acute anemia. Often adult Jehovah's Witnesses will carry cards with an advance directive; however, if questions arise, physicians should seek the guidance of their hospital ethics committees and legal advisors. An urgent application to the court system is appropriate in the case of minors or unconscious patients without decision-making capacity.[142,143]

In preparation for elective surgery for a Jehovah's Witness patient, the use of prohemostatic medications such as ESAs, antifibrinolytics, vitamin K, factor concentrates, and desmopressin should be considered, and should be available. In addition, the patient's preoperative hemoglobin should be optimized by stimulating erythropoiesis with recombinant erythropoietin, iron, and supplemental vitamin B_{12} and folate.[142,143] There is ongoing research into the clinical use of hemoglobin-based oxygen carriers that could revolutionize the treatment not only of Jehovah's Witnesses, but have yet to be approved in the United States.[142]

Disorders of Hemostasis: Diagnosis and Treatment

As discussed previously, hemostasis is a complex mechanism of checks and balances that aims to control bleeding from sites of vascular injury while maintaining blood flow throughout the rest of the body. It involves countless proteins, enzymes, ligands, and molecules to serve as activators, cofactors, regulators, and inhibitors in hemostasis. When the equilibrium of this process is disrupted, it results in abnormal bleeding or clotting, depending on the specific dysfunction or deficiency. Accordingly, disorders of hemostasis can be classified as those that facilitate hemorrhage and those that facilitate inappropriate thrombosis. The disorders are further separated by the involvement in primary hemostasis (the initial platelet plug) or secondary hemostasis (the clotting cascade and fibrin cross-linkage). Finally, hemostatic disorders are caused by either inherited genetic disease or acquired deficiencies.

Symptomatic disorders of primary hemostasis often present with superficial signs of bleeding on the skin or mucosa. Patients complain of petechiae, mucosal bleeding, and easy bruising. They often suffer from prolonged bleeding from minor injury, frequent epistaxis, and menorrhagia secondary to deficient or dysfunctional platelet activity. In contrast, disorders of secondary hemostasis involve qualitative or quantitative dysfunction of clotting factors and cause more severe and deep tissue bleeding. These patients present with spontaneous hemarthroses, hematomas, and excessive hemorrhage after traumatic injuries. Treatments depend on the specific cause of the disorder and often involve blood component therapy or pharmacologic agents that enhance, inhibit, or bypass specific sites in the hemostatic process.

Disorders of Primary Hemostasis

Primary hemostasis involves the initial recruitment of platelets at the site of vascular injury to form a fragile platelet plug. Once platelets bind to the injured subendothelium, they become activated, thereby exposing additional receptor sites and releasing factors involved in further platelet recruitment, activation, aggregation, and the initiation of secondary hemostasis.

Hereditary disorders of platelets are rare and usually associated with defective receptor binding. Bernard–Soulier syndrome is an autosomal recessive disorder that results from an abnormality of the GP Ib receptor. This qualitative and quantitative dysfunction impairs platelet adhesion to exposed vWF at the site of vascular injury.[149] Glanzmann thrombasthenia is an autosomal recessive genetic disorder that results from a defect in the platelet integrin αIIbβ3 receptor which, under normal circumstances, allows fibrinogen and other ligands to bind and facilitate platelet aggregation. Other inherited disorders of platelets generally involve ligand receptors or defects in the signaling cascade for molecules involved in platelet activation (e.g., thromboxane and adenine diphosphate).[149]

vWD is the most common hereditary bleeding disorder, with a prevalence of approximately 1% in the general population, although it is only reportedly symptomatic in 0.01%.[150] The clinical features and severity of vWD vary immensely, since it has several different types and classifications depending on the nature of the genetic mutation and its effect on the functionality of vWF (Table 17-12). Different genetic mutations affect various domains of vWF, causing different quantitative and functional deficiencies. Each type of vWD presents differently, and in fact there are several complex laboratory evaluations necessary to classify the exact type of disease for each patient. It is important to reach the correct diagnosis, since appropriate treatment and prophylaxis differs for each class of the disorder.[150]

vWF is produced in endothelial cells and megakaryocytes, and functions in primary platelet adhesion and aggregation at the site of vascular injury through interaction with the GP Ib receptor on the platelet surface. Once exposed, vWF facilitates the interaction of platelets with collagen within the subendothelium as well as platelet–platelet interactions. Both of these result in the initial platelet plug and subsequent platelet activation.[150] Furthermore, vWF circulates as a complex with FVIII, providing stability to the otherwise labile clotting factor until vWF binds to activated platelets via the GP IIb/IIIa receptor. This localizes FVIII to the site of injury.[150,151] The clinical features of vWD vary with differing levels of functionality that result from inherited disorders in protein synthesis, structure, function, and clearance. However, most types of vWD result from decreased levels or deficient function of vWF in primary hemostasis. Patients typically present with mucocutaneous bleeding (e.g., epistaxis), menorrhagia, and prolonged bleeding from minor wounds and dental extractions. Frequently, patients are not aware of the disorder until they undergo a bleeding questionnaire in anticipation of major surgery.

There are three types of vWD. Types 1 and 3 result from quantitative deficiencies of vWF, whereas type 2 occurs with various mutations causing qualitative dysfunction. Type 2 is further classified (A, B, M, and N) depending on the domain of the protein that is affected and the functional defect (Table 17-12).[150,152] Type 1 has an autosomal dominant inheritance pattern and results from a partial quantitative deficiency in vWF levels either from decreased synthesis and secretion or from accelerated proteolysis and clearance. It is the most common and mildest type of vWD.[150] Type 3 is the most severe, but also the rarest; it has a recessive pattern of inheritance and results in significantly depressed levels of vWF. This is the only type likely to cause spontaneous hemorrhage in joints and soft tissues.[150] Types 2A and 2M result in deficiencies in platelet adhesion and decreased activity of vWF relative to the factor levels within the plasma. Type 2B involves increased affinity of vWF for the GP Ib receptor on the platelet surface. This causes spontaneous binding of vWF to circulating platelets, thereby increasing the cleavage and clearance of vWF. This type of vWD can be associated with thrombocytopenia. DDAVP treatment is commonly used to increase cleavage from FVIII and overall availability.[150] Lastly, type 2N is characterized by decreased affinity for FVIII and deficiencies in secondary hemostasis. This type is often confused with hemophilia A, given the depressed levels of FVIII associated with significantly decreased factor half-life.[150,152]

The three primary criteria for diagnosis of vWD are (1) a history of mucosal bleeding or prolonged bleeding after dental extractions, surgical procedures, or postpartum hemorrhage; (2) a family history of bleeding disorders (understanding this can be unreliable or unavailable); and (3) reduced activity of vWF demonstrated by various assays designed to test platelet adhesion, aggregation, and levels of vWF or FVIII complexes (e.g., vWF:factor antigen, vWF:ristocetin cofactor activity, vWF:collagen-binding activity, and vWF:GP 1b binding activity).[152] The laboratory diagnosis and classification of vWD is complex and often requires a hematologist to correctly specify the type of disorder, and to prescribe the appropriate prophylaxis and treatment options. Overall, it is important to recognize that traditional coagulation profile tests such as PT and aPTT are often normal in patients with vWD.

There are two primary treatment options for patients with vWD—DDAVP and factor concentrates. DDAVP promotes the cleavage of vWF from FVIII and increases the availability of both. This is beneficial for most patients with type 1 partial deficiency and some type 2 subclassifications of vWD (with the exception of type 2B as discussed above). DDAVP may not be therapeutic by itself for patients with type 3 and severely depressed levels of vWF. Often these patients require treatment with additional hemostatic medications such as antifibrinolytics and/or factor replacement with plasma-derived vWF/FVIII concentrates (Heamate P/Humate P). These concentrates are only needed in approximately 20% of patients with vWD who do not respond to DDAVP, and may vary in efficacy. Accordingly, it is important to obtain the correct diagnosis in order to best manage each patient prophylactically before surgery and therapeutically in the event of uncontrolled bleeding.[153]

On rare occasions, vWD may be acquired in association with various disease processes such as lymphoproliferative or myeloproliferative disorders; autoimmune disease; cardiac dysfunction (e.g., aortic stenosis, ventricular assist devices), or medication-induced

Table 17-12	Classification of Inherited von Willebrand Disease	
Type	Pathophysiology	Comments
1	Partial quantitative deficiency of vWF	Mildest; most common; responds to DDAVP
2A	Dysfunction in platelet adhesion	May respond to DDAVP
2M	Dysfunction in platelet adhesion	May respond to DDAVP
2B	Increased platelet-binding affinity	Thrombocytopenia with DDAVP
2N	Decreased FVIII-binding affinity	Often confused with hemophilia A
3	Severe quantitative deficiency of vWF	Rarest; most severe; usually requires factor concentrates

vWF, von Willebrand factor; DDAVP, desmopressin; FVIII, factor VIII.

from quinolones, valproic acid, and hydroxyl ethyl starches. The pathophysiology of acquired vWD is multifactorial and may involve various mechanisms including immune-mediated clearance by ADAMTS-13–mediated cleavage of high–molecular-weight vWF, binding or absorption with large molecules such as the starches, or enhanced proteolysis secondary to shear stress.[151] Treatment starts with discontinuation of the offending agent or management of the underlying condition; however, adjunctive treatment with DDAVP and/or antifibrinolytics are helpful.

Disorders of Secondary Hemostasis

The Hemophilias

Hemophilia is a genetic disease that results from deficiencies or dysfunction of specific clotting factors. The most common form is hemophilia A, which accounts for about 85% of the disease and stems from deficiencies of FVIII. Hemophilia B (Christmas disease) involves a defect in the production of factor IX, and is the second most common type of hemophilia. Both hemophilia A and B are X-linked recessive disorders and are found almost exclusively in male patients, although new mutations are common and account for about a third of hemophilias in male and female patients without family history.[154] Hemophilia was originally called the "royal disease," since Queen Victoria of England was a carrier of hemophilia B and passed the disorder to the royal families of Spain, Germany, and Russia. Lastly, hemophilia C is very rare (1% of all hemophiliacs), and results from genetic mutations in FXI, and is the only form that has an autosomal recessive inheritance pattern.

Hemophilia A affects approximately 1 in 5,000 males worldwide. Clinically, these patients suffer from spontaneous bleeding into their joints, muscles, and internal organs, often requiring orthopedic surgery for long-term complications of hemarthroses. Central nervous system bleeding is rare, but can lead to severe disability and death.[154] Normal plasma concentrations of FVIII range between 100 and 200 ng/mL, and the severity of disease varies depending on the residual factor activity. Patients with mild disease maintain factor levels between 5% and 40% of normal, and account for about 50% of patients with hemophilia A. Approximately 10% of patients have moderate disease, with only 1% to 5% of residual FVIII activity. The most severely affected patients account for about 40% of the disease prevalence and have less than 1% of normal factor activity.[154,155] Carrier females generally maintain about 50% of FVIII activity with no clinical signs of bleeding. Homozygous females may present with hemophilia, but this is rare and often associated with Turner syndrome or X-chromosomal mosaicism. Diagnosis starts with patients reporting a personal and/or family history of bleeding disorders among male relations. Confirmatory laboratory evidence includes prolonged aPTT and low factor activity levels. Typically, the PT and bleeding times will be normal.[156]

Treatment for all hemophilia patients involves replacement of coagulation factor deficiencies, which can be accomplished with plasma transfusion or factor concentrates. Historically, hemophiliacs were exposed to several transfusion-related infectious risks prior to the availability of recombinant and virally inactivated factor concentrates. In the 1980s, a significant percentage of patients with hemophilia contracted AIDS from transfusion-transmitted HIV. Frequent transfusions for these patients are clearly associated with numerous infectious and noninfectious transfusion risks, including the development of factor inhibitors and alloantibodies. Up to 30% of patients with severe hemophilia develop inhibitor antibodies to FVIII by the time they reach adulthood, making them less responsive to factor concentrates. Patients with severe hemophilia are at highest risk for developing inhibitors, since they require frequent high-dose treatment and primary prophylaxis starting at younger ages.[157]

The goals of managing hemophilia continue to focus on prophylaxis against spontaneous bleeding, as well as aggressive blood conservation strategies for anticipated invasive procedures. Patients with mild hemophilia A and hemophilia C often benefit from treatment with DDAVP, to raise the circulating availability of FVIII by increasing dissociation from vWF.[154,158] However, those with more severe disease require treatment of spontaneous and traumatic bleeding episodes, as well as prophylaxis to avoid the long-term complications of hemarthroses. This is accomplished with transfusion of specific factor concentrates derived from virally inactivated plasma-derived or recombinant products.[155] Patients with inhibitors to FVIII or FIX often respond to bypass agents such as rFVIIa or PCCs.[158,159] Factor concentrates are given in anticipation of surgery or invasive procedures, and are dosed individually depending on severity of illness and risk of bleeding. The appropriate dosing regimen for prophylaxis is highly variable among patients, due to differing levels of disease severity and the impact of factor inhibitors. Titration of the dose of factor concentrates to trough levels of no less than 1 IU/dL (1% of normal) is recommended during long-term prophylaxis.[154,155]

Hemophilia B is clinically and pathophysiologically similar to hemophilia A, except it involves FIX and is much less common worldwide, affecting roughly 1 in 25,000 males. This form of hemophilia is treated with recombinant FIX concentrates, but requires less frequent dosing regimens than FVIII concentrates due to a longer half-life (18 hours as opposed to 12 hours). Fortunately, the development of factor inhibitors is much less prevalent in patients with hemophilia B than in patients with hemophilia A, and occurs in only 1% to 6% of severe patients. These patients are also generally responsive to bypass treatment with PCCs or rFVIIa in the case of urgent bleeding.[160]

Acquired hemophilia is a rare disease that usually develops in association with connective tissue disorders, pregnancy, or malignancy. It rarely occurs in young patients and stems from the development of antibodies to FVIII. The clinical symptoms of acquired hemophilia typically include subcutaneous bleeding episodes and soft tissue hematomas, as opposed to the hemarthroses common to congenital hemophilia.[156] Diagnostically, the aPTT is prolonged in conjunction and low FVIII levels do not correct in a mixing study due to the presence of inhibitors. The treatment for acquired hemophilia with acute bleeding depends on bypass agents such as rFVIIa or PCCs, although some patients with mild disease will respond to adjunctive therapies such as DDAVP and antifibrinolytics. Once hemostasis is achieved, long-term management involves immunosuppression with steroids or cytotoxic agents.[156]

Hereditary Hypercoagulability

The *FVL* genetic mutation causes resistance to the anticoagulant effects of APC on clotting factor V. It is the most common hereditary risk factor for hypercoagulability. Heterozygous patients have a fivefold increase in the risk of venous thromboembolism. This rises to 20- to 80-fold increased risk in homozygotes. Treatment involves lifelong therapeutic anticoagulation. The prevalence amongst Caucasians is approximately 5% throughout North America and Europe. Some investigators propose that the high prevalence in Caucasians stems from a protective genetic interplay against bleeding and mortality risk associated with hemophilia.[20]

Protein C and S deficiencies are autosomal dominant genetic diseases that result in increased risk of venous thromboembolism. Protein C inactivates factor V to curb the clotting cascade, and depends on protein S as a cofactor for appropriate function. Accordingly, deficiencies or dysfunction in either protein C or S result in a prothrombotic state. Clinically, patients present with venous thromboembolism in early adulthood, but arterial thrombosis is rare. Treatment of acute thrombosis requires therapeutic anticoagulation. Warfarin is indicated for long-term management, but should be started slowly once the patient is therapeutic on heparin, to avoid the risk of warfarin limb necrosis.[161]

Acquired Disorders of Hemostasis

Vitamin K Deficiency

Vitamin K is one of the essential fat-soluble vitamins required for the synthesis and final processing of several hemostatic factors, including factors II, VII, IX, X, and proteins C and S. Without vitamin K, these proteins do not undergo carboxylation and therefore cannot actively bind to the phospholipid membrane of platelets during secondary hemostasis. There are two sources of vitamin K—phylloquinone (K_1) is available in a number of foods such as leafy greens, whereas menaquinone (K_2) is synthesized in the GI tract by intestinal bacteria and accounts for the bulk of vitamin K stored in the liver. The absorption of both types occurs in the small intestine and depends on the availability of bile salts. Accordingly, liver insufficiency, the sterile gut in newborns, and oral antibiotic treatments are some of the leading causes of vitamin K deficiency.[162] Other causes include chronic kidney disease, total parenteral nutrition, intestinal obstruction, or hyperperistalsis.[162]

Vitamin K deficiency presents with prolonged PT and aPTT, but can also be diagnosed by low vitamin K levels or measures of noncarboxylated prothrombin. It is treated with vitamin K replacement, which can be administered parenterally, orally, or subcutaneously. Oral administration has the best bioavailability, but can take 24 hours for full effect. When rapid correction for a bleeding patient is needed, improvements in PT can be seen within 6 to 8 hours of intravenous administration, especially with high doses of 5 to 10 mg.[163]

Liver Disease

Patients with severe liver disease often present with bleeding complications, including central nervous system hemorrhage or gastrointestinal bleeding. They were traditionally managed with prophylactic transfusions and adjunctive hemostatic medications prior to surgical procedures or in response to a prolonged PT. However, new guidelines recommend against prophylaxis without clinical symptoms of bleeding. There are several etiologies of bleeding diathesis associated with liver disease, including endothelial dysfunction, portal hypertension, thrombocytopenia, and the procoagulant imbalance discussed in the following section. However, the hemostatic system in chronic liver disease often remains in balance, although fragile. Conventional laboratory tests such as the PT and aPTT overestimate the bleeding tendency of patients with liver disease and should not be used as the sole method for titrating plasma transfusion or treatment with hemostatic agents.[164,165]

Primary hemostasis was typically thought to be inefficient in chronic liver disease because of thrombocytopenia secondary to decreased production of thrombopoietin in the liver. However, the low platelet count is often balanced with increased circulating levels of vWF that result from a reduced presence of ADAMTS-13, the protease that regulates plasma concentrations of vWF.[164,165] This balance remains fragile, given that patients with severe liver disease and acute illness are also prone to endothelial and platelet dysfunction.

Secondary hemostasis is also affected because liver disease results in deficiencies of factors II, V, VII, IX, X, and XI that will prolong the PT and aPTT in vitro. However, the liver is also responsible for the synthesis of protein C, protein S, and AT, which are integral anticoagulant factors.[164] Furthermore, these patients have increased circulating levels of FVIII in association with the increases in vWF mentioned above. Thus, the decreased levels of procoagulant factors are offset by deficient amounts of anticoagulant factors and increased FVIII activity,[164,165] maintaining secondary hemostasis.

Although hemostatic equilibrium is generally maintained with chronic liver disease, the balance is not stable and can be tipped toward either hemorrhage or thrombosis by acute illness, malnutrition, renal injury, infection, or medications. Laboratory testing difficult because conventional PT and aPTT conducted in vitro do not mimic the in vivo compensation mechanisms associated with chronic liver disease. Thrombin generation by procoagulant factors is regulated in vivo by the anticoagulant activity of protein C and its main activator, thrombomodulin.[164,165] In contrast, in vitro thrombin generation only assesses activation by procoagulant factors and will misrepresent the actual bleeding tendency of the patient.

Lastly, fibrinolysis is also maintained in chronic liver disease. Although these patients are plasminogen deficient, they have higher than normal levels of tPA secondary to lower levels of TAFI. This maintains the normal ratio of plasminogen to plasmin.[164,165] However, the balance of fibrinolysis and antifibrinolysis can be disrupted by infection, trauma, surgery, and medications common to chronic liver patients.

As mentioned above, conventional hemostatic tests such as PT and aPTT assays do not reflect the bleeding or thrombotic tendencies of chronic liver disease. Patients with normal coagulation profiles can present with catastrophic gastrointestinal bleeding or prolonged PTs, yet develop venous, arterial, and portal thrombosis. The overall hemostatic state can be evaluated with viscoelastography, or by measuring thrombin generation in the presence and absence of thrombomodulin. The circumstances of these tests are more akin to the in vivo state of patients with liver disease than conventional PT and aPTT tests. Accordingly, it is no longer recommended to prophylactically transfuse plasma in response to PT times, elevated INR, or prior to minor procedures in such patients without clinical signs of bleeding. Furthermore, despite prolonged coagulation tests, patients with liver disease are still at significant risk for venous and arterial thrombosis and should be treated with appropriate prophylactic anticoagulation.[165]

Disseminated Intravascular Coagulopathy (DIC)

DIC is a disorder characterized by systemic activation of coagulation. It is always associated with a comorbid condition such as infection, inflammation, or malignancy, which causes widespread activation of the coagulation cascade.[166–168] Table 17-13 lists the medical diseases and syndromes known to cause DIC. Supportive care and treatment of the underlining disorder are the mainstays of DIC management. In severe cases of major hemorrhage or ischemic organ failure, DIC is treated with factor and fibrinogen replacement, anticoagulation, or pharmacologic therapies.[166,168]

The exact pathophysiology of DIC depends on the causative condition, but primarily involves uncontrolled activation of hemostatic mechanisms for thrombin generation with simultaneous inhibition of fibrinolysis. Thrombin generation in DIC is initiated by TF and activated factor VII in the extrinsic pathway for coagulation. The exposure of TF is facilitated by extensive vascular injury, expression on neoplastic cells, or the release of proinflammatory cytokines such as interleukin-6. DIC progresses as the regulation of thrombin generation is impaired secondary to decreased levels of naturally occurring anticoagulants including AT-III, protein C, and TFPI. Finally, impaired fibrinolysis from an inappropriate increase in circulating levels of PAI-1 facilitates the progression of vascular microthrombi.[167,168]

DIC is a catastrophic complication for many hospitalized patients with both chronic and acute illness. The clinical presentation of DIC ranges from thromboembolism and organ dysfunction to consumptive coagulopathy and major bleeding. The kidneys and lungs are particularly vulnerable to ischemia from microthrombi and may progress to acute renal failure and acute respiratory distress syndrome, especially in patients with DIC secondary to obstetric complications or sepsis.[168] The bleeding type of DIC results from widespread activation of hemostasis with consumption of coagulation factors and platelets. The primary diagnosis for these patients is often trauma or hematopoietic malignancy, who present with bleeding from sites of vascular injury, or spontaneous intracranial or intraperitoneal hemorrhage.[167,168] DIC with features of microthrombi, organ dysfunction, and consumption results in severe thrombocytopenia and often leads to massive hemorrhage with a poor overall prognosis.[167] However, major bleeding is rather infrequent with DIC and usually occurs only with platelets less than 50,000/μL or patients undergoing procedures. In fact, in a study of DIC with sepsis, transfusion for major bleeding was only required in 5% to 12% of patients.[167,168]

The diagnosis of DIC must consider the underlying disorder in conjunction with an abnormal hemostasis profile. Unfortunately, there is not a single laboratory finding indicative of DIC. High levels of fibrin split products are a sensitive marker, but carry very low specificity.[166-168] Rather, the compilation of prolonged PT and aPTT, thrombocytopenia, hypofibrinogenemia, and increasing fibrin degradation products in a patient with an associated condition leads to the clinical diagnosis of DIC. The International Society of Thrombosis and Hemostasis developed a scoring algorithm for the diagnosis of overt DIC that depends on these four laboratory findings (Table 17-14).[166-168] This algorithm is only one of several clinically used scoring systems worldwide, but was prospectively validated and found to have a sensitivity of 91% and a specificity of 97%.[167] Overall, DIC is a dynamic condition and most accurately diagnosed with repeated measures of coagulation tests showing progression of thrombocytopenia and hypofibrinogenemia, with increasing prolongation of PT and levels of fibrin degradation products.

The management for DIC primarily involves treatment of the causative condition and supportive measures to control progressive thrombosis and hemorrhage. Consumptive coagulopathy and thrombocytopenia with clinical signs of bleeding are treated with transfusion of plasma and platelets, respectively. There is no evidence for improved outcomes with transfusion of plasma or platelets unless thrombocytopenia is severe (platelet counts <10,000 to 20,000/μL) or moderate (<50,000/μL), with clinical signs of bleeding, or in preparation for invasive procedures.[166-168]

Plasma is the mainstay of replacement therapy for consumption of clotting factors in DIC; however, it often requires large volumes (10 to 15 mL/kg) to correct the coagulopathy.[166-168] In the past, rFVIIa and PCCs have been used for patients with active bleeding and consumptive coagulopathy; however, the administration of active factor concentrates in the preparations of rFVIIa and PCCs can lead to progressive thrombosis in patients with overt DIC and is not recommended. Rather, the use of specific factor concentrate is preferred for measured factor deficiencies in patients with active bleeding.[166-168] Cryoprecipitate is the product of choice for treatment of overt DIC with consumptive coagulopathy and major bleeding, because it contains FVIII and fibrinogen with a low overall volume of transfusion.[167,168]

Arterial and venous thromboembolisms are more concerning than hemorrhage in patients with DIC and evidence of acute organ dysfunction. Anticoagulation is indicated to inhibit further activation of hemostasis in patients with signs of microthrombi such as organ failure or diagnosed thromboembolism.[167,168] Studies of patients with DIC in sepsis proved the efficacy of heparin to halt thrombin generation, improve the coagulation profile, and reduce the risk of thrombosis. It is understandably difficult to initiate therapeutic anticoagulation on a patient with signs or risks of bleeding; however, maintaining chemoprophylaxis against venous thromboembolism is of utmost importance, especially early in the course of DIC in the absence of major bleeding. Literature support is limited, but LMWH alternatives to unfractionated heparin (UFH) may provide better efficacy with lower bleeding risks.[167,168]

AT-III levels decrease in DIC, and several animal studies have shown improved survival in DIC models after AT-III replacement. However, multiple studies failed to demonstrate survival benefit with AT-III treatment for patients with DIC secondary to sepsis, obstetric complications, liver disease, and burn injury.[166] Treatment with APC for septic patients with severe DIC was reported beneficial for morbidity and mortality, especially in patients with multiorgan dysfunction. In 2009, the BCSH recommended its use as standard treatment for patients with DIC

Table 17-13 Common Disorders Associated with Disseminated Intravascular Coagulation

Disorder	Average Incidence of DIC	Comments
Sepsis	30–50%	Highest with gram-negative bacilli
Trauma and burns	Rare	Associated with the degree of tissue injury
Malignancy	Up to 20%	Highest with adenocarcinoma or leukemia and lymphoma
Vascular disease	Rare	Higher with giant hemangiomas
Obstetric complication	Up to 50%	Including preeclampsia, placental abruption, or amniotic fluid embolism
Hemolysis	Rare	Higher with intravascular hemolysis
Severe organ dysfunction	Rare	Including pancreatitis, hepatitis, and end-stage renal failure

Table 17-14 Scoring Algorithm for the Diagnosis of Disseminated Intravascular Coagulation

Diagnostic Test	Score
Platelet count	>100,000/mm³ = 0 <100,000/mm³ = 1 <50,000/mm³ = 2
Prothrombin time prolongation	<3 s = 0 >3 s but <6 s = 1 >6 s = 2
Fibrin degradation products	No increase = 0 Moderate increase = 2 Strong increase = 3
Fibrinogen level	>1 g/L = 0 <1 g/L = 1

Score calculation:
If ≥5, consistent with overt DIC.
If <5, not likely overt DIC; repeat tests in 1–2 days.

Algorithm developed by the International Society of Thrombosis and Hemostasis.

in severe sepsis without pre-existing risks of bleeding or thrombocytopenia. However, subsequent reviews of treatment with APC failed to show consistent survival benefits, yet documented increased risks of bleeding complications. Consequently, in 2012, the BCSH changed its recommendation and APC concentrates were removed from the market.[169] Overall, the best therapy for overt DIC of any cause is to treat the underlying condition, continue to support organ function, and maintain control of hemostasis.

Anticoagulation and Pharmacologic Therapy

Anticoagulation Regimens and Associated Anesthetic Concerns

29 *Antiplatelet therapy* is indicated for patients at risk for cerebral vascular accident, myocardial infarction, or other vascular thrombosis complications. There are several mechanisms for platelet dysfunction including COX inhibition, PDE inhibition, ADP receptor antagonism, and GP IIb/IIIa receptor antagonism.

Cyclooxygenase Inhibitors

Aspirin and nonsteroidal anti-inflammatory drugs (NSAIDs) are the most notable members of this class. There are two forms of the COX enzyme with variable distribution throughout the body. COX-1 plays an integral part in maintaining the integrity of the gastric lining, renal blood flow, and initiating the formation of TxA_2, an important molecule for platelet aggregation. Inhibition of COX-1 puts the patient at risk for bleeding, as well as for gastrointestinal and renal morbidity. COX-2 is primarily responsible for synthesizing the prostaglandin mediators of pain and inflammation. Aspirin is a noncompetitive and irreversible inhibitor of both COX enzymes.[170] Consequently, the effects of aspirin therapy last the lifetime of the affected platelets and can only be fully reversed with platelet transfusion, although DDAVP is frequently used to improve platelet function in the presence of aspirin.[163]

NSAIDs are competitive antagonists whose effects last only as long as the drug's time to elimination. Most NSAIDs (naprosyn and ibuprofen) are nonselective COX inhibitors. However, the development of selective COX-2 antagonists such as celecoxib aimed to provide pain relief without the gastrointestinal bleeding complications. Unfortunately, the initial benefits of COX-2 inhibitors were not sustained in long-term outcome studies, and the decreased incidence of gastrotoxicity is clinically insignificant when patients are simultaneously taking aspirin.[170] Postmarket clinical trials with selective COX-2 antagonists reported increased risks for cardiovascular complications likely secondary to impaired vascular endothelial function. The mechanism for cardiovascular risk is thought to be unchecked inhibition of PGI_2 without antagonizing the synthesis of TxA_2 from COX-1 within platelets. This tips the balance in favor of a prothrombotic state.[170,171] In 2007, the American Heart Association (AHA) recommended a stepwise approach to prescribing NSAIDs in patients with cardiovascular disease, emphasizing the use of nonselective or partially selective COX inhibitors first. If selective COX-2 inhibitors, namely celecoxib, are needed they recommend the lowest effective dose in conjunction with a proton pump inhibitor and low-dose aspirin.[171]

Phosphodiesterase Inhibitors

PDE inhibitors are primarily used for stroke prophylaxis, since they increase the production of cAMP, an active inhibitor of platelet aggregation. These medications are rarely the drug of choice for patients with cerebrovascular disease, but rather used in conjunction with aspirin therapy. Dipyridamole is a reversible ADP reuptake inhibitor and the prime therapeutic agent in this class, but caffeine, aminophylline, and theophylline also result in reversible platelet dysfunction.[163]

ADP Receptor Antagonists

$P2Y_{12}$ *ADP receptor antagonists*, such as clopidogrel, prasugrel, and ticagrelor, prevent the expression of GP IIb/IIIa on the surface of activated platelets, thereby inhibiting platelet adhesion and aggregation. These drugs are indicated for patients with coronary artery disease to prevent myocardial infarction and in-stent thrombosis, or for patients with cerebrovascular or peripheral artery disease to inhibit thromboembolism. Clopidogrel is the most commonly prescribed agent in this class and is a noncompetitive and irreversible antagonist. It is an inactive prodrug that requires oxidation to its active metabolite.[73,172] Recently, a genetic polymorphism was discovered that results in the inability to metabolize clopidogrel, making it ineffective and putting patients at risk for cardiovascular morbidity and mortality. The FDA put a black box warning on the medication to remind clinicians to monitor the activity. Platelet function studies are insensitive and unreliable for clopidogrel, but tests are now available to measure the inhibition of the $P2Y_{12}$ ADP receptor.[73,172,173] Patients who are resistant to clopidogrel may be converted to prasugrel or ticagrelor for increased antiplatelet effects.[173] Prasugrel is also an irreversible $P2Y_{12}$ ADP inhibitor indicated for primary prevention of acute coronary syndrome, but not recommended by the AHA for immediate use in patients presenting with acute myocardial ischemia. Ticagrelor is a reversible inhibitor with similar mechanism of action, with AHA endorsement for use in acute coronary syndrome. Both ticagrelor and prasugrel are associated with higher bleeding risk than clopidogrel and should not be used with aspirin doses over 100 mg/day.[73]

GP IIb/IIIa Receptor Antagonists

GP IIb/IIIa receptor blockers inhibit the cross-linkage of fibrinogen, the final step in the common hemostatic pathway for platelet aggregation. They include the monoclonal antibody abciximab, and two other molecules which simulate the binding sight of fibrinogen, tirofiban, and eptifibatide. These agents are administered intravenously and primarily used for management of acute coronary syndrome. Their effects are monitored with ACTs and reversed by clearance of the drug. Most of these agents are renally excreted, with half-lives around 20 to 40 minutes, except for abciximab which has a significantly longer context-sensitive half-time secondary to protein binding (24 to 48 hours).[163] All of these drugs cause thrombocytopenia, but the effect is strongest with abciximab with an incidence of about 2.5%, as opposed to 0.5% with the other receptor antagonists.[174] Vorapaxar, a *PAR-1 antagonist,* is a reversible agent with a very long half-life (3 to 4 days) that clinically inhibits thrombin activity for significantly longer than its partner agents in this class of anticoagulants. Vorapaxar's clinical usefulness is limited, but it is available for patients with significant renal insufficiency.[163,174]

Vitamin K Antagonists

Warfarin is an oral anticoagulant therapy frequently used for management of hypercoagulable disorders, venous thromboembolism, and stroke prophylaxis in patients with atrial fibrillation, artificial heart valves, or mechanical assist devices. Mechanistically, it competes with vitamin K for carboxylation-binding sites and inhibits the synthesis of vitamin K–dependent clotting factors II, VII, IX, and X. Proteins C and S are also dependent on vitamin K, and thus are inhibited with warfarin therapy. In fact, patients may be hypercoagulable during the initial phase of treatment, since proteins C and S have shorter half-lives than most clotting factors and will be inhibited first, thereby leaving thrombin generation unregulated. Accordingly, patients at high risk for thromboembolism must be bridged with another anticoagulation regimen until the target INR is achieved.[175] Warfarin therapy is monitored with the INR (see section on laboratory interpretation). Therapeutic targets generally range between 2.0 and 3.0, and will vary depending on the disease and the patient's bleeding risk.[175]

There is a significant risk of bleeding with any anticoagulation regimen, which demands appropriate protocols for reversal of the specific drug effects. The management protocol for warfarin reversal depends on the patient's symptoms and the urgency. Because warfarin inhibits the synthesis of vitamin K–dependent clotting factors II, VII, IX, and X, the most logical and appropriate reversal agent is replacement of vitamin K. Guidelines for the administration and reversal of warfarin were written and updated by the BCSH in 2011.[175] For patients with INR higher than 5.0 and no signs or symptoms of bleeding, warfarin administration should be held for one to two doses. Oral vitamin K should be administered if the INR is over 8.0. Patients who present with high INR and nonmajor bleeding should be reversed with 1 to 3 mg of intravenous vitamin K; this usually corrects the INR within 6 to 8 hours. Emergency reversal for patients with major bleeding or those who require immediate surgery can be achieved with PCCs. Four-factor PCCs (II, VII, IX, X) are generally preferred to three-factor PCCs because the three-factor formulations lack sufficient amounts of factor VII to reliably reverse the effects of warfarin. Furthermore, patient-centered protocols that include weight-based dosing and consideration for the INR and clinical bleeding risks are preferred.[163,175] The half-life of most PCCs is short, and vitamin K should be given simultaneously for sustained results. Historically, emergency reversal of warfarin was achieved with plasma; however, this requires large volumes of transfusion (10 to 30 mL/kg) and provides unreliable results with inherent delay in treatment secondary to the time needed to type and screen the patient, thaw, prepare, and administer multiple units of plasma.[163] rFVIIa has also been used to reverse warfarin, but the supporting literature is retrospective. Although it reliably corrects the INR, it does not consistently correct clinical bleeding likely secondary to the ongoing inhibition of other vitamin K–dependent clotting factors, and is no longer an appropriate reversal agent for warfarin toxicity.[175] Consequently, the BCSH, SCCM, and Neurocritical Care Society recommend the use of plasma only when PCCs are not available, especially for patients with warfarin-related intracranial hemorrhage.[163,175]

Anticoagulation regimens using oral vitamin K antagonists can be difficult to regulate within the target range. Warfarin has a long onset and offset of action that puts patients at risk for thrombosis and bleeding, especially in the perioperative period. It also has many food and drug interactions, and its metabolism is subject to pharmacogenomics that make dosing highly variable. Warfarin is hepatically metabolized by the P450 CYP2 enzymes and will interact with other commonly used medications such as antibiotics, barbiturates, phenytoin, and proton pump inhibitors. Alterations in dietary intake of vitamin K will also vary the clinical effect of maintenance dosages. Furthermore, there are genetic polymorphisms for the CYP2 enzymes that decrease the metabolism of warfarin and increase bleeding risk.[176] For these reasons, alternative oral anticoagulant agents have been pursued for many years, with a new focus on oral DTIs and FXa inhibitors.

New Oral Anticoagulants

Dabigatran (a DTI), and the FXa inhibitors, rivaroxaban, apixaban, and edoxaban have completed phase III trials and passed FDA approval for stroke prophylaxis and therapeutic anticoagulation for patients with history of venous thromboembolism.[177] Thrombin and factor X are at the end of the common pathway for clot formation and stabilization, and play an integral part in secondary hemostasis. Consequently, they are highly desirable targets for antagonism of anticoagulation. These agents are significantly easier to manage than warfarin. They have short half-lives and rapid onsets of action that negate the need for bridging therapy. They are also reliably bioavailable and have little interindividual variability. Thus, coagulation monitoring is unnecessary, although efficacy can be measured with diluted thrombin times or anti-Xa assays.[177] Lastly, new oral anticoagulants (NOACs) have few drug or dietary interactions. All of these agents have a wide therapeutic window, making dosing simple and universal with the exception of patients on dialysis. Dabigatran and rivaroxaban in particular rely on renal excretion for clearance. Dabigatran may be cleared with dialysis; however, both carry FDA warnings against use in patients with end-stage renal disease (Table 17-15).[177,178]

The Re-Ly investigators, the ARISTOTLE group, and the EINSTEIN, ENGAGE-AF, and ROCKET-AF trials, all compared dabigatran, apixaban, rivaroxaban, and edoxaban to warfarin, in large, multicenter, randomized controlled trials.[179–182] These trials were mostly noninferiority studies documenting the efficacy of NOACs compared to warfarin for treatment of venous thromboembolism, and stroke prevention in valvular and nonvalvular atrial fibrillation. Recent trials demonstrate their usefulness for prevention of venous thromboembolism in perioperative orthopedic patients undergoing knee and hip arthroplasty.[177,183] Their full clinical potential has yet to be determined, especially

Table 17-15	Oral Anticoagulation Medications				
	Warfarin	**Dabigatran**	**Apixaban**	**Rivaroxaban**	**Edoxaban**
Target	Vitamin K	Thrombin	Factor Xa	Factor Xa	Factor Xa
Time to peak (h)	72–96	0.5–2	3–4	2–4	1.5
Half-life (h)	36–42	14–17	12	5–13	6–11
Protein binding (%)		35	87	95	55
Monitoring test	INR	Thrombin time	Anti-Xa	Anti-Xa	Anti-Xa
Renal excretion (%)	None	85	54	73	56
Metabolism	CYP2C9	minimal	CYP3A4	CYP3A4	CYP3A4

in the perioperative setting. Unfortunately, there is currently no reliable coagulation test to monitor the clinical effects of these agents. They may prolong the aPTT, thrombin time, or the ECT, but these are not sensitive monitors for increased risk of bleeding. This is an active area for research at this time.[177]

In an emergency, there is limited evidence to guide therapeutic reversal of the NOACs. Various societies drafted recommendations for the use of activated PCCs, and a monoclonal antibody (idarucizumab) was recently FDA approved for reversal of dabigatran after favorable results were published in the interim analysis of the RE-VERSE AD study.[184] Furthermore, dabigatran can be cleared with dialysis.[178] However, no reliable regimen for drug reversal exists for the direct FXa inhibitors at this time. Because NOACs are competitive inhibitors of thrombin and FXa, PCCs containing factors II, VII, IX, and X can reverse the antagonistic effects. Current guidelines from the SCCM and the Neurocritical Care Society recommend activated PCCs, PCCs, or rFVIIa to reverse the clinical bleeding risks associated with direct FXa inhibitors, and idarucizumab for reversal of dabigatran.[163] Perioperatively, these agents should be discontinued 24 hours before minor surgery or diagnostic procedures, and 48 hours before major surgery or procedures involving the eye, spine, or brain. The half-lives of these agents are approximately 12 hours; thus, assuming normal hepatic and renal function, more than four half-lives ensure significant drug clearance. However, further research is needed to document the best method for reversing the clinical effects of NOACs.

Heparin Therapy

Heparin therapy is one of the oldest and most common anticoagulation regimens. There are two main forms of heparin, UFH and LMWH. UFH indirectly inhibits thrombin and FXa by binding to AT-III, causing a conformational shape change which significantly increases its activity. Although the use of UFH for prophylaxis against venous thromboembolism has decreased in favor of LMWH and indirect FXa inhibitors, it is still used for immediate anticoagulation with acute coronary syndrome, pulmonary embolism, and during cardiopulmonary bypass or vascular surgery. The clinical effects of heparin therapy are monitored with the aPTT or ACT. Patients may be resistant to UFH if they have a hereditary insufficiency of AT-III or an acquired deficiency from prolonged heparin administration. AT-III is replenished with plasma transfusion. UFH is given parenterally and its clinical effects are fully reversible with protamine.[163] The main complication is HIT, discussed later.

LMWH is a fractionated form of heparin with similar mechanism of action, but with more specific inhibition of FXa. Several agents are currently available, including enoxaparin, dalteparin, and reviparin. LMWH is preferred over UFH for both DVT prophylaxis and treatment because laboratory monitoring is unnecessary, and its longer half-life allows for once- or twice-daily dosing. Treatment can be monitored with FXa levels, but this is only necessary for obese patients and those with renal insufficiency, which prolongs elimination. Reversal with protamine is unpredictable and not likely to completely resolve bleeding tendencies.[163]

Indirect Factor Xa Antagonists

Fondaparinux is the principal agent used in this class. It is a highly specific antagonist for free FXa that also acts via binding with AT-III. Like LMWH, it is popular for DVT treatment and prophylaxis because it has a long half-life and requires only once-daily dosing, and highly reliable absorption that negates the need for coagulation monitoring. However, fondaparinux undergoes renal elimination, necessitating a lower dose or coagulation monitoring with FXa levels in patients with renal insufficiency. There is no available antidote in the event of bleeding or the need for emergency procedures. Fortunately, the incidence of HIT is relatively low for this class of agents, although they are not approved for use in patients with a history of HIT.[185]

Heparin-Induced Thrombocytopenia

HIT is a clinical disorder that develops after extended heparin therapy. It occurs in approximately 1 in 5,000 hospitalized patients, with the highest incidence of 1% to 3% in patients recovering from cardiac surgery. It is associated with significant organ failure, vascular compromise, and mortality from thromboembolic complications.[25,186,187] There are two types: HIT1 describes mild thrombocytopenia, is benign and does not involve immune complexes. HIT2 is an immune-mediated response and carries a significant risk of hypercoagulability. IgG antibodies bind to heparin–PF4 complexes on the surface of platelets, thereby initiating primary hemostasis and thrombin generation.[25,187] HIT2 can occur in any patient receiving heparin therapy. Typically, 5 to 10 days are required to mount a significant immune response, but patients who have recent exposure to heparin or a history of HIT can present with clinical symptoms immediately. Any form of heparin therapy can initiate HIT; however, UFH is more likely than LMWH to lead to immune complexes because the fractionated form is less antigenic with a weaker bond to heparin–PF4.[25,187]

There are no specific laboratory tests for the clear diagnosis of HIT, and clinical signs can be clouded by alternative causes of thrombocytopenia and thrombosis. Guidelines from the American College of Chest Physicians and the national European guidelines recommend a diagnostic scoring algorithm to determine the pretest probability of clinical HIT. Variables to consider include the degree of thrombocytopenia (defined as a fall in platelet count of 30% to 50%), the timing of platelet decrease (typically day 5 to 10 of heparin therapy), any thromboembolic complications, and the likelihood of alternative diagnoses. Intermediate to high clinical suspicion of HIT is then confirmed with laboratory tests. The enzyme-linked immunosorbent assay (ELISA) for heparin–PF4 IgG antibodies is sensitive, but not as specific as the serotonin release functional assay, which is currently the gold standard test.[25,187] Patients suspected of having HIT should be managed with therapeutic anticoagulation and immediate discontinuation of all heparin therapy including heparin-coated indwelling catheters. The most commonly used agents are the parenteral DTIs such as bivalirudin and argatroban. Oral vitamin K antagonists are contraindicated for HIT treatment because the decreased synthesis of proteins C and S enhances the patient's prothrombotic state. Furthermore, warfarin has been shown to cause gangrenous thrombosis of the limbs in patients with HIT.[25,186] Platelet transfusion should also be held unless the patient is severely thrombocytopenic (<20,000/μL) with signs of bleeding.

Parenteral Direct Thrombin Inhibitors

Argatroban and bivalirudin are synthetic agents that directly inhibit thrombin in its free and fibrin-bound states. They are not immunogenic and there is no risk of HIT.[185] The half-lives of these agents vary. Furthermore, there are currently no known antidotes to the DTIs; therefore, reversal depends upon clearance. Clinical effects can be monitored with ACT or aPTT measurements. They are both approved for use in the United States for treatment of HIT. Argatroban is metabolized by the liver, with variable clearance in patients with hepatic dysfunction. It is commonly used for patients with HIT, who suffer from concurrent renal failure. Argatroban will prolong the INR as well as the aPTT, which can complicate clinical titration of warfarin therapy for long-term anticoagulation. Bivalirudin is a short-acting DTI with rapid onset of action and renal excretion. It is the drug of choice for patients with both renal and hepatic dysfunction, and its clinical versatility makes it a good agent for use during cardiopulmonary bypass in patients with HIT.[25]

Recombinant Activated Factor VII

Recombinant activated factor VII (rFVIIa) was originally FDA approved for prophylaxis and treatment of patients with hemophilia A or B complicated by inhibitors to FVIII and factor IX concentrates. It is now also indicated for the treatment of acquired hemophilia and factor VII deficiency.[188] However, most of its use is off-label for the prevention and treatment of coagulopathy and major blood loss in patients with postpartum hemorrhage, trauma, reversal of various anticoagulants, and high-risk cardiac surgery. The supporting data for these uses stem from retrospective reports, observational studies, and case series. There are few randomized controlled trials showing improved clinical outcomes and no trials that report definitive mortality benefits.[134] In fact, a recent meta-analysis demonstrated an increased risk of arterial thromboembolism, especially in elderly patients with use of high doses of rFVIIa (>120 μg/kg).[188] The current guidelines for the reversal of NOACs recommend PCCs as the drugs of choice; however, if activated PCCs are not available, low dose rFVIIa (15 to 20 μg/kg) should be considered for life-threatening hemorrhage. Overall, the lack of consistent dosing protocols and definitive evidence leaves one without clear indications for the use of rFVIIa for critical bleeding.[134]

The mechanism for rFVIIa remains unclear, but likely involves more than the physiologic role of factor VII in secondary hemostasis. Theoretically, rFVIIa will only act with TF exposed from the vascular endothelial lining at a site of injury. However, certain hemorrhagic disorders such as DIC or polytrauma can initiate systemic release of TF. Furthermore, rFVIIa can directly activate factor X and platelets, generating a thrombin burst for procoagulant activity.[134] These mechanisms explain why arterial and venous thromboembolism are the major adverse effects of rFVIIa, and why DIC and high thromboembolism risk are the main contraindications.[134,188]

Prothrombin Complex Concentrates

PCCs have been available for treatment of patients with hemophilia B for several decades. They were first used as a source of factor IX in the 1970s prior to the advent of specific factor concentrates. Subsequently they provided bypass treatment for hemophiliacs with factor inhibitors. Over the years, the safety and efficacy of PCCs have improved dramatically, and they are now FDA approved for use in hemophilia and reversal of vitamin K antagonists. PCCs are also the first-line agents for reversal of NOACs, although evidence is limited and their use for this indication remains off label.[134]

There are several commercially available formulations of PCCs, containing varying amounts of three to four coagulation factors, as well as one or more type of anticoagulant. The compositions include the vitamin K–dependent factors (II, VII, IX, and X), although not all products contain significant concentrations of factor VII. Some PCCs are "three-factor" concentrates lacking factor VII, but most formulations contain all four factors, with the addition of a natural anticoagulant such as heparin or AT to decrease the thrombogenic risks. Activated PCCs such as the Factor Eight Inhibitor Bypass Agent (FEIBA) are frequently used for bypass therapy in hemophilia patients with inhibitors, or for reversal of direct antifactor Xa antagonists.[134]

PCCs are now the drug of choice for immediate reversal of oral anticoagulants in place of rFVIIa and FFP, although in phase III trials, rFVIIa failed to show significant outcome improvements for warfarin-related intracerebral hemorrhage.[134] This is likely because it only replaces one of the vitamin K–dependent factors and, although the INR and PT decrease, this did not translate to meaningful survival benefits. PCCs are now preferred over plasma for several reasons. First, they provide faster correction of coagulopathy. The factors in plasma are relatively dilute, and a large volume (10 to 15 mL/kg) is required for clinical reversal of oral anticoagulants. It takes additional time to match the patient's blood type and thaw the plasma, putting the patient at risk for volume overload. Furthermore, PCCs stem from human plasma, but they are treated with at least one viral reduction process, whereas transfusion of several units of plasma carries a significant risk of infectious and noninfectious transfusion reactions. It is important to remember that although PCCs provide factor replacement for thrombin generation, their action still depends on adequate concentrations of platelets and fibrinogen.

The potential for PCCs to generate a significant thrombin burst puts patients at risk for thrombotic complications. The exact pathogenesis for thrombosis remains unclear, but animal models indicate that the accumulation of prothrombin, inactive factor II, and/or factor X after PCC administration correlates with thrombogenesis. Furthermore, this risk is associated with patients having thrombotic tendencies, such as those on anticoagulation and elderly patients who have a history of stroke. There are very few outcome studies evaluating their safety, but thus far no significant thrombotic complications have been reported with PCCs for critical bleeding.[189]

The thromboembolic risk can be minimized by avoiding repeat dosing. The factors within PCCs have varied half-lives, with prothrombin remaining active in plasma for up to 60 hours and factor X present for 30 hours. This is in contrast to labile factor VII, whose half-life is only approximately 6 hours. Consequently, factors II and X, which are thought to be primarily responsible for thrombotic complications, have the potential to accumulate with repeat doses of PCCs. The need for repeat dosing can be avoided by the coadministration of vitamin K in patients treated for oral anticoagulant toxicity. This allows for increased synthesis of coagulation factors. Furthermore, PCC dosing should be guided by the appropriate coagulation profile test. PT and INR only measure the procoagulant half of the hemostatic mechanism, and ignore the presence of anticoagulant activity such as AT or proteins C and S. In patients with severe liver disease or dilutional coagulopathy, the PT and INR times may be prolonged, but the concentrations of anticoagulants are also decreased, leaving hemostasis balanced. Thrombin generation times or thromboelastography are more appropriate measures of the patient's risk of bleeding and better indicators of the efficacy of PCC. These tests should be considered before redosing, since these patients may require simultaneous treatment with AT, platelets, or fibrinogen. The only absolute contraindications to PCC administration are in patients at high risk for thrombosis, such as those in DIC or with active HIT.[134,189]

Desmopressin

Desmopressin (DDAVP) is a synthetic analogue for the endogenous antidiuretic hormone, vasopressin. It acts at the V2 receptor found in the nephron and within endothelial cells. DDAVP was originally introduced for treatment of diabetes insipidus, but it was also found to improve hemostasis and platelet function. Consequently, it is one of the drugs of choice for treatment of mild bleeding in patients with vWD and mild hemophilia A, as discussed earlier.[134] Mechanistically, it causes the release of FVIII and vWF from within vascular endothelial cells, thereby improving platelet function. The appropriate dose for hemostasis is 0.3 μg/kg intravenously over 20 to 30 minutes, with therapeutic effects lasting for approximately 6 to 8 hours. Clinical benefits have been demonstrated for high-risk surgery, especially in patients with aspirin-induced platelet dysfunction.[134,190] Hypotension is the most commonly reported side effect, presumably secondary to arterial vasodilation from the release of NO; it is best avoided with slower infusion rates. Hyponatremia and water retention are rare complications, but have been reported in pediatric patients. As with all prothrombotic agents, DDAVP should be avoided in patients at high risk for thromboembolism, although the most recent meta-analysis did not report a significant incidence of thromboembolic complications.[134,190]

The hemostatic potential for DDAVP has been carefully studied for patients with critical bleeding from cardiac or spine surgery, uremia, antiplatelet agents, and liver disease. Several meta-analyses of randomized controlled trials report mild decreases in blood loss (80 mL per patient), but fail to translate into significant outcome improvements. There is no apparent effect on the number of patients transfused or the incidence of postoperative complications (including reoperation). The only consistent clinical benefit of DDAVP is improved bleeding times for patients with congenital or acquired platelet dysfunction from cardiopulmonary bypass, chronic renal failure, or aspirin therapy.[134,190]

Antifibrinolytic Therapy

Antifibrinolytic agents have been used to prevent and treat surgical blood loss for several decades. There are two types—the lysine analogues EACA and TXA, and a serine protease inhibitor, aprotinin. Aprotinin was reported to have superior efficacy for reducing blood loss, minimizing transfusions, and preventing reoperations in cardiac surgery. However, it was removed from the market after observational studies raised concern for relative risk of renal failure, myocardial infarction, and death. These findings were confirmed by the Blood Conservation Using Antifibrinolytics in a Randomized Trial (BART), which was stopped early due to significantly higher mortality associated with aprotinin when compared to EACA and TXA.[191–193] However, the risks may have been exaggerated with mechanistic concerns in the BART trial. Aprotinin is currently available in Canada and worldwide. Both the lysine derivatives are widely used throughout the United States. Today, they are commonly administered as part of a multimodal approach to perioperative blood conservation strategies.

Aprotinin is a nonspecific serine protease inhibitor. It prevents the action of several proteins involved in coagulation and fibrinolysis, including trypsin, plasmin, and kallikrein. It may also have an indirect effect on platelets to preserve their function, especially during extracorporeal circulation. The clinical efficacy of aprotinin to reduce perioperative blood loss, transfusions, and reoperations is clear; however, there is also much evidence reporting the negative association with renal failure and mortality.[134,192,193] Overall, aprotinin remains an option for perioperative blood conservation, but it is perhaps not worth the increased risks of adverse reactions.

Lysine Analogues

EACA and TXA are synthetic derivatives of the amino acid, lysine. They competitively inhibit the binding site on plasminogen, thereby preventing cleavage to plasmin and the resultant fibrinolysis. Both agents are excreted by the kidney and may be administered intravenously or topically. Although there is more evidence to support the use of TXA, these agents appear to have equivalent efficacy and have been shown to moderately decrease perioperative blood loss in cardiac surgery, as well as liver transplantation, orthopedic operations, and spine fusions.[134,192,193] Active research continues to focus on clarifying the appropriate dosing regimens and patient population to determine effects on rates of transfusion, reoperation, length of stay, morbidity, and mortality. The lysine analogues are inexpensive compared to aprotinin, and there have been no reports of increased risk of thrombotic complications or renal failure. The only documented adverse effects are possible seizure risk with TXA at high doses.[134,192,193] Besides perioperative indications, antifibrinolytics were recently studied for their potential to minimize critical bleeding in trauma patients. The CRASH II multinational randomized controlled trial compared TXA with placebo in trauma patients with major hemorrhage and documented a reduced all-cause mortality and risk of death due to bleeding.[190] Overall, the lysine analogues are inexpensive and low-risk adjunctive agents that should be considered for use in major surgery or critical bleeding as part of a multimodal approach to blood conservation.

Conclusions

Clinical anesthesiology is a perioperative specialty that aims to maintain the patient's health and wellness throughout the course of surgery. This requires a clear understanding of how a person's pre-existing comorbid status and anticipated surgical procedure can best be managed to gain the most therapeutic benefits from interventions with the least incurred risk. The anesthesiologist must remain vigilant in order to anticipate the possibility of derangements to coagulation and hemostasis that may occur with surgery, trauma, or critical illness. They must also know the best methods for avoiding and treating hemorrhagic or thrombotic complications of surgery while limiting the risks of transfusion therapy and hemostatic pharmacologic agents.

Overall, understanding the hemostatic mechanisms and the specifics of transfusion therapy is integral to the practice of anesthesia.

REFERENCES

1. Brown CH, Savage WJ, Masear CG, et al. Odds of transfusion for older adults compared to younger adults undergoing surgery. *Anesth Analg.* 2014;118(6):1168–1178.
2. Frank SM, Savage WJ, Rothschild JA, et al. Variability in blood and blood component utilization as assessed by an anesthesia information management system. *Anesthesiology.* 2012;117(1):99–106.
3. Rivera J, Lozano ML, Navarro-Nunez L, et al. Platelet receptors and signaling in the dynamics of thrombus formation. *Haematologica.* 2009;94(5):700–711.
4. Brass L. Understanding and evaluating platelet function. *Hematology Am Soc Hematol Educ Program.* 2010;2010:387–396.
5. Brass LF, Tomaiuolo M, Stalker TJ. Harnessing the platelet signaling network to produce an optimal hemostatic response. *Hematol Oncol Clin North Am.* 2013;27(3):381–409.
6. Metharom P, Berndt MC, Baker RI, et al. Current state and novel approaches of antiplatelet therapy. *Arterioscler Thromb Vasc Biol.* 2015;35(6):1327–1338.
7. Mann KG. Thrombin generation in hemorrhage control and vascular occlusion. *Circulation.* 2011;124(2):225–235.
8. The 2011 national blood collection and utilization survey report. Bethesda, MD: US Department of Health and Human Services and the American Association of Blood Banks; 2011.
9. Chapin JC, Hajjar KA. Fibrinolysis and the control of blood coagulation. *Blood rev.* 2015;29(1):17–24.
10. Orfanakis A, Deloughery T. Patients with disorders of thrombosis and hemostasis. *Med clin North Am.* 2013;97(6):1161–1180.
11. Harrison P, Lordkipanidze M. Testing platelet function. *Hematol Oncol Clin North Am.* 2013;27(3):411–441.
12. Matthews DC. Inherited disorders of platelet function. *Pediatr Clin North Am.* 2013;60(6):1475–1488.
13. Stone ME, Mazzeffi M, Derham J, et al. Current management of von Willebrand disease and von Willebrand syndrome. *Curr Opin Anaesthesiol.* 2014;27(3):353–358.
14. Tiede A. Diagnosis and treatment of acquired von Willebrand syndrome. *Thromb Res.* 2012;130 Suppl 2:S2–S6.
15. Sborov DW, Rodgers GM. How I manage patients with acquired haemophilia A. *Br J Haematol.* 2013;161(2):157–165.
16. Lison S, Spannagl M. Monitoring of direct anticoagulants. *Wien Med Wochenschr.* 2011;161(3–4):58–62.
17. Whiting D, DiNardo JA. TEG and ROTEM: technology and clinical applications. *Am J Hematol.* 2014;89(2):228–232.
18. Karon BS. Why is everyone so excited about thromboelastography (TEG)? *Clin Chim Acta.* 2014;436:143–148.
19. MacCallum P, Bowles L, Keeling D. Diagnosis and management of heritable thrombophilias. *BMJ.* 2014;349:g4387.
20. Franchini M. Utility of testing for factor V Leiden. *Blood Transf.* 2012;10(3):257–259.
21. Previtali E, Bucciarelli P, Passamonti SM, et al. Risk factors for venous and arterial thrombosis. *Blood Transf.* 2011;9(2):120–138.
22. Ng VL. Anticoagulation monitoring. *Clin Lab Med.* 2009;29(2):283–304.
23. Pirmohamed M, Kamali F, Daly AK, et al. Oral anticoagulation: a critique of recent advances and controversies. *Trends pharmacol sci.* 2015;36(3):153–163.
24. Harter K, Levine M, Henderson SO. Anticoagulation drug therapy: a review. *West J Emerg Med.* 2015;16(1):11–17.
25. Greinacher A. Heparin-induced thrombocytopenia. *N Engl J Med.* 2015;373(3):252–261.
26. Fenger-Eriksen C, Munster AM, Grove EL. New oral anticoagulants: clinical indications, monitoring and treatment of acute bleeding complications. *Acta Anaesthesiol Scand.* 2014;58(6):651–659.
27. Gehrie E, Tormey C. Novel oral anticoagulants: efficacy, laboratory measurement, and approaches to emergent reversal. *Arch Pathol Lab Med.* 2015;139(5):687–692.
28. Crowther M, Crowther MA. Antidotes for novel oral anticoagulants: current status and future potential. *Arterioscl Thromb Vasc Biol.* 2015;35(8):1736–1745.
29. Eder A, Muniz, MDLA. Allogeneic and autologous blood donor selection. In: Fung MK GB, Hillver CD, et al, eds. *Technical Manual.* 18th ed. Bethesda, MD: American Association of Blood Banks; 2014:117–134.
30. Nascimento B, Goodnough LT, Levy JH. Cryoprecipitate therapy. *Br J Anaesth.* 2014;113(6):922–934.
31. Katus MC, Szczepiorkowski ZM, Dumont LJ, et al. Safety of platelet transfusion: past, present and future. *Vox Sang.* 2014;107(2):103–113.
32. Leparc GF. Safety of the blood supply. *Cancer Contr.* 2015;22(1):7–15.
33. Vamvakas EC, Blajchman MA. Transfusion-related immunomodulation (TRIM): an update. *Blood Rev.* 2007;21(6):327–348.
34. Kopolovic I, Ostro J, Tsubota H, et al. A systematic review of transfusion-associated graft-versus-host disease. *Blood.* 2015;126(3):406–414.
35. Dunbar. NM hospital storage, monitoring, pretransfusion processing, distribution, and inventory management of blood components. In: Fung MK GB, Hillver CD, et al, eds. *Technical Manual.* Bethesda, MD: American Association of Blood Banks; 2014:213–229.
36. Brunskill SJ, Wilkinson KL, Doree C, et al. Transfusion of fresher versus older red blood cells for all conditions. *Cochrane Database Syst Rev.* 2015;5:CD010801.
37. Lacroix J, Hebert PC, Fergusson DA, et al. Age of transfused blood in critically ill adults. *N Engl J Med.* 2015;372(15):1410–1418.
38. Salunkhe V, van der Meer PF, de Korte D, et al. Development of blood transfusion product pathogen reduction treatments: a review of methods, current applications and demands. *Transfus Apher Sci.* 2015;52(1):19–34.
39. Ramsey G. Hemostatic efficacy of pathogen-inactivated blood components. *Semin Thromb Hemost.* 2015;42(2):172–182.
40. Tao Z, Ghoroghchian PP. Microparticle, nanoparticle, and stem cell-based oxygen carriers as advanced blood substitutes. *Trends biotechnol.* 2014;32(9):466–473.
41. Palmer AF, Intaglietta M. Blood substitutes. *Annu Rev Biomed Eng.* 2014;16:77–101.
42. Thon JN, Medvetz DA, Karlsson SM, et al. Road blocks in making platelets for transfusion. *J Thromb Haemost.* 2015;13(suppl 1):S55–S62.
43. Hart S, Cserti-Gazdewich CM, McCluskey SA. Red cell transfusion and the immune system. *Anaesthesia.* 2015;70(suppl 1):38–45, e13–e16.
44. American Society of Anesthesiologists Task Force on Perioperative Blood Management. Practice guidelines for perioperative blood management: an updated report by the American Society of Anesthesiologists Task Force on Perioperative Blood Management*. *Anesthesiology.* 2015;122(2):241–275.
45. Carson JL, Terrin ML, Noveck H, et al. Liberal or restrictive transfusion in high-risk patients after hip surgery. *N Engl J Med.* 2011;365(26):2453–2462.
46. Hajjar LA, Vincent JL, Galas FR, et al. Transfusion requirements after cardiac surgery: the TRACS randomized controlled trial. *JAMA.* 2010;304(14):1559–1567.
47. Hebert PC, Wells G, Blajchman MA, et al. A multicenter, randomized, controlled clinical trial of transfusion requirements in critical care. Transfusion Requirements in Critical Care Investigators, Canadian Critical Care Trials Group. *N Engl J Med.* 1999;340(6):409–417.
48. Villanueva C, Colomo A, Bosch A, et al. Transfusion strategies for acute upper gastrointestinal bleeding. *N Engl J Med.* 2013;368(1):11–21.
49. Napolitano LM, Kurek S, Luchette FA, et al. Clinical practice guideline: red blood cell transfusion in adult trauma and critical care. *Critical care medicine.* 2009;37(12):3124–3157.
50. Carson JL, Duff A, Poses RM, et al. Effect of anaemia and cardiovascular disease on surgical mortality and morbidity. *Lancet.* 1996;348(9034):1055–1060.
51. Ferraris VA, Brown JR, Despotis GJ, et al. 2011 update to the Society of Thoracic Surgeons and the Society of Cardiovascular Anesthesiologists blood conservation clinical practice guidelines. *Ann Thorac Surg.* 2011;91(3):944–982.
52. Carson JL, Guyatt G, Heddle MN, et al. Clinical Practice Guidelines from the AABB Red Blood Cell Transfusion Thresholds and Storage. *JAMA.* 2016; E1-11.
53. Kozek-Langenecker SA, Afshari A, Albaladejo P, et al. Management of severe perioperative bleeding: guidelines from the European Society of Anaesthesiology. *Eur J Anaesthesiol.* 2013;30(6):270–382.
54. Retter A, Wyncoll D, Pearse R, et al. Guidelines on the management of anaemia and red cell transfusion in adult critically ill patients. *Br J Haematol.* 2013;160(4):445–464.
55. Kramer AH, Zygun DA. Anemia and red blood cell transfusion in neurocritical care. *Crit Care.* 2009;13(3):R89.
56. Naidech AM, Jovanovic B, Wartenberg KE, et al. Higher hemoglobin is associated with improved outcome after subarachnoid hemorrhage. *Crit care med.* 2007;35(10):2383–2389.
57. Robertie PG, Gravlee GP. Safe limits of isovolemic hemodilution and recommendations for erythrocyte transfusion. *Int Anesthesiol Clin.* 1990;28(4):197–204.
58. Wang JK, Klein HG. Red blood cell transfusion in the treatment and management of anaemia: the search for the elusive transfusion trigger. *Vox sanguinis.* 2010;98(1):2–11.

59. Yuruk K, Milstein DM, Bezemer R, et al. Transfusion of banked red blood cells and the effects on hemorrheology and microvascular hemodynamics in anemic hematology outpatients. *Transfusion.* 2013;53(6):1346–1352.
60. Metivier F, Marchais SJ, Guerin AP, et al. Pathophysiology of anaemia: focus on the heart and blood vessels. Nephrology, dialysis, transplantation: official publication of the European Dialysis and Transplant Association. *ERA.* 2000;15(suppl 3):14–18.
61. Carson JL, Brooks MM, Abbott JD, et al. Liberal versus restrictive transfusion thresholds for patients with symptomatic coronary artery disease. *Am Heart J.* 2013;165(6):964–971.e1.
62. Cooper HA, Rao SV, Greenberg MD, et al. Conservative versus liberal red cell transfusion in acute myocardial infarction (the CRIT Randomized Pilot Study). *Am J Cardiol.* 2011 Oct 15;108(8):1108–1111.
63. British Committee for Standards in Haematology, Blood Transfusion Task Force. Guidelines for the use of platelet transfusions. *Br J Haematol.* 2003;122(1):10–23.
64. Goodnough LT, Levy JH, Murphy MF. Concepts of blood transfusion in adults. *Lancet.* 2013;381(9880):1845–1854.
65. Stainsby D, MacLennan S, Thomas D, et al. Guidelines on the management of massive blood loss. *Br J Haematol.* 2006;135(5):634–641.
66. Estcourt LJ, Stanworth SJ, Doree C, et al. Comparison of different platelet count thresholds to guide administration of prophylactic platelet transfusion for preventing bleeding in people with haematological disorders after myelosuppressive chemotherapy or stem cell transplantation. *Cochrane Database Syst Rev.* 2015;11:CD010983.
67. Kaufman RM, Djulbegovic B, Gernsheimer T, et al. Platelet transfusion: a clinical practice guideline from the AABB. *Ann Intern Med.* 2015;162(3):205–213.
68. Levy JH, Welsby I, Goodnough LT. Fibrinogen as a therapeutic target for bleeding: a review of critical levels and replacement therapy. *Transfusion.* 2014;54(5):1389–1405; quiz 8.
69. Roback JD, Caldwell S, Carson J, et al. Evidence-based practice guidelines for plasma transfusion. *Transfusion.* 2010;50(6):1227–1239.
70. Zeller MP, Al-Habsi KS, Golder M, et al. Plasma and plasma protein product transfusion: A Canadian blood services centre for innovation symposium. *Transfus Med Rev.* 2015;29(3):181–194.
71. O'Shaughnessy DF, Atterbury C, Bolton Maggs P, et al. Guidelines for the use of fresh-frozen plasma, cryoprecipitate and cryosupernatant. *Br J Haematol.* 2004;126(1):11–28.
72. Stanworth SJ, Walsh TS, Prescott RJ, et al. A national study of plasma use in critical care: clinical indications, dose and effect on prothrombin time. *Crit Care.* 2011;15(2):R108.
73. Yang L, Stanworth S, Hopewell S, et al. Is fresh-frozen plasma clinically effective? An update of a systematic review of randomized controlled trials. *Transfusion.* 2012;52(8):1673–1686; quiz
74. Holcomb JB, del Junco DJ, Fox EE, et al. The prospective, observational, multicenter, major trauma transfusion (PROMMTT) study: comparative effectiveness of a time-varying treatment with competing risks. *JAMA surgery.* 2013;148(2):127–136.
75. Nascimento B, Callum J, Tien H, et al. Effect of a fixed-ratio (1:1:1) transfusion protocol versus laboratory-results-guided transfusion in patients with severe trauma: a randomized feasibility trial. *CMAJ.* 2013;185(12):E583–E589.
76. de Biasi AR, Stansbury LG, Dutton RP, et al. Blood product use in trauma resuscitation: plasma deficit versus plasma ratio as predictors of mortality in trauma (CME). *Transfusion.* 2011;51(9):1925–1932.
77. Ho AM, Dion PW, Yeung JH, et al. Prevalence of survivor bias in observational studies on fresh frozen plasma: Erythrocyte ratios in trauma requiring massive transfusion. *Anesthesiology.* 2012;116(3):716–728.
78. Holcomb JB, Tilley BC, Baraniuk S, et al. Transfusion of plasma, platelets, and red blood cells in a 1:1:1 vs a 1:1:2 ratio and mortality in patients with severe trauma: the PROPPR randomized clinical trial. *JAMA.* 2015;313(5):471–482.
79. Novak DJ, Bai Y, Cooke RK, et al. Making thawed universal donor plasma available rapidly for massively bleeding trauma patients: experience from the Pragmatic, Randomized Optimal Platelets and Plasma Ratios (PROPPR) trial. *Transfusion.* 2015;55(6):1331–1339.
80. Lang T, Johanning K, Metzler H, et al. The effects of fibrinogen levels on thromboelastometric variables in the presence of thrombocytopenia. *Anesth Analg.* 2009;108(3):751–758.
81. Sorensen B, Bevan D. A critical evaluation of cryoprecipitate for replacement of fibrinogen. *Br J Haematol.* 2010;149(6):834–843.
82. Karkouti K, Callum J, Crowther MA, et al. The relationship between fibrinogen levels after cardiopulmonary bypass and large volume red cell transfusion in cardiac surgery: an observational study. *Anesth Analg.* 2013;117(1):14–22.
83. Spahn DR, Bouillon B, Cerny V, et al. Management of bleeding and coagulopathy following major trauma: an updated European guideline. *Crit Care.* 2013;17(2):R76.
84. Chung KW, Harvey A, Basavaraju SV, et al. How is national recipient hemovigilance conducted in the United States? *Transfusion.* 2015;55(4):703–707.
85. Harvey AR, Basavaraju SV, Chung KW, et al. Transfusion-related adverse reactions reported to the National Healthcare Safety Network Hemovigilance Module, United States, 2010 to 2012. *Transfusion.* 2015;55(4):709–718.
86. Tinegate H, Birchall J, Gray A, et al. Guideline on the investigation and management of acute transfusion reactions. Prepared by the BCSH Blood Transfusion Task Force. *Br J Haematol.* 2012;159(2):143–153.
87. Allain JP, Stramer SL, Carneiro-Proietti AB, et al. Transfusion-transmitted infectious diseases. *Biologicals.* 2009;37(2):71–77.
88. Kramer K, Verweij MF, Zaaijer HL. An inventory of concerns behind blood safety policies in five Western countries. *Transfusion.* 2015;55(12):2816–2825.
89. Lindholm PF, Annen K, Ramsey G. Approaches to minimize infection risk in blood banking and transfusion practice. *Infect Disord Drug Targets.* 2011;11(1):45–56.
90. Zou S, Stramer SL, Dodd RY. Donor testing and risk: current prevalence, incidence, and residual risk of transfusion-transmissible agents in US allogeneic donations. *Transfus Med Rev.* 2012;26(2):119–128.
91. Dwyre DM, Fernando LP, Holland PV. Hepatitis B, hepatitis C and HIV transfusion-transmitted infections in the 21st century. *Vox sanguinis.* 2011;100(1):92–98.
92. Kleinman SH, Lelie N, Busch MP. Infectivity of human immunodeficiency virus-1, hepatitis C virus, and hepatitis B virus and risk of transmission by transfusion. *Transfusion.* 2009;49(11):2454–2489.
93. Dorsey KA, Moritz ED, Steele WR, et al. A comparison of human immunodeficiency virus, hepatitis C virus, hepatitis B virus, and human T-lymphotropic virus marker rates for directed versus volunteer blood donations to the American Red Cross during 2005 to 2010. *Transfusion.* 2013;53(6):1250–1256.
94. Sandler SG, Zantek ND. Review: IgA anaphylactic transfusion reactions. Part II. Clinical diagnosis and bedside management. *Immunohematology/American Red Cross.* 2004;20(4):234–238.
95. Seed CR, Wong J, Polizzotto MN, et al. The residual risk of transfusion-transmitted cytomegalovirus infection associated with leucodepleted blood components. *Vox sanguinis.* 2015;109(1):11–17.
96. Simancas-Racines D, Osorio D, Marti-Carvajal AJ, et al. Leukoreduction for the prevention of adverse reactions from allogeneic blood transfusion. *Cochrane Database Syst Rev.* 2015;12:CD009745.
97. Faddy HM, Flower RL, Seed CR, et al. Detection of emergent strains of West Nile virus with a blood screening assay. *Transfusion.* 2015.
98. Administration FUSFaD. Fatalities reported to FDA following blood collection and transfusion: Annual summary for fiscal year 2012. 2012.
99. Jenkins C, Ramirez-Arcos S, Goldman M, et al. Bacterial contamination in platelets: incremental improvements drive down but do not eliminate risk. *Transfusion.* 2011.
100. Hong H, Xiao W, Lazarus HM, et al. Detection of septic transfusion reactions to platelet transfusions by active and passive surveillance. *Blood.* 2016;127(4):496–502.
101. Marti-Carvajal AJ, Sola I, Gonzalez LE, et al. Pharmacological interventions for the prevention of allergic and febrile non-haemolytic transfusion reactions. *Cochrane Database Syst Rev.* 2010(6):CD007539.
102. Sandler SG, Eder AF, Goldman M, et al. The entity of immunoglobulin A-related anaphylactic transfusion reactions is not evidence based. *Transfusion.* 2015;55(1):199–204.
103. Anani W, Triulzi D, Yazer MH, et al. Relative IgA-deficient recipients have an increased risk of severe allergic transfusion reactions. *Vox sanguinis.* 2014;107(4):389–392.
104. Flegel WA. Pathogenesis and mechanisms of antibody-mediated hemolysis. *Transfusion.* 2015;55(suppl 2):S47–S58.
105. Berseus O, Boman K, Nessen SC, et al. Risks of hemolysis due to anti-A and anti-B caused by the transfusion of blood or blood components containing ABO-incompatible plasma. *Transfusion.* 2013;53(suppl 1):114S–123S.
106. Cata JP, Wang H, Gottumukkala V, et al. Inflammatory response, immunosuppression, and cancer recurrence after perioperative blood transfusions. *Br J Anaesth.* 2013;110(5):690–701.
107. Rohde JM, Dimcheff DE, Blumberg N, et al. Health care-associated infection after red blood cell transfusion: a systematic review and meta-analysis. *JAMA.* 2014;311(13):1317–1326.
108. Shaw RE, Johnson CK, Ferrari G, et al. Blood transfusion in cardiac surgery does increase the risk of 5-year mortality: results from a contemporary series of 1714 propensity-matched patients. *Transfusion.* 2014;54(4):1106–1113.
109. Long K, Woodward J, Procter L, et al. In vitro transfusion of red blood cells results in decreased cytokine production by human T cells. *J Trauma Acute Care Surg.* 2014;77(2):198–201.
110. Muszynski JA, Bale J, Nateri J, et al. Supernatants from stored red blood cell (RBC) units, but not RBC-derived microvesicles, suppress monocyte function in vitro. *Transfusion.* 2015;55(8):1937–1945.
111. Dhabangi A, Ainomugisha B, Cserti-Gazdewich C, et al. Effect of transfusion of red blood cells with longer vs shorter storage duration on elevated blood lactate levels in children with severe anemia: The TOTAL randomized clinical trial. *JAMA.* 2015;314(23):2514–2523.
112. Fergusson DA, Hebert P, Hogan DL, et al. Effect of fresh red blood cell transfusions on clinical outcomes in premature, very low-birth-weight infants: the ARIPI randomized trial. *JAMA.* 2012;308(14):1443–1451.
113. Steiner ME, Ness PM, Assmann SF, et al. Effects of red-cell storage duration on patients undergoing cardiac surgery. *N Engl J Med.* 2015;372(15):1419–1429.

114. Zimring JC, Welniak L, Semple JW, et al. Current problems and future directions of transfusion-induced alloimmunization: summary of an NHLBI working group. *Transfusion.* 2011;51(2):435–441.
115. Nickel RS, Hendrickson JE, Fasano RM, et al. Impact of red blood cell alloimmunization on sickle cell disease mortality: a case series. *Transfusion.* 2016;56(1):107–114.
116. Schonewille H, Honohan A, van der Watering LM, et al. Incidence of alloantibody formation after ABO-D or extended matched red blood cell transfusions: a randomized trial (MATCH study). *Transfusion.* 2016;56(2):311–320.
117. Bolton-Maggs PH, Cohen H. Serious hazards of transfusion (SHOT) haemovigilance and progress is improving transfusion safety. *Br J Haematol.* 2013;163(3):303–314.
118. Clifford L, Jia Q, Subramanian A, et al. Characterizing the epidemiology of postoperative transfusion-related acute lung injury. *Anesthesiology.* 2015;122(1):12–20.
119. Sachs UJ, Wasel W, Bayat B, et al. Mechanism of transfusion-related acute lung injury induced by HLA class II antibodies. *Blood.* 2011;117(2):669–677.
120. Muller MC, van Stein D, Binnekade JM, et al. Low-risk transfusion-related acute lung injury donor strategies and the impact on the onset of transfusion-related acute lung injury: a meta-analysis. *Transfusion.* 2015;55(1):164–175.
121. Roubinian NH, Looney MR, Kor DJ, et al. Cytokines and clinical predictors in distinguishing pulmonary transfusion reactions. *Transfusion.* 2015;55(8):1838–1846.
122. Silliman CC. The two-event model of transfusion-related acute lung injury. *Crit Care Med.* 2006;34(5 Suppl):S124–S131.
123. Neves JF, Marques A, Valente R, et al. Nonlethal, attenuated, transfusion-associated graft-versus-host disease in an immunocompromised child: case report and review of the literature. *Transfusion.* 2010;50(11):2484–2488.
124. Demir T, Sahin M, El H, et al. Post-transfusion purpura following cardiac surgery. *J Cardiac Surg.* 2015;30(3):253–255.
125. Clifford L, Jia Q, Yadav H, et al. Characterizing the epidemiology of perioperative transfusion-associated circulatory overload. *Anesthesiology.* 2015;122(1):21–28.
126. Lieberman L, Maskens C, Cserti-Gazdewich C, et al. A retrospective review of patient factors, transfusion practices, and outcomes in patients with transfusion-associated circulatory overload. *Transfus Med Rev.* 2013;27(4):206–212.
127. Murphy EL, Kwaan N, Looney MR, et al. Risk factors and outcomes in transfusion-associated circulatory overload. *Am J Med.* 2013;126(4):357.e29–e38.
128. Sihler KC, Napolitano LM. Complications of massive transfusion. *Chest.* 2010;137(1):209–220.
129. Porter JB, Garbowski M. The pathophysiology of transfusional iron overload. *Hematol Oncol Clin North Am.* 2014;28(4):683–701, vi.
130. Vassallo R, Goldman M, Germain M, et al. Preoperative autologous blood donation: Waning indications in an era of improved blood safety. *Transfus Med Rev.* 2015;29(4):268–275.
131. Singbartl G, Held AL, Singbartl K. Ranking the effectiveness of autologous blood conservation measures through validated modeling of independent clinical data. *Transfusion.* 2013;53(12):3060–3079.
132. Grant MC, Resar LM, Frank SM. The efficacy and utility of acute normovolemic hemodilution. *Anesth Analg.* 2015;121(6):1412–1414.
133. Zhou X, Zhang C, Wang Y, et al. Preoperative acute normovolemic hemodilution for minimizing allogeneic blood transfusion: A meta-analysis. *Anesth Analg.* 2015;121(6):1443–1455.
134. Goodnough LT, Shander A. Current status of pharmacologic therapies in patient blood management. *Anesth Analg.* 2013;116(1):15–34.
135. So-Osman C, Nelissen RG, Koopman-van Gemert AW, et al. Patient blood management in elective total hip- and knee-replacement surgery (Part 1): a randomized controlled trial on erythropoietin and blood salvage as transfusion alternatives using a restrictive transfusion policy in erythropoietin-eligible patients. *Anesthesiology.* 2014;120(4):839–851.
136. Ashworth A, Klein AA. Cell salvage as part of a blood conservation strategy in anaesthesia. *Br J Anaesth.* 2010;105(4):401–416.
137. Carey PA, Schoenfeld AJ, Cordill RD, et al. A comparison of cell salvage strategies in posterior spinal fusion for adolescent idiopathic scoliosis. *J Spinal Disord Tech.* 2015;28(1):1–4.
138. Liang J, Shen J, Chua S, et al. Does intraoperative cell salvage system effectively decrease the need for allogeneic transfusions in scoliotic patients undergoing posterior spinal fusion? A prospective randomized study. *Eur Spine J.* 2015;24(2):270–275.
139. Vonk AB, Meesters MI, Garnier RP, et al. Intraoperative cell salvage is associated with reduced postoperative blood loss and transfusion requirements in cardiac surgery: a cohort study. *Transfusion.* 2013;53(11):2782–2789.
140. So-Osman C, Nelissen RG, Koopman-van Gemert AW, et al. Patient blood management in elective total hip- and knee-replacement surgery (part 2): a randomized controlled trial on blood salvage as transfusion alternative using a restrictive transfusion policy in patients with a preoperative hemoglobin above 13 g/dL. *Anesthesiology.* 2014;120(4):852–860.
141. van Bodegom-Vos L, Voorn VM, So-Osman C, et al. Cell salvage in hip and knee arthroplasty: A meta-analysis of randomized controlled trials. *J Bone Joint Surg Am.* 2015;97(12):1012–1021.
142. Lawson T, Ralph C. Perioperative Jehovah's Witnesses: a review. *Br J Anaesth.* 2015;115(5):676–687.
143. Mason CL, Tran CK. Caring for the Jehovah's Witness Parturient. *Anesth Analg.* 2015;121(6):1564–1569.
144. Salaria ON, Barodka VM, Hogue CW, et al. Impaired red blood cell deformability after transfusion of stored allogeneic blood but not autologous salvaged blood in cardiac surgery patients. *Anesth Analg.* 2014;118(6):1179–1187.
145. Goucher H, Wong CA, Patel SK, et al. Cell salvage in obstetrics. *Anesth Analg.* 2015;121(2):465–468.
146. Munoz M, Slappendel R, Thomas D. Laboratory characteristics and clinical utility of post-operative cell salvage: washed or unwashed blood transfusion? *Blood Transfus.* 2011;9(3):248–261.
147. Xie J, Feng X, Ma J, et al. Is postoperative cell salvage necessary in total hip or knee replacement? A meta-analysis of randomized controlled trials. *Int J Surg.* 2015;21:135–144.
148. Vermeijden WJ, Hagenaars JA, Scheeren TW, et al. Additional postoperative cell salvage of shed mediastinal blood in cardiac surgery does not reduce allogeneic blood transfusions: a cohort study. *Perfusion.* 2015.
149. Israels SJ, El-Ekiaby M, Quiroga T, et al. Inherited disorders of platelet function and challenges to diagnosis of mucocutaneous bleeding. *Haemophilia.* 2010;16(suppl 5):152–159.
150. de Jong A, Eikenboom J. Developments in the diagnostic procedures for von Willebrand disease. *J Thromb Haemost.* 2016;14(3):449–460.
151. Jilma-Stohlawetz P, Quehenberger P, Schima H, et al. Acquired von Willebrand factor deficiency caused by LVAD is ADAMTS-13 and platelet dependent. *Thromb Res.* 2016;137:196–201.
152. Favaloro EJ, Mohammed S. Evaluation of a von Willebrand factor three test panel and chemiluminescent-based assay system for identification of, and therapy monitoring in, von Willebrand disease. *Thromb Res.* 2016;141:202–211.
153. Berntorp E. Prophylaxis in von Willebrand disease. *Haemophilia.* 2008;14(suppl 5):47–53.
154. Srivastava A, Brewer AK, Mauser-Bunschoten EP, et al. Guidelines for the management of hemophilia. *Haemophilia.* 2013;19(1):e1–e47.
155. Mahlangu J, Powell JS, Ragni MV, et al. Phase 3 study of recombinant factor VIII Fc fusion protein in severe hemophilia A. *Blood.* 2014;123(3):317–325.
156. Kessler CM, Knobl P. Acquired haemophilia: an overview for clinical practice. *Eur J Haematol.* 2015;95(suppl 81):36–44.
157. Dargaud Y, Pavlova A, Lacroix-Desmazes S, et al. Achievements, challenges and unmet needs for haemophilia patients with inhibitors: Report from a symposium in Paris, France on 20 November 2014. *Haemophilia.*2016;22(suppl 1):1–24.
158. Franchini M, Zaffanello M, Lippi G. The use of desmopressin in mild hemophilia A. *Blood Coagul Fibrinolysis.* 2010;21(7):615–619.
159. Matino D, Makris M, Dwan K, et al. Recombinant factor VIIa concentrate versus plasma-derived concentrates for treating acute bleeding episodes in people with haemophilia and inhibitors. *Cochrane Database Syst Rev.* 2015;12:CD004449.
160. Giangrande P. Haemophilia B: Christmas disease. *Expert Opin Pharmacother.* 2005;6(9):1517–1524.
161. Thomas RH. Hypercoagulability syndromes. *Archives of internal medicine.* 2001 Nov 12;161(20):2433–9.
162. Willems BA, Vermeer C, Reutelingsperger CP, et al. The realm of vitamin K dependent proteins: shifting from coagulation toward calcification. *Mol Nutr Food Res.* 2014;58(8):1620–1635.
163. Frontera JA, Lewin III JJ, Rabinstein AA, et al. Guideline for reversal of antithrombotics in intracranial hemorrhage: A statement for healthcare professionals from the Neurocritical Care Society and Society of Critical Care Medicine. *Neurocrit Care.* 2016;24(1):6–46.
164. Kujovich JL. Coagulopathy in liver disease: a balancing act. *Hematology Am Soc of Hematol Educ Program.* 2015;2015(1):243–249.
165. Tripodi A, Mannucci PM. The coagulopathy of chronic liver disease. *N Engl J Med.* 2011;365(2):147–156.
166. Di Nisio M, Baudo F, Cosmi B, et al. Diagnosis and treatment of disseminated intravascular coagulation: guidelines of the Italian Society for Haemostasis and Thrombosis (SISET). *Thromb Res.* 2012;129(5):e177–e184.
167. Levi M, Toh CH, Thachil J, et al. Guidelines for the diagnosis and management of disseminated intravascular coagulation. British Committee for Standards in Haematology. *Br J Haematol.* 2009;145(1):24–33.
168. Wada H, Matsumoto T, Yamashita Y. Diagnosis and treatment of disseminated intravascular coagulation (DIC) according to four DIC guidelines. *J Intensive Care.* 2014;2(1):15.
169. Thachil J, Toh CH, Levi M, et al. The withdrawal of Activated Protein C from the use in patients with severe sepsis and DIC [Amendment to the BCSH guideline on disseminated intravascular coagulation]. *Br J Haematol.* 2012;157(4):493–494.
170. Vardeny O, Solomon SD. Cyclooxygenase-2 inhibitors, nonsteroidal anti-inflammatory drugs, and cardiovascular risk. *Cardiol Clin.* 2008;26(4):589–601.
171. Pham TT, Miller MJ, Harrison DL, et al. Cardiovascular disease and non-steroidal anti-inflammatory drug prescribing in the midst of evolving guidelines. *J Eval Clin Pract.* 2013;19(6):1026–1034.
172. Smock KJ, Saunders PJ, Rodgers GM, et al. Laboratory evaluation of clopidogrel responsiveness by platelet function and genetic methods. *Am J Hematol.* 2011;86(12):1032–1034.

173. Mikkelsson J, Paana T, Lepantalo A, et al. Personalized ADP-receptor inhibition strategy and outcomes following primary PCI for STEMI (PASTOR study). *Int J Cardiol.* 2016;202:463–466.
174. Giordano A, Musumeci G, D'Angelillo A, et al. Effects of glycoprotein IIb/IIIa antagonists: Anti platelet aggregation and beyond. *Current drug metabolism.* 2016;17(2):194–203.
175. Keeling D, Baglin T, Tait C, et al. Guidelines on oral anticoagulation with warfarin - fourth edition. *Br J Haematol.* 2011;154(3):311–324.
176. Bauer KA. Recent progress in anticoagulant therapy: oral direct inhibitors of thrombin and factor Xa. *J Thromb Haemost.* 2011;9(suppl 1):12–19.
177. Gomez-Outes A, Suarez-Gea ML, Lecumberri R, et al. Direct-acting oral anticoagulants: pharmacology, indications, management, and future perspectives. *Eur J Haematol.* 2015;95(5):389–404.
178. Chan KE, Edelman ER, Wenger JB, et al. Dabigatran and rivaroxaban use in atrial fibrillation patients on hemodialysis. *Circulation.* 2015;131(11):972–979.
179. Agnelli G, Buller HR, Cohen A, et al. Oral apixaban for the treatment of acute venous thromboembolism. *N Engl J Med.* 2013;369(9):799–808.
180. Buller HR, Decousus H, Grosso MA, et al. Edoxaban versus warfarin for the treatment of symptomatic venous thromboembolism. *N Engl J Med.* 2013;369(15):1406–1415.
181. Buller HR, Prins MH, Lensin AW, et al. Oral rivaroxaban for the treatment of symptomatic pulmonary embolism. *N Engl J Med.* 2012;366(14):1287–1297.
182. Ruff CT, Giugliano RP, Braunwald E, et al. Comparison of the efficacy and safety of new oral anticoagulants with warfarin in patients with atrial fibrillation: a meta-analysis of randomised trials. *Lancet.* 2014;383(9921):955–962.
183. Rachidi S, Aldin ES, Greenberg C, et al. The use of novel oral anticoagulants for thromboprophylaxis after elective major orthopedic surgery. *Exp Rev Hematol.* 2013;6(6):677–695.
184. Pollack CV Jr, Reilly PA, Eikelboom J, et al. Idarucizumab for dabigatran reversal. *N Engl J Med.* 2015;373(6):511–520.
185. Levy JH, Key NS, Azran MS. Novel oral anticoagulants: implications in the perioperative setting. *Anesthesiology.* 2010;113(3):726–745.
186. Augoustides JG. Update in hematology: heparin-induced thrombocytopenia and bivalirudin. *J Cardiothorac Vasc Anesth.* 2011;25(2):371–375.
187. Bambrah RK, Pham DC, Zaiden R, et al. Heparin-induced thrombocytopenia. *Clin Adv Hematol Oncol.* 2011;9(8):594–599.
188. Levi M, Levy JH, Andersen HF, et al. Safety of recombinant activated factor VII in randomized clinical trials. *N Engl J Med.* 2010;363(19):1791–800.
189. Sorensen B, Spahn DR, Innerhofer P, et al. Prothrombin complex concentrates: evaluation of safety and thrombogenicity. *Crit Care.* 2011;15(1):201.
190. Crescenzi G, Landoni G, Biondi-Zoccai G, et al. Desmopressin reduces transfusion needs after surgery: a meta-analysis of randomized clinical trials. *Anesthesiology.* 2008;109(6):1063–1076.
191. Fergusson DA, Hebert PC, Mazer CD, et al. A comparison of aprotinin and lysine analogues in high-risk cardiac surgery. *N Engl J Med.* 2008;358(22):2319–2331.
192. Ortmann E, Besser MW, Klein AA. Antifibrinolytic agents in current anaesthetic practice. *Br J Anaesth.* 2013;111(4):549–563.
193. Simmons J, Sikorski RA, Pittet JF. Tranexamic acid: from trauma to routine perioperative use. *Curr Opin Anaesthesiol.* 2015;28(2):191–200.

Section 4
ANESTHETIC DRUGS AND ADJUVANTS

18 Inhaled Anesthetics

THOMAS J. EBERT • SAWYER A. NAZE

Introduction and Overview
Pharmacokinetic Principles
    Unique Features of Inhaled Anesthetics
    Physical Characteristics of Inhaled Anesthetics
    Gases in Mixtures
    Gases in Solution
    Anesthetic Transfer: Machine to Central Nervous System
    Uptake and Distribution
    Distribution (Tissue Uptake)
    Metabolism
    Overpressurization and the Concentration Effect
    Second Gas Effect
    Ventilation Effects
    Perfusion Effects
    Ventilation–Perfusion Mismatching
    Elimination
Clinical Overview of Current Inhaled Anesthetics
    Isoflurane
    Desflurane
    Sevoflurane
    Xenon
    Nitrous Oxide
Neuropharmacology of Inhaled Anesthetics
    Minimum Alveolar Concentration
    Other Alterations in Neurophysiology
The Circulatory System
    Hemodynamics
    Myocardial Contractility
    Other Circulatory Effects
    Coronary Steal, Myocardial Ischemia, and Cardiac Outcome
    Cardioprotection from Volatile Anesthetics
    Autonomic Nervous System
The Pulmonary System
    General Ventilatory Effects
    Ventilatory Mechanics
    Response to Carbon Dioxide and Hypoxemia
    Bronchiolar Smooth Muscle Tone
    Mucociliary Function
    Pulmonary Vascular Resistance
Hepatic Effects
Neuromuscular System and Malignant Hyperthermia
Genetic Effects, Obstetric Use, and Effects on Fetal Development
Anesthetic Degradation by Carbon Dioxide Absorbers
    Compound A
    Carbon Monoxide and Heat
    Generic Sevoflurane Formulations
Anesthetic Metabolism
    Fluoride-induced Nephrotoxicity
Clinical Utility of Volatile Anesthetics
    For Induction of Anesthesia
    For Maintenance of Anesthesia

KEY POINTS

1. At equilibrium, the CNS partial pressure of inhaled anesthetics equals their arterial partial pressure, which in turn equals their alveolar partial pressure if cardiopulmonary function is normal.
2. The inspired concentration and the blood:gas solubility of an inhaled anesthetic are the major determinants of the speed of induction. Solubility alone determines the rate of elimination, provided there is normal cardiopulmonary function.
3. Isoflurane is the most potent of the volatile anesthetics in clinical use, desflurane is the least soluble, and sevoflurane is the least irritating to the airways.
4. Nitrous oxide (N_2O) can expand a pneumothorax to double or triple its size in 10 to 30 minutes, and washout of N_2O can lower alveolar concentrations of oxygen and carbon dioxide, a phenomenon called *diffusion hypoxia*.
5. Minimum alveolar concentration (MAC) is the alveolar concentration of an inhaled anesthetic at one atmosphere that prevents movement in response to a surgical stimulus in 50% of patients. Concentrations of inhaled anesthetics that provide loss of awareness and recall are about 0.4 to 0.5 MAC.
6. MAC decreases approximately 6% per decade.
7. Volatile anesthetics depress cerebral metabolic rate and increase cerebral blood flow (CBF) in a dose-dependent manner. The latter effect may increase intracranial pressure in patients with a mass-occupying lesion of the brain.

8. Hypocapnia may blunt or abolish volatile anesthetic-induced increases in coronary blood flow depending on when the hypocapnia is produced and the nature of the cerebral disease process.
9. Volatile anesthetics produce dose-dependent depression of the electroencephalogram, sensory-evoked potentials, and motor-evoked potentials.
10. Volatile anesthetics in current use decrease arterial blood pressure, systemic vascular resistance, and myocardial function comparably and in a dose-dependent fashion.
11. Volatile anesthetics decrease tidal volume, decrease ventilatory response to hypercarbia and hypoxia, increase respiratory rate, and relax airway smooth muscle in a dose-dependent fashion.
12. Unlike halothane, volatile anesthetics in current use have minimal adverse effects on the liver and might afford some protection for hepatocytes from ischemic and/or hypoxic injury.
13. Volatile anesthetics are potent triggers for malignant hyperthermia in genetically susceptible patients.
14. CO_2 absorbents degrade sevoflurane, desflurane, and isoflurane to carbon monoxide when the normal water content of the absorbent (13% to 15%) is markedly decreased (<5%).

Introduction and Overview

Inhalation anesthetics are the most common drugs used for the provision of general anesthesia. Adding only a fraction of a volatile anesthetic to the inspired oxygen results in a state of unconsciousness and amnesia. When combined with intravenous adjuvants, such as opioids and benzodiazepines, a balanced technique is achieved that results in analgesia, further sedation/hypnosis, and amnesia. Inhaled anesthetics for surgical procedures are popular because of their ease of administration and the clinician's ability to reliably monitor their effects with both clinical signs and end-tidal concentrations. In addition, the volatile anesthetic gases are relatively inexpensive in terms of overall cost.

Sevoflurane, desflurane, and isoflurane are the most popular potent inhaled anesthetics used in adult surgical procedures (Fig. 18-1). Although there are many similarities in terms of the overall effects of the volatile anesthetics (e.g., they all have a dose-dependent effect to decrease blood pressure [BP]), there are some unique differences that might influence the clinician's selection process depending on the patient's age, health, and the surgical procedure. For example, sevoflurane is the most commonly used anesthetic in the pediatric population based on its relative lack of pungency when inhaled and its relative speed of emergence. These beneficial attributes outweigh the emergence agitation associated with the use of sevoflurane in pediatric patients. Discussion of the attributes of the three most popular inhaled anesthetics provides the major emphasis of this chapter. For the sake of completeness and for historical perspective related to metabolism and toxicity, comments on halothane and enflurane are also included.

Pharmacokinetic Principles

Kety[1] in 1950 was the first to examine the pharmacokinetics of inhaled agents in a systematic fashion. Eger[2] accomplished much of the early research in the field, leading to his landmark text on the subject in 1974. The inhaled anesthetics differ substantially from nearly all other therapeutic drugs because they are gases given via inhalation. Drug pharmacology is classically divided into two disciplines, pharmacodynamics and pharmacokinetics. *Pharmacodynamics* can be defined as what drugs do to the body. It describes the desired and undesired effects of drugs, as well as the cellular and molecular changes leading to these effects. *Pharmacokinetics* can be defined as how the body handles drugs. It describes where drugs are distributed, how they are transformed, and the cellular and molecular mechanisms underlying these processes.

Tissues are often grouped into hypothetical *compartments* based on perfusion. An important implication of different compartments and perfusion rates is the concept of redistribution. After a given amount of drug is administered, it reaches highly perfused tissue compartments first, where it can equilibrate rapidly and exert its effects. With time, however, compartments with lower perfusion rates receive sufficient drug to reach equilibrium between blood and tissue. As the tissues with lower perfusion rates absorb the drug, maintenance of equilibria throughout the body requires drug transfer from highly perfused compartments back into the bloodstream. This lowering of drug concentration in one compartment by delivery into another compartment is called *redistribution*.

In discussions of the inhaled anesthetics, the absorption phase is usually called *uptake*, the metabolic phase is usually called *biotransformation*, and the excretion phase is usually called *elimination*.

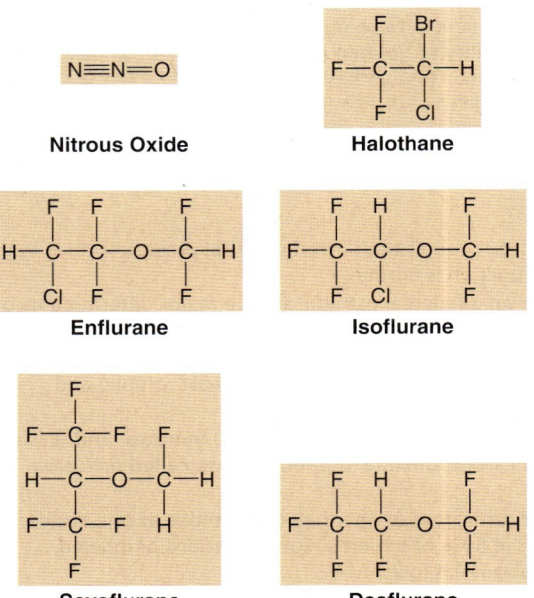

Figure 18-1 Chemical structure of inhaled anesthetics. Halothane is an alkane, a halogen-substituted ethane derivative. It is no longer available commercially. Isoflurane and enflurane are isomers that are methyl ethyl ethers. Desflurane differs from isoflurane in the substitution of a fluorine for a chlorine atom and sevoflurane is a methyl isopropyl ether.

Unique Features of Inhaled Anesthetics

Speed, Gas State, and Route of Administration

The inhaled anesthetics are among the most rapidly acting drugs in existence, and when used for general anesthesia, this speed provides a margin of safety. The ability to quickly increase or decrease anesthetic levels as necessary can mean the difference between an anesthetic state and an anesthetic misadventure. Speed also means efficiency. Rapid induction and recovery may lead to faster operating room turnover times, shorter recovery room stays, and earlier discharge times to home.

Only N_2O and xenon are true gases, while the so-called *potent anesthetics* are the vapors of volatile liquids. But for simplicity, all of them are referred to as gases because they are all in the gas phase when administered via the lungs. As gases, none deviate significantly from ideal gas behavior. These anesthetics are all nonionized and have low molecular weights. This allows them to diffuse rapidly without the need for facilitated diffusion or active transport from bloodstream to tissues. The other advantage of gases is that they can be delivered to the bloodstream via a unique route available in all patients: the lungs.

Speed, gaseous state, and route of administration combine to form the major beneficial feature of the inhaled anesthetics: the ability to decrease plasma concentrations as easily and as rapidly as they are increased.

Physical Characteristics of Inhaled Anesthetics

The physical characteristics of inhaled anesthetics are shown in Table 18-1. The goal of delivering inhaled anesthetics is to produce the anesthetic state by establishing a specific concentration of anesthetic molecules in the central nervous system (CNS), which is done by establishing the specific partial pressure of the agent in the lungs that ultimately equilibrates with the brain and spinal cord.[1] At equilibrium, CNS partial pressure equals blood partial pressure, which in turn equals alveolar partial pressure:

$$P_{CNS} = P_{blood} = P_{alveoli} \quad (18\text{-}1)$$

where P is partial pressure. Equilibration is a result of three factors:

1. Inhaled anesthetics are gases rapidly transferred bidirectionally via the lungs to and from the bloodstream and subsequently to and from CNS tissues as partial pressures equilibrate.
2. Plasma and tissues have a low capacity to absorb the inhaled anesthetics relative to the amount we can deliver to the lungs, allowing us to quickly establish or abolish anesthetizing concentrations of anesthetic in the bloodstream and ultimately the CNS.
3. Metabolism, excretion, and redistribution of the inhaled anesthetics are minimal relative to the rate at which they are delivered or removed from the lungs. This permits easy maintenance of blood and CNS concentrations.

The so-called permanent gases, such as oxygen and nitrogen, exist only as gases at ambient temperatures. Gases such as N_2O can be compressed into liquids under high pressure at ambient temperature. *Potent volatile anesthetics* with the exception of desflurane are liquids at ambient temperature and pressure. If volatile liquids reside in a closed container, molecules of the substance will equilibrate between the liquid and gas phases. At equilibrium, the pressure exerted by molecular collisions of the gas against the container walls is the *vapor pressure*. One important property of vapor pressure is that as long as *any* liquid remains in the container, the vapor pressure is independent of the volume of that liquid. As with any gas, however, vapor pressure is proportional to temperature.

At room temperature, most of the potent agents have a vapor pressure that is below atmospheric pressure. If the temperature is raised, the vapor pressure increases. The *boiling point* of a liquid is the temperature at which its vapor pressure exceeds atmospheric pressure in an open container. Desflurane is bottled in a special container because its boiling point of 23.5°C makes it

Table 18-1 Physiochemical Properties of Volatile Anesthetics

Property	Sevoflurane	Desflurane	Isoflurane	Enflurane	Halothane	N_2O
Boiling point (°C)	59	24	49	57	50	–88
Vapor pressure at 20°C (mmHg)	157	669	238	172	243	38,770
Molecular weight (g)	200	168	184	184	197	44
Oil:gas partition coefficient	47	19	91	97	224	1.4
Blood:gas partition coefficient	0.65	0.42	1.46	1.9	2.50	0.46
Brain:blood solubility	1.7	1.3	1.6	1.4	1.9	1.1
Fat:blood solubility	47.5	27.2	44.9	36	51.1	2.3
Muscle:blood solubility	3.1	2.0	2.9	1.7	3.4	1.2
MAC in O_2 30–60 years, at 37°C P_B 760 (%)	1.8	6.6	1.17	1.63	0.75	104
MAC in 60–70% N_2O (%)	0.66	2.38	0.56	0.57	0.29	—
MAC, >65 years (%)	1.45	5.17	1.0	1.55	0.64	—
Preservative	No	No	No	No	Thymol	No
Stable in moist CO_2 absorber	No	Yes	Yes	Yes	No	Yes
Flammability (%) (in 70% N_2O/30% O_2)	10	17	7	5.8	4.8	
Recovered as metabolites (%)	2–5	0.02	0.2	2.4	20	

MAC, minimum alveolar concentration; N_2O, nitrous oxide.

boil at typical room temperatures. Boiling does not occur within the bottle because it is countered by buildup of vapor pressure within the bottle, but once opened to air, the desflurane would quickly boil away.

Gases in Mixtures

For any mixture of gases in a closed container, each gas exerts a pressure proportional to its *fractional mass*. This is its *partial pressure*. The sum of the partial pressures of each gas in a mixture of gases equals the total pressure of the entire mixture (Dalton's law):

$$P_{total} = P_{gas1} + P_{gas2} + \ldots + P_{gasN} \qquad (18\text{-}2)$$

Another way to state this is that each gas in a mixture of gases at a given volume and temperature has a partial pressure, that is, the pressure it would have *if it alone* occupied the volume. The entire mixture behaves just as if it were a single gas according to the ideal gas law.

Gases in Solution

Partial pressure of a gas in solution is a bit complex because pressure can only be measured in the gas phase, while in solution the amount of gas is measured as a concentration. Partial pressure of a gas in solution refers to the pressure of the gas in the gas phase (if it were present) in equilibrium with the liquid. However, it is important to talk of partial pressures, because gases equilibrate based on partial pressures, not concentrations.

Gas molecules within a liquid interact with solvent molecules to a much larger extent than do molecules in the gas phase. *Solubility* is the term used to describe the tendency of a gas to equilibrate with a solution, hence determining its concentration in solution. Henry's law expresses the relationship of concentration of a gas in solution to the partial pressure of the gas with which the solution is in equilibrium:

$$C_g = kP_g \qquad (18\text{-}3)$$

where C_g is concentration of gas in solution, k is a solubility constant, and P_g is the partial pressure of the gas. From Eq. 18-3 one can see that doubling the pressure of a gas doubles its concentration in solution. A more clinically useful expression of solubility is the solubility coefficient, λ:

$$\lambda = V_{dissolved\ gas}/V_{liquid} \text{ at } 37°C \qquad (18\text{-}4)$$

where V = volume. This equation states that for any gas in equilibrium with a liquid, a certain volume of that gas dissolves in a given volume of liquid.

The principles of partial pressures and solubility apply in mixtures of gases in solution. That is, the concentration of any one gas in a mixture of gases in solution depends on two factors: (1) its partial pressure in the gas phase in equilibrium with the solution, and (2) its solubility within that solution.

The implications of these properties are that anesthetic gases administered via the lungs diffuse into blood until the partial pressures in alveoli and blood are equal. The concentration of anesthetic in the blood depends on the partial pressure at equilibrium and the blood solubility. Likewise, transfer of anesthetic from blood to target tissues also proceeds toward equalizing partial pressures, but at this interface there is no gas phase. A partial pressure still exists to force anesthetic molecules out of solution and into a gas phase but there is no gas phase because blood (outside the lungs) and tissues are like closed, liquid-filled containers. Remember the principle: The partial pressure of a gas in solution represents the pressure that the gas in equilibrium with the liquid *would* have if a gas phase existed in contact with the liquid phase.

The concentration of anesthetic in target tissue depends on the partial pressure at equilibrium and the target tissue solubility. Because inhaled anesthetics are gases, and because partial pressures of gases equilibrate throughout a system, *monitoring the alveolar concentration of inhaled anesthetics provides an index of their effects in the brain.*

In summary:
1. Inhaled anesthetics equilibrate based on their partial pressures in each tissue (or tissue compartment), not based on their concentrations.
2. The partial pressure of a gas in solution is defined by the partial pressure in the gas phase with which it is in equilibrium. Where there is no gas phase the partial pressure reflects a force to move out of solution.
3. The concentration of anesthetic in a tissue depends on its partial pressure and the tissue solubility of the anesthetic.

Finally, the particular terminology used when referring to gases in the gas phase or absorbed in plasma or tissues is important. Inspired concentrations or fractional volumes of inhaled anesthetic are typically used rather than partial pressure. Partial pressure is expressed in millimeters of mercury (mmHg) or Torr (1 Torr = 1 mmHg) or kilopascals (kPa). For most drugs, concentration is expressed as mass (milligram [mg]) per volume (milliliter [mL]), but it can also be expressed in percent by weight or volume. Since volume of a gas in the gas phase is directly proportional to mass according to the ideal gas law, it is easier to express this fractional concentration as a percent by volume. In the gas phase, fractional concentration is equal to the partial pressure divided by ambient pressure, usually atmospheric, or:

$$\text{Fractional volume} = P_{anesthetic}/P_{barometric} \qquad (18\text{-}5)$$

Anesthetic Transfer: Machine to Central Nervous System

When the fresh gas flow (FGF) and the vaporizer are turned on, fresh gas with a fixed fractional concentration of anesthetic leaves the fresh gas outlet and mixes with the gas in the circuit—the bag, tubing, absorbent canister, and piping. It is immediately diluted to a lower fractional concentration, then slowly rises as this compartment equilibrates with the delivered flow. With spontaneous patient ventilation by mask, the anesthetic gas passes from circuit to airways. The fractional concentration of anesthetic leaving the circuit is designated as F_I (fraction inspired). In the lungs the gas comprising the dead space in the airways (trachea, bronchi) and the alveoli further dilutes the circuit gas. The fractional concentration of anesthetic present in the alveoli is F_A (fraction alveolar). The anesthetic then passes across the alveolar–capillary membrane and dissolves in pulmonary blood according to the partial pressure of the gas and its blood solubility. It is further diluted and travels via bulk blood flow throughout the vascular tree. The anesthetic then passes via simple diffusion from blood to tissues as well as between tissues.

The vascular system delivers blood to three physiologic tissue groups: the vessel-rich group (VRG), the muscle group, and the fat group. The VRG includes the brain, heart, kidney, liver, digestive tract, and glandular tissues. The percent of body mass and perfusion of each group are shown in Table 18-2. The CNS tissues of the VRG are referred to as *tissues of desired effect.* The other tissues of the VRG that comprise the compartment are

Table 18-2 Distribution of Cardiac Output by Tissue Group			
Group	% Body Mass	% Cardiac Output	Perfusion (mL/min/100 g)
Vessel-rich	10	75	55–500
Muscle	50	19	3
Fat	20	6	1

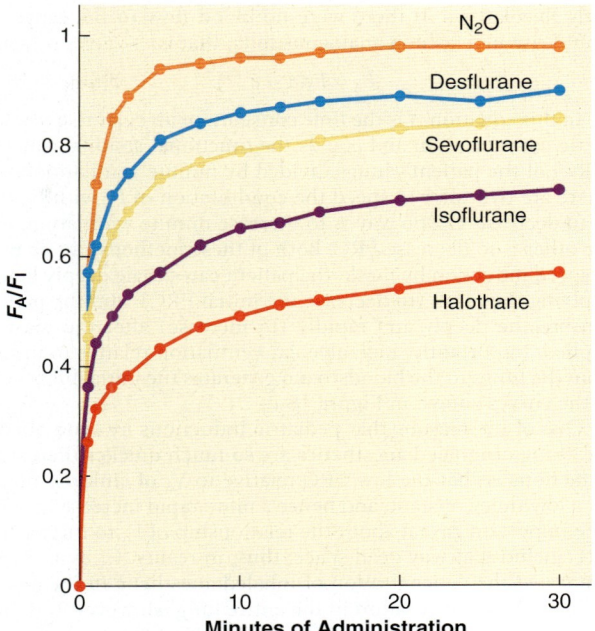

Figure 18-2 The rise in alveolar (F_A) anesthetic concentration toward the inspired (F_I) concentration is most rapid with the least soluble anesthetics, N_2O (nitrous oxide), desflurane, and sevoflurane. It rises most slowly with the more soluble anesthetics, such as halothane. All data are from human studies.[181,182]

referred to as *tissues of undesired effects*. The tissues of the muscle and fat groups comprise the *tissues of accumulation*.

Anesthetic is delivered most rapidly to the VRG because of high blood flow. Here it diffuses according to partial pressure gradients. CNS tissue takes in the anesthetic according to the tissue solubility, and at a high enough tissue concentration, unconsciousness and anesthesia are achieved. Increasing CNS tissue concentrations cause progressively deeper stages of anesthesia. As this is occurring, anesthetic is also distributing to other VRG tissues. Also coincident with delivery to the CNS, anesthetic is being delivered—albeit more slowly because of lower perfusion—to muscle and fat, where it accumulates and may affect the speed of emergence from the anesthetic. In reality, the fat solubilities provide little influence on emergence in cases lasting more than 4 hours since the delivery of anesthetic to fat tissue is extremely slow as a result of low blood flow. The concentration of inhaled anesthetic in a given tissue at a particular time during the administration depends not only on tissue blood flow, but also on tissue solubility, which governs how the inhaled anesthetics partition themselves between blood and tissue. Partitioning depends on the relative solubilities of the anesthetic for each compartment. These relative solubilities are expressed by a partition coefficient, δ, which is the ratio of dissolved gas (by volume) in two-tissue compartments at equilibrium. Some of the partition coefficients for the inhaled anesthetics are shown in Table 18-1.

Uptake and Distribution

F_A/F_I

A simple, common way to assess anesthetic uptake is to follow the ratio of fractional concentration of alveolar anesthetic to inspired anesthetic (F_A/F_I) over time. Experimentally derived data for F_A/F_I versus time during induction are shown in Figure 18-2. The faster F_A rises relative to F_I, the faster the speed of induction since F_A is proportional to P_A ($F_A = P_A/P_{barometric}$) and $P_A = P_{blood} = P_{CNS}$; that is, the alveolar fraction is directly proportional to the partial pressure of anesthetic in the CNS.

As fresh gas carrying anesthetic begins to flow into the air-filled circuit (assuming complete mixing), the concentration in the circuit (F_I) will rise according to first-order kinetics:

$$F_I = F_{FGO}(1 - e^{-T/\tau}) \quad (18\text{-}6)$$

F_{FGO} is the fraction of inspired anesthetic in the gas leaving the fresh gas outlet (i.e., the vaporizer setting), T is time, and τ is a time constant. The time constant is simply the volume or "capacity" of the circuit (V_C) divided by the FGF or $\tau = V_C/FGF$. For example, if the bag, tubing, absorbent canister, and piping comprise 8 L, and the FGF is 2 L, the time constant $\tau = 8/2 = 4$. One of the characteristics of first-order kinetics is that 95% of maximum is reached after three time constants—in this case, $3 \times 4 = 12$ minutes.

Since 12 minutes is relatively long, starting with a higher F_{FGO} can increase the rate of rise of F_I. Using the earlier example with $\tau = 4$, by first-order kinetics 63% of maximum is reached after one time constant, or 4 minutes. To attain an F_I of 2% at 4 instead of 12 minutes, the F_{FGO} can be set to 3.2% (2% divided by 0.63) and then lowered to 2% at the 4-minute mark.

Other ways to speed the increase in F_I include increasing the FGF, thus decreasing τ. Furthermore, the rebreathing bag can be collapsed prior to starting the FGF, such that the capacity in the circuit (V_C) is less, which also decreases τ. Finally, at high flows (>4 L/min) there is far less mixing because fresh gas pushes "old" gas out of the circuit via the pop-off valve before complete mixing occurs, causing F_I to increase at a greater rate; this is the most important factor in rapidly increasing F_I to the desired concentration.

One factor that delays the rate of rise of F_I is that CO_2 absorbent can adsorb and decompose the inhaled anesthetics. From a practical standpoint, this does not affect the rate of rise in F_I to a significant extent compared with other factors. Another factor that delays the rate of rise of F_I is solubility of the inhaled anesthetics in some of the plastic and rubber parts of the anesthesia circuit. This absorption has been quantified, but plays only a small role in decreasing the rate of rise of F_I.

Rise in F_A in the Absence of Uptake

The rate of rise in F_I discussed earlier assumes that no anesthetic is mixing with gas in the patient's lungs. In reality, circuit gas mixes with exhaled gases from the lung with each breath, thus lowering F_I within the circuit. If high FGFs (>4 L/min), which produce a high volume of gas at the desired concentration, are used, little mixing with exhaled air occurs and F_I is relatively fixed. In this situation, circuit gas enters the lungs where it mixes with alveolar gas. If there were no blood flow to the lungs, F_A would rise in a fashion analogous to F_I; that is:

$$F_A = F_I(1 - e^{-T/\tau}) \quad (18\text{-}7)$$

In this equation, τ is the time constant for alveolar rise in anesthetic concentration and equals the functional residual capacity (FRC) of the patient's lungs divided by minute ventilation ($\dot{V}_A$). There are two ways to speed the equilibration of F_A with F_I, that is, to decrease τ. One way is to increase minute ventilation, and the other is to decrease FRC. Both of these methods can be used to speed induction by mask; the patient can exhale deeply before applying the mask (to decrease the initial FRC), and the patient can breathe deeply and rapidly (to increase) after the mask is applied. Importantly, high alveolar ventilation relative to uptake from the lungs to the bloodstream generates the initial high slope to the curves shown in Figure 18-2.

One of the reasons that pediatric inductions by spontaneous breathing of inhaled anesthetics are so much quicker than adult inductions is that the low FRC relative to $\dot{V}_A$ of children makes for a low time constant, and hence a more rapid increase in F_A/F_I. One important caveat about the relationship of F_A to FRC is that FRC includes airway dead space; thus, in reality, F_A by Eq. 18-7 is not just the concentration of inhaled anesthetic in the alveoli but also the concentration in the entire lung. However, it is simply called the alveolar concentration because the dead space in the airways is relatively insignificant and only the alveolar gas is exchanging anesthetic with the blood.

Rise in F_A in the Presence of Uptake

Anesthetics *are* soluble in tissues, thus uptake of anesthetic from alveoli to blood is again characterized by first-order kinetics:

$$P_{bl}\text{ (blood)} = P_A\text{ (alveoli)} \times (1 - e^{-T/\tau}),$$

where

$$P_A = F_A \times P_B \text{ (barometric)} \quad (18\text{-}8)$$

Here, P_B is the barometric pressure and the time constant, τ, equals "capacity" (volume of anesthetic dissolved in blood at the desired alveolar partial pressure) divided by flow (volume of anesthetic delivered per unit time). For any given flow of anesthetic into the system, this capacity for the more soluble halothane is greater than the capacity for the less soluble desflurane; thus, τ for halothane is greater than that for desflurane. The more soluble the inhaled anesthetic, the larger the capacity of the blood and tissues for that anesthetic, and the longer it takes to saturate at any given delivery rate.

The most important factor in the rate of rise of F_A/F_I is uptake of anesthetic from the alveoli into the bloodstream. The rate of rise of F_A/F_I (especially the position of the "knees" in the curves of Fig. 18-2) reflects the speed at which alveolar anesthetic (F_A) equilibrates with that being delivered to the lungs (F_I). Since there is uptake from alveoli to blood, F_A is not solely a function of F_I and time. The greater the uptake, the slower the rate of rise of F_A/F_I, and vice versa. Since uptake is proportional to tissue solubility, the less soluble the anesthetic (such as desflurane), the lesser its uptake and the faster it reaches equilibrium, $P_A = P_{blood} = P_{CNS}$.

Consider a hypothetical example. Suppose that halothane and desflurane are soluble in blood, but insoluble in all other tissues. Suppose further that total lung capacity and blood volume were both 5 L. If a fixed volume of anesthetic is delivered to the lungs (by asking the patient to take one deep breath and hold it), according to the blood:gas partition coefficients for halothane (2.5) and desflurane (0.42), 71.4% of the delivered halothane will be transferred to the blood while 28.6% remains in the alveoli (71.4/28.6 = 2.5). In contrast, 29.6% of the desflurane will be transferred to the blood while 70.4% remains in the alveoli (29.6/70.4 = 0.42). Therefore, 2.4 times (71.4/29.6) more halothane than desflurane (by volume or number of molecules) will be transferred from alveoli to bloodstream before partial pressures equilibrate. At equilibrium, the alveolar partial pressures of halothane and desflurane are 28.6% and 70.4% of their inhaled values, respectively. This means that F_A rises faster with desflurane than halothane, as does F_A/F_I.

Blood uptake of anesthetic is expressed by the equation:

$$\dot{V}_B = \delta_{b/g} * Q \times ((P_A - P_V))/P_B \quad (18\text{-}9)$$

where $\dot{V}_B$ is blood uptake, $\delta_{b/g}$ is the blood:gas partition coefficient, Q is cardiac output, P_A is alveolar partial pressure of anesthetic, P_V is mixed venous partial pressure of anesthetic, and P_B is barometric pressure. This is the Fick equation applied to blood uptake of inhaled anesthetics. *The greater the value of $\dot{V}_B$, the greater the uptake from alveoli to blood, and the slower the rise in F_A/F_I.*

From the preceding paragraphs, the parameters that increase or decrease the rate of rise in F_A/F_I during induction can now be clearly delineated and these important factors have been substantiated in experimental models.

Distribution (Tissue Uptake)

The maximum F_A/F_I at a given inspired concentration of anesthetic, cardiac output, and minute ventilation depends entirely on the solubility of that drug in the blood as characterized by the blood:gas partition coefficient $\delta_{b/g}$. This can be seen in the time curves for the rise in F_A/F_I during induction for the various inhalation anesthetics shown in Figure 18-2. The first "knee" in each curve in Figure 18-2 represents the point at which the rapid rise in P_V begins to taper off; that is, when significant inhaled anesthetic concentrations begin to build up in the bloodstream because of distribution to and equilibration with the various tissue compartments.

As blood is equilibrating with alveolar gas, it also begins to equilibrate with the VRG, muscle, and, more gradually, the fat compartments based on perfusion. Muscle is not that different from the VRG, having partition coefficients that range from 1.2 (N_2O) to 3.4 (halothane), just under a threefold difference; and for each anesthetic except N_2O, the muscle partition coefficient is approximately double that for the VRG. Although both VRG and muscle are lean tissues, the muscle compartment equilibrates far more slowly than the VRG. The explanation comes in part due to the mass of the compartments relative to perfusion. The perfusion of the VRG is about 75 mL/min/100 g of tissue, whereas it is only 3 mL/min/100 g of tissue in the muscle (Table 18-2). This 25-fold difference in perfusion between VRG (especially brain) and muscle means that even if the partition coefficients were equal, the muscle would still take 25 times longer to equilibrate with blood.

Fat is perfused to a lesser extent than muscle and its time for equilibration with blood is considerably slower because the partition coefficients are so much greater. All of the potent agents are highly lipid-soluble. Partition coefficients range from 27 (desflurane) to 51 (halothane). On average, the solubility for these agents is about 25 times greater in fat than in the VRG group. Thus, fat equilibrates far more slowly with the blood and does not play a significant role in determining speed of induction. After long anesthetic exposures (>4 hours), the high saturation of fat tissue may play a role in delaying emergence.

Nitrous oxide represents an exception. Its partition coefficients are fairly similar in each tissue: It does not accumulate to any great extent and is not a very potent anesthetic. Its utility lies as an adjunct to the potent agents, and as a vehicle to speed induction.

Metabolism

Data suggest that enzymes responsible for biotransformation of inhaled anesthetics become saturated at less than anesthetizing doses of these drugs, such that metabolism plays little role in opposing induction. It may, however, have some significance to recovery from anesthesia, as discussed later.

Overpressurization and the Concentration Effect

There are several ways to speed uptake and induction of anesthesia with the inhaled anesthetics. The first is *overpressurization*, which is analogous to an intravenous bolus. This is the administration of a higher partial pressure of anesthetic than the alveolar concentration (F_A) actually desired for the patient. Inspired anesthetic concentration (F_I) can influence both F_A and the *rate of rise* of F_A/F_I. The greater the inspired concentration of an inhaled anesthetic, the greater the rate of rise. This concentration effect has two components: the concentrating effect and an augmented gas inflow effect.

For example, consider the administration of 10% anesthetic (10 parts anesthetic and 90 parts other gas) to a patient in whom 50% of the anesthetic in the alveoli is absorbed by the blood. In this case, five parts (0.5 × 10) anesthetic remain in the alveoli, five parts enter the blood, and 90 parts remain as other alveolar gas. The alveolar concentration is now 5/(90 + 5) = 5.3%. Consider next administering 50% anesthetic with the same 50% uptake. Now 25 parts anesthetic remain in alveoli, 25 parts pass into blood, and 50 parts remain as other alveolar gas. The alveolar concentration becomes 25/(50 + 25) = 33%. Giving five times as much anesthetic will lead to a 33%/5.3% = 6.2 times greater alveolar concentration. The higher the F_I, the greater the effect. Thus N_2O, typically given in concentrations of 50% to 70%, has the greatest concentrating effect. This is why the F_A/F_I versus time curve in Figure 18-2 rises the most quickly with N_2O, even though desflurane has a slightly lower blood:gas solubility.

This is not the complete picture; there is yet another factor to consider. As gas is leaving the alveoli for the blood, new gas at the original F_I is entering the lungs to replace that which is taken up by the blood. This other aspect of the concentration effect has been called *augmented gas inflow*. Again, take the example of 10% anesthetic delivered with 50% uptake into the bloodstream. The five parts anesthetic absorbed by the bloodstream are replaced by gas in the circuit that is still 10% anesthetic. The five parts anesthetic and 90 parts other gas left in the lungs mix with five parts replacement gas, or 5 × 0.10 = 0.5 parts anesthetic. Now the alveolar concentration is (5 + 0.5)/(100) = 5.5% (as compared to 5.3% without augmented inflow). For 50% anesthetic and 50% uptake, 25 parts of anesthetic removed from the alveoli are replaced with 25 parts of 50% anesthetic, giving a new alveolar concentration of (25 + 12.5)/(100) = 37.5% (as compared to 33% without augmented inflow). Thus, 5 times the F_I leads to 37.5/5.5 = 6.8 times greater F_A (compared to 6.2 times without augmented gas inflow). Of course, this cycle of absorbed gas being replaced by fresh gas inflow is continuous and has a finite rate, so our example is a simplification.

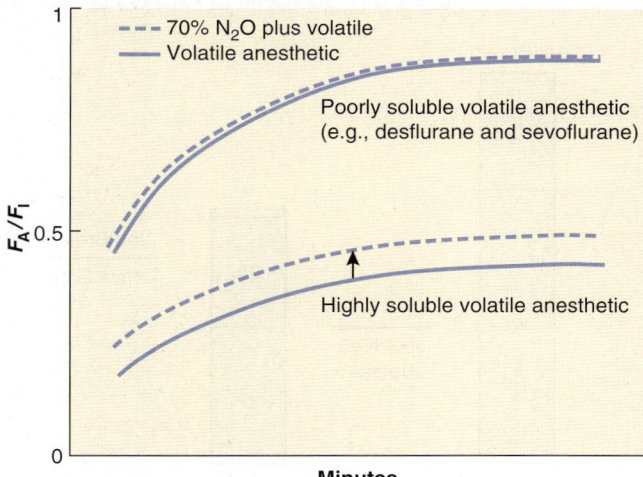

Figure 18-3 The second gas effect is demonstrated in the graphs. The F_A/F_I ratio for a more soluble gas such as halothane rises more rapidly when given with 70% N_2O than when given with 10% N_2O. This effect is less with less soluble gases. (Adapted from Epstein RM, Rackow H, Salanitre E, et al. Influence of the concentration effect on the uptake of anesthetic mixtures: the second gas effect. *Anesthesiology.* 1964;25:364.)

Second Gas Effect

A special case of concentration effect applies to administration of a potent anesthetic with N_2O, that is, two gases simultaneously. Along with the concentration of potent agent in the alveoli via its uptake, there is further concentration via the uptake of N_2O, a process called the *second gas effect*. The principle is simple (Figs. 18-3 and 18-4). Consider, for example, administering 2% of a potent anesthetic in 70% N_2O and 28% oxygen. In this case, N_2O, with its extremely high partial pressure (despite low solubility), partitions into the blood more rapidly than the potent anesthetic, decreasing the alveolar N_2O concentration by some amount (e.g., by 50%). Ignoring uptake of the potent anesthetic, the uptake of N_2O is 35 parts, leaving 35 parts N_2O, 28 parts O_2, and two parts potent agent in the alveoli. The anesthetic gas is now present in the alveoli at a concentration of 2/(2 + 35 + 28) = 3.1%. The potent agent has been concentrated and F_A is increased.

Ventilation Effects

As indicated by Figure 18-2, inhaled anesthetics with very low tissue solubility have an extremely rapid rise in F_A/F_I with induction. This suggests that there is very little room to improve this rate by increasing or decreasing ventilation, which is demonstrated in Figure 18-5. The greater the solubility of an inhaled anesthetic, the more rapidly it is absorbed by the bloodstream, such that anesthetic delivery to the lungs may be rate limiting to the rise in F_A/F_I. Therefore, for more soluble anesthetics, augmentation of anesthetic delivery by increasing minute ventilation also increases the rate of rise in F_A/F_I.

However, spontaneous minute ventilation is not static, and to the extent that the inhaled anesthetics depress spontaneous ventilation with increasing inspired concentration, $\dot{V}_A$ will decrease and

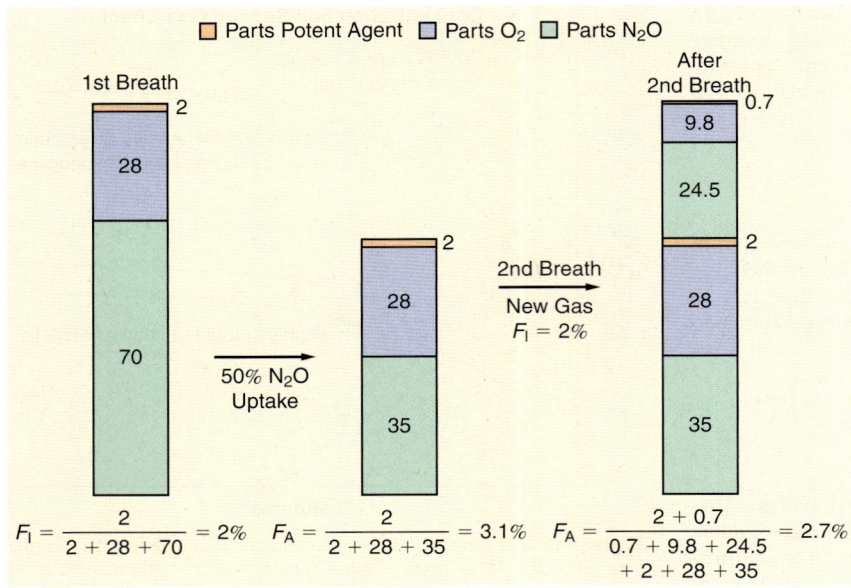

Figure 18-4 A graphic and relative equation to demonstrate the second gas effect. In this hypothetical example, the second gas is set at 2% of a potent anesthetic and the model is set for 50% uptake of the first gas (N_2O [nitrous oxide]) in the first inspired breath. The second gas is concentrated because of the uptake of N_2O **(middle panel)**. On replenishing the inspired second gas ($F_I = 2\%$) in the next breath, the second gas has been concentrated to be 2.7% because of the uptake of N_2O in the previous breath.

so will the rate of rise of F_A/F_I. This is demonstrated in Figure 18-5. This negative feedback should not be considered a drawback of the inhaled anesthetics because the respiratory depression produced at high anesthetic concentrations essentially slows the rise in F_A/F_I. This might arguably add a margin of safety in preventing an overdose. Controlled ventilation does not offer this margin of safety.

Perfusion Effects

As with ventilation, cardiac output is not static during the course of induction. For the less soluble agents, changes in cardiac output do not affect the rate of rise of F_A/F_I to a great extent, but for the more soluble agents the effect is noticeable (Figure 18-5). However, as inspired concentration increases, greater cardiovascular depression reduces anesthetic uptake and actually increases the rate of rise of F_A/F_I. This positive feedback can rapidly lead to profound cardiovascular depression.

Ventilation–Perfusion Mismatching

Ventilation and perfusion are normally fairly well matched in healthy patients, such that P_A (alveolar partial pressure)/P_I and P_a (arterial partial pressure)/P_I are the same curve. However, if significant intrapulmonary shunt occurs, as in the case of inadvertent bronchial intubation, the rate of rise of alveolar and arterial anesthetic partial pressures can be affected (Fig. 18-6). Ventilation of the intubated lung is dramatically increased while perfusion increases slightly. The nonintubated lung receives no ventilation, while perfusion decreases slightly. For the less-soluble anesthetics, increased ventilation of the intubated lung cannot appreciably increase alveolar partial pressure relative to inspired concentration on that side, but alveolar partial pressure on the nonintubated side is essentially zero. Pulmonary mixed venous blood, therefore, comprises nearly equal parts of blood containing normal amounts of anesthetic and blood containing no anesthetic; that is, diluted relative to normal. Thus the rate of rise in P_a (arterial) relative to P_I is significantly reduced. There is less total anesthetic uptake, so the rate of rise of P_A (alveolar) relative to P_I increases even though induction of anesthesia is slowed because CNS partial pressure equilibrates with P_a. For the more soluble anesthetics, increased ventilation of the intubated lung *does* increase the alveolar partial pressure relative to inspired concentration on that side. Pulmonary venous blood from the intubated side contains a higher concentration of anesthetic that lessens the dilution by blood from the nonintubated side. Thus, the rate of rise of P_a/P_I is not as reduced and induction of anesthesia is less delayed relative to normal.

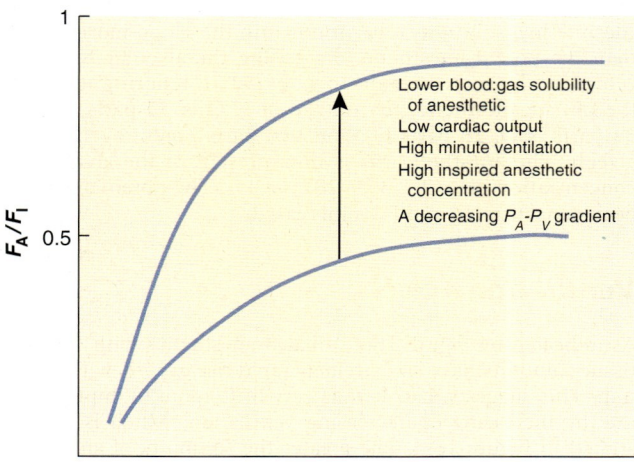

Figure 18-5 The F_A/F_I ratio rises more rapidly if ventilation and the anesthetic concentration are increased. A decreasing P_A-P_V gradient that occurs shortly after anesthetic induction, slows anesthetic uptake and increases the rate of rise of F_A/F_I. A low CO and low blood:gas solubility slow anesthetic uptake (Equation 18-9) and increases the rate of rise of F_A/F_I. The influence of CO and ventilation on F_A/F_I are magnified for the more soluble anesthetics.

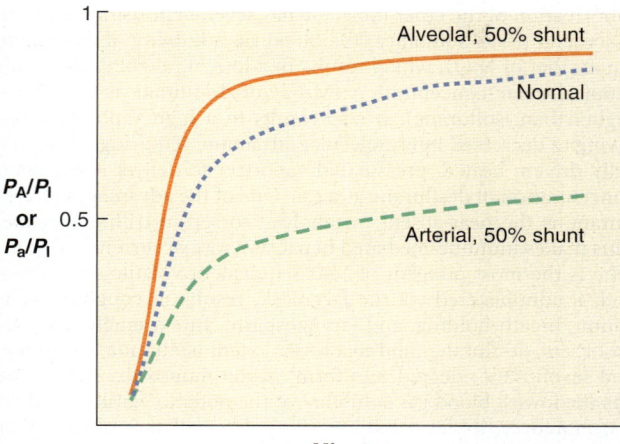

Figure 18-6 When no ventilation/perfusion abnormalities exist, the alveolar (P_A) and arterial (P_a) anesthetic partial pressures rise together (dotted blue lines) toward the inspired partial pressure (P_I). When 50% of the cardiac output is shunted through the lungs, such as with a mainstem intubation, the rate of rise of the alveolar partial pressure, P_A (orange lines) is accelerated while the rate of rise of the arterial partial pressure, P_a (dotted green lines) is slowed, resulting in a slower induction of anesthesia. The greatest effect of shunting is found with the least soluble anesthetics, e.g., sevoflurane and desflurane.

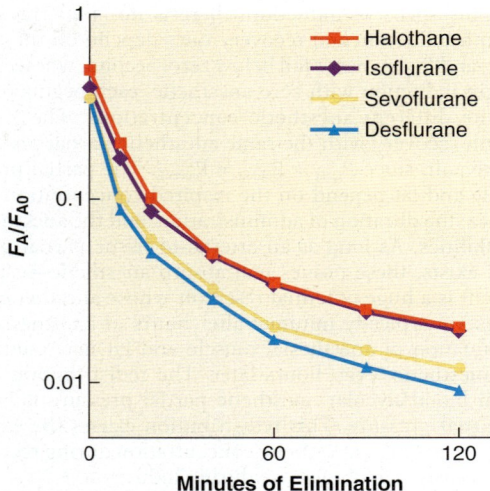

Figure 18-7 Elimination of anesthetic gases is defined as the ratio of end-tidal anesthetic concentration (F_A) to the last F_A during administration and immediately before the beginning of elimination (F_{A0}). During the 120-minute period after ending the anesthetic delivery, the elimination of sevoflurane and desflurane is 2 to 2.5 times faster than isoflurane or halothane (note logarithmic scale for the ordinate).[181,182]

Elimination

Percutaneous and Visceral Loss

Although the loss of inhaled anesthetics via the skin is very small, it does occur and the loss is the greatest for N_2O. These anesthetics also pass across gastrointestinal viscera and the pleura. During open abdominal or thoracic surgery there is some anesthetic loss via these routes. Relative to losses by all other routes, losses via percutaneous and visceral routes are insignificant.

Diffusion Between Tissues

Using more elaborate mathematical modeling of inhaled anesthetic pharmacokinetics than presented here, several laboratories have derived a five-compartment model that best describes tissue compartments. These compartments are the alveoli, the VRG, the muscle, the fat, and one additional compartment. Current opinion is that this fifth compartment represents adipose tissue adjacent to lean tissue that receives anesthetic via intertissue diffusion. This transfer of anesthetic is not insignificant, and may account for up to one-third of uptake during long administration.

Exhalation and Recovery

Recovery from anesthesia, like induction, depends on anesthetic solubility, cardiac output, and minute ventilation. Solubility is the primary determinant of the rate of fall of F_A (Fig. 18-7). The greater the solubility of inhaled anesthetic, the larger the capacity for absorption in the bloodstream and tissues. The "reservoir" of anesthetic in the body at the end of administration depends on tissue solubility (which determines the capacity) and the dose and duration of anesthetic (which determine how much of that capacity is filled). Recovery from anesthesia, or "washout," is usually expressed as the ratio of expired fractional concentration of anesthetic (F_A) to the expired concentration at time zero (F_{A0}) when the anesthetic was discontinued (or F_A/F_{A0}). One of the arguments for using sevoflurane and desflurane has been their relative speed in terms of emergence from anesthesia. This argument has been tempered somewhat by the basic knowledge that downward titration of volatile anesthetics can speed emergence times. Even the more soluble drug, isoflurane, can be titrated downward guided by clinical experience and/or a processed EEG monitor, permitting fast wake-ups. However, in general the use of the less-soluble drugs in the longest surgical cases makes awakening a simpler and expedient process (Fig. 18-8).[3]

There are two major pharmacokinetic differences between recovery and induction. First, whereas overpressurization can

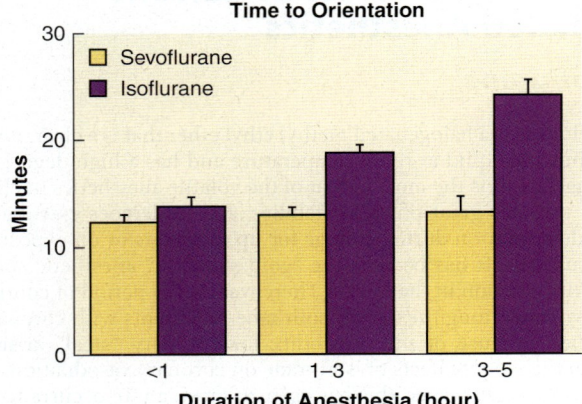

Figure 18-8 The recovery times to orientation after anesthesia of varying durations. With the less soluble anesthetic sevoflurane, the time to orientation was independent of the anesthetic duration. In contrast, long anesthetic durations with isoflurane were associated with delayed times to orientation. (Adapted from Ebert TJ, Robinson BJ, Uhrich TD, et al. Recovery from sevoflurane anesthesia: a comparison to isoflurane and propofol anesthesia. *Anesthesiology*. 1998;89:1524.)

increase the speed of induction, there is no "underpressurization." Both induction and recovery rates depend on the P_A to P_v gradient, and P_A can never fall below zero. Second, whereas all tissues begin induction with zero anesthetic, each begins recovery with quite different anesthetic concentrations. The VRG tissues begin recovery with the same anesthetic partial pressure as that in alveoli, since $P_{CNS} = P_{blood} = P_{alveoli}$. The partial pressures in muscle and fat depend on the inspired concentration during anesthesia, the duration of administration, and the anesthetic tissue solubilities. As long as an arterial-to-tissue partial pressure gradient exists, these tissues will absorb anesthetic—especially fat, since it is a huge potential reservoir whose anesthetic partial pressures are typically minimal after hours of anesthesia. After discontinuation of anesthesia, muscle and fat may continue to absorb anesthetic, even hours later. The redistribution continues until blood/alveolar anesthetic partial pressure falls below tissue partial pressure. This redistribution causes the early rate of decline in alveolar anesthetic concentration during recovery to exceed its early rate of increase during induction.

Because VRG tissues are highly perfused and washout of anesthetic is mostly via elimination from these tissues early in recovery, all anesthetics, regardless of duration of administration, have approximately the same rate of elimination to 50% of F_{A0}. Unfortunately, halving the CNS concentration of anesthetic is rarely sufficient for waking the patient. More commonly, 80% to 90% of inhaled anesthetic must be eliminated before emergence. At these amounts of washout, the more soluble anesthetics are eliminated more slowly than less soluble agents.

Diffusion Hypoxia

During recovery from anesthesia, washout of high concentrations of N_2O can lower alveolar concentrations of oxygen and carbon dioxide, a phenomenon called *diffusion hypoxia*. The resulting alveolar hypoxia can cause hypoxemia, and alveolar hypocarbia can depress respiratory drive, which may exacerbate hypoxemia. It is therefore appropriate to initiate recovery from N_2O anesthesia with 100% oxygen rather than less concentrated O_2/air mixtures.

Clinical Overview of Current Inhaled Anesthetics

Isoflurane

Isoflurane is a halogenated methyl ethyl ether that is a clear, nonflammable liquid at room temperature and has a high degree of pungency. It is the most potent of the volatile anesthetics in clinical use, has great physical stability, and undergoes essentially no deterioration during storage for up to 5 years or on exposure to sunlight. It has become the "gold standard" anesthetic since its introduction in the 1970s. There was a brief period of controversy concerning the use of isoflurane in patients with coronary disease because of the possibility for coronary "steal" arising from the potent effects of isoflurane on coronary vasodilation. In clinical use, however, this has been, at most, a rare occurrence.

Desflurane

Desflurane is a fluorinated methyl ethyl ether that differs from isoflurane by just one atom: A fluorine atom is substituted for a chlorine atom on the α-ethyl component of isoflurane (Fig. 18-1). Fluorination of the ether molecule has several effects. It decreases blood and tissue solubility (the blood:gas solubility of desflurane equals that of N_2O), which results in a loss of potency (the minimum alveolar concentration [MAC] of desflurane is five times higher than isoflurane). It also results in a high vapor pressure owing to decreased intermolecular attraction, requiring an electrically driven, heated, pressurized vaporizer to deliver a regulated concentration of desflurane as a gas. One of the advantages of desflurane is the near-absent metabolism to serum trifluoroacetate. This makes immune-mediated hepatitis a rare occurrence. Desflurane is the most pungent of MAC-equivalent volatile anesthetics and, if administered via the facemask, results in coughing, salivation, breath holding, and laryngospasm. In extremely dry CO_2 absorbers, desflurane (and to a lesser extent isoflurane, enflurane, and sevoflurane) degrades to form carbon monoxide. Desflurane has the lowest blood:gas solubility of the potent volatile anesthetics; moreover, its fat solubility is roughly half that of the other volatile anesthetics. Thus, desflurane requires less downward titration in long surgical procedures to achieve a rapid emergence by virtue of decreased tissue saturation. This may be particularly advantageous in the morbidly obese patient.[4] Desflurane has been associated with tachycardia and hypertension when used with minimal opioids and, in select cases, myocardial ischemia when used in high concentrations or when rapidly increasing the inspired concentration.

Sevoflurane

Sevoflurane is a sweet smelling, completely fluorinated methyl isopropyl ether (Fig. 18-1). Its vapor pressure is roughly one-fourth that of desflurane and it can be used in a conventional vaporizer. The blood:gas solubility of sevoflurane is second only to desflurane in terms of potent volatile anesthetics. Sevoflurane is approximately half as potent as isoflurane, and some of the preservation of potency, despite fluorination, is because of the bulky propyl side chain on the ether molecule. Its pleasant odor, lack of pungency, and potent bronchodilating characteristics make sevoflurane administration via the facemask for induction of anesthesia in both children and adults a reasonable alternative to IV anesthetics. Sevoflurane is half as potent a coronary vasodilator as isoflurane, but is 10 to 20 times more vulnerable to metabolism than isoflurane. The metabolism of sevoflurane results in inorganic fluoride but has not been associated with renal-concentrating defects. Unlike other potent volatile anesthetics, sevoflurane is not metabolized to trifluoroacetate; rather, it is metabolized to an acyl halide (hexafluoroisopropanol). This does not stimulate formation of antibodies associated with hepatitis.

Sevoflurane exposed to purposely dried absorbent can form carbon monoxide and can cause high heat and fire via an exothermic reaction. New generic versions of sevoflurane have the potential to break down to hydrogen fluoride when exposed to metal compounds because of their lack of adequate water in the formulation. Sevoflurane also breaks down in the presence of the carbon dioxide absorber to form a vinyl halide called *compound A*. Compound A has been shown to be a dose-dependent nephrotoxin in rats, but has not been associated with renal injury in human volunteers or patients, with or without renal impairment, even when FGFs are 1 L/min or less.

Xenon

Xenon is an inert gas occurring naturally in air at 0.05 parts per million (ppm). Xenon has received considerable interest in the last few years because it has many characteristics approaching those of an "ideal" inhaled anesthetic.[5] It has a quick onset and offset, minimal effects on the cardiovascular and neural systems, and it is not a trigger for malignant hyperthermia (MH). It is not a pollutant or an occupational hazard, and does not add to global warming or the greenhouse gas effect. Its blood:gas partition coefficient is 0.115, and unlike the other potent volatile anesthetics (except methoxyflurane), xenon provides some degree of analgesia. This action is likely due to N-Methyl-d-aspartate (NMDA) receptor inhibition. The MAC of xenon in humans is 71%, which might prove to be a limitation. It is nonexplosive, nonpungent, and odorless, and thus can be inhaled with ease. In addition, it does not produce significant myocardial depression or alter coronary blood flow.[6] Because of its scarcity and high cost related to extraction by fractional distillation of the atmosphere, its role as a replacement for current lower cost anesthetics remains uncertain. It may have potential for neuroprotection in select settings via its inhibitory action of the NMDA receptor glycine site.

Nitrous Oxide

Nitrous oxide is a sweet-smelling, nonflammable gas of low potency (MAC = 104%), and is relatively insoluble in blood. It is most commonly administered as an anesthetic adjuvant in combination with opioids or volatile anesthetics during the conduct of general anesthesia. At room temperature it is a gas; its boiling point is −88.48°C (Table 18-1). It is stored in cylinders and condensed to 50 atmospheres, leading to a pressure of 745 psi. Only cylinder weight is a reliable indicator of the volume of N_2O in storage tanks since psi is maintained until no liquid remains. Although not flammable, N_2O will support combustion. Unlike the potent volatile anesthetics in clinical use, N_2O does not produce significant skeletal muscle relaxation, but it does have modest analgesic effects. Despite a long track record of use, controversy has surrounded N_2O in four areas:[7] its role in postoperative nausea and vomiting; its potential toxic effects on cell function via inactivation of vitamin B_{12}; its adverse effects related to absorption and expansion into air-filled structures and bubbles; and lastly, its effect on embryonic development. The most valid and most clinically relevant concern is the ability of N_2O to expand air-filled spaces because of its greater solubility in blood compared to nitrogen. This might explain the increased postoperative nausea and vomiting (PONV) associated with N_2O use since closed gas spaces reside in the middle ear and bowel. Other closed spaces may occur as a result of disease or surgery, such as a pneumothorax. Since nitrogen in air-filled spaces cannot be removed readily via the bloodstream, N_2O delivered to a patient diffuses from the blood into these closed gas spaces quite easily until the partial pressure equals that of the blood and alveoli. Compliant spaces will continue to expand until sufficient pressure is generated to oppose further N_2O flow into the space. The higher the inspired concentration of N_2O, the higher the partial pressure required for equilibration.

Seventy-five percent N_2O can expand a pneumothorax to double or triple its size in 10 and 30 minutes, respectively. Air-filled cuffs of pulmonary artery catheters and endotracheal tubes also expand with the use of N_2O, possibly causing tissue damage via increased pressure in the pulmonary artery or trachea, respectively. Accumulation of N_2O in the middle ear can diminish hearing postoperatively[8] and is contraindicated for tympanoplasty because the increased pressure can dislodge a tympanic graft.

Neuropharmacology of Inhaled Anesthetics

Minimum Alveolar Concentration

Pharmacodynamic effects of anesthetics are based on their dosing. In the case of inhaled agents, we describe dose as the *minimum alveolar concentration* or MAC. MAC is the alveolar concentration of an anesthetic at one atmosphere (in volume%) that prevents movement in response to a surgical stimulus in 50% of patients. It is analogous to the ED_{50} expressed for intravenous drugs and can be used to compare anesthetic potency, that is, the lower the MAC the more potent the agent. Movement to a surgical stimulus, commonly abdominal incision, has been used to establish the MAC for each inhaled anesthetic. MAC values for humans for the inhaled anesthetics are shown in Table 18-1.

The 95% confidence ranges for MAC are approximately ±25% of the listed MAC values. Manufacturer's recommendations and clinical experience establish 1.2 to 1.3 times MAC as a dose that will often prevent patient movement during a surgical stimulus. Loss of consciousness typically precedes the absence of stimulus-induced movement by a wide margin.

Concentrations of inhaled anesthetics that provide loss of self-awareness and recall are about 0.4 to 0.5 MAC barring other conditions that increase MAC in a given patient (Table 18-3). Several lines of reasoning support the assertion. First, most patients receiving only 50% N_2O (approximately 0.4 to 0.5 MAC), as in a typical dentist's office, will have no recall of their procedure during N_2O administration. Second, various studies have shown that a shift in electroencephalogram (EEG) dominance to the anterior leads, that is, the shift from self-aware to non–self-aware, accompanies loss of consciousness, and in primates, the EEG shift and loss of consciousness occur at 0.5 MAC.[9] Third, in dogs, loss of consciousness accompanies a sudden nonlinear fall in cerebral metabolic rate ($CMRO_2$) at approximately 0.5 MAC (Fig. 18-9).

MAC values can be established for any measurable response. For example, MAC-awake and MAC-BAR. MAC-awake is the alveolar concentration of anesthetic at which a patient opens his or her eyes to command, and it varies from 0.15 to 0.5 MAC. Interestingly, transition from awake to unconscious and back typically shows some hysteresis in that it quite consistently takes 0.4 to 0.5 MAC to lose consciousness, but less than that (as low as 0.15 MAC) to regain it. This may be because of the speed of alveolar wash-in versus wash-out.[10] MAC-BAR is the alveolar concentration of anesthetic that blunts adrenergic responses to noxious stimuli. It has been approximated at 50% higher than standard MAC.[11] MAC values also have been established for discreet levels of EEG activity, such as onset of burst suppression or isoelectricity.

Standard MAC values are roughly additive. Administering 0.5 MAC of a potent agent and 0.5 MAC of N_2O is equivalent to 1 MAC of potent agent in terms of preventing *patient movement*,

Table 18-3 Factors that Increase Minimum Alveolar Concentration
Increased central neurotransmitter levels (monoamine oxidase inhibitors, acute dextroamphetamine administration, cocaine, ephedrine, levodopa)
Hyperthermia
Chronic ethanol abuse (determined in humans)
Hypernatremia

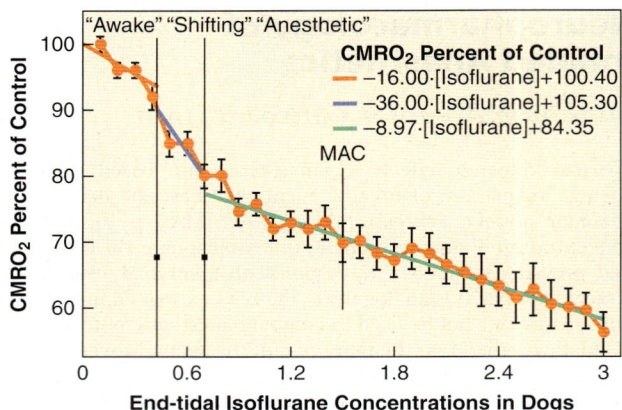

Figure 18-9 The effects of isoflurane on cerebral metabolic rate of oxygen consumption ($CMRO_2$) as a percentage of control ("awake"). $CMRO_2$ is plotted versus end-tidal isoflurane concentration. Regression lines for changes in $CMRO_2$ are drawn for each electroencephalogram-determined area. The pattern depicted here is characteristic of all of the anesthetics examined (enflurane, halothane, and isoflurane). MAC, minimum alveolar concentration. (Adapted from Stullken EH Jr, Milde JH, Michenfelder JD, et al. The nonlinear responses of cerebral metabolism to low concentrations of halothane, enflurane, isoflurane and thiopental. *Anesthesiology.* 1977;46:28.)

Table 18-4 Factors that Decrease Minimum Alveolar Concentration

Increasing age
Metabolic acidosis
Hypoxia (PaO_2, 38 mmHg)
Induced hypotension (mean arterial pressure <50 mmHg)
Decreased central neurotransmitter levels (α-methyldopa, reserpine, chronic dextroamphetamine administration, levodopa)
$α_2$-agonists
Hypothermia
Hyponatremia
Lithium
Hypo-osmolality
Pregnancy
Acute ethanol administration[a]
Ketamine
Pancuronium[a]
Physostigmine (10 times clinical doses)
Neostigmine (10 times clinical doses)
Lidocaine
Opioids
Opioid agonist-antagonist analgesics
Barbiturates[a]
Chlorpromazine[a]
Diazepam[a]
Hydroxyzine[a]
Δ-9-Tetrahydrocannabinol
Verapamil
Anemia (<4.3 mL O_2/dL blood)

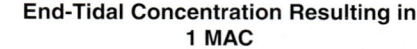
[a]Determined in humans.

although this does not hold over the entire range of N_2O doses. MAC effects for other response parameters such as cardiovascular or respiratory measures, are not necessarily additive. For example, combining 0.6 MAC of N_2O with 0.6 MAC of isoflurane produces less hypotension than 1.2 MAC of isoflurane alone because isoflurane is a more potent vasodilator and myocardial depressant at equivalent MAC than N_2O.

Various factors increase (Table 18-3) or decrease (Table 18-4) MAC. Unfortunately, no single mechanism explains these alterations, supporting the view that anesthesia is the net result of numerous and widely varying physiologic alterations. In general, those factors that increase CNS metabolic activity, neurotransmission, and CNS neurotransmitter levels increase MAC; upregulated CNS responses to chronically depressed neurotransmitter levels (as in chronic alcoholism) also seem to increase MAC. Conversely, those factors that decrease CNS metabolic activity, neurotransmission, and CNS neurotransmitter levels, as well as downregulated CNS responses to chronically elevated neurotransmitter levels all seem to decrease MAC. Many notable factors do not alter MAC, including duration of administration, gender, type of surgical stimulation, thyroid function, hypo- or hypercarbia, metabolic alkalosis, hyperkalemia, and magnesium levels. However, there may be a genetic component influencing MAC. Red-haired females may have altered pain thresholds, perhaps explaining the 19% increase in MAC compared with dark-haired females.[12] Studies suggest involvement of mutations of the melanocyte stimulating hormone receptor (*MC1R*) allele. MAC also can vary in relationship to genotype and chromosomal substitutions as shown in rats.[13]

The Effect of Age on MAC

The MAC for each of the potent anesthetic gases shows a clear, age-related change (Fig. 18-10). MAC decreases with age and there are similarities between agents in the decline in MAC and age. There is a linear model that describes a change in MAC of approximately 6% per decade, a 22% decrease in MAC

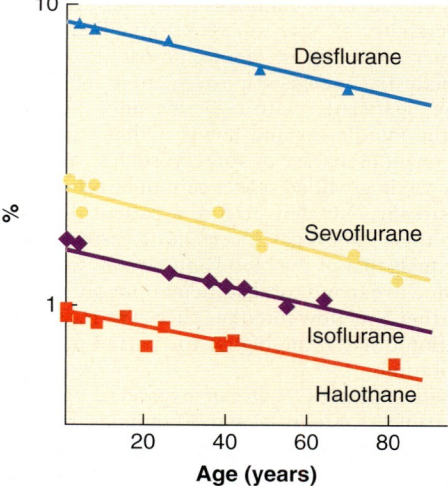

Figure 18-10 Effect of age on minimum alveolar concentration (MAC) is plotted. Regression lines are fitted to published values from separate studies. Data are from patients' ages 1 to 80 years. (Adapted from Mapleson WW. Effect of age on MAC in humans: a meta-analysis. *Br J Anaesth.* 1996;76:179.)

from age 40 to 80 years, and a 27% decrease in MAC from age 1 to 40 years.[14]

Other Alterations in Neurophysiology

The modern potent anesthetics, isoflurane, desflurane, and sevoflurane, all have reasonably similar effects on a wide range of parameters including $CMRO_2$, the EEG, cerebral blood flow (CBF), and flow–metabolism coupling. There are notable differences in effects on intracerebral pressure (ICP), CO_2 vasoreactivity, CBF autoregulation, and cerebral protection. Nitrous oxide departs from the potent agents in several important respects, and is therefore discussed separately.

Although neuroprotection from volatile anesthetics is a well-defined concept, the volatile anesthetics can cause injury in certain conditions via cerebral vasodilation and increases in intracranial pressure. A full understanding of the anesthetic effects on cerebral physiology helps prevent adverse cerebral events in clinical practice.

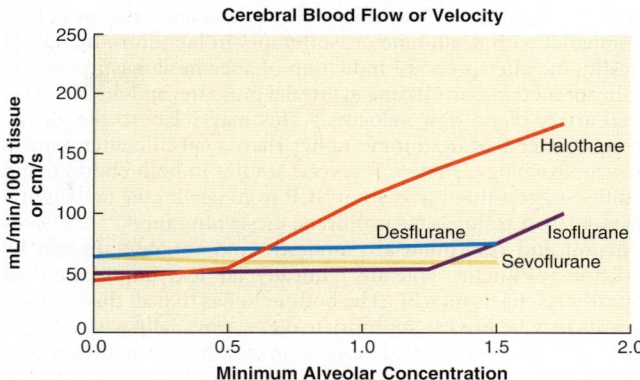

Figure 18-11 Cerebral blood flow (and velocity) measured in the presence of normocapnia and in the absence of surgical stimulation in volunteers receiving halothane or isoflurane.[188,189] At light levels of anesthesia, halothane (but not isoflurane) increased cerebral blood flow. At 1.6 minimum alveolar concentration (MAC), isoflurane also increased cerebral blood flow. Cerebral blood flow velocity measured before and during sevoflurane and desflurane anesthesia up to 1.5 MAC showed no change in cerebral blood flow and velocity.

Cerebral Metabolic Rate and Electroencephalogram

For most of the potent agents, $CMRO_2$ is decreased only to the extent that spontaneous cortical neuronal activity (as reflected on the EEG) is decreased. Once this activity is absent (an isoelectric EEG), no further decreases in $CMRO_2$ are generated. (Historically, halothane was the exception.) Isoflurane causes a larger MAC-dependent depression of $CMRO_2$ than halothane, and because of this, can abolish EEG activity at clinical doses that are usually well tolerated from a hemodynamic standpoint.[15] Desflurane and sevoflurane both cause decreases in $CMRO_2$ similar to isoflurane.[16,17] Interestingly, while both desflurane and sevoflurane depress the EEG and abolish activity at clinically tolerated doses of approximately 2 MAC[16,17] in *dogs*, desflurane-induced isoelectric EEG reverts to continuous activity with time despite an unchanging MAC, a property unique to desflurane.[16]

Sevoflurane has no noteworthy adverse effects on cerebral physiology at normal CO_2 and BP.[18] During sevoflurane use combined with extreme hyperventilation to decrease CBF by half, brain lactate levels can increase. High, long-lasting concentrations of sevoflurane (1.5 to 2.0 MAC), a sudden increase in cerebral sevoflurane concentrations, especially in females, and/or hypocapnia can trigger EEG abnormalities that have resulted in increases in heart rate (HR) in both adults and children.[19,20] These data question the appropriateness of sevoflurane in patients with epilepsy,[21] but it remains uncertain if sevoflurane truly has a proconvulsant effect.

Cerebral Blood Flow, Flow–Metabolism Coupling, and Autoregulation

All of the potent agents increase CBF in a dose-related manner. Isoflurane, sevoflurane, and desflurane cause far less cerebral vasodilation per MAC-multiple than halothane (Fig. 18-11). Desflurane and sevoflurane both influence CBF in a manner similar to isoflurane, with minimal changes in CBF at concentrations less than 1.5 MAC.[16,17,22] An initial dose-dependent increase in CBF with halothane and isoflurane administration to animals subsequently recovers to preinduction levels in approximately 2 to 5 hours. The mechanism of this recovery is unclear.

The increase in CBF with increasing anesthetic dose occurs despite decreases in $CMRO_2$. This phenomenon has been called *uncoupling*, but from a mechanistic standpoint, true uncoupling of flow from metabolism may not occur. That is, as $CMRO_2$ is depressed by the volatile anesthetics, there still is a coupled decline in CBF opposed by a coincident direct vasodilatory effect on the cerebral blood vessels. The net effect on the cerebral vessels depends on the sum of indirect vasoconstricting and direct vasodilating influences.

Autoregulation is the intrinsic myogenic regulation of vascular tone. In normal brain, the mechanisms of autoregulation of CBF over a range of mean arterial pressures from 50 to 150 mmHg are incompletely understood. Because the volatile anesthetics are direct vasodilators, all are considered to diminish autoregulation in a dose-dependent fashion such that at high anesthetic doses CBF is essentially pressure-passive. Sevoflurane preserves autoregulation up to approximately 1 MAC.[17] At 1.5 MAC, the dynamic rate of autoregulation (change in middle cerebral artery blood flow after a rapid transient decrease in BP) is better preserved with sevoflurane than isoflurane.[23] This may be result in a lesser direct vasodilator effect of sevoflurane, preserving the ability of the vessel to respond to changes in BP at 1.5 MAC. Based on a similar model but a separate study of dynamic autoregulation of CBF, both desflurane and isoflurane reduced autoregulation in a dose-dependent manner.[24]

Intracerebral Pressure

For most anesthesiologists, the area of greatest clinical interest is the effect of volatile anesthetics on ICP. In general, ICP will increase or decrease in proportion to changes in CBF. Isoflurane increases ICP minimally in animals both with and without brain pathology, including those with an already elevated ICP.[25] In human studies there usually are mild increases in ICP with isoflurane administration that are blocked or blunted by hyperventilation or barbiturate coadministration.[26] However, there are some contradictory data. In one human study, hypocapnia did not prevent elevations in ICP with isoflurane administration in patients with space-occupying brain lesions.[27]

Like isoflurane, both sevoflurane and desflurane greater than 1 MAC produce mild increases in ICP, paralleling their mild increases in CBF.[16,17,28,29] One potential advantage of sevoflurane is that its lower pungency and airway irritation may lessen the risk of coughing and bucking and the associated rise in ICP as compared with desflurane or isoflurane. In fact, introduction of desflurane after propofol induction of anesthesia has led to significant increases in HR, mean arterial pressure, and middle cerebral artery blood flow velocity.[30] This may relate to the airway irritant effects of desflurane rather than a specific alteration in neurophysiology. However, several studies in both children and adults suggest that increases in ICP from desflurane are slightly greater than from either isoflurane or sevoflurane.[30,31] CSF production and resorption are modestly and variably affected by volatile anesthetics and are clinically far less important than anesthetic effects on CBF. The bottom line is that all three potent agents may be used at appropriate doses, especially with adjunctive and compensatory therapies, in nearly any neurosurgical procedure.

Cerebral Blood Flow Response to Hypercapnia and Hypocapnia

Significant hypercapnia is associated with dramatic increases in CBF whether or not volatile anesthetics are administered. As discussed earlier, hypocapnia can blunt or abolish volatile anesthetic-induced increases in CBF depending on when the hypocapnia is produced. This vasoreactivity to CO_2 may be somewhat altered by the volatile anesthetics as compared with normal. Isoflurane does not abolish hypocapnic vasoconstriction.[32] Similarly, CO_2 vasoreactivity under desflurane anesthesia is normal up to 1.5 MAC,[25] and CO_2 vasoreactivity for sevoflurane is preserved at 1 MAC.[33]

Cerebral Protection

When isoflurane is used to lower BP and cerebral perfusion, tissue oxygen content is improved as compared to a similar BP effect created by other pharmacologic means. The improvement is most likely due to the beneficial effect of isoflurane to decrease $CMRO_2$.[34] Both sevoflurane and desflurane have been shown to improve neurologic outcome after incomplete cerebral ischemia in a rat model.[35,36] In piglets undergoing low-flow cardiopulmonary bypass, desflurane improved neurologic outcome compared with a fentanyl/droperidol-based anesthetic.[37]

In humans, desflurane has been shown to increase brain tissue PO_2 during administration, and to maintain PO_2 to a greater extent than thiopental during temporary cerebral artery occlusion during cerebrovascular surgery.[38] Neuroprotection and clinical outcome studies for sevoflurane and desflurane have not been published.

Postoperative Cognitive Dysfunction

Postoperative cognitive dysfunction (POCD) is defined as impairment to the mental processes of perception, memory, and information processing. These alterations are associated with increased morbidity and mortality in the first year after surgery from causes such as decubiti, pneumonia, and deep vein thrombosis.[39] In the elderly in particular, subtle cognitive dysfunction can persist long after expected drug clearance.

The effect of isoflurane on POCD has been more widely investigated than that of the other potent agents. As early as 1992, Tsai et al.[40] reported that desflurane was superior to isoflurane in both emergence characteristics and the recovery of cognitive function. Chen et al.[41] have demonstrated that sevoflurane and desflurane have similar profiles when it comes to cognitive recovery, and multiple other studies have further confirmed this. These results seem to be in conflict with those produced by Kanbak et al.[42] who demonstrated in cardiopulmonary bypass patients that isoflurane promoted better neurocognitive function than either sevoflurane or desflurane. It is clear from the wide variations in the results available in the literature that more research is required into this important topic. Further, while the mechanisms involved in the development of POCD are not well delineated, it seems clear that all modern anesthetics are associated with its development to one degree or another.

As with the potent inhalational anesthetics, use of N_2O is also associated with POCD and delirium, and high doses of N_2O seem to be associated with interference with many cognitive functions.[43] Interestingly, the development of postoperative delirium after exposure to N_2O in a mixed anesthetic has a similar incidence to that when not exposed, suggesting that the mechanisms, while possibly different, are not additive.[44]

Processed Electroencephalograms and Neuromonitoring

All of the volatile anesthetics produce dose-dependent effects on the EEG, sensory-evoked potentials (SEPs), and motor-evoked potentials (MEPs). EEGs recorded on the scalp can be processed to quantify the amount of activity in each of four frequency bands: δ (0 to 3 Hz), θ (4 to 7 Hz), α (8 to 13 Hz), and β (>13 Hz). All three currently used agents at greater than 1 MAC and N_2O at 30% to 70% can produce shifts to increasing frequencies. Between 1 and 2 MAC the potent agents produce shifts to decreasing frequencies and increases in amplitude. At greater than 2 MAC, all of the potent agents can produce burst suppression or electrical silence. These are important factors to remember because EEG changes during administration of general anesthesia can also be caused by hypoxia, hypercarbia, and hypothermia. The EEG must always be interpreted within the appropriate clinical context.

All of the volatile agents cause a dose-dependent increase in latency and decrease in amplitude in all cortical SEP modalities. In subcortical modalities, such as brainstem auditory evoked potentials, these agents are associated with negligible effects. In general, visual evoked potentials are somewhat more sensitive to the effects of the volatile anesthetics than somatosensory evoked potentials. Like EEGs, these effects from anesthetics must be kept in mind when changes during SEPs occur, and appropriate doses of the volatile agents must be used. Sudden changes in the anesthetic regimen (>0.5 MAC) also seem to have greater effects on SEPs than more gradual changes.

MEPs evaluate the functional integrity of descending motor pathways. The evoked response is most commonly recorded as a muscle potential or a peripheral nerve signal. The trigger is typically transosseous activation via electrical or magnetic stimulation. MEPs are exquisitely sensitive to depression by volatile anesthetics, which are usually avoided in these cases.

Nitrous Oxide

The effects of N_2O on cerebral physiology are not clear. Both the MAC for N_2O and its effects on $CMRO_2$ vary widely depending on species. The difference in $CMRO_2$ effects may in part be accounted for by differences in MAC, but MAC-equivalent effects on $CMRO_2$ also differ. Several studies in dogs, goats, and swine found that N_2O increases $CMRO_2$ and CBF, while in rodents no such increases or only slight increases occur. In human studies, N_2O administration preserved CBF but decreased $CMRO_2$.[15]

Another problem is that N_2O is a co-anesthetic used to supplement potent agents, not a complete anesthetic in itself, and $CMRO_2$ effects may differ depending on the presence or absence of potent agent as well as the particular agent and dose. Addition of N_2O to 1 MAC isoflurane does not alter $CMRO_2$, but it does increase CBF.

Barbiturates, narcotics, or a combination of the two appear to decrease or eliminate the increases in $CMRO_2$ and CBF produced by N_2O. N_2O administration increases ICP, but as is the case for $CMRO_2$ and CBF, changes in ICP are decreased or eliminated by a variety of co-anesthetics and, more importantly, by hypocapnia.

Nitrous oxide may be neuroprotective in rat models of cerebral ischemia, but other work suggests it is neurotoxic.[45] Given the conflicting data on the effects of N_2O on $CMRO_2$, CBF, ICP, and neuroprotection during ischemia, avoidance or discontinuation of its use should be considered in surgical cases with a high likelihood of elevated ICP or significant cerebral ischemia.

The Circulatory System

Hemodynamics

The cardiac, vascular, and autonomic effects of the volatile anesthetics have been defined through a number of studies carried out in human volunteers not undergoing surgery.[46–50] In general, the information from these volunteer studies has translated well to the patient population commonly exposed to these anesthetics during elective and emergent surgeries.

A common effect of the potent volatile anesthetics has been to decrease BP in a dose-related fashion with essentially no differences noted between the volatile anesthetics at equianesthetic concentrations (Fig. 18-12). Their primary mechanism to decrease BP is via a potent effect to relax vascular smooth muscle leading to decreases in regional and systemic vascular resistance (Fig. 18-13). They have only minimal effects on cardiac output.

In volunteers, sevoflurane up to about 1 MAC does not change HR while isoflurane and desflurane result in 5% to 10% increases in HR from baseline (Fig. 18-12). Both desflurane and, to a lesser extent, isoflurane have been associated with transient and significant increases in HR during rapid increases in the inspired concentration of either anesthetic.[51,52] The mechanism(s) underlying these transient HR surges is likely due to the relative pungency of these anesthetics, which stimulates airway receptors to elicit a reflex tachycardia.[53] The tachycardia can be lessened with opioid or α_2-agonist pretreatment.[54–56]

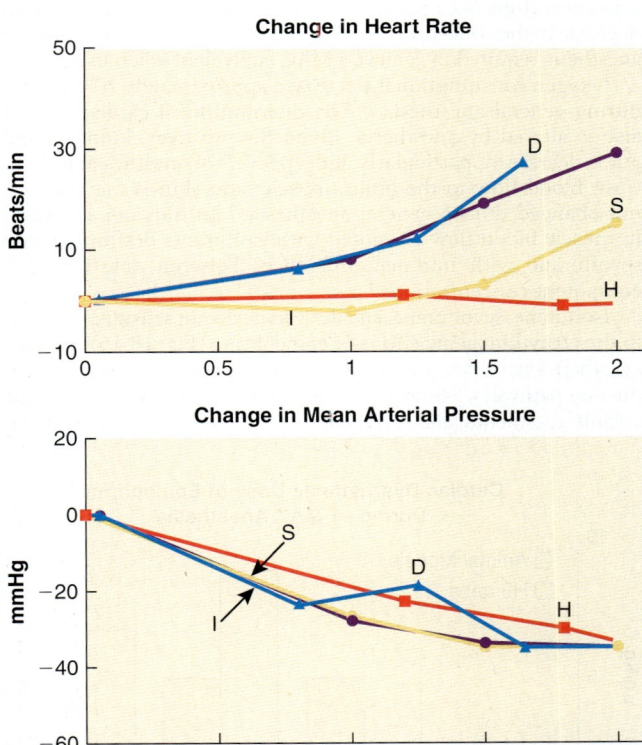

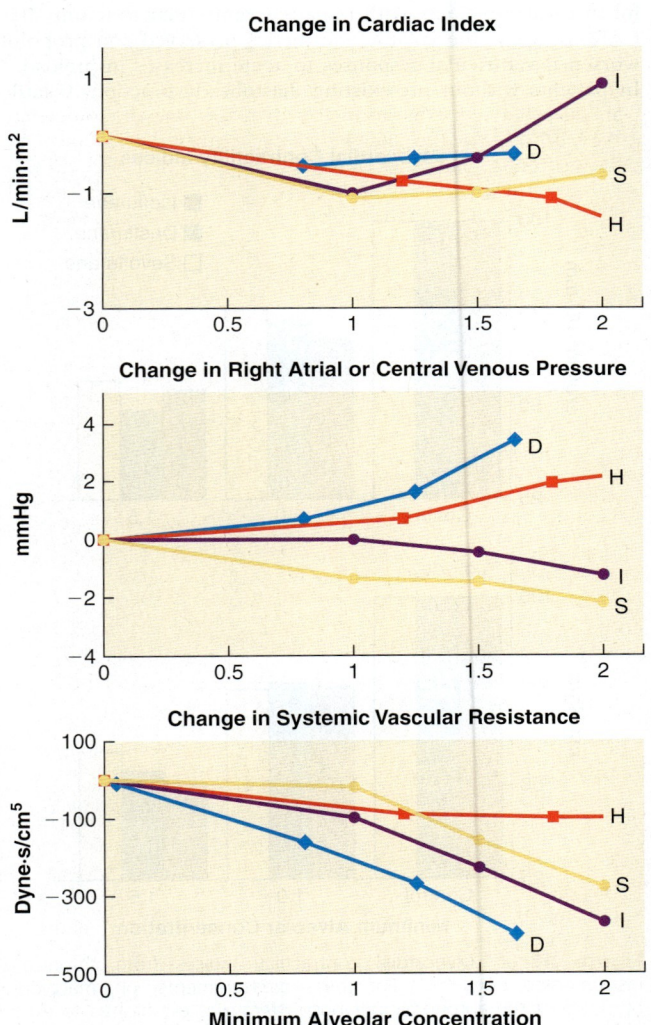

Figure 18-12 Heart rate and blood pressure changes (from awake baseline) in volunteers receiving general anesthesia with isoflurane (I), desflurane (D), or sevoflurane (S). Sevoflurane produced little or no change in heart rate below 1.5 minimum alveolar concentration.[47,60] All anesthetics caused similar decreases in blood pressure. Halothane (H) is presented for historical perspective.

Figure 18-13 Cardiac index, central venous pressure (or right atrial pressure), and systemic vascular resistance changes (from awake baseline) in volunteers receiving general anesthesia with isoflurane (I), desflurane (D), or sevoflurane (S).[47,60] Increases in central venous pressure from desflurane might be due to venoconstriction. Halothane (H) is presented for historical perspective.

Myocardial Contractility

Myocardial contractility indices have been directly evaluated in animals and indirectly evaluated in human volunteers during the administration of each of the volatile anesthetics. Isoflurane, desflurane, and sevoflurane produced similar dose-dependent reductions in indices of myocardial function in an autonomically denervated dog model (Fig. 18-14). Echocardiographic-determined indices of myocardial function in healthy humans, including the more noteworthy measurement of the velocity of circumferential fiber shortening have not been diminished by isoflurane, desflurane, or sevoflurane.[47–49] However, in cardiac patients with ejection fractions above 40%, 1 MAC sevoflurane and desflurane reduced contractility, assessed as dp/dt_{max}. Despite the small reduction in baseline contractility, the anesthetics did not affect the ability of the myocardium to respond to an acute increase in cardiac preload. Thus, functional reserve of the heart was not impaired by the volatile anesthetics.[57] In addition, when comparing sevoflurane and desflurane to propofol in cardiac patients with impaired ventricular function after CABG surgery, the volatile anesthetics preserved and propofol worsened ventricular responses to acute increases in preload.[58] In patients without pre-existing diastolic dysfunction, volatile anesthetics do not have any clinically relevant negative effect on early diastolic relaxation, although resultant decrease in global atrial function may impact late diastolic left ventricular filling.[59]

Other Circulatory Effects

Most of the volatile anesthetics have been studied during both controlled and spontaneous ventilation.[47,49,60] The process of spontaneous ventilation reduces the high intrathoracic pressures from positive pressure ventilation. The negative intrathoracic pressure during the inspiratory phase of spontaneous ventilation augments venous return and cardiac filling and improves cardiac output and BP. Spontaneous ventilation is associated with higher $PaCO_2$, causing cerebral and systemic vascular relaxation. This contributes to an improved cardiac output via afterload reduction. Spontaneous ventilation in theory would improve the safety of volatile anesthetic administration because the anesthetic concentration that produces cardiovascular collapse exceeds the concentration that results in apnea.

Nitrous oxide is commonly combined with potent volatile anesthetics to maintain general anesthesia. Nitrous oxide has unique cardiovascular actions. It increases sympathetic nervous system activity and vascular resistance when given in a 40% concentration.[50] When N_2O is combined with volatile anesthetics, systemic vascular resistance and BP are greater than when equipotent concentrations of the volatile anesthetics are evaluated without N_2O.[47,61] These effects might not be due solely to sympathetic activation from N_2O per se, but may be partially attributed to a decrease in the concentration of the coadministered potent volatile anesthetic required to achieve a MAC equivalent when using N_2O.

Oxygen consumption is decreased approximately 10% to 15% during general anesthesia.[62] The distribution of cardiac output also is altered by anesthesia. Blood flow to liver, kidneys, and gut is decreased, particularly at deep levels of anesthesia. In contrast, blood flow to the brain, muscle, and skin is increased or not changed during general anesthesia.[63] In humans, increases in muscle blood flow are noted with isoflurane, desflurane, and sevoflurane with minimal differences between anesthetics at equipotent concentrations.[64]

Isoflurane, sevoflurane, and desflurane do not sensitize the heart to the arrhythmogenic effects of epinephrine (Fig. 18-15). Volatile anesthetics have direct effects on cardiac pacemaker cells and conduction pathways.[65] Sinoatrial node discharge rate is slowed by the volatile anesthetics, and conduction in the His–Purkinje system and

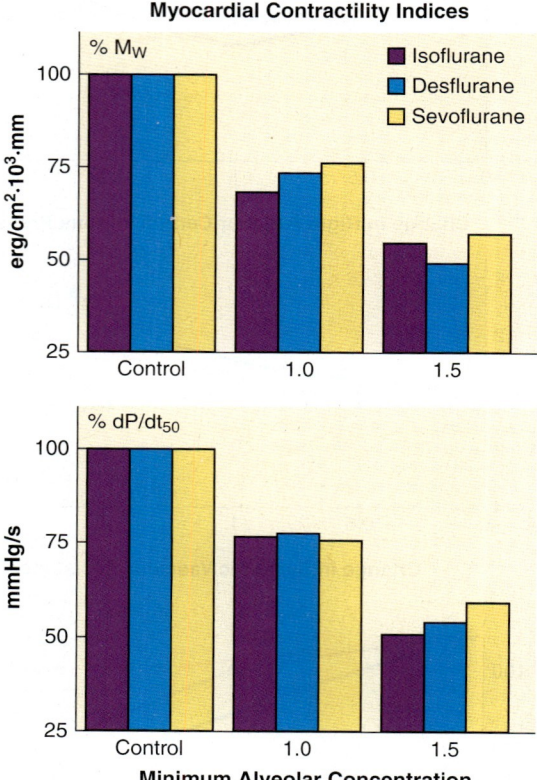

Figure 18-14 Myocardial contractility indices from chronically instrumented dogs.[183,184] For these measurements, pharmacologic blockade of the autonomic nervous system was established to eliminate neural or circulating humoral influences on the inotropic state of the heart. The conscious control data were assigned 100%, and subsequent reductions in the inotropic state are depicted for both 1 and 1.5 minimum alveolar anesthetic concentrations of sevoflurane, desflurane, and isoflurane. There were no differences between these three volatile anesthetics. M_w, slope of the regional preload recruitable stroke work relationship; dP/dt_{50}, change in pressure per unit of time.

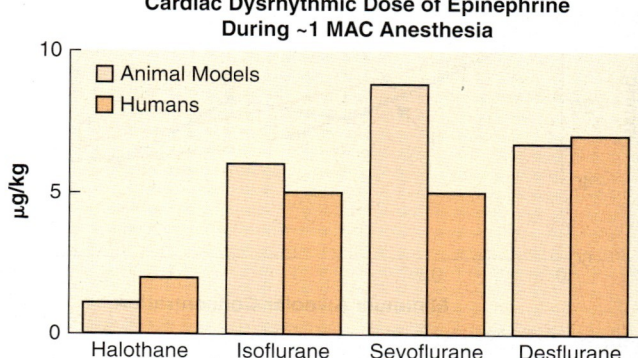

Figure 18-15 The dose of epinephrine associated with cardiac arrhythmias in animal and human models was least with halothane. The ether-based anesthetics—isoflurane, desflurane, and sevoflurane—required three- to sixfold greater doses of epinephrine to cause arrhythmias.

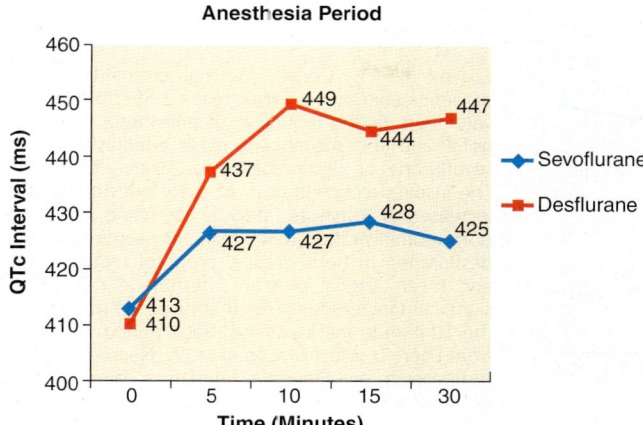

Figure 18-16 Mean QTc intervals in children, age 1 to 14 years, after inhalation of 2% sevoflurane or 6% desflurane, both in 66% N_2O/O_2. (Adapted from Aypar E, Karagoz AH, Ozer S, et al. The effects of sevoflurane and desflurane anesthesia on QTc interval and cardiac rhythm in children. *Pediatr Anaesth.* 2007;17:563-567.)

conduction pathways in the ventricle also is prolonged by the volatile anesthetics. The volatile anesthetics prolong QT_c interval and in theory, especially with a baseline prolongation in myocardial repolarization, may predispose to ventricular tachyarrhythmias including *torsade de pointes*. Such an effect has been noted in a child with congenital prolonged QT syndrome.[66] In children studied at steady state 1 MAC, QT_c was more prolonged with desflurane than sevoflurane (Fig. 18-16).[67] When the effects of sevoflurane, propofol, and desflurane on QT interval dispersion and p dispersion were evaluated in adults, only desflurane prolonged intervals, although no increase in cardiac dysrhythmias was noted.[68]

Coronary Steal, Myocardial Ischemia, and Cardiac Outcome

Isoflurane (and most other potent volatile anesthetics) increases coronary blood flow beyond that of the myocardial oxygen demand, thereby creating potential for "steal." Steal is the diversion of blood from a myocardial bed with limited or inadequate perfusion to a bed with more adequate perfusion; especially one that has a remaining element of autoregulation.

Despite early worries that the potent vasodilation from isoflurane might cause coronary steal, clinical outcome studies have been unable to find an association between the use of isoflurane in patients undergoing coronary artery bypass graft (CABG) operations with an increased incidence of myocardial infarction or perioperative death.[69,70] This is in agreement with findings in a chronically instrumented dog model of multivessel coronary artery obstruction where neither isoflurane, sevoflurane, or desflurane at concentrations up to 1.5 MAC resulted in abnormal collateral coronary blood flow redistribution (steal), whereas adenosine, a potent coronary vasodilator, clearly resulted in abnormal flow distribution.[71–73]

Several studies in patients with coronary artery disease undergoing either noncardiac or CABG surgery have demonstrated that myocardial ischemia and outcome from sevoflurane was no different from isoflurane.[74,75] Desflurane also appears to result in similar outcome effects as isoflurane in cardiac patients having CABG[76] with one exception. In a study in which desflurane was given without opioids to patients with coronary artery disease requiring CABG surgery, significant ischemia mandating the use of β-blockers was noted.[77] Desflurane has not been evaluated in terms of ischemia and outcome in a patient population with coronary disease undergoing noncardiac surgery. Most studies would suggest that determinants of myocardial oxygen supply and demand, rather than the anesthetic, are of far greater importance to patient outcomes.

Cardioprotection from Volatile Anesthetics

A preconditioning stimulus such as brief coronary occlusion and ischemia initiates a signaling cascade of intracellular events that helps protect the cardiac myocyte and reduce reperfusion myocardial injury following subsequent ischemic episodes. Ischemic preconditioning consists of early and late phase protection. The early phase, lasting approximately 2 hours, is mediated by the release of adenosine, inducing a protective signal through the activation of mitochondrial potassium channels (K_{ATP}) and opioid and bradykinin receptors.[78,79] The late phase, while not as strong as the early phase, provides additional myocardial protection for 24 to 72 hours. This delayed effect relates to induction of nitric oxide synthase, superoxide dismutase, and heat-shock proteins. The volatile anesthetics given before (preconditioning) or immediately after (postconditioning) mimic ischemic preconditioning and trigger a similar cascade of intracellular events resulting in reduced myocardial injury and myocardial protection that lasts beyond the elimination of the anesthetic.[79,80] Numerous factors may be involved in the protection, including the sodium:hydrogen exchanger, activation of opioid, bradykinin or adenosine receptors (particularly $α_1$ and $α_2$ subtypes), inhibitory G proteins, protein kinase C, tyrosine kinase, and potassium (K_{ATP}) channel opening. Pharmacologic blockade of these factors reduces or eliminates the cardioprotective effect of ischemic or volatile anesthetic preconditioning.[80,81] Alternatively, administration of certain drugs can mimic ischemic or volatile anesthetic preconditioning. These include adenosine, opioid agonists, and K_{ATP} channel openers.

Lipophilic volatile anesthetics diffuse through myocardial cell membranes and alter mitochondrial electron transport, leading to reactive oxygen species formation.[81] This may be the trigger for preconditioning via protein kinase C activation of K_{ATP} channel opening.[82,83] Approximately 30% to 40% of the cardioprotection from the volatile anesthetics appears to be related to a reduced loading of calcium into the myocardial cells during ischemia. This reduction in calcium accumulation improves the recovery of contractile function following reperfusion and makes the mitochondrial membrane more permeable to ATP precursors.[78] Preconditioned hearts may tolerate ischemia for 10 minutes longer than nonconditioned hearts.[84]

While these findings generally derive from animal models, there now is increasing evidence in cardiac patient populations that anesthetic cardioprotection lessens myocardial damage and improves cardiac outcomes during "on and off pump" cardiac surgery.[85,86] One meta-analysis of 22 trials including nearly 2,000 patients undergoing CABG surgery found that sevoflurane and desflurane compared to a TIVA technique were associated with a 50% reduction in MI, reductions in cardiac troponin I peak levels, inotropic support, and all cause mortality, and shorter periods of mechanical ventilation and ICU stay.[87] Preconditioning effects of sevoflurane are noted at a minimum of 1 MAC with a dose of 1.5 MAC needed for full efficacy.[78] Sulfonylurea oral hyperglycemic drugs close K_{ATP} channels, abolishing anesthetic preconditioning. They should be discontinued 24 to 48 hours prior to elective surgery in high-risk patients.[80] But hyperglycemia also prevents preconditioning, so insulin therapy should be started when holding

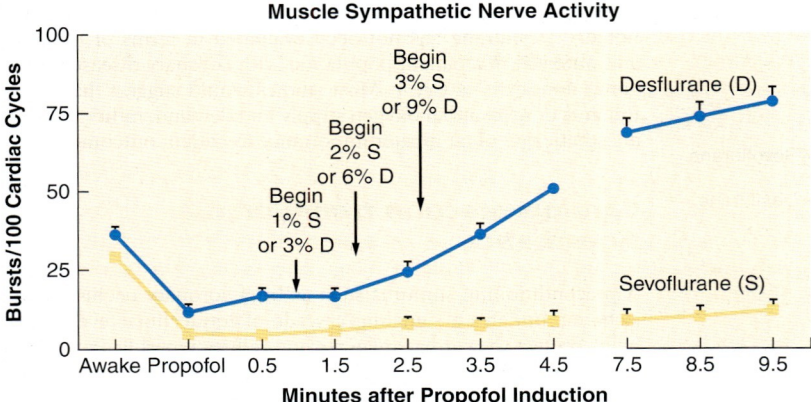

Figure 18-17 Consecutive measurements of sympathetic nerve activity (SNA; mean ± SE) from human volunteers during induction of anesthesia with propofol and the subsequent mask administration of sevoflurane or desflurane for a 10-minute period. The inspired concentration of these anesthetics was increased at 1-minute intervals beginning after propofol administration (0.41 MAC of sevoflurane and desflurane). In both groups, propofol reduced SNA and mean arterial pressure. Desflurane resulted in significant increases in SNA that persisted throughout the 10-minute mask administration period. (Adapted from Ebert TJ, Muzi M, Lopatka CW. Neurocirculatory responses to sevoflurane in humans: a comparison to desflurane. *Anesthesiology*. 1995;83:88.)

oral agents.[88] Recent evidence suggests that volatile anesthetics as well as xenon may protect other organs from ischemic injury, including kidney, liver, and brain.[89–92]

Autonomic Nervous System

The autonomic nervous system is modulated by baroreceptor reflex mechanisms. Studies have examined the behavior of the arterial baroreflex system during a hypotensive or hypertensive stimulus by evaluating changes in HR and sympathetic nerve activity in humans. Anesthetic mediated, dose-dependent decreases in reflex control of sympathetic output are most prominent at the 1 MAC or greater of the volatile anesthetics.[93–96] At these concentrations, there is a greater reduction in the reflex response to hypovolemia than at normovolemia. This may lead to earlier recognition of blood loss intraoperatively, as there is less masking of hypovolemia by sympathetic regulation of vasoconstriction and tachycardia.

Desflurane has a unique and prominent effect on sympathetic outflow in humans, which is not apparent in animal models. With increasing steady state concentrations of desflurane, there is a progressive increase in resting sympathetic nervous system activity and plasma norepinephrine levels.[97] Despite this increase in tonic sympathetic outflow, BP decreases similarly to sevoflurane and isoflurane (Fig. 18-12). This raises the question as to whether desflurane has the ability to uncouple neuroeffector responses. In addition, when the inspired concentration of desflurane is increased, especially to concentrations above 5% to 6%, it can cause substantial activation of the sympathetic nervous system leading to hypertension and tachycardia (Fig. 18-17).[97] Furthermore, the endocrine axis is activated as evidenced by 15- to 20-fold increases in plasma antidiuretic hormone, epinephrine, and norepinephrine (Fig. 18-18). The hemodynamic response persists for 4 to 5 minutes and the endocrine response persists for up to 30 minutes.[46,51,52] Adequate concentrations of opioids or clonidine given prior to increasing the concentration of desflurane have been shown to attenuate these responses.[54–56] The source of the neuroendocrine activation is likely from receptors in both the upper and lower airways that initiate the sympathetic activation.[53]

The Pulmonary System

General Ventilatory Effects

All volatile anesthetics decrease tidal volume and increase respiratory rate such that there are only minor effects on decreasing

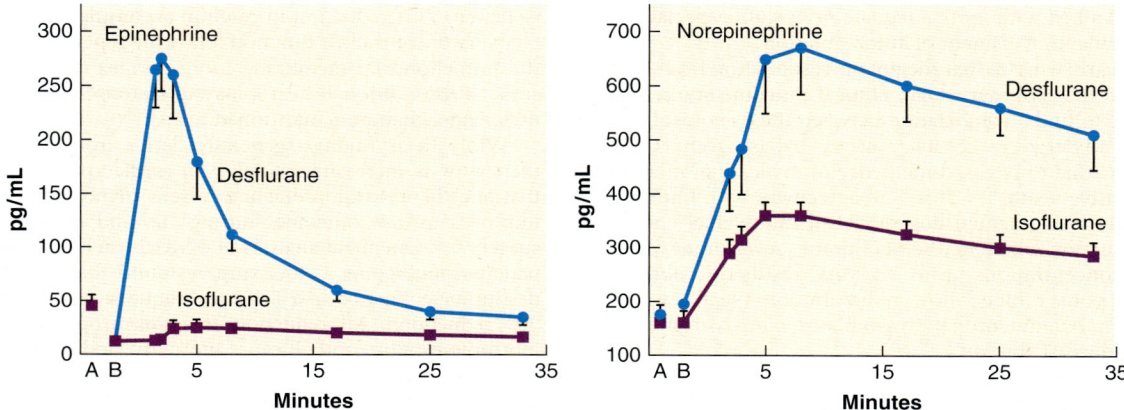

Figure 18-18 Stress hormone responses to a rapid increase in anesthetic concentration, from 4% to 12% inspired. Volunteers given desflurane showed a larger increase in plasma epinephrine and norepinephrine concentrations than when given isoflurane. Data are mean ± SE. A = awake value; B = value after 32 minutes of 0.55 minimum alveolar concentration; time represents minutes after the first breath of increased anesthetic concentration. (Adapted from Weiskopf RB, Moore MA, Eger EI II, et al. Rapid increase in desflurane concentration is associated with greater transient cardiovascular stimulation than with rapid increase in isoflurane concentration in humans. *Anesthesiology*. 1994;80:1035.)

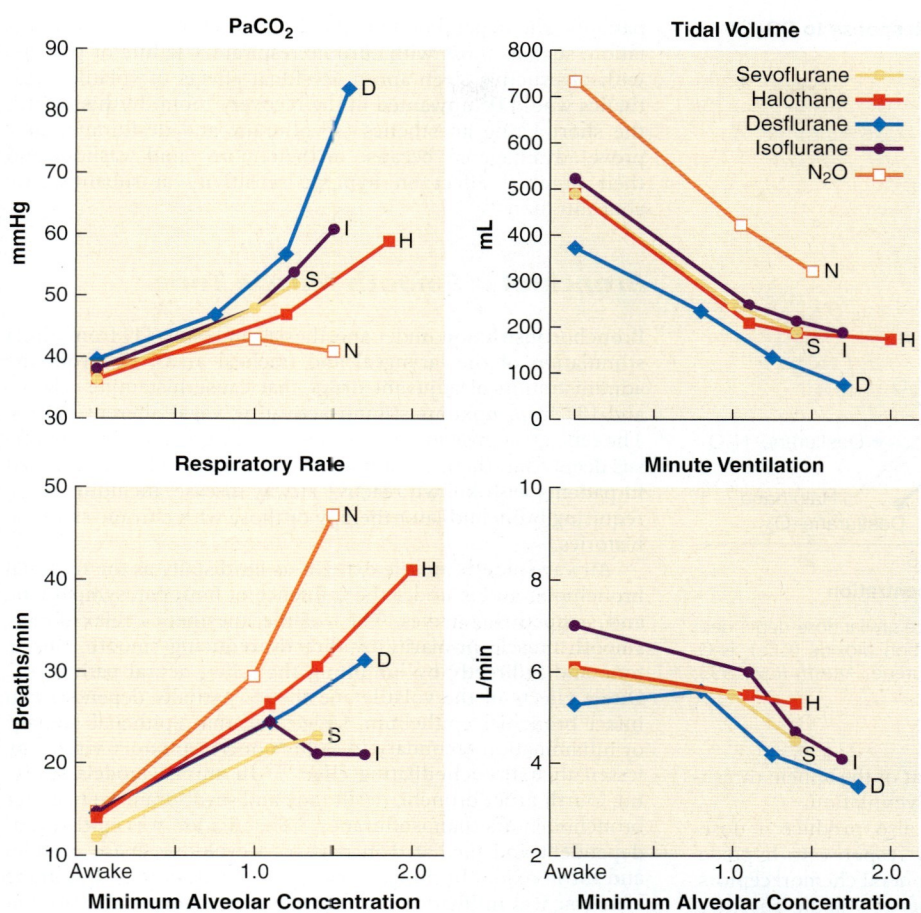

Figure 18-19 Comparison of mean changes in resting PaCO$_2$, tidal volume, respiratory rate, and minute ventilation in patients anesthetized with isoflurane, sevoflurane, desflurane, or N$_2$O(N).[185-187] Anesthetic-induced tachypnea compensates in part for the ventilatory depression caused by all volatile anesthetics (decrease in minute ventilation and tidal volume, and concomitant increase in PaCO$_2$). Desflurane results in the greatest increase in PaCO$_2$ with corresponding reductions in tidal volume and minute ventilation. Isoflurane, like all other inhaled agents, increases respiratory rate, but does not result in dose-dependent tachypnea.

minute ventilation (Fig. 18-19). The ventilatory effects are dose-dependent, with higher concentrations of volatile anesthetics resulting in greater decreases in tidal volume and greater increases in respiratory rate, with the exception of isoflurane, which does not increase respiratory rate above 1 MAC. Their net effect of a gradual decrease in minute ventilation has been associated with increasing resting PaCO$_2$. The respiratory depression can be partially antagonized during surgical stimulation where respiratory rate and tidal volume have been shown to increase, resulting in a decrease in the PaCO$_2$. Nitrous oxide increases respiratory rate as much or more than the inhaled anesthetics. When N$_2$O is added to sevoflurane or desflurane, resting PaCO$_2$ decreases relative to equi-MAC concentrations of sevoflurane or desflurane in O$_2$.

Ventilatory Mechanics

FRC is decreased during general anesthesia; this has been explained by a number of mechanisms including a decrease in the intercostal muscle tone, alteration in diaphragm position, changes in thoracic blood volume, and the onset of phasic expiratory activity of respiratory muscles. About 40% of the muscular work of breathing is via intercostal muscles and about 60% is from the diaphragm. During anesthesia, the diaphragmatic muscle function is relatively spared when contrasted to the parasternal intercostal muscles. However, inspiratory rib cage expansion is reasonably well maintained during anesthesia because of preserved activity of the scalene muscles. Expiration is generally considered a passive function mediated by the elastic recoil of the lung. The process of applying a resistance or load to expiration typically results in a slowing of respiration, but under anesthesia, further responses include a substantial asynchrony of the thoracic movements with respiration. This suggests that in patients with pulmonary disease associated with increased expiratory resistance, the act of spontaneous ventilation during general anesthesia might be poorly tolerated.

Response to Carbon Dioxide and Hypoxemia

In conscious humans, the central chemoreceptors respond vigorously to changes in arterial carbon dioxide tension such that minute ventilation increases 3 L/min per a 1 mmHg increase in PaCO$_2$. All of the inhaled anesthetics produce a dose-dependent depression of the ventilatory response to hypercarbia (Fig. 18-20). The addition of N$_2$O to a volatile anesthetic has been thought to diminish PaCO$_2$ responses less than an equi-MAC dose of the anesthetic alone. The threshold where respiratory drive ceases is called the apneic threshold. It is generally 4 to 5 mmHg below the prevailing resting PaCO$_2$ in a spontaneously breathing patient. It is unrelated to the slope of the CO$_2$ response curves or to the level of the resting PaCO$_2$. The clinical relevance of this threshold may be realized when assisting ventilation in an anesthetized patient who is breathing spontaneously. This only

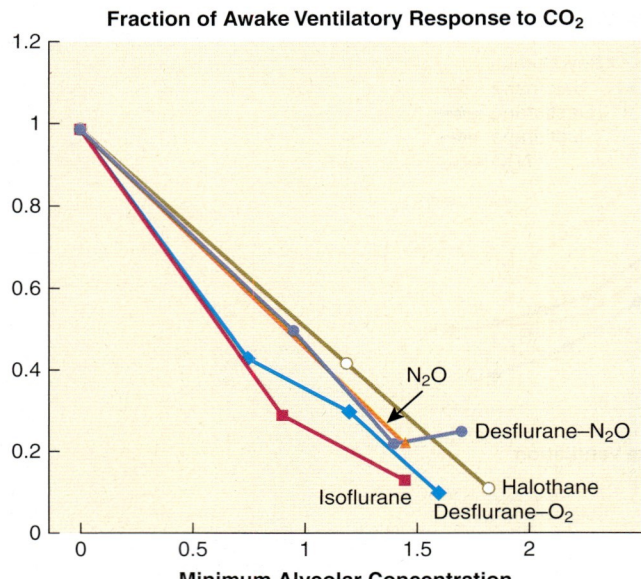

Figure 18-20 All inhaled anesthetics produce similar dose-dependent decreases in the ventilatory response to carbon dioxide (CO_2). N_2O, nitrous oxide. (Adapted from Eger EI II. Desflurane. *Anesth Rev.* 1993;20:87.)

serves to lower the $PaCO_2$ to approach that of the apneic threshold, therefore mandating more control of ventilation.

Inhaled anesthetics, including N_2O, also produce a dose-dependent attenuation of the ventilatory response to hypoxia. This action appears to depend on the peripheral chemoreceptors. In fact, even subanesthetic concentrations of volatile anesthetics (0.1 MAC) elicit anywhere from a 25% to 75% depression of the ventilatory drive to hypoxia (Fig. 18-21). The extreme sensitivity of the volatile anesthetics to inhibit ventilatory responses to hypoxia has important clinical implications, especially in patients who depend on hypoxic drive to set their level of ventilation, such as those with chronic respiratory failure or patients with obstructive sleep apnea. Residual effects of volatile anesthetics would be unwanted in the recovery room. In this regard, the short-acting anesthetics (sevoflurane and desflurane) may prove advantageous because of their more rapid washout and their minimal effect on hypoxic sensitivity at subanesthetic concentrations.

Bronchiolar Smooth Muscle Tone

Bronchoconstriction under anesthesia can result: (1) from direct stimulation of the laryngeal and tracheal areas, (2) from the administration of adjuvant drugs that cause histamine release, and (3) from noxious stimuli activating vagal afferent nerves. The reflex response to these stimuli may be greater in lightly versus deeply anesthetized patients.[98] The response also is enhanced in patients with known reactive airway disease, including those requiring bronchodilator therapy or those with chronic smoking histories.

Airway smooth muscle extends as far distally as the terminal bronchioles and is under the influence of both parasympathetic and sympathetic nerves. The volatile anesthetics relax airway smooth muscle primarily by directly reducing smooth muscle tone and indirectly by inhibiting the reflex neural pathways.[99] Direct effects of the volatile anesthetics partially depend on an intact bronchial epithelium, suggesting that epithelial damage or inflammation secondary to asthma or a respiratory virus may lessen their bronchodilating effect.[100] In animal models studying fourth order bronchi, desflurane and sevoflurane were better bronchodilators than isoflurane.[100] The dilation was epithelium-dependent and mediated in part by a cyclooxygenase product and nitric oxide. In humans, early administration of desflurane after tracheal intubation and high concentrations (1.5 MAC) at steady state lessen the decrease in respiratory system resistance seen with sevoflurane (Fig. 18-22).[101,102] This may be attributed to a direct effect on bronchial smooth muscle from the pungency of desflurane. Volatile anesthetics have been used effectively to treat status asthmaticus when other conventional treatments have failed, and appear to bronchodilate in patients with COPD.[103,104]

Mucociliary Function

Ciliated respiratory epithelium extends from the trachea to the terminal bronchioles. Cells and glands in the tracheobronchial tree secrete mucus that captures surface particles for transport via ciliary action. There are a number of factors involved in diminished mucociliary function, particularly in the mechanically ventilated patient where dried, inspired gases impair ciliary movement, thicken the protective mucus, and reduce the ability of mucociliary function to transport surface particles out of the airway. Volatile anesthetics and N_2O reduce ciliary movement and alter the characteristics of mucus.[105] Smokers have impaired mucociliary function, and the combination of a volatile anesthetic in a smoker who is mechanically ventilated sets up a scenario for inadequate clearing of secretions, mucus plugging, atelectasis, and hypoxemia.

Pulmonary Vascular Resistance

Although systemic vascular smooth muscle is notably affected by the volatile anesthetics, the pulmonary vascular relaxation

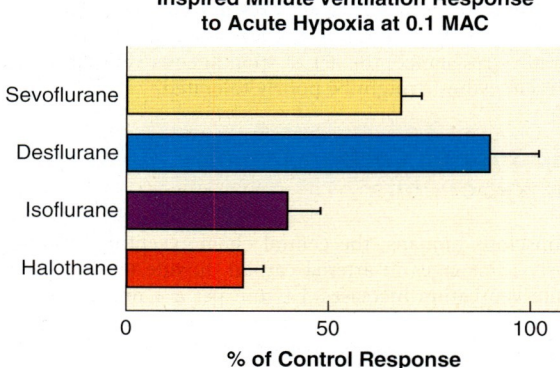

Figure 18-21 Influence of 0.1 minimum alveolar concentration (MAC) of four volatile anesthetic agents on the ventilatory response to a step decrease in end-tidal oxygen concentration. Values are mean ± SD. Subanesthetic concentrations of the volatile anesthetics, except desflurane and sevoflurane, profoundly depress the response to hypoxia. (Adapted from Sarton E, Dahan A, Teppema L, et al. Acute pain and central nervous system arousal do not restore impaired hypoxic ventilatory responses during sevoflurane sedation. *Anesthesiology.* 1996;85:295.)

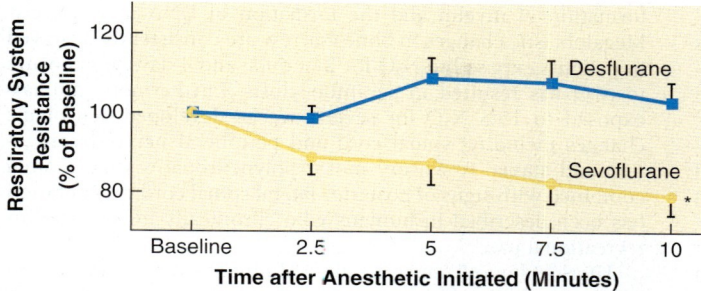

Figure 18-22 Changes in respiratory system resistance expressed as a percentage of the baseline recorded after tracheal intubation but prior to administration of sevoflurane or desflurane to the inspired gas mixture. Airway resistance responses to sevoflurane were significantly different from desflurane (*$p < 0.05$). (Adapted from Goff MJ, Arain SR, Ficke DJ, et al. Absence of bronchodilation during desflurane anesthesia: a comparison to sevoflurane and thiopental. *Anesthesiology*. 2000;93:404.)

from clinically relevant concentrations of inhaled anesthetics is minimal. The small amount of pulmonary vasodilation from volatile anesthetics is offset by anesthetic-related decreases in cardiac output, resulting in little or no change in pulmonary artery pressures and pulmonary blood flow. Even N_2O, which has little effect on cardiac output and pulmonary blood flow, has at most a small effect to increase pulmonary vascular resistance. However, pulmonary vascular constriction from N_2O may be magnified in patients with resting pulmonary hypertension.[106]

Perhaps more important in terms of volatile anesthetics and pulmonary blood flow is their potential to attenuate hypoxic pulmonary vasoconstriction (HPV). During periods of hypoxemia, HPV reduces blood flow to underventilated areas of the lung, thereby diverting blood flow to areas of the lung with greater ventilation. The net effect is to improve the V/Q matching, resulting in a reduced amount of venous admixture and improved arterial oxygenation. Although all of the modern inhaled anesthetics in high concentrations have been shown to attenuate HPV in animal models, the situation is less clear in patient studies. This may reflect the multifactorial effects of the volatile anesthetics on factors involved in pulmonary blood flow, including their cardiovascular, autonomic, and humoral actions. Furthermore, nonpharmacologic variables impair HPV, including surgical trauma, temperature, pH, $PaCO_2$, size of the hypoxic segment, and intensity of the hypoxic stimulus. One-lung ventilation (OLV) serves as a model where HPV should lessen the expected decrease in PaO_2 and intrapulmonary shunt fraction (Qs/Qt). In patients undergoing OLV during thoracic surgery, volatile anesthetics have had minimal effects on PaO_2 and Qs/Qt when changing from two-lung ventilation to OLV (Fig. 18-23).[107]

Hepatic Effects

Unlike most intravenous anesthetic drugs, modern-day volatile anesthetics undergo minimal liver metabolism, and because they are excreted primarily via the lungs, it is not surprising that they minimally affect hepatic function. The various factors that are known to affect drug metabolism, such as age, disease, genetics, and enzyme-inducing agents, have minor effects on the excretion of the volatile anesthetics.

There are two distinct mechanisms by which anesthetics have caused hepatitis; both discussed in Chapter 46: The Liver: Surgery and Anesthesia, on hepatic anatomy, function, and physiology.

Another consideration is convincing evidence that volatile anesthetics can infer organ protection from ischemic injury (discussed earlier in the chapter). When sevoflurane was compared to propofol anesthesia in a prospective, randomized study of 320 patients undergoing CABG surgery, postoperative biochemical markers of hepatic dysfunction were lower after the sevoflurane-based anesthetic.[91]

Neuromuscular System and Malignant Hyperthermia

The inhaled anesthetics have two important actions on neuromuscular function: (1) they directly relax skeletal muscle through a dose-dependent effect and (2) they potentiate the action of neuromuscular blocking drugs.[108,109] Relaxation of skeletal muscle is most prominent for potent volatile anesthetics above 1.0 MAC, with an effect enhanced by 40% in patients with myasthenia gravis.[110] Conversely, nitrous oxide does not affect skeletal muscle relaxation.

Volatile anesthetic potentiation of neuromuscular blockade has been well documented. For example, the infusion rate of rocuronium required to maintain neuromuscular blockade is 30% to 40% less during isoflurane, desflurane, and sevoflurane administration compared with propofol, with a similar effect

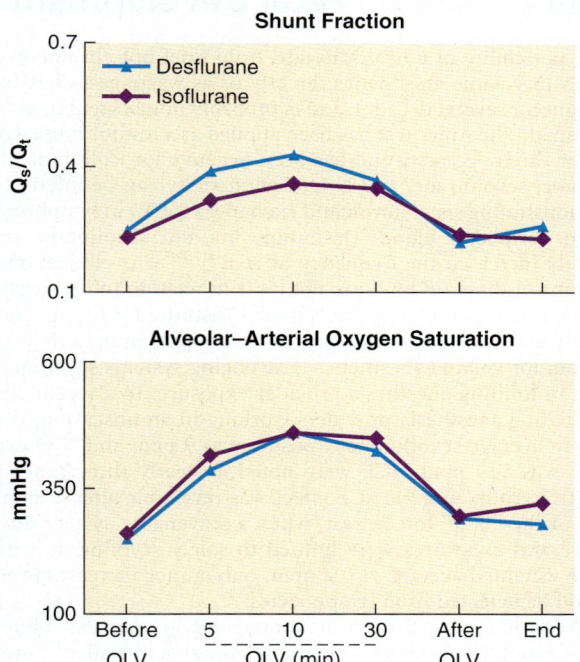

Figure 18-23 Shunt fraction **(top panel)** and the alveolar–arterial oxygen gradient **(bottom)** immediately before, during, and after one-lung ventilation (OLV) in patients anesthetized with desflurane or isoflurane. Data are means. (Adapted from Pagel PS, Fu JL, Damask MC, et al. Desflurane and isoflurane produce similar alterations in systemic and pulmonary hemodynamics and arterial oxygenation in patients undergoing one-lung ventilation during thoracotomy. *Anesth Analg*. 1998;87:800.)

observed with cisatracurium.[109,111] While the mechanism of volatile anesthetic potentiation of the neuromuscular blocking drugs is not entirely clear, it appears to be largely because of a postsynaptic effect at the nicotinic acetylcholine receptor located at the neuromuscular junction. Specifically, at the receptor level, the volatile anesthetics act synergistically with the neuromuscular blocking drugs to enhance their action.[112] The degree of enhancement is related to their aqueous concentration so that at equi-MAC concentrations, the less potent anesthetics (e.g., desflurane and sevoflurane vs. isoflurane) should have a greater inhibitory effect on neuromuscular transmission.[113] However, at equipotent concentrations, desflurane, sevoflurane, and isoflurane acted similarly to enhance the effect of cisatracurium on neuromuscular function.[109] This may relate to structural differences of the benzylisoquinolines versus aminosteroid neuromuscular blocking drugs.

Malignant hyperthermia is a clinical syndrome of acute, uncontrolled, increased skeletal muscle metabolism resulting in heightened oxygen consumption, lactate formation, heat production, and rhabdomyolysis. The hallmark findings of MH are a rapidly rising temperature, increasing up to 1°C every 5 minutes along with increasing end-tidal CO_2, arrhythmias, mixed respiratory/metabolic acidosis, and skeletal muscle rigidity.[114] Susceptibility to MH is an inherited autosomal dominant genetic disorder with reduced penetrance and variable expression. While N_2O and xenon are considered safe in MH-susceptible patients, all volatile anesthetics serve as triggers for MH in these patients.[115,116]

Genetic Effects, Obstetric Use, and Effects on Fetal Development

The possibility of a health hazard from brief but chronic exposures to volatile anesthetics directly or as waste gases has been sought for several decades, and is probably nonexistent or at best minimal. The Ames test has been applied as a test for mutagenicity or carcinogenicity and has been negative for isoflurane, desflurane, sevoflurane, and N_2O. Genotoxicity can be inferred by demonstrating sister chromatid exchanges (SCE) in lymphocytes from peripheral blood. Desflurane but not sevoflurane transiently increased the frequency of SCE.[117,118] The clinical implications of these findings are not clear in relation to the negative Ames test. Nonetheless, the National Institute for Occupational Safety and Health has set exposure limits of 25 ppm for N_2O and 2 ppm for volatile anesthetics. Scavenging systems seem important in limiting anesthesia provider exposure. In a recent study evaluating anesthesia providers working in an unscavenged OR where average sevoflurane exposure was 9 ppm and N_2O exposure was 119 ppm, SCE were noted at nearly three times the control group, and the SCE effect was reversible after 2 months out of the OR.[119] In contrast, when a scavenging system was in place and exposures were limited to solely sevoflurane with a time weighted average of 0.2 ppm, only minor increases in SCE could be detected from lymphocytes.[120]

Volatile anesthetics can be teratogenic in animals,[121] but do not cause teratogenicity in humans. Mazze and Källén[122] evaluated 5,405 surgeries in 2 million patients and found no increase in teratogenicity. Nitrous oxide decreases the activity of vitamin B_{12}-dependent enzymes, methionine synthetase (MS) and thymidylate synthetase. The mechanism appears to be an irreversible oxidation of the cobalt atom of vitamin B_{12} by N_2O; for example, there is a 50% inactivation of MS after exposure to 46 minutes of 70% N_2O. This might affect the rapidly developing embryo/fetus because MS and thymidylate synthetase are involved in the formation of myelin and the formation of DNA, respectively. Megaloblastic changes in bone marrow are consistently observed in patients exposed to N_2O for 24 hours, and 4 days of exposure to N_2O has resulted in agranulocytosis. Furthermore, animals exposed to 15% N_2O for several weeks developed neurologic changes including spinal cord and peripheral nerve degeneration and ataxia. A sensory motor polyneuropathy that is often combined with signs of posterior lateral spinal cord degeneration has been described in humans who chronically inhale N_2O for recreational use.[123]

Uterine smooth muscle tone is diminished by volatile anesthetics in similar fashion to the effects of volatile anesthetics on vascular smooth muscle. There is a dose-dependent decrease in spontaneous myometrial contractility that is consistent among the volatile anesthetics. Desflurane and sevoflurane also inhibit the frequency and amplitude of myometrial contractions induced by oxytocin in a dose-dependent manner.[124] Uterine relaxation/atony can become problematic at concentrations of volatile anesthesia greater than 1 MAC, and might delay the onset time of newborn respiration.[125] Consequently, a common technique used to provide general anesthesia for urgent cesarean sections is to administer low concentrations of the volatile anesthetic, such as 0.5 to 0.75 MAC, combined with N_2O. This decreases the likelihood of uterine atony and blood loss, especially at a time after delivery when oxytocin responsiveness of the uterus is essential. In some situations, uterine relaxation may be desirable, such as to remove a retained placenta. In this case, a brief, high concentration of a volatile anesthetic may be advantageous.

There has been an ongoing concern about the incidence of spontaneous abortions in operating room personnel chronically exposed to trace concentrations of inhaled anesthetics, especially N_2O.[126] Early epidemiologic studies suggested that operating room personnel had an increased incidence of spontaneous abortions and congenital abnormalities in offspring. However, subsequent analysis of the data suggests that inaccurate study design, confounding variables, and nonresponders might have led to flawed conclusions.[127] In prospective studies, no causal relationship has been shown between exposure to waste anesthetic gases and adverse health effects, regardless of the presence or absence of scavenging systems. Despite the unproven influence of trace concentrations of the volatile anesthetics on fetal development and spontaneous abortions, concerns for an adverse influence have resulted in the use of scavenging systems to remove anesthetic gases from operating and recovery rooms and have led to the establishment of standards for waste gas exposure.

In terms of neonatal effects from general anesthesia, Apgar scores and acid–base balance are not affected by anesthetic technique, such as spinal versus general.[128] More sensitive measures of neurologic and behavioral function, such as the Scanlon Early Neonatal Neurobehavioral Scale and the Neurologic and Adaptive Capacities Score (NACS) indicate some transient depression of scores following general anesthesia that resolves at 24 hours after delivery.[128,129]

Neonatal brain development is a complicated yet intricate process of excess neuron generation followed by apoptosis (selective cell death).[130] The "threshold effect" for neurotoxicity has been established in in vivo neonatal murine models, with accelerated neuronal apoptosis and degenerative effects noted in the temporal/somatosensory cortices, frontal cortex, and hippocampus related to increasing anesthetic exposure.[130,131] Observed cognitive and behavioral deficits in these models have been associated with disturbances in neuronal circuitry, mitochondrial morphology, and dendritic spine development. In addition, sevoflurane has been demonstrated to produce the least neurodegeneration compared to equipotent exposures of isoflurane and desflurane.[130,132] It is unclear if the findings in rodents can be extrapolated to humans, as the period of peak vulnerability with rapid synaptogenesis in rodents is very brief and easily exposed to an anesthetic. The equivalent period in humans extends from mid-gestation to several years after birth.[133,134] Human retrospective observational studies have demonstrated higher rates of learning disorders and behavioral impairment among children with multiple exposures to anesthesia.[135] Interpretation of these studies is limited by the ability to distinguish between anesthetic-induced neurotoxicity and confounders such as comorbidity, and the stresses of surgery and hospitalization. Prospective trials are currently ongoing and may impact future practice.[136,137]

Anesthetic Degradation by Carbon Dioxide Absorbers

Compound A

Sevoflurane undergoes base-catalyzed degradation in carbon dioxide absorbers to form a vinyl ether called *compound A*. The production of compound A is enhanced in low flow or closed circuit breathing systems and by warm or very dry CO_2 absorbents.[138,139] Dessicated barium hydroxide lime produces more compound A than soda lime and this can be attributed to slightly higher absorbent temperature during CO_2 extraction.[140] Desiccated barium hydroxide lime also has been implicated in the heat and fires associated with sevoflurane, discussed later. This absorbent has been removed from the US market.

In patients and volunteers receiving sevoflurane in closed circuit or low-flow delivery systems, inspired compound A concentrations averaged 8 to 24 ppm and 20 to 32 ppm with soda lime and barium hydroxide lime, respectively.[141-144] Total exposures as high as 320 to 400 ppm/hr have had no clear effect on clinical markers of renal function.[145-147] In randomized and prospective volunteer and patient studies, no adverse renal effects from low-flow (0.5 to 1.0 L/min) or closed circuit sevoflurane anesthesia were detected using both standard clinical markers of renal function (serum creatinine and blood urea nitrogen concentrations) and experimental markers of renal function and structural integrity (proteinuria, glucosuria, and enzymuria).[142-144,146,148-150] In a prospective, multicenter, randomized study in patients with preexisting renal disease, there were no adverse renal effects of long duration, low-flow sevoflurane.[151,152] The majority of countries that have approved sevoflurane for clinical use have no flow restriction, perhaps because of the proven safety of sevoflurane in scientific studies. Pharmacovigilance supports the science; there has not been a single case report of renal injury directly attributable to sevoflurane after nearly two decades of use.

One explanation for the inconsistency between the early rat studies and human studies in terms of renal injury from compound A may be related to species differences in the metabolism of compound A. The biodegradation of compound A to a cysteine conjugates and the further action of a renal enzyme called β-lyase on the conjugates can result in formation of a potentially toxic thiol. The β-lyase-dependent metabolism pathway in humans is far less extensive than the β-lyase pathway in rats (8 to 30 times less active).[153] Thus, compared with rats, humans (1) receive markedly lower doses of compound A, (2) metabolize a lower fraction of compound A via the renal β-lyase pathway, and (3) have not suffered renal injury.

Carbon Monoxide and Heat

Carbon dioxide (CO_2) absorbents degrade sevoflurane, desflurane, and isoflurane to carbon monoxide (CO) when the normal water content of the absorbent (13% to 15%) is markedly decreased to less than 5%.[154-156] The degradation is the result of an exothermic reaction of the anesthetics with the absorbent. There are no clinically useful humidification detectors in current systems that house the CO_2 absorbents on modern day anesthetic machines. Formation of CO is dependent on both the anesthetic molecular structure and the presence of a strong base in the carbon dioxide absorbent.[155] Desflurane and isoflurane contain a difluoromethoxy moiety that is essential for the formation of CO. When studies are conducted with dry CO_2 absorbents maintained at or just above room temperature, desflurane given at just under 1 MAC produced up to 8,000 ppm of CO versus 79 ppm with nearly 2 MAC sevoflurane.[156] In desiccated barium hydroxide, CO production from desflurane was nearly threefold higher than with soda lime. Instances of CO poisoning of patients have been reported in situations where the CO_2 absorbent presumably has been desiccated because an anesthetic machine had been left on with a high FGF passing through the CO_2 absorbent over an extended period of time.[157-160] In an experimental setting, drying of barium hydroxide with 10 L/min FGF for 24 hours resulted in significant CO production from desflurane, whereas 14 hours of drying did not result in CO production from desflurane.[161]

Higher temperatures of the CO_2 absorbents can promote CO formation. Lower FGFs increase the normal (25 to 45°C) canister temperature. In a laboratory setting where sevoflurane was administered through desiccated barium hydroxide, the exothermic reaction increased canister temperature above 80°C, resulting in significant CO production.[154] Although desflurane produces the most CO with desiccated CO_2 absorbers, the reaction with sevoflurane produces the most heat.[162] The strong exothermic reaction with significant heat production has caused fires and patient injuries.[163-165] Although sevoflurane is not flammable at up to 11% concentrations, other heat-induced degradation products, for example, formaldehyde, methanol, and formate have been identified,[166] and these alone or in combination with oxygen might be flammable at high canister temperatures. An important safety initiative in the United States has led to the removal of barium hydroxide as a CO_2 absorbent from the anesthesia marketplace.

There are newer CO_2 absorbents that do not degrade anesthetics (to either compound A or CO), and they reduce exothermic reactions (Figure 18-24).[167] Although they have a lower CO_2 absorptive capacity than soda lime, their benefit may be substantial. Adoption of these new absorbents into routine clinical practice is consistent with the patient safety goals of our anesthesia society.

Generic Sevoflurane Formulations

Generic formulations of sevoflurane were introduced into the clinical market in 2006. The methods for synthesizing sevoflurane differ between manufacturers.[168] Although the active ingredient of sevoflurane from different manufacturers is chemically equivalent, the water content in the formulations differs and this accounts for their different resistances to degradation when exposed to a Lewis acid (metal halides and metal oxides that are present in modern-day vaporizers). Adding water to the formulation inhibits the action of Lewis acids to degrade sevoflurane to hydrofluoric acid. Shortly after Abbott Labs introduced sevoflurane to the US market in 1995, the formulation of sevoflurane

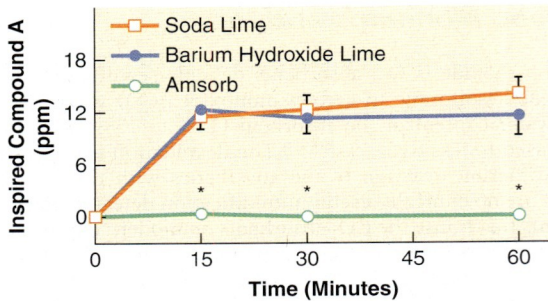

Figure 18-24 Compound A levels produced from three non-dessicated carbon dioxide absorbents during 1 minimum alveolar concentration sevoflurane anesthesia delivered to volunteers at 1 L/min fresh gas flow (mean ± SE). Gas samples were taken from the inspired limb of the anesthesia circuit. *Different from barium hydroxide lime or soda lime ($p < 0.05$). (Adapted from Mchaourab A, Arain SR, Ebert TJ. Lack of degradation of sevoflurane by a new carbon dioxide absorbent in humans. *Anesthesiology.* 2001;94:1007.)

was changed to contain 300 to 400 ppm of water, based on an adverse experience with hydrofluoric acid formation from their original low water formulation. One generic formulation with a low water content has been shown in clinical and laboratory studies to degrade to toxic and corrosive hydrogen fluoride.[169] Whether these differences in formulation lead to patient safety issues remains to be determined.

Anesthetic Metabolism

Fluoride-induced Nephrotoxicity

The metabolism of anesthetic gases has the potential to adversely affect organs via toxicity from the metabolite. For example, enflurane metabolism results in a well-described injury to renal collecting tubules.[170,171] The nephrotoxicity has been attributed to an increase in plasma fluoride and presents as a renal concentrating defect that is unresponsive to vasopressin and is characterized by dilute polyuria, dehydration, serum hypernatremia, hyperosmolality, elevated blood urea nitrogen, and creatinine. The traditional "fluoride toxicity" hypothesis stated that both the duration of the high systemic fluoride concentrations (area under the fluoride-time curve) and the peak fluoride concentration (peaks above 50 μM appear to represent the toxic threshold) were related to nephrotoxicity. Sevoflurane undergoes 5% metabolism leading to transient increases in serum fluoride concentrations without a renal-concentrating defect. The safety of sevoflurane may be the result of a rapid decline in plasma fluoride concentrations because of less availability of the anesthetic for metabolism from a fast elimination compared with enflurane.[172] In addition, renal defluorination of sevoflurane is minimal and may add to the absence of an adverse renal-concentrating effect.[173]

Clinical Utility of Volatile Anesthetics

For Induction of Anesthesia

The appeal of mask induction in the adult population centers on the potential safety and utility of this technique.[174–176] Sevoflurane is potent, poorly soluble in blood, nonpungent, and therefore inhaled easily. Spontaneous ventilation is preserved with a gas induction since patients essentially regulate their own depth of anesthesia (too much sevoflurane would suppress ventilation). Clinical studies indicate that stage two excitation is avoided with high concentrations of sevoflurane. The typical time to loss of consciousness is 60 seconds when delivering 8% sevoflurane via the face mask. Sevoflurane also has been administered by mask as an approach to the difficult adult airway because it preserves spontaneous ventilation and does not cause salivation.[177] Laryngeal mask placement can be successfully achieved 2 minutes after administering 7% sevoflurane via the face mask.[176] The addition of N_2O to the inspired gas mixture does not add significantly to the induction sequence. The gas induction technique is improved by pretreatment with benzodiazepines and worsened with opioid pretreatment because of apnea.[175] Importantly, patient acceptance of this technique has been relatively high, exceeding 90%.[174]

For Maintenance of Anesthesia

The volatile anesthetics are clearly the most popular drug used to maintain anesthesia. They are easily administered via inhalation, they are readily titrated, they have a high safety ratio in terms of preventing recall, and the depth of anesthesia can be quickly adjusted in a predictable way while monitoring tissue levels via end-tidal concentrations. They are effective regardless of age or body habitus. They have some properties that prove beneficial in the operating room, including relaxation of skeletal muscle, preservation of cardiac output and CBF, relatively predictable recovery profiles, and organ protection from ischemic injury. Some of the drawbacks to the use of the current volatile anesthetics are the absence of analgesic effects, their association with postoperative nausea and vomiting, their potential for carbon monoxide poisoning and hepatitis, their ability to induce neuroapoptosis leading to memory deficits in neonatal animal models, and greenhouse gas effects adding to the potential for global warming.[178–180]

REFERENCES

1. Kety SS. The physiological and physical factors governing the uptake of anesthetic gases by the body. *Anesthesiology.* 1950;11:517.
2. Eger EI. *Anesthetic Uptake and Action.* Baltimore, MD: Williams & Wilkins; 1974.
3. Ebert TJ, Robinson BJ, Uhrich TD, et al. Recovery from sevoflurane anesthesia: a comparison to isoflurane and propofol anesthesia. *Anesthesiology.* 1998;89(6):1524–1531.
4. McKay RE, Malhotra A, Cakmakkaya OS, et al. Effect of increased body mass index and anaesthetic duration on recovery of protective airway reflexes after sevoflurane vs desflurane. *Br J Anaesth.* 2010;104(2):175–182.
5. Law LS, Lo EA, Gan TJ. Xenon anesthesia: A systematic review and meta-analysis of randomized controlled trials. *Anesth Analg.* 2016;122:678–697.
6. Schaefer W, Meyer PT, Rossaint R, et al. Myocardial blood flow during general anesthesia with xenon in humans: a positron emission tomography study. *Anesthesiology.* 2011;114(6):1373–1379.
7. Schallner N, Goebel U. The perioperative use of nitrous oxide: renaissance of an old gas or funeral of an ancient relic? *Curr Opin Anaesthesiol.* 2013;26(3):354–360.
8. Waun JE, Sweitzer RS, Hamilton WK. Effect of nitrous oxide on middle ear mechanics and hearing acuity. *Anesthesiology.* 1987;28:846–850.
9. Tinker JH, Sharbrough FW, Michenfelder JD. Anterior shift of the dominant EEG rhythm during anesthesia in the Java monkey: correlation with anesthetic potency. *Anesthesiology.* 1977;46:252–259.
10. Katoh T, Suguro Y, Kimura T, et al. Cerebral awakening concentration of sevoflurane and isoflurane predicted during slow and fast alveolar washout. *Anesth Analg.* 1993;77:1012–1017.
11. Roizen MF, Horrigan RW, Frazer BM. Anesthetic doses blocking adrenergic (stress) and cardiovascular responses to incision–MAC BAR. *Anesthesiology.* 1981;54(5):390–398.
12. Liem EB, Lin C, Suleman M, et al. Anesthetic requirement is increased in redheads. *Anesthesiology.* 2004;101:279–283.

13. Stekiel TA, Contney SJ, Bosnjak ZJ, et al. Reversal of minimum alveolar concentrations of volatile anesthetics by chromosomal substitution. *Anesthesiology*. 2004;101:796–798.
14. Mapleson WW. Effect of age on MAC in humans: a meta-analysis. *Br J Anaesth*. 1996;76:179–185.
15. Smith AL, Wollman H. Cerebral blood flow and metabolism: Effects of anesthetic drugs and techniques. *Anesthesiology*. 1972;36:378–400.
16. Lutz LJ, Milde JH, Milde LN. The cerebral functional, metabolic, and hemodynamic effects of desflurane in dogs. *Anesthesiology*. 1990;73:125–131.
17. Scheller MS, Nakakimura K, Fleischer JE, et al. Cerebral effects of sevoflurane in the dog: Comparison with isoflurane and enflurane. *Br J Anaesth*. 1990; 65(3):388–392.
18. Fujibayashi T, Sugiura Y, Yanagimoto M, et al. Brain energy metabolism and blood flow during sevoflurane and halothane anesthesia: effects of hypocapnia and blood pressure fluctuations. *Acta Anaesthesiol Scand*. 1994;38:413–418.
19. Yli-Hankala A, Vakkuri A, Särkelä M, et al. Epileptiform electroencephalogram during mask induction of anesthesia with sevoflurane. *Anesthesiology*. 1999;91:1596–1603.
20. Julliac B, Guehl D, Chopin F, et al. Risk factors for the occurrence of electroencephalogram abnormalities during induction of anesthesia with sevoflurane in nonepileptic patients. *Anesthesiology*. 2007;106(2):243–251.
21. Hisada K, Morioka T, Fukui K, et al. Effects of sevoflurane and isoflurane on electrocorticographic activities in patients with temporal lobe epilepsy. *J Neurosurg Anesthesiol*. 2001;13:333–337.
22. Algotsson L, Messeter K, Nordström CH, et al. Cerebral blood flow and oxygen consumption during isoflurane and halothane anesthesia in man. *Acta Anaesthesiol Scand*. 1988;32:15–20.
23. Summors AC, Gupta AK, Matta BF. Dynamic cerebral autoregulation during sevoflurane anesthesia: a comparison with isoflurane. *Anesth Analg*. 1999;88:341–345.
24. Strebel S, Lam A, Matta B, et al. Dynamic and static cerebral autoregulation during isoflurane, desflurane, and propofol anesthesia. *Anesthesiology*. 1995;83:66–76.
25. Lutz LJ, Milde JH, Milde LN. The response of the canine cerebral circulation to hyperventilation during anesthesia with desflurane. *Anesthesiology*. 1991; 74:504–507.
26. Adams RW, Cucchiara RF, Gronert GA, et al. Isoflurane and cerebrospinal fluid pressure in neurosurgical patients. *Anesthesiology*. 1981;54(2):97–99.
27. Grosslight K, Foster R, Colohan AR, et al. Isoflurane for neuroanesthesia: risk factors for increases in intracranial pressure. *Anesthesiology*. 1985;63: 533–536.
28. Talke P, Caldwell JE, Richardson CA. Sevoflurane increases lumbar cerebrospinal fluid pressure in normocapnic patients undergoing transsphenoidal hypophysectomy. *Anesthesiology*. 1999;91:127–130.
29. Talke P, Caldwell J, Dodsont B, et al. Desflurane and isoflurane increases lumbar cerebrospinal fluid pressure in normocapnic patients undergoing transsphenoidal hypophysectomy. *Anesthesiology*. 1996;85:999–1004.
30. Muzzi DA, Losasso TJ, Dietz NM, et al. The effect of desflurane and isoflurane on cerebrospinal fluid pressure in humans with supratentorial mass lesions. *Anesthesiology*. 1992;76:720–724.
31. Sponheim S, Skraastad Ø, Helseth E, et al. Effects of 0.5 and 1.0 MAC isoflurane, sevoflurane and desflurane on intracranial and cerebral perfusion pressures in children. *Acta Anaesthesiol Scand*. 2003;47:932–938.
32. Drummond JC, Todd MM, Toutant SM, et al. Brain surface protrusion during enflurane, halothane, and isoflurane anesthesia in cats. *Anesthesiology*. 1983;59(4):288–293.
33. Bundgaard H, von Oettingen G, Larsen KM, et al. Effects of sevoflurane on intracranial pressure, cerebral blood flow and cerebral metabolism. *Acta Anaesthesiol Scand*. 1998;42:621–627.
34. Seyde WC, Longnecker DE. Cerebral oxygen tension in rats during deliberate hypotension with sodium nitroprusside, 2-chloroadenosine, or deep isoflurane anesthesia. *Anesthesiology*. 1986;64:480–485.
35. Engelhard K, Werner C, Reeker W, et al. Desflurane and isoflurane improve neurological outcome after incomplete cerebral ischaemia in rats. *Br J Anaesth*. 1999;83:415–421.
36. Werner C, Möllenberg O, Kochs E, et al. Sevoflurane improves neurological outcome after incomplete cerebral ischaemia in rats. *Br J Anaesth*. 1995; 75:756–760.
37. Loepke AW, Priestley MA, Schultz SE, et al. Desflurane improves neurologic outcome after low-flow cardiopulmonary bypass in newborn pigs. *Anesthesiology*. 2002;97:1521–1527.
38. Hoffman WE, Charbel FT, Edelman G, et al. Thiopental and desflurane treatment for brain protection. *Neurosurgery*. 1998;43(5):1050–1053.
39. Engelhard K, Werner C. Postoperative cognitive dysfunction. *Anaesthesist*. 2005;54(6):588–594.
40. Tsai SK, Lee C, Kwan W, et al. Recovery of cognitive functions after anaesthesia with desflurane or isoflurane and nitrous oxide. *Br J Anaesth*. 1992;69: 255–258.
41. Chen X, Zhao M, White PF, et al. The recovery of cognitive function after general anesthesia in elderly patients: a comparison of desflurane and sevoflurane. *Anesth Analg*. 2001;93:1489–1494.
42. Kanbak M, Saricaoglu F, Akinci SB, et al. The effects of isoflurane, sevoflurane, and desflurane anesthesia on neurocognitive outcome after cardiac surgery: a pilot study. *Heart Surg Forum*. 2007;10(1):E36–E41.
43. Mahoney FC, Moore PA, Baker EL, et al. Experimental nitrous oxide exposure as a model system for evaluating neurobehavioral tests. *Toxicology*. 1988; 49(2–3):449–457.
44. Leung JM, Sands LP, Vaurio LE, et al. Nitrous oxide does not change the incidence of postoperative delirium or cognitive decline in elderly surgical patients. *Br J Anaesth*. 2006;96(6):754–760.
45. Bracco D, Hemmerling TM. Nitrous oxide: from neurotoxicity to neuroprotection? *Crit Care Med*. 2008;36(9):2705–2706.
46. Ebert TJ, Muzi M, Lopatka CW. Neurocirculatory responses to sevoflurane in humans: a comparison to desflurane. *Anesthesiology*. 1995;83:88–95.
47. Malan TP Jr, DiNardo JA, Isner RJ, et al. Cardiovascular effects of sevoflurane compared with those of isoflurane in volunteers. *Anesthesiology*. 1995; 83:918–928.
48. Weiskopf RB, Cahalan MK, Eger EI, II, et al. Cardiovascular actions of desflurane in normocarbic volunteers. *Anesth Analg*. 1991;73:143–156.
49. Stevens WC, Cromwell TH, Halsey MJ, et al. The cardiovascular effects of a new inhalation anesthetic, Forane, in human volunteers at a constant arterial carbon dioxide tension. *Anesthesiology*. 1971;35:8–16.
50. Ebert TJ, Kampine JP. Nitrous oxide augments sympathetic outflow: direct evidence from human peroneal nerve recordings. *Anesth Analg*. 1989;69:444–449.
51. Ebert TJ, Muzi M. Sympathetic hyperactivity during desflurane anesthesia in healthy volunteers: a comparison with isoflurane. *Anesthesiology*. 1993;79: 444–453.
52. Weiskopf RB, Moore MA, Eger EI, II, et al. Rapid increase in desflurane concentration is associated with greater transient cardiovascular stimulation than with rapid increase in isoflurane concentration in humans. *Anesthesiology*. 1994;80:1035–1045.
53. Muzi M, Ebert TJ, Hope WG, et al. Site(s) mediating sympathetic activation with desflurane. *Anesthesiology*. 1996;85:737–747.
54. Yonker-Sell AE, Muzi M, Hope WG, et al. Alfentanil modifies the neurocirculatory responses to desflurane. *Anesth Analg*. 1996;82:162–166.
55. Pacentine GG, Muzi M, Ebert TJ. Effects of fentanyl on sympathetic activation associated with the administration of desflurane. *Anesthesiology*. 1995;82:823–831.
56. Devcic A, Muzi M, Ebert TJ. The effects of clonidine on desflurane-mediated sympatho-excitation in humans. *Anesth Analg*. 1995;80:773–779.
57. De Hert SG, Van der Linden PJ, ten Broecke PW, et al. Effects of desflurane and sevoflurane on length-dependent regulation of myocardial function in coronary surgery patients. *Anesthesiology*. 2001;95(2):357–363.
58. De Hert SG, Cromheecke S, ten Broecke PW, et al. Effects of propofol, desflurane, and sevoflurane on recovery of myocardial function after coronary surgery in elderly high-risk patients. *Anesthesiology*. 2003;99:314–323.
59. Bolliger D, Seeberger MD, Kasper J, et al. Different effects of sevoflurane, desflurane, and isoflurane on early and late left ventricular diastolic function in young healthy adults. *Br J Anaesth*. 2010;104(5):547–554.
60. Weiskopf RB, Cahalan MK, Ionescu P, et al. Cardiovascular actions of desflurane with and without nitrous oxide during spontaneous ventilation in humans. *Anesth Analg*. 1991;73:165–174.
61. Cahalan MK, Weiskopf RB, Eger EI,II, et al. Hemodynamic effects of desflurane/nitrous oxide anesthesia in volunteers. *Anesth Analg*. 1991;73:157–164.
62. Theye RA, Michenfelder JD. Whole-body and organ VO_2 changes with enflurane, isoflurane, and halothane. *Br J Anaesth*. 1975;47(8):813–817.
63. Crawford MW, Lerman J, Pilato M, et al. Haemodynamic and organ blood flow responses to sevoflurane during spontaneous ventilation in the rat: a dose-response study. *Can J Anaesth*. 1992;39(3):270–276.
64. Ebert TJ, Harkin CP, Muzi M. Cardiovascular responses to sevoflurane: a review. *Anesth Analg*. 1995;81:S11–S22.
65. Atlee J.L. III, Bosnjak ZJ. Mechanisms for cardiac dysrhythmias during anesthesia. *Anesthesiology*. 1990;72(2):347–374.
66. Saussine M, Massad I, Raczka F, et al. Torsade de pointes during sevoflurane anesthesia in a child with congenital long QT syndrome. *Paediatr Anaesth*. 2006;16(1):63–65.
67. Aypar E, Karagoz AH, Ozer S, et al. The effects of sevoflurane and desflurane anesthesia on QTc interval and cardiac rhythm in children. *Paediatr Anaesth*. 2007;17(6):563–567.
68. Kazanci D, Unver S, Karadeniz U, et al. A comparison of the effects of desflurane, sevoflurane and propofol on QT, QTc, and P dispersion on ECG. *Ann Card Anaesth*. 2009;12(2):107–112.
69. Slogoff S, Keats AS, Dear WE, et al. Steal-prone coronary anatomy and myocardial ischemia associated with four primary anesthetic agents in humans. *Anesth Analg*. 1991;72:22–27.
70. Tuman KJ, McCarthy RJ, Spiess BD, et al. Does choice of anesthetic agent significantly affect outcome after coronary artery surgery? *Anesthesiology*. 1989;70:189–198.
71. Hartman JC, Pagel PS, Kampine JP, et al. Influence of desflurane on regional distribution of coronary blood flow in a chronically instrumented canine model of multivessel coronary artery obstruction. *Anesth Analg*. 1991;72: 289–299.

72. Hartman JC, Kampine JP, Schmeling WT, et al. Steal-prone coronary circulation in chronically instrumented dogs: isoflurane versus adenosine. *Anesthesiology.* 1991;74:744–756.
73. Kersten JR, Brayer AP, Pagel PS, et al. Perfusion of ischemic myocardium during anesthesia with sevoflurane. *Anesthesiology.* 1994;81:995–1004.
74. Ebert TJ, Kharasch ED, Rooke GA, et al. Myocardial ischemia and adverse cardiac outcomes in cardiac patients undergoing noncardiac surgery with sevoflurane and isoflurane. *Anesth Analg.* 1997;85:993–999.
75. Searle NR, Martineau RJ, Conzen P, et al. Comparison of sevoflurane/fentanyl and isoflurane/fentanyl during elective coronary artery bypass surgery. *Can J Anaesth.* 1996;43:890–899.
76. Thomson IR, Bowering JB, Hudson RJ, et al. A comparison of desflurane and isoflurane in patients undergoing coronary artery surgery. *Anesthesiology.* 1991;75:776–781.
77. Helman JD, Leung JM, Bellows WH, et al. The risk of myocardial ischemia in patients receiving desflurane versus sufentanil anesthesia for coronary artery bypass graft surgery. *Anesthesiology.* 1992;77:47–62.
78. Swyers T, Redford D, Larson DF. Volatile anesthetic-induced preconditioning. *Perfusion.* 2014;29(1):10–15.
79. Lotz C, Kehl F. Volatile anesthetic-induced cardiac protection: molecular mechanisms, clinical aspects, and interactions with nonvolatile agents. *J Cardiothorac Vasc Anesth.* 2015;29(3):749–760.
80. Riess ML, Stowe DF, Warltier DC. Cardiac pharmacological preconditioning with volatile anesthetics: from bench to bedside? *Am J Physiol.* 2004;286: H1603–H607.
81. Stowe DF, Kevin LG. Cardiac preconditioning by volatile anesthetic agents: a defining role for altered mitochondrial bioenergetics. *Antioxid Redox Signal.* 2004;6:439–448.
82. Novalija E, Kevin LG, Camara AK, et al. Reactive oxygen species precede the epsilon isoform of protein kinase C in the anesthetic preconditioning signaling cascade. *Anesthesiology.* 2003;99:421–428.
83. Kwok WM, Martinelli AT, Fujimoto K, et al. Differential modulation of the cardiac adenosine triphosphate-sensitive potassium channel by isoflurane and halothane. *Anesthesiology.* 2002;97:50–56.
84. Kevin LG, Katz P, Camara AK, et al. Anesthetic preconditioning: effects on latency to ischemic injury in isolated hearts. *Anesthesiology.* 2003;99:385–391.
85. De Hert SG, Turani F, Mathur S, et al. Cardioprotection with volatile anesthetics: mechanisms and clinical implications. *Anesth Analg.* 2005;100(6):1584–1593.
86. Yu CH, Beattie WS. The effects of volatile anesthetics on cardiac ischemic complications and mortality in CABG: a meta-analysis. *Can J Anaesth.* 2006; 53(9):906–918.
87. Landoni G, Biondi-Zoccai GG, Zangrillo A, et al. Desflurane and sevoflurane in cardiac surgery: a meta-analysis of randomized clinical trials. *J Cardiothorac Vasc Anesth.* 2007;21(4):502–511.
88. Gu W, Pagel PS, Warltier DC, et al. Modifying cardiovascular risk in diabetes mellitus. *Anesthesiology.* 2003;98:774–779.
89. Clarkson AN. Anesthetic-mediated protection/preconditioning during cerebral ischemia. *Life Sci.* 2007;80(13):1157–1175.
90. Lee HT, Ota-Setlik A, Fu Y, et al. Differential protective effects of volatile anesthetics against renal ischemia-reperfusion injury in vivo. *Anesthesiology.* 2004;101(6):1313–1324.
91. Lorsomradee S, Cromheecke S, Lorsomradee S, et al. Effects of sevoflurane on biomechanical markers of hepatic and renal dysfunction after coronary artery surgery. *J Cardiothorac Vasc Anesth.* 2006;20(5):684–690.
92. Ma D, Lim T, Xu J, et al. Xenon preconditioning protects against renal ischemic-reperfusion injury via HIF-1alpha activation. *J Am Soc Nephrol.* 2009;20(4):713–720.
93. Muzi M, Ebert TJ. A randomized, prospective comparison of halothane, isoflurane and enflurane on baroreflex control of heart rate in humans. In: Bosnjak Z, Kampine JP, eds. *Advances in Pharmacology. Vol. 31: Anesthesia and Cardiovascular Disease.* San Diego, CA: Academic Press; 1994:379–387.
94. Muzi M, Ebert TJ. A comparison of baroreflex sensitivity during isoflurane and desflurane anesthesia in humans. *Anesthesiology.* 1995;82:919–925.
95. Ebert TJ, Perez F, Uhrich TD, et al. Desflurane-mediated sympathetic activation occurs in humans despite preventing hypotension and baroreceptor unloading. *Anesthesiology.* 1998;88(5):1227–1232.
96. Tanaka M, Nishikawa T. Arterial baroreflex function in humans anaesthetized with sevoflurane. *Br J Anaesth.* 1999;82:350–354.
97. Muzi M, Lopatka CW, Ebert TJ. Desflurane-mediated neurocirculatory activation in humans: Effects of concentration and rate of change on responses. *Anesthesiology.* 1996;84:1035–1042.
98. Hirshman CA, Bergman NA. Factors influencing intrapulmonary airway calibre during anaesthesia. *Br J Anaesth.* 1990;65:30–42.
99. Hirshman CA, Edelstein G, Peetz S, et al. Mechanism of action of inhalational anesthesia on airways. *Anesthesiology.* 1982;56:107–111.
100. Park KW, Dai HB, Lowenstein E, et al. Epithelial dependence of the bronchodilatory effect of sevoflurane and desflurane in rat distal bronchi. *Anesth Analg.* 1998;86:646–651.
101. Goff MJ, Arain SR, Ficke DJ, et al. Absence of bronchodilation during desflurane anesthesia: A comparison to sevoflurane and thiopental. *Anesthesiology.* 2000;93:404–408.
102. Nyktari V, Papaioannou A, Volakakis N, et al. Respiratory resistance during anaesthesia with isoflurane, sevoflurane, and desflurane: a randomized clinical trial. *Br J Anaesth.* 2011;107(3):454–461.
103. Ng D, Fahimi J, Hern HG. Sevoflurane administration initiated out of the ED for life-threatening status asthmaticus. *Am J Emerg Med.* 2015;33(8):1110. e3–1110.e6.
104. Volta CA, Alvisi V, Petrini S, et al. The effect of volatile anesthetics on respiratory system resistance in patients with chronic obstructive pulmonary disease. *Anesth Analg.* 2005;100(2):348–353.
105. Ledowski T, Manopas A, Lauer S. Bronchial mucus transport velocity in patients receiving desflurane and fentanyl vs. sevoflurane and fentanyl. *Eur J Anaesthesiol.* 2008;25(9):752–755.
106. Reiz S. Nitrous oxide augments the systemic and coronary haemodynamic effects of isoflurane in patients with ischaemic heart disease. *Acta Anaesthesiol Scand.* 1983;27:464–469.
107. Pagel PS, Fu JL, Damask MC, et al. Desflurane and isoflurane produce similar alterations in systemic and pulmonary hemodynamics and arterial oxygenation in patients undergoing one-lung ventilation during thoracotomy. *Anesth Analg.* 1998;87:800–807.
108. Kurahashi K, Maruta H. The effect of sevoflurane and isoflurane on the neuromuscular block produced by vecuronium continuous infusion. *Anesth Analg.* 1996;82:942–947.
109. Wulf H, Kahl M, Ledowski T. Augmentation of the neuromuscular blocking effects of cisatracurium during desflurane, sevoflurane, isoflurane or total i.v. anaesthesia. *Br J Anaesth.* 1998;80:308–312.
110. Nitahara K, Sugi Y, Higa K, et al. Neuromuscular effects of sevoflurane in myasthenia gravis patients. *Br J Anaesth.* 2007;98:337–341.
111. Bock M, Klippel K, Nitsche B, et al. Rocuronium potency and recovery characteristics during steady-state desflurane, sevoflurane, isoflurane or propofol anaesthesia. *Br J Anaesth.* 2000;84:43–47.
112. Paul M, Fokt RM, Kindler CH, et al. Characterization of the interactions between volatile anesthetics and neuromuscular blockers at the muscle nicotinic acetylcholine receptor. *Anesth Analg.* 2002;95:362–367.
113. Wright PMC, Hart P, Lau M, et al. The magnitude and time course of vecuronium potentiation by desflurane versus isoflurane. *Anesthesiology.* 1995; 82:404–411.
114. Rosenberg H, Pollock N, Schiemann A, et al. Malignant hyperthermia: a review. *Orphanet J Rare Dis.* 2015;10:93.
115. Wappler F. Anesthesia for patients with a history of malignant hyperthermia. *Curr Opin Anaesthesiol.* 2010;23(3):417–422.
116. Carlomagno M, Esposito C, Marra A, et al. Xenon anaesthesia in a patient with susceptibility to malignant hyperthermia: a case report. *Eur J Anaesthesiol.* 2016;33(2):147–150.
117. Krause T, Scholz J, Jansen L, et al. Sevoflurane anaesthesia does not induce the formation of sister chromatid exchanges in peripheral blood lymphocytes of children. *Br J Anaesth.* 2003;90:233–235.
118. Akin A, Ugur F, Ozkul Y, et al. Desflurane anaesthesia increases sister chromatid exchanges in human lymphocytes. *Acta Anaesthesiol Scand.* 2005;49: 1559–1561.
119. Eroglu A, Celep F, Erciyes N. A comparison of sister chromatid exchanges in lymphocytes of anesthesiologists to nonanesthesiologists in the same hospital. *Anesth Analg.* 2006;102:1573–1577.
120. Wiesner G, Schiewe-Langgartner F, Lindner R, et al. Increased formation of sister chromatid exchanges, but not of micronuclei, in anaesthetists exposed to low levels of sevoflurane. *Anaesthesia.* 2008;63(8):861–864.
121. Mazze RI, Wilson AI, Rice SA, et al. Fetal development in mice exposed to isoflurane. *Teratology.* 1985;32(3):339–345.
122. Mazze RI, Källén B. Reproductive outcome after anesthesia and operation during pregnancy: a registry study of 5405 cases. *Am J Obstet Gynecol.* 1989; 161(5):1178–1185.
123. Layzer RB, Fishman RA, Schafer JA. Neuropathy following use of nitrous oxide. *Neurology.* 1978;28:504–506.
124. Yildiz K, Dogru K, Dalgic H, et al. Inhibitory effects of desflurane and sevoflurane on oxytocin-induced contractions of isolated pregnant human myometrium. *Acta Anaesthesiol Scand.* 2005;49:1355–1359.
125. Abboud TK, Zhu J, Richardson M, et al. Desflurane: a new volatile anesthetic for cesarean section: maternal and neonatal effects. *Acta Anaesthesiol Scand.* 1995;39:723–726.
126. Lane GA, Nahrwold ML, Tait AR. Anesthetics as teratogens: nitrous oxide is fetotoxic, xenon is not. *Science.* 1980;210:899–901.
127. McGregor DG. Occupational exposure to trace concentrations of waste anesthetic gases. *Mayo Clinic Proceedings.* 2000;75:273–277.
128. Abboud TK, Nagappala S, Murakawa K, et al. Comparison of the effects of general and regional anesthesia for cesarean section on neonatal neurologic and adaptive capacity scores. *Anesth Analg.* 1985;64:996–1000.
129. Warren TM, Datta S, Ostheimer GW, et al. Comparison of the maternal and neonatal effects of halothane, enflurane, and isoflurane for cesarean delivery. *Anesth Analg.* 1983;62(5):516–520.
130. Liang G, Ward C, Peng J, et al. Isoflurane causes greater neurodegeneration than an equivalent exposure of sevoflurane in the developing brain of neonatal mice. *Anesthesiology.* 2010;112(6):1325–1334.

131. Amrock LG, Starner ML, Murphy KL, Baxter MG. Long-term effects of single or multiple neonatal sevoflurane exposures on rat hippocampal ultrastructure. *Anesthesiology.* 2015;122(1):87–95.
132. Kodama M, Satoh Y, Otsubo Y, et al. Neonatal desflurane exposure induces more robust neuroapoptosis than do isoflurane and sevoflurane and impairs working memory. *Anesthesiology.* 2011;115(5):979–991.
133. Cheek TG, Baird E. Anesthesia for nonobstetric surgery: maternal and fetal considerations. *Clin Obstet Gynecol.* 2009;52(4):535–545.
134. Reitman E, Flood P. Anaesthetic considerations for non-obstetric surgery during pregnancy. *Br J Anaesth.* 2011;107(Suppl 1):i72–i78.
135. Gano D, Andersen SK, Glass HC, et al. Impaired cognitive performance in premature newborns with two or more surgeries prior to term-equivalent age. *Pediatr Res.* 2015;78(3):323–329.
136. Rappaport B, Mellon RD, Simone A, et al. Defining safe use of anesthesia in children. *N Engl J Med.* 2011;364(15):1387–1390.
137. Gleich S, Nemergut M, Flick R. Anesthetic-related neurotoxicity in young children: an update. *Curr Opin Anaesthesiol.* 2013;26(3):340–347.
138. Ruzicka JA, Hidalgo JC, Tinker JH, et al. Inhibition of volatile sevoflurane degradation product formation in an anesthesia circuit by a reduction in soda lime temperature. *Anesthesiology.* 1994;81:238–244.
139. Fang ZX, Kandel L, Laster MJ, et al. Factors affecting production of compound A from the interaction of sevoflurane with Baralyme and soda lime. *Anesth Analg.* 1996;82:775–781.
140. Frink EJ Jr, Malan TP, Morgan SE, et al. Quantification of the degradation products of sevoflurane in two CO_2 absorbents during low-flow anesthesia in surgical patients. *Anesthesiology.* 1992;77:1064–1069.
141. Ebert TJ, Arain SR. Renal responses to low-flow desflurane, sevoflurane, and propofol in patients. *Anesthesiology.* 2000;93:1401–1406.
142. Kharasch ED, Frink EJ Jr, Zager R, et al. Assessment of low-flow sevoflurane and isoflurane effects on renal function using sensitive markers of tubular toxicity. *Anesthesiology.* 1997;86:1238–1253.
143. Bito H, Ikeuchi Y, Ikeda K. Effects of low-flow sevoflurane anesthesia on renal function: comparison with high-flow sevoflurane anesthesia and low-flow isoflurane anesthesia. *Anesthesiology.* 1997;86:1231–1237.
144. Bito H, Ikeda K. Closed-circuit anesthesia with sevoflurane in humans. Effects on renal and hepatic function and concentrations of breakdown products with soda lime in the circuit. *Anesthesiology.* 1994;80:71–76.
145. Eger EI II, Koblin DD, Bowland T, et al. Nephrotoxicity of sevoflurane versus desflurane anesthesia in volunteers. *Anesth Analg.* 1997;84:160–168.
146. Ebert TJ, Messana LD, Uhrich TD, et al. Absence of renal and hepatic toxicity after four hours of 1.25 minimum alveolar concentration sevoflurane anesthesia in volunteers. *Anesth Analg.* 1998;86:662–667.
147. Eger EI II, Gong D, Koblin DD, et al. Dose-related biochemical markers of renal injury after sevoflurane versus desflurane anesthesia in volunteers. *Anesth Analg.* 1997;85:1154–1163.
148. Ebert TJ, Frink EJ Jr, Kharasch ED. Absence of biochemical evidence for renal and hepatic dysfunction after 8 hours of 1.25 minimum alveolar concentration sevoflurane anesthesia in volunteers. *Anesthesiology.* 1998;88(3):601–610.
149. Groudine SB, Fragen RJ, Kharasch ED, et al. Comparison of renal function following anesthesia with low-flow sevoflurane and isoflurane. *J Clin Anesth.* 1999;11:201–207.
150. Bito H, Ikeda K. Renal and hepatic function in surgical patients after low-flow sevoflurane or isoflurane anesthesia. *Anesth Analg.* 1996;82:173–176.
151. Conzen PF, Kharasch ED, Czerner SFA, et al. Low-flow sevoflurane compared with low-flow isoflurane anesthesia in patients with stable renal insufficiency. *Anesthesiology.* 2002;97(3):578–584.
152. Litz RJ, Hübler M, Lorenz W, et al. Renal responses to desflurane and isoflurane in patients with renal insufficiency. *Anesthesiology.* 2002;97:1133–1136.
153. Spracklin D, Kharasch ED. Evidence for the metabolism of fluoromethyl-1, 1-difluoro-1-(trifluoromethyl)vinyl ether (compound A), a sevoflurane degradation product, by cysteine conjugate b-lyase. *Chem Res Toxicol.* 1996;9:696–702.
154. Holak EJ, Mei DA, Dunning MB III, et al. Carbon monoxide production from sevoflurane breakdown: modeling of exposures under clinical conditions. *Anesth Analg.* 2003;96:757–764.
155. Baxter PJ, Garton K, Kharasch ED. Mechanistic aspects of carbon monoxide formation from volatile anesthetics. *Anesthesiology.* 1998;89:929–941.
156. Fang ZX, Eger EI II, Laster MJ, et al. Carbon monoxide production from degradation of desflurane, enflurane, isoflurane, halothane, and sevoflurane by soda lime and baralyme. *Anesth Analg.* 1995;80:1187–1193.
157. Berry PD, Sessler DI, Larson MD. Severe carbon monoxide poisoning during desflurane anesthesia. *Anesthesiology.* 1999;90(2):613–616.
158. Woehlck HJ. Severe intraoperative CO poisoning. *Anesthesiology.* 1999;90:353–354.
159. Woehlck HJ, Dunning M III, Gandhi S, et al. Indirect detection of intraoperative carbon monoxide exposure by mass spectrometry during isoflurane anesthesia. *Anesthesiology.* 1995;83:213–217.
160. Woehlck HJ, Dunning M, Connolly LA. Reduction in the incidence of carbon monoxide exposures in humans undergoing general anesthesia. *Anesthesiology.* 1997;87:228–234.
161. Woehlck HJ, Dunning M III, Raza T, et al. Physical factors affecting the production of carbon monoxide from anesthetic breakdown. *Anesthesiology.* 2001;94:453–456.
162. Wissing H, Kuhn I, Warnken U, et al. Carbon monoxide production from desflurane, enflurane, halothane, isoflurane and sevoflurane with dry soda lime. *Anesthesiology.* 2001;95:1205–1212.
163. Castro BA, Freedman LA, Craig WL, et al. Explosion within an anesthesia machine: Baralyme®, high fresh gas flows and sevoflurane concentration. *Anesthesiology.* 2004;101:537–539.
164. Wu J, Previte JP, Adler E, et al. Spontaneous ignition, explosion, and fire with sevoflurane and barium hydroxide lime. *Anesthesiology.* 2004;101:534–537.
165. Fatheree RS, Leighton BL. Acute respiratory distress syndrome after an exothermic Baralyme®-sevoflurane reaction. *Anesthesiology.* 2004;101:531–533.
166. Hanaki C, Fujii K, Morio M, et al. Decomposition of sevoflurane by sodalime. *Hiroshima J Med Sci.* 1987;36:61–67.
167. Kharasch ED. Putting the brakes on anesthetic breakdown. *Anesthesiology.* 1999;91:1192–1193.
168. Baker MT. Sevoflurane: are there differences in products?. *Anesth Analg.* 2007;104(6):1447–1451.
169. Kharasch ED, Subbarao GN, Cromack KR, et al. Sevoflurane formulation water content influences degradation by Lewis acids in vaporizers. *Anesth Analg.* 2009;108(6):1796–1802.
170. Frink EJ, Jr, Malan TP Jr, Isner RJ, et al. Renal concentrating function with prolonged sevoflurane or enflurane anesthesia in volunteers. *Anesthesiology.* 1994;80:1019–1025.
171. Mazze RI, Calverley RK, Smith NT. Inorganic fluoride nephrotoxicity: Prolonged enflurane and halothane anesthesia in volunteers. *Anesthesiology.* 1977;46:265–271.
172. Mazze RI. The safety of sevoflurane in humans. *Anesthesiology.* 1992;77:1062–1063.
173. Kharasch ED, Hankins DC, Thummel KE. Human kidney methoxyflurane and sevoflurane metabolism: intrarenal fluoride production as a possible mechanism of methoxyflurane nephrotoxicity. *Anesthesiology.* 1995;82:689–699.
174. Thwaites A, Edmends S, Smith I. Inhalation induction with sevoflurane: a double-blind comparison with propofol. *Br J Anaesth.* 1997;78:356–361.
175. Muzi M, Colinco MD, Robinson BJ, et al. The effects of premedication on inhaled induction of anesthesia with sevoflurane. *Anesth Analg.* 1997;85:1143–1148.
176. Muzi M, Robinson BJ, Ebert TJ, et al. Induction of anesthesia and tracheal intubation with sevoflurane in adults. *Anesthesiology.* 1996;85:536–543.
177. Mostafa SM, Atherton AMJ. Sevoflurane for difficult tracheal intubation. *Br J Anaesth.* 1997;79:392–393.
178. Ryan SM, Nielsen CJ. Global warming potential of inhaled anesthetics: application to clinical use. *Anesth Analg.* 2010;111(1):92–98.
179. Sulbaek Andersen MP, Nielsen OJ, Karpichev B, et al. Atmospheric chemistry of isoflurane, desflurane, and sevoflurane: kinetics and mechanisms of reactions with chlorine atoms and OH radicals and global warming potentials. *J Phys Chem A.* 2012;116(24):5806–5820.
180. Sulbaek Andersen MP, Sander SP, Nielsen OJ, et al. Inhalation anaesthetics and climate change. *Br J Anaesth.* 2010;105(6):760–766.
181. Yasuda N, Lockhart SH, Eger EI II, et al. Comparison of kinetics of sevoflurane and isoflurane in humans. *Anesth Analg.* 1991;72:316.
182. Yasuda N, Lockhart SH, Eger EI II, et al. Kinetics of desflurane, isoflurane, and halothane in humans. *Anesthesiology.* 1991;74:489.
183. Pagel PS, Kampine JP, Schmeling WT, et al. Influence of volatile anesthetics on myocardial contractility in vivo: Desflurane versus isoflurane. *Anesthesiology.* 1991;74:900.
184. Harkin CP, Pagel PS, Kersten JR, et al. Direct negative inotropic and lusitropic effects of sevoflurane. *Anesthesiology.* 1994;81:156.
185. Lockhart SH, Rampil IJ, Yasuda N, et al. Depression of ventilation by desflurane in humans. *Anesthesiology.* 1991;74:484.
186. Doi M, Ikeda K. Respiratory effects of sevoflurane. *Anesth Analg.* 1987;66:24.
187. Fourcade HE, Stevens WC, Larson CP Jr, et al. The ventilatory effects of Forane, a new inhaled anesthetic. *Anesthesiology.* 1971;35:26.
188. Eger EI II. *Isoflurane (Forane): a compendium and reference.* Madison, OH:Ohio Medical Products; 1985.
189. Bedforth NM, Hardman JG, Nathanson MH. Cerebral hemodynamic response to the introduction of desflurane: a comparison with sevoflurane. *Anesth Analg.* 2000;91:152.

19 Intravenous Anesthetics

RAMON ABOLA • SOFIA GERALEMOU • MARTIN SZAFRAN • TONG J. GAN

Pharmacokinetics: General Principles for Intravenous Anesthetics
Propofol
  Pharmacokinetics
  Pharmacodynamics
  Clinical Uses
  Side Effects
Etomidate
  Pharmacokinetics
  Pharmacodynamics and Clinical Uses
  Side Effects
Ketamine
  Pharmacokinetics
  Pharmacodynamics
  Clinical Uses
  Side Effects
Dexmedetomidine
  Pharmacokinetics
  Pharmacodynamics

  Clinical Uses
  Side Effects
Benzodiazepines
  Pharmacokinetics
  Pharmacodynamics and Clinical Uses
  Side Effects
Barbiturates
  Pharmacokinetics
  Pharmacodynamics
  Clinical Uses
  Side Effects
New Intravenous Anesthetics
  Remimazolam
  Propofol Formulations
  Fospropofol
  Cyclopropyl-methoxycarbonyl metomidate
  Sedasys

KEY POINTS

1. The ideal intravenous anesthetic would cause hypnosis and amnesia with a rapid onset, minimal cardiovascular and respiratory effects, and rapid metabolism.
2. Context-sensitive half-time is defined as the time to achieve a 50% reduction in concentration after stopping a continuous infusion. Context-sensitive half-time demonstrates the influence of the distributive process in governing drug disposition.
3. The mechanism by which the unconscious state is attained by propofol is complicated, but primarily occurs via enhancement of GABA inhibitory pathways.
4. The rapid and smooth induction and emergence from anesthesia helped transform propofol into an intravenous sedative-hypnotic that is a viable alternative to standard inhalational agents and other intravenous drugs.
5. Etomidate is a hemodynamically stable induction medication with a relatively large safety margin. Adrenocortical suppression is a recognized adverse effect of etomidate.
6. Ketamine causes "dissociative anesthesia" acting through the N-methyl-D-aspartate (NMDA) receptor, and is associated with nystagmus, significant analgesia, and unconsciousness.
7. Dexmedetomidine, an α_2 agonist, has been used for ICU sedation in mechanically ventilated patients, for procedural sedation, and as an adjunct to general anesthesia. Dexmedetomidine is unique as a sedative in that it has limited respiratory depressant effects.
8. Benzodiazepines are frequently used to produce several clinically desirable effects: anxiolysis, anterograde amnesia, sedation, and hypnosis.
9. The mechanism of action of barbiturates involves cortical and brainstem GABA inhibitory pathways, leading to loss of consciousness, as well as respiratory and cardiovascular depression.
10. New drugs are being developed in an effort to achieve the ideal intravenous anesthetic with a short duration of action, a short context-sensitive half-time that allows for infusion administration, and minimal adverse effects.

Pharmacokinetics: General Principles for Intravenous Anesthetics

Traditionally, intravenous anesthetics have been utilized for the induction of anesthesia. Thiopental was introduced into clinical practice in 1934 and was the gold standard for intravenous anesthetics for 50 years. Thiopental had a rapid, smooth onset of sedative and hypnotic effects, predictable pharmacokinetics, and a rapid and smooth emergence. However, thiopental has a long context-sensitive half-time that made it less ideal for use as an infusion. A review article from 1989 stated that the use of intravenous anesthetics for maintenance was unpopular because bolus administration resulted in swings in hemodynamics and anesthetic level.[1] The introductions of anesthetics with shorter durations (midazolam, propofol, remifentanil) and the development of variable rate infusion pumps allowed for routine use of intravenous anesthetics for maintenance. Combination of these modalities with a depth of anesthesia monitor has been utilized

Table 19-1 Properties of the Ideal Intravenous Anesthetic Agent
Pharmacodynamic/pharmacokinetic properties
Hypnosis and amnesia
Rapid onset (time of one arm–brain circulation)
Rapid metabolism to inactive metabolites
Minimal cardiovascular and respiratory depression
No histamine release or hypersensitivity reactions
Nontoxic, nonmutagenic, noncarcinogenic
No untoward neurologic effects, such as seizures, myoclonus, antanalgesia, neurotoxicity
Other beneficial effects: analgesia, antiemetic, neuroprotection, cardioprotection
Pharmacokinetic-based models to guide accurate dosing
Ability to continuously monitor delivery
Physiochemical properties
Water-soluble
Stable formulation, nonpyrogenic
Nonirritating: painless on intravenous injection
Small volume needed for induction
Inexpensive to prepare and formulate
Antimicrobial preparation

From Hemmings HC. The pharmacology of intravenous anesthetic induction agents: a primer. *Anesthesiol News*. 2010;October:9–16.

to create a closed-loop automated anesthesia delivery system. Intravenous anesthetics are now a key component of modern anesthesia practice.

No single anesthetic agent is perfect. The characteristics of the ideal intravenous anesthetic agent were described by Hemmings and are outlined in Table 19-1.[2] The ideal intravenous anesthetic would cause hypnosis and amnesia with a rapid onset (time of one arm–brain circulation), minimal cardiovascular and respiratory effects, and rapid metabolism. Propofol has become the new "gold standard" in anesthesia practice, with a rapid onset, rapid recovery after bolus administration from redistribution, and utility as a continuous infusion. Propofol is remarkable for how patients are awake and oriented after administration with lack of "hangover" effect that was associated with older anesthetics. Added benefits of propofol include its antiemetic properties. Propofol has been used in multiple different settings: (1) induction of anesthesia, (2) maintenance of anesthesia, either with volatile anesthetics or as a component of total intravenous anesthesia (TIVA), and (3) monitored anesthesia care (MAC) sedation for minor procedures. Propofol is not without its problems. It causes hypotension, respiratory depression, pain with injection, and has a prolonged duration with continuous infusion. Prolonged infusion can cause propofol infusion syndrome (PRIS) (association with doses of 4 mg/kg/hr for >48 hours).[3] Future medications will likely improve on our currently available anesthetics.

Intravenous anesthetics have a rapid onset after administration. They rapidly distribute to higher perfused and vessel-rich tissues. Their lipophilicity allows for rapid crossing of the blood–brain barrier. The slight delay between target blood concentration and effect organ (brain) response is known as hysteresis. This delay occurs because of differences between peak plasma concentration and peak drug concentration in the brain. The action of a single bolus injection is terminated by redistribution of the anesthetic to lean tissues such as muscle. This property of intravenous anesthetics is key to understanding their pharmacokinetics in relation to continuous infusion and maintenance. An initial bolus or loading dose of an anesthetic establishes the desired blood concentration of the drug. Redistribution of intravenous anesthetics to nonactive tissues accounts for part of their initial clearance; however, this becomes less important as those tissues equilibrate with the blood. Therefore, the rate of infusion of an intravenous anesthetic for maintenance of anesthesia decreases over the duration of an infusion to maintain the desired blood concentration.

An understanding of the pharmacokinetics of intravenous anesthetics is important to understanding their administration. Following a bolus of an intravenous drug, the plasma concentration over time resembles the curve in Figure 19-1. This graph

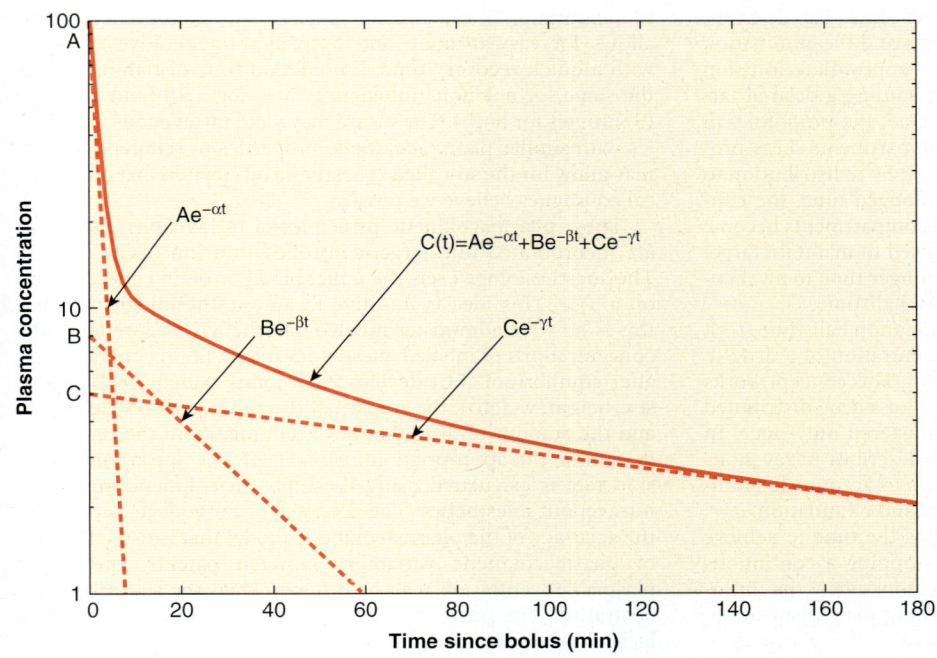

Figure 19-1 Plasma concentration after bolus injection of an intravenous anesthetic. Decreases in blood concentration occur in three components corresponding to rapid distribution (*A*), slow distribution (*B*), and elimination (*C*). The individual lines associated with each component term are also shown. The triexponential curve represents the algebraic sum of the individual exponential functions. The y-axis intercepts of the curve peel are shown as A, B, and C. These are present as coefficients of the triexponential equation. (Adapted with permission from Struys MMRF, De Smet T, Glen JB, et al. The history of target-controlled infusion. *Anesth Analg*. 2016;122(1):56–69.)

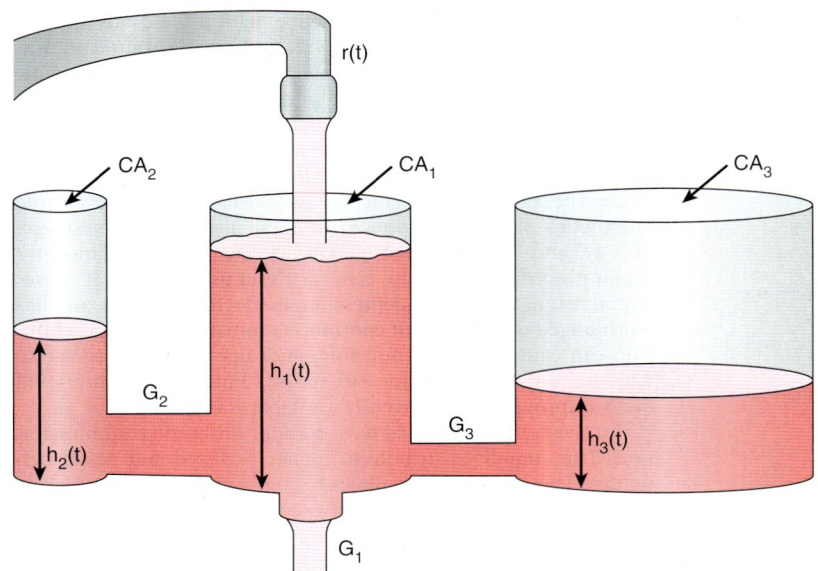

Figure 19-2 Hydraulic depiction of a three-compartment model. r(t) represented a drug infusion via a syringe pump adding drug to the blood. CA_1 represents the central compartment (blood). Administered medication will distribute to the peripheral compartments (CA_2, CA_3), which affects the drug's concentration in the blood. Ultimately the drug is eliminated by the body, depicted as G_1. (Adapted with permission from Hughes MA, Glass PS, Jacobs JR. Context-sensitive half time in multicompartment pharmacokinetic models for intravenous anesthetic drugs. *Anesthesiology.* 1992;76:334–341.)

shows the blood concentration of an intravenous anesthetic (i.e., propofol) after bolus injection. The curve can be explained by a triexponential equation. Essentially, there are three phases that occur after a bolus injection of propofol.[4] The first phase is a rapid distribution phase; propofol rapidly distributes from the plasma to peripheral tissues. The second phase is a slow distribution phase; propofol continues to distribute to other tissues concurrent with return of drug to the plasma from the rapid distribution tissue. The last phase is the terminal phase, or elimination phase, where propofol is removed from the body.

The three-compartment model is used to describe the behavior of an intravenous anesthetic. Figure 19-2 depicts a hydraulic version of the three-compartment model. We will use this model to understand the behavior of a propofol infusion. When propofol is first administered, it fills the central compartment (blood, CA_1). The propofol then distributes to peripheral compartments (CA_2, CA_3), one rapid and the other slow. The distribution of drug to the peripheral compartments and the elimination of propofol (G_1) can be matched with an appropriate infusion rate (r(t)) that would then allow for maintaining a desired target blood concentration. However, over time, the propofol will begin to accumulate in the peripheral compartments. Less propofol is removed from the central circulation by redistribution to these peripheral compartments. With prolonged time, the contributions of propofol from the peripheral compartments become greater, thus requiring less drug to be infused to maintain target blood concentration. This also leads to a longer time to awakening, and to the concept of context-sensitive half-time.

A concept most are familiar with is elimination half-time ($t_{1/2}$). It is the time it takes for the plasma concentration of a drug to decrease to 50% of its original concentration. This concept works well to describe a one-compartment model for a drug distributed only to the blood, or if the drug is administered only once. In contrast, pharmacokinetic modeling that describes intravenous anesthetics administered by infusion needs to account for multiple compartments, phases of distribution and elimination.

Context-sensitive half-time is defined as the time to achieve a 50% reduction in concentration after stopping a continuous infusion. Context-sensitive half-time demonstrates the influence of the distributive process in governing drug disposition. This refers to both the transfer of drug out of the plasma into peripheral compartments and the reverse process when there is a net transfer of drug back to the central compartment. Figure 19-3 shows the context-sensitive half-time of several anesthetic drugs. In comparison to thiopental, propofol has a much lower context-sensitive half-time. Although the elimination of propofol is prolonged with longer infusions, it is not to the same magnitude as with thiopental. It is the low context-sensitive half-time that allows for propofol to be used as a continuous infusion. Thiopental by comparison has a much longer context-sensitive half-time and is a poor choice to be used for continuous infusion.

The medication that best illustrates the concept of context-sensitive half-time is remifentanil. Remifentanil is an ultrashort opioid agonist. It has an ester component in its chemical structure and is eliminated rapidly because of metabolism by nonspecific plasma esterases. Because of these properties, remifentanil has a context-sensitive half-time that is essentially independent of the duration of the infusion (Fig. 19-4). The brevity of action allows for easy titration and optimal intraoperative analgesia with a quick recovery time. Elimination time of remifentanil is the same for a 1-hour infusion as it is for a 10-hour infusion (3 minutes for both). The future may yield intravenous anesthetics with similar pharmacokinetic properties to remifentanil that may allow for the so-called "anesthesia off" switch that our surgical colleagues believe we possess.

These pharmacokinetic principles of intravenous anesthesia are incorporated into target-controlled infusion (TCI) devices. The anesthesiologist sets the target blood or brain concentration on a TCI. This idea is intuitive to an anesthesiologist because this is how we administer inhaled anesthetics because end-tidal concentrations of inhaled anesthetics reflect brain concentration after equilibrium. TCI devices incorporate patient factors (age, sex, height, weight), the amount of drug that has been delivered, and the amount of drug that has accumulated in the tissues, to determine the appropriate infusion rate.[4] The appropriate infusion rate is calculated using these pharmacokinetic models of intravenous anesthetics. The accuracy of these devices relies on the accuracy of the pharmacokinetic model that is used. Because of pharmacokinetic variability between patients, the actual plasma concentration may be different than the set target concentration. The Food and Drug Administration (FDA) cited this lack of precision as an unacceptable risk. These concerns were

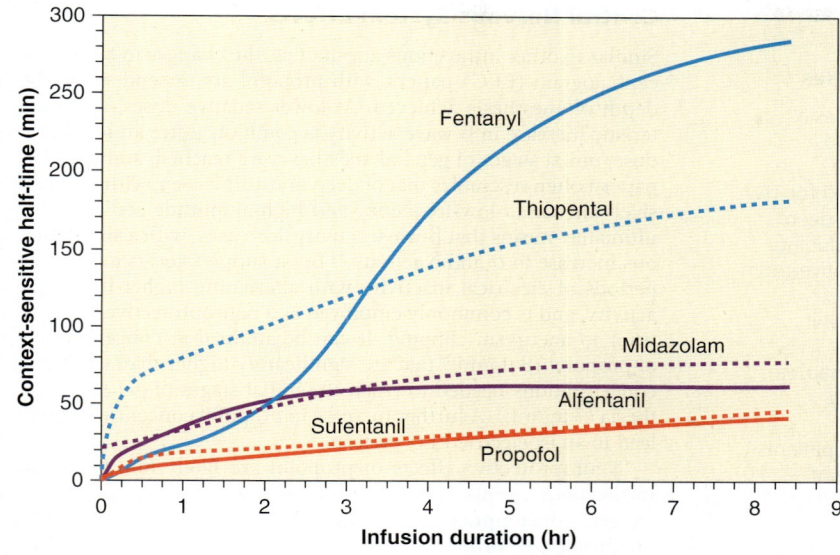

Figure 19-3 Context-sensitive half-time of intravenous anesthetics. (Adapted with permission from Hughes MA, Glass PS, Jacobs JR. Context-sensitive half-time in multi-compartment pharmacokinetic models for intravenous anesthetic drugs. *Anesthesiology.* 1992;76:334–341.)

raised despite extensive use of TCI systems outside the United States with a good safety record.[5]

Propofol

Propofol (2,6-diisopropylphenol) has become one of the most frequently used intravenous anesthetics on the market today (Fig. 19-5; Table 19-2). Its pharmacokinetic profile presents a desirable rapid onset, a predictable context-sensitive half-time, and a rapid emergence from anesthesia. Additionally, a favorable side-effect profile and antiemetic property allow for a wide spectrum of uses, including induction and maintenance of general anesthesia, intensive care unit (ICU) sedation, and as a sedative-hypnotic in a variety of outpatient procedures.

Derivation of the appropriate propofol formulation has always centered around the challenge of managing its lipophilicity and relative insolubility in aqueous solutions. After its introduction in the 1970s in Cremophor EL formulation,[6] it was rapidly withdrawn from the market due to concern for anaphylactic reactions.[7] Nearly a decade later it was reintroduced in its more current form consisting of 1% propofol, 10% soybean oil, 2.25% glycerol, and 1.2% egg phospholipid emulsifier. In the 1990s ethylenediaminetetraacetic acid (EDTA) was added to this formulation to deter microbial growth within the emulsion. The lipid emulsion comes in a familiar milky white consistency, and can be stored at room temperature without any significant degradation.

Pharmacokinetics

Propofol is primarily metabolized by the liver, and subsequently its inactive and water-soluble metabolites are excreted by the kidneys. A small amount of unmetabolized propofol is excreted in both urine and feces, but that is considered negligible (<3%). Despite the primary mechanism of metabolism, liver and kidney disease have not been noted to alter pharmacokinetics of propofol significantly. Also the clearance rate for propofol has been reported to be 20 to 30 mL/kg/min (≈1.5 L/min), exceeding average hepatic blood flow (15 mL/kg/min), suggesting that other forms of metabolism and elimination play a significant role. The most common extrahepatic sites of metabolism are the kidneys and lungs, both responsible for up to 30% of the common propofol metabolites, explaining why pharmacokinetics of propofol are relatively consistent across patient populations with different comorbid states.

To truly understand the kinetic properties of propofol, evaluation of multicompartment models is crucial. The distribution of propofol after an initial bolus dose has been described in a variety of kinetic models. In a simple two-compartment model, the blood concentration of propofol drops rapidly with the initial

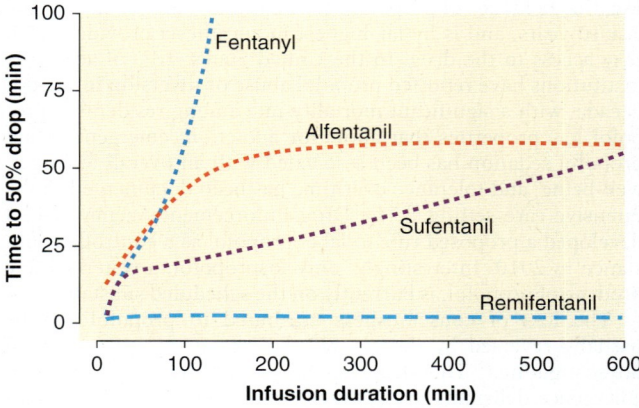

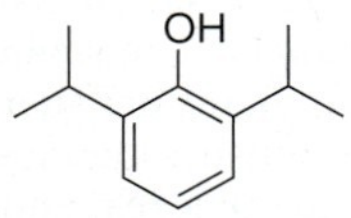

Figure 19-4 A simulation of the time necessary to achieve a 50% decrease in drug concentration in the blood after variable length intravenous infusions of remifentanil, fentanyl, alfentanil and sufentanil. Note that the context-sensitive half-time for remifentanil is independent of infusion duration. (Adapted with permission from Egan TD, Lemmens HJ, Fiset P, et al. The pharmacokinetics of the new short-acting opioid remifentanil (GI87084B) in healthy adult male volunteers. *Anesthesiology.* 1993;79:881–892.)

Figure 19-5 Propofol. 2,6-diisopropylphenol.

Table 19-2 Propofol

Key Pharmacology	Key Clinical Uses
Primary mechanism: GABA-A receptor agonist	General anesthesia induction and maintenance
Predictable context-sensitive half-time across various comorbidities	Commonly used for TIVA
CNS depressant, neuroprotective, anticonvulsant, decreases $CMRO_2$, CBF, and ICP	Conscious and deep sedation, including out-of-operative-room settings
Can be used for EEG burst suppression	Intensive care unit sedation
Cardiovascular: significant decreases in systemic vascular resistance, stroke volume, and cardiac output	Postoperative nausea and vomiting prophylaxis
Pulmonary: respiratory depressant and potent bronchodilator	Safe for use in patients with malignant hyperthermia
Addiction potential: may elicit feelings of well-being or euphoria during emergence	
Side effects: associated pain with injection, propofol infusion syndrome	

$CMRO_2$, cerebral metabolic oxygen consumption rate; CBF, cerebral blood flow; ICP, intracranial pressure; EEG, electroencephalogram; TIVA, total intravenous anesthesia.

distribution half-life of 2 to 4 minutes. In a three-compartment model propofol has the initial distribution half-life estimated to be 1 to 8 minutes and the secondary slow distribution half-life listed as 30 to 70 minutes. Elimination half-lives for both models are significantly slower, reported in a wider range from 2 to 24 hours. As noted in Figure 19-3, infusion duration of up to 8 hours maintains a reliable context-sensitive half-life of 40 minutes or less, allowing clinicians to take advantage of the predictable kinetic properties that yield a rapid recovery after initial bolus administration and continuous infusion.

Pharmacodynamics

[3] The mechanism by which the unconscious state is attained by induction doses of propofol is complicated and not fully understood. Primarily, it occurs via enhancement of GABA inhibitory pathways.[7] Other neuroreceptors have been linked to propofol activity, including α-adrenergic receptors and N-methyl-D-aspartate (NMDA) receptors. Alteration of the central cholinergic transmission by propofol may also play a role in achieving a state of unconsciousness.[8] The neurotransmission target is the vast array of interneurons involved within the cerebral cortex, brain stem, and thalamus that ultimately play a critical role in arousal.[9,10]

Initial low doses of propofol produce sedation, but at increased doses a state of paradoxical excitation may occur, where a patient is disinhibited, has unpredictable movement, broken speech, and is not readily arousable.[11] A further increase in dose of propofol leads to loss of consciousness, apnea, relative relaxation of muscles, loss of brainstem reflexes, and subsequently necessitates airway support.

Central Nervous System Effects

Similar to other intravenous anesthetics, the changes in electroencephalogram (EEG) pattern with propofol are dependent on the depth of anesthesia achieved. At lower sedative doses, a characteristic increase in β-wave activity is common. After an induction dose, initial stages of general anesthesia are reached, and the EEG pattern often resembles that of deep non-REM sleep, with progressively increased low-frequency and high-amplitude activity. This ultimately means that β-wave activity decreases, with a simultaneous increase in α and δ activity.[12] Burst suppression is marked by periods of electrical inactivity with alternating higher-frequency activity, and is commonly employed as a neuroprotective measure prior to aneurysm clipping. It can be attained at concentrations of propofol (8 μg/mL) that are significantly higher than the blood concentrations needed to reach the initial stages of general anesthesia (3 μg/mL). A further increase in propofol concentration will lead to an isoelectric EEG pattern.

Neuroprotective effects of propofol are likely multifactorial. Intravenous agents such as propofol lower cerebral metabolic oxygen consumption rate ($CMRO_2$) and decrease intracranial pressure (ICP) primarily by lowering cerebral blood flow (CBF). At the same time, cerebral perfusion pressure (CPP) may also be lowered, thus this benefit is not without limitations and should be employed carefully. Propofol has specific antioxidant properties, and its function as a free radical scavenger has been hypothesized to play a role in preventing injury during neurodegenerative processes such as stroke and trauma.[13] Other protective mechanisms have been hypothesized, including attenuation of excitotoxic glutamate pathways[14] that lower the likelihood of programmed neuronal apoptosis,[15] and its overall anti-inflammatory effects (e.g., decreasing TNF-α).[16]

Propofol is generally considered an anticonvulsant. At induction doses that reach burst suppression, EEG epileptiform activity is limited.[17] These results have not been reproduced in patients with epilepsy at lower sedative doses.[18] It has also been used successfully to treat status epilepticus, thus it is rarely the anesthetic of choice during induction of anesthesia for ECT because it shortens seizure duration. Contradictory case reports of propofol anesthetics associated with grand mal seizures do exist, but the proconvulsant effects are not well elucidated.

Although not traditionally considered a drug for recreational use, the incidence of propofol abuse has likely increased over the last 10 years, and is by far highest in anesthesia providers with easy access to the drug. In the United States, 18% of academic institutions have reported propofol abuse or diversion in the last decade, with a significant mortality rate among residents.[19] Propofol has properties that allow for addiction; emergence from propofol sedation has been associated with an overall feeling of well-being, and tolerance over time has been documented in the intensive care setting.[20] The Drug Enforcement Agency (DEA) developed a proposed rule to label propofol as a controlled substance in 2010. Interestingly, only fospropofol, a water-soluble prodrug of propofol, is currently on the scheduled substance list.

The loss of consciousness attributed to propofol can be partially reversed by the central cholinomimetic properties of physostigmine.[21] This drug has been used in the treatment of emergence delirium, and presumably the mechanism of propofol reversal is similar. Activation of central cholinergic pathways leads to an overall state of arousal, and likely alters propofol-induced state of unconsciousness (Fig. 19-6).

Cardiovascular Effects

The hemodynamic effects of propofol are dose-dependent and more significant after an induction dose than during a continuous

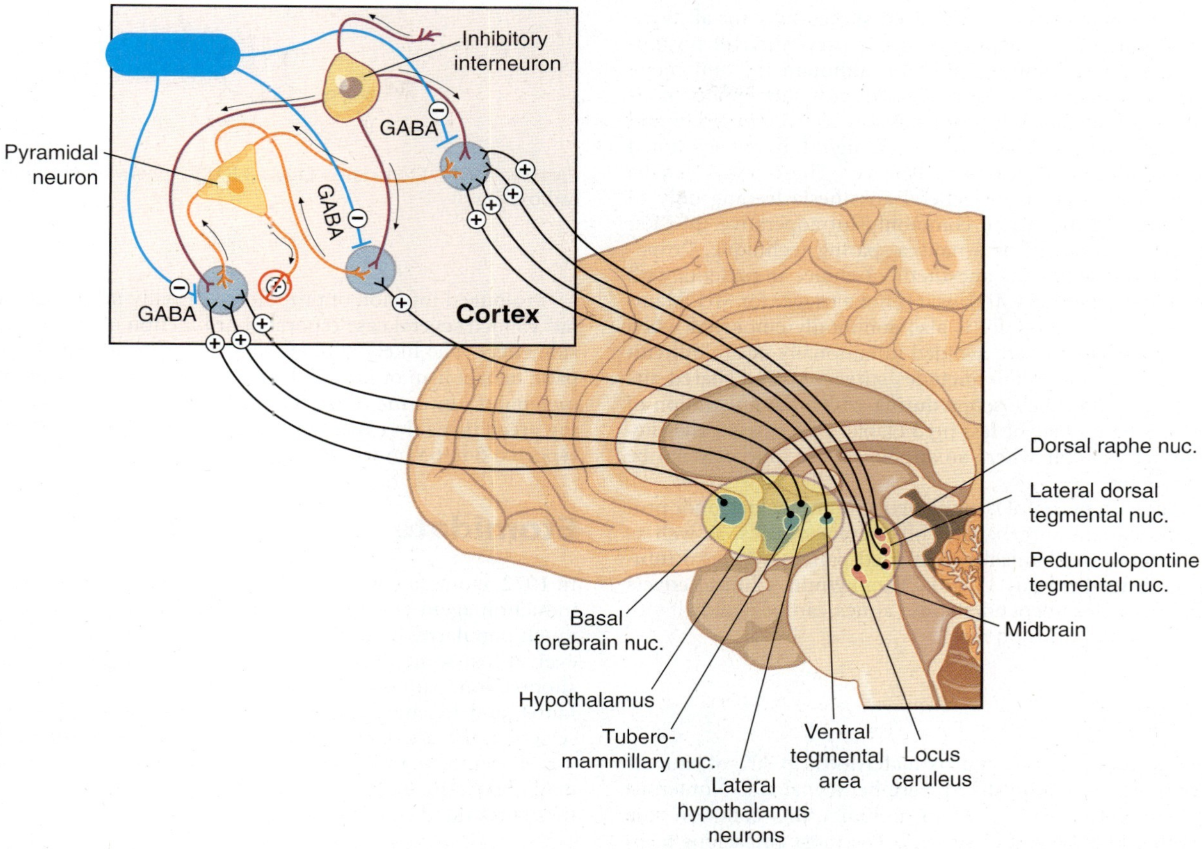

Figure 19-6 Propofol's proposed mechanism of action in the central nervous system. Ascending arousal pathways arise from both the thalamus and the midbrain to send excitatory inputs to a pyramidal neuron (*orange*). A GABAergic inhibitory interneuron (*purple*) synapses onto this pyramidal neuron. Propofol binds post-synaptically and enhances GABAergic inhibition. Unconsciousness occurs as this enhanced GABAergic inhibition counteracts ascending arousal inputs to the pyramidal neuron and decreases excitatory activity.

infusion. There is a characteristic drop in systolic and diastolic blood pressure without the expected increase in heart rate. The observed blood pressure drop results from a decrease in cardiac output, stroke volume, and systemic vascular resistance (SVR). Propofol decreases sympathetic activity and leads to indirect arterial vasodilation and venodilation. This effect is enhanced by direct effects on smooth muscle and depressant effects on the myocardium, affecting intracellular calcium balance and influx.[22] The decreased sympathetic tone is also coupled with direct inhibition of the baroreceptor response, leading to a diminished reflex increase in heart rate and a more pronounced hemodynamic effect. Suppression of supraventricular tachycardia has also been reported, and may be a direct result of propofol effects on the heart conduction system.[23]

Respiratory System Effects

The respiratory depressant effects of propofol are also dose-dependent. Apnea is relatively common with a higher induction dose, while a typical maintenance dose of propofol results in diminished tidal volumes and increased respiratory rate. There is also a blunted response to hypoxia that may be a direct effect on chemoreceptors, as well as decreased respiratory response to hypercarbia. Propofol is a potent bronchodilator, primarily because of its direct effects on intracellular calcium homeostasis.

Clinical Uses

The rapid and smooth induction and emergence from anesthesia helped transform propofol into an intravenous sedative-hypnotic that is a viable alternative to standard inhalational agents and other intravenous drugs. The induction dose in a healthy adult is approximately 1 to 2.5 mg/kg, and loss of consciousness is commonly achieved at corresponding blood concentration close to 3 µg/kg. Induction dose requirement variability is tremendous among patients with different characteristics and comorbidities. Elderly patients typically have prolonged effects and increased sensitivity to propofol because of decreased cardiac output and clearance.[24] On the opposite end of the spectrum, children typically have a larger than average volume of distribution and quicker clearance, resulting in increased propofol requirement on a per kilogram basis.[25] Morbidly obese patients should have lean body weight used when calculating propofol dosing.[26] Patients with chronic alcohol abuse, as expected, have an increased induction dose requirement. An exaggerated hemodynamic response is likely after induction of propofol in patients with cardiovascular disease. Thus, determination of the appropriate propofol induction dose requires careful assessment of premedication administration, patient history, and comorbidity.

Maintenance of general anesthesia with propofol can commonly be achieved with infusions between 100 and 200 µg/kg/min. TIVA with propofol alone—or together with opioids as part of a balanced anesthetic—has been utilized successfully for all types of surgery. One of the major benefits is prevention of postoperative nausea and vomiting (PONV), although the antiemetic properties of propofol can be replicated with subhypnotic concentrations. Maintenance infusions as low as 10 µg/kg/min and blood concentration levels as low as 350 ng/mL have been noted to cause significant decreases in PONV.[27] These levels can be reached after recovery from general anesthesia leading only to minimal sedation, but more commonly intraoperative infusion of propofol is employed as a nausea-sparing technique. Propofol can also be used as the anesthetic of choice in patients with malignant hyperthermia (MH), as it is not a trigger for MH. Maintenance infusion of propofol is also commonly employed when inhalational anesthetics are avoided intentionally or are difficult to administer. One example includes surgery with a shared airway such as rigid bronchoscopy during which administration of inhaled anesthetics may be less predictable. Office based anesthesia is another example where an anesthesia machine may not be readily available.

Sedation with propofol is employed commonly for minor procedures, outpatient surgery, and off-site anesthetics, as well as ICU sedation of mechanically ventilated patients. Typical infusion doses range between 25 and 75 µg/kg/min. Clinical effects of propofol are dose-dependent, and apnea can be avoided with careful titration of infusion rate.

Side Effects

Pain on injection occurs in approximately 60% to 70% of patients when propofol is administered peripherally alone. Numerous interventions have been tested to minimize this common side effect, with varying levels of success. The most efficacious technique is pretreatment with a local anesthetic such as lidocaine in conjunction with venous occlusion using a tourniquet, or in essence a modified Bier block.[28] Antecubital vein use as an alternative to smaller peripheral vein sites (e.g., hand) has proved to be the most important nondrug technique for minimizing pain on injection.[29] Addition of lidocaine to propofol, or pretreatment with lidocaine without the use of a tourniquet has also been shown to be beneficial. Pretreatment with opioids is commonly performed prior to induction with propofol, and it decreases pain on injection. Techniques to lower free propofol concentration, such as diluting the emulsion and changing the lipid solvent have shown some improvement. Pretreatment with other drugs has shown limited success, including non-steroidal anti-inflammatory drugs (NSAIDs), ketamine, steroids, and β-blockers.[29]

PRIS is an extremely rare, but potentially deadly side effect of propofol that was first described in children in the 1990s and subsequently in adults after its use for sedation in the ICU setting.[30,31] The key clinical characteristics include unexplained metabolic acidosis, hyperkalemia, hyperlipidemia, rhabdomyolysis, hepatomegaly, renal failure and most importantly ECG changes, arrhythmias, and progression to cardiac failure. The pathophysiology of PRIS is not well understood, but may involve mitochondrial toxicity and uncoupling of the intracellular respiration chain, although other hypotheses such as inhibition of fatty acid oxidation have been suggested. Development of clinical symptoms of PRIS is likely dependent on both the infusion dose and duration, but short-duration infusions have been associated with cardiac failure. In 2006, the FDA altered the recommended maximum propofol infusion dose to 4 mg/kg/hr, but it is unclear if the recommendations have altered the frequency of PRIS, and currently the rate of mortality from PRIS is still close to 50%.[32]

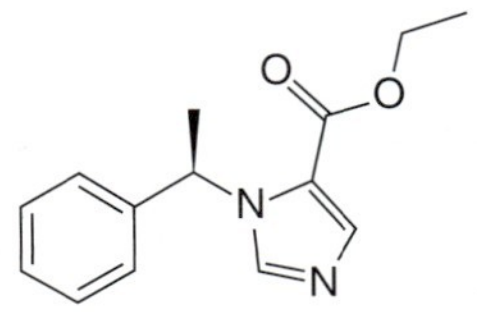

Figure 19-7 Etomidate. Ethyl 3-[(1R)-1-phenylethel)]imidazole-5-carboxylate.

Prolonged infusion of propofol, especially in the ICU setting, has yielded several case reports of production of green urine as a side effect. The likely etiology may be due to increased extrahepatic metabolism of propofol, and subsequent excretion of these metabolites in urine. Case reports of single-dose propofol causing green urine do exist, but are less common than the typically reported 6 to 64 hours after infusion has started.[33]

Etomidate

In 1972, etomidate was introduced into anesthetic practice as an induction agent (Fig. 19-7; Table 19-3). It subsequently gained much popularity because of its safe hemodynamic profile. However, it lost some proponents with increased reports of adrenal suppression, pain on injection, thrombophlebitis, PONV, myoclonus, and hiccups. Like most other decisions regarding drug selection, the use of etomidate is the result of a risk/benefit analysis. If hemodynamic stability is of paramount importance, one may choose to induce with etomidate and prepare to manage these unwanted side effects.

Pharmacokinetics

Etomidate is an imidazole derivative (the D(+) enantiomer) and is not stable in neutral pH solutions. The solvents in its formulation, namely propylene glycol, contribute to veno-irritation and phlebitis that occur frequently. Similar to other induction agents, etomidate has a quick onset of action ("vein to brain"), fast resolution of effect secondary to redistribution, and follows the three-compartment kinetic model. Etomidate's use as a continuous infusion is limited by its association with adrenal suppression. Etomidate is metabolized in the liver and excreted predominantly by the kidney (approximately 80%) and in bile (approximately 20%). It is largely protein bound (approximately 75%) and thus affected by pathologic conditions and/or drugs that alter serum proteins. Other pharmacokinetic values of etomidate are found in Table 19-4.

Table 19-3	Etomidate
Key Pharmacology	
GABA-A receptor agonist	
Hemodynamically stable	
Adrenocortical suppression	
Postoperative nausea and vomiting	
Key Clinical Uses	
Hemodynamically stable induction	
Cardiac, trauma, and hypovolemic patients	

Table 19-4	Etomidate Pharmacokinetics
Initial distribution half-life	2.7 minutes
Redistribution of half-life	29 minutes
Elimination half-life	2.9–5.3 hours
Volume of distribution	2.5–4.5 L/kg
Induction dose	0.2–0.3 mg/kg

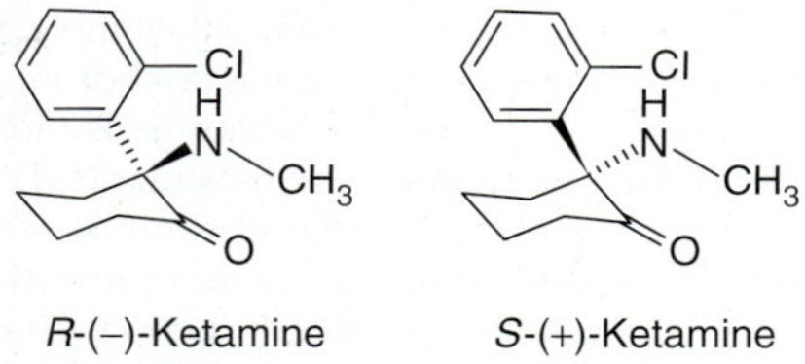

Figure 19-8 Ketamine. (RS)-2-2-chlorophenyl-2-(methylamino) cyclohexanone.

Pharmacodynamics and Clinical Uses

Etomidate binds as an agonist to the GABA-A receptor and thus has an inhibitory influence on the brain. It is a potent vasoconstrictor that reduces CBF, ICP, and $CMRO_2$. Because of etomidate's minimal effect on the mean arterial pressure (MAP), CPP is either maintained or increased. Unlike benzodiazepines, etomidate can achieve burst suppression with a concomitant decrease in ICP. However, despite its neurodepressant properties at high doses, etomidate is often associated with epileptogenic activity (excitatory spikes) on EEG. This alone may render etomidate an undesirable induction agent for patients undergoing neurosurgical procedures. The epileptogenic EEG activity is not to be confused with the observable seizure-like, myoclonic movements that often follow an induction dose of etomidate (although excitatory EEG spikes may also be present during this time). Similar to other maintenance intravenous anesthetics, etomidate will increase the latency intervals measured on somatosensory-evoked potentials (SSEPs). Paradoxically, etomidate increases the amplitude of SSEPs, in contrast to the typical effect of other anesthetics. Etomidate is used frequently for electroconvulsive therapy. Unlike the barbiturates (except methohexital), etomidate is proconvulsant and lowers the seizure threshold.

Etomidate is often touted as a hemodynamically stable induction medication with a relatively large safety margin. Etomidate has a minimal or nonexistent effect on MAP, pulmonary artery (PA) pressure, pulmonary artery wedge pressure, central venous pressure (CVP), stroke volume, cardiac index, SVR, and pulmonary vascular resistance (PVR).[34] Etomidate is frequently used for induction of anesthesia in cardiac operating rooms. Etomidate is also used for trauma patients who are hemodynamically unstable and are often hypovolemic.

There are mixed data regarding etomidate's effect on the respiratory system. It is widely believed that etomidate depresses airway reflexes less than propofol (unless co-administered with another sedative/analgesic agent). Etomidate also relaxes the smooth musculature of the pulmonary vasculature system to a similar degree as propofol.

Etomidate is a reasonable choice for MAC sedation because of the preservation of airway reflexes.

Side Effects

Adrenocortical suppression may be the most significant adverse effect of etomidate. Etomidate inhibits the activity of the enzyme 11β-hydroxylase and prevents the conversion of cholesterol to cortisol. It has been postulated that one dose is sufficient to transiently suppress the adrenocortical axis. Some suggest pretreatment with dexamethasone to curtail this effect.[35] Although many studies conclude that there are no direct adverse outcomes following a bolus of etomidate, even in the septic population,[36] other studies propose the opposite.[37] However, most practitioners, in an effort to limit this possibility, will not administer repeat doses or continuous infusions.

Ketamine

Phencyclidine (PCP; angel dust) was long ago noted to have remarkable analgesic and anesthetic effects. Ketamine was discovered in the search for a phencyclidine derivative with similar anesthetic and analgesic properties, but with fewer psychomimetic effects (Fig. 19-8; Table 19-5). Ketamine was described as causing "dissociative anesthesia" in human volunteers in 1965, acting through the NMDA receptor.[38] Key features associated with ketamine administration included marked nystagmus, significant analgesia, and unconsciousness. Emergence from ketamine anesthesia was associated with emergence delirium, hallucinations, and alterations in mood and affect. The use of ketamine as an anesthetic has been limited by its cardiovascular stimulating properties and the disturbing emergence reactions. Interestingly, the NMDA receptor has been found to play a key role in nociception, and low-dose ketamine has an opiate sparing effect in the management of acute pain. The effects of ketamine related to pain can be best described as antihyperalgesic, antiallodynic, or tolerance-protective.[39] More recently, ketamine has gained interest in the treatment of major depression, however its clinical effects are of short duration.[40]

Pharmacokinetics

Ketamine is an analog of phencyclidine that is a chiral compound and is a racemic mixture of S and R enantiomers. The S(+)

Table 19-5	Ketamine

Key Pharmacology

NMDA receptor antagonist
Cardiovascular stability; increases heart rate and blood pressure
Mild respiratory depression
Side effects: Emergence delirium, hallucinations, nystagmus, increased salivation
Trance-like cataleptic unconscious state ("dissociative anesthesia")

Key Clinical Uses

Anesthesia—intravenous and intramuscular induction
Analgesia
Chronic pain
Depression
Bronchodilator
Procedural sedation, especially in pediatric and burn patients

enantiomer of ketamine is three to four times more potent than the R-enantiomer. The S-enantiomer has a shorter duration of action and is cleared more rapidly.[41] Ketamine is bioavailable by multiple routes of administration. Intramuscular (IM) administration has a 93% bioavailability, transnasal administration has 25% to 50% bioavailability, and rectal or oral administration has 16% bioavailability.[42] The high lipid solubility and low protein binding (20%) allow for a rapid uptake of ketamine in the brain, as well as a fairly rapid redistribution. The onset of anesthesia after intravenous administration of ketamine is 30 to 60 seconds, with duration of 10 to 15 minutes. The induction dose of ketamine is 0.5 to 2 mg/kg for intravenous administration and 4 to 6 mg/kg for intramuscular administration. Peak plasma levels averaged 0.75 mg/mL and CSF levels were about 0.2 mg/mL 1 hour after dosing.[43]

After intravenous bolus administration, ketamine shows a bi- or triexponential pattern of elimination. The α-elimination phase (redistribution of ketamine from the central nervous system [CNS] to peripheral tissues) is 11 minutes, and the β-elimination phase is 2.5 hours.[44] Ketamine is metabolized primarily in the liver by cytochrome P-450 enzymes (CYP 3A4 > CYP 2C9 > CYP 2B6). The liver extensively metabolizes ketamine by demethylation to its principal metabolite norketamine. Norketamine is biologically active but only has one-third to one-fifth the activity of racemic ketamine. Norketamine is eliminated by renal excretion. Due to its lipophilicity, ketamine is only partially removed by dialysis.

Pharmacodynamics

The neuropharmacology of ketamine is complex. Antagonism of the NMDA receptor is primarily responsible for ketamine's specific clinical effects. However, ketamine also has clinical effects at opioid, noradrenergic, cholinergic, nicotinic, and muscarinic receptors.

Ketamine binds preferentially to the NMDA receptors on inhibitory interneurons in the cortex, limbic system, and hippocampus that promote uncoordinated increase in neuronal activity and an active EEG pattern, and produce unconsciousness.[45] Ketamine has been shown to increase the bispectral index (BIS) from 40 to 63 with higher doses of ketamine (0.5 mg/kg) under general anesthesia with propofol and fentanyl.[46]

There are NMDA receptors present on nearly all CNS cells, and especially those cells involved with nociception such as primary afferent nociceptors in the spinal dorsal horn. Ketamine binds to an interchannel site of the NMDA receptor called the phencyclidine (PCP) binding site and decreases channel opening time. Ketamine decreases the amplification of repeated stimulation of the NMDA receptor ("wind up") that is considered an elementary form of CNS sensitization. Antagonism of the channel is more profound if the NMDA channel has been previously opened by glutamate.[47]

Functional MRI has provided some insight into the analgesic pharmacodynamics of ketamine. Volunteers who were subjected to painful heat stimulation showed a typical pattern of pain activation from the thalamus to the insula, to the cingulate, and ultimately to the prefrontal cortex. There was a dose-dependent reduction in these cerebral activation pathways when volunteers were given ketamine. Ketamine has also been found to block signals from the spinoreticular pathway. Activity of the medial thalamic nuclei and medial reticular formation—important relays in nociceptive transmission between the spinal and supraspinal levels—are both depressed.[47]

Ketamine has been found to bind to opioid, noradrenergic, and cholinergic receptors (Fig. 19-9). Ketamine binds to μ, δ, and κ opioid receptors; however this does not account for its analgesic effects.[47] The primary analgesic mechanism of ketamine is believed to be in the prevention of developing hyperalgesia.[48] Ketamine causes stimulation of CNS noradrenergic neurons and inhibition of catecholamine uptake, which provokes a hyperadrenergic state (with increased release of norepinephrine, dopamine, and serotonin). Ketamine's effect on noradrenergic neurons is partly responsible for the hypnotic, psychic, and analgesic effects observed. Ketamine also affects CNS cholinergic neurons, and the anticholinergic physostigmine can antagonize the hypnotic effects of ketamine.

Clinical Uses

Anesthesia

Ketamine administration has been described as causing a dissociative amnestic state. Patients are unconscious with eyes open, maintain spontaneous respiration, and do not react to painful or noxious stimuli.[38] EEG shows a depression of the thalamocortical pathways and concomitant activation of the limbic system. Despite this increased epileptiform activity, there is no clinical evidence of seizure activity or spread of the epileptiform activity to cortical areas. Therefore, ketamine is less likely to cause a seizure and may in fact have CNS protective properties. Ketamine anesthesia is associated with profound analgesia that occurs at subanesthetic levels.

Induction doses of ketamine are 1 to 2 mg/kg, with an onset of 1 minute and a duration of 10 to 20 minutes. Ketamine administration is associated with an increase in heart rate and blood pressure. Ketamine is therefore a good choice for anesthetic induction in the hemodynamically unstable patient. Ketamine has been compared to etomidate in the unstable patient and has the advantage of not causing adrenal suppression.[49] The increased blood pressure and heart rate associated with ketamine may make it unsuitable for some cardiac patients (critical coronary artery disease). An increase in PVR associated with ketamine may make it an unsuitable choice in patients with severe right heart dysfunction.

Sedation

Ketamine has been used to provide sedation to burn patients during wound care. Benefits of ketamine in this patient population include analgesia as well as maintenance of spontaneous respiration and airway reflexes. Ketamine can be administered via intramuscular injection and has been used to provide sedation or anesthesia in uncooperative or hostile patients. Ketamine has also been used in pediatric patients for painful procedures such as reduction and casting of bone fractures in the emergency department.[42]

Analgesia

Ketamine has been extensively studied for its role as an analgesic in the management of acute postoperative pain. Ketamine has been shown to lower pain scores and decrease opiate requirements in postoperative patients. Administration of both a ketamine bolus prior to surgical incision and a ketamine infusion postoperatively has been found to be the most effective use of ketamine for acute pain. The analgesic effects of ketamine are achieved at subanesthetic blood concentrations. Ketamine reduces opiate requirements for postsurgical pain, but it cannot replace opiates altogether. Ketamine is useful in patients who

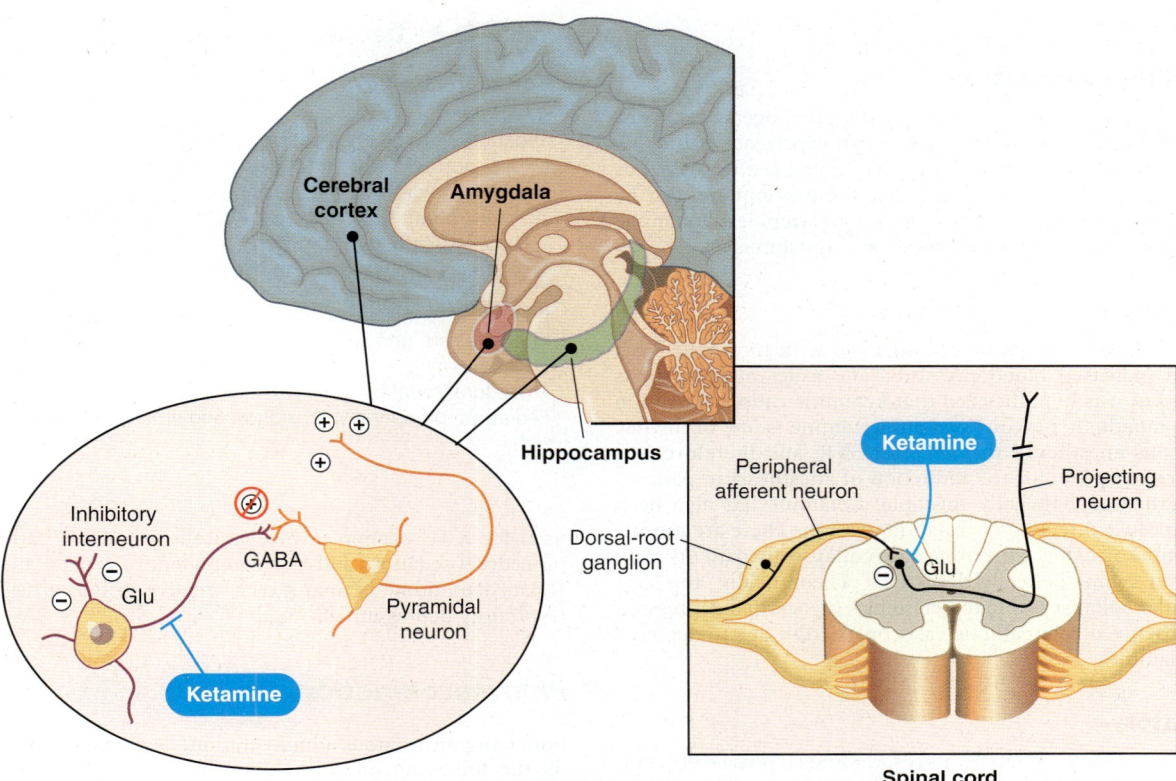

Figure 19-9 Ketamine's mechanism of action in the central nervous system. Ketamine binds preferentially to the *N*-methyl-D-aspartate (NMDA) receptors on inhibitory interneurons in the cortex, amygdala, and hippocampus. Unconsciousness results from an uncoordinated increase in neural activity. In the spinal cord, ketamine decreases arousal by blocking NMDA glutamate-mediated nociceptive signals from peripheral afferent neurons in the dorsal-root ganglion to projecting neurons.

will require high doses of opiates, such as patients on chronic opiate therapy or patients with a history of opiate abuse.[50]

The exact mechanism of analgesia provided by ketamine is unclear. The NMDA receptor has been found to be associated with central sensitization and winds up at the spinal cord associated with chronic pain. Studies have suggested that ketamine analgesia occurs by the prevention of hyperalgesia and decreases in central nervous system sensitization that occur with acute pain.[39]

Chronic Pain

Due to the NMDA receptor role in preventing hyperalgesia, ketamine has also been investigated for the management of chronic pain. Ketamine has been most extensively studied in patients with chronic regional pain syndrome (CRPS). Ketamine administration to patients with CRPS yields a decrease in pain scores and opiate consumption.[51] Unfortunately, these effects are only of limited duration after ketamine administration. Future studies are required to determine the most effective regimen for ketamine administration in patients with chronic pain. Ketamine has also been used in cancer patients with severe pain. Ketamine is associated with a decrease, but not elimination, of opiate requirements. Unfortunately, the CNS side effects and lack of oral administration limit the application of ketamine in patients with chronic pain.

Intranasal ketamine has been investigated for use in chronic pain. Intranasal ketamine was found to significantly lower the intensity of breakthrough pain in patients with chronic pain when compared with placebo.[52] Intranasal ketamine also decreased pain scores in patients with chronic neuropathic pain.[53] Both studies reported no serious side effects. Intranasal ketamine, in combination with intranasal midazolam, has been used in the management of acute postoperative pain, showing similar efficacy to morphine patient-controlled analgesia (PCA) after spine surgery.[54] Further studies are needed to determine the utility of intranasal ketamine.

Depression

Ketamine has been evaluated as a possible treatment for major depression. Ketamine decreased depression symptoms and suicidal ideation within 1 hour of administration.[55,56] Ketamine as an antidepressant represents a possible novel treatment, and has generated excitement because of poor results with current treatments of depression (slow onset, poor efficacy). The mechanism of ketamine's antidepressant effects remains unclear. Investigations using memantine, an NMDA antagonist, failed to improve depressive symptoms.[57] Therefore, the antidepressant effects of ketamine may not be related to its NMDA antagonism, but to its effect on other CNS receptors (dopamine, adrenergic). Unfortunately, the duration of ketamine's antidepressant effect is short after single administration. Further investigation is required to determine the best regimen in use of ketamine as an antidepressant.[41] Understanding the mechanism of action of ketamine in depression may yield new targets for the treatment of major depression.

Side Effects

Central Nervous System

The major side effect of ketamine is the psychogenic reactions seen with its administration. Patients can experience hallucinations and out-of-body experiences that have been described as frightening. Studies have shown that these symptoms can be reduced with coadministration of benzodiazepines. Ketamine also causes patients to have a lateral gaze nystagmus.[38]

Cardiovascular

Administration of ketamine is associated with increased heart rate and increased blood pressure. The exact mechanism is unclear, but it is hypothesized that ketamine causes activation of the sympathetic nervous system. Ketamine is one of the few intravenous anesthetics that increase SVR, and therefore it is an attractive option for the induction of anesthesia in patients who are hemodynamically unstable. Ketamine has also been found to cause direct myocardial depression. There are reports of ketamine causing cardiovascular collapse in patients who have been sympathetically depleted.[58] Theoretically, this cardiovascular collapse is due to ketamine's myocardial depression in the absence of sympathetic vasoconstriction due to depleted catecholamines.

Respiratory

Ketamine maintains spontaneous respiration. Hypoxia can occur, but it is easily treated with supplemental oxygen. Ketamine is also a bronchodilator, although it is not effective as a sole agent for the treatment of bronchospasm.[59] Rather, it is a secondary agent to consider for the management of severe bronchospasm or status asthmaticus. Ketamine does cause increased salivation that may result in laryngospasm.

Intracranial Pressure/Seizure Issues

Historically ketamine was not recommended in patients with elevated ICP. The excitatory CNS effects of ketamine would increase $CMRO_2$ and CBF. However, studies have found that ICPs remain normal with ketamine administration in neurosurgical patients with controlled ventilation. In fact, ketamine may be neuroprotective.[60] Ketamine is associated with epileptiform activity on EEG; however, these excitement waveforms are not seen in the cortex, and therefore ketamine seems unlikely to precipitate a seizure.

Dexmedetomidine

Dexmedetomidine is an α_2-adrenergic agonist similar to clonidine (Fig. 19-10; Table 19-6). It has seven to eight times greater affinity for the α_2-adrenergic receptor than clonidine. Introduced into clinical practice in 1999, dexmedetomidine has been

Table 19-6 Dexmedetomidine

Key Pharmacology
α_2-Adrenergic agonist
Sedation with minimal respiratory depression
Mimics normal sleep pattern on electroencephalogram
Provides analgesia at the spinal cord level
Administration: Bolus 0.5–1 µg/kg over 15 minutes, followed by 0.3–0.7 µg/kg/hr infusion
Side effects: bradycardia and hypotension

Key Clinical Uses
Intensive care unit sedation in mechanically ventilated patients
Procedural sedation
Pediatrics: preoperative anxiolysis and emergence delirium

used for ICU sedation in mechanically ventilated patients, for procedural sedation, and as a component of general anesthesia. Dexmedetomidine is unique as a sedative in that it has limited respiratory depressant effects.

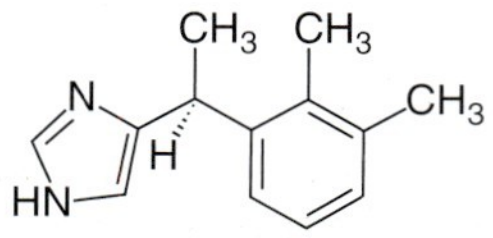

Pharmacokinetics

Following intravenous administration, dexmedetomidine exhibits the following pharmacokinetic parameters: a rapid distribution phase with a distribution half-life of approximately 6 minutes; a terminal elimination half-life of approximately 2 hours, and a steady state volume of distributions of approximately 118 L. Dexmedetomidine exhibits linear pharmacokinetics in the dose range from 0.2 to 0.7 µg/kg/hr when administered by intravenous infusion for up to 24 hours.[61] The average protein binding is 94% and constant across different plasma concentrations. The fraction of dexmedetomidine bound to plasma protein is significantly decreased in subjects with hepatic impairment compared to healthy subjects.

Dexmedetomidine undergoes almost complete biotransformation with very little unchanged dexmedetomidine in the urine and feces. Biotransformation involves both direct glucuronidation and cytochrome P450-mediated metabolism. The terminal elimination half-life is approximately 2 hours and clearance is estimated to be approximately 39 L/hr. Clearance values for dexmedetomidine are lower in patients with varying degrees of hepatic impairment. Dexmedetomidine pharmacokinetics are not significantly different in patients with severe renal impairment compared to healthy subjects.[62]

Pharmacodynamics

Dexmedetomidine acts on the α_2-adrenergic receptors in the spinal cord and brain (Fig. 19-11). Its effects are primarily at the locus coeruleus that activates sleep centers in the brain. Interestingly, the EEG pattern observed in patients receiving dexmedetomidine resembles that of non-REM sleep. Clinically, patients are sedated but easily arousable, and able to follow commands with minimal respiratory depression.[63]

The cardiovascular effects of dexmedetomidine are as expected for an α_2 agonist: bradycardia and hypotension. Compared to placebo, dexmedetomidine causes a 7 mmHg decrease in systolic blood pressure and a decrease in mean heart rate of 1 to 8 bpm.[61]

Figure 19-10 Dexmedetomidine. (S)-4-[1-(2,2-Dimethylphenyl)ethyl]-3-H-imidazole.

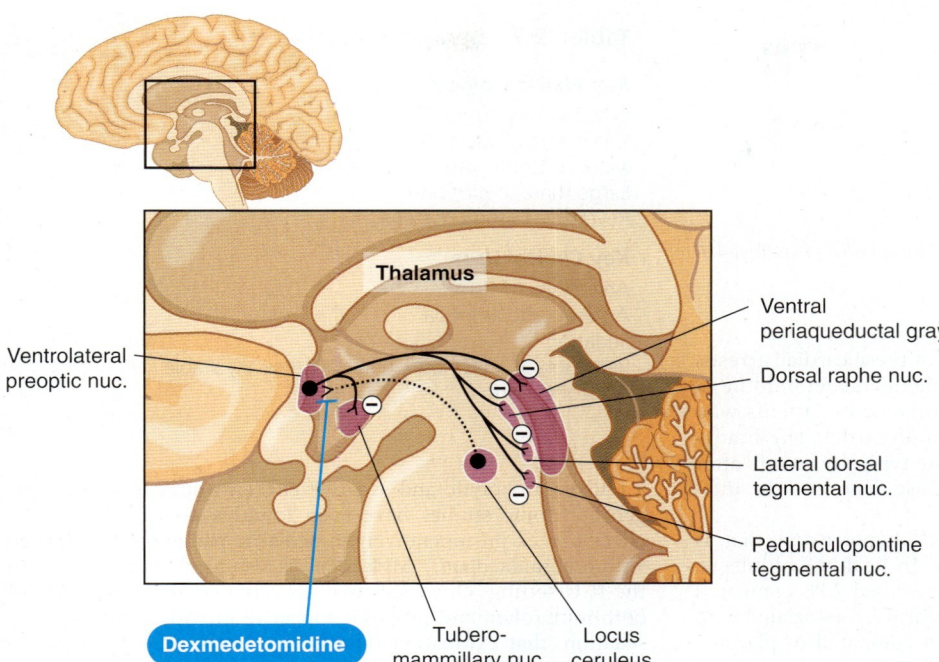

Figure 19-11 Dexmedetomidine's mechanism of action in the central nervous system. Dexmedetomidine activates the sleep centers in the brain. Dexmedetomidine binds to α_2 receptors on neurons from the locus ceruleus, inhibiting norepinephrine release (dashed line) in the ventrolateral preoptic nucleus. The disinhibited ventrolateral preoptic nucleus reduces arousal of the midbrain, hypothalamic, and pontine arousal nuclei.

Clinical Uses

7 Dexmedetomidine has been used to provide sedation for mechanically ventilated patients in the ICU. Patients receiving dexmedetomidine required less rescue sedation with midazolam or morphine versus placebo.[61] Maintenance of spontaneous respiration allows for ICU patients to be extubated while receiving a dexmedetomidine infusion. Dexmedetomidine is also attractive for ICU sedation in neurosurgery, as patients can participate in neurologic examinations while receiving this medication. Dexmedetomidine has been found to have analgesic properties, and can reduce opiate requirements in ICU patients who are mechanically ventilated. However, a systematic review of controlled trials failed to find sedation superiority when comparing dexmedetomidine to midazolam for ICU sedation.[64]

Dexmedetomidine can also be used for procedural sedation. Dexmedetomidine has been studied as an agent for sedation during awake fiberoptic intubation.[61] Maintenance of spontaneous ventilation makes this drug useful for this very purpose. Dexmedetomidine can also be used to provide MAC sedation alone or in combination with other medications. Typical administration involves at 0.5 to 1 µg/kg loading dose over 15 minutes, followed by an infusion of 0.3 to 0.7 µg/kg/hr.

Several studies have compared the efficacy of dexmedetomidine to propofol for procedural sedation. In the operating room, dexmedetomidine provided adequate sedation compared to propofol with less hypotension, and better pain scores in the post anesthesia care unit (PACU). However, the onset of sedation was longer with dexmedetomidine, and patients had prolonged sedation and more hypotension in the PACU when compared to propofol.[65,66] Two studies found dexmedetomidine to be inferior to propofol for sedation for upper endoscopy procedures.[67,68]

Although not approved for use in pediatrics, many investigators have evaluated its off-label use in children.[62] Intranasal dexmedetomidine (1 µg/kg) has been used for preoperative anxiolysis, with an onset of 25 minutes and duration of 85 minutes. Dexmedetomidine was found to be superior to oral midazolam in ensuring satisfactory levels of sedation; however, its long onset time limits this application. Because it preserves spontaneous respiration, dexmedetomidine has been used in airway procedures such as rigid bronchoscopy. Dexmedetomidine has been used as an adjunct to TIVA during posterior spine fusion surgery, and lowers both propofol and sevoflurane requirements. Dexmedetomidine has been found to have minimal effect on SSEPs and motor evoked potentials (MEPs) during spine surgery.[69]

Dexmedetomidine has been investigated for the prevention of emergence delirium. A meta-analysis found that α_2 agonists (clonidine or dexmedetomidine) decrease emergence delirium when given via the oral, intravenous, or caudal route. Dexmedetomidine given by intravenous bolus or infusion has been shown to decrease emergence delirium, but the optimal dose is unknown. Compared to placebo, dexmedetomidine (0.5 to 1 µg/kg) decreases the incidence of emergence delirium from 47% to 2.8%, with slightly prolonged emergence time.[70]

Dexmedetomidine has been investigated as a local anesthetic adjuvant for regional anesthesia. Dexmedetomidine was found to prolong both motor and sensory blocks when administered intrathecally in combination with local anesthetic. Perineural injection of dexmedetomidine as part of a brachial plexus block did extend the duration of the block, but this was not found to be statistically significant. Further studies are needed to define the potential benefit of dexmedetomidine as a local anesthesia adjuvant.[71]

Side Effects

The main adverse reactions of dexmedetomidine are hypotension, bradycardia, dry mouth, nausea, and hypertension. The incidence of bradycardia is reported as high as 40%, and can be managed with atropine, ephedrine, or volume administration.[72] There are case reports of patients who have developed severe bradycardia and cardiac arrest with dexmedetomidine administration.[73] However, in these reports, dexmedetomidine is

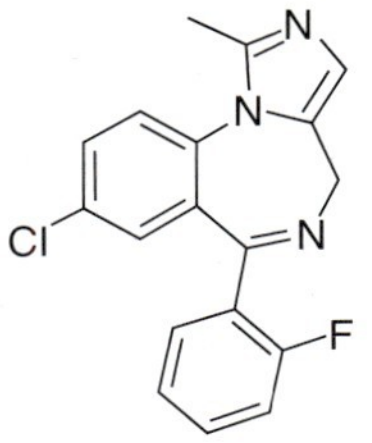

Figure 19-12 Midazolam. 8-chloro-6-(2-fluorophenyl)-1-methyl-4H-imidazo[1,5-a][1,4]benzodiazepine.

Table 19-7	Benzodiazepines

Key Pharmacology
GABA-A receptor agonist
Minimal respiratory depression
Minimal cardiovascular depression
Large therapeutic window
Reversible with flumazenil

Key Clinical Uses
Anxiolysis
Anterograde amnesia
Sedation
Induction of anesthesia, hemodynamically stable
Anticonvulsant

unlikely to be the only causative agent of these cardiac arrests. Therefore, care should be taken in using dexmedetomidine in patients who will not tolerate bradycardia, or in patients who are receiving medications that cause bradycardia. The bradycardia associated with dexmedetomidine typically occurs after a loading dose. Omitting the loading dose decreases the incidence of bradycardia.[72]

Dexmedetomidine is associated with hypotension that is expected with an α_2-adrenergic agonist. In healthy volunteers, after a 1 µg/kg bolus, blood pressure decreased 23% compared to baseline. Infusions of 0.2 to 0.7 µg/kg/hr were associated with larger decreases in blood pressure when compared to placebo. Blood pressure returns to baseline within 6 hours of treatment cessation without any apparent rebound effects. There are case reports of dexmedetomidine overdose. Two patients received infusions of 2 or 4 µg/kg/hr (instead of 0.2 to 0.4 µg/kg/hr), which caused excess sedation but had minimal effect on hemodynamics.[74] In a 3-year-old child who received an unintentional bolus of 9 µg/kg of dexmedetomidine, the heart rate, blood pressure, and oxygen saturation were all decreased. However, the child was managed with supplemental oxygen, fluid bolus, and epinephrine infusion, and recovered to baseline after 7 hours.[75]

Benzodiazepines

Benzodiazepines—midazolam in particular—are frequently used by anesthesiologists to produce several clinically desirable effects: anxiolysis, anterograde amnesia, sedation, and hypnosis. They can also be used as muscle relaxants and anticonvulsants. Benzodiazepines have a favorable safety profile and can be reversed by flumazenil to manage excessive sedation or respiratory depression.

Midazolam was first discovered in 1976 and is the most widely used benzodiazepine in the perioperative period (Fig. 19-12; Table 19-7). Its use as a premedication and anesthetic is largely due to its quick onset, short elimination half-life, anterograde amnestic effect, and minimal side-effect profile.[76] Midazolam can be administered intravenously, intranasally, orally, rectally, and intramuscularly. This flexibility in route of administration also contributes to its popularity. A 0.5-mg/kg dose of oral midazolam given 30 minutes preoperatively in children yields a reliable anxiolytic and sedative effect without delayed emergence.[77] Some studies have even found a positive behavioral effect 1 week postoperatively in pediatric patients premedicated with oral midazolam.[78] Midazolam is also used as an infusion in the ICU setting. One meta-analysis reported that "infusions of both midazolam and propofol appear to provide similar quality sedation, that extubation time and recovery time is shorter in patients sedated with propofol, and that hemodynamic complications related to either drug regimen are not usually clinically significant."[79]

Pharmacokinetics

Benzodiazepines are highly protein-bound and highly lipophilic (Tables 19-8 and 19-9). High protein binding renders a smaller free fraction of the drug available to cross the blood–brain barrier, and high lipophilicity results in a larger volume of distribution. Clinically, less drug is free to cross the blood–brain barrier, but the high lipophilicity results in a rapid-onset of action (the peak effect of intravenous midazolam is within 2 to 3 minutes).[80] Only a fraction of the available CNS binding sites need to be occupied to produce clinical effects. Midazolam's high lipid solubility, short duration of action, and short context-sensitive half-time allow this drug to be administered as a continuous infusion,[81] unlike other benzodiazepines.

Metabolism of benzodiazepines occurs largely in the hepatic cytochrome P450 system via oxidation and glucuronic conjugation. The metabolized drug is then renally excreted. Some drugs, such as diazepam, have pharmacologically active metabolites (i.e., desmethyldiazepam, 3-hydroxydiazepam) with long elimination half-lives that lead to a prolonged duration of action, especially in patients with renal failure. Drugs that inhibit the cytochrome P450 system can result in prolonged duration of benzodiazepines.

Favorable properties of midazolam are its high rate of hepatic clearance and relatively short elimination half-life. Midazolam has

Table 19-8	Benzodiazepine Metabolism and Clearance		
Drug	**Duration**	**Metabolites**	**Hepatic Clearance**
Midazolam	Short	1-Hydroxymidazolam (mild CNS depressant)	High
Diazepam	Intermediate	Oxazepam and desmethyldiazepam	Slow
Lorazepam	Long	Inactive	Intermediate

Table 19-9 Benzodiazepine Pharmacokinetics

Drug	Induction Dose (mg/kg)	Duration of Action (min)	Half-Life (min)	Protein Binding (%)	Volume of Distribution (L/kg)	Clearance (mL/kg/min)	Elimination Half-Life (hr)
Midazolam	0.1–0.3	15–20	7–15	94	1–3.1	6.4–11	1.8–2.6
Diazepam	0.3–0.6	15–30	10–15	98	0.7–1.7	0.2–0.5	20–50
Lorazepam	0.03–0.1	60–120	3–10	98	0.8–1.3	0.8–1.8	11–22

a volume of distribution of 1 to 3.1 L/kg after a single bolus dose, an elimination half-life of 1.8–2.6 to hours (mean approximately 3 hours), and a total clearance of 6.4–11 mL/kg/min.[82] Midazolam's active metabolite (1-hydroxymidazolam) contributes minimally to its clinical effects (approximately 20% of midazolam's potency). These properties are influenced by the patient's age and comorbidities, particularly kidney and liver dysfunction. With continuous infusions of midazolam, the metabolite will accumulate and exert a more pronounced and prolonged effect. Rather than metabolism, redistribution of midazolam results in the termination of its effects.

Pharmacodynamics and Clinical Uses

The three most commonly used parenteral benzodiazepines are lorazepam, diazepam, and midazolam. Lorazepam and diazepam are not soluble in water and often cause vein irritation due to the propylene glycol admixture. Alternative formulations are available as a lipid emulsion, but with a decrease in bioavailability. Midazolam is water-soluble and undergoes conformational change in the bloodstream, becoming more lipophilic. Midazolam is manufactured as an acidic formulation that may produce mild local tissue and vein irritation.

Benzodiazepines bind to specific receptor sites that are part of the GABA-A receptor complex. This binding augments the effect of the GABA-A receptor/chloride channel coupling, resulting in increased frequency of chloride channel opening. The resultant hyperpolarization of the cell ultimately leads to neural inhibition. It is this enhanced affinity of the GABA-A receptor for the GABA molecule, and subsequent decreased unbinding that produces the so-called ceiling effect.[83] Benzodiazepines thus have a dose-dependent CNS depressant effect (Table 19-10). For example, at 30% to 50% receptor occupancy, sedation is often produced, while at 20% occupancy one usually only achieves anxiolysis.[84]

The high density of GABA-A receptors in the cerebral cortex helps explain the sedative/hypnotic, anxiolytic, and amnestic capabilities of these drugs. Benzodiazepines also decrease both the $CMRO_2$ and CBF, while maintaining carbon dioxide responsiveness. They exert little if any effect on ICP. Because of the ceiling effect of benzodiazepines, an isoelectric EEG or burst suppression is not attained. This is in direct contrast to propofol and thiopental, each of which can achieve burst suppression. Thus, the neuroprotectant effect of benzodiazepines is quite limited, but likely not entirely absent. Some investigators have demonstrated that activation of GABA-A receptors, including the specific binding subunits for propofol and midazolam, play a role in the inhibition of neuronal death induced by brain ischemia.

Additionally, benzodiazepines are anticonvulsants and are a first-line therapy in the management of seizures. They can also be used as muscle relaxants, but this spinal cord–mediated response typically requires supratherapeutic doses.

Benzodiazepines can also have a profound effect on the respiratory system. Upper airway reflexes may be decreased and central respiratory drive is depressed. In the usual premedication dosage, respiratory depression is rarely an issue.; however, if the patient has other comorbidities and/or concurrent opioid use, then adverse respiratory events are more likely to occur.

Benzodiazepines, especially in induction doses, depress the SVR and decrease blood pressure. This effect is quite minimal as there is some preservation of homeostatic reflexes. This response may be more pronounced in the hypovolemic patient. Benzodiazepines are overall regarded as hemodynamically stable induction agents.

Side Effects

Aside from their previously discussed systemic effects, benzodiazepines are associated with limited adverse events. Anaphylaxis is extremely rare following the administration of a benzodiazepine. More frequently described is pain or thrombophlebitis that ensues following intravenous injection, especially diazepam. Propylene glycol is the organic solvent for diazepam and causes the pain associated with injection. In contrast, midazolam is water-soluble, but may also cause burning with injection secondary to its acidic formulation.

Barbiturates

Thiopental is one of the earliest intravenous anesthetics used, discovered in the 1930s and first used on human patients in 1934. It has withstood the test of time as an induction agent because of its favorable pharmacokinetic profile (Fig. 19-13; Table 19-11). In 2011, production of thiopental in the United States ceased, leading to a drastic decrease in intraoperative use. Two major classes of barbiturates, oxybarbiturates and thiobarbiturates, are of anesthetic clinical and historical relevance. Both classes contain a pyrimidine center, and either an oxygen or sulfur molecule at position 2. Used in clinical practice are the thiobarbiturates thiopental (2.5%) and thiamylal (2%), and the oxybarbiturate methohexital (1%). The thiobarbiturate solutions are produced

Table 19-10 Midazolam Dosing by Clinical Use

Premedication: anxiolysis, anterograde amnesia	0.02–0.04 mg/kg IV/IM; 0.4–0.8 mg/kg PO
Induction: hypnosis, amnesia sedation	0.1–0.2 mg/kg IV
Infusion (in conjunction with volatile anesthetics): hypnosis, amnesia	0.25–1 µg/kg/min

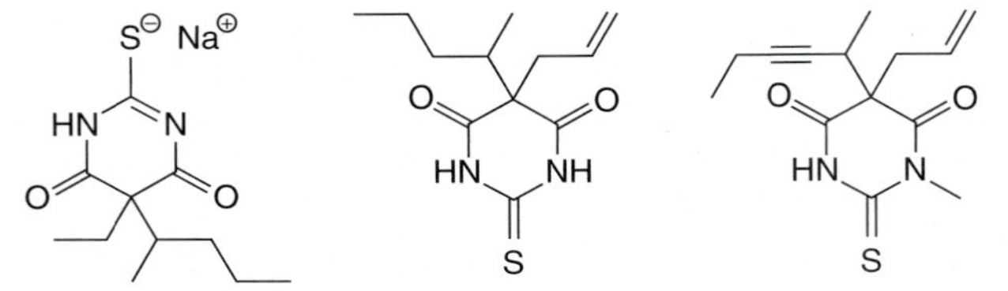

Figure 19-13 Thiopental: (RS)-[5-ethyl-4,6-dioxo-5-(pentan-2-yl)-1,4,5,6-tetrahydropyrimidin-2-yl]sulfanide sodium. Thiamylal: 5-Allyl-5-(1-methylbutyl)-2-thioxodihydropyrimidine-4,6(1H,5H)-dione. Methohexital: 5-hex-3-yn-2-yl-1- methyl-5-prop-2-enyl-1, 3-diazinane-2,4,6-trione.

as racemic mixtures, despite unequal potency between their two stereoisomers. Methohexital has two chiral centers and four potential stereoisomers, but not all isomers are included in the final product. Barbiturate solutions are highly alkaline, allowing for formation of water-soluble salts. Addition or reconstitution in acidic solutions leads to precipitation of these salts, preventing intravenous use. Unlike propofol, barbiturates cannot be stored for an extended period of time at room temperature after reconstitution in solvent. In alkaline solution, thiobarbiturates can be stored up to 2 weeks, and methohexital up to 6 weeks.

Pharmacokinetics

Primary metabolism of both barbiturate classes is hepatic, yielding water-soluble inactive metabolites that are subsequently eliminated in urine and bile. Oxidation of thiopental and methohexital to their respective hydroxyl derivatives is the most common form of metabolism.[85] Thiopental has a relatively long elimination half-life (12 hours), and its clearance rate (3 mL/kg/min) is 10-fold longer than that of propofol. Methohexital elimination half-life (4 hours) is also shorter than thiopental, secondary to a more efficient hepatic extraction of the drug (clearance rate 11 mL/kg/min). A negligible percentage of barbiturates is eliminated without metabolism in the urine.

Table 19-11 Barbiturates

Key Pharmacology
GABA-A receptor agonist
Prolonged context-sensitive half-time
CNS depressant, neuroprotective, anticonvulsant, decreases $CMRO_2$, CBF, and ICP
EEG burst suppression (thiopental)
Cardiovascular: decreases mean arterial pressure, venous vascular tone, and cardiac output
Pulmonary: Dose-dependent respiratory depression, does not cause bronchodilation

Key Clinical Uses
Induction of general anesthesia
Methohexital used for sedation, premedication, and electroconvulsive therapy
Barbiturate coma (thiopental)
Thiopental intra-arterial injection can lead to tissue necrosis

$CMRO_2$, cerebral metabolic oxygen consumption rate; CBF, cerebral blood flow; ICP, intracranial pressure; EEG, electroencephalogram.

Multicompartment pharmacokinetic models of barbiturates after administration of an induction dose have been described. Similar to other intravenous agents, rapid redistribution into highly perfused compartments accounts for the rapid termination of drug action after a single induction dose. After an extended infusion of thiopental, accumulation in poorly perfused compartments and slow elimination play larger pharmacokinetic roles, resulting in a prolonged context-sensitive half-time and delayed recovery. The long context-sensitive half-time of thiopental after high doses is explained by the drug exhibiting zero-order kinetics. The elimination of thiopental becomes independent of both drug plasma concentration and level of compartmental saturation, and remains constant and defined by the slow rate of clearance.

Pharmacodynamics

The mechanism of action of barbiturates involves cortical and brainstem GABA inhibitory pathways, leading to loss of consciousness, as well as respiratory and cardiovascular depression. Hypnotic effects of barbiturates are likely enhanced by the inhibition of central excitatory pathways, specifically those mediated by glutamate via NMDA receptors and acetylcholine.

Central Nervous System Effects

The progression of EEG changes after administration of barbiturates is dose-dependent. Initial low doses can generate a light level of anesthesia often associated with a high-frequency and low-amplitude EEG pattern. With higher doses, both burst suppression and an isoelectric EEG can be attained.[86] Thiopental is generally considered an anticonvulsant, having been used successfully for treatment of status epilepticus. At smaller concentrations thiopental has been noted to have proconvulsant properties. Methohexital is considered to have significant proconvulsant effects in patients with epilepsy, and is often the agent of choice for induction of anesthesia prior to electroconvulsive therapy.[87,88] The excitatory effects of methohexital are commonly exhibited muscle twitches that occur after an induction dose of the drug.

Barbiturates cause a decrease in $CMRO_2$ that is dose-dependent, eventually leading to an isoelectric EEG that is associated with up to a 50% decrease in oxygen consumption.[89] A concomitant increase in cerebral vascular resistance leads to decreased CBF and ICP. CPP is often unchanged or even improved, as the decrease in MAP is typically less than the decrease in ICP. Barbiturate CNS effects are considered neuroprotective and in part explained by the decrease in $CMRO_2$, although $CMRO_2$ decreases are not directly proportional to levels of ischemic neuroprotection.[90] Other neuroprotective mechanisms likely play a role, including barbiturate anticonvulsant properties, improved blood flow to ischemic parts of the brain (reverse steal effect), free-radical scavenging, attenuation of excitatory neurotransmitter release and pathways, and membrane stabilization. The reverse steal effect is a result of flow-metabolism coupling. At higher doses, the reduction in oxygen consumption in well perfused areas of the brain leads to decreased flow, with subsequent diversion of blood flow to ischemic areas.

Historically, barbiturate-induced "brain relaxation" has been utilized as a protective strategy during neurosurgery and after head trauma. The clinical benefit after barbiturate administration has been reproduced by other techniques, including cooling (to lower $CMRO_2$) and antihypertensive strategies. Barbiturate neuroprotection is generally considered more effective for focal and incomplete ischemia, rather than global injury. In the setting of comatose cardiac arrest survivors, thiopental loading after cardiac arrest has not been shown to significantly improve outcome.[91] In contrast, thiopental-induced burst suppression and isoelectric EEG prior to potential focal ischemic insult during cardiopulmonary bypass and carotid surgery have been shown to have clinical benefit.

Cardiovascular Effects

The most prominent cardiovascular changes after an induction dose of thiopental are decreases in both MAP and cardiac output. The primary mechanism is reduction of venous vascular tone, followed by peripheral pooling of venous blood and a decrease in venous return.[92] Thiopental also has negative inotropic effects, directly by altering intracellular calcium homeostasis and indirectly by diminishing sympathetic tone. Baroreceptor-mediated heart rate increase may be impaired by thiopental administration, but a reflex elevation in heart rate of 10% to 30% is still typically present. The negative hemodynamic effects after a thiopental bolus are more pronounced in patients with underlying cardiovascular disease and in hypovolemic states. Induction doses of methohexital are typically associated with a smaller decrease in MAP and larger increase in heart rate than what is described for thiopental.[93]

Respiratory System Effects

Barbiturates cause respiratory depression in a dose-dependent manner, leading to central apnea at deeper stages of anesthesia. After a typical induction dose, apnea is commonly noted after 1 to 1.5 minutes, with ventilatory response to carbon dioxide returning to baseline in approximately 6 minutes. The time course to recovery from respiratory depression is shorter with thiopental than with propofol.[94] Thiopental does not cause as much bronchodilation as propofol or inhalational anesthetics.[95,96] Case reports of laryngospasm and bronchospasm after induction of anesthesia with thiopental exist, and airway reflexes are generally considered to be more preserved compared to induction with propofol.

Clinical Uses

Rapid onset and emergence from a bolus dose of thiopental have made it an ideal induction agent. The typical induction dose is 2.5 to 5 mg/kg, resulting in light stages of anesthesia in 15 to 30 seconds, and deeper stages in 30 to 40 seconds that last for approximately 1 minute. Premedication may decrease the required induction dose by as much as 50%, and nitrous oxide may decrease the required plasma concentration of thiopental by 67%.[97] Patient variability will affect the required induction dose. Unpremedicated healthy children may require a 5- to 6-mg/kg induction dose, and infants may have an even higher requirement.[98] Elderly patients have a lower induction dose requirement, although no significant age-specific difference in plasma concentrations of thiopental were noted to achieve a given hypnotic effect.[99] The necessary reduction in dose is likely due to variation in pharmacokinetic profile of elderly patients, including decreased volume of distribution and slower redistribution times. Obesity also has been noted to lower thiopental induction requirement on a per kilogram basis,[100] but similar to elderly patients, the use of lean body mass to determine induction dose corrects the difference. Numerous comorbid states have been associated with a decrease in induction dose requirement, including liver disease, heart failure, shock, and severe anemia. Methohexital can also be used for induction of anesthesia, with the typical intravenous induction dose of 1 to 2 mg/kg. It has also been administered rectally in solution form as a sedative in the pediatric population, with the recommended dose of 25 mg/kg.[101]

Thiopental is rarely used as an intravenous infusion for maintenance of general anesthesia because higher doses lead to zero-order kinetics and a slow plasma clearance. The context-sensitive half-time of thiopental is relatively high and results in unpredictable and prolonged recovery from infusion. Methohexital has a shorter elimination half-life than thiopental, and at infusion doses of 50 to 150 µg/kg/min has been used for maintenance of sedation and general anesthesia. Concern for seizure activity after prolonged infusions in susceptible patient populations has minimized this utility. As noted, thiopental infusion for maintenance of barbiturate coma has been utilized in patients with elevated ICP after acute brain injury, although the efficacy of thiopental in preventing long-term brain injury and improving outcomes has been questioned.

Side Effects

Intravenous administration of thiopental is typically not irritating or painful, but if injected outside the vein into subcutaneous tissue it can cause discomfort. Methohexital-induced pain on injection is much more prevalent. Inadvertent arterial administration of thiopental has to be managed promptly, as formation of crystals can lead to decreased flow due to vasospasm and thrombus formation, pain at the arterial site, and possible tissue necrosis. Management includes arterial administration of papaverine, heparinization, and potential arteriodilation by appropriate regional anesthetic technique. Barbiturates are contraindicated in patients with acute intermittent porphyria, as an exacerbation of symptoms may be augmented by their direct effects on hepatic enzymes.

New Intravenous Anesthetics

New drugs are constantly being developed in an effort to achieve the ideal intravenous anesthetic with a short duration of action, a short context-sensitive half-time that allows for infusion administration, and minimal adverse effects.

Remimazolam

This investigational drug is a benzodiazepine with a structure and onset time similar to midazolam (Fig. 19-14), and it binds as an agonist to the GABA receptor. It has a rapid offset that follows first-order kinetics at the recommended doses due to metabolism

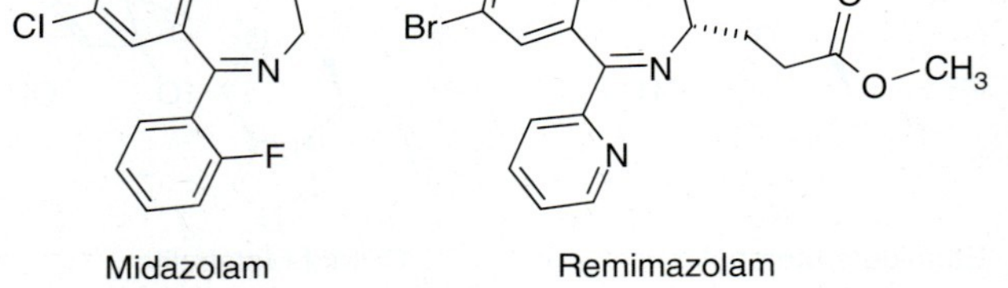

Figure 19-14 Structural comparison between midazolam and remimazolam.

by tissue esterases (similar to remifentanil), and thus does not result in accumulation of drug. In addition to organ-independent metabolism, this drug is reversible with flumazenil, further adding to the safety profile. The quick onset and offset offer the potential for use as an infusion. Remimazolam is initially being developed for procedural sedation during procedures such as colonoscopy.[102] It is also being considered for ICU sedation, as many critically ill patients have end-organ dysfunction and would benefit from the organ-independent metabolism of this drug. This drug provides an alternative to propofol by avoiding PRIS and accumulation of drug leading to prolonged sedation. To summarize, remimazolam takes advantage of the hypnotic and amnestic effects of midazolam with a speed and mode of metabolism similar to remifentanil.[103]

Propofol Formulations

Propofol is a hydrophobic oil that requires a lipid emulsion as a vehicle of administration. This emulsion, comprised largely of egg yolk lecithin, soybean oil, and glycerol, has several drawbacks. The most common complaint is pain on injection. More serious adverse effects include anaphylaxis, sepsis secondary to microbial contamination of an open vial (despite antimicrobial additives), and PRIS.[104] Many attempts have been made to develop a formulation of propofol that reduces these problems, including (1) to reduce the percentage of lipid in the emulsion, (2) to eliminate the lipid, and (3) to create a prodrug. One major challenge with tailoring the current formulation is that the drug's pharmacokinetics may also be altered.

Fospropofol

Fospropofol is a prodrug of propofol that was produced to reduce or eliminate the adverse effects of the current propofol emulsion. Fospropofol is a water-based solution that yields less pain on injection, less hyperlipidemia, and less risk for bacteremia. Its clinical application as a sedative-hypnotic has been approved for MAC sedation, but not for general anesthesia. A major deterrent to its use is its delayed onset time and longer elimination time. Although hypotension and respiratory depression may occur less frequently, these reactions still do occur. Fospropofol is also associated with an increase in pruritus and paresthesias.[105] Fospropofol was initially developed as a drug to be used by nonanesthesia medical providers. However, fospropofol is associated with similar respiratory depression as propofol, and practitioners must be able to rescue patients from unintended deep sedation or general anesthesia.

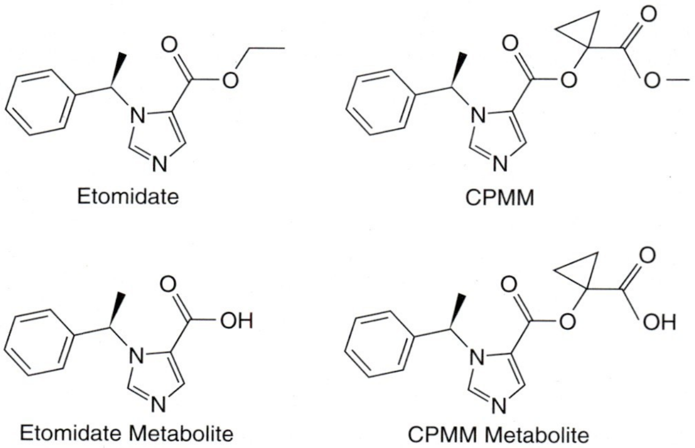

Cyclopropyl-methoxycarbonyl Metomidate

Cyclopropyl-methoxycarbonyl metomidate (CPMM), also known as AB700, is an analogue of etomidate that has shown promise in animal studies (Fig. 19-15). It causes less adrenal suppression compared with etomidate. It also is less potent and has a shorter duration of action than etomidate. The investigators of this drug purport its use as a bolus or infusion medication for both sedation and general anesthesia.[106] Although its structure is a derivative of etomidate, its clinical application seems to be more consistent with that of propofol. Some studies have even demonstrated that compared to propofol, CPMM has less drug accumulation and therefore more rapid recovery after prolonged infusion.[106]

THRX-918661/AZD-3043

The search for a sedative/hypnotic agent whose effects are terminated in a predictable and consistent time frame regardless of dose or duration of infusion has led to the development of THRX-918661/AZD-3043. This medication is a metabolically-labile, positive allosteric modulator of the GABA-A receptor. This investigational drug is water-soluble and rapidly hydrolyzed by blood and tissue esterases to an inactive carboxylate metabolite.[107] A Phase I clinical trial showed no serious adverse events and a rapid recovery after infusion administration. Further studies will be required to evaluate the potential of THRX-918661/AZD-3043 to provide rapid recovery regardless of duration of anesthesia.[108]

Sedasys

In May 2013, the FDA approved Sedasys, a computer-assisted patient-controlled sedation system that administers propofol for colonoscopies/endoscopies. Patients are monitored with electrocardiography, pulse oximetry, noninvasive blood pressure monitoring, and end-tidal carbon dioxide. Sedation is also further monitored via an earpiece through which the computer tells the patient to squeeze a handset. Based on these parameters, Sedasys will algorithmically adjust the infusion rate of propofol.

An early study of one thousand patients, ASA class 1–3, who used the Sedasys system found fewer episodes of desaturation and improved patient and physician satisfaction.[109] Sedasys affords nonanesthesia providers the ability to conduct procedures that require minimal to moderate sedation with propofol. Healthcare cost savings might theoretically result from removing the anesthesiologist from the cost of the procedure. However, many physicians, especially anesthesiologists, are skeptical of the safety of this patient-controlled system. For example, there are times when deeper planes of anesthesia are needed, yet cannot be provided by Sedasys. Patients may cough or buck or obstruct their airway during the procedure, and nonanesthesia providers may not be sufficiently trained or skilled in airway management. Furthermore, sampling of the end-tidal carbon dioxide may not be accurate secondary to the endoscope physically being near the airway.[110] Interestingly, in March, 2016 the device manufacturer has exited the market for this product.

Figure 19-15 Etomidate, cyclopropyl-methoxycarbonyl metomidate (CPMM), and their metabolites.

REFERENCES

1. White PF. Clinical uses of intravenous anesthetic and analgesic infusions. *Anesth Analg.* 1989;68:161–171.
2. Hemmings HC. The pharmacology of intravenous anesthetic induction agents: a primer. *Anesthesiology News.* October 8, 2010:9–16.
3. Kam PC, Cardone D. Propofol infusion syndrome. *Anaesthesia.* 2007;62(7):690–701.
4. Gepts E. Pharmacokinetic concepts for TCI anaesthesia. *Anaesthesia.* 1998;53:4–12.
5. Struys MM, De Smet T, Glen JI, et al. The history of target-controlled infusion. *Anesth Analg.* 2016;122(1):56–69.
6. Kay B, Rolly G. I.C.I. 35868, a new intravenous induction agent. *Acta Anaesthesiol Belg.* 1977;28(4):303–316.
7. Krasowski MD, Koltchine VV, Rick CE, et al. Propofol and other intravenous anesthetics have sites of action on the gamma-aminobutyric acid type A receptor distinct from that for isoflurane. *Mol Pharmacol.* 1998;53(3):530–538.
8. Kikuchi T, Wang Y, Sato K, et al. In vivo effects of propofol on acetylcholine release from the frontal cortex, hippocampus and striatum studied by intracerebral microdialysis in freely moving rats. *Br J Anaesth.* 1998;80(5):644–648.
9. Alkire MT, Hudetz AG, Tononi G. Consciousness and anesthesia. *Science.* 2008;322(5903):876–880.
10. Fiset P, Paus T, Daloze T, et al. Brain mechanisms of propofol-induced loss of consciousness in humans: a positron emission tomographic study. *J Neurosci.* 1999;19(13):5506–5513.
11. Bevan JC, Veall GR, Macnab AJ, et al. Midazolam premedication delays recovery after propofol without modifying involuntary movements. *Anesth Analg.* 1997;85(1):50–54.
12. Feshchenko VA, Veselis RA, Reinsel RA. Propofol-induced alpha rhythm. *Neuropsychobiology.* 2004;50(3):257–266.
13. Stratford N, Murphy P. Antioxidant activity of propofol in blood from anaesthetized patients. *Eur J Anaesthesiol.* 1998;15(2):158–160.
14. Lingamaneni R, Birch ML, Hemmings HC, Jr. Widespread inhibition of sodium channel-dependent glutamate release from isolated nerve terminals by isoflurane and propofol. *Anesthesiology.* 2001;95(6):1460–1466.
15. Engelhard K, Werner C, Eberspacher E, et al. Influence of propofol on neuronal damage and apoptotic factors after incomplete cerebral ischemia and reperfusion in rats: a long-term observation. *Anesthesiology.* 2004;101(4):912–917.
16. Liu J, Gao XF, Ni W, et al. Effects of propofol on P2x7 receptors and the secretion of tumor necrosis factor-alpha in cultured astrocytes. *Clin Exp Med.* 2012;12(1):31–37.
17. Ebrahim ZY, Schubert A, Van Ness P, et al. The effect of propofol on the electroencephalogram of patients with epilepsy. *Anesth Analg.* 1994;78(2):275–279.
18. Samra SK, Sneyd JR, Ross DA, et al. Effects of propofol sedation on seizures and intracranially recorded epileptiform activity in patients with partial epilepsy. *Anesthesiology.* 1995;82(4):843–851.
19. Wischmeyer PE, Johnson BR, Wilson JE, et al. A survey of propofol abuse in academic anesthesia programs. *Anesth Analg.* 2007;105(4):1066–1071.
20. Fulton B, Sorkin EM. Propofol. An overview of its pharmacology and a review of its clinical efficacy in intensive care sedation. *Drugs.* 1995;50(4):636–657.
21. Meuret P, Backman SB, Bonhomme V, et al. Physostigmine reverses propofol-induced unconsciousness and attenuation of the auditory steady state response and bispectral index in human volunteers. *Anesthesiology.* 2000;93(3):708–717.
22. Samain E, Bouillier H, Marty J, et al. The effect of propofol on angiotensin II-induced Ca(2+) mobilization in aortic smooth muscle cells from normotensive and hypertensive rats. *Anesth Analg.* 2000;90(3):546–552.
23. Pires LA, Huang SK, Wagshal AB, et al. Electrophysiological effects of propofol on the normal cardiac conduction system. *Cardiology.* 1996;87(4):319–324.
24. Kirkpatrick T, Cockshott ID, Douglas EJ, et al. Pharmacokinetics of propofol (diprivan) in elderly patients. *Br J Anaesth.* 1988;60(2):146–150.
25. Marsh B, White M, Morton N, et al. Pharmacokinetic model driven infusion of propofol in children. *Br J Anaesth.* 1991;67(1):41–48.
26. Ingrande J, Brodsky JB, Lemmens HJ. Lean body weight scalar for the anesthetic induction dose of propofol in morbidly obese subjects. *Anesth Analg.* 2011;113(1):57–62.
27. Gan TJ, Glass PS, Howell ST, et al. Determination of plasma concentrations of propofol associated with 50% reduction in postoperative nausea. *Anesthesiology.* 1997;87(4):779–784.
28. Picard P, Tramer MR. Prevention of pain on injection with propofol: a quantitative systematic review. *Anesth Analg.* 2000;90(4):963–969.
29. Jalota L, Kalira V, George E, et al. Prevention of pain on injection of propofol: systematic review and meta-analysis. *BMJ.* 2011;342:d1110.
30. Parke TJ, Stevens JE, Rice AS, et al. Metabolic acidosis and fatal myocardial failure after propofol infusion in children: five case reports. *BMJ.* 1992;305(6854):613–616.
31. Cremer OL, Moons KG, Bouman EA, et al. Long-term propofol infusion and cardiac failure in adult head-injured patients. *Lancet.* 2001;357(9250):117–118.
32. Krajcova A, Waldauf P, Andel M, et al. Propofol infusion syndrome: a structured review of experimental studies and 153 published case reports. *Crit Care.* 2015;19:398.
33. Tan CK, Lai CC, Cheng KC. Propofol-related green urine. *Kidney Int.* 2008;74(7):978.
34. Gooding JM, Corssen G. Effect of etomidate on the cardiovascular system. *Anesth Analg.* 1977;56(5):717–719.
35. Meyanci Koksal G, Erbabacan E, Tunali Y, et al. The effect of single dose etomidate during emergency intubation on hemodynamics and adrenal cortex. *Turk J Trauma Emerg Surg.* 2015;21(5):358–365.
36. Gu WJ, Wang F, Tang L, et al. Single-dose etomidate does not increase mortality in patients with sepsis: a systematic review and meta-analysis of randomized controlled trials and observational studies. *Chest.* 2015;147(2):335–346.
37. Chan CM, Mitchell AL, Shorr AF. Etomidate is associated with mortality and adrenal insufficiency in sepsis: a meta-analysis. *Crit Care Med.* 2012;40(11):2945–2953.
38. Domino E, Chodoff P, Corssen G. Pharmacologic effects of CI-581, a new dissociative anesthetic, in man. *Clin Pharmacol Ther.* 1965;6:279–291.
39. Visser E, Schug SA. The role of ketamine in pain management. *Biomed Pharmacother.* 2006;60(7):341–348.
40. Fond G, Loundou A, Rabu C, et al. Ketamine administration in depressive disorders: a systematic review and meta-analysis. *Psychopharmacology.* 2014;231(18):3663–3676.
41. Potter DE, Choudhury M. Ketamine: repurposing and redefining a multifaceted drug. *Drug Discov Today.* 2014;19(12):1848–1854.
42. Marland S, Ellerton J, Andolfatto G, et al. Ketamine: use in anesthesia. *CNS Neurosci Ther.* 2013;19(6):381–389.
43. Clements J, Nimo W, Grant I. Bioavailability, pharmacokinetics, and analgesics activity of ketamine in humans. *J Pharm Sci.* 1982;71(5):539–42.
44. Clements J, Nimmo W. Pharmacokinetics and analgesics effects of ketamine in man. *Br J Anaesth.* 1981;53:27–30.
45. Brown EN, Lydic R, Schiff N. General anesthesia, sleep and coma. *N Engl J Med.* 2010;363:2638–2650.
46. Sengupta S, Ghosh S, Rudra A, et al. Effect of ketamine of bispectral index during propofol-fentanyl anesthesia: a randomized controlled study. *Middle East J Anaesthesiol.* 2011;21(3):391–395.
47. Mion G, Villevieille T. Ketamine pharmacology: an update (pharmacodynamics and molecular aspects, recent findings). *CNS Neurosci Ther.* 2013;19(6):370–380.
48. Hirota K, Lambert DG. Ketamine: new uses for an old drug? *Br J Anaesth.* 2011;107(2):123–126.
49. Jabre P, Combes X, Lapostolle F, et al. Etomidate versus ketamine for rapid sequence intubation in acutely ill patients: a multicentre randomised controlled trial. *Lancet.* 2009;374(9686):293–300.
50. Schmid RL, Sandler AN, Katz J. Use and efficacy of low-dose ketamine in the management of acute postoperative pain: a review of current techniques and outcomes. *Pain.* 1999;82:111–125.
51. Niesters M, Martini C, Dahan A. Ketamine for chronic pain: risks and benefits. *Br J Clin Pharmacol.* 2014;77(2):357–367.
52. Carr DB, Goudas LC, Denman WT, et al. Safety and efficacy of intranasal ketamine in a mixed population with chronic pain. *Pain.* 2004;110(3):762–764.
53. Huge V, Lauchart M, Magerl W, et al. Effects of low-dose intranasal (S)-ketamine in patients with neuropathic pain. *Eur J Pain.* 2010;14(4):387–394.
54. Riediger C, Haschke M, Bitter C, et al. The analgesic effect of combined treatment with intranasal S-ketamine and intranasal midazolam compared with morphine patient-controlled analgesia in spinal surgery patients: a pilot study. *J Pain Res.* 2015;8:87–94.
55. Newport DJ, Carpenter LL, McDonald WM, et al. Ketamine and other NMDA antagonists: early clinical trials and possible mechanisms in depression. *Am J Psychiatry.* 2015;172(10):950–966.
56. Murrough JW, Iosifescu DV, Chang LC, et al. Antidepressant efficacy of ketamine in treatment-resistance major depression: a two-site randomized controlled trial. *Am J Psychiatry.* 2013;170:1134–1142.
57. Zarate CA, Singh JB, Quiroz JA, et al. A double-blind, placebo controlled study of memantine in the treatment of major depression. *Am J Psychiatry.* 2006;163(1):153–155.
58. Lippmann M, Appel PL, Mok MS, et al. Sequential cardiorespiratory patterns of anestheic induciton with ketamine in critically ill patients. *Crit Care Med.* 1983;11(9):730–734.
59. Allen JY, Macias CG. The efficacy of ketamine in pediatric emergency department patients who present with acute severe asthma. *Ann Emerg Med.* 2005;46(1):43–50.
60. Mayberg TS, Lam AM, Matta BF, et al. Ketamine does note increase cerebral blood flow velocity or intracranial pressure during isoflurane/nitrous oxide anesthesia in patients undergoing craniotomy. *Anesth Analg.* 1995;81:84–89.
61. Hoy SM, Keating GM. Dexmedetomidine: a review of its use for sedation in mechanically ventilated patients in an intensive care setting and for procedural sedation. *Drugs.* 2011;71(11):1481–1501.
62. Tobias JD. Dexmedetomidine: applications in pediatric critical care and pediatric anesthesiology. *Pediatr Crit Care Med.* 2007;8(2):115–131.
63. Gertler R, Brown HC, Mitchell DH, et al. Dexmedetomidine: a novel sedative-analgesic agent. *Proc (Bayl Univ Med Cent).* 2001(14):13–21.

64. Adams R, Brown GT, Davidson M, et al. Efficacy of dexmedetomidine compared with midazolam for sedation in adult intensive care patients: a systematic review. Br J Anaesth. 2013;111(5):703–710.
65. Arain SR, Ebert TJ. The efficacy, side effects and recovery characteristics of dexmedetomidine versus propofol when used for intraoperative sedation. Anesth Analg. 2002;95:461–466.
66. Kaygusuz K, Gokce G, Gursoy S, et al. A comparison of sedation with dexmedetomidine or propofol during shockwave lithotripsy: a randomized controlled trial. Anesth Analg. 2008;106(1):114–119.
67. Muller S, Borowics SM, Fortis EA, et al. Clinical efficacy of dexmedetomidine alone is less than propofol for conscious sedation during ERCP. Gastrointest Endosc. 2008;67(4):651–659.
68. Eberl S, Preckel B, Bergman JJ, et al. Satisfaction and safety using dexmedetomidine or propofol sedation during endoscopic oesophageal procedures: a randomised controlled trial. Eur J Anaesthesiol. 2016;33:631–637.
69. Mahmoud M, Mason KP. Dexmedetomidine: review, update, and future considerations of paediatric perioperative and periprocedural applications and limitations. Br J Anaesth. 2015;115(2):171–182.
70. Pickard A, Davies P, Birnie K, et al. Systematic review and meta-analysis of the effect of intraoperative alpha(2)-adrenergic agonists on postoperative behaviour in children. Br J Anaesth. 2014;112(6):982–990.
71. Abdallah FW, Brull R. Facilitatory effects of perineural dexmedetomidine on neuraxial and peripheral nerve block: a systematic review and meta-analysis. Br J Anaesth. 2013;110(6):915–925.
72. Piao G, Wu J. Systematic assessment of dexmedetomidine as an anesthetic agent: a meta-analysis of randomized controlled trials. Arch Med Sci. 2014;10(1):19–24.
73. Ingersoll-Weng E, Manecke GR, Thitlethwaite P. Dexmedetomidine and Cardiac arrest. Anesthesiology. 2004;2004(100):738–739.
74. Jorden V, Pousman R, Sanford M, et al. Dexmedetomidine overdose in the perioperative setting. Ann Pharmacother. 2004;38(5):803–807.
75. Nath SS, Singh S, Pawar ST. Dexmedetomidine overdosage: an unusual presentation. Indian J Anaesth. 2013;57(3):289–291.
76. Kanto J, Allonen H. Pharmacokinetics and the sedative effect of midazolam. Int J Clin Pharmacol Ther Toxicol. 1983;21(9):460–463.
77. Cote CJ, Cohen IT, Suresh S, et al. A comparison of three doses of a commercially prepared oral midazolam syrup in children. Anesth Analg. 2002;94(1):37–43.
78. Kain ZN, Mayes LC, Wang SM, et al. Postoperative behavioral outcomes in children: effects of sedative premedication. Anesthesiology. 1999;90(3):758–765.
79. Magarey JM. Propofol or midazolam: which is best for the sedation of adult ventilated patients in intensive care units? Aust Crit Care. 2001;14(4):147–154.
80. Fragen RJ. Pharmacokinetics and pharmacodynamics of midazolam given via continuous intravenous infusion in intensive care units. Clin Ther. 1997;19(3):405–419.
81. Hughes MA, Glass PS, Jacobs JR. Context-sensitive half-time in multicompartment pharmacokinetic models for intravenous anesthetic drugs. Anesthesiology. 1992;76(3):334–341.
82. Cunha JP. Midazolam injection 2015. RxList website. http://www.rxlist.com/midazolam-injection-drug/clinical-pharmacology.htm. Accessed October 25, 2016.
83. Bianchi MT, Botzolakis EJ, Lagrange AH, et al. Benzodiazepine modulation of GABA(A) receptor opening frequency depends on activation context: a patch clamp and simulation study. Epilepsy Res. 2009;85(2–3):212–220.
84. Amrein R, Hetzel W, Hartmann D, Lorscheid T. Clinical pharmacology of flumazenil. Eur J Anaesthesiol Suppl. 1988;2:65–80.
85. Dundee JW. Biotransformation of thiopental and other thiobarbiturates. Int Anesthesiol Clin. 1974;12(2):121–133.
86. Paul R, Harris R. A comparison of methohexitone and thiopentone in electrocorticography. J Neurol Neurosurg Psych. 1970;33(1):100–104.
87. Rampton AJ, Griffin RM, Stuart CS, et al. Comparison of methohexital and propofol for electroconvulsive therapy: effects on hemodynamic responses and seizure duration. Anesthesiology. 1989;70(3):412–417.
88. Modica PA, Tempelhoff R, White PF. Pro- and anticonvulsant effects of anesthetics (Part II). Anesth Analg. 1990;70(4):433–444.
89. Baughman VL. Brain protection during neurosurgery. Anesthesiol Clin North Am. 2002;20(2):315–327.
90. Warner DS, Takaoka S, Wu B, et al. Electroencephalographic burst suppression is not required to elicit maximal neuroprotection from pentobarbital in a rat model of focal cerebral ischemia. Anesthesiology. 1996;84(6):1475–1484.
91. Randomized clinical study of thiopental loading in comatose survivors of cardiac arrest. Brain Resuscitation Clinical Trial I Study Group. N Engl J Med. 1986;314(7):397–403.
92. Chamberlain JH, Seed RG, Chung DC. Effect of thiopentone on myocardial function. Br J Anaesth. 1977;49(9):865–870.
93. Bernhoff A, Eklund B, Kaijser L. Cardiovascular effects of short-term anaesthesia with methohexitone and propanidid in normal subjects. Br J Anaesth. 1972;44(1):2–7.
94. Blouin RT, Conard PF, Gross JB. Time course of ventilatory depression following induction doses of propofol and thiopental. Anesthesiology. 1991;75(6):940–944.
95. Wu RS, Wu KC, Sum DC, et al. Comparative effects of thiopentone and propofol on respiratory resistance after tracheal intubation. Br J Anaesth. 1996;77(6):735–738.
96. Goff MJ, Arain SR, Ficke DJ, et al. Absence of bronchodilation during desflurane anesthesia: a comparison to sevoflurane and thiopental. Anesthesiology. 2000;93(2):404–408.
97. Becker KE Jr. Plasma levels of thiopental necessary for anesthesia. Anesthesiology. 1978;49(3):192–196.
98. Cote CJ, Goudsouzian NG, Liu LM, et al. The dose response of intravenous thiopental for the induction of general anesthesia in unpremedicated children. Anesthesiology. 1981;55(6):703–705.
99. Homer TD, Stanski DR. The effect of increasing age on thiopental disposition and anesthetic requirement. Anesthesiology. 1985;62(6):714–724.
100. Jung D, Mayersohn M, Perrier D, et al. Thiopental disposition in lean and obese patients undergoing surgery. Anesthesiology. 1982;56(4):269–274.
101. Rodriguez E, Jordan R. Contemporary trends in pediatric sedation and analgesia. Emerg Med Clin North Am. 2002;20(1):199–222.
102. About remimzolam. PAION website. http://www.paion.com/pipeline/portfolio/remimazolam/. Accessed October 25, 2016.
103. Goudra BG, Singh PM. Remimazolam: the future of its sedative potential. Saudi J Anaesth. 2014;8(3):388–391.
104. Egan TD. Exploring the frontiers of propofol formulation strategy: is there life beyond the milky way? Br J Anaesth. 2010;104(5):533–535.
105. Bengalorkar GM, Bhuvana K, Sarala N, et al. Fospropofol: clinical pharmacology. J Anaesthesiol Clin Pharmacol. 2011;27(1):79–83.
106. Campagna JA, Pojasek K, Grayzel D, et al. Advancing novel anesthetics: pharmacological and pharmacokinetic studies of cyclopropyl-methoxycarbonyl metomidate in dogs. Anesthesiology. 2014;121(6):1203–1216.
107. Egan TD, Shafer SL, Jenkins TE, et al. The pharmacokinetics and pharmacodynamics of THRX-918661, a novel sedative/hypnotic agent field. Anesthesiology 2003; A516. Available from www.asaabstracts.com
108. Norberg A, Koch P, Kanes SJ, Bjornsson MA, et al. A bolus and bolus followed by infusion study of AZD3043, an investigational intravenous drug for sedation and anesthesia: safety and pharmacodynamics in healthy male and female volunteers. Anesth Analg. 2015;121(4):894–903.
109. Pambianco DJ, Vargo JJ, Pruitt RE, et al. Computer-assisted personalized sedation for upper endoscopy and colonoscopy: a comparative, multicenter randomized study. Gastrointest Endosc. 2011;73(4):765–772.
110. Goudra BG, Singh PM. SEDASYS, sedation, and the unknown. J Clin Anesth. 2014;26(4):334–336.

20 Opioids

ALBERT DAHAN • MARIEKE NIESTERS • TERRY SMITH • FRANK OVERDYK

Introduction
  History
  The Endogenous Opioid System
  Simultaneous Targeting of Multiple Opioid and Nonopioid Receptors
Opioid Mechanisms
  Central Opioid Analgesia
  Peripheral Opioid Analgesia
  Opioid-induced Hyperalgesia and Tolerance
Opioid Pharmacokinetics and Pharmacodynamics
  Classification of Exogenous Opioids
  Opioid Pharmacokinetics
  Metabolism: Which Pathways and Metabolites Are Clinically Relevant?
  PKPD Models of Opioid Effect: Which End Point Serves the Clinician Best?

Pharmacodynamics: Pain Relief
Pharmacogenetics
Opioid-induced Respiratory Depression
  Mechanisms of Opioid-induced Respiratory Depression
  Incidence and Risk of Opioid-induced Respiratory Depression
  Opioid-induced Respiratory Depression versus Opioid Analgesia
  Reversal of Opioid-induced Respiratory Depression
  Monitoring
Other Opioid-related Side Effects
  Nausea and Vomiting
  Smooth Muscle Effects
  Cardiovascular Effects
Remifentanil for Labor Pain
Gender Differences

KEY POINTS

1. Opioids produce analgesia as well as serious side effects. All physicians who prescribe opioids for relief of acute or chronic pain need to know how to use these drugs safely. This requires an in-depth understanding of the pharmacokinetics and pharmacodynamics of opioids as well as the acquisition of sufficient clinical experience in their use.

2. Opioids can be classified according to strength or potency based on the plasma concentrations at which they exert their effects (C_{50} or the plasma concentration causing a 50% effect). Strong opioids include fentanyl, sufentanil, and remifentanil. Weak opioids include codeine and tramadol. An intermediate group includes morphine, methadone, oxycodone, and buprenorphine.

3. Opioids act through specific opioid receptors on neuronal tissues such as peripheral nerves and neurons in the spinal cord and brain. The most important receptors include the μ-opioid receptor (MOR), δ-opioid receptor (DOR), and κ-opioid receptor (KOR). For anesthesia and pain relief, the MOR is most important. Opioids also act through nonneuronal pathways, such as those affecting the immune system, which may be of relevance in the treatment of inflammatory pain.

4. Endogenous opioid pathways are activated in cases of stress-induced analgesia, placebo-induced analgesia, and conditioned pain modulation (CPM). CPM occurs when pain arising from one focus is decreased by application of a second painful stimulus (pain inhibits pain).

5. Opioid-induced hyperalgesia (OIH) is a paradoxical opioid effect whereby pain sensitivity increases during or following escalating opioid treatment. It is also observed postoperatively following the use of a remifentanil infusion during anesthesia. Greater and more frequent doses of morphine are required to treat postoperative pain. OIH may be treated and prevented by administration of a low dose of ketamine, an *N*-methyl-D-aspartate (NMDA) receptor antagonist.

6. The pharmacokinetic characteristics of a drug determine its behavior in the body of a patient. One important pharmacokinetic concept is that of context-sensitive half-time (CSt½). This is the time needed for the drug's plasma concentration to decrease by 50% from a steady-state concentration. For most opioids, this value is dependent on the duration of drug infusion. For example, for fentanyl the CSt½ increases rapidly with the infusion duration. In contrast, the CSt½ of remifentanil is independent of the infusion duration due to its rapid elimination from plasma.

7. Opioid metabolism is affected by drugs that interfere with metabolizing cytochrome P450 enzymes, most importantly CYP3A4. Opioid metabolites can be active or inactive. Active metabolites need to be considered when treating patients. For example, the active metabolite of morphine, morphine-6-glucuronide, can accumulate in patients with renal impairment. Genetic variability in the CYP system can have important clinical implications, especially in case of variations in the copies of a gene coding for the metabolizing enzyme. An example is the enzyme CYP2D6, which catalyzes the conversion of codeine into morphine. Patients with multiple copies of the CYP2D6 gene and who receive codeine will have large plasma morphine concentrations with all related beneficial and adverse side effects.

8. Opioid effects are variable among patients. Dosing is optimum when opioids are titrated to the effect. It is also important to take into account the delay between the administration of an opioid and its effect, which is defined as the blood–effect site equilibration half-life, or t½k_{e0}. This will allow proper and timely dosing particularly when

anticipating a stressful event (laryngoscopy, intubation, skin incision, etc.) and administering opioids to prevent the occurrence of a large hemodynamic response to these stimuli. Since the t½k_{e0} of morphine is about 90 minutes, it is important to give an initial bolus dose or morphine at least 60 minutes before the end of surgery when using the drug for postoperative pain relief.

9. Opioids reduce the requirement of inhalational anesthetics and propofol during anesthesia, which makes rapid awakening from anesthesia possible. Using known pharmacokinetic and pharmacodynamic data it can be determined what doses and plasma concentrations will permit the shortest time to awakening. For example, termination of drug infusions at plasma concentrations of propofol 1.5 μg/mL and remifentanil 9.0 ng/mL will lead to patient awakening within 6.5 minutes.

10. In the perioperative setting careful, slow, infusion of opioids allows the gradual accumulation of arterial CO_2, which serves as a respiratory stimulant at the chemoreceptors and lowers the probability of apnea.

11. Administration of opioids can potentially lead to life-threatening respiratory depression. The incidence of serious perioperative respiratory events is approximately 0.5% (1 in every 200 patients). In the acute setting risk factors include sleep-disordered breathing, obesity, renal impairment, pulmonary disease, neurologic disorders, and CYP450 enzyme polymorphism. In the pediatric population risk factors include morphine administration in patients with renal impairment, adenotonsillectomy for recurrent tonsillitis, and/or obstructive sleep apnea and codeine use in patients with CYP2D6 gene polymorphism associated with the ultrarapid metabolizer phenotype. In chronic pain patients risk factors included renal failure, sensory deafferentation, and drug–drug interactions.

12. The nonspecific opioid receptor antagonist, naloxone, is currently the drug of choice to reverse opioid-induced respiratory depression. The required dose of naloxone depends on the pharmacokinetic and pharmacodynamic properties and the dose of the opioid that needs reversal. Postoperatively, when there is persistent apnea, opioid concentrations are often just above the threshold for respiratory depression. Intravenous administration of naloxone using incremental doses of 40 to 80 μg, to a cumulative dose of less than 400 μg, may be sufficient for breathing to resume.

13. New drugs are being developed that reverse or prevent opioid-induced respiratory depression without affecting analgesia. These drugs include blockers of potassium-channels expressed on oxygen-sensing cells of the carotid bodies and drugs that increase respiratory drive through action at α-amino-3-hydroxy-5-methyl-4-isoxazolepropionic acid receptors in brainstem respiratory centers involved in rhythmogenesis.

14. Apart from respiratory depression, opioids cause a large number of side effects that require attention: nausea, smooth muscle spasms, skeletal muscle rigidity, histamine release, pruritus (especially after spinal administration), miosis, sedation, and dizziness. The cardiovascular side effects of opioids include bradycardia and hypotension but are generally mild at usual clinical doses. However, when combined with anesthetics, even at usual clinical doses, or in severely ill patients, opioids may produce hemodynamic instability, which requires treatment.

Introduction

Opioids are the most potent painkillers available in modern medicine. Traditionally opioids are used in perioperative care by anesthesiologists and other anesthesia care providers to attenuate autonomic responses to noxious (surgical) stimulation and treat acute postoperative pain. In recent years, however, there has been an exponential increase in the prescription of opioid analgesics by pain specialists and other health-care providers, such as primary care doctors, for treatment of chronic (cancer and noncancer) pain. Consequently, a significant number of patients in developed countries are exposed to these potent drugs that not only produce pain relief but also cause a variety of side effects that range from dizziness, orthostatic hypotension, nausea, and constipation to harmful and potentially lethal effects such as addiction and critical respiratory depression. The "epidemic" of opioid use by nonsurgical patients, coupled with an emphasis on aggressive and effective postoperative pain management for patients undergoing surgery, has resulted in increasingly complex postoperative pain management problems for surgical patients,[1] and an increase in opioid-related complications for patients with pain in general.[2,3] Consequently, expertise in the use of opioids is not only required in the operating room and following surgery in the postanesthesia care unit (PACU) and on the ward, but also when caring for patients with chronic pain in nonsurgical settings. The expertise should cover all aspects of opioid effects such as pharmacokinetics (PK), pharmacodynamics (PD), and the side effect profile associated with opioid use.

History

Opium is among the oldest drugs in the world. Fossilized opium poppies have been found in Neanderthal excavation sites dating back to 30000 BC. Many old civilizations, including the Sumerians, Egyptians, Greeks, Romans, and Chinese, used opium for nutritional, medicinal, euphoric, spiritual, and religious purposes. The first written reference to the medicinal use of the opium poppy is described in a Sumerian text dated near 4000 BC. Just over 200 years ago, the German pharmacist and chemist Friedrich Sertürner isolated a stable alkaloid crystal from the opium sap and named it morphine after the Greek god of dreams, Morpheus.[4,5] Morphine was 10-fold more potent than opium and soon replaced it not only for the treatment of severe pain, but also for a myriad of other purposes such as cough and diarrhea. After the invention of the hypodermic syringe in 1853, the Englishman Alexander Wood was the first to inject morphine in a controlled

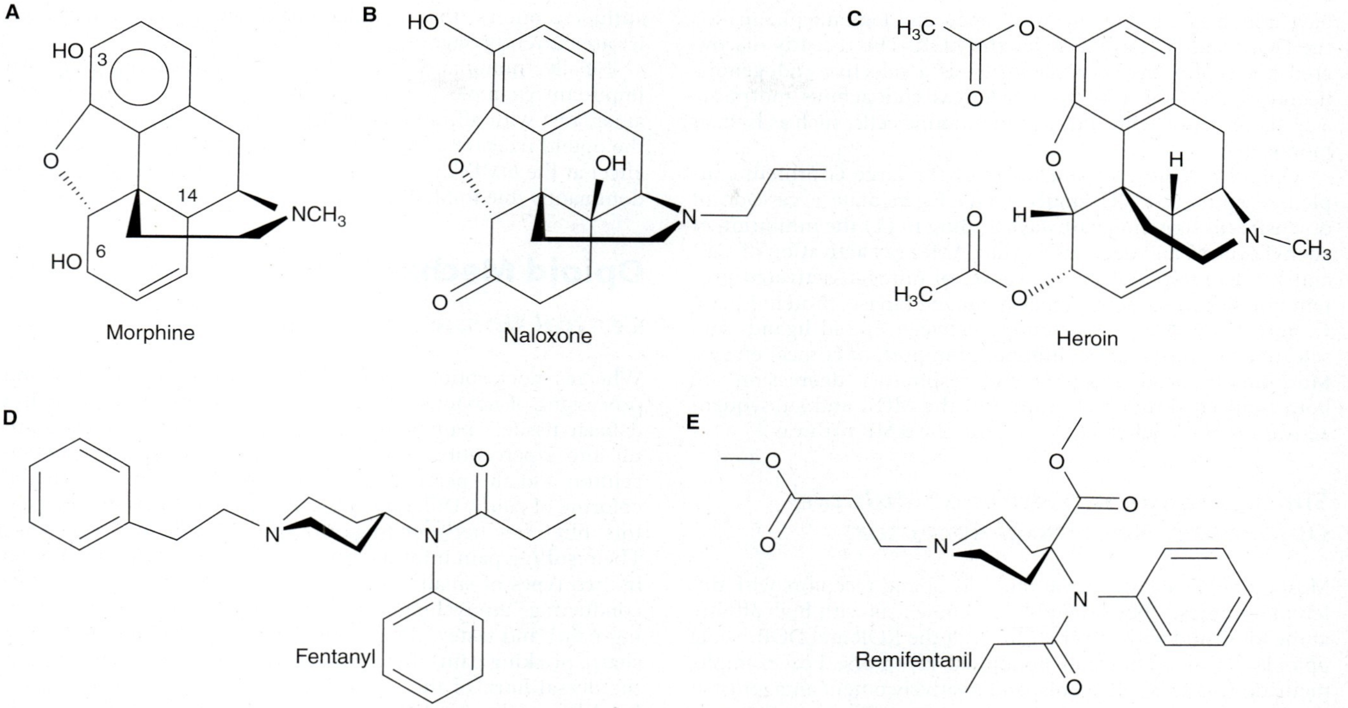

Figure 20-1 Chemical structure of commonly used opioids.

fashion into a patient producing more than a day's sleep.[6] The first reported casualty from morphine occurred shortly thereafter when Wood injected his wife with morphine resulting in a fatal overdose from respiratory depression. Morphine revolutionized the treatment of the wounded in battlefield medicine, but euphoric and addictive properties led to the addiction of thousands of soldiers to morphine during the American Civil War. The synthesis of heroin in 1874 was based on the empirical finding that boiling morphine with specific acids caused the replacement of the two morphine –OH groups by –OCOH$_3$ producing diamorphine or heroin (Fig. 20-1).

After the structure of morphine was determined in the 1920s, the synthesis of new morphine-like opioid compounds was based on chemical principles rather than empirical discoveries. In 1937, meperidine (or pethidine) became the first synthetic opioid synthesized on the basis of the central structure of morphine. Since then many synthetic and semisynthetic opioids have been produced, including the clinically important opioid antagonists naloxone and naltrexone, by replacing the N-methyl substituent in morphine with allyl and cyclopropylmethyl groups, respectively (Fig. 20-1).[7]

For clinical use during anesthesia the most important opioids are the fenylpiperidines: fentanyl, sufentanil, alfentanil, and remifentanil. These opioids produce potent analgesia and suppression of cardiovascular responses to noxious stimulation from surgery with predictable PK and PD.

Recently developed opioids include tapentadol and cebranopadol.[8,9] These opioids act simultaneously at multiple receptor systems. Tapentadol activates the μ-opioid receptor (MOR) and inhibits the neuronal uptake of noradrenaline.[8] Cebranopadol is an opioid with similar affinities for the MOR and nociception/orphanin FQ receptor (NOP, also known as opioid receptor-like receptor type 1).[9] The continued development of opioids with complex simultaneous actions at multiple target sites is driven by concerns that the side effect profile of potent opioids, which presents a serious risk to patients, needs to be minimized.

The Endogenous Opioid System

A major breakthrough in the understanding of opioid pharmacology came from a series of discoveries of opioid receptors, endogenous opioid peptides, their encoding genes, and endogenous opioid alkaloids. The endogenous opioid system is composed of a family of structurally related endogenous peptides that act at a four-member opioid receptor family consisting of the MOR, κ-opioid receptor (KOR), δ-opioid receptor (DOR), and NOP receptor.[10,11] This opioid system is involved in a variety of regulatory functions including important roles in nociceptive, stress, emotional, and hedonic responses, as well as modulation of thermoregulation, breathing, neuroendocrine function, gastrointestinal (GI) motility, and immune responses.

In rodents, various subtypes of opioid receptors have also been identified, with different pharmacologic functions. For example, at least three MOR subtypes have been described: $μ_1$ is predominantly involved in opioid analgesia, $μ_2$ is involved in opioid-induced respiratory depression, and $μ_3$ is involved in opioid-induced immune suppression.[12,13] The functional validation of most opioid receptor subtypes awaits the development of antagonists with sufficient selectivity to allow a clear differentiation by effect. The endogenous opioid peptides include endorphins, enkephalins, and dynorphins, each of which displays different affinities for MOR, KOR, and DOR.[14] β-endorphins have a high affinity for the MOR, met- and leu-enkephalins for the DOR, and Dynorphin A for the KOR. The recently discovered nociceptin has been identified as a selective endogenous ligand of the NOP receptor,[11] whereas endogenous morphine acts via the μ_3-receptor located on immune cells, such as human monocytes.[15]

Opioid receptors are members of the large G-protein-coupled receptor (GPCR) family.[16] GPCRs mediate a cascade of downstream signaling pathways leading to (1) the inhibition of adenyl cyclase and decreased cyclic AMP, (2) activation of Ca^{2+} and K^+ channels, and (3) activation of mitogen-activated protein kinase/extracellular signal-regulated kinase, protein kinase C, and P13 K/Akt.[17] Interactions between opioid ligands and selective receptors have a number of important clinical effects. Morphine-induced analgesia and respiratory depression are both induced through activation of the MOR and subsequent activation of the adenylate cyclase/cyclic AMP pathway.[18]

Simultaneous Targeting of Multiple Opioid and Nonopioid Receptors

Most opioid analgesics act at multiple opioid receptors with different affinities.[19] For example, morphine acts with high affinity at the MOR and with lower affinities at the KOR and DOR. Some opioids act at opioid and nonopioid receptors. For example, methadone is an MOR agonist and relatively potent antagonist at the N-methyl-D-aspartate (NMDA) receptor.[20,21] Antagonism of the NMDA receptor is clinically useful in reducing opioid tolerance and opioid-induced hyperalgesia (OIH) and in chronic pain states leading to pain hypersensitivity.[22]

Tramadol is an analgesic that produces pain relief through MOR agonism and inhibition of the neuronal reuptake of serotonin and noradrenaline,[23] which activate descending controls. Tramadol is a racemic mixture and its opioid action results from the (+)-enantiomer and the active metabolite O-desmethyltramadol (M1), which has a higher affinity for the MOR than its parent compound. The monoaminergic activity is related to the (−)-enantiomer. Since the metabolism of tramadol into its active compound M1 is dependent on the cytochrome P450 system, patients with a reduced CYP2D6 activity will require higher tramadol doses for analgesia.

Tapentadol is a new analgesic agent.[8] In contrast to tramadol, it is one molecule that has a dual mechanism of action. It is active at the MOR at spinal and supraspinal sites. It is also a norepinephrine reuptake inhibitor in the spinal cord, activating α_2-adrenergic receptors in the spinal cord dorsal horn. The affinity of tapentadol for the MOR is 50-fold lower than that of morphine. However, due to synergy between the two mechanisms of action, tapentadol produces potent analgesia and is useful in the treatment of moderate-to-severe acute and chronic pain. Tapentadol differs from tramadol due to its lack of serotonergic activity resulting in a lower incidence of nausea and vomiting. Tapentadol's low affinity for the MOR may limit its undesirable side effects although its respiratory side effects have not yet been fully studied. Tapentadol produces analgesic effects in chronic neuropathic pain patients by (re)activation of descending inhibitory pathways. In diabetic polyneuropathy patients, conditioned pain modulation (CPM, see below) increased significantly during tapentadol treatment, and was correlated strongly with its analgesic effect.[24]

Cebranopadol is a novel opioid and, like tapentadol, is a single molecule acting at multiple receptor systems, most importantly the MOR and NOP receptors.[9] In various animal models of acute and chronic (neuropathic) pain, cebranopadol produces potent antinociception with a favorable side effect profile. Human studies are currently ongoing.

Finally, nonopioids may also act at opioid receptors. An important example is ketamine, which is an NMDA receptor antagonist with affinity for multiple receptor systems including the opioid receptors.[25] Its anesthetic properties are related to its effect at the NMDA receptors while its analgesic effects are predominantly due to MOR activation.

Opioid Mechanisms

Central Opioid Analgesia

Whereas nociception is the neural process of encoding and processing of noxious stimuli that can potentially (or actually) damage tissue,[26] pain is the subjective translation of these stimuli into a perception or sensation. Opioids modify both nociception and the perception of a noxious stimulus (emotional coloring of pain). Different types of peripheral sensory nociceptors, often free nerve endings, are stimulated by tissue damage. The resulting pain information is transmitted to the spinal cord by two types of small diameter peripheral afferent fibers: slow conducting, unmyelinated C-fibers (which cause a dull burning pain) and faster, thinly myelinated Aδ fibers (which cause sharp, pricking pain). Both types of primary afferent fibers enter the dorsal horn of the spinal cord and terminate in its superficial layers (lamina I-II). Projection neurons from these laminae give rise to the ascending pathways of the spinothalamic tract. Thalamic nuclei receive the nociceptive inputs and pass the information to key brain pain reception sites such as the periaqueductal gray (PAG), amygdala, and somatosensory cortex. Activation of the MORs extensively located in these higher brain centers stimulates analgesia by activating *descending inhibitory pathways* from the PAG and rostroventral medulla (RVM) that inhibit nociceptive dorsal horn neuron firing in the spinal cord (Fig. 20-2A).[27,28] Opioids also exert actions in the cortex and limbic systems affecting cholinergic systems that lead to changes in arousal and pain perception.[29] Opioid receptors are further abundantly present in the spinal cord dorsal horn at pre- and postsynaptic locations. In the superficial laminae of the dorsal horn, local neuronal circuits process both ascending and descending pain pathways and are regulated by local endogenous opioid circuits.

MOR-induced analgesia and descending inhibitory pathways may be activated not only by exogenous opioids, but also by activation of endogenous opioid systems. Direct electrical stimulation of the PAG and RVM induces analgesia that is reversed by opioid antagonists.[30] The electrically stimulated sites overlap with the opioid receptor sites and with opioid-containing interneurons, linking together the actions of exogenously applied analgesic stimuli and endogenous opioid systems. Three major examples of analgesia driven by the endogenous opioid system are (1) stress-induced analgesia[31]; (2) placebo-induced analgesia[32]; and (3) conditioned pain modulation (CPM).[33]

1. *Stress-induced analgesia.* The endogenous opioid system is activated under stressful conditions, as demonstrated by the delayed onset of pain by soldiers wounded in battle.[34] The same higher brain centers bearing MORs are involved in the implementation of stress-induced analgesia.
2. *Placebo-induced analgesia.* The endogenous opioid system also mediates placebo-induced analgesia, a reduction of pain resulting from an expectation of pain relief. Studies using fMRI and PET show activation of the endogenous

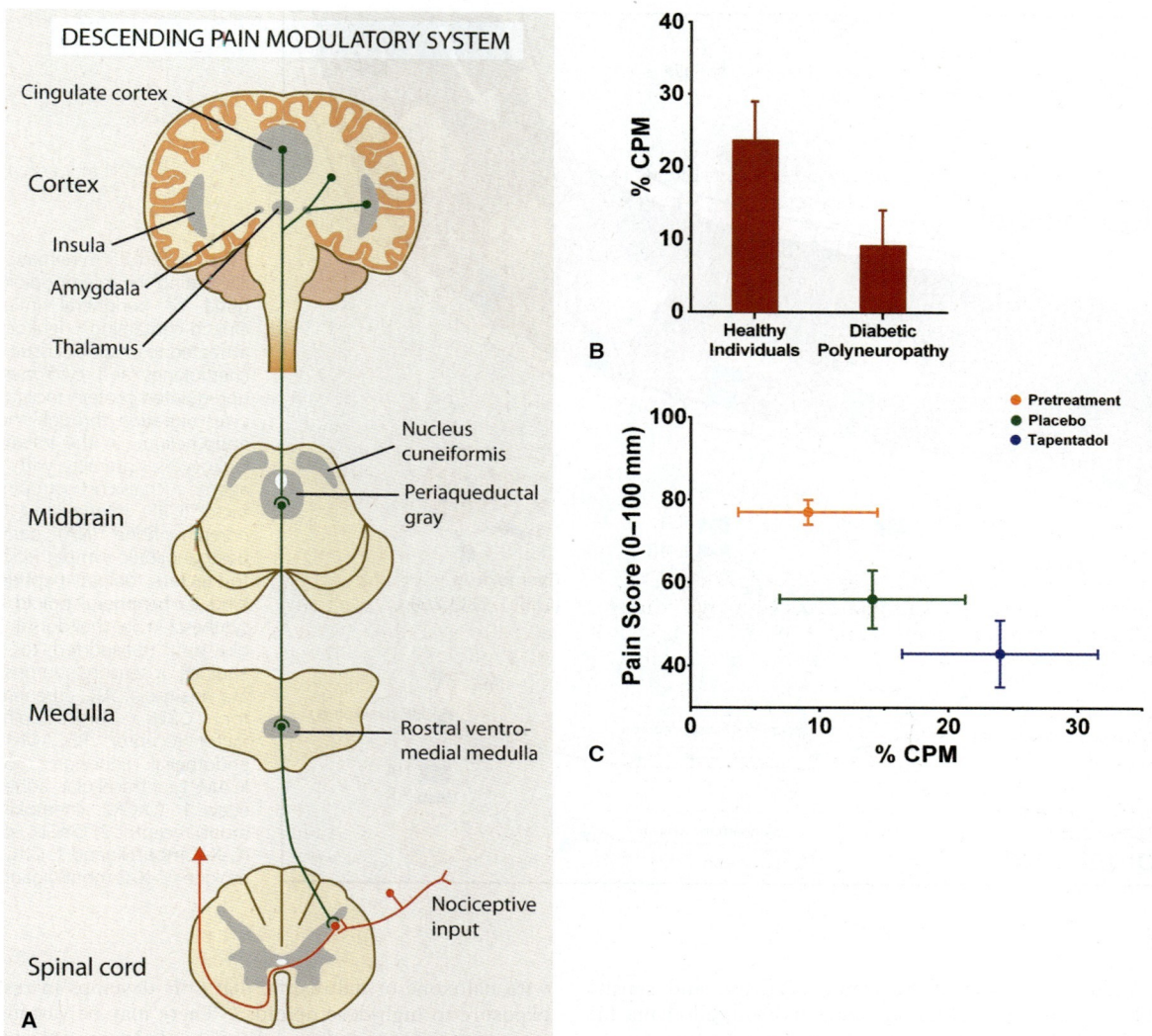

Figure 20-2 **A:** Simplified diagram of activated descending inhibitory pathways (*green lines*) in response to afferent nociceptive input (*red lines*). Descending inhibition is activated in various higher brain centers, including the rostral ventromedial medulla, periaqueductal gray, amygdala, cingulate cortex, insula, and orbitofrontal cortex. These same areas are involved in Conditioned Pain Modulation (CPM). (From Dahan A, Niesters M, Sarton E. Endogenous modulation of pain is visible in the brain. *Clin Neurophysiol.* 2012;123:642–643). **B:** Reduced or absent CPM responses are present in patients with diabetic polyneuropathy, reflecting inactive descending inhibitory pathways. **C:** Effect of 4-week treatment with the opioid/norepinephrine reuptake inhibitor tapentadol and placebo on CPM and pain scores in patients with diabetic polyneuropathy. (Data from Niesters M, Niesters M, Aarts L, et al. Tapentadol potentiates descending pain inhibition in chronic pain patients with diabetic polyneuropathy. *Br J Anaesth.* 2014;113:148–156.)

opioid systems and MORs in the brains of subjects receiving placebo described as an analgesic.[35,36]

3. *CPM.* Formerly known as diffuse noxious inhibitory control, CPM is a condition in which pain arising from a noxious stimulus applied to one part of the body is decreased by application of a second remote noxious stimulus (pain inhibits pain).[24,37,38] CPM is due to activation of descending inhibitory pathways by higher brain centers. An example of CPM from animal physiology is the observation that an imposed nose twitch in a horse attenuates the increase in heart rate induced by painful stimuli.[39] Since naloxone blocks this effect it is assumed that endogenous opioids are released during the nose twitch. In humans, tapentadol is an example of an opioid that induces analgesia through activation of descending pathways (Fig. 20-2B and C).[24]

Peripheral Opioid Analgesia

Opioids are also involved in peripheral analgesia by acting directly on sensory neurons (Aδ and C-fibers) to inhibit pain signal transmission. This is especially important in inflammatory pain. However, the immune system is also widely involved in peripheral analgesia.[40] Opioid receptors are located not only on neurons, but also on immune cells, such as human leukocytes.[41] An insult to a peripheral tissue triggers the local release of many proinflammatory mediators that generate an inflammatory

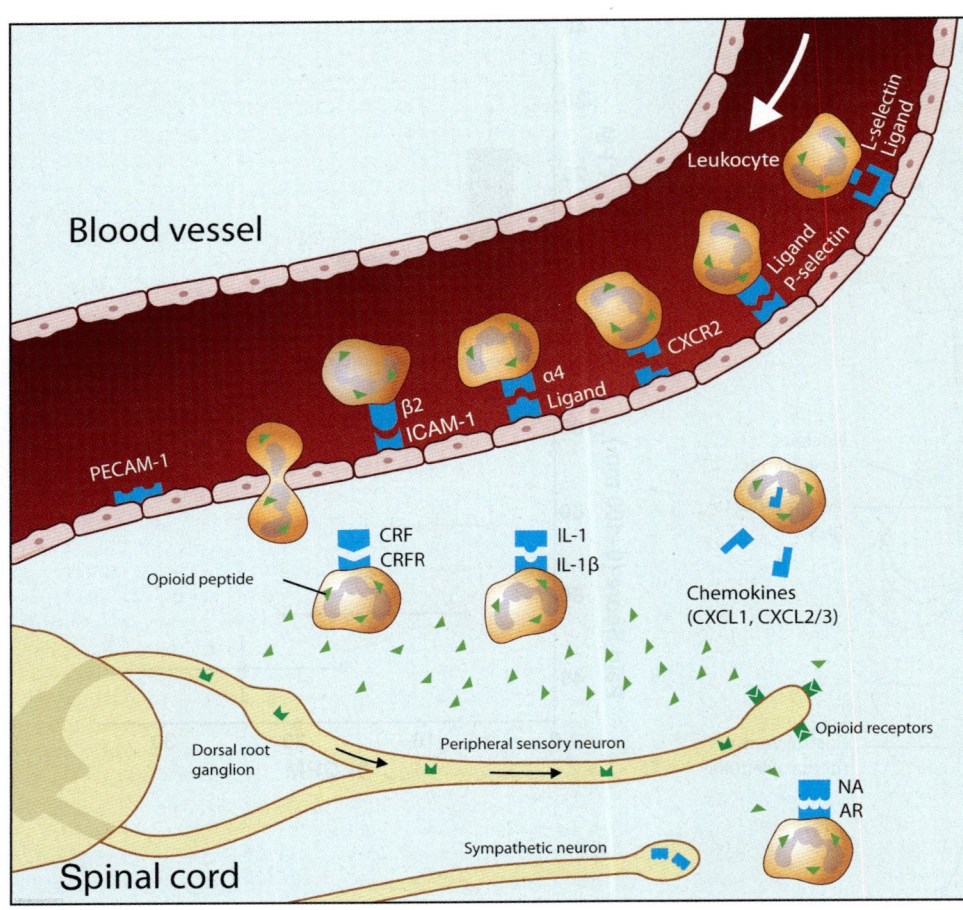

Figure 20-3 Schematic diagram illustrating the role of opioids in analgesia of peripheral inflammation. Opioid-containing leukocytes are attracted to inflamed tissue by various chemokines and cytokines. Specific upregulated protein facilitates leukocyte migration through the vascular endothelium. In the inflamed tissue leukocytes interact with releasing agents such as corticotropin-releasing factor (CRF), interleukin-1 (IL-1), and norepinephrine (NA) derived from postganglionic sympathetic neurons, to secrete opioid peptides. These bind to peripheral opioid receptors, synthesized in the dorsal root ganglia and transported to peripheral endings of sensory neurons, to mediate analgesia. AR, adrenergic receptor; CRFR, corticotropin-releasing factor receptor; PECAM-1, platelet endothelial adhesion molecule 1; ICAM-1, intracellular adhesion molecule 1; CXCR2, chemokine (C-X-C motif) receptor 2; CXCL1, chemokine (C-X-C motif) ligand 1; CXCL2/3, chemokine (C-X-C motif) ligand 1/2.

cascade, induce spontaneous nociceptor activity, and sensitize sensory neurons to induce spontaneous pain, allodynia (a nonpainful stimulus is perceived as painful), and hyperalgesia (increased pain sensitivity). Early in the inflammatory process there is an influx of leukocytes into the inflamed area and these cells are a major source of opioid peptides to inflamed sites. Opioid peptides released locally interact with the opioid neuronal receptors to induce analgesia (Fig. 20-3).[42] The inflammatory process also stimulates further opioid receptor upregulation and thereby increases the antinociceptive action of opioid peptides released by immune cells. In aggregate, the inflammatory process not only promotes inflammation and its painful sequelae, but also initiates and sustains a counteracting analgesia driven by endogenous opioids.[43]

Opioid-induced Hyperalgesia and Tolerance

Opioids can induce the paradoxical effect of OIH or an increase in pain sensitivity.[44] OIH may limit the analgesic effects of opioids. During long-term and/or high-dose opioid treatment, rapid opioid dose escalation, or administration of an opioid with rapid onset/offset (e.g., remifentanil), a paradoxical increase in pain accompanies the treatment escalation.[45,46] The MOR is not a prerequisite for OIH, because there is ample evidence from knockout mice studies (mice devoid of MORs) or studies in mice treated with naloxone or naltrexone that OIH develops in response to exposure to high-dose opioids.[47] There may be various mechanisms for OIH, including activation of the central glutaminergic system, central nitric oxide production, and facilitation of descending pronociceptive systems.

Postoperative patients who have received remifentanil infusions intraoperatively can have a higher incidence of OIH and need greater doses of morphine for control of postoperative pain than patients receiving nonremifentanil-based anesthesia. Although animal and human data indicate that all μ-opioids may cause OIH there seems to be a gradual difference in prevalence, with most observation of OIH following administration of rapid-acting opioids, such as remifentanil. In addition, this high incidence of exaggerated pain in surgical patients following remifentanil infusions may be related to its rapid offset of analgesia. In order to prevent severe pain responses following remifentanil-based anesthesia, administration of morphine (0.1 to 0.25 mg/kg) 45 to 60 minutes before the end of surgery is advisable, and adding a low-dose ketamine infusion may prevent the development of OIH (dose range: 10 to 30 mg/hr) due to ketamine's NMDA antagonistic properties.

OIH is not the same phenomenon as opioid tolerance. *Acute opioid tolerance* due to tachyphylaxis requires increasing doses of the opioid to reach a specific analgesic end point during the initial hours of opioid treatment. *Chronic tolerance*, often seen in opioid abusers, occurs over days and manifests as a decreasing analgesic effect, resulting in dose escalation and increasing the likelihood of OIH. In contrast to OIH, opioid receptor–related and postactivation intracellular processes play an important role in the development of tolerance (including β-arrestin–dependent receptor desensitization and internalization, and G-receptor uncoupling).[48,49] Finally, *pseudotolerance* is a phenomenon seen in chronic pain patients due to progression of disease with an increase in the level of nociception often due to destruction of nerves in the tumor region, resulting in neuropathic pain, which is poorly responsive to opioid dose escalation.

Opioid Pharmacokinetics and Pharmacodynamics

Classification of Exogenous Opioids

Opioids may be classified on the basis of their synthesis, chemical structure, potency, receptor binding, and effect at the opioid receptors. There are *natural* (opiates including morphine), *semisynthetic* (buprenorphine, codeine, etorphine, heroin, hydromorphone, oxycodone, and oxymorphone), and *synthetic* opioids (piperidines: loperamide, meperidine, alfentanil, fentanyl, sufentanil, remifentanil; methadones: methadone, dextro-propoxyphene). Opioid potency ranges from *weak opioids* such as codeine, dextro-propoxyphene, tramadol, and hydrocodone to *strong opioids*, which include etorphine, fentanyl, sufentanil, alfentanil, and remifentanil. Medium potency opioids include morphine, methadone, oxycodone, hydromorphone, and buprenorphine. Irrespective of the "strength" of these agents, all of these agents may potentially produce serious and potentially life-threatening side effects including sedation and respiratory depression, hypotension, and bradycardia. During surgery *strong* opioids are used in high doses while in the postoperative phase medium strength opioids such as morphine or methadone are used for treatment of acute pain. In 1986, the World Health Organization designed a stepwise approach for treatment of chronic cancer pain in which *weak* opioids are prescribed before *strong* opioids (www.who.int/cancer/palliative/painladder/en/). Opioids may be *full agonists*, which cause the maximum possible effect when activating their receptors. Opioid full agonists at the MOR include morphine, piperidines, and methadone. Opioid *partial agonists*, such as buprenorphine, activate their receptor but cause only a partial or reduced effect. Naloxone and naltrexone are opioid *antagonists*. It is more practical to classify opioids with a rapid onset and offset of action (e.g., remifentanil and alfentanil) versus agents with a slow onset/offset of action (e.g., morphine and buprenorphine). The concept of onset/offset of action will be discussed below.

Opioid Pharmacokinetics

When injected intravenously opioids are rapidly transported to the heart and pulmonary vessels from where they are dispersed to the various organs and tissues. After a standard dose of opioid, the inter-patient variability in plasma concentrations is large (at least 30-fold) and related to various factors including weight-related parameters (lean and fat body mass), organ function (hepatic and renal function), and cardiac output. This variability is manifest in the distribution and elimination constants that describe the PK profile of these drugs, which is also related to their physicochemical properties, such as molecule size, pK_a (affects the degree of ionization of the molecule and depends on the plasma pH), protein binding (to albumin and α_1-acid glycoprotein), and lipid solubility. These factors affect the passage of the drug into the brain across the blood–brain barrier, and thereby affect both the opioid's PK and PD characteristics. For example, a small increase in pH seen with respiratory alkalosis will increase the nonionized form of morphine, fentanyl, sufentanil, and remifentanil, which subsequently crosses the blood–brain barrier. Different drugs may also affect the blood–brain barrier's active transport systems that eliminate opioids from the brain. For example, cyclosporine enhances morphine's analgesic effect but not that of methadone, suggesting that cyclosporine selectively interferes with morphine's efflux from the brain via specific transporter proteins.

When an opioid is injected into the venous system, there is an initial rapid peak in plasma concentration. Next, the drug rapidly enters multiple organ systems with high blood flow (such as the brain, liver, kidney) from which the plasma drug concentration rapidly drops followed by a slower drop due to redistribution to organs (such as the muscles and later tissues with high fat content) that are less well perfused. These concentration changes over time are often described by noncompartmental PK models. Such models describe the drug's PK behavior in terms of volume of distribution (V_D = drug dose/steady-state plasma drug concentration), rapid and slow distribution half-lives, and elimination half-life ($t^{1/2}_{elim}$). A high V_D is observed for lipophilic opioids with low protein-binding affinity such as fentanyl (V_D = 300 L), whereas a low V_D is observed for remifentanil and alfentanil, due to a high clearance (remifentanil) and/or high protein binding. When V_D is small, clearance is responsible for the drop in plasma concentration and consequently the loss of analgesia, whereas redistribution accounts for loss of analgesic effect in drugs with a high V_D.

The time needed for the drug's plasma concentration to decrease by 50%, from a steady-state plasma concentration after the drug infusion has stopped, is called the context-sensitive half-time (CSt½) (Fig. 20-4).[50,51] A drug has not just one, but many such half-times, depending on the duration of the infusion, which is the context to which the term applies. For fentanyl, the context-sensitive half-time increases with the duration of the infusion,[50] while for remifentanil the half-time is independent of the duration because of its rapid clearance (50% drop in plasma concentration is 2 minutes, 75% drop is 8 minutes).[51] In clinical practice, the time to the loss of analgesia depends on the opioid dose, neuronal and receptor kinetic processes, the transport of the opioids from brain

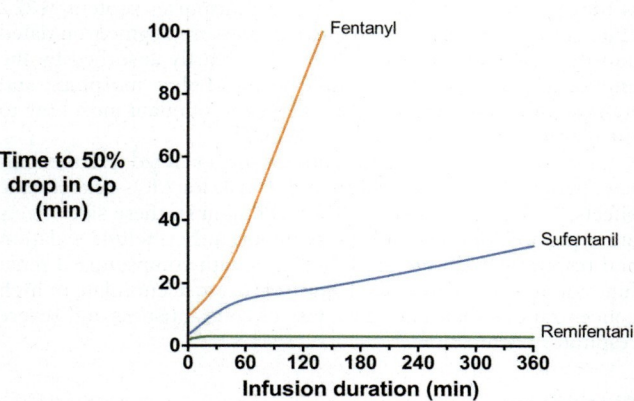

Figure 20-4 Context-sensitive half-times, or the time to a 50% drop in plasma concentration (Cp) versus infusion duration for remifentanil, fentanyl, and sufentanil.

to plasma, and the context-sensitive half-time. The time course of a specific effect is difficult to predict for individual patients. For some side effects such as opioid-induced respiratory depression, the prediction of onset or offset of effect is even more complicated due to counteracting forces, such as the respiratory stimulant effects of increased arterial carbon dioxide (CO_2) and the presence of pain.[52]

Metabolism: Which Pathways and Metabolites Are Clinically Relevant?

7 Most opioids are metabolized in the liver through either phase I (oxidative and reductive reactions catalyzed by the cytochrome P450 enzyme system) or phase II reactions (conjugation to a specific substrate). Metabolism may occur at other sites as well, such as in the enterocytes of the GI tract, the kidney, or the brain. Excretion of the parent drug and/or metabolites occurs via the kidney and/or via the biliary tract into the gut where some opioids (morphine, buprenorphine) may undergo reuptake of the compound into the bloodstream.

Three aspects of opioid metabolism have clinical importance:
1. Medications that inhibit or induce the CYP450 system may increase or decrease the clinical effect of opioids, respectively, by interfering with their metabolism (Table 20-1).[53]
2. Opioid metabolites may be either active or inactive, which applies not only to their analgesic effect but also to their unwanted side effects.[54–56]
3. Genetic variability in the CYP system has clinical implications that are discussed in the pharmacogenetics section.

Morphine

Morphine undergoes rapid metabolism (by UGT2B7, a phase II reaction) in the liver. Within minutes after its administration the two most important hydrophilic metabolites appear in plasma: morphine-3-glucuronide (M3G) and morphine-6-glucuronide (M6G).[54] M3G is the major metabolite and about 60% of morphine is converted into M3G, while just 5% to 10% is converted to M6G. In humans M3G has no analgesic or antianalgesic action. M6G is a full MOR agonist, but at the concentrations observed following morphine administration in a patient with normal renal function its contribution to the overall analgesic effect is minimal.[54] Due to its low lipophilicity, passage of M6G across the blood–brain barrier is slow and consequently limited. In the hepatocytes both M3G and M6G are transported back into the bloodstream via transporter protein MRP3, while a small part is transported into the bile ducts via transporter protein MRP2 (Fig. 20-5).[54] In the gut both glucuronides are deglucuronidated and the resultant morphine molecule is partly absorbed by the enterocytes. Enterocytes are able to metabolize morphine and transport the resultant M3G and M6G and remnant morphine to the bloodstream (the enterohepatic cycle).

Since the morphine-glucuronides are excreted via the kidney, patients with renal failure are at risk for M6G-related side effects.[54,55] Because M6G is a full MOR agonist, these side effects are typical of opioids and, most importantly, include sedation and respiratory depression. In patients with compromised renal function morphine treatment causes M6G to accumulate in high concentrations that may cause loss of consciousness and severe respiratory depression.[54]

Piperidines

Fentanyl, alfentanil, sufentanil, and remifentanil are lipophilic opioids that rapidly cross the blood–brain barrier. Fentanyl, alfentanil, and sufentanil are metabolized by the liver, catalyzed by the cytochrome P450 enzyme system.[57,58] *Fentanyl* has a high hepatic extraction ratio with clearance approaching liver blood flow (1.5 L/min). The major metabolite of fentanyl is the inactive compound norfentanyl. *Sufentanil* also has a high hepatic extraction ratio with a clearance of 0.9 L/min. *Alfentanil* is metabolized by CYP3A4 and 3A5 forming the inactive compounds noralfentanil and N-phenylpropionamide. The polymorphic expression of the CYP3A5 gene accounts for the great variability in alfentanil metabolism and clearance.[58] *Remifentanil* contrasts with the other piperidines in that it is not metabolized in the liver.[59]

Table 20-1 Inhibitors and Inducers of CYP3A and Inhibitors of CYP2D6

CYP3A Inhibitors

Antibiotics
- Erythromycin
- Clarithromycin

Calcium channel blockers
- Diltiazem
- Verapamil

Anti-HIV agents
- Delavirdine
- Indinavir
- Ritonavir
- Saquinavir

Antifungal agents
- Itraconazole
- Ketoconazole

Other
- Grapefruit juice

CYP3A Inducers

Antibiotics
- Rifampicin

Anticonvulsants
- Carbamazepine
- Phenytoin
- Phenobarbital

Anti-HIV agents
- Efavirenz
- Nevirapine

Others
- St. John's wort
- Dexamethasone

CYP2D6 Inhibitors

Antidepressants
- Clomipramine
- Fluoxetine
- Paroxetine

Antipsychotics
- Haloperidol

Antidysrhythmics
- Quinidine

Other
- Cimetidine

Data from Wilkinson GR. Drug metabolism and variability among patients in drug response. *N Engl J Med.* 2005;352:2211.

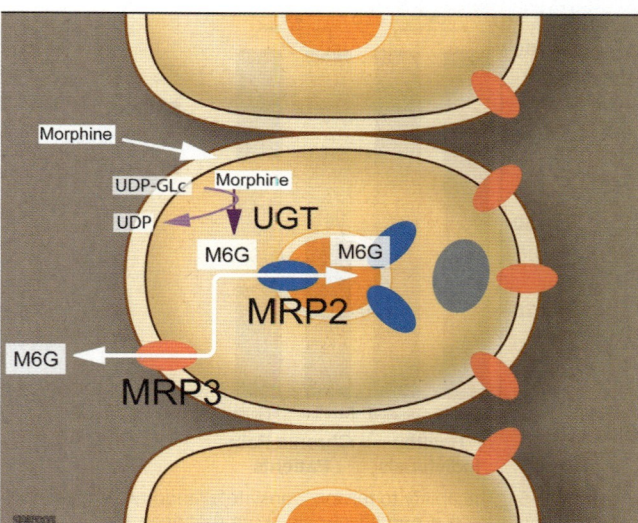

Figure 20-5 Morphine metabolism in the liver and transport of its metabolites into the bloodstream and bile system. Morphine enters the hepatocyte, where it undergoes metabolism by UGT2B7 (a phase II reaction) into morphine-3-glucuronide (not shown) and morphine-6-glucuronide (M6G). These two glucuronides are transported via transporter protein MRP3 (red) back into the systemic circulation and via transporter protein MRP2 (blue) back into the biliary duct system.

Remifentanil contains a methyl ester side chain (Fig. 20-1) that is metabolized by blood (within the erythrocyte) and tissue nonspecific esterases. This causes a rapid clearance of the drug (context sensitive half-life of 2 minutes) making it the most rapidly acting opioid currently available. Clearance of remifentanil is 3 to 5 L/min, which exceeds liver blood flow affirming its extrahepatic clearance. Remifentanil is usually administered as a continuous infusion since its plasma level decreases by 50% in as little as 40 seconds.[50,59]

Methadone

Methadone is extensively metabolized to an inactive form by CYP2B6, which is also affected by pharmacogenetic variability.[60] Methadone has a 60% to 95% oral bioavailability, high potency, and a long duration of action. Furthermore, there is considerable variation among recipients in the response to the drug. While methadone has properties which make it attractive for use intravenously as a perioperative analgesic, in a controlled and well-monitored environment, these same properties may prove hazardous when methadone is administered orally for treatment of patients with chronic pain. Large numbers of patient deaths have been attributed to the long, and often unpredictable, duration of action of methadone when administered orally.

Naloxone

Naloxone is the most valuable and popular nonspecific MOR antagonist.[61] Since it has a low and unpredictable bioavailability after oral intake due to an extensive (>95%) first-pass effect, naloxone is best given via the intravenous route. The most important metabolic pathway of naloxone is glucuronidation into the inactive naloxone-3-glucuronide. Its duration of effect is short, ranging from 15 to 45 minutes, which requires it to be redosed or administered as a continuous infusion when antagonism is required for long-acting opioids or for patients experiencing an opioid overdose.

PKPD Models of Opioid Effect: Which End Point Serves the Clinician Best?

The PK of a drug describes the time course of dose to concentration; the PD describes the concentration-to-effect relationship; the effect can be any of the desired or undesired drug effects. Pharmacokinetic–pharmacodynamic (PKPD) models are constructed for each drug to enable the clinician to understand and predict the clinical implication of a given dose to a desired effect.[62] These models allow dosing regimens to be constructed on the basis of patient characteristics such as total or lean body weight, gender, age, and other characteristics, making them particularly helpful when treating individual patients. The PK part of such models describes the drug distribution kinetics. This relates to both the parent drug and the possible metabolites. In compartmental models, the concentration–time profiles are described by drug transfer between interconnected hypothetical compartments, mimicking drug absorption, distribution, elimination, and metabolism. The PD part of the model describes the drug concentration–effect relationship. This hypothetical effect compartment is made infinitely small so that it does not influence the drug's disposition (PK) and is located at the drug's target organ, such as the muscle endplate for muscle relaxants and the brain for hypnotic drugs. For most opioid effects (such as analgesia, sedation, and respiratory depression) the effect site is located within the central nervous system (CNS) while the effect site for constipation is the GI tract. The delay between the peak drug concentration in the plasma and the peak concentration at the effect site is described by the plasma–effect site equilibration constant k_{e0} (or its half-life $t_{1/2}k_{e0} = \ln 2/k_{e0}$),[63,64] which is commonly referred to as hysteresis. For the analgesic and respiratory depressive effects of opioids, the hysteresis is determined by the drug's passage across the blood–brain barrier (the more lipophilic an opioid, the faster the transfer into the brain compartment), receptor kinetics, and neuronal dynamics. The effect site concentration–effect relationship is described by a sigmoid E_{max} model[62–64]:

$$Effect = (C_E/C_{50})^\gamma / [1 + (C_E/C_{50})^\gamma]$$

where C_E is the drug concentration in the hypothetical effect site, C_{50} is the measure of drug potency or the effect site or steady-state concentration causing 50% of the effect, and γ is the Hill or steepness parameter. In summary, any PKPD analysis using the above-mentioned descriptions yields PK parameters (volumes of distribution and clearances), as well as PD parameters related to drug potency (C_{50}) and the onset/offset times of the drug ($t_{1/2}k_{e0}$). It is important to understand that PK (volumes of distribution and rate constant) and PD (potency) values vary largely among patients. This is related to differences in physiology, underlying disease, age, weight, ethnicity, and other factors. Thus the clinician should choose a PK/PD set derived from a population of subjects whose characteristics are most similar to the individual they are treating. For example, due to changes in PK and PD behavior, elderly patients display a greater opioid sensitivity[65]; patients with liver or renal insufficiency require adaptation to their dosing; and patients with certain genetic abnormalities may experience unusual responses to opioids (see below).

For most opioids, the target effect when constructing PKPD models has traditionally been the slowing of the frequency components of the electroencephalogram (EEG), quantified by a shift in the 95th percentile of the power spectrum (95% spectral edge frequency). The C_{50} and $t_{1/2}k_{e0}$ derived from these studies are useful to

Table 20-2		Estimates of Analgesic $t\frac{1}{2}k_{e0}$ for Clinically Relevant End Points of Pain Relief and Respiratory Depression
Drug	$t\frac{1}{2}k_{e0}$	End Point Measured
Morphine	1.5 h	Postoperative analgesia
Ibuprofen	0.5 h	Postoperative analgesia
Acetaminophen	1 h	Postoperative analgesia
Morphine (men)	1.5 h	Relief of experimental pain
Morphine (women)	5 h	Relief of experimental pain
Fentanyl	20–40 min	Relief of experimental pain
Alfentanil	1–10 min	Relief of experimental pain
Remifentanil	1–1.5 min	Relief of experimental pain
Buprenorphine	2.5 h	Relief of experimental pain
S-ketamine	<1 min	Relief of experimental pain
Morphine	1.2 h	Respiratory depression
Buprenorphine	1.5 h	Respiratory depression
Fentanyl	15 min	Respiratory depression
Remifentanil	0.5 min	Respiratory depression
Naloxone	5–8 min	Relief of respiratory depression

Data from Martini C, Olofsen E, Yassen A, et al. Pharmacokinetic-pharmacodynamic modeling in acute and chronic pain: an overview of the recent literature. *Exp Rev Pharmacother*. 2011;4:719.

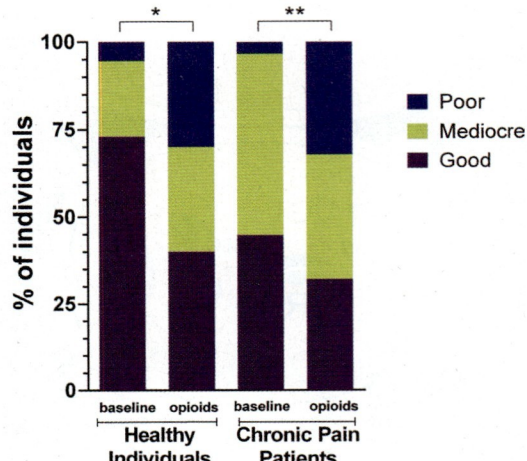

Figure 20-6 The ability to reliably translate a randomly applied nociceptive stimulus into a numerical pain score (between pain threshold and pain tolerance) is shown in healthy individuals and chronic pain patients, to demonstrate the effects of opioid treatment. Scores are divided into good, mediocre, and poor, reflecting the amount of deviation from an expected pain score. *p = 0.015, **p = 0.016. (Data from Oudejans LCJ, van Velzen M, Olofsen E, et al. Translation of random painful stimuli into numerical responses in fibromyalgia and perioperative patients. *Pain*. 2016;157:128–136.)

compare the potency and onset/offset of opioids. However, since the C_{50} for EEG effects occurs beyond the normal clinical dose range of opioids, more clinically useful C_{50} values would include those for the analgesic, respiratory depressive, and sedative effect of opioids. For alfentanil and fentanyl C_{50} values range from 75 and 1 ng/mL for sedation to 150 and 2 ng/mL for analgesia, respectively.[66,67] This indicates that these clinically relevant effects occur at lower doses than their effects on the EEG. For fentanyl it is of further interest that $t\frac{1}{2}k_{e0}$ values for analgesia (20 to 40 minutes) and respiratory depression are much longer (15 minutes) than those observed for EEG-slowing (5 to 6 minutes). In Table 20-2 values of $t\frac{1}{2}k_{e0}$ for the end points of pain relief and respiratory depression are given for various analgesics currently in use.

Pharmacodynamics: Pain Relief

In postoperative patients following major orthopedic surgery under general anesthesia, it has been observed that some patients require a morphine dose of 0.02 mg/kg to obtain a visual analog pain score of 30 mm (on a scale from 0, no pain, to 100 mm, most intense pain) or less while others require a dose 40 times as large (0.8 mg/kg).[68] Younger (<40 years) healthy volunteers of normal weight (BMI <25 kg/m²) had analgesic responses to a fixed dose of morphine that varied by a factor of 20.[69] This variability is not restricted to morphine, but is observed for all opioids used for treatment of acute, perioperative, and chronic pain, including strong opioids such as fentanyl and remifentanil. These data suggest that the variability in opioid effect is related to both variability in PK-related parameters (which in turn are attributable to differences in age, weight, body fat and muscle content, renal/liver function, cardiac output, genetic polymorphism in metabolic pathways, and co-medication) and variability in PD-related parameters. These PD differences of opioid sensitivity and pain perception most likely have a genetic origin. To date, no clear genetic basis for variability in morphine or any other opioid PD effect has been demonstrated (for exceptions see the pharmacogenetics section). Recently it was shown that the ability to score pain in a consistent and reliable fashion depends on various factors, including the presence of chronic pain and prior opioid administration (Fig. 20-6).[70,71] This may be related to changes in brain areas involved in the translation of nociceptive stimuli into a verbal numeric response (a complex cognitive process that requires many steps, including number sensing). In chronic pain patients these changes may be due to neuroplastic changes in the frontal and parietal cortices. Opioids may cause transient effects on cognition and signal processing.[71]

These data indicate that the safest approach to opioid analgesia is one of careful titration to analgesic effect during surgery and in the postoperative period, with acute awareness of the undesirable dose-related side effects. This admonition to carefully titrate the administration of opioids is perhaps even more crucial when administering long-acting opioids orally for the treatment of chronic pain.

During surgery opioids are titrated in doses sufficient to dampen and prevent exaggerated hemodynamic responses to painful surgical stimuli. In the postoperative period (and in chronic pain patients) opioids are usually titrated to the patient's verbal response to pain. This distinction requires not only a difference in administration, but also a difference in vigilance with respect to opioid side effects. During surgery, potent high-dose piperidines (e.g., fentanyl, remifentanil) are the opioids of choice, while in the postoperative period medium strength opioids (morphine, methadone) are often chosen. During anesthesia one should be aware of hypotension and bradycardia, a common side effect of strong opioids. In contrast, in the postoperative period the most important side effects to avoid are respiratory depression and severe sedation, while other non–life-threatening side effects impacting patient satisfaction and health costs are nausea/vomiting and loss of bowel motility.

Morphine

In two studies on the postoperative effects of morphine following major surgery, the average intravenous dose of morphine to reach 50% pain relief was 20 mg. This dose resulted in a plasma concentration of 34 ng/mL and a t½k_{e0} of about 2 hours, although the initial onset of analgesia occurred between 15 and 30 minutes.[72,73] Thus, there is a 1- to 2-hour delay between peak plasma morphine concentration and peak analgesic effect (i.e., hysteresis). Surprisingly, these parameters are not influenced by the patient's age, weight, and gender. Given the long time to peak analgesia, a practical strategy for dosing morphine in adults is to give an initial morphine bolus dose (0.15–0.2 mg/kg) at least 60 minutes before the end of surgery. When the patient is in pain in the postanesthesia care unit (PACU), 2 mg bolus doses at 5- to 10-minute intervals may be given until visual analog pain scores decrease to 30 or less (on a scale from 0 to 100) (Fig. 20-7). At that point, the patient can be started on a patient-controlled analgesia (PCA) pump.

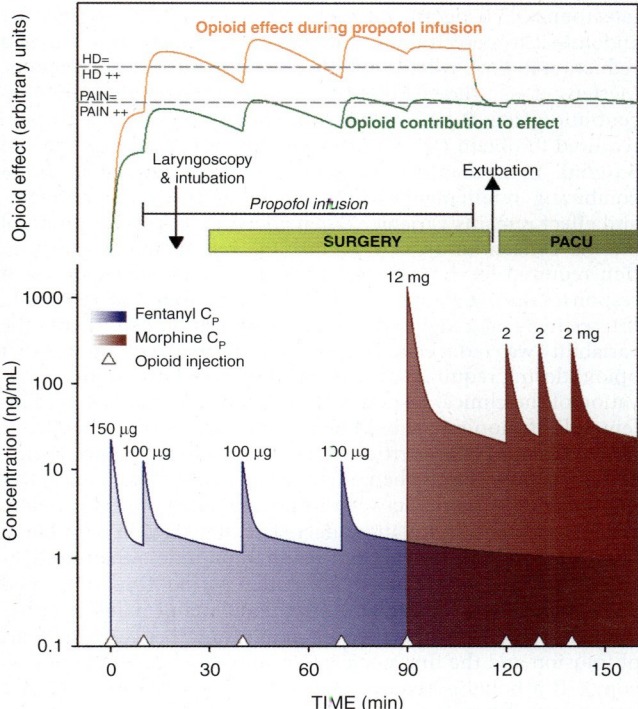

Figure 20-7 Simulated effect of multiple bolus doses of fentanyl (100 to 150 µg) during anesthesia, and morphine during and following anesthesia, on the analgesic and hemodynamic state of the patient. **Bottom:** An initial dose of morphine (12 mg) is given 30 minutes before the end of surgery followed by three 2-mg doses (at the end of this titration phase the patient can be set on PCA morphine). The *blue* and *red lines* are the simulated fentanyl and morphine plasma concentration (Cp). **Top:** The effect profile induced by the two opioids. During anesthesia fentanyl dosing is based predominantly on hemodynamic and other autonomic parameters; in the PACU morphine dosing is based on pain rating. During anesthesia, the combination of fentanyl and propofol (orange line) provides greater analgesia than opioids alone (*green line*). When propofol infusion is terminated the analgesic profile reverts to a lower level (from *orange* via *orange-green* to *green* line). HD indicates that hemodynamic and other autonomic responses are in the normal range, HD++ indicates increased responses (such as high blood pressure, tachycardia, and sweating) due to the surgical stress; PAIN indicates adequate analgesia, PAIN++ indicates pain. The *dotted lines* are the arbitrary divisions between adequate anesthesia and inadequate anesthesia, and adequate analgesia and inadequate analgesia.

Two considerations must accompany every postoperative acute pain plan. First, the postoperative analgesic regimen should be multimodal with morphine (or any other opioid), and combined with opioid-sparing drugs such as acetaminophen and nonsteroidal anti-inflammatory drugs such as diclofenac. Second, some patients require large doses of morphine, yet their pain appears unresponsive to morphine. The cause of such reduced opioid sensitivity is unclear. Irrespective of the cause, it is wise not to continue dosing (see Opioid-induced Respiratory Depression versus Opioid Analgesia) but to add an adjuvant such as the NMDA receptor antagonist ketamine (0.125 mg/kg), or an α_2-adrenergic receptor agonist, such as clonidine (75 µg). Both drugs are analgesics in their own right and enhance morphine's analgesic effect.[74,75] A practical morphine PCA regimen may consist of a 1-mg dose, a 5-minute lockout, and a maximum of 24 mg per 4 hours.

Fentanyl

Fentanyl is about 100 times more potent than morphine. Like all opioids the analgesic response to intravenous fentanyl is highly variable. Fentanyl's lipophilic structure means it rapidly crosses the blood–brain barrier, as is evident from a characteristic δ-wave appearing on the EEG (t½k_{e0} 6.5 minutes). However, fentanyl's t½k_{e0} for analgesic effect is longer with values ranging between 10 and 20 minutes[66]; fentanyl's potency (C_{50}) for analgesia ranges from 1 to 2 ng/mL.[66] Fentanyl is used during anesthesia to dampen cardiovascular responses to noxious stimulation from laryngoscopy, intubation, skin incision, and surgical stress. On average, the requirements for inhalational anesthetics and propofol are reduced by about 50% when administering 1.5 to 3 µg/kg IV fentanyl.[76–78] In fact, by combining fentanyl (or any other potent opioid) with propofol the requirement of both drugs to prevent movement and hemodynamic responses to laryngoscopy and surgical stress is reduced (Fig. 20-7).[77,78] Fentanyl dosing should be repeated at regular intervals in order to maintain a comfortable analgesic state (the dose and frequency are dependent on the patient's weight, dose, type of surgery, etc.). Be aware that a continuous infusion leads to the accumulation of the drug in the body as its 50% context-sensitive half-time increases rapidly with the duration of infusion (Fig. 20-4).[50,51] Similarly, frequent dosing of the drug may cause accumulation. Taking into account the drug's t½k_{e0} fentanyl should be administered 5 to 10 minutes prior to an anticipated painful/stressful event such as laryngoscopy or skin incision (Fig. 20-7).

In the 1980s, high-dose fentanyl was often used in combination with nitrous oxide to provide both analgesia and suppression of consciousness. Although this combination provided excellent hemodynamic stability, it could not assure amnesia. Hence, it is not surprising that this technique has been replaced by the technique of "balanced anesthesia" or total intravenous anesthesia (TIVA) where opioids are combined with sedatives, intravenous anesthetics, and muscle relaxants to assure amnesia, as well as analgesia.

Fentanyl is also used in the treatment of chronic pain. For example, the fentanyl patch is used in a large number of cancer and noncancer chronic pain patients. The transcutaneous delivery of fentanyl ranges from 12 to 100 µg/hr, although absorption depends on a variety of factors such as skin thickness, subcutaneous fat layer, and subcutaneous perfusion. Peak analgesic effect is reached only after 10 to 12 hours and the effect of one patch lasts 3 to 4 days. Other methods of administration include intranasal fentanyl, sublingual fentanyl, fentanyl lozenges (a solid preparation in the form of a lollipop), mucosal patch—all four methods are used for treatment of breakthrough pain—and iontophoretic transdermal fentanyl applications. The home use of fentanyl in chronic pain patients comes with the danger of misuse and abuse by the patients or by family members or friends. This is a major concern as it leads to an increasing number of opioid fatalities.

Sufentanil

Sufentanil is a thienyl derivate of fentanyl and about 10 times more potent than fentanyl; its lipophilicity is two times greater than that of fentanyl. Sufentanil acts selectively at the MOR with a C_{50} for analgesia of 30 pg/mL and t½k_{e0} similar to that of fentanyl. Sufentanil is metabolized in the liver to various inactive and one active compound, desmethylsufentanil. The latter has 10% of the activity of sufentanil, and since it is produced in minute quantities has no clinical relevance. Sufentanil is used predominantly as an analgesic during anesthesia, as it produces stable hemodynamics and cardiac output. A sublingual sufentanil PCA system for postoperative pain relief has also been introduced. Compared to other clinically available opioids, sufentanil has a high therapeutic index (= LD_{50}/ED_{50} where LD_{50} is the lethal dose in 50% of animals tested, and ED_{50} the effective dose in 50% of animals tested).

Remifentanil

Remifentanil, the newest piperidine available for use in humans, differs from the other strong opioids in its rapid onset/offset for all clinical effects including respiration (Fig. 20-8).[79] Indications for its use include anesthesia/surgery, PCA analgesia and sedation in the ICU, diagnostic procedures, and the treatment of obstetric labor pain. The use of remifentanil in spontaneous breathing patients at relatively low infusion rates (<0.1 to 0.2 µg/kg/min) is feasible[52,79] but requires adequate monitoring and skilled personnel to detect and manage an adverse respiratory event.

Remifentanil is 100 to 200 times more potent than morphine. Like other opioids, remifentanil displays large variability in effect among patients. For example, Drover and Lemmens[80] showed that the remifentanil plasma concentration causing a 50% probability (C_{P50}) of no clinical response to stimulation (laryngoscopy, intubation, skin incision, and skin closures) varies 50-fold, from 1.5 to 79 ng/mL, during abdominal surgery in patients anesthetized with a nitrous oxide and remifentanil combination. In that study, a clear gender difference in potency of remifentanil was found (C_{P50} men 4.1 ng/mL, women 7.5 ng/mL). This difference can be accounted for by the difference in surgical stimulation of the prostatectomies versus hysterectomies. Different surgeries produce differences in nociception (i.e., pain) and hemodynamic stress responses, and hence require different dosages to suppress pain and stress. The C_{P50} varied from 3.8 ng/mL for prostatectomies, 5.6 ng/mL for nephrectomies, and 7.5 ng/mL for abdominal hysterectomies. Like fentanyl, remifentanil causes a reduction in both volatile anesthetic and propofol requirements. Mertens et al.[81] showed that by increasing the remifentanil concentration from 0 to 2 ng/mL the mean propofol concentration required to obtain C_{P50} for laryngoscopy was reduced from 7 to 3 µg/mL, more than 60% reduction in dose requirement. When combining remifentanil with propofol (TIVA), the remifentanil effect remains variable. When added to a constant propofol plasma concentration of 2 µg/mL, the remifentanil concentration required for suppression of hemodynamic and movement responses during abdominal surgery varies from 3 to 15 ng/mL. Interestingly, at a higher propofol concentration of 4 µg/mL, the variability was reduced to 0 to 5 ng/mL. These data reinforce that opioid dosing requires titration to effect based on careful observation of the clinical response of the patient. Variations in remifentanil infusion rate should be based on an a priori knowledge of the PK and PD properties of the drug, patient characteristics, and, most importantly, hemodynamic responses and nociceptive input during surgery. Between intubation and surgical incision, when there is no stimulation, decreases of 30% to 40% in blood pressure and heart rate are not uncommon unless the remifentanil infusion dose is reduced during that period. Due to its rapid PK activity, the need for an initial remifentanil bolus is rather limited especially when there is ample time between the start of infusion and the first nociceptive stimulus (such as laryngoscopy). If a bolus is required, a slow infusion (given in 1 to 2 minutes) of 0.5 to 1 µg/kg can be used.

The minimum alveolar concentration (MAC) reduction observed with remifentanil use and its very short CSt½ (Fig. 20-4) make rapid awakening possible at the end of surgery.[82] For example, after a 3-hour infusion of propofol and remifentanil for abdominal surgery, the shortest time to awakening (≈7 minutes) was observed after constant propofol and remifentanil concentrations of 2.5 and 4.8 ng/mL, respectively (Fig. 20-9).[81] At higher propofol concentrations, but lower remifentanil concentrations, the time to awakening increases. The occurrence of postoperative pain following remifentanil "fast-track" anesthesia is frequently reported.[45,46] Postoperative pain scores are higher after a remifentanil-based anesthesia, and requirements for morphine are increased. This is due to the rapid decrease in opioid concentration causing a rapid decline in analgesic state, possibly combined with OIH. Strategies to counteract this problem include starting morphine administration 30 to 45 minutes before the end of surgery, or a single fentanyl bolus of 50 µg or ketamine 0.125 mg/kg at the end of surgery.[45]

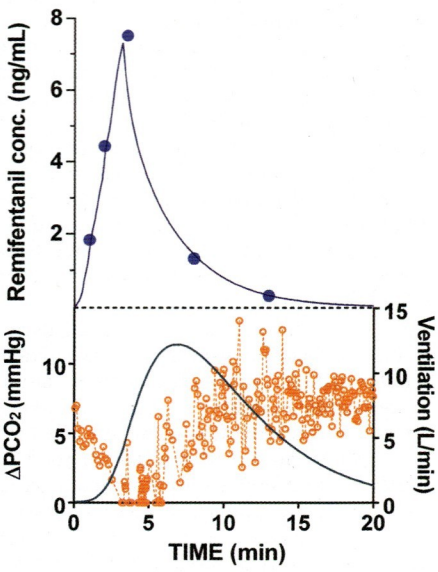

Figure 20-8 Effect of a short remifentanil infusion on breathing. **Top:** The measured remifentanil plasma concentration (*blue dots*) and the pharmacokinetic data fit (*blue line*). **Bottom:** The increase in end-tidal PCO_2 (ΔPCO_2, *green line*), the measured inspired ventilation (*orange dots*, each dot is one breath). Note the absence of a delay between the remifentanil plasma concentration and ventilation, and the short delay between changes in the plasma concentration and the end-tidal PCO_2. (Data from Olofsen E, Boom M, Nieuwenhuijs D, et al. Modeling the non-steady-state respiratory effects of remifentanil in awake and propofol sedated healthy volunteers. *Anesthesiology.* 2010;212:1382–1395.)

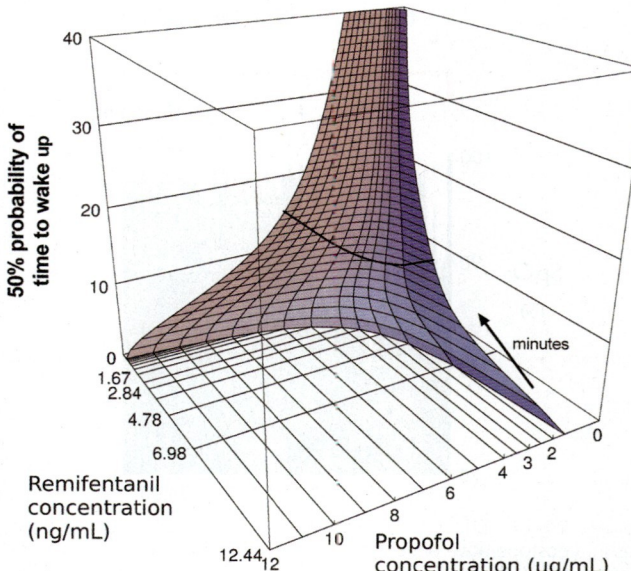

Figure 20-9 Propofol–remifentanil interaction on "time to wake up" following anesthesia. Remifentanil–propofol interaction causing 50% probability of no response to surgical stimulation are given at t = 0 minutes. Next the infusion pumps are switched off causing the decreasing effect site concentrations. The bold line on top of the 3D surface represents the 50% probability of return of consciousness. The lowest point represents the optimal propofol–remifentanil concentration during surgery that gives the minimal recovery time after the pumps are switched off. Note that this occurs at steady-state concentrations of 4.78 ng/mL remifentanil and 2 μg/mL propofol, and 50% probability of waking up occurs after 7 minutes. (Data from Vuyk J, Mertens MJ, Olofsen E, et al. Propofol anesthesia and rational opioid selection. Anesthesiology. 1997;87:1549–1562.)

Pharmacogenetics

Pharmacogenetics describes the relationship between genetic variations and drug response. Variations occur in genes that code for components of the metabolic pathways and transport of the drug across the blood–brain barrier (affecting PK behavior), and in genes that code for the opioid receptor or proteins in downstream signaling pathways (affecting PD behavior). The existence of a pharmacogenetic effect on PK is well established in opioid pharmacology, whereas an effect of genetic makeup on PD is less certain. For example, the literature on the significance of a specific mutation in the gene coding for MOR, $OPRM1:c.118\ A > G$ (dbSNP1799971), is equivocal.[83] Some examples of pharmacogenetic variations that influence opioid analgesia are given below.

The gene that codes for the melanocortin-1 receptor, the $MC1r$ gene, is involved in the regulation of skin and hair pigmentation and immunomodulation. Sixty percent of redheads have at least two variant alleles of the gene. Animal and human studies indicate that specific mutations in this gene cause a phenotype of red hair, a fair, freckled skin, and an increase in μ-opioid analgesia (Fig. 20-10).[84] The exact mechanism by which the $MC1r$ gene influences pain pathways and interacts with the opioidergic system remains unknown. Possibly, the inactive MC1r causes a reflex increase in α-melanocyte-stimulating hormone (αMSH) and ACTH, which may act as the endogenous ligands to MC1r and which may induce neurobehavioral changes. Interestingly, redheads require more midazolam and inhalational anesthetics compared to otherwise pigmented (either blond or dark) individuals.[85]

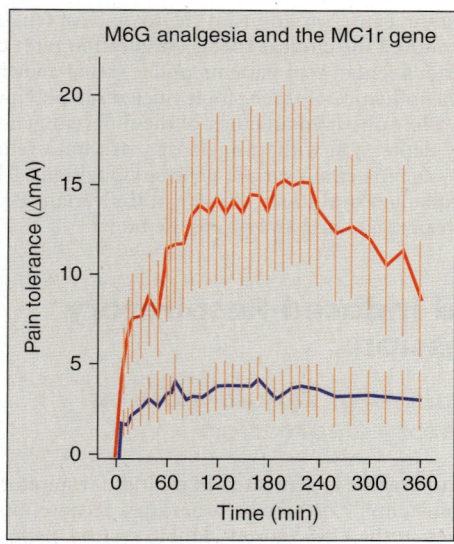

Figure 20-10 Analgesic response to morphine-6-glucuronide in volunteers with loss of functional mutations in the melanocortin-1-receptor gene (red line) compared to volunteers with an intact gene and blond or dark hair (blue). The greater opioid sensitivity is apparent in red heads. (Data from Mogil J, Ritchie J, Smith SB, et al. Melanocortin-1 receptor gene variants affect pain and mu-opioid analgesia in mice and humans. J Med Genet. 2005;42:583–587.)

While most CYP isoenzymes display polymorphisms, the genetic variability in the gene coding for CYP2D6 is clinically most important.[58,86] The CYP2D6 isoenzyme of the cytochrome P450 system is highly polymorphic with large variations between individuals in the number of gene copies in their DNA.[86] The rate of metabolism of opioids depends on the number of copies a subject expresses, ranging from ultrarapid metabolizing individuals with multiple copies of the CYP2D6 gene to poor metabolizing individuals with two nonfunctional alleles of the gene. The more copies of the gene the greater the metabolic power within the CYP2D6 pathway; the reverse is true for individuals without an active copy of the gene.[86] This is important for drugs that rely on CYP2D6 to convert an inactive precursor (prodrug), such as codeine, into the active component of pain therapy (for codeine this is morphine).[87] Patients without an active gene will have no benefit from treatment with codeine. Dangerous circumstances may occur when a patient is an extensive metabolizer and produces large amounts of the active component. There are multiple case reports showing codeine intoxication due to ultrarapid CYP2D6 metabolism (see below). A tragic example reported by Koren et al.[88] describes a normal full-term breastfed neonate that developed lethargy on postnatal day 7 and was found dead 6 days later. His mother had been prescribed 30 mg codeine combined with 500 mg acetaminophen for episiotomy pain (two tablets every 12 hours, reduced to 1 tablet per 12 hours after day 2 because of somnolence and constipation). Postmortem morphine plasma concentrations were 70 ng/mL (normal values for children breastfed by mothers receiving codeine is 0.2 to 2 ng/mL). The mother's milk contained 87 ng/mL morphine (typical mother milk concentrations after repeated codeine dosing is 2 to 20 ng/mL). Genotype analysis revealed that the mother had a 2 × 2 CYP2D6 gene duplication and was classified as an ultrarapid CYP2D6 metabolizer. The clinical picture is that of death due to morphine-induced respiratory depression.

Variations in the $ABCB1$ gene, the gene coding for P-glycoprotein, a protein involved in the efflux of xenobiotics from the brain, cause variations in the toxicity of fentanyl. Park et al.[89] monitored the clinical effects (respiration rate) of 2.5 µg/kg intravenous fentanyl in patients under spinal anesthesia and assessed the influence of three single nucleotide polymorphisms in *ABCB1*. They observed an effect of the different genotypes on respiratory depression with an increased risk for a reduction in respiratory rate in certain variant gene combinations. These data are best explained by a lesser efficacy of the variant P-glycoprotein to transport fentanyl away from the brain.

Opioid-induced Respiratory Depression

Mechanisms of Opioid-induced Respiratory Depression

The drive to breathe is generated in multiple respiratory centers in the brainstem.[90,91] Respiratory neurons receive inputs from various sites in the CNS (cortex, limbic system, hypothalamus, spinal cord), a set of receptors located in the brainstem (central chemoreceptors), and in the carotid bodies (peripheral chemoreceptors). These sensors send information (changes in pH, PCO_2, and PO_2 of the cerebrospinal fluid and arterial blood) to the brainstem respiratory centers, which appropriately adjust breathing rate and pulmonary tidal volume. For example, acidosis, hypercapnia, and hypoxia will cause hyperventilation, while hypocapnia and alkalosis will reduce minute ventilation. Opioids that activate MORs expressed on respiratory neurons cause a reduction in respiratory rate,[92] while a reduction in tidal volume is caused by the opioid-induced decreased afferent input into the brainstem from peripheral chemosensors.

When an opioid is administered to a patient and the injection rate is sufficiently slow (over minutes) that the depression of the respiratory neurons in the brainstem coincides with the accumulation of arterial CO_2, the stimulatory effect of the increased CO_2 at the peripheral and central chemoreceptors will offset the decrease in tidal volume and reduced respiratory rate.[52] When just monitoring respiratory rate and oxygen saturation it appears that the opioid injected has no effect on the ventilatory system, but when also monitoring end-tidal (or arterial) CO_2 the opioid effect becomes visible. When a strong opioid that rapidly crosses the blood-brain barrier is injected, a rapid depression of respiratory neurons occurs and there will be no time for gradual CO_2 accumulation, resulting in an apneic patient. An example is given in Figure 20-8, which shows that a rapid short-term infusion of remifentanil causes apnea and hypercapnia.[52] Breathing is restored by a high arterial CO_2 level combined with the rapid drop in brain (effect site) remifentanil concentration. Slowing the speed of injection of this strong opioid allows the accumulation of arterial CO_2, and apnea will be prevented and the patient will continue to breathe, albeit at a higher arterial PCO_2.

Apart from their effect on brainstem respiratory neurons (causing central apnea), opioids may increase the collapsibility of the upper airways due to suppression of neurons in the brainstem involved in maintaining the upper airway muscle tone or from the loss of muscle tone related to sedation.[90] Opioids combined with anesthetics do not increase the incidence of upper airway obstruction, but do increase the number of central apneic events.[93] However, any dose of opioid that produces a generalized state of sedation and/or reduced muscle tone will give rise to upper airway collapse, even when the patient is considered awake.[93] Furthermore, depression of the chemo- and arousal reflexes by opioids will cause a delayed and less forceful response

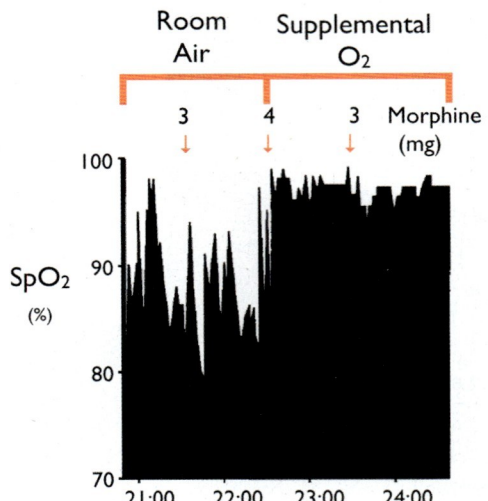

Figure 20-11 Effect of supplemental oxygen on pulse oximeter values in a postoperative patient on PCA morphine. (Data from Stone JG, Cozine KA, Wald A. Nocturnal oxygenation during patient-controlled analgesia. *Anesth Analg.* 1999;89:104–110.)

to upper airway obstruction.[90] Recent data indicate that most patients receiving opioids, whether diagnosed with obstructive sleep apnea syndrome or not, develop both central and obstructive apneic events resulting in recurrent hypoxemia during the first three to five nights postoperatively.[94–95] Stone et al.[96] showed that patients on PCA morphine without supplemental oxygen develop recurrent and deep hypoxic events during the first few postoperative nights (Fig. 20-11). While supplemental oxygen results in fewer hypoxic events, it has a serious disadvantage as it masks hypoventilation and early detection of an obstructive respiratory event because the lungs are primed with supplemental oxygen. Use of a pulse oximeter, especially in the presence of supplemental oxygen administration, is not a valid measure of the adequacy of ventilation. An example of the inability to detect an apneic event using pulse oximetry while on supplemental oxygen is given in Figure 20-12. A subject received a remifentanil bolus causing rapid respiratory depression and a reduction in respiratory rate, both during air and oxygen breathing. Desaturations were detected during air breathing only.[79]

Finally, strong, high-dose opioids, especially when given rapidly, cause skeletal muscle rigidity in thoracic, abdominal, and pharyngeal muscles, all of which can contribute to respiratory insufficiency.[97]

Incidence and Risk Factors of Opioid-induced Respiratory Depression

The incidence of respiratory depression from opioid treatment, acute or chronic, is poorly documented. The metrics in the literature defining respiratory depression are inconsistent, the data are predominantly retrospective, and most studies rely on intermittent sampling of data.[90] Thus, a significant number of respiratory depression events from which the patient recovers spontaneously or is rescued by other means are likely missed. A recent systematic review of the literature on postoperative opioid-induced respiratory depression estimates an average incidence of 0.5% with a range of 0.2% to 2%.[90] This would suggest that only one in 200 patients develops a respiratory event

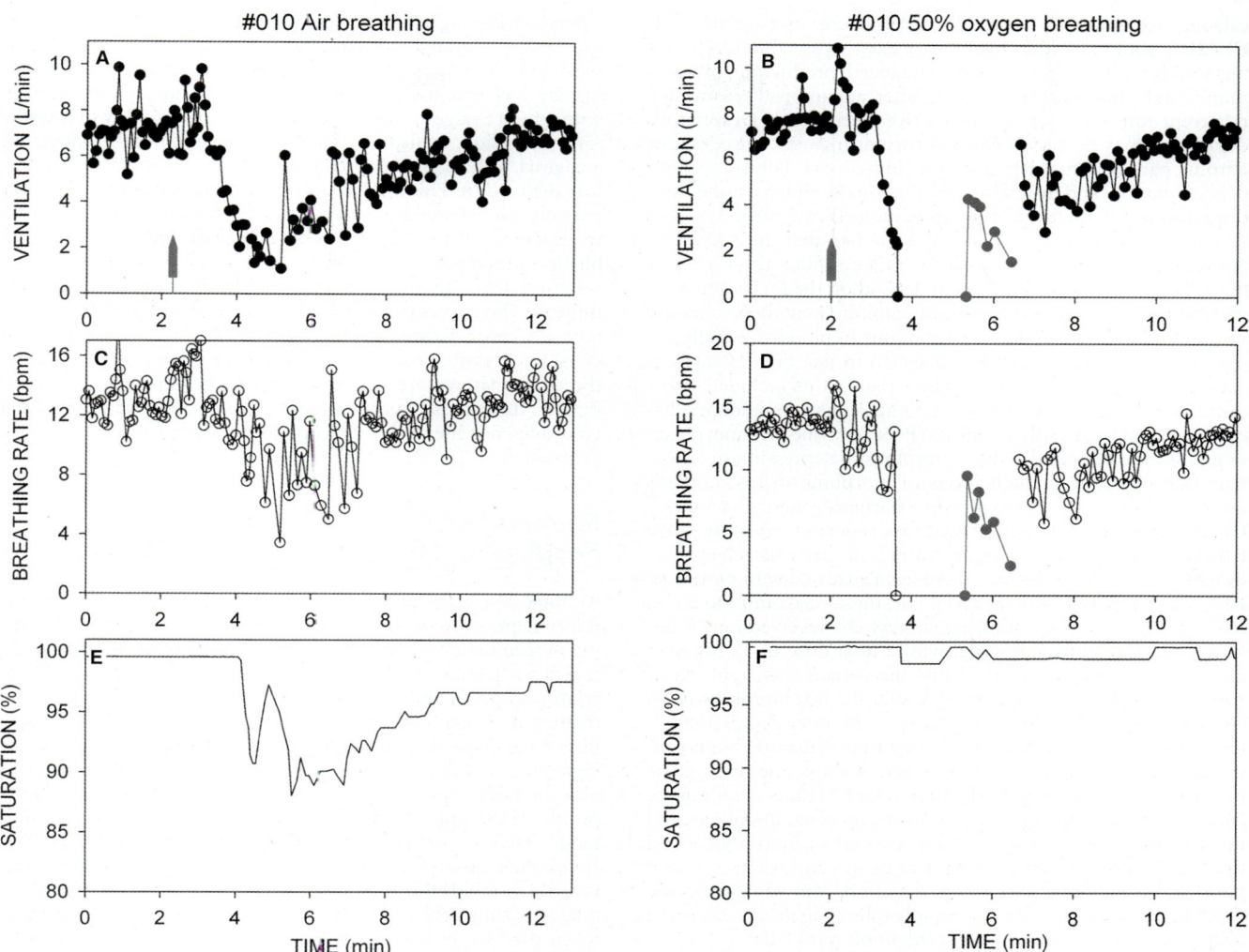

Figure 20-12 Effect of the administration of 50 μg remifentanil on ventilation in one subject during air breathing (**A**, **C**, and **E**) and during inhalation of 50% oxygen (**B**, **D**, and **F**). During air breathing the depression in ventilation is apparent from the reduced oxygen saturation (apart from the reduction in ventilation and respiratory rate). During administration of supplemental oxygen the pulse oximeter does not detect the apneic event. Mask ventilation is shown in red. The syringe indicates the time of remifentanil administration. (Data from Niesters M, Mahajan RP, Aarts L, et al. High-inspired oxygen concentration further impairs opioid-induced respiratory depression. *Br J Anaesth.* 2013;110:837–841.)

from opioids that requires an intervention such as the administration of naloxone. In the case of randomized controlled trials where morphine is used as positive control, the incidence of morphine-induced respiratory depression is many times higher, with hypoventilation (a respiratory rate <8 breaths/minute) occurring in as high as 30% of patients during PCA morphine treatment.[90,98] This suggests that the respiratory depression from opioids frequently goes undetected, and is therefore underreported. The same applies to opioid treatment for chronic pain. Accidental deaths from opioids in chronic cancer pain patients are often falsely attributed to the progression of the underlying disease. Recently, there has been an alarming increase in deaths from accidental opioid overdose among patients being treated for chronic noncancer pain. Unfortunately, no valid data are available on the incidence of opioid-induced respiratory depression in chronic pain patients on strong opioids.

Various patient groups are at higher risk for development of opioid-related respiratory depression. These include obese patients, patients with (central or peripheral) hypopneic and apneic periods during sleep, patients with neuromuscular disorders, (premature) neonates, chronic opioid users, and elderly patients.[90] Identification of these high-risk groups may be challenging. For instance, patients with undiagnosed sleep-related breathing disorders often present to the preoperative assessment clinic. A careful history (e.g., looking for daytime somnolence) and physical examination are required to uncover potential heightened opioid-associated respiratory risks. Furthermore specific questionnaires, such as the STOP-BANG questionnaire for obstructive sleep apnea, should be part of the screening routine in the obese and aging patient population.[99]

Recently, three independent analyses were published on all published cases of respiratory depression related to opioid administration in the pediatric population and in adults in acute and chronic pain.[100–102] From these data specific risk factors could be determined. In the pediatric population risk factors included[100]: morphine administration in patients with renal impairment, causing accumulation of M6G; codeine use in patients with CYP2D6 gene polymorphism associated with the ultrarapid metabolizer phenotype, causing enhanced production of morphine; and opioid use in patients after adenotonsillectomy for recurrent tonsillitis and/or obstructive sleep apnea (respiratory depression may be enhanced by recurrent hypoxic episodes). In chronic pain patients risk factors included renal failure, sensory deafferentation, and drug–drug interactions in which a nonopioid drug affects the metabolism of the opioid through the CYP450 system. One example of the latter is the fact that the polycyclic aromatic hydrocarbons in tobacco smoke induce the CYP system. Patients who use opioids that depend on the CYP system for metabolism and who suddenly quit smoking may then suddenly be exposed to high opioid concentrations in blood.[100] Finally, an underlying risk factor could be detected in just 60% of cases in acute and perioperative pain.[102] These risk factors included sleep-disordered breathing, obesity, renal impairment, pulmonary disease, neurologic disorders, and CYP450 enzyme polymorphism (e.g., the case of opioid-induced respiratory depression in a neonate that died due to high levels of morphine in his mother's milk has been given above; see the pharmacogenetics section).[88] One particularly well-documented case report of a postoperative lethal opioid-induced respiratory event is given by Lötsch et al.,[103] describing a healthy 26-year, 51-kg female treated with morphine after knee surgery under balanced anesthesia (sevoflurane 2% to 3%, 200-μg fentanyl). Following surgery she received four intravenous injections of morphine, with a total dose of 35 mg over 2 hours (almost 0.7 mg/kg). While the patient was comfortable and in no apparent distress directly after the last morphine dose, 40 minutes later the patient had "deep respiratory depression followed by a fatal cardiac arrest." At that time estimated brain concentrations were about 150 nM, which is above the toxic range for morphine, and highlight the importance of understanding the PK and PD of any opioid. The physicians involved in this case did not take into account the very slow passage of morphine across the blood–brain barrier causing a peak in central effect 1 to 2 hours following peak plasma concentration. And while the onset of analgesia occurred relatively rapidly following the last dose, the fatal respiratory depression occurred 40 minutes later.

Opioid-induced Respiratory Depression versus Opioid Analgesia

In general, when comparing opioid analgesics it is important to not only anticipate their side effects (respiratory depression), but also assess side effects relative to their analgesic properties. One way to compare opioids in this respect is by constructing so-called safety or utility functions (UFos).[104,105] UFos are constructed by estimating *the difference* in probability of analgesia and respiratory depression from PKPD analyses. The UFo is context-sensitive, that is, it may be defined for various end points, typically analgesia 50% or more, and respiratory depression 50% or less. A negative UFo value indicates that the probability for respiratory depression is larger than the probability for analgesic efficacy (Fig. 20-13A). In Figure 20-13B morphine and fentanyl UFos are compared. For low-dose morphine the probability for respiratory depression exceeds that of analgesia, whereas at higher doses resulting in a plasma concentration (C_P) more than 5 ng/mL the probability for analgesia is greater. At high morphine concentrations no difference in probability is apparent as the value of the UFo approaches zero. For fentanyl, an initial positive value at low doses (<0.5 ng/mL) is followed by a negative effect over the C_P range 0.5 to 3.0 ng/mL. For these reasons morphine is a better drug for postoperative PCA than fentanyl, when considering analgesia versus respiratory depression. In Figure 20-13C fentanyl UFos are given for individuals who display high fentanyl potency (C_{50} 250 ng/mL) versus individuals who display low fentanyl potency (C_{50} 1,500 ng/mL).[105] Individuals with a high analgesic efficacy display a low probability of respiratory depression, while individuals that respond poorly to fentanyl analgesia have a greater probability of development of respiratory depression. This is an important observation and implies that patients who show limited analgesic effect in response to opioid treatment are better off with other analgesic options (e.g., nerve blocks, intravenous ketamine).

These UFo curves are constructed from data in healthy volunteers. The curves of patients in pain will have a different form, typically more skewed to the left. However, since pain is not a constant in postoperative pain patients or chronic pain patients, the curves shown are still applicable to postoperative patients. Finally, it remains important to stress that a positive value of the UFo does not mean that the opioid does not cause respiratory depression.

Reversal of Opioid-induced Respiratory Depression

As noted above, the drug of choice in case of life-threatening respiratory depression or the inability to resume spontaneous breathing is naloxone.[61,106] Naloxone is a competitive MOR antagonist causing a parallel rightward shift of the opioid dose–response relationship. An oral MOR antagonist, naltrexone, is used in the treatment of alcoholism and opioid dependence.[61] Both antagonists are nonspecific, meaning that they antagonize all pharmacologic effects of opioids. The magnitude and duration of reversal of respiratory depression by naloxone depends on the PK and PD profile of the opioid that needs reversal and the administration mode of naloxone (bolus injections vs. continuous infusion).[106,107] Naloxone's onset time ($t\frac{1}{2}k_{e0}$) is 6.5 minutes, indicating that reversal is rapid. But the rate of decay of naloxone in plasma is relatively short ($t\frac{1}{2}_{elim}$ 30 minutes), resulting in "renarcotization" when used to reverse effects from opioids with a longer plasma half-life than naloxone. However, opioid concentrations are often just above the threshold for respiratory depression, and intravenous titration of naloxone 40 to 80 μg bolus doses to cumulative doses of less than 400 μg is often sufficient to restore spontaneous breathing.[90] Respiratory depression from opioids occurs at higher receptor occupancy rates than analgesia. Therefore, analgesia is not compromised with careful titration of naloxone to respiratory effect. Large doses of naloxone, as commonly used in resuscitation, will reverse analgesia immediately and may predispose patients to pain and catecholamine-associated hypertension and cardiac ischemia, if not monitored properly.[61]

The naloxone titration opioid reversal approach is adequate for most opioids, with the exception of opioids with a high affinity for the MOR, such as buprenorphine.[107] In that case, a continuous naloxone infusion (2 to 4 mg/hr) will cause a slow but steady resumption of breathing activity. For remifentanil the use of bolus naloxone doses in case of respiratory depression is unnecessary. The termination of the infusion will provide a rapid return of spontaneous breathing.

In recent years various drugs have been developed that reverse opioid-induced respiratory depression without affecting analgesia. These drugs stimulate the respiratory system at central (brainstem) and peripheral (carotid body) sites. One of the oldest respiratory stimulants used in clinical practice is doxapram.[108] It inhibits background K^+ channels (TASK1, TASK3 and the TASK1/2 heterodimer) on oxygen sensing cells in the carotid

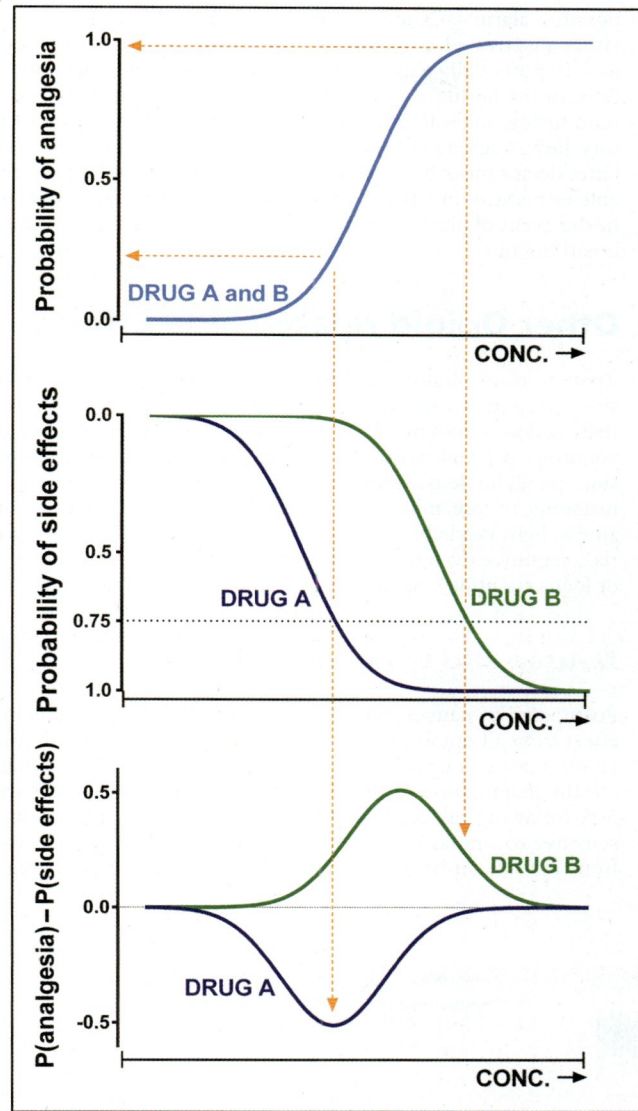
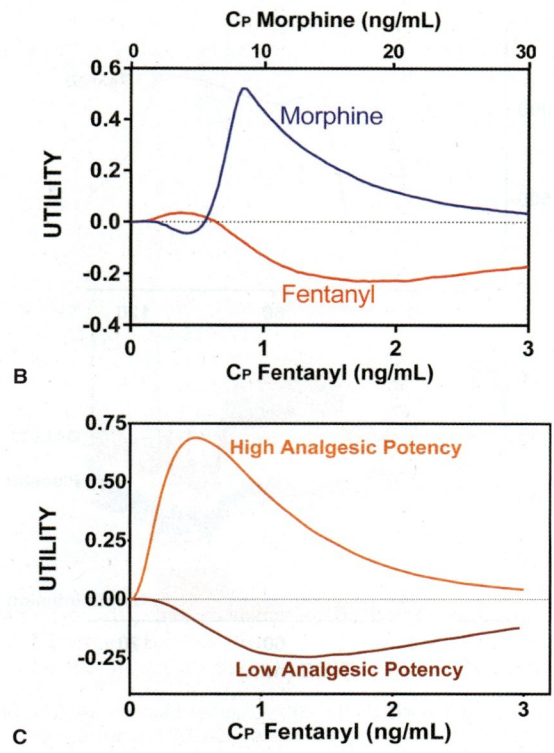

Figure 20-13 Safety or utility functions. **A:** Construction of two utility functions. Two drugs A and B have similar analgesic potencies (**top**), but differ in their potency to induce side effects (**middle**). The simplified utility is the difference between the probability for analgesia, P(analgesia), and the probability for side effects, P(side effects). The utility is negative for drug A, but positive for drug B. **B:** Utility functions for morphine and fentanyl. The probability of an analgesic effect greater than 50% minus the probability of side effects greater than 50% is given for the two opioids. **C:** Fentanyl utility functions in individuals with a high and low analgesic response to fentanyl. A high efficacy for analgesia is coupled to a low probability for respiratory depression and vice versa. (Data from C Pharmacotherapy for pain: efficacy and safety issues examined by subgroup analyses. *Pain.* 2015;156:S119–S126.)

body. However, doxapram produces various side effects (anxiety/panic attacks, hypertension, tachycardia, sweating, convulsions). A novel K+-channel blocker, GAL021, acting at BK_{Ca}-channels, is currently being developed for reversal/prevention of opioid-induced respiratory depression (Fig. 20-14) and possibly sleep-related upper airway obstructions.[109,110] Initial studies show that it does not produce doxapram-like side effects. A respiratory stimulant that acts at central sites is the ampakine CX717.[111] It increases respiratory drive by its action at the AMPA receptor in brainstem respiratory centers involved in rhythmogenesis.

Monitoring

On the ward, patients are monitored less comprehensively than in the operating room or PACU. On the ward "spot" oxygen saturation measurements by regular nurse visits are insufficient to detect or predict the occurrence of life-threatening respiratory events. A recent study in 833 patients recovering from noncardiac surgery in which continuous oxygen saturation was measured up to 48 hours after surgery showed that hypoxia was common and prolonged. The saturation values recorded in medical records seriously underestimated the presence, duration, and severity of postoperative hypoxemia (21% of patients had oxygen saturation levels <90% for 10 minutes or more per hour; 8% had saturation levels <85% for 5 minutes or more per hour, Fig. 20-15).[112] Apart from cardiopulmonary causes such as ventilation–perfusion mismatch, significant drops in oxygen saturation and tachydysrhythmias do occur when the patient's breathing system has been compromised for an appreciable period by recurrent central or obstructive apneas (or both) and no arousal occurs. Arousal is a "wake-up" from a state of sleep or sedation, and allows the patient to open his or her throat and hyperventilate to overcome the preceding period of hypoxemia. Arousal is triggered by hypoxia, and depressed by opioids and sedatives. Postoperative respiratory events are often episodic, with arousals and hyperventilation in-between events. This will cause repetitive triggering of the oxygen saturation monitoring alarm and

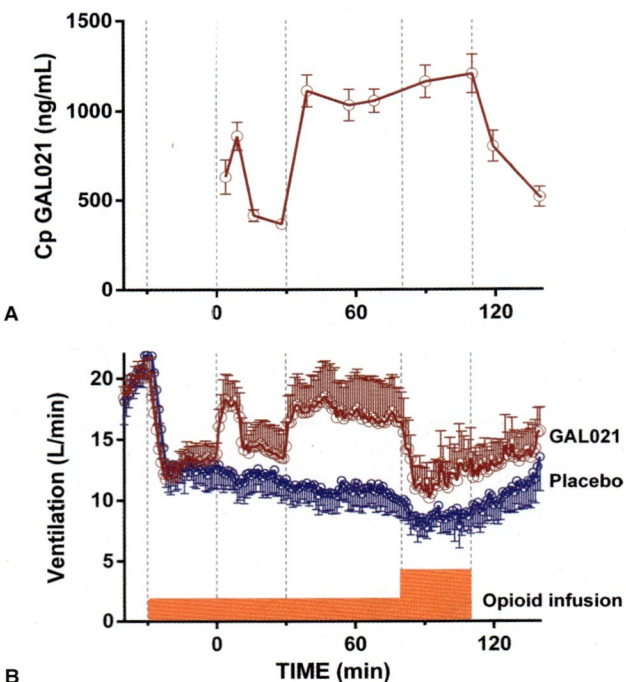

Figure 20-14 Influence of the BK$_{Ca}$-channel blocker GAL021 on opioid-induced respiratory depression. **A:** GAL021 plasma concentrations. **B:** The reduced ventilation induced by the opioid alfentanil (*orange*), along with the stimulatory effect of GAL021 are both clearly visible. (Data from Roozekrans M, Olofsen E, van der Schrier R, et al. Reversal of opioid-induced respiratory depression by BK-channel blocker GAL021: a pharmacokinetic-pharmacodynamic modelling study in healthy volunteers. *Clin Pharmacol Ther*. 2015;97:641–649.)

possibly alarm fatigue of the nursing staff. When the alarm is either inactivated or unattended, an arousal failure may occur and is potentially fatal (Fig. 20-16).[113] Monitors that directly indicate breathing activity are preferable to oxygen saturation monitoring, including monitors that indirectly measure expiratory flow, such as end-tidal carbon dioxide and humidity. The latter device measures the exhaled water content and gives a reliable estimate of breathing frequency.[114] Both monitors will alarm in the event of airway obstruction (flow rate is zero) or reduced breathing rates.

Other Opioid-related Side Effects

Apart from respiratory depression, opioids produce many other side effects that can cause patient discomfort, as well as potentially serious consequences. Common side effects are nausea and vomiting, delayed gastric emptying, constipation, bowel distension, paralytic ileus, sphincter of Oddi spasm, urinary retention, histamine release, miosis, muscle rigidity, diffuse CNS effects (dizziness, light headedness, sedation, drowsiness, euphoria, dysphoria), cognitive dysfunction (memory loss, inability to concentrate or focus attention), hallucinations, and cardiovascular effects.

Nausea and Vomiting

Postoperative nausea and vomiting (PONV) is a serious side effect from all opioids used in perioperative care. Although inhalation anesthetics contribute significantly to this effect, opioids are the major cause of PONV with an incidence of greater than 50% following balanced anesthesia.[115] Female patients seem more sensitive to opioid-induced PONV (see below). Patient distress from PONV can be so severe that patients may prefer being in

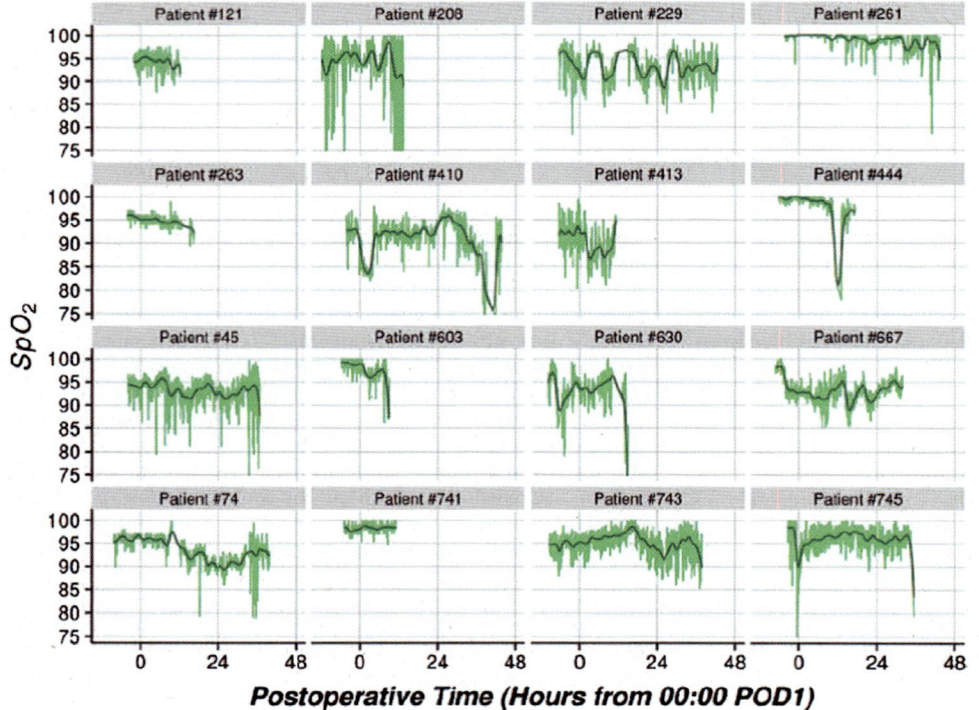

Figure 20-15 Oxygen saturation tracings of 16 patients following noncardiac surgery. The raw saturation data are shown (*light green*), along with the smoothed estimates (*black lines*). POD is postoperative day. (Data from Sun Z, Sessler DI, Dalton JE, et al. Postoperative hypoxemia is common and persistent: a prospective blinded observational study. *Anesth Analg*. 2014;121:709–715.)

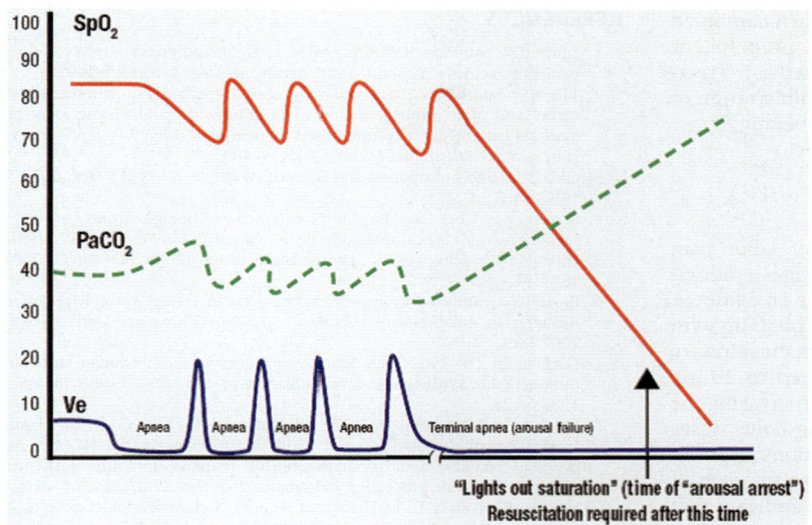
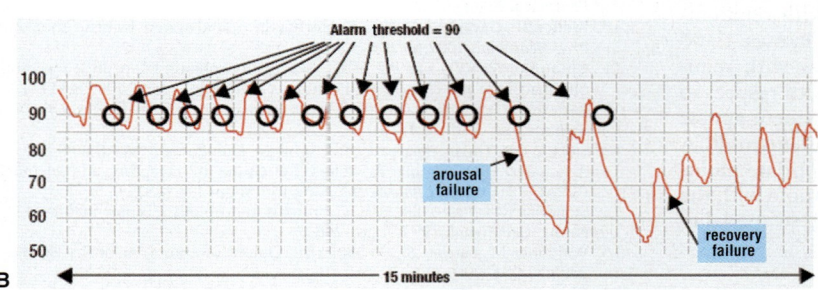

Figure 20-16 A: Episodic breathing pattern in a hypothetical patient with recurrent obstructive apneic events as might occur during sleep. SpO$_2$, oxygen saturation; PaCO$_2$, arterial carbon dioxide concentration; Ve, expired minute ventilation. **B:** Recurrent activation of the saturation alarm in a patient with sleep apnea (alarm threshold set at 90% oxygen saturation). This could possibly lead to alarm fatigue (y-axis = SpO$_2$). (Reprinted with permission from Curry JP, Lynn LA. Threshold monitoring, alarm fatigue, and the patterns of unexpected hospital death. *APSF Newsletter* Fall 2011;26:32. Copyright © 2011 Anesthesia Patient Safety Foundation.)

pain than being nauseated.[116] Furthermore, retching and vomiting will induce severe pain from the stress it places on recent surgical wounds. Opioids cause PONV by their effects on the chemoreceptor trigger zone (CTZ) in the area postrema of the brainstem, as well as by direct effects on the GI tract.[117] Movement effects (e.g., transport of the patient from the operating room to the PACU) may also contribute to PONV because opioids cause an increased sensitivity of the vestibular system. The CTZ contains opioid, serotonin (5HT$_3$), histamine, dopamine (D$_2$), and muscarinic acetylcholine receptors.[117] The CTZ, vagal nerve, and vestibular organs all send neural projections to the vomiting center in the medulla. Drugs used in the treatment of PONV include dopamine antagonists (e.g., droperidol), 5HT-antagonists (e.g., ondansetron), and corticosteroids.[115,117] In patients with a known history of PONV or those undergoing surgeries with a known high incidence of PONV, aggressive prevention strategies are used. Such strategies include the use of propofol rather than inhalation anesthetics, the use of regional postoperative analgesia rather than intravenous opioids, and multimodal pharmacologic therapy, including a 5HT-antagonist, a dopamine antagonist, and a steroid given prior to the end of surgery.

Smooth Muscle Effects

Opioid receptors are present in the enteric plexus within the smooth muscle layers of the GI tract. Opioids inhibit intestinal and pancreatic secretion, increase bowel tone, and decrease intestinal propulsive activity.[118] Consequently, opioids cause delayed gastric emptying, constipation, bowel distension, and paralytic ileus. Although opioids affect GI motility from central sites as well, blockade of opioid receptors with opioid antagonists that do not cross the blood–brain barrier (such as methylnaltrexone) will have a favorable effect on GI motility.[119]

Due to spasms of the sphincter of Oddi and common bile duct, opioids may cause acute upper abdominal pain and colic-like complaints.[120] Opioids may also contribute to misinterpretation of perioperative cholangiograms. Naloxone or glucagon can be used for treatment as both cause relaxation of the sphincter muscle.

Activated opioid receptors present in the wall of the bladder and ureters can cause acute urine retention.[121] It is most often seen after epidural or spinal opioid administration, with a higher incidence in men than in women. Urine retention is related to the inability of the urethral sphincter muscle to relax while the bladder tone increases. Opioid-induced bladder dysfunction can be treated with opioid antagonists.[122]

Cardiovascular Effects

Opioids affect the cardiovascular system at both central and peripheral sites.[123] Central effects include the activation of vagal nuclei and depression of vasomotor centers in the brainstem. Peripheral effects occur predominantly at high (supraclinical) doses and include direct myocardial depression and both arterial and venous dilatation. Morphine may cause additional cardiovascular effects via the release of histamine. The physiologic consequences are typically mild at clinical doses and include orthostatic hypotension, mild bradycardia, and a moderate reduction of systemic and pulmonary resistance. However, opioids at these doses can induce hemodynamic instability when combined with other drugs such as inhalation anesthetics, propofol, or benzodiazepines, and in severely ill patients (e.g., sepsis). Treatment of hemodynamic instability includes the administration of atropine and vasopressors and intravascular fluid therapy.

Remifentanil for Labor Pain

The primary indications for remifentanil PCA for labor pain are the presence of a condition which contraindicates epidural analgesia, or the unavailability of personnel to place an epidural. One approach is to use remifentanil at bolus doses of 30 μg with a 3-minute lockout period. In case of side effects (respiratory depression, nausea) the bolus dose may be reduced to 20 μg, whereas insufficient pain relief can be managed by increasing the bolus dose to 40 μg. An infusion scheme of 30 μg bolus doses at 3-minute intervals results in plasma concentrations between 2 and 4 ng/mL, and is typically sufficient to relieve the pain of the uterine contraction. Historical clinical studies indicate that while pain scores are not greatly reduced when compared to epidural analgesia, patient satisfaction is higher with remifentanil PCA.[124,125] However, a recent study performed in over 1,400 parturients showed that patient satisfaction is less with remifentanil PCA compared to epidural analgesia.[126] With respect to the technique' safety,[126] a recent study reported frequent apneic events and deeper desaturations in women on remifentanil PCA compared to epidural analgesia.[127] Still, with appropriate monitoring from personnel continuously present in the room with the patient, PCA remifentanil may be a safe labor analgesic modality in these selected clinical indications.

Gender Differences

A recent meta-analysis showed that women experience greater effects from opioids than men. This effect is attributed to enhanced opioid sensitivity in women; however, PK differences are equally important.[128] In studies following major abdominal or orthopedic surgery, women demonstrate a greater analgesic effect from PCA opioids than do men, and consequently consume fewer opioids postoperatively. Interestingly, in the first minutes postoperatively, greater morphine opioid efficacy is observed in men; however, this effect is reversed after 30 to 90 minutes. These data are best explained by a sex-related difference in morphine potency (greater in women), coupled with a slower onset/offset of the drug in women (i.e., greater value for t½k_{e0} in women).[69] The slower onset/offset times may be related to a slower passage across the blood–brain barrier or differences in receptor distribution and kinetics between men and women. As a consequence, morphine will take longer to induce adequate analgesia in women, while a speedier effect is observed in men. Due to the lower potency in men, they require multiple additional morphine administrations while women require fewer additional doses. This gender difference persists in older patients (>65 years), although in both sexes the opioid requirements for adequate analgesia are significantly reduced with age due to both PK and PD factors.[65]

Similar to analgesia, there are gender-related differences in opioid-induced respiratory depression and nausea and vomiting, with greater effects observed in women compared to men.[129,130] In a recent study of children undergoing outpatient tonsillectomy, a greater morphine effect was observed in girls compared to boys, including a higher incidence of respiratory depression, nausea, and prolonged stay in the PACU.[131]

REFERENCES

1. Dunn KM, Saunders KW, Rutter CM, et al. Opioid prescriptions for chronic pain and overdose: a cohort study. Ann Intern Med. 2010;152:85–92.
2. Vila H Jr, Smith RA, Augustyniak MJ, et al. The efficacy of pain management before and after implementation of hospital-wide pain management standards: is patient safety compromised by treatment solely based on numerical pain ratings? Anesth Analg. 2005;101:474–480.
3. Okie S. A flood of opioids, a rising tide of deaths. N Engl J Med. 2010;363:1981–1985.
4. Sertürner F. Uber das Morphium, eine neue salzfähige Grundlage, und die Mekonsäure, als Hauptbestandtheile des Opiums. Ann Physik. 1917;5:56.
5. Huxtable RJ, Schwartz SK. The isolation of morphine. Mol Interv. 2001;1:189–191.
6. Bovill JG. Opium: a drug ancient and modern. In: Dahan A, van Kleef JW, eds. Advances in Anesthesia and Analgesia. Leiden: University Medical Center; 2007;1:13.
7. Garfield E. The 1982 John Scott Award goes to Jack Fishman and Harold Blumberg for synthesis and investigation of naloxone. Essays Inform Sci. 1983;6:121.
8. Tzschentke TM, Christoph T, Kögel B, et al. (−)-(1R,2R)-3-(3-dymethylamino-1-ethyl-2-methyl-propyl)-phenol hydrochloride (tapentadol HCl): a novel μ-opioid receptor agonist/norepinephrine reuptake inhibitor with broad-spectrum analgesic properties. J Pharmacol Exp Ther. 2007;323:265–276.
9. Linz K, Christoph T, Tzschentke TM, et al. Cebranopadol: a novel potent analgesic nociception/orphanin FQ peptide and opioid receptor agonist. J Pharmacol Exp Ther. 2014;349:535–548.
10. Kieffer BL, Gavériaux-Ruff C. Exploring the opioid system by gene knockout. Prog Neurobiol. 2002;66:285–306.
11. Chiou LC, Liao YY, Fan PC, et al. Nociceptin/orphanin FQ peptide receptors: pharmacology and clinical implications. Curr Drug Targets. 2007;8:117–135.
12. Pasternak GW. Pharmacological mechanisms of opioid analgesics. Clin Neuropharmacol. 1993;16:1–18.
13. Stefano GB. The μ_3 opiate receptor subtype. Pain Forum. 1999;8:206–209.
14. Alexander SPH, Mathie A, Peters JA. Guide to receptors and channels (GRAC), 4th ed. Br J Pharmacol. 2009;158(Suppl 1):S1–S254.
15. Standifer KM, Pasternak GW. G proteins and opioid receptor-mediated signaling. Cell Signal. 1997;9:237–248.
16. Waldhoer M, Bartlett SE, Whistler JL. Opioid receptors. Annu Rev Biochem. 2004;73:953–990.
17. Chen YL, Law PY, Loh HH. The other side of the opioid story: Modulation of cell growth and survival signaling. Curr Med Chem. 2008;15:772–778.
18. Eguchi M. Recent advances in selective opioid receptor agonists and antagonists. Med Res Rev. 2004;24:182–212.
19. Bird MF, Lambert DG. Simultaneous targeting of multiple opioid receptor types. Curr Opin Supprt Palliat Care. 2015;9:98–102.
20. Callahan RJ, Au JD, Paul M, et al. Functional inhibition by methadone of N-methyl-D-aspartate receptors expressed in Xenopus oocytes: stereospecific and subunit effects. Anesth Analg. 2004;98:653–659.
21. Dykstra LA, Fischer FB, Balter RE, et al. Opioid antinociception, tolerance and dependence: Interactions with the N-methyl-D-aspartate system in mice. Behav Pharmacol. 2011;22:540–547.
22. Kissin I, Bright CA, Bradley L. The effect of ketamine on opioid-induced acute tolerance: can it explain reduction of opioid consumption with ketamine-opioid analgesic combinations? Anesth Analg. 2000;91:1483–1488.
23. Reeves RR, Burke RS. Tramadol: Basic pharmacology and emerging concepts. Drugs Today. 2008;44:827–836.
24. Niesters M, Martini M, Proto P, et al. Tapentadol potentiates descending pain inhibition in chronic pain patients with diabetic polyneuropathy. Br J Anaesth. 2014;113:148–156.
25. Sarton E, Teppema L, Olievier C, et al. Involvement of μ-opioid receptor in ketamine-induced respiratory depression and antinociception. Anesth Analg. 2001;93:1495–1500.
26. Loeser JD, Treede RD. The Kyoto protocol of IASP basic pain terminology. Pain. 2008;137:473–477.
27. Millan MJ. Descending control of pain. Prog Neurobiol. 2002;66:355–474.
28. Ossipov MH, Dussor GO, Porreca F. Central modulation of pain. J Clin Invest. 2010;120:3779–3787.
29. Brown EN, Purdon PL, Van Dort CJ. General anesthesia and altered states of arousal: a systems neuroscience analysis. Annu Rev Neurosci. 2011;34:601–628.
30. Akil H, Mayer DJ, Liebeskind JC. Antagonism of stimulation-produced analgesia by naloxone, a narcotic antagonist. Science. 1976;191:961–962.
31. Butler RK, Finn DP. Stress-induced analgesia. Prog Neurobiol. 2009;88:184–202.
32. Eipert F, Bingel U, Schoell ED, et al. Activation of opioidergic descending pain control system underlies placebo analgesia. Neuron. 2009;63:533–543.
33. Pud D, Granovsky Y, Yarnitsky D. The methodology of experimentally-induced diffuse noxious inhibitory (DNIC)-line effects in humans. Pain. 2009;144:16–19.
34. Beecher HK. Pain in men wounded in battle. Ann Surg. 1946;123:96–105.
35. Zubieta J-K, Bueller JA, Jackson LR, et al. Placebo effects mediated by endogenous opioid activity on μ-opioid receptors. J Neurosci. 2005;25:7754–7762.

36. Petrovic P, Kalso E, Petersson KM, et al. Placebo and opioid analgesia: imaging a shared neuronal network. *Science*. 2002;295:1737–1740.
37. Moont R, Pud D, Sprecher E, et al. "Pain inhibits pain" mechanisms: is pain modulation simply due to distraction. *Pain*. 2010;150:113–120.
38. Niesters M, Dahan A, Swartjes M, et al. Effect of ketamine on endogenous pain modulation in healthy volunteers. *Pain*. 2010;152:656–663.
39. Lagerwij E, Nelis P, Wiegant VM, et al. The twitch in horses: a variant of acupuncture. *Science*. 1984;225:1172–1174.
40. Scholz J, Woolf CJ. The neuropathic pain triad, neurons, immune cells and glia. *Nature Neurosci*. 2007;10:1361–1368.
41. Kapitzke D, Vetter I, Cabot PJ. Endogenous opioid analgesia in peripheral tissues and the implications for pain control. *Ther Clin Risk Manag*. 2005;1:279–297.
42. Stein S, Halina M. Modulation of peripheral sensory information by the immune system: Implication for pain therapy. *Pharmacol Rev*. 2011;63:860–881.
43. Busch-Dienstfertig M, Stein C. Opioid receptors and opioid peptide-producing leucocytes in inflammatory pain: basic and therapeutic aspects. *Brain Beh Immun*. 2010;24:683–694.
44. Bekhit MH. Opioid-induced hyperalgesia and tolerance. *Am J Ther*. 2010;17:498–510.
45. Bruno G, Bossard AE, Coste C, et al. Acute opioid tolerance: Intraoperative remifentanil increases postoperative pain and morphine requirement. *Anesthesiology*. 2000;93:409–417.
46. Joly V, Richebe P, Guignard B, et al. Remifentanil-induced postoperative hyperalgesia and its prevention with small-dose ketamine. *Anesthesiology*. 2005;103:147–155.
47. van Dorp EL, Kest B, Kowalczyk WJ, et al. Morphine-6-glucuronide rapidly increases pain sensitivity independently of opioid receptors in mice and humans. *Anesthesiology*. 2009;110:1356–1363.
48. Bohn LM, Lefkowitz RJ, Gainetdinov RR, et al. Enhanced morphine analgesia in mice lacking beta-arrestin 2. *Science*. 1999;286:2495–2498.
49. Zuo Z. The role of opioid receptor internalization and beta-arrestins in the development of opioid tolerance. *Anesth Analg*. 2005;101:728–734.
50. Hughes MA, Glass PSA, Jacobs JR. Context-sensitive half-time in multicompartment: pharmacokinetic models for intravenous anesthetic drugs. *Anesthesiology*. 1992;76:334–341.
51. Kapila A, Glass PSA, Jacobes JR, et al. Measured context-sensitive half-times of remifentanil and alfentanil. *Anesthesiology*. 1995;83:968–975.
52. Olofsen E, Boom M, Nieuwenhuijs D, et al. Modeling the non-steady-state respiratory effects of remifentanil in awake and propofol sedated healthy volunteers. *Anesthesiology*. 2010;212:1382–1395.
53. Wilkinson GR. Drug metabolism and variability among patients in drug response. *N Engl J Med*. 2005;352:2211–2221.
54. van Dorp E, Romberg R, Sarton E, et al. Morphine-6-glucuronide: morphine's successor for postoperative pain relief? *Anesth Analg*. 2006;102:1789–1797.
55. Romberg R, Olofsen E, Sarton E, et al. Pharmacokinetic/pharmacodynamic modeling of morphine-6-glucuronide-induced analgesia in healthy volunteers: absence of sex differences. *Anesthesiology*. 2004;100:120–133.
56. Dahan A, Lötsch J. Morphine is not a prodrug. *Br J Anaesth*. 2015;114:1005–1006.
57. Tateishi T, Krivoruk Y, Ueng YF, et al. Identification of liver cytochrome P-450 3 A as the enzyme responsible for fentanyl and sufentanil N-dealkylation. *Anesth Analg*. 1996;82:167–172.
58. Smith HS. The metabolism of opioid agents and the clinical impact of their active metabolites. *Clin J Pain*. 2011;27:824–838.
59. Scott LJ, Perry CM. Spotlight on remifentanil for general anesthesia. *CNS Drugs*. 2005;19:1069–1074.
60. Kharasch E. Intraoperative methadone: rediscovery, reappraisal and reinvigoration. *Anesth Analg*. 2011;112:13–16.
61. van Dorp E, Yassen A, Dahan A. Naloxone treatment in opioid addiction: the risks and benefits. *Exp Opin Drug Safe*. 2007;6:125–132.
62. Martini C, Olofsen E, Yassen A, et al. Pharmacokinetic-pharmacodynamic modeling in acute and chronic pain: an overview of the recent literature. *Exp Rev Pharmacother*. 2011;4:719–728.
63. Segre G. Kinetics of interaction between drugs and biological systems. *Farmaco Sci*. 1968;23:907–918.
64. Sheiner L, Stanski LB, Vozeh S, et al. Simultaneous modeling of pharmacokinetics and pharmacodynamics: application to d-tubocurarine. *Clin Pharmacol Ther*. 1979;25:358–371.
65. Aubrun F, Salvi N, Coriat P, et al. Sex- and age-related differences in morphine requirements for postoperative pain relief. *Anesthesiology*. 2005;103:156–160.
66. Dahan A, Boom M, Olofsen E. Differences in onset/offset times for different end-points: pain relief, pupil size and respiratory depression. *Anesthesiology*. 2011;A1569.
67. Olofsen E, Romberg R, Bijl H, et al. Alfentanil and placebo analgesia: absence of sex differences. *Anesthesiology*. 2005;103:130–139.
68. Aubrun F, Langeron O, Quesnel C, et al. Relationships between measurement of pain using visual analog score and morphine requirements during postoperative intravenous morphine titration. *Anesthesiology*. 2003;98:1415–1421.
69. Sarton E, Olofsen E, Romberg R, et al. Sex differences in morphine analgesia: An experimental study in healthy volunteers. *Anesthesiology*. 2000;93:1245–1254.
70. Wolrich J, Poots AJ, Kuehler BM, et al. Is number sense impaired in chronic pain patients? *Br J Anaesth*. 2014;113:1024–1031.
71. Oudejans LCJ, van Velzen M, Olofsen E, et al. Translation of random painful stimuli into numerical responses in fibromyalgia and perioperative patients. *Pain*. 2016;157:128–136.
72. Abou Hammoud H, Simon N, Urien S, et al. Intravenous morphine titration in immediate postoperative pain management: population kinetic-pharmacodynamic and logistic regression analysis. *Pain*. 2009;144:139–146.
73. Mazoit JX, Btscher K, Samii K. Morphine in postoperative patients: pharmacokinetics and pharmacodynamics of metabolites. *Anesth Analg*. 2007;105:70–78.
74. Tallarida RJ, Stone DJ, McCary JD, et al. Response surface analysis of synergism between morphine and clonidine. *J Pharmacol Exp Ther*. 1999;289:8–13.
75. Schulte H, Sollevi A, Sgerdahl M. The synergistic effect of combined treatment with systematic ketamine and morphine on experimentally induced wind-up pain in humans. *Anesth Analg*. 2004;98:1574–1580.
76. Daniel M, Weiskopf RB, Noorani M, et al. Fentanyl augments the blockade of the sympathetic response to incision (MAC-BAR) produced by desflurane and isoflurane. *Anesthesiology*. 1998;88:43–49.
77. Kazama T, Ikeda K, Morita K. The pharmacodynamic interaction between propofol and fentanyl with respect to suppression of somatic or hemodynamic responses to skin incision, peritoneum incision, and abdominal wall retraction. *Anesthesiology*. 1998;89:894–906.
78. Sebel PS, Glass PSA, Fletcher JE, et al. Reduction of the MAC of desflurane with fentanyl. *Anesthesiology*. 1992;88:52–59.
79. Niesters M, Mahajan RP, Aarts L, et al. High-inspired oxygen concentration further impairs opioid-induced respiratory depression. *Br J Anaesth*. 2013;110:837–841.
80. Drover D, Lemmens HJM. Population pharmacodynamics and pharmacokinetics of remifentanil as a supplement to nitrous oxide anesthesia for elective abdominal surgery. *Anesthesiology*. 1998;89:869–877.
81. Vuyk J, Mertens MJ, Olofsen E, et al. Propofol anesthesia and rational opioid selection. *Anesthesiology*. 1997;87:1549–1562.
82. Lang E, Kapila A, Schlugman D, et al. Reduction of isoflurane minimal alveolar concentration by remifentanil. *Anesthesiology*. 1996;85:721–728.
83. Klepstad P, Fladvad T, Skorpen F, et al. Influence from genetic variability on opioid use for cancer pain: a European genetic association study of 2294 pain patients. *Pain*. 2011;152:1139–1145.
84. Mogil J, Ritchie J, Smith SB, et al. Melanocortin-1 receptor gene variants affect pain and mu-opioid analgesia in mice and humans. *J Med Genet*. 2005;42:583–587.
85. Liem EB, Lin CM, Suleman MI, et al. Anesthetic requirement is increased in redheads. *Anesthesiology*. 2004;101:279–283.
86. Weinshilboum R. Inheritance and drug response. *N Engl J Med*. 2003;348:529–537.
87. Ciszkowski C, Madadi P, Phillips MS, et al. Codeine, ultrarapid-metabolism genotype, and postoperative death. *N Engl J Med*. 2009;361:827–828.
88. Koren G, Cairns J, Gaedigk A, et al. Pharmacogenetics of morphine poisoning in a breastfed neonate of a codeine-prescribed mother. *Lancet*. 2006;368:704.
89. Park HJ, Shinn HK, Ryu SH, et al. Genetic polymorphism in the ABCB1 gene and the effects of fentanyl in Koreans. *Clin Pharmacol Ther*. 2007;81:539–546.
90. Dahan A, Aarts L, Smith TW. Incidence, reversal and prevention of opioid-induced respiratory depression. *Anesthesiology*. 2010;112:226–238.
91. Pattinson KTS. Opioids and the control of breathing. *Br J Anaesth*. 2008;106:347–349.
92. Smith JC, Ellenberger HH, Ballanyi K, et al. Pre-Bötzinger complex: a brainstem region that may generate respiratory rhythm in humans. *Science*. 1991;254:726–729.
93. Bernards CM, Knowlton SL, Schmidt DF, et al. Respiratory and sleep effects of remifentanil in volunteers with moderate obstructive sleep apnea. *Anesthesiology*. 2009;110:41–49.
94. Wu A, Drummond GB. Sleep arousal after lower abdominal surgery and relation to recovery from respiratory obstruction. *Anesthesiology*. 2003;99:1295–1302.
95. Chung F, Liao P, Yang Y, et al. Postoperative sleep-disordered breathing in patients without preoperative sleep apnea. *Anesth Analg*. 2015;120:1214–1224.
96. Stone JG, Cozine KA, Wald A. Nocturnal oxygenation during patient-controlled analgesia. *Anesth Analg*. 1999;89:104–110.
97. Bennet JA, Abrams JT, Van Riper DF, et al. Difficult or impossible ventilation after sufentanil-induced anesthesia is caused primarily by vocal cord closure. *Anesthesiology*. 1997;87:1070–1074.
98. Overdyk F. Continuous oximetry/capnometry monitoring reveals frequent desaturations and bradypnea during patient-controlled analgesia. *Anesth Analg*. 2007;105:412–418.
99. Chung F, Yegneswaran B, Liao P, et al. Stop questionnaire: a tool to screen for obstructive apnea. *Anesthesiology*. 2008;108:812–821.
100. Niesters M, Overdyk F, Smith T, et al. Opioid-induced respiratory depression in peadiatrics: a review of case reports. *Br J Anaesth*. 2013;110:175–182.
101. Dahan A, Overdyk F, Smith T, et al. Pharmacovigilance: a systematic review on opioid-induced respiratory depression (OIRD) in chronic pain patients. *Pain Physician*. 2013;16:E85–E94.
102. Overdyk F, Dahan A, Roozekrans M, et al. Opioid-induced respiratory depression: a compendium of case reports. *Pain Manage*. 2014;4:317–325.

103. Lötsch J, Dudziak R, Freynhagen R, et al. Fatal respiratory depression after multiple intravenous morphine injections. *Clin Pharmacokinet.* 2006;45:1051–1060.
104. Boom M, Olofsen E, Neukirchen M, et al. Fentanyl utility function: a risk-benefit composite of pain relief and breathing responses. *Anesthesiology.* 2013;119:663–674.
105. Dahan A, Olofsen E, Niesters M. Pharmacotherapy for pain: efficacy and safety issues examined by subgroup analyses. *Pain.* 2015;156:S119–S126.
106. Olofsen E, van Dorp E, Teppema L, et al. Naloxone reversal of morphine and morphine-6-glucuronide-induced respiratory depression. *Anesthesiology.* 2010;112:1417–1427.
107. van Dorp E, Yassen A, Sarton E, et al. Naloxone-reversal of buprenorphine-induced respiratory depression. *Anesthesiology.* 2006;105:51–57.
108. Yost CS. A new look at the respiratory stimulant doxapram. *CNS Drug Rev.* 2006;12:236–249.
109. Roozekrans M, van der Schrier R, Okkerse P, et al. Two studies on reversal of opioid-induced respiratory depression by BK-channel blocker GAL021 in human volunteers. *Anesthesiology.* 2014;121:459–468.
110. Roozekrans M, Olofsen E, van der Schrier R, et al. Reversal of opioid-induced respiratory depression by BK-channel blocker GAL021: a pharmacokinetic-pharmacodynamic modelling study in healthy volunteers. *Clin Pharmacol Ther.* 2015;97:641–649.
111. Oertel B, Felden L, Trans P, et al. Selective antagonism of opioid-induced ventilatory depression by an ampakine molecule in humans without loss of opioid analgesia. *Clin Pharmacol Ther.* 2010;87:204–211.
112. Sun Z, Sessler DI, Dalton JE, et al. Postoperative hypoxemia is common and persistent: a prospective blinded observational study. *Anesth Analg.* 2014;121:709–715.
113. Curry JP, Lynn LA. A critical assessment of monitoring practices, patient deterioration, and alarm fatigue on inpatient wards: a review. *Pat Saf Surg.* 2014;8:29.
114. Niesters M, Mahajan R, Olofsen E, et al. Validation of a novel respiratory rate monitor based on exhaled humidity. *Br J Anaesth.* 2012;109:981–989.
115. Apfel CC, Korttila K, Abdalla M, et al. A factorial trial of six interventions for the prevention of postoperative nausea and vomiting. *N Engl J Med.* 2004;350:2441–2451.
116. Macario A, Weinger N, Truong P, et al. Which clinical anesthesia outcomes are both common and important to avoid? *Anesth Analg.* 1999;88:1085–1091.
117. Gan TJ. Mechanisms underlying postoperative nausea and vomiting and neurotransmitter receptor antagonist-based pharmacotherapy. *CNS Drugs.* 2007;21:813–833.
118. Panchal SJ, Müller-Schwefe P, Wurzelmann JI. Opioid-induced bowel dysfunction: Prevalence, pathophysiology and burden. *Int J Clin Pract.* 2007;61:1181–1187.
119. Thomas J. Opioid-induced bowel dysfunction. *J Pain Symptom Manage.* 2008;35:103–113.
120. Thompson DR. Narcotic analgesic effects on the sphincter of Oddi: A review of the data and therapeutic implications in treating pancreatitis. *Am J Gastroenterol.* 2001;96:1266–1272.
121. Verhamme KM, Strurkenboom MC, Stricker BH, et al. Drug-induced urinary retention: Incidence, management and prevention. *Drug Saf.* 2008;31:373–388.
122. Rosow CE, Gomery P, Chen TY, et al. Reversal of opioid-induced bladder dysfunction by intravenous naloxone and methylnaltrexone. *Clin Pharmacol Ther.* 2007;82:48–53.
123. DeSouza G, Lewis MC, TerRiet MF. Severe bradycardia after remifentanil. *Anesthesiology.* 1997;87:1019–1020.
124. Douma M, Middeldorp A, Dahan A, et al. A comparison of remifentanil patient-controlled analgesia with epidural analgesia during labour. *Int J Obstet Anesth.* 2011;20:118–123.
125. Volmanen PVE, Akural EI, Raudaskoski T, et al. Timing of intravenous patient-controlled remifentanil bolus during early labor. *Acta Anaesthesiol Scand.* 2011;55:486–494.
126. Freeman L, Bloemenkamp W, Franssen MT, et al. Remifentanil patient controlled analgesia versus epidural analgesia in labour: a randomised multicentre equivalence trial. *BMJ.* 2015;350:h846.
127. Douma M, Stienstra R, Middeldorp JM, et al. Differences in maternal temperature during labour with remifentanil patient-controlled analgesia or epidural analgesia: a randomised controlled trial. *Int J Obst Anesth.* 2015;24:313.
128. Niesters M, Dahan A, Kest B, et al. Do sex differences exist in opioid analgesia? A systematic review and meta-analysis of human experimental and clinical studies. *Pain.* 2010;151:61–68.
129. Dahan A, Sarton E, Olievier C. Sex-related differences in the influence of morphine on ventilatory control in humans. *Anesthesiology.* 1998;88:903–913.
130. Cepeda MS, Farra JY, Baumgarten M, et al. Side effects of opioids during short-term administration: effects of age, gender and race. *Clin Pharmacol Ther.* 2003;74:102–112.
131. Sadhasivam S, Chidambaran V, Olbrecht VA, et al. Opioid-related side-effects in children undergoing surgery: Unequal burden on younger girls with higher doses of opioids. *Pain Med.* 2015;16:985–997.

21 Neuromuscular Blocking Agents

SORIN J. BRULL

Physiology and Pharmacology
   Morphology of the Neuromuscular Junction
   Nerve Stimulation
   Presynaptic Events: Mobilization and Release
      of Acetylcholine
   Postsynaptic Events
   Receptor Up- and Downregulation
Pharmacologic Characteristics
Depolarizing Neuromuscular Blocking Drugs:
   Succinylcholine
   Neuromuscular Effects
   Characteristics of Depolarizing Blockade
   Pharmacology of Succinylcholine
   Side Effects
   Clinical Uses
   Contraindications
Nondepolarizing Neuromuscular Blocking Agents
   Characteristics
   Pharmacology

   Onset and Duration of Action
   Individual Nondepolarizing Agents
Drug Interactions
Altered Responses to Neuromuscular Blocking Agents
Monitoring Neuromuscular Blockade
   Monitoring and Risk–Benefit Ratio
   Stimulator Characteristics
   Monitoring Modalities
   Testing and Recording the Response
   Differential Muscle Sensitivity
   Electrode Placement
   Monitoring and Clinical Applications
Reversal of Neuromuscular Blockade
   Anticholinesterase Agents
   Drug Shortages and Clinical Impact
   Selective Relaxant Binding Agents
Conclusion

KEY POINTS

1. Neuromuscular blocking agents (NMBAs) improve conditions for tracheal intubation and protect against vocal cord damage, improve surgical conditions, and facilitate mechanical ventilation in the operating room and intensive care unit.
2. All NMBAs (depolarizing and nondepolarizing) interact with specific sites (α subunits) of the nicotinic cholinergic receptors and block muscle membrane depolarization, leading to flaccid paralysis.
3. Neuromuscular function can be measured (monitored) using neurostimulation. A train of four stimuli at 2 Hz (train-of-four [TOF]) will have four equal muscle contractions at baseline, indicated by a TOF ratio of 1.0 (fourth twitch, T4, equal in amplitude to first twitch, T1). With an increase in nondepolarizing block, the TOF ratio will decrease from 1.0 to 0. This ratio will return to normal with offset of block (recovery). The threshold for minimal recovery is TOF ratio 0.90 or higher.
4. Subjective (visual, tactile) evaluation of fade is unreliable, particularly when the TOF ratio is 0.40 or greater. Clinical testing (such as 5-second head-lift, grip strength, vital capacity, tidal volume) is notoriously inaccurate, and despite its wide clinical use, does not exclude residual neuromuscular block. When using subjective and clinical methods of assessment, the incidence of postoperative residual paralysis is 30% to 40%.
5. Objective methods of monitoring such as acceleromyography, mechanomyography, or electromyography can eliminate the incidence of residual paralysis and avoid postoperative critical respiratory events.
6. Monitoring of facial muscles instead of the adductor pollicis muscle in the hand generally leads to overestimation of neuromuscular function, and increases the incidence of postoperative residual paralysis and postoperative pulmonary complications.
7. Upper airway muscles (e.g., genioglossus) are very sensitive to minimal levels of neuromuscular block, and patients may be unable to protect the airway against aspiration even when TOF = 0.90.
8. Cholinesterase inhibitors prevent acetylcholine breakdown, and allow competition with nondepolarizing NMBAs for receptor sites. This restores normal neuromuscular transmission, but the reversal of nondepolarizing block is limited (cholinesterase inhibitors have a ceiling effect).
9. New selective relaxant binding agents such as sugammadex encapsulate aminosteroid NMBAs and quickly and reliably reverse nondepolarizing block of any depth if administered in sufficient doses that are based on neuromuscular monitoring data.
10. The combination of rocuronium (for rapid onset) and sugammadex (for emergent reversal of block) in a failed rapid-sequence induction scenario can be more rapid than spontaneous recovery from succinylcholine (as long as recovery from induction drugs is sufficient and airway patency is restored).

The neuromuscular junction (NMJ) is one of the most comprehensively studied models of neural function.[1] Neuromuscular blocking agents (NMBAs), also called "muscle relaxants" or "paralytics," have been used in the clinical setting for almost 75 years. Unlike many other classes of drugs used in medicine today, the list of NMBAs is relatively short, and they belong to only two classes: aminosteroidal and isoquinolinium (tetrahydroisoquinoline) compounds. A third class, quaternary amines (gallamine), is no longer in clinical use. Experience with these drugs has taught us the clinical usefulness of NMBAs, and the literature continues to remind us about the huge variability in responses to these drugs among patients. A thorough understanding of the concepts of neuromuscular transmission, of the effects of NMBAs in the normal individual and how these effects might be altered by certain disease states, electrolyte imbalances and interactions with other drugs, and knowledge of how best to monitor the effects of NMBAs, are of paramount importance in providing optimal, safe patient care.

Physiology and Pharmacology

Morphology of the Neuromuscular Junction

Lower motor neurons, whose cell bodies are located in the ventral horn of the spinal cord and the motor nuclei of cranial nerves, project their axons via the ventral roots to control effector organs (muscles and glands). The somatic motor neurons are typically large-diameter, myelinated, and fast conducting; as the axons approach their endings, they lose their myelin sheaths before branching into terminal fibers. Each terminal fiber supplies a muscle fiber via a specialized connection, the NMJ (or gap). The *NMJ* consists of the presynaptic motor neuron, the postsynaptic muscle fiber, and the intervening 50- to 70-nm gap (synaptic cleft) between the two, which contains the enzyme acetylcholinesterase (Fig. 21-1).

The NMJ has a highly ordered mechanism that converts the electrical signal of the motor nerve (the action potential) into a chemical signal (effected by the release of acetylcholine [ACh]), which in turn is converted into an electrical event (muscle membrane depolarization), leading to a mechanical response (muscle contraction). The *motor unit* consists of the motor neuron and the muscle fiber it innervates. The number of muscle fibers that each neuron innervates (innervation ratio) determines the precision of the muscle contraction: for muscle groups that require very fine control (e.g., eye or facial muscles), the innervation ratio is close to 1:2 (i.e., 1 nerve innervating 2 fibers). For large muscles that require coarse, powerful movement (thigh or back muscles), the innervation ratio approaches 1:2,000.

Nicotinic muscle-type Ach receptors (muscle-type nAChRs) are located in folds of the postsynaptic muscle membrane in very high concentrations and are not normally found extrasynaptically (see later). More than 90% of all nAChRs in a muscle fiber are located at the synapse, an area that represents less than 0.1% of the total muscle membrane surface area. At birth, the nAChRs are termed "fetal" or "immature" and are comprised of five protein subunits (two α subunits, one β, one γ, and one δ subunit—denoted as $\alpha_2\beta\gamma\delta$), arranged in a rosette with a central transmembrane channel (Fig. 21-2). The initial fetal receptor density is relatively low, approximately 1,000 receptors/μm². After birth, the fetal nAChRs become "mature" or "adult" nAChRs by replacing the fetal γ subunit with an ε subunit (denoted as $\alpha_2\beta\delta\epsilon$), and the receptor density increases substantially (10,000 receptors/μm²) (Fig. 21-3). The two α subunits of the receptor contain the ACh-binding sites (the α-recognition site).[2] The nAChRs are found preferentially at the endplate, on the crest of the membrane invaginations (folds), and their density decreases markedly outside the junctional area.[3]

Nerve Stimulation

ACh mediates transmission of an impulse from nerve to muscle. When depolarization of the motor nerve reaches the nerve terminal, voltage-gated Ca^{2+} channels open, and the vesicles (quanta) that contain ACh are released by exocytosis from the nerve terminal into the cleft. This release of ACh quanta (each containing 5,000 to 10,000 ACh molecules) is antagonized by hypocalcemia and hypermagnesemia. The K^+ channels in the nerve terminal

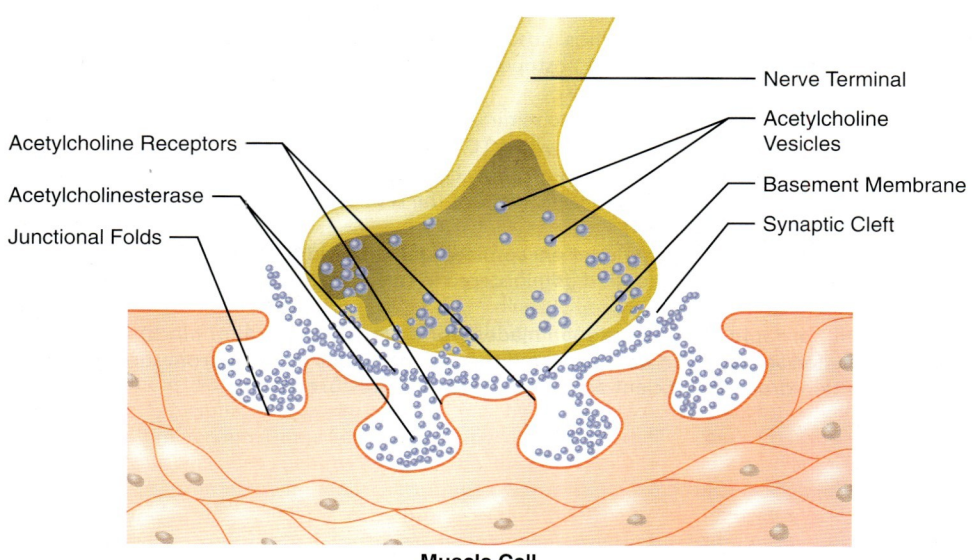

Figure 21-1 Schematic representation of the neuromuscular junction (not drawn to scale).

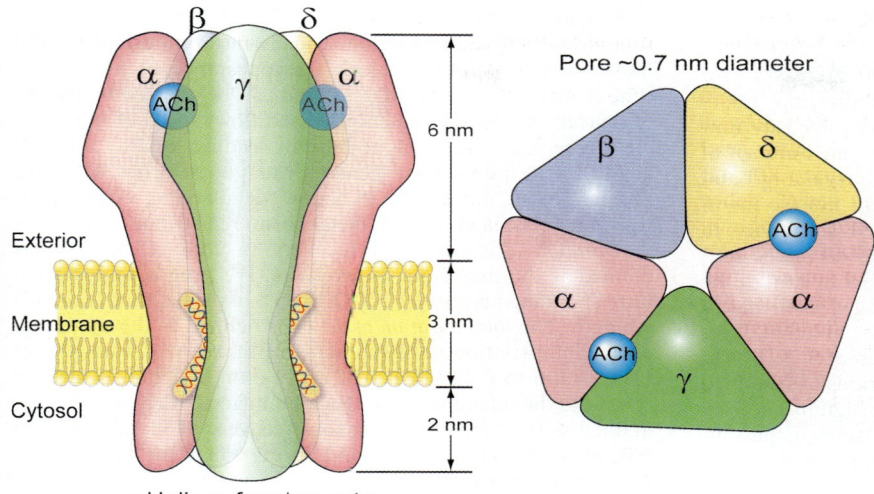

Figure 21-2 Nicotinic acetylcholine receptors (nAChRs) termed "fetal" (due to their expression early in development) consist of five subunits: two α subunits, as well as one β, one γ, and one δ subunit (denoted as $α_2βγδ$). During the first 2 postnatal weeks, each postsynaptic motor site is innervated by multiple presynaptic nerve terminals. The α subunits contain the recognition site for ACh and all neuromuscular blocking agents. (Reprinted with permission from Brull S, Naguib M. Review of neuromuscular junction anatomy and function. In: Mashour GA, Lydic R, eds. *The Neuroscientific Foundations of Anesthesiology.* New York, NY: Oxford University Press; 2011:205–210.)

area limit the extent of Ca^{2+} entry into the terminal, and regulate the transmitter quantal release, initiating nerve membrane repolarization.

Presynaptic Events: Mobilization and Release of Acetylcholine

ACh is synthesized in the presynaptic nerve terminal from acetate and choline, and is divided into two functional pools: the "*immediately available pool*" consists of a small fraction of all ACh available in the nerve terminal. Most of the ACh is contained in the "*reserve pool*" that first must be transported (mobilized) to the area adjacent to the membrane (the *active zone*) and become part of the immediately available pool before it can be released into the cleft. Once nerve depolarization occurs and the intracellular Ca^{2+} concentration increases, ACh quanta are released into the synaptic cleft. Released ACh can then bind to the postsynaptic nAChRs to initiate muscle contraction (see later), followed by rapid hydrolysis by acetylcholinesterase into choline and acetic acid; choline then re-enters the presynaptic nerve terminal. ACh can also bind to presynaptic neuronal nAChRs to facilitate ACh mobilization (feedback mechanism).

Postsynaptic Events

Small quantities of ACh are released spontaneously into the cleft, resulting in small depolarizations (5 mV) of the muscle membrane. These miniature end-plate potentials (MEPPs) may represent the membrane effects of a single ACh quantum. When sufficient ACh quanta are released (200 to 400 quanta, representing 1 to 4 million ACh molecules), the postjunctional muscle membrane depolarization reaches an end-plate potential (EPP) and the excitation–contraction sequence is activated: ACh binds to both recognition sites of the α subunits of the nAChRs, inducing a conformational change of the receptor that results in the opening of a central channel (pore). The central channel allows Na^+ influx and K^+ efflux, resulting in muscle cell membrane depolarization. Voltage-gated Na^+ channels on the muscle membrane propagate the action potential across the membrane, leading to the development of muscle tension (excitation–contraction coupling).

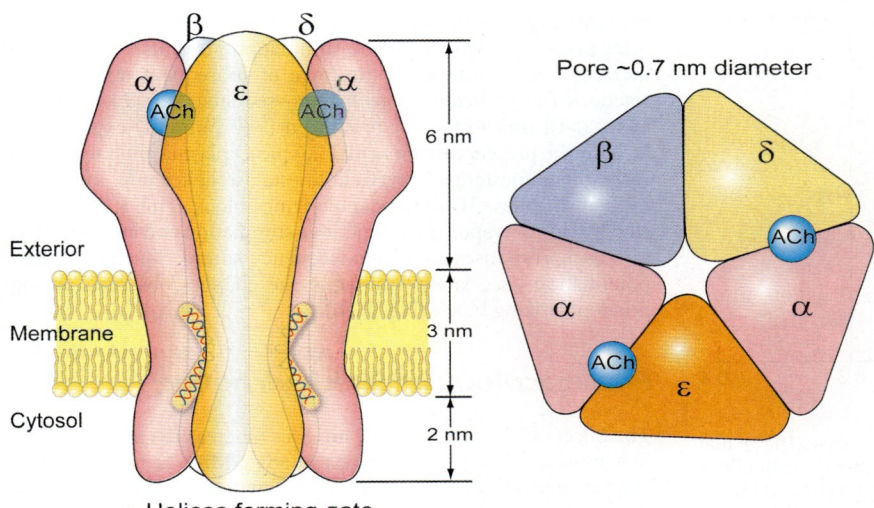

Figure 21-3 Nicotinic acetylcholine receptors (nAChRs) termed "adult" (due to their expression later in development) consist of five subunits: two α subunits, as well as one β, one δ, and one ε subunit (denoted as $α_2βδε$). Each postsynaptic adult motor site receives neuronal input from a single motor axon, and the adult nAChRs are restricted in high concentrations (10,000/μm²) in the postsynaptic membrane, but are virtually absent extrasynaptically. As with fetal nAChRs, the α subunit contains the recognition site for ACh and all neuromuscular blocking agents. (From Brull S, Naguib M. Review of neuromuscular junction anatomy and function. In: Mashour GA, Lydic R, eds. *The Neuroscientific Foundations of Anesthesiology.* New York, NY: Oxford University Press; 2011:205–210.)

Receptor Up- and Downregulation

When the frequency of stimulation at the NMJ decreases over days (or longer) due to severe burns, immobilization, infection/sepsis, prolonged use of NMBAs in the intensive care unit (ICU), or cerebrovascular accidents (CVAs), the number of immature (fetal) nAChRs increases (*receptor upregulation*) and they extend beyond the NMJ into the adjacent muscle membrane. The immature nAChRs have increased sensitivity to agonists (ACh and succinylcholine [SCh]), and decreased sensitivity to nondepolarizing NMBAs. The channel opening time of the immature nAChRs is up to 10-fold longer than that of mature receptors and may allow systemic release of lethal doses of intracellular K^+ in response to administration of SCh. *Downregulation* of mature nAChRs occurs during periods of sustained agonist stimulation; for instance, chronic neostigmine use (in patients with myasthenia gravis) or organophosphorus poisoning leads to resistance to SCh but extreme sensitivity to nondepolarizing NMBAs.

Pharmacologic Characteristics

NMBAs can be classified based on their mode of action: *depolarizing* NMBAs (e.g., SCh) produce muscle relaxation by directly depolarizing the nAChRs. This occurs because SCh (made up of two ACh molecules joined end to end) acts as a "false transmitter," mimicking ACh. *Nondepolarizing* NMBAs compete with ACh for the two α-subunits' (apostrophe) recognition sites, preventing normal nAChR function. Nondepolarizing agents can be classified further according to their chemical structure (benzylisoquinolinium or steroidal) or to their duration of action (short-, intermediate, or long-duration; see later).

Potency of a drug is determined by the dose required to produce a certain effect and is calculated from the dose-response sigmoidal curve (Fig. 21-4). For NMBAs, the effect (response) is depression of normal muscle contraction. Thus, a dose that depresses the baseline twitch height by 50% is termed "50% effective dose" or ED_{50}. Most NMBA potencies are expressed as the dose required for 95% depression of the baseline twitch height during nerve stimulation, or ED_{95}.

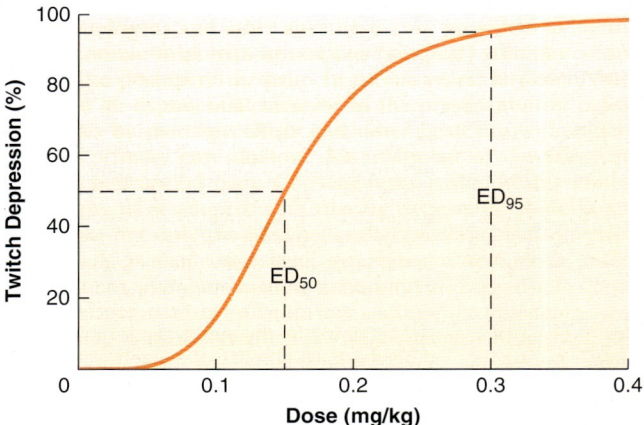

Figure 21-4 Example of a dose–response relationship. The actual numbers are approximately those for rocuronium. The ED_{50} is the dose that produces 50% depression of the control twitch height and ED_{95} is the dose that produces 95% depression of the control twitch height.

Onset of action (onset time) for all NMBAs is defined as the time from their administration (usually intravenously, IV) until maximal neuromuscular block (disappearance of ST). Onset time is inversely related to dose, and can be affected by its rate of delivery to the site of action (blood flow, speed of injection, etc.), receptor affinity (higher affinity leading to faster onset of action), drug potency (in general, less potent drugs will have a faster onset), mechanism of action (depolarizing vs. competitive), and plasma clearance (metabolism, redistribution).

Duration of action until recovery to 25% (DUR 25%) is defined as the time from intravenous (IV) drug administration until spontaneous recovery of ST to 25% of the baseline (normal) strength. The *total duration of action* is defined as the time from drug administration until spontaneous recovery of train-of-four (TOF) ratio to 0.90 (DUR 0.90). Duration of action is directly related to the total dose of NMBA administered. *Recovery index* is defined as the time of spontaneous recovery of ST from 25% to 75% of control (RI_{25-75}), a period during which the spontaneous recovery is relatively linear and is not affected significantly by the NMBA dose.

Depolarizing Neuromuscular Blocking Drugs: Succinylcholine

Neuromuscular Effects

SCh is the only depolarizing NMBA available clinically (Table 21-1). It has the fastest onset, the shortest duration, and greatest reliability (i.e., narrowest onset variability around the mean) of any NMBA. Because of its molecular similarity to ACh, SCh depolarizes both postsynaptic and extrajunctional receptors, but since it is not degraded by acetylcholinesterases, it depolarizes the muscle membrane for a longer period of time, leading to membrane hyperpolarization and desensitization. This desensitization then leads to flaccid paralysis after the initial receptor activation (which is manifested clinically as muscle "fasciculations").

Characteristics of Depolarizing Blockade

As with all NMBAs, increasing the dose of SCh leads to a progressive decrease in the force of muscle contraction (ST). However, the response to repetitive stimulation (TOF and tetanus patterns—see later) is maintained (*no fade*) because of progressive but equivalent decrease in the force of contractions. Additionally, after a brief period of high-frequency stimulation (tetanus), there is no increase (amplification) in the force of subsequent muscle contractions (*no posttetanic potentiation*—see later; Fig. 21-5). Large doses (>10 times ED_{95}) or prolonged (>30 minutes) exposure to SCh, or the presence of abnormal (atypical) plasma cholinesterases (pseudocholinesterase/butyrylcholinesterase deficiency), may lead to dual (or phase II, or nondepolarizing) block. This is characterized by fade of responses to repetitive stimulation and amplification of muscle responses after high-frequency stimulation (posttetanic potentiation—see later), similar to the changes observed during nondepolarizing block (Fig. 21-6).

Pharmacology of Succinylcholine

The onset of SCh at peripheral muscles (such as the adductor pollicis muscle [APM]) is the fastest of any NMBA (1 to 2 minutes) at equivalent doses. Its ED_{95} is approximately 0.30 mg/kg, and at doses of 1.0 to 1.5 mg/kg (3 to 5 × ED_{95}), the DUR 25% of SCh is

Table 21-1 Pharmacokinetic and Pharmacodynamic Properties of the Depolarizing Neuromuscular Blocking Agent Succinylcholine

Agent[a]	Succinylcholine
Type (structure)	Depolarizing
Type (duration)	Ultrashort
Potency—ED$_{95}$ (mg/kg)	0.25–0.30
Intubating dose (mg/kg)	1.0–1.5
Onset time (min)	1.0–1.5
Clinical duration (min)	7–12
Recovery index (RI$_{25–75}$) (min)	2–4
Volume of distribution (L/kg)	0.04
Clearance (mL/kg/min)	35
Elimination half-life (minutes)	
• Normal organ function	<1
• Renal impairment	<1
• Hepatic impairment	<1
Maintenance dose (mg/kg)	N/A
Infusion dose (μg/kg/min)	Titrate to ST muscle response
Elimination route/metabolism	Plasma cholinesterase
Active metabolites	No active metabolites (succinylmonocholine has minimal activity)
Side effects	Myalgia; bradycardia/asystole in children or with repeated dosing; dual (phase II) block; anaphylaxis
Contraindications (other than specific allergy)	High K$^+$; MH; muscular dystrophy; children; ACh receptor upregulation pseudocholinesterase deficiency
Comments	Fastest onset, most reliable NMBA for rapid tracheal intubation

[a]Agent in current clinical use. The data are averages obtained from published literature and assume there is no potentiation from other coadministered drugs (such as volatile inhalational anesthetics), and the effects are measured at the adductor pollicis muscle. Other factors, such as muscle temperature, mode of evoked response monitoring, type/site of muscle monitoring, etc., will affect the data.
NMBA, neuromuscular blocking agents; ED$_{95}$, effective dose to achieve 95% effect in 50% of patients; K$^+$, potassium; MH, malignant hyperthermia; ST, single twitch; ICU, intensive care unit.

10 to 12 minutes, but is prolonged beyond 15 minutes with larger doses. Despite paralysis at the APM, the diaphragm (and other central muscles) may start to contract, and spontaneous breathing may resume as fast as 5 minutes after 1 mg/kg SCh administration. SCh is most commonly administered intravenously, but intraosseous, intralingual, and intramuscular routes have been reported if an IV cannot be established. Onset is delayed, particularly with intramuscular administration. Hydrolysis of SCh by pseudocholinesterase (also known as butyrylcholinesterase or plasma cholinesterase) occurs in the plasma, where almost 90% of the IV dose of SCh is hydrolyzed before reaching the NMJ.

Side Effects

SCh can induce significant *bradycardia and asystole*, particularly in children, and in any patient after readministration. *Premature ventricular escape beats* are also common; cardiac effects can be

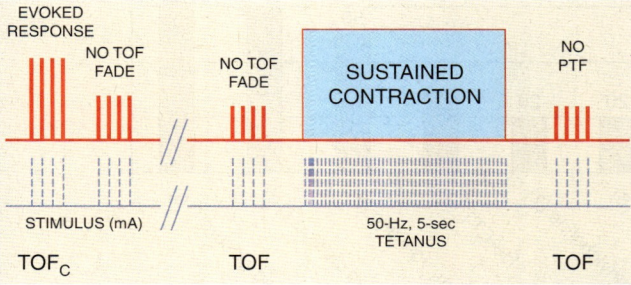

Figure 21-5 Characteristics of depolarizing block. Left: decrease in train-of-four (TOF) amplitude without fade in response to depolarizing agent administration. Right: lack of posttetanic (5 second) potentiation of evoked response. TOF, train-of-four; TOFc, control (baseline) TOF; PTF, posttetanic facilitation.

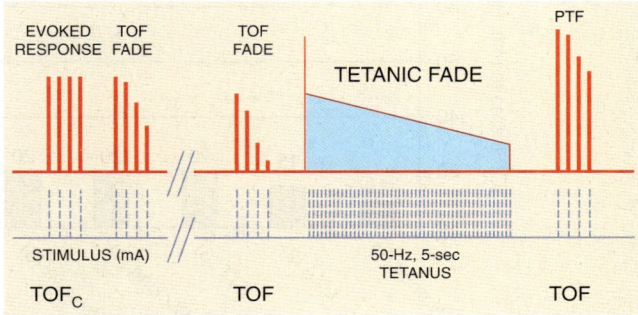

Figure 21-6 Characteristics of nondepolarizing block. Left: progressive decrease in train-of-four (TOF) ratio in response to non-depolarizing agent administration. Right: significant TOF fade and tetanic (5-sec) fade, followed by potentiation of evoked responses (increased amplitude, decreased fade). TOF, train-of-four; TOFc, control (baseline) TOF; PTF, posttetanic facilitation.

attenuated by pretreatment with anticholinergics. Disorganized muscle contractions (*fasciculations*) after SCh are very common (80% to 90% of patients). *Myalgias* are also very common 1 to 2 days postoperatively and can occur in 50% to 60% of patients. Fasciculations have been considered a possible etiology for postoperative myalgia, but systematic reviews have not established a clear relationship. A "defasciculating" pretreatment with a small dose of nondepolarizing NMBA (10% ED_{95}) is sometimes used to decrease the incidence of fasciculations and myalgia. However, this technique may render susceptible patients at risk of *regurgitation* and *pulmonary aspiration* because of partial paralysis of pharyngeal muscles. Alternatively, because of large interindividual variability, pretreatment may be ineffective in some patients. If pretreatment is used, the dose requirement for SCh is increased (up to 2 mg/kg). Defasciculation also may be achieved by administering 5 to 10 mg of SCh prior to administering the full SCh dose—this has been termed a "self-taming" dose of SCh, but is rarely used in modern practice. The most effective prophylaxis for myalgia without using nondepolarizing NMBAs is pretreatment with nonsteroidal anti-inflammatory drugs (e.g., aspirin or diclofenac), with a number needed to treat (NNT) of 2.5.[4] Lidocaine and rocuronium pretreatment also decrease the incidence of postoperative myalgia (NNT = 3), but the risk of untoward side-effects such as blurred vision, diplopia, inability to speak, and difficulty in breathing and swallowing likely do not justify this practice (number needed to harm [NNH] <3.5 patients).[4]

Although SCh may *increase intragastric pressure*, the lower esophageal sphincter tone is also increased, such that the intragastric-esophageal pressure gradient remains the same; thus, there is no increase in the risk of aspiration from the use of SCh. Normal *intraocular pressure* (IOP) is 12 to 20 mmHg with a diurnal variation of 2 to 3 mmHg, whereas changes in position may induce increases of up to 6 mmHg. In fact, otherwise innocuous settings, such as the Valsalva maneuver while playing wind instruments, can significantly (+9.2 mmHg) increase IOP (Fig. 21-7).[5] IOP also increases after administration of SCh (up to 15 mmHg increase), but these changes are transient (5 minutes).[6] Pretreatment with an NMBA does not attenuate this increase; lidocaine and sufentanil have been reported to decrease IOP by a mean of 5 mmHg, thus attenuating the IOP increases after SCh.[7]

Despite fears that this SCh-induced increase in IOP may induce extrusion of ocular contents in patients with an "open-globe" injury, clinical practice in thousands of patients has not reported this complication.[8,9] It should be noted that increases in IOP can be significant in the context of inadequate anesthesia and neuromuscular block that allows the patient to cough and perform Valsalva, particularly during laryngoscopy and tracheal intubation. Such settings generate much larger increases in IOP than those associated with SCh administration and must be avoided, particularly in the patient with an open-globe injury.[10]

Elevation in intracranial pressure (ICP) from SCh may occur, and this increase is attenuated by defasciculation. Inadequate levels of anesthesia during laryngoscopy and tracheal intubation, however, are much more likely to increase ICP. In a group of patients with head injury, a hypertensive response to laryngoscopy and tracheal intubation was observed in 80% of patients; importantly, in 11% of patients, the increase in ICP was 100% or more.[11]

SCh administration induces a mild elevation in the plasma level of potassium of 0.5 mEq/L; however, severe *hyperkalemia* with attendant cardiac arrest has been reported in cases in which there is proliferation of immature nAChRs (see earlier, Receptor Upregulation). Rare case reports have also associated administration of SCh with fatal hyperkalemia in children receiving oral β-blocker therapy (propranolol).[12] Other settings in which the use of SCh has been associated with hyperkalemia include chronic denervation states (spinal cord injury, prolonged bed rest), major burns, acute renal failure, sepsis, encephalitis, and severe trauma. Pretreatment with a nondepolarizing NMBA prior to SCh administration has not been shown to attenuate the hyperkalemic response. Treatment of hyperkalemia generally consists of hyperventilation, IV calcium chloride, and glucose/insulin to shift potassium intracellularly.

Particularly important is the association between pediatric myotonia and muscle dystrophies, and SCh administration, leading to rhabdomyolysis and fatal hyperkalemia. For this reason, the U.S. Food and Drug Administration (FDA) has a "black box" warning on the use of SCh and, in the pediatric population, SCh should only be used for emergency tracheal intubation. SCh may also trigger lethal *malignant hyperthermia* (MH), especially in patients anesthetized with volatile anesthetics. Some patients (both adults and children) may exhibit *masseter muscle spasm*

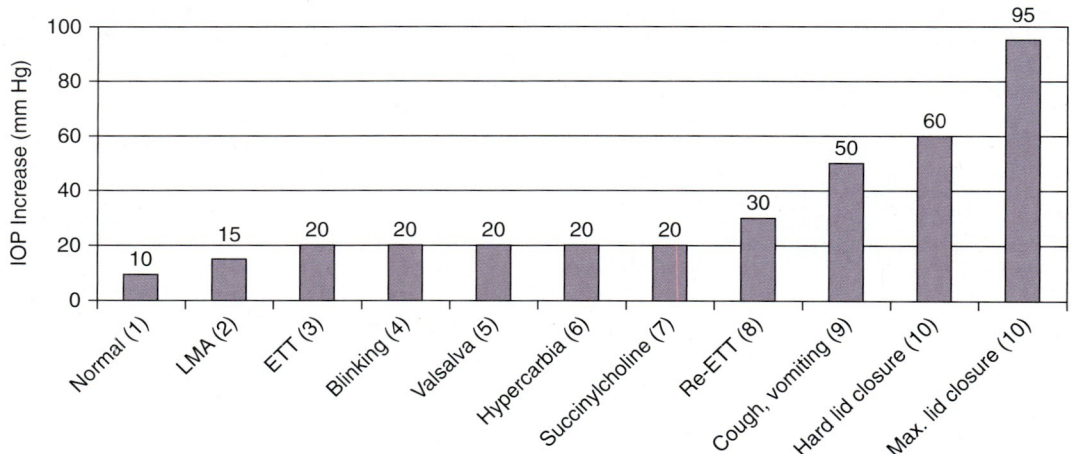

Figure 21-7 Mean increase in intraocular pressure (IOP) from baseline in response to various procedures and maneuvers. Normal IOP is 10 mmHg. LMA, laryngeal mask airway; ETT, endotracheal tube. (Adapted with permission from Aniskevich S, Brull S, Naguib M. Neuromuscular blocking agents. In: Johnson KB, ed. *Clinical Pharmacology for Anesthesiology*. New York, NY: McGraw-Hill Education, 2015.)

after SCh, making intubating conditions difficult. In some cases, particularly in pediatrics, masseter spasm is associated with malignant hyperthermia (MH). SCh can produce *allergic reactions (anaphylaxis)* in about 1 out of 10,000 administrations.

Patients receiving statin therapy may be particularly susceptible to muscle injury from administration of SCh, resulting in high plasma concentrations of myoglobin and creatine kinase, as well as hyperkalemia. However, these changes are likely of limited clinical significance.[13]

Clinical Uses

SCh is indicated for rapid attainment of optimal intubating conditions and prevention of regurgitation and pulmonary aspiration of gastric contents in patients at risk (those unfasted, with gastroparesis or gastrointestinal obstruction) in the "rapid sequence induction and intubation" (RSII) scenario. In this setting, SCh is the drug closest to the "ideal" NMBA. It has the shortest clinical duration (5 to 10 minutes at 1 mg/kg dose), so most patients will resume some diaphragmatic function before significant apnea-induced hypoxia occurs; it has the shortest onset time (1 minute at 1.5 mg/kg); and it has the highest reliability, with the fewest outliers (patients whose intubating conditions are poor at the time of intubation; Fig. 21-8). In obese individuals who need RSII, the dose of SCh should be calculated on the basis of actual body weight rather than ideal body weight. Children are more resistant than adults to the actions of SCh, and the usual dose (see Side Effects) is 1.5 to 2.0 mg/kg (up to 3 mg/kg in infants). In the 2015 Cochrane Database systematic review, the authors found there were no statistically significant differences in intubation conditions between SCh and rocuronium (1.2 mg/kg), but concluded that SCh "was clinically superior as it has a shorter duration of action."[14]

Contraindications

In the surgical population, the relative risk of MH with SCh administration (vs. without SCh) is 20 times higher when combined with volatile anesthetics.[15] Use of SCh is contraindicated in patients (and their relatives) with a history of MH. Other settings in which SCh is contraindicated include states of receptor upregulation (see earlier) due to potential for lethal hyperkalemia, critical care patients or those immobilized for prolonged periods (e.g., weeks), and patients with pseudocholinesterase deficiency. Patients with pseudocholinesterase (butyrylcholinesterase) deficiency are at risk of unintended intraoperative awareness and recall if they are awakened while paralyzed and neuromuscular monitoring is not used.[16] Approximately 1 in 25 patients may be heterozygous and 1 in 2,500 individuals may be homozygous for the "atypical" deficiency gene, and may require prolonged (hours) postoperative mechanical ventilation after SCh administration. In patients with renal failure, SCh may be administered if the plasma K^+ is not elevated. Lethal hyperkalemia following administration of SCh has been reported in severely acidotic and hypovolemic patients, and, in these settings, its use is contraindicated. In the intensive care setting, patients can be at increased risk of significant hyperkalemia (>6.5 mmol/L) after receiving SCh because of nicotinic receptor upregulation, particularly if their ICU length of stay at the time of SCh administration was greater than 16 days.[17] Succinylcholine has the potential to induce acute rhabdomyolysis and hyperkalemia followed by ventricular dysrhythmias, cardiac arrest and death after administration to pediatric patients who were subsequently found to have undiagnosed skeletal muscle myopathy, most frequently Duchenne's. For this reason, the U.S. Food and Drug Administration (FDA) has issued a black box warning for the use of succinylcholine in pediatric patients.

Nondepolarizing Neuromuscular Blocking Agents

Characteristics

Nondepolarizing NMBAs compete with ACh for binding to one or both of the α subunits of the nAChRs. With repetitive stimulation at frequencies between 0.1 and 2.0 Hz during partial block, muscle contraction fatigue (fade) develops (Fig. 21-6). The degree of fade can be determined with a sequence of four stimuli delivered at a 2-Hz frequency (TOF) by calculating the ratio of the amplitude (strength) of the fourth response (T4) to the amplitude of the first response (T1) of the TOF. This ratio is termed the TOF ratio, or T4/T1. Normal (baseline) TOF ratio is 1.0 (100%).

Another characteristic of nondepolarizing block is the transient amplification of responses that follows a 5-second period of tetanic stimulation (posttetanic potentiation [PTP], or facilitation [PTF]) that lasts about 2 to 3 minutes following tetanic stimulation (see PTP). Unlike depolarizing blockade, which is potentiated by the administration of anticholinesterases, the nondepolarizing block can be antagonized by these agents as long as the depth of block at the time of reversal is not excessive.

Pharmacology

Nondepolarizing NMBAs can be classified as long-, intermediate-, and short-acting, and their duration of action depends on metabolism, redistribution, and elimination (Tables 21-2 and 21-3). They also

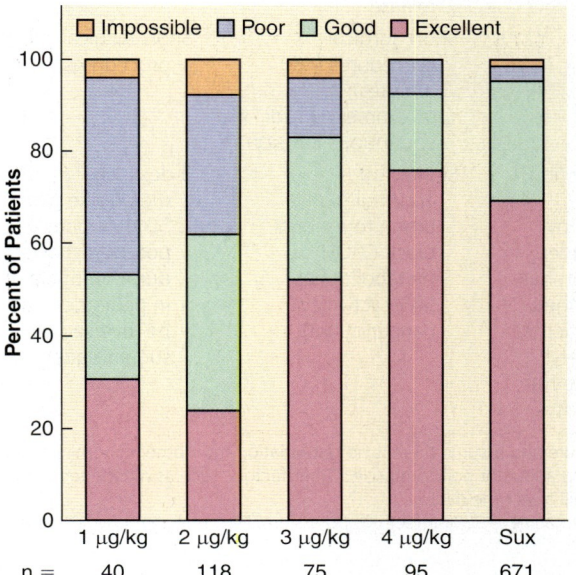

Figure 21-8 Neuromuscular blocking agents provide better intubating conditions than high doses of opioids, without hypotension. Hypnotic agent was propofol or thiopental. Intubating conditions are plotted against dose of remifentanil (in micrograms per kilogram). Results for succinylcholine (Sux), 1 mg/kg (with little opioid) are given for comparison. Hypotension was seen with remifentanil, 4 μg/kg.

Table 21-2 Pharmacokinetic and Pharmacodynamic Properties of Aminosteroid Nondepolarizing Neuromuscular Blocking Agents

Agent[a]	Vecuronium	Rocuronium	Pancuronium	Pipecuronium
Type (structure)	Nondepolarizing	Nondepolarizing	Nondepolarizing	Nondepolarizing
Type (duration)	Intermediate	Intermediate	Long	Ultralong
Potency—ED_{95} (mg/kg)	0.05	0.3	0.07	0.045
Intubating dose (mg/kg)	0.1	0.6	0.1	0.1
Onset time (minutes)	3–4	1.5–3.0	2–4	4–6
Clinical duration (minutes)	25–50	30–70	60–120	80–140
Recovery index (RI_{25-75}) (minutes)	10–25	8–13	30–45	60
Volume of distribution (L/kg)	0.4	0.3–0.7	0.2–0.3	0.25–0.30
Clearance (mL/kg/min)	5.0	3.0	1.8	2.5
Elimination half-life (min)				
• Normal organ function	65–75	100–250	90–160	90–220
• Renal impairment	Mild increase	100–300	Increased ×2	120–480
• Hepatic impairment	Significant increase	120–400	Increased ×2	—
Maintenance dose (mg/kg)	0.01	0.1	0.02	0.01
Infusion dose (μg/kg/min)	1–2	5–12	20–40 (not recommended)	NA (not recommended)
Elimination route/metabolism	Renal 10%–50%; Hepatic 30%–50%	Renal 30%; Hepatic 70%	Renal 40%–70%; Hepatic 20%	Renal 45%–60%; unchanged 40%
Active metabolites	3-desacetyl-vecuronium	17-desacetyl-rocuronium (minimal)	3-OH-pancuronium; 17-OH-pancuronium	3-desacetyl metabolite
Side effects	Vagal blockade with large doses	Minimal	Vagal block (tachycardia), catecholamine release	Minimal
Contraindications (other than specific allergy)	None	None	Short surgical procedures (<60 minutes); not recommended for continuous infusion	Short surgical procedures
Comments	Not for prolonged ICU administration (myopathy); reversible by sugammadex; elimination half-life halved in late pregnancy; 3-desacetyl metabolite has 60% of the parent compound potency	Pain on injection; easily reversible by sugammadex; elimination half-life prolonged in ICU patients; 17-desacetyl metabolite has 20% activity	Significant accumulation, prone to residual block (3-OH metabolite has 50% activity of pancuronium)	3-desacetyl metabolite has 50% of parent potency; shorter duration of action in pediatrics; can be reversed by sugammadex

[a]Agents in current clinical use. The data are averages obtained from published literature and assume there is no potentiation from other coadministered drugs (such as volatile inhalational anesthetics), and the effects are measured at the adductor pollicis muscle. Other factors, such as muscle temperature, mode of evoked response monitoring, and type/site of muscle monitoring, will affect the data.

NA, data not available; NMBA, neuromuscular blocking agents; ED_{95}, effective dose to achieve 95% effect; K^+, potassium; MH, malignant hyperthermia; ST, single twitch; ICU, intensive care unit.

can be classified based on their chemical structure as aminosteroid (vecuronium, rocuronium, pancuronium, pipecuronium) or benzylisoquinolinium (mivacurium, atracurium, cisatracurium, doxacurium) compounds. Nondepolarizing NMBAs are almost always administered IV, because intramuscular delivery leads to very slow and variable absorption and onset of action. Because they are positively charged, nondepolarizing NMBAs are distributed mostly in the extracellular fluid (ECF). Thus, in patients with renal or hepatic failure (who have increased ECF), and in burn patients, who exhibit shorter elimination half-life, larger initial doses may be required.[18]

Table 21-3 Pharmacokinetic and Pharmacodynamic Properties of Benzylisoquinolinium Nondepolarizing Neuromuscular Blocking Agents

Agent[a]	Mivacurium[b]	Atracurium	Cisatracurium	Doxacurium
Type (duration)	Short	Intermediate	Intermediate	Ultralong
Potency—ED_{95} (mg/kg)	0.08	0.25	0.05	0.020–0.033
Intubation dose (mg/kg)	0.2	0.5	0.15–0.20	0.050–0.080
Onset time (min)	3–4	3–5	4–7	3–10
Clinical duration (min)	15–20	30–45	35–50	80–160
Recovery index (RI_{25-75}) (min)	7–9	10–15	12–15	50–60
Volume of distribution (L/kg)	0.05	0.14	0.12–0.26	0.22
Clearance (mL/kg/min)	30–45	5.5	5.0–6.5	2.7
Elimination half-life (min)				
• Normal organ function	2.0–2.5	21	23–30	90–100
• Renal impairment	3–4	21	Mild increase	220
• Hepatic impairment	3–6	21	23–30	120
Maintenance dose (mg/kg)	0.1	0.1	0.01	0.01
Infusion dose (μg/kg/min)	5–8	10–20	1–3	NA (not recommended)
Elimination route/metabolism	Plasma cholinesterase (70% of succinylcholine rate)	Renal 10%; Hoffman 30%; ester hydrolysis 60%	Hoffman 30%; ester hydrolysis 60%	No metabolism; unchanged excretion in urine (30%–40%) and bile
Active metabolites	No active metabolites	No active metabolites	No active metabolites	No active metabolites
Side effects	Histamine release	Histamine release; laudanosine and acrylates production	None; histamine release at high doses	None
Contraindications (other than specific allergy)	Pseudocholinesterase deficiency	Hemodynamically unstable patients due to histamine release	None	None
Comments	Reversal by cholinesterase inhibitors; mixture of 3 isomers (cis-cis minimal); edrophonium for antagonism more effective during deep block	Organ-independent elimination	Trivial histamine release; minimal plasma laudanosine and acrylate levels	No accumulation; children more resistant, require higher doses; no histamine release; no cardiac effects at 3 × ED_{95} dose

[a]Agents in current and [b]anticipated clinical use. The data are averages obtained from published literature and assume there is no potentiation from other coadministered drugs (such as volatile inhalational anesthetics), and the effects are measured at the adductor pollicis muscle. Other factors, such as muscle temperature, mode of evoked response monitoring, and type/site of muscle monitoring, will affect the data.
NA, data not available; ED_{95}, effective dose to achieve 95% effect.

Onset and Duration of Action

Onset of nondepolarizing NMBAs generally depends on potency; less potent agents such as rocuronium (ED_{95} of 0.30 mg/kg) have more molecules per equivalent dose than a potent NMBA such as vecuronium (ED_{95} of 0.05 mg/kg); thus, an ED_{95} dose of (the less potent) rocuronium will have six times more molecules than an equipotent dose of vecuronium, and the plasma concentration of rocuronium will be greater than that of vecuronium. This greater concentration difference between the plasma and the biophase partly explains the more rapid onset of rocuronium (and SCh), as the rate of equilibration between blood and the effect compartment (the keO) will be faster (Fig. 21-9). A similar plasma/biophase concentration gradient might be achieved by administering, for instance, six times the ED_{95} of vecuronium; although this dose increase will speed up the onset, the much larger dose will also markedly prolong the total duration of action. Typically, a dose of 2 to 3 × ED_{95} of a nondepolarizing NMBA is used to facilitate tracheal intubation, whereas only 10% of the ED_{95} of a drug will be necessary to re-establish an existing deeper level of block.

Individual Nondepolarizing Agents

Aminosteroid Compounds

Pancuronium (Table 21-2) is one of the oldest nondepolarizing NMBAs. It is considered a long-acting agent with high predilection

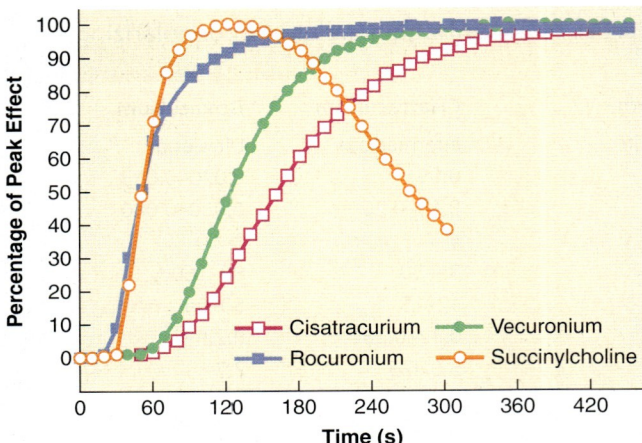

Figure 21-9 Neuromuscular blockade as a function of time for four neuromuscular blocking agents. Onset is faster for the less potent succinylcholine and rocuronium than for the more potent vecuronium and cisatracurium. (Adapted with permission from Kopman AF, Klewicka MM, Kopman DJ, et al. Molar potency is predictive of the speed of onset of neuromuscular block for agents of intermediate, short, and ultrashort duration. *Anesthesiology.* 1999;90:425.)

for significant accumulation because its main metabolite, 3-OH pancuronium, has 50% of the parent compound potency. DUR 25% is often more than 1 to 2 hours, but it can be prolonged further in renal or hepatic failure, or with repeated administration. Pancuronium has vagolytic effects as well as direct sympathomimetic effects; it blocks norepinephrine presynaptic reuptake. Because of its high potency, it is slow in onset so doses greater than $2 \times ED_{95}$ are usually needed for intubation in less than 5 minutes. It has traditionally been used in cardiac surgery, because its vagolytic effects counteract the bradycardic effects associated with high-dose opioid techniques. Anticholinesterase reversal of pancuronium-induced block is much less effective, but the reversal of shallow pancuronium block by the new agent sugammadex (see Selective Relaxant Binding Agents) appears to be effective.[19] Today, many clinicians find pancuronium obsolete because of the significant risk of postoperative residual neuromuscular weakness.

Pipecuronium (Table 21-2) is a long-acting aminosteroid NMBA that is currently not used in the United States, but it is still in use in Europe and Asia. It is structurally similar to pancuronium and vecuronium, and its antagonism of residual block by neostigmine is more effective than by edrophonium.[20] Recent data indicate that sugammadex is able to adequately and rapidly reverse pipecuronium-induced moderate block within 5 minutes.[21]

Vecuronium (Table 21-2) is an intermediate-duration NMBA that is devoid of cardiovascular effects; because it is more potent than rocuronium, its onset of action is slower. Vecuronium metabolism produces three byproducts (3-OH, 17-OH, and 3,17-(OH)$_2$ metabolites). The 3-OH (3-desacetyl) metabolite has 60% of the parent compound potency, and its accumulation with large and/or repeated doses in ICU patients likely is responsible for persistent paralysis in the critically ill patient (see Altered Responses to Neuromuscular Blocking Agents). Vecuronium precipitates in the IV tubing if administered immediately after thiopental, but does not precipitate after propofol. It has been reported that vecuronium recovery time may be prolonged significantly in patients with diabetes mellitus.[22] Since the introduction of rocuronium, vecuronium is no longer recommended for RSII.

Rocuronium (Table 21-2) is structurally similar to pancuronium and vecuronium. Because of its low potency, the high plasma concentration achieved after bolus administration decreases rapidly, such that its duration of action in patients with normal renal and hepatic function is determined mostly by its redistribution, and not its elimination. Unlike vecuronium, rocuronium metabolites are minimal, with very low neuromuscular blocking activity (17-OH rocuronium), so the risk of accumulation is minimal. In many cases, rocuronium has replaced the use of SCh in the RSII sequence. At doses of 3.5 to $4 \times ED_{95}$ (1.0 to 1.2 mg/kg), the onset rivals that of SCh, with similar intubating conditions.[23] The DUR 25%, however, at these doses averages 50 to 70 minutes (with a very wide range).

Similar to vecuronium, rocuronium does not cause significant hemodynamic perturbations and releases no histamine. Allergic reactions have been documented, and the rates of anaphylaxis (in Australia and New Zealand) are higher with rocuronium and SCh than any other NMBAs, whereas cisatracurium has the lowest rate of IgE-mediated anaphylaxis even in patients with previous anaphylaxis to rocuronium or vecuronium.[24,25] Reports from Europe also suggest that the incidence of anaphylaxis following rocuronium may be higher than with other NMBAs—this propensity having been ascribed in part to sensitization to an antitussive medication, pholcodine, that was previously available in some European countries. A similar increase in the incidence of IgE-mediated sensitization to NMBAs has been described in hairdressers, likely because of repetitive exposure to quaternary ammonium compounds used in cosmetics and hair products.[26] In the pediatric population, whereas both cisatracurium (see Nondepolarizing Neuromuscular Blocking Agents) and rocuronium have been shown to induce mild decreases in pulmonary function, these changes (maximum expiratory flow rate at 10%, MEF10) were more pronounced in patients receiving rocuronium.[27] Interestingly, anaphylaxis to rocuronium has been treated successfully with the new selective relaxant binding agent (SRBA) sugammadex.[28]

Potency of rocuronium appears to be greater in women, in older (60 to 75 years) patients, and in North American than in European patients. In laparoscopic procedures, the duration of neuromuscular block produced by rocuronium is increased by approximately 25%; this increase is attributed to the effects of pneumoperitoneum on hepatic perfusion and blood flow, which may alter the pharmacokinetics of rocuronium.[29] Patients with type II diabetes also have been reported to be at increased risk of residual neuromuscular block following rocuronium exposure.[30] In children, onset is faster and duration of action is shorter, although dose requirements are slightly increased. In patients aged 60 years and older, preadministration of magnesium may shorten its onset without significantly prolonging the duration of action.[31] The ability of sugammadex to reverse rocuronium-induced neuromuscular block, however, is not affected significantly by magnesium administration.[32]

Because of its rapid onset, rocuronium can be used in high doses (1.2 mg/kg) in the RSII setting, particularly in those patients in whom the use of SCh is contraindicated. It must be noted, however, that although the mean onset time at this dose approaches that of SCh (60 seconds), the variability of onset is greater with rocuronium, such that it is more likely that some rare outliers may have poor intubating conditions at the time of attempted laryngoscopy. It also must be borne in mind that after large doses, the DUR 25% is significantly prolonged (>60 minutes), and spontaneous (diaphragmatic) ventilation cannot be relied upon for maintenance of oxygenation in the "cannot-intubate, cannot-oxygenate" (CICO) scenario. In such emergencies, the administration of a large dose (16 mg/kg) of sugammadex may be life-saving, as long as the spontaneous ventilatory drive has not been blocked by the administration of opioids or anesthetics. Administration of high doses ($4 \times ED_{95}$) of rocuronium has no effect on the corrected QT interval in cardiac patients.[33]

Tetrahydroisoquinolinium ("Benzylisoquinolinium") Derivatives

These compounds, ubiquitously called "isoquinolinium" NMBAs, are tetrahydroisoquinolinium derivatives.

Doxacurium (Table 21-3) is a long-acting bisquaternary benzylisoquinolinium nondepolarizing NMBA. It is very potent (ED_{95} is 0.025 mg/kg), so it is the least rapid in onset (3 to 10 minutes), and also the longest acting (77 to 164 minutes) nondepolarizing NMBA.[34] Doxacurium releases no histamine in doses up to 2.7 times its ED_{95}, so is very stable from a cardiovascular standpoint.[35] Its elimination is primarily renal, and its duration of action is prolonged in renal failure[36] and elderly[37] patients. It was used preferentially during long surgical procedures, particularly in cardiac surgery, and in the ICU. Doxacurium is no longer available for clinical use in the United States.

Atracurium (Table 21-3) is a bis-benzylisoquinolinium compound of the curare family and is made up of a mixture of 10 optical isomers. It shares, with most of the isoquinolinium compounds, a unique, dual metabolic pathway: a nonenzymatic degradation that is directly proportional with temperature and pH (Hoffman reaction), and a secondary pathway that involves hydrolysis by nonspecific plasma esterases (same enzymes that degrade esmolol, remifentanil, and oseltamivir). At the usual dose for tracheal intubation (2 × ED_{95}), atracurium has a relatively long onset (3 to 5 minutes). Onset can be shortened by increasing the dose, but above 0.5 mg/kg, atracurium induces histamine release, resulting in skin flushing, tachycardia, and hypotension. DUR 25% is intermediate (30 to 45 minutes) and similar to the other intermediate-duration agents, but it is slightly more predictable, likely because of the dual metabolic pathway. Unlike aminosteroid NMBAs, atracurium potency is similar between men and women, and is not affected appreciably by age or organ failure. Allergic reactions have been reported with the same frequency as the other benzylisoquinolinium compounds. The breakdown products, such as laudanosine and acrylates, have no clinical significance at the doses of atracurium used in the clinical setting.

Cisatracurium (Table 21-3) was developed in an attempt to reduce atracurium's propensity for histamine release. It is a potent cis-cis isomer of atracurium, and its onset time is longer than that of atracurium. Because five times less cisatracurium is administered than atracurium at equipotent (ED_{95}) doses, cisatracurium does not induce histamine release. For this reason, the plasma concentrations of the metabolite laudanosine are similarly lower when cisatracurium is used.[38] Metabolism is largely independent of liver function, and because the organ-independent Hoffman elimination is the predominant pathway for its elimination, cisatracurium is preferred for use in the ICU setting. The incidence of anaphylactic reactions is similar to that of atracurium and lower than that of rocuronium and SCh.

Mivacurium (Table 21-3) was developed initially as the "ideal nondepolarizing neuromuscular blocking agent" that promised to achieve rapid onset with a duration of action significantly shorter than that of intermediate-duration agents. It consists of three stereoisomers (cis-trans, trans-trans, cis-cis). The cis-cis isomer has a much longer half-life (30 minutes) than the other two isomers (2 to 3 minutes), but it represents only 6% of the mixture, so its overall contribution to the drug's duration of action is limited. Mivacurium is rapidly hydrolyzed in plasma by butyrylcholinesterases, giving it a duration of action almost twice that of SCh (15 to 20 minutes). Because of its high potency, large doses (3 to 4 × ED_{95}) are needed for good intubating conditions and rapid onset, but at these doses, histamine release is observed. In smaller doses of 0.2 mg/kg (2.5 × ED_{95}), even when combined with propofol and remifentanil, mivacurium resulted in optimal intubating conditions in only 20% of patients.[39] In order to avoid histamine release when large doses are administered, some have suggested a "split-dose" technique in which a dose of 0.15 mg/kg is followed 30 seconds later by 0.10 mg/kg.[40] Even with this split administration, however, histamine release can still occur, and clinicians have not adopted the technique widely. When mivacurium is administered for tracheal intubation, four factors increase the probability of achieving excellent conditions: increasing mivacurium dose; opioid coadministration; delaying time to intubation (from 1 minute to 2 minutes); and patient age (>70 years).[41] Because of its rapid metabolism, the differential onset between the central (laryngeal) and peripheral (adductor pollicis) muscles is exaggerated. Thus, if the timing of tracheal intubation is guided by neuromuscular responses of peripheral muscles (e.g., APM), intubating conditions may not be ideal since the central muscles (e.g., the diaphragm) may have started recovering already.

Reversal of mivacurium-induced neuromuscular block is either spontaneous or pharmacologic, using anticholinesterases. Neostigmine also inhibits plasma cholinesterases (that should slow mivacurium metabolism), but these effects are less than the inhibition of acetylcholinesterases, resulting in a "net" reversal of nondepolarizing block. In patients with homozygous butyrylcholinesterase deficiency, the use of mivacurium (and SCh) will result in prolonged neuromuscular paralysis of 2 to 6 hours, so monitoring of neuromuscular function, mechanical ventilation, and appropriate sedation/amnesia are necessary to prevent unintended patient awareness and recall.[42] Administration of whole blood or fresh frozen plasma (each of which contains pseudocholinesterase) is not recommended unless there is another primary indication for the transfusion. Although mivacurium had been withdrawn from the United States market, it recently (2017) has been re-introduced into clinical use.

Drug Interactions

Nondepolarizing NMBAs may have either additive or synergistic effects when combined. Usually, combining two chemically similar drugs with similar duration of action (e.g., atracurium and cisatracurium) results in an additive potency interaction with no effect on total duration. When drugs of different classes are combined (e.g., cisatracurium plus rocuronium), the effects in term of total dose are synergistic, in which, for instance, ED_{25} of rocuronium plus ED_{25} of cisatracurium may have an ED_{95} effect.[43] Combining different drugs with different duration of action is a special case of interaction: when a short-duration drug (mivacurium) is added at the end of a vecuronium-based block, recovery will follow the intermediate (vecuronium) block. In contrast, when vecuronium is added during recovery from mivacurium, the vecuronium recovery will be shorter, similar to that of mivacurium. This apparent paradox is due to the fact that recovery will always follow that of the drug that blocked the majority (70% to 90%) of the receptors (the loading dose drug); the additional, maintenance drug dose is in comparison very small, and only blocks a small proportion (10% to 15%) of the free receptors. Thus, the predominant characteristics of recovery will be those of the loading drug.

Adding *depolarizing and nondepolarizing NMBAs* results in mutual antagonism. For instance, defasciculating doses of a nondepolarizing NMBA prior to administration of SCh will increase the SCh dose requirement and shorten the SCh duration of action.

Inhalational anesthetic agents potentiate neuromuscular block (desflurane > sevoflurane > isoflurane > halothane > nitrous oxide), likely by direct effects at the postjunctional receptors.

Higher concentration (minimum alveolar concentration [MAC]) and longer agent exposure will potentiate the neuromuscular block to a greater extent. The intravenous agent *propofol* has minimal effect on neuromuscular transmission, although the potency of rocuronium is enhanced after a 30-minute propofol infusion.[44]

Local anesthetics can potentiate the effects of both depolarizing and nondepolarizing NMBAs, but are insufficient to significantly shorten the onset time; NMBAs' duration of action can be prolonged due to both pre- and postsynaptic effects in animal studies.[45] In humans, epidurally administered levobupivacaine can significantly prolong the recovery time of vecuronium,[46] but a continuous infusion of IV lidocaine has no impact on the time course of rocuronium-induced neuromuscular block.[47] It is likely that these apparently contradictory effects of local anesthetics on neuromuscular transmission depend more on their plasma concentration rather than the type of local anesthetic.

The new generation of *antibiotics* has little, if any, propensity for prolonging the effects of NMBAs. Older antibiotics, such as streptomycin and neomycin, that were known to depress neuromuscular function, are used rarely today; the aminoglycosides have limited effects, but they may be involved in the process of ACh release.[48] Hypercarbia, acidosis, or hypothermia, however, may further potentiate the depressant effects of antibiotics in the critically ill patient.

In patients receiving acute administration of *anticonvulsants* (phenytoin, carbamazepine), neuromuscular block is potentiated, whereas chronic administration significantly decreases the duration of action of aminosteroids while having little effect on benzylisoquinolinium compounds. *Calcium channel antagonists* have clinically insignificant effects on NMBAs; *β-receptor antagonists* appear to delay the onset of rocuronium, whereas *ephedrine* has been shown to hasten the onset of rocuronium, likely by increasing cardiac output.[49]

Corticosteroids, particularly when administered in critical illness for prolonged periods in conjunction with neuromuscular blockade, will markedly increase the risk of myopathy (up to 50% of mechanically ventilated patients who receive both drugs may develop myopathy).

Altered Responses to Neuromuscular Blocking Agents

The use of NMBAs in the *ICU* setting is commonplace. Multiple reports have documented their benefits in facilitating tracheal intubation and maintenance of mechanical ventilation, particularly in patients requiring prone positioning for acute respiratory distress.[50] Short-term infusion of nondepolarizing NMBAs (cisatracurium) in the ICU has been shown in systematic reviews to reduce in-hospital mortality and barotrauma from mechanical ventilation, although not having any effect on the incidence of ICU-acquired weakness, as long as patients are not hyperglycemic and do not receive corticosteroids.[51,52] Similarly, continuous short-term neuromuscular blockade (<24 hours) after cardiac arrest was associated with improved lactate clearance, functional outcome, and survival.[53] However, when using NMBAs in the ICU, it is critical to remember that sedation is paramount in order to provide comfort and amnesia and avoid unintended patient awareness and recall. In addition, continuous neuromuscular block for prolonged periods (days) should be avoided, particularly in patients who receive steroid therapy concurrently. Although initially most reports of persistent paralysis involved aminosteroidal NMBAs, similar complications have been reported after benzylisoquinolinium compounds as well.[54]

Patients with *neuromuscular disease* may present a particular challenge to the anesthesiologist because of their increased risk of perioperative events, such as pulmonary and cardiovascular complications, residual neuromuscular weakness after administration of NMBAs, and metabolic syndromes such as MH.[55] In general, neuromuscular diseases can be classified into disorders of neuromuscular transmission, disorders of muscle and muscle membrane, disorders of lipid or glycogen storage, peripheral neuropathies, and disorders of the central nervous system with neuromuscular manifestations (Table 21-4). Patients with neuromuscular disorders have increased sensitivity to depolarizing, and variable sensitivity to nondepolarizing, NMBAs. In addition, because of the increased association with MH and rhabdomyolysis in many of the disorders, the use of SCh should be avoided, whereas the use of nondepolarizing NMBAs should always be guided by objective monitoring, not by subjective or clinical evaluation.

Multiple factors affect the pharmacokinetics of all drugs, including NMBAs. Intraoperative *hypothermia* prolongs the duration of NMBAs by decreasing receptor sensitivity and ACh mobilization, decreasing the force of muscle contraction, reducing renal and hepatic metabolism, and the Hoffman degradation pathway (and therefore prolonging the action of benzylisoquinolinium drugs, such as atracurium and cisatracurium). *Aging* results in decreased total body water and serum albumin concentration, reducing the volume of distribution of NMBAs; decreased cardiac function, glomerular filtration rate, and liver blood flow decrease the rate of NMBA elimination (especially the steroidal compounds). *Acid–base and electrolyte imbalance* affect the duration of action of NMBAs and their metabolism and elimination. Hypokalemia potentiates nondepolarizing block and decreases the effectiveness of anticholinesterases (neostigmine) in antagonizing nondepolarizing block. Hypermagnesemia prolongs the duration of action of NMBAs by inhibition of Ca^{2+} channels (both pre- and postsynaptically). Acidosis interferes with the effects of anticholinesterases in reversing a nondepolarizing block. *Hypercarbia* also leads to acidosis and interferes with NMBA antagonism. *Organ dysfunction* (aside from changes induced by aging) affects all NMBAs. All drugs with significant hepatic and renal metabolism (aminosteroids) will be affected and their duration of action prolonged by liver and kidney dysfunction. For this reason, benzylisoquinolinium-class NMBAs are preferred in patients with organ dysfunction (such as critically ill patients in the ICU), since the nonenzymatic Hoffman degradation is less dependent on normal organ function.

Monitoring Neuromuscular Blockade

Monitoring and Risk–Benefit Ratio

The introduction of NMBAs into clinical medicine (curare in 1942 and SCh in 1949) has facilitated major advances in medicine. Despite the tremendous advances afforded by NMBAs, these agents have their own set of complications. Allergic reactions and anaphylaxis, although rare, are significant problems; use of NMBAs without the ability to secure the airway may be lethal; and a substantial minority (30–40%) of patients who receive NMBAs has significant postoperative residual neuromuscular weakness (mistermed, "residual curarization" since curare is no longer used). Given that there are over 230 million major surgeries performed every year worldwide,[56] the number of patients exposed to potential complications is huge, and appropriate monitoring is a major

Table 21-4 Sensitivity of Patients with Neuromuscular Disease to Neuromuscular Blocking Agents and Association with Malignant Hyperthermia

Disorder Type	Depolarizing NMBA Sensitivity	Nondepolarizing NMBA Sensitivity	Other Considerations
Neuromuscular transmission disorders[a]	Increased (myasthenia) Avoid use (Lambert–Eaton)	Increased	No increased risk of MH
Muscle and muscle membrane disorders[b]	Avoid use	Increased	No increased risk of MH (myotonic dystrophy, inflammatory myopathy, mitochondrial myopathy, Brody) Increased risk (Duchenne and Becker muscular dystrophy; central core and multiminicore disease; nemaline rod myopathy; King-Denborough and hyperCKemia)
Storage disorders (lipid, glycogen)[c]	Avoid use	Variable, avoid use if possible	Evidence of increased susceptibility to MH
Peripheral neuropathies[d]	Avoid use	Variable, avoid use if possible	No increased risk of MH
Central nervous system disorders with neuromuscular manifestations[e]	Avoid use	Increased	No increased risk of MH

[a]Myasthenia gravis; Lambert–Eaton syndrome.
[b]Duchenne, Becker muscular dystrophy; myotonic dystrophy; central core and multiminicore disease; nemaline rod myopathy; inflammatory myopathy (dermatomyositis, polymyositis); mitochondrial myopathy; King-Denborough syndrome; hypercreatinekinasemia (hyperCKemia); Brody disease.
[c]Carnitine palmitoyltransferase II (CPT II) deficiency; myophosphorylase deficiency (McArdle disease).
[d]Guillain–Barré syndrome; Charcot–Marie–Tooth disease; chronic inflammatory demyelinating and critical illness polyneuropathy; critical illness myopathy.
[e]Postpolio syndrome; Friedreich ataxia; amyotrophic lateral sclerosis.
NMBA, neuromuscular blocking agent; MH, malignant hyperthermia; CK, creatine kinase.

patient safety issue. Aside from the cost of the monitors and related disposables (electrodes), there are no significant potential complications from monitoring neuromuscular function, so the risk–benefit ratio is heavily in favor of monitoring.[57] Several anesthesiology organizations around the world have recently published best-practice guidelines that recommend neuromuscular monitoring when neuromuscular blocking drugs are administered.[58,59]

Stimulator Characteristics

Monitoring involves the stimulation of a peripheral nerve and evaluation of the response (contraction, or twitch) of the innervated muscle. *Nerve stimulators* (also named peripheral nerve stimulators [PNSs]; Fig. 21-10A) have been in use for over 60 years; they are generally battery-operated, handheld units that provide the stimulus via wires connected to surface (skin) electrodes. Nerve stimulators should not be confused with *neuromuscular monitors* (Fig. 21-10B–E); the monitors not only provide nerve stimulation but also measure the evoked muscle response by using different technologies (see later). Neuromuscular monitors either are battery-operated, handheld devices (Fig. 21-10B,C) or can be incorporated into the anesthesia workstations as modular units (Fig. 21-10D). Nerve stimulators (and the stimulation units of the neuromuscular monitors) deliver a range of currents between 0 and 70 milliamperes (mA). The impulse generated by the nerve stimulator should have a square-wave pattern (i.e., should be monophasic and rectangular), as biphasic pulses may induce repetitive nerve stimulation.[60] The intensity of neurostimulation (charge, in Coulombs, Q) is a product of current (in amperes, A) and the duration of stimulation (pulse width, in seconds).[61] For instance, a charge of 4 µC can be achieved by either using a current stimulus of 20 mA with a pulse width of 200 µsec or a current stimulus of 10 mA with a pulse width of 400 µsec. The current should be constant over the duration of the impulse (which is at least 100 µsec to ensure depolarization of all nerve endings, but less than 300 to 400 µsec to avoid exceeding the nerve refractory period).

The current is delivered via surface (skin) *stimulating electrodes* that have a silver–silver chloride interface with the skin, reducing its resistance. Surface electrodes are preferred to the invasive, transcutaneous needle electrodes. The optimal conducting surface area is circular, with a diameter of 7 to 8 mm; this area provides sufficient current density to depolarize peripheral nerves. Skin can have very high resistance (up to 100,000 Ohms), and "curing" the skin (i.e., placing the electrodes over the abraded, cleansed skin and allowing at least 15 minutes for the silver chloride gel to penetrate the dermis) will decrease skin resistance to below 5,000 Ohms and will ensure delivery of a constant, maximal current.

Monitoring Modalities

The first nerve stimulators delivered single repetitive stimuli at frequencies between 0.1 and 10.0 Hz. The muscle response was an *ST* to each stimulus (Fig. 21-11A). The frequency of ST stimulation should not exceed 0.1 Hz (1 stimulus every 10 seconds), because muscle fatigue may occur with higher stimulation rates. To measure the degree of neuromuscular block, the current intensity is increased progressively (prior to NMBA administration) from 0 mA in 5-to 10-mA steps. The amplitude of the evoked muscle response is plotted over time,

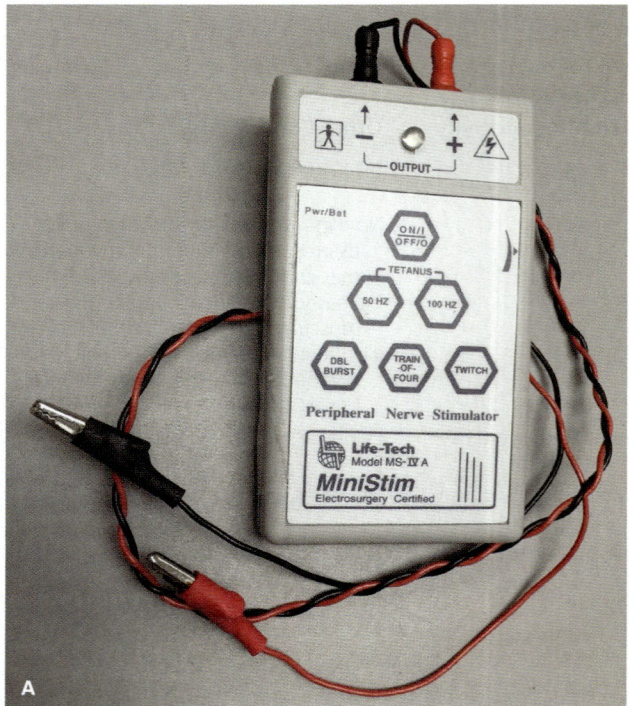
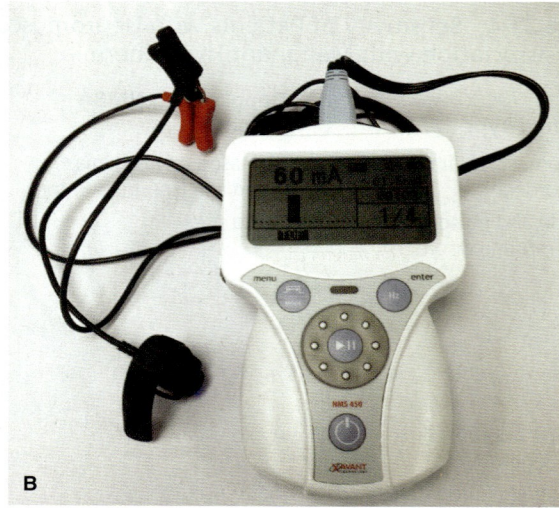
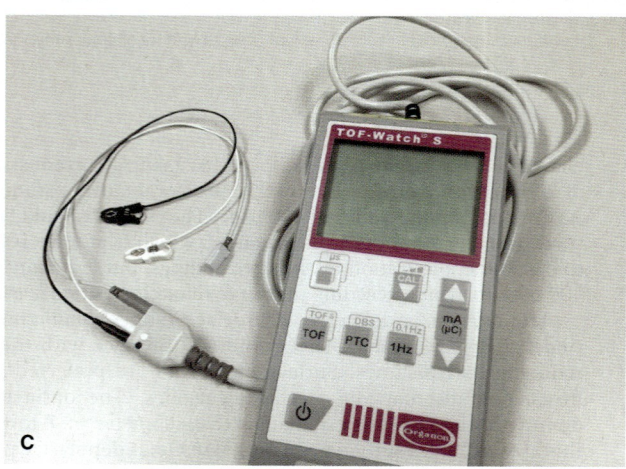
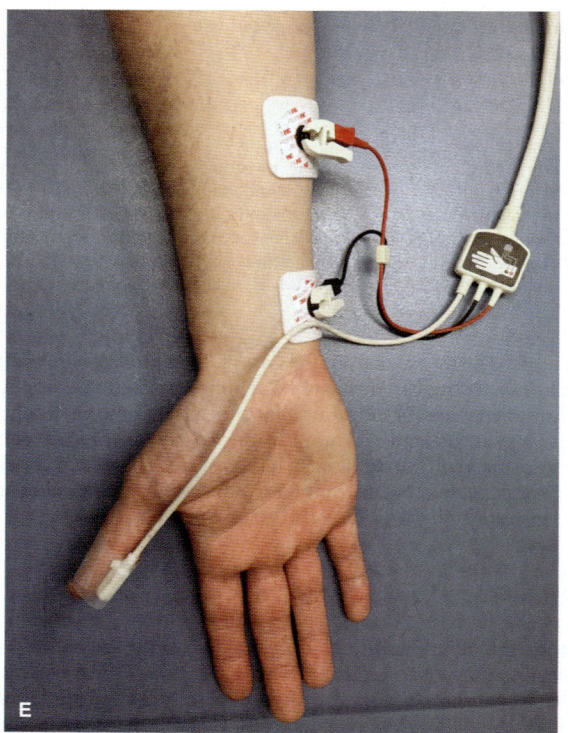
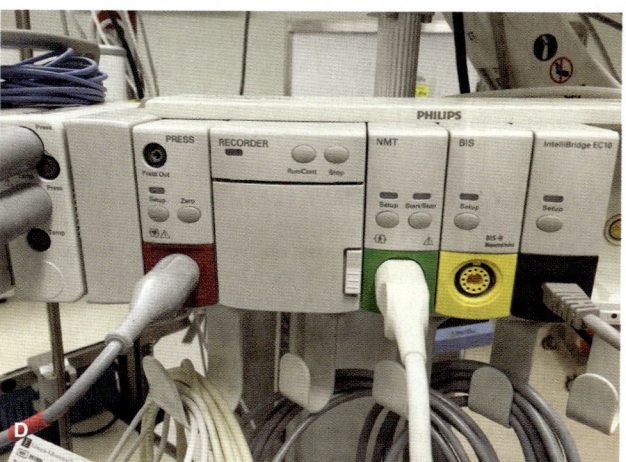

Figure 21-10 **A:** Peripheral nerve stimulator—MiniStim (Life-Tech, now Kimberly-Clark, Irving, TX). **B:** Acceleromyographic neuromuscular monitor—StimPod (Xavant Technologies, Pretoria, South Africa). **C:** Acceleromyographic neuromuscular monitor—TOF-Watch S (Organon Ltd, Swords, Co. Dublin, Ireland). The TOF-Watch accelerograph recently has been discontinued from manufacture and is no longer available. **D:** Philips NMT Modular Unit (Philips Healthcare, Amsterdam, The Netherlands). **E:** Philips acceleromyographic NMT monitor (Philips Healthcare, Amsterdam, The Netherlands). Electrodes are placed along the ulnar nerve, with the negative (*black*) electrode distal to the positive (*red*) electrode. The accelerometer is taped to the thumb, with the sensor perpendicular to the direction of thumb adduction.

and has a sigmoidal shape. Once the amplitude of the muscle response no longer increases as current intensity increases, the response is maximal, and the current required is called "maximal current." Increasing the current value by 20% above maximal level ensures that all fibers in the innervated nerve will depolarize despite changes in skin resistance over time; this is termed "supramaximal current." Because a baseline control value is needed in order to compare the force of contraction over time, ST modality is used clinically to determine onset of neuromuscular block, not its recovery. The characteristics of

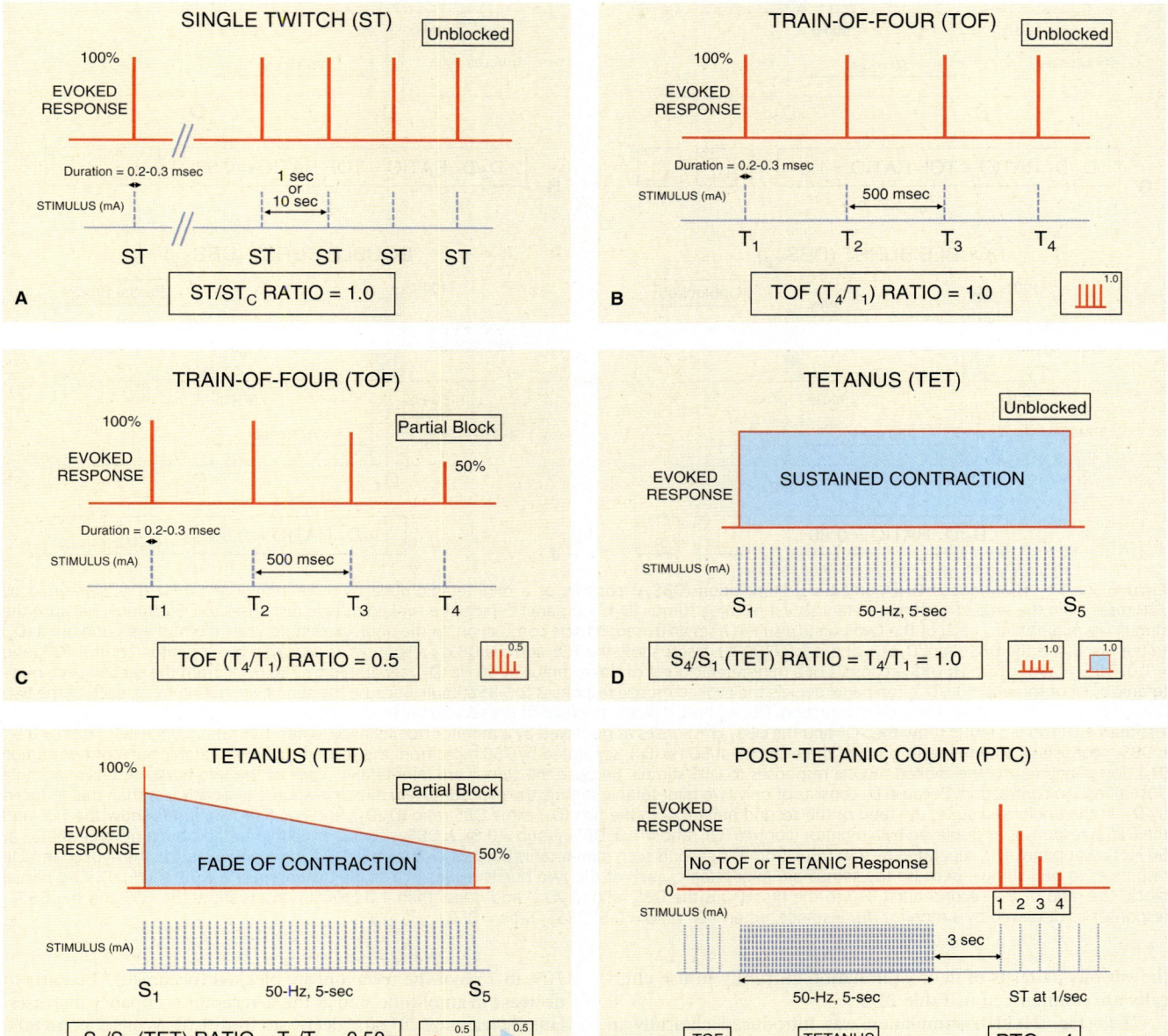

Figure 21-11 **A:** Single twitch (ST) stimulation. Following establishment of a baseline (control) ST amplitude at supramaximal current (STc), subsequent ST amplitudes are compared to STc (ST/STc ratio). ST is delivered at a frequency of 1 Hz or 0.1 Hz. **B:** Train-of-four (TOF) stimulation pattern. Unblocked state, TOF ratio = 1.0 (100%). Inset shows the TOF as displayed by a monitor. T_1 = first stimulus in the sequence; T_2 = second stimulus in the sequence; T_3 = third stimulus in the sequence; T_4 = fourth stimulus in the sequence. **C:** TOF stimulation pattern. Partial block, TOF ratio = 0.5 (50%). Inset shows the TOF as displayed by a monitor (TOF ratio = 0.5). **D:** Tetanic stimulation. Unblocked state, no fade between tension at the beginning of the 5-second stimulation (S_1) and the end of the stimulation (S_5). The ratio of tension at the end of the 5-second stimulation to that at the beginning is the tetanic ratio (S_5/S_1 ratio). Insets show the TOF and the TET as displayed by a monitor (TOF ratio = 1.0; TET ratio = 1.0). S_1 = tetanic tension at the beginning of 5-second TET; S_5 = tetanic tension at the end of 5-second TET; S_5/S_1 = TET ratio. **E:** Tetanic stimulation. Partial blockade, with fade of tension from S_1 to S_5. The ratio of tension at the end of the 5-second stimulation to that at the beginning is the tetanic ratio (S_5/S_1 ratio). Insets show the TOF and the TET as displayed by a monitor (TOF ratio = 0.5; TET ratio = 0.5). **F:** When there is no muscle response to TOF stimulation, a 5-second tetanic (50 Hz) stimulus is followed, 3 seconds later, by a series of ST stimuli at a frequency of 1 Hz. The number of rapidly fading twitches is counted; the resulting number of twitches is the posttetanic count. A lower posttetanic count (PTC) denotes deeper block. *(continued)*

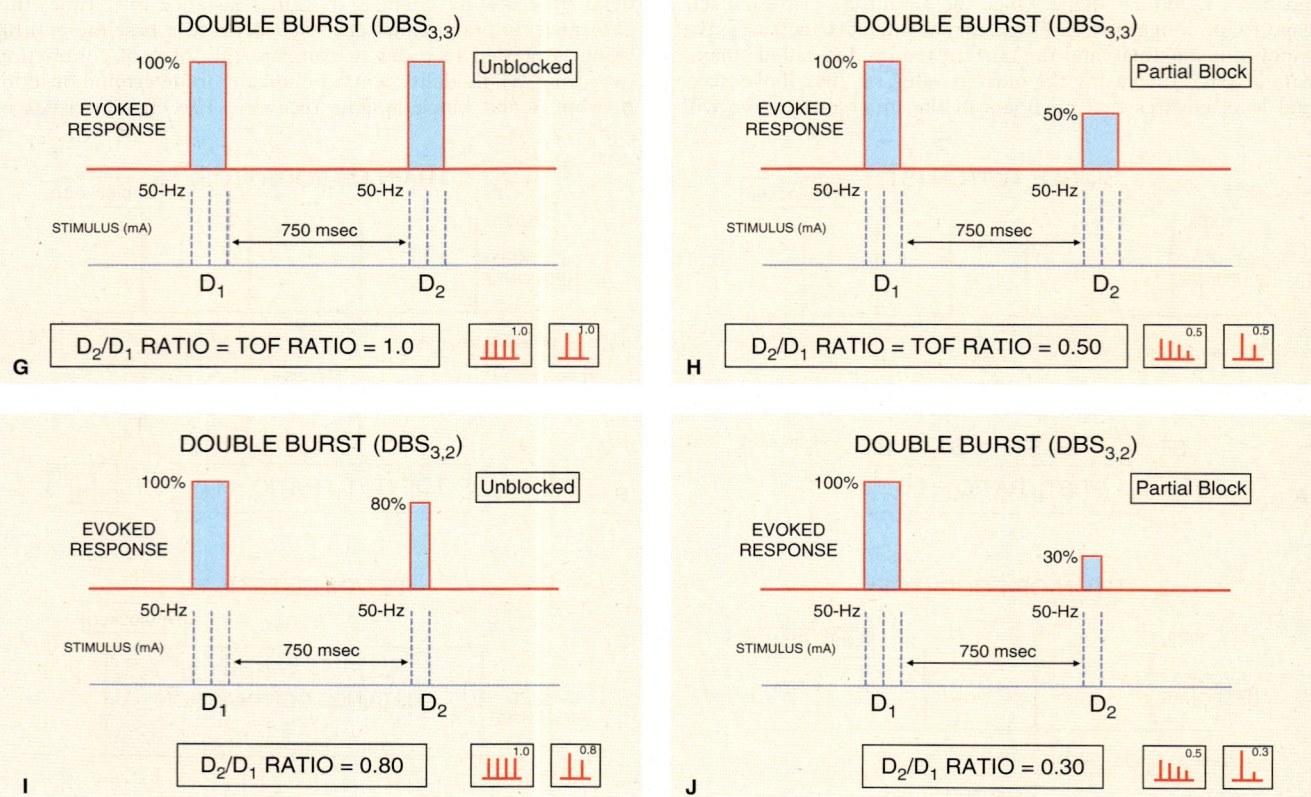

Figure 21-11 (*Continued*) **G:** Double-burst stimulation (DBS$_{3,3}$) consists of a mini-tetanic burst of three stimuli at 50 Hz (D$_1$), separated by 750 msec from the second such mini-tetanic burst of three stimuli (D$_2$). Top panel depicts the evoked muscle responses to DBS stimuli. Because the stimuli are mini-tetanic, each of the two bursts result in a single (fused) muscle contraction. In the unblocked state, the ratio of the second burst (D$_2$) to the first (D$_1$) is the DBS ratio (D$_2$/D$_1$), and is 1.0 (100%). Insets show the TOF and the DBS$_{3,3}$ responses as displayed by a monitor (control TOF ratio = 1.0; DBS$_{3,3}$ ratio = 1.0). **H:** DBS$_{3,3}$ consists of a mini-tetanic burst of three stimuli at 50 Hz (D$_1$), separated by 750 msec from the second such mini-tetanic burst of three stimuli (D$_2$). Top panel depicts the evoked muscle responses to DBS stimuli. Because the stimuli are mini-tetanic, each of the two bursts result in a single (fused) muscle contraction. During partial block, the ratio of the second burst (D$_2$) to the first (D$_1$) is the DBS ratio (D$_2$/D$_1$), and is less than 1.0 (100%). Insets show the TOF and the DBS$_{3,3}$ responses as displayed by a monitor (for instance, when TOF ratio = 0.5; DBS$_{3,3}$ ratio = 0.5). **I:** DBS$_{3,2}$ consists of a mini-tetanic burst of three stimuli at 50 Hz (D$_1$), separated by 750 msec from the second such mini-tetanic burst of two stimuli (D$_2$). Top panel depicts the evoked muscle responses to DBS stimuli. Because the stimuli are mini-tetanic, each of the two bursts results in a single (fused) muscle contraction. Because D$_2$ consists of only two mini-tetanic stimuli, the evoked (fused) muscle response is slightly less than that induced by D$_1$. In the unblocked state, the ratio of the second burst (D$_2$) to the first (D$_1$) is the DBS ratio (D$_2$/D$_1$), and is 0.8 (80%). Insets show the TOF and the DBS$_{3,2}$ responses as displayed by a monitor (control TOF ratio = 1.0; DBS$_{3,2}$ ratio = 0.8). **J:** DBS$_{3,2}$ consists of a mini-tetanic burst of three stimuli at 50 Hz (lower panel, D$_1$), separated by 750 msec from the second such mini-tetanic burst of two stimuli (D$_2$). Upper panel depicts the evoked muscle responses to DBS stimuli. Because the stimuli are mini-tetanic, each of the two bursts result in a single (fused) muscle contraction. During partial block, the ratio of the second burst (D$_2$) to the first (D$_1$) is the DBS ratio (D$_2$/D$_1$), and is less than 1.0 (100%). Insets show the TOF and the DBS$_{3,2}$ responses as displayed by a monitor (for instance, when TOF ratio = 0.5; DBS$_{3,2}$ ratio = 0.3).

the various patterns of neurostimulation currently in use clinically are summarized in Table 21-5.

TOF (Fig. 21-11B) stimulation was introduced clinically in 1971, and consists of four sequential ST stimuli (named T1, T2, T3, and T4) delivered at a frequency of 2 Hz.[62,63] Each train is delivered no more frequently than every 15 to 20 seconds to avoid facilitation of subsequent muscle responses. The TOF ratio is calculated by dividing the T4 amplitude by the T1 amplitude. The control TOF ratio (before administration of NMBA) is 1.0 (100%). During a partial nondepolarizing block, the ratio decreases (fades) as the degree of block increases (Fig. 21-11C). There is a well-described relationship between TOF fade and percent (%) postsynaptic receptor occupancy by nondepolarizing NMBAs.[64] Up to 65% to 70% of the nAChRs can be blocked without any apparent fade in the TOF ratio; these receptors make up the "margin of safety" of neuromuscular transmission.[65,66] Once approximately 70% to 75% of the receptors are blocked (occupied), T4 starts to decrease in amplitude, and as the % receptor occupancy increases, fade increases (TOF ratio decreases from 1.0). When 75% to 80% of the receptors are blocked, T4 disappears, so the TOF ratio (T4/T1) becomes 0; at this point, the TOF count (TOFC) is 3, meaning that there are three discernible muscle responses. As the % receptor occupancy increases to 80% to 85%, the TOFC becomes 2, and at 85% to 90% occupancy, T2 disappears (TOFC = 1). Once over 95% of the receptors are blocked, TOFC becomes 0 (Table 21-6).

TOF has multiple benefits over ST monitoring: at supramaximal stimulation, T1 and ST amplitudes are the same, so TOF does not require a baseline measurement—all subsequent responses are then measured as a fraction of T1. By eliciting four responses, the clinician sometimes is able to assess the degree of fade subjectively by visual or tactile means, or, more reliably, by counting the number of evoked responses (twitches) of TOF (TOFC).

Table 21-5 Characteristics of Various Patterns of Neurostimulation

Pattern	Characteristics
Single twitch (ST)	• A "control" ST needs to be established by determining maximal response to increasing stimulus current • Pulse duration is 0.1–0.3 msec (0.2 msec most common) • An increase in maximal current by 20%–30% is needed to establish "supramaximal" current and ensure activation of all muscle fibers and consistent recruitment over time • A single, supramaximal stimulus delivered at a frequency of 1/sec (1 Hz) or 1/10 sec (0.1 Hz) • Frequency higher than 1 Hz affects subsequent muscle response • Range of receptor occupancy detected by ST is narrow, ~75%–95% • Unable to differentiate depolarizing from nondepolarizing block
Train-of-four (TOF)	• Four ST stimuli at a frequency of 2 Hz • No "control" (prerelaxant) muscle response needed • Ratio of fourth to first response is T4/T1 or TOF ratio • "Fade" defined as a weaker fourth response (T4) than the first (T1) • Trains delivered at 15- to 20-second intervals do not induce potentiation of subsequent muscle responses • TOF ratios >0.40 cannot be detected subjectively • Able to differentiate depolarizing from nondepolarizing block • Less painful to measure in awake patients than tetanic (or DBS) stimulation • Can detect degree of block in the range of surgical relaxation, ~70%–100% receptor occupancy
Double burst stimulation (DBS)	• Two mini-tetanic bursts (two or three impulses at 50 Hz in each burst) separated by 750 msec • DBS delivered at 20-second intervals to avoid potentiation of subsequent muscle responses • $DBS_{3,3}$ contains 3 mini-tetanic bursts followed by 3 mini-tetanic bursts • $DBS_{3,2}$ contains 3 mini-tetanic bursts followed by 2 mini-tetanic bursts • No "control" (prerelaxant) muscle response needed • Ratio of 2nd to 1st muscle response is D2/D1 or DBS ratio • "Fade" defined as a weaker second response (D2) than the first (D1) • Fade of TOF is identical to fade of $DBS_{3,3}$ • TOF ratios >0.60 cannot be detected subjectively • Able to differentiate depolarizing from nondepolarizing block • Less painful to measure in awake patients than tetanic stimulation, but more painful than TOF • Subjective evaluation of DBS fade superior to TOF fade
Train-of-four count (TOFC)	• Available once T4 of TOF becomes 0 • At disappearance of T4, the TOFC = 3 • At disappearance of T3, the TOFC = 2 • At disappearance of T2, the TOFC = 1 • At disappearance of T1, the TOFC = 0 • There is a relationship between TOFC and receptor occupancy (blockade)
Tetanic stimulation (TET)	• Common frequency is 50 Hz for 5 seconds • Alternative more demanding TET is 100 Hz for 5 seconds • The 100-Hz TET may be supraphysiologic and can induce fade in normal controls • Able to differentiate depolarizing from nondepolarizing block • May induce direct muscle stimulation • Painful to awake patients • TET fade over 5 seconds is equivalent to TOF fade • TET at intervals less than 3 minutes will enhance (potentiate) subsequent muscle responses
Posttetanic count (PTC)	• TET at 50 Hz for 5 seconds followed 3 seconds later by ST at 1 Hz • More PTC responses indicate less block • Allows assessment of profound block (TOFC = 0) • When PTC = 0, further NMBA administration is not recommended • PTC at intervals less than 3 minutes will potentiate subsequent muscle responses

Additionally, the TOF ratio remains consistent over a range of stimulating currents, as long as the stimulating current intensity is at least 10 mA above the threshold current (Table 21-7).[67] This TOF consistency at varying stimulating currents allows this pattern to be used to measure the degree of neuromuscular recovery in patients recovering from anesthesia, as currents of 20 to 30 mA are not associated with the high degree of discomfort of supramaximal 60- to 70-mA stimulation.[68]

Tetanic stimulation (tetanus; Fig. 21-11D) describes repetitive stimulation at a frequency above 30 Hz. Below this threshold, repetitive nerve stimuli result in individual, rapid contractions. At frequencies above 30 Hz, the muscle responses become fused into a sustained contraction without fade (tetanic ratio = 1.0). During partial nondepolarizing block, the tetanic contraction gets weaker (fades; Fig. 21-11E). The maximal voluntary muscle contraction is approximately 60 Hz, so frequencies above this level are supraphysiologic and may result in muscle contraction fade even in the absence of NMBAs.[69] The fade of TOF in response to nondepolarizing NMBAs corresponds to the fade of tetanic stimulation. Tetanus has been studied extensively for

Table 21-6 Relationship between % Receptor Occupancy and Train-of-Four Ratio during Nondepolarizing Block

Percent Receptor Occupancy (%)	First TOF Twitch (T_1) (% Baseline)	Fourth Twitch (T_4) (% Baseline)	TOF Ratio (T1–T4 Responses)	TOF COUNT (TOFC)
100	0%	0%	0	TOFC = 0
90–95	0%	0%	0 (T_1 = 0)	TOFC = 0
85–90	10%	0%	0 (T_2 = 0)	TOFC = 1
	20%	0%	0 (T_3 = 0)	TOFC = 2
80–85	25%	0%	0 (T_4 = 0)	TOFC = 3
	80%–90%	48%–58%	0.60–0.70	TOFC = 4
	95%	69%–79%	0.70–0.75	TOFC = 4
70–75	100%	75%–100%	0.75–1.00	TOFC = 4
	100%	100%	0.9–1.0	TOFC = 4
50	100%	100%	1.0	TOFC = 4
25	100%	100%	1.0	TOFC = 4

TOF, train-of-four; T_1, first twitch of TOF; T_2, second twitch of TOF; T_3, third twitch of TOF; T_4, fourth twitch of TOF; TOFC, train-of-four count.

durations of 5 seconds, so clinicians should always use 5-second durations to evaluate neuromuscular function—decisions based on tetanic durations shorter than 5 seconds will undoubtedly be inaccurate. When tested during partial nondepolarizing block, the high frequency of tetanic stimulation will cause a temporary increase in the amount of ACh released such that subsequent responses will be increased transiently (period of PTP; Fig. 21-6). Depending on the tetanic frequency, this period of potentiated responses may last 1 to 2 minutes after a 5-second, 50-Hz tetanus, or up to 3 minutes after 100-Hz tetanus.[70,71] The response to stimulation during the period of PTP can be used to evaluate the degree of block when there are no responses to TOF stimulation (i.e., when the TOFC = 0).

Posttetanic count (PTC; Fig. 21-11F), used during periods of profound neuromuscular block, consists of a 5-second, 50-Hz tetanic stimulus, followed 3 seconds later by a series of 15 to 30 ST at a frequency of 1 Hz.[72] The number of posttetanic twitches is inversely proportional to the depth of block: the fewer posttetanic twitches there are, the deeper the block. From a depth of block of PTC = 1 until recovery to a TOFC of 1, intermediate-acting NMBAs require 20 to 30 minutes. PTC can also be used for dosing of sugammadex (See Selective Relaxant Binding Agents).

Studies have shown that visual and tactile (subjective) evaluation of fade to TOF stimulation fail to identify significant degrees of residual block (when the TOF ratio is >0.40).[73] By delivering two (instead of four) intense stimuli (mini-tetanic bursts) separated by 0.75 second, the two fused responses can be evaluated as a direct comparison, instead of comparing the fourth response of TOF to the first. This modality is termed *double burst stimulation* ($DBS_{3,3}$; Fig. 21-11G). The numbers 3,3 signify that each burst contains three stimuli at a frequency of 50 Hz.[74] Because the two individual bursts are tetanic in frequency, a longer recovery period between successive stimulations is necessary (20 seconds). Using DBS subjectively, clinicians are able to detect fade (Fig. 21-11H) when the TOF is less than 0.60, an improvement over the subjectively detected TOF fade (<0.40). The relationship between TOF ratio and $DBS_{3,3}$ ratio is linear and identical between 0.0 and 1.0. In order to further increase the ability to detect small degrees of fade, another pattern of DBS only uses two mini-tetanic stimuli in the second burst—this is called $DBS_{3,2}$, and the baseline control $DBS_{3,2}$ ratio is 0.8 when the TOF ratio and $DBS_{3,3}$ ratio is 1.0 (Fig. 21-11I).[75] This offset of 0.2 units is maintained as fade progresses (e.g., $DBS_{3,3}$ ratio of 0.5 corresponds to a $DBS_{3,2}$ of 0.3; Fig. 21-11J).

Testing and Recording the Response

There are different *modalities* to assess the degree of neuromuscular block, including subjective and objective evaluation and assessment of *clinical criteria*.[76] There are also different *technologies* for measuring the evoked response (objective evaluation). When assessing the degree of block (or state of neuromuscular recovery), it is important to note that most clinicians even today evaluate responses subjectively: by *visual* or *tactile* means.

Table 21-7 Consistency of the Train-of-Four Ratio in Response to Neurostimulation at Varying Current Intensity at Three Depths of Neuromuscular Block

Depth of Block Classification at 50 mA	TOF Ratio at 20 mA	TOF Ratio at 30 mA	TOF Ratio at 50 mA
TOF ≤ 0.70 (n = 28)	0.500 ± 0.180	0.506 ± 0.170	0.513 ± 0.160
TOF > 0.70, < 0.95 (n = 25)	0.915 ± 0.100	0.906 ± 0.080	0.894 ± 0.070
TOF ≥ 0.95 (n = 30)	0.972 ± 0.060	0.972 ± 0.040	0.995 ± 0.020

TOF, train-of-four; mA, milliamperes; n, number of assessments.
Data from Brull SJ, Ehrenwerth J, Silverman DG. Stimulation with submaximal current for train-of-four monitoring. *Anesthesiology.* 1990;72:629–632.

Table 21-8 Reliability in Correctly Identifying Presence of Fade in Response to Train-of-Four and Double-Burst Stimulation using Subjective (Visual or Tactile) Methods during Minimal Neuromuscular Block (TOF Ratio = 0.40–0.70).

True-Positives (Correct Identification of Presence of Fade)			
	TOF	$DBS_{3,3}$	$DBS_{3,2}$
Engbaek et al.[74]	—	64%	96%
Drenck et al.[78]	16%	78%	—
Viby-Mogensen et al.[73]	36%	—	—
Gill et al.[79]	16%	69%	—
Ueda et al.[75]	—	73%	96%
Brull et al.[80]	42%	67%	72%

TOF, train-of-four; DBS, double-burst stimulation.

Subjective evaluation of neuromuscular function may consist of feeling (tactilely) or observing (visually) the degree of fade to TOF stimulation. Such subjective assessments however are inaccurate (Table 21-8); when the TOF recovers to more than 0.40, clinicians are unable to detect TOF fade reliably. Evaluation of fade to 50-Hz tetanic stimulation is no more precise than evaluation of TOF fade. Subjective detection of fade to DBS or 100-Hz tetanic stimulation may be closer (when TOF <0.70) to the threshold of adequate recovery (defined as TOF ≥0.90), but such evaluations cannot be performed in awakening patients awaiting tracheal extubation due to the pain associated with DBS and tetanic stimulation. The ability to detect fade is not influenced by the observers' experience, and there is also no difference in the ability to detect fade between visual and tactile means.[73] Therefore, clinical decisions based on subjective (qualitative) evaluation of fade likely are incorrect, and do not decrease the risk of oxygen desaturation or need for tracheal re-intubation.[77] This fact is borne out by numerous studies for the past 40 years that continue to document the inability of clinicians to detect TOF fade, leading to a significant incidence of residual postoperative paralysis (Table 21-9).

Table 21-9 Selected Reports of Postoperative Residual Paralysi, 1979–2016

Study	Long-Acting NMBA	Intermediate-Acting NMBA	Reversal	TOF Threshold	Monitoring Modality	Residual Paralysis	Comments
Viby-Mogensen *Anesthesiology* 1979;50:539	d-TC Panc Gallam		Yes	0.7	None	42%	The first report to highlight the RNMB problem
Bevan *Anesthesiology* 1988;69:272	Panc	Atrac Vec	Yes Yes Yes	0.7	Subjective	36% 4% 9%	Less residual paralysis after intermediate-acting NMBAs
Brull *Can J Anaesth* 1991;38:164	Panc	Vec	Yes Yes	0.7	Subjective	45% 8%	Testing with low current to decrease discomfort
Fawcett *Acta Anaesthesiol Scand* 1995;39:288		Atrac/Vec Bolus Infusion	Yes Yes	0.7 0.7	Subjective	12% 24%	More RNMB after infusion than bolus
Berg *Acta Anaesthesiol Scand Suppl* 1997;110:156	Panc	Atrac/Vec	Yes Yes	0.7 0.7	Subjective	26% 5%	Atelectasis associated with RNMB
Debaene *Anesthesiology* 2003;98:1042		Atrac Vec Roc	No	0.7 0.9	None	16% 45%	RNMB present >4 hrs after single dose
Murphy *Anesth Analg* 2003;96:1301	Panc	Roc	No No	0.8 0.8	Optional	82% 0%	Postcardiac surgery
Murphy *Anesth Analg* 2004;98:193	Panc	Roc	Yes Yes	0.7 0.9 0.7 0.9	Subjective	40% 83% 5.9% 29%	Delayed PACU discharge
Baillard *Br J Anaesth* 2005;95:622		Atrac/Vec/Roc	Yes – in 42% of patients	0.9	60% of patients	3.5%	Less RNMB with reversal and when monitoring was used
Cammu *Anesth Analg* 2006;102:426		Atrac/Cis/Miv/ Roc Outpatients Inpatients	In 26% In 25%	0.9	Clinical (49% of cases)	38% 47%	One of 320 inpatients required reintubation in PACU; subjective assessment did not decrease incidence of residual paralysis
Murphy *Anesthesiology* 2008;109:389		Roc	Yes	0.9	AMG Subjective	5% 30%	AMG lowers RNMB risk
Butterly *Br J Anaesth* 2010;105:304		Vec/Cis	Yes	0.9	Subjective	22%	Less RNMB with cisatrac

(continued)

Table 21-9 Selected Reports of Postoperative Residual Paralysi, 1979–2016 (CONTINUED)

Study	Long-Acting NMBA	Intermediate-Acting NMBA	Reversal	TOF Threshold	Monitoring Modality	Residual Paralysis	Comments
Murphy *Anesthesiology* 2011;115:946		Roc	Yes	0.9 0.9	AMG Subjective	15% 50%	AMG monitoring lowers RNMB
De Souza *Rev Bras Anestesiol* 2011;61:145		Roc Atrac	Yes Yes	0.9 0.9	Clinical	10% 10%	Pediatric population (3 mos–12 yo); improper reversal (too deep or too shallow) in 46% of roc and 25% of atrac patients
Cammu *Anaesth Intensive Care* 2012;40:999		Atrac/Roc/Miv	None Neo Sgx	0.9	Subjective (38% of cases)	15% 15% 2%	Body mass index was an independent predictor of desaturation in PACU
Norton *Rev Esp Anestesiol Reanim* 2013;60:190		Roc/Cis	Yes	0.9	Optional	30%	CRE present in 51% of patients with RNMB; airway obstruction, severe hypoxemia, and respiratory failure all higher in RNMB patients
Ledowski *Indian J Anaesth* 2013;57:46		Not specified	None Neo Sgx	0.9	Subjective	16% 13% 3%	RNMB associated with atelectasis and pneumonia
Esteves *Eur J Anaesthesiol* 2013;30:243		Atrac/Cis/Roc/Vec	Yes (67% of patients)	0.9	Subjective	26%	Incomplete recovery more frequent after reversal than no reversal (31% vs. 17%)
Kotake *Anesth Analg* 2013;117:345		Roc	None Neo Sgx	0.9	Clinical	13% 24% 4%	RNMB as high as 9% with Sgx without monitoring
Pietraszewski *Anaesthesiol Intensive Ther* 2013;45:77		Roc	None	0.9	Not used	44%	Incidence of RNMB was 44% in elderly and 20% in young patients
Fortier *Anesth Analg* 2015;121:366		Roc	Yes	0.9	Optional	64%	Incidence of RNMB was 56% on PACU arrival
Xara *Arch Bronconeumol* 2015;51:69		NMBAs used in 66% of patients	Yes	0.9	Optional	18%	CRE more common (46%) in patients with RNMB
Ledowski *Anesthesiol Res Pract* 2015;2015:410		Atrac/Roc/Vec	Yes (48% of patients)	0.9	Optional (used in 23% of patients)	28%	RNMB after neo reversal was twice as high as no reversal in pediatric patients
Brueckmann *Br J Anaesth* 2015;115:743		Roc	Yes—Neo Yes- Sgx	0.9 0.9	Subjective	43% 0%	OR discharge shorter in Sgx-treated patients
Aytac *Braz J Anesthesiol* 2016;66:55		Atrac/Roc/Vec	Yes—Neo (66% of patients)	0.7 0.9	Clinical	15% 43%	82% of patients with $SpO_2 \leq 90\%$ had a TOF ≤ 0.90; 43% of patients with TOF < 0.70 required airway support

NMBA, neuromuscular blocking agent; TOF, train-of-four; d-TC, d-tubocurarine; Panc, pancuronium; Gallam, gallamine; RNMB, residual neuromuscular block; Atrac, atracurium; Cis, cisatracurium; Vec, vecuronium; Roc, rocuronium; Miv, mivacurium; PACU, postanesthesia care unit; AMG, acceleromyography; CRE, critical respiratory events; Sgx, sugammadex; OR, operating room.

The limitations of subjective evaluation extend to intraoperative management of the depth of block. Clinicians may consider that intraoperative management based on subjective evaluation of the depth of block (determined by the TOFC) may be more reliable than the evaluation of residual block (determined by TOF fade) performed prior to tracheal extubation. Unfortunately, such subjective evaluation of TOFC also is prone to significant overestimation of the degree of neuromuscular recovery (and underestimation of the depth of block).[81,82] All available data support the conclusion that subjective evaluation of neuromuscular function is inadequate in guiding intraoperative NMBA management or in detecting sufficient neuromuscular recovery to prevent residual neuromuscular paralysis and the occurrence of critical respiratory events.

Clinical testing has been advocated for decades; tests such as grip strength, vital capacity, tidal volume, head-lift, or leg-lift (despite their continued use) are notoriously poor at detecting residual fade. It should be noted that none of the currently used clinical signs require sufficient muscle function to allow clinicians to identify residual neuromuscular weakness. The negative inspiratory force (NIF) of −20 cm H_2O often (and incorrectly) used as an indicator of neuromuscular recovery[83] is less than 25% of the normal NIF of 90 cm H_2O (Table 21-10). In fact, none of the clinical tests has a sensitivity above 0.35 (general weakness); specificity above 0.89 (5-second sustained grip); a positive predictive value above 0.52 (sustained tongue depressor test); or negative predictive value above 0.66 (general weakness).[84] Even the often-used test of 5-second head-lift has the same poor predictive value: a majority of volunteers were able to maintain head lift for more than 5 seconds at a TOF ratio of 0.5. The best clinical test, the ability to resist removal of a tongue blade from clenched teeth, cannot be used in patients whose tracheas are still orally intubated.[85]

For decades, investigators have shown that regardless of the NMBA used, over 40% of patients managed intraoperatively by clinical criteria or subjective evaluation had residual paralysis (TOF <0.90) when tested objectively in the PACU (Table 21-9). This is significant, since postoperative mortality was increased 90-fold if patients who had residual paralysis required unplanned tracheal reintubation and ICU care postoperatively.[77] Given that postoperative pulmonary complications are relatively common in patients with residual neuromuscular block, objective monitoring of adequacy of reversal prior to tracheal extubation is strongly recommended.

Objective evaluation involves the actual recording, processing, and measurement of responses (electrical or mechanical) of muscles-to-nerve stimulation. *Electromyography (EMG)* is one of the oldest methods of measuring neuromuscular transmission. For EMG monitoring, a peripheral nerve (usually the ulnar nerve) is stimulated via surface (skin) electrodes, and the action potential generated at the innervated muscle (the APM) is measured. Measurement of the evoked response may involve the area under the curve of the muscle action potential, the peak-to-baseline, or the peak-to-peak amplitude of the signal. The stimulating electrodes should be placed along a peripheral nerve to avoid direct muscle stimulation (that is not subject to NMBA-induced blockade). One of the recording electrodes is placed on the belly of the monitored muscle (close to the location of the NMJ), and the second on the muscle's insertion point. Clinically, the ulnar nerve/APM combination is used most frequently because APM is the sole hand muscle on the radial side of the hand that is innervated by the ulnar nerve—decreasing the chance of direct muscle stimulation. Other muscles of the hand that can be monitored include the first dorsal interosseous (FDI) and the abductor digiti minimi (ADM) muscles. Although there are minor differences in the time course of relaxation and recovery between the hand muscles, the differences are clinically insignificant. A limitation of EMG is that the response is very sensitive to electrical interference (e.g., diathermy).

Mechanomyography (MMG), like EMG, is one of the standards of measurement of neuromuscular function that records the force of muscle contraction. With MMG (and EMG), the ulnar nerve is innervated, and the force of thumb (APM) adduction is measured via an interfaced force transducer. Although a majority of studies have used MMG for research, MMG monitors are no longer available clinically because of their cost, large size, and difficulty of use. In order to obtain accurate and consistent results, the monitored arm has to be immobilized, pre-tension has to be measured and applied as a control value, and strict temperature parameters have to be maintained, as MMG is sensitive to temperature fluctuation.

Acceleromyography (AMG) has been the most commonly used method of measuring muscle function in the past two decades. AMG consists of an accelerometer mounted to a moving muscle (usually the thumb) that measures the acceleration in response to nerve stimulation (the ulnar nerve; Fig. 21-10B,C,E). The technology is based on Newton's Second Law of Motion, $F = m \cdot a$, in which the force of APM contraction is proportional to the thumb acceleration (since mass remains unchanged). Although it is the most commonly used monitor, it has several major limitations that prevent it from becoming the "gold standard of care." The AMG setup can be simple, but is relatively time consuming, if performed properly; the thumb must be allowed to move freely throughout surgery—any arm or hand movement may change the direction of thumb adduction or the baseline, necessitating recalibration, because calibrated and noncalibrated measurements are not interchangeable[86]; AMG monitors cannot be used in procedures that require the patient's arms to be tucked under the surgical drapes unless the arm is protected in a specifically designed tube[87]; and during recovery from neuromuscular block, AMG-derived TOF values are less precise than EMG values and overestimate the extent of EMG-derived recovery.[88,89] Baseline (prerelaxant) TOF values measured with AMG are generally greater than 1.0 (100%), and may in fact be as high as 147%.

Table 21-10 Relationship between Various Clinical Signs and Peak Inspiratory Force in Healthy Awake Volunteers during Partial Neuromuscular Block

Parameter	Peak Inspiratory Force (cm H_2O)
Control (no neuromuscular block)	−90
5-second head lift	−53
Effective swallowing	−43
Patent airway without jaw lift	−39
Glottic closure against Valsalva maneuver	−30
Vital capacity > 33% of control	−20

At baseline, volunteers could generate a peak inspiratory force of −90 cm H_2O and perform all maneuvers. Following partial paralysis, the ability to maintain a patent airway (−39 cm H_2O) and swallow effectively (−43 cm H_2O) was not assured even when the peak inspiratory force was −30 cm H_2O.

Zwiers A, van den Heuvel M, Smeets J, et al. Assessment of the potential for displacement interactions with sugammadex: a pharmacokinetic-pharmacodynamic modelling approach. *Clin Drug Investig.* 2011;31:101–111; data from Pavlin EG, Holle RH, Schoene RB. Recovery of airway protection compared with ventilation in humans after paralysis with curare. *Anesthesiology.* 1989;70:381–385.

This overshoot necessitates "normalization"—or calculation of the percent recovery of the TOF as a function of the higher TOF ratio prior to tracheal extubation.[90] Newer AMG-based monitors employ three-dimensional accelerometers to improve consistency and reliability, but most of the rest of the limitations remain.

Measurement of displacement (*kinemyography [KMG]*) is a form of mechanomyography in which an electrical current is generated by bending of a mechanosensor (metallic strip). The molded strip is placed in the groove between the thumb and index finger; ulnar nerve stimulation produces APM contraction and bends the strip, generating a current. KMG is simple to use, but the results obtained are not interchangeable with those obtained with other technologies. For instance, a TOF ratio of 0.90 measured with KMG is equivalent to an EMG-obtained TOF ratio of 0.80. The limits of agreement between the two technologies, moreover, can be as low as 0.65 or as high as 1.0.[91] Another limitation is that KMG (similar to AMG) needs a freely moving thumb, and is very susceptible to arm or hand movement that will change the baseline and therefore introduce inaccuracy in subsequent measurements. Nevertheless, KMG is accepted as a valuable monitor in daily clinical practice.

Differential Muscle Sensitivity

It has long been appreciated that NMBAs do not affect all muscles at the same time, nor produce the same depth of relaxation. It is also important to note that NMBAs are administered in order to produce good intubating conditions, vocal cord paralysis, abdominal muscle relaxation, or diaphragmatic immobility. Yet, clinicians do not monitor laryngeal muscles, abdominal muscles, or the diaphragm. Understanding the relationship between the response of the different muscles to the effects of NMBAs is therefore clinically important.

The APM is monitored most commonly (subjectively or objectively). Being a peripheral muscle, the onset time at the APM is delayed compared to centrally located muscles, where blood flow (and thus drug delivery) is greater. However, the APM is more sensitive to nondepolarizing NMBAs, so recovery is delayed in comparison to central muscles (diaphragm, laryngeal muscles; Fig. 21-12). Even monitoring of similar peripheral muscles can induce error: stimulation of the ulnar nerve produces flexion of the fifth finger as well as APM contraction. However, the recovery of the fifth finger contraction occurs more rapidly than at the APM, so making clinical decisions based on recovery of the fifth finger will overestimate the degree of recovery at other muscles (Table 21-11).

When the patient's arms are not available for intraoperative monitoring, clinicians will often monitor facial muscles: innervation of the facial nerve and evaluation of contractions of the eye muscles, either the orbicularis oculi or the corrugator supercilii. However, the time course of recovery is not the same for these two facial muscles: the orbicularis oculi moves the eyelid and have a recovery time course similar to the APM. In contrast, the eyebrow muscle, the corrugator supercilii, has a time course similar to the central muscles, the laryngeal adductors (Fig. 21-12).

Less commonly, monitoring of neuromuscular blockade takes place using the flexor hallucis brevis in the lower extremity, which produces contraction of the great toe. The time course of this muscle is similar to that of the APM.

Electrode Placement

For monitoring the APM, stimulating electrodes are placed along the ulnar nerve, on the volar surface of the forearm. The distal (negative) electrode is placed 2 cm proximal to the wrist crease, and the proximal (positive) electrode is placed along the ulnar nerve, 3 to 4 cm proximal to the negative electrode (Fig. 21-10E).

A common clinical practice is to place the stimulating electrodes on the face and to monitor the eyelid (orbicularis oculi) muscle. Improper placement of electrodes on the temple and lower jaw may lead to direct muscle stimulation and false assessment of neuromuscular recovery. In fact, current clinical practice of monitoring "eye muscles" has been shown to result in a fivefold increased risk of postoperative residual paralysis.[92] Placement of the stimulating electrodes just lateral to the eye or along the zygomatic arch, as done most commonly in the clinical setting, may activate other facial muscles and confound assessment. The facial nerve is best stimulated at the anterior portion of the mastoid process, as the nerve exits the cranial vault, with the second electrode in front of the ear. Even with optimal electrode positioning, however, muscle responses can be elicited despite complete block due to direct muscle stimulation. Neurostimulation of the posterior tibial nerve along the medial malleolus produces flexion contraction of the great toe. The time course of neuromuscular block monitored at the great toe is similar to that at the APM.

Monitoring and Clinical Applications

Knowledge of time course for onset, duration, and recovery of neuromuscular block of NMBAs is important for optimal patient care. A current definition of "adequate" recovery is also important, as the *threshold of adequate recovery* has changed over the past 30 years. Currently, the recovery of a calibrated, normalized TOF ratio to 0.90 or more is considered the threshold (minimum requirement) for full recovery of neuromuscular function. At this level of recovery, most of the respiratory and other motor functions have returned to the prerelaxant state. Conversely, postoperative pulmonary function test (PFT) values (forced vital capacity and peak expiratory flow) can be decreased by 20% in patients who experience residual neuromuscular block.[93] Similarly, impairment in the ability to swallow and resultant aspiration of pharyngeal fluids can be observed in healthy volunteers who had achieved TOF ratios as high as 0.90 (Fig. 21-13).[94] Respiratory muscle weakness (measured by maximum inspiratory and expiratory pressures, forced vital capacity, and forced expiratory volume in 1 second) was noted following major abdominal

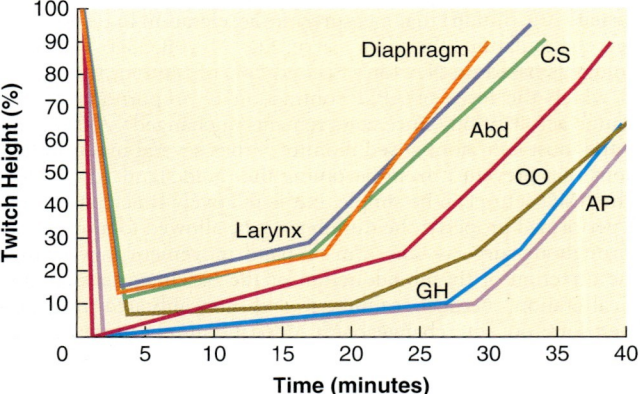

Figure 21-12 Approximate time course of twitch height after rocuronium, 0.6 mg/kg, at different muscles. Larynx, laryngeal adductors (vocal cords); CS, corrugator supercilii muscle (eyebrow); Abd, abdominal muscles; OO, orbicularis oculi muscle (eyelid); GH, geniohyoid muscle (upper airway); AP, adductor pollicis muscle (thumb).

Table 21-11 Suggested Management of Neuromuscular Blockade According to Monitoring

Site	Modality	Response	Interpretation	Comments
Prediction of Tracheal Intubating Conditions				
Any site	Single twitch, TOF	Present	Adequate conditions not met	Deep blockade is required for intubation
Corrugator supercilii	Single twitch, TOF	Absent	Adequate conditions likely	Corrugator supercilii reflects vocal cords and diaphragm
Adductor pollicis	Single twitch, TOF	Absent	Adequate conditions likely only if high dose given	Adductor pollicis is more sensitive than vocal cords and diaphragm
Flexor hallucis (foot)	Single twitch, TOF	Absent	Adequate conditions likely only if high dose given	Foot muscles are sensitive and block late
Intraoperative Conditions				
Adductor pollicis	PTC	1–2	Deep blockade	Return of diaphragm movements possible, no TOF response at adductor pollicis
Corrugator supercilii	TOF	1–2	Deep blockade	Return of abdominal tone possible, no TOF response at adductor pollicis
Adductor pollicis	TOF	1–2	Moderate blockade	Usually sufficient for most procedures
Corrugator supercilii	TOF	4, with or without fade	Moderate to shallow blockade	Difficult to interpret without adductor pollicis data
Adductor pollicis	TOF	4, with or without fade	Shallow blockade	Additional relaxation might be needed
Management of Recovery				
Adductor pollicis	PTC	0	Wait or sugammadex 16 mg/kg	Sugammadex after rocuronium or vecuronium only
Adductor pollicis	PTC	1–2	Wait or sugammadex 4 mg/kg	
Corrugator supercilii	TOF	1–2	Wait or sugammadex 4 mg/kg	
Adductor pollicis	TOF	2	Wait or sugammadex 2 mg/kg	
Corrugator supercilii	TOF	4, with or without fade	Wait or correlate with adductor pollicis or sugammadex 4 mg/kg	Corrugator supercilii recovers early. Correlation with adductor pollicis preferable
Hypothenar eminence (fifth finger)	TOF	4, with or without fade	Observe thumb motion	Adductor pollicis recovers later
Adductor pollicis	TOF, visual or tactile	4, with fade	Wait or neostigmine 0.04–0.05 mg/kg or sugammadex 2 mg/kg	Neostigmine: After any nondepolarizing agent
Adductor pollicis	TOF, visual or tactile	4, without fade	Wait or neostigmine 0.020 mg/kg	
Adductor pollicis	DBS, visual or tactile	Fade	Wait or neostigmine 0.02–0.05 mg/kg	Less neostigmine needed if no TOF fade
Adductor pollicis	DBS, visual or tactile	No fade	Wait or neostigmine 0.020 mg/kg	DBS fade detected when TOF ratio = 0.6
Adductor pollicis	TOF, quantitative	TOF ratio <0.90	Wait or neostigmine	Neostigmine 0.04–0.05 mg/kg if TOF ratio <0.4; 0.02 mg/kg if TOF ratio >0.4
Adductor pollicis	100 Hz TET	No fade	No reversal necessary	100 Hz TET fade detected when TOF ratio = 0.8–0.9
Adductor pollicis	TOF, quantitative	TOF ratio ≥0.9	No reversal necessary	Full recovery

TOF, train of four; PTC, posttetanic count; DBS, double burst stimulation; TET, 5-sec tetanic stimulation.
Actual management depends on patient, surgical procedure, and previous response to neuromuscular blocking agents. *See Table 21-12 for classification of depth of neuromuscular block.

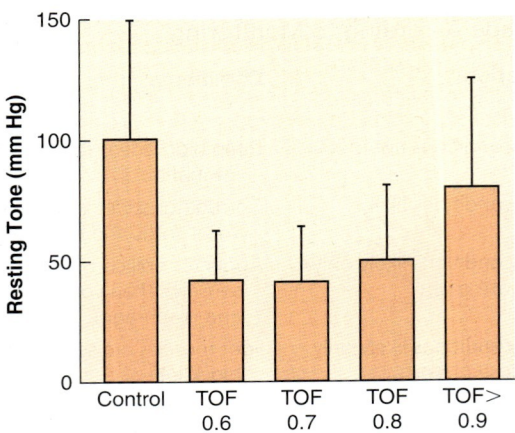

Figure 21-13. Upper esophageal resting tone in volunteers given vecuronium. Train-of-four (TOF) ratio was measured at the adductor pollicis muscle. Statistically significant decreases compared with control were found at all levels of paralysis until TOF ratio >0.9. (Adapted from Eriksson LI, Sundman E, Olsson R, et al. Functional assessment of the pharynx at rest and during swallowing in partially paralyzed humans: Simultaneous videomanometry and mechanomyography of awake human volunteers. *Anesthesiology.* 1997;87:1035.)

surgery, and the presence of residual neuromuscular paralysis was not ruled out until an acceleromyographic TOF ratio threshold of at least 1.0.[95] For these reasons, this threshold (TOF ≥0.90) should be the minimum accepted level of neuromuscular function, particularly in the elderly, in patients with pulmonary disease, or patients at risk of pulmonary aspiration.[96]

For assessing the quality of intubating conditions, monitoring of central muscles (or peripheral muscles with time course similar to central muscles) is paramount. When the dose of nondepolarizing NMBA is sufficiently large to offset the relative resistance of central muscles, onset at the laryngeal muscles will be faster than at the APM because of greater blood flow (and drug delivery; Fig. 21-12 and Table 21-11).

A special clinical challenge presents when surgery requires an *intense (profound)* or *deep level of intraoperative block* (see Reversal of Intense (Profound) Neuromuscular Block) (Table 21-12). This can be accomplished with larger doses of nondepolarizing NMBAs, but at the expense of markedly prolonging the duration of block, and increasing the likelihood of residual neuromuscular block and its complications. If a level of block that prevents diaphragmatic movement is required, the depth of block can be monitored with PTC—a PTC of 1 or 2 should be sufficient for most surgeries. At this level of block, reversal may be achieved with a medium dose of sugammadex (4 mg/kg). In contrast, spontaneous recovery of at least a TOFC of 2 or 3 should have occurred before attempting pharmacologic reversal with anticholinesterases (see Reversal of Neuromuscular Blockage). Patients managed with deep intraoperative block are at particular risk for postoperative residual paralysis, which is associated with an increased risk of silent aspiration, hypoxemia, need for reintubation, and prolonged stay in the postanesthesia care unit (PACU).[76]

It should also be noted that *monitoring of the depth of anesthesia* using the bispectral index (BIS monitor) may be affected by muscle activity. The BIS monitor is sensitive to changes in EMG activity, and the BIS values in awake, paralyzed volunteers decreased in response to neuromuscular paralysis to levels associated with general anesthesia (BIS values of 44 to 47).[97] The effect of NMB on depth of anesthesia monitors, however, remains controversial. Although one report suggested that both BIS and the spectral entropy levels (Entropy) may remain unchanged after sugammadex reversal of rocuronium block,[98] others have reported increases in the numerical values of BIS and Entropy during reversal of rocuronium-induced block by sugammadex (and neostigmine).[99,100]

Reversal of Neuromuscular Blockade

Anticholinesterase Agents

Blocking or inhibiting the breakdown of ACh at the NMJ results in an increase in the available pool of ACh at the synaptic cleft and better chances of competing with the nondepolarizing NMBA for binding to the receptor's α-subunit; this binding of ACh to nAChR results in normal transmission. There are three clinically available acetylcholinesterase inhibitors (anticholinesterase agents) in clinical use today: neostigmine, edrophonium, and pyridostigmine. These cholinesterase inhibitors are quaternary compounds and do not cross the blood–brain barrier in sufficient concentrations to have central effects. Their duration of action, at equivalent doses, is similar (60 to 120 minutes), but onset of action is fastest for edrophonium, intermediate for neostigmine, and longest for pyridostigmine. Physostigmine, another cholinesterase inhibitor, is a tertiary amine, but because it crosses the blood–brain barrier (and has central effects), it is not used for pharmacologic reversal of neuromuscular block. Edrophonium, similar to all cholinesterase inhibitors, is ineffective in reversing

Table 21-12 Classification of Depth of Nondepolarizing Neuromuscular Block Based on Subjective and Objective Criteria

Depth of Block	Posttetanic Count (PTC)	Train-of-Four Count (TOFC)	Subjective Train-of-Four (TOF) Ratio	Measured (Actual) Train-of-Four (TOF) Ratio
Intense (profound) block	0	0	0	0
Deep block	≥1	0	0	0
Moderate block	NA	1–3	0	0
Light (shallow) block	NA	4	Fade present	0.1–0.4
Minimal block	NA	4	No fade	>0.4 but <0.90
Full recovery	NA	4	No fade	≥0.90–1.00

NA, data not available.
Modified from Fuchs-Buder T, Claudius C, Skovgaard LT, et al. 8th International Neuromuscular Meeting: Good clinical research practice in pharmacodynamic studies of neuromuscular blocking agents II: the Stockholm revision. *Acta Anaesthesiol Scand.* 2007;51:789–808.

deep block, and it is used infrequently as a first-line agent, unless other agents are unavailable (see Drug Shortages and Clinical Impact). Because of its longer onset time than neostigmine, pyridostigmine is used rarely in anesthesia practice to antagonize neuromuscular block; it is used most often as an oral cholinesterase inhibitor for the treatment of myasthenia gravis. Neostigmine is the most frequently used anticholinesterase agent today, although a new, more effective agent recently has been approved in the United States (see Selective Relaxant Binding Agents).

Neostigmine

All cholinesterase inhibitors, including neostigmine, block acetylcholinesterases and result in increased concentrations of ACh at the NMJ, increasing the size and duration of EPPs, and facilitating normal neuromuscular transmission. Neostigmine's inhibitory effects are concentration dependent, and at higher concentrations ($>2.5 \times 10^{-5}$ M) it may have a direct action to block the ACh receptor.[101] Because acetylcholinesterase is blocked at all cholinergic synapses, all cholinesterase inhibitors have significant parasympathomimetic effects. For this reason, they are generally coadministered with either glycopyrrolate (which has a slower onset of action similar to neostigmine) or atropine (which has a more rapid onset of action similar to edrophonium). Neostigmine as a reversal agent has a ceiling effect, and may be limited in its ability to antagonize the neuromuscular block beyond neuromuscular function equivalent to a TOF ratio of 0.6. Increasing the dose beyond 70 μg/kg is not recommended, as this dose may induce neuromuscular dysfunction. Similarly, administration of even small doses of neostigmine (30 μg/kg) at a time when recovery of neuromuscular function is almost complete may produce upper airway collapse and may decrease the activity of the genioglossus muscle.[102]

In the pediatric population, residual neuromuscular block can be associated with serious complications, and NMBA reversal with neostigmine is routine in many settings. However, there are currently few if any data on the effectiveness or safety of routine neostigmine use in the pediatric population.[103]

Factors Affecting Reversal

The rate of cholinesterase inhibitor-aided recovery depends on several factors: *depth of neuromuscular block* at the time of pharmacologic reversal; *dose of cholinesterase inhibitor; type of NMBA* (long-acting vs. intermediate-acting); *patient age; anesthesia type* (total intravenous anesthesia [TIVA] vs. inhalational anesthesia). When administered at a *deep degree of block,* such as PTC of 1 or 2, duration of neostigmine-induced reversal (to a TOF ≥0.90) may be over 50 to 60 minutes, with a very wide range of recovery times of 46 to 312 minutes.[104] When administered at this level of deep block (PTC of 1 to 2), 23% of patients receiving neostigmine required more than 60 minutes for full recovery.[105] The literature suggests that reversal should not be attempted at a deep level of block for at least two reasons. First, studies have shown that "early" reversal (5 minutes after vecuronium or rocuronium administration when the TOF count is 0) does not confer any advantage over reversal at TOF count of 3 or 4: total recovery time was similar and independent of the timing of neostigmine administration.[106] Second, it is known that neostigmine-induced recovery is characterized by an initial rapid (and partial) recovery, followed by a later slower recovery (Fig. 21-14). If neostigmine is administered at a deep block, the initial rapid recovery will occur during a blind period, when no responses are possible (or visible), followed by a slow and prolonged recovery at shallower depths of block. The time course of this slower phase will occur during recovery of TOF ratio when subjective evaluation of residual fade is inadequate (TOF of 0.4 to 0.9), and when the patient is at increased risk of critical respiratory events due to premature tracheal extubation. On the other hand, if neostigmine reversal is administered later (or is effected with sugammadex), once spontaneous recovery progresses to a TOFC of 3 or 4, the initial rapid recovery from neostigmine will effect a return of TOF ratio toward normal, followed by a slower and later recovery to TOF of 1.0.[107]

It should also be mentioned that clinical practice sometimes differs from what scientific data show. Attempts at pharmacologic reversal using doses of neostigmine larger than 70 μg/kg or using a combination of cholinesterase inhibitors (e.g., neostigmine plus edrophonium) in an attempt to hasten pharmacologic reversal should be avoided. Cholinesterase inhibitors inhibit cholinesterases, and once they are 100% inhibited, no additional dose or type of inhibitor will be able to further increase the concentration of ACh at the NMJ to facilitate normal neuromuscular transmission. At this point, additional cholinesterase inhibitors may actually block the ACh receptors, leading to neuromuscular weakness.[101]

Most *inhalational anesthetic agents* potentiate neuromuscular block to varying degrees (desflurane > sevoflurane > isoflurane > halothane > nitrous oxide), whereas intravenous anesthetic techniques (for instance, based on propofol and/or opioid) will have minimal, if any, NMBA potentiation effects. When neostigmine 70 μg/kg is administered to antagonize a *moderate* degree of block (tactilely determined TOFC of 1), a dose of $2 \times ED_{95}$ of rocuronium requires an average of 8.6 minutes (range 5 to 19 minutes) for recovery to TOF of 0.9 during propofol-maintained anesthesia; the same dose of rocuronium requires 28.6 minutes (range 9 to 76 minutes) during sevoflurane-based anesthesia.[108] However, even during anesthetic techniques that do not potentiate NMBAs (such as nitrous oxide/propofol-based anesthesia), neostigmine reversal from a tactile-guided TOFC of 3 to recovery of TOF = 0.9 may require 17 minutes (range 8 to 46 minutes).[109]

The speed of reversal from *light* and *minimal* nondepolarizing block is markedly increased by neostigmine, as is the effectiveness of this reversal. Reversal of atracurium (during nitrous oxide/enflurane anesthesia) from T1 values of 40% to 50% of control (TOFC of 4 with fade) to TOF at least 0.70 using neostigmine 20 μg/kg required 4.5 minutes (range 3 to 8 minutes). When the neostigmine dose was increased to 40 μg/kg and 80 μg/kg (a dose that is currently not recommended for use, regardless of the depth of neuromuscular block), the recovery times were 3.0 (range 2 to 5) minutes and 2.3 (range 1 to 4) minutes, respectively, a statistically (and clinically) insignificant change.[110] The authors concluded that neostigmine 20 μg/kg is the optimum dose when atracurium-induced *light* (shallow) block is antagonized. A similar dose of neostigmine (20 μg/kg) was found effective in reversing rocuronium-induced *minimal* block.[111]

These data emphasize that the time from neostigmine (or any cholinesterase inhibitor) administration until full recovery (TOF ≥0.90) depends on the number of molecules of nondepolarizing NMBA in the body, the NMBA duration (long- vs. short-acting), factors affecting the NMBA elimination from the body, and the dose of neostigmine administered. In turn, the number of NMBA molecules in the body at the time of reversal depends on the total dose of NMBA administered during the case; the total duration of continuous (or intermittent) NMBA administration; and the time between the last NMBA dose and neostigmine administration. These factors underscore and explain why neostigmine-induced reversal of deep block may take upwards of 300 minutes, as recovery from this depth of block is mostly driven by spontaneous recovery.

Reversal of *minimal* neuromuscular block (TOF ratio of 0.40 and 0.60) to a TOF of 0.9 using neostigmine 10, 20, and 30 μg/kg during TIVA was reported to be shorter than spontaneous recovery.[112] Reduced doses of neostigmine (20 μg/kg) were required to

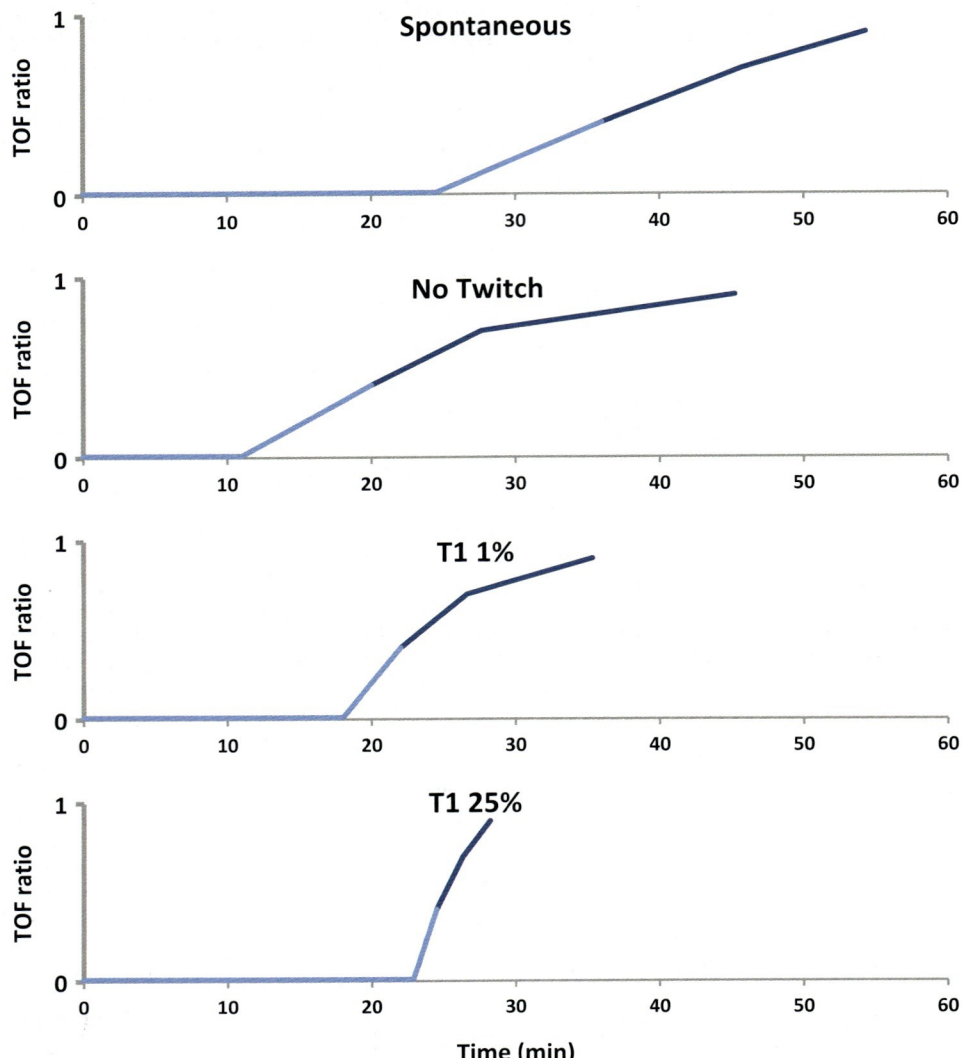

Figure 21-14 Time from injection of rocuronium until recovery to train of-four (TOF) ratio of 0.9 in adults. Reversal with neostigmine was either spontaneous or neostigmine was administered 5 minutes after rocuronium (no twitch), or at 1% twitch recovery (T1 1%), or at 25% twitch recovery (T1 25%). The TOF ratio is indicated against time until a TOF ratio of 0.9 was reached (end of the line). Time is shorter when neostigmine is given at T1 25%, than it is at reappearance of T1. This strategy also minimizes duration of blind paralysis (*dark blue segment*), when the TOF ratio is between 0.4 and 0.9 and fade is difficult to detect by visual or tactile means. (Data from Bevan JC, Collins L, Fowler C, et al. Early and late reversal of rocuronium and vecuronium with neostigmine in adults and children. *Anesth Analg.* 1999;89:333–339.)

reach reversal (TOF of ≥0.90) from a TOF ratio of either 0.4 or 0.6 with a 100% probability in the setting of atracurium-induced block during TIVA anesthetic.[112]

The TOF data were nonnormalized acceleromyographic ratios.[112] The AMG-based recovery times to a TOF ratio of 1.0 (complete recovery) are equivalent with the measurements obtained with MMG or EMG monitors to a TOF ratio of 0.90.[113] Similar results were reported using rocuronium; during TIVA-based anesthetic and EMG monitoring, a rocuronium-induced block was antagonized from a TOF ratio of 0.50 with various doses of neostigmine. The recovery time to a TOF ratio of 0.90 was 2.0 minutes (range 2 to 4 minutes) after neostigmine 40 μg/kg.[114] Low-dose neostigmine (10 μg/kg) administered to antagonize shallow atracurium block (TOF 0.6 to 0.9) during desflurane anesthesia required 5 minutes (range 3 to 8 minutes).[115] Compared with spontaneous recovery, neostigmine 10 μg/kg effected a faster recovery to TOF of 0.9. It should be pointed out, however, that the conclusion that neostigmine 10 μg/kg is effective in antagonizing this level of block is based on data from 12 patients; outlier patients who might require significantly longer recovery times are likely. For instance, a 2016 study found that even at a threshold TOFC of 4 (TOF ratio ≥0.20), neostigmine was not a 100% reliable antagonist of rocuronium-induced nondepolarizing block.[116]

Given the well-known variability in patient responses to NMBAs, we must ensure that there are no outlier patients who require unexpectedly long times for adequate neuromuscular recovery. Since there are no data to unequivocally demonstrate the reliability of a 10 μg/kg dose of neostigmine for reversal of light or minimal neuromuscular block, neostigmine doses of less than 20 μg/kg cannot be recommended.

Regardless of when administered, neostigmine-induced reversal is always faster than spontaneous recovery. Larger doses of neostigmine will also be more effective than lower doses in effecting neuromuscular block reversal—within the dose ranges in which neostigmine is effective (i.e., at doses less than the maximum 60 to 70 μg/kg). Although there is no difference in the speed of recovery induced by neostigmine among the intermediate-acting nondepolarizing NMBAs, reversal is prolonged when used with long-acting agents such as pancuronium.[117,118] Age also affects neostigmine-induced speed of reversal, being faster (and likely more complete) in children than in adults, and slower in the elderly.[106] Finally, drugs and conditions that potentiate the effect of nondepolarizing NMBAs will also prolong neostigmine-induced recovery: volatile anesthetics, aminoglycoside antibiotics, magnesium, opioids (because of the hypercarbia and acidosis they induce), and hypothermia.

Other Effects

Neostigmine (and the other anticholinesterases) induce vagal stimulation, so anticholinergic agents are usually coadministered. Atropine is faster in onset than glycopyrrolate, produces more tachycardia, and crosses the blood–brain barrier. For these reasons, glycopyrrolate is generally preferred. It is slower in onset and induces less tachycardia; for these reasons, it is preferred especially in patients with coronary artery disease. Neostigmine has been associated with prolongation of cardiac repolarization (prolonged corrected QT interval, QTc), which may trigger malignant ventricular arrhythmias (torsade de pointes).[119] Other side effects of neostigmine include increased salivation and bowel motility; although the anticholinergic agents are effective in preventing salivation, their effects on bowel motility are limited. Several recent meta-analyses of the effects of neostigmine on postoperative nausea and vomiting (PONV) in adult patients have not been able to conclusively show a connection.[120,121] When sugammadex- and neostigmine-induced pharmacologic reversal of neuromuscular block were compared with regard to incidence of PONV in adults, avoidance of neostigmine only slightly and transiently reduced PONV, but antiemetic and analgesic consumption was similar.[120] In the pediatric population, a recent systematic review of the literature has found no study that satisfied the inclusion criteria to determine whether neostigmine should be used routinely to reverse neuromuscular blockade, or to determine whether the use of neostigmine is associated with an increased incidence of nausea and vomiting.[103]

As previously noted, halogenated anesthetics potentiate neuromuscular block, and when continued after administration of neostigmine, they will prolong time to full reversal (TOF >0.90). Similarly, treatment with magnesium sulfate will slow neostigmine-induced spontaneous recovery.[122]

It is well known that administration of neostigmine to subjects who had not received any nondepolarizing NMBA may result in a significant reduction in the peak tetanic muscle contraction and severe tetanic fade; these effects persist for about 20 minutes, while the ST is slightly potentiated.[123] Similarly, an atracurium-induced neuromuscular block that corresponded to a TOF ratio of either 0.50 or 0.90 was established, followed by the administration of two doses of neostigmine 2.5 mg each, given 5 minutes apart. The effect of neostigmine on the depth of block was monitored with TOF and tetanic stimuli.[124] The first neostigmine dose antagonized the block, whereas the second 2.5-mg dose diminished tetanic height and increased tetanic fade, although it had minimal effects on the TOF measurement.

More significant effects on respiratory function were reported when neostigmine was administered after full recovery from neuromuscular block; there was a significant impairment of the upper airway dilator ability as a result of impaired genioglossus muscle and diaphragmatic function.[102,125,126] It should be noted that the preceding should not be interpreted as an argument in favor of omitting pharmacologic reversal; neostigmine-induced recovery is always faster than spontaneous recovery. The only remaining variable is the appropriateness of neostigmine administration as it relates to timing and dose.[127] The typical recovery curve for NMBAs (or any drug) is depicted in Figure 21-15. After administration of an intubating dose of a nondepolarizing NMBA, the depth of block may be profound (Table 21-12). At this depth of block, neostigmine will be ineffective, and should not be administered.

At the other extreme of this recovery curve, once the objectively measured TOF ratio is above 0.9 (full neuromuscular recovery), neostigmine reversal is unnecessary; in fact, if administered, it may induce respiratory muscle and diaphragmatic weakness. Full reversal (doses of neostigmine of 60 to 70 μg/kg) should be administered once the TOFC is at least 3 (preferably, 4) and when the TOF ratio is less than 0.4 (fade is present on subjective evaluation). In the absence of quantitative monitoring to ensure full recovery, even TOFCs of 4 without fade (determined subjectively) should prompt pharmacologic reversal. However, in these circumstances, doses of neostigmine of 20 to 30 μg/kg are sufficient to reliably assure satisfactory return of neuromuscular function within approximately 10 minutes (Fig. 21-15). While these guidelines may offer the clinician some broad parameters for improving the efficacy of pharmacologic reversal using cholinesterase inhibitors based on subjective evaluation of neuromuscular function, an optimal reversal strategy can only be assured if clinical decisions are based on quantitative assessment of the depth of neuromuscular block (see Monitoring Neuromuscular Blockade). As already noted, subjective (tactile, visual) assessment and clinical testing are inadequate substitutes for objective (quantitative) monitoring.

Drug Shortages and Clinical Impact

Drug shortages have existed for decades, but the number of drugs on the shortage list and the duration of shortages have increased significantly in the last decade.[128] There are several reasons for drug shortages, including the scarcity of raw materials, industry consolidation that trims redundant manufacturers, inconsistent and variable manufacturing quality control, and discontinuation of older drugs by manufacturers in favor of newer, more profitable alternatives. In 2011, the U.S. Food and Drug Administration (FDA) published revised guidance on "marketing of unapproved drugs" and established "an orderly approach

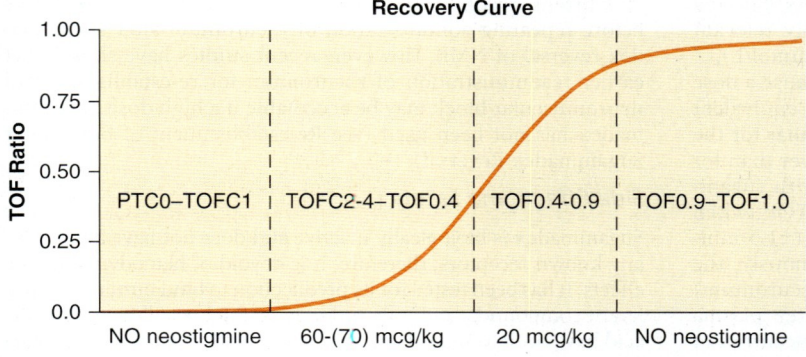

Figure 21-15 Neuromuscular blocking agent recovery curve and recommendations for pharmacologic (neostigmine) reversal of neuromuscular block. Typical recovery curve for a nondepolarizing neuromuscular blocking agent (NMBA), from maximal depth of block (PTC = 0) to full recovery (TOF ratio = 1.0). Dosing recommendations for administration of cholinesterase antagonism (neostigmine) are shown on the x-axis at four depths of neuromuscular block. TOF, train-of-four; PTC, posttetanic count; PTC0, posttetanic count of 0; TOFC, train-of-four count; TOFC1, train-of-four count of 1.

for removing unapproved drugs from the market." Neostigmine was one of the drugs that had not been FDA approved. A proprietary, FDA-approved preparation of neostigmine methylsulphate was later marketed as Bloxiverz (Eclat Pharmaceuticals, Chesterfield, MO). Following FDA approval, the manufacturing company requested that the FDA remove all unapproved (generic and much cheaper) neostigmine formulations from the market; currently, Bloxiverz is the only available neostigmine preparation, at a price at least six times as much as its "unapproved" predecessors. Other pharmaceutical companies are authorized distributors of Bloxiverz. In many clinical settings, the disappearance from the market of generic (and much less expensive) neostigmine has forced clinicians to seek alternative cholinesterase inhibitors, including edrophonium.

Edrophonium

Edrophonium is an anticholinesterase agent that is used clinically for reversal of nondepolarizing neuromuscular block. It is much faster in onset and to peak antagonism (1 to 2 minutes) than neostigmine (7 to 11 minutes) or pyridostigmine (12 to 16 minutes).[129] Edrophonium is also less effective as an antagonist than neostigmine, as it forms ionic (and much weaker) bonds with the acetylcholinesterase enzyme, rather than the stronger, covalent bonds that neostigmine forms.[130] Its elimination half-life is 33 to 110 minutes, and 67% of the dose is excreted renally. Because of its lower affinity for acetylcholinesterases, edrophonium should only be used to antagonize a shallow block (TOFC of 4). The usual dose of edrophonium is 0.50 mg/kg (approximately $4 \times ED_{95}$).

Edrophonium's duration of antagonism (66 minutes) is similar to that of neostigmine (76 minutes), but shorter than that of pyridostigmine.[129] Doses of 0.75 mg/kg provide minimal increases in efficacy over the 0.5 mg/kg dose.[131] Because of its propensity to induce bradycardia and its more rapid onset of action than neostigmine, edrophonium is usually administered in conjunction with atropine (as Enlon-Plus). The administration of the combination drug in divided doses over several minutes, as opposed to rapid bolus administration, will result in a lower peak plasma concentration of both agents, and will minimize the potential for bradycardia (from edrophonium) or tachycardia (from atropine).

Selective Relaxant Binding Agents

Sugammadex

Sugammadex is an FDA-approved gamma-cyclodextrin that has been developed as an selective relaxant binding agent (SRBA).[132,133] It is an eight-membered ring with a central cavity that perfectly encapsulates the steroid nucleus of steroidal intermediate-acting NMBAs (rocuronium>vecuronium >>pancuronium/pipecuronium)[21]—but has no affinity for any of the other depolarizing or nondepolarizing NMBAs. Binding to rocuronium is extremely tight, with no clinically relevant dissociation (dissociation constant estimate of 0.055 μmol/L).[134] Binding to vecuronium is one-third as tight, but because a dose of vecuronium has 6 times fewer molecules than an equivalent rocuronium dose, the effectiveness of reversal is similar for the two drugs. The affinity for pancuronium may be lower than for other aminosteroids, although successful reversal with sugammadex (4 mg/kg) from reappearance of the second TOF twitch (T2) has been accomplished in less than 3 minutes (±1.5 minutes).[19] Once sugammadex is administered intravenously, the rapid and complete binding to rocuronium (and vecuronium) occurs in the plasma, and the concentration of free plasma NMBA decreases rapidly. This decrease in plasma concentration of free NMBA leads to an increased concentration gradient between the biophase (NMJ) and plasma, resulting in movement of free NMBA back into the plasma. This movement of free NMBA from the NMJ back into plasma will occur as long as the concentration of free (unbound) sugammadex is sufficiently high. When this occurs, there is normalization of neuromuscular function (pharmacologic reversal).

Pharmacology

Sugammadex is highly water soluble and initial studies have shown it to be devoid of the side effects associated with the use of cholinesterase inhibitors and muscarinic antagonists.[135] The molecular weight of sugammadex is 2,178 daltons (Da), while that of rocuronium is 610 Da. Because the sugammadex/rocuronium complex occurs in a 1:1 molar ratio, 3.57 mg of sugammadex is required to bind to 1 mg of rocuronium. The 1:1 tight binding properties confer sugammadex significant advantages. The speed of reversal is dose dependent, and in general, larger sugammadex doses will hasten recovery. In doses of 2 mg/kg, sugammadex will antagonize both rocuronium and vecuronium from a TOFC of 2 to TOF of 0.9 in 2 to 4 minutes, a recovery that is significantly shorter than that induced by neostigmine.[136-139] When the level of neuromuscular block is deep (Table 21-12), larger sugammadex doses of 4 mg/kg are needed for recovery to TOF of 0.9, and the recovery time for sugammadex (geometric mean of 2.9 minutes) is significantly faster than the recovery following neostigmine (geometric mean of 50.4 minutes).[105] Reversal from profound block, such as that encountered during a failed RSII scenario in which mask ventilation is not possible (cannot-intubate-cannot-oxygenate [CICO]) requires doses of 16 mg/kg of sugammadex.[140] In this emergent situation, reversal of high-dose rocuronium with high-dose sugammadex is faster than spontaneous recovery from SCh for failed RSII (Fig. 21-16).[141] The rescue from CICO events can be effected as long as the induction agents and opioids administered do not interfere with spontaneous ventilation, and airway instrumentation has not caused airway swelling. Sugammadex (in rhesus monkey) also rapidly and effectively antagonizes the main metabolite of vecuronium, 3-desacetyl vecuronium, at a dose (0.5 to 1.0 mg/kg) that is lower than that required for reversal of vecuronium.[142]

Pharmacokinetics

The volume of distribution in adults approximates the ECF compartment. Metabolism of sugammadex is very limited, and it is eliminated primarily via renal excretion.[143] The sugammadex/rocuronium (or vecuronium) complex is also almost completely excreted by the renal route; its elimination half-life is approximately 100 minutes. In patients with severe renal impairment, both sugammadex and the sugammadex/rocuronium complex may be effectively removed with hemodialysis using a high-flux dialysis method.[144]

Current recommendations suggest waiting for 24 hours before repeating administration of rocuronium after sugammadex reversal of NMB. However, recent studies have shown that earlier readministration of rocuronium for re-establishment of neuromuscular block may be acceptable if a high dose of sugammadex has not been used (see Re-establishment of Block after Sugammadex Reversal).

Side Effects and Safety

Sugammadex is biologically inactive and does not have affinity for any known receptors; therefore, it is devoid of hemodynamic side effects. It has been tested for its predilection to bind hundreds of different compounds, and only toremifene, flucloxacillin, and fusidic acid have been found to bind to sugammadex.[134] *Oral contraception*

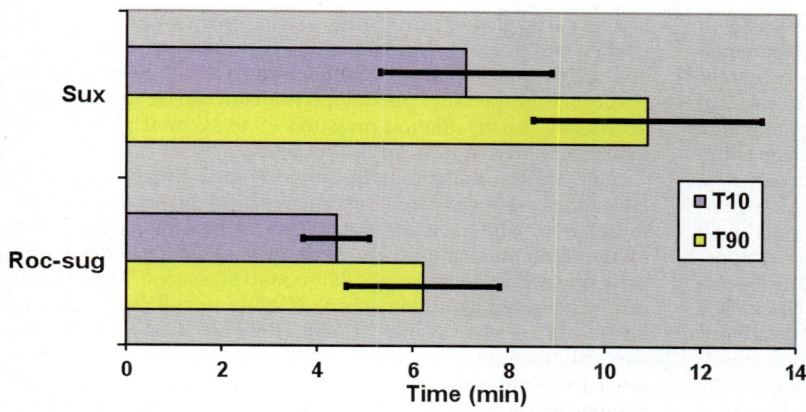

Figure 21-16 Duration of action of neuromuscular blockade with succinylcholine 1 mg/kg (Sux), and rocuronium 1.2 mg/kg followed 3 minutes later by sugammadex 16 mg/kg (Roc-sug). T10 and T90: Duration to 10% and 90% first twitch recovery, respectively. Bars indicate standard deviation. (Data from: Lee C, Jahr JS, Candiotti KA, et al. Reversal of profound neuromuscular block by sugammadex administered three minutes after rocuronium. *Anesthesiology*. 2009;110:1020–1025.)

may be affected, equivalent to missing one daily oral dose, and alternative means of birth control are recommended for a week after exposure to sugammadex. While the use of most cholinesterase antagonists (neostigmine, pyridostigmine) has been associated with prolongation of the QTc interval and with an increased risk of malignant arrhythmias (torsade de pointes), such an effect has not been associated with use of sugammadex, even in high doses.[119]

One of the major side effects associated with sugammadex administration has been the potential for *hypersensitivity reactions*. The perioperative prevalence of anaphylactic reactions is estimated to be between 1:3,500 and 1:20,000 procedures, with an associated mortality of up to 9%.[145] The main agents responsible for perioperative anaphylaxis are NMBAs, latex, antibiotics, hypnotics, opioids, and colloids. In a 2014 review, 15 cases of hypersensitivity to sugammadex were identified. In 93.3% of these cases, most of which met the World Anaphylaxis Organization criteria for anaphylaxis, the reactions occurred within the first 4 minutes after sugammadex administration.[146] For diagnosis of hypersensitivity reactions during general anesthesia, an elevated acute serum tryptase level is highly predictive of immunoglobulin-E (IgE)-mediated anaphylaxis.[147] Cardiovascular collapse following administration of sugammadex has been treated successfully with high-dose epinephrine and fluid resuscitation.[148]

The effects of sugammadex on *coagulation* have been investigated, and bleeding events within 24 hours of surgical procedures were reported in 2.9% of patients receiving sugammadex, compared with an incidence of postoperative bleeding of 4.1% in patients not exposed to the drug.[149] Compared with patients not exposed to sugammadex, increases of 5.5% in activated partial thromboplastin time (aPTT) and 3.0% in prothrombin time (PT) were observed 10 minutes after sugammadex administration; these values returned to baseline within 60 minutes.[149] In patients with a history of *pulmonary disease*, bronchospasm has an incidence similar to other drugs. Administered at a TOFC of 2, sugammadex 2 mg/kg rapidly and effectively reverses rocuronium in *renal failure* patients (creatinine clearance <30 mL/min) as quickly as in control patients (2 ± 0.7 minutes vs. 1.65 ± 0.63 minutes, respectively).[150] Deep neuromuscular block (PTC of 1 to 2) induced by rocuronium was reversed with sugammadex 4 mg/kg to full recovery (TOF >0.9) within a median of 3.1 minute (95% CI of 2.4 to 4.6 minutes) in renal patients (creatinine clearance <30 mL/min) versus patients with normal renal function (1.9 minutes, 95% CI of 1.6 to 2.8 minutes).[151] During mild intraoperative *hypothermia* (34.5°C to 35.0°C), sugammadex reversal of rocuronium-induced block was prolonged minimally (<1 minute).[152] Although certain antibiotics may potentiate postoperative neuromuscular block, administration of antibiotics prior to sugammadex reversal did not affect recovery time from rocuronium-induced block.[153]

Sugammadex has been marketed in Europe since 2009 without changes in its safety profile.

Clinical Use

Sugammadex is indicated for reversal of steroidal NMBAs, particularly rocuronium and vecuronium. Because it binds to the NMBA in a 1:1 molecular ratio, the recommended sugammadex dose is dependent on the depth of neuromuscular block. For immediate reversal of profound block (PTC = 0; Table 21-12), such as that achieved with 1.2 mg/kg rocuronium in the RSII scenario, a dose of sugammadex 16 mg/kg is recommended; for reversal of deep block (PTC = 1 to 2), a dose of 4 mg/kg is recommended; and for reversal of moderate block (TOFC of 1 to 2), the recommended dose is 2 mg/kg. In a dose of 1.0 mg/kg, sugammadex reverses rocuronium block from a TOFC of 4 in 2 minutes, whereas a dose of 0.5 mg/kg from the same depth of block requires 8 minutes.[154] In all these scenarios, reversal of block is typically accomplished in 2 to 3 minutes, as long as the sugammadex dose is sufficient to bind all of the free NMBA molecules in the plasma. In the morbidly obese patient, the dose of sugammadex has been calculated based on ideal body weight plus 40%. Alternatively, pooled analyses have indicated that recommended sugammadex doses based on actual body weight (in patients with BMI ≥30 kg/m^2) provided rapid and reliable recovery from neuromuscular block, and that no dosing adjustments were required.[155]

High-dose rocuronium for RSII and sugammadex-induced reversal may currently provide "near-ideal" neuromuscular block management without significant side effects: optimal intubating conditions with rocuronium, and rapid and effective reversal of block with sugammadex. In addition, such a drug combination may be preferable in clinical scenarios of CICO, as reversal of rocuronium with sugammadex may be quicker than waiting for spontaneous recovery of SCh.[141]

The *reliability* of sugammadex in reversing aminosteroid NMBA blockade has been documented, provided that sugammadex is administered in sufficient doses to encapsulate all NMBA molecules (see Sugammadex Pharmacology). However, as with any drug, there is a small but significant variability in patient response to sugammadex. A recent literature review[156] has documented that rare prolonged recovery times may occur after reversal with low doses (2 mg/kg) of sugammadex (up to 12 minutes,[157] with intermediate (4 mg/kg) doses (up to 22.3 minutes,[158] and even after high (16 mg/kg) doses (up to 16.6 minutes).[159] In special population groups such as the elderly (patients ≥75 years old); those with pulmonary, cardiac or renal disease; or those with body mass index (BMI) 40 or more–reversal to TOF 0.90 or more also can be prolonged.[139,144,157,160,161]

When used in the obese patient in suboptimal doses of 1 to 2 mg/kg, reparalysis has been reported.[162] In pediatric patients, a suboptimal dose of sugammadex also can lead to recurrent or residual paralysis.[163] Similar reports of reoccurrence of rocuronium-induced block (recurarization) after sugammadex reversal have been reported with administration of magnesium (60 mg/kg) for treatment of atrial fibrillation.[164] In contrast, when administered in adequate doses, the efficacy of sugammadex in reversing moderate and deep neuromuscular block was not affected by the administration of magnesium.[165] Importantly, if no neuromuscular monitoring is used intraoperatively, there is a significant risk of residual weakness (incidence of TOF < 0.9 as high as 9.4% of patients) even with administration of sugammadex 2 to 4 mg/kg.[166,167] Therefore, monitoring neuromuscular function to determine the appropriate dose of sugammadex and minimize the risk of residual block is strongly recommended.

The *effectiveness* of sugammadex-induced reversal of neuromuscular block was compared with that of neostigmine. The EMG activity of the diaphragm (EMGdi), as well as the tidal volume and oxygen saturation (PaO_2) were increased after sugammadex reversal compared with neostigmine, suggesting a more complete and faster recovery of the diaphragmatic ACh receptors.[168] A similar advantage of sugammadex over neostigmine reversal is reported as improved physiologic and nociceptive postoperative recovery, as well as superior patient satisfaction with recovery and anesthetic care.[169] Sugammadex-induced reversal was also associated with a lower incidence of PONV and with a reduced risk of pulmonary complications in elderly patients.[170]

One of the limiting factors to the wide adoption of sugammadex into routine clinical practice has been its relatively high acquisition cost; as of 2010, approximately $85, $170, and $506, for the 2 mg/kg, 4 mg/kg, and 16 mg/kg dose, respectively, for a typical 75-kg patient.[171] The cost of the drug in relation to the increased OR efficiency gained with its use (anesthesia OR time decreased from 144 minutes to 120 minutes) remains to be determined.[172]

Special Clinical Situations

Reversal in Patients with Neuromuscular Disorders

It is well known that patients with neuromuscular disorders may be at increased risk of complications from residual neuromuscular block. The use of sugammadex may be advantageous in such clinical situations, given its pharmacology and its rapid and predictable effects. Rapid and effective reversal of rocuronium-induced block without block reoccurrence has been reported in myotonic dystrophy and spinal muscular atrophy patients.[173] In patients with myasthenia gravis, judicious use of NMBAs is advocated; patients are generally resistant to the effects of SCh, although they are more sensitive to the effects of nondepolarizing NMBAs, particularly in more advanced disease states. For this reason, neuromuscular blocking drugs are generally avoided, and a deep inhalation anesthetic plus a regional anesthetic block are preferred. Since the introduction of sugammadex, multiple reports have documented the safety of NMBA reversal in patients with myasthenia gravis, both in elective and in emergency surgery that required RSII.[174-176]

Reversal of Intense (Profound) Neuromuscular Block

Laparoscopic and robotic surgical procedures present a particular challenge for both surgeons and anesthesiologists. Insufflation of the abdomen with carbon dioxide (pneumoperitoneum) facilitates the surgical procedure by allowing the surgeon a better field of vision. However, high pneumoperitoneum pressures (12 to 15 mmHg) that improve surgical exposure are associated with greater physiologic derangements (hypotension, tachycardia) and increase postoperative shoulder pain.[177] The hemodynamic effects of high-pressure pneumoperitoneum can be attenuated by decreasing the insufflation pressures (8 to 10 mmHg), but such maneuvers may worsen surgical exposure.

One way to address both surgical need (better exposure) and anesthesiologist need (maintenance of hemodynamic stability) is to achieve a profound level of neuromuscular block of the abdominal musculature, thereby allowing better surgical exposure at lower intra-abdominal pressures. These goals can be achieved by administering NMBAs in sufficient doses to obtain a PTC of 0 (Table 21-12). However, at the end of the surgical procedure, recovery from such an intense block is prolonged (60 minutes or more), and pharmacologic reversal with cholinesterase inhibitors (neostigmine) is contraindicated. Theoretically, all the ideal goals could be achieved by establishing intraoperative profound neuromuscular block (PTC of 0) with an aminosteroid NMBA (rocuronium) that would maximize surgical exposure at low intra-abdominal pressure (8 to 10 mmHg), followed by rapid (<5 minutes) and complete neuromuscular reversal with sugammadex. The literature on the actual benefits of such an approach, however, remains divided (Table 21-13). Some authors have shown that the enlargement of the surgical space (measured as the distance from the sacral promontory to the trocar) achieved with deep block was minor, and of "unknown clinical significance."[178] Others have shown that deep neuromuscular block reduced the intra-abdominal pressure requirements by up to 25%, particularly in younger females.[179] Deep neuromuscular block improved surgical conditions during laparoscopic hysterectomy, improved surgical field scores (rated by the surgeon), and prevented unacceptable surgical conditions.[180] Similar benefits of improved surgical conditions (scored on a five-point surgical rating scale) were described during retroperitoneal laparoscopies performed with deep neuromuscular block, and without adversely affecting the patients' perioperative cardiopulmonary conditions.[181] Although deep block facilitated surgical field visibility and prevented involuntary patient movement,[182] the benefits of deep block do not appear to be significant during low-pressure pneumoperitoneum.[183] Finally, the utility of moderate neuromuscular block (Table 21-12) in optimizing surgical conditions also has been investigated. A recent systematic review found that moderate block improved surgical conditions during open radical retropubic prostatectomy as well as laparoscopic cholecystectomy, nephrectomy, and prostatectomy.[184]

Until a clear and reproducible definition of surgical field exposure/visibility is developed, the interaction between intra-abdominal pressure and depth of block will likely remain controversial (Table 21-13).

Re-establishment of Block after Sugammadex Reversal

A specific clinical situation may occur when rapid re-establishment of neuromuscular block is needed after the patient has already received sugammadex. The drug's package insert recommends that at least 24 hours lapse before an aminosteroid NMBA is administered to patients who received sugammadex-induced reversal of neuromuscular block. Such a period would allow sufficient elimination of sugammadex via the renal route. In a recent report, rocuronium 1.0 mg/kg was administered 19 minutes after reversal with sugammadex; 3.5 minutes later, T1 was still present, and an additional 30 mg resulted in good intubating conditions. At the end of surgery, recovery was again facilitated with sugammadex,

(text continued on page 560)

Table 21-13 Summary of Randomized Trials Investigating the Relationship between Depth of Neuromuscular Block, Pneumoperitoneal (Intra-abdominal) Pressure and Outcome

Author	Surgery Type (number of patients)	NMBA Used	Depth of Block	IAP	Surgical Field Assessment	Results	Comments
Chassard *Anesth Analg* 1996;82:525	Laparoscopy (porcine model)	Atrac	No NMB vs. NMB	0–15 mmHg (incrementally)	Measured abdominal wall elastance	Elastance 3.98 ± 1.6 (no NMBA) vs. 3.86 ± 1.4 mmHg (with NMBA)	High intrathoracic pressures not affected by NMBA
Williams *Anaesthesia* 2003;58:574	Laparoscopic gynecologic surgery (n = 40)	Atrac	None (spontaneous breathing) vs. NMB	15 mmHg	End point was ease of trocar insertion in spontaneously breathing LMA vs. ETT + NMBA patients	IAP was higher in the LMA group	Surgical duration was greater in the ETT/NMBA group
Lindekaer *J Vis Exp* 2013	Laparoscopic surgery (n = 15, pilot study)	Roc	Deep NMB vs. no NMB	8 mmHg vs. 12 mmHg	Measured intra-abdominal space as distance from the promontory to skin at the 8 and 12 mmHg pressures with no NMB and with deep NMB	Intra-abdominal space at 8 mmHg IAP with NMB was comparable to space at 12 mmHg without NMB	Using NMB to maintain steady surgical conditions while reducing IAP with deep NMB "may improve patient outcome."
Dubois *Eur J Anaesthesiol* 2014;31:430	Laparoscopic hysterectomy (n = 102)	Roc	Deep NMB (TOFC ≤2) vs. shallow NMB (spontaneous recovery)	Stable at 13 mmHg	Surgeon subjective rating on 1 (excellent) to 4 (unacceptable) scale	"A trend towards higher scores was demonstrated in shallow NMB group"	21 patients in shallow NMB and 34 patients in deep NMB group had excellent surgical field
Martini *Br J Anaesth* 2014;112:498	Retroperitoneal laparoscopy (n = 24)	Atrac/mivac Roc	Moderate NMB (TOF 1–2) vs. deep NMB (PTC 1–2)	Standard	Subjective assessment by surgeon, SRS (1–5 scale), with 1 = extremely poor conditions and 5 = optimal conditions. Video images of working space evaluated post-hoc by anesthesiologists and surgeons.	In moderate NMB, 18% of SRS scores were 1–3; in deep NMB, 99% of SRS scores were 1–3. Mean SRS = 4.0 in moderate NMB, and 4.7 in deep NMB.	Deep NMB improves quality of surgical conditions over moderate NMB. Poor agreement between surgeons and anesthesiologists in scoring video images.

(*continued*)

Table 21-13 Summary of Randomized Trials Investigating the Relationship between Depth of Neuromuscular Block, Pneumoperitoneal (Intra-abdominal) Pressure and Outcome (CONTINUED)

Author	Surgery Type (number of patients)	NMBA Used	Depth of Block	IAP	Surgical Field Assessment	Results	Comments
Staehr-Rye *Anesth Analg* 2014;119:1084	Laparoscopic cholecystectomy (n = 48)	Roc	Moderate (spontaneous recovery) vs. deep (PTC = 0–1)	8 mmHg	4-point scale (1 = best) and surgical space conditions at dissection of gallbladder (0–100, where 0 = optimal and 100 = unacceptable)	Optimal conditions in 7/25 (28%) of deep NMB and 1/23 (4%) of moderate NMB	Deep NMB associated with marginal improvement in surgical space.
Blobner *Surg Endosc* 2015;29:627	Laparoscopic cholecystectomy (n = 57)	Roc	No NMB vs. "deep" NMB (TOFC = 0)	—	Assessed with Visual Analogue Scale (VAS)	In no NMB group, 48% of patients had events that impaired procedure. Only 4% of patients in deep NMB had events.	Surgeons requested additional roc in 40% of no NMB group patients, and 0% in deep NMB group.
Vlot *Surg Endosc* 2015;29:2210	Laparoscopy (porcine model) (n = 16)	—	Not specified	0 mmHg 5 mmHg 10 mmHg 15 mmHg	Working-space dimensions evaluated objectively using computed tomography (CT)	NMB had no effect on abdominal dimensions and laparoscopic working space.	Prestretching improved surgical condition.
Van Wijk *Acta Anaesthesiol Scand* 2015;59:434	Laparoscopic cholecystectomy (n = 20)	Roc	Lowest IAP that provided adequate surgical conditions in: no NMB vs. deep NMB (PTC <2)	No NMB IAP = 12.75 ± 4.5 vs. deep NMB IAP = 7.20 ± 2.5 mmHg	Not specified	25% lower IAP in deep NMB patients	Younger patients and females benefit more from deep NMB.
Vlot *J Pediatr Surg* 2015;50:465	Laparoscopy (porcine model)	Not specified	Not specified (block vs. no block)	8–10 mmHg	Working-space volume, anterior-posterior distance, and symphysis-to-diaphragm distance	Increasing IAP to 8 mmHg (from 0 mmHg) increased all surgical field parameters.	Prestretching the abdominal wall by a first insufflation improved surgical field. NMB had no effect on working space.
Madsen *Acta Anaesthesiol Scand* 2015;59:441	Gynecologic laparoscopy (n = 14, cross-over study)	Not specified	Deep NMB vs. no NMB	8 mmHg 12 mmHg	Surgical field: distance from sacral promontory to trocar (objective assessment)	At 12 mmHg, deep NMB increased surgical space by 0.33 cm; at 8 mmHg, surgical space increased by 0.3 cm.	Deep NMB had better surgical rating of surgical conditions during suturing of fascia.

Author	Surgery Type (number of patients)	NMBA Used	Depth of Block	IAP	Surgical Field Assessment	Results	Comments
Yoo *PLoS ONE* 2015;10:e0135412	Robot-assisted radical prostatectomy (n = 67)	Atrac Roc	Moderate NMB (TOFC 1–2) vs. deep NMB (PTC 1–2)	8 mmHg	Subjective assessment by surgeon (1–5 scale)	Highest IOP after 1 hr of steep head-down position: 23.3 mmHg in moderate NMB vs. 19.8 mmHg in deep NMB group	IOP was the primary parameter of interest.
Madsen *Eur J Anaesthesiol* 2016;33:341	Laparoscopic hysterectomy (n = 99)	Roc	8 mmHg and deep NMB (PTC 0–1) vs. standard 12 mmHg and moderate NMB	Low (8 mmHg) vs. standard (12 mmHg)	Not specified	Deep NMB and low pressure reduce postoperative pain.	Shoulder pain more frequent in moderate NMB group (60%) than deep NMB + low IAP (28.6%)
Kim *Medicine (Baltimore)* 2016;95:e2920	Laparoscopic colorectal surgery (n = 61)	Roc	Deep NMB (PTC 1–2) vs. moderate NMB (TOFC 1–2)	Titrated to maintain "operative field" by surgeon	Subjective by surgeon	Deep NMB IAP lower (9.3 mmHg) than moderate NMB (12 mmHg)	VAS pain scores lower, bowel function recovery faster in deep NMB group
Gurusamy *Cochrane Database Syst Rev* 2014:CD006930[a]	Laparoscopic cholecystectomy (21 studies, n = 1,092 patients)			Low pressure (<12 mmHg) vs. standard pressure (12–16 mmHg)		Laparoscopic cholecystectomy can be performed successfully in 90% of low pressure group.	No evidence is currently available to support the use of low pressure pneumoperitoneum in low-risk patients undergoing laparoscopic cholecystectomy.
Madsen *Acta Anaesthesiol Scand* 2015;59:1[a]	Abdominal and gynecologic surgery (15 studies, n = 998 patients)		Deep NMB vs. moderate NMB			Good to excellent surgical conditions can be achieved without NMB. Deep NMB is recommended in laparoscopic cholecystectomy, nephrectomy, and prostatectomy.	Good evidence that optimized surgical conditions can be achieved with deep NMB in laparoscopic cholecystectomy, hysterectomy, nephrectomy, prostatectomy.

[a]These studies are systematic reviews of the literature investigating the effects of intra-abdominal pressure or depth of neuromuscular block on surgical conditions and patient outcome.
NMBA, neuromuscular blocking agent; IAP, intra-abdominal pressure; SRS, surgical rating scale; NMB, neuromuscular block; atrac, atracurium; roc, rocuronium; LMA, laryngeal mask airway; ETT, endotracheal intubation; TOF, train-of-four; TOFC, train-of-four count.

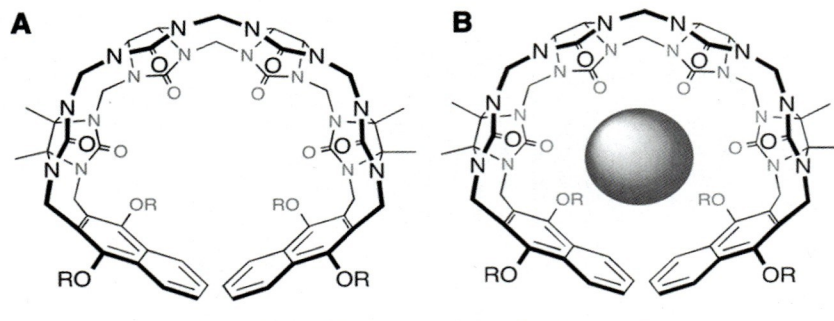

Figure 21-17 Calabadion 2 **(A)**, the second-generation cucurbituril receptor, features a cavity with naphthalene walls and binds with high affinity to steroidal (**B;** Ka = 0.53–3.4 × 10^9 M-1) and benzylisoquinoline (Ka = 4.8 × 10^6 M-1) neuromuscular-blocking agents. (Adapted from Haerter F1, Simons JC, Foerster U, et al. Comparative effectiveness of calabadion and sugammadex to reverse nondepolarizing neuromuscular-blocking agents. *Anesthesiology.* 2015;123(6):1337–1349.)

with return of normal neuromuscular function.[185] Similarly, a total dose of rocuronium between 0.6 and 1.2 mg/kg was sufficient to re-establish neuromuscular block when administered 12 to 465 minutes after sugammadex reversal.[186] Alternatively, depolarizing (succinylcholine) or nondepolarizing (benzylisoquinolinium) agents can be administered in usual doses to re-establish neuromuscular block after sugammadex.

Calabadion

A cucurbit[n]uril derivative, calabadion-1 has been reported to inactivate both steroidal and benzylisoquinoline nondepolarizing NMBAs by encapsulation.[187] However, its binding affinity toward rocuronium is less than that of sugammadex. A new compound, calabadion 2, was developed that has 89 times greater affinity for rocuronium than sugammadex, and a higher molar potency (Fig. 21-17).[188] In vivo experiments (in rats) report that calabadion 2 also has a very high affinity for cisatracurium, a property that sugammadex lacks. Interestingly, SCh can be administered safely and effectively after administration of calabadion 2 if rapid reparalysis is required.[188] Similar to sugammadex, the calabadion-NMBA complex is eliminated unchanged via the renal route.

Conclusion

After a relatively long period in which few pharmacologic advances were made with regard to NMBAs or their antagonists, the last decade has witnessed the introduction of a new and much more effective antagonist of aminosteroidal NMBAs, sugammadex. Current work suggests that newer, and even more effective, broad-spectrum encapsulating agents are being developed that could potentially reverse the actions of all NMBAs, aminosteroids and benzylisoquinolinium compounds alike. It is hoped that these advances in pharmacology will be paralleled by similar advances in perioperative monitoring that will increase the anesthesiologist's ability to provide optimal care and improve patient safety.

REFERENCES

1. Zong Y, Jin R. Structural mechanisms of the agrin-LRP4-MuSK signaling pathway in neuromuscular junction differentiation. *Cell Mol Life Sci*. 2013; 70:3077–3088.
2. Naguib M, Flood P, McArdle JJ, et al. Advances in neurobiology of the neuromuscular junction: implications for the anesthesiologist. *Anesthesiology.* 2002;96:202–231.
3. Martyn JAJ, Fagerlund MJ, Eriksson LI. Basic principles of neuromuscular transmission. *Anaesthesia.* 2009;64(Suppl 1):1–9.
4. Schreiber J-U, Lysakowski C, Fuchs-Buder T, et al. Prevention of succinylcholine-induced fasciculation and myalgia: a meta-analysis of randomized trials. *Anesthesiology.* 2005; 103:877–884.
5. Kappmeyer K, Lanzl IM. [Intra-ocular pressure during and after playing high and low resistance wind instruments]. *Ophthalmol Z Dtsch Ophthalmol Ges.* 2010;107:41–46.
6. Kelly RE, Dinner M, Turner LS, et al. Succinylcholine increases intraocular pressure in the human eye with the extraocular muscles detached. *Anesthesiology.* 1993;79:948–952.
7. Moeini HA, Soltani HA, Gholami AR, et al. The effect of lidocaine and sufentanil in preventing intraocular pressure increase due to succinylcholine and endotracheal intubation. *Eur J Anaesthesiol.* 2006;23:739–742.
8. Libonati MM, Leahy JJ, Ellison N. The use of succinylcholine in open eye surgery. *Anesthesiology.* 1985;62:637–640.
9. Vachon CA, Warner DO, Bacon DR. Succinylcholine and the open globe. Tracing the teaching. *Anesthesiology.* 2003;99:220–3.
10. Cunningham AJ, Barry P. Intraocular pressure—physiology and implications for anaesthetic management. *Can Anaesth Soc J.* 1986;33:195–208.
11. Perkins ZB, Wittenberg MD, Nevin D, Lockey DJ, O'Brien B. The relationship between head injury severity and hemodynamic response to tracheal intubation. *J Trauma Acute Care Surg.* 2013;74:1074–1080.
12. Ganigara A, Ravishankar C, Ramavakoda C, et al. Fatal hyperkalemia following succinylcholine administration in a child on oral propranolol. *Drug Metab Pers Ther.* 2015;30:69–71.
13. Turan A, Mendoza ML, Gupta S, et al. Consequences of succinylcholine administration to patients using statins. *Anesthesiology.* 2011;115:28–35.
14. Tran DTT, Newton EK, Mount VAH, et al. Rocuronium versus succinylcholine for rapid sequence induction intubation. *Cochrane Database Syst Rev.* 2015;10:CD002788.
15. Dexter F, Epstein RH, Wachtel RE, et al. Estimate of the relative risk of succinylcholine for triggering malignant hyperthermia. *Anesth Analg.* 2013;116:118–122.
16. Thomsen JL, Nielsen CV, Palmqvist DF, et al. Premature awakening and underuse of neuromuscular monitoring in a registry of patients with butyrylcholinesterase deficiency. *Br J Anaesth.* 2015;115 Suppl 1:i89–94.
17. Blanie A, Ract C, Leblanc P-E, et al. The limits of succinylcholine for critically ill patients. *Anesth Analg.* 2012;115:873–879.
18. Vega-Villa KR, Kaneda K, Yamashita S, et al. Vecuronium pharmacokinetics in patients with major burns. *Br J Anaesth.* 2014;112:304–310.
19. Decoopman M, Cammu G, Suy K, et al. Reversal of pancuronium-induced block by the selective relaxant binding agent sugammadex. (ABSTRACT). *Eur J Anaesthesiol.* 2007:110 (9AP2–1).
20. Naguib M, Abdulatif M. Dose-response relationships for edrophonium and neostigmine antagonism of pipecuronium-induced neuromuscular block. *Anesth Analg.* 1994;78:306–311.
21. Tassonyi E, Pongracz A, Nemes R, et al. Reversal of pipecuronium-induced moderate neuromuscular block with sugammadex in the presence of a sevoflurane anesthetic: A randomized trial. *Anesth Analg.* 2015;121:373–380.
22. Nitahara K, Sugi Y, Shigematsu K, et al. Recovery of train-of-four ratio to 0.70 and 0.90 is delayed in type 2 diabetes with vecuronium-induced neuromuscular block. *Eur J Anaesthesiol.* 2013;30:80–84.
23. Andrews JI, Kumar N, van den Brom RH, et al. A large simple randomized trial of rocuronium versus succinylcholine in rapid-sequence induction of anaesthesia along with propofol. *Acta Anaesthesiol Scand.* 1999;43:4–8.
24. Reddy JI, Cooke PJ, Schalkwyk JM, et al. Anaphylaxis is more common with rocuronium and succinylcholine than with atracurium. *Anesthesiology.* 2015;122:39–45.

25. Sadleir PHM, Clarke RC, Bunning DL, et al. Anaphylaxis to neuromuscular blocking drugs: incidence and cross-reactivity in Western Australia from 2002 to 2011. Br J Anaesth. 2013;110:981–987.
26. Dong S, Acouetey DS, Gueant-Rodriguez R-M, et al. Prevalence of IgE against neuromuscular blocking agents in hairdressers and bakers. Clin Exp Allergy J Br Soc Allergy Clin Immunol. 2013;43:1256–1262.
27. Yang CI, Fine GF, Jooste EH, et al. The effect of cisatracurium and rocuronium on lung function in anesthetized children. Anesth Analg. 2013;117:1393–1400.
28. Conte B, Zoric L, Bonada G, et al. Reversal of a rocuronium-induced grade IV anaphylaxis via early injection of a large dose of sugammadex. Can J Anaesth. 2014;61:558–562.
29. Wang T, Huang S, Geng G. Comparison of the duration of neuromuscular blockade following a single bolus dose of rocuronium during laparoscopic gynaecological surgery vs conventional open surgery. Anaesthesia. 2014;69:854–859.
30. Armendariz-Buil I, Lobato-Solores F, Aguilera-Celorrio L, et al. Residual neuromuscular block in type II diabetes mellitus after rocuronium: a prospective observational study. Eur J Anaesthesiol. 2014;31:411–416.
31. Rotava P, Cavalcanti IL, Barrucand L, et al.: Effects of magnesium sulphate on the pharmacodynamics of rocuronium in patients aged 60 years and older: A randomised trial. Eur J Anaesthesiol. 2013;30:599–604.
32. Germano Filho PA, Cavalcanti IL, Barrucand L, et al. Effect of magnesium sulphate on sugammadex reversal time for neuromuscular blockade: a randomised controlled study. Anaesthesia. 2015;70:956–961.
33. Ozturk T, Agdanli D, Bayturan O, et al. Effects of conventional vs high-dose rocuronium on the QTc interval during anesthesia induction and intubation in patients undergoing coronary artery surgery: a randomized, double-blind, parallel trial. Braz J Med Biol Res. 2015;48:370–376.
34. Mirakhur RK. Newer neuromuscular blocking drugs. An overview of their clinical pharmacology and therapeutic use. Drugs. 1992;44:182–199.
35. Basta SJ, Savarese JJ, Ali HH, et al. Clinical pharmacology of doxacurium chloride. A new long-acting nondepolarizing muscle relaxant. Anesthesiology. 1988;69:478–486.
36. Cashman JN, Luke JJ, Jones RM. Neuromuscular block with doxacurium (BW A938U) in patients with normal or absent renal function. Br J Anaesth. 1990;64:186–192.
37. Martlew RA, Harper NJ. The clinical pharmacology of doxacurium in young adults and in elderly patients. Anaesthesia. 1995;50:779–782.
38. Fodale V, Santamaria LB. Laudanosine, an atracurium and cisatracurium metabolite. Eur J Anaesthesiol. 2002;19:466–473.
39. Dieck T, Steffens J, Sander B, et al. Propofol, remifentanil and mivacurium: fast track surgery with poor intubating conditions. Minerva Anestesiol. 2011;77:585–591.
40. Ali HH, Lien CA, Witkowski T, et al. Efficacy and safety of divided dose administration of mivacurium for a 90-second tracheal intubation. J Clin Anesth. 1996;8:276–281.
41. Vanlinthout LEH, Mesfin SH, Hens N, et al. A systematic review and meta-regression analysis of mivacurium for tracheal intubation. Anaesthesia. 2014;69:1377–1387.
42. Cassel J, Staehr-Rye AK, Nielsen CV, et al. Use of neuromuscular monitoring to detect prolonged effect of succinylcholine or mivacurium: three case reports. Acta Anaesthesiol Scand. 2014;58:1040–1043.
43. Naguib M, Samarkandi AH, Ammar A, et al. Comparative clinical pharmacology of rocuronium, cisatracurium, and their combination. Anesthesiology. 1998;89:1116–1124.
44. Stäuble CG, Stäuble RB, Schaller SJ, et al. Effects of single-shot and steady-state propofol anaesthesia on rocuronium dose-response relationship: a randomised trial. Acta Anaesthesiol Scand 2015;59:902–911.
45. Braga A de F de A, Carvalho VH, et al. Influence of local anesthetics on the neuromuscular blockade produced by rocuronium: effects of lidocaine and 50% enantiomeric excess bupivacaine on the neuromuscular junction. Rev Bras Anestesiol. 2009;59:725–734.
46. Sahin SH, Colak A, Sezer A, et al. Effect of epidural levobupivacaine on recovery from vecuronium-induced neuromuscular block in patients undergoing lower abdominal surgery. Anaesth Intensive Care. 2011;39:607–610.
47. Czarnetzki C, Lysakowski C, Elia N, et al. Intravenous lidocaine has no impact on rocuronium-induced neuromuscular block. Randomised study. Acta Anaesthesiol Scand. 2012;56:474–481.
48. Paradelis AG, Triantaphyllidis C, Giala MM. Neuromuscular blocking activity of aminoglycoside antibiotics. Methods Find Exp Clin Pharmacol. 1980;2:45–51.
49. Szmuk P, Ezri T, Chelly JE, et al. The onset time of rocuronium is slowed by esmolol and accelerated by ephedrine. Anesth Analg. 2000;90:1217–1219.
50. Arroliga A, Frutos-Vivar F, Hall J, et al, International Mechanical Ventilation Study Group. Use of sedatives and neuromuscular blockers in a cohort of patients receiving mechanical ventilation. Chest. 2005;128:496–506.
51. Alhazzani W, Alshahrani M, Jaeschke R, et al. Neuromuscular blocking agents in acute respiratory distress syndrome: a systematic review and meta-analysis of randomized controlled trials. Crit Care. 2013;17:R43.
52. Hraiech S, Forel J-M, Papazian L. The role of neuromuscular blockers in ARDS: benefits and risks. Curr Opin Crit Care. 2012;18:495–502.
53. Salciccioli JD, Cocchi MN, Rittenberger JC, et al. Continuous neuromuscular blockade is associated with decreased mortality in post-cardiac arrest patients. Resuscitation. 2013;84:1728–1733.
54. Rubio ER, Seelig CB. Persistent paralysis after prolonged use of atracurium in the absence of corticosteroids. South Med J. 1996;89:624–626.
55. Romero A, Joshi GP. Neuromuscular disease and anesthesia. Muscle Nerve. 2013;48:451–460.
56. Weiser TG, Regenbogen SE, Thompson KD, et al. An estimation of the global volume of surgery: a modelling strategy based on available data. Lancet. 2008;372:139–144.
57. Todd MM, Hindman BJ, King BJ. The implementation of quantitative electromyographic neuromuscular monitoring in an academic anesthesia department. Anesth Analg. 2014;119:323–331.
58. Checketts MR, Alladi R, Ferguson K, et al. Recommendations for standards of monitoring during anaesthesia and recovery 2015 : Association of Anaesthetists of Great Britain and Ireland. Anaesthesia. 2016;71:85–93.
59. Anonymous: Indications of neuromuscular blockade in anaesthesia. Short text. Ann Fr Anesth Reanim. 2000;19(Suppl 2):352s–355s.
60. Kelly D, Brull SJ. Monitoring of neuromuscular function in the clinical setting. Yale J Biol Med. 1993;66:473–489.
61. Brull SJ, Silverman DG. Pulse width, stimulus intensity, electrode placement, and polarity during assessment of neuromuscular block. Anesthesiology. 1995;83:702–709.
62. Ali HH, Utting JE, Gray TC. Quantitative assessment of residual antidepolarizing block. I. Br J Anaesth. 1971;43:473–477.
63. Ali HH, Utting JE, Gray TC. Quantitative assessment of residual antidepolarizing block. II. Br J Anaesth. 1971;43:478–485.
64. O'Hara DA, Fragen RJ, Shanks CA. Comparison of visual and measured train-of-four recovery after vecuronium-induced neuromuscular blockade using two anaesthetic techniques. Br J Anaesth. 1986;58:1300–1302.
65. Waud BE, Waud DR. The margin of safety of neuromuscular transmission in the muscle of the diaphragm. Anesthesiology. 1972;37:417–422.
66. Waud BE, Waud DR. The relation between the response to "train-of-four" stimulation and receptor occlusion during competitive neuromuscular block. Anesthesiology. 1972;37:413–416.
67. Silverman DG, Connelly NR, O'Connor TZ, et al. Accelographic train-of-four at near-threshold currents. Anesthesiology. 1992;76:34–38.
68. Brull SJ, Ehrenwerth J, Silverman DG. Stimulation with submaximal current for train-of-four monitoring. Anesthesiology. 1990;72:629–632.
69. Merton PA. Voluntary strength and fatigue. J Physiol. 1954;123:553–564.
70. Brull SJ, Connelly NR, O'Connor TZ, et al. Effect of tetanus on subsequent neuromuscular monitoring in patients receiving vecuronium. Anesthesiology. 1991;74:64–70.
71. Silverman DG, Brull SJ. The effect of a tetanic stimulus on the response to subsequent tetanic stimulation. Anesth Analg. 1993;76:1284–1287.
72. Viby-Mogensen J, Howardy-Hansen P, Chraemmer-Jørgensen B, et al. Posttetanic count (PTC): a new method of evaluating an intense nondepolarizing neuromuscular blockade. Anesthesiology. 1981;55:458–461.
73. Viby-Mogensen J, Jensen NH, Engbaek J, et al. Tactile and visual evaluation of the response to train-of-four nerve stimulation. Anesthesiology. 1985;63:440–443.
74. Engbaek J, Ostergaard D, Viby-Mogensen J. Double burst stimulation (DBS): a new pattern of nerve stimulation to identify residual neuromuscular block. Br J Anaesth. 1989;62:274–278.
75. Ueda N, V-Mogensen J, V-Olsen N, et al. The best choice of double burst stimulation pattern for manual evaluation of neuromuscular transmission. J Anesth. 1989;3:94–99.
76. Brull SJ, Murphy GS. Residual neuromuscular block: lessons unlearned. Part II: methods to reduce the risk of residual weakness. Anesth Analg. 2010;111:129–140.
77. Grosse-Sundrup M, Henneman JP, Sandberg WS, et al. Intermediate acting non-depolarizing neuromuscular blocking agents and risk of postoperative respiratory complications: prospective propensity score matched cohort study. BMJ. 2012;345:e6329.
78. Drenck NE, Ueda N, Olsen NV, et al. Manual evaluation of residual curarization using double burst stimulation: a comparison with train-of-four. Anesthesiology. 1989;70:578–581.
79. Gill SS, Donati F, Bevan DR. Clinical evaluation of double-burst stimulation. Its relationship to train-of-four stimulation. Anaesthesia. 1990;45:543–548.
80. Brull SJ, Silverman DG. Visual and tactile assessment of neuromuscular fade. Anesth Analg. 1993;77:352–355.
81. Vincent RDJ, Brockwell RC, Moreno MC, et al. Posttetanic count revisited: are measurements more reliable using the TOF-Watch accelerographic peripheral nerve stimulator? J Clin Monit Comput. 2004;18:33–37.
82. Bhananker SM, Treggiari MM, Sellers BA, et al. Comparison of train-of-four count by anesthesia providers versus TOF-Watch® SX: a prospective cohort study. Can J Anaesth. 2015;62:1089–1096.
83. Murphy GS, Szokol JW, Marymont JH, et al. Residual paralysis at the time of tracheal extubation. Anesth Analg. 2005;100:1840–1845.

84. Cammu G, De Witte J, De Veylder J, et al. Postoperative residual paralysis in outpatients versus inpatients. Anesth Analg. 2006;102:426–429.
85. Kopman AF, Yee PS, Neuman GG. Relationship of the train-of-four fade ratio to clinical signs and symptoms of residual paralysis in awake volunteers. Anesthesiology. 1997;86:765–771.
86. Schreiber J-U, Mucha E, Fuchs-Buder T. Acceleromyography to assess neuromuscular recovery: is calibration before measurement mandatory? Acta Anaesthesiol Scand. 2011;55:328–331.
87. Dubois PE, De Bel M, Jamart J, et al. Performance of acceleromyography with a short and light TOF-tube compared with mechanomyography: a clinical comparison. Eur J Anaesthesiol. 2014;31:404–410.
88. Kopman AF, Chin W, Cyriac J. Acceleromyography vs. electromyography: an ipsilateral comparison of the indirectly evoked neuromuscular response to train-of-four stimulation. Acta Anaesthesiol Scand. 2005;49:316–322.
89. Liang SS, Stewart PA, Phillips S. An ipsilateral comparison of acceleromyography and electromyography during recovery from nondepolarizing neuromuscular block under general anesthesia in humans. Anesth Analg. 2013;117:373–379.
90. Suzuki T, Fukano N, Kitajima O, et al. Normalization of acceleromyographic train-of-four ratio by baseline value for detecting residual neuromuscular block. Br J Anaesth. 2006;96:44–47.
91. Stewart PA, Freelander N, Liang S, et al. Comparison of electromyography and kinemyography during recovery from non-depolarising neuromuscular blockade. Anaesth Intensive Care. 2014;42:378–384.
92. Thilen SR, Hansen BE, Ramaiah R, et al. Intraoperative neuromuscular monitoring site and residual paralysis. Anesthesiology. 2012;117:964–972.
93. Kumar GV, Nair AP, Murthy HS, et al. Residual neuromuscular blockade affects postoperative pulmonary function. Anesthesiology. 2012;117:1234–1244.
94. Eriksson LI, Sundman E, Olsson R, et al. Functional assessment of the pharynx at rest and during swallowing in partially paralyzed humans: simultaneous videomanometry and mechanomyography of awake human volunteers. Anesthesiology. 1997;87:1035–1043.
95. Piccioni F, Mariani L, Bogno L, et al. An acceleromyographic train-of-four ratio of 1.0 reliably excludes respiratory muscle weakness after major abdominal surgery: a randomized double-blind study. Can J Anaesth. 2014;61:641–649.
96. Cedborg AIH, Sundman E, Boden K, Hedstrom HW, et al. Pharyngeal function and breathing pattern during partial neuromuscular block in the elderly: effects on airway protection. Anesthesiology. 2014;120:312–325.
97. Schuller PJ, Newell S, Strickland PA, et al. Response of bispectral index to neuromuscular block in awake volunteers. Br J Anaesth. 2015;115 Suppl 1:i95–i103.
98. Illman H, Antila H, Olkkola KT. Reversal of neuromuscular blockade by sugammadex does not affect EEG derived indices of depth of anesthesia. J Clin Monit Comput. 2010;24:371–376.
99. Aho AJ, Kamata K, Yli-Hankala A, et al. Elevated BIS and Entropy values after sugammadex or neostigmine: an electroencephalographic or electromyographic phenomenon? Acta Anaesthesiol Scand. 2012;56:465–473.
100. Dahaba AA, Bornemann H, Hopfgartner E, et al. Effect of sugammadex or neostigmine neuromuscular block reversal on bispectral index monitoring of propofol/remifentanil anaesthesia. Br J Anaesth. 2012;108:602–606.
101. Fiekers JF. Concentration-dependent effects of neostigmine on the end-plate acetylcholine receptor channel complex. J Neurosci Off J Soc Neurosci. 1985;5:502–514.
102. Herbstreit F, Zigrahn D, Ochterbeck C, et al. Neostigmine/glycopyrrolate administered after recovery from neuromuscular block increases upper airway collapsibility by decreasing genioglossus muscle activity in response to negative pharyngeal pressure. Anesthesiology. 2010;113:1280–1288.
103. Yang L, Yang D, Li Q, et al. Neostigmine for reversal of neuromuscular block in paediatric patients. Cochrane Database Syst Rev. 2014;5:CD010110.
104. Lemmens HJ, El-Orbany MI, Berry J, et al. Reversal of profound vecuronium-induced neuromuscular block under sevoflurane anesthesia: sugammadex versus neostigmine. BMC Anesth. 2010;10:15.
105. Jones RK, Caldwell JE, Brull SJ, et al. Reversal of profound rocuronium-induced blockade with sugammadex: a randomized comparison with neostigmine. Anesthesiology. 2008;109:816–824.
106. Bevan JC, Collins L, Fowler C, et al. Early and late reversal of rocuronium and vecuronium with neostigmine in adults and children. Anesth Analg. 1999;89:333–339.
107. Illman HL, Laurila P, Antila H, et al. The duration of residual neuromuscular block after administration of neostigmine or sugammadex at two visible twitches during train-of-four monitoring. Anesth Analg. 2011;112:63–68.
108. Kim KS, Cheong MA, Lee HJ, et al. Tactile assessment for the reversibility of rocuronium-induced neuromuscular blockade during propofol or sevoflurane anesthesia. Anesth Analg. 2004;99:1080–1085.
109. Kirkegaard H, Heier T, Caldwell JE. Efficacy of tactile-guided reversal from cisatracurium-induced neuromuscular block. Anesthesiology. 2002;96:45–50.
110. Harper NJ, Wallace M, Hall IA. Optimum dose of neostigmine at two levels of atracurium-induced neuromuscular block. Br J Anaesth. 1994;72:82–85.
111. Sauer M, Stahn A, Soltesz S, et al. The influence of residual neuromuscular block on the incidence of critical respiratory events. A randomised, prospective, placebo-controlled trial. Eur J Anaesthesiol. 2011;28:842–848.
112. Fuchs-Buder T, Meistelman C, Alla F, et al. Antagonism of low degrees of atracurium-induced neuromuscular blockade: dose-effect relationship for neostigmine. Anesthesiology. 2010;112:34–40.
113. Capron F, Alla F, Hottier C, et al. Can acceleromyography detect low levels of residual paralysis? A probability approach to detect a mechanomyographic train-of-four ratio of 0.9. Anesthesiology. 2004;100:1119–1124.
114. Schaller SJ, Fink H, Ulm K, et al. Sugammadex and neostigmine dose-finding study for reversal of shallow residual neuromuscular block. Anesthesiology. 2010;113:1054–1060.
115. Fuchs-Buder T, Baumann C, De Guis J, et al. Low-dose neostigmine to antagonise shallow atracurium neuromuscular block during inhalational anaesthesia: A randomised controlled trial. Eur J Anaesthesiol. 2013;30:594–598.
116. Kaufhold N, Schaller SJ, Stäuble CG, et al. Sugammadex and neostigmine dose-finding study for reversal of residual neuromuscular block at a train-of-four ratio of 0.2 (SUNDRO20). Br J Anaesth. 2016;116:233–240.
117. Beattie WS, Buckley DN, Forrest JB. Continuous infusions of atracurium and vecuronium, compared with intermittent boluses of pancuronium: dose requirements and reversal. Can J Anaesth. 1992;39:925–931.
118. Baurain MJ, Hoton F, D'Hollander AA, et al. Is recovery of neuromuscular transmission complete after the use of neostigmine to antagonize block produced by rocuronium, vecuronium, atracurium and pancuronium? Br J Anaesth. 1996;77:496–499.
119. Staikou C, Stamelos M, Stavroulakis E. Impact of anaesthetic drugs and adjuvants on ECG markers of torsadogenicity. Br J Anaesth. 2014;112:217–230.
120. Koyuncu O, Turhanoglu S, Ozbakis Akkurt C, et al. Comparison of sugammadex and conventional reversal on postoperative nausea and vomiting: a randomized, blinded trial. J Clin Anesth. 2015;27:51–56.
121. Cheng C-R, Sessler DI, Apfel CC. Does neostigmine administration produce a clinically important increase in postoperative nausea and vomiting? Anesth Analg. 2005;101:1349–1355.
122. Fuchs-Buder T, Ziegenfuss T, Lysakowski K, et al. Antagonism of vecuronium-induced neuromuscular block in patients pretreated with magnesium sulphate: dose-effect relationship of neostigmine. Br J Anaesth. 1999;82:61–65.
123. Payne JP, Hughes R, Al Azawi S. Neuromuscular blockade by neostigmine in anaesthetized man. Br J Anaesth. 1980;52:69–76.
124. Goldhill DR, Wainwright AP, Stuart CS, et al. Neostigmine after spontaneous recovery from neuromuscular blockade. Effect on depth of blockade monitored with train-of-four and tetanic stimuli. Anaesthesia. 1989;44:293–299.
125. Eikermann M, Zaremba S, Malhotra A, et al. Neostigmine but not sugammadex impairs upper airway dilator muscle activity and breathing. Br J Anaesth. 2008;101:344–349.
126. Eikermann M, Fassbender P, Malhotra A, et al. Unwarranted administration of acetylcholinesterase inhibitors can impair genioglossus and diaphragm muscle function. Anesthesiology. 2007;107:621–629.
127. McLean DJ, Diaz-Gil D, Farhan HN, et al. Dose-dependent association between intermediate-acting neuromuscular-blocking agents and postoperative respiratory complications. Anesthesiology. 2015;122:1201–1213.
128. De Oliveira GS, Theilken LS, McCarthy RJ. Shortage of perioperative drugs: implications for anesthesia practice and patient safety. Anesth Analg. 2011;113:1429–1435.
129. Cronnelly R, Morris RB, Miller RD. Edrophonium: duration of action and atropine requirement in humans during halothane anesthesia. Anesthesiology. 1982;57:261–266.
130. Barber HE, Calvey TN, Muir KT. The relationship between the pharmacokinetics, cholinesterase inhibition and facilitation of twitch tension of the quaternary ammonium anticholinesterase drugs, neostigmine, pyridostigmine, edrophonium and 3-hydroxyphenyltrimethylammonium. Br J Pharmacol. 1979;66:525–530.
131. Kopman AF, Mallhi MU, Justo MD, et al. Antagonism of mivacurium-induced neuromuscular blockade in humans. Edrophonium dose requirements at threshold train-of-four count of 4. Anesthesiology. 1994;81:1394–1400.
132. Schaller SJ, Fink H. Sugammadex as a reversal agent for neuromuscular block: an evidence-based review. Core Evid. 2013;8:57–67.
133. Bom A, Clark JK, Palin R. New approaches to reversal of neuromuscular block. Curr Opin Drug Discov Devel. 2002;5:793–800.
134. Zwiers A, van den Heuvel M, Smeets J, et al. Assessment of the potential for displacement interactions with sugammadex: a pharmacokinetic-pharmacodynamic modelling approach. Clin Drug Investig. 2011;31:101–111.
135. Shields M, Giovannelli M, Mirakhur RK, et al. Org 25969 (sugammadex), a selective relaxant binding agent for antagonism of prolonged rocuronium-induced neuromuscular block. Br J Anaesth. 2006;96:36–43.
136. Flockton EA, Mastronardi P, Hunter JM, et al. Reversal of rocuronium-induced neuromuscular block with sugammadex is faster than reversal of cisatracurium-induced block with neostigmine. Br J Anaesth. 2008;100:622–630.
137. Blobner M, Eriksson LI, Scholz J, et al. Reversal of rocuronium-induced neuromuscular blockade with sugammadex compared with neostigmine during sevoflurane anaesthesia: results of a randomised, controlled trial. Eur J Anaesthesiol. 2010;27:874–881.

138. Khuenl-Brady KS, Wattwil M, Vanacker BF, et al. Sugammadex provides faster reversal of vecuronium-induced neuromuscular blockade compared with neostigmine: a multicenter, randomized, controlled trial. *Anesth Analg.* 2010;110:64–73.
139. McDonagh DL, Benedict PE, Kovac AL, et al. Efficacy, safety, and pharmacokinetics of sugammadex for the reversal of rocuronium-induced neuromuscular blockade in elderly patients. *Anesthesiology.* 2011;114:318–329.
140. Lee C, Jahr JS, Candiotti KA, et al. Reversal of profound neuromuscular block by sugammadex administered three minutes after rocuronium: a comparison with spontaneous recovery from succinylcholine. *Anesthesiology.* 2009;110:1020–1025.
141. Sorensen MK, Bretlau C, Gatke MR, et al. Rapid sequence induction and intubation with rocuronium-sugammadex compared with succinylcholine: a randomized trial. *Br J Anaesth.* 2012;108:682–689.
142. Staals LM, Egmond J van, Driessen JJ, et al. Sugammadex reverses neuromuscular block induced by 3-desacetyl-vecuronium, an active metabolite of vecuronium, in the anaesthetised rhesus monkey. *Eur J Anaesthesiol.* 2011;28:265–272.
143. Peeters P, Passier P, Smeets J, et al. Sugammadex is cleared rapidly and primarily unchanged via renal excretion. *Biopharm Drug Dispos.* 2011;32:159–167.
144. Cammu G, Van Vlem B, van den Heuvel M, et al. Dialysability of sugammadex and its complex with rocuronium in intensive care patients with severe renal impairment. *Br J Anaesth.* 2012;109:382–390.
145. Galvao VR, Giavina-Bianchi P, Castells M. Perioperative anaphylaxis. *Curr Allergy Asthma Rep.* 2014;14:452.
146. Tsur A, Kalansky A. Hypersensitivity associated with sugammadex administration: a systematic review. *Anaesthesia.* 2014;69:1251–1257.
147. Krishna MT, York M, Chin T, et al. Multi-centre retrospective analysis of anaphylaxis during general anaesthesia in the United Kingdom: aetiology and diagnostic performance of acute serum tryptase. *Clin Exp Immunol.* 2014;178:399–404.
148. Jeyadoss J, Kuruppu P, Nanjappa N, et al. Sugammadex hypersensitivity-a case of anaphylaxis. *Anaesth Intensive Care.* 2014;42:89–92.
149. Rahe-Meyer N, Fennema H, Schulman S, et al. Effect of reversal of neuromuscular blockade with sugammadex versus usual care on bleeding risk in a randomized study of surgical patients. *Anesthesiology.* 2014;121:969–977.
150. Staals LM, Snoeck MMJ, Driessen JJ, et al. Multicentre, parallel-group, comparative trial evaluating the efficacy and safety of sugammadex in patients with end-stage renal failure or normal renal function. *Br J Anaesth.* 2008;101:492–497.
151. Panhuizen IF, Gold SJA, Buerkle C, et al. Efficacy, safety and pharmacokinetics of sugammadex 4 mg kg-1 for reversal of deep neuromuscular blockade in patients with severe renal impairment. *Br J Anaesth.* 2015;114:777–784.
152. Lee HJ, Kim KS, Jeong JS, et al. The influence of mild hypothermia on reversal of rocuronium-induced deep neuromuscular block with sugammadex. *BMC Anesthesiol.* 2015;15:7.
153. Hudson ME, Rietbergen H, Chelly JE. Sugammadex is effective in reversing rocuronium in the presence of antibiotics. *BMC Anesthesiol.* 2014;14:69.
154. Pongracz A, Szatmari S, Nemes R, et al. Reversal of neuromuscular blockade with sugammadex at the reappearance of four twitches to train-of-four stimulation. *Anesthesiology.* 2013;119:36–42.
155. Monk TG, Rietbergen H, Woo T, et al. Use of sugammadex in patients with obesity: a pooled analysis. *Am J Ther.* 2015. doi:10.1097/MJT.0000000000000305.
156. Van Gestel L, Cammu G. Is the effect of sugammadex always rapid in onset? *Acta Anaesthesiol Belg.* 2013;64:41–47.
157. Amao R, Zornow MH, Cowan RM, et al. Use of sugammadex in patients with a history of pulmonary disease. *J Clin Anesth.* 2012;24:289–297.
158. White PF, Tufanogullari B, Sacan O, et al. The effect of residual neuromuscular blockade on the speed of reversal with sugammadex. *Anesth Analg.* 2009;108:846–851.
159. Puhringer FK, Rex C, Sielenkamper AW, et al. Reversal of profound, high-dose rocuronium-induced neuromuscular blockade by sugammadex at two different time points: an international, multicenter, randomized, dose-finding, safety assessor-blinded, phase II trial. *Anesthesiology.* 2008;109:188–197.
160. Dahl V, Pendeville PE, Hollmann MW, et al. Safety and efficacy of sugammadex for the reversal of rocuronium-induced neuromuscular blockade in cardiac patients undergoing noncardiac surgery. *Eur J Anaesthesiol.* 2009;26:874–884.
161. Gaszynski T, Szewczyk G, Gaszynski W. Randomized comparison of sugammadex and neostigmine for reversal of rocuronium-induced muscle relaxation in morbidly obese undergoing general anaesthesia. *Br J Anaesth.* 2012;108:236–239.
162. Le Corre F, Nejmeddine S, Fatahine C, et al. Recurarization after sugammadex reversal in an obese patient. *Can J Anaesth.* 2011;58:944–947.
163. Iwasaki H, Takahoko K, Otomo S, et al. A temporary decrease in twitch response following reversal of rocuronium-induced neuromuscular block with a small dose of sugammadex in a pediatric patient. *J Anesth.* 2014;28:288–290.
164. Unterbuchner C, Ziegleder R, Graf B, et al. Magnesium-induced recurarisation after reversal of rocuronium-induced neuromuscular block with sugammadex. *Acta Anaesthesiol Scand.* 2015;59:536–540.
165. Czarnetzki C, Tassonyi E, Lysakowski C, et al. Efficacy of sugammadex for the reversal of moderate and deep rocuronium-induced neuromuscular block in patients pretreated with intravenous magnesium: a randomized controlled trial. *Anesthesiology.* 2014;121:59–67.
166. Kotake Y, Ochiai R, Suzuki T, et al. Reversal with sugammadex in the absence of monitoring did not preclude residual neuromuscular block. *Anesth Analg.* 2013;117:345–351.
167. Ledowski T, Hillyard S, O'Dea B, et al. Introduction of sugammadex as standard reversal agent: Impact on the incidence of residual neuromuscular blockade and postoperative patient outcome. *Indian J Anaesth.* 2013;57:46–51.
168. Schepens T, Cammu G, Saldien V, et al. Electromyographic activity of the diaphragm during neostigmine or sugammadex-enhanced recovery after neuromuscular blockade with rocuronium: a randomised controlled study in healthy volunteers. *Eur J Anaesthesiol.* 2015;32:49–57.
169. Amorim P, Lagarto F, Gomes B, et al. Neostigmine vs. sugammadex: observational cohort study comparing the quality of recovery using the Postoperative Quality Recovery Scale. *Acta Anaesthesiol Scand.* 2014;58:1101–1110.
170. Ledowski T, Falke L, Johnston F, et al. Retrospective investigation of postoperative outcome after reversal of residual neuromuscular blockade: sugammadex, neostigmine or no reversal. *Eur J Anaesthesiol.* 2014;31:423–429.
171. Chambers D, Paulden M, Paton F, et al. Sugammadex for reversal of neuromuscular block after rapid sequence intubation: a systematic review and economic assessment. *Br J Anaesth.* 2010;105:568–575.
172. Watts RW, London JA, van Wijk RM, et al. The influence of unrestricted use of sugammadex on clinical anaesthetic practice in a tertiary teaching hospital. *Anaesth Intensive Care.* 2012;40:333–339.
173. Stewart PA, Phillips S, De Boer HD. Sugammadex reversal of rocuronium-induced neuromuscular blockade in two types of neuromuscular disorders: Myotonic dystrophy and spinal muscular atrophy. *Rev Esp Anestesiol Reanim.* 2013;60:226–229.
174. Casarotti P, Mendola C, Cammarota G, et al. High-dose rocuronium for rapid-sequence induction and reversal with sugammadex in two myasthenic patients. *Acta Anaesthesiol Scand.* 2014;58:1154–1158.
175. de Boer HD, Shields MO, Booij LH Reversal of neuromuscular blockade with sugammadex in patients with myasthenia gravis: a case series of 21 patients and review of the literature. *Eur J Anaesthesiol.* 2014;31:715–721.
176. Vymazal T, Krecmerova M, Bicek V, et al. Feasibility of full and rapid neuromuscular blockade recovery with sugammadex in myasthenia gravis patients undergoing surgery—a series of 117 cases. *Ther Clin Risk Manag.* 2015;11:1593–1596.
177. Madsen MV, Istre O, Staehr-Rye AK, et al. Postoperative shoulder pain after laparoscopic hysterectomy with deep neuromuscular blockade and low-pressure pneumoperitoneum: a randomised controlled trial. *Eur J Anaesthesiol.* 2016;33:341–347.
178. Madsen MV, Gatke MR, Springborg HH, et al. Optimising abdominal space with deep neuromuscular blockade in gynaecologic laparoscopy—a randomised, blinded crossover study. *Acta Anaesthesiol Scand.* 2015;59:441–447.
179. Van Wijk RM, Watts RW, Ledowski T, et al. Deep neuromuscular block reduces intra-abdominal pressure requirements during laparoscopic cholecystectomy: a prospective observational study. *Acta Anaesthesiol Scand.* 2015;59:434–440.
180. Dubois PE, Putz L, Jamart J, et al. Deep neuromuscular block improves surgical conditions during laparoscopic hysterectomy: a randomised controlled trial. *Eur J Anaesthesiol.* 2014;31:430–436.
181. Martini CH, Boon M, Bevers RF, et al. Evaluation of surgical conditions during laparoscopic surgery in patients with moderate vs deep neuromuscular block. *Br J Anaesth.* 2014;112:498–505.
182. Blobner M, Frick CG, Stauble RB, et al. Neuromuscular blockade improves surgical conditions (NISCO). *Surg Endosc.* 2015;29:627–636.
183. Staehr-Rye AK, Rasmussen LS, Rosenberg J, et al. Surgical space conditions during low-pressure laparoscopic cholecystectomy with deep versus moderate neuromuscular blockade: a randomized clinical study. *Anesth Analg.* 2014;119:1084–1092.
184. Madsen MV, Staehr-Rye AK, Gatke MR, et al. Neuromuscular blockade for optimising surgical conditions during abdominal and gynaecological surgery: a systematic review. *Acta Anaesthesiol Scand.* 2015;59:1–16.
185. Matsuki G, Takahata O, Iwasaki H: Repeat dosing of rocuronium after reversal of neuromuscular block by sugammadex. *Can J Anaesth.* 2011;58:769–770.
186. Iwasaki H, Sasakawa T, Takahoko K, et al. A case series of re-establishment of neuromuscular block with rocuronium after sugammadex reversal. *J Anesth.* 2016;30:534–537.
187. Hoffmann U, Grosse-Sundrup M, Eikermann-Haerter K, et al. Calabadion: A new agent to reverse the effects of benzylisoquinoline and steroidal neuromuscular-blocking agents. *Anesthesiology.* 2013;119:317–325.
188. Haerter F, Simons JCP, Foerster U, et al. Comparative effectiveness of calabadion and sugammadex to reverse non-depolarizing neuromuscular-blocking agents. *Anesthesiology.* 2015;123:1337–1349.

22 Local Anesthetics

YI LIN • SPENCER S. LIU

Mechanisms of Action of Local Anesthetics
   Anatomy of Nerves
   Electrophysiology of Neural Conduction and Voltage-gated Sodium Channels
   Molecular Mechanisms of Local Anesthetics
   Mechanism of Nerve Blockade
Pharmacology and Pharmacodynamics
   Chemical Properties and Relationship to Activity and Potency
   Additives to Increase Local Anesthetic Activity
Pharmacokinetics of Local Anesthetics
   Systemic Absorption
   Distribution
   Elimination
   Clinical Pharmacokinetics
Clinical Use of Local Anesthetics
Toxicity of Local Anesthetics
   Systemic Toxicity of Local Anesthetics
   Treatment of Systemic Toxicity from Local Anesthetics
   Neural Toxicity of Local Anesthetics
   Transient Neurologic Symptoms after Spinal Anesthesia
   Allergic Reactions to Local Anesthetics
Future Therapeutics and Modalities

KEY POINTS

1. Local anesthetics provide anesthesia and analgesia by blocking the transmission of pain sensation along nerve fibers.
2. The key target of local anesthetics is the voltage-gated sodium channel. The binding is intracellular and is mediated by hydrophobic interactions.
3. The degree of nerve blockade depends on both drug concentration and volume.
4. Most clinically relevant agents contain a lipid-soluble benzene ring connected to an amide group and are categorized as either aminoesters or aminoamides based on their chemical linkage.
5. Potency is related to lipid solubility and physiochemical properties of the agent. In general, more potent agents are more lipid-soluble.
6. Clinical use of local anesthetics may be increased by addition of epinephrine, opioids, and α_2-adrenergic agonists. The value of alkalinization of local anesthetics appears to be debatable as a clinically useful tool to improve anesthesia.
7. The rate of local anesthetic system absorption depends on the site of injection, the dose, the drug's intrinsic pharmacokinetic properties, and the addition of a vasoactive agent.
8. Systemic toxicity from the clinical use of local anesthetics is an uncommon occurrence. Patients with cardiovascular collapse from bupivacaine, ropivacaine, and levobupivacaine may be especially difficult to resuscitate; however, intravenous lipid infusion is an effective new therapy.

Local anesthetics block the conduction of impulses in electrically excitable tissues. One of the important uses is to provide anesthesia and analgesia by blocking the transmission of pain sensation along nerve fibers. The molecular target of these agents is specific and the interaction has been extensively studied. Existing clinical applications are numerous and continue to expand. A comprehensive understanding of the mechanisms and the physiochemical properties of these agents will optimize the therapeutic potential and avoid complications associated with inadvertent systemic toxicity.

Mechanisms of Action of Local Anesthetics

Anatomy of Nerves

Local anesthetics are used to block nerves in the peripheral nervous system (PNS) and central nervous system (CNS). In the PNS, nerves contain both afferent and efferent fibers, which are bundled into one or more fascicles and organized within three tissue layers.[1] Individual nerve fibers within each fascicle are surrounded by the *endoneurium*, a loose connective tissue containing glial cells, fibroblasts, and blood capillaries. A dense layer of collagenous connective tissue called the *perineurium* surrounds each fascicle. A final layer of dense connective tissue, the *epineurium*, encases groups of fascicles into a cylindrical sheath (Fig. 22-1). These layers of tissue offer protection to the surrounded nerve fibers and act as barriers to passive diffusion of local anesthetics.[2]

Nerves in both the CNS and PNS are differentiated by the presence or absence of myelin sheath. Myelinated nerve fibers are surrounded by Schwann cells in the PNS and by oligodendrocytes in the CNS. The cells form a concentrically wrapped lipid bilayer sheath around the axons that cover the length of the nerve.[3] The myelin sheath is interrupted at short regular intervals by specialized regions called *nodes of Ranvier*, which contain densely clustered protein elements essential for transmission of neuronal signals (Fig. 22-2).[4] As electrical signals are renewed at each node, nerve impulses move in myelinated fibers by saltatory conduction. In contrast, there are no nodes of Ranvier in nonmyelinated nerve fibers. Although these nerve fibers are similarly encased in Schwann cells, the plasma membrane does not wrap around the axons concentrically. Several nerve fibers may be simultaneously embedded within a single Schwann cell (Fig. 22-3).[1]

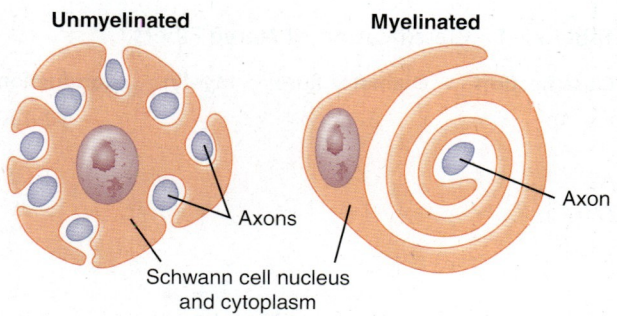

Figure 22-3 Schwann cells form myelin around one myelinated axon or encompass several unmyelinated axons. (Adapted from Carpenter RL, Mackey DC. Local anesthetics. In: Barash PG, Cullen BF, Stoelting RF, eds. *Clinical Anesthesia*. 3rd ed. Philadelphia, PA: Lippincott-Raven; 1996:413.)

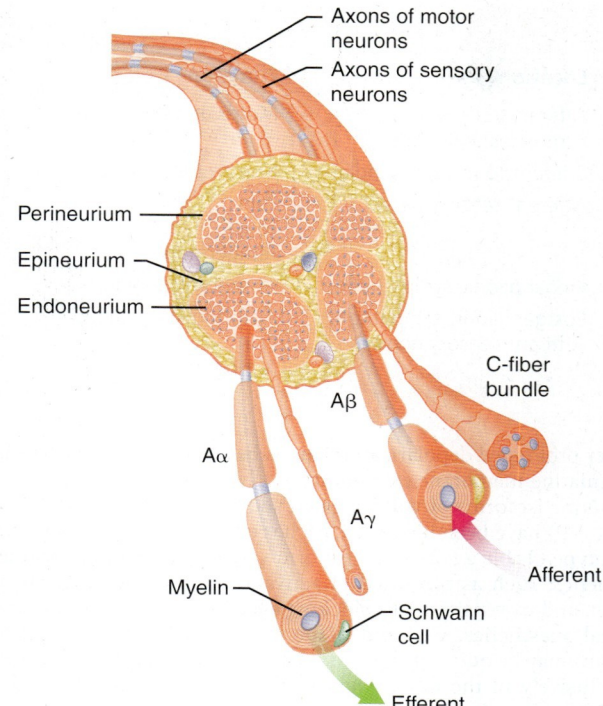

Figure 22-1 Schematic cross-section of a typical peripheral nerve. The epineurium, consisting of collagen fibers, is oriented along the long axis of the nerve. The perineurium is a discrete cell layer, whereas the endoneurium is a matrix of connective tissue. Both afferent and efferent axons are shown. Sympathetic axons (not shown) are also present in mixed peripheral nerves. (Adapted with permission from Strichartz GR. Neural physiology and local anesthetic action. In: Cousins MJ, Bridenbaugh PO, eds. *Neural Blockade in Clinical Anesthesia and Management of Pain*. Philadelphia, PA: Lippincott-Raven; 1998:35.)

Nerve fibers are commonly classified according to their size, conduction velocity, and function (Table 22-1). In general, nerve fibers with cross-sectional diameter greater than 1 μm are myelinated. Both a larger nerve size and the presence of myelin sheath are associated with faster conduction velocity.[5] Nerve fibers with large diameters have better intrinsic electric conductance. Myelin improves the electrical insulation of nerve fibers

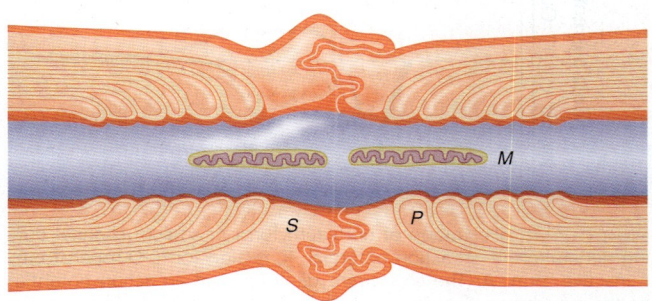

Figure 22-2 Diagram of node of Ranvier displaying mitochondria (*M*), tight junctions in paranodal area (*P*), and Schwann cell (*S*) surrounding node. (Adapted with permission from Strichartz GR. Mechanisms of action of local anesthetic agents. In: Rogers MC, Tinker JH, Covino BG, et al., eds. *Principles and Practice of Anesthesiology*. St. Louis, MO: Mosby Year Book; 1993:1197.)

and permits more rapid impulse transmission via saltatory conduction. Large-diameter myelinated fibers, many of which are classified as A fibers, are typically involved in motor and sensory functions in which speed of nerve transmission is critical. In contrast, small-diameter nonmyelinated C fibers have slower conduction velocity and relay sensory information such as pain, temperature, and autonomic functions.

Electrophysiology of Neural Conduction and Voltage-gated Sodium Channels

Transmission of electrical impulses along the cell membrane forms the basis of signal transduction along nerve fibers. Energy necessary for the propagation and maintenance of the electric potential is maintained on the cell surface by ionic disequilibria across the semipermeable cell membrane.[6] The resting membrane potential, approximately −60 to −70 mV in neurons (the extracellular electric potential is, by convention, defined as zero, and the intracellular potential is thus negative relative to it), is derived predominantly from a difference in the intracellular and extracellular concentrations of potassium and sodium ions. Neurons at rest are more permeable to potassium ions than sodium ions because of potassium leak channels; therefore, membrane potential is closer to the equilibrium potential of potassium (E_K −80 mV) than that of sodium (E_{Na} +60 mV). The ion gradient is continuously regenerated by protein pumps, cotransporters, and channels via an adenosine triphosphate–dependent process.

Electrical impulses are conducted along nerve fibers as action potentials. They are brief, localized spikes of positive charge, or depolarizations, on the cell membrane caused by rapid influx of sodium ions down its electrochemical gradient.[7] An action potential is initiated by local membrane depolarization, such as at the cell body or nerve terminal by a ligand–receptor complex. When a certain charge threshold is reached, an action potential is triggered and further depolarization occurs in an "all-or-none" fashion.[8] The spike in membrane potential peaks around +50 mV, at which point the influx of sodium is replaced with an efflux of potassium, causing a reversal of membrane potential, or repolarization. The passive diffusion of membrane depolarization triggers other action potentials in either adjacent cell membranes in *nonmyelinated* nerve fibers or adjacent nodes of Ranvier in *myelinated* nerve fibers, resulting in a wave of action potential being propagated along the nerve. A short *refractory period* that ensues after each action potential prevents

Table 22-1 Classification of Nerve Fibers

Classification	Diameter (μm)	Myelin	Conduction (m/s)	Location	Function
Aα, Aβ	6–22	+	30–120	Afferents/efferents for muscles and joints	Motor and proprioception
Aγ	3–6	+	15–35	Efferent to muscle spindle	Muscle tone
Aδ	1–4	+	5–25	Afferent sensory nerve	Pain Touch Temperature
B	<3	+	3–15	Preganglionic sympathetic	Autonomic function
C	0.3–1.3	−	0.7–1.3	Postganglionic sympathetic Afferent sensory nerve	Autonomic function Pain Temperature

the retrograde spread of action potential on previously activated membranes.[7]

The flow of ions responsible for action potentials is mediated by a variety of channels and pumps, the most important of which are the voltage-gated sodium channels. They are essential for the influx of sodium ions during the rapid depolarization phase of the action potential and belong to a family of channel proteins that also includes voltage-gated potassium and voltage-gated calcium channels. Each voltage-gated sodium channel is a complex made up of one principal α-subunit and one or more auxiliary β-subunits.[9] The α-subunit is a single-polypeptide transmembrane protein that contains most of the key components of the channel function. They include four homologous α-helical domains (D1 to D4) that form the channel pore and control ion selectivity, voltage-sensing regions that regulate gating function and inactivation, and phosphorylation sites for modulation by protein kinases. β-subunits are short polypeptide proteins with a single transmembrane domain. They are linked to α-subunits by either noncovalent or disulfide bonds; although they are dispensable for channel activity, evidence suggests that they perhaps play a role in modulation of channel expression, localization, and function.

In the absence of a stimulus, voltage-gated sodium channels exist predominantly in the resting or closed state (Fig. 22-4). On membrane depolarization, positive charges on the membrane interact with charged amino acid residues in the voltage-sensing regions (S4).[10] This induces a conformational change in the channel, converting it to the open state. Sodium ions rush through the opened pore, which is lined with negatively charged residues. Ion selectivity is determined by these amino acid residues; changes in their composition can lead to increased permeability for other cations, such as potassium and calcium.[11] Within milliseconds after opening, channels undergo a transition to the inactivated state. Depending on the frequency and voltage of the initial depolarizing stimulus, the channel may undergo either fast or slow inactivation. Slow or fast inactivation refers to the duration in which the channel remains refractory to repeat depolarization before resetting to the closed state. Fast inactivation completes within a millisecond and is sensitive to the action of local anesthetics. It is mediated by a short mobile intracellular polypeptide loop connecting domains D3 and D4 that closes the channel from inside the cell via a hinge-lid mechanism.[12] A triad of highly hydrophobic amino acids (isoleucine, phenylalanine, and methionine [IFM]) appears to be an important structural determinant of fast activation; disrupting the loop or changing the hydrophobicity of the amino acids abrogates fast inactivation.[13,14] Slow activation, lasting seconds to minutes, is distinct from fast activation. It is resistant to the action of local anesthetics and its mechanism is less well understood. It often occurs after prolonged depolarization and is believed to be important in regulating membrane excitability.

Nine isoforms of voltage-gated sodium channels (Na_V 1.1 to Na_V 1.9) have been identified; each relates to a unique α-subunit subtype (Table 22-2). Each isoform varies slightly in its channel kinetics, such as threshold of activation and mode of inactivation, and its sensitivity to blocking agents like tetrodotoxins and local anesthetics. Cell and tissue expression of individual isoforms may be quite specific; for instance, Na_V 1.2 is found almost exclusively in the CNS, whereas Na_V 1.6 is restricted to nodes of Ranvier in both CNS and PNS.[15] Likewise, several isoforms could be present on a single cell type; both Na_V 1.8 and Na_V 1.9 have been found in small- to medium-sized neurons in dorsal root ganglia that are connected to Aδ and C fibers. Whether individual isoforms each have a separate and defined role remains to

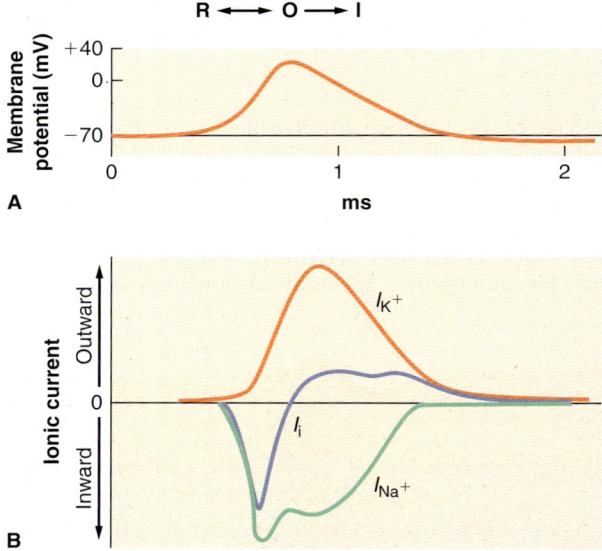

Figure 22-4 Illustration of dominant form of sodium channel during generation of an action potential. R, resting form; O, open form; I, inactive form. **A:** The concurrent generation of an action potential as the membrane depolarizes from resting potential. **B:** The concurrent changes in ion flux, as inward sodium current ($I_{NA}+$) and outward potassium current (I_K+) together yield the net ionic current across the membrane (I_i). (Adapted with permission from Strichartz GR. Neural physiology and local anesthetic action. In: Cousins MJ, Bridenbaugh PO, eds. *Neural Blockade in Clinical Anesthesia and Management of Pain.* Philadelphia, PA: Lippincott-Raven; 1998:35.)

Table 22-2 Voltage-Gated Sodium Channels

Name	Tissue Expression	Tetrodotoxin	Associated Channelopathies
Na_V 1.1	CNS, heart	Sensitive	Inherited febrile epilepsy
Na_V 1.2	CNS nonmyelinated axons	Sensitive	Inherited febrile epilepsy
Na_V 1.3	Fetal DRG	Sensitive	None known
Na_V 1.4	Skeletal muscle	Sensitive	Hyperkalemic periodic paralysis, paramyotonia congenital
Na_V 1.5	Heart, embryonic neurons	Insensitive	Brugada syndrome, long QT syndrome
Na_V 1.6	Nodes of Ranvier	Sensitive	None known
Na_V 1.7	CNS, DRG, sympathetic neurons	Sensitive	Erythromelalgia, paroxysmal extreme pain disorder, congenital insensitivity to pain
Na_V 1.8	Small DRG neurons	Insensitive	None known
Na_V 1.9	Small DRG neurons	Insensitive	None known

CNS, central nervous system; DRG, dorsal root ganglion.
Data adapted from Benarroch EE. Sodium channels and pain. *Neurology*. 2007:68:233; and Koopmann TT, Bezzina CR, Wilde AA. Voltage-gated sodium channels: Action players with many faces. *Ann Med*. 2006:38:472.

be seen; however, clues to their function may be inferred from studies of several inherited diseases that have been associated with sodium channelopathies. Hyperexcitability of Na_V 1.7 has been implicated in several painful disease states, such as primary erythromelalgia and paroxysmal extreme pain disorder.[16,17] Conversely the null mutation of Na_V 1.7 is linked to a rare genetic condition in which otherwise normal individuals have severely impaired perception to pain.[18,19]

Molecular Mechanisms of Local Anesthetics

Local anesthetics block the transmission of nerve impulses by targeting the function of voltage-gated sodium channels. Several local anesthetics can also bind to other receptors like voltage-gated potassium channels and nicotinic acetylcholine receptors and their amphipathic nature may enable them to interact with plasma membranes. However, it is widely accepted that local anesthetics induce anesthesia and analgesia through direct interactions with the sodium channels. Other molecules with local anesthetic properties, such as tricyclic antidepressants and anticonvulsants, may likewise interact with voltage-gated sodium channels; however, it is unclear if they act through similar mechanisms. Therefore, the following discussion is limited to the "traditional" set of local anesthetic molecules.

Local anesthetics reversibly bind the intracellular portion of voltage-gated sodium channels (Fig. 22-5). Early experiments with giant squid axons demonstrated that a derivative of lidocaine with a permanent positive charge and that cannot cross the plasma membrane (QX-314) blocks ion current through voltage-gated sodium channels only with intra-axoplasmic injections, but not with external application.[20] Subsequent mutational analyses have supported this observation and identified specific sites on the channel involved in drug recognition.[21] Several hydrophobic aromatic residues (a phenylalanine at position 1,764 and a tyrosine at position 1,771 in Na_V 1.2) located within an α-helix (S6) of domains 1, 3, and 4 are essential for drug binding (Fig. 22-6). They line an inner cavity within the intracellular portion of the channel pore and span a region about 11 Å apart, roughly the size of a local anesthetic molecule. Changes in either residue severely reduce the binding affinity. Another hydrophobic amino acid (an isoleucine at position 1,760), located near the outer pore opening, also influences the dissociation of local anesthetics from the channel by antagonizing the release of drugs through the channel pore.

Application of local anesthetics typically produces a concentration-dependent decrease in the peak sodium current.[22,23] Termed *tonic blockade*, this refers to the reduction in the number of sodium channels for a given drug concentration present in the open state at equilibrium. In contrast, repetitive stimulation of the sodium channels often leads to a shift in the steady-state equilibrium, resulting in a greater number of channels being blocked at the same drug concentration. This is termed *use-dependent blockade*—its exact mechanism is incompletely understood and has been the subject of many competing hypotheses. One popular

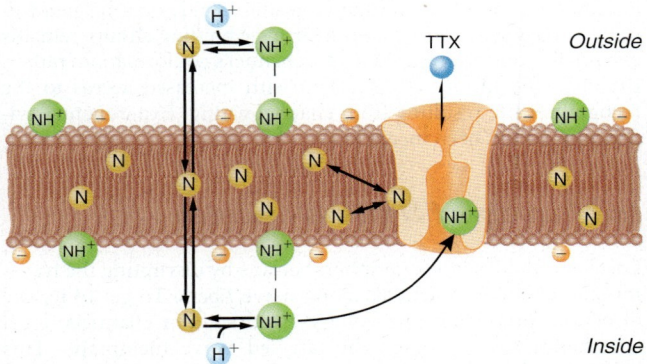

Figure 22-5 Diagram of the bilayer lipid membrane of conductive tissue with the sodium channel spanning the membrane. Tertiary amine local anesthetics exist as both neutral base (N) and protonated, charged form (NH^+) in equilibrium. The neutral base (N) is more lipid soluble, preferentially partitions into the lipophilic membrane interior, and easily passes through the membrane. The charged form (NH^+) is more water soluble and binds to the sodium channel at the negatively charged membrane surface. Both forms can affect the function of the sodium channel. The N form can cause membrane expansion and closure of the sodium channel. The NH^+ form will directly inhibit the sodium channel by binding with a local anesthetic receptor. The natural "local anesthetic" tetrodotoxin (TTX) binds at the external surface of the sodium channel and has no interaction with the clinically used local anesthetics. (Adapted with permission from Strichartz GR. Neural physiology and local anesthetic action. In: Cousins MJ, Bridenbaugh PO, eds. *Neural Blockade in Clinical Anesthesia and Management of Pain*. Philadelphia, PA: Lippincott-Raven; 1998:35.)

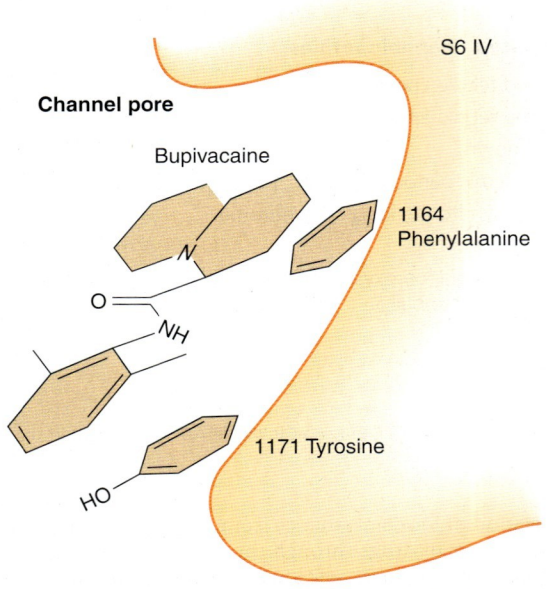

Figure 22-6 Diagram of the local anesthetic binding site, depicting a hydrophobic pocket within the sodium channel pore. (Adapted with permission from Ragsdale DS, McPhee JC, Scheuer T, et al. Molecular determinants of state-dependent block of Na+ channels by local anesthetics. *Science*. 1994;265:1724.)

the potency of the local anesthetics and the intrinsic conduction properties of nerve fibers, which in turn likely depend on the drug's binding affinity to the ion channels and the degree of drug saturation necessary to halt the transmission of action potentials. Accordingly, individual types of nerve fibers differ in their minimal blocking concentration, such that some A fibers are blocked by lower drug concentrations than C fibers.[25] Likewise, the pattern of stimulation (tonic vs. use-dependent blockade) influences the degree of conduction failure; repetitive stimulations, which can lead to a shift in steady-state equilibrium of blocked sodium channels, are associated with higher conduction failure than tonic stimulation at a given drug concentration.[26]

Of equal importance as drug concentration is the local anesthetic volume. A sufficient volume is needed to suppress the regeneration of nerve impulse over a critical length of nerve fiber. According to the model of decremental conduction (Fig. 22-7), as membrane depolarization from an action potential passively decays with distance along nerve fibers, the presence of local anesthetics decreases the ability of adjacent membrane or successive nodes of Ranvier to regenerate the impulse.[27] Transmission stops once the membrane depolarization falls below the threshold for action potential activation. If the exposure distance is inadequate, action potentials can "skip" over blocked segments and resume nerve conduction. In contrast, exposure over a long segment of nerve to even a relatively low drug concentration can still result in gradual extinction of impulse by decremental decay.

Not all sensory and motor modalities are blocked equally by local anesthetics. It has long been observed that application of local anesthetics produces an ordered progression of sensory and motor deficits, starting commonly with the disappearance of temperature sensation, followed in order by proprioception, motor function, sharp pain, and finally light touch. Termed *differential blockade*, historically this had been thought to be related simply to the diameter of the nerve fibers, with the smaller fibers inherently more susceptible to drug blockade than larger fibers.[28] However, although the "size principle" of differential blockade is consistent with many experimental findings, it is not universally true. Larger, myelinated Aδ fibers (believed to mediate sharp pain) are preferentially blocked over small, nonmyelinated

theory, the *modulated-receptor theory*, proposes that local anesthetics bind to the open or the inactivated channels more avidly than the resting channels, suggesting that drug affinity is a function of a channel's conformational state. An alternate theory, the *guarded-receptor theory*, assumes that the intrinsic binding affinity remains essentially constant regardless of a channel's conformation; rather, the apparent affinity is associated with increased access to the recognition site resulting from channel gating. Experimental evidence so far has been inconclusive.

Mechanism of Nerve Blockade

Local anesthetics block peripheral nerves by disrupting the transmission of action potentials along nerve fibers. To get to its site of action, principally the voltage-gated sodium channels, local anesthetics have to reach the targeted nerve membrane. This entails the diffusion of drugs through tissues and the generation of a concentration gradient. Even with close proximity of deposition, only about 1% to 2% of injected local anesthetics ultimately penetrate into the nerve.[24] As discussed earlier, the perineural sheath encasing nerve fibers appears to be an important determinant; nerves that have been desheathed in vitro require about a 100-fold lower local anesthetic concentration (in the 0.7–0.9 mM range for lidocaine) than nerves in vivo (the typical 2% lidocaine used clinically is equivalent to 75 mM concentration). Although it may vary with anatomic location and nerve physiology, functional block typically occurs within 5 minutes of injection in rat sciatic nerves, and this time course corresponds to the peak in the intraneural drug absorption.

The degree of nerve blockade depends on the local anesthetic concentration and volume. For a given drug, a minimal concentration is necessary to effect complete nerve blockade. It reflects

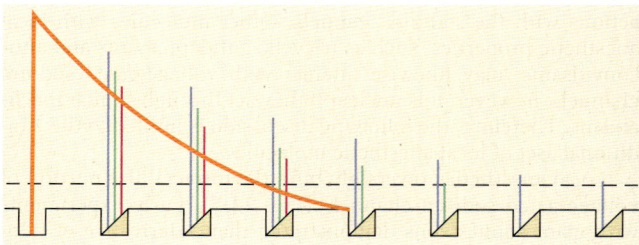

Figure 22-7 Diagram illustrating the principle of decremental conduction block by local anesthetic at a myelinated axon. The first node of Ranvier at left contains no local anesthetic and gives rise to a normal action potential (*solid curve*). If the nodes succeeding the first are occupied by a concentration of local anesthetic high enough to block 74% to 84% of the sodium conductance, then the action potential amplitudes decrease at successive nodes (amplitudes are indicated by *interrupted bars* representing three increasing concentrations of local anesthetic). Eventually, the impulse decays to below-threshold amplitude if the series of local anesthetic–containing nodes is long enough. Propagation of the impulse is then blocked by decremental conduction, even though none of the nodes are completely blocked. Concentrations of local anesthetics that block more than 84% of the sodium conductance at three successive nodes prevent any impulse propagation at all. (Adapted with permission from Fink BR. Mechanisms of differential axial blockade in epidural and spinal anesthesia. *Anesthesiology*. 1989;70:851.)

C fibers (dull pain). Furthermore, within the C fibers are fast and slow components of impulse transmission, each with distinct susceptibilities to drug blockade.[29] These observations argue against a purely pharmacokinetic mechanism as the sole explanation for differential blockade.

More likely, explanations may additionally be found in the intrinsic excitatory properties of the nerve fibers, namely, the patterned expression of ion pores and channels on the cellular membrane. Indeed, sodium channel isoforms Na_v 1.7 and Na_v 1.8 are highly expressed on the dorsal root ganglia, and have been shown to have distinct sensitivities to lidocaine.[30] Similarly, experiments with large pore, nonspecific cation channels, the transient receptor potential channel subfamily V (TRPV1) and member A1 (TRPA1), suggest that they can be activated by lidocaine and other local anesthetics.[31,32] Because these transient receptor potential channels are found predominantly on sensory neurons mediating specific stimulus modalities, their activation may selectively facilitate entry of local anesthetics, thereby resulting in the observed progression of sensory, autonomic, and motor blockade.

Pharmacology and Pharmacodynamics

Chemical Properties and Relationship to Activity and Potency

Most clinically relevant local anesthetics consist of a lipid-soluble, aromatic benzene ring connected to an amide group via either an amide or an ester moiety. The type of linkage broadly defines them into two categories, the *aminoesters* and the *aminoamides*, and affects how they are metabolized. Aminoesters are hydrolyzed by plasma cholinesterases and aminoamides are degraded by hepatic carboxylesterases. Some metabolites of aminoesters, such as *para*-aminobenzoic acid, can induce immunologic reactions and are responsible for the slightly greater incidence of severe allergic reactions associated with aminoesters. Other than these characteristics, physiochemical properties of both aminoesters and aminoamides are similar and are mainly determined by their dissociative constant, lipophilic makeup, and spatial arrangement of the molecule.

The tertiary amide on local anesthetics can accept a proton at low affinity; thus, these compounds are classified as weak bases. In aqueous solution, local anesthetics are in constant equilibrium between the protonated cationic form and the lipid-soluble neutral form. The ratio of the two forms depends on the pK_a or the dissociation constant of the local anesthetics and the surrounding pH (Table 22-3). A ratio with high concentration of the lipid-soluble form favors intracellular entry, as the cellular membrane restricts passage of the cationic form, but not the lipid soluble form.[2] Clinically, the proportion of the lipid-soluble form can be increased by alkalization of local anesthetic solution and thus accelerate the onset of action. Once inside the cell, equilibrium is reestablished between the cationic and the neutral forms, and experimental findings have shown that the cationic form is principally responsible for blockade of sodium channels.[33]

By far the most important physiochemical property of local anesthetics is their lipophilicity. Lipid solubility of local anesthetics is conferred by the composition of alkyl substitution on the amide and the benzene groups. In the laboratory, lipid solubility is measured by the partition coefficient in a hydrophobic solvent, octanol, and compounds with high octanol:buffer partition coefficient are more lipid soluble.[34] A positive correlation exists between the potency of the local anesthetics and their octanol:buffer partition coefficient; highly lipid-soluble agents are more potent and tend to have a longer duration of action than ones that are less lipid soluble.[35] The lipophilic property of local anesthetics may act at two levels. The first is at the level of cellular entry as greater lipid solubility facilitates passage through the lipid membrane barriers. The second is at the level of binding to the sodium channels. Detailed crystallographic findings show that local anesthetics bind to a hydrophobic pocket within the sodium channels and suggest that ligand binding may be mediated primarily by hydrophobic and van der Waals interactions (Fig. 22-6).[21]

The correlation between local anesthetic potency and lipophilicity is generally observed in vitro; however, it may be less exact in vivo. Compared with experimental setups using isolated nerves, many other factors may influence the potency of local anesthetics on nerves in situ.[36] Highly lipid-soluble agents may be sequestered into surrounding adipose cells and myelin sheaths. Local anesthetics cause vasodilation, which in turn could alter regional drug redistribution.[37,38] Finally, mounting evidence suggests that some local anesthetics can enter certain

Table 22-3 Physicochemical Properties of Clinically Used Local Anesthetics

Local Anesthetic	pK_a	Percent Ionized (at pH 7.4)	Partition Coefficient (Lipid Solubility)	Percent Protein Binding
Amides				
Bupivacaine[a]	8.1	83	3,420	95
Etidocaine	7.7	66	7,317	94
Lidocaine	7.9	76	366	64
Mepivacaine	7.6	61	130	77
Prilocaine	7.9	76	129	55
Ropivacaine	8.1	83	775	94
Esters				
Chloroprocaine	8.7	95	810	N/A
Procaine	8.9	97	100	6
Tetracaine	8.5	93	5,822	94

[a]Levobupivacaine has same physicochemical properties as racemate.
N/A, not available.
Data from Liu SS. Local anesthetics and analgesia. In: Ashburn MA, Rice LJ, eds. *The Management of Pain*. New York: Churchill Livingstone; 1997:141.

Table 22-4 Relative Potency of Local Anesthetics for Different Clinical Applications

	Bupivacaine	Chloroprocaine	Lidocaine	Mepivacaine	Prilocaine	Ropivacaine
Peripheral nerve	3.6	N/A	1	2.6	0.8	3.6
Spinal	9.6	1	1	1	1	N/A
Epidural	4	0.5	1	1	1	4

N/A, not available.

neurons via nonspecific cation channels, thereby circumventing the membrane barrier altogether.[31] Hence, relative potency of local anesthetics has been determined clinically for different applications, and these values are listed in Table 22-4.

Finally, anesthetic activity and potency are affected by the stereochemistry of the local anesthetic molecules. Many older drug preparations exist as racemic mixtures; that is, enantiomeric stereoisomers are in equal proportion. Newer agents, namely, ropivacaine and levobupivacaine, are available as specific enantiomers. They were initially developed as less cardiotoxic alternatives to bupivacaine. Although the desired improvement in the safety index has been generally supported in clinical studies, this is at the expense of a slight decrease in potency overall and shorter duration of action compared with racemic mixtures.[39,40] The underlying mechanism has not been defined. Topographic features at the channel-binding site are likely to play a key role in stereoselectivity of local anesthetics.

6 Additives to Increase Local Anesthetic Activity

Epinephrine

Reported benefits of epinephrine include prolongation of local anesthetic block, increased intensity of block, and decreased systemic absorption of local anesthetic.[41] Epinephrine's vasoconstrictive effects augment local anesthetics by antagonizing inherent vasodilating effects of local anesthetics, decreasing systemic absorption and intraneural clearance, and perhaps by redistributing intraneural local anesthetic.[41,42]

Direct analgesic effects from epinephrine may also occur via interaction with α_2-adrenergic receptors in the brain and spinal cord,[43] especially because local anesthetics increase the vascular uptake of epinephrine.[44] The clinical effects of the use of epinephrine are listed in Table 22-5. The smallest dose is suggested because epinephrine combined with local anesthetics may have toxic effects on tissue,[45] the cardiovascular system,[46] peripheral nerves, and the spinal cord.[41]

Alkalinization of Local Anesthetic Solution

Local anesthetic solutions are alkalinized in order to hasten onset of neural block.[47] The pH of commercial preparations of local anesthetics ranges from 3.9 to 6.5 and is especially acidic if prepackaged with epinephrine.[48] Because the pK_a of commonly used local anesthetics ranges from 7.6 to 8.9 (Table 22-3), less than 3% of the commercially prepared local anesthetics exist as the lipid-soluble neutral form. As previously discussed, the neutral form is believed to be important for penetration into the neural cytoplasm, whereas the charged form primarily interacts with the local anesthetic receptor within the sodium channel. Therefore, the rationale for alkalinization was to increase the ratio of local anesthetic existing as the lipid-soluble neutral form.

Table 22-5 Effects of Addition of Epinephrine to Local Anesthetics

	Increase Duration	Decrease Blood Levels (%)	Dose/Concentration of Epinephrine
Nerve Block			
Bupivacaine	+/−	10–20	1:200,000
Lidocaine	++	20–30	1:200,000
Mepivacaine	++	20–30	1:200,000
Ropivacaine	− −	0	1:200,000
Epidural			
Bupivacaine	+/−	10–20	1:300,000–1:200,000
Levobupivacaine	+/−	10	1:200,000–1:400,000
Chloroprocaine	++		1:200,000
Lidocaine	++	20–30	1:600,000–1:200,000
Mepivacaine	++	20–30	1:200,000
Ropivacaine	− −	0	1:200,000
Spinal			
Bupivacaine	+/−		0.2 mg
Lidocaine	++		0.2 mg
Tetracaine	++		0.2 mg

++, overall supported; − −, overall not supported; +/−, inconsistent.
Data from Liu SS. Local anesthetics and analgesia. In: Ashburn MA, Rice LJ, eds. *The Management of Pain*. New York: Churchill Livingstone; 1997:141; and Kopacz DJ. A comparison of epidural levobupivacaine 0.5% with or without epinephrine for lumbar spine surgery. *Anesth Analg*. 2001;93:755.

However, clinically used local anesthetics cannot be alkalinized beyond a pH of 6.05 to 8 before precipitation occurs[48] and these pH values will only increase the neutral form to about 10%.

Clinical studies on the association between alkalinization of local anesthetics and hastening of block onset have shown an improvement of less than 5 minutes compared with commercial preparations.[47,49] Furthermore, results from a study in rats indicate that alkalinization of lidocaine may also decrease the duration of peripheral nerve blocks if the mixture contained no epinephrine.[50] Together, alkalinization of local anesthetics appears limited as a clinically useful adjuvant to improving anesthesia.

Opioids

Opioids have multiple central and peripheral mechanisms of analgesic action (see Chapter 20). Spinal administration of opioids provides analgesia primarily by attenuating C-fiber nociception[51] and is independent of supraspinal mechanisms.[52] Coadministration of opioids with central neuraxial local anesthetics results in synergistic analgesia.[53] An exception to this analgesic synergy is chloroprocaine, which appears to decrease the effectiveness of opioids coadministered epidurally.[54] The reason is unclear, but the mechanism does not seem to involve direct antagonism of opioid receptors.[55] Nonetheless, clinical studies support the practice of central neuraxial coadministration of local anesthetics and opioids for prolongation and intensification of analgesia and anesthesia.[53]

The discovery of peripheral opioid receptors initially generated much interest in the use of opioids as adjuvants to local anesthetics for peripheral nerve blockade.[56] However, although some studies have reported favorable outcomes for such coadministration, others have failed to demonstrate any increased efficacy.[57] A problem that has plagued many studies is the lack of adequate controls for differentiating the analgesic effects of opioids acting peripherally versus a more central mechanism resulting from systemically absorbed opioids. Nonetheless, recent carefully designed trials have shown that some opioids, namely, buprenorphine, may enhance and prolong postoperative analgesia better than either local anesthetics alone or local anesthetics administered with intramuscular buprenorphine.[58,59] Finally, cumulative evidence does not support the use of intra-articular coadministration of local anesthetic and opioid for postoperative analgesia.[60]

β₂-Adrenergic Agonists

α₂-Adrenergic agonists can be a useful adjuvant to local anesthetics. α₂-Specific agonists such as clonidine produce analgesia via supraspinal and spinal adrenergic receptors.[61] Clonidine also has direct inhibitory effects on peripheral nerve conduction (A and C nerve fibers).[62] Thus, addition of clonidine may have multiple mechanisms of action depending on the type of application. Preliminary evidence suggests that coadministration of an α₂-agonist and local anesthetic results in central neuraxial and peripheral nerve analgesic synergy,[63] whereas systemic (supraspinal) effects are additive.[64] On average, clonidine improves the duration of analgesia by about 2 hours, regardless of whether an intermediate- or long-acting local anesthetic is used.[65] Overall, results from clinical trials indicate that clonidine can enhance local anesthetic effects when used for intrathecal and epidural anesthesia and peripheral nerve blocks.[65,66]

Steroids

Potent glucocorticoid injections have been widely used for the treatment of chronic low back pain caused by radiculopathy. Experiments in animals using extended-release preparations of local anesthetics have found that addition of dexamethasone to the mixture prolongs the conduction block after peripheral nerve application.[67,68] The duration of the blockade is associated with the potency of the glucocorticoid activity and appears to be steroid receptor dependent and locally mediated.[69] Clinical reports of the use of dexamethasone as an adjuvant to local anesthetics have shown similar prolongation of anesthesia after brachial plexus blockades[70,71] and intravenous regional anesthesia.[72] Combined with intermediate- to long-acting local anesthetics, dexamethasone extends the duration of analgesia by approximately 50% after supraclavicular[70] or interscalene approaches[71] to the brachial plexus block (Fig. 22-8). Although initial laboratory data show no evidence of increased neurotoxicity from use of dexamethasone as compared with other adjuvants, our current understanding of its mechanism of action and potential side effects remains incomplete.[73]

Liposomes

Commercially available preparations of liposomal bupivacaine are designed to provide sustained release of encapsulated bupivacaine after a single administration. Currently, such preparations are approved for local infiltration of surgical wounds after bunionectomy and hemorrhoidectomy.[74,75] Compared with placebo controls, liposomal bupivacaine reduced cumulative pain score, increased time to first opioid use, and required less rescue analgesia. However, in trials with active comparators (i.e., plain bupivacaine), there was no statistically significant difference among the cumulative pain scores across the treatment groups.[76,77] A direct comparison based on equivalent content of the bupivacaine (1.33%) showed that the addition of a liposomal formulation extends the

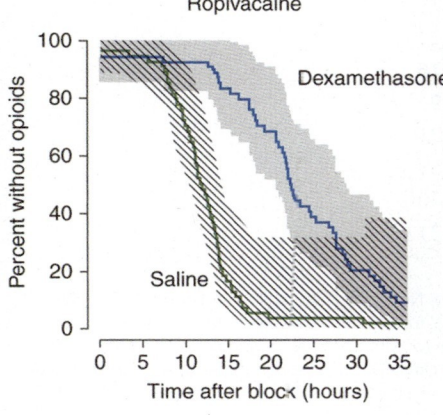
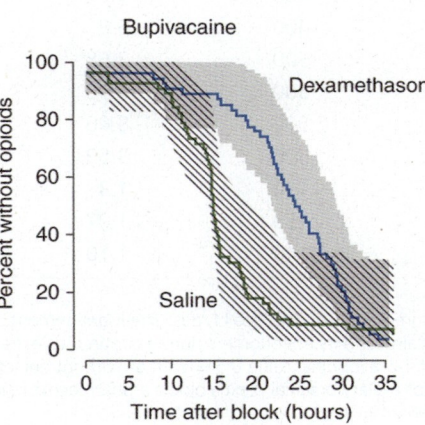

Figure 22-8 Addition of dexamethasone to either ropivacaine or bupivacaine increases the duration of analgesia after interscalene brachial plexus block. Data are shown as the Kaplan–Meier survival density estimates, with the shaded region representing the 95% confidence interval. (Reprinted with permission from Cummings KC, Napierkowski DE, Parra-Sanchez I, et al. Effect of dexamethasone on the duration of interscalene nerve blocks with ropivacaine or bupivacaine. Br J Anaesth. 2011;107:446.)

block duration by a modest 14% (240 minutes vs. 210 minutes for liposomal bupivacaine and 1.33% bupivacaine, respectively).[78]

In animal models, perineural infiltration of liposomal bupivacaine was associated with tissue inflammation and myotoxicity.[78] The degree of myotoxicity was comparable to that of 0.5% bupivacaine, although the inflammation due to liposomal bupivacaine persisted for much longer duration. There was no evidence of local neurotoxicity or CNS or cardiac toxicity.[79] Clinically, most frequently reported untoward effects of liposomal bupivacaine were nausea and pyrexia.[80]

Pharmacokinetics of Local Anesthetics

Plasma concentration of local anesthetics is a function of the dose administered and the rates of systemic absorption, tissue distribution, and drug elimination. Elevated levels may produce unintended effects in other electric-sensitive systems, most importantly, the cardiovascular system and the CNS. Having a thorough understanding of the factors involved would enable one to maximize the local anesthetic potential while avoiding possible complications arising from systemic local anesthetic toxicity.

Systemic Absorption

Decreasing systemic absorption of local anesthetics increases their safety margin in clinical uses. The rate and extent of systemic absorption depends on the site of injection, the dose, the drug's intrinsic pharmacokinetic properties, and the addition of a vasoactive agent. The vascularity of the tissue markedly influences the rate of drug absorption, such that deposition of local anesthetics in vessel-rich tissues results in higher peak plasma levels in a shorter period of time. Accordingly, the rate of systemic absorption is greatest with intercostal nerve blocks, followed in decreasing order by caudal and epidural injections, brachial plexus block, and femoral and sciatic nerve blocks (Table 22-6). Thus, the same amount of local anesthetics injected would result in unequal peak plasma levels depending on the site of drug delivery.

For a given site of injection, the rate of systemic absorption and the peak plasma level are directly proportional to the dose of local anesthetic deposited. This relationship is nearly linear (Fig. 22-9) and independent of the drug concentration and the speed of injection.[81]

The rate of systemic absorption differs with individual local anesthetics. In general, more potent lipid-soluble agents are associated with a slower rate of absorption than less lipid-soluble compounds (Fig. 22-10). Sequestration into lipid-rich compartments may not be the only explanation. Local anesthetics exert direct effects on vascular smooth muscles in a concentration-dependent manner. At low concentrations, more potent agents appear to cause more vasoconstriction than less potent agents, thereby decreasing the rate of vascular absorption.[38] At high concentrations, vasodilatory effects seem to predominate for most local anesthetics.

Distribution

Systemic absorption of local anesthetics leads to rapid distribution throughout the body. The steady-state drug concentration

Table 22-6 Typical C_{max} after Regional Anesthesia with Commonly Used Local Anesthetics

Local Anesthetic	Technique	Dose (mg)	C_{max} (μg/mL)	T_{max} (min)	Toxic Plasma Concentration (μg/mL)
Bupivacaine	Brachial plexus	150	1.0	20	3
	Celiac plexus	100	1.50	17	
	Epidural	150	1.26	20	
	Intercostal	140	0.90	30	
	Lumbar sympathetic	52.5	0.49	24	
	Sciatic/femoral	400	1.89	15	
Levobupivacaine	Epidural	75	0.36	50	4
	Brachial plexus	250	1.2	55	
Lidocaine	Brachial plexus	400	4.00	25	5
	Epidural	400	4.27	20	
	Intercostal	400	6.8	15	
Mepivacaine	Brachial plexus	500	3.68	24	5
	Epidural	500	4.95	16	
	Intercostal	500	8.06	9	
	Sciatic/femoral	500	3.59	31	
Ropivacaine	Brachial plexus	190	1.3	53	4
	Epidural	150	1.07	40	
	Intercostal	140	1.10	21	

C_{max}, peak plasma levels; T_{max}, time until C_{max}.
Data from Liu SS. Local anesthetics and analgesia. In: Ashburn MA, Rice LJ, eds. *The Management of Pain*. New York: Churchill Livingstone; 1997:141; Berrisford RG. Plasma concentrations of bupivacaine and its enantiomers during continuous extrapleural intercostal nerve block. *Br J Anaesth*. 1993;70:201; Kopacz DJ. A comparison of epidural levobupivacaine 0.5% with or without epinephrine for lumbar spine surgery. *Anesth Analg*. 2001;93:755; and Crews JC. Levobupivacaine for axillary brachial plexus block: a pharmacokinetic and clinical comparison in patients with normal renal function or renal disease. *Anesth Analg*. 2002;95:219.

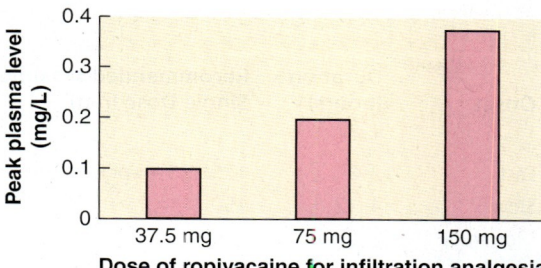

Figure 22-9 Increasing doses of ropivacaine used for wound infiltration result in linearly increasing maximal plasma concentrations (C_{max}). (Data from Mulroy MF, Burgess FW, Emanuelsson B-M. Ropivacaine 0.25% and 0.5%, but not 0.125%, provide effective wound infiltration analgesia after outpatient hernia repair, but with sustained plasma drug levels. *Reg Anesth Pain Med.* 1999;24:136.)

in plasma can be readily derived from the apparent volume of distribution (VD_{ss}; Table 22-7); however, regional differences in local anesthetic concentrations are seen among individual organ systems. The pattern of distribution is largely dependent on organ perfusion, the partition coefficient between compartments, and plasma protein binding.[82] Organs that are well perfused, such as the heart and the brain, have higher drug concentrations. Unfortunately, they are also the organs most seriously affected by local anesthetic toxicity.

Elimination

The metabolic pathway for clearance of local anesthetics is primarily determined by their chemical linkage. Aminoesters are hydrolyzed by plasma cholinesterases and aminoamides are transformed by hepatic carboxylesterases and cytochrome P450 enzymes. Severe liver disease may slow the clearance of

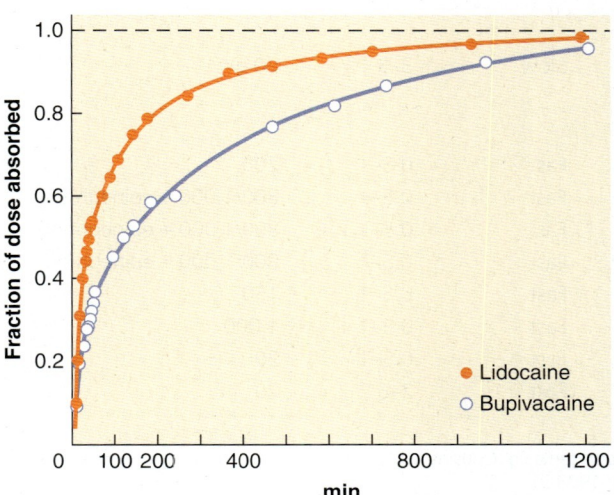

Figure 22-10 Fraction of dose absorbed into the systemic circulation over time from epidural injection of lidocaine or bupivacaine. Bupivacaine is a more lipid-soluble and more potent agent with less systemic absorption over time. (Adapted from Tucker GT, Mather LE. Properties, absorption, and disposition of local anesthetic agents. In: Cousins MJ, Bridenbaugh PO, eds. *Neural Blockade in Clinical Anesthesia and Management of Pain*. Philadelphia, PA: Lippincott-Raven; 1998:55.)

Table 22-7 Pharmacokinetic Parameters of Clinically Used Local Anesthetics

Local Anesthetic	VD_{ss} (L/kg)	CL (L/kg/h)	$T_{1/2}$ (hours)
Bupivacaine	1.02	0.41	3.5
Levobupivacaine	0.78	0.32	2.6
Chloroprocaine	0.50	2.96	0.11
Etidocaine	1.9	1.05	2.6
Lidocaine	1.3	0.85	1.6
Mepivacaine	1.2	0.67	1.9
Prilocaine	2.73	2.03	1.6
Procaine	0.93	5.62	0.14
Ropivacaine	0.84	0.63	1.9

VD_{ss}, volume of distribution at steady state; CL, total body clearance; $T_{1/2}$, terminal elimination half-life.
Data from Denson DD. Physiology and pharmacology of local anesthetics. In: Sinatra RS, Hord AH, Ginsberg B, et al., eds. *Acute Pain: Mechanisms and Management*. St. Louis, MO: Mosby Year Book; 1992:124; and Burm AG, van der Meer AD, van Kleef JW, et al. Pharmacokinetics of the enantiomers of bupivacaine following intravenous administration of the racemate. *Br J Clin Pharmacol.* 1994;38:125.

aminoamide local anesthetics and significant drug levels may therefore accumulate.[83]

Clinical Pharmacokinetics

The primary benefit of understanding the systemic pharmacokinetics of local anesthetics is the ability to predict the peak plasma level (C_{max}) after the agents are administered, thereby avoiding the administration of toxic doses (Tables 22-6, 22-8, and 22-9).

Table 22-8 Relative Potency for Systemic Central Nervous System Toxicity by Local Anesthetics and Ratio of Dosage Needed for Cardiovascular System: Central Nervous System (CVS:CNS) Toxicity

Agent	Relative Potency for CNS Toxicity	CVS:CNS
Bupivacaine	4.0	2.0
Levobupivacaine	2.9	2.0
Chloroprocaine	0.3	3.7
Etidocaine	2.0	4.4
Lidocaine	1.0	7.1
Mepivacaine	1.4	7.1
Prilocaine	1.2	3.1
Procaine	0.3	3.7
Ropivacaine	2.9	2.0
Tetracaine	2.0	

Data from Liu SS. Local anesthetics and analgesia. In: Ashburn MA, Rice LJ, eds. *The Management of Pain*. New York: Churchill Livingstone; 1997:141; and Groban L. Central nervous system and cardiac effects from long-acting amide local anesthetic toxicity in the intact animal model. *Reg Anesth Pain Med.* 2003;28:3.

Table 22-9 Clinical Profile of Local Anesthetics

Local Anesthetic	Concentration (%)	Clinical Use	Onset	Duration (hours)	Recommended Maximum Single Dose (mg)
Amides					
Bupivacaine	0.25	Infiltration	Fast	2–8	175/225 + epinephrine
Levobupivacaine	0.25–0.5	Peripheral nerve block	Slow	4–12	150
	0.5–0.75	Epidural anesthesia	Moderate	2–5	150
	0.03–0.25	Epidural analgesia	N/A	N/A	N/A
	0.5–0.75	Spinal anesthesia	Fast	1–4	20
Etidocaine	0.5	Infiltration	Fast	2–8	300/400 + epinephrine
	0.5–1	Peripheral nerve block	Fast	3–12	300/400 + epinephrine
	1–1.5	Epidural anesthesia	Fast	2–4	300/400 + epinephrine
Lidocaine	0.5–1	Infiltration	Fast	1–4	300/500 + epinephrine
	0.25–0.5	IV regional anesthesia	Fast	0.5–1	300
	1–1.5	Peripheral nerve block	Fast	1–3	300/500 + epinephrine
	1.5–2	Epidural anesthesia	Fast	1–2	300/500 + epinephrine
	1.5–5	Spinal anesthesia	Fast	0.5–1	100
	4	Topical	Fast	0.5–1	300
Mepivacaine	0.5–1	Infiltration	Fast	1–4	400/500 + epinephrine
	1–1.5	Peripheral nerve block	Fast	2–4	400/500 + epinephrine
	1.5–2	Epidural anesthesia	Fast	1–3	400/500 + epinephrine
	2–4	Spinal anesthesia	Fast	1–2	100
Prilocaine	0.5–1	Infiltration	Fast	1–2	600
	0.25–0.5	IV regional anesthesia	Fast	0.5–1	600
	1.5–2	Peripheral nerve block	Fast	1.5–3	600
	2–3	Epidural	Fast	1–3	600
Ropivacaine	0.2–0.5	Infiltration	Fast	2–6	200
	0.5–1	Peripheral nerve block	Slow	5–8	250
	0.5–1	Epidural anesthesia	Moderate	2–6	200
	0.05–0.2	Epidural analgesia	N/A	N/A	N/A
Mixture					
Lidocaine + prilocaine	2.5/2.5	Skin topical	Slow	3–5	20 g
Esters					
Benzocaine	Up to 20	Topical	Fast	0.5–1	200
Chloroprocaine	1	Infiltration	Fast	0.5–1	800/1,000 + epinephrine
	2	Peripheral nerve block	Fast	0.5–1	800/1,000 + epinephrine
	2–3	Epidural anesthesia	Fast	0.5–1	800/1,000 + epinephrine
Cocaine	4–10	Topical	Fast	0.5–1	150
Procaine	10	Spinal anesthesia	Fast	0.5–1	1,000
Tetracaine	2	Topical	Fast	0.5–1	20
	0.5	Spinal anesthesia	Fast	2–6	20

IV, intravenous; N/A, not available.
Adapted from Covino BG, Wildsmith JAW. Clinical pharmacology of local anesthetic agents. In: Cousins MJ, Bridenbaugh PO, eds. *Neural Blockade in Clinical Anesthesia and Management of Pain*. Philadelphia, PA: Lippincott-Raven; 1998:97.

Nonetheless, pharmacokinetics are difficult to predict in any given circumstance because both physical and pathophysiologic characteristics will affect the individual pharmacokinetics. There is some evidence for increased systemic plasma levels of local anesthetics in the very young and in the elderly owing to decreased clearance and increased absorption[84]; however, the correlation of systemic blood levels between the dose of local anesthetic and weight is often inconsistent (Fig. 22-11).[85] Effects of gender on clinical pharmacokinetics of local anesthetics have not been well defined,[86] although pregnancy may decrease clearance.[87] Pathophysiologic states such as cardiac and hepatic disease will alter expected pharmacokinetic parameters (Table 22-10),

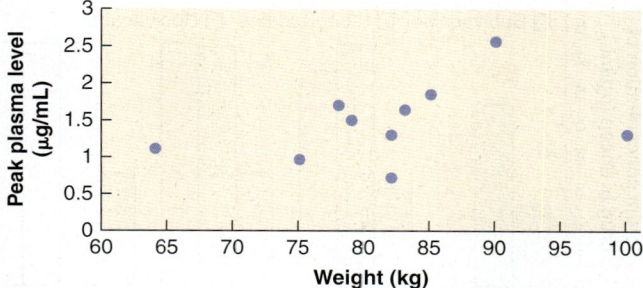

Figure 22-11 Lack of correlation between patient weight and peak plasma concentration after epidural administration of 150 mg of bupivacaine. (Data from Sharrock NE, Mather LE, Go G, et al. Arterial and pulmonary concentrations of the enantiomers of bupivacaine after epidural injection in elderly patients. *Anesth Analg.* 1998;86:812.)

and lower doses of local anesthetics should be used for these patients. As expected, renal disease has little effect on pharmacokinetic parameters of local anesthetics (Table 22-10). All of these factors should be considered when using local anesthetics and minimizing systemic toxicity, the commonly accepted maximal dosages (Table 22-9) notwithstanding.

Clinical Use of Local Anesthetics

There are a myriad of uses of local anesthetics in the modern practice of anesthesia. They all take advantage of their ability to attenuate or block pain and other noxious stimuli. When applied topically to the skin, a eutectic mixture of lidocaine and prilocaine reduces the sharp, painful sensation associated with needle insertion and intravenous catheter placement, particularly in the pediatric population. In the awake patient, aerosolized benzocaine and viscous lidocaine directed at the mucosal surface can help blunt the protective reflex responses associated with airway instrumentation (see Chapter 28). In addition, lidocaine can be given intravenously to decrease the incidence and the severity of pain associated with propofol administration (see Chapters 19, 31). Likewise, intravenous lidocaine may also help to reduce the hemodynamic response to tracheal intubation and extubation.[88,89]

By far the most common application, local infiltration of the dermis, provides quick onset of anesthesia suitable for a broad variety of minor superficial procedures. The clinical profile of some commonly used agents is listed in Table 22-9. For a wider and greater area of coverage, a regional anatomic approach to anesthesia and analgesia can be used. This can be accomplished either by intravenous administration of local anesthetics to a limb under pneumatic compression (Bier block) or by direct application of local anesthetics to individual peripheral nerves (nerve blocks). Local anesthetics can be deposited centrally near the nerve roots, either intrathecally in the lumbar cistern or epidurally in the thoracic, lumbar, and caudal regions of the spine (see Chapter 35). Alternatively, injections can be made peripherally at the plexus, such as at the brachial or lumbar plexus block or on the nerve fibers (see Chapter 36). The duration of the anesthesia and analgesia is dependent on the type of local anesthetics used, though it can be extended with continuous infusion through an indwelling catheter.

Toxicity of Local Anesthetics

Systemic Toxicity of Local Anesthetics

Central Nervous System Toxicity

Local anesthetics readily cross the blood–brain barrier and, as a result, CNS toxicity can occur with systemic absorption or inadvertent intravascular injections. The effects on the CNS are determined by the plasma concentration of the local anesthetics (Table 22-11). At low plasma concentration, mild disturbances to the sensory systems appear. As the plasma concentration increases, CNS excitation and seizure activities predominate. If the plasma concentration is sufficiently large or the increase is rapid, the CNS excitation may progress to generalized CNS depression and coma, leading to respiratory depression and arrest.[90]

The potential for CNS toxicity correlates directly with the potency of local anesthetics (Tables 22-4 and 22-8).[90] Highly potent lipid-soluble agents such as bupivacaine can cause CNS toxicity at doses that are a fraction of those of less potent agents. The potential for CNS toxicity is further modified by other factors. For example, a decrease in protein binding and clearance of local anesthetics, systemic acidosis, hypercapnia, and hypercarbia can all increase the risk for CNS toxicity. Conversely, coadministration of CNS depressive agents, such as barbiturates and benzodiazepines, may decrease the likelihood for seizures.[91]

Clinical reports suggest that CNS toxicity associated with the use of local anesthetics in regional anesthesia is uncommon. Surveys from France and the United States of over 280,000 cases involving regional anesthesia show an incidence of seizures of

Table 22-10 Effects of Cardiac, Hepatic, and Renal Disease on Lidocaine Pharmacokinetics

	VD_{ss} (L/kg)	CL (mL/kg/min)	$T_{1/2}$ (hours)
Normal	1.32	10.0	1.8
Cardiac failure	0.88	6.3	1.9
Hepatic disease	2.31	6.0	4.9
Renal disease	1.2	13.7	1.3

VD_{ss}, volume of distribution at steady state; CL, total body clearance; $T_{1/2}$, terminal elimination half-life.
Data from Thomson PD. Lidocaine pharmacokinetics in advanced heart failure, liver disease, and renal failure in humans. *Ann Intern Med.* 1973;78:499.

Table 22-11 Dose-Dependent Systemic Effects of Lidocaine

Plasma Concentration (µg/mL)	Effect
1–5	Analgesia
5–10	Lightheadedness Tinnitus Numbness of tongue
10–15	Seizures Unconsciousness
15–25	Coma Respiratory arrest
>25	Cardiovascular depression

approximately 1/10,000 with epidural injections and 7/10,000 with peripheral nerve blocks.[92,93] The higher incidence of CNS toxicity resulting from peripheral nerve blocks may be due to differences in practice or, perhaps, decreased clinical awareness. Nonetheless, in an analysis of closed malpractice claims in the United States from 1980 to 1999, epidural anesthesia (primarily obstetrical) constituted all of the cases of death or brain damage resulting from unintentional intravenous injection of local anesthetic.[94]

Cardiovascular Toxicity of Local Anesthetics

8 In general, systemic cardiovascular toxicity is seen at a plasma concentration far greater than that for CNS toxicity. The potential for cardiovascular toxicity, like that for CNS toxicity, correlates closely with the potency, or lipid solubility, of local anesthetics (Tables 22-4 and 22-8). However, although all local anesthetics can cause hypotension, dysrhythmias, and myocardial depression, more potent agents (bupivacaine, ropivacaine, and levobupivacaine) are predisposed to devastating outcomes, such as fatal cardiovascular collapse and complete heart block (Fig. 22-12).[95]

Among the potent long-acting agents, ropivacaine and levobupivacaine may have a safer cardiovascular toxicity profile than bupivacaine. In animal models, both ropivacaine and levobupivacaine appear to exhibit 30% to 40% less cardiovascular toxicity than bupivacaine on a milligram-to-milligram basis (Fig. 22-13)[34,90,96]; however, in human studies, that difference appears less striking (Fig. 22-14).[97,98] Detailed electrophysiologic studies with isolated heart muscles and cultured cardiomyocytes support the view that S(−)-bupivacaine (levobupivacaine) is generally less potent than R(+)-bupivacaine in blocking both the cardiac action potential[99] and binding of voltage-gated sodium channels during the inactivated stage.[100] Likewise for ropivacaine, evidence suggests that the propyl side chain renders it less cardiodepressive than the larger butyl side chain of bupivacaine.[101]

The underlying pathophysiology responsible for local anesthetic–induced cardiovascular collapse has not been fully established. Although local anesthetics can directly cause major disturbances to the heart, their effects on other components of cardiovascular systems may be just as important. For example, systemic bupivacaine has been shown to impair regulation by the CNS of the cardiovascular system. Disruption to the arterial baroreflex in the brainstem by bupivacaine can lead to attenuation of the heart rhythm response to changes in blood pressure.[102,103] Local anesthetics also act on smooth muscle endothelium surrounding blood vessels. In the periphery, vasoconstriction occurs at subclinical doses and vasodilation at higher doses.[104] In the pulmonary vasculature, however, increasing local anesthetic

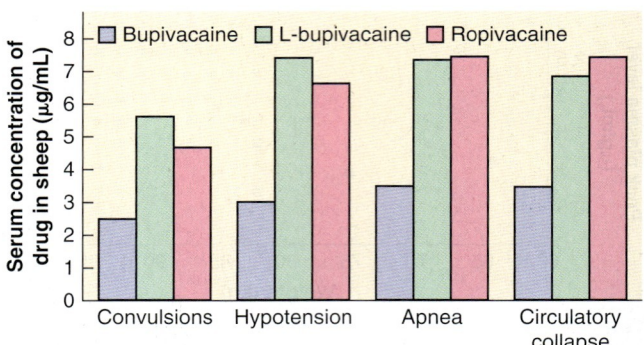

Figure 22-13 Serum concentrations in sheep at each toxic manifestation for bupivacaine, levo (L)-bupivacaine, and ropivacaine. Both levobupivacaine and ropivacaine required significantly greater serum concentrations than bupivacaine. (Data from Santos AC, DeArmas PI. Systemic toxicity of levobupivacaine, bupivacaine, and ropivacaine during continuous intravenous infusion to nonpregnant and pregnant ewes. *Anesthesiology*. 2001;95:1256.)

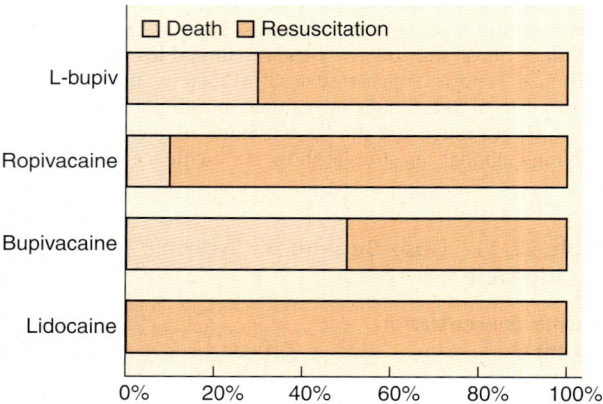

Figure 22-12 Success of resuscitation of dogs after cardiovascular collapse from intravenous infusions of lidocaine, bupivacaine, levobupivacaine (L-bupiv), and ropivacaine. Success rates were greater for lidocaine (100%) compared to ropivacaine (90%), levobupivacaine (70%), and bupivacaine (50%). Required doses to induce cardiovascular collapse were greater for lidocaine (127 mg/kg) compared to ropivacaine (42 mg/kg), levobupivacaine (27 mg/kg), and bupivacaine (22 mg/kg). (Data from Groban L, Deal DD, Vernon JC, et al. Cardiac resuscitation after incremental overdosage with lidocaine, bupivacaine, levobupivacaine, and ropivacaine in anesthetized dogs. *Anesth Analg*. 2001;92:37.)

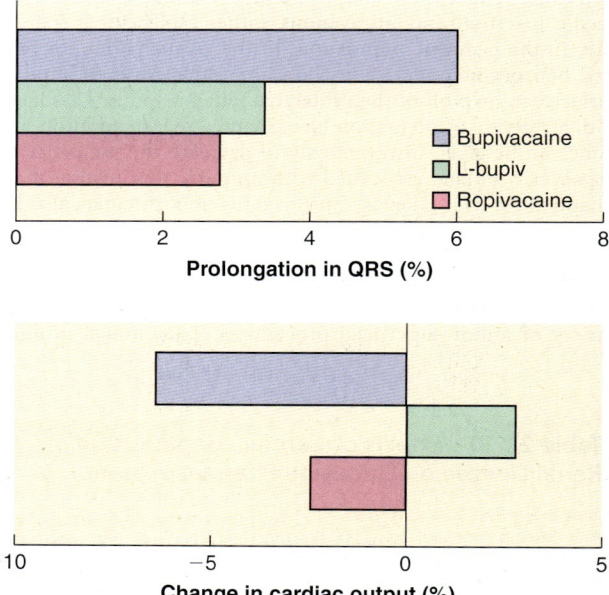

Figure 22-14 Mild prolongation in QRS interval and change in cardiac output after intravenous infusions of bupivacaine (103 mg), levobupivacaine (L-bupiv; 37 mg), and ropivacaine (115 mg) in healthy volunteers. (Data from Knudsen K, Beckman Suurkula M, Blomberg S, et al. Central nervous and cardiovascular effects of i.v. infusions of ropivacaine, bupivacaine and placebo in volunteers. *Br Anaesth*. 1997;78:507; and Stewart J, Kellett N, Castro D. The central nervous system and cardiovascular effects of levobupivacaine and ropivacaine in healthy volunteers. *Anesth Analg*. 2003;97:412.)

concentrations produce marked pulmonary artery hypertension.[105] The increase in the pulmonary vascular resistance occurs prior to any significant decrease in the cardiac output, suggesting that the result is a primary effect of local anesthetic intoxication, rather than secondary to a decline in cardiac contractility.

Elevated concentrations of local anesthetics have been shown to delay cardiac electrical conductivity and decrease cardiac contractility. Although all local anesthetics disturb the cardiac conduction system via a dose-dependent block of sodium channels (seen clinically as a prolongation of the PR interval and duration of the QRS complex), several features unique to bupivacaine seem to potentiate its cardiotoxicity. First, bupivacaine has an inherently greater affinity for binding resting and inactivated sodium channels than lidocaine.[106] Second, although all local anesthetics bind sodium channels during cardiac systole and dissociate during diastole (Fig. 22-15), the dissociation of bupivacaine during diastole occurs more slowly than lidocaine. This slow rate of dissociation prevents a complete recovery of the channels at the end of each cardiac cycle (at the physiologic heart rate of 60 to 80 beats/min), thereby leading to an accumulation and worsening of the conduction defect. In contrast, lidocaine fully dissociates from sodium channels during diastole and little accumulation of conduction delay occurs (Fig. 22-16).[106,107] Finally, bupivacaine exerts a greater degree of direct myocardial depression than less potent agents (Fig. 22-17).[90,101]

Current understanding of the molecular mechanisms underlying local anesthetic cardiac toxicity is limited. It is widely accepted that local anesthetics bind and disrupt the normal function of the heart-specific voltage-gated sodium channel, $Na_v1.5$, in cardiac myocytes; however, there appear to be other intracellular targets as well. Local anesthetics have been shown to antagonize the currents of other cations, primarily calcium and potassium.[106] The degree of antagonism between bupivacaine

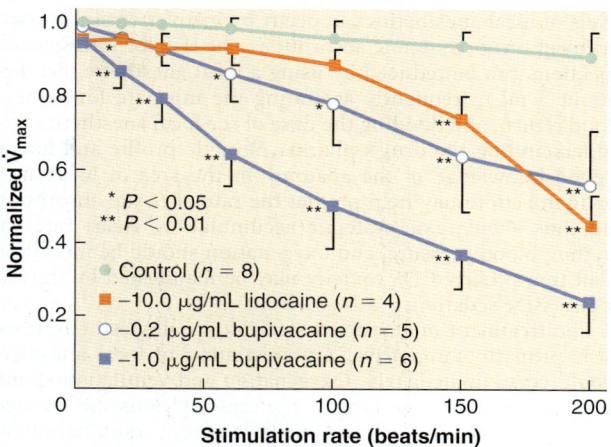

Figure 22-16 Heart rate–dependent effects of lidocaine and bupivacaine on velocity of the cardiac action potential ($\dot{V}_{max}$). Bupivacaine progressively decreases $\dot{V}_{max}$ at heart rates above 10 beats/min because of accumulation of sodium channel block, whereas lidocaine does not decrease $\dot{V}_{max}$ until heart rate exceeds 150 beats/min. (Adapted with permission from Clarkson CW, Hondeghem LM. Mechanisms for bupivacaine depression of cardiac conduction: Fast block of sodium channels during the action potential with slow recovery from block during diastole. *Anesthesiology*. 1985;62:396.)

and less potent agents appears to differ, and that difference may contribute to the severity in the disturbance of the cardiac membrane potentials. Lastly, individuals and experimental animal models with L-carnitine deficiency exhibit an increased susceptibility to local anesthetic–associated cardiac toxicity, suggesting that local anesthetics can affect mitochondrial function and fatty acid metabolism.[108,109]

Treatment of Systemic Toxicity from Local Anesthetics

The best practice for managing systemic local anesthetic intoxication starts with vigilance and prevention. Elevated plasma

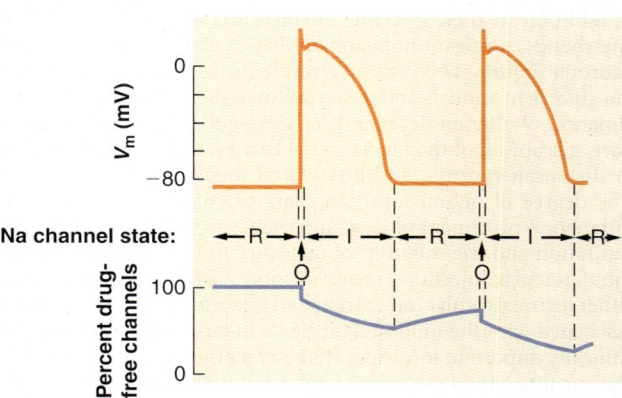

Figure 22-15 Diagram illustrating the relationship between cardiac action potential (*top*), sodium channel state (*middle*), and block of sodium channels by bupivacaine (*bottom*). Sodium channels are predominantly in the resting form during diastole, open transiently during the action potential upstroke, and are in the inactive form during the action potential plateau. Block of sodium channels by bupivacaine accumulates during the action potential (systole), with recovery occurring during diastole. Recovery of sodium channels results from dissociation of bupivacaine and is time-dependent. Recovery during each diastolic interval is incomplete and results in accumulation of sodium channel block with successive heartbeats. R, resting form; O, open form; I, inactive form. (Adapted with permission from Clarkson CW, Hondeghem LM. Mechanisms for bupivacaine depression of cardiac conduction: fast block of sodium channels during the action potential with slow recovery from block during diastole. *Anesthesiology*. 1985;62:396.)

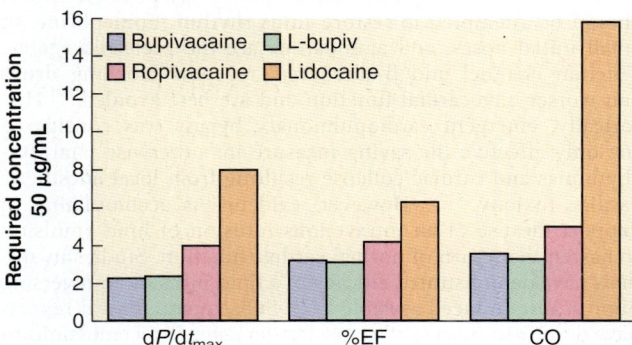

Figure 22-17 Plasma concentrations required to induce myocardial depression in dogs administered bupivacaine, levobupivacaine (L-bupiv), ropivacaine, and lidocaine. dP/dt_{max}, 35% reduction of inotropy from baseline measure; %EF, 35% reduction in ejection fraction from baseline measure; CO, 25% reduction in cardiac output from baseline measure. (Data from Groban L, Deal DD, Vernon JC, et al. Does local anesthetic stereoselectivity or structure predict myocardial depression in anesthetized canines? *Reg Anesth Pain Med*. 2002;27:460.)

levels of local anesthetics can occur by inadvertent intravascular injections or systemic absorption. The risk for intravascular injections can be reduced by using a local anesthetic test dose (about 3 mL), frequently aspirating the injectate for signs of blood return, and dividing the dose of the local anesthetics.[91,110] Understanding the drug's pharmacokinetic profile and having a good knowledge of the anatomy in the area of local anesthetic injection may help predict the rate of tissue absorption, and thus avoid toxic systemic accumulation. Heart rate and rhythm, blood pressure, and oxygenation should be monitored at all times. Early CNS toxicity may be manifested by tinnitus or excessive sedation.

The treatment of suspected systemic local anesthetic toxicity is primarily supportive. Administration of local anesthetic should cease immediately. Oxygenation and ventilation should be maintained and the airway, if necessary, must be secured. This is necessary not only as a standard part of resuscitation but also to prevent further exacerbation of local anesthetic toxicity by hypoxemia, hypercapnia, and acidemia.[91] In many cases, with proper airway management and reversal of acidosis, more serious complications of local anesthetic intoxication can be avoided, especially in cases involving less potent agents.

Local anesthetic–induced seizure activity can vastly increase the body's metabolism and the resultant metabolic acidosis may make resuscitation more difficult. Prolonged seizures should therefore be suppressed. Benzodiazepines, such as midazolam or diazepam, have been shown to raise the seizure threshold in animals and are the preferred agents for preventing and terminating seizures. Hypnotic agents, such as propofol and thiopental, may not be best suited for terminating local anesthetic–induced seizures, because at significant doses, they can potentiate the myocardial depression exerted by the causative agent.[110] If seizure activity is prolonged, succinylcholine or other neuromuscular blockers can be administered not only to facilitate pulmonary ventilation but also to disrupt muscular activity and reduce the consequent metabolic demand. However, it is important to note that muscle relaxants do not reduce the electrical excitation in the CNS and cerebral metabolic stress may continue unabated.

Mild myocardial depression and systemic vasodilation can be corrected with sympathomimetic agents such as ephedrine or epinephrine. Pending cardiovascular collapse from severe cardiac dysrhythmias should prompt immediate initiation of cardiopulmonary resuscitation. For ventricular fibrillation and cardiac arrest, electrocardioversion and pharmacologic means should be attempted to restore sinus rhythm. Epinephrine, in small initial doses, and amiodarone are the preferred agents. Calcium channel and β-adrenergic receptor blocking drugs can worsen myocardial function and are best avoided.[110] Historically, emergent cardiopulmonary bypass was considered the only effective life-saving measure for otherwise fatal dysrhythmias and cardiac collapse resulting from local anesthetic cardiac toxicity.[111,112] However, evidence is accumulating to support the use of an intravenous infusion of lipid emulsion to hasten the return of normal cardiac function. Studies in animals have demonstrated efficacy of a lipid infusion in reversing bupivacaine-induced asystole.[113,114] Subsequent clinical reports have described successful resuscitation using lipid emulsions in individuals with local anesthetic–induced cardiac arrest.[115,116] The lipid emulsion may act as a plasma "sink" to absorb tissue-bound local anesthetics via partition principles.[117] Alternatively, the lipids may provide a usable energy source to bypass the impediment on the cardiac mitochondria.[118] A summary of the American Society of Regional Anesthesia and Pain Medicine practice advisory on treatment of local anesthetic systemic toxicity is listed in Table 22-12.

Table 22-12 Practice Advisory on Treatment of Local Anesthetic Systemic Toxicity

For Patients Experiencing Signs or Symptoms of Local Anesthetic Systemic Toxicity

1. **Get Help**
2. **Initial Focus**
   Airway management: ventilate with 100% oxygen
   Seizure suppression: benzodiazepines are preferred
   Basic and advanced cardiac life support
3. **Infuse 20% Lipid Emulsion**
   Initiate intravenous bolus of 1.5 mL/kg over 1 minute
   Continue infusion at 0.25 mL/kg/min for at least 10 minutes after the return of cardiac function
   If cardiovascular instability continues, consider repeating the bolus and increasing the infusion to 0.5 mL/kg/min
   Up to 10 mL/kg over 30 minutes is the recommended upper limit for initial dosing
4. **Avoid** vasopressin, calcium channel blockers, beta blockers, or local anesthetics
5. **Alert** the nearest facility having cardiopulmonary bypass capability
6. **Avoid** propofol in patients having signs of cardiovascular instability

Adapted from Neal JM, Bernards CM, Butterworth JF, et al. ASRA practice advisory on local anesthetic systemic toxicity. *Reg Anesth Pain Med*. 2010:35;152.

Neural Toxicity of Local Anesthetics

In addition to their systemic effects, direct application of local anesthetics can result in histopathologic changes consistent with neuronal injury. The causative mechanisms remain speculative, but studies in animals and tissue cultures show evidence of demyelination, Wallerian degeneration, dysregulation of axonal transport, disruption of the blood–nerve barrier, decreased blood flow to the vasanervorum, and loss of cell membrane integrity.[119,120] The degree of neural injury appears to correlate with possible intraneural placement of local anesthetic, as well as the drug concentration and the duration of exposure to the local anesthetics. Intrafascicular injections result in more histologic changes than either extrafascicular or extraneural placement, with the latter associated with the mildest damage.[121] In large concentrations, all clinically important local anesthetics can produce dose-dependent abnormalities in nerve fibers; however, in clinically relevant concentrations, they appear generally safe.[122,123]

The significance of these experimental findings is unclear, because clinical injury is rare. A systematic review of approximately 2.7 million centrally administered local anesthetic neuraxial blocks determined an occurrence of radiculopathy at approximately 0.03% and of paraplegia at approximately 0.0008%.[124] Furthermore, direct intraneural injections of local anesthetics per se do not invariably lead to detectable neurologic symptoms.[125] Nonetheless, there have been clinical scenarios in which a greater propensity for nerve injury has been described. The use of microcatheters with a high concentration of lidocaine for continuous spinal anesthesia has been associated with an increased incidence of radiculopathy and cauda equina syndrome.[126] Likewise, chloroprocaine, used until the early 1980s for epidural and intrathecal injections, has been linked to prolonged sensory and motor deficits, possibly due to toxic effects of the preservative, sodium bisulfite.[127] Although the clinical use of local anesthetics appears to be safe, it behooves the practitioner to be mindful of their potential deleterious effects on nerves.

Transient Neurologic Symptoms after Spinal Anesthesia

Prospective randomized studies reveal a 4% to 40% incidence of transient neurologic symptoms (TNSs), including pain or sensory abnormalities in the lower back, buttocks, or lower extremities, after lidocaine spinal anesthesia[128,129] (see Chapter 35). These symptoms have been reported with other local anesthetics as well (Table 22-13), but have not resulted in permanent neurologic injury.[128] Increased risk of TNSs is associated with lidocaine, the lithotomy position, and ambulatory anesthesia, but not with baricity of solution or dose of local anesthetic.[128,129] The potential neurologic etiology of this syndrome coupled with known concentration-dependent toxicity of lidocaine led to concerns over a neurotoxic etiology for TNSs from spinal lidocaine.

However, evidence for a direct linear relation between nerve toxicity and symptoms is scant. Although the concentration of local anesthetics may be a strong factor for determining nerve injury, such as with cauda equina syndrome, there does not appear to be a dose relation in TNSs. The incidence of TNSs is similar when there is a 10-fold difference in the concentration of lidocaine utilized (0.5% and 5%).[130] Furthermore, a study comparing volunteers with and without TNSs after lidocaine spinal anesthesia shows no abnormalities detectable by routine electrophysiologic testing, such as electromyography, nerve conduction, or somatosensory-evoked potentials. Finally, effective treatment for TNS includes nonsteroidal anti-inflammatory agents and trigger point injections. These are regimens more effective for alleviating myofascial pain than for neuropathic pain.[128] Overall, there is little evidence to support a neurotoxic etiology for TNSs.[128] Other potential etiologies for TNSs include patient positioning, sciatic nerve stretch, muscle spasm, and myofascial strain.[128]

Myotoxicity of Local Anesthetics

As with neural toxicity, local anesthetics can also cause histopathologic changes in skeletal muscle. Myotoxicity can result from

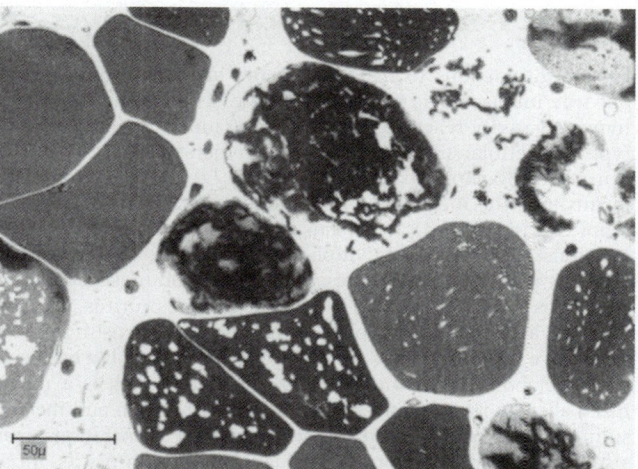

Figure 22-18 Skeletal muscle cross-section with characteristic histologic changes after continuous exposure to bupivacaine for 6 hours. A spectrum of necrobiotic changes can be encountered, ranging from slightly damaged vacuolated fibers and fibers with condensed myofibrils to entirely disintegrated and necrotic cells. The majority of the myocytes are morphologically affected. In addition, marked interstitial and myoseptal edema appears within the sections. However, scattered fibers remain intact. (Reprinted with permission from Zink W, Graf B. Local anesthetic myotoxicity. *Reg Anesth Pain Med*. 2004;29:333–340.)

most local anesthetic agents in clinically relevant concentrations[131] and manifest clinically as muscle pain and dysfunction. Histopathologic studies show hypercontracted myofibrils, followed by lytic degeneration of striated muscle sarcoplasmic reticulum, and diffuse myonecrosis (Fig. 22-18). The changes are drug-specific (tetracaine and procaine produce the least injury; bupivacaine the most) and both dose- and duration-dependent,[132] and seem to affect the young more than the old.[133] Experimental evidence points to disturbances in the oxidative function of mitochondria and dysregulation of intracellular calcium homeostasis as possible subcellular pathologic mechanisms.[134] In cell cultures, these disruptions appear to be diminished with coapplication with erythropoietin or N-acetylcysteine.[135,136] It remains to be seen if these agents may become clinically useful or necessary, because most myotoxic injuries are subclinical and appear entirely reversible.[132]

Table 22-13 The Incidence of Transient Neurologic Symptoms (TNSs) Varies with Type of Spinal Local Anesthetic and Surgery

Local Anesthetic	Concentration (%)	Type of Surgery	Approximate Incidence of TNSs (%)
Lidocaine	2–5	Lithotomy position	30–36
	2–5	Knee arthroscopy	18–22
	0.5	Knee arthroscopy	17
	2–5	Mixed supine position	4–8
Mepivacaine	1.5–4	Mixed	23
Procaine	10	Knee arthroscopy	6
Bupivacaine	0.5–0.75	Mixed	1
Levobupivacaine	0.5	Mixed	1
Prilocaine	2–5	Mixed	1
Ropivacaine	0.5–0.75	Mixed	1

Data from Pollock JE. Transient neurologic symptoms: Etiology, risk factors, and management. *Reg Anesth Pain Med*. 2002;27:581; and Breebaart MB. Urinary bladder scanning after day-case arthroscopy under spinal anaesthesia: Comparison between lidocaine, ropivacaine, and levobupivacaine. *Br J Anaesth*. 2003;90:309.

Allergic Reactions to Local Anesthetics

Untoward reactions to local anesthetics are relatively common, but true immunologic reactions are rare. The immune-mediated hypersensitivity reaction may be type I (immunoglobulin E) or type IV (cellular immunity). Type I hypersensitivity reactions can result in anaphylaxis and potentially be life-threatening, but fortunately, the incidence is estimated to be less than 1% of all reported cases. Type IV hypersensitivity reactions are delayed-type reactions mediated by T lymphocytes.[137,138] The symptoms can manifest within 12 to 48 hours of exposure and most commonly present as contact dermatitis (dermal erythema, pruritus, papules, and vesicles). The vast majority of reported hypersensitivity reactions have been associated with aminoester agents, likely due to their metabolism to *para*-aminobenzoic acid, which is a recognized allergen. Preservatives, such as methylparaben and metabisulfite that are present in many local anesthetic preparations, may also trigger allergic responses. Evaluation with skin-pricks, intradermal injections, or subcutaneous provocative dose challenges are recommended for individuals with suspected local anesthetic allergy (see also Chapter 9).[139]

Future Therapeutics and Modalities

Properties of ideal local anesthetics include selectivity for nociception, long duration of action, and absence of systemic and local tissue toxicities. Efforts to improve local anesthetics have benefitted from a better understanding of the molecular nature of pain. The identification of sodium channel isoforms and their associated channelopathies have focused much attention to developing molecules with specific channel selectivity.[140]

One of the new classes of molecules is the site 1 sodium channel blockers. They belong to a group of potent paralytic neurotoxins that reversibly antagonize voltage-gated sodium channels. In contrast to local anesthetics, they bind to the channel α subunit extracellularly and have select affinity for channel isoforms.[141] Neosaxitoxin is a well-characterized member of this group and shares the same binding region on the channel outer pore (designated as site 1) as tetrodotoxin. Injected subcutaneously, neosaxitoxin produced hypoesthesia of a modest duration.[142] However, in combination with bupivacaine and epinephrine, neosaxitoxin extended the duration of hypoesthesia almost fivefold compared to bupivacaine alone (median duration 50 vs. 10 hours, respectively, $p = 0.007$).[143] Systemic adsorption can result in a dose-dependent decrease in respiratory and skeletal muscle strength[144]; however, due to its relatively poor affinity for the cardiac sodium channel (Na_v 1.5), cardiac outputs were maintained and no significant cardiac arrhythmias or arrests were seen with systemic infusion.[144] Finally, there was scant evidence of either myotoxicity or neurotoxicity with local injections.[145]

Another promising development toward long-lasting, selective analgesia focuses on modulating large-pore TRPV1 and TRPA1 to facilitate entry of impermeant sodium channel blocker into nociceptor neurons.[146] As discussed previously, TRPV1 and TRPA1 are membrane channels belonging to the transient receptor potential family. In response to heat, capsaicins, or other noxious stimuli, these channels permit passage of large, nonspecific cationic molecules into the cell. The strategy exploits the finding that their presence is restricted to primary sensory nociceptor neurons. Application of membrane impermeable local anesthetic, such as the permanently charged lidocaine QX-314, results in selective blockade of those sensory, but not motor or autonomic, neurons.[147] In animal studies, coadministration of capsaicin and QX-314 on sciatic nerves produced a long-lasting sensory block with minimal motor deficit.[147] The addition of lidocaine further prolonged the duration of the block at the expense of an initial short and concomitant period of nonselective motor block.[148] However, the duration of the sensory block was much longer than the motor block, leading to a differential blockade of approximately 16 hours (Fig. 22-19). Many questions remain to be addressed before proceeding to volunteer studies. Nonetheless, if the laboratory findings are validated clinically, such combinations will be an invaluable addition to the use of local anesthetics for anesthesia and analgesia.

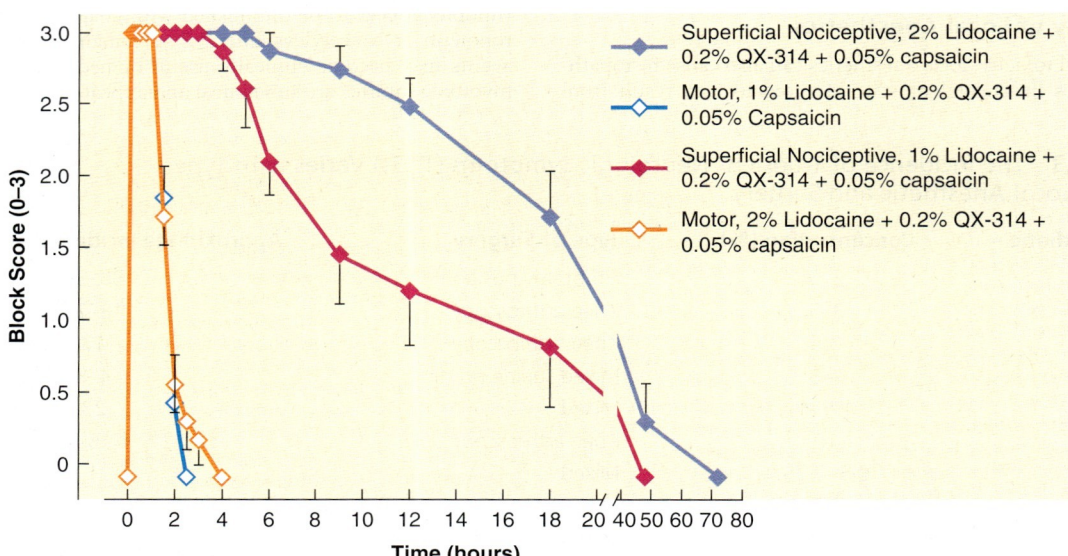

Figure 22-19 Comparison of the duration of nociceptive (*blue closed diamonds*) and motor (*blue open diamonds*) blockade produced by triple application of 1% lidocaine/capsaicin/QX-314 (*red diamonds*) or 2% lidocaine/capsaicin/QX-314 (*orange open diamonds*). Grading was as follows: 3, complete block; 2, partial block; 1, minimal block; 0, baseline. (Reprinted with permission from Binshtok AM, Gerner P, Oh SB, et al. Coapplication of lidocaine and the permanently charged sodium channel blocker QX-314 produces a long-lasting nociceptive blockade in rodents. *Anesthesiology*. 2009;111:127.)

REFERENCES

1. Wheater PR, Burkitt HG, Daniels VG. *Functional Histology*. 2nd ed. New York: Churchill Livingstone; 1987:95.
2. Ritchie JM, Ritchie B, Greengard P. The effect of the nerve sheath on the action of local anesthetics. *J Pharmacol Exp Ther*. 1965;150:160.
3. Coggeshall RE. A fine structural analysis of the myelin sheath in rat spinal roots. *Anat Rec*. 1979;194:201.
4. Waxman SG, Ritchie JM. Organization of ion channels in the myelinated nerve fiber. *Science*. 1985;228:1502.
5. Koester J. Passive membrane properties of the neuron. In: Kandel ER, Schwartz JH, Jessell TM. *Principles of Neuroscience*. 3rd ed. New York: Elsevier Science; 1991.
6. Hodgkin AL, Katz B. The effect of sodium ions on the electrical activity of the giant axon of the squid. *J Physiol*. 1949;108:37.
7. Hodgkin AL, Huxley AF. A quantitative description of membrane current and its application to conduction and excitation in nerve. *J Physiol*. 1952;117:500.
8. Sigworth FJ, Neher E. Single Na+ channel currents observed in cultured rat muscle cells. *Nature*. 1980;287:447.
9. Catterall WA. From ionic currents to molecular mechanisms: The structure and function of voltage-gated sodium channels. *Neuron*. 2000;26:13.
10. Hirschberg B, Rovner A, Lieberman M, et al. Transfer of twelve charges is needed to open skeletal muscle Na+ channels. *J Gen Physiol*. 1995;106:1053.
11. Heinemann SH, Terlau H, Stühmer W, et al. Calcium channel characteristics conferred on the sodium channel by single mutations. *Nature*. 1992;356:441.
12. Armstrong CM. Sodium channels and gating currents. *Physiol Rev*. 1981;61:644.
13. Stühmer W, Conti F, Suzuki H, et al. Structural parts involved in activation and inactivation of the sodium channel. *Nature*. 1989;339:597.
14. West JW, Patton DE, Scheuer T, et al. A cluster of hydrophobic amino acid residues required for fast Na(+)-channel inactivation. *Proc Natl Acad Sci USA*. 1992;89:10910.
15. Woods JN, Boorman JP, Okuse K, et al. Voltage-gated sodium channels and pain pathways. *J Neurobiol*. 2004;61:55.
16. Drenth JP, te Morsche RH, Guillet G, et al. SCN9A mutations define primary erythromelalgia as a neuropathic disorder of voltage gated sodium channels. *J Invest Dermatol*. 2005;124:1333.
17. Fertleman CR, Baker MD, Parker KA, et al. SCN9A mutations in paroxysmal extreme pain disorder: Allelic variants underlie distinct channel defects and phenotypes. *Neuron*. 2006;52:767.
18. Cox JJ, Reimann F, Nicholas AK, et al. An SCN9A channelopathy causes congenital inability to experience pain. *Nature*. 2006;444:894.
19. Goldberg Y, Macfarlane J, Macdonald M, et al. Loss-of-function mutations in the Na(v) 1.7 gene underlie congenital indifference to pain in multiple human populations. *Clin Genet*. 2007;71:311.
20. Frazier DT, Narahashi T, Yamada M. The site of action and active form of local anesthetics. II. Experiments with quaternary compounds. *J Pharmacol Exp Ther*. 1970;171:45.
21. Ragsdale DS, McPhee JC, Scheuer T, et al. Molecular determinants of state-dependent block of Na+ channels by local anesthetics. *Science*. 1994;265:1724.
22. Scholz A. Mechanisms of (local) anaesthetics on voltage-gated sodium and other ion channels. *Br J Anaesth*. 2002;89:52.
23. Ulbricht W. Sodium channel inactivation: Molecular determinants and modulation. *Physiol Rev*. 2005;85:1271.
24. Popitz-Bergez FA, Leeson S, Strichartz GR. Relation between functional deficit and intraneural local anesthetic during peripheral nerve block. A study in the rat sciatic nerve. *Anesthesiology*. 1995;83:583.
25. Fink BR, Cairns AM. Differential slowing and block of conduction by lidocaine in individual afferent myelinated and unmyelinated axons. *Anesthesiology*. 1984;60:111.
26. Fink BR, Cairns AM. Differential use-dependent (frequency-dependent) effects in single mammalian axons: Data and clinical considerations. *Anesthesiology*. 1987;67:477.
27. Fink BR. Mechanisms of differential axial blockade in epidural and subarachnoid anesthesia. *Anesthesiology*. 1989;70:851.
28. Gasser HS, Erlanger J. The role of fiber size in the establishment of a nerve block by pressure or cocaine. *Am J Physiol*. 1929;88:581.
29. Gokin AP, Philip B, Strichartz GR. Preferential block of small myelinated sensory and motor fibers by lidocaine: In vivo electrophysiology in the rat sciatic nerve. *Anesthesiology*. 2001;95:1441.
30. Chevrier P, Vijayaragavan K, Chahine M. Differential modulation of Nav 1.7 and Nav 1.8 peripheral nerve sodium channels by the local anesthetic lidocaine. *Br J Pharmacol*. 2004;142:576.
31. Leffler A, Fischer MD, Rehner D, et al. The vanilloid receptor TRPV1 is activated and sensitized by local anesthetics in rodent sensory neurons. *J Clin Invest*. 2008;118:763.
32. Leffler A, Lattrell A, Kronewald S, et al. Activation of TRPA1 by membrane permeable local anesthetics. *Molecular Pain*. 2011;7:62.
33. Narahashi T, Frazier DT, Yamada M. The site of action and active form of local anesthetics. I. Theory and pH experiments with tertiary compounds. *J Pharmacol and Exp Therap*. 1970;171:32.
34. Strichartz GR, Sanchez V, Arthur GR, et al. Fundamental properties of local anesthetics. II. Measured octanol: Buffer partition coefficients and pK_a values of clinically used drugs. *Anesth Analg*. 1990;71:158.
35. Bokesch PM, Post C, Strichartz G. Structure-activity relationship of lidocaine homologs producing tonic and frequency-dependent impulse blockade in nerve. *J Pharmacol Exp Ther*. 1986;237:773.
36. Gissen AJ, Covino BG, Gregus J. Differential sensitivity of fast and slow fibers in mammalian nerve. III. Effect of etidocaine and bupivacaine on fast/slow fibers. *Anesth Analg*. 1982;61:570.
37. Johns RA, DiFazio CA, Longnecker DE. Lidocaine constricts or dilates rat arterioles in a dose-dependent manner. *Anesthesiology*. 1985;62:141.
38. Johns RA, Seyde WC, DiFazio CA, et al. Dose-dependent effects of bupivacaine on rat muscle arterioles. *Anesthesiology*. 1986;65:186.
39. Foster RH, Markham A. Levobupivacaine: A review of its pharmacology and use as a local anaesthetic. *Drugs*. 2000;59:551.
40. McClellan KJ, Faulds D. Ropivacaine: An update of its use in regional anaesthesia. *Drugs*. 2000;60:1065.
41. Neal JM. Effects of epinephrine in local anesthetics on the central and peripheral nervous systems: Neurotoxicity and neural blood flow. *Reg Anesth Pain Med*. 2003;28:124.
42. Sinnott CJ, Cogswell III LP, Johnson A, et al. On the mechanism by which epinephrine potentiates lidocaine's peripheral nerve block. *Anesthesiology*. 2003;98:181.
43. Curatolo M, Petersen-Felix S, Arendt-Nielsen L, et al. Epidural epinephrine and clonidine: Segmental analgesia and effects on different pain modalities. *Anesthesiology*. 1997;87:785.
44. Ueda W, Hirakawa M, Mori K. Acceleration of epinephrine absorption by lidocaine. *Anesthesiology*. 1985;63:717.
45. Magee C, Rodeheaver GT, Edgerton MT, et al. Studies of the mechanisms by which epinephrine damages tissue defenses. *J Surg Res*. 1977;23:126.
46. Hall JA, Ferro A. Myocardial ischaemia and ventricular arrhythmias precipitated by physiological concentrations of adrenaline in patients with coronary artery disease. *Br Heart J*. 1992;67:419.
47. Lambert DH. Clinical value of adding sodium bicarbonate to local anesthetics. *Reg Anesth Pain Med*. 2002;27:328.
48. Ikuta PT, Raza SM, Durrani Z. pH adjustment schedule for the amide local anesthetics. *Reg Anesth*. 1989;14:229.
49. Neal JM, Hebl JR, Gerancher JC, et al. Brachial plexus anesthesia: essentials of our current understanding. *Reg Anesth Pain Med*. 2002;27:402.
50. Sinnott CJ, Garfield JM, Thalhammer JG. Addition of sodium bicarbonate to lidocaine decreases the duration of peripheral nerve block in the rat. *Anesthesiology*. 2000;93:1045.
51. Wang C, Chakrabarti MK, Galletly DC, et al. Relative effects of intrathecal administration of fentanyl and midazolam on A delta and C fibre reflexes. *Neuropharmacology*. 1992;31:439.
52. Niv D, Nemirovsky A, Rudick V. Antinociception induced by simultaneous intrathecal and intraperitoneal administration of low doses of morphine. *Anesth Analg*. 1995;80:886.
53. Walker SM, Goudas LC, Cousins MJ, et al. Combination spinal analgesic chemotherapy: A systematic review. *Anesth Analg*. 2002;95:674.
54. Karambelkar DJ, Ramanathan S. 2-chloroprocaine antagonism of epidural morphine analgesia. *Acta Anaesth Scand*. 1997;41:774.
55. Coda B, Bausch S, Haas M, et al. The hypothesis that antagonism of fentanyl analgesia by 2-chloroprocaine is mediated by direct action on opioid receptors. *Reg Anesth*. 1997;22:43.
56. Janson W, Stein C. Peripheral opioid analgesia. *Curr Pharm Biotechnol*. 2003;4:270.
57. Picard PR, Tramer MR, McQuay HJ, et al. Analgesic efficacy of peripheral opioids (all except intra-articular): A qualitative systematic review of randomised controlled trials. *Pain*. 1997;72:309.
58. Candido KD, Winnie AP, Ghaleb AH, et al. Buprenorphine added to the local anesthetic for axillary brachial plexus block prolongs postoperative analgesia. *Reg Anesth Pain Med*. 2002;27:162.
59. Candido KD, Hennes J, Gonzalez S, et al. Buprenorphine enhances and prolongs the postoperative analgesic effect of bupivacaine in patients receiving infragluteal sciatic nerve block. *Anesthesiology*. 2010;113:419.
60. Rosseland LA. No evidence for analgesic effect of intra-articular morphine after knee arthroscopy: A qualitative systematic review. *Reg Anesth Pain Med*. 2005;30:83.
61. Eisenach JC, De Kock M, Klimscha W. Alpha(2)-adrenergic agonists for regional anesthesia: A clinical review of clonidine (1984–1995). *Anesthesiology*. 1996;85:655.
62. Butterworth JF, Strichartz GR. The α_2-adrenergic agonists clonidine and guanfacine produce tonic and phasic block of conduction in rat sciatic nerve fibers. *Anesth Analg*. 1993;76:295.
63. Gaumann DM, Brunet PC, Jirounek P. Clonidine enhances the effects of lidocaine on C fiber action potential. *Anesth Analg*. 1992;74:719.
64. Pertovaara A, Hamalainen MM. Spinal potentiation and supraspinal additivity in the antinociceptive interaction between systemically administered α_2-adrenoreceptor agonist and cocaine in the rat. *Anesth Analg*. 1994;79:261.

65. Popping DM, Elia N, Marret E, et al. Clonidine as an adjuvant to local anesthetics for peripheral nerve and plexus blocks. *Anesthesiology.* 2009;111:406.
66. Colin JL, McCartney ED, Apatu E. Should we add clonidine to local anesthetic for peripheral nerve blockade? A qualitative systematic review of the literature. *Reg Anesth Pain Med.* 2007;32:330.
67. Curley J, Castillo J, Hotz J, et al. Prolonged regional nerve blockade: Injectable biodegradable bupivacaine/polyester microspheres. *Anesthesiology.* 1996; 84:140.
68. Drager C, Benziger D, Gao F, et al. Prolonged intercostal nerve blockade in sheep using controlled-release of bupivacaine and dexamethasone from polymer microspheres. *Anesthesiology.* 1998;89:969.
69. Castillo J, Curley J, Hotz J, et al. Glucocorticoids prolong rat sciatic nerve blockade in vivo from bupivacaine microspheres. *Anesthesiology.* 1996;85:1157.
70. Parrington SJ, O'Donnell DO, Chan V, et al. Dexamethasone added to mepivacaine prolongs the duration of analgesia after supraclavicular brachial plexus blockade. *Reg Anesth Pain Med.* 2010;35:422.
71. Cummings KC, Napierkowski DE, Parra-Sanchez I, et al. Effect of dexamethasone on the duration of interscalene nerve blocks with ropivacaine or bupivacaine. *Br J Anaesth.* 2011;107:446.
72. Bigat Z, Boztug N, Hadimioglu N, et al. Does dexamethasone improve the quality of intravenous regional anesthesia and analgesia? A randomized, controlled clinical study. *Anesth Analg.* 2006;102:605.
73. Williams BA, Hough KA, Tsui B, et al. Neurotoxicity of adjuvants used in perineural anesthesia and analgesia in comparison with ropivacaine. *Reg Anesth Pain Med.* 2011;36:225.
74. Golf M, Daniels SE, Onel E. A phase 3, randomized, placebo-controlled trial of DepoFoam bupivacaine (extended-release bupivacaine local analgesic) in bunionectomy. *Adv Ther.* 2011;28:776.
75. Gorfine SR, Onel E, Patou G, et al. Bupivacaine extended-release liposome injection for prolonged postsurgical analgesia in patients undergoing hemorrhoidectomy: a multicenter, randomized, double-blind, placebo-controlled trial. *Dis Colon Rectum.* 2011;54:1552.
76. Smoot JD, Bergese SD, Onel E, et al. The efficacy and safety of DepoFoam bupivacaine in patients undergoing bilateral, cosmetic, submuscular augmentation mammaplasty: a randomized, double-blind, active-control study. *Aesthet Surg J.* 2012;32:69.
77. Bramlett K, Onel E, Viscusi ER, et al. A randomized, double-blind, dose-ranging study comparing wound infiltration of DepoFoam bupivacaine, an extended-release liposomal bupivacaine, to bupivacaine HCl for postsurgical analgesia in total knee arthroplasty. *Knee.* 2012;19:530.
78. McAlvin JB, Padera RF, Shankarappa SA, et al. Multivesicular liposomal bupivacaine at the sciatic nerve. *Biomaterials.* 2014;35:4557.
79. Viscusi ER, Candiotti KA, Onel E et al. The pharmacokinetics and pharmacodynamics of liposome bupivacaine administered via a single epidural injection to healthy volunteers. *Reg Anesth Pain Med.* 2012;37:616.
80. Ilfeld BM, Viscusi ER, Hadzic A, et al. Safety and side effect profile of liposome bupivacaine (Exparel) in peripheral nerve blocks. *Reg Anesth Pain Med.* 2015;40:572.
81. Morrison LM, Emanuelsson BM, McClure JH, et al. Efficacy and kinetics of extradural ropivacaine: comparison with bupivacaine. *Br J Anaesth.* 1994; 72:164.
82. Tucker GT, Mather LE. Pharmacology of local anaesthetic agents: Pharmacokinetics of local anaesthetic agents. *Br J Anaesth.* 1975;47(suppl):213.
83. Thomson PD, Melmon KL, Richardson JA, et al. Lidocaine pharmacokinetics in advanced heart failure, liver disease, and renal failure in humans. *Ann Intern Med.* 1973;78:499.
84. Rosenberg PR, Veering BT, Urmey WF. Maximum recommended doses of local anesthetics: A multifactorial concept. *Reg Anesth Pain Med.* 2004;29:564.
85. Braid DP, Scott DB. Dosage of lignocaine in epidural block in relation to toxicity. *Br J Anaesth.* 1996;38:596.
86. Adinoff B, Devous Sr MD, Best SE, et al. Gender differences in limbic responsiveness, by SPECT, following pharmacologic challenge in healthy subjects. *Neuroimage.* 2003;18:697.
87. Tucker GT, Mather LE. Properties, absorption, and disposition of local anesthetic agents. In: Cousins MJ, Bridenbaugh PO, eds. *Neural Blockade in Clinical Anesthesia and Management of Pain.* 3rd ed. Philadelphia, PA: Lippincott-Raven Publishers; 1998:55.
88. Ugur B, Ogurlu M, Gezer E, et al. Effects of esmolol, lidocaine and fentanyl on haemodynamic responses to endotracheal intubation: a comparative study. *Clin Drug Investig.* 2007;27:269.
89. Adamzik M, Groeben H, Farahani R, et al. Intravenous lidocaine after tracheal intubation mitigates bronchoconstriction in patients with asthma. *Anesth Analg.* 2007;104:168.
90. Groban L. Central nervous system and cardiac effects from long-acting amide local anesthetic toxicity in the intact animal model. *Reg Anesth Pain Med.* 2003;28:3.
91. Weinberg GL. Current concepts in resuscitation of patients with local anesthetic cardiac toxicity. *Reg Anesth Pain Med.* 2002;27:568.
92. Brown DL, Ransom DM, Hall JA, et al. Regional anesthesia and local anesthetic-induced systemic toxicity: seizure frequency and accompanying cardiovascular changes. *Anesth Analg.* 1995;81:321.
93. Auroy Y, Benhamou D, Bargues L, et al. Major complications of regional anesthesia in France: the SOS Regional Anesthesia Hotline Service. *Anesthesiology.* 2002;97:1274.
94. Lee LA, Posner KL, Domino KB, et al. Injuries associated with regional anesthesia in the 1980s and 1990s: a closed claim analysis. *Anesthesiology.* 2004;101:143.
95. Butterworth JF. Models and mechanisms of local anesthetic cardiac toxicity. *Reg Anesth Pain Med.* 2010;35:167.
96. Mather LE, Copeland SE, Ladd LA. Acute toxicity of local anesthetics: underlying pharmacokinetic and pharmacodynamic concepts. *Reg Anesth Pain Med.* 2005;30:553.
97. Knudsen K, Beckman Suurkula M, Blomberg S, et al. Central nervous and cardiovascular effects of i.v. infusions of ropivacaine, bupivacaine and placebo in volunteers. *Br J Anaesth.* 1997;78:507.
98. Stewart J, Kellett N, Castro D. The central nervous system and cardiovascular effects of levobupivacaine and ropivacaine in healthy volunteers. *Anesth Analg.* 2002;97:412.
99. Vanhoutte F, Vereecke J, Verbeke N, et al. Stereoselective effects of the enantiomers of bupivacaine on the electrophysiological properties of the guinea-pig papillary muscle. *Br J Pharmacol.* 1991;103:1275.
100. Valenzuela C, Snyders D, Bennett PB, et al. Stereoselective block of sodium channels by bupivacaine in guinea pig ventricular myocytes. *Circulation.* 1995;92:3014.
101. Groban L, Deal DD, Vernon JC, et al. Does local anesthetic stereoselectivity or structure predict myocardial depression in anesthetized canines? *Reg Anesth Pain Med.* 2002;27:460.
102. Pickering AE, Waki H, Headley PM, et al. Investigation of systemic bupivacaine toxicity using the in situ perfused working heart-brainstem preparation of the rat. *Anesthesiology.* 2002;97:1550.
103. Chang KSK, Yang M, Andresen MC. Clinically relevant concentrations of bupivacaine inhibit rat aortic baroreceptors. *Anesth Analg.* 1994;78:501.
104. Newton DJ, McLeod GA, Khan F, et al. Vasoactive characteristics of bupivacaine and levobupivacaine with and without adjuvant epinephrine in peripheral human skin. *Br J Anaesth.* 2005;94:662.
105. Liu P, Feldman HS, Covina BM, et al. Acute cardiovascular toxicity of intravenous amide local anesthetics in anesthetized ventilated dogs. *Anesth Analg.* 1982;61:317.
106. Guo XT, Castle NA, Chernoff DM, et al. Comparative inhibition of voltage-gated cation channels by local anesthetics. *Ann N Y Acad Sci.* 1991;625:181.
107. Clarkson CW, Hondeghem LM. Mechanisms for bupivacaine depression of cardiac conduction: fast block of sodium channels during the action potential with slow recovery from block during diastole. *Anesthesiology.* 1985;62:396.
108. Nouette-Gaulain K, Forestier F, Malgat M, et al. Effects of bupivacaine on mitochondrial energy metabolism in heart of rats following exposure to chronic hypoxia. *Anesthesiology.* 2002;97:1507.
109. Wong GK, Crawford MW. Carnitine deficiency increases susceptibility to bupivacaine-induced cardiotoxicity in rats. *Anesthesiology.* 2011;114:1417.
110. Weinberg GL. Treatment of local anesthetic systemic toxicity (LAST). *Reg Anesth Pain Med.* 2010;35:188.
111. Long WB, Rosenblum S, Grady IP. Successful resuscitation of bupivacaine-induced cardiac arrest using cardiopulmonary bypass. *Anesth Analg.* 1989; 79:403.
112. Soltesz EG, van Pelt F, Byrne JG. Emergent cardiopulmonary bypass for bupivacaine cardiotoxicity. *J Cardiothorac Vasc Anesth.* 2003;17:357.
113. Weinberg GL, VadeBoncouer T, Ramaraju GA, et al. Pretreatment or resuscitation with a lipid infusion shifts the dose-response to bupivacaine-induced asystole in rats. *Anesthesiology.* 1998;99:1071.
114. Weinberg GL, Ripper R, Feinstein DL, et al. Lipid emulsion infusion rescues dogs from bupivacaine-induced cardiac toxicity. *Reg Anesth Pain Med.* 2003;28:198.
115. Rosenblatt MA, Abel M, Fischer GW, et al. Successful use of a 20% lipid emulsion to resuscitate a patient after a presumed bupivacaine-related cardiac arrest. *Anesthesiology.* 2006;105:217.
116. Litz RJ, Popp M, Stehr SN, et al. Successful resuscitation of a patient with ropivacaine-induced asystole after axillary plexus block using lipid infusion. *Anaesthesia.* 2006;61:800.
117. Weinberg GL, Ripper R, Murphy P, et al. Lipid infusion accelerates removal of bupivacaine and recovery from bupivacaine toxicity in the isolated rat heart. *Reg Anesth Pain Med.* 2006;31:296.
118. Weinberg GL, Palmer JW, VadeBoncouer TR, et al. Bupivacaine inhibits acyl-carnitine exchange in cardiac mitochondria. *Anesthesiology.* 2000;92:523.
119. Kitagawa N, Oda M, Totoki T. Possible mechanism of irreversible nerve injury caused by local anesthetics and membrane disruption. *Anesthesiology.* 2004;100:962.
120. Kalichman MW. Physiologic mechanisms by which local anesthetics may cause injury to nerve and spinal cord. *Reg Anesth.* 1993;18:448.
121. Whitlock EL, Brenner MJ, Fox IK, et al. Ropivacaine-induced peripheral nerve injection injury in the rodent model. *Anesth Analg.* 2010;111:214.
122. Selander D. Neurotoxicity of local anesthetics: animal data. *Reg Anesth.* 1993;18:461.

123. Kroin JS, Buvanendran A, Williams DK, et al. Local anesthetic sciatic nerve block and nerve fiber damage in diabetic rats. *Reg Anesth Pain Med.* 2010;35:343.
124. Brull R, McCartney CJ, Chan VW, et al. Neurological complications after regional anesthesia: contemporary estimates of risk. *Anesth Analg.* 2007;104:965.
125. Bigeleisen PE. Nerve puncture and apparent intraneural injection during ultrasound-guided axillary block does not invariably result in neurologic injury. *Anesthesiology.* 2006;105:779.
126. Rigler M, Drasner K, Krejcie T, et al. Cauda equina syndrome after continuous spinal anesthesia. *Anesth Analg.* 1991;72:275.
127. Reisner L, Hochman B, Plumer M. Persistent neurologic deficit and adhesive arachnoiditis following intrathecal 2-chloroprocaine injection. *Anesth Analg.* 1980;58:452.
128. Pollock JE. Transient neurologic symptoms: etiology, risk factors, and management. *Reg Anesth Pain Med.* 2002;27:581.
129. Zaric D, Christiansen C, Pace NL, et al. Transient neurologic symptoms after spinal anesthesia with lidocaine versus other local anesthetics: a systematic review of randomized, controlled trials. *Anesth Analg.* 2005;100:1811.
130. Pollock JE, Liu SS, Neal JM, et al. Dilution of lidocaine does not decrease the incidence of transient neurologic symptoms. *Anesthesiology.* 1999;90:445.
131. Hogan Q, Dotson R, Erickson S, et al. Local anesthetic myotoxicity: a case and review. *Anesthesiology.* 1994;80:942.
132. Zink W, Bohl JRE, Hacke N, et al. The long-term myotoxic effects of bupivacaine and ropivacaine after continuous peripheral nerve blocks. *Anesth Analg.* 2005;101:548.
133. Nouette-Gaulain K, Dadure C, Morau D, et al. Age-dependent bupivacaine-induced muscle toxicity during continuous peripheral nerve block in rats. *Anesthesiology.* 2009;111:1120.
134. Nouette-Gaulain K, Sirvent P, Canal-Raffin M, et al. Effects of intermittent femoral nerve injections of bupivacaine, levobupivacaine, and ropivacaine on mitochondrial energy metabolism and intracellular calcium homeostasis in rat psoas muscle. *Anesthesiology.* 2007;106:1026.
135. Nouette-Gaulain K, Bellance N, Prevost B, et al. Erythropoietin protects against local anesthetic myotoxicity during continuous regional anesthesia. *Anesthesiology.* 2009;110:648.
136. Galbes O, Bourret A, Nouette-Gaulain K, et al. N-Acetylcysteine protects against bupivacaine-induced myotoxicity caused by oxidative and sarcoplasmic reticulum stress in human skeletal myotubes. *Anesthesiology.* 2010;113:560.
137. Boren E, Teuber SS, Naguwa SM, et al. A critical review of local anesthetic sensitivity. *Clin Rev Allergy Immunol.* 2007;32:119.
138. Phillips JF, Yates AB, Deshazo RD. Approach to patients with suspected hypersensitivity to local anesthetics. *Am J Med Sci.* 2007;334:190.
139. McClimon B, Rank M, Li J. The predictive value of skin testing in the diagnosis of local anesthetic allergy. *Allergy Asthma Proc.* 2011;32:95.
140. Kwong K, Carr MJ. Voltage-gated sodium channels. *Curr Opin Pharmacol.* 2015;22:131.
141. Catterall WA: Neurotoxins that act on voltage-sensitive sodium channels in excitable membranes. *Annu Rev Pharmacol Toxicol.* 1980;20:15.
142. Rodriguez-Navarro AJ, Lagos N, Lagos M, et al. Neosaxitoxin as a local anesthetic: preliminary observations from a first human trial. *Anesthesiology.* 2007;106:339.
143. Lobo K, Donado C, Cornelissen L, et al. A phase 1, dose-escalation, double-blind, block-randomized, controlled trial of safety and efficacy of neosaxitoxin alone and in combination with 0.2% bupivacaine, with and without epinephrine for cutaneous anesthesia. *Anesthesiology.* 2015;123;873.
144. Wylie MC, Johnson VM, Carpino E, et al. Respiratory, neuromuscular, and cardiovascular effects of neosaxitoxin in isoflurane-anesthetized sheep. *Reg Anesth Pain Med.* 2012;37:152.
145. Templin JS, Wylie MC, Kim JD, et al. Improved therapeutic index using combinations with bupivacaine, with and without epinephrine. *Anesthesiology.* 2015;123;886.
146. Roberson DP, Binshtok AM, Blasl F, et al. Targeting of sodium channel blockers into nociceptors to produce long-duration analgesia: a systemic study and review. *Br J Pharmacol.* 2011;164:48.
147. Binshtok AM, Bean BP, Woolf CJ. Inhibition of nociceptors by TRPV1-mediated entry of impermeant sodium channel blockers. *Nature.* 2007;449;607.
148. Binshtok AM, Gerner P, Oh SB, et al. Coapplication of lidocaine and the permanently charged sodium channel blocker QX-314 produces a long-lasting nociceptive blockade in rodents. *Anesthesiology.* 2009;111:127.

Section 5

PREOPERATIVE ASSESSMENT AND PERIOPERATIVE MONITORING

23 Preoperative Patient Assessment and Management

TARA M. HATA • J. STEVEN HATA

Introduction
Changing Concepts in Preoperative Evaluation
Approach to the Healthy Patient
   Screening Patients Using a Systems Approach
Evaluation of the Patient with Known Systemic Disease
   Cardiovascular Disease
   Pulmonary Disease
   Endocrine Disease
   Renal Disease
   Liver Disease
   Other Diseases
Preoperative Laboratory Testing
   Defining Normal Values
   Risks and Costs versus Benefits

Summary of the Preoperative Evaluation
Preparation
   Smoking Cessation
   Continuing Current Medications/Treatment of Coexisting Diseases
   Prevention of Perioperative Pulmonary Aspiration
Psychological Preparation/Premedication
   Psychological Preparation
   Premedication
Antibiotic Prophylaxis
Summary of Patient Preparation

KEY POINTS

1. The goals of a preoperative evaluation are to reduce patient risk and morbidity associated with surgery and anesthesia, prepare the patient medically and psychologically, and also promote efficiency and reduce costs.

2. The anesthesiologist is responsible for assessing the medical condition of the patient and developing the anesthesia plan of care. The American Society of Anesthesiologists (ASA) published basic standards for preoperative care, as well as an updated practice advisory for preanesthesia evaluation that details evidence-supported recommendations.

3. It is important for the evaluation to be complete, accurate, and clear, not only to allow the information to be relayed to others who may care for the patient perioperatively but also for medicolegal purposes.

4. The preoperative evaluation serves as a screening tool to anticipate and avoid airway difficulties or problems with anesthetic drugs. In addition to the history and physical examination, previous anesthesia records should be reviewed and contraindications to specific drugs, such as succinylcholine, nitrous oxide, or volatile agents, should be sought.

5. A review of the patient's medication list, including over-the-counter and herbal preparations, should investigate potential drug interactions and potential indications for stress dose steroid coverage. The anesthesiologist should be aware of the patient's allergies and previous drug reactions, including the possibility of latex allergy.

6. When evaluating the patient with hypertension, diabetes mellitus, or obesity, it is important to determine the presence of end-organ damage, such as cardiovascular disease.

7. Exercise tolerance is a significant predictor of cardiac risk. Multiple specialty groups have contributed to formal guidelines for the perioperative cardiovascular evaluation and management of patients undergoing noncardiac procedures. The algorithms provide useful guides for further testing and evaluation.

8. Preoperative laboratory tests should be ordered on the basis of positive findings from the history and physical examination or from anticipated physiologic disturbances during surgery, such as blood loss.

9. Optimization of the patient's health status prior to surgery includes clear instruction regarding fasting times as well as which medications to continue until the time of surgery. In general, most medications for hypertension or cardiac disease should be continued, and consideration should be given to initiating β-blocker therapy before the day of surgery in appropriate patients who are at risk for cardiac adverse events. The need for subacute bacterial endocarditis prophylaxis should be anticipated. Likewise, drugs for asthma or chronic obstructive pulmonary disease should be continued or administered prophylactically. Medications taken for the treatment of esophageal reflux should be continued or initiated for those patients with untreated symptoms. For diabetic patients, oral hypoglycemic agents should often be held, but patients requiring insulin will need to continue to take adjusted doses.

10. Although preoperative sedation is generally limited to drugs given immediately prior to anesthesia, the administration must be carefully planned to allow optimal effect and avoid operating room delays.

Introduction

The goals of a preoperative evaluation are to reduce patient risk and morbidity associated with surgery and anesthesia, prepare the patient medically and psychologically, and promote efficiency and support cost-effectiveness. As we continue to expand our care at the extremes of age, we are held accountable for high-quality standards while we work to reduce costs. The Joint Commission (TJC) requires that all patients receive a preoperative anesthetic evaluation. The American Society of Anesthesiologists (ASA) web site contains the ASA Basic Standards for Preanesthetic Care that outline the minimum requirements for a preoperative evaluation, as well as the updated Practice Advisory for Preanesthesia Evaluation.[1] The most recent ASA Practice Guidelines can be found at https://www.asahq.org/quality-and-practice-management/standards-and-guidelines. Conducting a preoperative evaluation is based on the premise that it will modify patient care and improve outcome. Armed with such knowledge preoperatively, the anesthesiologist can prepare the patient as well as formulate an anesthetic plan that avoids dangers inherent in various disease states. Furthermore, preoperative evaluations may reduce both costs and surgery cancellation rates, increasing resource utilization in the operating room (OR).[2] This notion assumes that evaluations are done by anesthesiologists or other health care providers familiar with anesthesia, surgery, and perioperative events.

The preoperative evaluation has several components. It should include a review of the medical record as well as performance of a history and physical examination pertinent to the patient and planned procedure. On the basis of the history and physical examination, the appropriate diagnostic tests and preoperative consultations should be obtained. Through these, the anesthesiologist determines whether the patient's preoperative condition can be improved prior to surgery and develops the appropriate anesthetic care plan. Finally, the process is used to educate the patient about anesthesia and the perioperative period, answer all questions, and obtain informed consent.

The first part of this chapter outlines clinical risk factors pertinent to patients scheduled for anesthesia and surgery as well as the use of various tests to assess comorbid conditions. The second part discusses preoperative preparation. The chapter provides only an overview of the preoperative management process; for more details, the reader is referred to chapters focusing on specific organ systems.

Changing Concepts in Preoperative Evaluation

In the past, patients were typically admitted to the hospital a day prior to surgery, enabling the anesthesia team to perform the preoperative evaluation, order relevant laboratory tests or medications, and ensure that the patient was ready for surgery the next day. Currently, a minority of elective patients comes to the OR as inpatients. Older patients are increasingly scheduled for more complex procedures, and there also is more pressure on the anesthesiologist to reduce turnover time between cases. Although others may have seen the patient previously in a preoperative evaluation clinic, the first time that the anesthesiologist performing the anesthetic sees the patient may be just prior to surgery. Thus, only a short time may exist to develop the doctor–patient relationship, engender trust, and answer questions. Under such conditions, it is often impossible to alter medical therapy immediately preoperatively. However, preoperative screening clinics are becoming more effective and clinical practice guidelines are becoming more prevalent. Information technology helps the anesthesiologist to preview the upcoming patients who will be anesthetized. Preoperative questionnaires and computer-driven programs have become alternatives to traditional information retrieval. Finally, when anesthesiologists take responsibility for ordering preoperative laboratory tests, cost savings occur and cancellations of planned surgical procedures become less likely. In this setting, clear and efficient communication between the preoperative evaluation clinic and the anesthesiologist performing the anesthesia are critical.

Approach to the Healthy Patient

Standardization of best clinical practices may be enhanced by process control procedures. In this regard, the preoperative evaluation form can serve as the basis for formulating the best anesthetic plan tailored to the patient. It should aid the anesthesiologist in identifying potential complications, increase consistency in best-care practices, and serve as a medicolegal document. Because it is more common today for the preoperative evaluation to be completed in a clinic by another physician or health professional who may not personally perform the anesthesia and because regulatory agencies such as the TJC demand better documentation, the form's design must ensure that the information obtained is complete, concise, and legible. In hospitals with electronic medical records, legibility is rarely an issue. One report investigating the quality of preoperative evaluation forms across the United States rated them in three categories: informational content, ease of use, and ease of reading.[3] Their results revealed a surprisingly high percentage of forms missing important information. Table 23-1 offers one example of the pertinent areas of focus for a preoperative evaluation organized in a systems format.

Patient Diagnosis and Planned Procedure. One obviously important detail is the nature of the illness or injury necessitating surgery, as it will both determine the clinical urgency of the proposed operation and influence the available time and depth of the preoperative evaluation. True emergency procedures require

Table 23-1 Preanesthetic Evaluation Screen

Diagnosis/Procedure
Anesthetic/surgical history
   MH/adverse reactions
   Airway difficulty
Airway
Difficult airway, sleep apnea
Examination: Teeth, Mallampati class, mouth opening, chin length, neck size and mobility
	Age/Gender/Height/Weight
	Allergies/adverse reactions
	Medications
	   Over the counter/herbals, illicit drugs
	Cardiovascular
	Congenital heart disease, hypertension, coronary artery disease, heart failure, cardiomyopathy, valvular disease, syncope, dysrhythmia, pacemaker, vascular disease, angina, dyspnea, orthopnea, exercise tolerance
		Vital Signs
		NPO status
		   IV access/invasive monitors
		   Advance directives
		Pulmonary
		URI/bronchitis/pneumonia, tobacco, asthma, COPD, cough, dyspnea, sleep apnea, O_2/inhaler/steroid use, pneumothorax, ventilator settings, endotracheal tube size/depth

Central Nervous System Stroke, seizures, syncope, ↑intracranial pressure, altered mental status, headaches, neuromuscular disease, spinal cord injury, weakness, paresthesias, psych disorder	**GI/Hepatic** Liver disease, hepatitis, nausea/vomiting, reflux, bowel obstruction, EtOH use **Renal** Insufficiency, failure, dialysis	**Endocrine/Metabolic** Diabetes, thyroid disease, rheumatoid arthritis, steroid use
Infectious HIV, MRSA, VRE, influenza, TB, foreign travel	**Hematology** Anemia, coagulopathy, sickle cell, chemotherapy, transfusions	**Other** Pregnancy, weeks of gestation Trauma history

MH, malignant hyperthermia; NPO, nothing by mouth; IV, intravenous; URI, upper respiratory infection; COPD, chronic obstructive pulmonary disease; EtOH, ethanol; HIV, human immunodeficiency virus; MRSA, methicillin-resistant *Staphylococcus aureus*; VRE, vancomycin-resistant enterococci; TB, tuberculosis.

a more abbreviated evaluation and are associated with higher anesthetic morbidity and mortality. The approach to urgent procedures is less well defined. For example, ischemic limbs require surgery soon after presentation, but can usually be delayed for 24 hours for further evaluation. The anesthesiologist and surgeon must weigh the risk of morbidity of operative delay against the benefits of establishing associated diagnoses that can influence patient management. Table 23-2 shows one classification of operative urgency, though individual hospitals may have their own definitions. The indication for the surgical procedure may also have implications for other aspects of perioperative management. For example, the presence of a small bowel obstruction has implications regarding the risk of aspiration and the need for a rapid sequence induction. Similarly, the extent of a lung resection will dictate the need for further pulmonary testing and perioperative monitoring. Patients undergoing carotid endarterectomy may require a more extensive neurologic examination as well as additional testing to rule out coronary artery disease (CAD). The planned procedure also dictates patient positioning and whether blood products will be necessary. Frequently, obtaining such information will require communication with the surgeon and the OR team, enhancing both patient safety and OR efficiency.

Response to Previous Anesthetics. The ability to review previous anesthetic records is particularly helpful for detecting the presence of a difficult airway, a history of malignant hyperthermia (MH), and the individual's response to surgical stress and specific anesthetics. The patient should be questioned regarding any previous personal or familial difficulties with anesthesia. A patient's report of an "allergy" to anesthesia should raise suspicion for MH. A diagnosis of MH susceptibility will affect the anesthetic regimen and bring into question the appropriateness of outpatient surgery.

Although not life-threatening, persistent nausea and vomiting after a previous surgery may be the patient's most negative and lasting memory. There are multiple predictors of postoperative nausea and vomiting (PONV), including type of surgical procedure, anesthetic agents, and patient factors (Table 23-3). One

Table 23-2 Classification of Urgency of Surgical Procedures

Classification of Operation	Description	Optimal Timing	Example
Emergency	Life, limb, or organ-saving	<6 h	Ruptured aortic aneurysm Major trauma to thorax, abdomen Acute increase in intracranial pressure
Urgent	Conditions threaten life, limb, or organ	6–24 h	Perforated bowel Compound fracture Eye injury
Time sensitive	Stable, but requires intervention	Days to weeks	Tendon, nerve injuries Cancer procedures
Elective	Procedure planned at patient or surgeon convenience	Up to 1 yr	All other procedures that can be planned in advance

Adapted from Fleisher LA, Fleischmann KE, Auerbach AD, et al. ACC/AHA guideline on perioperative cardiovascular evaluation and management of patients undergoing noncardiac surgery. *Circulation*. 2014;130:e278–e333.

Table 23-3 Risk Factors for PONV in Adults

Evidence	Risk Factors
Positive overall	Female sex
	History of PONV or motion sickness
	Nonsmoking
	Younger age (<50 yr)
	General (vs. regional) anesthesia
	Volatile anesthetics and nitrous oxide
	Postoperative opioids
	Duration of anesthesia
	Type of surgery: cholecystectomy, laparoscopic, gynecologic
Conflicting	ASA status
	Menstrual cycle
	Anesthesia provider's experience
	Muscle relaxant reversal

PONV, postoperative nausea and vomiting; ASA, American Society of Anesthesiologists. Adapted from Gan TJ, Diemunsch P, Habib AS, et al. Consensus guidelines for the management of postoperative nausea and vomiting. *Anesth Analg.* 2014;118:85–113.

report predicting postoperative nausea and vomiting after *inhalation* anesthesia identified four risk factors: female gender, prior history of motion sickness or postoperative nausea, nonsmoking, and the use of postoperative opioids. The Apfel simplified risk score predicts PONV with 0, 1, 2, 3, or 4 risk factors as 10%, 20%, 40%, 60%, and 80%, respectively.[4] The investigators suggested prophylactic antiemetic therapy when two or more risk factors are present while using volatile anesthetics.[5] However, armed with this knowledge preoperatively, the anesthesiologist is also able to tailor the anesthetic or possibly avoid the most likely causes of PONV: volatile anesthetics, nitrous oxide, and postoperative opioids altogether.[6]

In children, Eberhart et al.[7] identified four independent predictors of postoperative vomiting (POV): duration of surgery longer than 30 minutes, age above 3 years, history of POV in patient or family, and strabismus surgery. Based on the presence of 0, 1, 2, 3, and 4 factors, the risk of POV was 9%, 10%, 30%, 55%, and 70%, respectively.

Medications/Allergies. The history should include a complete list of medications, including over-the-counter and herbal products (Table 23-4), to define a preoperative medication regimen, anticipate potential drug interactions, and provide clues to

Table 23-4 Herbal/Dietary Supplements and Drug Interactions

Brand Name	Common Uses	Pharmacologic Effects and Drug Interactions
Ephedra	Weight loss aid	Increased HR and BP, enhanced sympathomimetic effects with other sympathomimetics
	Bacteriostatic	
	Antitussive	Potential arrhythmias with digoxin or halothane, hypertension with oxytocin
Feverfew	Migraine prophylaxis	Inhibits platelet activity and increases bleeding
	Antipyretic	Rebound headache with sudden cessation
GBL, BD, GHB (γ-butyrolactone)	Bodybuilding	Illegally distributed drugs
	Weight loss aid	Death, seizures, unconsciousness
	Sleep aid	Bradycardia, slowed respirations
Garlic	Lower cholesterol, BP	Inhibition of platelet aggregation, potential for increased bleeding
	Antioxidant	
Ginger	Antinausea	Potent inhibitor of thromboxane synthetase; may increase bleeding time
	Antispasmodic	
Ginkgo	Blood thinner	May enhance bleeding in patients on anticoagulant or antithrombotic therapy
Ginseng	Energy level enhancer	May inhibit platelet aggregation and increase bleeding
	Antioxidant	Decreased blood glucose
Goldenseal	Diuretic	Functions as an oxytocic
	Anti-inflammatory	May worsen edema and/or hypertension
	Laxative	
Kava-kava	Anxiolytic	Potentiates sedative effects of anesthetics
		May cause hepatotoxicity
Licorice	Treats gastritis/ulcers	Glycyrrhizic acid in licorice may cause high blood pressure, hypokalemia, edema
	Treats cough/bronchitis	Contraindicated in many chronic liver conditions, renal insufficiency
St. John's wort	Treats depression, anxiety	May prolong effects of anesthesia
Valerian	Mild sedative, anxiolytic	May potentiate sedative effects of anesthetics
Vitamin E	Slow aging	May increase bleeding, particularly in conjunction with other anticoagulant and antithrombotic drugs
	Promotes wound healing	Can cause BP problems

HR, heart rate; BP, blood pressure; GBL, gamma butyrolactone; GHB, gamma-hydroxybutyrate. Adapted from the ASA Physician Brochure: What You Should Know About Your Patients' Use of Herbal Medicines and Other Dietary Supplements, 2003. www.ASAhq.org.

underlying disease. A complete list of drug allergies, including previous reactions, should be obtained, as well as an inquiry concerning reaction to latex.

If the patient presents on the day of surgery, the anesthesiologist should determine when the patient last ate and drank as well as note the sites of pre-existing intravenous cannulas and invasive monitors. Once the general issues are completed, the preoperative history and physical examination can focus on specific systems.

Screening Patients Using a Systems Approach

Airway

At the forefront of every anesthesiologist's mind is concern about the patient's airway. The anesthesiologist needs to recognize the potential for difficulty in maintaining a patent airway with a mask, a laryngeal mask airway, or in the ability to place an endotracheal tube when the patient is under general anesthesia. The ability to review previous anesthetic records is especially useful in uncovering an unsuspected "difficult airway" or to confirm previous uneventful tracheal intubations, noting whether the patient's body habitus or airway anatomy has changed in the interim. Patients should be questioned about their ability to breathe through their nose, whether there is suspected or diagnosed obstructive sleep apnea (OSA), and whether they have orthopnea. Evaluation of the airway involves examination of the oral cavity, including dentition, determination of the thyromental distance, assessment of the size of the patient's neck and potential tracheal deviation or masses, as well as evaluation of their ability to flex the base of the neck and extend the head. For trauma patients or patients with severe rheumatoid arthritis (RA) or Down syndrome, assessment of the cervical spine is critical. The presence of symptoms or signs of cervical cord compression should be assessed. In some instances, radiographic examination may also be required.

The Mallampati classification is the standard for assessing the relationship of the tongue size relative to the oral cavity (Table 23-5),[8] although by itself the Mallampati classification has a low positive predictive value in identifying patients who are difficult to intubate.[9,10] Intubation involves multiple steps: flexion of the lower neck, extension of the upper neck, opening the mouth to insert the laryngoscope, and displacing the tongue forward and down into the submandibular space to expose the glottis. Therefore, a multifactorial approach to predicting intubation difficulty, as shown in Table 23-6, has proven to be more helpful. One must distinguish factors that predict a difficult intubation and factors that predict a difficult mask airway. For example, the absence of teeth clearly makes laryngoscopy less difficult, but at the same time can make mask ventilation more challenging.

Table 23-5 Modified Mallampati Airway Classification System

Class	Direct Visualization, Patient Seated
I	Full view of soft palate, uvula, tonsillar pillars
II	Soft palate and upper portion of uvula
III	Soft palate
IV	Hard palate only

Modified with permission from Mallampati RS, Gatt SP, Gugino LD, et al. A clinical sign to predict difficult tracheal intubation: A prospective study. Can Anaesth Soc J. 1985;32:429–434.

Table 23-6 Components of the Airway Examination That Suggest Difficult Tracheal Intubation

1. Long upper incisors
2. Prominent "overbite"
3. Inability to protrude the mandibular incisors anterior to maxillary incisors
4. Distance between incisors is <3 cm when mouth is fully opened
5. Uvula not visible when tongue is protruded with patient sitting
6. Shape of palate highly arched or very narrow
7. Mandibular space noncompliant
8. Thyromental distance <3 fingerbreadths
9. Neck short or thick
10. Limited range of motion of head and neck

Clinical context and judgment determine which of the components apply to a particular patient.
Modified from the Task Force on Difficult Airway Management. Practice guidelines for management of the difficult airway: An updated report by the American Society of Anesthesiologist Task Force on Management of the Difficult Airway. Anesthesiology. 2003;98:1269–1277.

Pulmonary System

A screening evaluation should include questions regarding the history of tobacco use, dyspnea, exercise tolerance, cough, wheezing, bronchodilator or steroid use, recent upper respiratory tract infection, stridor, and snoring or sleep apnea. Physical examination should assess respiratory rate, chest excursion, use of accessory muscles, nail color, and the patient's ability to carry on a conversation or to walk without dyspnea. Auscultation can detect decreased breath sounds, wheezing, stridor, or crackles. For the patient with positive findings, see the section later on the preoperative evaluation of the patient with known pulmonary disease.

Cardiovascular System

When screening a patient for cardiovascular disease prior to surgery, the anesthesiologist is most interested in recognizing signs and symptoms of uncontrolled hypertension and unstable cardiac disease such as myocardial ischemia, congestive heart failure, valvular heart disease, and significant cardiac dysrhythmias. Symptoms of cardiovascular disease should be carefully sought, particularly the characteristics of dyspnea, chest pain, or syncope, as well as exercise tolerance. Certain populations of patients, such as the elderly, women, or diabetics, may present with more atypical features. The presence of unstable angina has been associated with a high perioperative risk of myocardial infarction (MI).[11] The perioperative period is associated with a hypercoagulable state and surges in endogenous catecholamines, both of which may exacerbate the underlying process in unstable angina, increasing the risk of acute infarction. The patient should be questioned about symptoms of clinically important valvular disease, such as angina, dyspnea, syncope, or congestive heart failure, that would require further evaluation. Importantly, the anesthesiologist must identify patients who have undergone placement of a coronary artery stent or an implantable cardiac device to be able to coordinate perioperative management with the cardiologist (see section on cardiovascular disease).

The anesthesiologist should also be familiar with the American Heart Association (AHA) web site (http://www.heart.org/) and its links to the latest AHA statements and guidelines for health professionals. Here one can find the most recent recommendations regarding the specific patients and procedures that require subacute bacterial endocarditis prophylaxis.[12]

The examination of the cardiovascular system should include blood pressure evaluation, measuring both arms when appropriate. The anesthesiologist should consider the effects of preoperative anxiety and review resting blood pressure measurements. However, according to one study, the admission blood pressure was the best predictor of heart rate and blood pressure response to laryngoscopy.[13] Auscultation of the heart is performed, specifically listening for a murmur radiating to the carotids suggestive of aortic stenosis, abnormal rhythms, or a gallop suggestive of heart failure. The presence of bruits over the carotid arteries warrants further workup to determine the risk of stroke. The extremities should be examined for peripheral pulses to exclude peripheral vascular disease or congenital cardiovascular disease.

Neurologic System

Neurologic system assessment in the apparently healthy patient can be accomplished through simple observation. The patient's ability to answer health history questions practically indicates a normal mental status. Questions can be directed regarding a history of stroke, symptoms of cerebrovascular disease, seizures, preexisting neuromuscular disease, or nerve injuries. The neurologic examination may be cursory in healthy patients or extensive in patients with coexisting disease. Testing of strength, reflexes, and sensation may be important in patients for whom the anesthetic plan or surgical procedure may result in a change in condition.

Endocrine System

Each patient should be questioned for a history or symptoms of endocrine diseases that may affect the perioperative course: diabetes mellitus, thyroid disease, parathyroid disease, endocrine-secreting tumors, and adrenal cortical suppression.

Evaluation of the Patient with Known Systemic Disease

Cardiovascular Disease

Recent clinical practice guidelines have established definitions applicable to the planned procedure and the perioperative risk of major adverse cardiac events (MACE), including death and MI. A low-risk procedure is defined as having a less than 1% incidence of MACE, whereas a high-risk procedure carries a risk of more than 1%. In the preoperative evaluation, a clinical history of cardiovascular disease, diabetes mellitus, and cerebrovascular disease support an elevated risk of MACE. Consistently, advanced age is independently associated with an increased risk of MACE and ischemic stroke. Prior MIs appear associated with both postoperative MI and 30-day mortality, which, in turn, are related to the timing of the initial MI.[14] Recent clinical practice guidelines support delaying noncardiac surgery at least 60 days after an MI in the absence of coronary intervention. Importantly, recent MI within 6 months of noncardiac surgery appears to be a risk factor for perioperative stroke.[15]

The preoperative evaluation of the patient with known or suspected cardiovascular disease is focused on two areas:

Table 23-7 American Society of Anesthesiologists (ASA) Physical Status (PS) Classification

ASA PS class 1	Normal healthy patient. No organic, physiologic, biochemical, or psychiatric disturbance
ASA PS class 2	Mild-to-moderate systemic disease that is well controlled and causes no organ dysfunction or functional limitation (e.g., treated hypertension)
ASA PS class 3	Severe systemic disease of at least one organ system that does cause functional limitation (e.g., stable angina)
ASA PS class 4	Severe systemic end-stage disease of at least one organ system that is life threatening with or without surgery (e.g., congestive heart failure or renal failure)
ASA PS class 5	Moribund patient who has little chance of survival but is submitted to surgery as a last resort (resuscitative effort; e.g., ruptured aortic aneurysm)
ASA PS class 6	A declared brain-dead patient whose organs are being removed for donor purposes
Emergency operation (E)	Any patient in whom an emergency operation is required

Modified from American Society of Anesthesiologists: New classification of physical status. *Anesthesiology*. 1963;24:111.

identification of clinical risk indices and preoperative cardiac testing. The goals are to define risk; identify which patients will benefit from further testing; determine whether perioperative β-blockade, interventional therapy, or even surgery would be beneficial before the planned procedure; and form an appropriate anesthetic plan. Multivariate risk indices, based on epidemiologic statistical methods, can add value in predicting MACE. Historically, these have included the ASA physical status index (Table 23-7) and the Goldman Cardiac Risk Index.

The Revised Cardiac Risk Index (RCRI) is an update of the Goldman Cardiac Risk Index and is a validated method to assign perioperative risk using readily available clinical variables.[16] In a population of 4,315 patients aged 50 years and older undergoing elective, major noncardiac procedures, six independent predictors of complications were identified and included in the RCRI: high-risk type of surgery, history of ischemic heart disease, history of congestive heart failure, history of cerebrovascular disease, preoperative treatment with insulin, and preoperative serum creatinine greater than 2 mg/dL. Cardiac complications rose with an increase in the number of risk factors present. Rates of major cardiac complications with 0, 1, 2, or 3 of these factors were 0.5%, 1.3%, 4%, and 9%, respectively, in the derivation cohort, and 0.4%, 0.9%, 7%, and 11%, respectively, among 1,422 patients in the validation cohort (Table 23-8). Figure 23-1 shows the rate of major cardiac complications for patients in each ASA class according to the type of procedure performed.

Surgical groups have also developed cardiac and surgical risk calculators. The American College of Surgeons (ACS) National Surgical Quality Improvement Program (NSQIP) Myocardial Infarction and Cardiac Arrest (MICA) risk-prediction calculator

Table 23-8	Revised Cardiac Risk Index (RCRI)	
Risk Factors	RCRI Risk Assessment	Event Rate (%)
Ischemic heart disease	Low (0 factor)	0.5
Congestive heart failure	Low (1 factor)	1.3
Cerebrovascular disease	Intermediate (2 factors)	3.6
Diabetes mellitus treated with insulin	High (3 or more factors)	9.1
Serum creatinine >2 mg/dL		
High-risk surgery (intraperitoneal, intrathoracic, or suprainguinal vascular)		

Modified from Lee TH, Marcantonio ER, Mangione CM, et al. Derivation and prospective evaluation of a simple index for prediction of cardiac risk of major noncardiac surgery. *Circulation.* 1999;100:1043–1049.

is a multivariate risk assessment tool for perioperative cardiac arrest and MI (http://www.surgicalriskcalculator.com/miorcardiacarrest).[17] The ACS NSQIP Surgical Risk Calculator uses current procedural terminology codes and 21 patient-specific variables for prediction of several groups of outcomes.[18]

Finally, the additional laboratory measurement of biomarkers (e.g., brain natriuretic peptide or N-terminal brain natriuretic peptide and C-reactive protein levels) may increase prediction accuracy.[19,20] For example, the preoperative measurement of elevated brain natriuretic peptide levels appears significantly associated with MACE in vascular patients within 30 days of surgery.[21]

Although all of these indices provide information to assess the probability of complications and provide an estimate of risk, the cardiovascular risk factors in any individual patient first need to be defined; then a plan for anesthesia and perioperative management can be prescribed.

In patients with symptomatic coronary disease, the preoperative evaluation may reveal a change in the frequency or pattern of anginal symptoms. Certain populations of patients—for example, the elderly, women, or diabetics—may present with more atypical features. The presence of unstable angina has been associated with a high perioperative risk of MI.[11]

In virtually all studies, the preoperative presence of active congestive heart failure is a major risk factor for increased perioperative cardiac morbidity.[22,23] Clinical evidence of heart failure includes symptoms of dyspnea, limited exercise tolerance, and orthopnea; as well as physical signs of jugular venous distention, crackles, third heart sound, and peripheral edema. A chest x-ray reveals pulmonary edema or vascular redistribution. Significantly reduced left ventricular ejection fraction (e.g., <30%) appears to be an independent risk factor for adverse perioperative outcome and long-term mortality.[24] Another study suggests that asymptomatic systolic or diastolic dysfunction is associated with increased 30-day cardiovascular perioperative risk.[25] Optimization of ventricular function and treatment of pulmonary edema are both important prior to elective surgery. Because the type of perioperative monitoring and treatment may be different, clarifying the cause of heart failure is important (e.g., nonischemic cardiomyopathy or cardiac valvular insufficiency and/or stenosis).

Patients with known valvular heart disease can be effectively managed during the perioperative period to limit morbidity. The 2014 AHA/ACC Guideline for the Management of Patients with Valvular Disease supports the use of preoperative echocardiography in patients with moderate or severe valvular stenosis or regurgitation with no echocardiography studies within 1 year, or worsening clinical status.[26] Valvular interventions (e.g., repair or replacement) may be indicated before elective noncardiac surgery depending on the symptoms or severity of disease. Understanding the severity of stenotic or regurgitant valvular disease, coupled with an intraoperative monitoring and management plan, may reduce the risk of perioperative congestive heart failure and respiratory failure.

Adults with a prior MI almost always have CAD. Traditionally, risk assessment for noncardiac surgery was based on the time interval between the MI and surgery, which was based on older data that demonstrated an increased incidence of reinfarction if the MI was within 6 months of surgery.[27] The importance of the intervening time interval may no longer be valid in the current era of interventional therapy and improvements in perioperative care. Although many patients with an MI may continue

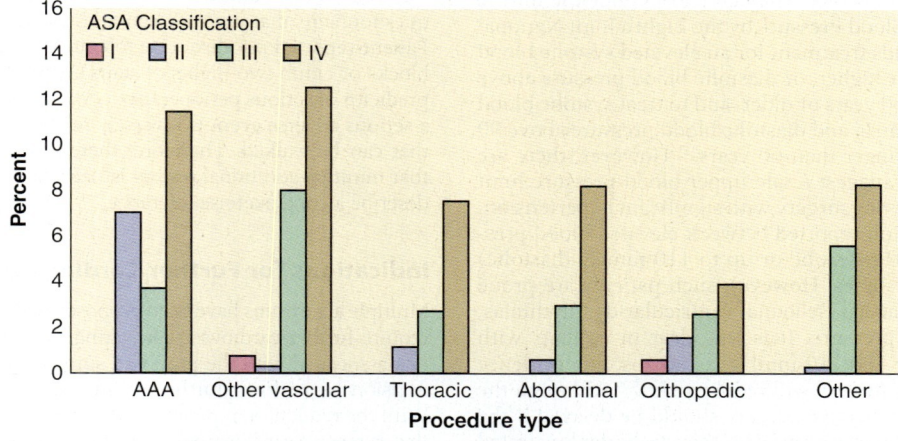

Figure 23-1 Cardiac risk (percent of patients expected to have major cardiac complications) by Revised Cardiac Risk Index (RCRI) class and type of surgical procedure. Bars represent rate of major cardiac complications in RCRI classes I to IV (based on patients with 0, 1, 2, or more risk factors, respectively) according to the type of procedure performed. Note that, by definition, patients undergoing abdominal aortic aneurysm (AAA), thoracic, and abdominal procedures were excluded from class I. In all subsets except patients undergoing AAA, there was a statistically significant trend toward greater risk with higher-risk class. See text for details. (Reproduced with permission from Lee TH, Marcantonio ER, Mangione CM, et al. Derivation and prospective validation of a simple index for prediction of cardiac risk of major noncardiac surgery. *Circulation.* 1999;100:1043.)

to have myocardium at risk for subsequent ischemia and infarction, other patients may have their critical coronary stenoses either totally occluded or widely patent, with no such risk. For example, the use of percutaneous transluminal coronary angioplasty, thrombolysis, and early coronary artery bypass grafting (CABG) has changed the natural history of the disease. Therefore, patients should be individually evaluated from the perspective of their risk for ongoing ischemia.

Identifying Patients at Risk for Atherosclerotic Cardiac Disease

For those patients without overt cardiac symptoms, the probability of CAD varies with the type and number of atherosclerotic risk factors present. Peripheral arterial disease has been shown to be associated with CAD in multiple studies.[28]

Diabetes Mellitus

Diabetes mellitus is a common disease with a pathophysiology that affects multiple organ systems. Complications of diabetes mellitus are frequently the cause of urgent or emergent surgery, especially in the elderly. Diabetes accelerates the progression of atherosclerosis, so it is not surprising that diabetics have a higher incidence of CAD than nondiabetics as well as a high incidence of both silent MI and myocardial ischemia.[29] Eagle et al.[30] demonstrated that diabetes is an independent risk factor for perioperative cardiac morbidity, and as mentioned earlier, diabetes requiring insulin treatment is a risk factor in the RCRI. The duration of the disease and presence of associated end-organ dysfunction may also alter the overall cardiac risk. Autonomic neuropathy has been reported as the best predictor of silent ischemia.[31] Because these patients are at very high risk for a silent MI, a preoperative electrocardiogram (ECG) should be obtained to examine for the presence of Q waves.

Hypertension

Hypertension has also been associated with an increased incidence of silent myocardial ischemia and infarction.[29] Hypertensive patients who have left ventricular hypertrophy and are undergoing noncardiac surgery are at a higher perioperative risk than nonhypertensive patients.[32] Investigators have suggested that the presence of a strain pattern on ECG suggests a chronic ischemic state.[33]

Aggressive treatment of blood pressure is associated with reduction in long-term MI risk. The new 2014 Guideline for the Management of High Blood Pressure by the Eighth Joint National Committee recommends treatment for an elevated systolic blood pressure 150 mmHg or higher, or diastolic blood pressure above 90 mmHg in patients 60 years or older, and to treat systolic blood pressure above 140 mmHg and diastolic blood pressure above 90 mmHg in patients younger than 60 years.[34] However, there are no such guidelines to suggest a safe upper blood pressure limit when a patient presents for surgery with significant hypertension. There is little association reported between elevated blood pressures (up to 180 mmHg systolic or up to 110 mmHg diastolic) and postoperative outcomes. However, such patients are prone to perioperative myocardial ischemia, ventricular dysrhythmias, and lability in blood pressure. It is less clear in patients with blood pressures above 180/110 mmHg, as no absolute evidence exists that postponing surgery will reduce risk.[35,36] Although the literature suggests that elective surgery should be delayed if the diastolic pressure is above 110 mmHg, this study demonstrated no major morbidity in that small group of patients.[37] Thus, in the absence of end-organ changes, such as renal insufficiency or left ventricular hypertrophy with strain, the benefits of optimizing blood pressure must be weighed against the risks of delaying surgery.

Metabolic Syndrome/Tobacco

"Metabolic syndrome" is a disorder comprising a group of risk factors that includes high blood pressure, atherogenic dyslipidemia (high triglyceride and low high-density lipoprotein cholesterol concentrations), high fasting glucose concentration, and central obesity. Metabolic syndrome has been associated with higher rates of cardiovascular, pulmonary, and renal perioperative events, as well as wound infections.[38]

Tobacco is also associated with the increased probability of developing CAD, although it has not been shown to independently increase perioperative cardiac risk.

Importance of Surgical Procedure

The surgical procedure influences the scope of required preoperative evaluation by suggesting the range of physiologic changes that may occur during the perioperative period. Few data exist defining the surgery-specific incidence of complications. Peripheral procedures are associated with an extremely low incidence of morbidity and mortality,[39] whereas major open vascular procedures are associated with the highest incidence of complications. Eagle et al.[40] published data from the Coronary Artery Surgery Study (CASS) on the incidence of perioperative MI and mortality by procedure for patients with known CAD treated preoperatively either medically or with CABG. Their data found that high-risk procedures included major vascular, abdominal, thoracic, and orthopedic surgery.

Importance of Exercise Tolerance

Exercise tolerance remains one of the most important predictors of perioperative risk for noncardiac surgery, and helps define the need for further testing and invasive monitoring. An excellent exercise tolerance, even in patients with stable angina, suggests that the myocardium can be stressed without failing. Alternatively, if patients experience dyspnea associated with chest pain during minimal exertion, the probability of extensive CAD is high, and is associated with greater perioperative risk. In addition, these patients are at risk for developing hypotension with ischemia and, therefore, may benefit from preoperative coronary intervention therapy, revascularization, or more intensive intraoperative monitoring.[41] Exercise tolerance can be assessed with formal treadmill testing or with a questionnaire that assesses activities of daily living (Table 23-9). Patient-reported poor exercise tolerance (i.e., inability to walk four blocks or climb two flights of stairs) appears to be an independent predictor of serious perioperative complications.[42] The likelihood of a serious adverse event is inversely related to the number of blocks that can be walked. Therefore, there is good evidence to suggest that minimal additional testing is necessary if the patient is able to describe a good exercise tolerance.

Indications for Further Cardiac Testing

Multiple algorithms have been proposed to determine which patients require further cardiovascular testing. As described previously, the risk associated with the proposed surgical procedure influences the decision to perform further diagnostic testing and interventions. With the reduction in perioperative morbidity, it has been suggested that extensive cardiovascular testing is not always necessary.

The algorithm to determine the need for testing in a patient at risk for CAD proposed by the ACC/AHA Task Force was updated in 2014[15] and is based on available evidence and expert opinion that integrates clinical history, surgery-specific risk, and exercise tolerance (Fig. 23-2). In the first step, the clinician evaluates

Table 23-9 Estimated Energy Requirement for Various Activities

1 MET	Daily self-care
	Eat, dress, or use the toilet
	Walk indoors around the house
	Walk a block or two on level ground at 2–3 mph or 3.2–4.8 km/h
	Do light work around the house, like dusting or washing dishes
4 METs	Climb a flight of stairs or walk up a hill
	Walk on level ground at 4 mph or 6.4 km/h
	Run a short distance
	Do heavy work around the house, like scrubbing floors or lifting or moving heavy furniture
	Participate in moderate recreational activities like golf, bowling, dancing, doubles tennis, or throwing a baseball or football
>10 METs	Participate in strenuous sports like swimming, singles tennis, football, basketball, or skiing

MET, metabolic equivalent.
Adapted from the Duke Activity Status Index and American Heart Association Exercise Standards. Reproduced from Eagle K, Brundage B, Chaitman B, et al. Guidelines for perioperative cardiovascular evaluation of the noncardiac surgery. A report of the American Heart Association/American College of Cardiology Task Force on Assessment of Diagnostic and Therapeutic Cardiovascular Procedures. *Circulation*. 1996;93:1278, with permission.

the urgency of the surgery and the appropriateness of a formal preoperative assessment. Next, one determines if the patient has undergone a recent revascularization procedure or coronary evaluation. Those patients with unstable coronary syndromes should be identified and appropriate treatment instituted. Finally, the decision to perform further testing depends on the interaction of the clinical risk factors, surgery-specific risk, and functional capacity. For patients at high risk, both exercise tolerance and the extent of the surgery are taken into account to determine the need for further testing. Most importantly, no preoperative cardiovascular testing should be performed if the results will not change perioperative management.

Electrocardiogram

A preoperative 12-lead ECG can provide important information about the patient's heart rhythm as well as evidence for left ventricular hypertrophy and prior MI. Abnormal Q waves in high-risk patients are highly suggestive of a past MI. It has been estimated that approximately 30% of MIs occur without symptoms ("silent infarctions") and can only be detected on screening ECGs, with the highest incidence occurring in patients with either diabetes or hypertension. The Framingham Study showed that long-term prognosis after MI is not improved by lack of symptoms at the time of MI.[29] The absence of Q waves on the ECG, however, does not exclude the occurrence of a Q-wave MI in the past.[43] Those patients in whom the ECG reverts to normal have improved survival compared to those with consistent abnormalities, with or without Q waves. The presence of Q waves on a preoperative ECG in a high-risk patient, regardless of symptoms, should alert the anesthesiologist to the increased perioperative risk and the potential for active ischemia.

The 2014 ACC/AHA Clinical Practice Guideline recommends a preoperative resting 12-lead ECG only for patients with known CAD or other structural heart disease (except for low-risk surgical procedures) and consideration in asymptomatic patients with clinical risk factors (except for low-risk procedures).[15]

Noninvasive Cardiovascular Testing

The exercise ECG stress test has been the traditional method for evaluating patients with suspected CAD. It represents the most cost-effective and least invasive method for detecting ischemia, with a sensitivity of 70% to 80% and a specificity of 60% to 75% for identifying CAD. A positive exercise stress test alerts the anesthesiologist that the patient is at risk for ischemia associated with increased heart rate, with the greatest risk in those who develop ischemia after only mild exercise. However, as discussed previously, the ability to exercise suggests that no further testing is necessary, and therefore exercise ECG stress testing is infrequently indicated.

Noninvasive pharmacologic stress testing before surgery can be used in high-risk patients who either are unable to exercise or have contraindications to exercise (e.g., claudication). These tests offer value in assessing risk in patients who have poor or indeterminate functional capacity (<4 METs), but should be performed only if their results will change management.[15] Testing options include the dobutamine stress echocardiogram (DSE), in which dobutamine is used to increase myocardial oxygen demand by increasing heart rate and blood pressure. The appearance of either new or more severe regional wall motion abnormalities by ECG with dobutamine represents areas at risk for myocardial ischemia and is considered a positive test. The advantage of a stress ECG is that it is a dynamic assessment of ventricular function. It is generally accepted that those at greatest risk demonstrate regional wall motion abnormalities at low heart rates.

Another noninvasive stress test is dipyridamole/adenosine/regadenoson myocardial perfusion imaging (MPI) with thallium-201 and/or technetium-99m and rubidium-82. Dipyridamole, adenosine, or regadenoson is administered as a coronary vasodilator to assess flow heterogeneity and the presence of a redistribution defect. The 2014 ACC/AHA Clinical Practice Guideline suggests that (1) a normal DSE or MPI supports a high negative predictive value for perioperative MI and/or cardiac death and (2) moderate to large areas of ischemia are associated with increased risk of perioperative MI and/or cardiac death. Findings of a fixed perfusion defect by MPI support a prior MI but offer limited predictive value, although this patient subset is at increased risk for long-term cardiac risk.[15]

The ambulatory ECG (e.g., Holter monitor) provides a means of continuously monitoring the ECG for significant ST segment changes. One study demonstrated that the presence of silent ischemia is a strong predictor of outcome, whereas its absence is associated with a favorable outcome in 99% of the patients studied.[44] Other investigators have demonstrated the value of ambulatory ECG monitoring, although the negative predictive values have not been as high.

Published meta-analyses of preoperative cardiac diagnostic tests have shown good predictive values for ambulatory ECG monitoring, dipyridamole thallium imaging, or DSE.[45,46] The studies demonstrated the superior value of DSE; however, there was significant overlap of the confidence intervals with other tests. The most important determinant with respect to the choice of preoperative testing is the testing expertise of the local institution.

Current recommendations are that patients with active cardiac conditions such as unstable angina, congestive heart failure, significant dysrhythmias, and severe valvular disease should undergo noninvasive stress testing before noncardiac surgery. For

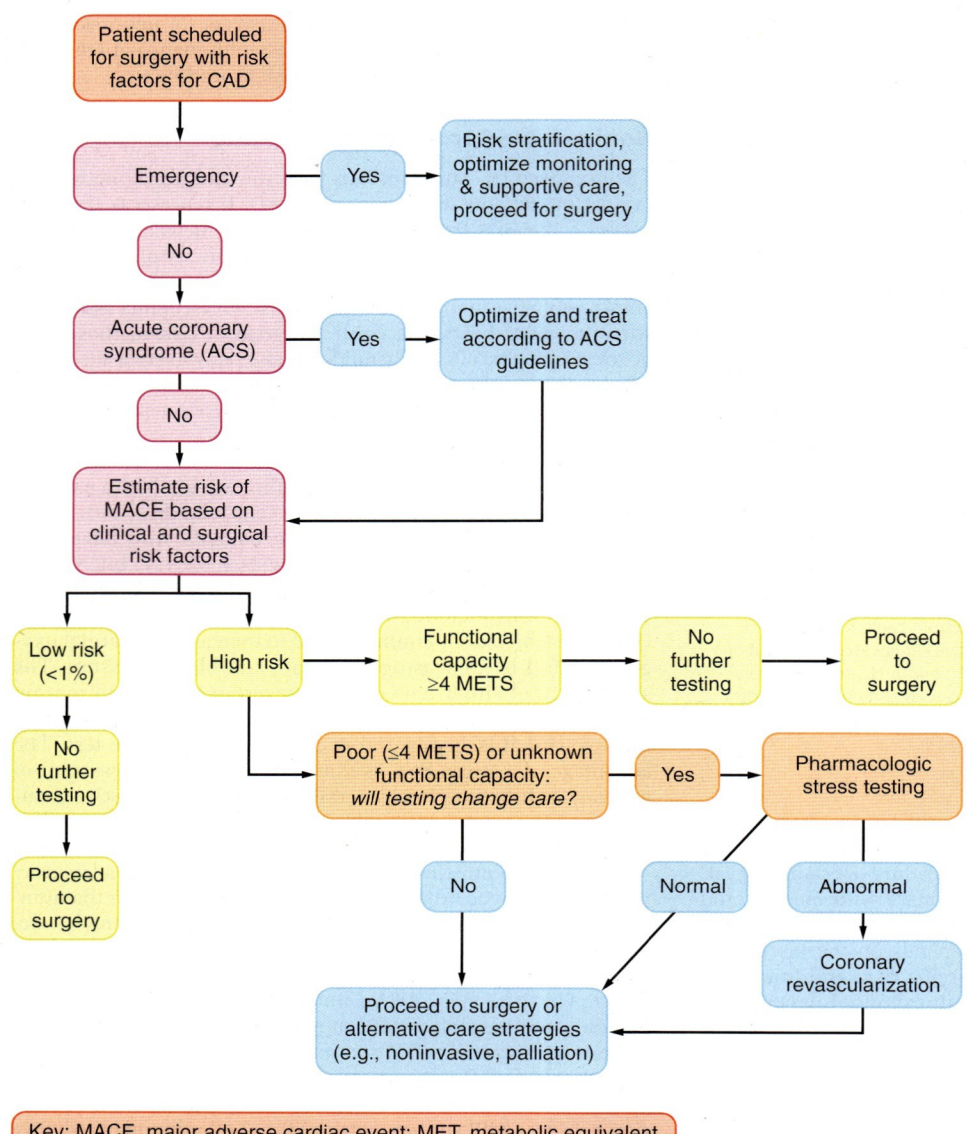

Figure 23-2 Approach to perioperative cardiac assessment for patients with coronary artery disease (CAD). (Modified with permission from Fleisher LA, Fleischmann KE, Auerbach AD, et al. ACC/AHA Guideline on Perioperative Cardiovascular Evaluation and Management of Patients Undergoing Noncardiac Surgery. *Circulation.* 2014;130:e278–e333. http://circ.ahajournals.org.)

patients who require vascular surgery and have multiple clinical risk factors and poor functional capacity, it is reasonable to undergo noninvasive stress testing if it will change management.[15]

Assessment of Ventricular and Valvular Function

Both echocardiography and radionuclide ventriculography can assess cardiac ejection fraction at rest and under stress. Echocardiography is less invasive and able to assess regional wall motion abnormalities, wall thickness, valvular function, and valve area. Pulse-wave Doppler can be used to determine the velocity time integral. Stroke volume can then be calculated by determining the cross-sectional area of the ventricle. Conflicting results exist with regard to the predictive value of the ejection fraction using either echocardiographic or radionuclide measurements. It is reasonable for those with dyspnea of unknown origin and for those with current or prior heart failure with worsening dyspnea or other change in clinical status to have preoperative evaluations of left ventricular function.

Echocardiography has the added advantage of assessing valvular function, which may have important implications for either cardiac or noncardiac surgery. Aortic stenosis has been associated with a poor prognosis in noncardiac surgical patients, and knowledge of valvular lesions may modify perioperative hemodynamic goals and therapy. As noted previously, the 2014 AHA/ACC Guideline for the Management of Patients with Valvular Disease supports the importance of preoperative echocardiography testing for moderate or severe degrees of valvular stenosis or regurgitation with no echocardiography studies within 1 year, or worsening clinical status.[26]

Coronary Angiography

Coronary angiography remains the best method for defining coronary anatomy and also assesses ventricular and valvular function.

Hemodynamic indices can be determined, such as atrial and ventricular pressures, as well as pressure gradients across valves. Although a critical coronary stenosis delineates an area of risk for developing myocardial ischemia, the functional response of that ischemia cannot be assessed by angiography alone. A critical stenosis may or may not be the underlying cause for a perioperative MI that occurs. In the ambulatory population, many infarctions are the result of acute thrombosis of a noncritical stenosis. The 2014 ACC/AHA Clinical Practice Guidelines do not recommend routine preoperative coronary angiography prior to noncardiac surgery without specific clinical indications.[15] Patients with restricted physical activity in whom functional capacity is difficult to determine may benefit from sophisticated imaging techniques, such as cardiac computed tomography (CT).[47] The role of coronary CT angiography with calcium scoring requires further validation as a preoperative assessment for noncardiac surgery.

Perioperative Coronary Interventions

Guidelines to reduce the perioperative risk of noncardiac surgery have recently been reviewed. There are several large studies suggesting that for patients who survive CABG, the risk of subsequent noncardiac surgery is low.[11,16] Although there are little data to support the notion of coronary revascularization solely for the purpose of improving perioperative outcome, it is true that for some patients scheduled for high-risk surgery, long-term survival may be enhanced by revascularization. Two studies used the Coronary Artery Surgery Study database and found that CABG significantly improved survival in those patients with both peripheral vascular disease and triple-vessel coronary disease, especially the group with depressed ventricular function.[48] After reviewing all available data, most clinicians believe the indication for CABG prior to noncardiac surgery remains the same as in other settings and is independent of the proposed noncardiac surgery.

The value of percutaneous transluminal coronary angioplasty is less well established, and current evidence does not support its use beyond established indications for nonoperative patients. In the recent ACC/AHA Clinical Practice Guideline, clinical factors that support percutaneous coronary interventions before noncardiac surgery included high-risk coronary anatomy (e.g., left main disease), unstable angina pectoris, MI, or life-threatening arrhythmias.[15]

Patients with Coronary Artery Stents

Early surgery after coronary stent placement has been associated with adverse cardiac events. A significant incidence of perioperative death and hemorrhage in patients after stent placement has been reported. The 2014 ACC/AHA Clinical Practice Guideline supports the delay of elective noncardiac surgery for 14 days after coronary balloon angioplasty and 30 days after bare metal stent (BMS) placement. The optimal waiting period for elective noncardiac surgery after drug-eluting stents (DESs) is 12 months; however, elective noncardiac surgery may be considered after 6 months based on comparative benefits of surgery compared with risk of stent thrombosis and myocardial ischemia.[15] This difference is because the incidence of stent thrombosis for DESs has been found to be similar to that of BMSs in the early phase after placement but is less well defined over a longer period of time. Dual antiplatelet therapy, for example, aspirin and clopidogrel, is often used after stent placement. A thienopyridine (ticlopidine or clopidogrel) is generally continued with aspirin for 1 month after BMA placement and for 12 months after DES placement (Fig. 23-3). Perioperative management must weigh the risk of bleeding versus stent thrombosis. The decision must

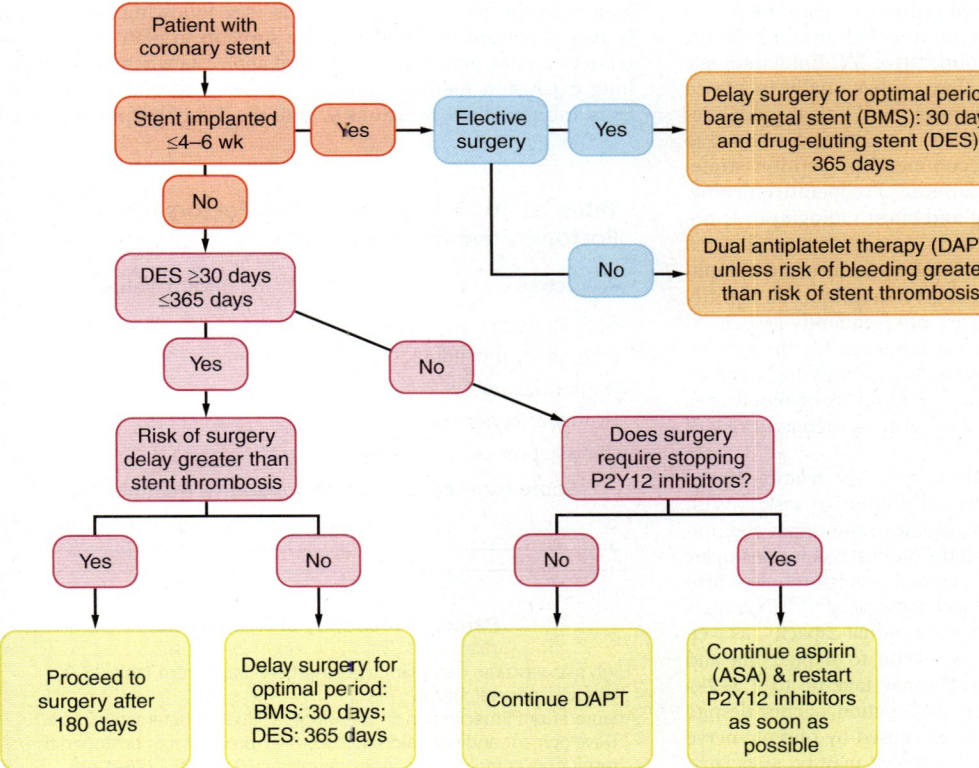

Figure 23-3 Approach to perioperative cardiac assessment for patients with coronary artery stent. P2Y12, Platelet receptor inhibitor (e.g., clopidogrel). (Modified with permission from Fleisher LA, Fleischmann KE, Auerbach AD, et al. ACC/AHA Guideline on perioperative cardiovascular evaluation and management of patients undergoing noncardiac surgery. *Circulation.* 2014;130:e278–e333. http://circ.ahajournals.org.)

involve the anesthesiologist, surgeon, cardiologist, and intensivist. For those patients who have a high risk for stent thrombosis, many advocate that at least aspirin be continued in the perioperative period. Also, the anesthesiologist must weigh the risk of regional versus general anesthesia when these patients are taking antiplatelet therapy. Surgery in patients with recent stent placement should probably only be considered in centers where interventional cardiologists are continuously available.[49,50]

Patients with Cardiovascular Implantable Electronic Devices

With the increasing prevalence of patients treated with pacemakers and implantable defibrillators, preoperative evaluation must address the management of cardiovascular implantable electronic devices (CIEDs) during the perioperative period. The function of these devices can be impaired by electromagnetic interference during surgery. It is important to understand the type of device, its programming, and its underlying clinical need. The cardiologist often needs to be involved in programming the CIED before and after surgery. The Heart Rhythm Society and the ASA have published clinical practice guidelines for perioperative management of patients with implantable defibrillators, pacemakers, and arrhythmia monitors (see Appendix).[51]

Pulmonary Disease

Postoperative pulmonary complications occur more frequently than cardiac complications in patients having major noncardiac surgeries. Perioperative pulmonary complications include atelectasis, pneumonia, exacerbation of chronic obstructive pulmonary disease, pulmonary edema, and respiratory failure requiring mechanical ventilation.[52] Postoperative respiratory failure is a major cause of morbidity and mortality, contributing to increased length of hospital stay and substantial economic cost. The risk of mortality with the development of respiratory failure is substantial and higher than the risk after a perioperative MI. Epidemiologic analyses of large clinical databases have substantially increased the understanding of clinical risk factors.[52,53] Clinical guidelines from the American College of Physicians have been developed to assess the preoperative risk and recommend prevention strategies to limit the risk of respiratory failure.[54] Preoperative testing, such as pulmonary function testing and chest radiograph, is not recommended on a routine basis, as it appears to have limited benefit in predicting perioperative respiratory failure and complication rate. Although a preoperative chest radiograph can identify structural lung abnormalities, these are not frequently associated with significant changes in clinical management for the general population. In contrast, laboratory studies identifying a reduction in serum albumin levels and increased levels of blood urea nitrogen (BUN) appear to be associated with an increased risk of perioperative pulmonary morbidity.[52]

Epidemiologic studies significantly support the relationship of the anatomic location of the surgery and pulmonary risk.[52] With regard to the surgical site, open aortic, thoracic, and upper abdominal surgeries have been associated with the highest risk for postoperative pulmonary morbidity. However, cranial procedures also carry an increased risk, as do vascular and neck surgeries.[52,55,56] Decreases in postoperative vital capacity, functional residual capacity, as well as diaphragmatic dysfunction can contribute to hypoxemia and atelectasis.[57] Functional residual capacity may take up to 2 weeks to return to baseline. Diaphragmatic dysfunction occurs despite adequate analgesia and is theorized to be caused by phrenic nerve dysfunction.[58] Neurosurgery and neck surgery may be associated with perioperative aspiration pneumonia, likely due to an altered sensorium or cranial nerve dysfunction leading to aspiration.

The need for emergency surgery and the need for general anesthesia are also associated with increased risk. Not only can the surgery affect pulmonary function, but general anesthesia also results in mechanical changes, such as a decrease in the functional residual capacity and reduced diaphragmatic function, leading to ventilation/perfusion abnormalities and atelectasis. General anesthesia also induces negative changes at the microscopic level, causing inhibition of mucociliary clearance, increased alveolar–capillary permeability, inhibition of surfactant production, increased nitric oxide synthetase, and increased sensitivity of the pulmonary vasculature to neurohumoral mediators. Subanesthetic levels of intravenous or volatile agents have the ability to blunt the ventilatory response to hypoxemia and hypercarbia as well. Duration of anesthesia is a well-established risk factor for postoperative pulmonary complications, with morbidity rates increasing after 2 to 3 hours.[59] However, when considering laparoscopic surgery, which is often longer in duration, the associated decrease in pulmonary complications compared with an open procedure usually outweighs the risk of increased anesthesia time.[60]

Brueckmann et al.[61] developed a simple scoring system using only preoperative variables to predict the risk of reintubation within the first 3 days after surgery, by examining the electronic records of over 33,000 adult patients who underwent inpatient surgery. The most common independent predictors for reintubation were: ASA Class 3 or greater, emergency surgery, high-risk surgical procedure (vascular, transplant, neurosurgery, thoracic, general, and burn surgery), history of congestive heart failure, and chronic pulmonary disease. A point value of 3, 3, 2, 2, and 1 were assigned to these predictors, respectively. They calculated the probability for reintubation as 0.12% with a score of 0, to 5.9% for scores of 7 to 11 (Table 23-10).

The preoperative evaluation is the time to identify pre-existing pulmonary disease and work with the patient and consultants to maximize the patient's health status (see following sections). It is also important to work with the surgeon to plan specific risk reduction strategies, such as epidural analgesia when appropriate, lung expansion methods, and deep venous thrombosis prophylaxis. Intraoperative measures to limit the risk of hospital-acquired

Table 23-10 Preoperative Risk Factors for Postoperative Reintubation

Predictors	Point Value
ASA score ≥3	3
Emergency procedure	3
[a]High risk surgery	2
History of congestive heart failure	2
Chronic pulmonary disease	1

Score for Prediction of Postoperative Reintubation

Score	0	1	2	3	4	5	6	7	8	9	10	11
Percent Probability of Reintubation	0.1			0.5		1.5			4.2			11.2

[a]High risk: vascular, transplant, neurosurgery graph from Table 23-9, thoracic, general, burns.
Adapted from Brueckmann B, Villa-Uribe JL, Brian T, Bateman BT, et al. Development and validation of a score for prediction of postoperative respiratory complications. *Anesthesiology*. 2013;118:1276–1285.

pneumonia have been proposed, largely focused on reducing the risk of bacterial contamination of the lung during the perioperative period. For high-risk patient groups, studies support preoperative oral antiseptic decontamination before tracheal intubation as well as the role of specialized endotracheal tubes to decrease the risk of nosocomial pneumonia.[62–64]

Tobacco Use

Smoking is an important risk factor, but one that usually is difficult to influence. Even among smokers who have not developed chronic lung disease, smoking is known to increase carboxyhemoglobin levels, decrease ciliary function, and increase sputum production, as well as cause stimulation of the cardiovascular system secondary to nicotine. Although cessation of smoking for 2 days can decrease carboxyhemoglobin levels, abolish the nicotine effects, and improve mucous clearance, prospective studies showed that smoking cessation for at least 4 to 8 weeks was necessary to reduce the rate of postoperative pulmonary complications.[65,66] Studies of nicotine transdermal patches used during the perioperative period have shown increased mortality and are best avoided.[67] Patients who smoke often show increased airway reactivity under general anesthesia; although without proven benefit, it may be useful to administer a bronchodilator, such as albuterol, preoperatively.

Asthma

Asthma is one of the most common coexisting diseases that confront the anesthesiologist. During the patient interview, it is important to elicit information regarding inciting factors, severity, reversibility, and current status. Frequent use of bronchodilators, hospitalizations for asthma, and requirement for systemic steroids are all indicators of more severe disease. After an acute exacerbation of asthma, airway hyperreactivity may persist for several weeks.[68] In addition to bronchodilators, perioperative steroids are worth considering as prophylaxis for the severe asthmatic. The possibility of adrenal insufficiency is also a concern in those patients who have received more than a "burst and taper" of steroids in the previous 6 months. This group of patients should be considered for "stress doses" of steroids perioperatively. Kabalin et al.[69] found there was a low complication rate for asthmatics treated with short-term steroids undergoing surgery. Significantly, they found no association with impaired wound healing or infections. For patients using inhaled steroids, they should be administered regularly, starting at least 48 hours prior to surgery for optimal effectiveness.

Obstructive Sleep Apnea

OSA is a syndrome defined by periodic obstruction of the upper airway during sleep, leading to episodic oxygen desaturation and hypercarbia. This episodic desaturation, in turn, causes episodic arousal, leading to chronic sleep deprivation with daytime hypersomnolence and even behavioral changes in children. Depending on the frequency and severity of events, it may lead to other changes, such as chronic pulmonary hypertension and right heart failure. It is estimated to be present in 26% of US adults between 30 and 70 years of age, and the incidence is climbing in association with the obesity epidemic.[70] Because of their propensity for airway collapse and sleep deprivation, patients with OSA are especially susceptible to the respiratory depressant and airway obstructive effects of sedatives, opioids, and inhaled anesthetics both intraoperatively and postoperatively.

In 2014, the ASA published updated practice guidelines for the perioperative management of patients with OSA.[71] Preoperative identification of those patients at risk is critical to formulate a safe perioperative plan.

Physical characteristics commonly associated with an increased risk of sleep apnea are:
- Obesity—body mass index 35 kg/m^2 or more, or at least 95th percentile in pediatric patients
- Increased neck circumference (men—17 inches, women—16 inches)
- Severe tonsillar hypertrophy
- Nasal obstruction
- Anatomic abnormalities of the upper airway.

Specific questions should be directed toward the patient and family regarding the presence of the following symptoms and signs of OSA:
- Does the patient snore loudly enough to be heard through a door or snore frequently?
- Have you observed pauses in the patient's breathing during sleep?
- Does the patient have frequent arousals from sleep or awakenings with a choking sensation?
- Does the patient experience frequent daytime somnolence and fatigue or fall asleep easily in a nonstimulating environment?
- Does your child appear restless when sleeping or have difficulty with breathing?
- Does your child have night terrors, sleep in unusual positions, or have new-onset enuresis?
- Is your child difficult to arouse at normal awake hours?
- Is your child overly aggressive or does he or she have trouble concentrating?

If a patient has positive signs or symptoms in two or more of the above, then there is a high probability for OSA and the anesthesiologist in conjunction with the surgeon should determine if the patient needs referral for a sleep study. If a sleep study is not warranted or not possible, the patient should be managed as if he or she has OSA.

The risk of perioperative complications in patients with OSA increases with the severity of sleep apnea, the invasiveness of surgery, and the amount of postoperative opioids required.[71]

There is general consensus that preoperative initiation of nasal mask continuous positive airway pressure (CPAP) reduces perioperative risk, perhaps by decreasing the sleep deprivation and secondary hypersomnolence. Importantly, OSA is also associated with difficult airway management, making it even more important to examine previous anesthesia records and to perform a thorough airway examination. Emergency airway equipment should be readily available at the surgical center.

There are multiple management decisions to make in coordination with the surgeon with respect to the OSA patient:
- Determine whether there are noninvasive ways of performing the operation that would decrease the need for opioids postoperatively.
- Discuss whether it is feasible to perform surgery under neuraxial, regional, or local anesthesia, decreasing the total amount of anesthesia or opioids needed.
- Determine whether nonsteroidal anti-inflammatory agents are acceptable for postoperative analgesia.
- Discuss whether outpatient surgery is a safe option.
- Determine whether the patient will be able to use CPAP postoperatively.
- Determine whether postoperative admission to an intensive care unit or monitored unit is required for the patient who is a first-time user of CPAP.

The ASA practice guidelines for OSA recommend hospitalization after uvulopalatoplasty surgery and after tonsillectomy for

OSA in children younger than 3 years. Postoperative hospitalization is also recommended for those OSA patients with other coexisting diseases.

Endocrine Disease

Diabetes Mellitus

Diabetes mellitus is the most common endocrinopathy, and according to the Centers for Disease Control and Prevention (CDC) Americans have an incidence of approximately 9% (almost 26% of those 65 years and older), with the highest rates in Native Americans, followed by Blacks, Hispanics, Asian Americans, then Whites (http://www.cdc.gov/diabetes). The incidence is expected to rise significantly for Americans born after 2000, largely because of the rise in obesity. Critical illness–induced hyperglycemia, defined as a blood glucose above 200 mg/dL in the absence of known diabetes, occurs most frequently in the elderly.[72] Diabetes mellitus has acute and chronic disease manifestations, making it more likely for diabetics to require surgery. The majority of diabetics develop secondary disease in one or more organ systems, which must be identified preoperatively so that an appropriate plan can be developed for perioperative management. Although long-term close control of glucose may limit some of the microvascular effects of diabetes (retinopathy, neuropathy, and nephropathy), macrovascular events such as myocardial ischemia, MI, or stroke may not be decreased. Diabetics have an increased risk of CAD, hypertension, congestive heart failure, and perioperative MI, with the incidence of silent ischemia increased due to associated autonomic neuropathy. The 2014 ACC/AHA Clinical Practice Guideline places diabetics, especially those receiving insulin, at an elevated risk.[15]

Diabetics are also more likely than the general population to have cerebral vascular, peripheral vascular, and renal vascular disease. Diabetes mellitus is the leading cause of renal failure requiring dialysis. Peripheral neuropathies and vascular disease make these patients more susceptible to positioning injuries both during and after surgery. Autonomic neuropathy may predispose the patient to hemodynamic instability during anesthesia and theoretically increase the risk of pulmonary aspiration because of the associated gastroparesis. These deficits should be documented prior to anesthesia and the anesthetic plan adjusted accordingly. Stiff joint syndrome due to glycosylation of proteins and abnormal collagen cross-linking may significantly affect the temporomandibular, atlanto-occipital, and cervical spine joints in patients with longstanding type 1 diabetes, resulting in difficulty with tracheal intubation. A thorough airway examination should be performed prior to anesthesia and a high index of suspicion maintained for a potentially difficult airway. Some suggest using the "prayer sign" as an evaluation tool; patients who are unable to completely oppose their hands (with no space between) should be suspected of also having changes in other joints potentially impacting airway manipulation.

Regimens for perioperative glycemic control vary enormously, not only between type 1 and type 2 diabetics but also within each group. Patients with type 1 diabetes have an absolute insulin deficiency usually due to destruction of pancreatic β cells. These patients must receive insulin to prevent diabetic ketoacidosis. Home glucose management most often relies on some combination of short, intermediate, and long-acting insulin regimens. Insulin pumps are increasingly common and are used to administer a continuous subcutaneous infusion of short-acting insulin, supplemented by boluses dictated by glucose levels, diet, and exercise. Type 2 diabetes accounts for the great majority of diabetics and is defined by variable degrees of insulin deficiency and resistance. Although most commonly associated with obesity, it may also be induced by corticosteroids or pregnancy. Ketoacidosis is uncommon in type 2 diabetics and the stress of severe infection or illness is more likely to provoke a nonketotic hyperosmolar state, which is characterized by severe dehydration, hyperglycemia, and hyperosmolarity. In type 2 diabetics, glucose control is most commonly achieved with diet, exercise, and oral hypoglycemic drugs. These agents primarily work by increasing endogenous insulin release, increasing insulin sensitivity, and/or decreasing hepatic gluconeogenesis. These drugs fall under the main categories of sulfonylureas, biguanides, thiazolidinediones, and meglitinides. If glycemic control is unsuccessful, then insulin is generally added to the regimen.

Ideally, both types 1 and 2 diabetic patients should be evaluated in the preoperative clinic as well as by the patient's endocrinologist 1 to 2 weeks before elective surgery. Questions should address the type, dose, and time of antidiabetic therapy as well as the frequency and manifestations of hypoglycemia and level at which symptoms occur.

In addition to a thorough history and physical examination, a judicious laboratory investigation should include determination of blood glucose, hemoglobin A1c, serum electrolytes, creatinine, and an ECG. If the patient's glycemic control is inadequate based on a hemoglobin A1c above the target range (<7.5% for type 1 diabetics and <7% for type 2 diabetics, as recommended by the American Diabetic Association), abnormal electrolytes, or ketonuria, then elective surgery should be delayed to allow optimization of preoperative glycemic control. Initiation of β-blockers prior to the day of surgery should be considered in diabetic patients with at least two other risk factors for an adverse cardiac event, as there is no evidence of worsened glucose intolerance or masking of hypoglycemic symptoms.[15]

Perioperative Glucose Management

Anesthesia and surgery interrupt the regular meal and insulin administration schedules in patients with diabetes mellitus. Perioperative stress may increase serum glucose concentrations secondary to the release of cortisol and catecholamines. The majority of available literature suggests that better glycemic control may limit morbidity (length of hospital/intensive care unit stay, infection rate, wound healing, outcomes after strokes/MIs) and mortality, particularly in cardiac surgery patients, carotid endarterectomy patients, and the critically ill.[72–75] Although a randomized trial found an increase in the incidence of death and perioperative stroke in cardiac surgery patients where an attempt was made to maintain the glucose between 80 and 100 mg/dL,[76] recent systematic reviews have found a reduction in morbidity and mortality associated with better glycemic control but recognize the increased risk of hypoglycemia.[77] More studies are needed to more closely define the target level for glucose control. There is general consensus that an attempt should be made to control the upper limit of glucose to less than 200 mg/dL, although some will argue that tighter control is warranted. Guidelines for ambulatory and hospitalized patients have been recently published.[78,79] The following recommendations can serve as a general guide:

Guide for Perioperative Glucose Control

- Plan with the surgeon to schedule the surgery as the first case of the day to prevent prolonged fasting.
- As a general rule, oral hypoglycemic agents are held on the day of surgery to avoid reactive hypoglycemia until oral intake is restarted.
- Insulin therapy should balance adequate glucose control with the avoidance of hypoglycemia. Insulin is usually continued through the evening before surgery.

- Schedule the patient to arrive in the early morning and check blood glucose on arrival.
- If patients develop symptoms or measurable hypoglycemia, they should be counseled to take a glucose tablet or clear juice.
- Type 1 diabetics should be continued on basal insulin administration even during preoperative fasting to prevent ketoacidosis. Administer half the usual morning dose of intermediate- or long-acting insulin after arrival to the surgery center, where a maintenance IV can be started. Hold the usual dose of rapid- or short-acting insulin.
- Use the patient's own sliding scale to administer short-acting insulin subcutaneously prior to the scheduled surgery and during short operations.
- Patients on insulin pumps may be managed by continuing the pump for short operations or changing over to an intravenous insulin infusion for longer or major operations.

This strategy, along with blood glucose determinations every 1 to 2 hours, may be all that is necessary for well-controlled diabetics undergoing short, noninvasive outpatient operations. In addition, it is important to prevent postoperative nausea and vomiting and to encourage the early resumption of diet, allowing return to their previous insulin regimen. For type 1 or 2 diabetics undergoing longer or major surgery, insulin is generally administered in the form of an intravenous infusion of regular insulin. Discontinuing the patient's own insulin pump will avoid problems with insulin preparations and pump technology.

There are several methods of administering an insulin infusion, none of which has proved superior. Concurrent separate infusions of insulin and glucose are more easily adjusted and may provide better glycemic control than combined glucose/insulin/potassium infusions. To increase safety, the insulin infusion (which is on a separate pump) is added via a side port to the same line delivering the glucose infusion. A separate nonglucose isotonic solution should be used to replace deficits and intraoperative fluid losses. All protocols rely on the frequent determination of a plasma glucose level at least every 1 to 2 hours to allow titration of insulin.[80-82]

Thyroid and Parathyroid Diseases

Thyroid and parathyroid diseases have clinical manifestations that are important to the preoperative evaluation. Although thyroid function tests are more sensitive, thyroid disease is usually adequately evaluated by clinical history, which should screen for signs and symptoms of hypothyroidism and hyperthyroidism. Hypothyroidism can lead to the development of hypothermia, hypoglycemia, hypoventilation, hyponatremia, and heart failure, as well as a susceptibility to anesthetics. Anesthesiologists should be alert to the possibility of the hypermetabolic state of thyroid storm in patients with hyperthyroidism. A large thyroid mass may distort the upper airway, producing inspiratory stridor or wheezing, especially evident in the supine position. In these cases, a chest x-ray should be obtained looking for evidence of tracheal deviation or narrowing. A CT scan of the upper airway and trachea will provide better detail of any airway compromise. Patients with hyperparathyroidism often have hypercalcemia, and a preoperative determination of a serum calcium level is warranted. Additional clinical manifestations of these conditions are shown in Table 23-11.

Adrenal Disorders

The classic clinical presentation of a patient with pheochromocytoma includes intermittent hypertension, headache, diaphoresis, and tachycardia. Patients with endocrine tumors have a higher incidence of multiple endocrine neoplasia syndrome and pheochromocytoma should be ruled out as the cause of unexplained hypertension. Over time, the mortality for surgical resection of a pheochromocytoma has decreased because of improvements in perioperative therapy for patients with the syndrome. A more important issue is preoperative identification of patients with a possible pheochromocytoma before they are scheduled for other types of surgery.

Adrenal–cortical suppression is a potential disorder in patients presenting for surgery; one should have a high index of suspicion in those patients taking long-term corticosteroids. Cushing syndrome is the most obvious manifestation of long-term high-dose steroid treatment, including moon facies, striations of the skin, truncal obesity, hypertension, easy bruisability, and hypovolemia. Preoperative preparation for patients with adrenal suppression includes correction of any fluid and electrolyte abnormalities, as well as steroid supplementation.

Many anesthesiologists believe that patients taking corticosteroids for long periods within the last 6 months require perioperative steroid supplementation to cover the stresses of anesthesia

Table 23-11 Clinical Manifestations of Thyroid and Parathyroid Diseases

	Hyperthyroidism	Hypothyroidism	Hyperparathyroidism
General	Weight loss; heat intolerance; warm, moist skin	Cold intolerance	Weight loss, polydipsia
Cardiovascular	Tachycardia, atrial fibrillation, congestive heart failure	Bradycardia, congestive heart failure, cardiomegaly, pericardial or pleural effusion	Hypertension, heart block
Neurologic	Nervousness, tremor, hyperactive reflexes	Slow mental function, minimal reflexes	Weakness, lethargy, headache, insomnia, apathy, depression
Musculoskeletal	Muscle weakness, bone resorption	Large tongue, amyloidosis	Bone pains, arthritis, pathologic fractures
Gastrointestinal	Diarrhea	Delayed gastric emptying	Anorexia, nausea, vomiting, constipation, epigastric pain
Hematologic	Anemia, thrombocytopenia		
Renal		Impaired free water clearance	Polyuria, hematuria

Adapted from Roizen MF. Anesthesia for the patient with endocrine disease, part 1. *Curr Rev Clin Anesth*. 1987;6:43.

and surgery, but not patients who have had only a short course of steroids more than 6 months prior. It is impossible to identify the specific duration of therapy or dose of steroids that produces clinically meaningful pituitary and adrenal suppression. Marked variability among patients exists, but one would expect more suppression in patients taking a higher dose for a longer duration. A conservative approach is to consider treatment in any patient who has received corticosteroid therapy for at least 1 month in the past 6 to 12 months and will be undergoing more than minor surgery. The dose and duration of supplemental steroid administration depend on an estimate of the stress of the surgical procedure in the perioperative period. The maximum dose of steroid given for coverage of the stress response is the patient's usual dosage the morning of surgery, followed by 100 mg of IV hydrocortisone before surgery and every 8 hours for the first day, followed by a taper. This dose is meant to approximate the maximum amount of steroid that the adrenal glands could produce during stress in a 24-hour period. Newer recommendations suggest giving 100 mg followed by 50 mg every 8 hours for the first day; for moderate procedures, it is recommended to decrease the hydrocortisone dose by 50%.[83] However, these various recommendations have been questioned and are not supported by studies.[83] The addition of supraphysiologic doses of steroids can increase the risk of acute side effects, such as hyperglycemia, hypertension, fluid retention, and an increased risk of infection. What experts do agree on is that patients should receive their usual daily glucocorticoid dose. Also, exogenous glucocorticoid administration should be considered in any patient who develops perioperative hypotension that is not responsive to standard resuscitative fluid administration or vasopressor therapy, and cannot be explained by other mechanisms, suggesting adrenal insufficiency.

Renal Disease

Renal disease has important implications for fluid and electrolyte management, as well as metabolism of drugs. The cause of renal failure has considerable impact on clinical management. Patients with primary renal disease are likely to be younger and have good cardiopulmonary reserve, whereas a significant percentage of older patients with renal failure secondary to diabetes mellitus or hypertension will also have diffuse atherosclerosis and heart disease. Chronic renal disease secondary to sickle cell anemia, systemic lupus erythematosus, or vasculitis implies multisystem involvement and dysfunction.[84] In those patients with renal failure, the timing of their most recent dialysis will determine whether they are hyper- or hypovolemic and hyper- or hypokalemic. It is important to assess the patient's electrolytes prior to surgery and to ensure they are euvolemic prior to induction of anesthesia. Some patients will require dialysis before surgery. Because renal failure is also associated with anemia and qualitatively deficient platelets, there should be a lower threshold for determining these laboratory results preoperatively.

Liver Disease

Liver disease is associated with decreased plasma protein production, thereby affecting drug binding, volume of distribution, metabolism and clearance. Coagulopathy accompanies liver failure and the etiology can be multifactorial; it can result from malnutrition (poor absorption of nutrients as a consequence of cholestasis), impaired synthesis of coagulation factors, or thrombocytopenia. The history should identify specific risk factors for liver disease, such as previous blood transfusions, illicit drug use, or excessive alcohol intake. The anesthesiologist should inquire about bruising, bleeding, or history of esophageal varices, the latter to potentially avoid esophageal instrumentation. Coagulation disorders may discourage the choice of regional anesthesia. The physical examination should screen for signs of underlying liver disease, such as jaundice, spider nevi, ascites, hepatosplenomegaly, or palmar erythema. Ascites, a more obvious physical finding of liver failure, may significantly affect the patient's respiratory mechanics and make it difficult to lie flat. In patients with chronic liver disease, perioperative risk increases with worsening severity of hepatic dysfunction as assessed by the Model for End-Stage Liver Disease (MELD) score. The MELD assigns the patient a score of 8 to 40 that is derived from a complex formula that incorporates three biochemical variables—the serum total bilirubin concentration, serum creatinine concentration, and international normalized ratio (INR). The MELD score has been prospectively validated as a prognostic marker of mortality in patients with cirrhosis, acute variceal bleeding, or acute alcoholic hepatitis.[85]

Other Diseases

Arthritis is becoming more prevalent in our aging population, worsened by our sedentary lifestyle. Osteoarthritis may result in difficulty positioning the head to facilitate tracheal intubation or difficulty in positioning for regional anesthesia. These are likewise problems in patients with RA; however, of particular importance is the potential for atlantoaxial instability or superior migration of the odontoid causing spinal cord compression. Involvement of the cervical spine in RA patients typically parallels the extent of peripheral disease and may warrant preoperative radiologic screening.[86] Although not as common, RA of the temporomandibular joint may impede mouth opening for tracheal intubation. RA is a multisystem disease, potentially leading to derangements in other organ systems, causing restrictive lung disease, pleural effusions, pericarditis, and anemia.

Finally, the anesthesiologist should inquire about infectious diseases, including questions about foreign travel, that will dictate the need for increased protective measures for OR personnel and equipment.

Preoperative Laboratory Testing

Defining Normal Values

In attempting to determine the optimal choice of preoperative tests, it is important to understand the interpretation of the results. Ideally, tests would either confirm or exclude the presence of a disease; however, most tests only increase or decrease the probability of disease. In determining reference ranges for diagnostic tests, values that fall outside the 95% confidence intervals for normal individuals are considered abnormal. Therefore, up to 5% of normal individuals can have "abnormal" test results. To determine its clinical relevance, a test must be interpreted within the context of the clinical situation. Performing tests in patients with no risk for having the pathophysiologic process of interest can yield a high number of false-positive results. For example, a low potassium value (3.0 mg/dL) in an otherwise healthy individual is most likely a normal result. Interpreting this test as abnormal, and initiating treatment, could lead to harm without any benefit.

Risks and Costs versus Benefits

8 The 2012 ASA Practice Advisory for Preanesthesia Evaluation[1] states that routine preoperative tests do not make an important contribution to preanesthetic evaluation of an asymptomatic patient. Selective preoperative tests should be ordered only after consideration of specific information obtained from the medical record, history and physical, and the type or invasiveness of the planned procedure and anesthesia.

Medical testing is associated with significant cost, both in real dollars and in potential harm. Routine preoperative testing has been estimated to cost billions of dollars annually in the United States. An "abnormal" test that is later determined to be a false result can lead to significant cost and real harm. For example, a positive exercise ECG stress test in a healthy 40-year-old woman may lead to coronary angiography. Coronary angiography is not a benign procedure and can lead to vascular injuries. On the basis of Bayesian analysis, a positive test result in this patient is most likely a false positive and the test was inappropriately used. Therefore, the woman and her physician would gain no additional information, thousands of dollars in medical costs would accrue, and she may sustain morbidity.

Several studies have evaluated the implications of reduced testing. Golub et al.[87] retrospectively reviewed the records of 325 patients who had undergone preadmission testing prior to ambulatory surgery. Of these, 272 (84%) had at least one abnormal screening test result, whereas only 28 surgeries were delayed or canceled. The authors estimated that only three patients potentially benefited from preadmission testing, including a new diagnosis of diabetes in one and nonspecific ECG changes in two, one of whom had known ischemic heart disease.

Narr et al.[88] demonstrated minimal benefits from routine testing and proposed that routine laboratory screening tests were not required in healthy patients. In a follow-up study, a cohort of patients who had no preoperative testing was reviewed and found to include no deaths or major perioperative morbidity.[89] The authors concluded that routine testing was not indicated in this healthy cohort.

Even if testing better defines a disease state, the risks of any intervention based on the results may outweigh the benefit. Cardiovascular testing is a classic example. If a noninvasive test is positive, coronary angiography may be performed. A positive angiogram may then result in CABG prior to the planned noncardiac surgery. Although cardiovascular morbidity and mortality may be reduced in patients with significant CAD who have undergone coronary revascularization, the morbidity associated with both the testing and the revascularization procedure may be greater than any potential benefit. Roizen and Cohn[90] have suggested a protocol for screening tests based on both the preoperative evaluation and proposed procedure using a risk–benefit analysis. The following protocol for laboratory testing is modified from their recommendations and the 2012 ASA Practice Advisory for Preanesthetic Evaluation[1]:

Clinical Considerations for Laboratory Testing

Blood Count
  Extremes of age
  Liver or kidney disease
  Anticoagulant use
  Bleeding/hematologic disorder
  Malignancy
  Type and invasiveness of procedure

Coagulation Studies
  Liver or kidney disease
  Bleeding disorder
  Anticoagulant use
  Chemotherapy

Serum Chemistries (glucose, electrolytes, renal and liver function)
  Liver or renal disease, or perioperative risk of dysfunction
  Diabetes
  Diuretic, digoxin, or steroid use
  Central nervous system disease
  Endocrine disorders
  Elderly
  Malnutrition
  Type and invasiveness of procedure

Chest X-ray
  Pulmonary disease or clinical manifestations
  Unstable cardiovascular disease
  Type and invasiveness of procedure

ECG
  Cardiovascular disease or clinical risk factors
  Pulmonary disease
  Type and invasiveness of procedure

Pregnancy Test
  Possible pregnancy

Complete Blood Count and Hemoglobin Concentration

A preoperative hemoglobin or hematocrit value has been suggested as the only test necessary in many patients prior to elective surgery; however, even this minimal standard has been questioned. Baron et al.[91] reviewed the records of 1,863 pediatric patients scheduled for elective outpatient procedures. In only 1.1% of patients was the hematocrit abnormal, and in none of these patients was the procedure canceled or the anesthetic plan modified. However, a baseline hematocrit is still indicated in any procedure with a risk of significant blood loss.

Both the standard for the lowest acceptable perioperative hematocrit and the indication for a preoperative transfusion have changed during the past decade. The current recommendations of the National Blood Resource Education Committee are that a hemoglobin level of 7 g/dL is acceptable in patients without systemic disease. In patients with systemic disease, signs of inadequate systemic oxygen delivery (tachycardia, tachypnea) are an indication for transfusion.

Coagulation Studies

Coagulation disorders can have a significant impact on the surgical procedure and perioperative management. In patients with hemophilia or von Willebrand disease, abnormal laboratory studies even in the absence of clinical abnormalities require preoperative preparation of the patient. Abnormal coagulation values may delay the surgery depending on the degree of abnormality and the procedure planned. For example, neurosurgery has little tolerance for values outside of the normal range due to the serious consequences if uncontrolled bleeding were to occur perioperatively. Surgery may be delayed for hours if fresh frozen plasma or platelets are needed to acutely correct a coagulopathy, or days if vitamin K is administered for correction.

Pregnancy Testing

Routine pregnancy testing in women of childbearing potential is a subject of considerable debate. The rationale is that surgery may be delayed or specific agents avoided if it is necessary to proceed. Information regarding the last menstrual period can help define the potential, but does not eliminate the possibility. A number of studies have evaluated the validity of history as a means of assessing pregnancy status in adolescents and yielded conflicting results. Current practice varies dramatically and may be a function of the population served.

Chest X-rays

A preoperative chest x-ray can identify abnormalities that may lead to either delay or cancellation of the planned surgical procedure or modification of perioperative care. For example, identification of pneumonia, pulmonary edema, pulmonary nodules, or a mediastinal mass could all lead to modification of care. However, routine testing in the population without risk factors can lead to more harm than benefit. Roizen and Cohn[90] have demonstrated substantial harm from additional procedures based on an abnormal routine preoperative chest x-ray.

The American College of Physicians suggests that a chest x-ray is indicated in the presence of active chest disease or an intrathoracic procedure but not on the basis of advanced age alone.[92] In a meta-analysis, Archer et al.[93] reviewed the published reports from 1966 to 1992 in the English, French, and Spanish literature. On average, abnormalities were reported in 10% of routine preoperative chest x-rays, of which only 1.3% were unexpected. These findings resulted in modification in management in only 0.1% of patients, with unknown influence on outcome. The authors estimated a cost of $23,000 for each finding that influenced management, concluding that routine chest x-rays without a clinical indication were not justified.

Pulmonary Function Tests

Consensus guidelines do not support routine use of pulmonary function studies to predict perioperative respiratory complications. Pulmonary function tests can be divided into two categories: spirometry and arterial blood gas analysis. Spirometry can provide information on forced vital capacity (FVC), forced expiratory volume in 1 second (FEV_1), ratio of FEV_1/FVC, and average forced expiratory flow from 25% to 75% (FEF 25% to 75%). Although each of these measures has a sound physiologic basis, their practical assessment can vary greatly among healthy persons and the tests rarely provide additional information beyond that obtained from history. For those patients considered for pulmonary resection, evaluation using spirometry, diffusion capacity measurements, radionucleotide lung perfusion scanning, and cardiopulmonary exercise testing may help to define those patients at high risk.[94]

With availability of the pulse oximeter, the use of preoperative arterial blood gas sampling has become less important. It may still be indicated in those with poor pulmonary function, since determining the baseline CO_2 is useful in managing perioperative ventilator settings and resting hypercapnia is associated with increased perioperative risk. One method of assessing the probability of CO_2 retention is evaluation of the serum bicarbonate. A normal serum bicarbonate value will virtually exclude the diagnosis of chronic CO_2 retention.

Summary of the Preoperative Evaluation

There are multiple factors that are associated with increased perioperative risk, as discussed within this chapter. Clinical judgment is necessary and requires addressing the following fundamental questions:
1. Are the risk factors modifiable?
2. Will delaying the procedure add to perioperative risk or patient morbidity?
3. What interventions during the preoperative period can be implemented to reduce risk?
4. Has the patient been provided enough information to make an informed decision?

An effective preoperative evaluation will address these concerns and recommend therapeutic interventions to limit risk. Finally, the anesthesiologist can play an important role in reducing inappropriate utilization of medical technology and in helping to coordinate the patient's care among the multiple physician specialties often required for patients with complex illnesses who require surgery.

Preparation

Smoking Cessation

The ASA is encouraging anesthesiologists to use the preoperative evaluation as a teachable moment to encourage patients to stop smoking, with educational resources for providers and patients available on the ASA website. Because patients will be unable to smoke in the hospital, such timing may help give them more incentive to quit. It should be explained to patients that they are at increased risk for pulmonary and cardiac complications as well as impaired wound healing and infection. The longer they are tobacco free before surgery the better, as their bodies will have more time for repair. Even only 12 hours of smoking cessation will reduce levels of nicotine and carbon monoxide, improving blood flow. The long-term benefits of quitting smoking include: addition of 6 to 8 years to their life, reduction in risk of lung cancer and heart disease, savings of at least $1400 per year (not including health-care costs), and reduced exposure of the family to secondhand smoke. Offer patients additional help to quit by referring them to 1-800-QUIT-NOW, a free, confidential counseling service (http://www.asahq.org/resources/clinical-information/asa-stop-smoking-initiative).

Continuing Current Medications/Treatment of Coexisting Diseases

It is the responsibility of the anesthesiologist to instruct patients regarding which medications to take or not take preoperatively. Occasionally, new medications will be prescribed or doses increased, such as steroids for adrenal insufficiency. Prescribed and over-the-counter medications may affect the anesthetic; anesthesiologists must be knowledgeable about their actions. As a general rule, patients may take their prescription medications with water on the day of surgery. Exceptions exist, particularly for the management of diabetes.

β-Blockers

The role of β-blockers during the perioperative period has evolved over time, based on clinical studies evaluating both effectiveness and the potential for risk. Historically, β-blockers in this setting have been felt to reduce the incidence of mortality and nonfatal MIs after surgery. Current guidelines recommend that β-blockers be continued in those receiving β-blockers to treat angina pectoris, symptomatic arrhythmias, and hypertension. Recent clinical studies, however, have questioned the decision to initiate perioperative β-blockers and have suggested that the decision be based on clinical judgment in evaluating the patient's risk factors for cardiovascular complications together with the type of surgery. The POISE trial, a large, multicenter, randomized controlled trial, compared preoperative β-blocker therapy with placebo.[95] Patients receiving β-blocker therapy had a lower risk of perioperative MI, but were at significantly increased risk for mortality and stroke. As potential mechanisms for enhanced risk, perioperative hypotension and bradycardia were significantly increased in patients receiving β-blockers. A meta-analysis evaluating perioperative β-blockade in noncardiac surgery in 33 randomized controlled trials with 12,306 patients found no difference in overall mortality, but decreased risk of perioperative MI.[96] Similar to the POISE trial, the risk of nonfatal stroke was increased with β-blockade. Recognizing the previous referenced studies and others addressing the benefits and risks of perioperative β-blocker therapy, national guidelines from the ACC/AHA have been updated.[97] The guidelines support, as a class I recommendation, the perioperative continuation of β-blockers for patients receiving β-blocker for appropriate conditions. They support the role for β-blocker therapy titrated to heart rate and blood pressure during vascular or intermediate-risk surgeries in patients with CAD, cardiac ischemia identified by preoperative testing, or more than one RCRI risk factor. Importantly, the ACC/AHA guidelines stress uncertainty for the role of β-blockade for vascular or intermediate-risk surgery in patients with only one risk factor without ischemic heart disease or in patients without risk factors who have not taken β-blocker therapy previously. On the basis of the POISE trial, there appears to be increased potential for perioperative risk associated with fixed, high-dose β-blocker therapy begun on the day of surgery. Initiation and titration of β-blockade prior to the day of surgery appears to offer a role in the reduction of risk for perioperative MI, but the optimal heart rate remains controversial.

Statins

There is growing evidence in the literature to suggest that perioperative statin therapy is safe and beneficial in reducing morbidity and mortality in the perioperative period. Statins work via several mechanisms: lowering lipids, enhancing nitric oxide–mediated pathways, reducing expression of cytokines and adhesion molecules, and lowering C-reactive protein levels with associated vasodilatory, anti-inflammatory, and antithrombotic effects. The greatest benefit occurs in patients at higher risk for cardiovascular complications. There is good evidence that the perioperative withdrawal of statins increases morbidity; both the ACC/AHA and the European Society of Cardiology (ESC) have made a class I recommendation that patients who are on a statin preoperatively should be restarted on a statin postoperatively as soon as possible. Patients with noncoronary atherosclerosis should be treated with statin therapy for secondary prevention, independent of noncardiac surgery. The ESC also recommends that statins be started in high-risk surgery patients, optimally between 30 days and at least 1 week before surgery. Guidelines from the ACC/AHA state that statin use is reasonable for patients undergoing vascular surgery with or without clinical risk factors, and statins may be considered for patients with at least one clinical risk factor who are undergoing intermediate-risk procedures.[98]

Prevention of Perioperative Pulmonary Aspiration

Many patients who present for anesthesia are at increased risk for aspiration. Research extrapolated from a study in monkeys led to the statement in 1974 that patients who had a 25 mL residual gastric volume with a pH lower than 2.5 were at risk. Using these guidelines in humans, some have estimated that 40% to 80% of patients scheduled for elective surgery may be at risk.[99,100] However, today, clinically significant pulmonary aspiration is very rare in healthy patients undergoing general anesthesia, quoted as occurring in 1 in 3,000 to 1 in 6,000 anesthetics. This increases to 1 in 600 for emergency anesthesia. Data presented on aspiration from the Australian Anaesthetic Incident Monitoring Study[101] found 133 cases of aspiration in 5,000 incidents reported. They rated the top 10 risk factors as shown in Table 23-12, although almost 25% of the patients had no risk factors. Errors in judgment, fault in airway management technique, and inadequate patient preparation were felt to be the most common factors contributing to the events.

ASA Fasting Guidelines

The ASA published updated Practice Guidelines for Preoperative Fasting and Pharmacologic Intervention for the Prevention of Perioperative Aspiration in 2011.[102] The guidelines specifically address healthy patients of all ages scheduled for elective procedures in which general anesthesia, regional anesthesia, or sedation will be administered. The purpose of the guidelines is not only to minimize the risk of pulmonary aspiration but also to avoid case delays as well as prolonged fasting leading to dehydration, hypoglycemia, and patient dissatisfaction.

Recommendations for Clear Liquids: At Least 2 Hours

The primary support for the task force recommendations comes from a meta-analysis of randomized controlled trials comparing fasting times for clear liquids of 2 to 4 hours versus more than 4 hours. Adult patients fasting for 2 to 4 hours had smaller gastric volumes and higher gastric pH values compared to those fasting more than 4 hours. The differences in gastric volumes were equivocal in children. Therefore, the task force recommendations

Table 23-12 Top 10 Factors Predisposing to Aspiration

1	Emergency surgery
2	Inadequate anesthesia
3	Abdominal pathology
4	Obesity
5	Opioid medication
6	Neurologic deficit
7	Lithotomy
8	Difficult intubation/airway
9	Reflux
10	Hiatal hernia

Adapted from Kluger MT, Short TG. Aspiration during anaesthesia: A review of 133 cases from the Australian Anaesthetic Incident Monitoring Study (AIMS). *Anaesthesia*. 1999;54:19–26.

are unchanged for healthy patients. Examples of clear liquids include, but are not limited to, water, fruit juices without pulp, carbonated beverages, clear tea, and black coffee (no alcohol). The type of liquid was more important than the volume.

Recommendations for Breast Milk: At Least 4 Hours

The fasting recommendations for breast milk are also unchanged, as the task force found only equivocal findings regarding gastric fluid volume and pH from observational studies in infants.[102]

Recommendations for Infant Formula, Nonhuman Milk, and Light Meal: At Least 6 Hours

Again, among the observational and randomized control studies, the task force found no evidence to support any change in the previous recommendations for at least a 6-hour fast before elective procedures.[102] They noted that the amount and type of food must be considered, and recommended at least 8 hours before elective procedures for fried or fatty food that typically delays gastric emptying time.

For a summary of the fasting guidelines, see Table 23-13.

Pharmacologic Agents to Reduce the Risk of Pulmonary Aspiration

Many different kinds of drugs have been used to decrease the volume and increase the pH of gastric fluid in an effort to reduce the risk of aspiration pneumonitis: Histamine-2 receptor antagonists, proton pump inhibitors (PPIs), antacids, antiemetics, and gastrokinetic agents. The ASA task force reviewed the literature and surveyed both experts and ASA members to arrive at their 2011 recommendations for pharmacologic agents. They found that the literature is insufficient to evaluate or support the effect of administering any of these classes of drugs on the perioperative incidence of emesis/reflux or pulmonary aspiration. Therefore, they could not recommend the routine preoperative use of such drugs for patients who have no apparent increased risk for pulmonary aspiration.[102] However, the drugs were found to be effective for their intended use and are more cost-effective when prescribed for patients with risk factors for pulmonary aspiration.

Histamine-2 (H-2) Receptor Antagonists

Meta-analyses of randomized placebo-controlled trials support the efficacy of the H-2 receptor antagonists cimetidine, ranitidine, and famotidine in reducing gastric volume and acidity.[102] They block the ability of histamine to induce secretion of gastric fluid with a high hydrogen ion concentration. Multiple-dose regimens may be more effective in increasing gastric pH than a single dose before operation on the day of surgery.

Cimetidine

Cimetidine is usually administered in 150- to 300-mg doses orally or parenterally. Administration of 300 mg of cimetidine orally 1 to 1.5 hours before surgery has been shown to increase the gastric fluid pH above 2.5 in 80% of patients.[103,104] Cimetidine can cross the placenta, but adverse fetal effects are unproved. The gastric effects of cimetidine last as long as 3 or 4 hours; thus, this drug is suitable for operations of that duration. Side effects of cimetidine include inhibition of the hepatic mixed-function oxidase enzyme system; therefore, it can prolong the half-life of many drugs, including diazepam, chlordiazepoxide, theophylline, propranolol, and lidocaine. The clinical significance of this after one or two preoperative doses of cimetidine is uncertain. Life-threatening cardiac dysrhythmias, hypotension, cardiac arrest, and central nervous system depression have been reported after cimetidine administration. These side effects may be especially likely to occur in critically ill patients after rapid intravenous administration. Cimetidine does not affect gastric fluid already present.

Ranitidine

Ranitidine is more potent, specific, and longer acting than cimetidine. The usual oral dose of 150 mg or 50 mg given parenterally will decrease gastric fluid pH within 1 hour. It is as effective in reducing the number of patients at risk for gastric aspiration as cimetidine and produces fewer cardiovascular or central nervous system side effects. The effects of ranitidine last up to 9 hours. Thus, it may be superior to cimetidine at the conclusion of lengthy procedures in reducing the risk of aspiration pneumonitis during emergence from anesthesia and extubation of the trachea.

Famotidine

Famotidine is another H-2 receptor blocker that is given preoperatively to raise gastric fluid pH. The pharmacokinetics are similar to those of cimetidine and ranitidine, with the exception of having a longer serum elimination half-life than the other two drugs. Famotidine in a dose of 40 mg orally 1.5 to 3 hours preoperatively has been shown to be effective in increasing gastric pH.

Proton Pump Inhibitors

PPIs suppress gastric acid secretion in a dose-dependent manner by binding to the proton pump of the parietal cell. Randomized controlled trials support their efficacy in reducing gastric volume and acidity.[102,105] For an adult patient, administering 40 mg of omeprazole intravenously 30 minutes before induction has been used. Oral doses of 40 mg to 80 mg must be given 2 to 4 hours before surgery to be effective. Effect on gastric pH may last as long as 24 hours.

Antacids

Antacids are used to neutralize the acid in gastric contents. Randomized controlled trials demonstrate their effectiveness.[102] A single dose of antacid given 15 to 30 minutes before induction

---

Table 23-13 Summary of Fasting Recommendations for All Ages to Reduce the Risk of Pulmonary Aspiration

Ingested Material	Minimum Fasting Period in hours
Clear liquids	2 h
Breast milk	4 h
Infant formula	6 h
Nonhuman milk	6 h
Light meal	6 h

This summary applies only to healthy patients who are undergoing elective procedures and is not intended for women in labor. Following the guidelines does not guarantee complete gastric emptying. Examples of clear liquids are water, fruit juices without pulp, carbonated beverages, clear tea, and black coffee.

Adapted from Practice guidelines for preoperative fasting and the use of pharmacologic agents to reduce the risk of pulmonary aspiration: Application to healthy patients undergoing elective procedures: An updated report by the American Society of Anesthesiologists Committee on Standards and Practice Parameters. *Anesthesiology.* 2011;114:495–511.

of anesthesia is almost 100% effective in increasing gastric fluid pH above 2.5. The nonparticulate antacid, 0.3 M sodium citrate, is commonly given before emergency operations. The nonparticulate antacids do not produce pulmonary damage themselves if aspiration should occur. Although colloid antacid suspensions may be more effective in increasing gastric fluid pH, aspiration of particulate antacids may cause significant and persistent pulmonary damage.

Withholding antacids because of concern about increasing gastric volume is not warranted, considering animal evidence documenting markedly increased mortality after aspiration of low volumes of acidic gastric fluid (0.3 mL/kg, pH 1) compared with aspiration of large volumes of buffered gastric fluid (1 to 2 mL/kg, pH > 1.8).[106] Complete mixing of the antacid with all gastric contents may be questionable in the immobile patient, and the effect of antacids on food particles within the stomach is unknown.

Gastrokinetic Agents: Metoclopramide

Metoclopramide is a dopamine antagonist that stimulates upper gastrointestinal motility, increases gastroesophageal sphincter tone, and relaxes the pylorus and duodenum to reduce gastric volume. A meta-analysis of randomized placebo-controlled trials supports the efficacy of metoclopramide to reduce gastric volume, but is equivocal regarding its effect on gastric acidity during the perioperative period.[102] It also has antiemetic properties. It may be administered orally or parenterally. A parenteral dose of 5 mg to 10 mg is usually given 30 minutes before induction. Administration intravenously over 3 to 5 minutes usually prevents the abdominal cramping that can occur from more rapid administration. An oral dose of 10 mg achieves onset within 30 to 60 minutes. The elimination half-life of metoclopramide is approximately 2 to 4 hours.

The clinical usefulness of the gastrokinetic agents is found in those patients who are likely to have large gastric fluid volumes, such as parturients, patients scheduled for emergency surgery, obese patients, trauma patients, and those with gastroparesis secondary to diabetes mellitus. However, it is not recommended for those patients diagnosed with bowel obstruction. The combination of metoclopramide with an H-2 receptor antagonist does not decrease the effect of either drug, and the effects may be additive.[102]

As reviewed earlier, the drugs used to decrease gastric fluid volume and acidity are effective and relatively free of side effects. The use of these agents is warranted in patients with decreased gastric emptying, reflux, and those presenting for emergency procedures. However, none of the drugs or combination of drugs is absolutely reliable in preventing the risk of aspiration in all patients all of the time. Therefore, their use does not eliminate the need for careful anesthetic techniques to protect the airway during induction, maintenance, and emergence from anesthesia.

Psychological Preparation/ Premedication

Anesthetic management for patients begins with preoperative psychological preparation and, if necessary, preoperative medication. The anesthesiologist should assess the patient's mental and physical condition during the preoperative visit. Because it is actually the beginning of the anesthetic, the decision to administer preoperative medication, and which one, should be based on the same considerations as the choice of anesthesia, including considerations of the patient's medical problems, requirements of the surgery, and recovery goals. Satisfactory preparation lessens the patient's (and family's) anxiety and smooths the anesthetic induction. No consensus exists on the choice of preoperative medications and, historically, their use was dominated by tradition. However, the ever-increasing number of outpatient procedures has led to a significant decrease in preoperative sedation.

Psychological Preparation

Psychological preparation of the patient involves a preoperative visit and interview with the patient and family members. The anesthesiologist should explain anticipated events and the proposed anesthetic management in an effort to reduce anxiety. Patients may perceive the day of surgery as the biggest, most threatening day in their lives; they do not wish to be treated impersonally in the OR. A growing number of patients receive their preanesthetic evaluations by others in preoperative evaluation clinics, such that their initial encounter with the anesthesiologist may be in the immediate preoperative period outside of the OR. Preoperative visits must be conducted efficiently, but they must also be informative and reassuring. Most of the anesthesiologist's time is spent with an unconscious or sedated patient; therefore, he or she must take time before the operation to earn the trust and confidence of that patient.

Studies show that, depending on the intensity of inquiry, 40% to 85% of patients are apprehensive before surgery. Most patients expect apprehension to be relieved before they arrive in the OR. An informative and comforting preoperative visit may replace many milligrams of a sedative medication. For example, the study by Egbert et al.[107] showed that more patients were adequately prepared for surgery after a preoperative interview than after 2 mg/kg of pentobarbital given intramuscularly 1 hour before surgery (Table 23-14). However, psychological preparation alone may not relieve all anxiety.

After the patient interview, the use of preoperative medication in selected patients serves to achieve sedation or amnesia as well as provide any needed analgesia. However, preoperative depressant drugs are not a substitute for a comforting and tactful preoperative visit.

Premedication

The ideal drug or combination of drugs for preoperative pharmacologic preparation is as elusive as is the ideal anesthetic

Table 23-14 Comparison of Preoperative Visit to Pentobarbital Premedication (% of patients)

	Felt Drowsy	Felt Nervous	Adequate Preparation
Control group	18	58	35
Pentobarbital group	30	61	48
Preoperative visit	26	40	65
Preoperative visit and pentobarbital	38	38	71

IM, intramuscularly.
Data from Egbert LD, Battit GE, Turndorf H, et al. The value of the preoperative visit by the anesthetist. *JAMA*. 1963;185:553–555.

technique and is not based on comprehensive or definitive data. In selecting the appropriate drug and dose for preoperative medication, the patient's psychological condition, physical status, age, and prior response to depressant drugs must be considered. Some patients should not receive depressant drugs before surgery. For example, those with little physiologic reserve, head injury, hypovolemia, or at the extremes of age may be harmed more than helped. Finally, the surgical procedure, expected duration, and postoperative discharge plan are important factors as well.

The goals to be achieved for each patient with preoperative medication should be tailored to the individual. Some goals, such as relief of anxiety, apply to almost every patient, whereas a goal to dry airway secretions may be reserved for the patient with a potentially difficult airway who may require fiberoptic tracheal intubation.

The timing and route of administration of the preoperative medications are important. Every attempt should be made to time the administration so that the premedication achieves its full effect before the patient's arrival in the OR. As a general rule, oral tablets should be given to the patient 60 minutes before arrival in the OR. Intravenous agents, on the other hand, produce effects after a few circulation times. The drug(s), doses, route of administration, and effects should be recorded on the anesthetic record. A list of common preoperative medications is presented in Table 23-15.

Benzodiazepines

Benzodiazepines are among the most popular preoperative medications because they produce anxiolysis, amnesia, and sedation (Table 23-16). Because the site of action of benzodiazepines is located on the GABA receptor in the central nervous system, there is relatively little depression of the ventilatory or cardiovascular systems with premedicant doses. Benzodiazepines have a wide therapeutic index and a low incidence of toxicity. Other than central nervous system depression, these drugs lack the side effects common to opioids, such as nausea and vomiting. Two caveats to keep in mind: these drugs are not analgesic agents, and benzodiazepines may not always produce a calming effect, but

Table 23-15 Common Preoperative Medications, Doses, and Administration Routes

Medication	Administration Route	Dose
Lorazepam	Oral, IV	0.5–4 mg
Midazolam	IV	1.0–2.5 mg doses
Fentanyl	IV	25–50 µg doses
Morphine	IV	1.0–2.5 mg doses
Meperidine	IV	10–25 mg doses
Cimetidine	Oral, IV	150–300 mg
Ranitidine	Oral	50–200 mg
Metoclopramide	IV	5–10 mg
Atropine	IV	0.2–0.4 mg
Glycopyrrolate	IV	0.1–0.2 mg

IV, Intravenous.
Modified from Stoelting RK, Miller RD, eds. *Basics of Anesthesia*. New York: Churchill Livingstone; 1984.

Table 23-16 Comparison of Pharmacologic Variables of Benzodiazepines

	Diazepam	Lorazepam	Midazolam
Dose equivalent (mg)	10	1–2	3–5
Time to peak effect after oral dose (h)	1–1.5	2–4	0.5–1
Elimination half-time (h)	20–40	10–20	1–4
Clearance (mL/kg/min)	0.2–0.5	0.7–1.0	6.4–11.1
Volume of distribution (L/kg)	0.7–1.7	0.8–1.3	1.1–1.7

Adapted from Reves JG, Fragen RJ, Vinick HR, et al. Midazolam: Pharmacology and uses. *Anesthesiology*. 1985;62:310–324; and Stoelting RK. *Pharmacology and Physiology in Anesthetic Practice*. Philadelphia, PA: JB Lippincott; 1987.

rarely can cause a paradoxical agitation, manifested as restlessness and delirium.

Midazolam

Midazolam has predominantly replaced lorazepam and diazepam for preoperative medication and moderate sedation (Fig. 23-4). It is common to administer sedative doses intravenously just prior to transfer to the OR. The physicochemical properties of the drug allow for its water solubility and rapid metabolism. As with other benzodiazepines, midazolam produces anxiolysis, sedation, and amnesia. It is 2 to 3 times more potent than diazepam because of its increased affinity for the GABA receptor. The usual incremental dose is 1 mg to 2 mg titrated intravenously. There is no irritation or phlebitis with injection of midazolam, as opposed to diazepam. The incidence of side effects after administration is low, although depression of ventilation and sedation may be greater than expected, especially in elderly patients or when the drug is combined with other central nervous system depressants. The onset after intravenous administration typically occurs after 1 to 2 minutes. In addition to quicker onset, more rapid recovery occurs after midazolam compared with diazepam. This more rapid onset and recovery is the result of the lipid solubility of midazolam and its rapid redistribution to the peripheral tissues and metabolic biotransformation. For these reasons, midazolam should usually be given within 1 hour of induction. Midazolam is metabolized by hepatic microsomal enzymes to essentially inactive hydroxylated metabolites. H-2 receptor antagonists do not interfere with its metabolism. The elimination half-life of midazolam is approximately 1 to 4 hours and may be extended in the elderly. Tests show that mental function usually returns to normal within 4 hours of administration, and amnesia may only last 20 to 30 minutes.[108] These properties make midazolam ideal for shorter procedures.

Lorazepam and Diazepam

Lorazepam is 5 to 10 times more potent than diazepam and can produce profound amnesia, anxiolysis, and sedation (Fig. 23-5).[109] Like diazepam, it has an extremely long half-life, but an even longer duration because of its affinity for the receptor.[110] Because of their duration, lorazepam and diazepam are not

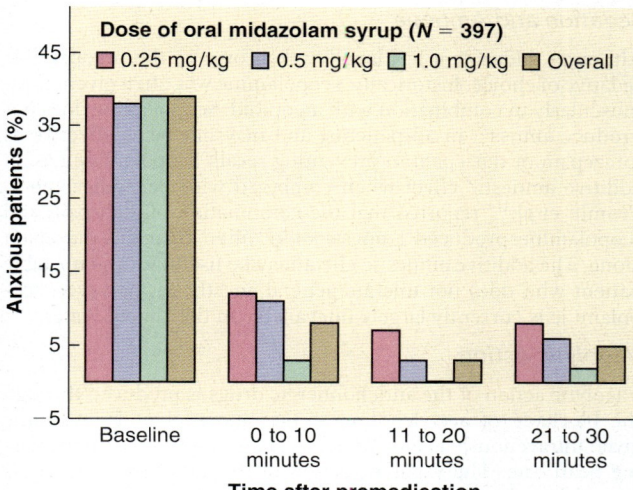

Figure 23-4 Percentage of patients exhibiting anxiety from baseline to time after oral midazolam. There was a positive association between dose and onset of anxiolysis ($p = 0.01$); a larger proportion of children achieved satisfactory anxiolysis within 10 minutes at the higher doses. (Reprinted with permission from Coté CJ, Cohen IT, Suresh S, et al. A comparison of three doses of a commercially prepared oral midazolam syrup in children. *Anesth Analg*. 2002;94:37.)

useful in instances in which rapid awakening is necessary, such as outpatient anesthesia. Their use may be more suited for those patients already taking chronic benzodiazepines for anxiety and who may need the anxiolysis prior to arrival in the preoperative area.

Although lorazepam is insoluble in water and requires a solvent such as polyethylene glycol or propylene glycol, intravenous administration is not associated with pain on injection or phlebitis. In addition to the intravenous route, lorazepam is reliably absorbed orally. Bradshaw et al.[111] demonstrated clinical effects 30 to 60 minutes after oral administration of lorazepam. Peak plasma concentrations may not occur until 2 to 4 hours after oral administration. Therefore, oral lorazepam must be given well before surgery so that the drug has time to be effective. Lorazepam also may be given sublingually at a dose of 25 to 50 µg/kg, not to exceed 4 mg.[109,110] With recommended doses, anterograde amnesia may be produced for as long as 4 to 6 hours without excessive sedation. Higher doses lead to prolonged and excessive sedation without more amnesia. There are no active metabolites of lorazepam and because its metabolism is not dependent on microsomal enzymes, there is less influence from age or liver disease. As with diazepam, little cardiorespiratory depression occurs with lorazepam.

Diphenhydramine

Diphenhydramine is a histamine-1 receptor antagonist, which blocks the peripheral effects of histamine. It also has sedative, anticholinergic, and antiemetic activity. A dose of 50 mg will last 3 to 6 hours in an adult. Diphenhydramine is not often used for preoperative sedation, but it is often used in combination with histamine-2 blockers and steroids for prophylaxis in patients with latex allergy as well as for prophylaxis before chemotherapy and radiologic studies using contrast.

Opioids

Morphine and meperidine were historically the most frequently used opioids for intramuscular preoperative medication during a time when the majority of patients were admitted the night before surgery. Currently, when analgesia is needed preoperatively, the administration of intravenous fentanyl, with its rapid onset and shorter duration, has become much more common. In a patient not experiencing pain, opioids may produce dysphoria. The opioids given in premedicant doses do not produce sedation or amnesia and are often combined with a benzodiazepine for these effects. Opioids are also useful to ameliorate the discomfort during regional anesthesia procedures or during the insertion of invasive monitoring catheters or large intravenous lines. The analgesic properties and respiratory depressant effects of opioids usually go hand in hand. The decrease in the CO_2 drive at the medullary respiratory center may be prolonged. Furthermore, there is a decrease in the responsiveness to hypoxia at the carotid body after injection of even low doses of opioids.[112] The anesthesiologist may consider supplemental oxygen for the patient receiving opioid premedication. A common side effect of all opioids is nausea and vomiting, due to effects on both the chemoreceptor trigger zone and the vestibular system.

Fentanyl is a synthetic opioid agonist structurally similar to meperidine. It is approximately 100 times more potent than morphine in its analgesia. The lipid solubility of fentanyl is greater than that of morphine, which contributes to its rapid onset of

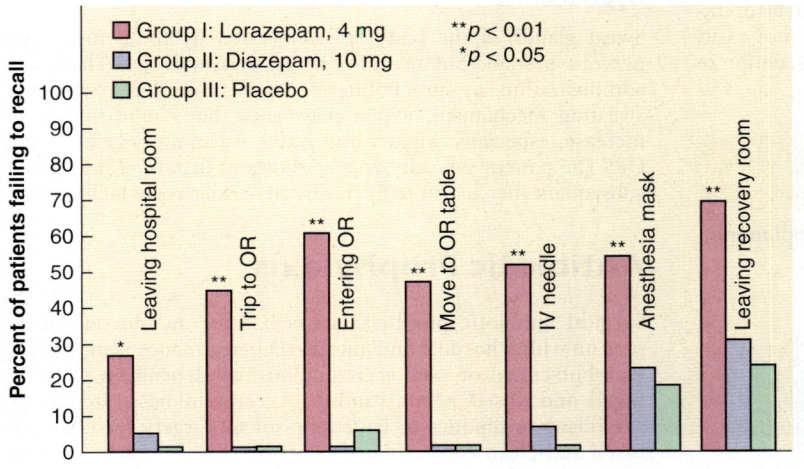

Figure 23-5 Percentage of patients in each group failing to recall specific events of the operative day. Medications were administered intramuscularly. OR, operating room; IV, intravenous. (Reprinted with permission from Fragen RJ, Caldwell N. Lorazepam premedication: Lack of recall and relief of anxiety. *Anesth Analg*. 1976;55:792.)

action. Peak plasma concentrations occur within 6 to 7 minutes following intravenous administration and its elimination half-time is 3 to 6 hours. The drug's much shorter duration of action is attributed to redistribution to inactive tissues, such as the lungs, fat, and skeletal muscle. Metabolism occurs primarily by N-demethylation to norfentanyl, which is a less potent analgesic. In doses of 1 to 2 μg/kg intravenously, fentanyl may be used to provide preoperative analgesia. Fentanyl causes neither myocardial depression nor histamine release, but may be associated with ventilatory depression and profound bradycardia. Elderly and debilitated patients can have an increased sensitivity to its effects. Synergistic effects with benzodiazepines warrant close observation when this combination is given in the preoperative period.

Opioid-dependent Patients

Withdrawal symptoms produced by drug cessation preoperatively are an issue for the patient who is opioid dependent. There should be an attempt to maintain opioid use at the usual level by continuing methadone or substituting other appropriate agents for methadone. The anesthesiologist should be cautioned about using agonist–antagonist drugs in these patients for fear of producing withdrawal.

Anticholinergics

Historically, anticholinergic drugs were widely used when inhalation anesthetics produced copious respiratory tract secretions and intraoperative bradycardia was a frequent danger. The advent of newer inhalation agents has markedly decreased the routine use of anticholinergic drugs for preoperative medication. Specific indications for an anticholinergic before surgery are (1) antisialogogue effect, (2) sedation and amnesia, and (3) vagolytic effect (Table 23-17). In the past, anticholinergics were also administered in an attempt to decrease gastric acid secretion, but research has shown them not to be effective for this purpose.[102]

Antisialagogue Effect

Anticholinergics have been prescribed in a selective fashion when drying of the upper airway is desirable. For example, when awake fiberoptic tracheal intubation or bronchoscopic examination is planned, conditions will be more satisfactory for visualization when an anticholinergic drug has been administered.[113] Anticholinergics are also felt to increase the effectiveness of topical anesthesia in the airway by preventing a dilutional effect from secretions and facilitating contact of the local anesthetic with the mucosa. Surgeons may also request an antisialagogue for intraoral operations. Glycopyrrolate is the most potent antisialagogue, with less likelihood of increasing heart rate than atropine. Because glycopyrrolate is a quaternary amine, it does not easily cross the blood–brain barrier and does not produce sedation or amnesia as seen with scopolamine, a tertiary amine.

Sedation and Amnesia

Although midazolam has largely taken over as the preoperative sedative of choice, historically, scopolamine was often given intramuscularly in combination with an opioid. Scopolamine does not produce amnesia in all patients, and may not be as effective as lorazepam or diazepam in preventing recall. Scopolamine has an additive amnestic effect when combined with benzodiazepines. Frumin et al.[114] reported that the combination of diazepam and scopolamine produced amnesia more often than did diazepam alone. The additive amnestic effect may be useful for the unstable patient who does not tolerate general anesthesia; however, scopolamine is currently largely unavailable in the United States.

Vagolytic Action

Vagolytic action of the anticholinergic drugs is produced through the blockade of acetylcholine at the sinoatrial node. Atropine given intravenously is more potent than glycopyrrolate in increasing heart rate. The vagolytic action of the anticholinergic drugs is useful in the prevention of reflex bradycardia that may result from traction on extraocular muscles or abdominal viscera, carotid sinus stimulation, or repeated doses of succinylcholine. As these bradycardic events occur intraoperatively, it is more effective to administer the drug during anesthesia.

Side Effects of Anticholinergic Drugs

Central Nervous System Toxicity

Scopolamine and atropine (tertiary amines) may cause central nervous system toxicity, the so-called central anticholinergic syndrome. This syndrome is most likely to occur after the administration of scopolamine, but can be seen after high doses of atropine and may include symptoms such as delirium, restlessness, confusion, and obtundation. Elderly patients and patients with pain appear to be particularly susceptible; the syndrome has been noted to be potentiated by inhalation anesthetics. The administration of 1 to 2 mg of physostigmine intravenously can successfully treat the syndrome.

Intraocular Pressure

Mydriasis and cycloplegia from anticholinergic drugs may place patients with glaucoma at risk for increased intraocular pressure. Atropine and glycopyrrolate may be less likely to increase intraocular pressure than scopolamine. In patients with glaucoma, it is generally safe to continue most glaucoma medications up until the time of surgery or use atropine or glycopyrrolate when necessary.

Hyperthermia

Sweat glands of the body are innervated by the sympathetic nervous system, but use cholinergic transmission. Therefore, administration of anticholinergic agents interferes with the sweating mechanism, which may cause body temperature to increase, especially when using active warming devices in the OR. The patient typically appears hot and dry. In children, the subsequent increase in temperature may exacerbate tachycardia.

Antibiotic Prophylaxis

Surgical antibiotic prophylaxis has become an outcome measure on which hospital and anesthesia performance is measured. Reimbursement or even accreditation may depend on properly timed and dosed administration. Anesthesiologists frequently administer antibiotics to patients prior to surgery for contaminated and clean-contaminated procedures or for clean surgical

Table 23-17 Comparison of Effects of Three Anticholinergic Drugs

	Atropine	Glycopyrrolate	Scopolamine
Increased heart rate	+++	++	+
Antisialagogue	+	++	+
Sedation	+	0	+++

0, no effect; +, small effect; ++, moderate effect; +++, large effect.
Adapted from Stoelting RK. *Pharmacology and Physiology in Anesthetic Practice*. Philadelphia, PA: JB Lippincott; 1991.

procedures when infection would be catastrophic, such as for device implants. Other indications for the use of prophylactic antibiotics include the prevention of endocarditis and the prevention of infection in immunocompromised patients.

Cephalosporins are the most popular antibiotics because they cover common skin microbes. For intestinal surgery, however, anaerobic and Gram-negative coverage is needed. The National Surgical Infection Project recommends that antibiotics be administered within 1 hour prior to incision.[115] There are two exceptions to this policy: (1) vancomycin should be given 2 hours prior to incision and (2) when a tourniquet is used, the antibiotics should be administered prior to its inflation. Furthermore, if the surgical procedure is prolonged, it is recommended that the antibiotic be redosed when two half-lives have elapsed. For example, cefazolin has a half-life of 2 hours; therefore, it should be redosed if the surgical procedure extends past 4 hours. Research on morbidly obese patients has shown that the dose required to achieve adequate tissue levels is twice that for normal-weight patients.[116] Those allergic to penicillin, cephalosporins, and related compounds (β-lactam allergy) may receive either vancomycin or clindamycin.

Summary of Patient Preparation

The anesthesiologist who takes the time to adequately prepare the patient medically and psychologically for anesthesia and surgery will find that his/her job of caring for the patient intraoperatively becomes easier, and is more likely to have both a positive clinical outcome and a satisfied patient.

REFERENCES

1. ASA Inc., Apfelbaum JL, Connis RT, Nickinovich DG. Practice advisory for preanesthesia evaluation: An updated report by the American Society of Anesthesiologists Task Force on Preanesthesia Evaluation. *Anesthesiology*. 2012;116(3):522–538. https://www.asahq.org/quality-and-practice-management/standards-and-guidelines.
2. Kash B, Cline K, Menser T, et al. *The Perioperative Surgical Home, A Comprehensive Literature Review for the American Society of Anesthesiologists*. 2014. https://www.asahq.org/psh.
3. Takata MN, Benumof JL, Mazzei WJ. The preoperative evaluation form: Assessment of quality from one hundred thirty-eight institutions and recommendations for a high-quality form. *J Clin Anes*. 2001;13:345–352.
4. Apfel CC, Läärä E, Koivuranta M, et al. A simplified risk score for predicting postoperative nausea and vomiting. *Anesthesiology*. 1999;91:693–700.
5. Apfel CC, Korttila K, Abdalla M, et al. A factorial trial of six interventions for the prevention of postoperative nausea and vomiting. *N Engl J Med*. 2004;350:2441–2451.
6. Gan TJ, Diemunsch P, Habib AS, et al. Consensus guidelines for the management of postoperative nausea and vomiting. *Anesth Analg*. 2014;118:85–113.
7. Eberhart LH, Geldner G, Kranke P, et al. The development and validation of a risk score to predict the probability of postoperative vomiting in pediatric patients. *Anesth Analg*. 2004;99:1630–1637.
8. Mallampati RS, Gatt SP, Gugino LD, et al. A clinical sign to predict difficult tracheal intubation: A prospective study. *Can Anaesth Soc J*. 1985;32:429–434.
9. Frerk CM. Predicting difficult intubation. *Anaesthesia*. 1991;46:1005–1008.
10. Savva D. Prediction of difficult tracheal intubation. *Br J Anaesth*. 1994;73:149–153.
11. Shah KB, Kleinman BS, Rao T, et al. Angina and other risk factors in patients with cardiac diseases undergoing noncardiac operations. *Anesth Analg*. 1990;70:240–247.
12. Wilson W, Taubert KA, Gewitz M, et al. Prevention of infective endocarditis: Guidelines from the American Heart Association: A Guideline from the American Heart Association Rheumatic Fever, Endocarditis, and Kawasaki Disease Committee, Council on Cardiovascular Disease in the Young, and the Council on Clinical Cardiology, Council on Cardiovascular Surgery and Anesthesia, and the Quality of Care and Outcomes Research Interdisciplinary Working Group. *Circulation*. 2007;116(15):1736–1754.
13. Bedford R, Feinstein B. Hospital admission blood pressure, a predictor for hypertension following endotracheal intubation. *Anesth Analg*. 1980;59:367–370.
14. Livhits M, Ko CY, Leonardi MJ, et al. Risk of surgery following recent myocardial infarction. *Ann Surg*. 2011;253:857–364.
15. Fleisher LA, Fleischmann KE, Auerbach AD, et al. ACC/AHA Guideline on perioperative cardiovascular evaluation and management of patients undergoing noncardiac surgery. *Circulation*. 2014;130:e278–e333. http://circ.ahajournals.org.
16. Lee TH, Marcantonio ER, Mangione CM, et al. Derivation and prospective validation of a simple index for prediction of cardiac risk of major noncardiac surgery. *Circulation*. 1999;100:1043–1049.
17. Gupta PK, Gupta H, Sundaram A, et al. Development and validation of a risk calculator for prediction of cardiac risk after surgery. *Circulation*. 2011;124:381–387.
18. Cohen ME, Ko CY, Bilimoria KY, et al. Optimizing ACS NSQIP modeling for evaluation of surgical quality and risk: patient risk adjustment, procedure mix adjustment, shrinkage adjustment, and surgical focus. *J Am Coll Surg*. 2013;217:336–346.
19. Karthikeyan G, Moncur RA, Levine O, et al. Is a pre-operative brain natriuretic peptide or N-terminal pro-B-type natriuretic peptide measurement an independent predictor of adverse cardiovascular outcomes within 30 days of noncardiac surgery? A systematic review and meta-analysis of observational studies. *J Am Coll Cardiol*. 2009;54:1599–1606.
20. Ryding AD, Kumar S, Worthington AM, et al. Prognostic value of brain natriuretic peptide in noncardiac surgery: A meta-analysis. *Anesthesiology*. 2009;111:311–319.
21. Rodseth RN, Buse GIL, Bollinger G, et al. The predictive ability of preoperative B-type natriuretic peptide in vascular patients for major adverse cardiac events. *J Am Coll Card*. 2011;58:522–529.
22. Goldman L, Caldera DL, Nussbaum SR, et al. Multifactorial index of cardiac risk in noncardiac surgical procedures. *N Engl J Med*. 1977;297:845–850.
23. Detsky A, Abrams H, McLaughlin J, et al. Predicting cardiac complications in patients undergoing non-cardiac surgery. *J Gen Intern Med*. 1986;1:211–219.
24. Healy KO, Waksmonski WA, Altman RK, et al. Perioperative outcome and long-term mortality for heart failure patients undergoing intermediate and high-risk noncardiac surgery: Impact of left ventricular ejection fraction. *Congest Heart Fail*. 2010;16:45–49.
25. Flu WJ, Van Kuijk JP, Hoeks SE, et al. Prognostic implications of asymptomatic left ventricular dysfunction in patients undergoing vascular surgery. *Anesthesiology*. 2010;112:1316–1324.
26. Nishimura RA, Otto CM, Bonow RO, et al. 2014 AHA/ACC guideline for the management of patients with valvular heart disease: A report of the American College of Cardiology/American Heart Association Task Force on Practice Guidelines. *Circulation*. 2014;129:e521–e643.
27. Shah KB, Kleinman BS, Sami H, et al. Reevaluation of perioperative myocardial infarction in patients with prior myocardial infarction undergoing noncardiac operations. *Anesth Analg*. 1990;71:231–235.
28. Hertzer NR, Bevan EG, Young JR, et al. Coronary artery disease in peripheral vascular patients: A classification of 1000 coronary angiograms and results of surgical management. *Ann Surg*. 1984;199:223–233.
29. Kannel W, Abbott R. Incidence and prognosis of unrecognized myocardial infarction: An update on the Framingham study. *N Engl J Med*. 1984;311:1144–1147.
30. Eagle KA, Coley CM, Newell JB, et al. Combining clinical and thallium data optimizes preoperative assessment of cardiac risk before major vascular surgery. *Ann Intern Med*. 1989;110:859–866.
31. Acharya DU, Shekhar YC, Aggarwal A, et al. Lack of pain during myocardial infarction in diabetics: Is autonomic dysfunction responsible? *Am J Cardiol*. 1991;68:793–796.
32. Hollenberg M, Mangano DT, Browner WS, et al. Predictors of postoperative myocardial ischemia in patients undergoing noncardiac surgery. The study of perioperative ischemia research. *JAMA*. 1992;268:205–209.
33. Pringle SD, MacFarlane PW, McKillop JH, et al. Pathophysiologic assessment of left ventricular hypertrophy and strain in asymptomatic patients with essential hypertension. *J Am Coll Cardiol*. 1989;13:1377–1381.
34. James PA, Oparil S, Carter BL, et al. 2014 Evidence-based guideline for the management of high blood pressure in adults: Report from the panel members appointed to the eighth joint national committee. *JAMA*. 2014;311(5):507–520.
35. Howell SJ, Sear JW, Foex P. Hypertension, hypertensive heart disease and perioperative cardiac risk. *Br J Anaesth*. 2004;92:570–583.
36. Wesker N, Klien M, Szendro G. The dilemma of immediate preoperative hypertension. *J Clin Anesth*. 2003;15:179–183.
37. Goldman L, Caldera DL. Risks of general anesthesia and elective operation in the hypertensive patient. *Anesthesiology*. 1979;50:285–292.
38. Tzimas P, Petrou A, Laou E, et al. Impact of metabolic syndrome in surgical patients. *Br J Anaesth*. 2015;115(2):194–202.
39. Warner MA, Shields SE, Chute CG. Major morbidity and mortality within 1 month of ambulatory surgery and anesthesia. *JAMA*. 1993;270:1437–1441.
40. Eagle KA, Rihal CS, Mickel MC, et al. Cardiac risk of noncardiac surgery: Influence of coronary disease and type of surgery in 3368 operations. CASS Investigators and University of Michigan Heart Care Program. *Circulation*. 1997;96:1882–1887.
41. Eagle K, Brundage B, Chaitman B, et al. Guidelines for perioperative cardiovascular evaluation of the noncardiac surgery. A report of the American

42. Reilly DF, McNeely MJ, Doerner D, et al. Self-reported exercise tolerance and the risk of serious perioperative complications. *Arch Intern Med.* 1999;159:2185–2192.
43. Kalbfleisch JM, Shudaksharappa KS, Conrad LL, et al. Disappearance of the Q deflection following myocardial infarction. *Am Heart J.* 1968;76:193–198.
44. Raby KE, Goldman L, Creager MA, et al. Correlation between perioperative ischemia and major cardiac events after peripheral vascular surgery. *N Engl J Med.* 1989;321:1296–1300.
45. Mantha S, Roizen MF, Barnard J, et al. Relative effectiveness of four preoperative tests for predicting adverse cardiac outcomes after vascular surgery: A meta-analysis. *Anesth Analg.* 1994;79:422–433.
46. Shaw LJ, Eagle KA, Gersh BJ, et al. Meta-analysis of intravenous dipyridamole–thallium-201 imaging (1985 to 1994) and dobutamine echocardiography (1991 to 1994) for risk stratification before vascular surgery. *J Am Coll Cardiol.* 1996;27:787–798.
47. Lavi R, Lavi S, Daghini E, et al. New frontiers in the evaluation of cardiac patients for noncardiac surgery. *Anesthesiology.* 2007;107:1018–1028.
48. Caplan RA, Connis RT, Nickinovich DG, et al. Practice alert for the perioperative management of patients with coronary artery stents: A report from the American Society of Anesthesiologists Committee on Standards and Practice Parameters. *Anesthesiology.* 2009;110(1):22–23.
49. Dupuis JY, Labinaz M. Noncardiac surgery in patients with coronary artery stent: What should the anesthesiologist know? *Can J Anesth.* 2005;52:356–361.
50. Schouten O, Jeroen JB, Poldermans D. Management of patients with cardiac stents undergoing noncardiac surgery. *Curr Opin Anaesthesiol.* 2007;20:274–278.
51. Crossley GH, Poole JE, Rozner MA, et al. The Heart Rhythm Society (HRS)/American Society of Anesthesiologists (ASA) expert consensus statement on the perioperative management of patients with implantable defibrillators, pacemakers and arrhythmia monitors. *Heart Rhythm.* 2011;8(7):1114–1154.
52. Arozullah AM, Daley J, Henderson WG, et al. Multifactorial risk index for predicting postoperative respiratory failure in men after major noncardiac surgery. The National Veterans Administration Surgical Quality Improvement Program. *Ann Surg.* 2000;232(2):242–253.
53. Johnson RG, Arozullah AM, Neumayer L, et al. Multivariable predictors of postoperative respiratory failure after general and vascular surgery: Results from the patient safety in surgery study. *J Am Coll Surg.* 2007;204(6):1188–1198.
54. Qaseem A, Snow V, Fitterman N, et al. Risk assessment for and strategies to reduce perioperative pulmonary complications for patients undergoing non-cardiothoracic surgery: A guideline from the American College of Physicians. *Ann Intern Med.* 2006;144(8):575–580.
55. Arozullah AM, Khuri SF, Henderson WG, et al. Development and validation of a multifactorial risk index for predicting postoperative pneumonia after major noncardiac surgery. *Ann Intern Med.* 2001;135:847–857.
56. Smetana GW. Preoperative pulmonary evaluation: Identifying and reducing risks for pulmonary complications. *Clev Clin J Med.* 2006;73:36–41.
57. Meyers JR, Lembeck L, O'Kane H, et al. Changes in functional residual capacity of the lung after operation. *Arch Surg.* 1975;110:576–583.
58. Dureuil B, Viires N, Cantineau JP, et al. Diaphragmatic contractility after upper abdominal surgery. *J Appl Physiol.* 1986;61:1775–1780.
59. Fisher BW, Majumdar SR, McAlistar FA. Predicting pulmonary complications after nonthoracic surgery: A systematic review of blinded studies. *Am J Med.* 2002;112:219–225.
60. Hall JC, Tarala RA, Hall JL. A case-control study of postoperative pulmonary complications after laparoscopic and open cholecystectomy. *J Laparoendosc Surg.* 1996;6:87–92.
61. Brueckmann B, Villa-Uribe JL, Brian T, et al. Development and validation of a score for prediction of postoperative respiratory complications. *Anesthesiology.* 2013;118:1276–1285.
62. Houston S, Hougland P, Anderson JJ, et al. Effectiveness of 0.12% chlorhexidine gluconate oral rinse in reducing prevalence of nosocomial pneumonia in patients undergoing heart surgery. *Am J Crit Care.* 2002;11(6):567–570.
63. Collard HR, Saint S, Matthay MA. Prevention of ventilator-associated pneumonia: An evidence-based systematic review. *Ann Intern Med.* 2003;138(6):494–501.
64. Kollef MH, Afessa B, Anzueto A, et al. Silver-coated endotracheal tubes and incidence of ventilator-associated pneumonia: The NASCENT randomized trial. *JAMA.* 2008;300(7):805–813.
65. Warner MA, Divertie MB, Tinker JH. Preoperative cessation of smoking and pulmonary complications in coronary artery bypass patients. *Anesthesiology.* 1984;60:609–616.
66. Rock P, Passannante A. Preoperative assessment: Pulmonary. *Anesthesiol Clin N Am.* 2002;22:77–91.
67. Paciullo CA, Short MR, Steinke DT, et al. Impact of nicotine replacement therapy on postoperative mortality following coronary artery bypass graft surgery. *Ann Pharmacother.* 2009;43(7):1197–1202.
68. Whyte MK, Choudry NB, Ind PW. Bronchial hyperresponsiveness in patients recovering from acute severe asthma. *Respir Med.* 1993;87:29–35.
69. Kabalin CS, Yarnold PR, Grammer LC. Low complication rate of corticosteroid-treated asthmatics undergoing surgical procedures. *Arch Intern Med.* 1995;155:1379–1384.
70. Peppard PE, Young T, Barnet JH, et al. Increased prevalence of sleep-disordered breathing in adults. *Am J Epidemiol.* 2013;177(9):1006–1014.
71. ASA Practice Guidelines for the Perioperative Management of Patients with Obstructive Sleep Apnea. Practice guidelines for the preoperative management of patients with obstructive sleep apnea: An updated report by the ASA task force on perioperative management of patients with obstructive sleep apnea. *Anesthesiology.* 2014;120(2):268–286.
72. Coursin DB, Connery LE, Ketzler JT. Perioperative diabetic and hyperglycemic management issues. *Crit Care Med.* 2004;32(4 Suppl):S116.
73. Furnary AP, Wu Y. Clinical effects of hyperglycemia in the cardiac surgery population: The Portland Diabetic Project. *Endocr Pract.* 2006;12(Suppl 3):22–26.
74. McGirt MJ, Woodworth GF, Brooke BS, et al. Hyperglycemia independently increases the risk of perioperative stroke, myocardial infarction, and death after carotid endarterectomy. *Neurosurgery.* 2006;58:1066–1073.
75. Blondet JJ, Beilman GJ. Glycemic control and prevention of perioperative infection. *Curr Opin Crit Care.* 2007;13:421–427.
76. Gandhi GY, Nuttall GA, Abel MD, et al. Intensive intraoperative insulin therapy versus conventional glucose management during cardiac surgery: A randomized trial. *Ann Intern Med.* 2007;146:233–243.
77. Gandhi GY, Murad MH, Flynn DN, et al. Effect of perioperative insulin infusion on surgical morbidity and mortality: Systematic review and meta-analysis of randomized trials. *Mayo Clin Proc.* 2008;83(4):418–430.
78. Joshi GP, Chung F, Vann MA, et al. Society for Ambulatory Anesthesia consensus statement on perioperative blood glucose management in diabetic patients undergoing ambulatory surgery. *Anesth Analg.* 2010;111(6):1378–1387.
79. Qaseem A, Humphrey LL, Chou R, et al. Use of intensive insulin therapy for the management of glycemic control in hospitalized patients: A clinical practice guideline from the American College of Physicians. *Ann Intern Med.* 2011;154(4):260–267.
80. Furnary AP, Cheek DB, Holmes SC, et al. Achieving tight glycemic control in the operating room: Lessons learned from 12 years in the trenches of a paradigm shift in anesthetic care. *Semin Thorac Cardiovasc Surg.* 2006;18:339–345.
81. Robertshaw HJ, Hall GM. Diabetes mellitus: Anaesthetic management. *Anaesthesia.* 2006;61:1187–1190.
82. Rhodes ET, Ferrari LR, Wolfsdorf JI, et al. Perioperative management of pediatric surgical patients with diabetes mellitus. *Anesth Analg.* 2005;101:986–999.
83. Garcia JE, Hill GE, Joshi GP. Perioperative stress dose steroids: Is it really necessary? *ASA Article.* 2013;77(11):32–35.
84. Sladen R. Anesthetic considerations for the patient with renal failure. *Anesthesiol Clin North America.* 2000;18(4):863–882.
85. Hanje AJ, Patel T. Preoperative evaluation of patients with liver disease. *Nat Clin Pract Gastroenterol Hepatol.* 2007;4(5):266–276.
86. Oda T, Fujiwara K, Yonenobu K, et al. Natural course of cervical spine lesions in rheumatoid arthritis. *Spine.* 1995;20(10):1128–1135.
87. Golub R, Cantu R, Sorrento JJ, et al. Efficacy of preadmission testing in ambulatory surgical patients. *Am J Surg.* 1992;163:565–570.
88. Narr BJ, Hansen TR, Warner MA. Preoperative laboratory screening in healthy Mayo patients: Cost-effective elimination of tests and unchanged outcomes. *Mayo Clin Proc.* 1991;66:155–159.
89. Narr BJ, Warner ME, Schroeder DR, et al. Outcomes of patients with no laboratory assessment before anesthesia and a surgical procedure. *Mayo Clin Proc.* 1997;72:505–509.
90. Roizen MF, Cohn S. Preoperative evaluation for elective surgery: What laboratory tests are needed? In: Stoelting RK, ed. *Advances in Anesthesia.* St. Louis, MO: Mosby Year Book; 1993:25.
91. Baron MJ, Gunter J, White P. Is the pediatric preoperative hematocrit determination necessary? *South Med J.* 1992;85:1187–1189.
92. Sox HCJ. *Common Diagnostic Tests: Use and Interpretation.* Philadelphia, PA: American College of Physicians; 1990.
93. Archer C, Levy AR, McGregor M. Value of routine preoperative chest x-rays: A meta-analysis. *Can J Anaesth.* 1993;40:1022–1027.
94. Colice GL, Shafazand S, Griffin JP, et al. Physiologic evaluation of the patient with lung cancer being considered for resectional surgery: ACCP evidenced-based clinical practice guidelines (2nd edition). *Chest.* 2007;132(3 Suppl):161S–177S.
95. Devereaux PJ, Yang H, Yusuf S, et al. Effects of extended-release metoprolol succinate in patients undergoing non-cardiac surgery (POISE trial): A randomized controlled trial. *Lancet.* 2008;371(9627):1839–1847.
96. Bangalore S, Wetterslev J, Pranesh S, et al. Perioperative beta blockers in patients having non-cardiac surgery: A meta-analysis. *Lancet.* 2008;372(9654):1962–1976.

97. Fleisher LA, Beckman JA, Brown KA, et al. ACCF/AHA focused update on perioperative beta blockade incorporated into the ACC/AHA 2007 guidelines on perioperative cardiovascular evaluation and care for noncardiac surgery. *J Am Coll Cardiol*. 2009;54(22):e13–e118.
98. Skrlin S, Hou V. A review of perioperative statin therapy for noncardiac surgery. *Semin Cardiothorac Vasc Anesth*. 2010;14(4):283–290.
99. Stoelting RK. Responses to atropine, glycopyrrolate and Riopan on gastric fluid pH and volume in adult patients. *Anesthesiology*. 1978;48:367–369.
100. Manchikanti L, Roush JR. The effect of preanesthetic glycopyrrolate and cimetidine in gastric fluid pH and volume in outpatients. *Anesth Analg*. 1984;63:40–46.
101. Kluger MT, Short TG. Aspiration during anaesthesia: A review of 133 cases from the Australian Anaesthetic Incident Monitoring Study (AIMS). *Anaesthesia*. 1999;54:19–26.
102. American Society of Anesthesiologists Committee. Practice guidelines for preoperative fasting and the use of pharmacologic agents to reduce the risk of pulmonary aspiration: Application to healthy patients undergoing elective procedures: An updated report by the American Society of Anesthesiologists Committee on Standards and Practice Parameters. *Anesthesiology*. 2011;114:495–511.
103. Stoelting RK. Gastric fluid pH in patients receiving cimetidine. *Anesth Analg*. 1978;57:675–677.
104. Maliniak K, Vahil AH. Pre-anesthetic cimetidine and gastric pH. *Anesth Analg*. 1979;58:309–313.
105. Haskins DA, Jahr JS, Texidor M, et al. Single-dose oral omeprazole for reduction of gastric residual acidity in adults for outpatient surgery. *Acta Anaesthesiol Scand*. 1992;36:513–515.
106. James CF, Modell JH, Gibbs CP, et al. Pulmonary aspiration: Effects of volume and pH in the rat. *Anesth Analg*. 1984;63:665–668.
107. Egbert LD, Battit GE, Turndorf H, et al. The value of the preoperative visit by the anesthetist. *JAMA*. 1963;185:553–555.
108. Reves JG, Fragen RJ, Vinick HR, et al. Midazolam: Pharmacology and uses. *Anesthesiology*. 1985;62:310–324.
109. Fragen RJ, Caldwell N. Lorazepam premedication: Lack of recall and relief of anxiety. *Anesth Analg*. 1976;55:792–796.
110. White PF. Pharmacologic and clinical aspects of preoperative medication. *Anesth Analg*. 1986;65:963–974.
111. Bradshaw EG, Ali AA, Mulley BA, et al. Plasma concentrations and clinical effects of lorazepam after oral administration. *Br J Anaesth*. 1981;53:517–522.
112. Weil JV, McCullough RE, Kline JS. Diminished ventilatory response to hypoxia and hypercapnia after morphine in man. *N Engl J Med*. 1975;292:1103–1106.
113. Falick YS, Smiler BG. Is anticholinergic premedication necessary? *Anesthesiology*. 1975;43:472–473.
114. Frumin MJ, Herekar VR, Jarvik ME. Amnesic actions of diazepam and scopolamine in man. *Anesthesiology*. 1976;45:406–412.
115. Bratzler DW, Houck PM. Antimicrobial prophylaxis for surgery: An advisory statement from the National Surgical Infection Prevention Project. *Am J Surg*. 2005;189:395–404.
116. Gorden SM. Antibiotic prophylaxis against postoperative wound infections. *Cleve Clin J Med*. 2006;73:S42–S45.

24 Rare Coexisting Diseases

STEPHEN F. DIERDORF • J. SCOTT WALTON • ANDREW F. STASIC • CHRISTOPHER L. HEINE

Musculoskeletal Diseases
   Muscular Dystrophy and Congenital Myopathy
   Myotonic Dystrophy
Skeletal Muscle Channelopathies
   Hyperkalemic Periodic Paralysis
   Hypokalemic Periodic Paralysis
   Andersen–Tawil Syndrome
   Myasthenia Gravis
   Myasthenic Syndrome (Lambert–Eaton Syndrome)
   Guillain–Barré Syndrome (Polyradiculoneuritis)
Central Nervous System Diseases
   Multiple Sclerosis
   Epilepsy
   Alzheimer Disease
   Parkinson Disease
   Huntington Disease
   Amyotrophic Lateral Sclerosis (ALS)
   Creutzfeldt–Jakob Disease

Other Inherited Disorders
   Malignant Hyperthermia
   Porphyria
   Cholinesterase Disorders
   Glycogen Storage Diseases
   Mucopolysaccharidoses
   Osteogenesis Imperfecta
Anemias
   Nutritional Deficiency Anemias
   Hemolytic Anemias
   Hemoglobinopathies
Connective Tissue Diseases
   Rheumatoid Arthritis
   Systemic Lupus Erythematosus
   Systemic Sclerosis (Scleroderma)
   Inflammatory Myopathies (Dermatomyositis/Polymyositis)
Skin Disorders
   Epidermolysis Bullosa
   Pemphigus

KEY POINTS

1. The cytoskeleton of the muscle membrane in patients with muscular dystrophy is fragile. Succinylcholine and/or halogenated anesthetics can cause the massive release of intracellular contents resulting in hyperkalemic cardiac arrest.
2. Myotonic dystrophy produces cardiac conduction delay that can manifest as third-degree atrioventricular block.
3. Patients with myasthenia gravis are exquisitely sensitive to nondepolarizing muscle relaxants. Short-acting muscle relaxants and objective monitoring of neuromuscular function are indicated.
4. Many types of cancer, in addition to small-cell carcinoma of the lung, can produce myasthenic syndrome.
5. Patients with multiple sclerosis can have an exacerbation of their neurologic symptoms despite a well-managed anesthetic.
6. An unexpected increase in end-tidal carbon dioxide is the most sensitive sign of malignant hyperthermia.
7. Hypoglycemia and metabolic acidosis are constant risks to patients with glycogen storage diseases.
8. The deposition of mucopolysaccharides in the upper airway of patients with mucopolysaccharidoses often complicates airway management during anesthesia.
9. Repeated episodes of sickling in patients with sickle cell disease cause pulmonary hypertension that increases perioperative risks.
10. Rheumatoid arthritis is a multisystem disease that causes subclinical cardiac and pulmonary dysfunction.
11. Patients with rheumatoid arthritis can have significant degeneration of the cervical spine with few neurologic symptoms. Cervical manipulation during laryngoscopy and tracheal intubation requires special precautions.
12. Esophageal dysfunction in patients with scleroderma and dermatomyositis increases the risk of aspiration pneumonitis.
13. Patients with epidermolysis bullosa can have undiagnosed dilated cardiomyopathy.

Musculoskeletal Diseases

Muscular Dystrophy and Congenital Myopathy

Muscular dystrophies and congenital myopathies are a heterogeneous group of progressive genetic muscle disorders characterized by skeletal muscle weakness (Table 24-1). There is variation in the muscle groups affected, severity of weakness, and age of onset. Cardiac and smooth muscle of the gastrointestinal tract are also affected. The pathology is the result of insufficient or abnormal proteins, such as dystrophin and sarcoglycans that form the cytoskeleton of the muscle membrane (Fig. 24-1). Skeletal muscle in the extremities, torso, and head is affected as well as muscles of the respiratory system, cardiac muscle, and smooth muscle of the gastrointestinal tract. An accurate classification of muscular dystrophies is complicated by the recent realization that similar phenotypes may be the result of mutations in different proteins and that allelic disorders on the same protein can result in different diseases (Fig. 24-2).[1]

> **Table 24-1** Types of Muscular Dystrophy and Congenital Myopathies
>
> **Muscular Dystrophies**
> Duchenne (DMD)
> Becker (BMD)
> Emery–Dreifuss
> Limb-girdle (LGMD)
> Facioscapulohumeral
> Oculopharyngeal
> Congenital muscular dystrophy
>
> **Congenital Myopathies**
> Nemaline myopathy
> Central core disease
> Minicore disease
> Centronuclear myopathy

Duchenne Muscular Dystrophy

Duchenne muscular dystrophy (DMD) is caused by the absence of dystrophin. Dystrophin is a large protein that plays a major role in stabilization of the muscle membrane and signaling between the cytoskeleton and extracellular matrix. DMD is the most common inherited muscle disease of childhood and is inherited as an X-linked recessive trait. Patients suffer from progressive proximal muscle weakness and wasting that produces symptoms in early childhood resulting in loss of ambulation by 12 years of age. DMD patients have elevated creatine kinase (CK) levels early in life. As the patient ages and more muscle atrophies, the CK level begins to decrease.

Even with recent improvements in supportive care, cardiorespiratory complications cause most of the mortality that occurs before the fourth decade of life. Typical ECG abnormalities include an R:S ratio greater than 1 in lead V1; deep Q waves in leads I, aVL, V5, and V6; right axis deviation; or a right bundle branch block. These ECG changes may precede other signs of cardiac dysfunction. Serial echocardiography reveals progressive left ventricular cavity expansion with impaired systolic and diastolic function. Contrast-enhanced MRI can identify early signs of myocardial damage and impending cardiac failure. Current recommendations call for cardiac evaluation every 2 years after diagnosis and each year after the age of 10 years. Early treatment with ACE inhibitors, diuretics, and β-adrenergic blockers may result in ventricular remodeling and functional improvement. Female carriers of DMD should be evaluated every 5 years, as they are prone to develop cardiomyopathy.[2]

Current treatment remains supportive and aimed at improving cardiorespiratory function. Noninvasive ventilation and cough assist techniques (manual and mechanical) can improve pulmonary function and reduce the risk of aspiration pneumonia. Gene therapies are under investigation.

Becker Muscular Dystrophy

A reduction in normal amounts of dystrophin results in Becker muscular dystrophy (BMD). Patients with BMD have a similar, but milder disease course than patients with DMD. The age of onset of BMD is 12 years although some patients will not be symptomatic until later in life. Causes of mortality are similar to those for DMD, but death does not occur until the fifth to sixth decade. It is recommended that patients with BMD have cardiac evaluation every 5 years if they are asymptomatic. More frequent evaluation is indicated when symptoms of cardiac disease develop. Female carriers can also have cardiac abnormalities.

Emery–Dreifuss Muscular Dystrophy

Emery–Dreifuss muscular dystrophy is caused by mutations in two proteins with different inheritance patterns. The X-linked form results from a mutation in the nuclear membrane protein emerin and the autosomal dominant form is the result of mutation in lamins A and C. Both forms typically present with contractures of the ankles, elbows, and neck. Progressive weakness of humeral and peroneal muscles and limb-girdle muscles develops. Cardiomyopathy and cardiac conduction abnormalities present by 30 years of age.[3]

Limb-Girdle Muscular Dystrophy

Limb-girdle muscular dystrophy (LGMD) is a progressive dystrophy subclassified by inheritance pattern and causative gene mutations. The autosomal dominant groups tend to be less severe. CK levels can be normal, mildly elevated, or significantly

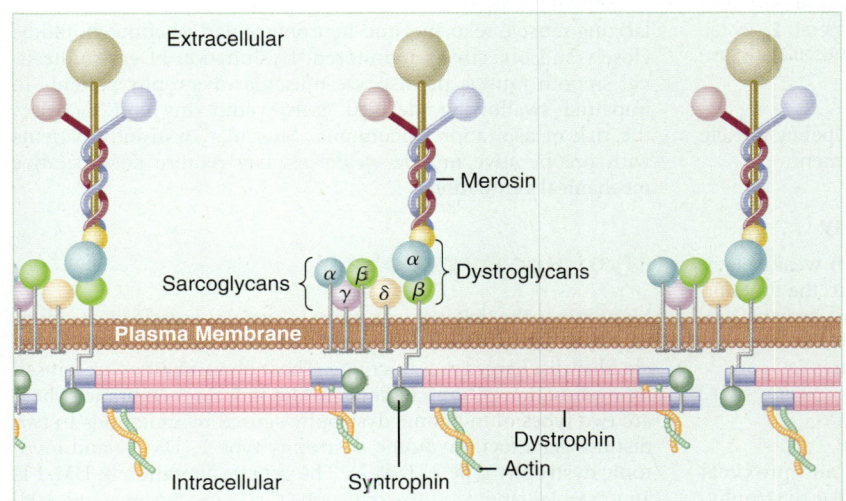

Figure 24-1 Muscle cell cytoskeleton. (Adapted from Duggan DJ, Gorospe JR, Fanin M, et al. Mutations in the sarcoglycan genes in patients with myopathy. *N Engl J Med.* 1997;336:618–624.)

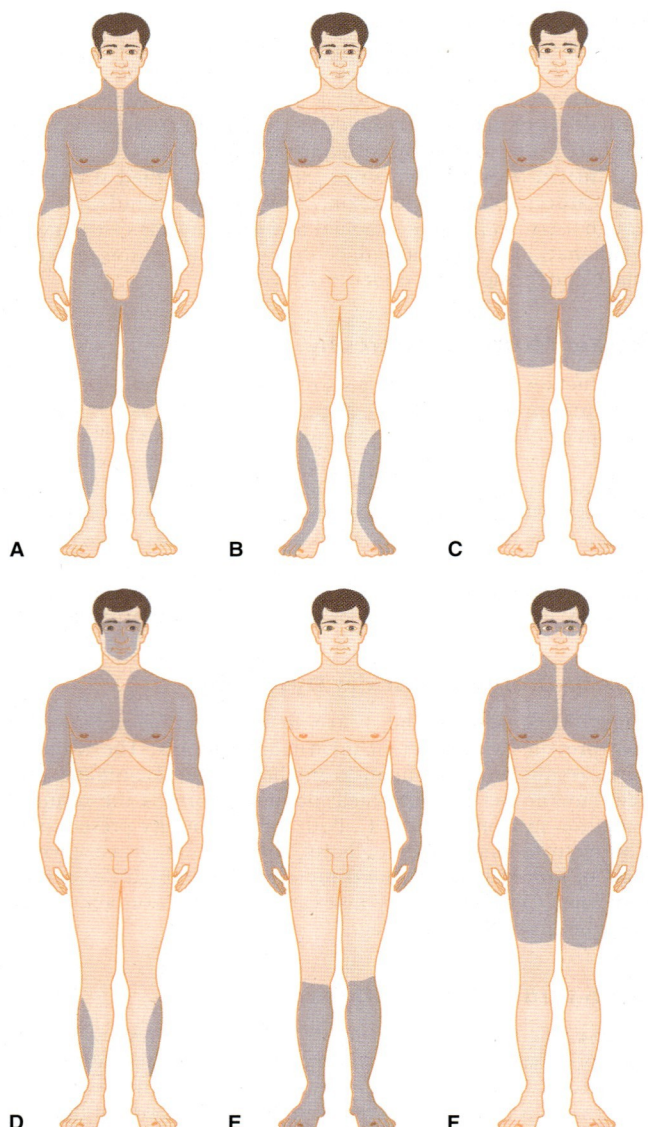

Figure 24-2 Distribution of predominant muscle weakness in different types of muscular dystrophy. **A:** Duchenne-type and Becker type. **B:** Emery–Dreifuss. **C:** Limb-girdle. **D:** Facioscapulohumeral. **E:** Distal. **F:** Oculopharyngeal. (Adapted from Emery AE. The muscular dystrophies. *BMJ.* 1998;317:991–995.)

elevated. LGMD patients suffer from shoulder and pelvic muscle weakness and can have significant cardiac involvement.

Facioscapulohumeral Muscular Dystrophy

This autosomal dominant dystrophy presents with weakness in the facial and shoulder muscles that later extends to the foot and pelvic girdle muscles. Retinal vascular disease and hearing loss may occur. Cardiac conduction abnormalities can develop, but cardiac muscle involvement does not usually occur.

Oculopharyngeal Muscular Dystrophy

Weakness in the extraocular, upper facial, neck, and proximal limb muscle characterizes oculopharyngeal muscular dystrophy. Ptosis and dysphagia are the usual presenting symptoms in the third decade of life and the reasons for seeking surgical therapy.

Congenital Muscular Dystrophy and Myopathy

Congenital muscular dystrophy (CMD) is characterized by onset of hypotonia during infancy, developmental delay, feeding difficulties, and respiratory dysfunction. There are three groups of diseases: collagenopathies (Ulrich CMD, Bethlem myopathy); merosinopathies; and dystroglycanopathies (Fukuyama CMD, muscle-eye-drain disease, Walker–Warburg syndrome). The congenital myopathies, now recognized as a class of diseases different from CMD, include nemaline myopathy, central core and minicore disease, and centronuclear myopathy. Although respiratory muscle dysfunction can be severe, cardiac involvement is not as prominent as in DMD or BMD. Patients with congenital myopathies may be susceptible to malignant hyperthermia (MH).[4,5]

Management of Anesthesia

The perioperative management of patients with muscular dystrophy is dependent of the particular disease and its progression. The complications of greatest concern are cardiac involvement and respiratory muscle weakness. Most recommendations for cardiac surveillance monitoring in the muscular dystrophies associated with heart failure or dysrhythmias call for echocardiograms and cardiac MRI. Preoperative review of these studies will assist in planning for anesthesia. Some patients with muscular dystrophy have very poor left ventricular function and will require advanced cardiac monitoring in the perioperative period.

Premedication can be administered for anxiolysis, unless there is a significant risk of respiratory dysfunction. Although muscular dystrophy was previously believed to be associated with an increased risk of MH, there is no evidence that the risk is greater than the general population. In contrast, patients with congenital myopathies such as central core disease or minicore disease should be considered to be at increased risk for MH.

Patients with muscular dystrophy, especially DMD, are at risk for rhabdomyolysis and severe hyperkalemia secondary to succinylcholine and possibly halogenated, inhaled anesthetics. The use of halogenated, inhaled anesthetics in patients with DMD is controversial.[6] A prudent approach would be to use halogenated, inhaled anesthetics only when necessary and for as brief a period of time as necessary. Succinylcholine should be avoided.

Patients with muscular dystrophy are sensitive to nondepolarizing muscle relaxants and neuromuscular function should be closely and objectively monitored. Dysfunction of gastrointestinal smooth muscle predisposes muscular dystrophy patients to impaired swallowing, delayed gastric emptying and increases the risk of aspiration pneumonia. Muscular dystrophy patients with preoperative muscle weakness may require postoperative mechanical ventilation.

Myotonic Dystrophy

Myotonia is the delayed relaxation of skeletal muscle after voluntary contraction. Electromyography demonstrates repetitive muscle fiber discharges that fluctuate. These abnormalities are caused by dysfunction of ion channels in the muscle membrane. There are two types of myotonic dystrophy caused by mutations in two distinct gene loci: myotonic dystrophy type 1 (DM-1) and myotonic dystrophy type 2 (DM-2). The genetic alteration in DM-1 is an unstable trinucleotide expansion (CTG) on chromosome 19q.

Table 24-2 Classification of Myotonic Dystrophy
Muscular Dystrophy Type 1
Congenital
Childhood-onset
Adult-onset
Late-onset
Muscular Dystrophy Type 2
Proximal myotonic dystrophy
Proximal myotonic myopathy
Proximal myotonic myopathy syndrome

DM-2 is caused by a quadnucleotide expansion (CCTG) on chromosome 3q. Both mutations cause RNA toxicity.

Myotonic Dystrophy Type 1

Myotonic dystrophy type 1 (DM-1) is the more common form and is subdivided by age of onset (Table 24-2). DM-1 is a multisystem disease that affects the musculoskeletal system, heart, respiratory system, central nervous system (CNS), and endocrine system.[7] Muscle weakness begins distally and progresses proximally with eventual muscle wasting. Pulmonary function studies demonstrate a restrictive pattern, mild arterial hypoxemia, and diminished ventilatory responses to hypoxia and hypercapnia. Respiratory muscle weakness diminishes cough effectiveness and may lead to pneumonia. Aspiration of gastric contents may occur because of gastric atony and pharyngeal muscle dysfunction. Myotonia of the respiratory muscles can cause intense dyspnea.

Cardiac manifestations include atrioventricular (AV) conduction delay, atrial tachydysrhythmias, diastolic dysfunction, mitral valve prolapse, and cardiomyopathy. Echocardiography may reveal subclinical evidence of left ventricular systolic and diastolic dysfunction.[8] Sudden death may be secondary to third-degree AV block or ventricular dysrhythmias.

Other clinical features of DM-1 include cataracts, premature balding, diabetes mellitus, thyroid dysfunction, adrenal insufficiency, and gonadal atrophy. Pregnancy may produce an exacerbation of myotonic dystrophy and congestive heart failure is more likely to occur during pregnancy. Cesarean section is often required because of uterine smooth muscle dysfunction. Infants of mothers with myotonic dystrophy may have hypotonia, feeding difficulty, and respiratory failure.

Myotonic Dystrophy Type 2

Patients with myotonic dystrophy type 2 (DM-2) may have similar clinical features (e.g., cataracts) as patients with DM-1. The clinical course in patients with DM-2 is, however, milder than that of patients with DM-1. AV conduction delay occurs in DM-2 patients, but sudden death is less likely. When compared to patients with DM-1, DM-2 patients are less likely to have diabetes and disability from chronic myopathy occurs much later in life. DM-2 patients are more likely to have myalgia, muscle strength variation, hypertrophy of the calf muscles, exacerbations during pregnancy, and a normal life expectancy.

There is no specific treatment for patients with DM-1 or DM-2. Mexiletine or flecainide may be effective for relief of muscle stiffness. Implantation of a defibrillating pacemaker is indicated for DM patients at risk for third-degree AV block or ventricular dysrhythmias.

Management of Anesthesia

Patients with DM-1 are more likely to have perioperative complications than patients with DM-2.[9,10] Considerations for anesthesia for patients with DM include the potential for cardiac and respiratory muscle disease and abnormal response to drugs used during anesthesia. Succinylcholine produces an exaggerated contracture and its use should be avoided. The myotonic response to succinylcholine can be so severe that ventilation and tracheal intubation are difficult. In theory neostigmine might provoke myotonia; however, patients with DM have received neostigmine without incident. The response to a peripheral nerve stimulator must be carefully evaluated because muscle stimulation may produce myotonia that could be misinterpreted as sustained tetanus when significant neuromuscular blockade still exists. Sugammadex has been used for reversal of rocuronium in patients with DM.

No specific anesthetic technique has been shown to be superior for patients with DM. Most postoperative complications reported in patients with DM are respiratory. Patients should be advised that postoperative ventilatory support may be required. Selection of short-acting inhaled and intravenous drugs is preferred. Patients with DM may be more susceptible to the respiratory depressant effects of opioids and sedatives. Sevoflurane and propofol have been successfully used. The high incidence of cardiac abnormalities in patients with DM mandates close monitoring of cardiac rhythm and function. Regional anesthesia has been used for both children and adults with DM. Patients with DM-2 are likely to have myalgia, weakness, and muscle cramps after surgery.[11]

Skeletal Muscle Channelopathies

Research in molecular biology and genetics has produced a reclassification of diseases with dissimilar clinical features (myotonia, periodic paralysis) but subcellular similarities. These diseases now constitute the group known as skeletal muscle channelopathies (Table 24-3). Disorders previously classified with myotonias but are now known to be channelopathies are myotonia congenita, sodium channel myotonia, and paramyotonia congenita. Diseases with periodic paralysis secondary to ion channel mutations are hyperkalemic periodic paralysis, hypokalemic periodic paralysis, thyrotoxic periodic paralysis, and Andersen–Tawil syndrome (ATS). The features that these disorders share are mutations in ion channels of the muscle membranes that affect muscle excitability or excitation-coupling.[12] The ion channels affected include chloride, sodium, calcium, and potassium channels.

Hyperkalemic Periodic Paralysis

Hyperkalemic periodic paralysis (hyperPP) is caused by a sodium ion channel mutation that causes prolonged muscle membrane depolarization and flaccid paralysis. Attacks can be provoked

Table 24-3 Skeletal Muscle Channelopathies
Hyperkalemic periodic paralysis
Hypokalemic periodic paralysis
Sodium channel myotonia
Thyrotoxic periodic paralysis
Myotonia congenita
Paramyotonia congenita
Andersen–Tawil syndrome

Table 24-4 Clinical Features of Familial Periodic Paralysis

Hyperkalemic
Sodium channel defect
Potassium >5.5 mEq/L during symptoms
Precipitating factors
    Rest after exercise
    Potassium infusions
    Metabolic acidosis
    Hypothermia
Skeletal muscle weakness may be localized to tongue and eyelids

Hypokalemic
Calcium channel defect
Potassium level <3 mEq/L during symptoms
Precipitating factors
    High glucose meals
    Strenuous exercise
    Glucose-insulin infusions
    Stress
    Hypothermia
Chronic myopathy with aging

---

by potassium loading, rest after exercise, and cold (Table 24-4). Episodes of paralysis can last for minutes to hours. The respiratory muscles are generally spared. Fifty percent of patients with hyperPP also report episodes of myotonia.

Measures that reduce serum potassium such as consumption of carbohydrate meals and administration of thiazide or carbonic anhydrase diuretics may prevent attacks. Severe attacks may require treatment with insulin and glucose.[13]

Hypokalemic Periodic Paralysis

Hypokalemic periodic paralysis (hypoPP) is caused by mutations in calcium or sodium channels. Patients with hypoPP develop flaccid paralytic attacks after carbohydrate loading and rest after exercise. Diaphragmatic function is generally maintained during attacks. Chronic muscle weakness develops as the patient ages.

Thyrotoxic hypokalemic periodic paralysis occurs with hyperthyroidism in combination with hypokalemia. The paralysis resolves after treatment of the hyperthyroidism.

Andersen–Tawil Syndrome

ATS is caused by a mutation in the potassium ion channel of skeletal muscle. This potassium ion channel is also abundant in ventricular myocytes. Patients with ATS develop periodic paralysis that may be associated with hypokalemia, normokalemia, or hyperkalemia. Ten percent of patients with ATS suffer a cardiac arrest.[14]

Management of Anesthesia

The clinical features and ion channel mutations in patients with channelopathies are diverse and the reported anesthesia experience with patients with channelopathies is quite varied. Many of the adverse events in patients with channelopathies are triggered by changes in potassium. Preoperative electrolyte abnormalities should be corrected before surgery. An effort should be made to monitor serum potassium levels and to maintain normokalemia during the perioperative period for both hyperPP and hypoPP. Metabolic changes (acidosis, alkalosis) and medications that cause changes in potassium levels (diuretics, insulin) may cause weakness or paralysis. Succinylcholine should be avoided as it may cause potassium flux. Avoidance of glucose loading, normocapnia, and normothermia are indicated for patients with hypoPP. The ECG should be continuously monitored for evidence of potassium-related dysrhythmias. Patients with channelopathies may develop a chronic myopathy and can be sensitive to nondepolarizing muscle relaxants.[15]

There are reports of perioperative hypermetabolic crises in patients with hypoPP. Whether these are true episodes of MH is controversial. There are so many possible gene mutations that some patients may be susceptible to MH.

Myasthenia Gravis

Myasthenia gravis (MG) is an autoimmune disease with autoantibodies directed against acetylcholine receptors (AChRs) or other proteins in the postsynaptic membrane of the neuromuscular junction. Eighty-five percent of patients with MG have anti-AChR antibodies. Other patients with MG have autoantibodies against muscle-specific tyrosine kinase (MuSK) or lipoprotein-related protein 4 (LRP4). Five percent of MG patients have no detectable antibodies. It is likely that these seronegative MG patients have low autoantibody titers that cannot be measured with current techniques. Autoantibodies damage the muscle membrane by activation of complement, lysis of the postsynaptic membrane, and loss of synaptic folds.[16] The thymus may play a central role in the pathogenesis of MG as 90% of MG patients have a thymoma, thymic hyperplasia, or thymic atrophy.

The clinical hallmark of MG is skeletal muscle weakness that is aggravated by repetitive muscle use. There can be periods of exacerbation alternating with remission. Any skeletal muscle can be affected, although there is a predilection for muscles innervated by cranial nerves. Initial symptoms include diplopia, dysarthria, or limb muscle weakness. Twenty to thirty percent of patients with MG will experience a myasthenic crisis during their life. A myasthenic crisis can be precipitated by poor control of MG, emotional stress, hyperthermia, or pulmonary infections. Myasthenic crisis is characterized by severe muscle weakness and respiratory failure. Cardiac manifestations of MG include focal myocarditis, atrial fibrillation, AV conduction delay, and left ventricular diastolic dysfunction.

Some pregnant patients have a remission during pregnancy whereas others (20% to 40%) have increased symptoms during pregnancy. Acute postpartum respiratory failure can occur. Fifteen to twenty percent of babies born to mothers with MG have transient myasthenia from passive transfer of AChR antibodies. Neonatal myasthenia begins 12 to 48 hours after birth and may persist for weeks. Babies with mothers with MuSK-MG have more severe neonatal myasthenia.

Disease classification is based on skeletal muscle groups affected as well as age of onset (Table 24-5). The Osserman staging system is based on the severity of the disease (Table 24-6).

No single test for myasthenia is diagnostic and the diagnosis of MG can be difficult, especially in the early stages of the disease. Diagnosis is based on symptomatology, serologic antibody testing, and electrodiagnostic testing.[17]

Treatment of MG includes cholinesterase inhibitors (pyridostigmine), corticosteroids, immunosuppressants, intravenous

Table 24-5 Clinical Presentations of Myasthenia Gravis

Type	Etiology	Onset	Sex	Thymus	Course
Neonatal myasthenia	Passage of antibodies from myasthenic mothers across the placenta	Neonatal	Both sexes	Normal	Transient
Congenital myasthenia	Congenital end-plate pathology, genetic autosomal recessive pattern of inheritance	0–2 yr	Male > female	Normal	Nonfluctuating compatible with long survival
Juvenile myasthenia	Autoimmune disorder	2–20 yr	Female > male (4:1)	Hyperplasia	Slowly progressive, tendency to relapse and remission
Adult myasthenia	Autoimmune disorder	20–40 yr	Female > male thymoma	Hyperplasia > within 3–5 yr	Maximum severity
Elderly myasthenia	Autoimmune disorder	>40 yr	Male > female	Thymoma (benign or locally invasive)	Rapid progress, higher mortality

Reproduced from Baraka A. Anesthesia and myasthenia gravis. *Can J Anaesth*. 1992;39:476, with permission.

immunoglobulin (IVIG), and plasmapheresis. Cholinesterase inhibitors increase the concentration of acetylcholine (ACh) at the postsynaptic membrane. Consistent control with only pyridostigmine can be challenging. Underdosing will result in residual weakness and overdosing may produce a "cholinergic crisis" characterized by abdominal pain, salivation, bradycardia, and skeletal muscle weakness. Corticosteroids (prednisone) are nonspecific immunosuppressants used when pyridostigmine does not produce satisfactory control. Other immunomodulators that may be used include azathioprine, mycophenolate mofetil, rituximab, methotrexate, cyclosporine, and tacrolimus. The administration of IVIG and plasmapheresis can be used when rapid treatment is required. Thymectomy is recommended for patients with a thymoma and patients with early-onset MG.

Management of Anesthesia

The primary concern for anesthesia is the potential interaction between the disease, MG medications, and anesthetic drugs that may exacerbate muscle weakness. The uncontrolled MG patient is exquisitely sensitive to nondepolarizing muscle relaxants (Fig. 24-3). Small doses of nondepolarizing muscle relaxants can produce profound respiratory muscle weakness. An anesthetic technique that avoids the use of muscle relaxants would be preferred. Halogenated, inhaled anesthetics (isoflurane, sevoflurane, desflurane) that depress neuromuscular transmission may be adequate for tracheal intubation. If muscle relaxation is required, a small dose of a short-acting nondepolarizing muscle relaxant should be used. The successful use of rocuronium and reversal with sugammadex has been reported in patients with MG.[18] MG patients who are poorly controlled are resistant to succinylcholine; however, a dose of 1.5 to 2 mg/kg will be adequate for rapid tracheal intubation. Pyridostigmine may prolong the duration of action of succinylcholine. Close objective monitoring of neuromuscular function is necessary. Postoperative mechanical ventilation in an ICU should be done if there is any question about the ability of the patient to maintain adequate spontaneous ventilation.[19]

Exacerbations of MG should be anticipated during pregnancy. Epidural analgesia can be used during labor and delivery.[20] Amide local anesthetics may be better than ester local anesthetics as the metabolism of amides is not affected by cholinesterase activity.

Table 24-6 Osserman Staging System for Myasthenia Gravis

Type	Description
I	Ocular weakness only
IIA	Generalized muscle weakness
IIB	Generalized moderate weakness and/or bulbar dysfunction
III	Acute, fulminant presentation and/or respiratory dysfunction
IV	Severe, generalized weakness

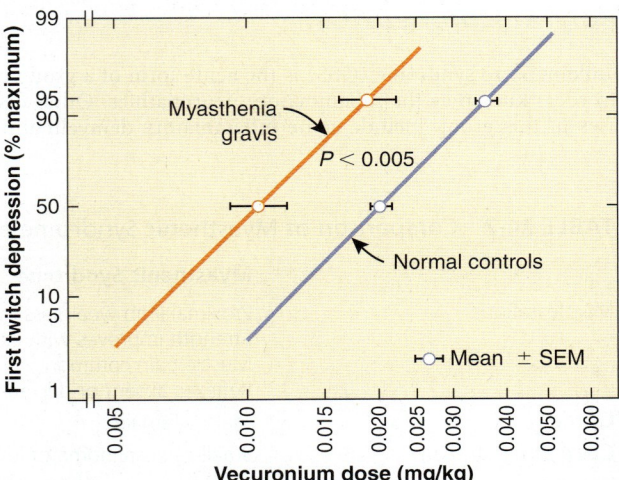

Figure 24-3 Dose–response for vecuronium in normal patients and patients with myasthenia gravis. (Adapted from Eisenkraft JB, Book WJ, Papatestas AE. Sensitivity to vecuronium in myasthenia gravis: a dose-response study. *Can J Anaesth*. 1990;37:3012–3016.)

Myasthenic Syndrome (Lambert–Eaton Syndrome)

The Lambert–Eaton syndrome (LEMS) is an autoimmune disease associated with cancer and is recognized as a paraneoplastic syndrome. Many tumors express onconeural antigens that resemble normal neural tissue components. Patients with LEMS have autoantibodies directed against presynaptic voltage-gated calcium ion channels. This results in a decreased release of acetylcholine and subsequent muscle weakness. Small-cell lung cancer is most frequently associated with LEMS and the weakness often precedes the discovery of the tumor. The typical LEMS patient is a male greater than 40 years of age with proximal muscle weakness (hip, shoulder) that affects gait and the ability to stand and climb stairs (Table 24-7). Autonomic dysfunction with dry mouth, constipation, erectile dysfunction, and reduced sweating often occurs. Paraneoplastic neurologic syndrome has also been reported with breast and ovarian cancer, lymphomas, testicular cancer, and neuroblastoma. The clinical diagnosis can be confirmed with electrophysiologic testing (repetitive nerve stimulation) and serologic testing for the autoantibody.[21]

Treatment of the underlying neoplasm may improve the neurologic condition. The most effective drug for the treatment of the muscle weakness is 3,4-diaminopyridine. 3,4-Diaminopyridine prolongs the presynaptic action potential and increases the release of acetylcholine. Side effects of 3,4-diaminopyridine include perioral tingling, digital paresthesias, seizures, and supraventricular tachycardia. If treatment with 3,4-diaminopyridine is inadequate, prednisone, azathioprine, IVIG, or plasmapheresis may be used.[22]

Management of Anesthesia

Patients with LEMS are sensitive to the effects of both depolarizing and nondepolarizing muscle relaxants. The most frequently reported perioperative complications are respiratory. The administration of 3,4-diaminopyridine should be continued until the time of surgery. Undiagnosed LEMS may be present in patients undergoing surgical procedures for cancer. This could be a cause of delayed recovery from muscle relaxants.[23]

Guillain–Barré Syndrome (Polyradiculoneuritis)

Guillain–Barré syndrome (GBS) is the acute form of a group of disorders known as the inflammatory neuropathies. Other diseases in this group include acute inflammatory demyelinating polyneuropathy (AIDP), acute motor axonal neuropathy (AMAN), acute motor–sensory axonal neuropathy, Miller-Fisher syndrome, and chronic inflammatory demyelinating polyneuropathy (CIDP).

GBS is an autoimmune disease triggered by a viral or bacterial infection and is an example of molecular mimicry and cross-reactivity. The infectious agent produces a substance that causes an immune reaction. That substance resembles a neural component of the host and autoantibodies develop that attack the host. Patients with GBS develop antibodies to gangliosides in the peripheral nerves.[24]

Most patients with GBS have a history of a respiratory or gastrointestinal infection within 4 weeks of the onset of neurologic symptoms. Infections with *Campylobacter jejuni*, *Haemophilus influenzae*, *Mycoplasma pneumoniae*, Epstein–Barr virus, and cytomegalovirus are most frequently associated with GBS. There are sporadic reports of GBS or a GBS-like syndrome presenting after surgical procedures, trauma, or some vaccinations. GBS is characterized by onset of skeletal muscle weakness or paralysis of the legs. Paresthesias may precede the weakness. The paralysis progresses cephalad to include the muscles of the trunk and arms with maximal weakness developing 2 to 4 weeks after the onset. A plateau phase develops before recovery begins. The most serious problem is ventilatory insufficiency and 25% of patients with GBS will require mechanical ventilation. Autonomic nervous system dysfunction can produce wide fluctuations in heart rate and blood pressure. In a manner similar to autonomic hyperreflexia, physical stimulation can precipitate hypertension, tachycardia, and cardiac dysrhythmias.

Plasma exchange and IVIG have been shown to be effective for patients with GBS.[25] Although 85% of GBS patients achieve a good recovery, 3% to 5% develop a chronic recurrent neuropathy.

Management of Anesthesia

Autonomic nervous system dysfunction may cause hypotension secondary to postural changes, blood loss, or positive pressure ventilation. Noxious stimuli such as laryngoscopy and tracheal intubation may produce exaggerated increases in heart rate and blood pressure.

Succinylcholine should be avoided because of the danger of hyperkalemia. This risk may persist after clinical recovery from GBS.[26] A short-acting nondepolarizing muscle with minimal cardiovascular effects (cisatracurium, rocuronium) would be a logical choice. The sensitivity to nondepolarizing muscle relaxants may vary from extreme sensitivity to resistance, depending on the phase of the disease.[27] It is likely that mechanical ventilation may be required in the immediate postoperative period. Patients

TABLE 24-7 Comparison of Myasthenic Syndrome and Myasthenia Gravis

	Myasthenic Syndrome	Myasthenia Gravis
Manifestations	Proximal limb weakness (arms > legs) Strength improves with exercise Muscle pain common Reflexes absent or decreased	Extraocular, bulbar, and facial muscle weakness Fatigue with exercise Muscle pain uncommon Reflexes normal
Gender	Male > female	Female > male
Coexisting pathology	Small-cell carcinoma of lung	Thymoma
Response to muscle relaxants	Sensitive to succinylcholine and nondepolarizing muscle relaxants Poor response to anticholinesterases	Resistant to succinylcholine Sensitive to nondepolarizing muscle relaxants Poor response to anticholinesterases

Reprinted from Stoelting RK, Dierdorf SF, eds. *Anesthesia and Co-Existing Disease*. 3rd ed. New York: Churchill Livingstone; 1993, with permission.

with GBS who have pronounced sensory disturbances may benefit from neuraxial opioids. There are reports of GBS developing after neuraxial anesthesia.[28]

Central Nervous System Diseases

Multiple Sclerosis

The features of multiple sclerosis (MS) are inflammation, demyelination, immune dysregulation, and failure of cell repair in the CNS. There is a complex interaction between genetics and environmental factors that lead to demyelination of CNS cells and peripheral nerves. An antigen-presenting dendritic cell crosses the blood–brain barrier and converts some T cells into inflammatory cells. These T cells induce macrophages that produce cytokines and oxygen radicals that cause demyelination and axonal decay. Demyelination interferes with neural transmission and CNS dysfunction ensues. As the disease progresses there is loss of brain volume and gray matter.[29]

The symptoms of MS depend on the sites of demyelination. Brainstem involvement can produce nystagmus, diplopia, ataxia, autonomic dysfunction, and alterations in ventilation that lead to respiratory failure. Lesions of the spinal cord produce weakness and paresthesias. The legs are affected more than the arms. Bowel retention and urinary incontinence are frequent complaints. Many patients with MS develop central neuropathic pain, trigeminal neuralgia, spasticity, and tonic seizures. The course of MS is characterized by exacerbation of symptoms at unpredictable intervals over years. Patients are classified during the early stages of the disease as relapsing-remitting (85%) or primary progressive MS (15%). Many patients with relapsing-remitting MS develop neurodegeneration and are then categorized as secondary progressive MS.

Clinical criteria for the diagnosis of MS include onset between 10 and 50 years of age, signs and symptoms of CNS white matter disease, two or more attacks separated by a month or more, and involvement of two or more noncontiguous anatomic areas. Elevated levels of IgG and albumin in the cerebrospinal fluid are characteristic of MS. Magnetic resonance imaging (MRI) is a sensitive diagnostic tool for MS and provides direct evidence of demyelinated plaques in the CNS. Pregnancy is generally associated with reduced risk of exacerbations whereas the postpartum period is notable for an increased risk of relapse.

Treatment of MS is directed at modulating the immunologic and inflammatory responses that damage the CNS. Most of the immunomodulating drugs do increase the patient's risk of infection and malignancy. Interferon preparations and glatiramer are self-injectable drugs with good safety profiles. Mitoxantrone is a general immunosuppressant that has limited use because of cardiotoxicity and treatment-related leukemia. Natalizumab has limited use because of the development of progressive multifocal leukoencephalopathy (PML). There are three oral disease-modifying drugs currently used for the treatment of relapsing MS: fingolimod, teriflunomide, and dimethyl fumarate. Side effects of fingolimod include bradycardia, macular edema, hypertension, and liver dysfunction. Teriflunomide can cause lymphopenia, hepatotoxicity, hypertension, and peripheral neuropathy. Dimethyl fumarate causes flushing, nausea, abdominal pain, and diarrhea. A number of monoclonal antibodies are under investigation for the treatment of MS.[30]

Management of Anesthesia

The effect of surgery and anesthesia on the course of MS is controversial. Some reports have suggested that general or regional anesthesia can exacerbate MS. Most reports, however, have found no influence of anesthesia on the course of the disease. It is likely that other factors such as infection, hyperpyrexia, and emotional stress could contribute to a perioperative exacerbation. Preoperatively, the patient should be advised that surgery and anesthesia could produce a relapse despite a well-managed anesthetic. Most of the old controversies concerning regional and epidural/spinal anesthesia and MS have been resolved by several studies supporting the use of these modalities in patients with MS.[31,32] There is no evidence that exposure to inhaled anesthetics, including nitrous oxide, increases the risk of MS to anesthesia providers.

The chronic effects of the neurologic dysfunction caused by MS and potent therapeutic drugs can be manifest during the perioperative period as autonomic dysfunction, myopathy, cardiotoxicity, and sensitivity or resistance to muscle relaxants. Succinylcholine could produce an exaggerated release of potassium. Respiratory muscle weakness and poor respiratory control increase the likelihood of postoperative respiratory support.

Epilepsy

A seizure is a common manifestation of many CNS diseases. A seizure is the result of an excessive discharge of large numbers of neurons depolarized in synchrony. Epilepsy (idiopathic seizures) begins in childhood. The onset of seizures in an adult may indicate focal brain disease (e.g., tumor). Onset of seizures after 60 years of age can be a result of cerebrovascular disease, head injury, tumor, infection, or metabolic abnormalities.

The most frequently encountered types of seizures are:
1. *Grand mal seizures* are characterized by generalized tonic–clonic activity. All respiratory effort ceases and arterial hypoxemia ensues. The tonic phase lasts 20 to 40 seconds and is followed by the clonic phase. In the postictal period, the patient is lethargic and confused.
2. *Focal cortical seizures* may be motor or sensory depending on the site of neuronal discharge. There is usually no loss of consciousness, although the focal seizure may induce a grand mal seizure.
3. *Absence seizures* (petit mal) are a sudden, brief loss of awareness (30 seconds). Additional features include staring, blinking, and rolling of the eyes. These seizures typically occur in children and young adults.
4. *Akinetic seizures* are a sudden loss of consciousness and postural tone. These types of seizures usually occur in children and can cause severe head injury from the fall.
5. *Status epilepticus* is defined as two consecutive tonic–clonic seizures without regaining consciousness or seizure activity that is unabated for 30 minutes. Grand mal status epilepticus can last for 48 hours with four or five seizures per hour and the mortality can be 20%.[33] As the seizure progresses, skeletal muscle activity diminishes and seizure activity may only be evident on the EEG. Respiratory effects of status epilepticus include respiratory center inhibition, impaired ventilation from uncoordinated skeletal muscle activity, and bronchoconstriction.

There are many antiepileptic drugs (AEDs) (Table 24-8). Most AEDs affect ion transfer, increase inhibitory neurotransmitters (GABA), or decrease levels of excitatory neurotransmitters. AEDs can be divided into two general categories: Broad-spectrum AEDs such as valproate, lamotrigine, topiramate, levetiracetam, and zonisamide are useful for generalized seizures. Narrow-spectrum AEDs such as carbamazepine, phenytoin, gabapentin, tiagabine, oxcarbazepine, and pregabalin are more appropriate

Table 24-8 Antiepileptic Drugs Classified by Mechanism of Action

Enhance GABAergic System
Barbiturates
Valproic acid
Tiagabine
Benzodiazepines
Primidone
Vigabatrin

Affect Cation Channels
Sodium channels
Carbamazepine
Felbamate
Lamotrigine
Phenytoin
Topiramate
Oxcarbazepine
Calcium channels
Gabapentin
Pregabalin
Ethosuximide
Potassium channels
Retigabine

Antagonists of Excitatory Amino Acids
Lacosamide
Talampanel
Levetiracetam

Unknown Mechanism of Action
Acetazolamide
sultiame

AEDs for Status Epilepticus
Propofol
Lorazepam
Fosphenytoin
Diazepam
Midazolam

for focal seizures.[34] Vagal nerve stimulators are often implanted for the treatment of medically refractory epilepsy.

The treatment of patients with status epilepticus requires airway protection and appropriate ventilatory assistance. Drug therapy for status epilepticus often requires combinations of lorazepam, midazolam, phenytoin, fosphenytoin, phenobarbital, pentobarbital, and propofol. On rare occasions, general anesthesia may be required.

Recent research has identified many genetic variations in patients with epilepsy. It is hoped that this research will result in highly effective, individualized therapy for epilepsy in the future.

Management of Anesthesia

Many anesthetics including halogenated inhaled anesthetics, nitrous oxide, etomidate, ketamine, and opioids have been reported to produce seizure activity. The clinical significance of these reports is unclear.[35] The degree of preoperative seizure control may be more important than the anesthetic agents.

Interruption of the patient's AED therapy should be minimized during the perioperative period.

Side effects of AEDs include leukopenia, anemia, hepatic dysfunction, pancreatitis, cardiotoxicity, hypothyroidism, and skin rash.[36] Vagal nerve stimulators can cause vocal cord paralysis, facial palsy, bradycardia/asystole, and airway obstruction.[37] AEDs can stimulate hepatic enzymes (cytochrome P450) that can lead to increased metabolism of other drugs.[38] In contrast, AEDs that are highly protein bound may increase blood concentrations of other drugs.

Alzheimer Disease

Alzheimer disease (AD) is the major cause of dementia in the United States. The incidence of AD increases progressively after 65 years of age and may be as high as 30% in persons over 85 years of age. Ninety-five percent of AD cases are sporadic and 5% have a genetic basis. The pathogenesis of AD is complex but appears to start with amyloid-β protein (Aβ), possibly years before clinical manifestations develop. Aβ most likely begins a cascade of events culminating in deposition of amyloid plaques, neurofibrillary tangles, and neuronal apoptosis (amyloid cascade). These changes cause a loss of cholinergic activity and a loss of glutamatergic neurons.

AD is characterized by loss of cognition, poor decision making, language deterioration, gait disturbances, seizures, agitation, and psychosis. Imaging studies show hippocampal atrophy (MRI) and glucose hypometabolism (PET scan). Medications currently approved for the treatment of AD include three acetylcholinesterase inhibitors (donepezil, rivastigmine, galantamine) and one NMDA inhibitor (memantine).[39] Cholinesterase inhibitors improve the patient's ability to perform daily living activities and may improve cognition. Side effects of cholinesterase inhibitors include nausea, emesis, bradycardia, syncope, and fatigue. Antidepressants, anticonvulsants, and antipsychotics are used for neuropsychiatric symptoms. Therapies under investigation are directed at early interruption of the amyloid cascade.

Management of Anesthesia

There is considerable concern that general anesthesia may cause postoperative cognitive dysfunction (POCD) and accelerate the processes that cause AD.[40] POCD is well known in elderly patients after surgery, but proof of cause has remained elusive.[41] Patients and their families should be advised that POCD may occur.

The selection of anesthetics will be influenced by the patient's physiologic condition and the degree of neurologic impairment. The patient's preoperative drug list should be reviewed for the possibility of interactions with anesthetics. Patients are likely to be confused and uncooperative because of dementia. Sedative premedication should be used with caution, if at all, as mental confusion may worsen. If an anticholinergic is required, glycopyrrolate, which does not cross the blood–brain barrier, is preferred rather than atropine or scopolamine. Patients receiving cholinesterase inhibitors may have a prolonged response to succinylcholine.

Parkinson Disease

Parkinson disease (PD) is a degenerative CNS disease caused by a loss of dopaminergic cells in the basal ganglia. The characteristic pathologic feature is the presence of Lewy bodies in the neurons of the substantia nigra. The etiology of PD is a complex interaction between a genetic predisposition and environmental factors such as pesticide exposure, agricultural occupation, rural living, prior head injury, and β-adrenergic blocker use.

The most characteristic features of PD are resting tremor, cogwheel rigidity of the upper extremities, bradykinesia, shuffling gait, stooped posture, and facial immobility. These features are secondary to diminished inhibition of the extrapyramidal motor system as a result of dopamine deficiency. Other clinical manifestations include seborrhea, sialorrhea, constipation, orthostatic hypotension, bladder dysfunction, diaphragmatic spasm, oculogyric crises, dementia, and depression.[42]

Current therapies for PD are directed at amelioration of symptoms. Current treatment research is aimed at prevention of underlying neurodegeneration. Levodopa is the most effective treatment available for PD. Levodopa is used in combination with drugs such as carbidopa (peripheral decarboxylase inhibitor) and entacapone (catechol-o-methyltransferase inhibitor) that prevent the adverse peripheral effects of dopamine. Other drugs that may improve function in patients with PD are the monoamine oxidase-B inhibitors, selegiline, and rasagiline. Dopamine agonists such as bromocriptine, pramipexole, ropinirole, pergolide, and cabergoline may also be effective. Pergolide and cabergoline are ergot-derived drugs that can cause cardiac valvular fibrosis and insufficiency. Implantation of deep-brain stimulators (DBS) may be quite effective for patients with advanced PD. The therapeutic regimen for PD is complex and requires a skilled neurologist to individualize therapy.[43]

Management of Anesthesia

The half-life of levodopa is short and interruption of therapy for more than 6 to 12 hours can result in severe skeletal muscle rigidity that interferes with ventilation. Consultation with the patient's neurologist and continuation of the patient's drug regimen may avert complications. Apomorphine is a dopamine agonist that can be administered subcutaneously or intravenously if oral levodopa cannot be given. Dopamine antagonists such as phenothiazines, droperidol, and metoclopramide should be avoided. Alfentanil and fentanyl may produce dystonic reactions when administered rapidly. The incidence of side effects from propofol is low. Although ketamine could produce an exaggerated sympathetic nervous system response with tachycardia and hypertension, it has been used without difficulty in patients with PD. There are no reports of adverse responses to isoflurane, sevoflurane, or desflurane. The likelihood of coexisting heart disease in elderly patients with PD will influence the selection of anesthetics and monitoring techniques.[44]

Anesthetics administered to patients who are receiving monoamine-B-oxidase inhibitors are generally uneventful. There are, however, reports of agitation, muscle rigidity, and hyperthermia in patients receiving selegiline and meperidine. Patients being treated with dopamine agonists may be at increased risk for neuroleptic malignant syndrome (NMS).

Autonomic dysfunction is common. The most consistent cardiovascular effect is orthostatic hypotension that may be aggravated by the vasodilatory effects of anti-Parkinson drugs and inhaled anesthetics. Excessive salivation and esophageal dysfunction are common and increase the risk of aspiration pneumonitis. Perioperative respiratory complications are common.[45] Upper airway obstruction may be a result of poor coordination of upper airway muscles secondary to neurotransmitter imbalance. Upper airway obstruction may respond favorably to anti-Parkinson drugs. Patients with PD are susceptible to postoperative confusion and hallucinations. These changes in mental function may not occur for 24 to 72 hours after surgery.

Anesthesia for PD patients undergoing implantation of DBS can be challenging. Awake techniques with sedation and local anesthesia are preferred so intraoperative testing of the stimulator can be performed. Agitated and uncooperative patients may require general anesthesia. Hypertension, seizures, and electrical interference with other devices can occur.[46]

Huntington Disease

Huntington disease (HD) is an autosomal dominant inherited disease characterized by progressive neurodegeneration. HD is one of the trinucleotide repeat disorders. An increase in cytosine, adenine, and guanine (CAG) sequences on chromosome 4 is the genetic defect that produces a mutant huntingtin protein. Huntingtin is found in all human cells, but most notably in brain cells. The role of huntingtin is not known, but it may prevent cell apoptosis. Neurons from patients with HD show abnormal inclusion bodies containing mutant huntingtin and polyglutamine. Associated with HD is atrophy of the caudate, putamen, and thalamus with cortical thinning. Recent evidence suggests that peripheral inflammatory mediators may gain access to the brain and trigger neurodegeneration. Identification of the huntingtin gene provides a reliable predictive test; however, the delayed nature of the clinical manifestations presents legal and ethical concerns about predictive testing.[47]

Onset of the clinical manifestations of HD typically begins between 35 and 40 years of age. Clinical features include choreiform movements, depression, and dementia. The disease continues to progress for several years and depression increases the possibility of suicide. Death occurs 17 to 20 years after diagnosis and is usually from malnutrition or aspiration pneumonitis. Hypothalamic atrophy can cause endocrine changes such as elevated cortisol levels, reduced testosterone levels, and diabetes. Hepatic dysfunction and skeletal muscle weakness are common.

There is no specific therapy for HD. Most therapy is palliative. Tetrabenazine is used for the treatment of chorea. Antiepileptics and antidepressants may be required for neuropsychiatric manifestations of HD.

Management of Anesthesia

The medical literature is sparse with regard to the anesthetic management of patients with HD. Many of the manifestations of HD are typical of patients with neurodegenerative disorders. As the disease progresses, the pharyngeal muscles become dysfunctional and the risk of aspiration pneumonitis increases.[48] Delayed emergence and an increased likelihood of respiratory complications must be anticipated after surgery.

Although there are no specific contraindications to the use of intravenous or inhaled anesthetics, recovery from propofol may be faster than with other intravenous hypnotics. Short-acting muscle relaxants are preferable to long-acting muscle relaxants. Decreased plasma cholinesterase activity may prolong the response to succinylcholine. Spinal anesthesia has been successfully used in patients with HD.

Amyotrophic Lateral Sclerosis

Amyotrophic lateral sclerosis (ALS, Lou Gehrig disease) is a degenerative disease of motor neurons: upper motor neuron (UMN) and lower motor neuron (LMN). Although the cause of ALS has not been discovered, glutamate excitotoxicity and/or oxidative stress may be important components. Degeneration of LMN and UMN may be dependent or independent processes. The end result is LMN degeneration and destruction of the neuromuscular junction. Progression of the disease is relentless—50% of patients die within 30 months of the onset of symptoms. Twenty percent may survive 5 to 10 years.

Signs and symptoms are influenced by the affected neurons. Initial symptoms are asymmetric limb weakness. Dysarthria and dysphagia are a result of bulbar atrophy. Pulmonary function testing demonstrates a decrease in vital capacity and maximal voluntary ventilation. Patients with ALS have autonomic dysfunction as evidenced by resting tachycardia, orthostatic hypotension, and elevated circulating levels of epinephrine and norepinephrine. Respiratory failure eventually develops and ventilatory support is required. The cause of death is respiratory failure or cardiovascular collapse.

Riluzole, a glutamate release inhibitor, is the only drug approved for the specific treatment of ALS. Improved survival, however, with riluzole is quite modest (3 to 6 months). Many other drugs may be employed to ameliorate the effects of ALS.[49] Treatment to avoid mechanical ventilation such as the use of diaphragmatic pacing is under investigation.

Management of Anesthesia

Surgical interventions for palliative care (gastrostomy, central venous catheter insertion, tracheostomy) are frequently required. Short-acting anesthetics such as propofol, remifentanil, sevoflurane, and desflurane are preferred. Neuromuscular transmission is abnormal and ALS patients may be very sensitive to nondepolarizing muscle relaxants. Succinylcholine should be avoided as it may provoke a massive release of potassium. The need for postoperative ventilatory support is likely.[50]

Creutzfeldt–Jakob Disease

Creutzfeldt–Jakob disease (CJD) is one of a group of diseases termed the transmissible spongiform encephalopathies. Pathologically, these diseases are characterized by vacuolation of brain cells and neuronal death. CJD is an infection caused by a prion, a small protein devoid of nucleic acid. PrP^c is a naturally occurring protein concentrated in neurons. A conformational change occurs in PrP^c and changes it to the pathologic form PrP^{sc}.[51] The structure of PrP^{sc} renders the protein resistant to conventional decontamination methods. There are four types of CJD: familial (fCJD), sporadic (sCJD), iatrogenic (iCJD), and variant (vCJD). CJD is a very rare cause of dementia, but the discovery of transmission of a prion disease from cows to humans (mad cow disease, 1996) catapulted CJD to international prominence. This form of CJD is the variant form (vCJD).

The clinical manifestations of sCJD are subacute dementia, myoclonus, and EEG changes. The EEG pattern is characteristic with diffuse slow activity and periodic complexes. Progressive loss of cognitive and neurologic function occurs. Patients with vCJD present with dysphoria, withdrawal, anxiety, and insomnia. Neurologic features develop 1 to 2 months after psychiatric changes commence. Transmission of vCJD is by ingestion of contaminated animal products. Iatrogenic transmission of iCJD has been linked to contaminated dural graft material, corneal transplants, contaminated surgical instruments, pooled human growth hormone, and blood. There is no specific treatment for CJD. Research has centered on therapies aimed at preventing prion transmission from the periphery to the CNS and neuronal regeneration.

Management of Anesthesia

CJD is a transmissible disease and appropriate precautions should be observed when administering anesthesia. Patient tissues with a high likelihood of contamination include brain, spinal cord, cerebrospinal fluid, lymphoid tissue, and blood. Single-use anesthesia supplies, including face masks, breathing circuits, laryngoscopes, and tracheal tubes offer the highest degree of protection.[52]

Patients with degenerative neurologic diseases are prone to aspiration pneumonitis because they have impaired swallowing function and decreased laryngeal reflexes. Lower motor neuron dysfunction occurs in patients with CJD and succinylcholine should be avoided. The autonomic and peripheral nervous systems are adversely affected and abnormal cardiovascular responses to anesthesia and vasoactive drugs should be expected.

Other Inherited Disorders

Malignant Hyperthermia

MH is a pharmacogenetic disorder of skeletal muscle that, when triggered, results in a hypermetabolic process associated with significant morbidity and mortality. MH is commonly triggered by succinylcholine or halogenated, inhaled anesthetics. It has also been associated with extreme physiologic stress or heat exhaustion. Individuals susceptible to MH have a mutation of the ryanodine receptor that permits the uncontrolled release of calcium (Ca^{+2}) from the sarcoplasmic reticulum (SR). This leads to sustained muscle contraction/rigidity, metabolic and respiratory acidosis, hypercarbia, tachycardia, hyperthermia, rhabdomyolysis, and hemodynamic instability.[53] Other mechanisms of calcium control may also be defective in patients with MH (Fig. 24-4).[54] The incidence of MH in adults varies from 1:40,00 to 1:250,000, but may be as high as 1:15,000 in children. Although the knowledge of the pathophysiology and genetics of MH has increased, mortality may still be as high as 9.5%.[55]

Management of the Acute Malignant Hyperthermia Episode

The earlier an episode of MH is identified and treated, the better the outcome. The first sign of an MH reaction is usually an increase in the end-tidal CO_2 ($ETCO_2$) that does not respond to an appropriate increase in ventilation. Nonspecific signs of MH include tachycardia, tachypnea (spontaneous ventilation), and hypertension. Muscle rigidity, masseter spasm, and respiratory and metabolic acidosis develop subsequently. Hyperthermia may occur early or late in the episode. Other conditions that may mimic MH are sepsis, hyperthyroidism, and NMS. If the presumptive diagnosis is an MH episode, any halogenated, inhaled anesthetic should be discontinued and hyperventilation with 100% oxygen initiated. A scoring system has been developed to assist the clinician with the diagnosis of a true MH reaction (Table 24-9).[56] The surgical team should be informed and the procedure aborted or terminated as quickly as possible under intravenous anesthesia. Charcoal filters placed in the anesthesia breathing system will rapidly purge the system of any halogenated anesthetic. The most definitive treatment for MH is dantrolene, a hydantoin derivative that inhibits the pathologic release of Ca^{+2}.[57] The initial intravenous dose of dantrolene is 2.5 mg/kg. Dantrolene should be repeated until the MH reaction has subsided. Some cases of acute MH may require 10 to 20 mg/kg of dantrolene. A newer formulation of dantrolene (Ryanodex, Eagle Pharmaceuticals, Woodcliff Lake, NJ) requires significantly

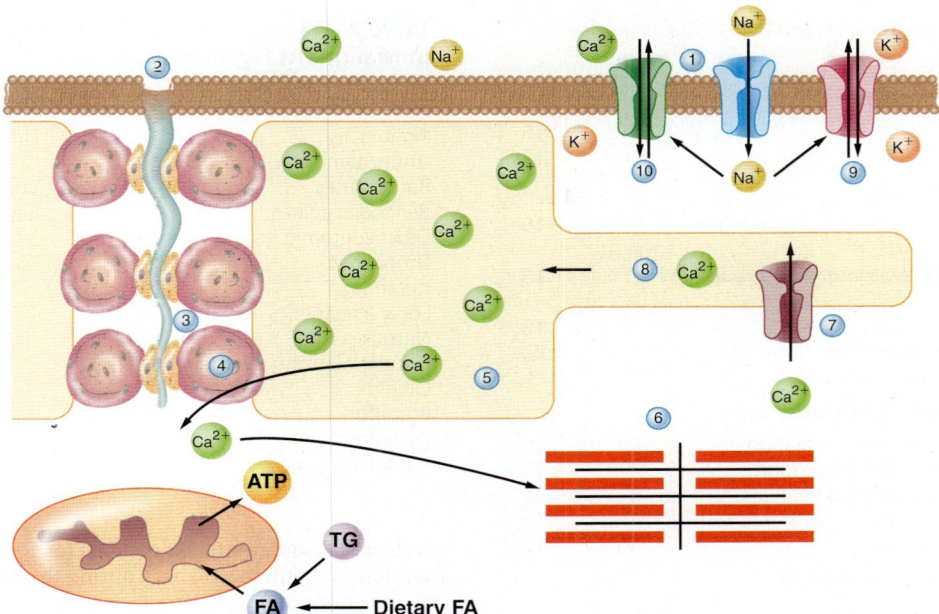

Figure 24-4 Excitation–contraction coupling and malignant hyperthermia. The action potential generated at the endplate region of the neuromuscular junction is propagated down the sarcolemma (muscle plasma membrane) by the opening of voltage-dependent Na^+ channels (1). The action potential continues down into the t-tubules (2) to the dihydropyridine receptors (3). The dihydropyridine receptors in skeletal muscle function as voltage sensors and are coupled to the Ca^{2+} release channels (4). Through this coupled signaling process, the Ca^{2+} release channels are opened, some of the available terminal cisternae Ca^{2+} stores (5) are released, and the levels of myoplasmic Ca^{2+} are elevated. The Ca^{2+} then diffuses to the myofibrils (6) and interacts with the troponin/tropomyosin complex associated with actin (*thin lines*) and allows interaction of actin with myosin (*thick lines*) for mechanical movement. The Ca^{2+} diffuses away from the myofibrils and this Ca^{2+} signal is terminated by an adenosine triphosphate (ATP)-driven Ca^{2+} pump (7), which pumps Ca^{2+} into the longitudinal sarcoplasmic reticulum (8). The Ca^{2+} diffuses from the longitudinal sarcoplasmic reticulum to the terminal cisternae, where it is concentrated for release by Ca^{2+} binding proteins. Na^+ entering during the action potential is subsequently extruded from the cell by the Na^+/K^+-ATPase (9) and possibly through Na^+/Ca^{2+} exchange (10). This latter process would elevate intracellular Ca^{2+} and could result from delayed inactivation of Na^+ currents. A major form of energy for supplying cellular ATP for the ion pumps and numerous other energy-consuming processes is fatty acids (FA) derived from the serum (dietary FA), or from intramuscular triglyceride (TG) stores. Therefore, a defect in the intracellular Ca^{2+} regulating processes (increased Ca^{2+} release or decreased Ca^{2+} uptake), or a defect in the sarcolemma could account for an increase in myoplasmic Ca^{2+}.

less time for reconstitution than the older preparation.[58] Serial arterial blood gas measurements are helpful for tracking the response to therapy. Supportive measures include hyperventilation, treatment of acidosis and hyperkalemia, active cooling, and maintenance of an adequate urinary output (Table 24-10).[59]

Management of the Malignant Hyperthermia Susceptible Patient

The most definitive test for MH susceptibility is the caffeine–halothane contracture test that must be performed at an experienced center. Supplemental genetic testing may detect an identifiable receptor mutation within the family.

Avoidance of known triggering agents is central to developing a plan for anesthesia for an MHS patient. Most intravenous agents such as propofol, benzodiazepines, opioids, nondepolarizing muscle relaxants, and nitrous oxide are safe for MHS patients (Table 24-11). Preparation of the anesthesia machine includes removal or closure of vaporizers, change of all disposable components, and flushing the machine with 100% oxygen (may require >2 hours). Charcoal filters attached to both limbs of the anesthesia breathing circuit before and during the procedure are effective for reducing halogenated anesthetics to less than trace amounts.[60] Preoperative administration of prophylactic dantrolene is not recommended. Dantrolene should, however, be readily available. The Malignant Hyperthermia Association of the United States (MHAUS) has detailed recommendations for management of MHS patients.

Porphyria

The porphyrias are caused by enzymatic deficiencies in the heme synthesis pathway. Heme is an essential component of hemoglobin, myoglobin, and cytochromes. Heme is synthesized in the liver and erythroid tissue from succinyl co-enzyme A and glycine in a process that requires eight enzymatic steps. Each of the porphyrias is caused by a deficiency of one of the eight enzymes that results in an accumulation of porphyrin precursors with toxic effects (δ-aminolevulinic acid, porphobilinogen). The four acute porphyrias that result in acute attacks are: (1) acute intermittent porphyria (AIP, most common), (2) hereditary coproporphyria (HCP), (3) variegate porphyria (VP), and (4) ALA-dehydratase-deficient porphyria (ADP, rarest) (Table 24-12).[61]

AIP typically occurs in young adults and is more common in women. The clinical features of AIP are fever, tachycardia, nausea, emesis, severe abdominal pain, weakness, seizures, confusion, and hallucinations. Muscle weakness can be so severe that respiratory failure ensues. Hyponatremia may occur secondary to inappropriate secretion of ADH. Rarely, severe hypertension and encephalopathy develop. The mental changes that occur during an acute attack are often misdiagnosed as a primary

Table 24-9 Malignant Hyperthermia Clinical Grading Scale

Process I: Muscle Rigidity
Generalized rigidity	15
Masseter rigidity	15

Process II: Myonecrosis
Elevated CK >20,000 (after succinylcholine administration)	15
Elevated CK >10,000 (without exposure to succinylcholine)	15
Cola-colored urine	10
Myoglobin in urine >60 mg/L	5
Blood/plasma/serum K+ >6 mEq/L	3

Process III: Respiratory Acidosis
PetCO$_2$ >55 with controlled ventilation	15
PaCO$_2$ >60 with controlled ventilation	15
PetCO$_2$ >60 with spontaneous ventilation	15
Inappropriate hypercarbia	15
Inappropriate tachypnea	10

Process IV: Temperature Increase
Rapid increase in temperature	15
Inappropriate temperature >38.8°C in perioperative period	10

Process V: Cardiac Involvement
Inappropriate tachycardia	3
Ventricular tachycardia or fibrillation	3

CK, creatine kinase.
See Larach, et al.[56] for full details of this scoring system. Briefly, a case may receive 15 points for the worst presentation in five of the first six categories. A sum of more than 50 points is termed *D6*, almost certainly a case of malignant hyperthermia (MH). A sum of 35 to 49 points is *D5*, very likely to be a case of MH.

Table 24-10 Treatment of an Acute Episode of Malignant Hyperthermia

Discontinue triggering agents
    Halogenated, inhaled anesthetics
    Succinylcholine
    Attach charcoal filters to the anesthesia breathing circuit
Hyperventilate with 100% oxygen
Administer dantrolene 2.5 mg/kg
    Titrate dantrolene to heart rate, temperature, and PaCO$_2$
    Serial monitoring of arterial blood gases
Correction of metabolic acidosis with NaHCO$_3$
Control of dysrhythmias
    Lidocaine
    Avoid calcium channel blockers
Active cooling
    Surface ice packs, body cavity lavage
    Cardiopulmonary bypass for severe cases
    Cease cooling when temperature decreases to 38°C
Correction of hyperkalemia
    Glucose, insulin, bicarbonate, hyperventilation
    Calcium if hyperkalemia causes cardiac dysfunction
After acute episode subsides, monitor for recrudescence of MH
    Disseminated intravascular coagulation (DIC)
    Myoglobinuria

Table 24-11 Safe versus Unsafe Drugs in Malignant Hyperthermia

Safe Drugs	Unsafe Drugs
Antibiotics	Halothane
Antihistamines	Isoflurane
Barbiturates	Enflurane
Benzodiazepines	Sevoflurane
Dexmedetomidine	Desflurane
Droperidol	Succinylcholine
Ketamine	
Local anesthetics	
Nitrous oxide	
Nondepolarizing muscle relaxants	
Opioids	
Propofol	
Propranolol	
Vasoactive drugs	

psychiatric disorder. Attacks may last for 1 to 2 weeks and can be triggered by hormone changes during the menstrual cycle, fasting, infections, and exposure to triggering drugs (Table 24-13). Treatment consists of removal of triggering agents, resolution of infection, and supportive care for skeletal muscle weakness. Specific therapy for an acute attack is the infusion of hemin solution that inhibits 5-aminolevulinic acid synthase and decreases the production of toxic intermediates. Liver transplantation has been effective for some patients with AIP.

The most common of the cutaneous porphyrias is porphyria cutanea tarda (PCT). Other porphyrias that develop skin lesions are congenital erythropoietic porphyria (CEP), erythropoietic protoporphyria (EPP), and X-linked erythropoietic protoporphyria (XLP). Sunlight can cause skin fragility, blisters, vesicles, and bullae.

Management of Anesthesia

The main goal for anesthesia is avoidance of drugs that may trigger acute porphyria. Susceptible patients, however, are rarely identified preoperatively and the triggering potential for many drugs is unknown. More than 300 mutations in the heme synthesis pathway have been identified and many variations in clinical response may occur. Barbiturates and etomidate should be avoided. Propofol, isoflurane, sevoflurane, desflurane, fentanyl, morphine, and ketamine have been administered without complications. Succinylcholine, cisatracurium, and rocuronium are acceptable for muscle relaxation. Regional anesthesia may be administered as well.

Table 24-12 Types of Porphyria

Acute
Acute intermittent porphyria (AIP)
Hereditary coproporphyria (HCP)
Variegate porphyria (VP)
ALA-dehydratase-deficient porphyria (ADP)

Nonacute
Porphyria cutanea tarda (PCT)
Congenital erythropoietic porphyria (CEP)
Erythropoietic protoporphyria (EPP)
X-linked erythropoietic protoporphyria (XLP)

Table 24-13 Drugs Known to Precipitate Acute Porphyria	
Sedatives	**Miscellaneous**
Barbiturates	Calcium channel blockers
Etomidate	Clonidine
Benzodiazepines	Aminophylline
Analgesics	Amiodarone
Pentazocine	Hydralazine
Antipyrine	Estrogens
Aminopyridine	Metoclopramide
Ropivacaine	
Ketorolac	
Ketamine	
Anticonvulsants	
Phenytoin	
Carbamazepine	
Valproic acid	
Oxcarbazepine	
Ethosuximide	
Antimicrobials	
Sulfonamides	
Chloramphenicol	
Erythromycin	
Fluconazole	
Griseofulvin	
Clindamycin	
Rifampin	
Nitrofurantoin	

Acute porphyria should be considered in patients with unexplained delayed emergence from anesthesia or postoperative muscle weakness.[62] Urinary porphobilinogen is markedly elevated during an acute attack and can be detected with a rapid test kit within 5 minutes.

Cholinesterase Disorders

Plasma cholinesterase (pseudocholinesterase, butyrylcholinesterase) is an enzyme synthesized in the liver. This enzyme hydrolyzes succinylcholine, mivacurium, procaine, chloroprocaine, tetracaine, and cocaine. The most significant complication for the anesthesiologist is prolonged apnea after succinylcholine. The molecular genetics of cholinesterase inheritance is not simple as 20 variants have been described. Some variants produce cholinesterase with very little activity and succinylcholine-induced paralysis may last for several hours. Individuals with other variants may have a prolongation of succinylcholine activity that is not clinically discernible. A few genetic variants produce a cholinesterase that accelerates the hydrolysis of succinylcholine, thereby producing a shorter duration of action. Individuals with genetically deficient cholinesterase are not known to have other pathologic conditions. There is some evidence that plasma cholinesterase variants in some ethnic groups may impart a protective effect against atherosclerosis.

Acquired deficiencies of cholinesterase are most notably caused by hepatic disease. Other diseases associated with decreased cholinesterase activity include carcinomas, uremia, connective tissue diseases, malnutrition, and myxedema. Plasma cholinesterase, however, must be decreased by more than 75% for there to be a clinically significant decrease in succinylcholine hydrolysis. Drugs that may interfere with succinylcholine metabolism include neostigmine, pyridostigmine, echothiophate, cyclophosphamide, chlorpromazine, and organophosphate insecticides.

Management of Anesthesia

Preoperative knowledge of a plasma cholinesterase abnormality allows the anesthesiologist to avoid the use of drugs that are hydrolyzed by cholinesterase and the course of anesthesia will be uneventful. The usual clinical presentation, however, of a cholinesterase abnormality is prolonged apnea after succinylcholine. Apnea can be very prolonged if additional succinylcholine is administered after tracheal intubation, or a nondepolarizing muscle relaxant is given followed by reversal with neostigmine.

A prudent clinical practice is to be certain that recovery from the initial dose of succinylcholine has occurred before administering more muscle relaxant. Mechanical ventilation and adequate sedation should be continued until full recovery of neuromuscular function is assured.

If prolonged apnea after succinylcholine occurs, laboratory testing should be performed after the patient has fully recovered. Inheritance of atypical cholinesterase is classic and there are three genotypes: normal (EuEu), heterozygous (EuEa), and homozygous abnormal (EaEa). The two tests that provide the most information are a cholinesterase activity level, and the dibucaine number (Table 24-14).

Glycogen Storage Diseases

The glycogen storage diseases (GSD) are inherited disorders caused by abnormal enzymes that regulate glycogen synthesis and breakdown (Fig. 24-5). These diseases have various manifestations and organ involvement (Table 24-15). There are, however, three common critical components: (1) *acidosis* related to fat and protein metabolism in metabolically active glycogen stores; (2) *hypoglycemia* is a constant risk and results from failure to metabolize glycogen to glucose; and (3) *cardiac and hepatic dysfunction* secondary to destruction and replacement of normal tissue by accumulated glycogen.

Many of the enzymes involved in glycogen metabolism have different isoforms controlled by many different genes. The clinical features can vary markedly within each type of GSD.

Management of Anesthesia

Type 1 (Von Gierke Disease; Glucose-6-phosphatase Deficiency)

Von Gierke disease is inherited as an autosomal recessive trait. Many patients survive to adulthood. Short stature and hepatomegaly are characteristic. Hypoglycemia, acidosis, and seizures

Table 24-14 Classic Cholinesterase Genotypes			
Genotype	Cholinesterase Activity	Dibucaine Number	Succinylcholine Apnea (min)
Normal (EuEu)	++++	78–86	5
Heterozygote (EuEa)	++	51–70	15
Homozygote (EaEa)	+	18–26	120–300

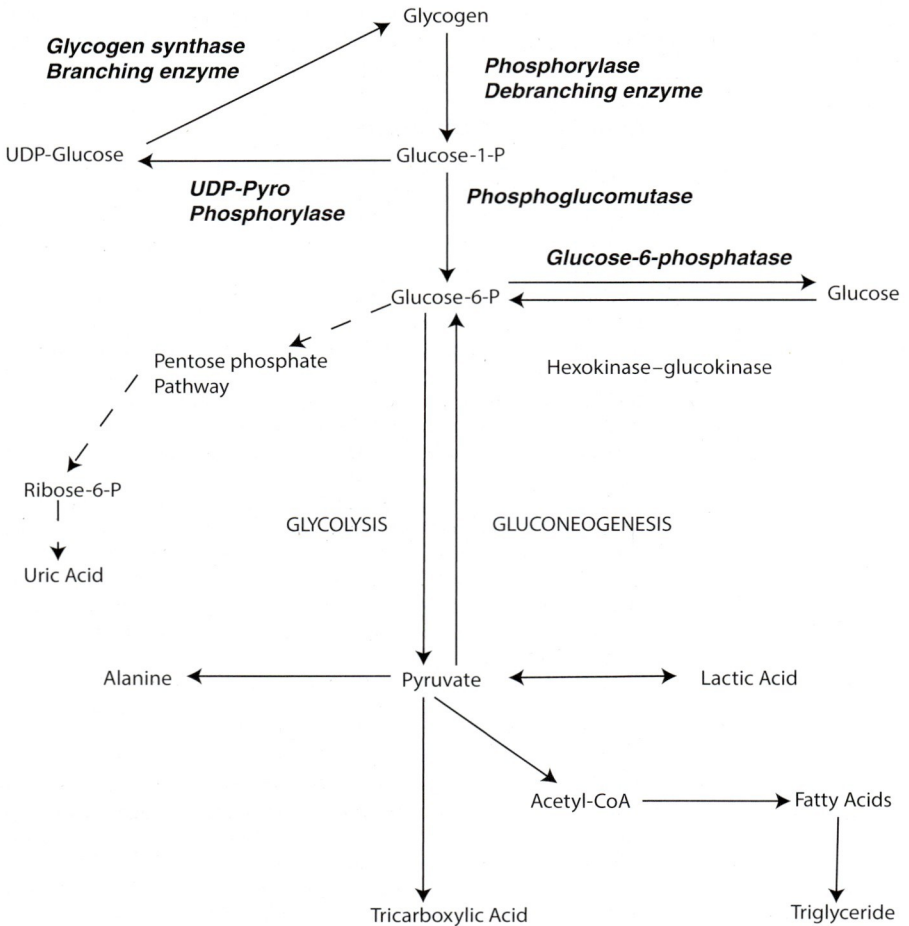

Figure 24-5 Simplified pathway of glycogen synthesis and degradation. (Adapted from Ozen H. Glycogen storage diseases: new perspectives. *World J Gastroenterol.* 2007;13:2541–2553.)

are common. Prolonged bleeding due to platelet dysfunction has been described. These patients do not tolerate fasting and should have preoperative intravenous glucose containing fluid therapy. Preoperative hyperalimentation is often used to reduce liver glycogen stores. Anesthesia and surgery cause release of counterregulatory hormones (epinephrine, norepinephrine) that can result in severe lactic acidosis. Cardiac dysrhythmias and cardiac arrest have occurred during anesthesia when acidosis develops. Preoperative intravenous glucose should be administered at 1.5 times the estimated hepatic production rate of glucose. This will reduce insulin secretion and minimize the effects of the stress response. If acidosis develops, a continuous infusion of bicarbonate should be administered. Portacaval shunting has been performed with limited success in patients with hepatic cirrhosis.

Type II (Pompe Disease; Lysosomal Acid Glucosidase Deficiency)

The infantile form is a devastating disease with a very poor prognosis. There is a deficiency of lysosomal acid glucosidase with an accumulation of glycogen in heart, liver, muscle, and CNS. Infants present with generalized weakness, hypotonia, and massive cardiomegaly. Glycogen infiltration of cardiac muscle leads to concentric hypertrophic cardiomyopathy. These patients are prone to tachydysrhythmias. If enzyme replacement therapy (ERT) is started by 9 months of age, it can decrease cardiac glycogen accumulation. Late-onset Pompe disease may manifest in older children or adults and has a milder clinical course.[63] The late onset form is characterized by a slow progressive myopathy culminating in respiratory failure. Preoperative evaluation should include an ECG, echocardiogram, and liver function tests. There are a significant number of reported cases of cardiac arrest during anesthesia in patients with the infantile form and mortality is high.[64] Induction of anesthesia with sevoflurane or high-dose propofol is more likely to result in adverse cardiac events, especially in patients with a left ventricular mass index (LVMI) greater than 350 g/m^2. A preoperative echocardiogram with measurement of LVMI is highly recommended.[65] If feasible, surgery should be performed with local or regional anesthesia.[66] If general anesthesia is required, a carefully monitored induction with ketamine is recommended.

Type III (Forbes or Cori Disease)

Type III GSD is due to a deficiency of amylo-1,6-glucosidase (glycogen debrancher). Symptoms are due to defective catabolism of glycogen and excessive glycogen deposition in the liver. Hepatomegaly and short stature are common. Mild hyperlipidemia and elevated serum transaminase concentrations are characteristic. Fasting induces ketotic hypoglycemia. Cirrhosis develops in the third and fourth decade of life. The enzyme deficiency in skeletal and cardiac muscle leads to weakness and cardiomyopathy. There are subgroups based on skeletal muscle involvement. Anesthetic concerns include macroglossia, hypotonia, sensitivity to nondepolarizing muscle relaxants, hypertrophic cardiomyopathy, and tachydysrhythmias. Hypoglycemia is a particular risk as it may

Table 24-15 Classification of Glycogen Storage Diseases

Type *Eponym*	Prevalence	Enzyme Defect	Main Clinical Features	Laboratory Abnormalities	Progressive Skeletal Muscle Deformities	Progressive Cardiac Involvement
Type I *Von Gierke*	1:200,000	Glucose-6-phophatase	Short stature, hepatomegaly, hepatic adenomas, seizures, developmental delay, failure to thrive, vomiting, xanthomata, nephromegaly, osteoporosis, inflammatory bowel disease	Symptomatic hypoglycemia, lactic acidosis, elevated triglycerides, platelet dysfunction, elevated uric acid, glucosuria, high urinary calcium	Muscle cramping, exercise intolerance	Severe cardiac arrhythmias, sudden death with fasting
Type II *Pompe, early onset*	1:400,000	Lysosomal acid glucosidase (acid maltase)	Growth delay, developmental delay, hepatomegaly, macroglossia, progressive hypotonia, death <1 yr of age	Markedly elevated creatinine kinase (CK) levels, elevated AST/ALT, LDH	Progressive cardiac, respiratory, skeletal muscle weakness	Massive cardiomegaly, concentric LV hypertrophy, outflow tract obstruction, cardiomyopathy, CHF, SVT, VT, VF, cardiorespiratory arrest with anesthesia
Type II *Pompe, late onset*	1:400,000	Lysosomal acid glucosidase (acid maltase)	Onset in second to seventh decade of life, progressive respiratory failure	Markedly elevated CK levels, elevated AST/ALT, LDH	Slowly progressive myopathy	None
Type IIIa1 *Forbes Cori's*	1:400,000	Amylo-1,6-glucosidase (glycogen debrancher)	Childhood-onset muscle weakness, hepatic dysfunction	Fasting hypoglycemia, mildly to moderately elevated ALT/AST, elevated CK, hyperlipidemia	Slowly progressive muscle weakness, gross motor delay	Concentric LV hypertrophy, rare cardiac dysfunction or arrhythmias
Type IIIa2 *Forbes*	1:400,000	Amylo-1,6-glucosidase (glycogen debrancher)	Hepatic dysfunction with onset in childhood and persistence in adulthood, adult-onset muscle weakness	Fasting hypoglycemia, mildly to moderately elevated ALT/AST, elevated CK, hyperlipidemia	Slowly progressive muscle weakness, gross motor delay	Concentric LV hypertrophy, rare cardiac dysfunction or arrhythmias
Type IIIa3 *Forbes*	1:400,000	Amylo-1,6-glucosidase (glycogen debrancher)	Hepatic dysfunction with onset in childhood and resolution in adulthood, adult-onset muscle weakness	Fasting hypoglycemia, mildly to moderately elevated ALT/AST, elevated CK, hyperlipidemia	Slowly progressive muscle weakness, gross motor delay	Concentric LV hypertrophy, rare cardiac dysfunction or arrhythmias
Type IIIa4 *Forbes*	1:400,000	Amylo-1,6-glucosidase (glycogen debrancher)	Adult-onset skeletal muscle symptoms	Fasting hypoglycemia, mildly to moderately elevated ALT/AST, elevated CK, hyperlipidemia	Slowly progressive muscle weakness, gross motor delay	Concentric LV hypertrophy, rare cardiac dysfunction or arrhythmias
Type IIIb *Forbes*	1:400,000	Amylo-1,6-glucosidase (glycogen debrancher)	Hepatic dysfunction	Fasting hypoglycemia, mildly to moderately elevated ALT/AST, elevated CK, hyperlipidemia	None	Rare cardiac dysfunction or arrhythmias

(continued)

Table 24-15 Classification of Glycogen Storage Diseases (CONTINUED)

Type Eponym	Prevalence	Enzyme Defect	Main Clinical Features	Laboratory Abnormalities	Progressive Skeletal Muscle Deformities	Progressive Cardiac Involvement
Type IV *Andersen*		Glycogen branching enzyme	Failure to thrive, hepatosplenomegaly, hypotonia, esophageal varices, portal hypertension, late hepatic cirrhosis/failure, neuropathy	Elevation of CK, moderate elevation of AST/ALT Myopathy, muscle weakness, exercise intolerance, exertional dyspnea, neuronal involvement	Two forms: stable and progressive	Dilated cardiomyopathy, CHF
Type V *McArdle*	1:100,000	Muscle glycogen phosphorylase	Muscle glycogenoses, exercise intolerance, *no* hepatic involvement	Episodic myoglobinuria	Muscle cramps	None
Type VI *Hers*	Very rare	Hepatic glycogen phosphorylase	Mild symptoms, short stature, hepatomegaly	Fasting ketotic hypoglycemia, mild hyperlipidemia, myoglobinuria, elevated AST/ALT, proximal renal tubular acidosis (rarely)	Hypotonia, muscle cramps	Usually none, rare cardiac failure with enzyme variant
Type VII *Tarui's*	Very rare	Muscle phosphofructokinase	Muscle glycogenoses, exercise intolerance, *no* hepatic involvement	Episodic myoglobinuria, hemolytic anemia	Muscle cramps	None
Type IX	Very rare	Glycogen phosphorylase kinase	Mild symptoms, short stature, hepatomegaly of X-linked variant	Fasting ketotic hypoglycemia, mild hyperlipidemia, myoglobinuria, elevated AST/ALT, proximal renal tubular acidosis (rarely)	Hypotonia, muscle cramps	Usually none, rare cardiac failure with enzyme variant
Type XI *Fanconi-Bickel*	Very rare	Glucose transporter	Hepatic glycogenosis, Fanconi renal syndrome	Short stature, hepatic glycogenosis, Fanconi renal syndrome	None	None
Type 0	Unknown	Hepatic glycogen synthase	Short stature, developmental delay (22%), seizures	Postprandial hyperglycemia and hyperlactatemia, recurring ketotic hypoglycemia, metabolic acidosis, fasting ketonuria	No skeletal muscle involvement	None

Data from: Weinstein DA, Wolfsdorf JI. Glycogen storages diseases: a primer for clinicians. *Endocrinologist.* 2002;12:531–538; Ozen H. Glycogen storage diseases: new perspectives. *World J Gastroenterol.* 2007;13:2541–2553; Chen M. Glycogen storage diseases. In: Monga SPS, ed. *Molecular Pathology of Liver Diseases.* New York: Springer; 2011:677–681; and Santer R, Schneppenheim R, et al. Fanconi-Bickel syndrome: the original patient and his natural history, historical steps leading to the primary defect, and a review of the literature. *Eur J Pediatr.* 1998;157:783–797.

occur within 4 to 6 hours of fasting. Continuous administration of intravenous glucose should be done in the preoperative period. Metabolic acidosis with ketoacids may occur even with careful management of anesthesia. Administration of lactate containing intravenous fluids is generally avoided. Succinylcholine should also be avoided because of the potential for rhabdomyolysis. Postoperative respiratory complications may occur due to respiratory muscle weakness, ineffective cough, poor clearance of secretions, and residual effects of anesthetics.[67,68]

Type IV (Andersen Disease, Amylopectinosis)

This is a very rare disorder caused by a deficiency of glycogen-branching enzyme (GBE). This leads to an accumulation of glycogen in liver, muscle, nerves, and cardiac muscle. Clinical manifestations are diverse depending on the affected tissues.[69] The severest form of the disease presents in infancy with hepatosplenomegaly, failure to thrive, and hypotonia. Esophageal varices, portal hypertension, and cirrhosis are common by 2 years of age. Muscle weakness with exercise intolerance and exertional dyspnea occur. Cardiac effects include dilated cardiomyopathy and congestive heart failure. The only effective treatment is liver transplantation. A neuromuscular variant presents in adults with sensory loss in the legs, gait disturbances, difficulty with urination, and cognitive dysfunction.

Type V (McArdle Disease)

McArdle disease is an autosomal recessive disorder due to a deficiency of glycogen phosphorylase in muscle. Skeletal muscle is unable to mobilize glycogen stores for sustained exercise and cramping with exercise is characteristic of this disorder. GSD type V is a multisystem disease that presents in adolescence with progressive muscle weakness, myalgia, and lack of endurance. Episodes of myoglobinuria with overexertion are due to rhabdomyolysis and may occur after administration of succinylcholine. Acute renal failure with rhabdomyolysis has been reported after cardiac surgery.[70] Tourniquets should not be used and frequent automated measurements of blood pressure should be done with caution. Whether patients with McArdle disease are susceptible to MH is controversial.[71] Dantrolene may, however, have a beneficial effect on non-MH rhabdomyolysis. Cardiac muscle is typically not affected in patients with McArdle disease.

Type VI (Hers Disease)

This relatively benign disorder is caused by a deficiency in a regulatory enzyme that controls hepatic glycogen phosphorylase. Symptoms include hepatomegaly, mild hypoglycemia, hyperlipidemia, and ketosis. A mild cardiomyopathy may develop with aging.[72] Lactic acidosis and hyperuricemia do not occur. Symptoms usually improve with age. Fever and acidosis after an anesthetic with ketamine, halothane, and succinylcholine have been reported. Liver transplantation has been performed in patients with more severe forms of Hers disease.

Type VII (Tarui Disease)

Tarui disease is caused by a deficiency of muscle phosphofructokinase. It is similar to McArdle disease and is characterized by muscle cramping. Patients with Tarui disease present with exercise intolerance and episodic myoglobinuria. There is usually no cardiac or hepatic involvement. The same enzyme defect in erythrocytes causes chronic hemolytic anemia. There are four forms of the disease: classic, late-onset, infantile (usually fatal), and hemolytic.[73]

Type IX

GSD type IX is caused by a deficiency of hepatic glycogen phosphorylase kinase and is clinically similar to Hers disease (type VI). There are several isoforms of the enzyme controlled by many genes. The clinical presentation can be very heterogeneous. Most patients have short stature, hypotonia, muscle cramps, exertional myoglobinuria, and hyperlipidemia.

Type XI (Fanconi–Bickel Syndrome)

Fanconi–Bickel syndrome is a rare autosomal recessive disorder caused by mutations of the glucose-transporting enzyme (Glut-2). These patients have short stature, hepatomegaly, glucose and galactose intolerance, fasting hypoglycemia, and a characteristic proximal renal tubular acidosis. They usually survive to adulthood.[74]

Type 0

Type 0 GSD is caused by a deficiency of the hepatic form of glycogen synthase that causes a decrease in liver glycogen. Hepatomegaly, consequently, does not occur. Clinical features include fasting ketotic hypoglycemia, short stature, and osteopenia. Many patients are asymptomatic and the disease is often diagnosed by the unsuspected discovery of hypoglycemia.[75] As preoperative fasting may cause hypoglycemia, intravenous administration of a glucose-containing solution may be necessary.

Mucopolysaccharidoses

The mucopolysaccharidoses (MPS) are rare familial diseases inherited as autosomal recessive disorders. The disorders are a result of a deficiency of a specific lysosomal enzyme that cleaves mucopolysaccharides. The result is an accumulation of mucopolysaccharides in the brain, heart, bone, liver, cornea, and tracheobronchial tree.[76]

There are eight types of MPS and several subtypes (Table 24-16). All forms of MPS are characterized by progressive craniofacial deformities, joint and skeletal anomalies, cardiac involvement, and early death from pulmonary infection or cardiac failure. The upper airway is characterized by a depressed nasal bridge, short neck, macroglossia, and tongue protrusion secondary to infiltration of mucopolysaccharides. Chronic rhinitis, enlarged tonsils and adenoids, and obstructive sleep apnea are typical. Clinical phenotypes within each MPS type range from severe to attenuated variants with longer life expectancy.

Hunter and Hurler syndromes are the best known of the MPS diseases. Respiratory infection and cardiac disease (valvular and ischemic) lead to death at an early age. MPS type IV (Morquio syndrome) is associated with the most significant skeletal deformities. Respiratory insufficiency with marked chest wall deformity is common. Severe dysplasia or absence of the odontoid process frequently leads to chronic or acute myelopathy. Neurologic manifestations such as developmental delay and hydrocephalus are due to MPS depositions in the CNS. Cardiac involvement occurs in most forms of MPS except the Sanfilippo variants (Type III). MPS infiltration of the myocardium, cardiac valves, and conducting system often lead to myocardial ischemia, cardiomyopathy, and dysrhythmias.

Patients with MPS develop coarse facial features (gargoylism), lumbar lordosis, stiff joints, chest deformities, small stature, corneal opacities, hepatomegaly, and splenomegaly. The diagnosis of MPS is based on detection of urinary glycosaminoglycans and measurement of enzyme activity in the serum, leukocytes, and fibroblasts. No definitive therapy exists for MPS. Depending on the specific enzyme defect, however, ERT may lessen the effects of the disease. ERT, however, does little to ameliorate the cardiac or neurologic effects of MPS.[77] The role of human stem cell transplantation (HSCT) for the treatment of MPS is controversial.

(text continued on page 632)

Table 24-16 Mucopolysaccharidoses

Type Eponym	Main Clinical Features	Prevalence	Enzyme Defect	Urinary Mucopolysaccharides	Progressive Craniofacial Deformities	Progressive Joint or Skeletal Deformities	Progressive Cardiac Involvement
Type I(H) *Hurler*	Severe Hurler phenotype, mental retardation, corneal clouding, death <14 yrs	1:100,000	α-L-Iduronidase	Dermatan sulfate Heparan sulfate	Macrocephaly, coarse facies, macroglossia, hydrocephalus	Stiff joints, thoracolumbar kyphosis, possible odontoid hypoplasia, short neck, short stature	Coronary intimal and valvular thickening, mitral regurgitation, cardiomegaly
Type I(S) *Scheie*	Corneal clouding, normal intelligence Survival to adulthood	1:500,000	α-L-Iduronidase	Dermatan sulfate	Mild to coarse facies, macroglossia, prognathia	Short neck, normal stature	Aortic regurgitation
Type I(H/S) *Hurler-Scheie*	Intermediate phenotype	1:111,000	α-L-Iduronidase	Dermatan sulfate Heparan sulfate	Macrocephaly, coarse facies, macroglossia, micrognathia	Diffuse joint limitation, short neck, short stature	Mitral and aortic valvular thickening or regurgitation
Type II *Hunter*	Variable course: severe to mild Survival to adulthood, possible mental retardation	1:162,000	Iduronidate-2-sulfatase	Dermatan sulfate	Macrocephaly, coarse facies, hydrocephalus	Diffuse joint limitation, short neck, short stature	Coronary intimal thickening, ischemic cardiomyopathy
Type IIIA *Sanfilippo*	Behavioral problems, aggression	1:114,000	Heparan-N-sulfatase	Heparan sulfate	Mildly coarse facies	Mildly stiff joints, lumbar vertebral dysplasia, short stature	Minimal to none
Type IIIB *Sanfilippo*	Progressive dementia, seizures Survival: 2nd to 3rd decade	1:211,000	α-N-acetyl-glucose-amidase	Heparan sulfate	Mildly coarse facies	Stiff joints that may not extend fully, ambulation difficulties	Minimal to none
Type IIIC *Sanfilippo*	Intrafamilial variability, mild dysmorphism	1:1,407,000	α-N-acetyl-glucose-amidase N-acetyltransferase	Heparan sulfate	Mildly coarse facies	Stiff joints that may not extend fully, walking problems	Minimal to none
Type IIID *Sanfilippo*	Coarse hair, clear cornea Normal height	1:1,056,000	N-acetyl-glucosamine-6-sulfatase	Heparan sulfate	Mildly coarse facies	Stiff joints that may not extend fully, walking problems	Minimal to none

Type	Incidence	Enzyme deficiency	Accumulated substrate	Physical features	Craniofacial features	Musculoskeletal features	Cardiac features
Type IVA Morquio	1:1,201,000	N-acetyl-galactosamine-6-sulfatase	Keratan sulfate	Short trunk type of dwarfism, fine corneal opacities, skeletal dysplasia spondyloepiphyseal dysplasia, final height <125 cm	Mildly coarse facies	Joint laxity, severe kyphoscoliosis, odontoid hypoplasia, short neck, C1–C2 subluxation possible, short stature	Aortic regurgitation
Type IVB Morquio	1:248,000	β-Galactosidase	Keratan sulfate	Same as MPS IVA but milder, final height >120 cm	Mildly coarse facies	Joint laxity, severe kyphoscoliosis, odontoid hypoplasia, short neck, C1–C2 subluxation possible, short stature	Aortic regurgitation
Type VI Maroteaux–Lamy	1:100,000	N-acetyl-galactosamine-4-sulfatase	Dermatan sulfate	Hurler phenotype with marked corneal clouding, normal intelligence	Macrocephaly, coarse facies, macroglossia	Mild joint stiffness, kyphoscoliosis, odontoid hypoplasia, short stature	Mitral and valvular thickening or regurgitation
Type VII Sly	1:2,111,000	β-Glucuronidase	Dermatan sulfate	Highly variable; dense inclusion in granulocytes	Macrocephaly, coarse facies	Mild joint stiffness, kyphoscoliosis, odontoid hypoplasia, short stature	Mitral and valvular thickening or regurgitation, aortic dissection

Data from Diaz JH, Belani KG. Perioperative management of children with mucopolysaccharidoses. *Anesth Analg.* 1993;77:1261–1270; Yeung AH, Cowan MJ, Horn B, et al. Airway management in children with mucopolysaccharidoses. *Arch Otolaryngol.* 2009;135:73–79; and Meikle PJ, Hopwood JJ, Clague AE, et al. Prevalence of lysosomal storage diseases. *JAMA.* 2011;281:249–254.

Management of Anesthesia

MPS patients have significant deformities of the upper airway and cardiorespiratory dysfunction and the risks of perioperative management must not be underestimated. The variability of clinical abnormalities in patients with MPS requires individualized treatment for each patient. Some types of MPS produce severe airway and cardiac effects, whereas other types have mild dysfunction.

Airway management can be extremely challenging. All options for airway management, including oropharyngeal airways, supraglottic airways, video laryngoscopes, and flexible fiberscopes should be readily available prior to induction of anesthesia. Careful positioning of the head and neck is required to minimize the risk of spinal cord damage. A slow, controlled inhalation induction with sevoflurane in oxygen is preferred. Mask ventilation, however, can become difficult and a supraglottic airway may be helpful during induction. Laryngoscopy is complicated by thick, noncompressible tissue of the upper airway, macroglossia, copious airway secretions, and bony deformities of the head and neck. Muscle relaxants should be avoided until the airway has been secured.[78,79] Postoperative respiratory complications are common.[80]

Careful preoperative evaluation with echocardiography is indicated for some types of MPS (e.g., Hurler syndrome). The presence of cardiac dysfunction will certainly influence the type of anesthesia and intraoperative monitoring.

Osteogenesis Imperfecta

Osteogenesis imperfecta (OI) is a heterogeneous group of diseases characterized by susceptibility to bone fractures due to a defect in collagen type I (Table 24-17). Type I collagen is the primary component of the extracellular matrix of bone and skin. Inheritance is autosomal dominant for most forms (type VI, autosomal recessive) and the incidence is 1 in 20,000 to 50,000 live births. OI is a multisystem disease characterized by brittle bones, osteoporosis, joint laxity, tendon weakness, cardiac anomalies, blue sclera,

Table 24-17 Anesthetic Considerations in Osteogenesis Imperfecta

Type	Clinical Severity	Inheritance	Mutant Gene	Manifestations	Anesthetic Considerations	Lifespan
I	Mild, nondeforming	Autosomal dominant	Col1A/2	Increased frequency of fractures; short stature; blue sclera; progressive hearing impairment	A: Normal dentition B: Dentinogenesis imperfecta	Long-term survival[a]
II	Perinatally lethal	Autosomal dominant	COL1A/2	Multiple fractures in utero; micromelia; bowed LEs; small thorax; respiratory failure		Death in utero or within first month of life
III	Progressively deforming	Autosomal dominant	COL1A/2	Growth retardation; multiple fractures; progressive kyphoscoliosis; vertebral compression; blue sclera; dentinogenesis imperfecta	Airway anomalies	Death in second to fourth decade
IV	Moderately deforming	Autosomal dominant	COL1A/2	In utero fractures; fractures with minor trauma; bowing of LEs with weight bearing	A: Normal dentition B: Dentinogenesis imperfecta; midface or mandibular deformity	Long-term survival[a]
V	Moderately deforming	Autosomal dominant	Unknown	In utero fractures; fractures with minor trauma; bowing of LEs with weight bearing	Potential for midface or mandibular deformity	Long-term survival[a]
VI	Moderately to severely deforming	Autosomal recessive	Unknown	In utero fractures; fractures with minor trauma; bowing of LEs with weight bearing	Potential for midface or mandibular deformity	Long-term survival[a]

[a]With appropriate medical care.
LEs, lower extremities.
Adapted from: Van Dijk FS, Pals G, Van Rijn RR, et al. Classification of osteogenesis imperfecta revisited. *Eur J Med Genet*. 2010;53(1):1–5; and Stynnowick GA, Tobias JD. Perioperative care of the patient with osteogenesis imperfect. *Orthopedics*. 2007;30(12):1043–1049.

platelet dysfunction, abnormal airway anatomy, and abnormal dentition. Pectus deformities of the chest and kyphoscoliosis may lead to restrictive pulmonary disease and respiratory failure.[81]

The most common cardiac lesion is aortic insufficiency. Aortic root dilation may lead to aortic dissection. Mitral valve prolapse and insufficiency can occur.[82] Central nervous manifestations include craniovertebral instability and atlantoaxial subluxation that can lead to quadriparesis. Hydrocephalus is common.

Management of Anesthesia

Patients with OI need to be carefully and gently positioned as minor trauma can cause fractures. The upper airway should be carefully examined and cervical range of motion determined. Megalocephaly and a short neck can make direct laryngoscopy difficult and alternative intubation techniques may be required. A preoperative echocardiogram may be beneficial if there is a history of valvular heart disease. Induction of anesthesia can be performed with inhalation or intravenous techniques. Regional anesthesia is generally avoided because of the risk of trauma to the spine and the potential for coagulopathy from platelet dysfunction. Caudal analgesia, however, has been used in selected patients.[83] Mild intraoperative temperature elevation can occur in patients with OI. There is no evidence that OI patients are at increased risk for MH.[84]

ANEMIAS

Anemia is a common finding among patients undergoing anesthesia. The absolute or relative deficiency of red blood cells (RBCs) is commonly due to blood loss, but can be due to inherited or acquired disorders of RBC production (Table 24-18). Several physiologic responses compensate for anemia. These responses include increased cardiac output, increased plasma volume, decreased blood viscosity, and increased levels of 2,3-diphosphoglycerate (Table 24-19).

It is estimated that one third of blood transfusions are administered for postoperative anemia. Many institutions have implemented some form of preoperative blood management that includes identification of preoperative anemia. The goal of these programs is to identify specific causes of anemia and institute appropriate therapy prior to elective surgery in order to reduce the need for perioperative blood transfusion.[85]

Table 24-18   Types of Anemia

Nutritional Deficiency
Iron
Vitamin B_{12}
Folate
Anemia of chronic illness

Hemolytic
Spherocytosis
Glucose-6-phosphate dehydrogenase deficiency
Pyruvate kinase deficiency
Immune mediated
Drug-induced ABO incompatibility

Hemoglobinopathies
Hemoglobin S (sickle cell)
Thalassemia major (Cooley anemia)
Thalassemia intermedia
Thalassemia minor

Table 24-19   Compensatory Mechanisms to Increase Oxygen Delivery with Chronic Anemia

Increased cardiac output
Increased RBC 2,3-diphophoglycerate
Increased P-50
Increased plasma volume
Decreased blood viscosity

Nutritional Deficiency Anemias

Deficiencies of iron, vitamin B_{12}, or folate (vitamin B_9) produce characteristic anemias. Nutritional anemia can be a result of decreased intake or the inability to absorb vital nutrients. Chronically ill patients may suffer a combination of these deficiencies with the added burden of a systemic inflammatory response that impairs the patient's ability to process nutrients and causes an *anemia of chronic illness*.

Iron deficiency anemia typically occurs because of a diet low in iron or chronic, slow blood loss. The hemogram of a person with iron deficiency anemia shows a low total hemoglobin, low mean corpuscular volume (MCV) (microcytosis), and a low mean corpuscular hemoglobin (MCH) (hypochromia).

Megaloblastic anemia is caused by a deficiency of vitamin B_{12} or folate. A critical deficiency of these vitamins inhibits cell division and maturation in the bone marrow. Vitamin B_{12} deficiency can be due to inadequate intake or poor absorption (pernicious anemia). Although the deficiency of either vitamin B_{12} or folate can cause megaloblastic anemia, neurologic deficits are associated with B_{12} deficiency. The neurologic changes are a result of patchy cerebral and spinal cord demyelination. The neurologic deficits may improve with vitamin B_{12} therapy. Regional anesthesia is relatively contraindicated if neurologic dysfunction is present. The administration of nitrous oxide is controversial. Nitrous oxide inactivates methionine synthetase, a B_{12}-based enzyme that catalyzes the conversion of homocysteine to methionine. Methionine synthetase deficiency causes megaloblastic cellular changes and neurologic deficits. The short exposure to nitrous oxide that occurs during a routine anesthetic is unlikely to have detrimental effects.[86] Prolonged or frequent exposure to nitrous oxide has caused confirmed instances of adverse hematologic and neurologic effects.

Folate deficiency is most frequently associated with alcoholism, pregnancy, or malabsorption.

Hemolytic Anemias

The normal lifespan of an RBC is 120 days and any cause of premature RBC destruction can cause anemia. The causes of premature RBC destruction can be due to fragility of the RBC cytoskeleton, immune mediated destruction, or a deficiency in a cytoplasmic enzyme.

Hereditary Spherocytosis

Hereditary spherocytosis and hereditary elliptocytosis are inherited conditions that cause misshapen and fragile RBCs. The abnormally shaped RBCs are removed from the circulation by the spleen and the severity of the anemia can be subclinical, mild, or severe. Other effects of premature RBC destruction include cholelithiasis, splenomegaly, and jaundice. Moderate to severe disease usually presents in infancy with hyperbilirubinemia. Splenectomy can be performed to alleviate the anemia.[87,88] Splenectomy is avoided in young children, if possible, as loss of the spleen can cause an overwhelming postsplenectomy infection (OPSI). OPSI is usually caused by encapsulated bacterial pathogens such as *Streptococcus pneumoniae, Haemophilus influenzae,* and *Neisseria meningitides.* Cholecystectomy due to cholelithiasis is commonly performed.

Glucose-6-Phosphate Dehydrogenase Deficiency

Glucose-6-phosphate dehydrogenase (G6PD) is the most common human enzymopathy. G6PD catalyzes the first step in the pentose phosphate shunt. NADPH is produced in this step and is deficient in the RBCs of affected individuals. NADPH deficiency increases the vulnerability of RBCs to oxidative stressors. Oxidative stress can result from the consumption of fava beans, exposure to drugs, infections, and metabolic derangements (e.g., diabetic ketoacidosis). The mechanism by which the "stressed" RBCs hemolyze is unknown. Many drugs and chemicals can cause hemolysis in patients with G6PD deficiency. Although anesthetic drugs are not likely to cause hemolysis, many common drugs can and should be avoided in the perioperative period (Table 24-20). Drugs that promote the formation of methemoglobin (prilocaine, nitroprusside) should also be avoided.[89]

Pyruvate Kinase Deficiency

Pyruvate kinase converts phosphoenolpyruvate to pyruvate and produces nearly half of the ATP in the RBCs. PK deficiency dramatically reduces the amount of ATP available to RBCs and shortens their lifespan. Clinical presentation is highly variable and may present in infancy with anemia and hyperbilirubinemia. Patients with PK deficiency can develop iron overload with or without blood transfusion and monitoring for signs of iron overload is necessary. Splenectomy may increase RBC lifespan. Pregnancy may be associated with increased hemolysis. Anesthesia care is directed at the degree of anemia and potential comorbidities.[90]

Immune Hemolytic Anemias

Immune hemolytic anemia may be classified at autoimmune, drug-induced, or alloimmune. Autoimmune hemolytic anemia occurs when autoantibodies are formed that attack antigens on the RBC. RBCs that are bound by the autoantibodies are damaged by activation of the complement cascade. The spectrum of illness caused by autoimmune hemolysis is broad. The autoantibodies may be further characterized as cold, warm, or mixed based on their range of activity at different temperatures. Autoimmune hemolytic anemia can be associated with infection, malignancy, lymphoma, organ transplantation, and connective tissue diseases.[91] Cold autoimmune hemolytic anemia is triggered in the perioperative period when a patient is exposed to a cold environment or receives cold intravenous solutions. Cooling during cardiopulmonary bypass could precipitate severe hemolysis unless a preoperative exchange transfusion is performed.

Drugs can act as haptens that bind to proteins on the RBC membrane forming a protein–hapten antigen that stimulates antibody production. The antibodies attack the antigen and lyse the RBC. Drugs that are frequently implicated in drug-induced hemolysis include penicillin, cephalosporins, and α-methyldopa. Anesthetic drugs have not been shown to induce hemolysis by this mechanism.[92]

Alloimmune hemolytic anemia occurs when a patient is transfused with incompatible donor blood. Hemolytic disease of the newborn is an example of this type of reaction. In this instance, appropriate pre-existing antibodies damage or destroy targeted "nonself" RBCs.

Hemoglobinopathies

Hemoglobinopathies occur when there is a genetic miscoding in the amino acid sequence of the hemoglobin. The end result is anemia and multisystem injury that can be severe. Normal hemoglobin (hemoglobin A) is comprised of four molecular subunits: two alpha (α-) globins, two beta (β-) globins, and ferrous iron. Normal and variant hemoglobins are listed in Table 24-21. Hemoglobinopathies are commonly found in areas of the world that are endemic for malaria. Individuals who are heterozygous for the hemoglobinopathy may have a resistance to malaria. Individuals who are homozygous for the hemoglobinopathy, however, have a broad spectrum of illnesses due to anemia, accumulation of excessive iron and hemoglobin precursors, immunocompromise, tissue ischemia, and inflammation. The most common hemoglobinopathies are sickle cell disease (SCD) and thalassemia. Together, these two hemoglobinopathies are the most severe genetic disorders in the world.

Sickle Cell Disease

SCD is transmitted as an autosomal recessive trait with an asymptomatic carrier state. In the United States, 1 in 600 African-Americans have SCD and 8% to 10% of the African-American population carries the trait.

Table 24-20 Drugs That Can Produce Hemolysis in Patients with Glucose-6-Phosphate Dehydrogenase Deficiency

Aspirin (high doses)	Penicillin
Chloramphenicol	Phenacetin
Dapsone	Phenazopyridine
Doxorubicin	Phenazopyridine
Furazolidone	Primaquine
Isoniazid	Quinidine
Methylene blue	Quinine
Nalidixic acid	Streptomycin
Naphthalene	Sulfacetamide
Niridazole	Sulfanilamide
Nitrofurantoin	Sulfapyridine

Table 24-21 Hemoglobin Variants

Hemoglobin	Globin Chains	Type
A	α2β2	Normal adult
A2	α2δ2	Normal adult (minor)
F	α2γ2	Normal fetal
S	α2S2	Sickle (HbS)
C	α2βC2	HbC (clinical illness)
E	α2βE2	HbE (clinical illness)
Bart's	γ4	α-Thalassemia (fetal demise)
H	β4	α-Thalassemia major

Table 24-22 Mechanisms of Cellular and Tissue Injury in Sickle Cell Disease

Capillary obstruction with tissue ischemia
RBC and platelet adhesion to the endothelium
Activation of coagulation with thrombosis and/or embolism
Reperfusion injury
Hemolysis and release of free hemoglobin
Leukocytosis and immune system activation
Free radical injury due to leukocyte superoxide release
Nitric oxide depletion due to superoxide release and uptake by free Hgb
Release of cytokines and inflammatory mediators
Endothelial injury
Iron accumulation

SCD is caused by a single amino acid substitution in the β-globin molecule. Valine is substituted for glutamine at the sixth amino acid position. The valine changes the physical characteristics of the affected hemoglobin under conditions of oxygen desaturation. When exposed to low oxygen tension, HbS polymerizes into fiber-like chains that distort the normal biconcave shape into the crescent or "sickle cell" shape. Sickled RBCs are relatively inflexible and have difficulty moving through capillaries. The spleen removes these abnormal cells from the circulation, reducing their lifespan to 12 to 17 days (normal = 120 days). The pathophysiology of SCD occurs because of microvascular obstruction, tissue ischemia, and chronic anemia. Less evident and insidious mechanisms cause other detrimental effects (Table 24-22).

Patients with SCD display a remarkable variability in the severity of the disease. Some patients experience severe complications and death at an early age whereas others have only mild symptoms. The severity of the symptoms has been correlated with the amount of fetal hemoglobin (HbF) that persists beyond the neonatal period. A higher concentration of HbF reduces symptoms and complications. The clinical manifestations of SCD affect almost all systems (Table 24-23).

Table 24-23 Complications of Sickle Cell Disease

Hematologic: hemolytic anemia, aplastic anemia, leukocytosis
Spleen: autoinfarction, hyposplenism, splenic sequestration
Central nervous system: stroke, hemorrhage, aneurysm, meningitis
Musculoskeletal: painful crisis, bone marrow hyperplasia, avascular necrosis, osteomyelitis, bone infarction, skeletal deformity, growth retardation, cutaneous ulceration
Cardiac: cardiomegaly, pulmonary hypertension, cor pulmonale, diastolic dysfunction, cardiomyopathy
Pulmonary: acute chest syndrome, asthma, fibrosis, pulmonary infarction, sleep apnea, pneumonia, hypoxemia, thromboembolism
Renal: papillary necrosis, glomerular sclerosis, renal failure
Genitourinary: priapism, infection
Hepatobiliary: jaundice, hepatitis, cirrhosis, cholelithiasis, cholestasis
Eye: retinopathy, hemorrhage, visual loss
Immune: immunosuppression, leukocytosis
Psychosocial: depression, anxiety, substance abuse, narcotic dependence

Several recurrent problems that cause significant morbidity and mortality afflict SCD patients. *Vaso-occlusive crisis (VOC)* is often the first and most frequent manifestation of SCD and is secondary to musculoskeletal ischemia. The pain of VOC ranges from mild to excruciating. Mild cases can be managed with oral analgesics, rest, and hydration. Severe VOC requires hospitalization, parenteral narcotics, intravenous hydration, supplemental oxygen, RBC transfusion, and in some cases regional analgesia. The incidence of VOC in the perioperative period is 10%. *Acute chest syndrome (ACS)* has a mortality of 1% to 20% and represents the single greatest threat to patients with SCD. Clinical manifestations of ACS are chest pain, dyspnea, cough, wheezing, hypoxemia, and chest infiltrates (radiography). ACS may be caused by thrombosis, embolism (clot, fat), and infection. The incidence of ACS is higher in children and may be due to infection. The treatment of ACS is supplemental oxygen, hydration, analgesia, and respiratory support. Antibiotics may be empirically administered pending the results of sputum culture. Severe ACS or ACS unresponsive to usual therapies may require RBC transfusion. The incidence of ACS after abdominal surgery is 10% to 20%. Factors that may contribute to postoperative ACS are pain, splinting, narcotics, and hypoventilation. The risk of postoperative ACS can be reduced by preoperative RBC transfusion and postoperative incentive spirometry. *Sequestration crisis* occurs when the splenic rate of RBC removal exceeds the rate of RBC production. Severe anemia and hemodynamic instability can occur rapidly. Sequestration may be an indication for splenectomy. Patients with SCD require a high and continuous rate of RBC production. Mild bone marrow suppression triggered by a viral infection (parvovirus B19) can precipitate an *aplastic crisis*. Asthma occurs in 50% of SCD patients and *pulmonary hypertension* occurs in 10% of SCD patients. Mortality is increased when either condition is present.[93]

Preventive treatment of SCD patients includes oral hydroxyurea to increase HbF production, pneumococcal vaccination to reduce the risk of sepsis, and daily penicillin in children less than 5 years of age. Transfusion of RBCs is performed when anemia is severe or as a preventive measure to reduce the amount of HbS. Bone marrow transplantation can be curative and is an option for severe SCD. Removal and genetic manipulation of the SCD patient's own bone marrow to increase HbF production is currently being investigated.[94]

Management of Anesthesia

Patients with SCD frequently require anesthesia and surgery. Patients enrolled in comprehensive sickle cell clinics are likely to have current surveillance evaluations by experienced hematologists. The clinic notes may provide important information. Preoperative evaluation is directed at identification of underlying organ dysfunction. Patients with a history of respiratory dysfunction, ECG abnormalities, functional limitations, or indicators of cor pulmonale should have a preoperative echocardiogram. Common echocardiographic findings include left ventricular hypertrophy, right ventricular dilation, atrial enlargement, and pulmonary hypertension.

Preoperative RBC transfusion to achieve a hemoglobin level of 10 g/dL can be performed and may reduce the likelihood of sickle cell complications (ACS, VOC). In most cases, a simple transfusion is preferable to an exchange transfusion. Exchange transfusion is indicated when preparing patients for cardiopulmonary bypass. There is a high incidence of alloimmunization among SCD patients and obtaining cross-matched RBCs can be time consuming.

Active measures to maintain normothermia and normovolemia should be employed in the perioperative period. Extremity tourniquets can be used in situations where the success of the surgery is dependent on their use. The complication rate after tourniquet use is 12%.

Administration of narcotics has been implicated as a cause of postoperative ACS. The use of regional analgesia and nonnarcotic analgesics to reduce the need for narcotics are encouraged. Spinal anesthesia for Cesarean section has been shown to decrease perioperative blood loss and reduce the need for postoperative narcotics.[95] If narcotics are required, careful monitoring of oxygenation and sedation should be performed. Early recognition of developing ACS and aggressive therapy may be critical to successful treatment.[96,97]

Thalassemia

Thalassemia is the result of deficient production of either the α- or β-globin components of hemoglobin. α-Thalassemia is caused by underproduction of α-globin and β-thalassemia from a deficit of β-globin. Anemia is caused by an inadequate amount of normal hemoglobin. The underproduction of one of the globin chains is not balanced by underproduction of the other globin chain. The globin that can be produced in normal amounts is overproduced. These excess globin chains are ineffective as they are not paired with the correct globin to form a functional tetramer. The excess unpaired globin chains cause cellular and tissue injury. Ineffective erythropoiesis causes severe bone marrow hyperplasia, skeletal deformity, and skeletal fragility. Multisystem injury is caused by many of the mechanisms that cause systemic injury in SCD.

The terms thalassemia major, intermedia, and minor are a reflection of the severity of the anemia that correlates with underproduction of the globin chain. Many patients with thalassemia minor do not require RBC transfusion. Routine transfusion of RBCs maintains an adequate hemoglobin level, suppresses bone marrow hyperplasia and extramedullary erythropoiesis. Routine transfusion, however, inevitably results in iron overload. Iron overload causes cardiac, hepatic, immune, and endocrine system dysfunction. Chelation therapy may reduce the amount of iron overload. Bone marrow transplantation may be considered for severely affected individuals.

Management of Anesthesia

Patients with thalassemia often require anesthesia for cholecystectomy, splenectomy, vascular access, and correction of skeletal abnormalities. The preoperative evaluation should include measurement of the hemoglobin and the search for evidence of cardiac, hepatic, and endocrine dysfunction from iron overload. There is a high incidence of alloimmunization and cross-matching blood can require considerable time.

Facial dysmorphism can cause difficulties with airway management.[98] Spontaneous hemorrhage from extramedullary bone marrow deposits has been reported. Although spinal anesthesia has been successfully used for Cesarean section, bone marrow deposits in the spinal canal can be considered to be a relative contraindication to neuraxial anesthesia.

Connective Tissue Diseases

The four most common connective tissues diseases are rheumatoid arthritis (RA), systemic lupus erythematosus (SLE), systemic sclerosis (SSc, scleroderma), and the inflammatory myopathies (dermatomyositis [DM]/polymyositis [PM]). Although many patients have well-defined diseases, many others have overlap syndromes with features of different connective tissue diseases.

The etiologies of the connective tissue diseases are unknown, although the immune system is clearly involved in the cascade of pathologic events that cause the clinical manifestations. Each of these diseases has effects on joints and diffuse systemic effects.

Rheumatoid Arthritis

RA is a chronic, autoimmune, and inflammatory disease characterized by symmetric polyarthropathy and diverse systemic effects. Although the etiology is unknown, research continues to unravel the pathogenesis. There are interactions between environmental factors and genetic susceptibility that initiates the process that causes RA. Smoking, exposure to silica, infection, and periodontal disease are associated with an increased risk of RA. Activated endothelial cells attract adhesion molecules that stimulate T cells and B lymphocytes. The release of cytokines (tumor necrosis factor [TNF], interleukins) accelerates the inflammatory cascade. B lymphocytes produce autoantibodies (rheumatoid factor) that further increase cytokine production.[99] Seventy-five percent of RA patients have measurable levels of rheumatoid factor. The pathologic effects of RA begin with cellular hyperplasia of the synovium followed by invasion of lymphocytes, plasma cells, macrophages, and fibroblasts. Cartilage and articular surfaces are ultimately destroyed.

The metacarpophalangeal and interphalangeal joints of the hands are involved first. The knee is the most frequently involved joint of the leg. The upper cervical spine is affected in 85% of patients with RA. Atlantoaxial and subaxial instability can lead to compression of the spinal cord. Plain radiography and CT of the cervical spine will demonstrate the bony changes. MRI is better suited to study the effects on the spinal cord. The degree of cord compression, however, may not correlate with symptoms. Although a very rare event, spinal cord damage after laryngoscopy and tracheal intubation has been reported.[100] Intradural cord compression secondary to rheumatoid nodules or pannus formation can occur. RA commonly affects the joints of the larynx, resulting in limitation of vocal cord movement and edema of the laryngeal mucosa that can progress to airway obstruction. The laryngeal effects and arthritic changes in the temporomandibular joint can complicate laryngoscopy and tracheal intubation.

Extra-articular and systemic effects of RA are diverse (Table 24-24). Cardiovascular disease is a common cause of mortality and there is a high incidence of subclinical cardiac dysfunction. Pericarditis occurs in 20% to 50% of RA patients and can produce restrictive pericarditis and cardiac tamponade. Other cardiovascular manifestations include coronary artery disease, myocarditis, aortitis (aortic root dilation, aortic valve insufficiency), diastolic dysfunction, dysrhythmias, and pulmonary hypertension.[101] Pulmonary changes include interstitial lung disease, reduced oxygen diffusing capacity, obstructive and restrictive lung disease, pulmonary nodules, and pleural effusions. Several of the antirheumatic drugs can cause or accentuate pulmonary damage.[102] Renal disease as a direct result of RA is uncommon, but glomerulonephritis and amyloidosis can cause kidney failure. Mild anemia is present in almost all patients with RA. The anemia may be secondary to decreased erythropoiesis or a side effect of drug therapy.

Neurologic complications of RA include peripheral nerve compression from joint destruction and noncompressive neuropathies (mononeuritis multiplex) secondary to vasculitis of the blood vessels supplying affected nerves (vasa nervorum). Cervical myelopathy may be secondary to cervical spine compression. Rheumatoid vasculitis can affect cerebral blood vessels resulting in headache, hemiparesis, aphasia, and confusion.

Table 24-24 Extra-articular Manifestations of Rheumatoid Arthritis

Skin	**Peripheral Nervous System**
Raynaud phenomenon	Compression syndromes
Digital necrosis	Mononeuritis
Eyes	**Central Nervous System**
Scleritis	Dural nodules
Corneal ulceration	Necrotizing vasculitis
Lung	**Liver**
Pleural effusions	Hepatitis
Pulmonary fibrosis	**Blood**
Heart	Anemia
Pericarditis	Leukopenia
Cardiac tamponade	
Coronary arteritis	
Aortic insufficiency	
Kidney	
Interstitial fibrosis	
Glomerulonephritis	
Amyloid deposition	

Table 24-25 Adverse Effects of Drugs Used to Treat Connective Tissue Diseases

Class of Drugs	Adverse Effects
Corticosteroids	Hypertension, osteoporosis, hyperglycemia
Immunosuppressants	
Methotrexate	Hepatotoxicity, anemia, leucopenia
Azathioprine	Biliary stasis, leucopenia
Cyclosporine	Nephrotoxicity, hypertension, hypomagnesemia
Cyclophosphamide	Hemorrhagic cystitis, cholinesterase inhibition
Leflunomide	Hepatotoxicity, weight loss, hypertension
Mycophenolate mofetil	Nausea, emesis, diarrhea
TNF Antagonists	
Etanercept	Infections, tuberculosis
Infliximab	Lymphoma, heart failure
Adalimumab	Infection, T-cell lymphoma, fatigue
Golimumab	Infection, lymphoma
Certolizumab	Infection, lymphoma
Interleukin-1 Antagonists	
Anakinra	Infection, skin irritation
Interleukin-6 Antagonists	
Tocilizumab	Infection, headache, stomatitis, fever
T-cell Inhibitors	
Abatacept	Infection
CD20 Monoclonal Antibody	
Rituximab	Infection, infusion reaction
Janus Kinase Inhibitors	
Tofacitinib	Infection, anemia, leucopenia
Antimalarials	
Hydroxychloroquine	Myopathy, retinopathy
Antibiotics	
Sulfasalazine	Nausea, neutropenia, hepatotoxicity
Heavy Metal Chelators	
Penicillamine	Autoimmune dermatoses, glomerulonephritis
Aspirin	Platelet dysfunction, peptic ulcers, sensitivity
NSAIDs	Peptic ulcer, leucopenia, coronary artery disease
COX-2 Inhibitors	Nephrotoxicity, cardiovascular dysfunction
Gold	Aplastic anemia, dermatitis, nephritis

The disease process of immunoinflammatory modulation that causes RA is complex and monotherapy is unlikely to be completely successful. There are four groups of antirheumatic drugs: nonsteroidal anti-inflammatory drugs (NSAIDs), corticosteroids, disease-modifying antirheumatic drugs (DMARDs), and biologic DMARD drugs. NSAIDs reduce pain and inflammation, but do little to affect the ultimate course of the disease. Corticosteroids are effective, but the side effects associated with long-term use limit their usefulness. DMARDs target T and B cells. Of the DMARDs, methotrexate has proven to be very effective and is often the initial drug of choice. Biologics target inflammatory mediators such as TNF, and interleukins. Potential side effects of biologic DMARDs are increased susceptibility to infection and cancer (Table 24-25).[103] Surgical procedures such as synovectomy, tenolysis, and joint replacement are performed to relieve pain and restore joint function.

Management of Anesthesia

RA is a multisystem disease with diverse clinical manifestations. Although the joint disabilities may be obvious, less evident are the effects of RA on the heart, lung, liver, CNS, and kidneys. The type and severity of systemic dysfunction must be considered when planning an anesthetic for the patient with RA.[104]

Arthritic changes in the temporomandibular joints, cricoarytenoid joints, and the cervical spine can complicate rigid, direct laryngoscopy, and tracheal intubation. The incidence of atlantoaxial subluxation may exceed 40% in RA patients and flexion of the neck can compress the spinal cord. Many patients with RA are asymptomatic with respect to cervical spine disease (Fig. 24-6). Preoperative imaging studies (radiography, CT, MRI) may be indicated if the degree of cervical involvement is unknown. An intubation technique that minimizes cervical movement is recommended. Awake intubation, video laryngoscopy, or flexible, fiberscope-assisted tracheal intubation should be considered. Cricoarytenoid arthritis produces edema of the larynx and may decrease the size of the glottis inlet, necessitating the use of a smaller than predicted tracheal tube.

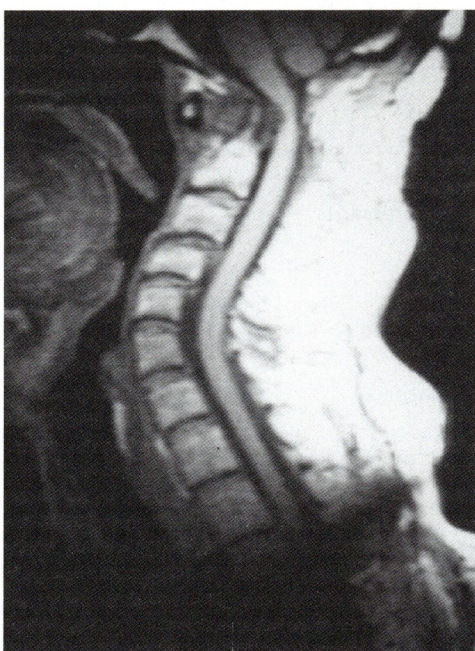

Figure 24-6 Magnetic resonance imaging of a cervical spine in a patient with rheumatoid arthritis. Although the patient had no neurologic symptoms, there was severe spinal stenosis in the upper cervical spine.

The degree of cardiopulmonary involvement by the rheumatoid process will influence the selection of anesthetics and level of intraoperative monitoring. The need for postoperative ventilatory support should be anticipated if severe pulmonary disease is present.

RA patients receiving corticosteroids may require corticosteroid supplementation during the perioperative period. Aspirin and other anti-inflammatory drugs interfere with platelet function and clotting may be abnormal. RA drugs that alter immune function can increase the risk of postoperative infection. Although methotrexate does not seem to increase the risk of infection, it is recommended that anti-TNF biologics be withheld before surgery.[105]

Restriction of joint mobility necessitates careful positioning of the patient during surgery. The extremities should be positioned to minimize the risk of neurovascular compression and further joint injury. Preoperative examination of joint motion will help determine how the extremities and head should be positioned. Regional anesthesia should be considered, but must be individualized. Factors such as technical impediments to nerve identification from joint deformity, potential for platelet dysfunction, and the patient's ability to tolerate positioning for a period of time must be factored into the decision for regional anesthesia.[106]

Systemic Lupus Erythematosus

SLE is a multisystem disease caused by complex interactions between genetic susceptibility, environmental factors, and alterations in innate and adaptive immunity. Deficiencies in the complement cascade, B-cell immunity, T-cell signaling, and apoptotic clearance have also been implicated. Anti-DNA antibodies, antiphospholipid antibodies, anticardiolipin antibodies, and lupus anticoagulant may be detected in many patients with SLE. The diverse clinical manifestations of SLE are undoubtedly secondary to many genes that influence the immune system.[107] Environmental influences include ultraviolet light exposure, vitamin D deficiency, and infection. Numerous drugs have been associated with lupus including clonidine, enalapril, captopril, hydralazine, methyldopa, isoniazid, and procainamide.

The clinical manifestations of SLE are varied and many can be life-threatening. The most common presenting features are polyarthritis and dermatitis. The arthritis is migratory and can involve any joint, including the cervical spine. The classic malar rash occurs in one third of SLE patients. Renal disease is present in 60% of SLE patients and is a common cause of morbidity. Lupus nephritis causes proteinuria, decreased creatinine clearance, and hypertension. Dialysis or renal transplantation is required for 10% to 20% of lupus patients. CNS manifestations of lupus are caused by vasculitis and include seizures, stroke, dementia, psychosis, myelitis, and peripheral neuropathy.

Cardiovascular manifestations of SLE include pericarditis, accelerated atherosclerosis, noninfectious endocarditis (Libman–Sacks), ventricular dysfunction, and dysrhythmias. Although pericardial effusions are common, cardiac tamponade is unusual. The pulmonary effects of SLE include serositis, interstitial disease, pulmonary embolism, pulmonary hemorrhage, and pulmonary hypertension. Pulmonary function studies typically reveal a restrictive disease pattern and a decreased diffusion capacity.[108] Hoarseness, stridor, and upper airway obstruction can be caused by cricoarytenoiditis. Gastrointestinal manifestations of SLE include esophageal dysmotility, peritonitis, pancreatitis, hepatitis, and bowel ischemia.

Despite the diverse effects of SLE and the lack of specific therapy, survival of SLE patients has significantly improved. The antimalarials hydroxychloroquine and chloroquine suppress production of cytokines and TNF-α and increase long-term survival. IVIG may induce remission in selected patients. Lupus nephritis has been treated with many drugs including corticosteroids, cyclophosphamide, azathioprine, tacrolimus, and methotrexate. More recently, monoclonal antibodies such as rituximab, belimumab, and epratuzumab have proven to be effective. The potential for side effects from any of the SLE drugs is significant (Table 24-25).[109]

Management of Anesthesia

Careful preoperative evaluation of the SLE patient is necessary because of the diverse effects of the disease.[110,111] Preoperative chest radiography, pulmonary function testing, and echocardiography may be indicated if the clinical history suggests cardiopulmonary dysfunction. Preoperative quantitation of renal function may be necessary. Although minor changes in hepatic function are common, these effects are generally not significant. Patients with SLE are at increased risk for infection.

Arthritic involvement of the cervical spine is unusual and tracheal intubation is generally not difficult. The potential for laryngeal involvement and upper airway obstruction does, however, require clinical evaluation of laryngeal function. Should postextubation laryngeal edema or stridor occur, intravenous corticosteroids are effective.

Drugs for the treatment of SLE will influence the choice of anesthetics. Patients receiving corticosteroids will usually require the administration of perioperative corticosteroids. Cyclophosphamide inhibits cholinesterase and may prolong the response to succinylcholine. Azathioprine can increase dose requirements for nondepolarizing muscle relaxants.

Systemic Sclerosis (Scleroderma)

SSc is characterized by changes in the microvasculature that cause inflammation and fibrosis of the skin, blood vessels, and internal organs. It appears that an environmental trigger when applied to genetically susceptible individuals initiates an autoimmune response that releases inflammatory mediators that cause edema and accelerated fibrosis of tissues.[112]

The skin becomes swollen and thickened and eventually becomes fibrotic and taut leading to joint immobility. Raynaud phenomenon occurs in 85% of SSc patients and may be the presenting symptom.

More than 80% of SSc patients develop interstitial lung disease that progresses to pulmonary fibrosis and pulmonary hypertension. The leading cause of death in patients with SSc is pulmonary hypertension and right ventricular failure.[113] Cardiac manifestations of SSc include myocardial fibrosis, fibrosis of the conduction system, and pericarditis. Echocardiography may reveal reduced systolic function and diastolic dysfunction.[114]

Renal dysfunction is common and secondary to renal vasculopathy. Five percent of SSc patients develop a scleroderma renal crisis with hypertension, retinopathy, and a rapid deterioration in renal function.[115] Gastrointestinal motility is decreased and frequent episodes of gastroesophageal reflux and aspiration pneumonitis exacerbate pulmonary dysfunction. Decreased small intestine and colonic motility can cause pseudo-obstruction.

Therapy is directed at immunomodulation with immunosuppressants such as cyclophosphamide, mycophenolate mofetil, azathioprine, and methotrexate. ACE inhibitors are commonly used to treat hypertension. Monoclonal antibodies directed at B-cells and cytokines are being investigated. Stem cell transplantation is effective in selected patients.[116]

Management of Anesthesia

SSC, like other connective tissue diseases is a multisystem disease with diverse manifestations. The type of anesthesia must be guided by the presence and severity of organ dysfunction.

Tracheal intubation can be quite difficult. Fibrotic and taut skin markedly reduces active and passive motion of the temporomandibular joint. Awake, fiberoptic-assisted tracheal intubation may be required. On some occasions, an awake tracheostomy may be necessary. Orotracheal intubation is preferred as fragility of the nasal mucosa increases the risk of severe nasal hemorrhage from nasotracheal intubation.

Esophageal dysmotility and gastroesophageal reflux increase the risk of aspiration pneumonitis during anesthesia. Chronic hypoxemia is common and is secondary to interstitial lung disease and pulmonary hypertension. Compromised myocardial function and coronary arteriosclerosis may necessitate invasive cardiovascular monitors and echocardiography during surgery. Venous access can be challenging and central venous cannulation may be required. Myopathy is present in most patients with SSc and an increased sensitivity to muscle relaxants can occur.

Regional anesthesia may be a suitable alternative to general anesthesia. The response to local anesthetics may be prolonged.[117] Anesthesiologists are frequently consulted for treatment of Raynaud phenomenon.

Inflammatory Myopathies (Dermatomyositis/Polymyositis)

Five diseases comprise the inflammatory myopathies: DM, PM, necrotizing autoimmune myositis (NAM), inclusion-body myositis (IBM), and overlap myositis. Although the clinical features of the five diseases are diverse, severe muscle weakness and noninfectious muscle inflammation are present in all five. Circulating autoantibodies are common.[118]

DM is the most common of the five and is the result of antibody-induced complement activation that causes muscle necrosis. Presenting features of DM are proximal muscle weakness and a characteristic skin rash. The skin rash consists of a purplish discoloration of the eyelids (heliotrope rash), periorbital edema, and scaly erythematous lesions on the knuckles (Gottron papules). DM occurs in children and adults. The presenting symptoms of PM are muscle pain and proximal muscle weakness that occur in the second decade of life. Fifty percent of patients with DM and PM have pulmonary disease. The pulmonary manifestations are interstitial pneumonitis, alveolitis, and bronchopneumonia. Aspiration pneumonia is very common.[119] Myocardial fibrosis can cause congestive heart failure and dysrhythmias.

Patients with NAM typically have an acute onset of severe proximal muscle weakness. IBM is characterized by the slow onset of proximal muscle weakness and frequent falls.

The treatment of DM, PM, and NAM is initially with corticosteroids, followed by immunosuppressants (azathioprine, methotrexate, cyclosporine, mycophenolate). IVIG and rituximab have also been used with success. No drugs have been shown to be effective for the treatment of IBM.

Management of Anesthesia

The reported experience with anesthesia in patients with inflammatory myopathies is very limited. Patients with DM have limited motion of the temporomandibular joint and decreased mouth opening. Rigid, direct laryngoscopy is usually difficult and alternative intubation techniques are often required. Tracheal intubation of patients with PM is generally not difficult. Dysphagia and gastroesophageal reflux are common and there is an increased risk of aspiration pneumonitis. Gastrointestinal perforations that require surgical intervention are common in patients with PM. Cardiac dysfunction may be subclinical and preoperative echocardiography may be informative.

It should be anticipated that the response to muscle relaxants will be varied. It would be prudent to avoid the use of succinylcholine as hyperkalemia may occur. Short-acting nondepolarizing muscle relaxants are preferred. Postoperative mechanical ventilation may be required for patients with significant muscle weakness and interstitial lung disease.

Skin Disorders

Most diseases of the skin are localized and cause few systemic effects or complications during the administration of anesthesia. Epidermolysis bullosa (EB) and pemphigus, two blistering skin diseases, can result in perioperative complications.

Epidermolysis Bullosa

EB is a rare skin disease that can be inherited or acquired. Patients with heritable forms have abnormalities in the anchoring systems of skin layers. The acquired forms are autoimmune disorders in which autoantibodies are produced that destroy the basement membrane of the skin and mucosa. The end result is the loss of normal intercellular bridges and separation of skin layers, intradermal fluid accumulation, and bullae formation (Fig. 24-7). Many gene mutations that contribute to abnormal skin structure

Figure 24-7 The ultrastructure of the zones of the skin. The diagram demonstrates where skin separation occurs in different types of epidermolysis bullosa (EB). (Adapted from Uitto J, Christiano AM. Molecular genetics of the cutaneous basement membrane zone. *J Clin Invest.* 1992;90:687–692.)

have been identified and there may be as many as 30 subtypes of EB. For clinical purposes there are four types depending on where skin separation occurs: epidermolysis simplex (EBS), separation within the epidermis; junctional epidermolysis (JEB), separation at the lamina lucida; epidermolysis bullosa dystrophica (DEB), separation beneath the lamina densa; and Kindler syndrome (mixed EB), separation at different levels.[120]

EBS is generally benign. Some types of JEB have marked involvement of the airway and are lethal by one year of age.[121]

DEB is caused by a defect in type VII collagen. Progressive blistering and scarring causes severe deformities of the fingers and toes with pseudosyndactyly formation (Fig. 24-8). Secondary infection and malignant degeneration of the skin are common. The esophagus is involved with resultant dysphagia, esophageal strictures, and poor nutrition. Dilated cardiomyopathy with ventricular dysfunction, aortic root dilation, and intracardiac thrombi can develop.[122] Anemia secondary to poor nutrition and recurrent infection is common. Streptococcal infection–induced glomerulonephritis with albuminuria occurs. Hypoplasia of tooth enamel often necessitates extensive dental restorations. Patients with DEB rarely survive beyond the third decade of life.

Medical therapy for DEB has not been very successful. Gene therapy, injection of fibroblasts, and bone marrow stem cell transplantation are under investigation. Surgical therapy is directed at improvement of hand function and improved nutrition.

Management of Anesthesia

Preoperative presence of an unrecognized cardiomyopathy should be considered as it will certainly influence the selection

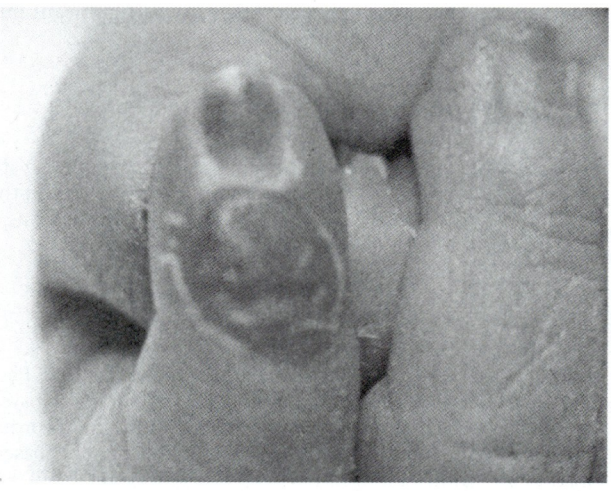
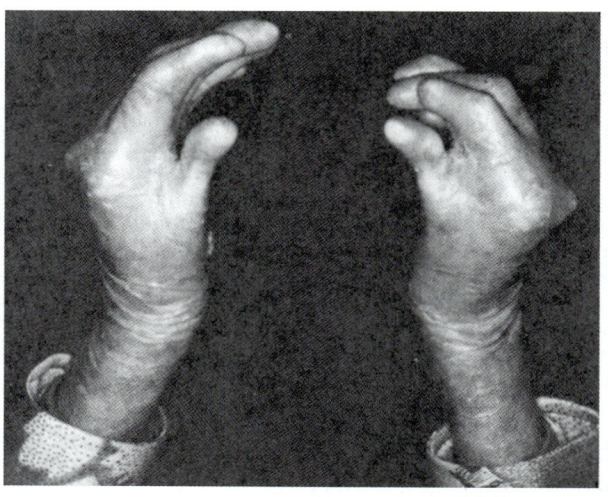

Figure 24-8 Epidermolysis bullosa. **A:** Bullous lesion of the finger in a neonate with epidermolysis bullosa. **B:** Hands of an older child with epidermolysis progression to produce severe scarring and pseudosyndactyly. (Courtesy of James E. Bennett, MD, Division of Plastic Surgery, Indiana University School of Medicine, Indianapolis, IN.)

of anesthesia and monitoring. Many patients with DEB have decreased physical activity from limb deformities and their history of exercise tolerance may not be an accurate reflection of cardiac function. Preoperative echocardiography may provide the best evaluation of cardiac function.

It is critical that trauma to the skin and mucous membrane be minimized during the intraoperative period. Movement should be minimized as much as possible. Lateral shearing forces applied to the tissue are especially damaging, whereas pressure applied perpendicular to the skin is not as hazardous. Gel pads (defibrillation pads) can be used for ECG monitoring. The blood pressure cuff can be padded with loose cotton dressings or PVC film. Intravenous lines can be secured with a nonadhesive material or sutured in place.

Despite the myriad of potential risks, anesthesia is generally well tolerated when care is rendered at centers with expertise in management of DEB patients. Surgical procedures that are commonly performed include hand reconstruction, dental restorations, esophageal dilation, and gastrostomy. Intravenous and inhalation induction have been used successfully in patients with DEB. Trauma from the face mask should be minimized with the use of a lubricated material. Frictional trauma to the oropharynx can cause large intraoral bullae and hemorrhage. All airway instruments must be well lubricated. Tracheal intubation is generally safe for patients with DEB; however, scarring of the oral cavity with microstomia and tongue immobility increases the difficulty of tracheal intubation. Fiberoptic-assisted tracheal intubation may be required. Nasotracheal intubation has been performed but its use is controversial. The laryngeal mask airway has been used for patients with DEB.[123]

Ketamine may be useful for superficial extremity procedures as it provides good analgesia and may not require supplementation with inhaled anesthetics. Regional anesthesia, including spinal, epidural, and brachial plexus block has been used successfully in patients with DEB.

Pemphigus

Pemphigus is an autoimmune blistering disease that involves extensive areas of the skin and mucous membranes. IgG autoantibodies attack desmosomal proteins, desmoglein 3 and desmoglein 1, leading to loss of cell adhesion and separation of epithelial layers. There are five types of pemphigus: pemphigus vulgaris (PV), pemphigus foliaceous, pemphigus erythematosus, drug-induced pemphigus, and paraneoplastic pemphigus. More than 50 drugs have been implicated as causes of pemphigus.[124]

PV is the most common type and is of most importance to the anesthesiologist because of the occurrence of oral lesions. Oral lesions develop in 50% to 70% of patients with PV. Oropharyngeal lesions can make eating so painful that malnutrition develops. Lesions of the pharynx, larynx, esophagus, urethra, conjunctiva, cervix, and anus can develop. Skin denudation and blister formation cause significant losses of fluid and protein and pose the risk of secondary infection.[125] As with EB, lateral shearing force is more likely to produce bullae than pressure applied perpendicularly to the skin. Systemic corticosteroids are the treatment of choice for pemphigus. Improvement may be seen within days of corticosteroid therapy. Immunosuppressants, immunomodulators, and IVIG can be used to reduce corticosteroid dosage.

Paraneoplastic pemphigus is associated with several malignant tumors, especially lymphomas and leukemias. IgG antibodies are produced that react to desmoglein 3 and desmoglein 1. Oral and cutaneous lesions occur. Obstructive respiratory failure may result from inflammation and sloughing of tracheal tissue.

Management of Anesthesia

Preoperative drug therapy and the extreme fragility of the mucous membranes are primary concerns for management of anesthesia. Corticosteroid supplementation will be necessary during the perioperative period for patients receiving chronic steroid therapy. Management of the airway and tracheal intubation should be performed as described for patients with DEB.[126]

There are no specific contraindications to the use of any intravenous or inhaled anesthetic. Regional anesthesia has been used for PV patients. Methotrexate may produce hepatorenal dysfunction and bone marrow suppression. Cyclophosphamide can prolong the action of succinylcholine by inhibition of cholinesterase.

REFERENCES

1. Mercuri E, Muntoni F. Muscular dystrophies. *Lancet*. 2013;381:845–860.
2. Yilmaz A, Sechtem U. Cardiac involvement in muscular dystrophy: advances in diagnosis and therapy. *Heart*. 2012;98:420–429.
3. Emery AE. The muscular dystrophies. *Lancet*. 2002;359:687–695.
4. Gilbreath HR, Castro D, Iannaccone ST. Congenital myopathies and muscular dystrophies. *Neurol Clin*. 2014;32:689–703.
5. Taylor A, Lachlan K, Manners RM, et al. A study of a family with the skeletal muscle RYR1 mutation (c.7354C>T) associated with central core myopathy and malignant hyperthermia susceptibility. *J Clin Neurosci*. 2012;19:65–70.
6. Veyckemans F. Can inhalation agents be used in the presence of a child with myopathy? *Curr Opin Anesthesiol*. 2010;23:348–355.
7. Meola G, Cardani R. Myotonic dystrophies: an update on clinical aspects, genetic, pathology, and molecular pathomechanisms. *Biochem Biophys Acta*. 2015;1852:594–606.
8. Bhakta D, Groh MR, Shen C, et al. Increased mortality with left ventricular systolic dysfunction and heart failure in adults with myotonic dystrophy type 1. *Am Heart J*. 2010;160:1137–1141.
9. Weingarten TN, Hofer RE, Milone M, et al. Anesthesia and myotonic dystrophy type 2: a case series. *Can J Anaesth*. 2010;57:248–255.
10. Kirzinger L, Schmidt A, Kornblum C, et al. Side effects of anesthesia in DM2 as compared to DM1: a comparative retrospective study. *Eur J Neurol*. 2010;17:842–845.
11. Veyckemans F, Scholtes JL. Myotonic dystrophies type 1 and 2: anesthetic care. *Paediatr Anaesth*. 2013;23:794–803.
12. Cannon SC. Channelopathies of skeletal muscle excitability. *Compr Physiol*. 2015;5:761–790.
13. Charles G, Zheng C, Lehmann-Horn F, et al. Characterization of hyperkalemic periodic paralysis: a survey of genetically diagnosed individuals. *J Neurol*. 2013;260:2606–2613.
14. Suetterlin K, Mannikko R, Hanna MG. Muscle channelopathies: recent advances in genetics, pathophysiology, and therapy. *Curr Opin Neurol*. 2014;27:583–590.
15. Bandschapp O, Iaizzo PA. Pathophysiologic and anesthetic considerations for patients with myotonia congenita or periodic paralyses. *Paediatr Anaesth*. 2013;23:824–833.
16. Gilhus NE, Verschuuren JJ. Myasthenia gravis: subgroup classification and therapeutic strategies. *Lancet Neurol*. 2015;14:1023–1036.
17. Berrih-Aknin S, Frenkian-Cuvelier M, Eymard B. Diagnostic and clinical classification of autoimmune myasthenia gravis. *J Autoimmun*. 2014;48–49:143–148.
18. Vymazal T, Krecmerova M, Bicek V, et al. Feasibility of full and rapid neuromuscular blockade recovery with sugammadex in myasthenia patients undergoing surgery—a series of 117 cases. *Ther Clin Risk Manag*. 2015:11:1593–1596.
19. Gritti P, Scarzi M, Carrara B, et al. A standardized protocol for the perioperative management of myasthenia gravis patients: experience with 110 patients. *Acta Anaesthesiol Scand*. 2012;56:66–75.
20. Blichfeldt-Lauridsen L, Hansen BD. Anesthesia and myasthenia gravis. *Acta Anaesthesiol Scand*. 2012;56:17–22.
21. Hulsbrink R, Hashemolhosseini S. Lambert-Eaton myasthenic syndrome-diagnosis, pathogenesis and therapy. *Clin Neurophysiol*. 2014;125:2328–2336.
22. Titulaer MJ, Lang B, Verschuuren JJGM. Lambert-Eaton myasthenic syndrome: from clinical characteristics to therapeutic strategies. *Lancet Neurol*. 2011;10:1098–1107.
23. Weingarten TN, Araka CN, Mogenson ME, et al. Lambert-Eaton myasthenic syndrome during anesthesia: a report of 37 patients. *J Clin Anesth*. 2014;26:648–653.
24. Yuki N, Hartung HP. Guillain-Barre syndrome. *N Engl J Med*. 2012;366:2294–2304.
25. Wong AH, Yuki N. Autoimmune inflammatory neuropathies: updates in pathogenesis, diagnosis, and treatment. *Curr Opin Neurol*. 2015;28:468–473.
26. Feldman JM. Cardiac arrest after succinylcholine in a pregnant patient recovered from Guillain-Barre syndrome. *Anesthesiology*. 1990;72:942–944.

27. Fiaccchino F, Gemma M, Bricchi M, et al. Hypo and hypersensitivity to vecuronium in a patient with Guillain-Barre syndrome. *Anesth Analg.* 1994;78: 187–189.
28. Mangar D, Sprenker C, Karinoski R, et al. Rapid onset of Guillain-Barre syndrome after an obstetric epidural block. *AA Case Rep.* 2013;1:19–22.
29. Grigoriadis N, van Pesch V. A basic overview of multiple sclerosis immunopathology. *Eur J Neurol.* 2015;22(Suppl 2):3–13.
30. Wingerchuk DM, Carter JL. Multiple sclerosis: current and emerging disease-modifying therapies and treatment strategies. *Mayo Clin Proc.* 2014;89:225–240.
31. Lirk P, Birmingham B, Hogan Q. Regional anesthesia in patients with preexisting neuropathy. *Int Anesthesiol Clin.* 2011;49:144–165.
32. McSwain JR, Doty JW, Wilson SH. Regional anesthesia in patients with pre-existing neurologic disease. *Curr Opin Anesthesiol.* 2014;27:538–543.
33. Betjemann JP, Lowenstein DH. Status epilepticus in adults. *Lancet Neurol.* 2015;14:615–624.
34. French JA, Pedley TA. Initial management of epilepsy. *N Engl J Med.* 2008; 359:166–176.
35. Kofke WA. Anesthetic management of the patient with epilepsy or prior seizures. *Curr Opin Anesthesiol.* 2010;23:391–399.
36. Bates K. Epilepsy. *Prim Care.* 2015;42:217–232.
37. Ramani R. Vagus nerve stimulator therapy for seizures. *J Neurosurg Anesthesiol.* 2008;20:29–35.
38. Perks A, Cheema S, Mohanraj R. Anaesthesia and epilepsy. *Br J Anaesth.* 2012;108:562–571.
39. Ehret MJ, Chamberlain KW. Current practices in the treatment of Alzheimer disease. Where is the evidence after the phase III trials? *Clin Ther.* 2015;37:1604–1616.
40. Chen CW, Lin CC, Chen KB, et al. Increased risk of dementia in people with previous exposure to general anesthesia. A nationwide population-based case-control study. *Alzheimers Dement.* 2014;10:196–204.
41. Berger M, Burke J, Eckenhoff R, et al. Alzheimer's disease, anesthesia, and surgery. A clinically focused review. *J Cardiothor Vasc Anesth.* 2014;28: 1609–1623.
42. Kalia LV, Lang AE. Parkinson's disease. *Lancet.* 2015;386:896–912.
43. Hickey P, Stacy M. Available and emerging treatments for Parkinson's disease: a review. *Drug Des Devel Ther.* 2011;5:241–254.
44. Kalenka A, Schwartz A. Anaesthesia and Parkinson's disease: how to manage with new therapies? *Curr Opin Anesthesiol.* 2009;22:419–424.
45. Galvez-Jimenez N, Lang AE. The perioperative management of Parkinson's revisited. *Neurol Clin.* 2004;22:367–377.
46. Poon CC, Irwin MG. Anaesthesia for deep brain stimulation and in patients with implanted neurostimulator devices. *Br J Anaesth.* 2009;103:152–165.
47. Roos RA. Huntington's disease: A clinical review. *Orphanet J Rare Dis.* 2010; 5:40–48.
48. Kivela JE, Sprung J, Southorn PA, et al. Anesthetic management of patients with Huntington disease. *Anesth Analg.* 2010;110:515–523.
49. Valadi N. Evaluation and management of amyotrophic lateral sclerosis. *Prim Care.* 2015;42:177–187.
50. Prabhakar A, Owen CP, Kaye AD. Anesthetic management of the patient with amyotrophic lateral sclerosis. *J Anesth.* 2013;27:909–918.
51. Kim MO, Geschwind MD. Clinical update of Jakob-Creutzfeldt disease. *Curr Opin Neurol.* 2015;28:302–310.
52. Telfer JM. Creutzfeldt-Jakob disease: Implications for anaesthetists in New Zealand. *Anaesth Intensive Care.* 2009;37:386–391.
53. Van Petegem F. Ryanodine receptors: Allosteric ion channel giants. *J Mol Biol.* 2015;427:31–53.
54. Hirshey Dirksen SJ, Larach MG, Rosenberg H, et al. Special article. Future directions in malignant hyperthermia research and patient care. *Anesth Analg.* 2011;113:1108–1119.
55. Larach MG, Brandom BW, Allen GC, et al. Malignant hyperthermia deaths related to inadequate temperature monitoring, 2007–2012: a report from the North American malignant hyperthermia registry of the malignant hyperthermia association of the United States. *Anesth Analg.* 2014;119:1359–1366.
56. Larach MG, Localio AR, Allen GC, et al. A clinical grading scale to predict malignant hyperthermia susceptibility. *Anesthesiology.* 1994;80:771–779.
57. Krause T, Gerbershagen MU, Fiege M, et al. Dantrolene: a review of its pharmacology, therapeutic use, and new developments. *Anaesthesia.* 2004;59:364–373.
58. Schutte JK, Becker S, Starosse A, et al. Comparison of the therapeutic effectiveness of a dantrolene sodium solution and a novel nanocrystalline suspension of dantrolene sodium in malignant hyperthermia normal and susceptible pigs. *Eur J Anaesthesiol.* 2011;28:256–264.
59. Glahn KP, Ellis FR, Halsall PJ, et al. Recognizing and managing a malignant hyperthermia crisis. *Br J Anaesth.* 2010;105:417–420.
60. Birgenheier N, Stoker R, Westenkow D, et al. Activated charcoal effectively removes inhaled anesthetics from modern anesthesia machines. *Anesth Analg.* 2011;112:1363–1370.
61. Karim Z, Lyoumi S, Nicolas G, et al. Porphyrias: A 2015 update. *Clin Res Hepatol Gastroenterol.* 2015;39:412–425.
62. Park EY, Kim YS, Lim KJ, et al. Severe neurologic manifestations in acute intermittent porphyria developed after spine surgery under general anesthesia. *Korean J Anesthesiol.* 2014;67:217–220.

63. Dasouki M, Jawdat O, Almadhoun O, et al. Pompe disease. *Neurol Clin.* 2014;32:751–776.
64. DeSena HC, Brumund MR, Superneau D, et al. Ventricular fibrillation in a patient with Pompe disease: A cautionary tale. *Congenit Heart Dis.* 2011;6: 397–401.
65. Wang LJ, Ross AK, Li JS, et al. Cardiac arrhythmias following anesthesia induction in infantile-onset Pompe disease: A case series. *Paediatr Anaesth.* 2007;17:738–748.
66. Walker RW, Briggs G, Bruce J, et al. Regional anesthetic techniques are an alternative to general anesthesia for infants with Pompe's disease. *Paediatr Anaesth.* 2007;17:697–702.
67. Kishnani PS, Austin SL, Arn P, et al. Glycogen storage type III diagnosis and management guidelines. *Genet Med.* 2010;12:446–463.
68. Mohart D, Russo P, Tobias JD. Perioperative management of a child with glycogen storage type III undergoing cardiopulmonary bypass and repair of an atrial septal defect. *Paediatr Anaesth.* 2002;12:649–654.
69. Ozen H. Glycogen storage diseases: New perspectives. *World J Gastroenterol.* 2007;13:2541–2553.
70. Lobato EB, Janelle GM, Urdaneta F, et al. Noncardiogenic pulmonary edema and rhabdomyolysis after protamine administration in a patient with unrecognized McArdle's disease. *Anesthesiology.* 1999;91:303–305.
71. Bollig G. McArdle's disease (glycogen storage disease type V) and anaesthesia-a case report and review of the literature. *Paediatr Anaesth.* 2013;23:817–823.
72. Roscher A, Patel J, Hewson S, et al. The natural history of glycogen storage disease type VI and IX. long term outcome from the largest metabolic center in Canada. *Mol Genet Metab.* 2014;113:171–176.
73. Wu PL, Yang YN, Tey SL, et al. Infantile form of muscle phosphofructokinase deficiency in a premature neonate. *Pediatr Int.* 2015;57:746–749.
74. Al-Haggar M. Fanconi-Bickel syndrome as an example of marked allelic heterogeneity. *World J Nephrol.* 2012;1:63–68.
75. Weinstein DA, Correia CE, Saunders AC, et al. Hepatic glycogen synthase deficiency: an infrequently recognized cause of ketotic hypoglycemia. *Mol Genet Metab.* 2006;87:284–288.
76. Muenzer J. Overview of the mucopolysaccharidoses. *Rheumatology (Oxford).* 2011;50:v4–v12.
77. Muenzer J. Early initiation of enzyme replacement therapy for mucopolysaccharidoses. *Mol Gen Metab.* 2014;115:63–72.
78. Walker R, Belani KG, Braunlin EA, et al. Anaesthesia and airway management in mucopolysaccharidoses. *J Inherit Metab Dis.* 2013;36:211–219.
79. Frawley G, Fuenzalida D, Donath S, et al. A retrospective audit of anesthetic techniques and complications in children with mucopolysaccharidoses. *Paediatr Anaesth.* 2012;22:737–744.
80. Megens JH, de Wit M, van Hasselt PM, et al. Perioperative complications in patients diagnosed with mucopolysaccharidosis and the impact of enzyme replacement followed by hematopoietic stem cell transplantation at early age. *Paediatr Anaesth.* 2014;24:521–527.
81. Forlino A, Marini JC. Osteogenesis imperfecta. *Lancet.* 2016;387:1657–1671.
82. Ashourina H, Johansen FT, Folkestad L, et al. Heart disease in patients with osteogenesis imperfect: a systematic review. *Int J Cardiol.* 2015;196:149–157.
83. Stynowick GA, Tobias JD. Perioperative care of the patient with osteogenesis imperfecta. *Orthopedics.* 2007;30:1043–1049.
84. Bojanic K, Kivela JE, Gurrieri C, et al. Perioperative course and intraoperative temperatures in patients with osteogenesis imperfecta. *Eur J Anaesthesiol.* 2011;28:370–375.
85. Munoz M, Gomez-Ramirez S, Kozek-Langeneker S. Pre-operative haematological assessment in patients scheduled for major surgery. *Anaesthesia.* 2016;71(Suppl 1):19–28.
86. Duma A, Cartmill C, Blood J, et al. The hematological effects of nitrous oxide anesthesia in pediatric patients. *Anesth Analg.* 2015;120:1325–1330.
87. Vecchio R, Intagliata E, Ferla F, et al. Laparoscopic splenectomy in patients with hereditary spherocytosis: Report on 12 consecutive cases. *Updates Surg.* 2013;65:277–281.
88. Donato H, Crisp RL, Rapetti MC, et al. Hereditary spherocytosis. Review. Part II. Symptomatology, outcome, complications, and treatment. *Arch Argent Pediatr.* 2015;113:168–176.
89. Cappellini MD, Fiorelli G. Glucose-6-phosphate dehydrogenase deficiency. *Lancet.* 2008;371:64–74.
90. Grace RF, Zanella A, Neufeld EJ, et al. Erythrocyte pyruvate kinase deficiency: 2015 status report. *Am J Hematol.* 2015;90:825–830.
91. Barcellini W. Immune hemolysis: Diagnosis and treatment recommendations. *Semin Hematol.* 2015;52:304–312.
92. Garratty G. Drug-induced immune hemolytic anemia. *Am Soc Hematol Educ Progr.* 2009;2009:73–79.
93. Abman SH, Hansmann G, Archer SL, et al. Pediatric pulmonary hypertension: Guidelines from the American Heart Association and American Thoracic Society. *Circulation.* 2015;132:2037–2099.
94. Eridani S, Mosca A. Fetal hemoglobin reactivation and cell engineering in the treatment of sickle cell anemia. *J Blood Med.* 2012;2:23–30.
95. Bakri MH, Ismail EA, Ghanem G, et al. Spinal versus general anesthesia for cesarean section in patients with sickle cell anemia. *Korean J Anesthesiol.* 2015;68:469–475.

96. Firth PG. Anesthesia and hemoglobinopathies. *Anesthesiol Clin.* 2009;27:321–336.
97. Hyder O, Yaster M, Bateman BT, et al. Surgical procedures and outcomes among children with sickle cell anemia. *Anesth Analg.* 2013;117:1192–1196.
98. Staikou C, Stavroulakis E, Karmaniolou I. A narrative review of peri-operative management of patients with thalassemia. *Anaesthesia.* 2014;69:494–510.
99. McInnes IB, Schett G. The pathogenesis of rheumatoid arthritis. *N Engl J Med.* 2011;365:2205–2219.
100. Yaszemski MJ, Shepler TR. Sudden death from cord compression associated with atlantoaxial instability in rheumatoid arthritis: A case report. *Spine (Phila Pa 1976).* 1990;15:338–341.
101. Sen D, Gonzalez-Mayda M, Brasington RD. Cardiovascular disease in rheumatoid arthritis. *Rheum Dis Clin North Am.* 2014;40:27–49.
102. Yunt ZX, Solomon JJ. Lung disease in rheumatoid arthritis. *Rheum Dis Clin North Am.* 2015;41:225–236.
103. Zampeli E, Vlachoyiannopoulos PG, Tzioufas AG. Treatment of rheumatoid arthritis. Unraveling the conundrum. *J Autoimmun.* 2015;65:1–18.
104. Krause ML, Matteson EL. Perioperative management of the patient with rheumatoid arthritis. *World J Orthop.* 2014;5:283–291.
105. Goodman SM. Rheumatoid arthritis: Perioperative management of biologics and DMARDs. *Semin Arthritis Rheum.* 2015;44:627–632.
106. Samanta R, Shoukrey K, Griffiths R. Rheumatoid arthritis and anaesthesia. *Anaesthesia.* 2011;66:1146–1159.
107. Lisnevskaia L, Murphy G, Isenberg D. Systemic lupus erythematosus. *Lancet.* 2014;384:1878–1888.
108. Goldblatt F, O'Neill SG. Clinical manifestations of autoimmune rheumatic diseases. *Lancet.* 2013;382:797–808.
109. Mirabelli G, Cannarile F, Bruni C, et al. One year in review 2015: Systemic lupus erythematosus. *Clin Exp Rheumatol.* 2015;33:414–425.
110. Ben-Menachem E. Systemic lupus erythematosus: A review for anesthesiologists. *Anesth Analg.* 2010;111:665–676.
111. Carrillo ST, Gantz E, Baluch AR, et al Anesthetic considerations for the patient with systemic lupus erythematosus. *Middle East J Anesth.* 2012;21:483–492.
112. Stern EP, Denton CP. The pathogenesis of systemic sclerosis. *Rheum Dis Clin North Am.* 2015;41:367–382.
113. Chaisson NF, Hassoun PM. Systemic sclerosis-associated pulmonary arterial hypertension. *Chest.* 2013;144:1346–1356.
114. Lambova S. Cardiac manifestations in systemic sclerosis. *World J Cardiol.* 2014;6:993–1005.
115. Hudson M. Scleroderma renal crisis. *Curr Opin Rheumatol.* 2015;27:549–554.
116. Antic M, Distler JH, Distler O. Treating skin and lung fibrosis in systemic sclerosis: A future filled with promise? *Curr Opin Pharmacol.* 2013;13:455–462.
117. Dempsey ZS, Rowell S, McRobert R. The role of regional and neuroaxial anesthesia in patients with systemic sclerosis. *Local Reg Anesth.* 2011;4:47–56.
118. Dalakas M. Inflammatory muscle diseases. *N Engl J Med.* 2015;372:1734–1747.
119. Miller SA, Glassberg MK, Ascherman DP. Pulmonary complications of inflammatory myopathy. *Rheum Dis Clin North Am.* 2015;41:249–262.
120. Shinkuma S. Dystrophic epidermolysis bullosa: A review. *Clin Cosmet Invest Dermatol.* 2015;8:275–284.
121. Ida JB, Livshitz I, Azizkhan RG, et al. Upper airway complications of junctional epidermolysis bullosa. *J Pediatr.* 2012;160:657–661.
122. Ryan TD, Lucky AW, King EC, et al. Ventricular dysfunction and aortic root dilation in patients with recessive dystrophic epidermolysis bullosa. *Br J Dermatol.* 2016;174:671–673.
123. Nandi R, Howard R. Anesthesia and epidermolysis bullosa. *Dermatol Clin.* 2010;28:319–324.
124. Stavropoulos PG, Soura E, Antoniou C. Drug-induced pemphigoid: a review of the literature. *J Eur Acad Dermatol Venereol.* 2014;28:1133–1140.
125. Venugopal SS, Murrell DF. Diagnosis and clinical features of pemphigus vulgaris. *Dermatol Clin.* 2011;29:373–380.
126. Takahashi M, Rhee AJ, Rakasi RR, et al. Cardiac surgery in a patients with pemphigus vulgaris: anesthetic and surgical considerations. *Semin Cardiothorac Vasc Anesth.* 2014;18:74–77.

25 The Anesthesia Workstation and Delivery Systems for Inhaled Anesthetics

KEVIN T. RIUTORT • JAMES B. EISENKRAFT

Anesthesia Workstation Standards and Preuse Procedures
Standards for Anesthesia Machines and Workstations
Failure of Anesthesia Equipment
Safety Features of Newer Anesthesia Workstations
Checkout of the Anesthesia Workstation
   Oxygen Analyzer Calibration
   Low-Pressure Circuit Leak Test
   Evaluation of the Circle System
   Workstation Self-tests
   Anesthesia Workstation Pneumatics
   Pipeline Supply Source
   Cylinder Supply Source
   Nitrous Oxide
   Machine Intermediate-Pressure System
   Oxygen Supply Pressure Failure Safety Devices
   Flowmeter Assemblies
   Electronic Flowmeters
   Proportioning Systems
   Oxygen Flush Valve
Web-based Anesthesia Software Simulation, the Virtual Anesthesia Machine
Vaporizers
   Physics
   Variable Bypass Vaporizers
   The Tec 6 and D-Vapor Vaporizers for Desflurane
   The GE-Datex-Ohmeda Aladin Cassette Vaporizer
   Maquet FLOW-i Electronic Injector Vaporizer

Anesthesia Breathing Circuits
   Mapleson Systems
   Circle Breathing Systems
CO_2 Absorbents
   The Absorber Canister
   Chemistry of Absorbents
   Absorptive Capacity
   Indicators
   Interactions of Inhaled Anesthetics with Absorbents
Anesthesia Ventilators
   Classification
   Operating Principles of Ascending Bellows Pneumatically Powered Ventilators
   Problems and Hazards
Anesthesia Workstation Variations
   Datex-Ohmeda S/5 ADU and GE Healthcare Aisys Carestation
   The Dräger Medical Narkomed 6000 Series, Fabius GS, and Apollo Workstations
   Maquet FLOW-i Workstation
Waste Gas Scavenging Systems
   Components
   Hazards
Appendix A
   FDA 1993 Anesthesia Apparatus Checkout Recommendations
Appendix B
   Recommendations for Preanesthesia Checkout Procedures (2008) Subcommittee of ASA Committee on Equipment and Facilities Guidelines for Preanesthesia Checkout Procedures
   ASA 2008 Guidelines for Developing Institution-Specific Checkout Procedures Prior to Anesthesia Delivery
Additional Notes

KEY POINTS

1. The most important (but often overlooked) item in the preuse checkout of the anesthesia workstation is to have immediately available a functioning self-inflating resuscitation bag (SIRB) and a full auxiliary tank of oxygen.
2. The low-pressure circuit (LPC) is the "vulnerable area" of the anesthesia workstation because it is most subject to breakage and leaks. The LPC is located downstream from all anesthesia machine safety features except the oxygen analyzer (or, in some cases, the ratio controller), and it is the portion of the machine where a leak is most likely to go unrecognized if an inappropriate LPC leak test is performed. Leaks in the LPC can cause delivery of a hypoxic or subanesthetic mixture, leading to patient hypoxic injury or awareness during anesthesia.
3. Because some GE Healthcare/Datex-Ohmeda anesthesia machines have a one-way check valve in the LPC, a negative-pressure leak test is required to detect leaks in the LPC. A positive-pressure leak test will not detect leaks in the LPC of a machine with an outlet check valve.
4. Before administering an anesthetic, the circle breathing system must be checked for leaks and for correct flow. To test for leaks, the circle system is pressurized to 30-cm water pressure, and the circle system airway pressure gauge is observed (static test). To check for appropriate flow to rule out obstructions and faulty valves, the ventilator and a test lung (breathing bag) are used (dynamic test). In addition, the manual/bag circuit must be actuated by compressing the reservoir bag, in order to rule out obstructions to flow in the manual/bag mode.
5. Internal vaporizer leaks can only be detected with the vaporizer turned to the "on" position. In the "off" position the vaporizer is excluded from the LPC.
6. Many new anesthesia workstation self-tests do not detect internal vaporizer leaks unless each vaporizer is individually turned on during repeated self-tests.

7. The oxygen failure cutoff valves (also known previously as "fail-safe" valves, "hypoxic guards," or "proportioning systems") help minimize the likelihood of delivery of a hypoxic gas mixture, but they are not foolproof. Delivery of a hypoxic mixture may still result from (1) the wrong supply gas, either in the cylinder or in the main pipeline; (2) a defective or broken safety device; (3) leaks downstream from the safety devices; (4) inert gas administration (e.g., helium); and (5) dilution of the inspired oxygen concentration by high concentrations of inhaled anesthetics.

8. In the event of a gas pipeline crossover, two actions must be taken. The backup oxygen cylinder must be turned on (since the tank valve should always be turned off when not in use), and the wall/pipeline supply sources must be disconnected.

9. Because of desflurane's low boiling point (22.8°C) and high vapor pressure (669 mmHg at 20°C), delivery of desflurane requires specially designed vaporizers, such as the GE Healthcare/Datex-Ohmeda Tec 6, the Dräger D-Vapor, and the GE Healthcare Aladin cassette vaporizing system.

10. Erroneous filling of an empty variable bypass vaporizer with desflurane could theoretically be catastrophic, resulting in delivery of a hypoxic mixture and a massive overdose of inhaled desflurane.

11. Inhaled anesthetics can interact with CO_2 absorbents and produce toxic compounds. During sevoflurane (only) anesthesia, compound A can be formed, particularly at low fresh gas flow (FGF) rates. Carbon monoxide may be produced when volatile anesthetics are utilized, particularly with desiccated absorbents.

12. Desiccated strong base absorbents (particularly barium hydroxide lime, Baralyme) can react with sevoflurane, producing extremely high absorber temperatures and combustible decomposition products. These, in combination with the oxygen- or nitrous oxide–enriched environment of the circle system, have produced very high temperatures and fires within the breathing system. For this reason, Baralyme is no longer available in the United States. Lithium-based absorbents are nonreactive.

13. Anesthesia ventilators with ascending bellows (bellows that ascend during the expiratory phase) were initially thought to be safer than descending bellows. This is because a breathing system disconnection would be obvious since the ascending bellows would not refill/rise during exhalation. Contemporary machines with descending bellows, however, have been carefully redesigned to address the initial limitations. Current descending bellows ventilators have featherlight bellows, an electric eye at the bottom of the bellows housing to detect bellows movement, and the bellows housing is subjected to PEEP, such that in case of a disconnect, the bellows would actually rise and stay up.

14. With older design machines, use of the oxygen flush valve during the inspiratory phase of mechanical ventilation could cause barotrauma, particularly in pediatric patients. The newer workstations have fresh-gas decouplers or peak-inspiratory pressure limiters that were designed to prevent these complications. Ventilators that use fresh gas decoupling (FGD) technology virtually eliminate the possibility of barotrauma by oxygen flushing during the inspiratory phase because FGF and oxygen flush flow are diverted to the reservoir bag. However, if the reservoir bag has a large leak or is absent altogether, patient awareness under anesthesia and delivery of a lower-than-expected oxygen concentration could occur due to entrainment of room air.

15. With newer GE Healthcare/Datex-Ohmeda anesthesia ventilators such as the 7900 series SmartVent, both the patient circuit gas and the drive gas are scavenged, resulting in substantially increased volumes of scavenged gas. Thus, the scavenging system flow removal must be set appropriately high to accommodate the increased volume; otherwise, undesired PEEP and contamination of the operating room environment could result.

16. Modern ventilators compensate for the changes in FGF, respiratory rate, and I:E ratio so that the delivered tidal volume does not change from that set to be delivered. This compensation is achieved either by "fresh gas decoupling" (in Dräger Fabius, Tiro, and Apollo workstations) or by "fresh gas compensation" (in GE Healthcare/Datex-Ohmeda workstations).

The anesthesia machine is, conceptually, a pump for delivering medical gases and inhalation agents to the patient's lungs. The function of the anesthesia machine is to (1) receive gases from the central supply and cylinders, (2) meter them and add anesthetic vapors, and finally, (3) deliver them to the patient breathing circuit.[1] The machine has evolved over the past 160 years from a rather simple ether inhaler to a complex device of valves, pistons, vaporizers, monitors, and electronic circuitry.

The "pump" in the modern anesthesia machine is either a mechanical ventilator or the lungs of the spontaneously breathing patient, or perhaps, a combination of the two. The anesthesia pump has a supply system: medical gases from either a pipeline supply or a gas cylinder, alongside vaporizers delivering potent inhaled anesthetic agents that are mixed with the medical gases. The anesthesia pump also has an exhaust system, the waste gas scavenging system, which removes excess gases from the patient's breathing circuit. The breathing circuit is a series of hoses, valves, filters, switches, and regulators that interconnect the supply system, the patient, and the exhaust system.

Modern anesthesia machines (Figs. 25-1 to 25-4) are now more properly referred to as *anesthesia workstations*. The anesthesia workstation, as defined by the International Standards Organization, is a system for administering anesthetics to patients consisting of *an anesthesia gas delivery system, an anesthetic breathing system and any required monitoring equipment, alarm systems, and protection devices.*[2] The protection device is designed to prevent the patient from hazardous output due to incorrect delivery of energy or substances; for example, the adjustable pressure-limiting (APL) valve prevents barotrauma.

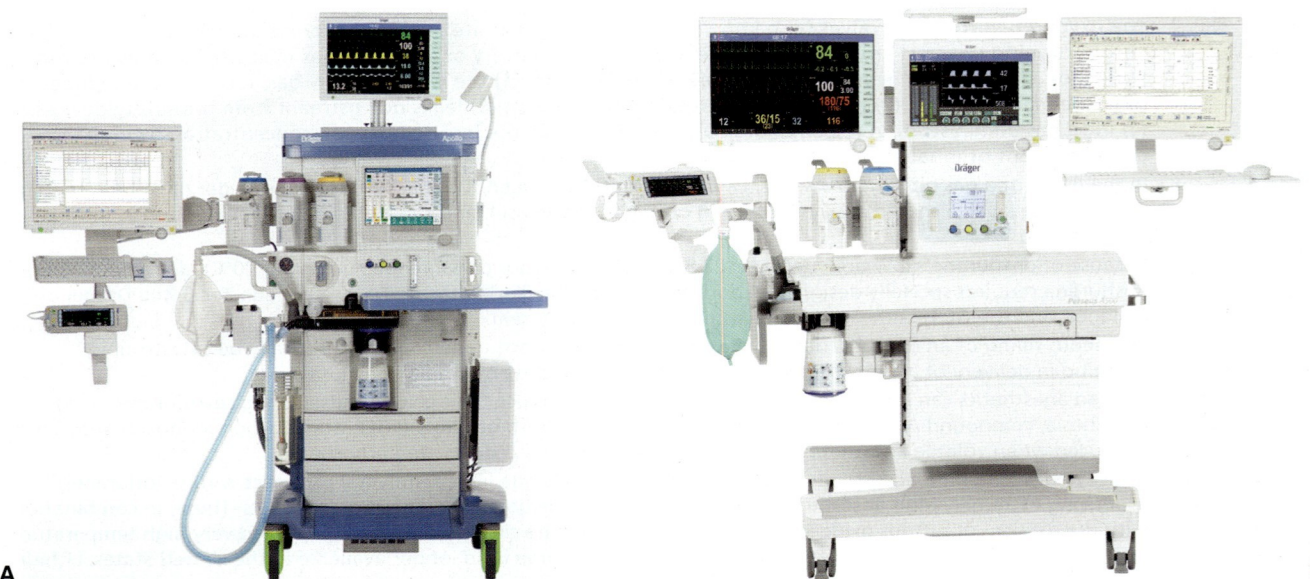

Figure 25-1 **A:** Dräger Apollo Workstation. **B:** Dräger Perseus A500 Workstation.

In this chapter, the anesthesia workstation is examined piece by piece. The normal operation, function, and integration of major anesthesia workstation subsystems are described. More importantly, the potential problems and hazards associated with the various components of the anesthesia delivery system, and the appropriate preoperative checks that may help to detect and prevent such problems, are illustrated.

Anesthesia Workstation Standards and Preuse Procedures

Years ago, a fundamental knowledge of the basic anesthesia machine pneumatics would have sufficed for most anesthesia providers. Today, a detailed understanding of pneumatics,

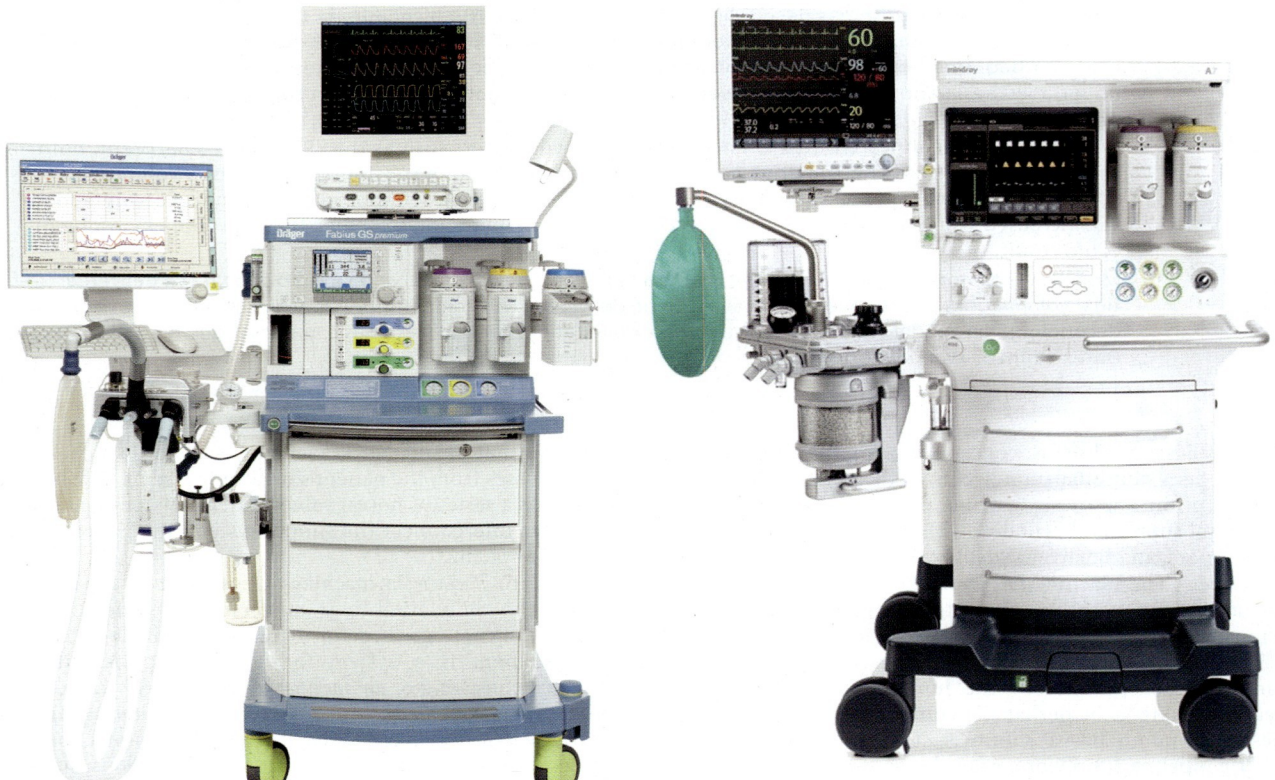

Figure 25-2 **A:** Dräger Fabius GS Workstation. **B:** Mindray A7 Workstation.

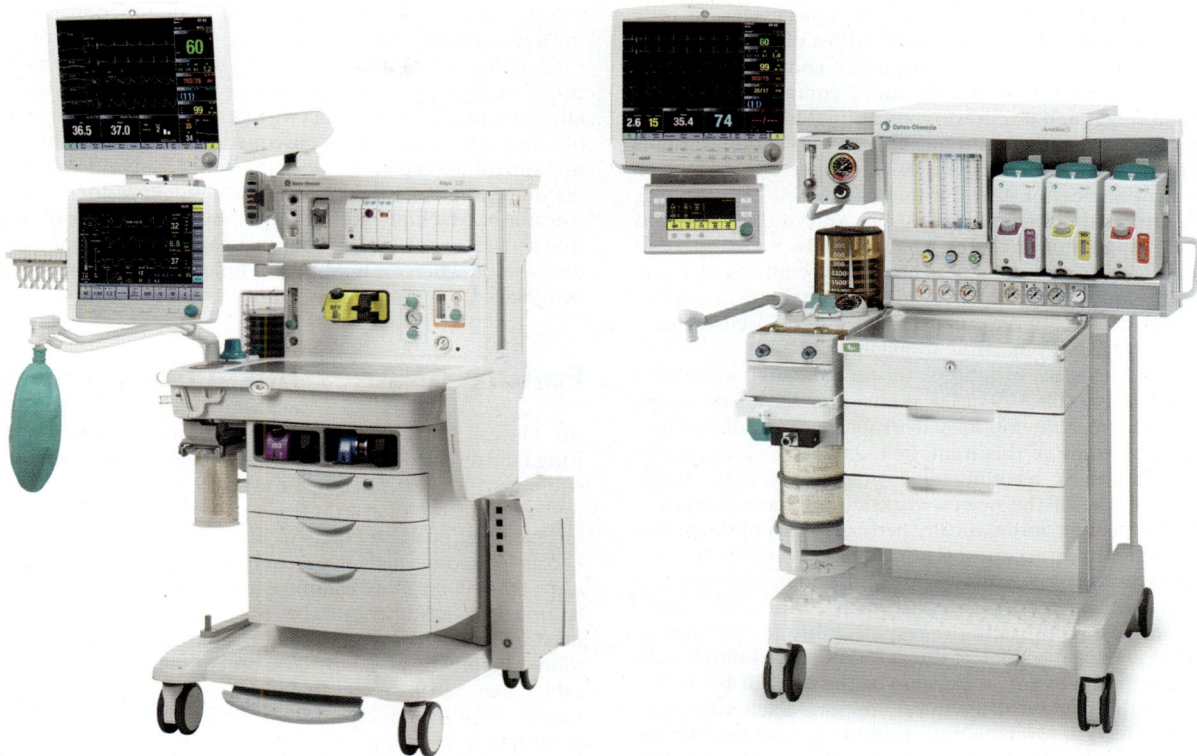

Figure 25-3 **A:** GE Aisys CS² Workstation. **B:** GE Aestiva Workstation. (Courtesy of GE Healthcare.)

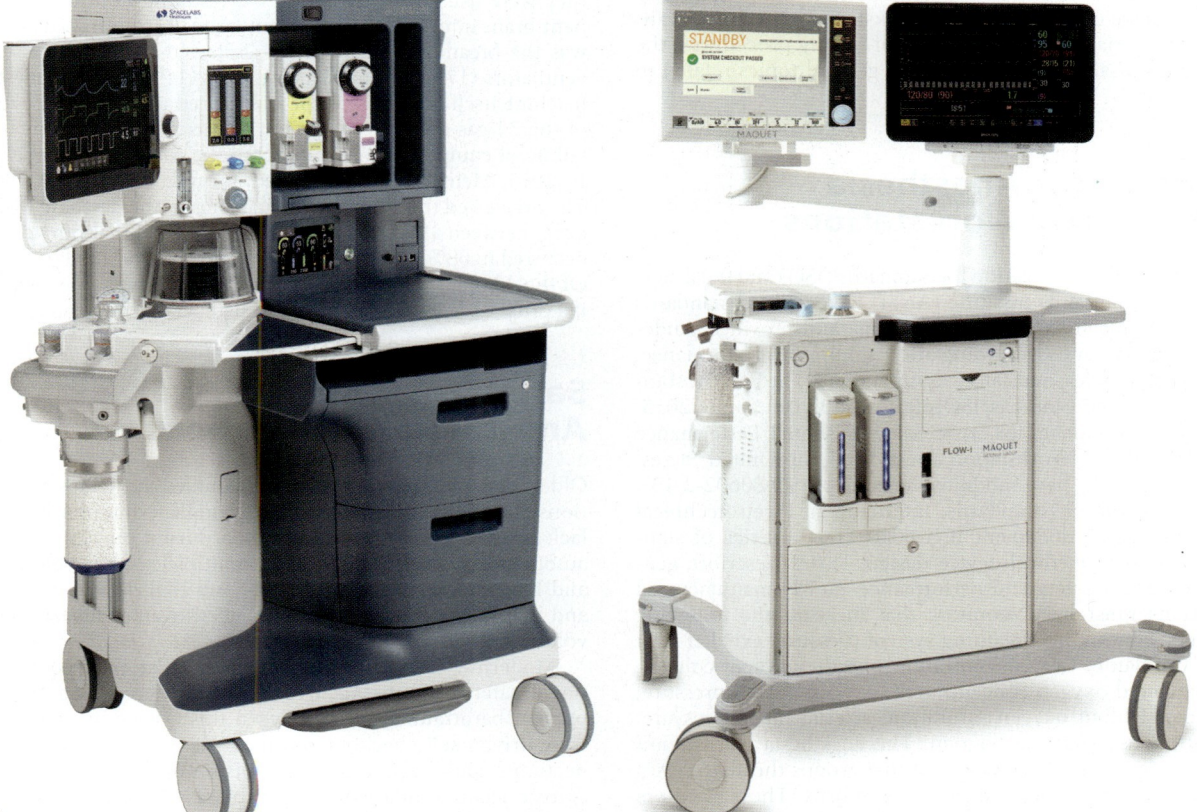

Figure 25-4 **A:** Spacelabs Healthcare ARKON workstation (courtesy Spacelabs Healthcare, Snoqualmie, Washington). **B:** Maquet FLOW-i C30 Workstation.

electronics, and even computer science is necessary to fully understand the capabilities and complexities of the anesthesia workstation. Along with the changes in the composition of the anesthesia workstation to include more complex ventilation systems and integrated monitoring, recently there has also been increasing divergence between anesthesia workstation designs from different manufacturers. In 1993, a joint effort between the American Society of Anesthesiologists (ASA) and the U.S. Food and Drug Administration (FDA) produced the 1993 FDA Anesthesia Apparatus Preuse Checkout Recommendations (Appendix A). This preuse checklist was versatile and could be applied to most commonly available anesthesia machines equally well and did not require users to vary the preuse procedure significantly from machine to machine.

Today, because of variations in fundamental anesthesia workstation design, the 1993 FDA preuse checklist is no longer applicable to many contemporary workstations. Anesthesia providers must be aware of this limitation, and the original equipment manufacturer's recommended preuse checklist should be followed. Some of the newer workstations have computer-assisted self-tests that automatically perform a part of the preuse machine checkout procedure. The availability of such automated checkout features further adds to the complexity of constructing a uniform preuse checklist such as the one utilized in the recent past. Ultimately the responsibility for performing an adequate preuse checkout of the anesthesia workstation falls to the individual operator, regardless of the level of his or her training and the quality of technical support. Each anesthesia care provider has the ultimate responsibility for proper function of all anesthesia delivery equipment that he or she uses. This includes an awareness of which anesthesia workstation components are checked out by automated self-tests and which ones are not. Because of the number of workstations currently available and the variability among their self-testing procedures, the following discussion will be limited to general topics related to these systems.

Standards for Anesthesia Machines and Workstations

The International Organization for Standards (ISO) and the American National Standards Institute (ANSI) have defined standards for anesthesia machines and workstations, and provided guidelines to manufacturers regarding their minimum performance, design characteristics, and safety requirements. The current standard in the United States is ISO 80601-2-13:2011/Amd1:2015, Particular Requirements for Basic Safety Essential Performance of and Anaesthetic Workstation (outside of the United States, other countries may have modified versions of ISO 80602-2-13). In addition to the ISO standards, International Electrotechnical Commission (IEC) document IEC 60601-1 is a series of standards that govern medical device design. Part 1 describes general standards for safety and performance. Newly manufactured workstations must have monitors that measure the following parameters: continuous breathing system pressure, exhaled tidal volume, ventilatory CO_2 concentration, anesthetic vapor concentration, inspired oxygen concentration, oxygen supply pressure, arterial hemoglobin oxygen saturation, arterial blood pressure, and continuous electrocardiogram. The anesthesia workstation must have a prioritized alarm system that groups the alarms into three categories: high, medium, and low priority. These monitors and alarms may be enabled automatically and made to function by turning on the anesthesia workstation, or the monitors and alarms can be enabled manually and made functional by following a preuse checklist.[2,3]

Perhaps just as important as the specifications for new anesthesia machines and workstations that are introduced into clinical care are the characteristics that render older machines obsolete. This is not an inconsequential issue, since the financial investment for replacing older machines is significant. The ASA document (dated June 22, 2004), "Guidelines for Determining Anesthesia Machine Obsolescence," addresses some of the absolute as well as relative criteria that can help institutions make a decision on when even otherwise functioning equipment should be replaced.[4]

Failure of Anesthesia Equipment

An 11-year study of 1,000 anesthesia incidents in the United Kingdom revealed that the most common failure was due to an equipment leak (61/1,000).[5] The authors stated the most likely underlying cause of system leaks was due to "design weakness"; for example, push-on tapers in breathing circuits that can easily become disconnected. Poor equipment maintenance and setup were the second most common underlying causes of equipment failure. The authors found that the pulse oximeter alarm was the most common principal monitor alerting the anesthesiologist to an equipment problem.[5] Equipment failure due to entrapped cables may result in the inability to ventilate (thus warranting careful attention to organization and tidiness of the anesthesia workstation environment).[6-8] In a 1997 review of the ASA "Closed Claims" database, Caplan et al.[9] found that although claims related to the medical gas-delivery system were rare, when they occurred they were usually severe, with 76% resulting in death or permanent brain injury. The most common malfunction in that review was the breathing circuit (39%), followed by vaporizers (21%), ventilators (17%), gas tanks or gas lines (11%), and the anesthesia machine itself (7%). Use error was judged to be the cause in 75% of the 72 gas delivery equipment claims reviewed, whereas pure failure of equipment was considered the cause in the remainder.[9] In 2013, Mehta et al.[10] published an update of the 1997 study. They reviewed the 40 most recent claims in the database (for incidents between 1990 and 2011) and concluded that provider error occurred in 68%, equipment failure only in 13%, and both in 18%. Of the 40 incidents, 35% were considered to have been avoidable if a proper preanesthesia checkout had been performed.

Safety Features of Newer Anesthesia Workstations

Older conventional anesthesia machines have design limitations that limit their safety. For example, some machines may lack features to prevent barotrauma during oxygen flush, lack automated preuse checkout, have multiple external connections, and have gas-driven ventilator bellows that do not fully empty and that may allow "breath stacking" as well as inaccurate tidal volume delivery.[11]

Modern workstations have designs that incorporate additional safety features such as fresh gas decoupling (FGD) to prevent barotrauma during oxygen flush, have integrated, software-driven self-checkout routines, have limited external connections, and have electronic, piston-driven ventilators that deliver accurate tidal volumes. Table 25-1 summarizes relevant safety features of newer anesthesia workstations.

(text continued on page 652)

Table 25-1 Comparison of Anesthesia Workstation Functions

Function	Narkomed AV2+	Ohmeda 7800	Dräger Narkomed 6400	Dräger Julian[a]	Dräger Fabius GS 1.3	GE/Datex-Ohmeda Aestiva/5	GE/Datex-Ohmeda ADU	GE/Datex-Ohmeda Aisys	GE/Datex-Ohmeda Avance CS²	Dräger Apollo	Mindray A3/A5	Spacelabs ARKON
Increase in fresh gas flow (FGF) increases tidal volume (Vt)	Yes	Yes	No	No	No	Initially	No	No	No	No	No	No
Preuse system leakage is measured	No	No	Yes	Yes	Yes	No	Yes	Yes	Yes	Yes	Yes	Yes
Proximal leak compensation	No	No	No	No	No	Yes	No	Yes	Yes	Yes	Yes	Yes
Leakage measurement during operation	No	No	Yes	No	No	No	No	Yes	Yes	No	Yes	Yes
Hose compliance compensation	No	No	Yes	Yes	Yes	No	Yes	Yes	Yes	Yes	Yes	Yes
System compliance compensation	No	No	Yes	Yes	Yes	Yes	Yes	Yes	Yes	Yes	Yes	Yes
The reported exhaled Vt is adjusted for hose compliance	No	No	Yes	No	Yes	No	No	Yes	Yes	Yes	Yes	Yes
The fresh gas inflow is distal to:	Absorber	Absorber	Absorber	Mid-absorber	Absorber	Absorber	Inspiratory valve	Absorber	Absorber/condenser	Absorber	Absorber	Absorber
The fresh gas inflow is proximal to:	Inspiratory valve	Inspiratory valve	Decoupling valve	Mid-absorber	Decoupling valve	Inspiratory valve	Y-piece	Inspiratory valve	Inspiratory valve	Decoupling valve	Inspiratory valve	Inspiratory valve
At low FGF, what gas fills the reservoir bag?	Exhaled	Exhaled	Scrubbed	Exhaled	Scrubbed	Exhaled	Exhaled	Exhaled	Exhaled	Exhaled	Exhaled	Exhaled
Mechanism of volume control ventilation (VCV)	Mechanical limit	Metered	Displacement	Metered	Displacement	Metered/servo	Metered/calculated	Metered, calculated	Metered, calculated	Metered	Metered	Metered, calculated

(continued)

Table 25-1 Comparison of Anesthesia Workstation Functions (CONTINUED)

Function	Narkomed AV2+	Ohmeda 7800	Dräger Narkomed 6400	Dräger Julian[a]	Dräger Fabius GS 1.3	GE/Datex-Ohmeda Aestiva/5	GE/Datex-Ohmeda ADU	GE/Datex-Ohmeda Aisys	GE/Datex-Ohmeda Avance CS²	Dräger Apollo	Mindray A3/A5	Spacelabs ARKON
Limiting of pressure control ventilation (PCV)	Pressure limited	None	Flow/pressure limited	Flow/pressure limited	Flow/pressure limited	Pressure limited	Flow/pressure limited	Flow/pressure limited	Flow/pressure limited with volume guarantee	Flow/pressure limited	Flow/pressure limited. Volume guarantee[b]	
FIO_2 compensated for volatile agent	No	No	No	No	No	No	Yes	Yes	Yes (0.15–15 L/m)	No	No	Yes
Synchronized intermittent mechanical ventilation (SIMV)	No	No	Yes	No	No	No	Yes	Yes	Yes	Yes	Yes	Yes
The manufacturer-specified minimum Vt	N/A	18	10	50	20	20	20	20	20	20	20	20
Fresh gas flow (FGF) control	Needle valve	Needle valve	Needle valve	Digital control	Needle valve	Needle valve	Needle valve	Digital control	Electronic gas mixer	Needle valve	Digital control	Digital control
Fresh gas flow (FGF) measurement	Flow tubes	Flow tubes	Flow tubes	Electronic	Electronic	Flow tubes	Electronic	Electronic	Electronic, multisensor	Electronic	Electronic	Electronic and flow tube
Backup flow tube	N/A	N/A	N/A	No	Yes	N/A	Yes	Yes (fail-safe mode)	Yes	Yes	Yes	Yes
Integrated capnography	No	No	Yes	Yes	No	No	Yes	Yes	Yes	Yes	Yes	Yes
Integrated anesthetic gas monitoring	No	No	Yes	Yes	No	No	Yes	Yes	Yes	Yes	Yes	Yes
Effect of lost oxygen pressure on FGF	No FGF	No FGF	No FGF	Auto air on	Air available	Air available	Air available	Air available	Air available	Air available	Air available	Air available
Sampled gas returned to circuit	No	No	No	No	No	No	Yes	No	Yes	Yes	No	Optional
Mechanical airway pressure gauge	Yes	Yes	No	No	Yes	Yes	No	No	No	Yes	Yes	Yes

650

Feature	1	2	3	4	5	6	7	8	9	10	11	12
Absorber removable during VCV	No	No	No	No	Yes	Yes	Yes	Yes (optional)	Yes (with optional EZchange canister)	Yes (optional)	Yes	Yes
Room air entrained during a circuit leak	No	No	Yes	Yes	Yes	No	No	No	No	No	No	No
Room air entrained with inadequate FGF	No	No	No	No	Yes	No	No	No	No	No	No	No
Effect of O$_2$ flush during VCV inspiration	>Vt, held at press. limit	>Vt at press. limit	None	>Vt, held at press. limit	None	>Vt, end at press. limit	>Vt, end at press. release	>Vt, end at press. release	None	None	None	Cycle to expiration
Fail-safe integrated with the ratio controller	No	No	No	Yes, electronic	Yes, pneumatic	No	Yes, electronic	Yes, electronic	Yes, electronic	Yes, electronic	Yes, electronic	Yes, electronic
Method to find a low-pressure/vaporizer leak	Positive pressure	Negative pressure	Automatic, vaporizer open	Automatic, vaporizer open	Automatic, vaporizer open	Negative pressure	Automatic	Automatic	Automatic; first with vaporizers closed, then with one open at a time[c]	Automatic, vaporizer open	Automatic; first with vaporizers closed, then with one open at a time	Automated checkout
Ventilator drive gas scavenging	No	No	N/A	Yes	N/A	Yes	Yes	Yes	Yes	N/A	Yes	No
Automated fresh gas flow optimization by workstation software	No	No	No	No	No	No	No	No	Yes (ecoFlow)	Yes (Low Flow Wizard)	No	No

Adapted from Olympio MA. Modern anesthesia machines offer new safety features. *APSF Newsletter.* 2003;18:17.

[a] Not available in the United States.
[b] A5 model only.
[c] If machine has optional auxiliary common gas outlet (ACGO) then a positive-pressure low-pressure system leak test may be performed at the ACGO in addition to the automated test.

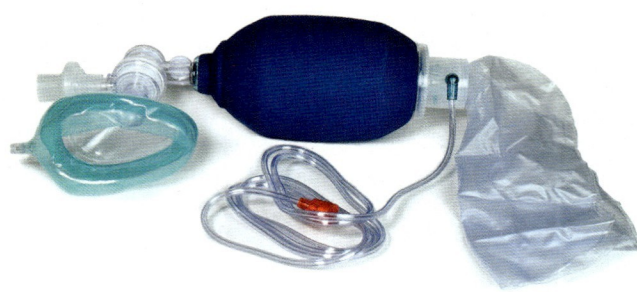

Figure 25-5 Self-inflating Resuscitation Bag (SIRB).

Checkout of the Anesthesia Workstation

A complete anesthesia apparatus checkout procedure must be performed each day prior to the first use of the anesthesia workstation. An abbreviated checkout procedure should be performed before each subsequent case. The 1993 FDA Anesthesia Apparatus Checkout Recommendations (reproduced in Appendix A) remain applicable to the majority of older anesthesia machines in use worldwide.[12–16]

In 2008, the ASA published recommendations for preanesthesia checkout of machines, taking into consideration newer workstations that perform automated checkout.[17] Since the design of newer workstations varies considerably, no single preuse procedure is applicable. These guidelines present a template for individual departments and practitioners to design preanesthesia checkout procedures specific to their needs and equipment (Appendix B). Sample checkout procedures are published on the ASA web site (www.asahq.org), and they encompass adult as well as pediatric equipment from major equipment manufacturers in the United States. The reader is strongly encouraged to review the checkout procedures reproduced in Appendices A and B at the end of this chapter and to understand the rationale for, and importance of, each step.

Perhaps the most important but often overlooked item in the preuse checkout of the anesthesia workstation is to have immediately available a functioning (tested) self-inflating resuscitation bag (SIRB) (Fig. 25-5) and a full auxiliary tank of oxygen. This is "plan B"—the backup plan. Many of the adverse outcomes associated with anesthesia equipment mishaps could have been averted if the SIRB had been used or used sooner. The SIRB is an item frequently missed in the preanesthesia setup.[18]

The next three most important preoperative checks are (1) oxygen analyzer calibration, (2) the low-pressure circuit (LPC) leak test, and (3) the circle system test. These are discussed in the following sections. Additional details regarding these systems are presented briefly in subsequent sections describing the anatomy of the anesthesia workstation; for a more comprehensive review, the reader is encouraged to consult the operator's manual of their own equipment manufacturer. For a simplified diagram of a two-gas anesthesia machine and the components described in the following discussion, please refer to Figure 25-6. A comprehensive discussion of Figure 25-6 can also be found in the Anesthesia Workstation Pneumatics section.

Oxygen Analyzer Calibration

The oxygen analyzer is one of the most important monitors on the anesthesia workstation. It is the only machine safety device that evaluates the integrity of the LPC in an ongoing fashion. Other machine safety devices, such as the oxygen supply pressure failure

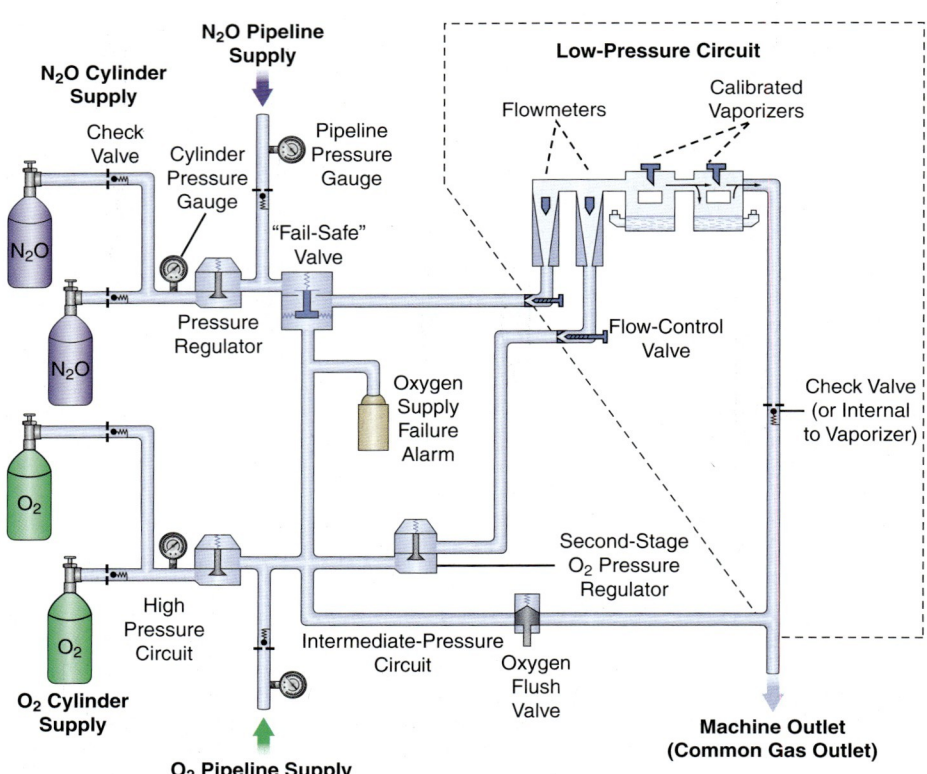

Figure 25-6 Diagram of a generic two-gas anesthesia machine. (Adapted from Check-Out, *A Guide for Preoperative Inspection of an Anesthesia Machine*. Schaumburg, IL: American Society of Anesthesiologists; 1987.)

cutoff ("fail-safe") valve, the oxygen supply pressure failure alarm, and the N₂O/O₂ proportioning system, are all upstream from the flow control valves. The only monitor that detects problems downstream from the flow control valves is the oxygen analyzer. Calibration of this monitor is described in Step 9 of Appendix A (Anesthesia Apparatus Checkout Recommendations, 1993). The actual procedure for calibrating the oxygen analyzer has remained reasonably similar over the recent generations of the anesthesia workstations (Guideline for Designing Preanesthesia Checkout Procedures, 2008, Item 10 in Appendix B). Generally, the oxygen concentration-sensing element (usually a fuel cell on traditional machines) must be exposed to room air (at sea level) for calibration to 21%. This may require manually setting a dial on older machines, but on newer ones, it usually only involves temporarily removing the sensor, selecting and then confirming that the oxygen calibration is to be performed from a set of menus on the workstation's display screen, and finally reinstalling the sensor. The function of the low oxygen concentration alarm should be verified by setting the alarm to trigger above the current oxygen reading. Some newer workstations use a side-stream sampling multigas monitoring module that incorporates a paramagnetic (fast) oxygen analyzer. These analyzers undergo automatic periodic oxygen calibration.[19] It should be noted that both the fuel cell and the paramagnetic oxygen analyzers actually measure PO_2 and express it as a percentage of 1 atmosphere at sea level. Thus, if a fuel cell were calibrated to 21% O_2 at sea level and then used at an altitude where the total air pressure is reduced, it would read less than 21% even though the composition of the atmosphere is unchanged (21%).

Low-Pressure Circuit Leak Test

The LPC leak test checks the integrity of the anesthesia machine from the flow control valves to the common gas outlet. It evaluates the portion of the machine that is downstream from all safety devices except the oxygen analyzer. The components located within this area are precisely the ones most subject to breakage and leaks. Leaks in the LPC can cause hypoxia or patient awareness.[20,21] Flow tubes, the most delicate pneumatic component of the machine, can crack or break. A typical three-gas anesthesia machine has 16 O-rings in the LPC. Leaks can occur at the interface between the glass flow tubes[22] and the manifold, and at the O-ring junctions between the vaporizer and its manifold. Loose filler caps on vaporizers are a common source of leaks, and these leaks can lead to delivery of subanesthetic doses of inhaled agents, causing patient awareness during general anesthesia.[23]

Several different methods have been used to check the LPC for leaks. They include the oxygen flush test, the common gas outlet occlusion test, the traditional positive-pressure leak test, the North American Dräger positive-pressure leak test, internal positive-pressure leak test, the GE Datex-Ohmeda negative-pressure leak test, the 1993 FDA universal negative-pressure leak test, and others. One reason for the large number of methods is that the internal design of various machines differs considerably. The most notable example is that many GE Healthcare/Datex-Ohmeda (hereafter frequently referred to as GE) machines/workstations have a check valve near the common gas outlet, whereas Dräger Medical workstations do not. The presence or absence of the outlet check valve profoundly influences which preuse check is indicated.

Several mishaps have resulted from application of the wrong leak test to the wrong machine.[24-27] Therefore, it is mandatory to perform the appropriate low-pressure system leak test each day. To do this, it is essential to understand the exact location and operating principles of the Datex-Ohmeda check valve. Many Datex-Ohmeda anesthesia workstations have a machine outlet check valve located in the LPC (Table 25-1). The check valve is located downstream from the vaporizers and upstream from the oxygen flush valve (Fig. 25-6). It is open in the absence of back pressure. Gas flow from the manifold moves the rubber flapper valve off its seat and allows gas to proceed freely to the common gas outlet. The valve closes when back pressure is exerted.[28] Back pressure sufficient to close the check valve may occur with the following conditions: use of the oxygen flush, peak breathing circuit pressures generated during positive-pressure ventilation, or use of a positive-pressure leak test.

Generally speaking, the LPC of anesthesia workstations without an outlet check valve can be tested using a positive-pressure leak test, and machines with outlet check valves must be tested using a negative-pressure leak test. When performing a positive-pressure leak test, the operator generates positive pressure in the LPC using flow from the anesthesia machine or from a positive-pressure squeeze bulb to detect a leak. When performing a negative-pressure leak test, the operator creates negative pressure in the LPC using a suction bulb to detect leaks. Two different LPC leak tests are described below.

Oxygen Flush Positive-Pressure Leak Test

Historically, older anesthesia machines did not have check valves in the LPC. Therefore, it was common practice to pressurize the breathing circuit and the LPC with the oxygen flush valve to test for internal anesthesia machine leaks by observing the breathing system pressure gauge. Because some modern GE-Datex-Ohmeda machines have check valves in the LPC, application of a positive-pressure leak test to these machines can be misleading or even dangerous (Fig. 25-7). Inappropriate use of the oxygen flush valve or the presence of a leaking flush valve may lead to inadequate evaluation of the LPC for leaks. In turn, this can lead the workstation user into a false sense of security despite the presence of large leaks.[29,30] Positive pressure from the breathing circuit results in closure of the outlet check valve, and the value on the breathing system pressure gauge will fail to decrease. The system appears to be gas-tight, but in actuality, only the circuitry downstream from the outlet check valve is leak-free.[31] Thus, a vulnerable area exists from the check valve back to the flow control valves because this area is not tested by a positive-pressure leak test.

Verifying the Integrity of the Gas Supply Lines between the Flowmeters and the Common Gas Outlet

The 1993 FDA Universal negative-pressure leak test (Appendix A, Step 5) was named "universal" because at that time it could be used to check all contemporary anesthesia machines regardless of the presence or absence of an outlet check valve in the LPC. It remains applicable for many older anesthesia machines, but for many newer machines this "universal" test is not applicable. Table 25-1 describes how newer workstations are tested for LPC and vaporizer leaks. Leaks in the gas supply lines between the flowmeters and the common gas outlet should be checked daily or whenever a vaporizer is changed (Appendix B, Item 8). The most thorough technique to check each vaporizer individually is by turning it on and then evaluating the low-pressure system for leaks. It is important to note that automated checkout procedures may not necessarily detect leaks at the vaporizer if the vaporizer is turned off during testing. In addition, vaporizers should be adequately filled and filler ports should be tightly closed (Appendix B, Item 7). As mentioned previously, the ASA

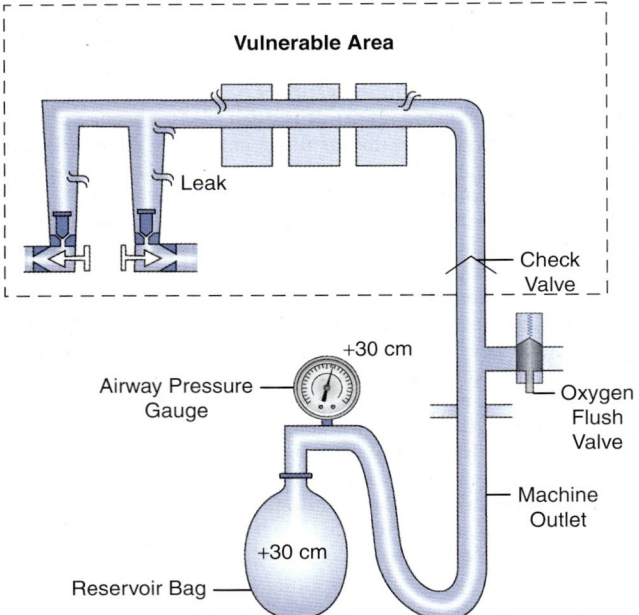

Figure 25-7 Inappropriate use of the oxygen flush valve to check the low-pressure circuit of a Datex-Ohmeda machine equipped with a check valve. The area within the rectangle is not checked by the inappropriate use of the oxygen flush valve. The components located within this area are precisely the ones most subject to breakage and leaks. Positive pressure within the patient circuit closes the check valve, and the value on the airway pressure gauge does not decrease despite leaks in the low-pressure circuit.

now recommends that individual institutions develop internal guidelines specific to their own equipment and needs.[17]

The 1993 FDA low-pressure system leak check is based on the Datex-Ohmeda negative-pressure leak test (Fig. 25-8). It is performed using a negative-pressure leak testing device, which is a simple suction 15-cc volume bulb that when evacuated generates a negative pressure of 65 mmHg. The machine main ON/OFF switch, the flow control valves, and the vaporizers are all turned off. The suction bulb is connected to the common gas outlet and squeezed repeatedly until it is fully collapsed. This action creates a vacuum in the low-pressure system circuitry. The machine is considered leak-free if the suction bulb remains collapsed for at least 10 seconds. A leak is present if the bulb reinflates during this period. The test is repeated with each vaporizer individually turned to the "on" position because internal vaporizer leaks can be detected only when the vaporizer is turned on and becomes part of the low-pressure system. Again, if the bulb reinflates in less than 10 seconds, a leak is present somewhere in the LPC.

Evaluation of the Circle System

The circle system tests (Appendix B, Items 12 and 13) evaluate the integrity of the circle breathing system, which spans from the machine common gas outlet to the Y-piece (Fig. 25-9). The test has two components: (1) breathing system pressure and leak testing and (2) verification that gas flows properly through the breathing circuit during both inspiration and exhalation. To thoroughly check the circle system for leaks, valve integrity, and obstruction, both tests must be performed preoperatively. The ASA 2008 recommendations call for performing the breathing system test and leak test before starting each case, such that pressure can be developed in the system during both manual/bag and automatic/mechanical ventilation.[17] Automated leak testing routines are implemented in modern workstations; system compliance is also calculated and used to adjust volume delivery during mechanical ventilation (Appendix B, Item 12). Because pressure and leak testing cannot identify all obstructions in the breathing circuit or confirm the function of the inspiratory and expiratory unidirectional valves, a test lung or second reservoir bag connected at the Y-piece can be used to confirm circuit integrity and function.[32,33] Visual inspection of the unidirectional valves should be performed daily, although subtle damage to these valves may be difficult to determine. Older 1993 FDA checkout procedures to identify valve incompetence that may not be visually obvious can be implemented, but are typically too complex for daily testing (Appendix B, Item 13).[34,35]

In the 1993 FDA Anesthesia Apparatus Checkout Recommendations, a *leak test* is performed by closing the APL (or pop-off) valve, occluding the Y-piece, and pressurizing the circuit to 30 cm H_2O pressure using the oxygen flush valve. The value on the pressure gauge will not decrease if the circle system is

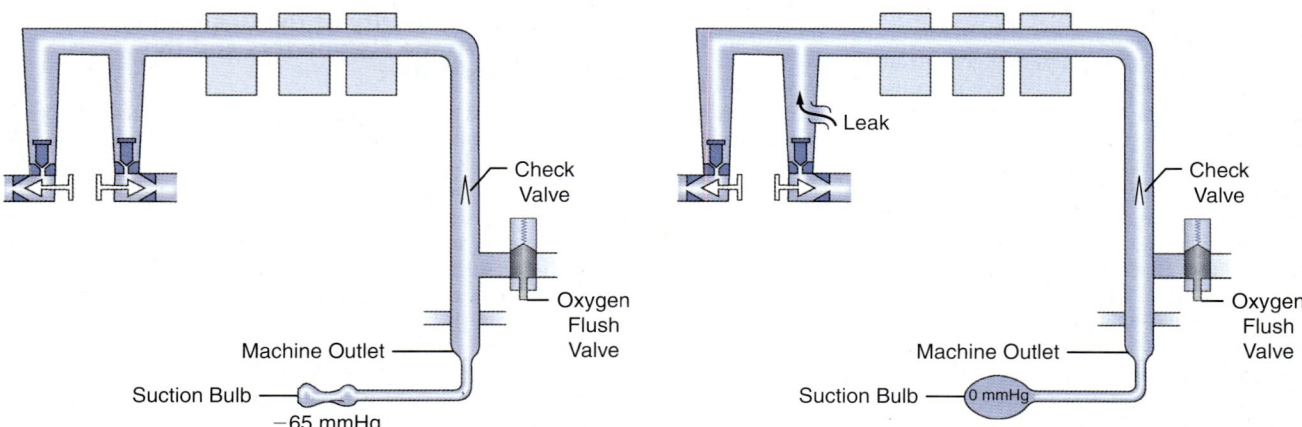

Figure 25-8 FDA negative-pressure leak test. A negative-pressure leak testing device is attached directly to the machine common gas outlet. Squeezing the bulb creates a vacuum in the low-pressure circuit and opens the check valve (*left*). When a leak is present in the low-pressure circuit, room air is entrained through the leak and the suction bulb inflates (*right*). (Adapted from Andrews JJ. Understanding anesthesia machines. In: 1988 Review Course Lectures, p. 78. Cleveland: International Anesthesia Research Society, 1988.)

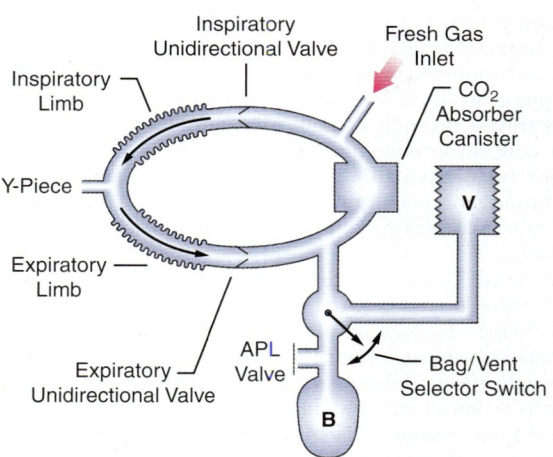

Figure 25-9 Components of the circle breathing system. B, reservoir bag; V, ventilator; APL, adjustable pressure-limiting (pop-off) valve. (Adapted from Brockwell RC. Inhaled anesthetic delivery systems. In: Miller RD, ed. *Anesthesia*. 6th ed. Philadelphia, PA: Churchill Livingstone; 2004:295.)

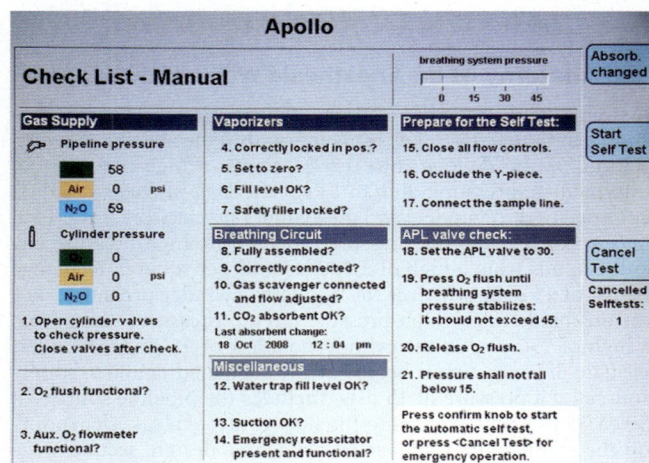

Figure 25-10 Apollo manual checklist screen.

leak-free, but this does not assure unidirectional valve integrity or function. The value on the pressure gauge will read 30 cm H_2O even if the unidirectional valves are stuck shut or are incompetent. In addition, a *flow test* checks the integrity of the unidirectional valves, and it detects obstruction in the circle system. It can be performed by removing the Y-piece from the circle system and breathing through the two corrugated hoses individually. The unidirectional valve leaflets should be present and should move appropriately. The operator should be able to inhale but not be able to exhale through the inspiratory limb. The operator should be able to exhale but not inhale through the expiratory limb. Needless to say, before performing this test, the operator must ensure there is no anesthetic gas in the circuit! The flow test can also be performed by using the ventilator and a reservoir bag connected to the "Y" piece as described in the 1993 FDA Anesthesia Apparatus Checkout Recommendations (Appendix A, Steps 11 and 12).[15]

Workstation Self-tests

Many new anesthesia workstations now incorporate technology that allows the machine to either automatically or manually guide the user through a series of self-tests to check for functionality of electronic, mechanical, and pneumatic components. Tested components commonly include the gas supply system, flow control valves, the circle system, ventilator, and integrated vaporizers. The comprehensiveness of these self-diagnostic tests varies from one model and manufacturer to another. If these tests are to be employed, users must be certain to read and strictly follow all manufacturer recommendations. Although a thorough understanding of what the particular workstation's self-tests include is very helpful, this information may be difficult to obtain and may vary greatly among devices. None of the preuse checkouts are fully automated; therefore, the user must perform certain functions for the checkout to be complete. It is important for the user to know what is in the automated checkout and even more important to know what is not. Figures 25-10 and 25-11 show screen shots from the Dräger Apollo workstation checkout procedures, manual and automated.

One particularly important point of caution with self-tests should be noted on systems with manifold-mounted vaporizers such as the Dräger Apollo and Dräger Fabius GS workstations. A manifold-mounted vaporizer does not become a part of an anesthesia workstation's low-pressure system until its concentration control dial is turned to the "on" position. Therefore, to detect internal vaporizer leaks in this type of a system, the "leak test" portion of the self-diagnostic must be repeated with each individual vaporizer turned to the "on" position. If this precaution is not taken, large leaks that could potentially result in patient awareness, such as those from a loose filler cap or cracked fill indicator, could go undetected.

A successful automated machine checkout does not necessarily preclude machine failure. In one example, a leak in an APL bypass valve of a Dräger Fabius GS Premium workstation was not detected by an automated checkout, resulting in a ventilator failure alarm. The authors concluded that a *functional test* of the ventilator and breathing circuit should be added to the checkout procedure. This may be performed by connecting a breathing bag to the circuit elbow. Activating the oxygen flush to inflate the bag will allow the bag to act as a model lung. The ventilator is now activated. Circuit pressure, tidal volume delivery, and bag inflation and deflation of the "lung" should be observed for proper function.[36]

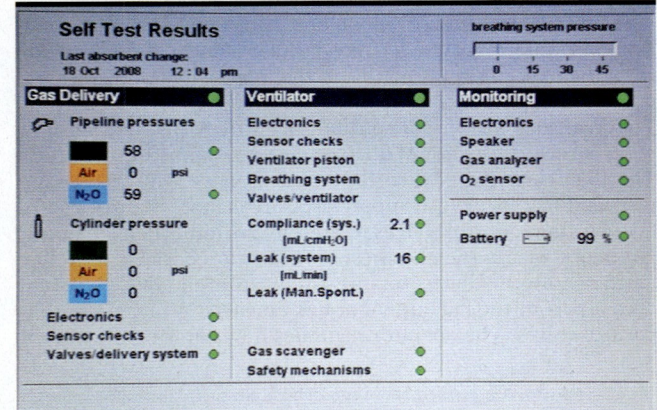

Figure 25-11 Apollo automated self-test screen.

Anesthesia Workstation Pneumatics

The Anatomy of an Anesthesia Workstation

A simplified diagram of a generic two-gas anesthesia machine is shown in Figure 25-6. The pressures within the anesthesia workstation can be divided into three circuits: a high-pressure, an intermediate-pressure, and an LPC. The *high-pressure circuit* is confined to the cylinders and the cylinder primary pressure regulators. For oxygen, the pressure range of the high-pressure circuit extends from a high of 2,200 pounds per square inch gauge (psig) to 45 psig, which is the regulated cylinder pressure.* For nitrous oxide in the high-pressure circuit, pressures range from a high of 750 psig in the cylinder to a low of 45 psig. The *intermediate-pressure circuit* begins at the regulated cylinder supply sources at a pressure of 45 psig, includes the pipeline sources at 50 to 55 psig and extends to the flow control valves. Depending on the manufacturer and specific machine design, second-stage pressure regulators may be used to decrease the pipeline supply pressures to the flow control valves to even lower pressures such as 14 psig or 26 psig within the intermediate-pressure circuit.[37,38] Finally, the LPC extends from the flow control valves to the common gas outlet. Therefore, the LPC includes the flow tubes, vaporizer manifold, vaporizers, and the one-way outlet check valve on most GE Healthcare/Datex-Ohmeda machines.

Both oxygen and nitrous oxide are supplied to the workstation from two sources: a pipeline supply source and a cylinder supply source. The pipeline supply source is the primary gas source for the anesthesia workstation. The hospital pipeline supply system provides gases to the machine at approximately 50 psig, which is the normal working pressure of most machines. The cylinder supply source serves as a backup if the pipeline supply fails or acts as the primary supply if the anesthesia workstation is being used in a location without the availability of pipeline supplied gases. As previously described, the oxygen cylinder source is regulated from 2,200 psig to approximately 45 psig, and the nitrous oxide cylinder source is regulated from 745 psig to approximately 45 psig.[39]

A safety device traditionally referred to as the *fail-safe* valve (and currently more appropriately termed the "*oxygen failure cutoff valve*") is located downstream from the nitrous oxide supply source. It serves as an interface between the oxygen and nitrous oxide supply sources. This valve shuts off, or proportionally decreases, the supply of nitrous oxide (and other gases) if the oxygen supply pressure decreases. Contemporary machines have an alarm device to monitor the oxygen supply pressure. A high-priority alarm is actuated when a decreasing oxygen supply pressure reaches a predetermined threshold, such as 30 psig.

Many GE Healthcare/Datex-Ohmeda machines have a second-stage pressure regulator for oxygen that is located downstream from the oxygen supply source in the intermediate-pressure circuit. It is adjusted to a precise pressure level, such as 14 psig. This regulator supplies a constant pressure to the oxygen flow control valve regardless of fluctuating oxygen pipeline pressures. The flow from the oxygen flow control valve will be constant provided that its oxygen supply pressure is more than 14 psig.

The flow control valves represent an important anatomic landmark within the anesthesia workstation because they separate the intermediate-pressure circuit from the LPC. The LPC is that part of the machine that lies downstream from the flow control valves. The operator regulates flow entering the LPC by adjusting the flow control valves. The oxygen and nitrous oxide flow control valves are linked mechanically or pneumatically by a proportioning system to help prevent unintended delivery of a hypoxic mixture. After leaving the flow tubes, the mixture of gases travels through a common manifold and may be directed to a concentration-calibrated vaporizer. Precise amounts of potent inhaled volatile anesthetic can be added, depending on vaporizer concentration control dial setting. The total FGF plus the anesthetic vapor then flow toward the common gas outlet.[40]

Some GE Datex-Ohmeda anesthesia machines have a one-way check valve located between the vaporizers and the common gas outlet in the mixed-gas line. Its purpose is to prevent back flow into the vaporizer during positive-pressure ventilation, therefore minimizing the effects of downstream intermittent pressure fluctuations on inhaled anesthetic concentration (see Vaporizers: Intermittent Back Pressure section). The presence or absence of this check valve *profoundly* influences which preoperative leak test is indicated (see Checking Your Anesthesia Workstation). The oxygen flush connection joins the mixed-gas line between the one-way check valve (when present) and the machine common gas outlet. Thus, when the oxygen flush valve is activated the pipeline oxygen flows directly to the common gas outlet at a rate of 35 to 75 L/min and potentially at a pressure of 55 psig.

Pipeline Supply Source

Most hospitals today have a central piping system to deliver medical gases including oxygen, nitrous oxide, air, and carbon dioxide to outlets in the operating room. The central piping system must supply the correct gases at the appropriate pressure for the anesthesia workstation to function properly. Unfortunately, this does not always occur. Even as recently as 2002, a large medical center with a huge cryogenic bulk oxygen storage system was not immune to component failures that contributed to a critical oxygen pipeline supply failure.[41] In this case, a faulty joint ruptured at the bottom of the primary cryogenic oxygen storage tank, releasing 8,000 gallons of liquid oxygen to flood the streets in the surrounding area and compromised oxygen delivery to the medical center.

In a 1976 survey of approximately 200 hospitals, 31% reported difficulties with pipeline systems.[42] The most common problem was inadequate oxygen pressure, followed by excessive pipeline pressures. The most devastating reported hazard, however, was accidental crossing of oxygen and nitrous oxide pipelines, which has led to many deaths. This problem caused 23 deaths in a newly constructed wing of a general hospital in Sudbury, Ontario, during a 5-month period.[43] In 2002, two hypoxic deaths were reported in New Haven, Connecticut. These resulted from a medical gas system failure in which an altered oxygen flowmeter was connected to a wall supply source for nitrous oxide.[44]

In the event that a pipeline crossover is suspected, the workstation user must immediately take two corrective actions. First, the backup oxygen cylinder should be turned on. Then, the pipeline supply must be disconnected. This second step is mandatory because the machine will preferentially use the (potentially) inappropriate 50 psig pipeline supply source instead of the lower-pressure (45 psig) oxygen cylinder source if the wall supply is not disconnected. Recent publications suggest that many anesthesia providers may not appreciate the importance of or reasons for these actions.[45,46]

The wall outlet connections for pipeline gases are gas-specific. If they are "quick connect" fittings then they are gas-specific within the same manufacturer. For example, a wall oxygen outlet

---

*Gauge pressure is the pressure above atmospheric pressure. Atmospheric pressure at sea level is 14.7 pounds per square inch absolute (psia). Thus in absolute pressure terms 45 psig would be 59.7 psia.

made by Ohmeda will not accept an oxygen connector made by Chemetron, even though the gas is the same. This can create problems if outlets and connectors by more than one manufacturer exist in the same facility.[47] Many institutions seeking to create uniformity are now using nationally standardized Diameter Index Safety System (DISS) threaded connections. The DISS provides threaded, noninterchangeable connections for medical gas lines, which minimizes the risk of misconnection. Regardless of which type of gas-specific connector (DISS or "quick connect") exists at the wall end of the hose conducting gas to the anesthesia machine, the gas enters the anesthesia machine through DISS inlet connections (Fig. 25-14A; arrows). A pressure gauge measures the pipeline gas pressure when the machine is connected to a pipeline supply. A check valve is located downstream from the inlet. It prevents reverse flow of gases from the machine to the pipeline or the atmosphere.

Cylinder Supply Source

Anesthesia workstations have E-cylinders for use when a pipeline supply source is not available or if the pipeline system fails. Anesthesia providers can easily become complacent and falsely assume that backup gas cylinders are, in fact, present on the anesthesia workstation, and further, if present, that they contain an adequate supply of compressed gas. The preuse checklist should contain steps that confirm both.

Medical gases supplied in E-cylinders are attached to the anesthesia machine via the hanger yoke assembly. The hanger yoke assembly orients and supports the cylinder, provides a gas-tight seal (using a washer called a Bodok seal between tank and hanger yoke), and ensures a unidirectional flow of gases into the machine. Each hanger yoke is equipped with the Pin Index Safety System (PISS). The PISS is a safeguard introduced to eliminate cylinder interchanging and the possibility of accidentally placing the incorrect gas on a yoke designed to accommodate another gas. Two metal pins on the yoke assembly are arranged so that that they project into corresponding holes in the cylinder valve (Fig. 25-12E). Each gas or combination of gases has a specific and unique pin arrangement.[48,49] It is generally assumed that in the United States all oxygen tanks are green in color and that the medical gas pin index system (PISS) will ensure that only an oxygen tank can be mounted in the hanger yoke for oxygen. In fact, there is no FDA standard for cylinder colors, so it is important to read the tank label.[50] A failure of the pin index system, and medical staff to properly identify E-cylinder contents, was the cause of an intraoperative fire during laparoscopy.[51] A mixture of CO_2 (14%) and oxygen (86%) was utilized rather than 100% CO_2. The wrong tank was able to be connected despite the PISS because all tanks containing more than 7% CO_2 have the same pin configuration.

Once the cylinders are turned on, compressed gases may pass from their respective high-pressure cylinder sources into the anesthesia machine (Fig. 25-6). A check valve is located downstream from each cylinder if a double-yoke assembly is used. This check valve serves several functions. First, it minimizes gas transfer from a cylinder at high pressure to one with a lower pressure. Second, it allows an empty cylinder to be exchanged for a full one while gas flow continues from the other cylinder into the machine with minimal loss of gas or supply pressure. Third, it minimizes leakage from an open cylinder to the atmosphere if one cylinder is absent. A cylinder supply pressure gauge is located downstream from the check valves. The gauge will indicate the pressure in the cylinder having the higher pressure when two reserve cylinders of the same gas are opened at the same time. In some electronic workstations, gas pressures are measured by transducers and displayed on the checkout screen (Fig. 25-10).

Each cylinder supply source has a pressure-reducing valve known as the cylinder pressure regulator. It reduces the high and variable storage pressure present in a cylinder to a lower, more constant pressure suitable for use in the anesthesia machine. The oxygen cylinder pressure regulator reduces the oxygen cylinder pressure from a high of 2,200 psig to approximately 45 psig. The nitrous oxide cylinder pressure regulator receives pressure of up to 745 psig and reduces it to approximately 45 psig.

The gas supply cylinder valves should be turned off when not in use, except during the preoperative machine preuse checkout. If the cylinder supply valves are left open, the reserve cylinder supply can be silently depleted whenever the pressure inside the machine decreases to a value lower than the regulated cylinder pressure. For example, oxygen pressure within the machine can decrease below 45 psig with oxygen flushing or possibly even during the use of a pneumatically driven ventilator, particularly at high inspiratory flow rates. In addition, the pipeline supply pressures of all gases can fall to less than 45 psig if problems exist in the central piping system. If the cylinders are left open when this occurs, they will eventually become depleted and no reserve supply may be available if a complete central pipeline failure were to occur.

The amount of time that an anesthesia machine can operate from the E-cylinder supply is important knowledge. This is particularly true now that anesthesia is being provided more frequently in office-based and in remote (outside the OR) hospital settings where pipeline oxygen may not be available. Oxygen can exist only in gaseous form at room temperature, and it obeys Boyle's law which states that for a fixed mass of gas at constant temperature, the product of pressure times volume is constant ($P1 \times V1 = P2 \times V2$).[52] The volume of oxygen available from the cylinder is directly proportional to the cylinder pressure.

An E-cylinder has an internal volume of 4.8 L and when "full" is pressurized to approximately 2,000 psig. Since psig is the pressure measured in excess of atmospheric pressure (14.7 psia, pounds per square inch absolute pressure), the cylinder pressure is 2,014.7 psia. Applying Boyle's Law:

$$2014.7 \times 4.8 = 14.7 \times V2.$$

Therefore, V2, the volume of oxygen in a "full" E-cylinder at 1 atm is:

$$(2014.7 \times 4.8)/14.7 = 658 \text{ L}.$$

The following equation has been proposed to help estimate the remaining time that oxygen can be delivered at a given flow rate[53]:

Approx. remaining time (hrs) = Oxygen cylinder pressure (psig)/(200 × oxygen flow rate [L/min])

For example, an E-cylinder of oxygen with a pressure of 1,000 psig, used at an oxygen flow rate of 5 L/min would be depleted in

$$[1000/(200 \times 5)] \approx 1 \text{ hour}$$

It should be noted that this calculation will provide only a gross estimate of remaining time and may not be exact. Furthermore, users should be cautioned that use of a pneumatically driven mechanical ventilator will dramatically increase oxygen utilization rates and decrease the remaining time until the cylinder is depleted.[54,55] Use of spontaneous or manual ventilation, with low FGF rates in a circle system with CO_2 absorption, will significantly reduce oxygen consumption from an E-cylinder if this is the only source of oxygen available. Because electrically

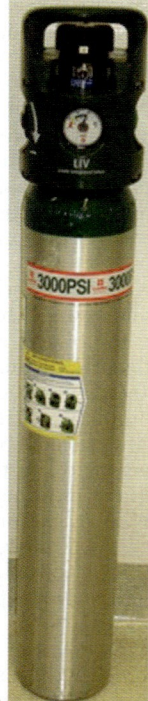
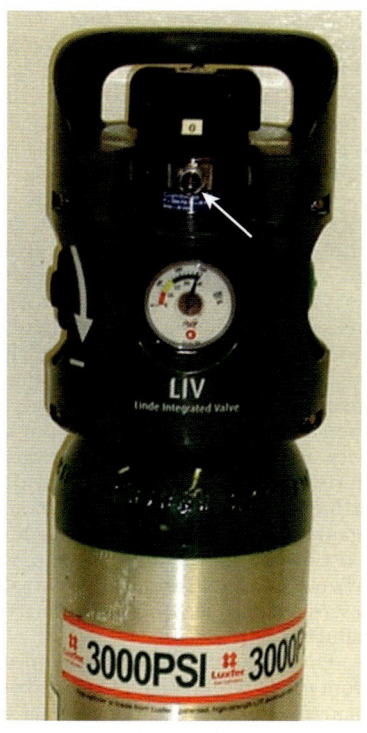
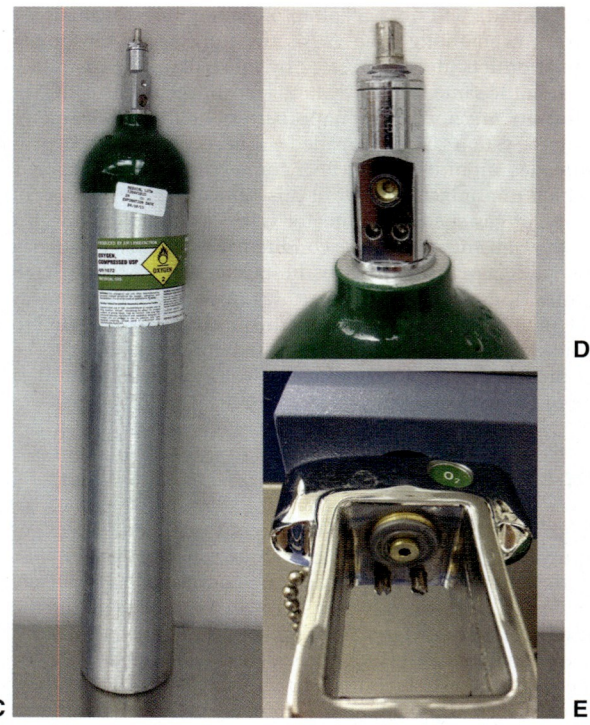

Figure 25-12 3,000 psig E-cylinder with Linde Integrated Valve, LIV (**A**). Linde Gas North America LLC that permits adjustable flows of ¼ to 25 L/min from the low-pressure nozzle (*arrow*) (**B**). There is also a high-pressure regulator that can supply oxygen at 50 psig via a DISS connector. Standard E-cylinder (**C**) showing pin-index safety system (**D**) and mating yoke (**E**).

powered piston-type anesthesia ventilators, such as found in the Dräger Fabius GS and Apollo workstations, do not impact oxygen usage rates they may be preferable to conventional gas-driven ventilators in practice settings where the supply of compressed gas cylinders may be limited.

An integrated valve and regulator for E-cylinders of oxygen is available that permits controlled delivery of oxygen via a nozzle at flows of 25 L/min or less for patient transport (Figs. 25-12 and 25-13). The tank regulator also permits delivery of oxygen at 50 psig from a DISS connection (Fig. 25-12B). If the oxygen hose from the anesthesia machine is connected to a central source (e.g., at the wall) via a DISS connector, and that central source becomes unavailable, then the machine hose can be easily connected to the tank's DISS connector and provide a backup supply of oxygen (Fig. 25-13). A conventional E cylinder with pin index safety system is shown in Figure 25-14.

Nitrous Oxide

Nitrous oxide (N_2O) can be supplied to the anesthesia machine from the pipeline system at a pressure of approximately 50 psig or from a backup E-cylinder in the N_2O hanger yoke. N_2O has a molecular weight of 44 atomic mass units (AMU) and a boiling point of −88°C at 760 mmHg (14.7 psia) pressure.[56] The critical temperature (CT) is the highest temperature at which a gas can exist in liquid form. The CT of N_2O is 36.5°C (critical pressure: 1,054 psig); therefore, N_2O can exist as a liquid at room temperature (20°C). E-cylinders of N_2O are factory-filled to 90% to 95% capacity with liquid N_2O. Above the liquid in the tank is N_2O vapor. Because the liquid agent is in equilibrium with its vapor or gas phase, the pressure exerted by the gaseous N_2O is its saturated vapor pressure (SVP) at the ambient temperature. At 20°C, the SVP of N_2O is 750 psig.

A full E-tank of N_2O generates approximately 1,600 L of gas at 1 atm pressure at sea level (14.7 psia). As long as some liquid N_2O is present in the tank and the ambient temperature remains at 20°C, the pressure in the N_2O tank will remain at 750 psig, which is the SVP of N_2O at 20°C. The volume of N_2O gas available from a tank therefore *cannot* be determined by reference to the N_2O tank pressure gauge. It is determined by weighing the tank and subtracting the weight of the empty tank (tare weight) to determine the weight of the contained N_2O. Once all the liquid N_2O has been used and the tank contains only vapor, the pressure in the tank will begin to decrease as nitrous oxide is used. However, because N_2O is a vapor and not a gas, it does not obey Boyle's law and the volume of nitrous oxide remaining in the tank cannot be calculated from the tank pressure gauge. When the last drop of liquid N_2O has just evaporated, nearly one-quarter of the full cylinder remains (i.e., ~400 L) in an E cylinder.[57] From then on, as N_2O continues to be utilized, the value on the tank pressure gauge will fall.

Nitrous oxide from the tank supply enters the N_2O hanger yoke at pressures of up to 750 psig (at 20°C) and then passes through a regulator that reduces this pressure to 40 to 45 psig (Fig. 25-6). The PISS is designed to ensure that only an N_2O tank may hang in an N_2O hanger yoke. As with oxygen, a check valve in each yoke prevents the back leakage of N_2O if no tank is hanging in the yoke.

The N_2O pipeline is supplied from a bulk storage container of liquid N_2O or from banks of large N_2O tanks, usually H-cylinders. (Each H-cylinder of N_2O evolves 16,000 L of gas at atmospheric pressure.) The pressure in the N_2O pipeline is regulated to approximately 50 psig to supply the outlets in the operating

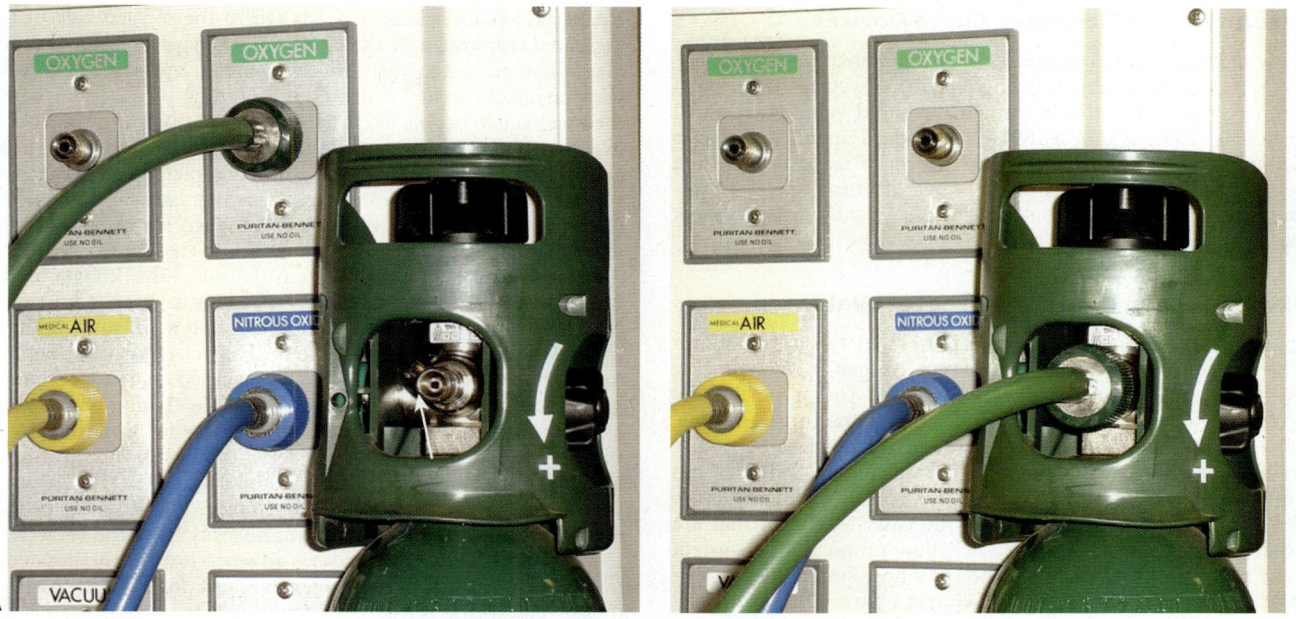

Figure 25-13 3,000 psig E-cylinder valve showing 50 psig DISS connection (*arrow*) (**A**) that could be connected to the machine oxygen hose if wall oxygen supply fails (**B**).

room. Having entered the anesthesia machine intermediate-pressure system, N_2O must flow past the "fail-safe" valve to reach the N_2O flow control.

Machine Intermediate-Pressure System

Having entered the anesthesia machine's intermediate-pressure system from the pipeline supply at approximately 50 psig, or from the tank supply at 45 psig, oxygen can take several paths:
1. To the DISS auxiliary oxygen takeoff, to which a Sanders type jet ventilating system can be connected
2. To supply a pneumatically powered bellows ventilator
3. Via a regulator and an auxiliary oxygen flowmeter to be connected to a nasal cannula, SIRB, and so forth
4. To the oxygen low-pressure alarm sensor
5. To the pressure sensitive shutoff ("fail-safe") valve
6. To the oxygen flush control valve
7. To the oxygen flowmeter (in some machines via a second-stage regulator)

Oxygen Supply Pressure Failure Safety Devices

The 2000 ASTM F1850–00 standard stated, "The anesthesia gas supply device shall be designed so that whenever oxygen supply pressure is reduced to below the manufacturer specified minimum, the delivered oxygen concentration shall not decrease below 19% at the common gas outlet." Contemporary anesthesia machines have a number of safety devices that act together in a cascade manner to minimize the risk of delivery of a hypoxic gas mixture as oxygen pressure decreases. Several of these devices are described in the following sections.

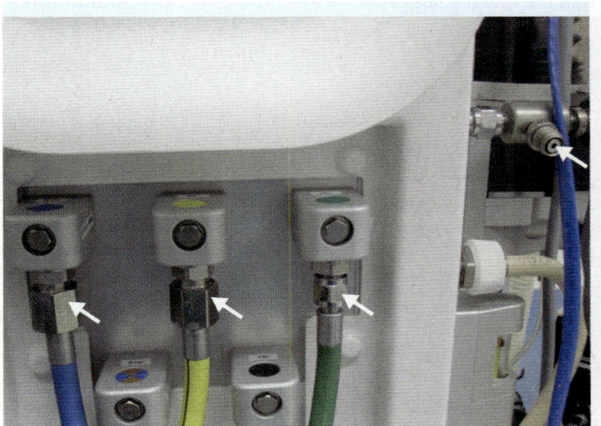 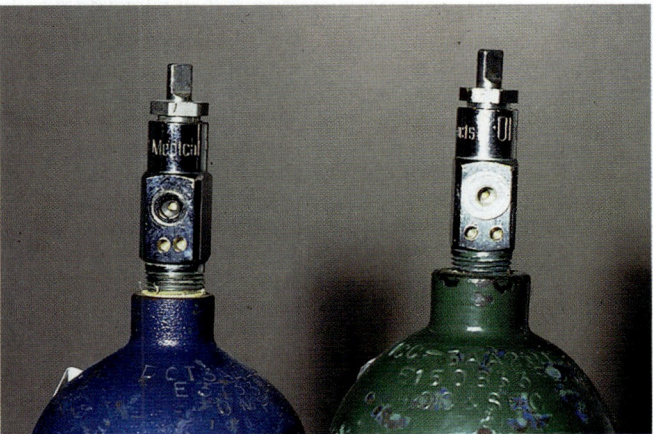

Figure 25-14   **A:** DISS connector. **B:** PISS connector.

Pneumatic and Electronic Alarm Devices

Many older anesthesia machines have a pneumatic alarm device that provides an audible warning when the oxygen supply pressure decreases to a predetermined threshold value such as 30 psig. The 2000 ASTM F1850–00 standard mandated that a medium priority alarm be activated within 5 seconds when the oxygen pressure decreases below a manufacturer-specific pressure threshold. Electronic alarm devices are now used to meet this requirement.

Oxygen Failure Cutoff ("Fail-Safe") Valves

An oxygen failure cutoff valve is present in the gas line supplying each of the flowmeters except oxygen. Controlled by oxygen supply pressure, the valve shuts off (or proportionally decreases) the supply pressure of all other gases (nitrous oxide, CO_2, helium, and in some machines, air) as the oxygen supply pressure decreases. Unfortunately, the misnomer "fail-safe" has led to the misconception that the valve prevents administration of a hypoxic mixture. This is not the case. Machines that are either not equipped with an N_2O/O_2 flow proportioning system (see Proportioning Systems section) or whose system may be disabled by the user can deliver a hypoxic mixture under normal working conditions. On such a system, the oxygen flow control valve can be closed intentionally or accidentally. Normal oxygen pressure will keep other gas lines open so that a hypoxic mixture could result.

Many GE-Datex-Ohmeda machines are equipped with a fail-safe valve known as the pressure-sensor shutoff valve. On older machines, this valve operates in a threshold manner and is either open or closed. Oxygen supply pressure opens the valve, and the valve return spring closes the valve. Figure 25-15 shows a nitrous oxide pressure-sensor shutoff valve with a threshold pressure of 20 psig. In Figure 25-15A, an oxygen supply pressure greater than 20 psig is exerted on the mobile diaphragm. This pressure moves the piston and pin upward and the valve opens. Nitrous oxide flows freely to the nitrous oxide flow control valve. In Figure 25-15B, the oxygen supply pressure is less than 20 psig, and the force of the valve return spring completely closes the valve. Nitrous oxide flow stops at the closed fail-safe valve, and it does not advance to the nitrous oxide flow control valve.

In the GE Datex Aestiva/5, which is a more recent model machine, the "fail-safe" valve is not of an "open or closed" design, rather it is a variable valve in a balance regulator. The balance regulator works as follows. The second-stage pressure regulator for oxygen reduces the pressure to about 30 psig in the intermediate-pressure system. The oxygen pressure is then piloted to the balance regulator where it is applied to the oxygen side of the regulated diaphragm. If the pressure of oxygen is sufficient, the diaphragm pushes against a mechanism that opens the flow pathway for nitrous oxide. If the oxygen piloting pressure decreases, the mechanism begins to close off the pathway for nitrous oxide in proportion to the decrease in piloted oxygen pressure. The balance regulator for nitrous oxide closes completely when the pressure of oxygen falls to 0.5 psig. Balance regulators for heliox and CO_2 interrupt the flows of these gases when the piloted oxygen pressure falls below 10 psig.

Dräger Medical uses a different fail-safe valve known as the Oxygen Failure Protection Device (OFPD) to interface the oxygen pressure with that of other gases, such as nitrous oxide or inert gases. Similar in principle to the balance regulator described in the previous paragraph, the OFPD is based on a proportioning principle rather than a threshold principle. The pressure of all gases controlled by the OFPD will decrease in proportion with the oxygen pressure. The OFPD consists of a seat–nozzle assembly connected to a spring-loaded piston (Fig. 25-16). The oxygen supply pressure in the left panel is 50 psig. This pressure pushes the piston upward, forcing the nozzle away from the valve seat. Nitrous oxide and/or other gases advance toward the flow control valve at 50 psig. The oxygen pressure in the right panel is 0 psig. The spring is expanded and forces the nozzle against the seat, preventing flow through the device. Finally, the center panel shows an intermediate oxygen pressure of 25 psig. The force of the spring partially closes the valve. The nitrous oxide pressure delivered to the flow control valve is 25 psig. There is a continuum of intermediate configurations between the extremes (0 to 50 psig) of oxygen supply pressure. These intermediate valve configurations are responsible for the proportional nature of the OFPD. An important concept to be understood with these particular fail-safe devices is that the older Datex-Ohmeda Pressure Sensor Shutoff Valve is threshold in nature (all-or-nothing), whereas the GE balance regulator and Dräger OFPD are variable flow type proportioning systems. It is important to recognize that the "fail-safe" valve is pressure sensitive and not flow sensitive. As long as the pressure in the intermediate pressure system for oxygen is adequate, nitrous oxide can flow to its flow control valve (Fig. 25-17).

Second-stage Oxygen Pressure Regulator

Most contemporary GE Datex-Ohmeda workstations have a second-stage oxygen pressure regulator set at a specific value, ranging from 12 to 19 psig. Output from the oxygen flowmeter is constant when the oxygen supply pressure exceeds the threshold (minimal)

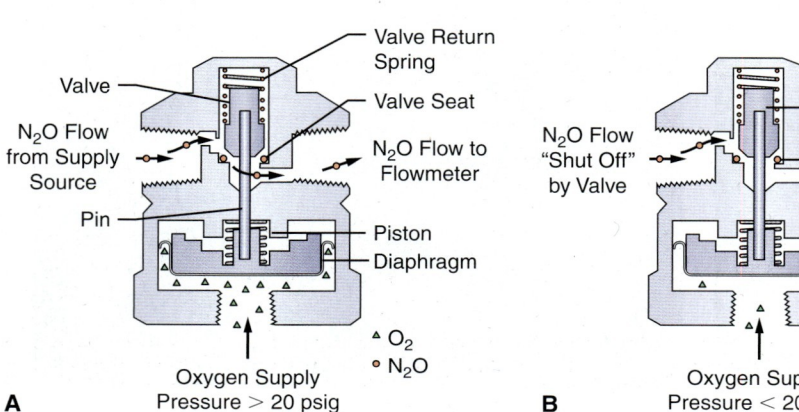

Figure 25-15 Pressure-sensor shutoff valve. **A:** The valve is open because the oxygen supply pressure is greater than the threshold value of 20 psig. **B:** The valve is closed because of inadequate oxygen pressure. (Adapted from Bowie E, Huffman LM. *The Anesthesia Machine: Essentials for Understanding.* Madison, WI, Ohmeda, a division of BOC Healthcare, Inc., 1985.)

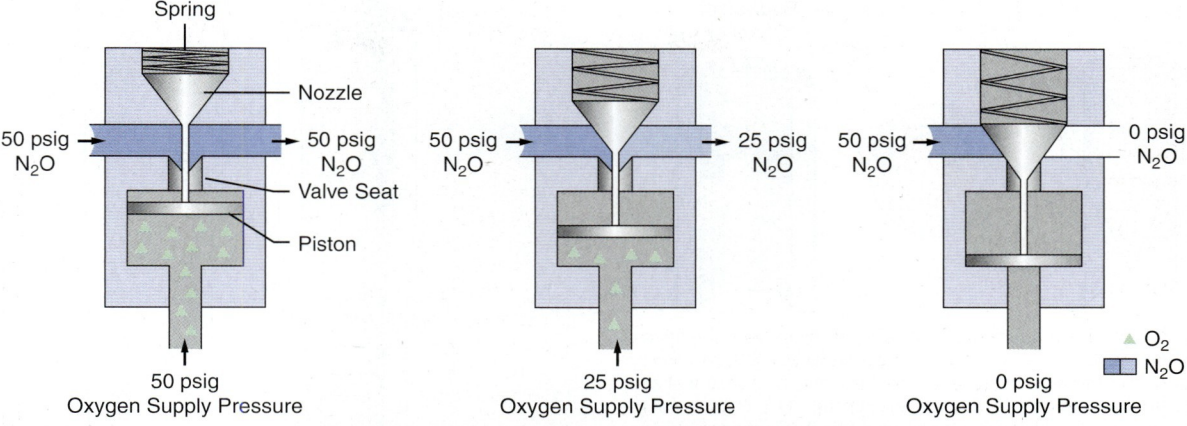

Figure 25-16 Oxygen Failure Protection Device/Sensitive Oxygen Ratio Controller (OFPD/S-ORC), which responds proportionally to changes in oxygen supply pressure. (Adapted from Narkomed 2A *Anesthesia System: Technical Service Manual.* 6th ed. Telford, PA: North American Dräger; 1985.)

value. The pressure-sensor shutoff valve of older Datex-Ohmeda machines is set at a higher threshold value (20 to 30 psig) to ensure that oxygen is the last gas flowing if oxygen pressure failure occurs.

Flowmeter Assemblies

The flowmeter assembly (Fig. 25-18) precisely controls and measures gas flow to the common gas outlet. With traditional glass flowmeter assemblies, the flow control needle valve regulates the amount of flow that enters a tapered, transparent flow tube known as a Thorpe tube. The tube is tapered such that it has a small cross-sectional area at its lower (low flow) end, and a larger cross-sectional area at its upper (high flow) end. A mobile indicator float inside the flow tube indicates the amount of flow passing through the associated flow control valve. The quantity of flow is indicated on a scale associated with the flow tube. Some newer anesthesia workstations have now replaced the conventional glass flow tubes with electronic flow sensors that measure the flow of the individual gases. The flow rate data are then presented in numerical format, graphical format, or a combination of the two on the workstation screen. The integration of these "electronic flowmeters" is an essential step in the evolution of the anesthesia workstation if it is to become fully integrated with anesthesia data-capturing systems, such as computerized anesthesia record keepers (or anesthesia information management systems, AIMS).

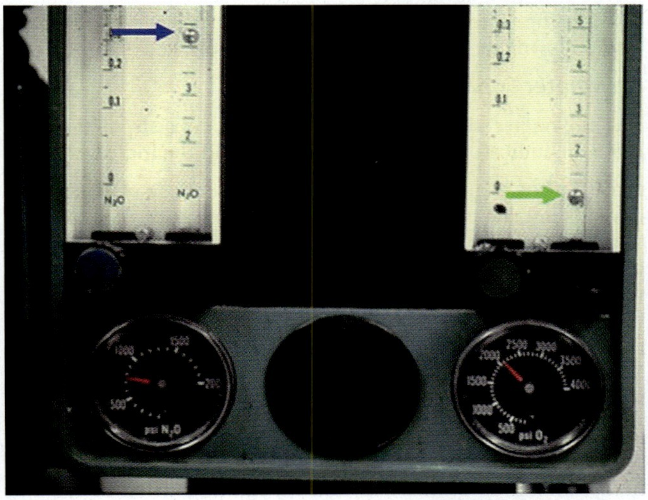

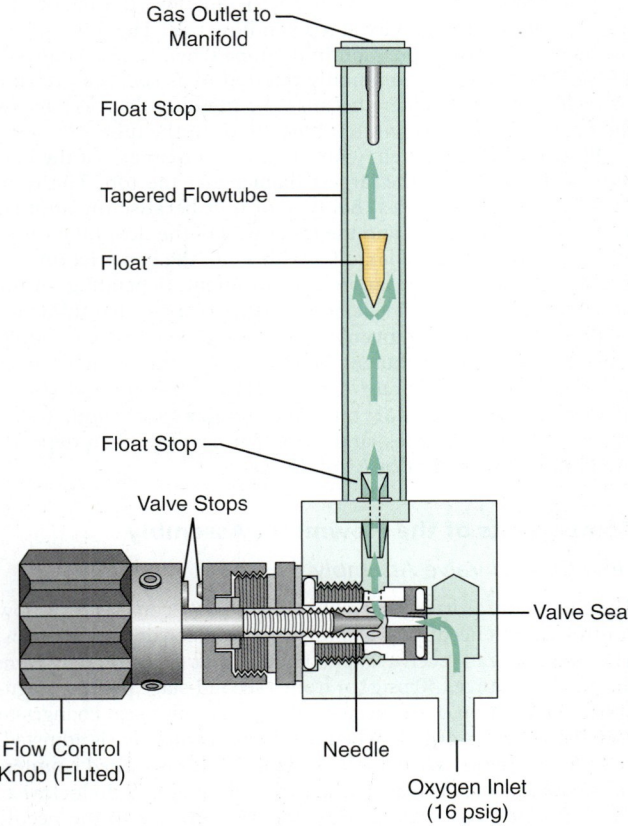

Figure 25-17 Failure of fail-safe valve to prevent a hypoxic mixture.

Figure 25-18 Oxygen flowmeter assembly. The oxygen flowmeter assembly is composed of the flow control valve assembly plus the flowmeter subassembly. Note that this is a GE Datex-Ohmeda design because in this figure oxygen is supplied to the flowmeter at 16 psig from a second-stage regulator. (Adapted from Bowie E, Huffman LM. *The Anesthesia Machine: Essentials for Understanding.* Madison, WI: Ohmeda, a division of BOC Healthcare, Inc., 1985.)

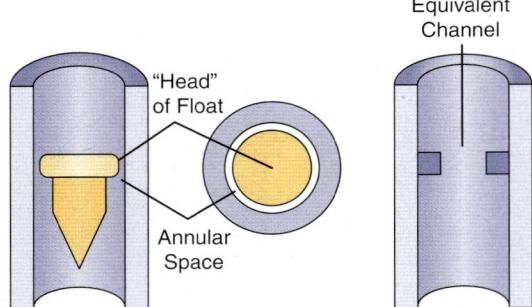

Figure 25-19 The annular space. The clearance between the head of the float and the flow tube is known as the annular space. It can be considered equivalent to a circular channel of the same cross-sectional area. (Adapted from Macintosh R, Mushin WW, Epstein HG. *Physics for the Anaesthetist*. 3rd ed. Oxford: Blackwell Scientific Publications; 1963.)

Operating Principles of Conventional Flowmeters

Opening the flow control needle valve allows gas to travel through the space between the float and the flow tube. This space is known as the annular space (Fig. 25-19). The indicator float hovers freely in an equilibrium position where the upward force resulting from gas flow equals the downward force on the float resulting from gravity at a given flow rate. The float moves to a new equilibrium position in the tube when flow is changed. These flowmeters are commonly referred to as *constant pressure variable orifice* flowmeters because the pressure decrease across the float remains constant for all positions in the tube.[58,59]

Flow tubes are tapered, with the smallest diameter at the bottom of the tube and the largest diameter at the top. The term *variable orifice* designates this type of unit because the annular space between the float and the inner wall of the flow tube varies with the position of the float. Flow through the constriction created by the float can be laminar or turbulent, depending on the flow rate (Fig. 25-20). The characteristics of a gas that influence its flow rate through a given constriction are viscosity (laminar flow) and density (turbulent flow). Because the annular space is tubular, at low flow rates laminar flow is present and *viscosity* determines the gas flow rate. The annular space simulates an orifice at high flow rates, and turbulent gas flow then depends predominantly on the *density* of the gas.

Components of the Flowmeter Assembly

Flow Control Valve Assembly

The flow control valve assembly (Fig. 25-18) consists of a flow control knob, a needle valve, a valve seat, and a pair of valve stops. The assembly can receive its pneumatic input either directly from the pipeline source (50 psig) or from a second-stage pressure regulator. The location of the needle valve in the valve seat changes to establish different orifices when the flow control valve is adjusted. Gas flow increases when the flow control valve is turned counterclockwise, and it decreases when the valve is turned clockwise. Extreme clockwise rotation may result in damage to the needle valve and valve seat. Therefore, flow control valves are equipped with valve "stops" to prevent this occurrence.

Safety Features. Flow control valve assemblies have numerous safety features. The oxygen flow control knob is physically distinguishable from other gas knobs. It is distinctively fluted, projects beyond the control knobs of the other gases, and is

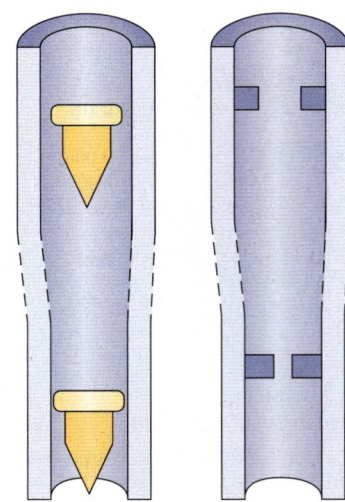

Figure 25-20 Flow tube constriction. The lower half of illustration represents the lower portion of a flow tube. The clearance between the head of the float and the flow tube is narrow. The equivalent channel is tubular because its diameter is less than its length. Viscosity is dominant in determining gas flow rate through this tubular constriction. The upper half of illustration represents the upper portion of a flow tube. The equivalent channel is orificial because its length is less than its width. Density is dominant in determining gas flow rate through this orificial constriction. (Adapted from Macintosh R, Mushin WW, Epstein HG. *Physics for the Anaesthetist*. 3rd ed. Oxford: Blackwell Scientific Publications; 1963.)

larger in diameter than the flow control knobs of other gases. All knobs are color coded for the appropriate gas, and the chemical formula or name of the gas is permanently marked on each. Flow control knobs are recessed or protected with a shield or barrier to minimize accidental change from a preset position. If a single gas has two flow tubes, the tubes are arranged in series and are controlled by a single flow control valve.

In many of the new anesthesia workstations, the flowmeters have been replaced by electronic control panels that contain "soft keys." To adjust any gas flow, the operator must perform the following steps: (1) select and press the "soft key" to identify the gas and anesthetic agent selected; (2) turn the selector knob to adjust the desired flow level; and (3) press the selector knob again to confirm the selected flow level and anesthetic agent (see Electronic Flowmeters section).

Flowmeter Subassembly

The flowmeter subassembly (Fig. 25-18) consists of the flow tube, the indicator float with float stops, and the indicator scale.

Flow Tubes. Contemporary flow tubes are made of glass. Most have a single taper in which the inner diameter of the flow tube increases uniformly from bottom to top. Manufacturers provide double flow tubes for oxygen and nitrous oxide to provide better visual discrimination at low flow rates. A fine flow tube indicates flow from approximately 200 mL/min to 1 L/min, and a coarse flow tube indicates flow from approximately 1 mL/min to 10 or 12 L/min. The two tubes are connected in series and supplied from a single flow control valve.

Indicator Floats and Float Stops. Anesthesia machines with traditional flowmeters use several different types of bobbins or floats, including plumb-bob floats, rotating skirted floats, and ball floats. Flow is read at the top of plumb-bob and skirted floats and at the center of the ball on the ball-type floats. Flow tubes are equipped with float stops at the top and bottom of the tube. The upper stop prevents the float from ascending to the top of the tube and plugging the outlet. It also ensures that the float will be visible at maximum flows instead of being hidden in the manifold. The bottom float stop provides a central foundation for the indicator when the flow control valve is turned off.

Scale. The flowmeter scale can be marked directly on the flow tube or located to the right of the tube. Gradations corresponding to equal increments in flow rate are closer together at the top of the scale because the annular space increases more rapidly than does the internal diameter from bottom to top of the tube. Rib guides are used in some flow tubes with ball-type indicators to minimize this compression effect. They are tapered glass ridges that run the length of the tube. There are usually three rib guides that are equally spaced around the inner circumference of the tube. In the presence of rib guides, the annular space from the bottom to the top of the tube increases almost proportionally with the internal diameter. This results in a nearly linear scale. Rib guides are employed on many Dräger Medical flow tubes.

Safety Features. The flowmeter subassemblies for each gas on the GE-Datex-Ohmeda and Aestiva models are housed in independent, color-coded, pin-specific modules. The flow tubes are adjacent to a gas-specific, color-coded backing. The flow scale and the chemical formula (or name of the gas) is permanently etched on the backing to the right of the flow tube. Flowmeter scales are individually hand-calibrated to provide a high degree of accuracy. The tube, float, and scale make an inseparable unit. The entire set must be replaced if any component is damaged.

Dräger Medical does not use a modular system for the flowmeter subassembly. The flow scale, the chemical symbol, and the gas-specific color codes are etched directly onto the flow tube.

Problems with Flowmeters

Leaks

Flowmeter leaks are a significant hazard because the flowmeters are located downstream from all machine safety devices except the oxygen analyzer.[60] Leaks can occur at the O-ring junctions between the glass flow tubes and the metal manifold or in cracked or broken glass flow tubes, the most fragile pneumatic component of the anesthesia machine. Even though gross damage to conventional glass flow tubes is usually apparent, subtle cracks and chips may be overlooked, resulting in errors of delivered flows.[61] The use of electronic flowmeters and the removal of conventional glass flow tubes from some newer anesthesia workstations (e.g., GE-Datex-Ohmeda S/5 ADU and the Dräger Fabius) may help to eliminate these potential sources of leaks (see Electronic Flowmeters section).

Eger et al.[62] demonstrated that, in the presence of a flowmeter leak, a hypoxic mixture is less likely to occur if the oxygen flowmeter is located downstream from all other flowmeters. Figure 25-21 is an updated version of the figure in Eger's original publication. The unused air flow tube has a large leak. Nitrous oxide and oxygen flow rates are set at a ratio of 3:1. A potentially dangerous arrangement is shown in Figure 25-21A and B because the nitrous oxide flowmeter is located in the downstream position. A hypoxic mixture can result because a substantial portion of oxygen flow passes through the leak, and all nitrous oxide is directed to the common gas outlet. Safer configurations are

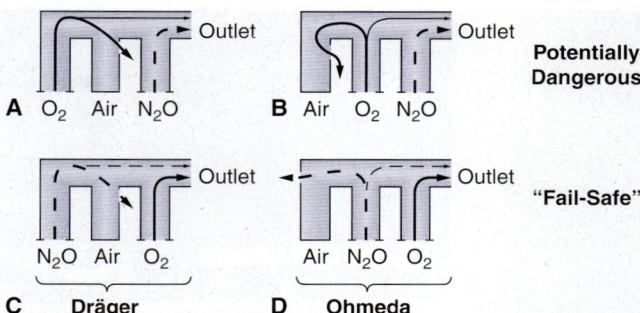

Figure 25-21 Flowmeter sequence—a potential cause of hypoxia. In the event of a flowmeter leak (in this example, air), a potentially dangerous arrangement exists when nitrous oxide is located in the downstream position (**A, B**). The safest configuration exists when oxygen is located in the downstream position (**C, D**). See text for details. (Adapted from Eger EI 2nd, Hylton RR, Irwin RH, et al. Anesthetic flowmeter sequence—a cause for hypoxia. *Anesthesiology.* 1963;24:396.)

shown in Figure 25-21C and D, where the oxygen flowmeter is located in the downstream position.

The above, preferred, arrangement is not infallible. A leak in the oxygen flow tube may result in creation of a hypoxic mixture even when oxygen is located in the downstream position (Fig. 25-22). Oxygen escapes through the leak and nitrous oxide continues to flow toward the common outlet, particularly at high ratios of nitrous oxide to oxygen flow.

Inaccuracy

Flow measurement error can occur even when flowmeters are assembled properly with appropriate components. Dirt or static electricity can cause a float to stick, and the actual flow may be higher or lower than that indicated. Sticking of the indicator float is more common in the low flow ranges because the annular space is smaller. A damaged float can cause inaccurate readings because the precise relationship between the float and the flow tube is altered. Back pressure from the breathing circuit can cause a float to drop so that it reads less than the actual flow. Finally, if flowmeters are not aligned properly in the vertical position (plumb), readings can be inaccurate because tilting distorts the annular space.

Ambiguous Scale

Before the standardization of flowmeter scales and the widespread use of oxygen analyzers, at least two deaths resulted from confusion created by ambiguous scales.[63] The operator read the float position beside an adjacent but erroneous scale in both

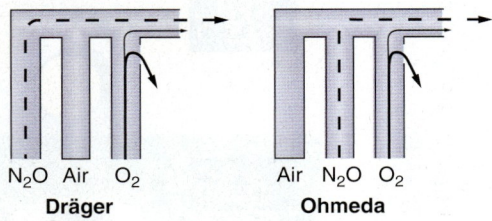

Figure 25-22 Oxygen flow tube leak. An oxygen flow tube leak can produce a hypoxic mixture regardless of flow tube arrangement. (Adapted from Brockwell RC. Inhaled anesthetic delivery systems. In: Miller RD, ed. *Anesthesia*. 6th ed. Philadelphia, PA: Churchill Livingstone; 2004:281.)

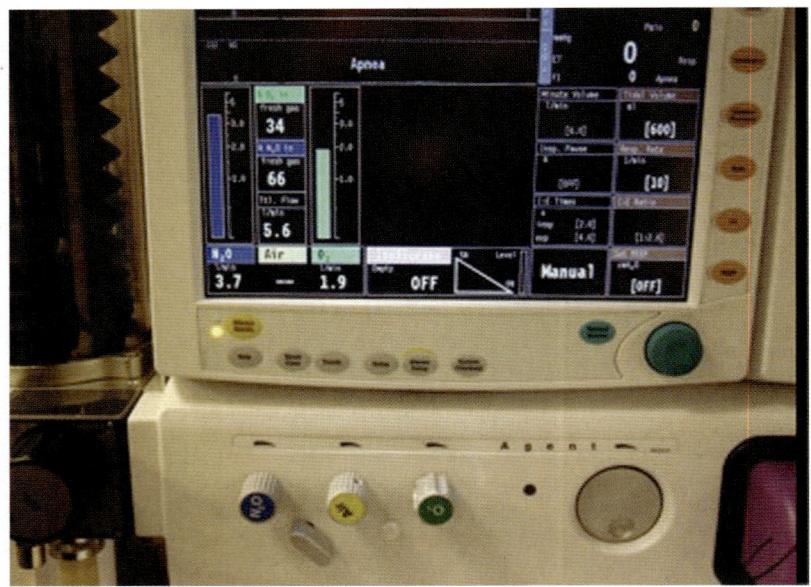

Figure 25-23 Datex S5/ADU. Note mechanical needle valve controls for the gas flows but electronic display of virtual flowmeter and digital readout.

cases. Today this error is less likely to occur because contemporary flowmeter scales are marked either directly onto the flow tube or immediately to the right of it.

Electronic Flowmeters

Many of the newer anesthesia workstations (e.g., the Dräger Apollo, Dräger Fabius GS, Spacelabs Healthcare's ARKON, and Datex S5/ADU; Figs. 25-23 and 25-1A, 25-2A, 25-4A) have conventional flow control knobs and flow control valves, but have electronic flow sensors and digital displays rather than glass flow tubes. The output from the flow control valve is represented graphically and/or numerically in liters per minute on the workstation's integrated user interface. These systems are dependent on electrical power to provide a precise display of gas flows. However, even when electrical power is totally interrupted, since the flow control valves themselves are mechanical (i.e., nonelectronic), the set gas flows will continue uninterrupted. Since these machines do not have individual flow tubes that physically quantify the flow of each gas, a small conventional pneumatic "fresh gas" or "total flow" indicator is also provided that gives the user an estimate of the total quantity of fresh gas flowing from all gas flow control valves to the anesthesia workstation's common gas outlet, and is functional even in the event of a total power failure (Fig. 25-24).

In the GE Aisys Carestation (Fig. 25-3A), the traditional needle valve gas flow controls and color-coded control knobs are

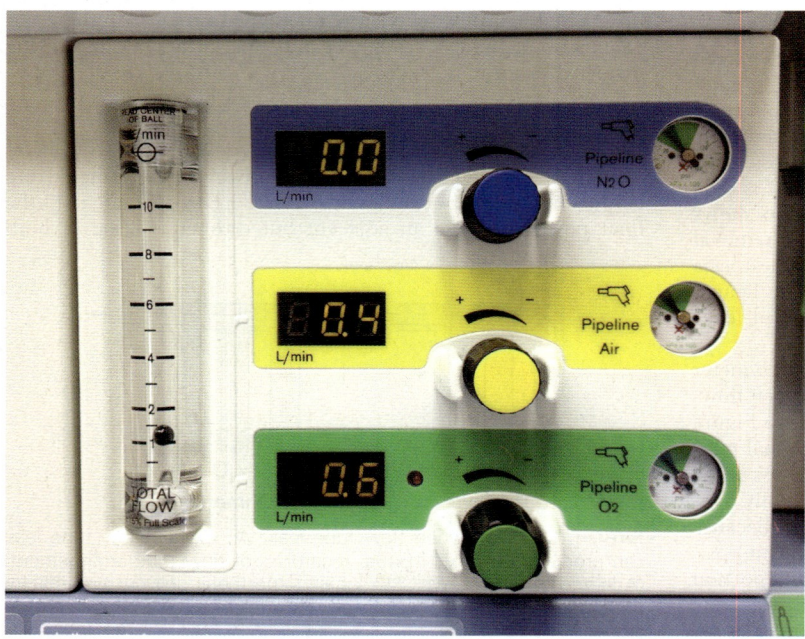

Figure 25-24 Dräger Fabius GS. Note needle valve controls, graphical and digital flow displays. The total gas flow rotameter continues to function if electrical power is lost.

replaced by an electronic control system that uses a gas mixer. In this model, the second gas, either N_2O or air is first selected, followed by the desired inspired oxygen concentration (FIO_2) and total FGF. Total flow and FIO_2 selections are made by pressing soft keys on the control panel, adjusting the settings using a "com wheel," and then pressing the com wheel to "confirm."

In the GE Aisys Carestation (Fig. 25-3A), the controls to increase or decrease flows (or agent concentration) represent a departure from the traditional. The traditional needle valve gas flow controls were designed by mechanical engineers so that one turns the flow control knob counterclockwise to increase flow (by opening the valve wider). The same applies to increasing agent concentration on a variable bypass vaporizer. The Aisys Carestation controls are designed by electrical engineers where the standard is to increase the output by rotating the dial (com wheel) in a clockwise direction. Thus, when learning to use the Aisys Carestation workstation, the operator must adapt to "clockwise to increase" and remember to confirm new settings; otherwise they are not implemented. In the event the gas mixer fails, the Aisys Carestation will switch to a backup system that permits delivery of oxygen to the breathing system via an alternate oxygen flowmeter, which is a traditional mechanical needle valve and rotameter flow tube.

Automated Fresh Gas Flow Optimization by Workstation Software

Anesthetic gas cost and environmental impact of excessive waste anesthetic gas are increasing concerns. The Dräger Apollo anesthesia workstation has an FGF optimization tool called the Low Flow Wizard (LFW). The LFW gives the user an indication of whether there is too much, too little, or the correct amount of FGF. It is important to understand how this tool works and to understand its limitations. Figure 25-25 shows the three possible recommendations from the LFW.

The LFW determines minimum FGF by calculating the difference between inspiratory and expiratory minute volume. In addition, anesthetic uptake is calculated using inspired and expired anesthetic gas concentrations as well as N_2O and CO_2 concentrations. This algorithm is designed to err on the side of overestimation of uptake. Oxygen uptake is calculated using CO_2 uptake because the gas analysis system is able to determine CO_2 concentrations with greater precision than oxygen concentrations. During laparoscopic surgery with CO_2 insufflation, if end-tidal CO_2 is increased, the calculated oxygen uptake will increase, thus the LFW will recommend higher FGF. In addition, application or removal of PEEP will transiently affect LFW calculations until gas flow dynamics reach a state of equilibrium.[64] A simulator-based study demonstrated that use of the LFW reduced isoflurane consumption by 53% during the maintenance phase of anesthesia.[65]

GE-Datex-Ohmeda has developed an optional software tool, called "ecoFLOW" to determine approximate minimum flow of O_2 required to maintain a preset FiO_2. This system (available on the Aisys CS^2 and Avance CS^2 models) also shows approximate amount of agent used and cost per hour. The minimum O_2 flow is calculated using patient O_2 uptake, the dilution effect of the delivered anesthetic agent, and the effects of the circle breathing system.[66]

Proportioning Systems

Manufacturers equip anesthesia workstations with N_2O/O_2 proportioning systems designed to prevent creation and delivery of a hypoxic mixture when nitrous oxide is administered. Nitrous oxide and oxygen are interfaced mechanically and/or pneumatically, or electronically (on the GE Aisys Carestation), so that the minimum oxygen concentration at the common gas outlet is between 23% and 25% depending on the manufacturer.

GE-Datex-Ohmeda Link-25 Proportion-Limiting Control System

Traditional GE-Datex-Ohmeda machines use the Link-25 System. The heart of the system is the mechanical integration of the nitrous oxide and oxygen flow control valves. It allows independent adjustment of either valve, yet automatically intercedes to maintain a minimum 25% oxygen concentration with a maximum nitrous oxide–oxygen flow ratio of 3:1. The Link-25 automatically increases oxygen flow to prevent delivery of a hypoxic mixture.

Figure 25-26 illustrates the GE-Datex-Ohmeda Link-25 System. A 14-tooth sprocket is attached to the nitrous oxide flow control valve, and a 29-tooth sprocket is attached to the oxygen flow control valve. A stainless steel chain physically links the sprockets. When the nitrous oxide flow control valve is turned through 2.09 revolutions the oxygen flow control valve will revolve once because of the gear ratio. The final 3:1 flow ratio results because the nitrous oxide flow control valve is supplied with nitrous oxide at a pressure of approximately 26 psig from a second-stage N_2O regulator, whereas the oxygen flow control valve is supplied by a second-stage regulator at 14 psig. The combination of the mechanical and pneumatic aspects of the system yields the final minimum 25% oxygen concentration. The GE-Datex-Ohmeda Link-25 proportioning system increases oxygen flow when nitrous oxide flow would be excessive by opening the O_2 needle valve more. Conversely, if the oxygen flow is decreased such that the nitrous oxide flow would be excessive, it acts to decrease the flow of N_2O by physically decreasing the opening of the nitrous oxide needle valve.

Several reports have described failures of the Link-25 system.[67-70] The authors of these reports describe failures that either

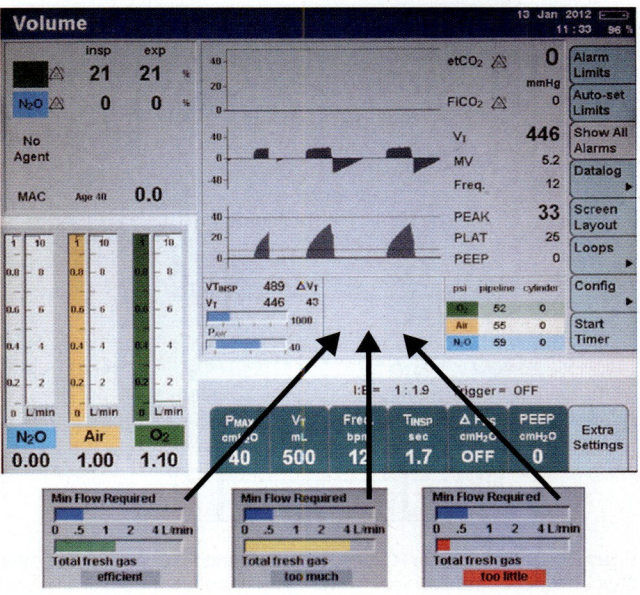

Figure 25-25 Low flow wizard of the Drager Apollo workstation.

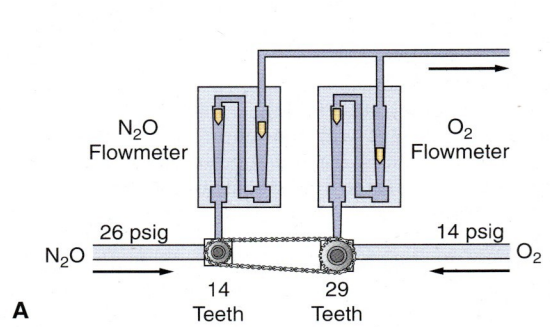 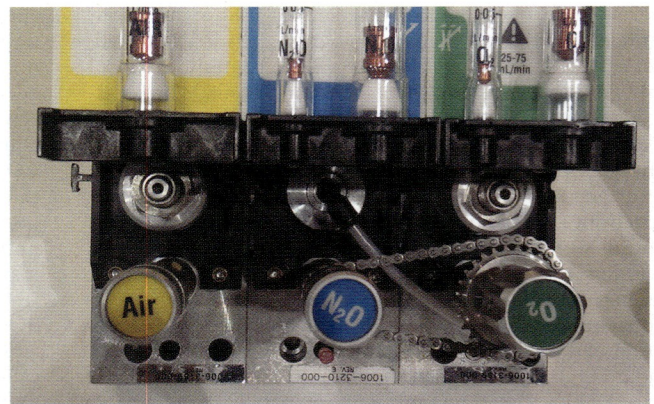

Figure 25-26 Schematic (**A**) and photo (**B**) of Ohmeda Link-25 Proportion-Limiting Control System. See text for details.

resulted in inability to administer oxygen without nitrous oxide or allowed creation of a hypoxic mixture.

Dräger Oxygen Ratio Monitor Controller/Sensitive Oxygen Ratio Controller System

The Oxygen Ratio Monitor Controller (ORMC) is the nitrous oxide:oxygen proportioning system used on older model North American Dräger anesthesia machines (e.g., Narkomed models 2B, 2C, 3, and 4). In the more recent model Dräger anesthesia workstations (e.g., Fabius GS, Apollo) the same ORMC is renamed the Sensitive Oxygen Ratio Controller (S-ORC). The ORMC/S-ORC is a pneumatic oxygen–nitrous oxide interlock system designed to maintain a fresh gas oxygen concentration of at least $25 \pm 3\%$ when nitrous oxide is used. It controls the fresh gas oxygen concentration to levels substantially greater than 25% when the oxygen flow rate is less than 1 L/min. The ORMC/S-ORC limits nitrous oxide flow to prevent delivery of a hypoxic mixture by decreasing the supply pressure of nitrous oxide to its flow control needle valve. This is unlike the GE-Datex-Ohmeda Link-25 system, in which the gas supply pressure to the nitrous oxide needle valve is held constant (by the second-stage regulator) and gas flow changes are made by physically changing the size of the needle valve opening.

A schematic of the ORMC/S-ORC is shown in Figure 25-27. It consists of an oxygen chamber, a nitrous oxide chamber, and a nitrous oxide slave control valve. All are interconnected by a mobile horizontal shaft. The pneumatic input into the device is from the oxygen and the nitrous oxide flowmeters. These flowmeters are unique because they have specific resistors located downstream from the flow control valves. When nitrous oxide and oxygen are flowing, these resistors create back pressures directed to the oxygen and nitrous oxide chambers. The value of the oxygen flow tube resistor is three to four times that of the nitrous oxide flow tube resistor, and the relative value of these resistors determines the value of the controlled fresh gas oxygen concentration. The back pressures in the oxygen and nitrous oxide chambers are applied against rubber diaphragms attached to the mobile horizontal shaft. Movement of the shaft adjusts the opening of the nitrous oxide slave control valve, which in turn adjusts the feed pressure to the nitrous oxide flow control needle valve.

If the oxygen flow, and therefore back pressure, is proportionally higher than the nitrous oxide back pressure, the nitrous oxide slave control valve opens more widely, increasing the pressure of nitrous oxide upstream of the nitrous oxide flow control needle valve, which results in an increase in nitrous oxide flow. As the nitrous oxide flow is increased manually, the nitrous oxide back pressure forces the shaft rightward toward the oxygen chamber. The nitrous oxide slave control valve opening becomes more restrictive and limits the nitrous oxide feed pressure to the flowmeter, which decreases the nitrous oxide flow. When the oxygen flow is less than 200 mL/min, the slave control valve closes completely, preventing any flow of nitrous oxide.

Figure 25-27 illustrates the action of a single ORMC/S-ORC under different sets of circumstances. The back pressure exerted on the oxygen diaphragm in the upper configuration is greater than that exerted on the nitrous oxide diaphragm. This causes the horizontal shaft to move to the left, opening the nitrous oxide slave control valve. Nitrous oxide is then able to proceed to its flow control valve and out through the flowmeter. In the lower configuration, the nitrous oxide slave control valve is closed because of inadequate oxygen back pressure. To summarize, in contrast to the GE-Datex-Ohmeda Link-25 System, which actively increases oxygen flow to maintain a fresh gas oxygen concentration 25% or higher, the Dräger ORMC/S-ORC

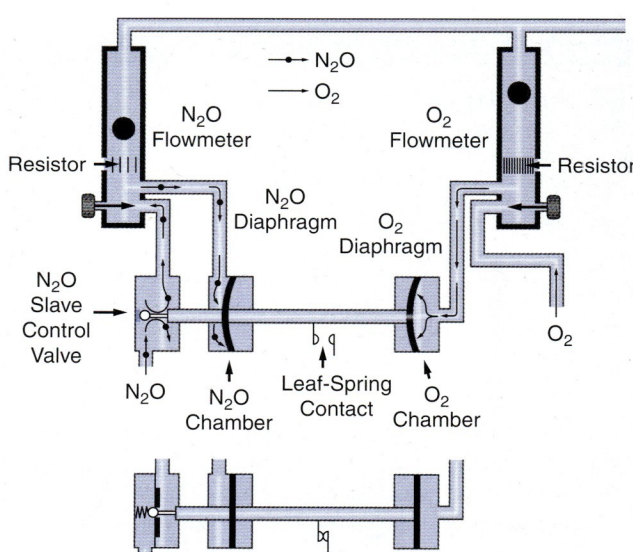

Figure 25-27 Dräger Oxygen Ratio Monitor Controller/Sensitive Oxygen Ratio Controller. See text for details. (Adapted from Schreiber P. *Safety Guidelines for Anesthesia Systems*. Telford, PA: North American Dräger; 1984.)

are systems that limit nitrous oxide flow to prevent delivery of a fresh gas mixture with an oxygen concentration no higher than 25%.

Limitations

N_2O/O_2 proportioning systems are not foolproof. Workstations equipped with these systems can still deliver a hypoxic mixture under certain conditions. The following is a description of some of the situations in which this may occur.

Wrong Supply Gas

Both the GE-Datex-Ohmeda Link-25 and the Dräger S-ORC will be defeated if a gas other than oxygen is present in the oxygen pipeline and will allow delivery of hypoxic gas mixtures. In the Link-25 System, the nitrous oxide and oxygen flow control valves will continue to be mechanically linked. Nevertheless, a hypoxic mixture can proceed to the common gas outlet. In the case of the Dräger S-ORC, the rubber diaphragm for oxygen will reflect adequate supply pressure on the oxygen side even though the incorrect gas is present, and flow of both the wrong gas plus nitrous oxide will result. The oxygen analyzer is the only workstation monitor besides an integrated multigas analyzer that would detect this condition in either system.

Defective Pneumatics or Mechanics

Normal operation of the Datex-Ohmeda Link-25 and the Dräger/S-ORC is contingent on pneumatic and mechanical integrity.[71] Pneumatic integrity in the Datex-Ohmeda system requires properly functioning second-stage regulators. A nitrous oxide:oxygen ratio other than 3:1 may result if the regulators are not precise. The chain connecting the two sprockets must be intact—if the chain is cut or broken, a 97% nitrous oxide concentration can result.[72] In the Dräger System, a functional OFPD is necessary to supply appropriate pressure to the S-ORC. The mechanical aspects of the S-ORC, such as the rubber diaphragms, the flow tube resistors, and the nitrous oxide slave control valve, must likewise be intact.

Leaks Downstream

The S-ORC and the Link-25 function at the level of the flow control valves. A leak downstream from these devices, such as a broken oxygen flow tube (Fig. 25-22), can result in delivery of a hypoxic mixture to the common gas outlet. In this situation, oxygen escapes through the leak and the predominant gas delivered is nitrous oxide. The oxygen monitor and/or integrated multigas analyzer are the only machine safety devices that can detect this problem. For the majority of anesthesia workstations a preuse positive or negative-pressure leak test (depending on the manufacturer) is recommended to detect such a leak (see Checking Your Anesthesia Workstation section).

Inert Gas Administration

Administration of a third inert gas, such as helium, nitrogen, or carbon dioxide, can cause a hypoxic mixture because contemporary proportioning systems link only nitrous oxide and oxygen.[73] Use of an oxygen analyzer to monitor the inspired oxygen concentration is mandatory (or a multigas analyzer when available) if the operator uses a third gas.

Dilution of Inspired Oxygen Concentration by Potent Inhaled Volatile Anesthetics

Volatile inhaled anesthetics are added to the mixed gases downstream from both the flowmeters and the proportioning system. High concentrations of less-potent inhaled anesthetics such as desflurane (MAC ~7%) may inadvertently be added downstream of the proportioning system, with a resulting gas/vapor mixture that may contain an inspired oxygen concentration that is below 21%. Awareness of this possibility, particularly when high concentrations of desflurane are used, is essential.

Oxygen Flush Valve

The oxygen flush valve allows direct communication between the oxygen intermediate-pressure circuit and the LPC (Fig. 25-6). Flow from the oxygen flush valve enters the LPC downstream from the vaporizers and, most importantly, downstream from any outlet check valve, if present. The spring-loaded oxygen flush valve remains closed until the operator opens it by depressing the oxygen flush button. Actuation of the valve delivers 100% oxygen at a flow of 35 to 75 L/min to the breathing circuit.

The oxygen flush valve can provide a "high pressure" oxygen source that might be used for jet ventilation under the following circumstances: (1) the anesthesia machine is equipped with a one-way check valve positioned between the vaporizers and the oxygen flush valve; and (2) when a positive-pressure relief valve exists downstream from the vaporizers. The pressure relief valve must be upstream of the outlet check valve. For example, because the Ohmeda Modulus II has such a one-way check valve and its low-pressure system positive-pressure relief valve is upstream from the outlet check valve, the entire oxygen flow of 35 to 75 L/min is delivered to the common gas outlet at a pressure of 45 to 50 psig. On the other hand, the Ohmeda Modulus II Plus and some GE-Datex-Ohmeda Excel machines are not capable of functioning as an appropriate oxygen source for jet ventilation. The Ohmeda Modulus II Plus, which does not have the check valve, provides only 7 psig at the common gas outlet because much of the oxygen flows retrograde into the LPC and out to atmosphere through an internal relief valve located upstream from the oxygen flush valve. The Ohmeda Excel 210, which does have a one-way check valve, also has a positive-pressure relief valve downstream from the check valve and therefore is unsuitable for jet ventilation. Older North American Dräger machines such as the Narkomed 2A (which also does not have the outlet check valve) produce a pressure of 18 psig at the common gas outlet because oxygen is vented to atmosphere through a pressure relief valve located in the Dräger Vapor vaporizers.[74]

It must be emphasized that use of the oxygen flush to drive a jet ventilation system connected at the machine's common gas outlet is an "off label" use of the machine, and is not recommended by the machine manufacturers. If jet ventilation is required, a purpose-built Sanders type system should be used, connected to a 50 psig oxygen source.

Several hazards have been reported with use of the oxygen flush valve. A defective or damaged valve can stick in the fully, or partially, open position, resulting in barotrauma,[75] or patient awareness during general anesthesia due to high oxygen flow diluting the inhaled anesthetic. Overzealous intraoperative oxygen flushing can also dilute inhaled anesthetics. Oxygen flushing during the inspiratory phase of positive-pressure ventilation can produce barotrauma in patients if the anesthesia machine does not incorporate fresh gas decoupling (FGD) or an appropriately adjusted inspiratory pressure limiter. Anesthesia systems, such as the Dräger Narkomed 6000 series, Julian, Fabius GS, or Apollo, use FGD which minimizes the chance of producing barotrauma from inappropriate oxygen flush valve use (see Fresh Gas Decoupling section).

With traditional anesthesia breathing circuits, excess volume cannot be vented during the inspiratory phase of mechanical ventilation because the ventilator pressure relief valve is closed and the APL valve is either out-of-circuit or closed. An alternative solution to this problem is used in the GE-Datex-Ohmeda S/5 ADU and GE-Aestiva. The breathing systems on these machines utilize an integrated adjustable pressure limiter. If this device is properly adjusted, it functions like the APL (or pop-off) valve to limit the maximum airway pressure to a safe level, thereby reducing the possibility of barotrauma.

Web-based Anesthesia Software Simulation, the Virtual Anesthesia Machine

The advances in web-based application technology, as well as trends to incorporate simulation into anesthesia training and education, have generated development of online anesthesia simulation resources. The Virtual Anesthesia Machine (VAM) is a web-based anesthesia simulation environment (Fig. 25-28) that provides information on the function of anesthesia machines along with tutorials and operational scenarios, including failure modes of new and traditional anesthesia workstations.[76] It is available for use free of charge but may not be available indefinitely due to limited funding. The authors of the VAM, in collaboration with the Anesthesia Patient Safety Foundation (APSF), have created the Anesthesia Machine Workbook (AMW). The AMW provides additional information and tutorials covering six anesthesia machine subsystems: the high-pressure system, the low-pressure system, the breathing circuit, manual ventilation, mechanical ventilation, and the scavenging system.[1] Some workstation manufacturers offer web-based interactive product trainers.[77–80]

Vaporizers

As dramatic as the evolution of the anesthesia workstation has been in recent years, vaporizers have also changed from rudimentary ether inhalers and the "Copper Kettle" to the temperature-compensated, computer-controlled, and flow-sensing devices in use today. In 1993, with the introduction into clinical use of desflurane, an even more sophisticated vaporizer was introduced to handle the unique physical properties of this agent. Now, a new generation of anesthesia vaporizers blending traditional technology and "new" computerized control technology has emerged in the GE-Datex Aladin cassette vaporizer system. Before proceeding with a discussion of variable bypass vaporizers, the Datex-Ohmeda Tec 6 desflurane vaporizer and the GE-Datex-Ohmeda Aladin cassette vaporizer, it is important to review certain physical principles to facilitate understanding of the operating principles, construction, and design of contemporary volatile anesthetic vaporizers.

Physics

The physical properties of potent inhaled volatile anesthetic agents that are pertinent to a discussion of vaporizers and vaporization are shown in Table 25-2.

Vapor Pressure

Contemporary inhaled volatile anesthetics exist in the liquid state at temperatures below 20°C. When a volatile liquid is in a closed container, molecules escape from the liquid phase to the vapor phase until the number of molecules in the vapor phase is constant. These molecules in the vapor phase bombard the wall of the container and create a pressure known as the *SVP*. As the temperature increases, more molecules enter the vapor phase, and the vapor pressure increases (Fig. 25-29). Vapor pressure is independent of atmospheric pressure and is dependent only on the temperature and physical characteristics of the liquid. The *boiling point* of a liquid is defined as that temperature at which the vapor pressure equals atmospheric pressure. At 760 mmHg, the boiling points for desflurane, isoflurane, halothane, enflurane, and sevoflurane are approximately 22.8°C, 48.5°C, 50.2°C, 56.5°C, and 58.5°C, respectively. Unlike other contemporary inhaled anesthetics, desflurane boils at temperatures that may be

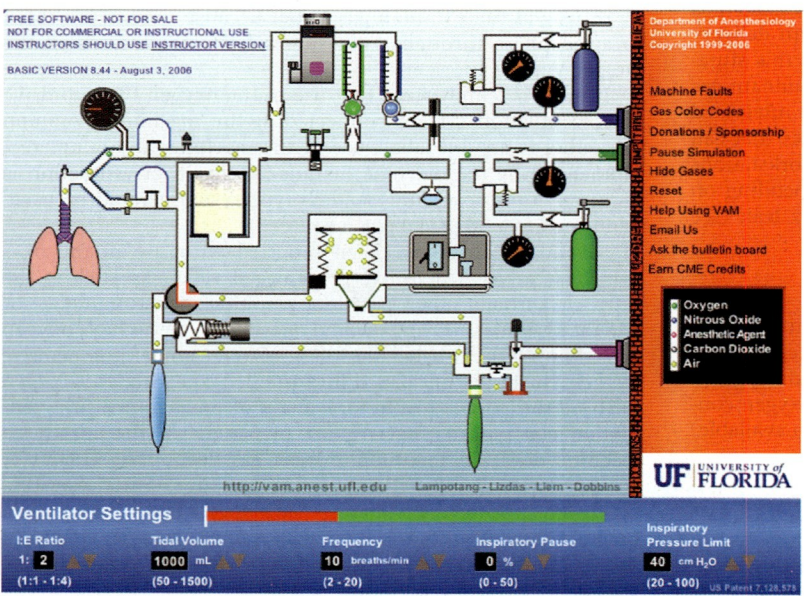

Figure 25-28 The Virtual Anesthesia Machine (VAM) simulator, an interactive model of an anesthesia machine. (With permission from Lampotang S, Lizdas DE; see http://vam.anest.ufl.edu/)

Table 25-2 Physical Properties of Potent Inhaled Volatile Anesthetic Agents

Parameter/Agent	Halothane	Enflurane	Isoflurane	Sevoflurane	Desflurane
Structure	$CHBrClCF_3$	$CHFClCF_2OCHF_2$	$CF_2HOCHClCF_3$	$CH_2FOCH(CF_3)_2$	$CH_2HOCFHCF_3$
Molecular weight	197.4	184.5	184.5	200	168
Boiling point at 769 mmHg (°C)	50.2	56.5	48.5	58.5	22.8
SVP at 20°C	243	175	238	160	669
Saturated vapor concentration at 20°C and 1 atmosphere absolute (vol%)	32	23	31	21	87
MAC at 1 atmosphere absolute (vol%)	0.75	1.68	1.15	1.7	6.0–7.25[a]
P_{MAC1} (mmHg)	5.7	12.8	8.7	12.9	46–55[a]
Specific gravity of liquid at 20°C	123	130	130	120	143
Vapor (mL) per liquid at 20°C	226	196	195	182	207

[a]Age-related.

encountered in particularly warm clinical settings such as pediatric and burn operating rooms. This unique physical characteristic alone mandates a special vaporizer design to control the delivery of desflurane. If agent-specific vaporizers are accidentally filled with incorrect liquid anesthetic agents, the resulting mixtures of volatile agents may demonstrate properties that differ from those of the individual component agents and may alter the anticipated output of the vaporizer (see section on Variable Bypass Vaporizers: Misfilling).[81]

Latent Heat of Vaporization

When a molecule is converted from a liquid to the gaseous phase, energy is consumed because the molecules of a liquid tend to cohere. The amount of energy that is consumed by a given liquid as it is converted to a vapor is referred to as the *latent heat of vaporization*. It is more precisely defined as the number of calories required to change 1 g of liquid into vapor without a temperature change. The thermal energy for vaporization must be derived from the liquid itself or from an external source. The temperature of the liquid itself will decrease during vaporization in the absence of an external energy source. This energy loss can lead to significant decreases in temperature of the remaining liquid and can greatly decrease subsequent vaporization.[82]

Specific Heat

The *specific heat* of a substance is the number of calories required to increase the temperature of 1 g of a substance by 1°C. The substance can be a solid, liquid, or gas. The concept of specific heat is important to the design, operation, and construction of vaporizers because it is applicable in two ways. First, the specific heat value for an inhaled anesthetic is important because it indicates how much heat must be supplied to the liquid to maintain a constant temperature when heat is being lost during vaporization. Second, manufacturers select vaporizer component materials that have a high specific heat to minimize temperature changes associated with vaporization.

Thermal Conductivity

Thermal conductivity is a measure of the rate at which heat flows through a substance. The higher the thermal conductivity, the better the substance conducts heat. Vaporizers are constructed of metals that have relatively high thermal conductivity, thus maintaining a uniform internal temperature.

Ambient Pressure Effects

These are discussed in the section titled GE-Datex-Ohmeda Tec 6 and Dräger D-Vapor Vaporizers for Desflurane: Factors that Influence Vaporizer Output: Varied Altitudes.

Variable Bypass Vaporizers

The GE-Datex-Ohmeda Tec 4, Tec 5, and Tec 7, as well as the Dräger Vapor 19.n, 2000, and 3000 series, vaporizers are classified as variable bypass, flow-over, temperature-compensated, agent-specific, out-of-breathing circuit vaporizers. *Variable bypass* refers to the method for regulating the anesthetic agent concentration output from the vaporizer. As fresh gas from the machine flowmeters enters the vaporizer inlet, the concentration control dial setting determines the ratio of incoming gas that flows through the bypass chamber to that entering the vaporizing chamber (sump). The gas channeled through the vaporizing chamber flows over a wick system saturated with the liquid anesthetic and subsequently also becomes saturated with vapor.

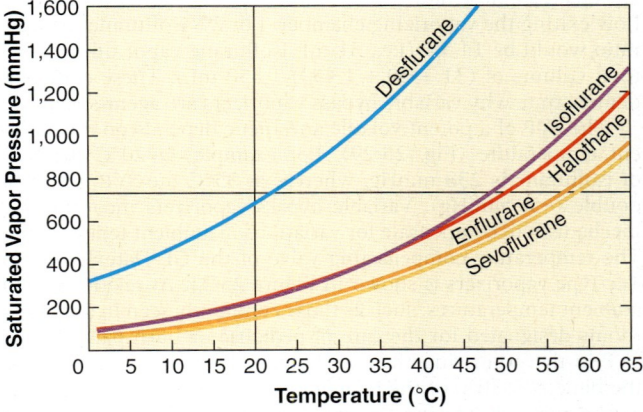

Figure 25-29 Saturated vapor pressure versus temperature curves for desflurane, isoflurane, halothane, enflurane, and sevoflurane. The vapor pressure curve for desflurane is both steeper and shifted to higher vapor pressures when compared with the curves for other contemporary inhaled anesthetics. (Adapted from inhaled anesthetic package insert equations and from Susay SR, Smith MA, Lockwood GG. The saturated vapor pressure of desflurane at various temperatures. *Anesth Analg.* 1996;83:864.)

Thus, *flow-over* refers to the method of vaporization and is in contrast to a *bubble-through* system that is used in now-obsolete measured flow vaporizers (e.g., Copper Kettle, Verni-Trol). The GE-Ohmeda Tec 4, Tec 5, and Tec 7, and the Dräger Vapor 19.n and Vapor 2000 and 3000 series are further classified as *temperature compensated*. Each is equipped with an automated temperature-compensating device that helps maintain a constant vapor concentration output for a given concentration dial setting, and over a wide range of operating temperatures. These vaporizers are *agent specific* because each is designed to accommodate a single anesthetic agent, and are *out-of-circuit*, that is, physically located outside of the breathing circuit. Variable bypass vaporizers are used to deliver halothane, enflurane, isoflurane, and sevoflurane, but not desflurane.

Basic Operating Principles

A diagram of a generic, variable bypass vaporizer is shown in Figure 25-30. In principle, it creates a saturated vapor concentration of the liquid agent in the vaporizing chamber and dilutes this to clinically usable concentrations by mixing it with fresh gas from the vaporizer bypass. For example, the SVP of sevoflurane is 160 mmHg at 20°C, at sea level. This corresponds to a vapor concentration of 160 mmHg/760 mmHg × 100 = 21%, which is too high for clinical use. Therefore, the vaporizer must dilute this 21% concentration to a clinically desirable value indicated on the vaporizer dial. Vaporizer components include the concentration control dial, the bypass chamber, the vaporizing chamber, the filler port, and the filler cap. Using the filler port, the operator fills the vaporizing chamber with liquid anesthetic. The maximum safe fill level is predetermined by the position of the filler port, which is designed to minimize the likelihood of overfilling. If a vaporizer is overfilled or tilted, liquid anesthetic can spill into the bypass via the inlet and outlet chambers. If this were to happen, both the vaporizing chamber flow and the bypass flow could potentially be carrying saturated anesthetic vapor, and an overdose would result. The concentration control dial is a variable restrictor, which controls gas flow through the bypass and through the outlet of the vaporizing chamber.[83]

FGF from the machine's flowmeters enters the inlet of the vaporizer. Most of the flow passes straight through the bypass chamber to the vaporizer outlet. A smaller fraction of the fresh gas inflow is diverted to the vaporizing chamber. Depending on the temperature and vapor pressure of the particular inhaled anesthetic, the fresh gas entering the vaporizing chamber entrains a specific flow of the anesthetic agent saturated vapor. The mixture that exits the vaporizer outlet comprises flow through the bypass chamber, flow through the vaporizing chamber, and flow of entrained anesthetic vapor. The final concentration of inhaled anesthetic (in volumes percent) is the ratio of the flow of the entrained anesthetic vapor to the total gas flow.[84] The quantity (mL) of liquid volatile anesthetic agent used by a typical vaporizer is proportional to the FGF rate and the concentration set on the dial. It can be approximated from the following formula[85]:

$$3 \times FGF \text{ (L/min)} \times vol\% = mL \text{ liquid volatile anesthetic/hr}$$

Figure 25-30 shows that the agent concentration emerging from the vaporizer is controlled by proportioning the vaporizing chamber outflow to the bypass flow. For example, assume that the vaporizing chamber outflow is 100 mL/min. The SVP of sevoflurane is 160 mmHg at 20°C (Table 25-2), the saturated vapor concentration of sevoflurane is 21% (i.e., 160/760); therefore, each 100 mL of gas exiting the vaporizing chamber contains 21 mL of sevoflurane vapor, the other 79 mL being the gas entering the vaporizing chamber. If the vaporizer dial is set to deliver 1% sevoflurane, the bypass flow will be 2,000 mL/min because 21 mL of sevoflurane vapor will be diluted in a total volume of 2,100 mL (21 + 79 + 2,000); 21/2,100 = 1% by volume. To achieve this the vaporizer concentration dial has created a flow ratio of 2,000:100 or 20:1 between the bypass flow and the flow exiting the vaporizing chamber. When the dial is set to deliver 2% sevoflurane, the vaporizer concentration dial creates a ratio of 950:100, or 9.5:1; i.e., 21 mL of sevoflurane vapor are diluted in a total volume of (21 + 79 + 950) 1,050 mL (21/1,050 = 2%).

In the case of an isoflurane vaporizer set to deliver 1% isoflurane, the concentration of isoflurane vapor in the vaporizing chamber will be 238/760 = 31% at 20°C (Table 25-2). Each 100 mL of gas leaving the vaporizing chamber will contain 31 mL of isoflurane vapor, the other 69 mL being the gas that entered the vaporizing chamber. The bypass flow must be 3,000 mL because now 31 mL of isoflurane vapor is diluted in a total volume of 3,100 (31 + 69 + 3,000). The vaporizer concentration dial has created a flow ratio of 30:1 between the bypass flow and the flow exiting the vaporizing chamber. For 2% isoflurane the flow ratio would be 14.5:1 (i.e., 31 mL isoflurane vapor diluted in a total volume of (31 + 69 + 1,450) 1,550 mL). These examples demonstrate why variable bypass vaporizers are agent-specific.

The SVP of a potent volatile anesthetic depends on the ambient temperature (Fig. 25-29). For example, at 20°C the SVP of isoflurane is 238 mmHg, whereas at 35°C the SVP is almost double (450 mmHg). Variable bypass vaporizers incorporate a mechanism to compensate for variations in ambient temperature. The temperature-compensating valve of the GE-Datex-Ohmeda Tec-type vaporizers is shown in Figure 25-31. At relatively high ambient temperatures, such as those commonly seen in operating rooms designated for the care of pediatric or burn patients, the SVP in the vaporizing chamber is high. To compensate for this, the bimetallic strip of the temperature-compensating valve leans to the right, decreasing the resistance to gas flow through the bypass chamber. This allows more flow to pass through the bypass chamber and less flow to pass through the vaporizing chamber. In contrast, in a cold environment, the SVP of the agent in the vaporizing chamber is decreased. To compensate for this decrease in SVP, the bimetallic strip leans to the left. This increases the resistance to flow through the bypass chamber, causing relatively more flow to pass through the vaporizing chamber and less flow

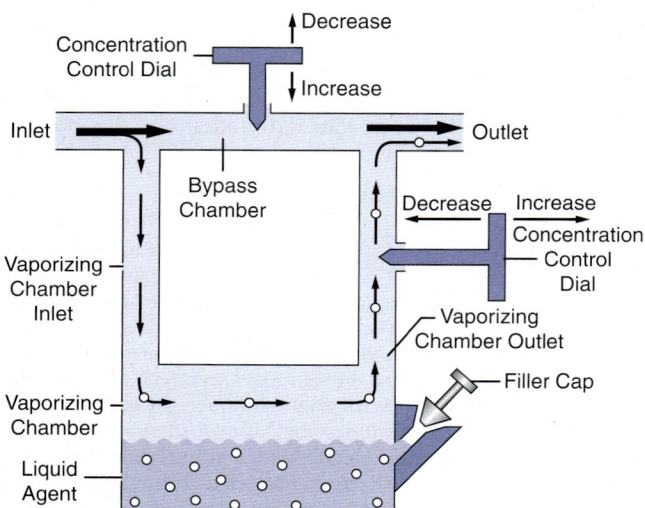

Figure 25-30 Generic variable bypass vaporizer. See text for details.

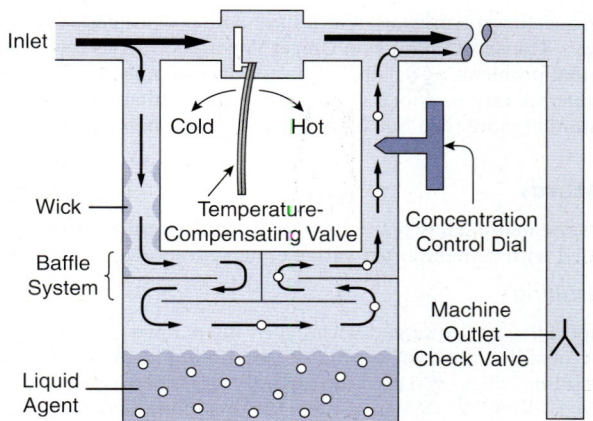

Figure 25-31 Simplified schematic of the GE-Ohmeda Tec Type Vaporizer. Note bimetallic strip temperature-compensating mechanism in the bypass chamber. See text for details.

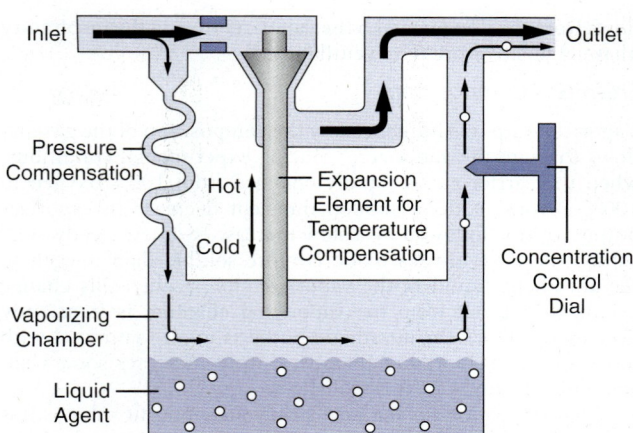

Figure 25-32 Simplified schematic of the Dräger Vapor 19.1 vaporizer. Here an expansion element performs the same function as the bimetallic strip in the previous figure. See text for details.

to pass through the bypass chamber. The net effect in both situations is maintenance of relatively constant vapor output concentration despite large swings in ambient temperature.

Factors That Influence Vaporizer Output

If an ideal vaporizer existed, for a given concentration dial setting, its output would be constant regardless of changes in FGF rate, temperature, back pressure, and fresh gas mixture composition and ambient pressure. Designing such a vaporizer is difficult because as ambient conditions change, the physical properties of gases and of the vaporizers themselves can change. Contemporary vaporizers approach ideal but still have some limitations. Even though some of the most sophisticated vaporizing systems now available use computer-controlled components and multiple sensors, they have yet to become significantly more accurate than conventional mechanical flow-splitting (variable bypass) vaporizers. Several factors that affect vaporizer performance in general are described below.

Fresh Gas Flow Rate

With a fixed dial setting, vaporizer output can vary with the rate of gas flowing through the vaporizer. This variation is particularly notable at extremes of flow rates. The output of all variable bypass vaporizers is less than the dial setting at low flow rates (<250 mL/min). This results from the relatively high density of volatile inhaled anesthetic vapors. At low flow rates, insufficient turbulence is generated in the vaporizing chamber to advance the vapor molecules upwardly. At extremely high flow rates, such as 15 L/min, the output of most variable bypass vaporizers is less than that set on the dial. This discrepancy is attributed to incomplete mixing and failure to saturate the carrier gas in the vaporizing chamber. In addition, the resistance characteristics of the bypass chamber and the vaporizing chamber can vary as flow increases.

Temperature

Because of improvements in design, the output of contemporary temperature-compensated vaporizers is almost linear over a wide range of temperatures. Automatic temperature-compensating mechanisms in the bypass chamber maintain a constant vaporizer output with varying temperatures. As previously described, a bimetallic strip (Fig. 25-31) or in Dräger Vapor vaporizers, an expansion element (Fig. 25-32), directs a greater proportion of gas flow through the bypass chamber as temperature increases. In addition, the wick systems are placed in direct contact with the metal wall of the vaporizer to help replace energy (heat) consumed during vaporization.

The materials from which vaporizers are constructed are chosen because they have a relatively high specific heat and high thermal conductivity. These factors help minimize the effect of cooling of the liquid anesthetic during vaporization. In addition, they should not react chemically with the liquid anesthetic agent.[86]

Intermittent Back Pressure

Intermittent back pressure that results from either positive-pressure ventilation or use of the oxygen flush valve may result in higher-than-expected vaporizer output. This phenomenon, known as the *pumping effect*, is more pronounced at low FGF rates, low concentration dial settings, and low levels of liquid anesthetic in the vaporizing chamber.[87,88] In addition, the pumping effect is increased by rapid respiratory rates, high peak inspired pressures, and rapid decreases in pressure during exhalation.[89] Modern variable bypass vaporizers are relatively immune from the pumping effect. One proposed mechanism for the pumping effect is dependent on retrograde pressure transmission from the patient circuit to the vaporizer during the inspiratory phase of positive-pressure ventilation. Gas molecules are compressed in both the bypass and vaporizing chambers. When the back pressure is suddenly released during the expiratory phase of positive-pressure ventilation, vapor exits the vaporizing chamber via both the vaporizing chamber outlet and retrograde through the vaporizing chamber inlet.

To decrease the pumping effect, the vaporizing chambers of contemporary variable bypass systems are smaller than those of older model vaporizers. Consequently, no substantial volumes of vapor can be discharged from the vaporizing chamber into the bypass chamber during the expiratory phase of ventilation. The Dräger Vapor 19.1 and 20.n (Fig. 25-32) have a long spiral tube that serves as the inlet to the vaporizing chamber. When the pressure in the vaporizing chamber is released, some of the vapor enters this tube but does not enter the bypass chamber because of the tube's length. The Tec 4 (Fig. 25-31) has an extensive baffle system in the vaporizing chamber, and a one-way check valve has been inserted at the common gas outlet (outlet check valve) to minimize the pumping effect. This check valve attenuates, but does not eliminate, the pressure increase because gas still flows from the flowmeters to the vaporizer during the inspiratory phase of positive-pressure ventilation.[90]

Fresh Gas Composition

Vaporizer output is influenced by the composition of the gas that flows through the vaporizer.[91] During experimental conditions, when the carrier gas is rapidly changed from 100% oxygen to 100% nitrous oxide, a sudden transient decrease in vaporizer output occurs, followed by a slow increase to a new steady-state value.[92] Because nitrous oxide is more soluble than oxygen in the anesthetic liquid in the vaporizer sump, when this change occurs the output from the vaporizing chamber is transiently decreased.[93] Once the anesthetic liquid is totally saturated with nitrous oxide, vaporizing chamber output increases somewhat, and a new steady state is established.

The explanation for the new steady-state output value is less well understood.[94,95] With contemporary vaporizers such as the Dräger Vapor 19.n and 20.n and the GE Tec-type vaporizers, the steady-state output value is less when nitrous oxide rather than oxygen is the carrier gas (Fig. 25-33). Conversely, the output of some older vaporizers is increased when nitrous oxide is the carrier gas instead of oxygen.[96,97] Factors that contribute to the characteristic steady-state response resulting when various carrier gases are used include the viscosity and density of the carrier gas (i.e., whether the flow is laminar or turbulent), the relative solubilities of the carrier gas in the anesthetic liquid, the flow-splitting characteristics of the specific vaporizer, and the concentration control dial setting.

Safety Features

Contemporary vaporizers (e.g., Dräger Vapor 19.n and Vapor 2000 series, and the GE-Datex-Ohmeda Tec 5, and Tec 7) have built-in safety features that have minimized or eliminated many of the hazards once associated with variable bypass vaporizers. Agent-specific, keyed filling devices help prevent filling a vaporizer with the wrong agent. Overfilling of vaporizers is minimized because the filler port is located at the maximum safe liquid level. Vaporizers are firmly secured to a vaporizer manifold on the anesthesia workstation and have antispill protection designs (e.g., "Transport" setting on Dräger Vapor 2000 series vaporizers) so that problems associated with vaporizer tipping are prevented. Contemporary interlock systems prevent simultaneous administration of more than one inhaled volatile anesthetic.

Hazards

Despite many safety features, some hazards continue to be associated with contemporary variable bypass vaporizers.

Misfilling

Vaporizers not equipped with keyed fillers have been occasionally misfilled with the wrong anesthetic liquid. A potential for misfilling exists even on contemporary vaporizers equipped with keyed fillers.[98–100] When a vaporizer misfilling occurs, patients can be rendered inadequately, or excessively, anesthetized depending on which "incorrect" agent is in the vaporizer.[101] The use of an anesthetic agent analyzer should alert the user to such a problem. In principle, if a vaporizer designed for an agent with a relatively low SVP (e.g., sevoflurane-160 mmHg at 20°C) is erroneously filled with an agent that has a relatively high SVP (e.g., isoflurane-238 mmHg at 20°C) the output concentration of isoflurane (in vol%) will be greater than that set on the concentration dial of the sevoflurane vaporizer. Conversely, an isoflurane vaporizer misfilled with sevoflurane will deliver a lower concentration of sevoflurane than that set on the concentration dial. In addition to considering the agent concentration output of a misfilled vaporizer, one must also consider the potency output. Thus, a sevoflurane vaporizer set to deliver 2% sevoflurane (1 MAC) that is misfilled with isoflurane will deliver about 3% isoflurane which would be more than double the potency (MAC multiple) expected!

Understanding the principles of operation of a variable bypass vaporizer (i.e., how gas flows are split between bypass and vaporizing chamber) makes it possible to predict the output of an erroneously filled vaporizer so that in certain situations (e.g., remote locations, impoverished countries) deliberate mismatch has been safely used.[102] But caution is required. Mismatching of inhaled agent and vaporizer is a dangerous practice and should not be performed unless it is absolutely necessary.

Contamination of anesthetic vaporizer contents has occurred by filling an isoflurane vaporizer with a contaminated bottle of isoflurane. A potentially serious incident was avoided because the operator detected an abnormal acrid odor.[103]

Tipping

Tipping of a vaporizer can occur when they are incorrectly "switched out" or moved. However, tipping is unlikely when a vaporizer is secured to the anesthesia workstation manifold short of the entire machine being turned over. Excessive tipping can cause the liquid agent to enter the bypass chamber and can cause an output with extremely high agent vapor concentration.[104]

One milliliter of liquid anesthetic produces approximately 200 mL of anesthetic vapor at 20°C and 1 atm pressure so that even a small quantity of liquid anesthetic in the bypass can produce a large amount of vapor (Table 25-2). If a vaporizer has been tipped, it should not be used clinically until it has been purged for 20 to 30 minutes using a high FGF rate from the machine's flowmeters. During this procedure, the vaporizer concentration control dial should be set at a high concentration which maximizes bypass chamber flow as well as vaporizing chamber inlet and outlet flows. Purging should continue until all spilled liquid anesthetic has been cleared. Following this procedure the accuracy of the vaporizer output must be confirmed using an agent analyzer

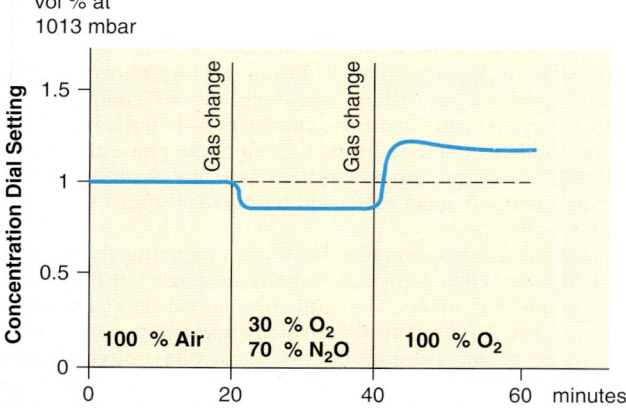

Figure 25-33 Influence of gas composition on delivered anesthetic concentration. A Dräger Vapor 2000 vaporizer is initially set at 1 vol% and 100% air. The concentration falls by 10% (not more than 0.4 vol%) of the set value after switching to a mixture of 30% O_2 and 70% N_2O. When 100% O_2 is used, the concentration rises by 10% of the set value (not more than 0.4 vol%). (Adapted from Schreiber P. *Anaesthetic Equipment: Performance, Classification, and Safety*. New York, NY: Springer; 1972.)

before placing the vaporizer back into clinical service. As mentioned above, the Dräger Vapor 2000 and 3000 series vaporizers have a transport ("T") dial setting that prevents tipping-related problems. When the dial is set to this position, the vaporizer sump is isolated from the bypass chamber, thereby reducing the likelihood of spillage (and a possible accidental overdose). In order to remove a Vapor 2000 or 3000 from the anesthesia workstation, the control dial must be set to the "T" position.

The design of the GE-Datex-Ohmeda Tec 6 and the Aladin cassette vaporizer systems has essentially eliminated the dangers of tipping. Since the Aladin vaporizer's bypass chamber is physically separated from the "cassette," and permanently resides in the anesthesia workstation, the possibility of tipping is virtually eliminated. Tipping of the Aladin cassettes themselves when they are not installed in the vaporizer is not problematic. Similarly, Dräger's D-Vapor (desflurane) vaporizer is hermetically tight and can be transported in any position before draining.

Improper Filling

Overfilling of a vaporizer combined with failure of the vaporizer sight glass can cause an anesthetic overdose. When liquid anesthetic enters the bypass chamber, up to 10 times the intended vapor concentration can be delivered to the common gas outlet.[105,106] Most modern vaporizers are now relatively immune to overfilling because of side-fill rather than top-fill designs.

Just as with overfilling, underfilling of anesthetic vaporizers may also be problematic. When a Tec 5 sevoflurane vaporizer is in a low-fill state and used under conditions of high FGF rates (>7.5 L/min) and high dial setting (such as seen during inhalational inductions), the vaporizer output may abruptly decrease to less than 2%. The causes of this problem are likely multifactorial. However, the combination of low vaporizer fill state (<25% full) in combination with the high vaporizing chamber flow can result in a clinically significant and reproducible decrease in vapor output.[107]

Simultaneous Inhaled Anesthetic Administration

Some older anesthesia machines, such as the Datex-Ohmeda with the Select-a-Tec three-vaporizer manifold, do not utilize a vapor-interlock system. Thus, two inhaled anesthetics potentially can be administered simultaneously. Newer anesthesia workstations have a built-in vapor-interlock or vapor-exclusion device that prevents this problem.

Leaks

Vaporizer leaks do occur frequently and can potentially result in patient awareness during anesthesia[108] or in contamination of the operating room environment. A loose filler cap is the most common source of vaporizer leaks. Leaks can also occur at the O-ring junctions between the vaporizer and its manifold. To detect a leak within a vaporizer, the concentration control dial must be in the "on" position. Even though vaporizer leaks in Dräger anesthesia systems can potentially be detected with a conventional positive-pressure low-pressure system leak test (because of the absence of an outlet check valve), a negative-pressure leak test is probably more sensitive. GE-Datex-Ohmeda recommends a negative-pressure leak testing device (suction bulb) to detect vaporizer leaks in the Modulus I, Modulus II, Excel, and the Aestiva workstations because of the check valve located just upstream of each machine's fresh gas outlet (see Checking Your Anesthesia Workstation section).

Many newer anesthesia workstations are capable of performing self-testing procedures that, in some cases, may eliminate the need for the conventional negative-pressure leak testing. However, it is of vital importance that anesthesia providers understand that these self-tests may not detect internal vaporizer leaks in systems with add-on vaporizers. For the self-tests to determine if an internal vaporizer leak is present, the leak test must be repeated for each vaporizer sequentially, while its concentration control dial is turned to the "on" position. Recall that when a vaporizer's concentration control dial is set in the "off" position, it may not be possible to detect even major internal leaks such as an absent or loose filler cap.

Vaporizers in the MRI Suite

The presence of a powerful magnetic field, the significant noise pollution, and limited access to the patient during an MRI procedure all complicate care in this setting. It is imperative that only nonferrous (MRI compatible) equipment be used. Some anesthesia vaporizers, although they may appear nonferrous by testing with a horseshoe magnet, may indeed contain substantial internal ferrous components. Inappropriate use of such a device in an MRI suite may potentially turn it into a dangerous missile if left unsecured.[109]

The Tec 6 and D-Vapor Vaporizers for Desflurane

Because of its unique physical characteristics, the controlled vaporization of desflurane requires a novel approach to vaporizer design. Ohmeda developed the Tec 6 vaporizer, the first such system, and introduced it into clinical use in the early 1990s. The Tec 6 vaporizer is an electrically heated, pressurized device specifically designed to deliver desflurane.[110,111] The vapor pressure of desflurane is three to four times that of other contemporary inhaled anesthetics, and it boils at 22.8°C which is slightly above normal room temperature (Fig. 25-29). Desflurane has a minimum alveolar anesthetic concentration (MAC) value of 6% to 7%.[112] It is valuable because it has a low blood:gas partition coefficient of 0.45 at 37°C, and recovery from anesthesia is more rapid than from other potent inhaled anesthetics. In 2004, Dräger Medical received FDA approval for its own version of the Tec 6 desflurane vaporizer, the D-Vapor. The operating principles described in the following discussion are applicable to both vaporizers, although reference is made to the Tec 6 specifically.

Unsuitability of Contemporary Variable Bypass Vaporizers for Controlled Vaporization of Desflurane

Desflurane's high volatility and moderate potency preclude its use with contemporary variable bypass vaporizers such as GE-Datex-Ohmeda Tec 4, Tec 5, and Tec 7, or the Dräger Vapor 19.n or 20.n for two primary reasons (Table 25-2):

1. At 20°C the SVP of desflurane is 669 mmHg (almost 1 atm pressure at sea level). The vapor pressures of sevoflurane, enflurane, isoflurane, halothane, and desflurane at 20°C are 160, 172, 240, 244, and 669 mmHg, respectively (Fig. 25-29; Table 25-2). Equal amounts of flow through a traditional vaporizer would vaporize many more volumes of desflurane than any other of these agents. For example, at 1 atm and 20°C, 100 mL/min passing through the vaporizing chamber would entrain 735 mL/min desflurane versus 25, 29, 46, and 47 mL/min of sevoflurane, enflurane, isoflurane, and halothane, respectively.[98] In addition, at temperatures of 22.8°C or higher at 1 atm, desflurane will boil. The amount of vapor produced would be uncontrolled and limited only by the heat energy available from the vaporizer.[98]

2. Contemporary variable bypass vaporizers lack an external heat source. The latent heat of vaporization for desflurane is approximately equal to those of the other potent agents but its MAC is four to nine times higher. Thus, the absolute amount of desflurane liquid vaporized over a given time period is considerably greater than that of the other anesthetic agents. To deliver desflurane via a conventional vaporizer in higher (equivalent MAC) concentrations would lead to excessive cooling of the vaporizer and would significantly reduce its output. In the absence of an external heat source, temperature compensation using traditional mechanical devices would be almost impossible. Because of the broad range of temperatures seen in the clinical setting, and because of desflurane's steep SVP versus temperature curve (Fig. 25-29), the delivery of desflurane in a conventional anesthetic vaporizer would be unpredictable.[113]

Operating Principles of the Tec 6 and D-Vapor

The physical appearance and operation of the Tec 6 are similar to other vaporizers, but some aspects of the internal design and operating principles are radically different. Functionally, the Tec 6's operation is more accurately described as a dual-gas blender than as a vaporizer. A simplified schematic of the Tec 6 is shown in Figure 25-34. The vaporizer has two independent gas circuits arranged in parallel. The fresh gas circuit is shown in darker gray, and the vapor circuit in light gray. The FGF from the machine's flowmeters enters at the fresh gas inlet, passes through a fixed restrictor (R1), and exits at the vaporizer gas outlet. The vapor circuit originates at the desflurane sump, which is electrically heated and thermostatically controlled to 39°C, a temperature well above desflurane's boiling point at 1 atm. The heated sump assembly creates a reservoir of desflurane vapor. At 39°C, the vapor pressure in the sump is approximately 1,500 mmHg, or 2 atm absolute (Fig. 25-29). Just downstream from the sump is the shutoff valve. After the vaporizer has warmed up to working temperature, the shutoff valve fully opens when the concentration control valve is turned to the "on" position.

A pressure-regulating valve located downstream from the shut-off valve regulates downward the pressure to approximately 1.1 atm absolute (74 mmHg gauge) at an FGF rate of 10 L/min. The operator controls desflurane output by adjusting the concentration control valve (R2), which is a variable restrictor. The vapor flow through R2 joins the FGF through R1 at a point downstream from the restrictors. Until this point, the two circuits are physically separated. They are interfaced pneumatically and electronically, however, through differential pressure transducers, a control electronics system, and a pressure-regulating valve. When a constant FGF encounters the fixed restrictor, R1, a specific back pressure, proportional to the FGF rate, pushes against the diaphragm of the control differential pressure transducer. The differential pressure transducer conveys the pressure difference between the fresh gas circuit and the vapor circuit to the control electronics system. The control electronics system regulates the pressure-regulating valve so that the pressure in the vapor circuit equals the pressure in the fresh gas circuit. This equalized pressure supplying R1 and R2 is the working pressure, and the working pressure is constant at a fixed FGF rate. If the operator increases the FGF rate, more back pressure is exerted upon the diaphragm of the control pressure transducer, and the working pressure of the vaporizer increases.

Table 25-3 shows the approximate correlation between FGF rate and working pressure for a typical vaporizer. At an FGF rate of 1 L/min, the working pressure is 10 millibars, or 7.4 mmHg gauge. At an FGF rate of 10 L/min, the working pressure is 100 millibars, or 74 mmHg gauge. Therefore, there is a linear relationship between FGF rate and working pressure. When the FGF rate is increased 10-fold, the working pressure increases 10-fold.[110]

The following are two examples to demonstrate the operating principles of the Tec 6 (and D-Vapor). Example A: Constant FGF rate of 1 L/min, with an increase in the dial setting.

With an FGF rate of 1 L/min, the working pressure of the vaporizer is 7.4 mmHg. That is, the pressure supplying R1 and R2 is 7.4 mmHg. As the operator increases the dial setting, the opening at R2 becomes larger, allowing more vapor to pass through R2. Specific vapor flow rates at different dial settings are shown in Table 25-4.

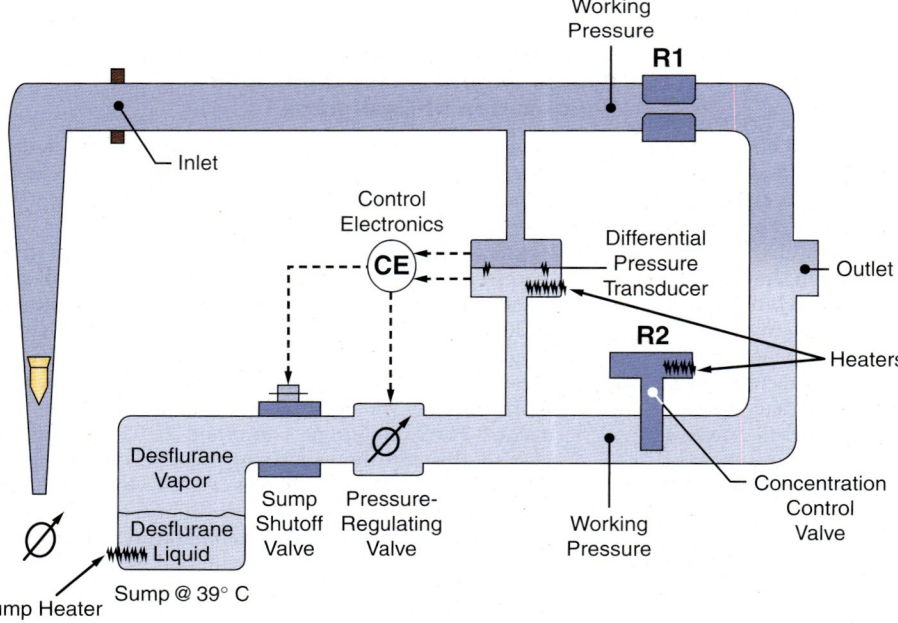

Figure 25-34 Simplified schematic of the Tec 6 desflurane vaporizer. (Modified from Andrews JJ. *Operating Principles of the Ohmeda Tec 6 Desflurane Vaporizer: A Collection of Twelve Color Illustrations.* Washington, DC: Library of Congress, Copyright 1996.)

Table 25-3 Fresh Gas Flow Rate versus Working Pressure

Fresh Gas Flow Rate (L/min)	Working Pressure at R1 and R2 (Gauge) (Gas Inlet Pressure)		
	mbar	cm Water	mmHg
1	10	10.2	7.4
5	50	51.0	37.0
10	100	102.0	74.0

Reprinted with permission from: Andrews JJ, Johnston RV Jr. The new Tec 6 desflurane vaporizer. *Anesth Analg.* 1993;76:1338.

Table 25-4 Dial Setting versus Flow through Restrictor R2

Dial Setting (vol%)[a]	Fresh Gas Flow Rate (L/min)	Approximate Vapor Flow Rate Through R2 (mL/min)
1	1	10
6	1	64
12	1	136
18	1	220

Reprinted with permission from: Andrews JJ, Johnston RV Jr. The new Tec 6 desflurane vaporizer. *Anesth Analg.* 1993;76:1338.
[a]vol% = [(vapor flow rate)/(fresh gas flow rate + vapor flow rate)] × 100%.

Example B: Constant dial setting with an increase in FGF from 1 to 10 L/min.

At an FGF rate of 1 L/min, the working pressure is 7.4 mmHg, and at a dial setting of 6% the vapor flow rate through R2 is 64 mL/min (Tables 25-3 and 25-4). With a 10-fold increase in the FGF rate, there is a concomitant 10-fold increase in the working pressure to 74 mmHg. The ratio of resistances of R2 to R1 is constant at a fixed dial setting of 6%. Because R2 is supplied by 10 times more pressure, the vapor flow rate through R2 increases 10-fold to 640 mL/min. Vaporizer output in volumes percent is constant because both the FGF and the vapor flow increase proportionally.

Altitude Can Influence Vaporizer Output

Changes in ambient pressure may significantly affect the output of older Tec-type vaporizers (i.e., those in which gas flow splitting occurs at the entrance to the vaporizing chamber rather than at the exit) in terms of volumes percent (i.e., concentration), but the effect on anesthetic potency (i.e., partial pressure of agent) is minimal. This effect is illustrated using the example of isoflurane shown in Table 25-5. With a constant dial setting of 0.89%, at 1 atm (760 mmHg), if perfectly calibrated, the volumes percent delivered would be 0.89% and the partial pressure of isoflurane would be 6.8 mmHg. Maintaining the same dial setting and lowering ambient pressure to 0.66 atm (roughly equivalent to 10,000 ft elevation) would result in an increase in the concentration output to 1.75% (almost double), but the partial pressure only increases to 8.77 mmHg (a 29% increase) because of the proportionate decrease in ambient pressure (Fig. 25-35).

It is generally considered that the partial pressure of the anesthetic agent in the central nervous system, not its concentration in volumes percent, is responsible for the anesthetic effect. To obtain a consistent depth of anesthesia when gross changes in barometric pressure occur, the concentration in volumes percent must be changed in inverse proportion to the barometric pressure.

In contemporary variable bypass vaporizers (e.g., GE Tec 5, Tec 7, Dräger Vapor 19.1 and Vapor 2000) the flow proportioning occurs as gas leaves the vaporizing chamber, so that for any given dial setting and FGF, the volume of gas saturated with vapor that leaves the vaporizing chamber remains constant, to be diluted by the bypass flow. Assume that gas leaves the vaporizing chamber of an isoflurane vaporizer at 100 mL/min. At 1 atm (760 mmHg) that gas would be 31.3% isoflurane by volume (238/760) and the partial pressure would be 31.3% × 760 = 238 mmHg. At a barometric pressure of 500 mmHg, the gas exiting the vaporizing chamber would be 47.6% isoflurane by volume (238/500) and the partial pressure would be 47.6% × 500 = 238 mmHg. By proportioning

Table 25-5 Performance of OLDER[a] Tec Type Vaporizers versus the Tec 6 Desflurane Vaporizer at Varying Ambient Pressures

Atmospheres	Ambient Pressure (mmHg)	Isoflurane Vaporizer with a Dial Setting of 0.89%			Tec 6 Desflurane Vaporizer with a Dial Setting of 6%
		Isoflurane Vapor Entrained by 100 cc O_2	Output Concentration (%)	Partial Pressure Output (mmHg)	Partial Pressure Output of Desflurane (mmHg)
0.66 (2/3)	500 (10,000 ft)	91	1.753	8.77	30
0.74	560	74	1.429	8.0	33.6
0.80	608 (6,564 ft)	64.32	1.25	7.6	36.5
1.0	760	46	0.89	6.8	45.6
1.5	1,140	26.4	0.515	5.87	68.4
2	1,520	19	0.36	5.5	91.2
3	2,280	11.65	0.228	5.198	136

The following were assumed: 5,000 cc bypass chamber flow, 100 cc vaporizing chamber flow—equivalent to an isoflurane dial setting of 0.89%.
[a]Variable bypass vaporizers in which the incoming gas flow is split before gas enters the vaporizing chamber.

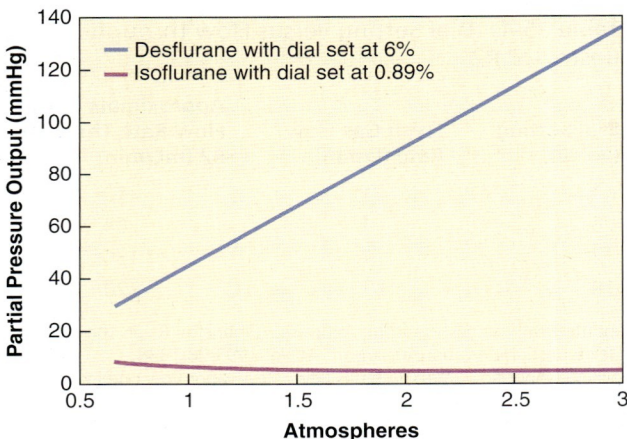

Figure 25-35 Performance of Tec type vaporizer versus the Tec 6 desflurane vaporizer at varying ambient atmospheric pressures (1 atm = 760 mmHg).

flow as gas leaves the vaporizing chamber, these vaporizers essentially become ambient pressure compensated.

The above examples should be considered in stark contrast to the response of the Tec 6 desflurane vaporizer at varied altitudes (Fig. 25-35 and Table 25-5). One must remember this device is more accurately described as a dual gas "blender" than a vaporizer. Regardless of the ambient pressure, the Tec 6 will maintain a constant concentration of vapor output (in vol%), not a constant partial pressure. This means that at high altitudes, the partial pressure of desflurane for any given dial setting will be decreased in proportion to the atmospheric pressure divided by the calibration pressure (normally 760 mmHg) according to the following formula:

Required dial setting = normal dial setting (v/v × 760 mmHg)/ ambient pressure (mmHg)

Consider a Tec 6 vaporizer that is set to deliver 10% desflurane at 1 atmosphere. The partial pressure of desflurane delivered from the vaporizer (Pdes) is 76 mmHg (i.e., 10% × 760). If used at an altitude at which the ambient pressure is 500 mmHg, the Tec 6 dial setting must be increased to 15% to maintain the same anesthetic potency (15% × 500 = Pdes 75 mmHg). Conversely, the Tec 6's maintenance of a constant vol% output under hyperbaric conditions could produce significant increases in partial pressure output and, if not accounted for, the potential for anesthetic overdose. Therefore, in hyperbaric situations the Tec 6 dial setting would need to be decreased to maintain the desired partial pressure output of desflurane.

Carrier Gas Composition Can Influence Vaporizer Output

Vaporizer output approximates the dial setting when oxygen is the carrier gas because the Tec 6 vaporizer is calibrated by the manufacturer using 100% oxygen. At low flow rates when a carrier gas other than 100% oxygen is used, however, a clear trend toward reduction in vaporizer output emerges. This reduction parallels the proportional decrease in viscosity of the carrier gas. Nitrous oxide has a lower viscosity than oxygen, so the back pressure generated by resistor R1 (Fig. 25-34) is less when nitrous oxide is the carrier gas, and the working pressure is reduced. At low flow rates using nitrous oxide as the carrier gas, vaporizer output is approximately 20% less than the dial setting. This suggests that, at clinically useful FGF rates, the gas flow across resistor R1 is laminar, and the working pressure is proportional to both the FGF rate and the viscosity of the carrier gas.[114]

Safety Features

Because desflurane's SVP at room temperature is near 1 atm, misfilling contemporary vaporizers with desflurane could theoretically result in both desflurane overdose and creation of a hypoxic gas mixture.[115] GE-Datex-Ohmeda has introduced a unique, anesthetic-specific filling system to minimize occurrence of this potential hazard. The agent-specific filler of the desflurane bottle known as the "Saf-T-Fill" adapter is intended to prevent its use with traditional vaporizers. The filling system also minimizes spillage of liquid or vapor anesthetic by maintaining a "closed system" during the filling process. Each desflurane bottle has a spring-loaded filler cap with an O-ring on the tip. The spring seals the bottle until it is engaged in the filler port of the vaporizer. Thus, this anesthetic-specific filling system interlocks the vaporizer and the dispensing bottle, preventing loss of anesthetic to the atmosphere. Despite these safety features designed to minimize filling errors, a case report described the misfilling of a Tec 6 desflurane vaporizer with sevoflurane. This error was possible because of similarities between a new type of keyed filler for sevoflurane and the desflurane Saf-T-Fill adapter. In this case, however, the desflurane vaporizer detected this error and automatically shut itself off.[98] Major vaporizer faults cause the shutoff valve located just downstream from the desflurane sump (Fig. 25-34) to close, producing a no-output situation. The valve is closed and a "no-output" alarm is activated immediately if any of the following conditions occur: (1) the anesthetic level decreases to <20 mL; (2) the vaporizer is tilted; (3) a power failure occurs; or (4) there is a disparity between the pressure in the vapor circuit versus the pressure in the fresh gas circuit exceeding a specified tolerance. Note the alarm panel on the front of the Tec 6 vaporizer (Fig. 25-36A) showing "No Output," "Low Agent," "Warm Up," and "Alarm Battery Low" indicators.

The Dräger D-Vapor vaporizer has similar alarms (Fig. 25-36B). The "No Output" alarm (flashes red) indicates that the vaporizer is unable to deliver anesthetic (i.e., the vaporizer is warming up) or there is a device failure. The "Delivery Low" alarm (flashes red) triggers when the vaporizer is unable to supply the output set by the concentration dial (only with FGF > 1.5 L/min), the reservoir is empty, or if there is an apparatus fault. The "Fill Up" alarm (glows amber) indicates the reservoir level has dropped below the refill mark (the reservoir contains <40 mL). The "Battery" alarm will indicate (1) *amber glow* if the vaporizer is not able to operate without power, (2) *amber flashing* if the vaporizer is currently operating on battery backup, (3) *flashing amber plus* "No Output" *flashing red* if the vaporizer battery is depleted after operating on battery backup and another method of anesthesia is required. The vaporizer will also provide an audible alarm along with visual alarms. Medium priority alarms (amber glowing and flashing) may be silenced; high-priority alarms (red flashing) cannot be silenced.[113]

The GE-Datex-Ohmeda Aladin Cassette Vaporizer

The vaporizer system used in the GE-Datex-Ohmeda S/5 ADU and GE Aisys Carestation is unique in that the single electronically controlled vaporizer is designed to deliver five different inhaled anesthetics including halothane, isoflurane, enflurane, sevoflurane, and desflurane (Figs. 25-37 and 25-38). The vaporizer consists of a permanent internal control unit housed within

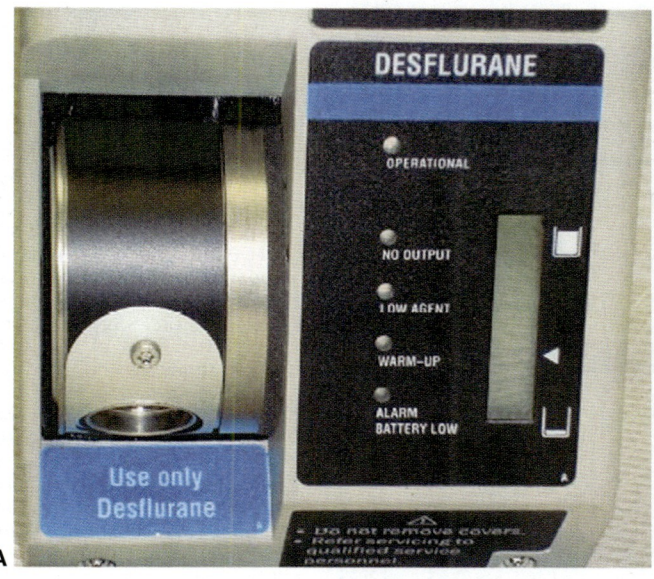
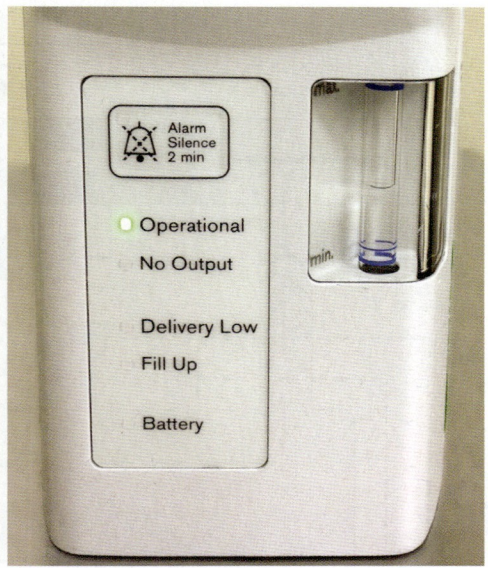

Figure 25-36 **A:** Tec 6 desflurane vaporizer alarm indicators. **B:** Dräger D-Vapor desflurane alarm indicators.

the workstation and an interchangeable Aladin agent-specific cassette that contains anesthetic liquid. The Aladin agent cassettes are color coded for each anesthetic agent, and they are also magnetically coded so that the workstation can identify which anesthetic cassette has been inserted. The cassettes are filled using agent-specific fillers.

Though very different in external appearance, the functional anatomy of the Aladin cassette vaporizer (Fig. 25-39) is very similar to that of the traditional variable bypass vaporizers because it is also made up of a bypass chamber and vaporizing chamber. A fixed restrictor is located in the bypass chamber, and flow measurement sensors are located both in the bypass chamber and in the outlet of the vaporizing chamber. The heart of the Aladin vaporizer is the electronically regulated flow control valve located in the vaporizing chamber outlet. This valve is controlled by a central processing unit (CPU). The CPU receives input from multiple sources including the concentration control dial, a pressure sensor located inside the vaporizing chamber (cassette), a temperature sensor located inside the vaporizing chamber, a flow measurement unit located in the bypass chamber, and a flow measurement unit located in the outlet of the vaporizing chamber. The CPU also receives input from the machine's flowmeters regarding the composition of the carrier gas. Using data from these multiple sources, the CPU is able to precisely regulate the flow control valve to attain the desired vapor concentration output. Appropriate electronic control of the flow control valve is essential to the proper function of this vaporizer.[116]

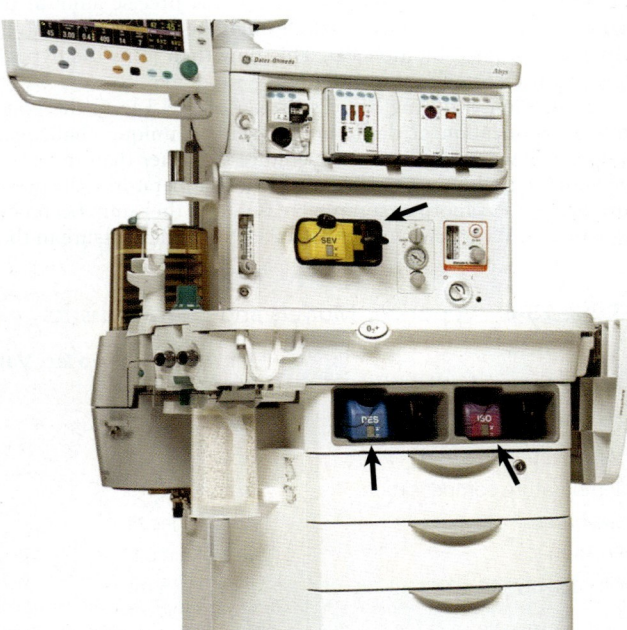

Figure 25-37 Aladin vaporizer sevoflurane cassette (courtesy of GE Healthcare).

Figure 25-38 Aladin cassette vaporizers (*arrows*) on a GE Datex-Ohmeda Aisys Carestation. Upper cassette is in use, lower cassettes are stored on workstation.

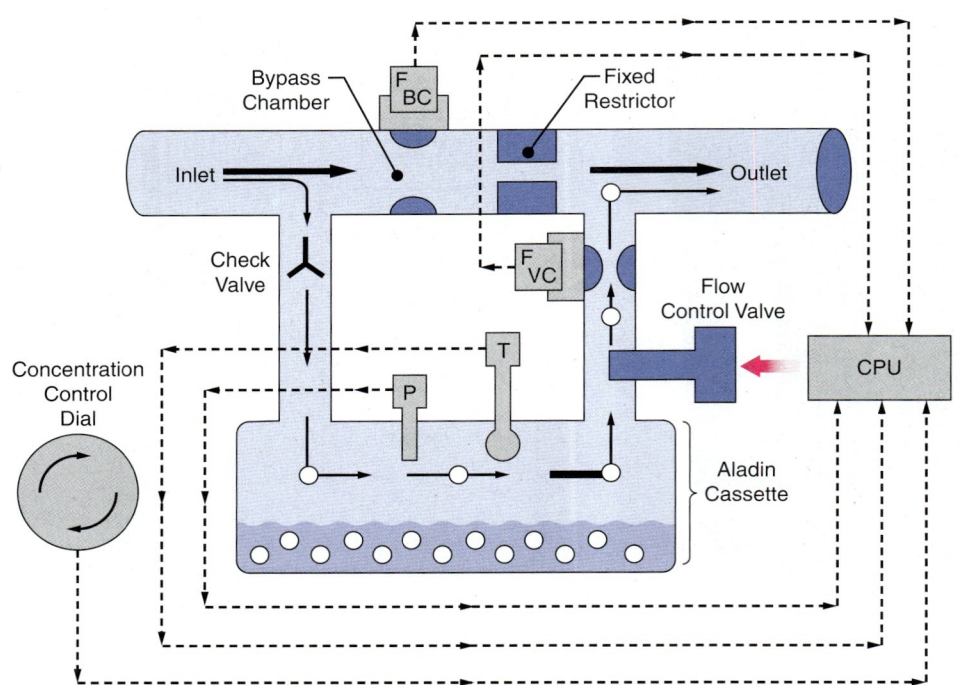

Figure 25-39 Simplified schematic of GE-Datex-Ohmeda Aladin Cassette Vaporizer. The *black arrows* represent flow from the flowmeters, and the *white circles* represent anesthetic vapor. The heart of the vaporizer is the electronically controlled flow control valve located in the outlet of the vaporizing chamber. CPU, central processing unit; FBC, flow measurement unit, which measures flow through the bypass chamber; FVC, flow measurement unit, which measures flow through the vaporizing chamber; P, pressure sensor; T, temperature sensor. (Modified from Andrews JJ. *Operating Principles of the Datex-Ohmeda Aladin Cassette Vaporizer: A Collection of Color Illustrations*. Washington, DC: Library of Congress; 2000.)

A fixed restrictor is located in the bypass chamber, and it causes flow from the vaporizer inlet to be split into two flow streams (Fig. 25-39). One stream passes through the bypass chamber, and the other portion enters the inlet of the vaporizing chamber and passes through a one-way check valve. The presence of this check valve is unique to the Aladin system. This one-way valve prevents retrograde flow of the anesthetic vapor back into the bypass chamber, and its presence is crucial when delivering desflurane if the room temperature is greater than the boiling point for desflurane (22.8°C). A precise amount of vapor-saturated carrier gas passes through the flow control valve, which is regulated by the CPU. This flow then joins the bypass flow and is directed to the outlet of the vaporizer.

As mentioned during the discussion of the Tec 6, the controlled vaporization of desflurane presents a unique challenge, particularly when the room temperature is greater than the boiling point of desflurane (22.8°C). At higher temperatures, the pressure inside the vaporizer sump increases, and the sump becomes pressurized. When the sump pressure exceeds the pressure in the bypass chamber, the one-way check valve located in the vaporizing chamber inlet closes preventing carrier gas from entering the vaporizing chamber. At this point, the carrier gas passes straight through the bypass chamber and its flow sensor. Under these conditions, the electronically regulated flow control valve simply meters in the appropriate flow of pure desflurane vapor needed to achieve the desired final concentration selected by the user.

During operating conditions in which high FGF rates and/or high dial settings are used, large quantities of anesthetic liquid are rapidly vaporized. The temperature of the remaining liquid anesthetic and the vaporizer itself decreases as a result of energy consumption of the latent heat of vaporization. To offset this cooling effect, the workstation (GE ADU and Aisys) is equipped with a fan that forces warmed air from an "agent heating resistor" across the cassette (vaporizer sump) to raise its temperature when necessary. The fan is activated during two common clinical scenarios: (1) desflurane induction and maintenance and (2) sevoflurane induction. A summary of the characteristics of various vaporizer models currently in use is found in Table 25-6.

Table 25-6 Vaporizer Models and Characteristics

Type of Vaporizer	Tec 4, Tec 5, SevoTec, Vapor 19.n, Vapor 2000, Aladin	Tec 6 (Desflurane), D-Vapor (Desflurane)
Carrier gas flow	Variable bypass	Dual circuit
Vaporization method	Flow-over	Gas/vapor blender
Temperature compensation	Automatic	Thermostatically controlled at 39°C
Calibration	Agent specific	Agent specific
Position	Out of circuit	Out of circuit
Fill capacity	Tec 4: 125 mL Tec 5: 300 mL Vapor 19.n: 200 mL Vapor 2000: 360 mL (dry wick) Aladin: 250 mL	Tec 6: 425 mL D-Vapor: 300 mL

Maquet FLOW-i Electronic Injector Vaporizer

The ability to calculate volume of vapor produced per mL of liquid agent (Table 25-2) is applied in the vaporizing system of the Maquet FLOW-i workstation (Fig. 25-4B). In principle, and somewhat analogous to fuel injection in an automobile engine, measured amounts of liquid anesthetic are injected into the FGF stream. An electronically controlled valve in the injector controls the amount of anesthetic that is delivered. The fresh gas flows through a chamber in which the anesthetic is injected. Various electronic controls and feedback mechanisms as well as continuous gas analysis ensure that the desired concentration of inhaled anesthetic is delivered in the fresh gas flowing to the patient.

Anesthesia Breathing Circuits

As the prescribed mixture of gases from the flowmeters and vaporizer exits the anesthesia workstation at the common gas outlet, it then enters an anesthetic breathing circuit. The function of the anesthesia breathing circuit is not only to deliver oxygen and anesthetic gases to the patient but also to eliminate CO_2. Carbon dioxide can be removed either by washout with adequate fresh gas inflow or by the use of CO_2 absorbent media (e.g., soda lime absorption).

Mapleson Systems

In 1954, Mapleson described and analyzed five different semi-closed anesthetic systems; these are now classically referred to as the Mapleson systems and are designated with letters A through E (Fig. 25-40).[117] Subsequently in 1975, Willis et al.[118] described the F system that was added to the original five. The Mapleson systems consist of several common components. These components commonly include a facemask, a spring-loaded pop-off valve, reservoir tubing, fresh gas inflow tubing, and a reservoir bag. Within the Mapleson systems, three distinct functional groups can be seen. They include the A; the B, C; and the D, E, F groups. The Mapleson A, also known as the Magill attachment, has a spring-loaded pop-off valve located near the facemask, and the FGF enters the opposite end of the circuit near the reservoir bag. In the B and C systems, the spring-loaded pop-off valve is located near the facemask, but the fresh gas inlet tubing is located near the patient. The reservoir tubing and reservoir bag serve as a blind limb where fresh gas, dead space gas, and alveolar gas can collect. Finally, in the Mapleson D, E, F group, or "T-piece" group, the fresh gas enters near the patient, and excess gas is released at the opposite end of the circuit.

Although the components and component arrangements are simple, functional analysis of the Mapleson systems can be complex. The amount of CO_2 rebreathing associated with each system is multifactorial, and variables that dictate the ultimate CO_2 concentration include (1) the fresh gas inflow rate, (2) the patient's minute ventilation, (3) the mode of ventilation (spontaneous or controlled), (4) the tidal volume, (5) the respiratory rate, (6) the I:E ratio, (7) the duration of the expiratory pause, (8) the peak inspiratory flow rate, (9) the volume of the reservoir tube, (10) the volume of the breathing bag, (11) ventilation by mask, (12) ventilation through an endotracheal tube, and (13) the CO_2 sampling site.

The performance of the Mapleson systems is best understood by studying the expiratory phase of the respiratory cycle.[119] Illustrations of the various Mapleson system component arrangements

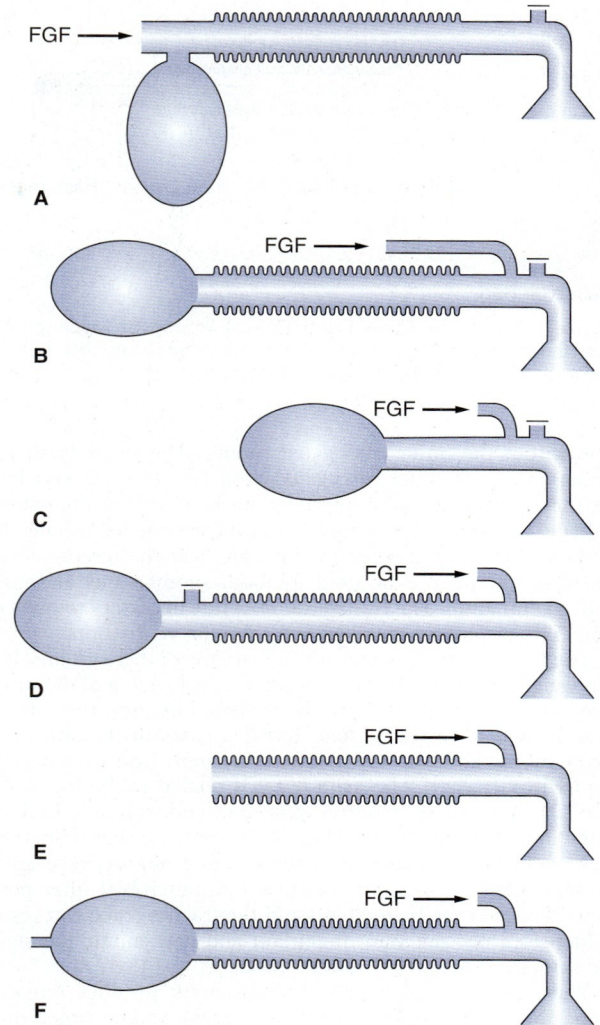

Figure 25-40 Mapleson breathing systems (**A–F**). (Adapted from Willis BA, Pender JW, Mapleson WW. Rebreathing in a T-piece: volunteer and theoretical studies of the Jackson-Rees modification of Ayre's T-piece during spontaneous respiration. *Br J Anaesth.* 1975;47:1239.)

are shown in Figure 25-40. During spontaneous ventilation, the Mapleson A has the best efficiency of the six systems requiring a fresh gas inflow rate of only one time the patient's minute ventilation to prevent rebreathing of exhaled CO_2. However, it has the least efficiency during controlled ventilation, requiring an FGF as high as 20 L/min to prevent rebreathing. Systems D, E, and F are slightly more efficient than systems B and C. To prevent rebreathing of CO_2, the D, E, and F systems require an FGF rate of approximately 2.5 times the minute ventilation, whereas the FGF rates required for B and C systems are somewhat higher.[120]

The Mapleson A, B, and C systems are rarely used today, but the D, E, F systems are still commonly employed. In the United States, the most popular representative from the D, E, F group is the Bain circuit.

Bain Circuit

The Bain circuit is a coaxial circuit and a modification of the Mapleson D system. The fresh gas flows through a narrow inner

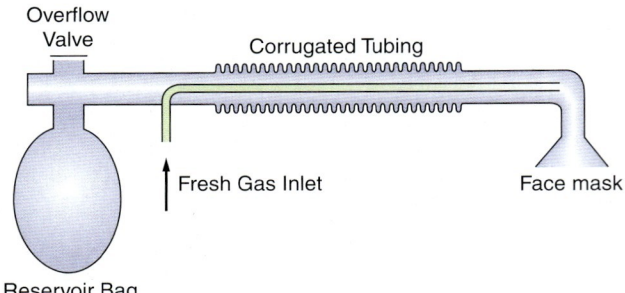

Figure 25-41 The Bain Circuit (Coaxial version of Mapleson D). (Adapted from Bain JA, Spoerel WE. A streamlined anaesthetic system. Can Anaesth Soc J. 1972;19(4):426–435.)

tube within the outer corrugated tubing. The inner fresh gas tubing enters the outer corrugated hose near the reservoir bag, but the fresh gas actually empties into the circuit at the patient end (Fig. 25-41). Exhaled gases enter the corrugated tubing and are vented through the expiratory valve near the reservoir bag. The Bain circuit may be used for both spontaneous and controlled ventilation. The fresh gas inflow rate necessary to prevent rebreathing is 2.5 times the patient's minute ventilation.

The Bain circuit has many advantages over other systems. It is lightweight, convenient, and disposable. Scavenging of the waste gases from the "pop-off" valve is facilitated because the valve is located away from the patient. Exhaled gases in the outer reservoir tubing add warmth by countercurrent heat exchange to inspired fresh gases. The main hazards related to the use of the Bain circuit are either an unrecognized disconnection or kinking of the inner fresh gas hose. These problems can cause hypercarbia from inadequate gas flow or increased respiratory resistance. As with other circuits, an obstructed antimicrobial filter positioned between the Bain circuit and the tracheal tube can result in increased resistance in the circuit and may mimic the signs and symptoms of severe bronchospasm.[121]

The outer corrugated tube is transparent to allow ongoing inspection of the inner tube. The integrity of the inner tube can be assessed as described by Pethick.[122] With his technique, high-flow oxygen is fed into the circuit while the patient end is occluded until the reservoir bag is filled. The patient end is opened, and oxygen is flushed into the circuit. If the inner tube is intact, the Venturi effect occurs at the patient end. This causes a decrease in pressure within the circuit, and as a result, the reservoir bag deflates. Conversely, a leak in the inner tube allows the fresh gas to escape into the expiratory limb, and the reservoir bag will remain inflated. This test is recommended as a part of the preanesthesia check if a Bain circuit is used.

Circle Breathing Systems

For many years, the overall design of the circle breathing system has undergone few changes. The individual components and the order in which they appear in the circle system were consistent across major platforms. More recently, however, with the increasing technologic complexity of the anesthesia workstation, the circle system has gone through some major changes as well. These changes have resulted in part from an effort to improve patient safety (as in the integration of Fresh Gas Decoupling and Inspiratory Pressure Limiters), but have also allowed the deployment of new technologic advances. Examples of major new technologies include (1) a return to the application of single-circuit piston-type ventilators and (2) use of new spirometry devices that are located at the Y-connector instead of at the traditional location in the expiratory limb of the circuit. The following discussion first focuses on the traditional circle breathing system, and then is followed by a brief discussion of some variations in the designs of newer circle systems.

The Traditional Circle Breathing System

The circle system remains the most popular breathing system in the United States. It is so named because its components are arranged in a circular manner (Fig. 25-9). A coaxial version of the traditional circle system, referred to as either a "Universal F" (King Systems, Noblesville, IN) or a "single limb circuit," has increased in popularity over recent years. Although these systems appear very different externally, they have the same overall functional layout as the traditional circle system and the following discussion is applicable to both the traditional circle system and the coaxial Universal F system.

The circle system prevents rebreathing of CO_2 by use of CO_2 absorbents, but allows partial rebreathing of other exhaled gases. The extent of rebreathing of the other exhaled gases depends on breathing circuit component arrangement and the FGF rate. A circle system can be semiopen, semiclosed, or closed, depending on the amount of FGF.[123] A *semiopen* system has no rebreathing and requires a very high FGF. A *semiclosed* system is associated with some rebreathing of exhaled gases and is the system that is most commonly used in the United States. A *closed* system is one in which the FGF exactly matches that being taken up, or consumed, by the patient. In a closed system, there is complete rebreathing of exhaled gases after absorption of CO_2, and the overflow (pop-off or APL) valve or ventilator pressure relief valve remains closed.

The circle system (Fig. 25-9) consists of seven primary components: (1) a fresh gas inflow source; (2) inspiratory and expiratory unidirectional valves; (3) inspiratory and expiratory corrugated tubes; (4) a Y-piece connector; (5) an overflow or pop-off valve, referred to as the APL valve; (6) a reservoir bag; and (7) a canister containing CO_2 absorbent. The inspiratory and expiratory valves that are placed in the system to ensure gas flow through the corrugated hoses remains unidirectional. The fresh gas inflow enters the circle by a connection from the common gas outlet of the anesthesia machine.

Numerous variations of the circle arrangement are possible, depending on the relative positions of the unidirectional valves, the APL valve, the reservoir bag, the CO_2 absorber, and the site of fresh gas entry. However, to prevent rebreathing of CO_2 *in a traditional circle system,* three rules must be followed[124]:

1. A unidirectional valve must be located between the patient and the reservoir bag on both the inspiratory and the expiratory limbs of the circuit.
2. The fresh gas inflow cannot enter the circuit between the expiratory valve and the patient.
3. The overflow (pop-off) valve cannot be located between the patient and the inspiratory valve.

If these rules are followed, any arrangement of the other components will prevent rebreathing of CO_2. Some newer anesthesia workstations now employ less traditional circle breathing systems. Two of these systems (the Datex-Ohmeda S/5 ADU breathing system and the Dräger Apollo and Fabius GS workstations breathing system) are discussed in greater detail (see the Anesthesia Workstation Variations section).

The most efficient circle system arrangement with the highest conservation of fresh gases is one in which the unidirectional valves are near the patient and the pop-off valve is located just downstream from the expiratory valve. This arrangement minimizes dead space gas and preferentially eliminates exhaled alveolar gases. A more practical arrangement, the one used on most conventional anesthesia machines (Fig. 25-9), is somewhat less efficient because it allows alveolar and dead space gases to mix before they are vented.[125]

The main advantages of the circle system over other breathing systems include its (1) maintenance of relatively stable inspired gas concentrations; (2) conservation of respiratory moisture and heat; and (3) prevention of operating room atmosphere contamination by waste gases. In addition, the circle system can be used as a semiclosed system or as a closed system with very low FGFs. The major disadvantage of the circle system stems from its complex design. Commonly, the circle system may have 10 or more different connections. These multiple connection sites set the stage for misconnections, disconnections, obstructions, and leaks. In the 1997 ASA closed claims analysis of adverse anesthetic outcomes arising from gas delivery equipment, more than onethird (25/72) of malpractice claims resulted from breathing circuit misconnections or disconnections.[9] Malfunction of the circle system's unidirectional valves can result in life-threatening problems. Rebreathing can occur if the valves stick in the open position, and total occlusion of the circuit can occur if they are stuck shut. If the expiratory valve is stuck in the closed position, breath-stacking and barotrauma or volutrauma can result. Obstructed filters located in the expiratory limb of the circle breathing system have caused increased airway pressures, hemodynamic collapse, and bilateral tension pneumothorax. Causes of circle system obstruction and failure include manufacturing defects, debris, patient secretions, and particulate obstruction from other odd sources such as albuterol nebulization.[126–129] Some systems, such as the GE Datex-Ohmeda 7900 SmartVent, use flow transducers located on both the inspiratory and the expiratory limbs of the circle system. In one report, cracks in the flow transducer tubing used by this system produced a leak in the circle system that was difficult to detect.[130]

CO_2 Absorbents

In the early 2000s, there were several reports of adverse chemical reactions between CO_2 absorbent materials and anesthetic agents. Some of these undesirable interactions were quite dramatic, such as sevoflurane interacting with desiccated Baralyme, resulting in fires within the breathing system and severe patient injury.[131,132] Although other sources of ignition and fire in the breathing system continue to be described, the Baralyme-sevoflurane problem is somewhat unique in that nothing "unusual" is added to or removed from the breathing system for this to occur.[133] In August 2004, the manufacturer of Baralyme (Allied Healthcare Products) discontinued the sale of this absorbent. Other reactions between agents such as desflurane or sevoflurane and desiccated strong base absorbents can produce more insidious patient morbidity and potentially even death from the release of byproducts such as carbon monoxide or compound A.[134] Although absorbent materials may be problematic, they still represent an important component of the circle breathing system.

Different anesthesia breathing systems eliminate CO_2 with varying degrees of efficiency. The closed and semiclosed circle systems both *require* that CO_2 be absorbed from the exhaled gases to avoid hypercapnia. If one could design an ideal CO_2 absorbent, its characteristics would include lack of reactivity with common anesthetics, lack of toxicity, low resistance to gas flow, low cost, ease of handling, and efficiency in CO_2 absorption.

The Absorber Canister

On many anesthesia machines, the absorber canister (Fig. 25-9) is composed of two clear plastic canisters arranged in series. The canisters can be filled either with loose bulk absorbent or with absorbent supplied by the factory in prefilled plastic disposable cartridges called prepacks. Free granules from bulk absorbent can create a clinically significant leak if they lodge between the clear plastic canister and the O-ring gasket of the absorber, or between other joints in the circuit.[135] Leaks have also been caused by defective prepacks, which were larger than factory specifications.[136] Prepacks can also cause total obstruction of the circle system if the clear plastic shipping wrapper is not removed prior to use.[137] Contemporary workstations from GE Healthcare and Dräger use proprietary CO_2 absorbent canisters that allow exchange of the canisters while maintaining the breathing circuit integrity.

Chemistry of Absorbents

Several formulations of CO_2 absorbents are available today, including soda lime, and calcium hydroxide lime (Amsorb). Of these agents, the most commonly used is soda lime.[138] All serve to remove CO_2 from the breathing circuit with varying degrees of efficiency.

By weight, the approximate composition of "high moisture" soda lime is 80% calcium hydroxide, 15% water, 4% sodium hydroxide, and 1% potassium hydroxide (an activator). Small amounts of silica are added to produce calcium and sodium silicate. This addition produces a harder and more stable pellet and thereby reduces dust formation. The efficiency of the soda lime absorption varies inversely with the hardness; therefore, little silicate is used in contemporary soda lime.[139,140] Sodium hydroxide is the catalyst for the CO_2 absorptive properties of soda lime. Calcium hydroxide lime is one of the newest clinically available CO_2 absorbents. It consists primarily of calcium hydroxide and calcium chloride and contains two setting agents: calcium sulfate and polyvinylpyrrolidone. The latter two agents serve to enhance the hardness and porosity of the agent.[141] The most significant advantage of calcium hydroxide lime over other agents is its lack of the strong bases, sodium and potassium hydroxide. The absence of these chemicals eliminates the undesirable production of carbon monoxide, the potentially nephrotoxic substance known as compound A, and may reduce or eliminate the possibility of a fire in the breathing circuit.[142] The most significant disadvantages of calcium hydroxide lime are less absorptive capacity, about 50% less than strong-base containing absorbents, and generally higher cost per unit than other absorbents.[143,144]

The size of the actual absorptive granules has been determined over time by trial and error. The current size particles represent a compromise between resistance to gas flow and absorptive efficiency. The smaller the granule size, the greater the surface area that is available for absorption. However, as particle size decreases, resistance to gas flow increases. The granular size of soda lime used in clinical practice is between 4 and 8 mesh, a size at which absorptive surface area and resistance to flow are optimized. Mesh size refers to the number of openings per linear inch in a sieve through which the granular particles can pass. The absorption of CO_2 by absorbents such as soda lime occurs by a series of chemical reactions; it is not a physical process like soaking water into a sponge. CO_2 combines with water to form carbonic acid. Carbonic acid reacts with the hydroxides to form sodium (or potassium) carbonate and water. Calcium hydroxide accepts the carbonate to form calcium carbonate and sodium (or potassium) hydroxide. The equations for the reactions are as follows:

1. $CO_2 + H_2O \Leftrightarrow H_2CO_3$
2. $H_2CO_3 + 2NaOH(KOH) \Leftrightarrow Na_2CO_3(K_2CO_3) + 2H_2O + Heat$
3. $Na_2CO_3(K_2CO_3) + Ca(OH)_2 \Leftrightarrow CaCO_3 + 2NaOH(KOH)$

Some CO_2 may react directly with $Ca(OH)_2$, but this reaction is much slower.

Absorptive Capacity

The maximum amount of CO_2 that can be absorbed by soda lime is 26 L of CO_2 per 100 g of absorbent. The absorptive capacity of calcium hydroxide lime is significantly less and has been reported at 10.2 L per 100 g of absorbent. However, as previously mentioned, absorptive capacity is the product of both available chemical reactivity and physical (granule) availability. As the absorbent granules stack up in the absorber canisters, small passageways inevitably form. These small passages channel gases preferentially through low resistance areas. Because of this phenomenon, functional absorptive capacity of either soda lime or calcium hydroxide lime may be substantially decreased.[145]

Indicators

Ethyl violet is the pH indicator added to soda lime to help assess the functional integrity of the absorbent. This compound is a substituted triphenylmethane dye with a critical pH of 10.3.[142] Ethyl violet changes from colorless to violet in color when the pH of the absorbent decreases as a result of CO_2 absorption. When the absorbent is fresh, the pH exceeds the critical pH of the indicator dye, and it exists in its colorless form. However, as absorbent becomes exhausted, the pH decreases below 10.3, and ethyl violet changes to its violet form because of alcohol dehydration. This change in color indicates that the absorptive capacity of the material has been consumed. Unfortunately, in some circumstances ethyl violet may not always be a reliable indicator of the functional status of absorbent. For example, prolonged exposure of ethyl violet to fluorescent lights can produce photodeactivation of this dye.[146] When this occurs, the absorbent appears white even though it may have a reduced pH and its absorptive capacity has been exhausted. Even in the absence of color changes, clinical signs that the CO_2 absorbent is exhausted include:

1. Increased spontaneous respiratory rate (requires that no neuromuscular blocking drug be used)
2. Initial increase in blood pressure and heart rate, followed later by a decrease in both
3. Increased sympathetic drive: skin flushing, sweating, tachydysrhythmia, hypermetabolic state (increased CO_2 production; must rule out malignant hyperthermia)
4. Respiratory acidosis as evidenced by arterial blood gas analysis
5. Increased surgical bleeding—due to both hypertension and coagulopathy

Although a diagnosis of depletion of CO_2 absorbent capability can be made by observation of clinical signs, the most sensitive indicator of this problem is capnography. If the end-expiratory level of exhaled CO_2 is increased, and the inspiratory level is greater than zero, then exhaustion of the CO_2 absorbent must be pursued as a possible cause.

Interactions of Inhaled Anesthetics with Absorbents

It is important and desirable to have CO_2 absorbents that neither release toxic particles or fumes nor produce toxic compounds when exposed to common anesthetics. Soda lime and Amsorb generally fit this description, but inhaled anesthetics do interact with all absorbents to some extent.

Sevoflurane has been shown to produce degradation products upon interaction with CO_2 absorbents.[147,148] The major degradation product produced is an olefin compound known as fluoromethyl-2, 2-difluoro-1-(trifluoromethyl) vinyl ether, or compound A. During sevoflurane anesthesia, factors apparently leading to an increase in the concentration of compound A include (1) low flow or closed circuit anesthetic techniques; (2) the use of Baralyme (now no longer available); (3) higher concentrations of sevoflurane in the anesthetic circuit; (4) higher absorbent temperatures; and (5) fresh absorbent.[149,150] Interestingly, the dehydration of Baralyme increased the concentration of compound A, but the dehydration of soda lime decreases the concentration of compound A.[151,152] Apparently, the degradation products released during clinical conditions do not commonly result in adverse effects in humans even during low flow anesthesia.[153-155] Hepatorenal function biomarkers using sevoflurane are unchanged in patients during low flow anesthesia when compared to high flow anesthesia.[156] Desiccated strong-base absorbents can also degrade contemporary inhaled anesthetics to clinically significant concentrations of carbon monoxide (CO) as well as trifluoromethane, which can interfere with anesthetic gas monitoring. Under certain conditions, this process can produce very high carboxyhemoglobin concentrations, reaching 35% or more.[157] Higher levels of carbon monoxide are more likely after prolonged contact between absorbent and anesthetics, and after disuse of an absorber for at least 2 days, especially over a weekend.[158] Thus, case reports describing carbon monoxide poisoning have been most common in patients anesthetized on Monday morning, presumably because continuous flow from the unused anesthesia machine desiccated the absorbents over the weekend. FGF rates of 5 L/min or more through the breathing system and absorbent (without a patient connected) are sufficient to cause critical drying of the absorbent material. This is even worse when the reservoir bag is left off the breathing circuit. Absence of the reservoir bag facilitates retrograde flow through the circle system (Fig. 25-9).

Several factors appear to increase the production of carbon monoxide and result in increased carboxyhemoglobin levels. They include (1) the inhaled anesthetic used (for a given MAC multiple, the magnitude of CO production from greatest to least is desflurane ≥ enflurane > isoflurane ≫ halothane = sevoflurane); (2) the absorbent dryness (completely dry absorbent produces more CO than hydrated absorbent); (3) the type of absorbent (at a given water content, Baralyme produced more CO than does soda lime); (4) the temperature (increased temperature increases CO production); (5) the anesthetic concentration (more CO is produced from higher anesthetic concentrations)[151]; (6) low FGF rates; and (7) reduced experimental animal (patient) size per 100 g of absorbent.[159]

Several interventions have been suggested to reduce the incidence of carbon monoxide exposure in patients undergoing general anesthesia. These interventions include (1) educating anesthesia personnel regarding the etiology of CO production; (2) turning off the anesthesia machine at the conclusion of the last case of the day to eliminate FGF that dries the absorbent; (3) changing CO_2 absorbent if fresh gas was found flowing during the morning machine preuse check; (4) rehydrating desiccated absorbent by adding water; (5) changing the chemical composition of soda lime to reduce or eliminate potassium hydroxide (such products now available include Drägersorb 800 plus, Sofnolime, and Spherasorb); and (6) using absorbent materials such as calcium hydroxide lime that are free of both sodium and potassium hydroxides. The elimination of sodium and potassium hydroxides from desiccated soda lime diminishes or eliminates degradation of desflurane to carbon monoxide and sevoflurane to compound A, but does not compromise CO_2 absorption.[160]

As a result of the increasing evidence that exposure of volatile anesthetics to desiccated CO_2 absorbents could be hazardous (Table 25-7), the Anesthesia Patient Safety Foundation convened in 2005 a conference on CO_2 absorption safety considerations. The conference experts agreed with the following recommendations[138]:

1. Turn off all gas flow when the machine is not in use
2. Change absorbents regularly (on Monday mornings, since the absorbent may have become desiccated over the weekend)
3. Change absorbent whenever the color change indicates exhaustion
4. Change BOTH canisters in a two-canister system
5. Change absorbent whenever the FGF has been left on for an extensive or indeterminate period of time
6. If compact canisters are used, consider changing them more frequently

One extremely rare but potentially life-threatening complication related to CO_2 absorbent use is the development of fires within the breathing system. Specifically, this can occur as the result of interactions between the strong-base absorbents (particularly with the now obsolete Baralyme) and the inhaled anesthetic, sevoflurane. When desiccated strong-base absorbents are exposed to sevoflurane, absorber temperatures of several hundred degrees may result from their interaction. The build-up of very high temperatures, the formation of combustible degradation by-products (formaldehyde, methanol, and formic acid), plus the oxygen- or nitrous oxide-enriched environment provide all the substrates necessary for a fire to occur.

New CO_2 absorbents that incorporate lithium have become available.[161] One example is Litholyme (Allied Healthcare, St. Louis, MO), which consists of calcium hydroxide, lithium chloride, and ethyl violet indicator. It is supplied as pellets (similar to soda lime granules). Litholyme contains a lithium catalyst to facilitate CO_2 absorption and does not use strong bases (NaOH or KOH). The lithium catalyst does not react with common inhaled anesthetic agents and therefore eliminates the potential for generation of CO or Compound A. Absorption of CO_2 is minimally exothermic. The indicator color change from off-white to violet is permanent and profound, indicating both exhaustion and/or desiccation and eliminating the possibility for unintentional use of expended absorbent.

Another absorbent that uses lithium is SpiraLith (Micropore Inc., Elkton, MD). It is supplied on a polymer matrix base and rolled up as a fixed spiral in a cylinder. It does not use an indicator to show exhaustion so that the anesthesiologist must monitor inspired CO_2. An advantage is that the exhausted absorbent can be recycled by the manufacturer.

Table 25-7 Absorbent Comparisons[138a]

Company	Product Name	H_2O%	NaOH%	KOH%	$Ca(OH)_2$%	Significant Other	US Availability
Allied Healthcare/Chemetron	Baralyme	11.0–16.0	0.0	<5	73	$Ba(OH)_2$	No longer
Allied Healthcare	Carbolime[b]	12.0–19.0	3	0.0	>75	—	Yes
W.R. Grace and Company	Sodasorb	15.0–17.0	3.7	—	50–100	—	Yes
Intersurgical Ltd.	Intersorb Plus	13.5–17.5	2.6	0.0	81	—	Yes
Intersurgical Ltd.	Spherasorb	13.5–17.5	1.3	0.0	78	4% Zeolite	Yes
Intersurgical Ltd.	LoFloSorb	13.5–17.5	0.0	0.0	78	6.5% Silica	Yes
Armstrong Medical Ltd.	Amsorb	13.5–16.5	0.0	0.0	79–82	$CaCl_2$	No Longer
Armstrong Medical Ltd.	Amsorb Plus	13.0–18.0	0.0	0.0	>80	$CaCl_2$	Yes
Dräger Medical, Inc.	Drägersorb 800	—	~2	~3	—	—	No longer
Dräger Medical, Inc.	Drägersorb 800 Plus	~16	1–3	NA	75–83	—	Yes
Dräger Medical, Inc.	Drägersorb Free	14–18	0.5–2	NA	74–82	$CaCl_2$	Yes
Airgas/Molecular Products	Sodalime	—	<3.5	2.6	>80	—	Yes
Molecular Products	Sofnolime	12–19	<3.5	0.0	—	—	No[d]
GE Medical[c]/Molecular Products	Medisorb	—	<3.5	0.0	—	—	Yes

[a]This table was formulated based on information supplied by the various manufacturers. The APSF assumes no responsibility for variations in, or deviations from, the formulations that are represented in this table. The table is supplied for educational and conceptual purposes.
[b]Manufactured by Molecular Products.
[c]Distributor of product manufactured by Molecular Products.
[d]Not available in US market as a medical product, although diving and military grades are available in the US. Medical grade is available outside the United States.
More than one manufacturer reported variable absorption capacity based on canister design, shape, volume FGF, hydration, and carbon dioxide concentration. Nearly all reported price variability dependent upon marketing and type of fill.
Reproduced with permission from Anesthesia Patient Safety Foundation (APSF) Newsletter, Volume 20, No. 2, Summer 2005.

Anesthesia Ventilators

The ventilator on the modern anesthesia workstation serves as a mechanized substitute for the manual squeezing of the reservoir bag of the circle system, the Bain circuit, or another breathing system. As recently as the late 1980s, anesthesia ventilators were mere adjuncts to the anesthesia machine. Today, in newer anesthesia workstations, they have attained a prominent central role. In addition to the near ubiquitous role of the anesthesia ventilator in today's anesthesia workstation, many advanced ICU-style ventilation features have also been integrated into anesthesia ventilators (Fig. 25-42). Although many similarities exist between today's anesthesia ventilator and ICU ventilator, some fundamental differences in ventilation parameters and control systems remain.

Classification

Ventilators can be classified according to their power source, drive mechanism, cycling mechanism, and bellows type.[162,163]

Power Source

The power source required to operate a mechanical ventilator is provided by compressed gas, electricity, or both. Older pneumatic ventilators required only a pneumatic power source to function properly. Contemporary electronic ventilators from Dräger Medical, GE Datex-Ohmeda, and others require either an electrical only or both an electrical and a pneumatic power source.

Drive Mechanism and Circuit Designation

Double-circuit ventilators (in which one circuit contains patient gas and the other circuit contains drive gas) are used most commonly in modern anesthesia workstations. Generally, these conventional ventilators are pneumatically driven. In a double-circuit ventilator, a driving force—pressurized gas—compresses a component analogous to the reservoir bag known as the ventilator bellows. The bellows then in turn delivers ventilation to the patient. The driving gas in the GE-Datex-Ohmeda ventilators is 100% oxygen. In the Dräger AV-E and AV-2+, a Venturi device mixes oxygen and air. Some newer pneumatic anesthesia workstations have the ability for the user to select whether compressed air or oxygen is used as the driving gas.

More recently, with the introduction of circle breathing systems that integrate fresh gas decoupling (FGD, as described in more detail below), resurgence has been seen in the utilization of mechanically driven anesthesia ventilators. These "piston"-type ventilators use a computer-controlled stepper motor instead of compressed drive gas to actuate gas movement in the breathing system. In these systems, rather than having dual circuits, a single patient gas circuit is present. Thus, they are classified as piston-driven, single-circuit ventilators. The piston operates much like the plunger of a syringe to deliver the desired tidal volume or airway pressure to the patient breathing circuit. Sophisticated computerized controls are able to provide advanced types of ventilatory support such as synchronized intermittent mandatory ventilation (S-IMV), pressure-controlled ventilation (PCV), and pressure support–assisted ventilation, in addition to the conventional volume and pressure control. Since the patient's mechanical breath is delivered without the use of compressed gas to actuate a bellows, these systems consume dramatically less compressed gas during ventilator operation than traditional pneumatic ventilators. This improvement in efficiency may have clinical significance when the anesthesia workstation is used in a setting where no pipeline gas supply is available (e.g., remote locations or office-based anesthesia practices).

Cycling Mechanism

Most anesthesia machine ventilators are time cycled and provide ventilator support in the control mode. Inspiratory phase is initiated by a timing device. Older pneumatic ventilators use a fluidic (fluid logic) timing device. Contemporary electronic ventilators use a solid-state electronic timing device and are thus classified as time cycled and electronically controlled. More advanced ventilation modes such as S-IMV, PCV, and modes that utilize a pressure-support option have an adjustable threshold pressure trigger as well. In these modes, pressure sensors provide feedback to the ventilator control system to allow it to determine when to initiate and/or terminate the respiratory cycle.

Bellows Classification

The direction of bellows movement during the expiratory phase determines the bellows classification. *Ascending (standing) bellows* ascend during the expiratory phase (Fig. 25-43B), whereas *descending (hanging) bellows* descend during the expiratory phase. Of the two configurations, the ascending bellows is generally thought to be safer. An ascending bellows will not fill if a total disconnection occurs. However, the bellows of a descending bellows ventilator will continue its upward and downward movement despite a patient disconnection. The driving gas pushes the bellows upward during the inspiratory phase. During the expiratory phase, room air is entrained into the breathing system at the site of the disconnection because gravity acts on the weighted bellows. The disconnection pressure monitor and the volume monitor may be fooled even if a disconnection is complete (see Problems and Hazards section). Some contemporary anesthesia workstation designs have returned to the descending bellows to integrate FGD (e.g., Mindray Anestar). An essential safety feature on any anesthesia workstation that utilizes a descending bellows is an integrated CO_2 apnea alarm that cannot be disabled while the ventilator is in use.

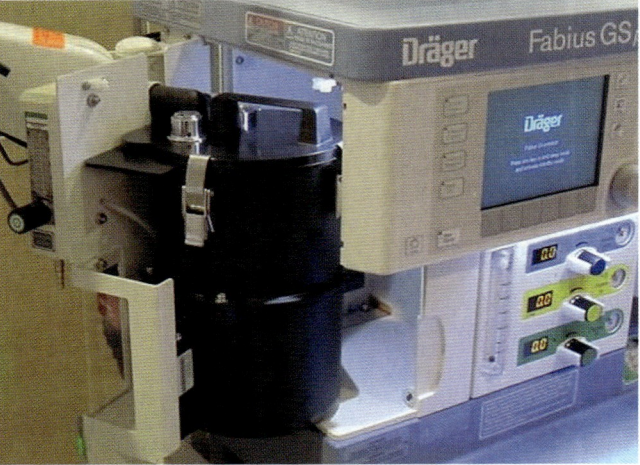

Figure 25-42 Dräger Fabius GS ventilator.

Operating Principles of Ascending Bellows Pneumatically Powered Ventilators

Contemporary examples of ascending bellows, double-circuit, electronic ventilators include the Dräger Medical AV-E, AV-2+, the GE-Datex-Ohmeda 7000, 7800, and 7900 series. A generic ascending bellows ventilator is illustrated in Figure 25-43. It may be viewed as a reservoir bag (bellows) located within a clear plastic box. The bellows physically separates the driving gas circuit from the patient gas circuit. The driving gas circuit is located outside the bellows, and the patient gas circuit is inside the bellows. During the inspiratory phase (Fig. 25-43A) the driving gas enters the bellows chamber, causing the pressure within it to increase. This increase in pressure is responsible for two events. First, the ventilator relief valve closes, preventing anesthetic gas from escaping into the scavenging system. Second, the bellows is compressed, and the anesthetic gas within the bellows is delivered to the patient's lungs. This compression action is analogous to the hand of the anesthesiologist squeezing the breathing bag.

During the expiratory phase (Fig. 25-43B), the driving gas exits the bellows housing. This produces a decrease to atmospheric pressure within both the bellows housing and the pilot line to the ventilator relief valve. The decrease in pressure to the ventilator relief valve causes the "mushroom valve" portion of the assembly to open. Exhaled patient gases refill the bellows before any scavenging can begin. The bellows refill first because a weighted ball (like those used in ball-type positive end-expiratory pressure [PEEP] valves) or similar device is incorporated into the base of the ventilator relief valve. This ball produces 2 to 3 cm H_2O of back pressure; therefore, flow to scavenging occurs only after the bellows fills completely and the pressure inside the bellows exceeds the pressure threshold of the "ball valve." This design causes all ascending bellows ventilators to produce 2 to 3 cm water pressure

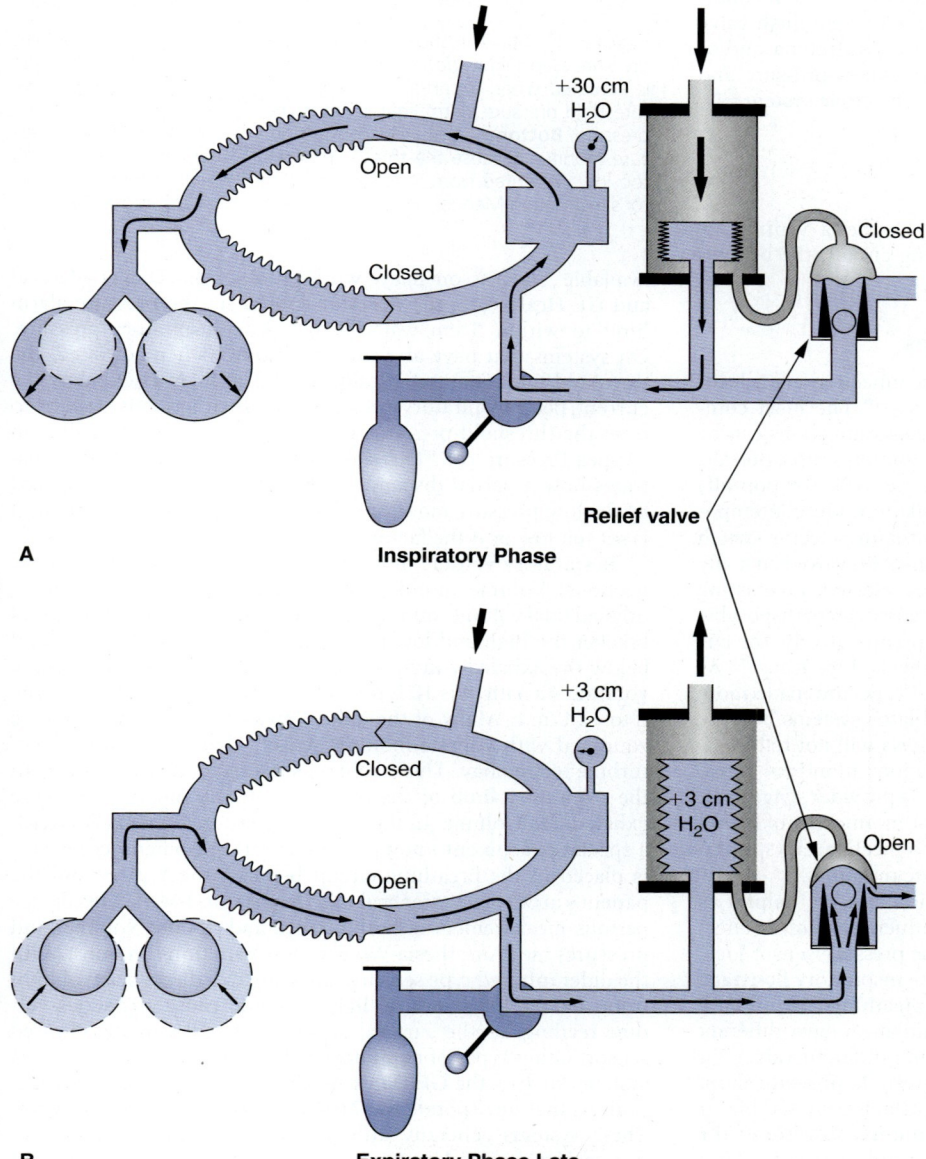

Figure 25-43 Inspiratory (**A**) and expiratory (**B**) phases of gas flow in a traditional circle system with an ascending bellows ventilator. The bellows physically separates the driving-gas circuit from the patient gas circuit. The driving-gas circuit is located outside the bellows, and the patient gas circuit is inside the bellows. During inspiratory phase (**A**), the driving gas enters the bellows chamber, causing the pressure within it to increase. This causes the ventilator relief valve to close, preventing anesthetic gas from escaping into the scavenging system, and the bellows to compress, delivering anesthetic gas within the bellows to the patient's lungs. During expiratory phase (**B**), pressure within the bellows chamber and the pilot line decreases to zero, causing the mushroom portion of the ventilator relief valve to open. Gas exhaled by the patient refills the bellows before any scavenging occurs, because a weighted ball is incorporated into the base of the ventilator relief valve. Scavenging occurs only during the expiratory phase, because the ventilator relief valve is only open during expiration. (Adapted from Andrews JJ. *The Circle System. A Collection of 30 Color Illustrations.* Washington, DC: Library of Congress; 1998.)

of PEEP within the breathing circuit when the ventilator is in use. Scavenging occurs only during the expiratory phase, as the ventilator relief valve is open only during expiration.

It is important to understand that on most older anesthesia workstations, gas flow from the anesthesia machine into the breathing circuit is continuous and independent of ventilator activity. During the inspiratory phase of mechanical ventilation, the ventilator relief valve is closed (Fig. 25-43A), and the breathing system's APL (pop-off) valve is most commonly out of circuit. Therefore, the patient's lungs receive the volume from the bellows plus that entering the circuit from the flowmeters during the inspiratory phase. Factors that influence the relationship between set tidal volume and exhaled tidal volume include the FGF settings, the inspiratory time, the compliance of the breathing circuit, external leakage, and the location of the tidal volume sensor. Usually, the volume gained from the flowmeters during inspiration is counteracted by the volume lost to compliance of the breathing circuit, and set tidal volume generally approximates the exhaled tidal volume. However, certain conditions such as inappropriate activation of the oxygen flush valve during the inspiratory phase can result in barotrauma and/or volutrauma to the patient's lungs because excess pressure and volume may not be able to be vented from the circle system.[164]

Problems and Hazards

Numerous hazards are associated with anesthesia ventilators. These include problems with the breathing circuit, the bellows assembly, and the control assembly.

Traditional Circle System Problems

Breathing circuit misconnections and disconnection are a leading cause of critical incidents in anesthesia.[165] The most common disconnection site is at the Y-piece. Disconnections can be complete or partial (leaks). In the past, a common source of leaks with older absorbers was failure to close the APL (or pop-off) valve upon initiation of mechanical ventilation. On contemporary anesthesia workstations, the bag/ventilator selector switch has virtually eliminated this problem, as the APL valve is usually out of circuit when the ventilator mode is selected. Preexisting undetected leaks can exist in compressed, corrugated, disposable anesthetic circuits. To detect such a leak preoperatively, the circuit must be fully expanded before it is checked for leaks.[166] As previously mentioned, disconnections and leaks are made more obvious with the ascending bellows ventilator systems because they result in a situation in which the bellows will not refill.

Several breathing system disconnection monitors exist, although none should replace the anesthesia provider's vigilance. Observation of chest wall excursion and/or monitoring of breath sounds should continue despite use of both mechanical (spirometers and pressure sensors) and physiologic monitors.

Pneumatic and electronic pressure monitors are helpful in detecting disconnections. Factors that influence monitor effectiveness include the disconnection site, the pressure sensor location, the threshold pressure alarm limit, the inspiratory flow rate, and the resistance of the disconnected breathing circuit.[167–169] Various anesthesia workstations and ventilators have different locations for the airway pressure sensor and different values for the threshold pressure alarm limit. The threshold pressure alarm limit may be preset at the factory or adjustable. An audible or visual alarm is actuated if the peak inspiratory pressure of the breathing circuit does not exceed the threshold pressure alarm limit. When an adjustable threshold pressure alarm limit is

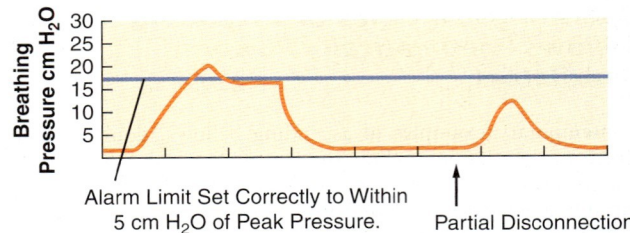

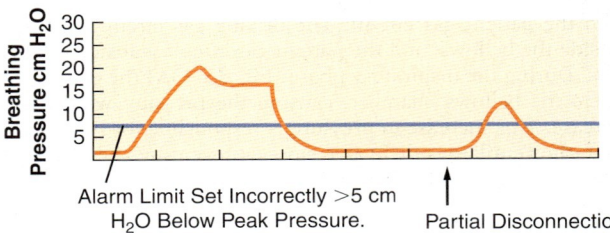

Figure 25-44 Threshold pressure alarm limit. **Top:** The threshold pressure alarm limit (*dotted line*) has been set appropriately. An alarm is actuated when a partial disconnection occurs (*arrow*) because the threshold pressure alarm limit is not exceeded by the breathing circuit pressure. **Bottom:** A partial disconnection is unrecognized by the pressure monitor because the threshold pressure alarm limit has been set too low. (Adapted from Baromed Breathing Pressure Monitor: Operator's Instruction Manual. Telford, PA: North American Dräger; 1986.)

available, such as on many workstations from Dräger Medical and GE Healthcare, the operator should set the pressure alarm limit to within 5 cm water of the peak inspiratory pressure. On systems that have an "autoset" feature, when activated, the threshold limit is automatically set at 3 to 5 cm H_2O below the current peak inspiratory pressure. On such systems, failure to reset the threshold pressure alarm limit may result in either an "Apnea Pressure" or "Threshold Low" alert. Figure 25-44 illustrates how a partial disconnection (leak) may be unrecognized by the low-pressure monitor if the threshold pressure alarm limit is set too low or if the factory preset value is relatively low.

Respiratory volume monitors are useful in detecting disconnections. Volume monitors may sense exhaled tidal volume, inhaled tidal volume, minute volume, or all three. The user should bracket the high and low threshold volumes slightly above and below the exhaled volumes. For example, if the exhaled minute volume of a patient is 10 L/min, reasonable alarm limits would be 8 to 12 L/min. Many of the older Datex-Ohmeda ventilators are equipped with volume monitor sensors that use infrared light/turbine technology. These volume sensors are usually located in the expiratory limb of the breathing circuit and thus measure exhaled tidal volume. In the case of the Datex-Ohmeda S/5 ADU, a special attachment known as the D-Lite spirometry connector is placed in the breathing circuit between the Y-piece and the patient's airway (i.e., tracheal tube connector, LMA). This device permits measurement of both inhaled and exhaled volumes and pressures (see Anesthesia Workstation Variations section). With the older infrared type sensors, exposure to a direct beam of light from the overhead surgical lighting could cause erroneous volume readings as the surgical beam interfered with the infrared sensor. Other types of expiratory volume sensors can be seen in systems such as the GE Datex Aestiva, Aespire, and other workstations that incorporate the 7100 ventilator or 7900 SmartVent. These systems generally utilize differential pressure transduction technology to determine inhaled and exhaled volumes and to measure airway pressures. Some Dräger workstations use an ultrasonic flow sensor located in the expiratory limb. Other systems from Dräger measure exhaled volume using "hot wire" sensor technology. With this type of sensor, a tiny array of two platinum wires is electrically heated to a high temperature. As gas flows past the heated wires, they tend to be cooled. The amount of energy required to maintain the temperature of the wire is proportional to the volume of gas flowing past it. This system, however, has been associated in at least one report of accidental fire in the breathing circuit.

Capnographs (CO_2 monitors) are probably the best devices for revealing circuit disconnections. CO_2 concentration is measured near the Y-piece either directly (mainstream) or by continuous aspiration of a gas sample to the analyzer instrument (sidestream). Either a sudden change in the differences between the inspiratory and end-tidal CO_2 concentrations or the acute absence of measured CO_2 indicates a disconnection, a nonventilated patient, or other problems. Importantly, an absence of exhaled CO_2 can also be an indication of low (or no) cardiac output rather than a mechanical equipment problem.

Misconnections of the breathing system are unfortunately relatively common. Despite the efforts of standards committees to eliminate this problem by assigning different diameters to various hoses and hose terminals, they continue to occur. Anesthesia workstations, breathing systems, ventilators, and scavenging systems incorporate many of these diameter-specific connections. The "ability" of anesthesia providers to outwit these "foolproof" systems has led to various hoses being cleverly adapted or forcefully fitted to inappropriate terminals and even to various other solid cylindrically shaped protrusions of the anesthesia machine.

Occlusion (obstruction) of the breathing circuit may occur. Tracheal tubes can become kinked. Hoses throughout the breathing circuit are subject to occlusion by internal obstruction or external mechanical forces, which can impinge on flow and have severe consequences. For example, blockage of a bacterial filter in the expiratory limb of the circle system has resulted in bilateral tension pneumothorax.[127] Incorrect insertion of flow direction–sensitive components can result in a no-flow state. Examples of these components include some PEEP valves and cascade humidifiers. Depending on the location of the occlusion relative to the pressure sensor, a high-pressure alarm may (or may not) alert the practitioner to the problem.

Excess inflow to the breathing circuit from the anesthesia machine during the inspiratory phase can cause barotrauma. The best example of this phenomenon is oxygen flushing. Excess volume cannot be vented from the system during inspiration because the ventilator relief valve is closed and the APL valve is out of circuit. A high-pressure alarm, if present, may be activated when the pressure becomes excessive. With many Dräger Medical systems, both audible and visual alarms are actuated when the high-pressure threshold is exceeded. The GE ventilators automatically switch from the inspiratory to the expiratory phase when the adjustable peak pressure threshold is exceeded.

On workstations equipped with adjustable inspiratory pressure limiters (such as the GE-Datex-Ohmeda S/5 ADU, Aestiva and Aisys, and Dräger Medical's Narkomed series, 2B, 2C, GS, Fabius GS, and Apollo) the maximal inspiratory pressure may be set by the user to a desired peak airway pressure. An adjustable pressure relief valve will open when the predetermined user-selected pressure threshold is exceeded. This should prevent generation of excessive airway pressure. Unfortunately, this feature is dependent on the user having preset the appropriate "pop-off" pressure. If the setting is too low, insufficient pressure for ventilation may be generated, resulting in inadequate minute ventilation; if set too high, the excessive airway pressure may still occur, resulting in barotrauma. The piston-driven ventilator in the Dräger Fabius GS and Apollo, as well as others may also include a factory preset peak inspiratory pressure safety valve that opens at a preset airway pressure such as 75 cm H_2O to minimize the risk of barotrauma.

Bellows Assembly Problems

Leaks can occur in the bellows assembly. Improper seating of the plastic bellows housing can result in inadequate ventilation because a portion of the driving gas leaks to the atmosphere. A hole in the bellows can lead to alveolar hyperinflation and possibly barotrauma in some ventilators because high-pressure driving gas can enter the patient circuit. The oxygen concentration of the patient gas may increase when the driving gas is 100% oxygen, or it may decrease if the driving gas is composed of an air–oxygen mixture.[170]

The ventilator relief valve can cause problems. Hypoventilation occurs if the valve is incompetent because the anesthetic gases are delivered to the scavenging system instead of to the patient during the inspiratory phase. Gas molecules preferentially exit into the scavenging system because it represents the path of least resistance, and the pressure within the scavenging system can be subatmospheric. Ventilator relief valve incompetency can result from a disconnected pilot line, a ruptured valve, or from a damaged flapper valve.[171,172] A ventilator relief valve stuck in the closed or partially closed position can produce either barotrauma or undesired PEEP.[173] Excessive suction from the scavenging system can draw the ventilator relief valve to its seat and close the valve during both the inspiratory and expiratory phases. In this case, breathing circuit pressure increases because excess anesthetic gas cannot be vented. It is worthwhile to note that during the expiratory phase, some newer machines from GE-Datex-Ohmeda (S/5 ADU, 7100 and 7900 SmartVent) scavenge both excess patient gases and the exhausted ventilator drive gas. That is, when the ventilator relief valve opens, and waste anesthetic gases are vented from the breathing circuit, the drive gas from the bellows housing joins with it to enter the scavenging system. Under certain conditions, the large volume of exhausted gases could overwhelm the scavenging system, resulting in contamination of the operating room atmosphere with waste anesthetic gases (see Scavenging Systems section). Other mechanical problems that can occur include leaks within the system, faulty pressure regulators, and faulty valves. Unlikely problems such as an occluded muffler on the Dräger AV-E ventilator can result in barotrauma. In this case, obstruction of driving gas outflow closes the ventilator relief valve, and excess patient gas cannot be vented.[174]

Control Assembly and Power Supply Problems

The control assembly can be the source of both electrical and mechanical problems. Electrical failure can be total or partial; the former is the more obvious. As anesthesia workstations are becoming increasingly dependent on integrated computer-controlled systems, power supply interruptions become more significant. Battery backup systems are designed to continue operation of essential electronics during brief outages. However, even with these systems, in the event of a failure, significant time may be required to reboot a computerized system after an electrical outage has occurred. During this time, the availability of certain workstation features such as manual or mechanical ventilation can be variable. One cluster of electrical failures that could have potentially resulted in operating room fires was attributed to the workstation's power supply printed circuit boards. This prompted a corrective recall action by the equipment manufacturer.[175]

Anesthesia Workstation Variations

With the introduction of new technology, often comes the need for adaptation of current technology to successfully allow its integration into existing systems. Otherwise, a more comprehensive redesign of an entire anesthesia system "from the ground up" could be necessary. One such example of adaptation in the anesthesia workstation can be seen with two new design variations of the circle breathing system. The first of these is found on the GE-Datex-Ohmeda S/5 ADU, and the second is incorporated into the Dräger Fabius GS and Apollo workstations. Since use of the circle system is fundamental to the day-to-day practice for most anesthesiologists, a comprehensive understanding of these new systems is crucial for their safe use.

Datex-Ohmeda S/5 ADU and GE Healthcare Aisys Carestation

15 The Datex-Ohmeda S/5 ADU debuted as the AS/3 ADU in 1998 (Fig. 25-45A). Along with its more comprehensive safety features and integrated design that eliminated glass flow tubes and conventional anesthesia vaporizers in exchange for a computer screen with digital FGF scales and the built-in Aladin Cassette vaporizer system, the machine had a radically different appearance in general. It is not until closer inspection that the other unique properties of the ADU begin to stand out. The principal difference in the ADU's circle system lies in the incorporation of the patented "D-Lite" flow and pressure transducer (Fig. 25-45B) inserted into the circle at the level of the Y-connector. The D-Lite spirometry module was redesigned to accommodate low-flow anesthesia and is currently an optional feature of the GE Healthcare Aisys workstation. On most traditional circle systems, exhaled tidal volume is measured by a spirometry sensor located in proximity to the expiratory unidirectional valve. The placement of the D-Lite fitting at the Y-connector provides a better location to perform exhaled volume measurement and allows airway gas composition and pressure monitoring to be done with a single adapter instead of with multiple fittings added to the breathing circuit. In addition, it provides the ability to assess both inspiratory and expiratory gas flows and therefore generation of complete flow-volume spirometry. The relocation of the spirometer sensor to the Y-connector also makes it necessary to move the location of the fresh gas inlet to the "patient" side of the inspiratory unidirectional valve without adversely affecting accuracy of exhaled tidal volume measurement. On the other hand, placement of the D-Lite sensor near the patient adds bulk and weight to the breathing circuit and may interfere with mask ventilation.

This atypical circle system arrangement with the fresh gas entering on the patient side of the inspiratory valve is advantageous for several reasons. It is likely to be more efficient in delivering fresh gas to the patient, while preferentially eliminating exhaled gases. It is also less likely to cause desiccation of the CO_2 absorbent (see Interactions of Inhaled Anesthetics with Absorbents section). Other notable changes on the S/5 ADU circle system include a compact proprietary CO_2 absorbent canister design that can be changed during ventilation without loss of circle system integrity, and the reorientation of the inspiratory and expiratory unidirectional valves from a horizontal position to a vertical position on the "compact block" assembly just below the absorbent canister.

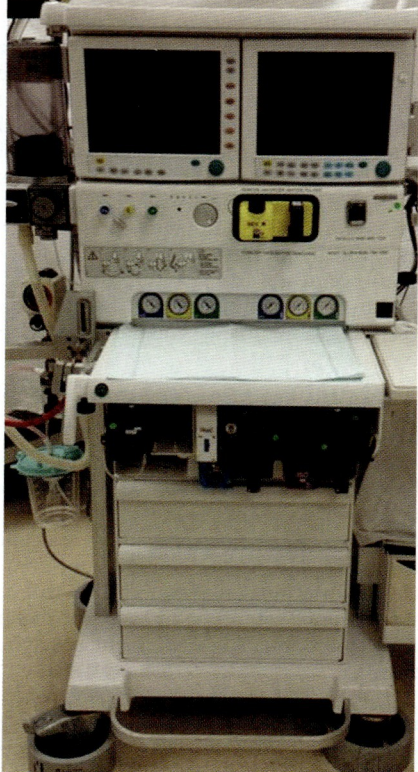
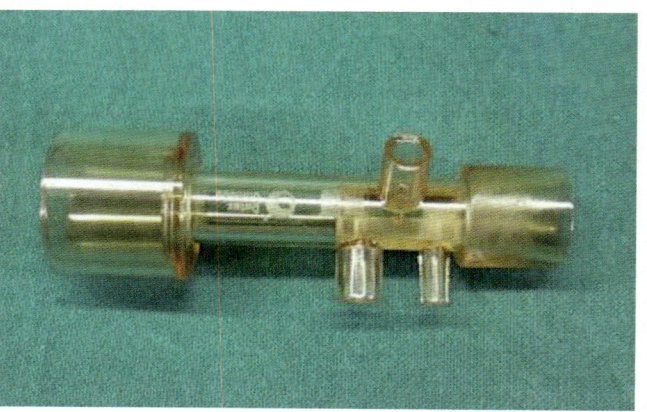

Figure 25-45 A: The GE Datex-Ohmeda AS/3 ADU workstation. **B:** D-Lite sensor. (Courtesy of GE Healthcare.)

The reorientation of the unidirectional valves reduces the breathing circuit resistance encountered by a spontaneously breathing patient. The vertically oriented unidirectional valves only have to be tipped away from the vertical position to be opened, unlike conventional horizontal valve discs, which have to be physically lifted off from the valve seat against gravity to be opened.

In the newest GE workstations (e.g., Aisys, Aespire, Avance) that use the Advanced Breathing System, the inspiratory and expiratory check valves are oriented horizontally and the circle system arrangement is such that fresh gas enters the circuit upstream from the inspiratory unidirectional valve.

The GE SmartVent 7900 is an electronically controlled, pneumatically driven ventilator. Sensors in the breathing circuit allow the ventilator to compensate for compression losses, fresh gas contribution, and small leaks. Delivered tidal volume is determined by differential pressure, variable orifice flow sensors on both the inspiratory and expiratory sides of the breathing circuit. The inspiratory flow sensor is located downstream of the gas system inspiratory check valve. Feedback from this sensor is used to calculate and supply tidal volume corrections for FGF and circuit compression losses. The expiratory flow sensor is located at the input to the gas system expiratory check valve. Breathing rate and expiratory tidal volume are determined by this sensor. Excess fresh gas from the bellows and ventilator drive gas is transferred to the scavenging system.

The Dräger Medical Narkomed 6000 Series, Fabius GS, and Apollo Workstations

Several important differences exist between the traditional circle breathing systems and those utilized in the more recent Dräger products. At first glance, the most notable difference lies in the appearance and design of the ventilators used with these systems. From the inconspicuous horizontally mounted Divan piston ventilator of the Dräger Narkomed 6000/6400 to the vertically mounted and visible piston ventilator of the Dräger Fabius GS with its electronic FGF indicators (virtual flowmeters displayed on the screen), these systems appear drastically different from traditional anesthesia systems. The piston ventilators of the Dräger Narkomed 6000 (Divan ventilator) and Dräger Fabius series (E-Vent ventilator) anesthesia systems are classified as electrically powered, piston driven, single circuit, electronically controlled with fresh gas decoupling (FGD). The ventilator found on the Dräger Apollo workstation, the E-Vent plus, is an electrically driven and electronically controlled, fresh gas decoupled, high-speed piston ventilator that requires no drive gas (unlike the traditional bellows ventilators). The E-Vent plus ventilator offers modes of ventilation previously found only on intensive care unit ventilators, including synchronized volume mode with adjustable flow trigger and pressure support.

The circle breathing systems utilized by these Dräger workstations incorporate a feature known as FGD. The incorporation of this patient safety enhancing technology has required a significant redesign of the traditional circle system. A functional schematic of a circle system similar to the one used by the Dräger Fabius GS series mechanical ventilation can be seen in Figure 25-46. To understand the operating principles of FGD, it is important to have a good understanding of gas flows in a traditional circle system both during inspiratory and expiratory phases of mechanical ventilation. A complete discussion of this was presented earlier in the section titled Operating Principles of Ascending Bellows Ventilators.

The key concept of the FGD breathing system can be illustrated during the inspiratory phase of mechanical ventilation. With the traditional circle system, several events are occurring: (1) continuous FGF from the flowmeters and/or the oxygen flush valve is entering the circle system at the fresh gas inlet; (2) the ventilator is delivering the prescribed tidal volume to the patient's lungs; and (3) the ventilator relief valve (ventilator exhaust valve) is closed, so no gas is escaping the circle system except into the patient's lungs.[176] In a traditional circle system, when these events coincide and fresh gas inflow is coupled directly into the circle system, the total volume delivered to the

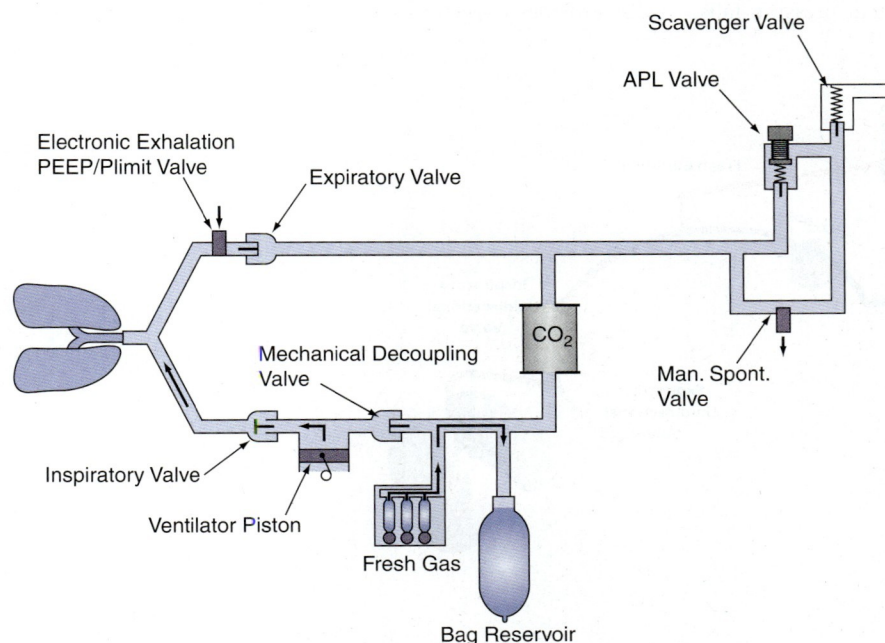

Figure 25-46 Dräger Fabius GS fresh gas decoupled (FDG) breathing system during inspiratory phase of mechanical ventilation. The figure demonstrates the path of fresh gas (and O_2 flush) into the reservoir bag during upstroke of the ventilator piston. Note the requirement here for a mechanical decoupling valve and electronic exhalation/PEEP/Plimit valve. A man./spont. valve is electronically opened during CMV, so that excess gas can escape through the low-pressure scavenger valve, which also allows preferential filling of the reservoir bag during the inspiratory phase. (Adapted from Olympio MA. Modern anesthesia machines offer new safety features. *APSF Newsletter*. 2003;18:17.)

patient's lungs is the sum of the volume delivered by the ventilator, plus the volume of gas that enters the circle via the fresh gas inlet minus the volume lost to breathing system compliance (usually 2 to 3 mL/cm H$_2$O pressure). In contrast, when FGD is used, during the inspiratory phase (Fig. 25-46) the fresh gas coming from the anesthesia workstation flowmeters via the fresh gas inlet is diverted into the reservoir bag by a decoupling valve that is located between the fresh gas source and the ventilator circuit. The reservoir (breathing) bag serves as an accumulator for fresh gas until the expiratory phase begins. During expiratory phase, the decoupling valve opens, allowing the accumulated fresh gas in the reservoir bag to be drawn into the circle system to refill the piston ventilator chamber (or descending bellows in the Mindray Anestar). Since the ventilator exhaust valve also opens during the expiratory phase, excess fresh gas and exhaled patient gases are allowed to escape to the scavenging system.

Contemporary fresh gas decoupled systems are designed with either piston-type (Dräger) or descending bellows–type ventilators. Since the bellows in either of these types of systems refills under slight negative pressure, it allows the accumulated fresh gas from the reservoir bag to be drawn into the ventilator for delivery to the patient during the next ventilator cycle.

The claimed advantages of circle systems using FGD include more accurate delivery of the set tidal volume and decreased risk of barotrauma and volutrauma. With a traditional circle system, increases in FGF from the flowmeters or from inappropriate use of the oxygen flush valve may contribute directly to tidal volume, which if excessive, may result in pneumothorax or other injuries. Since systems with FGD isolate fresh gas coming into the system from the patient while the ventilator exhaust valve is closed, the risk of barotrauma is greatly reduced.

Possibly the greatest disadvantage to the new anesthesia circle systems that utilize FGD is the possibility of entraining room air into the patient gas circuit. As previously discussed, in a fresh gas decoupled system the bellows or piston refills under slight negative pressure. If the volume of gas contained in the reservoir bag plus the returning volume of gas exhaled from the patient's lungs is inadequate to refill the bellows or piston chamber, negative patient airway pressures could develop. To prevent this, a negative-pressure relief valve is incorporated into the breathing system. If breathing system pressure falls below a preset value such as −2 cm H$_2$O, then the relief valve opens and ambient air is entrained into the patient gas circuit. If this goes undetected, the entrained atmospheric gases could lead to dilution of the inhaled anesthetic agents, the enriched oxygen mixture (resulting in a lowering of the enriched oxygen concentration toward 21%), or both. If unnoticed, this dilution of patient gases could lead to intraoperative patient awareness or hypoxia. High-priority alarms with both audible and visual alerts should notify the user that FGF is inadequate and room air is being entrained.

Another potential problem with an FGD system is its reliance on the reservoir bag to accumulate the incoming fresh gas. If the reservoir bag is removed during mechanical ventilation, or if it has a significant leak from poor fit on the bag mount or a perforation, room air may enter the breathing circuit as the ventilator piston unit refills during expiratory phase.[177] This may also result in dilution of the inhaled anesthetic agents, the enriched oxygen mixture, or both. Furthermore, this type of a disruption could lead to significant contamination of the operating room atmosphere with anesthetic gases as fresh gases would be allowed to escape into the atmosphere. Incompetence of the FGD valve leads to inability to ventilate the patient's lungs using the ventilator, but ability to ventilate using the reservoir bag in the circuit.[178] If there is a leak in the low pressure system of the workstation that permits air entry, mechanical ventilation is possible but not manual. The piston ventilator will continue to deliver the tidal volume as air. If the expiratory unidirectional valve is missing or incompetent, mechanical ventilation is possible but manual is not.[179]

Maquet FLOW-i Workstation

The Maquet FLOW-i workstation uses a novel breathing system that dispenses with the need for a bellows or piston to provide positive-pressure ventilation (Fig. 25-47).[180] The system incorporates a volume reflector (a 3.6-m–long plastic coil of internal volume 1.2 L) located between the circle system, and the reservoir bag and APL/PEEP valve (Fig. 25-48). Also connected directly to the volume reflector is the reflector oxygen module that provides oxygen as the drive gas during positive-pressure

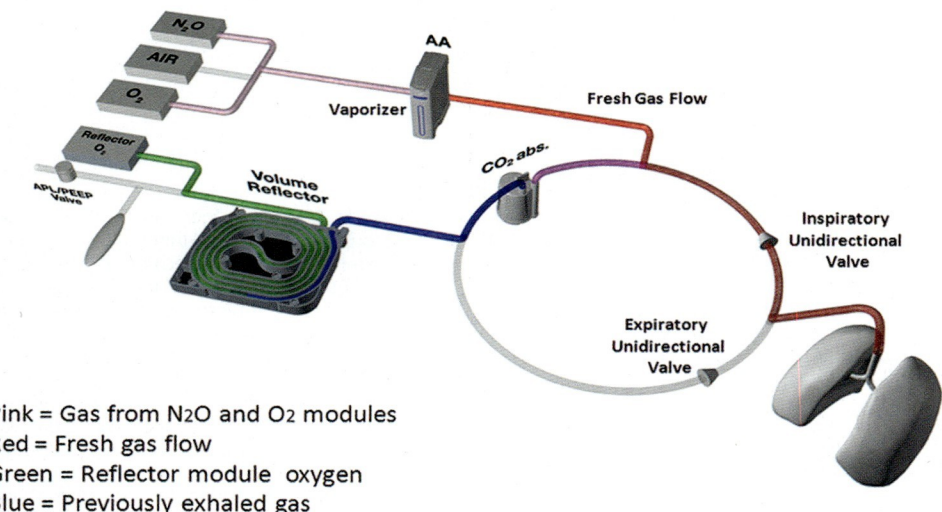

Figure 25-47 Maquet FLOW-i breathing and ventilator circuit during positive-pressure inspiration. For details, see text.

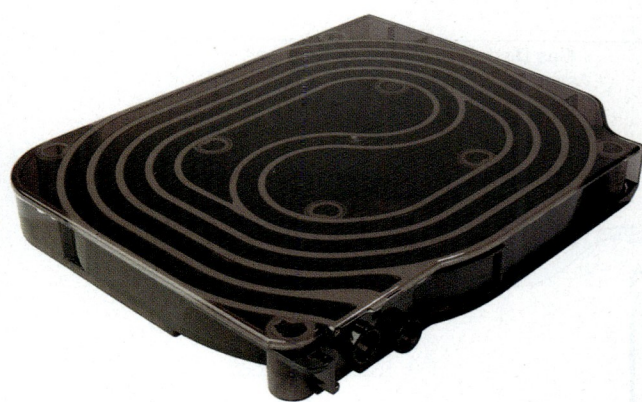

Figure 25-48 Maquet FLOW-i volume reflector.

ventilation. During exhalation, the patient exhales through the volume reflector. During positive-pressure inspiration, the APL/PEEP valve closes and the computer controlled reflector gas module delivers oxygen into the reflector, forcing the gas in the reflector back into the circle system through the absorber, past the inspiratory unidirectional valve to the patient's airway. FGF is added to the circuit during positive-pressure inspiration, combining with the reflector gas module oxygen flow to achieve the set FiO_2 and anesthetic agent concentration. The gas flows are electronically controlled using pressure and flow sensors to provide the set ventilation parameters (e.g., TV, MV, ventilator patterns). During exhalation, reflector gas module and FGFs cease, the PEEP valve (that was closed during positive-pressure inspiration) opens to the set PEEP, and exhaled gas flows via the volume reflector and on to the waste gas scavenging system.

The FLOW-i is purported to be more economical than bellows or piston ventilators during controlled ventilation because fresh gas enters the circuit only during inspiration. In the other systems described FGF enters the circuit continuously throughout the respiratory cycle. During spontaneous or manually assisted ventilation, however, the FLOW-i's economy is the same as other systems because in this mode FGF is continuous and the FLOW-i functions as a conventional circle breathing system.

Waste Gas Scavenging Systems

Scavenging is the collection and the subsequent removal of waste anesthetic gases from the operating room.[181] In most cases, the amount of gas used to anesthetize a patient for a given anesthetic far exceeds the minimal amount needed. Therefore, scavenging minimizes operating room contamination by removing this excess of gases. In 1977, the National Institute for Occupational Safety and Health (NIOSH) published a document entitled "Criteria for a Recommended Standard: Occupational Exposure to Waste Anesthetic Gases and Vapors."[182] Although a minimum safe level of exposure could not be defined, NIOSH made the recommendations shown in Table 25-8. The recommended ceiling for volatile anesthetics was established before desflurane and sevoflurane were introduced into clinical practice. However, this limit is likely to be similarly applicable for the newer volatile anesthetics.[183] The NIOSH recommendations have never promulgated into law and therefore are not enforceable. (For a more in-depth discussion of this topic, refer to the chapter on Occupational Health.)

In 1991, the ASTM released the ASTM F1343–91 standard titled "Standard Specification for Anesthetic Equipment–Scavenging Systems for Anesthetic Gases."[184] The document provided guidelines for devices that safely and effectively scavenge waste anesthetic gases to reduce contamination in anesthetizing areas. Because of lack of safety data on exposure to the newer halogenated anesthetic agents, in 2006 NIOSH requested comments and information relevant to the evaluation of health risks associated with occupational exposure to these agents in order to establish recommended maximum exposure levels (REL).[185] The ASA Task Force on Trace Anesthetic Gases developed a booklet entitled "Waste Anesthetic Gases: Information for Management in Anesthetizing Areas and the Postanesthesia Care Unit." This ASA publication addresses analysis of the literature, the role of regulatory agencies, scavenging and monitoring equipment, and recommendations.[186]

The two major causes of waste gas contamination in the operating room are the anesthetic technique employed and equipment issues.[186] Regarding the anesthetic technique, the following factors cause operating room atmosphere contamination: (1) failure to turn off gas flow control valves at the end of an anesthetic; (2) poorly fitting masks; (3) flushing the circuit; (4) filling anesthetic vaporizers; (5) use of uncuffed tracheal tubes; and (6) use of breathing circuits such as the Jackson-Rees (modification of Ayre's T-piece/Mapleson E rebreathing circuit), which are difficult to scavenge. Equipment failure or lack of understanding of proper equipment use can also contribute to operating room contamination. Leaks can occur in the high-pressure hoses, the nitrous oxide tank mounting, the high-pressure circuit and LPC of the anesthesia machine, or in the circle system, particularly at the CO_2 absorber assembly. The anesthesia provider must be certain that the scavenging system is operational and adjusted properly to ensure adequate scavenging. If sidestream CO_2 or multigas analyzers are used, the analyzed gas (withdrawn from the circuit at a rate of 50 to 250 cc/min) must be directed to the scavenging system or returned to the breathing system to prevent contamination of the operating room atmosphere.

Components

Scavenging systems generally consist of five components (Fig. 25-49): (1) the gas-collecting assembly, (2) the transfer means,

Table 25-8 NIOSH Recommendations for Maximum Levels for Exposure of Personnel to Trace Anesthesia Gases and Vapors

Anesthetic Gas	Maximum TWA[a] Concentration (ppm)
Halogenated agent alone	2
Nitrous oxide	25
Combination of halogenated agent plus nitrous oxide	—
Halogenated agent	0.5
Nitrous oxide	25
Dental facilities (nitrous oxide alone)	50

Reprinted from US Department of Health, Education, and Welfare. Criteria for a recommended standard: occupational exposure to waste anesthetic gases and vapors. March ed., Washington, DC; 1977.
Note: Despite being in clinical use for more than 15 years, isoflurane, desflurane, and sevoflurane have not been tested for maximum recommended trace gas levels.
[a]TWA, time-weighted average. Time-weighted average sampling, also known as time-integrated sampling, is a sampling method that evaluates the average concentration of anesthetic gas over a prolonged period of time, such as 1 to 8 hours.

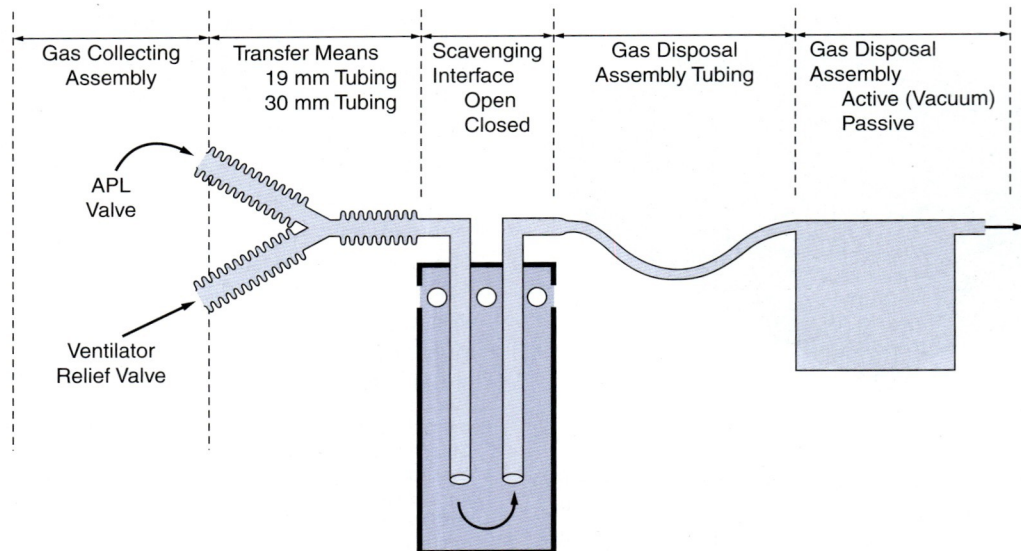

Figure 25-49 Components of a scavenging system. APL, adjustable pressure-limiting valve.

(3) the scavenging interface, (4) the gas-disposal assembly tubing, and (5) an active or passive gas-disposal assembly. An "active system" uses a central evacuation (vacuum) system to remove waste gases. The "weight" or pressure of the waste gas itself produces flow through a "passive system."

Gas-Collecting Assembly

The gas-collecting assembly captures excess anesthetic gas and delivers it to the transfer tubing. Waste anesthetic gases are vented from the anesthesia system either through the APL valve or through the ventilator relief valve. All excess patient gas either is vented into the room (e.g., from a poor facemask fit or tracheal tube leak) or exits the breathing system through one of these valves. Gas passing through these valves accumulates in the gas-collecting assembly and is directed to the transfer means. In some newer GE Healthcare systems (e.g., S5/ADU workstation) and others that incorporate either the 7100 or 7900 ventilators, the ventilator drive gas is also exhausted into the scavenging system. This is significant, because under conditions of high FGFs and high minute ventilation, the gases flowing into the scavenging interface may overwhelm the evacuation system. If this occurs, waste anesthetic gases may overflow the system via the positive-pressure relief valve (closed systems) or through the atmospheric vents (open systems) into the operating room atmosphere. In contrast, most other pneumatic ventilators from both Datex-Ohmeda and Dräger Narkomeds with AV-E ventilators exhaust their drive gas (oxygen or an oxygen/air mixture) into the operating room through a small vent on the back of the ventilator control housing.

Transfer Means

The transfer means carries excess gas from the gas-collecting assembly to the scavenging interface. The tubing diameter must be either 19 or 30 mm, as specified by the ASTM F1343–91 standard.[184] The tubing should be sufficiently rigid to prevent kinking, and as short as possible to minimize the chance of occlusion. Some manufacturers color code the transfer tubing with yellow bands to distinguish it from 22-mm diameter breathing system tubing. Many machines have separate transfer tubes for the APL valve and for the ventilator relief valve. The two tubes usually merge into a single hose before they enter the scavenging interface. Occlusion of the transfer means can be particularly problematic since it is upstream from the pressure-buffering features of the scavenging interface. If the transfer means is occluded, baseline breathing circuit pressure will increase and barotrauma can occur.

Scavenging Interface

The scavenging interface is the most important component of the system because it protects the breathing circuit or ventilator from excessive positive or negative pressures. The interface should limit the pressures immediately downstream from the gas collecting assembly to between −0.5 and +10 cm H_2O with normal working conditions. Positive-pressure relief is mandatory, irrespective of the type of disposal system used, to vent excess gas in case of occlusion downstream from the interface. If the disposal system is an "active system," negative-pressure relief is necessary to protect the breathing circuit or ventilator from excessive subatmospheric pressure. A reservoir is highly desirable with active systems, since it stores waste gases until the evacuation system can remove them. Interfaces can be open or closed, depending on the method used to provide positive- and negative-pressure relief.

Open Interfaces

An open interface contains no valves and is open to the atmosphere, allowing both positive- and negative-pressure relief. Open interfaces should be used only with active disposal systems that use a central evacuation system. Open interfaces require a reservoir because waste gases are intermittently discharged in surges, whereas flow from the evacuation system is continuous.

Many contemporary anesthesia machines are equipped with open interfaces like those in Figures 25-50A and B.[187] An open canister provides reservoir capacity. The canister volume should be large enough to accommodate a variety of waste gas flow rates. Gas enters the system at the top of the canister and travels through a narrow inner tube to the canister base. Gases are stored in the

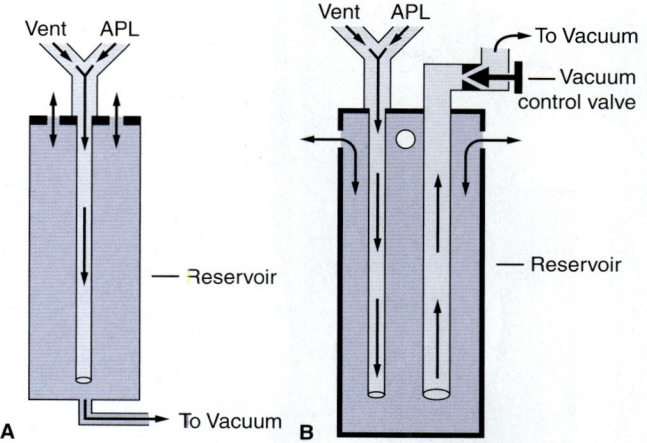

Figure 25-50 A, B: Two open reservoir scavenging interfaces. Each requires an active disposal system. APL, adjustable pressure-limiting valve. See text for details. (Adapted from Dorsch JA, Dorsch SE. Controlling trace gas levels. In: Dorsch JA, Dorsch SE, eds. *Understanding Anesthesia Equipment*. 4th ed. Baltimore, MD: Williams & Wilkins; 1999:355.)

rate per minute must equal or exceed the volume of excess gases to prevent spillage. The volume of the reservoir and the flow characteristics within the interface are important. Spillage will occur if the volume of a single exhaled breath exceeds the capacity of the reservoir. The flow characteristics of the system are important because gas leakage can occur long before the volume of waste gas equals the reservoir volume if significant turbulence occurs within the interface.[188]

Closed Interfaces

A closed interface communicates with the atmosphere through valves. All closed interfaces must have a positive-pressure relief valve to vent excess system pressure if obstruction occurs downstream from the interface. A negative-pressure relief valve is mandatory to protect the breathing system from subatmospheric pressure if an active disposal system is used. Two types of closed interfaces are commercially available. One has positive-pressure relief only; the other has both positive- and negative-pressure relief. Each type is discussed in the following sections.

Positive-Pressure Relief Only. This interface (Fig. 25-51, left) has a single positive-pressure relief valve and is designed to be used only with passive disposal systems. Waste gas enters the interface at the waste gas inlets. Transfer of the waste gas from the interface to the disposal system relies on the "weight" or pressure of the waste gas itself since a negative-pressure evacuation system is not used. The positive-pressure relief valve opens at a preset value such as 5 cm water if an obstruction between the interface and the disposal system occurs.[189,190] On this type of system, a reservoir bag is not required.

reservoir between breaths. Positive- and negative-pressure relief is provided by holes in the top of the canister. The open interface shown in Figure 25-50A differs somewhat from the one shown in Figure 25-50B. The operator can regulate the vacuum by adjusting the vacuum control valve shown in Figure 25-50B. The efficiency of an open interface depends on several factors. The vacuum flow

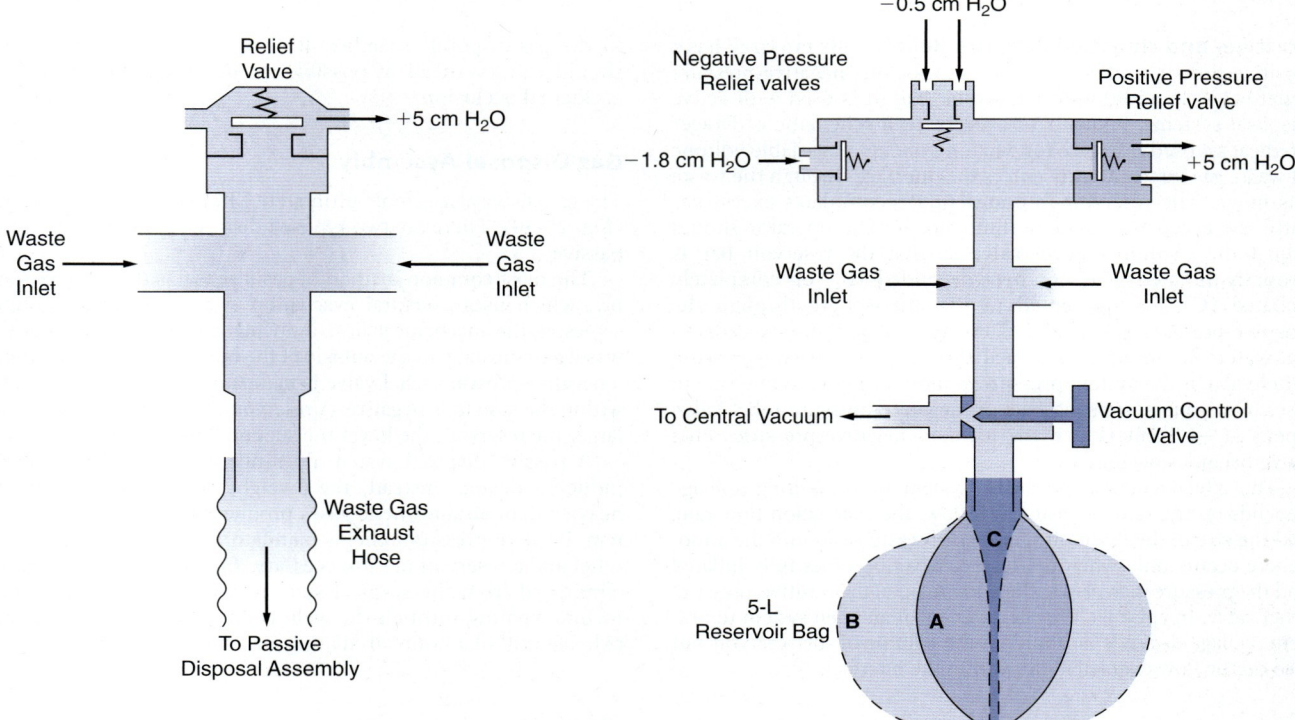

Figure 25-51 Closed scavenging interfaces. **Left:** Interface used with a passive disposal system. (Adapted from *Scavenger Interface for Air Conditioning: Instruction Manual*. Telford, PA: North American Dräger; 1984.) **Right:** Interface used with an active system. See text for details. (Adapted from *Narkomed 2A Anesthesia System: Technical Service Manual*. Telford, PA: North American Dräger; 1985.)

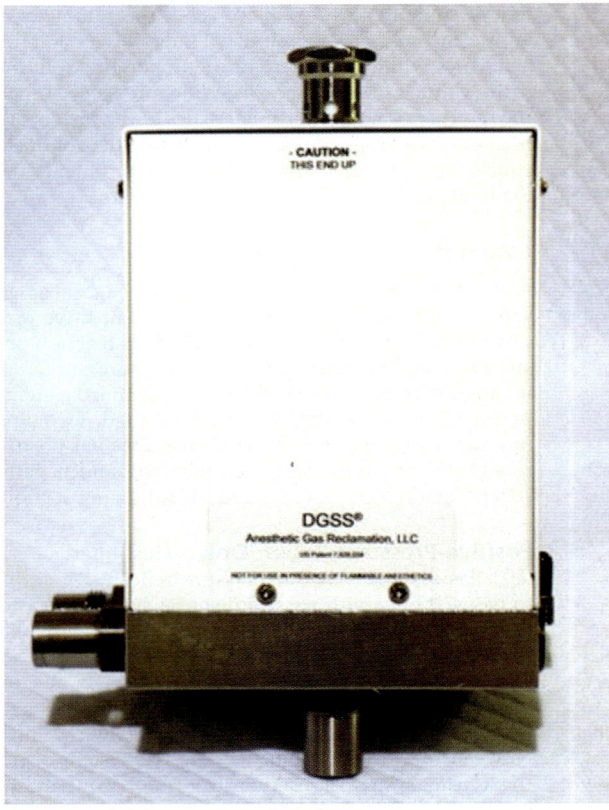
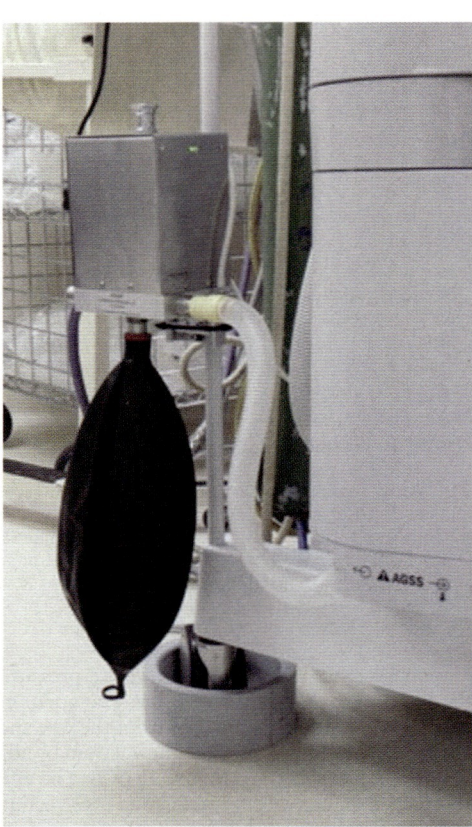

Figure 25-52 Dynamic Gas Scavenging System (DGSS). **A:** DGSS interface; **B:** Interface mounted on a GE anesthesia workstation. For details see text.

Positive- and Negative-Pressure Relief. This interface has a positive-pressure relief valve, and at least one negative-pressure relief valve, in addition to a reservoir bag. It is used with active disposal systems. Figure 25-51 (right) is a schematic of Dräger Medical's closed interface for suction systems. A variable volume of waste gas intermittently enters the interface through the waste gas inlets. The reservoir intermittently accumulates excess gas until the evacuation system eliminates it. The operator should adjust the vacuum control valve so that the reservoir bag is properly inflated (A), not over-distended (B), or completely deflated (C). Gas is vented to the atmosphere through the positive-pressure relief valve if the system pressure exceeds +5 cm water. Room air is entrained through the negative-pressure relief valve if the system pressure is more negative than −0.5 cm H_2O. On some systems, a backup negative-pressure relief valve opens at −1.8 cm H_2O if the primary negative-pressure relief valve becomes occluded.

The effectiveness of a closed system in preventing spillage depends on the rate of waste gas inflow, the evacuation flow rate, and the size of the reservoir. Leakage of waste gases into the atmosphere occurs only when the reservoir bag becomes fully inflated and the pressure increases sufficiently to open the positive-pressure relief valve. In contrast, the effectiveness of an open system to prevent spillage depends not only on the volume of the reservoir but also on the flow characteristics within the interface.

Gas-Disposal Assembly Conduit

The gas-disposal assembly conduit, or disposal assembly tubing (Fig. 25-49), conducts waste gas from the scavenging interface to the gas-disposal assembly. It should be collapse-proof and should run overhead, if possible, to minimize the chances of accidental occlusion.

Gas-Disposal Assembly

The gas-disposal assembly ultimately eliminates excess waste gas (Fig. 25-49). There are two types of disposal systems: active and passive.

The most common method of gas disposal is the active assembly, which uses a central evacuation system. A vacuum pump serves as the mechanical flow-inducing device that removes the waste gases usually to the outside of the building. An interface with a negative-pressure relief valve is mandatory because the pressure within the system is negative. A reservoir is very desirable, and the larger the reservoir, the lower the suction flow rate needed.

A passive disposal system does not use a mechanical flow-inducing device. Instead, the "weight" or pressure from the heavier-than-air anesthetic gases produces flow through the system. Positive-pressure relief is mandatory, but negative-pressure relief and a reservoir are unnecessary. Excess waste gases can be eliminated from the surgical suite in a number of ways. Some include venting through the wall, ceiling, floor, or to the room exhaust grill of a nonrecirculating air conditioning system.

Hazards

Scavenging systems minimize operating room atmosphere contamination, yet they add complexity to the anesthesia system.

A scavenging system functionally extends the anesthesia circuit all the way from the anesthesia machine to the ultimate disposal site. This extension increases the potential for problems. Obstruction of scavenging pathways can cause excessive positive pressure in the breathing circuit, and barotrauma can occur. Excessive vacuum applied to a scavenging system can result in undesirable negative pressures within the breathing system. For most contemporary anesthesia workstations, preuse checkout of the scavenging system is a function that must be performed manually by the operator according to the manufacturer's instructions. In the Spacelabs Healthcare's ARKON workstation the scavenger test is a component of the automated checkout.[191]

Another unusual problem is a report of fires in engineering equipment rooms that house the vacuum pumps used for waste anesthetic gas evacuation.[192] It seems that in some hospitals, waste gases are not directly vented outside, but may be vented into machine rooms that have vents that open to the outside. Since some anesthesia machines are designed such that ventilator drive gas (oxygen) is also scavenged, the environment in these machine rooms into which the scavenged gas is vented may become highly enriched with oxygen. These sites may contain equipment or materials such as petroleum distillates (pumps/oil/grease) that in the presence of an oxygen-enriched atmosphere could be excessively combustible and present a severe fire hazard.

Low-Flow Scavenging Systems

Active waste gas scavenging systems draw large volumes of gas—anesthetic waste plus entrained air in the range of 25 to 75 L/min—from each OR. This requires large and costly vacuum pumps that operate continuously, incurring a high-energy cost. In an effort to reduce the carbon footprint associated with running these pumps, a more efficient, low-flow scavenger interface has been designed and evaluated.[193] The Dynamic Gas Scavenging System (DGSS; Anesthetic Gas Reclamation, Nashville, TN) interface is a gas-tight metal container with a 3-L reservoir bag attached to ensure compliance with OSHA recommendations (Fig. 25-52). The design is such that scavenging outflow to the vacuum system remains closed until a pressure of 0.5 cm H_2O from the anesthesia workstation exhaust, via the APL or ventilator pressure relief valve, is sensed in the interface enclosure by a sensitive pressure transducer. A solenoid valve then opens and remains open until the internal pressure reaches −0.5 cm H_2O, thus emptying the interface reservoir bag. In this way the flow to the vacuum system is continuously titrated according to needs. An additional benefit is that by producing a more concentrated flow of waste gases, technologies designed to recover potent inhaled anesthetic agents from the waste-gas flow are facilitated. Such technologies are likely to become more important because the inhaled anesthetics are greenhouse gases with the potential to increase global warming.[194,195]

REFERENCES

1. Lampotang S, Lizdas DE, Liem EB, et al. *The Anesthesia Patient Safety Foundation Anesthesia Machine Workbook v1.1a*. 2011; http://vam.anest.ufl.edu/simulations/theAPSFworkbook.php
2. International Standards Organization. ISO 80601–2–13:2011(en) Medical electrical equipment. Part 2–13: Particular requirements for basic safety and essential performance of an anaesthetic workstation. 2011. Amended 2015.
3. American National Standards Institute. *Minimum Performance and Safety Requirements for Components and Systems of Continuous Flow Anesthesia Machines for Human Use (ANSI Z79.8–1979)*. New York, NY: American National Standards Institute; 1979.
4. American Society of Anesthesiologists. Guidelines for determining anesthesia machine obsolescence. In: *Manual for Anesthesia Department Organization and Management*. 2004. Available on ASA website (www.asahq.org).
5. James RH. 1000 anaesthetic incidents: experience to date. *Anesthesia*. 2003;58(9):856–863.
6. Robards C, Corda D. A potential hazard involving the gas sampling line and the adjustable pressure limiting valve on the Drager Apollo Anesthesia Workstation. *Anesth Analg*. 2010;111(2):578–580.
7. Vijayakumar A, Saxena DK, Sivan Pillay A, et al. Massive leak during manual ventilation: adjustable pressure limiting valve malfunction not detected by pre-anesthetic checkout. *Anesth Analg*. 2010;111(2):579–580.
8. Kibelbek MJ. Cable trapped under Dräger Fabius automatic pressure limiting valve causes inability to ventilate. *Anesthesiology*. 2007;106(3):639–640.
9. Caplan RA, Vistica MF, Posner KL, et al. Adverse anesthetic outcomes arising from gas delivery equipment. *Anesthesiology*. 1997;87:741–748.
10. Mehta SP, Eisenkraft JB, Posner KL, et al. Patient injuries from anesthesia gas delivery equipment. *Anesthesiology*. 2013;119:788–795.
11. Olympio MA. Modern anesthesia machines offer new safety features. *APSF Newslett*. 2003;18(2):17.
12. Cooper JB. Toward prevention of anesthetic mishaps. *Int Anesthesiol Clin*. 1984;22:167–183.
13. Emergency Care Research Institute. Avoiding anesthetic mishaps through pre-use checks. *Health Devices*. 1982;11:201.
14. Food and Drug Administration. *FDA Anesthesia Apparatus Checkout Recommendations*. 8th ed. Rockville, MD: Food and Drug Administration; 1986.
15. Food and Drug Administration. *Anesthesia Apparatus Checkout Recommendations*. Rockville, MD: Food and Drug Administration; 1993.
16. Spooner RB, Kirby RR. Equipment related anesthetic incidents. *Int Anesthesiol Clin*. 1984;22(2):133–147.
17. American Society of Anesthesiologists. *Guidelines for designing pre-anesthesia checkout procedures*. Park Ridge, IL; 2008. http://www.asahq.org/For-Members/Clinical-Information/2008-ASA-Recommendations-for-PreAnesthesia-Checkout.aspx.
18. Demaria S Jr, Blasius K, Neustein SM. Missed steps in the preanesthetic setup. *Anesth Analg*. 2011;113(1):84–88.
19. Eisenkraft JB, Jaffe MB. Respiratory gas monitoring. In: Ehrenwerth J, Eisenkraft JB, Berry JM, eds. *Anesthesia Equipment: Principles and Applications*. 2nd ed. New York, NY: Elsevier; 2013:191–222.
20. Lewis SE, Andrews JJ, Long GW. An unexpected Penlon sigma elite vaporizer leak. *Anesthesiology*. 1999;90:1221–1224.
21. Myers JA, Good ML, Andrews JJ. Comparison of tests for detecting leaks in the low-pressure system of anesthesia gas machines. *Anesth Analg*. 1997;84:179–184.
22. Eng TS, Durieux ME. Automated machine checkout leaves an internal gas leak undetected: the need for complete checkout procedures [case report]. *Anesth Analg*. 2012; 114:144–146.
23. Eisenkraft JB. Hazards of the anesthesia workstation. 2016 Refresher Courses in Anesthesiology. Shaumburg, Illinois, American Society of Anesthesiologists. Expected release date: May 2017.
24. Comm G, Rendell-Baker L. Back pressure check valves a hazard. *Anesthesiology*. 1982;56:327–328.
25. Rendell-Baker L. Problems with anesthetic and respiratory therapy equipment. *Int Anesthesiol Clin*. 1982;20:1–258.
26. Yasukawa M, Yasukawa K. Hypoventilation due to disconnection of the vaporizer and negative-pressure leak test to find disconnection. *Masui*. 1992;41:1345–1349.
27. Peters KR, Wingard DW. Anesthesia machine leakage due to misaligned vaporizers. *Anesth Rev*. 1987;14:36.
28. Datex-Ohmeda. *Explore the Anesthesia System*. Madison, WI: GE Healthcare; 2003.
29. Dodgson BG. Inappropriate use of the oxygen flush to check an anaesthetic machine. *Can J Anaesth*. 1988;35:436–437.
30. Mann D, Ananian J, Alston T. Oxygen flush valve booby trap. *Anesthesiology*. 2004;101:558.
31. Dorsch JA, Dorsch SE. Equipment checkout and maintenance. In: Dorsch JA, Dorsch SE, eds. *Understanding Anesthesia Equipment*. 5th ed. Baltimore, MD: Williams & Wilkins; 2007:931.
32. Olympio MA, Stoner J. Tight mask fit could have prevented "airway" obstruction. *Anesthesiology*. 1992;77:822–825.
33. Dosch MP. Automated checkout routines in anesthesia workstations vary in detection and management of breathing circuit obstruction. *Anesth Analg*. 2014;118:1254–1257.
34. Weigel WA, Murray WB. Detecting unidirectional valve incompetence by the modified pressure decline method. *Anesth Analg*. 2005;100(6):1723–1727.
35. Eappen S, Corn SB. The anesthesia machine valve tester: a new device and method for evaluating the competence of unidirectional anesthetic valves. *J Clin Monit*. 1996;12(4):305–309.
36. Paulson AW. Problems with automated anesthesia machine checkout. *Anesthesia Patient Safety Foundation Newsletter*. 2015;30:31.
37. Bowie E, Huffman LM. *The Anesthesia Machine: Essentials for Understanding*. Madison, WI: Ohmeda, The BOC Group Inc; 1985.
38. Dorsch JA, Dorsch SE. The anesthesia machine. In: Dorsch JA, Dorsch SE, eds. *Understanding Anesthesia Equipment*. 5th ed. Baltimore, MD: Williams & Wilkins; 2007:83.
39. Malayaman SN, Mychaskiw G, Ehrenwerth J. Medical gases: storage and supply. In: Ehrenwerth J, Eisenkraft JB, Berry JM, eds. *Anesthesia Equipment: Principles and Applications*. 2nd ed. New York, NY: Elsevier; 2013:3–24.

40. Eisenkraft JB. The anesthesia machine and workstation. In: Ehrenwerth J, Eisenkraft JB, Berry JM, eds. *Anesthesia Equipment: Principles and Applications*. 2nd ed. New York, NY: Elsevier; 2013:25–63.
41. Schumacher SD, Brockwell RC, Andrews JJ, et al. Bulk liquid oxygen supply failure. *Anesthesiology*. 2004;100:186–189.
42. Feeley TW, Hedley-Whyte J. Bulk oxygen and nitrous oxide delivery systems: design and dangers. *Anesthesiology*. 1976;44:301–305.
43. Pelton DA. Non-flammable medical gas pipeline systems. In: Wyant GM, ed. *Mechanical Misadventures in Anesthesia*. Toronto: University of Toronto Press; 1978:8.
44. Surgery mix-up causes 2 deaths. New Haven Register. January 20, 2002.
45. Mudumbai SC, Fanning R, Howard SK, et al. Use of medical simulation to explore equipment failures and human-machine interactions in anesthesia machine pipeline supply crossover. *Anesth Analg*. 2010;110(5):1292–1296.
46. Lorraway PG, Savoldelli GL, Joo HS, et al. Management of simulated oxygen supply failure: is there a gap in the curriculum? *Anesth Analg*. 2006;102(3): 865–867.
47. Ellett AE, Shields JC, Ifune C, et al. A near miss: a nitrous oxide-carbon dioxide mix-up despite current safety standards. *Anesthesiology*. 2009;110:1429–1431.
48. Adriani J. Clinical application of physical principles concerning gases and vapor to anesthesiology. In: Adriani J, ed. *The Chemistry and Physics of Anesthesia*. 2nd ed. Springfield, IL: Charles C Thomas; 1962:58.
49. Manual of the Compressed Gas Association. *Standards for Compressed Cylinder Valve Outlet and Inlet Connections*. Washington, DC; 1994.
50. Rose G, Durbin K, Eichhorn J. Gas cylinder colors ARE NOT an FDA Standard! *APSF Newsletter*, 2010;(Spring)25:16
51. Greilich PE, Greilich NB, Froelich EG. Intraabdominal fire during laparoscopic cholecystectomy. *Anesthesiology*. 1995;83:871–874.
52. Partbrook GD, Davis PD, Parbrook EO. Basic Physics and Measurement in Anesthesia. 2nd ed. Norwalk, CT: Appleton Century Crofts; 1986.
53. Atlas G. A method to quickly estimate remaining time for an oxygen E-cylinder. *Anesth Analg*. 2004;98:1190.
54. Klemenzson GK, Perouansky M. Contemporary anesthesia ventilators incur a significant "oxygen cost." *Can J Anaesth*. 2004;51:616–620.
55. Taenzer AH, Kovatsis PG, Raessler KL. E-cylinder-powered mechanical ventilation may adversely impact anesthetic management and efficiency. *Anesth Analg*. 2002;95:148–150.
56. Davis PD, Parbrook GD, Kenny GNC. *Basic Physics and Measurement in Anesthesia*. 4th ed. Boston: Butterworth-Heinemann; 1995.
57. Macintosh R, Mushin WW, Epstein HG. *Physics for the Anaesthetist*. Philadelphia: FA Davis Co, 1963:100.
58. Adriani J. Principles of physics and chemistry of solids and fluids applicable to anesthesiology. In: Adriani J, ed. *The Chemistry and Physics of Anesthesia*. 2nd ed. Springfield, IL: Charles C Thomas; 1962:7.
59. Macintosh R, Mushin WW, Epstein HG, eds. *Physics for the Anaesthetist*. 3rd ed. Oxford: Blackwell Scientific Publications; 1963:196.
60. Schreiber P. *Safety Guidelines for Anesthesia Systems*. Telford, PA: North American Dräger; 1984.
61. Eger EI, II, Epstein RM. Hazards of anesthetic equipment. *Anesthesiology*. 1964;24:490–504.
62. Eger EI, II, Hylton RR, Irwin RH, et al. Anesthetic flowmeter sequence—a cause for hypoxia. *Anesthesiology*. 1963;24:396.
63. Mazze RI. Therapeutic misadventures with oxygen delivery systems: the need for continuous in-line oxygen monitors. *Anesth Analg*. 1972;51:787–792.
64. Dräger Technical Engineering. *Explanation of Low Flow Wizard Function. Letter from Dräger Medical*. Telford, PA: Dräger Medical; 2015.
65. Luria I, Lampotang S, Schwab W, et al. Automated, real-time fresh gas flow recommendations alter isoflurane consumption during the maintenance phase of anesthesia in a simulator-based study. *Anesth Analg*. 2013;117(5):1139–1147.
66. Datex-Ohmeda, Inc. *Avance CS2 User's Reference Manual*. Madison, WI: GE Healthcare; 2015:11–23.
67. Mazze RI. Therapeutic misadventures with oxygen delivery systems: the need for continuous in-line oxygen monitors. *Anesth Analg*. 1972;51:787–792.
68. Cheng CJ, Garewal DS. A failure of the chain link mechanism of the Ohmeda Excel 210 anesthetic Machine. *Anesth Analg*. 2001;92:913–914.
69. Kidd AG, Hall I. Fault with an Ohmeda Excel 210 anesthetic machine [letter and response]. *Anaesthesia*. 1994;49:83.
70. Lohman G. Fault with an Ohmeda Excel 410 machine [letter and response]. *Anaesthesia*. 1991;46:695.
71. Richards C. Failure of a nitrous oxide–oxygen proportioning device. *Anesthesiology*. 1989;71:997–998.
72. Abraham ZA, Basagoitia B. A potentially lethal anesthesia machine failure. *Anesthesiology*. 1987;66:589–590.
73. Neubarth J. Another hazardous gas supply misconnection [letter]. *Anesth Analg*. 1995;80:206.
74. Gaughan SD, Benumof JL, Ozaki GT. Can an anesthesia machine flush valve provide for effective jet ventilation? *Anesth Analg*. 1993;76:800–808.
75. Anderson CE, Rendell-Baker L. Exposed O_2 flush hazard. *Anesthesiology*. 1982;56:328.
76. Lampotang S, Lizdas DE, Liem EB. The virtual anesthesia machine website. 2007; http://vam.anest.ufl.edu/.
77. Web based educational program. GE Healthcare, Madison, WI. http://www3.gehealthcare.com/en/education/product_education_-_technical/anesthesia_and_respiratory/
78. Fabius GS product trainer. Web based program. Dräger Medical http://static.draeger.com/trainer/fabius_gs_premium_en/flashpage.htm?lang=en#id=A1100.
79. Apollo Product Trainer. Dräger Medical. Web based program. http://static.draeger.com/trainer/apollo/apollo_trainer/start.html#id = A1100
80. EXPLORE Aestiva. *Web based program*. Madison, WI: GE Healthcare.
81. Korman B, Richie IM. Chemistry of halothane–enflurane mixtures applied to anesthesia. *Anesthesiology*. 1985;63:152–156.
82. Macintosh R, Mushin WW, Epstein HG, eds. *Physics for the Anaesthetist*. 3rd ed. Oxford: Blackwell Scientific Publications; 1963:26.
83. Schreiber P. *Anaesthesia Equipment: Performance, Classification, and Safety*. New York, NY: Springer; 1972.
84. Eisenkraft JB. Anesthesia vaporizers. In: Eisenkraft JB, Ehrenwerth J, Berry JM, eds. *Anesthesia Equipment: Principles and Applications*. 2nd ed. New York, NY: Elsevier; 2013.
85. *Dräger Vapor 2000 Anesthetic Vaporizer Operating Instructions*. Telford, PA: Dräger Medical; 2001:62.
86. Kharasch ED, Subbarao GN, Cromack KR, et al. Sevoflurane formulation water content influences degradation by Lewis acids in vaporizers. *Anesth Analg*. 2009;108:1796–1802.
87. Hill DW. The design and calibration of vaporizers for volatile anaesthetic agents. *Br J Anaesth*. 1968;40:648.
88. Hill DW, Lowe HJ. Comparison of concentration of halothane in closed and semi-closed circuits during controlled ventilation. *Anesthesiology*. 1962;23: 291–298.
89. Anonymous. Internal leakage from anesthesia unit flush valves. *Health Devices*. 1981:10.
90. Morris LE. Problems in the performance of anesthesia vaporizers. *Int Anesthesiol Clin*. 1974;12:199–219.
91. Diaz PD. The influence of carrier gas on the output of automatic vaporizers. *Br J Anaesth*. 1976;48:387–391.
92. Palayiwa E, Sanderson MH, Hahn CEW. Effects of carrier gas composition on the output of six anaesthetic vaporizers. *Br J Anaesth*. 1983;55: 1025–1038.
93. Gould DB, Lampert BA, MacKrell TN. Effect of nitrous oxide solubility on vaporizer aberrance. *Anesth Analg*. 1982;61:938–940.
94. Lin CY. Assessment of vaporizer performance in low-flow and closed-circuit anesthesia. *Anesth Analg*. 1980;59:359–366.
95. Scheller MS, Drummond JC. Solubility of N_2O in volatile anesthetics contributes to vaporizer aberrancy when changing carrier gases. *Anesth Analg*. 1986;65:88–90.
96. Nawaf K, Stoelting RK. Nitrous oxide increases enflurane concentrations delivered by ethrane vaporizers. *Anesth Analg*. 1979;58:30–32.
97. Stoelting RK. The effect of nitrous oxide on halothane output from Fluotec Mark 2 vaporizers. *Anesthesiology*. 1971;35:215–218.
98. Broka SM, Gourdange PA, Joucken KL. Sevoflurane and desflurane confusion. *Anesth Analg*. 1999;88:1194.
99. George TM. Failure of keyed agent-specific filling devices. *Anesthesiology*. 1984;61:228–229.
100. Riegle EV, Desertspring D. Failure of the agent-specific filling device [letter]. *Anesthesiology*. 1990;73.353–354.
101. Abel M, Eisenkraft JB. Performance of erroneously filled sevoflurane, enflurane and other agent specific vaporizers. *J Clin Monit*. 1996;12:119–125.
102. Adler AC, Connelly NR, Ankam A, et al. Technical communication: inhaled anesthetic agent-vaporizer mismatch: management in settings with limited resources: don't try this at home. *Anesth Analg*. 2013;116:1272–1275.
103. Lippmann M, Foran W, Ginsburg R, et al. Contamination of anesthetic vaporizer contents. *Anesthesiology*. 1993;78:1175–1177.
104. Munson WM. Cardiac arrest: a hazard of tipping a vaporizer. *Anesthesiology*. 1965;26:235.
105. Sinclair A, van Bergen J. Vaporizer overfilling. *Can J Anaesth*. 1993;40:1–2.
106. Hardy J-F. Vaporizer overfilling (Editorial). *Can J Anaesth*. 1993;40:1–2.
107. Seropian MA, Robins B. Smaller than expected sevoflurane concentrations using the SevoTec 5 vaporizer at low fill states and high fresh gas flows. *Anesth Analg*. 2000;91:834–836.
108. Meister GC, Becker KE, Jr. Potential fresh gas flow leak through Dräger Vapor 19.1 vaporizer with key-index fill port. *Anesthesiology*. 1993;78:211–212.
109. Zimmer C, Janssen M, Treschan T, et al. Near-miss accident during magnetic resonance imaging by a "flying sevoflurane vaporizer" due to ferromagnetism undetectable by handheld magnet. *Anesthesiology*. 2004;100:1329–1330.
110. Andrews JJ, Johnston RV Jr. The new Tec 6 desflurane vaporizer. *Anesth Analg*. 1993;76:1338–1341.
111. Weiskopf RB, Sampson D, Moore MA. The desflurane (Tec 6) vaporizer: design, design considerations and performance evaluation. *Br J Anaesth*. 1994; 72:474–479.
112. Eger EI 2nd. New inhaled anesthetics. *Anesthesiology*. 1994;80:906–922.
113. *D-Vapor Desflurane Vaporizer Instructions for Use*. Telford, PA: Dräger Medical; 2005.

114. Johnston RV Jr, Andrews JJ, Deyo DJ, et al. The effects of carrier gas composition on the performance of the Tec 6 desflurane vaporizer. *Anesth Analg.* 1994;79:548–552.
115. Andrews JJ, Johnston RV Jr, Kramer GC. Consequences of misfilling contemporary vaporizers with desflurane. *Can J Anaesth.* 1993;40:71–76.
116. Hendrickx JF, Carette RM, Deloof T, et al. Severe ADU desflurane vaporizing unit malfunction. *Anesthesiology.* 2003;99:1459–1460.
117. Mapleson WW. The elimination of rebreathing in various semiclosed anaesthetic systems. *Br J Anaesth.* 1954;26:323–332.
118. Willis BA, Pender JW, Mapleson WW. Rebreathing in a T-piece: volunteer and theoretical studies of the Jackson-Rees modification of Ayre's T-piece during spontaneous respiration. *Br J Anaesth.* 1975;47:1239–1246.
119. Sykes MK. Rebreathing circuits: a review. *Br J Anaesth.* 1968;40(9):666–674.
120. Froese AB, Rose DK. A detailed analysis of T-piece systems. In: Steward, ed. *Some Aspects of Paediatric Anaesthesia.* Amsterdam, The Netherlands: Elsevier North-Holland Biomedical Press; 1982:101.
121. Aarhus D, Sørredie E, Holst-Larsen H. Mechanical obstruction in the anaesthesia delivery-system mimicking severe bronchospasm. *Anaesthesia.* 1997;52:992–994.
122. Pethick SL. Letter to the editor. *Can Anaesth Soc J.* 1975;22:115.
123. Moyers J. A nomenclature for methods of inhalation anesthesia. *Anesthesiology.* 1953;14:609–611.
124. Eger EI II. Anesthetic systems: construction and function. In: Eger EI II, ed. *Anesthetic Uptake and Action.* Baltimore, MD: Williams & Wilkins; 1974:206.
125. Eger EI II, Ethans CT. The effects of inflow, overflow and valve placement on economy of the circle system. *Anesthesiology.* 1968;29:93–100.
126. Chacon AC, Kuczkowski KM, Sanchez RA. Unusual case of breathing circuit obstruction: plastic packaging revisited [letter to the editor]. *Anesthesiology.* 2004;100:753.
127. McEwan AI, Dowell L, Karis JH. Bilateral tension pneumothorax caused by a blocked bacterial filter in an anesthesia breathing circuit. *Anesth Analg.* 1993;76:440–442.
128. Smith CR, Otworth JR, Kaluszyk GSW. Bilateral tension pneumothorax due to a defective anesthesia breathing circuit filter. *J Clin Anesth.* 1991;3:229–234.
129. Walton JS, Fears R, Burt N, et al. Intraoperative breathing circuit obstruction caused by albuterol nebulization. *Anesth Analg.* 1999;89:650–651.
130. Dhar P, George I, Mankad A, et al. Flow transducer gas leak detected after induction. *Anesth Analg.* 1999;89:1587.
131. Kanno T, Aso C, Saito S, et al. A combustive destruction of expiration valve in an anesthetic circuit. *Anesthesiology.* 2003;98:577–579.
132. Laster M, Roth P, Eger E II. Fires from the interaction of anesthetics with desiccated absorbent. *Anesth Analg.* 2004;99:769–774.
133. Laudanski K, Schwab WK, Bakuzonis CW, et al. Thermal damage of the humidified ventilator circuit in the operating room: an analysis of plausible causes. *Anesth Analg.* 2010;111:1433–1436.
134. Holak EJ, Mei DA, Dunning MB III, et al. Carbon monoxide production from sevoflurane breakdown. *Anesth Analg.* 2003;96:757–764.
135. Kummar P, Korula G, Kumar S, et al. Unusual cause of leak in Datex Aisys. *Anesth Analg.* 2009;109(4):1350–1351; discussion 1351–1352.
136. Kshatri AM, Kingsley CP. Defective carbon dioxide absorber as a cause for a leak in a breathing circuit. *Anesthesiology.* 2004;84:475–476.
137. Norman PH, Daley MD, Walker JR, et al. Obstruction due to retained carbon dioxide absorber canister wrapping. *Anesth Analg.* 1996;83:425–426.
138. Olympio MA. Carbon dioxide absorbent desiccation safety conference convened by APSF. *APSF Newsletter.* 2005;20(2):25–29.
139. Adriani J. Carbon dioxide absorption. In: Adriani J, ed. *The Chemistry and Physics of Anesthesia.* 2nd ed. Springfield, IL: Charles C. Thomas; 1962:151.
140. Dewey Almy Chemical Division. *The Sodasorb Manual of CO_2 Absorption.* New York, NY: W.R. Grace & Co; 1962.
141. Murray JM, Renfrew CW, Bedi A, et al. A new carbon dioxide absorbent for use in anesthetic breathing systems. *Anesthesiology.* 1999;91:1342–1348.
142. Versichelen LF, Bouche MP, Rolly G, et al. Only carbon dioxide absorbents free of both NaOH and KOH do not generate compound—A during in vitro closed system sevoflurane. *Anesthesiology.* 2001;95:750–755.
143. Higuchi H, Adachi Y, Arimura S, et al. The carbon dioxide absorption capacity of Amsorb is half that of soda lime. *Anesth Analg.* 2001;93:221–225.
144. Sosis MB. Why not use Amsorb alone as the CO_2 absorbent and avoid any risk of CO production? [letter to the editor] *Anesthesiology.* 2003;98(5):1299.
145. Brown ES. Performance of absorbents: continuous flow. *Anesthesiology.* 1959;20:41–44.
146. Andrews JJ, Johnston RV Jr, Bee DE, et al. Photodeactivation of ethyl violet: a potential hazard of Sodasorb. *Anesthesiology.* 1990;72:59–64.
147. Kharasch ED, Powers KM, Artru AA. Comparison of Amsorb®, sodalime, Baralyme® degradation of volatile anesthetics and formation of carbon monoxide and compound A in swine in vivo. *Anesthesiology.* 2002;96:173–182.
148. Morio M, Fujii K, Satoh N, et al. Reaction of sevoflurane and its degradation products with soda lime. *Anesthesiology.* 1992;77:1155–1164.
149. Fang ZX, Kandel L, Laster MJ, et al. Factors affecting production of compound-A from the interaction of sevoflurane with Baralyme® and soda lime. *Anesth Analg.* 1996;82:775–781.
150. Frink EJ Jr, Malan TP, Morgan SE, et al. Quantification of the degradation products of sevoflurane in two CO_2 absorbents during low-flow anesthesia in surgical patients. *Anesthesiology.* 1992;77:1064–1069.
151. Eger EI II, Ionescu P, Laster MJ, et al. Baralyme dehydration increases and soda lime dehydration decreases the concentration of compound A resulting from sevoflurane degradation in a standard anesthetic circuit. *Anesth Analg.* 1997;85:892–898.
152. Steffey EP, Laster MJ, Ionescu P, et al. Dehydration of Baralyme® increases compound A resulting from sevoflurane degradation in a standard anesthetic circuit used to anesthetize swine. *Anesth Analg.* 1997;85:1382–1386.
153. Bito H, Ikeuchi Y, Ikeda K. Effects of low-flow sevoflurane anesthesia on renal function: comparison with high-flow sevoflurane anesthesia and low-flow isoflurane anesthesia. *Anesthesiology.* 1997;86:1231–1237.
154. Eger EI 2nd, Koblin DD, Bowland T, et al. Nephrotoxicity of sevoflurane versus desflurane anesthesia in volunteers. *Anesth Analg.* 1997;84:160–168.
155. Kharasch ED, Frink EJ Jr, Zager R, et al. Assessment of low-flow sevoflurane and isoflurane effects on renal function using sensitive markers of tubular toxicity. *Anesthesiology.* 1997;86:1238–1253.
156. Fukuda H, Kawamoto M, Yuge O, et al. A comparison of the effects of prolonged (>10 hour) low-flow sevoflurane, high-flow sevoflurane, and low-flow isoflurane anaesthesia on hepatorenal function in orthopaedic patients. *Anaesth Intensive Care.* 2004;32(2):210–218.
157. Berry PD, Sessler DI, Larson MD. Severe carbon monoxide poisoning during desflurane anesthesia. *Anesthesiology.* 1999;90:613–616.
158. Woehlck HJ, Dunning M III, Connolly LA. Reduction in the incidence of carbon monoxide exposures in humans undergoing general anesthesia. *Anesthesiology.* 1997;87(2):228–234.
159. Bonome C, Belda J, Alavarez-Refojo F, et al. Low-flow anesthesia and reduced animal size increase carboxyhemoglobin levels in swine during desflurane and isoflurane breakdown in dried soda lime. *Anesth Analg.* 1999;89:909–916.
160. Neumann MA, Laster MJ, Weiskopf RB, et al. The elimination of sodium and potassium hydroxides from desiccated soda lime diminishes degradation of desflurane to carbon monoxide and sevoflurane to compound A but does not compromise carbon dioxide absorption. *Anesth Analg.* 1999;89:768–773.
161. Zilberman P. The CO_2 absorber based on LiOH: a review. *Acta Med Marisiensis.* 2015;61:4–6.
162. McPherson SP, Spearman CB, eds. Introduction to ventilators. *Respiratory Therapy Equipment.* 3rd ed. St. Louis, MO: CV Mosby; 1985:230.
163. Modak RK, Olympio MA. Anesthesia ventilators. In: Ehrenwerth J, Eisenkraft JB, Berry JM, eds. *Anesthesia Equipment: Principles and Applications.* 2nd ed. New York, NY: Elsevier, 2013:148–178.
164. Scheller MS, Jones BR, Benumof JL, The influence of fresh gas flow and inspiratory/expiratory ratio on tidal volume and arterial CO_2 tension in mechanically ventilated surgical patients. *J Cardiothor Anesth.* 1989;3:564–567.
165. Cooper JB, Newbower RS, Kitz RJ. An analysis of major errors and equipment failures in anesthesia management: considerations for prevention and detection. *Anesthesiology.* 1984;60:34–42.
166. Reinhart DJ, Friz R. Undetected leak in corrugated circuit tubing in compressed configuration. *Anesthesiology.* 1993;78:218.
167. Raphael DT, Weller RS, Doran DJ. A response algorithm for the low-pressure alarm condition. *Anesth Analg.* 1988;67:876–883.
168. Slee TA, Pavlin EG. Failure of low pressure alarm associated with use of a humidifier. *Anesthesiology.* 1988;69:791–793.
169. Eisenkraft JB, Jaffe M. Respiratory gas monitoring. In: Ehrenwerth J, Eisenkraft JB, Berry JM, eds. *Anesthesia Equipment: Principles and Applications.* 2nd ed. New York, NY: Elsevier; 2013:191–222.
170. Feeley TW, Bancroft ML. Problems with mechanical ventilators. *Int Anesthesiol Clin.* 1982;20:83–93.
171. Khalil SN, Gholston TK, Binderman J, et al. Flapper valve malfunction in an Ohio closed scavenging system. *Anesth Analg.* 1987;66:1334–1336.
172. Sommer RM, Bhalla GS, Jackson JM, et al. Hypoventilation caused by ventilator valve rupture. *Anesth Analg.* 1988;67:999–1001.
173. Bourke D, Tolentino D. Inadvertent positive end-expiratory caused by a malfunctioning ventilator relief valve. *Anesth Analg.* 2003;97:492–493.
174. Roth S, Tweedie E, Sommer RM. Excessive airway pressure due to a malfunctioning anesthesia ventilator. *Anesthesiology.* 1986;65:532–534.
175. Usher A, Cave D, Finegan B. Critical incident with Narkomed 6000 anesthesia system [letter to the editor]. *Anesthesiology.* 2003;99:762.
176. Dorsch JA, Dorsch SE. Anesthesia ventilators. In: Dorsch JA, Dorsch SE, eds. *Understanding Anesthesia Equipment.* 5th ed. Baltimore, MD: Williams & Wilkins; 2007:310.
177. Sandberg WS, Kaiser S. Novel breathing circuit architecture: new consequences of old problems. *Anesthesiology.* 2004;100:755–756.
178. Ortega RA, Zambricki ER. Fresh gas decoupling valve failure precludes mechanical ventilation in a Draeger Fabius GS anesthesia machine. *Anesth Analg.* 2007;104:1000–1001.
179. Sims C. Absent expiratory valve missed by automated check in Dräger Primus anaesthesia workstation. *Anaesth Int Care.* 2013;41:681–682.
180. User's Manual FLOW-i 3.0. Anesthesia System, Maquet Critical Care AB, Solna, Sweden. 2012.

181. Eisenkraft JB, McGregor DG. Waste anesthetic gases and scavenging systems. In: Ehrenwerth J, Eisenkraft JB, Berry JM, eds. *Anesthesia Equipment: Principles and Applications*. 2nd ed. New York, NY: Elsevier; 2013:125–147.
182. US Department of Health Education and Welfare. *Criteria for a Recommended Standard: Occupational Exposure to Waste Anesthetic Gases and Vapors*. March ed. Washington, DC: US Department of Health Education and Welfare; 1977.
183. Sessler DI, Badgwell JM. Exposure of postoperative nurses to exhaled anesthetic gases. *Anaesth Analg*. 1998;87:1083–1088.
184. American Society for Testing and Materials. *Standard Specification for Anesthetic Equipment-Scavenging Systems for Anesthetic Gases (ASTM F1343–91)*. Philadelphia, PA: American Society for Testing and Materials; 1991.
185. Hall A. Request for information on waste halogenated anesthetic agents: isoflurane, desflurane, and sevoflurane. *Fed Regist*. 2006;71:8859–8860.
186. ASA Task Force on Trace Anesthetic Gases. *Waste Anesthetic Gases: Information for Management in Anesthetizing Areas and the Postanesthesia Care Unit*. Park Ridge, IL: American Society of Anesthesiologists; 1999.
187. Kanmura Y, Sakai J, Yoshinaka H, et al. Causes of nitrous oxide contamination in operating rooms. *Anesthesiology*. 1999;90:693–696.
188. *Open Reservoir Scavenger: Operator's Instruction Manual*. Telford, PA: North American Dräger; 1986.
189. Gray WM. Symposium on anaesthetic equipment: scavenging equipment. *Br J Anaesth*. 1985;57:685–695.
190. Brockwell RC, Andrews JJ. *Understanding your anesthesia machine*. In: Schwartz AJ, ed. *ASA Refresher Courses*. Philadelphia, PA: Lippincott Williams & Wilkins; 2002.
191. *ARKON Anesthesia System User Manual, Revision A*. Snoqualmie, WA: Spacelabs Healthcare, December 2015.
192. Allen M, Lees DE. Fires in medical vacuum pumps: do you need to be concerned? *ASA Newsletter*. 2004;68(10):22.
193. Barwise JA, Lancaster LJ, Michaels D, et al. Technical communication: an initial evaluation of a novel anesthetic scavenging interface. *Anesth Analg*. 2011;113:1064–1067.
194. Ryan SM, Nielsen CJ. Global warming potential of inhaled anesthetics: application to clinical use. *Anesth Analg*. 2010;111:92–98.
195. Feldman JM. Managing fresh gas flow to reduce environmental contamination. *Anesth Analg*. 2012;114:1093–1101.

Appendix A

FDA 1993 Anesthesia Apparatus Checkout Recommendations

This checkout, or a reasonable equivalent, should be conducted before administration of anesthesia. These recommendations are only valid for an anesthesia system that conforms to current and relevant standards and includes an ascending bellows ventilator and at least the following monitors: Capnograph, pulse oximeter, oxygen analyzer, respiratory volume monitor (spirometer), and breathing system pressure monitor with high- and low-pressure alarms. This is a guideline that users are encouraged to modify to accommodate differences in equipment design and variations in local clinical practice. Such local modifications should have appropriate peer review. Users should refer to the operator's manual for the manufacturer's specific procedures and precautions, especially the manufacturer's low-pressure leak test (Step 5).

Emergency Ventilation Equipment

1. *Verify Backup Ventilation Equipment is Available and Functioning

High-Pressure System

2. *Check Oxygen Cylinder Supply
    a. Open O_2 cylinder and verify at least half full (about 1,000 psi)
    b. Close cylinder
3. *Check Central Pipeline Supplies
    a. Check that hoses are connected and pipeline gauges read about 50 psi

Low-Pressure System

4. *Check Initial Status of Low-pressure System
    a. Close flow control valves and turn vaporizers off
    b. Check fill level and tighten vaporizers' filler caps
5. *Perform Leak Check of Machine Low-pressure System
    a. Verify that the machine master switch and flow control valves are OFF
    b. Attach "Suction Bulb" to common (fresh) gas outlet
    c. Squeeze bulb repeatedly until fully collapsed
    d. Verify bulb stays fully collapsed for at least 10 seconds
    e. Open one vaporizer at a time and repeat "c" and "d" as above
    f. Remove suction bulb and reconnect fresh gas hose
6. *Turn on Machine Master Switch and all other necessary electrical equipment
7. *Test Flowmeters
    a. Adjust flow of all gases through their full range, checking for smooth operation of floats and undamaged flow tubes
    b. Attempt to create a hypoxic O_2/N_2O mixture and verify correct changes in flow and/or alarm

Scavenging System

8. *****Adjust and Check Scavenging System**
   a. Ensure proper connections between the scavenging system and both APL (pop-off) valve and ventilator relief valve
   b. Adjust waste gas vacuum (if possible)
   c. Fully open APL valve and occlude Y-piece
   d. With minimum O_2 flow, allow scavenger reservoir bag to collapse completely and verify that absorber pressure gauge reads about zero
   e. With the O_2 flush activated, allow the scavenger reservoir bag to distend fully and then verify that absorber pressure gauge reads <10 cm H_2O

Breathing System

9. *****Calibrate O_2 Monitor**
   a. Ensure monitor reads 21% in room air
   b. Verify low O_2 alarm is enabled and functioning
   c. Reinstall sensor in circuit and flush breathing system with O_2
   d. Verify that monitor now reads greater than 90%
10. **Check Initial Status of Breathing System**
    a. Set selector switch to "Bag" mode
    b. Check that breathing circuit is complete, undamaged, and unobstructed
    c. Verify that CO_2 absorbent is adequate
    d. Install the breathing circuit accessory equipment (e.g., humidifier, PEEP valve) to be used during the case
11. **Perform Leak Check of the Breathing System**
    a. Set all gas flows to zero (or minimum)
    b. Close APL (pop-off) valve and occlude Y-piece
    c. Pressurize breathing system to about 30 cm H_2O with O_2 flush
    d. Ensure that pressure remains fixed for at least 10 seconds
    e. Open APL (pop-off) valve and ensure that pressure decreases

Manual and Automatic Ventilation Systems

12. **Test Ventilation Systems and Unidirectional Valves**
    a. Place a second breathing bag on Y-piece
    b. Set appropriate ventilator parameters for next patient
    c. Switch to automatic ventilation (Ventilator) mode
    d. Turn ventilator ON and fill bellows and breathing bag with O_2 flush
    e. Set O_2 flow to minimum, other gas flows to zero
    f. Verify that during inspiration bellows deliver appropriate tidal volume and that during expiration bellows fill completely
    g. Set fresh gas flow to about 5 L/min
    h. Verify that the ventilator bellows and simulated lungs fill and empty appropriately without sustained pressure at end expiration
    i. Check for proper action of unidirectional valves
    j. Exercise breathing circuit accessories to ensure proper function
    k. Turn ventilator OFF and switch to manual ventilation (bag/APL) mode
    l. Ventilate manually and assure inflation and deflation of artificial lungs and appropriate feel of system resistance and compliance
    m. Remove second breathing bag from Y-piece

Monitors

13. **Check, Calibrate, and/or Set Alarm Limits of All Monitors**
    a. Capnometer
    b. Oxygen Analyzer
    c. Pressure monitor with High- and Low-airway Pressure Alarms
    d. Pulse Oximeter
    e. Respiratory Volume Monitor (Spirometer)

Final Position

14. **Check Final Status of Machine**
    a. Vaporizers off
    b. APL valve open
    c. Selector switch to "Bag"
    d. All flowmeters to zero (or minimum)
    e. Patient suction level adequate
    f. Breathing system ready to use

---

*From Food and Drug Administration. Anesthesia Apparatus Checkout Recommendations. Rockville, MD: Food and Drug Administration; 1993.

Appendix B

Recommendations for Preanesthesia Checkout Procedures (2008)

Subcommittee of ASA Committee on Equipment and Facilities

Guidelines for Preanesthesia Checkout (PAC) Procedures

Background

Improperly checking anesthesia equipment prior to use can lead to patient injury and has also been associated with an increased risk of severe postoperative morbidity and mortality.[1,2] In 1993 a preanesthesia checkout (PAC) was developed and widely accepted to be an important step in the process of preparing to deliver anesthesia care.[3] Despite the accepted importance of the PAC, available evidence suggests that the current version is neither well understood nor reliably utilized by anesthesia providers.[4-6] Furthermore, anesthesia delivery systems have evolved to the point that one checkout procedure is not applicable to all anesthesia delivery systems currently on the market. For these reasons, a new approach to the PAC has been developed. The goal was to provide guidelines applicable to all anesthesia delivery systems so that individual departments can develop a PAC that can be performed consistently and expeditiously.

General Considerations

The following document is intended to serve not as a PAC itself, but rather as a template for developing checkout procedures that are appropriate for each individual anesthesia machine design. When using this template to develop a checkout procedure for systems that incorporate automated checkout features, items that are not evaluated by the automated checkout need to be identified, and supplemental manual checkout procedures included as needed.

Simply because an automated checkout procedure exists does not mean it can completely replace a manual checkout procedure or that it can be performed safely without adequate training and a thorough understanding of what the automated checkout accomplishes. An automated checkout procedure can be incomplete and/or misleading. For example, the leak test performed by some current automated checkouts does not test for leaks at the vaporizers. As a result, a loose vaporizer filler cap, or a leak at the vaporizer mount, could easily be missed.

Ideally automated checkout procedures should clearly reveal to the user the functions that are being checked, any deficient function that is found, and recommendations to correct the problem. Documentation of the automated checkout process should preferably be in a manner that can be recorded on the anesthesia record.

Operator's manuals, which accompany anesthesia delivery systems, include extensive recommendations for equipment checkout. Although these recommendations are quite extensive and typically not utilized by anesthesia providers, they are nevertheless important references for developing machine-specific and institution-specific checkout procedures.

Personnel Performing the PAC

The previously accepted Anesthesia Apparatus Checkout Recommendation placed all of the responsibility for preuse checkout on the anesthesia provider. Sole reliance on one individual to complete the checkout process may increase the likelihood that one or more steps will be omitted or performed improperly. This guideline identifies those aspects of the PAC that could be completed by a qualified anesthesia and/or biomedical technician. Utilizing technicians to perform some aspects of the PAC may improve compliance with the PAC. Steps completed by a technician may be part of the morning preuse check or part of a procedure performed at the end of each day. Critical checkout steps (e.g., availability of backup ventilation equipment) will benefit from intentional redundancy (i.e., having more than one individual responsible for checking the equipment). *Regardless of the level of training and support by technicians, the anesthesia care provider is ultimately responsible for proper function of all equipment used to provide anesthesia care.*

Adaptation of the PAC to local needs, assignment of responsibility for the checkout procedures, and training are the responsibilities of the individual anesthesia department. Training procedures should be documented. Proper documentation should include records of completed coursework (e.g., a manufacturer course) or for in-house training, a listing of the competency items taught and records of successful completion by trainees.

Objectives for a New PAC

- Outline the essential items that need to be available and functioning properly prior to delivering every anesthetic.
- Identify the frequency with which each of the items needs to be checked.
- Suggest which items may be checked by a qualified anesthesia technician, biomedical technician, or a manufacturer-certified service technician.

Basic Principles

- The anesthesia care provider is ultimately responsible for ensuring that the anesthesia equipment is safe and ready for use. This responsibility includes adequate familiarity with the equipment, following relevant local policies for performing and documenting the PAC and being knowledgeable about those procedures.

- Depending upon the staffing resources in a particular institution, anesthesia technicians and/or biomedical technicians can participate in the PAC. Biomedical technicians are often trained and certified by manufacturers to perform on-site maintenance of anesthesia delivery systems and therefore can be a useful resource for completing regular checkout procedures. Anesthesia technicians are not commonly trained to perform checkout procedures. Involving the anesthesia technicians is intended to enhance compliance with the PAC. Each department should decide whether the available technicians can or should be trained to assist with checkout procedures. Formal certification of anesthesia technicians by the American Society of Anesthesia Technicians and Technologists (ASATT) is encouraged but does not necessarily guarantee familiarity with checkout procedures.
- Critical items will benefit from redundant checks to avoid errors and omissions.
- When more than one person is responsible for checking an item, all parties should perform the check if intentional redundancy is deemed important, or either party may be acceptable, depending upon the available resources.
- Whoever conducts the PAC should provide documentation of successful performance. The anesthesia provider should include this documentation on the patient chart.
- Whenever an anesthesia machine is moved to a new location, a complete beginning-of-the-day checkout should be performed.
- Automated checks should clearly distinguish the components of the delivery system that are checked automatically from those which require manual checkout.
- Ideally, the date, time, and outcome of the most recent check(s) should be recorded and the information made accessible to the user.
- Specific procedures for preuse checkout cannot be prescribed in this document since they vary with the delivery systems. Clinicians must learn how to effectively perform the necessary preuse check for each piece of equipment they use.
- Each department or health-care facility should work with the manufacturer(s) of their equipment to develop preuse checkout procedures that satisfy both the following guidelines and the needs of the local department.
- Default settings for ventilators, monitors, and alarms should be checked to determine if they are appropriate
- These checkout recommendations are intended to replace the preexisting FDA-approved Anesthesia Apparatus Checkout Recommendations. They are not intended to be a replacement for required preventive maintenance.
- The PAC is essential to safe care but should not delay initiating care if the patient needs are so urgent that time taken to complete the PAC could worsen the patient's outcome.

ASA 2008 Guidelines for Developing Institution-Specific Checkout Procedures Prior to Anesthesia Delivery

These guidelines describe a basic approach to checkout procedures and rationale that will ensure that these priorities are satisfied. They should be used to develop institution-specific checkout procedures designed for the equipment and resources available. (Example of institution-specific procedures for current anesthesia delivery systems are published on the same web site as this document.)

Requirements for Safe Delivery of Anesthesia Care

- Reliable delivery of oxygen at any appropriate concentration up to 100%.
- Reliable means of positive-pressure ventilation.
- Backup ventilation equipment available and functioning.
- Controlled release of positive pressure from the breathing circuit.
- Anesthesia vapor delivery (if intended as part of the anesthetic plan).
- Adequate suction.
- Means to conform to standards for patient monitoring.[7,8]

Specific Items

The following items need to be checked as part of a complete PAC. The intent is to identify what to check, the recommended frequency of checking and the individual(s) who could be responsible for the item. For these guidelines, the responsible party would fall into one of four categories: Provider, Technician, Technician or Provider, or Technician and Provider. The designation "Technician and Provider" means that the provider must perform the check whether or not it has been completed by a technician. It is not intended to make the use of technician checks mandatory. The intent is not to specify how an item needs to be checked, as the specific checkout procedure will depend upon the equipment being used.

> **Item 1:** Verify whether auxiliary oxygen cylinder and self-inflating manual ventilation device are available and functioning.
> **Frequency:** Daily
> **Responsible Parties:** Provider and Technician
> **Rationale:** Failure to be able to ventilate is a major cause of morbidity and mortality related to anesthesia care. Because equipment failure with resulting inability to ventilate the patient can occur at any time, a self-inflating manual ventilation device (e.g., AMBU bag) should be present at every anesthetizing location for every case and should be checked for proper function. In addition, a source of oxygen separate from the anesthesia machine and pipeline supply, specifically an oxygen cylinder with regulator and a means to open the cylinder valve, should be immediately available and checked. After checking the cylinder pressure, it is recommended that the main cylinder valve be closed to avoid inadvertent emptying of the cylinder through a leaky or open regulator.

Item 2: Verify patient suction is adequate to clear the airway.
  Frequency: Prior to each use
  Responsible Parties: Provider and Technician
  Rationale: Safe anesthetic care requires the immediate availability of suction to clear the airway if needed.

Item 3: Turn on anesthesia delivery system and confirm that AC power is available.
  Frequency: Daily
  Responsible Parties: Provider or Technician
  Rationale: Anesthesia delivery systems typically function with backup battery power if AC power fails. Unless the presence of AC power is confirmed, the first obvious sign of power failure can be a complete system shutdown when the batteries can no longer power the system. Many anesthesia delivery systems have visual indicators of the power source showing the presence of both AC and battery power. These indicators should be checked and connection of the power cord to a functional AC power source should be confirmed.
  Desflurane vaporizers require electrical power and recommendations for checking power to these vaporizers should also be followed.

Item 4: Verify availability of required monitors and check alarms.
  Frequency: Prior to each use
  Responsible Parties: Provider or Technician
  Rationale: Standards for patient monitoring during anesthesia are clearly defined.[7,8] The ability to conform to these standards should be confirmed for every anesthetic. The first step is to visually verify that the appropriate monitoring supplies (BP cuffs, oximetry probes, etc.) are available. All monitors should be turned on and proper completion of power-up self-tests confirmed. Given the importance of pulse oximetry and capnography to patient safety, verifying proper function of these devices before anesthetizing the patient is essential. Capnometer function can be verified by exhaling through the breathing circuit or gas sensor to generate a capnogram, or verifying that the patient's breathing efforts generate a capnogram before the patient is anesthetized. Visual and audible alarm signals should be generated when this is discontinued. Pulse oximeter function, including an audible alarm, can be verified by placing the sensor on a finger and observing for a proper recording. The pulse oximeter alarm can be tested by introducing motion artifact or removing the sensor.
  Audible alarms have also been reconfirmed as essential to patient safety by the American Society of Anesthesiologists (ASA), American Association of Nurse Anesthetists (AANA), Anesthesia Patient Safety Foundation (APSF), and Joint Commission on the Accreditation of Healthcare Organizations (JCAHO). Proper monitor functioning includes visual and audible alarm signals that function as designed.

Item 5: Verify that pressure is adequate on the spare oxygen cylinder mounted on the anesthesia machine.
  Frequency: Daily
  Responsible Parties: Provider and Technician
  Rationale: Anesthesia delivery systems rely on a supply of oxygen for various machine functions. At a minimum, the oxygen supply is used to provide oxygen to the patient. Pneumatically powered ventilators also rely on a gas supply. Oxygen cylinder(s) should be mounted on the anesthesia delivery system and determined to have an acceptable minimum pressure. The acceptable pressure depends on the intended use, the design of the anesthesia delivery system and the availability of piped oxygen.
  - Typically, an oxygen cylinder will be used if the central oxygen supply fails.
  - If the cylinder is intended to be the primary source of oxygen (e.g., remote site anesthesia), then a cylinder supply sufficient to last for the entire anesthetic is required. If a pneumatically powered ventilator that uses oxygen as its driving gas will be used, a full "E" oxygen cylinder may provide only 30 minutes of oxygen. In that case, the maximum duration of oxygen supply can be obtained from an oxygen cylinder if it is used only to provide fresh gas to the patient in conjunction with manual or spontaneous ventilation. Mechanical ventilators will consume the oxygen supply if pneumatically powered ventilators that require oxygen to power the ventilator are used. Electrically powered ventilators do not consume oxygen so that the duration of a cylinder supply will depend only on total fresh gas flow.
  - The oxygen cylinder valve should be closed after it has been verified that adequate pressure is present, unless the cylinder is to be the primary source of oxygen (i.e., piped oxygen is not available). If the valve remains open and the pipeline supply should fail, the oxygen cylinder can become depleted while the anesthesia provider is unaware of the oxygen supply problem. Other gas supply cylinders (e.g., Heliox, CO_2, air, N_2O) need to be checked only if that gas is required to provide anesthetic care.

Item 6: Verify that piped gas pressures are 50 psig or higher.
  Frequency: Daily
  Responsible Parties: Provider and Technician
  Rationale: A minimum gas supply pressure is required for proper function of the anesthesia delivery system. Gas supplied from a central source can fail for a variety of reasons. Therefore, the pressure in the piped gas supply should be checked at least once daily.

Item 7: Verify that vaporizers are adequately filled and, if applicable, that the filler ports are tightly closed.
  Frequency: Prior to each use
  Responsible Parties: Provider. Technician if redundancy desired.
  Rationale: If anesthetic vapor delivery is planned, an adequate supply is essential to reduce the risk of light anesthesia or recall. This is especially true if an anesthetic agent monitor with a low agent alarm is not being used. Partially open filler ports are a common cause of leaks that may not be detected if the vaporizer control dial is not open when a leak test is performed. This

leak source can be minimized by tightly closing filler ports. Newer vaporizer designs have filling systems that automatically close the filler port when filling is completed.

High and low anesthetic agent alarms are useful to help prevent over- or underdosage of anesthetic vapor. Use of these alarms is encouraged and they should be set to the appropriate limits and enabled.

Item 8: Verify that there are no leaks in the gas supply lines between the flowmeters and the common gas outlet.
Frequency: Daily and whenever a vaporizer is changed
Responsible Parties: Provider or Technician
Rationale: The gas supply in this part of the anesthesia delivery system passes through the anesthetic vaporizer(s) on most anesthesia delivery systems. In order to perform a thorough leak test, each vaporizer must be turned on individually to check for leaks at the vaporizer mount(s) or inside the vaporizer. Furthermore, some machines have a check valve between the flowmeters and the common gas outlet, requiring a negative-pressure test to adequately check for leaks. Automated checkout procedures typically include a leak test but may not evaluate leaks at the vaporizer especially if the vaporizer is not turned on during the leak test. When relying upon automated testing to evaluate the system for leaks, the automated leak test would need to be repeated for each vaporizer in place. This test should also be completed whenever a vaporizer is changed. The risk of a leak at the vaporizer depends upon the vaporizer design. Vaporizer designs where the filler port closes automatically after filling can reduce the risk of leaks.

Technicians can provide useful assistance with this aspect of the machine checkout since it can be time-consuming.

Item 9: Test scavenging system function.
Frequency: Daily
Responsible Parties: Provider or Technician
Rationale: A properly functioning scavenging system prevents room contamination by anesthetic gases. Proper function depends upon correct connections between the scavenging system and the anesthesia delivery system. These connections should be checked daily by a provider or technician. Depending upon the scavenging system design, proper function may also require that the vacuum level is adequate, which should also be confirmed daily. Some scavenging systems have mechanical positive- and negative-pressure relief valves. Positive- and negative-pressure relief is important to protect the patient circuit from pressure fluctuations related to the scavenging system. Proper checkout of the scavenging system should ensure that positive- and negative-pressure relief is functioning properly. Due to the complexity of checking for effective positive- and negative-pressure relief, and the variations in scavenging system design, a properly trained technician can facilitate this aspect of the checkout process.

Item 10: Calibrate, or verify calibration of, the oxygen monitor and check the low oxygen alarm.
Frequency: Daily
Responsible Parties: Provider or Technician.
Rationale: Continuous monitoring of the inspired oxygen concentration is the last line of defense against delivering hypoxic gas concentrations to the patient. The oxygen monitor is essential for detecting adulteration of the oxygen supply. Most oxygen monitors require calibration once daily, although some are self-calibrating. For self-calibrating oxygen monitors, they should be verified to read 21% when sampling room air. This is a step that is easily completed by a trained technician. When more than one oxygen monitor is present, the primary sensor that will be relied upon for oxygen monitoring should be checked.

The low oxygen concentration alarm should also be checked at this time by setting the alarm above the measured oxygen concentration and confirming that an audible alarm signal is generated.

Item 11: Verify carbon dioxide absorbent is not exhausted.
Frequency: Prior to each use
Responsible Parties: Provider or Technician
Rationale: Proper function of a circle anesthesia system relies on the absorbent to remove carbon dioxide from rebreathed gas. Exhausted absorbent as indicated by the characteristic color change should be replaced. It is possible for absorbent material to lose the ability to absorb CO_2 yet the characteristic color change may be absent or difficult to see. Some newer absorbents do change color when desiccated. Capnography should be utilized for every anesthetic and, when using a circle anesthesia system, rebreathing carbon dioxide as indicated by an inspired CO_2 concentration above 0 can also indicate exhausted absorbent. (See Additional Note 2, below.)

Item 12: Breathing system pressure and leak testing.
Frequency: Prior to each use
Responsible Parties: Provider and Technician
Rationale: The breathing system pressure and leak test should be performed with the circuit configuration to be used during anesthetic delivery. If any components of the circuit are changed after this test is completed, the test should be performed again. Although the anesthesia provider should perform this test before each use, anesthesia technicians who replace and assemble circuits can also perform this check and add redundancy to this important checkout procedure. Proper testing will demonstrate that pressure can be developed in the breathing system during both manual and mechanical ventilation and that pressure can be relieved during manual ventilation by opening the APL valve.

Automated testing is often implemented in the newer anesthesia delivery systems to evaluate the system for leaks and also to determine the compliance of the breathing system. The compliance value determined during this testing will be used to automatically adjust the volume delivered by the ventilator to maintain a constant volume delivery to the patient. It is important that the circuit configuration that is to be used be in place during the test.

Item 13: Verify that gas flows properly through the breathing circuit during both inspiration and exhalation.
  Frequency: Prior to each use
  Responsible Parties: Provider and Technician
  Rationale: Pressure and leak testing does not identify all obstructions in the breathing circuit or confirm proper function of the inspiratory and expiratory unidirectional valves. A test lung or second reservoir bag can be used to confirm that flow through the circuit is unimpeded. Complete testing includes both manual and mechanical ventilation. The presence of the unidirectional valves can be assessed visually during the PAC. Proper function of these valves cannot be visually assessed since subtle valve incompetence may not be detected. Checkout procedures to identify valve incompetence that may not be visually obvious can be implemented but are typically too complex for daily testing. A trained technician can perform regular valve competence tests. (See Note 4 in Appendix.) Capnography should be used during every anesthetic and the presence of carbon dioxide in the inspired gases can help to detect an incompetent valve.

Item 14: Document completion of checkout procedures.
  Frequency: Prior to each use
  Responsible Parties: Provider and Technician
  Rationale: Each individual responsible for checkout procedures should document completion of these procedures. Documentation gives credit for completing the job and can be helpful if an adverse event should occur. Some automated checkout systems maintain an audit trail of completed checkout procedures that are dated and timed.

Item 15: Confirm ventilator settings and evaluate readiness to deliver anesthesia care. (ANESTHESIA TIME OUT)
  Frequency: Immediately prior to initiating the anesthetic
  Responsible Parties: Provider
  Rationale: This step is intended to avoid errors due to production pressure or other sources of haste. The goal is to confirm that appropriate checks have been completed and that essential equipment is indeed available. The concept is analogous to the "time out" used to confirm patient identity and surgical site prior to incision. Improper ventilator settings can be harmful especially if a small patient is following a much larger patient or vice versa. Pressure limit settings (when available) should be used to prevent excessive volume delivery from improper ventilator settings.
  Items to check:
  - Monitors functional?
  - Capnogram present?
  - Oxygen saturation by pulse oximetry measured?
  - Flowmeter and ventilator settings proper?
  - Manual/ventilator switch set to manual?
  - Vaporizer(s) adequately filled?

Additional Notes

1. *Testing the flowmeters:* This step is present in the 1993 Checkout Recommendation and is intended to check the oxygen/nitrous oxide proportioning system. It has been eliminated from the Preanesthesia Checkout in these guidelines because proper function is verified during the preventive maintenance and failures of this system in a properly maintained delivery system are rare.
2. *Desiccated carbon dioxide absorbent:* Carbon dioxide absorbents which contain sodium, potassium, or barium hydroxide may become dangerous when desiccated, producing carbon monoxide and/or excessive heat leading to fires. Unfortunately, it is not possible to reliably identify when the absorbent material has been desiccated. Some departments elect to change all absorbent material on Monday morning to eliminate the possibility of using absorbent exposed to continuous fresh gas flow throughout the weekend. Other departments elect to use absorbent materials that do not pose a risk when desiccated. It is important to have a strategy to prevent the hazards related to using absorbents containing the problematic hydroxides that have desiccated. There are no steps that could be included in the checkout recommendation that can reliably identify desiccated absorbent. If a department uses absorbent that may be hazardous when desiccated, it may be prudent to change the absorbent material whenever the duration of time exposure to high fresh gas flow cannot be determined and is likely to have been prolonged. A protocol for preventing absorbent hazards should be part of every department's risk management strategy.
3. *Anesthesia information systems and automated record keepers:* These systems are being adopted by an increasing number of anesthesia departments and are the mainstay of the recordkeeping process in those departments. Reliably functioning systems is therefore important to the conduct of an anesthetic, although not essential to patient safety in the same fashion as the anesthesia delivery system and patient monitors. For departments that rely upon these systems, it would be prudent to have a protocol for checking connections and the proper functioning of the associated computers, displays, and network function.
4. *Testing circle system valve competence:* As part of the test Item 13 (Verify that gas flows properly through the breathing circuit during both inspiration and exhalation), the inspiratory and expiratory valves are visually observed for proper cycling (opening and closing fully). Visual inspection will also detect a missing valve leaflet. Ascertaining full closure of the valve is subjective. Incompetence of the valve may also be detected during test Item 13 through spirometry at the expiratory limb. For expiratory valve malfunction, a spirometer with reverse flow detection will alarm when gas flows retrograde in the expiratory limb. For inspiratory valve malfunction, the measured exhaled tidal volume will be less than the expected value. Capnography may also help to detect incompetence of the unidirectional valves. Intraoperatively, an inspiratory valve malfunction may not be indicated by an elevation of the inspired CO_2 baseline. If the delivered tidal volume exceeds the volume of gas in the inspiratory limb containing CO_2, rebreathing will appear on the capnogram as a gradual, instead of sharp, downstroke. An expiratory valve malfunction is indicated by an elevated CO_2 baseline as there is typically a large volume of exhaled gas containing CO_2 that can return to the patient.

SUMMARY OF CHECKOUT RECOMMENDATIONS BY FREQUENCY AND RESPONSIBLE PARTY

To Be Completed Daily

Item to Be Completed	Responsible Party
Item 1: Verify whether auxiliary oxygen cylinder and self-inflating manual ventilation device are available and functioning.	Provider and Tech
Item 2: Verify patient suction is adequate to clear the airway.	Provider and Tech
Item 3: Turn on anesthesia delivery system and confirm that ac power is available.	Provider or Tech
Item 4: Verify availability of required monitors, including alarms.	Provider or Tech
Item 5: Verify that pressure is adequate on the spare oxygen cylinder mounted on the anesthesia machine.	Provider and Tech
Item 6: Verify that the piped gas pressures are ≥ 50 psig.	Provider and Tech
Item 7: Verify that vaporizers are adequately filled and, if applicable, that the filler ports are tightly closed.	Provider or Tech
Item 8: Verify that there are no leaks in the gas supply lines between the flowmeters and the common gas outlet.	Provider or Tech
Item 9: Test scavenging system function.	Provider or Tech
Item 10: Calibrate, or verify calibration of, the oxygen monitor and check the low oxygen alarm.	Provider or Tech
Item 11: Verify carbon dioxide absorbent is not exhausted.	Provider or Tech
Item 12: Breathing system pressure and leak testing.	Provider and Tech
Item 13: Verify that gas flows properly through the breathing circuit during both inspiration and exhalation.	Provider and Tech
Item 14: Document completion of checkout procedures.	Provider and Tech
Item 15: Confirm ventilator settings and evaluate readiness to deliver anesthesia care. (ANESTHESIA TIME OUT)	Provider

To Be Completed Prior to Each Procedure

Item to Be Completed	Responsible Party
Item 2: Verify patient suction is adequate to clear the airway.	Provider and Tech
Item 4: Verify availability of required monitors, including alarms.	Provider or Tech
Item 7: Verify that vaporizers are adequately filled and if applicable that the filler ports are tightly closed.	Provider
Item 11: Verify carbon dioxide absorbent is not exhausted	Provider or Tech
Item 12: Breathing system pressure and leak testing.	Provider and Tech
Item 13: Verify that gas flows properly through the breathing circuit during both inspiration and exhalation.	Provider and Tech
Item 14: Document completion of checkout procedures.	Provider and Tech
Item 15: Confirm ventilator settings and evaluate readiness to deliver anesthesia care. (ANESTHESIA TIME OUT)	Provider

REFERENCES TO APPENDIX B

1. Cooper JB, Newbower RS, Kitz RJ. An analysis of major errors and equipment failures in anesthesia management: considerations for prevention and detection. *Anesthesiology*. 1984;60:34–42.
2. Arbous MS, Meursing AE, van Kleef JW, et al. Impact of anesthesia management characteristics on severe morbidity and mortality. *Anesthesiology*. 2005;102:257–268.
3. Anesthesia Apparatus Checkout Recommendations, 1993. http://www.fda.gov/cdrh/humfac/anesckot.html.
4. March MG, Crowley JJ. An evaluation of anesthesiologists' present checkout methods and the validity of the FDA checklist. *Anesthesiology*. 1991;75:724–729.
5. Lampotang S, Moon S, Lizdas DE, et al. Anesthesia machine pre-use check survey: preliminary results. (abstracted) *Anesthesiology*. 2005:A1195.
6. Larson ER, Nuttall GA, Ogren, BD, et al. A prospective study on anesthesia machine fault identification. *Anesth Analg*. 2007;104(1):154–156.
7. American Society of Anesthesiologists. Standards for Basic Anesthetic Monitoring. October 28, 2015. http://www.asahq.org/publicationsAndServices/standards/02.pdf.
8. Scope and Standards for Nurse Anesthesia Practice, In: *The Professional Practice Manual for the Certified Registered Nurse Anesthetist*. Park Ridge, IL: American Association of Nurse Anesthetists; 2006.

26 Commonly Used Monitoring Techniques

CHRISTOPHER W. CONNOR • CHRISTOPHER M. CONLEY

Introduction
Monitoring of Inspired Oxygen Concentration
   Principles of Operation
   Proper Use and Interpretation
   Indications
   Contraindications
   Common Problems and Limitations
Monitoring of Arterial Oxygenation by Pulse Oximetry
   Principles of Operation
   Proper Use and Interpretation
   Indications
   Contraindications
   Common Problems and Limitations
Monitoring of Expired Gases
   Principles of Operation
   Proper Use and Interpretation
   Indications
   Contraindications
   Common Problems and Limitations
Invasive Monitoring of Systemic Blood Pressure
   Principles of Operation
   Proper Use and Interpretation
   Indications
   Contraindications
   Common Problems and Limitations
Intermittent Noninvasive Monitoring of Systemic Blood Pressure
   Principles of Operation
   Proper Use and Interpretation
   Indications
   Contraindications
   Common Problems and Limitations
Monitoring of Central Venous and Right-Heart Pressures
   Principles of Operation
   Proper Use and Interpretation
   Indications
   Contraindications
   Common Problems and Limitations
Monitoring of Cardiac Output by Pulmonary Arterial Catheter
   Principles of Operation
   Proper Use and Interpretation
   Indications
   Contraindications
   Common Problems and Limitations
Monitoring of Cardiac Output by Arterial Waveform Analysis
   Principles of Operation
   Proper Use and Interpretation
   Indications
   Contraindications
   Common Problems and Limitations
Monitoring of Body Temperature
   Principles of Operation
   Proper Use and Interpretation
   Indications
   Contraindications
   Common Problems and Limitations
Monitoring of Processed EEG Signals
   Principles of Operation
   Proper Use and Interpretation
   Indications
   Contraindications
   Common Problems and Limitations
Future Trends in Monitoring

KEY POINTS

1. The purpose of monitoring equipment is to augment the situational awareness of the anesthesiologist by providing clinical data either more rapidly than can be achieved manually or more precisely than can be achieved by direct examination of the patient. The value of any particular monitoring technique lies in its ability to inform the anesthesiologist so that the patient's physiologic condition can be maintained within satisfactory parameters. No monitoring technique, however sophisticated, can substitute for the judgment of the anesthesiologist.

2. It is mandatory to measure inspired oxygen concentration for patients receiving general anesthesia to prevent the inadvertent administration of a hypoxic gas mixture. However, inspired oxygen concentration monitoring cannot reliably detect disconnection of the circuit nor does it guarantee adequate arterial oxygenation.

3. Pulse oximetry provides a noninvasive means to detect the onset of hypoxemia rapidly. Modern pulse oximeters are noninvasive, continuous, autocalibrating, have quick response times, and are suitable for use during transport. However, pulse oximetry is a poor indicator of adequate ventilation; desaturation is a late sign of apnea or respiratory insufficiency.

4. Monitoring of expired carbon dioxide is now recommended for procedures involving moderate to deep sedation in addition to procedures performed under general anesthesia. Advances in infrared absorption spectroscopy have led to the production of conveniently portable devices for expired gas analysis.

5. During direct invasive arterial pressure monitoring, the fidelity of the system is optimized when the catheter and tubing are stiff, the mass of the fluid is small, and the length of the connecting tubing is not excessive.

6. Automated noninvasive blood pressure monitors use the oscillometric method to estimate arterial blood pressure. Pulsatile flow generates oscillations in the internal pressure of an inflated blood pressure cuff; these oscillations are greatest when the cuff is inflated to mean arterial pressure. During prolonged surgical cases, it may be prudent to relocate the blood pressure cuff every few hours to reduce the risk of neurapraxia or cutaneous injury.
7. On the basis of available evidence, it is difficult to draw meaningful conclusions regarding the effectiveness of pulmonary artery catheter (PAC) monitoring in reducing morbidity and mortality in critically ill patients. Expert opinion suggests that perioperative complications may be reduced if PACs are used in the appropriate patients and settings and if clinicians interpret and apply the data provided by the PAC correctly.
8. New noninvasive devices have been developed to generate similar cardiac output (CO) parameters to the PAC as well as potentially to be able to predict fluid responsiveness. However, certain common comorbidities can impair the accuracy of these devices; the PAC thermodilution technique remains the clinical gold standard for measuring CO.
9. Clinical studies have demonstrated that patients in whom intraoperative hypothermia develops are at a higher risk for development of postoperative myocardial ischemia and wound infection compared with patients who are normothermic in the perioperative period. Although liquid crystal skin temperature strips are convenient to apply, they do not correlate well with core temperature measurements.
10. Although the algorithms used by processed electroencephalogram (EEG) monitors are proprietary, the general features of the EEG that they use are well described. Processed EEG monitors have not been demonstrated to be superior to end-tidal agent concentration monitoring in the prevention of awareness under anesthesia, although neither technique is sufficient to avoid awareness with complete reliability.
11. The advent of "smarter" and more technically sophisticated monitoring devices does not relieve anesthesiologists of their obligation to employ their clinical judgment wisely. On the contrary, it requires anesthesiologists to understand the operation of these devices intimately so that they can be used safely, accurately, and appropriately.

Introduction

Historically, the foundation of anesthesia practice has been vigilance and ongoing clinical examination of the patient. The development of modern monitoring equipment does not replace these responsibilities. Automated monitoring equipment provides the anesthesiologist with the ability to acquire clinical information either more rapidly or more frequently than can be achieved through manual techniques or in a more quantitatively precise manner than can be achieved by physical examination alone. The purpose of monitoring equipment, then, is to augment the situational awareness of the anesthesiologist so that clinical problems can be recognized and addressed in a timely manner and to guide treatment. The value of any particular monitoring technique lies in its ability to inform the practice of the anesthesiologist so that the patient's physiologic condition can be maintained within satisfactory parameters. The term itself is derived from *monere*, which in Latin means to warn, remind, or admonish.

This chapter discusses the methods and biomedical devices through which anesthesiologists monitor the physiologic state of the patient during anesthesia care. The principles of operation for each of these devices are explained. These explanations are, by necessity, simplified, as the actual design of a biomedical device involves significant engineering complexity. However, the explanations are intended to be sufficient to allow the anesthesiologist to understand how the device acquires its clinical data and how that process might be compromised and the data made erroneous as well as to understand how the device works and how it may fail. There is little high-grade evidence that electronic monitors, by themselves, reduce morbidity and mortality. There is also controversy regarding the need for specific monitors in certain clinical situations, particularly in which use of the monitor in question may add significant cost or where the invasiveness of the monitoring technique may place the patient at risk of iatrogenic complications. Against these costs and risks, the anesthesiologist must balance the likely benefit from a particular monitoring technique when used and interpreted correctly. Therefore, alongside the science and engineering aspects of monitoring, there is also the clinical art of choosing how a patient should best be monitored intraoperatively. For each of the monitoring techniques, relative indications, contraindications, and common technical problems are discussed.

Standards for basic anesthetic monitoring have been established by the American Society of Anesthesiologists (ASA). Since 1986, these standards have emphasized the evolution of technology and practice. The current standards (which became effective on July 1, 2011) emphasize the importance of regular and frequent measurements, integration of clinical judgment and experience, and the potential for extenuating circumstances that can influence the applicability or accuracy of monitoring systems.[1]

Standard I requires qualified personnel to be present in the operating room during general anesthesia, regional anesthesia, and monitored anesthesia care to monitor the patient continuously and to modify anesthesia care based on clinical observations and the responses of the patient to dynamic changes resulting from surgery or drug therapy. Standard II focuses attention on continually evaluating the patient's oxygenation, ventilation, circulation, and temperature. Standard II specifically mandates the following:

1. Use of an inspired oxygen analyzer with a low concentration-limit alarm during general anesthesia.
2. Quantitative assessment of blood oxygenation during any anesthesia care.
3. Continuously ensuring the adequacy of ventilation by physical diagnostic techniques during all anesthesia care. Continual identification of expired carbon dioxide is performed unless precluded by the type of patient, procedure, or equipment.
4. Quantitative monitoring of tidal volume and capnography is strongly encouraged in patients undergoing general anesthesia.
5. When administering regional anesthesia or local anesthesia, ventilation sufficiency should be assessed by qualitative clinical signs. During moderate or deep sedation, ventilation shall be evaluated by continual evaluation of qualitative clinical signs as well as monitoring for the presence of exhaled carbon dioxide unless precluded by the type of patient, procedure, or equipment.

6. Ensuring correct placement of an endotracheal tube or laryngeal mask airway requires clinical assessment and qualitative identification of carbon dioxide in the expired gas.
7. When using a mechanical ventilator, use of a device that is able to detect a disconnection of any part of the breathing system.
8. The adequacy of circulation should be monitored by the continuous display of the electrocardiogram, and by determining the arterial blood pressure and heart rate (HR) at least every 5 minutes. During general anesthesia, circulatory function is to be continually evaluated by at least one of the following: palpation of a pulse, auscultation of heart sounds, monitoring of a tracing of intra-arterial pressure, ultrasound peripheral pulse monitoring, or pulse plethysmography or oximetry.
9. During all anesthetics, the means for continuously measuring the patient's temperature must be available. Every patient receiving anesthesia shall have temperature monitored when clinically significant changes in body temperature are intended, anticipated, or suspected.

Monitoring of Inspired Oxygen Concentration

Principles of Operation

Oxygen is a highly reactive chemical species, providing many chemical and physical opportunities to detect its presence. Three main types of oxygen analyzer are seen in clinical practice: paramagnetic oxygen analyzers, galvanic cell analyzers, and polarographic oxygen analyzers.

Paramagnetic gases are attracted to magnetic energy because of unpaired electrons in their outer shell orbits. Oxygen is a highly paramagnetic gas. Differential paramagnetic oximetry has been incorporated into a variety of operating room monitors. These instruments detect the change in sample line pressure resulting from the attraction of oxygen by switched magnetic fields. Signal changes during electromagnetic switching correlate with the oxygen concentration in the sample line.[2]

Galvanic cell analyzers meet the performance criteria necessary for operative monitoring. These analyzers measure the current produced when oxygen diffuses across a membrane and is reduced to molecular oxygen at the anode of an electrical circuit.[3] The electron flow (current) is proportional to the partial pressure of oxygen in the fuel cell. Galvanic cell analyzers require regular replacement of the galvanic sensor capsule. In the sensor, the electric potential for the reduction of oxygen results from a chemical reaction. Over time, the reactants require replenishment.[4]

Polarographic oxygen analyzers are commonly used in anesthesia monitoring. In this electrochemical system, oxygen diffuses through an oxygen-permeable polymeric membrane and participates in the following reaction: $O_2 + 2H_2O + 4e^- \rightarrow 4OH^-$. The current change is proportional to the number of oxygen molecules surrounding the electrode. Polarographic oxygen sensors are versatile and are important components of gas machine oxygen analyzers, blood gas analyzers, and transcutaneous oxygen analyzers.[5]

Proper Use and Interpretation

The concentration of oxygen in the anesthetic circuit must be measured. Anesthesia machine manufacturers place oxygen sensors on the inspired limb of the anesthesia circuit to detect and alarm in the event that hypoxic gas mixtures are delivered to the patient. Carbon dioxide may reduce the usable lifetime of a galvanic oxygen sensor, so it is preferable to place the oxygen sensor on the inspired limb. Oxygen monitors require a fast response time (2 to 10 seconds), accuracy (±2% of the actual level), and stability when exposed to humidity and inhalation agents.

The removable external oxygen sensors seen commonly on anesthesia machines, such as the Dräger Narkomed and Dräger Fabius (Dräger, Inc., Telford, PA) are of the galvanic type. These devices should be calibrated against room air (21% FiO_2) daily, and also after 8 hours of use. These devices may also infrequently require calibration against 100% FiO_2. As part of the preoperative checkout of the anesthesia machine, the clinician must confirm that the alarm limits of the inspired oxygen analyzer are set appropriately to alert to the presence of hypoxic mixtures. Inspired oxygen alarms cannot be relied upon to detect disconnection of the circuit.

Indications

According to the ASA Standards for Basic Anesthesia Monitoring,[1] Standard 2.2.1 states, "During every administration of general anesthesia using an anesthesia machine, the concentration of oxygen in the patient breathing system shall be measured by an oxygen analyzer with a low oxygen concentration limit alarm in use."

The careful monitoring of the inspired oxygen concentration is of particular significance during low-flow anesthesia, in which the anesthesiologist attempts to minimize the fresh gas flow to the amount of oxygen necessary to replace the patient's metabolic utilization. The gas mixture within the breathing circuit may become hypoxic if insufficient fresh gas flow is supplied, even if the fresh gas flow itself comprises pure oxygen.

Contraindications

The requirement to monitor inspired oxygen concentration may be waived by the responsible anesthesiologist under extenuating circumstances. There are no clinical contraindications to monitoring inspired oxygen concentration.

Common Problems and Limitations

Adequate inspiratory oxygen concentration does not guarantee adequate arterial oxygen concentration.[6] Consequently, ASA[1] Standard 2.2.2 mandates additional monitoring for blood oxygenation, including the provision of adequate lighting and exposure to assess the patient's color by direct observation. The practice of pediatric anesthesia merits additional vigilance to monitoring inspired oxygen concentration. Indications for altering inspired oxygen concentrations to facilitate anesthetics in children are common; for example, using a nitrous oxide–oxygen blend to facilitate inhalation inductions of anesthesia. Increased awareness of fire hazards in the operating room environment further reinforces the need for careful monitoring of FiO_2 in pediatric anesthesia. Tonsillectomy and adenoidectomy, among the most common of surgical procedures in the pediatric anesthesia population, carry an increased risk of airway fire. In addition to using of cuffed endotracheal tubes, careful monitoring and maintenance of a decreased inspired oxygen concentration whenever electrosurgical equipment is in use may decrease airway fire risk in these patients.[7,8]

Monitoring of Arterial Oxygenation by Pulse Oximetry

Principles of Operation

Pulse oximeters measure pulse rate and estimate the oxygen saturation of hemoglobin (SPO_2) on a noninvasive, continuous basis.[9] The oxygen saturation (SaO_2) of hemoglobin (as a percentage) is related to the oxygen tension (as a partial pressure, mmHg) by the oxyhemoglobin dissociation curve. On the steep part of the curve, a predictable correlation exists between SaO_2 and partial pressure of oxygen (PaO_2). In this range, the SaO_2 is a good reflection of the extent of hypoxemia and the changing status of arterial oxygenation. For PaO_2 greater than 75 mmHg, the SaO_2 reaches a plateau and no longer reflects changes in PaO_2. Coexisting medical conditions, such as hypercapnia, acidosis, and hyperthermia, cause the oxyhemoglobin dissociation curve to shift to the right and decrease the affinity of hemoglobin for oxygen. This change favors the unloading of oxygen from hemoglobin to peripheral tissues, as shown in Figure 26-1.

Pulse oximetry is based on the following premises:
1. The color of blood is a function of oxygen saturation.
2. The change in color results from the optical properties of hemoglobin and its interaction with oxygen.
3. The ratio of oxyhemoglobin (HbO_2) and hemoglobin (Hb) can be determined by absorption spectrophotometry.

Oxygen saturation is determined by spectrophotometry, which is based on the Beer–Lambert law. At a constant light intensity and hemoglobin concentration, the intensity of light transmitted through a tissue is a logarithmic function of the oxygen saturation of Hb. Two wavelengths of light are required to distinguish HbO_2 from Hb. Light-emitting diodes in the pulse sensor emit red (660 nm) and near infrared (940 nm) light. The percentage of HbO_2 is determined by measuring the ratio of infrared and red light sensed by a photodetector. Pulse oximeters perform a plethysmographic analysis to differentiate the pulsatile "arterial" signal from the nonpulsatile signal resulting from "venous" absorption and other tissues, such as skin, muscle, and bone. The absence of a pulsatile waveform during extreme hypothermia or hypoperfusion can limit the ability of a pulse oximeter to calculate the SPO_2.

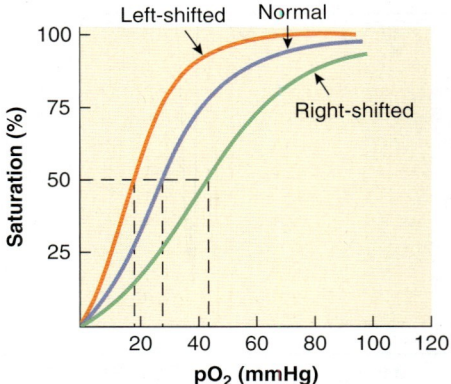

Figure 26-1 The oxyhemoglobin dissociation curve. The relationship between arterial saturation of hemoglobin and oxygen tension is represented by the sigmoid-shaped oxyhemoglobin dissociation curve. When the curve is left-shifted, the hemoglobin molecule binds oxygen more tightly. (Adapted from: Brown M, Vender JS. Noninvasive oxygen monitoring. *Crit Care Clin*. 1988;4:493–509.)

The SPO_2 measured by pulse oximetry is not the same as the arterial saturation (SaO_2) measured by a laboratory co-oximeter. Pulse oximetry measures the "functional" saturation, which is defined by the following equation:

$$SPO_2 = \frac{HbO_2}{HbO_2 + Hb} \times 100\%$$

Laboratory co-oximeters use multiple wavelengths to distinguish other types of Hb, such as carboxyhemoglobin (COHb) and methemoglobin (MetHb) by their characteristic absorption. Co-oximeters measure the "fractional" saturation, which is defined by the following equation:

$$SaO_2 = \frac{HbO_2}{HbO_2 + Hb + COHb + MetHb} \times 100\%$$

In clinical circumstances in which other Hb moieties are present, the SPO_2 measurement may not correlate with the actual SaO_2 reported by the blood gas laboratory. For example, MetHb absorbs red and infrared wavelengths of light in a 1:1 ratio corresponding to a SPO_2 of approximately 85%. Therefore, increases in MetHb produce an underestimation when $SPO_2 > 70\%$ and an overestimation when $SPO_2 < 70\%$. Similarly, COHb also produces artificially high and misleading results; one study showed that at 70% COHb, the SPO_2 still measured 90%. In most patients, MetHb and COHb are present in low concentrations so that the functional saturation approximates the fractional value.[10]

Proper Use and Interpretation

The assessment of arterial oxygenation is an integral part of anesthesia practice. Early detection and prompt intervention may limit serious sequelae of hypoxemia. The clinical signs associated with hypoxemia (e.g., tachycardia, altered mental status, cyanosis) are often masked or difficult to appreciate during anesthesia.

The appropriate use of pulse oximetry necessitates an appreciation of both physiologic and technical limitations. Despite the numerous clinical benefits of pulse oximetry, other factors affect its accuracy and reliability. Factors that may be present during anesthesia care and that affect the accuracy and reliability of pulse oximetry include dyshemoglobins, dyes (methylene blue, indocyanine green, and indigo carmine), nail polish, ambient light, light-emitting diode variability, motion artifact, and background noise. Electrocautery can interfere with pulse oximetry if the radiofrequency emissions are sensed by the photodetector. Surgical stereotactic positioning systems that make use of infrared position sensors may interfere with the infrared signals used by the pulse oximeter. Reports of burns or pressure necrosis exist but are infrequent. Inspecting the digits during monitoring can reduce these complications.

Recent developments in pulse oximetry technology reportedly may permit more accurate measurements of SPO_2 during patient movement, low-perfusion conditions, and in the presence of dyshemoglobins. Some of these instruments use complex signal processing of the two wavelengths of light to improve the signal-to-noise ratio and reject artifact. Studies in volunteers suggest that the performance of pulse oximeters incorporating this technology is superior to conventional oximetry during motion of the hand, hypoperfusion, and hypothermia.[11,12] Other pulse oximetry devices incorporate eight wavelengths of light to more accurately measure COHb and MetHb.[10]

Indications

Pulse oximetry has been used in all patient age groups to detect and prevent hypoxemia. The clinical benefits of pulse oximetry are enhanced by its simplicity. Modern pulse oximeters are noninvasive, continuous, and autocalibrating. They have quick response times and their battery backup provides monitoring during transport. The clinical accuracy is typically reported to be within ±2% to 3% at 70% to 100% saturation and ±3% at 50% to 70% saturation. Published data from numerous investigations support accuracy and precision reported by instrument manufacturers. Quantitative assessment of arterial oxygen saturation is mandated by the ASA monitoring standards,[1] and the convenience and safety of pulse oximetry has supplanted earlier techniques such as heated transcutaneous pO_2 electrodes.[13]

Pulse oximetry has wide applicability in many hospital and nonhospital settings. However, there are no definitive data demonstrating a reduction in morbidity or mortality associated with the advent of pulse oximetry. An older large randomized trial did not detect a significant difference in postoperative complications when routine pulse oximetry was used.[14] However, a reduction of anesthesia mortality, as well as fewer malpractice claims from respiratory events, coincident with the introduction of pulse oximeters suggests that the routine use of these devices may have been a contributing factor.

Contraindications

There are no clinical contraindications to monitoring arterial oxygen saturation with pulse oximetry.

Common Problems and Limitations

Arterial oxygen monitors do not ensure adequacy of oxygen delivery to, or utilization by, peripheral tissues and should not be considered a replacement for arterial blood gas measurements or mixed central venous oxygen saturation when more definitive information regarding oxygen supply and utilization is required.

Pulse oximetry is a poor indicator of adequate ventilation; patients who have been breathing supplemental oxygen may be apneic for several minutes before desaturation is detected by the pulse oximeter. Once the PaO_2 has fallen sufficiently to cause a detectable decrease in SPO_2, further desaturation may occur precipitously once the steep part of the oxyhemoglobin dissociation curve is reached.

Placing and obtaining reliable data from blood pressure cuffs and electrocardiogram leads may be challenging in an awake and vigorous child prior to inhalation induction. Therefore, at a minimum, efforts should be made to place a pulse oximetry device on the child or infant prior to induction of anesthesia. Pulse oximetry has also been shown to be a more sensitive monitor than capnography for unrecognized main-stem/endobronchial intubation in pediatric anesthesia.[15] Respiratory events leading to inadequate ventilation and oxygenation represent the majority of perianesthetic morbidity in the pediatric anesthesia population. In conjunction with vigilant clinical assessment of the child's airway and oxygenation, the pulse oximeter usually provides the most important indicator of patient well-being during pediatric anesthesia.[16] Stress caused by hypoxemia and respiratory acidosis in infants and young children triggers a vagal response and subsequent systemic hypoperfusion. Infants cannot adequately increase their cardiac stroke volume (SV) in compensation and so, according to the cardiac output (CO) equation:

$$\text{Cardiac Output} = \text{Heart Rate} \times \text{Stroke Volume}$$

Therefore, in infants, CO must be maintained with an increase over their baseline HR. A decline in the pitch or rapidity of pulse oximetry tones may be the first signs of impending cardiovascular collapse.

Monitoring of Expired Gases

Principles of Operation

The patient's expired gas is likely to be composed of a mixture of oxygen (O_2), nitrogen (NO_2), carbon dioxide (CO_2), and anesthetic gases such as nitrous oxide (N_2O) and highly potent halogenated agents (sevoflurane, isoflurane, or desflurane). Anesthesiologists have long sought to measure the composition of expired gases noninvasively and in real time; these measurements can provide vital information regarding the patient's respiratory condition and assist in the titration of volatile anesthetic agents. Early anesthetic gas detectors were based simply on the change in elastance of rubber strips exposed to the circulating gas.[17] Later methods made use of Raman scattering[18] or multiplexed mass spectrometry.[19]

These techniques have now all been supplanted in clinical practice by infrared absorption spectrophotometry (IRAS). Asymmetric, polyatomic molecules like CO_2 absorb infrared light at specific wavelengths. By transmitting light through a pure sample of a known gas over the range of infrared frequencies, a unique infrared transmission spectrum (like a fingerprint) can be created for the gas. CO_2, for example, strongly absorbs infrared light with a wavelength of 4.3 microns, as shown in Figure 26-2. At this wavelength, there is minimal interference from other gases that may also be present, such as water vapor, O_2, N_2O, and inhaled anesthetic agents. Infrared light at this wavelength can be passed through a sample of gas to an infrared detector. As the concentration of CO_2 increases, the intensity of the light that reaches the detector decreases in accordance with the Beer–Lambert law.

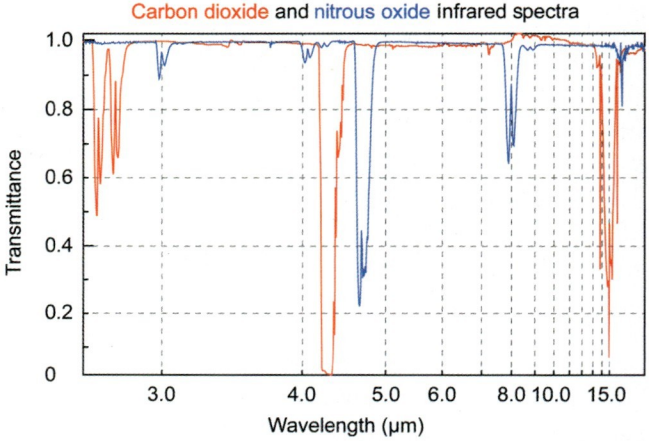

Figure 26-2 Gaseous-phase infrared transmission spectrum for carbon dioxide and nitrous oxide. (Modified from the National Institute of Standards and Technology (http://www.nist.gov); and Craver CD, Coblentz Society. The Coblentz Society desk book of infrared spectra. 2nd ed. Kirwood, MO: The Society; 1982.)

IRAS devices have five components: a multiple-wavelength infrared light source, a gas sampler, an optical path, a detection system, and a signal processor. Operating room IRAS devices can detect CO_2, N_2O, and the potent inhaled anesthetic agents as mixed together in a sample of the patient's expired gas. The gas mixture is passed through the optical path of multiple infrared beams whose wavelengths are chosen to correspond to key features in the transmission spectra of the gases of interest. By analyzing the combination of absorption of infrared light at these wavelengths, the presence and concentrations of all of these gases can be determined simultaneously.[20] The use of multiple wavelengths allows the gases to be identified automatically. Older IRAS devices used a hot electrical element to generate radiant infrared light over a broad range of wavelengths. An optical filter wheel was then used to cut out all but the desired wavelengths. Contemporary devices make use of small lasers and filters, designed such that they emit only at the desired wavelengths. This approach consumes much less electrical power, is physically less heavy, and has led to the development of conveniently portable handheld gas analyzers.[21]

Proper Use and Interpretation

Expired gas analysis allows the clinician to monitor inspired and expired concentrations of CO_2 and anesthetic gases simultaneously. These measurements require separate clinical interpretation. Critical events that can be detected by the analysis of respiratory gases and anesthetic vapors are listed in Table 26-1.

Interpretation of Inspired and Expired Carbon Dioxide Concentrations

Capnometry is the measurement and numeric representation of the CO_2 concentration during inspiration and expiration. A

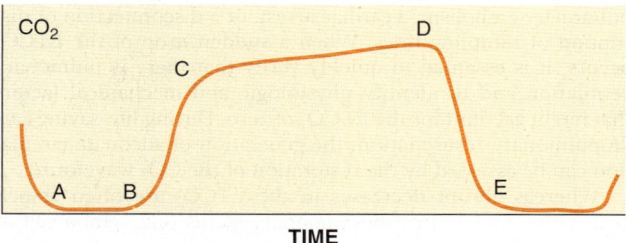

Figure 26-3 The normal capnogram. Point D delineates the end-tidal CO_2 (ETCO$_2$). ETCO$_2$ is the best reflection of the alveolar CO_2 partial pressure.

capnogram is a continuous concentration–time display of the CO_2 concentration sampled at a patient's airway during ventilation. The capnogram is divided into four distinct phases, as shown in Figure 26-3.

The first phase (A–B) represents the initial stage of expiration. Gas sampled during this phase occupies the anatomic dead space and is normally devoid of CO_2. At point B, CO_2-containing gas presents itself at the sampling site and a sharp upstroke (B–C) is seen in the capnogram. The slope of this upstroke is determined by the evenness of expiratory ventilation and alveolar emptying. Phase C–D represents the alveolar or expiratory plateau. At this phase of the capnogram, alveolar gas is being sampled. Normally, this part of the waveform is almost horizontal. However, when ventilation and perfusion are mismatched, Phase C–D may take an upward slope. Point D is the highest CO_2 value and is called the end-tidal CO_2 (ETCO$_2$). ETCO$_2$ is the best reflection of the alveolar CO_2 (P_ACO_2). As the patient begins to inspire, fresh gas is entrained and there is a steep downstroke (D–E) back to baseline. Unless rebreathing of CO_2 occurs, the baseline approaches zero. If the P_ACO_2–$PaCO_2$ gradient is constant and small, capnography provides a noninvasive, continuous, real-time reflection of ventilation. The ETCO$_2$–$PaCO_2$ gradient typically is around 5 mmHg during routine general anesthesia in otherwise healthy supine patients.

The size and shape of the capnogram waveform can provide additional clinical information.[22] A slow rate of rise of the second phase (B–C) is suggestive of either chronic obstructive pulmonary disease or acute airway obstruction as from bronchoconstriction (asthma) secondary to mismatch in alveolar ventilation and alveolar perfusion. A normally shaped capnogram with an increase in ETCO$_2$ suggests alveolar hypoventilation or an increase in CO_2 production. Transient increases in ETCO$_2$ are often observed during tourniquet release, aortic unclamping, or the administration of bicarbonate.

Capnography is an essential element in determining the appropriate placement of endotracheal tubes. The presence of a stable ETCO$_2$ for three successive breaths indicates that the tube is not in the esophagus. A continuous stable CO_2 waveform ensures the presence of alveolar ventilation but does not necessarily indicate that the endotracheal tube is properly positioned in the trachea. An endobronchial intubation, in which the tip of the tube is located in a main stem bronchus, cannot be ruled out until breath sounds are auscultated bilaterally. A continuous CO_2 tracing also does not guarantee that the endotracheal tube is placed securely; an endotracheal tube placed proximally to the vocal cords may still produce an otherwise satisfactory tracing until it becomes dislodged.

A sudden drop in ETCO$_2$ to near zero followed by the absence of a CO_2 waveform heralds a potentially life-threatening problem that could indicate malposition of an endotracheal tube into the pharynx or esophagus, sudden severe hypotension, massive

Table 26-1 Detection of Critical Events by Implementing Gas Analysis

Event	Gas Measured by Analyzer
Error in gas delivery	O_2, N_2, CO_2, agent analysis
Anesthesia machine malfunction	O_2, N_2, CO_2, agent
Disconnection	CO_2, O_2, agent analysis
Vaporizer malfunction or contamination	Agent analysis
Anesthesia circuit leaks	N_2, CO_2 analysis
Endotracheal cuff leaks	N_2, CO_2
Poor mask or LMA fit	N_2, CO_2
Hypoventilation	CO_2 analysis
Malignant hyperthermia	CO_2
Airway obstruction	CO_2
Air embolism	CO_2, N_2
Circuit hypoxia	O_2 analysis
Vaporizer overdose	Agent analysis

LMA, laryngeal mask airway.
Modified from Knopes KD, Hecker BR. Monitoring anesthetic gases. In: Lake CL, ed. *Clinical Monitoring*. Philadelphia, PA: WB Saunders; 1990:24, with permission.

pulmonary embolism, a cardiac arrest, or a disconnection or disruption of sampling lines. When a sudden drop of the $ETCO_2$ occurs, it is essential to quickly verify that there is pulmonary ventilation and to identify physiologic and mechanical factors that might account for the $ETCO_2$ of zero. During life-saving cardiopulmonary resuscitation, the generation of adequate circulation can be assessed by the restoration of the CO_2 waveform.

Whereas abrupt decreases in the $ETCO_2$ are often associated with an altered cardiopulmonary status (e.g., embolism or hypoperfusion), gradual reductions in $ETCO_2$ more often reflect decreases in $PaCO_2$ that occur when there exists an imbalance between minute ventilation and metabolic rate (i.e., CO_2 production), as commonly occurs during anesthesia at a fixed minute ventilation. Increases in $ETCO_2$ can be expected when CO_2 production exceeds ventilation, such as in hyperthermia or when an exogenous source of CO_2 is present. Capnographic waveforms that do not return to zero during inspiration indicate rebreathing of CO_2. This nonzero inspiration phase can occur if the CO_2 absorber in an anesthesia machine is chemically exhausted, if a valve in the ventilator circuit is not functioning properly, or if the flow of fresh gas is insufficient. An elevated baseline can also be seen if the device is calibrated incorrectly.

Alterations in ventilation, CO, distribution of pulmonary blood flow, and metabolic activity influence end-tidal CO_2 concentration and the capnogram obtained during quantitative expired gas analysis. Table 26-2 summarizes the common elements that may be reflected by changes in $ETCO_2$ during anesthesia care.

Interpretation of Inspired and Expired Anesthetic Gas Concentrations

Monitoring the concentration of expired anesthetic gases assists the anesthesiologist in titrating those gases to the clinical circumstances of the patient. At high fresh-gas flow rates, the concentration of an anesthetic gas in a circle breathing system will approximate the concentration set on the vaporizer. However, high fresh-gas flow rates lead to wasteful use of anesthetic vapor. As the fresh-gas flow rate is lowered, the concentration within the circuit and the concentration set at the vaporizer can become more decoupled. Inspired and expired gas concentration monitoring allows the anesthesiologist to maintain satisfactory and well-controlled agent levels in the circuit even when extremely low fresh-gas flows are used. In an ideal, leak-free anesthesia system, the fresh-gas flow can be minimized to only the amount of pure oxygen necessary to replace the patient's metabolic utilization—a practiced known as "closed-circuit anesthesia." This practice makes the most economic use of potent anesthetic vapor.[23]

Anesthetic gases have differing potencies; thus, their concentrations are often normalized against the concentration of that agent required to produce a predetermined clinical end point. The most commonly used end point is the minimum alveolar concentration (MAC) value, defined as the end-tidal gas concentration that when maintained constant for 15 minutes at a pressure of one atmosphere, inhibits movement in response to a midline laparotomy incision in 50% of patients.[24,25] Historically, MAC is an acronym for *minimum alveolar concentration*, although it is more accurately a median constant end-tidal partial pressure. Monitoring of end-tidal gas concentrations performed with reference to MAC values helps to prevent the occurrence of intraoperative awareness and in some studies was superior to the use of processed electroencephalogram (EEG) monitors.[26]

Indications

Monitoring of the partial pressure of expiratory CO_2 has evolved into an important physiologic and safety monitor. Capnography is the standard of care for monitoring the adequacy of ventilation in patients receiving general anesthesia. It is also now mandated for use in monitoring ventilation during procedures performed while the patient is under moderate or deep sedation.[1]

Contraindications

There are no contraindications to the use of capnography, provided that the data obtained are evaluated in the context of the patient's clinical circumstances. It is generally safe to use capnography for the monitoring of all patients.

Monitoring of expired anesthetic gases is only informative if detectable gases are used to maintain anesthesia. Infrared spectroscopy cannot detect Xenon, and is not informative if anesthesia is maintained using a total intravenous technique.

Common Problems and Limitations

The sampling lines or water traps of expired gas analyzers may become occluded with condensed water vapor during prolonged use. Disconnecting the sampling line and flushing it with air from a syringe can sometimes clear it, but it may be necessary to replace these components. Elevating the sidestream sampling line above the ventilator circuit helps prevent the entry of condensed water. A humidity barrier is also useful, although this will increase the response time of the capnogram.

Although mass spectroscopy and Raman scattering are no longer seen in clinical practice, these technologies are able to detect the concentration of N_2 directly. Nitrogen monitoring provides quantification of washout during preoxygenation. A sudden rise in N_2 in the exhaled gas indicates either introduction of air from leaks in the anesthesia delivery system or venous air embolism. Infrared gas analyzers do not detect N_2 directly and its concentration must be inferred as the amount remaining after other measurable gases are accounted for.

Although capnography provides a quantitative measurement of $ETCO_2$, it is not as accurate as blood gas analysis for the assessment of the partial pressure of arterial carbon dioxide. A gradient exists between the partial pressure of arterial carbon dioxide and $ETCO_2$; this gradient increases as the dead-space volume increases.

Table 26-2 Factors That May Change End-Tidal CO_2 ($ETCO_2$) during Anesthesia

Increases in $ETCO_2$	Decreases in $ETCO_2$
Elements that Change CO_2 Production	
Increases in metabolic rate	Decreases in metabolic rate
Hyperthermia	Hypothermia
Sepsis	Hypothyroidism
Malignant hyperthermia	
Shivering	
Hyperthyroidism	
Elements that Change CO_2 Elimination	
Hypoventilation	Hyperventilation
Rebreathing	Hypoperfusion
	Pulmonary embolism

In disease states characterized by increased dead space and ventilation–perfusion mismatch, such as emphysema or pulmonary embolism, or in iatrogenic single-lung ventilation or in very low CO states, an arterial blood gas analysis is necessary for an accurate determination of the partial pressure of arterial carbon dioxide.

Younger children desaturate rapidly following apnea, largely due to increased oxygen consumption and a smaller ratio of functional residual capacity (FRC) to closing volume.[27] Hypoxemia may precipitate a hypoperfusing bradycardic state, especially in neonates. Capnography's role in early recognition of apnea via a sudden drop or newly absent CO_2 signal makes it particularly valuable in pediatric anesthesia. Endotracheally intubated neonates, particularly very-low-birthweight infants in neonatal intensive care units, present unique challenges to accurate measurement of exhaled CO_2. These infants are typically intubated with cuffless endotracheal tubes. A cuffless tube permits a larger internal diameter, which reduces resistance to flow and work-of-breathing, but also allows leakage of expired gases. Capnography measurements therefore become more likely to underestimate actual end-tidal CO_2 levels.[28]

Sidestream capnography systems are the most commonly utilized in the operating room. Sidestream sampling units suction up to 200 mL/min out of the breathing circuit, diverting this to a remote sensor where the gas is analyzed.[29] Given that the neonatal minute ventilation is normally 200 to 300 mL/kg/min, sidestream sampling rates can approach and even surpass the minute ventilation of premature infants. In neonates, sidestream capnography systems may report erroneously low end-tidal CO_2 levels since the capnography system may be sampling gas that never actually participated in ventilation.[30] The true end-tidal CO_2 has been erroneously diluted by fresh gas. Newer, low-flow sidestream capnography systems have since been developed to address this problem.[31] Because most anesthesia machines in the operating room are used with common higher-flow sidestream capnography devices, additional care must be taken when providing general endotracheal anesthesia for infants. In a neonate, an apparently normal $ETCO_2$ on the monitor may in fact represent inadequate ventilation, which would predispose the patient to respiratory acidemia.

Invasive Monitoring of Systemic Blood Pressure

Principles of Operation

Indwelling arterial cannulation permits the opportunity to monitor arterial blood pressure continuously and to have vascular access for arterial blood sampling. Intra-arterial blood pressure monitoring uses fluid-filled tubing to transmit the force of the pressure pulse wave to a pressure transducer that converts the displacement of a silicon crystal into voltage changes. These electrical signals are amplified, filtered, and displayed as the arterial pressure trace. Intra-arterial pressure-transducing systems are subject to many potential errors based on the physical properties of fluid motion and the performance of the catheter–transducer–amplification system used to sense, process, and display the pressure pulse wave.

The behavior of transducers, fluid couplings, signal amplification, and display systems can be described by a complex second-order differential equation. Solving the equation predicts the output and characterizes the fidelity of the system's ability to faithfully display and estimate the arterial pressure over time. The fidelity of fluid-coupled transducing systems is constrained by two properties: *damping* (ζ) and *natural frequency* (f_n). Zeta (ζ) describes the tendency for fluid in the measuring system to extinguish motion and f_n describes the frequency at which the measuring system is most prone to resonance. The fidelity of the transduced pressure depends on optimizing ζ and f_n so that the system can respond appropriately to the range of frequencies contained in the pressure pulse wave. Analysis of high-fidelity recordings of arterial blood pressure indicates that the pressure trace contains frequencies from 1 to 30 Hz. The "fast flush" test is a method used at the bedside to determine the natural frequency and damping characteristics of the transducing system. This test examines the characteristics of the resonant waves recorded after the release of a flush tail. Damping is estimated by the amplitude ratio of the first pair of resonant waves and the natural frequency is estimated by dividing the tracing speed by the interval cycle.[32]

Proper Use and Interpretation

Multiple arteries can be used for direct measurement of blood pressure, including the radial, brachial, axillary, femoral, and dorsalis pedis arteries (Table 26-3). The radial artery remains the most popular site for cannulation because of its accessibility and the presence of a collateral blood supply. In the past, assessment of the patency of the ulnar circulation by performance of an Allen test has been recommended before cannulation. An Allen test is performed by compressing both radial and ulnar arteries while the patient tightens his or her fist. Releasing pressure on each respective artery determines the dominant vessel supplying blood to the hand. The prognostic value of the Allen test in assessing the adequacy of the collateral circulation has not been confirmed.[33,34]

Three techniques for cannulation are common: direct arterial puncture, guidewire-assisted cannulation (Seldinger technique), and the transfixion–withdrawal method.[35] A necessary condition for percutaneous placement is identification of the arterial pulse,

Table 26-3 Arterial Cannulation and Direct Blood Pressure Monitoring

Arterial Cannulation Site	Clinical Points of Interest
Radial artery	Preferred site for monitoring Nontapered catheters preferred
Ulnar artery	Complication similar to radial Primary source of hand blood flow
Brachial artery	Insertion site medial to biceps tendon Median nerve damage is potential hazard Can accommodate 18-gauge cannula
Axillary artery	Insertion site at junction of pectoralis and deltoid muscles Specialized kits available
Femoral artery	Easy access in low-flow states Potential for local and retroperitoneal hemorrhage Longer catheters preferred
Dorsalis pedis artery	Collateral circulation = posterior tibial artery Higher systolic pressure estimates

which may be enhanced by a Doppler flow detection device in patients with poor peripheral pulses.[36] Ultrasound imaging with Doppler color flowmetry can provide valuable further assistance when the pulse is difficult to locate or the caliber of the vessel appears to be small.[37]

Arterial blood pressure transduction systems must be "zeroed" before use. The transducer is positioned at the same level as the right atrium, the stopcock is opened to the atmosphere so that the pressure-sensing crystal senses only atmospheric pressure, and the "Zero Sensor" (or equivalent) option is selected on the monitoring equipment. This procedure establishes the calibration of the sensor and establishes the level of the right atrium as the datum reference point. For neurosurgical procedures in which the patient may be positioned in an upright or beach-chair position, it is common practice to zero the transducer at the level of the Circle of Willis so that the arterial pressure tracing provides a reading that is adjusted for the height of the fluid column between the heart and the brain; it represents the arterial pressure at the base of the brain.

Direct arterial pressure monitoring requires constant vigilance. The data displayed must correlate with clinical conditions before therapeutic interventions are initiated. Sudden increases in the transduced blood pressure may represent a hydrostatic error because the position of the transducer was not adjusted after change in the operating room table's height. Sudden decreases often result from kinking of the catheter or tubing. Before initiating therapy, the transducer system should be examined quickly and the patency of the arterial cannula verified. This ensures the accuracy of the measurement and avoids the initiation of a potentially dangerous medication error.

Traumatic cannulation has been associated with hematoma formation, thrombosis, and damage to adjacent nerves. Abnormal radial artery blood flow after catheter removal occurs frequently. Studies suggest that blood flow normalizes in 3 to 70 days. Radial artery thrombosis can be minimized by using small catheters, avoiding polypropylene-tapered catheters, and reducing the duration of arterial cannulation. Flexible guidewires may reduce the potential trauma associated with catheters negotiating tortuous vessels. After arterial cannulation has been performed, the tissues that are perfused by that artery should be examined intermittently for signs of thromboembolism or ischemia. During cannula removal, the potential for thromboembolism may be diminished by compressing the proximal and distal arterial segment while aspirating the cannula during withdrawal.

Indications

The standards for basic monitoring[1] stipulate that arterial blood pressure shall be determined and recorded at least every 5 minutes. This standard is usually met by intermittent, noninvasive blood pressure monitoring. However, continuous monitoring may be indicated by patient comorbidities or by the nature of the surgery to be performed.

Arterial catheters provide continuous monitoring of blood pressure and convenient vascular access to obtain blood samples for laboratory assays, including blood gas analysis to assess respiratory function. Placement of an arterial catheter can therefore be indicated by the need for any of these capabilities:

1. **Rapid changes in blood pressure or extremes of blood pressure are anticipated.**
   High-risk vascular surgeries, trauma surgeries, neurosurgical procedures, and intrathoracic and cardiac procedures are associated with the risk of sudden blood loss and rapid changes in blood pressure. These procedures may also involve periods of deliberate hypotension or hypertension.

2. **The ability of the patient to tolerate hemodynamic instability is impaired.**
   Patients with clinically significant cardiac disease, such as coronary artery disease, valvular disease, or heart failure, may require continuous monitoring in order to allow treatment for hypotension to be implemented rapidly and minimize the risk of coronary ischemia. Similar concerns apply to patients with a history of cerebrovascular disease. Procedures that involve potential compromise to the vascular supply of the spinal cord indicate the use of an arterial catheter to maintain adequate perfusion and decrease the risk of postoperative paraplegia from spinal cord infarction.[38]

   Critically ill patients may already be hemodynamically unstable at the time of presentation, and require the administration of inotropes and vasopressors. Continuous blood pressure monitoring is indicated to manage the titration of these agents.

3. **Compromise of the patient's respiratory function, oxygenation, or ventilation is anticipated.**
   Mismatch between pulmonary ventilation and perfusion will impair the ability of end-tidal CO_2 to predict P_ACO_2. This variance may arise iatrogenically during procedures that require single-lung ventilation. Patients may present with pulmonary comorbidities, such as ARDS, pulmonary embolism, and pulmonary hypertension with consequent ventilation–perfusion mismatch and impaired alveolar diffusion. Arterial catheters provide a means to obtain arterial blood gas samples frequently to assess changes in respiratory function.

4. **Metabolic derangements are anticipated.**
   Surgical procedures that are anticipated to produce large-volume fluid shifts may indicate the placement of an arterial catheter to enable laboratory samples to be drawn frequently and to allow electrolyte and acid–base disturbances to be detected and corrected.

Contraindications

Arterial cannulation is regarded as an invasive procedure with documented morbidity. Ischemia after radial artery cannulation resulting from thrombosis, proximal emboli, or prolonged shock has been described.[39] Contributing factors include severe atherosclerosis, diabetes, low CO, and intense peripheral vasoconstriction. Ischemia, hemorrhage, thrombosis, embolism, cerebral air embolism (retrograde flow associated with flushing), aneurysm formation, arteriovenous fistula formation, skin necrosis, and infection have reportedly occurred as the direct result of arterial cannulation, arterial blood sampling, or high-pressure flushing. Patients with compromised collateral arterial supply, such as those with Reynaud phenomenon or thromboangiitis obliterans (Buerger disease), are at increased risk for ischemic complications.[35]

Common Problems and Limitations

The fidelity of the transducer system is optimized when catheters and tubing are stiff, the mass of the fluid is small, the number of stopcocks is limited, and the connecting tubing is not excessive. Figure 26-4 demonstrates the effect of damping on the character of the arterial pressure trace. In clinical practice, underdamped transducer systems tend to overestimate the systolic pressure by 15 to 30 mmHg and amplify artifacts. Likewise, excessive increases in ζ reduce fidelity and underestimate systolic pressure.

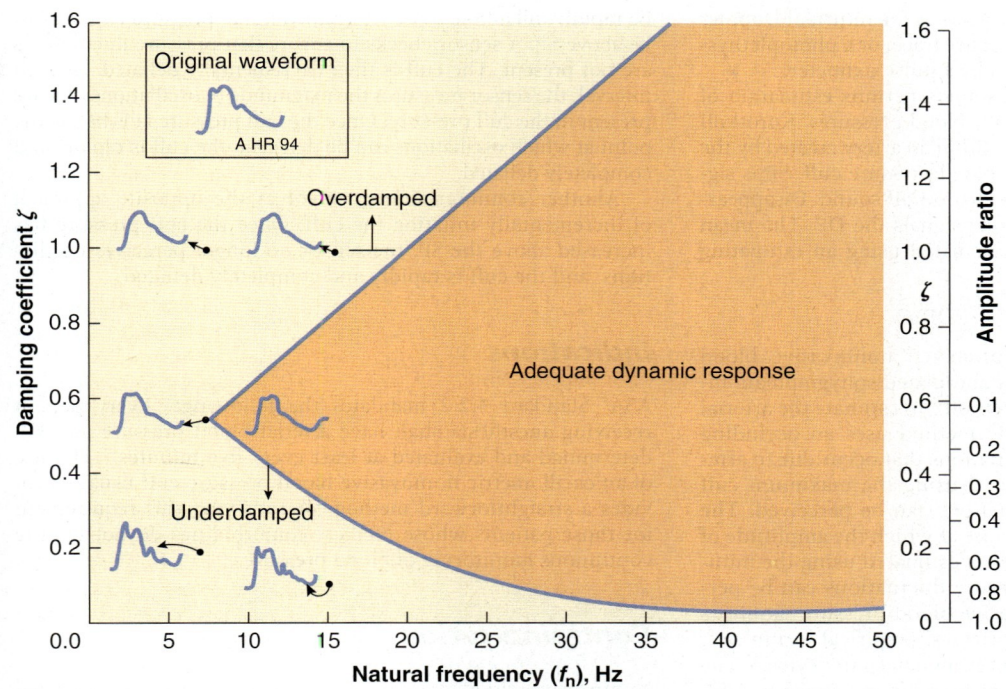

Figure 26-4 The relationship between the frequency of fluid-filled transducing systems and damping. The shaded area represents the appropriate range of damping for a given natural frequency (f_n). The size of the wedge also depends on the steepness of the arterial pressure trace and heart rate. (Adapted from Gardner RM. Direct blood pressure measurement–dynamic response requirements. *Anesthesiology*. 1981;54:227–236.)

Continuous-flush devices are incorporated into disposable transducer kits and infuse at 3 to 6 mL/hour. In neonates, the infusion volume may contribute to fluid overload. Continuous-flush devices have little effect on the blood pressure measurement. However, pressurized flush systems may serve as a source of an air embolism. Removing air from the pressurized infusion bag, stopcocks, and tubing minimizes the potential for air embolism.

A satisfactory Allen test does not rule out the possibility of formation of thrombus on the catheter and subsequent distal embolic complications. Although an intact palmar arch will provide some collateralization of arterial blood supply to the hand, this does not protect against emboli to the distal digital arteries.[40]

Invasive blood pressure monitoring in the pediatric population presents unique challenges for the anesthesiologist. Smaller-caliber arteries, lower circulating blood volume, and a closer anatomic proximity of peripheral vessels to the great vessels, the heart, and the cerebral circulation combine to make line placement more technically difficult and make line maintenance more hazardous. Three of the more common sites of arterial blood pressure monitoring in pediatric and neonatal anesthesia are the umbilical artery, the radial artery, and the femoral artery.

In critically ill newborn infants, the umbilical artery represents a convenient site for catheterization in order to measure arterial blood pressure and for blood sampling for laboratory values. Attaining access may require a cutdown procedure on the umbilical arteries.[41] Arterial catheters at this site carry a risk of aortic thrombosis and have been implicated in the development of other aortic complications, including coarctation; thus, these should be removed as soon as they are no longer necessary for patient care.[42,43]

The use of smaller catheters (i.e., 22 g, or even 24 g) for radial arterial catheterization in pediatric patients has been established as safe for invasive blood pressure monitoring in young patients, including children under 1 year of age. Preemptive use of ultrasound in radial artery cannulation may increase first-pass success and decrease iatrogenic injury in children.[44–46]

Femoral arterial lines have also been used extensively in critically ill infants and children, with high rates of success and low complication rates.[47] Though rare, complications including hematoma, minor bleeding, and AV fistula formation may occur.[48] Young children (age <3 years) are at increased risk of pediatric groin line complications requiring surgical intervention.[49] Routine use of ultrasound guidance in pediatric groin line placement decreases these risks.[50]

Practices commonly accepted in arterial line management and maintenance in adults may prove hazardous in pediatric patients. Arterial line flushing should be kept to a minimum, particularly in the care of smaller children and infants, to reduce the risk of volume overload and inadvertent hemodilution. High-pressure flushing should not be attempted in efforts to restore function to an apparently occluded indwelling arterial catheter. It is best to clear the line by hand with a small syringe, using the minimum pressure and volume necessary, as even small-volume flushes (0.5 to 1 mL) injected into the radial arteries of small infants using automated pressurizing systems may cause retrograde flow into the cerebral vessels.[51–55] Due to heightened risk of thromboembolism, blood removed in the process of arterial line sampling should only be returned to the patient intravenously (not arterially). Meticulous care must be taken to ensure that all arterial line tubing is tightened securely to prevent hemorrhage from line disconnection.

Intermittent Noninvasive Monitoring of Systemic Blood Pressure

Principles of Operation

The simplest method of blood pressure determination estimates systolic blood pressure by palpating the return of an arterial pulse while a more proximal occluding cuff is deflated. Modifications of this technique include the observance of the return of Doppler sounds, the transduced arterial pressure trace, or a photoplethysmographic pulse wave as produced by a pulse oximeter.

Auscultation of the Korotkoff sounds permits estimation of both systolic (SP) and diastolic (DP) blood pressures. Korotkoff sounds result from turbulent flow within an artery created by the mechanical deformation from the blood pressure cuff. SP is signaled by the appearance of the first Korotkoff sound. Disappearance of the sound or a muffled tone signals the DP. The mean arterial pressure (MAP) can be calculated using an estimating equation:

$$MAP = DP + (SP - DP)/3$$

In contemporary practice, automated noninvasive blood pressure monitors (also known as automated sphygmomanometers) employ the oscillometric method[56] to estimate the arterial blood pressure. The oscillometric method uses an occluding cuff to measure the pressure fluctuations that occur due to arterial pulsations. The SP is estimated using the maximum cuff pressure at which pressure oscillations can be perceived. The MAP is estimated by the cuff pressure at which the amplitude of the oscillations is greatest. The DP is estimated using the minimum cuff pressure at which pressure fluctuations can be perceived. Some automated noninvasive blood pressure monitors refine these estimates using proprietary, empirical formulae[57]; thus, results may not be consistent from device to device.[58] The operation of automated blood pressure cuffs is covered by US[59] and international[60] standards.

Proper Use and Interpretation

In the anesthetized patient, automated oscillometry is usually accurate and versatile. A variety of cuff sizes makes it possible to use oscillometry in all age groups. Different strategies of cuff inflation and deflation may be used to obtain blood pressure measurements. A common approach, as shown in Figure 26-5, is for the cuff to be rapidly inflated to a predetermined initial pressure expected to be above SP. A sensor checks to ensure that pressure fluctuations are not present. The cuff is then decrementally deflated. At each interval, the sensor measures the magnitude of oscillations that are present in the cuff pressure. Once the cuff pressure falls below the point at which oscillations can be detected, the cuff is rapidly and completely deflated.

Another common strategy involves the opposite approach of incrementally inflating the cuff. Once the cuff pressure has increased above the SP, the sensor no longer perceives oscillations, and the cuff is rapidly and completely deflated.

Indications

ASA[1] Standard 4.2.2 mandates the following: "Every patient receiving anesthesia shall have arterial blood pressure and HR determined and evaluated at least every five minutes." The use of an oscillometric noninvasive blood pressure cuff usually provides a straightforward method for satisfying this requirement for those patients whose medical comorbidities do not require continuous monitoring of blood pressure.

Contraindications

Noninvasive blood pressure cuffs apply force to the encircled limb that is sufficient to occlude blood flow. Contraindications to their use therefore exist in circumstances in which the patient is likely to sustain traumatic injury from this repeated mechanical process. Examples include local bone fracture (such as a humeral fracture), open injuries to the extremity, local presence of an arteriovenous dialysis fistula, or indwelling peripherally inserted central catheter (PICC) line. The site of measurement should also be carefully chosen in patients who have undergone axillary lymph node dissection, as these patients may have impaired lymphatic drainage from the associated limb and may be susceptible to limb edema from repeated vascular occlusion.

Noninvasive blood pressure cuffs can potentially become a source of iatrogenic injury even in normal use on a healthy limb. The repeated cycling of the blood pressure cuff during very prolonged surgical cases may lead to local skin abrasion or contusion; applying a light dressing underneath the cuff may mitigate these side effects. The radial nerve describes a spiraling path around the humerus and is also potentially susceptible to neurapraxia from mechanical compression.[61,62] During very prolonged surgical cases, it may be prudent to relocate the blood pressure cuff every few hours.

Common Problems and Limitations

The American Heart Association recommends that the bladder width for indirect blood pressure monitoring should approximate 40% of the circumference of the extremity. Bladder length should be sufficient to encircle at least 80% of the extremity. Falsely high estimates result when cuffs are too small, when cuffs are applied too loosely, or when the extremity is below heart level. Falsely low estimates result when cuffs are too large, when the extremity is above heart level, or after quick deflations.[63]

The detection of changes in Korotkoff sounds is subjective and prone to errors based on deficiencies in sound transmission or hearing. Cuff deflation rate also influences accuracy; quick deflations underestimate blood pressure. Noninvasive blood pressure

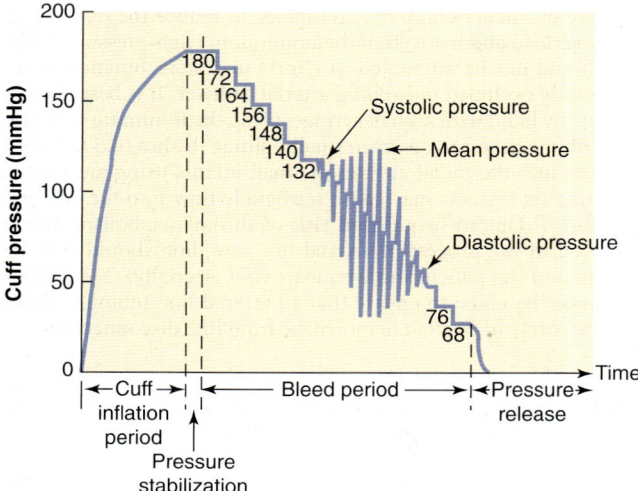

Figure 26-5 Sequence of oscillometric blood pressure determination. The pressure oscillations increase in magnitude, then decrease. The oscillations are analyzed to determine systolic, mean, and diastolic pressures as shown. (Adapted from Dorsch JA, Dorsch SE. *Understanding Anesthesia Equipment*. 4th ed. Baltimore, MD: Williams & Wilkins; 1999.)

cuffs are also subject to significant wear-and-tear from repeated use in the operating room. The development of a small air leak in the hose or cuff will often prevent the device from following its inflation strategy and render it inoperative.[64]

Palpation, auscultatory, and oscillometric techniques require pulsatile blood flow and may be unreliable during conditions of low flow or if the arterial walls are sufficiently sclerotic or stiffened such that pulsations are not readily transmitted.

Automated oscillometry has been demonstrated to correlate well with direct intra-arterial measurement of MAP and DP.[65–67] Oscillometry does require additional signal processing to smooth out pronounced respiratory variations or motion artifacts, but these events tend to occur at frequencies that are distinct from pulsatile variations in pressure. Cuff movement, erratic pulse transmission, arrhythmias, and inadvertent occlusion of the pressure tubing may influence accuracy. Periods of significant hemodynamic variability may require more frequent measurement of blood pressure to guide optimal intraoperative management.[68] This problem can be approached statistically by assessing the ability of a blood pressure measurement to predict the next blood pressure measurement, and hence the ability of the anesthesiologist to infer and intervene upon unacceptable trends in the blood pressure. Although Standard 4.2.2 mandates that blood pressure be measured only every 5 minutes, some evidence exists that this predictive ability may begin to decline for measurement intervals of greater than 3 minutes.[69]

Automated noninvasive blood pressure cuffs are usually placed around the upper arm, but it is usually acceptable to place the cuff around the forearm, wrist, or ankle if the upper arm is inaccessible or if the patient's body habitus is otherwise unfavorable.[70–72] As the site of measurement is moved more peripherally, the measured SP tends to increase, and the DP tends to decrease. An exception is the parturient undergoing cesarean section; the correlation between calf and upper arm blood pressures was found to be poor in this patient population.[73]

In pediatric patients, the upper extremity is generally the preferred site for blood pressure monitoring as it more closely correlates with cerebral perfusion. The greatest disparity between blood pressures measured in the upper versus lower extremity is found in patients weighing less than 1,000 g.[74] Premature infants, particularly those with pulmonary hypertension or respiratory distress, are at higher risk for having patent ductus arteriosus. Placing the blood pressure cuff on the right arm (preductal) gives the best approximation of cerebral perfusion in this patient population.[75]

Monitoring of Central Venous and Right-Heart Pressures

Principles of Operation

Central venous cannulas are important portals for intraoperative vascular access and for the assessment of changes in vascular volume. Central venous cannulas permit the rapid administration of fluids, insertion of pulmonary artery catheters (PACs) or central venous oximetry catheters, insertion of transvenous electrodes, monitoring of central venous pressure (CVP), and a site for observation and treatment of venous air embolism. The main value of monitoring central venous and right-heart pressures lies in their ability to approximate or trend in conjunction with the left ventricular end-diastolic pressure (LVEDP). The LVEDP predicts left-ventricular filling (i.e., left ventricular end-diastolic volume, LVEDV) through the Frank–Starling mechanism.

Figure 26-6 demonstrates the progression of pressures from CVP through LVEDP. Ideally, all proximal pressures reflect changes in LVEDP. The CVP is the easiest to measure as it does not require that any portion of the catheter to be placed within the heart. The CVP is essentially equivalent to right atrial pressure and serves as a reflection of right ventricular preload.[76] The output of the right ventricle and the output of the left ventricle must be approximately the same in a structurally normal cardiopulmonary system, notwithstanding a small amount of physiologic shunt. However, it has been well demonstrated that right-sided pressures in the heart often are poor indicators of left ventricular filling, either as absolute numbers or in terms of the direction of change in response to therapy. The correlation of these pressures as estimates of LVEDP (and, by extension, LVEDV) is directly related to their proximity to the left ventricle and the status of ventricular compliance. PACs therefore provide more clinical information than central venous monitoring

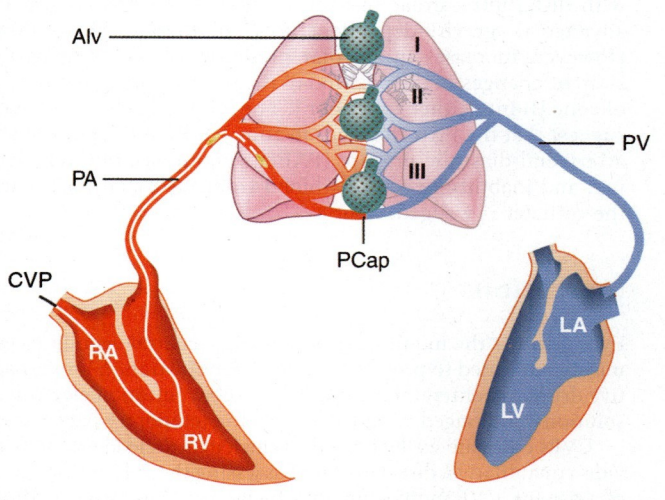

Figure 26-6 The progression of intracardiac pressures from central venous pressure to end-diastolic left ventricular pressure. The anatomic position of a pulmonary artery catheter in the pulmonary artery is shown. The dashed line shows the position of the inflated pulmonary artery catheter balloon in the "wedged" position. CVP, central venous pressure; RA, right atrium; RV, right ventricle; PA, pulmonary artery; Alv, alveolus; PCap, pulmonary capillary; PV, pulmonary vein; LA, left atrium; LV, left ventricle. I, II, and III characterize the relationship of $P_{aveolar}$, $P_{arterial}$, and P_{venous} as described by West et al.[77] The bottom of the figure shows a progressive correlation of vascular pressures. (Adapted from Vender JS. Invasive cardiac monitoring. *Crit Care Clin*. 1988;4:455–477.)

alone; PACs are able to separate the behavior of the right side of the heart, the lung parenchyma, and the left side of the heart. Pulsatile pressures in the pulmonary artery provide an assessment of right ventricular function. The *pulmonary capillary wedge pressure* (PCWP) provides the closest approximation to LVEDP. The PAC is allowed to wedge, with the balloon inflated, in the pulmonary vasculature. During end-diastole, there is cessation of forward blood flow and a static fluid column is presumed to exist from the left ventricle to the PAC tip with no pressure drop.

The measurement of right-heart pressures can therefore indirectly assess left ventricular preload, diagnose the existence of pulmonary hypertension, or differentiate cardiac and noncardiac causes of pulmonary edema.

Proper Use and Interpretation

Careful leveling and zeroing of the pressure transducers is essential, as described earlier for invasive arterial pressure monitoring. The normal CVP waveform, as shown in Figure 26-7, consists of three peaks (a, c, and v waves) and two descents (x, y), each resulting from the ebb and flow of blood in the right atrium. The character of the CVP trace depends on many factors, including HR, conduction disturbances, tricuspid valve function, normal or abnormal intrathoracic pressure changes, and changes in right ventricular compliance. In patients with atrial fibrillation, a waves are absent. When resistance to the emptying of the right atrium is present, large a waves are often observed. Examples include tricuspid stenosis, right ventricular hypertrophy as a result of pulmonic stenosis, or acute or chronic lung disease associated with pulmonary hypertension. Large a waves may also be observed when right ventricular compliance is impaired.

Tricuspid regurgitation typically produces giant v waves that begin immediately after the QRS complex. Large v waves are often observed when right ventricular ischemia or failure is present or when ventricular compliance is impaired by constrictive pericarditis or cardiac tamponade. A prominent v wave during CVP monitoring may suggest right ventricular papillary muscle ischemia and tricuspid regurgitation. When right ventricular compliance decreases, the CVP often increases with prominent a and v waves fusing to form an m or w configuration.

CVP monitoring can be unreliable for estimating left ventricular filling pressures, especially when cardiac or pulmonary parenchymal disease processes alter the normal cardiovascular pressure–volume relationships. However, CVP monitoring is

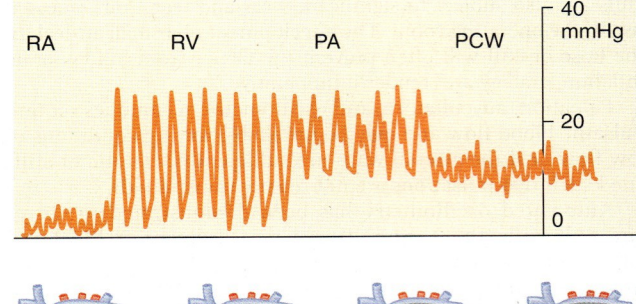
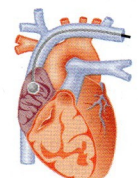 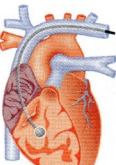 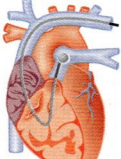 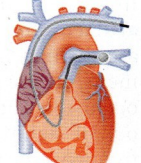

Figure 26-8 Pressure tracing observed during the flotation of a pulmonary artery catheter. RA, right atrium; RV, right ventricle; PA, pulmonary artery; PCW, pulmonary capillary wedge pressure. (Adapted from Dizon CT, Barash PG. The value of monitoring pulmonary artery pressure in clinical practice. *Conn Med.* 1977;41:622–625.)

less invasive and less costly than pulmonary artery monitoring and offers an understanding of right-sided hemodynamic events and the status of vascular volume. The validity of PAC monitoring depends on a properly functioning pressure monitoring system, correctly identifying the "true" PCWP and integration of the various factors that affect the relationship of PCWP, and the other cardiac pressures and volumes that are determinants of ventricular function. Figure 26-8 depicts the transduced pressure waves observed as a PAC is floated to the wedged position. Catheter placement is most commonly performed by observing the pressure waves as the catheter is floated from the CVP position through the right heart chambers into the pulmonary artery.

West et al.[77] described a gravity-dependent difference between ventilation and perfusion in the lung. The variability in pulmonary blood flow is a result of differences in pulmonary artery (P_A), alveolar (P_{alv}), and venous pressures (P_V) and is categorized into three distinct zones, as shown in Figure 26-6. Only Zone III ($P_A > P_V > P_{alv}$) meets the criteria for uninterrupted blood flow and for a continuous communication via a static fluid column with distal intracardiac pressures. Flow-directed PACs usually advance to gravity-dependent areas of highest blood flow. However, increases in alveolar pressure, decreases in perfusion, or changes in the position of the patient can convert areas of zone III into either zone II or I. The following characteristics suggest that the PAC tip is not in zone III: PCWP > pulmonary artery end-diastolic presure (PAEDP), nonphasic PCWP tracing, and inability to aspirate blood from the distal port when the catheter is wedged.

Indications

Even without the monitoring of pressures, central venous access may be indicated to provide a route of administration for vasoactive drugs, parenteral nutrition, higher-concentration electrolyte solutions, prolonged vascular access, or a temporary pacemaker.

CVPs correlate well with right ventricular preload and so provide a quantitative, direct means of assessing the volumetric status of a patient. CVP monitoring may be indicated in cases in which there are expected to be rapid or large shifts in intravascular

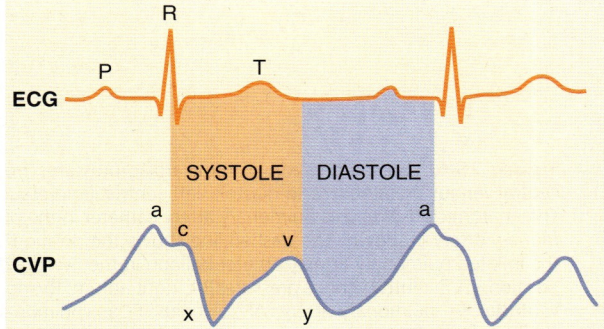

Figure 26-7 The normal central venous pressure (CVP) trace. ECG, electrocardiogram. (Adapted from Mark JB. Central venous pressure monitoring: Clinical insights beyond the numbers. *J Cardiothorac Vasc Anesth.* 1991;5:163–173.)

volume. CVP monitoring may also be useful in assessing volumetric status when other clinical signs of volumetric status, such as urine output, may be inaccurate or unavailable due either to the procedure or to the patient's comorbidities.

PACs have not been shown to improve outcomes.[78] The decision to place a PAC therefore requires careful individualization of patient care. There must be a specific question regarding the patient's management that can only be addressed with the data that the catheter will provide. This question should be of sufficient importance that the plan of management will potentially be altered depending on the results of PAC monitoring. The information that PACs provide may be particularly informative in the management of patients with severe pulmonary hypertension or to help differentiate noncardiogenic and cardiogenic shock.

Contraindications

Obstruction at the mitral valve from mitral stenosis, atrial myxoma, or clot can interfere with the ability of left atrial pressure to reflect LVEDP. Similarly, mitral regurgitation, a noncompliant left atrium, or left-to-right intracardiac shunting often is associated with large v waves. Decreases in left ventricular compliance, aortic regurgitation, or premature closure of the mitral valve may reverse the left atrial pressure–LVEDP pressure gradient. When these comorbidities occur, PCWP is not a valid reflection of LVEDP.

Central venous access represents an invasive process with inherent risks, some of which are rare but are potentially life-threatening. Adverse effects from CVP or PAC monitoring can be a result of accessing the central venous circulation, the catheterization procedure, or from use or presence of the catheter after placement. Unintentional puncture of nearby arteries, bleeding, neuropathy, and pneumothorax may result from needle insertion into adjacent structures. Air embolism may occur if a cannula is open to the atmosphere and air is entrained during or after catheter placement. Dysrhythmias are common during the catheterization procedure, with a reported incidence of 4.7% to 68.9%. Ventricular tachycardia or fibrillation may be induced during catheter advancement. Catheter advancement has been associated with right bundle-branch block and may precipitate complete heart block in patients with pre-existing left bundle-branch block. The most dreaded complication associated with PAC monitoring is pulmonary artery rupture. Pulmonary hypertension, coagulopathy, and heparinization are often present in patients who have died of pulmonary artery rupture. Perforations and subsequent hemorrhage can be avoided by restricting "overwedging," minimizing the number of balloon inflations, and using proper technique during balloon inflations. Table 26-4 summarizes the adverse effects as reported by the ASA Task Force on pulmonary artery catheterization.[79]

Common Problems and Limitations

The right internal jugular vein is the most common site for cannulation by anesthesiologists because it is accessible from the head of the operating table, has a predictable anatomy, and has a high success rate in both adults and children.[80] The left-sided internal jugular vein is also available but is less desirable because of the potential for damaging the thoracic duct or difficulty in maneuvering catheters through the jugular–subclavian junction. Accidental carotid artery puncture is a potential problem with either location. Use of an ultrasound-guided technique is now strongly recommended to reduce complications and improve first-attempt success rates.[81]

Alternatives to the internal jugular vein include the external jugular, subclavian, antecubital, and femoral veins. Although the Centers for Disease Control and Prevention suggests that the preferred site for central venous cannulation should be the subclavian site to potentially reduce bloodstream infections, this recommendation must be taken in the context of the particular clinical situation.[81] The internal jugular approach may be superior in those patients with coagulopathies (in whom bleeding at the subclavian site may be more difficult to stop) or patients with severe acute lung injury (for whom the risk of pneumothorax may be heightened). When comparing the subclavian approach with the femoral approach, the reported reduction in infection risk favors subclavian. However, there is a paucity of prospective randomized data when comparing subclavian to internal jugular.[82] Infection is a potential complication of the continued use of CVP catheters and PACs, although ongoing research suggests that this complication may be preventable with scrupulous attention to sterile technique.[83]

Femoral, subclavian, and internal jugular veins are all utilized for central venous access in infants and children. Physician experience and comfort is the primary determinant of insertion site and has the greatest impact on complication rates for each site.[84]

Table 26-4 Adverse Effects Associated with Pulmonary Artery Monitoring

Complication	Reported Incidence (%)
Central venous access	
Arterial puncture	0.1–13
Postoperative neuropathy	0.3–1.1
Pneumothorax	0.3–4.5
Air embolism	0.5
Flotation of pulmonary artery catheter	
Minor dysrhythmias	4–68.9
Ventricular tachycardia or fibrillation	0.3–62.7
Right bundle-branch block	0.1–4.3
Complete heart block (prior left bundle-branch block)	0–8.5
Complications associated with catheter residence	
Pulmonary artery rupture	0.03–1.5
Positive cultures from catheter tip	1.4–34.8
Sepsis secondary to catheter residence	0.7–11.4
Thrombophlebitis	6.5
Venous thrombosis	0.5–66.7
Pulmonary infarction	0.1–5.6
Mural thrombus	28–61
Valvular or endocardial vegetations	2.2–100
Deaths attributed to pulmonary artery catheter	0.02–1.5

Reprinted with permission from American Society of Anesthesiologists Task Force on Pulmonary Artery Catheter. Practice guidelines for pulmonary artery catheterization: an updated report by the American Society of Anesthesiologists Task Force on Pulmonary Artery Catheterization. *Anesthesiology*. 2003;99(4):988–1014.

At all three sites, routine use of ultrasound for central venous catheter placement may decrease risk of iatrogenic vascular injury.[85] Subclavian venous catheters in pediatric patients may have a lower risk of dislodgment as well as being less restrictive to patients' range of motion.[84] Disadvantages of subclavian lines include lower success rates of placement and increased rates of catheter malposition, inadvertent arterial puncture, and pneumothorax.[86] The femoral vein may be the preferential site of central venous access in critically ill pediatric patients.[87] As with femoral arterial line placement, the use of ultrasound guidance for femoral venous line placement in children may decrease risk of iatrogenic vascular injury.[50] Femoral venous lines in children do not appear to carry an increased risk of infection compared with subclavian and jugular venous catheters,[88] although there is a higher risk of line maintenance-related complications, particularly catheter thrombosis, and accidental dislodgment. Internal jugular catheterizations appear to have the highest placement success rate, though they may cause increased patient discomfort, as site dressings may limit neck mobility.[86]

Monitoring of Cardiac Output by Pulmonary Arterial Catheter

Principles of Operation

Provided that the heart is structurally normal, without septal defects and without a patent ductus so that no intracardiac recirculation or shunting of blood can occur, the time-averaged flow of blood through the right ventricular outflow tract (RVOT) will accurately approximate the CO. A small amount of venous return to the left side of the heart from the bronchial circulation and thebesian veins is neglected. Time averaging suppresses the effects of beat-to-beat pulsatility.

A properly positioned PAC passes through the RVOT. CO monitoring using a pulmonary arterial catheter therefore depends on assessing the rate of blood flow through the right side of the heart and using this as a measure of CO. Techniques to measure the flow rate are based upon the idea of measuring the dilution by the passing blood flow of some known quantity of an indicator.[89] This indicator could be a dye, O_2 content (Fick method), or CO_2 content (indirect Fick method).[90] However, the most commonly used technique in clinical practice is based upon thermodilution.[91] Thermodilution cardiac output (TCO) depends on the measurement of temperature near the tip of the PAC using a thermistor.

CO can be assessed intermittently by using a bolus injection of room-temperature or chilled fluid as the indicator. The thermistor on the pulmonary arterial catheter records the fall in temperature as this bolus is injected via a more proximal port on the PAC and mixes with the surrounding blood flow. The total flow through the RVOT, and hence the CO, can be estimated from the area under this blood temperature curve, combined with knowledge of the specific heat capacity and gravity of blood and the injectate, the volume of the injectate, and the size of the catheter. When performed properly, TCO measurements correlate well with direct Fick or dye dilution estimates of CO.[92]

Continuous CO monitoring offers the potential to identify acute changes in ventricular performance as they occur. Pulsed thermodilution uses a coiled filament that applies a low-power heating signal within the right atrium and ventricle in a cyclical manner based on a proprietary pseudorandom sequence. The thermistor at the tip of the PAC detects these changes in blood temperature and sends the temperature information to a microcomputer that uses stochastic analysis to create a thermodilution curve. CO is then computed in a similar fashion to the bolus technique, using a conservation of heat equation, although effectively using a warmed bolus rather than a chilled bolus.[93] Another technique applies heat to a thermistor located at the tip of a PAC. The blood flow through the right ventricular outflow subsequently cools the tip, and the temperature changes registered are proportional to the rate of blood flow. Although a time lag can exist, continuous CO monitoring compares favorably with bolus CO measurements, even under conditions of varying patient temperature and CO.

Proper Use and Interpretation

TCO estimates can vary with the respiratory cycle. Performing measurements at peak inspiration or end expiration can reduce this variability. Ensuring that the rate of injection and the volume are constant enhances precision. Most TCO computers require that repeat measurements be delayed for 30 to 90 seconds to stabilize the thermal environment of the PAC thermistor. The TCO computer displays the CO directly in L/min.

TCO measurements depend on the assumption that changes in thermal energy are carried forward to the thermistor; thus, the measurements depend on the correct positioning of the catheter. If the catheter is insufficiently advanced such that the port through which a bolus injectate is administered is still within the introducer sheath, then there will be reflux of the injectate within the introducer sheath. This will result in some of the change in thermal energy being "lost" into the sheath. A smaller-than-expected change in temperature will then be seen at the thermistor, appearing as if the injectate had been injected into a larger volume of blood flow. The TCO computer will interpret and present this as an erroneously high CO. Similarly erroneous readings may be produced if the catheter is advanced too far, such that the heating filament of a continuous TCO catheter lies beyond the pulmonic valve. Hypothermia and the rapid concurrent administration of unwarmed intravenous fluids may affect the accuracy of TCO measurements.

Indications

Measurement of CO is required to determine physiologic factors such as the rate of oxygen delivery to peripheral tissues. Possible clinical indications include severe sepsis, cardiogenic shock, and dependence on inotropes. An additional technologic refinement of the pulmonary arterial catheter is the *oximetric* PAC, which uses reflectance spectrophotometry to identify the saturation of the mixed venous blood surrounding the tip of the PAC, SvO_2. Three-wavelength in vivo systems correlate well with simultaneous samples measured by co-oximetry.[94] Knowledge of the SvO_2 allows the rate of extraction of oxygen by peripheral tissues ($\dot{\psi}o_2$) to be calculated. Neglecting the small amount of oxygen dissolved in blood:

$$\dot{\psi}o_2 = 13.8 \times [Hgb] \times CO \times (SaO_2 - SvO_2)$$

where [Hgb] is the concentration of hemoglobin, 13.8 is a conversion factor for the oxygen-carrying capacity of hemoglobin, CO is the cardiac output in L/min, and ($SaO_2 - SvO_2$) is the difference between the arterial and mixed venous oxygen saturations.

The use of PACs in practice has diminished over the last decade[95]; this may partly be due to the greater use of techniques such as transesophageal echocardiography and arterial waveform analysis that can estimate CO in a less-invasive manner.

However, thermodilution via a PAC remains the clinical gold standard for the determination of CO and should be considered when knowledge of the CO is necessary for the patient's management and when other comorbidities would render less invasive techniques inaccurate.

Contraindications

Measurement of CO requires a PAC that is designed for the purpose. There are no additional contraindications for CO monitoring.

Common Problems and Limitations

The intermittent TCO technique assumes that there is adequate mixing of the cooled injectate with the surrounding blood flow. It is necessary that the temperature of the injectate be distinct from the temperature of the blood in order to generate a change in the distal temperature measurement. Improved measurements can be obtained by using a cooler injectate, producing a greater temperature change to detect and hence an improved signal-to-noise ratio.[96]

The presence of intracardiac shunts or significant tricuspid regurgitation can invalidate the assumptions underlying TCO. Intracardiac shunts allow accessory blood flow paths, such that flow through the RVOT may no longer approximate CO accurately. Significant tricuspid regurgitation can compromise thermodilution methods by permitting retrograde blood flow, invalidating the assumption that all changes in thermal energy caused by the indicator are carried forward to the detecting thermistor.

Clinicians are unable to estimate the cardiac index in pediatric patients reliably, even using associated clinical indicators such as SV variation, blood pressure, and HR.[97,98] Nevertheless, continuous CO monitoring is rarely used in the perioperative management of pediatric patients. Femoral arterial thermodilution (FATD) has been validated as an alternative to pulmonary arterial thermodilution techniques in patients ranging from infancy to adolescence.[99,100] FATD correlates closely with Fick-based calculations while only minimally overestimating cardiac index.[100] When compared to pulmonary-arterial sampling methods, FATD monitoring systems are less hazardous to place, as they avoid the potential for pneumothorax and pulmonary arterial injury.[99]

Monitoring of Cardiac Output by Arterial Waveform Analysis

Principles of Operation

The use of a PAC remains the gold standard for the determination of CO, but the use of PACs in the management of patients requiring intensive care has not been demonstrated to be associated with reduced mortality.[101] PACs can be associated with a high rate of iatrogenic complications,[102] and the ASA recommends that only clinicians with regular ongoing experience of the procedure[79] should place pulmonary catheters. Nevertheless, the determination of CO allows more accurate assessment of the hemodynamic status of a critically ill patient than can be obtained by clinical assessment alone. This conundrum has created increasing interest in biomedical devices that can estimate CO in a less invasive manner; arterial waveform analysis is one such technique.[103]

There are three arterial waveform CO devices on the market that are based on peripheral arterial pressure readings from an invasive arterial cannula: FloTrac (Edwards Lifesciences, Irvine, CA), PiCCO (PULSION Medical Systems AG, Munich, Germany), and LiDCOrapid (LiDCO Ltd., London, UK).[104] These devices directly measure the fluctuations in arterial pressure and the HR, from which they estimate the beat-to-beat SV. The CO is given by the product of the HR and SV (CO = HR × SV).

A more recent device, ClearSight (Edwards Lifesciences, Irvine, CA) does not use an invasive arterial cannula, but instead uses a noninvasive finger blood-pressure cuff (Nexfin, Ultron, The Netherlands) that is dynamically inflated and deflated to attempt to track the blood pressure in the brachial artery. This means of inferring arterial blood pressure relies on a method originally described by Peñáz,[105] in which the fingertip is compressed by a pressure cuff while simultaneously being transilluminated by infrared light. Arterial pulsations cause the volume of blood within the fingertip to increase, increasing the absorption of infrared light by hemoglobin. The system rapidly changes the inflation pressure of the cuff to attempt to hold the absorption of infrared light constant. Because the infrared absorption is held constant, according to the Peñáz method, the volume of blood within the fingertip must be constant, which means that the pressures applied to the fingertip are exactly equal and opposed to the arterial pulsation. Consequently, the cuff pressures must equal the arterial pressures. This simple model has been subsequently refined to include compensation for pressure reflection in the vascular tree between the fingertip and brachial artery[106] and to reflect the variable vertical fluid column between the fingertip and the heart.[107] This noninvasive reconstruction of an arterial waveform also allows CO to be estimated by waveform analysis.

It is a straightforward matter to measure HR from an arterial waveform tracing; it is the estimation of beat-to-beat SV that presents the technical challenge. The first modern mathematical description of the shape of the arterial waveform was described by Otto Frank,[108] and gave rise to the "Windkessel" (German: *air chamber*) model for arterial behavior. Usually when considering the flow of an incompressible fluid, such as blood, in a section of tube, the assumption is made that the volume of the fluid entering the tube is the same as the volume of the fluid leaving the tube. This assumption allows a *continuity equation* to be created from which models of fluid flow can be derived. The basis of the Windkessel model is the realization that although blood is incompressible, the artery itself is distensible, and so the volumes of blood entering and leaving an arterial segment at any given moment may be different. There is storage of blood and distension of the artery during systole and ejection of blood and relaxation of the artery during diastole. The volumes of blood entering and leaving are only the same when averaged over the cardiac cycle, as shown in Figure 26-9.

This behavior is mathematically similar to that seen in the modeling of a compressible fluid, such as air, when flowing in rigid vessels, hence the name of the "Windkessel" model. The air may store and release energy through changes in pressure and compression. In arterial waveform analysis, it is the fluid that is incompressible, and it is the nonrigid arterial vessel that may store and release energy by elastic deformation. The behavior of the artery is dependent on its resistance to flow R and its compliance C; from cadaveric studies of the human aorta,[109] these values are known to be predictable.

The total SV must be equal to the forward flow in systole Q_s plus the forward flow in diastole Q_d, assuming the aortic valve is competent.

$$SV = Q_s + Q_d$$

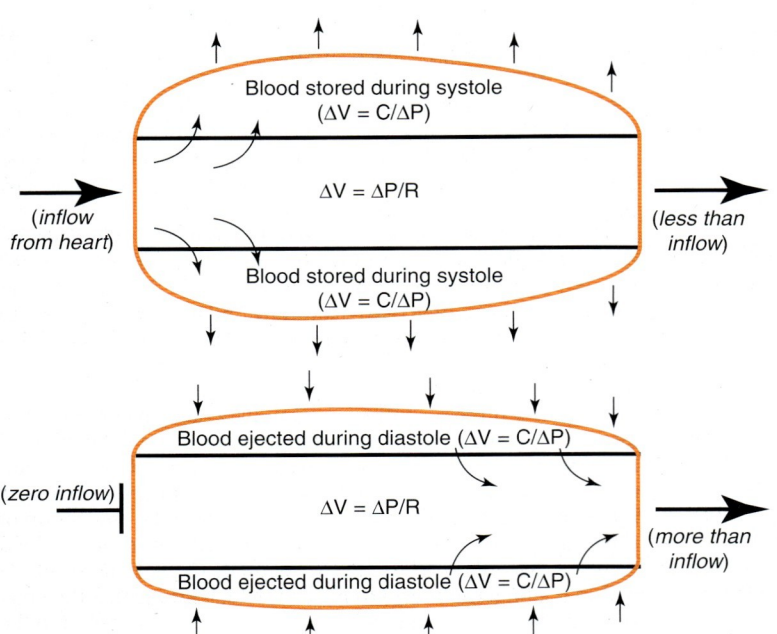

Figure 26-9 Depiction of blood flow into and out of a prototypical "Windkessel artery." Several points are to be noted: first, during systole, inflow into the artery is less than outflow because some of the blood is stored in the expanding compliant vessel. Second, during diastole, inflow into the artery is zero and outflow is enhanced by the contracting vessel. C, compliance; P, pressure; R, resistance; V, volume. (Adapted from Thiele RH, Durieux ME. Arterial waveform analysis for the anesthesiologist: Past, present, and future concepts. *Anesth Analg*. 2011; 113:766–776.)

At the beginning of diastole, there is no further inflow into the aorta, and so Q_d is proportional to the difference between the pressure in the aorta and the pressure in the arterial beds. This is described as the end-systolic mean distending pressure P_{md}, equivalent to the idea of a "pressure head." Therefore,

$$Q_d = k \times P_{md}$$

where k is a constant of proportionality dependent on the properties of resistance and compliance, as described earlier. As the peripheral vascular resistance should not change over a single cardiac cycle, the values of Q_s and Q_d should be proportional to A_s and A_d, the areas under the pressure curve during systole and diastole, respectively, as shown in Figure 26-10. Therefore,

$$Q_s/A_s = Q_d/A_d \quad \text{or, alternatively,} \quad Q_s = Q_d \frac{A_s}{A_d}$$

Rearranging these model equations:

$$SV = Q_d \left(1 + \frac{A_s}{A_d}\right) \quad \text{and so} \quad SV = kP_{md}\left(1 + \frac{A_s}{A_d}\right)$$

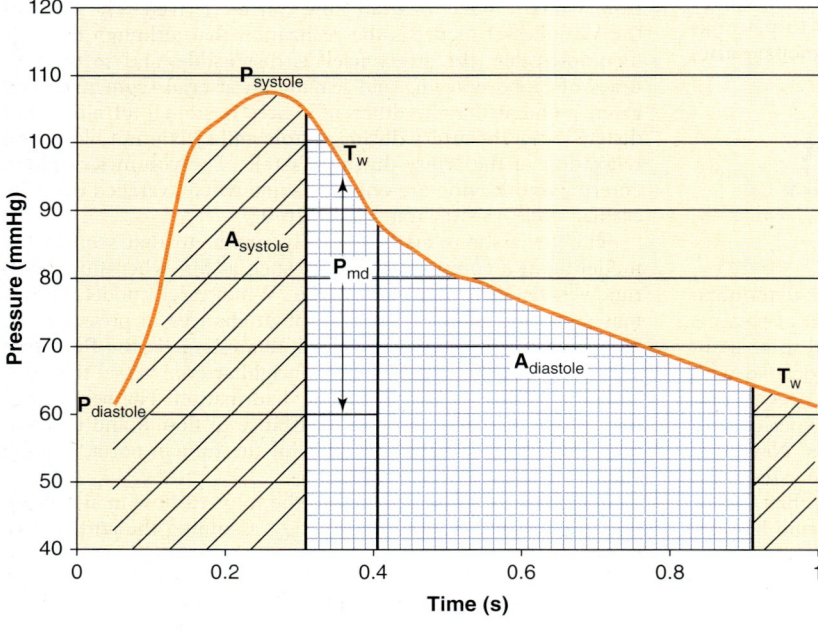

Figure 26-10 A graphical depiction of the components of the arterial waveform used by the Windkessel-based area under the curve method. Note that P_{md} represents the increment in mean pressure over the whole arterial bed at the end of systole[168] and that T_w represents the transmission time (from the aorta to the periphery). (Adapted from Thiele RH, Durieux ME. Arterial waveform analysis for the anesthesiologist: Past, present, and future concepts. *Anesth Analg*. 2011;113:766–776.)

This model demonstrates how, in principle, a beat-to-beat estimate of SV can be generated from measurements of the arterial waveform. The algorithms used by actual clinical devices are more complex and proprietary. Although the previous analysis is necessarily simplified, it nevertheless illustrates the fundamental principles and requirements of these devices. For instance, the model depends on an additional value k, which has to be determined either by calibrating the prediction of this model to another measurement of SV (such as transesophageal echocardiography [TEE] or thermodilution) or in an uncalibrated manner by estimating its value from biophysical models based on variables such as the patient's age, sex, height, and weight.[110] The PiCCO device makes use of an external calibration reading, whereas the FloTrac and LiDCOrapid devices use an uncalibrated biophysical model approach.

Proper Use and Interpretation

Arterial waveform CO monitors make use of standard equipment for arterial cannulation. A stiff arterial line, flushed from a pressurized fluid source, is attached to the arterial cannula in the usual fashion. However, in place of the usual piezoelectric pressure sensor with a single electrical connection, a specialized sensor is used with two connectors so that pressure information can be supplied simultaneously to the anesthesia monitor and to the CO monitor. The arterial line is zeroed in the usual fashion. The display of arterial pressures by the anesthesia monitor is unaffected by the presence of the CO monitor. It is possible to transduce arterial pressures alone without connecting the CO monitor. Uncalibrated devices, such as the FloTrac and LiDCOrapid, require information about the patient such as age, height, weight, and sex in order to estimate the physiologic properties of the patient's arterial system and estimated body surface area. The device may require a brief interval of time to gather initial arterial pressure data, but will shortly begin to report CO and other indices such as cardiac index, SV, stroke volume variation (SVV), and SV index. These indices represent various combinations of SV, HR, and body surface area. Further user intervention is not generally required. These values, in the manner estimated by the device, are most useful for assessing relative volume status and for assessing the response to fluid resuscitation.[111–114] The ability of the device to respond to changes in CO caused by inotropes or vasopressors[111,115] is uncertain; the limits of its reliability, accuracy, and utility in this setting are the subject of ongoing research and algorithmic refinement.

Indications

The use of an arterial waveform CO monitor is not mandated so the indications for use are at the discretion of the practitioner. The device is likely to be most helpful to the clinician in cases in which there are expected to be large fluid shifts and in which the patient's intravascular volume status may become difficult to determine by clinical assessment and usual monitoring techniques. It may be preferable, and less invasive, to guide fluid resuscitation with arterial waveform CO measurements rather than placing a central venous catheter or a PAC. This approach is particularly attractive if the patient already requires an arterial line for other indications or if the patient's comorbidities relatively contraindicate the placement of a central line or PAC. The FloTrac device has been demonstrated to show excellent concordance with TEE in measuring CO under conditions of changing fluid preload.[111]

It is possible to extract other indices from analysis of the arterial waveform, and measurements such as systolic pulse variation (SPV) and SVV may also be useful in predicting responsiveness to fluid resuscitation.[116,117]

Contraindications

Devices such as the FloTrac and LiDCOrapid that do not require additional calibration are no more invasive than the arterial line to which they are attached. The same contraindications that apply to arterial lines, such as poor or absent collateralization of arterial supply to the extremity, also apply to these devices.

Devices that estimate CO from the arterial waveform do so based upon a number of physiologic assumptions that were touched upon during the derivation of the simplified model. There are many disease states, some common, which violate these assumptions and can significantly compromise the accuracy of the device; these are discussed later.

Common Problems and Limitations

All arterial waveform CO monitors are dependent on accurate, high-fidelity measurement of arterial pressures. Satisfactory operation depends upon good arterial perfusion to the site of measurement and good peripheral arterial cannulation. The pressure transducer system must use appropriate tubing and be flushed and zeroed correctly so that bias, signal dampening, or flail are not seen in the arterial waveform. These artifacts corrupt the frequency spectrum of the arterial waveform, and impair accurate measurement. The use of an intra-aortic balloon pump may distort the arterial waveform to such an extent that the resulting waveform is uninterpretable, rendering the device inoperative.[118]

The simplified model of arterial waveform analysis made use of information obtained from only a single cardiac cycle. In contrast, all of the current monitors make use of algorithms that depend on information obtained over many cardiac cycles. The FloTrac monitor depends, for example, upon the standard deviation, skewness, and kurtosis of the statistical distribution of arterial pressures obtained over the preceding 20 seconds.[110] This implicitly assumes that the CO remains relatively beat-to-beat constant over the sampling interval. This assumption can be violated in the presence of irregular heart rhythms, in which the preload of the left ventricle and hence the SV can demonstrate significant beat-to-beat variability. Arterial waveform CO monitors are therefore known to be prone to inaccuracy in the setting of atrial fibrillation.[119]

In the simplified model, the properties of systemic vascular resistance (SVR) and arterial compliance (C) were subsumed into the parameter k, and it was proposed that k might be obtained from a population-based biophysical model. However, in the presence of sepsis[115,120] or some other high-output state, such as liver transplantation surgery,[114] the deviation of these values from the expected population norms can cause inaccuracy when compared to the measurement of CO by PAC. With ongoing research and refinement of the devices and their algorithms, this situation appears to be improving.[113] However, a similar problem applies to the iatrogenic reduction of the compliance of arterial vessels through the administration of vasopressors. Arterial waveform CO devices appear to be reliable at assessing changes in CO caused by fluid resuscitation, of some utility at detecting changes caused by inotropes,[111] but poor at assessing changes caused by alteration in vascular tone by agents such as phenylephrine[111] or norepinephrine.[112]

Finally, arterial waveform analysis depends upon the assumption that there is no further inflow into the arterial system at the end of systole, as used in the analysis based on the parameter P_{md}. This assumption is violated in the setting of aortic insufficiency, in which there is negative regurgitant flow to the left ventricle. Arterial waveform analysis is expected to demonstrate inaccuracy in this presentation.[118] Conversely, aortic stenosis does not appear to impair the accuracy of measurement of CO.

Use of the entirely noninvasive ClearSight/Nexfin system has so far been limited in clinical practice. In one published trial, the CO estimated by the device showed a satisfactory correlation with a different invasive arterial waveform CO monitor (PiCCO).[121] However, when compared directly to the gold standard of CO monitoring via a PAC, the absolute accuracy of the device appeared to be limited.[122]

In summary, arterial waveform analysis has been demonstrated in many studies to provide a reasonable estimate of CO and a reasonable approximation to more invasive techniques. The degree to which a new monitoring technique must agree with the gold standard to be clinically useful is a matter of clinical judgment and not a question that can be definitively addressed by statistics alone. Presently, these devices appear to be most useful as guides to fluid resuscitation and for trend monitoring rather than as guides to the administration of inotropes or vasopressors. There are a number of relatively common clinical scenarios in which the accuracy of these devices can be anticipated to be impaired based upon violation of the underlying physiologic assumptions on which their algorithms depend. The clinician must exercise caution in interpreting the measurements of CO obtained under those circumstances.

In the pediatric population, estimation of CO via arterial waveform analysis has proven more challenging. A technique called pressure recording analytical method (PRAM) has had only mixed results in its ability to reliably estimate pediatric CO despite the use of more advanced algorithms and higher sampling frequencies.[123–125] Moreover, pediatric studies of this technology have excluded children with hemodynamic instability, arguably the clinical circumstance in which CO monitoring would be most useful to the anesthesiologist.[123,124]

Monitoring of Body Temperature

Principles of Operation

Heat is produced as a consequence of cellular metabolism. In adults, thermoregulation involves the control of basal metabolic rate, muscular activity, sympathetic arousal, vascular tone, and hormone activation balanced against exogenous factors that determine the need for the body to create heat or to adjust the transfer of heat to the environment. Both general and regional anesthesia inhibit afferent and efferent control of thermoregulation.[126,127]

Heat losses may result from radiation, conduction, convection, and evaporation. Radiation refers to the infrared rays emanating from all objects above absolute temperature. Conduction refers to the transfer of heat from contact with objects. Convection refers to the transfer of heat from air passing by objects. Evaporation represents the heat loss that results when water vaporizes. For every gram of water evaporated, 0.58 kcal of heat is lost. Perioperative hypothermia predisposes patients to increases in metabolic rate (shivering) and cardiac work, decreases in drug metabolism and cutaneous blood flow, and creates impairments of coagulation. Anesthesiologists frequently monitor temperature and attempt to maintain central core temperature at near-normal values in all patients undergoing anesthesia. Clinical studies have demonstrated that patients in whom intraoperative hypothermia develops are at a higher risk for development of postoperative myocardial ischemia and wound infection compared with patients who are normothermic in the perioperative period.[128,129]

Proper Use and Interpretation

Central core temperatures can be estimated using probes that can be placed into the bladder, distal esophagus, ear canal, trachea, nasopharynx, or rectum.[130] Pulmonary artery blood temperature is also a good estimate of central core temperature. Thermoregulatory responses are based on a physiologically weighted average reflecting changes in the mean body temperature. Mean body temperature is estimated by the following equation:

$$T_{mean\ body} = 0.85\ T_{core} + 0.15\ T_{skin}$$

Indications

The ability to monitor body temperature is a standard of anesthesia care.[1] The continual observation of temperature changes in anesthetized patients allows for the detection of accidental heat loss or malignant hyperthermia.

Contraindications

There are no absolute contraindications to temperature monitoring. In patients whose thermoregulatory responses are intact, such as conscious patients or patients receiving light or moderate sedation, continuous temperature monitoring is usually uninformative.

Common Problems and Limitations

Skin temperature monitoring has been advocated to identify peripheral vasoconstriction but is not adequate to determine alterations in mean body temperature that may occur during surgery. Core temperature sites have been established as reliable indicators of changes in mean temperature. During routine noncardiac surgery, temperature differences between these sites are small. When anesthetized patients are being cooled, changes in rectal temperature often lag behind those of other probe locations, and the adequacy of rewarming is best judged by measuring temperature at several locations. Although liquid crystal skin temperature strips are convenient to apply, they do not correlate with core temperature measurements.[131]

Monitoring of Processed EEG Signals

Principles of Operation

EEG monitoring initially entered anesthetic practice as a highly sensitive and moderately specific means of monitoring for cerebral ischemia, and as such found use in carotid surgery. Occlusion of one of the carotid arteries for surgery makes the ipsilateral side of the brain dependent on perfusion from the contralateral carotid artery via the Circle of Willis, creating a risk of ipsilateral ischemia. In this form, a dedicated technician usually performs intraoperative EEG monitoring.

More recently, EEG monitoring has begun to gain acceptance as a means of estimating depth of anesthesia. Statistical signal-processing techniques have been developed and embodied as biomedical devices that are able to take an ensemble of EEG data and, in real time, display an estimate of "anesthetic depth." The two most commonly used processed EEG monitors are the bispectral index (BIS) (Covidien, King of Prussia, PA) and SedLine (Masimo Irvine, CA) The operation of these devices is similar. After first cleaning the patient's forehead, a single-use set of small adhesive electrical sensors are applied. The sensors are positioned to enable the device to detect EEG activity in the frontal lobes of the brain. The sensors are attached to the main device via a single connector. The device checks the quality of the electrical connection to the sensors, and checks that each of the sensors has made a good electrical contact with the patient's forehead and that the sensors are not in inadvertent electrical connection with each other. In the event that the configuration of the sensors is unacceptable, the device displays a pictorial indication of the problem so that the practitioner can attempt to remedy the problem. If the electrical connection between the sensor and the skin is poor, signal reception will be impaired and the device will warn that the sensor impedance (i.e., its electrical resistance) is too high. The sensors make use of a conductive electrical gel; this can often be remedied by applying firm but careful pressure to the affected sensor to produce a better electrical contact. However, too much pressure may cause the gel to leak out from under the sensor and cause a "gel bridge," an inadvertent direct electrical connection to a neighboring electrode. In this case, the surplus gel may be wiped away or a new set of sensors may be required. When all the electrical connections are satisfactory, the device will begin to acquire and process EEG data.

Although the algorithms used by processed EEG monitors are proprietary, the general features of the EEG that they use are well described.[132] Processed EEG monitors make use of the following statistical measures:

- Zero Crossing Frequency (ZXF). An estimate of the "average" frequency of the EEG, obtained by calculating the number of times the EEG voltage crosses the zero voltage level per second.[133]
- Burst Suppression Ratio (BSR). During periods of deep anesthesia, the EEG may demonstrate periods of low voltage or even zero (isoelectric) voltage, and bursts of higher voltage activity are no longer seen. Suppressed states are defined as those periods for which the EEG demonstrates a voltage of less than 5 mV for a period of at least 0.5 seconds, and the BSR is defined as that ration of that time fraction to the overall EEG recording. Profoundly burst suppressed (isoelectric) states are sometimes induced as part of neuroanesthesia,[134] as they may provide some protection against cerebral ischemia by reducing cellular metabolic demand. Burst suppression is also seen in unanesthetized comatose patients, although in these patients it carries a grave prognosis.[135]
- Median Power Frequency (MPF) and Spectral Edge Frequency (SEF): The EEG signal can be converted to a frequency spectrum using the Fast Fourier Transform,[136] making it possible to describe the amount of signal power present at various frequencies. The MPF is the frequency at which the power in the signal can be split into two equal frequency bands, above and below. The SEF is the frequency below which 95% of the total signal power can be found.[132]
- Beta (β)-Power Ratio: The β-power ratio describes the relative amount of β_2-wave activity in the EEG signal (signal power between 30 and 47 Hz) compared to the amount of β-wave activity (signal power between 11 and 20 Hz). Changes in this ratio appear to correlate clinically with the onset of light sedation.
- Bispectrum. The bispectrum is a second-order property of the frequency spectrum of the EEG signal.[137] The bispectrum can be used to calculate bicoherence, a mathematical property that describes the similarity in phase between signals at three different frequencies: f_1, f_2, and $f_1 + f_2$. A high level of bicoherence is suggestive that the signals may be generated from a common underlying rhythm. As sedation is increased, local cortical activity becomes suppressed and the EEG activity begins to demonstrate a greater underlying cortical synchronization, which can be detected as increased bicoherence in the EEG signal.

Proper Use and Interpretation

Both the BIS and SedLine devices display a unitless number in the range of 0 to 100, which is derived from the measured EEG data by the device's proprietary algorithms. A value of 0 corresponds to an absence of any discernable electrical activity. A value of 100 corresponds to the EEG activity seen in a fully awake and alert individual. The algorithms used in the devices specify a differing "optimal range" for general anesthesia: for the BIS it is defined as between 40 and 60, for the SedLine it is 25 to 50.

The algorithms used in the devices appear to correlate best with clinical assessment of the depth of anesthesia when anesthetic agents such as volatile gases or propofol are used, as shown in Figure 26-11, although increasing concentrations of these agents do not always reliably lower the reported number further[138–140] if the patient is already deeply anesthetized. This relationship between concentration and effect is not seen for all anesthetic agents.

Dissociative intravenous agents such as ketamine can actively confound processed EEG monitors through paradoxical cortical excitation; the monitor tends to misread the increased cortical activity as a sign of lessened anesthesia.[141] Lower doses of ketamine may be desirable as part of an overall anesthetic plan to reduce opioid administration; appropriate quantities of ketamine can be infused more slowly without apparently affecting the processed EEG reading.[142] Propofol and remifentanil are often used in combination for total intravenous anesthesia (TIVA), but processed EEG monitors can be insensitive to the administration of even high concentrations of opioids.[143] The monitor may therefore reflect mostly the action of the propofol on the anesthetic state.

Indications

The use of processed EEG monitors is not mandated; thus, the indications for use are at the discretion of the practitioner. Processed EEG monitors have not been demonstrated to be superior to end-tidal agent concentration monitoring in the prevention of awareness under anesthesia. However, the use of end-tidal agent concentration monitoring assumes that volatile anesthetic gases are used and that their end-tidal concentrations provide a reasonable surrogate for their action on consciousness. Processed EEG monitoring may be useful as a guide when a TIVA approach is planned, since it can provide some degree of feedback on the current pharmacodynamics effects of the administered agents when there is no end-tidal agent concentration to measure.

Patients with pre-existing cognitive deficits, sensory impairment,[144] or known risk of postoperative delirium may benefit

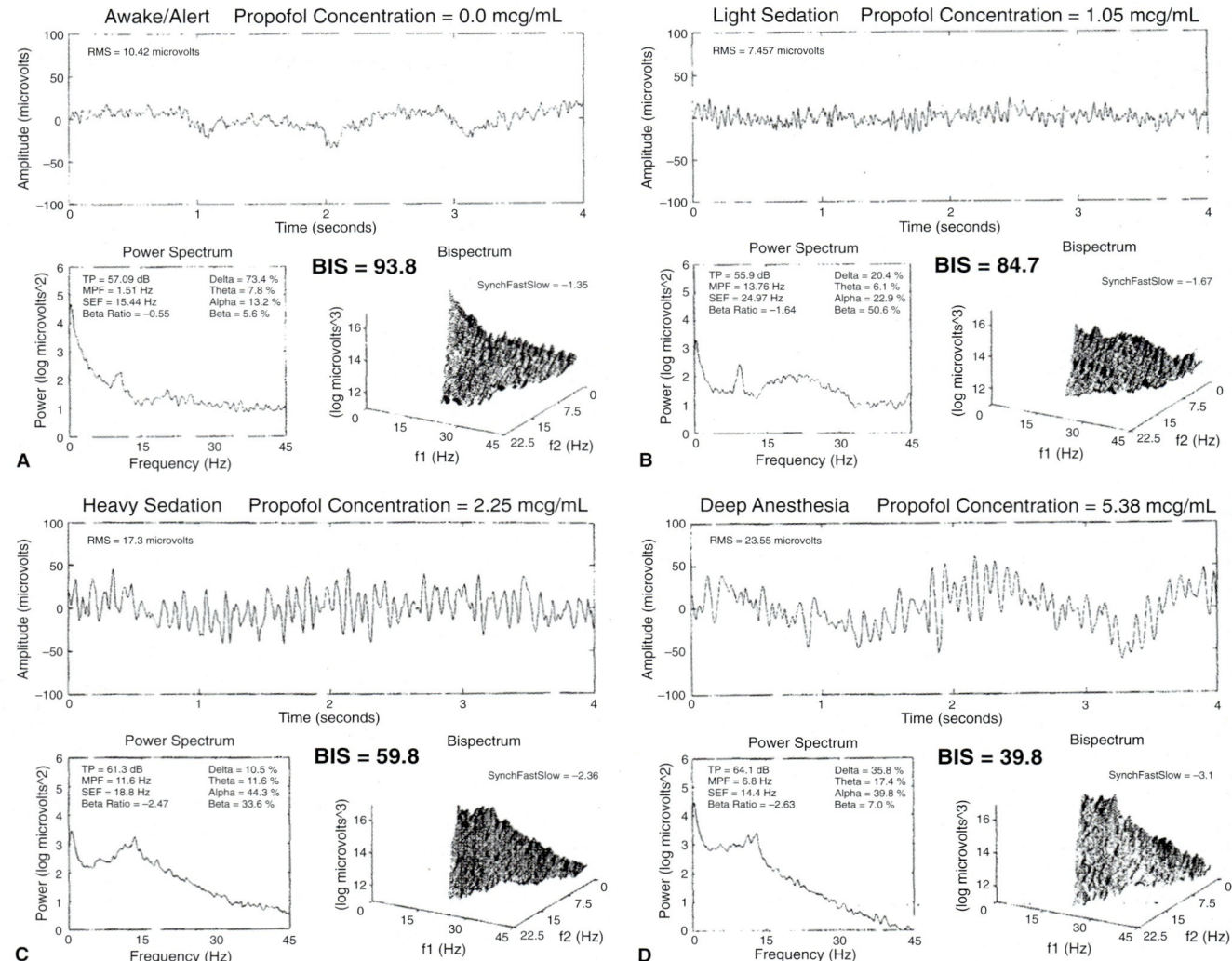

Figure 26-11 Representative data from a single human volunteer demonstrating changes in EEG with increasing serum concentrations of propofol. In each of the four concentrations, 4 seconds of raw EEG data is plotted in the top half of the figure. In the lower left is the corresponding power spectrum and spectral parameters computed from the same EEG epoch. The lower right quadrant displays the bispectrum for the same raw data. The final BIS score is shown. Figures **A, B, C,** and **D** represent increasingly deeper levels of anesthesia. (Adapted from Rampil IJ. A primer for EEG signal processing in anesthesia. *Anesthesiology.* 1998;89:980–1002.)

from the administration of less anesthesia than would be indicated by end-tidal agent monitoring alone.[145] Processed EEG monitoring may be useful in satisfactorily titrating their anesthetic plan to permit faster recovery from anesthesia.[146]

For types of emergent surgery, such as cesarean sections under general anesthesia,[147] trauma laparotomies, or surgery in the critically ill hemodynamically unstable patient, it may not be physiologically possible to administer the usual quantities of anesthesia, placing these patients at a greater risk of intraoperative awareness. Processed EEG monitoring may provide some assistance in titrating anesthesia in these vulnerable patients and some reassurance that explicit recall will be unlikely. A prior history of intraoperative awareness may therefore also be an indication.

Mechanically ventilated patients in the intensive care unit are usually assessed clinically for their level of sedation, but the use of the standard Sedation-Agitation Scale or the Richmond Agitation-Sedation Scale may be impossible in some patients due to therapeutic neuromuscular paralysis. Processed EEG monitors may provide some guidance to sedation management under these circumstances.[148,149]

Contraindications

Use of a processed EEG device may be contraindicated in a patient with significant craniofacial trauma, such that the physical pressure required to place the sensors cannot be safely applied. Placement may also be relatively contraindicated in patients with existing superficial injury to the forehead in the region where the sensors will be applied.

The use of processed EEG sensors for patients who will be in prone position for surgery is controversial and may be a relative contraindication. In prone position, the patient's head may rest such that excessive continuous pressure is applied to the skin underneath the sensors. Disfiguring injury to the forehead has been reported,[150] perhaps related to a combination of pressure and irritation from the conductive gel on the sensors. This can lead to a dilemma: prolonged spinal surgery performed using somatosensory or motor evoked potential monitoring can relatively contraindicate the use of volatile gases and neuromuscular blockers, and make a propofol–remifentanil TIVA technique attractive. This anesthetic technique provides an indication for processed EEG monitoring, but the prolonged prone positioning provides a relative contraindication. Prone positioning requires vigilant attention to facial features, such as the eyes and nose, to avoid injury by pressure and impingement. Therefore, if it is determined that processed EEG monitoring is to be applied to a prone patient, it is recommended that equally vigilant attention be paid to the condition of the forehead.

Common Problems and Limitations

It has been suggested that processed EEG monitoring devices may reduce the risk of intraoperative awareness.[151] However, subsequent studies have either failed to demonstrate a reduction[152] in intraoperative awareness or even, conversely, have found an increase in intraoperative awareness[26] when compared to anesthetic practice guided by the end-tidal agent concentrations[20] of anesthetic gases[25].

Cases of intraoperative awareness were found when using either end-tidal agent concentration monitoring or processed EEG monitoring; neither technique was sufficient to avoid awareness with complete reliability. This difficulty may relate to our lack of understanding of what "anesthetic depth" even means.[145,153] Intraoperative awareness as a phenomenon is dependent on the interaction of consciousness, memory, and the biologic action of anesthetic agents. These, even taken individually, are complex and incompletely understood processes.[154–156] It should not therefore be surprising that any device or algorithm that seeks to reduce these processes to a single numerical readout may prove to be fallible.

Compared to adults, pediatric patients have more than three times greater incidence of awareness under anesthesia.[157–159] At the same time, there is a conflicting pressure to reduce exposure to anesthetic agents in young children. An increasing body of evidence suggests that anesthetic agents harm early brain development, reinforced by recent studies demonstrating a decline in listening comprehension and performance IQ in young children following surgery with anesthesia.[160] A number of attempts have been made to investigate the utility of perioperative processed EEG monitoring to guide care in these younger patients. Some evidence supports the application of the adult BIS algorithm in children age above 12 months, but infant BIS values do not closely correlate with end-tidal sevoflurane concentrations.[161] As with adults, processed EEG may be a useful adjunct in this patient demographic, but is not a substitute for provider vigilance and contextual clinical judgment.

Future Trends in Monitoring

Anesthesiologists have been at the forefront of the incorporation of innovative biomedical devices and technologies into their practice. We will continue to adapt our practice to make use of new technologies to enhance patient safety. There are three trends in device design that appear most likely to lead to further improvements in our practice: greater automated marshaling of monitoring and clinical data, the dissemination of our current devices into wider hospital use, and the development of devices with greater algorithmic sophistication to obtain clinical data less invasively.

The Anesthesia Information Management Systems (AIMS) will continue to become more interconnected with patient monitoring devices, as well as with drug delivery systems such as infusion pumps and vaporizers. The AIMS will also begin to interface more deeply with hospital-wide Computerized Provider Order Entry (CPOE) systems, allowing patient clinical data and documentation to be available immediately to the anesthesiologist. The safety of the administration of intravenous medications will be enhanced by the routine use of machine-readable labels, whether by barcoding or radiofrequency identification (RFID), so that the intended administration of a medication will be known to the AIMS prior to the actual administration. The AIMS will make use of this information to alert to the potential for drug interactions and allergies during the case itself immediately prior to administration. The automatic availability of this data will allow the AIMS to provide decision support to the anesthesiologist, tracking the administration of intravenous medications and providing predictions of plasma and effect site concentrations to improve dose titration. Overall, improvements in the automated marshaling and display of patient data will assist the anesthesiologist with situational awareness. Further, using more intelligent alarm systems to decrease false-positive alerts will more accurately guide the anesthesiologist to aspects of the patient's management that require attention. The sophistication of AIMS user interfaces will continue to improve so that the interaction between the anesthesiologist and the tasks of computer-based monitoring and charting will become smooth, fast, natural, and efficient.

In the recent revision of the ASA Standards for Basic Monitoring,[1] the indications for capnography have been broadened to include the evaluation of ventilation during moderate or deep sedation. Moderate sedation may be performed by clinicians untrained in the practice of anesthesia; the effect of this standard will be the dissemination of capnographic equipment previously used only by anesthesiologists to the wider care environment. Anesthesiologists should be at the forefront of educational efforts to ensure that our medical colleagues use these devices appropriately, enhancing patient safety.

A trend in the development of biomedical devices is toward devices that use complex algorithmic models to infer clinical data in a less invasive or more rapid manner. Examples are arterial waveform CO monitors that produce an estimate of CO from the arterial pressure tracing alone, noninvasive hemoglobin monitors that estimate serum hemoglobin from infrared pulse oximetry, target-controlled infusion pumps that make use of population pharmacokinetic and pharmacodynamics data to estimate the redistribution and effect of a medication, and processed EEG monitors that attempt to reduce an ensemble of EEG data to a quantitated end point of consciousness. These devices are examples of incredible biomedical sophistication, usually the product of decades of scientific research and subsequent engineering refinement. However, the algorithms that these devices use are generally derived from the responses of healthy volunteers. The protocols used for the development of the algorithms are often seemingly simplistic or artificial when compared to the complexity of actual anesthetic practice. The result is that, during their initial introduction to practice, the functionality of the devices in the sickest of patients is not necessarily well characterized or understood. To put it more briefly: it may work, but does it *really* work? It is our sickest patients who have the most to gain from devices that allow us to assess their clinical condition more rapidly and less invasively, but it is our sickest patients who are the most vulnerable should the devices tend to become inaccurate under just those clinical conditions. The limits of the reliability and clinical applicability of these devices must be a matter of concern for the practicing anesthesiologist. Though devices are becoming "smarter," that knowledge does not excuse us of the knowledge to know how to employ them wisely.

REFERENCES

1. American Society of Anesthesiologists. *Basic Anesthetic Monitoring, Standards for 2015*. Schaumburg, IL: American Society of Anesthesiologists; 2015.
2. Merilainen PT. A differential paramagnetic sensor for breath-by-breath oximetry. *J Clin Monit.* 1990;6(1):65–73.
3. Roe PG, Tyler CK, Tennant R, et al. Oxygen analysers. An evaluation of five fuel cell models. *Anaesthesia.* 1987;42(2):175–181.
4. Meyer RM. Oxygen analyzers: Failure rates and life spans of galvanic cells. *J Clin Monit.* 1990;6(3):196–202.
5. Bageant RA. Oxygen analyzers. *Respir Care.* 1976;21(5):410–416.
6. Barker L, Webb RK, Runciman WB, et al. The Australian Incident Monitoring Study. The oxygen analyser: applications and limitations–an analysis of 200 incident reports. *Anaesth Intensive Care.* 1993;21(5):570–574.
7. Kaddoum RN, Chidiac EJ, Zestos MM, et al. Electrocautery-induced fire during adenotonsillectomy: report of two cases. *J Clin Anesth.* 2006;18(2):129–131.
8. Roy S, Smith LP. What does it take to start an oropharyngeal fire? Oxygen requirements to start fires in the operating room. *Int J Pediatr Otorhinolaryngol.* 2011;75(2):227–230.
9. Ortega R, Hansen CJ, Elterman K, et al. Videos in clinical medicine. Pulse oximetry. *N Engl J Med.* 2011;364(16):e33.
10. Barker SJ, Curry J, Redford D, et al. Measurement of carboxyhemoglobin and methemoglobin by pulse oximetry: a human volunteer study. *Anesthesiology.* 2006;105(5):892–897.
11. Barker SJ. "Motion-resistant" pulse oximetry: A comparison of new and old models. *Anesth Analg.* 2002;95(4):967–972.
12. Nishiyama T. Pulse oximeters demonstrate different responses during hypothermia and changes in perfusion. *Can J Anaesth.* 2006;53(2):136–138.
13. Eberhard P, Severinghaus JW. Measurement of heated skin O2 diffusion conductance and PO2 sensor induced O2 gradient. *Acta Anaesthesiol Scand Suppl.* 1978;68:1–3.
14. Moller JT, Johannessen NW, Espersen K, et al. Randomized evaluation of pulse oximetry in 20,802 patients: II. Perioperative events and postoperative complications. *Anesthesiology.* 1993;78(3):445–453.
15. Rolf N, Cote C. Diagnosis of clinically unrecognized endobronchial intubation in paediatric anaesthesia: which is more sensitive, pulse oximetry or capnography? *Pediatr Anesth.* 1992;2(1):31–35.
16. Murat I, Constant I, Maud'huy H. Perioperative anaesthetic morbidity in children: a database of 24,165 anaesthetics over a 30-month period. *Paediatr Anaesth.* 2004;14(2):158–166.
17. White DC, Wardley-Smith B. The "narkotest" anaesthetic gas meter. *Br J Anaesth.* 1972;44(10):1100–1104.
18. Westenskow DR, Smith KW, Coleman DL, et al. Clinical evaluation of a Raman scattering multiple gas analyzer for the operating room. *Anesthesiology.* 1989;70(2):350–355.
19. Jee GI, Roy RJ. Adaptive control of multiplexed closed-circuit anesthesia. *IEEE Trans Biomed Eng.* 1992;39(10):1071–1080.
20. Walder R, Lauber R, Zbinden AM. Accuracy and cross-sensitivity of 10 different anesthetic gas monitors. *J Clin Monit.* 1993;9(5):364–373.
21. Colman Y, Krauss B. Microstream capnograpy technology: a new approach to an old problem. *J Clin Monit Comput.* 1999;15(6):403–409.
22. Williamson JA, Webb RK, Cockings J, et al. The Australian incident monitoring study. The capnograph: applications and limitations–an analysis of 2000 incident reports. *Anaesth Intensive Care.* 1993;21(5):551–557.
23. Lockwood GG, White DC. Measuring the costs of inhaled anaesthetics. *Br J Anaesth.* 2001;87(4):559–563.
24. Eger EI, 2nd, Saidman LJ, Brandstater B. Minimum alveolar anesthetic concentration: A standard of anesthetic potency. *Anesthesiology.* 1965;26(6):756–763.
25. Eger EI, 2nd. Age, minimum alveolar anesthetic concentration, and minimum alveolar anesthetic concentration-awake. *Anesth Analg.* 2001;93(4):947–953.
26. Avidan MS, Jacobsohn E, Glick D, et al. Prevention of intraoperative awareness in a high-risk surgical population. *N Engl J Med.* 2011;365(7):591–600.
27. Patel R, Lenczyk M, Hannallah RS, et al. Age and the onset of desaturation in apnoeic children. *Can J Anaesth.* 1994;41(9):771–774.
28. Weiss M, Dullenkopf A, Fischer JE, et al. European Paediatric Endotracheal Intubation Study G. Prospective randomized controlled multi-centre trial of cuffed or uncuffed endotracheal tubes in small children. *Br J Anaesth.* 2009;103(6):867–873.
29. Jaffe MB. *Mainstream or Sidestream Capnography?* Wallingford CT: Respironics Novametrix, Inc., 2002.
30. Kugelman A, Zeiger-Aginsky D, Bader D, Bader, et al. A novel method of distal end-tidal CO2 capnography in intubated infants: Comparison with arterial CO2 and with proximal mainstream end-tidal CO2. *Pediatrics.* 2008;122(6):e1219–e1224.
31. Hagerty JJ, Kleinman ME, Zurakowski D, et al. Accuracy of a new low-flow sidestream capnography technology in newborns: a pilot study. *J Perinatol.* 2002;22(3):219–225.
32. Kleinman B, Powell S, Kumar P, et al. The fast flush test measures the dynamic response of the entire blood pressure monitoring system. *Anesthesiology.* 1992;77(6):1215–1220.
33. Slogoff S, Keats AS, Arlund C. On the safety of radial artery cannulation. *Anesthesiology.* 1983;59(1):42–47.
34. McGregor AD. The Allen test––an investigation of its accuracy by fluorescein angiography. *J Hand Surg Br.* 1987;12(1):82–85.
35. Tegtmeyer K, Brady G, Lai S, et al. Videos in clinical medicine. Placement of an arterial line. *N Engl J Med.* 2006;354(15):e13.
36. Maher JJ, Dougherty JM. Radial artery cannulation guided by Doppler ultrasound. *Am J Emerg Med.* 1989;7(3):260–262.
37. Levin PD, Sheinin O, Gozal Y. Use of ultrasound guidance in the insertion of radial artery catheters. *Crit Care Med.* 2003;31(2):481–484.
38. Hobai IA, Bittner EA, Grecu L. Perioperative spinal cord infarction in non-aortic surgery: report of three cases and review of the literature. *J Clin Anesth.* 2008;20(4):307–312.
39. Vender JS, Watts DR. Differential diagnosis of hand ischemia in the presence of an arterial cannula. *Anesth Analg.* 1982;61(5):465–468.
40. Mangano DT, Hickey RF. Ischemic injury following uncomplicated radial artery catheterization. *Anesth Analg.* 1979;58(1):55–57.
41. Clark JM, Jung AL. Umbilical artery catheterization by a cutdown procedure. *Pediatrics.* 1977;59 Suppl(6 Pt 2):1036–1040.
42. Goetzman BW, Stadalnik RC, Bogren HG, et al. Thrombotic complications of umbilical artery catheters: A clinical and radiographic study. *Pediatrics.* 1975;56(3):374–379.
43. Adelman RD, Morrell RE. Coarctation of the abdominal aorta and renal artery stenosis related to an umbilical artery catheter placement in a neonate. *Pediatrics.* 2000;106(3):E36.
44. Varga EQ, Candiotti KA, Saltzman B, et al. Evaluation of distal radial artery cross-sectional internal diameter in pediatric patients using ultrasound. *Paediatr Anaesth.* 2013;23(5):460–462.
45. Schwemmer U, Arzet HA, Trautner H, et al. Ultrasound-guided arterial cannulation in infants improves success rate. *Eur J Anaesthesiol.* 2006;23(6):476–480.
46. Ishii S, Shime N, Shibasaki M, et al. Ultrasound-guided radial artery catheterization in infants and small children. *Pediatr Crit Care Med.* 2013;14(5):471–473.
47. Venkataraman ST, Thompson AE, Orr RA. Femoral vascular catheterization in critically ill infants and children. *Clin Pediatr (Phila).* 1997;36(6):311–319.
48. Kelm M, Perings SM, Jax T, et al. Incidence and clinical outcome of iatrogenic femoral arteriovenous fistulas: Implications for risk stratification and treatment. *J Am Coll Cardiol.* 2002;40(2):291–297.
49. Lin PH, Dodson TF, Bush RL, et al. Surgical intervention for complications caused by femoral artery catheterization in pediatric patients. *J Vasc Surg.* 2001;34(6):1071–1078.
50. Iwashima S, Ishikawa T, Ohzeki T. Ultrasound-guided versus landmark-guided femoral vein access in pediatric cardiac catheterization. *Pediatr Cardiol.* 2008;29(2):339–342.
51. Butt WW, Gow R, Whyte H, et al. Complications resulting from use of arterial catheters: Retrograde flow and rapid elevation in blood pressure. *Pediatrics.* 1985;76(2):250–254.
52. Weiss M, Balmer C, Cornelius A, et al. Arterial fast bolus flush systems used routinely in neonates and infants cause retrograde embolization of flush solution into the central arterial and cerebral circulation. *Can J Anaesth.* 2003;50(4):386–391.
53. Murphy GS, Szokol JW, Marymont JH, et al. Retrograde air embolization during routine radial artery catheter flushing in adult cardiac surgical patients: An ultrasound study. *Anesthesiology.* 2004;101(3):614–619.
54. Murphy GS, Szokol JW, Marymont JH, et al. Retrograde blood flow in the brachial and axillary arteries during routine radial artery catheter flushing. *Anesthesiology.* 2006;105(3):492–497.
55. Cornelius A, Fischer J, Frey B, et al. Pressurized bag pump and syringe pump arterial flushing systems: An unrecognized hazard in neonates? *Intensive Care Med.* 2002;28(11):1638–1643.
56. Ng KG, Small CF. Survey of automated noninvasive blood pressure monitors. *J Clin Eng.* 1994;19(6):452–475.
57. Ramsey M, 3rd. Blood pressure monitoring: Automated oscillometric devices. *J Clin Monit.* 1991;7(1):56–67.
58. Kaufmann MA, Pargger H, Drop LJ. Oscillometric blood pressure measurements by different devices are not interchangeable. *Anesth Analg.* 1996;82(2):377–381.
59. Institute ANS. *Manual, Electronic or Automated Sphygmomanometers*. New York, NY: American National Standard Institute; 2002.
60. Commission IE. Part 2–30. *Particular Requirements for the Safety, Including Essential Performance, of Automatic Cycling Non-Invasive Blood Pressure Monitoring Equipment*. Geneva, Switzerland: International Electrotechnical Commission; 1999.

61. Swei SC, Liou CC, Liu HH, et al. Acute radial nerve injury associated with an automatic blood pressure monitor. *Acta Anaesthesiol Taiwan.* 2009;47(3):147–149.
62. Lin CC, Jawan B, de Villa MV, et al. Blood pressure cuff compression injury of the radial nerve. *J Clin Anesth.* 2001;13(4):306–308.
63. Jones DW, Appel LJ, Sheps SG, et al. Measuring blood pressure accurately: new and persistent challenges. *JAMA.* 2003;289(8):1027–1030.
64. Webb RK, Russell WJ, Klepper I, et al. The Australian incident monitoring study. Equipment failure: an analysis of 2000 incident reports. *Anaesth Intensive Care.* 1993;21(5):673–677.
65. Loubser PG. Comparing direct and indirect arterial blood pressures. *Anesthesiology.* 1985;63(5):566–567.
66. Nystrom E, Reid KH, Bennett R, et al. A comparison of two automated indirect arterial blood pressure meters: With recordings from a radial arterial catheter in anesthetized surgical patients. *Anesthesiology.* 1985;62(4):526–530.
67. van Egmond J, Hasenbos M, Crul JF. Invasive v. non-invasive measurement of arterial pressure. Comparison of two automatic methods and simultaneously measured direct intra-arterial pressure. *Br J Anaesth.* 1985;57(4):434–444.
68. Derrick JL, Bassin DJ. Sampling intervals to record severe hypotensive and hypoxic episodes in anesthetised patients. *J Clin Monit Comput.* 1998;14(5):347–351.
69. Harrison MJ, Connor CW. Statistics-based alarms from sequential physiological measurements. *Anaesthesia.* 2007;62(10):1015–1023.
70. Emerick DR. An evaluation of non-invasive blood pressure (NIBP) monitoring on the wrist: Comparison with upper arm NIBP measurement. *Anaesth Intensive Care.* 2002;30(1):43–47.
71. Singer AJ, Kahn SR, Thode HC, Jr., et al. Comparison of forearm and upper arm blood pressures. *Prehosp Emerg Care.* 1999;3(2):123–126.
72. Block FE, Schulte GT. Ankle blood pressure measurement, an acceptable alternative to arm measurements. *Int J Clin Monit Comput.* 1996;13(3):167–171.
73. Zahn J, Bernstein H, Hossain S, et al. Comparison of non-invasive blood pressure measurements on the arm and calf during cesarean delivery. *J Clin Monit Comput.* 2000;16(8):557–562.
74. Konig K, Casalaz DM, Burke EJ, et al. Accuracy of non-invasive blood pressure monitoring in very preterm infants. *Intensive Care Med.* 2012;38(4):670–676.
75. McEwan A. Anesthesia for children undergoing heart surgery. In: Cote CJ, Lerman J, Todres ID, ed. *A Practice of Anesthesia for Infants and Children.* 4th ed. Philadelphia, PA: Saunders/Elsevier; 2009:331–359.
76. Mark JB. Central venous pressure monitoring: Clinical insights beyond the numbers. *J Cardiothorac Vasc Anesth.* 1991;5(2):163–173.
77. West JB, Dollery CT, Naimark A. Distribution of blood flow in isolated lung; relation to vascular and alveolar pressures. *J Appl Physiol.* 1964;19:713–724.
78. Shah MR, Hasselblad V, Stevenson LW, et al. Impact of the pulmonary artery catheter in critically ill patients: Meta-analysis of randomized clinical trials. *JAMA.* 2005;294(13):1664–1670.
79. American Society of Anesthesiologists Task Force on Pulmonary Artery Catheterization. Practice guidelines for pulmonary artery catheterization: an updated report by the American Society of Anesthesiologists Task Force on Pulmonary Artery Catheterization. *Anesthesiology.* 2003;99(4):988–1014.
80. Ortega R, Song M, Hansen CJ, et al. Videos in clinical medicine. Ultrasound-guided internal jugular vein cannulation. *N Engl J Med.* 2010;362(16):e57.
81. O'Grady NP, Alexander M, Burns LA, et al. Summary of recommendations: Guidelines for the prevention of intravascular catheter-related infections. *Clin Infect Dis.* 2011;52(9):1087–1099.
82. Hamilton HC, Foxcroft DR. Central venous access sites for the prevention of venous thrombosis, stenosis and infection in patients requiring long-term intravenous therapy. *Cochrane Database Syst Rev.* 2007;(3):CD004084.
83. Pronovost P, Needham D, Berenholtz S, et al. An intervention to decrease catheter-related bloodstream infections in the ICU. *N Engl J Med.* 2006;355(26):2725–2732.
84. Citak A, Karabocuoglu M, Ucsel R, et al. Central venous catheters in pediatric patients—subclavian venous approach as the first choice. *Pediatr Int.* 2002;44(1):83–86.
85. Costello JM, Clapper TC, Wypij D. Minimizing complications associated with percutaneous central venous catheter placement in children: recent advances. *Pediatr Crit Care Med.* 2013;14(3):273–283.
86. Karapinar B, Cura A. Complications of central venous catheterization in critically ill children. *Pediatr Int.* 2007;49(5):593–599.
87. Stenzel JP, Green TP, Fuhrman BP, et al. Percutaneous femoral venous catheterizations: a prospective study of complications. *J Pediatr.* 1989;114(3):411–415.
88. Casado-Flores J, Barja J, Martino R, et al. Complications of central venous catheterization in critically ill children. *Pediatr Crit Care Med.* 2001;2(1):57–62.
89. Stewart GN. Researches on the Circulation Time and on the Influences which affect it. *J Physiol.* 1897;22(3):159–183.
90. Hamilton WF, Riley RL, et al. Comparison of the Fick and dye injection methods of measuring the cardiac output in man. *Am J Physiol.* 1948;153(2):309–321.
91. Fegler G. Measurement of cardiac output in anaesthetized animals by a thermodilution method. *Q J Exp Physiol Cogn Med Sci.* 1954;39(3):153–164.
92. Branthwaite MA, Bradley RD. Measurement of cardiac output by thermal dilution in man. *J Appl Physiol.* 1968;24(3):434–438.
93. Mihm FG, Gettinger A, Hanson CW, 3rd, et al. A multicenter evaluation of a new continuous cardiac output pulmonary artery catheter system. *Crit Care Med.* 1998;26(8):1346–1350.
94. Scuderi PE, MacGregor DA, Bowton DL, et al. A laboratory comparison of three pulmonary artery oximetry catheters. *Anesthesiology.* 1994;81(1):245–253.
95. Koo KK, Sun JC, Zhou Q, et al. Pulmonary artery catheters: evolving rates and reasons for use. *Crit Care Med.* 2011;39(7):1613–1618.
96. Pearl RG, Rosenthal MH, Nielson L, et al. Effect of injectate volume and temperature on thermodilution cardiac output determination. *Anesthesiology.* 1986;64(6):798–801.
97. Tibby SM, Hatherill M, Marsh MJ, et al. Clinicians' abilities to estimate cardiac index in ventilated children and infants. *Arch Dis Child.* 1997;77(6):516–518.
98. Egan JR, Festa M, Cole AD, et al. Clinical assessment of cardiac performance in infants and children following cardiac surgery. *Intensive Care Med.* 2005;31(4):568–573.
99. Tibby SM, Hatherill M, Marsh MJ, et al. Clinical validation of cardiac output measurements using femoral artery thermodilution with direct Fick in ventilated children and infants. *Intensive Care Med.* 1997;23(9):987–991.
100. McLuckie A, Murdoch IA, Marsh MJ, et al. A comparison of pulmonary and femoral artery thermodilution cardiac indices in paediatric intensive care patients. *Acta Paediatr.* 1996;85(3):336–338.
101. Connors AF, Jr., Speroff T, Dawson NV, et al. The effectiveness of right heart catheterization in the initial care of critically ill patients. SUPPORT Investigators. *JAMA.* 1996;276(11):889–897.
102. Harvey S, Harrison DA, Singer M, et al. Assessment of the clinical effectiveness of pulmonary artery catheters in management of patients in intensive care (PAC-Man): a randomised controlled trial. *Lancet.* 2005;366(9484):472–477.
103. Thiele RH, Durieux ME. Arterial waveform analysis for the anesthesiologist: Past, present, and future concepts. *Anesth Analg.* 2011;113(4):766–776.
104. Critchley LA. Validation of the mostcare pulse contour cardiac output monitor: Beyond the bland and altman plot. *Anesth Analg.* 2011;113(6):1292–1294.
105. Penaz J. Photoelectric measurement of blood pressure, volume and flow in the finger. Digest of the 10th International Conference on Medical and Biological Engineering; *Dresden*1973. 102–104.
106. Gizdulich P, Prentza A, Wesseling KH. Models of brachial to finger pulse wave distortion and pressure decrement. *Cardiovasc Res.* 1997;33(3):698–705.
107. Martina JR, Westerhof BE, van Goudoever J, et al. Noninvasive continuous arterial blood pressure monitoring with Nexfin(R). *Anesthesiology.* 2012;116(5):1092–1103.
108. Sagawa K, Lie RK, Schaefer J. Translation of Otto Frank's paper "Die Grundform des Arteriellen Pulses" Zeitschrift fur Biologie 37: 483–526 (1899). *J Mol Cell Cardiol.* 1990;22(3):253–254.
109. Langewouters GJ, Wesseling KH, Goedhard WJ. The static elastic properties of 45 human thoracic and 20 abdominal aortas in vitro and the parameters of a new model. *J Biomech.* 1984;17(6):425–435.
110. Maus TM, Lee DE. Arterial pressure-based cardiac output assessment. *J Cardiothorac Vasc Anesth.* 2008;22(3):468–473.
111. Meng L, Tran NP, Alexander BS, et al. The impact of phenylephrine, ephedrine, and increased preload on third-generation Vigileo-FloTrac and esophageal doppler cardiac output measurements. *Anesth Analg.* 2011;113(4):751–757.
112. Monnet X, Letierce A, Hamzaoui O, et al. Arterial pressure allows monitoring the changes in cardiac output induced by volume expansion but not by norepinephrine. *Crit Care Med.* 2011;39(6):1394–1399.
113. Biancofiore G, Critchley LA, Lee A, et al. Evaluation of a new software version of the FloTrac/Vigileo (version 3.02) and a comparison with previous data in cirrhotic patients undergoing liver transplant surgery. *Anesth Analg.* 2011;113(3):515–522.
114. Biais M, Nouette-Gaulain K, Cottenceau V, et al. Cardiac output measurement in patients undergoing liver transplantation: pulmonary artery catheter versus uncalibrated arterial pressure waveform analysis. *Anesth Analg.* 2008;106(5):1480–1486, table of contents.
115. Monnet X, Anguel N, Naudin B, et al. Arterial pressure-based cardiac output in septic patients: Different accuracy of pulse contour and uncalibrated pressure waveform devices. *Crit Care.* 2010;14(3):R109.
116. Michard F. Changes in arterial pressure during mechanical ventilation. *Anesthesiology.* 2005;103(2):419–428; quiz 49–55.
117. Biais M, Nouette-Gaulain K, Cottenceau V, et al. Uncalibrated pulse contour-derived stroke volume variation predicts fluid responsiveness in mechanically ventilated patients undergoing liver transplantation. *Br J Anaesth.* 2008;101(6):761–768.
118. Lorsomradee S, Cromheecke S, De Hert SG. Uncalibrated arterial pulse contour analysis versus continuous thermodilution technique: Effects of alterations in arterial waveform. *J Cardiothorac Vasc Anesth.* 2007;21(5):636–643.
119. Opdam HI, Wan L, Bellomo R. A pilot assessment of the FloTrac cardiac output monitoring system. *Intensive Care Med.* 2007;33(2):344–349.
120. Slagt C, Beute J, Hoeksema M, et al. Cardiac output derived from arterial pressure waveform analysis without calibration vs. thermodilution in septic shock: evolving accuracy of software versions. *Eur J Anaesthesiol.* 2010;27(6):550–554.
121. Ameloot K, Van De Vijver K, Van Regenmortel N, et al. Validation study of Nexfin(R) continuous non-invasive blood pressure monitoring in critically ill adult patients. *Minerva Anestesiol.* 2014;80(12):1294–1301.

122. Bubenek-Turconi SI, Craciun M, Miclea I, et al. Noninvasive continuous cardiac output by the Nexfin before and after preload-modifying maneuvers: A comparison with intermittent thermodilution cardiac output. *Anesth Analg.* 2013;117(2):366–372.
123. Urbano J, Lopez J, Gonzalez R, et al. Measurement of cardiac output in children by pressure-recording analytical method. *Pediatr Cardiol.* 2015;36(2):358–364.
124. Saxena R, Durward A, Puppala NK, et al. Pressure recording analytical method for measuring cardiac output in critically ill children: A validation study. *Br J Anaesth.* 2013;110(3):425–431.
125. Calamandrei M, Mirabile L, Muschetta S, et al. Assessment of cardiac output in children: A comparison between the pressure recording analytical method and Doppler echocardiography. *Pediatr Crit Care Med.* 2008;9(3):310–312.
126. Sessler DI. Central thermoregulatory inhibition by general anesthesia. *Anesthesiology.* 1991;75(4):557–559.
127. Ozaki M, Kurz A, Sessler DI, et al. Thermoregulatory thresholds during epidural and spinal anesthesia. *Anesthesiology.* 1994;81(2):282–288.
128. Kurz A, Sessler DI, Lenhardt R. Perioperative normothermia to reduce the incidence of surgical-wound infection and shorten hospitalization. Study of Wound Infection and Temperature Group. *N Engl J Med.* 1996;334(19):1209–1215.
129. Frank SM, Fleisher LA, Breslow MJ, et al. Perioperative maintenance of normothermia reduces the incidence of morbid cardiac events. A randomized clinical trial. *JAMA.* 1997;277(14):1127–1134.
130. Yamakage M, Kawana S, Watanabe H, et al. The utility of tracheal temperature monitoring. *Anesth Analg.* 1993;76(4):795–799.
131. Vaughan MS, Cork RC, Vaughan RW. Inaccuracy of liquid crystal thermometry to identify core temperature trends in postoperative adults. *Anesth Analg.* 1982;61(3):284–287.
132. Rampil IJ. A primer for EEG signal processing in anesthesia. *Anesthesiology.* 1998;89(4):980–1002.
133. Burch NR, Nettleton WJ Jr., Sweeney J, et al. Period analysis of the electroencephalogram on a general-purpose digital computer. *Ann N Y Acad Sci.* 1964;115:827–843.
134. Doyle PW, Matta BF. Burst suppression or isoelectric encephalogram for cerebral protection: Evidence from metabolic suppression studies. *Br J Anaesth.* 1999;83(4):580–584.
135. Brenner RP, Schwartzman RJ, Richey ET. Prognostic significance of episodic low amplitude or relatively isoelectric EEG patterns. *Dis Nerv Syst.* 1975;36(10):582–587.
136. Cooley JW, Tukey JW. An algorithm for machine calculation of complex Fourier series. *Math. Comp.* 1965;19(90):297–301.
137. Proakis JG. *Advanced Digital Signal Processing.* New York, NY: Maxwell Macmillan International; 1992:xiv, 610.
138. Kreuer S, Bruhn J, Larsen R, et al. Comparison of BIS and AAI as measures of anaesthetic drug effect during desflurane-remifentanil anaesthesia. *Acta Anaesthesiol Scand.* 2004;48(9):1168–1173.
139. Whitlock EL, Villafranca AJ, Lin N, et al. Relationship between bispectral index values and volatile anesthetic concentrations during the maintenance phase of anesthesia in the B-unaware trial. *Anesthesiology.* 2011;115(6):1209–1218.
140. Tirel O, Wodey E, Harris R, et al. Variation of bispectral index under TIVA with propofol in a paediatric population. *Br J Anaesth.* 2008;100(1):82–87.
141. Hans P, Dewandre PY, Brichant JF, et al. Comparative effects of ketamine on Bispectral Index and spectral entropy of the electroencephalogram under sevoflurane anaesthesia. *Br J Anaesth.* 2005;94(3):336–340.
142. Faraoni D, Salengros JC, Engelman E, et al. Ketamine has no effect on bispectral index during stable propofol-remifentanil anaesthesia. *Br J Anaesth.* 2009;102(3):336–339.
143. Yufune S, Takamatsu I, Masui K, et al. Effect of remifentanil on plasma propofol concentration and bispectral index during propofol anaesthesia. *Br J Anaesth.* 2011;106(2):208–214.
144. Brandes IF, Stuth EA. Use of BIS monitor in a child with congenital insensitivity to pain with anhidrosis. *Paediatr Anaesth.* 2006;16(4):466–470.
145. Crosby G. General anesthesia—minding the mind during surgery. *N Engl J Med.* 2011;365(7):660–661.
146. Gan TJ, Glass PS, Windsor A, et al. Bispectral index monitoring allows faster emergence and improved recovery from propofol, alfentanil, and nitrous oxide anesthesia. BIS Utility Study Group. *Anesthesiology.* 1997;87(4):808–815.
147. Chin KJ, Yeo SW. A BIS-guided study of sevoflurane requirements for adequate depth of anaesthesia in Caesarean section. *Anaesthesia.* 2004;59(11):1064–1068.
148. Fraser GL, Riker RR. Bispectral index monitoring in the intensive care unit provides more signal than noise. *Pharmacotherapy.* 2005;25(5 Pt 2):19S–27S.
149. Vivien B, Di Maria S, Ouattara A, et al. Overestimation of Bispectral Index in sedated intensive care unit patients revealed by administration of muscle relaxant. *Anesthesiology.* 2003;99(1):9–17.
150. Pousman RM, Eilers WA, 3rd, Johns B, et al. Irritant contact dermatitis after use of Bispectral Index sensor in prone position. *Anesth Analg.* 2002;95(5):1337–1338, table of contents.
151. Myles PS, Leslie K, McNeil J, et al. Bispectral index monitoring to prevent awareness during anaesthesia: The B-Aware randomised controlled trial. *Lancet.* 2004;363(9423):1757–1763.
152. Avidan MS, Zhang L, Burnside BA, et al. Anesthesia awareness and the bispectral index. *N Engl J Med.* 2008;358(11):1097–1108.
153. Sleigh JW. Depth of anesthesia: perhaps the patient isn't a submarine. *Anesthesiology.* 2011;115(6):1149–1150.
154. Dehaene S, Changeux JP. Experimental and theoretical approaches to conscious processing. *Neuron.* 2011;70(2):200–227.
155. Kandel ER. The biology of memory: A forty-year perspective. *J Neurosci.* 2009;29(41):12748–12756.
156. Brown EN, Lydic R, Schiff ND. General anesthesia, sleep, and coma. *N Engl J Med.* 2010;363(27):2638–2650.
157. Davidson AJ, Huang GH, Czarnecki C, et al. Awareness during anesthesia in children: A prospective cohort study. *Anesth Analg.* 2005;100(3):653–661, table of contents.
158. Malviya S, Galinkin JL, Bannister CF, et al. The incidence of intraoperative awareness in children: Childhood awareness and recall evaluation. *Anesth Analg.* 2009;109(5):1421–1427.
159. Davidson AJ, Smith KR, Blusse van Oud-Alblas HJ, et al. Awareness in children: A secondary analysis of five cohort studies. *Anaesthesia.* 2011;66(4):446–454.
160. Backeljauw B, Holland SK, Altaye M, et al. Cognition and brain structure following early childhood surgery with anesthesia. *Pediatrics.* 2015;136(1):e1–e12.
161. Davidson AJ, McCann ME, Devavaram P, et al. The differences in the bispectral index between infants and children during emergence from anesthesia after circumcision surgery. *Anesth Analg.* 2001;93(2):326–330, 2nd contents page.
162. Brown M, Vender JS. Noninvasive oxygen monitoring. *Crit Care Clin.* 1988;4(3):493–509.
163. Craver CD, Coblentz Society. *The Coblentz Society desk book of infrared spectra.* 2nd ed. Kirkwood, MO (P.O. Box 9952, Kirkwood 63122): The Society; 1982. iii, 538.
164. Gardner RM. Direct blood pressure measurement—dynamic response requirements. *Anesthesiology.* 1981;54(3):227–236.
165. Dorsch JA, Dorsch SE. *Understanding Anesthesia Equipment.* 4th ed. Baltimore, MD: Lippincott Williams & Wilkins; 1999:xii, 1066.
166. Vender JS. Invasive cardiac monitoring. *Crit Care Clin.* 1988;4(3):455–477.
167. Dizon CT, Barash PG. The value of monitoring pulmonary artery pressure in clinical practice. *Conn Med.* 1977;41(10):622–625.
168. Warner HR, Swan HJ, Connolly DC, et al. Quantitation of beat-to-beat changes in stroke volume from the aortic pulse contour in man. *J Appl Physiol.* 1953;5(9):495–507.

27 Echocardiography

ALBERT C. PERRINO JR • WANDA M. POPESCU • FARID JADBABAIE • NIKOLAOS J. SKUBAS

Principles and Technology of Echocardiography
- Physics of Sound
- Properties of Sound Transmission in Tissue
- Instrumentation
- Signal Processing
- Image Display
- Spatial versus Dynamic Image Quality

Two-dimensional and Three-dimensional Transesophageal Echocardiography Examination
- Probe Insertion
- Transesophageal Echocardiography Safety
- Contraindication to Transesophageal Echocardiography Probe Placement
- Probe Manipulation
- Orientation
- Goals of the Two-dimensional Examination
- Three-dimensional Echocardiography

Doppler Echocardiography and Hemodynamics
- Spectral Doppler
- Color-flow Doppler
- Hemodynamic Assessments

Echocardiographic Evaluation of Systolic Function
- Left Ventricular Walls
- Left Ventricular Cavity

Evaluation of Left Ventricular Diastolic Function
- Diastolic Physiology
- Echocardiographic Assessment of Left Ventricular Diastolic Function
- Pericardial Disease: Constrictive Pericarditis and Pericardial Tamponade

Evaluation of Valvular Heart Disease
- Aortic Stenosis
- Mitral Stenosis
- Aortic Regurgitation
- Mitral Regurgitation
- Tricuspid and Pulmonic Valve Regurgitation

Diseases of the Aorta
- Two-dimensional and Motion-mode Echocardiography

Cardiac Masses

Congenital Heart Disease

Echocardiography-assisted Procedures
- Ultrasound-guided Central Vein Cannulation

Epicardial and Epiaortic Echocardiography
- Epicardial Echocardiography
- Epiaortic Examination

Echocardiography Outside the Operating Room

Focused Transthoracic Cardiac Ultrasound
- Focused Exam Views
- Focused Assessed Transthoracic Echo

KEY POINTS

1. Understanding the principles of ultrasound and echocardiographic instrumentation is essential in optimizing image quality.
2. Two-dimensional and Doppler techniques have complementary roles in the assessment of cardiovascular function.
3. Global left ventricular systolic function is influenced by load and contractility alterations; regional wall motion grading is based on systolic endocardial excursion and myocardial thickening.
4. Doppler assessments of transmitral flow and myocardial tissue velocities provide accurate diastolic function assessment.
5. Severity of aortic stenosis is estimated based on maximal pressure gradient across the aortic valve and the aortic valve area calculated by the continuity equation.
6. The ratio of the width of the regurgitant jet to the diameter of the left ventricular outflow tract is useful in assessing the severity of aortic insufficiency. Diastolic flow reversal in the descending thoracic aorta is significant for severe aortic insufficiency.
7. Mitral regurgitation can be of structural or functional etiology. The vena contracta of the regurgitant jet is useful to grade severity.
8. Aortic atheromas larger than 4 mm are harbingers of thromboembolic events.
9. The false lumen of aortic dissection does not have diastolic flow.
10. Transthoracic-focused cardiac ultrasound provides rapid bedside assessment of cardiac pathology and potential causes of altered hemodynamics.

Echocardiography is the first imaging technique to enter the mainstream of intraoperative patient monitoring. A remarkably versatile tool, real-time echocardiography provides a comprehensive evaluation of myocardial, valvular, and hemodynamic performances. These capabilities attracted the attention of anesthesiologists and surgeons challenged by the unique difficulties of perioperative cardiovascular management. Over the 30 years following the first report of intraoperative echocardiography to assess ventricular function by Barash and colleagues in 1978, echocardiography has emerged as the technique of choice for a wide variety of intraoperative case challenges.[1]

The benefit of intraoperative echocardiography in both cardiac and noncardiac surgical populations is supported by several case series.[2-8] Applications range from guiding the placement of intracardiac and intravascular catheters and devices, to the assessment of the severity of valve pathology and immediate evaluation of a surgical intervention, to the rapid diagnosis of acute hemodynamic instability and directing appropriate therapies.[9-11] Consequently, expertise in intraoperative echocardiography is highly desired among anesthesiology practitioners. The National Board of Echocardiography has established a certification pathway in perioperative transesophageal echocardiography (TEE), http://www.echoboards.org/certification/certexpl.html. The American Society of Anesthesiologists in conjunction with the National Board of Echocardiography has established a second certification pathway in basic perioperative echocardiography, www.echoboards.org/content/basic-pteexam. These efforts are unique in intraoperative monitoring and attest to the critical role that accurate and thorough echocardiographic interpretation plays in current anesthetic practice.

Principles and Technology of Echocardiography

Echocardiography generates dynamic images of the heart from the reflections of sound waves. The echocardiography system transmits a brief pulse of high-frequency sound (i.e., ultrasound) that propagates through and is subsequently reflected from the cardiac structures encountered. The ultrasound transducer records the time delay and signal intensity for each returning reflection. Since the speed of sound in tissue is constant, the time delay allows the echo system to precisely calculate the location of cardiac structures and thereby create an image map of the heart.

Physics of Sound

Sound is the vibration of a physical medium. In clinical echocardiography, a mechanical vibrator, known as the *transducer*, is placed in contact with the esophagus (TEE), skin (transthoracic echocardiography [TTE]), or the heart (epicardial echocardiography) to create tissue vibrations. The resulting tissue vibrations create a longitudinal wave with alternating areas of *compression* and *rarefaction* (Fig. 27-1).

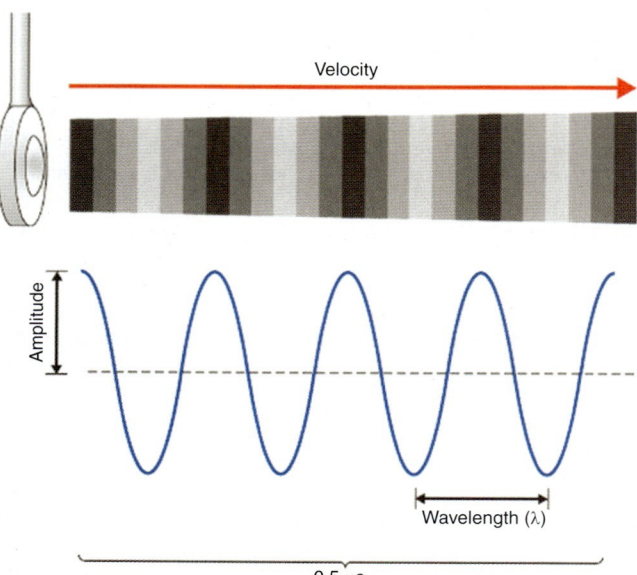

Figure 27-1 Sound wave. Vibrations of the ultrasound transducer create cycles of compression and rarefaction in the adjacent tissue. The ultrasound energy is characterized by its amplitude, wavelength, frequency, and propagation velocity. In this example, four sound waves are shown in a period of 0.5 μs. The frequency can be calculated as four cycles divided by 0.5 μs and equals 8 MHz.

The *amplitude* of a sound wave represents its peak pressure and is appreciated as loudness. The level of sound energy in an area of tissue is referred to as *intensity*. The intensity of the sound signal is proportional to the square of the amplitude and is an important factor regarding the potential for tissue damage with ultrasound. Since levels of sound pressure vary over a large range, it is convenient to use the logarithmic decibel (dB) scale:

$$\text{Decibels} = 10 \log_{10} I/I_r = 10 \log_{10} A^2/A_r^2 = 20 \log_{10} A/A_r$$

where A is the measured sound amplitude and A_r is a standard reference sound level; I is the intensity and I_r is a standard reference intensity. The Food and Drug Administration limits the intensity output of cardiac ultrasound systems to be below 720 W/cm² because of concerns of potential tissue injury.[12]

Sound waves are also characterized by their *frequency* (f), or pitch, expressed in cycles per second, or Hertz (Hz), and by their *wavelength* (λ). These attributes significantly impact the depth of penetration of a sound wave in tissue and the image resolution of the ultrasound system.

The propagation *velocity* of sound (v) is determined solely by the medium through which it passes. In soft tissue, the speed of sound is approximately 1,540 m/s. As the product of wavelength and frequency equals velocity: $V = \lambda \times f$, it becomes apparent that the wavelength and frequency are inversely related: $\lambda = v \times 1/f$ and that $\lambda = (1,540 \text{ m/s})f$. High-frequency, short-wavelength ultrasound is more easily focused and directed to a specific target location. Image resolution also increases with short-wavelength sound waves; for these reasons, ultrasonic frequencies of 2 to 10 MHz are preferred in clinical echocardiography.

Properties of Sound Transmission in Tissue

The propagation of a sound wave through the body is markedly affected by its interactions with the various tissues encountered. These interactions result in reflection, refraction, scattering, and attenuation of the ultrasound signal and determine the resulting appearance of the two-dimensional image.

Echocardiographic imaging relies on the transmission and subsequent reflection of ultrasound energy back to the transducer. A sound wave propagates smoothly through uniform tissue until it encounters the interface between two tissues varying in acoustic impedance (a property largely related to the *density* [ρ] of the tissue and the speed that ultrasound travels). A large interface oriented perpendicular to the sound beam will produce a mirror-like reflection of sound back toward the transducer with only a portion of the signal passing through the interface. Since cardiac structures are detected by their reflected echocardiography signal, echocardiographers adjust the position of the TEE transducer so that the direction of its beam is perpendicular to the cardiac structure of interest.

Refraction causes a change in direction of propagating sound and occurs when an interface lies oblique to the sound beam. Refraction is an important factor in the formation of artifacts as the transducer mistakenly interprets a reflection from the refracted beam as originating from a cardiac structure located within the *intended* scanning field.

Scattering reflections occur when an ultrasound beam encounters small or irregularly shaped surfaces, such as red blood cells. These reflectors scatter ultrasound energy in all directions so that far less energy is reflected back to the transducer. This type of reflection is the basis of the Doppler analysis of blood flow (see following).

Even when traveling through uniform tissue, sound undergoes a steady loss (i.e., *attenuation*) in intensity as a consequence of dispersion and absorption. Attenuation results in less energy returning to the transducer and low-quality images with poor signal-to-noise ratios. To combat attenuation, echocardiographers select better penetrating low-frequency signals (e.g., 2.5 instead of 7.5 MHz) and choose an imaging window that is close to the structure of interest. Adjusting the gain controls to amplify the weak returning signals makes their appearance brighter on the display. Unfortunately, this increases the brightness of artifactual noise, which negatively impacts the image appearance.

Instrumentation

Transducers

Ultrasound transducers use piezoelectric crystals to create a brief pulse of ultrasound. Alternating electrical current stimulates polarized particles within the crystal's matrix to rapidly vibrate, generating ultrasound. Conversely, when a sound reflection strikes the crystal, the impact vibrates the polarized particles and generates an electric current. This property allows the piezoelectric crystal to function as both a transmitter and a receiver of ultrasound.

The shorter the length of the sound pulses, the better the axial resolution of the system. High-resolution imaging transducers emit sound pulses of just two to four cycles of short-wavelength, high-frequency sound.

Beam Shape

The ultrasound transducer emits a three-dimensional ultrasound beam similar to a movie projection (Fig. 27-2). The beam is narrow in the near field and then diverges into the far field zone. Focusing of the beam is used to improve spatial resolution by narrowing the ultrasound beam at the desired depth. The dense, narrow beam is preferred because it provides improved spatial resolution, produces high-intensity reflections, and reduces artifact. Echocardiographers adjust focal depth and focus to optimize the image resolution.

Resolution

Three parameters are evaluated when assessing the resolution of an ultrasound system: the resolution of objects lying along the axis of the ultrasound beam (*axial resolution*), the resolution of objects horizontal to the beam's orientation (*lateral resolution*), and the resolution of objects lying vertical to the beam's orientation (*elevational resolution*).

Short pulses of high-frequency ultrasound offer the greatest axial resolution but have a decreased tissue penetration. As resolution is highest along the axial plane, echocardiographic measurements are most precise when taken parallel to the beam's axis. Accordingly, echocardiographers select transmitted frequency based on the particular imaging need.

Beam size determines the lateral and elevational resolution. Broad beams produce a "smeared" image of two nearby objects, whereas narrow beams can identify each object individually. Beam size is reduced by selecting high-signal frequencies and minimizing imaging depth.

Signal Processing

To convert echoes into images, the returning ultrasound pulses are received, electronically processed, and displayed. The oscillator repeatedly cycles the transducer from a brief transmission to a relatively long receive mode. During the receive phase, the reflected echocardiography signals are captured and converted to electrical signals by the piezoelectric crystal. The echocardiography system employs a series of controls, including system gain, time gain compensation, compression, and postprocessing settings (not unlike those available with digital imaging software) to optimize the signal for display. Adjustments are used, for example, to emphasize edge detection versus tissue texture or to improve the delineation of weaker reflectors. The choice of settings is dictated by the examination and preferences of the echocardiographer.

Image Display

Ultrasonic imaging is based on the amplitude and time delay of the reflected signals. Since the velocity in tissue is a relatively constant 1,540 m/s, only the distance of the structure from the transducer alters the time required for the ultrasound wave to travel to and from the reflected structure. So, by timing the interval between transmission and return of the reflections, the echocardiography system can precisely calculate the distance of a structure from the transducer.

Current imaging is based on brightness mode, or *B-mode technology*. With B-mode, the amplitude of the returning echoes from

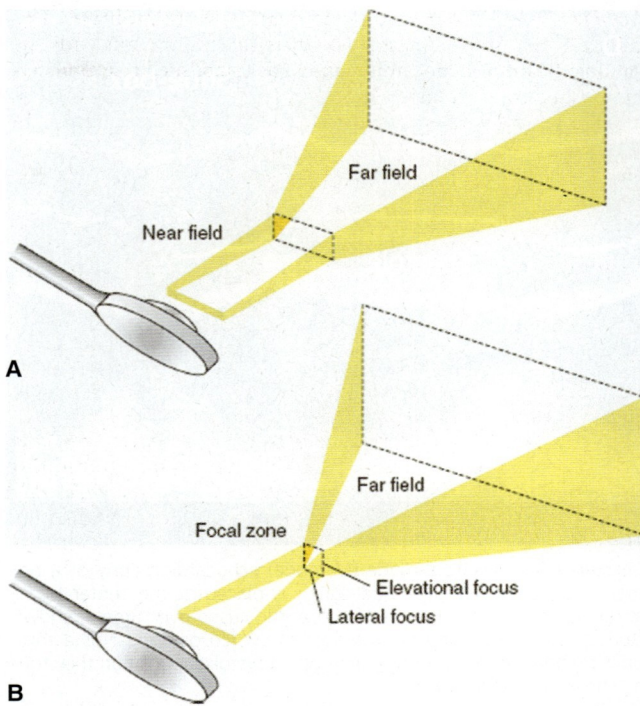

Figure 27-2 Three-dimensional beam. The ultrasound probe projects a three-dimensional beam. The dimensions of this projection have important effects on the imaging resolution and artifact. Typically, a narrow profile is preferred. **A**: Unfocused beam. The beam is narrow in the near field and then diverges in the far field. **B**: Focused beam. Focusing has resulted in a narrower beam in both the lateral and elevational planes so that the imaging resolution of structures in the focal zone is improved. Distal to the focal zone, the beam rapidly diverges and the images of structures in this area will be of lower quality.

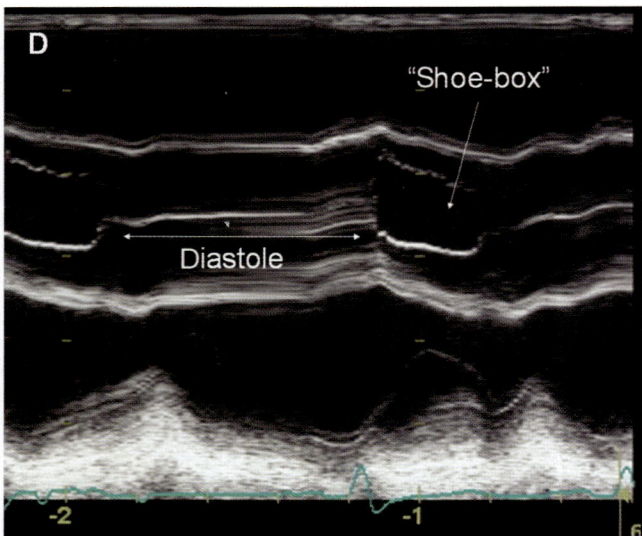

Figure 27-3 Method-mode (M-mode) echocardiography of a normal aortic valve. The M-mode cursor is placed at the center of the aortic valve and the motion of the aortic cusps over time is shown. During diastolic coaptation, the aortic valve cusps appear as a thick, bright white line (*long arrow*), whereas in systolic apposition they form a "shoe-box" (*short arrow*).

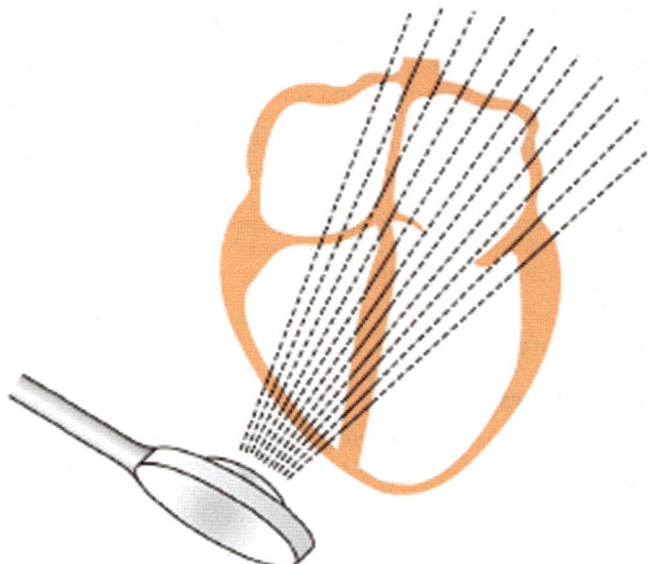

Figure 27-4 Scan lines. Illustration of the arced sector from a phased array two-dimensional echocardiogram. Each *dotted line* represents an individual brightness mode scan line. Any structure that interacts with a scan line will create reflections (*dark highlight*); however, structures that lie between the scan lines are not interrogated and the echocardiography system averages the neighboring signals to fill in this defect. Accordingly, the closer the scan lines, the better the image quality.

a single pulse determines the display brightness of the representative pixels. *M-mode*, or motion mode, adds temporal information to B-mode by displaying a series of sequentially collected B-mode images. M-mode echocardiography provides a one-dimensional, single-beam view through the heart but updates the B-mode images at a very high rate, providing dynamic real-time imaging. M-mode remains the best technique for examining the timing of cardiac events (Fig. 27-3).

Two-dimensional (2D) echocardiography is a modification of B-mode echocardiography and the mainstay of the echocardiographic examination. Instead of repeatedly firing ultrasound pulses in a single direction, the transducer in 2D echocardiography sequentially directs the ultrasound pulses across a sector of the cardiac anatomy. In this way, 2D imaging displays a tomographic section of the cardiac anatomy and, unlike M-mode, reveals the shape and lateral motion (Fig. 27-4).

Two-dimensional scanning is achieved using phased array technology, which sequentially activates each crystal in the array and thereby steers the beam without the transducer itself being moved. The two commonly used electronic scanning systems in medical ultrasound are the linear scanners and sector scanners.

The *linear scanner* uses a long linear array. Groups of crystals are activated sequentially from one end of the transducer to the other. The firing of each group of crystals creates an image of the structures directly in front of them. With sequential firing, the anatomic features from one end of the transducer to the other are imaged (Fig. 27-5). The disadvantage of this approach is that the transducer face must be large to cover a broad anatomic area. The linear array is commonly used to guide vascular access and regional anesthetic procedures.

The phased array *sector scanner* is the most commonly used in echocardiography. Here, the ultrasound scan is sequentially directed in a fan-like arc. The resulting sector image, known as a *frame*, is similar in shape to that covered by a windshield wiper. The 2D scanner then repeats the entire process to update the image and capture motion.

Spatial versus Dynamic Image Quality

Expert echocardiographers select machine settings to optimize particular image qualities for the examination at hand. As discussed in the following sections, these selections will determine whether sector size, spatial resolution, or dynamic motion is best displayed.

The *pulse repetition frequency* is the rate at which sound pulses are triggered. The greater the pulse repetition frequency, the greater the number of scan lines that are emitted in a given period of time. This enhances motion display. Unfortunately, sector depth must be reduced because pulse repetition frequency is inversely related to the sector depth, as a longer period of time is required for the ultrasound to travel the increased distances.

The *frame rate* is the frequency at which the sector is rescanned. A high frame rate improves the capture of movement.

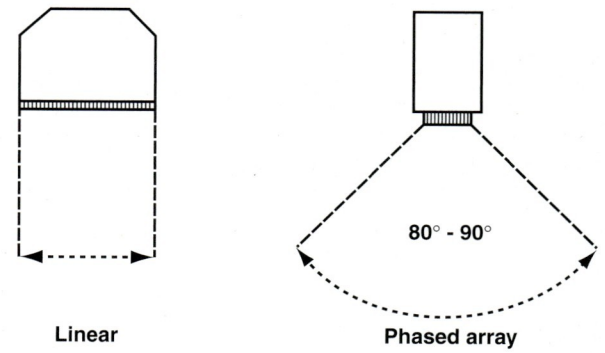

Figure 27-5 Linear scanners image a rectangular section of the anatomy compared with the arced sector imaged with phased array scanners.

Typically, frame rates greater than 30 per second are desired. The frame rate is critically dependent on the sector depth, which determines the time required for each scan line to be received, and the sector width, which increases the number of scan lines that must be transmitted. Consequently, increases in sector size and depth come at the cost of a decreased frame rate and poor motion imaging.

The number of scan lines per degree of the sector (*scan line density*) greatly affects the image resolution. Doubling the scan lines essentially doubles the lateral resolution. However, the cost is a decrease in the frame rate and motion imaging.

The echocardiographer must thoughtfully select among settings that will often have opposing effects between the size of the imaging field, the imaging resolution, and the frame rate. A common approach is to focus each part of the examination on a given structure of interest and select the imaging plane that best delineates the structure in the near field. Motion display can then be enhanced without costs in lateral resolution by decreasing the sector angle and depth. In situations in which the maximal frame rate is desired, M-mode is chosen.

Two-dimensional and Three-dimensional Transesophageal Echocardiography Examination

TEE is the favored approach to intraoperative echocardiography. Compared with TTE, TEE offers additional "windows" to view the heart, often with improved image quality from the anatomic proximity of the esophagus and heart. In the operating room (OR), TEE is useful because the probe does not interfere with the operative field and can be left in situ, providing continuous, real-time hemodynamic information used to diagnose and manage critical cardiac events. TEE is also useful in situations in which the transthoracic examination is limited by various factors (obesity, emphysema, surgical dressings, and prosthetic valves) and for examining cardiac structures not well visualized with TTE (left atrial appendage).

This section is designed to introduce TEE image orientation and the diagnostic utility of each view. In addition, examination sequences useful for obtaining a comprehensive or targeted examination are provided. Readers are referred to *A Practical Approach to Transesophageal Echocardiography*[13] for a more detailed description of the TEE examinations described in this section.

Probe Insertion

The TEE probe is inserted in the anesthetized patient in a manner similar to insertion of an orogastric tube. For improved image quality, the stomach is emptied of gastric contents and air prior to probe insertion. The jaw is lifted with the left hand and the TEE probe, well lubricated, is inserted with the right hand by applying gentle but constant pressure. If significant resistance is encountered, additional force should be strictly avoided as oropharyngeal or esophageal injury may result. Rather, a decrease in neck extension and/or use of a laryngoscope to visualize the oropharyngeal structures often will allow easy passage of the probe. The TEE probe is advanced beyond the larynx and the cricopharyngeal muscle (around 25–30 cm from teeth) until a loss of resistance is appreciated. At this point, the TEE probe lies in the upper esophagus and the first cardiovascular images are seen. Extrinsic compression of the esophagus (e.g., osteophytes or an aortic aneurysm) may impede probe placement.[9,10]

Transesophageal Echocardiography Safety

TEE is a semi-invasive procedure. When performed by qualified operators, TEE has a low incidence of complications. A retrospective study performed on 846 patients who underwent TEE described the following complications: three patients with pharyngeal abrasions, one patient with a chipped tooth, and few patients with transient vocal cord paresis.[14] Another retrospective study performed on a large case series of 7,200 patients showed that the morbidity associated with TEE placement is 0.2% and the mortality is 0%.[15] The most common complaint (0.1%) was postoperative odynophagia. Various studies have suggested an association between swallowing dysfunction after cardiac surgery and the use of intraoperative TEE.[16,17] This fact is important, as postoperative swallowing dysfunction is associated with pulmonary complications.[16]

Contraindication to Transesophageal Echocardiography Probe Placement

To maintain the safety profile of TEE, each patient should be evaluated before the procedure for signs, symptoms, or history of esophageal pathology. Among the most feared complications of TEE are esophageal or gastric perforation.[18] For skilled practitioners, this complication is extremely rare. Patients with extensive esophageal and gastric diseases are at highest risk of perforation. Contraindications to TEE probe placement are esophageal stricture, rings or webs, esophageal masses (especially malignant tumors), recent bleeding of esophageal varices, Zenker diverticulum, status postradiation to the neck, and recent gastric bypass surgery.[13,18] In the rare case in which TEE is essential and is the only alternative, placement of the TEE probe can be performed under direct visualization with a combined gastroscopic and echocardiographic examination.[13]

Probe Manipulation

Image acquisition depends on precise manipulation of the TEE probe. By advancing the shaft of the probe, the probe position can be moved from the upper esophagus to the midesophagus and into the stomach. The shaft can also be manually rotated to the left or to the right. By using the large knob on the probe handle, the head of the probe can be anteflexed (turning the knob clockwise) and retroflexed (turning the knob counterclockwise). The smaller knob, located on top of the large knob, is used to tilt the head of the probe to the right or to the left. Using the electronic switch on the probe handle, the operator can rotate the ultrasound beam from 0 (transverse plane) to 180 degrees in 1-degree increments.

Orientation

The previously mentioned controls allow experienced echocardiographers to perform comprehensive cardiac imaging. However, the diversity of imaging planes can confuse less experienced echocardiographers, leaving them unable to recognize the various anatomic structures presented. Thus, an understanding of the basic rules of imaging orientation is essential to echocardiographic interpretation.

The ultrasound beam is always directed perpendicular to the probe face. The 2D TEE image is displayed as a sector scan. The

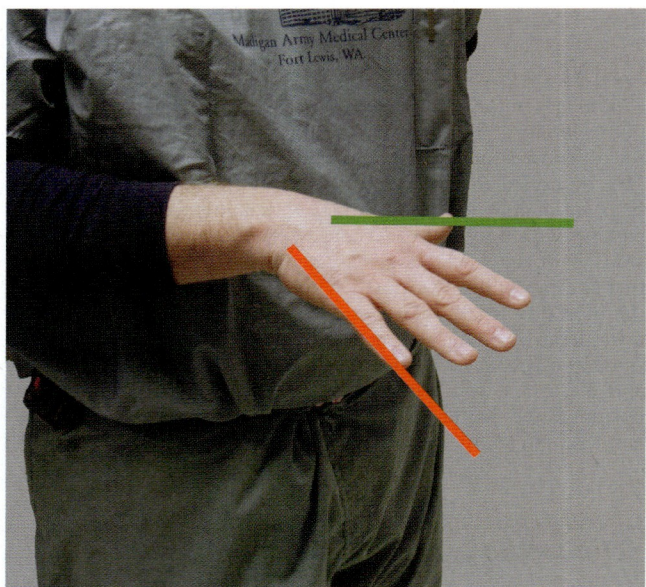

Figure 27-6 Orientation of the hand, as described in the text, for an imaging plane of 0 degrees. The imaging plane is projected like a wedge anteriorly through the heart. The image is created by multiple scan lines traveling back and forth from the patient's left (*green line*) to the patient's right (*red line*). The resulting image is displayed on the monitor as a sector with the green edge (*green line*) on the right side of the monitor and the red edge (*red line*) on the left.

apex of the sector is in close proximity to the TEE probe and the structures seen in this area will be the posterior ones (e.g., left atrium). The arc of the sector will display the more distal and thereby more anterior structures. The angle of rotation of the imaging array determines the right and left orientations. An easy way to understand this orientation is to place your right hand in front of your chest with the palm facing down, the thumb oriented left and the fingers oriented anterior right. The scan lines that generate the TEE image start at your fingers and sweep toward the thumb. Consequently, the right anatomic structures will be displayed on the left side of the monitor (similar to chest x-ray orientation; Fig. 27-6). Increasing the imaging plane angle produces clockwise rotation of the sector scan. This can be visualized by rotating your hand in a clockwise fashion. For example, at the 90-degree imaging plane, the left side of the screen now displays posterior structures (note position of fingers) and the right side of the screen anterior structures (note the position of the thumb; Fig. 27-7).

Goals of the Two-dimensional Examination

Each TEE examination is performed with the goal that no important diagnosis is missed. For this reason, a comprehensive evaluation is preferred with each cardiac chamber and valve imaged in at least two orthogonal planes. However, in an emergency situation, such examination may not be possible. In these cases, most echocardiographers will focus the TEE examination to those views most likely to provide a diagnosis, that is, in a hypotensive patient the transgastric short-axis view of the left ventricle is examined for diagnosing hypovolemia, coronary ischemia, or acute heart failure.

To achieve the goals of the intraoperative TEE examination, the Society of Cardiovascular Anesthesiologists together with the American Society of Echocardiography has published guidelines for performing a comprehensive intraoperative TEE examination.[19] These guidelines include 28 standardized 2D echocardiographic views. Each TEE examination should be recorded along with a detailed report of the examination. Miller et al.[20] proposed a shortened version of the comprehensive examination that would meet the goals established by these guidelines for basic intraoperative TEE proficiency and is particularly useful when time constraints preclude a more extensive examination. Additionally, guidelines for a basic perioperative transesophageal examination geared toward intraoperative monitoring and rapid delineation of the cause of hemodynamic instability has been established.[21] In the following section, we detail the acquisition and anatomic features of the 11 views composing the basic examination. The ultrasound appendix in the electronic version of this textbook provides video examples of the additional cross sections included in the comprehensive examination.[19]

1. **Midesophageal four-chamber view**
   This view is obtained at a multiplane angle between 0 and 20 degrees and slightly advancing the probe to the level of the mitral valve (MV). In this view, the four cardiac chambers and the TV and MV are visualized (Fig. 27-8). Slight withdrawal or anteflexion of the probe will visualize the LVOT and AV and represents the midesophageal five-chamber view. The midesophageal four-chamber view is one of the most recognizable and valuable diagnostic views. Its main uses are to evaluate the:
   a. Left atrium, right atrium, RV, and the LV (inferoseptal and anterolateral walls) size and function
   b. TV and MV structure and function; color-flow Doppler (CFD) will detect valvular pathology
   c. Diastolic function
   d. The presence of atrial or ventricular septal defect

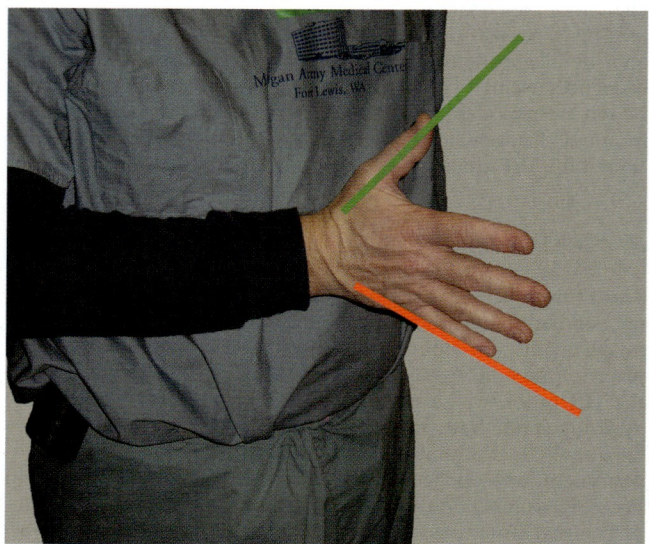

Figure 27-7 Orientation of the hand, as described in the text, for an imaging plane of 90 degrees. The imaging sector is rotated so that the green edge (*green line*) has moved clockwise and is now cephalad and the red edge is now caudad. As previously described, the green edge is displayed on the right side of the monitor and the red edge on the left.

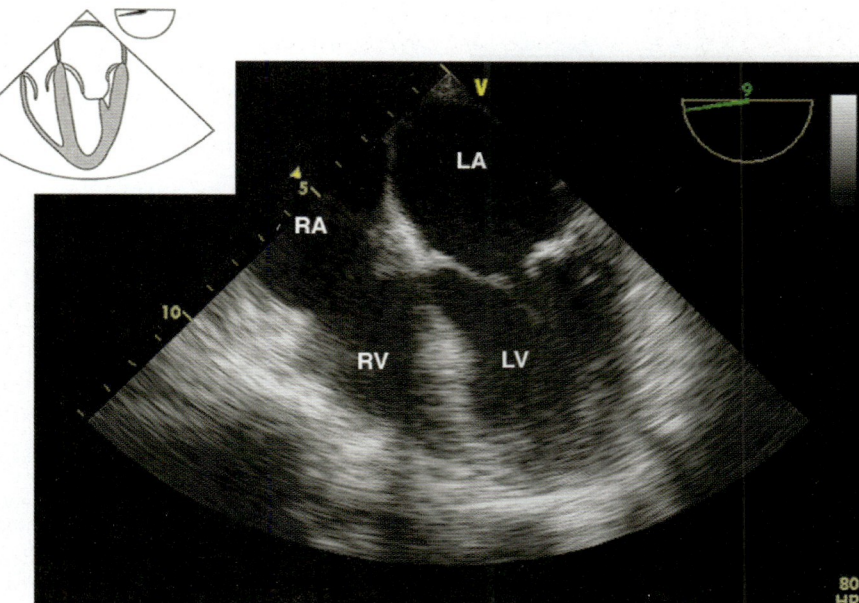

Figure 27-8 Midesophageal four-chamber view. RA, right atrium; RV, right ventricle; LA, left atrium; LV, left ventricle.

2. **Midesophageal two-chamber view**
   This view is obtained from the previous view by rotating the multiplane angle to 90 degrees. In this view, the left atrial appendage is examined for the presence of thrombus. Slight retroflexion is used to avoid a foreshortened view of the LV so as to visualize the LV apex (Fig. 27-9). The main uses of the midesophageal two-chamber view are to evaluate the following:
   a. LV anterior and inferior wall function
   b. LV apex as well as to diagnose apical thrombus
3. **Midesophageal long-axis view**
   This view is obtained from the previous view by rotating the multiplane angle to 120 to 135 degrees (Fig. 27-10). The main uses of the midesophageal long-axis view are to evaluate the following:
   a. LV anteroseptal and posterior wall function
   b. LV outflow tract (LVOT) pathology
   c. MV anatomy and function
4. **Midesophageal (ME) ascending aorta (AA) long-axis (LAX) view** (Fig. 27-11)
   This view is obtained by withdrawing the probe from the ME LAX view. The main uses of this view are to evaluate the following:
   a. Ascending aorta in the long axis (atheroma, dissection)
   b. Pulmonary artery in the short axis
5. **Midesophageal ascending aorta short-axis view**
   The view is obtained by advancing the probe from the upper esophagus until the AA is seen and then rotating the multiplane angle from 0 to 45 degrees to obtain a true short axis (Fig. 27-12). This "great vessel view" images

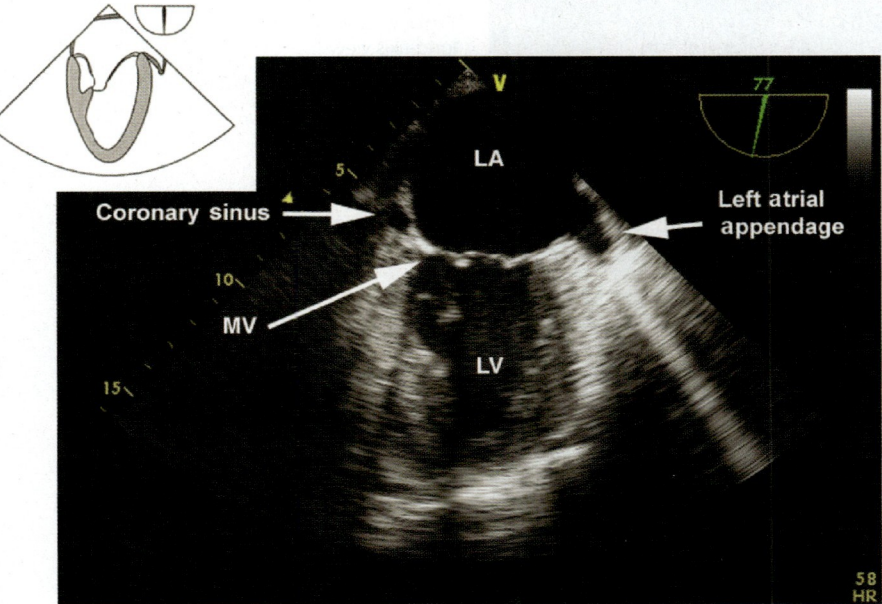

Figure 27-9 Midesophageal two-chamber view. LA, left atrium; MV, mitral valve; LV, left ventricle.

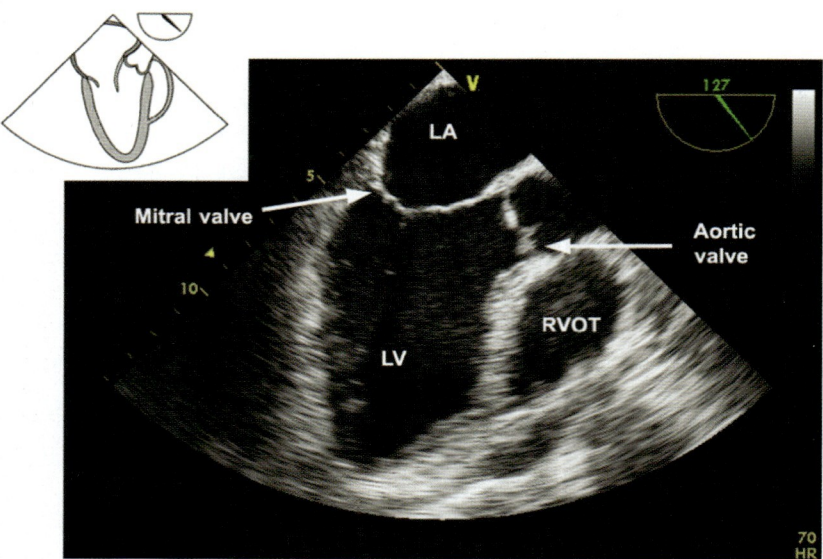

Figure 27-10 Midesophageal long-axis view. LA, left atrium; LV, left ventricle; RVOT, right ventricular outflow tract.

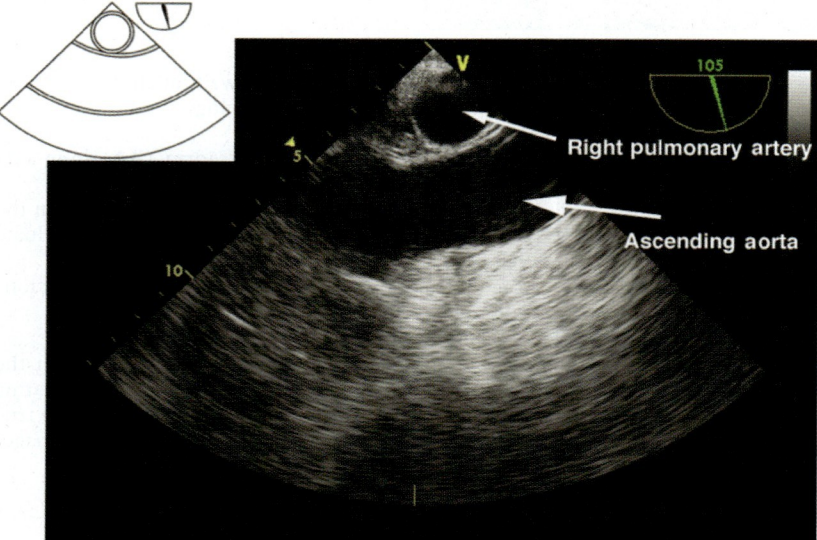

Figure 27-11 Midesophageal ascending aortic long-axis view.

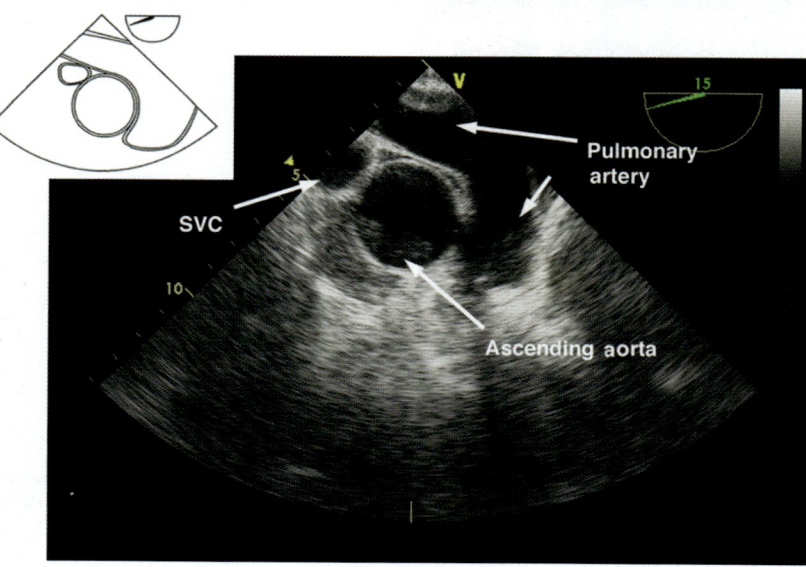

Figure 27-12 Midesophageal ascending aortic short-axis view. SVC, superior vena cava.

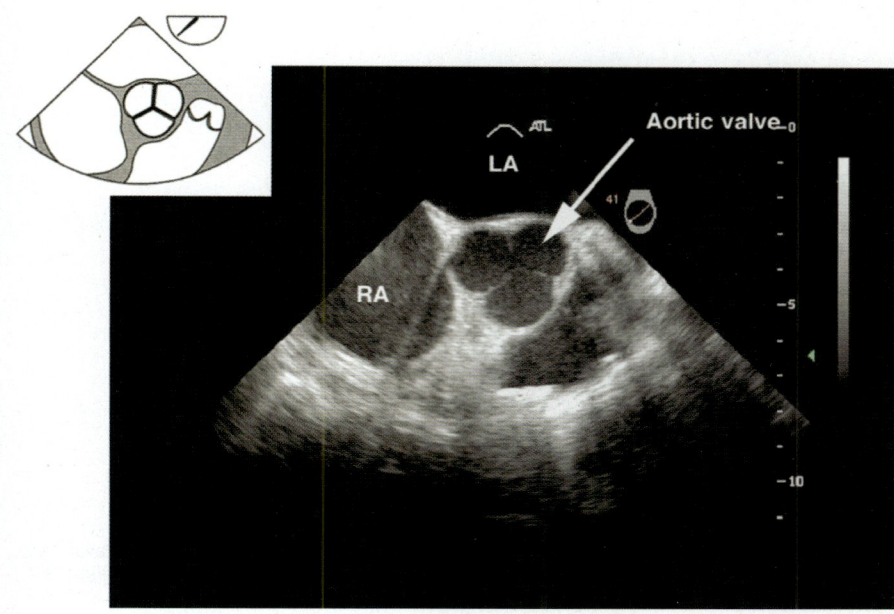

Figure 27-13 Midesophageal aortic valve short-axis view. RA, right atrium; LA, left atrium.

the ascending aorta and superior vena cava in short axis and the pulmonary artery in long axis. The view is used to:
a. Measure the AA dimensions and evaluate the presence of dissection flaps
b. Evaluate the PA (position of pulmonary artery catheter [PAC] or rule out thrombus)
c. Align the Doppler beam parallel to the blood flow in the main PA

6. **Midesophageal aortic valve short-axis view**
This view is obtained from the previous view by advancing the probe until the aortic valve (AV) is visible, and then rotating the multiplane angle between 30 and 60 degrees. In the closed position, the three cusps of the AV form what is known as the "Mercedes Benz" sign (Fig. 27-13). This view is used to:

a. Evaluate the size, number, appearance and motion of AV cusps
b. Measure the area of the AV orifice (planimetry)
c. Evaluate the presence of aortic insufficiency (AI) or aortic stenosis (AS) by applying CFD
d. Assess the interatrial septum for patent foramen ovale (PFO) or atrial septal defect (ASD)

7. **Midesophageal right ventricular inflow–outflow view**
This view is obtained from the previous view by decreasing the multiplane angle to approximately 60 to 90 degrees (Fig. 27-14). The main uses of the view are to evaluate the:
a. Pulmonic valve (PV) by measuring the Pulmonic annulus and to detect Pulmonic insufficiency by applying CFD

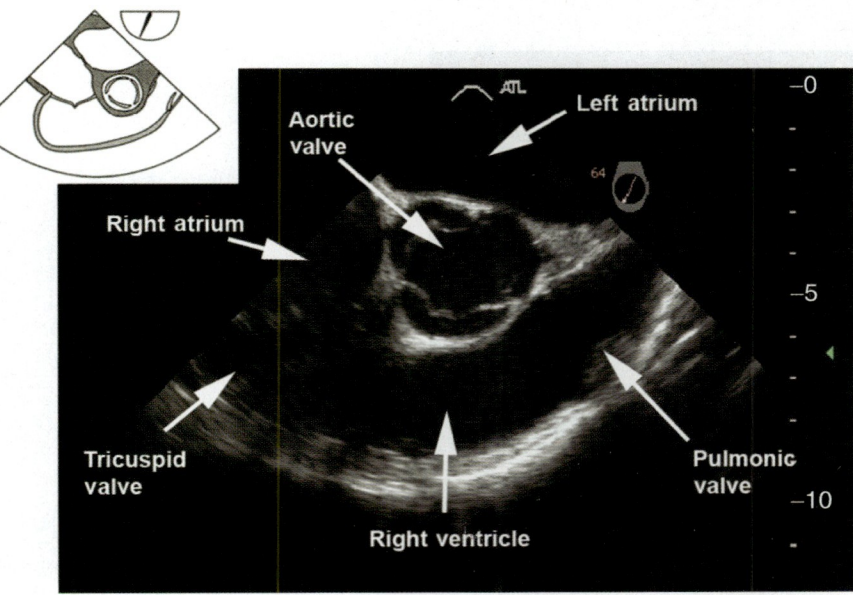

Figure 27-14 Midesophageal right ventricular inflow–outflow view.

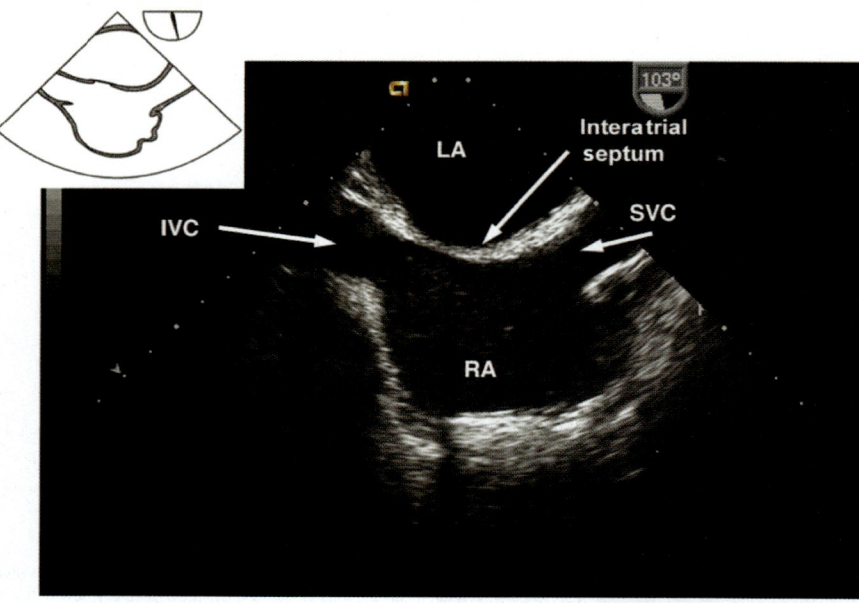

Figure 27-15 Midesophageal bicaval view. IVC, inferior vena cava; LA, left atrium; SVC, superior vena cava; RA, right atrium.

  b. RV and right ventricular outflow tract (RVOT) structure and function
  c. Tricuspid valve (TV) anatomy and function by aligning the Doppler beam with the RV diastolic blood inflow or a systolic regurgitation
  d. Passage of a PAC across the RV to the PA

8. **Midesophageal bicaval view**
   This view is obtained from the previous view by turning the probe shaft to the patient's right and decreasing the multiplane angle to 110 degrees (Fig. 27-15). The view is used to:
   a. Assess the interatrial septum (aided by CFD) to detect a PFO or ASD. Evaluate the passage of agitated saline across the interatrial septum following release of a Valsalva maneuver
   b. Guide placement of catheters, wires, and cannulae
   c. Examine for the presence of thrombus or tumors

9. **Transgastric midpapillary short-axis view**
   The view is obtained by advancing the TEE probe from the midesophageal four-chamber view into the stomach, anteflexing and then withdrawing until contact is made with the gastric wall. The LV is visualized as a doughnut in cross-section; both papillary muscles should be seen (Fig. 27-16). Additional anteflexion obtains the transgastric basal short-axis view, which allows for inspection of the anterior and posterior mitral valve leaflets. Advancement of the probe with anteflexion reveals the deep TG long axis view. The transgastric midpapillary short-axis view is unique in that it visualizes LV walls perfused by each of the three major coronary arteries. The view is

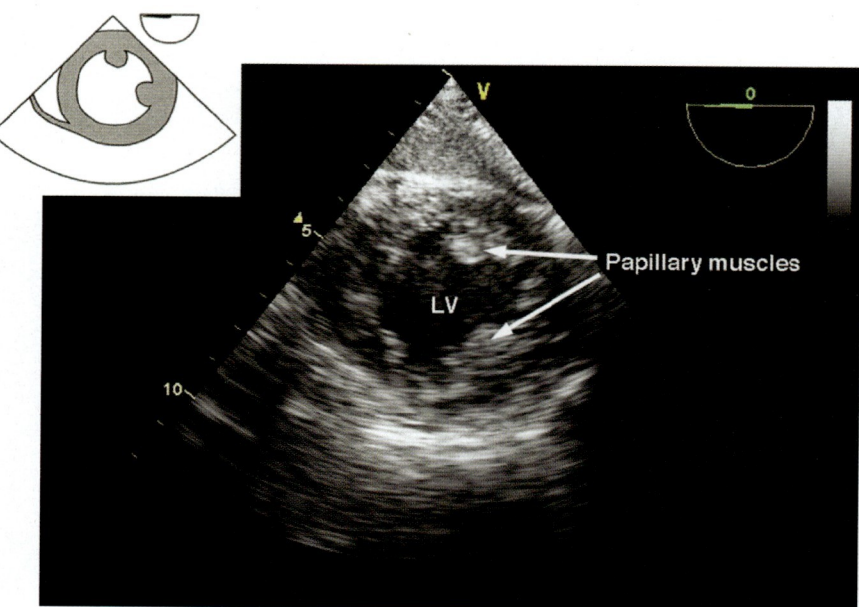

Figure 27-16 Transgastric short-axis view. LV, left ventricle.

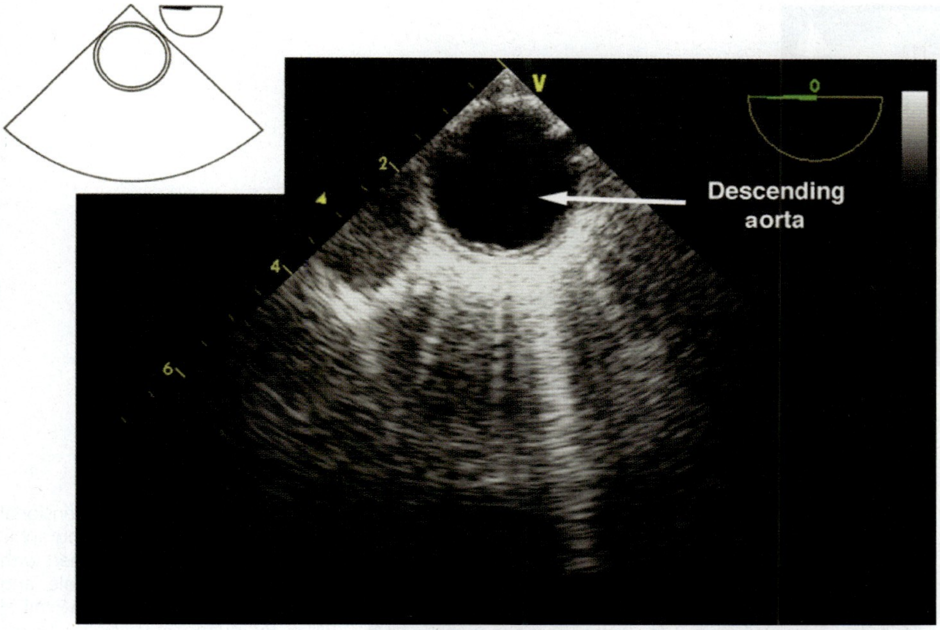

Figure 27-17 Descending aortic short-axis view.

considered to be the most useful one in situations of intraoperative hemodynamic instability, as it allows immediate diagnosis of hypovolemic state, contractile failure, or coronary ischemia.

The primary uses of the transgastric midpapillary short-axis view include assessment of the:
a. LV size (enlargement, hypertrophy) and cavity volume
b. Global ventricular systolic function and regional wall motion

10. **Descending aortic short- and long-axis views**
The descending aortic short-axis view is obtained from the midesophageal four-chamber view by turning the TEE probe to the left until the descending aorta in cross-section is seen as a circular structure (Fig. 27-17). Rotating the multiplane angle to 90 degrees visualizes the descending aorta in a longitudinal section as a tubular vascular structure (Fig. 27-18). To examine the entire descending aorta, the probe is gradually advanced and withdrawn in the esophagus. These views are used to:
a. Identify pathology of the descending aorta (atheroma, hematoma, dissection flaps, aneurysm)
b. Assist with placement of guide wires and cannulae (intra-aortic balloon pump [IABP], aortic cannula)

Three-dimensional Echocardiography

In order to better conceptualize the morphology and pathology of the heart, three-dimensional (3D) image presentation has

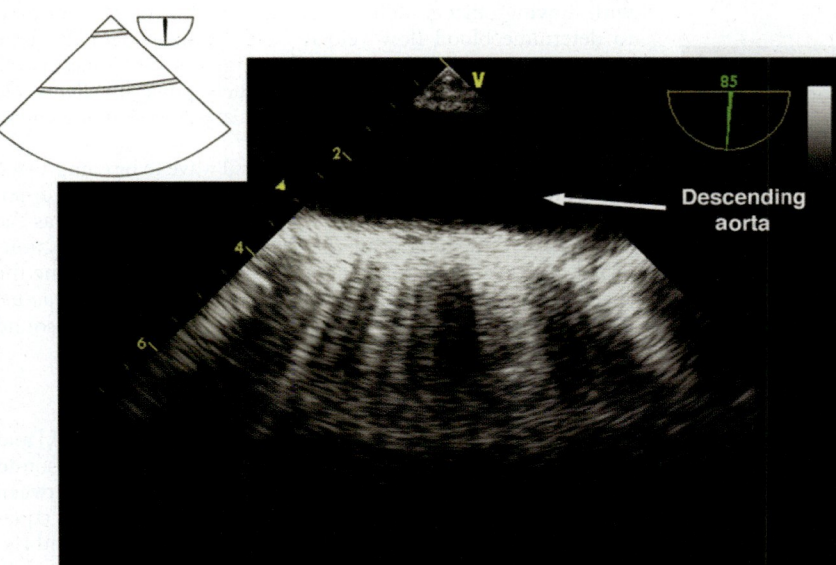

Figure 27-18 Descending aortic long-axis view.

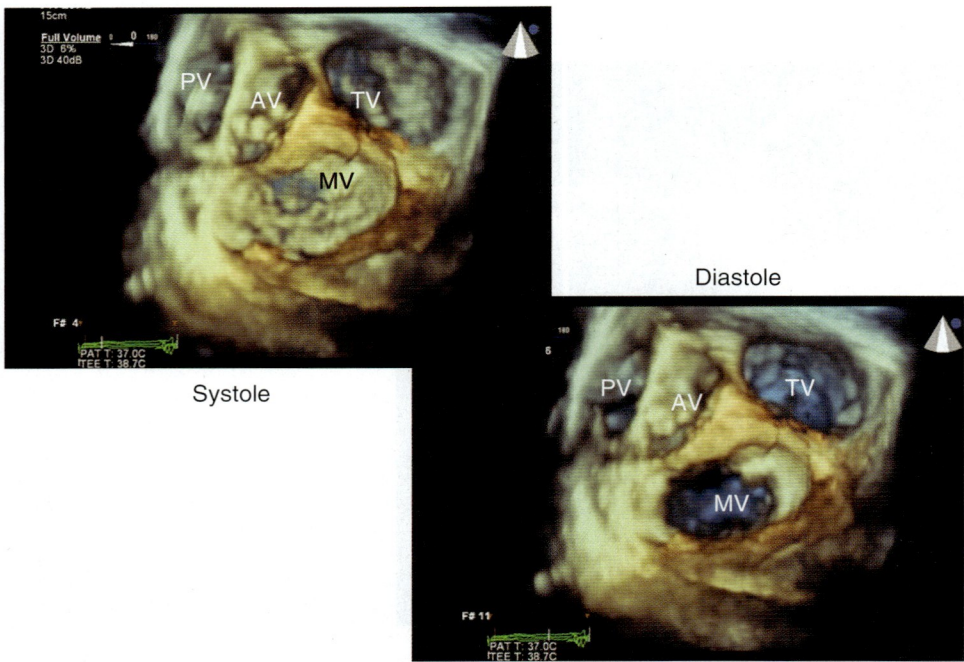

Figure 27-19 Three-dimensional transesophageal echocardiographic imaging of the base of the heart with the atria removed, in systole and diastole. AV, aortic valve; MV, mitral valve; PV, pulmonic valve; TV, tricuspid valve.

been developed. The recent introduction of a real-time 3D TEE probe makes this goal a reality for intraoperative echocardiographers. This technology is capable of acquiring full volumes of the left ventricle, of visualizing heart valves in three dimensions (Fig. 27-19), and assessing the synchrony of LV contraction.[22]

Uses of 3D TEE are continuing to emerge. The utility of 3D imaging of the MV in MV repair surgery is of particular interest (Fig. 27-20).[23] This technique allows assessment of LV contraction synchrony in patients undergoing resynchronization therapy with biventricular pacing and may offer a means to maximize their cardiac output. Additional intraoperative applications have emerged, involving percutaneous procedures (transcutaneous aortic valve insertion, noninvasive mitral repair, repair of paraprosthetic leaks, closure of ASD) and open surgical procedures.

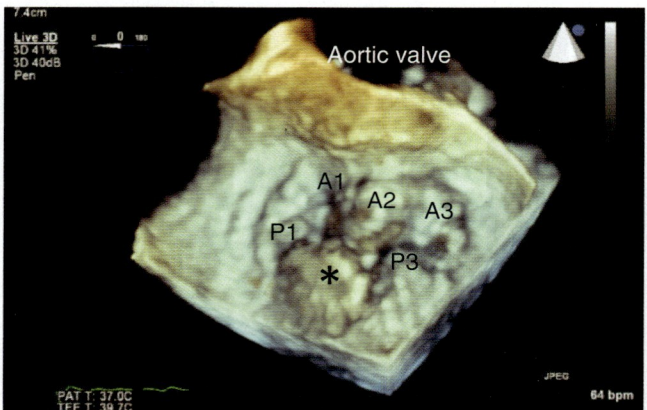

Figure 27-20 Three-dimensional imaging of prolapsing middle scallop of the posterior mitral valve leaflet (*asterisk*). A1–3, lateral, middle, and medial scallops of the anterior mitral valve leaflet; P1, lateral scallop of the posterior mitral valve leaflet; P3, medial scallop of the posterior mitral valve leaflet.

Guidelines on the use of 3D echocardiography have also been published.[24]

Doppler Echocardiography and Hemodynamics

The use of 2D echocardiography captures high-fidelity motion images of cardiac structures but not blood flow. Blood flow indices—such as blood velocities, stroke volume (SV), and pressure gradients—are the domain of Doppler echocardiography. Unlike 2D imaging, which relies on the time delay and amplitude of reflected ultrasound, Doppler technologies are based on the change in frequency that occurs when ultrasound interacts with moving objects. Reflections from red blood cells are used to determine blood flow velocity and calculate hemodynamic parameters. The combination of 2D images and quantitative Doppler measurements creates a uniquely powerful diagnostic tool. Accordingly, Doppler assessments are an essential element of the echocardiographic examination.[25]

The motion of an object causes a sound wave to be compressed in the direction of the motion and expanded in the direction opposite to the motion. This alteration in frequency is known as the *Doppler effect*. By monitoring the frequency pattern of reflections of red blood cells, Doppler echocardiography can determine the speed, direction, and timing of blood flow. The *Doppler equation* describes the relationship between the alteration in ultrasound frequency and blood flow velocity (Fig. 27-21):

$$\Delta f = v \times \cos \theta \times 2f_t/c$$

where Δf is the difference between transmitted frequency (f_t) and received frequency, v is blood velocity, c is the speed of sound in blood (1,540 m/s), and θ is the angle of incidence between the ultrasound beam and blood flow. Conceptually, the equation is simplified by observing that the change in ultrasound frequency is related to just two variables: blood velocity and $\cos \theta$.

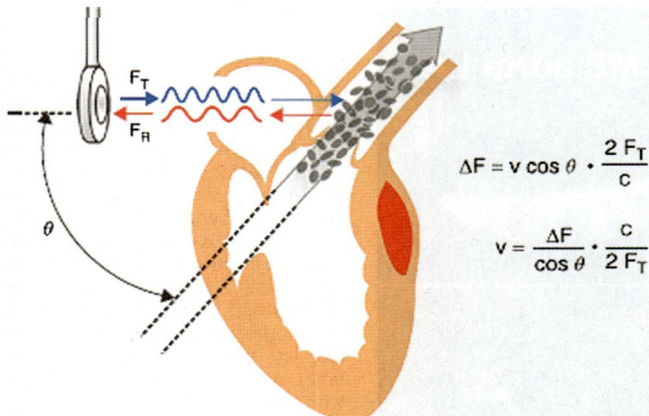

Figure 27-21 Calculating blood flow velocity. The Doppler equation calculates blood flow velocity based on two variables: The Doppler frequency shift (ΔF) and the cosine (cos) of the angle of incidence between the ultrasound beam and the blood flow. The Doppler frequency shift is measured by the echocardiographic system, but $\cos \theta$ is unknown, and manual entry by the echocardiographer is required for its estimation. v, flood flow velocity; F_T, transmitted signal frequency; F_R, reflected signal frequency; ΔF, difference between F_R and F_T; c, speed of sound in tissue; θ, angle of incidence between the orientation of the ultrasound beam and that of the blood flow.

$$\Delta F = v \cos \theta \cdot \frac{2 F_T}{c}$$

$$v = \frac{\Delta F}{\cos \theta} \cdot \frac{c}{2 F_T}$$

For this reason, the Doppler signal is shifted *only* by the component of the blood velocity that is in the direction of the beam path (i.e., $v \cos \theta$). When the beam angle divergence is greater than 30 degrees, the value of $\cos \theta$ decreases rapidly and the Doppler system will markedly underestimate blood velocity. The requirement of near-parallel orientation ($\cos \theta = 1$) for Doppler examinations contrasts with the near-perpendicular orientation preferred for 2D imaging. Consequently, the preferred imaging planes for Doppler will differ from those used for 2D imaging.

Spectral Doppler

Two Doppler techniques, *pulsed wave* (PW) and *continuous wave* (CW), are commonly used to evaluate blood flow. A thorough understanding of the advantages and disadvantages of each technique is critical in selecting the one most appropriate for the clinical setting at hand.[26,27] In clinical practice, PW and CW Dopplers are frequently used in conjunction with 2D imaging. The 2D image is used to identify the area of interest and guide the echocardiographer in precisely localizing the sampling volume in a PW study or in directing the beam in a CW study.

Pulsed-wave Doppler

PW Doppler offers the echocardiographer the ability to sample blood flow velocity from a particular location. The PW transducer uses a single crystal as both the emitter and the receiver of ultrasound waves. Like the pulsed echocardiography system described for 2D imaging, the PW Doppler system transmits a short burst of ultrasound toward the target and then switches to receive mode to interpret the returning echoes. Since the speed of sound (c) in tissue is constant, the time delay for a signal to reach its target and return to the transducer depends solely on the distance (d) to the target. Consequently, reflected signals from locations more distant from the transducer return after a greater time interval. By *time gating*, the electronic circuitry of the PW transducer interprets returning echoes only after a predetermined time delay following the transmission of an ultrasound pulse. In this way, only those signals associated with a location, referred to as the *sample volume*, are selected for evaluation.

The pulsed-Doppler system uses a repeating pattern of ultrasound transmission and reception. The rate at which the device repeatedly generates sound bursts is known as the *pulse repetition frequency*. Since the speed of sound through tissue is a constant, the pulse repetition frequency is directly related to the depth of the sample volume. The pulse repetition frequency is analogous to the frame rate of a movie camera. Like the multiple frames on a roll of movie film, each ultrasound pulse interacts with the blood flow for a brief period of time, and just as a series of movie frames displays motion, a series of pulsed cycles is consecutively analyzed to determine the blood flow. The Doppler data are frequently presented as a velocity–time plot known as the *spectral display* (Fig. 27-22B).

Since the pulsed-Doppler data are collected intermittently, the maximal frequency and blood flow velocity that can be accurately measured by PW Doppler are limited. The maximal frequency, which equals half the pulse repetition frequency, is known as the *Nyquist limit*. At blood velocities above the Nyquist limit, analysis of the returning signal becomes ambiguous, with the velocities appearing to be in the opposite direction. A similar effect is seen in movie animation, in which a rapidly spinning wheel appears to spin backward because of the slow frame rate. The ambiguous signal from frequencies above the Nyquist limit produces *aliasing* and the velocity signal may appear on the other side of the zero-velocity baseline, hence the term *wraparound*. The Nyquist limitation has led to an alternative approach for the assessment of high-velocity blood flows, continuous-wave Doppler (CW Doppler).

Continuous-wave Doppler

The CW Doppler technique avoids the maximal velocity limitation of PW systems by using two crystals, one continuously transmitting and the other continuously receiving the reflected ultrasound signal. With continuous reception of the Doppler signal, the Nyquist limit is not applicable, and blood flows with very high velocities are recorded accurately. The CW mode receives reflected signals from blood flow throughout its beam path because it is not time-gated like the PW technique (Fig. 27-22A). The inability to select blood flow from a specific location favors the selection of CW Doppler primarily for the detection of the highest velocities along the beam path, which is useful in applications such as determining the high-velocity jet of aortic stenosis.

Color-flow Doppler

CFD provides a dramatic display of both blood flow and cardiac anatomy by combining 2D echocardiography and Doppler (Fig. 27-23). The PW Doppler used for CFD differs from that previously discussed in two important ways. CFD performs *multiple* sample volume recordings along each scan line as the beam is swept through the sector. This approach provides flow data at each location in the sector, which can be overlaid on the structural data obtained by 2D imaging. The Doppler velocity data from each sample volume are color-coded and superimposed on top of the gray-scale 2D image. In the most widely accepted color code, red hues indicate flow toward the transducer and blue hues indicate flow away from the transducer. The ability to provide a real-time integrated display of flow and structural information makes CFD useful for assessing valvular function, aortic dissection, and congenital heart abnormalities.

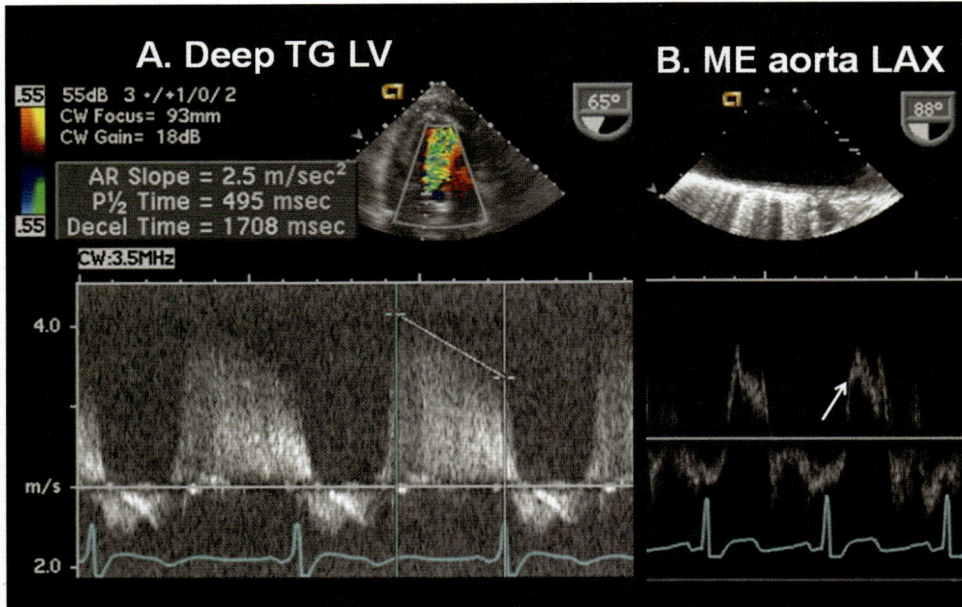

Figure 27-22 Doppler echocardiography in aortic insufficiency. **A**: The deep transgastric (deep TG) long-axis view is displayed. A color-Doppler sector is placed over the aortic valve and LV outflow tract and the aortic insufficiency (AI) jet is imaged. The continuous-wave (CW) Doppler cursor is positioned at the center of the AI flow and the spectral display of the AI jet is shown against time. The slope of the AI jet is used to calculate the pressure half-time (P½ time). A short P½ time is associated with severe AI. **B**: The descending aorta is imaged in long axis. The sample volume of pulsed-wave Doppler is placed upstream. There is a systolic wave above the baseline, as the blood moves toward the transesophageal echocardiography transducer, and a diastolic wave (arrow), indicating reversal of aortic flow because of severe AI. Decel, deceleration.

However, an important caveat to its use in the clinical setting must be noted. Since it relies on PW Doppler measurements, CFD is susceptible to alias artifacts. Aliasing in the color flow map is illustrated in Figure 27-24.

Hemodynamic Assessments

Doppler echocardiography's ability to quantitatively measure blood velocity yields a wealth of information on the hemodynamic state. Stroke volume, chamber pressures, valvular disease, pulmonary vascular resistance, ventricular function (systolic and diastolic), and anatomic defects are commonly assessed with perioperative Doppler echocardiography.[28]

Volumetric Flow Assessments

Measurements such as stroke volume and cardiac output express the volume of blood ejected by the heart over time. Volumetric parameters are calculated using the principle that volumetric

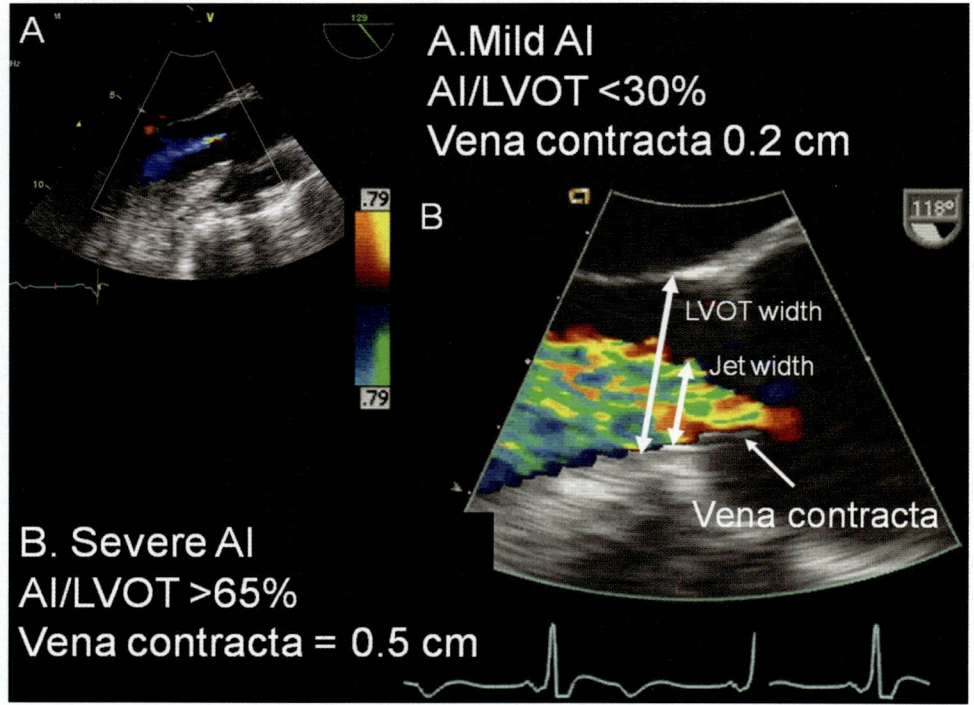

Figure 27-23 Evaluation of aortic insufficiency (AI). Color-flow Doppler of the aortic valve (AV) in the midesophageal long-axis view. AI is graded using (**A**) the relative ratio of the AI jet thickness to the diameter of left ventricular outflow tract (LVOT); both measurements are performed at the same site, usually within 0.5 to 1 cm proximal to the AV plane; and (**B**) the width of the AI jet as it crosses the AV cusps (vena contracta).

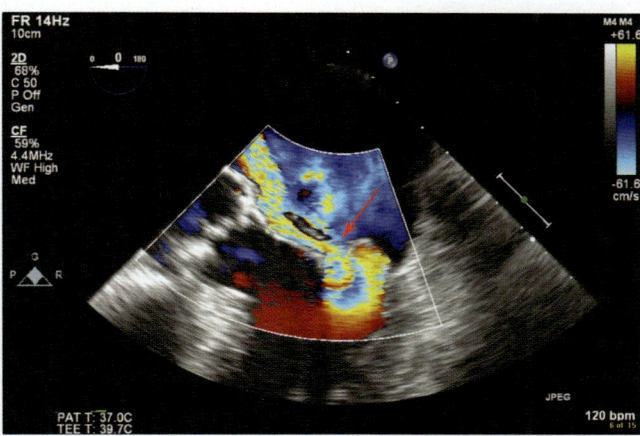

Figure 27-24 Doppler evaluation of mitral regurgitation (MR; midesophageal five-chamber view). Aliasing of the color signal and vena contracta (*arrow*) are visualized.

flow (Q) equals blood flow velocity (v) times the cross-sectional area (CSA) of the conduit, that is, Q = v × CSA. To determine volumetric flows with echocardiography, a Doppler measurement of the blood flow velocities and a 2D measurement of the CSA are recorded.

Stroke Volume and Cardiac Output

To calculate stroke volume, the instantaneous velocities during systole are traced from the spectral display and the echocardiographic system's software package calculates the time–velocity integral (VTI, in centimeters). In effect, the VTI represents the distance (v × t = d) blood traveled during systole (i.e., stroke distance). By multiplying the VTI by the CSA (in square centimeters) of the conduit (e.g., aorta, MV, PA) through which the blood traveled, the stroke volume (in cubic centimeters) is obtained: SV = VTI × CSA (Fig. 27-25).[29–31] Cardiac output (CO), which expresses volumetric flow in cubic centimeters per minute, is estimated from the product of SV and heart rate: CO = VTI × CSA × HR. Figure 27-26 demonstrates calculation of cardiac output and SV from the LVOT.

Valve Area

The Continuity Equation. The principle of conservation of mass is the basis of the *continuity equation*, which is commonly used to measure the aortic valve area.[32] The continuity equation simply states that the volume of blood passing through one site in the heart (e.g., the LVOT) is equal to the mass or volume of blood passing through another site (e.g., the aortic valve).

Volumetric flow$_1$ = volumetric flow$_2$; therefore:

$$CSA_1 \times VTI_1 = CSA_1 \times VTI_2 \text{ and}$$

$$CSA_1 = CSA_2 \times VTI_2/VTI_1$$

Figure 27-27 demonstrates calculation of AV area using this approach.

Pressure Assessment

The Bernoulli Equation. Pressure gradients are used to estimate intracavitary pressures and to assess conditions such as valvular disease (e.g., aortic stenosis), septal defects, outflow tract obstruction, and major vessel pathology (e.g., coarctation). As blood flows across a narrowed or stenotic orifice, blood flow velocity increases. The increase in velocities relates to the degree of narrowing. In the clinical situation, the *simplified Bernoulli equation* describes the relation between the increases in blood flow velocity and the pressure gradient across the narrowed orifice[11]:

$$\Delta P = 4V_{max}^2$$

where ΔP in millimeters of mercury is the pressure gradient across the narrowed orifice and V_{max} in meters per second is the maximum velocity across that orifice measured by Doppler.

Thus, in clinical echocardiography the pressure gradient is obtained by the straightforward process of measuring the peak velocity of blood flow across the lesion of interest.[33,34] The measured peak velocity is then entered into the simplified Bernoulli equation to estimate the pressure gradient.

The Bernoulli equation is commonly employed to measure the pressure gradient across a stenotic valve. In addition, the rate of decline in the pressure gradient across the valve is related to the severity of the disease.[35,36] This *pressure half-time* is the time required for the peak transvalvular pressure gradient to decrease

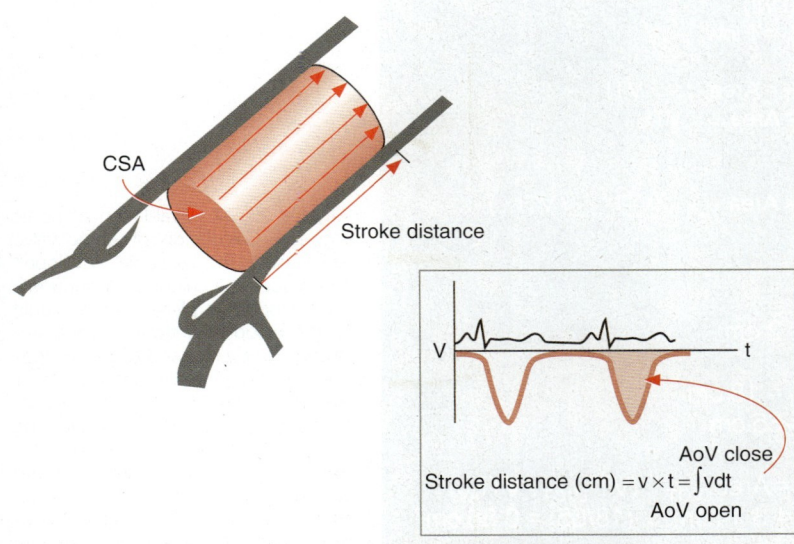

Figure 27-25 Determination of stroke volume. Volumetric flow can be determined from a combination of area and velocity measurements. In this example, the flow through the ascending aorta is used to determine the stroke volume. Integrating the Doppler-derived flow velocities over time (known as the time–velocity integral) during a single cardiac cycle calculates the stroke distance. The cross-sectional area measurement is obtained by two-dimensional echocardiography. The product of these two measurements, conceptualized as a cylinder, is the stroke volume. CSA, cross-sectional area; AoV, aortic valve.

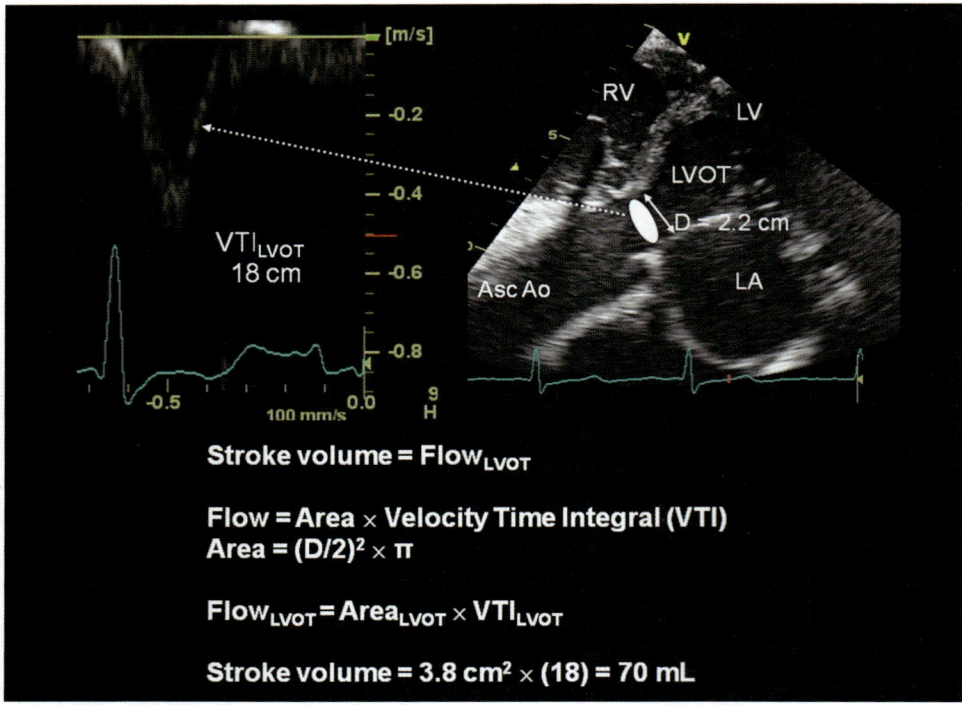

Figure 27-26 Stroke volume calculation. Stroke volume is equal to the blood flow crossing the left ventricular outflow tract (LVOT). In the deep transgastric long-axis view, the LVOT orifice (*large oval*) can be calculated from the LVOT diameter (D). The blood flow velocity across the LVOT is measured with pulsed Doppler and the velocity time integral (VTI) by tracing the velocity envelope. RV, right ventricle; LA, left atrium.

by 50%. Typically, a larger orifice will have a shorter pressure half-time, as pressures equalize faster.

Measurement of Intracavitary Pressures

Intracavitary and pulmonary arterial pressures are estimated from the pressure gradient across two adjacent chambers. The pressure gradient is defined as the difference in pressure from the "driving" chamber to the "receiving" chamber. Echocardiographically, the pressure gradient is calculated from the Doppler-derived velocities of the regurgitant jet into the receiving chamber.[37-39] Table 27-1 provides calculations of intracardiac and PA pressures.

Echocardiographic Evaluation of Systolic Function

Evaluation of LV systolic function is a primary component of every echocardiographic examination. Information about global

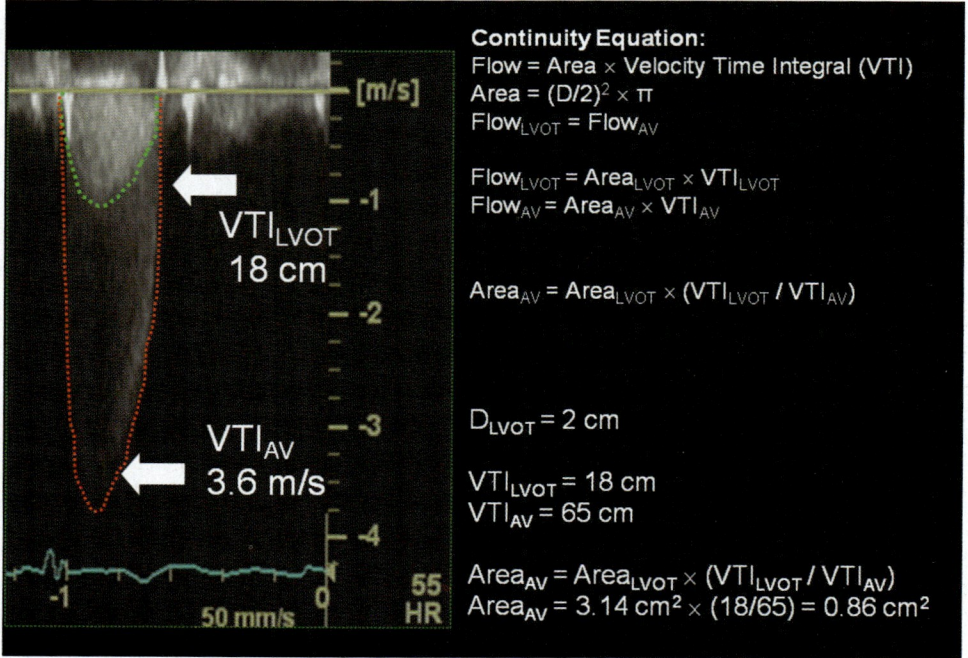

Figure 27-27 Evaluation of aortic stenosis. Calculation of aortic valve area using the "double envelope" technique. The cursor of continuous-wave Doppler is placed in the middle of the blood flow traversing the stenosed aortic valve, and two envelopes are identified. The one with the slower velocity is from the left ventricular outflow tract (LVOT) and the one with the fastest is from the aortic valve (AV). The envelopes of the velocities are traced to derive the respective velocity time integrals (VTI). The aortic valve area is calculated using the continuity equation. D, diameter.

Table 27-1 Calculation of Cardiopulmonary Pressures

Pressure	Equation
RVSP or PASP	$= 4(V_{TR})^2 + RAP$
PAMP	$= 4(V_{early\ PI})^2 + RAP$
PADP	$= 4(V_{late\ PI})^2 + RAP$
LAP	$= SBP - 4(V_{MR})^2$
LVEDP	$= DBP - 4(V_{AI\ end})^2$

RVSP, right ventricular systolic pressure; PASP, pulmonary artery systolic pressure; V, peak velocity; TR, tricuspid regurgitation; RAP, right atrial pressure; PAMP, pulmonary artery mean pressure; PI, pulmonic valve insufficiency; PADP, pulmonary artery diastolic pressure; LAP, left atrial pressure; SBP, systolic blood pressure; MR, mitral regurgitation; LVEDP, left ventricular end-diastolic pressure; DBP, diastolic blood pressure; AI, aortic insufficiency.

as well as regional LV performance is accomplished by assessing the size, shape, and LV contractile function. Both qualitative assessments (which are inherently subjective) and quantitative techniques (which produce hard numerical estimates) are useful: 2D and M-mode image the LV walls and cavity and Doppler echocardiography measures the velocity of blood flow and moving tissue.

Left Ventricular Walls

The LV cavity and walls at the basal, mid, and apical levels are evaluated in the midesophageal and transgastric views. From the midesophageal position, the TEE imaging array is rotated electronically in a clockwise fashion to scan the entire circumference of the LV cavity and walls in a longitudinal orientation.

Further advancement of the TEE probe to the transgastric position combined with anterior flexion (anteflexion) of the probe sequentially images the LV short axis from its base to apex. The echocardiographic imaging of blood and myocardium is based on their different acoustic properties: Muscle tissue is reflective and imaged in shades of gray, whereas ultrasound easily propagates through blood, resulting in the LV cavity appearing dark. Their interface is the endocardial surface, which typically produces the brightest signal. The evaluation focuses on the shape, size, and motion of LV walls.

Shape

The LV's longitudinal shape is evaluated in the midesophageal views (Fig. 27-28). It appears bullet-shaped with the mitral annulus and leaflets comprising its broad base, and the walls tapering toward its apex. In the midesophageal view at 0-degree rotation (midesophageal four-chamber, midesophageal five-chamber) the inferolateral wall of the LV appears on the right of the TEE monitor screen and the inferoseptal wall on the left. Clockwise rotation of the multiplane angle to about 90 degrees (midesophageal two-chamber) will image the long axis of the LV, with the anterior and inferior walls presented on the right and left sides of the monitor, respectively. Further rotation to approximately 135 degrees will image the LV anteroseptal and inferolateral walls on the right and left sides of the screen.

The echocardiographer must be careful to image the LV along the true long axis in the midesophageal views. Often, in the midesophageal four-chamber view, the imaging plane may cut obliquely in an anterior direction, which causes an increase in the apparent wall thickness and foreshortens the LV cavity. This is avoided by confirming that the LV long-axis measurement approximates that of the LV length (as measured from the mitral annular plane to the apex, typically in the midesophageal two-chamber view). In many cases, slight retroflection or rotation of the multiplane angle from 0 to 20 degrees is helpful to achieve

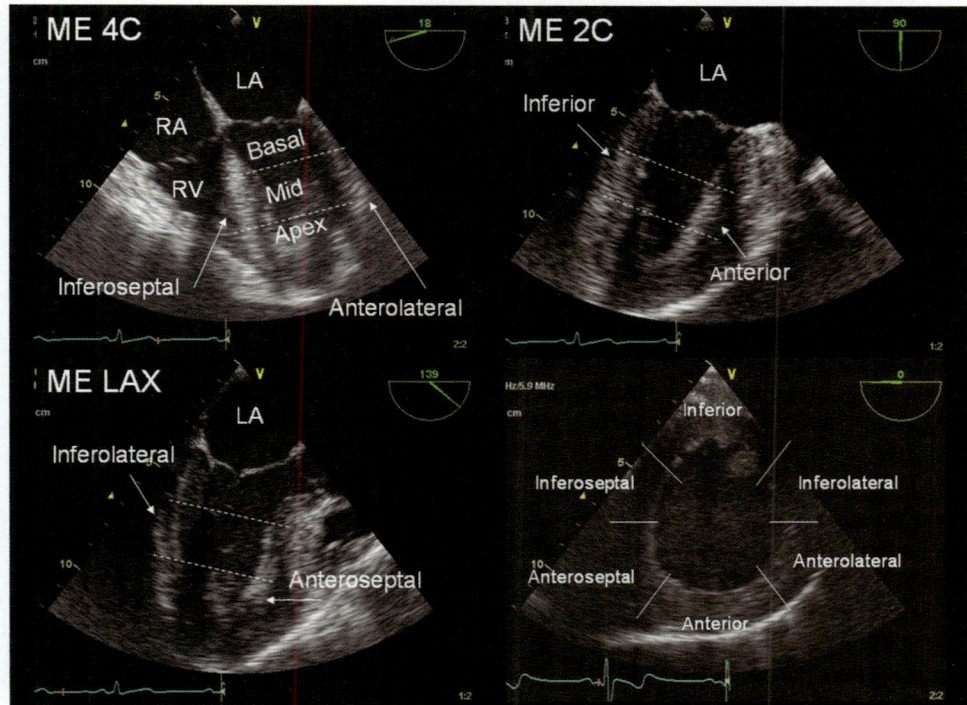

Figure 27-28 Left ventricular (LV) walls. In the esophagus, the transesophageal echocardiography (TEE) probe is rotated clockwise from 0 to 140 degrees to obtain the midesophageal (ME) views. Advancement of the TEE probe inside the stomach obtains the transgastric (TG) midpapillary short-axis view. In the ME views, the LV is divided in basal, mid, and apical segments. 4C, four-chamber; 2C, two-chamber; LA, left atrium; RA, right atrium; RV, right ventricle.

the best alignment. The LV walls are divided into three segments each—basal, mid, and apical—as defined by lines drawn perpendicular to the LV long axis at the tips and base of the papillary muscles.

From the transgastric position, the LV is seen along its short axis; its shape resembles a doughnut. The basal segments are imaged in the short axis with the TEE probe in the distal esophagus or very high up inside the stomach. At this depth, the mitral leaflets (base of heart) are seen "enface." Gradual advancement of the TEE probe into the stomach images the mid-LV segments (Fig. 27-16). Here, the anatomic landmark is the body of the papillary muscles at 2 o'clock (posteromedial) and 5 o'clock (anterolateral). Further advancement of the TEE probe will image the LV apex, much thicker and with a smaller cavity. In either midesophageal or transgastric imaging planes, the LV walls thicken in systole and thin in diastole. As seen in the midesophageal views, the LV base descends toward the LV apex and ascends at diastole.

Aneurysms

Aneurysms appear as a dilated part of the LV perimeter with thinned wall(s) and decreased motion. Aneurysms are always pathologic and usually due to ischemia-related necrosis and weakening of the LV wall. Aneurysms are separated into true and false. If all myocardial layers (epi-, mid-, and endocardium) are present in the wall of the aneurysm, it is called a *true aneurysm*. The "neck" of a true aneurysm is usually wide, and the aneurysmal cavity shallows with a smooth transition from normal to aneurysmal walls. An aneurysm is called *false* or "pseudo" if the LV wall contains only some of the myocardial layers (usually the epicardium and part of the midwall). False aneurysms are caused by necrosis of the LV wall, usually from myocardial infarction. Sometimes, the wall of a false aneurysm consists only of the attached pericardium. False aneurysms have a narrower neck and the transition between healthy and diseased wall segments is abrupt. A false aneurysm is prone to rupture and is treated surgically. Blood flow is sluggish within aneurysms. Red blood cells clump together, which increases echogenicity and creates spontaneous echocardiography contrast, a smoke-like appearance inside the LV cavity. Thrombus, appearing with brightness similar to that of myocardium but clearly separated from the LV wall, can also develop in aneurysms.

Texture

The *texture* of the LV walls may offer additional information in patients with infiltrative cardiomyopathies, such as amyloid, where the thickened myocardium has a speckled appearance.

Wall Thickness

LV hypertrophy is termed *concentric* if the cavity is not increased (usually resulting from increased pressure work) and *eccentric* when there is LV dilation (usually resulting from increased volume work). The diagnosis is made by summing the end-diastolic (ED) wall thickness of the anteroseptal and inferolateral LV segments in the basal transgastric short-axis view, just at the tips of the papillary muscles (Fig. 27-29). Normal values are 18 ± 2 mm (men) and 15.5 ± 1.5 mm (women).

Segments and Regional Function

Abnormal myocardial wall systolic thickening is a sensitive marker of myocardial ischemia that appears earlier than electrocardiographic and hemodynamic changes.[40–42] Regional LV systolic function reflects the regional myocardial blood flow.[43] The association of the regional LV wall motion with the underlying coronary artery distribution is used to diagnose local perfusion defects. The LV is divided into 17 regional segments (Fig. 27-28).[44] Along the longitudinal plane, each wall is divided into basal, mid, and apical levels. The basal and mid-levels are further divided into anterior, inferior, two septal (anteroseptal and

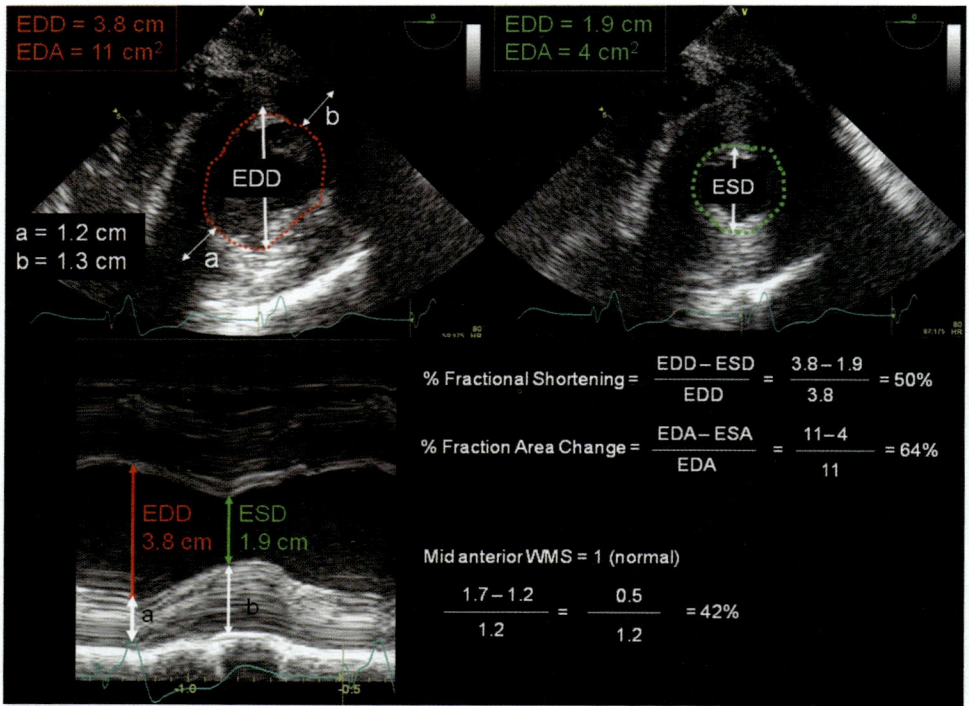

Figure 27-29 Two-dimensional evaluation of left ventricular (LV) global and regional functions. Regional and global evaluation of the LV using the transgastric short-axis view at the midpapillary level. Measurements are performed at end-diastole (ED) and end-systole (ES). **Top panels**: Measurement of diameters (D), areas (A), and wall thickness. Wall thickness is measured at ED in the anteroseptal and inferolateral wall segments. **Bottom panel**: Diameter and wall thickness measured using method mode with the cursor crossing the middle of inferior (**top**) and anterior (**bottom**) segments. The percent change of wall thickness of the midanterior wall segment can be used to grade its regional function. In this example, wall motion score (WMS) is 1 **(normal)** because the segment thickens >30%.

Left Ventricular Cavity

Diameters

The LV cavity is defined by its long and short axes. The LV major (or long) axis dimension is measured in the midesophageal two-chamber view, from the base of the mitral annulus to the LV apex (Fig. 27-30); the minor (or short) axis dimension is measured in either the midesophageal or transgastric two-chamber views, perpendicular to the long axis, at the height of the papillary muscle tips. The minor axis is equal to one-half of the long-axis measurement. Proper measurement of the LV minor axis is used to quantify the LV ED volume. Normal LV ED dimensions (EDDs) are 4.2 to 5.9 cm (men) and 3.9 to 5.3 cm (women). An increased LV EDD denotes LV dilation and volume overload, whereas a decreased LV EDD denotes hypovolemia and inadequate preload.

Global Systolic Function

Systolic function is responsible for delivering a sufficient amount of blood to the vessels at a high enough pressure to perfuse the tissues adequately. A variety of echocardiographic measurements are used to evaluate the components (preload, afterload, and contractility), which collectively define LV global systolic function. The techniques for LV evaluation are described in detail in references.[48,49]

Percent Fractional Shortening (%FS)

FS measures the relative change of the LV short-axis diameter between ED and end-systole (ES; Fig. 27-29). FS is a one-dimensional, unitless measurement of systolic function. Measurements are done in the transgastric midpapillary short-axis view, just above the papillary muscles. A larger number occurs when the LV has normal or increased systolic function. FS is not a substitute for ejection fraction (EF) and may overestimate systolic function if there is LV dilation or abnormal wall motion

Table 27-2 Grading of Wall Function

Regional Function	Grade	Inward Radial Motion (Systolic Wall Thickening)
Normal	1	>30% (marked)
Hypokinetic	2	>10% to <30% (reduced)
Akinetic	3	<10% (negligible)
Dyskinetic	4	Paradoxical systolic motion (systolic thinning)
Aneurysmal	5	Thin wall, no thickening

inferoseptal), and two lateral (anterolateral and inferolateral) segments. The apical level is divided into four segments (anterior, inferior, septal, and lateral) and the apical cap is the 17th segment. To limit misdiagnosis, evaluation of each segment is done in at least two different views, ensuring that both endocardium and epicardium are visible. A midesophageal or transgastric view is digitally stored and played over time. The segmental (or regional) function is evaluated by noticing the presence or absence of endocardial excursion (toward the LV cavity) and degree of systolic wall thickening during one or two consecutive cardiac cycles (Fig. 27-29). The electrocardiogram is used to define systole and diastole. The function of each wall segment is scored as shown in Table 27-2.[45] The wall motion score index is the sum of all scores divided by the number of segments evaluated. The evaluation of segmental wall motion to detect ischemia is not error-free. In addition to being a subjective assessment, wall motion may be affected by tethering, regional loading conditions, and stunning.[46] Epicardial pacing of the free wall of the RV (as in the post-bypass period) produces a left bundle block and induces septal wall motion abnormalities. Interobserver reproducibility is better for normally contracting segments than for dysfunctional segments.[47] Because of these issues, wall thickening is a more reliable marker of regional function.

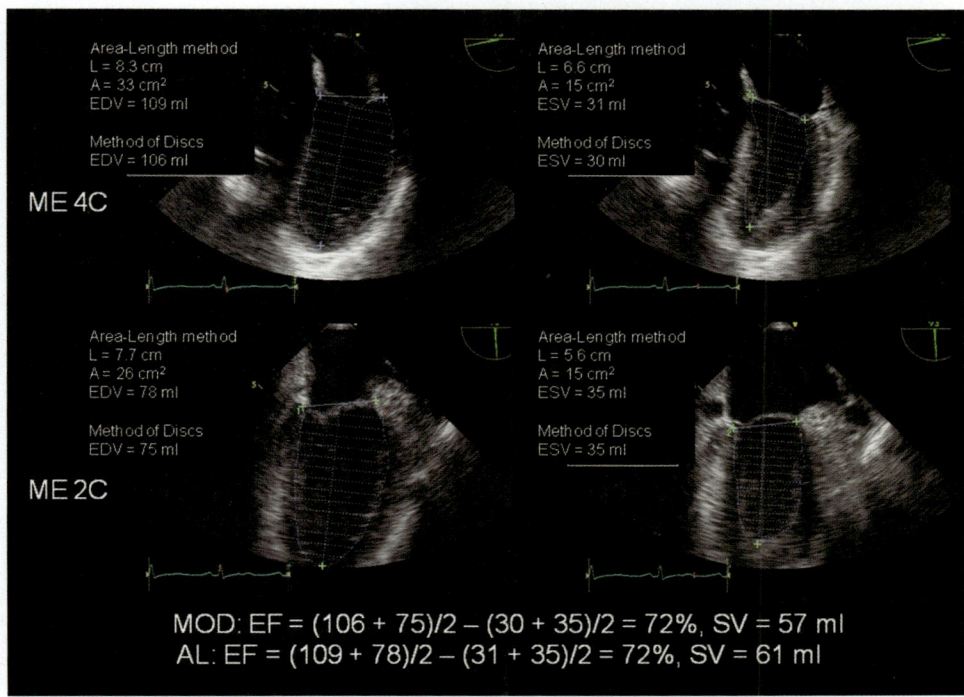

Figure 27-30 Quantitation of left ventricular (LV) systolic function. The midesophageal (ME) LV four-chamber (ME 4C) and two-chamber (ME 2C) views are obtained. The images are examined in end-diastole (ED) and end-systole (ES). The LV endocardium is traced. This automatically defines the LV area (A) and long axis (L). The system software will calculate LV volumes using either the method of discs (MOD) or the area–length method (AL). EF, ejection fraction; EDV, end-diastolic volume; ESV, end-systolic volume; SV, stroke volume.

at another level. %FS = (LV EDD − LV ESD)/(LV EDD) × 100 and is normally 27% to 45%.

Volumes

LV volume measurements are used to calculate preload (ED volume [EDV]) as well as SV and EF. The ED and ES LV volumes can be derived from manually tracing the endocardial border in ED and ES, respectively.

LV volume is commonly measured using the modified Simpson or the area length method. The biplane method of discs (or modified Simpson rule) conceives a series of disks inside the LV cavity, which have equal thickness and are stacked like coins along the LV long-axis dimension (Fig. 27-30). The diameter of each disk is the short-axis dimension as defined from the LV endocardium tracing. Measurements are performed in the midesophageal four- and two-chamber views. Alternatively, the area length method can be used to calculate LV volume: LV volume = 5/6 × ([area] × [length]). This approach is performed in one of the previous views and calculates the LV volume using the endocardial-enclosed area and the LV major axis (Fig. 27-30). In most adults, an ED area less than 12 cm^2 indicates hypovolemia.[50] Reliable and correct visualization of the endocardial border is paramount for accurate measurement of LV volumes with either method. The methods underestimate LV volume when the LV cavity is "foreshortened."

Percent Fractional Area Change

Fractional area change (FAC) is the percent difference between ED and ES LV areas (Fig. 27-29). The LV area is measured by manually tracing the endocardial border in the transgastric midpapillary short-axis view in ED and in ES. The papillary muscles are not traced. Unlike LVEF measurements, FAC does not take into account the presence of wall motion abnormalities at a different level: for example, the function of the LV apex, which is frequently involved in coronary artery disease. Therefore, caution is advised when interpreting FAC. Normal values are 56% to 65%.[51]

Visual Estimation of FAC

The most frequently used technique to evaluate global LV function as well as preload is visual estimation of FAC, often referred to as the *eyeball* EF. Although highly subjective, it is practiced widely and is accurate in experienced echocardiographers, especially in normally contracting ventricles.[52] With LV dysfunction, visual evaluations of FAC become less reproducible among different observers.[47]

Ejection Fraction

EF is the most frequently used estimate of LV systolic function. The evaluation of EF provides prognostic information about mortality and morbidity.[53] EF and SV are affected by factors such as preload, afterload, and heart rate, and thus are not always indicators of intrinsic systolic function. Typical clinical scenarios in which EF does not represent LV systolic function include the hypercontractile LV in mitral regurgitation (MR; where more than half of ED volume may regurgitate inside the left atrium) or the hypocontractile LV in aortic stenosis (where LV systolic performance is poor despite preserved contractility).

Stroke Volume

Stroke volume is calculated as the difference between EDV and ESV (end-systolic volume), and percent EF is calculated as %EF = SV/EDV × 100 = (EDV − ESV)/EDV × 100. Normal values are EDV, 67 to 155 mL (men), 56 to 104 mL (women); ESV, 22 to 58 mL (men) and 19 to 49 mL (women); %EF, greater than 55%.

Associated Findings

Sluggish flow will clump together red blood cells, producing spontaneous echocardiography contrast, which is imaged as "smoke." Thrombus is also found if there is blood stasis, such as inside an aneurysm or at the LV apex. These findings are often present when LV function is depressed.

Tissue Echocardiography—Myocardial Velocity

Tissue Doppler imaging (TDI) measures the velocity of myocardial motion along the longitudinal axis and is a sensitive measurement of regional and global functions and outcome.[54] The myocardial velocity is measured from the basal LV segments with the sample volume placed next to the mitral annulus. The velocities are comprised of a systolic (S′) followed by, in the opposite direction, two diastolic waves, one early (E′) and one following atrial contraction (A′). A reduced or delayed S′ velocity is associated with development of regional ischemia (Fig. 27-31).[55]

Evaluation of Left Ventricular Diastolic Function

An increased recognition of the impact of LV diastolic function on the overall cardiac function and outcome has driven efforts to both monitor and optimize diastolic performance in the perioperative period. The presence of preoperative asymptomatic ventricular dysfunction in patients undergoing vascular surgery is associated with increased short- and long-term morbidity and mortality.[56] Furthermore, there is a significant association between the presence of perioperative diastolic dysfunction and postoperative heart failure as well as increased hospital length of stay.[57] Several echocardiographic studies have suggested that patients with diastolic dysfunction presenting for cardiac surgery may be prone to intraoperative hemodynamic instability and worse outcomes.[58,59] These reasons support diastolic function assessment as part of the comprehensive perioperative echocardiographic examination.[60] Doppler echocardiography is the preferred technique to assess diastolic performance and grade the severity of the disease process.

Diastolic dysfunction is defined as the inability of the LV to fill at normal left atrial (LA) pressures and is characterized by a decrease in relaxation and/or LV compliance. Diastolic dysfunction may be present in the absence of clinical symptoms of heart failure. When these symptoms occur in the presence of diastolic dysfunction, then the diagnosis of diastolic heart failure is made.

Diastolic Physiology

Traditionally, the cardiac cycle has been divided into two phases: systole, comprising isovolumic contraction and ejection, and diastole, comprising isovolumic relaxation, rapid filling, diastasis, and atrial contraction. Rather than a passive phase of the cardiac cycle when filling of the heart occurs, diastole is currently regarded as being intimately coupled and interdependent with systole. In this respect, Nishimura and Tajik[61] have proposed dividing the cardiac cycle into three phases: contraction, relaxation, and filling. Contraction encompasses the isovolumic contraction and

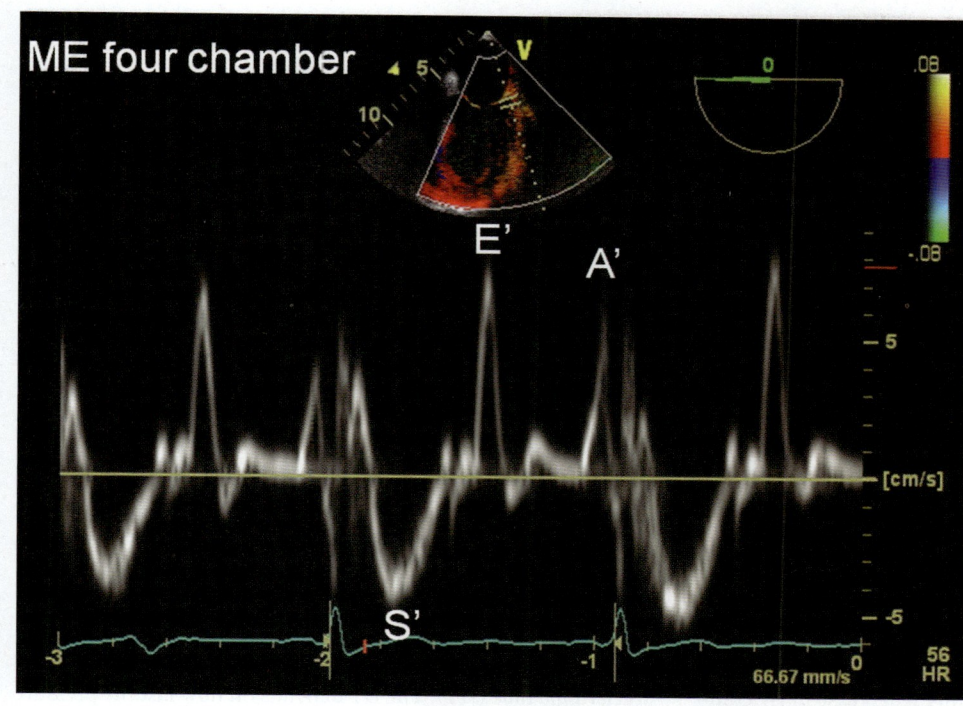

Figure 27-31 Tissue Doppler imaging. Myocardial velocity of basal anterolateral segment of left ventricle is measured with pulsed-wave tissue Doppler. ME, midesophageal; S', systolic velocity; E', early diastolic velocity; A', late diastolic velocity.

the first half of ejection. The critical insight into the proposal of Nishimura and Tajik is that relaxation begins during the second part of *ejection*, and then continues during the isovolumic relaxation and rapid filling phases, illustrating the interdependency of systole and diastole. The filling phase consists of the early rapid filling phase, diastasis, and atrial contraction.

Relaxation, the active phase of diastole, commences with the dissociation of actin–myosin cross-bridges and a lowering of the intracellular calcium. LV pressure begins to fall and eventually becomes lower than ascending aortic pressure, resulting in closure of the AV. As the ventricle continues to relax, the LV pressure falls below LA pressure, reaching its nadir, and promotes opening of the MV. At this point, the pressure gradient between the LA and LV is maximal and early rapid filling phase of the LV occurs. This phase coincides with and depends on the continuation of relaxation. The early filling phase is responsible for 80% to 90% of LV filling. As the ventricle fills, the LV pressure gradually rises and equates the pressure in the LA; thus, minimal flow or diastasis occurs. With commencement of the atrial contraction phase, the pressure gradient between the LA and LV rises once again and blood flows from the LA to the LV. At the end of the LA systole, the pressure in the LV rises above the LA pressure and promotes closure of the MV (Fig. 27-32).

Ventricular filling is affected by load factors (preload and afterload) as well as mechanical factors, such as ventricular relaxation and compliance, ventricular contraction, atrial contraction and MV dynamics, viscoelastic forces of the myocardium, and pericardial restraint.

The early manifestation of diastolic dysfunction is characterized by an impaired relaxation, implying that the rate and duration of decrease in LV pressure after systolic contraction is prolonged. This results in an inability of the LV to fill adequately during the rapid filling phase. A compensatory increase in filling occurs with atrial contraction. This stage of disease is known as *grade I diastolic dysfunction*. In more advanced stages of disease, grades II and III of diastolic dysfunction, a decrease in LV

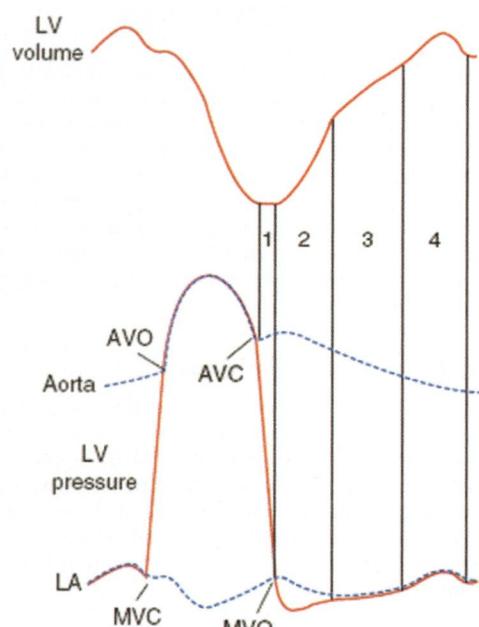

Figure 27-32 Diastolic phase of the cardiac cycle. During isovolumic relaxation (1) left ventricular (LV) pressure falls rapidly following aortic valve closure (AVC). When LV pressure decreases below left atrial (LA) pressure, the mitral valve opens (MVO), initiating early, rapid LV filling (2). Equilibration of LV and LA pressures results in diminished transmitral flow during diastasis (3) until atrial contraction (4). Diastole terminates with mitral valve closure (MVC). (Reproduced from Plotnick GD. Changes in diastolic function—difficult to measure, harder to interpret. *Am Heart J.* 1989;118:637, with permission.)

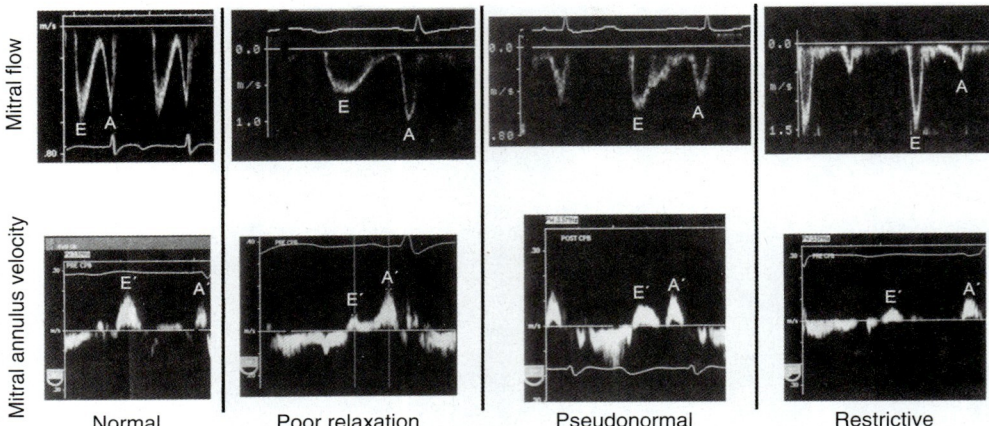

Figure 27-33 The impact of progressive left ventricular (LV) diastolic dysfunction on transmitral mitral flow (E, A) and mitral annular velocities (E′, A′). In the first stage, diastolic dysfunction both E and E′ are decreased. However, with progressing grades of disease, while the E velocity increases (due to LA pressure increases) the E′ velocity remains reduced. This supports the utility of E′ as a measure of LV relaxation as well as its relative load independence. (Reprinted with permission from Shernan SK. A practical approach to the echocardiographic evaluation of ventricular diastolic function. In: Perrino AC Jr, Reeves ST, eds. *A Practical Approach to Transesophageal Echocardiography.* 3rd ed. Philadelphia: Lippincott Williams & Wilkins; 2014:138–158.)

compliance ensues. Compliance is defined as a change of volume with respect to a change in pressure. Thus, a decrease in LV compliance will lead to a disproportionate increase in LV pressures and, ultimately, LA pressures.

Echocardiographic Assessment of Left Ventricular Diastolic Function

Echocardiography has become the diagnostic modality of choice for patients with diastolic dysfunction. Echocardiographic assessments have been validated by cardiac catheterization and correlate with clinical presentation.[62] The American Society of Echocardiography has issued recommendations for evaluating and grading left ventricular diastolic function using a combination of 2D echocardiography, pulsed-wave Doppler, M-mode color Doppler, and tissue Doppler.[60,63] This section is limited to the discussion of the two most commonly used methods: pulsed-wave Doppler of transmitral flow and TDI.

Imaging Views and Techniques

The echocardiographic acquisition of the diastolic parameters is best done when integrated in a standard examination. The typical view used for both transmitral flow (TMF) Doppler as well as for the TDI is the midesophageal four-chamber view. The interrogation volume sample should be placed at the tips of the MV for TMF assessment. For TDI of myocardial velocity profiles, the sample volume is typically placed at the junction of the mitral annulus and the lateral wall.

Interpretation of Pulsed-wave Doppler Velocity Curves

Doppler assessment of the TMF velocities reflects the instantaneous pressure gradient (see previous discussion of the Bernoulli principle). Therefore, the displayed velocity waveforms parallel the changes in pressure gradient occurring in the left heart. The TMF profile consists of two waves, the "E" and "A" waves. The peak E wave represents the peak early filling velocity. The rate of decrease of velocity following the peak E velocity is known as the *deceleration time* (DT). The DT depends on how fast the pressure rises in LV during the rapid filling phase and represents a direct measure of ventricular compliance. Thus, if the ventricular compliance decreases, the DT shortens. The peak A wave represents the peak blood velocity during atrial contraction. In a normal individual, the E wave is slightly larger than the A wave and the DT is 200 ± 40 ms (Fig. 27-33).

The mitral annular TDI technique assesses diastolic function by evaluating the myocardial velocities at the level of the mitral annulus. The myocardial motion produces high-amplitude low-velocity signals. A normal profile has a biphasic diastolic component: the early diastolic wave E′, which represents the myocardial elongation caused by early filling, and the late diastolic wave A′, which represents the myocardial distension generated by blood flow during atrial contraction (Fig. 27-31). In a healthy patient, the TDI pattern mirrors the TMF pattern, except with lower velocities. E′ reflects LV relaxation and values less than 10 cm/s are considered a sign of diastolic dysfunction.[64] Thus, in patients with pseudonormal or restrictive disease, in whom normal or elevated E wave TMF velocities occur despite advanced pathology, the TDI E′ wave remains reduced, making it a useful approach to diagnosis.

As diastolic dysfunction develops, the patterns of the flow velocity curves change in concordance with the pressure gradient changes in the pulmonary vein—LA–LV system. In grade I diastolic dysfunction, as the LV is incompletely relaxed when early ventricular filling occurs, the pressure gradient, and thus E wave velocity, is less than normal. The delayed relaxation prolongs LV filling late into diastole, and therefore the DT is prolonged. A compensatory increase in TMF during atrial contraction, due to the higher residual atrial preload, generates a high A wave velocity. Thus, the TMF curve of an individual with abnormal relaxation is represented by a low E, high A, and prolonged DT (Fig. 27-33).

Progression of diastolic disease leads to grade II diastolic dysfunction, which is marked by decreases in LV compliance. LA pressure rises as a compensatory mechanism to normalize the pressure gradient across the MV. In this scenario, the TMF velocities resemble the normal curve; thus, this stage is known as *pseudonormal* (Fig. 27-33).

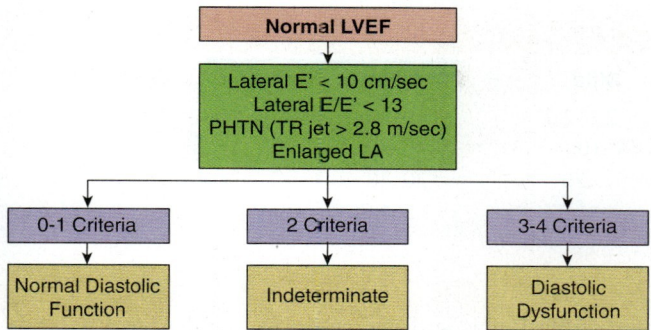

Figure 27-34 Algorithm for diagnosis of left ventricular diastolic dysfunction. LVEF, left ventricular ejection fraction; PHTN, pulmonary hypertension; TR, tricuspid regurgitation; LA, left atrium. Adapted from the 2016 Recommendations for evaluation of left ventricular diastolic dysfunction by echocardiography.[63]

Grade III diastolic dysfunction, known as the *restrictive phase*, is characterized by a significantly decreased LV compliance. The high LA–LV pressure gradient produces a fast acceleration of blood flow in the LV. A high E velocity on the TMF curve is representative for grade III diastolic dysfunction. LV pressure increases rapidly during filling because of the increased LV stiffness resulting in a short DT. The forward filling velocity at atrial contraction is low (small A wave) because of the decreased compliance (Fig. 27-33). One of the important caveats to assessing diastolic function using pulsed-wave Doppler is that the flow patterns depend on pressure gradients and therefore are affected by both preload and afterload. In settings in which the load conditions vary at a fast pace, such as the operating room, changes in TMF velocities may be difficult to interpret. TDI, which directly measures myocardial velocities, provides a more load-independent method of diastolic function assessment.[65] The updated guidelines utilize 4 criteria to diagnose diastolic dysfunction (Fig. 27-34).[63]

Pericardial Disease: Constrictive Pericarditis and Pericardial Tamponade

Diastolic filling is also impacted by pericardial restraint. Pericardial pathologies, such as constrictive pericarditis or pericardial tamponade, impede diastolic flow.[66] On TMF Doppler profiles, these diseases resemble the diastolic restrictive filling pattern. Two-dimensional echocardiography can be helpful in differentiating among these pathologies. In constrictive pericarditis, the pericardium appears thick, fibrotic, calcified, and thus echogenic; the inferior vena cava is dilated and the ventricular septum has an abnormal motion.

Pericardial effusions can be global, surrounding the entire heart, or loculated, as seen mostly after cardiac surgery (Fig. 27-35). Since the intrapericardial volume is constant, cardiac chambers are compressed when at their lowest pressure (atria in systole, ventricles in diastole). Pericardial tamponade is characterized by the presence of a large pericardial effusion seen as an echo-free (black) space, a "swinging motion" of the heart, early diastolic RV collapse, and late diastolic right atrium (RA) collapse.

In summary, diastolic filling is an active process and a major component of effective cardiac performance. The presence of diastolic dysfunction, whether resulting from loss in fluid volume, LV disease, or pericardial restraint, is associated with potential deleterious surgical outcomes. Doppler echocardiography, in particular TDI, provides the anesthesiologist the means to rapidly diagnose and guide therapy of such patients in the perioperative period.

Evaluation of Valvular Heart Disease

Two-dimensional echocardiography and Doppler are complementary methods in valve assessment. The 2D echocardiography

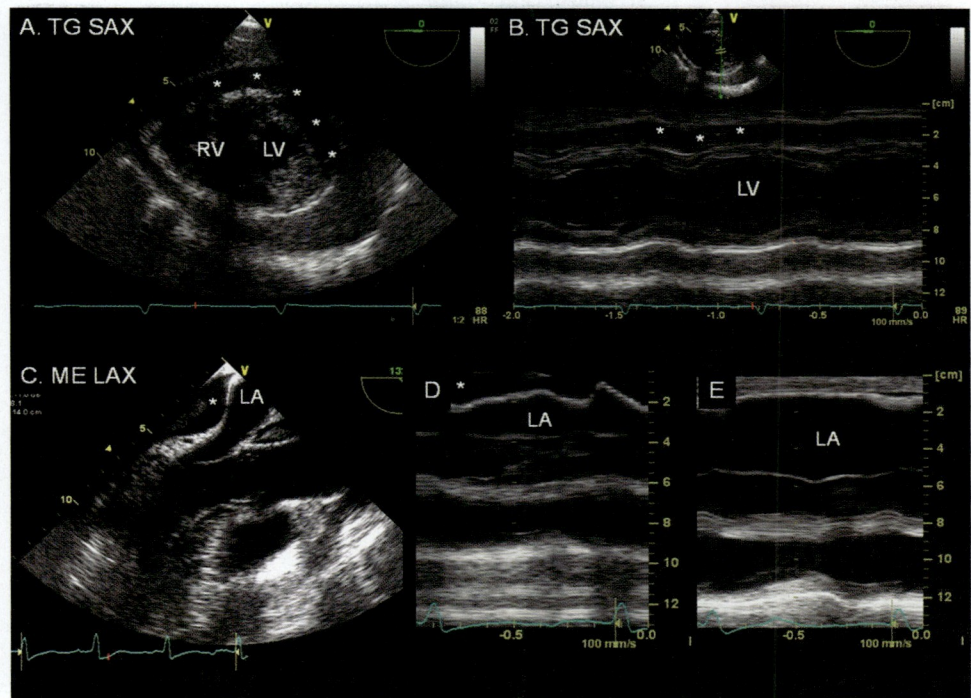

Figure 27-35 Echocardiographic findings in pericardial effusion. **A**: Global pericardial effusion (*asterisks*) surrounding both right ventricle (RV) and left ventricle (LV). Transgastric short-axis (TG SAX) view. **B**: M-mode echocardiography demonstrates separation of the epicardium from the pericardium (*asterisks*) from pericardial effusion. **C**: Regional pericardial effusion (*asterisk*) compressing the left atrium (LA), seen in the midesophageal long-axis (ME LAX) view. **D**: M-mode echocardiography reveals systolic compression (*asterisk*) of LA. **E**: After evacuation of the fluid collection, the LA size increases.

Table 27-3 Grading of Aortic Stenosis

	Aortic Sclerosis	Mild	Moderate	Severe	
Peak AV velocity (m/s)	≤2.5	2.6–2.9	3.0–4.0	>4	>4.0
LVOT/AV velocity ratio		>0.5	0.25–0.5	<0.25	
Mean transvalvular gradient (mmHg)		<20	20–40	>4	>40
AVA (cm²)		>1.5	1.5–1.0	<1	<1.0

AV, aortic valve; LVOT, left ventricular outflow tract; AVA, AV area.

provides evaluation of valve anatomy and function; Doppler assesses the physiologic consequences and severity of the lesion.

Aortic Stenosis

Two-dimensional and M-mode Echocardiography

The normal AV has three cusps, which open without restriction in systole, yielding an AV area 3 to 4 cm². The AV is imaged enface in the midesophageal aortic valve short-axis view (Fig. 27-13) and its profile in the midesophageal aortic valve long-axis view. With the TEE probe inside the stomach, the AV is imaged in the deep transgastric long-axis and transgastric long-axis views (see Ultrasound Appendix for examples of these views). Owing to the increased afterload, associated findings may include concentric hypertrophy of the LV, decreased EF, as well as MR and left atrial dilatation.

Doppler Echocardiography

Jet Velocity, Transvalvular Pressure Gradient. The transvalvular pressure gradient can be calculated from the CWD-measured velocity (V) using the modified Bernoulli equation: Δpressure.[67] The mean gradient, calculated from the VTI tracing, is commonly reported as it correlates well with the angiographically determined pressure gradient.[68] However, for any given valve area, the flow velocity and pressure gradient vary with changes in stroke volume and cardiac output. An LV with normal function will generate a large pressure gradient across a critically stenosed AV and a dysfunctional LV will not.[69]

Valve Area

5 Using the continuity equation, the flow across the LVOT equals the flow across the stenosed AV or $VTI_{LVOT} \times Area_{LVOT} = VTI_{AV} \times Area_{AV}$. By rearranging the equation, $Area_{AV} = (VTI_{LVOT} \times Area_{LVOT})/(VTI_{AV})$. The $Area_{LVOT}$ is calculated using the LVOT diameter at the site of the Doppler measurement (Fig. 27-27). An error in the LVOT diameter measurement is geometrically increased as $Area_{LVOT} = \pi \times (D/2)^2$. The VTI_{LVOT}/VTI_{AV} ratio is often calculated to avoid this error as flow changes will be reflected proportionally across both the AV and LVOT (Doppler dimensionless index). An index value less than 0.25% indicates an AV area less than 0.75 cm². The echocardiographic cut-off values for grading aortic stenosis are shown in Table 27-3.[70]

Mitral Stenosis

Two-dimensional Echocardiography

The MV is imaged in the midesophageal views and in the basal transgastric short-axis views. The leaflets can appear thickened and calcified (thus, strongly echogenic), and there may be fusion of the chordae and papillary muscles. The major and most striking finding in mitral stenosis (MS) is the inability of the two mitral leaflets to separate from each other in diastole. Instead, their tips remain opposed while the body of the leaflets bows toward the LV cavity because of the incoming blood (Fig. 27-36). The area of the MV orifice can be traced by planimetry in the transgastric basal short-axis view.[71] Associated findings in MS are a dilated left atrium and left atrial appendage (because of increased pressure) and the presence of thrombus or spontaneous echocardiographic contrast due to low flow in the LA. The LV cavity appears small, with a thickened and immobile interventricular septum. The right ventricle may be dilated and/or hypertrophied, with thickened walls, because of increased pressure work (Fig. 27-36 and Table 27-4).

Doppler Echocardiography

Transvalvular Pressure Gradient. The increased diastolic pressure gradient is measured with continuous Doppler in the midesophageal four-chamber or long-axis view.[67] The early diastolic velocity of the transmitral flow (E wave) is increased (usually >1.5 m/s). This is not specific to MS, as E velocity will also be elevated in the presence of increased blood flow, as in severe MR.[72] In severe MS, the mean pressure gradient is greater than 10 mmHg (Fig. 27-37).

Pressure Half-time (PHT)

The deceleration of E velocity is decreased, because in MS the equalization of transmitral valve pressures takes a longer time. PHT is the time required for the peak pressure to decrease to half its value. The decaying velocity is traced on the CWD signal obtained from across the MV in diastole and the analysis package calculates the PHT (Fig. 27-37B). MV area (MVA) is calculated as 220/PHT. A prolonged PHT greater than 220 ms is related to severe MS (calculated MVA <1 cm²) as smaller MV orifices will prolong the pressure decay across the valve.[73] When LV compliance is decreased or there is coexisting aortic regurgitation, the increased LV pressure results in a faster

Table 27-4 Grading of Mitral Stenosis

	Mild	Moderate	Severe
Mean pressure gradient (mmHg)	<6	5–10	>10
Pressure half time (ms)	≤100	100–220	>220
Mitral valve area (cm²)	>1.5	1.0–1.5	<1.0
Systolic pulmonary artery pressure (mmHg)	<30	30–50	>50

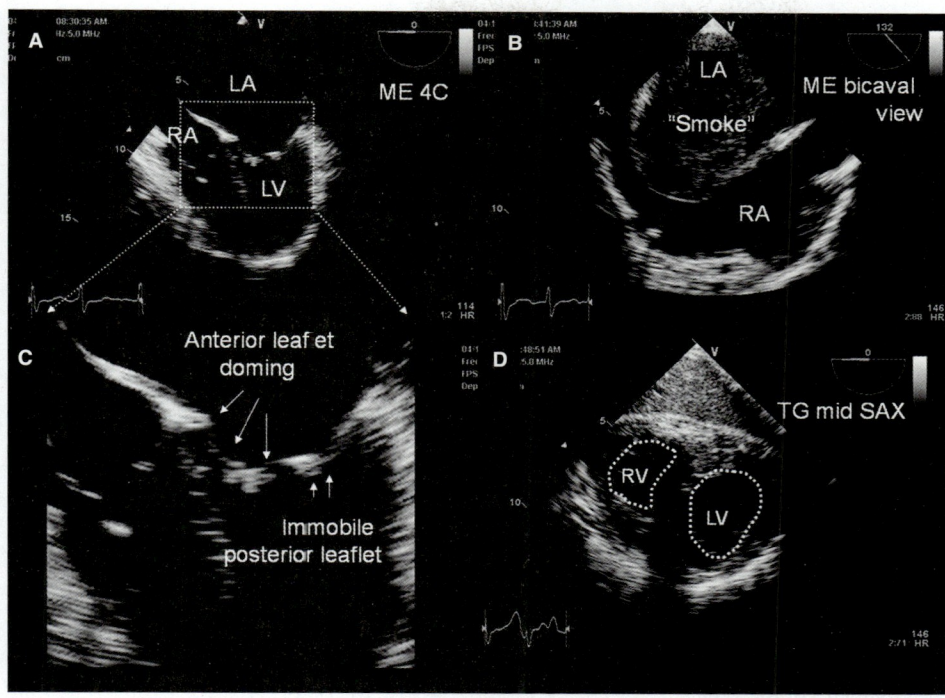

Figure 27-36 Two-dimensional echocardiographic findings in mitral stenosis. **A:** In the midesophageal four-chamber (ME 4C) view, echocardiographic signs of mitral stenosis include a dilated left atrium (LA) with a rightward displacement of the interatrial septum (indicating elevated LA pressure), and a small left ventricle (LV). **B:** In the midesophageal bicaval view, red blood cell clumping creates spontaneous echocardiography contrast. Note the rightward displacement of the interatrial septum toward the right atrium (RA). **C:** A zoom image of the mitral valve and neighboring structures in ME 4C view. The anterior mitral leaflet exhibits diastolic doming whereas the posterior mitral leaflet is immobile. **D:** In the transgastric midpapillary short-axis (TG mid-SAX) view, the LV cavity is relatively small as compared with the right ventricle (RV), and the interventricular septum appears thickened.

pressure equilibration across the stenosed MV. In such cases, PHT will be shortened, and the calculated MVA may be erroneously overestimated.[74]

Associated Findings

CFD will display a "rising sun" pattern of diastolic velocities inside the LA, indicating the high velocity (and increased pressure gradient) across the stenosed MV that exceeds the limits of the color scale (Fig. 27-37A). Associated findings include pulmonary insufficiency due to pulmonary hypertension and tricuspid regurgitation (TR).

Aortic Regurgitation

Two-dimensional and M-mode Echocardiography

The AV is imaged in the same views used for the assessment of aortic stenosis. Associated findings may include dilated aortic root (Marfan syndrome), endocarditis lesions, dilated ascending aorta, calcified AV, aortic dissection (may be associated with acute aortic AI), fluttering of the anterior mitral leaflet and

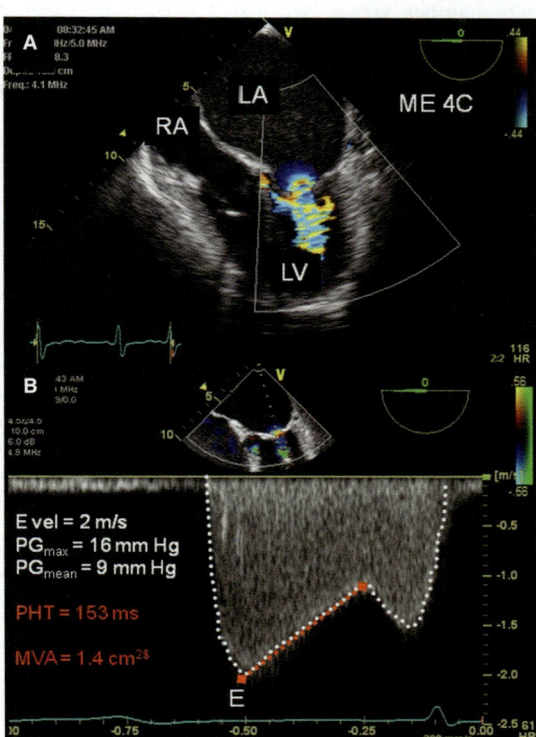

Figure 27-37 Doppler echocardiography findings in mitral stenosis. **A:** Diastolic blood acceleration upstream of the mitral valve is seen with color-flow Doppler ("rising sun"). **B:** Spectral display of the diastolic velocity decay is imaged with a pulsed-wave Doppler sample volume placed at the tips of the mitral valve. Tracing of the velocity envelope (white dots) calculates the maximum and mean pressure gradient (PG). The pressure half-time (PHT) is calculated from the deceleration of the peak velocity (Evel) (red dots). The mitral valve area (MVA) is derived from the empiric formula: MVA = 220/PHT.

Table 27-5	Grading of Aortic Insufficiency (AI)		
	Mild	Moderate	Severe
AI jet height/LVOT diameter (%)	<25	25–64	>65
Vena contracta (mm)	<0.3	0.3–0.6	>6
PHT (ms)	>500	200–500	<200
Aortic diastolic flow reversal	—	—	Holodiastolic

LVOT, left ventricular outflow tract; PHT, pressure half-time.

restricted diastolic opening of the MV from the AI jet, or a dilated LV in chronic AI (Table 27-5).

Doppler Echocardiography

Color Flow. In either the midesophageal or the transgastric views of the AV, a CFD sector over the AV and the LVOT will demonstrate the presence or absence of the AI regurgitant jet. CFD reveals the characteristics of the AI jet as it enters the LVOT in diastole. The following techniques are used to grade the severity of AI.

Ratio of Jet Height to LVOT Diameter

The maximal height of the AI jet (within <1 cm from the AV plane) is compared with the LVOT diameter at the same point. The recommended view is the midesophageal aortic valve long-axis view. A central jet usually is caused by aortic root dilation, whereas an eccentric jet implies an AV cusp lesion. The propagation of the jet into the LV does not correlate well with the angiographic degree of AI and should not be used to grade AI (Fig. 27-23).[75]

Vena Contracta

Vena contracta is the narrowest "neck" of the AI jet as it traverses the AV plane, usually best appreciated in the midesophageal aortic valve long-axis view. The largest diameter of the vena contracta in diastole is selected (Fig. 27-23). The size of vena contracta is relatively load-independent and provides a reliable way to quantitate AI intraoperatively in the presence of fluctuating hemodynamics.[75]

Pressure Half-time

PHT of the AI jet is recorded in the transgastric long-axis or deep transgastric long-axis view (see Ultrasound Appendix for examples of these views). PHT expresses the pressure equilibration of the diastolic blood pressure ("driving" pressure) and the diastolic LV pressure ("resistance" pressure). A short PHT (<200 ms) is associated with severe AI. Factors associated with decreased LV compliance (e.g., LV failure with restrictive filling pattern) will cause the transaortic pressure gradient to dissipate faster and will overestimate the severity of AI (Fig. 27-22A).

Aortic Diastolic Flow Reversal

Retrograde diastolic flow in the descending and abdominal aorta is sensitive and specific for severe AI. This is imaged with PWD in the midesophageal long-axis view of the distal descending aorta (Fig. 27-22B).[76]

Other Findings

Severe AI rapidly elevates LV diastolic pressure and shortens the early transmitral flow velocity, resulting in a *restrictive LV filling pattern*. The *regurgitant volume* is calculated using the continuity equation and equals the difference between LVOT flow and the diastolic transmitral flow. Values greater than 60 mL are consistent with severe AI.

Mitral Regurgitation

Two-dimensional Echocardiography

The normal MV anatomy consists of two leaflets (anterior and posterior), their coaptation surface, the fibrous mitral annulus,

Table 27-6 Carpentier Classification of Mitral Regurgitation (MR)

Carpentier Type	Motion Leaflet	Jet Direction
1	Normal	Central
2	Excessive (prolapse, flail)	Away from lesion
3a	Restricted, structure is abnormal	Variable
3b	Restricted, structure is normal	

the subvalvular apparatus with the two papillary muscles (anterolateral and posteromedial), and their chordae tendineae, which attach to the underside of the mitral leaflets. The competency of the MV depends on adequate coaptation between the D-shaped anterior leaflet and the crescent-shaped posterior leaflet. Common causes of MR are myxomatous valve degeneration, endocarditis, and ischemic, rheumatic, and congenital heart disease (CHD).

The TEE views for imaging of the MV include the midesophageal four-chamber (Fig. 27-8), midesophageal commissural, midesophageal two-chamber (Fig. 27-9), midesophageal aortic valve long-axis view, and the basal transgastric short-axis and two-chamber views (see also Ultrasound Appendix).[77] Echocardiographic findings may include any of the following: abnormal texture of leaflets (myxomatous degeneration), flail and/or prolapsing leaflet, ruptured chordae, papillary muscle dysfunction or rupture (secondary to ischemia), mitral annulus calcification, or endocarditis lesions. The leaflet motion is commonly reported using Carpentier classification as described in Table 27-6.

Doppler Echocardiography

CFD is commonly used as a screening tool for the detection of MR. It provides an easy, qualitative technique, but additional tests are advised to grade the severity of MR (Fig. 27-38). Despite its appearance, the color area associated with MR is not equivalent to regurgitant volume. CFD simply shows the area within the LA where blood has abnormal velocity and is dependent on the systolic pressure gradient between the LV (adequate LV systolic function) and the LA (chamber compliance). In acute MR, for example, the MR jet velocities are low because MR occurs in a noncompliant chamber. Eccentric jets that are in contact with the LA walls are underestimated (Coandă effect),[78] whereaas machine settings such as frame rate and color Doppler scale influence the appearance of the MR jet.

Vena Contracta

Vena contracta is the narrowest part of the MR jet, and reflects the effective or physiologic area of the MR jet (Fig. 27-24). MR is severe if vena contracta is 7 mm or greater.

Pulmonary Vein Inflow Pattern

The increased volume inside the LA will augment the transmitral diastolic pressure gradient and will produce a restrictive filling pattern in severe MR (E to A wave ratio >2). For the same reasons, the systolic filling of the LA via the pulmonary veins (S wave) will be decreased in moderate and severe MR (Table 27-7).

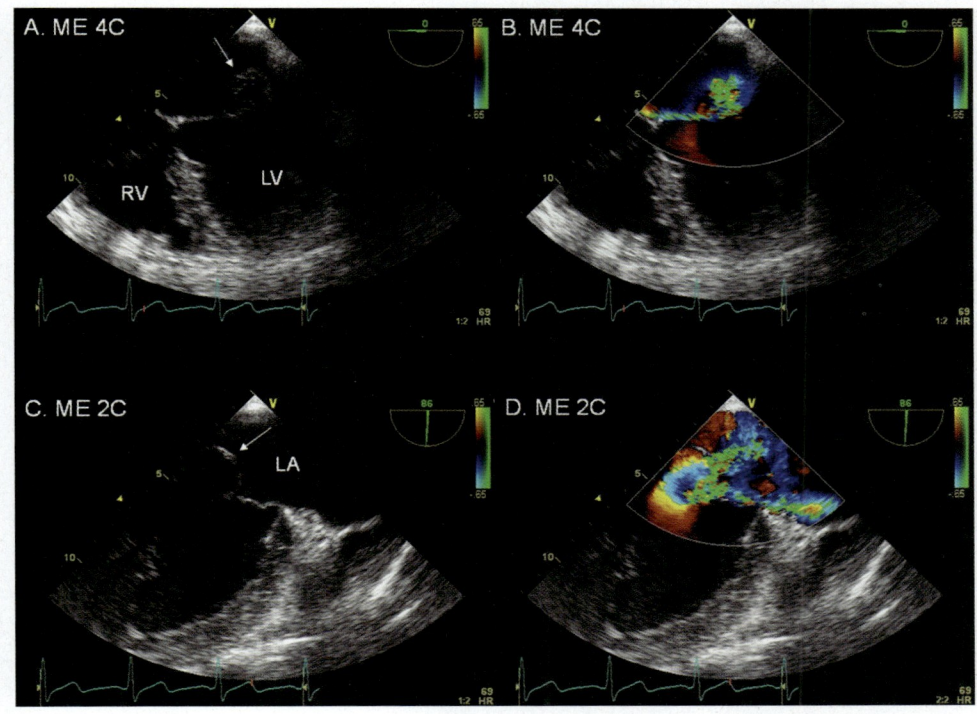

Figure 27-38 Mitral regurgitation. The anatomy of the mitral valve (MV) is depicted with two-dimensional (**A** and **C**) echocardiographic imaging, and the presence of mitral regurgitation (MR) is imaged with color Doppler (**B** and **D**). The MV is incompetent because of posterior leaflet prolapse inside the left atrium (LA) during systole (*arrows left* in **A** and **C**). Left ventricular (LV) systolic contraction generates an anterior-directed MR jet away from the MV lesion area. ME 4C, midesophageal four-chamber view; ME 2C, midesophageal two-chamber view.

Tricuspid and Pulmonic Valve Regurgitation

Similar approaches are used for the grading of severity of TR and PV regurgitation (Tables 27-8 and Table 27-9).

Diseases of the Aorta

The evaluation of the aorta is an important part of perioperative TEE. In routine cases, such as coronary artery bypass surgery, evaluation of the aorta may reveal previously unknown, significant atheromatous disease of the aorta and alter the surgical plan (off-pump bypass, alternative sites for cannulation). In emergencies, the diagnosis of aortic pathology (dissection, aneurysm, transection) may prove life-saving.

Table 27-7 Grading of Mitral Regurgitation

	Mild	Moderate	Severe
Qualitative Findings			
Jet area/LA area	<20%	—	>40%
Density of CW signal	—	—	Dense, complete envelope
Pulmonary blood flow	—	S blunted (S/D < 1)	S reversed (S < 0)
Quantitative Measurements			
Vena contracta (mm)	<3	3–7	≥7

LA, left atrium; CW, continuous wave; S, S wave; S/D, systolic wave of pulmonary vein flow to diastolic wave of pulmonary vein flow ratio; EROA, effective regurgitant orifice area.

Table 27-8 Grading of Tricuspid Regurgitation

Echocardiographic Parameter	Mild	Severe
TV morphology	Normal	Prolapse, malcoaptation, endocarditis lesion, mass
IVC/RA/RV size	Normal	Dilated/increased
TR jet area (cm²)	<5	>10
Vena contracta width (mm) (Nyquist limit 50–60 cm/s)	—	>7
TR jet features	Soft, parabolic	Dense, triangular, early peak
Hepatic vein flow pattern	S > D	Systolic wave below baseline

TV, tricuspid valve; IVC, inferior vena cava; RA, right atrium; RV, right ventricle; PISA, proximal isovelocity surface area; TR, tricuspid regurgitation; S, systolic wave of hepatic view flow; D, diastolic wave of hepatic vein flow.

Table 27-9 Grading of Pulmonary Regurgitation

Parameter	Mild	Severe
PV morphology	Normal	Abnormal
RV size	Normal	Dilated
PR jet size	Length <1 cm, narrow origin	Large, wide origin
PR jet features	Soft, slow deceleration	Dense, rapid deceleration

PV, pulmonary vein; RV, right ventricle; PR, pulmonary regurgitation.

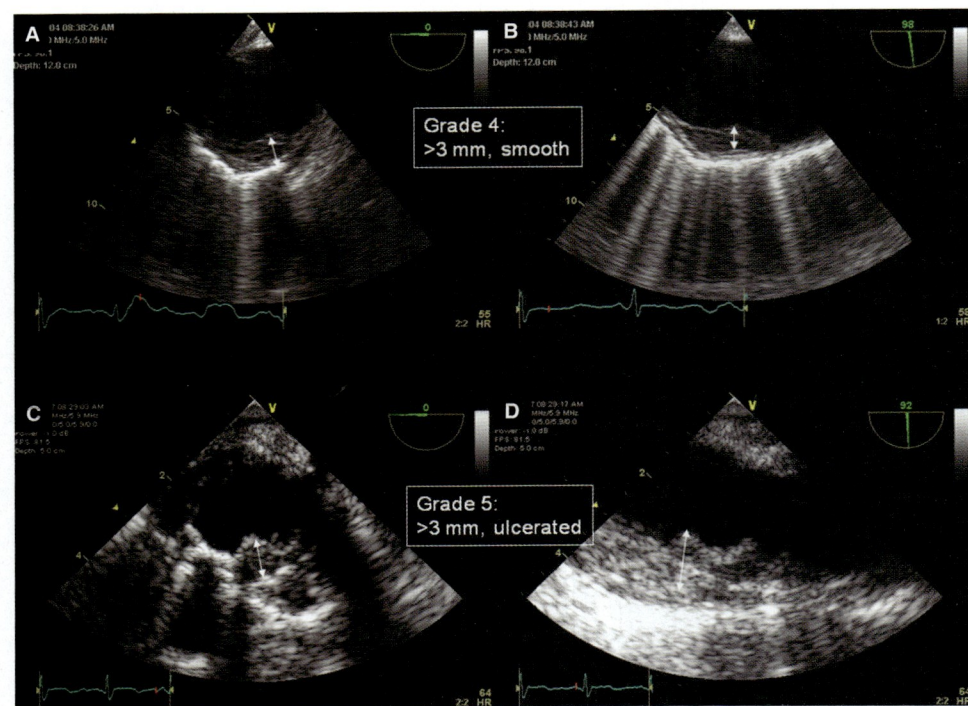

Figure 27-39 Aortic atheromas imaged in descending thoracic aorta short-axis (**A** and **C**) and long-axis (**B** and **D**) views.

Two-dimensional and Motion-mode Echocardiography

The entire thoracic aorta can be imaged with TEE, apart from the distal ascending and proximal arch segments, where the interposition of the left main bronchus between the esophagus and the left atrium prohibits the propagation of ultrasound. This blind spot can be imaged using epiaortic scanning.[79] The normal aorta has a smooth endothelial surface, and blood flow is laminar. Atherosclerotic plaques are irregularly shaped, sometimes mobile protrusions inside the aortic lumen. The search for atheromas should be done by imaging the entire circumference of the aortic lumen (short-axis views). Once a particular lesion is found, scanning in long-axis view should be performed (Fig. 27-39). Plaques thicker than 4 mm are more likely to cause an embolic event.[80,81]

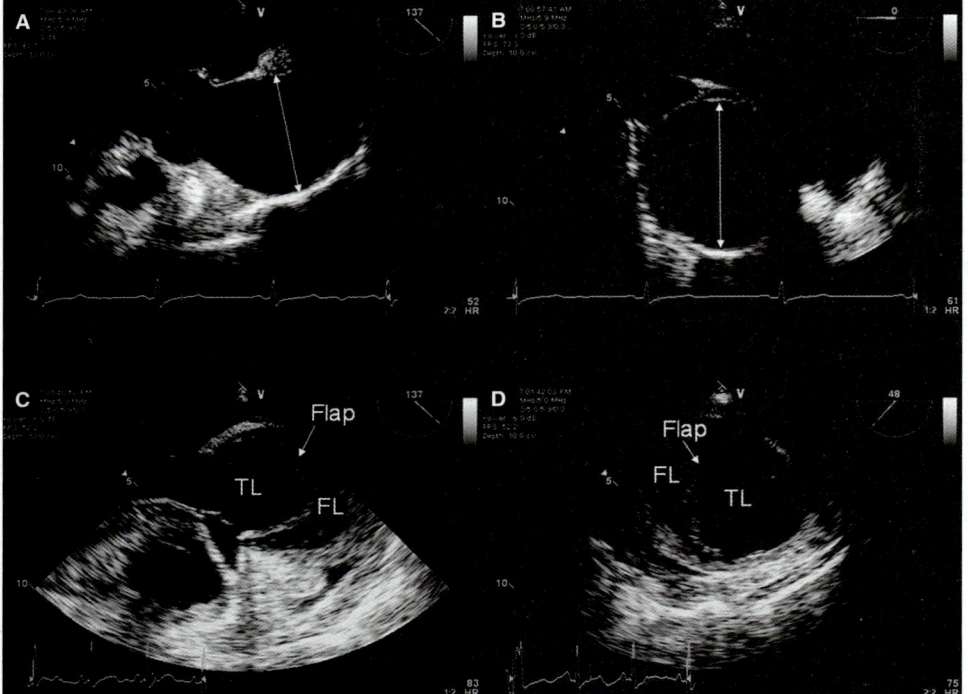

Figure 27-40 Aortic disease. Ascending aorta aneurysm distal to the sinotubular junction (midesophageal ascending aorta long-axis (**A**) and short-axis (**B**) views). The diameter of the aorta is 5 cm. **C:** Ascending aorta dissection (Stanford type A) originating from the sinotubular junction. The true lumen (TL) expands in systole and the flap is convex toward the false lumen (FL). **D:** Descending aorta dissection (DeBakey type III).

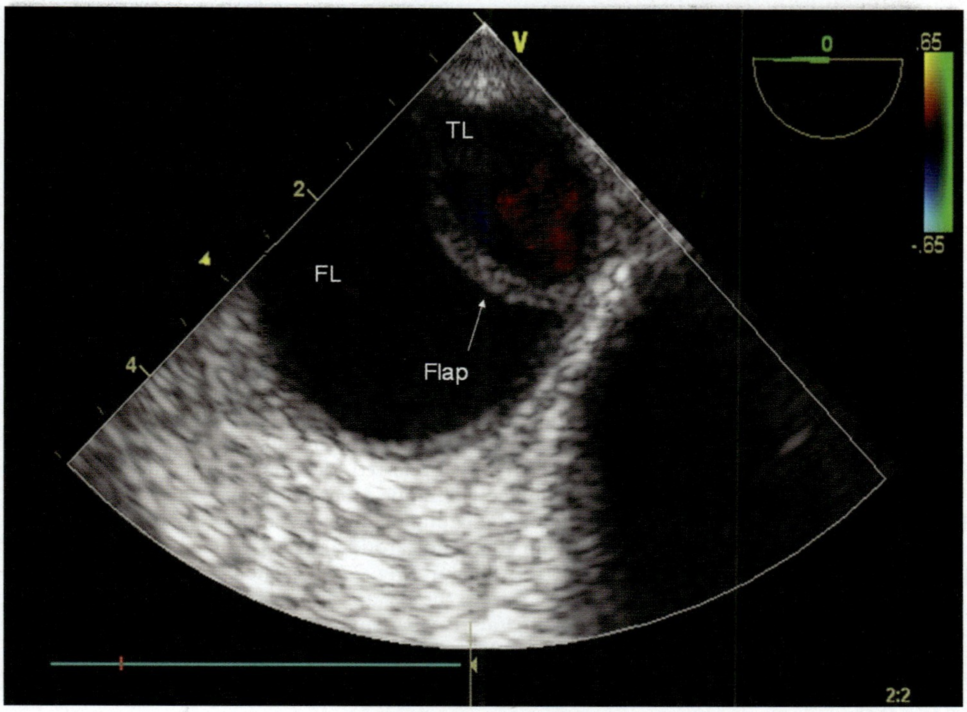

Figure 27-41 Aortic dissection. The descending aorta is seen in short axis. The aortic true lumen (TL) contains the aortic endothelium and has a smooth endoluminal surface. The intimal flap usually bows toward the false lumen (FL). Color-flow Doppler demonstrates blood flow inside the true lumen (which expands in systole) and the absence of flow inside the false lumen.

Aortic aneurysm is a dilatation of the aorta, usually greater than 4 cm. Once the aneurysm is greater than 5.5 cm, the probability of rupture increases (Fig. 27-40A,B). Dissection is a separation between the intimal and medial layers of the aortic wall, creating a false lumen for blood flow (Figs. 27-40C,D and 27-41).[82] Both the true and false lumens fill with blood during systole, but only the true lumen has blood flow during diastole. Intramural hematoma is considered a precursor of dissection and should be treated similarly.[83] Compared with an atheroma, an intramural hematoma has a smooth surface.

Cardiac Masses

Cardiac tumors either can originate from the heart or are metastases from other sites. They can embolize, cause arrhythmias, or

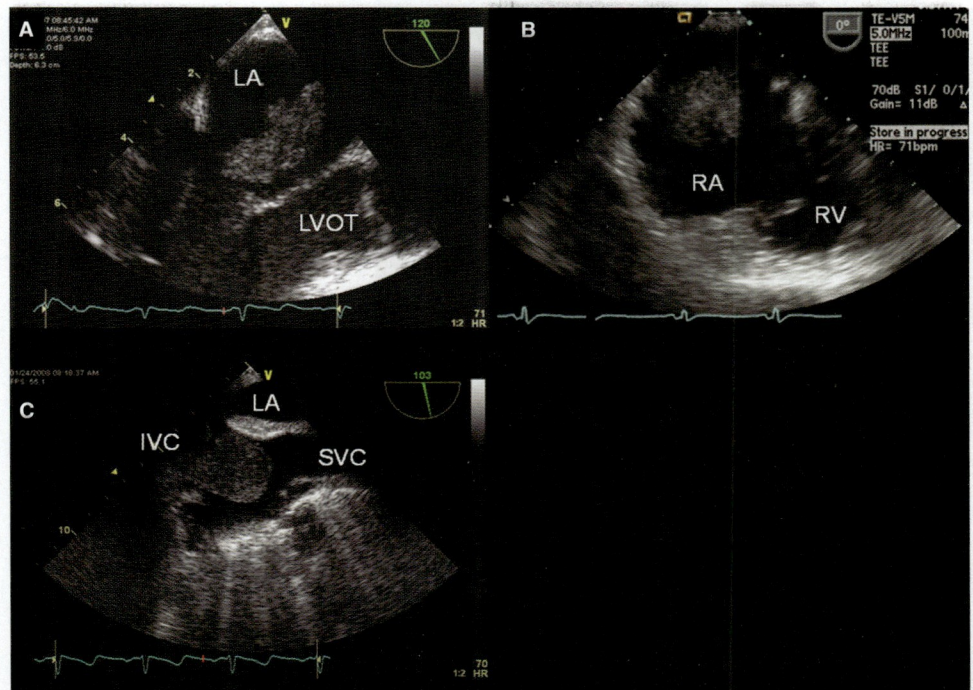

Figure 27-42 Cardiac masses. **A:** Left atrial (LA) myxoma seen in the midesophageal long-axis view. **B:** Right atrial myxoma seen inside the right atrium (RA) in the midesophageal four-chamber view. **C:** Renal cell tumor occupying the inferior vena cava (IVC) and extending inside the RA. LVOT, left ventricular outflow tract; RV, right ventricle; SVC, superior vena cava.

cause heart failure. The most common primary tumor is myxoma, which is located most frequently at the interatrial septum (Fig. 27-42). The potential of myxomas to obstruct the inflow or outflow region of a ventricle is demonstrated with Doppler echocardiography. The next most frequent tumor is fibroma of the ventricular wall. Fibromas are usually calcified and can decrease the ventricular volume. Renal cell tumors often extend into the inferior vena cava and right atrium (Fig. 27-42C). Pacemaker wires, thrombus, and normal anatomic structures that mimic the appearance of pathology (Eustachian valve, crista terminalis, Chiari network, or "Coumadin" ridge) should be differentiated from tumors.

Congenital Heart Disease

The spectrum of CHD seen in adults varies widely. Echocardiography is the primary imaging modality for diagnostic assessment of CHD. Advances in surgery have increased the survival rate of children with repaired CHD and, as a consequence, adults with repaired CHD are increasingly common in the OR. Common lesions evaluated with TEE include ASD, ventricular septal defect, patent ductus arteriosus, coarctation of the aorta, bicuspid AV, and repaired tetralogy of Fallot (Fig. 27-43).[84]

Echocardiography-assisted Procedures

In addition to its role in diagnostics, echocardiography is also employed to assist various procedures such as the placement of a central venous catheter, intra-aortic balloon pump (IABP) catheter, coronary sinus (CS) cannula, and guide wires for other venous or arterial cannulae.

Ultrasound-guided Central Vein Cannulation

The placement of central venous catheters is associated with complications including injury to vascular structures (carotid artery), pleura, nerve bundles, lymphatic system, and even the spinal canal. Historically, anatomic landmarks guided needle orientation during central venous access. However, multiple studies have demonstrated that the anatomic relationship between the internal jugular vein and the carotid artery varies and that even experienced physicians encounter complications.[85] Visual guidance by ultrasound provides real-time feedback, reducing the complication rate and the procedure time.[86] For patient safety reasons, the National Institute for Clinical Excellence and the Society of Cardiovascular Anesthesiologists have recommended that internal jugular central lines be placed under guidance of 2D ultrasound imaging.[87,88]

A linear array handheld transducer with high frequencies (7.5 to 12 MHz) is preferred for ultrasound-guided central line placement. The technique relies on placing the transducer over the traditional anatomic landmarks and identifying the internal jugular vein (IJV) and carotid artery (CA) in short axis and their anatomic relationship (Fig. 27-44). The 2D criteria of differentiating the CA from the IJV are distensibility (the IJV increases in size with the Valsalva maneuver and the Trendelenburg position) and compressibility (the IJV will decrease in size with pressure applied over it by the transducer). Applying CFD with the transducer oriented slightly caudad displays the CA with red pulsating flow and the IJV with a continuous blue flow (Fig. 27-44). If the transducer is oriented cephalad, the colors are reversed. The needle insertion and venous puncture is performed under ultrasound guidance. The longitudinal view (Fig. 27-45A) is then used to view the wire's placement in the vessel. TEE can confirm the guide wire's position in the superior vena cava (Fig. 27-45B).

For PAC placement, TEE is useful in guiding the catheter through the right heart and confirming proper position in the

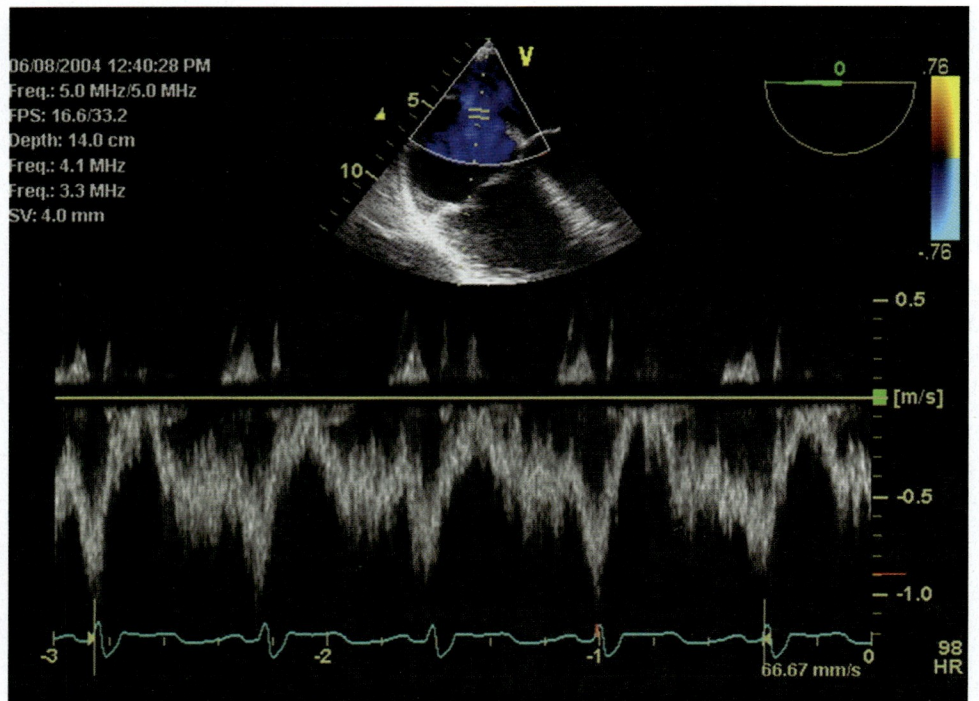

Figure 27-43 Atrial septal defect (ASD). In the midesophageal four-chamber view, a color-Doppler sector is positioned over the interatrial septum. An ASD with a left-to-right communication is shown in *blue*, as the blood moves away from the transducer (**top panel**). Pulsed-wave Doppler interrogation of the ASD measures a peak velocity gradient of 1 m/s.

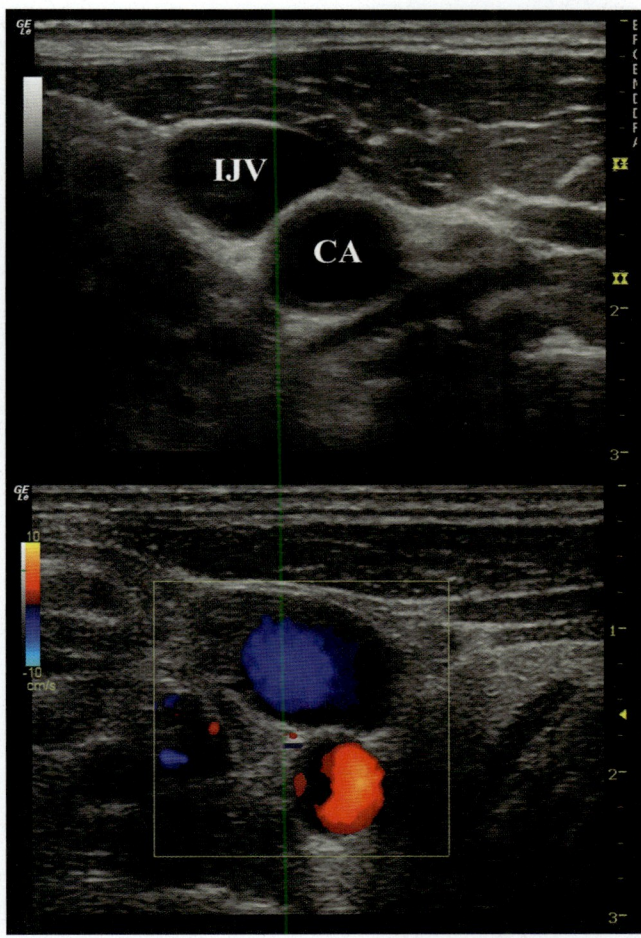

Figure 27-44 Internal jugular vein (IJV) and carotid artery (CA) and their anatomic relationship. **Top panel:** Two-dimensional examination, using a linear scanner, showing the IJV lateral to the CA. **Bottom panel:** Color-flow Doppler is applied showing continuous blue flow in the IJV and pulsating red flow in the CA (transducer oriented caudad).

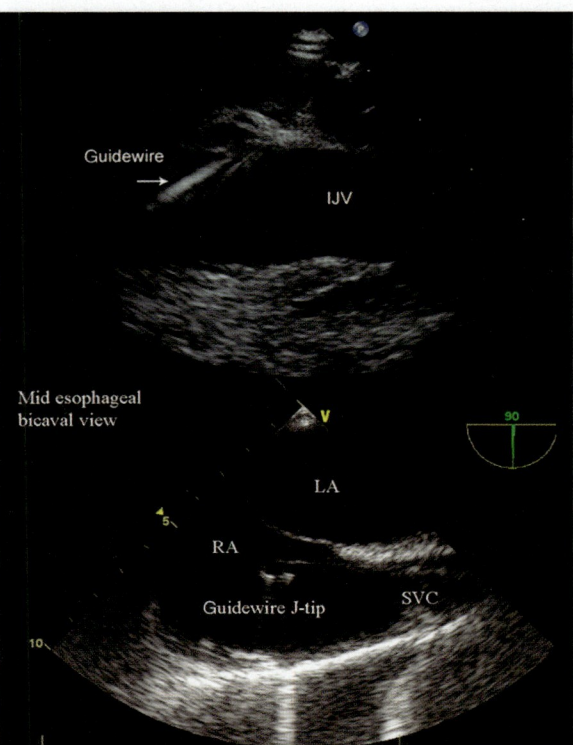

Figure 27-45 Top: Ultrasound confirmation of guide wire position. A sector scanner transducer is used to visualize the internal jugular vein (IJV) in long axis. The guide wire is seen as a thin echo-dense linear structure positioned in the lumen of the vein. **Bottom:** Transesophageal echocardiographic confirmation of guide wire position. The midesophageal bicaval view is used. The guide wire is seen in the superior vena cava (SVC), with the tip in the right atrium (RA). LA, left atrium.

PA. In the midesophageal right ventricular inflow–outflow view, the PAC can be followed from the RA, passing the TV into the RV, and then passing the PV into the PA. The midesophageal ascending aortic short-axis view may be used to position the PAC so that its tip lies in the right PA (if that is the desired position; some clinicians prefer positioning the PAC in the main PA).

Although ultrasound can be a valuable tool in decreasing the number of complications associated with central vein cannulation and PAC placement, it does not eliminate the risks.

Epicardial and Epiaortic Echocardiography

Epicardial Echocardiography

During surgeries performed via sternotomy or thoracotomy, epicardial echocardiography can be performed and is particularly valuable in those cases in which the TEE probe cannot be placed or is contraindicated. The epicardial views are similar to the ones obtained via TTE. The American Society of Echocardiography in collaboration with the Society of Cardiovascular Anesthesiologists has issued guidelines for the performance of epicardial echocardiography.[89] The epicardial probe uses high-frequency transducers (5 to 12 MHz) that may require a standoff device and/or saline in the mediastinum for best imaging. Epicardial imaging offers superior image quality as well as a better window to the anterior cardiac structures (aorta and AV, PA and PV).

Epiaortic Examination

Because of the interposition of the left bronchus, the distal aortic arch (AA) and the proximal AA cannot be visualized with TEE. The ascending and proximal AAs are of particular interest during cardiac surgeries, as they represent sites for aortic cannulation. Epiaortic scanning for atheroma is performed using a small footprint, linear array transducer. Guidelines for intraoperative epiaortic examination were published in 2007.[79]

Echocardiography Outside the Operating Room

An understanding of echocardiography is also relevant to anesthesiologists in that many patients with a history of heart disease will have undergone an echocardiographic examination prior to surgery. The echocardiography report from a preoperative examination is useful for assessing surgical risk and developing the anesthetic plan. Echocardiography has also established itself as particularly valuable in the assessment of postoperative hemodynamic instability. It offers rapid diagnosis by differentiating among the potential complications faced in postoperative care, such as hypovolemia, pericardial tamponade aortic dissection, myocardial infarction, endocarditis, and pulmonary embolism.

Focused Transthoracic Cardiac Ultrasound

A focused transthoracic cardiac ultrasound (FoCUS) is a collection of echocardiographic images often obtained in urgent or semiurgent settings where a complete echocardiogram may not be feasible. FoCUS is aimed toward a rapid, qualitative assessment of cardiac pathology and potential causes of altered hemodynamics.[90,91] For example, in a patient with a heart murmur heard during preoperative visit for urgent or same day surgery, FoCUS can identify aortic stenosis and trigger appropriate management (Fig. 27-46). Similarly, in a postoperative patient with unexplained hemodynamic instability, FoCUS can rapidly identify conditions such as pericardial effusion (Fig. 27-47) or severe LV dysfunction.

Advancements in portable ultrasound technology have led to the wide availability of these devices throughout the hospital. As such, focused exams are increasingly performed at the bedside as an adjunct to the clinical exam by anesthesiology and critical care physicians lacking advanced training in echocardiography.[92–94] The FoCUS exam is often obtained in urgent settings under time constraints, where image quality may be suboptimal. Because of the inherent procedural and diagnostic challenges to FoCUS, physicians must obtain appropriate didactic education as well as training in hands-on skills and image interpretation in order to avoid diagnostic pitfalls.

Training in FoCUS is increasingly being recognized as a fundamental for teaching curriculums in medical school and post-graduate training programs.[95,96] Such training applied to anesthesiology residency has been shown to enhance detection of new pathology and impact clinical decision making.[97,98] Importantly, FoCUS training should involve the institution's reference echocardiography laboratories, which can also provide oversight, quality control, and ensure maintenance of skills. The importance of structured training and maintenance of competencies has been recognized by professional societies as essential components to fully utilize the advantages and minimize drawbacks of this type of cardiac ultrasound examination.[90,99–101]

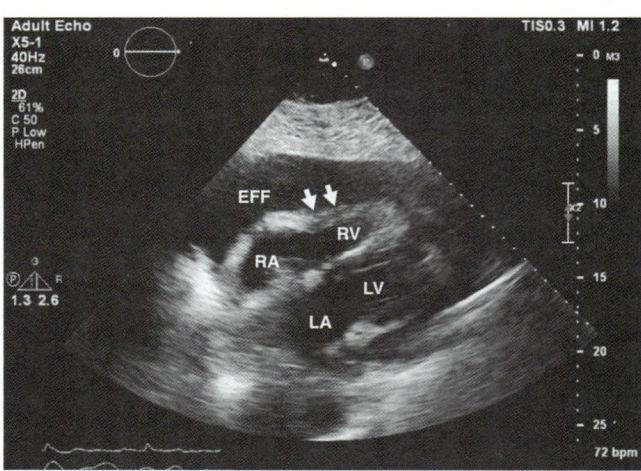

Figure 27-47 Subcostal four-chamber view of a patient with cardiac tamponade. Large circumferential pericardial effusion (EFF) is seen. Arrows point to diastolic collapse of the right ventricular (RV) free wall. LA, left atrium; RA right atrium; LV, left ventricle.

Focused Exam Views

A focused cardiac examination uses transthoracic echocardiographic images obtained from the parasternal, apical, and subcostal windows. At each window, the corresponding orthogonal views of the heart are obtained. For the purpose of FoCUS, the parasternal and subcostal windows are preferred, as they are the easiest to access in a supine patient with limited mobility. In addition, most of the cardiac abnormalities sought out can be easily recognized from these windows.

Parasternal views are obtained in the third intercostal space at the left sternal border with the patient in left lateral position. The parasternal long-axis view (PLAX) is obtained by holding the ultrasound probe notch or marker aligned toward the right shoulder (Fig. 27-48A). In this view, the LA, MV, LV, and a small portion of the RV are seen. The orthogonal parasternal short axis (PSAX) view is obtained by clockwise rotation of the probe (Fig. 27-48B).

Apical views are obtained at the point of maximal impulse (apex) with the patient in the left lateral position. The apical four-chamber view (A-4Ch) is obtained by aligning the probe notch to the left of the patient (Fig. 27-48C). In this view, the LA, LV, RA, and RV are seen together with mitral and tricuspid valves.

Subcostal views are obtained from below the xiphoid process with the patient in supine position. The subcostal four-chamber view is obtained by aligning the probe notch to the patient's left side (Fig. 27-48D). In this view, all four cardiac chambers can be seen. A counterclockwise rotation renders the subcostal short-axis view and visualization of RA and IVC.

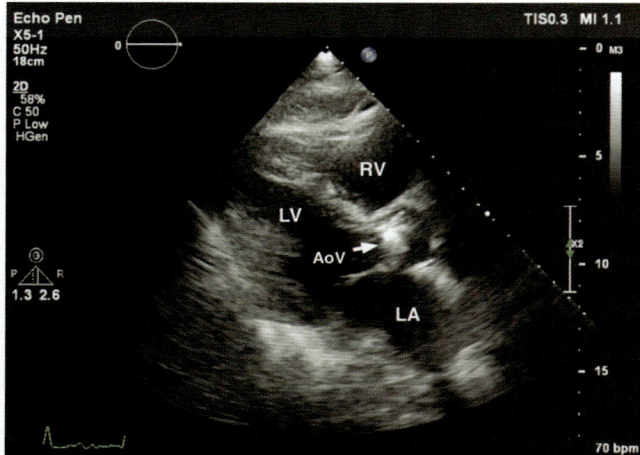

Figure 27-46 Parasternal long-axis view of a patient with aortic stenosis detected on preoperative echo. The aortic valve (*arrow*) is thickened and heavily calcified with restricted mobility. LA, left atrium; LV, left ventricle; RV, right ventricle.

Table 27-10 Common Clinical Conditions and Associated Focus Targets

Clinical Condition	Suspected Abnormality	FoCUS Targets	FoCUS Views	Findings
Heart Failure	Severe LV dysfunction, cardiomyopathy	LV	PLAX, PSAX, A-4Ch, Subcostal	Dilated poorly contracting LV
Hypotension	Hypovolemia	IVC	Subcostal	Small, collapsed
Acute Respiratory Compromise	Pulmonary hypertension, pulmonary emboli	RV	PSAX, A4Ch, subcostal	Markedly enlarged
Murmur	Aortic stenosis	Aortic valve	PLAX	Thickened with restricted mobility
Hypertension	Left ventricular hypertrophy	LV	PLAX, PSAX	Thickened walls
Post CT Surgery	Pericardial effusion	Pericardium	Subcostal, PLAX, A-4Ch	Echo-free space

LV, left ventricle; PLAX, parasternal long-axis view; PSAX, parasternal short-axis view; A-4Ch, apical four-chamber view; IVC, inferior vena cava; RV, right ventricle.

Focused Assessed Transthoracic Echo

Multiple focused ultrasound protocols have been proposed for detection of cardiac abnormalities at bedside.[102,103] One of the commonly used protocols among anesthesiologists, especially as a "rescue echo" during unexplained hemodynamic instability, is the Focused Assessed Transthoracic echo, or FATE exam.[103] This protocol involves rapidly obtaining a series of key transthoracic images to identify conditions such as pericardial effusion, hypovolemia, and severe chamber enlargement and dysfunction. In addition, this protocol involves lung ultrasound imaging which is useful to identify pleural effusions, lung edema, and pneumothorax. Table 27-10 shows the utility of the FoCUS exam in common clinical scenarios.

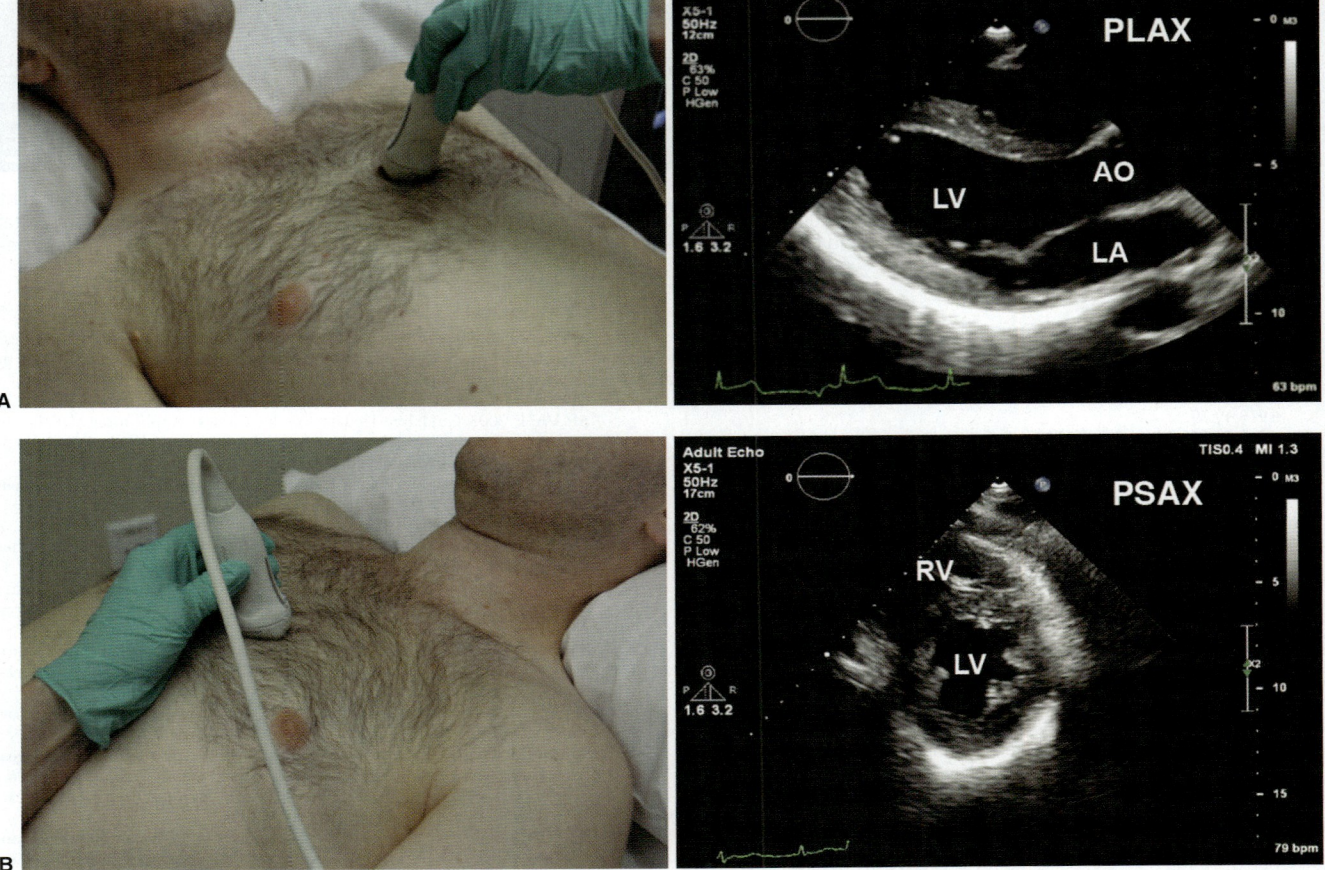

Figure 27-48 Standard transthoracic echo (TTE) images obtained during a FoCUS exam; each panel shows the ultrasound probe positioning and corresponding echo images: **Panel A:** Parasternal long-axis view (PLAX) obtained at parasternal window probe is positioned with the marker pointing toward the right shoulder; LA, left atrium; LV, left ventricle; Ao, Aorta. **Panel B:** Parasternal short axis (PSAX) view at the level of papillary muscles; LV, left ventricle; RV, right ventricle. (*continued*)

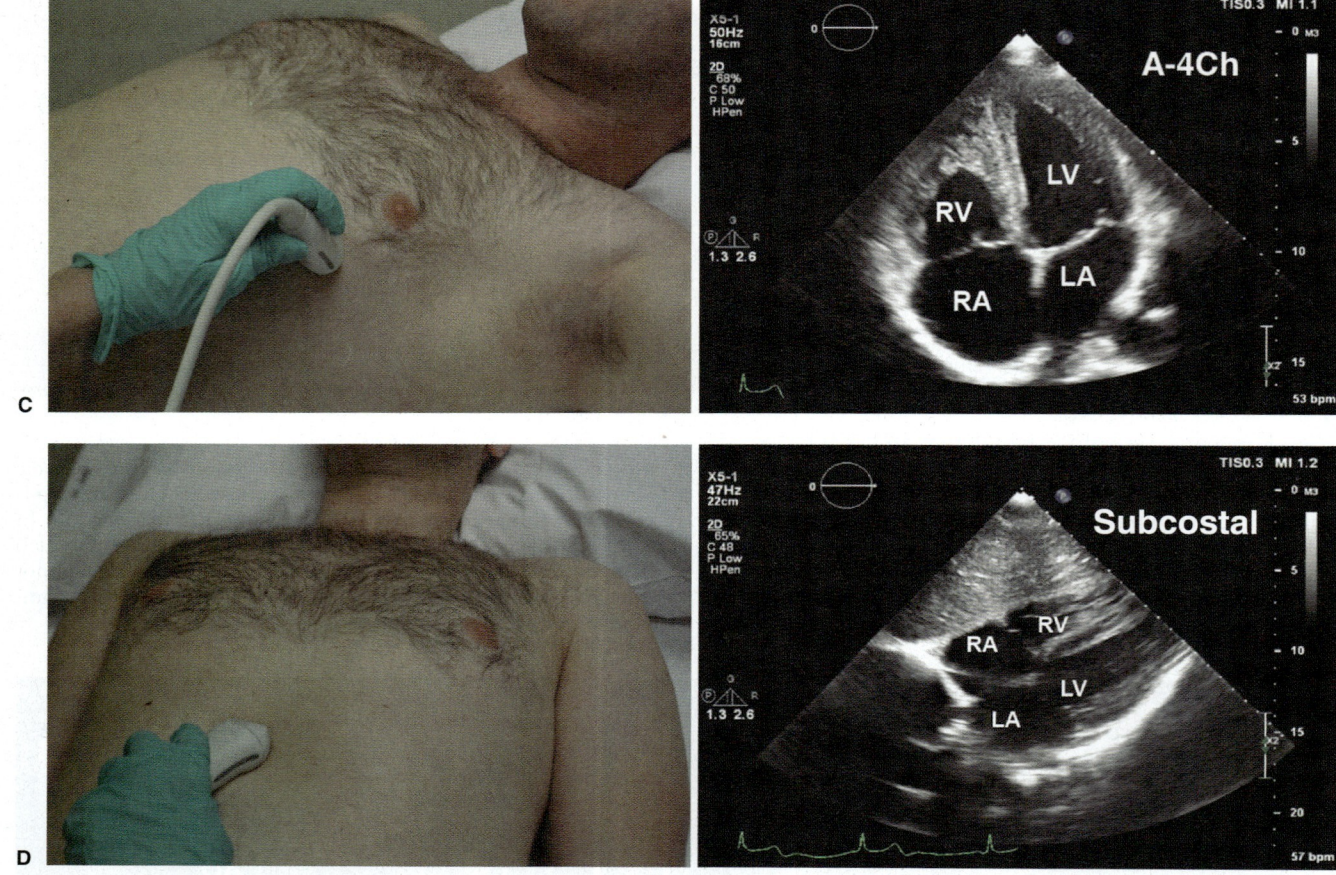

Figure 27-48 *(Continued)* **Panel C:** Apical four-chamber view (A-4Ch) obtained at apical window probe is positioned with the marker pointing toward the left flank; LA, left atrium; RA, right atrium; LV, left ventricle; RV, right ventricle. **Panel D:** Subcostal four-chamber view (Subcostal) obtained with the probe positioned below the xiphoid process and marker pointing toward the left flank. LA, left atrium; RA, Right atrium; LV, left ventricle; RV, right ventricle.

REFERENCES

1. Barash PG, Glanz S, Katz JD, et al. Ventricular function in children during halothane anesthesia: an echocardiographic evaluation. *Anesthesiology.* 1978;49:79.
2. Click RL, Abel MD, Schaff HV. Intraoperative transesophageal echocardiography: 5-year prospective review of impact on surgical management. *Mayo Clin Proc.* 2000;75:241.
3. Couture P, Denault AY, McKenty S, et al. Impact of routine use of intraoperative transesophageal echocardiography during cardiac surgery. *Can J Anaesth.* 2000;47:20.
4. Schmidlin D, Bettex D, Bernard E, et al. Transesophageal echocardiography in cardiac and vascular surgery: implications and observer variability. *Br J Anaesth.* 2001;86:497.
5. Perrino AC, Reeves ST. Echocardiographic assessment during non-cardiac surgery. In: Savage RM, Aronson S, eds. *Comprehensive Textbook of Intraoperative TEE.* Philadelphia, PA: Lippincott Williams & Wilkins; 2004.
6. Suriani RJ, Neustein S, Shore-Lesserson L, et al. Intraoperative transesophageal echocardiography during noncardiac surgery. *J Cardiothorac Vasc Anesth.* 1998;12:274.
7. Kolev N, Brase R, Swanvelder M, et al. The influence of transesophageal echocardiography on intra-operative decision making. *Anaesthesia.* 1998;53:767.
8. Denault AY, Couture P, McKenty S, et al. Perioperative use of transesophageal echocardiography by anesthesiologists: impact in noncardiac surgery and in the intensive care unit. *Can J Anaesth.* 2002;49:287.
9. American Society of Anesthesiologists and the Society of Cardiovascular Anesthesiologists Task Force on Transesophageal Echocardiography. Practice guidelines of perioperative transesophageal echocardiography. *Anesthesiology.* 1996;84:986.
10. American Society of Anesthesiologists, Society of Cardiovascular Anesthesiologists Task Force. Practice guidelines for perioperative transesophageal echocardiography: An update report by the American Society of Anesthesiologists and the Society of Cardiovascular Anesthesiologists Task Force on Transesophageal Echocardiography. *Anesthesiology.* 2010;112:1084.
11. Cheitlin MD, Armstrong WF, Aurigemma GP, et al. ACC. AHA. ASE. ACC/AHA/ASE 2003 Guideline Update for the Clinical Application of Echocardiography. Summary article: a report of the American College of Cardiology/American Heart. *Circulation.* 2003;108:1146–1162.
12. Center for Devices and Radiological Health. *Revised 510(k) Diagnostic Ultrasound Guidance for 1993.* Rockville, MD: US Food and Drug Administration; 1993.
13. Miller JP. Two-dimensional examination. In: Perrino AC, Reeves S, eds. *A Practical Approach to Transesophageal Echocardiography.* 3rd ed. Philadelphia, PA: Lippincott Williams & Wilkins; 2014:24.
14. Rafferty T, LaMantia KR, Davis E, et al. Quality assurance for intraoperative transesophageal echocardiography monitoring: a report of 846 procedures. *Anesth Analg.* 1993;76:228.
15. Kallameyer IJ, Collard CD, Fox JA, et al. The safety of intraoperative transesophageal echocardiography: a case series of 7200 cardiac surgical patients. *Anesth Analg.* 2001;92:1126.
16. Hogue CW, Lappas GD, Creswell LL, et al. Swallowing dysfunction after cardiac operations. *J Thorac Cardiovasc Surg.* 1995;110:517.
17. Rousou JA, Tighe DA, Garb JL, et al. Risk of dysphagia after transesophageal echocardiography during cardiac operations. *Ann Thorac Surg.* 2000;69:486.
18. Hilberath JN, Oakes DA, Shernan SK, et al. Safety of transesophageal echocardiography. *J Am Soc Echocardiogr.* 2010;23:1115.
19. Hahn RT, Abraham T, Adams MS, et al. Guidelines for performing a comprehensive intraoperative multiplane transesophageal echocardiographic examinations: recommendations of the American Society of Echocardiography and the Society of Cardiovascular Anesthesiologists. *J Am Soc Echocardiogr.* 2013;26:921.
20. Miller JP, Lambert AS, Shapiro WA, et al. The adequacy of basic intraoperative transesophageal echocardiography performed by experienced anesthesiologists. *Anesth Analg.* 2001;92:1103.

21. Reeves ST, Finlay AC, Skubas NJ, et al. Basic perioperative transesophageal echocardiography examination: a consensus statement of the American Society of Echocardiography and the Society of Cardiovascular Anesthesiologists. *J Am Soc Echocardiogr*. 2013;26:443.
22. Meineri M, Vegas A. Three-dimensional transesophageal echocardiography is a major advance for intraoperative clinical management of patients undergoing cardiac surgery: a core review. *Anesth Analg*. 2010;110:1548.
23. Ahmed S, Nanda NC, Miller AP, et al. Usefulness of transesophageal three-dimensional echocardiography in the identification of individual segment/scallop prolapse of the mitral valve. *Echocardiography*. 2003;20:203.
24. Lang RM, Badano LP, Tsang W, et al. EAE/ASE Recommendations for image acquisition and display using three-dimensional echocardiography. *J Am Soc Echocardiogr*. 2012;25:3.
25. Perrino AC. Doppler technology and technique. In: Perrino AC, Reeves S, eds. *A Practical Approach to Transesophageal Echocardiography*. 3rd ed. Philadelphia, PA: Lippincott Williams & Wilkins; 2014:102.
26. Quiñones MA, Otto CM, Stoddard M, et al. Recommendations for quantification of Doppler echocardiography: a report from the Doppler Quantification Task Force of the Nomenclature and Standards Committee of the American Society of Echocardiography. *J Am Soc Echocardiogr*. 2002;15:167.
27. Nishimura RA, Miller FA, Callahan MJ, et al. Doppler echocardiography: theory, instrumentation, technique, and application. *Mayo Clin Proc*. 1985;60:321.
28. Maslow A, Perrino AC. Quantitative Doppler and hemodynamics. In: Perrino AC, Reeves S, eds. *A Practical Approach to Transesophageal Echocardiography*. 3rd ed. Philadelphia, PA: Lippincott Williams & Wilkins; 2014:118.
29. Perrino AC, Harris SN, Luther MA. Intraoperative determination of cardiac output using multiplane transesophageal echocardiography: a comparison to thermodilution. *Anesthesiology*. 1998;89:350.
30. Harris SN, Luther MA, Perrino AC. Multiplane transesophageal echocardiography acquisition of ascending aortic flow velocities: a comparison with established techniques. *J Am Soc Echocardiogr*. 1999;12:754.
31. Muhiudeen IA, Kuecherer HF, Lee E, et al. Intraoperative estimation of cardiac output by transesophageal pulsed Doppler echocardiography. *Anesthesiology*. 1991;74:9.
32. Otto CM, Pearlman AS, Comess KA, et al. Determination of the stenotic aortic valve area in adults using Doppler echocardiography. *J Am Coll Cardiol*. 1986;7:509.
33. Currie PJ, Seward JB, Reeder GS, et al. Continuous-wave Doppler echocardiographic assessment of severity of calcific aortic stenosis: a simultaneous Doppler-catheter correlative study in 100 adult patients. *Circulation*. 1985;71:1162.
34. Hatle L, Brubakk A, Tromsdal A, et al. Noninvasive assessment of pressure drop in mitral stenosis by Doppler ultrasound. *Br Heart J*. 1978;40:131.
35. Stamm RB, Martin RP. Quantification of pressure gradients across stenotic valves by Doppler ultrasound. *J Am Coll Cardiol*. 1983;2:707.
36. Teague SM, Heinsimer JA, Anderson JL, et al. Quantification of aortic regurgitation utilizing continuous wave Doppler ultrasound. *J Am Coll Cardiol*. 1986;8:592.
37. Lee RT, Lord CP, Plappert T, et al. Prospective Doppler echocardiographic evaluation of pulmonary artery diastolic pressure in the medical intensive care unit. *Am J Cardiol*. 1989;64:1366.
38. Gorcsan J III, Snow FR, Paulsen W, et al. Noninvasive estimation of left atrial pressure in patients with congestive heart failure and mitral regurgitation by Doppler echocardiography. *Am Heart J*. 1991;11:858.
39. Nishimura RA, Tajik AJ. Determination of left-sided pressure gradients by utilizing Doppler aortic and mitral regurgitation signals: validation by simultaneous dual catheter and Doppler studies. *J Am Coll Cardiol*. 1988;11:317.
40. Leung JM, O'Kelly BF, Mangano DT. Relationship of regional wall motion abnormalities to hemodynamic indices of myocardial oxygen supply and demand in patients undergoing CABG surgery. *Anesthesiology*. 1990;73:802.
41. Hauser AM, Gangadharan V, Ramos RG, et al. Sequence of mechanical, electrocardiographic and clinical effects of repeated coronary artery occlusion in human beings: echocardiographic observations during coronary angioplasty. *J Am Coll Cardiol*. 1985;5:193.
42. Battler A, Froelicher VF, Gallagher KP, et al. Dissociation between regional myocardial dysfunction and ECG changes during ischemia in the conscious dog. *Circulation*. 1980;62:735.
43. Ross J Jr. Myocardial perfusion-contraction matching: Implications for coronary artery disease and hibernation. *Circulation*. 1991;83:1076.
44. Cerqueira MD, Weissman NJ, Dilsizian V, et al; American Heart Association Writing Group on Myocardial Segmentation and Registration for Cardiac Imaging. Standardized myocardial segmentation and nomenclature for tomographic imaging of the heart: a statement for healthcare professionals from the cardiac imaging committee of the Council on Clinical Cardiology of the American Heart Association. *Circulation*. 2002;105:539.
45. Lang RM, Bierig M, Devereux RB, et al. Recommendations for chamber quantification: a report from the American Society of Echocardiography's Guidelines and Standards Committee and the Chamber Quantification Writing group, developed in conjunction with the European Association of Echocardiography, a branch of the European Society of Cardiology. *J Am Soc Echocardiogr*. 2005;18:1440.
46. Lieberman AN, Weiss JL, Jugdutt BI, et al. Two-dimensional echocardiography and infarct size: relationship of regional wall motion and thickening to the extent of myocardial infarction in the dog. *Circulation*. 1981;63:739.
47. Bergquist BD, Leung JM, Bellows WH. Transesophageal echocardiography in myocardial revascularization. I. Accuracy of intraoperative real-time interpretation. *Anesth Analg*. 1996;82:1132.
48. Odell DH, Cahalan MK. Assessment of left ventricular global and segmental systolic function with transesophageal echocardiography. *Anesthesiol Clin*. 2006;24:755.
49. London MJ. Assessment of left ventricular global systolic function by transesophageal echocardiography. *Ann Card Anaesth*. 2006;9:157.
50. Cheung AT, Savino JS, Weiss SJ, et al. Echocardiographic and hemodynamic index of left ventricular preload in patients with normal and abnormal ventricular function. *Anesthesiology*. 1994;81:376.
51. Skarvan K, Lambert A, Filipovic M. Reference values for left ventricular function in subjects under general anesthesia and controlled ventilation assessed by two-dimensional transesophageal echocardiography. *Eur J Anaesthesiol*. 2001;18:713.
52. Swenson JD, Bull D, Stringham J. Subjective assessment of left ventricular preload using transesophageal echocardiography: corresponding pulmonary artery occlusion pressures. *J Cardiothorac Vasc Anesth*. 2001;15:580.
53. Ditooe N, Stultz D, Schwartz BP, et al. Qualitative left ventricular systolic function: From chamber to myocardium. *Crit Care Med*. 2007;35:S330.
54. Skubas N. Intraoperative Doppler tissue imaging is a valuable addition to the cardiac anesthesiologists' armamentarium: a core review. *Anesth Analg*. 2009;108:48–66.
55. Derumeaux G, Ovize M, Loufoua J, et al. Doppler tissue imaging quantitates regional wall motion during myocardial ischemia and reperfusion. *Circulation*. 1998;97:1970.
56. Flu WJ, van Kujik JP, Hoeks SE, et al. Prognostic implications of asymptomatic left ventricular dysfunction in patients undergoing vascular surgery. *Anesthesiology*. 2010;112:1316.
57. Matyal R, Hess PE, Subramaniam B, et al. Perioperative diastolic dysfunction during vascular surgery and its association with postoperative outcome. *J Vasc Surg*. 2009;50:70.
58. Bernard F, Denault A, Babin D, et al. Diastolic dysfunction is predictive of difficult weaning from cardiopulmonary bypass. *Anesth Analg*. 2001;92:291.
59. Swaminathan M, Nicoara A, Phillips-Bute B, et al. Utility of a simple algorithm to grade diastolic dysfunction and predict outcome after bypass graft surgery. *Ann Thorac Surg*. 2011;91:1844.
60. Matyal R, Skubas NJ, Shernan SK, et al. Perioperative assessment of diastolic dysfunction. *Anesth Analg*. 2011;113:449.
61. Nishimura RA, Tajik AJ. Evaluation of diastolic filling of left ventricle in health and disease: Doppler echocardiography is the clinician's Rosetta stone. *J Am Coll Cardiol*. 1997;30:8.
62. Gilman G, Nelson TA, Hansen WH. Diastolic function: A sonographer's approach to the essential echocardiographic measurements of left ventricular diastolic function. *J Am Soc Echocardiogr*. 2007;20:199.
63. Nagueh SF, Otto AS, Appleton CP, et al. Recommendations for evaluation of left ventricular diastolic function by echocardiography: an update from the American Society of Echocardiography and the European Association of Cardiovascular Imaging. *J Am Soc Echocardiogr*. 2016;29:277.
64. Pirracchio R, Cholley B, De Hert S, et al. Diastolic heart failure in anesthesia and critical care. *Br J Anaesth*. 2007;98:707.
65. Sutherland GR, Stewart MJ, Groundstroem KW, et al. Color Doppler myocardial imaging: a new technique for the assessment of myocardial function. *J Am Soc Echocardiogr*. 1994;7:441
66. Shernan SK. In: Perrino AC, Reeves S, eds. *A Practical Approach to Transesophageal Echocardiography*. 3rd ed. Philadelphia, PA: Lippincott Williams & Wilkins; 2014:138.
67. Baumgartner H, Hung J, Bermejo J, et al. Echocardiographic assessment of valve stenosis: EAE/ASE recommendations for clinical practice. *J Am Soc Echocardiogr*. 2009;22:1.
68. Baumgartner H, Stefenelli T, Niederberger J, et al. "Overestimation" of catheter gradients by Doppler ultrasound in patients with aortic stenosis: a predictable manifestation of pressure recovery. *J Am Coll Cardiol*. 1999;33:1655.
69. Burwash IG, Dickinson A, Teskey RJ. Aortic valve area discrepancy by Gorlin equation and Doppler echocardiography continuity equation: relationship to flow in patients with valvular aortic stenosis. *Can J Cardiol*. 2000;16:985.
70. Nishimura RA, Otto CA, Bonow RO, et al. 2014 AHA/ACC Guideline for the management of patients with valvular heart disease. *Circulation*. 2014;129:2440.
71. Henry WL, Griffith JM, Michaelis LL. Measurement of mitral orifice area in patients with mitral valve disease, by real-time, two-dimensional echocardiography. *Circulation*. 1975;51:827.
72. Bruce CJ, Nishimura RA. Clinical assessment and management of mitral stenosis, valvular heart disease. *Cardiol Clin*. 1998;16:375.
73. Libanoff AJ, Roadbard S. Atrioventricular pressure half-time: measure of mitral valve orifice area. *Circulation*. 1968;38:144.
74. Braverman AC, Thomas JD, Lee R. Doppler echocardiographic estimation of mitral valve area during changing hemodynamic conditions. *Am J Cardiol*. 1991;68:1485.

75. Perry GJ, Helmecke F, Nanda NC. Evaluation of aortic insufficiency by Doppler color flow mapping. *J Am Coll Cardiol*. 1987;9:952.
76. Takenaka K, Sakamoto T, Dabestani A. Pulsed Doppler echocardiographic detection of regurgitant blood flow in the ascending, descending and abdominal aorta of patients with aortic regurgitation. *J Cardiol*. 1987;17:301.
77. Lambert AS, Miller JP, Merrick SH. Improved evaluation of the location and mechanism of mitral valve regurgitation with a systemic transesophageal echocardiography examination. *Anesth Analg*. 1999;88:1205.
78. Schiller NB, Foster E, Redberg RF. Transesophageal echocardiography in the evaluation of mitral regurgitation: the twenty-four signs of severe mitral regurgitation. *Cardiol Clin*. 1993;11:399.
79. Glas KE, Swaminathan M, Reeves ST, et al. Guidelines for the performance of a comprehensive intraoperative epiaortic ultrasonographic examination: recommendations of the American Society of Echocardiography and the Society of Cardiovascular Anesthesiologists; endorsed by the Society of Thoracic Surgeons. *J Am Soc Echocardiogr*. 2007;20:1227.
80. Massachusetts Medical Society. Atherosclerotic disease of the aortic arch as a risk factor for recurrent ischemic stroke: the French study of aortic plaques in stroke groups. *N Engl J Med*. 1996;334:1216.
81. Weber A, Jones EF, Zavala JA, et al. Intraobserver and interobserver variability of transesophageal echocardiography in aortic arch atheroma measurement. *J Am Soc Echocardiogr*. 2008;21:127.
82. Vignon P, Spencer KT, Rambaud G, et al. Differential transesophageal echocardiographic diagnosis between linear artifacts and intraluminal flap of aortic dissection or disruption. *Chest*. 2001;119:1778.
83. Hiratzka LF, Bakris GL, Beckman JA, et al. 2010 ACCF/AHA/AATS/ACR/ASA/SCA/SCAI/SIR/STS/SVM guidelines for the diagnosis and management of patients with thoracic aortic disease: executive summary. *Anesth Analg*. 2010;111:279.
84. Russell IA, Rouine-Rapp K, Stratmann G, et al. Congenital heart disease in the adult: a review with Internet-accessible transesophageal echocardiographic images. *Anesth Analg*. 2006;102:694.
85. Denys BG, Uretsky BF. Anatomical variations of internal jugular vein location: impact on central venous access. *Crit Care Med*. 1991;19:1516.
86. Karakitsos D, Labropoulos N, De Groot E, et al. Real-time ultrasound-guided catheterization of the internal jugular vein: a prospective comparison with the landmark technique in critical care patients. *Crit Care*. 2006;10:R162.
87. National Institute for Clinical Excellence (NICE). *Guidance on the Use of Ultrasound Locating Devices for Placing Central Venous Catheters*. London, UK: National Institute for Clinical Excellence; 2002.
88. Troianos CA, Hartman GS, Glas KE, et al. Guidelines for performing ultrasound guided vascular cannulation: recommendations of the American Society of Anesthesiologists and the Society of Cardiovascular Anesthesiologists. *J Am Soc Echocardiogr*. 2011;24:1291.
89. Reeves ST, Glass KE, Eltzschig H, et al. Guidelines for performing a comprehensive intraoperative epicardial echocardiography examination: recommendations of the American Society of Echocardiography and the Society of Cardiovascular Anesthesiologists. *J Am Soc Echocardiogr*. 2007;20:427.
90. Spencer KT, Kimura BJ, Korcarz CE, et al. Focused cardiac ultrasound: recommendations from the American Society of Echocardiography. *J Am Soc Echocardiogr*. 2013;26:567.
91. Spencer KT. Focused cardiac ultrasound: where do we stand? *Curr Cardiol Rep*. 2015;17:567.
92. Bøtker MT, Vang ML, Grøfte T, et al. Routine pre-operative focused ultrasonography by anesthesiologists in patients undergoing urgent surgical procedures. *Acta Anaesthesiol Scand*. 2014;58:807.
93. Canty DJ, Royse CF, Kilpatrick D, et al. The impact of focused transthoracic echocardiography in the pre-operative clinic. *Anaesthesia*. 2012;67:618.
94. Cowie BS. Focused transthoracic echocardiography in the perioperative period. *Anaesth Intensive Care*. 2010;38:823.
95. Stokke TM, Ruddox V, Sarvari SI, et al. Brief group training of medical students in focused cardiac ultrasound may improve diagnostic accuracy of physical examination. *J Am Soc Echocardiogr*. 2014;27:1238.
96. Cawthorn TR, Nickel C, O'Reilly M, et al. Development and evaluation of methodologies for teaching focused cardiac ultrasound skills to medical students. *J Am Soc Echocardiogr*. 2014;27:302.
97. Ramsingh D, Rinehart J, Kain Z, et al. Impact assessment of perioperative point-of-care ultrasound training on anesthesiology residents. *Anesthesiology*. 2015;123:670.
98. Tanzola RC, Walsh S, Hopman WM, et al. Focused transthoracic echocardiography training in a cohort of Canadian anesthesiology residents: a pilot study. *Can J Anaesth*. 2013;60:32.
99. Via G, Hussain A, Wells M, et al; International Liaison Committee on Focused Cardiac UltraSound (ILC-FoCUS), International Conference on Focused Cardiac UltraSound (IC-FoCUS). International evidence-based recommendations for focused cardiac ultrasound. *J Am Soc Echocardiogr*. 2014;27:683.e1.
100. Neskovic AN, Edvardsen T, Galderisi M, et al. Focus cardiac ultrasound: the European Association of Cardiovascular Imaging viewpoint. *Eur Heart J Cardiovasc Imag*. 2014;15:956.
101. Labovitz AJ, Noble VE, Bierig M, et al. Focused cardiac ultrasound in the emergent setting: a consensus statement of the American Society of Echocardiography and American College of Emergency Physicians. *J Am Soc Echocardiogr*. 2010;23:1225.
102. Kennedy Hall M, Coffey EC, Herbst M, et al. The "5Es" of emergency physician-performed focused cardiac ultrasound: a protocol for rapid identification of effusion, ejection, equality, exit, and entrance. *Acad Emerg Med*. 2015;22:583.
103. Jensen MB, Sloth E, Larsen KM, et al. Transthoracic echocardiography for cardiopulmonary monitoring in intensive care. *Eur J Anaesthesiol*. 2004;21:700.

Section 6
BASIC ANESTHETIC MANAGEMENT

28 Airway Management

WILLIAM H. ROSENBLATT • RON O. ABRONS • WARIYA SUKHUPRAGARN

Perspectives on Airway Management
  Review of Airway Anatomy
  History of Airway Management
  Limitations of Patient History and Physical Examination
Clinical Management of the Airway
  Preoxygenation
  Support of the Airway with the Induction of Anesthesia
The Difficult Airway Algorithm
  The Airway Approach Algorithm
  Awake Airway Management
  Clinically Difficult Airway Scenarios

The Flexible Intubation Scope in Airway Management
  Elements of the Flexible Intubation Scope
  Use of the Flexible Intubation Scope
The SGA in the Failed Airway
  Other Devices
Conclusions

KEY POINTS

1. Management of the airway is paramount to safe perioperative care. A series of evaluation procedures favorably affects outcomes.
2. The anatomically complex airway undergoes growth and development, including significant changes in its size, shape, and relation to the cervical spine, from infancy into childhood.
3. The advent of the laryngeal mask airway, as well as other supraglottic airways, has revolutionized both routine and emergency airway management.
4. Airway management always begins with a thorough airway-relevant history and physical examination.
5. Preoxygenation (also commonly termed *denitrogenation*) should be practiced in all cases when time allows.
6. The goal of direct laryngoscopy is to produce a direct line of sight from the operator's eye to the larynx.
7. Videolaryngoscopy mimics the actions of direct laryngoscopy, but places an imaging device toward the distal end of the laryngoscope blade. This moves the provider's point of view past the tongue, avoiding the need for a direct line of sight to the glottis.
8. The technique of rapid-sequence induction is performed to gain control of the airway in the shortest period of time after the ablation of protective airway reflexes with the induction of anesthesia.
9. The period of extubation may be far more treacherous than that of induction of anesthesia and tracheal intubation.
10. In most instances, awake intubation can be accomplished successfully if approached with care and patience.
11. Awake airway management remains a mainstay of the American Society of Anesthesiologists' difficult airway algorithm.
12. An ever-increasing number of airway management devices are commercially available.
13. When intubation and mask and SGA ventilation fail, airway access via the extrathoracic trachea may be warranted.

Perspectives on Airway Management

In the nearly three decades since the publication of the first edition of this text, the field of airway management has undergone a vigorous revolution. Although many of the tools available in 1988 remain in use, the array of devices, algorithms, and pharmaceuticals in the modern airway armamentarium can be daunting. Fortunately, careful planning and expertise in a limited, albeit complementary, set of tools typically suffices. The final decade of the last century saw a resolute swing toward the application of supraglottic ventilation. More recently, the introduction of videolaryngoscopy (VL) has offered us yet another quantum leap that promises to address many of the failings of direct laryngoscopy, a technique that has been in use for more than 200 years.

Dedication: To the late Andranik Ovassapian, MD—his contributions appear so often in this chapter that he must be considered a co-author.

Along with offering the provider better tools, technology has also aided in the creation of large databases of airway-related records from which a wealth of information can be collected retrospectively. With databases as large as 2.9 million anesthetics,[1] we can begin to better understand the incidence of, and contributing factors to, even rare airway events.

Techniques and practices in airway management have long been an important concern of anesthesia societies, as illustrated by the publication and revision of various difficult airway guidelines.[2,3] Analysis of the American Society of Anesthesiologists' (ASA) Closed Claims Database in the periods before and after the 1993 publication of the ASA difficult airway guidelines reveals both encouraging and disturbing trends. A significant decrease in claims related to death/brain death at the induction of anesthesia is not matched with similar progress during emergence and in the postoperative period.[4] Although the closed claims data is useful, it has significant limitations, including its retrospective nature and the lack of a denominator.

Management of the airway is paramount to safe perioperative care. Difficult and failed airway management account for 2.3% to 16.6% of anesthetic deaths [5,6] and the following steps become necessary to favorably affect outcome: (1) thorough airway history and physical examination; (2) consideration of the ease of rapid tracheal intubation by direct or indirect laryngoscopy; (3) preinduction formation of a management plan, which includes the use of supraglottic ventilation (e.g., facemask supraglottic airway [SGA]); (4) aspiration risk assessment; and (5) estimation of the relative risk of failed airway maneuvers.[7] This chapter will reflect the need to consider these five factors when approaching any patient who requires or may require airway control. This text will focus on routine and rescue airway management techniques that are the fundamentals upon which all airway management is based. Specialty-specific techniques (e.g., elective suspension laryngoscopy) will not be addressed.

Review of Airway Anatomy

The term *airway* refers to the upper airway—consisting of the nasal and oral cavities, pharynx, larynx, trachea, and principal bronchi. The airway in humans is primarily a conducting pathway. Because the oroesophageal and nasotracheal passages cross each other, anatomic and functional complexities have evolved for protection of the sublaryngeal airway against aspiration of food passing through the pharynx. As are other bodily systems, the airway is not immune from the influence of genetic, nutritional, and hormonal factors. **The anatomically complex airway undergoes significant changes in its size, shape, and relationship to the cervical spine from infancy into childhood.**[8] Table 28-1 illustrates the anatomic differences in the larynx of infants and adults.

Table 28-1 Anatomic Differences between Infant and Adult Larynxes

Infant larynx proportionately smaller
Vertical location: C3–C5 in infant; C4–C6 in adult
Pliable laryngeal cartilage in the infant/child
Vocal folds: Anterior angle with respect to perpendicular axis of larynx in infant/child
Aryepiglottic folds closer to midline in infant/child
Epiglottis: Relatively longer, narrower, and stiffer in infant
Mucosa more vulnerable to trauma in infant

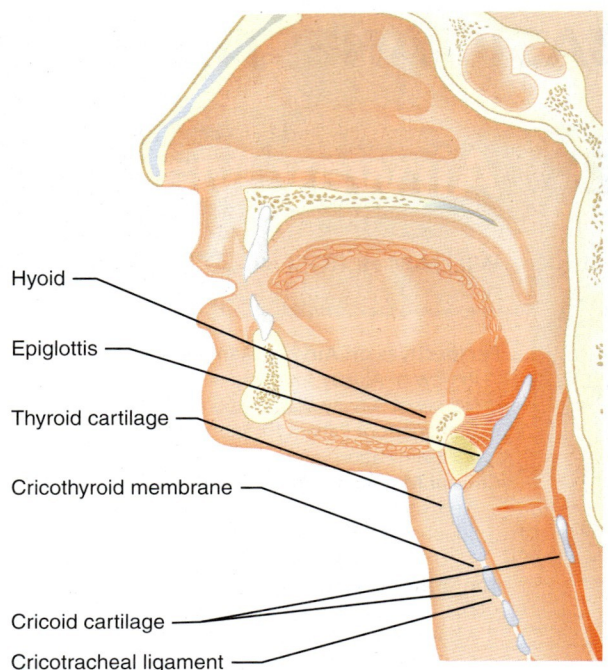

Figure 28-1 The major landmarks of the airway mechanism. Note that the cricoid cartilage is <1 cm in height in its anterior aspect, but may be 2 cm in height posteriorly.

The laryngeal skeleton consists of nine cartilages (three paired and three unpaired); together, these house the vocal folds, which extend in an anterior–posterior plane from the thyroid cartilage to the arytenoid cartilages. The shield-shaped thyroid cartilage acts as the anterior "protective housing" of the vocal mechanism (Fig. 28-1). Movements of the laryngeal structures are controlled by two groups of muscles: the extrinsic muscles, which move the larynx as a whole; and the intrinsic muscles, which move the various cartilages in relation to one another. The larynx is innervated by the superior and recurrent laryngeal nerves, which are branches of the vagus nerve. Because the recurrent laryngeal nerves supply all of the intrinsic muscles of the larynx (with the exception of cricothyroid muscle), trauma to these nerves can result in vocal cord dysfunction. With unilateral recurrent laryngeal nerve injury, hoarseness is the primary symptom, though the protective role of the larynx in preventing aspiration may be compromised. Bilateral injury can result in complete airway obstruction due to fixed cord adduction and may be a surgical emergency.

An important externally identifiable structure is the cricothyroid membrane (CTM), which joins the superior aspect of the cricoid cartilage and the inferior edge of the thyroid cartilage. In an adult, the membrane is typically 8 to 12 mm in width and 10.4 to 13.7 mm in height and is composed of a yellow elastic tissue that lies directly beneath the skin and a fascial layer. It can be identified 1 to 1.5 fingerbreadths below the laryngeal prominence (thyroid notch).[9] The membrane has a central portion known as the *conus elasticus* and two lateral thinner portions. Directly beneath the membrane is the laryngeal mucosa. Because of anatomic variability in the course of veins and arteries and the membrane's proximity to the vocal folds (which may be 0.9 cm above the ligaments' upper border), it is suggested that any incisions or needle punctures to the CTM be made in its inferior third and be directed posteriorly (a posterior probing

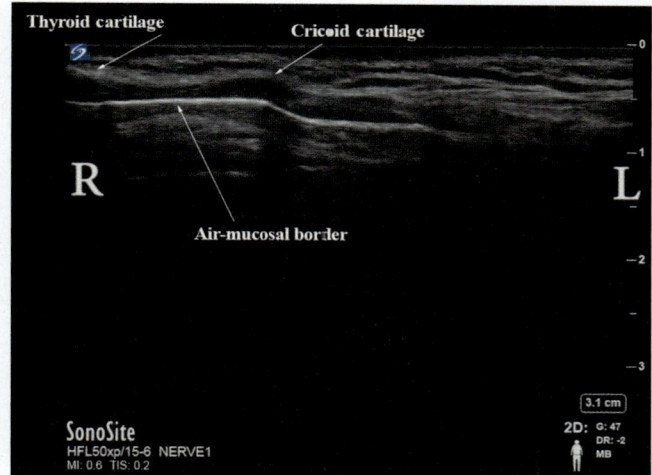

Figure 28-2 Ultrasound image of the cricothyroid membrane (CTM, midline sagittal).

needle will strike the back side of the ring-shaped cricoid cartilage). Identification of an appropriate incision or puncture site may be difficult. Campbell et al.[10] found that, though 80% of anesthesiologists were able to correctly identify the skin over the CTM in males, this number fell to 30% in females. The ASA difficult airway guidelines suggest that every patient be evaluated for difficult surgical airway.[2] This should lead to routine examination of laryngeal structures, including the marking of surface anatomy, and the use of ultrasound identification, especially in at-risk patients (Fig. 28-2).[11]

At the base of the larynx, suspended by the underside of the CTM, is the signet ring–shaped cricoid cartilage. This cartilage is approximately 1 cm in height anteriorly, but almost 2 cm in height in its posterior aspect as it extends in a cephalad direction (Fig. 28-1). The tracheal cartilages are interconnected by fibroelastic tissue, which allows for expansion of the trachea in both length and diameter with inspiration/expiration and flexion/extension of the thoracocervical spine. Inferiorly, the trachea is suspended from the cricoid cartilage by the cricotracheal ligament.

The trachea measures approximately 15 cm in adults and is circumferentially supported by 17 to 18 C-shaped cartilages, with a membranous posterior aspect overlying the esophagus. In adults, the first tracheal ring is anterior to the sixth cervical vertebra.

The trachea ends at the carina (opposite the fifth thoracic vertebra), where it bifurcates into the principal bronchi. The right principal bronchus is larger in diameter than the left and deviates from the sagittal plane of the trachea at a less acute angle. For these reasons, aspirated materials, as well as a deeply inserted endotracheal tube (ETT), tend to gain entry into the right principal bronchus, although left-sided positioning cannot be excluded. Cartilaginous ring support continues through the first seven generations of the bronchi.

History of Airway Management

Prior to 1874, mechanisms of airway obstruction were poorly understood. Opening the mouth with a wooden screw and drawing the tongue forward with a forceps or a steel-gloved finger was the height of nonsurgical airway management.[12] Not until 1880 was it recognized that most airway obstruction resulted from the tongue falling against the posterior pharyngeal wall. Though it is possible that similar devices were used toward the end of the first millennium, the first use of a SGA is credited to Joseph Thomas Clover (1825–1882), who used a nasopharyngeal tube for the delivery of chloroform anesthesia.[13] Over the next 50 years, several modifications of the basic oropharyngeal airway were described. In the 1930s, Ralph Waters introduced the now-familiar flattened tube oral airway. Arthur Guedel modified Waters' concept by fitting his airway within a stiff rubber envelope in an attempt to reduce mucosal trauma.

Tracheal intubation was first described in 1788 as a means of resuscitation of the "apparently dead,"[14] but was not used for the delivery of anesthesia until almost 100 years later. The forerunner of the modern oral ETT was designed by Joseph O'Dwyer in the 1880s. O'Dwyer cared for pediatric patients suffering airway obstruction secondary to diphtherial pseudomembrane formations. He was aware of the work of Emile Trousseau, a French physician who reported having performed over 200 tracheostomies in patients with diphtheria. O'Dwyer, hoping to provide his patients nonsurgical relief from airway obstruction, designed brass tracheal tubes that were placed in the larynx using blind digital intubation technique. Some 20 years later, German otolaryngologist Dr. Franz Kuhn (1866–1929) developed a flexometallic tube that resisted kinking and could be shaped to the patient's upper airway anatomy. Like O'Dwyer's tubes, it was inserted using blind digital technique. The patients were intubated awake and the hypopharynx was sealed with oiled gauze packing.

Sir Ivan Magill and Stanley Rowbotham are credited with the initial development of modern tracheal intubation. Performing anesthesia for reconstructive facial surgery during World War I, they developed a two-tube nasal system. One narrow tube (gum elastic design) was passed through the nares and guided into the larynx using a surgical laryngoscope. The other tube was blindly passed into the pharynx to provide for the escape of gases. During use of this "Magill" tube, the exhaust lumen would occasionally pass blindly into the larynx, leading Sir Ivan to describe "blind nasal intubation."[15]

Cuffed SGAs were initially described in the early part of the 20th century. Three factors led to the development of these devices: (1) the introduction of cyclopropane (which was explosive and required an airtight circuit for appropriate gas containment), (2) appreciation that blind and laryngoscope-guided tracheal intubation remained a difficult task, and (3) a need for protection of the lower airway from blood and surgical debris in the upper airway.[13] The Primrose cuffed oropharyngeal tube, the Shipway airway (a Guedel oropharyngeal airway fitted with a cuff and a circuit connector designed by Sir Ivan Magill), and the Lessinger airway were predecessors of the modern supraglottic devices. In 1937, Leech introduced a "pharyngeal bulb gasway" with a noninflatable cuff that fit snugly into the hypopharynx.

The use of SGAs remained dominant until the introduction of curare in 1942, and the mass training of anesthesiologists in tracheal intubation in anticipation of casualties during World War II. The description by Mendelson[16] of gastric-content aspiration in parturients managed with a mask airway (66 of 44,016 patients, with 2 deaths) furthered the shift toward tracheal intubation in most surgical procedures. Within a few years, proficiency in direct laryngoscopy and tracheal intubation became a mark of professionalism. The advent of succinylcholine in 1951 furthered the dominance of tracheal intubation by providing rapid and profound muscle relaxation.

By 1981, two types of airway management prevailed—tracheal intubation and facemask ventilation with or without a Guedel airway. Although time-tested, both had failings. Tracheal intubation was associated with dental and soft tissue injury as well as cardiovascular stimulation, and mask ventilation often required a prolonged hands-on-the-airway technique. These difficulties led to the reconsideration of SGAs.

3 The advent of the laryngeal mask airway (LMA) and other SGAs revolutionized both routine and emergency airway management. In 1981, Dr. Archie Brain conceived the idea of fitting a mask-like structure over the larynx. The motivation behind his early concepts and the evolution of his designs was the belief that airway control could be achieved less traumatically than with tracheal intubation and more reliably than with facemask ventilation. The first prototypes of the LMA were built from the Goldman dental mask, fitted with a tracheal tube. The LMA Classic (Teleflex, Research Triangle Park, NC) was introduced into practice in the United Kingdom in 1989 and approved by the U.S. Food and Drug Administration in 1991. The variety of advanced models that followed (e.g., with intubation and gastric drainage capabilities) will be discussed later in this chapter. With the expiration of the early patents and the introduction of other design concepts (e.g., non-inflatable masks), several additional devices applying the supraglottic concept were introduced.

Parallel to the development of SGAs, the concept of indirect laryngoscopy was increasingly being considered. Although fiberoptic devices were applied to the problem of difficult tracheal intubation in the late 1960s, this technology was expensive and required a unique skill set. It was not until the late 1980s, when the technology became readily available, that skill in flexible fiberoptic airway management was considered critical to safe practice.[17] Bullard introduced the use of a fiberoptic bundle to the rigid laryngoscope. The Bullard laryngoscope (ACMI/Circon, Southborough, MA) incorporated optical and light-transmitting fiberoptic bundles into an anatomically shaped blade. A detachable stylet held the tracheal tube near the optic objective, which could be placed proximal to the larynx with minimal movement of the head and neck. Though less commonly used today, the Bullard laryngoscope can be considered the vanguard of the modern videolaryngoscopes and optical and video stylets.[18] Fiberoptic elements were also incorporated into standard laryngoscope blades, such as the Storz Video-Macintosh blade (Karl Storz, Tuttlingen, Germany), which was developed by Dr. George Berci, an endoscopic surgery pioneer.

In the first years of the 21st century, the era of VL was born with the advent of inexpensive and miniaturized light-sensitive computer chip devices (e.g., complementary metal-oxide-semiconductors or CMOS). The Glidescope (Verathon, Bothell, WA) was the first of a generation of devices to use CMOS technology to visualize the larynx indirectly. The Glidescope's acutely angled blade placed the clinician's point of vision around the base of the tongue, obviating the need to establish a direct line of sight from the operator's eye to the larynx. Difficulty in placement of the ETT quickly led to the introduction of both specialized stylets and channeled-type laryngoscopes. Each of these advents will be discussed within this chapter.

Limitations of Patient History and Physical Examination

2

4 **Airway management always begins with a thorough airway-relevant history and physical examination**, including a search for documentation of previous airway-related anesthetic events. When a patient requires more than routine care (anticipated or unanticipated), the patient should be made aware of diagnostic evaluations and therapeutic interventions that were employed. It is becoming common practice for a dedicated "difficult airway note" to be incorporated into electronic medical records and for a "difficult airway letter" to be given to, and reviewed with,

patients and their families, describing critical and nonanticipated airway events. The patient may also be referred to difficult airway registries, such as the MedicAlert (http://www.medicalert.org/everybody/difficult-airwayintubation-registry). In the absence of such documentation, the clinician should seek the anesthetic records of past surgical visits, which in some cases may involve contacting other institutions. When this information is not available, adopting a low threshold for using a more conservative approach to airway management (e.g., awake intubation) will mitigate risk. This, though, assumes that the clinician is skilled in these techniques. It is not unusual for a patient to be referred to a different facility or practitioner due to airway management concerns. Signs and symptoms related to potentially difficult airway management, including aspiration risk, should be sought (Tables 28-2 and 28-3). Many congenital and acquired syndromes are associated with difficult airway management (Table 28-4).

Several physical evaluation measures have become popular (Table 28-5), although their reproducibility and predictability have been disputed. The difficulty in developing the perfect airway evaluation tool lies in two interrelated areas: simplicity and interdependency. Simple bedside evaluation tools are useful, but adequate evaluation may require endoscopic, radiologic, or other currently uncommon examinations.[19-21] Interdependency refers to the predictive value of one airway examination measure based on the findings of another. Details of the various examinations and their interdependency are discussed later in "Direct Laryngoscopy," under the topic of Functional Airway Assessment.

Historically, airway assessment has been synonymous with evaluation for the ease of direct laryngoscopy (DL), the end point being the anticipated degree of visualization of the larynx. The changing landscape of laryngoscopy (i.e., the rapid proliferation of indirect techniques, including VL) may make

Table 28-2 Physical Exam Features with Airway Management Implications

Physical Exam Feature	Significance
Mouth opening	Difficult blade insertion/tongue displacement if limited
Jaw protrusion	Difficult tongue displacement if limited
Dentition	Obstructed view (if large central incisors), increased risk of dental trauma (if poor or restored dentition), difficult mask ventilation (if edentulous)
Retrognathia	Difficult tongue displacement
Thyromental distance	Reflects neck mobility and degree of retrognathia
Mallampati grade	Describes the relationship between mouth opening, tongue size, and pharyngeal space
Presence of beard	Difficult mask seal
Airway pathology	Potential for difficult mask ventilation (obstructive masses/tissue, atypical facial contours) and laryngoscopy (friable tissue, atypical or absent landmarks, and limited mouth opening, jaw protrusion, tongue displacement, and neck mobility)

Table 28-3 Conditions with Airway Management Implications

Increased risk of difficult laryngoscopy, mask ventilation, or SGA ventilation	Increased aspiration risk

• History of failed or traumatic airway management
  • Dental damage or prolonged airway soreness after a previous anesthetic
• History of head/neck surgery or radiation therapy
• Various congenital and acquired syndromes (Table 28-4)
• Supraglottic pathology
  • Obstructive sleep apnea (BMI >35 kg/m^2, loud snoring, daytime somnolence, gasping or pauses in breathing during sleep)
  • Lingual tonsillar hyperplasia
• Acute airway pathology
  • Airway cyst or tumor
  • Airway bleeding
  • Stridor
Cervical spine disease or limited range of motion
Temporomandibular joint disease
	Recent meal
	Acute trauma
	Acute gastrointestinal pathology
	Acute narcotic therapy
	Significant gastroesophageal reflux
	Current intensive care unit admission
	Pregnancy (gestational age ≥12 weeks)
	Postpartum (before second postpartum day)
	Frequent pneumonia
	History of voice change, vocal cord polyp, or coughing after eating/drinking
	Systemic-disease associated with gastroparesis: diabetes mellitus, collagen vascular disease, advanced Parkinson disease, central nervous system tumors

Table 28-4 Syndromes Associated with Difficult Airway Management

Pathologic Condition	Features Affecting Airway Management
Congenital	
Pierre Robin sequence	Micrognathia, relative macroglossia, glossoptosis, cleft palate
Treacher Collins syndrome	Malar and mandibular hypoplasia, microstomia, choanal atresia
Down syndrome	Macroglossia, microcephaly, cervical spine abnormalities
Klippel–Feil syndrome	Congenital fusion of cervical vertebrae, decreased cervical range of motion
Cretinism	Macroglossia, compression or deviation of larynx/trachea by goiter
Cri du chat syndrome	Micrognathia, laryngomalacia, stridor
Alport syndrome	Maxillary hypoplasia, prognathism, cleft soft palate, tracheobronchial cartilaginous anomalies
Beckwith syndrome	Macroglossia
Cherubism	Mandibular and maxillary fibrous tissue overgrowth
Meckel syndrome	Microcephaly, micrognathia, cleft epiglottis
Neurofibromatosis type I (von Recklinghausen disease)	Tumors may occur in the larynx and right ventricle outflow tract. Increased incidence of pheochromocytoma
Hurler/Hunter syndrome	Stiff joints, upper airway obstruction due to infiltration of lymphoid tissue, abnormal tracheobronchial cartilages
Pompe disease	Muscle deposits, macroglossia
Acquired Infections	
Epiglottitis	Epiglottal edema
Croup	Laryngeal edema
Papillomatosis	Obstructive papillomas
Intraoral/retropharyngeal abscess	Airway distortion/stenosis, trismus
Ludwig angina	Airway distortion/stenosis, trismus
Arthritis	
Rheumatoid arthritis	Restricted cervical spine mobility, temporomandibular joint ankylosis, atlantoaxial instability
Ankylosing spondylitis	Ankylosis/immobility of cervical spine and temporomandibular joints
Tumors	
Cystic hygroma, lipoma, adenoma, goiter	Airway distortion or stenosis
Carcinoma of tongue/larynx/thyroid	Airway distortion or stenosis, fixation of larynx or adjacent tissues
Trauma	
Head/facial/cervical spine	Airway edema or hemorrhage, unstable facial or mandibular fractures, intralaryngeal damage
Miscellaneous Conditions	
History of head/neck radiation	Friable tissue, edema from impaired lymphatic drainage
Morbid obesity	Short, thick neck, large tongue and obstructive sleep apnea are likely
Acromegaly	Macroglossia, prognathism
Acute burns	Airway edema, bronchospasm, decreased apnea tolerance

Table 28-5 Techniques of Common Airway Indexes Measurement

Examination	
Thyromental distance	Measured from tip of mentum to thyroid notch in neck-extended position
Mouth opening	Interincisor distance (or interalveolar distance when edentulous) with the mouth maximally opened
Mallampati score	(See Fig. 28-8)
Head and neck mobility	Range of motion from full flexion to full extension
Ability to prognath	Capacity to bring lower incisors in front of upper incisors

Table 28-7 Simplified Risk Score for Difficult Intubation[27]

Number of Risk Factors[a]	Incidence of Difficult Intubation
0	0
1	2%
2	4%
3	8%
4 or 5	17%

[a]Presence of upper front teeth, history of a difficult intubation, Mallampati >1, Mallampati of 4, mouth opening <4 cm.

many evaluation indices irrelevant. Efforts to define attributes that identify patients who may be difficult to intubate by DL have been only modestly successful. In their meta-analysis of the physical predictors of difficult DL, Shiga et al.[22] concluded that, when interpreted as individual tests, currently used techniques of evaluation have only modest discriminative power (Table 28-6).

Despite the disappointing usefulness of these individual indexes, other authors have recognized that combinations of tests can provide improved predictability. El-Ganzouri et al.[23] designed a statistical model for stratifying risk of difficult DL in a large population. This multivariate index assigned relative weights to each physical examination or historical finding based on the odds of a high-grade laryngeal view being achieved with DL. The authors noted that with increasing multivariate index scores, positive predictive value increased, but sensitivity decreased (i.e., higher multivariate index scores occur when there are more positive physical findings, but not all difficult laryngoscopy patients will manifest multiple findings). Compared with the Mallampati classification alone, the multivariate composite index had improved positive predictive and specificity values at equal sensitivity. Of course, some pathology will only present with the induction of anesthesia and/or attempts at laryngoscopy.[24,25] Other groups have used similar regimens to increase the predictability of multivariate indexes by incorporating imaging technologies. In a small population of patients, Naguib et al.[26] were able to achieve high predictive accuracy (90% or higher) when physical examination and imaging scores (x-ray and three-dimensional computed tomography) were weighted. A simplified scoring system, studied on a multi-institution population of 3,763 patients, recognized both the difficulty of constructing a complex analysis in the preoperative holding area and the failure of any model to be completely predictive.[27] Accepting a discriminating power of 70%, this model found five attributes that could be used to predict difficult laryngoscopy (Table 28-7).

Until recently, there was limited data on external airway findings that may indicate failure of *indirect* laryngoscopy. Studies comparing DL with a Macintosh laryngoscope and VL with the Glidescope indicate that, though no single examination finding may predict the success or failure with each device, the failure to visualize the larynx with the Glidescope was characterized by higher multivariate risk scores of the same clinical finding.[28] Others have found that the following preoperative findings contribute to failure of VL: scarring, radiation, masses or thickness of the neck, thyromental distance of less than 6 cm, limited cervical motion, and operator experience.[29] In 2016, based on a secondary analysis of 1,100 VL intubations, Aziz et al.[30] identified four distinct predictors of difficult acute-angle VL. Of note, the "supine sniffing" position was associated with more difficult VL than the "supine neutral" position (Odds Ratio: 1.646), suggesting that this common position may be best avoided when initial plans include VL.

In general, tracheal intubation should be considered nonroutine under the following conditions: (1) the presence of equally important priorities to the management of the airway (such as a "full stomach" or emergency surgery); (2) abnormal airway anatomy; or (3) direct injury to the upper airway, larynx, spine, and/or trachea. Although the finding of abnormal anatomy is not synonymous with difficult airway management, it should kindle heightened suspicion.

Few studies have objectively determined findings that identify patients who will be difficult to mask ventilate as defined in Table 28-8(A). In a study of 1,502 patients, Langeron et al.[20] found 5% of patients to be difficult to mask ventilate, with only one patient in the series being impossible to mask ventilate. Table 28-8(B) describes the five independent clinical predictors found by Langeron, with the presence of two or more indicating a high likelihood of difficult mask ventilation. Kheterpal et al.,[31] using different criteria, found 0.15% of patients to be impossible to mask ventilate. The same study showed that high Mallampati score, male sex, the presence of a beard, and a history of sleep apnea or neck radiation were independent predictors of impossible mask ventilation.

Ultrasound (US) technology is widely used, portable, and provides rapid, real-time, dynamic images. Bedside US can confirm endotracheal intubation with both a sensitivity and specificity of 0.98[32] and can be used to identify the CTM, rule out esophageal intubation and verify ventilation in the absence of CO_2 detection (assuring bilateral lung excursion).[33] Subglottic hemangiomas, papillomas, and laryngeal cysts and stenosis have also been identified by US. Another use for US imaging is the estimation of ETT (including double lumen) size. Although it may be possible to

Table 28-6 Summary of Pooled Sensitivity and Specificity of Commonly Used Methods of Airway Evaluation[22]

Examination	Sensitivity (%)	Specificity (%)
Mouth opening	46	89
Mallampati classification	49	86
Thyromental distance	20	94
Sternomental distance	62	82

Table 28-8 Assessment and Predictability of Difficult Mask Ventilation[20]

(A) Criteria for Difficult Mask Ventilation

Inability for one anesthesiologist to maintain oxygen saturation >92%
Significant gas leak around facemask
Need for ≥4 L/min gas flow (or use of fresh gas flow button more than twice)
No chest movement
Two-handed mask ventilation needed
Change of operator required

(B) Independent Risk Factors for Difficult Mask Ventilation

Risk Factors	Odds Ratio
Presence of a beard	3.18
Body mass index >26 ng/m^2	2.75
Lack of teeth	2.28
Age >55 yr	2.26
History of snoring	1.84

examine the upper airway for changes such as hypertrophic lingual tonsils, the clinical relevancy (e.g., impact on laryngoscopy and ventilation) of ultrasonography has not been studied[33] and the applications of US in preoperative airway evaluation are still limited. When using ultrasound for airway evaluation, the linear high-frequency transducer is the most useful probe.

Predicting difficult DL remains, in large part, an enigma. As previously illustrated, the commonly used indexes may not only be less predictive than originally thought, but may also be misleading. The advent of VL may make these deficits irrelevant and new criteria would need to be explored.

Clinical Management of the Airway

Preoxygenation

Preoxygenation should be practiced in all cases when time allows.[34] This procedure entails the replacement of the nitrogen volume of the lung (as much as 95% of the functional residual capacity) with oxygen in order to provide an apneic oxygen reservoir. Under ideal conditions, a healthy patient breathing room air (F_{IO_2} = 0.21) will experience oxyhemoglobin desaturation to a level of less than 90% after approximately 1 to 2 minutes of apnea. In the same patient, several minutes of preoxygenation with 100% O_2 via a tight-fitting facemask may support at least minutes of apnea before desaturation occurs. Patients with pulmonary disease, obesity, or conditions affecting metabolism frequently evidence desaturation sooner, owing to decreased functional residual capacity, increased O_2 extraction, and/or right-to-left transpulmonary shunting. In one study, healthy obese patients breathing 100% O_2 preoperatively sustained oxygen saturation of greater than 90% for 6 ± 0.5 minutes, as opposed to 2.7 ± 0.25 minutes for obese patients under the same conditions.[35]

Time-sparing methods of preoxygenation have also been described. Using a series of four vital capacity breaths of 100% over a 30-second period, a high arterial Pa_{O_2} (339 mmHg) can be achieved, but the time to desaturation remains shorter than with traditional techniques.[34] A modified vital capacity technique, wherein the patient is asked to take eight deep breaths in a 60-second period, shows promise in terms of prolonging the time to desaturation.[34] The authors of the current chapter prefer the technique of applying a tight-fitting mask for 5 minutes or more of tidal volume breathing 100% oxygen at flows of 10 to 12 L/min. The mask is placed immediately after the patient has been made comfortable on the operating room (OR) table and remains in place during OR check-in and the application of monitors.

In the obese patient, bilevel positive airway pressure and reverse-Trendelenburg position have been advocated to reach maximal preinduction arterial oxygenation and to delay oxyhemoglobin desaturation.[34,36] Pharyngeal insufflation of oxygen can also delay the onset of oxyhemoglobin desaturation during apnea. In this technique, oxygen is insufflated at a rate of 3 to 15 L/min via a nasal cannula or nasal-only facemask upon induction of anesthesia.[34,37,38] This technique relies on the phenomenon of apneic oxygenation, a process by which gases are entrained into the alveolar space during apnea.

Transnasal Humidified Rapid-Insufflation Ventilatory Exchange (THRIVE) has recently been introduced not only as a method of preoxygenation but also for use during periods of unplanned or intentional apnea (e.g., failed tracheal intubation or suspension laryngoscopy, respectively).[39] Oxygen flows of 30 to 70 L/min of oxygen are delivered via specialized nasal cannulae (OptiFlow™, Fisher and Paykel Healthcare Limited, Panmure, Aukland, New Zealand) throughout the preinduction and intubation phases or during other apneic periods. Apneic durations of 55 minutes have been reported with this technique. Hypercapnia occurs to a limited degree as compared to traditional apnea, which is attributed to turbulent flow at the glottic opening.

Certain circumstances can limit the effectiveness of preoxygenation, as exemplified by the patient who experiences claustrophobia with the anesthesia facemask (which can almost always be overcome by having the patient hold the mask or by removing the mask and allowing the patient to breathe directly from the anesthesia machine circuit) or the use of self-inflating breathing bags (which do not deliver an F_{IO_2} of 100% during spontaneous breathing) or nasal-only masks. Likewise, leaks around the facemask can allow entrainment of air, thereby reducing the F_{IO_2}. Leaks as small as 4 mm (cross-sectional) can cause significant reductions in the inspired oxygen content.[40]

Support of the Airway with the Induction of Anesthesia

With the induction of anesthesia and the onset of apnea, ventilation and oxygenation must be supported. Traditional methods include the anesthesia facemask, SGA, and ETT. High-flow nasal oxygen, as noted earlier, has also been used.

The Anesthesia Facemask

With the induction of anesthesia, the patient's level of consciousness changes from the awake state, with a competent and protected airway, to the unconscious state, with an unprotected and potentially obstructed airway. This drug-induced central ventilatory depression, along with relaxation of the upper airway musculature, can lead rapidly to hypercapnia and hypoxia. The anesthesia facemask is the device most commonly used to deliver anesthetic gases and ventilate an apneic patient. Facemask ventilation is highly effective, minimally invasive, and

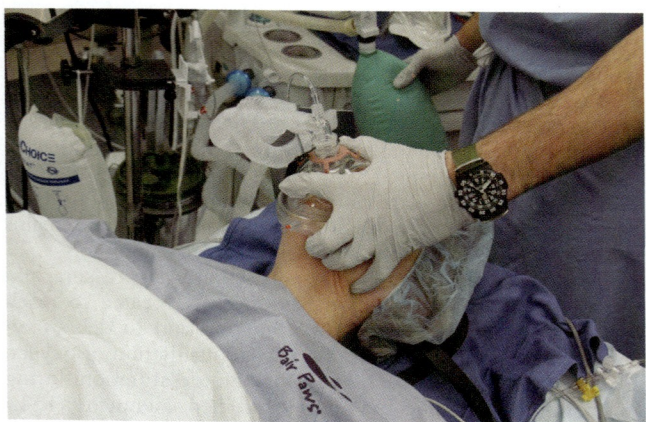

Figure 28-3 Holding the anesthesia mask on the face. The thumb and the first finger grip the mask in such a fashion that the anesthesia circuit (or self-inflating resuscitation bag) connection abuts the web between these digits. This allows the palm of the hand to apply pressure to the left side of the mask, while the tips of these two digits apply pressure over the right. The third finger helps to secure under the mentum, and the fourth finger is under the angle of the mandible or along the lower mandibular ridge. Mask straps (on pillow) may be used to complement the hand grip by securing the right side of the mask.

requires the least sophisticated equipment, making it critical to initial management of the airway and a mainstay in the delivery of anesthesia.

A facemask is gently held on the patient's face with the thumb and first finger of the operator's left hand, leaving the right hand free for other tasks (Fig. 28-3). Most modern masks can be distorted by the operator's fingers to form a seal around facial contours. Air leaks around the mask's edges can be prevented by gentle downward pressure with the awake patient or, if the patient is asleep, by pulling the mandible upward into the mask. A two-handed jaw-thrust technique has been shown to be superior to the classic one-handed grip for this maneuver.[41] Elastic "mask straps" may also be used and can be particularly helpful for the clinician with short fingers or for "hands-off" preoxygenation while other tasks are being performed. Gas leaks should be avoided, as the most common reason for suboptimal preoxygenation is a loose-fitting mask, which allows the entrainment of room air.[34]

Appropriate positioning of the patient is paramount for delivery of positive pressure ventilation via facemask. With the patient supine, "ramped," or in reverse Trendelenburg position, the head and neck are placed in the *sniffing* position, described later (see discussion of *tracheal intubation*). This position improves mask ventilation by anteriorizing the base of the tongue and the epiglottis.[42]

After induction of anesthesia, a tight fit of the facemask is achieved by upward displacement of the mandible into the mask, which is held in position by the thumb and first finger. This maneuver, commonly known as a *jaw thrust*, raises the soft tissues of the anterior airway off the pharyngeal wall and allows for improved ventilation. In patients who are obese, edentulous, or bearded, two hands or a mask strap may be required to ensure an adequate mask seal. When two hands are required for holding the facemask, a second operator may be required to squeeze the reservoir bag. If necessary, the second operator can improve the mask's fit by providing additional jaw-thrust and chin lift. If no help is available, the ventilator can be used to deliver the breaths.

One useful, albeit poorly characterized, maneuver that aids in facemask ventilation is the *expiratory chin drop*. When positive-pressure inspiration is successful, but is not followed by passive gas escape during expiration, allowing phasic head flexion and reducing chin/jaw lifting will often improve gas egress.

Well-secured dentures may improve the mask seal for an edentulous patient.[43] The advantage of this must be weighed against the risk of denture displacement or damage. Dentures may be removed when laryngoscopy is initiated.

A patient with normal lung compliance should require no more than 20 to 25 cm H_2O pressure for lung inflation, as measured on the anesthesia circle manometer. If more pressure is required, the adequacy of the mask technique should be reevaluated. This includes adjusting the mask fit, seeking aid with the mask hold, administering muscle relaxants, or considering adjuncts such as oral and nasal airways. Both oral and nasal airways can bypass upper airway obstruction by creating an artificial passage to the hypopharynx. Nasal airways are less likely to stimulate coughing, gagging, or vomiting in the lightly anesthetized patient but may cause epistaxis. For this reason, nasal airways are typically avoided in patients at high risk for bleeding (e.g., iatrogenic or pathologic coagulopathy, pregnancy, hereditary hemorrhagic telangiectasia, uncontrolled hypertension).

The nasal airway should be long enough to reach from the nare to the thyroid notch when placed alongside the patient's face. It is inserted along the floor of the nose, in an anterior–posterior direction, and should always be prepared with water-soluble lubricant to reduce trauma to the highly vascular nasal mucosa. A vasoconstrictor agent (e.g., oxymetazoline or phenylephrine) may be applied before insertion of the nasal airway to decrease this risk. Resistance to insertion should prompt repositioning of the airway bevel, reassessment of the direction of insertion, or change to a smaller airway or the contralateral nare.

The typical rounded oral airway is placed with its longitudinal concavity rotated in a rostrad direction. Once the distal end of the airway has been inserted to the level of the oropharynx, the device is rotated 180 degrees and insertion is continued to its ultimate position. This maneuver avoids displacement of the tongue into the hypopharynx and can be aided by caudad displacement of the tongue with a tongue depressor. A small oral aperture, intrapharyngeal mass or foreign body, intact gag reflex or otherwise light anesthesia may prevent oral airway placement. As will be discussed later, some intubating oral airways are large and have a rectangular cross-section. These devices tend to be too large for intraoral rotation and are inserted with the concavity facing caudally while the tongue is stabilized by a tongue depressor or held by the operator. Similar to nasal airway sizing, oral airways should reach from teeth (or alveolar ridge) to the mandibular angle.

Obstruction to mask ventilation may be caused by laryngospasm, a local reflex closure of the vocal folds. Laryngospasm may be triggered by a foreign body (e.g., oral or nasal airway), saliva, blood, or vomitus touching the glottis. It may also result from pain or visceral stimulation. Hypoxia as well as negative pressure) pulmonary edema can result from continued spontaneous ventilation against closed vocal cords (or other obstruction). Management of laryngospasm consists of removing the offending stimulus (if identified), administering oxygen with continuous positive airway pressure, deepening the plane of the anesthesia, and, if other maneuvers are unsuccessful, administering a rapid-acting muscle relaxant.

The practice of withholding muscle relaxants until establishment of facemask ventilation, which has been a mainstay of anesthetic teaching, has recently come into question. Objective evidence supports administration of depolarizing or non-depolarizing muscle relaxants simultaneously with induction agents[45] to facilitate mask ventilation, laryngoscopy, and tracheal intubation. This is discussed in detail in the cases later (case 4).

If there are no contraindications (e.g., increased aspiration risk), mask ventilation can be the primary ventilatory technique for anesthetic maintenance. Otherwise, it is commonly used to administer anesthetic gases and oxygen and to facilitate ventilation until the anesthetic state is adequate for use of another means of airway support, such as an SGA or ETT. This decision should be made after careful consideration of the patient's coexisting diseases and surgical requirements.

Supraglottic Airways

Devices that isolate the airway above the vocal cords are referred to as SGAs. Although initially approved as a substitute for face-mask ventilation and when tracheal intubation was not achievable, SGAs soon became widely used in surgical cases traditionally managed with tracheal intubation.[46,47] SGAs are associated with lower incidence of sore throat, coughing, and laryngospasm on emergence, as well with decreased reversible bronchospasm than seen with tracheal intubation.[48,49] With the expiration of the US patents on the original LMA in 2002, there was a proliferation of similar devices. Although older data suggest that 35% or more of general anesthetics in the United States are performed with SGAs, more recent data from the United Kingdom imply a 56% incidence.[46,50,51]

As the first device of its kind, a wealth of information exists on the LMA Classic and its subsequent iterations (Fig. 28-4). Much of this knowledge may be applied to newer SGAs as well. That this chapter devotes considerable text to the LMA family of devices is not meant to infer preference, but rather the availability of information.

The advent of the LMA as well as other SGAs has led some to question the relative safety of tracheal intubation.[52] This, along with the ASA Closed Claims Database information, lends support to the search for safe alternatives to tracheal intubation whenever possible.[53] Similarly, pharyngeal mucosa appears to be more resilient to trauma from SGAs than tracheal mucosa to damage from ETTs. In one animal study, mucosal injury from the LMA ProSeal (Teleflex, Research Triangle Park, NC) did not occur until more than 9 hours of continuous use.[54] The hemodynamic effects associated with airway management are also reduced with SGAs. Increases in heart rate, blood pressure, and intraocular pressure are all less during airway management with an SGA than with an ETT.[55,56]

The LMA Classic. The original SGA, the LMA Classic, is composed of a perilaryngeal mask and an airway barrel. The device is designed to sit in the hypopharynx with an anterior surface aperture overlying the laryngeal inlet. The mask has an inflatable cuff that fills the hypopharyngeal space, creating a seal that allows positive-pressure ventilation with up to 20 cm H_2O pressure. The adequacy of the seal depends on correct placement, appropriate size, and patient anatomy, and is less dependent on the cuff-filling pressure or volume. Attached to the posterior surface of the mask is a barrel (airway tube) which extends proximally from the mask's central aperture and can be connected to a self-inflating resuscitation bag or anesthesia circuit. While the LMA Classic is constructed of reusable silicone, several models constructed with silicone or polyvinyl chloride (PVC) are currently available from various manufacturers.

LMAs come in varying sizes, from neonatal to large adult, and selection is critical to both successful use and complication avoidance. The manufacturer recommends that the clinician choose the largest size that will fit comfortably within the oral cavity. LMA insertion technique mimics the processes of swallowing. Just as food intended for the esophageal opening is pressed cephalad and posteriorly against the palate, so is the tip of the LMA, as it shares the same destination. As with swallowing, head extension and neck flexion enlarge the space behind the tongue to allow passage into the hypopharynx. These functions allow the food bolus, or the LMA, to reach its mark while avoiding contact with the anterior pharyngeal structures or stimulation of protective airway reflexes.

The insertion of the LMA as described by its inventor, Dr. Archie Brain, has been modified by a number of writers. Discussion of these various alternatives is beyond the scope of this text. The principles of LMA insertion can be applied to many other SGAs, though the individual manufacturer's recommendations should be consulted. The currently recommended insertion technique, illustrated in Figure 28-5, has a 94% success rate.[57] In this technique, the mask is completely deflated and the palatal surface lubricated with a non-local anesthetic containing lubricant. The operator's nondominant hand is placed under the occiput to flex the neck on the thorax and extend the head at the atlanto-occipital joint (creating a space behind the larynx; this action also tends to open the mouth).[58] The index finger of the dominant hand is placed in the cleft between the mask and barrel. The hard palate is visualized and the superior (nonaperture) surface of the mask is placed against it. Force is applied by the index finger in an upward direction toward the top of the patient's head. This causes the mask to flatten and follow the contour of the palate into the pharynx and hypopharynx. The index finger continues along this arc, continually applying an outward pressure until resistance from the upper esophageal sphincter is met. The most common error made by clinicians is the application of pressure with a posterior vector, causing the LMA's tip to impact the posterior pharyngeal wall, often resulting in tip folding, device misplacement, and tissue trauma.

Prior to attachment of the anesthesia circuit, the LMA is inflated with the minimum amount of pressure that allows ventilation to 20 cm H_2O without an air leak. The manufacturer recommends keeping the intracuff pressure under 60 cm H_2O and evidence exists for keeping it under 44 mmHg.[59] When an adequate seal cannot be obtained with 60 cm H_2O cuff pressure, the LMA's positioning, sizing, or type should be re-evaluated. Light anesthesia and laryngospasm also may contribute to poor seal. With inflation, one should be able to observe a rising of the cricoid and thyroid cartilages and a lifting of the barrel out of the

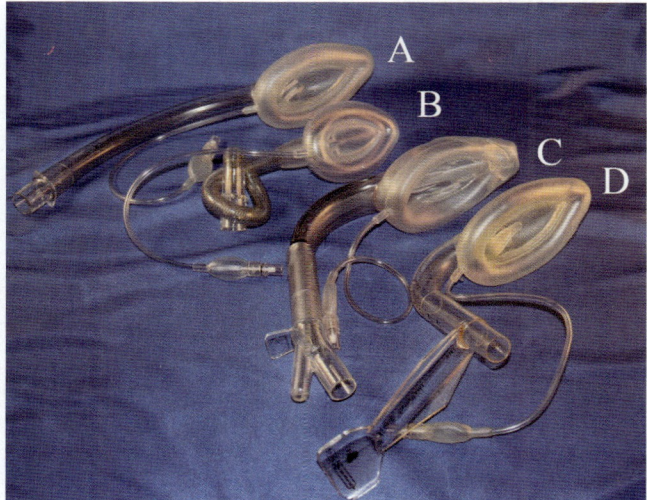

Figure 28-4 The family of aryngeal mask airways (from top): (**A**) Unique, (**B**) Flexible, (**C**) Supreme, (**D**) Fastrach.

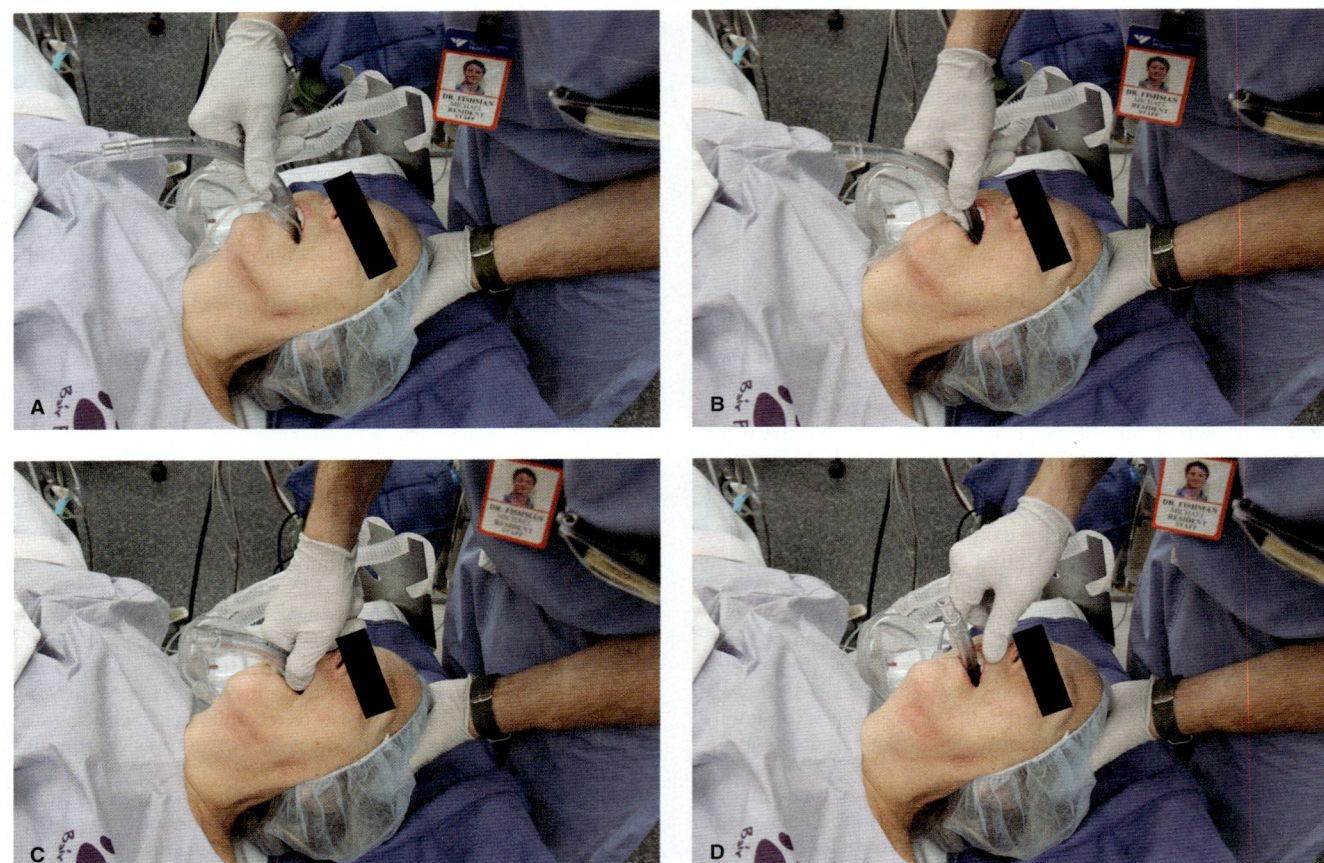

Figure 28-5 Insertion of the laryngeal mask airway (LMA). The LMA is inserted with the index finger of the dominant hand pressing with a force vector against the hard palate (**A** and **B**). The outward force vector is continued from the hard palate to the pharynx and hypopharynx (**C**) until the index finger meets resistance against the upper esophageal sphincter and is removed (**D**).

mouth by approximately 1 cm as the mask expands. If a midline position is not possible due to the patient's position or the surgical procedure, a flexible LMA (discussed later) should be considered. A bite block is recommended to prevent biting and occlusion of the LMA barrel. Cuff pressure should be measured after insertion and periodically monitored if nitrous oxide is being used.

Although the distal tip of the LMA mask sits in the esophageal inlet, it does not reliably seal it. The LMA was not designed to protect against the aspiration of gastric contents nor does it reliably do so. Despite this, when used in patients at low risk for regurgitation, the rate of aspiration during LMA use is similar to that in all non-LMA general anesthetics (approximately 2 in 10,000 cases).[60,61] The incidence of gastroesophageal reflux may be increased when compared with use of the facemask,[60] but when populations of patients considered to have a full stomach are studied (in controlled trials, prospective series, or anecdotally), there is still a low incidence of aspiration noted with elective or emergency LMA use. Reports have included safe use in patients who are morbidly obese or have experienced frequent gastroesophageal reflux, those undergoing elective cesarean section or airway rescue during labor, and those presenting to emergency departments or paramedic crews.[62,63] During cardiopulmonary resuscitation, the incidence of gastroesophageal regurgitation is four times greater with a bag-valve mask than with the LMA.[64]

If at any time gastric contents are noted in an SGA barrel, maneuvers similar to those applied when using an ETT should be instituted. The SGA should be left in place, the barrel suctioned, the patient placed in Trendelenburg position, and 100% oxygen administered.

Although first introduced for use with spontaneous ventilation, the LMA has proved useful and safe for cases in which positive-pressure ventilation is either desired or preferred.[56,65] There is no difference in gastric inflation with positive-pressure ventilation (<17 cm H_2O) when comparing an LMA to an ETT.[66] With the LMA Classic, tidal volumes are limited to 8 mL/kg and airway pressure to 20 cm H_2O. These devices have been used successfully with supine, prone, lateral, oblique, Trendelenburg, and lithotomy positions. Although the manufacturer recommends use for a maximum of 2 to 3 hours, reports of use for more than 24 hours exist.[67] In a porcine model, Goldmann et al.[54] saw no evidence of mucosal changes with up to 9 hours of LMA ProSeal use, though damage was consistently evident after 12 hours.

The LMA Flexible. The introduction of flexible barrel SGAs (e.g., the LMA Flexible, Teleflex, Research Triangle Park, NC; Fig. 28-4) has permitted extension of SGA use to a variety of cases in which the airway is within the surgical field or shared with the surgical team (e.g., ophthalmologic or otolaryngologic procedures). These devices differ in design from traditional SGAs by virtue of a thin-walled, small-diameter, wire-reinforced (kink-resistant) barrel, which can be positioned out of the midline without affecting the hypopharyngeal position of the mask. This device was designed to be paired with a tonsillar mouth gag commonly

> **Table 28-9** Advantages of the Laryngeal Mask Airway in Supraglottic Surgery
>
> Improved protection of the airway from blood and surgical debris
> Reduced cardiovascular responses
> Reduced coughing on emergence
> Reduced intraoperative bronchospasm
> Reduced laryngospasm after airway device removal
> Improved oxygen saturation after airway device removal
> Ability to administer oxygen until complete restoration of airway reflexes

used in oral and pharyngeal surgery.[68] Additionally, the LMA Flexible has proved useful when heavy drapes are placed over the airway (e.g., ophthalmic procedures), when there is movement of the head during surgery (e.g., tympanostomy tubes), or when the LMA barrel cannot be secured in the midline (e.g., mid or lateral facial surgery). The use of this mask in surgery above the level of the hypopharynx, including tonsillectomy, affords a number of clinically important advantages over tracheal intubation (Table 28-9). When correctly placed, LMAs protects the airway from blood, secretions, and surgical debris from above the level of the mask better than tracheal tubes, which do not protect the trachea from liquids instilled into the pharynx.[69,70]

The SGA and Bronchospasm. SGAs produce significantly less reversible bronchospasm than ETTs. For this reason, they appear to be well suited to the patient with a history of bronchospasm (e.g., chronic obstructive pulmonary disease) who is not at risk for reflux or aspiration.[49] Because the halogenated inhaled anesthetics are potent bronchodilators, bronchospasm is more likely to occur at the times of induction and emergence. SGAs present a unique opportunity for the clinician to conveniently and effectively control the airway without introducing a foreign body into the trachea and stimulating the sensitive bronchial tree. If uncontrollable bronchospasm does occur (e.g., from vagal stimuli), intubation can be performed through many SGAs or after SGA removal. When tracheal intubation is mandatory for the surgical procedure and bronchospasm concerns exist, the Bailey maneuver can be employed. In this maneuver, the deflated LMA is placed behind the *in situ* ETT. The ETT is removed, the LMA is inflated, and the patient is emerged on the LMA.[71] If an SGA was utilized as a conduit for tracheal intubation, the option exists to deflate the SGA cuff and leave the device *in situ*. When the ETT is no longer needed, it can be removed, leaving the SGA as the primary airway. This latter technique can be of great benefit in cases where an ETT is needed intraoperatively, but coughing or hypertension during emergence would be deleterious.

SGA Removal. The timing of SGA removal is critical.[72] An SGA should be removed either when the patient is deeply anesthetized or after protective airway reflexes have returned and the patient is able to open the mouth on command. Removal during excitation stages of emergence can be accompanied by coughing and/or laryngospasm. Many clinicians remove the LMA fully inflated so that it acts as a "scoop" for secretions above the mask, bringing them out of the airway.[73]

Contraindications to SGA Use. SGAs do not reliably prevent the aspiration of regurgitated gastric contents. Thus, SGAs are contraindicated in clinical scenarios with an increased risk of regurgitation (e.g., full stomach, hiatus hernia with significant gastroesophageal reflux, intestinal obstruction, delayed gastric emptying, unclear history), though their use as an airway salvage technique in these populations is acceptable. Other contraindications include high airway resistance, glottic or subglottic obstruction, and limited mouth opening (<1.5 cm).[74]

Complications of SGA Use. Apart from aspiration, reported complications include laryngospasm, coughing, gagging, and other events characteristic of airway manipulation. The incidence of SGA-induced postoperative sore throat varies from 4% to 50% and is highly dependent on the study methods. No single device shows a consistently lower rate of dysphagia. All appear to be better than tracheal intubation in this regard, with expected rates of 30% to 70%.[75] Rare reports exist of nerve injury associated with SGA use, including damage to the hypoglossal, lingual, and recurrent laryngeal nerves. These injuries typically manifest within 48 hours postoperatively and resolve spontaneously in 1 hour to 18 months. Predisposing factors include the use of small masks, lidocaine lubrication, and nitrous oxide, cuff overinflation, difficult or alternate insertion techniques, nonsupine positioning, and cervical bone or joint disease.[76] Pressure neuropraxia from the tube or cuff is the most common cause.

The King Laryngeal Tube (King LT, Ambu, Ballerup, Denmark) consists of a single-lumen tube with distal and proximal low-pressure cuffs that are inflated via a common pilot valve (Fig. 28-6). When positioned correctly, the distal cuff sits within and obstructs the upper esophageal sphincter and the proximal cuff seals the oral and nasal pharynx. In this position, apertures between the cuffs approximate the larynx and serve as orifices for spontaneous or positive-pressure ventilation. The King LT requires a mouth opening of at least 2.3 cm and is inserted either blindly or with the aid of a laryngoscope. The Laryngeal Tube Suction (King LTS-D, Ambu, Ballerup, Denmark) is a single-use device which adds a lumen terminating distal to the esophageal cuff, facilitating gastric drainage. One case report describes the successful use of the LTS-D as an emergency airway for a pregnant woman who underwent cesarean section but could not be intubated. The device improved oxygenation and facilitated drainage of gastric contents during the patient's emergence from a failed rapid-sequence intubation.[77]

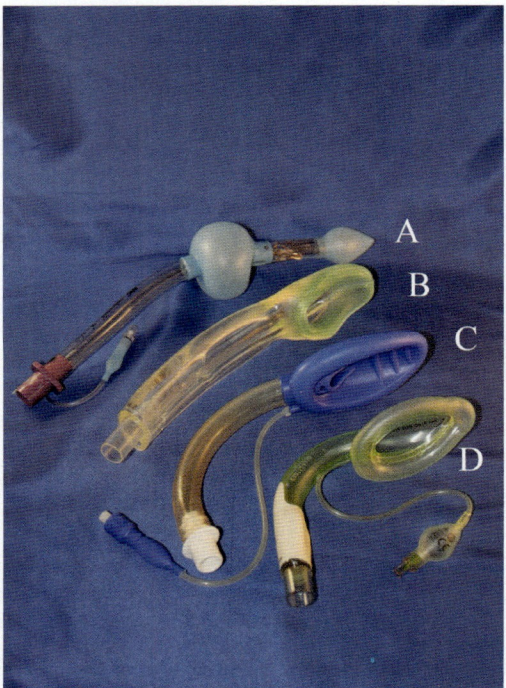

Figure 28-6 (**A**) The King LT, (**B**) I-Gel, (**C**) air-Q, and (**D**) Aura-I.

The Laryngeal Tube is available in six sizes (0 to 5) suitable for children to large adults. In children under 10 years old, the Laryngeal Tube is less effective than the LMA during spontaneous or assisted ventilation and for fiberoptic evaluation of the airway.[78] The Laryngeal Tube is not recommended for children weighing less than 10 kg, as it is associated with technical difficulties and inadequate ventilation.[79]

A cadaveric study demonstrated that mucosal pressures in the lateral pharynx, base of tongue, and posterior pharynx were similar between the Laryngeal Tube and LMA ProSeal. The pressure with the Laryngeal Tube was higher on the posterior hypopharynx, though, and the investigators expressed concern that this increased pressure might impede pharyngeal perfusion.[80] A case of acute tongue and uvula ulceration after using the Laryngeal Tube for hysteroscopy has been reported.[81]

Cookgas air-Q. Developed by Dr. Daniel Cook, the air-Q perilaryngeal airway (Cookgas LLC, St. Louis, MO; Fig. 28-6) can function both as an elective SGA and a conduit for blind or flexible scope-aided intubation (described later in this chapter). A cuff, grossly the shape of the LMA Classic cuff, seals the perilaryngeal space and has airway seal pressures of 25 to 30 cm H_2O, similar to that of the LMA ProSeal.[82] The device comes in sizes 0.5 to 4.5 and is inserted using a technique similar to that recommended for the LMA (see previous discussion). The inventor recommends filling the cuff with less than 10 mL of air, as a poor seal is often secondary to cuff *over*inflation. If, after insertion, the airway is obstructed, an up–down motion of the barrel often realigns the epiglottis. A recent innovation, the self-pressurizing air-Q sp, does not require cuff insufflation but rather varies intracuff pressure based on airway pressure.

Second-Generation Supraglottic Airways. The LMA ProSeal was the first SGA with a gastric port and thus the first "second-generation" SGA (Table 28-10). The original intent of the ProSeal's gastric drain was to aid the clinician in the diagnosis of SGA malposition. If the device's distal tip were not appropriately within the esophageal opening, then gas escape would be detected via the esophageal port with positive-pressure ventilation. Additional tests have subsequently been developed to verify device positioning.[83-86] The gastric port also allows passive (regurgitation) and active (gastric tube insertion) emptying of the stomach.[84,86-88] The design of the ProSeal cuff improves airway seal during positive-pressure ventilation as compared with other LMA devices (≥40 cm H_2O). These advanced capabilities allow its use in the care of obese patients, patients undergoing intra-abdominal procedures, and in airway resuscitation.[89-91] A single-use version of the ProSeal, the LMA Supreme (Teleflex, Research Triangle Park, NC), incorporates a fixed curvature, replicating the insertion ease of the LMA Fastrach[92] (Fig. 28-4). The Supreme also supports inspiratory pressures of greater than 35 cm H_2O, and has been used for intra-abdominal procedures.[93]

The i-gel. This uniquely designed SGA has a solid elastomer gel body mounted on a plastic barrel without an inflatable cuff (Intersurgical Inc., East Syracuse, NY, Fig. 28-6). A drain tube runs from the distal tip, which sits over the esophageal inlet, to an outlet lateral to the airway circuit connector. A gastric tube may be placed via this drain (the largest size accommodating a 14-French tube), which also serves as a passage for passively regurgitated gastric contents. Airway leak pressures have been reported as ranging from 24 to 30 cm of water in adults. The incidence of sore throat appears to be less than with the LMA[94] and some reports note a lower rate of visible blood on the device at time of removal. Success rates (first-time insertion, adequate seal pressure, etc.) are comparable to the LMA Classic and ProSeal.[95] Contrary to a widely held belief, the solid mask of the i-gel does not change shape as it is warmed by the pharyngeal mucosa (personal communication, Muhammed Nasir, MD).

Tracheal Intubation

Direct Laryngoscopy. The goal of direct laryngoscopy is to produce a direct line of sight from the operator's eye to the larynx. This requires the creation of a new nonanatomic visual axis, achieved via maximal alignment of the axes of the oral and pharyngeal cavities, and displacement of the tongue. Unanticipated failure of DL is primarily a problem of tongue displacement, as inability to align the axes typically can be predicted by physical examination. As pointed out in the ASA Difficult Airway Practice Guidelines, no one measure may be adequate to determine difficulty of DL and multiple measures must be integrated in order to make sensible airway management decisions.[2] Shiga et al.[22] published a meta-analysis of studies regarding airway physical examination scores and cautioned on the poor sensitivity and modest specificity of all routine tests.

In 1944, Bannister and MacBeth proposed a three-axis model to explain the anatomic relationships involved in airway axis alignment.[96] Based on this model, alignment of the laryngeal, pharyngeal, and oral axes would result in adequate glottic view. This model explains the rationale of the intubation sniffing position (SP) in which the neck is flexed by 35 degrees and the head extended by 15 degrees. This positioning is achieved by placing a support (around 7 cm in the adult) under the patient's occiput. The three-axis explanation has been challenged by Adnet et al.[97] who noted that, although extension at the atlanto-occipital joint maximally facilitated an oral cavity/pharyngeal alignment, no significant improvement was achieved with flexion of the cervical spine on the thorax.

Chou and Wu[98] proposed a two-axes/tongue-displacement model. This model does not depend on the alignment of all axes to create an in-line view of the larynx but rather maximizes the spaces between the alveolar ridge and laryngeal aperture through oropharyngeal alignment and tongue displacement. This concept

Table 28-10 Features of the LMA ProSeal

Feature	Clinical Impact
Gastric drain	Confirmation of device positioning • Suprasternal notch test[a,85] • No gas leak via gastric port[b,84]
	Gastric tube placement • Active and passive gastric emptying Protection from gastric-content aspiration
Posterior cuff	Increased seal pressure
Bite block	Prevention of obstruction from biting Confers rotational stability Confirmation of device positioning—50% or more of the bite block should be within the oral cavity[85]
Placement	First insertion less successful than LMA Classic
Size choice	Size down from LMA Classic

[a]When a small amount of lubricant is used to occlude the gastric drain, gentle pressure on the suprasternal notch is reflected in movement of the lubricant meniscus.
[b]If the lubricant meniscus does not move with positive-pressure ventilation, there is no connection between the esophageal and laryngeal ports and ventilation is unlikely to cause gastric insufflation.

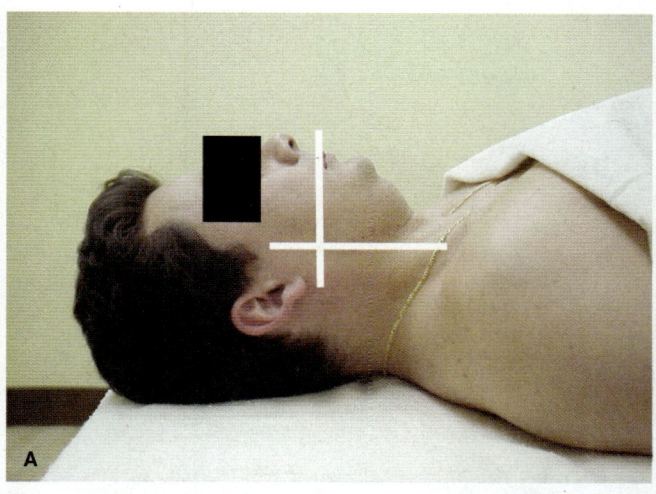 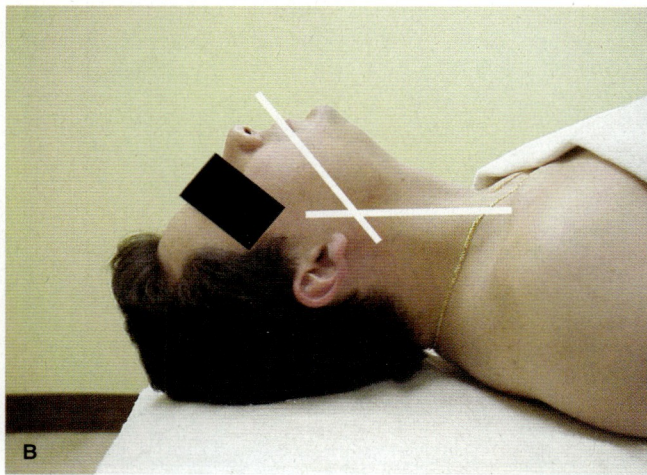

Figure 28-7 A: With the patient supine, the oral and pharyngeal axes do not overlap. **B:** Extension at the atlanto-occipital joint maximally overlaps the oral and pharyngeal axes.

may explain difficulties with DL as well as why common methods of airway assessment lack predictive power. This concept has been described as Functional Airway Assessment (FAA).[99]

FAA is a method of examining the functional nature of each of the anatomic correlates of the commonly used airway assessment indices. FAA places an emphasis on the interdependence of these anatomic characteristics rather than on their individual size or functional integrity. As explained by Chou and Wu,[98] when the head and neck are in the neutral position, the oral and pharyngeal axes are perpendicular to each other. With maximal extension of a normal atlanto-occipital joint, 35 degrees or more of motion is attained (Fig. 28-7). This brings the angle between the oral and pharyngeal axes to 125 degrees. Although an improvement, it is certainly not the 180 degrees required for creating a line of sight to the glottis. Additional space must be created, which is accomplished by displacement of the tongue with the laryngoscope. Although atlanto-occipital extension cannot by itself allow direct laryngeal vision, it does provide anterior displacement of the mass of the tongue and bring the alveolar ridge into an improved position relative to the tongue and larynx. The extension of the atlanto-occipital joint also provides an advantage in mouth opening; Calder et al.[58] showed that maximal mouth opening is 26% greater in full atlanto-occipital extension as compared with the neutral head position. Mandibular mobility also facilitates displacement of the tongue away from the required visual axis—rotation and translation of the temporomandibular joint result in relaxation of the tongue insertion as well as creation of the aperture width needed for instrumentation.

Using the FAA approach to airway evaluation also helps to explain the value of the popular, yet highly criticized, Mallampati and thyromental distance indices.[100] These two measures have historically been considered important because they approximate the relative mass of the tongue (Mallampati) and the anterior–posterior borders of space into which it will be displaced by the laryngoscope (Fig. 28-8). As noted elsewhere, these indices have shown to have poor and/or variable predictive power. Two groups have studied the interrelated nature of these measures in a way that reveals why they perform poorly when considered individually. Ayoub et al.[101] found a high Mallampati score to be predictive of difficult DL when the thyromental distance was less than 4 cm. When the thyromental distance was more than 4 cm, relative tongue size, as determined by the Mallampati classification,

was not predictive. Iohom et al.[9] found similar results using a thyromental distance cutoff of 6 cm. The finding that the predictive power of the Mallampati improves when the mandible is short is consistent with the concept of FAA: when the mandibular space is restricted, tongue size is important. When the space is large, a tongue of any nonpathologic size should be accommodated easily. An exception to this may be a hypopharyngeal tongue, as described by Chou and Wu,[102] although, according to those authors, measurement of the mandibular hyoid distance should help in diagnosing this.

As noted earlier, a common cause of difficulty in DL is a pathologic increase in tongue size. Ovassapian et al.[104] identified lingual tonsil hyperplasia as the most common cause of *unanticipated* difficult DL. In a review of all cases of unanticipated difficult DL in their institution from 1999 to 2000, 33 patients were identified. All patients were found, on fiberoptic examinations, to have lingual tonsil hyperplasia (Fig. 28-9).

Devices that aid in obtaining a sniffing position are commercially available. These include the Sniff Position Pillow (Popitz Pillow, Alimed, Dedham, MA) and Pi's Pillow (American Eagle Medical, Holbrook, NY), which can be configured for the awake (neutral position) then asleep (functional position) patient. Some have suggested positioning the patient with the external auditory meatus level with the patient's sternal notch (EAM-SN position). This is especially helpful in obese patients[105] to move the mass of the chest away from the airway and allow space for manipulation of the laryngoscope handle. This may require placing a wedge-shaped lift (e.g., the Troop Elevation Pillow, Mercury Medical, Clearwater, FL) under the scapula, shoulders, and nape of neck. This raises the head and neck above the thorax, producing the EAM-SN position and allowing gravity to pull the pannus away from the airway.

After the head and neck have been positioned, the mouth is opened by one of two techniques. The first method encourages extension of the atlanto-occipital joint by the use of the right hand under the occiput. This maneuver is reserved for patients with stable cervical spines and leads to passive opening of the mouth, which can be accentuated by using the fourth finger of the left hand (holding the laryngoscope) to apply pressure over the chin in a caudad direction. In the second technique, which tends to be more effective but requires contact of the (gloved) hand with the teeth and/or gums, the right thumb applies caudad

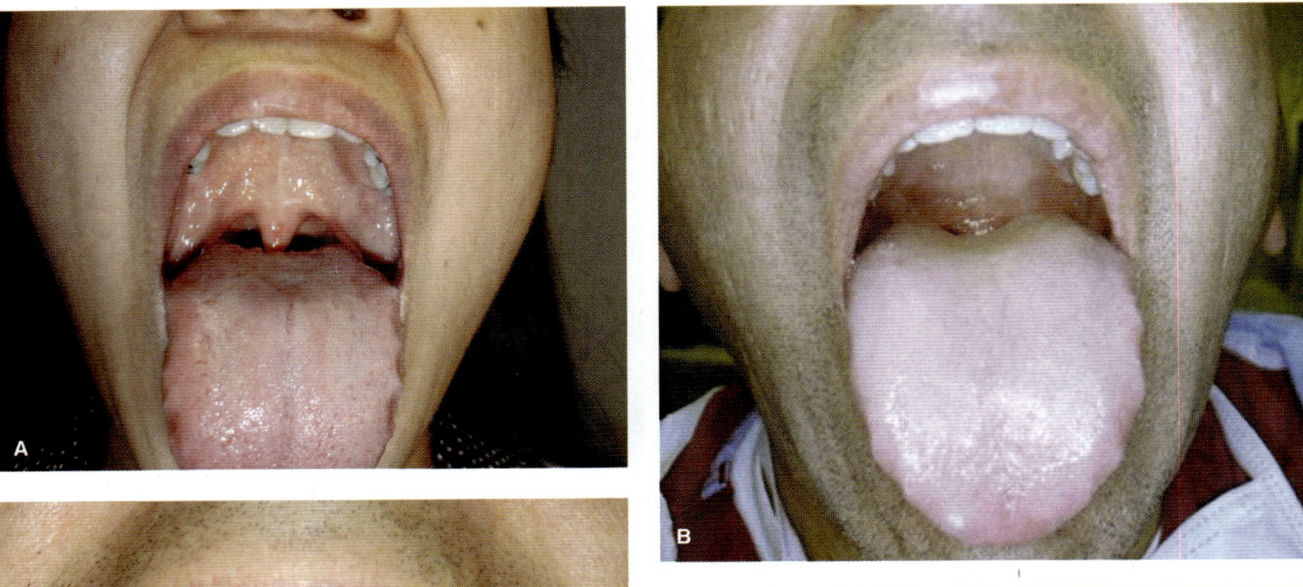

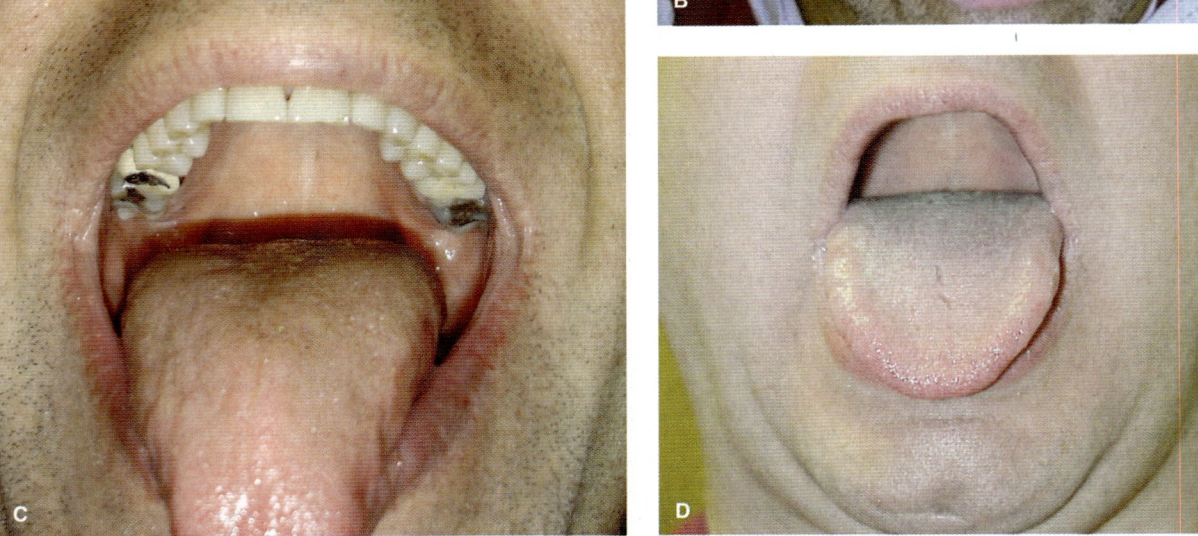

Figure 28-8 Mallampati/Samsoon–Young classification of the oropharyngeal view.[103] **A:** Class I: Uvula, faucial pillars, soft palate visible. **B:** Class II: Faucial pillars, soft palate visible. **C:** Class III: Soft and hard palate visible. **D:** Class IV: Only hard palate visible (added by Samsoon and Young).

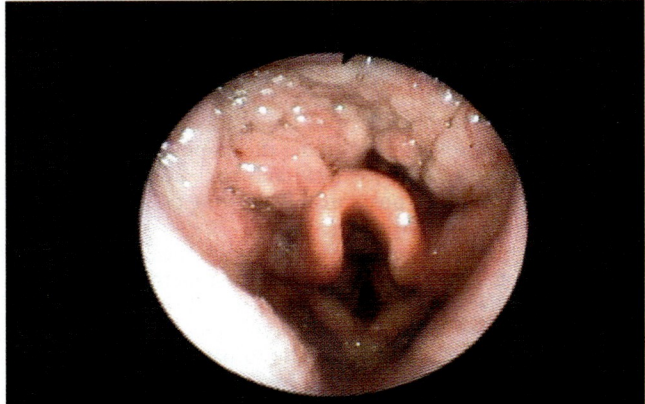

Figure 28-9 Lingual tonsil hyperplasia. The vallecula is filled with hyperplastic lymphoid tissue in a patient who had an unanticipated difficult direct laryngoscopy.

pressure to the mandibular canine/bicuspids on the patient's same side while the first or second finger, crossed below the thumb, applies cephalad pressure to the ipsilateral maxillary canine/bicuspid. The ultimate goal of both techniques is rotation and translation of the temporomandibular joint to maximize the interincisor gap.

Direct Laryngoscope Blades. Two blades, each with a unique manner of application, are in common use. Many other blades are described in the literature but will not be discussed here. There are some excellent reviews detailing these.[106]

The Macintosh (curved) blade is used to displace the epiglottis out of the line of sight by placement of the distal tip in the vallecula and tensing of the glossoepiglottic ligament. The Miller (straight) blade reveals the glottis by compressing the epiglottis against the base of the tongue (Fig. 28-10). Both blades include a flange along the left side of their length which is used to sweep the tongue to the left. Blades with a right-sided flange are available for the left-handed practitioner, but are not found in common practice.

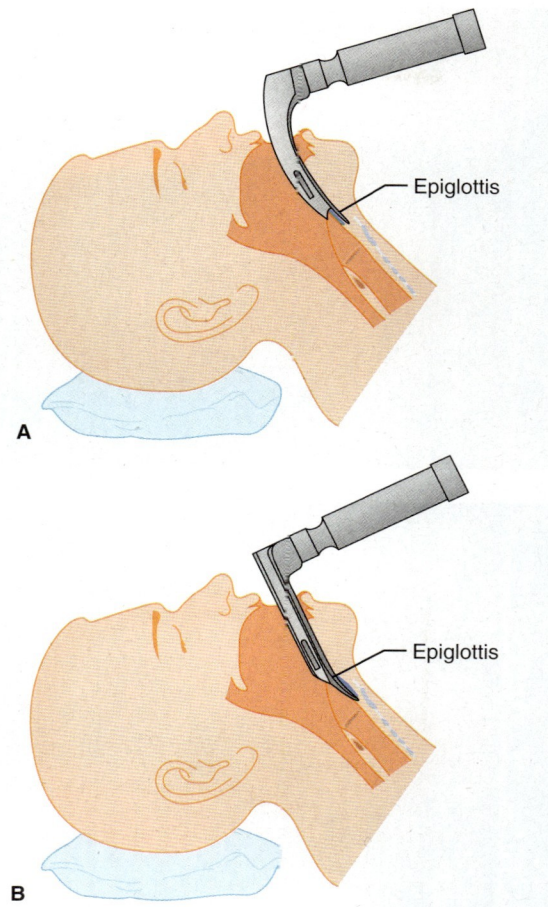

Figure 28-10 **A:** When a curved laryngoscope blade is used, the tip of the blade is placed in the vallecula, the space between the base of the tongue and the pharyngeal surface of the epiglottis. **B:** The tip of a straight blade is advanced beneath the epiglottis.

Blade size needs to be chosen appropriately and, on occasion, exchanged after a failed attempt at laryngoscopy. As a generalization, the Macintosh blade is regarded as advantageous whenever there is little room to pass an ETT (e.g., small mouth), whereas the Miller blade is considered better in the patient who has a small mandibular space, large incisors, or a large epiglottis.[44] Ultimately, the optimal blade tends to be the one with which the provider has the most experience

For laryngoscopy, the laryngoscope handle is held in the left hand and the mouth opened, as described earlier. The blade is inserted into the right side of the mouth, with care taken to avoid unnecessary contact with the lips or teeth. As the blade is advanced toward the epiglottis, the tongue is swept leftward and compressed into the mandibular space. Once reaching the base of the tongue (with the Macintosh blade in the vallecula or the Miller blade compressing the epiglottis against the base of the tongue), the operator's arm and shoulder lift in an anterior–caudad direction.

With either blade, the laryngoscopist must avoid rotating the laryngoscope in a cephalad direction, bringing the blade into contact with the upper incisors. Inserting either blade style too deeply can result in the tip of the blade resting under the larynx itself such that forward pressure lifts the airway from view.

Special considerations apply to the technique of laryngoscopy and intubation in the infant and child. Because of the relatively larger size of the occiput in children, elevation of the head is not required to achieve a sniffing position.[44] In fact, on occasion, the practitioner may need to elevate the thorax instead. Hyperextension at the atlanto-occipital joint, as done in adults, may cause airway obstruction from the relative pliability of the trachea and should be avoided. The comparatively short neck of a child gives the impression of an anterior position of the larynx and external laryngeal manipulation is often required to move the laryngeal inlet into view. A straight blade often is chosen, as it is helpful in displacing the stiff, omega-shaped epiglottis. Because the cricoid cartilage is the most rigid portion of the airway until 6 to 8 years of age, the intubator must be sensitive to resistance to advancement of an ETT that has easily passed the vocal folds. Due to the short length of the trachea, there is a higher risk of endobronchial intubation or accidental extubation with head movement. Continuous close attention should always be paid to the depth of the tube in pediatric patients.

A laryngeal view scoring system that has won general acceptance was developed by Cormack and Lehane,[107] who described four grades of laryngeal view. Grade 1 includes visualization of the entire glottic aperture, grade 2 includes visualization of only the posterior aspects of the glottic aperture, grade 3 is visualization of the tip of the epiglottis, and grade 4 is visualization of no more than the soft palate (Fig. 28-11). A Cormack–Lehane grade 3 or 4 is expected in 1.5% to 8.5% of adult laryngoscopies.[108] A modification of the Cormack and Lehane score was proposed by Yentis and Lee,[48] who noted that when a partial vocal cord view (2A) is achieved, tracheal intubation was significantly easier than when only the arytenoids and epiglottis were visualized (2B). A finer classification of a Cormack and Lehane grade 3 view has also been described. When the epiglottis can be manipulated with repositioning or an intubating bougie, it is referred to as a "3a" view and a nonmovable epiglottis constitutes a "3b" view.[109] The Cormack and Lehane grades are used to describe the view at laryngoscopy and have never been validated as a correlate of successful tracheal intubation.

Another view scoring system is based on the clinician's estimate of the percent of glottic opening (POGO) seen during laryngoscopy, for example, 0% to 100% of the span from anterior commissure to the interarytenoid notch. The POGO score has improved interexaminer reliability when compared to the Cormack and Lehane system and has been adopted by many researchers in the comparative evaluation of video laryngoscopy.[110]

If a satisfactory laryngeal view is not achieved, the backward–upward–rightward pressure (BURP) maneuver may be applied. In this maneuver, the larynx is displaced backward (B) against the cervical vertebrae, upward (U, superiorly) and to the patient's right (R), using pressure (P) over the thyroid cartilage. The BURP maneuver has been shown to improve the laryngeal view, decreasing the rate of difficult intubation in a study of 1,993 patients from 4.7% to 1.8%.[111] Similarly, Benumof and Cooper describe "optimal external laryngeal manipulation," which consists of pressing posteriorly and cephalad over the thyroid, hyoid, and cricoid cartilages.[112]

Once the larynx is visualized, the tracheal tube is inserted from the right-hand side, care being taken not to obstruct the view of the vocal cords. Whenever possible, the action of the ETT passing through the vocal cords should be witnessed by the laryngoscopist. This decreases the possibility of accidental esophageal placement or trauma to paraglottic structures. The tracheal tube cuff should be advanced at least 2 cm past the glottic opening to approximate a midtracheal placement. This should correlate to depths of 21 and 23 cm at the teeth for the typical adult female

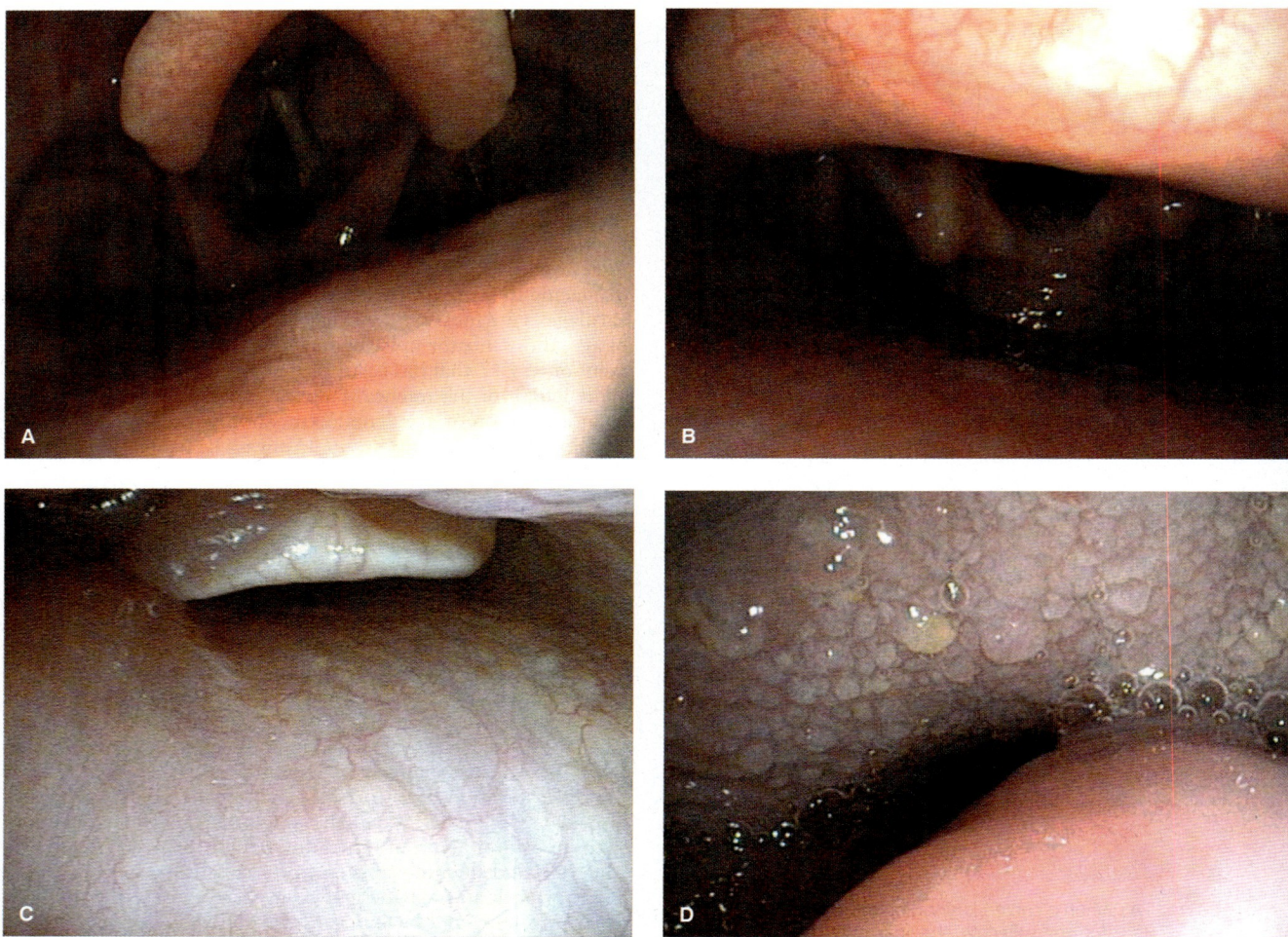

Figure 28-11 The Cormack–Lehane laryngeal view scoring system: grade 1 (**A**), grade 2 (**B**), grade 3 (**C**), and grade 4 (**D**).

and male, respectively. Though allowances should be made for individual circumstances, a size 7 to 7.5 ID tracheal tube is typically used in the adult female and size 7.5 to 8 ID in the adult male. Larger tracheal tubes may be desirable if pulmonary toilet or diagnostic or therapeutic bronchoscopy is to be part of the clinical course. Pediatric tracheal tube sizes are presented in detail in Table 28-11 (see also Chapter 42).

An alternative approach to DL has been described by Henderson.[113] In this "paraglossal" approach, a straight-bladed laryngoscope is introduced into the right side of the mouth and advanced between the tongue and palatine tonsil. The blade passes below the epiglottis, which is then elevated. This approach subjects the tongue to less compressive forces and may improve the view of the larynx in the presence of lingual tonsil hyperplasia.

The gold standard for verification of tracheal intubation is sustained detection of exhaled carbon dioxide. Additional verification techniques include visualization of tube placement through the vocal folds, auscultation over the chest and abdomen, visualization of chest excursion, observation of humidity in the ETT, full return of tidal volume during expiration, use of a self-inflating bulb (TubeChek-B, Ambu, Ballerup, Denmark), flexible scope identification of tracheal anatomy, and ultrasound or chest x-ray.[33]

Although DL remains the most common method for tracheal intubation, it is far from successful in all cases and not always benign when successful. DL may be difficult (Cormack and Lehane grade 3 or 4 view) or impossible in 4.4 and 0.3% to 0.43% of attempts, respectively.[114–116] Analysis of the ASA Closed Claims Database reveals that claims for laryngeal injury during

Table 28-11 Size and Length of Pediatric Tracheal Tubes Relative to Airway Anatomy

Age	Internal Diameter (mm)	Distance from Lips to Midtrachea[a] (cm)
Premature	2.5	8
Full term	3	10
1–6 months	3.5	11
6–12 months	4	12
2 years	4.5	13
4 years	5	14
6 years	5.5	15
8 years	6.5	16

[a]Add 2 to 3 cm for nasal tubes.

DL arise more often in "easy" as opposed to difficult laryngoscopies.[53] Among the 4,460 cases in the database, 87 instances of laryngeal trauma were recorded. Of these, 80% occurred during routine (nondifficult) tracheal intubation in which no injury was suspected. This has led some to question whether routine tracheal intubation is as safe as assumed.[52]

Image-guided laryngoscopy promises to dominate modern airway management. The first decade of the 21st century saw a proliferation of optical and video-transmitting devices primarily as the result of the availability of inexpensive CMOS technology. The unifying characteristics of these laryngoscopes is that a direct line of sight is no longer needed from the provider's eye to the glottis. A large variety of these devices exist, some of which are detailed later.

Optical Stylets. Optical stylets incorporate both optical and light source elements into a single stylet-like shaft. Some examples of these are the Shikani Seeing Stylet (Clarus Medical, LLC, Minneapolis, MN) and the Bonfils Intubation Fiberscope (BIF, Karl Storz, Tuttlingen, Germany; Fig. 28-12). Both require less cervical spine motion than direct laryngoscopy.[117,118]

The BIF is a long rigid tubular device with conventional optical and light-transmitting fiberoptic elements.[119] The distal end has a 40-degree angulation and the objective lens allows a 100-degree field of view. A proximal-end eyepiece can be used with the naked eye or fitted with a standard endoscopy camera. A cable (or battery-powered attachment) brings illumination from an external light source and suction may be applied through a working channel. Laryngoscopy technique replicates the paraglossal approach discussed previously in this chapter and sizes with external diameters of 2, 3.5, and 5 mm are available.

The Shikani Seeing Optical Stylet (SOS) has a similar configuration to the BIF, with the exception that the distal half of the stylet is malleable (Fig. 28-13). The light source may be cabled or self-contained with a proprietary handle or a green line laryngoscope handle (Rusch Medical, Duluth, GA). Unlike the BIF, the SOS uses a midline approach. Although the SOS can be used as an independent intubating device, it can also be employed as an adjunct to direct laryngoscopy when a high Cormack and Lehane score is achieved. While the SOS is primarily an oral intubation device, it has been used also for nasal intubation. The pediatric and adult SOSs can accommodate tracheal tubes as small as 2.5 and 5.5-mm ID, respectively.

The Levitan First Pass Success Scope (FPS, Clarus Medical, LLC, Minneapolis, MN) is a shorter (30-cm) version of the SOS designed to be used as an adjunct to DL when a poor laryngeal

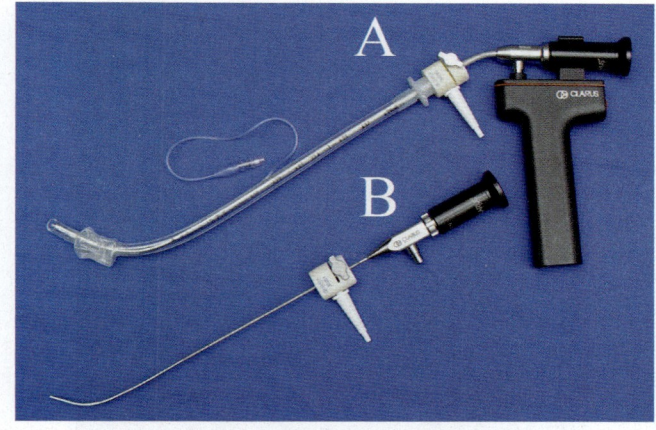

Figure 28-13 **A:** The Shikani Seeing Optical Stylet (*Clarus* Medical, LLC, Minneapolis, MN). **B:** The Levitan FPS.

view is encountered (Fig. 28-13). The shorter length allows easier positioning by the laryngoscopist,[120] but standard tracheal tubes (6-mm ID or larger can be used) should be trimmed in length so that the objective lens is within the bevel.[121,122] The hypothetical benefits of using the device in this manner are the reduction of unanticipated difficult intubations and the maintenance of alternative technique skills by incorporating this or similar devices into daily practice.[122]

The Clarus Video System (Clarus Medical, LLC, Minneapolis, MN; Fig. 28-14) marries the malleable stylet concept of the SOS with CMOS technology. A 4-inch adjustable-angle LED screen is mounted on the handle and has a proprietary video-out port. The device also supports intubation via transillumination technique by incorporating a distal, anteriorly positioned red diode that may be visible through the skin when the tip of the device is in the larynx.

Videolaryngoscopy

VL mimics the operator actions of direct laryngoscopy but places an imaging device toward the distal end of the laryngoscope blade. This moves the provider's point of view past the tongue, avoiding the need for a direct line of sight to the glottis. The ASA Difficult Airway Taskforce recommends that a

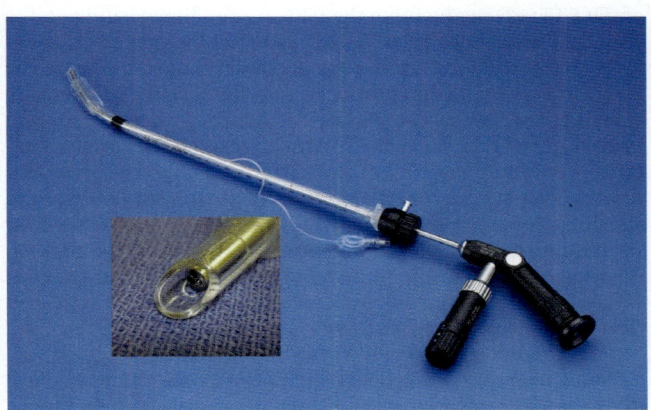

Figure 28-12 The Bonfils (Karl Storz, Tuttlingen, Germany). Inset: Objective end within tracheal tube.

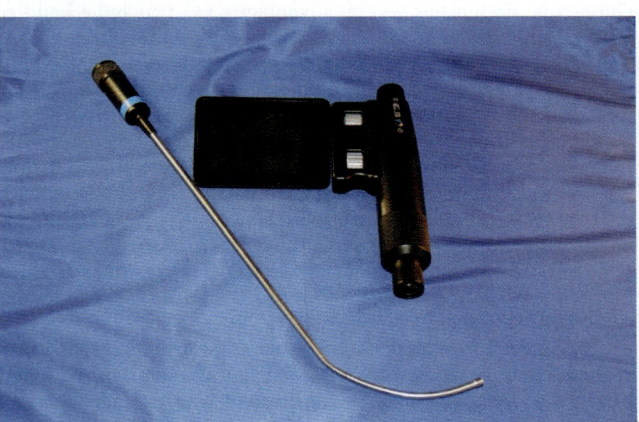

Figure 28-14 The Clarus Video System (Clarus Medical, LLC, Minneapolis, MN).

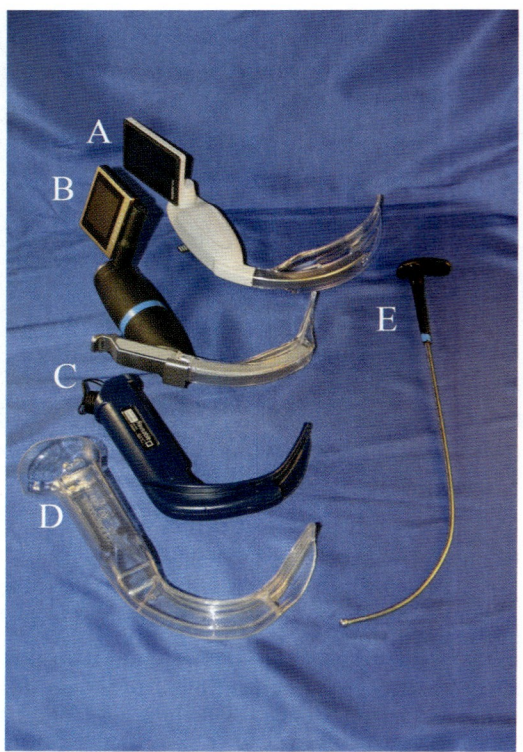

Figure 28-15 (**A**) McGrath Mac and (**B**) Mcgrath Series 5 (Medtronic, Dublin, Ireland), (**C**) Glidescope Multiuse blade and (**D**) Glidescope Cobalt single-use blade (Verathon, Bothell, WA), and (**E**) Gliderite rigid stylet (Verathon, Bothell, WA).

videolaryngoscope be available as a first attempt or rescue device for all patients being intubated.[2] VL improves the ability to visualize the larynx, and intubation success approaches 97% to 98%. An added benefit is decreased cervical motion when compared with DL, which appears to be more pronounced with the channeled devices.

The first widely available videolaryngoscope was the Glidescope (Verathon, Bothell, WA; Fig. 28-15). The Glidescope blade has both a light-emitting diode and a CMOS chip and is cabled to an LCD monitor.[123] The distal portion of the blade has a 60-degree angulation, making it an "acute-angle" videolaryngoscope. The Glidescope design has several advantages: (1) It may be handled with a skill set similar to that used with conventional DL. (2) As the video apparatus is positioned close to the distal end of the blade, the operator "sees" from a position beyond the base of the tongue and tongue displacement is not as critical as it is with DL. Similarly, with the optics positioned distal to the lingual tonsils, tonsillar hyperplasia should not affect the visual axis as it does with conventional DL. (3) The video apparatus eliminates fragile fiberoptic elements. (4) The airway image is displayed on a portable screen, allowing for observation by more than one individual (e.g., aid, mentor, and student). (5) The 60-degree distal angulation reduces cervical spine motion by 50% at the C2–5 segments compared with Macintosh DL.[124]

When used by inexperienced operators, the Glidescope provides a better glottic view than DL (Cormack–Lehane grade 1 view in 85.7% vs. 48.9% of patients) and can obtain a Cormack–Lehane grade 1 or 2 view in 77% of patients in whom no glottic exposure was achieved by DL.[123] A large prospective, nonrandomized study of 1,755 patients showed a 98% intubation success rate with the Glidescope, including 96% success in patients predicted to be difficult by DL, and 94% success in airway rescue after failed DL.[29] Although achieving an adequate laryngeal view with the Glidescope appears relatively easy, ETT manipulation into the larynx appears to be more difficult. In one study, placement of the ETT required an additional 16 seconds (on average) when compared to DL.[123,125] This is likely due to difficulty in maneuvering the ETT around the acute angle of the blade. For this reason, the use of a stylet is advised.[126,127] A dedicated, nonmalleable stylet, the Gliderite Rigid Stylet (Verathon, Bothell, WA), has a 90-degree distal bend and may be used with various videolaryngoscopes. A study by Jones et al.[128] suggests that the angle of the ETT has greater impact on time to intubation than the Cormack and Lehane grade of the image. Because the stylet is rigid and its distal tip faces anteriorly, it may get caught on the anterior tracheal rings. A 1 to 2 cm withdrawal of the stylet as the glottis is entered may facilitate advancement into the larynx as well as counterclockwise rotation of the tracheal tube as it is advanced off the stylet. Insertion of the stylet into the larynx should be minimal, if any.

Theoretically, the airway axes do not need to be aligned to achieve adequate glottic visualization with VL. Manipulation of the Glidescope to the position needed for adequate image can cause cervical segment extension, though.[129] Care must be taken in that regard, especially if the cervical spine is unstable. The Glidescope has been successfully used to achieve tracheal intubation in patients with limited cervical spine movement because of ankylosing spondylitis and cervical spine trauma, but it may be difficult to use in patients with limited mouth opening.[130,131]

The classic Glidescope insertion technique follows the midline approach. After the uvula is visualized, the blade is advanced in the midline into the vallecula or is passed posterior to the epiglottis.[123] For patients with a limited mouth aperture, the blade can be inserted like a Guedel airway, with the Glidescope blade concavity facing rostrad and rotated 180 degrees counterclockwise once the distal tip is in the oropharynx. This maneuver displaces the tongue to the left and minimizes neck movements.

Practitioners must visualize, to completion, insertion of both the blade and the ETT into the oropharynx. Traumatic complications associated with the use of the Glidescope videolaryngoscope have been related to blind manipulation of the ETT as it enters the airway but is not yet visualized on the video screen. Traumatic events, which appear to be more likely with the use of a rigid stylet, have been reported relating primarily to the soft palate, palatoglossal arch, right palatopharyngeal arch, and right anterior tonsillar pillar (Fig. 28-16).[132,133] Steps to avoid soft tissue trauma include (1) assuring that the stylet is within the bevel of the ETT; (2) maintaining the ETT in a midline position and as close to the blade as possible; (3) focusing the operator's attention on the patient's oral cavity (as is done during DL) as the blade and then ETT are advanced into the mouth, occasionally glancing at the VL monitor—full attention is turned to the video image only when the distal ETT can be seen on the image monitor; (4) avoiding levering of the blade inward, as this increases the "blind spot" inferiorly; (5) using the least force necessary to advance the ETT; and (6) practicing "reverse loading" of the ETT (as described later).[134] The potential for trauma to the oropharyngeal soft tissues, due to the above-described "blind spot," is similar for all videolaryngoscopes listed later, unless true direct laryngoscopic technique is used.

Control studies have shown no significant advantage of the Glidescope in preventing hemodynamic responses to orotracheal intubation as compared with the Macintosh direct laryngoscope, although others have shown cardiovascular responses similar to intubation with a flexible intubation scope.[135] The Glidescope

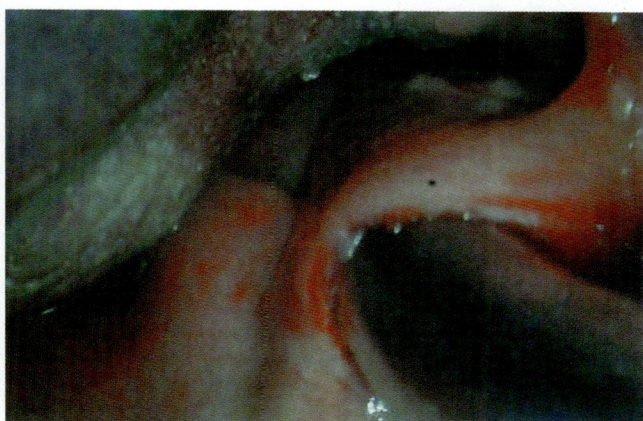

Figure 28-16 Passage of a tracheal tube through the right palatoglossal arch due to a blind spot created with videolaryngoscopy.

has also been used to facilitate nasotracheal intubation with a reduced time to intubation when compared with DL and a high first-time success rate. Reverse loading technique and use of a gum elastic bougie have also been described. Reverse loading entails bending the distal tip of the stylet in the opposite direction of the natural ETT curvature. This promotes a more posteriorly directed delivery of the ETT and decreases the chance of impingement on the anterior commissure or tracheal rings.[136]

A newer version of the Glidescope, the Glidescope Titanium (Verathon, Bothell, WA), is available. Functioning like the original, the new design is made of titanium and has two standard curved blades (MAC T3 and T4) as well as two low-profile acute-angle blades (LoPro T3 and T4). Plastic, single-use versions are also available (LoPro/Mac P3 and P4). The mouth openings needed for commonly used indirect laryngoscopes are listed in Table 28-12.

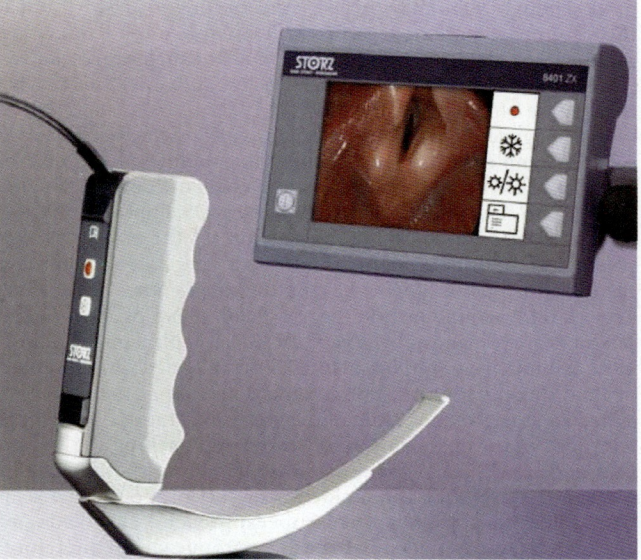

Figure 28-17 The Storz C-MAC (Reprinted with permission from Karl Storz, Tuttlingen, Germany).

The C-MAC system (Karl Storz, Tuttlingen, Germany; Fig. 28-17) consists of an electronic laryngoscope handle with exchangeable metal blades. One of these, the D-Blade, is an acute-angle blade similar in angulation to the Glidescope, designed for when difficult DL is anticipated. A large multicenter prospective randomized trial of 1,100 patients showed no difference in intubation success rate (with two attempts) between the Glidescope and C-MAC D-Blade in patients with anticipated difficult laryngoscopy.[137]

The C-MAC platform also works with blades that are identical to standard Macintosh and Miller blades but with integrated illumination and CMOS optics. This allows the device to be used as either a videolaryngoscope or a standard direct laryngoscope. Although the image projected from the C-MAC closely resembles that seen with the naked eye, ETT placement is facilitated because the video image obviates the need to maintain an unobstructed line of sight to the glottis. Use of the C-MAC is identical to standard DL, making the video facility uniquely valuable during supervised instruction. A comparison study of direct and video-assisted views of the larynx revealed significant improvement of the glottic view with C-MAC video assistance.[138]

The McGrath Series 5 videolaryngoscope (Medtronic, Dublin, Ireland, Fig. 28-15) incorporates a blade, handle, power source, and LCD screen into a self-contained device. Unique design features include an acute-angle blade of adjustable length and disposable blade covers. As with the Glidescope, the acute-angle blade improves laryngeal view but has the drawback of more awkward tracheal tube placement, and use of a rigid or semi-malleable ETT stylet is advised. In one uncontrolled series, tracheal intubation with the McGrath was successful in 98% of 150 elective surgery patients.[139]

The McGrath Mac (Medtronic, Dublin, Ireland) is the newer-generation McGrath videolaryngoscope with a reduced blade curvature and a slimmer blade design (11.9 mm). Compared to the acute-angle blade of the Series 5, the reduced curvature allows easier use as a direct laryngoscope and an improved screen allows shared viewing. The "blind spot" noted with the Glidescope and McGrath Series 5 is reduced if a DL approach is

Table 28-12 Mouth Opening Needed for Commonly Used Indirect Laryngoscopes

Device	Mouth Opening Needed
Glidescope	17.4 mm
Glidescope Ranger*	
Glidescope Titanium*	
Glidescope LoPro	12.4 mm
Storz C-MAC (Mac 3)*	
Storz C-MAC (D-Blade)*	
Airtraq SP (size 0)	11 mm
Airtraq SP (size 1)	12 mm
Airtraq SP (size 2)	15 mm
Airtraq SP (size 3)	16 mm
Airtraq AVANT (sizes 2 and 3)	17 mm
McGrath Mac*	
McGrath Mac X*	
King Vision (size 1)	10 mm (nonchanneled)
King Vision (size 2)	10 mm (nonchanneled), 13 mm (channeled)
King Vision (size 3)	13 mm (nonchanneled), 18 mm (channeled)

*Company stated "No available data."

used. Though there may be less concern for soft tissue trauma, the cautions mentioned earlier still apply. Another McGrath product, the McGrath X blade, has an acute angle tip for anticipated difficult airways, a slimmer design, and a portrait display to decrease blind-spot.

A new generation of videolaryngoscopes, termed "channeled scopes," employ a J-shaped channel that follows the course of the optical elements from the viewing element (optical or video imaging) to the distal objective lens or CMOS chip. Whereas DL accommodates for the right-angle nature of the airway by displacing the anterior structures and VL accommodates by placing the operator's point of view beyond the tongue, the "channeled" devices replicate the near 90-degree relationship of the oral and pharyngeal axes, limiting the need for tissue displacement and cervical manipulation. A lubricated ETT is preloaded into the channel and therefore guided in the same trajectory as the objective. When adequate visualization of the glottis is achieved, the ETT is advanced in the channel until observed approaching the larynx. In theory, as the tracheal tube is never in a blind-spot, this technique should reduce the incidence of soft tissue trauma seen with the classic videolaryngoscope approach. The blades of channeled devices typically have an anatomic shape; therefore, a neutral head and neck position tends to result in improved glottic alignment. Minor manipulations of the videolaryngoscope (anterior, posterior, caudad, rostrad, and rotational) may be needed to align the ETT and facilitate passage through the glottis.

The Airtraq optical laryngoscope (Prodol Meditec S.A., Vizcaya, Spain; Fig. 28-18) is a single-use, anatomically shaped, channeled laryngoscope with periscopic optics. The device has a built-in antifog system and a low-temperature light that facilitates the laryngeal view. The Airtraq has been used successfully as a rescue device in patients after failed intubation with DL.[140] Anterior forces (e.g., those applied to the tongue) are reduced compared to that found with DL, but some cervical spine movement still occurs.[129] Reports of its use in awake patients, patients with cervical spine disease, and after failed DL have been published as well.[141] One study showed the need for fewer maneuvers to improve glottic exposure and fewer alterations in blood pressure and heart rate when compared with DL.[142] Reduced cervical spine movement in patients with midline axial stabilization also has been demonstrated. The Airtraq AVANT (Prodol Meditec S.A., Vizcaya, Spain), functions similarly, but with reusable prismatic optics sheathed in a disposable blade. A study of 100 patients showed better glottic visualization with the AVANT than with DL utilizing a Macintosh blade.[143]

The Airway Scope (Pentax AWS, AWS-S100; Hoya-Pentax, Tokyo, Japan) is a reusable, channeled device with a CMOS camera cord fitted into a single-use blade (Fig. 28-18). The handle incorporates a 2.4-inch LCD monitor, the angle of which can be adjusted for easier viewing. The channel on the disposable blades accepts ETTs with internal diameters between 6.5 and 8.0 mm and incorporates a working channel that can be used for placement of a small suction catheter, injection of lidocaine, or insufflation of oxygen. Unlike the Airtraq, the manufacturer of the AWS recommends using the blade to lift the epiglottis (similar to using a Miller blade) prior to ETT insertion. The difference in technique appears to be related to the ETT being closer to the device tip during tube extrusion with the AWS than with the Airtraq.[144] In one small, nonblinded, noncrossover study, the AWS produced less of a hemodynamic response and had a higher intubation success rate than the Glidescope (100% vs. 96%) in patients predicted to be difficult by DL.[145] As with other channeled devices, the AWS has a higher success rate than the Glidescope in normal volunteers with restricted neck mobility.[29]

The KingVision Video Laryngoscope (Ambu, Ballerup, Denmark) includes a reusable, battery-operated OLED display and disposable channeled and nonchanneled blades. The device can therefore be used as a classic VL or as a channeled scope. The on-handle display gives a higher-quality image than most other VLs and includes a composite video-out port.

NPO Status and Rapid-Sequence Induction

Aspiration of gastric contents trails only failed intubation in frequency amongst reported adverse events.[1] Induction of anesthesia profoundly depresses intrinsic reflexes that protect the airway from the entrance of foreign bodies, including regurgitated material. In addition, manipulation of the upper esophageal inlet reduces the closing pressure of the lower esophageal sphincter. Many patients will present in situations in which aspiration is a significant risk (Table 28-13A) and rapid-sequence induction (RSI), as described, is practiced. If, in addition, difficult airway management is anticipated, awake intubation is often chosen (see Airway Approach Algorithm below). When aspiration is of concern, pharmacologic therapy can help mitigate risk, with the goal of reducing both the volume and acidity of gastric contents. Obesity has long been considered a risk factor for gastric-content aspiration and preoperative treatment with gastric emptying and acid-reducing agents has been recommended,[146] though this remains controversial. Although initial studies touted the increased volume and decreased pH of gastric secretions in the obese fasting patient, others have refuted this claim.[147,148]

Control of Gastric Contents

Preventing pulmonary aspiration of gastric contents is a primary concern during airway management. Control of gastric contents involves (1) minimizing intake, (2) increasing gastric emptying, and (3) reducing gastric volume and acidity (Table 28-13B). Altered physiologic states (e.g., pregnancy and diabetes mellitus) and gastrointestinal pathology (e.g., bowel obstruction and peritonitis) adversely affect the rate of gastric emptying, thereby increasing aspiration risk. The extent of delayed gastric emptying with diabetes mellitus correlates well with the presence of autonomic neuropathy but not with age, duration of disease, HbA_{1C}, or peripheral neuropathy. The difference in the gastric emptying times between healthy patients and those with type I diabetes ranges from 30 minutes to 2 hours.[150] Human breast milk is cleared more rapidly than other

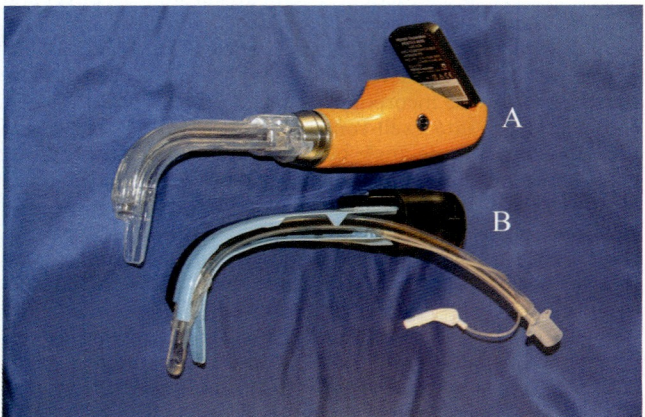

Figure 28-18 (**A**) The Pentax Airway Scope (Hoya-Pentax, Tokyo, Japan). (**B**) The Airtraq laryngoscope (Prodol Meditec S.A., Vizcaya, Spain).

Table 28-13 Pulmonary Aspiration: Patients at Risk for Aspiration, Methods to Reduce Aspiration Risk, and ASA Recommended Fasting Guidelines

(A) Patients at Risk of Aspiration
- Full stomach (recent ingestion)
- Diabetes mellitus (with peripheral neuropathy)
- Clinically significant gastroesophageal reflux/hiatal hernia
- Pregnancy
- Acute pain/acute opioid therapy, renal colic
- Bowel obstruction/intra-abdominal process
- Trauma/unknown timing of last meal

(B) Methods to Reduce Aspiration Risk
- Minimize intake: adequate preoperative fasting, clear liquids only if necessary
- Increase gastric emptying: prokinetics (e.g., metoclopramide)
- Reduce gastric volume and acidity: preinduction nasogastric tube, nonparticulate antacid (e.g., sodium citrate), H_2-receptor antagonists, proton pump inhibitors
- Airway protection: rapid placement of cuffed ETT after induction, cricoid pressure (controversial)

(C) Summary of Preoperative Fasting Recommendations[149]

Ingested material:	Minimum fasting period:
Clear liquids	2 hours
Breast milk	4 hours
Infant formula	6 hours
Nonhuman milk	6 hours
Light meal	6 hours
Meal containing fatty foods or meat	≥8 hours

milk products[151] and the ASA recommends a fasting period of 4 hours for breast milk and 6 hours for nonhuman milk, infant formula, and a light solid meal. Clear liquids can be administered to children up to 2 hours, and adults up to 3 hours, prior to anesthesia without increased risk for regurgitation and aspiration (Table 28-13C).[149]

Reduction of gastric acidity can be achieved with the aid of H_2-receptor antagonists and proton pump inhibitors (PPIs), which also reduce gastric volume. Famotidine given a few hours before surgery effectively reduces gastric volume and increases gastric pH better than ranitidine.[152] The PPIs rabeprazole, lansoprazole, and omeprazole are most effective when given in two successive doses: one the evening before and one the morning of anesthesia.[153,154] When given in a single dose, rabeprazole and lansoprazole should be administered on the morning of anesthesia, as they are not sufficiently effective when given the night before. This is in contrast to single-dose therapy with omeprazole, which is most effective when administered the night before.[153–155] Sodium citrate oral solution increases gastric pH and is best administered within 1 hour preoperatively in a dose of 15 to 30 mL. When combined with metoclopramide (10 mg IV), sodium citrate (15 mL PO) reduces gastric volume by 33% and increases gastric pH by 38% versus unmedicated controls.[156] A nasogastric (NG) tube can also be used to reduce gastric volume prior to induction of anesthesia in patients at high risk of regurgitation. An NG in situ provides a passage for passive drainage of gastric contents and does not diminish the effectiveness of cricoid pressure.[157] NGs are best left in place and open to freely drain during induction of anesthesia. The presence of an NG tube does not guarantee an empty stomach, though, and may impair the function of the lower and upper esophageal sphincters.

Rapid-Sequence Induction. RSI is indicated when there is increased risk of gastric content aspiration. The goal of RSI is to gain control of the airway in the shortest amount of time after the ablation of protective airway reflexes with the induction of anesthesia. In the RSI technique, an intravenous anesthetic induction agent is administered and immediately followed by a rapidly acting neuromuscular blocking drug. Historically, mask ventilation is omitted for fear of gastric insufflation. Laryngoscopy and intubation are performed as soon as muscle relaxation is confirmed. Classically, cricoid pressure is applied (Sellick maneuver), which entails the posterior displacement of the cricoid cartilage against the vertebral bodies, and is held from the beginning of induction until confirmation of ETT placement. In this manner, it was presumed that the lumen of the esophagus was ablated while the circumferential structure of the cricoid cartilage maintained the tracheal lumen.

Early cadaveric studies showed that correctly applied cricoid pressure was effective in preventing gastric fluids from leaking into the pharynx. Recently, MRI studies have suggested that the esophagus is laterally displaced in a majority of normal patients[158]; thus, the adequacy of esophageal ablation has been questioned. In addition, cricoid pressure may worsen the laryngoscopic view[159] and is contraindicated during active vomiting (risk of esophageal rupture), and with cervical spine or laryngeal fracture. There is also little evidence that omission of mask ventilation provides any clinical benefit, especially in patients with poor pulmonary reserve. In fact, if oxyhemoglobin desaturation occurs, gentle positive-pressure ventilation (<25 cm H_2O) is recommended as is, in the instance of poor laryngeal view, the release of cricoid pressure.[160] For these reasons, and the lack of randomized controlled trials evaluating outcomes in regard to cricoid pressure,[161] some practitioners have altogether abandoned classic RSIs in favor of gentle mask ventilation, without cricoid pressure, while waiting for fast-acting paralytics to work.[162] If mask ventilation is omitted, high-flow oxygen via nasal cannula can be used to increase apnea tolerance via apneic oxygenation, as discussed earlier.

Another, more insidious, mode of aspiration is "microaspiration," which occurs when ETT cuff occlusion of the tracheal lumen is imperfect. Leakage of liquids past the cuff may be related to an underinflated cuff or channeling secondary to cuff folding and can be worsened by negative intrathoracic pressure in the spontaneously breathing patient.[163] For these reasons, ETTs with subglottic suction ports are recommended for patients who will likely stay intubated past the immediate postoperative period.[70]

The Intubating Supraglottic Airways. Blind, flexible scope-aided, stylet-guided, and laryngoscopy-directed tracheal intubation via SGAs has been widely reported, but many limitations have been described. In an effort to overcome these limitations, Brain et al. introduced a version of the LMA, the LMA (Teleflex, Research Triangle Park, NC), designed specifically as a conduit to intubation (Fig. 28-4). Other manufacturers have introduced similar devices including the Aura-I (Ambu, Ballerup, Denmark) and the air-Q (Fig. 28-6). Most non-Fastrach devices require guided tracheal intubation (e.g., with a flexible intubation scope) during the intubation process. Expert groups, such as the Difficult Airway Society of the United Kingdom, recommend this visually guided approach.[3]

The mask of the LMA Fastrach differs from Dr. Brain's original LMA design with the incorporation of a vertically oriented, semirigid bar fixed at the proximal end of the bowl aperture. This "epiglottic elevating bar" sits beneath the epiglottis in the average-sized adult and guides the ETT toward the larynx. A handle at the proximal end of the barrel is used for insertion, repositioning, and removal of the device. Originally made of stainless steel and silicone, a plastic single-use version is available. The LMA Fastrach barrel can accommodate up to an 8-mm ID-cuffed ETT, which can be inserted blindly or over a fiberscope or other flexible stylet device. The Fastrach is designed to be used with a wire-reinforced tracheal tube, although the use of both standard and Parker Flex-Tip (Parker Medical, Englewood, CO) PVC tracheal tubes has been described.[164] The LMA Fastrach is available in sizes with cuffs equivalent to the size 3, 4, and 5 LMA Classics. Experience suggests that most adults between 40 and 70 kg are best managed with a size 4 Fastrach and heavier persons require a size 5.

A large study has shown the utility of the LMA Fastrach. Ferson et al.[92] successfully intubated 234 patients with this device, including patients for whom they anticipated difficult intubation. Successful blind intubation via the LMA Fastrach occurred in 97% of these patients; the remaining intubations were facilitated with adjunct use of a fiberoptic intubation scope. A modification of the LMA Fastrach design, the LMA CTrach (introduced in 2004 but no longer commercially available), incorporated into the device bowl a CMOS camera connected to a handle-mounted monitor.

Prior to insertion, the mask of the LMA Fastrach cuff is tested, deflated, and lubricated as described for the LMA Classic. With the patient's head in neutral position, the device is inserted into the mouth so that the mask lies flat against the palate. Gentle pressure on the handle and barrel reproduces the palatal pressure described earlier for LMA Classic insertion. A smooth backward rotation of the handle toward the top of the head seats the tip of the mask in the hypopharynx, posterior to the cricoid cartilage. Once seated, the mask of the Fastrach is inflated and ventilation is attempted. The position of the device can be optimized by lateral and anterior–posterior manipulation of the handle, known as the *Chandy maneuver* (after Dr. Chandy Verghese, Redding, UK).[165] A seemingly common cause of airway obstruction with the LMA Fastrach is down-folding of the epiglottis. This can be relieved with a smooth rotational movement of the inflated LMA Fastrach out of the airway (6 cm along the axis of the insertion) and immediate replacement (the "up–down maneuver").

Blind tracheal intubation is undertaken only if the airway is clear and the patient is muscle relaxed and/or sufficiently anesthetized. After adequate ventilation and anesthesia are achieved, the ETT is advanced though the barrel. As the ETT exits the bowl aperture of the LMA Fastrach, the elevating bar is pushed anteriorly, carrying the epiglottis out of the way. If positioned correctly, the ETT can freely enter the glottis.

When blind intubation fails (esophageal insertion or inability to advance the ETT) and flexible intubation scopes or stylets are not available, several maneuvers may be performed.[165] As early obstruction is typically caused by a down-folded epiglottis, an up–down maneuver, as described earlier, can be employed and intubation attempts repeated. If unsuccessful, a second part of the Chandy maneuver may be attempted in which the handle is used to gently lift (without rotation) the device anteriorly, sealing the bowl against the larynx. Early resistance may also signify vallecular entrapment secondary to an LMA Fastrach size. The operator may remove the LMA Fastrach and place a smaller one. Later obstruction may signify entrapment or too small a device and, again, a change may be indicated.

When intubation fails despite these maneuvers and/or a change in the device size, the clinician should recall that ventilation typically will be adequate despite failure to intubate. At this juncture, the clinician can (1) continue with short surgical procedures using the Fastrach as a simple SGA (procedures longer than 15 minutes may be ill advised because of the pressure exerted by the LMA Fastrach on pharyngeal tissues), (2) change to a different SGA, (3) diagnose the intubation impediment with the aid of another device (e.g., flexible intubation scope), (4) remove the SGA and employ an alternate technique of tracheal intubation, or (5) perform a surgical airway while continuing ventilation via the SGA. This last procedure may be an underappreciated facility of all the SGAs, as these devices may serve as bridges while invasive airway procedures are performed.

Once successful intubation is confirmed by capnography and physical exam, an intubating SGA may be removed. Though this is typically a requirement of the rigid devices (e.g., LMA Fastrach), some intubating SGAs (e.g., the Aura-I or air-Q) may be left *in situ*. For removal, the ETT circuit adapter is removed and the intubating SGA is withdrawn over the ETT. During this removal, the ETT is stabilized either coaxially by a stabilizing rod (supplied by the manufacturer) or by Magill forceps holding the proximal tip of the ETT (as described by Rosenblatt et al.).[166] In the midremoval position, a finger is placed in the mouth to stabilize the ETT while the SGA is fully retreated.

The precurved Aura-I intubating SGA lacks the rigid components as well as the epiglottic lifting bar concept of the LMA Fastrach. Because it does not apply as much pressure to pharyngeal mucosa, it can be left *in situ* after intubation or used for long periods as a simple SGA. When using an Aura-I for tracheal intubation, a flexible intubation scope should be used.

The air-Q SGA also foregoes the rigid components and epiglottic lifting bar. Unlike the devices discussed earlier, it lacks the 90-degree precurvature of the barrel. The air-Q barrel will accept a tracheal tube from 4.5 to 8.0 mm internal diameter (ID) and the keyhole-shaped airway outlet is designed to steer the ETT toward the larynx. For blind intubation, the ETT cuff is deflated, lubricated, and inserted into the device barrel. If the larynx is entered, advancement past 12 to 15 cm should occur with little resistance. If resistance is met, the air-Q can be repositioned and ETT advancement attempted again. Once tracheal intubation is confirmed, the device can be removed with the help of a specialized stylet provided by the manufacturer. In a study comparing like devices, the LMA Fastrach had a higher blind intubation success rate than the air-Q (99% vs. 77%, respectively, with two attempts), though greater than 95% of patients could be intubated with either device if flexible optical guidance was utilized.[167] Unlike the other intubating SGAs, a range of pediatric-sized air-Qs are available and intubation success rates of 95% have been achieved in infants.[168]

Extubation of the Trachea

Although a wealth of literature is focused on the field of tracheal intubation, few reviews have intensely contemplated the area of extubation after completion of surgery or prolonged ventilatory support.[169] Indeed, the period of extubation may be far more treacherous than that of intubation.[1]

Routine Extubation

Extubation of the trachea must not be considered a benign procedure, as it is fraught with its own set of potential complications (Table 28-14). As planning, preparation, and a back-up plan are needed for safe intubation, they are also needed for the procedure of extubation. Appropriately trained personnel and equipment

Table 28-14 Complications of Tracheal Extubation

Respiratory drive failure (e.g., residual anesthetic, decreased response to high CO_2/low O_2)
Hypoxia (e.g., atelectasis)
Upper airway obstruction (e.g., edema, residual anesthetic or paralytic, reduced upper airway tone)
Vocal fold–related obstruction (e.g., laryngospasm, vocal cord edema or paralysis)
Tracheal obstruction (e.g., subglottic edema or tracheomalacia from prolonged intubation)
Bronchospasm (airway irritation from endotracheal tube)
Aspiration (from decreased gag and swallow reflexes)
Hypertension
Increased intracranial pressure
Increased ocular pressure
Increased pulmonary artery pressure
Increased bronchial stump pressure (e.g., after pulmonary resection)
Increased abdominal wall pressure (risk of wound dehiscence)

should be immediately available at the time of extubation. This may range from a postanesthetic care unit nurse or respiratory therapist with a set of laryngoscopes to a surgeon prepared to perform an emergency tracheostomy. An excellent reference exists in the Difficult Airway Society Extubation Guidelines, which outline a strategic stepwise approach to decision making before, during, and after both routine and "at risk" extubations.[170]

Most adult patients are extubated after the return of spontaneous respiration, the resolution of neuromuscular block, and the demonstration of the ability to follow simple commands (Table 28-15). After the patient is asked to open their mouth, a suction catheter is used to remove supraglottic secretions or blood. The airway pressure is allowed to rise to 5 to 15 cm of H_2O to facilitate a "passive cough" and the ETT is removed after the cuff (if present) is deflated.[44] If coughing or straining is contraindicated or hazardous (e.g., increased intracranial pressure), extubation may be performed while the patient is in a surgical plane of anesthesia and breathing spontaneously ("deep" extubation). The three requirements for deep extubation are (a) easy mask ventilation following induction, (b) non-airway surgery, and (c) empty stomach. If deep extubation is desired and the patient is at risk of gastric content aspiration (e.g., full stomach) or upper airway obstruction (e.g., obstructive sleep apnea), the clinician needs to assess the relative risk of each potential morbidity (e.g., coughing vs. aspiration vs. obstruction).

Laryngospasm upon ETT removal accounts for 23% of all critical postoperative respiratory events in adults.[44] The mechanism of laryngospasm is the contraction of the lateral cricoarytenoids, the thyroarytenoid, and the cricothyroid muscles in response to stimulation of the vagus nerve. Potential stimuli include secretions, vomitus, blood, or foreign body in the airway, pelvic or abdominal visceral stimulation, and pain. Management of laryngospasm consists of the immediate removal of the offending stimulus (if identifiable), administration of oxygen with CPAP and, if other maneuvers are unsuccessful, the use of a small dose of short-acting induction agent or muscle relaxant.[44]

Patients who are not fully recovered from neuromuscular relaxation are also at risk of airway obstruction and aspiration at the time of extubation.[171] This is, in part, due to the fact that pharyngeal function is hindered when the train-of-four (TOF) ratio remains less than 0.9.[172] Fortier et al.[173] found that 65% of patients who received nondepolarizing neuromuscular blocker and had been reversed with neostigmine still had residual neuromuscular blockade (TOF <0.9) at the time of extubation and 60% had residual neuromuscular blockade on arrival to the postanesthesia care unit (PACU). This data suggests that neostigmine alone cannot be relied on for adequate reversal and vigilance is needed during intraoperative titration of neuromuscular blockers. Though cholinesterase antagonists have historically been used to reverse nondepolarizing neuromuscular blockers, a new class of agents has been introduced. Cyclodextrins are hollow-structure molecules capable of trapping other molecules within their core. The lipophilic core of the agent sugammadex (Merck & Co., Whitehouse Station, NJ) so tightly encapsulates rocuronium or vecuronium molecules that it can remove blocking agents that are already bound to the neuromuscular junction. The trapped neuromuscular blocker is unavailable to bind elsewhere and excreted in the urine. This is discussed more thoroughly in Chapter 21.

Mechanical airway obstruction may also result in extubation failure and the risk is higher in patients with obstructive sleep apnea. Obstruction may result from trauma related to intubation (e.g., multiple failed attempts), surgical manipulation (e.g., lingual edema caused by mouth gags), and impaired lymphatic (e.g., after radiation therapy) and venous (e.g., with extreme neck flexion) drainage. Palatopharyngeal edema associated with anterior cervical spine procedures or hematomas (e.g., following endarterectomy) may also result in postextubation airway failure.

Unilateral vocal cord paralysis may result from trauma to the recurrent laryngeal nerve. If the contralateral nerve has been damaged previously, airway obstruction can occur due to unopposed vocal cord adduction. This may occur following neck or intrathoracic surgery or even after internal jugular line placement or endotracheal intubation. Transient vocal cord and swallowing dysfunction has been demonstrated in absence of injury, placing even healthy patients at risk of aspiration after general anesthesia. Many patients will undergo preoperative nasopharyngoscopy to assess the state of laryngeal function prior to one of these high-risk procedures.

Pharmacologic agents used during maintenance and emergence of anesthesia may also affect the success of extubation. Though low concentrations of potent inhalation anesthetics

Table 28-15 Criteria for Routine "Awake" Postsurgical Extubation

Subjective clinical criteria:
- Breathing spontaneously
- Following commands
- Five-second sustained head lift
- Intact gag reflex
- Airway clear of debris
- Adequate pain control
- Minimal end-expiratory concentration of inhaled anesthetics

Objective criteria:
- Vital capacity ≥10 mL/kg
- Peak voluntary negative inspiratory pressure > –20 cmH_2O
- Tidal volume >6 mL/kg
- Sustained tetanic contraction (5 seconds)
- T1/T4 ratio >0.7–0.8
- Alveolar–arterial Pa_{O_2} gradient <350 mmHg (on F_{IO_2} of 1)[a]
- Dead space to tidal volume ratio ≤0.6[a]

[a]Used during weaning from mechanical ventilation in the intensive care setting.

(e.g., 0.2 Minimal Alveolar Concentration [MAC]) do not alter the respiratory response to CO_2, they may blunt hypoxic drive. Opiates and, to a lesser extent, benzodiazepines affect both hypercarbic and hypoxic respiratory drives. Some nondepolarizing muscle relaxants also reduce the hypoxic ventilatory drive secondary to their effect on cholinergic receptors in the carotid body.[169,171]

A randomized control trial revealed that multiple-dose dexamethasone effectively reduced incidence of postextubation stridor in adult patients at high risk for postextubation laryngeal edema. In contrast, single-dose injection of dexamethasone given 1 hour before extubation did not reduce the number of patients requiring reintubation.[174]

Identification of Patients at Risk for Complications after Extubation

All patients should be evaluated for potentially difficult extubation just as they are evaluated for potentially difficult intubation. A number of well-known clinical situations may place patients at increased risk for difficulty with oxygenation or ventilation at the time of extubation (Table 28-16).

A popular test used to predict postextubation airway competency is the detection of a leak on deflation of the ETT cuff. A meta-analysis showed that the absence of a cuff leak is associated with a higher risk of reintubation, but the presence of a detectable leak has low predictive value.[175]

When mask ventilation and intubation are without difficulty and there is no substantial reason to believe that an interim insult to the airway has occurred, extubation may be accomplished in a routine fashion. Even under these circumstances, one must always be prepared for emergent reintubation.

Approach to the Difficult Extubation

When there is a suspicion that a patient may have difficulty with oxygenation or ventilation after tracheal extubation, the clinician may choose from a number of management strategies. These range from continued ventilation, to the preparation of standby reintubation equipment, to the active establishment of a bridge or guide for reintubation or oxygenation.

A number of obturators, which may be left in the airway for extended periods, are available for use in trial extubation. These devices are generally referred to as airway exchange catheters (AECs). The success of first-pass reintubation is significantly higher, and the incidence of hypoxia is lower, in patients with a retained AEC.[176]

There are many commercially available AECs. Two examples of these are the Cook Airway Exchange Catheters (Cook Critical Care, Bloomington, IN) and the CardioMed Endotracheal Ventilation Catheter (CardioMed, Gromley, Ontario, Canada). Both of these are available in multiple sizes and have a central lumen and rounded, atraumatic ends. The proximal ends are fitted with a Luer-lock adapter that with an oxygen source can be used to provide insufflated or jet-ventilated oxygen. These adapters are helpful if the patient fails extubation or reintubation attempts and can be quickly decoupled for ETT removal or exchange.

Despite their advantages, AECs have been associated with significant morbidity, and complication rates of up to 60% have been reported.[177] Complications have included loss of airway control, mucosal trauma, esophageal intubation, pneumothorax (even in the absence of gas insufflation), and death.[178] Specific cautions are often exercised to reduce complications with AECs, though little empiric literature is available.

Prior to placement of an AEC, the patient should meet extubation criteria and, in most cases, be fully preoxygenated. An AEC with an external diameter closest to the internal diameter of the ETT that would be used for reintubation should be chosen to prevent "hang-up" (see later under Use of the Flexible Intubation Scope).

When the patient is ready for extubation, the ventilator is disconnected and the distal end of the lubricated AEC is placed to the depth of the tracheal tube bevel. Most AECs have depth markings that may be matched with the markings on the ETT (Fig. 28-19). If care was taken with the initial tracheal tube positioning, this will result in a midtracheal positioning of the AEC and reduce the chance of endobronchial placement. As the ETT is removed, careful attention is paid to maintaining the AEC's position. If tracheal reintubation is required and the ETT will not pass through the glottis, lifting the tongue with a laryngoscope may facilitate reintubation. A 2 or 3 cm withdrawal of the ETT, counterclockwise tracheal tube rotation (90 degrees), and reinsertion will often overcome "hang-up."

If jet insufflation of oxygen via the AEC is required, the patient should be flaccid or muscle relaxed and an oral airway or other device should be used to maintain an open upper airway. In addition, inspiratory pressure and duration must be carefully titrated to observe chest expansion and recoil. These precautions are designed to limit chest-wall resistance and facilitate gas egress.

During removal of the ETT, a flexible intubation scope may be used to view tracheal structures. If extubation is tolerated,

Table 28-16 Clinical Situations Presenting Increased Risk for Complications at Time of Extubation

Edema (local, generalized or angioneurotic)	Airway narrowing
Thyroid surgery	Recurrent laryngeal nerve injury
Laryngoscopy (diagnostic)	Edema, laryngospasm (especially after biopsy)
Uvulopalatoplasty	Palatal and oropharyngeal edema
Obstructive sleep apnea	Upper airway obstruction
Carotid endarterectomy	Wound hematoma, glottic edema, nerve palsies
Maxillofacial trauma	Laryngeal fracture, mandibular/maxillary wires
Cervical vertebrae decompression/fixation	Supraglottic and hypopharyngeal edema
Anaphylaxis	Laryngotracheal narrowing
Upper cervical fracture	Prevertebral/retropharyngeal hematoma
Hypopharyngeal infections	Laryngotracheal narrowing
Hypoventilation syndromes	(e.g., residual anesthetic, central sleep apnea, myasthenia gravis, morbid obesity, severe chronic obstructive pulmonary disease)
Hypoxemic syndromes	(e.g., ventilation–perfusion mismatch, increased oxygen consumption, impaired alveolar oxygen diffusion, severe anemia)
Inadequate airway-protective reflexes	Increased aspiration risk

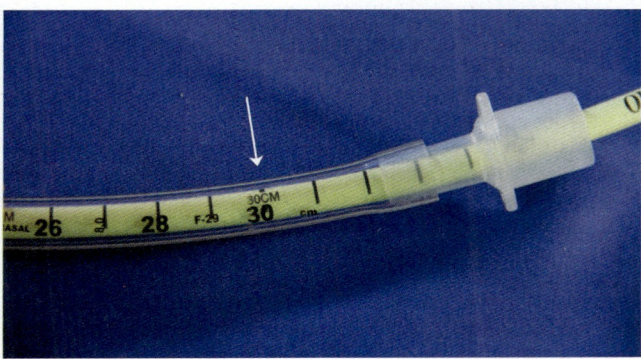

Figure 28-19 Markings of an airway exchange catheter (AEC) are aligned with the markings on the *in situ* tracheal tube. Aligning these marks as the AEC is inserted prevents bronchial trauma.

the bronchoscope can be slowly withdrawn into the subglottic region and the vocal folds and other structures visualized and evaluated.

The Difficult Airway Algorithm

Difficult and failed airway management accounts for 2.3% of anesthetic deaths in the United States.[5] The ASA defines the difficult airway as the situation in which the "conventionally trained anesthesiologist experiences difficulty with intubation, mask ventilation or both." In 1993, to address such a scenario, the ASA Task Force on the Difficult Airway first published an algorithm that has become a staple of modern airway management. This algorithm was reissued in 2003 and again in 2013.[2] The most significant change in the ASA difficult airway algorithm (ASA-DAA) has been the repositioning of the SGA from the emergency to the non-emergency management pathway and the inclusion of VL as an option for both initial airway management and after failed tracheal intubation (Fig. 28-20).

Though the ASA-DAA is a staple in the United States and much of the world, several groups worldwide have written their own airway algorithms emphasizing techniques and approaches native to their practice; the reader is encouraged to explore these as well.[3,108,179,180]

The text of the ASA-DAA succinctly states the challenge of recommending practices for management of the difficult airway: "The difficult airway represents a complex interaction between patient factors, the clinical setting, and the skills of the practitioner."[2] Although the algorithm largely speaks for itself, its salient features are discussed here.

Entry into the algorithm begins with physical evaluation of the airway. Although there is some debate as to the value of particular evaluation methods, the clinician must use all available data and his or her own clinical experience to reach a general impression as to the likelihood of difficulty in terms of laryngoscopy (e.g., DL or VL), intubation, and supraglottic ventilation. The risk of aspiration and the likely degree of apnea tolerance must also be weighed.

This evaluation should direct the clinician to enter the ASA-DAA at one of its two root points: awake intubation (Fig. 28-20A) or intubation attempts after the induction of general anesthesia (Fig. 28-20B). The decision to enter the algorithm via either approach is made after a thorough preoperative evaluation.

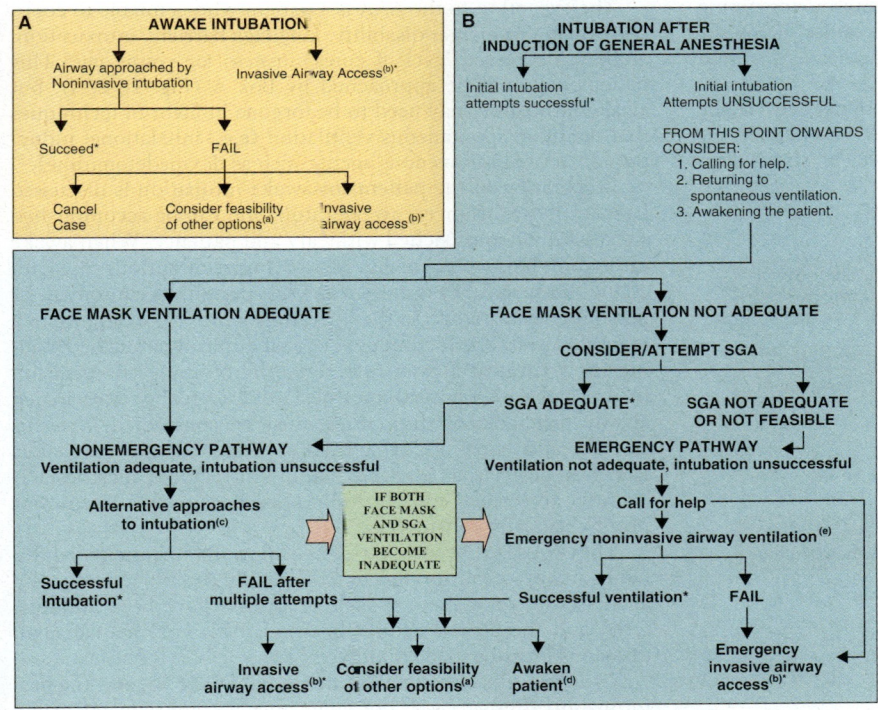

*Confirm ventilation, tracheal intubation, or SGA placement with exhaled CO_2.

a. Other options include (but are not limited to): surgery utilizing face mask or supraglottic airway (SGA) anesthesia (e.g., LMA, ILMA, laryngeal tube), local anesthesia infiltration or regional nerve blockade. Pursuit of these options usually implies that mask ventilation will not be problematic. Therefore, these options may be of limited value if this step in the algorithm has been reached via the Emergency Pathway.

b. Invasive airway access includes surgical or percutaneous airway, jet ventilation, and retrograde intubation.

c. Alternative dificult intubation approaches include (but are not limited to): video-assisted laryngoscopy, alternative laryngoscope blades, SGA (e.g., LMA or ILMA) as an intubation conduit (with or without fiberoptic guidance), fiberoptic intubation, intubating stylet or tube changer, light wand, and blind oral or nasal intubation.

d. Consider re-preparation of the patient for awake intubation or canceling surgery.

e. Emergency non-invasive airway ventilation consists of a SGA.

Figure 28-20 The American Society of Anesthesiologists Difficult Airway Algorithm. **A:** Awake intubation. **B:** Intubation attempts after induction of anesthesia.

Box A is chosen when difficulty is anticipated with either ventilation or intubation that will place the patient at jeopardy. Box B is for the setting in which difficulty may be anticipated but no uncorrectable situations are expected.

The Airway Approach Algorithm

These decisions have been further defined in a preoperative decision tree by Rosenblatt[7] known as the *Airway Approach Algorithm* (AAA). Figure 28-21 outlines the AAA, a simple one-pathway algorithm for entering into the ASA-DAA based on five fundamental questions. Movement through the AAA is dependent on the clinician's skill and experience. Details of the AAA can be found elsewhere and are summarized here.[7,181]

1. **Is airway control necessary?** Can regional, neuraxial, or infiltrative anesthesia be applied? Periodic analysis of the closed claims database illustrates that a plan for airway control is always needed independent of the choice of anesthetic technique. This concept was highlighted in the 2013 iteration of the ASA-DAA.[2] However routine the practices of sedation or general anesthesia becomes, whether or not to make a patient apneic should always be considered and alternatives contemplated.
2. **Could tracheal intubation be (at all) difficult?** If there is no indication that rapid tracheal intubation (e.g., by DL, VL, or other means familiar to the operator) will be difficult, the clinician may proceed as clinically appropriate. If there is an indication, based on history or physical examination, that there may be difficulty with rapid tracheal intubation, the AAA is followed to the next question. By choosing to continue down the algorithm, the clinician is not assuming that tracheal intubation will be difficult; rather, he or she is anticipating the viability of rescue maneuvers should difficulty occur.
3. **Can supraglottic ventilation be used if needed?** If the clinician identifies a reason that SGA ventilation (by facemask or SGA) could be difficult, he or she is projecting the possibility that a juncture of "cannot intubate (Question 2)—cannot ventilate (Question 3)" could be reached. Because this is a preoperative algorithm, Box A (awake intubation) of the ASA-DAA may be the preferred root entry point.
4. **Is there an aspiration risk?** The patient at risk for aspiration is not a candidate for elective SGA use. Because the AAA is a preoperative algorithm, and therefore allows the luxury of discretionary paths, the juncture of "cannot intubate/should not ventilate" can be avoided by entering the ASA-DAA at Box A.
5. a. **Will the patient tolerate an apneic period?** Should intubation fail and facemask and SGA ventilation prove inadequate, will the patient rapidly desaturate? Factors such as age, pregnancy, pulmonary status, abnormal oxygen consumption (e.g., fever), and choice of induction agents will influence this. If time to oxyhemoglobin desaturation is limited, Box A may be prophylactically chosen.
   b. **Can hypoxia be rapidly corrected through other means?** This question requires the operator to consider percutaneous emergency airway access (PEAA),[182] including the availability of equipment and the knowledge and experience of the operator and support personnel. For example, if an error in judgment is made and the operator is in a "cannot intubate/cannot ventilate" scenario, will these conditions allow for the use of PEAA to temporize the situation? All conditions may be right, but if the patient is morbidly obese or has had scarring or radiation changes over the larynx/trachea, this option may not be available. These factors have been discussed in detail elsewhere.[7,181]

The exception to the AAA is a patient who is unable to cooperate owing to mental disability, language barriers, intoxication, anxiety, depressed level of consciousness, or young age. This patient may still be approached by Box A (Fig. 28-20A), but awake intubation may need to be forgone in favor of techniques that maintain spontaneous ventilation (e.g., inhalational induction or titrated intravenous agents such as dexmedetomidine).

Preparation of the patient for awake intubation is discussed later. In most instances, awake intubation can be accomplished successfully if approached with care and patience. When awake intubation fails, the clinician has a number of options: (1) canceling the surgical case and arranging specialized equipment or personnel for a return to the operating room; (2) changing to a regional anesthetic technique; or (3) if clinically indicated, calling for a surgical airway (e.g., cricothyrotomy). The decision to proceed with regional anesthesia due to real or anticipated airway management difficulties must be considered in terms of risks and benefits (Table 28-17). The ASA Closed Claims Database project has identified failure of regional anesthesia as a source of serious complication when no airway strategy was prophylactically considered.[2,4]

The ASA-DAA becomes truly useful in the unanticipated difficult airway scenario (Box B in Fig. 28-20). When induction agents (with or without muscle relaxants) have been administered and the airway cannot be controlled, vital management decisions must be made rapidly.

Typically, the clinician has attempted DL or VL and tracheal intubation after successful or failed anesthesia mask ventilation. Even if the patient's oxygen saturation remains adequate, the number of laryngoscopy attempts should be limited.[183,184] The exact number of attempts allowed is unclear and will depend on the clinical scenario, but the authors recommend limiting the number of DL or VL attempts to two (or potentially three if the initial attempts were performed under suboptimal

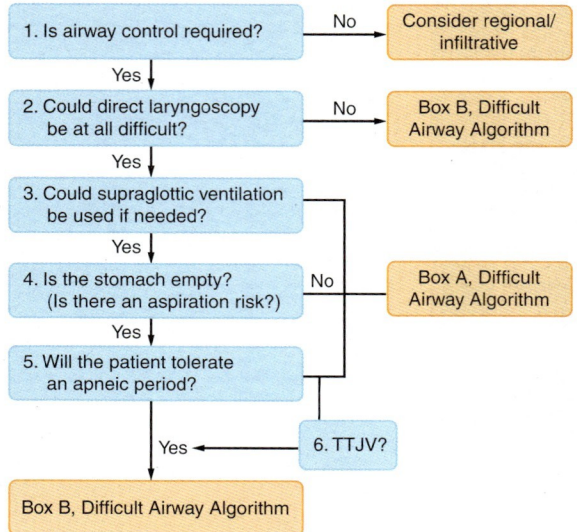

Figure 28-21 The Airway Approach Algorithm: a decision tree approach to entry into the American Society of Anesthesiologists Difficult Airway Algorithm. TTJV: transtracheal jet ventilation.

Table 28-17 Regional Anesthesia (RA) for Patients with Likely Difficult Airways	
May Consider RA	**Should Not Consider RA**
Superficial surgery	Cavity-invading surgery
Minimal sedation needed	Moderate or heavy sedation needed
Local infiltration adequate	Large-volume local anesthetic required or high risk of intravascular injection/absorption
Easy access to the airway	Poor access to the airway
Surgery can be halted at any time	Surgery cannot be stopped once started

Table 28-18 The Vortex Approach: Maneuvers and Alterations between Noninvasive Airway Attempts
Manipulation: head, neck, larynx
Change in device or device size
Change in operator
Airway adjuncts: oral/nasal airways, bougie, suction
Pharmacologic adjuncts: muscle relaxants, reversal agents

conditions or by an inexperienced provider). This emphasizes the importance of optimizing the first attempt, as significant soft tissue trauma can result from laryngoscopy, especially after multiple attempts, which may diminish the efficacy of a rescue facemask or SGA.

If two to three attempts at laryngoscopy fail, mask ventilation should be instituted and, if adequate, the ASA-DAA nonemergency pathway is entered. The clinician may then turn to the most convenient and/or appropriate technique for establishing tracheal intubation, if needed. This might include, but is not limited to, the use of a flexible intubation scope; an SGA or intubating SGA; or a bougie, lighted stylet, or retrograde wire. A surgical airway will sometimes be the most appropriate approach. (The most widely applied of these procedures, as well as new techniques, will be discussed within the clinical scenarios presented later.)

When mask ventilation fails, the algorithm suggests supraglottic ventilation via an SGA. If successful, the nonemergency pathway of the ASA-DAA has again been entered and alternative techniques of tracheal intubation may be used, if needed. Should SGA ventilation fail to sustain the patient adequately, the emergency pathway is entered and the ASA-DAA suggests use of percutaneous emergency airway access (e.g., via the CTM or a surgical airway. At any juncture, the decision to awaken the patient should be considered based on the adequacy of ventilation, the risk of aspiration, and the risk of proceeding with intubation attempts or the surgical procedure.

A nonalgorithmic approach to the failed and critical airway has also been suggested. The Vortex Approach is a simple cognitive aid to be used during the critical cannot intubate/cannot oxygenate (CICO) scenario (Fig. 28-22).[179] The Vortex Approach is not a substitute for the emergency pathway of the ASA-DAA or any other published recommendation, but rather is a simple visual clue to the steps that may be taken during an airway emergency.

The Vortex Approach assumes that there are three categories of noninvasive techniques available during an airway "code": mask ventilation, SGA ventilation, and tracheal intubation. Up to three attempts with devices from each of these categories may be attempted prior to pursuing invasive (surgical) airway access. The limitation placed on the number of attempts is because repeated attempts are unlikely to be successful and are likely to incur trauma and waste time, as discussed earlier. Attempts with the three noninvasive techniques can be made in any order that is clinically relevant, but, if a second or third attempt is needed with devices from any given category, a change must be instituted between attempts (e.g., different device, method of insertion, patient positioning, and so on) (Table 28-18).

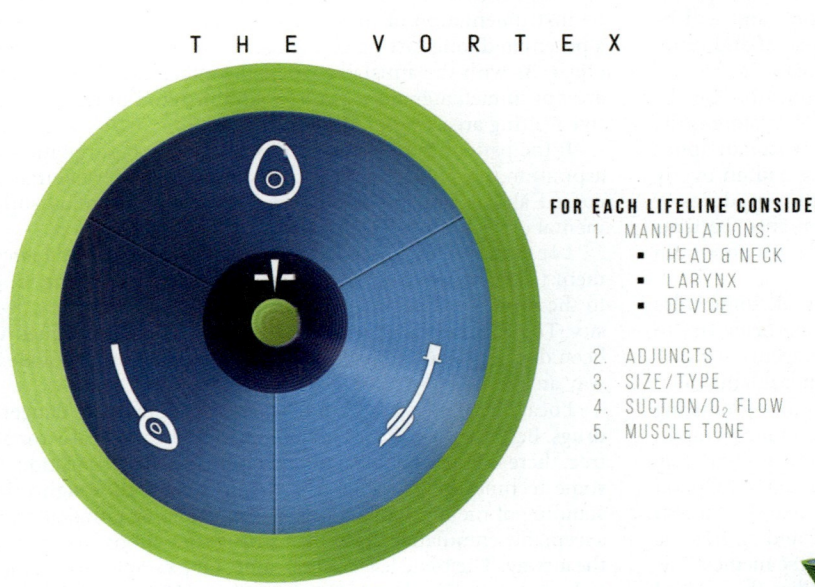
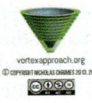

Figure 28-22 The Vortex Approach. The Vortex is a cognitive aid for use during failed airway exercises. (Reproduced with permission from Chrimes N, Fritz P. The Vortex Approach: Management of the Unanticipated Difficult Airway. Smashwords Edition, 2013. Available at: http://www.vortexapproach.org.)

After exhaustion of the allowed nine noninvasive attempts, a surgical airway is immediately sought. The choice of invasive airway management technique is dependent on operator experience and equipment availability. As a consequence of this approach, an invasive airway will ideally be initiated prior to oxyhemoglobin desaturation. This is contrary to traditional teaching, in which an invasive airway is not attempted until oxyhemoglobin desaturation has begun. Because more than three attempts at noninvasive techniques are unlikely to be successful,[180] an early approach to an invasive airway should allow for a more controlled technique and lower risk of hypoxic damage.

Awake Airway Management

Awake airway management remains a mainstay of the American Society of Anesthesiologists' difficult airway algorithm. Awake techniques provide maintenance of spontaneous ventilation in the event that the airway cannot be secured rapidly. Other benefits include increased size and patency of the pharynx, relative forward placement of the base of the tongue, posterior placement of the larynx, and the ability of the patient to cooperate with procedures.[185] Additionally, the awake state confers some maintenance of upper and lower esophageal sphincter tone, thus reducing the risk of regurgitation. In the event of regurgitation, the patient can expel aspirated foreign bodies by cough to the extent that these reflexes have not been obtunded by local anesthesia.[186] Finally, patients at risk for neurologic sequelae (e.g., patients with unstable cervical spine pathology) may undergo active sensory–motor testing after tracheal intubation and positioning. In an emergent situation, there may be cautions (e.g., cardiovascular stimulation in the presence of cardiac ischemia or ischemic risk, bronchospasm, increased intraocular or intracranial pressure) but no absolute contraindications to awake intubation. Contraindications to elective awake intubation include patient refusal or inability to cooperate (e.g., child, profound mental disability, dementia, intoxication) and allergy to local anesthetics.

Once the clinician has decided to proceed with awake airway management, the patient must be prepared both physically and psychologically. Most adult patients will appreciate an explanation of the need for an awake airway examination and will be more cooperative once they realize the importance of and rationale for, any potentially uncomfortable procedures.

Along with an appropriate explanation, medication can be used to reduce anxiety. If sedatives are to be administered, the clinician must keep in mind that producing obstruction or apnea in the difficult airway patient can be devastating and an overly sedated patient may not be able to cooperate with procedures or protect the airway from regurgitated gastric contents. Patients with sleep apnea may be particularly prone to obstruction, even with minimal sedation.

Although almost any sedative agent can be used, some rules should apply to all: dose judiciously, avoid polypharmacy (try to use no more than two agents), and have reversal agents at hand. Small doses of benzodiazepines (e.g., diazepam, midazolam, lorazepam) are commonly used to alleviate anxiety without producing significant respiratory depression (when used as a monotherapy). These drugs may be given in intravenous or oral forms and may be reversed with specific antagonists (e.g., flumazenil). Opioid receptor agonists (e.g., fentanyl, alfentanil, remifentanil) can also be used in small, titrated doses for their sedative and antitussive effects. Extreme caution must be exercised with these medications as (1) their respiratory-depressant effects contradict the goal of maintenance of spontaneous ventilation and (2) when administered with other sedative (e.g., benzodiazepines), their respiratory depressant effect is accentuated. A specific antagonist (e.g., naloxone) should always be immediately available if opiates are administered. If adequately topicalized, little (or no) systemic analgesic should be needed.

Ketamine, droperidol, and dexmedetomidine have also been popular among clinicians. Dexmedetomidine is a highly selective centrally acting α_2-adrenergic agonist. When combined with topical anesthesia, sedation with dexmedetomidine provides for a smooth intubation without significant respiratory depression. Dexmedetomidine has been used as a mono-agent for awake intubation in patients with local anesthetic allergy. The success of this technique is likely due to the combined anxiolytic, sedative, and analgesic properties of the drug.[187] A typical loading dose of dexmedetomidine is 1 µg/kg intravenously over 10 minutes followed by a maintenance infusion of 0.2 to 0.7 µg/kg/h.[44] Dexmedetomidine, especially with boluses, may cause bradycardia and both hypo- and hypertension. Bradycardia is reliably treated with atropine or glycopyrrolate, which is often given as a pretreatment for bradycardia prophylaxis as well as its antisialagogue effect. Hypotension can be corrected with phenylephrine or ephedrine and hypertension is treated by decreasing the rate of or stopping, the dexmedetomidine infusion. Deep sedation with any agent should not be confused with awake intubation, during which the patient remains responsive to verbal commands.

Administration of an antisialagogue is important to the success of awake intubation techniques, as even small amounts of liquid can obscure the objective lens of indirect optical instruments (e.g., flexible or rigid intubating scopes and videolaryngoscopes). Antisialagogues have the secondary benefit of increasing the effectiveness of topical anesthetics by limiting secretions that may act as a barrier to mucosal contact. Additionally, copious salivary secretions will act as an intra-airway foreign body and may cause cough or laryngospasm. The commonly used antisialagogues are atropine (0.5–1 mg intramuscularly or intravenously) and glycopyrrolate (0.2–0.4 mg intramuscularly or intravenously). As the drying effects of these medications may take some time (approximately 15 minutes), they are often administered in the preoperative waiting area.

Vasoconstriction of the nasal passages is required if there is to be instrumentation of this part of the airway. Oxymetazoline is a potent and long-lasting vasoconstrictor commonly used to this effect. As with the antisialagogues, the effects of this medication are not immediate and it is often administered in the preoperative waiting area.

If the patient is at increased risk for gastric regurgitation and aspiration, prophylactic measures should be undertaken as discussed above. Patients should also receive continuous supplemental oxygen until ETT placement is confirmed.

Local anesthetics are a cornerstone of awake airway management (see Chapter 22). The airway, from the base of the tongue to the bronchi, is exquisitely sensitive as an evolutionary necessity. Topical anesthesia and injected nerve block techniques have been developed to blunt the protective reflexes and provide airway analgesia.

Local anesthetics are both effective and potentially dangerous drugs. Because these agents are used within the tracheal–bronchial tree, there is potential for significant intravascular absorption with some techniques. The clinician should have a thorough understanding of the mechanism of action, metabolism, toxicities, and acceptable cumulative doses of any drug they choose to employ in the airway. The toxic level of lidocaine, for example, is considered to be 4 µg/mL. In a human study, 400 or 800 mg of lidocaine gel was applied topically to the upper airway. Serial blood lidocaine levels were measured, peaking 60 to 70 minutes later at 0.57 and

1.39 μg/mL, respectively.[188] In another human study, using nebulized lidocaine of the same dose, serum levels of 2.8 and 6.5 μg/mL were measured within 10 minutes of dose completion, respectively.[189] This underscores the need for vigilance and forethought with local anesthetic dosing, especially when applied to the subglottic airways, as with nebulization.

Despite the myriad of local anesthetics available, only those most commonly used in airway preparation will be discussed here. In reality, the choice of local anesthetic employed has little to do with success of the technique of awake intubation; ignoring the other aspects of preparation leads to failure just as readily.[181]

Lidocaine, an amide local anesthetic, is available in a wide variety of preparations and doses. Topically applied, peak analgesia occurs within 15 minutes. This relatively rapid onset and breadth of preparations (e.g., liquid, gel, ointment) make it a common choice for airway topicalization.

Benzocaine, an ester local anesthetic, is popular among some clinicians because of its very rapid onset (<1 minute) and short duration (approximately 10 minutes). It is available in 10%, 15%, and 20% solutions and has been combined with tetracaine in some preparations to prolong the duration of action. A 0.5-second aerosol administration of benzocaine can deliver as much as 30 mg of benzocaine. With the toxic dose being 100 mg, caution must be taken not to spray too liberally. Benzocaine may also produce methemoglobinemia (especially in children) which is treated with methylene blue (1–2 mg intravenously over several minutes).[190]

Tetracaine, another ester local anesthetic, has a longer duration of action than lidocaine or benzocaine and is available in solutions of 0.5%, 1%, and 2%. Absorption of this drug from the respiratory and gastrointestinal tracts is rapid. Toxicity after nebulized application has been reported with doses as low as 40 mg, although the acceptable safe dose in adults is 100 mg by other routes of application.[191]

Among otolaryngologists, cocaine is a popular topical agent. Not only is it a highly effective local anesthetic, but it is also the only local anesthetic that is a potent vasoconstrictor. Cocaine is commonly available in a 4% solution and the total dose applied to the mucosa should not exceed 200 mg in the adult. Cocaine should not be used in patients with known cocaine hypersensitivity, hypertension, ischemic heart disease, preeclampsia, or those taking monoamine oxidase inhibitors. Because cocaine is metabolized by pseudocholinesterase, it is also contraindicated in patients who are deficient in this enzyme.

For awake airway management, local anesthetic therapy is directed to three anatomic areas: the nasal cavity/nasopharynx, the pharynx/base of the tongue, and the hypopharynx/larynx/trachea (Fig. 28-23).

In the authors' experience, the nasal passages should always be included in the preparation for awake intubation for two reasons. First, if during the course of the awake intubation the plan is changed from the oral to the nasal route, preparation is complete. Second, much of the preparation of the nose with local anesthesia will also affect the pharyngeal airway. The nasal cavity is innervated by the greater and lesser palatine nerves (innervating the nasal turbinates and most of the nasal septum) and the anterior ethmoidal nerve (innervating the nares and anterior third of the nasal septum), which are distal branches of the trigeminal nerve (CN V). The palatine nerves arise from the sphenopalatine ganglion located posterior to the middle turbinate. Two techniques for palatine nerve block have been described. In the noninvasive nasal approach, cotton-tipped applicators soaked in local anesthetic are passed along the lower border of the middle turbinate until the posterior wall of the nasopharynx is reached and left there for 5 to 10 minutes. In the invasive

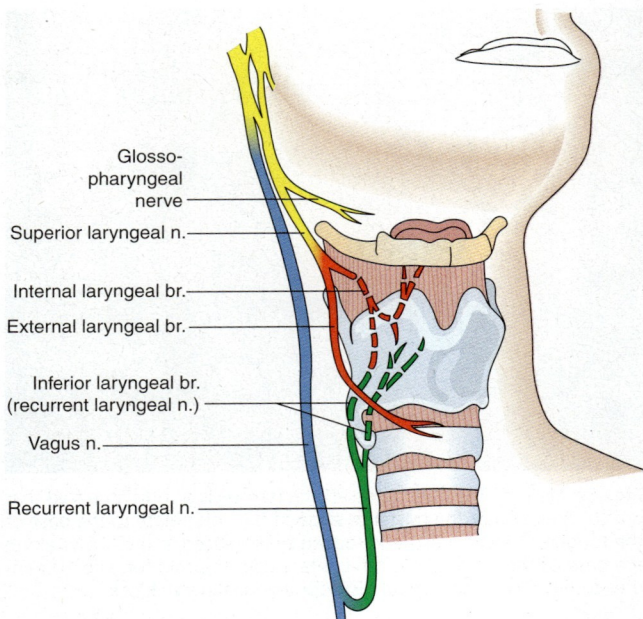

Figure 28-23 Airway innervation.

oral approach, a needle is introduced into the greater palatine foramen, which can be palpated in the posterior-lateral aspect of the hard palate 1 cm medial to the second and third maxillary molars. A spinal needle inserted in a superior/posterior direction to a depth of 2 to 3 cm and anesthetic solution (1 to 2 mL) is injected, taking care to avoid intravascular (sphenopalatine artery) injection. The anterior ethmoidal nerve can be blocked by cotton-tipped applicators soaked in local anesthetic and placed along the dorsal surface of the nose until the anterior cribriform plate is reached. The applicators are left in place for 5 to 10 minutes.

The oropharynx is innervated by branches of the vagus, facial, and glossopharyngeal nerves. A wide variety of techniques may be used to anesthetize this part of the airway. The simplest techniques involve aerosolized local anesthetic solution, or a voluntary local anesthetic "swish and swallow."

The glossopharyngeal nerve (CN IX) travels anteriorly along the lateral surface of the pharynx and supplies sensory innervation to the posterior third of the tongue, walls of the pharynx (pharyngeal branch), tonsils (tonsillar branch), vallecula, and anterior surface of the epiglottis (lingual branch). As it also supplies the afferent limb for the pharyngeal (gag) reflex, anesthesia of the glossopharyngeal nerve is key to comfortable awake airway management. Even after local anesthetic topicalization, some patients may still require a glossopharyngeal nerve block for complete ablation of the gag reflex.

The branches of the glossopharyngeal nerve are most easily accessed as they transverse the palatoglossal folds. These folds are seen as soft tissue ridges that extend from the posterior aspect of the soft palate to the base of the tongue bilaterally (Fig. 28-24). A noninvasive technique employs anesthetic-soaked cotton-tipped applicators held gently against the inferior most aspect of the contralateral folds for 5 to 10 minutes. When this noninvasive technique proves inadequate, local anesthetic can be injected in a similar manner. Standing on the contralateral side, the operator displaces the extended tongue and a 25-gauge spinal needle is inserted into the fold near the floor of the mouth and

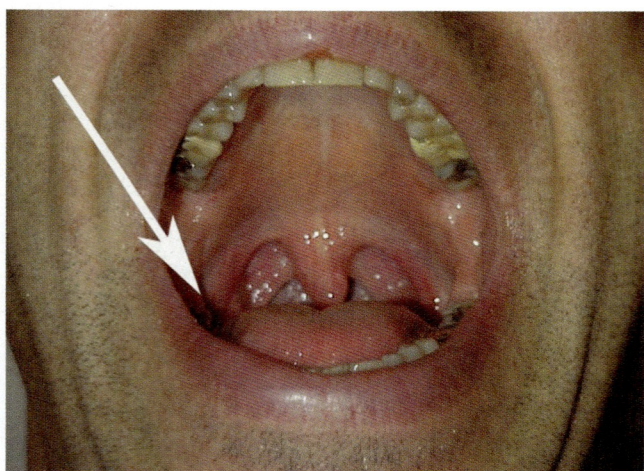

Figure 28-24 The palatoglossal arch (*arrow*) is a soft tissue fold that is a continuation of the posterior edge of the soft palate to the base of the tongue. A local anesthetic-soaked swab placed in the gutter along the base of the tongue is left in contact with the fold for 5 to 10 minutes to produce an ipsilateral glossopharyngeal nerve block.

an aspiration test is performed. If air is aspirated, the needle has passed through-and-through the membrane and is withdrawn slightly prior to injection. If blood is aspirated, the needle tip is redirected more medially. The lingual branch is most readily blocked in this manner, but retrograde tracking of the injectate has also been demonstrated.[186] Even though it provides a reliable block, this more invasive technique is reported to be painful and may result in a bothersome and persistent hematoma.[192] A posterior approach to the glossopharyngeal nerve has also been described in the otolaryngologic literature. As the site of needle insertion is behind the palatopharyngeal arch where it is difficult to see, and in close proximity to the carotid artery, this advanced technique will not be described here and the reader is referred to a more authoritative text.[44]

The superior laryngeal nerve is a branch of the vagus nerve (CN X). The internal branch of the superior laryngeal nerve provides sensory innervation to the base of the tongue, posterior surface of the epiglottis, aryepiglottic folds, and arytenoids. This branch originates lateral to the cornu of the hyoid bone, pierces the thyrohyoid membrane and travels under the mucosa in the pyriform recess. The external branch of the superior laryngeal nerve supplies motor innervation to the cricothyroid muscle and has no sensory component.

Several blocks of the internal branch have been described. In many instances, topical application of anesthetics in the pharyngeal/hypopharyngeal cavities will provide adequate analgesia. For a targeted noninvasive technique, the patient is asked to open their mouth widely and the tongue is grasped with a gauze pad. Right-angled forceps (e.g., Jackson–Krause forceps) with anesthetic-soaked cotton swabs are slid over the lateral tongue and into the pyriform sinuses bilaterally. The swabs are held in place for 5 minutes. An invasive block may be performed with the patient supine with the head extended and the clinician standing on the side of the nerve to be blocked. The clinician identifies the greater cornu of the hyoid bone beneath the angle of the mandible. Using one hand, medially directed pressure is applied to the contralateral hyoid cornu, displacing the hyoid toward the clinician. Caution must be taken to locate the carotid artery and displace it if necessary. The needle can then be inserted directly over the ipsilateral greater cornu and "walked" off the bone in an inferomedial direction until it can be passed through the thyrohyoid ligament to a depth of 1 to 2 cm. Before injecting local anesthetic, an aspiration test should be performed to ensure that one has not entered the pyriform sinus or a vascular structure. Local anesthetic (1.5 to 2 mL) is injected in the space between the thyrohyoid membrane and pharyngeal mucosa.

Sensory innervation of the vocal folds and the trachea is provided by the recurrent laryngeal nerve, another branch of the vagus nerve. Transtracheal injection of local anesthetic is a simple technique that can produce adequate analgesia of these structures. A syringe with a fine needle and filled with a local anesthetic solution (e.g., 2–4 mL of 2% or 4% lidocaine) is inserted through the CTM perpendicular to the plane of the cervical spine. In this orientation, a needle advanced too far will likely impact the posterior aspect of the cricoid cartilage instead of puncturing the esophagus. In addition, this angle will help to avoid trauma to the near-lying vocal folds. Constant retraction on the syringe plunger will result in air aspiration when the trachea is entered. Upon entry into the trachea, the anesthetic agent is injected. Coughing is likely to occur; thus, the needle should be stabilized to prevent mucosal abrasions. Coughing can be advantageous for spread of local anesthesia; by having the patient exhale fully prior to injection, a breath will need to be taken prior to coughing, spreading the medication proximally before being spread distally by the cough.

Another effective technique of tracheal and vocal cord topicalization is to inject local anesthetic through the working channel of the flexible intubation scope. A disadvantage of this technique is that the local anesthetic can obscure the objective lens. This can be overcome by use of an epidural catheter inserted through the working channel, as described by Ovassapian.[193] Not only does this prevent the obscuring of the view but it also allows "aiming" of the anesthetic stream. For this procedure, multiorifice catheters should be trimmed in length so that only a single distal orifice exists.

Clinically Difficult Airway Scenarios

The clinician approaching the patient with a difficult airway has a vast armamentarium of instruments and techniques available.[194] Although this array can be confusing, textbook authors cannot dictate specific approaches in every situation; moreover, the variability of patient presentation makes specific recommendations difficult. Thus, in order to discuss management, the following section presents a number of brief clinical scenarios and the authors' own approach. Major alternative airway management techniques are discussed in this manner. All of the clinical cases described herein have been managed by the authors or a colleague. Other techniques that might be applied in each situation are also discussed. In these cases, as in actual practice, the first technique applied may not have been the best one. The principle of flexibility (and the willingness to change course quickly) will be emphasized repeatedly—the clinician must be prepared to alter their approach as the situation demands.

Case 1: Preoperative Endoscopy

A 52-year-old man presents for DL, esophagoscopy, and biopsy of a base of the tongue tumor. The patient had sought otolaryngologic consultation after 6 months of progressive difficulty in swallowing and the sensation of fullness in his throat. Aside from sleep apnea requiring CPAP, he had no other medical issues and denied voice change or gastroesophageal reflux disease. Physical examination revealed a left neck mass and a 3-cm base of the tongue mass. In the preoperative holding area, oxymetazoline was applied to both nares, followed by 50 mg of 2% lidocaine viscous solution. A 3.2-mm diameter flexible intubation scope was then inserted via the more patent nare. The scope's objective was positioned in the nasopharynx and, on flexion, the epiglottis and glottis could be visualized. The patient was then taken to the operating room where general anesthesia was induced and the trachea intubated using a videolaryngoscope.

Modeled on the airway exam employed by otolaryngologists in office consultations, Preoperative Endoscopic Airway Evaluation (PEAE) can help guide airway management decisions.[21] In the case described, pathology of the hypopharyngeal airway complicated preoperative decision making—an airway mass might compromise tracheal intubation or facemask or SGA ventilation. As discussed earlier in the Airway Approach Algorithm, with only routine information available, an awake intubation might have been the best approach but, as was observed in this case, was unnecessary. By using PEAE to confirm the airway as nonthreatening, the decision could be made to proceed with routine induction of anesthesia. PEAE was studied in 148 patients presenting for intra-airway surgery. In 24% of patients, PEAE resulted in a modification of the initial clinically decided airway plan. Though clinical assessment dictated awake intubation in 44 patients, only 16 were judged to need awake intubation after PEAE. More importantly, 8 of 94 patients who were to have asleep airway management were switched to an awake technique after a concerning preoperative endoscopic exam.[21] PEAE typically requires less than 5 minutes to complete. During the exam, the clinician asks three key questions: (1) is there an obstruction to rapid intubation of the trachea, (2) is there a lesion that could interfere with the placement or function of an SGA, and (3) is there a lesion that routine laryngoscopy (direct or indirect) might dislodge or otherwise traumatize? An affirmative answer to any of these questions encourages awake intubation. As noted earlier, PEAE most often serves to reassure the clinician that lesions, otherwise invisible on physical examination, will not be a hindrance to routine airway management. Likewise, PEAE can often reveal unexpectedly compromising lesions for which the clinician might have been otherwise unprepared.

Case 2: Flexible Intubation Scope-aided Intubation

A 50-year-old man with symptomatic cervical vertebral disc herniation presents for disc resection and spinal fixation. His past medical history includes tobacco use, alcohol consumption, and gastroesophageal reflux. In the preoperative holding area, 0.4 mg of intravenous glycopyrrolate and bilateral nasal oxymetazoline are administered. Five percent lidocaine ointment (50 mg) is applied to the nares via long cotton-tipped applicators. Fifteen minutes later, in the operating room, when the patient reports a dry mouth, he receives 2 mg of intravenous midazolam and topical anesthesia is administered to the remainder of the airway as described earlier. An intubating oral airway is placed which does not elicit a gag reflex. A flexible intubation scope, preloaded with a 7.0-ID ETT, is advanced into the hypopharynx. The vocal ligaments are visualized and 4 mL of 4% lidocaine solution is injected toward the laryngeal and sublaryngeal structures through the accessory lumen of the fiberscope (Ovassapian catheter technique).[193] The distal end of the fiberscope is then advanced into the larynx and trachea until the carina is identified. The ETT is advanced and the fiberscope removed, leaving behind the ETT, which is observed to remain above the carina. The anesthesia circuit is attached to the tracheal tube and a steady output of carbon dioxide is detected by capnography. A brief sensory and motor neurologic examination is performed by the attending surgeon and general anesthesia is induced.

The Flexible Intubation Scope in Airway Management

In 1967, the technique of fiberoptic-aided intubation was first performed using a choledochoscope in a patient with Still disease (idiopathic, adult-onset arthritis).[195] By the late 1980s, it was recognized by experts that the use of the flexible fiberoptic bronchoscope represented such a significant advancement in the management of the patient with a difficult airway that no anesthesiologist could afford not to be facile with the technique.[17] With advancements in imaging technology, the fragile optical strands of fiberoptic scopes are now giving way to video imaging via distally mounted cameras on the same flexible shafts. These flexible (fiberoptic and video) intubation scopes are the most versatile tool available for situations when it is difficult or dangerous to create a line of sight to the glottis.[194]

There is no firm indication for flexible scope-aided intubation. There are, however, many clinical situations in which the flexible intubation scope can be of unparalleled aid in securing the airway.[193] These include anticipated difficult intubation by history or physical examination findings, unanticipated difficult intubation (in which other techniques have failed), lower and upper airway obstruction, unstable or fixed cervical spine disease, mass effect in the upper or lower airways, dental risk or damage, and awake intubation.[193] Unlike the other devices used to intubate the trachea, the flexible intubation scope also allows visualization of structures below the level of the vocal folds. This is useful in verifying single- and double-lumen ETT placement, identifying subglottic pathology and facilitating pulmonary toilet (Fig. 28-25).

Unfortunately, clinicians rarely employ alternative techniques until a difficult situation arises. As with any critical competency, mastery of these techniques involves gaining and maintaining skills through use in *routine* airway management.[122] As an example, Heidegger et al. introduced a simple algorithm for incorporating flexible fiberoptic-aided tracheal intubation into daily practice as a routine alternative to DL. Their incidence of difficult intubation was 6 in 1,324 cases, or 0.049%, markedly lower than reported previously.[122]

Contraindications to flexible scope-aided intubation are relative (Table 28-19). Although flexible scope-aided intubation is a versatile and vital technique, there are several pitfalls, the most common of which are listed in Table 28-20. Because the optical elements are small (the objective lens is typically 2 mm in diameter or smaller), minute amounts of airway secretions, blood, or traumatic debris can hinder visualization. Care must be taken to remove these obstacles from the airway beforehand. Administration of an antisialogogue (as discussed earlier) will produce a drying effect, but caution should be taken in patients who may not be able to tolerate an increase in heart rate. Vasoconstriction of the nose using topical oxymetazoline, phenylephrine, or cocaine reduces the chances of nasal bleeding if this route is chosen. If an awake flexible scope intubation is planned, the patient must be able to cooperate—a "quiet" airway, with little motion of the head, neck, tongue, and larynx, is vital to success. Finally, because flexible scope-aided intubation can require significant time (especially if the clinician is not facile with the device), hypoxia or impending airway loss is a contraindication and a more rapid method of securing an airway (e.g., SGA or surgical airway) should be considered.

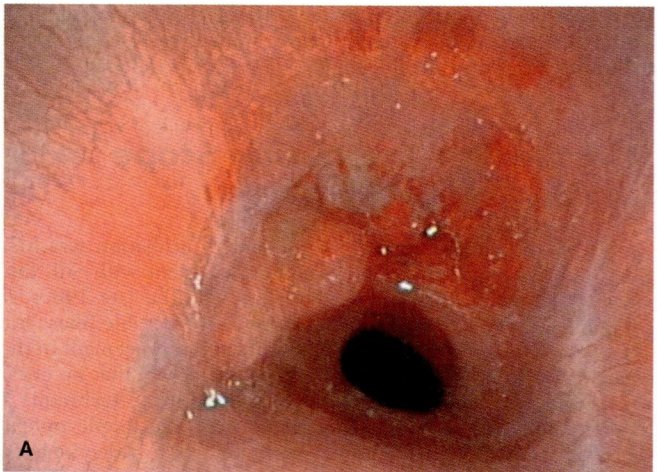 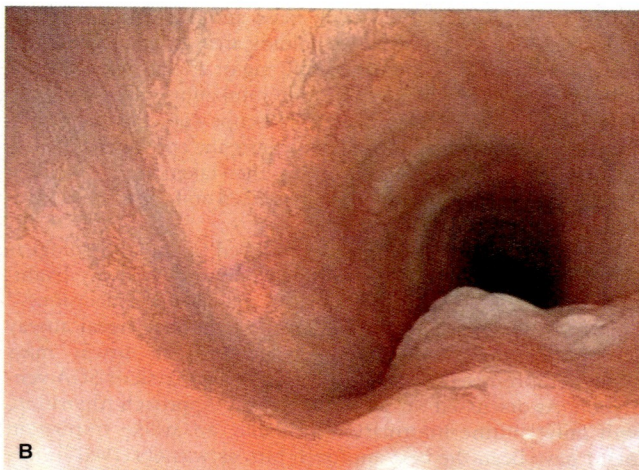

Figure 28-25 The flexible intubation scope may be useful for diagnosis and therapy below the level of the vocal ligaments, including examination of bronchial segments and pulmonary toilet. **A:** Laryngeal web found in an asymptomatic patient who had had one previous tracheal intubation. **B:** Tracheal mass in a patient with thyroid cancer.

It should also be mentioned that any methods used for tracheal intubation in the asleep patient can also be employed for awake intubation. The authors have used the following devices and techniques for awake intubation: Glidescope, KingVision, McGrath, and C-MAC VLs; Unique and Fastrach LMAs; retrograde wire and blind and bougie-aided nasal intubation techniques.

Elements of the Flexible Intubation Scope

The classic fiberoptic bronchoscope is an innately fragile device with both optical and nonoptical elements. The fundamental element consists of a 60-cm-long glass–fiber bundle (10,000–30,000 fibers per bundle) running the length of the insertion cord. Each fiber is 8 to 12 microns in diameter and is coated with a secondary glass layer termed *cladding*. Broken fibers, which can easily occur with bending of the insertion cord, entrapping of the cord in other equipment, or dropping the fiberoptic bronchoscope, are readily apparent as missing pixels in the image. These are typically just a nuisance until the number of broken fibers interferes with the visual field. The new generation of video-based flexible scopes employ a light-sensitive CMOS chip in the distal insertion cord. This technology offers high-definition images at reduced production costs. A single-use version of this technology is available (aScope 3, Ambu, Ballerup, Denmark; Fig. 28-26).

Along with imaging elements, the insertion cord contains an *accessory lumen* or "working channel": a lumen, up to 2 mm in diameter, which travels from the distal tip to the handle. This can be used for applying suction, administering oxygen or medications (e.g., local anesthetics) or placing a wire for wire-guided airway exchange techniques (e.g., the Arndt Airway Exchange Catheter Kit, Cook Critical Care, Bloomington, IN). In general, flexible intubation scopes that are less than 2 mm in external diameter (e.g., pediatric) do not have a working channel.

The distal end of the insertion cord is hinged for movement. Two wires, traveling from the control lever in the handle down the length of the insertion cord, control the movement of the distal tip in the sagittal plane. Coronal plane movement is accomplished by a combined use of the control lever and rotation of the *entire* flexible intubation scope (from handle to distal end). It is key to keep the insertion cord completely straight as this maximizes rotational control by ensuring that rotation of the hand piece translates to identical rotation of the distal tip.

The final element of the flexible scope is the light source. In the fiberoptic devices, illumination of the objective is provided by one or two noncoherent bundles of glass fibers that transmit light from the handle to the distal tip. The light is provided either by a cord that emerges from the handle and is inserted into an endoscopic light source or may be provided by a portable battery-operated light source on the handle. CMOS-based flexible scopes are fitted with an LED light source in the distal tip, obviating the need for glass bundles in the insertion cord.

Table 28-19 Contraindications to Flexible Scope Intubation

Hypoxia
Significant airway secretions not relieved with antisialagogues and suction
Airway bleeding not relieved with suctioning
Local anesthetic allergy (for awake attempts)
Inability to cooperate (for awake attempts)

Table 28-20 Common Reasons for Failure of Flexible Scope Intubation

Lack of provider experience
Failure to adequately dry the airway: antisialagogue underdose, rushed technique
Failure to adequately anesthetize the airway (awake patient)
Nasal cavity bleeding: inadequate vasoconstriction/lubrication, rushed technique
Obstructing base of tongue: insufficient tongue displacement (may require jaw thrust/tongue extrusion)
Hang-up: ETT/scope diameter ratio too large
Flexible scope fogging: suction or oxygen not attached to working channel, cold bronchoscope

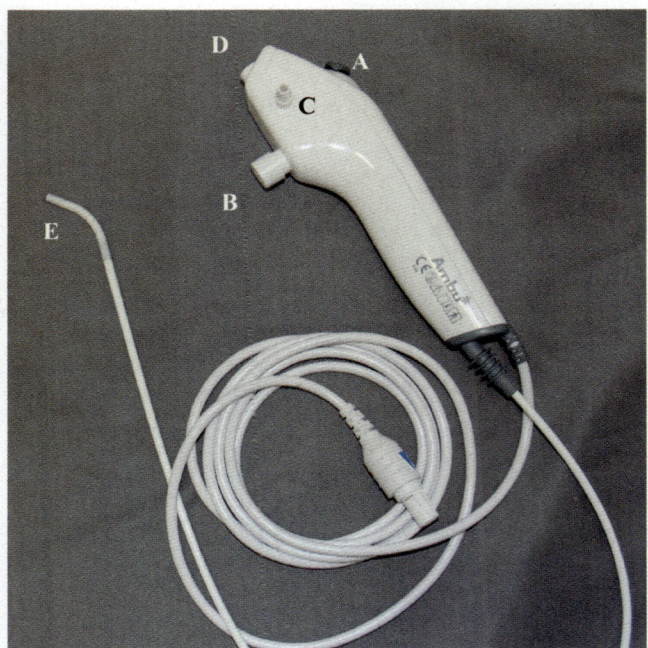

Figure 28-26 The Ambu aScope 3 single-use flexible intubation scope. (Ambu, Ballerup, Denmark). **A:** Directional control. **B:** Suction/oxygen activator valve. **C:** Suction/oxygen attachment port. **D:** Working channel access. **E:** Articulating objective end.

Flexible bronchoscope-aided intubation is a technology-intense technique. Apart from the delicate optics, there are cameras, recorders, light sources, and a variety of disposable adjuncts that are typically required. Dedicated wheeled carts, designed to carry equipment in a functional arrangement, are often utilized.

Use of the Flexible Intubation Scope

The flexible intubation scope is held with the thumb over the control lever and the index finger poised over the working channel valve. The contralateral hand is used to steady and hold the insertion cord at the level of the patient. An experienced endoscopist will recognize that the fine control required for steadying the bronchoscope while making minute directional adjustments and advancing it through the airway is where the art of endoscopy lies.

The flexible scope insertion cord is lubricated with a medical-grade lubricant and threaded through the lumen of an ETT with the objective end emerging from the main ETT orifice. A clinically appropriate ETT should be chosen, as the greater the difference between the internal diameter of the ETT and the external diameter of the insertion cord, the greater the risk of "hang-up" on airway structures.

"Hang-up" occurs when a cleft exists between the ETT and intubating guide (e.g., AEC, flexible scope insertion cord, gum-elastic bougie, retrograde wire, lighted stylet) because of the difference in their sizes (Fig. 28-27). This is most thoroughly described with flexible scope-aided intubation, for which it occurs in 20% to 30% of attempts.[193] Hang-up most commonly involves the right vocal cord, but may involve entrapment of the epiglottis, corniculate/arytenoid cartilages, or aryepiglottic folds. If hang-up occurs, rotation of the ETT 90 degrees counterclockwise places the bevel cleft posteriorly and improves passage.

During nasotracheal intubation, the epiglottis may be entrapped and a bevel-up position (rotation of the ETT 90 degrees clockwise) may facilitate passage.[196]

Tracheal tube design may also affect hang-up. It has been suggested that the Parker Flex-Tip tracheal tube may pass the airway structures more easily than a standard ETT bevel.[196] The use of soft-tipped ETTs, asking the patient to inspire deeply during the ETT advancement, and the "double setup," which uses a small ETT within a clinically adequate ETT (e.g., a 5.0 ID inside a 7.5 ID) to overcome the size differentials, have been described as well.[197]

The route of intubation, either oral or nasal, is based on surgical needs, patient anatomy and clinical condition, operator experience, and other techniques available should primary attempts fail. The nasal route is considered anatomically easier by many clinicians, although cautions apply: the turbinates may obstruct ETT passage, bleed, be avulsed, or be painful when traumatized.[198] Nasal vasoconstrictors should be applied to reduce bleeding and promote nasal patency. An ETT of the smallest size clinically acceptable should be chosen. The nasal tube is softened in warm saline or water[199] and well lubricated prior to insertion.

While mandibular advancement and/or tongue extraction typically suffice, a variety of oral airways designed to facilitate flexible scope orotracheal intubation are commercially available. These devices function to provide a clear visual path from the oral aperture to the hypopharynx, keep the bronchoscope and tracheal tube midline, prevent the patient from biting the insertion cord, and provide a clear airway for spontaneous or mask ventilation. The common characteristic of all intubating oral

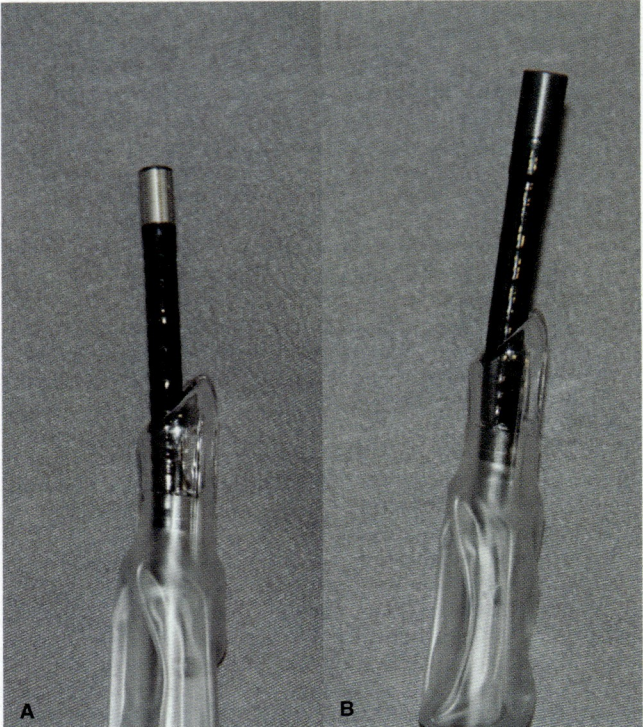

Figure 28-27 Size discrepancy between an airway exchange catheter or flexible intubation scope and a tracheal tube can create clefts that can trap tissues and hinder intubation. **A:** A 6.5-ID tracheal tube inserted over a 3.2-mm Storz Endovision F.I.V.E. scope (Karl Storz, Tuttlingen, Germany) with a notable cleft. **B:** The same tracheal tube inserted over a 5.5-mm Storz Endovision F.I.V.E. scope with near-complete obliteration of the cleft.

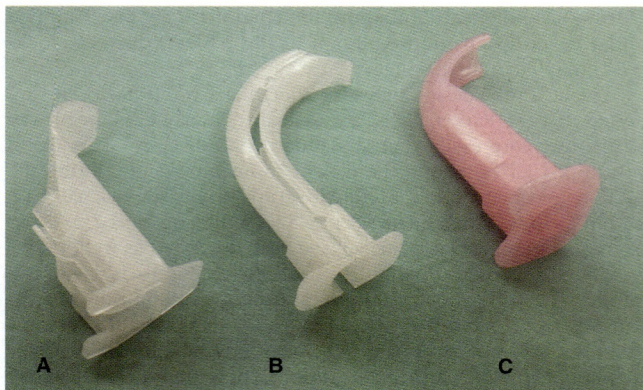

Figure 28-28 Intubating oral airways: (**A**) Ovassapian, (**B**) Berman and (**C**) Williams intubating oral airways.

airways is a channel along the length of the airway that accommodates passage of an ETT.

The Ovassapian intubating oral airway (Fig. 28-28) provides two sets of semicircular, incomplete flexible flanges that stabilize the ETT (up to size 9 ID) in the midline and allow easy disengagement from the ETT after successful intubation. The flat lingual surface of the airway affords lateral and rotational stability. Both the Williams and the Berman airways were designed for blind orotracheal intubation. Both are molded plastic with circular internal lumens that guide the ETT toward the larynx. These airways have a smaller profile than the Ovassapian airway, but tend to have less rotational stability. Because its internal lumen is a complete circle, the ETT circuit adapter must be removed prior to withdrawing a Williams airway. This may pose difficulty if the ETT has a fused circuit adapter. The Berman airway addresses this problem with a split along the length of one side. If the interincisor gap is adequate, malleable plastic seams on the contralateral side allow the airway to be removed laterally from around the ETT.

After successful navigation past the tongue (whether facilitated by tongue extraction, mandibular advancement, or an intubating oral airway), the endoscopist visualizes the vocal folds. If glottic closure, gag, or coughing occurs, the operator can choose to apply local anesthetic through the working channel, administer more intravenous sedation, withdraw the scope and reinforce airway analgesia, or advance the scope into the larynx without further preparation. The action taken must be dictated by the individual clinical situation. In the elective scenario, there is likely to be time for additional airway preparation, whereas in the face of impending respiratory arrest, patient discomfort may need to be tolerated.

Once the larynx is entered, the flexible scope is advanced until the carina is visualized. The ETT is then advanced off the insertion cord and into the trachea. Simply having the flexible scope enter the trachea does not guarantee that the intubation will be successful; hang-up and accidental scope withdrawal (via coughing or inattention) may still occur. Therefore, a patient with a critical airway should not be induced with a general anesthetic until intratracheal tube placement is confirmed. The distance between the ETT and carina can be readily determined by advancing the scope to the carina and measuring how far it can be withdrawn before the objective reenters the ETT bevel.

The primary literature contains a number of variations and adjuncts to flexible scope-aided intubation. Table 28-21, which is not meant to be exhaustive, lists several of these techniques.

Table 28-21 Flexible Scope-aided Intubation Techniques

Technique	Advantage
Endoscopy mask	Controlled (or assisted) ventilation maintained during or between attempts at flexible scope-aided intubation
Laryngeal mask	Excellent view of the larynx and ability to ventilate during or between attempts
Flexible scope-aided retrograde intubation	Guiding of the flexible intubating scope with a wire known to be in the trachea
Retrograde fiberoptic intubation	Changing a tracheostomy to an oral or nasal tracheal tube when antegrade intubation is difficult or impossible
Flexible scope intubation with the aid of a rigid laryngoscope	Helpful with an obstructing mass or large epiglottis

Case 3: Failed Rapid-sequence Induction and the SGA

A 39-year-old man who is healthy aside from obstructive sleep apnea (apnea-hypopnea index of 15) and has no surgical history presents for elective uvulopharyngopalatoplasty. His maximal interincisor gap is 5 cm, thyromental distance is 7 cm, and his oropharyngeal view is a Samsoon–Young class 2.[103] There is no limitation in neck flexion or extension. The patient has significant gastroesophageal reflux; thus, an RSI is planned. As cricoid pressure is held (Sellick maneuver), a hypnotic and succinylcholine are administered. DL with a Macintosh 3 blade is made difficult by significant base of tongue hyperplasia and all that can be visualized is a large epiglottis (Cormack–Lehane grade 3 view). The BURP maneuver does not improve glottic visualization. Macintosh 4 and Miller 3 blades are utilized without improvement of the glottic view. Oxygen saturation has fallen from 100% to 92% and facemask ventilation is initiated with maintenance of cricoid pressure. Complete obstruction to ventilation is encountered. Placement of an oral airway, chin and jaw lift, two-person ventilation, and reduction in the degree of cricoid pressure do not result in adequate mask ventilation. The oxygen saturation falls to 85% and a size 5 LMA Classic (which had been prepared prior to induction) is inserted with maintenance of cricoid pressure. A clear airway is immediately noted. A second dose of hypnotic is administered and the patient is intubated by the blind passage of an Aintree Intubation Catheter (Cook Critical Care, Bloomington, IN), guided into position with a flexible intubation scope. The LMA and flexible scope are removed and the Aintree catheter is used to guide a tracheal tube into position.

The SGA in the Failed Airway

Kheterpal et al. found that 0.4% of patients presented difficulty in both mask ventilation and DL[114] and there have been many reports of cases in which the airway was rescued with an SGA.[200,201] A wealth of literature describes the use of the various SGAs, in both awake and unconscious patients, in anticipated and unanticipated difficult airway situations, cervical spine injury, and pediatric dysmorphic syndromes.[89,90,176]

The characteristics of the SGAs that underlie their superiority as a tool in the management of the difficult airway are numerous: Their placement follows an intrinsic pathway (swallowing) which, unlike laryngoscopy, requires minimal tissue distortion; they can be utilized as part of a blind technique not hindered by blood, secretions, debris, and edema from previous attempts at laryngoscopy[202]; and, as the anatomic issues that result in difficult laryngoscopy do not necessarily result in difficult SGA placement, they are an excellent choice for airway rescue when laryngoscopy has failed. Because the success of SGA placement does not fully depend on anatomy that can be assessed on routine physical examination, many typical airway assessment measures do not apply.[203]

The major disadvantage of SGA use during cardiopulmonary resuscitation is the lack of mechanical protection from aspiration.[204–206] Cricoid pressure is effective with an LMA in situ, but may prevent proper seating in a minority of instances[207]—this may require the brief removal of cricoid pressure until the LMA has been properly seated. Despite these drawbacks, the rate of regurgitation during cardiopulmonary resuscitation with an LMA (3.5%) has been shown to be less than with bag-valve-mask ventilation (12.4%).[64] Even in cases of regurgitation, pulmonary aspiration is a rare event[60] and a secondary concern to life-threatening hypoxemia. Had one been available, an intubating SGA would have been an excellent choice in this case scenario.

Case 4: Deviation from the Difficult Airway Algorithm

Thirteen hours after admission to the intensive care unit, a 76-year-old woman with head, neck, and facial trauma from a motor vehicle accident is noted to have progressive decline in her level of consciousness and respiratory effort. On examination, there appears to be an adequate interincisor gap and thyromental distance, but the oropharyngeal view and cervical range of motion cannot be evaluated. Because of the inability to evaluate her airway fully with respect to ease of intubation, an awake technique is chosen. Oropharyngeal blood from continued epistaxis suggests that adequate drying and analgesia of the airway may be difficult and that the use of a flexible intubation device may not be prudent. Techniques requiring significant patient preparation are not considered due to the rapid progression of the patient's respiratory failure. Blind nasal intubation is contraindicated based on the obvious facial trauma and the risk of cribriform plate disruption. Neither an esophageal tube nor equipment for retrograde intubation is readily available. Although the patient's altered mental status is believed to reflect an intracranial process, the risk of airway loss is considered to be the primary clinical hazard. Awake DL is attempted with manual in-line axial stabilization of the neck. After clearing fresh blood from the pharynx, a Cormack–Lehane grade 3 laryngeal view is obtained. Due to significant patient resistance (head and neck movement and biting of the laryngoscope), tracheal intubation is not achieved. The decision is made to proceed with RSI and intubation, with emergency tracheostomy as the back-up plan. After surgical preparation of the neck, application of manual in-line stabilization, and preoxygenation, intravenous etomidate and succinylcholine are administered, DL is undertaken, the larynx is easily visualized, and the trachea is intubated.

Muscle Relaxants and Direct Laryngoscopy

In the case described, the use of muscle relaxants significantly improved laryngeal visualization. In one study, the use of muscle relaxants for DL increased intubation success rate and was associated with fewer intubation attempts, incidents of airway trauma, esophageal intubations, aspiration events, and even deaths.[208] A retrospective study in the pediatric population also found an increased rate of airway complications in patients intubated without the aid of a paralytic.[209] There are few well-controlled trials investigating the effects of muscle relaxants on intubating conditions, though, as the superior conditions achieved with these medications have discouraged inclusion of control groups. Muscle relaxation improves laryngoscopic view by facilitating temporomandibular joint relaxation, relaxation of the supraglottic larynx, and anterior movement of the epiglottis.[210] Muscle relaxants also tend to fix the vocal folds in a neutral open position. Neuromuscular blockade tends to facilitate facemask ventilation and is often utilized in cases in which facemask ventilation is unexpectedly difficult. The classic teaching of withholding muscle relaxants until facemask ventilation has been demonstrated is rapidly being abandoned.

Leaving the Algorithm

The scenario described in case 4 is unusual in that the clinical situation necessitated deviation from the ASA-DAA. The conditions described were more akin to the "crash" airway described by Walls.[211] In this case, the administration of a muscle relaxant, which might be considered contraindicated in the assumed difficult-to-intubate patient, allowed for full visualization of the larynx. Knowing that failure to intubate would likely result in loss of the airway, the clinical team was wisely prepared for cricothyrotomy. Although the ASA-DAA is a valuable tool in the management of the difficult airway, the clinician must be prepared for cases that do not fit the mold. As stated earlier, adaptability in rapidly changing clinical scenarios is critical to the success of airway management.

Other Devices

An ever-increasing number of airway management devices are commercially available. Although encyclopedic coverage of these tools is beyond the scope of this chapter, a review of the more established equipment follows.

Esophageal Tubes with Laryngeal Openings. Esophageal tubes with laryngeal openings are SGAs with designs based on the propensity for blindly inserted oral tubes to enter the esophagus. They can be of single-lumen (King LT, Ambu, Ballerup, Denmark) and double-lumen (Combitube, Covidien, Mansfield, MA, and EasyTube, Teleflex, Research Triangle Park, NC) design with distal esophageal and proximal pharyngeal cuffs on either side of the laryngeal apertures, which act as ventilation ports (Fig. 28-29). When properly inflated, the cuffs prevent esophageal and oral leakage of gasses, making the larynx the route of least resistance for inspired gasses. These devices are quicker and easier for inexperienced providers to place than are ETTs.[212] This, combined with data showing the deleterious effects of repeat laryngoscopy,[183,184] has led to frequent use of these devices by prehospital emergency providers who may have limited or infrequent experience with laryngoscopy.

Airway Bougie

Airway bougies are semimalleable stylets that may be blindly manipulated through the glottis when a poor laryngeal view is obtained (Cormack-Lehane grade 3 or 4). An ETT is then "threaded" over the bougie and into the trachea. These bougies are generally low cost and highly portable. The Eschmann introducer (Eschmann Health Care, Kent, England) is a 60-cm long,

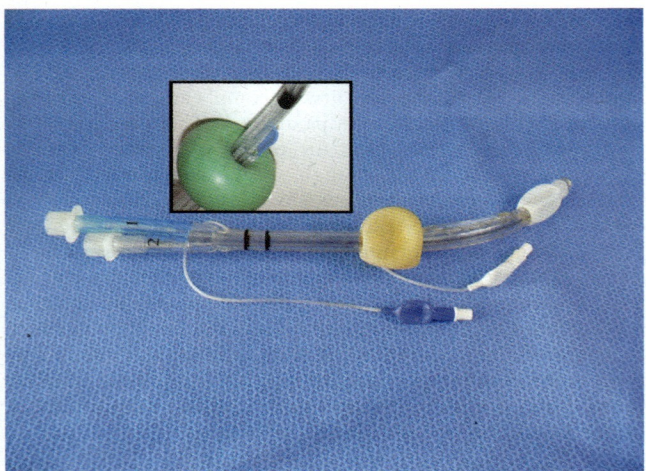

Figure 28-29 The Esophageal Tracheal Combitube. Inset: The fiberoptic port of the EasyTube.

Table 28-23 Equipment for Retrograde Wire Intubation

Angiocatheter (18 gauge or larger)
Luer-lock syringe (3 mL or larger)
Guide wire:
- Type: J-type end preferable
- Length: at least 2.5 times the length of a standard ETT (typically 110–120 cm)
- Diameter: capable of passing via chosen angiocatheter

Other: scalpel blade, nerve hook, Magill forceps, silk suture

15 French bougie with a 40 degree coudé tip 3.5 cm from its distal end. This introducer (also known as the *gum elastic bougie*) can be manipulated under the epiglottis, its angled segment directed anteriorly toward the larynx. Once it has entered the larynx and trachea, the operator often feels "clicks" as the bougie's tip passes over the cartilaginous structures of the anterior trachea. A similar device, the Frova Intubating Introducer (Cook Critical Care, Bloomington, IN) is a disposable device with a narrow internal lumen. The lumen allows for the insufflation of oxygen, detection of carbon dioxide, and use of a self-inflating bulb to detect inadvertent esophageal placement. An optional "stiffening" stylet can be placed through the lumen to increase device rigidity.

Transtracheal Procedures. When intubation and mask and SGA ventilation fail, airway access via the extrathoracic trachea may be warranted (Table 28-22). Though the noninvasive tools of the modern airway armamentarium can manage most situations, the clinician must be familiar with these alternative techniques of intubation, oxygenation, and ventilation for both elective and emergency airway access. This text will focus on percutaneous techniques, as surgical tracheostomy and cricothyrotomy are beyond the scope of this chapter.

Retrograde Wire-Aided Tracheal Intubation

In 1993, the technique of retrograde wire intubation (RWI) was included in the ASA's Difficult Airway Algorithm, but removed in the 2013 update. The technique involves the antegrade passage of an ETT into the airway using a wire that has been passed into the larynx via a percutaneous puncture through the cricothyroid or cricotracheal membrane. This wire is blindly passed in the cephalad direction into the hypopharynx, pharynx, and out of the mouth or nose and then used as an intubating conduit. The basic equipment used for retrograde intubation is listed in Table 28-23.

RWI has been described in a number of clinical situations as a primary intubation technique (both elective and urgently) and for use after failed attempts at DL, fiberoptic-aided intubation, and LMA-guided intubation.[44] The most common indication for RWI is the inability to visualize the vocal folds owing to blood, secretions, unstable cervical spine or anatomic variations (e.g., upper airway malignancy, mandibular fracture, massive airway trauma). Contraindications include lack of access to the CTM or cricotracheal ligament (such as with severe neck deformity, obesity, or overlying mass), laryngotracheal disease (stenosis, malignancy, infection), coagulopathy, and overlying skin infection.

Common complications reported with RWI include bleeding, subcutaneous emphysema, pneumomediastinum, pneumothorax, breath-holding, a caudally traveling wire, and trigeminal nerve trauma.

Cricothyrotomy

Cricothyrotomy, cricothyroidotomy, coniotomy, and minitracheostomy are synonyms for establishing an air passage through the CTM. The CTM is a fibroelastic membrane that overlays the tracheal mucosa and is attached to the inferior border of the thyroid cartilage and superior edge of the cricoid cartilage. Although cricothyrotomy is the procedure of choice in an emergency situation, it may also be of use in elective situations when there is limited access to the trachea (e.g., severe cervical kyphoscoliosis). Cricothyrotomy is contraindicated in children younger than 6 years of age and in patients with laryngeal fractures. Otolaryngologists and other surgical services prefer transtracheal airway access caudad to the cricoid cartilage whenever feasible due to the high incidence of long-term complications after surgical cricothyrotomy.

Percutaneous Emergency Airway Access (PEAA), as a form of cricothyrotomy, is the most familiar to anesthesiologists. The ASA-DAA lists PEAA as an option in the "cannot mask ventilate/cannot intubate" (CNV/CNI) situation. PEAA is a simple and relatively safe means to sustain the patient's life in this critical situation.[44] Three techniques are commonly used for PEAA: narrow-bore catheter over a needle, large-bore cannula over a wire or trochar, and surgical cutdown[182] with or without a tube guide.[213] Success rates of these techniques vary greatly and are highly dependent on operator experience and the clinical scenario. As an example, the success rate of cannula cricothyrotomy performed by an anesthesia provider is roughly 50%,[1] while the success rate of an emergency surgical airway performed by a surgeon or trained prehospital provider is 90% to 100%.[1,214] This is not to suggest that PEAA be avoided by the anesthesia provider,

Table 28-22 Criteria for Performing Emergent Invasive Airway Management

When all five criteria are met, an emergent invasive airway is indicated
- Cannot intubate
- Cannot ventilate
- Cannot awaken patient
- Supraglottic airway has failed
- Clinically significant hypoxemia

but rather to advise that, if available, a surgeon experienced in cricothyrotomy may be the better choice for the initial attempt at surgical airway management.

A body of literature exists detailing the jerry-rigging of conveyance systems for PEAA and the use of intravenous catheters for transtracheal puncture. These systems have proven to be faulty, inadequate, and dangerous.[215] Catheters designed for intravenous infusion are known to kink in the airway.[216] Experts in the field recommend that all anesthetizing locations have access to both manufactured high-pressure oxygen conveyance devices and percutaneous transtracheal jet ventilation (PTJV), also known as Percutaneous Transtracheal Volume Ventilation–specific translaryngeal catheters). Dedicated devices, such as the Cook TTJV Catheter (Cook Critical Care, Bloomington, IN), are made of kink-resistant materials and designed specifically for this task. The Ravussin translaryngeal catheter (VBM Medizintechnik, Sulz am Neckar Germany) is precurved to reduce kinking.

Before contemplating PEAA, the location of the CTM will need to be identified. Campbell et al.[10] have cast doubt on the ability of anesthesiologists to locate the CTM in elective, let alone emergency, situations. Obesity, cervical kyphosis, female gender, therapeutic radiation, and surgical or traumatic scarring may hinder CTM identification. A careful reading of the ASA-DAA should lead the airway manager to identify the CTM in every patient, and applying this examination in all instances should improve familiarity with the surface landmarks.[182] Bedside ultrasound in the sagittal plane can reveal the CTM as a lucent shadow between opaque cartilaginous structures and may be useful in emergency situations if immediately available.

When performing PEAA, the patient is positioned supine with the head midline or extended on the neck and thorax (if not contraindicated by the clinical situation). After aseptic preparation, local anesthetic may be injected over the CTM (if the patient is awake and time permits). The clinician stands to the side of the patient with one's dominant hand cephalad and can use the nondominant hand to stabilize the larynx. A large-bore translaryngeal catheter (14 gauge or larger) attached to a 5- to 10-mL empty or fluid-filled (saline or local anesthetic) syringe is used. The catheter-needle is advanced at right angles to the plane of the cervical spine through the caudad third of the CTM. From the moment of skin puncture, there should be constant aspiration on the syringe plunger. Free aspiration of air confirms entrance into the trachea (air-contrast technique) but does not indicate the direction that the catheter travels in the larynx; this is important, as cephalad advancement will not provide adequate oxygenation. Unless there is significant pulmonary fluid (e.g., blood or aspirated liquid), the aspiration of tracheal air should be incontrovertible. The needle–catheter assembly should be advanced slightly prior to threading of the catheter into the airway.

Once the catheter has been successfully placed, a high-pressure oxygen source should be attached. A 50-psi oxygen source with a metered and adjustable hand-controlled valve and a Luer-lock connector (Fig. 28-30) is down-regulated to 15 to 30 psi (central hospital supply or regulated cylinder) and delivered through the catheter. Insufflations should last 1 to 1.5 seconds at a rate of 12 insufflations per minute. Insufflation and expiration ratios, as well as driving pressure, are adjusted to provide visible chest excursion and recoil. If a 14-gauge catheter has been placed, this system will deliver a tidal volume of 400 to 700 mL. Low-pressure systems cannot provide enough flow to expand the chest adequately for oxygenation and ventilation (e.g., Ambu bag, 6 psi; anesthesia machine common gas outlet, 20 psi). Critically, systems delivering pressurized oxygen require a path for gas egress.[217] Standard high-pressure regulating valves, as described earlier, are unidirectional and generally contraindicated when the upper airway is

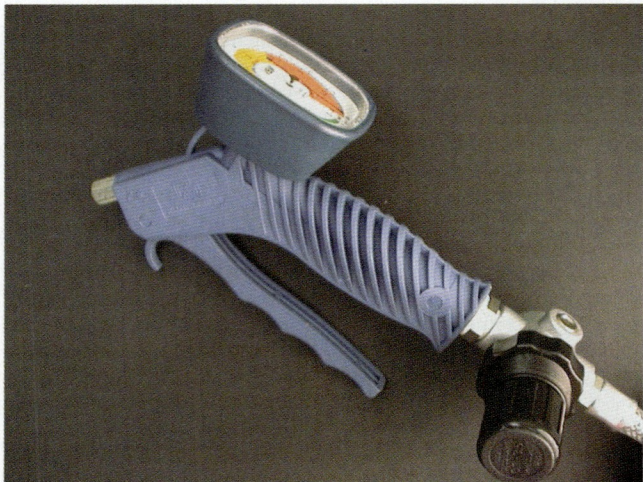

Figure 28-30 System for regulation of a high-pressure oxygen source for transtracheal jet ventilation.

completely obstructed. Fortunately, this tends to be an uncommon situation. In any case, the clinician employing any type of translaryngeal oxygenation must strive to maintain upper airway patency with devices such as oral airways, nasal airways, or SGAs.

PEAA can also be accomplished using low-flow oxygen delivery meters, which are common in the hospital environment. These systems are capable of delivering a constant flow of 15 L/min and have been shown to be effective for resuscitation. Generally, these devices utilize "flow interruption." Flow is directed to the patient during the inspiratory phase, then diverted during expiration. As discussed earlier, jerry-rigged devices often fail to function as desired. For example, using a standard three-way stopcock as a flow diverter is potentially hazardous, as forward flow (inspiration) is never fully stopped.[218] The Enk flow modulator (Cook Critical Care, Bloomington, IN) is a simple hand-operated flow diverter that not only stops forward gas flow during the expiratory phase but also acts as a pathway for passive expiratory flow (Fig. 28-31). The Enk flow modulator has been used successfully in models of near and complete upper airway obstruction.[215]

A new concept in PEAA is "expiratory ventilatory assistance."[219] Using the Bernoulli principle, the Ventrain (Ventinova Medical B.V., Eindhoven, The Netherlands; Fig. 28-31) is

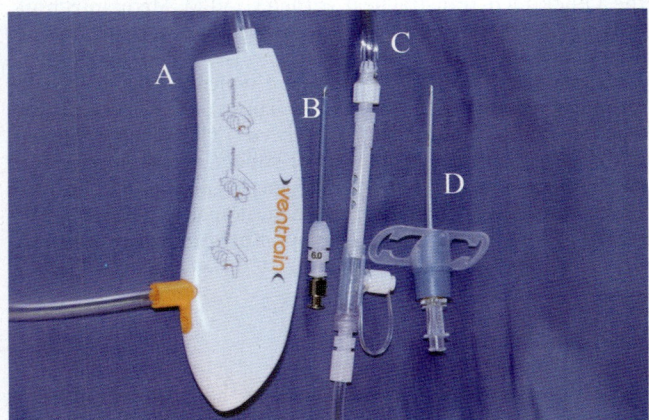

Figure 28-31 (**A**) Ventrain. (**B**) Cook Transtracheal Catheter. (**C**) Enk flow modulator. (**D**) Ravussin needle.

capable of *active* gas removal from a rescue catheter during the expiratory phase of PEAA. The clear benefit is the avoidance of air trapping in the lungs, especially when the upper airway is completely obstructed. The device can achieve physiologic minute ventilation via a 2-mm ID transtracheal catheter[219] and has been effective in oxygenation and carbon dioxide removal in two large animal models.[220,221] In the first of these studies, the upper airways were critically or completely obstructed and the animals ventilated for 15 minutes via the Ventrain or a commercially available jet ventilation system. While both devices facilitated reoxygenation, the Ventrain was associated with superior minute ventilation (4.7 vs. 0.1 L/min), a lesser degree of acidosis (pH of 7.34 vs. 7.01) and decreased peak airway pressure on rescue (16 vs. 40 cm H_2O).[220] In the latter study, in a complete upper airway obstruction model, the peak airway pressure was significantly less with the Ventrain using an I:E of 1:1 (30 mbar) than with the commercial jet ventilator at a ratio of 1:4 (50 mbar),[221] highlighting the benefit of expiratory ventilatory assistance. The Ventrain has also proven effective in both elective and emergent human airway management.[222,223]

Specialized percutaneous cricothyrotomy systems have been developed to improve the ease of transtracheal ventilation. These devices generally provide large-bore access adequate for oxygenation and ventilation with low-pressure systems. The Melker emergency cricothyrotomy catheter set (Cook Critical Care, Bloomington, IN) is placed using Seldinger technique and comes in a variety of cannula sizes (3.5-, 4-, and 6-mm ID, both cuffed and uncuffed). Preparation and positioning of the patient are the same as with needle cricothyrotomy. A 1- to 1.5-cm vertical incision, through the skin only, is made over the lower third of the CTM. Aiming 45 degrees caudally, a percutaneous puncture of the CTM is made with the provided 18-gauge needle–catheter assembly and syringe. After air is aspirated, the catheter is advanced into the trachea as described earlier. The provided guidewire is inserted through the catheter and into the trachea. The catheter is removed and the large-bore tracheal cannula, fitted internally with a curved dilator, is threaded onto the wire. The dilator is advanced through the CTM using firm pressure. Significant resistance on advancement typically indicates that the skin incision needs to be extended. Once the cannula–dilator assembly has been fully inserted, the dilator and wire are removed. The cannula's 15-mm circuit adapter is attached to a self-inflating resuscitation bag or anesthesia circuit and ventilation is initiated.

Other percutaneous needle systems include the Portex Cricothyroidotomy Kit (Smiths Medical, Minneapolis, MN) and the Quicktrach transtracheal catheter (VBM Medizintechnik, Sulz am Neckar, Germany). Nonneedle puncture techniques are beyond the scope of this text.

Severe complications of PEAA are typically related to barotrauma. Analysis of the ASA Close Claims Database reveals that 89% of patients reported who received TTJV developed pneumothorax, pneumomediastinum, or subcutaneous emphysema,[4] and bilateral tension pneumothorax has been reported.[224] Causes of air insufflation into the paratracheal spaces include a misplaced cannula, multiple tracheal punctures, and cannula migration due to patient coughing.

Conclusions

Apart from monitoring, management of the "routine" airway is the most common task of the anesthesia provider. Even during the administration of regional anesthesia, the airway must be monitored and possibly supported. The consequences of a lost airway are so devastating that the clinician can never afford a lackadaisical approach.

Although the ASA's taskforce on the difficult airway has given the medical community an immensely valuable tool in the approach to the patient with the difficult airway, the ASA's algorithm must be viewed as a starting point only. Judgment, experience, the clinical situation, and available resources all affect the appropriateness of the chosen pathway through, or divergence from, the algorithm.

Whereas one may argue that the last decade of the 20th century was the decade of the SGA, the first decades of the 21st century have brought the application of digital imaging to airway management. Although an increasingly vast array of devices exists, the clinician does not need to be expert in all the equipment and techniques, and no single device can be considered superior to another when viewed in isolation. Rather, a broad range of approaches should be mastered so that the failure of one does not preclude safe airway management and emergency rescue. The clinician's judgment and resources, both equipment and personnel, determine the effectiveness of any technique. When managing the difficult airway, flexibility, not rigidity, prevails.

REFERENCES

1. Cook TM, Woodall N, Frerk C, et al. Major complications of airway management in the UK: results of the Fourth National Audit Project of the Royal College of Anaesthetists and the Difficult Airway Society. Part 1: anaesthesia. *Br J Anaesth.* 2011;106:617–631.
2. Apfelbaum JL, Hagberg CA, Caplan RA, et al. Practice guidelines for management of the difficult airway: an updated report by the American Society of Anesthesiologists Task Force on Management of the Difficult Airway. *Anesthesiology.* 2013;118:251–270.
3. Frerk C, Mitchell VS, McNarry AF, et al. Difficult Airway Society 2015 guidelines for management of unanticipated difficult intubation in adults. *Br J Anaesth.* 2015;115:827–848.
4. Peterson GN, Domino KB, Caplan RA, et al. Management of the difficult airway: a closed claims analysis. *Anesthesiology.* 2005;103:33–39.
5. Li G, Warner M, Lang BH, et al. Epidemiology of anesthesia-related mortality in the United States, 1999–2005. *Anesthesiology.* 2009;110:759–765.
6. Hove LD, Steinmetz J, Christoffersen JK, et al. Analysis of deaths related to anesthesia in the period 1996–2004 from closed claims registered by the Danish Patient Insurance Association. *Anesthesiology.* 2007;106:675–680.
7. Rosenblatt WH. The Airway Approach Algorithm: a decision tree for organizing preoperative airway information. *J Clin Anesth.* 2004;16:312–316.
8. Westhorpe RN. The position of the larynx in children and its relationship to the ease of intubation. *Anaesth Intensive Care.* 1987;15:384–388.
9. Iohom G, Ronayne M, Cunningham AJ. Prediction of difficult tracheal intubation. *Eur J Anaesthesiol.* 2003;20:31–36.
10. Campbell M, Shanahan H, Ash S, et al. The accuracy of locating the cricothyroid membrane by palpation—an intergender study. *BMC Anesthesiol.* 2014;14:108.
11. Kristensen MS, Teoh WH, Graumann O, et al. Ultrasonography for clinical decision-making and intervention in airway management: from the mouth to the lungs and pleurae. *Insights Imaging.* 2014;5:253–279.
12. Sykes W, ed. *Essays on the First Hundred Years of Anesthesia.* London: Churchill Livingstone; 1982.
13. Brimacombe J, ed. *Laryngeal Mask Anesthesia: Principles and Practice.* Philadelphia, PA: Saunders; 2005.
14. Brandt L. The first reported oral intubation of the human trachea. *Anesth Analg.* 1987;66:1198–1199.
15. Magill IW. Technique in endotracheal anaesthesia. *Proc R Soc Med.* 1928;22:
16. Mendelson CL. The aspiration of stomach contents into the lungs during obstetric anesthesia. *Am J Obstetr Gynecol.* 1946;52:191–205.
17. Ovassapian A, Yelich SJ, Dykes MH, et al. Learning fibreoptic intubation: use of simulators v. traditional teaching. *Br J Anaesth.* 1988;61:217–220.
18. Kaplan MB, Ward DS, Berci G. A new video laryngoscope-an aid to intubation and teaching. *J Clin Anesth.* 2002;14:620–626.
19. Breitmeier D, Wilke N, Schulz Y, et al. The lingual tonsillar hyperplasia in relation to unanticipated difficult intubation: is there any relationship between lingual tonsillar hyperplasia and tonsillectomy? *Am J Forensic Med Pathol.* 2005;26:131–135.
20. Langeron O, Masso E, Huraux C, et al. Prediction of difficult mask ventilation. *Anesthesiology.* 2000;92:1229–1236.
21. Rosenblatt W, Ianus AI, Sukhupragarn W, et al. Preoperative endoscopic airway examination (PEAE) provides superior airway information

and may reduce the use of unnecessary awake intubation. *Anesth Analg.* 2011;112:602–607.
22. Shiga T, Wajima Z, Inoue T, et al. Predicting difficult intubation in apparently normal patients: a meta-analysis of bedside screening test performance. *Anesthesiology.* 2005;103:429–437.
23. el-Ganzouri AR, McCarthy RJ, Tuman KJ, et al. Preoperative airway assessment: predictive value of a multivariate risk index. *Anesth Analg.* 1996;82:1197–1204.
24. Wilson ME, Spiegelhalter D, Robertson JA, et al. Predicting difficult intubation. *Br J Anaesth.* 1988;61:211–216.
25. Patel SK, Whitten CW, Ivy R, 3rd, et al. Failure of the laryngeal mask airway: an undiagnosed laryngeal carcinoma. *Anesth Analg.* 1998;86:438–439.
26. Naguib M, Malabarey T, AlSatli RA, et al. Predictive models for difficult laryngoscopy and intubation. A clinical, radiologic and three-dimensional computer imaging study. *Can J Anaesth.* 1999;46:748–759.
27. Eberhart LH, Arndt C, Aust HJ, et al. A simplified risk score to predict difficult intubation: Development and prospective evaluation in 3763 patients. *Eur J Anaesthesiol.* 2011;27:935–940.
28. Cortellazzi P, Minati L, Falcone C, et al. Predictive value of the El-Ganzouri multivariate risk index for difficult tracheal intubation: a comparison of Glidescope videolaryngoscopy and conventional Macintosh laryngoscopy. *Br J Anaesth.* 2007;99:906–911.
29. Aziz MF, Healy D, Kheterpal S, et al. Routine clinical practice effectiveness of the Glidescope in difficult airway management: an analysis of 2,004 Glidescope intubations, complications, and failures from two institutions. *Anesthesiology.* 2011;114:34–41.
30. Aziz MF, Bayman EO, Van Tienderen MM, et al. Predictors of difficult videolaryngoscopy with Glidescope or C-MAC with D-blade: secondary analysis from a large comparative videolaryngoscopy trial. *Br J Anaesth.* 2016;117:118–123.
31. Kheterpal S, Martin L, Shanks AM, et al. Prediction and outcomes of impossible mask ventilation: a review of 50,000 anesthetics. *Anesthesiology.* 2009;110:891–897.
32. Das SK, Choupoo NS, Haldar R, et al. Transtracheal ultrasound for verification of endotracheal tube placement: a systematic review and meta-analysis. *Can J Anaesth.* 2015;62:413–423.
33. Kristensen MS. Ultrasonography in the management of the airway. *Acta Anaesthesiol Scand.* 2011;55 1155–1173.
34. Tanoubi I, Drolet P, Donati F. Optimizing preoxygenation in adults. *Can J Anaesth.* 2009;56:449–466.
35. Jense HG, Dubin SA, Silverstein PI, et al. Effect of obesity on safe duration of apnea in anesthetized humans. *Anesth Analg.* 1991;72:89–93.
36. Boyce JR, Ness T, Castroman P, et al. A preliminary study of the optimal anesthesia positioning for the morbidly obese patient. *Obes Surg.* 2003;13:4–9.
37. Ramachandran SK, Cosnowski A, Shanks A, et al. Apneic oxygenation during prolonged laryngoscopy in obese patients: a randomized, controlled trial of nasal oxygen administration. *J Clin Anesth.* 2010;22:164–168.
38. Weingart SD, Levitan RM. Preoxygenation and prevention of desaturation during emergency airway management. *Ann Emerg Med.* 2012;59:165–175 e161.
39. Patel A, Nouraei SA. Transnasal Humidified Rapid-Insufflation Ventilatory Exchange (THRIVE): a physiological method of increasing apnoea time in patients with difficult airways. *Anaesthesia.* 2015;70:323–329.
40. Kwei P, Matzelle S, Wallman D, et al. Inadequate preoxygenation during spontaneous ventilation with single patient use self-inflating resuscitation bags. *Anaesth Intensive Care.* 2006;34:685–686.
41. Joffe AM, Hetzel S, Liew EC. A two-handed jaw-thrust technique is superior to the one-handed "EC-clamp" technique for mask ventilation in the apneic unconscious person. *Anesthesiology.* 2010;113:873–879.
42. Isono S, Tanaka A, Ishikawa T, et al. Sniffing position improves pharyngeal airway patency in anesthetized patients with obstructive sleep apnea. *Anesthesiology.* 2005;103:489–494.
43. Conlon NP, Sullivan RP, Herbison PG, et al. The effect of leaving dentures in place on bag-mask ventilation at induction of general anesthesia. *Anesth Analg.* 2007;105:370–373.
44. CA H, ed. *Benumof's Airway Management: Principles and Practice.* Philadelphia, PA: Mosby; 2007.
45. Joffe AM, Ramaiah R, Donahue E, et al. Ventilation by mask before and after the administration of neuromuscular blockade: a pragmatic non-inferiority trial. *BMC Anesthesiology.* 2015;15:134.
46. Rosenblatt WH, Ovassapian A, Eige S. Use of the Laryngeal Mask Airway in the United States: A Randomized Survey of ASA Members. In: *ASA Annual Meeting,* Orlando, FL; October 1998.
47. Halaseh BK, Sukkar ZF, Hassan LH, et al. The use of ProSeal laryngeal mask airway in caesarean section—experience in 3000 cases. *Anaesth Intensive Care.* 2010;38:1023–1028.
48. Yentis SM, Lee DJ. Evaluation of an improved scoring system for the grading of direct laryngoscopy. *Anaesthesia.* 1998;53:1041–1044.
49. Kim ES, Bishop MJ. Endotracheal intubation, but not laryngeal mask airway insertion, produces reversible bronchoconstriction. *Anesthesiology.* 1999;90:391–394.
50. Ezri T, Szmuk P, Warters RD, et al. Difficult airway management practice patterns among anesthesiologists practicing in the United States: have we made any progress? *J Clin Anesth.* 2003;15:418–422.
51. Woodall NM, Cook TM. National census of airway management techniques used for anaesthesia in the UK: first phase of the Fourth National Audit Project at the Royal College of Anaesthetists. *Br J Anaesth.* 2011;106:266–271.
52. Maktabi MA, Smith RB, Todd MM. Is routine endotracheal intubation as safe as we think or wish? *Anesthesiology.* 2003;99:247–248.
53. Domino KB, Posner KL, Caplan RA, et al. Airway injury during anesthesia: a closed claims analysis. *Anesthesiology.* 1999;91:1703–1711.
54. Goldmann K, Dieterich J, Roessler M. Laryngopharyngeal mucosal injury after prolonged use of the ProSeal LMA in a porcine model: a pilot study. *Can J Anaesth.* 2007;54:822–828.
55. Lamb K, James MF, Janicki PK. The laryngeal mask airway for intraocular surgery: effects on intraocular pressure and stress responses. *Br J Anaesth.* 1992;69:143–147.
56. Idrees A, Khan FA. A comparative study of positive pressure ventilation via laryngeal mask airway and endotracheal tube. *J Pak Med Assoc.* 2000;50:333–338.
57. McCrirrick A, Ramage DT, Pracilio JA, et al. Experience with the laryngeal mask airway in two hundred patients. *Anaesth Intensive Care.* 1991;19:256–260.
58. Calder I, Picard J, Chapman M, et al. Mouth opening: a new angle. *Anesthesiology.* 2003;99:799–801.
59. Seet E, Yousaf F, Gupta S, et al. Use of manometry for laryngeal mask airway reduces postoperative pharyngolaryngeal adverse events: a prospective, randomized trial. *Anesthesiology.* 2010;112:652–657.
60. Brimacombe JR, Berry A. The incidence of aspiration associated with the laryngeal mask airway: a meta-analysis of published literature. *J Clin Anesth.* 1995;7:297–305.
61. Warner MA, Warner ME, Weber JG. Clinical significance of pulmonary aspiration during the perioperative period. *Anesthesiology.* 1993;78:56–62.
62. Yardy N, Hancox D, Strang T. A comparison of two airway aids for emergency use by unskilled personnel. The Combitube and laryngeal mask. *Anaesthesia.* 1999;54:181–183.
63. Han TH, Brimacombe J, Lee EJ, et al. The laryngeal mask airway is effective (and probably safe) in selected healthy parturients for elective Cesarean section: a prospective study of 1067 cases. *Can J Anaesth.* 2001;48:1117–1121.
64. Stone BJ, Chantler PJ, Baskett PJ. The incidence of regurgitation during cardiopulmonary resuscitation: a comparison between the bag valve mask and laryngeal mask airway. *Resuscitation.* 1998;38:3–6.
65. Verghese C, Brimacombe JR. Survey of laryngeal mask airway usage in 11,910 patients: safety and efficacy for conventional and nonconventional usage. *Anesth Analg.* 1996;82:129–133.
66. Brimacombe JR, Brain AI, Berry AM, et al. Gastric insufflation and the laryngeal mask. *Anesth Analg.* 1998;86:914–915.
67. Brimacombe J, Shorney N. The laryngeal mask airway and prolonged balanced regional anaesthesia. *Can J Anaesth.* 1993;40:360–364.
68. Williams PJ, Bailey PM. Comparison of the reinforced laryngeal mask airway and tracheal intubation for adenotonsillectomy. *Br J Anaesth.* 1993;70:30–33.
69. Kaplan A, Crosby GJ, Bhattacharyya N. Airway protection and the laryngeal mask airway in sinus and nasal surgery. *Laryngoscope.* 2004;114:652–655.
70. Dezfulian C, Shojania K, Collard HR, et al. Subglottic secretion drainage for preventing ventilator-associated pneumonia: a meta-analysis. *Am J Med.* 2005;118:11–18.
71. Nair I, Bailey PM. Use of the laryngeal mask for airway maintenance following tracheal extubation. *Anaesthesia.* 1995;50:174–175.
72. Goldmann K, Kuhlmann S, Gerlach M, et al. [Removal of the laryngeal mask airway in the post-anesthesia care unit. A means of process optimization?]. *Der Anaesthesist.* 2011;60:1002–1008.
73. Deakin CD, Diprose P, Majumdar R, et al. An investigation into the quantity of secretions removed by inflated and deflated laryngeal mask airways. *Anaesthesia.* 2000;55:478–480.
74. Brimacombe JR. Advanced uses: Clinical situations. In: Brimacombe JR, Brain AIJ. *The Laryngeal Mask Airway: A Review and Practical Guide.* London: WB Saunders; 2004.
75. Turkstra TP, Smitheram AK, Alabdulhadi O, et al. The Flex-Tip tracheal tube does not reduce the incidence of postoperative sore throat: a randomized controlled trial. *Can J Anaesth.* 2011;58:1090–1096.
76. Brimacombe J, Clarke G, Keller C. Lingual nerve injury associated with the ProSeal laryngeal mask airway: a case report and review of the literature. *Br J Anaesth.* 2005;95:420–423.
77. Zand F, Amini A. Use of the laryngeal tube-S for airway management and prevention of aspiration after a failed tracheal intubation in a parturient. *Anesthesiology.* 2005;102:481–483.
78. Bortone L, Ingelmo PM, De Ninno G, et al. Randomized controlled trial comparing the laryngeal tube and the laryngeal mask in pediatric patients. *Paediatr Anaesth.* 2006;16:251–257.
79. Richebe P, Semjen F, Cros AM, et al. Clinical assessment of the laryngeal tube in pediatric anesthesia. *Paediatr Anaesth.* 2005;15:391–396.
80. Keller C, Brimacombe J, Kleinsasser A, et al. Pharyngeal mucosal pressures with the laryngeal tube airway versus ProSeal laryngeal mask airway. *Anasthesiol Intensivmed Notfallmed Schmerzther.* 2003;38:393–396.
81. Banchereau F, Delaunay F, Herve Y, et al. [Oropharyngeal ulcers following anaesthesia with the laryngeal tube S]. *Ann Fr Anesth Reanim.* 2006;25:884–887.

82. Galgon RE, Schroeder KM, Han S, et al. The air-Q((R)) intubating laryngeal airway vs the LMA-ProSeal(TM): a prospective, randomised trial of airway seal pressure. Anaesthesia. 2011;66:1093–1100.
83. O'Connor CJ, Jr., Borromeo CJ, Stix MS. Assessing ProSeal laryngeal mask positioning: the suprasternal notch test. Anesth Analg. 2002;94:1374–1375; author reply 1375.
84. Brain AI, Verghese C, Strube PJ. The LMA 'ProSeal'—a laryngeal mask with an oesophageal vent. Br J Anaesth. 2000;84:650–654.
85. Stix MS, O'Connor CJ, Jr. Depth of insertion of the ProSeal laryngeal mask airway. Br J Anaesth. 2003;90:235–237.
86. Brimacombe J, Keller C, Fullekrug B, et al. A multicenter study comparing the ProSeal and Classic laryngeal mask airway in anesthetized, nonparalyzed patients. Anesthesiology. 2002;96:289–295.
87. Evans NR, Llewellyn RL, Gardner SV, et al. Aspiration prevented by the ProSeal laryngeal mask airway: a case report. Can J Anaesth. 2002;49:413–416.
88. Su BC, Yang MW, Lee HC, et al. Protection against large-volume regurgitated fluid aspiration by the ProSeal laryngeal mask airway. Acta Anaesthesiol Taiwan. 2008;46:34–38.
89. Rosenblatt WH. The use of the LMA-ProSeal in airway resuscitation. Anesth Analg. 2003;97:1773–1775.
90. Awan R, Nolan JP, Cook TM. Use of a ProSeal laryngeal mask airway for airway maintenance during emergency Caesarean section after failed tracheal intubation. Br J Anaesth. 2004;92:144–146.
91. Lu PP, Brimacombe J, Yang C, et al. ProSeal versus the Classic laryngeal mask airway for positive pressure ventilation during laparoscopic cholecystectomy. Br J Anaesth. 2002;88:824–827.
92. Ferson DZ, Rosenblatt WH, Johansen MJ, et al. Use of the intubating LMA-Fastrach in 254 patients with difficult-to-manage airways. Anesthesiology. 2001;95:1175–1181.
93. Belena JM, Gracia JL, Ayala JL, et al. The Laryngeal Mask Airway Supreme for positive pressure ventilation during laparoscopic cholecystectomy. J Clin Anesth. 2011;23:456–460.
94. de Montblanc J, Ruscio L, Mazoit JX, et al. A systematic review and meta-analysis of the i-gel((R)) vs laryngeal mask airway in adults. Anaesthesia. 2014;69:1151–1162.
95. Shin WJ, Cheong YS, Yang HS, et al. The supraglottic airway I-gel in comparison with ProSeal laryngeal mask airway and classic laryngeal mask airway in anaesthetized patients. Eur J Anaesth. 2010;27:598–601.
96. Bannister FB, Macbeth RG. Direct laryngoscopy and Tracheal Intubation. Lancet. 1944;1:651–654.
97. Adnet F, Borron SW, Lapostolle F, et al. The three axis alignment theory and the "sniffing position": perpetuation of an anatomic myth? Anesthesiology. 1999;91:1964–1965.
98. Chou HC, Wu TL. Rethinking the three axes alignment theory for direct laryngoscopy. Acta Anaesthesiol Scand. 2001;45:261–262.
99. Rosenblatt WH. Preoperative planning of airway management in critical care patients. Critical Care Medicine. 2004;32:S186–192.
100. Mallampati SR, Gatt SP, Gugino LD, et al. A clinical sign to predict difficult tracheal intubation: a prospective study. Can J Anaesth. 1985;32:429–434.
101. Ayoub C, Baraka A, el-Khatib M, et al. A new cut-off point of thyromental distance for prediction of difficult airway. Middle East J Anaesthesiol. 2000;15:619–633.
102. Chou HC, Wu TL. Thyromental distance and anterior larynx: misconception and misnomer? Anesth Analg. 2003;96:1526–1527.
103. Samsoon GL, Young JR. Difficult tracheal intubation: a retrospective study. Anaesthesia. 1987;42:487–490.
104. Ovassapian A, Glassenberg R, Randel GI, et al. The unexpected difficult airway and lingual tonsil hyperplasia: a case series and a review of the literature. Anesthesiology. 2002;97:124–132.
105. El-Orbany M, Woehlck H, Salem MR. Head and neck position for direct laryngoscopy. Anesth Analg. 2011;113:103–109.
106. Levitan RM. Advanced concepts in laryngoscope blade design. In: Levitan RM. The Airway Cam Guide to Intubation and Practical Emergency Airway Management. Exton, PA: AirWay Cam Technologies; 2004.
107. Cormack RS, Lehane J. Difficult tracheal intubation in obstetrics. Anaesthesia. 1984;39:1105–1111.
108. Crosby ET, Cooper RM, Douglas MJ, et al. The unanticipated difficult airway with recommendations for management. Can J Anaesth. 1998;45:757–776.
109. Cook TM. A new practical classification of laryngeal view. Anaesthesia. 2000;55:274–279.
110. Ochroch EA, Hollander JE, Kush S, et al. Assessment of laryngeal view: percentage of glottic opening score vs Cormack and Lehane grading. Can J Anaesth. 1999;46:987–990.
111. Ulrich B, Listyo R, Gerig HJ, et al. [The difficult intubation. The value of BURP and 3 predictive tests of difficult intubation]. Der Anaesthesist. 1998;47:45–50.
112. Benumof JL, Cooper SD. Quantitative improvement in laryngoscopic view by optimal external laryngeal manipulation. J Clin Anesth. 1996;8:136–140.
113. Henderson JJ. The use of paraglossal straight blade laryngoscopy in difficult tracheal intubation. Anaesthesia. 1997;52:552–560.

114. Kheterpal S, Healy D, Aziz MF, et al. Incidence, predictors, and outcome of difficult mask ventilation combined with difficult laryngoscopy: a report from the multicenter perioperative outcomes group. Anesthesiology. 2013;119:1360–1369.
115. Rose DK, Cohen MM. The airway: problems and predictions in 18,500 patients. Can J Anaesth. 1994;41:372–383.
116. Burkle CM, Walsh MT, Harrison BA, et al. Airway management after failure to intubate by direct laryngoscopy: outcomes in a large teaching hospital. Can J Anaesth. 2005;52:634–640.
117. Turkstra TP, Pelz DM, Shaikh AA, et al. Cervical spine motion: a fluoroscopic comparison of Shikani Optical Stylet vs Macintosh laryngoscope. Can J Anaesth. 2007;54:441–447.
118. Rudolph C, Schneider JP, Wallenborn J, et al. Movement of the upper cervical spine during laryngoscopy: a comparison of the Bonfils intubation fibrescope and the Macintosh laryngoscope. Anaesthesia. 2005;60:668–672.
119. Halligan M, Charters P. A clinical evaluation of the Bonfils Intubation Fibrescope. Anaesthesia. 2003;58:1087–1091.
120. Greenland KB, Liu G, Tan H, et al. Comparison of the Levitan FPS Scope and the single-use bougie for simulated difficult intubation in anaesthetised patients. Anaesthesia. 2007;62:509–515.
121. Levitan RM. Design rationale and intended use of a short optical stylet for routine fiberoptic augmentation of emergency laryngoscopy. Am J Emerg Medic. 2006;24:490–495.
122. Heidegger T, Gerig HJ, Ulrich B, et al. Validation of a simple algorithm for tracheal intubation: daily practice is the key to success in emergencies—an analysis of 13,248 intubations. Anesth Analg. 2001;92:517–522.
123. Cooper RM, Pacey JA, Bishop MJ, et al. Early clinical experience with a new videolaryngoscope (GlideScope) in 728 patients. Can J Anaesth. 2005;52:191–198.
124. Turkstra TP, Craen RA, Pelz DM, et al. Cervical spine motion: a fluoroscopic comparison during intubation with lighted stylet, GlideScope, and Macintosh laryngoscope. Anesth Anal. 2005;101:910–915.
125. Sun DA, Warriner CB, Parsons DG, et al. The GlideScope Video Laryngoscope: randomized clinical trial in 200 patients. Br J Anaesth. 2005;94:381–384.
126. Kramer DC, Osborn IP. More maneuvers to facilitate tracheal intubation with the GlideScope. Can J Anaesth. 2006;53:737.
127. Doyle DJ, Zura A, Ramachandran M. Videolaryngoscopy in the management of the difficult airway. Can J Anaesth. 2004;51:95; author reply 95–96.
128. Jones PM, Turkstra TP, Armstrong KP, et al. Effect of stylet angulation and endotracheal tube camber on time to intubation with the GlideScope. Can J Anaesth. 2007;54:21–27.
129. Hindman BJ, Santoni BG, Puttlitz CM, et al. Intubation biomechanics: laryngoscope force and cervical spine motion during intubation with Macintosh and Airtraq laryngoscopes. Anesthesiology. 2014;121:260–271.
130. Gunaydin B, Gungor I, Yigit N, et al. The Glidescope for tracheal intubation in patients with ankylosing spondylitis. Br J Anaesth. 2007;98:408–409.
131. Easker DD, Policeni BA, Hindman BJ. Lateral Cervical Spine Radiography to Demonstrate Absence of Bony Displacement After Intubation in a Patient with an Acute Type III Odontoid Fracture. A & A Case Reports. 2015;5:25–28.
132. Raja J, Clyne S, Levine J, et al. Otorhinolaryngology management of seven patients with iatrogenic penetrating injuries from GlideScope™: our experience. Clin Otolaryngol. 2014;39:251–254.
133. Cooper RM. Complications associated with the use of the GlideScope videolaryngoscope. Can J Anaesth. 2007;54:54–57.
134. Dupanovic M. Maneuvers to prevent oropharyngeal injury during orotracheal intubation with the GlideScope video laryngoscope. J Clin Anesth. 2010;22:152–154.
135. Xue FS, Zhang GH, Li XY, et al. Comparison of hemodynamic responses to orotracheal intubation with the GlideScope videolaryngoscope and the Macintosh direct laryngoscope. J Clin Anesth. 2007;19:245–250.
136. Dow WA, Parsons DG. 'Reverse loading' to facilitate Glidescope intubation. J Clin Anesth. 2007;54:161–162.
137. Aziz MF, Abrons RO, Cattano D, et al. First-attempt intubation success of video laryngoscopy in patients with anticipated difficult direct laryngoscopy: a multicenter randomized controlled trial comparing the C-MAC D-blade versus the GlideScope in a mixed provider and diverse patient population. Anesth Analg. 2016;122(3):740–750.
138. Kaplan MB, Hagberg CA, Ward DS, et al. Comparison of direct and video-assisted views of the larynx during routine intubation. J Clin Anesth. 2006;18:357–362.
139. Shippey B, Ray D, McKeown D. Case series: the McGrath videolaryngoscope–an initial clinical evaluation. Can J Anaesth. 2007;54:307–313.
140. Maharaj CH, Costello JF, McDonnell JG, et al. The Airtraq as a rescue airway device following failed direct laryngoscopy: a case series. Anaesthesia. 2007;62:598–601.
141. Suzuki A, Toyama Y, Iwasaki H, et al. Airtraq for awake tracheal intubation. Anaesthesia. 2007;62:746–747.
142. Maharaj CH, Buckley E, Harte BH, et al. Endotracheal intubation in patients with cervical spine immobilization: a comparison of Macintosh and Airtraq laryngoscopes. Anesthesiology. 2007;107:53–59.
143. Ueshima H, Kitamura A. Use of the new Airtraq "Airtraq AVANT" in clinical settings. J Clin Anesth. 2015;27:441–442.

144. Suzuki A, Abe N, Sasakawa T, et al. Pentax-AWS (Airway Scope) and Airtraq: big difference between two similar devices. *J Clin Anesth.* 2008;22:191–192.
145. Malik MA, Subramaniam R, Maharaj CH, et al. Randomized controlled trial of the Pentax AWS, Glidescope, and Macintosh laryngoscopes in predicted difficult intubation. *Br J Anaesth.* 2009;103:761–768.
146. Mahajan V, Hashmi J, Singh R, et al. Comparative evaluation of gastric pH and volume in morbidly obese and lean patients undergoing elective surgery and effect of aspiration prophylaxis. *J Clin Anesth.* 2015;27:396–400.
147. Juvin P, Fevre G, Merouche M, et al. Gastric residue is not more copious in obese patients. *Anesth Analg.* 2001;93:1621–1622.
148. Harter RL, Kelly WB, Kramer MG, et al. A comparison of the volume and pH of gastric contents of obese and lean surgical patients. *Anesth Analg.* 1998;86:147–152.
149. American Society of Anesthesiologists Committee. Practice guidelines for preoperative fasting and the use of pharmacologic agents to reduce the risk of pulmonary aspiration: application to healthy patients undergoing elective procedures: an updated report by the American Society of Anesthesiologists Committee on Standards and Practice Parameters. *Anesthesiology.* 2011;114:495–511.
150. Merio R, Festa A, Bergmann H, et al. Slow gastric emptying in type I diabetes: relation to autonomic and peripheral neuropathy, blood glucose, and glycemic control. *Diabetes Care.* 1997;20:419–423.
151. Van Den Driessche M, Peeters K, Marien P, et al. Gastric emptying in formula-fed and breast-fed infants measured with the 13C-octanoic acid breath test. *J Pediatr Gastroenterol Nutr.* 1999;29:46–51.
152. Kulkarni PN, Batra YK, Wig J. Effects of different combinations of H2 receptor antagonist with gastrokinetic drugs on gastric fluid pH and volume in children—a comparative study. *Int J Clin Pharmacol Ther.* 1997;35:561–564.
153. Nishina K, Mikawa K, Takao Y, et al. A comparison of rabeprazole, lansoprazole, and ranitidine for improving preoperative gastric fluid property in adults undergoing elective surgery. *Anesth Analg.* 2000;90:717–721.
154. Nishina K, Mikawa K, Maekawa N, et al. A comparison of lansoprazole, omeprazole, and ranitidine for reducing preoperative gastric secretion in adult patients undergoing elective surgery. *Anesth Analg.* 1996;82:832–836.
155. Escolano F, Castano J, Lopez R, et al. Effects of omeprazole, ranitidine, famotidine and placebo on gastric secretion in patients undergoing elective surgery. *Br J Anaesth.* 1992;69:404–406.
156. Manchikanti L, Grow JB, Colliver JA, et al. Bicitra (sodium citrate) and metoclopramide in outpatient anesthesia for prophylaxis against aspiration pneumonitis. *Anesthesiology.* 1985;63:378–384.
157. Vanner RG, Asai T. Safe use of cricoid pressure. *Anaesthesia.* 1999;54:1–3.
158. Smith KJ, Dobranowski J, Yip G, et al. Cricoid pressure displaces the esophagus: an observational study using magnetic resonance imaging. *Anesthesiology.* 2003;99:60–64.
159. Levitan RM, Kinkle WC, Levin WJ, et al. Laryngeal view during laryngoscopy: a randomized trial comparing cricoid pressure, backward-upward-rightward pressure, and bimanual laryngoscopy. *Ann Emerg Med.* 2006;47:548–555.
160. Alstrom HB, Belhage B. [Cricoid pressure a.m. Sellick in rapid sequence intubation?]. *Ugeskrift For Laeger.* 2007;169:2305–2308.
161. Algie CM, Mahar RK, Tan HB, et al. Effectiveness and risks of cricoid pressure during rapid sequence induction for endotracheal intubation. *Cochrane Database Syst Rev.* 2015;11:CD011656.
162. Brown JP, Werrett G. Bag-mask ventilation in rapid sequence induction. *Anaesthesia.* 2009;64:784–785.
163. Rosenblatt J, Reitzel R, Jiang Y, et al. Insights on the role of antimicrobial cuffed endotracheal tubes in preventing transtracheal transmission of VAP pathogens from an in vitro model of microaspiration and microbial proliferation. *BioMed Res Int.* 2014;2014:120468.
164. Kundra P, Sujata N, Ravishankar M. Conventional tracheal tubes for intubation through the intubating laryngeal mask airway. *Anesth Analg.* 2005;100:284–288.
165. Gerstein NS, Braude DA, Hung O, et al. The Fastrach Intubating Laryngeal Mask Airway: an overview and update. *Can J Anaesth.* 2010;57:588–601.
166. Rosenblatt WH, Murphy M. The intubating laryngeal mask: use of a new ventilating-intubating device in the emergency department. *Ann Emerg Med.* 1999;33:234–238.
167. Karim YM, Swanson DE. Comparison of blind tracheal intubation through the intubating laryngeal mask airway (LMA Fastrach) and the Air-Q. *Anaesthesia.* 2011;66:185–190.
168. Sinha R, Chandralekha, Ray BR. Evaluation of air-Q intubating laryngeal airway as a conduit for tracheal intubation in infants—a pilot study. *Paediatr Anaesth.* 2012;22:156–160.
169. Miller KA, Harkin CP, Bailey PL. Postoperative tracheal extubation. *Anesth Analg.* 1995;80:149–172.
170. Difficult Airway Society Extubation Guidelines Group, Popat M, Mitchell V, et al. Difficult Airway Society Guidelines for the management of tracheal extubation. *Anaesthesia.* 2012;67:318–340.
171. Murphy GS, Brull SJ. Residual neuromuscular block: lessons unlearned. Part I: definitions, incidence, and adverse physiologic effects of residual neuromuscular block. *Anesth Analg.* 2010;111:120–128.
172. Eriksson LI, Sundman E, Olsson R, et al. Functional assessment of the pharynx at rest and during swallowing in partially paralyzed humans: simultaneous videomanometry and mechanomyography of awake human volunteers. *Anesthesiology.* 1997;87:1035–1043.
173. Fortier LP, McKeen D, Turner K, et al. The RECITE Study: A Canadian Prospective, Multicenter Study of the Incidence and Severity of Residual Neuromuscular Blockade. *Anesth Analg.* 2015;121:366–372.
174. Lee CH, Peng MJ, Wu CL. Dexamethasone to prevent postextubation airway obstruction in adults: a prospective, randomized, double-blind, placebo-controlled study. *Critical Care.* 2007;11:R72.
175. Ochoa ME, Marin Mdel C, Frutos-Vivar F, et al. Cuff-leak test for the diagnosis of upper airway obstruction in adults: a systematic review and meta-analysis. *Intensive Care Med.* 2009;35:1171–1179.
176. Mort TC. Continuous airway access for the difficult extubation: the efficacy of the airway exchange catheter. *Anesth Analg.* 2007;105:1357–1362.
177. Mort TC ME, Waberski WM. Exchanging a tracheal tube in the ICU patient: A comparison of two exchangers with direct laryngoscopy. *Anesthesiology.* 1997;87:240A.
178. Harris K, Chalhoub M, Maroun R, et al. Endotracheal tube exchangers: should we look for safer alternatives? *Heart & Lung.* 2012;41:67–69.
179. Chrimes NC. The Vortex: striving for simplicity, context independence and teamwork in an airway cognitive tool. *Br J Anaesth.* 2015;115:148–149.
180. Petrini F, Accorsi A, Adrario E, et al. Recommendations for airway control and difficult airway management. *Minerva Anestesiol.* 2005;71:617–657.
181. Rosenblatt WH. Awake intubation made easy! In: ASA refresher course in anesthesiology. In., vol. 37; 2009: 167–172.
182. Kristensen MS, Teoh WH, Baker PA. Percutaneous emergency airway access; prevention, preparation, technique and training. *Br J Anaesth.* 2015;114:357–361.
183. Mort TC. Emergency tracheal intubation: complications associated with repeated laryngoscopic attempts. *Anesth Analg.* 2004;99:607–613.
184. Sakles JC, Chiu S, Mosier J, et al. The importance of first pass success when performing orotracheal intubation in the emergency department. *Acad Emerg Med.* 2013;20:71–78.
185. Nandi PR, Charlesworth CH, Taylor SJ, et al. Effect of general anaesthesia on the pharynx. *Br J Anaesth.* 1991;66:157–162.
186. Benumof JL. Management of the difficult adult airway. With special emphasis on awake tracheal intubation. *Anesthesiology.* 1991;75:1087–1110.
187. Madhere M, Vangura D, Saidov A. Dexmedetomidine as sole agent for awake fiberoptic intubation in a patient with local anesthetic allergy. *J Anesth.* 2011;25:592–594.
188. Nydahl PA, Axelsson K. Venous blood concentration of lidocaine after nasopharyngeal application of 2% lidocaine gel. *Acta Anaesthesiologica Scandinavica.* 1988;32:135–139.
189. Wieczorek PM, Schricker T, Vinet B, et al. Airway topicalisation in morbidly obese patients using atomised lidocaine: 2% compared with 4%. *Anaesthesia.* 2007;62:984–988.
190. McEvoy GK. Methylene Blue. In: *AHFS Drug Information 2007.* Bethesda, MD: American Society of Health-System Pharmacists; 2007.
191. Weisel W, Tella RA. Reaction to tetracaine (pontocaine) used as topical anesthetic in bronchoscopy; study of 1,000 cases. *J Am Med Assoc.* 1951;147:218–222.
192. Sitzman BT, Rich GF, Rockwell JJ, et al. Local anesthetic administration for awake direct laryngoscopy. Are glossopharyngeal nerve blocks superior? *Anesthesiology.* 1997;86:34–40.
193. Ovassapian A, ed. *Fiberoptic Endoscopy and the Difficult Airway.* Vol. 47. Philadelphia, PA: Lippincott-Raven; 1996.
194. Rosenblatt WH, Wagner PJ, Ovassapian A, et al. Practice patterns in managing the difficult airway by anesthesiologists in the United States. *Anesth Analg.* 1998;87:153–157.
195. Murphy P. A fibre-optic endoscope used for nasal intubation. *Anaesthesia.* 1967;22:489–491.
196. Kristensen MS. The Parker Flex-Tip tube versus a standard tube for fiberoptic orotracheal intubation: a randomized double-blind study. *Anesthesiology.* 2003;98:354–358.
197. Rosenblatt WH. Overcoming obstruction during bronchoscope-guided intubation of the trachea with the double setup endotracheal tube. *Anesth Analg.* 1996;83:175–177.
198. Ovassapian A, Yelich SJ, Dykes MH, et al. Fiberoptic nasotracheal intubation–incidence and causes of failure. *Anesth Analg.* 1983;62:692–695.
199. Lu PP, Liu HP, Shyr MH, et al. Softened endotracheal tube reduces the incidence and severity of epistaxis following nasotracheal intubation. *Acta Anaesthesiol Sin.* 1998;36:193–197.
200. Martin SE, Ochsner MG, Jarman RH, et al. Laryngeal mask airway in air transport when intubation fails: case report. *J Trauma.* 1997;42:333–336.
201. Brimacombe JR, De Maio B. Emergency use of the laryngeal mask airway during helicopter transfer of a neonate. *J Clin Anesth.* 1995;7:689–690.
202. Asai T, Latto IP. Role of the laryngeal mask in patients with difficult tracheal intubation and difficult ventilation. In: Latto IP Vaughan RS, eds. *Difficulties in Tracheal Intubation.* Philadelphia: WB Saunders; 1997:177.
203. Brimacombe JR, Berry AM. Mallampati grade and laryngeal mask placement. *Anesth Analg.* 1996;82:1112–1113.

204. Agro F, Frass M, Benumof JL, et al. Current status of the Combitube: a review of the literature. *J Clin Anesth.* 2002;14:307–314.
205. Verghese C, Prior-Willeard PF, Baskett PJ. Immediate management of the airway during cardiopulmonary resuscitation in a hospital without a resident anaesthesiologist. *Eur J Emerg Med.* 1994;1:123–125.
206. Keller C, Brimacombe J, Bittersohl J, et al. Aspiration and the laryngeal mask airway: three cases and a review of the literature. *Br J Anaesth.* 2004;93:579–582.
207. Aoyama K, Takenaka I, Sata T, et al. Cricoid pressure impedes positioning and ventilation through the laryngeal mask airway. *Can J Anaesth.* 1996;43:1035–1040.
208. Li J, Murphy-Lavoie H, Bugas C, et al. Complications of emergency intubation with and without paralysis. *Am J Emerg Med.* 1999;17:141–143.
209. Gnauck K, Lungo JB, Scalzo A, et al. Emergency intubation of the pediatric medical patient: use of anesthetic agents in the emergency department. *Ann Emerg Med.* 1994;23:1242–1247.
210. Sivarajan M, Joy JV. Effects of general anesthesia and paralysis on upper airway changes due to head position in humans. *Anesthesiology.* 1996;85:787–793.
211. Walls RM. Management of the difficult airway in the trauma patient. *Emerg Med Clin N A.* 1998;16:45–61.
212. Ruetzler K, Roessler B, Potura L, et al. Performance and skill retention of intubation by paramedics using seven different airway devices—a manikin study. *Resuscitation.* 2011;82:593–597.
213. Reardon R, Joing S, Hill C. Bougie-guided cricothyrotomy technique. *Acad Emerg Med.* 2010;17:225.
214. Hubble MW, Wilfong DA, Brown LH, et al. A meta-analysis of prehospital airway control techniques part II: alternative airway devices and cricothyrotomy success rates. *Prehosp Emerg Care.* 2010;14:515–530.
215. Hamaekers AE, Borg PA, Enk D. A bench study of ventilation via two self-assembled jet devices and the Oxygen Flow Modulator in simulated upper airway obstruction. *Anaesthesia.* 2009;64:1353–1358.
216. Sukhupragarn W, Rosenblatt WH. Kinking of catheters during translaryngeal jet ventilation: a bench model investigation of eight devices. *J Med Assoc Thailand.* 2011;94:972–977.
217. Hamaekers A, Borg P, Enk D. The importance of flow and pressure release in emergency jet ventilation devices. *Paediatr Anaesth.* 2009;19:452–457.
218. Lenfant F, Pean D, Brisard L, et al. Oxygen delivery during transtracheal oxygenation: a comparison of two manual devices. *Anesth Analg.* 2010;111:922–924.
219. Hamaekers AE, Borg PA, Enk D. Ventrain: an ejector ventilator for emergency use. *Br J Anaesth.* 2012;108:1017–1021.
220. Berry M, Tzeng Y, Marsland C. Percutaneous transtracheal ventilation in an obstructed airway model in post-apnoeic sheep. *Br J Anaesth.* 2014;113:1039–1045.
221. Paxian M, Preussler NP, Reinz T, et al. Transtracheal ventilation with a novel ejector-based device (Ventrain) in open, partly obstructed, or totally closed upper airways in pigs. *Br J Anaesth.* 2015;115:308–316.
222. Borg PA, Hamaekers AE, Lacko M, et al. Ventrain(R) for ventilation of the lungs. *Br J Anaesth.* 2012;109:833–834.
223. Willemsen MG, Noppens R, Mulder AL, et al. Ventilation with the Ventrain through a small lumen catheter in the failed paediatric airway: two case reports. *Br J Anaesth.* 2014;112:946–947.
224. Bellemain A, Ghimouz A, Goater P, et al. [Bilateral tension pneumothorax after retrieval of transtracheal jet ventilation catheter]. *Ann Fr Anesth Reanim.* 2006;25:401–403.

29 Patient Positioning and Potential Injuries

MARY E. WARNER • REBECCA L. JOHNSON

General Principles
Supine Positions
   Variations of Supine Positions
   Complications of Supine Positions
Lateral Positions
   Variations of Lateral Positions
   Complications of Lateral Positions
Prone Positions
   Full Prone
   Complications of Prone Positions
Head-elevated Positions
   Variations of Head-elevated Positions
   Complications of Head-elevated Positions
Head-down Positions
   Complications of Head-down Positions
Summary

KEY POINTS

1. The etiologies of peripheral neuropathies are often not clear. Although there are potential anatomic and neurophysiologic reasons, perioperative inflammation, resulting in microvasculitis, may be an important etiologic factor.
2. Stretching nerves 5% or more beyond their resting lengths may kink feeding arterioles and result in ischemia.
3. Padding provided by any number of different materials (e.g., gel or foam pads, blankets) should be used to widely disperse point pressure on body parts and soft tissues.
4. Sedated or anesthetized patients should be placed in positions that are comfortable while they are awake.
5. Permanent loss of vision can occur after nonocular surgical procedures, especially those performed in a prone position.

Positioning a patient for a surgical procedure is frequently a compromise between what the anesthetized patient can tolerate, both structurally and physiologically, and what the surgical team requires for access to its anatomic target. Establishment of the intended surgical posture may need to be modified to match the patient's tolerance. This chapter presents the significance of various positions in which a patient may be placed during an operation, briefly describes the techniques of establishing the positions, and discusses the potential complications of each posture. It also will present data that suggest perioperative inflammatory responses may play an important role in the development of peripheral, and potentially central, neuropathies.

It is very important for clinicians to understand the physiologic and potential pathologic consequences of patient positioning. A number of studies of large surgical populations have provided information on the frequency and natural history of rare perioperative events such as neuropathies and vision loss. However, these studies frequently have provided insufficient data to allow speculation as to potential mechanisms of injury. Based on the findings of these studies, investigators are seeking to confirm mechanisms of injury and the efficacy of novel interventions to decrease the frequency of these perioperative events. Until these investigations are complete, the etiologic mechanisms for many potential positioning-related complications remain unknown.

The lack of solid scientific information on basic mechanisms of positioning-related complications often leads to medicolegal entanglements. Notations on anesthesia and operating room records may be absent or uninformative. Careful descriptive notations about positions used during anesthesia and surgery, as well as brief comments about special protective measures such as eye care and pressure-point padding, are useful to include on the anesthesia record. In potentially complicated or contentious circumstances, a separate brief description of care documented in the patient's record is advisable. Only in this manner can subsequent inquiries be properly answered on behalf of either the patient or the anesthesiologist. When credible expanded knowledge that further delineates mechanisms of positioning-related complications is available, these issues and the care of patients will be improved.

General Principles

Without doubt, direct compression of neural and soft tissue may result in ischemia and tissue damage. Many efforts have been directed at provider education over the years to reduce direct tissue trauma from compression. Most anesthesia providers are taught from the start of their training that various maneuvers, pads, and positioning devices are useful to reduce point pressure on neural and soft tissues. Despite these efforts, neuropathies and soft tissue damage still occur. Is it a failure of education, the incorrect application of this information, or other issues that contribute to the continued presence of perioperative positioning injuries? Or perhaps, are there etiologic mechanisms at work that we do not yet understand?

Recent studies and editorials suggest that we do not yet fully understand the etiologic mechanisms of positioning issues.[1-4] These studies reported inflammatory neuropathies in patients who developed severe postsurgical peripheral neuropathies. Surprisingly, the majority of these patients had widespread microvasculitic neuropathies, and many were responsive to immunologic modulation with high doses of corticosteroids. The inflammatory response may be dramatically altered in the perioperative period, and microvasculitic neuropathy appears to be a previously unrecognized cause of peripheral neuropathy.

For example, anesthetic drugs and transfusion of blood products are known to promote systemic inflammation.[5,6] Large epidemiologic studies will eventually help determine the role that this new etiology plays in the origin of perioperative neuropathies of all sorts. In the meantime, these reports serve as evidence that a number of perioperative neuropathies may, in fact, have no relationship to intraoperative positioning or management of physiologic factors.[4]

Viruses have been associated with central as well as peripheral neuropathies that develop in the perioperative period. As noted earlier, immunosuppression is present in a fairly significant proportion of patients undergoing major surgical procedures. This immunosuppression may provide opportunities for existing viruses or newly introduced viruses to activate, particularly in neural tissues. For example, the onset of shingles may be more frequent in surgical compared to general populations.[7]

Positioning can, of course, cause tissue damage. Stretch of neural tissue may be an important factor in the development of peripheral and central neuropathies. Stretch of many mammalian nerves to 5% greater than their normal resting length has

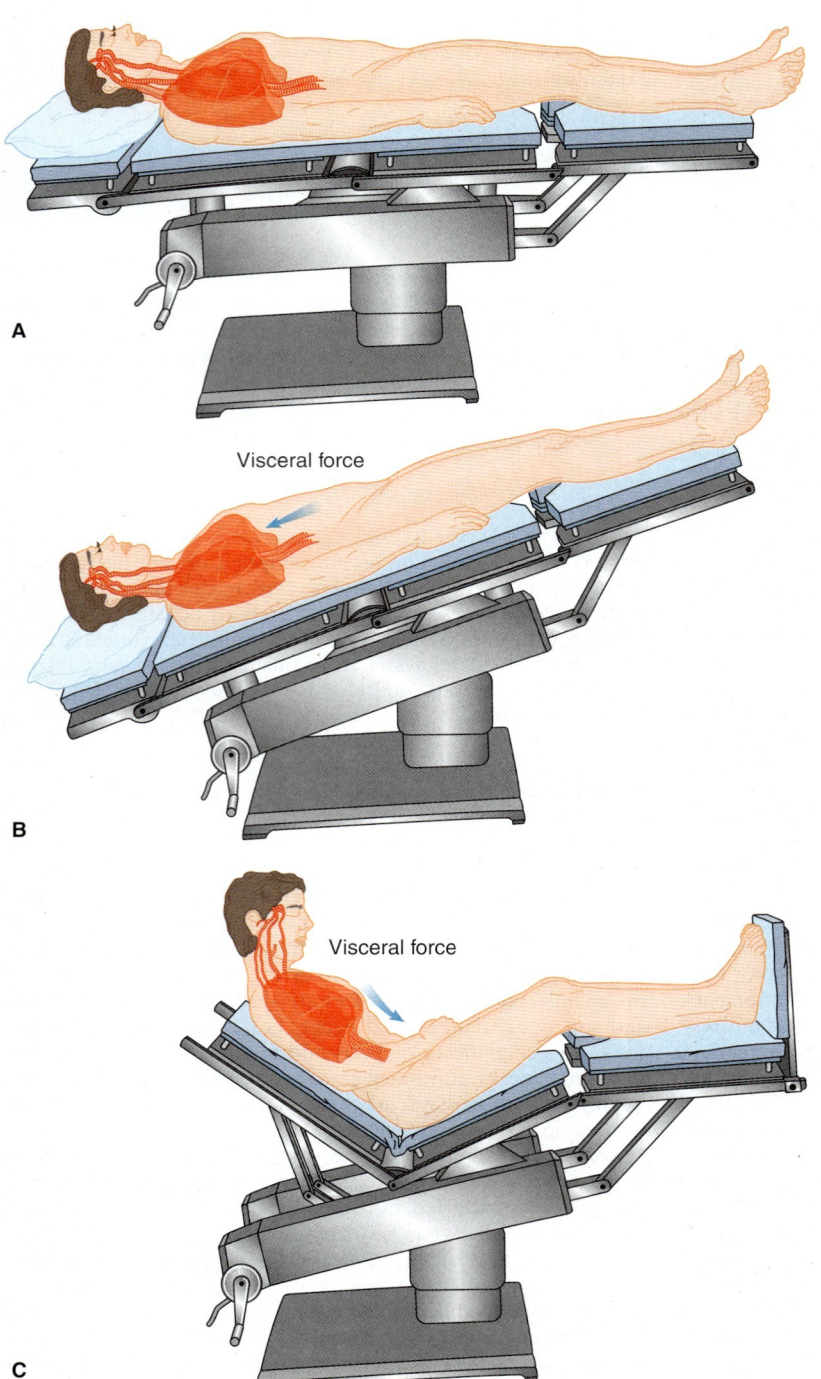

Figure 29-1 A: Supine adult with minimal gradients in the horizontal vascular axis. Pulmonary blood volume is greatest dorsally. Viscera displace the diaphragm cephalad. Cerebral circulation is slightly above heart level if the head is on a small pillow. **B:** Head-down tilt aids blood return from lower extremities but encourages reflex vasodilation, congests vessels in the poorly ventilated lung apices, and increases intracranial blood volume. **C:** Elevation of the head shifts abdominal viscera away from the diaphragm and improves ventilation of the lung bases. According to the gradient above the heart, pressure in arteries of the head and neck decreases; pressure in accompanying veins may become subatmospheric.

been shown repeatedly to lead to ischemia by reducing both arteriole and venule blood flow. The kinking of the arterioles and venules associated with neuronal stretch leads to ischemia.[8] If the ischemia is prolonged, it may result in permanent neural damage. The impact of stretch on other soft tissues is less well documented and would be highly dependent on the type of tissue and amount of stretch.

Point pressure on any soft tissue may reduce local blood flow and cause ischemia. There are many ways to reduce point pressure, but the most commonly used involve padding. Although there may be distinct differences in mechanical properties of various padding materials (e.g., gels, foam, textiles, and others), none have been proven to be significantly better than the others in reducing the frequency or severity of nerve or soft tissue damage perioperatively. The basic principle is to use any of these materials to protect nerves and soft tissues from point pressure.

Supine Positions

Variations of Supine Positions

Horizontal

In the traditional supine position, the patient lies on his or her back with a small pillow beneath the head (Fig. 29-1A). The arms are either comfortably padded and restrained alongside the trunk or abducted on well-padded arm boards. Either arm (or both) may be extended ventrally and the flexed forearm secured to an elevated frame in such a way that perfusion of the hand is not compromised, no skin-to-metal contact exists to cause electrical burns if cautery is used, and the brachial neurovascular bundle is neither stretched nor compressed at the axilla. The lumbar spine may need padded support to prevent a postoperative backache (see "Complications of Supine Positions"). Bony contact points at the occiput, elbows, and heels should be padded. Fortunately, most modern surgical tables have mattress pads that are sufficiently buoyant and thick to allow dispersion of point pressure.

Although the horizontal supine posture has a long history of widespread use, it does not place hip and knee joints in neutral positions and is poorly tolerated for prolonged periods by an immobilized, awake patient.

Contoured

A contoured supine posture (Fig. 29-2) has been termed the *lawn chair position*. It is established by arranging the surface of the operating table so that the trunk–thigh hinge is angulated approximately 15 degrees and the thigh–knee hinge is angulated a similar amount in the opposite direction. Alternatively, a rolled towel, pillow, or blanket can be placed beneath the patient's knees to keep them flexed. The patient of average height then lies comfortably with hips and knees flexed gently.

Lateral Uterine or Abdominal Mass Displacement

With a patient in the supine position, a mobile abdominal mass, such as a very large tumor or a pregnant uterus, can rest on the great vessels of the abdomen and compromise circulation. This is known as the *aortocaval syndrome* or the *supine hypotensive syndrome*. A significant degree of perfusion can be restored if the compressive mass is rolled toward the left hemiabdomen by leftward tilt of the tabletop or by a wedge under the right hip.

Lithotomy

Standard

In the standard lithotomy position (Fig. 29-3), the patient lies supine, typically with one or both arms extended laterally to less than 90 degrees on arm boards. Each lower extremity is flexed at the hip and knee, and both limbs are simultaneously elevated and separated so that the perineum becomes accessible to the surgeon. For many gynecologic and urologic procedures, the patient's thighs are flexed approximately 90 degrees on the trunk and the knees are bent sufficiently to maintain the lower legs nearly parallel to the floor. More acute flexion of the knees or hips can threaten to angulate and compress major vessels at either joint. In addition, hip flexion to greater than 90 degrees on the trunk has been shown to increase stretch of the inguinal ligaments.[8] Branches of the lateral femoral cutaneous nerves often pass directly through these ligaments and can be impinged and become ischemic within the stretched ligament.

Numerous devices are available to hold legs that are elevated during obstetric delivery or perineal operations. Each device should be fitted to the stature of the individual patient. Care should be taken to ensure that angulations or edges of the padded

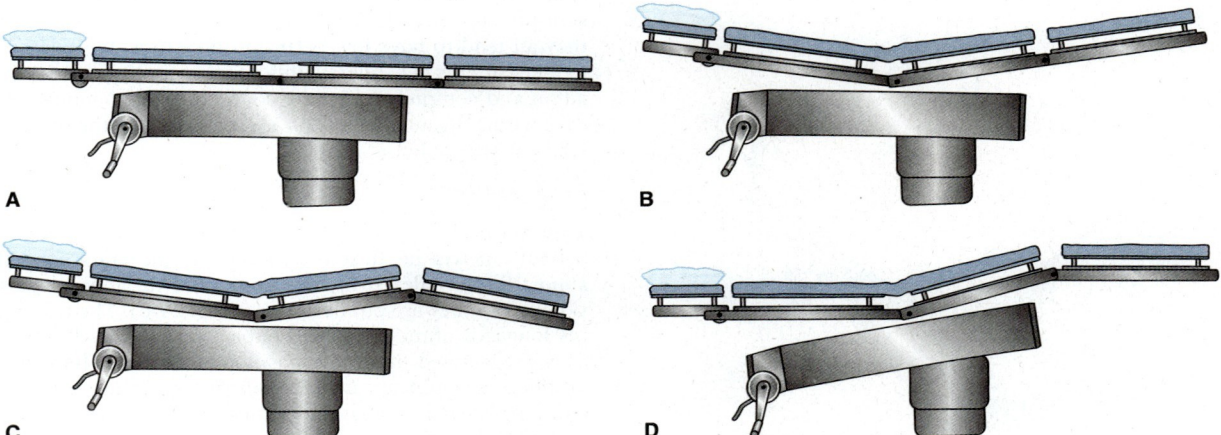

Figure 29-2 Establishment of the contoured supine (lawn chair) position. **A:** Traditional flat supine tabletop. **B:** Thighs flexed on trunk. **C:** Knees gently flexed in final body position. **D:** Trunk section leveled to stabilize floor-supported arm board.

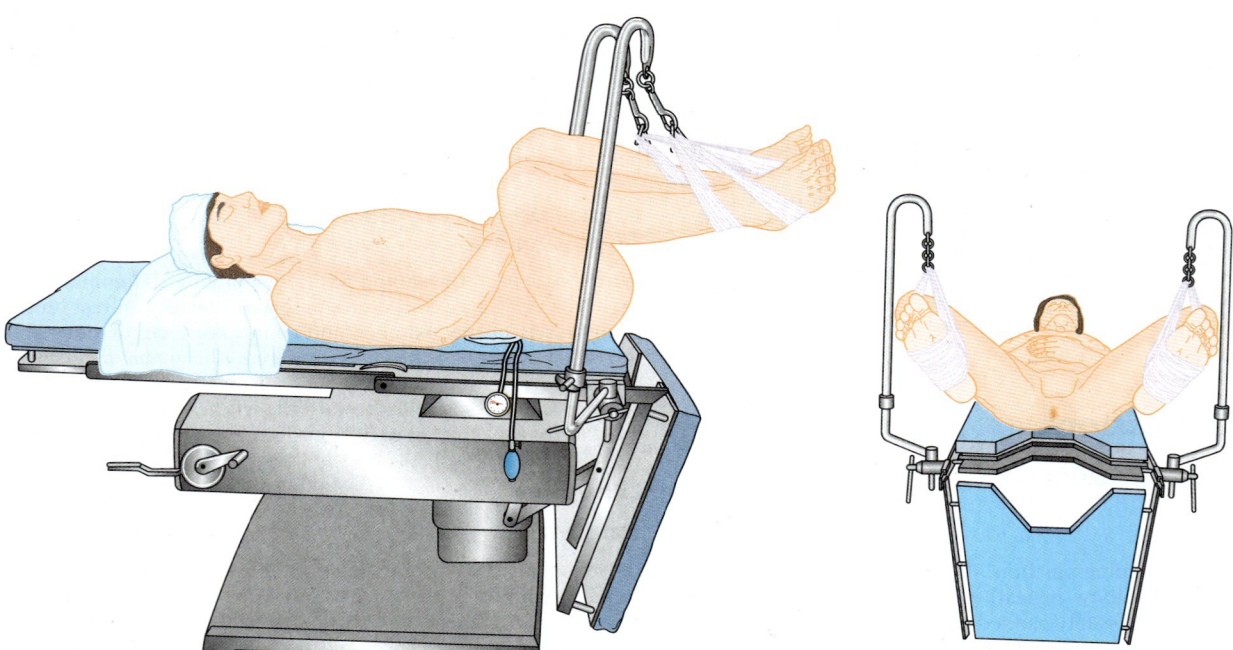

Figure 29-3 Standard lithotomy position with "candy cane" extremity support. Thighs are flexed approximately 90 degrees on the abdomen; knees are flexed enough to bring the lower legs grossly parallel to the torso section of the tabletop. Arms are retained on the boards, crossed on the abdomen, or snugged at the sides of patient.

holder do not compress the popliteal space or the upper dorsal thigh. Compartment syndromes of one or both lower extremities have resulted from prolonged use of the lithotomy position with various types of support devices.

Low

For most urologic procedures and for many procedures that require simultaneous access to the abdomen and perineum, the degree of thigh elevation in the lithotomy position is only approximately 30 to 45 degrees (Fig. 29-4). This reduces perfusion gradients to and from the lower extremities and improves access to a perineal surgical site for members of the operating team who may need to stand at the lateral aspect of either leg.

High

Some surgeons prefer to improve access to the perineum by suspending the patient's feet from high poles. The effect is to have the patient's legs almost fully extended on the thighs (Fig. 29-5) and the thighs flexed 90 degrees or more on the trunk. The posture produces a significant uphill gradient for arterial perfusion into the feet, requiring careful avoidance of systemic hypotension. There is considerable variation in lower extremity perfusion pressure in volunteers placed in high lithotomy positions; they all tend to have low perfusion pressures, however.[9,10] Less mobile patients may tolerate this posture poorly because of angulation and compression of the contents of the femoral canal by the inguinal ligament (Fig. 29-5A), or stretch of the sciatic nerve (Fig. 29-5B), or both.

Exaggerated

Transperineal access to the retropubic area requires that the patient's pelvis be flexed ventrally on the spine, the thighs almost forcibly flexed on the trunk, and the lower legs aimed skyward so they are out of the way (Fig. 29-6). The result places the long axis of the symphysis pubis almost parallel to the floor. This exaggerated lithotomy position stresses the lumbar spine, produces a significant uphill gradient for perfusion of the feet, and may restrict ventilation because of abdominal compression by bulky thighs. If pre-existing painful lumbar spine disease is present, an alternative surgical position may need to be chosen beforehand to avoid severely accentuating the lumbar distress

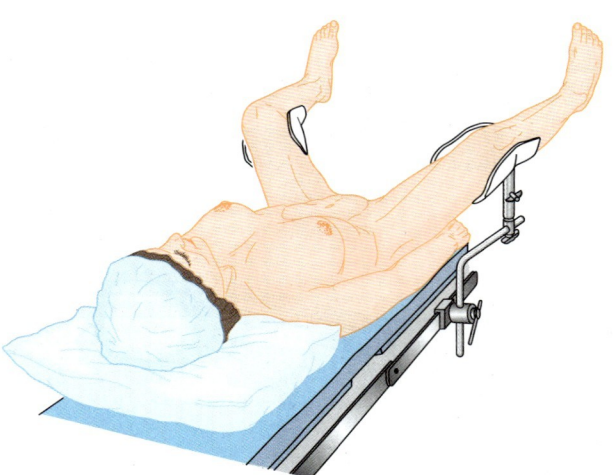

Figure 29-4 Low lithotomy position for perineal access, transurethral instrumentation, or combined abdominoperineal procedures.

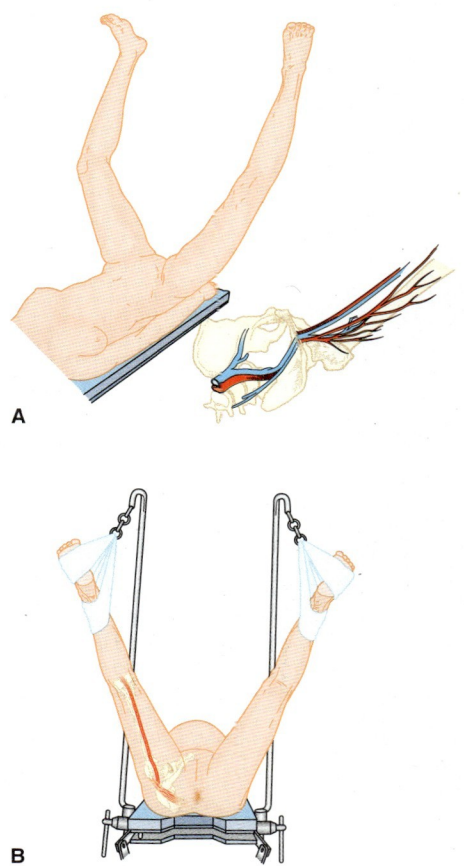

Figure 29-5 High lithotomy position. Note potential for angulation and compression/obstruction of contents of femoral canal (**A**, *inset*) or stretch of sciatic nerve (**B**). (**A**) Adapted from McLeskey CH, ed. *Geriatric Anesthesiology*. Baltimore, MD: Williams & Wilkins; 1997:146.

after surgery. This position has been associated with a very high frequency of lower extremity compartment syndrome.[11] Maintenance of adequate perfusion pressure in the legs is important.

Complications of Supine Positions

Brachial Plexus Neuropathy

Root Injuries

Shoulder braces placed tight against the base of the neck can compress and injure the roots of the brachial plexus when steep head-down positions are used. Braces, if needed at all, are considered less harmful when placed more laterally over the acromioclavicular joint. In general, the use of shoulder braces should be discouraged. The same is true of straps or tape crisscrossed from above the shoulders to keep patients from sliding cephalad.

Supine positions do not usually threaten structures in the patient's neck unless considerable lateral displacement of the head occurs or if steep head-down tilt is added. When lateral displacement of the head occurs, the roots of the brachial plexus on the side of the obtuse head–shoulder angle can be stretched and damaged. If the upper extremity is fixed to the operating table at the wrist (e.g., by wrist wrap or a sheet or towel used to tuck the arm), the stretch injury of the plexus can be accentuated as the head moves laterally away from the anchoring point of the wrist. Similarly, exaggerated rotation of the head away from an extended arm may be associated with a brachial plexus injury.

Sternal Retraction

Frequently, the patient undergoing a median sternotomy has both arms padded and secured alongside the torso. An alternative is to have both arms abducted.[12] Vander Salm et al.[13,14] described first-rib fractures and brachial plexus injuries associated with median sternotomies. They related the extent of the injury to the amount of retractor displacement of the rib, with the most severe injury being caused by displacement sufficient to produce a first-rib fracture. Roy et al.,[15] in a study of 200 consecutive adults scheduled for cardiac surgery via a median sternotomy, positioned the left arm either abducted and padded on an arm board with the palm supinated or secured by a draw sheet alongside the trunk; the right arm was always placed alongside the trunk. They found a 10% incidence of upper extremity nerve injury that was not influenced by internal mammary artery harvest, internal jugular vein catheterization, or left arm position. Surgical manipulation was more contributory than extremity positioning in producing trauma to the brachial plexus. Jellish et al.[12] reported that there is less slowing of somatosensory evoked potentials (SSEPs) of the ulnar nerve during sternotomy when both arms are abducted instead of tucked at the sides. However, they found no differences in perioperative symptoms between patients in the arm-abducted versus arm-at-side groups.

Long Thoracic Nerve Dysfunction

A number of lawsuits have centered on postoperative serratus anterior muscle dysfunction and winging of the scapula (Fig. 29-7)

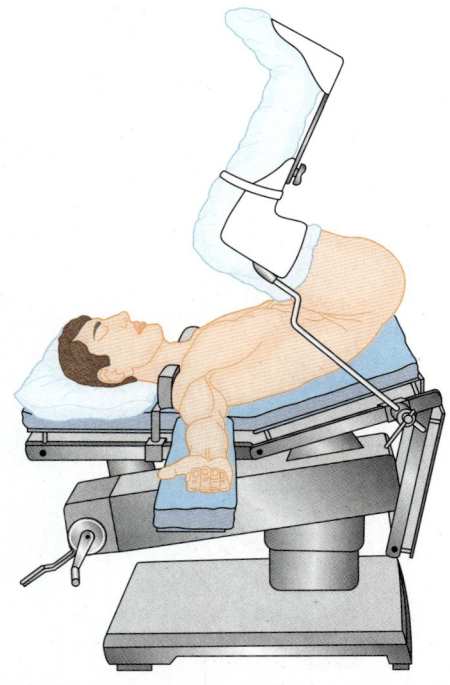

Figure 29-6 The exaggerated lithotomy position. Shoulder support may be needed to stabilize the torso. If used, it should be placed over the acromioclavicular area to minimize compression of the brachial plexus and adjacent vessels.

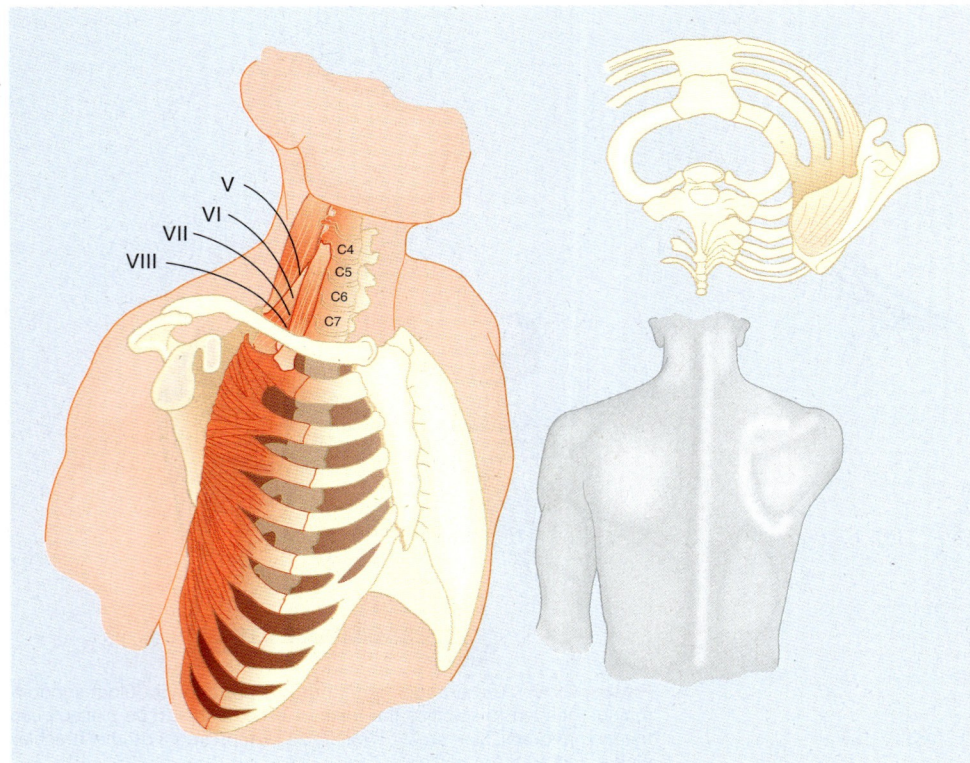

Figure 29-7 Scapular winging. The serratus anterior muscle (*upper right*) is supplied solely by the long thoracic nerve that branches immediately from C5, C6, C7, and sometimes C8 (*left figure*). Arising on the lateral ribs and inserting on the deep surface of the scapula, the muscle keeps the shoulder girdle approximated to the dorsal rib cage. Long thoracic nerve palsy allows dorsal protrusion of the scapula (*lower right*). See text for details.

alleged to be the result of position-related injuries to the long thoracic nerve, a nerve arising from nerve roots C5, C6, and C7. Because C5 and C6 fibers of the nerve course through the middle scalene muscle and emerge from its lateral border to join the fibers from C7, it has been proposed that neuropathies of the long thoracic nerve are traumatic in origin.[16,17] Because the nerve is not routinely involved in a stretch injury of the brachial plexus and because the plexus is not routinely involved when long thoracic nerve dysfunction occurs, the relationship between postoperative long thoracic neuropathy and patient positioning remains speculative. Based on evidence of Foo and Swann[18] plus data from various litigations, Martin[17] concluded that in the absence of demonstrable trauma, postoperative dysfunctions of the long thoracic nerve were quite likely the result of coincidental neuropathies, possibly of viral or inflammatory origin.

Axillary Trauma from the Humeral Head

Abduction of the arm on an arm board to greater than 90 degrees may thrust the head of the humerus into the axillary neurovascular bundle. This bundle typically lies on the flexion side of the shoulder joint. However, when the arm is abducted to greater than 90 degrees, the bundle is now on the extension side of the joint. The bundle is both compressed and stretched at that point, and its neural structures may be damaged. In the same manner, vessels can be compressed or occluded and perfusion of the extremity can be jeopardized.

Radial Nerve Compression

The radial nerve, arising from roots C6–8 and T1, passes dorsolaterally around the middle and lower portions of the humerus in the musculospiral groove. At a point on the lateral aspect of the arm, approximately three fingerbreadths proximal to the lateral epicondyle of the humerus, the nerve can be compressed against the underlying bone and injured. Pressure from the vertical bar of an anesthesia screen or a similar device against the lateral aspect of the arm, excessive cycling of an automatic blood pressure cuff, and compression at the midhumerus level by restrictive sheets or towels used to tuck the arms have been implicated in causing damage to the radial nerve. Other support devices, including arm boards and slings used when patients are positioned laterally, can directly compress the radial nerve as it wraps around the musculospiral groove.

Median Nerve Dysfunction

Isolated perioperative injuries to the median nerve are uncommon and the mechanism is usually obscure.[19,20] A potential source of injury is iatrogenic trauma to the nerve during access to vessels in the antecubital fossa, as might occur during venipuncture. Anecdotally, this problem appears to occur primarily in men 20 to 40 years of age who cannot easily extend their elbows completely. Forced elbow extension after administration of muscle relaxants and while positioning the arms, with resultant stretch of the median nerve, has been suggested as one potential mechanism for this problem.

Ulnar Neuropathy

Improper anesthetic care and patient malpositioning have been implicated as causative factors in the development of ulnar neuropathies since reports by Büdinger[21] and Garriques[22] in the 1890s. These factors likely play an etiologic role for this problem in some surgical patients. Other factors, however, may contribute to the development of postoperative ulnar neuropathies. In a series of 12 inpatients with newly acquired ulnar neuropathy, Wadsworth and Williams[23] determined that external compression of an ulnar nerve during surgery was a factor in only two patients. Ulnar neuropathies develop in medical as well as surgical patients.[24] Thus, the mechanisms of ulnar neuropathy are unclear.

Typically, anesthesia-related ulnar nerve injury is thought to be associated with external nerve compression or stretch caused by malpositioning during the intraoperative period. Although this implication may be true for some patients, three findings suggest that other factors may contribute. First, patient characteristics (e.g., male gender, high body mass index, and prolonged postoperative bed rest) are associated with these ulnar neuropathies.[25] Various reports suggest that 70% to 90% of patients who have this problem are men.[19,20,23–25] Second, many patients with perioperative ulnar neuropathies have a high frequency of contralateral ulnar nerve conduction dysfunction.[26] This finding suggests that many of these patients likely have asymptomatic but abnormal ulnar nerves before their anesthetics, and these abnormal nerves may become symptomatic during the perioperative period. Finally, many patients do not notice or complain of ulnar nerve symptoms until more than 48 hours after their surgical procedures.[25,26] A prospective study of ulnar neuropathy in 1,502 surgical patients found that none of the patients had symptoms of the neuropathy during the first 2 postoperative days.[27] It is not clear whether onset of symptoms indicates the time that an injury has occurred to the nerve. Prielipp et al.[28] found that 8 of 15 awake volunteers who had notable alterations in their ulnar nerve SSEP signals from direct ulnar nerve pressure did not perceive a paresthesia, even when the SSEP waveforms decreased as much as 72%.

Elbow flexion can cause ulnar nerve damage by several mechanisms. In some patients, the ulnar nerve is compressed by the aponeurosis of the flexor carpi ulnaris muscle and cubital tunnel retinaculum when the elbow is flexed by greater than 110 degrees (Fig. 29-8).[29,30] In other patients, this fibrotendinous roof of the cubital tunnel is poorly formed and can lead to anterior subluxation or dislocation of the ulnar nerve over the medial epicondyle of the humerus during elbow flexion. This displacement has been observed in approximately 16% of cadavers in whom the flexor muscle aponeurosis and supporting tissues have not been dissected.[31,32] Ashenhurst[32] has speculated that the ulnar nerve may be chronically damaged by recurrent mechanical trauma as the nerve is in subluxation over the medial epicondyle.

External compression in the absence of elbow flexion also may damage the ulnar nerve.[33,34] Although compression within the medial epicondylar groove may be possible if the groove is shallower than normal, the bony groove usually is deep and the nerve is well protected from external compression.[35] External compression may occur distal to the medial epicondyle, where the nerve and its associated artery are relatively superficial. In an anatomic study, Contreras et al.[36] observed that the ulnar nerve and posterior recurrent ulnar artery pass posteromedially to the tubercle of the coronoid process, where they are covered only by skin, subcutaneous fat, and a thin distal band of the aponeurosis of the flexor carpi ulnaris.

There are several anatomic differences between men and women that may increase the likelihood of perioperative ulnar neuropathy developing in men. First, two anatomic differences may increase the chance of ulnar nerve compression in the region of the elbow. The tubercle of the coronoid process is approximately 1.5 times larger in men than women.[36] In addition, there is less adipose tissue over the medial aspect of the elbow of men

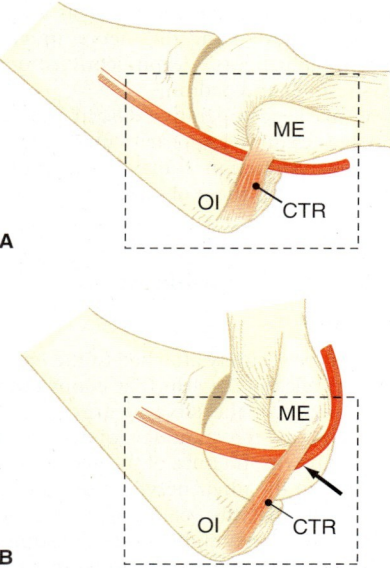

Figure 29-8 Medial-to-lateral view of right elbow. The cubital tunnel retinaculum (CTR) is lax in extension (**A**) as it stretches from the medial epicondyle (ME) to the olecranon (Ol). The retinaculum tightens in flexion (**B**) and can compress the ulnar nerve (*arrow*). (Adapted from O'Driscoll SW, Horii E, Carmichael SW, et al. The cubital tunnel and ulnar neuropathy. *J Bone Joint Surg Br*. 1991;73:615.)

compared with women of similar body fat composition.[36–38] Second, men may be more likely to have a well-developed cubital tunnel retinaculum than women, and the retinaculum, if present, is thicker. A thicker cubital tunnel retinaculum may increase the risk of ulnar nerve compression in the cubital tunnel when the elbow is flexed.

Clinical manifestations of ulnar nerve dysfunction vary with the location and extent of the lesion.[39] Nearly all patients have numbness, tingling, or pain in the sensory distribution of the ulnar nerves once they become symptomatic. However, there can be considerable ulnar nerve dysfunction before symptoms appear. Prielipp et al.[28] found that only 8 of 15 male volunteers with significant ulnar nerve conduction slowing noted any symptoms. More studies are needed to better understand the mechanism and natural history of ulnar neuropathy.

Perioperative ulnar neuropathy is relatively common.[19,20,27] Also, a significant proportion of patients have symptoms of bilateral ulnar nerve dysfunctions both before and after surgery.[27] Therefore, some have speculated that it might be helpful during the preanesthetic interview to inquire about a history of ulnar neuropathies ("crazy bone" problems) or previous surgery at the elbow. If such a history is indicated, the finding must be recorded and a discussion with the patient or family should present the possibility of a postoperative recurrence despite special precautions of padding and positioning.

The time of recognition of digital anesthesia associated with ulnar nerve dysfunction may be quite important in establishing the origin of the postoperative syndrome. If ulnar hypesthesia or anesthesia is noted promptly after the end of anesthesia, as in the recovery facility, the condition is likely to be associated with events that occurred during anesthesia or surgery. If the recognition is delayed for many hours, the likelihood of cause shifts from the intra-anesthetic period to postoperative events. In a review of closed claims, Cheney et al.[20] commented that postoperative ulnar dysfunction can occur as a result of events in the postanesthetic period and that nerve injury may develop in certain susceptible patients "despite conventionally accepted methods of positioning and padding."

Opioids may mask postoperative dysesthesias and pain, but even strong analgesics do not appear to mask a loss of sensation as a result of nerve dysfunction. It may be helpful to assess ulnar nerve function and record these observations before discharging the patient from the recovery room.

Other Supine Position Problems

Arm Complications

Arm boards should be securely attached to the operating table to prevent accidental release. An arm that is not properly secured can slip over the edge of the table or arm board, resulting in injury to the capsule of the shoulder joint by excessive dorsal extension of the humerus, fracture of the neck of an osteoporotic humerus, or injury to the ulnar nerve at the elbow. Conversely, in the unlikely event that the retaining strap or other holding device or cloth is excessively tight across the supinated forearm (Fig. 29-9), the potential exists for pressure to compress the anterior interosseous nerve, a branch of the median nerve in the upper forearm that courses with its artery along the volar surface of the tough interosseous membrane. The result is an ischemic injury to the distribution of the nerve and artery that resembles a compartment syndrome in the lower extremity and may require prompt surgical decompression.[40–42]

Backache and Paraplegia

Lumbar backache can be worsened by the ligamentous relaxation that occurs with general, spinal, or epidural anesthesia. Loss of normal lumbar curvature in the supine position is apparently the issue. As a general rule, when possible prior to induction of anesthesia, patients should be placed in positions that are comfortable while they are awake. Padding placed under the lumbar spine before the induction of anesthesia may help retain lordosis and make a patient with known lumbar distress more comfortable. Hyperlordosis should be avoided, however. Hyperextension of the lumbar spine, especially to an angulation of greater than 10 degrees at the L2–3 apex of the lumbar spine, may result in ischemia of the spinal nerves.[43] Multiple patients undergoing pelvic procedures have been reported to have developed paraplegia. In these patients, hyperlordosis was induced by retroflexing the operating room tables maximally, elevating

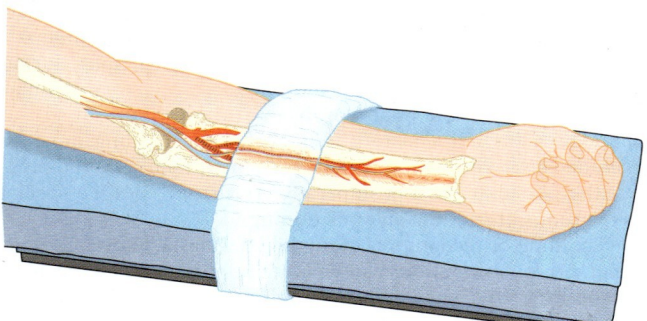

Figure 29-9 Arm restraint, if excessively tight, can compress the anterior interosseous nerve and vessel against the interosseous membrane in the volar forearm to produce an ischemic neuropathy. (Adapted from McLeskey CH, ed. *Geriatric Anesthesiology.* Baltimore, MD: Williams & Wilkins; 1997:155.)

kidney rests fully, and adding padding (e.g., towels, rolls, pillows, and even liter bags of crystalloid) under the lumbar spine to maximize hyperlordosis.

Compartment Syndrome

If, for whatever reason, perfusion to an extremity is inadequate, a compartment syndrome may develop. Characterized by ischemia, hypoxic edema, elevated tissue pressure within fascial compartments of the leg, and extensive rhabdomyolysis, the syndrome produces extensive and potentially lasting damage to the muscles and nerves in the compartment.

Causes of a compartment syndrome that may be associated with positioning factors while a patient is in any of the dorsal decubitus positions include (1) systemic hypotension and loss of driving pressure to the extremity (augmented by elevation of the extremity); (2) vascular obstruction of major leg vessels by intrapelvic retractors, by excessive flexion of knees or hips, or by undue popliteal pressure from a knee crutch; and (3) external compression of the elevated extremity by straps or leg wrappings that are too tight, by the inadvertent pressure of the arm of a surgical assistant, or by the weight of the extremity against a poorly supportive leg holder. A tight strap on an arm as well as tight "draw sheets" for maintaining arms at the patient's sides may compress the anterior interosseous neurovascular bundle and may be associated with an anterior interosseous neuropathy or a forearm or hand compartment syndrome.[41,42]

Several clinical characteristics seem to be associated with perioperative compartment syndrome. Prolonged lithotomy posture in excess of 5 hours has been a common factor in literature anecdotes of postlithotomy compartment syndromes. For lengthy procedures in the lithotomy position, well-padded holders that immobilize the limb by supporting the foot without compressing the calf or popliteal fossa seem to be the least threatening choice. There is considerable variability in the perfusion pressure of the lower extremity in elevated legs. Halliwill et al.[9] and Pfeffer et al.[10] found significant blood pressure variation at the ankle in volunteers placed in various lithotomy positions. Several volunteers had mean pressures of greater than 20 mmHg when positioned in the high lithotomy position. This pressure is less than intracompartment pressures commonly measured in many lithotomy positions.

Warner et al.[44] have shown that perioperative compartment syndromes occur in patients in positions other than lithotomy. The frequency of this problem appears to occur as often (approximately 1 in 9,000 patients studied retrospectively) in anesthetized patients who are positioned laterally as in similar patients who are positioned in lithotomy. The difference between compartment syndromes in these two groups is that patients in a lateral decubitus position tend to have compartment syndromes of either arm, whereas those in a lithotomy position have compartment syndromes of the lower extremities.

Lateral Positions

There are several general positioning concepts to consider when placing a patient into a lateral decubitus position. Wrapping the legs and thighs in compressive bandages has been commonly used to combat venous pooling. Marked flexion of the lower extremities at knees and hips can partially or completely obstruct venous return to the inferior vena cava either by angulation of vessels at the popliteal space and inguinal ligament or by thigh compression against an obese abdomen. A small support placed just caudad of the downside axilla can be used to lift the thorax enough to relieve pressure on the axillary neurovascular bundle and prevent disturbed blood flow to the arm and hand. However, this chest support (inappropriately called an *axillary roll* by some) has not been proven to reduce the frequency of ischemia, nerve damage, or compartment syndrome to the downside upper extremity. It may, however, decrease shoulder discomfort postoperatively. Any padding should support only the chest wall and it should be periodically observed to ensure that it does not impinge on the neurovascular structures of the axilla.

Variations of Lateral Positions

Standard Lateral Position

In the standard lateral position (Fig. 29-10), the patient is rolled onto one side on a flat table surface and stabilized in that posture by flexing the downside thigh. The downside knee is bent to retain the leg on the table and improve stabilization of the trunk. The common peroneal nerve of that side is padded to minimize compression damage caused by the weight of the legs. The upside thigh and leg are extended comfortably, and pillows are placed between the lower extremities. The head is supported by pillows or a headrest so that the cervical and thoracic spines are properly aligned. A small pad, thick enough to raise the chest wall and prevent excessive compression of the shoulder or entrapment/compression of the neurovascular structures of the axilla, is placed just caudad to the downside axilla. This padding may support adequate perfusion of the downside hand and minimize circumduction of the dependent shoulder, which might stretch its suprascapular nerve.

Arms may be extended ventrally and retained on a single arm board with suitable padding between them, or they may be individually retained on a padded two-level arm support that can also help to stabilize the thorax. An alternate method of arm arrangement is to flex each elbow and place the arms on suitable padding on the table in front of the patient's face.

The patient is stabilized in the lateral position by the use of one or more retaining tapes or straps stretched across the hip and fixed to the underside of the tabletop. Care must be taken to see that the hip tapes or straps lie safely between the iliac crest and the head of the femur rather than over the head of the femur. An additional restraining tape or strap may be used across the thorax or shoulders if needed. Other methods, such as the use of "bean bag" or vacuum-supported retention devices, are commonly used. As with any such devices, it is essential to ensure that point pressure on bony prominences is minimized and body structures are appropriately supported.

Semisupine and Semiprone

Semi-lateral postures are designed to allow surgeons to reach anterolateral (semisupine) and posterolateral (semiprone) structures of the trunk. In the semisupine position, the upside arm must be carefully supported so that it is not hyperextended and no traction or compression is applied to the brachial and axillary neurovascular bundles (Fig. 29-11). The supporting bar should be well wrapped to prevent electrical grounding contact (Fig. 29-11A). Sufficient noncompressible padding should be placed under the torso and hip to prevent the patient from rolling supine and stretching the anchored extremity. The pulse of the restrained wrist should be checked to ensure adequate circulation in the elevated arm and hand (Fig. 29-11B).

Flexed Lateral Positions

Lateral Jackknife

The lateral jackknife position places the downside iliac crest over the hinge between the back and thigh sections of the table (Fig. 29-12). The tabletop is angulated at that point to flex the thighs on the trunk laterally. After the patient has been suitably positioned and restrained, the chassis of the table is tipped so that the uppermost surface of the patient's flank and thorax becomes essentially horizontal. As a result, the feet are below the level of the atria, and significant amounts of blood may pool in distensible vessels in each leg.

The lateral jackknife position is usually intended to stretch the upside flank and widen intercostal spaces as an asset to a thoracotomy incision. However, in terms of lumbar stress, restriction by the taut flank of upside costal margin motion, and pooling of blood in depressed lower extremities, the position has the potential to impose a significant physiologic insult. Actually, its usefulness to the surgeon is brief, and its use should be limited. Once the rib-spreading retractor is placed in the incision, the position has reduced value for the rest of the operation.

Kidney

The kidney position (Fig. 29-13) resembles the lateral jackknife position, but it adds the use of an elevated rest (the *kidney rest*) under the downside iliac crest to increase the amount of lateral flexion and improve access to the upside kidney under the overhanging costal margin. Unlike the lateral jackknife position, the kidney position does not have a useful alternative for a flank approach to the kidney. Thus, the physiologic insults associated with the posture need to be limited by vigilant anesthesia and, hopefully, rapid surgery. Strict stabilizing precautions should be taken to prevent the patient from subsequently shifting caudad on the table in such a manner that the elevated rest relocates into the downside flank and becomes a severe impediment to ventilation of the dependent lung.

Complications of Lateral Positions

Eyes and Ears

Injuries to the dependent eye are unlikely if the head is properly supported during and after the turn from the supine to the

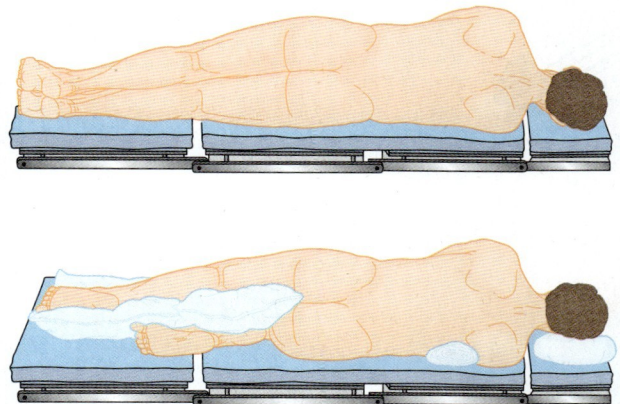

Figure 29-10 The standard lateral decubitus position. Proper head support, chest support, and leg pillow arrangements are shown on the *lower figure*. The downside leg is flexed at the hip and knee to stabilize the torso. Retaining straps and pad for the downside peroneal nerve are not shown.

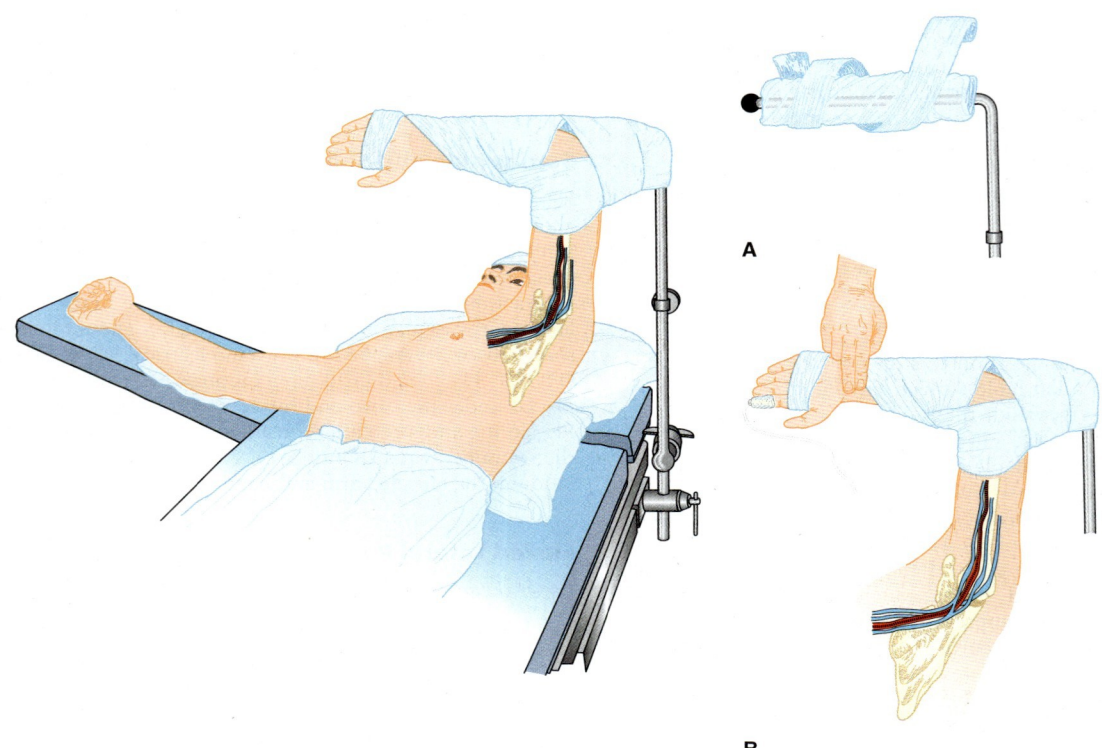

Figure 29-11 The semisupine position with dorsal pads supporting the torso, the extended arm padded at the elbow, and the elevated arm restrained on a well-cushioned, adjustable overhead bar (**A**). Axillary contents (**B**) are not under tension and are not compressed by the head of the humerus, and a pulse oximeter ensures that the digital circulation is not compromised. The position is safe only if the arm does not become a hanging mechanism to support the torso. (Adapted from Collins VJ, ed. *Principles of Anesthesiology*, 3rd ed. Philadelphia, PA: Lea & Febiger; 1993:176.)

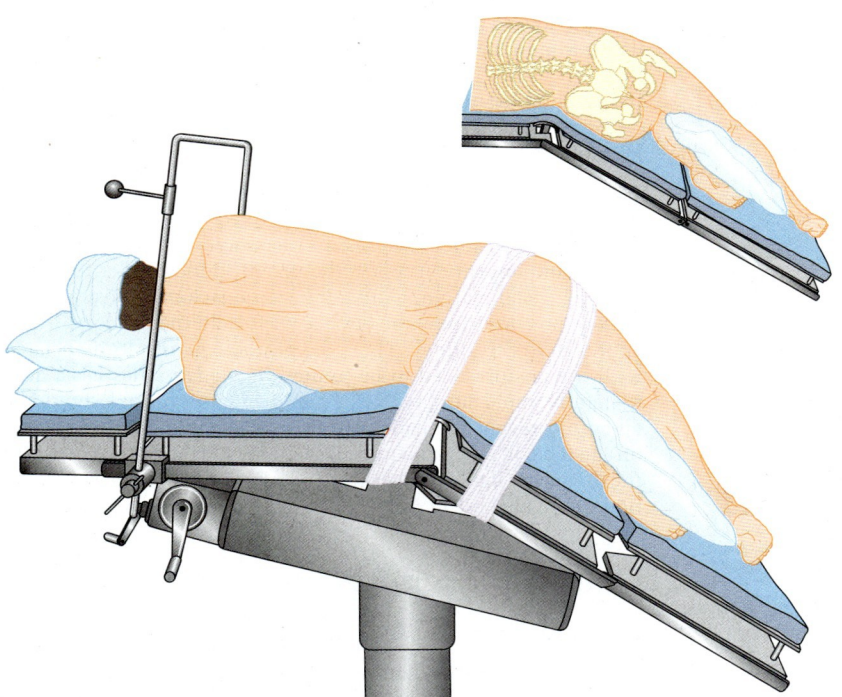

Figure 29-12 The lateral jackknife position, intended to open intercostal spaces. Note the properly placed restraining tapes (*large figure*) thrusting cephalad to retain the iliac crest at the flexion point of the table and prevent caudad slippage, which compresses the downside flank (*inset*).

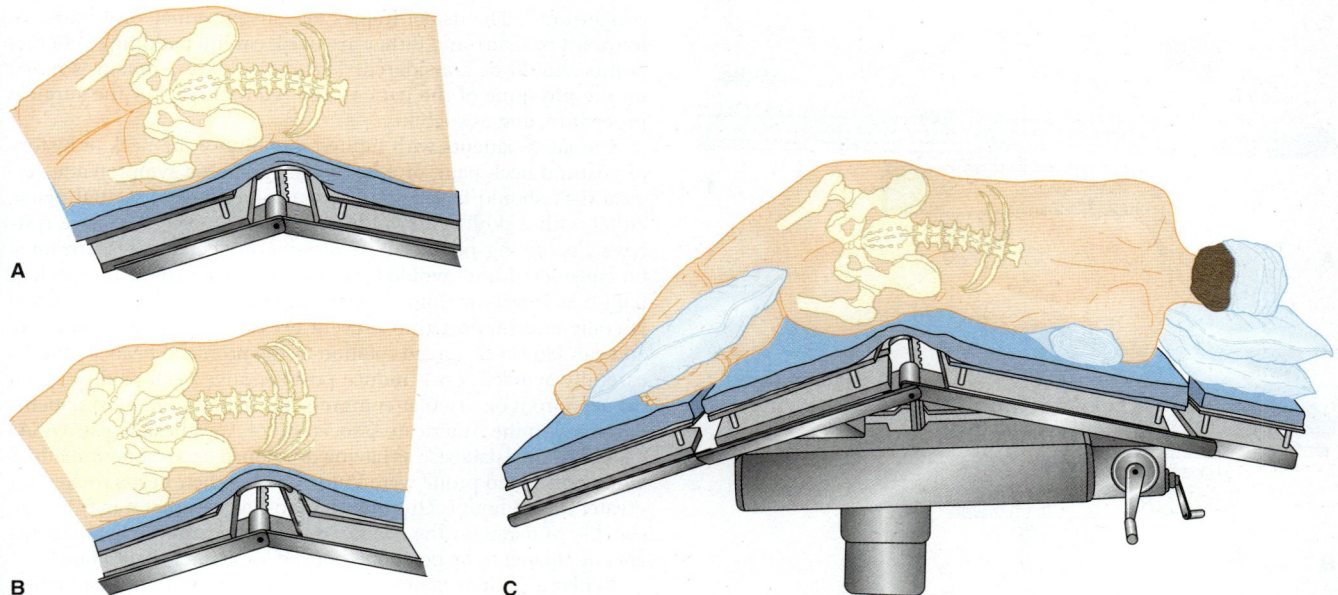

Figure 29-13 The flexed lateral (kidney) position. Upper panels show improper locations of the elevated transverse rest, the flexion point of the table, in the flank (**A**) or at the lower costal margin (**B**) to impede ventilation of the downside lung. The iliac crest at the proper flexion point (**C**), allowing the best possible expansion of the downside lung. Restraining tapes deleted for clarity.

lateral position. If the patient's face turns toward the mattress, however, and the lids are not closed or the eyes otherwise protected, abrasions of the ocular surface can occur. Direct pressure on the globe can displace the crystalline lens, increase intraocular pressure or, particularly if systemic hypotension is present, cause ischemia.

In the lateral position, the weight of the head can press the downside ear against a rough or wrinkled supporting surface. Careful padding with a pillow or a foam sponge is usually sufficient protection against contusion of the ear. The external ear should also be palpated to ensure that it has not been folded over in the process of placing support beneath the head.

Neck

Lateral flexion of the neck is possible when the head of a patient in the lateral position is inadequately supported. If the cervical spine is arthritic, postoperative neck pain can be troublesome. Pain from a symptomatic protrusion of a cervical disk can be intensified unless the head is carefully positioned so that lateral or ventral flexion, extension, or rotation is avoided.

Suprascapular Nerve

Ventral circumduction of the dependent shoulder can rotate the suprascapular notch away from the root of the neck (Fig. 29-14). Because the suprascapular nerve is fixed both paravertebrally and at the notch, circumduction can stretch the nerve and produce troublesome, diffuse, dull shoulder pain. The diagnosis is established by blocking the nerve at the notch and producing pain relief. Treatment may require resecting the ligament over the notch to decompress the nerve. A supporting pad placed under the thorax caudad of the axilla and thick enough to raise the chest off the shoulder may prevent a circumduction stretch injury to the nerve.

Prone Positions

Full Prone

In the so-called *full prone position* (Fig. 29-15), the requirement to elevate the trunk off the supporting surface so that the ventral abdominal wall is freed of compression almost always results in the head and lower extremities being below the level of the spine. If the tabletop is angulated at the trunk–thigh hinge to remove the lumbar lordosis and separate the lumbar spinous processes, and if the chassis is then rotated head-up sufficiently to level the patient's back, a significant perfusion gradient may develop between the legs and the heart. Wrapping the legs in compressive

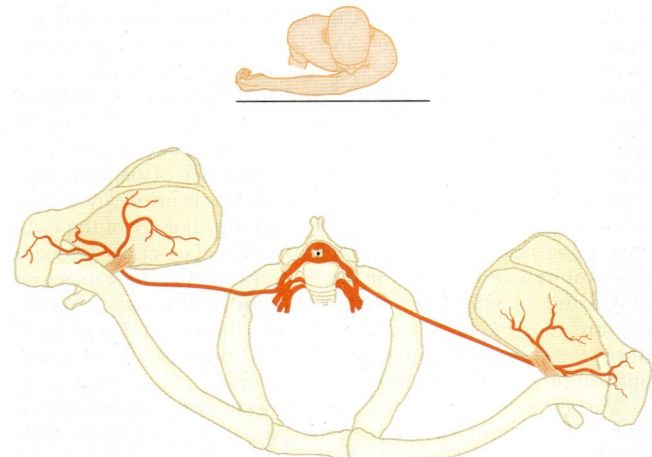

Figure 29-14 Circumduction of the arm displacing the scapula and stretching the suprascapular nerve between its anchoring points at the cervical spine and the suprascapular notch.

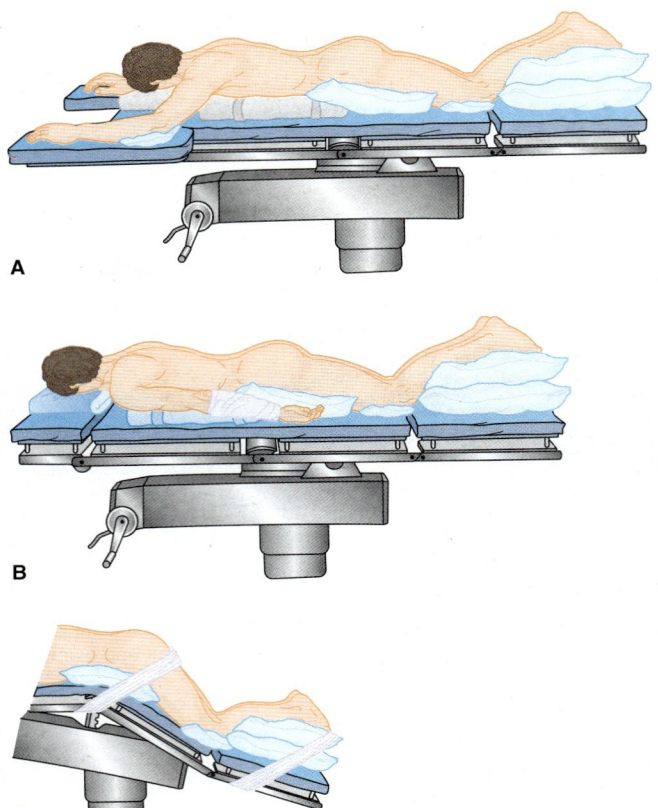

Figure 29-15 The classic prone position. **A:** Flat table with relaxed arms extended alongside the patient's head. Parallel chest rolls extended from just caudad of the clavicle to just beyond the inguinal area, with a pillow over the pelvic end. Elbows and knees are padded, and legs are bent at the knees. The head is turned onto a C-shaped pad, gel, or foam sponge that frees the downside eye and ear from compression. **B:** The same posture with arms snugly retained alongside the torso. **C:** Table flexed to reduce lumbar lordosis; subgluteal area straps placed after the legs are lowered to provide cephalad thrust and prevent caudad slippage.

bandages, or the use of full-length elastic hosiery, minimizes pooling of blood in distensible vessels and supports venous return.

When this position results in the head being lower than the heart, the pressure gradient can result in venous and lymphatic stasis in the head. This position may result in facial and airway edema, making extubation of intubated patients challenging, especially after prolonged procedures such as spine fusions. In addition, over the past decade or two, long spine surgical procedures have resulted in a surprising number of patients who experience severe vision loss. This vision loss is primarily related to ischemic optic neuropathy. Although the etiology of the ischemic optic neuropathy is not entirely clear, Lee et al.[45] suggest that prone positions with the head lower than the heart may lead to venous and lymphatic congestion in the optic canal. This congestion, added to the effect of gravity on the suspended globe of the eye, can result in optic nerve stretch and possibly the development of ischemic neuropathy (see later).[46]

Various pelvic, abdominal, and chest supports, including parallel rolls of tightly packed sheets, gels, padded and adjustable metal frames, and four-pillar frames, have been devised to free the abdomen from compression. Of these, the Wilson frame is particularly concerning in that its use results in the head being lower than the heart, potentially contributing to optic nerve congestion.[45] The use of frames may also produce opportunities for point pressure and if they are used, careful padding of contact points should be considered. The choice of equipment is based on the physique of the patient, the requirements of the surgical procedure, and availability.

Pronated patients with limited mobility of the neck, a history of postural neck pain, or a history suggesting a symptomatic cervical disk should have their heads retained in the sagittal plane, either with a skull-pin head clamp or with a face rest. Face rests have fluctuating popularity. Excessive periocular pressure must be considered and avoided if a face rest is used. If the neck is pain-free and its mobility is satisfactory, the head can be turned laterally and supported to prevent pressure on the downside eye and ear. However, forced rotation of the pronated head should be carefully avoided lest it induce postoperative neck pain or cervical nerve root or vascular compression. In addition, most patients described in the American Association of Anesthesiologists (ASA) Closed Claims database as having developed cervical neuropathies while positioned prone were found to have their heads rotated for greater than 3 hours. This information suggests that it may be reasonable to maintain the head in a neutral position when patients are anticipated to be positioned prone for greater than 3 hours.

When a patient is scheduled to be pronated after induction of anesthesia, it is worthwhile during the preanesthetic interview to obtain and record information about any limitations that may exist in his or her ability to raise the arms overhead during work or sleep. If the patient is symptomatic, it may be prudent to place the arms alongside the torso after pronation (see Thoracic Outlet Syndrome). If the arms are placed alongside the head (i.e., extended ventrally at the shoulder, flexed at the elbow, and abducted onto arm boards; the "surrender" position), the musculature about the shoulders should be under no tension, neither humeral head should stretch or compress its axillary neurovascular bundle (i.e., shoulders should be abducted <90 degrees), ulnar nerves at the elbow should be padded, and the pulses at the wrists should remain full. Anterior (forward) flexion of the shoulders may reduce tension on the neurovascular structures of the axilla.

Complications of Prone Positions

Eyes and Ears

The eyes and ears may sustain injury in the prone position. The eyelids should be closed, and each eye should be protected in some manner so that the lids cannot be accidentally separated and the cornea scratched. Instillation of lubrication in the eyes should be considered, although the value of this treatment is being debated. The eyes should also be protected against the head turning after positioning and pressure being exerted on the globe. Monitoring wires and intravenous tubing should be checked after pronation to see that none has migrated beneath the head. If the head is retained in the sagittal plane, the eyes should be checked after positioning to ensure that they are safe from compression by any headrest.

Conjunctival edema usually occurs in the eyes of the pronated patient if the head is at or below the level of the heart. It is usually transient, inconsequential, and requires only reestablishment of the normal tissue perfusion gradients of the supine position, or of a slight amount of head-up tilt, to be redistributed. There does not appear to be any connection between this edema and the occurrence of posterior ischemic optic neuropathy.

Blindness

Permanent loss of vision can occur after nonocular surgical procedures, especially those performed in a prone position.[45] The occurrence of this devastating complication is associated particularly with extensive surgical procedures done in the prone position, such as reconstructive spine surgery, where there is associated blood loss, anemia, and hypotension.

Lee et al.[43] used data from the American Society of Anesthesiologists Visual Loss Registry to study ischemic optic neuropathy in spine fusion patients. Using a 1:4 case-control methodology, the authors found six risk factors, half of which strongly support their speculation that acute venous congestion of the optic canal is a potential etiology of ischemic optic neuropathy in this setting. The use of a Wilson surgical bed frame with its elevated curvature resulting in the head being lower than the heart, obesity with its potential elevation of intra-abdominal pressure in prone-positioned patients, and long anesthetic durations can all contribute to elevated venous congestion in the optic canal and potentially reduce optic nerve perfusion pressure. The authors also found that increased estimated blood loss, male gender, and lower percent of colloid administration were independently associated with the development of ischemic optic neuropathy after spinal fusion surgery.

These results suggest that the ASA's 2012 Practice Advisory on this issue is relevant.[46] Basically, it is prudent to attempt to reduce venous congestion in the optic canal. That is, consideration should be given to using positions that allow the patients' heads to be level with or higher than their hearts. It may be helpful to use colloids as well as crystalloids to maintain intravascular volume. Intraoperative positioning that helps reduce intra-abdominal pressure and, therefore, venous congestion, may be useful. The use of the Wilson frame and other positioning devices should be assessed carefully, with a goal to reduce pressure on the abdomen and to keep the head level with or higher than the heart. Since the authors found duration of anesthesia to be an independent risk factor for ischemic optic neuropathy in this population, it may be prudent to work with the spine surgeons to determine if there is merit to limiting the duration of surgeries that are anticipated to be prolonged, especially 6 hours or longer. Staging these procedures may be helpful.

Neck Problems

Anesthesia impairs reflex muscle spasm that protects the skeleton against motion that would be painful if the patient were alert. Lateral rotation of the head and neck of an anesthetized, pronated patient, particularly one with an arthritic cervical spine, can stretch relaxed skeletal muscles and ligaments and injure articulations of cervical vertebrae. Postoperative neck pain and limitation of motion can result. The arthritic neck is usually best managed by keeping the head in the sagittal plane when the patient is prone.

Extremes of head and neck rotation can also interfere with flow in either the ipsilateral or contralateral vessels to and from the head. Excessive head rotation can reduce flow in both the carotid[47] and vertebral systems.[48] Impaired cerebral perfusion is the obvious consequence.

Brachial Plexus Injuries

Stretch injuries to the roots of the brachial plexus (Fig. 29-16A) on the side contralateral to the turned face are possible if the contralateral shoulder is held firmly caudad by a wrist restraint. If an arm is placed on an arm board alongside the head, care must be taken to ensure that the head of the humerus is not stretching and compressing the axillary neurovascular bundle (Fig. 29-16B,C).

When an arm is placed on an arm board alongside the head, the forearm naturally pronates. As a result, the ulnar nerve, lying in the cubital tunnel (the groove between the olecranon process and the medial epicondyle of the humerus), is vulnerable to being compressed by the weight of the elbow (Fig. 29-16D). Consequently, the medial aspect of the elbow must be well padded and its weight borne across a large area to avoid point pressure.

Asking patients about their ability to work or sleep with arms elevated overhead may identify patients with *thoracic outlet obstruction*. A useful preoperative test if the history is in question is to have the patient clasp hands behind the occiput during the interview. If the patient describes dysesthesias, it may be prudent to keep the arms alongside the trunk in the prone position. Agonizing, debilitating, and unremitting postoperative pain has been known to follow overhead arm placement in pronated patients who have had prior discomfort in their arms in that position.

Breast Injuries

The breasts of a pronated woman, if forced laterally or medially by chest and abdominal wall supports, can be stretched and injured along their sternal borders. Direct pressure on breasts (particularly if breast prostheses are present) can cause ischemia to breast tissue and should be avoided. Multiple cases of breast tissue ischemia have been reported, often resulting in mastectomy and the need for reconstruction.

Abdominal Compression

Compression of the abdomen by the weight of the prone patient's trunk can cause viscera to force the diaphragm cephalad enough

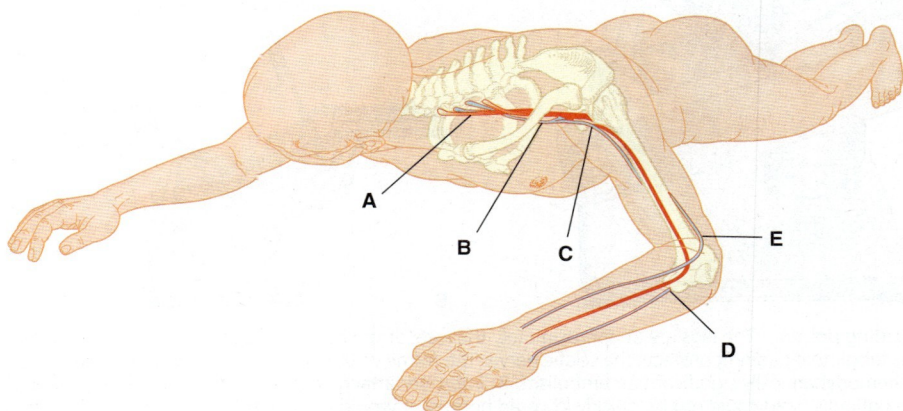

Figure 29-16 Sources of potential injury to the brachial plexus and its peripheral components when the patient is in the prone position. **A:** Neck rotation, stretching roots of the plexus. **B:** Compression of the plexus and vessels between the clavicle and first rib. **C:** Injury to the axillary neurovascular bundle from the head of the humerus. **D:** Compression of the ulnar nerve before, beyond, and within the cubital tunnel. **E:** Area of vulnerability of the radial nerve to lateral compression proximal to the elbow.

to impair ventilation. If intra-abdominal pressure approaches or exceeds venous pressure, return of blood from the pelvis and lower extremities is reduced or obstructed. Because the vertebral venous plexuses communicate directly with the abdominal veins, increased intra-abdominal pressure is transmitted to the perivertebral and intraspinal surgical field in the form of venous distention and increased difficulty with hemostasis. All of the various supportive pads and frames, when properly used, are designed to remove pressure from the abdomen and avoid these problems.

Stoma and Genitals

Stoma that drain visceral contents through the abdominal wall are at risk in the prone position if they lie against a part of any supporting frame or pad. Compressive ischemia of the stomal orifice can cause it to slough. The same issue is present for genitals, especially the penis and scrotum of men turned prone.

Head-elevated Positions

Variations of Head-elevated Positions

Sitting

The classic *sitting position* for surgery places the patient in a semi-reclining posture on an operating table, with the legs elevated to approximately the level of the heart and the head flexed ventrally on the neck (Fig. 29-17). Head flexion should not be sufficient to force the chin into the suprasternal notch (see "Midcervical Tetraplegia"). Elastic stockings or compressive wraps around the legs reduce pooling of blood in the lower extremities. The head often is held in place by some type of a face rest or by a three-pin skull fixation frame.

Supine—Tilted Head Up

A supine recumbent position with the head of the patient elevated is used for many operations involving the ventral and lateral aspects of the head (Fig. 29-18) and neck, and occasionally with the neck flexed, for transcranial access to the top of the brain. Its purpose is to improve access to the surgical target for the operating team as well as to drain blood and irrigation solutions away from the wound. The back section of the surgical table can be elevated as needed to produce a low sitting position (Fig. 29-18A) or the entire table can be rotated head-high with the patient's extended legs supported by a foot rest (Fig. 29-18B). Although the degree of tilt typically is not great, small pressure gradients are created along the vascular axis that can pool blood in the lower extremities or entrain air in patulous vessels that are incised above the level of the heart.

For operations around the shoulder joint, the patient may be placed in a head-elevated semisupine position (Fig. 29-19). The upper trunk typically is moved laterally until the raised surgical shoulder extends beyond the edge of the operating table. The torso is supported so that the hips are on the table, the surgical shoulder is off and above the table edge, and the head rests on either a pillow (Fig. 29-19A) or a headrest (Fig. 29-19B). Access is thereby provided to both the dorsal and ventral aspects of the shoulder girdle. The surgical arm remains on the front of the torso and is prepared and draped to be mobile in the surgical field.

Lateral—Tilted Head Up

The lateral position with the head somewhat elevated, a means of access to occipitocervical lesions, has also been referred to as the *park bench position*. All the stabilizing requirements needed for the usual lateral position apply. The head may be held firmly in a three-pin skull fixation holder, which can be readjusted as needed

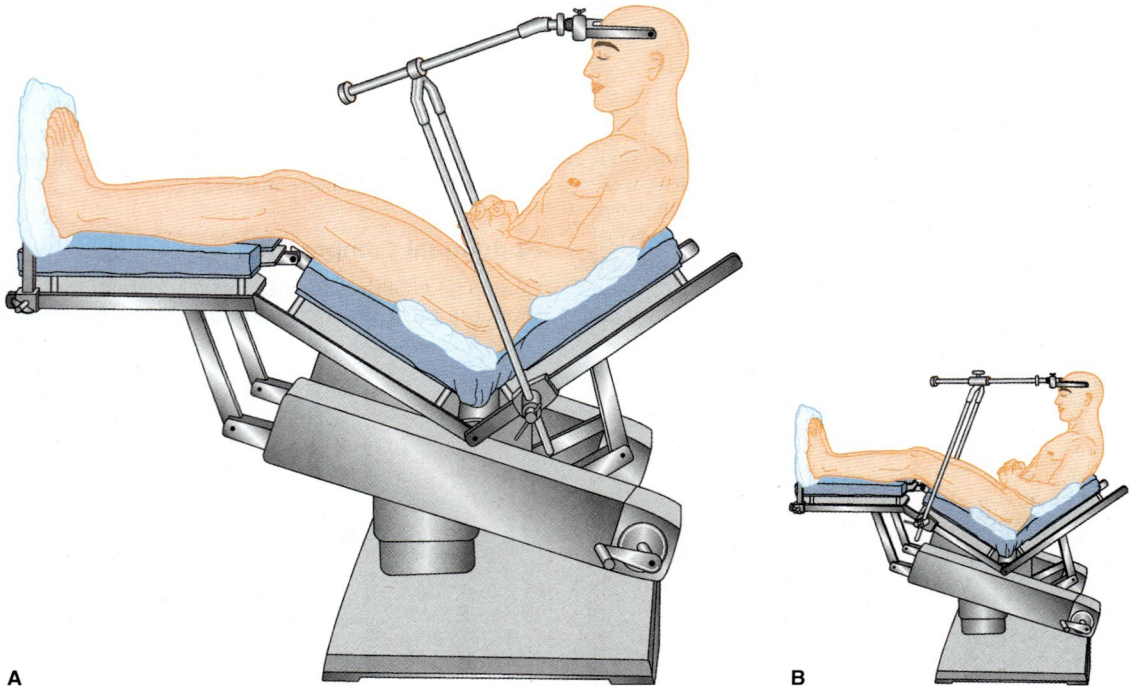

Figure 29-17 **A:** Conventional neurosurgical sitting position. The legs are at approximately the level of the heart and gently flexed on the thighs; the feet are supported at right angles to the legs; subgluteal padding protects the sciatic nerve. The frame of the head holder is *properly* clamped to the side rails of the back section in the event of hemodynamically significant air embolism. **B:** *Improper* attachment of the head frame to the table side rails at the thigh section. In this position, the patient's head could not be quickly lowered because it would require disengaging the skull clamp.

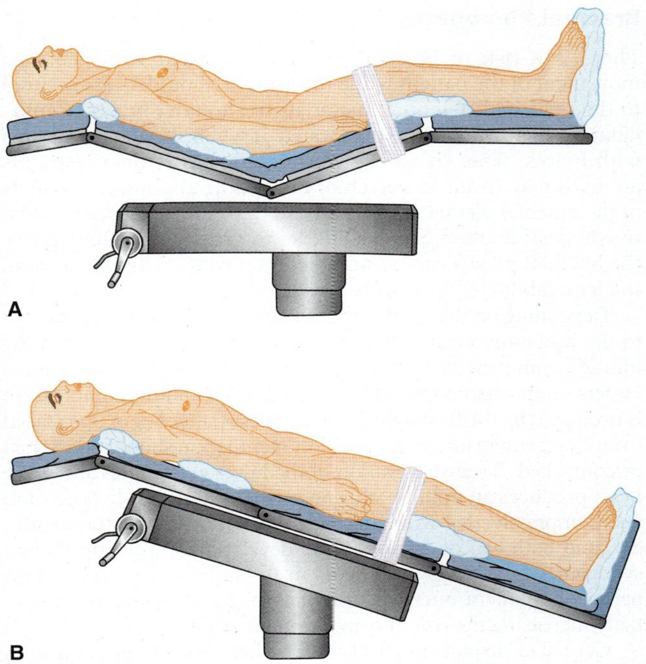

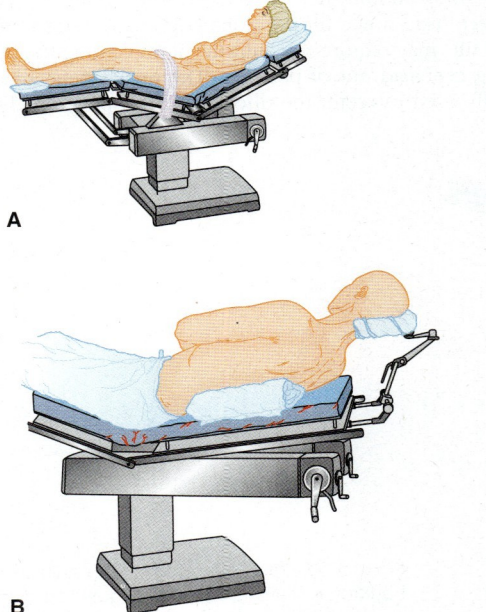

Figure 29-18 Head-elevated positions often used for operations about the ventral and ventrolateral aspects of the head, face, neck, and cervical spine. **A:** The legs are at approximately heart level and the gradient into the head is appreciable but slight. **B:** The flat table and foot rest are useful when a thyroidectomy is planned under regional anesthesia.

during surgery, or supported by pillows or padding. Although the degree of head elevation used typically is less than 15 degrees, the position does not completely remove the threat of air embolization. The anesthesiologist has good access to the patient's face and thorax for purposes of monitoring, manipulation, and resuscitation. Considerable attention should be directed to avoiding compression of neck veins, which can lead to an increase in intracranial pressure and to edema of the tongue.

Complications of Head-elevated Positions

Postural Hypotension

In the anesthetized patient, establishing any of the head-elevated positions is frequently accompanied by some degree of reduction in systemic blood pressure. The normal protective reflexes are inhibited by drugs used during anesthesia. Measuring mean arterial pressures at the level of the circle of Willis is recommended by many to assess cerebral perfusion pressures more accurately. This recommendation, however, is controversial.[49–53]

Air Embolus

Air embolization is potentially lethal. In the bloodstream, air migrates to the heart, where it creates a compressible foam that destroys the propulsive efficiency of ventricular contraction and irritates the conduction system. Air can also move into the pulmonary vasculature, where bubbles obstruct small vessels and compromise gas exchange, or it can cross through a patent foramen ovale to the left side of the heart and the systemic circulation.

The potential for venous air embolization increases with the degree of elevation of the operative site above the heart. Although the occurrence of air emboli is a relatively frequent phenomenon in head-elevated positions, most of the emboli are small in volume, clinically silent, and recognizable only by sophisticated Doppler detection or echocardiographic (e.g., transesophageal) techniques. Nevertheless, the potential for dangerous accumulations of entrained air requires immediate detection of the embolization, a careful search for its portal of entry, and prompt treatment of its clinical effects.

Edema of the Face, Tongue, and Neck

Severe postoperative macroglossia, apparently because of venous and lymphatic obstruction, can be caused by prolonged, marked neck flexion. Postoperative need for a tracheostomy has been reported. Try to avoid placing the patient's chin firmly against the chest and use an oral airway to protect the endotracheal tube. Extremes of neck flexion, with or without head rotation, have been widely used to gain access to structures in the posterior fossa and cervical spine, but their potential for damage should be understood and excessive flexion–rotation avoided if possible. Moore et al.[54] have suggested that the primary mechanism may be neurologically determined rather than being the result of either vascular obstruction or local trauma. This problem also has been described with the use of transesophageal echocardiography probes.

Midcervical Tetraplegia

This devastating injury occurs after hyperflexion of the neck, with or without rotation of the head, and is attributed to stretching of the spinal cord with resulting compromise of its vasculature in the midcervical area. An element of spondylosis or a spondylotic bar may be involved.[55,56] The result is paralysis below the general level of the fifth cervical vertebra. Although most reports in the literature have described the condition as occurring after the use of the sitting position, midcervical tetraplegia has also occurred after prolonged, nonforced head flexion for intracranial surgery in the supine position.

Figure 29-19 **A:** The lawn chair position for surgery around the shoulder joint. **B:** The upper torso is rotated toward the nonsurgical shoulder and supported with a firm roll or pad.

Sciatic Nerve Injury

Stretch injuries of the sciatic nerve can occur in some seated patients if the hips are markedly flexed without bending the knees. Prolonged compression of the sciatic nerve as it emerges from the pelvis is possible in a thin seated patient if the buttocks are not suitably padded. Foot drop may be the result of injuries to either the sciatic nerve or the common peroneal nerve and can be bilateral.

Head-down Positions

The introduction of robotic procedures has resulted in an increased use of head-down positions. The great majority of robotic procedures early in the introduction of the technology have involved prostatectomies, colorectal, and gynecologic procedures. Thus, most of these initial procedures and the experience gained with robotic procedures have been performed in the pelvis and lower abdomen. As with any introduction of new technology, there is a steep learning curve for the operators. Typically, early adopters of robotic technology have requested steep head-down positions of supine patients. These steep head-down positions have resulted in a variety of complications that challenge anesthesia providers and patients.

Complications of Head-down Positions

Head and Neck Injury

During the years coincident with the introduction of robotic surgery techniques, several patients have suffered severe injury and have even died from body shifts on operating room tables that have been tilted severely head-down. There are several anecdotes from medicolegal actions involving patients who slid off operating tables with resulting neck injuries. In one instance, a patient in a supine and very steep head-down position apparently somersaulted heels over head off of the operating room table and subsequently died from a massive intracranial bleed. Steep head-down tilt is not often warranted and should be actively discouraged when appropriate. Skilled operators often find that they need less steep head-down tilt as they gain experience and expertise with robotic procedures.

Brachial Plexopathy

There is a risk of brachial injuries associated with cephalad movement of the patient while the arms or shoulders are secured to the table with retention materials or shoulder braces. Cephalad movement when arms are fixated or when shoulder restraints with braces, tape, "bean bag" devices, or other torso restraints are used may result in stretch of the middle and lower divisions of the brachial plexus. If the cephalad movement results in a relative hyperabduction of the shoulder to greater than 90 degrees, the brachial plexus can be stretched as it courses distally around the hyperabducted head of the humerus.

Depending on the degree of head depression, the addition of tilt to the lithotomy position combines the worst features of both the lithotomy and the head-down postures. The weight of abdominal viscera on the diaphragm adds to whatever abdominal compression is produced by the flexed thighs of an obese patient or of one placed in an exaggerated lithotomy position. Ventilation should be assisted or controlled. Because elevation of the lower extremities above the heart produces an uphill perfusion gradient, systemic hypotension and compressive leg wrapping may limit perfusion to the periphery, and both can be factors in the development of compartment syndromes in the legs of patients in the lithotomy position. This perfusion gradient often is unpredictable and exaggerated, potentially increasing the risk of compartment syndrome.[9,10]

Cephalad displacement of the diaphragm and obstruction of its caudad inspiratory stroke accompany a head-down position because of gravity-shifted abdominal viscera. Consequently, the work of spontaneous ventilation is increased for an anesthetized patient in a posture that already worsens the ventilation–perfusion ratio by gravitational accumulation of blood in the poorly ventilated lung apices. During controlled ventilation, higher inspiratory pressures are needed to expand the lung.

Cranial vascular congestion and increased intracranial pressure can be expected to result from head-down tilt. For patients with known or suspected intracranial disease, the position should be used only in those rare instances in which a surgically useful alternate posture cannot be found. Maintenance of the position should then be as brief as possible.[57,58]

Steep head-down tilt positions (e.g., 30 to 45 degrees of head-down tilt) may require some means of preventing the patient from sliding cephalad out of position. The use of bent knees is occasionally used to retain the tilted patient in position (Fig. 29-20).

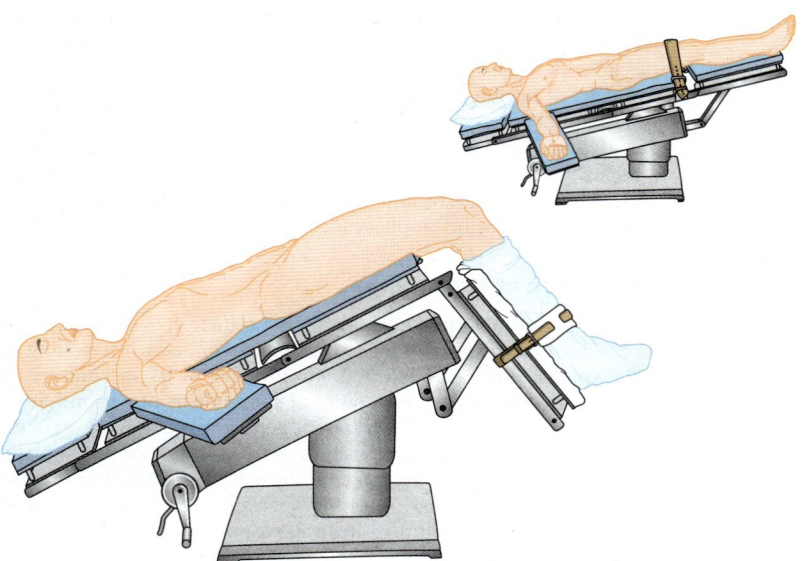

Figure 29-20 Head-down tilt. *Lower figure* shows traditional steep (30- to 45-degree) tilt. Leg restraints and knee flexion stabilize the patient, avoiding the need for wristlets or shoulder braces that threaten the brachial plexus. *Upper figure* shows 10 to 15 degrees of head-down tilt.

Historically, shoulder braces, straps, or tape also have been used to prevent cephalad sliding in steep head-down tilt positions. These are best tolerated if placed over the acromioclavicular joints, but care must be taken to see that the shoulder is not forced sufficiently caudad to trap and compress the subclavian neurovascular bundle between the clavicle and the first rib. If they are placed medially against the root of the neck, they may easily compress neurovascular structures that emerge from the area of the scalene musculature. For these and other reasons, the use of shoulder braces and other retaining approaches have waned in popularity. In general, the use of steep head-down positions should be limited to only those portions of procedures in which their use is most important.[57,58]

Summary

There are many ways that patients can be injured during surgical procedures. Careful consideration of intraoperative and postoperative positioning may help reduce the frequency and severity of perioperative positioning-related events. Although many problems that appear to be related to perioperative positioning may seem simple and preventable, the etiologic mechanisms of many of these problems are not readily apparent. Much work still remains to determine the role of other potential etiologies, such as perioperative inflammatory responses, immunosuppression, and virus activation, on the development of these problems.

REFERENCES

1. Staff NP, Engelstad J, Klein CJ, et al. Post-surgical inflammatory neuropathy. *Brain*. 2010;133:2866–2880.
2. Staff NP, Dyck PJ, Warner MA. Post-surgical inflammatory neuropathy should be considered in the differential diagnosis of diaphragm paralysis after surgery. *Anesthesiology*. 2014;120:1057.
3. Laughlin RS, Dyck JB, Watson JC, et al. Ipsilateral inflammatory neuropathy after hip surgery. *Mayo Clin Proc*. 2014;89:454–461.
4. Warner ME, Warner MA. Inflammatory neuropathy: a potentially treatable etiology of perioperative neuropathies. *Mayo Clin Proc*. 2014;89:434–436.
5. Hunter JD. Effects of anaesthesia on the human immune system. *Hosp Med*. 1999;60:658–663.
6. Brand A. Immunological aspects of blood transfusions. *Transplant Immunol*. 2002;10:183–190.
7. Gilden DH, Katz RI. Surgical induction of zoster in a contralateral homologous dermatomal distribution. *Arch Neurol*. 2003;60:616–617.
8. Martin JT. Compartment syndromes: Concepts and perspectives for the anesthesiologist. *Anesth Analg*. 1992;75:275–283.
9. Halliwill JR, Hewitt SA, Joyner MJ, et al. Effects of various lithotomy positions on lower extremity blood pressures. *Anesthesiology*. 1999;89:1373–1376.
10. Pfeffer SD, Halliwill JR, Warner MA. Effects of lithotomy position and external compression on lower leg muscle compartment pressure. *Anesthesiology*. 2001;95:632–636.
11. Angermeier KW, Jordan GH. Complications of the exaggerated lithotomy position: A review of 177 cases. *J Urol*. 1994;151:866–868.
12. Jellish WS, Blakeman B, Warf P, et al. Hands-up positioning during asymmetric sternal retraction for internal mammary artery harvest: A possible method to reduce brachial plexus injury. *Anesth Analg*. 1997;84:260–265.
13. Vander Salm TJ, Cereda J-M, Cutler BS. Brachial plexus injury following median sternotomy. *J Thorac Cardiovasc Surg*. 1980;80:447–452.
14. Vander Salm TJ, Cutler BS, Okike ON. Brachial plexus injury following median sternotomy: Part II. *J Thorac Cardiovasc Surg*. 1982;83:914–917.
15. Roy RC, Stafford MA, Charlton JE. Nerve injury and musculoskeletal complaints after cardiac surgery: Influence of internal mammary artery dissection and left arm position. *Anesth Analg*. 1988;67:277–279.
16. Gregg JR, Labosky D, Harty M, et al. Serratus anterior paralysis in the young athlete. *J Bone Joint Surg Am*. 1979;61:825–832.
17. Martin JT. Postoperative isolated dysfunction of the long thoracic nerve: A rare entity of uncertain etiology. *Anesth Analg*. 1989;69:614–619.
18. Foo CL, Swann M. Isolated paralysis of the serratus anterior. *J Bone Joint Surg Br*. 1983;65:552–556.
19. Kroll DA, Caplan RA, Posner K, et al. Nerve injury associated with anesthesia. *Anesthesiology*. 1990;73:202–207.
20. Cheney FW, Domino KB, Caplan RA, et al. Nerve injury associated with anesthesia. *Anesthesiology*. 1999;90:1062–1069.
21. Büdinger K. Ueber Lähmungen nach Chloroform-Narkosen. *Archiv für Klinische Chiruque*. 1894;47:121.
22. Garriques HJ. Anaesthesia-paralysis. *Am J Med Sci*. 1897;113:81–89.
23. Wadsworth TG, Williams JR. Cubital tunnel external compression syndrome. *BMJ*. 1973;1:662–666.
24. Warner MA, Warner DO, Harper CM, et al. Ulnar neuropathy in medical patients. *Anesthesiology*. 2000;92:613–615.
25. Warner MA, Warner ME, Martin JT. Ulnar neuropathy: Incidence, outcome, and risk factors in sedated or anesthetized patients. *Anesthesiology*. 1994;81:1332–1340.
26. Alvine FG, Schurrer ME. Postoperative ulnar-nerve palsy: Are there predisposing factors? *J Bone Joint Surg Am*. 1987;69:255–259.
27. Warner MA, Warner DO, Matsumoto JY, et al. Ulnar neuropathy in surgical patients. *Anesthesiology*. 1999;90:54–59.
28. Prielipp RC, Morell RC, Walker FO, et al. Ulnar nerve pressure: Influence of arm position and relationship to somatosensory evoked potentials. *Anesthesiology*. 1999;91:345–354.
29. Campbell WW, Pridgeon RM, Riaz G, et al. Variations in anatomy of the ulnar nerve at the cubital tunnel: Pitfalls in the diagnosis of ulnar neuropathy at the elbow. *Muscle Nerve*. 1991;14:733–738.
30. O'Driscoll SW, Horii E, Carmichael SW, et al. The cubital tunnel and ulnar neuropathy. *J Bone Joint Surg Am*. 1991;73:613–617.
31. Childress HM. Recurrent ulnar nerve dislocation at the elbow. *J Bone Joint Surg*. 1956;38:978–984.
32. Ashenhurst EM. Anatomical factors in the etiology of ulnar neuropathy. *CMAJ*. 1962;87:159–163.
33. Macnicol MF. Extraneural pressures affecting the ulnar nerve at the elbow. *Hand*. 1982;14:5–11.
34. Morell RC, Prielipp RC, Harwood TN, et al. Men are more susceptible than women to direct pressure on unmyelinated ulnar nerve fibers. *Anesth Analg*. 2003;97:1183–1188.
35. Pechan J, Julis I. The pressure measurement in the ulnar nerve: A contribution to the pathophysiology of the cubital tunnel syndrome. *J Biomech*. 1975;8:75–79.
36. Contreras MG, Warner MA, Charboneau WJ, et al. The anatomy of the ulnar nerve at the elbow: Potential relationship of acute ulnar neuropathy to gender differences. *Clin Anat*. 1998;11:372–378.
37. Shimokata H, Tobin JD, Muller DC, et al. Studies in the distribution of body fat: I. Effects of age, sex, and obesity. *J Gerontol*. 1989;44:M66–M73.
38. Hattori K, Numata N, Ikoma M, et al. Sex differences in the distribution of subcutaneous and internal fat. *Hum Biol*. 1991;63:53–63.
39. Chusid JG. *Correlative Neuroanatomy and Functional Neurology*. Los Altos, CA: Lange Medical Publications; 1985:149.
40. Hill NA, Howard FM, Huffer BR. The incomplete anterior interosseous nerve syndrome. *J Hand Surg [Am]*. 1985;10:4–16.
41. Kies SJ, Danielson DR, Dennison DJ, et al. Perioperative compartment syndrome of the hand. *Anesthesiology*. 2004;101:1232–1234.
42. Contreras MG, Warner MA, Carmichael SW, et al. Perioperative anterior interosseous neuropathy. *Anesthesiology*. 2002;96:243–245.
43. Amoiridis G, Wöhrle JC, Langkafel M, et al. Spinal cord infarction after surgery in a patient in the hyperlordotic position. *Anesthesiology*. 1996;84:228–230.
44. Warner ME, LaMaster LM, Thoeming AK, et al. Compartment syndrome in surgical patients. *Anesthesiology*. 2001;94:705–708.
45. The Postoperative Visual Loss Study Group. Risk factors associated with ischemic optic neuropathy after spinal fusion surgery. *Anesthesiology*. 2012;116:15–24.
46. American Society of Anesthesiologists Committee on Standards and Practice Parameters. Practice advisory for perioperative visual loss associated with spine surgery. *Anesthesiology*. 2012;116:274–285.
47. Sherman DD, Hart RG, Easton JD. Abrupt change in head position and cerebral infarction. *Stroke*. 1981;12:2–6.
48. Toole JF. Effects of change of head, limb and body position on cephalic circulation. *N Engl J Med*. 1968;279:307–311.
49. Cullen DJ, Kirby RR. Beach chair position may decrease cerebral perfusion. *APSF Newsletter*. 2007;22:25.
50. Cucchiara RF. Hazards of beach chair position explored. *APSF Newsletter*. 2008;22:8.
51. Munis J. The problems of posture, pressure, and perfusion. *APSF Newsletter*. 2008;22:82.
52. Drummond JC, Hargens AP, Patel PM. Hydrostatic gradient is important – blood pressure should be corrected. *APSF Newsletter*. 2009;24:6.
53. Lanier WL. Cerebral perfusion: err on the side of caution. *APSF Newsletter*. 2009;24:1.
54. Moore JK, Chaudhri S, Moore AP, et al. Macroglossia and posterior fossa disease. *Anaesthesia*. 1988;43:382–385.
55. Hitselberger WE, House WF. A warning regarding the sitting position for acoustic tumor surgery. *Arch Otolaryng*. 1980;106:69.
56. Wilder BL. Hypothesis: The etiology of midcervical quadriplegia after operation with the patient in the sitting position. *Neurosurgery*. 1982;11:530–531.
57. Mills JT, Burris MB, Warburton DJ, et al. Positioning injuries associated with robotic assisted urologic surgery. *J Urol*. 2013;190:580–584.
58. Pridgeon S, Bishop CV, Adshead J. Lower limb compartment syndrome as a complication of robot-assisted radical prostatetectomy: the UK experience. *BJ Urol International*. 2013;112:485–488.

30 Monitored Anesthesia Care

MELISSA M. MASARACCHIA • KYLENE E. HALLORAN • AARON J. MANCUSO • SIMON C. HILLIER

Terminology
Preoperative Assessment
Techniques of Monitored Anesthesia Care
Pharmacologic Basis of Monitored Anesthesia Care Techniques: Optimizing Drug Administration
Distribution, Elimination, Accumulation, and Duration of Action
   Elimination Half-life
   Context-Sensitive Half-time
Drug Interactions
Specific Drugs Used for Monitored Anesthesia Care
   Propofol
   Fospropofol
   Benzodiazepines
   Opioids
   Remifentanil
   Ketamine
   Dexmedetomidine
   Amnesia during Sedation with Dexmedetomidine or Propofol
   Patient-controlled Sedation and Analgesia

Respiratory Function and Sedative–Hypnotic Drugs
   Sedation and Upper Airway Patency
   Sedation and Protective Airway Reflexes
   Sedation and Respiratory Control
Supplemental Oxygen Administration
   Head and Neck Fires with the Use of Supplemental Oxygen
Monitoring during Monitored Anesthesia Care
   American Society of Anesthesiologists Standards
   Communication and Observation
   Auscultation
   Pulse Oximetry
   Capnography
   Cardiovascular System
   Temperature Monitoring and Management during Monitored Anesthesia Care
   Bispectral Index Monitoring during Monitored Anesthesia Care
   Preparedness to Recognize and Treat Local Anesthetic Toxicity
   Sedation and Analgesia by Nonanesthesiologists
   Computer-assisted Personalized Sedation—SEDASYS
Conclusion

KEY POINTS

1. The standards for preoperative evaluation, intraoperative monitoring, and the continuous presence of a member of the anesthesia care team are no different from those for general or regional anesthesia.
2. As a general principle, to avoid excessive levels of sedation, drugs should be titrated in small increments or by adjustable infusions rather than administered in larger doses according to predetermined notions of efficacy.
3. At the present time, no single drug can provide all the components of monitored anesthesia care (i.e., analgesia, anxiolysis, and hypnosis) with an acceptable margin of safety or ease of titratability.
4. Excessive sedation leading to respiratory compromise is the most common cause of death or central nervous system injury during MAC.
5. The important mechanisms whereby respiratory function may be compromised during monitored anesthesia care include the effects of sedatives and opioids on respiratory drive, upper airway patency, and protective airway reflexes.
6. Burns, particularly around the head and neck, are an important cause of patient injury during MAC. The combination of electrocautery, supplemental oxygen, alcohol prep, and flammable drapes is particularly dangerous.
7. If anesthesiologists are not willing or able to provide MAC or sedation/analgesia services, others, who are less qualified, are prepared to assume that role.

Monitored anesthesia care is a specific anesthesia service in which an anesthesiologist has been requested to participate in the care of a patient undergoing a diagnostic or therapeutic procedure and includes all the usual aspects of anesthetic care—a preprocedure evaluation, intraprocedure care, and postprocedure management. *Monitored anesthesia care does not describe the continuum of depth of sedation.* During monitored anesthesia care, the continuous attention of the anesthesiologist is directed at optimizing patient comfort and safety. Monitored anesthesia care usually (but not always) involves the administration of drugs with anxiolytic, hypnotic, analgesic, and amnestic properties, either alone or as a supplement to a local or regional technique. Monitored anesthesia care is provided by a Physician Anesthesiologist, thus can safely encompass the complete spectrum of sedation from light sedation/analgesia to conversion to general anesthesia if required. The American Society of Anesthesiologists (ASA) has published several position statements, guidelines, and advisories on various topics that relate to monitored anesthesia care and moderate sedation. These are listed in Table 30-1 and are a well worth reviewing.

Terminology

It is important to distinguish between the terms "monitored anesthesia care" and "moderate sedation/analgesia." In October 2013, the ASA House of Delegates reaffirmed the statement titled "Distinguishing Monitored Anesthesia Care from Moderate Sedation/Analgesia."[1]

Moderate sedation/analgesia is the term used by the ASA in their published *Practice Guidelines for Sedation and Analgesia by Non-Anesthesiologists*.[2] During moderate sedation (conscious

Table 30-1 American Society of Anesthesiologists Statements, Guidelines, and Practice Advisories Related to Monitored Anesthesia Care and Sedation/Analgesia.

Title of ASA Statement, Guideline, or Advisory	Date of Publication
Position on Monitored Anesthesia Care	October 2013
Statement on Anesthesia Care for Endoscopies	October 2014
Statement on Granting Privileges to Non-anesthesiologist Physicians for Personally Administering or Supervising Deep Sedation	October 2012
Statement on Granting Privileges for Administration of Moderate Sedation to Practitioners who are not Anesthesiologists	October 2011
Advisory on Granting Privileges for Deep Sedation to Non-anesthesiologist Sedation Practitioners	October 2010
Practice Guidelines for Sedation and Analgesia by Non-Anesthesiologists	April 2002
Continuum of Depth of Sedation: Definition of General Anesthesia and levels of Sedation/Analgesia	October 2014
Statement on Safe Use of Propofol	October 2014
Distinguishing Monitored Anesthesia Care (MAC) from Moderate Sedation/Analgesia (Conscious Sedation)	October 2013
Guidance for Directors of Anesthesia Services for Computer-Assisted Personalized Sedation Devices	January 2014

sedation), care need not be provided by an anesthesiologist and a full anesthetic preoperative evaluation is typically not performed. Sedation/analgesia provided by nonanesthesia providers should not intend to attain a level of sedation in which the patient is unresponsive. Monitored anesthesia care implies the potential for a deeper level of sedation than that provided by sedation/analgesia and is always administered or medically directed by an anesthesiologist. The provider of MAC is prepared and qualified to convert to a general anesthetic if and when necessary. The standards for preoperative evaluation, intraoperative monitoring, and the continuous presence of a member of the anesthesia care team are no different from those for general or regional anesthesia.[3]

Conceptually, monitored anesthesia care utilizing sedation rather than general anesthesia is attractive because it should invoke less physiologic disturbance and allow a more rapid recovery than general anesthesia. It is instructive to review the ASA position statement that defines monitored anesthesia care[3]:

> Monitored anesthesia care is a specific anesthesia service for a diagnostic or therapeutic procedure. Indications for monitored anesthesia care include the nature of the procedure, the patient's clinical condition, and/or the potential need to convert to a general or regional anesthetic.
>
> Monitored anesthesia care includes all aspects of anesthesia care—a preprocedure visit, intraprocedure care, and postprocedure anesthesia management. During monitored anesthesia care, the anesthesiologist provides or medically directs a number of specific services, including but not limited to:
> - Diagnosis and treatment of clinical problems that occur during the procedure
> - Support of vital functions
> - Administration of sedatives, analgesics, hypnotics, anesthetic agents, or other medications as necessary for patient safety
> - Psychological support and physical comfort
> - Provision of other medical services as needed to complete the procedure safely.
>
> Monitored anesthesia care may include varying levels of sedation, analgesia, and anxiolysis as necessary. The provider of monitored anesthesia care must be prepared and qualified to convert to general anesthesia when necessary. If the patient loses consciousness and the ability to respond purposefully, the anesthesia care is a general anesthetic, irrespective of whether airway instrumentation is required.
>
> Monitored anesthesia care is a physician service provided to an individual patient. It should be subject to the same level of payment as general or regional anesthesia. Accordingly, the ASA Relative Value Guide provides for the use of proper base procedural units, time units, and modifier units as the basis for determining payment.*

The ASA also states that monitored anesthesia care should be requested by the attending physician and be made known to the patient, in accordance with accepted procedures of the institution. In addition, the ASA states that the service must include the following:
- Performance of a preanesthetic examination and evaluation
- Prescription of anesthetic care
- Personal participation in, or medical direction of, the entire plan of care
- Continuous physical presence of the anesthesiologist or, in the case of medical direction, of the resident or nurse anesthetist being medically directed
- Proximate presence, or in the case of medical direction, availability of the anesthesiologist for diagnosis and treatment of emergencies

Furthermore, the ASA states that all institutional regulations pertaining to anesthesia services shall be observed, and all the usual services performed by the anesthesiologist shall be furnished, including but not limited to:
- Usual noninvasive cardiocirculatory and respiratory monitoring
- Oxygen administration, when indicated
- Administration of sedatives, tranquilizers, antiemetics, narcotics, other analgesics, β-blockers, vasopressors, bronchodilators, antihypertensives, or other pharmacologic therapy as may be required in the judgment of the anesthesiologist

Preoperative Assessment

The preoperative evaluation is an essential prerequisite to monitored anesthesia care and should be as comprehensive as that performed prior to any general or regional anesthetic (see Chapter 23). However, in addition to the usual evaluation for the

---

*Excerpt from the American Society of Anesthesiologists, 1601 American Lane, Schaumburg, Illinois 60173–4973 or online at www.asahq.org.

patient who is scheduled to undergo general anesthesia, there are additional considerations unique to the monitored anesthesia care that may ultimately determine the success or failure of the procedure. It is important to evaluate the patient's ability to remain motionless and, if necessary, actively cooperate throughout the procedure. Thus, it is important to evaluate the patient's psychological preparation for the planned procedure. It is also important to elicit the presence of coexisting sensorineural or cognitive deficits. These factors or the inability to communicate with the patient may occasionally make general anesthesia a more appropriate alternative. Verbal communication between physician and patient is very important for three reasons: as a monitor of the level of sedation and cardiorespiratory function, as a means of explanation and reassurance for the patient, and as a mechanism of communication when the patient is required to actively cooperate. Although cardiorespiratory disease is often cited as an indication to perform a procedure using monitored anesthesia care rather than general anesthesia, there are occasions when cardiorespiratory disease may reduce the utility of monitored anesthesia care. For example, the presence of a persistent cough may make it very difficult for the patient to remain immobile, which can be particularly dangerous during ophthalmologic or awake neurosurgical procedures. Attempts to attenuate coughing with sedation techniques are likely to be unsuccessful and potentially harmful because a significant level of anesthesia is required to abolish the cough reflex. Similarly, some patients with significant cardiovascular or pulmonary disease may be unable to lie flat for an extended period.

Techniques of Monitored Anesthesia Care

A variety of medications are commonly administered during monitored anesthesia care with the desired end points to provide patient comfort, maintain cardiorespiratory stability, improve operating conditions, and prevent recall of unpleasant perioperative events. It is helpful to delineate and individualize the goals for each patient in order to formulate an appropriate regimen, which frequently involves the administration of either individual or combinations of analgesic, amnestic, and hypnotic drugs. There should be a minimal incidence of side effects, such as cardiorespiratory depression, nausea and vomiting, delayed emergence, and dysphoria, and there should be a rapid and complete recovery. Ideally, the patient should be able to communicate during the procedure. Clinical experience suggests that a level of sedation that allows verbal communication is optimal for the patient's comfort and safety. If the level of sedation is deepened to the extent that verbal communication is lost, the risks of the technique approach those of general anesthesia with an unprotected and uncontrolled airway. However, because monitored anesthesia care is provided by anesthesiologists, the range of sedation may include deeper sedation techniques than those provided by nonanesthesiologists during sedation/analgesia.

The preanesthetic evaluation and plan should identify specific causes and provide specific therapy for pain, anxiety, and agitation. Pain may be treated by local or regional analgesia, systemic analgesics, or removal of the painful stimulus. Anxiety may be reduced by the use of an anxiolytic such as a benzodiazepine and reassurance by the anesthesiologist. Patient agitation may be a result of pain or anxiety or life-threatening factors such as hypoxia, hypercarbia, impending local anesthetic toxicity, and cerebral hypoperfusion. Other causes of pain and agitation include a distended bladder, hypothermia, hyperthermia, pruritus, nausea, positional discomfort, uncomfortable oxygen masks and nasal cannulae, intravenous (IV) cannulation site infiltration, a member of the surgical team leaning on the patient, and prolonged pneumatic tourniquet inflation.

Pharmacologic Basis of Monitored Anesthesia Care Techniques: Optimizing Drug Administration

The ability to predict the effects of the drugs in our armamentarium demands an understanding of their pharmacokinetic and pharmacodynamic properties. This understanding is a fundamental prerequisite for the design of an effective sedation regimen and greatly increases the probability of producing the desired therapeutic effect. Context-sensitive half-time, effect site equilibration time, and anesthetic/sedative drug interactions are fundamental concepts that are particularly useful in the context of monitored anesthesia care and are discussed in more detail in other chapters of this book.

The ultimate objective of any dosing regimen is to deliver a therapeutic concentration of drug to its site of action, which is determined by the unique pharmacokinetic properties of that drug in that particular patient. The therapeutic response to a particular drug concentration is described by the pharmacodynamics of that particular patient–drug combination. There is a large degree of pharmacokinetic and pharmacodynamic variability, producing a significant variability in the dose–response relationship in clinical practice. Excessive sedation may result in cardiac or respiratory depression. Inadequate sedation may result in patient discomfort and potential morbidity from lack of cooperation. As a general principle, to avoid excessive levels of sedation, drugs should be titrated in small increments or by adjustable infusions rather than administered in larger doses according to predetermined notions of efficacy.[4] In an ideal dosing regimen, an effective concentration of drug is achieved and then adjusted according to the magnitude of the noxious stimulus. If the noxious stimulus is increased or decreased, the concentration is increased or decreased accordingly. By the end of the procedure, the drug concentration should have decreased to a level compatible with rapid recovery. This approach requires the easily titratable drugs such as propofol. When using drugs such as propofol, adjustable-rate continuous infusions are the most logical method of maintaining a desired therapeutic concentration. If intermittent bolus administration is used, significant fluctuations in drug concentration occur. Under these circumstances, the plasma concentrations are either above or below the desired therapeutic range for a significant proportion of the procedure (Fig. 30-1). Continuous infusions are generally superior to intermittent bolus dosing because they produce less fluctuation in drug concentration, thus reducing the number of episodes of inadequate or excessive sedation. Administration of drugs by continuous infusion rather than by intermittent dosing also reduces the total amount of drug administered and facilitates a more prompt recovery.[5]

Distribution, Elimination, Accumulation, and Duration of Action

Following the administration of IV anesthetic drugs, the immediate distribution phase causes a brisk decrease in plasma levels as the drug is transported to the rapidly equilibrating vessel-rich group of tissues. There is a simultaneously occurring distribution

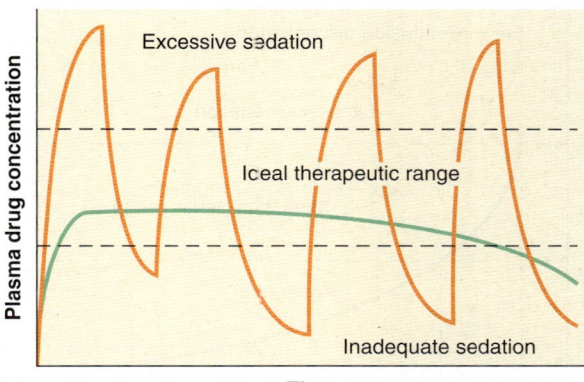

Figure 30-1 The changes in drug concentration during differing administration techniques. The *green line* represents a continuous infusion of a drug. In this situation the drug is maintained within the therapeutic range for most of the procedure. The *orange line* represents the drug concentration resulting from intermittent bolus administration. The drug concentration is significantly above or below the desired therapeutic level for most of the procedure.

of drug to the less well-perfused tissues such as muscle and skin. Over time, the drug is also distributed to the poorly perfused tissues such as bone and fat. Although the latter compartments are poorly perfused, they may accumulate significant amounts of lipophilic drugs during prolonged administration. This peripheral depot may contribute to a delayed recovery when the drug is eventually released back into the central compartment after its administration is discontinued. Redistributive factors are important determinants of drug effect and influence the plasma concentration of a drug in a time-dependent fashion.

Elimination Half-life

Until recently, the elimination half-time was the predominant pharmacokinetic parameter used as the predictor of an anesthetic drug's duration of action. In everyday clinical practice, however, this parameter does not greatly enhance our ability to predict anesthetic drug disposition. Only in single-compartment models does the elimination half-time actually represent the time required for a drug to reach half of its initial concentration after administration. In a single-compartment model, elimination is the only process that can alter drug concentration. Intercompartmental distribution cannot occur because there are no other compartments for the drug to be distributed to and from. Most drugs in the anesthesiologist's armamentarium are lipophilic and are, therefore, more suited to multicompartmental modeling than single-compartment modeling. Similarly, other pharmacokinetic parameters, such as distribution half-time, distribution volume, intercompartmental rate constants, and so forth, do not provide us with a practical means of predicting drug disposition. In multicompartmental models, the metabolism and excretion of some IV anesthetic drugs may have only a minor contribution to the changes in plasma concentration when compared with the effects of intercompartmental distribution.

Context-sensitive Half-time

The concept of context-sensitive half-time was developed to improve the description and understanding of anesthetic drug disposition.[6] This concept has greatly improved our understanding of anesthetic drug disposition and is clinically applicable. The effect of distribution on plasma drug concentration varies in magnitude and direction over time and depends on the drug concentration gradients that exist between the various compartments. For example, during the early part of an infusion of a lipophilic drug, distributive factors will tend to decrease plasma concentrations as the drug is transported to the unsaturated peripheral tissues. Later, after the infusion is discontinued, drug will return from the peripheral tissues and re-enter the central circulation. The relative effect on plasma concentrations of distributive processes versus elimination varies over time and from drug to drug. The context-sensitive half-time describes the time required for the plasma drug concentration to decline by 50% after terminating an infusion of a particular duration.[7] This parameter is calculated by using computer simulation of multicompartmental models of drug disposition (Fig. 30-2). The context-sensitive half-time reflects the combined effects of distribution and metabolism on drug disposition. There are several interesting aspects of these data. First, the data confirm the clinical impression that as the infusion duration increases, the context-sensitive half-time of all the drugs increases; this phenomenon is not described in any way by the elimination half-life. The increase in context-sensitive half-time is particularly marked with fentanyl and thiopental. In the case of fentanyl, drug that is irreversibly eliminated from the plasma by hepatic clearance is immediately replaced by drug returning from the peripheral compartments. Thus, although fentanyl has a shorter *elimination* half-life than that of sufentanil (462 vs. 577 minutes), its *context-sensitive* half-time is much greater than that of sufentanil after an infusion of longer than 2 hours. The storage and later release of fentanyl from peripheral binding sites delay the decline in plasma concentration that would otherwise occur. *The context-sensitive half-times of all the drugs bear no constant relationship to their elimination half-times.* For example, compare also the context-sensitive half-times of propofol and thiopental (Fig. 30-2). Although the context-sensitive half-times

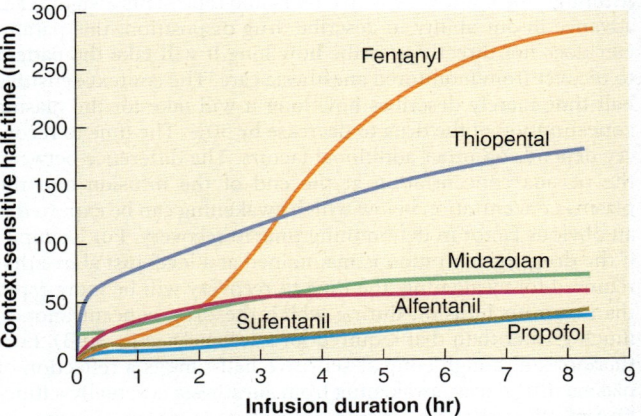

Figure 30-2 Context-sensitive half-time as a function of infusion duration. These data were generated from the computer model of Hughes et al.[5] It can be seen that the context-sensitive half-time of propofol demonstrates a minimal increase as the duration of the infusion increases. Also note that for infusions of short duration, sufentanil has a shorter half-time than alfentanil. (Reproduced with permission from Hughes MA, Glass PSA, Jacobs JR. Context-sensitive half-time in multicompartment pharmacokinetic models for intravenous anesthetic drugs. *Anesthesiology*. 1992;76:334, with permission.)

of propofol and thiopental are comparable following a brief infusion, the context-sensitive half-time of thiopental increases rapidly following all but the shortest infusions. This finding confirms the clinical impression that thiopental is not an ideal drug for continuous infusion during ambulatory procedures. The context-sensitive half-time of propofol is prolonged to a minimal extent as the infusion duration increases. After an infusion of propofol, the drug that returns to the plasma from the peripheral compartments is rapidly cleared by metabolic processes and is, therefore, not available to retard the decay in plasma levels. This difference between thiopental and propofol is attributable to (1) the high metabolic clearance of propofol compared with thiopental, and (2) the relatively slow rate at which propofol returns to the plasma from peripheral compartments.

Alfentanil is the opioid that was, until the introduction of remifentanil, frequently studied, described, and promoted in the context of ambulatory techniques. Alfentanil has a very short elimination half-time, one-fifth that of sufentanil (111 vs. 577 minutes). However, despite the longer elimination half-time of sufentanil, its context-sensitive half-time is actually less than that of alfentanil for infusions up to 8 hours in duration. This phenomenon is explained in part by the huge distribution volume of sufentanil. After termination of a sufentanil infusion, the decay in plasma drug concentrations is accelerated not only by elimination but also by the continued redistribution of sufentanil into peripheral compartments. On the other hand, the small distribution volume of alfentanil equilibrates rapidly; therefore, peripheral distribution of drug away from the plasma is not a significant contributor to the decay in plasma concentration after an infusion. The data derived from computer simulation by Hughes et al.[6] show that the plasma decay of alfentanil is slower than that of sufentanil following infusions of similar duration to those used during conscious sedation. Thus, despite its short elimination half-time, alfentanil may not necessarily be superior to sufentanil.[8]

How Does the Context-sensitive Half-time Relate to the Time to Recovery?

Although the context-sensitive half-time represents a significant advance in our ability to describe drug disposition, this parameter does not directly describe how long it will take the patient to recover from monitored anesthesia care. The context-sensitive half-time merely describes how long it will take for the plasma concentration of the drug to decrease by 50%. The time to recovery depends on other additional factors. The difference between the plasma concentration at the end of the infusion and the plasma concentration below which awakening can be expected is an obvious factor in determining time to recovery. For example, if the drug concentration is maintained at a level just above that required for awakening, the time to recovery will be more rapid than after an infusion during which the drug concentration is much greater than that required for awakening (Fig. 30-3). Furthermore, although context-sensitive half-time is a reflection of plasma drug decay, awakening from anesthesia is actually a function of effect site (i.e., brain) concentration decay. Changes in effect site concentration demonstrate a variable time lag behind changes in plasma drug concentration. Effect site equilibration is a concept that is particularly relevant to IV sedation. When a drug is administered intravenously by bolus or infused rapidly, there is a delay before the onset of clinical effect. This delay occurs because the plasma is not usually the site of action but is merely the route by which the drug reaches its effect site. If some parameter of drug effect can be measured (e.g., power spectrum electroencephalographic [EEG] analysis in the case of opioids),

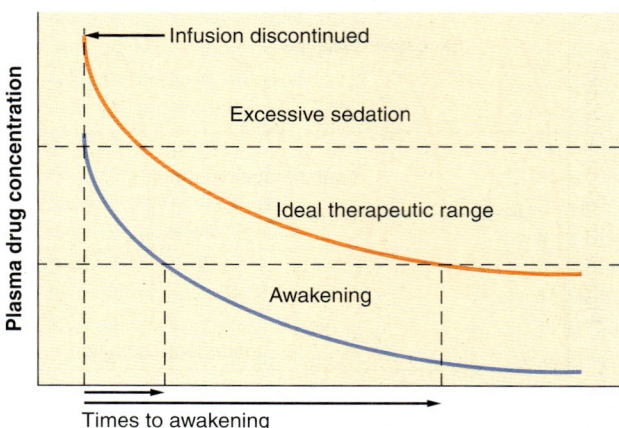

Figure 30-3 The context-sensitive half-time is not the sole determinant of the time it takes for the patient to awaken. This parameter merely reflects the time taken for the plasma concentration of a drug to decrease by 50%. The time to awakening is determined in addition by the difference in concentration at the end of the procedure and the concentration below which awakening will occur.

the half-time of equilibration between drug concentration in the blood and the drug effect can then be determined.[9] This parameter is abbreviated $t_{1/2}k_{e0}$. Drugs with a short $t_{1/2}k_{e0}$ will equilibrate rapidly with the brain and have a shorter delay in onset than drugs that have a longer $t_{1/2}k_{e0}$. Thiopental, propofol, and alfentanil have short $t_{1/2}k_{e0}$ values compared with midazolam, sufentanil, and fentanyl.

The $t_{1/2}k_{e0}$ allows predictions to be made of the time course of equilibration of the drug between the blood and the brain. A distinct time lag between the peak serum fentanyl concentration and the peak EEG slowing can be seen. In contrast, following alfentanil administration, the EEG changes closely parallel serum concentrations. The $t_{1/2}k_{e0}$ for fentanyl is 6.4 minutes compared with a $t_{1/2}k_{e0}$ of 1.1 minutes for alfentanil. Therefore, if an opioid is required to blunt the response to a single brief stimulus, alfentanil might represent a logical choice over fentanyl. The $t_{1/2}k_{e0}$ is an important determinant of bolus spacing when titrating drugs to clinical effect. In the case of drugs like midazolam and propofol, boluses of drug should be spaced far enough apart to allow the full peak effect to be clinically appreciated before further drug administration in order to avoid inadvertent overdosing.[10–12] For example, even if the shortest quoted equilibration half-time for midazolam (0.9 minutes) is used, it will take 2.7 (i.e., three half-times) minutes for effect site concentrations to be 87.5% equilibrated. Other factors are also important determinants of bolus size and spacing. For example, a low cardiac output will markedly delay drug arrival at the site of action. If sufficient time is not given for the drug to take effect before giving additional drug increments, significant cardiorespiratory compromise may occur. Furthermore, the effects of initial doses of most drugs in anesthetic practice are terminated by redistribution, which depends on blood flow to redistribution sites. If there is reduced blood flow to redistribution sites because of pre-existing and iatrogenic decreases in cardiac output, the dangerous adverse effects of these drugs are likely to be both delayed and markedly prolonged. An example of this scenario is the patient with a hemodynamic compromise caused by a tachydysrhythmia who requires sedation for cardioversion. Careful, well-spaced, small boluses of drug should be given to induce the appropriate level of sedation, bearing in mind that it may take several minutes for the full effect of a small bolus dose to become apparent.

Drug Interactions

At the present time, no single drug can provide all the components of monitored anesthesia care (i.e., analgesia, anxiolysis, and hypnosis) with an acceptable margin of safety or ease of titratability. Therefore, patient comfort is usually maintained with a combination of drugs. By acting synergistically, combinations of drugs enable reductions in the dose requirements of individual drugs. For example, the combination of propofol and fentanyl by infusion has been shown to produce a more rapid recovery and better stress response abolition than the use of propofol alone.[13–15] In addition, lower doses of each drug may reduce the untoward side effects associated with higher doses leading to increased patient satisfaction and decreased times to discharge. However, synergistic interaction may also extend to the undesirable interactions of the drugs such as cardiorespiratory depression.

Drug interactions may have both a pharmacodynamic and a pharmacokinetic basis and may vary depending on the combination of drugs being coadministered, the dose range over which these drugs are administered, and the specific clinical effect that is measured. For example, because fentanyl is primarily an analgesic rather than a hypnotic, it reduces propofol requirements for suppression of response to skin incision to a much greater degree than it reduces propofol requirements for induction of anesthesia.[16] On the other hand, because midazolam has significant hypnotic properties, it displays significant synergism with propofol or thiopental when used to induce hypnosis for prevention of movement in response to a painful stimulus.[17–19]

The plasma concentration of a drug at steady state that is required to abolish purposeful movement at skin incision in 50% of patients ($Cp_{ss}50$) is a measure of potency that is analogous to the familiar parameter of minimum alveolar concentration (MAC) of the volatile inhaled anesthetics. IV anesthetic interactions may be evaluated by their effect on the $Cp_{ss}50$ in a manner analogous to the expression of the effects of opioids on volatile anesthetic requirements in terms of MAC reduction.[20] For example, during general anesthesia, opioid requirements to suppress the responses to noxious stimuli are tenfold higher when used as the sole agent compared with when they are used in conjunction with a nitrous oxide/potent inhaled vapor technique. This interaction persists at the lighter levels of anesthesia encountered during monitored anesthesia care. Therefore, it is likely that a rapid recovery would be facilitated by using opioids in combination with other agents (e.g., propofol/midazolam) rather than as the sole drug.

Drug interactions are dose dependent. For example, when fentanyl is combined with isoflurane, the greatest reduction in isoflurane MAC occurs within the analgesic concentration range of fentanyl (i.e., 1 to 2 ng/mL). At a fentanyl concentration of 1.7 ng/mL, the MAC of isoflurane is reduced by 50%.[21] Once the fentanyl concentration is increased beyond 3 ng/mL, there appears to be minimal further reduction with the largest MAC reduction of 80%. Likewise, the MAC of desflurane is reduced by approximately 50%, 25 minutes after a 3-μg/kg IV bolus of fentanyl.[22] However, when the fentanyl bolus is increased to 6 μg/kg, there is no significant further decrease in the MAC of desflurane. Studies with other opioids have yielded similar results.[23–25] The interactions between propofol and opioids are important because these agents are frequently used during monitored anesthesia care. When analgesic concentrations of fentanyl (0.6 ng/mL) are used in combination with propofol for anesthesia, the $Cp_{ss}50$ of propofol is reduced by 50% compared with when propofol is used as the sole agent.[17] However, when the dose of fentanyl is increased, there is no significant further reduction of the $Cp_{ss}50$ for propofol beyond a fentanyl concentration of 3 ng/mL.

Although the data presented here pertain to patients under general anesthesia, these findings have important implications for monitored anesthesia care. These studies demonstrate that the potentiating effects of opioids on coadministered sedatives are pronounced within the dose range commonly used during monitored anesthesia care. Furthermore, the data suggest that the dose–response curve is likely to be steep within this dose range, thus supporting the clinical impression that significant increases in depth of sedation can occur with only modest increments in opioid or hypnotic/sedative dosage. The following clinical recommendations can be made: During monitored anesthesia care, the maximum benefit of opioid supplementation, in terms of potentiation of other administered sedatives, will accrue when the opioid is used in the analgesic dose range. Within this dose range there is great potential for adverse cardiorespiratory interaction.

Opioid and benzodiazepine combinations are frequently used to achieve the components of hypnosis, amnesia, and analgesia. This drug combination displays marked synergism in producing hypnosis. Approximately 25% of the median effective dose for each individual drug is required in combination to induce hypnosis in 50% of patients.[26] If the combination were simply additive, hypnosis would be induced in only approximately 25% of patients. Even subanalgesic doses of alfentanil (3 μg/kg) produce a profound reduction in midazolam requirements for hypnosis.[27] This synergism also extends to the unwanted effects of these drugs, producing the life-threatening complications of respiratory and cardiac depression. Several fatalities have been reported after the use of midazolam, the majority of these being related to adverse respiratory events.[28] In many of these cases, midazolam was used in combination with an opioid. The effects of midazolam and fentanyl on respiratory function in healthy volunteers have been examined by Bailey et al.[29] Whereas midazolam produced no significant respiratory effects alone, and fentanyl alone produced hypoxemia (oxyhemoglobin saturation ≤95%) in half of the subjects, the combination of midazolam 0.05 μg/kg and fentanyl 2 μg/kg resulted in hypoxemia in 11 of 12 subjects and apnea (no spontaneous respiratory effort for 15 seconds) in 6 of 12 subjects. The combination of midazolam and fentanyl places patients at high risk for developing hypoxemia and apnea. The respiratory depressant effects of this drug combination are likely to be even more significant in the patient with coexisting respiratory or central nervous system disease or at the extremes of age. In clinical practice, the clinical advantages of the synergy between opioids and benzodiazepines for the maintenance of patient comfort should be carefully weighed against the disadvantages of the potentially adverse effect of this drug combination on the cardiovascular and respiratory systems.

Specific Drugs Used for Monitored Anesthesia Care

Propofol

Propofol has become a popular choice for monitored anesthetic care due to its side effect profile and ease of titratability. Propofol has many of the ideal properties of a sedative–hypnotic for use in monitored anesthesia care. Its pharmacokinetic profile, that is, a context-sensitive half-time that remains short even after infusions of prolonged duration and a short effect site equilibration time, makes it an easily titratable drug with an excellent recovery profile. The quality of recovery and the low incidence of nausea and vomiting make propofol particularly well suited to ambulatory monitored anesthesia care procedures. A significant body of experience with the use of propofol for monitored anesthesia care has emerged.

Propofol has significant advantages compared with benzodiazepines when used as the hypnotic component of a monitored anesthesia care technique. Although midazolam has a relatively short elimination half-time, its context-sensitive half-time is approximately twice that of propofol. Whereas propofol is noted for the rapid return to clear-headedness, midazolam is often associated with prolonged postoperative sedation and psychomotor impairment, particularly in the elderly. Propofol in typical moderate sedation doses (25 to 75 μg/kg/min) has minimal analgesic properties. On the other hand, the use of propofol as a component of general anesthesia has been associated with less postoperative pain and narcotic use when compared to isoflurane.[30] However, the unique advantages of propofol can be exploited to the maximum when propofol is used to provide sedation when the analgesic component is provided by a local or regional analgesic technique. The use of propofol (50 to 70 μg/kg/min) to provide sedation (defined as sleep with preservation of the eyelash reflex and purposeful reaction to verbal or mild physical stimulation) as an adjunct to spinal anesthesia for lower limb surgery has been examined.[31–33] After termination of infusions of approximately 100 minutes, patients regained consciousness in approximately 4 minutes. The authors also noted the ease with which general anesthesia could be induced if necessary by increasing the propofol infusion. The same group also compared propofol (60.5 μg/kg/min) with midazolam (4.3 μg/kg/min) as an adjunct to spinal anesthesia. The propofol group had faster immediate recovery than the midazolam group (2.3 vs. 9.2 minutes to spontaneous eye opening). Furthermore, psychomotor function was comparable with baseline values following propofol sedation but did not return to baseline until 2 hours after midazolam administration. Several studies comparing propofol and midazolam sedation for local and regional anesthesia demonstrated that propofol produced less postoperative sedation, drowsiness, confusion, and clumsiness than midazolam but the discharge times varied.[34,35]

General anesthesia with propofol is generally associated with less nausea and vomiting than most other anesthetic techniques.[36–41] There is growing evidence that even subhypnotic doses of propofol also possess direct antiemetic properties particularly when combined with an antiemetic in patients at risk for nausea and vomiting.[42–45] Thus, it is likely that the beneficial effects of propofol upon nausea and vomiting will be a feature of monitored anesthesia care techniques using this drug. On the other hand, even during low-dose infusions used for sedation, pain during injection of propofol may be troublesome in 33% to 50% of patients.[35–46] Several strategies for reducing the pain of propofol administration are described in Table 30-2.[47]

Fospropofol

Fospropofol, a prodrug of propofol, was approved in 2008 by the FDA for use during monitored anesthetic care in adults; however, this drug was not extensively used or studied and has now been withdrawn from the market in the United States. This phosphate ester prodrug is metabolized by endothelial cell alkaline phosphatases to propofol, formaldehyde, and phosphate.[48–55] The major advantage of fospropofol was a reduction in pain on injection compared to propofol. Other purported advantages were the lack of need for an infusion pump and avoidance of the lipid-emulsion related drug shortages seen with propofol. Theoretically, during a propofol shortage, fospropofol could be used for MAC sedation cases in adults, thus preserving the limited propofol supply for other cases. Unfortunately, the metabolism of fospropofol to its active metabolite, propofol, takes several minutes, resulting in a prolonged time to peak effect (1 to 8 minutes) compared to propofol and a slower recovery, making the optimal dosing technique somewhat different to that of propofol. The standard dosing regimen recommended by the manufacturer was an initial IV bolus dose of 6.5 mg/kg followed by supplemental doses of 1.6 mg/kg as needed. The initial dose should not exceed 16.5 mL; no supplemental bolus should exceed 4 mL. Supplemental doses should only be administered after patients can demonstrate movement upon command (verbal or tactile stimulation) and not more frequently than every 4 minutes to avoid dose stacking. The most common adverse effects reported included paresthesias described as a burning sensation in the perineal and perianal area, pruritus, hypoxemia, hypotension, and abdominal pain. These side effects occurred approximately 4 minutes after administration and may have been related to the phosphate metabolite.

Benzodiazepines

Benzodiazepines are commonly used during monitored anesthesia care for their anxiolytic, amnestic, and hypnotic properties. Patients presenting for diagnostic and surgical procedures frequently request some form of anxiolytic. Midazolam is usually administered prior to the start of the surgical or diagnostic procedures to facilitate amnesia and reduce the patient's level of anxiety. Compared to other benzodiazepines, midazolam's relatively short elimination half-life and decreased likelihood of concomitant drug interactions makes this a superior choice to other benzodiazepines. The important differences between midazolam and diazepam are listed in Table 30-3.[56] Although midazolam has a short elimination half-time, there is often significant and prolonged psychomotor impairment following sedation techniques using midazolam as a significant component. With the recent availability of propofol, midazolam may be better used in a modified role by using lower doses prior to the start of a propofol infusion to provide the specific amnestic and perhaps anxiolytic

Table 30-2 Published Strategies for Reducing the Pain on Intravenous Injection of Propofol

Using larger veins in antecubital fossa
Decreasing the speed of injection
Injection into a fast-running intravenous line
Diluting with 5% glucose or 10% intralipid
Adding lidocaine to propofol
Pretreating with lidocaine and venous occlusion
Pretreatment with opioid
Pretreatment with pentothal
Cooling propofol to 4°C prior to injection
Injecting cooled saline (4°C) prior to injection
Discontinuing intravenous fluid administration during injection
Formulation in medium chain rather than long chain triglyceride

Table 30-3 Comparison of the Important Properties of Midazolam and Diazepam	
Midazolam	**Diazepam**
Water-soluble, does not require propylene glycol for solubilizing	Lipid-soluble, requires propylene glycol for solubilizing
Nonvenoirritant, usually painless	Venoirritant, pain on injection
Thrombophlebitis rare	Thrombophlebitis common
Short elimination half-time (1–4 h)	Long elimination half-time (>20 h)
Clearance unaffected by H_2 antagonists	Clearance reduced by H_2 antagonists
Inactive metabolites (1-hydroxymidazolam)	Active metabolites (desmethyldiazepam, oxazepam)
Resedation unlikely	Resedation more likely

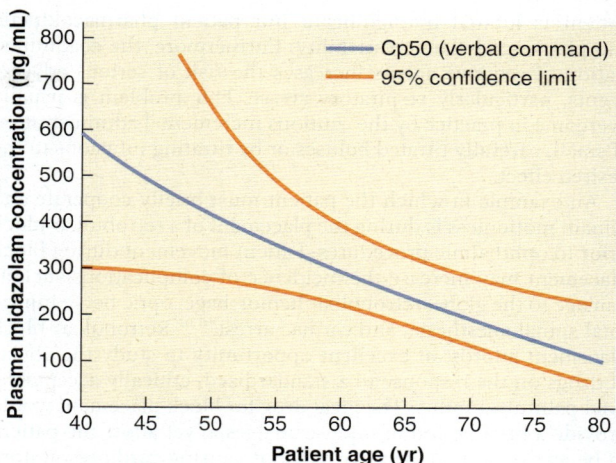

Figure 30-4 Midazolam Cp50 (the concentration at which 50% of subjects will fail to respond to a verbal command) as a function of age. There is a marked decrease in midazolam requirements as patient age increases. (Reproduced with permission from Jacobs JR, Reves JG, Marty J, et al. Aging increases pharmacodynamic sensitivity to the hypnotic effects of midazolam. *Anesth Analg.* 1995;80:143, with permission.)

component of a "balanced" sedation technique rather than as the major hypnotic component.[57] A study in healthy volunteers demonstrated that propofol reduced the distribution and clearance of midazolam in a concentration-dependent manner. The group reported increased plasma levels of midazolam ranging from 5% to 25% during increasing doses of propofol for monitored anesthesia care. This strategy allows the more evanescent and titratable propofol to provide the desired level of deep sedation in an adjustable manner according to the specific stimulus. The analgesic component, if required, of a balanced monitored anesthesia care technique may be provided by regional/local techniques or opioids. Again, when using opioids with benzodiazepines, the potential for significant respiratory impairment should be considered.

The age of the patient should be taken into consideration when administering benzodiazepines. The dose of a particular benzodiazepine required to reach a desired clinical end point is reduced in elderly compared with younger patients.[58] This difference in dosing requirements in elderly patients is mainly related to pharmacodynamic factors. As demonstrated by the threefold decrease in plasma concentration of midazolam, 50% of patients would be expected not to respond to verbal command (Cp50) in an 80-year-old patient compared with a 40-year-old patient (Fig. 30-4).[59]

Benzodiazepines are valuable components of monitored anesthesia care techniques because they enhance patient comfort, improve operating conditions, and provide amnesia. However, recovery of psychomotor and cognitive function may be significantly prolonged following benzodiazepine sedation, especially when compared with sedative–hypnotic techniques using propofol as the major component.[60] The specific benzodiazepine antagonist flumazenil provides the potential to improve the recovery profile of benzodiazepines by permitting the active termination of their sedative and amnestic effects without invoking adverse side effects. However, the potential for resedation remains an obstacle to the routine use of benzodiazepine reversal, particularly in patients undergoing ambulatory procedures. The effects of midazolam may recur up to 90 minutes following the administration of flumazenil.[46] Thus, it is possible that patients could be discharged prematurely to a less well-monitored area, or even out of the hospital in the case of ambulatory surgery, and later experience recurrence of benzodiazepine effects. Typical dose requirements for use of flumazenil are listed in Table 30-4.

Opioids

Opioids are administered in the context of monitored anesthesia care to provide the specific analgesic component of a "balanced" technique. Opioids are indicated when regional or local anesthetic techniques are inappropriate or ineffective, and are typically administered immediately prior to the painful or invasive portion of the procedure. In addition, opioids may be indicated to blunt untoward hemodynamic and physiologic responses, a desirable effect in patients with significant cardiac disease. Pain relief may be required for factors other than the procedure itself, such as uncomfortable positioning, propofol injection, pneumatic tourniquet pain, or other pain not relieved by the local anesthetic technique. The choice of a particular opioid depends on several factors including cost, availability, time of onset, duration, and potential side effects. Opioids frequently administered during monitored anesthesia care include alfentanil, fentanyl, and remifentanil. Their adverse effects include respiratory depression, muscle rigidity, and nausea and vomiting, all of which are undesirable in the spontaneously breathing patient with an unprotected airway. A complicating issue is that the ability to predict the effect of a given dose of opioid in a particular

Table 30-4 Recommended Regimen for the Use of Flumazenil to Antagonize Benzodiazepine Effects

Initial recommended dose of 0.2 mg
If desired level of consciousness is not achieved in 45 sec, repeat 0.2-mg dose
0.2-mg doses may need to be repeated every 60 sec until a maximum of 1 mg is administered
Be aware of the potential for resedation

patient is limited by significant interpatient pharmacokinetic and pharmacodynamic variability. Furthermore, the coadministration of sedative agents increases the risk of serious adverse events, particularly respiratory arrest. This problem is usually overcome in practice by the cautious incremental administration of small, carefully titrated boluses or by titrating infusions to the desired effect.

An example in which the patient must briefly cooperate and remain motionless is during the placement of a retrobulbar block prior to ophthalmic procedures. Patient movement during block placement may increase the incidence of complications such as damage to the globe, retrobulbar hemorrhage, optic nerve injury, total spinal anesthesia, and cardiac arrest.[61,62] Retrobulbar block placement affords an excellent opportunity to study the effects of drugs on the response to a standardized, ethically acceptable, brief painful stimulus. The ideal drug for block placement would provide a brief period of intense analgesia, yet allow the patient to be awake and cooperative without causing cardiorespiratory depression or nausea and vomiting. Alfentanil appears to have a pharmacokinetic advantage for the treatment of discrete stimuli because of its short effect site equilibration time, which allows rapid access of the drug to the brain and facilitates titration. Yee et al.[63] studied the effect of the addition of alfentanil to propofol for sedation during placement of a retrobulbar block. The authors found that the addition of alfentanil improved the conditions of block placement although increased doses of alfentanil were associated with oxygen desaturation. In addition, the total amount of propofol for sedation decreased proportional to the increasing concentration of alfentanil. Other opioids, including fentanyl and remifentanil, have been successfully administered for ophthalmic surgery without significant side effects.[64–66] In a study conducted by Ahmad et al.,[67] a bolus of 1 µg/kg of remifentanil over 30 seconds was administered 90 seconds prior to block placement. More than three-quarters of patients receiving remifentanil did not report any pain during subsequent block placement. However, 15% of the patients given a single bolus alone had significant respiratory depression (respiratory rates <8 breaths per minute), and 19% of those given a bolus followed by an infusion had significant respiratory depression. The group also noted that remifentanil provided superior analgesia compared to alfentanil administered at a dose of 7 µg/kg.

The well-described phenomenon of patient awareness and subsequent recall of intraoperative events following high-dose opioid anesthesia is taken as evidence that opioids lack significant amnestic properties. However, when the effects of low-dose fentanyl on memory were specifically examined in volunteers, it was found that although the subjects appeared to be awake during the fentanyl infusion, there was significant memory impairment.[68] In this study, the degree of stimulation was probably less than that experienced by a patient undergoing a painful surgical procedure. Recall for a painful stimulus during an invasive procedure may not be impaired to the same degree as recall for the less noxious stimuli experienced by the subjects of this study. Aydin et al.[69] noted that the addition of fentanyl to local anesthesia during cataract surgery provided a significant difference in sedation levels; however, it was of brief duration. If amnesia is desired as part of a balanced technique, a sedative–hypnotic agent should be administered and the dose of both agents decreased to avoid any cardiorespiratory events.

Remifentanil

Remifentanil is a potent, ultrashort-acting opioid used during monitored anesthesia care to provide analgesia during brief, painful procedures. Remifentanil is typically administered by a bolus to achieve therapeutic analgesia followed by a continuous infusion. If the situation permits, the bolus should be avoided to decrease the incidence of adverse cardiorespiratory effects. It has been suggested that the administration of continuous infusions during monitored anesthesia care improves the operative conditions for the proceduralist.[70,71]

Remifentanil has pharmacodynamic properties similar to those of other potent µ-opioid receptor agonists such as fentanyl and alfentanil. However, remifentanil is predominantly metabolized by nonspecific esterases, generating an extremely rapid clearance and termination of effect and making it an attractive choice for patients with significant hepatic or renal disease.[72,73] Another major advantage is the intense analgesia of limited duration, which is advantageous to prevent respiratory depression after the stimulating portion of the procedure is completed. The context-sensitive half-time of remifentanil is consistently short, 3 to 5 minutes, increasing to a minimal degree with the duration of the infusion.[74,75] Furthermore, remifentanil has a short effect site equilibration time ($t_{1/2}k_{e0}$) of 1 to 1.5 minutes. This $t_{1/2}k_{e0}$ is slightly longer than that of alfentanil (0.6 to 1.2 minutes) but much shorter than that of fentanyl (4 to 5 minutes) and morphine (approximately 20 minutes), and makes the onset of effect after drug administration very rapid, thus facilitating titration of effect during monitored anesthesia care.

In clinical practice, remifentanil has been used successfully as the analgesic component of sedation techniques for regional and local anesthesia. Its unique pharmacokinetic profile makes it well suited for monitored anesthesia care techniques. Published experience with the use of remifentanil suggests that it is possible to titrate remifentanil administration to provide effective analgesia with minimal respiratory depression. The published data can be used to generate some practical clinical guidelines,[76] which are discussed here.

1. The most desirable therapeutic end point for remifentanil administration is effective analgesia and patient comfort rather than sedation. Sedative drugs such as propofol or midazolam can be used in combination with remifentanil to provide the hypnotic–amnestic component of the sedation technique, remembering that the concomitant administration of midazolam decreases remifentanil dose requirements by up to 50%.[77]
2. Published data suggest that bolus administration of remifentanil is associated with an increased incidence of respiratory depression and chest wall rigidity. Because these side effects are likely to be related to high peak concentrations of drugs, it is recommended that remifentanil boluses be administered slowly (over 30 to 90 seconds) or avoided completely by using a pure infusion technique. If respiratory depression is promptly recognized and the remifentanil administration is reduced or discontinued, it should resolve within approximately 3 minutes. Despite the pharmacokinetic advantages of remifentanil, the level of vigilance required for its administration should be no different from that for any other potent opioid. Although the offset time of remifentanil is rapid, it still requires the recognition of respiratory depression to trigger a downward adjustment in dosage. Similarly, the short $t_{1/2}k_{e0}$ of remifentanil suggests that sudden respiratory depression may occur in response to upward adjustments in dosage. Despite the potential for respiratory depression, the efficacy of remifentanil boluses during monitored anesthesia care has been investigated by several groups.[66,78–80]
3. The effects of coadministration of benzodiazepines and opioids are well documented. The addition of midazolam

to provide the anxiolytic–sedative and amnestic components of a sedation technique has been shown to increase patient satisfaction and significantly reduce remifentanil dose requirements. Even relatively low-dose midazolam (2 mg IV) produces significant reductions in remifentanil requirements and patient anxiety. During breast or lymph node biopsy, remifentanil infusion requirements were 0.065 µg/kg/min when preceded by midazolam compared with 0.123 µg/kg/min when used alone.[77] The advantages of coadministration of small doses of midazolam include increased patient satisfaction, increased amnesia, decreased nausea and vomiting, and decreased anxiety. The disadvantages include a tendency toward increased respiratory depression, apnea, and excessive sedation.

4. Because most painful stimuli are of unpredictable duration and because the risk of adverse respiratory events is increased following bolus administration, the most logical method for the administration of remifentanil during monitored anesthesia care is by an adjustable infusion. This should ideally be preceded by a small bolus of midazolam. Most investigators have used infusion rates that start at 0.1 µg/kg/min approximately 5 minutes prior to the first painful stimulus. This initial "loading" infusion is then weaned to approximately 0.05 µg/kg/min to maintain patient comfort. The maintenance infusion is adjusted upward in response to pain or hemodynamic response or downward in response to excessive sedation, respiratory depression, or apnea. A typical incremental change in infusion rate is 0.025 µg/kg/min. The use of remifentanil infusions of 0.2 µg/kg/min is associated with an increased incidence of respiratory depression that is not necessarily associated with superior analgesia. As in the case of propofol administration, inadvertent interruption of remifentanil administration will result in abrupt offset of effect, which may result in patient discomfort, hemodynamic instability, and even morbidity due to patient movement. It is therefore very important to ensure that the drug delivery system is monitored carefully during the procedure. Remifentanil is supplied as a powder that must be reconstituted prior to use. It is particularly important when administering this drug to patients with an unsecured airway to ensure that there are no errors in drug dilution that would result in inadvertent dosing errors.

Typical adult dose recommendations for opioids and other drugs discussed in the text are listed in Table 30-5.

Ketamine

Ketamine, a phencyclidine derivative, is an intense analgesic frequently used as a component of pediatric sedation techniques and is rapidly gaining popularity in the adult population, particularly in the opioid tolerant patient.[81–83] When used in small doses (0.25 to 0.5 mg/kg), its use is associated with minimal respiratory and cardiovascular depression. Ketamine produces a dissociative state in which the eyes remain open with a nystagmic gaze. However, as the dose of ketamine increases, or when used in combination with other sedatives, a state of deep sedation and/or general anesthesia may be inadvertently achieved. It is often stated that increased oral secretions make laryngospasm more likely. The fear of laryngospasm is the underlying rationale for the frequent administration of an antisialagogue such as atropine or glycopyrrolate. Ketamine is frequently combined with a benzodiazepine to reduce the incidence of hallucinations associated with its use. However, this practice is controversial.[84]

Table 30-5 Typical Dose Ranges of Sedative, Hypnotic, and Analgesic Drugs

Drug	Typical Adult Intravenous Dose Range (Titrated to Effect in Small Increments)
Benzodiazepines	
Midazolam	1–2 mg prior to propofol or remifentanil infusion
Diazepam	2.5–10 mg as the major component of sedation technique
Opioid Analgesics	
Alfentanil	5–20 µg/kg bolus 2 min prior to stimulus
Fentanyl	0.5–2 µg/kg bolus 2–4 min prior to stimulus
Remifentanil	Infusion 0.1 µg/kg/min 5 min prior to stimulus Wean to 0.05 µg/kg/min as tolerated Adjust up or down in increments of 0.025 µg/kg/min Reduce dose accordingly when co-administered with midazolam or propofol Avoid boluses
Hypnotics	
Propofol	250–500 µg/kg boluses 25–75 µg/kg/min infusion
Dexmedetomidine	Loading infusion: 0.5–1 µg/kg over 10–20 min Maintenance infusion: 0.2–0.7 µg/kg/h

There are increasing reports in the emergency medicine literature of replacing benzodiazepines and/or opioids with propofol when ketamine is administered for sedation. Advantages of the administration of "ketofol" are predominantly due to the ability of these drugs to balance the negative side effects of the other. For example, the analgesic effect of ketamine reduces the dosage of propofol required in order to complete an invasive or painful procedure. Frequent advantages cited included preserved hemodynamic stability, decreased nausea and vomiting, improved procedural conditions, and decreased airway complications.[85–89] Problems may arise when repeated doses or prolonged administration of the drug combinations are required due to differences in half-life. The effect of ketamine may outlast the effects of propofol under these conditions. Patient movement may make ketamine less than ideal for procedures requiring a completely motionless patient. Ketamine can elevate intracranial and intraocular pressure and is thus relatively contraindicated in patients with increased intracranial pressure and with glaucoma or open-globe injuries.[90] Although it has been suggested that airway reflexes are relatively preserved with ketamine, there is no convincing evidence to support this notion.

Ketamine can be also administered orally or intramuscularly. The oral dose of ketamine is 4 to 6 mg/kg. The onset of action typically occurs within 20 to 30 minutes and the duration of effect is between 60 and 90 minutes. The intramuscular dose is 2 to 4 mg/kg with an onset of action of 5 to 10 minutes and typically has a duration of effect of 30 to 120 minutes. When administered via the IV route, ketamine should be given in small (0.25 to 1 mg/kg) increments, titrating to effect with an onset of action of 1 to 2 minutes and an approximate duration of 20 to 60 minutes.

Dexmedetomidine

Dexmedetomidine is a selective α_2-receptor agonist that depresses central sympathetic function and produces sedation and analgesia. The α_2-agonists potentiate opioid-induced analgesia, benzodiazepine-induced hypnosis, and have potent MAC-sparing effects when administered with volatile agents.

Compared with other sedative and analgesic drugs, dexmedetomidine appears to have relatively minor effects on respiratory function when used in the typical dose range.[91–93] Of note, unlike during opioid-induced sedation, the hypercapnic arousal response, a feature of natural sleep, appears to be preserved during dexmedetomidine sedation. When compared to propofol, use of dexmedetomidine to facilitate sedation may be associated with improved airway patency,[94] particularly in patients with suspected obstructive sleep apnea. This consideration is ever important given the increasing prevalence of obesity and associated sleep disordered breathing in our current practice. However, occasional airway intervention to relieve obstruction and apnea may be required during dexmedetomidine administration, particularly when used in combination with other respiratory depressants.[95] Dexmedetomidine has been used for sedation during instrumentation of the difficult airway. Patients undergoing fiberoptic intubation who are sedated using dexmedetomidine are generally comfortable yet cooperative.[96–100] Administration of α_2-agonist is associated with a reduction of sympathetic outflow and an increase in cardiac vagal activity; therefore, it is not surprising that hypotension and bradycardia may occur during dexmedetomidine administration. Clinically significant episodes of bradycardia and sinus arrest have been associated with dexmedetomidine administration in young, healthy volunteers with high vagal tone, particularly during rapid IV or bolus administration.[101,102] The α_2-agonists do have peripheral vasoconstrictive effects that can occasionally precipitate hypertension. Despite this phenomenon, the incidence of hypertensive episodes requiring intervention is lower when compared with an equivalent propofol-based technique.[103]

Dexmedetomidine has been used successfully in both adult and pediatric patients for monitored anesthesia care during the awake portions of craniotomies requiring patient cooperation for cortical speech mapping.[104,105] Dexmedetomidine has been used as sedative supplementation to regional anesthesia during carotid endarterectomy. Under these circumstances, there were fewer fluctuations from the desired sedation level when compared with the combination of midazolam, fentanyl, and propofol.[106] Dexmedetomidine tends to decrease cerebral blood flow both directly via α_2-mediated constriction of cerebral blood vessels and indirectly via its effect on systemic pressure. However, there appears to be a concomitant decrease in cerebral metabolic rate.[107] To add further reassurance, the use of dexmedetomidine does not appear to be associated with an increase in the need for intracarotid shunting in patients undergoing awake carotid endarterectomy.[108]

The lack of pain on injection and its analgesic and minimal adverse respiratory properties would seem to make dexmedetomidine a useful alternative to propofol in certain circumstances. However, when compared with propofol, the target sedation level takes longer to achieve with dexmedetomidine (25 vs. 10 minutes).[109] Furthermore, if loading boluses of dexmedetomidine are used to accelerate the onset of sedation, bradycardia and hypotension may occur. Although the use of dexmedetomidine may result in greater sedation, lower blood pressure, and improved analgesia in the recovery room when compared with propofol, the time to postanesthesia care unit discharge is not significantly different.[110] Dexmedetomidine is most often delivered as an initial bolus followed by a continuous infusion. Initial bolus doses range from 0.5 to 1 µg/kg over 10 to 20 minutes, followed by a continuous infusion of 0.2 to 0.7 µg/kg/hr.

Two large retrospective observational studies from a single children's hospital suggest that dexmedetomidine may be used for sedation for pediatric magnetic resonance imaging and computed tomography studies.[110,111] In these studies, the loading dose of dexmedetomidine was 2 to 3 µg/kg over 10 minutes, followed by an infusion of between 1 and 2 µg/kg/hr. However, approximately 15% of patients required a second bolus in order to achieve satisfactory conditions to complete the scan. The analgesic properties of dexmedetomidine may make it a useful alternative to the use of propofol as a sole agent during painful procedures. However, the time taken to deliver the loading dose, the occasional need to rebolus, hypotension, bradycardia, and the relatively long recovery time may limit the utility of dexmedetomidine for very brief procedures such as computed tomography studies. On the other hand, the pain on injection of propofol and the legislative constraints on the administration of propofol by nonanesthesia-trained providers may make dexmedetomidine advantageous in certain circumstances.

Amnesia during Sedation with Dexmedetomidine or Propofol

Drugs with sedative–hypnotic properties reduce attention to stimuli as a direct consequence of depression of consciousness. Therefore, all sedative–hypnotics have the potential to impair memory formation because attention to stimuli is a crucial element of explicit memory formation. However, like benzodiazepines, propofol has significant amnestic effects at subhypnotic doses, suggesting an additional amnestic mechanism that is separate from its sedative effect.[112] In the case of propofol, drug-induced amnesia appears to be a consequence of lack of retention of information that was already successfully stored into long-term memory.[113] In contrast to propofol and benzodiazepines, it is unlikely that dexmedetomidine has amnestic properties at subhypnotic doses.[114] If amnesia is desired for a procedure performed during dexmedetomidine administration, loss of consciousness would be necessary if dexmedetomidine is used as the sole agent. Alternatively, amnestic doses of propofol or a benzodiazepine may be used to supplement dexmedetomidine. The properties of propofol and dexmedetomidine are compared in Table 30-6.

Patient-controlled Sedation and Analgesia

Techniques that allow the direct patient control of the level of sedation may positively affect patient satisfaction.[115] The degree of sedation desired by the patient varies significantly and the individual response to drugs is variable. Patient-controlled sedation appears to be an attractive solution to this problem. One approach to patient-controlled sedation has been to use a conventional patient-controlled analgesia (PCA) delivery system set to deliver 0.7-mg/kg boluses of propofol with a 3-minute lockout period.[116] Other approaches include fixed-dose combinations of 0.5-mg midazolam and 25-µg fentanyl with a 5-minute

Table 30-6 A Comparison of Some Important Properties of Propofol and Dexmedetomidine

	Propofol	Dexmedetomidine
Pain on injection	Yes	Minimal
Analgesic properties in subhypnotic doses	Minimal	Yes
Amnestic properties in subhypnotic doses	Significant	Insignificant
Time of onset with typical administration	Rapid	5–10 min
Restrictive regulations on use by nonanesthesia-trained providers	Yes	No
Potential for significant bradycardia	Minimal	Significant

lockout interval between doses.[117] The pharmacokinetic profile of alfentanil is ideal for the treatment of short, discrete episodes of pain. These properties have been exploited during vaginal ovum retrieval procedures, when ultrasonically guided needles are passed through the vaginal wall under monitored anesthesia care. To this end, Zelcer et al.[118] used a PCA delivery system to allow self-administration of alfentanil during this procedure. After midazolam premedication and a loading dose of alfentanil, patients received 5-μg/kg boluses of alfentanil via the PCA pump with a mandatory 3-minute lockout period. Patient acceptability, alfentanil dosage, respiratory variables, and pain scores were similar to those obtained with physician-controlled analgesia. From the limited data that are available, intraoperative PCA during monitored anesthesia care appears to be an effective alternative to physician-administered analgesia.

Respiratory Function and Sedative–Hypnotic Drugs

During monitored anesthesia care, there is significant potential for respiratory compromise, as highlighted by the American Society of Anesthesiologists Closed Claims Database Study that examined claims related to MAC.[119,120] In that study, excessive sedation leading to respiratory compromise was the most common cause of death or central nervous system injury during MAC. An accompanying editorial noted that MAC is no less risky than general anesthesia in terms of occurrences of permanent brain injury and death for patients undergoing predominantly elective procedures in outpatient settings. The adverse respiratory effects of sedation administration include adverse effects on respiratory drive, airway patency, and loss of airway protective reflexes. These effects result either directly as a result of sedative–hypnotic or opioid administration or indirectly as a consequence of brain stem hypoperfusion resulting from hypotension. There may also be a marked increase in the work of breathing because of increased upper airway resistance[121] and adverse effects on respiratory system mechanics resulting from a decline in functional residual capacity.[122,123]

Sedation and Upper Airway Patency

The upper airway is located outside the thorax. During inspiration, the pressure within the upper airway is subatmospheric; thus, there is a tendency for the upper airway to collapse under the influence of the surrounding atmospheric pressure. However, in the normal subject this tendency for airway collapse is opposed by upper airway dilator muscle tone. These muscles increase the diameter and reduce the compliance of the upper airway. An increase in upper airway dilator muscle tone occurs during inspiration, commencing just prior to diaphragmatic contraction.[124] The coordinated activation of the diaphragmatic and upper airway respiratory muscles are critical in maintaining airway patency. However, upper airway dilator muscle control appears to be extremely sensitive to sedative–hypnotic drug administration.[125] For example, sedative doses of benzodiazepines have been reported to increase inspiratory subglottic airway resistance by three- to fourfold[126] and to selectively suppress genioglossal muscle activity to a greater degree than diaphragmatic activity; furthermore, this effect is exaggerated in elderly patients. The response to this obstruction is a significant increase in intercostal and accessory muscle activity. However, this response is only partially effective because the increase in inspiratory force will further decrease intraluminal upper airway pressure, thus predisposing to further airway collapse. It is likely that these effects will be of greatest significance in patients with pre-existing respiratory compromise, such as elderly patients or those with chronic obstructive pulmonary disease. These patients often have limited respiratory reserve and are unable to increase their respiratory muscle activity in response to the increased work of breathing induced by sedation and may become hypercarbic, acidotic, and hypoxic. Not surprisingly, the aforementioned ASA Closed Claims Database Study showed that MAC-related adverse respiratory outcomes were overrepresented in the elderly and ASA class 3 and 4 populations.

Sedation and Protective Airway Reflexes

Competent laryngeal and upper airway reflexes are required to protect the lower airway from aspiration. Protective laryngeal and pharyngeal reflexes are depressed by anesthesia and sedation. Furthermore, it is also well documented that protective airway reflexes are compromised by advanced age and debilitation. Therefore, it is likely that significant further impairment of airway reflexes occurs during sedation in the elderly or debilitated patient. Aspiration of gastric contents can potentially occur any time during the perioperative period, particularly if oral intake is allowed before the return of adequate upper airway protective reflexes. The time required for the return of protective reflexes varies considerably. Complete recovery of the swallowing reflex occurs approximately 15 minutes after the return of consciousness following propofol anesthesia.[127] However, the IV administration of 15 mg of diazepam has been shown to depress the swallowing reflex for up to 4 hours.[128] The swallowing reflex is significantly depressed for up to 2 hours following the administration of midazolam despite the return to a normal state of consciousness.[129] In otherwise healthy adult male volunteers, the inhalation of 50% nitrous oxide was associated with marked depression of the swallowing reflex.[130]

It is apparent from the sources previously quoted that the protective airway reflexes alone cannot be relied on to protect the lower airway from aspiration during sedation. Thus, patients who are deemed to be at risk from aspiration of gastric contents should be maintained at the lightest level of sedation possible. Ideally, the patient should be awake enough to recognize the regurgitation of gastric contents and be able to protect his or her own airway. If the ability of the patient to protect his or her own airway cannot be reliably guaranteed and regurgitation/aspiration is thought to be a significant risk, placement of a cuffed endotracheal tube under general anesthesia should be seriously considered. Propofol has a particularly potent suppressive effect upon upper airway protective reflexes.[131] This property of propofol is exploited by anesthesiologists in our daily clinical practice. We use propofol to facilitate LMA insertion, to prevent and treat laryngospasm, and to facilitate endotracheal intubation without the use of muscle relaxants. However, the obvious downside to propofol-induced protective reflex suppression is that propofol-based techniques with an unprotected airway might be associated with a greater likelihood of aspiration. There is some evidence to support this supposition. A large Medicare database–based study (>100,000 patients) retrospectively examined whether receiving anesthesia for screening colonoscopy was associated with an increase in complications, including aspiration pneumonia, requiring hospitalization within 30 days of colonoscopy.[132] Aspiration occurred more frequently in those patients receiving anesthesia services versus those who did not (0.14% vs. 0.1%).

Sedation and Respiratory Control

Clinical experience would lead most anesthesiologists to predict that the administration of sedative–hypnotic drugs is associated with the depression of respiratory drive. However, the findings of scientific studies in this area are often conflicting and confusing. On occasion they show minimal effects of sedative drugs, if any,[134–136] on ventilatory responsiveness. However, it is important to note that in many cases the methods used to measure respiratory drive may affect the outcome of the study by stimulating the subject, thus attenuating the negative effect of the drug on respiratory drive. In clinical practice, it is likely that during regional anesthesia there is a degree of deafferentation that will potentiate the respiratory depressant effects of sedative–hypnotic drugs.[137] Most studies have demonstrated that opioids depress the ventilatory response to hypercapnia and hypoxia.[138–142] Reports of the effects of sedative doses of benzodiazepines on carbon dioxide responsiveness have shown variable results, including no significant effect and clinically significant depression.[143–146] However, when opioids and benzodiazepines are used in combination, there appears to be a consistent and marked negative effect on respiratory responsiveness.[142] Although the addition of sedative doses of propofol to opioids showed little potentiation of the respiratory effects of opioids, caution is still warranted when combinations of sedative–hypnotics are used.

Supplemental Oxygen Administration

Hypoxia as a result of alveolar hypoventilation is a relatively common occurrence following the administration of sedatives, analgesics, and hypnotics. In the absence of significant lung disease, the administration of only modest concentrations of supplemental oxygen is frequently effective in restoring the patient's oxygen saturation to an acceptable level. This concept is well illustrated by reference to the familiar alveolar gas equation. An extreme example illustrates the point: An otherwise healthy adult male breathing room air receives a dose of an opioid that causes marked alveolar hypoventilation such that his alveolar PCO_2 is increased to 80 mmHg. The alveolar gas equation predicts that his arterial PO_2 will fall to approximately 40 mmHg as shown here:

$$PAO_2 = PiO_2 - PACO_2/R$$
$$PiO_2 = FiO_2 \times (P_B - P_{H_2O})$$
$$PiO_2 = 0.21 \times (760 - 47) = 150 \text{ mmHg}$$
$$PAO_2 = 150 - 80/0.8$$
$$PAO_2 = 50 \text{ mmHg}$$

where PAO_2 is alveolar partial pressure of oxygen, PiO_2 is inspired partial pressure of oxygen, $PACO_2$ is alveolar partial pressure of carbon dioxide, R is respiratory quotient, P_B is barometric pressure, and P_{H_2O} is water vapor pressure at body temperature.

Assuming a normal alveolar to arterial (A–a) gradient, his PAO_2 will be 40 mmHg, corresponding to an arterial oxygen saturation of 75%. If while initiating definitive therapy for hypoventilation this patient were to receive only a modest increase in inspired oxygen, a marked improvement in arterial saturation would be achieved:

$$FiO_2 \text{ increased to } 28\%$$
$$PiO_2 = 0.28 \times (760 - 47) = 200 \text{ mmHg}$$
$$PAO_2 = 200 - 80/0.8$$
$$PAO_2 = 100 \text{ mmHg}$$

This theoretical example serves to highlight an important point. First, in isolated hypoventilation modest increases in inspired oxygen are remarkably effective at restoring oxygen saturation to acceptable levels. On the other hand, *a patient who is receiving minimal supplemental oxygen and has an acceptable oxygen saturation may have significant undetected alveolar hypoventilation.* The necessity to administer oxygen supplementation is controversial. Deitch et al.[143] reported that the use of supplemental oxygen (2 L/min) during sedation with midazolam and fentanyl did not reduce the occurrence of hypoxia compared to patients on room air. The investigators conducted a similar study evaluating the effect of 3 L/min of oxygen in patients receiving propofol and reported that patients on oxygen had a lower incidence of desaturations compared to patients on room air (18% vs. 28%, respectively) although it was not found to be significant.[144] The authors claimed that physician recognition and correction of an obstructed airway was of greater significance than supplemental oxygen. It should be noted that the data from the ASA closed claims analysis shows that respiratory depression associated with monitored anesthesia care accounted for over one-third of closed-claim injuries in remote locations.[145] We recommend that before discharging patients, it is useful to measure their oxygen saturation while breathing room air.

Head and Neck Fires with the Use of Supplemental Oxygen

From the ASA closed-claims study of Bhananker et al.,[119] we learned that the leading cause of death and severe nervous system injury during MAC is hypoxia due to suppression of spontaneous respiration by sedative-hypnotic drugs. Although administration of supplemental oxygen is generally prudent, the authors of that study also note the surprising finding that the second most common cause of injury was cautery fires, particularly around the head and neck. Thus, caution should be used when supplemental oxygen is administered to patients undergoing surgery in

Table 30-7 Recommendations to Prevent Burn Injuries during MAC
Open face draping techniques; that is, avoiding tent of drapes
Supplemental oxygen at lowest acceptable flows guided by SpO_2
Use of compressed air rather than oxygen to prevent CO_2 accumulation
Stopping oxygen flow 60 sec prior to use of electrocautery
Avoidance of alcohol-based prep solutions
Awareness of the causes and prevention of surgical fires

Adapted from Bhananker SM, Posner KL, Cheney FW, et al. Injury and liability associated with monitored anesthesia care – A closed claims analysis. Anesthesiology. 2006;104:228–234.

the head and neck. The combination of supplemental oxygen, electrocautery, alcoholic prep solution, and flammable drapes is particularly dangerous, especially when a tent of drapes around the patient's head creates a pocket of increased oxygen concentration. Recommendations to prevent fires in this situation are listed in Table 30-7.

Monitoring during Monitored Anesthesia Care

American Society of Anesthesiologists Standards

The ASA standards for basic anesthetic monitoring are applicable to all levels of anesthesia care, including monitored anesthesia care. It is useful to review the components of the ASA standards that are pertinent to monitored anesthesia care as approved by the House of Delegates in October 2010.[146]

Communication and Observation

A conscientious and well-trained anesthesia caregiver is the single most vital monitor in the operating room. However, his or her effectiveness will be markedly enhanced by the use of the basic quantitative and qualitative monitoring devices, which should be readily available in all operating rooms. It is important that the anesthesiologist continually evaluates the patient's response to verbal stimulation to effectively titrate the level of sedation and to allow the earlier detection of neurologic or cardiorespiratory dysfunction. Continuous visual, tactile, and auditory assessment of physiologic function could include observation of the rate, depth, and pattern of respiration; palpation of the arterial pulse; and assessment of peripheral perfusion by extremity temperature and capillary refill. In addition, the patient should be continually observed for diaphoresis, pallor, shivering, cyanosis, and acute changes in neurologic status.

Auscultation

Auscultation of heart and breath sounds has long been a vital component of monitoring during anesthesia. Placement of a precordial stethoscope near the sternal notch of a nonintubated patient provides important information concerning upper airway patency as well as a continuous monitor of heart sounds and ventilation. Continuous precordial auscultation is an inexpensive, effective, and essentially risk-free process that serves as an additional important purpose by bringing the anesthesia care provider closer to the patient.

Pulse Oximetry

No monitor of oxygen transport has had a greater impact on the practice of anesthesiology than the pulse oximeter.[147] Pulse oximetry is noninvasive, safe, and comfortable to the awake patient; it is also technically simple to apply and interpret, and allows continuous real-time monitoring of arterial oxygenation. The use of a quantitative measure of oxygenation is specifically mandated by the ASA standards for intraoperative monitoring. The important mechanisms whereby respiratory function may be compromised during monitored anesthesia care include the effects of sedatives and opioids on respiratory drive, upper airway patency, and protective airway reflexes. Additional important risk factors for arterial desaturation include obesity, pre-existing upper airway obstruction and respiratory disease, increased metabolic rate, general anesthesia, the extremes of age, surgical site, and patient positioning.[148-150] The fundamental importance of monitoring oxygenation during monitored anesthesia care can be appreciated from the closed-claim study of Caplan et al.[133] who examined 14 cases of sudden cardiac arrest in otherwise healthy patients who received spinal anesthesia. These major anesthetic mishaps occurred before the routine adoption of pulse oximetry. One of the major findings of this study was that cyanosis frequently heralded the onset of cardiac arrest, suggesting that unappreciated respiratory insufficiency may have played an important role. Further support for the use of pulse oximetry comes from the ASA Committee on Professional Liability analysis of closed anesthesia claims, which reveals that respiratory events constitute the single largest source of adverse outcome. Furthermore, review of these cases suggests that pulse oximetry in combination with capnometry would have prevented the adverse outcome in most cases.

Capnography

Although capnography is most effective in the intubated patient, useful information may be obtained from a spontaneously breathing, nonintubated patient. Capnography may be used to monitor respiratory rate and aid in the detection and management of airway obstruction. There are numerous methods to monitor end-tidal carbon dioxide. In addition, it may be able to detect hypoventilation during the administration of supplemental oxygen.[151] Sidestream capnographs have been adapted for use with face masks, nasal airways, and nasal cannulae and have been used successfully during monitored anesthesia care.[152,153] Nasal cannulae for oxygen delivery have been modified to provide an integral port for respiratory gas sampling and are available commercially. Alternatively, capnograph sampling lines can be attached to shortened IV catheters and inserted inside nasal oxygen probes. There is growing evidence that capnography may reduce risk associated with sedation/analgesia or monitored anesthesia care in both the pediatric and adult population.[151,154,155] Waugh et al.[156] conducted a meta-analysis to determine if the addition of capnography identified more respiratory complications than standard monitoring alone. They reported that cases of respiratory depression were 17.6 times more likely to be detected if monitored with capnography. Currently, capnography is not a standard of care; however, because of the low cost and enhanced patient safety, we recommend routine use for all patients receiving sedation/analgesia or monitored anesthesia care.

Cardiovascular System

At a minimum, the electrocardiogram must be continually displayed and the blood pressure measured and recorded at least every 5 minutes during monitored anesthesia care. The pulse should be monitored by palpation, oximetry, or auscultation. The selection of additional hemodynamic monitoring is usually determined more by the cardiovascular status of the patient than the magnitude of the procedure. Most procedures performed under monitored anesthesia care do not involve major hemorrhage, fluid shifts, or major physiologic trespass. Decisions concerning choice of monitoring for myocardial ischemia and other adverse hemodynamic events will need to be individualized on a case-by-case basis.

Temperature Monitoring and Management during Monitored Anesthesia Care

The value of temperature monitoring is well established during general anesthesia, the perioperative period being frequently complicated by hypothermia and hyperthermia. Although sedation techniques used during monitored anesthesia care do not generally trigger malignant hyperthermia, there is potential for significant inadvertent hypothermia, particularly during neuraxial anesthesia. Even monitored anesthesia care techniques unaccompanied by regional anesthesia are associated with hypothermia at the extremes of age, both the old and very young having impaired thermoregulatory mechanisms. The elderly also have markedly reduced muscle mass and therefore basal heat production. Although the anesthesiologist may be able to exert some control over the ambient temperature in the operating room, he or she may be unable to influence the temperature at remote anesthetizing locations. Radiology suites are often maintained at lower temperatures to accommodate the computer systems that are used to reconstruct images. Radiant heating lamps, forced-air heaters, fluid warmers, or warming blankets, all common items in operating rooms, may be unavailable and unsuitable for use at remote locations. Forced-air heating has been shown to be an effective means of maintaining normothermia, and can be combined with IV fluid warming.[157,158] Even mild perioperative hypothermia (i.e., 1°C to 2°C) accompanying general anesthesia is associated with adverse myocardial outcomes, increased bleeding tendency and transfusion requirements, wound infections, and delayed wound healing and hospital discharge.[159-164] At this time, there is no evidence suggesting that the morbidity associated with perioperative hypothermia is any less during monitored anesthesia care than during general anesthesia. The morbidity associated with perioperative hypothermia is well described in high-risk patients; this is a group of patients who are very likely to undergo procedures under monitored anesthesia care. When hypothermia is significant, shivering may interfere with the planned procedure and markedly increase oxygen requirements and predispose susceptible patients to myocardial ischemia or respiratory insufficiency. The major thermoregulatory defenses against hypothermia include vasoconstriction, shivering, and behavior. Vasoconstriction and shivering are impaired during major conduction anesthesia. Behavioral thermoregulation is impaired even in the conscious patient. Regional anesthesia has major effects on thermoregulation.[165] Lower extremity vasodilatation causes central cooling via a redistribution of heat from the core to the periphery. Afferent input to the hypothalamus from the warm peripheral compartment counteracts conflicting input from the cooling central compartment, thus delaying the initiation of compensatory thermoregulation. In the absence of reliable temperature monitoring, it is possible that the first indication of hypothermia would be the onset of shivering, by which time considerable central cooling may have occurred.

Frank et al.[166] have examined the issue of temperature monitoring and management during neuraxial anesthesia and found that temperature monitoring is significantly underused, with only one-third of patients being monitored. Furthermore, the method that was most frequently used to monitor temperature may not accurately reflect core temperature, the most important determinant of thermoregulatory response and perioperative morbidity. Forehead skin surface was the most commonly monitored site. The accuracy of these devices for perioperative temperature monitoring remains controversial; they do not reliably detect malignant hyperthermia and are not sufficiently accurate for fever screening purposes in children.[167] Sessler[168] recommends the use of a properly positioned axillary probe or intermittent oral temperature monitoring during neuraxial anesthetics.

Patients will frequently complain of feeling too warm when covered by heavy drapes. Although malignant hyperthermia is rare during monitored anesthesia care, hyperthermia is still possible as a result of thyroid storm or malignant neuroleptic syndrome. The subjective sensation of hyperthermia may also be the first indicator of important adverse events in evolution such as hypoxia, hypercarbia, cerebral ischemia, local anesthetic toxicity, and myocardial ischemia.

Bispectral Index Monitoring during Monitored Anesthesia Care

The bispectral index (BIS) is a processed EEG parameter that was developed specifically to evaluate patient response during drug-induced anesthesia and sedation. Sedation monitoring is attractive because of the potential to titrate drugs more accurately, avoiding the adverse effects of both over- and underdosing. BIS monitoring has some potential advantages over conventional intermittent techniques of patient assessment. Conventional assessment involves patient stimulation at frequent intervals to determine the level of consciousness, requires patient cooperation, and is subject to testing fatigue. An example of a conventional assessment tool is the Observer's Assessment of Alertness/Sedation Scale (Table 30-8)[169] and the ASA Continuum of Depth of Sedation Definition (Table 30-9).[170] The BIS has been shown to be a useful monitor of drug-induced sedation and recall in volunteers and has been shown to correlate with Observer's Assessment of Alertness/Sedation Scale scores during propofol-induced sedation in patients undergoing surgery with regional anesthesia.[169] An increasing depth of sedation was associated with a predictable decrease in the BIS. Absence of recall was associated with BIS values below 80. These findings correspond with those of Kearse et al.[171] who found no intraoperative recall at BIS values below 79 during midazolam-, isoflurane-, and propofol-induced sedation. However, the inability to recall a nonnoxious stimulus such as a picture, as used in the previously mentioned studies, may not necessarily correspond to amnesia to noxious events such as surgical stimulation. Despite this caveat, Liu et al.[172] suggest that using a combination of propofol and midazolam to achieve a BIS value below 80 will minimize the possibility of intraoperative

Table 30-8 Observer's Assessment of Alertness/Sedation Scale

Responsiveness	Speech	Facial Expression	Eyes	Composite Score
Responds readily to name spoken in normal tone	Normal	Normal	Clear, no ptosis	5 (alert)
Lethargic response to name spoken in normal tone	Mild slowing or thickening	Mild relaxation	Glazed or mild ptosis (less than half the eye)	4
Responds only after name is called loudly or repeatedly	Slurring or prominent slowing	Marked relaxation (slack jaw)	Glazed and marked ptosis (half the eye or more)	3
Responds only after mild prodding or shaking	Few recognizable words			2
Does not respond to mild prodding or shaking				1 (asleep)

recall. Although the use of BIS to monitor sedation is appealing, conventional assessment of sedation is an important mechanism whereby continuous patient contact is maintained. Ideally, BIS monitoring will be employed in the future as an adjunct to clinical evaluation rather than as the primary monitor of consciousness.

Preparedness to Recognize and Treat Local Anesthetic Toxicity

Monitored anesthesia care is often provided in the context of regional or local anesthetic techniques. It is vitally important that the anesthesiologist responsible for the patient have a high index of suspicion and be fully prepared to recognize and treat local anesthetic toxicity immediately (see Chapter 22). This point deserves special emphasis, particularly in view of the fact that monitored anesthesia care is often provided to the elderly or debilitated patient who has been deemed "unfit" for general anesthesia; these are the patients most likely to suffer adverse reactions to local anesthetic drugs. Even if the anesthesiologist does not perform the block personally, he or she is in a unique position to fulfill an important "preventive" role by advising the surgeon about the most appropriate volume, concentration, and type of local anesthetic drug or technique to be used.

Systemic local anesthetic toxicity occurs when plasma concentrations of drug are excessively high. Plasma concentrations will increase when the rate of entry of drug into the circulation exceeds the rate of drug clearance from the circulation. The clinically recognizable effects of local anesthetics on the central nervous system are concentration dependent. At low concentrations, sedation and numbness of the tongue and circumoral tissues and a metallic taste are prominent features. As concentrations increase, restlessness, vertigo, tinnitus, and difficulty focusing may occur. Higher concentrations result in slurred speech and skeletal muscle twitching, which often herald the onset of tonic–clonic seizures.

The conduct of monitored anesthesia care may modify the individual's response to the potentially toxic effects of local anesthetic administration and adversely affect the margin of safety of a regional or local technique. For example, a patient with compromised cardiovascular function may experience a further decline in cardiac output during sedation. The resultant reduction in hepatic blood flow will reduce the clearance of local anesthetics that are metabolized by the liver and have a high hepatic extraction ratio, thereby increasing the likelihood of achieving toxic plasma concentrations. A patient receiving sedation may experience respiratory depression and a subsequent increase in arterial carbon dioxide concentration. Hypercarbia adversely affects the margin of safety in several ways. By increasing cerebral blood flow, hypercarbia will increase the amount of local anesthetic that is delivered to the brain, thereby increasing the potential for neurotoxicity. By reducing neuronal axoplasmic pH, hypercarbia

Table 30-9 Continuum of Depth of Sedation

	Minimal Sedation Anxiolysis	Moderate Sedation/Analgesia ("Conscious Sedation")	Deep Sedation/Analgesia	General Anesthesia
Responsiveness	Normal response to verbal stimulation	Purposeful[a] response to verbal or tactile stimulation	Purposeful response following repeated or painful stimulation	Unarousable, even with a painful stimulus
Airway	Unaffected	No intervention required	Intervention may be required	Intervention often required
Spontaneous ventilation	Unaffected	Adequate	May be inadequate	Frequently inadequate
Cardiovascular function	Unaffected	Usually maintained	Usually maintained	May be impaired

[a]Reflex withdrawal from a painful stimulus is not considered a purposeful response.
Adapted with permission from ASA House of Delegates. Continuum of depth of sedation: Definition of General Anesthesia and Levels of Sedation/Analgesia, 2014. A copy of the full text can be obtained from ASA, 1061 American Lane, Schaumburg, IL 60173–4973 or online at www.asahq.org.

increases the intracellular concentration of the charged, active form of local anesthetic, thus also increasing its toxicity. In addition, hypercarbia, acidosis, and hypoxia all markedly potentiate the cardiovascular toxicity of local anesthetics. Furthermore, the administration of sedative–hypnotic drugs may interfere with the patient's ability to communicate the symptoms of impending neurotoxicity. However, the anticonvulsant properties of benzodiazepines and barbiturates may attenuate the seizures associated with neurotoxicity. In both of these circumstances, it is possible that the symptoms of cardiotoxicity will be the first evidence that an adverse reaction has occurred. Thus, appropriate treatment is delayed or inadvertent intravascular injection is continued because of the absence of any clinical evidence of neurotoxicity. Cardiovascular toxicity usually occurs at a higher plasma concentration than neurotoxicity, but when it does occur, it is usually much more difficult to manage than neurotoxicity. Although cardiotoxicity is usually preceded by neurotoxicity, it may on occasion be the initial presenting feature.

Sedation and Analgesia by Nonanesthesiologists

Although anesthesiologists have specific training and expertise to provide sedation and analgesia, in clinical practice minimal and moderate sedation services are frequently provided by nonanesthesiologists. Deep sedation is occasionally delivered by trained specialists, including emergency department physicians and intensivists. The specific reasons for nonanesthesiologist involvement differ from institution to institution and from case to case and include convenience, availability, and scheduling issues; perceived lack of anesthesiologist availability; perceived increased cost; and a perceived lack of benefit concerning patient satisfaction and safety when sedation and analgesia are provided by anesthesiologists. Despite our frequent noninvolvement in these cases, anesthesiologists are indirectly involved in the care of these patients by being required to participate in the development of institutional policies and procedures for sedation and analgesia, as mandated by the Joint Commission. To assist anesthesiologists in this process, an ASA task force has developed practice guidelines for sedation and analgesia by nonanesthesiologists.[173,174]

Four levels of sedation are defined in the ASA practice guidelines and include minimal sedation, moderate sedation, deep sedation, and general anesthesia. The practice guidelines emphasize that sedation and analgesia represent a continuum of sedation wherein patients can easily pass into a level of sedation deeper than intended. The ASA House of Delegates issued a statement on this continuum of depth of sedation originally in October 1999, and most recently amended it in October 2014. This statement contains a chart representing the clinical progression along this continuum (Table 30-9).[172] When monitoring a sedated patient during a procedure, it is important to recognize when a patient becomes more deeply sedated than intended so that the care team can act appropriately to prevent cardiorespiratory compromise.

The sedation guidelines emphasize the importance of preprocedure patient evaluation, patient preparation, and appropriate fasting periods. The importance of continuous patient monitoring is discussed—in particular, the response of the patient to commands as a guide to the level of sedation. The appropriate monitoring of ventilation, oxygenation, and hemodynamics is also discussed, and recommendations are made for the contemporaneous recording of these parameters. The task force strongly suggests that an individual other than the person performing the therapeutic or diagnostic procedure be available to monitor the patient's comfort and physiologic status. Education and training of providers is recommended. Specific educational objectives include the potentiation of sedative-induced respiratory depression by concomitantly administered opioids, adequate time intervals between doses of sedative/analgesics to avoid cumulative over-dosage, and familiarity with sedative/analgesic antagonists. The routine administration of supplemental oxygen is recommended. At least one person with Basic Life Support training should be available during moderate sedation, with immediate availability (1 to 5 minutes) of personnel trained in Advanced Life Support. For procedures requiring Deep Sedation, the ASA recommends ACLS trained personnel be present in the procedure room. This individual should have the ability to recognize airway obstruction, establish an airway, and maintain oxygenation and ventilation. The practice guidelines recommend that appropriate patient-size emergency equipment be readily available, specifically including equipment for establishing an airway and delivering positive pressure ventilation with supplemental oxygen, emergency resuscitation drugs, and a working defibrillator. The presence of reliable IV access until the patient is no longer at risk for cardiorespiratory depression will improve safety. Adequate postprocedure recovery care with appropriate monitoring must be provided until discharge. Certain high-risk patient groups (e.g., unco-operative patients, extremes of age, severe cardiac, pulmonary, hepatic, renal, or central nervous system disease, morbid obesity, sleep apnea, pregnancy, and patients who abuse drug or alcohol) will be encountered, and the guidelines recommend that preprocedure consultation with anesthesiologists, cardiologists, pulmonologists, and so forth be performed *before* administration of sedation and analgesia by nonanesthesiologists.

Controversy exists regarding the level of training required for nonanesthesiologists to be credentialed to provide moderate and deep sedation. The ASA released a statement in October 2005, amended in 2011, suggesting a framework for granting privileges that will help ensure competence of individuals who administer or supervise the administration of moderate sedation.[174] This statement suggests that the practitioner should complete formal training in (1) the safe administration of sedative and analgesic drugs used to establish a level of moderate sedation, and (2) rescue of patients who exhibit adverse physiologic consequences of a deeper-than-intended level of sedation. The ASA released an advisory in October 2010 on granting privileges for deep sedation to nonanesthesiologist sedation practitioners.[174]

Recently, the Centers for Medicare and Medicaid Services (CMS) published revised hospital anesthesia services interpretive guidelines requiring hospitals to establish policies and procedures that address whether specific clinical situations involve "anesthesia" versus "analgesia" services. The CMS document places general anesthesia, monitored anesthesia care, deep sedation, and regional anesthesia under "anesthesia" services. These "anesthesia" services must be provided by: A qualified anesthesiologist; a doctor of medicine or osteopathy, a dentist, oral surgeon, or podiatrist who is qualified to administer anesthesia under state law; an appropriately supervised Certified Registered Nurse Anesthetist or Anesthesia Assistant, all who are separate from the practitioner performing the procedure. Moderate sedation and minimal sedation fall under "analgesia" services.[175] The statement released by the ASA on the safe use of propofol, most recently amended in 2014, is explicit that the drug should be administered only by "persons trained in the administration of general anesthesia, who are not simultaneously involved in these surgical or diagnostic procedures.... Failure to follow these recommendations could put patients at increased risk of significant injury or death."[176]

Computer-assisted Personalized Sedation—SEDASYS

Although the SEDASYS device has now been withdrawn from the US market, it is worthwhile to briefly review the circumstances prompting its development and its design features. In December 2009, the American College of Gastroenterology (ACG) released a position statement which suggested that non-anesthesiologist administered propofol is more cost-effective than standard sedation for routine endoscopic GI procedures; and that the utilization of anesthesiologist-administered sedation for "healthy, low risk patients results in higher cost with no proven benefit in terms of patient safety."[177] Although the professional cost of anesthesia services is only a small fraction (3%) of the total physician services, the recent increase in spending on monitored anesthesia care for esophagogastroduodenoscopy and colonoscopy is significant. Given the ACG stance on the cost-effectiveness of nonanesthesiologist administered propofol, the cost associated with anesthesiologist-administered sedation, and the increasing demand for large numbers of patients to receive sedation for endoscopic procedures, it is not surprising that alternatives to anesthesiologist-administered sedation might be considered attractive. Recent advances in technology have allowed the development of computer-assisted personalized sedation (CAPS) devices. These devices integrate patient monitoring variables with the programmed delivery of propofol. The most publicized of these systems, SEDASYS (SEDASYS Computer-Assisted Personalized Sedation System, Ethicon Endo-Surgery, Inc. Cincinnati, Ohio) integrated information extracted from standard ASA monitors (including pulse oximetry, capnography, electrocardiography, and blood pressure surveillance) with dosing algorithms to deliver a titratable infusion of propofol in order to achieve and maintain minimal-to-moderate sedation. The manufacturer of this system required that it should only be used in facilities where an anesthesia professional is immediately available to assist or consult as needed. The ASA recommends that in this particular context, that at a minimum, "immediate availability" could be a code or rapid response team that includes an anesthesia professional.

SEDASYS primarily achieved sedation with propofol. However, the device worked in conjunction with a single administered dose of fentanyl given 3 minutes prior to the start of a propofol infusion in an attempt to yield some analgesic effect.[2,3] Patients less than 65 years of age received a 50 to 100 µg IV bolus of fentanyl, whereas patients 65 years of age and older were limited to 25 to 50 µg. Initial propofol infusion rates varied between 25 and 75 µg/kg/min. After a maintenance infusion rate escalation, further increases were limited by a 3-minute lockout period.[178,179] If patient variables suggested a need for increased sedation, a maximum infusion rate of 200 µg/kg/min could be achieved over the course of 12 minutes. There were several safety mechanisms in place to ensure both adequate depth of sedation, and prevention of oversedation. An automated responsiveness monitor actuated by the patient assessed his/her responsiveness by requiring interaction with a hand-held device when prompted by vibratory or auditory stimulation. Oxygen delivery was also automatically titrated as determined by oxygen saturation measurement. There were alarm systems to alert the provider to low respiratory rate, low oxygen saturation or apnea events. Triggering these alarms resulted in the discontinuation of the propofol infusion. Although the aforementioned safety features were effective in generally healthy adults, some patients were not considered to be suitable candidates for sedation with SEDASYS, including age under 18 years, ASA IV or V classification, BMI over 35, abnormal airway anatomy or evidence of obstructive sleep apnea, chronic pain patient utilizing a fentanyl patch, gastroparesis, patients undergoing both colonoscopy and EGD in the same procedure, emergent colonoscopy or EGD. Although SEDASYS was withdrawn from the market, it seems likely that other CAPS devices will be developed. In 2014, the ASA issued a guidance document with recommendations on sedation with regard to the integration of CAPS devices into medical practices in the safest and most efficient way. The ASA statement notes that it is important when working with new technology to investigate ways to ensure it is used safely. Highlights of the recommendations are that Directors of Anesthesia Services should be familiar with the manufacturer's recommendations and the FDA labeling information on the operation and safe use of the device, and that quality and safety programs in procedural sedation should be revised to include data collection on all sedation including these devices. The Anesthesia Quality Institute (AQI) publishes guidelines for quality metrics for procedural sedation. These guidelines now include metrics for patients receiving sedation via CAPS.[180]

Conclusion

Through the use of monitored anesthesia care, an often terrifying and painful procedure can be made safe and comfortable for the patient. Monitored anesthesia care presents an opportunity for our patients to observe us at work. For the anesthesiologist, monitored anesthesia care presents an opportunity to provide a more prolonged and intimate level of care and reassurance to our patients that is in contrast to the more limited exposure that occurs during and after general anesthesia. Our airway management skills and our daily practice of applied pharmacology make us uniquely qualified to provide this service. Monitored anesthesia care presents us with an opportunity to display these skills and increase our recognition in areas outside the operating room. The availability of drugs with a more favorable pharmacologic profile allows us to tailor our techniques to provide the specific components of analgesia, sedation, anxiolysis, and amnesia with minimal morbidity and to facilitate a prompt recovery. As the population ages, increasing numbers of patients will become candidates for monitored anesthesia care. Significant advances in nonsurgical fields (e.g., interventional radiology) will increase the number of procedures that are ideally performed under monitored anesthesia care. It is our responsibility to clearly demonstrate to our nonanesthesia colleagues that anesthesiologist-provided monitored anesthesia care contributes to the best outcome for our patients. If anesthesiologists are not willing or able to provide these services, others, who are less well qualified, are prepared to assume that role.

REFERENCES

1. American Society of Anesthesiologists. Distinguishing monitored anesthesia care ("MAC") from moderate sedation/analgesia (conscious sedation). www.asahq.org. Accessed May 26, 2016.
2. American Society of Anesthesiologists. Practice guidelines for sedation and analgesia by non-anesthesiologists. *Anesthesiology*. 2002;96:1004–1017.
3. American Society of Anesthesiologists. Position on monitored anesthesia care. www.asahq.org. October 2013. Accessed May 26, 2016.
4. Miner JR, Huber D, Nichols S, et al. The effect of the assignment of a pre-sedation target level on procedural sedation using propofol. *J Emerg Med*. 2007;32:249–255.

5. Ausems ME, Vuyk J, Hug CC, et al. Comparison of a computer-assisted infusion versus intermittent bolus administration of alfentanil as a supplement to nitrous oxide for lower abdominal surgery. *Anesthesiology*. 1988;68:851–861.
6. Hughes MA, Glass PS, Jacobs JR. Context-sensitive half-time in multicompartment pharmacokinetic models for intravenous anesthetic drugs. *Anesthesiology*. 1992;76:334–341.
7. Bailey JM. Context-sensitive half-times: What are they and how valuable are they in anaesthesiology? *Clin Pharmacokinet*. 2002;41:793–799.
8. Shafer SL, Varvel JR. Pharmacokinetics, pharmacodynamics, and rational opioid selection. *Anesthesiology*. 1991;74:53–63.
9. Scott JC, Ponganis KV, Stanski DR. EEG quantitation of narcotic effect: the comparative pharmacodynamics of fentanyl and alfentanil. *Anesthesiology*. 1985;62:234–241.
10. Avramov MN, White PF. Use of alfentanil and propofol for outpatient monitored anesthesia care: Determining the optimal dosing regimen. *Anesth Analg*. 1997;85:566–572.
11. Mandema JW, Sansom LN, Dios-Vièitez MC, et al. Pharmacokinetic-pharmacodynamic modeling of the electroencephalographic effects of benzodiazepines. Correlation with receptor binding and anticonvulsant activity. *J Pharmacol Exp Ther*. 1991;257:472–478.
12. Newson C, Joshi GP, Victory R, et al. Comparison of propofol administration techniques for sedation during monitored anesthesia care. *Anesth Analg*. 1995;81:486–491.
13. Smith C, McEwan AI, Jhaveri R, et al. The interaction of fentanyl on the Cp50 of propofol for loss of consciousness and skin incision. *Anesthesiology*. 1994;81:820–828; discussion 26A.
14. Kazama T, Ikeda K, Morita K. Reduction by fentanyl of the Cp50 values of propofol and hemodynamic responses to various noxious stimuli. *Anesthesiology*. 1997;87:213–227.
15. Kazama T, Ikeda K, Morita K. The pharmacodynamic interaction between propofol and fentanyl with respect to the suppression of somatic or hemodynamic responses to skin incision, peritoneum incision and abdominal wall retraction. *Anesthesiology*. 1998;89:894–906.
16. Smith C, McEwan AI, Jhaveri R, et al. Reduction of propofol Cp50 by fentanyl. *Anesthesiology*. 1992;77:A340.
17. Short TG, Plummer JL, Chui PT. Hypnotic and anaesthetic interactions between midazolam, propofol and alfentanil. *Br J Anaesth*. 1992;69:162–167.
18. Short TG, Chui PT. Propofol and midazolam act synergistically in combination. *Br J Anaesth*. 1991;67:539–545.
19. Teh J, Short TG, Wong J, et al. Pharmacokinetic interactions between midazolam and propofol: An infusion study. *Br J Anaesth*. 1994;72:62–65.
20. Hillier SC. Achieving control of anesthetic administration: The infusion pump versus the vaporizer. *Anesthesiol Clin North America*. 1996;14:265–280.
21. McEwan AI, Smith C, Dyar O, et al. Isoflurane minimum alveolar concentration reduction by fentanyl. *Anesthesiology*. 1993;78:864–869.
22. Sebel PS, Glass PSA, Fletcher JE, et al. Reduction of the MAC of desflurane with fentanyl. *Anesthesiology*. 1992;76:52–59.
23. Lang E, Kapila A, Shlugman D, et al. Reduction of isoflurane minimal alveolar concentration by remifentanil. *Anesthesiology*. 1996;85:721–728.
24. Westmoreland CL, Sebel PS, Gropper A. Fentanyl or alfentanil decreases the minimum alveolar anesthetic concentration of isoflurane in surgical patients. *Anesth Analg*. 1994;78:23–28.
25. Brunner MD, Braithwaite P, Jhaveri R, et al. MAC reduction of isoflurane by sufentanil. *Br J Anaesth*. 1994;72:42–46.
26. Vinik HR, Bradley EL, Kissin I. Midazolam-alfentanil synergism for anesthetic induction in patients. *Anesth Analg*. 1989;69:213–217.
27. Kissin I, Vinik HR, Castillo R, et al. Alfentanil potentiates midazolam-induced unconsciousness in subanalgesic doses. *Anesth Analg*. 1990;71:65–69.
28. Food and Drug Administration. Midazolam Black Box Warning. *Drug Bulletin*. 1988;18:15–16.
29. Bailey PL, Pace NL, Ashburn MA, et al. Frequent hypoxemia and apnea after sedation with midazolam and fentanyl. *Anesthesiology*. 1990;73:826–830.
30. Cheng SS, Yeh J, Flood P. Anesthesia matters: Patients anesthetized with propofol have less postoperative pain than those anesthetized with isoflurane. *Anesth Analg*. 2008;106:264–269.
31. Mackenzie N, Grant IS. Propofol for intravenous sedation. *Anaesthesia*. 1987;42:3–6.
32. Wilson E, David A, Mackenzie N, et al. Sedation during spinal anaesthesia: Comparison of propofol and midazolam. *Br J Anaesth*. 1990;64:48–52.
33. Wilson E, Mackenzie N, Grant IS. A comparison of propofol and midazolam by infusion to provide sedation in patients who receive spinal anaesthesia. *Anaesthesia*. 1988;43:91–94.
34. Smith I, Monk TG, White PF, et al. Propofol infusion during regional anesthesia. *Anesth Analg*. 1994;79:313–319.
35. White PF, Negus JB. Sedative infusions during local and regional anesthesia: a comparison of midazolam and propofol. *J Clin Anesth*. 1991;3:32–39.
36. Gecaj-Gashi A, Hashimi M, Sada F, et al. Propofol vs isoflurane anesthesia-incidence of PONV in patients at maxillofacial surgery. *Adv Med Sci*. 2010;55:308–312.
37. Gauger PG, Shanks A, Morris M, et al. Propofol decreases early postoperative nausea and vomiting in patients undergoing thyroid and parathyroid operations. *World J Surg*. 2008;32:1525–1534.
38. Tan T, Bhinder R, Carey M, et al. Day-surgery patients anesthetized with propofol have less postoperative pain than those anesthetized with sevoflurane. *Anesth Analg*. 2010;111:83–85.
39. Vari A, Gazzanelli S, Cavallaro G, et al. Post-operative nausea and vomiting (PONV) after thyroid surgery: A prospective, randomized study comparing totally intravenous versus inhalational anesthetics. *Am Surg*. 2010;76:325–328.
40. Apfel CC, Korttila K, Abdalla M, et al. A factorial trial of six interventions for the prevention of postoperative nausea and vomiting. *N Engl J Med*. 2004;350:2441–2451.
41. Tramèr M, Moore A, McQuay H. Propofol anaesthesia and postoperative nausea and vomiting: Quantitative systematic review of randomized controlled studies. *Br J Anaesth*. 1997;78:247–255.
42. Fujii Y, Itakura M. Comparison of propofol, droperidol, and metoclopramide for prophylaxis of postoperative nausea and vomiting after breast cancer surgery: A prospective, randomized, double-blind, placebo-controlled study in Japanese patients. *Clin Ther*. 2008;30:2024–2029.
43. Fujii Y, Itakura M. Low-dose propofol to prevent nausea and vomiting after laparoscopic surgery. *Int J Gynaecol Obstet*. 2009;106:50–52.
44. Arslan M, Demir ME. Prevention of postoperative nausea and vomiting with a small dose of propofol combined with dexamethasone 4 mg or dexamethasone 8 mg in patients undergoing middle ear surgery: a prospective, randomized, double-blind study. *Bratisl Lek Listy*. 2011;112:332–336.
45. Borgeat A, Wilder-Smith OHG, Saiah M, et al. Subhypnotic doses of propofol possess direct antiemetic properties. *Anesth Analg*. 1992;74:539–541.
46. Ghouri AF, Ramirez Ruiz MA, White PF. Effect of flumazenil on recovery after midazolam and propofol sedation. *Anesthesiology*. 1994;81:333–339.
47. Smith I, White PF, Nathanson M, et al. Propofol. An update on its clinical use. *Anesthesiology*. 1994;81:1005–1043.
48. Sneyd JR, Rigby-Jones AE. New drugs and technologies, intravenous anaesthesia is on the move (again). *Br J Anaesth*. 2010;105:246–254.
49. Levitzky BE, Vargo JJ. Fospropofol disodium injection for the sedation of patients undergoing colonoscopy. *Ther Clin Risk Manag*. 2008;4:733–738.
50. Garnock-Jones KP, Scott LJ. Fospropofol. *Drugs*. 2010;70:469–477.
51. Struys MMRF, Fechner J, Schuttler J, et al. Erroneously published fospropofol pharmacokinetic-pharmacodynamic data and retraction of the affected publications. [Retraction of Fechner J, Ihmsen H, Hatterscheid D, Schiessl C, Vornov JJ, Burak E, Schwilden H, Schuttler J. Anesthesiology. 2003 Aug;99(2):303–13; PMID: 12883403]. [Retraction of Fechner J, Ihmsen H, Hatterscheid D, Jeleazcov C, Schiessl C, Vornov JJ, Schwilden H, Schuttler J. Anesthesiology. 2004 Sep;101(3):626–39; PMID: 15329587]. [Retraction of Shah A, Mistry B, Gibiansky E, Gibiansky L. Anesthesiology. 2008 Nov;109(5):937; discussion 937; PMID: 18946316]. [Retraction of Struys MM, Vanlunche AL, Gibiansky E, Gibiansky L, Vornov J, Mortier EP, Van Bortel L. Anesthesiology. 2005 Oct;103(4):730–43; PMID: 16192765]. [Retraction of Gibiansky E, Struys MM, Gibiansky L, Vanluchene AL, Vornov J, Mortier EP, Burak E, Van Bortel L. Anesthesiology. 2005 Oct;103(4):718–29; PMID: 16192764]. *Anesthesiology*. 2010;112:1056–1057.
52. Shah A, Mistry B, Gibiansky E, et al. Fospropofol assay issues and impact on pharmacokinetic and pharmacodynamic evaluation. [Erratum appears in Anesthesiology. 2008 Nov;109(5):940]. [Retraction in Struys MM, Fechner J, Schuttler J, Schwilden H. Anesthesiology. 2010 Apr;112(4):1056–7; PMID: 20177373]. *Anesthesiology*. 2008;109:937; discussion.
53. Shah A, Mistry B, Gibiansky E, et al. Fospropofol assay issues and impact on pharmacokinetic and pharmacodynamic evaluation. *Anesth Analg*. 2009;108:382; author reply 383.
54. Cohen LB. Clinical trial: A dose-response study of fospropofol disodium for moderate sedation during colonoscopy. *Aliment Pharmacol Ther*. 2008;27:597–608.
55. Cohen LB, Cattau E, Goetsch A, et al. A randomized, double-blind, phase 3 study of fospropofol disodium for sedation during colonoscopy. *J Clin Gastroenterol*. 2010;44:345–353.
56. Stoelting RKHS. *Benzodiazepines, Pharmacology and Physiology in Anesthetic Practice*. 4th ed. Philadelphia, PA: JB Lippincott; 2006.
57. Taylor E, Ghouri AF, White PF. Midazolam in combination with propofol for sedation during local anesthesia. *J Clin Anesth*. 1992;4:213–216.
58. Ekstein M, Gavish D, Ezri T, et al. Monitored anaesthesia care in the elderly: Guidelines and recommendations. *Drugs Aging*. 2008;25:477–500.
59. Jacobs JR, Reves JG, Marty J, et al. Aging increases pharmacodynamic sensitivity to the hypnotic effects of midazolam. *Anesth Analg*. 1995;80:143–148.
60. Pratila MG, Fischer ME, Alagesan R, et al. Propofol versus midazolam for monitored sedation: A comparison of intraoperative and recovery parameters. *J Clin Anesth*. 1993;5:268–274.
61. Tognetto D, di Lauro M, Fanni D, et al. Iatrogenic retinal traumas in ophthalmic surgery. *Graefes Arch Clin Exp Ophthalmol*. 2008;246:1361–1372.
62. Hamilton RC. Complications of ophthalmic regional anesthesia. In: Finucane BT, ed. *Complications of Regional Anesthesia*. New York, NY: Springer; 2007:87–101.

63. Yee JB, Burns TA, Mann JM, et al. Propofol and alfentanil for sedation during placement of retrobulbar block for cataract surgery. *J Clin Anesth.* 1996;8:623–626.
64. Inan UU, Sivaci RG, Ermis SS, et al. Effects of fentanyl on pain and hemodynamic response after retrobulbar block in patients having phacoemulsification. *J Cataract Refract Surg.* 2003;29:1137–1142.
65. McHardy FE, Fortier J, Chung F, et al. A comparison of midazolam, alfentanil and propofol for sedation in outpatient intraocular surgery. *Can J Anaesth.* 2000;47:211–214.
66. Ryu JH, So YM, Hwang JW, et al. Optimal target concentration of remifentanil during cataract surgery with monitored anesthesia care. *J Clin Anesth.* 2010;22:533–537.
67. Ahmad S, Leavell ME, Fragen RJ, et al. Remifentanil versus alfentanil as analgesic adjuncts during placement of ophthalmologic nerve blocks. *Reg Anesth Pain Med.* 1999;24:331–336.
68. Veselis RA, Reinsel RA, Feshchenko VA, et al. Impaired memory and behavioral performance with fentanyl at low plasma concentrations. *Anesth Analg.* 1994;79:952–960.
69. Aydın ON, Ugur B, Kir E, et al. Effect of single-dose fentanyl on the cardiorespiratory system in elderly patients undergoing cataract surgery. *J Clin Anesth.* 2004;16:98–103.
70. Akcaboy ZN, Akcaboy EY, Albayrak D, et al. Can remifentanil be a better choice than propofol for colonoscopy during monitored anesthesia care? *Acta Anaesthesiol Scand.* 2006;50:736–741.
71. Keidan I, Berkenstadt H, Sidi A, et al. Propofol/remifentanil versus propofol alone for bone marrow aspiration in paediatric haemato-oncological patients. *Paediatr Anaesth.* 2001;11:297–301.
72. Glass PSA, Hardman D, Kamiyama Y, et al. Preliminary pharmacokinetics and pharmacodynamics of an ultra-short-acting opioid. *Anesth Analg.* 1993;77:1031–1040.
73. Westmoreland CL, Hoke JF, Sebel PS, et al. Pharmacokinetics of remifentanil (GI87084B) and its major metabolite (GI90291) in patients undergoing elective inpatient surgery. *Anesthesiology.* 1993;79:893–903.
74. Egan TD, Lemmens HJ, Fiset P, et al. The pharmacokinetics of the new short-acting opioid remifentanil (GI87084B) in healthy adult male volunteers. *Anesthesiology.* 1993;79:881–892.
75. Kapila A, Glass PSA, Jacobs JR, et al. Measured context-sensitive half-times of remifentanil and alfentanil. *Anesthesiology.* 1995;83:968–975.
76. Servin F, Desmonts JM, Watkins WD. Remifentanil as an analgesic adjunct in local/regional anesthesia and in monitored anesthesia care. *Anesth Analg.* 1999;89:S28–S32.
77. Avramov MN, Smith I, White PF. Interactions between midazolam and remifentanil during monitored anesthesia care. *Anesthesiology.* 1996;85:1283–1289.
78. Ryu JH, Kim JH, Park KS, et al. Remifentanil-propofol versus fentanyl-propofol for monitored anesthesia care during hysteroscopy. *J Clin Anesth.* 2008;20:328–332.
79. Sa Rego MM, Inagaki Y, White PF. Remifentanil administration during monitored anesthesia care: Are intermittent boluses an effective alternative to a continuous infusion? *Anesth Analg.* 1999;88:518–522.
80. Smith I, Avramov MN, White PF. A comparison of propofol and remifentanil during monitored anesthesia care. *J Clin Anesth.* 1997;9:148–154.
81. Green SM. Research advances in procedural sedation and analgesia. *Ann Emerg Med.* 2007;49:31–36.
82. Green SM, Klooster M, Harris T, et al. Ketamine sedation for pediatric gastroenterology procedures. *J Pediatr Gastroenterol Nutr.* 2001;32:26–33.
83. McCarty E, Mencio G, Green N. Anesthesia and analgesia for the ambulatory management of fractures in children. *J Am Acad Orthop Surg.* 1999;7:81–91.
84. Sherwin TS, Green SM, Khan A, et al. Does adjunctive midazolam reduce recovery agitation after ketamine sedation for pediatric procedures? A randomized, double-blind, placebo-controlled trial. *Ann Emerg Med.* 2000;35:229–238.
85. Akin A, Esmaoglu A, Guler G, et al. Propofol and propofol-ketamine in pediatric patients undergoing cardiac catheterization. *Pediatr Cardiol.* 2005;26:553–557.
86. Akin A, Guler G, Esmaoglu A, et al. A comparison of fentanyl-propofol with a ketamine-propofol combination for sedation during endometrial biopsy. *J Clin Anesth.* 2005;17:187–190.
87. Aouad MT, Moussa AR, Dagher CM, et al. Addition of ketamine to propofol for initiation of procedural anesthesia in children reduces propofol consumption and preserves hemodynamic stability. *Acta Anaesthesiol Scand.* 2008;52:561–565.
88. Erden IA, Pamuk AG, Akinci SB, et al. Comparison of two ketamine-propofol dosing regimens for sedation during interventional radiology procedures. *Minerva Anestesiol.* 2010;76:260–265.
89. Phillips W, Anderson A, Rosengreen M, et al. Propofol versus propofol/ketamine for brief painful procedures in the emergency department: Clinical and bispectral index scale comparison. *J Pain Palliat Care Pharmacother.* 2010;24:349–355.
90. Nagdeve NG, Yaddanapudi S, Pandav SS. The effect of different doses of ketamine on intraocular pressure in anesthetized children. *J Pediatr Ophthalmol Strabismus.* 2006;43:219–223.
91. Hsu Y-W, Cortinez LI, Robertson KM, et al. Dexmedetomidine pharmacodynamics: part I: Crossover comparison of the respiratory effects of dexmedetomidine and remifentanil in healthy volunteers. *Anesthesiology.* 2004;101:1066–1076.
92. Shukry M, Miller JA. Update on dexmedetomidine: Use in nonintubated patients requiring sedation for surgical procedures. *Ther Clin Risk Manag.* 2010;6:111–121.
93. Ebert TJ, Hall JE, Barney JA, et al. The effects of increasing plasma concentrations of dexmedetomidine in humans. *Anesthesiology.* 2000;93:382–394.
94. Mahmoud M, Gunter J, Donnelly LF. A comparison of dexmedetomidine with propofol for magnetic resonance imaging sleep studies in children. *Anesth Analg.* 2009;109:745–753.
95. Ho AM-H, Chen S, Karmakar MK. Central apnoea after balanced general anaesthesia that included dexmedetomidine. *Br J Anaesth.* 2005;95:773–775.
96. Ramsay MA, Luterman DL. Dexmedetomidine as a total intravenous anesthetic agent. *Anesthesiology.* 2004;101:787–790.
97. Jooste EH, Ohkawa S, Sun LS. Fiberoptic intubation with dexmedetomidine in two children with spinal cord impingements. *Anesth Analg.* 2005;101:1248.
98. Maroof M, Khan R, Jain D, et al. Dexmedetomidine is a useful adjunct for awake intubation. *Can J Anaesth.* 2005;52:776–777.
99. Stamenkovic DM, Hassid M. Dexmedetomidine for fiberoptic intubation of a patient with severe mental retardation and atlantoaxial instability. *Acta Anaesthesiol Scand.* 2006;50:1314–1315.
100. Abdelmalak B, Makary L, Hoban J, et al. Dexmedetomidine as sole sedative for awake intubation in management of the critical airway. *J Clin Anesth.* 2007;19:370–373.
101. Videira RLR, Ferreira RMV. Dexmedetomidine and asystole. *Anesthesiology.* 2004;101:1479.
102. Ingersoll-Weng E, Manecke GRJ, Thistlethwaite PA. Dexmedetomidine and cardiac arrest. *Anesthesiology.* 2004;100:738–739.
103. Talke P, Richardson CA, Scheinin M, et al. Postoperative pharmacokinetics and sympatholytic effects of dexmedetomidine. *Anesth Analg.* 1997;85:1136–1142.
104. Bekker AY, Kaufman B, Samir H, et al. The use of dexmedetomidine infusion for awake craniotomy. *Anesth Analg.* 2001;92:1251–1253.
105. Ard J, Doyle W, Bekker A. Awake craniotomy with dexmedetomidine in pediatric patients. *J Neurosurg Anesthesiol.* 2003;15:263–266.
106. Bekker AY, Basile J, Gold M, et al. Dexmedetomidine for awake carotid endarterectomy: Efficacy, hemodynamic profile, and side effects. *J Neurosurg Anesthesiol.* 2004;16:126–135.
107. Drummond JC, Dao AV, Roth DM, et al. Effect of dexmedetomidine on cerebral blood flow velocity, cerebral metabolic rate, and carbon dioxide response in normal humans. *Anesthesiology.* 2008;108:225–232.
108. Bekker A, Gold M, Ahmed R, et al. Dexmedetomidine does not increase the incidence of intracarotid shunting in patients undergoing awake carotid endarterectomy. *Anesth Analg.* 2006;103:955–958.
109. Arain SR, Ebert TJ. The efficacy, side effects, and recovery characteristics of dexmedetomidine versus propofol when used for intraoperative sedation. *Anesth Analg.* 2002;95:461–466.
110. Mason KP, Zgleszewski SE, Prescilla R, et al. Hemodynamic effects of dexmedetomidine sedation for CT imaging studies. *Paediatr Anaesth.* 2008;18:393–402.
111. Mason KP, Zurakowski D, Zgleszewski SE, et al. High dose dexmedetomidine as the sole sedative for pediatric MRI. *Paediatr Anaesth.* 2008;18:403–411.
112. Veselis RA, Reinsel RA, Feshchenko VA, et al. Information loss over time defines the memory defect of propofol: A comparative response with thiopental and dexmedetomidine. *Anesthesiology.* 2004;101:831–841.
113. Robert AV. Memory: A guide for anaesthetists. *Best Pract Res Clin Anaesthesiol.* 2007;21:297–312.
114. Veselis RA, Reinsel RA, Feshchenko VA, et al. The comparative amnestic effects of midazolam, propofol, thiopental, and fentanyl at equisedative concentrations. *Anesthesiology.* 1997;87:749–764.
115. Perry F, Parker RK, White PF, et al. Role of psychological factors in postoperative pain control and recovery with patient-controlled analgesia. *Clin J Pain.* 1994;10:57–63; discussion 82–85.
116. Rudkin GE, Osborne GA, Finn BP, et al. Intra-operative patient-controlled sedation. *Anaesthesia.* 1992;47:376–381.
117. Park WY, Watkins PA. Patient-controlled sedation during epidural anesthesia. *Anesth Analg.* 1991;72:304–307.
118. Zelcer J, White PF, Chester S, et al. Intraoperative patient-controlled analgesia. *Anesth Analg.* 1992;75:41–44.
119. Bhananker SM, Posner KL, Cheney FW, et al. Injury and liability associated with monitored anesthesia care. *Anesthesiology.* 2006;104:228–234.
120. Hug CC. MAC should stand for maximum anesthesia caution not minimal anesthesia care. *Anesthesiology.* 2006;104:221–223.
121. Morel DR, Forster A, Bachmann M, et al. Effect of intravenous midazolam on breathing pattern and chest wall mechanics in human. *J Appl Physiol.* 1984;57:1104–1110.
122. Prato F, Knill R. Diazepam sedation reduces functional residual capacity and alters the distribution of ventilation in man. *Can J Anaesth.* 1983;30:493–500.
123. Cohen M. Phrenic and recurrent laryngeal discharge patterns and the Hering-Breuer reflex. *Am J Physiol.* 1975;228:1489–1496.

124. Gottfried SB, Strohl KP, Van de Graaff W, et al. Effects of phrenic stimulation on upper airway resistance in anesthetized dogs. *J Appl Physiol*. 1983;55: 419–426.
125. Leiter JC, Knuth SL, Krol RC, et al. The effect of diazepam on genioglossal muscle activity in normal human subjects. *Am Rev Respir Dis*. 1985;132:216–219.
126. Montravers P, Dureuil B, Desmonts JM. Effects of I.V. midazolam on upper airway resistance. *Br J Anaesth*. 1992;68:27–31.
127. Rimaniol JM, D'Honneur G, Duvaldestin P. Recovery of the swallowing reflex after propofol anesthesia. *Anesth Analg*. 1994;79:856–859.
128. Groves ND, Rees JL, Rosen M. Effects of benzodiazepines on laryngeal reflexes. *Anaesthesia*. 1987;42:808–814.
129. Lambert Y, D'Honneur G, Abhay K, et al. Depression of swallowing reflex two hours after midazolam. *Anesthesiology*. 1991;75:A891.
130. Nishino T, Takizawa K, Yokokawa N, et al. Depression of the swallowing reflex during sedation and/or relative analgesia produced by inhalation of 50% nitrous oxide in oxygen. *Anesthesiology*. 1987;67:995–998.
131. Sundman E, Witt H, Sandin R, et al. Pharyngeal function and airway protection during subhypnotic concentrations of propofol, isoflurane, and sevoflurane. *Anesthesiology*. 2001;95:1125–1132.
132. Cooper G, Kou TD, Rex DK. Complications following colonoscopy with anesthesiology assistance. *JAMA*. 2013;173:551–556.
133. Caplan RA, Ward RJ, Posner K, et al. Unexpected cardiac arrest during spinal anesthesia: A closed claims analysis of predisposing factors. *Anesthesiology*. 1988;68:5–11.
134. Weil JV, McCullough RE, Kline JS, et al. Diminished ventilatory response to hypoxia and hypercapnia after morphine in normal man. *N Engl J Med*. 1975;292:1103–1106.
135. Santiago TV, Johnson J, Riley DJ, et al. Effects of morphine on ventilatory response to exercise. *J Appl Physiol*. 1979;47:112–118.
136. Rigg JRA. Ventilatory effects and plasma concentration of morphine in man. *Br J Anaesth*. 1978;50:759–765.
137. Pattinson KTS. Opioids and the control of respiration. *Br J Anaesth*. 2008; 100:747–758.
138. Power SJ, Morgan M, Chakrabarti MK. Carbon dioxide response curves following midazolam and diazepam. *Br J Anaesth*. 1983;55:837–842.
139. Alexander CM, Gross JB. Sedative doses of midazolam depress hypoxic ventilatory responses in humans. *Anesth Analg*. 1988;67:377–382.
140. Jordan C, Lehane JR, Jones JG. Respiratory depression following diazepam: Reversal with high-dose naloxone. *Anesthesiology*. 1980;53:293–298.
141. Yaster M, Nichols DG, Deshpande JK, et al. Midazolam-fentanyl intravenous sedation in children: Case report of respiratory arrest. *Pediatrics*. 1990;86: 463–467.
142. White JM, Irvine RJ. Mechanisms of fatal opioid overdose. *Addiction*. 1999;94: 961–972.
143. Deitch K, Chudnofsky CR, Dominici P. The utility of supplemental oxygen during emergency department procedural sedation and analgesia with midazolam and fentanyl: A randomized, controlled trial. *Ann Emerg Med*. 2007;49:1–8.
144. Deitch K, Chudnofsky CR, Dominici P. The utility of supplemental oxygen during emergency department procedural sedation with propofol: A randomized, controlled trial. *Ann Emerg Med*. 2008;52:1–8.
145. Metzner J, Posner KL, Domino KB. The risk and safety of anesthesia at remote locations: The US closed claims analysis. *Curr Opin Anaesthesiol*. 2009;22: 502–508.
146. American Society of Anesthesiologists. Standards for basic anesthesia monitoring. www.asahq.org 2011.
147. KK BST. *Pulse Oximetry, Anesthetic Equipment: Principles and Applications*. St. Louis: Mosby; 1993:249.
148. Moller JT, Johannessen NW, Berg H, et al. Hypoxaemia during anaesthesia—an observer study. *Br J Anaesth*. 1991;66:437–444.
149. Motoyama EK, Glazener CH. Hypoxemia after general anesthesia in children. *Anesth Analg*. 1986;65:267–272.
150. Xue FS, Li BW, Zhang GS, et al. The influence of surgical sites on early postoperative hypoxemia in adults undergoing elective surgery. *Anesth Analg*. 1999;88:213–219.
151. Lightdale JR, Goldmann DA, Feldman HA, et al. Microstream capnography improves patient monitoring during moderate sedation: A randomized, controlled trial. *Pediatrics*. 2006;117:e1170–e1178.
152. Bowe EA, Boysen PG, Broome JA, et al. Accurate determination of end-tidal carbon dioxide during administration of oxygen by nasal cannulae. *J Clin Monit Comput*. 1988;5:105–110.
153. Pressman MA. A simple method of measuring ETCO2 during MAC and major regional anesthesia. *Anesth Analg*. 1988;67:905–906.
154. Soto RG, Fu ES, Vila H, et al. Capnography accurately detects apnea during monitored anesthesia care. *Anesth Analg*. 2004;99:379–382.
155. Vargo JJ, Zuccaro G Jr, Dumot JA, et al. Automated graphic assessment of respiratory activity is superior to pulse oximetry and visual assessment for the detection of early respiratory depression during therapeutic upper endoscopy. *Gastrointest Endosc*. 2002;55:826–831.
156. Waugh JB, Epps CA, Khodneva YA. Capnography enhances surveillance of respiratory events during procedural sedation: A meta-analysis. *J Clin Anesth*. 2011;23:189–196.
157. Kurz A, Kurz M, Poeschl G, et al. Forced-air warming maintains intraoperative normothermia better than circulating-water mattresses. *Anesth Analg*. 1993; 77:89–95.
158. Hynson JM, Sessler DI. Intraoperative warming therapies: A comparison of three devices. *J Clin Anesth*. 1992;4:194–199.
159. Kurz A, Sessler DI, Lenhardt R. Perioperative normothermia to reduce the incidence of surgical-wound infection and shorten hospitalization. *N Engl J Med*. 1996;334:1209–1216.
160. Sessler DI. Complications and treatment of mild hypothermia. *Anesthesiology*. 2001;95:531–543.
161. Frank SM, Fleisher LA, Breslow MJ, et al. Perioperative maintenance of normothermia reduces the incidence of morbid cardiac events. *JAMA*. 1997;277: 1127–1134.
162. Frank SM, Higgins MS, Breslow MJ, et al. The catecholamine, cortisol, and hemodynamic responses to mild perioperative hypothermia: A randomized clinical trial. *Anesthesiology*. 1995;82:83–93.
163. Schmied H, Reiter A, Kurz A, et al. Mild hypothermia increases blood loss and transfusion requirements during total hip arthroplasty. *Lancet*. 1996;347: 289–292.
164. Lenhardt R, Marker E, Goll V, et al. Mild intraoperative hypothermia prolongs postanesthetic recovery. *Anesthesiology*. 1997;87:1318–1323.
165. Arkiliç CF, Akça O, Taguchi A, et al. Temperature monitoring and management during neuraxial anesthesia: An observational study. *Anesth Analg*. 2000;91:662–666.
166. Frank SM, Nguyen JM, Garcia CM, et al. Temperature monitoring practices during regional anesthesia. *Anesth Analg*. 1999;88:373.
167. Scholefield JH, Gerber MA, Dwyer P. Liquid crystal forehead temperature strips: A clinical appraisal. *Am J Dis Child*. 1982;136:198–201.
168. Sessler DI. Temperature monitoring and management during neuraxial anesthesia. *Anesth Analg*. 1999;88:243.
169. Chernik DA, Gillings D, Laine H, et al. Validity and reliability of the observer's assessment of alertness/sedation scale: Study with intravenous midazolam. *J Clin Psychopharmacol*. 1990;10:244–251.
170. American Society of Anesthesiologists. Continuum of depth of sedation, definition of general anesthesia and levels of sedation/analgesia. www.asahq.org 2014.
171. Kearse LA, Manberg P, Chamoun N, et al. Bispectral analysis of the electroencephalogram correlates with patient movement to skin incision during propofol/nitrous oxide anesthesia. *Anesthesiology*. 1994;81:1365–1370.
172. Liu J, Singh H, White PF. Electroencephalographic bispectral index correlates with intraoperative recall and depth of propofol-induced sedation. *Anesth Analg*. 1997;84:185–189.
173. American Society of Anesthesiologists. Statement on granting privileges for administration of moderate sedation to practitioners who are not anesthesia professionals. www.asahq.org 2011.
174. American Society of Anesthesiologists. Advisory for granting privileges for administration of moderate sedation to practitioners who are not anesthesia professionals. www.asahq.org 2010.
175. Centers for Medicare and Medicaid Services. Revised hospital anesthesia interpretive guidelines. www.asahq.org 2011.
176. American Society of Anesthesiologists. Statement of the safe use of propofol. www.asahq.org 2009.
177. American Society for Gastrointestinal Endoscopy. "Position Statement: Non-anesthesiologist administration of propofol for GI endoscopy." *Gastrointest Endosc*. 2009;70(6):1053–1059.
178. Pambianco DJ, Vargo JJ, Pruitt RE, et al. Computer-assisted personalized sedation for upper endoscopy and colonoscopy: a comparative, multicenter randomized study. *Gastrointest Endosc*. 2011;73(4):765–772.
179. Ethicon Endo-Surgery, Inc. Computer-Assisted Personalized Sedation System: Clinical User Guide/Operator's Manual, Cincinnati: pp. 1-17, 2-1, 2-2. *Retrieved from*: http://www.accessdata.fda.gov/cdrh_docs/pdf8/P080009c.pdf.
180. www.aqihq.org/files/Procedural-Sedation-Metrics.docx. Accessed May 23, 2016.

31 Ambulatory Anesthesia

J. LANCE LICHTOR • PETER MANCINI

Place, Procedures, and Patient Selection
Preoperative Screening
   Upper Respiratory Tract Infection
   Restriction of Food and Liquids Prior to Ambulatory Surgery
   Anxiety Reduction
Managing the Anesthetic: Premedication
   Benzodiazepines
   Opioids and Nonsteroidal Analgesics
Intraoperative Management: Choice of Anesthetic Method
   Regional Techniques
   Spinal Anesthesia

Epidural and Caudal Anesthesia
Nerve Blocks
Sedation and Analgesia
General Anesthesia
Management of Postanesthesia Care
   Reversal of Drug Effects
   Nausea and Vomiting
   Pain
   Preparation for Discharging the Patient
Acknowledgments

KEY POINTS

1. Procedures appropriate for ambulatory surgery are those associated with low rates of postoperative complications that do not require intensive physician or nursing management.
2. Medically stable ASA physical status III or IV patients may be appropriate candidates for ambulatory surgical procedures.
3. ASA, Society for Ambulatory Anesthesia, and American College of Chest Physicians agree that a procedure typically performed as an ambulatory procedure with local or regional anesthesia can also be performed as an ambulatory procedure in patients with obstructive sleep apnea (OSA).
4. Airflow obstruction in adults may persist for up to 6 weeks after viral infections. For that reason, many agree that surgery should be delayed for 6 weeks. For children, whether surgery should be delayed for that length of time is questionable.
5. The most recent ASA revised practice guidelines for preoperative fasting was published in 2011. The guidelines allow a light meal up to 6 hours before an elective procedure and support a fasting period for clear liquids of 2 hours for all patients.
6. Most premedicants do not prolong recovery when given in appropriate doses for appropriate indications, although drug effects may be apparent even after discharge.
7. Regional and general anesthesia in the ambulatory setting are equally safe. However, even for experienced anesthesiologists, there is a failure rate associated with regional anesthesia.
8. Nerve blocks improve postoperative patient satisfaction and decrease postoperative nausea and vomiting (PONV) and postoperative pain.
9. Two primary concerns for ambulatory anesthesia are speed of wake-up and incidence of PONV.
10. It is important to distinguish between wake-up time and discharge time. Patients may emerge from anesthesia with desflurane and nitrous oxide significantly faster than after propofol or sevoflurane and nitrous oxide, though the ability to sit up, stand, and tolerate fluids and the time to fitness for discharge may be no different.
11. Nausea, with or without vomiting, is probably the most important factor contributing to a delay in discharge and an increase in unanticipated admissions after ambulatory surgery.
12. In addition to the postanesthesia care unit (PACU), most ambulatory surgery centers (ASCs) in the United States have Phase II Recovery, which may be located within or separate from the PACU. Patients remain in Phase II Recovery until they are able to tolerate liquids, walk, and (depending on the operation) void.

Ambulatory anesthesia for ambulatory surgery may seem to be a recent phenomenon, although it has been around for over 100 years. The Society for Ambulatory Anesthesia (SAMBA) in the United States and the British Association of Day Surgery roughly 30 years ago helped to bring together those who practice ambulatory anesthesia to provide education and stimulate research. The International Association for Ambulatory Surgery (http://www.iaas-med.com) was formed in 1995, is designed to promote worldwide development of ambulatory surgery, has a peer reviewed journal, *Ambulatory Surgery*, and currently has members from 18 nations.

The U.S. National Library of Medicine (USNLM) defines the term "ambulatory surgical procedure" as "Surgery performed on an outpatient basis. It may be hospital-based or performed in an office or surgicenter." USNLM groups office-based and ambulatory surgery together. Hospital-based ASCs in the United States and Canada can receive accreditation through The Joint Commission (TJC), DNV-GL, and Healthcare Facilities Accreditation Program (HFAP). In the United States, they can be accredited through a state survey agency or the Centers for Medicare and Medicaid Services. Freestanding US ASCs and offices receive accreditation through the Accreditation Association for Ambulatory Health

Care, Inc., The American Association for Accreditation of Ambulatory Surgery Facilities, Inc., or TJC.

Place, Procedures, and Patient Selection

Place: Ambulatory surgery occurs in a variety of settings. Some centers are within a hospital or in a freestanding satellite facility affiliated with or independent from a hospital. The independent facilities are often for-profit and not located in rural or inner-city areas. Some private companies acquire or build ambulatory facilities and then work with local surgeons who become the company's affiliated staff. Procedures might also be performed in a physician's office (see also Chapter 32). Freestanding, independent facilities continue to grow in number and popularity, although some consumers prefer care in units affiliated with hospitals or health-care systems.

A major concern of freestanding ambulatory surgery growth is that the surgery centers may force some hospitals out of business. This issue can be particularly problematic in areas in which population density or median income are low. Freestanding ambulatory facilities usually do not provide charity or government-subsidized care. Some surgeons may work exclusively in a freestanding facility and not be on the staff of a hospital since a requirement for hospital staff privileges frequently is that a physician provides coverage for the hospital's emergency department. Some hospitals have lost emergency department coverage for an entire surgical specialty because that surgical specialty works exclusively in a freestanding facility.

Costs are lower for ASCs. Scheduling can be more predictable because the variety of cases is low. Turnaround times are also usually lower. The profits, particularly for freestanding facilities, do not have to subsidize more costly areas of the hospital. Yet some hospitals own ASCs. ASCs also tend to serve mostly insured patients. Medicare pays ASCs at a lower percent than what they pay hospitals for the same procedure. Medicare can then save money, though the payment system may force some ambulatory facilities to decide whether they accept Medicare patients.

Procedures: What case is appropriate for an ambulatory surgical procedure? Some centers use maximum duration of surgery time, for example, 4 hours, as a criterion for allowing a procedure to take place in an ambulatory care facility. Others consider an ambulatory procedure as one that does not pose a significant safety risk or require an overnight stay. Generally, procedures appropriate for ambulatory surgery are those associated with postoperative care that is easily managed at home, have low rates of postoperative complications, and do not require intensive physician or nursing management. Establishing a low rate of postoperative complication depends on the relative aggressiveness of the facility, surgeon, patient, and payer. For example, procedures that postoperatively result in intense pain may be treated with continuous regional techniques that are continued at home, whereas in other settings, the same procedures are limited to inpatients. Quite a bit of variability exits between facilities concerning rates of postoperative complications after ambulatory surgery (Fig. 31-1).[1]

Patients undergoing longer procedures should have their operations earlier in the day, primarily because resources are more efficiently managed during regular working hours. The need for transfusion is also not a contraindication for ambulatory procedures. Some patients undergoing outpatient liposuction, for example, receive autologous blood. Because of blood bank proximity, procedures that require the use of a blood bank are more commonly performed in larger facilities. Freestanding dialysis facilities commonly receive blood shipped from a blood bank located elsewhere and the same can be set up with freestanding ambulatory surgery facilities. The key is to have proper procedures established.

Some have questioned the safety of office-based procedures, in part because of reports of deaths in Florida (see also Chapter 32). A 2012 analysis revealed 46 deaths and 263 procedure-related complications and hospital transfers in Florida, and 3 deaths and 49 complications or hospital transfers in Alabama over several years.[2] An accompanying editorial notes that liposuction on awake patients using tumescent local anesthesia is safe; however, liposuction performed in conjunction with abdominoplasty under general anesthesia is problematic and should be avoided.[3]

Patient selection: Age is an important consideration in patient selection. Term infants whose postconceptual age is less than

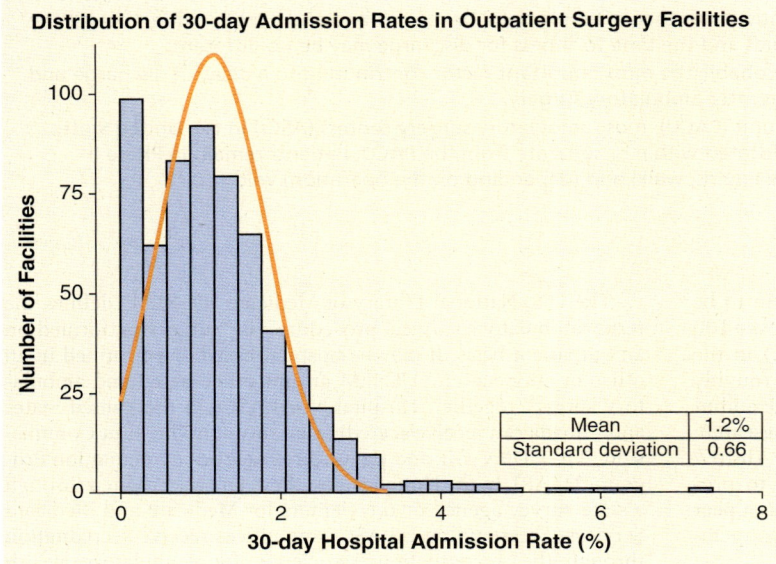

Figure 31-1 Admission rates after ambulatory surgery among 635 California outpatient surgery facilities, studied between 2005 and 2015. On average, 30-day admission rate was 1.2%; 18 facilities were statistically significant outliers; and 79 facilities had no patients that needed hospital admission. (Adapted with permission from Parina R, Chang D, Saad AN, et al. Quality and safety outcomes of ambulatory plastic surgery facilities in California. *Plast Reconstr Surg.* 2015;135:791–797.)

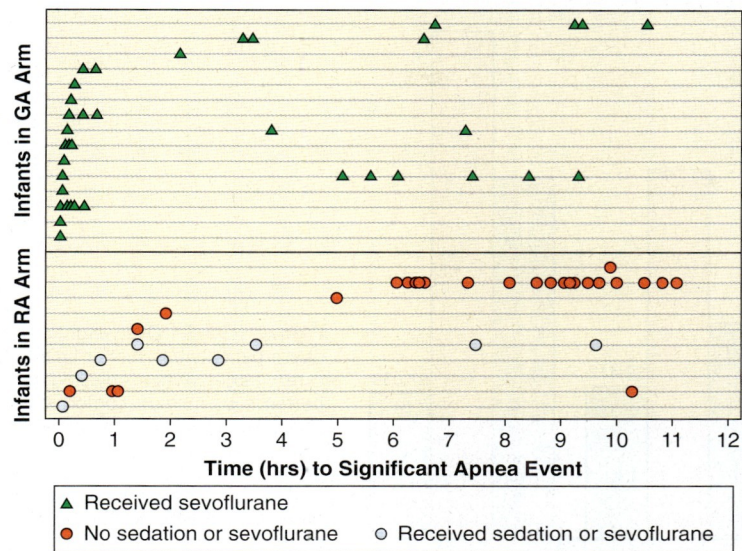

Figure 31-2 Apnea after regional and general anesthesia in infants. Regional anesthesia (RA) group further divided into those who received only regional anesthesia without sedation or general anesthesia (*closed circles*) and those who received spinal anesthesia and sedation or general anesthesia (*closed squares*). (Adapted with permission from Davidson AJ, Morton NS, Arnup SJ, et al. General anesthesia compared to spinal anesthesia (GAS) consortium: apnea after awake regional and general anesthesia in infants: the general anesthesia compared to spinal anesthesia study-comparing apnea and neurodevelopmental outcomes, a randomized controlled trial. *Anesthesiology*. 2015. Copyright © 2015, Wolters Kluwer Health.)

46 weeks, or preterm infants whose postconceptual age (PCA) is less than 60 weeks should be monitored for 12 hours after their procedure. They are at risk of developing postoperative apnea even without a history of apnea (Fig. 31-2; Table 31-1).[4] In one series of over 700 patients who underwent inguinal hernia surgery, the overall incidence of postoperative apnea was 6.1% in prematurely born infants and 0.3% in full-term infants. There was no difference in the incidence of apnea in patients who received either regional or general anesthesia.[4] However, the incidence and severity of apnea, 0 to 30 minutes in the postanesthesia care unit (PACU), was less in those infants who received regional anesthesia. Two infants in that study experienced apnea 6 to 7 hours after their procedures; they were 29 weeks of gestation and 43 weeks PCA, and 30 weeks of gestation and 42 weeks PCA.

At the other extreme of life, advanced age alone is not a reason to disallow surgery in an ambulatory setting. In a study of over 500 patients, postoperative outcome was no different when patients 65 years and older undergoing inguinal hernia repair were compared to patients less than 54 years old.[5] Based on another series, older patients had less chronic post herniorrhaphy pain.[6] Increasing age, however, does affect the pharmacokinetics of drugs (see also Chapter 11). Even short-acting drugs such as midazolam and propofol have decreased clearance in older individuals. Increased age may increase the likelihood of unanticipated admission, but, by itself, does not contraindicate ambulatory surgery.

Hospital admission is not necessarily a failure if it results in a better quality of care. With proper patient selection for typically elective ambulatory procedures, the incidence of hospital admission should be very low. Most medical problems that older individuals experience after ambulatory procedures are not related to patient age, but to specific organ dysfunction. For that reason, all individuals, whether young or old, should receive a careful preoperative history and physical examination.

Patients of ASA physical status III or IV are appropriate candidates for some ambulatory surgical procedures if their systemic diseases are medically stable. In a review of over 10,000 patients who underwent ambulatory orthopedic surgical procedures between June 1993 and June 2012, no major complications were reported. Of the 14 patients who needed overnight admission, the majority were ASA III.[7] That very low rate of major complications resulted from selecting patients whose medical problems were well controlled.

Obese patients represent a special situation. Obese patients are more likely to have adverse outcomes, and they have a higher incidence of obstructive sleep apnea (OSA). One review of over 47,000 discharges from almost 1,000 ASCs for patients undergoing outpatient blepharoplasty, abdominoplasty, breast reduction, and liposuction included 4.3% who were obese. The obese patients more often had at least one hospital-based, acute care encounter within 30 days of discharge and because of that had higher health-care charges (Fig. 31-3).[8] In a meta-analysis of patients undergoing nonupper airway surgery, patients with or at high risk of OSA were more prone to adverse perioperative outcomes including respiratory, cardiac, and neurologic complications, and unplanned ICU transfer. Further, patients with sleep apnea had higher risk of hypoxemia postoperatively.[9] Some feel that patients with OSA who need more opioids may be at greater risk for apnea and should be observed for a longer period after their procedure. The ASA, SAMBA, and American College

Table 31-1 Guide to Determine Length of Stay for Infants after Surgery

Born (Weeks Postconception)	Age at Time of Surgery (Weeks Postconception)	Other Factors	Disposition
<37	<60		Admit overnight
>36	<46		Admit overnight
	<60	Still in PACU @ 9 PM	Admit overnight

PACU, postanesthesia care unit

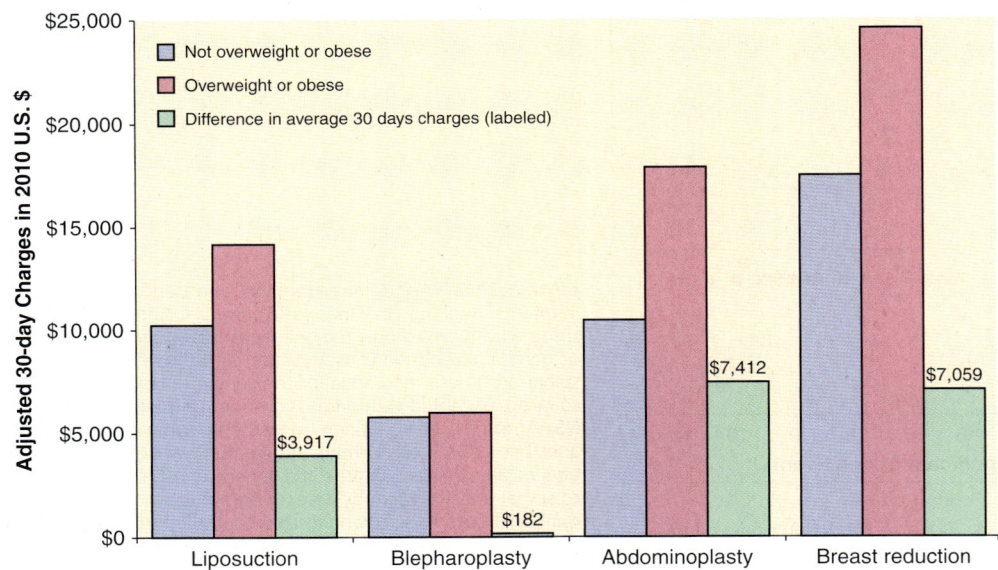

Figure 31-3 Overweight or obese patients had higher healthcare charges, when adjusted for presence of medical comorbidity. (Adapted with permission from Sieffert MR, Fox JP, Abbott LE, et al. Obesity is associated with increased health care charges in patients undergoing outpatient plastic surgery. *Plast Reconstr Surg.* 2015;135:1396–1404.)

of Chest Physicians published practice guidelines for the perioperative management of patients with OSA.[10–12] For patients with OSA, if a procedure is typically performed as an outpatient procedure and local or regional anesthesia is used, the procedure can also be performed as an ambulatory procedure. Conversely, those patients with OSA who are undergoing major surgery, or who are undergoing a procedure with an increased risk for perioperative complications, should not have their procedure performed as an ambulatory procedure (Table 31-2).

Patients who undergo ambulatory surgery should have an adult take them home and stay with them afterward until the next morning to provide care. Before the procedure, the patient should receive information about the procedure, where it will be performed, laboratory studies that will be ordered, and dietary

Table 31-2 An Example of a Scoring System That Can Be Used to Determine Whether a Patient Is at Increased Risk for Complications due to OSA

	Points
A. Severity of sleep apnea based on a sleep study or clinical indicators:	
None	0
Mild	1
Moderate	2
Severe	3
Mild or moderate OSA (obstructive sleep apnea) has resting $PaCO_2$ > 50 mmHg	1
Uses CPAP (continuous positive airway pressure) or NIPPV (noninvasive positive pressure ventilation) before surgery and will continue the appliance consistently postoperatively	−1
B. Invasiveness of surgery and type of anesthesia:	
Superficial surgery, local or peripheral block, no sedation	0
Superficial surgery with moderate sedation or general anesthesia	1
Peripheral surgery, spinal or epidural anesthesia, at most moderate sedation	1
Peripheral surgery with general anesthesia	2
Airway surgery with moderate sedation	2
Major surgery, general anesthesia	3
Airway surgery, general anesthesia	3
C. Postoperative opioid requirement:	
None	0
Low-dose oral opioids	1
High-dose oral opioids, parenteral or neuraxial opioid	3

Perioperative risk: A plus (B or C, whichever greater).
Score = 4: increased perioperative risk from OSA
Score = 5: significantly increased perioperative risk from OSA
Reprinted with permission from American Society of Anesthesiologists Task Force on Perioperative Management of patients with obstructive sleep apnea. Practice guidelines for the perioperative management of patients with obstructive sleep apnea: an updated report by the American Society of Anesthesiologists Task Force on Perioperative Management of patients with obstructive sleep apnea. *Anesthesiology.* 2014;120:268–286. Copyright © 2014, Wolters Kluwer Health.

restrictions. The patient must understand before the procedure that an overnight stay is not intended. The patient, or some responsible person, must ensure all instructions are followed. Once at home, the patient must be able to tolerate the pain from the procedure, assuming adequate pain therapy is provided. The majority of patients are satisfied with early discharge, although a few prefer a longer stay in the facility. Patients for certain procedures such as laparoscopic cholecystectomy or transurethral resection of the prostate should live close to the ambulatory facility because postoperative complications may require their prompt return. "Reasonable" distance and time for the patient to get care if problems arise are not easily defined. This issue must be addressed by each facility for individual patients based on the planned procedure.

Preoperative Screening

Each outpatient facility should develop its own method of preoperative screening. The patient may visit the facility, or the staff members may telephone to obtain necessary information about the patient, including a complete medical history of the patient and family, the medications the patient is taking, and the problems the patient or the patient's family may have had with previous anesthetics. At some facilities, experienced nurses make those telephone calls. Regardless of who performs screening, screened patients are less likely to cancel surgery.[13] Screening may uncover the need for transportation to the facility or the need for childcare. The process also provides the staff with an opportunity to remind patients of arrival time, suitable attire, and dietary restrictions (e.g., when to stop eating and drinking, no jewelry or makeup). Staff members can determine whether a responsible person is available to escort the patient to and from the facility and care for the patient at home after surgery. The screening is the ideal time for the anesthesiologist to talk to the patient, but if that is not possible, the anesthesiologist may review the screening record to determine whether additional evaluation by other consultants is necessary and whether laboratory tests are needed.

Upper Respiratory Tract Infection

Following viral upper respiratory infections (URIs) in adults, airflow obstruction persists for up to 6 weeks. For that reason, many agree that surgery should be delayed if an adult presents with an URI until 6 weeks have elapsed. In the case of children, whether surgery should be delayed for that length of time is questionable. In a year-long survey of almost 10,000 children who underwent surgery, URI was associated with an increased risk for perioperative respiratory adverse events only when symptoms were present or had occurred within the 2 weeks before the procedure.[14] This Swiss study included children who were febrile or who had mucopurulent airway secretions and nevertheless had surgery. Of interest, children with these symptoms in the United States would have had their operations cancelled. Although a case may be cancelled because a child is symptomatic, the child may develop another URI when the procedure is rescheduled. Independent risk factors for adverse respiratory events in children with URIs include use of an endotracheal tube (vs. use of a laryngeal mask airway [LMA] or face mask), history of prematurity, history of reactive airway disease, history of parental smoking, surgery involving the airway, presence of copious secretions, and nasal congestion. Generally, if a patient with a URI has a normal appetite, does not have a fever or an elevated respiratory rate, and does not appear toxic, it is probably safe to proceed with the planned procedure.

Restriction of Food and Liquids Prior to Ambulatory Surgery

To decrease the risk of aspiration of gastric contents, we routinely ask patients not to eat or drink anything (*non per os* [NPO] or "nothing by mouth") for at least 6 to 8 hours before surgery. Prolonged fasting could be detrimental to a patient. Yet, hydration, as measured by urine osmolality, does not correlate with intraoperative hypotension.[15] In children, there is no correlation between hunger, thirst, and gastric volume; nor do hunger and thirst correlate with duration of fasting.[16] Shorter fasting times are correlated with increased patient satisfaction.[17] The most recent ASA revised practice guidelines for preoperative fasting were published in 2011 (Table 31-3).[18] The guidelines allow a patient to eat a nonfat meal up to 6 hours before an elective procedure and support a fasting period for clear liquids of 2 hours for all patients. Coffee and tea are considered clear liquids. Coffee and tea drinkers should follow fasting guidelines but should be encouraged to drink coffee prior to their procedure because physical signs of caffeine withdrawal (headache) can occur. It is not clear if the more liberal NPO guidelines should apply to patients with diabetes or dyspepsia. There is some evidence that shorter periods of preoperative fasting are accompanied by less postoperative nausea and vomiting (PONV).

To ensure patients are optimally medically managed before their outpatient surgery, patients should have clear instructions concerning what chronic medications they should take before surgery and when (Table 31-4).

Anxiety Reduction

Most patients are anxious before scheduled surgery, and they are probably anxious long before they come to the outpatient area. Anxiety may begin as soon as the surgeon states the

Table 31-3 Fasting Guidelines before Surgery	
Food/Drink	Time to Fast Prior to Surgery (h)
Clear liquids (e.g., water, fruit juices without pulp, carbonated beverages, clear tea, and black coffee)	2
Breast milk	4
Infant formula	6
Nonhuman milk	6
Light meal (toast and clear liquids)	6
Meals that include fried or fatty foods or meat	8

Reprinted with permission from American Society of Anesthesiologists Committee. Practice guidelines for preoperative fasting and the use of pharmacologic agents to reduce the risk of pulmonary aspiration: application to healthy patients undergoing elective procedures: an updated report by the American Society of Anesthesiologists Committee on Standards and Practice Parameters. *Anesthesiology*. 2011;114:495–511. Copyright © 2011, Wolters Kluwer Health.

Table 31-4 A Guide to Medications Appropriate to Take Prior to Surgery

Medications that should be taken on the day of surgery:
β-Blockers
Statins
Antiarrhythmics
Antihypertensives (except ACE I, ARB, diuretics)
Pulmonary inhalers
Pain medications (except NSAIDs)
Antiseizure medications
Hyperthyroid medications

Medications that should be avoided on the day of surgery:
ACE I/ARB (angiotensin-converting-enzyme inhibitor/angiotensin II receptor blockers)—risk of profound hypotension unresponsive to traditional treatments
Diuretics—hypokalemia and dehydration
Anticoagulants/antiplatelet—depending on surgery, surgeon and underlying medical conditions—we leave these decisions up to surgeon and prescribing physician
Oral hypoglycemic agents
Vitamins which affect platelets (vitamin E)
Herbal supplements which may affect bleeding

Nonessential medications that can be continued on the day of surgery:
Hypothyroid medications
Antidepressants

Source: Jill Zafar, Yale University Department of Anesthesiology.

patient needs an operation and may not end even after discharge from the outpatient facility. Reasons for anxiety include concerns about family, worry about pain after the procedure, fear of complications, and lack of social support. Preoperative reassurance from nonanesthesia staff, use of booklets or audiovisual instruction with information about the procedure, or a preoperative visit by the anesthesiologist can all help reduce preoperative anxiety. However, not all outpatients are anxious and whether it is necessary to give every patient a preoperative drug to decrease anxiety is not clear. If in doubt about patient anxiety, ask the patient; do not assume every patient needs a drug to reduce anxiety.

Like adults, children should have some idea of what to expect during a procedure. Certainly some of a child's anxiety before surgery concerns separation from a parent or parents. A child is more likely to demonstrate problematic behavior from the time of separation from parents to induction of anesthesia if the procedure has not been explained preoperatively. Parents and children need to be involved in some preoperative discussions together so that the parents do not transmit their anxiety to the child. If the parents are calm and can effectively manage the physical transfer to a warm and playful anesthesiologist or nurse, premedication is not necessary.

Whether having the parent present during induction reduces a child's anxiety is unclear, though the practice of parental presence during anesthesia induction is widespread. Certain parental behaviors are more helpful than are others. Some parents can become upset when they see their anesthetized child, who appears to be dead, albeit breathing, and with a beating heart. Separation anxiety on the part of the parents is probably no different if the child is awake or asleep.

Managing the Anesthetic: Premedication

The outpatient is not that different from the inpatient undergoing surgery. In both, premedication is useful to control anxiety, postoperative pain, nausea and vomiting, and to reduce the risk of aspiration during induction of anesthesia. Because the outpatient is going home on the day of surgery, the drugs given before anesthesia should not hinder recovery. Most premedicants do not prolong recovery when given in appropriate doses for appropriate indications, although drug effects may be apparent even after discharge.

Benzodiazepines

Midazolam, a benzodiazepine, is currently the drug most commonly used to reduce preoperative anxiety and induce sedation. It can be administered intravenously and orally. In adults, it can be used to control preoperative anxiety and, during a procedure alone or in combination with other drugs, for intravenous sedation. For children, oral midazolam in doses as small as 0.25 mg/kg produces effective sedation and reduces anxiety (Fig. 31-4).[19] With this dose, most children can be effectively separated from their parents after 10 minutes and satisfactory sedation can be maintained for 45 minutes. Some children, particularly younger and more anxious children, even when they receive midazolam 0.5 mg/kg, show signs of distress.[20] Discharge may be delayed when midazolam is given before a short procedure. Oral diazepam is useful to control anxiety in adult patients, either the day before surgery or the day of surgery and before intravenous line insertion.

Sleepiness associated with the effects of anxiolytics may delay or prevent the discharge of patients on the day of surgery, although more frequently patients are admitted because of the effects of the operation. With regard to anesthesia effects, patients more frequently stay in the facility not because they are too sleepy but because they are nauseous. In adults, particularly when midazolam is combined with fentanyl, patients can remain

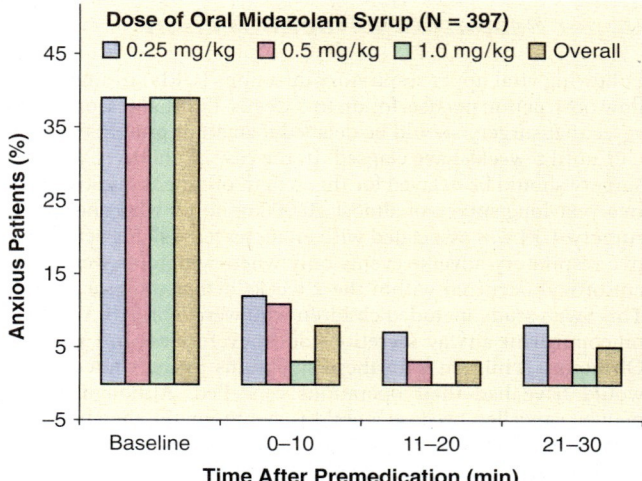

Figure 31-4 The very smallest dose (0.25 mg/kg) of oral midazolam syrup was equally as effective as the two higher doses when commercially prepared oral midazolam syrup was used. Onset was faster with the larger dose. (Adapted with permission from Coté CJ, Cohen IT, Suresh S, et al. A comparison of three doses of a commercially prepared oral midazolam syrup in children. *Anesth Analg.* 2002;94:37–43.)

sleepy for up to 8 hours. Although children may be sleepier after oral midazolam, discharge times are not affected.

At proper doses, neither midazolam nor diazepam place patients at any additional risk for cardiovascular and respiratory depression. Decreased oxygen saturation has been reported after injection of midazolam. Routine administration of supplemental oxygen with or without continuous monitoring of arterial oxygenation is recommended whenever benzodiazepines are given intravenously. This precaution is important not only when midazolam is given as a premedicant but also when it is used alone or with other drugs for conscious sedation. The potential for amnesia after premedication is another concern, especially for patients undergoing ambulatory surgery. Anterograde but probably not retrograde amnesia occurs. For benzodiazepines, the effects on memory are separate from the effects on sedation. In addition, amnesia is not simply an effect of drug administration but, among other factors, it is also a function of stimulus intensity.

Opioids and Nonsteroidal Analgesics

Opioids can be administered preoperatively to sedate patients, control hypertension during tracheal intubation, and decrease pain before surgery. Meperidine (but not morphine or fentanyl) is sometimes helpful in controlling shivering in the OR or the PACU. Treatment for shivering is usually instituted at the time of shivering, not in anticipation of the event. Other drugs, including clonidine, tramadol, and ketamine can also help control shivering.[21]

Opioids are useful in controlling hypertension during tracheal intubation. Opioid premedication prevents increases in systolic pressure in a dose-dependent fashion. After tracheal intubation, systolic, diastolic, and mean arterial blood pressures sometimes decrease below baseline values.

It would seem that preoperative administration of opioids or nonsteroidal anti-inflammatory drugs (NSAIDs) may be useful for controlling pain in the early postoperative period. The term "preventive analgesia" (as opposed to "preemptive analgesia") is used to mean treatment of postoperative pain for a longer duration than the effect of the target drug (e.g., at least 5.5 half-lives of the drug), so that the effect of the drug is more than its analgesic effect.[22,23] The drug then does not necessarily have to be administered before surgery. Laparoscopic cholecystectomy is less painful than open cholecystectomy, though patients undergoing the laparoscopic procedure also have postoperative pain. Based on a Cochrane review, pain is less after NSAIDs plus opioids, and anticonvulsant analgesics, 4 to 8 hours and 9 to 24 hours, respectively after surgery. Anticonvulsant analgesics are more effective than NSAIDs plus opioids though it is unclear if pain control is any different if the drugs are given pre- or intraoperatively.[24] Children undergoing cleft-lip repair who received acetaminophen before surgery had similar pain relief postoperatively as compared to patients who received the acetaminophen intraoperatively.[25] Ibuprofen or acetaminophen can be given orally preoperatively, or administered rectally to children around the time of induction. In children, an initial rectal loading dose of 40 mg/kg is appropriate. When preoperative rectal acetaminophen is combined with an NSAID, particularly for more painful procedures, postoperative pain is less than when either drug is given alone.[26]

Not every patient needs preoperative sedation. However, for those whose anxiety is not relieved by a reassuring preoperative clinic visit, we recommend oral diazepam 2 to 5 mg/70 kg body weight, prescribed for the night before and at 6 AM on the day of surgery (even if surgery is scheduled for 1 PM or later). For patients seen for the first time in the preoperative holding area,

Table 31-5 A Guide to Premedication

A patient is seen least 24 hours before a scheduled procedure, expresses a desire for medication to relieve anxiety or has anxiety that cannot be relieved with comforting: oral diazepam, 2 to 5 mg per 70 kg body weight the night before and at 6 AM on the day of surgery, even if surgery is scheduled for 1 PM or later.

A patient is seen for the first time in the preoperative holding area and seems to need medication: midazolam, 0.01 mg/kg intravenously, or in the OR, propofol, 0.7 mg/kg, intravenously.

For an anxious child, oral midazolam, 0.25 mg/kg, administered in the preoperative holding area.

midazolam 0.01 mg/kg is administered intravenously. For anxious children, oral midazolam, 0.25 mg/kg, can be administered in the preoperative holding area (Table 31-5).

Intraoperative Management: Choice of Anesthetic Method

There are several choices among anesthetic methods: general anesthesia, regional anesthesia, and local anesthesia. Regional and local anesthesia can be used with or without sedation. Except for obstetric cases, for which regional anesthesia may be safer than general anesthesia, all three types are otherwise equally safe. However, even for experienced anesthesiologists, there is a failure rate associated with regional anesthesia.

Certainly, some procedures are possible only with a general anesthetic. For others, the preference of patients, surgeons, or anesthesiologists may determine selection. The cost of sedation is usually less than the cost of a general or regional anesthetic. In one study using New York's ambulatory surgery databases, the authors analyzed patients undergoing inguinal hernia repair. They found that hospital cost was less if open inguinal hernia repair with local/regional anesthesia was used ($6,845) compared to general anesthesia ($7,839) and laparoscopic repair ($11,340).[27] The different types of anesthesia and surgery, though, are not an option for all operations. Another study that compared groin hernia repair after either general, regional, or local infiltration, found that medical complications were more common, particularly in patients of 65+ years after regional versus general anesthesia and urologic complications were more common after regional versus local infiltration.[28] Lower cost may not always accompany improved quality. In a retrospective study, authors compared spinal anesthesia to general anesthesia for patients undergoing hip or knee replacement procedures. They found that hospital treatment costs and length of stay were less for patients who received spinal anesthesia.[29]

The choice of anesthetic method may also influence time to recovery. In a review of peripheral regional anesthesia and outcome, the authors note that outcome studies of peripheral regional analgesia have yet to be published. However, postoperative mobilization and upper limb analgesia are generally better following regional anesthesia.[30] In one retrospective study of patients undergoing ambulatory surgery at a large tertiary center, regional anesthesia use was associated with shorter PACU length of stay compared to general anesthesia; in addition, when regional anesthesia was used in conjunction with general anesthesia, PACU length of stay was shorter than when general anesthesia was used alone.[31] Patients who receive spinal anesthesia for ambulatory surgery may take longer to be discharged if micturition is required, though discharge instructions do not necessarily have to require a patient to micturate prior to discharge. Generally, pain and PONV are greater after general anesthesia compared to regional anesthesia. When applying studies of regional anesthesia to everyday practice, remember that the studies arise from centers where the authors are experienced in performing regional anesthesia and there are good systems to support the practice. Note also that anesthesiologists who are more experienced performing regional anesthesia are more likely to provide regional anesthesia.

With regional anesthesia or sedation, some of the side effects of general anesthesia can be avoided. Whenever drugs that affect memory are given, patients might complain that they do not remember events that occurred after the procedure. Performing a block may take longer than inducing general anesthesia, and the incidence of failure is higher. However, performing the block beforehand in a preoperative holding area can obviate unnecessary delays that may prompt surgeons to discourage regional anesthetics for their cases despite the evidence that postoperative pain control is best with regional techniques. Surgeons might feel that regional anesthesia is beneficial, but the potential delay in establishing a block and perceived unpredictable success might detract from their enthusiasm for regional anesthesia.

One adverse effect associated with spinal anesthesia is postdural puncture headache, although patients also experience headaches after general anesthesia. The incidence of headache after either technique is similar when smaller spinal needles are used. Patients may experience backache after spinal anesthesia, but sore throat and nausea are higher after general anesthesia than spinal anesthesia.

Regional Techniques

Local anesthesia and regional anesthesia have long been used for ambulatory surgery. As early as 1963, for example, 56% of ambulatory procedures were performed with the use of these techniques.[32] Regional techniques commonly used for ambulatory surgery, in addition to spinal and epidural anesthesia, include local infiltration, brachial plexus and other peripheral nerve blocks, and intravenous regional anesthesia. General anesthesia can also be supplemented with regional nerve blocks.

An occasional patient may experience syncope when the needle for the regional block is inserted. This event is alarming to patient and providers. Needle phobia can be minimized by using oral premedication with benzodiazepines or intravenous sedation before starting the block, monitoring patients during the procedure, and having available atropine and vasopressors.[33] After a regional block, patients may still have a numb extremity (e.g., after a brachial plexus block) but otherwise meet all criteria for discharge. In such instances, the extremity must be well protected (e.g., with a sling for an upper extremity procedure) and patients must be cautioned to protect against injury because they are without normal sensations that would warn them of vulnerability. Reassurance that sensation will return should be provided.

Spinal Anesthesia

Children

Some centers use spinal anesthesia most commonly for ex-premature infants undergoing hernia repair because the risk of postoperative apnea is reduced and because neurodevelopmental outcome is likely less affected by spinal anesthesia compared to general. When planning spinal anesthesia, general anesthesia should be available as a backup because spinal anesthesia failure rates for this population is as high as 20%.[4] The authors found that though apnea in the immediate postoperative period may be lower with spinal anesthesia, it does not reduce the risk of apnea seen up to 12 hours after surgery. Furthermore, premature infants and those who have postoperative apnea within 30 minutes after surgery are more likely to have apnea up to 12 hours after surgery. A bloody tap on the first attempt at lumbar puncture is the only predictor of spinal anesthesia failure.[34] Interestingly, in that study, such factors as experience of the anesthesiologist were not predictive of success.

Adults

Spinal anesthesia is suitable for pelvic, lower abdominal, lower extremity, and even laparoscopic cholecystectomy surgery. Motor block of the legs may delay a patient's ability to walk. However, the use of a short-acting local anesthetic will minimize this problem. Nausea is much less frequent after epidural or spinal anesthesia than after general anesthesia. Though not a comparison of patients receiving general anesthesia, in one Danish study of patients undergoing total hip or knee arthroplasty, more than 85% of patients who received low-dose spinal anesthesia were ready for discharge from the PACU 15 minutes after arrival, and the median PACU stay was 25 minutes.[35]

Different drugs and drug concentrations have been used for spinal anesthesia. Though any intrathecal local anesthetic can cause transient neurologic symptoms, lidocaine use is particularly problematic because of its high association with transient neurologic symptoms. Bupivacaine can be problematic for ambulatory surgical procedures because of its longer duration of action. In one study where spinal anesthesia was compared with either 0.75% hyperbaric bupivacaine 7.5 mg (n = 53) or 2% preservative-free 2-chloroprocaine 40 mg (n = 53), discharge readiness was 76 minutes faster with chloroprocaine.[36]

Although headache is a common complication of lumbar puncture, smaller-gauge needles result in a lower incidence of postdural puncture headache. For those patients who do receive spinal anesthesia, it is incumbent on the anesthesiologist and the facility to have follow-up with telephone calls to ensure no disabling symptoms of headache have developed (see also Chapter 35). If the headache does not respond to bed rest, analgesics, and oral hydration, the patient must return to hospital for a course of intravenous caffeine therapy or an epidural blood patch. Instructions regarding postdural puncture headache should be included in the preoperative consent process.

Spinal anesthesia should not be avoided in ambulatory surgery patients simply because they may be more active postoperatively than inpatients. Bed rest does not reduce the frequency of headache. Indeed, early ambulation may decrease the incidence.

Epidural and Caudal Anesthesia

Epidural anesthesia (see also Chapter 35) takes longer to perform than spinal anesthesia. Onset with spinal anesthesia is more rapid, although recovery may be the same with either technique. When spinal anesthesia and epidural anesthesia are combined, the initial onset of block is faster than with epidural anesthesia alone. Epidural anesthesia is particularly advantageous for procedures where duration of surgery is unclear. Another advantage of the epidural block is that it can be performed outside the OR and avoids the problem of postdural puncture headache provided there is no "wet tap."

Caudal anesthesia is a form of epidural anesthesia commonly used in children having infraumbilical operations as a supplement to general anesthesia and to control postoperative pain. In a 2012 review of patients recorded in the Pediatric Regional Anesthesia Network (PRAN) database, almost 19,000 received a caudal block. The authors found that the incidence of complications, consisting mostly of block failure, blood aspiration, and intravascular injection, was about 2% and there were no permanent sequelae.[37] Nearly 25% of patients in the database received bupivacaine higher than 2 mg/kg, a seemingly large dose, though it was unclear if the larger doses included epinephrine in the caudal drug mix. Two patients who had signs of systemic toxicity received a bupivacaine dose lower than 2 mg/kg. Different adjuvants have been used to increase the duration of analgesia such as opioids, ketamine, and clonidine, though the potential toxicity of different additives is not clear. *Anesthesia & Analgesia* (*A&A*) includes a link in their Guide for Authors concerning the status of drugs for neuraxial or perineural administration (Table 31-6).[38] *A&A* will not publish studies that involve the administration of drugs not included on the list in neuraxial or perineural locations. Caudal blocks may be more difficult in children, particularly those who weigh more than 10 kg and in obese children if landmarks for the block are difficult to locate. The block is usually administered after the induction of general anesthesia. After the caudal block, the depth of general anesthesia can be reduced. Because of better pain control after a caudal block, children can usually ambulate earlier and be discharged sooner than without a caudal block. Pain control and discharge times are no

Table 31-6 Status of Drugs Used for the Neuraxial or Perineural Human Research

Drug	Intrathecal Status	Epidural Status	Perineural	Notes
Adenosine	IND required	IND required	—	—
Alfentanil	IND required	IND required	—	—
Baclofen	Approved	—	"50 µg, 500 µg, or 2,000 µg/mL"	—
Buprenorphine	IND required	IND required	—	—
Chloroprocaine	IND required	Approved	2–3%	—
Clonidine	Widely accepted	Approved	100 µg/mL or 500 µg/mL	—
Dexamethasone	IND required	Widely accepted	IND required	—
Diazepam	IND required	IND required	—	—
Droperidol	IND required	IND required	—	—
Ephedrine	IND required	IND required	—	—
Epinephrine	Approved	Approved	—	—
Fentanyl	Widely accepted	—	Widely accepted	50 µg/mL
Hydromorphone	Widely accepted	—	Widely accepted	2 mg/mL
Ketamine	IND required	IND required	—	—
Ketorolac	IND required	IND required	—	—
Lidocaine	Approved	—	Approved	5%
Liposomal morphine	Not approved	Approved	—	10 mg/mL
Magnesium	IND required	IND required	IND required	—
Meperidine	—	Widely accepted	—	50 mg/mL
Midazolam	IND required	IND required	—	—
Morphine	Approved	Approved	"0.5 mg/mL, 1 mg/mL, 10 mg/m, 25 mg/mL"	—
Neostigmine	IND required	IND required	—	—
Parecoxib	IND required	IND required	—	—
Phenylephrine	IND required	IND required	—	—
Remifentanil	IND required	IND required	—	—
Sufentanil	—	Widely accepted	Approved	50 µg/mL
Tramadol	IND required	IND required	—	—
Triamcinolone	IND required	IND required	—	—

Notes
1. Use of approved agents is based on the use of concentrations approved for human use.
2. No intrathecal agent should be considered if it contains preservative or other adjuvants not prescribed for human intrathecal use.
3. None of these agents have been officially approved for neonatal or pediatric use.
4. Blank entries indicate drugs and routes of delivery that have not been considered. It should be assumed that they are not approved.
5. Triamcinolone is no longer acceptable for epidural injection, as particulates have caused injury if intra-arterial injection.

Reprinted with permission from *Anesthesia & Analgesia Guide for Authors* 2011. Version: February 22, 2011 (Accessed November, 2015, at www.aaeditor.org/Neuraxial.Perineura.Drugs.xls). Copyright © 2011 International Anesthesia Research Society. Original author: Dr. Steven Shafer.
IND, investigational new drug

different whether the caudal block is administered before or after the operation.

Nerve Blocks

8 Nerve blocks are an important technique in ambulatory anesthesia (see also Chapter 36). They improve patient satisfaction and reduce both PONV and postoperative pain. In a study of patients undergoing arthroscopic rotator cuff repair surgery, most patients in the continuous interscalene brachial plexus block group had pain scores less than 4 compared to patients in the single injection interscalene brachial plexus block group or the general anesthesia group whose pain scores were more than 4. These findings were observed on postoperative days 1, 2, and 7.[39] A designated room where regional anesthesia can be performed far enough in advance of the OR such that the block is effective by the time the patient enters the OR will reduce turnover time.[40] Counterintuitively, there was no difference in PACU times between with regional anesthesia and with or without general anesthesia; but PACU length of stay was shorter with regional anesthesia compared to general anesthesia alone.[31]

Certain procedures can be quite painful, and hospitalization may be required to control pain. Nerve blocks with catheters intended to provide postoperative analgesia can be placed preoperatively. Recent examples of their use in ambulatory surgery include posterior insertion of transverse abdominis blocks kept in place for 2 days after inguinal hernia repair,[42] use of a continuous infraclavicular nerve block with a portable infusion pump for patients undergoing total elbow arthroplasty,[43] continuous popliteal sciatic nerve block for outpatient foot surgery in adults[44] and children,[45] and paravertebral somatic nerve block for breast surgery, followed by a continuous perineural infusion of local anesthetic at home for 24 to 48 hours.[46] Femoral nerve catheters left in for 2 days after discharge following anterior cruciate ligament reconstruction had decreased postoperative pain up to 4 days after surgery (Fig. 31-5).[47] Interscalene perineural catheters, kept in for 4 days after surgery, have been used for patients undergoing moderately painful shoulder surgery.[48] Patients who are discharged with interscalene perineural catheters and ropivacaine infusion pumps are discharged earlier on the first postoperative day and require less opioids at home than those treated with single-shot regional techniques. The same techniques have been used in children and adolescents; except for two patients who required hospital readmission, over 1,200 patients remained comfortable at home with only oral opioids after major orthopedic surgery (Fig. 31-6).[49]

Patients who go home with catheters inserted must be taught about pump function, understand signs of local anesthesia toxicity, and have someone else at home who can provide assistance. Patients must be able to communicate with someone by phone. There should also be a catheter removal protocol. The number of patients who have been sent home with catheters is increasing but

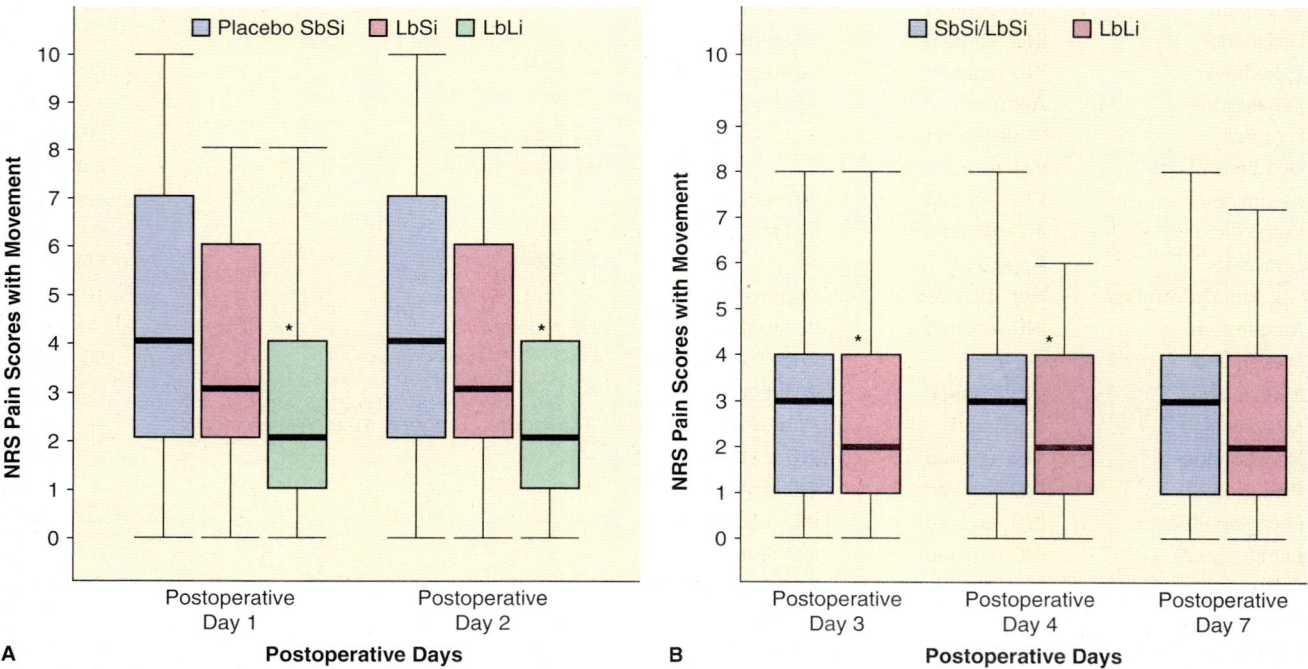

Figure 31-5 When a continuous femoral perineural infusion, spinal anesthesia, and multimodal analgesia, are used together, pain scores are less, when compared with the same spinal anesthetic technique and multimodal analgesia plan coupled with a placebo femoral nerve catheter. Box plots show numeric pain score differences (NRS) after anterior cruciate ligament reconstruction. The *thick black line* inside the box represents the median NRS value; the lowest bar on the y-axis represents the 10th percentile, the bottom and top of the boxes represent the interquartile range (25th and 75th percentiles), and the top bar represents the 90th percentile. Placebo SbSi is the placebo treatment group receiving a saline bolus and saline infusion through the femoral nerve block catheter, whereas treatment group LbSi received a levobupivacaine bolus and saline infusion, and LbLi received both a bolus and infusion containing levobupivacaine. **A:** On both days 1 and 2, the LbLi treatment group had significantly lower pain scores when compared with the other two nerve block treatment groups (*). **B:** On postoperative days 3 and 4, the LbLi treatment group had significantly lower pain scores when compared with the other two nerve block treatment groups (*) but by day 7, no differences are seen. (Adapted with permission from Williams BA, Kentor ML, Vogt MT, et al. Reduction of verbal pain scores after anterior cruciate ligament reconstruction with 2-day continuous femoral nerve block: a randomized clinical trial. *Anesthesiology*. 2006;104:315–327.)

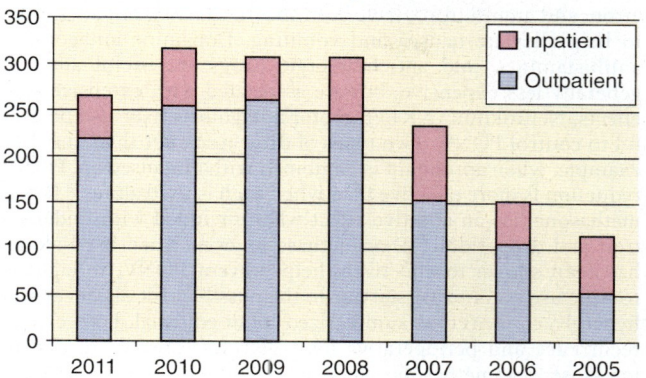

Figure 31-6 Number of patients with a continuous peripheral nerve block (CPNB) per year by discharge status (inpatient vs. outpatient) placed at one children's hospital from 2005 to 2011. Shown in each column are patients discharged home with a CPNB versus patients who stayed in the hospital until the CPNB was removed. During the last 5 years, the percentage of patients discharged home with a CPNB has increased to approximately 80%. (Adapted with permission from Gurnaney H, Kraemer FW, Maxwell L, et al. Ambulatory continuous peripheral nerve blocks in children and adolescents: a longitudinal 8-year single center study. *Anesth Analg.* 2014;118:621–627.)

is not large. More study is needed in order to demonstrate patient safety. The use of these catheters has recently been reviewed.[50]

Sedation and Analgesia

Many patients who undergo surgery with local or regional anesthesia prefer to be sedated and to have no recollection of the procedure. Sedation is important, in part, because injection with local anesthetics can be painful and lying on a hard OR table can be uncomfortable. Levels of sedation vary from light, during which a patient's consciousness is minimally depressed, to very deep, in which protective reflexes are partially blocked and response to physical stimulation or verbal command may not be appropriate.

General Anesthesia

The drugs selected for general anesthesia determine how long patients stay in the PACU after surgery, and for some patients, whether they can be discharged to go home.

Induction

Though in previous editions of this chapter, propofol and Pentothal has been compared, Pentothal is no longer available for use in humans in this country. Though the effect of drugs given for induction may seem to be transient, they can depress psychomotor performance for several hours. Propofol's half-life is 1 to 3 hours, and after an induction dose of propofol, impairment is apparent for only 1 hour compared to methohexital which has a half-life of 6 to 8 hours.

Pain on injection can be a problem with propofol. Pain is more likely when injected into dorsal hand veins and is minimized if forearm or larger antecubital veins are used. Some individuals, though, experience pain if the drug is injected into proximal larger veins. Nonetheless, thrombophlebitis does not appear to be a problem after intravenous administration of this agent. As noted in one meta-analysis, the most effective technique to decrease pain related to propofol injection is to use IV lidocaine (0.5 mg/kg), given with a rubber tourniquet on the forearm, 30 to 120 seconds before injection of propofol.[51] As the authors of a review published in 2014 noted, when comparing manuscripts published after the review by Picard et al.,[51] "Firstly, although the systematic review had identified a simple, effective, and low cost intervention and strongly suggested that additional trials on this specific issue were no longer necessary, the publication of trials has not decreased. Secondly, although the systematic review provided a clear research agenda, its influence on the design of further trials has remained poor. Thirdly, the proportion of subsequently published trials that could have had an impact on clinical practice has remained low. Finally, citing the systematic review had no clear influence on the design or relevance of subsequently published research."[52] Whether patients remember the pain of injection with propofol after the procedure is unclear.

Most children and some adults prefer not to have an intravenous catheter inserted before the start of anesthesia. Sevoflurane has a relatively low blood–gas partition coefficient and the speed of induction is only slightly slower than propofol. Induction with sevoflurane can be hastened when the patient is told to breathe out to residual volume, take a vital capacity breath through a primed anesthesia circuit, and then hold the breath.

For short procedures, some patients may not require neuromuscular-blocking drugs; others may need brief paralysis (e.g., with succinylcholine) to facilitate tracheal intubation. Nondepolarizing drugs can be used to facilitate intubation and for paralysis during the procedure. Large doses of rocuronium have rapid onset times that are similar to those with succinylcholine. Of course, paralysis is not needed to insert an endotracheal tube; drug combinations such as propofol, alfentanil, or remifentanil, with or without lidocaine obviate the need for paralysis. Succinylcholine should be used with caution in children because of the possibility of cardiac arrest related to malignant hyperthermia or unsuspected muscular dystrophy, particularly Duchenne disease. Indeed, patients can experience painful myalgias after receiving succinylcholine.

Maintenance

Although many factors affect the choice of agents for maintenance of anesthesia, two primary concerns for ambulatory anesthesia are speed of wake-up and incidence of PONV.

Anesthesia Maintenance and Wake-up Times

Time to recovery may be measured by various criteria; however, for an ambulatory center, a patient may be considered awake only when he or she is able to leave the center. Actual discharge from an ambulatory center, though, may depend on administrative issues such as a written order from a surgeon or anesthesiologist. The time necessary before a patient can be taken from the OR after completion of surgery, or a patient's ability to skip the PACU and go directly to Phase II recovery (see also Chapter 54), may be directly related to the anesthetic and may result in cost savings for an institution.

Does choice of maintenance agent affect recovery after anesthesia? Propofol, desflurane, and sevoflurane have characteristics that make them ideal for maintenance of anesthesia for ambulatory surgery. Propofol has a short half-life and, when used as a maintenance agent, results in rapid recovery and few side effects. Desflurane and sevoflurane, halogenated ether anesthetics with low blood–gas partition coefficients, seem to be ideal for general anesthesia for ambulatory surgery. Sevoflurane, unlike desflurane, facilitates a smooth inhalation induction of anesthesia and is the preferred technique to ensure rapid recovery of children in ASCs.

It is important to distinguish between wake-up time and discharge time. Patients may emerge from anesthesia with desflurane and nitrous oxide significantly faster than after propofol or sevoflurane and nitrous oxide, although the ability to sit up, stand, and tolerate fluids and the time to fitness for discharge may be no different. Fast wake-up times may translate to bypass of phase I, which can result in cost savings.

Intraoperative Management of Postoperative Nausea and Vomiting

Nausea, with or without vomiting, is probably the most important factor contributing to a delay in discharge of patients and an increase in unanticipated admissions of both children and adults after ambulatory surgery. Patients often fear PONV more than postoperative pain. Reducing risk factors can significantly decrease the incidence of PONV (Table 31-7). To decrease the risk of PONV:

- Use regional anesthesia.
- If general anesthesia is necessary, use a propofol infusion instead of an inhalation agent (propofol is now generic so the decision to use the drug should not be based on cost).
- Avoid nitrous oxide.
- Minimize use of perioperative opioids.
- Try to avoid paralysis.
- Provide adequate hydration.

The incidence of emesis may be greater after nitrous oxide than after potent inhalation agents. Although many studies have shown that nitrous oxide can be used successfully for ambulatory anesthesia, there is evidence that when nitrous oxide is used for less than 1 hour, the risk of PONV is not increased.[53]

Women have a higher incidence of PONV as do those with a previous history of PONV or motion sickness. Patients who undergo certain procedures, such as laparoscopy; lithotripsy; major breast surgery; and ear, nose, or throat surgery are at increased risk for PONV. The greater the number of risk factors, the greater the risk for nausea or vomiting after surgery.

There are also specific genotypes that are associated with more susceptibility to PONV. A recent review suggests that there may be a genetic relationship to PONV since some patients have resistance to antiemetic prophylaxis and/or therapy, some patients have PONV in several generations of families, and there is PONV concordance in monozygotic twins.[54] Pharmacogenetic research focused on 5HT3 receptor antagonists, metabolic pathways of 5HT3 antagonists, and other genes associated with PONV and chemotherapy-induced nausea and vomiting. Sensitivity is probably multifactorial and may include several genomic pathways; more study relating genetic makeup and possible treatment implications is needed.

PONV treatment has been based on sites and pathways in the brain that are associated with PONV. Receptor antagonists, specifically selective serotonin antagonists (ondansetron, dolasetron, and granisetron), have been shown to have similar efficacy to help alleviate nausea and vomiting. Dopamine antagonists, antihistamines, and anticholinergic drugs are useful and are generally less expensive, but are associated with extensive side effects. Neurokinin (NK1) receptor antagonists may also be useful to control PONV. Two types of drug are better than one. For example, when aprepitant is combined with ondansetron, PONV reduction is more effective than when each is used alone.[55] Dexamethasone has an additive effect when included with ondansetron and droperidol.[56] Dexamethasone, even when used alone, has been shown to effectively help prevent PONV, though its routine use is controversial due to the possible risk of cancer and hyperglycemia. Yet, as summarized in an editorial, both cancer recurrence and perioperative hyperglycemia are not related to low-dose dexamethasone when used to help prevent PONV.[57] Other therapies useful in controlling PONV include acupuncture or acupressure,[58] supplemental fluid therapy, and clonidine (perhaps in part because it decreases anesthesia requirement). If, intraoperatively, leads to monitor patient paralysis are placed at the P6 acupuncture point and tetanus monitoring is used as the neuromuscular monitoring mode, PONV is reduced.[59]

Though much work has been focused on PONV, postdischarge nausea and vomiting (PDNV) is also an issue. In one study, the overall incidence of PDNV was almost 60%, and PDNV continued until day 7 for 2% of patients. Those who had a history of motion sickness, previous PONV, migraine headaches, and pain on activity postdischarge were more likely to have PDNV. Nitrous oxide and the use of a regional block as an adjunct to inhalation anesthesia was not associated with PDNV.[60] Another group found a relationship between patients with high pain and PDNV for all of the first 6 postoperative days. It was not until postoperative day 6 that PDNV scores in the high and low pain groups were the same (Fig. 31-7).[61]

Paralysis

Muscle paralysis for ambulatory anesthesia extends beyond the time of paralysis for intubation, particularly when nondepolarizing drugs are used. The duration of action of rocuronium, vecuronium, rapacuronium, and cisatracurium ranges from 25 to 40 minutes. Reversal agents must be used unless there is no doubt that muscle relaxation is fully reversed. Patient safety is optimized when acceleromyography is used to monitor the extent of paralysis and the adequacy of reversal.[62] Furthermore, when quantitative monitoring of neuromuscular block depth guides neostigmine dosing, respiratory complications can be minimized (Fig. 31-8).[63]

Intraoperative Management of Postoperative Pain

Intraoperative opioid administration provides analgesia for both the intraoperative and postoperative course. Fentanyl is probably the most popular drug, although all other available opioids have been tried. All opioids can cause nausea, sedation, and dizziness, which can delay a patient's discharge. Nonsteroidal analgesics are not effective as supplements during general anesthesia, although they are useful in controlling postoperative pain, particularly when given before skin incision. To control postoperative pain, combination therapy is most useful. (See also the earlier discussion on opioids and nonsteroidal analgesics in this chapter.)

Airway Adjuncts

The use of supraglottic airways, such as the LMA, provides several advantages for allowing a patient to return to baseline status quickly. Muscle relaxants are generally avoided. Coughing is less than with tracheal intubation. Anesthetic requirements, hoarseness, and sore throat are all reduced. Overall, cost savings result with the use of LMAs. Because of gastric insufflation, though,

---

Table 31-7 Techniques to Decrease Postoperative Nausea and Vomiting Risk

Use regional anesthesia alone if possible
If general anesthesia is needed, use a propofol infusion instead of an inhalation agent (propofol is now generic so the decision to use the drug should not be based on cost)
Avoid use of nitrous oxide for anesthesia maintenance, particularly for procedures longer than 1 hour
Minimize use of perioperative opioids
Try to avoid paralysis if clinically indicated
Consider adequate hydration

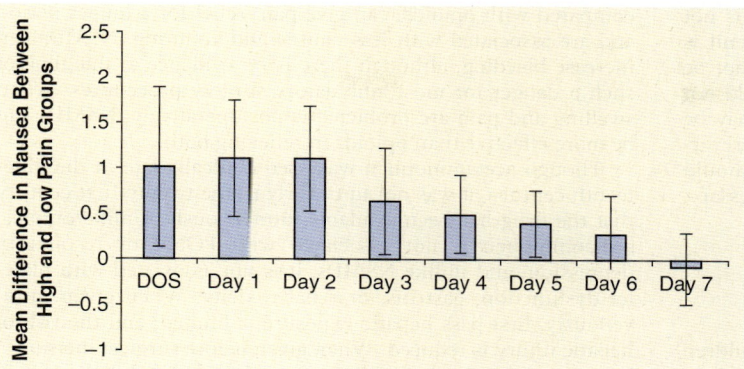

Figure 31-7 Mean differences in daily nausea scores between high-pain and low-pain groups, with 95% confidence intervals from day of surgery (DOS) to postoperative day 7. The largest difference was seen on the second day after surgery, followed by a gradual decrease. Differences on days 6 and 7 were not significant. (Adapted with permission from Odom-Forren J, Rayens MK, Gokun Y, et al. The relationship of pain and nausea in postoperative patients for 1 week after ambulatory surgery. *Clin J Pain*. 2015;31:845–851.)

nausea and vomiting may be greater. After an LMA is inserted, there is a 1% failure rate requiring endotracheal tube insertion.[64] In the study of almost 16,000 patients, risk factors for failure included surgical table rotation, male gender, poor dentition, and increased body mass index. Patients for whom LMA failed had a three-fold increase of difficult mask ventilation, unplanned admission rate was almost 14%, and almost 6% needed ICU admission due to persistent hypoxemia.

Management of Postanesthesia Care

Many recovery challenges are part of patient selection and perioperative management and must be considered before the patient enters the PACU (see also Chapter 54). Managing common problems in the PACU quickly and effectively is as important as appropriate patient selection and choice of anesthetic technique if the patient is to return home on the day of surgery. The three most common reasons for delay in patient discharge from the PACU are drowsiness, nausea and vomiting, and pain. All three are a function of intraoperative management, but nausea, vomiting, and pain can be treated in the PACU.

Reversal of Drug Effects

Reversal of muscle relaxants is not unique to the ambulatory surgery patient and is not discussed here (see also Chapter 21). Reversal of opioids may sometimes be necessary. Flumazenil, a benzodiazepine receptor antagonist, has primarily been used to reverse the effects of sedation after endoscopy and spinal anesthesia. Reversal of psychomotor impairment with flumazenil is

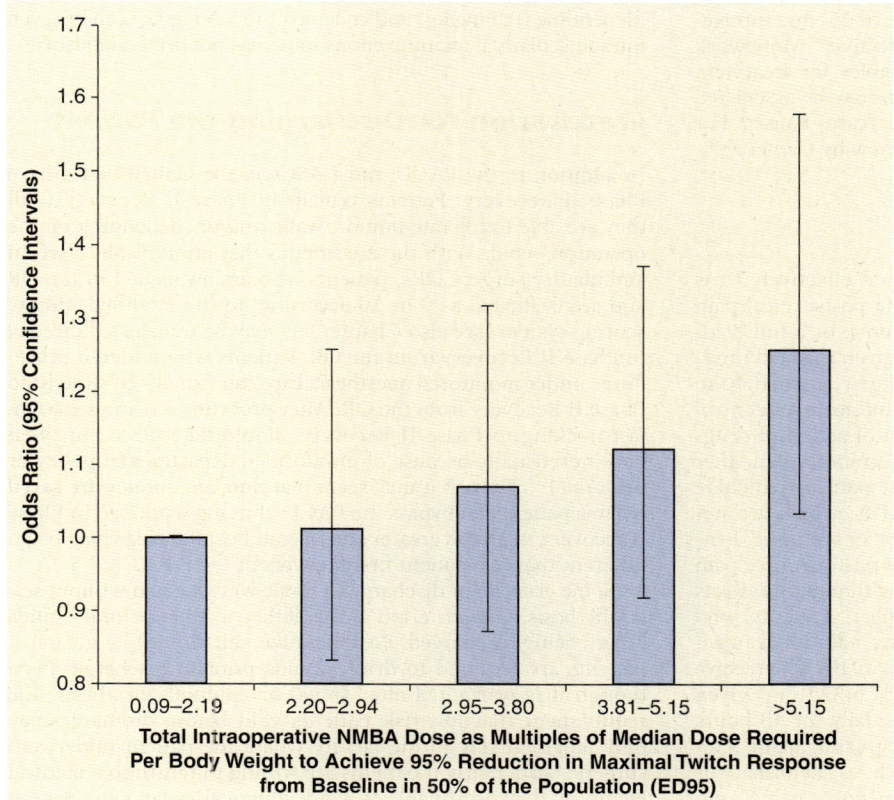

Figure 31-8 As the dose of neuromuscular blocking agent (intraoperative dose of atracurium, cisatracurium, rocuronium, or vecuronium) increases, the likelihood of respiratory complications increases. (Adapted with permission from McLean DJ, Diaz-Gil D, Farhan HN, et al. Dose-dependent association between intermediate-acting neuromuscular-blocking agents and postoperative respiratory complications. *Anesthesiology*. 2015;122:1201–1213.)

not complete, and the subjective experience of sedation is not necessarily attenuated. Reversal of amnesia with flumazenil is only partial, and the duration of the reversal effect may not be long enough to be clinically significant. Flumazenil should not be used routinely as a benzodiazepine antagonist, but may be used when sedation appears to be excessive. In addition, reversal of benzodiazepine-induced sedation by flumazenil should not replace appropriate ventilation assistance and, if necessary, placement of an endotracheal tube.

Nausea and Vomiting

Nausea and vomiting are the most common reasons both children and adults have protracted stays in the PACU or unexpected hospital admission due to anesthesia. Nausea and vomiting are also the most common adverse effect in patients in the PACU. Much research has been undertaken to study prophylactic treatment of this problem before surgery, as well as techniques in the OR that can minimize nausea and vomiting in the PACU. The treatment of this problem, once it occurs in the PACU, has not received as much study. Yet, there are a variety of drugs that are effective in treating the problem. The 5-HT3 antagonists seem particularly effective. Dexamethasone, 8 mg, given with other antiemetics can enhance treatment of established PONV in the PACU.[56]

Midazolam and propofol, although more commonly used for sedation, have antiemetic effects that are longer in duration than their effects on sedation. Acupressure bands or acupressure stimulation in the region of the P6 acupuncture point can help reduce PONV. If patients have already received ondansetron prophylaxis in the OR, and then are nauseous in the PACU, another dose might not be effective. Based on a retrospective analysis of patients with nausea after receiving prophylactic ondansetron, established PONV was more effectively treated with promethazine than ondansetron; and promethazine, 6.25 mg intravenously, rather than higher doses was most effective.[65] More work is obviously needed to study effective therapies for treatment of PONV in the PACU. Finally, because pain may be associated with nausea, treatment of pain frequently decreases nausea. For a more complete discussion, consider the review by Gan et al.[66]

Pain

Postsurgical pain must be treated quickly and effectively. It is important for the practitioner to differentiate postsurgical pain from the discomfort of hypoxemia, hypercapnia, or a full bladder. Medications for pain control should be given in small intravenous doses (e.g., morphine 1 to 3 mg/70 kg or fentanyl 10 to 25 µg/70 kg). Intramuscular injection of opioid for pain control in the PACU is usually not necessary. Onset of action of drugs is faster after intravenous catheter administration than after oral administration. Control of postoperative pain may include administration of opioid analgesics or NSAIDs, which are not associated with respiratory depression, nausea, or vomiting. Fentanyl is the opioid frequently used to control postoperative pain that ambulatory surgery patients experience, although the effects of morphine and hydromorphone last longer. Patients who receive fentanyl for pain control may require additional injections and go home no sooner compared with patients who receive morphine. Oral tramadol/paracetamol (TP 37.5/325 mg) given after surgery and then as 1 tablet four times daily for 48 hours is an effective fixed drug combination for treating pain after discharge.[67] Nonsteroidal medications, such as ketorolac or ibuprofen, can also effectively control postoperative pain[68] and, compared with opioids, can give pain relief for a longer period and are associated with less nausea and vomiting. NSAIDs can increase bleeding, although there is no evidence at this time of such a danger for most ambulatory surgery procedures. When swelling and pain are problematic postoperatively, NSAIDs can be more effective than opioids in relieving both.

Though acetaminophen was used clinically late in the nineteenth century, it was not until early in the twenty-first century that the drug has been available intravenously. Unlike opioids, acetaminophen is not associated with PONV or respiratory depression, and unlike NSAIDs, it is not associated with platelet dysfunction, gastritis, or renal toxicity. When given intravenously, first-pass hepatic exposure is limited, and the risk of hepatic injury is reduced. When given before surgical incision,[69] or postoperatively,[70] opioid need is reduced. Total daily dose of acetaminophen should not exceed 4 g/day and 2 g/day or less for patients with impaired liver or kidney function.

We manage pain in both adults and children initially either with a short-acting opioid analgesic such as fentanyl (25 µg/70 kg for pain on a scale of 3-5 out of 10 and 50 µg/70 kg for pain on a scale of 6-10 out of 10), or with an injection of ketorolac, 30 to 60 mg/70 kg intravenously or acetaminophen 650 mg (12.5 mg/kg for children 2 to 12 years or adults <50 kg). Fentanyl is repeated at 5-minute intervals until pain is controlled. For children, we also use an elixir of acetaminophen containing codeine (120 mg acetaminophen and 12 mg codeine, in each 5 mL of solution). Five milliliters is administered to children between the ages of 3 and 6, and 10 mL to children between the ages of 7 and 12. Children are returned to parental care as soon as they are awake. We find frequently that infants younger than 6 months of age usually need to be reunited with their mothers for nursing or bottle feeding after a procedure not associated with severe pain. For older infants and young children in the PACU, acetaminophen, 60 mg per year of age (given orally or rectally), is commonly used to relieve mild pain. Meperidine (0.5 mg/kg) and codeine (1 to 1.5 mg/kg) can be given intramuscularly if an intravenous route has not been established.

Preparation for Discharging the Patient

In addition to the PACU, most ASCs in the United States have Phase II Recovery. Patients remain in Phase II Recovery until they are able to tolerate liquids, walk, and/or (depending on the operation) void. With the anesthetics that are typically used in ambulatory surgery ORs, patients who are awakened in the OR and are evaluated as 9 or 10 according to the modified Aldrete scoring system (see also Chapter 54) may be transferred directly to Phase II Recovery from the OR. Patients who undergo procedures under monitored anesthesia care can usually go straight to Phase II Recovery from the OR. After procedures using sedation, fast-tracking to Phase II Recovery should take place but often does not, usually because of uninformed departmental policy or personnel.[71] Though it may seem that time and money are saved when a patient can bypass the PACU, nursing workload in Phase II recovery might be greater and overall hospital costs may be no different than if a patient first recovers in the PACU.

Some criteria for discharge to home were created without scientific basis. One criterion is the ability to tolerate oral liquids before being discharged. Postoperative nausea may be greater if patients are required to drink liquids prior to discharge. Even though it is warranted after spinal or epidural anesthesia, the requirement that low-risk patients void before discharge may only lengthen stay in the facility where the patient underwent surgery, particularly if patients are willing to return to a medical facility if they are unable to void. Practical criteria for patient discharge from the OR, from the PACU, and from Phase II Recovery are needed such that there is no compromise in patient safety. The value of psychomotor tests to measure different phases of recovery, except for research purposes, is questionable.

Although scoring systems may be used to guide transfer from the PACU to the Phase II Recovery and from Phase II Recovery to home, they do little to test higher levels of function, such as the ability to use one's hands, to drive a car, or to remain alert long enough to drive. Patients may feel fine after they leave the hospital, but they should be advised against driving for at least 24 hours after a procedure. Patients and responsible parties should be reminded that the patient should not operate power tools or be involved in major business decisions for up to 24 hours. Once the patient leaves the medical facility, supervision may not be as good as it was in the hospital. Therefore, before a patient is discharged, dressings should be checked. It is wise to include the responsible person in all discharge instructions.

Patients should also be informed that they may experience pain, headache, nausea, vomiting, or dizziness and, if succinylcholine was used, muscle aches and pains apart from the incision for at least 24 hours. A patient will be less stressed if the described symptoms are expected in the course of a normal recovery. Written instructions are important. The addition of written and oral education techniques at discharge has a significant impact on improving compliance.

When discussing discharge planning, it is also important to consider where a patient should return in case of a problem. Unlike a hospital, most ambulatory centers are not open around the clock. As ambulatory procedures are becoming more prevalent, patients are traveling farther distances.[72] Whether this is associated with increased risk is yet to be determined.

For patients with a language barrier, consent forms, procedural explanation, and discharge information may have to be written in languages other than English and the services of an interpreter may be necessary. Nursing staff should assess the adult who will take the patient home to determine whether he or she is a responsible person. A responsible person is someone who is physically and intellectually able to take care of the patient at home. Facilities should develop a method of follow-up after the patient has been discharged. At some facilities, staff members telephone the patient the next day to determine the progress of recovery; others use follow-up postcards.

Whenever we become innovative in the management of our outpatients, we must assess how a cost-effective, "no frills" approach to care affects patient safety. We must determine what we can do for the patient who lives alone, for the patient whose responsible person is unable to manage his or her needs, for the patient without means of transportation, and for the patient with limited insurance coverage. Hospital beds can be set aside for patients who require observation. Patients in these beds after an ambulatory surgical procedure are still considered outpatients. They are charged for the hours spent in the observation area. Some hospitals have joined with management firms to build a hospital hotel or medical motel close to the hospital itself. The hotel, usually a nonmedical facility, offers the outpatient a comfortable, inexpensive, and convenient place to recuperate while being cared for by family or nurses. Home health-care nursing may be appropriate after surgical procedures such as reduction mammoplasty, abdominoplasty, vaginal hysterectomy, and major open ligament repairs of the knee. The various services for management and/or observation of outpatients after surgery stand today where techniques for management of outpatients during surgery stood in the health-care delivery system 20 years ago. Prospective studies are needed to assess the quality of care and the effect that these innovative approaches have on patient safety.

Patient, procedure, availability and quality of aftercare, and anesthetic technique must be individually and collectively assessed to determine acceptability for ambulatory surgery. A delicate balance must be maintained between the physical status of the patient, the proposed surgical procedure, and the appropriate anesthetic technique, to which must be added the expertise level of the anesthesiologist caring for a patient.

Anesthesia for ambulatory surgery is a rapidly evolving specialty. Patients who were once believed to be unsuitable for ambulatory surgery are now considered appropriate candidates. Operations once believed unsuitable for outpatients are now routinely performed in the morning, so patients can be discharged in the afternoon or evening. The appropriate anesthetic management before these patients come to the OR, during their operation, and then afterward is the key to success. The availability of both shorter-acting anesthetics and longer-acting analgesics and antiemetics enables us to care for patients in ambulatory centers effectively.

Acknowledgments

Thanks to Yale University, Department of Anesthesiology.

REFERENCES

1. Parina R, Chang D, Saad AN, et al. Quality and safety outcomes of ambulatory plastic surgery facilities in California. *Plast Reconstr Surg.* 2015;135:791–797.
2. Starling J, 3rd, Thosani MK, Coldiron BM. Determining the safety of office-based surgery: what 10 years of Florida data and 6 years of Alabama data reveal. *Dermatol Surg.* 2012;38:171–177.
3. Hanke CW. Commentary: Advocating for mandatory adverse event reporting. *Dermatol Surg.* 2012;38:178–179.
4. Davidson AJ, Morton NS, Arnup SJ, et al. Apnea after awake regional and general anesthesia in infants: The general anesthesia compared to spinal anesthesia study-comparing apnea and neurodevelopmental outcomes, a randomized controlled trial. *Anesthesiology.* 2015;123(1):38–54.
5. Pierides G, Mattila K, Vironen J. Quality of life change in elderly patients undergoing open inguinal hernia repair. *Hernia.* 2013;17:729–736.
6. Poobalan AS, Bruce J, King PM, et al. Chronic pain and quality of life following open inguinal hernia repair. *Br J Surg.* 2001;88:1122–1126.
7. Martin-Ferrero MA, Faour-Martin O, Simon-Perez C, et al. Ambulatory surgery in orthopedics: experience of over 10,000 patients. *J Orthop Sci.* 2014;19:332–338.
8. Sieffert MR, Fox JP, Abbott LE, et al. Obesity is associated with increased health care charges in patients undergoing outpatient plastic surgery. *Plast Reconstr Surg.* 2015;135:1396–1404.
9. Gaddam S, Gunukula SK, Mador MJ. Post-operative outcomes in adult obstructive sleep apnea patients undergoing non-upper airway surgery: a systematic review and meta-analysis. *Sleep Breath.* 2014;18:615–633.
10. American Society of Anesthesiologists Task Force on Perioperative Management of patients with obstructive sleep apnea. Practice guidelines for the perioperative management of patients with obstructive sleep apnea: an updated report by the American Society of Anesthesiologists Task Force on Perioperative Management of patients with obstructive sleep apnea. *Anesthesiology.* 2014;120:268–286.
11. Stierer TL, Collop NA. Perioperative assessment and management for sleep apnea in the ambulatory surgical patient. *Chest.* 2015;148:559–565.
12. Joshi GP, Ankichetty SP, Gan TJ, et al. Society for ambulatory anesthesia consensus statement on preoperative selection of adult patients with obstructive sleep apnea scheduled for ambulatory surgery. *Anesth Analg.* 2012;115:1060–1068.
13. Dexter F, Maxbauer T, Stout C, et al. Relative influence on total cancelled operating room time from patients who are inpatients or outpatients preoperatively. *Anesth Analg.* 2014;118:1072–1080.
14. von Ungern-Sternberg BS, Boda K, Chambers NA, et al. Risk assessment for respiratory complications in paediatric anaesthesia: a prospective cohort study. *Lancet.* 2010;376:773–783.
15. Osugi T, Tatara T, Yada S, et al. Hydration status after overnight fasting as measured by urine osmolality does not alter the magnitude of hypotension during general anesthesia in low risk patients. *Anesth Analg.* 2011;112:1307–1313.
16. Buehrer S, Hanke U, Klaghofer R, et al. Hunger and thirst numeric rating scales are not valid estimates for gastric content volumes: a prospective investigation in healthy children. *Paediatr Anaesth.* 2014;24:309–315.
17. Brady M, Kinn S, Ness V, et al. Preoperative fasting for preventing perioperative complications in children. *Cochrane Database Syst Rev.* 2009;(4):CD005285. doi:CD005285.

18. American Society of Anesthesiologists Committee. Practice guidelines for preoperative fasting and the use of pharmacologic agents to reduce the risk of pulmonary aspiration: application to healthy patients undergoing elective procedures: an updated report by the American Society of Anesthesiologists Committee on Standards and Practice Parameters. *Anesthesiology.* 2011;114:495–511.
19. Coté CJ, Cohen IT, Suresh S, et al. A comparison of three doses of a commercially prepared oral midazolam syrup in children. *Anesth Analg.* 2002;94:37–43.
20. Kain ZN, MacLaren J, McClain BC, et al. Effects of age and emotionality on the effectiveness of midazolam administered preoperatively to children. *Anesthesiology.* 2007;107:545–552.
21. Park SM, Mangat HS, Berger K, et al. Efficacy spectrum of antishivering medications: meta-analysis of randomized controlled trials. *Crit Care Med.* 2012;40:3070–3082.
22. Katz J, Clarke H, Seltzer Z. Review article: Preventive analgesia: quo vadimus? *Anesth Analg.* 2011;113:1242–1253.
23. Kissin I. A call to reassess the clinical value of preventive (preemptive) analgesia. *Anesth Analg.* 2011;113:977–978.
24. Gurusamy KS, Vaughan J, Toon CD, et al. Pharmacological interventions for prevention or treatment of postoperative pain in people undergoing laparoscopic cholecystectomy. *Cochrane Database Syst Rev.* 2014;3:CD008261.
25. Nour C, Ratsiu J, Singh N, et al. Analgesic effectiveness of acetaminophen for primary cleft palate repair in young children: a randomized placebo controlled trial. *Paediatr Anaesth.* 2014;24:574–581.
26. Kraglund F. Acetaminophen plus a nonsteroidal anti-inflammatory drug decreases acute postoperative pain more than either drug alone. *J Am Dent Assoc.* 2014;145:966–968.
27. Bourgon AL, Fox JP, Saxe JM, et al. Outcomes and charges associated with outpatient inguinal hernia repair according to method of anesthesia and surgical approach. *Am J Surg.* 2015;209:468–472.
28. Bay-Nielsen M, Kehlet H. Anaesthesia and post-operative morbidity after elective groin hernia repair: a nation-wide study. *Acta Anaesthesiol Scand.* 2008;52:169–174.
29. Chen WH, Hung KC, Tan PH, et al. Neuraxial anesthesia improves long-term survival after total joint replacement: a retrospective nationwide population-based study in Taiwan. *Can J Anaesth.* 2015;62:369–376.
30. Kessler J, Marhofer P, Hopkins PM, et al. Peripheral regional anaesthesia and outcome: lessons learned from the last 10 years. *Br J Anaesth.* 2015;114:728–745.
31. Corey JM, Bulka CM, Ehrenfeld JM. Is regional anesthesia associated with reduced PACU length of stay? A retrospective analysis from a tertiary medical center. *Clin Orthop Relat Res.* 2014;472:1427–1433.
32. Cohen DD, Dillon JB. Anesthesia for outpatient surgery. *JAMA.* 1966;196:1114–1116.
33. Sokolowski CJ, Giovannitti JA, Jr, Boynes SG. Needle phobia: etiology, adverse consequences, and patient management. *Dent Clin North Am.* 2010;54:731–744.
34. Frawley G, Bell G, Disma N, et al. Predictors of failure of awake regional anesthesia for neonatal hernia repair: Data from the general anesthesia compared to spinal anesthesia study-comparing apnea and neurodevelopmental outcomes. *Anesthesiology.* 2015;123:55–65.
35. Lacasse MA, Roy JD, Forget J, et al. Comparison of bupivacaine and 2-chloroprocaine for spinal anesthesia for outpatient surgery: a double-blind randomized trial. *Can J Anaesth.* 2011;58:384–391.
36. Suresh S, Long J, Birmingham PK, et al. Are caudal blocks for pain control safe in children? an analysis of 18,650 caudal blocks from the Pediatric Regional Anesthesia Network (PRAN) database. *Anesth Analg.* 2015;120:151–156.
37. Walker SM, Yaksh TL. Neuraxial analgesia in neonates and infants: a review of clinical and preclinical strategies for the development of safety and efficacy data. *Anesth Analg.* 2012;115:638–662.
38. Anesthesia & Analgesia Guide for Authors. 2011. (Accessed November, 2015, at http://www.aaeditor.org/Neuraxial.Perineural.Drugs.xls).
39. Salviz EA, Xu D, Frulla A, et al. Continuous interscalene block in patients having outpatient rotator cuff repair surgery: a prospective randomized trial. *Anesth Analg.* 2013;117:1485–1492.
40. Mercereau P, Lee B, Head SJ, et al. A regional anesthesia-based "swing" operating room model reduces non-operative time in a mixed orthopedic inpatient/outpatient population. *Can J Anaesth.* 2012;59:943–949.
41. Lunn TH, Kristensen BB, Gaarn-Larsen L, et al. Post-anaesthesia care unit stay after total hip and knee arthroplasty under spinal anaesthesia. *Acta Anaesthesiol Scand.* 2012;56:1139–1145.
42. Heil JW, Ilfeld BM, Loland VJ, et al. Ultrasound-guided transversus abdominis plane catheters and ambulatory perineural infusions for outpatient inguinal hernia repair. *Reg Anesth Pain Med.* 2010;35:556–558.
43. Ilfeld BM, Wright TW, Enneking FK, et al. Total elbow arthroplasty as an outpatient procedure using a continuous infraclavicular nerve block at home: a prospective case report. *Reg Anesth Pain Med.* 2006;31:172–176.
44. Zaric D, Boysen K, Christiansen J, et al. Continuous popliteal sciatic nerve block for outpatient foot surgery—a randomized, controlled trial. *Acta Anaesthesiol Scand.* 2004;48:337–341.
45. Dadure C, Bringuier S, Nicolas F, et al. Continuous epidural block versus continuous popliteal nerve block for postoperative pain relief after major podiatric surgery in children: a prospective, comparative randomized study. *Anesth Analg.* 2006;102:744–749.
46. Buckenmaier CC,3rd, Klein SM, Nielsen KC, et al. Continuous paravertebral catheter and outpatient infusion for breast surgery. *Anesth Analg.* 2003;97:715–717.
47. Williams BA, Kentor ML, Vogt MT, et al. Reduction of verbal pain scores after anterior cruciate ligament reconstruction with 2-day continuous femoral nerve block: a randomized clinical trial. *Anesthesiology.* 2006;104:315–327.
48. Ilfeld BM, Vandenborne K, Duncan PW, et al. Ambulatory continuous interscalene nerve blocks decrease the time to discharge readiness after total shoulder arthroplasty: a randomized, triple-masked, placebo-controlled study. *Anesthesiology.* 2006;105:999–1007.
49. Gurnaney H, Kraemer FW, Maxwell L, et al. Ambulatory continuous peripheral nerve blocks in children and adolescents: a longitudinal 8-year single center study. *Anesth Analg.* 2014;118:621–627.
50. Machi AT, Ilfeld BM. Continuous peripheral nerve blocks in the ambulatory setting: an update of the published evidence. *Curr Opin Anaesthesiol.* 2015;28:648–655.
51. Picard P, Tramer MR. Prevention of pain on injection with propofol: a quantitative systematic review. *Anesth Analg.* 2000;90:963–969.
52. Habre C, Tramer MR, Popping DM, et al. Ability of a meta-analysis to prevent redundant research: systematic review of studies on pain from propofol injection. *BMJ.* 2014;348:g5219.
53. Peyton PJ, Wu CY. Nitrous oxide-related postoperative nausea and vomiting depends on duration of exposure. *Anesthesiology.* 2014;120:1137–1145.
54. Janicki PK, Sugino S. Genetic factors associated with pharmacotherapy and background sensitivity to postoperative and chemotherapy-induced nausea and vomiting. *Exp Brain Res.* 2014;232:2613–2625.
55. Vallejo MC, Phelps AL, Ibinson JW, et al. Aprepitant plus ondansetron compared with ondansetron alone in reducing postoperative nausea and vomiting in ambulatory patients undergoing plastic surgery. *Plast Reconstr Surg.* 2012;129:519–526.
56. Ormel G, Romundstad L, Lambert-Jensen P, et al. Dexamethasone has additive effect when combined with ondansetron and droperidol for treatment of established PONV. *Acta Anaesthesiol Scand.* 2011;55:1196–1205.
57. Colin B, Gan TJ. Cancer recurrence and hyperglycemia with dexamethasone for postoperative nausea and vomiting prophylaxis: more moot points? *Anesth Analg.* 2014;118:1154–1156.
58. Lee A, Fan LT. Stimulation of the wrist acupuncture point P6 for preventing postoperative nausea and vomiting. *Cochrane Database Syst Rev.* 2009;(2):CD003281. doi:CD003281.
59. Kim YH, Kim KS, Lee HJ, et al. The efficacy of several neuromuscular monitoring modes at the P6 acupuncture point in preventing postoperative nausea and vomiting. *Anesth Analg.* 2011;112:819–823.
60. Odom-Forren J, Jalota L, Moser DK, et al. Incidence and predictors of postdischarge nausea and vomiting in a 7-day population. *J Clin Anesth.* 2013;25:551–559.
61. Odom-Forren J, Rayens MK, Gokun Y, et al. The relationship of pain and nausea in postoperative patients for 1 week after ambulatory surgery. *Clin J Pain.* 2015;31:845–851.
62. Brull SJ, Prielipp RC. Reversal of neuromuscular blockade: "identification friend or foe". *Anesthesiology.* 2015;122:1183–1185.
63. McLean DJ, Diaz-Gil D, Farhan HN, et al. Dose-dependent association between intermediate-acting neuromuscular-blocking agents and postoperative respiratory complications. *Anesthesiology.* 2015;122:1201–1213.
64. Ramachandran SK, Mathis MR, Tremper KK, et al. Predictors and clinical outcomes from failed Laryngeal Mask Airway Unique: a study of 15,795 patients. *Anesthesiology.* 2012;116:1217–1226.
65. Habib AS, Reuveni J, Taguchi A, et al. A comparison of ondansetron with promethazine for treating postoperative nausea and vomiting in patients who received prophylaxis with ondansetron: a retrospective database analysis. *Anesth Analg.* 2007;104:548–551.
66. Gan TJ, Diemunsch P, Habib AS, et al. Consensus guidelines for the management of postoperative nausea and vomiting. *Anesth Analg.* 2014;118:85–113.
67. Alfano G, Grieco M, Forino A, et al. Analgesia with paracetamol/tramadol vs. paracetamol/codeine in one day-surgery: a randomized open study. *Eur Rev Med Pharmacol Sci.* 2011;15:205–210.
68. White PF, Tang J, Wender RH, et al. The effects of oral ibuprofen and celecoxib in preventing pain, improving recovery outcomes and patient satisfaction after ambulatory surgery. *Anesth Analg.* 2011;112:323–329.
69. De Oliveira GS, Jr, Castro-Alves LJ, McCarthy RJ. Single-dose systemic acetaminophen to prevent postoperative pain: a meta-analysis of randomized controlled trials. *Clin J Pain.* 2015;31: 86–93.
70. Dahl JB, Nielsen RV, Wetterslev J, et al Postoperative Pain Alliance (ScaPAlli): Post-operative analgesic effects of paracetamol, NSAIDs, glucocorticoids, gabapentinoids and their combinations: a topical review. *Acta Anaesthesiol Scand.* 2014; 58: 1165–1181.
71. Twersky RS, Sapozhnikova S, Toure B. Risk factors associated with fast-track ineligibility after monitored anesthesia care in ambulatory surgery patients. *Anesth Analg.* 2008;106:1421–1426, table of contents.
72. Neuman MD, David G, Silber JH, et al. Changing access to emergency care for patients undergoing outpatient procedures at ambulatory surgery centers: evidence from Florida. *Med Care Res Rev.* 2011;68:247–258.

32 Office-based Anesthesia

LAURENCE M. HAUSMAN • MEG A. ROSENBLATT

Brief Historical Perspective of OBA
Advantages and Disadvantages of Office-based
  Surgery and Anesthesia
Office Safety
Patient Selection
Surgeon Selection
Office Selection and Requirements
  Accreditation
Procedure Selection
  Specific Procedures
Anesthetic Techniques
  Anesthetic Agents
Postanesthesia Care Unit
Regulations
  Business and Legal Aspects
Conclusions

KEY POINTS

1. An office-based anesthetic is one that is performed in an outpatient venue such as a freestanding medical or surgical office or procedure room that is not accredited as either an ambulatory surgery center (ASC) or a hospital.
2. Cost containment and patient convenience are the two major advantages of office-based procedures over traditional hospital-based procedures.
3. The disadvantages of office-based procedures are related to patient safety, reporting, quality improvement, and peer review. Thus, great care must be taken concerning these issues.
4. Office-based morbidity and mortality are usually the result of inadequate perioperative patient monitoring, oversedation, and thromboembolic events.
5. The injuries that occur in offices tend to be of greater severity than those that occur in ambulatory surgical centers. Twenty-one percent of the reported injuries sustained in offices were temporary and nondisabling in nature and 64% were permanent or led to death, whereas 62% of the injuries sustained in ambulatory surgical centers were temporary and nondisabling and only 21% were permanent or led to death.
6. The American Society of Plastic Surgeons acknowledged that the ideal patient for an office-based procedure has an ASA physical status of 1 or 2. They recommended that American Society of Anesthesiology (ASA) physical status 3 patients undergo an office-based procedure only after an anesthesia consultation and only have an office-based procedure performed under local anesthesia without sedation.
7. Pulmonary embolism arising from deep vein thrombosis remains an important risk of an office-based procedure.
8. When formulating a quality improvement program, there should be random chart reviews as well as key sentinel events that trigger a case review.
9. The anesthesiologist should function as a zealous patient advocate in assuring that an anesthetic only is performed in a safe anesthetizing location. Issues that must be sorted out and codified include equipment, monitoring in conformance with ASA standards, emergency drugs and equipment, controlled substance handling and storage, medical director and governance, plan for hospital admission if needed, fire prevention and preparedness, and accreditation.
10. Nonfatal injuries occurring during monitored anesthesia care were more likely to be permanent than the nonfatal injuries occurring during general anesthesia, which were more frequently temporary. Of all injuries occurring during monitored anesthesia care, 34% were fatalities.
11. In terms of smooth operation of an office-based anesthesia practice and patient satisfaction, prevention of postoperative nausea and vomiting and pain are paramount.

Office-based anesthesia (OEA) is a subset of both nonoperating room anesthesia (NORA) and ambulatory anesthesia. NORA refers to any anesthetic that takes place outside of the traditional operating room (OR) but often performed within a fully licensed hospital. NORA locations include endoscopy suites, invasive radiology suites, magnetic resonance imaging (MRI) machine or an area in which electroconvulsive therapy (ECT) takes place. An ambulatory anesthetic is defined as one in which the patient arrives to the surgical venue on the day of the procedure, is anesthetized, and is discharged home later that same day.

An office-based anesthetic is one that is performed in an outpatient venue such as a freestanding medical or surgical office or procedure room that is not accredited as either an ambulatory surgery center (ASC) or a hospital. The surgical/medical office often provides practitioners with the space for other activities such as consultation with new patients, the performance of routine history and physicals, and office administration. Office-based practices are generally confined to one specialty such as urology, gastroenterology, plastic surgery, or dentistry,[1,2] but some surgical offices provide OR space for a number of surgical and procedural subspecialties.

Although an OBA practice may be an exciting alternative to the traditional hospital-based one, it requires the anesthesiologist to expand his or her role within the health-care delivery system. Along with providing safe anesthetics across the spectrum of young to old, and healthy to medically challenged patients undergoing increasingly complex procedures, the anesthesiologist must understand office safety and policy, legal and financial issues such as antitrust laws, state laws or regulations that may exist, the need for possible accreditation and billing and collection issues.[3,4] These are relatively new responsibilities for the anesthesiologist, who historically has worked as a member within a hospital department either in the private or academic setting, where these responsibilities are given to hospital administrators, lawyers, nurses, and other medical professionals. A further challenge to the office-based practitioner is that presently he or she has received little to no training in OBA within the anesthesia residency curriculum.[5]

Brief Historical Perspective of OBA

There have been reports of office-based surgery and anesthesia since the mid-nineteenth century. In 1856, John Snow documented his experience in providing anesthesia with chloroform for 867 dental patients, and approximately 3,021 teeth were extracted in private dental offices under his care.[6] In addition to dental care, the family physician often performed house calls where numerous small surgical procedures such as the lancing of boils and repair of wounds were conducted within the comfort of the patient's home. The physician's private medical office was, likewise, utilized in the service of this type of surgical care.

As surgery became more invasive, the need for intensive perioperative physiologic monitoring became increasingly necessary. The capacity to administer blood products and the development of an extensive array of pharmaceutical agents began to play a role in patient care, fostering the growth of larger health-care delivery teams to assist in patient care. Thus, over time, the inpatient hospital became the primary setting in which surgery would be performed.

Over the past several decades, as a result of both surgical and anesthetic advances, the surgical experience has again changed. Through innovations such as laparoscopic and endoscopic surgical capabilities, surgery has become increasingly less invasive and less painful. In addition, newer anesthetics have the benefit of a "fast-acting" profiles (associated with quick onsets and rapid termination of effect) and with fewer hemodynamic side effects, lending increasing numbers and types of procedures to be suitable for performance in outpatient venues.[7–9]

During the 1970s, less than 10% of all surgical and diagnostic procedures were performed on an ambulatory basis and, virtually all of these were performed in hospitals. By 1987, approximately 25 million, or 40% of all procedures, were performed on an ambulatory basis. In the United States, between 1984 and 1990, the number of office-based procedures increased from 400,000 to 1.2 million, and by 1994, 8.5% of all procedures were performed in offices.[10] In 1994, a landmark survey of the membership of the American Society of Plastic Surgeons (ASPS) revealed that 55% of the respondents performed the majority or all of their procedures in an office.[11] By the year 2000, approximately 75% of all procedures were performed on an outpatient basis; 17% in freestanding ASCs, and 14% to 25% (approximately 8 to 10 million) in physicians' offices.[12–16] By 2005, the American Hospital Association reported that although 82% of all procedures were performed on an ambulatory basis, 16% of all these ambulatory procedures were performed in private offices.[17] Even more recent data confirm that presently, 17% to 24% of all surgical procedures (approximately 10,000,000 procedures) are performed in private surgical offices annually.[18]

Advantages and Disadvantages of Office-based Surgery and Anesthesia

There are many advantages to an office-based procedure when compared to a traditional hospital-based one, with one of the most obvious being cost containment.[19] Several components make up the actual cost of a given surgical procedure. In addition to the professional fees of both the proceduralist and the anesthesiologist (which are usually negotiated prior to an elective procedure), there is a facility fee charged by the hospital or ASC. This fee generally covers the associated costs to the specific site, and includes overhead such as maintenance, equipment, and staffing. It often constitutes a large component of the patient's overall charge. In an office, this amount can easily be predicted and is often significantly less. The reason for this discrepancy is that although the overhead costs in a small office are usually quite reasonable and managed, the comparable costs in a large tertiary care hospital can be both enormous and unforeseen.[12,13,20,21]

To get a historical perspective of cost analysis, in 1994, Schultz determined the cost of an inhospital laparoscopic inguinal hernia repair to be $5,494. When the same procedure was performed in an office, the price was decreased to $1,534. Similarly, the average cost of an inhospital open inguinal hernia repair that same year was found to be $2,237, whereas only $894.79 when performed in a private office.[22] More recently, it has been reported that office-based ocular surgeries, performed under monitored anesthesia care (MAC), can cost 70% less than similar procedures performed in a hospital.[23] A recent study, found that when dental rehabilitation is performed in an office the cost is approximately 13 times less than when done in a hospital.[21] This change resulted in an average savings of $6,800 per case. It is understandable that insurance companies now offer incentives to surgeons who utilize an office location as their preferred surgical venue.[24]

Other clear advantages of office-based procedures include ease of scheduling (often with less paperwork), patient and surgeon convenience, decreased patient exposure to nosocomial infections, and both improved patient privacy and continuity of care, since an office is usually staffed by a small consistent group of personnel.[3,13,25,26]

There are potential disadvantages to an office-based procedure. These usually relate to patient safety, reporting, quality improvement, and peer review.[27] In some parts of the country, no regulations governing office-based surgery and OBA exist. Therefore, there may be little to no oversight regarding the certification/qualification of either the surgeon or anesthesiologist to perform the intended procedures, the surgical office's policy regarding peer review, performance and quality improvement, documentation, general policies and procedures, and the reporting of adverse outcomes. However, the number of such states without regulation and oversight is rapidly decreasing (Table 32-1).[28] It is therefore

Table 32-1 States That Have Regulations Regarding Office-based Surgery and Anesthesia

Alabama	New Hampshire
Arizona	New Jersey
California	New Mexico
Colorado	New York
Connecticut	North Carolina
Delaware	Ohio
District of Columbia	Oklahoma
Florida	Oregon
Georgia	Pennsylvania
Illinois	Rhode Island
Indiana	South Carolina
Kansas	Tennessee
Montana	Texas
Nebraska	Utah
Nevada	Virginia

imperative that the practicing anesthesiologist be familiar with all and any regulations that may be in place in his/her state.[29]

Office Safety

Media reports and newspaper articles raised the earliest questions regarding the safety of office-based procedures.[30] These exposés in the lay press may be legitimate. In fact, the remote location of an office may specifically confer an increased risk of injury during an office-based anesthetic.[31]

Data reveal that injuries and deaths occurring in offices are often multifactorial in causation. Reasons include toxicity of local anesthetics; prolonged surgery with occult blood loss; pulmonary embolism; and accumulation of multiple anesthetics resulting in oversedation, hypovolemia, hypoxemia, and the use of reversal drugs with short half-lives.[32-34] Both the Anesthesia Patient Safety Foundation and the American Society of Anesthesiologists (ASA) have emerged as leaders in the field of OBA safety and have advocated that the quality of care in office-based practice be no less than that of a hospital or ASC.[35,36] Thus, it is imperative to ensure that all safety precautions one may take for granted in a hospital be present in the surgical office.

In 1990, the mortality rate from anesthesia was approximately 1/100,000. By the year 2000, the rate had decreased to 1/250,000 in hospitals and 1/400,000 in freestanding ASCs.[37] Although the interpretation of these figures is open to debate, the decrease in mortality can be attributed, in part, to improvements in the training of the anesthesia providers, the safety profiles of the newer anesthetics, enhanced perioperative monitoring capabilities, and intrinsic safety mechanisms in place within the anesthetizing location. Since the majority of office-based patients are young and healthy, one would expect that anesthetics performed in offices would be at least equally as safe as those performed in hospitals, if not safer. However, reports of morbidity and mortality within office-based practices exist. In 1997, Morello et al. conducted a survey querying 418 accredited plastic surgeons' offices. They had a 57% response rate and found that over a 5-year period, 400,675 office procedures were performed; of these, 63.2% were cosmetic and 36.8% were reconstructive. Several outcomes were reviewed including hemorrhage, hypertension, hypotension, wound infection, and need for hospital admission and reoperation. There was an overall complication rate of 0.24%, and seven mortalities occurred, which were secondary to both surgery and anesthesia. They included two myocardial infarctions (MI) (one following an augmentation mammaplasty, the other 4 hours after a rhinoplasty), one case of cerebral hypoxia during an abdominoplasty, one tension pneumothorax during a breast augmentation, one cardiac arrest during carpal tunnel surgery, one stroke 3 days after a rhytidectomy and brow lift, and one unexplained death.[38] This information represented an overall mortality rate of 1 in 57,000. A later report by Hoefflin et al.,[39] however, found no complications after 23,000 plastic surgical procedures that occurred in a single office under general anesthesia (GA). Similarly, Sullivan et al. retrospectively reviewed the results in an office performing over 5,000 surgical procedures by five independent plastic surgeons. The primary anesthetic technique during this time period consisted of deep sedation in conjunction with local anesthesia or regional block, which was performed by an anesthesiologist supervising a certified registered nurse anesthetist (CRNA). No mortalities occurred over the 5-year period.[40] Bitar et al. retrospectively studied adverse outcomes in 3,615 consecutive patients undergoing 4,778 plastic surgery procedures in offices between 1995 and 2000. The anesthetics were MAC with midazolam, propofol, and an opioid, and again, no deaths were reported. Dyspnea occurred in 0.05% of patients, nausea and vomiting in 0.2%, and there was a 0.05% rate of hospital admissions.[41] When analyzing these outcomes, it must be appreciated that since the mortality rate from anesthesia is so low, an extremely large cohort group would be necessary to provide real data regarding the relative risk of an office-based anesthetic.

A close look at the more recent data again supports the supposition that an office-based procedure is as safe as a procedure done in a more traditional setting. Keyes et al. looked at adverse events in offices accredited by the American Association for Accreditation of Ambulatory Surgical Facilities (AAAASF) between 2001 and 2002. This group found no increase in morbidity and mortality in patients who had procedures with OBA, when compared to those having surgery in a freestanding ASC.[42,43] The group then analyzed the charts of 1,000,000 patients undergoing ambulatory procedures between 2001 and 2006. They found an overall mortality rate of 0.002% (with more than half the deaths being caused by a pulmonary embolism). They concluded that there is no increase in mortality for an ambulatory setting when compared to a freestanding hospital.[43] Similar results were reported by Soltani et al.[44] when looking at 5,500,000 patients undergoing outpatient surgery.

One important caveat when looking at safety records for office-based surgery is that there are no prospective randomized studies. All data are from retrospective chart reviews. When examining the literature, it becomes clear that there have been several studies that report a poor outcome for patients undergoing office-based procedures. According to closed malpractice claims in Florida, Rao et al. reported 830 deaths and 4,000 injuries associated with OBA between 1990 and 1999. These claims accounted for 30% of all malpractice claims in that state. Some more recent data have shown that office-based morbidity and mortality are usually the result of inadequate perioperative patient monitoring, oversedation, and thromboembolic events.[31,33,45] The challenge of acquiring accurate morbidity and mortality data for OBA is complicated by the fact that many offices are not required to report adverse events. In addition, although an anesthesiologist may not even be administering the anesthetic in an office, many complications may still be reported as anesthetic-related.

Why should the surgical venue affect the safety of a particular procedure? Again, the difference may be multifactorial. For example, traditional credentialing procedures, such as board certification and the granting or renewing of hospital privileges based on competency and proof of continuing medical education, may not be required or enforced in an office. Within and among offices, providers of anesthesia may also have varying degrees of both education and expertise. The provider may be an anesthesiologist, a nurse anesthetist, a dental anesthetist, or a surgeon with little or no training in anesthesia. Furthermore, safety within an anesthetizing location also depends on the perioperative patient monitoring capabilities. Although hospital patients are mandated by the accrediting organizations to have defined standards of care for monitoring in the ORs and postanesthesia care units (PACUs), these may be lacking in inadequately prepared and nonaccredited surgical offices.[41] There have been patient injuries reported during office-based procedures resulting from the use of obsolete and/or malfunctioning anesthesia machines, as well as from alarms that have not been serviced and/or are not functioning properly.[46] The ASA created guidelines for defining obsolete anesthesia machines which prohibit the use of any anesthesia machine that lacks essential safety features (e.g., oxygen ratio device, oxygen pressure failure alarm), has the presence of unacceptable features (e.g., copper kettles, or vaporizers with rotary concentration dials that increase vapor concentration when the dial is turned clockwise), or for which routine maintenance is no longer possible.[46]

Without prospective data regarding injuries occurring during office-based surgery, anesthesia databases offer the most reliable approximation. A review of ASA Closed Claims Project data, which incorporates information from the 35 liability insurers that indemnify approximately 50% of the practicing anesthesiologists in the United States, reveals safety concerns in office-based practices are more than theoretical.[32,47] As of 2001 there were 753 (13.7%) claims for ambulatory procedures and 14 (0.26%) for office-based ones. This small number of claims is most likely due to the 3- to 5-year time lag in reporting to the database.[37] ASA physical status 1 or 2 females who had undergone elective surgery under GA make up most of the claims filed. This statistic parallels the profiles of trends seen in ORs and freestanding ASCs. The injuries that occur in offices tend to be of greater severity than those that occur in ASCs. Twenty-one percent of the reported injuries sustained in offices were temporary and nondisabling in nature and 64% were permanent or led to death, while 62% of the injuries sustained in ASCs were temporary and nondisabling and only 21% were permanent or led to death.[37] A study by Coté et al.[48,49] concluded that the causes for injuries in offices ranged from human error to machine and equipment malfunction (Table 32-2).

The Closed-Claims Project database reveals that injuries during office-based procedures occur throughout the perioperative period, and are multifactorial in etiology. The majority, 64%, occurred intraoperatively, while 14% occurred in the PACU and 21% after discharge.[37] Half of these adverse events were respiratory and included airway obstruction, bronchospasm, inadequate oxygenation and ventilation, and unrecognized esophageal intubation. The second most common group of events were considered to be drug-related, occurring 25% of the time. These included incorrect agents or doses, allergies, and malignant hyperthermia (MH). Cardiovascular and equipment-related injuries each occurred in 8% of incidents.[37]

An important point to consider when looking at adverse events is whether or not they were preventable. Again, according to the information in the Closed-Claims Project database, only 13% of the events that occurred in ASCs were considered preventable, whereas 46% of the office-based ones were deemed so. Furthermore, all of the adverse respiratory events that occurred in the PACUs of offices could have been prevented, had pulse oximetry, and capnography been used. Care was considered to be substandard in 50% of OBA claims and in 34% of ASC ones. In 2001, claims originating from an office-based procedure resulted in a monetary award 92% of the time, with a median payment of $200,000 (ranging between $10,000 and $2,000,000), whereas claims originating from ASC-based procedures were compensated only 59% of the time with a median payout of $85,000 (ranging between $34 and $14,700,000).[37]

Table 32-2 Causes of Injury in the Office-based Practice[48,49]

- Inadequate resuscitation equipment
- Inadequate monitoring (most commonly lack of pulse oximetry)
- Inadequate preoperative or postoperative evaluation
- Human error
  - Slow recognition of an event
  - Slow response to an event
  - Lack of experience
  - Drug overdosage

Ensuring office-based practice safety is critical. After several highly publicized office liposuction injuries and deaths in August 2000, the State of Florida attempted to address this problem by placing a 90-day moratorium on all office-based procedures that utilized anesthetic depths greater than conscious sedation. During that time a safety panel comprised of surgeons, anesthesiologists, and other health-care professionals was formed and charged with the task of developing recommendations to improve the safety record of office-based procedures. The panel's recommendations focused on factors including patient selection, preoperative evaluation and testing, procedures to be excluded, surgeon qualification, and facility standards.[26,50] Other major organizations that played a leading role in developing standards for the office-based practitioner include the ASA, ASPS, the American Association of Nurse Anesthetists (AANA), and the American Medical Association (AMA).[35,50–52]

Patient Selection

Prior to presenting for an office-based procedure, the patient's medical condition should be optimally managed.[53] He or she should have a preoperative history and physical examination documented within 30 days prior to the procedure, and all pertinent laboratory tests as well as any medically indicated specialist consultation(s) must be readily available. Consent for the procedure and the anesthetic must also be in the chart. The anesthesiologist should have access to all of this information preoperatively and, when possible, contact the patient prior to the scheduled procedure. If a patient's ASA physical status is 1 or 2, the surgeon's office should arrange the surgery as per office protocol. However, if a patient has significant comorbid conditions, a preoperative anesthesiology consultation should be obtained before scheduling the patient for office-based surgery. A protocol regarding the scheduling of patients with significant comorbidities has become increasingly important in OBA. As OBA has become more commonplace, the medical/surgical community began to include older and sicker patients in this venue. There are many office-based practices that perform procedures on ASA 3 patients and several on ASA physical status 4 patients.[54]

Patient selection has always been a controversial topic among anesthesiologists practicing OBA because little morbidity and mortality data exist to support the inclusion or exclusion of specific populations. In 1982, Meridy[55] reported that patients should not be excluded from undergoing ambulatory procedures based solely on their age, the type of procedure, or the duration of the planned procedure. Conflicting recommendations do exist. The ASPS acknowledged that the ideal patient for an office-based procedure has an ASA physical status of 1 or 2. They recommended that ASA physical status 3 patients undergo an office-based procedure only after an anesthesia consultation and only have an office-based procedure performed under local anesthesia without sedation. The ASA also has developed recommendations regarding patient selection.[56] It is important to realize that the office is often remote, and the anesthesiologist may be unable to get assistance should it be required. Thus, groups of patients in whom anticipated anesthetic problems may develop should be avoided (Table 32-3). Individual anesthesiologists should therefore consider excluding certain patients with significant comorbid conditions in order to avoid unanticipated problems. Again, these are recommendations that are not based on evidence.

Morbidly obese patients and those with obstructive sleep apnea (OSA) syndrome present unique and increasingly frequent challenges to the office-based practitioner.[57] Indeed, they are usually the same population, with estimates of 60% to 90% of all

Table 32-3 Unsuitable Candidates for an Office-Based Procedure
• Poorly controlled diabetes
• History of substance abuse
• Seizure disorder
• Malignant hyperthermia susceptibility
• Potential difficult airway
▪ Morbid obesity
▪ Severe obstructive sleep apnea syndrome
• NPO (solid foods) < 8 h
• No escort
• Previous adverse outcome from anesthesia
• Significant drug allergies
• Aspiration risk

Table 32-4 Risk Factors for the Development of Deep Vein Thrombosis (DVT)
• Age > 40
• Antithrombin III deficiency
• Central nervous system disease
• Family history of DVT
• Heart failure
• History of a DVT
• Hypercoagulable states
• Lupus anticoagulant
• Malignancy
• Obesity
• Oral contraceptive use
• Polycythemia
• Previous miscarriage
• Radiation therapy for pelvic neoplasms
• Severe infection
• Trauma
• Venous insufficiency

OSA patients being obese (body mass index ≥30 kg/m^2).[58,59] Confounding this problem is that the majority of the patients with OSA syndrome have yet to be formally diagnosed.[60,61] In patients who have not been diagnosed with OSA syndrome, the STOP-Bang (snoring, tiredness, observed apnea, high blood pressure, BMI, age, neck circumference, male gender) questionnaire is a helpful and highly sensitive tool.[62–64]

Patients with OSA syndrome are often difficult to ventilate and intubate. One of the first steps in the ASA algorithm for management of the difficult intubation is to call for help, which, in an office, is usually not possible. Assuming an airway is secured during surgery, patients with OSA syndrome are likely to experience major anesthetic problems after extubation of the trachea.[65] These patients tend to be exquisitely sensitive to the respiratory depressant effects of even small dosages of sedation and/or narcotics.[51] They are prone to respiratory distress after extubation or may suffer from respiratory arrest with postoperative sedation or analgesia.[49,66] Although perhaps clinically unimportant, transient hypoxia is often seen during the recovery phase of patients with OSA syndrome.[67] Furthermore, respiratory depression may not be reversible with pharmacologic antagonism.[68] Some recommend that a postoperative observational unit with close monitoring of oxygen saturation or an intensive care unit setting be used for monitoring the OSA syndrome patient postoperatively.[69] It may thus be prudent to avoid performing GA in which narcotics are required during the perioperative period on any patient with severe OSA syndrome in an office-based venue.[70] An alternative would be to completely avoid administering any anesthetic in an office to a patient with severe OSA syndrome.

Pulmonary embolism has long been known to be a significant cause of perioperative morbidity and mortality from office-based surgical procedures.[71,72] Recent studies have revealed that this risk has not dissipated with time.[43,44] Even in 1998, Reinisch found that 0.39% (37/9,493) of patients who underwent rhytidectomy developed a deep vein thrombosis (DVT). Of these, 40.5% (15/37) went on to form a pulmonary embolism. Although GA had only accounted for 43% of the anesthetic techniques used for the procedure, 83.7% of the embolic events were associated with the patient having received a general anesthetic.[73] Studies by Keyes et al.[43] and Soltani et al.[44] confirm that pulmonary embolism (PE), in 2014, remains an important risk of an office-based procedure. Risk factors for the development of DVT appear in Table 32-4.[74] The ASPS recommends that patients be stratified according to risk and the prophylactic treatment be guided by risk (Table 32-5).

As more subspecialties begin to perform office-based procedures, and as the population ages, older and sicker patients will present for surgery and anesthesia.[75] The anesthesiologist must be the patient's advocate in the matter of safety. This advocacy can only result from a true understanding of how to adequately select appropriate patients for this unique surgical venue.

Surgeon Selection

The relationship between the surgeon and anesthesiologist must be one of mutual trust and understanding. Since the surgeon performing the procedure may also own the office, he or she must not put pressure on the anesthesiologist to perform an

Table 32-5 Recommended Treatment for Prevention of Deep Vein Thrombosis in Patients, Stratified by Risk[73,74]	
Cohort	Treatment
Low Risk	
No risk factors
Uncomplicated surgery
Short duration	• Comfortable position
• Knees flexed at 5 degrees
• Avoid constriction and external pressure
Moderate Risk	
Age >40 with no other risks
Procedure >30 min
Oral contraceptive use	• Proper positioning
• Intermittent pneumatic compression of calf or ankle (prior to sedation and continued until patient is awake and moving)
• Frequent alterations of the OR table
High Risk	
Age >40 with concomitant risk factors
Procedure >30 min	• Treatment as per patients with moderate risk
• Preoperative hematology consultation with consideration of perioperative antithrombotic therapy

anesthetic if he or she believes that the patient or procedure is not appropriate.

The surgeon must have a valid medical license, registration, and Drug Enforcement Administration (DEA) certificate. He or she should be either board eligible or board certified by a recognized member of the American Board of Medical Specialties, and either have privileges to perform the proposed procedure in a local hospital, or have training and documented competency comparable to a practitioner who does have such privileges in a hospital. Although this requirement may sound intuitive, there have been cases reported of surgeons performing procedures for which they have little or no training.[13] In addition, the surgeon must have adequate liability insurance, at least equal to that carried by the anesthesiologist. If a lawsuit should arise and the surgeon is inadequately insured, the anesthesiologist may be held financially responsible and become the "deep pocket." Similarly, the facility itself should have adequate liability insurance.

In addition, there should be a system in place for monitoring continuing medical education as well as peer review and ongoing quality improvement for the surgeon/proceduralist, anesthesiologist, and nursing staff. This provision is often not the case in an office-based practice.[13] If an anesthesia group provides care at more than one office, an overall peer review for the practice may be used; it need not be specific to each individual office-site. Solo anesthesia practitioners should not be exempt from this process. Anesthesiologists should only align themselves with the offices which have ongoing processes, or help organize one. The peer review committee should include surgeons, anesthesiologists, and nursing staff. It should meet regularly and maintain a written record of minutes and recommendations. Similarly, continuing medical education should also be documented and at a minimum should be sufficient to meet relicensing requirements.

When formulating a quality improvement program, there should be random chart reviews as well as key sentinel events that trigger a case review (Table 32-6). It is imperative that this review be an open forum to ensure continued quality improvement of care, and not be biased or hindered by fear of litigation. Legal counsel should be sought to determine whether information disclosed at these meetings is discoverable in a court of law, should a malpractice claim arise.

Office Selection and Requirements

The anesthesiologist should function as a zealous patient advocate in assuring that an anesthetic only is performed in a safe anesthetizing location. The office needs to be appropriately equipped, stocked, and maintained to perform GA (Table 32-7). All supplies must be age and size appropriate for the patient population. If an anesthesia machine or ventilator is present, it must be regularly serviced and calibrated. If potent inhaled volatile agents or N_2O is used, there must be a functioning waste gas scavenging system. This system may be exhausted via a window or roof vent. However, the exhaust must not be situated such that there is a possibility that it will be vented back into the office or into any other inhabited space. Further, it must be in accordance with Occupational Safety and Health Administration (OSHA), as well as state and federal standards. Portable scavenging systems presently available can be safely used. Air testing should be done on a regular basis. In an office without an exhaust system, total intravenous anesthesia (TIVA) techniques should be employed.

All offices, even those without ventilators or anesthesia machines, require a means to deliver positive pressure ventilation to the patient's lungs. This ventilation can be achieved by using a self-inflating resuscitation device. An adequate supply of compressed oxygen must be present as well as a back-up supply for use in an emergency. In offices that do not have a pipeline supply of oxygen, H cylinders are usually used and several E cylinders should be available in reserve. A policy must be in place describing the transport, storage, and disposal of medical gases, consistent with state and local laws. All equipment described in the ASA algorithm for management of the difficult airway should

Table 32-6 Sentinel Events That Should Trigger a Case Review and Be Presented at a Performance Improvement/Quality Assurance Meeting

- Death
- Neurologic injury
- Perioperative MI or stroke
- Aspiration
- Reintubation/unanticipated intubation postop
- Return to the operating room
- Peripheral nerve injury
- Adverse drug reaction
- Uncontrolled pain or nausea/vomiting
- Unexpected hospital admission
- Cardiac arrest
- Dental injury
- Incomplete charts
- Controlled substance discrepancy
- Patient complaints
- Corneal abrasion

Table 32-7 Equipment Required for Safe Delivery of Office-based Anesthesia

Monitors
    Noninvasive blood pressure with an assortment of cuff sizes
    Heart rate/electrocardiogram
    Pulse oximeter
    Temperature
Capnography
Airway supplies
    Nasal cannulas
    Oral airways
    Face-masks
    Self-inflating bag–mask ventilation device
    Laryngoscopes multiple sizes and styles (Mac and Miller)
    Handles
    Various sizes of tracheal tubes
    Stylettes
Emergency airway equipment (laryngeal mask airways, cricothyrotomy kit, transtracheal jet ventilation equipment)
A video laryngoscope
Suction catheters and suction equipment
Cardiac defibrillator
Emergency drugs
    Advanced cardiac life support drugs
    Dantrolene and malignant hyperthermia supplies
    Intravenous lipid infusion if nerve blocks are being performed
Anesthetic drugs
Vascular cannulation and IV equipment

be present.[76] A readily available means to create an emergency surgical airway and jet ventilation capability may be lifesaving.

Perioperative monitoring must adhere to the ASA standards for basic anesthetic monitoring.[77] These monitors include continuous monitoring of heart rate and oxygen saturation, intermittent noninvasive blood pressure monitoring, end-tidal carbon dioxide ($EtCO_2$) monitoring and the capacity for both temperature monitoring and continuous ECG. Monitors must be routinely serviced, calibrated and repaired as per manufacturers' recommendations (preventive maintenance is usually performed annually). All monitors should have a back-up battery supply and there should be an extra monitor available for an emergency. It is of interest to note that the ASA only requires $EtCO_2$ monitoring to be used if sedation is performed by an anesthesiologist; if sedation is performed by a nonanesthesiologist, the ASA has no such requirement. However, in 2014, the American Association of Oral and Maxillofacial Surgeons Board of Trustees mandated the use of capnography by all of its members for deep sedation and GA.[78]

All emergency drugs appearing on the American Heart Association Advanced Cardiac Life Support (ACLS) protocol should be immediately available. The expiration dates for these agents should be checked on a regular basis, and outdated drugs replaced. A cardiac defibrillator with a battery back-up must be immediately available and routinely checked and maintained, as should a source of suction including pharyngeal suction catheters. Having an "MH" cart containing at least 12 bottles of dantrolene is a requirement, if triggering agents are stocked in an office. A complete listing of MH supplies is available online at www.mhaus.org.[79] The office-based anesthesiologist should be familiar with the signs and symptoms of MH and be prepared to initiate treatment. It is recommended that the published MH algorithm be displayed in all areas where triggering agents are used. The office staff should undergo MH drills at least annually.

A protocol for the delivery and secure storage of controlled substances must be in place. A licensed anesthesiologist may supply these drugs in accordance with DEA regulations, as can any licensed physician with a current DEA registration certificate. Instead of transporting drugs, it is often more convenient to store them in the surgical office. In this situation, they must be stored in a double-locked storage cabinet installed in a secure location, in accordance with state and local regulations. The office in which the controlled substances will be dispensed must also be properly registered with the DEA. Drug accounting must be performed in accordance with state and federal regulations. Individual states have different provisions and regulations regarding the dispensing of controlled substances, and it is the responsibility of the dispensing physician to assure that the office-based practice is in compliance.

A medical director and a governing body, responsible for overall operations and ensuring high quality patient care, should be identified for every office. This provision even applies to solo practitioner offices. The governing body should meet regularly and amongst other duties, be responsible for the credentialing and privileging of all health-care providers. There must also be a policy and procedures manual that outlines the responsibilities of the governing body, each staff member including nurses (circulating/scrub and postop), physician assistants, surgical technicians, and office staff and administrators. The manual should include a description of the infection control policy, risk management, safety issues, anesthesia policies, and so forth. All nurses should be licensed by the state and have training and education consistent with their responsibilities. Basic cardiac life support (BCLS) certification should be mandatory and ACLS certification is preferable for nurses. In addition, either the anesthesiologist or the physician who supervises the anesthesia care provider must be ACLS or pediatric advanced life support (PALS) certified, depending on the patient population. There should always be at least one member of the health-care team with ACLS/PALS certification present in the office until the last patient has been physically discharged from the unit.

Emergencies such as cardiac arrest, earthquakes, hurricanes, and fires can and do occur in office-based settings (Table 32-8). Each office must have a plan in place delineating the responsibilities of each staff member, in the event of such an occurrence. The physical structure of the office is an important consideration. There should be a clear egress that would easily accommodate a stretcher carrying a mechanically ventilated patient. Adequate clearance and room for transport in an elevator must also be considered.

Destinations for a patient in need of hospital admission must be identified. Developing an office-hospital relationship is challenging, as hospitals may be reluctant to be involved in office mishaps. However, it is of utmost importance to have a formal written transfer agreement in place with a local hospital. Telephoning the emergency services number (911) is an acceptable plan for transportation, provided the response time is rapid. If 911 is unavailable in a specific city, or has a slow response time, the office should have a contractual agreement with a local ambulance company.

The office must be prepared to respond to an intraoperative fire. The ASA has published an advisory on the prevention and management of such an emergency.[80] Fire requires three components known as the "fire triad": an oxidizer (oxygen and nitrous oxide [N_2O]), an ignition source (electrocautery, laser, drill, etc.), and fuel (sponges, drapes, endotracheal tubes, solutions containing alcohol or other volatile compounds, etc.). The modern OR contains all three in great supply. The first step in fire prevention is education. All members of the surgical and anesthesia team must be educated on how fires are started, sustained, and prevented. There must be regularly scheduled fire drills that include all employees, even those with nonclinical duties. These drills should highlight the responsibilities of each staff member. A yearly meeting with the local fire marshal is often helpful.

Fire prevention is of the utmost importance. The ASA recommends that if flammable materials are used to prep the skin they should be allowed to completely dry prior to draping the surgical field. The field should then be draped in a manner that does not allow for oxygen to accumulate. These accumulated pockets of oxygen may flow into the surgical field, where there is a source of ignition such as electrocautery. There must be communication

Table 32-8 Emergencies That Require Contingency Plans

- Fire
- Bomb/bomb threat
- Power loss
- Equipment malfunction
- Loss of oxygen supply pressure
- Cardiac or respiratory arrest in the waiting room, operating room, or postanesthesia care unit
- Earthquake
- Hurricane
- External disturbance such as a riot
- Malignant hyperthermia
- Massive blood loss
- Emergency transfer of patient to a hospital

between the surgeon and anesthesiologist when an oxygen-rich environment is being created near a surgical site. This scenario is common during facial plastic surgery. Medical air insufflation or suctioning can be used to reduce oxygen accumulation and the use of N_2O avoided. When using an ignition source in an oxygen-rich environment, the ASA recommends reducing the oxygen flow as low as possible without creating hypoxia, and waiting several minutes to allow the oxygen to dissipate.[74]

The management of a fire will require recognizing the early signs, stopping the procedure and ignition source, extinguishing the fire, and delivering care to the patient. It may even be necessary to evacuate the building. In any case, it is imperative that all these steps be reviewed regularly and drills performed. The office should have at least a 1-hour firewall present to help prevent in the spread of the fire.

There must be contingency plans in the event of a power supply interruption or electrical failure. Each office should have an emergency generator capable of running necessary equipment and monitors; monitors should have battery back-up power that is routinely checked. Battery reserve power will usually last for 1.5 hours, but this duration needs to be verified for each piece of electrically powered equipment.

The office should keep patient records (including anesthesia records) in accordance with local laws, which is usually for a minimum of 5 to 7 years. Clinical records must be stored in a secure location, with access limited to medical professionals who are privileged to review these records. Similarly, the anesthesiologist should maintain his or her own records, which include the preanesthesia history and physical, informed consent, intraoperative documentation and postoperative care record, as well as discharge orders.

Accreditation

One way to objectively evaluate an office is to have it be accredited by a nationally recognized accrediting agency. The ASA has developed a classification of offices that stratifies them by the level of anesthetic depth that may be administered (Table 32-9).[56] Presently many states require offices to be accredited and more are following suit. In states that do not require accreditation, there are benefits to voluntarily obtaining it. Often accreditation will allow the facility fee to be reimbursed by a third-party payer in medically necessary procedures.[81] It should be noted that presently Medicare and Medicaid will not pay a facility fee for an office-based procedure. Another benefit of accreditation is that the patient may feel more comfortable undergoing a procedure in an office that has been accredited. Finally, as more states require accreditation, if a surgeon's office proactively becomes accredited in a state that subsequently requires it, there would be no interruption of services.

Currently there are three major accrediting bodies for office-based surgery offices, although several other agencies are also recognized. The Accreditation Association for Ambulatory Health Care (AAAHC) was the first major accrediting body, offering certification since 1998. The AAAASF, originally the Accreditation Association for Ambulatory Plastic Surgical Facilities (AAAAPSF), was the second, followed by The Joint Commission (TJC). To date, the most active organization in the accreditation of surgical offices is the AAAASF. Although its requirements are similar to those of AAAHC and TJC, the accreditation process is occasionally less expensive. Changes are currently underway to allow AAAHC and TJC to be more competitive.[3] Each agency has different criteria for eligibility and different accreditation cycles pertaining to the time limit of a certificate.[82] The agencies deal with the entire perioperative spectrum of running a surgical office, ranging from the actual facility through patient issues, governance, risk management, safety, infection, clinical record keeping, and administration (Table 32-10). Each agency has a workbook available to the practitioners to review all

Table 32-10 Factors Considered in Accrediting an Office for Surgical Procedures

- Governance
- Administration
- Clinical records
- Credentialing and privileging
- Safety
- Infection control
- Physical layout of the office
- Laboratory values
- Quality improvement
- Personnel records
- Surgeon qualification
  - Training
  - Local hospital privileges (surgical and admission)
- Peer review
- Anesthesiologist requirements
- Staffing intraoperatively and postoperatively
- Monitoring capabilities both intraoperatively and postoperatively
- Ancillary care
- Equipment
- Drugs (emergency, controlled substances, routine medications)
- Basic, advanced cardiac, and pediatric life support certification
- Temperature
- Neuromuscular functioning
- Patient positioning
- Pre- and postanesthesia care/documentation
- Quality assurance/peer review
- Liability insurance
- Postanesthesia care unit evaluation
- Discharge evaluation
- Emergency preparedness (fire/admission/transfer, etc.)
- A complete listing of criteria can be obtained from the individual agencies

Table 32-9 American Society of Anesthesiology Classification of Surgical Procedures[56]

Class A
Minor surgical procedures
Local, topical, or infiltration of local anesthetic
No sedation preoperatively or intraoperatively

Class B
Minor or major surgical procedures
Sedation via oral, rectal, or intravenous sedation
Analgesic or dissociative drugs

Class C
Minor or major surgical procedures
General anesthesia
Major conduction block anesthesia

requirements of accreditation. Of note, the AAAHC can accredit not only the surgical office but also an anesthesia group that provides OBA.

The accrediting agencies were developed, in part, to reduce some of the variability that exists among offices in regard to safety and administrative issues. Several professional societies are encouraging their members to perform procedures only in accredited facilities. The Society for Aesthetic Plastic Surgeons mandates that all of its members perform procedures only in offices that have been accredited by one of the nationally recognized accrediting agencies, or have been certified to participate in the Medicare program under title XVIII, or are licensed by the state. The actual improvement in safety conferred by performing surgery in an accredited office has yet to be determined, and there are those who suggest that it provides no advantage.[83] As long as there is no mandatory reporting system in place, it will be impossible to determine true incidence of morbidity associated with office-based practice. Presently, the only accrediting agency that requires reporting of all adverse outcomes in the AAAASF. In addition, several states have similar reporting mandates. Clearly though, safety in an office depends upon more than just accreditation; there must be constant vigilance by all members of the health-care team.

Procedure Selection

Early in the development of office-based surgery, procedures were generally noninvasive and of short duration. However, as newer surgical and anesthetic techniques have evolved, longer and more invasive procedures have been successfully performed.[84–91] Suitable office-based procedures range the gamut from superficial incision and drainage of abscesses to more invasive microlaparoscopies.

Duration of procedure has long been correlated with the need for hospital admission, with procedures lasting more than 1 hour being associated with a higher incidence of unplanned admission.[92] Other data have shown that longer procedures are also often associated with an increased incidence of postoperative nausea and vomiting (PONV), postoperative pain, and bleeding,[93,94] which may warrant hospital admission. For these reasons the ASPS has recommended that procedures be limited to 6 hours and be completed by 3 PM, thus allowing for a full patient recovery with maximum office staffing.[50] In addition, when determining the suitability of a procedure one must consider the possibility of hypothermia, blood loss, or significant fluid shifts.[50]

Specific Procedures

Liposuction

Liposuction is the most commonly performed cosmetic procedure performed primarily by plastic surgeons and dermatologists.[95,96] It is accomplished by inserting hollow rods into small incisions in the skin, and suctioning subcutaneous fat into an aspiration canister. Superwet and tumescent techniques, introduced in the mid-1980s, utilize large volumes (1 to 4 mL) of infiltrate solution (0.9% saline or Ringer lactate with epinephrine 1:1,000,000 and lidocaine 0.025% to 0.1%) for each 1 cc of fat to be removed. Blood loss is generally 1% of the aspirate with these techniques.[97] The peak serum levels of lidocaine occur 12 to 14 hours after injection and decline over the subsequent 6 to 14 hours.[98,99] Although the maximum dose of lidocaine has been traditionally limited to 7 mg/kg, 35- to 55-mg/kg doses have been used safely because the tumescent technique results in a single compartment clearance similar to that of a sustained-release medication.[100]

Liposuction is not a benign procedure.[101] In 2000, a census survey of the 1,200 members of the ASAPS, revealed an overall mortality rate of 19.1 per 100,000 liposuction procedures, with pulmonary embolism the diagnosis in 23.1% of deaths. Other etiologies of mortality included abdominal viscous perforation, anesthesia causes, fat embolism, infection, and hemorrhage; 28.5% of all deaths in this study were reported as of unknown or confidential etiology.[102] Risk factors identified included the use of multiliter wetting solution infiltration, mega-volume aspiration causing massive third spacing, multiple concurrent procedures, anesthetic sedative effects yielding hypoventilation, and permissive discharge policies. The management of the postoperative period, with attention to fluid and electrolyte balance and pain control, is critical to an optimal outcome after liposuction. The patient's fluid deficit, maintenance, intraoperative loss, and third spacing should guide fluid management throughout the perioperative period. Generally, an office liposuction should be limited to 5,000 mL of total aspirant which includes supernatant fat and fluid.[50] It is also recommended that large volume liposuction not be performed in conjunction with other procedures.

Iverson et al. developed the following considerations and recommendations regarding office-based liposuction[26,50]:

- Plastic surgeons should follow the current ASA Guidelines for Sedation and Analgesia.
- GA can be used safely in the office setting.
- GA has advantages for more complex liposuction procedures that include precise dosing of sedatives, controlled patient movement, and airway management.
- Epidural and spinal anesthesia in the office setting are discouraged because of the possibility of vasodilatation, hypotension, and fluid overload.
- Moderate sedation/analgesia augments the patient's comfort and is an effective adjunct to the anesthetic infiltrate solutions.

In 2002, 261 respondents to a survey sent to the membership of The American Society for Dermatologic Surgery reported no mortalities among 66,570 liposuction procedures performed in hospitals, ASCs, and offices. The authors reported adverse events, which mirrored those of the ASAPS. They found that serious adverse events occurred more frequently with procedures performed in hospital and ASCs than in offices. This difference may be due to the fact that, in hospitals, liposuction is performed on sicker patients or that the procedures are associated with removal of a larger amount of fat. Interestingly, 71% of the offices surveyed were nonaccredited. Further, the authors reported that morbidity correlated better with the area of the body suctioned (abdomen and buttocks as compared to extremities, which has lower associated morbidity), than the facility in which the procedure took place.[103]

Aesthetics

Many facial aesthetic procedures such as blepharoplasty, rhinoplasty, and meloplasty are routinely performed offices, usually under varying depths of MAC, but occasionally with GA. Facial plastic procedures that require use of a laser or even routine electrocautery, pose a problem for the anesthesiologist. Supplemental nasal oxygen in patients receiving sedation presents a fire hazard. Any supplemental oxygen must be turned off during periods of laser or electrocautery use about the face, and this requires vigilance by the anesthesiologist who must be in constant communication with the surgeon. Methods for delivering supplemental oxygen to a patient having a facial procedure include nasal cannula, an oxygen hood, or placement of oxygen tubing in an oral/nasal airway. The latter usually requires a deeper level of sedation. The avoidance of supplemental oxygen when medically appropriate is ideal.

Breast

Procedures such as breast biopsy or augmentation, implant exchange, or completion of transverse rectus abdominal muscle (TRAM) flap (i.e., nipple construction or revisions) are routinely performed in office settings. Breast augmentation entails separating the pectoralis muscles from the chest wall, which is painful and usually requires GA and can be accomplished by using either a laryngeal mask airway (LMA) or tracheal tube. The use of regional anesthesia with paravertebral nerve blocks has also been reported.[104] Breast surgery is associated with a high incidence of PONV; thus, it is likely that patients undergoing breast surgery will require antiemetic medication in addition to postoperative analgesics.[105]

Gastrointestinal Endoscopy

Procedures performed by gastroenterologists include esophageal, gastric and duodenal endoscopies (EGD) and colonoscopies. This patient population tends to be older, with significant comorbid conditions. Upper GI procedures rarely require endotracheal intubation because, although many of these patients have gastroesophageal reflux, the stomach is emptied under direct visualization. The endoscopist requires patient participation to aid in insertion of the endoscope, which can usually be accomplished with sedation using small doses of propofol with or without midazolam.

Colonoscopy is uncomfortable secondary to the insertion and manipulation of the endoscope, and may be associated with cardiovascular effects, including dysrhythmias, bradycardia, hypotension, hypertension, myocardial infarction, and death. The mechanism of these cardiovascular effects is not known, but there is evidence that they may be mediated by the autonomic nervous system when stimulated by anxiety or discomfort.[106] Adding an opioid to midazolam during colonoscopy has been shown to improve patient tolerance of the procedure and decrease pain without increasing the frequency of respiratory events.[107] Interestingly, anesthetic techniques consisting of midazolam,[108] remifentanil/propofol, and fentanyl/propofol/midazolam[109] lower the number of episodes of heart rate variability which reflects sympathetic activation as seen on continuous electrocardiography, and may contribute to the number of cardiovascular events that occur during colonoscopy.

Recently the gastroenterology community has sought to be able to provide moderate or even deep sedation with propofol without the assistance of a trained anesthesiologist.[110] However, due to safety concerns propofol may still only be given by an anesthesiologist as indicated in the product insert. In addition, the Institute for Safe Medical Practices has indicated that propofol may only be administered by individuals who are "trained in the administration of drugs that cause deep sedation and GA," dedicated to only providing the sedation (not also performing the procedure) and proficient at tracheal intubation.[111] The AAAASF has, likewise, indicated that anesthesia professionals are best qualified to administer propofol sedation. Every office should clearly delineate who is privileged and credentialed to administer propofol.

Dentistry and Oral and Maxillofacial Surgery

N$_2$O has been used for most of the world's office-based dental anesthetics since 1884, when Horace Wells, himself a dentist, had N$_2$O administered for a wisdom tooth extraction by a colleague. It was Harry Langa, another dentist, who pioneered the concept of using lower concentrations of N$_2$O in combination with local anesthetics. This idea of "relative analgesia" was the forbearer of "conscious sedation."[112]

The American Association of Oral and Maxillofacial Surgeons studied a prospective cohort of patients who underwent oromaxilofacial surger (OMS) surgery between January and December 2001. Of the 34,191 patients included, 71.9% received deep sedation or GA, 15.5% conscious sedations, and 12.6% local anesthesia. The operating surgeon provided anesthesia services in 96% of cases, and anesthesia-specific hospitalization rate was 4 per 100,000, with no reported mortalities. The authors attributed this safety level to the use of pulse oximetry, blood pressure and ventilation monitoring, as well as administration of supplemental oxygen.[113] Newer studies found that most patients are satisfied with the use of office-based sedation and GA.[115] Patients' biggest concerns and reason for dissatisfaction continue to be pain, nausea and vomiting, or being "awake" during the procedure.[114] Because office-based OMS procedures are so commonplace and patients are presenting with more comorbidities, it is likely that anesthesiologists will increase their presence in this arena.

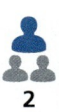

Orthopedics and Podiatry

Orthopedic offices provide excellent locations for anesthesiologists who practice regional anesthesia. Although knee arthroscopies can be performed with intra-articular local anesthesia and MAC, an adductor canal block with bupivacaine or ropivacaine, supplementing the intra-articular local anesthetic in an arthroscopically assisted anterior cruciate ligament repair will provide long-acting postoperative analgesia. Interscalene, supraclavicular, infraclavicular, and axillary blocks avoid airway manipulations in patients undergoing upper extremity procedures, whereas ankle blocks or blocks of the sciatic nerve in the popliteal fossa provide anesthesia for operations on the lower extremity. All of these blocks can be supplemented with short-acting anxiolytic agents.

Spinal anesthetics in the office-based setting must be of short duration secondary to limited PACU space. Lidocaine, which provides reliable short-acting analgesia, may be associated with an increased risk of transient neurologic symptoms in the ambulatory patient population,[115] whereas using procaine–fentanyl spinals are associated with nausea and vomiting as well as pruritus.[116] When the neuraxial anesthetic wears off, postoperative pain may arise; therefore, the patient must be discharged with oral analgesics as well as contact information for both the surgeon and the anesthesiologist.

Gynecology and Genitourinary

Many procedures, such as cervical dilation and curettage, vasectomy, and cystoscopy have been routinely performed in offices, often with local anesthesia and no sedation.[117] Recently there has been an increase in more invasive procedures (on older patients) such as minilaparoscopies, ovum retrieval, prostate biopsies, and lithotripsy, necessitating an anesthesiologist's expertise.[118] A variety of anesthetic options are available for these procedures and the anesthetic choice is dependent upon the surgeon, patient, and anesthesiologist's preferences.

Ophthalmology and Otolaryngology

Ophthalmologic procedures suitable for the office include cataract extractions, lacrimal duct probing, and ocular plastics.

Topical anesthesia and periorbital or retrobulbar blocks are frequently used to provide analgesia. Supplemental sedation may be required. Otolaryngology procedures include endoscopic sinus surgery, turbinate resection, septoplasty, and myringotomy.[119] Again, combinations of topical and regional nerve blocks with supplemental sedation are commonly employed, but occasionally GA is used.[120,121]

Pediatrics

Although no minimum age requirement for a child to undergo an office-based anesthetic has been established, patients greater than 6 months of age and ASA physical status 1 or 2 may be reasonable candidates.[20] Appropriate OBA pediatric cases are usually dental, and chloral hydrate with N_2O has historically been the anesthetic choice of many dentists. The use of these agents is however associated with significant morbidity. Ross et al.[20] found that in children between the ages of 1 and 9 years, 70 mg/kg of chloral hydrate with 30% N_2O resulted in hypoventilation in 94% of patients, which increased to 97% of patients when the chloral hydrate was combined with 50% N_2O. This increase is significant in view of the findings of Coté et al., who reviewed 95 adverse sedation-related events in pediatric patients. In the 93% of these cases that resulted in permanent neurologic injury or death, the anesthetic was delivered by an oral surgeon, periodontist, or CRNA supervised by a dentist.[48,49]

There are increasing numbers of ophthalmologic (examination under anesthesia, lacrimal duct probing), otolaryngology (myringotomy), cast/dressing changes, and minor plastics procedures being performed on children in offices. The American Academy of Pediatrics, Section on Anesthesiology has developed guidelines for the pediatric perioperative environment, which should be adhered to in the office setting (Table 32-11).[122]

Table 32-11 Considerations for the Pediatric Perioperative Anesthesia Environment

Patient Care Facility and Medical Staff Policies
Designation of operative procedures
Categorization of pediatric patients undergoing anesthesia
Annual minimal case volume to maintain clinical competence

Clinical Privileges of Anesthesiologists
Regular privileges
Special clinical privileges
Pain management

Patient Care Units
Preoperative evaluation and preparation units
Operating room
Anesthesiologists
Other health-care providers involved in perioperative care
Clinical laboratory and radiologic services availability and capabilities
Pediatric anesthesia equipment and drugs including resuscitation cart
PACU
  Nursing staff
  Anesthesiologist/physician staff
  Pediatric anesthesia equipment and drugs

Postoperative Intensive Care
Availability of transfer to local hospital intensive care unit, with arranged admissions through the emergency department

Anesthetic Techniques

The ASA recommends that anesthetics be provided or supervised by a fully licensed anesthesiologist.[56] If an anesthesiologist is directing anesthesia care, he or she must be immediately available throughout the entire perioperative period. Regulations in several states have questioned the need for this level of anesthesia training in the delivery of OBA. Some states allow for an anesthetic to be performed by a nonphysician anesthesia provider supervised by a licensed physician. In this situation, the supervising physician must be qualified to perform a preanesthetic focused history and physical examination as well as be immediately available throughout the perioperative period. He or she must know how to handle anesthetic-related emergencies and complications. The supervising physician must be ACLS certified.

OBA requires many levels of anesthesia ranging from moderate sedation through regional and GA.[123] Anesthesia is, however, a continuum and it is often impossible to predict how a patient will react. The ASA has developed definitions regarding depths of anesthesia (Table 32-12). Patients will routinely drift between the anesthetic depths; thus it is imperative that the anesthesia provider or supervisor be able to rescue a patient from a deeper level of anesthetic than was anticipated.

Table 32-12 Definitions of Levels of Sedation/Analgesia by the American Society of Anesthesiology

Minimal Sedation (Anxiolysis)
Drug-induced sedation
Patient responds normally to verbal commands
Cognitive and motor function may be impaired
Ventilatory and cardiovascular function maintained normally

Moderate Sedation/Analgesia (Conscious Sedation)
Drug-induced sedation
Patient responds purposefully to verbal commands either alone or with light tactile stimulation
Patient maintains a patent airway and spontaneous ventilation
Cardiovascular function maintained

Deep Sedation/Analgesia
Drug-induced sedation
Patient cannot be easily aroused but can respond purposefully to repeated or painful stimulation
Ventilatory function may be impaired, requiring assistance in maintaining a patent airway, and spontaneous ventilation may be inadequate
Cardiovascular function is usually maintained

General Anesthesia
Drug-induced loss of consciousness
Patients are not arousable by painful stimulation
Ventilatory function is often impaired; patient may require assistance in maintaining a patent airway
Spontaneous ventilation may be impaired as well as neuromuscular functioning
Positive pressure ventilation is often required
Cardiovascular function may be impaired

Adapted from American Society of Anesthesiologists. Continuum of depth of sedation: definition of general anesthesia and levels of sedation/analgesia. Blue Cross and Blue Shield of Tennessee website. http://www.bcbst.com/mpmanual/American_Society_of_Anesthesiologists_Definitions_.htm. Accessed June 6, 2106.

Table 32-13 Distribution of Types of Patient Injury during MAC Recorded in ASA Closed Claims Project Database during 1990s[125]

Injury	Occurrence
Death	34%
Brain damage	19%
Nerve damage	7%
Eye damage	12%
Myocardial infarction	4%
Stroke	4%
Burn	4%
Emotional distress	4%
Aspiration	4%

When formulating an anesthetic plan, one must consider that all agents and techniques used should be short acting, and patients should be ready for discharge home soon after the completion of the procedure. Furthermore, any agents used should have a high safety profile, few side effects, and be cost-effective. One must not be under the false impression that sedation is inherently safer than GA. Cohen et al.[124] reviewed the data from 100,000 anesthetics and found that the group with the greatest number of mortalities had undergone procedures with sedation, whereas sedation constituted only 2% of all cases. The complication rate related to MAC anesthetics is increasing, as its use expands.

The ASA Closed Claims Project database reveals that in the 1970s sedation (often referred to as MAC) cases accounted for 1.6% of the claims; in the 1980s, 1.9%; and by the 1990s, 6% of the cases were MAC. The injuries sustained in patients receiving MAC ranged from emotional distress to death (Table 32-13). The percentage of claims resulting from mortality was identical for both MAC and GA cases. In the 1990s, when injuries other than death occurred during MAC anesthetics, they were more likely to be permanent, whereas injuries occurring during GA were more frequently temporary.[125] MAC anesthetics also tend to lead to litigation. Suits were filed in 90% of the MAC claims; 65% were settled, 20% went to judgment, and 15% were discontinued. The range of payout was $2,000 to $6,300,000, with a median of $75,000.[125]

Anesthetic Agents

Intravenous sedation (propofol, barbiturates, midazolam, fentanyl) is the most often used anesthetic technique in the OBA setting. When selecting an anesthetic for an office-based procedure, one must consider factors such as duration of action, cost-effectiveness, and safety/side effects profile; drugs should have a short half-life, be inexpensive, and not be associated with undesirable side effects such as nausea and vomiting.

Because of its desirable pharmacokinetics and pharmacodynamics, propofol, a di-isopropyl phenol molecule, has long been a mainstay of ambulatory anesthesia. It has a rapid onset (approximately 1 arm-brain circulation time), and because of rapid redistribution, has a short clinical duration of action (approximately 15 minutes). Its short context-sensitive half-time causes propofol's clinical effect to be terminated relatively quickly, even after relatively long infusion times (8 hours).[126] In addition to its hypnotic properties, it has an intrinsic antiemetic effect. Propofol may cause a burning sensation on injection or elicit an allergic reaction. It is also associated with bradycardia and respiratory depression, and it supports microbial growth. It can be used alone or in combination with other agents by intermittent boluses or continuous infusion.

Fentanyl has long been the gold standard for "short-acting" narcotics, but recently the use of remifentanil has also increased in popularity. Remifentanil, an ultra–short-acting opioid, when combined with propofol for conscious sedation, has been shown to provide discharge readiness within 15 minutes after colonoscopy. This time frame is a marked reduction from the 48 to 80 minutes reported after the traditional meperidine/midazolam technique.[127] Remifentanil is also an ideal drug for use during many office-based procedures such as facial cosmetic procedures, which can be quite painful while the local anesthetic is being injected after which are relatively painless. An important caveat to the use of remifentanil is that it may cause nausea and vomiting as well as apnea. Infusions of remifentanil are also associated with acute tolerance and hyperalgesia during the recovery phase, which may limit its utility.[128–131] In addition, it often requires the use of an infusion pump.

Ketamine, a phencyclidine derivative, has experienced a resurgence in popularity over the past several years in the OBA practice. The use of ketamine–propofol sedation has been described as an excellent way to provide a relaxed surgical field in a quiet, immobile patient, often eliminating the need for supplemental oxygen.[132] Ketamine functions as both an anesthetic and an analgesic. It does not depress respiration, and will increase laryngeal reflexes, thus decreasing the risk of aspiration. Furthermore, it is not associated with nausea and vomiting. Ketamine can, however, cause an increase in secretions as well as cause hallucinations. The latter can be decreased or eliminated by adding propofol or midazolam.[133–136] Glycopyrrolate can be used as an antisialagogue. Another advantage of ketamine is that it is relatively inexpensive.

Clonidine has been found to be useful in an office. Since it is an α_2-agonist, clonidine will help control blood pressure throughout the perioperative period, thus potentially minimizing blood loss.[137,138] In addition it may decrease the total propofol usage.[113] Its use may however precipitate hypotension and oversedation.

Dexmedetomidine has also recently become a mainstay infusion drug for an office-based anesthetic.[139] It is a short-acting, α_2-adrenergic receptor agonist with sedative qualities. Dexmedetomidine permits patients to retain their respiratory drive and does not cause nausea and vomiting. It is however associated with hypotension.

TIVA is a common choice for non-OR anesthetics. TIVA usually consists of propofol as the hypnotic component used in conjunction with fentanyl, remifentanil, or ketamine as the analgesic component. All of these drugs can be given by intermittent bolus or infusion. Mathews found that remifentanil 0.085 μg/kg/min can substitute for 66% N_2O.[140] Advantages of TIVA over inhalation anesthesia include the avoidance of the need for gas scavenging and a reduced incidence of PONV. Since the availability of the newer less soluble inhalation agents (e.g., desflurane and sevoflurane), many authors have compared recovery times from these agents with the recovery time after a total intravenous anesthetic using a propofol infusion.[141,142] Recently, Gupta conducted a meta-analysis of all such publications and reported an overall more rapid recovery from desflurane when compared to either isoflurane- or propofol-based anesthetics. Recovery was also found to be faster with sevoflurane when compared to isoflurane. However, there was more PONV as well as postdischarge nausea and vomiting in the isoflurane groups as compared to the propofol ones; for these considerations isoflurane may not be the best choice of inhalation agent in non-OR locations. Overall, the inhalation agent groups required more antiemetic treatment than did the propofol groups.[143]

Depth of anesthesia monitoring has been shown to decrease the time to extubation and discharge readiness.[144–146] A depth of anesthesia monitor has been described as useful in the office during MAC procedures, resulting in a possible decrease in total propofol usage.[147] Whether this type of monitoring will prove to be cost-effective or not, in office-based settings, remains to be seen.

Any type of anesthesia from sedation through GA and regional anesthesia can be administered in an office setting safely but it is vital that the office be adequately equipped and staffed to rescue a patient from a deeper stage of anesthesia. Thus, if MAC is planned, GA must be anticipated.

Postanesthesia Care Unit

Following an office-based procedure, a patient should be able to sit in a chair, or ambulate to an examination room to dress almost immediately postoperatively, and be free of pain and PONV. All vital signs should be within 10% of baseline. A formal PACU may not be present, and the patient may be required to recover in the surgical suite. Regardless of where the patient recovers, it is important to adhere to all the ASA standards for monitoring and documentation throughout the postoperative period. Staffing in the recovery area must be adequate, and the use of a pulse oximeter is imperative.[148] It is recommended that there be at least one ACLS/PALS certified member of the health-care team present until the last patient has left the office.

Since PACU space in an office is often limited and the anesthesiologist may have multiple locations to attend in a single day, patient satisfaction and prevention of PONV and pain are paramount. The effect of these physiologic occurrences may also have a profound economic impact on an office surgical unit.[149] It is imperative that every anesthetic administered be designed to maximize postoperative patient alertness and mobility and minimize the risks of the need for a prolonged PACU stay. Twersky has recommended that the postanesthesia discharge scoring system and clinical discharge criteria used in ambulatory surgery also be used in the office-based setting.[150] Interestingly, there is a trend to discharge patients, particularly after colonoscopy, without escorts. This practice has been sanctioned in some states. In New York, regulations require that all patients undergoing a procedure with anesthesia be "discharged in the company of a responsible adult, unless exempted by a physician."[151] Specific data confirming the enhanced safety of this practice do not exist.

Local anesthesia alone, minimal to moderate and deep sedation supplemented by wound infiltration with local anesthetics, or peripheral nerve blocks, often form the basis for a multimodal strategy for postoperative pain management. These effective pain relief techniques not only decrease the anesthetic and analgesic requirements during surgery but also reduce the need for opioid analgesics in the postoperative period, thus facilitating the recovery process.[152] Nonopicid analgesics (e.g., acetaminophen) and nonsteroidal anti-inflammatory drugs (e.g., ketorolac) are routinely used. Ketorolac decreases the incidence of PONV and patients tolerate oral fluids and meet discharge criteria sooner than those receiving opioids.[153] In an effort to minimize the potential for postoperative bleeding and risk of gastrointestinal (GI) complications, more specific COX-2 inhibitors are being increasingly used as nonopioid adjuvants for minimizing postoperative pain.[154]

An optimal antiemetic regimen for OBA has yet to be established. However, since the etiology of PONV is multifactorial, combination prophylactic therapies may be beneficial in high-risk patients.[155] Many of the older first-line therapies are associated with sedation, drowsiness, and extrapyramidal side effects, and have been supplanted by $5-HT_3$ antagonists such as ondansetron, dolasetron, and granisetron.[156] Dexamethasone has been shown to improve the efficacy of both $5-HT_3$ antagonists[157] as well as dopamine antagonists when used for the prevention of PONV.[156] Dexamethasone has no utility as a rescue drug for PONV.[158] Routine prophylaxis of all patients, though, has not been shown to offer any advantage over symptomatic treatment[159] and has associated costs. Prophylaxis should be considered for all patients with a high risk of PONV. Such patients include, young women having breast or gynecologic surgery, nonsmokers, or patients with a history of PONV. Ensuring adequate hydration (up to 20 mL/kg of crystalloid), to avoid orthostatic hypotension and, thus, to prevent the release of emetogenic chemicals by decreasing blood flow to the midbrain emetic centers is an intervention that may be successful in the prevention of PONV.[156]

Regulations

Governmental oversight of office-based surgery varies among states; currently regulations exist in the majority of states with others following. A complete list of regulations in each of the states is available online.[28] Whereas accreditation is often a voluntary certification of an office, in some states, regulations, which are governmental mandates imposed by the local or state government, exist. It is imperative that anesthesiologists embarking on an office-based practice familiarize themselves with any rules and regulations that govern practice in his/her particular state.

In 1994, California was the first state to adopt legislation regarding OBA, and was soon followed by New Jersey. A closer look at these two states provides an example of the varied requirements being enforced by states throughout the country. California's regulations pertain to patients undergoing a GA, and do not address procedures performed under local, peripheral nerve block, or sedation/anxiolysis administered in doses that do not affect a patient's life-preserving reflexes.[160] The regulations deal with issues ranging from office policy and mandatory reporting of adverse outcomes, to surgeon and anesthesia provider qualifications.[160] California Health and Safety Code 1248-1248.85 mandates that surgical procedures occur only in offices that have been accredited or have been certified to participate in the Medicare Program under Title XVIII (42 U.S.C. Sec. 1395 et seq.), with very few exceptions.[161] In addition, offices must have a written plan in place that deals with issues regarding emergency admissions. Surgeons must have admitting privileges at a local licensed or accredited acute care hospital or have a written transfer agreement with a physician who does have such privileges. Offices must have an agreement with the hospital for the admission, in accordance with the hospital's system of quality assurance and peer review. California law also requires that offices have adequate patient monitoring throughout the perioperative period, and have a system in place for the storage and maintenance of patient records. Any office that fails to comply with these regulations risks sanctions ranging from reprimand with or without monetary penalties to criminal prosecution.

New Jersey's administrative Code 13:35-4A.1-13:35-4A.18 develops criteria for patient selection. Only ASA physical status

1 and 2 patients may undergo GA or regional anesthesia. ASA physical status 3 patients can undergo only conscious sedation. Providers of GA must be credentialed to do so by a hospital, and only appropriately credentialed physicians may supervise CRNAs. New Jersey law establishes guidelines regarding mandatory monitoring, emergency supplies that must be present, physician credentialing, and peer review. In contrast to California, New Jersey's regulations pertain to all patients undergoing surgical procedures regardless of the anesthetic depth. However, similar to California, violations may result in fines ranging from reprimand to license revocation and criminal prosecution.[162]

In states that have no regulations regarding office-based surgical procedures any physician who holds a valid medical license may perform any procedure that he/she so chooses, within his/her office without oversight. A surgeon may perform a procedure for which he/she may have had little to no training, and may sedate a patient without any training in anesthesia or airway management. In fact, there have been reported cases of patients undergoing procedures without any preoperative evaluation, pertinent laboratory tests, informed consent, intraoperative or postoperative monitoring or operative report, and without regard for sterile technique.[13] It is therefore imperative that the anesthesiologist continues to maintain the role of a zealous patient advocate, and help to educate the surgeon as to what constitutes a safe anesthetizing location.

Business and Legal Aspects

It is in the anesthesia provider's best interest to seek legal counsel and to create a valid business model before embarking on a career in OBA. This model must consider the overhead costs associated with staffing and running a safe surgical office as well as the potential and probable case load and patient insurance mix. An OBA division within a department may provide benefits to an academic practice, in addition to the monetary ones. There may be an intangible benefit to the community it serves, as well enhancing the anesthesia training program.[5] It would however become necessary to involve the American Board of Anesthesiology (ABA) as well as the American College of Graduate Education (ACGME) to ensure that any resident rotation outside the ACGME-approved hospital setting is acceptable.

Many OBA groups have formed either professional corporations or limited liability companies. Although not eliminating the need for liability insurance, both of these arrangements serve to protect the private assets of the anesthesiologists in the case of a malpractice claim.[3] Legal counsel may also prove to be beneficial in creating business plans that follow all state and federal laws regarding billing/collection and antitrust.[163]

It is imperative to have an aboveboard and legal relationship with every office in which anesthesia services are being delivered. Billing strategies must be legal and ethical. In this complex environment of third-party payers it is quite easy to make legal errors. Ignorance of the law offers no protection or excuse, and one should seek the advice of expert billing agencies, even if one chooses not to outsource this responsibility. In calculating pricing one must include all overhead charges such as drugs, equipment, time, and business expenses including malpractice insurance. A pricing structure with the surgeon must exist before embarking on a clinical relationship. One must outline specifically what will be provided by the office (intravenous equipment, antibiotics, monitors, etc.) and what the anesthesiologist will supply. These decisions take on further legal implications when the office is receiving a facility fee.

Conclusions

OBA continues to rapidly expand and pose unique challenges to anesthesiologists, who must not only provide medical care in remote environments but also have a solid business sense and an extensive understanding of OR management. Although regulations have not kept pace with the growth of OBA, it is imperative that anesthesiologists make it their responsibility to help ensure that every possible safety measure is afforded to their patients. Decisions about appropriate patient/procedure selection and equipping anesthetizing locations must be made in conjunction with surgeons. All clinical decisions and anesthetic choices must take into consideration the need for rapid turnover and limited PACU availability. Any depth of anesthesia from minimal sedation through regional anesthesia and GA may be delivered as long as the proper safeguards are in place.

The many advantages afforded by office-based surgery are fueling its evolution and as more complex procedures are performed on patients with increasing numbers of comorbidities. The anesthesiologist's role in providing care and serving as their patients' advocate is both complex and vital.

REFERENCES

1. Twersky R, Saad M. Office-based anesthesia: successes and challenges. *ASA Refresher Courses Anesthesiol*. 2013;41:125–134.
2. Office based anesthesia and surgery. American Society of Anesthesiologists website. http://www.asahq.org/lifeline/types%20of%20anesthesia/office%20based%20anesthesia%20and%20surgery. Accessed June 2, 2016.
3. Koch ME, Dayan S, Barinholtz D. Office-based anesthesia: an overview. *Anesthesiol Clin North Am*. 2003;21:417–443.
4. Federation of State Medical Boards. Office-based surgery: states N–Z. FSMB website. https://www.fsmb.org/Media/Default/PDF/FSMB/Advocacy/GRPOL_Office_Based_Surgery_N-Z.pdf. Accessed June 2, 2016.
5. Hausman LM, Levine AI, Rosenblatt MA. A survey evaluating the training of anesthesiology residents in office-based anesthesia. *J Clin Anesth*. 2006;18:499–503.
6. Snow J. *On Chloroform and Other Anesthetics*. London, UK: John Churchill; 1858:314–315.
7. Tang J, White PF, Wender RH, et al. Fast-track office-based anesthesia: A comparison of propofol versus desflurane with antiemetic prophylaxis in spontaneously breathing patents. *Anesth Analg*. 2001;92(1):95–99.
8. White PF, Song D. New criteria for fast-tracking after outpatient anesthesia: A comparison with the modified Aldrete's scoring system. *Anesth Analg*. 1999;88(5):1069–1072.
9. Cullen KA, Hall MJ, Golosinsky A. *Ambulatory surgery in the United States, 2006. National Health Statistics Report, No. 11*. Hyattsville, MD: National Center for Health Statistics; 2009.
10. Lazarov SJ. Office-based surgery and anesthesia: Where are we now? *World J Urol*. 1998;16:384–385.
11. Courtiss EH, Goldwyn RM, Joffe JM, et al. Anesthetic practices in ambulatory surgery. *Plast Reconstr Surg*. 1994;93:792–801.
12. Wetchler BV. Online shopping for ambulatory surgery: Let the buyer beware! *Ambul Surg*. 2000;8:111.
13. Quattrone MS. Is the physician office the wild, wild west of health care? *J Ambul Care Manage*. 2000;23:64–73.
14. Laurito CE. Report of educational meeting: The Society for Office-Based Anesthesia, Orlando, Florida, March 7, 1998. *J Clin Anesth*. 1998;10:445–448.
15. American Hospital Association (AHA). Trendwatch chartbook 2007: trends affecting hospitals and health systems, April 2007. Chart 2.5: percentage of outpatient surgeries by facility type, 1981-2005. http://www.aha.org/research/reports/tw/chartbook/2007chartbook.shtml
16. Kurrekk MM, Twersky RS. Office-based anesthesia: How to start an office-based practice. *Anesthesiol Clin*. 2010;28:253–267.
17. American Hospital Association website. http://www.aha.org/research/reports/tw/05econcontribwithtax.pdf. Accessed June 2, 2016.
18. Kurrek MM, Twersky RS. Office-based anesthesia, how to start an office-based practice. *Anesthesiol Clin*. 2010;28(2):353–367.
19. Shapiro FE, Punwani N, Rosenberg NM, et al. Office-based anesthesia: safety and outcomes. *Anesth Analg*. 2014;119(2):276–285.
20. Ross AK, Eck JB. Office-based anesthesia for children. *Anesthesiol Clin North Am*. 2002;20:195–210.
21. Rashewsky S, Parameswaran A, Sloane C, et al. Time and cost analysis: pediatric dental rehabilitation with general anesthesia in the office and the hospital setting. *Anesth Prog*. 2012;59(4):147–153.

22. Schultz LS. Cost analysis of office surgery clinic with comparison to hospital outpatient facilities for laparoscopic procedures. *Int Surg*. 1994;79:273–277.
23. Bartamian, M, Meyer DR. Site of service, anesthesia, and postoperative practice patterns for oculoplastic and orbital surgeries. *Ophthalmology*. 1996;103:1628–1633.
24. Way JC, Culham BA. Establishment and cost analysis of an office surgical suite. *Can J Surg*. 1996;39:379–383.
25. Anello S. Office-based anesthesia: advantages, disadvantages and the nurse's role. *Plast Surg Nurs*. 2002;22:107–111.
26. Iverson RE, Lynch DJ. ASPS Task Force on Patient Safety in Office-Based Surgery Facilities: Patient safety in office-based surgery facilities: II. Patient selection. *Plast Reconstr Surg*. 2002;110:1785–1790.
27. Metzner J, Posner KL, Domino KB. The risk and safety of anesthesia at remote locations: The US closed claims analysis. *Curr Opin Anesthesiol*. 2009;22:502–508.
28. State requirements for accreditation. Accreditation Association for Ambulatory Health Care website. https://www.aaahc.org/en/news/Federal-and-State-Regulations/State-Laws-and-Regulations/. Accessed June 2, 2016.
29. Legislative reference. American Association for the Accreditation of Ambulatory Surgical Facilities website. http://www.aaaasf.org/pub/asc_legislative_reference.pdf. Accessed June 5, 2016
30. Arens J. Anesthesia for office-based surgery: are we paying too high a price for access and convenience? *Mayo Clin Proc*. 2000;75:225–228.
31. Missant C, Velde M. Morbidity and mortality related to anesthesia outside the operating room. *Curr Opin Anesthesiol*. 2004;17:323–327.
32. Vila H, Soto R, Cantor AB, et al. Comparative Outcomes analysis of procedures performed in physician offices and ambulatory surgery centers. *Arch Surg*. 2003;138:991–995.
33. Clayman MA, Caffee HH. Office surgery safety and the Florida moratoria. *Ann Plast Surg*. 2006;56:78–81.
34. Melloni C. Morbidity and mortality related to anesthesia outside the operating room. *Minerva Anestesiol*. 2005;325–334.
35. American Society of Anesthesiologists. *Directory of Members*. Park Ridge, IL: ASA; 2000:480.
36. Anesthesia Patient Safety Foundation. Office based anesthesia growth provokes safety fears. *APSF*. 2000;15:1.
37. Domino KB. Office-based anesthesia: Lessons learned from the closed-claims project. *ASA Newslett*. 2001;65:9.
38. Morello DC, Colon GA, Fredricks S, et al. Patient safety in accredited office surgical facilities. *Plast Reconstr Surg*. 1997;99:1496–1500.
39. Hoefflin SM, Bornstein JB, Gordon M. General anesthesia in an office-based plastic surgical facility: a report on more than 23,000 consecutive office-based procedures under general anesthesia with no significant anesthetic complications. *Plast Reconstr Surg*. 2001;107:243–251.
40. Sullivan PK, Tattini CD. Office-based operatory experience: an overview of anesthetic technique, procedures and complications. *Med Health RI*. 2001;84:392.
41. Bitar G, Mullis W, Jacobs W, et al. Safety and efficacy of office-based surgery with monitored anesthesia care/sedation in 4778 consecutive plastic surgery procedures. *Plast Reconstr Surg*. 2003;111:157–158.
42. Keyes GR, Singer R, Iverson RE, et al. Analysis of outpatient surgery center safety using an internet based quality improvement and peer review program. *Plast Reconstr Surg*. 2004; 113(6):1760–1770.
43. Keyes GR, Singer R, Iverson RE, et al. Mortality in outpatient surgery. *Plast Reconstr Surg*. 2008;122(1):245–250.
44. Soltani AM, Keyes GR, Singer R, et al. Outpatient surgery and sequelae: An analysis of the AAAASF internet-based quality assurance and peer review database. *Clin Plast Surg*. 2013;40(3):465–473.
45. McDevitt NB. Deep vein thrombosis prophylaxis. *Plast Reconstr Surg*. 1999;104:1923–1928.
46. Dorsch JA. Guidelines published for determining anesthesia machine obsolescence. Anesthesia Patient Safety Foundation website. http://www.apsf.org/newsletters/html/2004/winter/05guidelines.htm. Accessed June 6, 2016.
47. Robbertze, R, Posner KL, Domino K. Closed claims review of anesthesia for procedures outside the operating room. *Curr Opin Anesthesiol*. 2006;19:436–442.
48. Coté CJ, Karl HW, Notteman DA, et al. Adverse sedation events in pediatrics: analysis of medications used for sedation. *Pediatrics*. 2000;106:663–644.
49. Coté CJ, Notteman DA, Karl HW, et al. Adverse sedation events in pediatrics: a critical incident analysis of contributing factors. *Pediatrics*. 2000;105:8–15.
50. Iverson R, ASPS Task Force on Patient Safety in Office-Based Surgery Facilities: Patient safety in office-based surgery facilities. I. Procedures in the office-based surgery setting. *Plast Reconstr Surg*. 2002;110:1337–1342.
51. Tunajek SK. Office based procedure standards. *AANA J*. 1999;67:115–120.
52. American Medical Association House of Delegates at the I-01 Meeting. Office-based surgery core principles. *Am Soc Anesthesiol Newslett*. 2004;68:14.
53. Haeck PC, Swanson JA, Iverson RE, et al. Evidence-based patient safety advisory: patient selection and procedures in ambulatory surgery. *Plast Reconstr Surg*. 2009;124:6S–38S.
54. Shapiro FE, Jani SR, Liu X, et al. Initial results from the national anesthesia clinical outcomes registry and overview of office-based anesthesia. *Anesth Clin*. 2014;32:431–444.
55. Meridy HW. Criteria for selection of ambulatory surgical patients and guidelines for anesthetic management: a retrospective of 1553 cases. *Anesth Analg*. 1982;61:921–926.
56. American Society of Anesthesiologists Committee on Ambulatory Surgical Care and the American Society of Anesthesiologists Task Force on Office-Based Anesthesia. *Office-Based Anesthesia: Considerations for Anesthesiologists in Setting Up and Maintaining a Safe Office Anesthesia Environment*. Park Ridge, IL: American Society of Anesthesiologists; 2000.
57. Haeck PC, Swanson JA, Iverson RE, et.al. Evidence-based patient safety advisory: patient assessment and prevention of pulmonary side effects in surgery. Part 1. Obstructive sleep apnea and obstructive lung disease. *Plast Reconstr Surg*. 2009;124S:45S–56S.
58. Benumof JL. Obstructive sleep apnea in the adult obese patient: Implications for airway management. *J Clin Anesth*. 2001;13:144–156.
59. Boushra NN. Anaesthetic management of patients with sleep apnea syndrome. *Can J Anaesth*. 1996;43:599–616.
60. Benumof JL. Policies and procedures needed for sleep apnea patients. *APSF Newslett*. 2002–3; Winter 57.
61. Young T, Evans L, Finn L, et al. Estimation of the clinically diagnosed proportion of sleep apnea syndrome in middle-aged men and women. *Sleep*. 1997;20:705–706.
62. Chung F, Abdullah HR, Liao P. STOP-Bang questionnaire: a practical approach to screen for obstructive sleep apnea. *Chest*. 2016;149(3):631–638.
63. Chung F, Liao P, Farney R. Correlation between the STOP-Bang score and the severity of obstructive sleep apnea. *Anesthesiology*. 2015;122(6):1436–1437.
64. Chung F, Yang Y, Brown R, et al. Alternative scoring models of STOP-Bang questionnaire improve sensitivity to detect undiagnosed obstructive sleep apnea. *J Clin Sleep Med*. 2014;10(9):951–958.
65. Lofsky A. Sleep apnea and narcotic postoperative pain medication: A morbidity and mortality risk. *APSF Newslett*. 2002;17:24.
66. Xara D, Mendonca J, Pereira H, et al. Adverse respiratory events after general anesthesia in patients at high risk of obstructive sleep apnea. *Braz J Anesthesiol*. 2015;65(5)359–366.
67. Kurrek MM, Cobourn C, Wojtasik Z, et al. Morbidity in patients with or at high risk for obstructive sleep apnea after ambulatory laparoscopic gastric banding. *Obes Surg*. 2011;21(10):1494–1498.
68. Samuels SI, Rabinov W. Difficulty reversing drug-induced coma in a patient with sleep apnea. *Anesth Analg*. 1986;65:1222–1224.
69. Benumof JL. Creation of observational unit may decrease sleep apnea risk. *APSF Newslett*. 2002;17:39.
70. Ankichetty S, Chung F. Considerations for patients with obstructive sleep apnea undergoing ambulatory surgery. *Curr Opin Anesthesiol*. 2011;24(6):605–611.
71. Coldiron B, Shreve E, Balkrishnan R. Patient injuries from surgical procedures performed in medical offices: Three years of Florida data. *Dermatol Surg*. 2004;30:1435–1443.
72. Claymen MA, Seagle BM. Office surgery safety: The myths and truths behind the Florida moratoria—six years of Florida data. *Plast Reconstr Surg*. 2006;118:777–785.
73. Reinisch JF, Russo RF, Bresnick SD. Deep vein thrombosis and pulmonary embolism following face lift: A study of incidence and prophylaxis. *Plastic Surg For*. 1998;21:159.
74. Davison SP, Venturi ML, Attinger CE, et al. Prevention of venous thromboembolism in the plastic surgery patient. *Plast Reconstr Surg*. 2004;114;43E–51E.
75. Galway U, Borkowski R. Office-based anesthesia for the urologist. *Urol Clin North Am*. 2013;40:497–515.
76. American Society of Anesthesiologists. Practice guidelines for management of the difficult airway: An updated report. *Anesthesiology*. 2003;98:1269–1277.
77. American Society of Anesthesiologists. *Standards for Basic Anesthetic Monitoring*. Park Ridge, IL: American Society of Anesthesiologists; 2001:493.
78. Matin MB, Gonzalez ML, Dodson TB. What factors influence community oral and maxillofacial surgeons' choice to use capnography in the office-based ambulatory anesthesia setting. *J Oral Maxillofac Surg*. 2015;73:1484e1–e1510.
79. Gurunluoglu R, Swanson JA, Haeck PC, et al. Evidence-based patient safety advisory: malignant hyperthermia. *Plast Reconstr Surg*. 2009;124:68S–81S.
80. American Society of Anesthesiologists Task Force on Operating Room Fires. Practice advisory for the prevention and management of operating room fires. *Anesthesiology*. 2008;108:786–801.
81. Moss E. MD office regs stalled in New Jersey. *APSF Newslett*. 1997; Winter 37.
82. Yates JA; American Society of Plastic Surgeons. Office-based surgery accreditation crosswalk. *Plast Surg Nurs*. 2002;22:125–132.
83. Coldiron B. Office surgical incidents: 19 months of Florida data. *Dermatol Surg*. 2002;28:710–712.
84. Bing J, McAuliffe MS, Lupton JR. Regional anesthesia with monitored anesthesia care for dermatologic laser surgery. *Dermatol Clin*. 2002;20:123–134.
85. Morris KT, Pommier RF, Vetto JT. Office-based wire-guided open breast biopsy under local anesthesia is accurate and cost effective. *Am J Surg*. 2000;179:422–425.
86. Jones JS, Streem SB. Office-based cystoureteroscopy for assessment of the upper urinary tract. *J Endourol*. 2002;16:307–309.

87. Friedman O, Deutsch ES, Reilly JS, et al. The feasibility of office-based laser-assisted tympanic membrane fenestration with tympanostomy tube insertion: The duPont Hospital experience. *Int J Pediatr Otorhinolaryngol.* 2002; 62:31–35.
88. Jones JS, Oder M, Zippe CD. Saturation prostate biopsy with periprostatic block can be performed in the office. *J Urol.* 2002;168:2108–2110.
89. Goldrath MH, Sherman AI. Office hysteroscopy and suction curettage: can we eliminate the hospital diagnostic dilatation and curettage? *Am J Obstet Gynecol.* 1985;152:220–229.
90. Armstrong M. Office-based procedures in rhinosinusitis. *Otolaryngol Clin North Am.* 2005;38:1327–1338.
91. Siegel GJ, Seiberling KA, Aguado AS. Office CO_2 laser turbinoplasty. *Ear Nose Throat J.* 2008;87:386–391.
92. Mingus ML, Bodian CA, Bradford CN, et al. Prolonged surgery increases the likelihood of admission of scheduled ambulatory surgery patients. *J Clin Anesth.* 1997;9:446–450.
93. Fortier J, Chung F, Su J. Unanticipated admission after ambulatory surgery: A prospective study. *Can J Anaesth.* 1997;45:612–619.
94. Gold BS, Kitz DS, Lecky JH, et al. Unanticipated admission to the hospital following ambulatory surgery. *JAMA.* 1989;262:3008–3010.
95. American Society of Plastic Surgeons. 2007 quick facts: Cosmetic and reconstructive plastic surgery trends. http://www.plasticsurgery.org/media/statistics/loader.cfm?url=/commonspot/security/getfile.cfm&pageID=29285.
96. American Society of Plastic Surgeons. 2013 Plastic Surgery statistics report. http://www.plasticsurgery.org/Documents/news-resources/statistics/2013-statistics/plastic-surgery-statistics-full-report-2013.pdf. Accessed June 2, 2016.
97. Iverson RE, Lynch DJ; American Society of Plastic Surgeons Committee on Safety. Practice advisory on liposuction. *Plast Reconstr Surg.* 2004;113: 1478–1490.
98. Fodor PB, Watson JP. Wetting solutions in ultra-sound assisted lipoplasty: A review. *Clin Plast Surg.* 1999;26:289–293.
99. Klein JA. Tumescent technique for regional anesthesia permits lidocaine doses of 35 mg/kg. *J Dermatol Surg Oncol.* 1990;16:248–263.
100. Ostad A, Kageyama N, Moy RL. Tumescent anesthesia with lidocaine dose of 55 mg/kg is safe for liposuction. *Dermatol Surg.* 1996;22:921.
101. Martinez MA, Ballesteros S, Segura LJ, et al. Reporting a fatality during tumescent liposuction. *Forens Sci Intl.* 2008;178:e11–e16.
102. Grazer FM, deJong RH. Fatal outcome from liposuction: census survey of cosmetic surgeons. *Plast Reconstr Surg.* 2000;105:436–446.
103. Housman TS, Lawrence N, Mellen BG, et al. The safety of liposuction: Results of a national survey. *Dermatol Surg.* 2002;28:971–978.
104. Conveney E, Weltz CR, Greengrass R, et al. Use of paravertebral block anesthesia in the surgical management of breast cancer: Experience in 156 cases. *Ann Surg.* 1998;227:496–501.
105. Jaffe SM, Campbell P, Bellman M, et al. Postoperative nausea and vomiting in women following breast surgery: An audit. *Eur J Anaesth.* 2000;17:261–264.
106. Vawter M, Vicaroi MD, Moorthy K, et al. Electrocardiographic monitoring during colonoscopy. *Am J Gastroenterol.* 1975;63:115.
107. Radaelli F, Meucci G, Terruzzi V, et al. Single bolus of midazolam versus bolus midazolam plus meperidine for colonoscopy: A prospective, randomized trial. *Gastrointest Endosc.* 2003;57:329.
108. Ristikankare M, Julkunen R, Laitinen T. Effect of conscious sedation on cardiac autonomic regulation during colonoscopy. *Scand J Gastroenterol.* 2000;9: 990–996.
109. Petelenz M, Gonciarz M, Macfarlane P, et al. Sympathovagal balance fluctuates during colonoscopy. *Endoscopy.* 2004;36:508–514.
110. Chutkan R, Cohen M, Abedi M, et al. Training guideline for use of propofol in gastrointestinal endoscopy. *Gastrointest Endosc.* 2004;60:167–172.
111. Propofolsedation. Who should administer? Institute for Safe Medication Practices website. http://www.ismp.org/Newsletters/acutecare/articles/20051103.asp. Published November 3, 2005; accessed June 2, 2016.
112. Finder RL. The art and science of office-based anesthesia in dentistry: a 150-year history. *Int Anesthesiol Clin.* 2003;41:1–12.
113. Perrott DH, Yuen JP, Andresen RV, et al. Office-based ambulatory anesthesia: outcomes of clinical practices of oral and maxillofacial surgeons. *J Oral Maxillofac Surg.* 2003;61:983–995.
114. Coyle TT, Helfrick JF, Gonzalez ML, et al. Office-based ambulatory anesthesia: factors that influence patient satisfaction with deep sedation/general anesthesia. *J Oral Maxillofac Surg.* 2005;63:163–172.
115. Freedman JM, Li DK, Drasner K, et al. Transient neurologic symptoms after spinal anesthesia: an epidemiologic study of 1,873 patients. *Anesthesiology.* 1998;89:633–641.
116. Mulroy MF, Larkin KL, Siddiqui A. Intrathecal fentanyl-induced pruritus is more severe in combination with procaine than with lidocaine or bupivacaine. *Reg Anesth Pain Med.* 2001;26:252–256.
117. Sardo ADS, Bettocchi S, Spinelli M, et al. Review of new office-based hysteroscopic procedures 2003–2009. *J Min Invas Gynecol.* 2010;17:436–448.
118. Wortman M. Instituting an office-based surgery program in the gynecologists office. *J Min Invas Gynecol.* 2010;17:673–683.
119. Jourdy DN, Kacker A. Regional anesthesia for office-based procedures in otorhinolaryngology. *Anesthesiol Clin.* 2010;28:457–468.
120. Woo P. Office-based laryngeal procedures. *Otolaryngol Clin North Am.* 2006; 39;111–133.
121. Lan MC, Hsu YB, Chang SY, et al. Office-based treatment of vocal cord polyp with flexible laryngovideostroboscopic surgery. *J Otolaryngol Head Neck Surg.* 2010;39:90–95.
122. Hackel A, Badgwell JM, Binding RR, et al. Guidelines for the pediatric perioperative environment. American Academy of Pediatrics Section on Anesthesiology. *Pediatrics.* 1999;103:512–515.
123. Tang J, Chen L, White PF, et al. Use of propofol for office-based anesthesia: Effect of nitrous oxide on recovery. *J Clin Anesth.* 1999;11:226–230.
124. Cohen MM, Duncan PG, Tate RB. Does anesthesia contribute to operative mortality? *JAMA.* 1988;260:2859–2863.
125. Domino KB. Trends in anesthesia litigation in the 1990's: monitored anesthesia care claims. *ASA Newslett.* 1997;61:17.
126. Hughes MA, Glass PS, Jacobs JR. Context sensitive half-time in multicompartment pharmacokinetic models for intravenous anesthetic drugs. *Anesthesiology.* 1992;76:334–341.
127. Rudner R, Jalowiecki P, Kawecki P, et al. Conscious analgesia/sedation with remifentanil and propofol versus total intravenous anesthesia with fentanyl, midazolam, and propofol for outpatient colonoscopy. *Gastrointest Endosc.* 2003;57:657–663.
128. Angst MS. Intraoperative use of remifentanil for TIVA: postoperative pain, acute tolerance, and opioid-induced hyperalgesia. *J Cardiothor Vasc Anesth.* 2015;29(1):S16–S22.
129. Thomas B. Remifentanil versus fentanyl in total intravenous anesthesia for lumbar spine surgery: A retrospective cohort study. *J Clin Anesth.* 2015;27: 391–395.
130. Guignard B, Bossard AE, Coste C, et al. Acute opioid tolerance: Intraoperative remifentanil increases postoperative pain and morphine requirement. *Anesthesiology.* 2000;93:409–417.
131. Liu Y, Zheng Y, Ga X, et al. The efficacy of NMDA receptor antagonists for preventing remifentanil-induced increase in postoperative pain and analgesic requirement: A meta-analysis. *Minerva Anesthesiol.* 2012;78:653–667.
132. Friedberg BL. Facial laser resurfacing with the propofol-ketamine technique: Room air, spontaneous ventilation (RASV) anesthesia. *Dermatol Surg.* 1999;25:569–572.
133. Friedberg BK. Propofol-ketamine technique: dissociative anesthesia for office surgery (a five year review of 1,264 cases). *Aesthet Plast Surg.* 1999;23: 70–75.
134. Friedberg BL. Propofol-ketamine technique. *Aesthet Plast Surg.* 1993;17: 297–300.
135. Friedberg BL. Hypnotic doses of propofol block ketamine-induced hallucinations. *Plast Reconstr Surg.* 1993;91:196–197.
136. Friedberg BL, Sigl JC. Clonidine premedication decreases propofol consumption during bispectral index (BIS) monitored propofol-ketamine technique for office-based surgery. *Dermatol Surg.* 2000;26:848–852.
137. Man D. Premedication with oral clonidine for facial rhytidectomy. *Plast Reconstr Surg.* 1994;94:214–215.
138. Baker TM, Stuzin JM, Baker TJ, et al. What's new in aesthetic surgery? *Clin Plast Surg.* 1996;23:16.
139. Kumar P, Priya K, Kirti S, et al. Dexmedetomidine supported office based genioplasty: A pilot study. *J Maxillofac Oral Surg.* 2015;14(3):750–753.
140. Mathews DM, Gaba V, Zaku B, et al. Can remifentanil replace nitrous oxide during anesthesia for ambulatory orthopedic surgery with desflurane and fentanyl? *Anesth Analg.* 2008;106:101–108.
141. Nathan N, Peyclit A, Lahrimi A, et al. Comparison of sevoflurane and propofol for ambulatory anaesthesia in gynaecological surgery. *Can J Anaesth.* 1998;45:1148–1150.
142. Song D, Joshi GP, White PF. Fast-track eligibility after ambulatory anesthesia: A comparison of desflurane, sevoflurane and propofol. *Anesth Analg.* 1998;86:267–273.
143. Gupta A, Stierer T, Zuckerman R, et al. Comparison of recovery profile after ambulatory anesthesia with propofol, isoflurane, sevoflurane and desflurane: A systematic review. *Anesth Analg.* 2004;98:632–641.
144. Drover DR, Lemmens JH, Pierce ET, et al. Patient state index: Titration of delivery and recovery from propofol, alfentanil, and nitrous oxide anesthesia. *Anesthesiology.* 2002;97:82–89.
145. Gan TJ, Glass PS, Windsor A, et al. Bispectral index monitoring allows faster emergence and improved recovery from propofol, alfentanil, and nitrous oxide anesthesia. *Anesthesiology.* 1997;87:808–815.
146. Song D, Joshi GP, White PF. Titration of volatile anesthetics using bispectral analysis index facilitates recovery after ambulatory anesthesia. *Anesthesiology.* 1997;87:842–848.
147. Friedberg B, Sigl JC. Bispectral index (BIS) monitoring decreases propofol usage during propofol-ketamine office based anesthesia. *Anesth Analg.* 1999;88:54.
148. Singer R, Thomas PE. Pulse oximeter in the ambulatory aesthetic surgical facility. *Plast Reconstr Surg.* 1988;82:111–115.

149. Tang J, Chen X, White PF, et al. Antiemetic prophylaxis for office-based surgery-are the 5-HT3 receptor antagonists beneficial? *Anesthesiology.* 2003;98:293–298.
150. Chung FF, Chan VW, Ong D. A postanesthetic discharge scoring system for home readiness after ambulatory surgery. *J Clin Anesth.* 1995;7:500–506.
151. Title 10 NYCRR. Section 755.6.f; Volume D. https://www.health.ny.gov/regulations/nycrr/title_10/
152. White PF. The role of non-opioid analgesic techniques in the management of pain after ambulatory surgery. *Anesth Analg.* 2002;94:577–585.
153. Ding Y, White PF. Comparative effects of ketorolac, dezocine and fentanyl as adjuvants during outpatient anesthesia. *Anesth Analg.* 1992;75:566–571.
154. Desjardins PJ, Shu VS, Recker DP, et al. A single preoperative oral dose of valdecoxib, a new cyclooxygenase-2 specific inhibitor, relieves post-oral surgery or bunionectomy pain. *Anesthesiology.* 2002;97:565–573.
155. Gan TJ, Meyer TA, Apfel CC, et al. Society for ambulatory anesthesia guidelines for the management of postoperative nausea and vomiting. *Anesth Analg.* 2007;105:1615–1628.
156. Kovac AL. Prevention and treatment of postoperative nausea and vomiting. *Drugs.* 2000;59:213–243.
157. Henzi I, Walder B, Tramer MR. Dexamethasone for prophylaxis of postoperative nausea and vomiting: a quantitative systematic review. *Anesth Analg* 2000;90:186–194.
158. Eberhart LH, Morin AM, Georgieff M. Dexamethasone for prophylaxis of postoperative nausea and vomiting: a meta-analysis of randomized controlled studies. *Anaesthetist.* 2000;49:713–720.
159. Scuderi PE, James RL, Harris L, et al. Antiemetic prophylaxis does not improve outcomes after outpatient surgery when compared to symptomatic treatment. *Anesthesiology.* 1999;90:360–371.
160. California Codes, Business & Professions Code, Division 2. Healing Arts. Chapter 5. Medicine: Article 11.5. Surgery in certain outpatient settings. 2003; 2215–2240.
161. California Health and Safety Code, Division 2. *Licensing Provisions. Chapter 1.3. Outpatient settings.* §1248.1. Required settings. 2003.
162. New Jersey Administrative Code. *Title 13. Law and public safety: Chapter 35. Board of medical examiners: Subchapter 4A. Surgery, special procedures, and anesthesia services performed in an office setting.* 2003.
163. Manchikanti L, McMahon EB. Physician refer thyself: is stark II, phase III the final voyage? *Pain Physician.* 2007;10:725–741.

33 Nonoperating Room Anesthesia

KAREN J. SOUTER • ANDREW J. PITTAWAY • CARLY PETERSON

General Principles
Three-step Approach to Nonoperating Room Anesthesia
    The Patient
    The Procedure
    The Environment
Patient Safety in Nonoperating Room Anesthesia
    Adverse Events
    Preprocedural Checklists
    Standards of Care for Nonoperating Room Anesthesia
Sedation and Anesthesia
    Definition of Sedation and Anesthesia
    The Continuum of Anesthesia
Environmental Considerations for Nonoperating Room Anesthesia
    X-rays and Fluoroscopy
    Intravenous Contrast Agents

Specific Nonoperating Room Procedures
    Angiography
    Interventional Neuroradiology
    Computed Tomography
    Radiofrequency Ablation
    Transjugular Intrahepatic Portosystemic Shunt
    Magnetic Resonance Imaging
    Pediatric Sedation and Anesthesia for MRI and CT Scans
    Radiation Therapy
    Positron Emission Tomography
    Gastroenterology
    Cardiology and Interventional Cardiology
    Electroconvulsive Therapy
Summary

KEY POINTS

1. Nonoperating room (NOR) locations are remote from a hospital's main operating room sites.
2. A three-step approach that considers the patient, the procedure, and the environment is useful in considering any anesthetic in the NOR setting.
3. All significant patient comorbidities must be carefully assessed, and the appropriate level of sedation, general anesthesia, and level of monitoring determined by the anesthesiologist caring for the patient.
4. Procedural considerations are both general (e.g., duration, position, and level of discomfort) and specific to individual specialties.
5. Patients must receive the same standard of care at a NOR site as they do in the operating room and the American Society of Anesthesiologists (ASA) has defined guidelines to be applied to the administration of anesthesia in NOR locations.[1]
6. The anesthetic and monitoring equipment used for nonoperating room anesthesia (NORA) must meet the same standards as equipment provided in the operating room.
7. Following NORA, the patient should be transported to an appropriate postanesthesia care unit, accompanied and monitored by anesthesia-trained personnel.
8. Environmental considerations in NOR locations include hazards such as radiation, magnetic resonance imaging, and the side effects of intravenous contrast agents.

General Principles

Nonoperating room anesthesia (NORA) refers to anesthesia that is provided at any location remote from the traditional operating room.[1] These locations include radiology departments, endoscopy suites, magnetic resonance imaging (MRI), and computerized tomography (CT) scanners. This chapter will consider the care of the patient undergoing procedures in these locations. Discussion of anesthesia in stand-alone ambulatory centers, or offices, is addressed in Chapters 31 and 32. Anesthesia and analgesia provided for labor and delivery is discussed in Chapter 41.

Examination of data from the National Anesthesia Clinical Outcomes Registry (NACOR)[2] between 2010 and 2013 has estimated that NORA accounts for about 30% of anesthesia cases, and although the number of OR anesthesia cases remains static, the number of NORA cases has steadily increased recently, the highest rate of increase being in gastroenterologic procedures.[3]

Three-step Approach to Nonoperating Room Anesthesia

Away from the operating room, the anesthesiologist may lack familiar equipment and staff experienced in the care of the anesthetized patient. NORA therefore presents unique challenges and a systematic approach using the simple three-step paradigm "the PATIENT, the PROCEDURE, and the ENVIRONMENT" is recommended (Fig. 33-1).

The Patient

Patients presenting for NOR procedures tend to be older (above 50 years) and in the case of gastroenterologic, cardiology, and radiologic procedures, of higher ASA status than patients cared for in the standard operating rooms. Patients presenting for NOR procedures are also more likely to receive monitored anesthesia

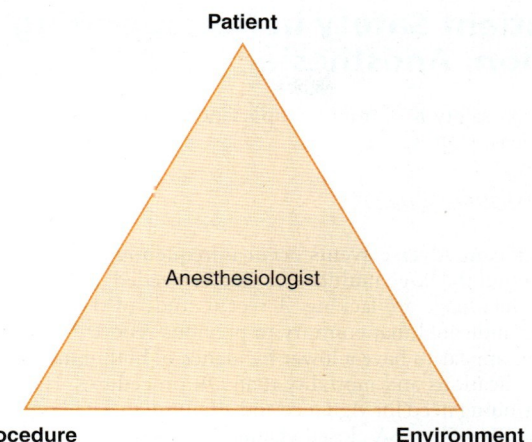

Figure 33-1 A three-step paradigm for nonoperating room anesthesia.

care (MAC) or sedation than those undergoing OR procedures.[3] Patients may require sedation or anesthesia to tolerate NOR procedures for a number of reasons (Table 33-1). Children commonly require sedation or anesthesia for diagnostic and therapeutic procedures.[4] Palliative, less-invasive procedures are increasingly being offered to patients too ill to tolerate a major surgical procedure representing a continuing challenge for the NOR anesthesiologist. All patients presenting for NORA require a thorough preanesthetic assessment, standard preanesthesia care,[5] the development of a sound anesthetic plan with appropriate levels of monitoring,[6] and the appropriate postanesthesia care.[7]

The Procedure

Common NOR procedures for which the patient may require anesthesia or sedation are listed in Table 33-2. The anesthesiologist must understand the nature of the procedure, including the position of the patient, how painful the procedure will be, and how long it will last. The optimum anesthesia plan provides safe patient care and facilitates the procedure. Discussions with the proceduralist must include contingencies for emergencies and adverse outcomes.

The Environment

The American Society of Anesthesiologists (ASA) has developed standards for NORA.[1] Prior to the anesthetic, the presence and

Table 33-1 Patient Factors Requiring Sedation or Anesthesia for Nonoperating Room Procedures

Claustrophobia, anxiety, and panic disorders
Cerebral palsy, developmental delay, and learning difficulties
Seizure disorders, movement disorders, and muscular contractures
Pain, both related to the procedure and other causes
Acute trauma with unstable cardiovascular, respiratory, or neurologic function
Raised intracranial pressure
Significant comorbidity and patient frailty (American Society of Anesthesiology physical status III, IV)
Children, especially those below 10 years

Table 33-2 Common Nonoperating Room Anesthesia Procedures

	Procedure
Radiologic imaging	Computed tomography Magnetic resonance imaging Positron emission tomography
Interventional radiology[a]	Vascular imaging, stenting, and embolization procedures Biopsy and/or drainage of lesions, tumors, cysts Radiofrequency ablation Transjugular intrahepatic portosystemic shunt
Interventional neuroradiology[a]	Occlusive ("closing") procedures • Embolization of cerebral aneurysm • Embolization of arteriovenous malformations • Embolization of vascular tumors "Opening" procedures in acute thromboembolic stroke, cerebral atherosclerosis, or cerebral vasospasm • Angioplasty • Stenting • Thrombolysis
Radiotherapy	Radiation therapy Intraoperative radiotherapy
Interventional cardiology[a]	
Cardiac catheterization laboratory	Diagnostic cardiac catheterization Percutaneous coronary interventions Percutaneous ventricular assist devices Percutaneous closure of septal defects Alcohol septal ablation Structural heart procedures • Transcatheter aortic valve replacement • Mitral valve repair for mitral regurgitation ("MitraClip") • Left atrial appendage occlusion
Electrophysiology laboratory (EPL)	Cardiac implantable electronic devices Electrophysiology studies with ablation Laser lead extraction
Other cardiac procedures	Cardioversion Diagnostic transesophageal echocardiography
Gastroenterology[a]	Upper gastroenterology endoscopy Esophageal dilatation or stenting Percutaneous endoscopic gastrostomy tube placement Endoscopic retrograde cholangiopancreatography Colonoscopy Liver biopsy
Psychiatry	Electroconvulsive therapy

[a]Diagnostic and therapeutic procedures.

Table 33-3 American Society of Anesthesiology Standards for Nonoperating Room Anesthetizing Locations[1]

1. Oxygen-reliable source—ideally piped and full backup E-cylinder
2. Suction-adequate and reliable
3. Scavenging system if inhalational agents are administered
4. Anesthetic equipment
   - Backup self-inflating bag capable of delivering at least 90% oxygen by positive-pressure ventilation
   - Adequate anesthetic drugs, supplies, and equipment for intended anesthesia care
   - Adequate monitoring equipment to allow adherence to the ASA standards for basic monitoring[6]
   - Anesthesia machine with equivalent function to those in the operating rooms and maintained to the same standards
5. Electrical outlets
   - Sufficient for anesthesia machine and monitors
   - Isolated electrical power or ground fault circuit interrupters if "wet location"
6. Adequate illumination of patient, anesthesia machine, and monitoring equipment; battery-operated backup light source
7. Sufficient space for:
   - Personnel and equipment
   - Easy and expeditious access to patient, anesthesia machine, and monitoring equipment
8. Resuscitation equipment immediately available
   - Defibrillator/emergency drugs/cardiopulmonary resuscitation equipment
9. Adequately trained staff to support the anesthesiologist and a reliable means of two-way communication
10. All building and safety codes and facility standards should be observed
11. Postanesthesia care facilities[7]
    - Adequately trained staff to provide postanesthesia care
    - Appropriate equipment to allow safe transport to main postanesthesia care unit

proper functioning of all equipment needed for safe patient care must be established; this is described in Table 33-3. The location of immediately available resuscitation equipment should be noted and protocols developed with the local staff for dealing with emergencies, including cardiopulmonary resuscitation and the management of anaphylaxis.

Anesthesia Equipment and Monitors

Anesthesia machines and monitors may or may not be provided in NOR locations. Small, portable anesthesia machines and monitors are available if a site does not offer a permanent anesthesia work station. Anesthesia machines and monitors that remain in a NOR location need to undergo routine maintenance. Infrequent use may result in degradation of equipment and the use of preprocedural checks, preferably with a standardized checklist, cannot be overemphasized before embarking on NORA. If more advanced monitors (e.g., an arterial line, central venous pressure, or intracranial pressure [ICP] monitoring) are required, these devices should be readily available. A preprepared cart containing essential equipment that is checked and restocked after each case is recommended.

Patient Safety in Nonoperating Room Anesthesia

Patient safety is of utmost importance in all types of anesthesia, not least NORA.

Adverse Events

Significant adverse events occur infrequently in NOR locations, although the large multicenter studies needed to determine their true incidence are lacking. A recent study of the NACOR database[3] indicated that contrary to previous reports,[8] NORA procedures appear to have a lower incidence of both minor and major complications and mortality than OR procedures. However, the continuing need for vigilance and attention to detail remains high in NORA. The ASA closed claims database has identified NORA as an area of liability for the anesthesiologist.[8] The gastroenterology suite, cardiac laboratory, and the emergency department are sites where adverse events are likely to occur and the elderly, medically complex patients have been determined to be more at risk by both the closed claims and the NACOR analyses.[3,9] Respiratory depression secondary to oversedation was the most common type of adverse event in the closed claims study.[8,9] Capnography provides an early monitor of impending respiratory depression during sedation and is recommended.[6,10,11] Adverse events associated with NORA have been divided into minor and major and appear to be more frequent in patients undergoing radiology procedures and in cardiology locations (Table 33-4).[3]

Preprocedural Checklists

The use of checklists and pre- and postprocedural team briefings has been broadly embraced in operating room practice and

Table 33-4 Complications of Nonoperating Room Anesthesia[3]

Minor Complications (in order of frequency)
Postoperative nausea and vomiting
Inadequate postoperative pain control
Hemodynamic instability
Minor neurologic complications such as postdural puncture headache (cardiology and radiologic locations)
Minor respiratory complications (cardiology and radiologic locations)
Complications related to central/intravenous lines (cardiology locations)
Need for opioid reversal (cardiology and radiologic locations)

Major Complications
Unintended patient awareness (gastroenterologic locations)
Anaphylaxis (radiology procedures and cardiology locations)
Need for upgrade of care
Serious hemodynamic instability
Respiratory complications
Need for resuscitation
Central and peripheral nervous system injury (radiology procedures and cardiology locations)
Vascular access-related complications (radiology procedures and cardiology locations)
Wrong patient/wrong site (radiology procedures and cardiology locations)
Fall or burn (radiology procedures and cardiology locations)

emerging evidence points toward improved patient outcomes when checklists are employed.[12,13] Similar systems should be adopted in NOR sites and recently a checklist has been proposed for use in interventional radiology suites.[14]

Standards of Care for Nonoperating Room Anesthesia

Patient Transfer

Sick, unstable patients may be transferred back and forth between the intensive care unit, the operating rooms, and NOR locations for imaging, therapeutic, or diagnostic procedures. During transport the patient should be accompanied by skilled personnel to evaluate, monitor, and support the patient's medical condition. A specialized transport team may contribute to reducing the number of critical incidents that occur during the transport of ventilated and critically ill patients.[15] Patients are often mechanically ventilated and receiving a number of drug infusions for both sedation and hemodynamic support. Portable ventilators are useful for transport; these are often oxygen powered, and adequate supplies of oxygen must be available for the transfer. A manual self-inflating bag is essential in the event of ventilator failure. Infusion pumps and portable monitors should have adequate battery power for transit. The transport team should carry spare anesthetic and emergency drugs, equipment for intubation or reintubation, portable suction, and if the patient's condition requires, a portable defibrillator. It is vital to notify the destination area that the patient is in transit, so that appropriate preparations to receive the patient can be made in advance. It is also useful to send personnel ahead to secure the elevators to prevent delays during transfer.

Sedation and Anesthesia

Definition of Sedation and Anesthesia

Many NOR procedures are performed under sedation and MAC for which the ASA developed guidelines.[16] A consistent definition of these terms is essential for clear communications between the various stakeholders involved in provision of NORA. On January 14, 2011, the Centers for Medicare and Medicaid Services (CMS) issued a revision to Interpretive Guideline (IG) for Hospitals No. 482.52 concerning anesthesia services. This revised guideline places the responsibility and oversight for all anesthesia services under the direction of one suitably qualified individual, the "director of anesthesia services."[17] IG 482.52 defines "anesthesia," to mean general anesthesia, regional anesthesia, deep sedation/analgesia, or MAC. "Analgesia/sedation" is defined as local/topical anesthesia, minimal sedation, and moderate sedation/analgesia ("conscious sedation").

The Continuum of Anesthesia

Anesthesia exists along a continuum and the transition from minimal sedation to general anesthesia is not clear-cut (Table 33-5).[16–19] As sedation deepens, it is important to recognize the progressive blunting and loss of airway reflexes and patency, together with depression of spontaneous ventilation and cardiovascular function. The individual responsiveness of patients to different sedative agents varies, as do the levels of stimulation during the course of a procedure. Consequently, during the course of an NOR procedure under sedation, the patient may drift to a deeper level than the one intended, including transitioning into general anesthesia with loss of airway reflexes and possibly airway obstruction. In any circumstances where a particular level of sedation is being provided, services must be immediately available to rescue a patient from a deeper than intended level of sedation or general anesthesia.[18]

Environmental Considerations for Nonoperating Room Anesthesia

X-rays and Fluoroscopy

X-rays are produced when electrons are accelerated through a high voltage in a vacuum tube and collide with a metal target. In medical x-ray tubes, the target is usually tungsten or a more crack-resistant alloy of rhenium (5%) and tungsten (95%). X-ray production is determined by, and directly proportional to, the tube current and the voltage. Fluoroscopy is a technique used to obtain real-time moving images of the internal structures. The patient is positioned between the x-ray source and a fluorescent screen. By coupling the fluoroscope to an x-ray image intensifier and a video camera, the images can be recorded and played on a monitor. Fluoroscopy is widely and increasingly used in NOR locations including interventional radiology, cardiac catheterization, and electrophysiologic procedures and in the gastroenterology suite. Large, C-shaped, mobile fluoroscopy devices (C-arms) are used to provide images in multiple dimensions. The C-arm moves back and forth around the patient during the procedure,

Table 33-5 Definition of General Anesthesia and Levels of Sedation/Analgesia[18]

	Minimal Sedation (Anxiolysis)	Moderate Sedation/Analgesia (Conscious Sedation)	Deep Sedation/Analgesia	General Anesthesia
Responsiveness	Normal response to verbal stimulation	Purposeful[a] response to verbal or tactile stimulation	Purposeful[a] response after repeated or painful stimulation	Unarousable, even with painful stimulus
Airway	Unaffected	No intervention required	Intervention may be required	Intervention often required
Spontaneous ventilation	Unaffected	Adequate	May be inadequate	Frequently inadequate
Cardiovascular function	Unaffected	Usually maintained	Usually maintained	May be impaired

[a]Reflex withdrawal from a painful stimulus is *not* considered a purposeful response.

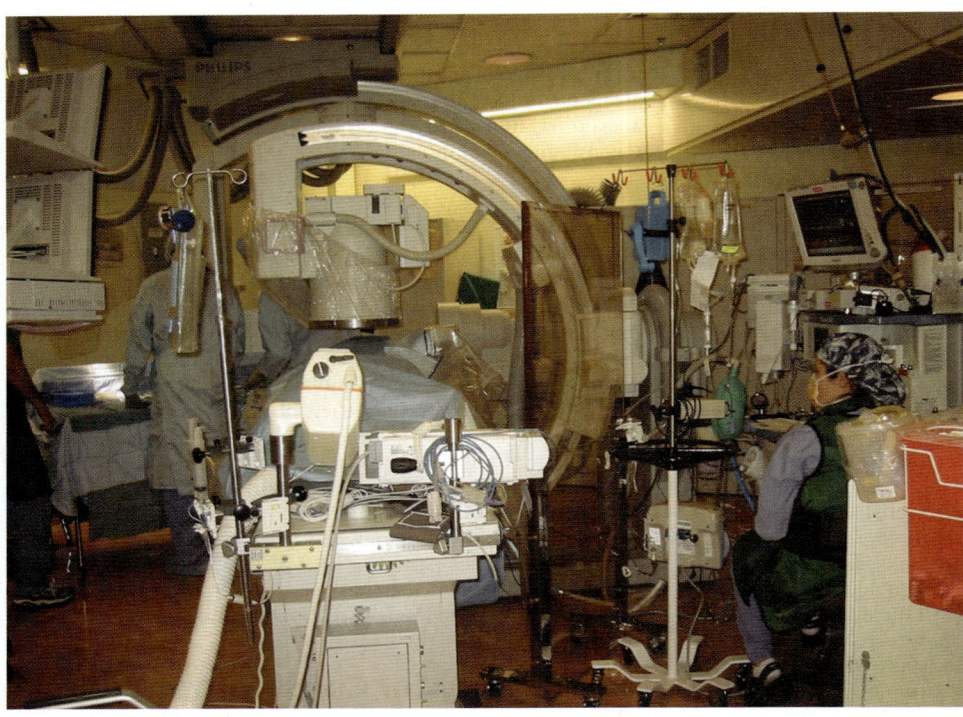

Figure 33-2 A radiology suite showing a C-arm and the high density of equipment that may separate the anesthesiologist from the patient.

taking up large amounts of space, limiting access to the patient, and serving as a means of dislodging intravenous lines and endotracheal tubes (Fig. 33-2).

Hazards of Ionizing Radiation

The effects of ionizing radiation on biologic tissues are classified as deterministic (dose related causing cell death and tissue damage) and stochastic (the development of cancer from direct DNA ionization or the creation of hydroxyl radicals from x-ray interactions with water molecules). Patient exposure to radiation during imaging and treatment varies depending on the type of procedure as well as patient- and operator-related factors.[20] For example, the radiation a patient receives from a simple chest x-ray is 0.02 millisieverts (mSv), and between 20 and 40 mSv for pulmonary angiography.[21] Exposure from fluoroscopy is 100 and 1,000 greater than from simple x-rays. Standard procedures exist to minimize patient exposure to radiation and efforts to reduce occupational exposure for staff including anesthesiologists working in radiology suites are an important consideration. A number of terms are used to define exposure to radiation[22]; these are summarized in Table 33-6.

Table 33-6 Common Terms Used in Radiation Exposure[22]

Term	Units	Definition	Notes
Exposure	Roentgen (R)—defined as 2.58×10^{-4} coulombs (C)/kg (SI units).	Quantity of x-radiation or gamma radiation required to produce an amount of ionization (electric charge) in air at standard temperature and pressure	Ionization measurements are often made in exposure rate, i.e., amount of exposure per unit time, e.g., fluoroscopy is measured in R/min
Absorbed dose	Rad (radiation absorbed dose) or Gray (Gy, the SI unit)	Amount of ionizing radiation absorbed by the body	Depends on exposure to x-ray beam and the tissue type A Gray represents 100 times more radiation than a Rad
Dose equivalent	Sievert (Sv) or roentgen equivalent in man (rem)	Absorbed dose multiplied by a radiation quality factor specific for the type of radiation	Measures the "harmfulness" of any radiation-absorbed dose
Effective dose	Sievert (Sv)	Dose equivalent to the entire body caused by irradiating only a localized area. Calculated by multiplying the dose equivalent by a weighting factor specific for the irradiated organ	Takes into account the differing radiosensitivity of different organs Used to estimate cancer risk for patients (stochastic effects) and to calculate equivalent whole body exposure in staff wearing personal dosimeters for comparison with annual personnel dose limits

Staff, including the anesthesiologists, must be aware of the hazards of occupational exposure to ionizing radiation and take appropriate measures to protect themselves.[23] Exposure to ionizing radiation may come from direct exposure and scatter. Patients are subjected to direct exposure where the beam enters the skin, whereas staff members working in fluoroscopy suites are more at risk from scattered radiation. As a general rule the exposure to staff is 1/1,000th the entrance skin exposure at 1 m from the fluoroscopy tube. A recent study of radiation exposure to operating room personnel during fluoroscopic-guided endovascular repair of thoracoabdominal aortic aneurysms using fenestrated endografts (FEVAR) identified that anesthesiologists were likely to receive 15 times the dose of radiation compared to the scrub nurses even though both types of practitioners were at the same distance (7 feet) from the C-arm.[24] This finding was attributed to anesthesiologists being less likely to use the protective shielding during their patient care activities. Another recent study demonstrated that anesthesiologists working in the neurointerventional suite were at equal risk of developing cataracts as neuroradiologists, and that the radiation may even be directed away from the neuroradiologists and toward the anesthesiologist.[25] These studies highlight the need for anesthesiologists to be aware of the risks and the means to protect themselves from radiation, especially in areas where fluoroscopy is used.

Staff exposure to radiation can be minimized by a number of precautions[22,23]:

1. *Limiting the time of exposure to radiation.*
2. *Increasing the distance from the source of radiation.* (Dose rates increase or decrease according to the inverse square of the distance from the source.)
3. *Using protective shielding* (lead-lined garments and fixed and/or movable shields).

    Lead aprons, thyroid shields, and leaded eyeglasses are recommended despite being bulky and contributing to staff fatigue. Anesthesiology staff should consider using movable or fixed lead-lined glass shields so that they can gain easy access to their patients while protecting themselves from radiation.

4. *Measuring occupational exposure to radiation.*

    The dose limits for occupational exposure to radiation established by the International Commission on Radiological Protection (IRCP) have been adopted in most countries.[26] In the United States, the National Council on Radiation Protection and Measurements (NCRP) recommends an occupational limit of 50 mSv in any 1 year and a lifetime limit of 10 mSv multiplied by the individual's age in years.[23,27] Health-care workers including anesthesiologists should be issued individual dosimeter badges to monitor their cumulative exposure to radiation. These data should be regularly reviewed by the facility's radiation safety section or medical physics department.

Intravenous Contrast Agents

Intravenous contrast agents are commonly used in radiologic and MRI to enhance vascular imaging. Radiologic contrast media are iodinated compounds classified according to their osmolarity (high, low, or iso-osmolar), their ionicity (ionic or nonionic), and the number of benzene rings (monomer or dimer). Nonionic contrast agents cause less discomfort on injection and have a lower incidence of adverse reactions.[28] MRI contrast agents are also divided into ionic and nonionic compounds. They are chelated metal complexes containing gadolinium, iron, or manganese.

Adverse reactions to contrast agents may be divided into renal adverse reactions and hypersensitivity reactions.[29]

Renal Adverse Reaction

Contrast agents are eliminated via the kidneys, and contrast-induced nephropathy (CIN) associated with their use is estimated to account for nearly 10% of hospital-acquired acute renal failure.[30] CIN is defined as an increase in serum creatinine of 0.5 mg/dL or a 25% increase from the baseline within 48 to 72 hours after iodinated contrast medium administration. Chronic kidney disease is the most important predictor of CIN, increasing the risk by 20 times[30]; other risk factors for CIN include history of renal disease, prior renal surgery, proteinuria, diabetes mellitus, hypertension, gout, and use of nephrotoxic drugs. Preventative measures to avoid CIN include adequate hydration, maintaining a good urine output, and using sodium bicarbonate infusions to improve elimination of the contrast agent. Nephrotoxic medications such as nonsteroidal anti-inflammatory drugs, aminoglycosides, and diuretics should be avoided for 24 to 48 hours before and after the use of intravenous contrast agents. The efficacy of N-acetylcysteine and other agents such as fenoldopam, dopamine, calcium-channel blockers, atrial natriuretic peptide, and L-arginine in mitigating CIN has not been proven.[31]

Hypersensitivity Reactions

Hypersensitivity reactions to contrast media are divided into immediate (<1 hour) and nonimmediate (>1 hour) reactions.[28,29] Mild immediate reactions occur in about 0.5% to 3% and severe reactions occur in 0.01% to 0.04%. Fatal hypersensitivity reactions may occur in about 1 per 100,000 contrast administrations. The frequency of nonimmediate reactions is much more variable (0.5% to 23%) related partly to difficulty in determining whether symptoms relate to contrast agents or not. The clinical manifestations of various hypersensitivity reactions to contrast media are outlined in Table 33-7.[32] Although widely used, the effectiveness of corticosteroids and antihistamines in preventing hypersensitivity reactions to contrast agents in unselected patients is doubtful.[33] Treatment of severe hypersensitivity reactions includes discontinuing the causative agent and supportive therapy, oxygen, intubating the trachea, cardiovascular support with fluids, vasopressors, and inotropes, and if required, bronchodilators.[29] Reactions to gadolinium-based contrast agents used for MRI are less frequent than to iodinated contrast agents. Hypersensitivity to gadolinium-containing agents occurs in 5.9 per 10,000 injections and the rate is higher (13 per 10,000) in patients undergoing abdominal MRI examinations. Severe reactions occur 1:10,000 to 1:40,000 and the mortality rate is 1 in a million injections.[34] Gadolinium-containing compounds have been associated with nephrogenic systemic fibrosis (NSF), a disease manifesting fibrosis of the skin and internal organs with some similarities to scleroderma in patients with renal insufficiency.[29,35]

Specific Nonoperating Room Procedures

Angiography

Angiography causes minimal discomfort and may be performed under local anesthesia with or without light sedation. Patients are required to remain completely motionless during these procedures, which may be lengthy, particularly spinal angiography. Neurologic disorders such as recent subarachnoid hemorrhage,

Table 33-7 Clinical Manifestations of Immediate and Nonimmediate Hypersensitivity Reactions to Radiocontrast Agents[a,32]

Immediate Reactions
Pruritus
Urticaria
Angioedema/facial edema
Abdominal pain, nausea, diarrhea
Rhinitis (sneezing, rhinorrhea)
Hoarseness, cough
Dyspnea (bronchospasm, laryngeal edema)
Respiratory arrest
Hypotension, cardiovascular shock
Cardiac arrest

Nonimmediate Reactions
Pruritus
Exanthema (mostly macular or maculopapular drug eruption)
Urticaria, angioedema
Erythema multiforme minor
Fixed drug eruption
Stevens–Johnson syndrome
Toxic epidermal necrolysis
Graft-versus-host reaction
Drug-related eosinophilia with systemic symptoms (DRESS)
Symmetrical drug-related intertriginous and flexural exanthema (SDRIFE)
Vasculitis

[a]Most frequent are in italics.

stroke, and depressed level of consciousness or raised ICP may necessitate anesthesia with intubation for airway protection. Angiography is often performed via the femoral artery; the femoral vein may also be accessed when imaging arteriovenous malformations (AVMs) or dural venous abnormalities. Liberal use of local anesthetic at the puncture site precludes the need for intravenous analgesia. The injection of contrast media into the cerebral arteries may cause discomfort, burning, or pruritus around the face and eyes. Hypotension and bradycardia may also occur and discomfort from a full bladder as a result of fluid and IV contrast administration is a consideration in nonanesthetized patients. During angiography and other interventional radiologic procedures, the patient is placed on a moving gantry and the radiologist positions the patient to track catheters as they pass from the groin into the vessels of interest. It is vital to have extensions on all anesthesia breathing circuits, infusion lines, and monitors to prevent these implements from being accidentally dislodged as the radiologist swings the x-ray table back and forth. Care should be taken with positioning of radiopaque pieces of equipment. The electrocardiogram electrodes and metallic coils in the cuffs of endotracheal tubes may cause interesting and annoying artifacts if they lie over the area being imaged.

Interventional Neuroradiology

A variety of neurosurgical conditions especially neurovascular diseases are effectively managed by interventional neuroradiology.[36] These procedures may be subdivided as "occlusive" and "opening" procedures (Table 33-2).

Cerebral aneurysms and AVMs are particularly amenable to occlusive endovascular treatments.[37] A commonly employed technique is to insert detachable platinum coils into the abnormal vessel(s). Other occlusive agents include cyanoacrylates, "Onyx liquid embolic system" (Micro therapeutics Inc., USA), a biocompatible liquid embolic agent, and polyvinyl alcohol particles. These particles may also be used to produce temporary occlusion of blood vessels for preoperative embolization of vascular tumors, particularly meningiomas. In 2009, a large multicenter study, the International Subarachnoid Aneurysm Trial (ISAT) reported better outcomes in patients with ruptured anterior and posterior circulation aneurysms undergoing interventional neuroradiology compared to surgical clipping.[38] The benefits of coiling appear to be prolonged with the most recent follow-up of ISAT reporting the probability of disability-free survival to be significantly greater in the endovascular group compared to the neurosurgical group at 10 years.[39] The World Federation of Neurosurgical Societies' (WFNS's) poor grade for cerebral aneurysms in elderly patients did not clearly establish the superiority of one treatment or the other.[40,41] The management of an unruptured intracranial aneurysm depends on many factors including aneurysm size, shape, location, and patient comorbidity. In 2015, the American Heart Association and American Stroke Association jointly published guidelines for management of unruptured intracranial aneurysms.[42]

"Opening" procedures include the management of acute thromboembolic stroke and postsubarachnoid hemorrhage vasospasm. In the case of acute ischemic stroke, early (within 6 hours of symptoms) intervention to recanalize the occluded vessel by superselective intra-arterial thrombolytic therapy has been shown to improve outcome.[43,44] Specialized centers have developed various "stroke code protocols"[45] to manage these patients with the NOR anesthesiologist forming a key member of the team.

Procedural and Anesthetic Technique Considerations in Interventional Neuroradiology

For most interventional neuroradiologic procedures, arterial access is gained using a 6 or 7 French gauge sheath via the femoral or, rarely, the carotid or axillary artery. The umbilical vessels are an alternative route in neonates. Anticoagulation is required during and up to 24 hours after interventional radiologic procedures to prevent thromboembolism. Heparin, between 3,000 and 5,000 IU (50 to 70 IU/kg), followed by an infusion is used to keep the activated clotting time (ACT) between two and three times the patient's baseline.[43] At the end of the procedure or in case of hemorrhage heparin may be reversed with protamine. General anesthesia and conscious sedation are both suitable techniques for interventional neuroradiology depending on the complexity of the procedure, the need for blood pressure manipulation, and the need for intraprocedural assessment of neurologic function.[36,43] The anesthetic management of patients undergoing endovascular treatment for acute ischemic stroke received much attention recently.[46,47]

Cases performed under general anesthesia and associated with hypotension have been related to poorer neurologic outcome compared to cases performed under local anesthesia and no hypotension. General anesthesia for interventional neuroradiology is usually conducted with endotracheal intubation and intermittent positive-pressure ventilation, although the laryngeal mask airway (LMA) is a suitable alternative in selected cases.[48] Sedation techniques vary; propofol infusions are widely used, as are combinations of a benzodiazepine (usually midazolam) and opioid (usually fentanyl). The anesthesiologist may facilitate the procedure by manipulating systemic blood pressure and controlling end-tidal carbon dioxide tension.

Controlled hypotension is often requested to facilitate embolization of AVMs and moderate hypertension may help reduce cerebral ischemia by maintaining cerebral perfusion. Certain procedures require patients to be awake for part of the procedure. The Wada test (injection of a small dose of a barbiturate or other anesthetic drug directly into one) is used to determine the dominant side for cognitive functions such as speech and memory. This procedure may be used prior to surgery for non–life-threatening conditions such as epilepsy. Permanent neurologic deficits follow embolization of AVMs in approximately 10% of cases.[49] The superselective anesthesia functional examination (SAFE), an extension of the Wada test, may be performed prior to permanent embolization by injecting anesthetic into the vessels to identify angiographically occult vessels that supply normal brain tissue.[50] The worldwide unavailability of amobarbital has led to the use of other agents in these tests including propofol[50,51] and etomidate.

Major complications of interventional neuroradiology are hemorrhagic, such as aneurysm rupture, intracranial vessel injury, or dissection; occlusive, such as displacement or fragmentation of embolic materials or vasospasm; or non-CNS complications, such as contrast hypersensitivity, anaphylaxis, CIN, and hemorrhage at the peripheral vessel puncture site causing groin or retroperitoneal hematoma.[36,43]

Computed Tomography

Computed tomography (CT) scanners obtain a cross-sectional image in a few seconds, and spiral scanners can image a slice of the body in less than 1 second, minimizing problems with motion artifacts. The procedure is painless and most adults do not require sedation or anesthesia. There is an absolute requirement for the patient to remain motionless while the study is being performed and children or adults with psychologic or neurologic disorders preventing immobility may require sedation or anesthesia (Table 33-1). Contrast agents for CT imaging may be administered orally and the anesthesiologist needs to be aware of the possibility of a full stomach. CT scanning may be employed to facilitate invasive procedures such as abscess localization and drainage, ablation of bony metastases, and radiofrequency ablation (RFA) of malignancies. Patients with acute thoracic, abdominal, and cerebral trauma often require urgent imaging to facilitate diagnosis. These patients may develop hemorrhagic shock, raised ICP, depression of consciousness, and cardiac arrest in the CT scanner and must be adequately resuscitated and stabilized before transportation to the radiology department.

Radiofrequency Ablation

Percutaneous RFA is carried out in the radiology suite for treatment of primary and metastatic tumors in the liver, lung, adrenal gland, breast, thyroid, prostate, kidney, and spleen. A high-frequency alternating current is used to generate a localized heat source directly into the tumor causing coagulative necrosis and tumor cell death while avoiding injury to the surrounding tissues. The majority of these procedures are tolerated without sedation. If an anesthesiologist does become involved in the care of these patients, careful evaluation is required; patients may be in the later stages of their disease, have often failed surgical treatment, and may have undergone extensive radiation therapy and/or chemotherapy. Recently, high-frequency jet ventilation (HFJV) has been evaluated in patients undergoing anesthesia for RFA of liver tumors.[52] Positioning of the probe is critical and excursions of the diaphragm in ventilated or spontaneously ventilating patients may cause excessive movement; HFJV minimizes liver motion during these procedures. A variety of anesthesia techniques have been described for percutaneous RFA of hepatic tumors including general anesthesia, sedation, thoracic epidural, and thoracic paravertebral block.[53]

Transjugular Intrahepatic Portosystemic Shunt

The transjugular intrahepatic portosystemic shunt (TIPS) is a connection between the hepatic portal and systemic circulations created via a percutaneous catheter inserted in the internal jugular vein and directed into the liver. The TIPS functions to decompress the portal circulation in patients with portal hypertension. Beneficial effects include reduction in bleeding from varices and control of refractory cirrhotic ascites. The TIPS is often performed in patients who have failed to respond to medical therapy and may be used as a bridge to transplant in patients with poor liver function. The procedure causes minimal stimulation, lasts between 2 and 3 hours, and may be performed under sedation or general anesthesia.[54] Patients presenting for a TIPS procedure, in general, have significant hepatic dysfunction, and require careful preoperative assessment and intraoperative management. The considerations are outlined in Table 33-8 (see also Chapter 46 The Liver: Surgery and Anesthesia).

Table 33-8 Considerations in Patients Presenting for the Transjugular Intrahepatic Portosystemic Shunt Procedure

Airway—risk of aspiration	Recent gastrointestinal bleeding
	Raised intragastric pressure due to ascites
	Decreased level of consciousness due to hepatic encephalopathy
CNS	Hepatic encephalopathy
	Altered mental status
	Variable response to anesthetic agents
Respiratory system	Decreased functional residual capacity due to ascites
	Pleural effusion
	Intrapulmonary shunts
	Pneumonia
Cardiovascular system	Associated alcoholic cardiomyopathy
	Altered volume status
	Acute hemorrhage from esophageal varices
	Intraperitoneal hemorrhage
Hematologic system	Coagulopathy
	Thrombocytopenia
Fluid balance	Ascites
	Risk of hepatorenal syndrome
Endocrine system	Tendency to hypoglycemia
Pharmacokinetics	Increased volume of distribution
	Decreased protein binding, drug metabolism, and elimination

Magnetic Resonance Imaging

Physical Principles

The physical principles of MRI are well described in detail elsewhere.[55] Briefly, when atoms with an odd number of protons in their nuclei, notably hydrogen, are subjected to a powerful static magnetic field, they align themselves with the magnetic field. If they are then intermittently exposed to a radiofrequency wave, the nuclei change their alignment. As the radiofrequency pulses are discontinued, the protons return to their original alignment ("relax") within the magnetic field and, as they do, they release energy. The release of energy over time (the relaxation time) is specific for given tissues and is used to generate the MRI signal. Magnetic field strengths are expressed in Gauss (G) and Tesla (T) (1 T = 10,000 G). The earth's magnetic field is approximately 0.3 to 0.7 G. MRI scanners used for clinical purposes generate a field of 1.5 to 3 T, and machines generating magnetic fields from 4 to 9.4 T are used in research.

Hazards of MRI

MRI is devoid of the risks related to ionizing radiation; however, peripheral nerve stimulation (PNS) has been reported in biologic tissues exposed to radiofrequencies greater than 60 Hz. PNS results in sensory phenomena ranging from mild tingling to intolerable pain. MRI workers may experience transient vertigo-related symptoms and a metallic taste in the mouth when working in high (>3 T) magnetic fields.[56] Ferromagnetic implantable medical devices may move in the magnetic field with disastrous consequences. This issue is a particular concern in patients with cardiac pacemakers, which may also malfunction, and cerebral aneurysm clips.[57] Before entering the vicinity of the magnet, patients and staff need to complete a rigorous checklist to ensure that they have no ferrometallic objects in their bodies. The magnetic field takes several days to establish and is constantly present, decreasing in strength with distance from the center of the magnet. Ferromagnetic equipment such as IV poles, gas cylinders, laryngoscopes, and pens become potentially lethal projectiles if brought too close.

Considerable noise is generated by the rapidly alternating currents of the MRI scanner; this may exceed the occupational exposure limits, defined as a weekly average exposure of 99 dB and peak exposure of 140 dB.[58] Patients and staff should wear ear protection and staff should minimize time spent in the scanner. Cables and wires wound in loops may cause induction-heating effects and thermal injury may also occur in skin with large tattoos, especially those with ferromagnetic inks. Patient monitors, ventilator equipment, and electrical infusion pumps may all malfunction when they come too close to the magnetic field. The electrocardiogram is sensitive to the changing magnetic signals, and it is nearly impossible to eliminate all artifacts. The electrodes should be placed close together and toward the center of the magnetic field and the leads insulated from the patient's skin to avoid causing thermal injury. MRI-compatible devices have been developed; however, in the absence of MRI-compatible monitors, tube extensions can be used to keep standard infusion pumps and monitors at a distance.[55] An MRI sequence takes upward of 30 minutes and many patients find it difficult to stay still for long periods. It may become very warm within the coil of the magnet, often reaching 80°F, adding to patient discomfort and is of particular concern in children whose temperatures should be monitored. Once a scan sequence is initiated, no one may enter or leave the scan room. In the case of an emergency, the MRI technicians should be notified, the scan sequence stopped, and the patient rapidly removed. Resuscitation attempts should take place outside the scanner because equipment such as laryngoscopes, oxygen cylinders, and cardiac defibrillators cannot be taken close to the magnet.

Anesthetic Technique

Claustrophobia is a real concern for up to 15% of all adult patients undergoing MRI necessitating sedation or even general anesthesia for them to complete the imaging studies.[59] Sedation may be provided by the oral route with benzodiazepines, as intravenous sedation or MAC. Interventions including the design of the MRI scanner, cognitive-behavioral strategies, prone positioning, and fragrance administration have also been reported to reduce anxiety during MRI scan.[60] Anesthesiologists may become involved with more complex patients such as those with obesity, obstructive sleep apnea, raised ICP, movement disorders, developmental delay, and when there is a potential for a difficult airway.

Pediatric Sedation and Anesthesia for MRI and CT Scans

In children, a combination of incomprehension, separation anxiety, and fear can result in noncooperation and intolerance of relatively brief periods of immobility. Most children younger than 5 years and some as old as 11 years, particularly those with developmental delay, require sedation or general anesthesia for successful acquisition of MRI or CT images.[61] There is ongoing debate about the optimal care and techniques for these cases.[62,63] The benefits of a "sedation-only" approach include ease of medication administration (oral, rectal, or sometimes intravenous), lower cost (a sedation-trained nurse rather than an anesthesiologist), and more rapid wakening and discharge home. Disadvantages include a higher failure rate than general anesthesia, airway complications arising from oversedation, unpredictable onset of enteral sedatives causing schedule delays, and inadequate analgesia during painful procedures. The choice of sedation or general anesthesia for a particular child is multifactorial and has been obfuscated in the past by the use of imprecise terms to describe the different clinical states.[64] As with all NORA, the standards of care for pediatric patients undergoing sedation and/or general anesthesia for MRI and CT imaging are the same as those in the operating room; a useful acronym "SOAPME" (Suction, Oxygen, Airway equipment, appropriate Pharmaceuticals, Monitoring, and special Equipment) has been coined before embarking upon any pediatric sedation or anesthetic.[65]

Sedative Agents

Older sedation practices in pediatric patients included the use of oral chloral hydrate, "lytic cocktails," barbiturates, and the "feed, wrap, and scan" technique in otherwise healthy neonates avoiding sedation or anesthesia altogether. These techniques, however, are being superseded by the use of short-acting agents including propofol, remifentanil, and dexmedetomidine[4] which provide more reliable pharmacologic profiles and have preferable track records for adverse events.[66]

Radiation Therapy

External beam radiation is a common treatment for children with malignancies, making use of either highly tissue-targeted or total

> **Table 33-9** Common Radiosensitive Tumors in Children
>
> Primary CNS tumor—neuroblastoma, medulloblastoma
> Acute leukemia—CNS leukemia
> Radiosensitive ocular tumors—retinoblastoma
> Intra-abdominal tumors—Wilms tumor
> Rhabdomyosarcoma
> Other tumors—Langerhans cell histiocytosis

body irradiating (TBI) doses of x-rays. Proton beam therapy is a newer modality of this therapy, which has less potential for collateral injury to adjacent or beam-traversed tissues, a factor of utmost importance in pediatric patients at risk of long-term complications of radiation exposure.[67,68] Radiosensitive malignancies occurring in children are shown in Table 33-9. Tumors commonly involve vital structures such as the airway, thorax, mediastinum, heart, and central nervous system (CNS). Thorough preoperative assessment is essential, including assessment for raised ICP in children with CNS tumors. Many children receive concurrent cytotoxic or immunosuppressive chemotherapy and are at increased risk of sepsis, thrombocytopenia, and anemia. The challenges of anesthesia for children undergoing radiation therapy have recently been reviewed.[68–70] Patients are typically scheduled for a series of daily treatments, which can last upward of 45 minutes, over a 6-week period. Radiation doses in the range of 180 to 250 centiGray (cGy) are employed, so interfaced systems of closed-circuit television and telemetric microphones are used with standard monitoring to prevent staff being exposed to high levels of radiation. In the event of a problem, shutdown of the radiation beam and immediate access to the patient (within 20 to 30 seconds) is crucial. Children older than 6 or 7 years can sometimes tolerate repeated treatment sessions without sedation or anesthesia using behavioral techniques,[70] although most require general anesthesia or deep sedation techniques with propofol.[71,72] Absence of movement is crucial to ensure treatment beam accuracy and immobilization devices, especially those applied to the face and head, are unpleasant for the child and may cause airway concerns for the anesthesiologist. Most children will have indwelling central venous access, avoiding the need for repeated intravenous puncture or inhalational induction. Radiation treatments are also used in adults who have a greater capacity than children to remain still without sedation or general anesthesia.

Positron Emission Tomography

Positron emission tomography (PET) scanning is a newer imaging modality using radiolabeled isotopes to measure tissue glucose uptake thereby estimating tumor extent. Anesthesia concerns are those for CT; studies typically take longer to complete which may affect choice of technique/agent. Patients are typically exposed to greater ionizing radiation from both isotope and CT sources.[55]

Gastroenterology

Procedures commonly performed in the gastrointestinal (GI) endoscopy suite are described in Table 33-2. Procedures may be performed under general anesthesia or sedation.[73] The American Gastroenterological Association reports that 98% of patients for upper and lower endoscopies receive sedation.[74] Of these, over one-third are performed in ambulatory surgery centers and only 29% of these procedures involve anesthesia care providers.[74,75] Controversy surrounds the administration of sedation for GI procedures both in the United States[74] and world-wide.[76] A wide variety of sedation techniques are practiced and gastroenterologists are increasingly advocating for the use of propofol sedation by nonanesthesiologists, citing the safety and efficacy of these techniques (nonanesthesiologist administered propofol "NAAP" or nurse-administered propofol sedation "NAPS").[77,78] However, the use of propofol by those without expert airway skills remains controversial in the anesthesiology community.[79] It should, however, be noted that in recently published guidelines, gastroenterologists do universally agree that patients in ASA classes III or IV, for complex procedures, or with histories of adverse or inadequate responses to sedation require the involvement of an anesthesiologist.[76,80]

Upper Gastrointestinal Endoscopy

Upper GI endoscopy is performed for diagnostic procedures, such as biopsy, and for therapeutic procedures, such as retrieval of foreign bodies, treatment of esophageal varices with sclerotherapy or band ligation, dilation of esophageal strictures, and placement of a percutaneous endoscopic gastrostomy. Patients may have a number of comorbidities, or a risk of gastroesophageal reflux, hepatic dysfunction, coagulopathy, and ascites. Sedation techniques or general anesthesia may be used after careful patient assessment and discussion with the endoscopist. Under general anesthesia, tracheal intubation is the gold standard to protect the airway and facilitate passage of the endoscope; however, a-LMA may serve as an alternative device for airway management.[81] Local anesthetic is sprayed into the oropharynx to facilitate passage of the endoscope, which can abolish the gag reflex, increasing the risk of aspiration. A bite block is inserted to prevent the patient from biting down on the endoscope and damaging both the teeth and the endoscope. Procedures are performed in the prone or semiprone position with the patient's head rotated to the side, making the airway less accessible. Care and attention should also be paid to pressure areas, particularly the eyes, lips, and teeth, and extreme rotation of the neck should be avoided. Most procedures are brief, lasting 10 to 30 minutes, and are generally painless.

Endoscopic Retrograde Cholangiopancreatography

Endoscopic retrograde cholangiopancreatography (ERCP) is important in the diagnosis and treatment of both biliary and pancreatic diseases. During the procedure, the biliary and pancreatic duct systems are identified, instrumented, and therapeutic maneuvers such as the passage of stents or removal of stones carried out. The complication rate during ERCP is reported as between 5% and 10% with a mortality of 0.1% to 1%. Complications include acute pancreatitis, hemorrhage, and perforation.[82,83] Patients usually experience discomfort during ERCP and general anesthesia or deep sedation techniques are recommended for the procedure, which usually lasts between 20 and 80 minutes. The airway and patient positioning considerations are similar to those for GI endoscopy. Sphincter of Oddi manometry may be performed in which case drugs that affect sphincter pressure such as atropine, glycopyrrolate, glucagon, and various opioids should be avoided. Patients presenting for ERCP may have significant comorbidities including acute cholangitis with septicemia, jaundice with liver dysfunction and coagulopathy, bleeding from esophageal varices resulting in hypovolemia, or biliary stricture following major hepatobiliary surgery, including liver transplantation. Transient bacteremia may occur during endoscopy, and antibiotic prophylaxis is recommended for patients with cardiac valvular abnormalities. Gastroenterologists frequently use antispasmodics such as glucagon and intravenous hyoscyamine to reduce duodenal motility and improve operating conditions during endoscopy[84]; sinus tachycardia may occur.

Cardiology and Interventional Cardiology

The number of interventional cardiology and electrophysiology (EP) procedures has dramatically increased in most institutions over the last decade, with approximately 400,000 pacemakers and implantable cardiac defibrillators (ICDs) being placed each year in the United States.[85] As volumes and patient complexity increase anesthesiologists are playing a much more significant role in the EP and cardiac catheterization laboratories. Hybrid operating rooms with fluoroscopy capability are becoming more common in the design plans for new ORs and these are usually designed with the anesthesiologist in mind. Cardiac catheterization laboratories and EP laboratories are often simply modified to accommodate anesthesia providers. This retrofit can make for frequent territorial and ergonomic constraints.

Percutaneous Intervention

For patients with evidence of myocardial ischemia, cardiac catheterization and coronary angiography is an essential step in the diagnosis of coronary artery disease. Often this step is followed by coronary angioplasty with stenting for intracoronary luminal obstructions that are more than 70%.[86] The procedures are usually done with mild sedation administered by the catheterization laboratory team: blood pressure, EKG, and pulse oximetry are monitored and the patient breathes spontaneously with oxygen administered by nasal prongs or a facemask. However, the care of an anesthesiologist may be required for patients who are hemodynamically unstable or in cardiogenic shock either before or during the procedure. Early recognition of at-risk patients allows for coordination between the anesthesiologist and cardiologists to avoid hypoxia and hypercarbia. Certain percutaneous interventions (PCIs) have a higher level of complexity and can involve patients with significant comorbidities. Coronary atherectomy for chronic total occlusion can be time consuming and technically difficult due to complex anatomy and general anesthesia is usually required. The anesthesiologist should prepare for potential hemodynamic instability with routine anesthetic monitors, possible arterial blood pressure monitoring, and good peripheral or central IV access. Cardiologists are often working through the femoral veins and in an emergency situation it is possible to link sterile intravenous tubing to the access sites for administration of inotropes and vasopressors.

Percutaneous Ventricular Assist Devices

Patients in cardiogenic shock or having high-risk PCI or EP procedures may benefit from the hemodynamic support provided by percutaneous ventricular assist devices. The TandemHeart (Cardiac Assist, Inc., Pittsburg, Pennsylvania) is a left atrial to femoral bypass system that offers flow rates up to 4.0 L/min through an external centrifugal pump. It is designed for short duration support (14 to 162 hours for cardiogenic shock and 1 to 24 hours for high-risk PCIs).[87] The Impella Recover 2.5 and 5.0 (Abiomed Inc., Danvers, MA, USA) are similar devices but allow for easier implantation as there is no requirement for a transseptal puncture and the device is smaller. A microaxial pump supports either 2.5 or 5.0 L/min.[88] Patients who are unable to keep still or lie flat will require general anesthesia; the rest can be managed with light sedation using agents such as dexmedetomidine or propofol. Transesophageal echocardiography (TEE) guidance may also be required to guide cannula positioning.

Percutaneous Closure of Septal Defects

A number of different devices have been introduced for the closure of patent foramen ovales (PFOs) and atrial septal defects (ASDs). These devices are placed by the cardiologist under the guidance of fluoroscopy and ultrasound. The introduction of intracardiac echocardiography (ICE) has lessened the need for general anesthesia to facilitate TEE guidance[89]; however, general anesthesia is still useful to ensure patient comfort and safety while the devices are deployed. Special attention should be paid to avoiding air in any intravenous tubing as left to right shunts can be reversed with the drop in systemic vascular resistance that accompanies many anesthetic agents.

Alcohol Septal Ablation

Alcohol septal ablation offers an alternative to open heart myomectomy for patients with hypertrophic cardiomyopathy with equivalent mortality outcomes.[90] Specific septal perforator vessels are identified using coronary angiography and injection of approximately 3 mL of absolute ethanol into these vessels causes a controlled infarction of the hypertrophic septum.[91] This infarction can be visualized in real time on live echocardiography. Although the majority of the procedure requires only minimal sedation the alcohol injection can be very painful. A controlled myocardial infarction feels very much like an uncontrolled one so deep sedation will be necessary for the injection portion of the procedure.

Structural Heart Procedures

Transcatheter Aortic Valve Replacement

Calcific aortic stenosis affects almost 5% of adults over the age of 65.[92] Once symptoms of syncope and heart failure begin, 50% of patients will die within 3 years; however, surgical aortic valve replacement (SAVR) in elderly patients with multiple comorbidities can carry a mortality rate of up to 20%.[93] Transcatheter aortic valve replacements (TAVRs) use a sophisticated catheter delivery system to deploy a folded replacement valve through a sheath in the common femoral artery, subclavian artery, or via a minithoracotomy directly into the aorta or left ventricular apex.[92] Rapid ventricular pacing is used to minimize left ventricular ejection so that the new valve can be deployed into the correct position. Initially TAVR was only offered to extremely high-risk surgical patients; however, ongoing studies show potential benefit to intermediate surgical risk patients.[93]

The CoreValve ReValving System (Medtronic, Inc., Minneapolis, MN) is self-expanding and is made of bioprosthetic porcine pericardial tissue sutured into a malleable metal stent that is rigid at body temperature.[92] The compressed CoreValve is slowly deployed as its delivery system is pulled back and allows for some repositioning before the valve is fully released. The Edwards SAPIEN XT transcatheter heart valve (Edwards Lifesciences, Irvine, CA) is a bovine pericardial tissue valve in a cobalt chromium alloy stent, which has a smaller diameter delivery system. This valve expands with a balloon within the native valve with the goal of displacing the native leaflets.[93]

Research and development in structural heart procedures is ongoing and new and improved TAVR devices will be available for clinical use soon. Initial experience with TAVR procedures required general anesthesia and TEE for all patients; however, many institutions are using sedation with transthoracic echo (TTE) standby.[94] These patients are at high risk for cardiac death during the procedure and experience frequent hemodynamic instability during the rapid ventricular pacing that is required for balloon valvuloplasty and for valve deployment.[94,95] Cardiopulmonary bypass standby is present for many patients. Given the physiologic sequelae of aortic stenosis, all patients undergoing TAVR procedures should have preinduction arterial line blood pressure monitoring. Central access in the neck or groin is essential for inotrope and vasopressor administration and large bore IV access is necessary for fluid resuscitation if blood loss is significant. The large cannulae that are exchanged in and out of the groin during the procedure can result in a surprising drop in hematocrit which should be checked frequently during the procedure. One-lung ventilation may be helpful for both the transapical approach and when directly cannulating the ascending aorta, which can be accomplished with either a double lumen tube or a bronchial blocker. The goal for most of these procedures is to extubate the patient in the procedure room or shortly thereafter. Many of the patients are elderly and at high risk for delirium; thus, benzodiazepines and long-acting opioids should be avoided if possible.

MitraClip

Mitral regurgitation (MR) is the most common valvular disorder in the aging population in the United States.[96] Cardiac surgical mitral valve repair should be offered to all surgical candidates with symptomatic MR.[97] In North America, the MitraClip (Evalve, San Francisco, California) is intended to treat patients with moderately severe to severe symptomatic degenerative MR who are considered too high risk for open heart surgery.[96] In Europe, these guidelines expand to also include those with severe symptomatic functional MR.[98] The MitraClip delivers a clip device percutaneously that mimics the Alfieri edge-to-edge repair to create a double orifice mitral valve (Figs. 33-3 and 33-4).[99]

Recent evaluations have shown that the MitraClip is effective in reducing MR and improving LV remodeling. As well, mortality associated with the MitraClip is less than with surgery using the predicted outcomes surgical risk predictors.[96] Patients

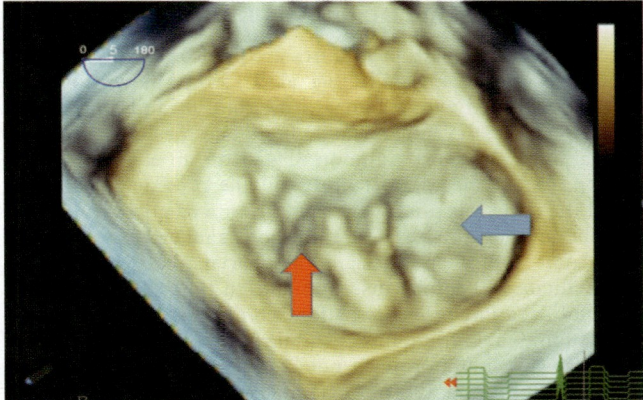

Figure 33-3 Three dimensional en face view of mitral valve. *Blue arrow* points to A3 portion of anterior mitral leaflet. *Red arrow* points between P1 (left) and P2 prolapsing segments of the posterior leaflet with flail chordae visible. (Courtesy of Dr G.B. Mackensen MD, PhD, FASE.)

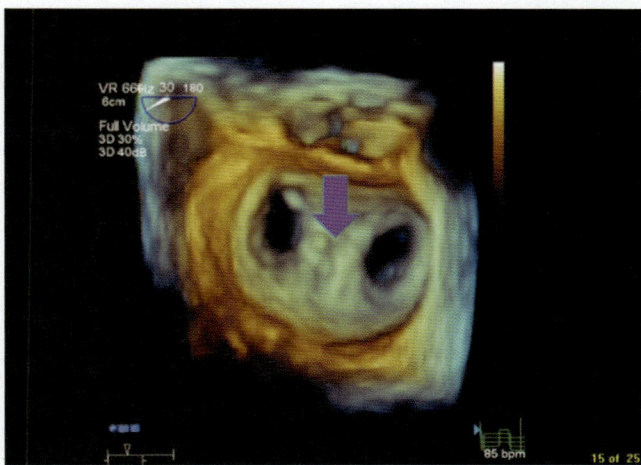

Figure 33-4 Three dimensional en face view of mitral valve after two MitraClips deployed. *Purple arrow* shows where the two clips have been placed between A2 and P2 segments of the mitral valve. (Courtesy of Dr G.B. Mackensen MD, PhD, FASE.)

undergoing the MitraClip procedure receive a general anesthetic with invasive monitors and TEE.

Left Atrial Appendage Occlusion

The left atrial appendage (LAA) is a source of clot formation in patients with atrial fibrillation and patients require lifelong anticoagulation to prevent this source of embolism. If the LAA can be removed, then anticoagulation is no longer necessary. Traditionally LAA closures have been performed through median sternotomy; however, the Watchman (Boston Scientific, Minneapolis, MN) is a novel device that can be deployed directly into the LAA via a transfemoral catheter.[100] Presently the Watchman is offered to patients with nonvalvular atrial fibrillation and at least one risk factor (age >75 years, hypertension, diabetes, or prior stroke/transient ischemic attack).[101] An additional indication for this device is patients who have a major contraindication to long-term anticoagulation. The device has been shown to reduce hemorrhagic stroke and cardiovascular death when compared to warfarin although there is an increased incidence of ischemic stroke as a periprocedural event.[102] The procedure requires meticulous evaluation of the LAA by TEE to ensure proper device is selected. Arterial catheters should be used to measure arterial blood pressure for most of these procedures.

Electrophysiology

Like many catheterization laboratory procedures, sedation for EP procedures can sometimes be managed by cardiologists; however, both patient and procedure complexity often necessitate general anesthesia to facilitate a safe and comfortable experience for the patient. EP studies can be divided into cardiac implantable electronic devices (CIEDs) and EP studies with ablation.[103]

Cardiac Implantable Electronic Devices

CIEDs include pacemakers for symptomatic bradycardia and for chronic resynchronization therapy (CRT) and implantable cardioverter defibrillators (ICDs). These devices are usually implanted in the left pectoral area with one to three transvenous leads inserted into the axillary, subclavian, or cephalic veins.[104] Pacemakers can generally be placed under light sedation with local anesthetic to the skin for the pacemaker pocket; if significant patient comorbidities exist it may be necessary to administer general anesthesia for this procedure. ICDs decrease the risk of sudden cardiac death by both primary and secondary prevention of ventricular tachycardia and ventricular fibrillation.[105] Primary prevention ICDs are indicated for those with an EF less than 35%, with NYHA class II–III symptoms who are on optimal heart failure medical therapy.[106] Secondary prevention ICDs are for patients who have had a documented ventricular fibrillation cardiac arrest or an episode of sustained ventricular tachycardia.[107] The implantation of the device is similar to the process for placing a pacemaker; however, the defibrillation threshold testing requires much deeper sedation. General anesthesia may be necessary for threshold testing in patients with left ventricular dysfunction.[85] CRT pacemakers are indicated for those with cardiomyopathy, an EF less than 35%, a left bundle branch block (LBBB), QRS duration less than 120 milliseconds, and NYHA class II–IV symptoms.[108] A lead is placed transvenously into the coronary sinus which allows for simultaneous pacing of the left and right ventricles: this reduces mortality and improves quality of life.[109] Many patients in heart failure are unable to lie flat for the duration of the procedure and placing a lead into the coronary sinus in someone with ventricular dilatation and valvular regurgitation can be challenging with sedation alone.[85]

EP Studies with Ablations

EP studies can be performed for risk stratification or to evaluate specific symptoms that suggest an arrhythmia[105]; however, it is uncommon to not pair these with concurrent ablation procedures, especially if the ablation is to treat tachyarrhythmias (Table 33-10).

The most common ablation procedures performed currently are for narrow complex tachycardias such as atrial fibrillation or atrial flutter and for wide complex tachycardias like polymorphic ventricular tachycardia. Patients with atrial fibrillation should be effectively anticoagulated or have a TEE assessment preablation to rule out an LAA thrombus. Ablation catheters are inserted via the femoral veins into the right heart to try to induce arrhythmias. Complex mapping techniques localize the source of the arrhythmia and an energy source is applied to ablate this source. Ablations can be performed with either radiofrequency or cryothermy with the former being much more stimulating for the patient.[110] Saline irrigation is used to cool the energy delivery system and therefore can result in significant volume administration during long procedures.[111] The phrenic nerve lies close to the right upper pulmonary veins and is at risk during ablation. Avoidance of neuromuscular blockade will alert the electrophysiologist to phrenic irritation when this area is being ablated.[109] Although drugs that affect the sympathetic and parasympathetic systems can influence the sinus and atrioventricular nodes, there is little evidence to support the notion that general anesthesia affects inducibility of specific arrhythmias.[85,112] The duration of ablation procedures can be lengthy (4 to 8 hours) and mapping requires minute catheter adjustments that are sensitive to patient movement. The ablation process can also be painful and general anesthesia may be required. Invasive arterial blood pressure monitoring is helpful in these patients, especially for those with reduced ejection fractions in whom hemodynamically unstable arrhythmias might be induced.

Laser Lead Extractions

As pacemakers and ICDs become more widespread, so does the need for lead extractions. Device infections, lead endocarditis, thrombosis or venous stenosis, chronic pain due to leads/device, and nonfunctional leads are all reasons for lead removal.[113] Leads become well adhered to the subclavian vein and/or the endocardium which makes this particular procedure very anxiety provoking for all involved. Vascular injury causing significant blood loss and cardiac tamponade is rare but the involved clinicians should be prepared for it. General anesthesia with large bore intravenous access and invasive blood pressure monitoring is essential; TEE is usually advisable for prompt evaluation of hemodynamic changes. As expected, centers with higher lead extraction volume have a lower probability of complications and death.[114]

Cardioversions and Diagnostic TEEs

Cardioversion and TEE procedures are brief procedures but are exquisitely stimulating. Elective electrical cardioversions are ideally performed with a bolus of propofol on fully monitored patients under the supervision of an anesthesiologist. Atrial fibrillation is the most common reason for an elective cardioversion, so it is necessary to rule out the presence of an LAA clot if the patient is not on therapeutic anticoagulation to avoid embolic complications.[115] TEE is the gold standard for evaluating the LAA.[116] Topical anesthesia in the pharynx with 4% lidocaine can facilitate TEE probe insertion and an infusion of low-dose propofol sedation provides patient comfort with spontaneous ventilation. Standard monitors should be applied, and although end-tidal CO_2 monitoring is not completely necessary, it can be very helpful. Many of the patients presenting for cardioversion and elective TEE have compromised cardiac function; thus, resuscitation drugs should be readily available.

The anesthesiologist may also be involved in elective TEEs for specific indications under the American Society of Echocardiography (ASE) guidelines including evaluation of suspected

Table 33-10 Arrhythmia Classification

Bradyarrhythmias
Sick sinus syndrome
Atrioventricular block
    First-degree heart block
    Second-degree heart block (Mobitz type I and II)
    Third-degree heart block

Tachyarrhythmias
Regular rhythm, normal QRS
    Sinus tachycardia
    Atrioventricular nodal reentrant tachycardia
    Atrioventricular reciprocating tachycardia—orthodromic
    Junctional tachycardia
    Atrial flutter
Irregular rhythm, narrow QRS
    Atrial fibrillation
    Multifocal atrial tachycardia
    Frequent premature atrial contractions
Regular rhythm, wide QRS
    Monomorphic ventricular tachycardia
    Atrioventricular reciprocating tachycardia, antidromic
    Regular supraventricular tachycardias with bundle branch block
Irregular rhythm, wide QRS
    Polymorphic ventricular tachycardia
    Ventricular fibrillation
    Frequent premature ventricular contractions
    Irregular supraventricular tachycardias with bundle branch block

Table 33-11 Anesthetic Consideration for Electroconvulsive Therapy

Anesthetic Requirements	Comments
Amnesia	With induction agent of choice
Airway management	Usually with bag–mask ventilation, although the laryngeal mask has been used with success[122]
Moderate hypocapnia	Improves the quality and duration of seizures[123]
Protection of the teeth and tongue during the seizure	Using a soft bite block
Prevention of seizure-related injuries (fractures and dislocations)	Small doses of muscle relaxant, e.g., succinic choline (0.75–1.5 mg/kg) are most commonly used unless there are contraindications
Control of hemodynamic responses	Labetalol; esmolol; and the calcium channel antagonists nifedipine, diltiazem, and nicardipine all attenuate the hemodynamic responses to ECT. Dexmedetomidine (1 μg/kg administered over 10 minutes just before induction of anesthesia) has been shown to be effective in controlling blood pressure without affecting seizure duration.[124]
Control or prevention of the parasympathetic effects of ECT (salivation, transient bradycardia, and asystole)	Can be prevented with glycopyrrolate or atropine
Analgesia to relieve postseizure myalgia	Ketorolac 15–30 mg is effective in younger patients Acetaminophen or aspirin may be used in older patients or where NSAIDs are contraindicated

aortic dissection, determining suitability for valve repair, diagnosis of endocarditis, evaluation of persistent fever with an intracardiac device, and evaluation for LAA thrombus.[117] Anesthesiologists caring for these patients should ensure that there are no contraindications to TEE related to known esophageal pathology (strictures, varices, malignancy, recent ulcer or hemorrhage, Zenker diverticulum) or those with a history of unevaluated dysphagia.[117] Although topical anesthesia and sedation are usually sufficient, uncooperative patients and those with a potentially difficult airway should be prophylactically intubated and maintained on TIVA. In these situations, the anesthesiologist can help facilitate passage of the TEE probe using a laryngoscope.

Electroconvulsive Therapy

Electroconvulsive therapy (ECT) has had an important role in the management of depression, mania, and affective disorders since the 1930s.[118] Typically it is performed three times a week for 6 to 12 treatments, followed by weekly or monthly maintenance therapy to prevent relapses.[119]

Physiologic Response to Electroconvulsive Therapy

The physiologic response to ECT includes generalized motor seizures and an acute cardiovascular response. The seizure usually lasts several minutes and minimum seizure duration of 25 seconds is recommended to ensure adequate antidepressant efficacy.[120] The cardiovascular response includes transient bradycardia and occasional asystole giving way to more prominent hypertension and tachycardia. Increased cerebral blood flow, raised ICP and cardiac dysrhythmias, myocardial ischemia, infarction, or neurologic vascular events may be precipitated. Short-term memory loss is also common following ECT. Other sequelae include myalgias, bone fractures, joint dislocations, headache, emergence agitation, status epilepticus, and sudden death.

Anesthetic Considerations for ECT

Scalp electrodes are placed to monitor the electroencephalogram and a blood pressure cuff is applied to an extremity and inflated before muscle relaxant is administered to monitor the seizure. Patients presenting for ECT are often elderly, with a number of coexisting conditions.[121] Patients may be taking antidepressant medications which include tricyclic antidepressants, monoamine oxidase inhibitors, and selective serotonin-reuptake inhibitors. Of these drugs, the monoamine oxidase inhibitors have the most significant interactions with anesthetic agents. The anesthetic requirements for ECT are described in Table 33-11.

Most of the intravenous induction agents have been used for ECT,[121] despite their anticonvulsant effects. Methohexital (1 to 1.5 mg/kg), historically considered the "gold standard," appears to have less anticonvulsant activity than the other agents. Etomidate (0.15 to 0.3 mg/kg) is generally associated with longer seizure duration and is the preferred agent of some psychiatrists, despite a slightly longer recovery and associated myoclonus. Propofol is more effective at attenuating the acute hemodynamic responses than etomidate and in small doses (0.75 mg/kg) seizure duration is usually acceptable.[125] Short-acting opioids, such as remifentanil, can be used to decrease the dose of induction agent and prolong seizure duration without reducing the depth of anesthesia.[126] Recently ketamine, either alone or in combination, has been attributed intrinsic antidepressant effects when used as an anesthetic agent for ECT, although its effects are far from certain.[127]

Summary

The number and complexity of NOR procedures is steadily increasing. This increase has resulted in an expansion of anesthesia services in areas remote from the operating room that may not be familiar to anesthesia providers. In preparing to administer anesthesia or sedation in a NOR site, a simple three-step approach can be followed. This approach involves giving careful consideration to the evaluation and the needs of the *patient*, the particular challenges posed by the *procedure*, and the hazards and limitations of the *environment*. In all cases, the standards of anesthesia care and monitoring should be no different than those provided in the conventional operating room.

REFERENCES

1. Committee of Origin: Standards and Practice Parameters. Statement on non-operating room anesthetizing locations. Approved by the ASA House of Delegates on October 19, 1994, and last amended on October 16. 2013. https://www.asahq.org/quality-and-practice-management/standards-and-guidelines. Accessed December 18, 2015.
2. Anesthesia Quality Institute. https://www.aqihq.org. National Anesthesia Clinical Outcomes Registry (NACOR). Accessed December 3, 2015.
3. Chang B, Kaye AD, Diaz JH, et al. Complications of non-operating room procedures: outcomes from the National Anesthesia Clinical Outcomes Registry. *J Patient Saf.* 2015 Apr 7 [Epub ahead of print].
4. Tobias JD. Sedation of infants and children outside of the operating room. *Curr Opin Anaesthesiol.* 2015;28(4):478–485.
5. Care Committee of Origin: Standards and Practice Parameters. Basic standards for preanesthesia. (Approved by the ASA House of Delegates on October 14, 1987, and last affirmed on October 28, 2015). https://www.asahq.org/quality-and-practice-management/standards-and-guidelines. Accessed December 18, 2015.
6. Committee of Origin: Standards and Practice Parameters. Standards for basic anesthetic monitoring. Approved by the ASA House of Delegates on October 21, 1986, and last amended on October 20, 2010, and last affirmed on October 28, 2015. http://www.asahq.org/quality-and-practice-management/standards-and-guidelines. Accessed December 18, 2015.
7. Committee of Origin: Standards and Practice Parameters. Standards for post-anesthesia care. Approved by the ASA House of Delegates on October 27, 2004, and last amended on October 15, 2014. http://www.asahq.org/quality-and-practice-management/standards-and-guidelines. Accessed December 18, 2015.
8. Metzner J, Posner KL, Domino KB. The risk and safety of anesthesia at remote locations: the US closed claims analysis. *Curr Opin Anaesthesiol.* 2009; 22(4):502–508.
9. Metzner J, Domino KB. Risks of anesthesia or sedation outside the operating room: the role of the anesthesia care provider. *Curr Opin Anaesthesiol.* 2010;23(4):523–531.
10. Metzner J, Posner KL, Lam MS, et al. Closed claims' analysis. *Best Pract Res Clin Anaesthesiol.* 2011;25(2):263–276.
11. Waugh JB, Epps CA, Khodneva YA. Capnography enhances surveillance of respiratory events during procedural sedation: a meta-analysis. *J Clin Anesth.* 2011;23(3):189–196.
12. Semel ME, Resch S, Haynes AB, et al. Adopting a surgical safety checklist could save money and improve the quality of care in U.S. hospitals. *Health Aff (Millwood).* 2010;29(9):1593–1599.
13. Hill MR, Roberts MJ, Alderson ML, et al. Safety culture and the 5 steps to safer surgery: an intervention study. *Br J Anaesth.* 2015;114(6):958–962.
14. Lee MJ, Fanelli F, Haage P, et al. Patient safety in interventional radiology: a CIRSE IR checklist. *Cardiovasc Intervent Radiol.* 2012;35(2):244–246.
15. Kue R, Brown P, Ness C, et al. Adverse clinical events during intrahospital transport by a specialized team: a preliminary report. *Am J Crit Care.* 2011; 20(2):153–161.
16. Position on monitored anesthesia care. Committee of Origin: Economics. Approved by the House of Delegates on October 25, 2005, and last amended on October 16, 2013. https://www.asahq.org/search?q=position on monitored anesthesia care. Accessed December 18, 2015.
17. ASA interpretive guidelines templates. Approved by the ASA Committee on Quality Management and Departmental Administration on May 19, 2011, and last amended on October 8, 2014. https://www.asahq.org/quality-and-practice-management/quality-improvement/qmda-toolkit/interpretive-guidelines-templates. Accessed December 18, 2015.
18. Committee of Origin: Quality Management and Departmental Administration. Continuum of depth of sedation: definition of general anesthesia and levels of sedation/analgesia. Approved by the ASA House of Delegates on October 13, 1999, and last amended on October 15, 2014. https://www.asahq.org/quality-and-practice-management/standards-and-guidelines. Accessed December 18, 2015.
19. Martel JP, Barnett SR. Sedation: definitions and regulations. *Int Anesthesiol Clin.* 2015;53(2):1–12.
20. Miller DL. Overview of contemporary interventional fluoroscopy procedures. *Health Phys.* 2008;95(5):638–644.
21. Semelka RC, Armao DM, Elias J, et al. Imaging strategies to reduce the risk of radiation in CT studies, including selective substitution with MRI. *J Magn Reson Imaging.* 2007;25(5):900–909.
22. Mitchell EL, Furey P. Prevention of radiation injury from medical imaging. *J Vasc Surg.* 2011;53(1 Suppl):22S–27S.
23. Miller DL, Vañó E, Bartal G, et al. Occupational radiation protection in interventional radiology: a joint guideline of the Cardiovascular and Interventional Radiology Society of Europe and the Society of Interventional Radiology. *J Vasc Interv Radiol.* 2010;21(5):607–615.
24. Mohapatra A, Greenberg RK, Mastracci TM, et al. Radiation exposure to operating room personnel and patients during endovascular procedures. *J Vasc Surg.* 2013;58(3):702–709.
25. Anastasian ZH, Strozyk D, Meyers PM, et al. Radiation exposure of the anesthesiologist in the neurointerventional suite. *Anesthesiology.* 2011;114(3): 512–520.
26. ICRP, 2007. The 2007 Recommendations of the International Commission on Radiological Protection. ICRP Publication 103. *Ann. ICRP.* 37:2–4.
27. National Council on Radiation Protection and Measurements. *Limitation of exposure to ionizing radiation. NCRP Report No. 116.* Bethesda, MD: National Council on Radiation Protection and Measurements; 1993.
28. Thomsen HS. Contrast media safety-an update. *Eur J Radiol.* 2011;80(1):77–82.
29. Beckett KR, Moriarity AK, Langer JM. Safe use of contrast media: what the radiologist needs to know. *Radiographics.* 2015;35(6):1738–1750.
30. Nicola R, Shaqdan KW, Aran K, et al. Contrast-induced nephropathy: identifying the risks, choosing the right agent, and reviewing effective prevention and management methods. *Curr Probl Diagn Radiol.* 2015;44(6):501–504.
31. McCullough PA. Radiocontrast-induced acute kidney injury. *Nephron Physiol.* 2008;109(4):61–72.
32. Brockow K. Immediate drug hypersensitivity: epidemiology, clinical features, triggers and management. *Hautarzt.* 2014;65(5):409–414.
33. Davenport MS, Cohan RH, Ellis JH. Contrast media controversies in 2015: imaging patients with renal impairment or risk of contrast reaction. *AJR Am J Roentgenol.* 2015;204(6):1174–1181.
34. Prince MR, Zhang H, Zou Z, et al. Incidence of immediate gadolinium contrast media reactions. *AJR Am J Roentgenol.* 2011;196(2):W138–W143.
35. Zou Z, Zhang HL, Roditi GH, et al. Nephrogenic systemic fibrosis: review of 370 biopsy-confirmed cases. *JACC Cardiovasc Imaging.* 2011;4(11):1206–1216.
36. Guercio JR, Nimjee SM, James ML, et al. Anesthesia for interventional neuroradiology. *Int Anesthesiol Clin.* 2015;53(1):87–106.
37. Fusco MR, Ogilvy CS. Surgical and endovascular management of cerebral aneurysms. *Int Anesthesiol Clin.* 2015;53(1):146–165.
38. Molyneux AJ, Kerr RS, Birks J, et al. Risk of recurrent subarachnoid haemorrhage, death, or dependence and standardised mortality ratios after clipping or coiling of an intracranial aneurysm in the International Subarachnoid Aneurysm Trial (ISAT): long-term follow-up. *Lancet Neurol.* 2009;8(5):427–433.
39. Molyneux AJ, Birks J, Clarke A, et al. The durability of endovascular coiling versus neurosurgical clipping of ruptured cerebral aneurysms: 18 year follow-up of the UK cohort of the International Subarachnoid Aneurysm Trial (ISAT). *Lancet.* 2015;385(9969):691–697.
40. Schulenburg E, Matta B. Anaesthesia for interventional neuroradiology. *Curr Opin Anaesthesiol.* 2011;24(4):426–432.
41. Ryttlefors M, Enblad P, Kerr RS, et al. International subarachnoid aneurysm trial of neurosurgical clipping versus endovascular coiling: subgroup analysis of 278 elderly patients. *Stroke.* 2008;39(10):2720–2726.
42. Thompson BG, Brown RD, Amin-Hanjani S, et al. Guidelines for the management of patients with unruptured intracranial aneurysms: a guideline for healthcare professionals from the American Heart Association/American Stroke Association. *Stroke.* 2015;46(8):2368–2400.
43. Lee CZ, Young WL. Anesthesia for endovascular neurosurgery and interventional neuroradiology. *Anesthesiol Clin.* 2012;30(2):127–147.
44. Furlan A, Higashida R, Wechsler L, et al. Intra-arterial prourokinase for acute ischemic stroke. The PROACT II study: a randomized controlled trial. Prolyse in Acute Cerebral Thromboembolism. *JAMA.* 1999;282(21):2003–2011.
45. Jauch EC, Saver JL, Adams HP, et al. Guidelines for the early management of patients with acute ischemic stroke: a guideline for healthcare professionals from the American Heart Association/American Stroke Association. *Stroke.* 2013;44(3):870–947.
46. Davis MJ, Menon BK, Baghirzada LB, et al. Anesthetic management and outcome in patients during endovascular therapy for acute stroke. *Anesthesiology.* 2012;116(2):396–405.
47. Abou-Chebl A, Yeatts SD, Yan B, et al. Impact of general anesthesia on safety and outcomes in the endovascular arm of Interventional Management of Stroke (IMS) III Trial. *Stroke.* 2015;46(8):2142–2148.
48. See JJ, Manninen PH. Anesthesia for neuroradiology. *Curr Opin Anaesthesiol.* 2005;18(4):437–441.
49. The Arteriovenous Malformation Study Group. Arteriovenous malformations of the brain in adults. *N Engl J Med.* 1999;340(23):1812–1818.
50. González JA, Llibre Guerra JC, Prince López JA, et al. Feasibility of the superselective test with propofol for determining eloquent brain regions in the endovascular treatment of arteriovenous malformations. *Interv Neuroradiol.* 2013;19(3):320–328.
51. Mikuni N, Takayama M, Satow T, et al. Evaluation of adverse effects in intracarotid propofol injection for Wada test. *Neurology.* 2005;65(11):1813–1816.
52. Raiten J, Elkassabany N, Gao W, et al. Medical intelligence article: novel uses of high frequency ventilation outside the operating room. *Anesth Analg.* 2011;112(5):1110–1113.

53. Piccioni F, Fumagalli L, Garbagnati F, et al. Thoracic paravertebral anesthesia for percutaneous radiofrequency ablation of hepatic tumors. *J Clin Anesth.* 2014;26(4):271–275.
54. Scher C. Anesthesia for transjugular intrahepatic portosystemic shunt. *Int Anesthesiol Clin.* 2009;47(2):21–28.
55. Veenith T, Coles JP. Anaesthesia for magnetic resonance imaging and positron emission tomography. *Curr Opin Anaesthesiol.* 2011;24(4):451–458.
56. Institute of Physics. *MRI and the physical agents (EMF) directive.* Institute of Physics Report; 2008. http://www.iop.org/publications/iop/2008/page_38214.html. Accessed November 3, 2015.
57. Farling PA, Flynn PA, Darwent G, et al. Safety in magnetic resonance units: an update. *Anaesthesia.* 2010;65(7):766–770.
58. United States Department of Labor. Occupational Safety and Health Administration (OSHA) Technical manual section III: Chapter 5. Noise. https://www.osha.gov/dts/osta/otm/new_noise/index.html-standards. Accessed December 18, 2015.
59. Dewey M, Schink T, Dewey CF. Claustrophobia during magnetic resonance imaging: cohort study in over 55,000 patients. *J Magn Reson Imaging.* 2007;26(5):1322–1327.
60. Munn Z, Jordan Z. Interventions to reduce anxiety, distress and the need for sedation in adult patients undergoing magnetic resonance imaging: a systematic review. *Int J Evid Based Healthc.* 2013;11(4):265–274.
61. Kannikeswaran N, Mahajan PV, Sethuraman U, et al. Sedation medication received and adverse events related to sedation for brain MRI in children with and without developmental disabilities. *Paediatr Anaesth.* 2009;19(3):250–256.
62. Krauss B, Green SM. Training and credentialing in procedural sedation and analgesia in children: lessons from the United States model. *Paediatr Anaesth.* 2008;18(1):30–35.
63. Arthurs OJ, Sury M. Anaesthesia or sedation for paediatric MRI: advantages and disadvantages. *Curr Opin Anaesthesiol.* 2013;26(4):489–494.
64. American Academy of Pediatrics; American Academy of Pediatric Dentistry, Coté CJ, Wilson S; Work Group on Sedation. Guidelines for monitoring and management of pediatric patients during and after sedation for diagnostic and therapeutic procedures: an update. *Paediatr Anaesth.* 2008;18(1):9–10.
65. American Academy of Pediatrics; American Academy of Pediatric Dentistry, Coté CJ, Wilson S; Work Group on Sedation. Guidelines for monitoring and management of pediatric patients during and after sedation for diagnostic and therapeutic procedures: an update. *Pediatrics.* 2006;118(6):2587–2602.
66. Cravero JP. Risk and safety of pediatric sedation/anesthesia for procedures outside the operating room. *Curr Opin Anaesthesiol.* 2009;22(4):509–513.
67. Alonso-Basanta M, Lustig RA, Kennedy DW. Proton beam therapy in skull base pathology. *Otolaryngol Clin North Am.* 2011;44(5):1173–1183.
68. Chalabi J, Patel S. Radiation therapy in children. *Int Anesthesiol Clin.* 2009;47(3):45–53.
69. McFadyen JG, Pelly N, Orr RJ. Sedation and anesthesia for the pediatric patient undergoing radiation therapy. *Curr Opin Anaesthesiol.* 2011;24(4):433–438.
70. Harris EA. Sedation and anesthesia options for pediatric patients in the radiation oncology suite. *Int J Pediatr.* 2010;2010:870921.
71. Buehrer S, Immoos S, Frei M, et al. Evaluation of propofol for repeated prolonged deep sedation in children undergoing proton radiation therapy. *Br J Anaesth.* 2007;99(4):556–560.
72. Anghelescu DL, Burgoyne LL, Liu W, et al. Safe anesthesia for radiotherapy in pediatric oncology: St. Jude Children's Research Hospital Experience, 2004–2006. *Int J Radiat Oncol Biol Phys.* 2008;71(2):491–497.
73. Bryson EO, Sejpal D. Anesthesia in remote locations: radiology and beyond, international anesthesiology clinics: gastroenterology: endoscopy, colonoscopy, and ERCP. *Int Anesthesiol Clin.* 2009;47(2):69–80.
74. Cohen LB, Wecsler JS, Gaetano JN, et al. Endoscopic sedation in the United States: results from a nationwide survey. *Am J Gastroenterol.* 2006;101(5):967–974.
75. Goulson DT, Fragneto RY. Anesthesia for gastrointestinal endoscopic procedures. *Anesthesiol Clin.* 2009;27(1):71–85.
76. Dumonceau JM, Riphaus A, Schreiber F, et al. Non-anesthesiologist administration of propofol for gastrointestinal endoscopy: European Society of Gastrointestinal Endoscopy, European Society of Gastroenterology and Endoscopy Nurses and Associates Guideline. Updated June 2015. *Endoscopy.* 2015;47(12):1175–1189.
77. Rivera M. The current status of nurse-administered propofol sedation in endoscopy: an evidence-based Practice Nurse Fellowship Project. *Gastroenterol Nurs.* 2015;38(4):297–304.
78. Birk J, Bath RK. Is the anesthesiologist necessary in the endoscopy suite? A review of patients, payers and safety. *Expert Rev Gastroenterol Hepatol.* 2015;9(7):883–885.
79. Werner C, Smith A, Van Aken H. Guidelines on non-anaesthesiologist administration of propofol for gastrointestinal endoscopy: a double-edged sword. *Eur J Anaesthesiol.* 2011;28(8):553–555.
80. Cohen LB, Ladas SD, Vargo JJ, et al. Sedation in digestive endoscopy: the Athens international position statements. *Aliment Pharmacol Ther.* 2010;32(3):425–442.
81. Osborn IP, Cohen J, Soper RJ, et al. Laryngeal mask airway: a novel method of airway protection during ERCP: comparison with endotracheal intubation. *Gastrointest Endosc.* 2002;56(1):122–128.
82. Garewal D, Powell S, Milan SJ, et al. Sedative techniques for endoscopic retrograde cholangiopancreatography. *Cochrane Database Syst Rev.* 2012;6:CD007274.
83. Garewal D, Vele L, Waikar P. Anaesthetic considerations for endoscopic retrograde cholangio-pancreatography procedures. *Curr Opin Anaesthesiol.* 2013;26(4):475–480.
84. Lynch CR, Khandekar S, Lynch SM, et al. Sublingual L-hyoscyamine for duodenal antimotility during ERCP: a prospective randomized double-blinded study. *Gastrointest Endosc.* 2007;66(4):748–752.
85. Buch E, Boyle NG, Belott PH. Pacemaker and defibrillator lead extraction. *Circulation.* 2011;123(11):e378–e380.
86. Faillace RT, Kaddaha R, Bikkina M, et al. The role of the out-of-operating room anesthesiologist in the care of the cardiac patient. *Anesthesiol Clin.* 2009;27(1):29–46.
87. Kar B, Adkins LE, Civitello AB, et al. Clinical experience with the TandemHeart percutaneous ventricular assist device. *Tex Heart Inst J.* 2006;33(2):111–115.
88. Windecker S, Meier B. Impella assisted high-risk percutaneous coronary intervention. *Karddiovask Med.* 2005;27(3):157–162.
89. Praz F, Wahl A, Schmutz M, et al. Safety, feasibility, and long-term results of percutaneous closure of atrial septal defects using the Amplatzer septal occluder without periprocedural echocardiography. *J Invasive Cardiol.* 2015;27(3):157–162.
90. Singh K, Qutub M, Carson K, et al. A meta analysis of current status of alcohol septal ablation and surgical myectomy for obstructive hypertrophic cardiomyopathy. *Catheter Cardiovasc Interv.* 2015 Nov 3. [Epub ahead of print].
91. Alam M, Dokainish H, Lakkis NM. Hypertrophic obstructive cardiomyopathy-alcohol septal ablation vs. myectomy: a meta-analysis. *Eur Heart J.* 2009;30(9):1080–1087.
92. Horne A, Reineck EA, Hasan RK, et al. Transcatheter aortic valve replacement: historical perspectives, current evidence, and future directions. *Am Heart J.* 2014;168(4):414–423.
93. Stolker JM, Patel AY, Lim MJ, et al. Estimating the adoption of transcatheter aortic valve replacement by US interventional cardiologists and clinical trialists. *Clin Cardiol.* 2013;36(11):691–697.
94. Mayr NP, Michel J, Bleiziffer S, et al. Sedation or general anesthesia for transcatheter aortic valve implantation (TAVI). *J Thorac Dis.* 2015;7(9):1518–1526.
95. Mahajan A, Chua J. Pro: a cardiovascular anesthesiologist should provide services in the catheterization and electrophysiology laboratory. *J Cardiothorac Vasc Anesth.* 2011;25(3):553–556.
96. Velazquez EJ, Samad Z, Al-Khalidi HR, et al. The MitraClip and survival in patients with mitral regurgitation at high risk for surgery: a propensity-matched comparison. *Am Heart J.* 2015;170(5):1050–1059.e3.
97. Bonow RO, Carabello BA, Chatterjee K, et al. 2008 Focused update incorporated into the ACC/AHA 2006 guidelines for the management of patients with valvular heart disease: a report of the American College of Cardiology/American Heart Association Task Force on Practice Guidelines (Writing Committee to Revise the 1998 Guidelines for the Management of Patients With Valvular Heart Disease): endorsed by the Society of Cardiovascular Anesthesiologists, Society for Cardiovascular Angiography and Interventions, and Society of Thoracic Surgeons. *Circulation.* 2008;118(15):e523–e661.
98. Deuschl F, Schofer N, Lubos E, et al. MitraClip-data analysis of contemporary literature. *J Thorac Dis.* 2015;7(9):1509–1517.
99. Mauri L, Foster E, Glower DD, et al. 4-year results of a randomized controlled trial of percutaneous repair versus surgery for mitral regurgitation. *J Am Coll Cardiol.* 2013;62(4):317–328.
100. Holmes DR, Kar S, Price MJ, et al. Prospective randomized evaluation of the Watchman Left Atrial Appendage Closure device in patients with atrial fibrillation versus long-term warfarin therapy: the PREVAIL trial. *J Am Coll Cardiol.* 2014;64(1):1–12.
101. Reddy VY, Doshi SK, Sievert H, et al. Percutaneous left atrial appendage closure for stroke prophylaxis in patients with atrial fibrillation: 2.3-year follow-up of the PROTECT AF (Watchman left atrial appendage system for embolic protection in patients with atrial fibrillation) trial. *Circulation.* 2013;127(6):720–729.
102. Holmes DR, Doshi SK, Kar S, et al. Left atrial appendage closure as an alternative to warfarin for stroke prevention in atrial fibrillation: a patient-level meta-analysis. *J Am Coll Cardiol.* 2015;65(24):2614–2623.
103. Peterson C, Prutkin JM, Robinson M, et al. Echocardiography for electrophysiology procedures. *Curr Anesthesiol Rep.* 2015;5(4):429–437.
104. Khazanie P, Hammill BG, Qualls LG, et al. Clinical effectiveness of cardiac resynchronization therapy versus medical therapy alone among patients with heart failure: analysis of the ICD Registry and ADHERE. *Circ Heart Fail.* 2014;7(6):926–934.
105. Epstein AE, DiMarco JP, Ellenbogen KA, et al. 2012 ACCF/AHA/HRS focused update incorporated into the ACCF/AHA/HRS 2008 guidelines for device-based therapy of cardiac rhythm abnormalities: a report of the American College of Cardiology Foundation/American Heart Association Task Force on Practice Guidelines and the Heart Rhythm Society. *J Am Coll Cardiol.* 2013;61(3):e6–e75.

106. Moss AJ, Zareba W, Hall WJ, et al. Prophylactic implantation of a defibrillator in patients with myocardial infarction and reduced ejection fraction. *N Engl J Med*. 2002;346(12):877–883.
107. Jiménez-Candil J, Hernández J, Martín A, et al. Differences in ventricular tachyarrythmias and antitachycardia pacing effectiveness according to the ICD indication (primary versus secondary prevention): an analysis based on the stored electrograms. *J Interv Card Electrophysiol*. 2015;44(2):187–195.
108. Chung ES, Leon AR, Tavazzi L, et al. Results of the predictors of response to CRT (PROSPECT) trial. *Circulation*. 2008;117(20):2608–2616.
109. Leyva F, Nisam S, Auricchio A. 20 years of cardiac resynchronization therapy. *J Am Coll Cardiol*. 2014;64(10):1047–1058.
110. Lowe MD, Meara M, Mason J, et al. Catheter cryoablation of supraventricular arrhythmias: a painless alternative to radiofrequency energy. *Pacing Clin Electrophysiol*. 2003;26:500–503.
111. Haddy S. Anesthesia for structural heart interventions. *Cardiol Clin*. 2013;31(3):455–465.
112. Mountantonakis SE, Elkassabany N, Kondapalli L, et al. Provocation of atrial fibrillation triggers during ablation: does the use of general anesthesia affect inducibility? *J Cardiovasc Electrophysiol*. 2015;26(1):16–20.
113. Tanawuttiwat T, Gallego D, Carrillo RG. Lead extraction experience with high frequency excimer laser. *Pacing Clin Electrophysiol*. 2014;37(9):1120–1128.
114. Di Monaco A, Pelargonio G, Narducci ML, et al. Safety of transvenous lead extraction according to centre volume: a systematic review and meta-analysis. *Europace*. 2014;16(10):1496–1507.
115. Priester R, Bunting T, Usher B, et al. Role of transesophageal echocardiography among patients with atrial fibrillation undergoing electrophysiology testing. *Am J Cardiol*. 2009;104(9):1256–1258.
116. Wasmer K, Eckardt L. Management of atrial fibrillation around the world: a comparison of current ACCF/AHA/HRS, CCS, and ESC guidelines. *Europace*. 2011;13(10):1368–1374.
117. Flachskampf FA, Badano L, Daniel WG, et al. Recommendations for transoesophageal echocardiography: update 2010. *Eur J Echocardiogr*. 2010;11(7):557–576.
118. UK ECT Review Group. Efficacy and safety of electroconvulsive therapy in depressive disorders: a systematic review and meta-analysis. *Lancet*. 2003;361(9360):799–808.
119. Ding Z, White PF. Anesthesia for electroconvulsive therapy. *Anesth Analg*. 2002;94(5):1351–1364.
120. American Psychiatric Association. *The Practice of Electroconvulsant Therapy: Recommendations for Treatment, Training and Privileging*. Washington, DC: American Psychiatric Press; 2000.
121. MacPherson RD. Which anesthetic agents for ambulatory electro-convulsive therapy? *Curr Opin Anaesthesiol*. 2015;28(6):656–661.
122. Nishihara F, Ohkawa M, Hiraoka H, et al. Benefits of the laryngeal mask for airway management during electroconvulsive therapy. *J ECT*. 2003;19(4):211–216.
123. Sawayama E, Takahashi M, Inoue A, et al. Moderate hyperventilation prolongs electroencephalogram seizure duration of the first electroconvulsive therapy. *J ECT*. 2008;24(3):195–198.
124. Begec Z, Toprak HI, Demirbilek S, et al. Dexmedetomidine blunts acute hyperdynamic responses to electroconvulsive therapy without altering seizure duration. *Acta Anaesthesiol Scand*. 2008;52(2):302–306.
125. Patel AS, Gorst-Unsworth C, Venn RM, et al. Anesthesia and electroconvulsive therapy: a retrospective study comparing etomidate and propofol. *J ECT*. 2006;22(3):179–183.
126. Chen ST. Remifentanil: a review of its use in electroconvulsive therapy. *J ECT*. 2011;27(4):323–327.
127. McGirr A, Berlim MT, Bond DJ, et al. A systematic review and meta-analysis of randomized controlled trials of adjunctive ketamine in electroconvulsive therapy: efficacy and tolerability. *J Psychiatr Res*. 2015;62:23–30.

34 Anesthesia for the Older Patient

ITAY BENTOV • G. ALEC ROOKE

Demographics and Economics of Aging
The Process of Aging
   Functional Reserve and the Concept of Frailty
   Physiologic Age
The Physiology of Organ Aging
   Changes in Body Composition, and Liver and Kidney Aging
   Central Nervous System Aging
   Drug Pharmacology and Aging

Cardiovascular Aging
Pulmonary Aging
Thermoregulation and Aging
Conduct of Anesthesia
   The Preoperative Visit
   Intraoperative Management
   Postoperative Care
   Perioperative Complications
The Future

KEY POINTS

1. The aging of America presents a medical and economic challenge to the entire health-care system as older patients present for surgery in ever-increasing numbers.
2. The aging process affects connective tissue and cellular function, including the mitochondria, and inevitably leads to decreased function and, ultimately, frailty.
3. The rate at which diminished function and frailty develop is highly variable and lends credence to the concept of physiologic age.
4. Decreased organ reserve and increased sensitivity to anesthetic agents result from generalized body composition changes such as connective tissue stiffening and decreased muscle mass, plus impaired autonomic reflexes, and increased sensitivity to drugs.
5. Preoperative preparation will more often involve evaluation of how best to enhance recovery of function after surgery, and discussions surrounding informed consent, living wills, and ethical treatment of the older patient.
6. Intraoperative management must take into account the increased sensitivity to drugs in the elderly patient, as well as an increased likelihood of hemodynamic, pulmonary, and thermoregulatory instability.
7. Analgesia is an important component of postoperative care, but is made more difficult by the increased likelihood of adverse consequences from the analgesic regimen.
8. Perioperative complications, most notably pulmonary, cardiac, and central nervous system complications such as delirium or cognitive decline, occur more commonly in the elderly patient because of an interaction between comorbid disease and the decreased physiologic reserve of aging.

Age is not a particularly interesting subject. Anyone can get old. All you have to do is live long enough.

—Don Marquis

This quote suggests that aging is dull. To many medical practitioners, it is far worse than "dull." It is high risk due to the complexity of care, and discouraging in its monetary reimbursement. To those concerned with the federal budget and personal expenses, medical care for the aged threatens to bankrupt the nation. Nevertheless, the impact of aging on the practice of medicine is far-reaching and profound, and therefore cannot be ignored. Just as children are not "little adults," the older patient is truly different from the younger adult counterpart. All caregivers, including anesthesiologists, should be knowledgeable of at least some aspects of aging in order to provide intelligent deviation from their standard practice. Basic information is more available than ever before, much of it electronically from the American Society of Anesthesiologists (www.asahq.org), the Society for the Advancement of Geriatric Anesthesia (www.sagahq.org), and the American Geriatrics Society (www.americangeriatrics.org). In reality, caring for an older patient is rarely dull, if for no other reason than their diverse and fascinating lives. Anyone with a passing interest in physiology should enjoy the application of aging physiology to anesthetic management. Yes, their care is often time-consuming, stressful, and requires extra effort, but more often than not it provides the anesthesia caregiver the opportunity to truly practice medicine and make a positive impact on a vulnerable patient's life. Furthermore, the older patient is likely to be a prime candidate for the benefits provided by the perioperative surgical home (PSH).

Demographics and Economics of Aging

I advise you to go on living solely to enrage those who are paying your annuities. It is the only pleasure I have left.

—Voltaire

When Social Security was initiated in 1935, only 6.1% of the US population was older than 65 years.[1] By 2010 that percentage had grown to 13.0% and represented 40 million people.[2] By 2040 it is expected to be nearly 20% of the US population and represent 71 million people.[3] The percentage of the US population older than 85 is expected to more than double from 2010 to 2040 (from 1.8% to an estimated 4.5%).[3] The growth of the US population and its older subgroups is shown in Figure 34-1. The impact of these statistics is enormous with respect to medical care. In 2010, patients over 65 represented 13% of the population but accounted for 45% of the 167 million total US inpatient days, a rate per capita more than five times greater than for those under 65.[4] On the examination of the 2006 inpatient and ambulatory procedure data, there were an estimated 73 million surgical and nonsurgical procedures performed in the United States

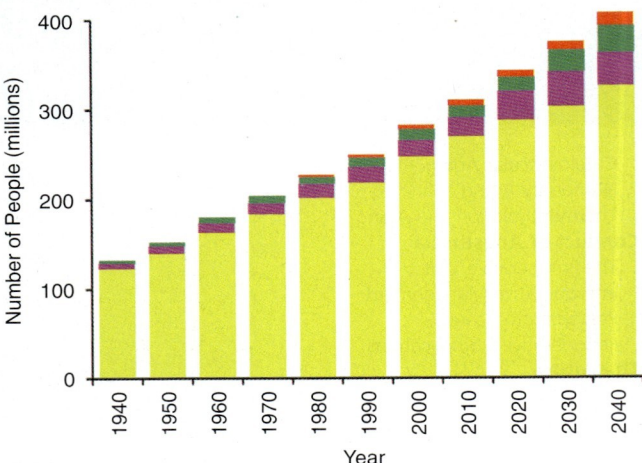

Figure 34-1 The actual and estimated US population from 1940 to 2040 is shown broken down by age range. *Yellow bar* = age above 65; *purple bar* = age 65 to 74; *green bar* = age 75 or above for years 1940 to 1970, and age 75 to 84 from 1980 on; *red bar* = age 85 or above. (From http://www2.census.gov/library/publications/2011/compendia/statab/131ed/tables/pop.pdf. Accessed December 3, 2015.)

after exclusion of procedures that were unlikely to have involved anesthesia services.[5,6] Of these, 28% were on patients older than 65 years. Thus it appears that people over age 65 have surgery 2.7 times more often than people under age 65.

Federal spending for Medicare in 2015 was $546 billion or 14.8% of the federal budget. This amount is approximately twice what was spent in 2000 after adjusting for inflation, and represents an approximate 50% increase per enrollee.[7] As impressive as Medicare expenditures may be, federal spending grossly underestimates the total cost of all health-care spending for people over age 65. It is estimated that people over age 65 account for nearly half of the nation's health-care costs, which totaled $3.1 trillion in 2014, or approximately 17.8% of the gross national product.[8,9] In consequence, there is considerable pressure to contain health-care costs in this country, including physician reimbursement, by both private insurance companies and the federal government. Unfortunately, federal reimbursement to anesthesiologists is especially poor. In 2004, Medicare reimbursed anesthesia care at approximately 33% of what commercial insurance companies paid.[7] This percentage is in sharp contrast to all other specialties, for which Medicare reimbursement is approximately 83% of commercial rates.[10] The average conversion factor has improved considerably in the last few years. Nevertheless, the 2015 national average value of $22.61 has barely matched inflation since the nadir of $16.60 in 2002.[11] Although Medicare will reimburse at the 50% level for up to four concurrent medically directed procedures, academic programs had been at a disadvantage since faculty are not permitted to staff more than two procedures simultaneously if residents were involved. Fortunately, as of 2010, Medicare now reimburses academic institutions at 100% for two concurrent cases.

The Process of Aging

You can't help getting older, but you don't have to get old.
—George Burns

Aging involves a gradual, cumulative process of damage and deterioration. The question could be posed: Why is such a process allowed in nature? Classical evolutionary teleologic explanations would suggest that aging confers an advantage to the survival of the species. In the end of the nineteenth century, August Weismann theorized (and later abandoned his theory) that older members of a species need to remove themselves to sustain the turnover that is essential for evolution. Newer theories arose in the second part of the twentieth century, such as mutation accumulation, which suggests that the random, detrimental mutations that do not cause mortality early in life will ultimately accumulate and lead to deterioration later in life. Another proposal was antagonistic pleiotropy, meaning that a single gene has more than one phenotype (effect or trait). The phenotypes may prove beneficial in early life but detrimental in old age. Lastly, the disposable soma theory suggested that the organism must allocate energy to bodily functions and resources that are focused upon early survival, growth, and reproduction while compromising repair functions that would prevent deterioration with age. The existence of mechanisms that promote death (e.g., apoptosis, cellular senescence, and telomerase shortening) are used by some to support the classical evolutionary theories, and by others to criticize them.

A new, hierarchical approach to aging groups the mechanisms of aging into three tiers. The first tier is primary mechanisms, all of which are clearly negative. Examples of the first tier mechanisms include: DNA damage and mitochondrial DNA mutations, and telomere loss. Telomeres are stretches of DNA at the ends of chromosomes, analogous to plastic tips on shoelaces. Without them the chromosome would unravel and stick to each other, which could scramble the DNA. Each time a cell divides, the telomeres get shorter, and when they become too short, the cell can no longer divide.

Another first tier mechanism is epigenetic drift: nongenetic DNA changes that influence gene expression. The most studied epigenetic phenomenon is the addition of methyl groups (methylation) of DNA. Most of the genome undergoes gradual demethylation while other, specific regions undergo hypermethylation, leading to disrupted transcription. Lastly, the production, folding, and degradation of proteins within the cell regulate their functionality. These pathways or homeostasis of proteins are referred to as proteostasis. Defective proteostasis has been implicated in several diseases like diabetes and Alzheimer's, as well as the aging process.

The second tier includes antagonistic mechanisms that are primarily beneficial and protect the younger individual from damage or nutrient shortage. After prolonged use, however, these mechanisms themselves produce damage. Mechanisms in the second tier include senescence, a state in which the cell is alive and metabolically active but is not capable of dividing. Oxygen is important to providing large amounts of energy; however, reactive oxygen species such as peroxides and superoxides cause damage to DNA and proteins. Another second tier mechanism is disrupted nutrient-sensing; for example, the mammalian target of rapamycin (mTOR) is a protein that senses cellular nutrient, oxygen, and energy levels. Activation of mTOR supports cell growth, proliferation, and survival. However, activation of mTOR is not without a price. Reduction in mTOR activity (e.g., due to a restrictive diet) has been found to increase life span in several animal models.[12] The last mechanism in the second tier is mitochondrial dysfunction; age is correlated not only with the accumulation of mitochondrial DNA mutations but also with a decline in respiratory chain function which may contribute to inefficient use of energy in the cell and reduced exercise capacity.

The third tier consists of integrative mechanisms which operate when the accumulated damage caused by the primary and antagonistic hallmarks cannot be compensated by tissue homeostatic mechanisms: stem cell numbers decline with age, suggesting that there has been a failure to replace damaged cells. Another mechanism is altered intercellular communication. Examples of intercellular communication are neurohormonal signaling processes such as renin–angiotensin, adrenergic, or insulin-IGF1 signaling pathways. Deregulated neurohormonal signaling in the aged is implicated in development of diseases such as hypertension, heart failure, diabetes, and malignancies.

The newly coined term "geroscience" refers to an interdisciplinary field which aims to understand the relationship between aging and age-related diseases.[15] A fundamental concept of geroscience is that numerous human diseases arise, at least in part, from aging itself. Aging is the major risk factor for diseases like Alzheimer's, Parkinson's, and numerous malignancies. Studying aging mechanisms across a wide variety of pathologies raises an important question: are aging and disease different processes or are they, at least to some degree, inseparable? Elucidating each one of these processes could provide not just insight but potential solutions for the other.

Most of the gains in average human life span have been as the result of reducing those factors that cause premature death: predation, accidents, and disease. The inability to thwart aging entirely implies that the human life span is limited, and that if everyone died only of "old age," the age at death would end up being a bell-shaped curve centered at a certain value, probably around age 85.[14] Nevertheless, it is possible that the bell-shaped curve could be shifting to a higher value, but how far it can be shifted is unclear. The focus of research has transitioned from just extending the number of years lived (life span) to extending the period during which one is generally healthy and free from serious comorbidities (healthspan). Several interventions (smoking cessation, weight loss, and exercise) have been shown to improve both life span and healthspan.[15,16]

Functional Reserve and the Concept of Frailty

Old age is no place for sissies.
—Bette Davis

Functional reserve represents the degree to which organ function can increase above the level necessary for basal activity. For healthy individuals, reserve peaks at approximately age 30, gradually declines over the next several decades, and then experiences more rapid decline beginning around the eighth decade. Assessment of reserve is something anesthesiologists perform all the time. For example, the ability to achieve a minimum of four metabolic equivalents appears to confer enough cardiovascular reserve to tolerate the stress of most surgical procedures.[17] As age advances, there emerges an extreme form of decreased reserve and limited resistance to stressors. This biologic syndrome is often referred to as frailty. Frailty is a result of cumulative declines across multiple physiologic systems, and causing vulnerability to adverse outcomes. Frailty, disability, and comorbidity overlap but are not synonymous (Fig. 34-2). Although the diagnosis of frailty is often intuitive, there are two classical ways to define it. The first method is the frailty phenotype which is defined as a clinical syndrome in which three or more of the following criteria are present: unintentional weight loss (10 lb in past year), self-reported exhaustion, weakness (grip strength), slow walking speed, and low physical activity.[18] The second definition of frailty is the frailty index which considers frailty in relation to deficit accumulation. A list of symptoms, signs, diseases, and disabilities are surveyed and scored in a binomial fashion (yes/no), and the fraction of the positive deficits from the total number surveyed is calculated (e.g., 10 positive out of 40 surveyed equals a frailty index of 0.25).[19] Although the frailty phenotype and the

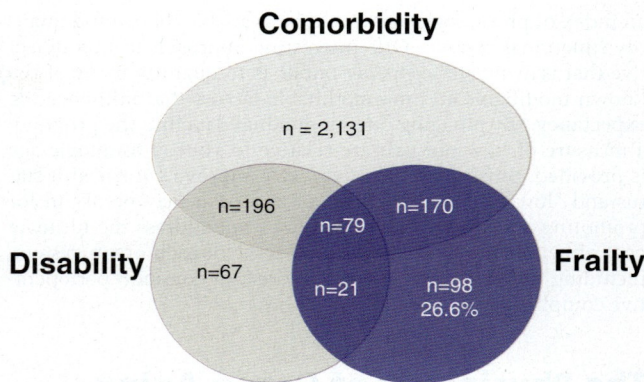

Figure 34-2 Overlap of frailty with disability and comorbidity. 2,762 community dwelling adults (age >65) who had comorbidity (defined as two or more out of the following nine diseases: myocardial infarction, angina, congestive heart failure, claudication, arthritis, cancer, diabetes, hypertension, COPD) and/or disability (defined by inability to perform one or more activities of daily living [ADL] tasks) and/or frailty. Of 368 frail subjects, 98 (26.6%) were not identified by assessment of disability or comorbidity. (Reproduced with permission from Fried LP, Tangen CM, Walston J, et al. Frailty in older adults: evidence for a phenotype. *J Gerontol A Biol Sci Med Sci*. 2001;56:M146–M157.)

frailty index do not necessarily identify the same patients,[20] both predict mortality and institutionalization in community dwelling elderly. Numerous studies that used a range of assessment tools to determine frailty status have shown that frail patients undergoing surgical procedures had a higher likelihood than nonfrail patients of experiencing mortality, morbidity, complications, increased hospital length of stay, and discharge to an institution.[21] A population-based retrospective cohort study that examined over 200,000 community dwelling adults older than 65 years undergoing elective, major, noncardiac surgery from 2002 to 2012 found that while preoperative frailty appears to impact some surgical procedures more than others, overall it is associated with an increased risk of 1-year mortality that was particularly notable in the early postoperative period.[22] It is tempting to hypothesize that once frailty is identified, could a preoperative habilitation program potentially reverse frailty and improve surgical outcomes? In the general nonsurgical population, trials of exercise (resistance training, aerobic training, balance, and flexibility), nutritional supplements, and pharmaceutical agents show limited success at reversing frailty and improving outcomes.[23] For patients scheduled for elective surgery, it seems that interventions provided before surgery (prehabilitation) were superior to similar interventions provided after surgery (rehabilitation).[24] A meta-analysis of eight RCT studies that examined preoperative conditioning to improve physiologic function and clinical outcomes suggested that a major obstacle is the low adherence to the prehabilitation programs.[25] A trial is currently underway that will compare preoperative, interdisciplinary exercise and health promotion intervention in a population of frail patients undergoing elective cardiac surgery to determine if the intervention improves 3- and 12-month clinical outcomes (The PREHAB trial).[26]

Physiologic Age

If you didn't know how old you were, how old would you be?
—James Hubert 'Eubie' Blake

The aging process is highly variable from one individual to the next. The older we get, the more different we become. Ideally, an index of physiologic age would be available that would quantify functional reserve. One interesting approach to this objective that is available to the lay public is to quantify many of the known modifiable and nonmodifiable factors that influence life expectancy.[7] By plugging one's individual data into the program, a measure of how old you are relative to your chronologic age is provided, plus tips on how you can improve your health status and "lower" your age. Such an approach may be useful for promoting a healthy lifestyle, but does not address the ultimate goal of being able to quantify the reserve of each organ system, including the brain, and predict the risk of common perioperative complications.

The Physiology of Organ Aging

If I'd known I was going to live this long, I'd have taken better care of myself.

—James Hubert 'Eubie' Blake, age 100

Defining what constitutes "normal aging" is difficult. Is it what happens under the best of circumstances, or what happens to the "average" person? Comparisons of young and elderly subjects may not strictly reflect aging, as the elderly subjects may have experienced a much different diet, lifestyle, and environmental exposure than what the young group will have experienced by the time they become old. Following a group of healthy subjects over a long period is more likely to define the effects of aging, but not all available data come from such longitudinal studies. Studies that examine only the very old may actually underestimate the typical effects of aging because individuals generally do not achieve old age unless there is something intrinsically robust about them. Lastly, the reader is reminded to keep two principles in mind. The effect of aging varies considerably from one patient to another, and, disease will interact with aging to further diminish functional organ reserve.

Changes in Body Composition, and Liver and Kidney Aging

I have everything I had twenty years ago, only it's all a little bit lower.

—Gypsy Rose Lee

Changes in body composition are primarily characterized by a gradual loss of skeletal muscle and an increase in body fat, although the latter is more prominent in women (Fig. 34-3). Basal metabolism declines with age, with most of the decline accounted for by the change in body composition.[27] There is a reduction in total body water that reflects the reduction in cellular water that is associated with a loss of muscle and an increase in adipose tissue.[28] Aging causes a small decrease in plasma albumin levels; however, there is a small increase in α_1-acid glycoprotein.[29] However, the effect of these changes on drug protein binding and drug delivery appear to be minimal.

Liver mass decreases with age, and accounts for most, but not all, of the 20% to 40% decrease in liver blood flow.[30] There is also a modest reduction in phase I drug metabolism and bile secretion with age. Other than the effect of aging on drug metabolism, liver reserve should be more than adequate even in the very old in the absence of disease.

Renal cortical mass also decreases by 20% to 25% with age, but the most prominent effect of aging is the loss of up to half of the glomeruli by age 80.[31] The decrease in the glomerular filtration

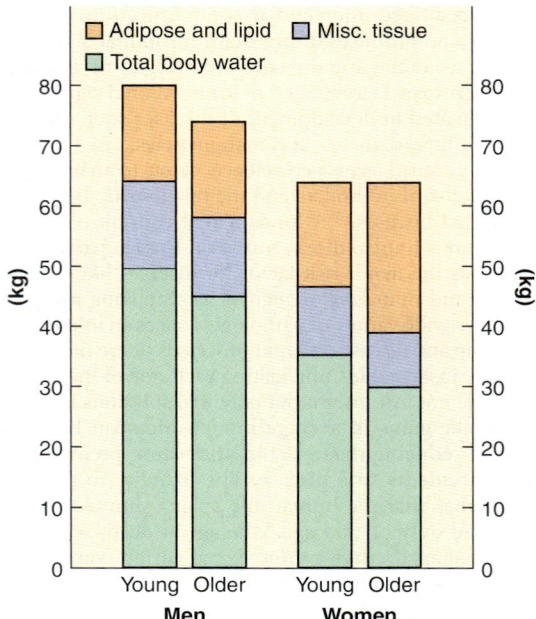

Figure 34-3 Age-related changes in body composition are gender-specific. In women, total body mass remains constant because increases in body fat (*upper shaded segment*) offset bone loss (*middle segment*) and intracellular dehydration (*lower shaded segment*). In men, body mass declines despite maintenance of body lipid and skeletal tissue elements because accelerating loss of skeletal muscle and other components of lean tissue mass produces marked contraction of intracellular water (*lower shaded segment*).

rate of approximately 1 mL/min/yr after age 40 typically reduces renal excretion of drugs to a level where drug dosage adjustment becomes a progressively important consideration beginning at approximately age 60. Nevertheless, the degree of decline in glomerular filtration rate is highly variable and is likely to be much less than predicted in many individuals, especially those who avoid excessive dietary protein.[32]

The aged kidney does not eliminate or retain sodium when necessary as effectively as that of a young adult.[32] Part of the failure to conserve sodium when appropriate may be because of reduced aldosterone secretion. Similarly, the aged kidney does not retain or eliminate free water as rapidly as young kidneys when challenged by water deprivation or free water excess. Lastly, the sensation of thirst declines with age. In short, fluid and electrolyte homeostasis is more vulnerable in the older patient, particularly when an older patient suffers acute injury or disease and eating and drinking becomes more of a chore.

For the most part, functional endocrine decline does not interact with anesthetic management to any significant degree. However, aging is associated with decreased insulin secretion in response to a glucose load, and also increased insulin resistance, particularly in skeletal muscle.[33] Thus, even healthy elderly patients may require perioperative insulin therapy more often than young adults. Aging also results in decreases in testosterone, estrogen, and growth hormone production.[34] The use of hormonal therapy to reduce sarcopenia, frailty in general, and cognitive decline and dementia is controversial, and does not have any current relevance to anesthetic management.

Central Nervous System Aging

By the time you're eighty years old you've learned everything. You only have to remember it.

—George Burns

Brain mass begins to decrease slowly beginning at approximately age 50 and declines more rapidly later, such that an 80-year-old brain has typically lost 10% of its weight.[35] Neurotransmitter functions suffer more significantly, including dopamine, serotonin, γ-aminobutyric acid, and especially the acetylcholine system.[36] The latter is especially important because of its connection to Alzheimer disease. Response times increase, and learning is more difficult, but vocabulary, "wisdom," and past knowledge are better preserved.[35] Nevertheless, of those individuals aged 85 and older, nearly half have significant cognitive impairment. In addition, some degree of atherosclerosis appears to be inevitable. Fortunately, and contrary to prior belief, the aged brain does make new neurons and is capable of forming new dendritic connections.[37]

The major effect of brain aging on anesthetic management is the increased sensitivity to many anesthetic agents. Perhaps the best-known example is the approximately 6% decrease in minimum alveolar concentration (MAC) per decade.[38] However, many intravenous agents also demonstrate an enhanced response in the older brain. These effects of aging are relatively simple to deal with in the clinical arena. More difficult to manage is the potential interaction of anesthesia, the stress of surgery, and a brain with minimal reserve. Age is a major risk factor for postoperative delirium and/or cognitive decline (see "Perioperative Complications").

Drug Pharmacology and Aging

I don't do alcohol anymore. I get the same effect just standing up fast.
—Unknown

Drugs typically have a more pronounced effect in an older patient. The cause can be either pharmacodynamic, in which case the target organ (often the brain) is more sensitive to a given drug tissue level, or pharmacokinetic, in which case a given dose of drug commonly produces higher blood levels in older patients.

Most intravenous anesthetic drugs are highly lipid soluble and so begin to enter tissue even before fully mixed in the blood. The rate of transfer depends on the rate of delivery (concentration times blood flow per gram of tissue), the concentration gradient of the drug between the blood and the tissue (obviously a high gradient initially), the ease with which the drug crosses the blood and tissue membranes, and the solubility of the drug in the tissue. Thus, the vessel-rich group (brain, heart, kidney, muscle) will acquire drug much more rapidly than the vessel-poor group (fat, bone). Protein binding may affect transfer, with drugs that are highly protein-bound having a lower free concentration and a slower rate of transfer.

Given the preceding, there are many ways for a drug bolus to have a more pronounced initial effect on older patients. During the drug redistribution phase the blood concentration typically is higher in older patients, partly because of a mildly contracted blood volume and partly because the reduction in muscle mass limits the rate and amount of drug removal by muscle. By keeping drug blood levels higher for a longer time, more drug will be driven into the other organs of the vessel-rich group such as the brain (often the target organ) or heart. A prime example of this phenomenon is sodium pentothal, and to a lesser degree, propofol.[39]

Despite the fact that drugs typically have a greater effect on older patients, there is a general impression that bolus drugs take longer to achieve that greater effect. It is not entirely clear why this is so. Slower circulation is sometimes hypothesized, but total blood flow to any organ does not appear to decrease beyond that expected from the decrease in organ mass. Another possibility is a slower rate of transfer into the target organ. Drug effects are the result of tissue, not plasma concentrations. Brain–plasma equilibration is not instantaneous, and for at least some drugs (e.g., remifentanil), the equilibration half-life is prolonged in older brains.[40] Why crossing the blood–brain barrier should take longer with age is not understood.

Ultimately, though, the drug will distribute throughout the body based on tissue mass and solubility. Because most intravenous drugs used in anesthesia are highly lipid-soluble, most of the drug will end up in fat. How completely the drug is dispersed out of the blood and into the tissue is reflected by Vd_{ss}, the drug's volume of distribution at steady state. This variable is expressed as the liters of plasma that would be necessary to dilute the amount of drug administered down to the concentration observed in the plasma. As such, drugs that are very fat-soluble can have a value for Vd_{ss} that is several times greater than total body water. After the initial redistribution into vessel-rich group tissue, the drug will slowly diffuse back into the plasma as it continues to be absorbed into fat. In so doing, the target organ (e.g., brain) drug level will fall because the target organ is always in the vessel-rich group. Once a single therapeutic dose of a drug has fully distributed throughout the body, the blood and target organ drug levels are typically too low to have a meaningful clinical effect. However, very large doses, repeated doses, or infusions will eventually deliver enough drug to yield residual drug levels that produce therapeutic effects. At this point, the only way to decrease blood and target organ levels and eliminate the drug's effects is through metabolism. The elimination or metabolic half-life of a drug in the blood equals the volume of distribution at steady state (Vd_{ss}) divided by the clearance, where clearance represents the amount of blood from which drug is eliminated per minute.

The most prominent and consistent pharmacokinetic effect of aging is a decrease in drug metabolism, typically due to both a decrease in clearance and an increase in Vd_{ss} (Fig. 34-4).

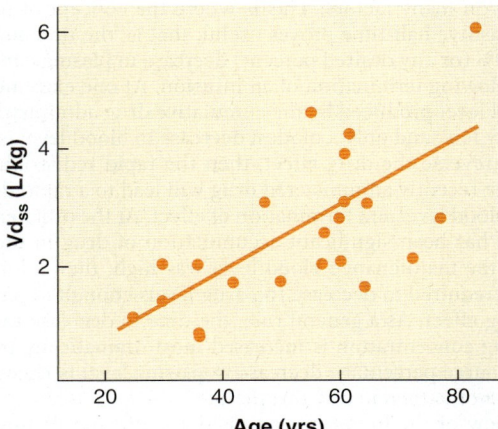

Figure 34-4 The effect of age on the volume of distribution at steady state (Vd_{ss}) for pentothal in women. (Reproduced with permission from Jung D, Mayersohn M, Perrier D, et al. Thiopental disposition as a function of age in female patients undergoing surgery. *Anesthesiology.* 1982;56:263.)

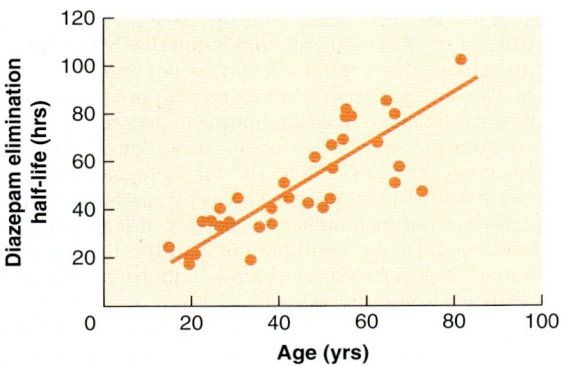

Figure 34-5 The effect of age on the elimination half-life of diazepam. The half-life in hours is equal to approximately the patient's age in years. (Reproduced with permission from Klotz U, Avant GR, Hoyumpa A, et al. The effects of age and liver disease on the disposition and elimination of diazepam in adult men. *J Clin Invest*. 1975;55:347.)

The increase in Vd_{ss} with age is likely due to the increase in body fat. Clearance decreases with age for any drug metabolized by the liver or kidney. When drug metabolism is via the liver, decreased liver mass and blood flow will decrease clearance for both high and low extraction drugs. In addition, elderly patients are often on a host of chronic medications, a setup for drug interactions as well as for inhibition of drug metabolism. Drugs with primarily renal elimination will experience decreased metabolism because of reductions in glomerular filtration rate with aging. The net effect on drug metabolism is typically a doubling of the elimination half-life between old and young adults. However, with some drugs, the effect on half-life can be dramatic. In the case of diazepam, the half-life in hours is roughly equal to the patient's age (Fig. 34-5).[41] For a 72-year-old person, it would therefore require 3 days to metabolize half of a dose of diazepam. Such pharmacokinetics clearly illustrate why there is no place in modern medicine for the chronic use of diazepam and other drugs with similar half-lives when the desired effect is supposed to be transient (e.g., as a sleeping aid).

When dealing with infusions—or for that matter a series of bolus injections—the time it takes to decrease the blood and target organ drug levels to below the therapeutic threshold will depend on many factors. This is where the concept of the context-sensitive half-time proves useful; that is, the time necessary for a 50% (or any desired percent) decrease in plasma concentration following termination of an infusion. At one extreme, if the residual level produced by the cumulative drug administration is still very low, and only a modest decrease in blood level is necessary to reverse the drug effect, then the rapid redistribution of the most recently administered drug will lead to a rapid decrease in the blood level and termination of effect. At the other extreme, if there has been significant accumulation of drug in the body, and/or the maintenance blood level was high, then a long time may be required to decrease the drug levels enough to terminate the drug effect. As a general rule, the time to decrease the effect site drug concentration is increased most dramatically by aging when a large percentage decrease in plasma level is necessary to dip below the therapeutic threshold.[42]

Review of the literature can yield a confusing picture when trying to sort out what pharmacologic variable is responsible for a given clinical effect. Fortunately, one does not need to know such details in order to use anesthetic drugs in an intelligent fashion with older patients. Table 34-1 summarizes some of this information for many of the common anesthetic drugs.[42–45] The effect of aging on sedative–hypnotic agents variably involves both pharmacodynamic and pharmacokinetic changes. For the opioids, the older brain appears to be more sensitive than that of young adults, whereas the pharmacokinetics of opioids are largely unaffected by age.

Despite the loss of muscle and motor neurons with age, muscle relaxants do not appear to be more potent in the older patient when steady-state blood levels for a given level of paralysis are compared.[45] Muscle relaxants often have a decreased initial volume of distribution, but this pharmacokinetic change does not seem to translate into smaller doses. The most commonly used relaxants, vecuronium and rocuronium, have modestly slowed metabolism with aging, so an increased duration of effect should be expected, especially with repetitive dosing. As such, the older patient is at greater risk for residual neuromuscular blockade (see section on Intraoperative Management).

Cardiovascular Aging

A man is as old as his arteries.

—Thomas Sydenham

Virtually all components of the cardiovascular system are affected by aging. The major changes include (1) decreased response to β-receptor stimulation; (2) stiffening of the myocardium, arteries, and veins; (3) changes in the autonomic nervous system with increased sympathetic activity and decreased parasympathetic activity; (4) conduction system changes; and (5) defective ischemic preconditioning. Although atherosclerosis appears to affect everyone by virtue of the fact that the mechanisms of aging contribute to the development of atherosclerosis, it is not clear that it inevitably leads to functional impairment or disease.

With age, there is increased sympathetic activity at rest and there is typically an exaggerated response to stimuli that increase sympathetic activity.[46] Although there is decreased responsiveness of α-receptors with age, the swings in sympathetic activation during surgery can still produce significant changes in vascular resistance during anesthesia. These changes in vascular resistance contribute to the lability in blood pressure in the aged, as well as to a decrease in blood pressure when anesthesia removes the sympathetic tone.[47,48]

The efficacy of baroreflex control of blood pressure decreases with age.[49] The mechanism is primarily a decrease in the heart rate response and not a decrease in the baroreflex control of vascular tone. The decreased heart rate response to changes in blood pressure is in part due to lesser vagal tone at rest but the major mechanism is a decrease in the cardiac response to β-receptor stimulation.[48] The mechanism does not appear to be a downregulation of β-receptors on the heart, but a defect in the intracellular coupling. Both heart rate and contractility increase less in response to endogenous release or exogenous administration of catecholamines. The increase in heart rate with exercise is therefore also diminished, as is maximal heart rate (often quoted as 220 minus age), and the decrement contributes to the decreased exertional capacity with age, even in trained individuals. The decrease in resting vagal tone may limit the increase in heart rate after administration of atropine or glycopyrrolate.

Conductance artery (aorta to arterioles) stiffening typically leads to systolic hypertension via two mechanisms.[50,51] First, approximately half of the stroke volume remains in the thoracic aorta after ejection. Pressure must increase more to stretch out a stiffened aorta to accommodate that volume. Secondly, generalized arterial stiffening causes the pressure wave to transmit more rapidly. In everyone, the pressure wave reflects off the arterial walls and branch points and returns to the thoracic aorta. The

Table 34-1 Effect of Age on Drug Dosing

Drug	Bolus Administration	Multiple Boluses or Infusion	Comments[a]
Propofol	20–60% reduction, dose on lean body mass, 1 mg/kg in very old	50% reduction, infusions beyond 50 min progressively increase the time required to decrease the blood level by 50% (but effect site levels may decrease faster in elderly)	↑ brain sensitivity (by some reports), decreased V_{cen}, slowed redistribution
Dexmedetomidine	Consider reduction	Consider reduction	Higher incidence of bradycardia and hypotension
Thiopental	20% reduction	20% reduction	= brain sensitivity, decreased V_{cen}, slowed redistribution
Etomidate	25–50% reduction	—	= brain sensitivity
Midazolam	Compared to age 20, modest reduction at age 60, 75% reduction at age 90	Similar to bolus (metabolic $t_{½}$ longer, but not meaningful unless very large doses are used)	↑↑ brain sensitivity
Morphine	Probably 50% reduction. Peak morphine effect is 90 min (though half of peak effect at 5 min)	Long effect site equilibration time translates into very slow reduction in effect on termination of infusion (4 hrs for 50% reduction)	Metabolite morphine-6-glucoronide build-up requires prolonged morphine use, but its renal excretion will make it very long acting
Fentanyl	50% reduction	50% reduction	↑ brain sensitivity, minimal changes in pharmacokinetics; delayed absorption from fentanyl patch
Alfentanil, sufentanil	50% reduction	50% reduction	Probably ↑ brain sensitivity, minimal changes in pharmacokinetics
Remifentanil	50% reduction	50% reduction	Slower blood–brain equilibration, suggesting slower onset and offset, modest decreased V_{cen}
Hydromorphone	No studies on aging exist, but assume increased potency in elderly	Assume 50% reduction	Compared with morphine, no active metabolite, faster onset
Methadone	No studies on aging exist, but assume increased potency in elderly	Assume 50% reduction	—
Meperidine	Use only for postoperative shivering	Do not use	Toxic metabolite normeperidine, whose renal excretion decreases with age
Vecuronium	Slower onset (≈ 33%)	Slower recovery times	Slightly greater liver metabolism than renal, age nearly doubles metabolic $t_{½}$
Mivacurium	Equally fast onset in young and old	Modest dose reduction for infusion, longer recovery time on repeated bolus	Elimination by plasma cholinesterase, modest prolongation of metabolic $t_{½}$ by age
Cisatracurium	Slower onset (≈ 33%)	No significant changes with age	Mostly Hoffmann elimination, modest prolongation of metabolic $t_{½}$ by age
Rocuronium	Minimally slower onset	—	Liver metabolism slightly greater than renal, modest increase in metabolic $t_{½}$ by age
Pancuronium	—	—	Primarily renal elimination, aging doubles metabolic $t_{½}$
Pipecuronium	Slower onset (≈ 50%), elderly may be *less* sensitive	—	Primarily renal elimination, no apparent change in metabolic $t_{½}$
Succinylcholine	Slower onset (≈ 40%)	—	
Edrophonium	Similar dosing and onset	—	↑ V_{cen}, primarily renal elimination, modest increase in metabolic $t_{½}$ by age
Neostigmine	Despite pharmacokinetic changes, some studies indicate need for increased dose with age	—	↑ V_{cen}, hepatic elimination, modest increase in metabolic $t_{½}$ by age

[a]V_{cen}, central volume of distribution or initial volume of distribution. Although V_{cen} does not have an anatomic correlate, a smaller V_{cen} will increase initial plasma levels and enhance transfer of the drug in the target organ (e.g., brain, muscle).

reflected waves return more rapidly in an older person because of the stiffer vessels. In young people, the reflected waves do not return to the heart until after ejection is complete. These waves are responsible for the modest bump in pressure in the aortic root just after the dicrotic notch. But in older people, the reflected waves return to the heart by late ejection and increase the pressure against which the left ventricle must pump to complete the stroke volume. At the end of ejection the ventricular contraction weakens, so ideal coupling would have the ventricle pushing against an ever-decreasing pressure. Since in the older person the ventricle must now pump against a higher pressure, this increased stress to the muscle stimulates hypertrophy.

Hypertrophy in and of itself stiffens the ventricle, but even worse, hypertrophy slows diastolic relaxation that, in turn, impairs ventricular filling in early diastole. The left ventricle now becomes more dependent on the atrial kick and requires an increase in left atrial pressure in order to preserve diastolic filling. The increase in atrial pressure is present at rest, but can be quite dynamic with acute increases during stress such as tachycardia. This phenomenon, termed diastolic dysfunction, increases in severity with age. The majority of cases of congestive heart failure in very old persons are due to diastolic dysfunction and occur in the absence of clinically significant systolic dysfunction.[48,52]

Adequate ventricular filling becomes more critical with age. The decreased response to β-receptor stimulation requires the ventricles to depend more on an adequate end-diastolic volume to generate enough contractile strength via the length–tension (Frank–Starling) relationship. The diastolic dysfunction requires an increase in central and pulmonary venous pressure to maintain that end-diastolic volume. The range in acceptable filling pressures ends up becoming narrower with age because too low a pressure results in inadequate filling. Since the normal pressure is already elevated, any further increase is that much closer to a pressure that results in fluid extravasation and adverse consequences such as pulmonary edema.

Unfortunately, aging also decreases the ability to maintain filling pressures in the acceptable range. In everyone, the veins serve as a reservoir for blood and serve to buffer changes in blood volume in order to maintain ventricular filling at an appropriate level. However, veins stiffen with age.[53] Venous stiffening impairs this buffering capacity and creates a situation where modest changes in venous blood volume may produce more dramatic changes in venous pressures and cardiac filling. In short, the system has become inherently more unstable as illustrated by the development of postural hypotension in elderly persons but not in young adults with mild hypovolemia (Fig. 34-6).[54]

Rhythm disturbances may develop with age. Fibrosis of the conduction system may lead to conduction blocks, and loss of sinoatrial node cells may make the older patient more prone to sick sinus syndrome. The prevalence of atrial fibrillation climbs exponentially with age, perhaps in part because of atrial enlargement.

Aging appears to diminish or even eliminate any protective effect of ischemic preconditioning, a phenomenon whereby a brief period of myocardial ischemia will lessen the adverse effects of a subsequent, more prolonged ischemic event. "Warm-up angina" is the ability to achieve a higher level of exertion after first exercising to the point of angina. Starting around age 65 the increment in the level of exertion progressively diminishes with age.[48] In younger adults, death or heart failure is a less frequent complication of a myocardial infarction if the patient had been experiencing angina within 2 weeks of the myocardial infarction. This protective effect of angina is not present in older adults.[48]

This section began with a quote from Thomas Sydenham. Evidence is mounting that the quote is truly prophetic: arterial

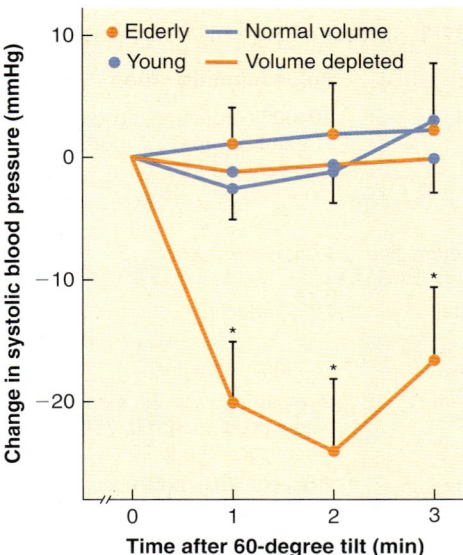

Figure 34-6 Young and elderly adults are subjected to a passive tilt test in their euvolemic state and after an approximate 2 kg of water and 100 mEq of sodium loss. With tilt, blood pools in the legs. Although young subjects tolerate tilt under both circumstances, the combination of hypovolemia and tilt exceeds the compensatory mechanisms of the older subjects. (Reproduced with permission from Shannon RP, Wei JY, Rosa RM, et al. The effect of age and sodium depletion on cardiovascular response to orthostasis. *Hypertension.* 1986;8:438.)

stiffening may indeed be a marker of physiologic age. One of the manifestations of arterial stiffening is a widened pulse pressure. Once the difference between systolic and diastolic pressure reaches 80 mmHg or more, there is a clear association with all-cause mortality; cardiovascular mortality; and a variety of morbidities including stroke, coronary disease, and renal failure.[50,55] Increased pulse pressure is also associated with increased morbidity and mortality after coronary artery bypass grafting.[50]

Pulmonary Aging

The most prominent effects of aging on the pulmonary system are increased stiffness of the chest wall and a decreased stiffness of the lung parenchyma.[56,57] With aging, the thorax becomes more barrel-shaped which leads to flattening of the diaphragm. Less diaphragmatic curvature provides a mechanical disadvantage for the generation of negative pressure in the intrapleural space. The stiffened chest wall and flattened diaphragm increase the work of breathing. Combined with an age-related loss of muscle mass, it is easy to understand how the older patient will be more prone to fatigue when challenged by an increase in minute ventilation, and thus more likely to experience respiratory failure.

The decrease in lung tissue stiffness is due to a loss of elastin with age. Unlike elsewhere in the body, the elastin is not replaced with collagen and so older lungs become easier to inflate. There are several adverse effects of this increase in compliance. Small airways do not have enough inherent stiffness and so depend on tethering by the surrounding tissue to remain open. The degree of outward pull by the tissue depends on the stiffness of the tissue and the degree of stretch of the tissue. As the tissue loses its

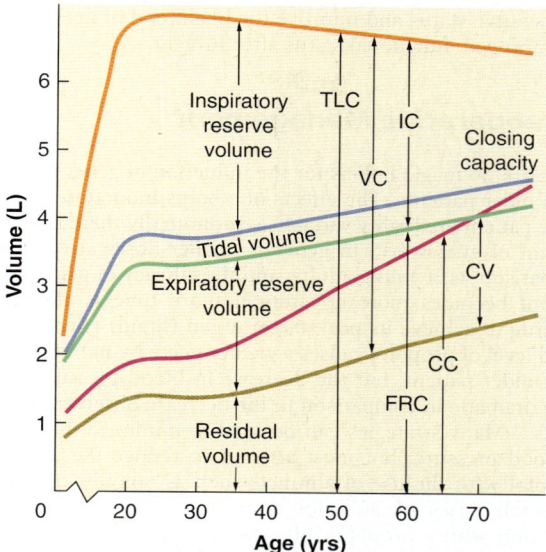

Figure 34-7 Effect of aging on lung volumes. With age, inspiratory capacity (IC) is compromised because of the combined effect of modest decreases in total lung capacity (TLC) and modest increase in functional residual capacity (FRC). Vital capacity (VC) decreases because of the decrease in IC and the increase in residual volume. However, the most dramatic change with aging is the increase in closing volume (CV) and closing capacity (CC) such that in very old persons, closing capacity exceeds functional residual capacity. (Adapted from Smith TC. Respiratory system: aging, adversity, and anesthesia. In: McLeskey CH, ed. *Geriatric Anesthesiology*. Baltimore, MD: Williams & Wilkins; 1997:85.)

springiness, greater lung inflation is needed to produce the same amount of outward pull on the airways. The need for greater lung inflation to prevent small airway collapse is reflected by the increase in closing capacity with age (Fig. 34-7). Closing capacity typically exceeds functional residual capacity in the mid-60s, and will eventually exceed the tidal volume at some later age. Decreased lung tissue stiffness also increases ventilation–perfusion mismatch as each piece of lung tissue is less tethered to its neighbor, making ventilation less uniform. These changes, plus a modest reduction in alveolar surface area with age, contribute to a modest decline in resting PaO_2 with age.[58]

Less-effective small airway tethering also leads to greater limitations during forced exhalation. At all ages, forced exhalation produces positive pressures in the intrapleural space that tends to compress intrathoracic airways. Only the airway connective tissue and lung tissue tethering oppose that compression. With less lung tissue tethering, airways compress at a larger lung volume in older subjects and produce a limitation in air flow during exhalation over a much larger percentage of the exhalation (e.g., the last 45% in a 70-year-old person) than in a younger subject (e.g., 20% in a 30-year-old person).[59]

Changes within the nervous system further influence the respiratory system. Aging leads to an approximate 50% decrease in the ventilatory response to hypercapnia, and an even greater decrease in the response to hypoxia, especially at night.[60] Generalized loss of muscle tone with age applies to the hypopharyngeal and genioglossal muscles and predisposes elderly persons to upper airway obstruction. A high percentage, perhaps even 75%, of people over age 65 have sleep-disordered breathing, a phenomenon that may or may not be the same as sleep apnea, but certainly places the elderly people at increased risk of hypoxia postoperatively.[61] Aging also results in less-effective coughing and impaired swallowing. Aspiration is a significant cause of community-acquired pneumonia and may well play a role in the development of postoperative pneumonia.[62]

Thermoregulation and Aging

In the past two decades there has been heightened awareness of the adverse consequences of perioperative hypothermia as well as improved methods to prevent hypothermia. Even outside the operating room, elderly individuals are prone to hypothermia when stressed by modestly cold environments that would not affect younger individuals. The initial response to a cold environment is vasoconstriction, and if that response is insufficient and the subject becomes colder, then shivering is the second response. Both mechanisms are triggered by decreases in core and/or skin temperature. The two temperatures interact such that a decrease in skin temperature of 1° is equivalent to a decrease in core temperature of approximately 0.2°.[63] Although there is great variability among the elderly over the degree to which vasoconstriction and shivering are impaired, one should anticipate that elderly patients will have not only impaired vasoconstriction but also decreased heat production due to a lower metabolism.[64]

At all ages, both inhalational and some intravenous agents (e.g., propofol and alfentanil but not midazolam) alter the regulatory thresholds such that body temperature must fall by as much as 4°C (7°F) before initiation of vasoconstriction or shivering. Aging further impairs the thresholds, by approximately 1°C (2°F), not only during general anesthesia but during spinal anesthesia as well.[63]

Given the impaired temperature regulation and decreased heat production of the elderly, it is not surprising that hypothermia occurs more frequently in older patients.[65] The risks of hypothermia include myocardial ischemia, surgical wound infection, coagulopathy with increased blood loss, and impaired drug metabolism.[63] Shivering places a significant metabolic stress on a patient and may not be well tolerated by a patient with borderline cardiac or pulmonary reserve. The prevention and treatment of hypothermia in an elderly patient does not appear to be any different than for younger adults.

Conduct of Anesthesia

We've put more effort into helping folks reach old age than into helping them enjoy it.

—Frank A. Clark

The Preoperative Visit

The preoperative visit can be extremely important in the care of the elderly patient. Although the goals of the visit are no different than for any other patient, there are issues more common among the elderly population that should be raised. For example, will the patient's living situation provide the support necessary for a successful recovery? An aged spouse may not be physically capable of helping the patient dress, bath, or perform some other activity of daily living (ADL) that the surgery temporarily prevents the patient from performing. Furthermore, elderly patients may require a long time to return to their preoperative level of function, assuming full recovery is even possible.

For example, after major abdominal surgery, most older patients require at least 3 months for ADLs and independent ADLs to return to baseline.[66] Persistent disability at 6 months varies with the task. Although there is only a 9% incidence of persistent ADL deficits, there is a 19% incidence of deficit in independent ADLs, and a 52% incidence of diminished grip strength.

Older patients often recognize that the end of their lives is no longer the theoretical consideration of youth, so they are more likely to have living wills, health-care proxies, and health-care directives in place at the time of surgery. Yet they often have surgery near the end of life. A retrospective cohort survey of elderly Medicare beneficiaries found that almost a third undergo surgery in their last year of life and that over 18% undergo surgery in the last month of their lives.[67] The older patient's expectations from surgery may be much different than that of their younger counterparts, and medical practitioners must be careful not to judge a patient's decision-making based on the practitioner's values or expectations. The prospect of functional impairment may be more worrisome to the older patient than even death. Such personal values are particularly important when questions of competence arise and the physician could be tempted to question competence if the patient's decision does not coincide with the opinion of the physician.[68] A discussion of risks and benefits needs to include the probable degree of functional recovery and the speed with which that recovery is likely to occur. If healthcare directives prohibit various life-sustaining or resuscitative procedures, the patient/proxy and anesthesiologist must come to a mutual understanding of what will or will not be performed if an untoward event occurs in the perioperative period.

Polypharmacy and drug interactions are a huge problem for the elderly. As much as 30% of ambulatory older adults require medical care for adverse drug events, and upward of 30% of hospitalizations in the elderly are related to drug effects.[69] In fact, one of the major goals of geriatric consult services to surgical patients is to pare down those medications whenever possible. The anesthesiologist can help by alerting the primary care team to this issue and suggest a geriatric consult. In the very old, dehydration, elder abuse, and malnutrition are all more common than generally appreciated. In the case of malnutrition, the deficit may be limited to isolated deficiencies such as vitamin D or B_{12}, or it may be more global and include inadequate caloric intake from poor oral hygiene or the "anorexia of aging," in which neuroendocrine changes lead to early satiety and diminished sense of taste.[70] Nutritional status is an underappreciated risk factor for surgery. In fact, the Veterans Affairs National Surgical Quality Improvement Program found albumin to be as sensitive an index for mortality or morbidity as any other single indicator, including the American Society of Anesthesiologists status.[71]

Clearly there are many issues surrounding surgery in the elderly that are rarely present with younger patients. Integration of the patient's medical status, the impact of surgery, and the patient's goals require a comprehensive approach that encompasses both preoperative optimization and potentially prolonged postoperative recovery. For these reasons the aged are an important opportunity for the potential advances offered by the PSH.[72] The ASA supported initiative of PSH is a patient-centered, physician-led, interdisciplinary, and team-based care model, that strives to achieve better health, better health care, and reduced expenditures by implementing multidisciplinary interventions as soon as need for surgery or procedure is identified.[73] In the preoperative period coordination of care, cost-effective testing and consultation and development of discharge and transition plans are started immediately leading to identification of patients who need specialized care and interventions to optimize preoperative status and improve the likelihood of maintained, if not improved, functional status after surgery.

Intraoperative Management

There are no magic bullets for the induction of general anesthesia in older patients. The effects of a bolus induction dose on a single patient are highly variable, so admittedly there is a certain amount of guesswork. In general, smaller doses are needed in comparison with young adults, and the efficacy of using a lesser amount becomes more apparent if more time is allowed for the drug to achieve its peak target organ (brain) effect. A given blood level of propofol causes a greater decrease in brain activity in an older patient, but the decrease in blood pressure is even more dramatic in comparison to the decrease observed in young adults.[74] Many strategies can be used to minimize the decrease in blood pressure, but most attempt to reduce the amount of propofol with the use of adjuncts such as opioids, or combining small doses of propofol with etomidate. Some advocate induction with a propofol infusion of 400 µg/kg/min until the bispectral index (BIS) reaches 60 to lessen the risk of overdose.[43] Etomidate has been observed to produce less hypotension than propofol in older patients.[75] Care must be taken, though, not to underdose at induction. It can be argued that an excessive hypertensive response to intubation may be more harmful than a brief period of hypotension. One must expect that significant changes in blood pressure, up or down, will occur, and the sooner the practitioner recognizes those changes, the quicker the aberration can be treated. Cycling the blood pressure cuff every minute should alert the practitioner to these changes sooner than would less frequent cycling. Although swings in blood pressure may not be desirable, there is little evidence that even major, but brief, changes in blood pressure lead to adverse outcomes.

Whether general or neuraxial anesthesia is used, the maintenance phase of anesthesia will commonly result in a significant decrease in systemic blood pressure, more so than typically occurs in younger patients.[76] Although decreases in both systemic vascular resistance and cardiac output likely occur, the decrease in vascular resistance is probably the largest contributor, although this observation has really been confirmed only during spinal anesthesia.[47] Figure 34-8 demonstrates this large decrease in vascular resistance and further shows that venous pooling is responsible for a decrease in preload that in turn decreases cardiac output. However, the afterload reduction from the decrease in blood pressure presumably allowed the ejection fraction to increase, thereby ameliorating the effect the decrease in end-diastolic volume had on stroke volume. Because vascular resistance contributes significantly to the decrease in blood pressure during anesthesia, it has been argued that the use of α-agonists is an appropriate therapy and may be more effective than volume alone.[48] α-Agonists also tend to promote venoconstriction, thereby shifting blood back to the central circulation and reducing the decrease in ventricular preload by venous pooling, and presumably reducing the need for at least some volume administration. Although no one would advocate vasoconstriction as a treatment for hypovolemia (except as a stopgap measure), the ventricle can only get so big; therefore, it is impossible for volume administration alone to raise cardiac output enough to compensate for a large decrease in vascular resistance. Furthermore, when sympathetic nervous system activity returns postoperatively, blood will shift from the periphery to the central circulation. Excess peripheral volume now becomes excess central volume and could push an elderly heart into diastolic heart failure. In short, volume administration to an older patient

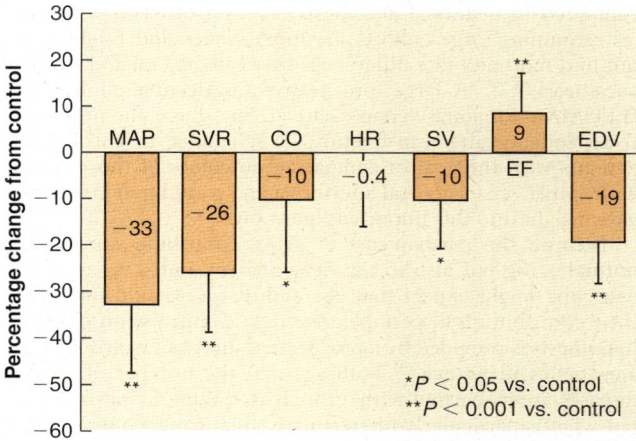

Figure 34-8 The response to total sympathectomy from spinal anesthesia as illustrated in older men with cardiac disease. Over 70% of the decrease in mean arterial blood pressure (MAP) was due to a decrease in systemic vascular resistance (SVR). Cardiac filling (EDV, end-diastolic volume) was markedly diminished, but its effect on stroke volume (SV) and cardiac output (CO) was ameliorated by an increase in ejection fraction (EF). Although heart rate (HR) increased in some subjects and decreased in others, the overall effect was no change. (Reproduced with permission from Rooke GA, Freund PR, Jacobson AF. Hemodynamic response and change in organ blood volume during spinal anesthesia in elderly men with cardiac disease. *Anesth Analg.* 1997;85:99. Copyright © 1997 International Anesthesia Research Society.)

may be problematic, with a very fine line between too much and too little, and what was "just right" in a deeply anesthetized state may become "too much" later on.

The choice between an endotracheal tube and a laryngeal mask airway involves many considerations, including body habitus, apparent frailty, surgical positioning, risk of regurgitation, and duration of surgery (see Chapter 29). An endotracheal tube will likely have more adverse effects than a laryngeal mask on mucociliary clearance and possibly on swallowing. The advantage of an endotracheal tube is in the ability to guarantee control of ventilation and thereby greater ability to prevent hypercarbia and intraoperative atelectasis.

If positive-pressure ventilation is utilized, one important goal is to have the lung volume exceed closing capacity during the respiratory cycle in order to prevent atelectasis. Two approaches have been advocated: high tidal volumes versus modest tidal volumes (generally accompanied by positive end-expiratory pressure [PEEP]). Initial studies found that the low tidal volume strategy tended to be associated with lower levels of inflammatory markers.[77] More recently, studies have appeared that document a decreased incidence of perioperative pulmonary complications with the use of modest tidal volumes, a conclusion best summarized in a meta-analysis.[78] Consequently, the modest tidal volume strategy plus PEEP as needed appears to be the preferred approach.

Another aspect of anesthetic management that is likely deleterious to the aging pulmonary system is the presence of residual neuromuscular blockade. Initially observed with pancuronium, intermediate acting neuromuscular blocking agents have also been implicated and the phenomenon is associated with adverse respiratory events such as hypoxia and airway obstruction.[79] Further complicating this picture is the observation that the use of neostigmine reversal may actually worsen residual blockade.[80,81] The adverse effect of neostigmine may be ameliorated by the use of neuromuscular transmission monitoring, presumably by permitting selection of an appropriate dose of neostigmine,[82] but even this observation is controversial.[81] Nevertheless, at least one study has shown that older patients (average age 75) are at almost double the risk of residual neuromuscular blockage and adverse respiratory events in comparison to middle-aged adults.[83] This observation argues for very careful use of nondepolarizing muscle relaxants in older patients.

Postoperative Care

The goals of emergence and the immediate postoperative period are no different for an elderly than a young patient; they are just more difficult to achieve. Analgesia is a major goal, and it should be stated up front that there is no evidence that pain is any less severe or any less detrimental in an older patient than in young patients. Less drug may be required (or not), but given that the standard approach to analgesia is to titrate to the desired effect, the outcome should be good pain relief for patients of any age. However, there are impediments to achieving adequate analgesia in an older patient.[84] Elderly patients sometimes underreport their pain level and may be more tolerant of their acute pain, perhaps partly because of the existence of chronic pain in their life. Older patients have more difficulty with visual analog scoring systems than verbal or numeric systems. If the patient is cognitively impaired, communication of pain is further impaired; indeed, demented patients often experience severe pain after hip surgery, but even mild cognitive impairment can lead to problems with pain assessment or with use of a patient-controlled analgesia machine.

Failure to achieve adequate levels of analgesia is associated with numerous adverse outcomes, including sleep deprivation, respiratory impairment, ileus, suboptimal mobilization, insulin resistance, tachycardia, and hypertension. The apparent paradox of adequate analgesia is that opioids are the mainstay of postoperative analgesia, and opioids are capable of producing many of those same adverse outcomes. Therefore, as with all medical care of elderly patients, good judgment, caution, and frequent monitoring of analgesia and adverse effects are essential. Adjunctive medications such as nonsteroidal anti-inflammatory drugs have been shown to reduce opioid requirements and some of the opioid adverse effects, but often carry their own risks such as renal damage or gastrointestinal toxicity.[84] Epidural analgesia is well known to provide analgesia that is superior to intravenous therapy, a finding that has been specifically replicated in the elderly.[85,86] Although improved cardiopulmonary outcomes were equivocal, more rapid return of bowel function, earlier mobilization, and nutritional status were better with epidural analgesia.

Although many aspects of postoperative care are more likely to be the purview of the surgeon or the internist, there are some things that the anesthesiologist could and probably should be watchful for when performing a postoperative visit on an older patient. If a patient had a surgery with major fluid requirements, it is important to look for signs of fluid overload, including rales, dyspnea, tachypnea, and orthopnea, particularly around postoperative day 2 when third space fluid tends to mobilize. A timely administration of a diuretic may prevent the development of overt pulmonary edema and the accompanying escalation of therapy and risk. Feel the pulse: atrial fibrillation is often intermittent and the more often someone looks for it, the more likely it will be detected. Delirium often goes undetected in older patients, in part because it may come and go. Take the time to chat with the patient for a few minutes. It should not be difficult to become suspicious if the patient demonstrates waxing and waning alertness, is inattentive or distractible, displays rambled or incoherent speech, is disoriented, or has perceptual disturbances. It has been demonstrated that overall recovery and avoidance of complications, including delirium, pneumonia, uncontrolled pain, infection, and length of stay, can be enhanced by comprehensive evaluation and management of risk factors.[87,88] Anesthesiologists should be prepared to support such programs as much as possible.

Perioperative Complications

My diseases are an asthma and a dropsy and, what is less curable, seventy-five.

—*Samuel Johnson*

The older patient is at increased risk for complications in the perioperative period, in part from comorbid disease and in part from the reduction in organ system reserve due to the aging process. Whether the aging process can be thought of as mere decreased reserve or subclinical disease is a matter of semantics. The result is the same: the elderly are at increased risk for almost every possible perioperative complication including cardiovascular, pulmonary, renal, central nervous system, wound infection, and death.[89–91]

There is increasing evidence that anesthetic management may influence long-term outcomes. The elderly are particularly sensitive to the effect of anesthetics and thus may be more susceptible to the detrimental effects of anesthesia. Although specific sensitivity to anesthesia is difficult to define, several lines of evidence suggest that it can be attained by clinically available modalities. For example, an intraoperative state of "triple low" (low concentrations of volatile anesthetics that is accompanied by low blood pressure and a deep hypnotic level as defined by a BIS monitor) is associated with longer hospital stay and increased 1-month mortality.[92] Although association does not imply causation and the "triple low" state may merely be a marker of low physiologic reserve, it is possible that identification of sensitivity may lead to improved outcomes. Additional studies show an association between intraoperative hypotension and other 1-month adverse outcomes including cardiac events, kidney dysfunction, and possibly stroke.[93–96] Age above 68 was an independent risk factor in one of these studies.[94] Another study that looked at 1-year mortality found no relation to intraoperative hypotension in the younger adult population, but found that the elderly subjects had a higher 1-year mortality that corresponded to the duration of the intraoperative hypotension.[97] Again, whether the hypotension is causal or just a marker is not clear, but these studies do suggest that permitting prolonged hypotension may not be a good idea.

Anesthesiologists who care for the elderly frequently face a worrisome query: does the choice of anesthetic technique (regional vs. general) or depth of anesthesia, affect outcome? With an estimated annual incidence of more than 1.5 million cases worldwide, operative fixation of hip fractures is the classical case in question. Hip fractures carry an ominous inhospital and 30-day mortality (roughly 5% to 10%) with high rates of cardiovascular and pulmonary complications and substantial postoperative disability. Any potential improvement for this vulnerable group has far reaching social and economic implications. Initially a meta-analysis of 141 clinical trials prompted the use of regional anesthesia as it found a reduction in postoperative mortality compared to general anesthesia.[98] However, some of the quoted studies were small, some had methodologic flaws and some were conducted over three decades ago. Although a large retrospective observational study from Taiwan found more adverse outcomes in patients who had general anesthesia when compared to neuraxial anesthesia,[99] recent observational studies examining large cohorts in United States and England did not find mortality rate differences between general and regional anesthesia.[100–102] A large, prospective multicenter clinical trial (REGAIN—REgional versus General Anesthesia for promoting INdependence after hip fracture) is scheduled to enroll 1,600 patients with the goal of comparing outcomes of those treated with spinal versus general anesthesia and would potentially provide insight into this important question.

Because the mechanisms of aging contribute not only to normal aging but also to the development and severity of disease, one might expect that age and disease would interact in their contribution to perioperative risk. Confirmation of such a hypothesis is provided by a prospective survey of nearly 200,000 anesthetics in France.[103] Both age and the number of chronic diseases are associated with an increased rate of complications, but what is particularly interesting is an apparent interaction of these two factors. Figure 34-9 demonstrates that, for any given age group, the number of complications increases with the number of comorbid diseases. To be young and sick likely represents a special case as suggested by the point representing the no more than 34-year-old group with three or more comorbid diseases. Ignoring that outlier, connecting the dots of equal number of comorbid disease reveals a modest increase in risk with age for patients with zero comorbid disease, but examination of points for one, two, or three or more diseases reveals an effect of age that becomes increasingly larger. In other words, age appears to interact with comorbid disease to increase risk.

Complications of the cardiovascular and pulmonary systems are associated with the greatest perioperative mortality. The best database is provided by the Veterans Affairs National Surgical Quality Improvement Project, and much of the database involves examination of patients older than 80 (Table 34-2).[90] Although the perioperative complications of myocardial infarction or cardiac arrest carry higher associated mortality rates than pneumonia, prolonged intubation, or reintubation, the higher incidences of the pulmonary complications suggest that greater mortality results from pulmonary complications than from cardiac

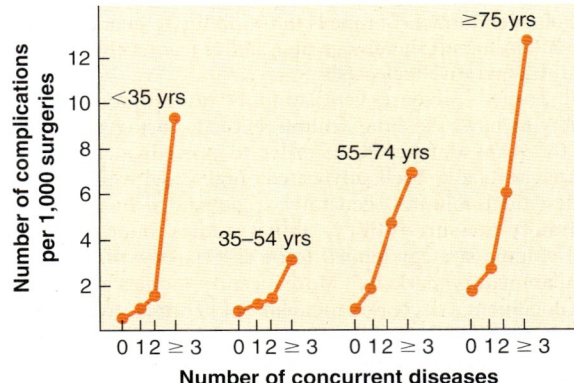

Figure 34-9 The interaction between age and comorbid disease. For each age bracket, as comorbid disease increases, so does the rate of complications. The effect of age on the complication rate is best visualized by examining points of equal comorbid disease. At zero disease, only a modest increase in complications is observed with increasing age. At ever-increasing degrees of comorbid disease, however, the increase in complications with age becomes more and more pronounced. (Reproduced with permission from Tiret L, Desmonts JM, Hatton F, et al. Complications associated with anaesthesia: a prospective survey in France. *Can Anesth Soc J.* 1986;33:336. With kind permission from Springer Science+Business Media.)

Table 34-2 Effect of Age on Selected Perioperative Complications and Associated Mortality[a]

Complication	Complication Rate		Mortality Rate from the Complication	
	Age <80	Age ≥80	Age <80	Age ≥80
Myocardial infarction	0.4	1.0	37.1	48.0
Cardiac arrest	0.9	2.1	80.0	88.2
Pneumonia	2.3	5.6	19.8	29.2
>48 hrs on ventilator	2.1	3.5	30.1	38.5
Required reintubation	1.6	2.8	32.3	44.0
Cerebrovascular accident	0.3	0.7	26.1	39.3
Coma >24 hrs	0.2	0.3	65.9	80.9
Prolonged ileus	1.2	1.7	9.2	16.0

[a]All differences between patients less than 80 versus 80 and older are significant at $p < 0.001$, except for coma mortality ($p = 0.004$).
Modified from Hamel MB, Henderson WG, Khuri SF, et al. Surgical outcomes for patients aged 80 and older: morbidity and mortality from major noncardiac surgery. J Am Geriat Soc. 2005;53:424.

complications. That pulmonary complications are so significant underscores the need for a better understanding of the mechanism of postoperative pneumonia, particularly the likely contribution of silent aspiration.[104]

Central nervous system complications are also a major source of morbidity and mortality. The most burdensome problems appear to be stroke, postoperative delirium, and postoperative cognitive decline. All have the potential to cause debilitating morbidity and an adverse impact on the patient's quality of life, their families, and the cost of medical care. Postoperative cognitive dysfunction (POCD) is a highly controversial topic in geriatric anesthesia, primarily because of the concern that general anesthesia may play an etiologic role.

In a nonsurgical elderly population, there is an annual stroke incidence of approximately 1%. The incidence of perioperative stroke in the older general surgical population is approximately 0.5% (Table 34-2).[90,105–107] Risk factors include age, atrial fibrillation (odds ratio 2.0), history of a prior stroke or TIA (odds ratio at least 1.6), recent myocardial infarction, COPD or current smoking, acute renal dysfunction or chronic dialysis, the type of surgery, and a variety of comorbid diseases including diabetes and renal or cardiovascular disease.[105–109] A particularly interesting risk factor, at least for cardiac surgery patients is an elevated arterial pulse pressure.[110] This finding supports the concept that age-related changes can influence perioperative risk just as it appears to influence morbidity in the general population. The PeriOperative ISchemic Evaluation study (POISE) raised the issue of perioperative β-blockade increasing the risk of stroke, but when chronic, less intense β-blockade is used that risk is not present.[111,112] Strokes typically occur well after surgery, on average 7 days later, although upward of half occur within 24 hours.[105,107] Most perioperative strokes are ischemic and presumably from thromboembolism originating in the heart or arteries. The contribution of hypotension to focal stroke is questionable, although the POISE study could be cited as evidence that hypotension increases stroke risk.[107] Mortality after a perioperative stroke is approximately twice that of a stroke in the general population, and overall mortality from perioperative stroke is at least 20%.[105,109]

Postoperative delirium is an acute confusional state manifested by an acute onset (hours to days) and vacillating levels of attention and cognitive skill.[113–115] Disorientation, perceptual disturbances (from situational misinterpretation to overt hallucinations), disorganized thinking, and problems with memory may be manifested. Emergence delirium alone does not qualify as postoperative delirium, but may be a risk factor.[116] Although most often short-lived (24 hours), delirium can be persistent and extend beyond hospital discharge.[113]

Delirium is most often diagnosed using Confusion Assessment Method, at least in research studies.[113,117] The mini-mental status examination can also be helpful, but its utility is higher for the identification of patients with pre-existing dementia. The risk of postoperative delirium after major surgery in older patients is approximately 10%; however, the risk varies with the surgical procedure.[114] Highest risk is emergent hip surgery, with an incidence of some 35%. The etiology of delirium is multifactorial. Risk factors include age, baseline low cognitive function (including dementia), depression, overall frailty, and general debility including dehydration or visual/auditory impairment.[113,115,118,119] The more risk factors present, the fewer perioperative stressors are required to push the patient over the edge to delirium.[114] Those additional stressors can include virtually any drug with central nervous system effects, including narcotics (especially meperidine), benzodiazepines (especially lorazepam), and drugs that possess anticholinergic properties (except perhaps glycopyrrolate). Other factors that likely contribute to delirium include sleep deprivation, being in an unfamiliar environment, and perioperative blood loss. The role of absolute intraoperative hypotension in the development of postoperative delirium is controversial, yet delirium is associated with fluctuations in blood pressure.[120]

The effect of anesthetic depth in general anesthesia on particularly neurologic outcomes is highly controversial. It is the routine practice of many anesthesiologists to provide adequate anesthetic depth to not only ensure there is no recall but also control increases in blood pressure. Perhaps it is the latter goal that accounts for what appears to be a tendency to provide higher levels of volatile anesthesia to the elderly when anesthetic dosing is adjusted for age.[121] A new body of evidence from different types of anesthetic techniques for hip, major noncardiac and cardiac surgery suggests that using a BIS-guided strategy to reduce anesthetic exposure and depth reduces the risk of postoperative delirium.[122–124] Similar findings demonstrated that using processed EEG, cumulative time of burst suppression was correlated with the risk of postoperative delirium.[125] Furthermore, in a study that employed BIS-guided sedation with propofol in patients having hip fracture repair under spinal anesthesia, it was found that in the sicker patients (Charlson comorbidity index >4), light sedation was associated with lower 1-year mortality than deep sedation.[126] An international trial (BALANCED) looking at general anesthesia with inhaled anesthetics titrated to BIS, planning to recruit 6,500 patients, will potentially answer the question of whether anesthetic depth is associated with poor outcomes in the aged.

Narcotic administration represents a fine line between too much and too little, as inadequate pain control is also associated with delirium.[127] Analgesia with meperidine should be avoided, except perhaps in small doses for shivering, as it is clearly a risk factor for delirium, but there appears to be no superior choice among fentanyl, hydromorphone, and morphine.[128] Nevertheless, multimodal analgesia to reduce opiate use is considered a rational approach. Disappointingly, the selection of epidural analgesia over IV opioid analgesia does not appear to reduce the incidence of delirium.[128] Similarly, the use of regional instead of general anesthesia does not seem to reduce delirium, but this result may be due to the use of inappropriate drugs and/or heavy sedation in conjunction with the regional technique. Controlled sedation along with regional anesthesia does appear to reduce the incidence of delirium.[114,124] This is an important concept, as patients with diminished cognitive function have lower drug requirements for the same level of sedation.[113,129] Dexmedetomidine may be a better choice than benzodiazepines for ICU sedation.[113,130]

Delirium often goes undiagnosed in the elderly patient as it is typically hypoactive. The patient does not demonstrate behavior that draws attention. This characteristic is unfortunate because delirium is associated with an increased duration of hospitalization and its attendant costs, poorer long-term functional recovery, and increased mortality.[113,114,131] Outcomes are worst when the delirium is persistent. Once detected, management focuses on reversible risk factors such as current medications, pain management, and a better sleep environment. Special care programs designed to limit the reversible risk factors appear to reduce the incidence of delirium by up to 50%.[88,132] In the event the delirium is agitated, haloperidol in doses no greater than 1.5 mg can be helpful.[113] Prophylactic haloperidol in hip surgery reduced the severity and duration of delirium but not its incidence,[133] whereas in critically ill elderly patients after noncardiac surgery, haloperidol (0.5 mg intravenous bolus injection followed by continuous infusion at a rate of 0.1 mg/hr for 12 hours administered at ICU admission) reduced the incidence of delirium.[134] The use of a subanesthetic dose of intraoperative ketamine to decrease the incidence of postoperative delirium is currently being examined in the PODCAST (Prevention of Delirium and Complications Associated with Surgical Treatments) study.[135] To summarize, effective approaches for prevention and treatment of postoperative delirium include targeting reversible risk factors with preemptive assessment and multifactorial interventions, limiting use of sedatives (especially benzodiazepines), avoiding drugs with atropinic properties (except glycopyrrolate), judicious treatment of postoperative pain, and, perhaps, careful use of antipsychotics.[136] The National Institute for Health and Clinical Excellence in United Kingdom (NICE) and the American Geriatric Society recently published guidelines on how to recognize, prevent, and treat delirium.[137,138]

POCD is characterized by a long-term decrease in mental abilities after surgery. Other than the rare patient who suffers obvious impairment, POCD is inherently more difficult to diagnose than delirium because it usually requires sophisticated neuropsychologic testing, including baseline tests prior to surgery. Selection of tests, their timing, and what deficits are required to qualify as cognitive decline have proven problematic in the literature.[115] The question is whether anesthesia contributes to POCD, and if so, to what degree?

Animal studies provide the most evidence for anesthetic CNS toxicity. Many studies of animals (typically rodents) exposed to volatile anesthesia demonstrate impaired memory and diminished learning ability that persists for at least months after exposure.[139] Volatile anesthesia increases brain production of β-amyloid and abnormal τ protein (leads to neurofibrillary tangles), both of which are associated with Alzheimer disease, and also cell apoptosis.[139,140] However, other studies found that memory impairment and CNS chemical change only occurred in animals that had surgery plus anesthesia. Anesthesia without surgery was no different than control animals.[139] Curiously, the anesthetics in these latter studies were fentanyl, droperidol, and chloral hydrate, thereby raising the possibility that not all anesthesia agents yield similar results. In addition to the potential neurodegenerative mechanism described above, cognitive decline could also result from a neuroinflammatory stress response to surgery and/or anesthesia.[141]

A seminal study not only examined surgical patients before and after surgery but included control subjects who were tested over time as well, but did not have surgery. At 3 months, a 10% incidence of POCD was observed in the patients who had surgery, in comparison to a 3% incidence who did not.[142] Risk factors for POCD at 3 months after surgery include age, lower levels of education, prior history of stroke even in the absence of residual deficit, and POCD at hospital discharge.[143] Increased mortality at 1 year is associated with patients who demonstrate cognitive decline at both hospital discharge and at 3 months postoperatively.[143] A study that examined the association between exposure to surgery and anesthesia and cognitive function in 8,503 pairs of middle aged and elderly twins identified 87 monozygotic and 124 dizygotic same-sexed twin pairs in whom one had major surgery and the other did not. A statistically significant but clinically negligible difference was found. For example, when participants were asked to provide as many names of animals as possible in 1 minute, the mean number of animals named was 23.5 in those that were exposed to surgery versus 24.2 in those that were not.[144]

Regarding the first few days after surgery, a few observations have been made that are neither surprising nor particularly worrisome. First of all, there is a similar degree of cognitive deficit in all age groups, not just the elderly.[145] Secondly, greater cognitive impairment can be observed with general anesthesia than with regional anesthesia.[146] Lastly, for the first few days the choice of general anesthesia makes a difference with propofol < desflurane < sevoflurane in degree of cognitive decline.[147,148] By 3 months, however, the presence of POCD is almost exclusively a problem in older patients.[145] Furthermore, no differences can be detected between general and regional anesthetic options.[146–148] By 1 year, even the best controlled studies suggest little or no demonstrable cognitive decline.[115,149] A longitudinal analysis of an Alzheimer disease database of patients who started with none to mild dementia showed the same overall rate of cognitive decline whether or not they had surgery or suffered a major illness.[150] Using before and after neuropsychologic testing, the incidence of POCD was compared for patients who underwent coronary angiography, total hip arthroplasty, or coronary artery bypass grafting.[151] At 1 week postoperatively, POCD was documented in 43% of the bypass graft patients and 17% for the hip replacement patients (angiography patients not tested at 1 week). At 3 months postprocedure, the incidence of POCD was 16% for both surgical groups and 21% for the angiography group (differences not significant). These two studies suggest there is no overall long-term adverse cognitive impact on patients, and that it is not the anesthetic which is to blame for whatever changes do occur. Effective treatment strategies for POCD are still absent and therefore the best treatment seems to be prevention. Small limited trials have assessed different strategies to reduce the incidence of POCD in animal models[152] and in humans,[122,153–155] but guidelines or recommendations that are supported by rigorous science are unavailable.

Delirium and POCD are often inappropriately perceived as a single entity along a time continuum. There may be an association between delirium and POCD, but if there is, the relationship has not been fully elucidated. Predictors of postoperative delirium such as hypoxemia[156] were not found to be risk factors for POCD.[142] Furthermore, postoperative delirium has not been found to be a risk factor for cognitive dysfunction at 3 months.[118]

So what do we tell our patients about stroke, delirium, and POCD? This is not an easy question to answer, especially for cognitive decline. However, patients are usually satisfied to know the facts and are willing to accept the unknown, including the fact that there does not seem to be any clear evidence that basic anesthetic techniques differ in their impact on outcome. Furthermore, at least for POCD, some believe that the accumulated evidence does not support the concept of long-term POCD as a clinical problem and that patients can be reassured that surgery and anesthesia are unlikely to be implicated in causing persistent cognitive decline or dementia.[157]

Nevertheless, there are a few specific points about the conduct of anesthesia that can be made. Besides the obvious caveats ("avoid hypotension and hypoxia"), the basic approach to an anesthetic for an elderly patient can be described as cautious. Since stroke is likely a thromboembolic phenomenon, there may be little that can be done beyond standard, good anesthetic care. However, it is not clear that antiplatelet therapy needs to be discontinued for surgery as much as currently occurs. The efficacy of statins has also not been adequately assessed. As previously discussed, drug choices and dosage have a potentially major impact on delirium. Pain control with multimodal therapy to reduce opioid consumption is probably a good thing, but poor pain control may be as bad as too much opioid. Finally, it is not clear what the relationship is between anesthesia and cognitive decline, if there is one at all. Given that unsatisfactory statement, it seems reasonable to choose the anesthetic technique based on the other factors germane to the patient and surgery.

The Future

I will never be an old man. To me, old age is always 15 years older than I am.

—*Francis Bacon*

Improvements in surgical and anesthetic techniques that reduce the overall stress to the patient are permitting more surgeries to be performed on older and sicker patients than ever before. Nevertheless, the older patient will continue to experience the majority of perioperative adverse outcomes. Much remains to be accomplished in the quest to find ways to decrease the incidence and severity of those adverse outcomes.[104] The most pressing issues are arguably the prevention of postoperative delirium, cognitive decline, pneumonia, respiratory failure, and cardiovascular complications. Improved pain-control techniques that also diminish side effects, especially to the brain and bowels, would be welcome. However, other realms of care are just in their infancy, most notably whether preoperative improvement in the functional status of frail patients is helpful. For example, can short courses of better nutrition, exercise regimens, or even dietary supplements reduce complications, speed recovery, or improve functional recovery? When caring for the elderly, especially the frail elderly, the overriding goal should be to produce as little stress to the patient as possible during both surgery and the subsequent hospitalization and recovery. Complete care will be multidisciplinary out of necessity. No single specialty possesses the total perspective, and the anesthesiologist's expertise is an important component of that care.

REFERENCES

1. Lerner W. Historical statistics of the United States. http://www.census.gov/history/pdf/histstats-colonial-1970.pdf. Accessed December 30, 2015.
2. Werner CA. The older population: 2010. November 2011; http://www.census.gov/prod/cen2010/briefs/c2010br-09.pdf. Accessed December 30, 2015.
3. Statistics on the growth, distribution, and characteristics of the U.S. population. 2012; http://www2.census.gov/library/publications/2011/compendia/statab/131ed/tables/pop.pdf. Accessed December 30, 2015.
4. Number, rate, and average length of stay for discharges from short-stay hospitals, by age, region, and sex: United States. 2010; http://www.cdc.gov/nchs/data/nhds/1general/2010gen1_agesexalos.pdf. Accessed December 30, 2015.
5. Buie VC, Owings MF, DeFrances CJ, et al. National hospital discharge survey: 2006 annual summary. *Vital Health Stat*. 2010(168):1–79.
6. Cullen KA, Hall MJ, Golosinskiy A, Statistics NCfH. *Ambulatory surgery in the United States, 2006*. US Department of Health and Human Services, Centers for Disease Control and Prevention, National Center for Health Statistics; 2009.
7. Chantrill C. Medicare Spending Analysis. http://www.usgovernmentspending.com/medicare_spending_by_year. Accessed December 30, 2015.
8. National Health Expenditure Projections 2014–2024. https://www.cms.gov/Research-Statistics-Data-and-Systems/Statistics-Trends-and-Reports/NationalHealthExpendData/downloads/proj2014.pdf. Accessed December 30, 2015.
9. GDP at market prices (current US$). http://data.worldbank.org/indicator/NY.GDP.MKTP.CD. Accessed December 30, 2015.
10. Medicare and Private Payment Differences for Anesthesia Services July 2007. http://www.gao.gov/new.items/d07463.pdf. Accessed December 30, 2015.
11. Anesthesiologists Center. https://www.cms.gov/Center/Provider-Type/Anesthesiologists-Center.html?redirect=/center/anesth.asp. Accessed December 30, 2015.
12. Bishop NA, Guarente L. Genetic links between diet and lifespan: shared mechanisms from yeast to humans. *Nature Rev Genet*. 2007;8(11):835–844.
13. Hayden EC. Age research: a new angle on 'old'. *Nature*. 2007;450(7170):603–605.
14. Fries JF. Aging, natural death, and the compression of morbidity. *N Engl J Med*. 1980;303(3):130–135.
15. Mercken EM, Carboneau BA, Krzysik-Walker SM, et al. Of mice and men: the benefits of caloric restriction, exercise, and mimetics. *Ageing Res Rev*. 2012;11(3):390–398.
16. Kennedy BK, Berger SL, Brunet A, et al. Geroscience: linking aging to chronic disease. *Cell*. 11/6/ 2014;159(4):709–713.
17. Fleisher LA, Fleischmann KE, Auerbach AD, et al. 2014 ACC/AHA Guideline on perioperative cardiovascular evaluation and management of patients undergoing noncardiac surgery: a report of the American College of Cardiology/American Heart Association Task Force on Practice Guidelines. *J Am Coll Cardiol*. 2014;64(22):e77–e137.
18. Fried LP, Tangen CM, Walston J, et al. Frailty in older adults: evidence for a phenotype. *J Gerontol A Biol Sci Med Sci*. 2001;56(3):M146–M157.
19. Rockwood K, Mitnitski A. Frailty in relation to the accumulation of deficits. *J Gerontol A Biol Sci Med Sci*. 2007;62(7):722–727.
20. Rockwood K, Andrew M, Mitnitski A. A comparison of two approaches to measuring frailty in elderly people. *J Gerontol A Biol Sci Med Sci*. 2007;62(7):738–743.
21. Beggs T, Sepehri A, Szwajcer A, et al. Frailty and perioperative outcomes: a narrative review. *Can J Anaesth*. 2015;62(2):143–157.
22. McIsaac DI, Bryson GL, van Walraven C. Association of frailty and 1-year postoperative mortality following major elective noncardiac surgery: A population-based cohort study. *JAMA Surg*. 2016;151(6):538–545.
23. Bibas L, Levi M, Bendayan M, et al. Therapeutic interventions for frail elderly patients. Part I. Published randomized trials. *Prog Cardiovasc Diss*. 2014;57(2):134–143.
24. Gillis C, Li C, Lee L, et al. Prehabilitation versus rehabilitation: a randomized control trial in patients undergoing colorectal resection for cancer. *Anesthesiology*. 2014;121(5):937–947.
25. Lemanu D, Singh P, MacCormick A, et al. Effect of preoperative exercise on cardiorespiratory function and recovery after surgery: a systematic review. *World J Surg*. 2013;37(4):711–720.
26. Fairhall N, Kurrle SE, Sherrington C, et al. Effectiveness of a multifactorial intervention on preventing development of frailty in pre-frail older people: study protocol for a randomised controlled trial. *BMJ*. 2015;5(2):e007091.
27. Fukagawa NK, Bandini LG, Young JB. Effect of age on body composition and resting metabolic rate. *Am J Physiol Endocrinol Metab*. 1990;259(2):E233–E238.
28. Doherty TJ. Invited review: aging and sarcopenia. *J Appl Physiol*. 2003;95(4):1717–1727.
29. Grandison MK, Boudinot FD. Age-related changes in protein binding of drugs. *Clin Pharmacokinet*. 2000;38(3):271–290.
30. Schmucker DL. Age-related changes in liver structure and function: implications for disease? *Exp Gerontol*. 2005;40(8):650–659.
31. Mühlberg W, Platt D. Age-dependent changes of the kidneys: pharmacological implications. *Gerontology*. 1999;45(5):243–253.
32. Epstein M. Aging and the kidney. *J Am Soc Nephrol*. 1996;7(8):1106–1122.
33. Scheen A. Diabetes mellitus in the elderly: insulin resistance and/or impaired insulin secretion? *Diabetes Metab*. 2005;31:5S27–25S34.
34. Paganelli R, Di Iorio A, Cherubini A, et al. Frailty of older age: the role of the endocrine-immune interaction. *Curr Pharmaceut Design*. 2006;12(24):3147–3159.
35. Drachman DA. Aging of the brain, entropy, and Alzheimer disease. *Neurology*. 2006;67(8):1340–1352.
36. Mrak RE, Griffin WST, Graham DI. Aging-associated changes in human brain. *J Neuropathol Exp Neurol*. 1997;56(12):1269–1275.
37. Shors TJ, Miesegaes G, Beylin A, et al. Neurogenesis in the adult is involved in the formation of trace memories. *Nature*. 2001;410(6826):372–376.
38. Mapleson W. Effect of age on MAC in humans: a meta-analysis. *Br J Anaesth*. 1996;76(2):179–185.

39. Jung D, Mayersohn M, Perrier D, et al. Thiopental disposition as a function of age in female patients undergoing surgery. *Anesthesiology.* 1982;56(4):263–268.
40. Minto CF, Schnider TW, Egan TD, et al. Influence of age and gender on the pharmacokinetics and pharmacodynamics of remifentanil. I. Model development. *Anesthesiology.* 1997;86(1):10–23.
41. Klotz U, Avant G, Hoyumpa A, et al. The effects of age and liver disease on the disposition and elimination of diazepam in adult man. *J Clin Invest.* 1975;55(2):347.
42. Shafer SL. Pharmacokinetics and pharmacodynamics of the elderly. In: Charles McLeshey, ed. *Geriatric Anesthesiology.* Baltimore, MD: Williams & Wilkins; 1997:123–142.
43. McEvoy MD, Reves J. Intravenous hypnotic anesthetics. In: Silverstein JH, Rooke GA, Reves JG, et al. eds. *Geriatric Anesthesiology.* 2nd ed. New York, NY: Springer; 2008:229–245.
44. Shafer SL, Flood P. The pharmacology of opioids. In: Silverstein JH, Rooke GA, Reves JG, et al. eds. *Geriatric Anesthesiology.* 2nd ed. New York, NY: Springer; 2008:209–228.
45. Lien CA, Suzuki T. Relaxants and their reversal agents. In: Silverstein JH, Rooke GA, Reves JG, McLeskey CH, eds. *Geriatric Anesthesiology.* 2nd ed. New York, NY: Springer; 2008:266–277.
46. Folkow B, Svanborg A. Physiology of cardiovascular aging. *Physiol Rev.* 1993;73:725–764.
47. Rooke GA, Freund PR, Jacobson AF. Hemodynamic response and change in organ blood volume during spinal anesthesia in elderly men with cardiac disease. *Anesth Analg.* 1997;85(1):99–105.
48. Rooke GA. Cardiovascular aging and anesthetic implications. *J Cardiovasc Vasc Anesth.* 2003;17(4):512–523.
49. Ebert TJ, Morgan BJ, Barney JA, et al. Effects of aging on baroreflex regulation of sympathetic activity in humans. *Am J Physiol Heart Circ Physiol.* 1992; 263(3):H798–H803.
50. Barodka VM, Joshi BL, Berkowitz DE, et al. Implications of vascular aging. *Anesth Analg.* 2011;112(5):1048.
51. Nichols WW, O'Rourke MF, Avolio AP, et al. Effects of age on ventricular-vascular coupling. *Am J Cardiol.* 1985;55(9):1179–1184.
52. Lakatta EG. Cardiovascular aging in health. *Clin Geriatr Med.* 2000;16(3):419–443.
53. Bouissou H, Julian M, Pieraggi M-T, et al. Structure of healthy and varicose veins. In: Vanhoutte PM, ed. *Return Circulation and Norepinephrine: An Update.* Paris: John Libbey Eurotext; 1991:139–150.
54. Shannon RP, Wei JY, Rosa RM, et al. The effect of age and sodium depletion on cardiovascular response to orthostasis. *Hypertension.* 1986;8(5):438–443.
55. Domanski MJ, Davis BR, Pfeffer MA, et al. Isolated systolic hypertension prognostic information provided by pulse pressure. *Hypertension.* 1999;34(3):375–380.
56. Crapo R. The aging lung. *Lung Biol Heal Dis.* 1993;63:1–25.
57. Wahba W. Influence of aging on lung function-clinical significance of changes from age twenty. *Anesth Analg.* 1983;62(8):764–776.
58. Zaugg M, Lucchinetti E. Respiratory function in the elderly. *Anesthesiol Clin North Am.* 2000;18(1):47–58.
59. DeLorey DS, Babb TG. Progressive mechanical ventilatory constraints with aging. *Am J Respir Crit Care Med.* 1999;160(1):169–177.
60. Kronenberg RS, Drage CW. Attenuation of the ventilatory and heart rate responses to hypoxia and hypercapnia with aging in normal men. *J Clin Invest.* 1973;52(8):1812–1819.
61. Ancoli-Israel S, Coy T. Are breathing disturbances in elderly equivalent to sleep apnea syndrome? *Sleep.* 1994;17(1):77–83.
62. Marik PE, Kaplan D. Aspiration pneumonia and dysphagia in the elderly. *Chest.* 2003;124(1):328–336.
63. Sessler DI. Perioperative thermoregulation. In: Silverstein JH, Rooke GA, Reves JG, et al, eds. *Geriatric Anesthesiology.* 2nd ed. New York, NY: Springer; 2008:107–122.
64. Kenney WL, Munce TA. Invited review: aging and human temperature regulation. *J Appl Physiol (1985).* 2003;95(6):2598–2603.
65. Vaughan MS, Vaughan RW, Cork RC. Postoperative hypothermia in adults: relationship of age, anesthesia, and shivering to rewarming. *Anesth Analg.* 1981;60(10):746–751.
66. Lawrence VA, Hazuda HP, Cornell JE, et al. Functional independence after major abdominal surgery in the elderly. *J Am Coll Surg.* 2004;199(5):762–772.
67. Kwok AC, Semel ME, Lipsitz SR, et al. The intensity and variation of surgical care at the end of life: a retrospective cohort study. *Lancet.* 2011;378(9800):1408–1413.
68. Rosenthal RA, Kavic SM. Assessment and management of the geriatric patient. *Crit Care Med.* 2004;32(4 Suppl):S92–S105.
69. By the American Geriatrics Society Beers Criteria Update Expert Panel. American Geriatrics Society 2015 Updated Beers Criteria for potentially inappropriate medication use in older adults. *J Am Geriatr Soc.* 2015;63(11):2227–2246.
70. Rosenthal RA. Nutritional concerns in the older surgical patient. *J Am Coll Surg.* 2004;199(5):785–791.
71. Gibbs J, Cull W, Henderson W, et al. Preoperative serum albumin level as a predictor of operative mortality and morbidity: results from the National VA Surgical Risk Study. *Arch Surg.* 1999;134(1):36–42.
72. Englesbe MJ, Lussiez AD, Friedman JF, et al. Starting a surgical home. *Ann Surg.* 2015;262(6):901–903.
73. Mello MT, Azocar RJ, Lewis MC. Geriatrics and the perioperative surgical home. *Anesthesiol Clin.* 2015;33(3):439–445.
74. Kazama T, Ikeda K, Morita K, et al. Comparison of the effect-site k(eO)s of propofol for blood pressure and EEG bispectral index in elderly and younger patients. *Anesthesiology.* 1999;90(6):1517–1527.
75. Reich DL, Hossain S, Krol M, et al. Predictors of hypotension after induction of general anesthesia. *Anesth Analg.* 2005;101(3):622–628.
76. Forrest JB, Rehder K, Cahalan MK, et al. Multicenter study of general anesthesia. III. Predictors of severe perioperative adverse outcomes. *Anesthesiology.* 1992;76(1):3–15.
77. Guldner A, Kiss T, Serpa Neto A, et al. Intraoperative protective mechanical ventilation for prevention of postoperative pulmonary complications: a comprehensive review of the role of tidal volume, positive end-expiratory pressure, and lung recruitment maneuvers. *Anesthesiology.* 2015;123(3):692–713.
78. Serpa Neto A, Hemmes SN, Barbas CS, et al. Protective versus conventional ventilation for surgery: a systematic review and individual patient data meta-analysis. *Anesthesiology.* 2015;123(1):66–78.
79. Grosse-Sundrup M, Henneman JP, Sandberg WS, et al. Intermediate acting non-depolarizing neuromuscular blocking agents and risk of postoperative respiratory complications: prospective propensity score matched cohort study. *BMJ.* 2012;345:e6329.
80. Esteves S, Martins M, Barros F, et al. Incidence of postoperative residual neuromuscular blockade in the postanaesthesia care unit: an observational multicentre study in Portugal. *Eur J Anaesthesiol.* 2013;30(5):243–249.
81. Meyer MJ, Bateman BT, Kurth T, et al. Neostigmine reversal doesn't improve postoperative respiratory safety. *BMJ.* 2013;346:f1460.
82. Hunter JM. Antagonising neuromuscular block at the end of surgery. *BMJ.* 2012;345:e6666.
83. Murphy GS, Szokol JW, Avram MJ, et al. Residual neuromuscular block in the elderly: incidence and clinical implications. *Anesthesiology.* 2015; 123(6):1322–1336.
84. Aubrun F. Management of postoperative analgesia in elderly patients. *Region Anesth Pain Med.* 2005;30(4):363–379.
85. Mann C, Pouzeratte Y, Boccara G, et al. Comparison of intravenous or epidural patient-controlled analgesia in the elderly after major abdominal surgery. *Anesthesiology.* 2000;92(2):433–441.
86. Carli F, Mayo N, Klubien K, et al. Epidural analgesia enhances functional exercise capacity and health-related quality of life after colonic surgery: results of a randomized trial. *Anesthesiology.* 2002;97(3):540–549.
87. Harari D, Hopper A, Dhesi J, et al. Proactive care of older people undergoing surgery ('POPS'): designing, embedding, evaluating and funding a comprehensive geriatric assessment service for older elective surgical patients. *Age Ageing.* 2007;36(2):190–196.
88. Marcantonio ER, Flacker JM, Wright RJ, et al. Reducing delirium after hip fracture: a randomized trial. *J Am Geriatr Soc.* 2001;49(5):516–522.
89. Turrentine FE, Wang H, Simpson VB, et al. Surgical risk factors, morbidity, and mortality in elderly patients. *J Am Coll Surg.* 2006;203(6):865–877.
90. Hamel MB, Henderson WG, Khuri SF, et al. Surgical outcomes for patients aged 80 and older: morbidity and mortality from major noncardiac surgery. *J Am Geriatr Soc.* 2005;53(3):424–429.
91. Bentov I, Reed MJ. Anesthesia, microcirculation, and wound repair in aging. *Anesthesiology.* 2014;120(3):760–772.
92. Sessler DI, Sigl JC, Kelley SD, et al. Hospital stay and mortality are increased in patients having a "triple low" of low blood pressure, low bispectral index, and low minimum alveolar concentration of volatile anesthesia. *Anesthesiology.* 2012;116(6):1195–1203.
93. Bijker JB, Persoon S, Peelen LM, et al. Intraoperative hypotension and perioperative ischemic stroke after general surgery: a nested case-control study. *Anesthesiology.* 2012;116(3):658–664.
94. Kheterpal S, O'Reilly M, Englesbe MJ, et al. Preoperative and intraoperative predictors of cardiac adverse events after general, vascular, and urological surgery. *Anesthesiology.* 2009;110(1):58–66.
95. Walsh M, Devereaux PJ, Garg AX, et al. Relationship between intraoperative mean arterial pressure and clinical outcomes after noncardiac surgery toward an empirical definition of hypotension. *Anesthesiology.* 2013;119(3):507–515.
96. van Waes JA, van Klei WA, Wijeysundera DN, et al. Association between intraoperative hypotension and myocardial injury after vascular surgery. *Anesthesiology.* 2016;124(1):35–44.
97. Bijker JB, van Klei WA, Vergouwe Y, et al. Intraoperative hypotension and 1-year mortality after noncardiac surgery. *Anesthesiology.* 2009;111(6):1217–1226.
98. Rodgers A, Walker N, Schug S, et al. Reduction of postoperative mortality and morbidity with epidural or spinal anaesthesia: results from overview of randomised trials. *BMJ.* 2000;321(7275):1493.
99. Chu CC, Weng SF, Chen KT, et al. Propensity score-matched comparison of postoperative adverse outcomes between geriatric patients given a general or a neuraxial anesthetic for hip surgery: a population-based study. *Anesthesiology.* 2015;123(1):136–147.

100. Patorno E, Neuman MD, Schneeweiss S, et al. Comparative safety of anesthetic type for hip fracture surgery in adults: retrospective cohort study. BMJ. 2014;348:g4022.
101. Neuman MD, Rosenbaum PR, Ludwig JM, et al. Anesthesia technique, mortality, and length of stay after hip fracture surgery. JAMA. 2014;311(24):2508–2517.
102. White SM, Moppett IK, Griffiths R. Outcome by mode of anaesthesia for hip fracture surgery: an observational audit of 65 535 patients in a national dataset. Anaesthesia. 2014;69(3):224–230.
103. Tiret L, Desmonts JM, Hatton F, et al. Complications associated with anaesthesia—a prospective survey in France. Can Anaesth Soc J. 1986;33(3 Pt 1):336–344.
104. Cook DJ, Rooke GA. Priorities in perioperative geriatrics. Anesth Analg. 2003;96(6):1823–1836.
105. Kam PC, Calcroft RM. Peri-operative stroke in general surgical patients. Anaesthesia. 1997;52(9):879–883.
106. Bateman BT, Schumacher HC, Wang S, et al. Perioperative acute ischemic stroke in noncardiac and nonvascular surgery: incidence, risk factors, and outcomes. Anesthesiology. 2009;110(2):231–238.
107. Ng JL, Chan MT, Gelb AW. Perioperative stroke in noncardiac, nonneurosurgical surgery. Anesthesiology. 2011;115(4):879–890.
108. Kaatz S, Douketis JD, Zhou H, et al. Risk of stroke after surgery in patients with and without chronic atrial fibrillation. J Thromb Haemost. 2010;8(5):884–890.
109. Mashour GA, Shanks AM, Kheterpal S. Perioperative stroke and associated mortality after noncardiac, nonneurologic surgery. Anesthesiology. 2011;114(6):1289–1296.
110. Benjo A, Thompson RE, Fine D, et al. Pulse pressure is an age-independent predictor of stroke development after cardiac surgery. Hypertension. 2007;50(4):630–635.
111. Group PS, Devereaux PJ, Yang H, et al. Effects of extended-release metoprolol succinate in patients undergoing non-cardiac surgery (POISE trial): a randomised controlled trial. Lancet. 2008;371(9627):1839–1847.
112. van Lier F, Schouten O, Hoeks SE, et al. Impact of prophylactic beta-blocker therapy to prevent stroke after noncardiac surgery. Am J Cardiol. 2010;105(1):43–47.
113. Rudolph JL, Marcantonio ER. Review articles: postoperative delirium: acute change with long-term implications. Anesth Analg. 2011;112(5):1202–1211.
114. Sieber FE. Postoperative delirium in the elderly surgical patient. Anesthesiol Clin. 2009;27(3):451–464.
115. Silverstein JH, Timberger M, Reich DL, et al. Central nervous system dysfunction after surgery and anesthesia in the elderly. Anesthesiology. 2007;106(3):622–628.
116. Sharma PT, Sieber FE, Zakriya KJ, et al. Recovery room delirium predicts postoperative delirium after hip-fracture repair. Anesth Analg. 2005;101(4):1215–1220.
117. Inouye SK, van Dyck CH, Alessi CA, et al. Clarifying confusion: the confusion assessment method: a new method for detection of delirium. Ann Intern Med. 1990;113(12):941–948.
118. Jankowski CJ, Trenerry MR, Cook DJ, et al. Cognitive and functional predictors and sequelae of postoperative delirium in elderly patients undergoing elective joint arthroplasty. Anesth Analg. 2011;112(5):1186–1193.
119. Leung JM, Tsai TL, Sands LP. Brief report: preoperative frailty in older surgical patients is associated with early postoperative delirium. Anesth Analg. 2011;112(5):1199–1201.
120. Hirsch J, DePalma G, Tsai TT, et al. Impact of intraoperative hypotension and blood pressure fluctuations on early postoperative delirium after non-cardiac surgery. Br J Anaesth. 2015;115(3):418–426.
121. Van Cleve WC, Nair BG, Rooke GA. Associations between age and dosing of volatile anesthetics in 2 academic hospitals. Anesth Analg. 2015;121(3):645–651.
122. Chan MT, Cheng BC, Lee TM, et al. BIS-guided anesthesia decreases postoperative delirium and cognitive decline. J Neurosurg Anesthesiol. 2013;25(1):33–42.
123. Whitlock EL, Torres BA, Lin N, et al. Postoperative delirium in a substudy of cardiothoracic surgical patients in the BAG-RECALL clinical trial. Anesth Analg. 2014;118(4):809–817.
124. Sieber FE, Zakriya KJ, Gottschalk A, et al. Sedation depth during spinal anesthesia and the development of postoperative delirium in elderly patients undergoing hip fracture repair. Mayo Clin Proc. 2010;85(1):18–26.
125. Fritz BA, Kalarickal PL, Maybrier HR, et al. Intraoperative electroencephalogram suppression predicts postoperative delirium. Anesth Analg. 2015;22(1):234–242.
126. Brown CH, Azman AS, Gottschalk A, et al. Sedation depth during spinal anesthesia and survival in elderly patients undergoing hip fracture repair. Anesth Analg. 2014;118(5):977–980.
127. Vaurio LE, Sands LP, Wang Y, et al. Postoperative delirium: the importance of pain and pain management. Anesth Analg. 2006;102(4):1267–1273.
128. Fong HK, Sands LP, Leung JM. The role of postoperative analgesia in delirium and cognitive decline in elderly patients: a systematic review. Anesth Analg. 2006;102(4):1255–1266.
129. Laalou FZ, Egard M, Guillot M, et al. Influence of preoperative cognitive status on propofol requirement to maintain hypnosis in the elderly. Br J Anaesth. 2010;105(3):342–346.
130. Riker RR, Shehabi Y, Bokesch PM, et al. Dexmedetomidine vs midazolam for sedation of critically ill patients: a randomized trial. JAMA. 2009;301(5):489–499.
131. Zakriya K, Sieber FE, Christmas C, et al. Brief postoperative delirium in hip fracture patients affects functional outcome at three months. Anesth Analg. 2004;98(6):1798–1802, table of contents.
132. Bjorkelund KB, Hommel A, Thorngren KG, et al. Reducing delirium in elderly patients with hip fracture: a multi-factorial intervention study. Acta Anaesthesiol Scand. 2010;54(6):678–688.
133. Kalisvaart KJ, de Jonghe JF, Bogaards MJ, et al. Haloperidol prophylaxis for elderly hip-surgery patients at risk for delirium: a randomized placebo-controlled study. J Am Geriatr Soc. 2005;53(10):1658–1666.
134. Wang W, Li H-L, Wang D-X, et al. Haloperidol prophylaxis decreases delirium incidence in elderly patients after noncardiac surgery: a randomized controlled trial. Crit Care Med. 2012;40(3):731–739.
135. Avidan MS, Fritz BA, Maybrier HR, et al. The Prevention of Delirium and Complications Associated with Surgical Treatments (PODCAST) study: protocol for an international multicentre randomised controlled trial. BMJ. 2014;4(9):e005651.
136. Marcantonio ER. Postoperative delirium: a 76-year-old woman with delirium following surgery. JAMA. 2012;308(1):73–81.
137. Young J, Murthy L, Westby M, et al; Guideline Development Group. Diagnosis, prevention, and management of delirium: summary of NICE guidance. BMJ. 2010;341:c3704.
138. American Geriatrics Society Expert Panel on Postoperative Delirium in Older Adults. American Geriatrics Society abstracted clinical practice guideline for postoperative delirium in older adults. J Am Geriatr Soc. 2015;63(1):142–150.
139. Bittner EA, Yue Y, Xie Z. Brief review: anesthetic neurotoxicity in the elderly, cognitive dysfunction and Alzheimer's disease. Can J Anaesth. 2011;58(2):216–223.
140. Tang J, Eckenhoff MF, Eckenhoff RG. Anesthesia and the old brain. Anesth Analg. 2010;110(2):421–426.
141. Hudson AE, Hemmings HC, Jr. Are anaesthetics toxic to the brain? Br J Anaesth. 2011;107(1):30–37.
142. Moller JT, Cluitmans P, Rasmussen LS, et al. Long-term postoperative cognitive dysfunction in the elderly ISPOCD1 study. ISPOCD investigators. International Study of Post-Operative Cognitive Dysfunction. Lancet. 1998;351(9106):857–861.
143. Monk TG, Weldon BC, Garvan CW, et al. Predictors of cognitive dysfunction after major noncardiac surgery. Anesthesiology. 2008;108(1):18–30.
144. Dokkedal U, Hansen TG, Rasmussen LS, et al. Cognitive functioning after surgery in middle-aged and elderly Danish twins. Anesthesiology. 2016;124(2):312–321.
145. Crosby G, Culley DJ. Surgery and anesthesia: healing the body but harming the brain? Anesth Analg. 2011;112(5):999–1001.
146. Wu CL, Hsu W, Richman JM, et al. Postoperative cognitive function as an outcome of regional anesthesia and analgesia. Reg Anesth Pain Med. 2004;29(3):257–268.
147. Royse CF, Andrews DT, Newman SN, et al. The influence of propofol or desflurane on postoperative cognitive dysfunction in patients undergoing coronary artery bypass surgery. Anaesthesia. 2011;66(6):455–464.
148. Rortgen D, Kloos J, Fries M, et al. Comparison of early cognitive function and recovery after desflurane or sevoflurane anaesthesia in the elderly: a double-blinded randomized controlled trial. Br J Anaesth. 2010;104(2):167–174.
149. Ancelin ML, de Roquefeuil G, Scali J, et al. Long-term post-operative cognitive decline in the elderly: the effects of anesthesia type, apolipoprotein E genotype, and clinical antecedents. J Alzh Dis. 2010;22 Suppl 3:105–113.
150. Avidan MS, Searleman AC, Storandt M, et al. Long-term cognitive decline in older subjects was not attributable to noncardiac surgery or major illness. Anesthesiology. 2009;111(5):964–970.
151. Evered L, Scott DA, Silbert B, Maruff P. Postoperative cognitive dysfunction is independent of type of surgery and anesthetic. Anesth Analg. 2011;112(5):1179–1185.
152. Kawano T, Eguchi S, Iwata H, et al. Impact of preoperative environmental enrichment on prevention of development of cognitive impairment following abdominal surgery in a rat model. Anesthesiology. 2015;123(1):160–170.
153. Ballard C, Jones E, Gauge N, et al. Optimised anaesthesia to reduce post operative cognitive decline (POCD) in older patients undergoing elective surgery, a randomised controlled trial. PLoS One. 2012;7(6):e37410.
154. Hudetz JA, Iqbal Z, Gandhi SD, et al. Ketamine attenuates post-operative cognitive dysfunction after cardiac surgery. Acta Anaesthesiol Scand. 2009;53(7):864–872.
155. Wang Y, Sands LP, Vaurio L, et al. The effects of postoperative pain and its management on postoperative cognitive dysfunction. Am J Geriatr Psych. 2007;15(1):50–59.
156. Kazmierski J, Kowman M, Banach M, et al. Incidence and predictors of delirium after cardiac surgery: results from The IPDACS Study. J Psychosom Res. 2010;69(2):179–185.
157. Avidan MS, Evers AS. The fallacy of persistent postoperative cognitive decline. Anesthesiology. 2016;124(2):255–258.

35 Neuraxial Anesthesia

MARK C. NORRIS

Introduction
Indications and Contraindications
Neuraxial Anesthesia and Outcome
Anatomy
    Vertebrae
    Ligaments
    Epidural Space
    Meninges
    Cerebrospinal Fluid
    Spinal Cord
    Ultrasound Anatomy of the Spine
Technique
    Patient Preparation
    Needles
    Approach
    Technique
    Choice of Technique
    Efficiency and Neuraxial Anesthesia

Pharmacology
    Subarachnoid Anesthesia
    Epidural Anesthesia
Physiology
    Central Nervous System
    Cardiovascular System
    Respiratory System
    Gastrointestinal System
    Temperature Homeostasis
Complications
    Backache
    Headache
    Hearing Loss
    High Block/Total Subarachnoid Spinal Block
    Systemic Toxicity
    Neurologic Injury

KEY POINTS

1. A growing body of evidence suggests that spinal and epidural anesthesia are associated with less morbidity and mortality than general anesthesia. This association is strongest in patients undergoing major hip or knee surgery.
2. The epidural space is not a homogeneous, continuous cylinder surrounding the subarachnoid space. Instead, discrete pockets of epidural fat lie in the posterior and lateral epidural space. Epidural veins pass through the anterior and lateral space. Blood in an epidural needle or catheter suggests that you are not in the midline.
3. Develop a mental model of spinal anatomy that will allow you to systematically locate the spinal or epidural space.
4. The hemodynamic effects of spinal and epidural anesthesia are proportional to the extent of local anesthetic block.
5. Patient variables (age, height, weight, etc.) minimally effect the spread of intrathecal and epidural medications.
6. Unrecognized *intrathecal (subarachnoid)* injection of local anesthetics is a common cause of morbidity during epidural block. Early signs of unintended intrathecal local anesthetic injection can be subtle and easily missed. Commonly used intrathecal test doses can produce excessive levels of sensory and motor block.
7. *Intravenous* injection of local anesthetics can produce seizures and cardiac arrest. Test doses and incremental injection are key safety steps to prevent this complication.
8. Patients receiving antithrombotic or thrombolytic medications are at increased risk of developing spinal or epidural hematoma. Refer to the American Society of Regional Anesthesia and Pain Medicine Regional Guidelines for Antithrombotic and Thrombolytic Therapy for current information.

Introduction

Subarachnoid spinal and epidural anesthesia are key techniques that every anesthesiologist should master. Subarachnoid or intrathecal anesthesia is commonly referred to as spinal anesthesia. Some use the term peridural instead of epidural. Caudal block refers to injection into the caudal epidural space via the sacral hiatus. Neuraxial includes both subarachnoid and epidural injection.

Subarachnoid injection of a small dose of local anesthetic can rapidly produce dense surgical anesthesia. Subarachnoid injection is almost always done in the lumbar region, below the termination of the spinal cord. Subarachnoid anesthesia can provide excellent operating conditions for lower abdominal, pelvic, and lower extremity surgery. Most subarachnoid anesthetics are single injections and have a finite duration. Single injection subarachnoid anesthesia will last 2 to 3 hours at most. It is not a good choice for prolonged or unpredictable surgeries.

Continuous subarachnoid anesthesia with a catheter can provide extended duration block. However, continuous subarachnoid anesthesia requires a large-gauge dural puncture. Such needles can produce an unacceptably high incidence of headache, especially in younger patients (see "Complications"). Micro subarachnoid catheters, which could be inserted through a 25-gauge needle were associated with permanent neurologic injury and are no longer available. In addition, subarachnoid catheters can be mistaken for epidural catheters. Dangerous levels of block can occur if a larger epidural dose of medication is accidentally injected into a continuous subarachnoid catheter. Still, continuous subarachnoid anesthesia allows careful titration of medication, which may provide better hemodynamic stability in fragile patients. In addition, subarachnoid catheters can be redosed as needed during prolonged surgeries.

Epidural anesthesia requires larger doses of local anesthetic and takes more time to establish. However, when a catheter is in the epidural space, local anesthetic can be injected repeatedly and anesthesia can be prolonged to match the duration of the surgery. Epidural injection can safely be performed in the lumbar, thoracic, and even cervical regions. Lumbar epidural anesthesia and subarachnoid anesthesia can be used for many of the same procedures. Thoracic epidural anesthesia is a useful adjunct to general anesthesia for upper abdominal and thoracic surgeries. Cervical epidural injection is rarely used for surgery; however, it is commonly used to treat pain associated with cervical disc disease. See Chronic Pain chapter for further discussion of cervical epidural injection.

The caudal canal is the lower extension of the epidural space. Caudal anesthesia and analgesia are uncommon in adults but can be useful for pediatric surgeries.

Epidural injection of medications also can provide analgesia. Dilute mixtures of local anesthetic and opioid can provide postoperative analgesia with minimal motor block. Epidural analgesia is a key element of many enhanced recovery protocols. The flexibility of continuous epidural block makes it an excellent choice for labor pain relief. Dilute local anesthetic and opioid solutions can provide labor *analgesia* with minimal maternal motor block and negligible effects on the progress and outcome of labor. Should surgical delivery be required, the epidural catheter can be dosed with more concentrated local anesthetics to provide operative *anesthesia* (see OB anesthesia chapter).

In some settings, the anesthesiologist may combine subarachnoid and epidural injections. This approach offers the rapid onset of dense anesthesia produced by subarachnoid injection of local anesthetic and the flexibility of an epidural catheter.

Indications and Contraindications

There are no absolute indications for subarachnoid or epidural anesthesia. Their use is determined by a combination of patient, surgeon, and anesthesiologist preferences. Contraindications to neuraxial anesthesia include patient refusal, coagulopathy, hemodynamic instability, and infection at the site of injection.

Neuraxial Anesthesia and Outcome

Many investigators have compared patient outcomes associated with neuraxial and general anesthesia. Small randomized controlled trials examining major morbidity and mortality after high-risk and vascular surgeries yielded conflicting results.[1,2] By 2012, 40 studies including over 3,000 patients were available for meta-analysis.[3] Subarachnoid and epidural anesthesia were associated with a lower risk of death within 30 days of surgery (risk ratio [RR] 0.71). Neuraxial anesthesia also reduced the risk of postoperative pneumonia (RR 0.45), but not the risk of myocardial infarction (RR 1.17). Interestingly, adding neuraxial anesthesia to general anesthesia did not reduce the risk of death or myocardial infarction compared to general anesthesia alone. However, the combination of neuraxial and general anesthesia was associated with a reduced risk of postoperative pneumonia (RR 0.69).

Large, multi-institutional databases allow robust comparisons of neuraxial and general anesthesia. In more than 18,000 patients undergoing hip fracture surgery, neuraxial anesthesia was associated with a decreased risk of in-hospital death and pulmonary complications.[4] However, the same authors reported a follow-up study of more than 50,000 patients and did not find any decreased mortality after neuraxial anesthesia.[5] In contrast, neuraxial anesthesia was associated with lower 30-day mortality and fewer prolonged hospital stays in nearly 400,000 patients undergoing hip or knee replacement.[6]

Neuraxial anesthesia also may improve outcomes in some subgroups of patients. A small retrospective review from a single institution found fewer postoperative pulmonary complications and arrhythmias as well as shorter intensive care unit stays among patients receiving regional instead of general anesthesia for lower extremity amputation.[7] A review of more than 5,000 patients with chronic obstructive pulmonary disease (COPD) found that regional anesthesia (subarachnoid, epidural, or peripheral nerve block) was associated with fewer adverse respiratory events (postoperative pneumonia, prolonged ventilator dependence, and unplanned postoperative intubation) than general anesthesia.[8] There were fewer wound infections, blood transfusions, pneumonias, and total infections associated with neuraxial versus general anesthesia among more than 14,000 patients undergoing total knee arthroplasty.[9] Hospital length of stay was also shorter in the neuraxial anesthesia patients.[10] In contrast, a different review of more than 7,000 hip fracture patients found no anesthesia-related differences in mortality but an *increased* risk of superficial wound infection and urinary tract infection among patients receiving subarachnoid anesthesia.[11]

Some investigators have reported a lower risk of thromboembolism in patients receiving neuraxial anesthesia.[12] However, not all studies have confirmed this benefit.[6] There are insufficient data to determine if regional anesthesia improves outcomes for patients undergoing major vascular surgery.[13] One retrospective study of 822 patients found that regional anesthesia does *not* improve graft patency after lower extremity revascularization.[14]

An intriguing advantage of epidural anesthesia and analgesia might be improved survival after cancer surgery. Regional anesthesia and analgesia avoid the immunosuppression associated with general anesthesia and postoperative opioid analgesia. In a recent meta-analysis, epidural anesthesia and analgesia was associated with longer survival but no difference in cancer recurrence after surgery.[15]

Anatomy

Subarachnoid and epidural anesthesia are exercises in applied anatomy. The anesthesiologist must have a thorough grasp of the relationships between surface landmarks and deeper structures. Text and two-dimensional images are a useful, but imperfect, way to learn vertebral anatomy. Careful examination of skeletal models can help. Recently, investigators have used high-resolution magnetic resonance images to construct interactive virtual three-dimensional models of bony, ligamentous, and nervous structures of the spine (http://hdl.handle.net/2445/44844).[16]

Vertebrae

The spine is comprised of 33 vertebrae: 7 cervical, 12 thoracic, 5 lumbar, 5 fused sacral, and 4 fused coccygeal. All vertebrae have the same structural components but with varying shapes and sizes at different levels. The vertebrae surround and protect the vertebral canal, which contains the spinal cord, cerebrospinal fluid (CSF), meninges, spinal nerves, and epidural space. Each vertebra has a body anteriorly, two pedicles that project posteriorly from the body, and laminae that connect the two pedicles (Fig. 35-1). The transverse processes arise laterally from the junction of the pedicle and lamina, and the spinous process projects posteriorly from the union of the bilateral laminae. The paraspinous muscles and ligaments attach to these bony projections.

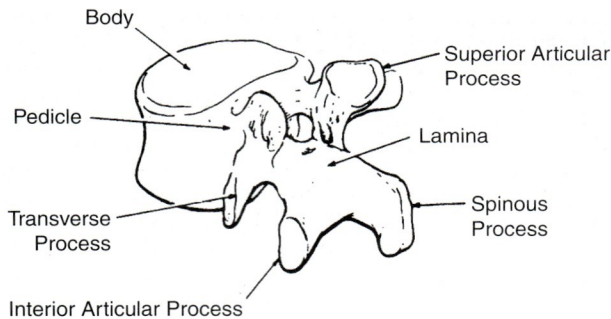

Figure 35-1 The vertebral body. (From Norris MC, ed. *Obstetric Anesthesia*. 2nd ed. Philadelphia: Lippincott Williams & Wilkins; 1999:286.)

The pedicles form the superior and inferior vertebral notches, through which the spinal nerves exit the vertebral canal. The lamina and pedicles meet at the superior and inferior articular processes, which form the joints that connect the adjacent vertebrae. The first and second cervical vertebrae, also referred to as the atlas and dens, have a unique appearance in that C1 lacks a vertebral body or spinous process and C2 has a large articulating process (dens).

Five fused vertebrae form the sacrum. In 0.9% to 6.4% of the population, sacralization (fusion of the L5 and S1 vertebrae) occurs.[17] Up to 60% of those with this variation have only unilateral fusion, known as hemisacralization.[17] The fifth sacral vertebra does not fuse posteriorly, forming the sacral hiatus, which provides access to the most caudal point of the epidural space. The sacral hiatus is usually open in children but its patency varies in adults. The four coccygeal vertebrae fuse to form the coccyx, which represents a vestigial tail and serves as an anchor for the attachment of tendons, ligaments, and muscles.

In surgical and obstetric patients, neuraxial block is usually accomplished without the aid of imaging. Attaining the desired level for neuraxial block and avoiding complications requires familiarity with surface landmarks. Commonly identified landmarks include the C7 spinous process (vertebra prominens), the twelfth rib, and the iliac crests. Many anesthesiologists use the line between the iliac crests (Tuffier line) to identify the L4–L5 interspace. However, this landmark commonly misleads even experienced anesthesiologists.[18] When possible, locating the L5–S1 interspace and counting up is a more reliable way to identify a specific lumbar interspace. In obese patient, a midline skin crease and the gluteal cleft can help local the midline.

Ligaments

Several ligaments serve to stabilize the vertebral column. The anterior and posterior longitudinal ligaments link the ventral surfaces of the vertebral bodies. Dorsally, the supraspinous and interspinous ligaments, as well as the dense ligamentum flavum, connect the vertebrae. The supraspinous ligament covers the tips of the spinous processes between C7 and the sacrum; from C7 to the external occipital protuberance it continues as the ligamentum nuchae. The supraspinous ligament thins in the lower lumbar region, allowing greater flexion of the spine. The intraspinous ligament runs between spinous processes. It may contain slit-like, fat-filled cavities that can create a false loss of resistance during attempts to identify the epidural space. The intraspinous ligament merges with both supraspinous ligament and ligamentum flavum. The ligamentum flavum (yellow ligament) is a pair of dense trapezoid-shaped structures made mostly of elastin. The two ligaments fuse in the midline at an 80- to 90-degree angle. This fusion is often incomplete. Lumbar midline gaps occur in approximately 10% of patients (Fig. 35-2).[19] When attempting to locate the epidural space, try to appreciate the "snap" of the supraspinous ligament, the "mushy" intraspinous ligament, and the "gritty" ligamentum flavum.

Epidural Space

The epidural space lies within the vertebral canal but outside the dural sac. It extends from the foramen magnum to the sacral hiatus. The epidural space is bound anteriorly by the posterior longitudinal ligament and posteriorly by the lamina and ligamentum flavum. Laterally the epidural space extends to the pedicles where it communicates with the paravertebral space via the intervertebral foramina.[20] The epidural space is often absent because the dural intermittently abuts the bony and ligamentous structures of the spine. The remainder of the space consists of discontinuous, fat-filled pockets that open readily upon injection of air or liquid.[20] The cervical level contains no epidural fat. In the lumbar region, fat in the anterior and posterior aspects of the epidural space forms multiple, metameric, discrete collections (Fig. 35-3).[20,21] This fat may play an important role in the kinetics of epidural medications.[22]

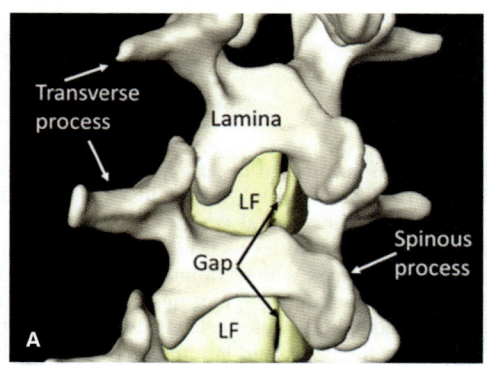
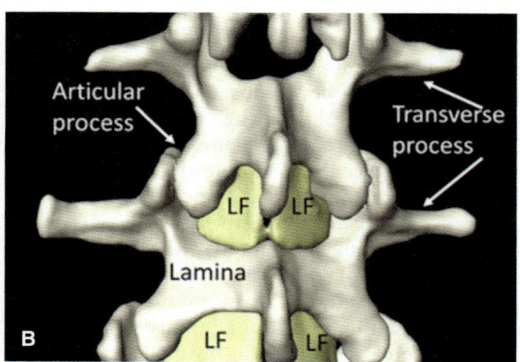

Figure 35-2 Three-dimensional reconstruction of human lumbar ligamentum flavum (LF). **A:** Posterior-lateral view. **B:** Posterior view. Note the gap (*arrow*) between the two halves of the ligamentum flavum. (Adapted from Reina MA, Lirk P, Puigdellívol-Sánchez A, et al. Human lumbar ligamentum flavum anatomy for epidural anesthesia: reviewing a 3D MR-based interactive model and postmortem samples. *Anesth Analg.* 2016;122:903–907. ©2016 International Anesthesia Research Society.)

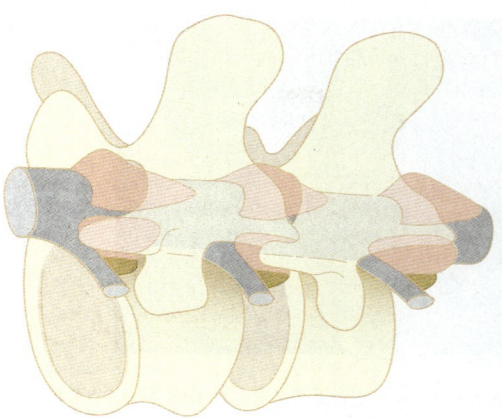

Figure 35-3 The compartments of the epidural space (*grey*) are discontinuous. Areas in between are a potential space where the dural mater normally abuts the sides of the vertebral canal. (Adapted from Hogan Q. Lumbar epidural anatomy: a new look by cryomicrotome section. *Anesthesiology*. 1991;75:767–775.)

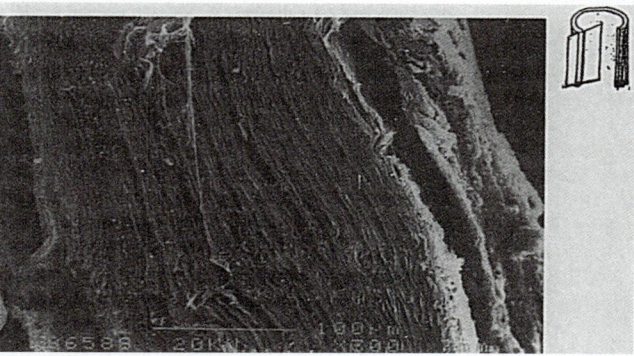

Figure 35-5 Scanning electron microscopic image of a radial longitudinal section of human dura mater. Total thickness is a composite of all concentric layers. (Adapted from Reina MA, Dittmann M, Lopez Garcia A, et al. New perspectives in the microscopic structure of human dura mater in the dorsolumbar region. *Reg Anesth*. 1997;22:161–168.)

Epidural veins are located mostly in the anterior epidural space. The intervertebral foramina allow transmission of intra-abdominal pressure into the epidural space. Conditions that increase intra-abdominal pressure (i.e., pregnancy) can cause engorgement of epidural veins, leading to more frequent venous cannulation and possibly enhancing the spread of injected medications.

Meninges

The meninges surround and protect the spinal cord, cerebral spinal fluid (CSF), and nerve roots until they exit the foramina. The dura, arachnoid, and pia mater form three structurally distinct meningeal layers (Fig. 35-4).

Dura

The dura mater (hard mother) is the thickest, outermost meningeal layer. It is 270 to 280 μm thick and consists mostly of collagen fibers arranged in about 80 layers of very fine lamellae (Fig. 35-5). The external (epidural surface) contains bands of collagen fibers running in different directions. The dura also contains thick elastic fibers and fine granular material. The inner (subarachnoid) surface includes fine fibers that fuse with the arachnoid mater.[23] A potential subdural space exists between the dura and arachnoid mater. Drugs, needles, or catheters intended for the epidural or subarachnoid spaces rarely may end up there (Fig. 35-6).

The dura is a continuation of the spinal meninges, extending from the foramen magnum to approximately S2, where it fuses with the filum terminale. It extends laterally with individual nerve roots and fuses with the epineurium near the intervertebral foramina.

Arachnoid

The arachnoid mater (spider mother) lies within the dura. It has two portions. A compact laminar layer of flattened epithelial-like

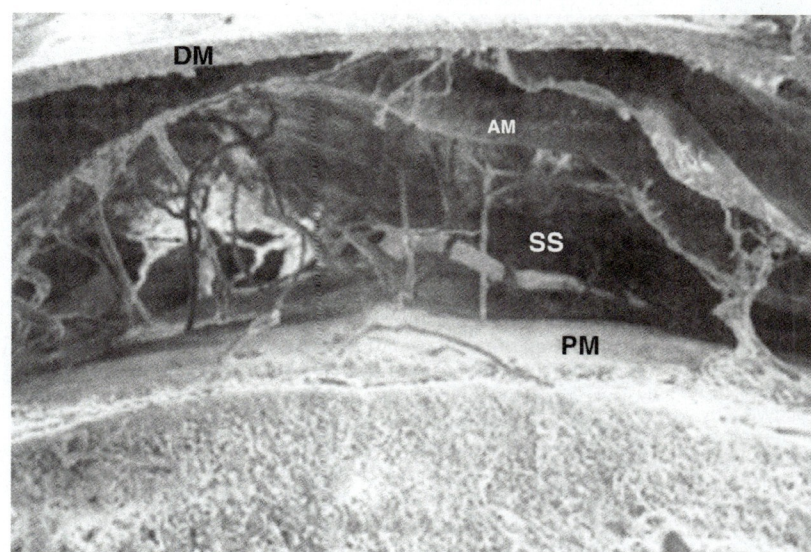

Figure 35-4 The spinal meninges of a dog, showing the pia mater (PM) in apposition to the spinal cord, the subarachnoid space (SS), the arachnoid mater (AM) with trabeculae stretching from the arachnoid mater to the pia mater, and the dura mater (DM). The separation between the arachnoid mater and the dural mater is the subdural space, which was created here as an artifact of preparation. (Adapted from Peters A, Palay SL, Webster H, eds. *The Fine Structure of the Nervous System: The Neurons and Supporting Cells*. Philadelphia, PA: WB Saunders; 1976.)

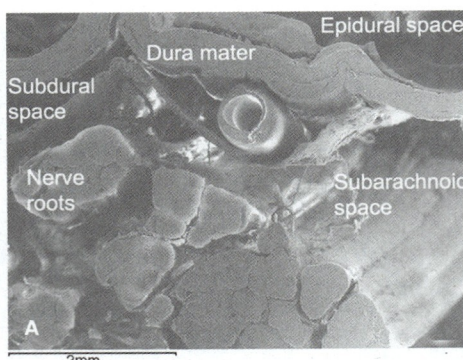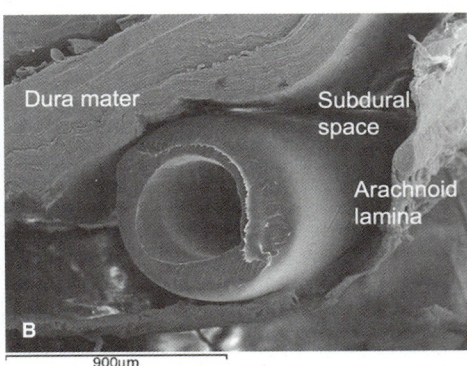

Figure 35-6 Human spinal dural sac. **A:** Enhanced view (×20) of an epidural catheter inside a subdural space. **B:** Detail (×60) of **A**. Sample was obtained from a cadaver under scanning electron microscopy. (Adapted from Reina MA, Collier CB, Prats-Galino A, et al. Unintentional subdural placement of epidural catheters during attempted epidural anesthesia: an anatomic study of spinal subdural compartment. *Reg Anesth Pain Med*. 2011;36:537–541.)

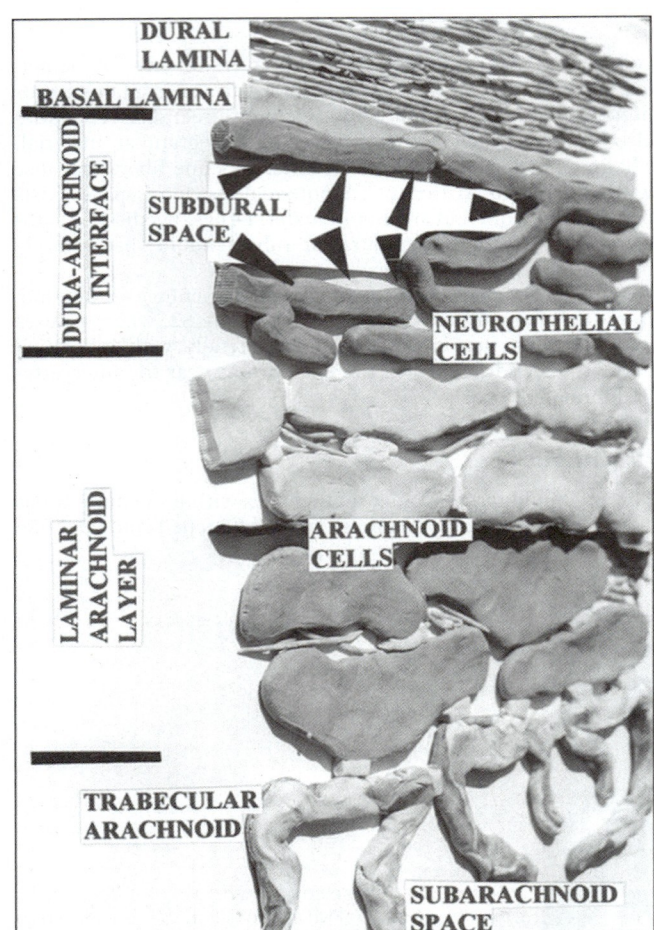

Figure 35-7 Dura–arachnoid interface model. From the top: the dural lamina (dura mater's most internal portion) is followed by the dura–arachnoid interface; the interface is filled with neurothelial cells, and forms the subdural space. Below are the laminar and trabecular portions of the arachnoid mater. (Adapted from Reina MA, De Leon Casasola O, Lopez A, et al. The origin of the spinal subdural space: ultrastructure findings. *Anesth Analg*. 2002;94: 991–995.)

cells that are tightly connected to one another covers the inner surface of the dura. Then, a trabecular web-like portion extends to the pia mater (Fig. 35-7).[24] Because of this cellular architecture, the arachnoid, not the dura, hinders drug movement through meninges. The low permeability of the arachnoid mater keeps the CSF in the subarachnoid, not the subdural space.[25] Specialized intercellular junctions within the internal portion of the arachnoid mater explain its selective permeability.[26]

The spinal nerve roots traverse the dura and arachnoid membranes as they exit the vertebral foramina. Here, the arachnoid mater herniates through the dura and forms arachnoid granulations. These granulations provide an exit for material leaving the central nervous system.

Pia

The innermost layer of the spinal meninges is the pia mater (soft mother). The pia consists of flat overlapping cells that coat the spinal cord and nerve roots. The pial cells contain numerous fenestrations along the lumbar spinal cord and nerve roots (Fig. 35-8). Any role these fenestrations might play in the action of subarachnoid or epidural medications is speculative.[27]

Cerebrospinal Fluid

CSF is an aqueous solution consisting of 99% water. Multiple minor components include protein, glucose, electrolytes, and neurotransmitters. In adult humans, the volume of CSF is 100 to 160 mL. For many years, we thought that CSF was primarily produced in the choroid plexus and then flowed from the ventricles to the subarachnoid space, where it was absorbed by arachnoid granulations. This hypothesis is incomplete and probably incorrect. The choroid plexus is not the sole site of CSF production and the arachnoid granulations are not its primary absorption sites. CSF and interstitial fluid (IF) are closely related. They are both mainly produced and absorbed in the parenchymal capillaries of the brain and spinal cord. The lymphatic system also absorbs a considerable amount of CSF and IF.[28] CSF movement is not unidirectional flow. Instead, transmitted cardiac oscillations produce local mixing, whereas other drugs spread slowly by diffusion. Solutes are reabsorbed across capillary membranes into the bloodstream.[29]

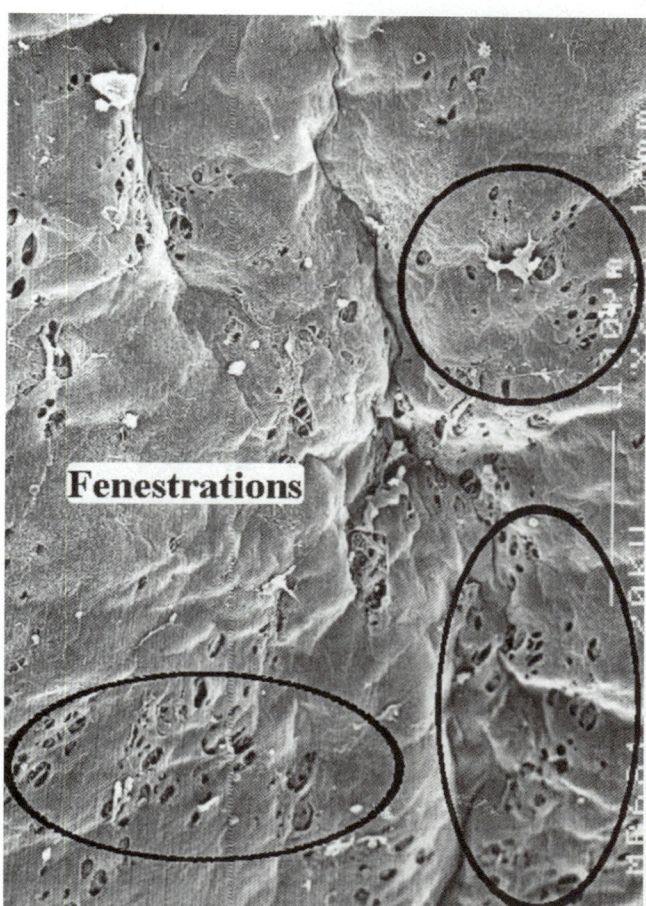

Figure 35-8 Fenestrations in the pial cellular layer at the level of the spinal cord. Numerous fenestrations appear in this scanning electron micrograph. (Adapted from Reina MA, De Leon Casasola O, Villanueva MC, et al. Ultrastructural findings in human spinal pia mater in relation to subarachnoid anesthesia. *Anesth Analg.* 2004;98:1479–1485.)

Spinal Cord

In the first trimester fetus, the spinal cord extends to the end of the sacrum. The vertebral column grows faster than the spinal cord and at birth the cord usually ends at the level of the third lumbar vertebra. In adults, the cord most often ends at around L1. However, there is considerable interindividual variation. The cord ends at T12 in some but may extend to L3 in up to 10% of adults.

There are 31 pairs of spinal nerves, each with an anterior motor root and a posterior sensory root. These nerve roots arise from individual spinal cord segments. Each posterior sensory root innervates a specific dermatome (Fig. 35-9). The sympathetic nervous system arises from the intermediolateral grey matter of the T1 to L2 spinal cord segments. This grey matter contains the cell bodies of the preganglionic sympathetic neurons, which travel with the corresponding spinal nerve through the intervertebral foramen. They then diverge and join the sympathetic chain ganglia.

The spinal nerves and their corresponding dermatomes are named for the foramina through which they exit the vertebral column. In the cervical region, spinal nerves are named after the lower vertebrae (i.e., C5 exits between C4 and C5). Elsewhere, the roots are named by the upper vertebrae (L2 emerges between L2 and L3). Since the vertebral column is longer than the spinal cord, the thoracic, lumbar, and sacral nerve roots traverse progressively greater distances from their originating spinal cord segment to their exiting foramina. The lumbar and sacral spinal nerves that extend beyond the tip of the cord are called the cauda equina. These nerve roots, covered only by pia mater, may be more susceptible to chemical injury than more proximal roots.

In one study examining magnetic resonance images of seven adults, the dural sac volume from S1 to T12 was 43 mL. The average CSF volume was 34 mL. The remaining 9 to 10 mL consisted of conus medullaris and nerve roots. The percentage of nerve volume to dural sac volume increased from 7% to 14% at L5, to 25% at L4, to 30% to 43% at T12. Not only do upper lumbar punctures risk contact with the conus medullaris, but the cauda equina also is vulnerable to contact with lower punctures.[30]

Ultrasound Anatomy of the Spine

There has been increasing interest in using ultrasound to complement clinical examination when performing neuraxial blocks. Ultrasound examination of the lumbar spine can establish the depth of the epidural space, identify the intervertebral level, and locate the midline and interspinous/interlaminar spaces. This information can help guide subsequent needle insertion. Systematic reviews suggest that ultrasound increases the success and reduces the technical difficulty of lumbar neuraxial blocks. Ultrasound may reduce the risk of traumatic procedures, and may contribute to the safety of lumbar neuraxial blocks.[31]

Although real-time, ultrasound-guided approaches have been described,[32] most experts use ultrasound before attempted neuraxial block to locate landmarks. Once mastered, a preprocedure ultrasound examination can quickly identify the exact lumbar interspace, the midline, the skin puncture point, the angle of needle insertion, and the depth of the epidural space.[33]

The basic ultrasound examination of the lumbar spine consists of two scans: a paramedian longitudinal scan and a transverse or axial scan. The paramedian longitudinal approach can identify specific interspace levels by scanning through interlaminar windows. Place the transducer longitudinally along the spine, parallel to it, 2 to 3 cm lateral to the midline, and directed toward the center of the spinal canal. Multiple vertebral levels can be seen in one scanned image. The structures seen in this view include sacrum, lamina, ligamentum flavum, and dorsal dura mater (Fig. 35-10).[33] The ligamentum flavum and dorsal dura mater appear as a single bright line in the interlaminar window. A deeper bright reflection emanates from the ventral dura/posterior longitudinal ligament/vertebral body complex. Once the desired puncture level is identified in the paramedian longitudinal plane, turn the transducer perpendicular to the axis of the spine to view the entire interspace. The structures that can be seen in the axial plane include the ligamentum flavum and dorsal dura mater, the ventral dura/posterior longitudinal ligament/vertebral body complex, the articular processes, and the transverse processes (Fig. 35-11).[33]

After acquiring the best image of interspace structure and ligamentum flavum/dura, center the target interspace on the screen of the ultrasound machine. Then, holding the probe steady, mark the skin at the midline of both the vertical and horizontal edges of the probe. Remove the probe and connect the marks to make a cross. With a transverse probe, this cross will identify a midline puncture site (Fig. 35-12). With a longitudinal probe, the cross identifies a paramedian insertion site. By freezing the image on the ultrasound machine, one can also measure the depth of the ligamentum flavum/dura and estimate the best angle for needle insertion.[33]

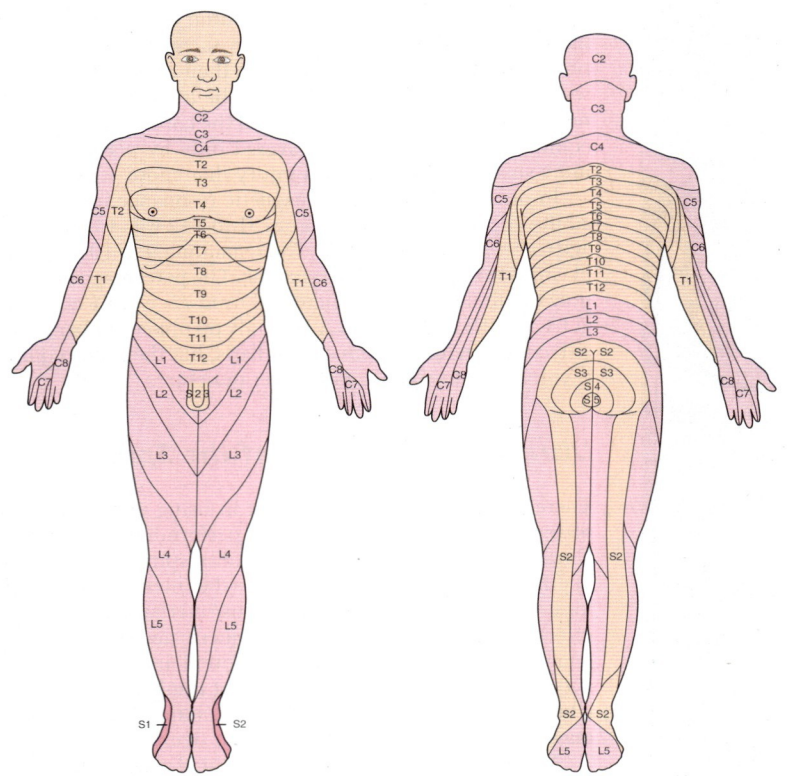

Figure 35-9 Human sensory dermatomes.

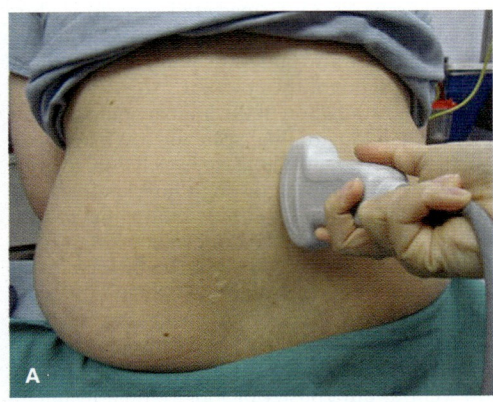
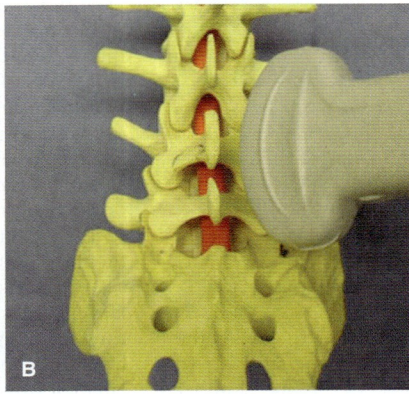
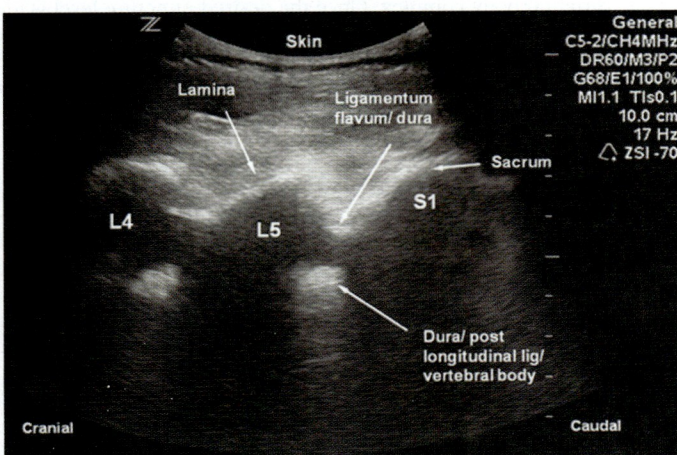

Figure 35-10 A: Scanning in the paramedian longitudinal plane. **B:** Probe oriented parallel to the axis of spine model. **C:** Ultrasound image with a typical saw-tooth sign: hyperechoic flat band on the right represents sacrum, saw-teeth indicate lamina, and the two parallel bands between saw-teeth correspond to the interspace containing the ligamentum flavum–dorsal dura unit (*upper*) and the ventral dura posterior longitudinal ligament–vertebral body complex (*lower*). (Adapted from Balki M. Locating the epidural space in obstetric patients—ultrasound a useful tool: continuing professional development. *Can J Anesth.* 2010;57:1111–1126.)

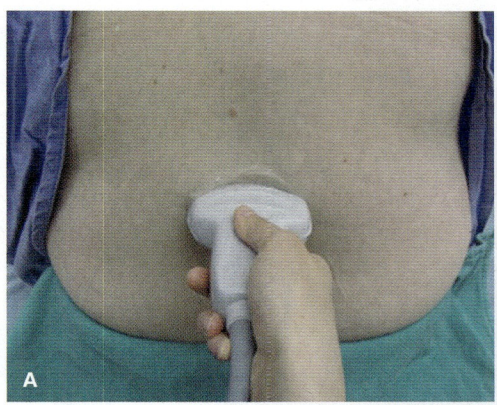
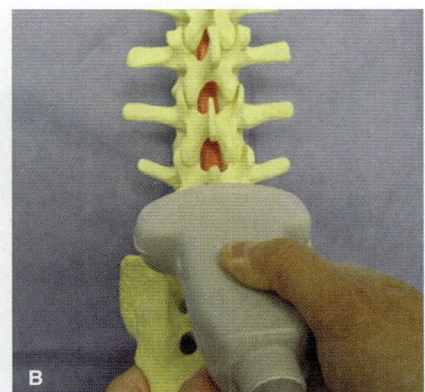
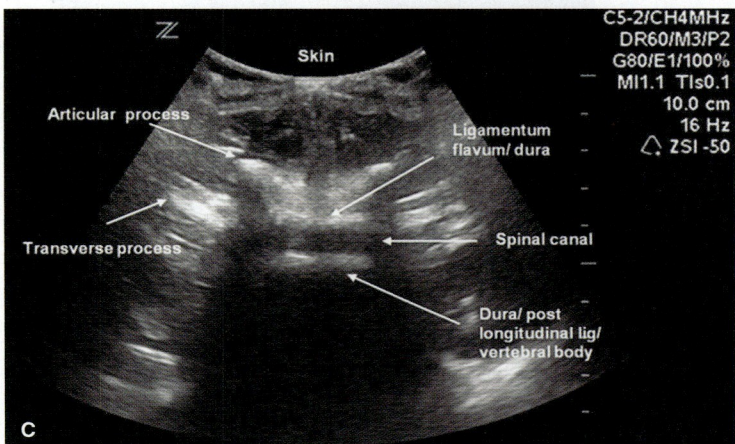

Figure 35-11 **A:** Scanning in the transverse plane. **B:** Probe oriented perpendicular to the axis of spine model. **C:** Typical sonogram of a lumbar interspace: midline hyperechoic structures represent the ligamentum flavum–dorsal dura unit (*upper*) and the ventral dura posterior longitudinal ligament–vertebral body complex (*lower*); bilateral symmetrical hyperechoic structures indicate articular and transverse processes with their acoustic shadows. (Adapted from Balki M. Locating the epidural space in obstetric patients—ultrasound a useful tool: continuing professional development. *Can J Anesth.* 2010;57:1111–1126.)

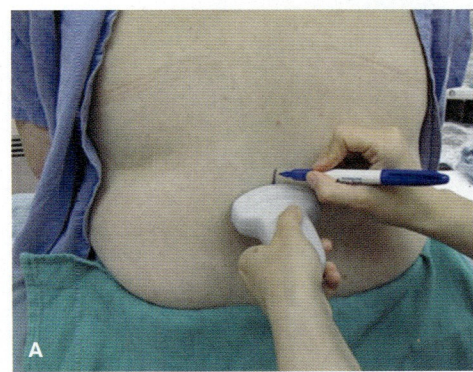
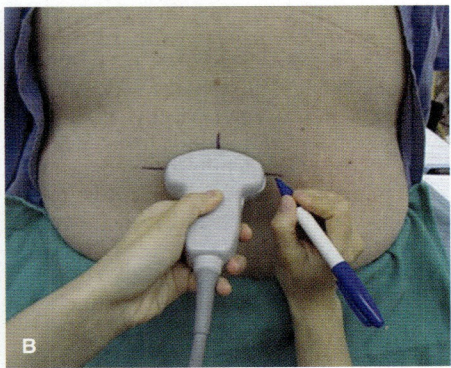
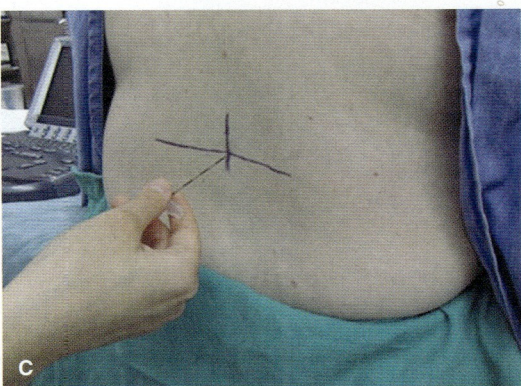

Figure 35-12 Marking skin insertion point in the transverse plane. **A:** Vertical line marking the midline. **B:** Horizontal line marking the interspace. **C:** Skin insertion point at the intersection of these lines. (Adapted from Balki M. Locating the epidural space in obstetric patients—ultrasound a useful tool: continuing professional development. *Can J Anesth.* 2010;57:1111–1126.)

Technique

Patient Preparation

Equipment

Before inducing subarachnoid or epidural anesthesia, assemble all of the equipment you might need. This list includes both the supplies needed to perform the block and the emergency equipment required to treat rare, but potentially catastrophic complications. Always monitor at least blood pressure and pulse oximetry. Subarachnoid anesthesia is usually induced in an operating room or nearby procedure room. The needed supplies and equipment should be readily available. Epidural anesthesia can be induced in a labor room or in the preoperative holding area. A dedicated cart can hold the needed supplies (Table 35-1).

Positioning

Most patients will either sit or lie on one side during induction of neuraxial anesthesia. Inserting a spinal needle with the patient in the prone jackknife position has been described, but is rarely used in contemporary practice. Still, a recent report describes a real-time ultrasound-guided approach to the L5–S1 interspace in prone patients.[32] The choice between sitting and lateral position depends on the provider, the patient, and the procedure. Many providers prefer the sitting position.[34] Thin patients (BMI <25) report being more comfortable in the lateral position. Obese patients (BMI >30) may prefer sitting.[35] Some clinical situations dictate the lateral position (i.e., hip fractures, labor analgesia in rapidly progressing patients, and certain emergency cesarean sections). You should be comfortable inserting spinal and epidural needles with patients in either position so you can choose the most suitable approach for each patient and procedure.

When sitting, place the patient squarely on the operating table with back and buttocks at the near edge. Have the patient relax his shoulders and curl to flex the lumbar spine (Fig. 35-13). Tilting the operating table may help flex the patient's hips and lumbar spine, further opening the lumbar interspaces (Fig. 35-14).[36] Having obese patients, and those with poorly palpable landmarks, sitting can make it easier to identify the subarachnoid or epidural space. When positioned properly, a line from the C7 vertebral prominence to the gluteal cleft identifies the midline.

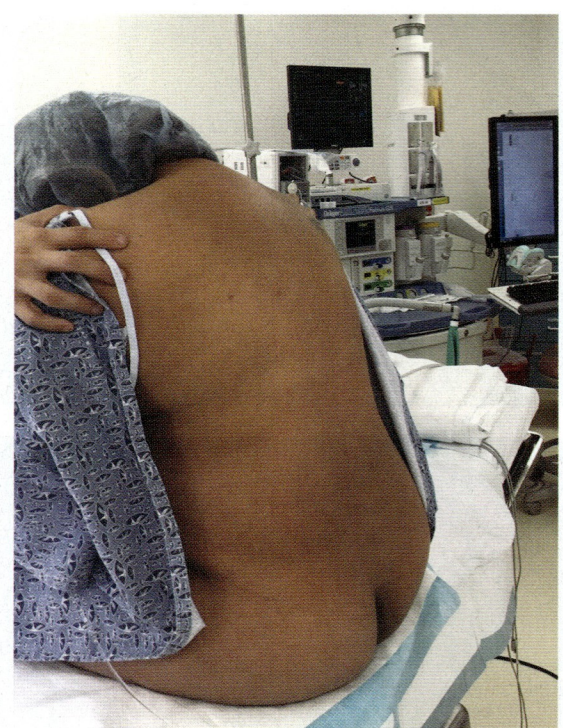

Figure 35-13 Sitting position for neuraxial block. Position the patient squarely on the bed or operating table with the buttocks at the edge near the operator. The patient's legs can be supported by the table, a stool, or (in Labor and Delivery) flexed on the bed. An assistant should provide support. Instruct the patient to relax their shoulders and flex their lumbar spine. ("Arch your back like a rainbow.")

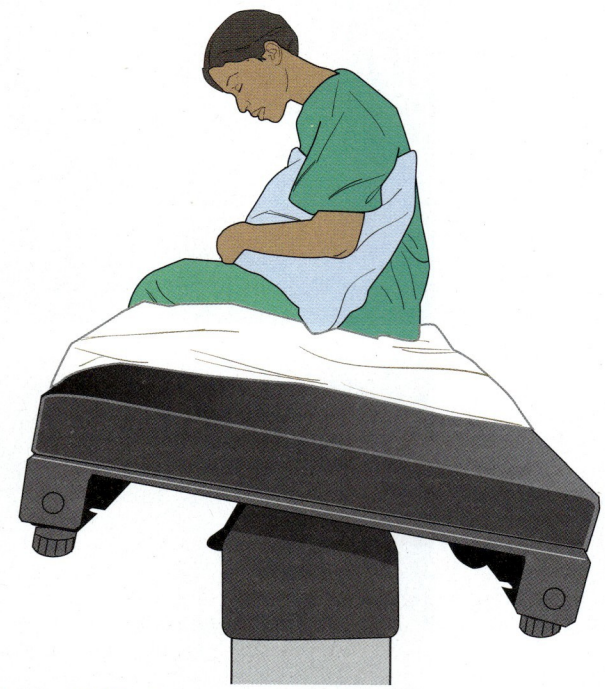

Figure 35-14 Tilting the operating table can encourage the patient to flex her hips and lumbar spine.

Table 35-1 Suggested Contents for an Epidural Cart

Epidural Supplies
- Epidural trays
- Sterile gloves
- Sterile prep sticks
- Extra epidural needles/catheters
- Extra loss of resistance syringes
- Sterile dressings
- Tape

Emergency Equipment
- Self-inflating bag–valve mask
- Oral airways
- Working laryngoscope and blade
- Endotracheal tubes/supraglottic airways
- 20% lipid emulsion

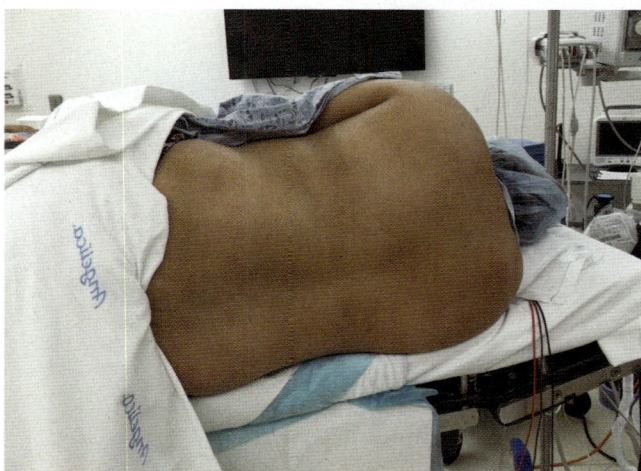

Figure 35-15 Lateral position for neuraxial block. The patient's hips and shoulders are even with the edge of the bed. The head and neck are supported to remain even with the spine.

When using the lateral position, bring the patient's back to the edge of the table. Position the hips and shoulders perpendicular to the bed (Fig. 35-15). Place a pillow under the patient's head. An assistant can help the patient bend her knees and hips and flex her lumbar spine. The site of surgery and baricity of the local anesthetic will determine the choice of side. With hyperbaric drug, position the operative side down. With isobaric/hypobaric drug, put the operative side up. When inducing subarachnoid anesthesia for cesarean section using either hyperbaric or isobaric drug, place the patient on her *right* side, then turn supine, and provide *left* uterine displacement.[37]

In either position, keep in mind patient comfort. Use blankets and pillows to make sure the patient is warm, comfortable, and appropriately covered. Light sedation with midazolam or fentanyl may sometimes be appropriate. Patients with painful fractures may need deeper sedation to allow appropriate positioning. Here, use small doses of ketamine or propofol. Although skilled pediatric anesthesiologists have a good record of safely inducing neuraxial anesthesia after induction of general anesthesia in children,[38] this approach does not seem prudent in adults.[39,40]

Skin Preparation

Pay close attention to aseptic technique. The American Society of Anesthesiologists (ASA) recommends removing jewelry (e.g., rings and watches), hand washing, sterile gloves, caps, and masks.[41] Use individual antiseptic packets to cleanse the skin. (Previously opened, multiple-use bottles of povidone–iodine can be contaminated).[42] Both chlorhexidine with alcohol and povidone–iodine with alcohol provide effective skin decontamination.[43]

Needles

Spinal and epidural needles are categorized by the design of their tips (Fig. 35-16). Spinal needles may have a beveled, cutting tip or a pencil-point, noncutting tip. Pencil-point needles produce fewer postdural puncture headaches (PDPHs) than cutting tip needles. Most anesthesiologists use thin (≤24-gauge) needles to limit the risk of headache. A shorter introducer needle helps puncture the skin and guide the flimsier spinal needle toward the subarachnoid space.

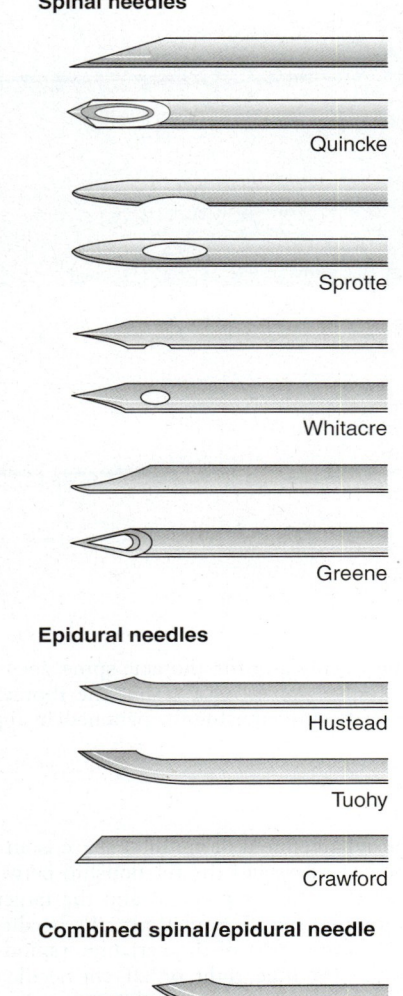

Figure 35-16 Some spinal and epidural needles. Needles are distinguished by their tip designs.

Epidural needles are usually larger than spinal needles (Fig. 35-16). This larger diameter improves the tactile feel as the needle advances through the ligamentum flavum and into the epidural space. In addition, an 18-gauge needle will allow passage of a 20-gauge catheter. Epidural needles usually have a curved tip to help guide the catheter in the epidural space. Curved tip epidural needles, as well as the straight-tipped Crawford needle, also can be used for caudal block.

Combined subarachnoid epidural block can be performed sequentially with regular needles or as a needle-through-needle technique. The needle-through-needle technique can be done most simply with an extra long spinal needle and a regular epidural needle (Fig. 35-17). Here, the spinal needle should protrude at least 1.5 cm beyond the tip of the epidural needle. Specialized needle-through-needle, or needle-beside-needle combinations are also available (Fig. 35-16).

Approach

Lumbar neuraxial block can be performed with either a midline or paramedian approach (Fig. 35-18). The thoracic spinous

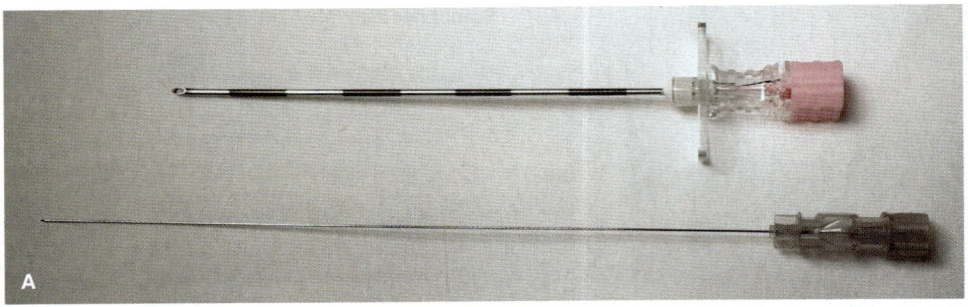

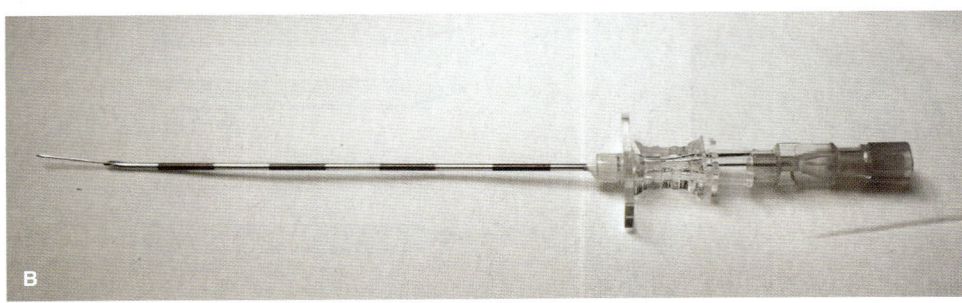

Figure 35-17 Combined spinal epidural using standard needles. **A:** An 18-gauge, 90-mm Tuohy needle and 27-gauge, 127-mm Whitacre needle side by side. **B:** Whitacre needle inserted through Tuohy needle.

processes slope steeply and the thoracic spine does not flex as much as the lumbar spine. As a result, the thoracic epidural space is more easily entered using the paramedian approach.

Technique

3 Identifying the subarachnoid or epidural space is an exercise in applied anatomy. Understand the relationship between surface landmarks (i.e., the spinous process) and the target (the subarachnoid or epidural space). Sometimes, the needle will strike bone. Recognize which part of the vertebrae (spinous process, lamina) and where (midline, right, or left) the needle is touching and make an informed choice to redirect the needle toward the target (Fig. 35-19).

2 The midline approach is the most straightforward. After positioning the patient, identify the midline by palpating the spinous processes. In obese patients, estimate the midline by imagining a line between the C7 prominence and the intergluteal cleft. Insert the needle in the middle to upper part of the desired interspace. In patients with poor landmarks, insert the needle in the presumed midline and explore. If the needle strikes bone, assess your location (spinous process: intermediate or shallow depth; lamina: deeper) and adjust your approach accordingly.

The paramedian approach requires some applied geometry. The insertion site is approximately 1 cm lateral to the superior edge of the inferior spinous process (Fig. 35-18). Angle the needle slightly cephalad and slightly medial, aiming for the midline at the estimated depth of the epidural or subarachnoid space. A bony obstruction at the estimated depth of the subarachnoid or epidural space is usually lamina. Most often, the needle strikes the upper edge of the lateral, lower lamina. Gradually walk the needle cephalad until you enter the epidural or subarachnoid space. When attempting thoracic epidural needle placement, many experts intentionally contact the lamina of the vertebral body below the target interspace. This contact provides an estimation of the depth of the epidural space. The epidural needle can then be walked up the lamina and into the desired epidural space (Fig. 35-20).

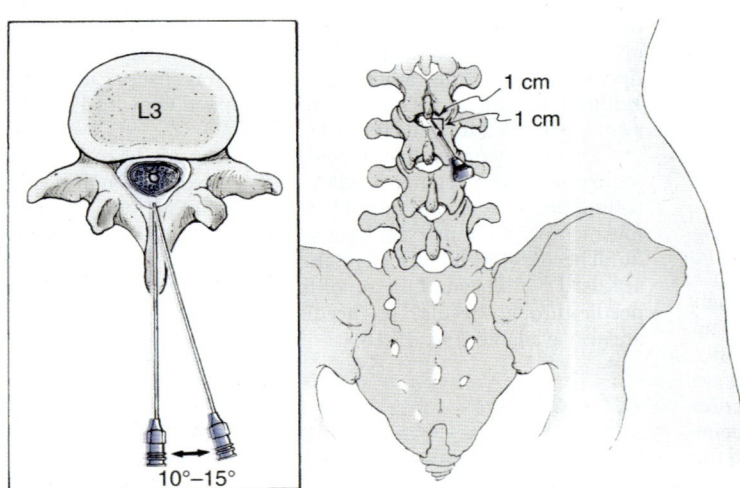

Figure 35-18 Vertebral anatomy of the lumbar midline and paramedian approaches. The midline approach requires anatomic projection in only two planes: sagittal and horizontal. The paramedian approach adds the oblique plane. The paramedian approach requires less lumbar flexion. The paramedian needle insertion site is 1 cm lateral and slightly below the cephalad edge of the more caudal spinous process. The needle is inserted 10 to 15 degrees off both sagittal and horizontal planes (inset). (Adapted from Chestnut DH, Wong CA, Tsen LC, et al., eds. *Chestnut's Obstetric Anesthesia: Principals and Practice.* 5th Ed. Philadelphia, PA: WB Saunders; 2014:239.)

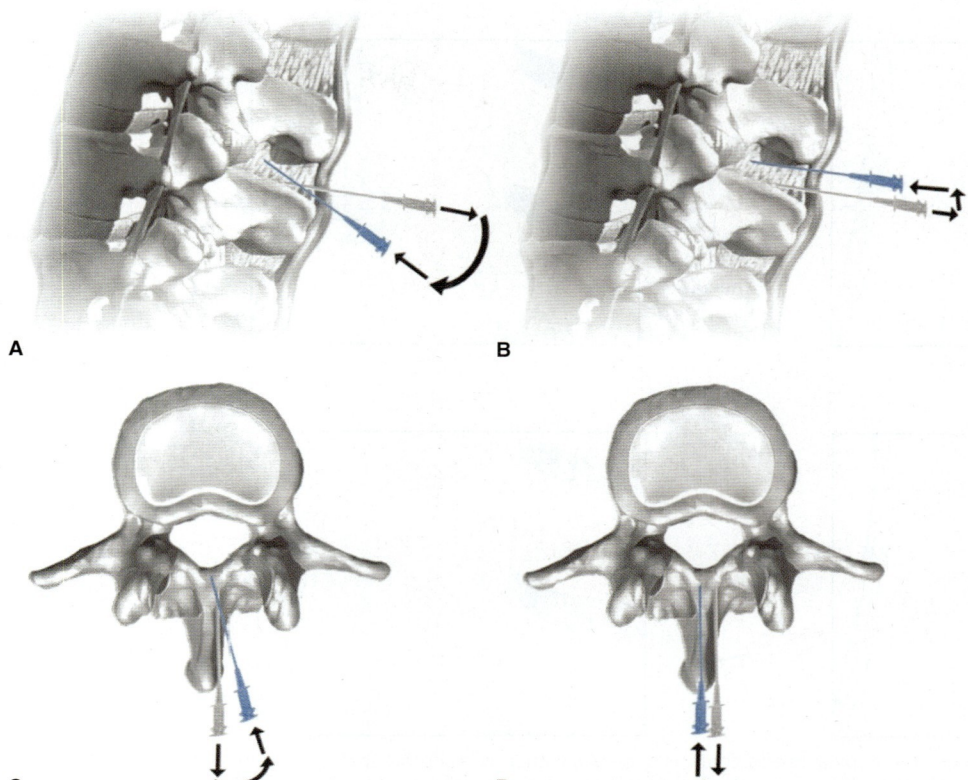

Figure 35-19 Troubleshooting contact with bones. The *gray* needle is the initial approach; the *blue* needle is the adjusted approach. **A:** If the needle is midline, redirect slightly more cephalad. **B:** Or, lift the needle after withdrawing into the subcutaneous tissues. **C:** If the needle is off midline and contacting lamina, redirect as in **A**. **D:** Or, withdraw the needle into the subcutaneous tissue and shift as in **B**. (Adapted from Chestnut DH, Wong CA, Tsen LC, et al. eds. *Chestnut's Obstetric Anesthesia: Principals and Practice*. 5th Ed. Philadelphia: WB Saunders; 2014:239.)

Subarachnoid Spinal Anesthesia

After positioning the patient, preparing the skin, and applying a sterile drape, infiltrate the skin with a small amount of local anesthetic. A single pass with a finder needle may help identify

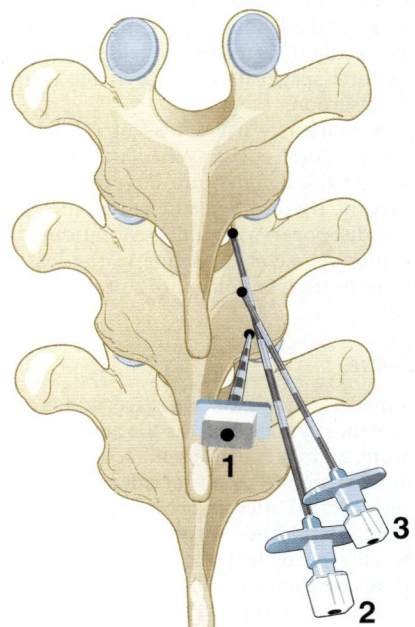

Figure 35-20 Thoracic epidural insertion: use the lamina as a depth marker and "walk" the needle into the epidural space.

the interspace. Injecting too much local anesthetic can obscure landmarks and make things more difficult. Using either a midline or paramedian approach, insert the introducer needle. Note that the introducer needle has a beveled tip. In the occasional thin or small patient, the introducer needle may accidentally enter the subarachnoid space. To limit the risk of PDPH in this situation, always insert the introducer needle as you would a cutting tip spinal needle with the bevel oriented parallel to the longitudinal axis of the back. Next, pass the spinal needle through the shaft of the introducer needle and advance toward the subarachnoid space. Hold the hub of the spinal needle with your fingertips and appreciate the "clicks" and "pops" as the needle traverses the ligamentum flavum and the dura. Remove the stylet from the spinal needle after each pop. Look for CSF. If the patient is sitting, CSF should appear promptly. If the patient is lying on her side (or prone), or if the spinal needle tip is angled downward, CSF may appear more slowly. If the spinal needle contacts bone, withdraw it into the shaft of the introducer needle and *pivot* the introducer slightly and reinsert the spinal needle (Fig. 35-21). If a midline introducer needle is inserted in the center of an interspace and the spinal needle contacts bone, it is most likely lamina of the lower vertebra (Fig. 35-19). By slowly redirecting the needle cephalad, you should be able to "walk" off the lamina and into the subarachnoid space. The spinal needle should advance a little deeper with each redirection. If you still do not enter the subarachnoid space, remove the spinal needle, palpate the back, and reassess the insertion site of your introducer needle.

Patients will occasionally report a transient paresthesia during spinal needle insertion. These paresthesias may be from needle to nerve root contact within the subarachnoid space[44] or they may emanate from the dura. Should a transient paresthesia occur, stop advancing the spinal needle, and withdraw the stylet.

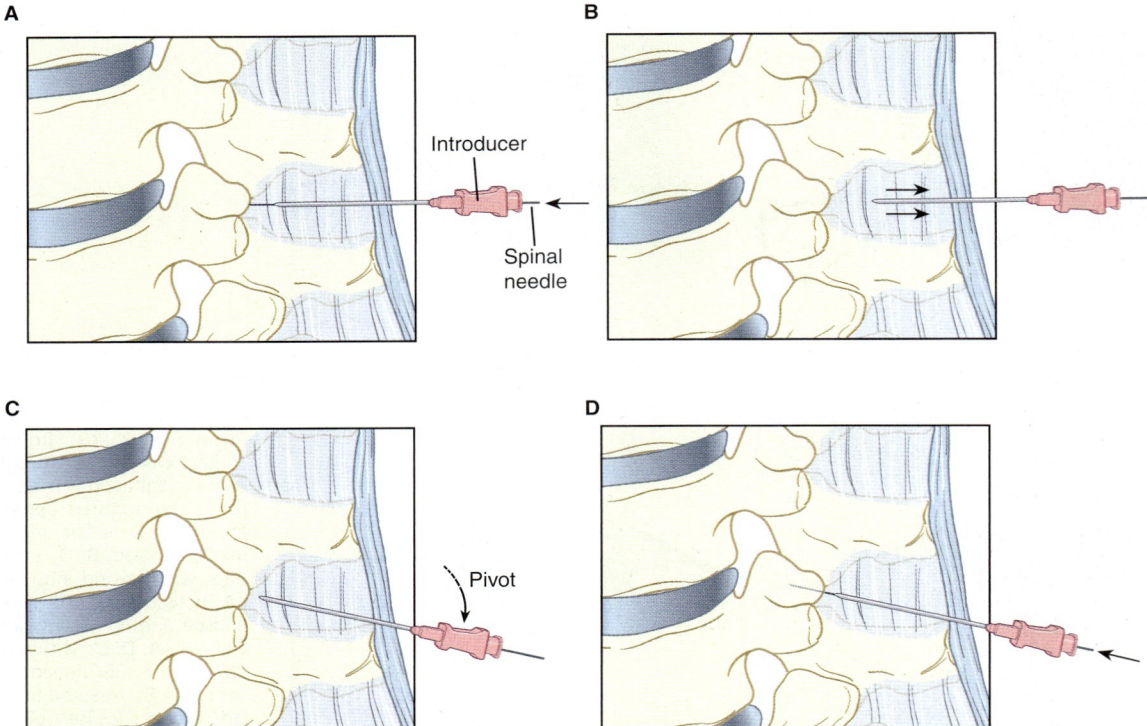

Figure 35-21 Using an introducer needle. If the spinal needle contacts bone (**A**), withdraw it into the shaft of the introducer needle (**B**). Otherwise, the spinal needle will merely bend, not change direction. After withdrawing the spinal needle, *pivot* the introducer (**C**) and reinsert the spinal needle (**D**).

If you see CSF, inject the medication into the subarachnoid space. Do not inject if the paresthesia persists or recurs. Instead, remove and reposition the spinal needle.

Once clear CSF appears in the hub of the spinal needle, fix the needle in position with your nondominant hand and attach the syringe containing the medication. Aspirate gently. If using a hyperbaric solution, you will see birefringence (Schlieren lines), which indicates the mixing of solutions of differing baricities. Some experts recommend rotating the spinal needle 360 degrees to confirm free flow of CSF in four quadrants. This step is unnecessary.

Drug emerges directly from the tip of cutting point needles, so needle bevel orientation has no effect on the subsequent level of subarachnoid block. Pencil-point needles have side holes, which produce directional flow of injected drug. Side-hole orientation, especially caudal versus cephalad, influences the distribution of both hyperbaric and isobaric local anesthetics.[45,46] In most cases, orient the side-hole toward the head to ensure adequate sensory block and to minimize the risks of local anesthetic pooling around the cauda equina (see toxicity, below).

Continuous Subarachnoid Spinal Anesthesia

After identifying the subarachnoid space with a large-gauge needle, insert an appropriate sized catheter 2 to 3 cm into the subarachnoid space. The catheter will advance more easily and be more likely to lie cephalad to the insertion site if the bevel or orifice of the needle is directed toward the patient's head. Caudally directed catheters may cause pooling and maldistribution of local anesthetic, which has been associated with permanent neurologic injury (see Complications).

Epidural Anesthesia

The epidural space can be identified with either the hanging drop or loss of resistance technique. With the hanging drop technique, place a drop of saline at the hub of the epidural needle. As the needle enters the epidural space, the drop of liquid will be pulled into the needle. This technique relies on negative pressure within the epidural space. It is more reliable for thoracic than lumbar needle insertion.

Most anesthesiologists use a loss of resistance technique to identify the epidural space. When the tip of the epidural needle lies within the ligamentum flavum, there is resistance to injection. As the tip of the needle enters the epidural space, this resistance disappears. Common variations of the loss of resistance technique use air or saline in the loss of resistance syringe and intermittent or continuous pressure to advance the epidural needle.

Air versus Saline

Anesthesia providers often have a preference for air or saline in the loss of resistance syringe. Air has the advantage of simplicity. In addition, using air makes it easier to recognize an accidental or intentional dural puncture or an intrathecal catheter. However, intracranial air, injected after an accidental dural puncture, will produce an instant headache.[47] In addition, large amounts of epidural air, especially in smaller patients, may interfere with the distribution of local anesthetic. Possible advantages of saline include fewer dural punctures, fewer PDPHs, easier insertion of the epidural catheter, fewer paresthesias, fewer intravascular catheters, better analgesia, and fewer unblocked segments after epidural local anesthetic injection. *But,* a recent meta-analysis found no

1

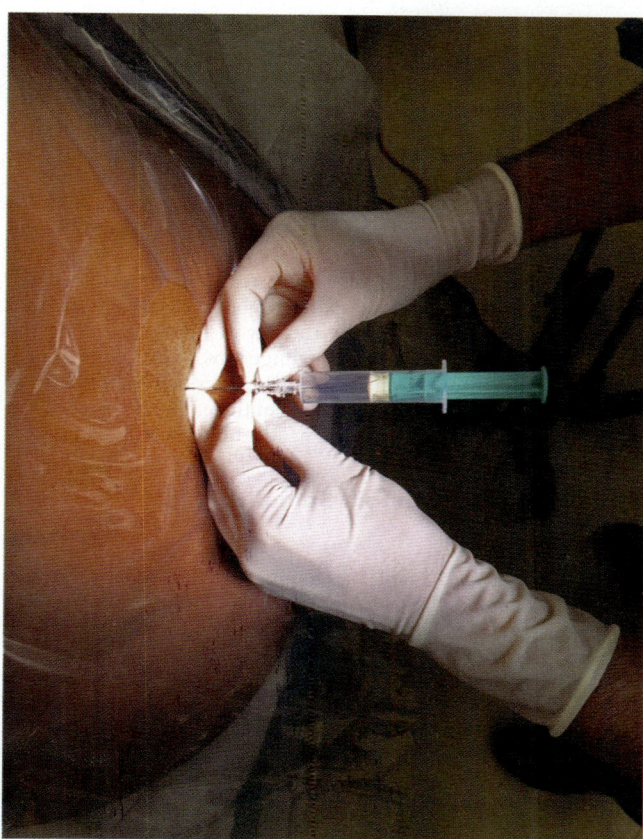

Figure 35-22 Hand positions for intermittently advancing a needle toward the epidural space using a winged needle. Grasping the wings with your index fingers and thumb, place your long fingers alongside the shaft at the site of insertion. Your thumb and index fingers advance the needle while the middle fingers control the needle's forward movement.

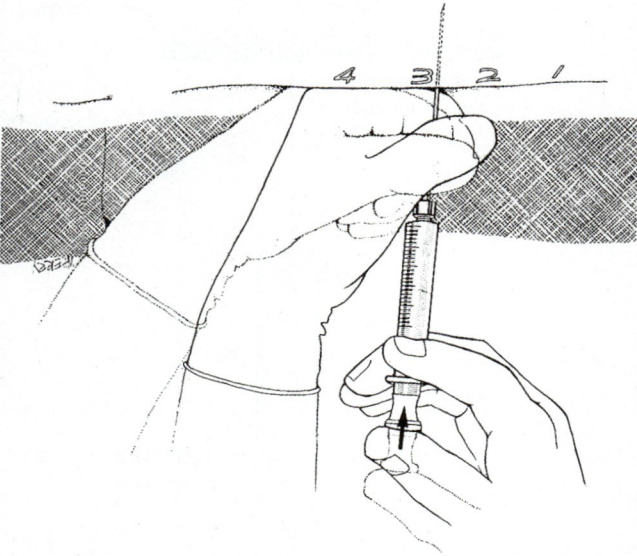

Figure 35-23 The Bromage technique for identifying the epidural space. (From Norris MC, ed. *Obstetric Anesthesia*. 2nd ed. Philadelphia: Lippincott Williams & Wilkins; 1999:302.)

advantages of saline versus air.[48] Clinical outcomes are similar when anesthesiologists use the technique of their choice.[49]

Intermittent versus Continuous

The epidural needle can be advanced intermittently or continuously. In the United States, the intermittent, or "stop go," technique is probably more common. Grasp the epidural needle firmly with both hands (Fig. 35-22) and advance it millimeter by millimeter. The intraspinous ligament will present little resistance, whereas the ligamentum flavum will feel firm and gritty. In between each advance, firmly tap the plunger of the loss of resistance syringe. If using saline in the syringe, include a bubble of air that can be compressed with each tap. When the needle is in the ligamentum flavum, the plunger will recoil. Once the tip of the needle enters the epidural space, the plunger will collapse.

Continuous pressure techniques have been described by Bromage[50] and Doughty.[51] For the Bromage technique, make a fist with your nondominant hand and place your carpal–metacarpal joints on the patient's back. Firmly grasp the shaft of the epidural needle between your thumb and forefinger. Advance the needle slowly by rolling your fist into the patient's back. Meanwhile, use your dominant hand to apply continuous pressure to the plunger of the loss of resistance syringe, which can contain either air or saline. Stop advancing the needle when the plunger collapses (Fig. 35-23).

In the Doughty technique, the roles of the hands are reversed. Now, *brace* the epidural needle with your nondominant hand to control its advance. Grasp the barrel of the loss of resistance syringe with your dominant hand so the metacarpal head of your index finger is positioned on the end of the plunger (Fig. 35-24). Slowly advance the needle by balancing the driving pressure from your dominant hand with resistance from your bracing hand. Use the metacarpal head of the dominant index finger to exert pressure on the end of the plunger; you will perceive the loss of resistance immediately upon entering the epidural space.[51]

More common today are various "son-of-Doughty" techniques. Here, the driving pressure is applied directly to the plunger of a saline-filled loss of resistance syringe (Fig. 35-25).[52] When the tip of the needle enters the epidural space, the plunger collapses and the needle stops advancing.

As with the choice between air and saline, any technique done well is better than the best technique done poorly.

The Epidural Catheter

After identifying the epidural space, you can inject local anesthetic through either the needle or a catheter. Injecting through the needle will provide slightly faster onset but risks complications if drug is accidentally injected intrathecally or intravenously. Inserting a catheter into the epidural space encourages more careful injection of the initial dose of medication and allows the provision of epidural anesthesia or analgesia for as long as needed. Most epidural catheters are made of nylon or polyamide. Some are wire reinforced. Catheters can have a single orifice at the tip or multiple orifices along the distal end. Multiorifice catheters allow wider distribution of injected medication and, in laboring women, are associated with more extensive block and better analgesia. Nylon and polyamide catheters can be flimsy and kink at the hub of the epidural needle. Many come with "threading assist devices" that seat in the hub of the epidural needle and ease catheter insertion. Try to insert about 5 cm of catheter into the epidural space. Inserting less increases the chances that the catheter will become dislodged. Inserting

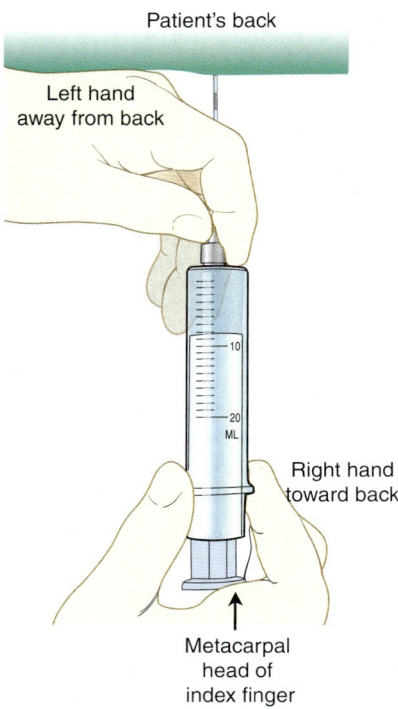

Figure 35-24 The Doughty technique: the nondominant (*left*) hand braces the needle against the patient's back. The dominant (*right*) hand advances the needle by grasping the hub while applying pressure to the plunger with the metacarpal head of the index finger. The right hand will feel the loss of resistance as soon as it occurs.

more makes it more likely that the catheter will enter a blood vessel.[53] Although the orientation of the epidural needle bevel will determine the initial direction of the epidural catheter, it does not reliably aim the catheter in a cephalad or caudad direction. Most epidural catheters curl on themselves at the level of insertion. If you meet resistance while inserting the catheter, *do not* withdraw and try to reinsert. Some epidural needles have a sharp inner bevel that can shear the tip of a catheter. Instead, remove both needle and catheter together and reidentify the epidural space.

Once the epidural catheter is inserted, it is time to remove the needle. Hold the epidural catheter about 1 cm from the hub of the needle. Gently withdraw the needle, sliding it along the catheter until the hub meets your fingertips. Move your fingers back another centimeter and repeat the process. When the tip of the needle comes out of the skin, grasp the catheter between the needle and the skin and slide the needle off the catheter.

Combined Subarachnoid Spinal Epidural

Technique

The needle-through-needle technique is the most common method of combined subarachnoid spinal epidural (CSE) block. Because the conus medullaris sometimes extends to L2 or even L3, it is safest to perform CSE block at the L3–L4 or L4–L5 interspaces (see Complications, below). First, identify the epidural space with your usual technique. Using air in the loss of resistance syringe will assure that any liquid flowing through the spinal needle is indeed CSF. After identifying the epidural space, insert a long, small-gauge spinal needle. You should feel some resistance as the tip of the spinal needle passes the tip of the epidural needle. Then

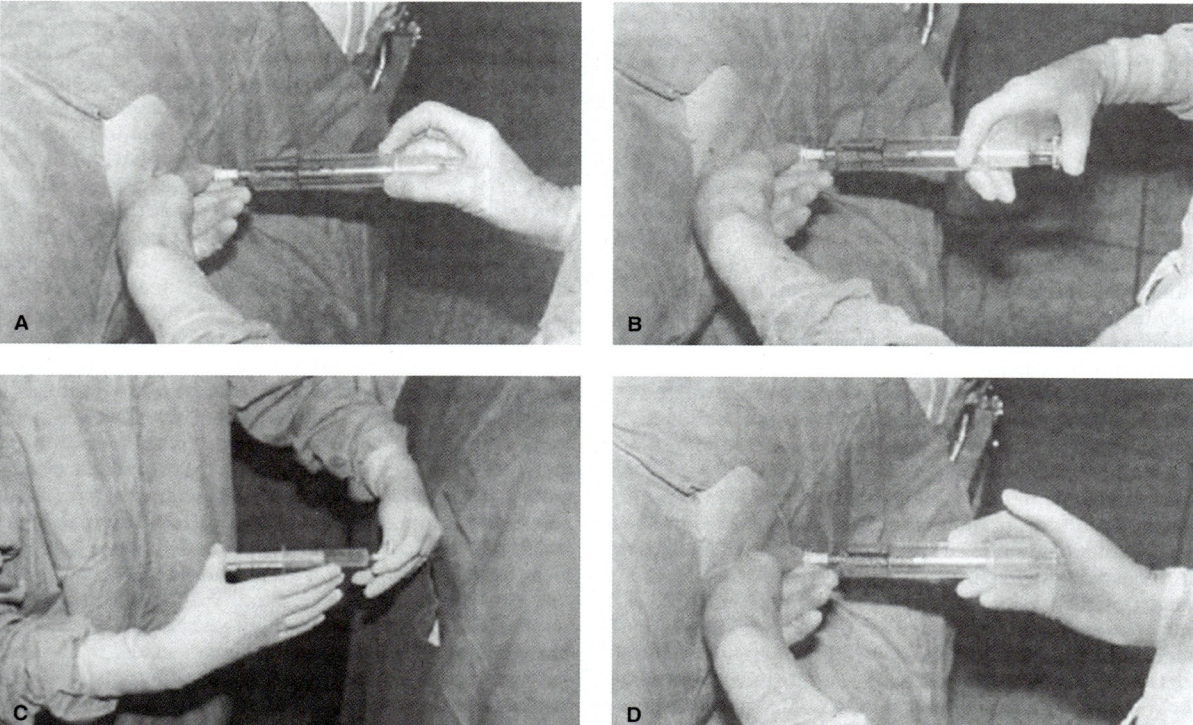

Figure 35-25 Hand positions for (**A**) the original Doughty technique and (**B**), (**C**), and (**D**) various "son-of-Doughty" techniques. (**A, B,** and **D** from Russell R, Porter J, Scrutton M. In: Reynolds F, ed. *Pain Relief in Labour*. London: BMJ Publishing, 1997, with permission; **C** from Reynolds F. Hand positions and the 'son-of-Doughty' technique. *Anaesthesia*. 2005;60:717–718. ©2016 Association of Anaesthetists of Great Britain & Ireland.)

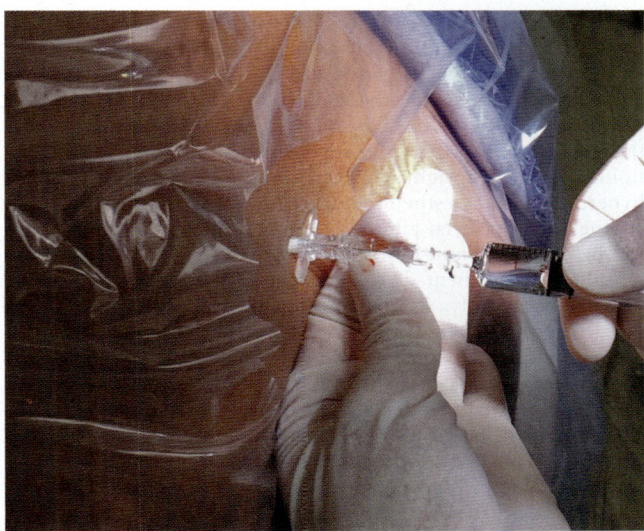

Figure 35-26 Hand position for stabilizing CSE needles. The thumb and index finger pinch the hubs of both spinal and epidural needles to fix the position of the spinal needle.

you will feel a subtle pop as the spinal needle pierces the dura. Stabilize the spinal needle by pinching the hubs of both needles between your thumb and finger (Fig. 35-26). Withdraw the stylet from the spinal needle and look for CSF. Carefully inject the subarachnoid medication, withdraw the spinal needle, and insert the epidural catheter.

Troubleshooting

The most common problem encountered with the needle-through-needle technique is failure to see CSF in the hub of the spinal needle (Fig. 35-27). Most often, the spinal needle has not entered the subarachnoid space. The epidural needle may not be in the epidural space or it may be directed laterally. Sometimes the needle does not extend far enough to penetrate the dura. This problem is more likely to occur if the patient is in the lateral position instead of sitting. Sometimes, rotating the spinal needle 360 degrees will be enough to enter the subarachnoid space. Otherwise, consider proceeding with an epidural technique or reidentifying the epidural space.

Drug Dosing

The CSE technique can alter the behavior of both intrathecal and epidural medications. Because the epidural catheter can be used to supplement the subarachnoid block, it is possible to use smaller doses of subarachnoid medication. Less intrathecal local anesthetic may limit the hemodynamic effects of subarachnoid anesthesia. Epidural injection of local anesthetic or saline can raise the level of sensory block even after the level of subarachnoid anesthesia has stabilized (Fig. 35-28). The presence of a small-gauge dural hole also may enhance the spread of subsequent epidural medications. This effect may be responsible for the improved labor epidural analgesia reported after previous 25-gauge needle dural puncture.[54]

Choice of Technique

Subarachnoid anesthesia, with its rapid onset of dense sensory block is often the best choice for surgeries of known duration

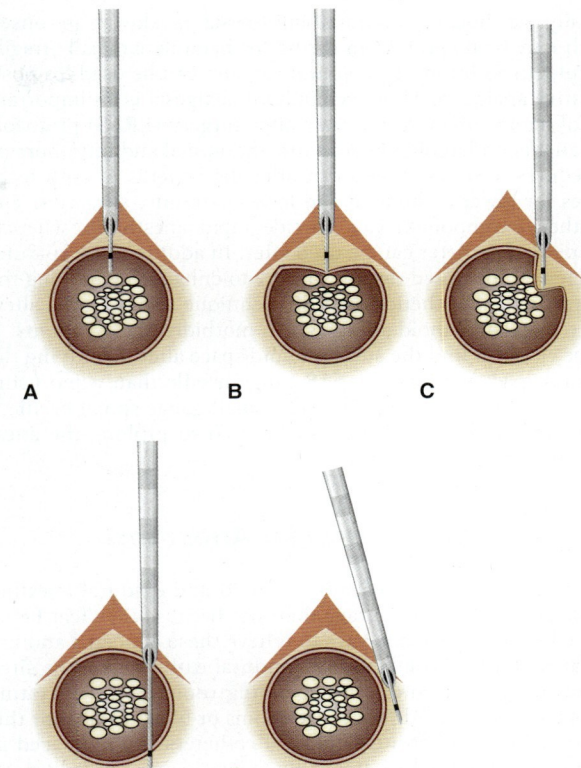

Figure 35-27 Different positions of epidural and spinal needles with the needle-through-needle CSE technique. **A:** The ideal position; a midline epidural needle guides the spinal needle into the subarachnoid space. **B:** Spinal needle too short; it indents but does not pierce the dura. **C:** Spinal needle too short and too lateral. **D:** Spinal needle too long; it has passed through the subarachnoid space. **E:** Spinal needle too lateral; the epidural needle is in the epidural space but it guides the spinal needle away from the dural sac. (Adapted from Norris MC, ed. *Obstetric Anesthesia*. 2nd ed. Philadelphia, PA: Lippincott Williams & Wilkins; 1999:307.)

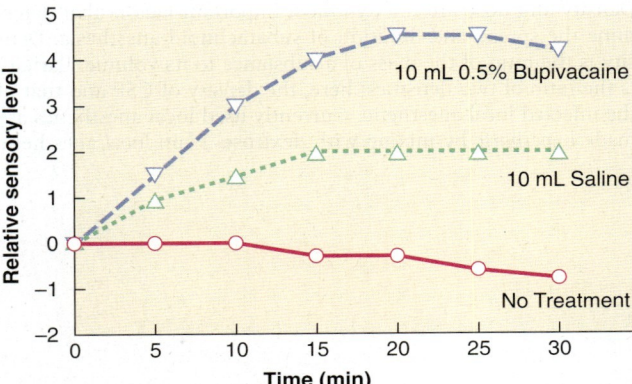

Figure 35-28 Spread of sensory block with CSE. Nonpregnant patients received 10 mg 0.5% bupivacaine intrathecally. After the maximum level of sensory block had been achieved, patients received nothing (○), 10 mL epidural saline (△), or 10 mL epidural bupivacaine (▽). (Adapted from Norris MC, ed. *Obstetric Anesthesia* 2nd ed. Philadelphia, PA: Lippincott Williams & Wilkins; 1999:309.)

(usually <2 hours). Epidural anesthesia is slower in onset, which may be helpful when caring for hemodynamically fragile patients. In addition, the epidural catheter can be used for postoperative analgesia. Thoracic epidural analgesia is an important part of many enhanced recovery after surgery (ERAS) protocols for patients undergoing major intra-abdominal and intrathoracic procedures. CSE anesthesia can offer the benefits of both techniques for lower abdominal and lower extremity surgeries. The intrathecal component can provide rapid anesthesia, whereas the epidural catheter can be used later. In addition, the epidural catheter can be dosed during surgery to enhance or prolong the subarachnoid anesthetic. The CSE technique also is a good alternative to subarachnoid anesthesia in morbidly obese patients. It can be easier to find the subarachnoid space after identifying the epidural space with a 17- or 18-gauge needle than when using just a short introducer needle and a small-gauge spinal needle.[55] Again, the epidural catheter can be used to prolong the anesthetic for longer operations.

Efficiency and Neuraxial Anesthesia

Despite the advantages of subarachnoid and epidural anesthesia, surgeons often discourage their use because they fear being delayed. There are many ways to relieve these concerns and use neuraxial anesthesia efficiently. Epidural catheters can be sited before the patient enters the operating room. Some operating suites have designated procedure rooms or block rooms for this purpose. In other settings, epidural catheters can be placed in the preoperative holding area. Subarachnoid anesthesia kits can be opened in advance. Drugs can be drawn up into appropriately labeled sterile syringes. The kit can then be rewrapped and set aside, ready to use as soon as the patient enters the OR. Lastly, performing subarachnoid and epidural blocks regularly will improve skills and build confidence, both yours and your surgeon's.

Pharmacology

Subarachnoid Anesthesia

Spread and Duration

Density and dose are the two most important factors that determine the spread and duration of subarachnoid anesthesia. Density is the ratio of the mass of a substance to its volume. Baricity is the ratio of two densities; here, the density of CSF and that of the injected local anesthetic. Currently used local anesthetics are made *hyperbaric* by mixing with dextrose. Plain local anesthetic solutions are isobaric or slightly *hypobaric*. Table 35-2 offers suggestions for dose and baricity when performing subarachnoid anesthesia for various surgeries.

Hyperbaric local anesthetics are denser than CSF and will flow with gravity to the dependent areas of the spine, usually the upper thoracic region in supine patients (Fig. 35-29). Positioning patients upright or lateral can limit the initial spread of hyperbaric local anesthetic. But, when the patient returns to the supine position, even after 20 to 30 minutes, the sensory level reaches the usual mid-thoracic dermatomes.

Bulk displacement determines the initial spread of isobaric drug. Subsequently, movement of CSF by either transmission of cardiac pulsations[56] or gross patient movements (i.e., turning from lateral to supine position[57]) will determine the ultimate spread of block.

In nonpregnant patients, hyperbaric local anesthetics produce more consistent levels of sensory block than isobaric drug (Fig. 35-30).[58] Isobaric drugs produce longer blocks.[59] When used for subarachnoid anesthesia for cesarean section, there is little difference between equal doses of isobaric or hyperbaric bupivacaine.[60]

Patient Variables

Height, weight, body mass index, and vertebral column length have no clinically significant effect on the spread of subarachnoid anesthesia. Increasing age is associated with slower onset and longer duration but no change in extent of subarachnoid block.[61] Both female gender and pregnancy increase motor block produced by intrathecal isobaric bupivacaine.[62] One small study reported that CSF volume correlated with the spread of subarachnoid anesthesia.[63] Pregnant patients will develop higher levels of sensory block than nonpregnant patients when given the same dose of intrathecal local anesthetic. This enhanced sensitivity disappears shortly after delivery.[64] In nonpregnant adults, increasing abdominal girth correlates with increasing extent of sensory block after intrathecal injection of isobaric bupivacaine.[65] Increases in intra-abdominal and consequently epidural space pressure associated with both pregnancy and obesity may enhance sensory spread by decreasing lumbar CSF volume.

Local Anesthetic Dose

Within commonly used ranges (i.e., 7.5 to 12 mg hyperbaric bupivacaine), increasing the dose of local anesthetic does not significantly increase the level of block.[61] At some point (i.e., 15 mg hyperbaric bupivacaine) a higher sensory level will develop.[66] Larger doses of both hyperbaric and isobaric local anesthetics do produce denser and longer lasting anesthesia.

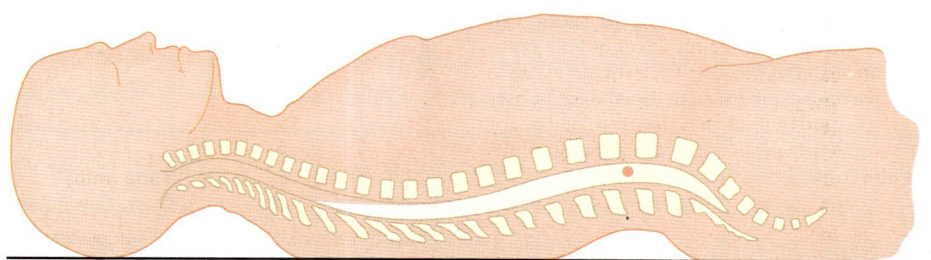

Figure 35-29 In the supine position, hyperbaric local anesthetics injected at the apex of the lumbar lordosis (*circle*) flow with gravity and pool in the sacrum and thoracic kyphosis. Thoracic pooling may be why hyperbaric solutions typically produce mid-thoracic levels of sensory block. (From Barash PG, Cullen BF, Stoelting RK, et al., eds. *Clinical Anesthesia*. 7th ed. Philadelphia, PA: Wolters Kluwer; 2015;917.)

Table 35-2 Some Common Surgical Procedures That Can Be Done with Subarachnoid Spinal Anesthesia

Procedure	Level	Local Anesthetic	Comments
Obstetrics			
Cesarean section	≥ T6	12–15 mg hyperbaric bupivacaine[a]	Lower doses may produce less hypotension but should be used as part of a combined subarachnoid epidural technique. Adding a lipophilic opioid may improve intraoperative analgesia.
Postpartum tubal ligation (mini laparotomy)	≥ T8	10–12 mg hyperbaric bupivacaine	
Cervical cerclage	≥ T10	5–7.5 mg hyperbaric bupivacaine	Faster discharge with smaller doses
Orthopedics			
Hip fracture or replacement	≥ T12	15–20 mg isobaric[b] bupivacaine	Sitting or lateral position with the operative side *up*
Knee replacement	≥ T12	12–15 mg hyperbaric bupivacaine	Higher level if tourniquet used
Knee arthroscopy	≥ T12	5–7.5 mg either isobaric or hyperbaric bupivacaine	Faster discharge with smaller dose. Lipophilic opioid may help with tourniquet pain. Some use 40 mg preservative-free 2-chloroprocaine for outpatient procedures.
Ankle surgery	≥ T12	At least 7.5 mg hyperbaric bupivacaine	Dose depends on expected duration of procedure. Combined subarachnoid epidural can add postoperative analgesia.
Urology			
Cystoscopy	≥ T10	2.5–5.0 mg isobaric or hyperbaric bupivacaine	Faster discharge with smaller dose
Trans urethral resection of bladder tumor or prostate	≥ T10	At least 7.5 mg isobaric or hyperbaric bupivacaine	Adjust dose according to expected duration of surgery.
Penile prosthesis	≥ T10	12–15 mg hyperbaric bupivacaine	
General Surgery			
Inguinal hernia repair/open appendectomy	≥ T8	12–15 mg hyperbaric bupivacaine	
Perianal/perirectal	Sacral	5–7.5 mg hyperbaric bupivacaine (lithotomy position)	Smaller doses of isobaric bupivacaine (2.5–5 mg) can be used if the patient will be prone.

[a]In the United States: 0.75% bupivacaine with 8.25% dextrose.
[b]Preservative-free 0.5% bupivacaine.

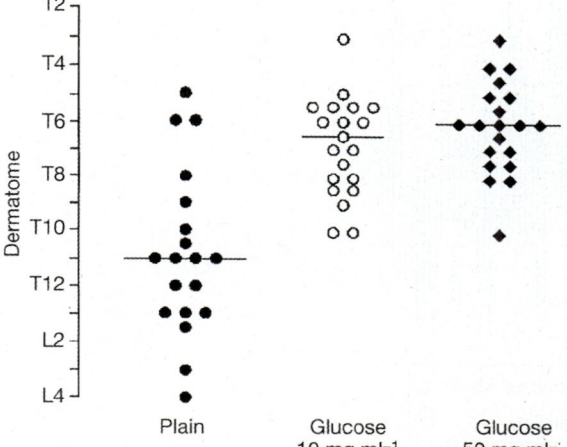

Figure 35-30 Range of sensory block after intrathecal injection of two different solutions of 0.5% tetracaine. Solutions containing dextrose, which are hyperbaric, produce more consistent levels of block than plain (isobaric) solutions. (From Whiteside JB, Burke D, Wildsmith JA. Spinal anesthesia with ropivacaine 5 g·mL^{-1} in glucose 10 mg·mL^{-1} or 50 mg·mL^{-1}. *Br J Anaesth*. 2001;86:241–244.)

Adjuvants

Many drugs have been studied for their ability to prolong or improve subarachnoid anesthesia. Vasoconstrictors, such as epinephrine or phenylephrine may prolong the intrathecal block by inhibiting absorption of intrathecal local anesthetics or by acting directly on spinal cord α-receptors. Vasoconstrictors prolong the duration of intrathecal tetracaine. They have no clinically significant effects on the duration of intrathecal lidocaine or bupivacaine.

The $α_2$-agonists clonidine and dexmedetomidine prolong the duration of subarachnoid anesthesia and analgesia. Associated bradycardia may require atropine.[67] Larger doses of intrathecal clonidine also can cause hypotension and sedation.[68]

Lipid soluble opioids (fentanyl or sufentanil) can enhance intraoperative anesthesia and provide a few hours of postoperative analgesia. Small doses of fentanyl (5 to 10 μg) are as effective as larger doses and may produce less itching. Intrathecal morphine can provide prolonged (12 to 24 hours) postoperative analgesia but side effects, including itching and nausea and vomiting, are common and challenging to treat. Rarely, intrathecal morphine can produce delayed respiratory depression.

Epidural Anesthesia

Lumbar epidural anesthesia can be used interchangeably with subarachnoid anesthesia in most cases. One exception is procedures involving the S1 dermatome (i.e., ankle surgery). S1 is the largest nerve root in the body and the onset of epidural block can be slow and incomplete. Thoracic epidural injection can provide segmental block, which can supplement general anesthesia for upper abdominal and intrathoracic surgeries (Table 35-3).

Spread of Block

Patient variables, drug dose, and site of injection are the main determinants of the spread of epidural block.[69] A given dose of local anesthetic will spread farther in older compared to younger patients. As a result, the risk of hypotension associated with epidural local anesthetics may be greater in older patients. Height, weight, and BMI have no clinically significant effects on the extent of epidural block. Pregnant patients will develop more extensive block after a fixed dose of local anesthetic than non-pregnant patients.[70]

The extent of epidural block is proportional to the dose of local anesthetic injected. Mass of drug, not the volume injected, mostly determines the extent of sensory block. However, the relationship is not linear. A smaller dose produces a relatively greater spread (dermatomes/dose) than a larger dose.[69]

Site of injection has a major impact on the spread of epidural block. Small doses of local anesthetic (5 to 10 mL) will produce a band of block around the injection site. Lumbar injection spreads more cephalad than caudad, whereas upper thoracic drug blocks more dermatomes below than above the injection site (Fig. 35-31).[71]

Table 35-3 Recommendations for Epidural Anesthesia

Type of Surgery	Insertion Site	Typical Spread of Block
Thoracic	T2–T6	T2–T6 (5–10 mL local anesthetic)
Abdominal	T6–L1	T1–L4 (10–20 mL local anesthetic)
Lower extremity Pelvic Peripheral vascular	Lumbar L2–L5	T8–S5 (20 mL local anesthetic)
Obstetric		C8–T8 (upper level of sensory block)

Modified from Visser WA, Lee RA, Gielen MJM. Factors affecting the distribution of neural blockade by local anesthetics in epidural anesthesia and a comparison of lumbar versus thoracic epidural anesthesia. *Anesth Analg.* 2008;107:708–721.

Onset and Duration

Onset and duration of epidural anesthesia depend largely on the choice of anesthetic (Table 35-4). Some sign of sensory block should be detectable at the dermatomal level of injection within 5 to 10 minutes. The full extent of block usually develops within 20 to 30 minutes. Differences in onset time between local anesthetics are small and rarely clinically significant.[72] 2-Chloroprocaine has the shortest duration followed by lidocaine and mepivacaine. The more potent drugs, bupivacaine and ropivacaine have the

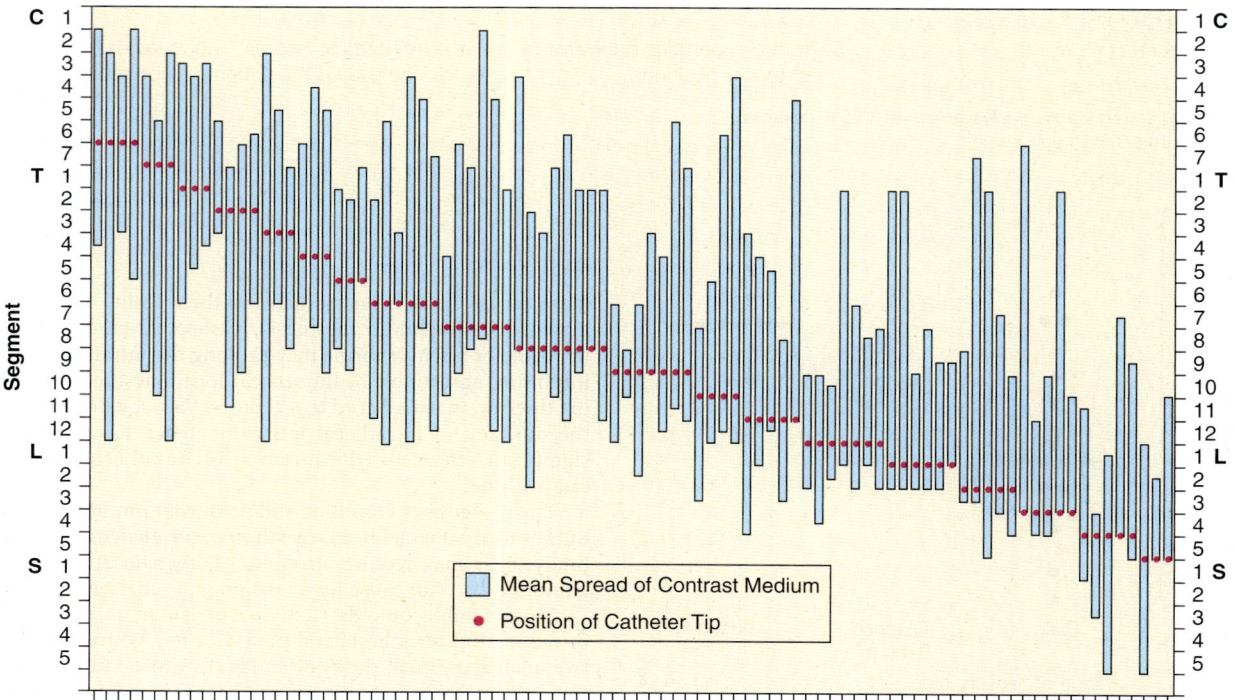

Figure 35-31 Mean radiographic spread after epidural injection of 5 mL iotrolan, 240 mg I/mL, in 90 patients. C, cervical segment; L, lumbar segment; S, sacral segment; T, thoracic segment. Cervical injection spreads more caudally, whereas lumbar injection spreads more cranially. (Adapted from Yokoyama M, Hanazaki M, Fujii H, et al. Correlation between the distribution of contrast medium and the extent of blockade during epidural anesthesia. *Anesthesiology.* 2004;100:1504–1510.)

Table 35-4 Local Anesthetics Used for Surgical Epidural Block

Drug	Duration		Prolongation by Epinephrine (%)
	Two-dermatome Regression (min)	Complete Resolution (min)	
2-Chloroprocaine 3%	45–60	100–160	40–60
Lidocaine 2%	60–100	160–200[a]	40–80[b]
Mepivacaine 2%	60–100	160–200	40–80
Ropivacaine 0.5%–1.0%	90–180	240–420	No
Bupivacaine 0.5–0.75%[c]	120–240	300–460	No

[a]Motor block can outlast sensory block.
[b]Epinephrine also improves quality of sensory block.
[c]Use only 0.5% bupivacaine in obstetric patients.

slowest onset but the longest durations. Lidocaine produces relatively more motor block than sensory block. Postoperative patients may have pain before the motor block has completely regressed. Sensory block usually outlasts motor block with mepivacaine, ropivacaine, and bupivacaine.

Surgery often outlasts the duration of the initial epidural injection. Injecting half the initial dose once the block has regressed by two dermatomes should maintain an adequate level of block. Another way to maintain surgical anesthesia is to inject a fixed dose of drug at regular intervals. For lumbar epidural catheters, inject 5 mL 0.5% ropivacaine or bupivacaine every 60 minutes. Use the same approach with thoracic epidural catheters, but inject a smaller dose (2.5 mL).

Adjuvants

Adjuvants can speed the onset, improve the quality, and prolong the duration of epidural block.[69]

Sodium Bicarbonate

Sodium bicarbonate raises the pH of commercially prepared local anesthetics, increasing the amount of nonionized, active, drug. Adding sodium bicarbonate speeds the onset and increases the density of epidural local anesthetic block. These effects are most pronounced with lidocaine. Bupivacaine readily precipitates in the presence of sodium bicarbonate.

Epinephrine and α₂-Agonists

Epinephrine-induced vasoconstriction decreases systemic absorption of local anesthetics. In addition, stimulation of spinal cord α_2-receptors produces analgesia. Adding α_2-agonists (epinephrine, clonidine, or dexmedetomidine) to local anesthetic speeds the onset and improves the quality of epidural anesthesia. Clinically, adding epinephrine, 5 μg/mL to lidocaine markedly improves the quality of epidural anesthesia for cesarean section. Patients who receive lidocaine with epinephrine are about half as likely to experience intraoperative pain or need conversion to general anesthesia compared with women who receive plain lidocaine.[73] Epidural clonidine or dexmedetomidine intensify and prolong the effects of epidural local anesthetics.[74] These drugs also provide postoperative analgesia.[75] Sedation is common.

Opioids

Epidural opioids also speed the onset and improve the quality of block produced by local anesthetics. Fentanyl, sufentanil, and morphine are the most commonly used opioids. These drugs also can provide postoperative analgesia. Itching, nausea, and vomiting are common side effects, especially with epidural morphine.[76]

Test Doses

Currently, most clinicians use a blind technique to identify the epidural space and insert a catheter. Intended epidural catheters may be subarachnoid, subdural, intravascular, or elsewhere. Misplaced injection of drugs intended for the epidural space can have serious adverse consequences. To minimize these risks, all epidural catheters should be tested *throughout* their use. The purpose of these tests is twofold: to prove that the catheter is not in an unintended place (i.e., intrathecal or intravenous) *and* to prove that the catheter is indeed in the epidural space.

The most common cause of significant anesthetic-related morbidity and mortality in laboring women is unrecognized *intrathecal* injection of local anesthetics.[77,78] When inducing epidural anesthesia or analgesia, first inject a small dose of local anesthetic (i.e., 30 to 45 mg lidocaine or 5 to 10 mg bupivacaine) through the catheter and look for signs of subarachnoid anesthesia. Within 2 to 3 minutes of intrathecal local anesthetic injection, patients will note warmth and tingling in their legs or feet. Sensory block to cold and pinprick can be detected.[79] In parturients, intrathecal lidocaine will also produce motor block by 3 minutes. In laboring women, rapid onset of analgesia should also alert to intrathecal injection. Pay close attention to the intrathecal test dose. Positive findings can be subtle and easily overlooked on a busy labor and delivery floor.

Be aware of two limitations of lidocaine as an intrathecal test dose in pregnant women. First, some women will report warmth in their legs and motor weakness after *epidural* injection of 30 to 45 mg lidocaine. As a result, a positive intrathecal test dose should be evaluated carefully to avoid removing an appropriately placed epidural catheter. Second, these small doses of lidocaine can produce extensive sensory and sympathetic block (Fig. 35-32). Dangerously high subarachnoid anesthesia can occur.[80] In a recent report, unplanned intrathecal injection of 45 mg lidocaine produced clinically significant complications in 60% of patients (Table 35-5).[81]

Intravascular local anesthetic injection can produce seizures and even cardiac arrest. The most widely used intravenous test dose is lidocaine with epinephrine. Intravenous injection of epinephrine 15 μg will increase heart rate by at least 10 beats per minute and systolic blood pressure by at least 15 mmHg.[82] Unfortunately, sedation, general anesthesia, β-blockade, advancing age, and pre-existing neuraxial block can blunt this response. In laboring women, pain-induced tachycardia can be confused with a

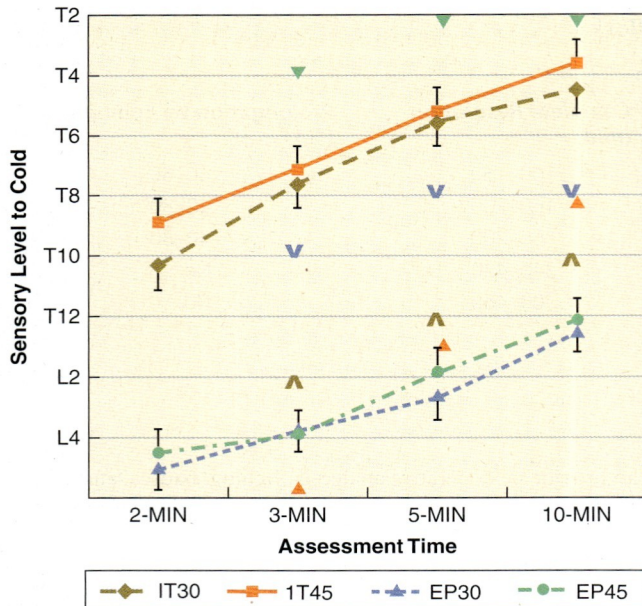

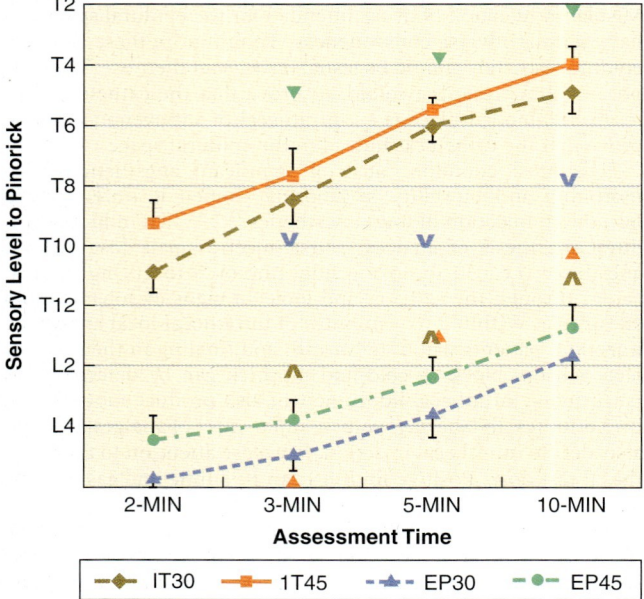

Figure 35-32 Spread of sensory block after intrathecal (IT) or epidural (EP) injection of 30 or 45 mg lidocaine. Both intrathecal doses produced significantly higher block than both epidural doses ($P < 0.01$ for each). IT30 = intrathecal injection of 30 mg lidocaine; IT45 = intrathecal injection of 45 mg lidocaine; EP30 = epidural injection of 30 mg lidocaine; EP45 = epidural injection of 45 mg lidocaine. The maximum and minimum outliers for each dose are added to demonstrate the overlap in sensory levels between epidural and intrathecal dosing. Maximum epidural outliers are represented by the *blue open triangle* for 30-mg dose, and *green solid triangle* for 45-mg dose. Minimum intrathecal outliers are represented by *black open triangle* for the 30-mg dose, and *red solid triangle* for the 45-mg dose. (Adapted from Pratt S, Hess P, Vasudevan A. A prospective randomized trial of lidocaine 30 mg versus 45 mg for epidural test dose for intrathecal injection in the obstetric population. *Anesth Analg.* 2013;116:125–132.)

Table 35-5 Complications of Unintended Intrathecal Injection of 45 mg of Lidocaine in Parturients	
Number of Patients (%)	**Complication**
8 (32%)	Hypotension prompting vasopressors (only)
3 (12%)	Cesarean delivery for nonreassuring fetal status (also received vasopressors)
4 (16%)	High spinal (shortness breath, sensory level above T4, vasopressors)
10 (40%)	No complication

Data from Bolden N, Gebre E. Accidental dural puncture management: 10-year experience at an academic tertiary care center. *Reg Anesth Pain Med.* 2016;41:169–174.

positive epinephrine response. In one study, the epinephrine test dose produced more false positive than true positive responses.[83]

In pregnant women, observation and aspiration will detect almost all intravascular catheters. It is tempting to withdraw an intravascular catheter until blood can no longer be aspirated. Unfortunately, these catheters are often still in a blood vessel.[83]

Rarely, a catheter may be subdural (inside the dura mater but outside of the arachnoid mater) (Fig. 35-6).[84] Subdural catheters can present with varying degrees of sensory, motor, and sympathetic block. The subdural space may extend as far as the floor of the third ventricle. Unrecognized subdural injection may be the cause of excessive epidural block. (The epidural space ends at the base of the skull and the cervical epidural space is very narrow. Lumbar *epidural* injection of local anesthetics should not produce cervical or higher levels of sensory block.)

The best test of an epidural catheter is to obtain a level and density of block that are consistent with the local anesthetic injected. Thus, a laboring woman should develop bilateral sensory change and effective analgesia 20 to 30 minutes after receiving 10 to 15 mL of dilute local anesthetic or dilute local anesthetic opioid solution. A surgical patient should notice warmth and numbness 5 to 10 minutes after receiving 2-chloroprocaine or lidocaine and 15 to 30 minutes after bupivacaine or ropivacaine. However, even a properly sited epidural catheter can migrate into a blood vessel or penetrate the dura.

Because no test dose is foolproof and even working epidural catheters can migrate, inject *all* drugs in increments small enough that they will not cause harm if misplaced (i.e., every dose is a "test" dose). Incremental injection may not detect intravascular catheters, but it should prevent systemic toxicity. If an epidural catheter does not behave as expected, do not inject more drug. Instead, remove and replace it.

Physiology

Central Nervous System

Site of Action

The exact site of action of subarachnoid and epidural anesthesia remains unknown. Local anesthetic can be detected throughout the spinal nerve rootlets and spinal cord after intrathecal injection. Local anesthetic injected into the epidural space diffuses through the dura and arachnoid and also can be identified in the nerve rootlets and spinal cord.

Intrathecal local anesthetics reduce, but do not routinely eliminate, somatosensory evoked potentials (SSEPs). Cortical evoked potentials from direct spinal cord stimulation diminish but persist. These results suggest that some block of spinal cord conduction occurs but that subarachnoid anesthesia occurs mostly within the spinal nerve roots.[85]

In monkeys, epidural local anesthetics alter evoked potentials in the nerve roots, dorsal root entry zone, and the long tracts of the spinal cord white matter.[36] In humans, epidural local anesthetics decrease SSEPs in areas of sensory block but not in dermatomes above or below,[87] suggesting a peripheral, but not spinal cord site of action.

Although intrathecal and epidural local anesthetics do not reach the brain, extensive neuraxial anesthesia does produce sedation. Neuraxial block also potentiates the effects of sedatives and decreases the minimum alveolar concentration of potent inhaled agents.[88,89]

Differential Nerve Block

Neuraxial local anesthetics have different potencies on motor, sensory, and sympathetic nerves. This differential block is largely related to the size of different nerves. Large motor nerves (and larger lumbar and sacral nerve roots) are most resistant to local anesthetic block. Sensory nerves have intermediate sensitivity. Preganglionic sympathetic fibers are the smallest and most sensitive to local anesthetics. These differences occur with both subarachnoid and epidural anesthesia. Analgesia (loss of sensation of sharpness to pinprick) extends two or more segments more cephalad than anesthesia (loss of sensation to touch).[90] Sympathetic block (as measured by increase skin temperature) may extend as many as six spinal segments higher than the upper limit of sensory block.[91]

Cardiovascular System

Subarachnoid

Intrathecal injection of local anesthetics produces extensive sympathetic block. Earlier investigators argued that venodilation and the subsequent fall in venous return led to lower cardiac output and hypotension. Intravenous fluids should help prevent or treat hypotension by this mechanism. Unfortunately, multiple studies have shown that increasing intravascular volume with infusions of crystalloid or colloid have little effect on the incidence of subarachnoid anesthesia-related hypotension. Recent studies monitoring cardiac output have clearly and consistently shown that cardiac output **increases** after induction of subarachnoid anesthesia and that a fall in systemic vascular resistance leads to lower blood pressures (Fig. 35-33).[92,93] The degree of hypotension varies widely among patients. Risk factors include pregnancy, hypovolemia, advanced age, obesity, concurrent general anesthesia, and sensory level above T6.[94]

Heart rate may increase, decrease, or remain unchanged. Thoracic levels of anesthesia can produce cardiac sympathetic block (T1–T4). The resultant vagal predominance can decrease heart rate. A decrease in cardiac filling pressures may also stimulate vagally mediated bradycardia via the Bezold–Jarisch reflex. This bradycardia is usually benign, but can occasionally be profound. Cardiac arrest has been reported.[95] A review of 14 closed anesthesia malpractice claims from the 1970s found that prompt treatment with ephedrine, atropine, and chest compressions, but delayed administration of epinephrine produced uniformly poor neurologic outcomes after subarachnoid anesthesia-associated cardiac arrest.[96] Unrecognized hypoxemia may have contributed to the earlier adverse outcomes. Recent cases with pulse oximetry monitoring report better outcomes.[95,97]

Epidural

Hypotension and bradycardia can also occur during epidural anesthesia. The major risk factors for hypotension are the extent and onset of sensory block: Faster onset and more extensive block increase the frequency of hypotension.[98] Bradycardia (heart rate ≤ 45 beats per minute) is more common in males. Genetics also may alter the risk of hypotension after epidural anesthesia. One study, using phenylephrine requirement as a marker, found that β_2-adrenoreceptor gene variants altered vasopressor requirements during thoracic epidural anesthesia. These authors also reported that women required more vasopressors than men.[99]

Prevention and Treatment

Volume

Intravenous fluids have long been used to prevent or treat hypotension associated with neuraxial anesthesia. However, even large volumes of crystalloid (2 L) do not reliably prevent maternal hypotension at cesarean section.[100] Colloid infusion is more effective, but hypotension is still common.[101] Fluids infused after the induction of epidural anesthesia increase both blood pressure and plasma volume. However, they are no more effective than vasopressors and, when given in excess, cause complications of their own.[102] In parturients, rapid infusion of 750 mL crystalloid slightly increased cardiac output and decreased systemic vascular resistance. It also significantly increased markers of endothelial glycocalyx destruction.[103] (The endothelial glycocalyx is an intricate meshwork of proteoglycans and glycoproteins that line the vascular endothelium. An intact glycocalyx prevents extravasation of intravascular fluid by maintaining an oncotic gradient.)

Vasopressors

Ephedrine and phenylephrine are the most commonly used vasopressors for hypotension associated with neuraxial anesthesia. In parturients during cesarean section, ephedrine raises blood pressure primarily by increasing stroke volume and cardiac output. Phenylephrine increases systemic vascular resistance and decreases cardiac output (Fig. 35-34).[104] However, since cardiac output increases with induction of subarachnoid anesthesia, it usually remains above baseline even after phenylephrine.[104] Changes in heart rate parallel the changes in cardiac output. Ephedrine usually increases heart rate, whereas phenylephrine causes a reflex slowing.[104]

Norepinephrine also can be used to prevent or treat maternal hypotension associated with subarachnoid anesthesia. Unlike phenylephrine, norepinephrine maintains heart rate and cardiac output.[105] The clinical implications of these findings remain to be seen. Vasopressin may be a treatment of last resort in severe hypovolemic hypotension or for patients taking medications that impair the renin–angiotensin system.

The Bezold–Jarisch reflex is an alternate explanation for the bradycardia that often accompanies hypotension after neuraxial anesthesia. This reflex is mediated by 5HT-3 serotonin receptors located in the vagus nerve and in ventricular myocardium. Activation of these receptors in response to systemic hypotension increases efferent vagal signaling, producing bradycardia, reduced cardiac output, and worsened hypotension.[106] Several groups have studied the effects of HT-3 receptor antagonists like ondansetron on the hemodynamic effects of neuraxial

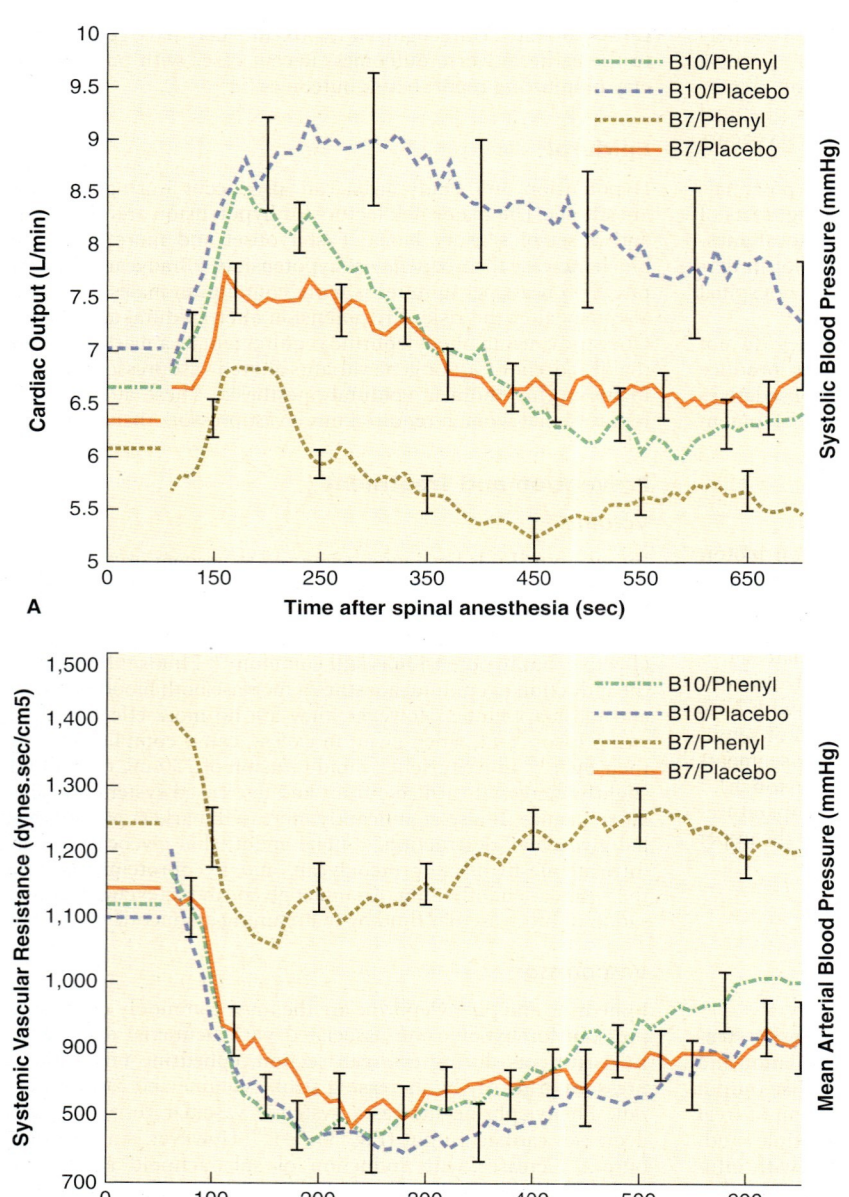

Figure 35-33 Mean differences in cardiac output (**A**) and systemic vascular resistance (**B**) in term parturients after intrathecal injection of 7 (B7) or 10 (B10) mg isobaric bupivacaine. Placebo patients received a normal saline intravenous infusion after injection. Phenyl patients received an intravenous infusion of phenylephrine after injection. (Adapted from Langesaeter E, Rosseland LA, Shubhaug A. Continuous invasive blood pressure and cardiac output monitoring during cesarean delivery. *Anesthesiology.* 2008;109:856–863.)

anesthesia. Meta-analysis of these results suggests that ondansetron may halve the risk of subarachnoid anesthesia-induced hypotension.[107] Ondansetron also limited the risk of bradycardia, nausea, and vomiting. Unfortunately, the small number of patients studied to date and the high likelihood publication bias limits the strength of these conclusions.[108]

Respiratory System

Subarachnoid and epidural anesthesia have little effect on pulmonary function. Although patients often note chest tightness and dyspnea with thoracic levels of sensory block, respiratory function is usually unchanged. One study reported decreased forced vital capacity (FVC) and one second forced expiratory volume (FEV(1)) only in patients over 60 years old with subarachnoid block above T6.[109] Cervical levels neuraxial block can impair diaphragmatic function and produce significant respiratory compromise.

Gastrointestinal System

Neuraxial anesthesia-induced sympathetic block leads to unopposed vagal stimulation of the gastrointestinal system. Secretions increase, sphincters relax and the bowel constricts. Many patients experience nausea and vomiting. Risk factors for nausea and vomiting include: female gender, opioid premedication and high level of block.[94] At cesarean section, nausea and vomiting are strongly associated with maternal hypotension.

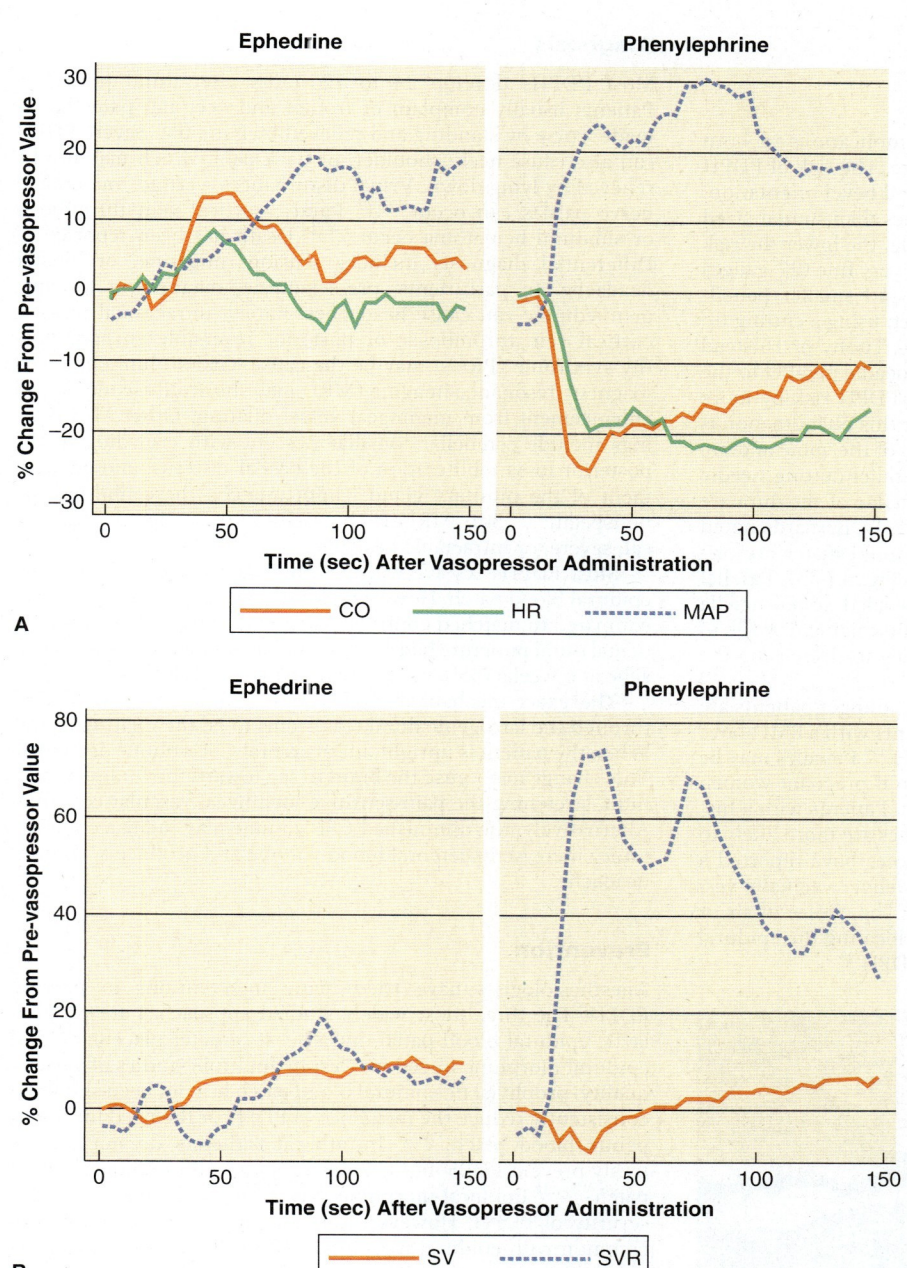

Figure 35-34 **A:** Percentage changes from prevasopressor values in cardiac output (CO), heart rate (HR), and mean arterial pressure (MAP) after the administration of phenylephrine or ephedrine. **B:** Percentage changes from prevasopressor values, in stroke volume (SV), and systemic vascular resistance (SVR) after the administration of phenylephrine or ephedrine. (Adapted from Dyer RA, Reed AR, van Dyk D, et al. Hemodyamic effects of ephedrine, phenylephrine, and the coadministration of phenylephrine with oxytocin during spinal anesthesia for elective cesarean delivery. Anesthesiology. 2009;111:753–765.)

Temperature Homeostasis

Hypothermia occurs routinely. Neuraxial anesthesia inhibits central thermoregulatory control. More importantly, block of peripheral sympathetic and motor nerves prevents vasoconstriction and shivering. As with general anesthesia, body temperature initially falls because heat redistributes from the core to the periphery. Heat loss continues through convection, radiation, and evaporation. Eventually, shivering may arise in the upper extremities, but this response does little to maintain body temperature.[110] Forced air warming, fluid warming, or both may limit the fall in maternal temperature after induction of subarachnoid anesthesia for cesarean section.[111]

Complications

Backache

Back pain is common after pregnancy. A poorly controlled, retrospective study published in 1990 suggested that labor epidural analgesia was associated with an increased risk of long-term backache.[112] Multiple subsequent studies have failed to confirm this association.[113] However, this concern may persist in some communities.[114] A recent case series reported that women who suffered an accidental dural puncture were more likely to report persistent backache at 6 weeks postpartum than women who had uncomplicated labor epidural analgesia (58% vs. 4%).[115]

Headache

Risk Factors

Headache is one of the most common complications of both intentional and unintentional dural puncture. The risk of PDPH correlates with the needle tip design, size, and bevel orientation. Pencil-point needles produce fewer headaches than similar sized cutting-point needles. The smaller the needle, the lower the risk of PDPH. This relationship persists down to very fine (27-gauge) cutting tip needles.[116] Twenty-four–gauge and smaller pencil-point needles carry similar PDPH risks. When using a cutting tip needle (i.e., Quincke point spinal needle or Tuohy or Hustead epidural needle), orienting the bevel of the needle parallel to the longitudinal axis of the back decreases the PDPH risk by more than half.[117,118] The common explanation for this phenomenon is that dural fibers run parallel to the long axis of the spine and are separated, not sliced when entered by a parallel cutting needle bevel. However, the collagen fibers and lamellae of the dura are oriented randomly, making this reason unlikely. Bernards noted that the cells of lamellar layer of the arachnoid mater are oriented parallel to the long axis of the spine (Fig. 35-35). Parallel puncture of the arachnoid mater with a beveled spinal needle results in a narrow slit-like hole. Perhaps minimizing damage to the arachnoid, not the dura mater, is the key to decreasing the frequency of PDPH.[25]

Other risk factors for PDPH include age; younger patients are *more* likely to develop PDPH and BMI; patients with a BMI above 30 kg/m² may be *less* likely to develop PDPH.[119] Females may be more susceptible to PDPH.[120] It is unknown if pregnant women are at greater risk than nonpregnant women. Patients with a history of PDPH or those with chronic headaches are more likely to develop a new PDPH.[121] Observational studies have reported a higher incidence of PDPH in women who deliver vaginally versus those who have a cesarean section.[81,119] The choice of air or saline for detecting loss of resistance while locating the epidural space does not influence the incidence of PDPH.[48]

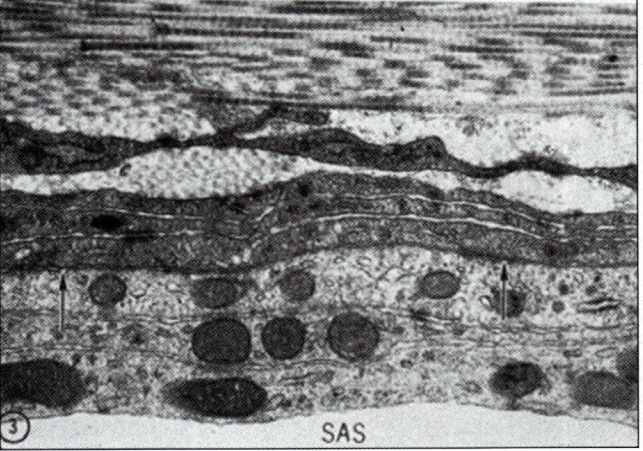

Figure 35-35 Transmission electron micrograph of the acellular dura mater (collagen bundles in the top one-third of the micrograph) and the cellular arachnoid mater (bottom two-thirds of the micrograph). *Arrows* indicate tight junctions, SAS indicates subarachnoid space, and *circled 3* identifies a mitochondrion. Note that the collagen bundles of the dura mater course in multiple planes (parallel, perpendicular, and oblique to the plane of section), whereas the arachnoid cells lie in a single plane oriented cephalocaudad. (Adapted from Bernards CM. Sophistry in medicine: lessons from the epidural space. *Reg Anesth Pain Med*. 2005;30:56–66.)

Diagnosis

Most PDPHs develop 24 to 72 hours after dural puncture. Patients usually complain of frontal and occipital pain that is made worse by standing and relieved by lying flat. Severe PDPH can also cause neck, shoulder, or back pain, which may not be relieved by lying down. Visual disturbances, vertigo, and cranial nerve palsies can occur.[122,123] Rarely, cortical vein thrombosis or subdural hematoma occur.[124,125] Death has been reported.[126] Differential diagnosis includes tension, migraine, or cluster headache. In parturients, pre-eclampsia, magnesium therapy, or nifedipine can cause headaches. Rarely, intracranial masses, cortical vein thrombosis, or posterior reversible encephalopathy syndrome (PRES) may be the cause. Gadolinium-enhanced magnetic resonance imaging (MRI) may show diffuse meningeal enhancement from meningeal vessel dilation. Other MRI findings include cerebellar tonsillar descent with crowding of the posterior fossa, obliteration of the basilar cisterns, and enlargement of the pituitary gland. Unfortunately, these findings are nonspecific.[121] Still, MRI may be useful in the patient with atypical, severe, or intractable headache.

Most PDPHs resolve within 5 to 7 days or after therapeutic epidural blood patch. However, two recent case series report that, compared to matched controls, parturients who suffered an accidental dural puncture had an increased incidence of chronic headache at 6 weeks (35% vs. 2%) and 24 months (28% vs. 5%).[115,127]

The exact mechanism of PDPH is unknown. Loss of CSF through the iatrogenic dural tear seems to be the inciting factor. When the patient is upright, intracerebral CSF volume decreases. This change may cause the brain to sag toward the foramen magnum, stretching the pain-sensitive meningeal vascular covering. Alternatively, the diminished CSF volume may incite a compensatory increase in cerebral blood volume and produce a vascular headache.

Prevention

Anesthesiologists have tried many interventions to prevent PDPH. The three most widely studied approaches are prophylactic epidural blood patch, intrathecal catheter placement, and epidural morphine injection. Despite multiple studies of varying quality, prophylactic epidural blood patch has not been shown to consistently reduce the incidence of PDPH or the need for therapeutic blood patch.[128,129] Intrathecal catheters do not consistently prevent PDPH but may lower the need for epidural blood patch.[130–132] Epidural morphine may decrease the frequency and severity of PDPH. However, itching, nausea, and vomiting are common with epidural morphine.[133] Two small case series have reported that intrathecal injection of 10 mL saline, either immediately after accidental dural puncture or just before removing an intrathecal catheter, is associated with a decreased need for epidural blood patch.[81,134]

Treatment/Epidural Blood Patch

Once PDPH develops, most therapy is symptomatic. Bed rest will often relieve PDPH pain but does not shorten its duration.[135] Neither oral nor intravenous hydration has any effect on PDPH.[135] Patients with PDPH should have access to adequate analgesics. Acetaminophen, nonsteroidal anti-inflammatory drugs (NSAIDs), and opioids can be effective. Caffeine may relieve the symptoms of PDPH but the data supporting its use are weak.

Epidural blood patch is the definitive therapy for PDPH. The efficacy of epidural blood patch has clearly been established in small, but well-conducted, randomized prospective trials.[136]

Most authors report that a single epidural blood patch cures 75% to 90% of PDPHs.[121,137] A second blood patch is usually effective for patients with incomplete relief or recurrent symptoms. However, a recent study reported a significantly lower success rate.[138] Only 67% of women reported headache relief after a single epidural blood patch. Fewer than 20% reported permanent relief. PDPH often recurred 4 to 5 days after the original blood patch. Twenty one percent of the women received a second epidural blood patch.[138] Eleven percent of women in a series of 917 epidural blood patches collected from 30 hospitals in the United States received a second blood patch.[77]

Unresolved questions about epidural blood patch include the timing of the procedure in relation to the original dural puncture and the volume of blood that should be injected. Several retrospective chart reviews have suggested that epidural blood patch is more likely to provide headache relief if it is performed at least 72 hours after dural puncture compared with less than 24 hours after puncture.[137,138] However, these types of studies cannot control for headache severity. A more severe PDPH may have both a more rapid onset and be more difficult to cure with an epidural blood patch.

The initial reports of epidural blood patch used very small volumes (2 to 3 mL) of blood. Since then, the volume of blood injected has steadily increased. Most authors now recommend around 20 mL.[138] Patients often report back pain as blood is being injected into the epidural space. This pain usually recedes if the injection is halted. More blood can be injected after a moment or two. Stop trying to add more blood if the back pain returns immediately after resuming injection. Mild back pain is common after epidural blood patch. Serious complications are rare. However, epidural hematoma requiring surgical decompression has been reported.[139] Another patient with idiopathic intracranial hypertension developed acute vision loss after rapid epidural injection of 25 mL autologous blood.[140]

Hearing Loss

Transient, low frequency hearing loss can occur after subarachnoid anesthesia.[141] This complication may be more common in the elderly.[142] Hearing loss is presumably due to the effects of decreased CSF pressure on inner ear function. The risk of hearing loss is lower with smaller-gauge versus larger-gauge spinal needles.[141] Although hearing usually returns to normal in about 1 month, permanent loss has been reported.[143]

High Block/Total Subarachnoid Spinal Block

Subarachnoid and epidural anesthesia have enviable safety records. However, high levels of sensory block can occur. If unrecognized or not managed properly, high levels of block can produce respiratory compromise and cardiac arrest.[144] The exact frequency of these events is unknown. High neuraxial block (otherwise undefined) complicated approximately 1 in 4,000 obstetric neuraxial anesthetics.[77] Suggested, but unproven, risk factors for high block included obesity, short stature, subarachnoid block after failed epidural, repeat epidural after unintended dural puncture, and spinal deformity. A disturbing cause of high block in laboring women is unrecognized intrathecal injection during attempted labor epidural analgesia.[77,78,81]

High neuraxial block can produce both cardiac and respiratory instability. Extensive sympathetic block can lead to hypotension and bradycardia. Extensive sympathetic block combined with moderate to deep sedation (and presumed hypoxemia) can lead to sudden cardiac arrest, even in otherwise healthy young patients. In a series of 14 such arrests, prompt treatment with ephedrine, atropine, and chest compressions, but delayed administration of epinephrine produced uniformly poor neurologic outcomes. More rapid treatment with epinephrine might help counter the subarachnoid anesthesia-induced sympathetic block and lead to better results.[96] High neuraxial block can also produce significant respiratory compromise. Although patients often note chest tightness and dyspnea with thoracic levels of sensory block, respiratory function is usually unchanged. As the block ascends into the cervical regions, handgrip will weaken. Lastly, blocks to C3–C5 will impair diaphragmatic function. These patients will only be able to whisper. They should be ventilated promptly and intubated if needed. When faced with a high level of sensory block after intrathecal injection of hyperbaric local anesthetic, you may be tempted to limit the rising block by placing the patient in reverse Trendelenburg position. Don't! This position may decrease the cephalad spread of sensory block but it will cause the patient's blood to pool in the legs, exacerbating the hypotensive effects of subarachnoid anesthesia. Reverse Trendelenburg position will also decrease blood flow to the brain, further hampering respiration. Instead, flex the patient's head at the neck. This may help prevent further cervical spread of the local anesthetic. Continue to monitor the patient's respiratory and cardiovascular status and intervene as needed.

Systemic Toxicity

Systemic local anesthetic toxicity can follow absorption from the epidural space or unrecognized intravascular injection. Signs and symptoms range from tinnitus and metallic taste to seizures and cardiac arrest. Important safety steps to prevent local anesthetic toxicity include incremental injection, limiting the total dose of local anesthetic and using a test dose that contains a marker in intravascular injection.[82] Incremental injection of 3 to 5 mL of local anesthetic every 90 to 120 seconds is probably the most effective of these steps. Treatment of local anesthetic toxicity is discussed in Chapter 22.

Neurologic Injury

Neurologic injury is a rare, but potentially catastrophic complication of neuraxial block. Serious or permanent neurologic harm may occur after 1:20,000 to 35,000 neuraxial blocks.[77,145] Direct trauma, mass effect, and physiologic damage can cause neurologic injury.[146]

Needle Trauma

Spinal and epidural needles can damage both the spinal cord and nerve roots (Fig. 35-36). Although the spinal cord typically ends at L1–L2 in adults, the exact termination varies and the cord extends farther caudad in children. In addition, anesthesiologists using palpation often misidentify the lumbar interspaces and end up inserting needles at a higher level than intended.[18] Permanent damage to the conus medullaris has been reported after attempted subarachnoid or CSE anesthesia at the presumed L2–L3 vertebral interspace.[147] In parturients, using the space just below, instead of above, the palpated intercristal line can decrease the frequency of inserting the spinal or epidural needle at or above L2–L3.[148] Lateral deviation of the needle may injure

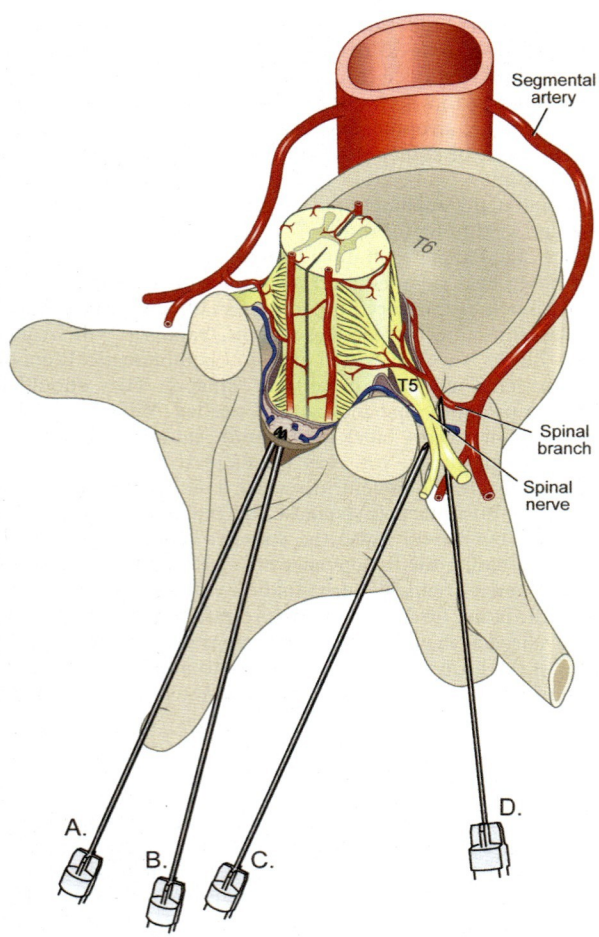

Figure 35-36 Midline or paramedian approaches (needles *A* and *B*) may directly traumatize the spinal cord, whereas unintentional lateral deviation of the needle (*C*) may contact the spinal nerve or the anterior or posterior primary ramus outside the foramen. Intentional lateral approaches, for example, transforaminal approach (needle *D*), have the potential to come in close proximity to the spinal nerve or a spinal artery. Note that transforaminal approaches are typically at the cervical or lumbar levels, not the T6 level as illustrated. (Illustration by Gary J. Nelson. From Neal JM, Kopp SL, Pasternak JJ, et al. Anatomy and pathophysiology of spinal cord injury associated with regional anesthesia and pain medicine: 2015 update. *Reg Anesth Pain Med.* 2015;40:506–525.)

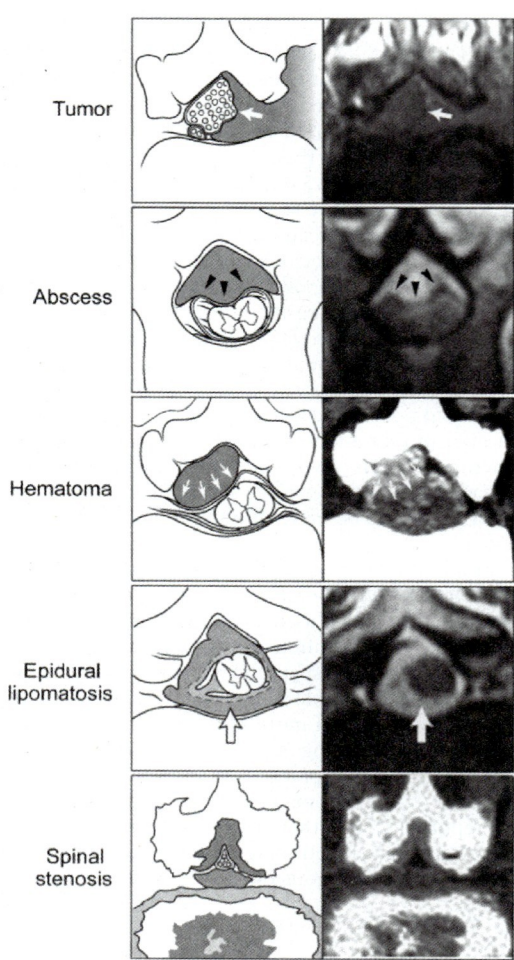

Figure 35-37 Extradural mass lesions. Note how various conditions can reduce spinal canal cross-sectional area and either directly compress the spinal cord or the cauda equina (*arrows*) or increase epidural space or CSF pressures through their mass effect.

the spinal nerve or the anterior or posterior primary ramus outside the foramen (Fig. 35-36).[146]

The risk of direct spinal cord injury is highest with cervical epidural injection. The cervical epidural space is narrow and the underlying spinal cord is vulnerable to needle trauma. Injury associated with cervical epidural injection was the most common damaging event in a recent review of pain medicine malpractice claims. Cervical epidural injections represent fewer than one-quarter of epidural injections but generate two-thirds of epidural injection related claims.[149]

Mass Lesions

Mass lesions also can injure the spinal cord (Fig. 35-37). These lesions can compress the spinal cord and decrease perfusion pressure. Spinal cord ischemia or infarction can follow. Abscess and hematoma are the most widely studied compressive complications of neuraxial block. Significant hematoma may occur as often as 1:3,600 blocks or as rarely as 1:260,000.[145] Patients undergoing orthopedic procedures and those taking medications that interfere with coagulation are at greatest risk.[144,145,150,151] Hematoma is more common after epidural than subarachnoid block.[152] Hematoma also can occur after removing an epidural catheter. The American Society of Regional Anesthesia has a regularly updated guideline (www.asra.com/advisory-guidelines) that provides recommendations for the safe use of neuraxial block in patients taking antithrombotic or thrombolytic medications.

Epidural abscess is less common, complicating approximately 1:100,000 neuraxial blocks. Rarely, the combination of neuraxial local anesthetics and other mass lesions (tumors, lipomas, cysts, or granulomas) can produce compressive symptoms (Fig. 35-37).[146]

Patients with mass lesions may present with severe back pain. Other worrisome signs are persistent or recurrent sensory or motor block and bowel or bladder dysfunction. MRI provides more useful information about soft tissues and spinal canal pathology than computed tomography (CT). However, if MRI is not immediately available, CT can detect space-occupying lesions that

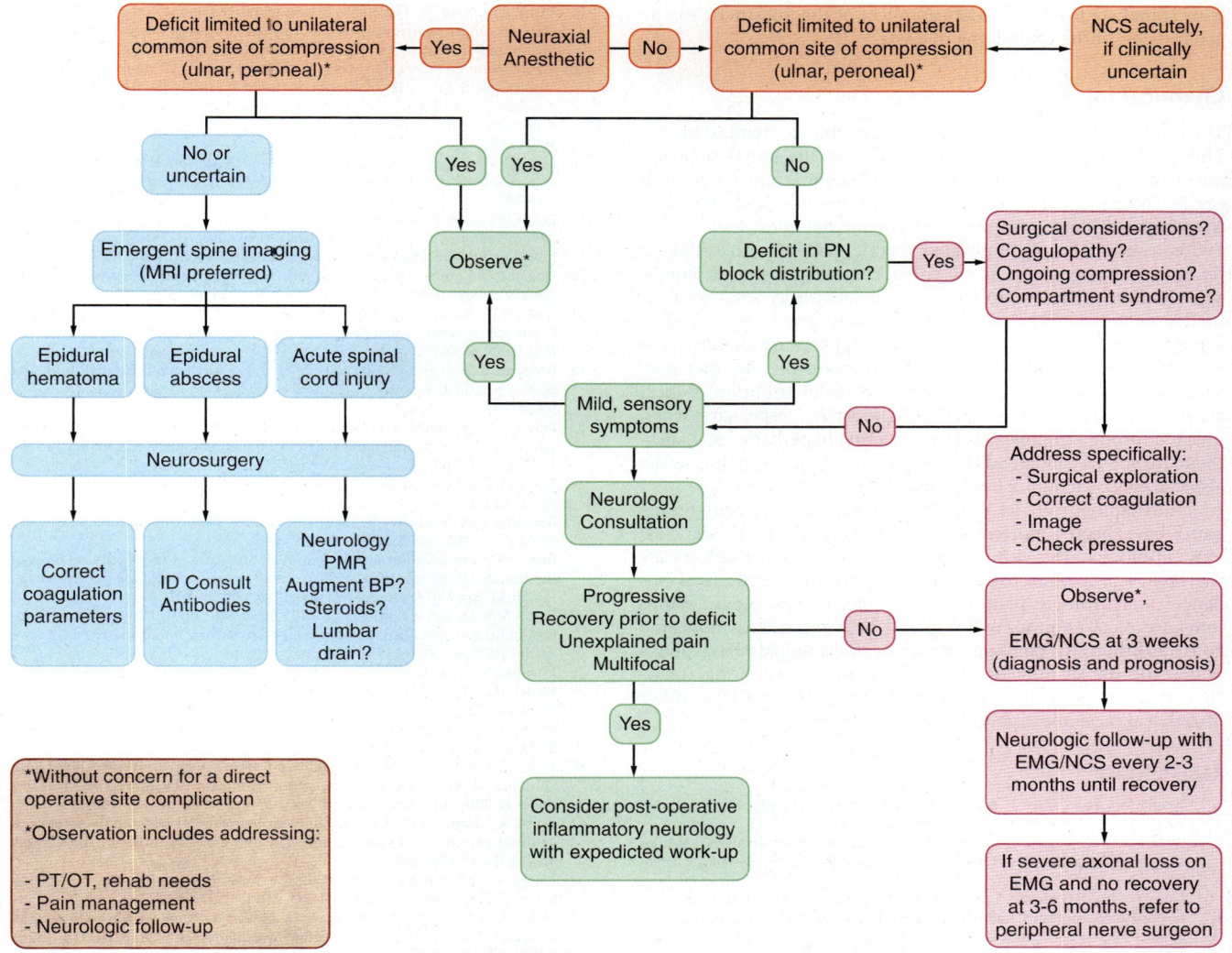

Figure 35-38 Approach to perioperative nerve injury. BP, blood pressure; EMG, electromyography; NCS, nerve conduction studies; PMR, physical medicine rehabilitation specialty consultation; PN, peripheral nerve. (Adapted from Watson JC, Huntoon MA. Neurologic evaluation and management of perioperative nerve injury. Reg Anesth Pain Med. 2015;40:491–501.)

may require immediate surgical intervention. Complete or partial neurologic recovery seems most likely if surgical decompression occurs within 8 to 12 hours of symptom onset.[146] However, complete recovery may occur even after a longer delay.[151] Figure 35-38 shows a systematic approach to the evaluation and treatment of a patient with suspected perioperative nerve injury.[153]

Hypoperfusion

Other potential causes of spinal cord ischemia include direct needle trauma to the spinal cord vasculature, prolonged hypoperfusion related to systemic hypotension, and spinal stenosis. Direct needle trauma to spinal vessels is extremely rare. Spinal cord ischemia or infarction related to systemic hypotension also is unusual. However, there are cases of ischemic spinal cord injury attributed to a prolonged period of hypotension.[146] Risks may include spinal stenosis, anemia (reduced oxygen-carrying capacity), hypocapnia, raised intrathoracic pressure (e.g., during mechanical ventilation in lung-injured patients), extremes of patient position, chronic hypertension, unrecognized vascular abnormalities, and variation in the lower level autoregulation of cerebral blood flow. Current guidelines, based only on expert opinion, suggest keeping blood pressure within 20% to 30% of baseline.[146] However, rare, uniquely susceptible patients may suffer spinal cord ischemia during an otherwise routine subarachnoid anesthetic.[154]

Spinal Stenosis

Pre-existing spinal stenosis also may increase the risk of neurologic injury after neuraxial block. Osteoporosis can cause degenerative spinal stenosis. Also, hypertrophy of the ligamentum flavum and bony elements of the spinal canal can reduce spinal canal cross-sectional area, limiting space for the spinal cord and nerve roots. Spinal stenosis, combined with degenerative narrowing of the intervertebral foramina, may lead to increased vertebral canal pressure and decreased spinal cord blood flow after neuraxial injection of local anesthetics. Currently, it is unclear if worsening neurologic symptoms after neuraxial block in patients with spinal stenosis represents an effect of the anesthetic or the progression of the underlying disease.[152,155]

Chemical Injury

The cauda equina may be especially susceptible to chemical injury. These nerve roots travel long distances within the spinal canal and are not extensively myelinated.[146] Direct chemical injury can cause cauda equina syndrome, adhesive arachnoiditis and, possibly, transient neurologic symptoms after neuraxial anesthesia. In the 1980s, a series of cases implicated unrecognized intrathecal injection of 2-chloroprocaine as a cause of cauda equina syndrome or adhesive arachnoiditis. Most, but not all, laboratory studies attributed this complication to the sodium bisulfate preservative. Today, some centers use preservative-free 2-chloroprocaine for subarachnoid anesthesia without reported complications.[156] Another possible cause of cauda equina syndrome is maldistribution of local anesthetics, most often hyperbaric lidocaine, especially when injected through a spinal catheter. Injecting hyperbaric local anesthetic through a caudally directed, side-holed, pencil-point needle also can cause sacral pooling of drug.[45]

Transient neurologic symptoms (persistent low back and leg pain) have been reported after subarachnoid anesthesia. The exact etiology of this complication is unclear. Some think it may represent subtle neurologic toxicity.[146] But, there is no firm evidence of neurologic pathology.[157] Transient neurologic symptoms are most commonly associated with intrathecal lidocaine and the lithotomy position. Most anesthesiologists have abandoned the use of lidocaine for subarachnoid anesthesia. Transient neurologic symptoms are much less common after other intrathecal local anesthetics.[146,157]

REFERENCES

1. Yeager M, Glass D, Neff R, et al. Epidural anesthesia and analgesia in high-risk surgical patients. *Anesthesiology*. 1987;66:729–736.
2. Bode R, Lewis KP, Zarach SW, et al. Cardiac outcome after peripheral vascular surgery. Comparison of general and regional anesthesia. *Anesthesiology*. 1996; 84:3–13.
3. Guay J, Choi PT, Suresh S, et al. Neuraxial anesthesia for the prevention of postoperative mortality and major morbidity: an overview of Cochrane Systematic Reviews. *Anesth Analg*. 2014;119:716–725.
4. Neuman MD, Silber JH, Elkassabany NM, et al. Comparative effectiveness of regional versus general anesthesia for hip fracture surgery in adults. *Anesthesiology*. 2012;117:72–92.
5. Neuman MD, Rosenbaum PR, Ludwig JM, et al. Anesthesia technique, mortality, and length of stay after hip fracture surgery. *JAMA*. 2014;311:2508–2517.
6. Memtsoudis SG, Sun X, Chiu YL, et al. Perioperative comparative effectiveness of anesthetic technique in orthopedic patients. *Anesthesiology*. 2013; 118:1046–1058.
7. Chery J, Semaan E, Darji S, et al. Impact of regional versus general anesthesia on the clinical outcomes of patients undergoing major lower extremity amputation. *Ann Vasc Surg*. 2014;28:1149–1156.
8. Hausman MS, Jewell ES, Engoren M. Regional versus general anesthesia in surgical patients with chronic obstructive pulmonary disease: Does avoiding general anesthesia reduce the risk of postoperative complications? *Anesth Analg*. 2015;120:1405–1412.
9. Liu J, Ma C, Elkassabany N, et al. Neuraxial anesthesia decreases postoperative systemic infections risk compared with general anesthesia in knee arthroplasty. *Anesth Analg*. 2013;117:1010–1016.
10. Pugely AJ, Martin CT, Gao Y, et al. Differences in short-term complications between spinal and general anesthesia for primary total knee arthroplasty. *J Bone Joint Surg Am*. 2013;95(3):193–199.
11. Whiting PS, Molina CS, Greenberg SE, et al. Regional anaesthesia for hip fracture surgery is associated with significantly more peri-operative complications compared with general anaesthesia. *Int Orthopaedics*. 2015;39:1321–1327.
12. Modig J, Borg T, Karlstrom G, et al. Thromboembolism after total hip replacement: role of epidural and general anesthesia. *Anesth Analg*. 1983;62:174–180.
13. Barbosa FT, Jucá MJ, Castro AA, et al. Neuraxial anaesthesia for lower-limb revascularization (Review). *Cochrane Database Syst Rev*. 2013;7:CD007083.
14. Wiis JT, Jensen-Gadegaard P, Altintas U, et al. One-week postoperative patency of lower extremity in situ bypass graft comparing epidural and generalanesthesia: retrospective study of 822 patients. *Ann Vasc Surg*. 2014;28:295–300.
15. Sun Y, Li T, Gan TJ. The effects of perioperative regional anesthesia and analgesia on cancer recurrence and survival after oncology surgery. A systematic review and meta-analysis. *Reg Anesth Pain Med*. 2015;40:589–598.
16. Prats-Galino A, Reina MA, Mavar Haramija M, et al. 3D interactive model of lumbar spinal structures of anesthetic interest. *Clin Anat*. 2015;28:205–212.
17. Avrahami E, Cohn DF, Yaron M. Computerized tomography, clinical and X-ray correlations in the hemisacralized fifth lumbar vertebra. *Clin Rheumatol*. 1986;5:332–337.
18. Lee AJ, Ranasinghe JS, Chehade JM, et al. Ultrasound assessment of the vertebral level of the intercristal line in pregnancy. *Anesth Analg*. 2011;113: 559–564.
19. Reina MA, Lirk P, Puigdellívol-Sánchez A, et al. Human lumbar ligamentum flavum anatomy for epidural anesthesia: reviewing a 3D MR-based interactive model and postmortem samples. *Anesth Analg*. 2016;122:903–907.
20. Hogan QH. Lumbar epidural anatomy, a new look by cryomicrotome section. *Anesthesiology*. 1999;75:767–775.
21. Reina, MA, Franco, CD, Lopez A, et al. Clinical implications of epidural fat in the spinal canal. A scanning electron microscopic study. *Acta Anaesthesiol Belg*. 2009;60:7–17.
22. Bernards CM, Shen DD, Sterling ES, et al. Epidural, cerebrospinal fluid, and plasma pharmacokinetics of epidural opioids (Part 1). *Anesthesiology*. 2003; 99:455–465.
23. Reina MA, Dittmann M, Lopez Garcia A, et al. New perspectives in the microscopic structure of human dura mater in the dorsolumbar region. *Reg Anesth*. 1997;22:161–166.
24. Reina MA, de Leon Casasola O, Lopez A, et al. The origin of the spinal subdural space: ultrastructure findings. *Anesth Analg*. 2002;94:991–995.
25. Bernards CM. Sophistry in medicine: lessons from the epidural space. *Reg Anesth Pain Med*. 2005;30:56–66.
26. Reina MA, Prats-Galino A, Sola RG, et al. Structure of the arachnoid layer of the human spinal meninges: a barrier that regulates dural sac permeability]. [Spanish]. *Rev Esp Anestesiol Reanim*. 2010;57:486–492.
27. Reina MA, De Leon Casasola O, Villanueva MC, et al. Ultrastructural findings in human spinal pia mater in relation to subarachnoid anesthesia. *Anesth Analg*. 2004;98:1479–1485.
28. Miyajima M, Arai H. Evaluation of the production and absorption of cerebrospinal fluid. *Neurol Med Chir (Tokyo)*. 2015;55:647–656.
29. Bulat M, Lupret V, Orehkovic D, et al. Transventricular and transpial absorption of cerebrospinal fluid into cerebral microvessels. *Coll Antropol*. 2008;32:43–50.
30. Prats-Galino A, Reina MA, Puigdellivol-Sanchez A, et al. Cerebrospinal fluid volume and nerve root vulnerability during lumbar puncture or spinal anaesthesia at different vertebral levels. *Anaesth Intensive Care*. 2012;40:643–647.
31. Perlas A, Chaparro LE, Chin KJ. Lumbar neuraxial ultrasound for spinal and epidural anesthesia: A systematic review and meta-analysis. *Reg Anesth Pain Med*. 2016;41:251–260.
32. Lee PJ, Tang R, Sawka A, et al. Real-time ultrasound-guided spinal anesthesia using Taylor's approach. *Anesth Analg*. 2011;112:1236–1238.
33. Balki M. Locating the epidural space in obstetric patients—ultrasound a useful tool: Continuing professional development. *Can J Anesth*. 2010;57:1111–1126.
34. Polley LS. Neuraxial techniques for labor analgesia should be placed in the lateral position (Con). *Int J Obstet Anesth*. 2008;17:149–152.
35. Vincent RD, Chestnut DH. Which position is more comfortable for the parturient during induction of epidural anesthesia? *Int J Obstet Anesth*. 1991;1:9–11.
36. Jones AR, Carle C, Columb M. Effect of table tilt on ligamentum flavum length measured using ultrasonography in pregnant women. *Anaesthesia*. 2013;68: 27–30.
37. Kapur D, Grimsehl K. A comparison of cerebrospinal fluid pressure and block height after spinal anaesthesia in the right and left lateral position in pregnant women undergoing cesarean section. *Eur J Anaesth*. 2001;18:668–672.
38. Taenzer AH, Walker BJ, Bosenberg AT, et al. Asleep versus awake: Does it matter? Pediatric regional block complications by patient state: A report from the Pediatric Regional Anesthesia Network. *Reg Anesth Pain Med*. 2014;39: 279–283.
39. Bromage PR, Benumof JL. Paraplegia following intracord injection during attempted epidural anesthesia under general anesthesia. *Reg Anesth Pain Med*. 1998;23:104–107.
40. Bernards CM, Hadzic A, Suresh S, et al. Regional anesthesia in anesthetized or heavily sedated patient. *Reg Anesth Pain Med*. 2008;33:449–460.
41. American Society of Anesthesiologists Task Force on infectious complications associated with neuraxial techniques. Practice Advisory for the prevention, diagnosis, and management of infectious complications with neuraxial techniques. *Anesthesiology*. 2010;112:530–545.
42. Birnbach DJ, Stein DJ, Murray O, et al. Providone iodine and skin disinfection before initiation of epidural anesthesia. *Anesthesiology*. 1998;88:668–672.
43. Birnbach DJ, Meadows W, Stein DJ, et al. Comparison of povidone iodine and DuraPrep, an iodophor-in-isopropyl alcohol solution, for skin disinfection prior to epidural catheter insertion in parturients. *Anesthesiology*. 2003; 98:164–169.
44. Pong, RP, Gmelch BS, Bernards CM. Does a paresthesia during spinal needle insertion indicate intrathecal needle placement? *Reg Anesth Pain Med*. 2009;34:29–32.

45. Holman SJ, Robinson RA, Beardsley D, et al. Hyperbaric dye solution distribution characteristics after pencil-point needle injection in a spinal cord model. *Anesthesiology.* 1997;86:966–973.
46. Stroumpoulis K, Stamatakis E, Koutroumanis P, et al. Pencil-point needle bevel direction influences ED50 of isobaric ropivacaine with fentanyl in spinal anesthesia for cesarean delivery: a prospective, double-blind sequential allocation study. *Int J Obstet Anesth.* 2015;24:225–229.
47. Aida S, Taga K, Yamakura T, et al. Headache after attempted epidural block: the role of intrathecal air. *Anesthesiology.* 1998;88:76–81.
48. Antibas PL, do Nascimento P Jr, Braz LG, et al. Air versus saline in the loss of resistance technique for identification of the epidural space. [Review]. *Cochrane Database Syst Rev.* 2014;7:CD008938.
49. Segal S, Arendt KW. A retrospective effectiveness study of loss of resistance to air or saline for identification of the epidural space. *Anesth Analg.* 2010;110:558–563.
50. Bromage PR. *Epidural Analgesia.* Philadelphia, PA: WB Saunders; 1978.
51. Doughty A. Paternity of the Doughty technique. *Anaesthesia.* 2005;60:1242–1243.
52. Reynolds F. Hand positions and the 'son-of-Doughty' technique. *Anaesthesia.* 2005;60:717–718.
53. Beilin Y, Bernstein HH, Zucker-Pinchoff B. The optimal distance that a multiorifice epidural catheter should be threaded into the epidural space. *Anesth Analg.* 1995;81:301–304.
54. Capiello E, O'Rourke N, Segal S, et al. A randomized trial of dural puncture epidural technique compared with the standard epidural technique for labor analgesia. *Anesth Analg.* 2008;107:1646–1651.
55. Ross VH, Dean LS, Thomas JA, et al. Techniques in morbidly obese parturients undergoing cesarean delivery: time for initiation of anesthesia. *Anesth Analg.* 2014;118:168–172.
56. Hsu Y, Hettiarachchi M, Zhu DC, et al. The frequency and magnitude of cerebrospinal fluid pulsations influence intrathecal drug distribution: Key factors for interpatient variability. *Anesth Analg.* 2012;115:386–394.
57. Xu F, Qian M, Wei Y, et al. Postural change from lateral to supine is an important mechanism enhancing cephalic spread after injection of intrathecal 0.5% plain bupivacaine for cesarean section. *Int J Obstet Anesth.* 2015;24:308–312.
58. Whiteside JB, Burke D, Wildsmith JA. Spinal anaesthesia with ropivacaine 5 mg/mL or 50 mg/L. *Br J Anaesth.* 2001;86:241–244.
59. Malinovsky JM, Renaud G, Le Corre P, et al. Intrathecal bupivacaine in humans: Influence of volume and baricity of solutions. *Anesthesiology.* 1999;91:1260–1266.
60. Sia AT, Tan KH, Sng BL, et al. Use of hyperbaric versus isobaric bupivacaine for spinal anaesthesia for caesarean section. [Review]. *Cochrane Database Syst Rev.* 2013;5:CD005143.
61. Hocking G, Wildsmith JAW. Intrathecal drug spread. *Br J Anaesth.* 2004;93:568–578.
62. Camorcia M, Capogna G, Columb MO. Effect of sex and pregnancy on the potency of intrathecal bupivacaine: determination of ED50 for motor block with the up–down sequential allocation method. *Eur J Anaesthesiol.* 2011;28:240–244.
63. Carpenter RL, Hogan QH, Liu SS, et al. Lumbosacral cerebrospinal fluid volume is the primary determinant of sensory block extent and duration during spinal anesthesia. *Anesthesiology.* 1998;89:4–9.
64. Teoh WH, Ithnin F, Sia AT. Comparison of an equal-dose spinal anesthetic for cesarean section and for post partum tubal ligation. *Int J Obstet Anesth.* 2008;17:228–232.
65. Zhou QH, Xiao WP, Shen YY. Abdominal girth, vertebral column length, and spread of spinal anesthesia in 30 minutes after plain bupivacaine 5 mg/mL. *Anesth Analg.* 2014;119:203–206.
66. De Simone CA, Leighton BL, Norris MC. Spinal anesthesia for cesarean section: A comparison of two doses of hyperbaric bupivacaine. *Reg Anesth.* 1995;20:90–94.
67. Abdallah FW, Abrishami A, Brull R. The facilitatory effects of intravenous dexmedetomidine on the duration of spinal anesthesia: a systematic review and meta-analysis. [Review]. *Anesth Analg.* 2013;117:271–278.
68. De Kock M, Gautier P, Fanard L, et al. Intrathecal ropivacaine and clonidine for ambulatory knee arthroscopy. *Anesthesiology.* 2001; 94:574–578.
69. Visser WA, Lee RA, Gielen MJM. Factors affecting the distribution of neural blockade by local anesthetics in epidural anesthesia and a comparison of lumbar versus thoracic epidural anesthesia. *Anesth Analg.* 2008;107:708–721.
70. Arakawa M. Does pregnancy increase the efficacy of lumbar epidural anesthesia? *Int J Obstet Anesth.* 2004;13:86–90.
71. Yokoyama M, Hanazaki M, Fujii H, et al. Correlation between the distribution of contrast medium and the extent of blockade during epidural anesthesia. *Anesthesiology.* 2004;100:1504–1510.
72. Hillyard SG, Bate TE, Corcoran TB, et al. Extending epidural analgesia for emergency caesarean section: a meta-analysis. *Br J Anaesth.* 2011;107:668–678.
73. Kinsella SM. A prospective audit of regional anaesthesia failure in 5080 Caesarean sections. *Anaesthesia.* 2008;63:822–832.
74. Eisenach JC, De Kock M, Klimscha W. Alpha2-adrenergic agonists for regional anesthesia. A clinical review of clonidine (1984–1995). *Anesthesiology.* 1996;85:655–674.
75. Tong Y, Ren H, Ding X, et al. Analgesic effect and adverse events of dexmedetomidine as additive for pediatric caudal anesthesia: a meta-analysis. [Review]. *Paediatr Anaesth.* 2014;24:1224–1230.
76. Youssef N, Orlov D, Alie T, et al. What epidural opioid results in the best analgesia outcomes and fewest side effects after surgery? A meta-analysis of randomized controlled trials. *Anesth Analg.* 2014;119:965–977.
77. D'Angelo R, Smiley R, Riley ET, et al. Serious complications related to obstetric anesthesia. The serious complication repository project of the Society for Obstetric Anesthesia and Perinatology. *Anesthesiology.* 2014;120:1505–1512.
78. Davies JM, Posner KL, Lee LA, et al. Liability associated with obstetric anesthesia. A closed claims analysis. *Anesthesiology.* 2009;110:131–139.
79. Pratt S, Vasudevan A, Hess P. A prospective randomized trial of lidocaine 30 mg versus 45 mg for epidural test dose for intrathecal injection in the obstetric population. *Anesth Analg.* 2013;116:125–132.
80. Richardson MG, Lee AC, Wissler RN. High spinal anesthesia after epidural test dose administration in five obstetric patients. *Reg Anesth.* 1996;21:119–123.
81. Bolden N, Gebre E. Accidental dural puncture management. 10-Year experience at an academic tertiary care center. *Reg Anesth Pain Med.* 2016;41:169–174.
82. Guay J. The epidural test dose: A review. *Anesth Analg.* 2006;102:921–929.
83. Norris MC, Ferrenbach D, Dalman H, et al. Does epinephrine improve the diagnostic accuracy of aspiration during labor epidural analgesia? *Anesth Analg.* 1999;88:1073–1076.
84. Reina MA, Collier CB, Prats-Galino A, et al. Unintentional subdural placement of epidural catheters during attempted epidural anesthesia. An anatomic study of spinal subdural compartment. *Reg Anesth Pain Med.* 2011;36:537–541.
85. Boswell MV, Iacono RP, Guthkelch AN. Sites of action of subarachnoid lidocaine and tetracaine: observations with evoked potential monitoring during spinal cord stimulator implantation. *Reg Anesth.* 1992;17:37–42.
86. Cusick JF, Myklebust JB, Abrams SE. Differential neural effects of epidural anesthetics. *Anesthesiology.* 1980;53:299–306.
87. Dahl JB, Rosenberg J, Lund C, et al. Effect of thoracic epidural bupivacaine 0.75% on somatosensory evoked potentials after dermatomal stimulation. *Reg Anesth.* 1990; 15:73–75.
88. Hodgson P, Liu SS, Gras TW. Does epidural anesthesia have general anesthetic effects? A prospective, randomized, double-blind, placebo-controlled trial. *Anesthesiology.* 1999;91:1687–1692.
89. Reinoso-Barbero F, Martinez-Garcia E, Hernandez-Gancedo C, et al. The effect of epidural bupivacaine on maintenance requirements of sevoflurane evaluated by bispectral index in children. *Eur J Anaesthesiol.* 2006;23:460–464.
90. Brull SJ, Greene NM. Zones of differential sensory block during extradural anaesthesia. *Br J Anaesth.* 1991;66:651–655.
91. Chamberlain DP, Chamberlain BD. Changes in the skin temperature of the trunk and their relationship to sympathetic blockade during spinal anesthesia. *Anesthesiology.* 1986;65:139–143.
92. Langesaeter E, Rosseland LA, Shubhaug A. Continuous invasive blood pressure and cardiac output monitoring during cesarean delivery. *Anesthesiology.* 2008;109:856–863.
93. Langesaeter E, Dyer RA. Maternal haemodynamic changes during spinal anaesthesia for caesarean section. *Curr Opin Anaesthesiol.* 2011;24:242–248.
94. Tarkkila P, Isola J. A regression model for identifying patients at high risk of hypotension, bradycardia and nausea during spinal anesthesia. *Acta Anaesthesiol Scand.* 1992;36:554–558.
95. Kumari A, Gupta R, Bajwa SJ, et al. Unanticipated cardiac arrest under spinal anesthesia: An unavoidable mystery with review of current literature. *Anesth Essays Res.* 2014;8:99–102.
96. Caplan RA, Ward RJ, Posner K, et al. Unexpected cardiac arrest during spinal anesthesia: A closed claims analysis of predisposing factors. *Anesthesiology.* 1988;68:5–11.
97. Dyamanna DN, Bs SK, Zacharia BT. Unexpected bradycardia and cardiac arrest under spinal anesthesia: case reports and review of literature. *Middle East J Anaesthesiol.* 2013;22:121–125.
98. Curatolo M, Scaramozzin P, Venuti FS, et al. Factors associated with hypotension after epidural blockade. *Anesth Analg.* 1996;83:1033–1040.
99. Frey UH, Karlik J, Herbstreit F, et al. B2-adrenoreceptor gene variants vasopressor requirements in patients after thoracic epidural anaesthesia. *Br J Anaesth.* 2011;112:477–484.
100. Norris MC. Hypotension during spinal anesthesia for cesarean section: Does it affect neonatal outcome? *Reg Anesth.* 1997;12:191–194.
101. Mercier FJ, Diemunsch P, Ducloy-Bouthors A-S, et al. 6% Hydroxyethyl starch (130/0.4) vs. Ringer's lactate preloading before spinal anaesthesia for Caesarean delivery: the randomized, double-blind, multicentre CAESAR trial. *Br J Anaesth.* 2014;113:459–467.
102. Holte K, Foss NB, Svensen C, et al. Epidural anesthesia, hypotension and changes in intravascular volume. *Anesthesiology.* 2004;100:281–286.
103. Powell M, Mathru M, Brandon A, et al. Assessment of endothelial glycocalyx disruption in term parturients receiving a fluid bolus before spinal anesthesia: a prospective observational study. *Int J Obstet Anesth.* 2014;23:330–334.
104. Dyer RA, Reed AR, van Dyk D, et al. Hemodynamic effects of ephedrine, phenylephrine, and the coadministration of phenylephrine with oxytocin during spinal anesthesia for elective cesarean delivery. *Anesthesiology.* 2009;111:753–765.

105. Ngan Kee WD, Lee SWY, Ng FF, et al. Randomized double-blinded comparison of norepinephrine and phenylephrine for maintenance for blood pressure during spinal anesthesia for cesarean delivery. *Anesthesiology.* 2015;122:736–745.
106. Watts SW, Morrison SF, Davis RP, et al. Serotonin and blood pressure regulation. *Pharmacol Rev.* 2012;64:359–388.
107. Gao L, Zheng L, Han J, et al. Effects of prophylactic ondansetron on spinal anesthesia-induced hypotension: a meta-analysis. *Int J Obstet Anesth.* 2015;24:335–343.
108. Terkawi AS, Mavridis D, Flood P, et al. Does ondansetron modify sympathectomy due to subarachnoid anesthesia? Meta-analysis, meta-regression, and trial sequential analysis. *Anesthesiology.* 2016;124:846–869.
109. Ogurlu M, Sen S, Polatli M, et al. The effect of spinal anesthesia on pulmonary function tests in old patients. *Tuberk Toraks.* 2007;55:64–70.
110. Sessler DI. Perioperative heat balance. *Anesthesiology.* 2000;92:578–596.
111. Sultan P, Habib AS, Cho Y, et al. The effect of patient warming during caesarean delivery on maternal and neonatal outcomes: a meta-analysis. *Br J Anaesth.* 2015;115:500–510.
112. MacArthur C, Lewis M, Knox EG, et al. Epidural anaesthesia and long term backache after childbirth. *BMJ.* 1990;301:9–12.
113. Reynolds F. Obstetric problems? Blame the epidural! *Reg Anest Pain Med.* 2008;33:472–476.
114. Orejuela FJ, Garcia T, Green C, et al. Exploring factors influencing patient request for epidural analgesia on admission to labor and delivery in a predominantly Latino population. *J Immigr Minor Health.* 2012;14:287–291.
115. Ranganathan P, Golfeiz C, Phelps AL, et al. Chronic headache and backache are long-term sequelae of unintentional dural puncture in the obstetric population. *J Clin Anesth.* 2015;27:201–206.
116. Lambert DH, Hurley RJ, Hertwig L, et al. Role of needle gauge and tip configuration in the production of lumbar puncture headache. *Reg Anesth.* 1997;22:66–72.
117. Norris MC, Leighton BL, DeSimone CA. Needle bevel direction and headache after inadvertent dural puncture. *Anesthesiology.* 1989;70:729–731.
118. Richman JM, Joe EM, Cohen SR, et al. Bevel direction and postdural puncture headache: a meta-analysis. *Neurologist.* 2006;12:224–228.
119. Peralta F, Higgins N, Lange E, et al. The relationship of body mass index with the incidence of postdural puncture headache in parturients. *Anesth Analg.* 2015;121:451–456.
120. Wu CL, Rowlingson AJ, Cohen SR, et al. Gender and post-dural puncture headache. *Anesthesiology.* 2006;105:613–618.
121. Baysinger CL. Accidental dural puncture and postdural puncture headache management. *Int Anesthesiol Clin.* 2014;52:18–39.
122. Loures V, Savoldelli G, Kern K, et al. Atypical headache following dural puncture in obstetrics. *Int J Obstet Anesth.* 2014;23:246–252.
123. Hofer JE, Scavone BM. Cranial Nerve VI palsy after dural-arachnoid puncture. *Anesth Analg.* 2015;120:644–646.
124. Nepomuceno R, Herd A. Bilateral subdural hematoma after inadvertent dural puncture during epidural analgesia. *J Emerg Med.* 2013;44:e227–e230.
125. Cuypers V, Van d Velde, Devroe S. Intracranial subdural haematoma following neuraxial anaesthesia in the obstetric population: a literature review with analysis of 56 reported cases. *Int J Obstet Anesth.* 2015;25:58–65.
126. Freedman RL, Lucas DN. MBRACE-UK: Saving lives, improving mothers' care – implications for anesthetists. *Int J Obstet Anesth.* 2015;24:161–173.
127. Webb CAJ, Weyker PD, Zhang L, et al. Unintentional dural puncture with a Tuohy needle increases risk of chronic headache. *Anesth Analg.* 2012;115:124–132.
128. Bradbury CL, Singh SI, Badder SR, et al. Prevention of post-dural puncture headache in the parturients: a systematic review and meta-analysis. *Acta Anaesthsiol Scand.* 2013;57:417–430.
129. Kaddoum R, Motlani F, Kaddoum RN, et al. Accidental dural puncture, postdural puncture headache, intrathecal catheters, and epidural blood patch: revisiting the old nemesis. *J Anesth.* 2014;28:628–630.
130. Verstraete S, Walters MA, Devroe S, et al. Lower incidence of post-dural puncture headache with spinal catheterization after accidental dural puncture in obstetric patients. *Acta Anaesthiol Scand.* 2014;58:1233–1239.
131. Heesen M, Klohr S, Rossaint R, et al. Insertion of an intrathecal catheter following accidental dural puncture: a meta-analysis. *Int J Obstet Anesth.* 2013;22:26–30.
132. Jagannathan DK, Arrianga AF, Elterman KG, et al. Effect of neuraxial technique after dural puncture on obstetric outcomes and anesthetic complications. *Int J Obstet Anesth.* 2015;25:23–29.
133. Al-metwalli RR. Epidural morphine injections for prevention of post dural puncture headache. *Anaesthesia.* 2008;63:847–850.
134. Charsley MM, Abram SE. The injection of intrathecal normal saline reduces the severity of post dural puncture headache. *Reg Anesth Pain Med.* 2001;26:301–305.
135. Arevalo-Rodriguez I, Ciapponi A, Munoz L, et al. Posture and fluids for preventing post-dural puncture headache (Review). *Cochrane Database Syst Rev.* 2013;7:CD009199.
136. van Kooten F, Oedit R, Bakker SLM, et al. Epidural blood patch in post dural puncture headache: a randomised, observer-blind, controlled clinical trial. *J Neurol Neurosurg Psychiatry.* 2008;79:553–558.
137. Kokki M, Sjovall S, Keinanen M, et al. The influence of timing on the effectiveness of epidural blood patches in parturients. *Int J Obstet Anesth.* 2013;22:303–309.
138. Paech MJ, Doherty DA, Christmas T, et al. The volume of blood for epidural blood patch in obstetrics: A randomized, blinded clinical trial. *Anesth Analg.* 2011;113:126–133.
139. Mehta SP, Keogh BP, Lam AM. An epidural blood patch causing acute neurologic dysfunction necessitating a decompressive laminectomy. *Reg Anesth Pain Med.* 2014;39:78–80.
140. Pagani-Estavez GI, Chen JJ, Watson JC, et al. Acute vision loss secondary to epidural blood patch. *Reg Anesth Pain Med.* 2016;41:164–168.
141. Cosar A, Yetiser S, Sizlan A, et al. Hearing impairment associated with spinal anesthesia. *Acta Oto-Laryngologica.* 2004;124:1159–1164.
142. Ok G, Tok D, Erbuyun K, et al. Hearing loss does not occur in young patients undergoing spinal anesthesia. *Reg Anesth Pain Med.* 2004;29:430–433.
143. Kilickan L, Gurkan Y Ozkarakas H. Permanent sensorineural hearing loss following spinal anesthesia. *Acta Anaesthesiol Scand.* 2002;46:1155–1157.
144. Lee LA, Posner KL, Domino KB, et al. Injuries associated with regional anesthesia in the 1980s and 1990s. A closed claims analysis. *Anesthesiology.* 2004;101:143–152.
145. Moen V, Dahlgren N, Irestedt L. Severe neurological complications after central neuraxial blockades in Sweden 1990–1999. *Anesthesiology.* 2004;101:950–959.
146. Neal JM, Kopp SL, Pasternak JJ, et al. Anatomy and pathophysiology of spinal cord injury associated with regional anesthesia and pain medicine. 2015 update. *Reg Anesth Pain Med.* 2015;40:506–525.
147. Reynolds F. Damage to the conus medullaris following spinal anaesthesia. *Anaesthesia.* 2001;56:238–234.
148. Srinivasan KK, Deighan M, Crowley L, et al. Spinal anaesthesia for caesarean section: an ultrasound comparison of two different landmark techniques. *Int J Obstet Anesth.* 2014;23:206–212.
149. Pollak KA, Stephens LS, Posner KL, et al. Trends in pain medicine liability. *Anesthesiology.* 2015;123:1133–1141.
150. Pumberger M, Memtsoudis SG, Stundner O, et al. An analysis of the safety of epidural and spinal neuraxial anesthesia in more than 100,000 consecutive major lower extremity joint replacements. *Reg Anesth Pain Med.* 2013;38:515–519.
151. Bateman BT, Mhyre JM, Ehrenfeld J, et al. The risk and outcomes of epidural hematomas after perioperative and obstetric epidural catheterization: A report from the multicenter perioperative outcomes group research consortium. *Anesth Analg.* 2013;116:1380–1385.
152. Neal JM, Barrington MJ, Brull R, et al. The second ASRA practice advisory on neurologic complications associated with regional anesthesia and pain medicine. Executive summary 2015. *Reg Anesth Pain Med.* 2015;40:401–430.
153. Watson JC, Huntoon MA. Neurologic evaluation and management of perioperative nerve injury. *Reg Anesth Pain Med.* 2015;40:491–501.
154. Zaphiratos V, McKeen DM, Macaulay B, et al. Persistent paralysis after spinal anesthesia for cesarean delivery. *J Clin Anesth.* 2015;27:68–72.
155. Kopp SL, Peters SM, Rose PS, et al. Worsening of neurologic symptoms after spinal anesthesia in two patients with spinal stenosis. *Reg Anesth Pain Med.* 2015;40:502–505.
156. Goldblum E, Atchabahian A. The use of 2-chloroprocaine for spinal anaesthesia. *Acta Anaesthesiol Scand.* 2013;57:545–552.
157. Zaric D, Pace NL. Transient neurologic symptoms (TNS) following spinal anaesthesia with lidocaine versus other local anaesthetics. *Cochrane Database Syst Rev.* 2009:CD003006.

area should have sufficient lighting. In addition, cardiovascular resuscitation equipment (e.g., crash cart) should be readily available.
- A practically organized equipment storage cart (Fig. 36-1) is desirable and should contain all of the necessary equipment (including that required for emergency procedures), supplies, local anesthetics, needles, nerve stimulators, block trays, dressings, and resuscitation drugs. A US machine should also be present.
- It is ideal to have a prepared specialty tray that includes items for sterile skin preparation and draping, a marking pen and ruler for landmark identification, needles and syringes for skin infiltration, and specific block needles and catheters.
- A selection of sedatives, hypnotics, and intravenous anesthetics should be immediately available to prepare patients for regional anesthesia. These drugs should be titrated to maximize benefits and minimize adverse effects (high therapeutic index); short-acting drugs with a high safety margin are desirable.
- Emergency drugs should include atropine, epinephrine, phenylephrine, ephedrine, propofol, midazolam, succinylcholine, and Intralipid. In addition, guidelines for resuscitation in the event of local anesthetic toxicity should be laminated and kept with the Intralipid.

Monitoring

When performing regional anesthesia, skilled personnel should be present at all times to monitor the patient. At a minimum, standard monitoring should include electrocardiogram (ECG), noninvasive blood pressure (NIBP), and pulse oximetry. In addition, the patient's level of consciousness should be gauged frequently with verbal contact since vasovagal episodes are common during many regional procedures. Although there are currently no practical or effective devices to detect rising blood levels of local anesthetic, the addition of pharmacologic markers, such as epinephrine, in appropriate concentrations to the local anesthetic can provide an indirect indication of increasing systemic local anesthetic dose. Close observation for systemic toxicity secondary to rapid intravenous injection (within 2 minutes) as well as delayed (~20 minutes) absorption is essential. The patient should be monitored for at least 30 minutes following a regional block.
- Standard ECG, blood pressure monitoring, and pulse oximetry are essential when performing regional anesthesia.
- Careful monitoring of the patient's heart rate (along with ECG measurement) is important to detect tachycardia seen with epinephrine when it is included in a test dose. It is also useful as an indicator of systemic toxicity with bupivacaine and other potent local anesthetics.
- Prior to performing blocks with significant sympathetic effects, a baseline blood pressure reading should be obtained. Once the regional anesthesia procedure is complete, monitors should remain attached. In conscious patients, end-tidal carbon dioxide monitoring is not required; however, there are special nasal prongs available for monitoring patients when this is considered necessary.
- At a minimum, stable vital signs following regional anesthesia must be present to fulfill discharge criteria from the recovery area. If the block has not begun to regress, appropriate protection for the anesthetized limb and complete instructions should be provided to the patient and their family before discharge. For inpatients, appropriate orders should be written to assure limb protection.
- Patients receiving perineural local anesthetic infusions should be visited regularly by a qualified physician or member of the Acute Pain Service postoperatively with ongoing documentation of their condition in the medical record.
- The same monitoring procedures apply to pediatric patients undergoing regional anesthesia; however, due to their generally uncooperative nature and reduced ability to communicate pain clearly, nerve blocks in children are commonly performed under general anesthesia or deep sedation. As such, monitoring to reduce the risk of nerve damage (e.g., US, NS, and injection pressure) is especially important in pediatric practice. In addition, the use of muscle relaxants is contraindicated in anesthetized children receiving nerve blocks with NS guidance.

Premedication and Sedation

The best preparation for a regional technique is careful patient selection and ensuring that the patient is adequately educated and informed about the anesthetic and surgical procedures. Supplemental medication is often helpful. Appropriate sedation and analgesia is an essential part of successful regional anesthesia in order to produce maximum benefit with minimal side effects. Effective sedation can be achieved with a variety of medications, including but not limited to propofol, midazolam, fentanyl, ketamine, remifentanil, alfentanil, or a combination of these drugs. The medications should be titrated to reach an appropriate level of sedation for the individual patient, specific nerve block procedure, and length of surgery. Some examples are listed next.

Bolus

- Midazolam 1 to 2 mg (titrated up to 0.07 mg/kg)
- Fentanyl 0.5 to 1 µg/kg
- Alfentanil 7 to 10 µg/kg
- Ketamine 0.1 to 0.5 mg/kg

In addition to the general comments about premedication discussed in earlier chapters, regional anesthesia techniques have special requirements. Sedation must be adjusted to the required level of patient cooperation. In the case of elicitation of a paresthesia (as during several blocks in the head and neck region) or electrical stimulation techniques, the level of sedation must be sufficient to allow the patient to identify and report nerve contact. Although a low dose of opioid (50 to 100 µg of fentanyl or equivalent) will help ease the discomfort of nerve localization, patient responsiveness must be maintained. This does not preclude the use of an amnestic agent, and small doses of propofol or midazolam may provide excellent amnesia while maintaining levels of consciousness that still allow cooperation.

Documentation

Creation of a preblock checklist is a key step in ensuring correct block performance in the correct location on the patient's body. The list should include documentation of relevant preoperative conditions, discussion of risks and benefits, and obtaining consent. In contrast to general and neuraxial anesthesia, no formal documentation guidelines exist for PNB, even though they are now considered routine and are associated with the same medicolegal implications as other forms of anesthesia. Documentation of PNB procedures is especially recommended in order to have a record of the procedure in case the information is required for quality assurance, research, or medicolegal reasons.

Block Performance Stage

Common Techniques: Nerve Stimulation

Basics of Technique and Equipment

Electrical stimulation of nerve structures was introduced to regional anesthesia in the late 1960s to 1970s.[9,10] A low-current electrical impulse applied to a peripheral nerve produces stimulation of motor fibers and theoretically indicates proximity to the nerve without actual needle contact or related patient discomfort. When NS techniques are used, actual contact with the nerve is unnecessary (in contrast to the paresthesia method). In theory, this implies that risk of nerve injury should be less when using NS methods, although this has not yet been proven. The concept of using NS to guide accurate placement was also applied to catheters, and stimulating catheters were introduced in an attempt to increase our ability to accurately advance catheters over greater distances.[11,12]

The main limitations with NS are related to the technique's inconsistent results[13,14] and the variance in electrical properties of different nerve stimulators.[15] In addition, many other variables affect the ability to stimulate nerves, including conductive area of the electrode (needle or stimulating catheter tip), electrical impedance of the tissues, electrode-to-nerve distance, current flow, and pulse duration.[16] Ultimately, NS relies on the physiologic responses of neural structures to the stimulating current, which is subject to considerable interindividual variation.

Today's nerve stimulators have features to improve ease-of-use and success, such as maintaining a constant current with adjustable frequency, pulse width, and current intensity (milliamperes [mA]). This enables a stable current output (an important safety feature) in the presence of varied resistances from the needle, tissues, and connectors. A clear digital display indicating the actual current delivery is important, as is regular calibration and testing. Some nerve stimulators are equipped with low (up to 6 mA) and high (up to 80 mA) current output ranges. The lower range is primarily for localizing peripheral nerves, whereas the higher range is mainly used for monitoring neuromuscular blockade. Recently, higher ranges have been used for transcutaneous NS techniques[17] (2 to 5 mA), including percutaneous electrode guidance[18] and surface nerve mapping,[11,19] and the epidural stimulation test (1 to 10 mA).[20,21] Most nerve stimulators deliver an electrical pulse width of 100 or 200 microseconds for stimulating motor nerves. Similar to current amplitude, the length of time over which the current is delivered (pulse width) is usually considered important, as shorter duration currents can selectively stimulate motor components of mixed nerves while sparing the discomfort caused by stimulation of sensory components. Some sophisticated devices allow variable pulse widths from 50 microseconds to 1 millisecond in an attempt to provide such selective stimulation. The general rule is to use short-duration current of no longer than 100 microseconds for peripheral NS, although there is some evidence that duration does not impact patient discomfort[22] and that intensity (mA) of the stimulation is perhaps the most important variable.[23]

Practical Guidelines

When using NS as the sole nerve-seeking device, the nerve stimulator should be set to deliver a current of 1 to 2 mA in order to gauge the approximate distance to the nerve during initial advancement of the needle. Depolarization of the nerve can also be improved by using the positive (red) pole of the stimulator as the ground (reference or surface electrode) electrode and the negative (black) lead as the connection to the needle itself (known as cathodal preference). The actual location of the ground electrode is of little importance with the use of constant-current nerve stimulators.[23] Generally, the needle is in proximity to the nerve when the threshold for motor response is between 0.3 and 0.5 mA; placing the needle to the point where a motor response only requires 0.1 to 0.2 mA may increase the chance of intraneural injection and should be avoided.[24] Once a low threshold response is obtained, 2 to 3 mL of local anesthetic is injected, and the operator watches for disappearance of the motor twitch, signaling to inject the remainder of the proposed dose in divided aliquots. This so-called "Raj test"[25] was originally thought to result from physical displacement of the targeted nerve by the injectate, but this response has also been attributed to a change in the electrical field at the needle–tissue interface. Electrically conducting solutions (e.g., local anesthetic or saline) reduce the current density at the needle tip, thereby increasing the current threshold for motor response, whereas solutions (e.g., dextrose 5% in water; D5W) increase the current density and maintain or augment the twitch response (Fig. 36-2).[26]

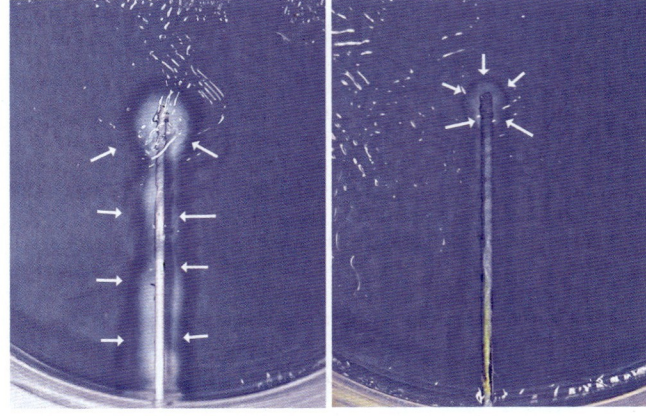

Figure 36-2 Current density is localized to the needle tip when using nonconducting solutions (e.g., D5W), thereby maintaining the motor response to the threshold current level during nerve stimulation.

Following nerve localization with a stimulating needle, continuous analgesia can be delivered via stimulating catheter with continuous stimulation of the nerve. Similar current thresholds are applicable with the use of stimulating catheters. Use of an appropriate pulse width is critical for different applications during PNB and neuraxial block. Motor peripheral nerves can be stimulated with currents greater than 0.3 mA at a pulse width of 0.1 milliseconds. With a pulse width of 0.2 milliseconds, different threshold currents can be used to differentiate the epidural (1 to 15 mA) and intrathecal (<1 mA) spaces. Stimulation in the epidural space can also be performed with a pulse width of 1 millisecond and a threshold current of 6 mA. If it is desirable to dilate the perineural space, injection of D5W is preferable in order to maintain the motor response to stimulation.[27] The reader is referred to the section on Other Related Equipment for optimal features of stimulating catheters.

Common Techniques: Ultrasound Imaging

Basics of Technique and Equipment

US imaging has emerged as a valuable regional anesthesia tool, given that the size, depth, and precise location of many nerves in

36 Peripheral Nerve Blockade

BAN C. H. TSUI • RICHARD W. ROSENQUIST

Introduction
General Principles and Equipment
   Preblock Stage
   Premedication and Sedation
   Block Performance Stage
   Other Related Equipment
   Postblock Stage
   Avoiding Complications
Clinical Anatomy
   Head and Neck
   Spine
   Upper Extremity
   Trunk
   Lower Extremity
Specific Techniques
   Head and Neck
   Upper Extremity
   Trunk Nerve Blocks
   Penile Block
   Lower Extremity
   Techniques
   Continuous Catheter Technique
Acknowledgments

KEY POINTS

1. Peripheral nerve blocks (PNBs) provide effective anesthesia and analgesia in a site-specific manner with the potential for long-lasting effects.
2. Safety and success of PNBs depends on accurate identification of target nerves and precise and adequate placement of local anesthetic.
3. Ultrasound imaging allows visualization of needle movement toward nerve structure(s) in real time, minimizing the risk of needle contact with critical structures and potentially reducing complications. Although highly desirable as an aid to performing regional anesthesia, ultrasound technology requires considerable training and thorough knowledge of both the equipment and cross-sectional anatomy relevant to regional nerve blocks.
4. Peripheral nerve stimulators are useful tools to facilitate nerve blocks, but they do not eliminate the risk of nerve injury. In the adult patient, maintenance of responsiveness may allow reporting of nerve contact or pain during injection.
5. Nerve blocks associated with bony or vascular landmarks are more reliable and easier to perform than those dependent on surface landmarks alone.
6. Larger volumes of local anesthetic may increase the potential success of PNBs; however, total milligram dosage must be limited to avoid systemic toxicity. Higher concentrations of local anesthetics increase the degree of motor block. Ultrasound imaging, through increased accuracy of nerve localization and visualization of local anesthetic spread, may enable successful blocks to be performed with reduced volumes of local anesthetics, but this has yet to be proven.
7. Pediatric nerve block procedures are generally similar to those for adults but often require special considerations, the most important of which is that nerve blocks are routinely performed under general anesthesia or heavy sedation in children.

Introduction

Regional anesthesia enables site-specific, long-lasting, and effective anesthesia and analgesia. It is suitable for many surgical patients and can improve analgesia[1] and reduce morbidity, mortality, and the need for reoperation after major surgical procedures.[2] Peripheral nerve blocks (PNBs) can be used alone as the sole "surgical" anesthetic, as a supplement to provide analgesia and muscle relaxation together with general anesthesia, or as the initial step in providing prolonged postoperative analgesia, as with brachial plexus blocks or continuous peripheral nerve catheters. Compared to parenteral analgesics, single-injection or continuous PNB can provide superior analgesia and reduce the incidence of side effects.[3-5] Optimal pain relief and minimal side effects (e.g., nausea and vomiting) following surgery have a major impact on patient outcome, including patient satisfaction and earlier mobilization, as well as fulfilling the need for streamlined surgical services with lower costs.[6] Nevertheless, the safety and success of PNB techniques are highly dependent on accurate delivery of the correct dose of local anesthetic. Even in experienced hands, there is an inherent failure rate associated with regional anesthesia[7] with the potential—albeit rare—for systemic toxicity, infection, bleeding, permanent nerve injury, or other physical injury. In addition to the benefits of PNB, advances in knowledge (e.g., physiologic characteristics of solutions during electrical nerve stimulation [NS]) and technology (e.g., the introduction of anatomically based ultrasound [US] imaging) have encouraged many anesthesiologists and surgeons to use PNB on a more frequent basis.

Advancements in medical knowledge and techniques are being made constantly and, whereas new advancements provide an opportunity for improved patient care, they need to be studied and compared to currently accepted techniques to evaluate their safety and utility. In contrast, anatomic structures are static, and an understanding of basic anatomy cannot be replaced by excellent technical skills and knowledge of the technique when performing regional anesthesia. This chapter provides an in-depth discussion of regional anatomy, while providing an overview of two current techniques for nerve localization and block performance: NS and US imaging. Specific techniques are described in sections grouped by body location. Special considerations for nerve blocks in pediatric patients will be specifically addressed where appropriate.

General Principles and Equipment

Regional anesthesia has long been regarded as an "art," and, until recently, real success with these techniques was confined to a few gifted individuals. The introduction of NS, which relies on physiologic responses of neural structures to electrical impulses, was the first step toward transforming regional anesthesia into a "science." There is considerable interindividual variation in physiologic response to NS. Furthermore, other factors, including injectates, physiologic solutions (e.g., blood), and disease, influence responses to NS. Despite these limitations, NS was one of the first objective methods available in regional anesthesia to guide needle placement in proximity to a target nerve with some reliability.

One of the most exciting recent advances in regional anesthesia technology has been the introduction of anatomically based US imaging. Since the beginning of regional anesthesia practice, this is the first time that the target nerve can be visualized. This is a quantum leap in technology for those in the field, and the realization of its potential benefits may encourage those anesthesiologists who had previously abandoned regional anesthesia techniques to resume or increase their use of them. Despite initial excitement over this advancement, US images are subject to individual interpretation depending on experience, training, and where that experience and training was obtained. Importantly, there is a substantial learning curve associated with US-guided regional anesthesia. It is therefore prudent in many situations to combine NS and US imaging in order to try to achieve 100% block success. Used alone, US may allow good visualization of the needle and nerve as well as a reasonable estimate of the spread of the full dose of the local anesthetic, although the identity of the nerve may be unknown, especially for novice ultrasonographers.[8] By stimulating the nerve, its identity may be determined objectively by observing the motor response to NS or in some cases, the anatomic distribution of a paresthesia-like sensation in response to NS for a sensory nerve.

Patient monitoring and other factors related to optimizing patient care and prevention of complications are similar to those for general anesthesia, with some important differences. Safe and successful performance of PNB requires careful selection of patients and administration of an appropriate type and dose of local anesthetic in the correct location. In addition, the patient must be monitored during the procedure and prior to discharge, and ambulatory patients with home-going catheters should be monitored remotely with either telephone follow-up or home health-care team visits until the catheter has been removed and the block has resolved completely.

Preblock Stage

Setup

Regional blocks can be performed in the operating room setting, although it is preferable and desirable to administer them in a designated room or area outside the immediate operating room environment (Fig. 36-1) for adult patients. This is a consequence of what is commonly referred to as "soak time," which is the time it takes for local anesthetics to cross the cell membrane, block action potentials, and produce either analgesia or surgical anesthesia. The designated area must contain the necessary equipment for safe monitoring and resuscitation but must also contain all of the supplies and equipment to perform common and sophisticated regional block techniques. Some important considerations for this "block room" are described here:

- All supplies located in this area must be readily identifiable and accessible to the anesthesiologist.
- The area should be of ample size to allow block performance, patient monitoring, and resuscitation.
- There should be equipment for monitoring, oxygen delivery, emergency airway management and suction, and the

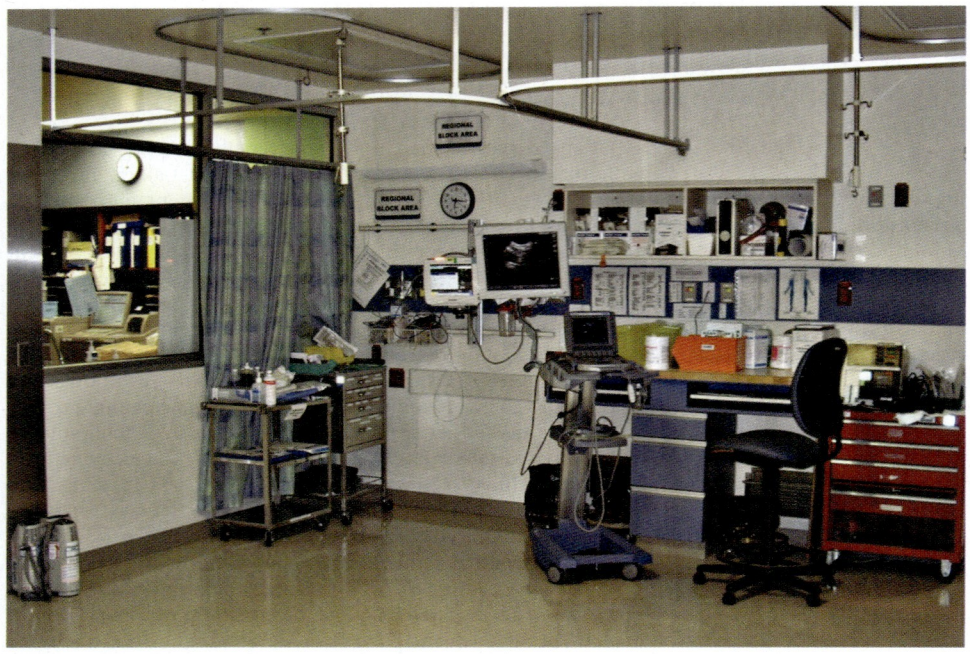

Figure 36-1 Designated regional block room with labeled storage cart.

their surrounding environment can be determined upon correct interpretation of the visual image. Visualization of the moving needle, once inserted at an appropriate angle and within the plane of the US probe, as well as the spread of local anesthetic, provides assistance to the anesthesiologist performing regional anesthesia. With US-guided PNB techniques, the operator can adjust needle or catheter placement under direct vision, which may lead to fewer needle attempts and ultimately improved motor and sensory blocks. Furthermore, visibility of vital structures (e.g., blood vessels and pleura) is advantageous in order to avoid complications. Today, technologic advances have led to the development of US systems that can deliver high frequency (≥10 MHz) sound waves, offering the high axial resolution required for visualization of nerves and the ability to distinguish them from surrounding anatomic structures (e.g., tendons, muscles). Compared to NS, the proposed benefits of US guidance for upper extremity blocks include improved block success[28] and completeness,[29] reduced block performance and onset times,[28–31] prolonged block duration,[30] and reduction in complications.[32] Although the cumulative evidence may appear convincing, many of the studies show conflicting results for certain parameters, and the large variability in trial methodologies and application of different outcome measures account for many of the discrepancies. Indeed, the various end points used in regional anesthesia research may bias outcomes when comparing multiple regional techniques. Marhofer et al.[33,34] have published an excellent review of the current status of US and its use in regional anesthesia. They emphasize that adequate training in US-guided techniques is essential and suggest that education and proper technique can help ensure safe blocks. In addition, current advantages of using US in regional anesthesia, including direct visualization of subcutaneous structures, identification of anatomic variation, ability to use less local anesthetic, and improvement in block quality and patient satisfaction, are discussed.

US is defined as any sound with a frequency above 20 kHz, although medical imaging generally requires between 3 and 15 MHz. Within the body, US scanners emit sound waves that produce an echo when they encounter a tissue interface. Therefore, US images reflect contours, including those of anatomic structures, based on differing acoustic impedances of tissue or fluids. Significant reflection of sound waves occurs at interfaces between substances of different acoustic impedance, resulting in good contour definition between different tissues. High US beam reflection from high impedance/dense structures (e.g., bone, connective tissue) results in a bright (hyperechoic) image, often with dorsal shadowing underneath; low impedance structures reflect beams to a smaller extent and appear gray (hypoechoic); minimal impedance structures/spaces (e.g., fluid in vessels) appear black (anechoic).

Higher frequencies offer the best spatial resolution at superficial locations (e.g., brachial plexus at supraclavicular fossa), whereas lower frequencies are often required for structure delineation at deep locations (e.g., sciatic nerve in the subgluteal region). Block location and depth of target nerve structures determine which transducer offers the best imaging and resolution. It is important to have familiarity with several functions of the US system, including field and gain functions as well as Doppler Effect. Doppler Effect is useful for identifying blood vessels during nerve localization using US guidance since many nerves are situated in proximity to vascular structures.

Practical Guidelines

Both the probe and skin of the patient should be prepared for maximum sterility and optimal imaging. Probe sterility is paramount if performing real-time, or dynamic, US guidance during block performance. This can be maintained by standard sleeve covers (Fig. 36-3A), but these can be expensive and cumbersome. For single-injection blocks, it is practical to use a sterile transparent dressing (e.g., Tegaderm; 3M Health Care, St Paul, MN) without the full cover of a sterile sleeve (Fig. 36-3B).[35] An issue when using standard long covers is the potential for air to track between the probe and the skin, which reduces image quality. The target area should be scanned using a generous amount of US gel (water soluble conductivity gel is optimal) prior to sterile preparation to identify the target structures. One of the most common reasons for poor visualization is lack of sufficient gel for skin-probe contact.

For nerve localization during US-guided PNB, it is helpful to first identify one or more reliable anatomic landmarks (bone or vessel) with a known relationship to the nerve structure. The operator can then localize the nerve at a location near the landmark, and proceed to follow, or "trace," the nerve to the optimal block location (Table 36-1).[36] Generally, nerve structures are most visible when the angle of incidence is approximately 90 degrees to the US beam. Obtaining a transverse axis view of the nerve usually allows the best appreciation of the anatomic relationship of the nerve with its surrounding structures. To obtain the best possible view of the shaft and tip of the needle, it is imperative to align the needle shaft to the longitudinal axis ("in-plane" [IP]) of the US transducer (probe) (Fig. 36-3C). The nerve structure is often placed at the edge of the US screen to ensure adequate viewing distance for the needle shaft. An alternative approach uses a transverse or tangential ("out-of-plane" [OOP]) alignment, which only allows appreciation of the needle in cross-section (Fig. 36-3D). The nerve structure is often placed in the center of the screen to guarantee that aligning the needle puncture with the center of the probe will ensure close needle tip–nerve alignment. This approach can be beneficial in certain block locations (compact areas) and for inserting catheters (e.g., at the subgluteal area) but should never be used in areas where needle tip visibility in relation to vital structures is critical (e.g., supraclavicular fossa near the pleura).

After the needle is seen to be close to the nerve(s), a 1- to 2-mL test dose of D5W can be injected to visualize the spread. The solution will be seen as a hypoechoic expansion and will often illuminate the surrounding area, enabling better visibility of the nerves and block needle. If NS is being used to confirm nerve identity, D5W should be used in order to maintain accurate motor responses.[27] This will be especially important during catheter introduction and advancement. If the test shows undesired injection near or within vessels or cavities, subsequent injection of local anesthetic should be postponed until better needle localization is achieved. If suboptimal spread of injectate is observed, the needle can be repositioned to allow another injection.

There can be a steep learning curve for US-guided nerve blocks, and techniques to improve needle and catheter visibility during advancement are important in order to improve training to use the technology. Two such approaches have been described experimentally:

The "walk-down" approach,[37] used during OOP needling, involves calculating the required depth of puncture (with measurement to the desired neural structure recorded using US prior to the block) and using trigonometry with the shaft angle and length to calculate a "reasonable" location to place the initial needle puncture site. The initial shallow puncture will be seen easily as a bright dot on the screen, and the needle tip can be followed as it is "walked down" to the final calculated depth. For example, if the final depth of penetration for the block is 2 cm, the needle will ultimately be at a 45-degree angle if the initial puncture site is 2 cm from the probe and the needle is incrementally angled to this level.

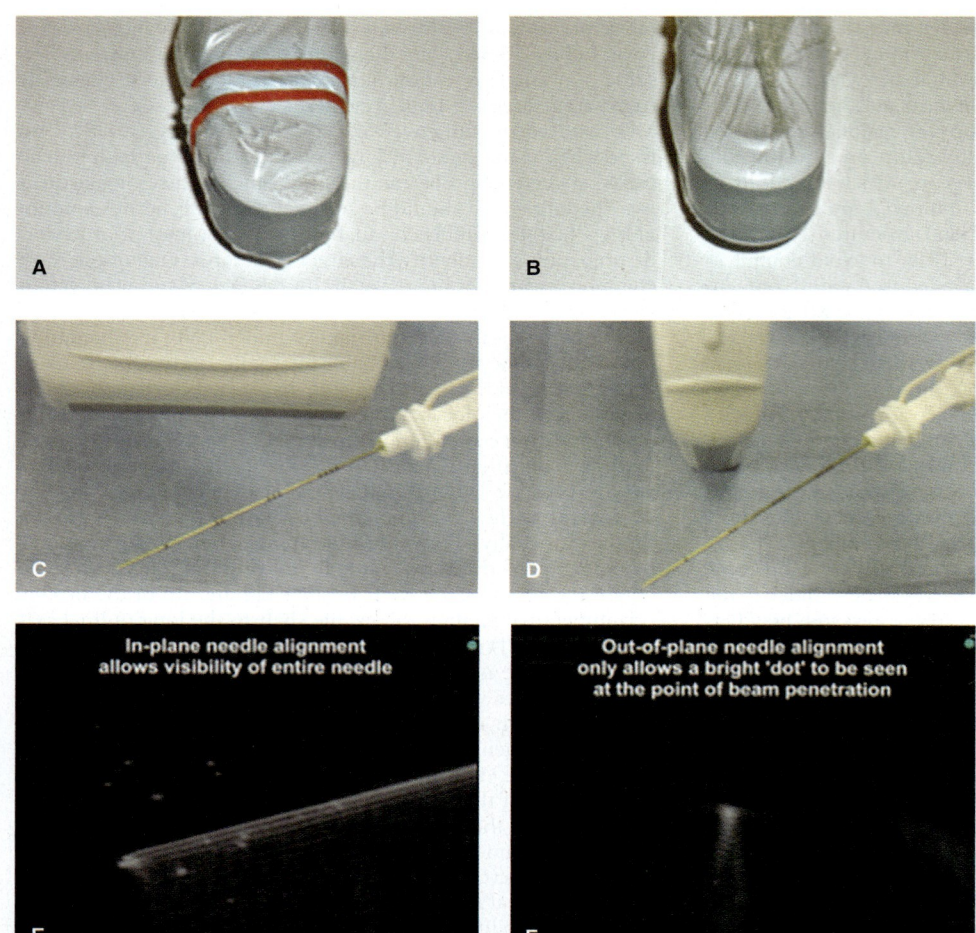

Figure 36-3 Probe sterility using the full cover of a sterile sleeve (**A**) and a sterile transparent dressing (e.g., Tegaderm; 3M Health Care, St Paul, MN) (**B**). In-plane (**C, E**) and out-of-plane (**D, F**) needle alignment and needle visibility on ultrasound.

A method of needle–probe alignment using a laser attachment for the probe has also been reported; the laser line will project onto both the needle shaft and the midline of the probe, indicating an IP position.[38] Aligning the visible optical laser line with the longitudinal axis of the US probe will mimic the "invisible" beam from the US probe and allow improvements with IP needle alignment. With the laser-unit attachment, any misalignment of the needle to the US beam can be easily detected and adjusted in real-time. Recently, commercially available GPS guidance systems intended to guide the needle tip location have been developed, but the merit of these devices remains to be determined.

Most experts recommend the use of combined US and NS techniques. Using this approach, a typical setup will feature the nerve stimulator set at 0.3 to 0.5 mA, whereas the nerve is sought primarily using visualization under US guidance. The goal of nerve stimulator is to serve as an alert when the insulated needle tip is too close to nerve (i.e., contacting or inside the nerve).

Other Related Equipment

Needles

Needles used for regional techniques are often modified from standard injection needles. Although reports may speculate that needle design is a determinant of nerve or other tissue injury, there is insufficient evidence to fully substantiate this claim. For PNB, the "short bevel" (i.e., 30 to 45 degrees) or "B bevel" is often used to reduce the potential for injury to nerves.[39] Other modifications, such as the "pencil-point" needle, have been introduced in attempts to reduce nerve injury. Single-injection PNB techniques generally require 22- to 24-gauge insulated needles with short bevels. If superficial and field blocks are performed, smaller gauge (e.g., 25- to 26-gauge) sharp needles can be utilized. Continuous blocks require larger-bore needles to facilitate catheter introduction (e.g., 18-gauge needles for 20-gauge catheters) when using a catheter-through-needle technique. Blunt-tipped Tuohy needles are commonly used for continuous PNB with success.[40] Short-bevel and Tuohy needles offer more resistance and give a better "feel" when traversing different tissues. Desired needle length will depend on each specific block and individual patient characteristics. One must keep in mind that longer needles are more prone to bending upon insertion and may therefore benefit from the strength offered by a larger gauge. Clear markings throughout the entire length of the needle are important for measuring depth of penetration, particularly for correspondence to US measurements. A variety of echogenic needles are available for use with US; these needles possess special coatings, grooves, or "Cornerstone" reflectors that enhance echogenicity, allowing easier visualization when performing US-guided blocks.

Table 36-1 Useful Anatomic Landmarks for Localizing Nerves during Common Ultrasound-guided Peripheral Nerve Blocks

Peripheral Nerve Block Location	Anatomic Landmark(s)	Approach for Ultrasound Imaging
Interscalene	Subclavian artery and scalene muscles	Locate the plexus trunks/divisions superolateral to the artery at the supraclavicular fossa, and trace proximally to where the roots/trunks lie between the scalenus anterior and medius muscles (Fig. 36-19).
Supraclavicular	Subclavian artery	Scan from lateral to medial on the superior aspect of the clavicle to locate the pulsatile artery; the plexus trunks/divisions lie lateral and often superior to the artery (Fig. 36-20). Color Doppler is useful.
Infraclavicular	Subclavian/axillary artery and vein	Place the artery at the center of the field and locate the brachial plexus cords surrounding the artery (Fig. 36-21).
Axillary	Axillary artery	The terminal nerves surround the artery (Fig. 36-22).
Peripheral nerves		
Radial nerve at anterior elbow	Humerus at spiral groove and deep brachial artery	To confirm the nerve's identity at the elbow, trace the nerve proximally and posteriorly toward the spiral groove of the humerus, just inferior to the deltoid muscle insertion. The nerve is located here adjacent to the deep brachial artery and can be followed back to the anterior elbow (Fig. 36-23).
Median nerve at forearm	Brachial artery	The large anechoic artery lies immediately lateral to the nerve (Fig. 36-25).
Ulnar nerve at forearm	Ulnar artery	Scan at the anteromedial surface of the forearm approximately at the junction of its distal third and proximal two-thirds, to capture the ulnar nerve as it approaches the ulnar artery on its medial aspect (Fig. 36-25).
Lumbar plexus	Transverse processes	The plexus lies between and just deep to the lateral aspect (tips) of the processes (Fig. 36-34).
Femoral	Femoral artery	The nerve lies lateral to the artery (vein most medial) (Fig. 36-35). Insert the needle above the branching of the deep femoral artery.
Sciatic		
Classical/Labat	Ischial bone and inferior gluteal or pudendal vessels	The nerve lies lateral to the thinnest aspect of the ischial bone. The inferior gluteal artery generally lies medial to and at the same depth as the nerve (Fig. 36-39).
Subgluteal	Greater trochanter and ischial tuberosity	The nerve lies between the two bone structures (Fig. 36-40).
Popliteal	Popliteal artery	Trace the tibial and common peroneal nerves from the popliteal crease to where they form the sciatic nerve. At the crease, the tibial nerve lies adjacent to the popliteal artery. Scanning proximally to the sciatic bifurcation, the artery becomes deeper and at a greater distance from the nerve (Fig. 36-41).
Ankle		
Tibial (posterior tibial)	Posterior tibial artery	The nerve lies posterior to the artery (Fig. 36-43).
Deep peroneal	Anterior tibial artery	The nerve lies lateral to the artery (Fig. 36-44).

Practical Tips

Techniques and devices have been proposed to limit injection pressure since considerable variation exists among anesthesiologists with regard to the amount of pressure they apply during injections.[41] High-pressure injections into the nerve (especially intrafascicular) are associated with damage in animals.[42,43] Disposable, in-line injection pressure monitors are available, although their ability to prevent long-term injury is not well documented. Alternatively, a compressed air injection technique (CAIT) has been described to limit generation of excessive pressure during injection. With this method, air is drawn into the syringe and compressed by 50% during the entire injection to maintain pressures of approximately 760 mmHg (Boyle law: Pressure × volume = constant) (Fig. 36-4), which is well below the 1,300 mmHg threshold considered to be an associated risk factor for clinically significant nerve injury.[44]

Catheters

Continuous-infusion catheter kits suitable for PNB are available that include a standard polyamide catheter, such as those previously used for epidural analgesia, combined with an insulated Tuohy needle with NS capability. Recently, catheters have been developed that are amenable to stimulation (an electrode is placed into the catheter tip), thereby enabling more accurate advancement of catheters over substantial distances to provide continuous analgesia. Some studies have suggested that it may be helpful to inject a solution to dilate the perineural compartment to

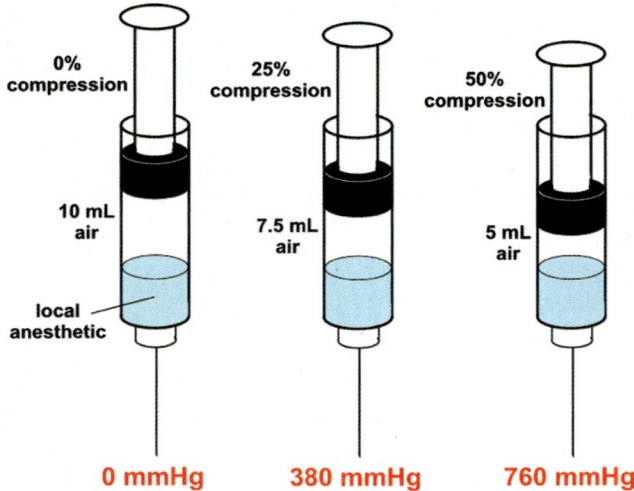

Figure 36-4 Compressed air injection technique (CAIT) used to avoid high injection pressure; 50% compression of air volume within the syringe corresponds to an injection pressure of 760 mmHg.

facilitate advancement of the catheter. The reader is referred to the discussion of practical guidelines of NS in the section Common Techniques: Nerve Stimulation and Ultrasound Imaging for discussion of injection solutions for perineural dilation. The recent reintroduction of catheter-over-needle assemblies allows for the needle and catheter to be inserted as a single unit, avoiding the potential problems associated with threading the catheter through the needle. In theory, a catheter introduced over the needle is more stable in the skin and can be targeted to the desired location with good accuracy. These assemblies are discussed in more detail at the end of the chapter. There are a number of continuous-infusion devices now available for both inpatient and outpatient use, which allow delivery of dilute local anesthetic concentrations for as long as 72 hours after surgery. Standard precautions are required to maintain sterility of the catheter and the insertion site, but complications have been rare with these techniques and new devices.

Postblock Stage

Block Assessment and Monitoring

Following administration of a PNB, progression of the block should be monitored, and the patient's sensory and motor response in the blocked region should be assessed closely. Traditional block monitoring tools, which rely on application of cold stimuli (ice, alcohol swab) or touch (pinprick, pinch, monofilament), are generally subjective. More objective tools, such as infrared thermal imaging of the block area[45,46] and current perception threshold measurement[47] have also been studied. The latter has been shown to be a reliable method of monitoring block progression in a clinical setting.[48]

Sensory assessment relies primarily on collecting feedback directly from the patient using validated pain rating scales. The most popular of these are variations on the 0 to 10 scale, with 0 indicating "no pain" and 10 indicating "worst pain imaginable." Other pain scales consist of or incorporate cartoons representing a series of faces in progressing severity of pain; these scales are useful for children and individuals who cannot otherwise communicate their pain verbally. Pain rating scales for individuals with dementia or other cognitive impairments are also available and rely on the assessor's judgment of pain based on various physical and verbal cues.

Assessment of motor blockade is commonly performed by collecting a Bromage score[49] or equivalent score based on a graded scale where the lowest score indicates full range of movement and the highest score indicates complete blockade/no movement. As with sensory assessment, this method is subjective and relies on the assessor's ability to differentiate differing degrees of motor ability. A more objective tool is strength testing using a force transducer. The patient exerts force against a transducer to test the body part that has been blocked (e.g., shoulder abduction for axillary nerve assessment), and the force (or lack thereof) can be recorded over time to assess block onset or resolution.

Discharge Criteria

Stable vital signs are a must in order to fulfill criteria for discharge from the recovery area. In some cases, acceptable evidence of regressing sensory and motor blocks should be present. However, if a long-lasting local anesthetic was used to perform the block or a continuous catheter with an infusion of local anesthetic is used, the block may not show evidence of regression at the time of discharge. Postoperative follow-up is important to confirm that neurologic function has returned to normal. If a deficit is suspected, early neurologic assessment is critical to determine the appropriate course of management.

Patients should have well-controlled pain upon discharge. Incorporating a standard level of pain relief (e.g., on a verbal rating scale) prior to discharge home or to the ward is prudent. Specific common risks for certain blocks should be discussed with the patient prior to discharge. When discharging patients from postanesthesia care units while an extremity is still anesthetized (e.g., the block was performed to provide extended analgesia), it is absolutely necessary to provide in-depth instruction related to potential risks and their prevention (e.g., risk of burns to anesthetized areas will require avoidance of certain forms of cooking, and the potential for developing pressure neuropathies). A clear understanding of the information provided is important for both the patient and their caregivers. Written instructions including expected course, common side effects, and 24-hour contact information should be provided.

Avoiding Complications

In general, regional anesthesia has an excellent safety record. Complication rates are as low as 8 per 10,000 for seizures[2] and lower than 0.1% to 1% for nerve injury.[7,50] Only rare cases of severe chronic pain syndromes following regional anesthesia have been reported.[51] Nevertheless, the incidence of some complications is often higher in PNB than other regional anesthesia/analgesia techniques, and the results can be devastating. Choosing a suitable patient and applying the right dose of local anesthetic in the correct location are the primary considerations. Careful attention to any unusual responses or reports of pain during block performance, as well as follow-up prior to and after discharge, is equally important, although often overlooked.

Patient Selection

Patient selection is a critical element for the performance of safe and effective PNB. Not all patients are suitable candidates for PNB. In general, patients scheduled for extremity, thoracic, abdominal, or perineal surgery should be considered potential candidates for peripheral regional anesthetic techniques. Adamant refusal of regional anesthesia by a patient or, in the case of children, a parent/guardian, is an absolute contraindication to the procedure.

Other contraindications include local infection, systemic anticoagulation, and severe systemic coagulopathy. In most cases, schizophrenic patients should only receive regional techniques if general anesthesia is also performed. The presence of pre-existing neurologic disease is a controversial topic and, although limited data are available in the case of spinal anesthesia, the safety with respect to PNB is unclear. One must be cognizant of the potential to compound existing neurologic deficits; therefore, clear documentation of the deficits prior to the procedure and a careful discussion of the potential risks and benefits are critical. For every clinical situation, the use of regional anesthesia must be evaluated carefully as a matter of risk versus benefit. It is imperative to follow applicable national and international guidelines, such as those set by the American Society of Anesthesiologists (ASA) for patient monitoring and those in place for anticoagulated patients, as provided by the American Society of Regional Anesthesia and Pain Medicine (ASRA).

Local Anesthetic Drug Selection, Toxicity, and Doses

This section will provide an overview of drug selection and toxicity during PNB. For a more detailed discussion of the pharmacology and toxicity of local anesthetics, the reader is referred to Chapter 21.

Rates of systemic and local toxicity and nerve injury with PNB are generally low, but the use of available methods to reduce inadvertent intravascular and intraneural injection is clearly warranted. It is important to note that lower concentrations of local anesthetic (e.g., 1% to 1.5% lidocaine, 0.125% to 0.5% bupivacaine) compared to those used for epidural anesthesia are appropriate for peripheral nerves. Neural toxicity of these anesthetics appears to be concentration-dependent.[52] The use of highly concentrated solutions may be useful to increase motor block, but it also increases the total milligram dose of local anesthetic. To limit total drug dose, lower concentrations are usually indicated when larger volumes are required to anesthetize poorly localized peripheral nerves or to block a series of nerves. Nevertheless, no clinical evidence exists to suggest that prolonged exposure (as with continuous PNB) of nerves to local anesthetic solutions of appropriate concentration predisposes to neurotoxic injury.[53]

Systemic toxicity is most often related to accidental intravascular injection and rarely to the administration of an excessive quantity of local anesthetic to an appropriate site. The risk of systemic toxic reactions is often related to the drug used. Ropivacaine (generally at 0.5%) is an example of a drug introduced into clinical practice in order to reduce central nervous system and cardiovascular toxicity through its physiochemical and stereoselective properties.[54,55] Nevertheless, there are examples of ropivacaine toxicity during PNB.[56-59] One potential strategy to achieve successful block while keeping local anesthetic volume and concentration low is US imaging, which allows more accurate needle positioning in proximity to the nerve and visualization of local anesthetic spread to ensure adequate exposure.[60,61] Of greatest importance is the ability to avoid intravascular injection. This risk may be reduced when using US, especially if combined with color Doppler for vessel localization.

The degree of systemic drug absorption and duration of anesthesia can also vary depending on the site of injection (i.e., level of local vascularity) and addition of vasoconstrictors. The highest blood levels of local anesthetic occur after intercostal blocks, followed by caudal, epidural, brachial plexus, intravenous regional, and lower extremity blocks. Equivalent doses of local anesthetic may produce only 3 to 4 hours of anesthesia when placed in the epidural space but 12 to 14 hours in the arm and 24 to 36 hours when injected along the sciatic nerve. Many believe that the addition of epinephrine (1:200,000 to 1:400,000) is advantageous in prolonging the duration of block and in reducing systemic blood levels of local anesthetic, although this has more relevance to local anesthetics like lidocaine and less to ones like bupivacaine. Its use is not appropriate in the vicinity of "terminal" blood vessels, such as in the digits, penis, or ear or when using an intravenous regional technique. Using significant quantities of local anesthetic during PNB should not be performed unless oxygen, suction, monitoring, and appropriate resuscitation equipment is immediately available. However, even small doses of local anesthetic may produce significant side effects when injected into susceptible regions such as the neck. When performing PNB, a test dose of an epinephrine-containing solution and small incremental injections are recommended to reduce the risk of unrecognized intravascular injection. Toxicity can also occur from peripheral absorption of excessive doses of local anesthetic. Patients should be observed carefully for at least 30 minutes following injection since peak blood levels may occur at this time.

Animal studies[62] and case reports[63,64] have shown successful resuscitation from local anesthetic toxicity by intravenous administration of Intralipid 20% (not the 10% lipid of propofol), using one or more boluses (each of 1 to 2 mL/kg or 100 mL) followed by a 30-minute infusion (0.5 mL/kg/min). It is important to use this strategy as an acute resuscitation agent only after standard measures have proven ineffective.

Nerve Damage and Other Complications

Peripheral nerve injury in humans may result from intraneural injection[65,66] or direct needle trauma,[67] although there are other causes, including those related to the surgical procedures (e.g., patient positioning, proximity of nerve to surgical site, and tourniquet application).[68] Needle-related trauma without injection may result in injury of lesser magnitude than that from injection injury.[69] In animal studies, nerve injury appears to occur when high injection pressures are applied intrafascicularly and particularly when highly concentrated local anesthetic solutions or their preservatives are used.[42,43,70] One major sequela from intrafascicular injection is endoneurial ischemia.[71] Although in some cases these syndromes resolve uneventfully, full recovery of some peripheral injuries may never occur or may require several months, a result of slow regeneration of injured peripheral nerves.[65]

Other minor complications that have been reported following PNB include pain at the site of injection and local hematoma formation, but these are self-limiting side effects and are best dealt with by communication with the patient and reassurance by the anesthesiologist. A hematoma around a peripheral nerve is not of the same significance or risk as that occurring in the epidural or subarachnoid space. It is important to address concerns expressed by patients and to make every effort to relieve any pain or discomfort resulting from various interventions.

Clinical Anatomy

Anatomical descriptions of major nerve structures, including plexuses and terminal/peripheral nerves are discussed in this section. The section is divided on the basis of regions of the body: head and neck, spine, upper extremity, trunk, and lower extremity.

Head and Neck

Trigeminal Nerve

Sensory and motor innervation of the face is provided by the branches of the fifth cranial (trigeminal) nerve. The roots of this nerve arise from the base of the pons and send sensory branches to the large semilunar (trigeminal or Gasserian) ganglion, which lies on the dorsal surface of the petrous bone. Its anterior margin gives rise to three main branches: The ophthalmic, maxillary, and mandibular nerves (Fig. 36-5). A smaller motor fiber nucleus lies behind the main trigeminal ganglion and sends motor branches to the terminal mandibular nerve. The three major branches of the trigeminal nerve each have a separate exit from the skull:

- The uppermost ophthalmic branch passes through the sphenoidal fissure into the orbit. The main terminal fibers of this sensory nerve, the *frontal nerve*, run to behind the center of the orbital cavity and bifurcate into the supratrochlear and supraorbital nerves. The *supratrochlear* branch traverses the orbit along the superior border and exits on the front of the face in the easily palpated supraorbital notch; the *supraorbital nerve* runs in a medial direction toward the trochlea.

- The *maxillary* nerve contains only sensory fibers. It exits the skull through the round foramen (foramen rotundum), passes beneath the skull anteriorly, and enters the sphenopalatine fossa. At this point, it lies medial to the lateral pterygoid plate on each side. At the anterior end of this channel, it again moves superiorly to re-enter the skull in the infraorbital canal in the floor of the orbit. It branches to form the zygomatic nerve, which extends to the orbit, the short sphenopalatine (pterygopalatine) nerves, and the posterior dental branches. The anterior dental nerves arise from the main trunk as it passes through the infraorbital canal. The terminal infraorbital nerve penetrates through the inferior orbital fissure to the base of the orbit, to the infraorbital groove and canal (just below the eye and lateral to the nose), and reaches the facial surface of the maxilla. It then divides into the palpebral (lower eyelid), nasal (wing of the nose), and labial nerves (upper lip).

- The *mandibular* nerve is the third and largest branch of the trigeminal nerve and the only one to receive motor fibers. It exits the skull posterior to the maxillary nerve through the foramen ovale, forms a short thick trunk, and then divides into anterior and posterior trunks, which are mainly motor and sensory, respectively. The main branch (posterior trunk) continues as the inferior alveolar nerve medial to the ramus of the mandible and innervates the molar and premolar teeth. This nerve curves anteriorly to follow the mandible and exits as a terminal branch (mental nerve) through the mental foramen. The *mental* nerve provides sensation to the lower lip and chin. Other terminal nerves include the lingual nerve (floor of mouth and anterior two-thirds of tongue) and the auriculotemporal nerve (ear and temple).

Cervical Plexus

Sensory and motor fibers of the neck and posterior scalp arise from the anterior rami (branches) of the first four cervical (C1–C4) spinal nerves (Fig. 36-6). The cervical plexus is unique in that it divides early into cutaneous branches (penetrating the cervical fascia) and muscular branches (deeper branches that innervate the muscles and joints), which can be blocked separately (see Specific Techniques section). The dermatomes of the cervical nerves C2–C4 are illustrated in Figure 36-7.

- Classic cervical plexus anesthesia along the tubercles of the vertebral body produces both motor and sensory blockade. The transverse processes of the cervical vertebrae form elongated troughs for the emergence of their nerve roots (Fig. 36-8). These troughs lie immediately lateral to a medial opening for the cephalad passage of the vertebral artery. The trough at the terminal end of the transverse process divides into an anterior and a posterior tubercle, which can often be easily palpated.

- These tubercles also serve as the attachments for the anterior and middle scalene muscles, which form a compartment for the cervical plexus as well as the brachial plexus immediately below. The compartment at this level is less developed than the one formed around the brachial plexus.

- The deep muscular branches curl anteriorly around the lateral border of the anterior scalene and then proceed caudally and medially. Many branches serve the deep anterior neck muscles, but other branches include the inferior descending cervical nerve, the trapezius branch of the plexus, and the phrenic nerve, which give anterior branches to the sternocleidomastoid muscle as they pass behind it.

- The sensory fibers emerge behind the anterior scalene muscle but separate from the motor branches and continue

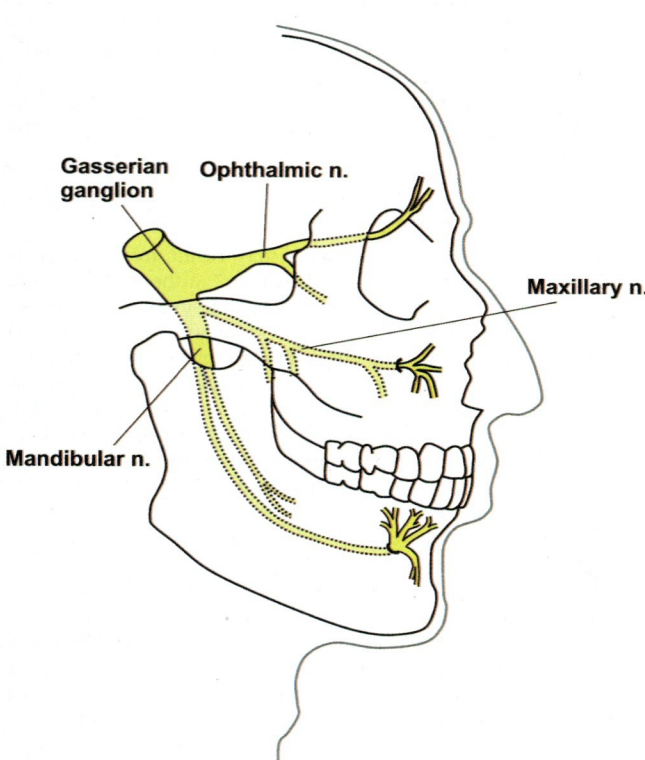

Figure 36-5 Major branches of the trigeminal nerve. The roots of the trigeminal nerve arise from the pons and form the large Gasserian (or semilunar) ganglion. The three major branches have separate exits from the skull. The main terminal fibers of the ophthalmic nerve—the frontal nerve—terminate as the supraorbital and supratrochlear nerves and exit their respective foramina. The maxillary and mandibular branches emerge from the skull medial to the lateral pterygoid plate. The maxillary nerve terminates as the infraorbital nerve (through the infraorbital foramen), and the mandibular nerve provides the inferior alveolar nerve (as well as motor branches), which exits at the mental foramen as the mental nerve.

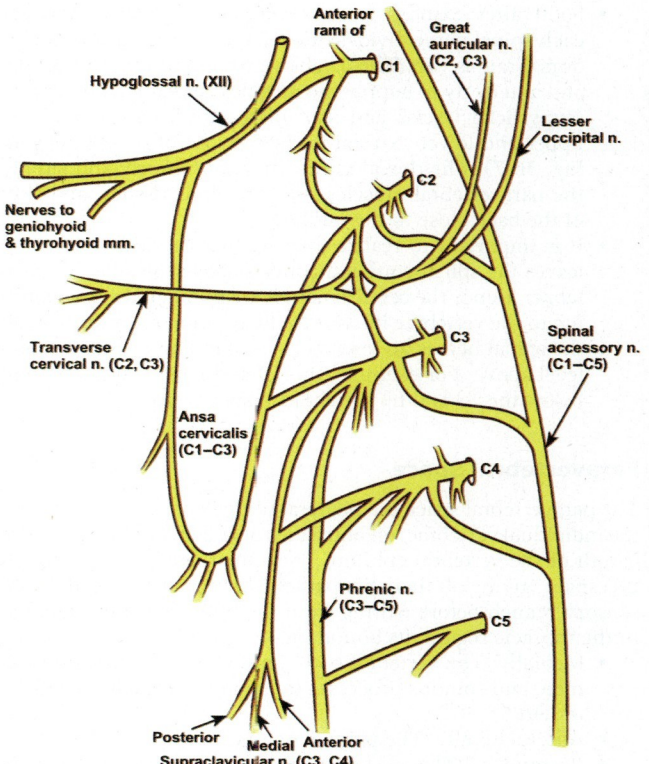

Figure 36-6 Schematic diagram of the cervical plexus, which arises from the anterior primary rami of C2–C4. The motor branches (including the phrenic nerve) curl anteriorly around the anterior scalene muscle and travel caudally and medially to supply the deep muscles of the neck. The sensory branches exit at the lateral border of the sternocleidomastoid muscle to supply the skin of the neck and the shoulder.

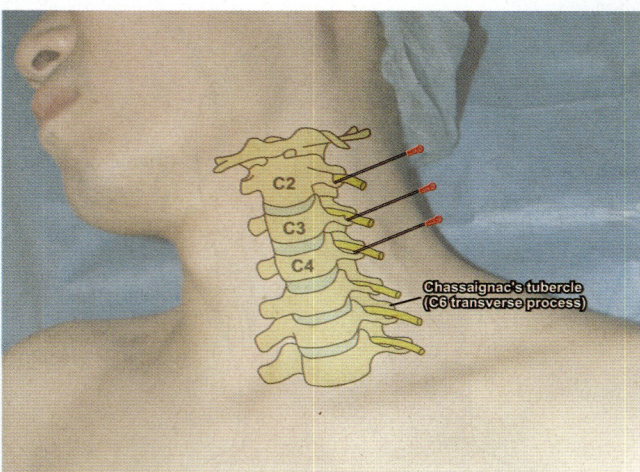

Figure 36-8 Needle insertion points and angles for deep cervical plexus block. The nerve roots exit the vertebral column via troughs formed by the transverse processes. Using caudad and posterior angulation, the needle is inserted to contact the articular pillars of C2–C4.

laterally to emerge superficially under the posterior border of the sternocleidomastoid muscle. The branches, including the lesser occipital nerve, great auricular nerve, transverse cervical nerve, and the supraclavicular nerves (anterior, medial, and posterior branches), innervate the anterior and posterior skin of the neck and shoulder.

Occipital Nerve

The ophthalmic branch of the trigeminal nerve provides sensory innervation to the forehead and anterior scalp. The remainder of

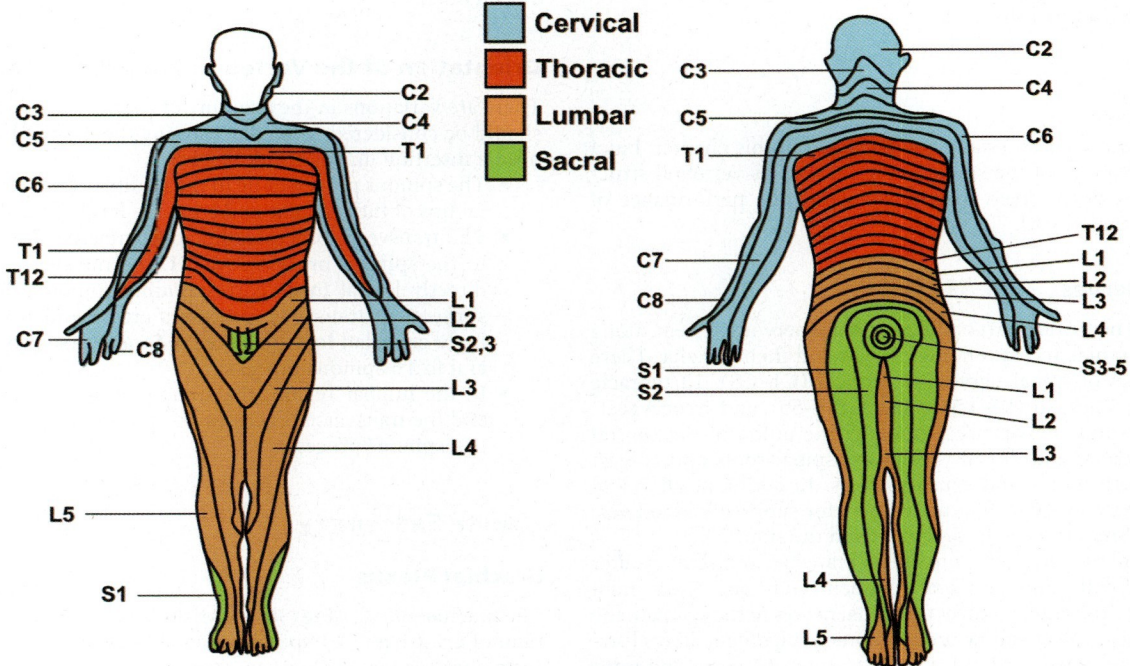

Figure 36-7 The cervical, thoracic, lumbar, and sacral dermatomes of the body.

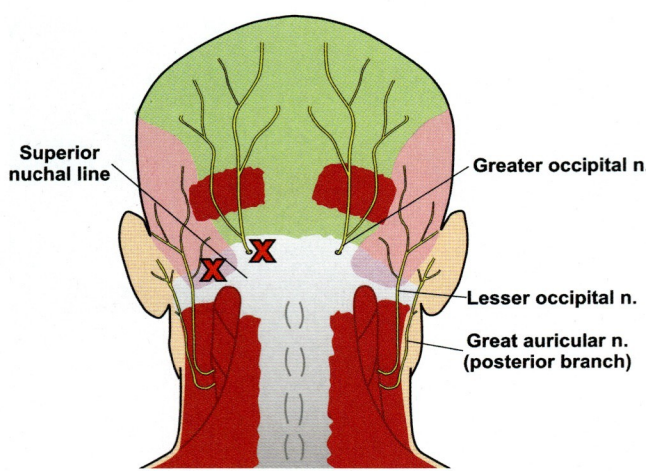

Figure 36-9 Greater and lesser occipital nerve anatomy, supply (*green*, greater occipital nerve; *pink*, lesser occipital nerve), and block needle insertion sites (*X*).

the scalp is innervated by fibers of the greater and lesser occipital nerves (Fig. 36-9).

- The *lesser occipital nerve* arises from the superficial (cutaneous) cervical plexus (Fig. 36-6), traverses cephalad from the posterior edge of the sternocleidomastoid muscle toward the top of the head, and divides into several branches. The *greater occipital nerve* arises from the posterior ramus of the second cervical spinal nerve (the cervical plexus arises from the anterior rami) and travels in a cranial direction to reach the skin in the area of the superior nuchal line while giving branches to supply the head and laterally toward the ear.
- These nerves can be blocked by superficial injection at the point on the posterior skull where they emerge from below the muscles of the neck.

Spine

Spinal/epidural anesthesia is not discussed in this chapter, but a basic description of the spinal nerves as well as vertebral structures is provided, given their relevance to the performance of other regional blocks.

Spinal Nerves

The spinal nerves are part of the peripheral nervous system, along with the cranial and autonomic nerves and their ganglia. There are 31 pairs of spinal nerves—8 cervical (C1–C8), 12 thoracic (T1–T12), 5 lumbar (L1–L5), 5 sacral (S1–S5), and 1 coccygeal.

- The spinal nerves are formed by the union of the ventral (anterior) and dorsal (posterior) spinal roots and consist of both motor and sensory fibers. In addition, all spinal nerves contain sympathetic fibers for supplying blood vessels, smooth muscle, and glands in the skin.
- The nerves give off sympathetic branches immediately after leaving the intervertebral foramen. Gray and white rami communicantes connect the spinal nerves to the sympathetic chain ganglia to allow preganglionic sympathetic fibers leaving the spinal cord (T1–L2/L3) to enter the chain and leave it again to be distributed with spinal nerves at all levels.
- Soon after exiting the intervertebral (spinal) foramina, each spinal nerve divides into a larger ventral and a smaller dorsal ramus (branches). The ventral rami course laterally and anteriorly to supply the muscles, subcutaneous tissues (superficial fascia) and skin of the neck, trunk, and the upper and lower extremities (see layout of dermatomes in Fig. 36-7). The dorsal rami course posteriorly and supply the paravertebral muscles, subcutaneous tissues, and skin of the back close to the midline.
- It is important to realize that the first cervical (C1) nerve leaves the spinal cord and courses above the atlas (C1 vertebra). Hence the cervical nerves are numbered corresponding to the vertebrae inferior to them. From this point on, all the spinal nerves are named corresponding to the vertebral level above. For example, the T3 and L4 spinal nerves exit below the T3 and L4 vertebrae, respectively.

Paravertebral Space

The paravertebral space is a bilateral wedge-shaped area between the individual vertebrae, on both sides of and extending the entire length of the vertebral column. The spinal nerves pass through this space, giving off their sympathetic branch and a small dorsal sensory branch before exiting from the intervertebral foramina. In the thoracic region, its boundaries are as follows:

- Medially: The vertebral body, intervertebral disc and foramen, and spinous processes (angulation decreases from T1 to L4/L5).
- Anterolaterally: The parietal pleura.
- Posteriorly: The costotransverse process, approximately 2.5 cm from the tip of the spinous process, often in a slightly caudad orientation.

The intervertebral foramina at each level lie between the transverse processes and approximately 1 to 2 cm anterior to the plane formed by the transverse processes in their associated fasciae. At this point, the sympathetic ganglia lie close to the somatic nerves, and coincidental sympathetic blockade is usually attained.

Orientation of the Vertebral Body Processes

There are variations in the anatomy of the vertebral column that should be considered when determining the desired location for needle insertion during trunk blocks.

- The spinous processes lie in the midline, with T7 at the distal tips of the scapulae and L4 at the level of the iliac crests.
- The transverse processes lie approximately 2.5 cm lateral to the spinous processes: at T1, the transverse process is directly lateral to its corresponding spinous process, but subsequent transverse processes are extended to increasingly cephalad locations (i.e., T7 transverse process is lateral to T6 spinous process).
- In the lumbar region, the spinous processes are straight, and the transverse processes lie opposite their own respective spinous process.

Upper Extremity

Brachial Plexus

The brachial plexus (Fig. 36-10) arises from the anterior primary rami of C5–C8 and T1 spinal nerves. The plexus consists of five *roots*, three *trunks*, six *divisions* (two per trunk), three *cords*, and five major terminal nerves.

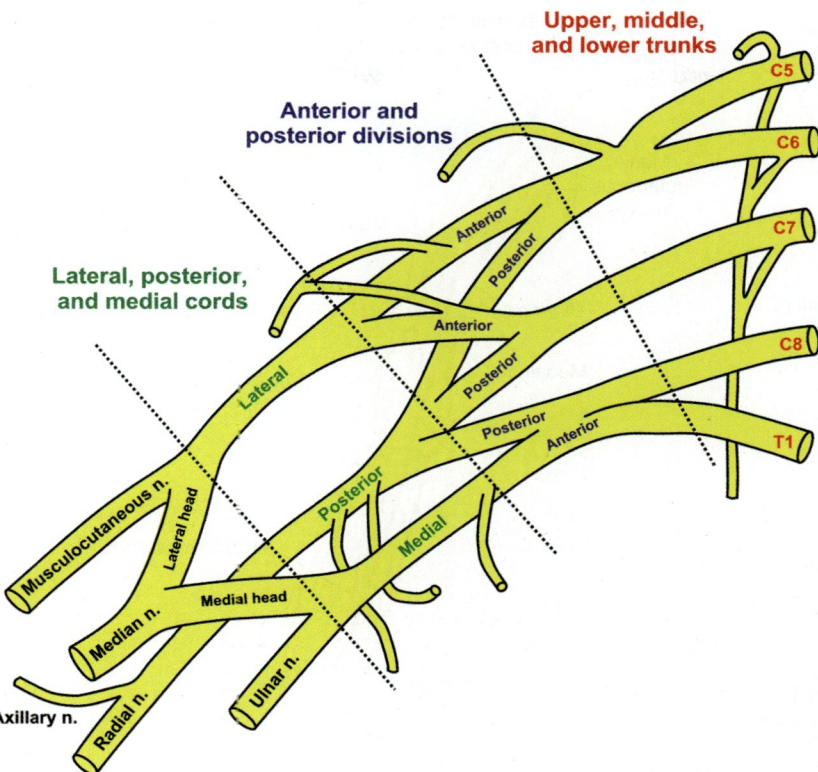

Figure 36-10 Schematic diagram of the brachial plexus. Not shown are the many branches, including the medial cutaneous nerves of the forearm and arm, which arise from the medial cord.

- The C5–T1 nerve roots emerge from their corresponding intervertebral foramina and then travel along the grooves between the anterior and posterior tubercles of the corresponding transverse process. They finally emerge between the scalenus anterior and medius muscles, above the second part of subclavian artery and posterior to vertebral artery.
- The C5 and C6 nerve roots unite to form the *upper (superior) trunk*, C7 continues as the *middle trunk*, and C8 and T1 converge into the *lower (inferior) trunk*.
- Fibrous sheaths (as part of the prevertebral fascia) surround the anterior and posterior parts of the plexus and continue to envelope the plexus between the scalene muscles more distally (called the *interscalene fascial sheath* proximally and the *axillary sheath* distally).
- The three trunks travel inferolaterally and cross the base of the posterior triangle of the neck (superficial) and the first rib (upper and middle trunks above the subclavian artery and lower trunk behind or below the artery). At the lateral border of first rib, each trunk bifurcates into *anterior* and *posterior* divisions.
- Approximately at the level where the nerves course under the pectoralis minor muscle, the divisions converge to form three *cords*: *Lateral cord*—anterior divisions of upper and middle trunks (C5–C7); *medial cord*—anterior division of lower trunk (C8, T1); *posterior cord*—posterior divisions of all three trunks (C5–T1).
- The cords are grouped around the second part of the axillary artery (within 2.5 cm from its center).[72] There are three parts of the axillary artery named for their positions above (medial to), behind, and below (lateral to) the pectoralis minor muscle. Typically, with a US probe placed to view the transverse axis of the cords, the medial cord lies inferior, the lateral cord superior, and the posterior cord posterior to the first part of the axillary artery.
- Immediately beyond the pectoralis minor muscle, the three cords diverge into the terminal branches, including the median, ulnar, radial, axillary, and musculocutaneous nerves.
- The phrenic nerve normally descends anterior to the scalenus anterior muscle and crosses the muscle from lateral to medial as it descends and passes under the clavicle and through the superior thoracic aperture into the superior mediastinum, just medial to the external jugular vein. However, there is anatomic variation of the course of the phrenic nerve, and it is not always anterior to the scalenus anterior muscle.

Terminal Nerves of the Brachial Plexus

The anatomy of the peripheral nerves is outlined here, although the clinically related innervation patterns are included in the discussion of each block's technique. Figure 36-11 illustrates the courses of these nerves within the upper extremity. Figure 36-12 illustrates the cutaneous innervation of the terminal nerves of the upper extremity. The axillary nerve is an additional terminal nerve of the upper extremity, but the anatomy and blockade of this nerve will not be discussed here.

Radial Nerve (Originates from C5–C8 and T1 Roots, Upper and Middle Trunks, Posterior Divisions, and Posterior Cord)

- This nerve originates deep (often posteromedial)[73] to the axillary artery, descends within the axilla (giving off branches to long head of the triceps brachii), passes between the medial and lateral heads of the triceps, and then descends obliquely across the posterior aspect of the humerus along the spiral (radial) groove at the level of the deltoid insertion.

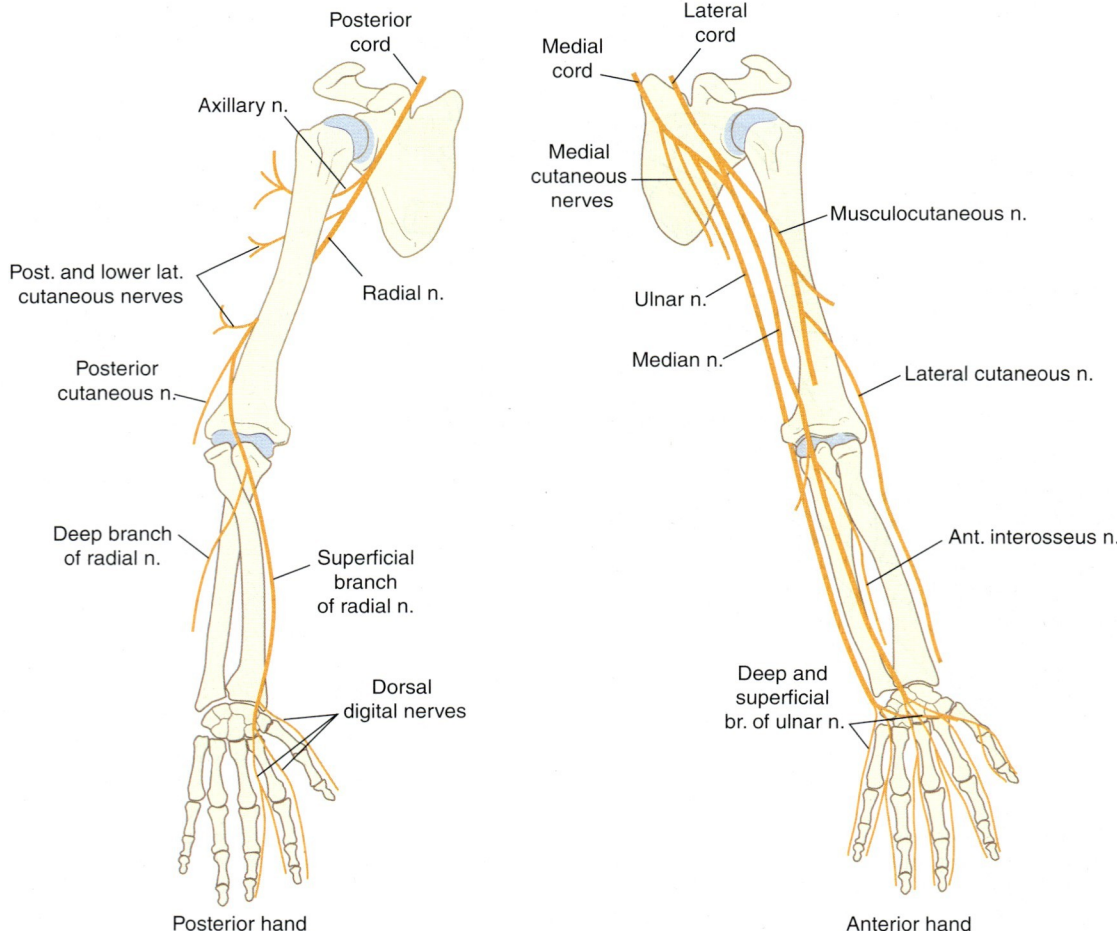

Figure 36-11 Courses of the terminal nerves of the upper extremity. The anterior view shows branches from the lateral (musculocutaneous and median nerves) and medial (median and ulnar nerves) cords, whereas the posterior view shows branches from the posterior cord (axillary and radial nerves).

- The nerve travels posterior and medial to the deep brachial artery of the arm and reaches the lateral margin of the humerus 5 to 7 cm above the elbow before crossing over the lateral epicondyle and entering the anterior compartment of the arm.

- In front of the elbow, the nerve divides and continues as the superficial radial (sensory) and the deep posterior interosseous (motor) nerves.

Median Nerve (Originates from C5–C8, T1, All Trunks, and Lateral and Medial Cords)

- In the axilla, this nerve often lies anterolateral to the axillary artery.[73,74] The nerve descends along the medial aspect of the arm lateral to the brachial artery and crosses the artery, usually anteriorly, at the midpoint of the arm at the insertion of the coracobrachialis muscle.
- The nerve crosses the elbow lying medially on the brachialis muscle and just medial to the brachial artery and vein (all of these are medial to the biceps brachii tendon).
- Distal to the antecubital fossa, the nerve gives off the anterior interosseous nerve and cutaneous sensory branches.

Musculocutaneous Nerve (Originates from C5–C7 Roots, Upper and Middle Trunks, Anterior Divisions, and Lateral Cord)

- This nerve leaves the fascial sheath of the plexus approximately at the level of the coracoid process; thus, the infraclavicular location for brachial plexus block is the most distal block for this nerve.

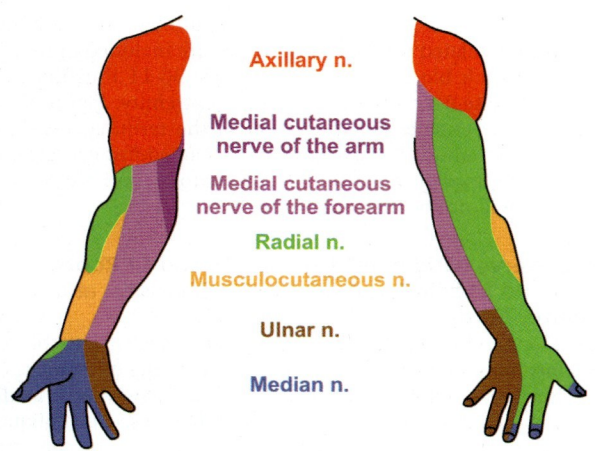

Figure 36-12 Cutaneous innervation of the upper extremity.

- Just distal (2 to 3 cm) to the pectoralis major muscle attachment, the nerve usually pierces the coracobrachialis muscle, after which it exits and comes to lie between the coracobrachialis muscle and the short and long heads of the biceps brachii muscle.
- Although it is difficult to observe using US, the nerve continues as the lateral cutaneous nerve of the forearm at the antecubital fossa and courses along the lateral aspect of the forearm providing subsequent anterior and posterior branches.

Ulnar Nerve (Originates from C7–C8, T1 Roots, Lower Trunk, Anterior Division, and Medial Cord)

- Initially, the nerve often courses between the axillary artery and vein (it may lie anteromedial to the artery and vein) and then along the medial aspect of the brachial artery to the midpoint of the humerus before passing posteriorly and following the anterior surface of the medial head of the triceps
- The nerve then passes behind the medial epicondyle of the humerus (in the condylar groove), divides between the humeral and ulnar heads of the flexor carpi ulnaris, and lies on the medial aspect of the elbow joint.
- During its descent through the forearm, the nerve courses anteriorly to approach the ulnar artery directly anterior to the ulna at the junction of the lower third and upper two-thirds of the forearm.
- At the wrist, it crosses superficial to the flexor retinaculum and divides into superficial and deep branches. The ulnar artery lies anterolateral to the nerve at the wrist.

Anatomic Variation

There are many variations in the anatomy of the brachial plexus[75] and in the course of the terminal nerves and vascular elements. Some of these variations may contribute to difficulty performing PNB since there may be unexpected NS responses (e.g., if two nerves are conjoined) or poor localization by NS or by US imaging (e.g., if the nerve follows a substantially different path). Some examples are described here:

- The plexus may include anterior rami from C4 to C8 ("prefixed") or, less commonly, from C5 to T2 ("postfixed").
- The existence and/or characteristics of the connective tissue sheath that invests the plexus at various regions are controversial. A continuous, tubular sheath has been shown unlikely, especially in the axillary region. A more convoluted and septated structure may be the cause of nonuniform distribution of local anesthetic in many cases, which supports the findings that multiple injection techniques may be superior.[76] US guidance can be valuable in this location to ensure circumferential spread of local anesthetic around the nerves.
- The interscalene groove may have variation in the relationship between the plexus roots and trunks and the muscles. For example, the C5 and/or C6 nerve roots may traverse either through or anterior to the anterior scalene muscle.[77]
- In many cadaver specimens, no inferior trunk exists.[78] A single cord or a pair of cords may develop. It has been observed that no discrete posterior cord forms in some cases, with the posterior divisions diverging to form terminal nerves.[75]
- The terminal nerves may lie in various relations to the axillary vessels. The use of combined NS- and US-guided technique to both confirm the nerve localization (NS) and obtain circumferential spread of local anesthetic around each of the nerves (US) may improve block success.[8] The musculocutaneous nerve may fuse to or have communications with the median nerve, which can result in the absence of the former from within the coracobrachialis muscle.[79,80] Communication between the median and ulnar nerves in the forearm are common, with the median nerve replacing the innervation to various muscles normally supplied by the ulnar nerve.[81]
- There may also be variations with respect to the vessels within the arm, with aberrant formations including double axillary veins, high origin of the radial artery, and double brachial arteries.[82-84]

Trunk

Intercostal Nerves and Articulations

Intercostal Nerves

- At the thoracic level, each anterior primary ramus enters a neurovascular bundle with its respective artery and vein and travels along the intercostal groove on the ventral caudad surface of each rib.
- The fasciae of the internal and external intercostal muscles provide the borders of the intercostal groove.
- As the intercostal nerves travel beyond the mid-axillary line, they give off a lateral sensory branch, whereas the main trunk continues on to the anterior abdominal wall to provide sensory and motor innervation for the trunk and abdomen down to the level of the pubis.
- The intercostal groove becomes less well defined anterior to the mid-axillary line, and the nerves begin to move away from their protected position. The lowermost intercostal nerve (subcostal; 12th) is less proximal to its accompanying rib and is not as easy to identify and anesthetize using a classic intercostal blockade technique.

Costovertebral Articulations

- The ribs articulate through two synovial joints with the vertebral column, each enclosed in fibrous capsules that are reinforced by ligaments:

Costovertebral joint is a synovial articulation of the head of the rib with the demi-facets on the adjacent thoracic vertebral bodies and the corresponding intervertebral disc of the upper vertebral joint (except for 1st, 10th, 11th, and 12th ribs, which articulate with a single vertebral facet).

Costotransverse joint is a synovial joint between the articular facets on the tubercles of the ribs and the transverse processes of the thoracic vertebrae (the 11th and 12th ribs lack this articulation since they do not possess tubercles). Penetration of the costotransverse ligament may occur during paravertebral block.

Lumbar Spinal Nerves and Plexus

The spinal nerves at the lumbar level follow the same course as those of the thoracic level when leaving the intervertebral foramen, yet the anterior (ventral) rami form the lumbar plexus instead of continuing as intercostal nerves. The lumbar plexus (Fig. 36-13) is formed by the union of the anterior primary rami of L1–L3 and part of L4.

- The upper nerve roots emerge from their foramina into a compartment lined by the fasciae of muscles anterior and posterior to it. In this case, the quadratus lumborum is posterior, whereas the posterior fascia of the psoas muscle

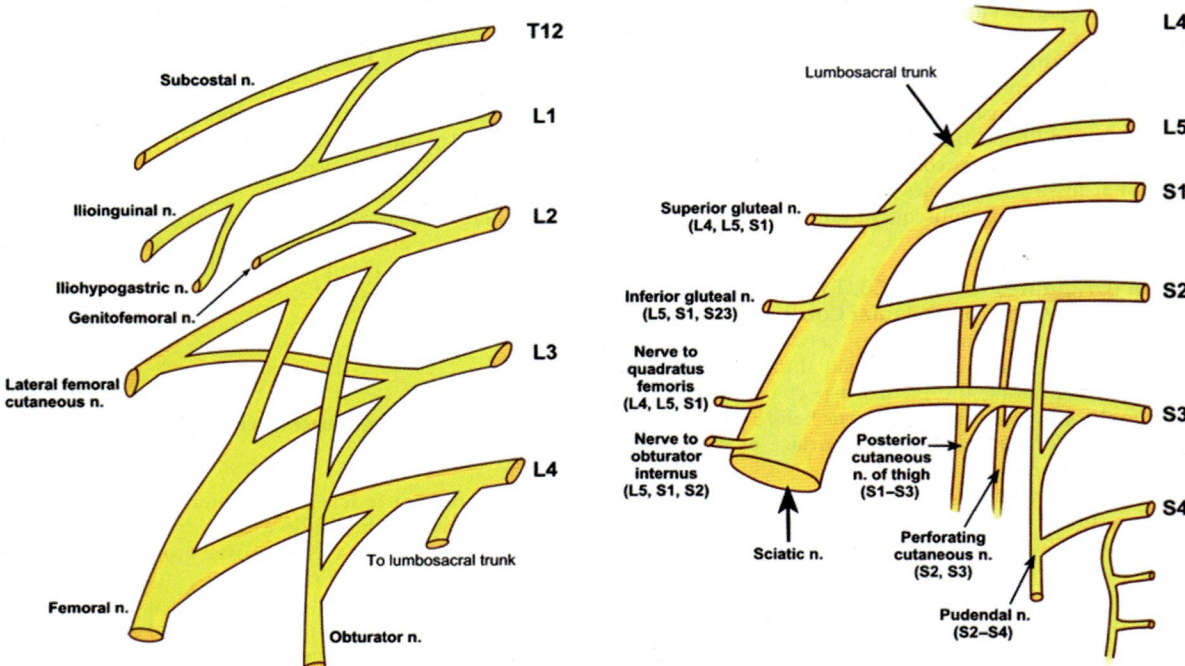

Figure 36-13 Schematic diagrams of the lumbar (left; L1–L4) and sacral (right; L4–S4) plexuses.

provides the anterior border of the compartment before the nerves move into the body of the muscle.
- The lumbar plexus supplies the skin and muscles of the lower part of the anterior abdominal wall (including the external genitalia) and the skin and muscles of the anterior and medial compartments of the thigh. L1 bifurcates into an *upper* part (iliohypogastric and ilioinguinal nerves) and *a lower* part, which joins with a branch from L2 to form the genitofemoral nerve. L3, with portions of L2 and L4, divides into *anterior* and *posterior divisions;* the anterior division forms the obturator (L2–L4) and accessory obturator (L3, L4, when present) nerves, whereas the posterior division forms the lateral (femoral) cutaneous nerve of the thigh (L2–L3) and the femoral nerve (L2–L4).

In anatomic relation to the psoas major muscle, the obturator (L2–L4) and accessory obturator nerves emerge from its medial border, the genitofemoral (L1, L2) pierces the muscle to lie on its anterior surface, and all others emerge from its lateral border.

Terminal nerves of the lumbar plexus are discussed in the Lower Extremity section.

Inguinal Nerves

The iliohypogastric nerve penetrates the transverse abdominis muscle just above the iliac crest, supplies the muscle, and divides into anterior and lateral cutaneous branches:
- The anterior branch pierces and supplies the internal oblique muscle just 2 cm medial to the anterior superior iliac spine. It then courses deep to the external oblique muscle and superior to the inguinal canal and pierces the external oblique aponeurosis about 2 to 3 cm above the superficial inguinal ring, terminating subcutaneously in the skin of the suprapubic region.
- The lateral cutaneous branch supplies the anterolateral portion of the gluteal skin after piercing both the oblique muscles. The ilioinguinal nerve pierces and supplies the internal oblique muscle and then enters the inguinal canal, where it traverses outside the spermatic cord to emerge through the superficial (external) inguinal ring (the external oblique aponeurosis), providing cutaneous innervation to the skin of the scrotum (or labium majus) and adjacent thigh.

Lower Extremity

Together, the lumbar and sacral plexuses (Fig. 36-13) supply the lower limb. The formation of the lumbar plexus is discussed in the section above. Important landmarks that contain the plexus during its course include the psoas compartment, bordered posteriorly by the quadratus lumborum muscle and anteriorly by the posterior fascia of the psoas muscle, and, more distally, the substance of the psoas major muscle. The anatomy of the terminal nerves is examined later, as are the formation and branches of the sacral plexus. Cutaneous innervation in the lower extremity is shown in Figure 36-14. The lower extremity dermatomes are shown in Figure 36-7.

Sacral Plexus: Formation and Branches

At the medial border of the psoas major muscle, the lumbosacral trunk is formed by the union of a branch of L4 and the anterior ramus of L5. After exiting through the anterior sacral foramina, the anterior primary rami of S1–S4 join the lumbosacral trunk to form the sacral plexus (Fig. 36-13). The nerves of the plexus converge toward the greater sciatic foramen anterior to the piriformis muscle on the posterior pelvic wall. The main terminal nerves are the sciatic nerve (continuation of the plexus) and the pudendal nerves ("terminal branches"). Several other small branches are given off, including muscular branches (e.g., inferior and superior gluteal nerves and nerves to the quadratus

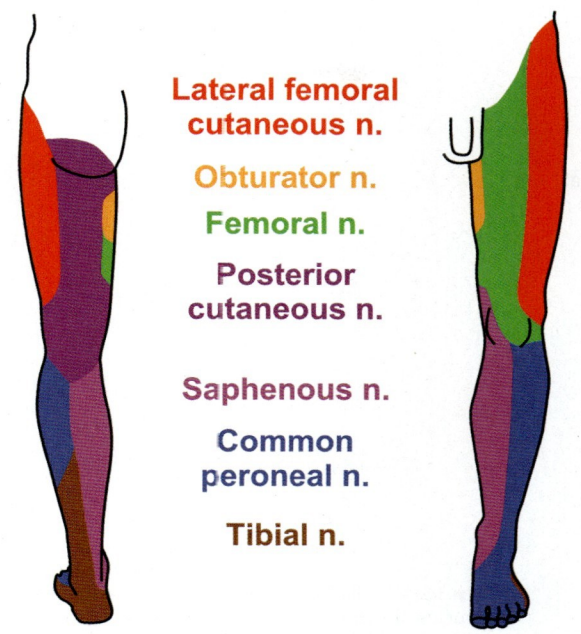

Figure 36-14 Cutaneous innervation of the lower extremity by terminal nerves.

femoris, piriformis, obturator internus, and external sphincter muscles), cutaneous branches (e.g., posterior cutaneous nerve of the thigh), and visceral branches (pelvic splanchnic nerves). The gluteal vessels (superior and inferior) generally follow the course of the sacral nerves in the anterior plane and can be used to help identify the sciatic nerve at its proximal course. Additional vascular structures that may be identified under US imaging are the pudendal vessels, which pass from the greater to lesser sciatic foramen between the sciatic and pudendal nerves.

Sciatic, Tibial, and Common Peroneal Nerves

The sciatic nerve—the largest nerve of the body—is usually the conjunction of two trunks initially enveloped in a common sheath: A lateral trunk (L4–S2), which eventually emerges as the common peroneal nerve and a medial trunk (L4–S3), which later becomes the tibial nerve. These combined nerves exit through the sciatic notch and pass anteriorly to the piriformis muscle to then lie between the ischial tuberosity and the greater trochanter of the femur. They curve caudally and descend in the posterior thigh adjacent to the femur. At a variable distance within the posterior thigh (often high in the popliteal fossa), the sciatic nerve bifurcates into the tibial and common peroneal nerves. The common peroneal nerve descends along the medial border of the biceps femoris muscle and then on the lateral border of the gastrocnemius muscle. At the fossa, it gives off the lateral sural nerve, which forms the lateral sural cutaneous nerve by joining the medial sural nerve supplied by the tibial nerve. It winds around neck of the fibula and terminates as the deep and superficial peroneal nerves. In the posterior thigh, the tibial nerve is covered medially by the semitendinosus and semimembranosus muscles and laterally by the biceps femoris muscle. Beyond the knee joint, it is covered by both heads of the gastrocnemius muscle and then deep to the soleus muscle, before coming to an end on the tibialis posterior muscle and finally on the posterior surface of the tibial shaft medial to the medial malleolus. Within the fossa, it gives off muscular branches (gastrocnemius, soleus, popliteus, and plantaris muscles) as well as the medial sural nerve (to join its lateral counterpart from the common peroneal nerve). In the lower leg and foot, it gives off muscular, articular (ankle), and cutaneous branches and terminates as the medial and lateral plantar nerves. The nerve is often called the posterior tibial nerve in the lower leg.

Terminal Nerves of the Lumbar Plexus

Genitofemoral Nerve (L1, L2)

This nerve leaves the lumbar plexus at the lower border of the L3 vertebra. It pierces and then lies anterior to the psoas major muscle before descending subperitoneally and behind the ureter, where it divides into two branches (genital and femoral) at a variable distance above the inguinal ligament. The genital branch crosses the external iliac artery and traverses the inguinal canal. It supplies the cremaster muscle and skin over the scrotum and adjacent thigh (males) or the skin over anterior part of labium majus and mons pubis (females). The femoral branch descends lateral to the external iliac artery, passes under the inguinal ligament, enters the femoral sheath lateral to the femoral artery, and pierces the anterior layer of the femoral sheath and fascia lata. It innervates the skin immediately below the crease of the groin anterior to the upper part of the femoral triangle.

Lateral Cutaneous Nerve of Thigh (aka, Lateral Femoral Cutaneous Nerve) (L2, L3)

This nerve passes obliquely from the lateral border of the psoas major muscle over the iliacus to enter the thigh below or through the inguinal ligament, variably medial to the anterior superior iliac spine (Fig. 36-15). On the right side of the body, the nerve passes posterolateral to the cecum, and on the left it traverses behind the lower part of the descending colon. The nerve lies on top of the sartorius muscle before dividing into anterior (supplies skin over the anterolateral aspect of the thigh) and posterior (supplies skin on the lateral aspect of thigh from the greater trochanter to the mid-thigh) branches. Occasionally, this nerve is a branch of the femoral nerve rather than its own nerve.

Femoral Nerve (L2–L4)

The femoral nerve is the largest nerve of the lumbar plexus, supplying muscles and skin on the anterior aspect of the thigh. It descends through the psoas major muscle and emerges low at its lateral border, coursing inferiorly between the iliacus and psoas major muscles to enter the thigh under the inguinal ligament (Fig. 36-15). At the inguinal ligament (line running between anterior superior iliac spine and the medial pubic tubercle) and just distal to it (in the femoral triangle), the nerve lies slightly deeper (0.5 to 1 cm) and lateral (approximately 1.5 cm) to the femoral artery; the vein is medial to the artery ("VAN" is the mnemonic for the anatomic relationship, starting medially). At the femoral (inguinal) crease (a few centimeters caudad to the inguinal ligament), the nerve lies underneath the fascia iliaca (iliopectineal fascia), deep to the fascia lata. Beyond the femoral triangle, the nerve branches into anterior (quite proximally) and posterior divisions. The anterior division gives muscular branches to the pectineus and sartorius muscles and cutaneous branches (intermediate and medial cutaneous nerves of thigh) to the skin on the anterior aspect of the thigh. The posterior division sends muscular branches to the quadriceps femoris muscle and gives rise to the *saphenous nerve*, its largest cutaneous branch. The saphenous nerve follows the femoral artery, lying lateral to it within the adductor (Hunter's, subsartorial) canal and then crossing it

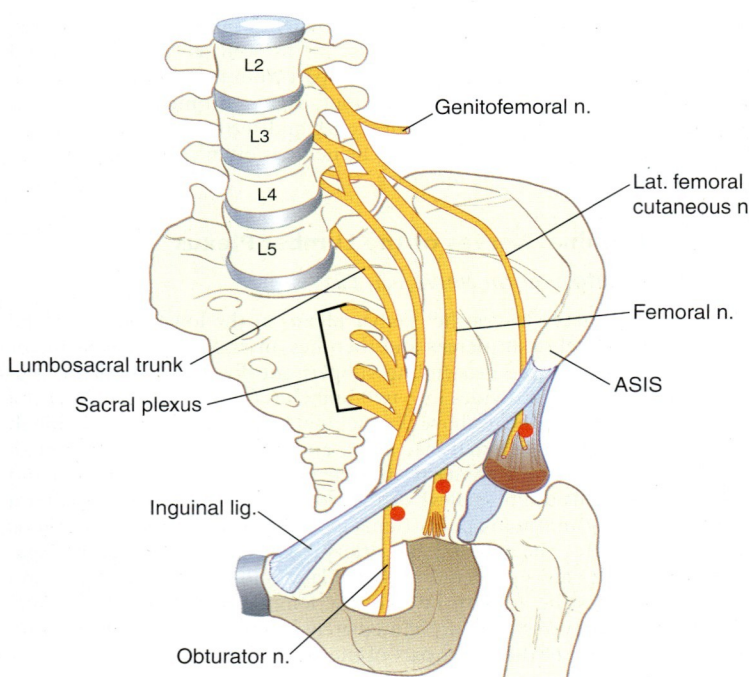

Figure 36-15 Illustration of the anterior pelvic area showing courses of major branches of the lumbar plexus. Needle insertion sites (●) for blocking the lateral femoral cutaneous, femoral, and obturator nerves are shown. ASIS, anterior superior iliac spine.

anteriorly to lie medial to the artery. Distal to the canal, the saphenous nerve leaves the artery to lie superficial at the medial aspect of the knee; the nerve then continues inferiorly (subcutaneously) with the long (great) saphenous vein along the medial aspect of the leg down to the tibial aspect of the ankle. The saphenous branch supplies the skin on the medial aspect of the leg below the knee and on the medial aspect of the foot; it provides articular branches to the hip, knee, and ankle joints.

Obturator Nerve (L2–L4)

The obturator nerve emerges from the medial border of the psoas major muscle at the pelvic brim to pass behind the common iliac vessels and lateral to the internal iliac vessels. It then courses inferiorly and anteriorly along the lateral wall of the pelvic cavity on the obturator internus muscle toward the obturator canal, through which it enters the upper part of the medial aspect of the thigh above and anterior to the obturator vessels. The nerve divides into its anterior and posterior branches near the obturator foramen (Fig. 36-15); the anterior branch passes into the thigh anterior to the obturator externus, descends in front of the adductor brevis, and behind the pectineus and adductor longus muscle, with its terminal cutaneous branches emerging as it courses alongside the femoral artery. It supplies the adductor longus, gracilis, adductor brevis (usually), and pectineus (often) muscles. Cutaneous branches supply the skin on the medial aspect of the thigh and perhaps to the medial knee. The nerve's posterior branch pierces the obturator externus muscle anteriorly and supplies it, then passes behind the adductor brevis muscle (sometimes supplies it) to descend on the anterior aspect of the adductor magnus muscle (medial to the anterior branch), which it supplies. There is no apparent cutaneous supply from this nerve. It then traverses the adductor canal with the femoral artery and vein to enter the popliteal fossa, where it terminates as an articular branch to the back of the knee joint capsule (oblique popliteal ligament).

Accessory Obturator Nerve (L3, L4)

This nerve is present in about 30% of individuals. It descends along the medial border of the psoas major muscle, crosses the superior pubic ramus behind the pectineus muscle, supplies the muscle, and gives articular branches to the hip joint.

Nerves at the Ankle

By the time the femoral, tibial, and common peroneal nerves reach the ankle, there are five branches that cross this joint to provide innervation for the skin and muscles of the foot.

Deep Peroneal Nerve (L5, S1)

This nerve lies anterior to the tibia and interosseus membrane and lateral to the anterior tibial artery and vein at the ankle. It travels deep to and between the tendons of the extensor hallucis longus and extensor digitorum longus muscles. Beyond the extensor retinaculum, it branches into medial and lateral terminal branches; the medial branch passes over the dorsum of the foot and supplies the first web space through two terminal digital branches, and the lateral branch traverses laterally and terminates as the second, third, and fourth dorsal interosseus nerves.

Tibial Nerve (aka, Posterior Tibial Nerve; S1–S3)

On the posterior aspect of the knee joint, the tibial nerve joins the posterior tibial artery and then runs deep through to the lower third of the leg where it emerges at the medial border of the calcaneal tendon (Achilles tendon). Behind the medial malleolus it lies beneath several layers of fascia and is separated from the Achilles tendon only by the tendon of the flexor hallucis longus muscle. The nerve is posteromedial to the posterior tibial artery and vein, which are, in turn, posteromedial to the tendons of the flexor digitorum longus and tibialis posterior muscles. Just below the medial malleolus, the nerve divides into the lateral and medial plantar nerves. The nerve innervates the ankle joint through its articular branches and the skin over the medial malleolus, the inner aspect of the heel (including Achilles tendon), and the dorsum of the foot (through the medial and lateral plantar nerves) with its cutaneous branches.

Superficial Peroneal Nerve

The superficial peroneal nerve lies lateral to the deep peroneal nerve in the upper leg. In the anterolateral aspect of lower leg, it becomes superficial about 7 to 8 cm above the lateral malleolus and divides into medial and lateral dorsal cutaneous nerves to supply the dorsum of the foot.

Sural Nerve

This nerve arises from tibial (medial sural nerve) and common peroneal (lateral sural nerve) nerves. It emerges to the superficial compartment at a similar but posterior level to the superficial peroneal nerve, 7 to 8 cm above the lateral malleolus. It then curves around the malleolus at some distance (1 to 1.5 cm) to enter and innervate the lateral aspect of the dorsal surface of the foot.

Saphenous Nerve

The saphenous nerve is the superficial terminus of the femoral nerve and supplies the skin over the medial lower leg (Fig. 36-14). It leaves the femoral nerve proximally in the femoral triangle (Scarpa triangle), descends within the adductor canal, and courses beneath the sartorius muscle with the femoral artery (beginning lateral of the vessel at first and then crossing to the medial side superior to the artery just proximal of the lower end of the adductor magnus muscle). Further distally, the femoral artery departs away from the sartorius muscle, traveling deep to continue as the popliteal artery at the adductor hiatus. At this location, the saphenous nerve continues its course under the sartorius muscle, traveling adjacent to the saphenous branch of the descending genicular artery. It runs superficial at the medial surface of the lower leg and in front of the heel.

Specific Techniques

The remainder of this chapter is devoted to the procedural details of specific blocks, arranged by regions of the body. In the sections for Upper Extremity, Trunk, and Lower Extremity, details for using NS and US imaging during the blocks are included. The nerve stimulator is set to deliver variable currents with a frequency of 2 Hz and pulse width of 0.1 millisecond unless stated otherwise. The volumes of local anesthetic included are those suggested for blocks during which NS was used for nerve localization; US guidance may reduce the required volume in some instances. The figures in these sections will focus predominantly on using combined US- and NS-guided technique, although procedures for blind techniques using NS are also described. The figures also include cadaveric sections obtained from the Visible Human Visualization Software which show anatomic arrangement of structures relevant to each of the blocks. It is important to note that the figures illustrating techniques in humans are representative of the clinical scenario, but without any of the sterile preparation required so as to facilitate observation of proper probe and needle handling. The description of each technique is accompanied by practical tips and evidence-based recommendations. In addition, most of the suggestions related to volume of local anesthetic are based on conventional technique. More detailed descriptions of US- and NS-guided nerve block procedures can be found in Dr. Tsui's textbooks, *Atlas of Ultrasound- and Nerve Stimulation-Guided Regional Anesthesia*[85] and *Pediatric Atlas of Ultrasound- and Nerve Stimulation-Guided Regional Anesthesia*.[86]

Head and Neck

Regional anesthesia for the head and neck is diverse, and many head and neck surgical procedures are amenable to some form of regional block. A regional technique may be the sole mode of anesthesia or may be incorporated into a balanced general anesthetic offering optimal postsurgical analgesia. Blocks can be used for ophthalmic, neurologic, ENT, plastic, and endocrine surgeries. Regional anesthesia techniques, such as trigeminal or occipital nerve block, may also be used for diagnostic and therapeutic purposes in acute and chronic pain syndromes. Block techniques range from local infiltration to field block to specific nerve blocks. Since intraoperative airway control can be challenging, the absence of definitive airway control is a frequent source of concern with regional techniques.

Regional anesthesia of the head and neck depends primarily on local infiltration and/or specific nerve blocks placed with reliable anatomic landmarks. Elicitation of paresthesia is the primary method for nerve localization, and neither NS nor US imaging have been performed or reported to any extent for these blocks. Therefore, the description of techniques in this section will deviate from other areas where there is greater reliance on nerve localization modalities using NS and US imaging.

Trigeminal Nerve Blocks

For every procedure, prepare the needle insertion site and other applicable skin areas with an antiseptic solution, and use sterile equipment. All of the blocks described here use the extraoral route, although alternative intraoral routes may be suitable in many cases.

Semilunar (Gasserian) Ganglion Block

The most comprehensive blockade of the trigeminal nerve targets the central ganglion (Fig. 36-5). This block is usually performed by neurosurgeons under fluoroscopic guidance for treatment of disabling trigeminal neuralgia. Few anesthesiologists perform this technically difficult block, and it will not be described in detail here.

Superficial Trigeminal Nerve Branch Block

Trigeminal block can be performed easily by injection of the three individual terminal superficial branches (supraorbital, infraorbital, mental nerves). Each nerve is associated closely with their respective foramina, and all foramina lie in the same sagittal plane on each side of the face (approximately 2.5 cm lateral to the mid-facial line passing through the pupil) (Fig. 36-16) and are easily located by US.[87] These foramina are readily palpable, and the nerves can be blocked with superficial injections of small quantities of local anesthetic. The bony landmarks are usually sufficient themselves for routine anesthetic purposes. However, paresthesias are desirable when performing neurolytic blocks with alcohol. An additional block of the supratrochlear nerve is required if the field of anesthesia is to cross the midline. Generally, fine, short needles (e.g., 24 to 26 gauge, 25 to 40 mm) and small syringes (1 to 5 mL) will be suitable for these blocks. The block is usually performed with the patient in the supine position.

Procedure
- *Supraorbital nerve (terminal nerve of ophthalmic branch).* The supraorbital notch can be easily palpated at the medial upper angle of the orbit or located by US as shown in Figure 36-16. The needle is inserted, and local anesthetic (see Clinical Pearls) is injected slowly after aspiration,

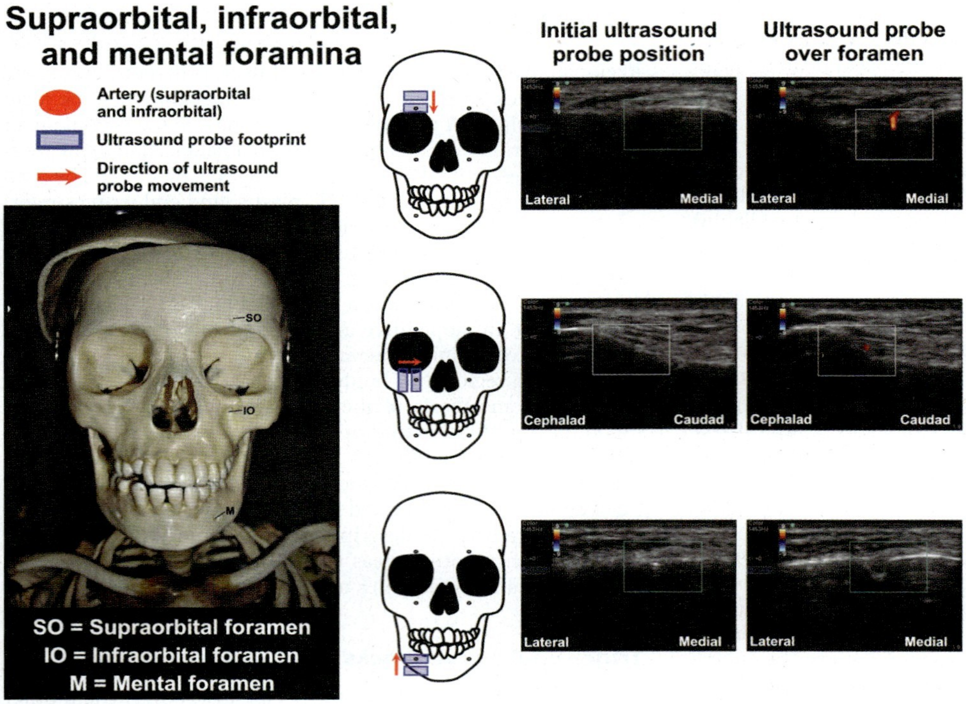

Figure 36-16 Ultrasound scanning of the supraorbital, infraorbital, and mental foramina. Discontinuation of the hyperechoic bony line indicates the position of the foramen.

slightly outside the notch, producing anesthesia of the ipsilateral forehead.
- *Supratrochlear nerve (terminal nerve of ophthalmic branch).* Anesthesia of the supratrochlear nerve is obtained with superficial infiltration of the upper internal angle of the orbital rim. This is needed if the field of anesthesia is to cross the midline.
- *Infraorbital nerve (terminal branch of maxillary nerve).* The infraorbital foramen lies about 1 cm below the middle of the lower orbital margin. If the foramen cannot be palpated directly, it can be identified by locating the discontinuity of the hyperechoic line on US (Fig. 36-16).[87] The needle should be introduced in a cranial direction through a skin wheal approximately 0.5 cm below the expected opening. After making contact with the bone and withdrawing slightly, injection of a small quantity of local anesthetic is performed. This block produces anesthesia of the middle third of the ipsilateral face.
- *Mental nerve (sensory terminal branch of mandibular nerve).* The mental nerve emerges from its foramen, which lies inferior to the outer lip at the level of the second premolar, midway between the upper and lower borders of the mandible. The mental canal angles medially and inferiorly; therefore, needle insertion should start approximately 0.5 cm above and 0.5 cm lateral to the anticipated location of the orifice if it cannot be palpated directly. Again, the use of US can aid identification of the foramen (Fig. 36-16). Slow injection after aspiration at the opening of the canal produces anesthesia of the mandibular area. Injection directly into the canal should be avoided to reduce the risk of neural injury.

Clinical Pearls
- Choice of local anesthetic for all blocks will depend on the purpose of the block and the duration of anesthesia required (e.g., 1% mepivacaine for shorter procedures and 0.75% ropivacaine for longer procedures). For surgical anesthesia, 2 to 5 mL of local anesthetic may be used, whereas diagnostic or therapeutic volumes or volumes for infants will be much smaller (0.5 to 1 mL).
- Blocks should be followed by local compression to prevent hematoma formation.
- PNB of the terminal branches of the trigeminal nerve offers a safe and effective alternative to local infiltration for soft-tissue injury of the face. Despite this, local infiltration is often required to rectify incomplete anesthesia, especially of the supraorbital and infraorbital nerves.[88]
- Infraorbital nerve block may be performed for postoperative analgesia after cleft lip repair. Palpating anatomic landmarks for this block can be difficult in the neonate due to the developing facial configuration.
- Skull nerve blocks can be used for craniotomy procedures and are also recommended to attenuate postoperative pain.[89] The nerves blocked to achieve successful anesthesia for craniotomy include the supraorbital and supratrochlear nerves, the greater and lesser occipital nerves, the auriculotemporal nerves, and the great auricular nerve.
- Supraorbital nerve blocks often require supplementation, perhaps due to the anatomic variation of the nerve. The nerve may exit the skull undivided, or its medial and lateral branches may exit separately. For frame pin placement during stereotactic neurosurgery, failure to block the lateral branch may account for inadequate coverage.[90]
- During mental nerve block in older patients, resorption of the superior margin of the mandible will make the foramen appear to lie more superiorly along the ramus.

Maxillary Nerve Block

This block should be performed by practitioners with related and adequate experience. It is required when superficial block of the infraorbital nerve does not produce adequate anesthesia or when anesthesia of the more proximal superior dental nerves is required. This can be performed by a lateral approach to the sphenopalatine fossa.

Procedure

- The patient either sits with the mouth slightly open or lies supine with a small towel under the occiput and the head turned slightly away from the side to be blocked.
- Above the zygomatic arch: The center of the upper zygomatic arch is marked. A 60- to 90-mm needle is introduced at 45 degrees caudally and medially, toward the contralateral molar teeth. After paresthesia is elicited at the nostril, upper lip, and cheek, the needle is withdrawn slightly, and local anesthetic is injected slowly and incrementally and with frequent aspiration.
- Below the zygomatic arch (Fig. 36-17): The zygomatic arch is marked along its course, and the patient is asked to open and close the mouth slowly so that the curved upper border of the mandible can be identified. The mandibular fossa is palpated between the condylar and coronoid processes. The lowest point of the mandibular notch is palpated, and an "X" is marked at this spot, which is usually at the midpoint of the zygoma. A local anesthetic skin wheal is raised at the "X" after appropriate skin preparation.
- With the patient's jaw in the open position, a 60- to 90-mm needle is introduced through the "X" at a 45-degree angle toward the dorsal part of the eyeball (cephalad and slightly anterior).
- The needle should contact the lateral portion of the pterygoid process (pterygoid plate) at a depth of 4 to 5 cm. The needle is then withdrawn and redirected slightly cephalad and anteriorly until it passes beyond the pterygoid plate and enters the pterygopalatine fossa at an additional depth of no more than 1 cm. A paresthesia in the nose or the upper teeth confirms nerve localization. The pterygopalatine fossa is highly vascular, so care must be exercised to avoid intravascular injection.
- Anesthesia can be achieved by injecting 5 mL into the pterygopalatine fossa, either upon obtaining the paresthesia or blindly by advancing 1 cm beyond the plate.

Clinical Pearls

- One concern during this block is spread of local anesthetic to adjacent structures, especially to the nerves in the orbit. If pain occurs in the region of the orbit during the procedure, the injection should be stopped, and the needle should be withdrawn.
- Although the mainstay of treatment for trigeminal neuralgia continues to be pharmacologic or neuroablative, maxillary nerve block with extraoral mandibular nerve block has been reported to provide relief in some settings.[91]

Mandibular Nerve Block

This nerve can be blocked for dental and maxillary surgery or for inferior dental pain, trigeminal neuralgia in the third branch, or temporomandibular joint dysfunction. It is the only branch of the trigeminal nerve where anesthesia carries the risk of loss of motor (mastication) function.

Procedure

- The patient lies supine with the face in profile. Landmarks for location of the mandibular fossa are the same as those described for maxillary nerve blockade.
- A 60- to 90-mm needle is introduced through the skin wheal and directed perpendicularly to the skin, without the cephalad angulation required for maxillary nerve anesthesia.
- When the pterygoid plate is contacted, the depth should be noted. The needle is then redirected posteriorly until it passes beyond the pterygoid plate. It should contact the nerve 0.5 to 1 cm deep from the point where the pterygoid plate was contacted (Fig. 36-17).
- Paresthesia of the lower jaw, lower lip, and lower incisors at a depth of approximately 4 to 4.5 cm confirms proximity to the nerve. Gentle exploration in a cephalad and caudad direction, from the initial point where the needle passes posterior to the plate, may be required. After slight needle withdrawal, 5 to 10 mL of solution is injected incrementally with repeated aspiration to avoid intravascular injection. As with maxillary blockade, paresthesias can be painful to the patient.

Clinical Pearls

- Anesthesia of the auriculotemporal nerve is often delayed.
- Facial nerve anesthesia can occasionally be seen when large volumes are injected to block the mandibular nerve. This is of little consequence unless neurolytic agents are used.
- A more serious complication is the possibility of intravascular injection in this highly vascular area. Injection should be performed incrementally with small quantities, and there should be constant observation for signs of toxicity.
- For patients with abnormal anatomy or accessory innervation to the mandible, alternatives to the standard mandibular block include the Gow-Gates and Akinosi–Vazirani blocks.[92]

Cervical Plexus Blocks

Anesthesia of either the deep or superficial cervical plexus or both can be used for procedures of the lateral or anterior neck such as parathyroidectomy and carotid endarterectomy. During carotid surgery, local infiltration of the carotid bifurcation may be necessary to block reflex hemodynamic changes associated with glossopharyngeal stimulation.

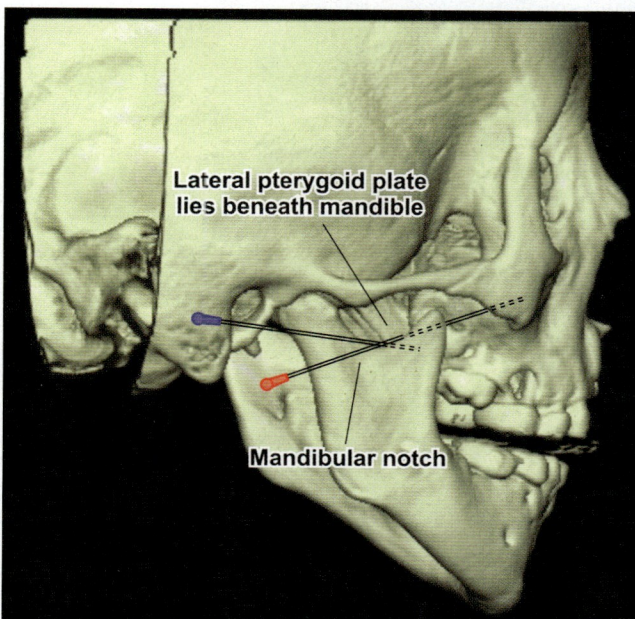

Figure 36-17 Lateral view of a computed tomography-scanned skull showing the bony landmarks and final needle insertion angles for the maxillary (*red needle*) and mandibular (*blue needle*) nerves. Each block procedure involves first reaching the lateral pterygoid plate (see text for details).

Deep Cervical Plexus Block

Procedure
- The patient is placed supine with a small towel under the head, which is turned 45 degrees to the opposite side with slight neck extension.
- Landmarks include the posterior edge of the sternocleidomastoid muscle, the caudal portion of the mastoid process, the angle of the jaw, and the transverse processes of cervical vertebrae C2–C5 (about 1.5 cm apart). If all transverse processes cannot be palpated, the most prominent tubercle of C6 (Chassaignac's) is marked. A line is drawn from the mastoid process along the sternocleidomastoid muscle to reach the transverse process of C6. Each transverse process of C2–C5 is marked approximately 0.5 to 1 cm behind the line; the transverse process of C2 lies about 1.5 cm inferior to the mastoid process.
- Skin infiltration is carried out at the "X" marks of C2–C4, and three needles (22 gauge, 3.5 to 5 cm) are introduced perpendicular to the skin and advanced about 30 degrees caudally with a slight posterior orientation (Fig. 36-8).
- After confirming contact with the transverse process, the needle is withdrawn slightly and a syringe is connected to the needle. Two to three milliliters of local anesthetic solution are injected per segment for therapeutic or diagnostic purposes or for blocks in children, whereas 5 to 10 mL per segment may be sufficient for surgical block (limiting the total to approximately 20 mL if superficial blocks are also performed).

Clinical Pearls
- The deep block may be performed by single injection at C3 or C4 as originally described by Winnie et al.[93] or by a standard three-injection technique.
- A recent anatomic study demonstrated that the longus capitis muscle is a suitable landmark for US-guided deep cervical plexus block.[94] With this approach, both the deep cervical plexus and sympathetic trunk can be blocked.
- Paresthesia occurring during these blocks has been associated with more effective anesthesia.[95]
- Anesthesia for carotid endarterectomy may involve performing combined superficial and deep cervical plexus blocks, yet the benefit of combined over superficial block alone has been questioned.[96,97] There appears to be no difference between these two approaches in the amount of supplemental local anesthesia required.
- There are several life-threatening complications that may arise from deep cervical plexus block; in fact, this block is administered rarely. Injection may occur into the vertebral artery, and subarachnoid or epidural injections are possible if the needle is advanced too far medially into the vertebral foramen. This is more likely in the cervical region because of the longer dural sleeves that accompany these nerve branches. Careful monitoring of the patient should continue for 60 minutes after the block has been performed.
- Phrenic nerve palsy leading to hemidiaphragmatic paresis is a common occurrence with deep cervical plexus block.[98] This block is not indicated in any patient who depends on the diaphragm for tidal ventilation, nor is bilateral blockade ever recommended.
- Other well-described side effects include Horner syndrome (if the superior cervical or cervicothoracic ganglion is blocked),[99] stellate ganglion block,[100] and hoarseness due to recurrent laryngeal nerve block.

Superficial Cervical Plexus Block

This block is performed in a position similar to deep cervical plexus block and results in anesthesia only of the sensory fibers of the plexus.

Procedure
- An "X" is made at the midpoint of the posterior border of the sternocleidomastoid muscle.
- Local skin infiltration is performed with a fan-like injection using 10 to 20 mL of local anesthetic (0.1 to 0.2 mL/kg for children) along the posterior border of the sternocleidomastoid muscle 4 cm above and below the level of the midpoint (Fig. 36-18).

Clinical Pearls
- The most common approach for minimally invasive parathyroidectomy (involving a small unilateral incision rather than bilateral neck exploration) includes a combination of C2–C4 superficial cervical plexus block, infiltration along the incision line and infiltration of the upper thyroid pedicle.[101] This approach can result in shorter anesthetic and operative times, leading to earlier hospital discharge, as well as significantly better postoperative pain relief.[101,102]
- Initial studies of US-guided superficial cervical plexus block showed no added benefit over the blind technique,[103] although US guidance may be helpful in emergency situations.[104]
- Using a modified surgical approach, thyroid surgery has been performed under superficial cervical plexus block in combination with anterior field block.[105]
- Minimally invasive surgery may require conversion to general anesthesia when there is difficulty ensuring adequate protection of the recurrent laryngeal nerve or when

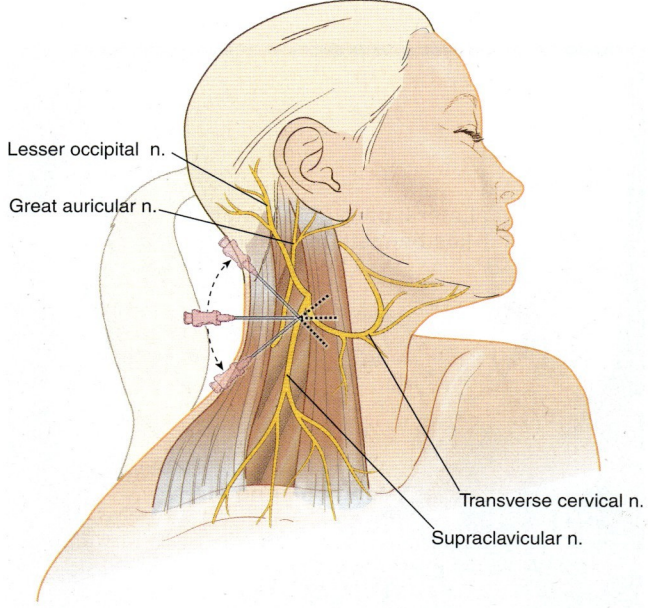

Figure 36-18 Lateral view of the head and neck, showing block needle insertion angles needed to perform superficial cervical plexus block. Initially, the needle is inserted perpendicular to the skin at the midpoint of the lateral border of the sternocleidomastoid muscle (where it is crossed by the external jugular vein). The needle can then be repositioned to superior and inferior angulations to reach the entire cervical plexus.

intraoperative diagnosis of parathyroid carcinoma or multiglandular parathyroid hyperplasia occurs.
- Phrenic nerve paralysis leading to diaphragmatic dysfunction,[95] vagus nerve block with resultant recurrent nerve paralysis,[106] and inadvertent intravascular injection[107] have all been reported.

Occipital Nerve Blocks

The greater and lesser occipital nerves can be blocked by superficial injection at the points on the posterior skull where they emerge from below the muscles of the neck. This block is rarely used for surgical procedures and is more often applied as a diagnostic step in evaluating head and neck pain complaints.

Procedure

- The patient sits with their head tilted forward slightly to expose the prominent nuchal ridge of bone at the posterior base of the skull.
- The inferior nuchal line is palpated at one-third of the distance between the external occipital protuberance and the foramen magnum. A mark is placed on the nuchal line at the lateral border of the insertion of the erector muscles of the neck, usually 2.5 cm from the midline. At this point, the branches of the greater occipital nerve usually pass laterally from behind the muscle to cross the nuchal line. The nerve is located directly lateral to the easily palpated occipital artery. During its ascent along the posterior skull, the lesser occipital nerve can be located an additional 2.5 cm away from the greater occipital nerve along the inferior nuchal line; a mark should be placed here as well (Fig. 36-9).
- A short, fine needle (e.g., 25 mm 25 gauge) is introduced with a slight cranial angulation at each mark to the depth of the skull itself. After slight withdrawal, local anesthetic is injected (e.g., 0.5 to 1 mL of 1% lidocaine for diagnostic procedures or 1 to 3 mL of 0.75% ropivacaine for therapeutic procedures). Paresthesias are occasionally encountered but are not essential for obtaining simple skin anesthesia.
- If more anterior anesthesia of the scalp is required, the lesser occipital nerve branches can also be blocked by advancing the needle subcutaneously from this point in an anterior direction toward the mastoid process. A band of anesthetic solution is deposited along the line between skin entry and the mastoid process using 2 to 3 mL of local anesthetic.

Clinical Pearls

- Blockade of the lesser occipital and great auricular nerves (both blocked by subcutaneous injection from the angle of the mandible to the mastoid process) has been successful in providing postoperative analgesia after otoplasty.[108] Reducing the requirement for opioid analgesia (with its associated nausea and vomiting) is essential due to the high incidence of pain and vomiting on the first postoperative day related to the surgical procedure alone.
- Greater occipital nerve block is commonly used for primary headache syndromes. For chronic syndromes, the anterior region involving the trigeminal nerve is also blocked.[109] It has been reported for use with cervicogenic headache, occipital neuralgia, migraine, and cluster headache.[110]
- Complications with this technique are rare. Care must be taken not to advance the needle anteriorly under the skull, as the foramen magnum might be entered unintentionally with a long needle. Local hematoma may be produced with superficial injection, but this is only a temporary problem.

Upper Extremity

Although many approaches to the brachial plexus have been described, there are traditionally four anatomic locations where local anesthetics are placed: (1) the interscalene groove near the cervical transverse processes, (2) the subclavian sheath at the first rib, (3) near the coracoid process in the infraclavicular fossa, and (4) surrounding the axillary artery in the axilla. The introduction of US imaging has increased the use of blocks at the supraclavicular fossa, as visualization of the subclavian artery and lung make these critical structures easier to avoid. It is important to stress that clear visibility of the needle is essential for this block (and generally for all blocks of the brachial plexus). The appropriate choice of approach depends not only on the patient's anatomy but also on the site of surgery and the method used to locate nerve structures.

The terminal branches of the brachial plexus can also be anesthetized by local anesthetic injection along their peripheral course as they cross joint spaces, where they lie proximal to easily identifiable structures (Table 36-1), or by injection of a dilute local anesthetic solution intravenously below a pneumatic tourniquet on the upper arm ("intravenous regional" or Bier block). The use of US may increase the number of locations where the terminal nerves can be successfully blocked. For example, the ulnar nerve can be blocked effectively at the medial surface of the midforearm, which may reduce the risk of ulnar nerve palsy posed by block at the elbow near the cubital tunnel. As stated in the introduction to Specific Techniques, the use of combined US- and NS-guided technique is stressed in the figures, and, for simplicity of viewing, the necessary sterile precautions are not shown.

Brachial Plexus Block

Interscalene Block

This block, as described by Winnie[111] in 1970, is indicated mostly for surgical anesthesia of the shoulder, upper arm, and forearm but is often insufficient for the hand. Frequently, it spares the lowest branches of the plexus, the C8 and T1 fibers, which innervate the caudad (ulnar) border of the forearm. Nevertheless, recent reports provide evidence that a low interscalene block (below C6, just superior to the clavicle) may provide sufficient anesthesia and analgesia for procedures on the lower arm.[112,113] The patient is positioned supine, with their head faced slightly to the contralateral side. The main surface landmark used for this block—the sternocleidomastoid muscle—can be accentuated by asking the patient to reach for the ipsilateral knee and by rotating the head approximately 45 degrees to the nonoperative side. The head should also be elevated slightly, and the patient should be instructed to take a deep breath since contraction of the scalenus muscles accentuates the interscalene groove. This groove lies immediately behind the lateral border of the clavicular head of the sternocleidomastoid muscle at the level of the cricoid cartilage (C6). As for all procedures of the upper extremity, prepare the needle insertion site and other applicable skin areas with an antiseptic solution and, if using US imaging, ensure sterility of the US probe with a standard sleeve cover or transparent dressing.

Procedure Using Nerve Stimulation Technique

- Landmarks: Using the maneuvers described earlier, the interscalene groove is palpated by rolling the fingers posteriorly off the lateral border of the sternocleidomastoid muscle; mark the groove as high as possible. After the patient relaxes, the prominent transverse process of C6 can often be felt directly in the groove and should be marked.
- Needling: A skin wheal is raised in the interscalene groove at the level of the cricoid. A 22-gauge, 36- to 50-mm

insulated needle (shorter for pediatric patients) is introduced through the wheal. The needle is directed medially, caudally, and slightly posteriorly in the direction of the C6 transverse process. The caudad tilt of the needle is important to avoid either entering the neural foramen or injection into the dural nerve root sheath, increasing the risk of high-spinal anesthesia or spinal cord injury.[114] Avoiding medial placement by using a mostly caudad and posterior direction may reduce the risks even more. The superficial structures of the plexus have been shown to be located at an average, shallow depth of 5.5 mm.[115] Due to compact arrangement of neck anatomy in children, an angled insertion may be needed (as opposed to perpendicular in adults) to avoid puncture of the vertebral artery or epidural/subarachnoid space.

- Nerve localization: Applying an initial current of 0.8 mA is sufficient for stimulation of the plexus (usually at a depth of 1 to 3 cm), and the current is reduced to aim for a threshold current of 0.4 mA before injection after obtaining an appropriate motor response. Diaphragmatic or trapezius twitches should be avoided, as they are associated with cervical plexus stimulation. A diaphragmatic response indicates that the phrenic nerve is being stimulated and that the needle is too anterior.
- Injection: After careful aspiration, 25- to 30-mL local anesthetic is injected in small increments to detect intraneural or intravascular placement of the needle.

Procedure Using Ultrasound Guidance (Fig. 36-19)
- Scanning: Two scanning techniques are recommended for viewing the brachial plexus at the interscalene level: (1) beginning anteriorly at the cricoid cartilage level (C6) with movement from anterior and medial to posterior and lateral toward the interscalene groove, and (2) scanning proximally from the supraclavicular fossa to the interscalene location.
- Appearance: At the supraclavicular fossa, the brachial plexus (trunks/divisions) can be seen in short axis as a tightly enclosed cluster (i.e., honeycomb-like), superior and lateral to the subclavian artery (Fig. 36-20). After tracing the nerves in a proximal fashion toward the interscalene groove, the nerve structures (roots/trunks) are visualized in a sagittal oblique section as three (usually) or up to five round or oval-shaped hypoechoic (see Common Techniques: Nerve Stimulation and Ultrasound Imaging section) structures, sometimes with a few internal punctate echoes, lying between the scalenus anterior and medius muscles. The C8 and T1 roots may be difficult to identify because of their depth.[116,117]
- Needling: After infiltration of local anesthetics to the skin at the anticipated needle puncture site, a 22-gauge, 50-mm needle (insulated is recommended) is introduced either OOP (see Common Techniques section) or IP to the probe (Fig. 36-19) and advanced to a maximum of 3 cm for most patients. For OOP needle insertion technique, the clinician stands beside or cephalad to the probe and places the initial needle puncture site cranial to the probe. The needle is typically angled somewhat caudally toward the US beam plane. For IP needle insertion technique, the needle is moved from lateral to medial (still slightly caudad) and will first penetrate the scalenus medius muscle before entering the interscalene groove. It is recommended to use NS to enable further nerve localization. Note that, in children, the brachial plexus roots are located relatively superficial at the interscalene level compared to adults. In infants, the roots may be only millimeters below the skin surface.
- Local anesthetic spread: A test injection of D5W is recommended and will help further confirm nerve localization with NS and estimate the pattern of local anesthetic spread. Local anesthetic should be deposited in the midst of the neural structures so that it spreads to surround the nerves circumferentially. Local anesthetic distention in this compartment can be seen by US as a hypoechoic (fluid) expansion.

Clinical Pearls
- The use of long-acting local anesthetics may provide analgesia for 10 to 12 hours. For longer analgesia, insertion of a continuous catheter is effective for procedures such as total shoulder replacement, although securing the catheters in the mobile neck tissues is a challenge.

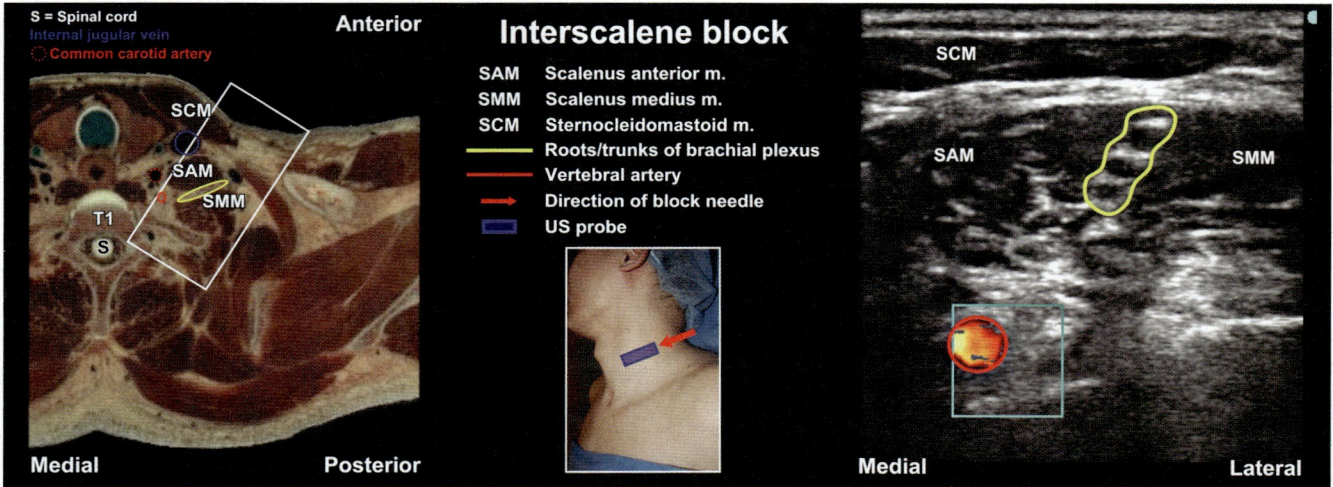

Figure 36-19 Arrangement of relevant anatomy for ultrasound-guided interscalene brachial plexus block. The block is performed using an IP needle alignment to a linear, high frequency probe. The needle is directed lateral medial with slight caudal angulation to avoid the intervertebral foramen. The roots/trunks of the plexus are usually seen as three or more round or oval-shaped hypoechoic structures sandwiched between the scalenus anterior and medius muscles in the interscalene groove. Note that the vertebral artery lies medial and deep to the brachial plexus.

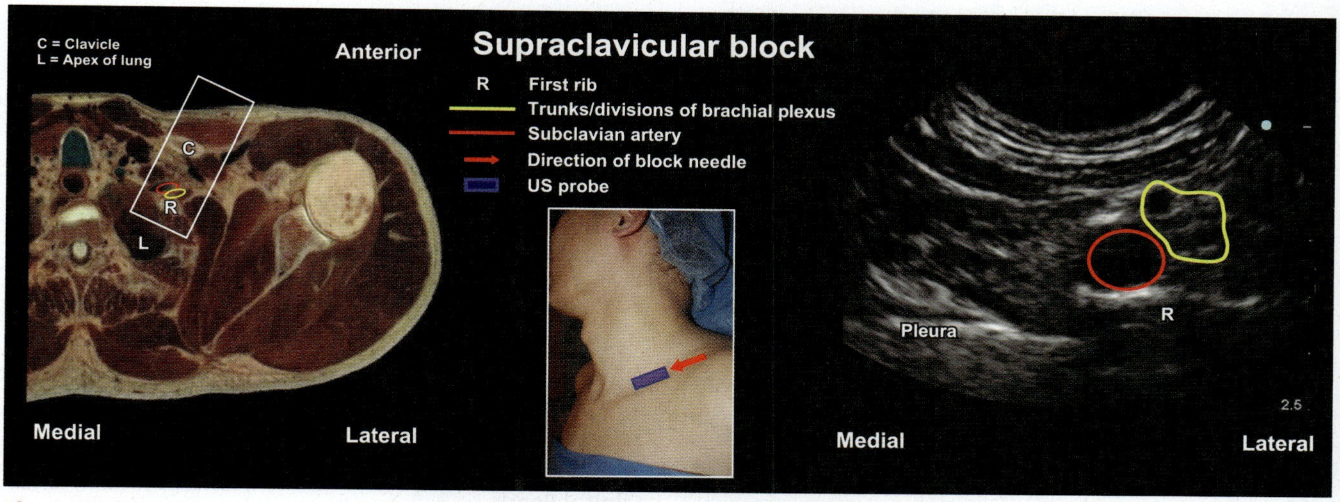

Figure 36-20 Arrangement of relevant anatomy for ultrasound-guided supraclavicular brachial plexus block. The block is performed using IP needle alignment to a small footprint curved probe with the needle inserted lateral to medial in a slightly sagittal plane. Color Doppler can be valuable to quickly locate the subclavian artery inferomedial to the plexus trunks/divisions.

- Equal success has been achieved when any of the appropriate muscle responses are elicited as a positive stimulating test. Palpation of the muscle may confirm the motor response.
- Despite the fact that subarachnoid or intraneural injection can occur even when the threshold current is more than 0.4 mA, it is advisable to avoid injecting when the current responses are less than 0.4 mA.
- If a continuous block is indicated, the needle entry point may be moved a centimeter cephalad for the OOP approach, making the corresponding angle of insertion a little steeper and more tangential to the course of the plexus. The bevel of the introducing needle should be directed laterally. Placement of a stimulating catheter may be aided by dilating the perineural space with D5W, which will allow the user to monitor the catheter's advancement to a location where motor response is maintained at less than 0.5 mA.
- Securing catheters in the freely mobile neck is a challenge. Some prefer to secure the catheter by tunneling 3 to 4 cm below the skin by passing it back through an intravenous catheter that has been introduced subcutaneously near the entry site.
- During OOP US-guided technique, more than 45-degree needle angulation should be avoided, as the needle may be inserted too deep and directed toward the spinal cord.
- Complications from this approach are related to the structures located in the vicinity of the tubercle. The cupola of the lung is close, particularly on the right side, and can be contacted if the needle is directed too far caudally. Pneumothorax should be considered if cough or chest pain is produced while exploring for the nerve. If the needle is allowed to pass directly medially, it may enter the intervertebral foramen, and injection of local anesthetic may produce spinal or epidural anesthesia. The vertebral artery passes posteriorly at the level of the sixth vertebra to lie in its canal in the transverse process that can be seen as a pulsatile structure deep to the plexus; direct injection into this vessel can rapidly produce central nervous system toxicity and convulsions. Careful aspiration and incremental injections are important to help avoid both of these potential problems.
- Even with appropriate injection, local anesthetic solution can spread to contiguous nerves. It may produce cervical plexus block, including motor fibers to the diaphragm, which may be a problem in patients with respiratory insufficiency. A case report described an optimal spread of local anesthetic and the possibility of using saline dilution technique should phrenic nerve block occur.[118]
- Horner syndrome is common because of spread to the sympathetic chain on the anterior vertebral body.
- Neuropathy of the C6 root is a potential problem because the needle may unintentionally pin the nerve root against the tubercle and predispose to intraneural injection. The needle should be withdrawn slightly if the first injection produces the characteristic "crampy" pain sensation.
- An alternative technique for blocking the roots of the brachial plexus is to perform a cervical paravertebral block,[119] which can utilize the bony landmarks of the vertebral column. This is a high quality but advanced block and should be performed using US guidance. A lateral US view of the brachial plexus at the level of C6 allows visualization of the needle as it passes lateral to the C6 transverse process and into the interscalene space. This view avoids the challenges of attempting to view the brachial plexus from a posterior approach, where the bony structures may obscure the view of the needle and plexus.

Supraclavicular Block

The supraclavicular block targets the trunks and/or divisions of the brachial plexus, depending on the location of the injection site and the patient's anatomy. Similar to the interscalene block, the patient is positioned supine with the head turned approximately 45 degrees to the contralateral side. Prepare the needle insertion site and other applicable skin areas with an antiseptic solution, and ensure sterility of the US probe with a standard sleeve cover or transparent dressing.

Procedure Using Nerve Stimulation Technique (Note that most clinicians prefer to perform this block under US guidance to minimize potential complications; some may use NS as an adjunct method with US.)

- Landmarks: The outline of the clavicle is drawn on the skin, and the midpoint of the clavicle is marked. An "X" is placed posterior to this midpoint in the interscalene groove,

usually 1 cm behind the clavicle. Since the plexus lays immediately cephaloposterior to the subclavian artery, its pulse serves as a reliable landmark in thinner individuals.
- Needling: Local infiltration is performed at the site of the nerve, and a 2.5- to 5-cm, 22-gauge needle is introduced in the parasagittal plane at the superior border of the clavicle at the lateral edge of the sternocleidomastoid muscle insertion. An initial insertion angle of 45 degrees cephalad is recommended, with subsequent reductions in angle as necessary,[120] although an angle of less than 20 degrees may lead to the needle contacting the pleura and/or subclavian vein prior to the plexus. The rib may be contacted, with subsequent anteroposterior needle adjustment to contact the plexus, but avoiding rib contact may be most prudent. Careful lateral or medial exploration may be needed, but probing too medially increases the risk of contacting the pleura. For children, a weight-dependent guide can help in determining needle insertion depth. In general, for a 10-kg child, the needle is inserted 10 mm; depth of insertion increases 3 mm for every 10 kg increase in weight until 50 kg. For children above this weight, insertion advances 1 mm for every 10 kg increase in weight (maximum depth should not be >35 mm). However, it would be much preferable to use US as a guide.
- Nerve localization: Responses to NS can be useful for confirmation of needle proximity to the separate trunks. Twitches of pectoralis, deltoid, biceps (upper trunk), triceps (upper/middle trunk), forearm (upper/middle trunk), and hand (lower trunk) muscles with current intensity of 0.4 mA (0.1 to 0.3 milliseconds) are acceptable. Distal responses (hand or wrist flexion or extension) are best to confirm placement within the fascia. Multiple nerve responses are not required.
- Injection: If a nerve response is produced during the course of exploration, the anesthetic solution can be injected while the needle is fixed in position. Twenty-five to forty milliliters of local anesthetic will produce adequate analgesia. In children, the fascia surrounding the nerve trunks is less adherent than in adults, which may lead to greater spread of local anesthetic.

Procedure Using Ultrasound Imaging (Fig. 36-20)
- Scanning: The probe is first placed in a coronal oblique plane at the lateral end and just above the upper border of the clavicle. It is then moved medially until an image of the subclavian artery appears on the screen. Some dorsal and ventral rotations of the probe may be necessary. With the subclavian artery in the middle of the screen, the plexus is located superolateral to the artery, and the neurovascular structures lie above the first rib. Small-footprint probes are generally used for scanning children since they offer better needle movement around the probe.
- Appearance: The subclavian artery is anechoic, hypodense, pulsatile, and round; its identity can be further confirmed by color Doppler. Trunks/divisions of the brachial plexus appear as a cluster of hypoechoic "grape-like" structures consisting of usually three (more as one moves distally) hypoechoic nodules, all surrounded by a hyperechoic lining (presumably the connective tissues). With the probe in a coronal oblique plane, the plexus depth has been shown with MRI to equal 1.65 cm in males and 1.45 cm in females.[120,121] Medial and deep to the artery, the rib may be seen as a hyperechoic line with dorsal shadowing. The anechoic subclavian vein may be seen inferomedial to the artery.
- Needling: The selected needle insertion site is often more lateral with the US-guided technique than when using NS techniques. The skin is infiltrated with local anesthetic, and a 22-gauge, 50-mm (or less) needle (insulated is recommended) is introduced with IP needle alignment to a curved, small footprint (Fig. 36-20) or linear probe. The needle is inserted immediately above the clavicle in a lateral-to-medial direction with a slight cephalad angle. It is recommended to have the concurrent use of NS for additional confirmation of nerve localization and as an additional monitor to prevent intraneural injection by having the threshold stimulation more than 0.2 mA. See earlier for acceptable motor responses to NS.
- Local anesthetic spread: It is best to deposit a local anesthetic next to the nerve structures immediately lateral to the subclavian artery on top of the first rib. Injection in this location will often lift the nerve structures superiorly away from the first rib and subclavian artery. The hypoechoic spread of local anesthetic surrounding the nerves may be seen on the US screen.

Clinical Pearls
- It is recommended to use US imaging combined with NS technique during this block to help avoid puncturing the pleura. When using US, it is critical to be able to visualize both the first rib and the pleura and to optimize the image such that the first rib covers the pleura, especially just lateral to the subclavian artery where the target of the needle tip is. It is critical to measure and be aware of the skin–pleura distance with US prior to needle insertion. The responses to NS can be useful for confirmation of needle proximity to the separate trunks.
- The major challenge with US imaging in this region is the presence of a bony prominence (clavicle) and curved soft tissue contour that can interfere with imaging of the brachial plexus in short axis. Despite the advantages of commercially available, low to moderate frequency curved array probes (e.g., C11, Titan or MicroMaxx, Sonosite Inc., Bothell, WA), a curved array probe with a small footprint is extremely useful in this compact area.
- The lateral-to-medial IP needle approach will ensure that the needle approaches the nerve structures before reaching the subclavian artery (i.e., less chance of inadvertent vascular puncture). However, using a slightly sagittal plane (Fig. 36-20) may reduce the risk of pleural puncture. The needle should be viewed at all times when using a lateral-to-medial approach.
- The greatest risk when using this technique is pneumothorax, as the cupola of the lung lies just medial to the first rib, not far from the plexus. The risk of pneumothorax is greater on the right side as the cupola of the lung is higher on that side. The risk is also greater in tall, thin patients. In children, the brachial plexus at this level is relatively superficial and close to the pleura; careful needle insertion must be exercised to avoid the risk of pneumothorax.
- This method does not introduce any more complications than other methods of brachial plexus block.
- When using a catheter-over-needle method, a medial-to-lateral approach is indicated to reduce the risk of dislodgement.[122] This approach will place the needle tip in the corner immediately lateral to the subclavian artery and above the first rib.

Infraclavicular Block

Infraclavicular block targets the cords of the brachial plexus, and the nerves can be blocked next to the second part of the axillary artery at the level of the coracoid process. Brachial plexus block in the infraclavicular area offers excellent analgesia of the entire arm and allows introduction of continuous catheters to provide prolonged postoperative pain relief. The infraclavicular approach blocks the musculocutaneous and axillary nerves more consistently because they often branch off high in the axilla and can be missed with the axillary block approach. However, multiple injections may be required for successful infraclavicular and axillary blocks.

Infraclavicular blocks are indicated for forearm, elbow, and hand surgeries. The patient is supine with the head turned approximately 45 degrees to the nonoperative side, and their arm may be either at their side with hand on the abdomen or abducted with their palm placed behind their head. When preparing for this block, it is common to have the patient's elbow flexed and the hand resting on the abdomen to facilitate observation of motor responses generated with NS. Alternatively, externally rotating the arm and placing the hand behind the head stretches the cords and brings the nerves closer around the axillary artery, which may facilitate local anesthetic spread around the nerves. As always, prepare the needle insertion site and other applicable skin areas with an antiseptic solution and ensure sterility of the US probe with a standard sleeve cover or transparent dressing.

Procedure Using Nerve Stimulation Technique

Several approaches have been described for infraclavicular block, all with various needle puncture sites and angles of insertion.[123–128] Here we describe a lateral approach,[124] which may improve plexus cord localization and reduce risk of puncture to both the pleura and axillary artery.[129,130]

- Landmarks: With the patient's arm adducted and their hand resting on their abdomen, the medial aspect of the coracoid process is palpated as one slips their finger off the clavicle.
- Needling: After skin preparation and skin wheal, a 50- to 90-mm, 18- to 22-gauge needle is inserted where the clavicle meets the medial aspect of the coracoid process, generally directed 0 to 15 degrees posterior to the horizontal plane (Fig. 36-21 illustrates this needle insertion when using US guidance). The 15-degree trajectory will likely increase the chances of contacting the more posteriorly located posterior or medial cords which may improve analgesia. A greater angle may be required to achieve adequate responses to NS, since local anesthetic injection at more than one cord may be beneficial. The cords should be approximately 4 to 6 cm deep (insertion of more than 7.5 cm may risk pleural puncture).[124] The needle puncture site may be adjusted slightly caudad to this location, as with the technique of Kapral et al.[123] If the needle is placed 2.5 cm caudad to the coracoid process, a laterally projected needle directed toward the axillary artery may be effective.[124]
- Nerve localization: The first response (elbow flexion) obtained is usually the musculocutaneous nerve arising from the lateral cord. For complete anesthesia of the hand, a separate distal response needs to be obtained from the medial (distal flexors) and posterior (distal and proximal extensors) cords.[131] A simplified approach to determining the specific cord distal responses during infraclavicular block has been described.[132] A close examination of the movements of the fifth digit (pinkie) can be useful to differentiate the cords, with lateral movement (i.e., pronation) representing the lateral cord, medial movement (i.e., flexion) representing the medial cord, and dorsal movement (i.e., extension) representing the posterior cord.[132] Some practitioners also advocate that eliciting a forearm response (pronation via the lateral cord) is essential for a complete block.[133] The artery may be punctured easily at this point, and careful aspiration is required to prevent intravascular injection.
- Injection: If a musculocutaneous nerve response is obtained, the nerve or lateral cord can be blocked by an injection of 5 to 10 mL of local anesthetic. Once responses in the hand are obtained, a further 25 mL of local anesthetic can be injected along the posterior and medial cords.

Procedure Using Ultrasound Imaging (Fig. 36-21)

- Scanning: Immediately medial and inferior to the coracoid process, position a linear or curved lower frequency transducer (4 to 7 MHz), depending on body habitus, in a parasagittal plane, and capture the best possible short-axis view of the brachial plexus cords and axillary vessels. If the patient is quite thin or if using a more medial location (not described here) where the nerves are more superficial, a higher frequency probe may be used.
- Appearance: The pectoralis major and minor muscles are separated by a hyperechoic lining (perimysium); the

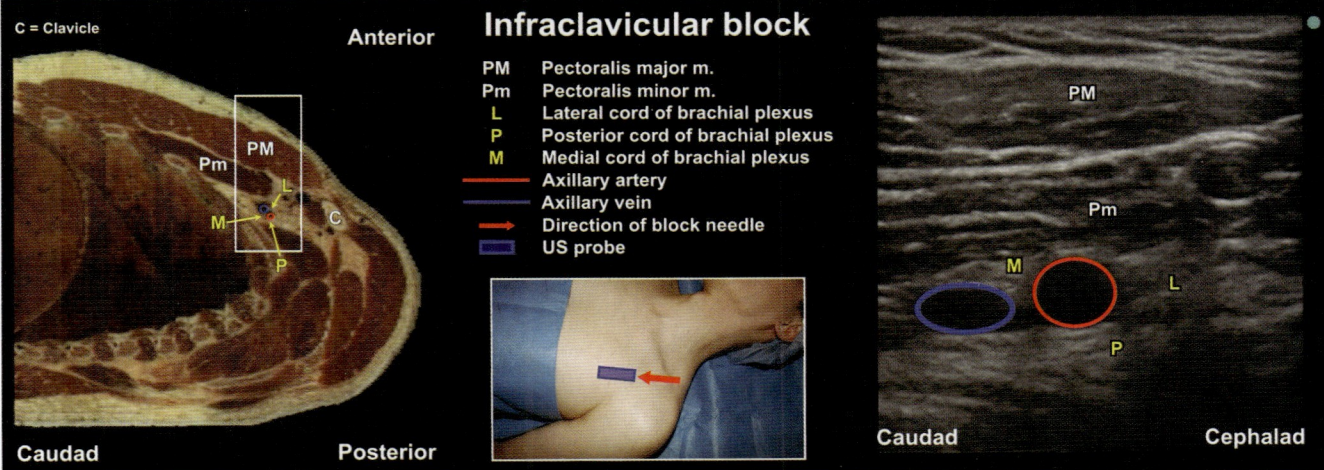

Figure 36-21 Arrangement of relevant anatomy for ultrasound-guided infraclavicular brachial plexus block. The block is performed using IP needle alignment to a linear probe and directing the needle 15 degrees posteriorly in a cephalad-to-caudad direction. In contrast to the more proximal blocks, the nerves (cords) appear hyperechoic due to higher fascial content and the relatively hyperechoic surrounding tissue (muscle).

pectoralis major lies superficial and lateral to the pectoralis minor. Approximately 4 to 5 cm deeper lies the axillary neurovascular bundle. The large axillary vein lies medial and caudad to the artery. The lateral cord of the plexus is often readily visualized as a hyperechoic oval structure, although the medial and posterior cords may not be easily identified since the medial cord lies between the axillary artery and vein, whereas the posterior cord can be hidden deep to an axillary artery acoustic shadow. In addition, the medial cord can be posterior or even slightly cephalad to the axillary artery. It is important to realize that there is a great deal of individual anatomic variation in cord location around the artery. The nerve structures now appear hyperechoic, rather than hypoechoic as seen more proximally, presumably due to an increase in the number of fascicles and amount of (hyperechoic-appearing) connective tissue.[75]

- Needling: The skin is infiltrated with local anesthetic. For single-injection technique, a 50- to 90-mm, 18- to 22-gauge insulated needle is suitable if using NS, whereas a 90-mm, 17- to 20-gauge needle can be used for catheter placement. Using an IP needle alignment will be most suitable in most cases; however, in young children, this may be difficult due to the limited space between the clavicle and US probe. The block needle is inserted cephalad to the probe and is then advanced caudally and posteriorly at approximately 30 degrees to the skin (IP insertion caudad to the probe is acceptable for young children in whom there is limited space cephalad to the probe). The cords should be found at a depth of 4 to 6 cm.[134] It is recommended to combine US with NS for accurate nerve localization (e.g., musculocutaneous nerve or specific cord), due to the high variability of cord location.
- Local anesthetic spread: Aim to place the needle and local anesthetic posterior to the axillary artery next to the posterior cord (spread from this location is optimal for complete block success). Performing a test dose with D5W is recommended prior to local anesthetic injection to visualize spread and confirm nerve localization. Inject 20 to 25 mL of local anesthetic around the posterior cord. If local anesthetic spread is deemed inadequate to surround all cords, reposition the needle before injecting any additional local anesthetic.

Clinical Pearls

- In the past, numerous techniques were developed with modifications to localize nerves and avoid vessel and pleural punctures. Real-time guidance with US addresses some of these issues, although US-guided blocks are still undergoing a rapid development process to determine the safest and most successful approaches.
- Techniques that incorporate multiple injections may be easier and potentially safer under combined US and NS guidance, which provides direct visualization of the anatomic structures.
- If a catheter is to be threaded, the aim should be to elicit motor responses in the hand itself. The tip of the Tuohy needle (90 mm, 17 to 20 gauge) should be directed laterally to allow the catheter to run in the direction of the nerves.
- Compared to blocks at more proximal locations, the infraclavicular block has the advantage of lower risk of blocking the phrenic nerve or stellate ganglion. However, in some cases, continuous catheters may lie along one cord and fail to provide complete anesthesia and analgesia of the entire brachial plexus with small volume infusions. This may be overcome to some degree by intermittent boluses of larger volumes of local anesthetic.
- Vessel puncture is a potential complication; therefore, frequent aspiration should be performed. Lateral needle insertion will help avoid the risk of pneumothorax.

Axillary Block

The nerves targeted for axillary block course distally with the axillary artery and vein along the humerus from the apex of the axilla (Fig. 36-11). This block is useful for surgery of the elbow, forearm, and hand. The ulnar, median, and radial nerves are the primary targets. The musculocutaneous nerve often leaves the plexus (via the lateral cord) proximal to this point and may be blocked separately during the axillary block (in the coracobrachialis muscle) or at mid-humeral locations (along its diagonal course through or beyond the coracobrachialis muscle). Relative to the third part of the axillary artery, the usual course of the terminal nerves is as follows: the median nerve lies anterior and medial, the ulnar nerve lies posterior and medial, the musculocutaneous nerve lies anterior and lateral, and the radial nerve lies posterior and lateral. Because the single sheath may be broken up into separate compartments by fascial septa surrounding individual nerves in the axilla, some practitioners advocate that local anesthetic should be injected at multiple sites in the axilla, in contrast to the single injections possible with proximal approaches. The patient is positioned supine with the arm abducted at 70 to 80 degrees and externally rotated with the elbow flexed at 90 degrees.

Procedure Using Nerve Stimulation Technique

- Landmarks: The axillary artery is marked as high in its course through the axilla as is practical. It is usually felt in the intramuscular groove between the coracobrachialis and the triceps muscles. It also passes between the insertions of the pectoralis major and the latissimus dorsi muscles on the humerus.
- Needling: A 30- to 50-mm, 22-gauge insulated needle is suitable for this block. After aseptic preparation, a skin wheal is raised over the proximal portion of the artery. The index and middle fingers of the nondominant hand straddle the artery just below this point, both locating the pulsation and compressing the neurovascular bundle below the intended site of injection. The needle is inserted in a slight cephalad direction, followed by a two-step, four-injection process with puncture at locations just superior and inferior to the artery.
- Nerve localization: With NS technique, ideally, the nerves serving the area of proposed surgery are sought first. The median and the musculocutaneous nerves lie on the superior aspect of the artery (as viewed by the operator), whereas the ulnar and radial nerves lie below and behind the vessel. Obtaining a direct musculocutaneous nerve response (elbow flexion) indicates localization of this particular nerve but not necessarily all nerves.
- Injection: Experience has shown that a multiple injection technique around each individual nerve is the most reliable approach (10 to 15 mL at each nerve location). Less volume may be required, but the minimum required dose/volume per nerve is currently unknown.

Procedure Using Ultrasound Imaging (Fig. 36-22)

- Scanning: High-frequency, linear probes are generally recommended (10 to 15 MHz) for imaging since the nerves are superficial (1 to 2 cm) below the skin. Small footprint probes are recommended for young children. The most proximal location at the apex of the axilla may be the best

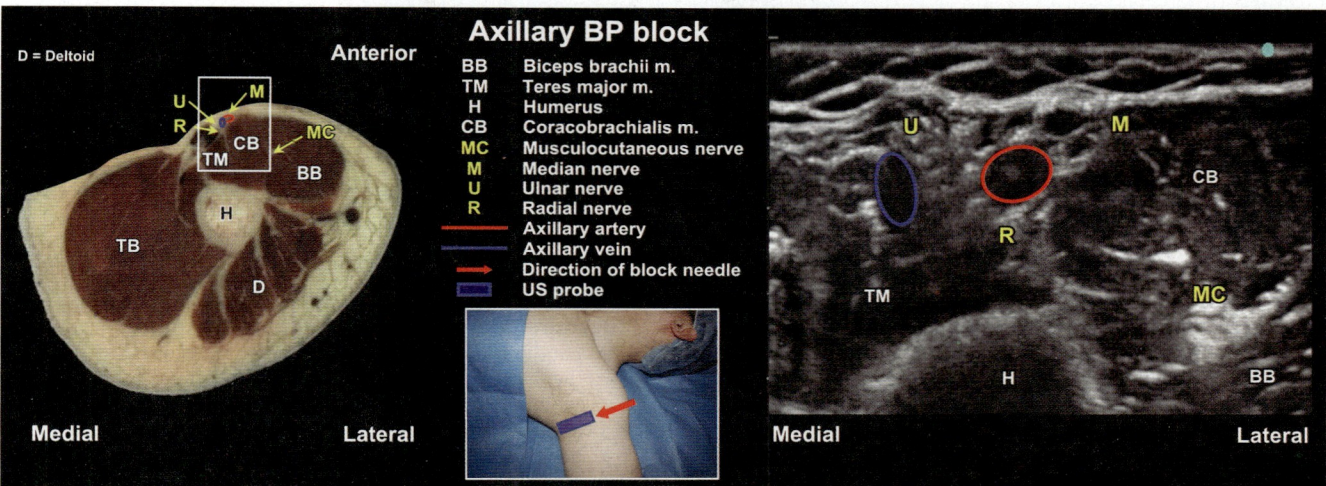

Figure 36-22 Arrangement of relevant anatomy for ultrasound-guided axillary brachial plexus block. The block is performed using IP needle alignment to a linear, high frequency probe. Typically, the block needle is advanced in sequence to reach each of the median, ulnar, and radial nerves.

for viewing all of the terminal branches of the brachial plexus. The probe is positioned perpendicular to the anterior axillary fold and in cross-section to the humerus at the bicipital sulcus (and at the level of the axillary pulse) to capture the transverse, or short-axis, view of the neurovascular bundle.

- Appearance: In cross-section:
  - The coracobrachialis and the biceps brachii muscles are seen laterally; the teres major and the triceps brachii muscles lay medially, the latter being deeper than the biceps brachii muscle.
  - The anechoic and circular axillary artery lies centrally, adjacent to both the biceps brachii and coracobrachialis muscles and is surrounded by the nerves.
  - The nerves appear round-to-oval in short axis, generally appearing as hyperechoic masses due to the large amount of connective tissue (epi- and perineurium) interspersed within the hypoechoic nerve fascicles.
  - The *median* nerve is often located superficial and between the artery and the biceps brachii muscle; the *ulnar* nerve is usually located medial and superficial to the artery; the *radial* nerve lies deep to the artery at the midline (clock-wise: median, ulnar, radial—but there are many variations).
  - The *musculocutaneous* nerve is commonly located in the hyperechoic plane between the biceps brachii and coracobrachialis muscles.
- Needling: A 50-mm, 22-gauge insulated needle (combined US and NS technique is recommended) is suitable. Both IP and OOP needle approaches can be used for axillary block. An OOP approach, with the needle distal to the probe and in transverse axis to the nerve, is similar to the traditional blind procedure, except that the needle will be aligned at an angle rather than perpendicularly to optimize its visibility. An angle of 30 to 45 degrees from the skin, with the needle placed approximately 1 to 2 cm caudad to the probe, may allow optimal needle visibility (see description of the walk-down technique in the section on Common Techniques: Nerve Stimulation and Ultrasound Imaging). The IP approach involves inserting the needle at an acute angle (20 to 30 degrees) to the skin in a lateral-to-medial direction (Fig. 36-22). Typically, the block needle is advanced to contact the median nerve. It is then crossed over the axillary artery to contact the ulnar nerve superficially and then finally behind the artery to the deeper radial nerve. Follow NS procedure if using this technique.
- Local anesthetic spread: Performing a test dose with D5W is recommended prior to local anesthetic application to visualize spread and confirm nerve localization. A proper injection is indicated by fluid spread completely around the nerve structure, with nerve movement away from the needle tip. Improper injection (e.g., injection outside the sheath) appears as partial asymmetrical fluid expansion not immediately adjacent to the nerve structure.

Clinical Pearls
- Although a multiple-injection NS technique has been used extensively for this and other blocks, it is important to consider that some spread of the local anesthetic solution will occur, and hypesthesia can occur in an unpredictable fashion, limiting the identification of subsequent nerves. A recent evaluation of a two-injection technique—with one injection posterior to the axillary artery and the other to the musculocutaneous nerve—demonstrated that this approach may be as effective as blocking each of the ulnar, median, radial, and musculoskeletal nerves separately,[135] potentially minimizing unwanted spread to adjacent nerves.
- If forearm anesthesia is required and the musculocutaneous nerve was not localized previously, supplementary anesthesia of the musculocutaneous nerve should be attained using some reliable means of nerve localization (i.e., NS and/or US guidance) rather than blind injection into the coracobrachialis muscle. US imaging 1 to 2 cm distal to the axillary block location can identify the muscle and usually the nerve.
- Intercostobrachial and medial brachial cutaneous nerve blocks can be achieved by subcutaneous injections (5 mL in total) on the medial surface of the upper arm all the way from the biceps to triceps muscles. Both of these nerves are relatively small and can be difficult to visualize under US; however, local anesthetics can be infiltrated superficially above the median nerve toward the triceps.

- Perivascular infiltration and transarterial approaches are also traditionally performed for axillary block, although these techniques have been replaced by advanced technologies such as NS and US.
- For continuous nerve blocks, a 17- to 18-gauge Tuohy needle is required to facilitate catheter placement. Securing the catheter in the axilla may be challenging and may require a short tunnel to stabilize the catheter.
- Axillary approaches to the brachial plexus are associated with minimal complications compared to more proximal brachial plexus blocks. Neuropathy from needle puncture or intraneural injection of local anesthetic is the foremost consideration, although this may be reduced with US imaging and careful attention to injection pressures during the block. Hematoma can occur if the axillary artery is punctured, but this is a self-limiting complication.

Terminal Upper Extremity Nerve Blocks

Upper extremity PNBs are of particular value as rescue blocks to supplement incomplete surgical anesthesia and to provide long-lasting selective analgesia in the postoperative period. The peripheral nerves may be individually blocked at upper mid-humeral, elbow, or wrist locations, depending on the specific nerve. If using US guidance, the elbow and forearm regions appear to be the most suitable block regions, and blocks at these sites may improve the accuracy of nerve localization and local anesthetic spread. The wrist is highly populated with tendons and fascial tissues (e.g., flexor and extensor retinacula) which, on US, can be difficult to distinguish from nerves and which may also obscure visualization of nerves. With the help of color Doppler, US can be used to identify the nerves at many desirable locations, as they are often situated near blood vessels (Table 36-1). This chapter will focus on blocks for which NS and US imaging are most amenable but will also comment on nerve blocks at the wrist. Musculocutaneous nerve block at the upper mid-humeral level is discussed in the section on Axillary Block. Figures 36-11 and 36-12 illustrate the courses and cutaneous innervation of the terminal nerves of the upper extremity.

Radial Nerve

The radial nerve can be blocked at the anterosuperior aspect of the lateral epicondyle of the humerus. The radial nerve supplies the posterior compartments of the arm and forearm, including the skin and subcutaneous tissues. It also innervates skin on the posterior aspect of the hand laterally near the base of the thumb and the dorsal aspect of the index and the lateral half of the ring finger up to the distal interphalangeal crease. For radial nerve blocks, the patient is positioned supine with their arm slightly abducted and laterally rotated and with the elbow extended.

Procedure Using Nerve Stimulation Technique

- Landmarks: A line is drawn on the anterior elbow between the medial and lateral epicondyles of the humerus. The radial nerve is located beneath this intercondylar line, approximately 1 to 2 cm lateral to the biceps tendon. This position should be marked with an "X."
- Needling: A 30- to 50-mm, 22- to 24-gauge insulated needle is used and a skin wheal is raised at the "X." The needle is then inserted perpendicular to the plane passing through the humeral epicondyles.
- Nerve localization: The correct response to radial NS at this location is extension (dorsiflexion) of the wrist and digits on the operative side. Elbow extension should not be elicited since the branch to the long head of the triceps has diverged proximally.
- Injection: Approximately 5 mL of local anesthetic are injected under low pressure.

Procedure Using Ultrasound Imaging (Fig. 36-23)

- Scanning: A linear probe in the frequency range of 5 to 10 MHz is suitable for scanning in most cases, although high frequency (10 to 15 MHz) probes are recommended for children due to the short distance between the skin and the nerve. The radial nerve can first be located proximally at the level of the spiral (radial) groove of the humerus where it lies immediately adjacent to the humerus and posteromedial to the deep brachial (profunda brachii) artery of the arm. The patient's arm should be internally rotated and placed with the hand over the abdomen on the opposite

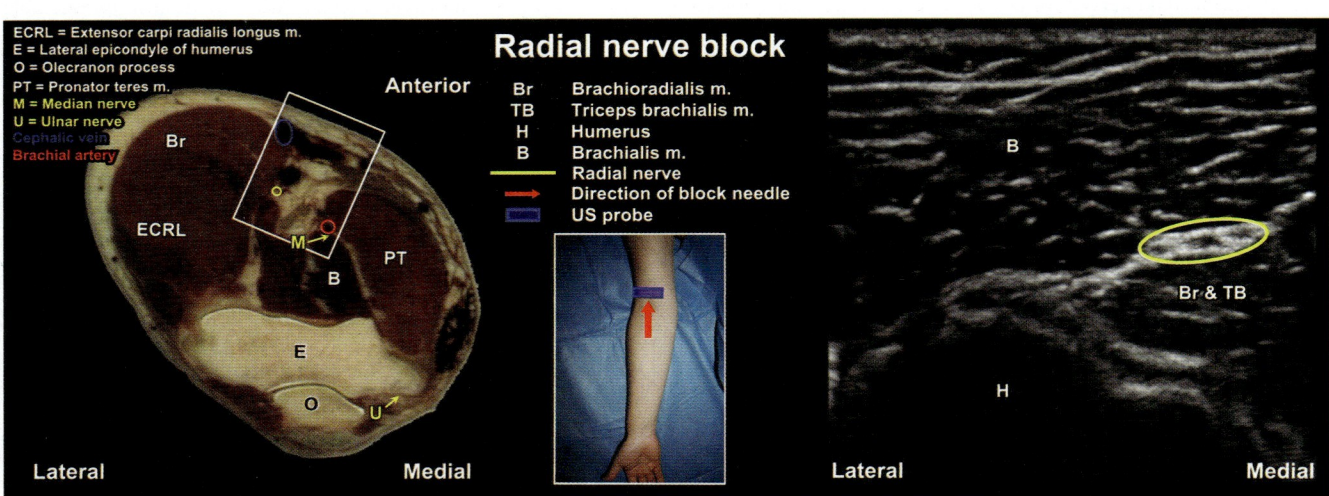

Figure 36-23 Arrangement of relevant anatomy for ultrasound-guided radial nerve block. The block is performed using an OOP needle alignment to a linear probe at the anterolateral elbow. The ideal placement will be a few centimeters above the elbow where the nerve has not yet divided into superficial and deep branches.

side of the body. The spiral groove lies immediately distal and posterior to the deltoid tubercle. Subsequent tracing of the nerve from this humeral location to the anterolateral elbow may facilitate its precise localization. The probe can be rotated slowly to scan the nerve both in the longitudinal and transverse planes at the elbow for confirmation of its location.
- Appearance: At the spiral groove of the humerus, the bone is quite superficial and appears deep to the hypoechoic triceps brachii muscle as a clearly demarcated hyperechoic oval shape with dark shadowing in its interior (not shown). The nerve appears oval and predominantly hyperechoic and is located in the posterior aspect of the humerus and immediately adjacent to the small, pulsatile deep brachial (profunda brachii) artery (as verified with Doppler). At a point just proximal to the anterior compartment of the elbow, the humerus appears to have changed shape and appears smaller and almost rectangular in cross-section. The hyperechoic radial nerve now lies at some distance from the humerus, is sandwiched between the brachialis and brachioradialis muscles, and appears oval-shaped.
- Needling: A 30- to 50-mm, 22-gauge insulated needle is suitable if using NS. The needle can be aligned using both IP and OOP (Fig. 36-23) approaches to block the nerve at the anterosuperior aspect of the lateral epicondyle of the humerus. The nerve should be blocked slightly above the elbow since it divides into deep and superficial branches approximately 2 cm above the elbow. The block needle is advanced to approach the target nerve on its side, preferably avoiding direct needle contact with the nerve.
- Local anesthetic spread: Performing a test dose with D5W is recommended prior to local anesthetic application to visualize spread and confirm nerve localization. The aim is to inject approximately 5 mL of local anesthetic and observe spread around the nerve circumferentially.

Clinical Pearls
- Needle contact with the humerus indicates that the needle is too deep, whereas deep needle penetration without bone contact indicates that the needle is lateral to the humerus (beyond the bone).
- The radial nerve can be blocked at the wrist or even lateral distal forearm adjacent to the radial artery. At the wrist, 3 mL of solution is injected into the "anatomic snuffbox" formed by the tendons of the extensor pollicis longus and extensor pollicis brevis tendons. A subcutaneous wheal is then raised from this point, extending over the dorsum of the wrist 3 to 4 cm onto the back of the hand. This approach is suboptimal for most procedures since the nerve divides immediately beyond the elbow and continues as the superficial radial (sensory) and deep posterior interosseous (motor) nerves.

Median Nerve

The median nerve can be blocked at the midline of the anterior elbow or at the mid-to-distal aspect of the anterior forearm (Fig. 36-24). The nerve is located adjacent (medial) to the brachial artery at the elbow, facilitating its localization here. In the forearm, the nerve can be located at its position lateral to the ulnar nerve. The median nerve supplies the skin anteriorly on the medial surface of the thumb, palm, and digits two to four, and posteriorly on the distal third of the second to fourth digits. It causes flexion at the metacarpophalangeal joints and extension at the interphalangeal joints of digits two and three. The nerve innervates muscles which produce flexion and opposition of the thumb, middle, and index fingers and pronation and flexion of the wrist. For blocks at the anterior wrist or anterior distal forearm, the patient's arm should be positioned next to the torso, with the elbow flexed slightly and the hand free to allow a wrist or thumb flexion response elicited by NS.

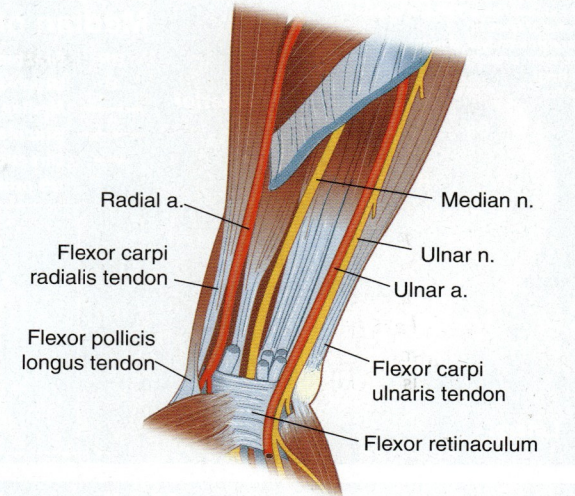

Figure 36-24 Illustration of the anterior forearm showing the courses of the median and ulnar nerves. The ulnar artery is a reliable landmark to localize the ulnar nerve when using ultrasound imaging.

Procedure Using Nerve Stimulation Technique
At the elbow:
- Landmarks: As with radial nerve block, an intercondylar line is drawn, and the nerve is located where this line crosses the pulsation of the brachial artery, usually 1 cm to the ulnar side of the biceps brachii tendon.
- Needling: Using a 30- to 50-mm insulated needle, a skin wheal is raised at the point identified with landmarks (see earlier), and the needle is introduced perpendicularly at this point.
- Nerve localization: Nerve responses to electrical stimulation are sought immediately adjacent to the artery. The optimal NS response for median nerve block at the elbow location is any one of the following or a combination thereof: flexion and opposition of the thumb, middle, and index fingers; flexion of the wrist; and pronation of the forearm.
- Injection: Injection of 5 mL local anesthetic should be sufficient to block this nerve. Care should be taken to avoid intravascular and intraneural injection.

In the forearm:
- It may be difficult to locate this nerve blindly in the forearm using NS, although the technique of transcutaneous electrical stimulation[17] or, similarly, percutaneous electrode guidance[18,136] can be used to locate the nerve with a probe placed on or indenting the skin's surface. Once the nerve has been localized, an insulated needle is inserted perpendicular to the plane of the forearm and NS responses are sought. A similar volume of local anesthetic should suffice.

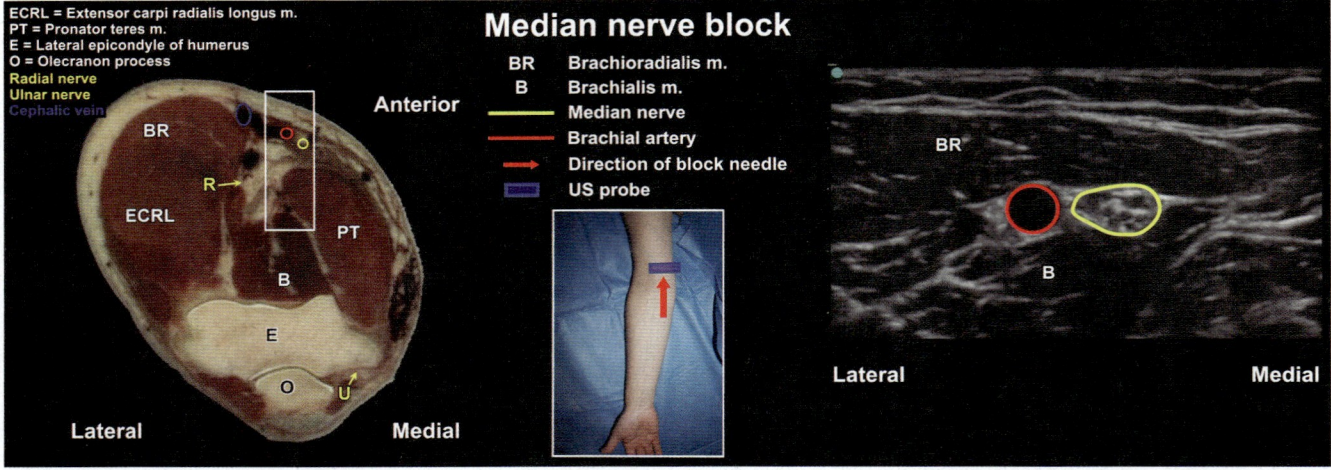

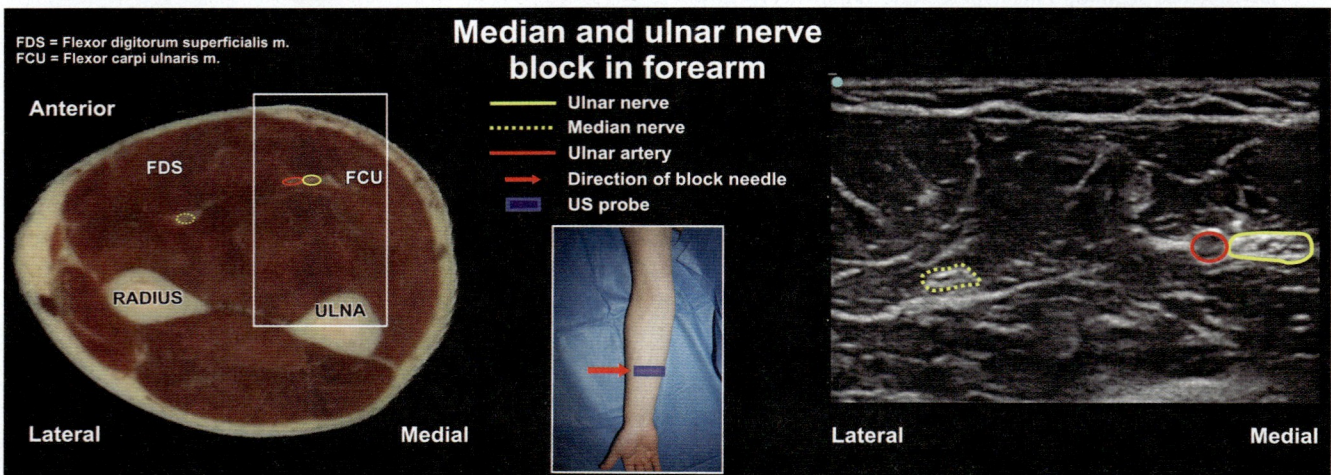

Figure 36-25 Arrangement of relevant anatomy for ultrasound-guided median and ulnar nerve block. **Top:** Ultrasound-guided median nerve block at the medial aspect of the elbow using an OOP approach. **Bottom:** Ultrasound-guided ulnar nerve block in the mid-distal forearm using an IP needle aligned to a small footprint, linear ("hockey stick") probe. For ulnar nerve block, the ideal location to avoid arterial puncture is where the nerve has yet to fully approach the ulnar artery.

Procedure Using Ultrasound Imaging (Fig. 36-25)

- Scanning: A high-frequency (10 to 15 MHz) linear probe can be used to capture a transverse view of the nerve and to localize the brachial artery, both at the elbow, where the nerve lies medial to both the artery and then the tendon of the biceps brachii muscle. At the anterolateral forearm, the nerve lies lateral to the ulnar nerve and artery (localizing the ulnar nerve first will help identify the median nerve). Color Doppler may be used to confirm the location of the above-named arteries.
- Appearance: At the elbow, the median nerve can be identified at approximately 1 to 2 cm in depth as a hyperechoic yet distinctly honeycomb-like structure, lying medial to the anechoic pulsatile brachial artery. Deep to the neurovascular structures lies the musculature of the superior aspect of the elbow (pronator teres and brachialis muscles) as a hypoechoic homogeneous mass. At the forearm, the nerve appears oval-shaped and lateral to the ulnar artery.
- Needling: Both OOP and IP techniques can be used for either block location. For OOP needling at the elbow (not shown), after adjusting the US image to place the nerve in the middle of the screen, insert a 30- to 50-mm insulated needle perpendicular to the transversely placed probe at a 45- to 60-degree angle. If using combined technique, NS procedure should be followed. An IP technique with the needle in a medial to lateral direction may be advantageous at the elbow to allow easy tracking of the needle to ensure it avoids puncturing the brachial artery.
- Local anesthetic spread: After performing a test dose with D5W, the aim is to spread approximately 5 mL of local anesthetic around the nerve in a circular fashion, avoiding nerve contact and obtaining complete blockade.

Clinical Pearls

- The median nerve lies deep to the flexor retinaculum at the wrist, and there is always the potential risk of causing carpal tunnel syndrome due to elevated pressure within the tunnel following injection. For this reason, the elbow or forearm locations for blocking the median nerve are the more logical choices.
- At the wrist, the median nerve lies between the tendons of the palmaris longus and the flexor carpi radialis muscles. If

only the palmaris longus muscle can be felt, the nerve lies just to the radial side of its tendon. A skin wheal is raised, and a needle is inserted until it pierces the deep fascia. An injection of 3 to 5 mL of local anesthetic is sufficient to produce anesthesia.
- Aspiration of blood into the tubing during elbow block indicates brachial artery puncture. In this case, the needle should be reinserted after applying pressure to the puncture site until hemostasis is achieved. Contact with the humerus indicates that the needle is too deep. Localized contraction of the arm muscles (e.g., elbow flexion and/or forearm pronation) indicates stimulation of the local muscles and also that the needle is likely too deep.

Ulnar Nerve

In the periphery, the ulnar nerve can be blocked at the elbow, forearm, or wrist. Ulnar nerve block may be used for rescue analgesia or surgical anesthesia for surgery on the fifth digit. At the junction of the distal third and proximal two-thirds of the medial forearm, the nerve is commonly located just medial to the pulsatile ulnar artery (Fig. 36-24). US-guided technique is advised when using this block location in order to avoid the artery and localize the nerve accurately. The ulnar nerve supplies muscles that produce flexion of the ring (fourth) and little (fifth) fingers and ulnar deviation of wrist. It innervates the skin over the medial surface (anterior and posterior) of the hand and digits four and five. Before performing the block, the patient's arm should be flexed at the elbow by 30 degrees and the forearm supinated. The forearm can rest on an arm board with an additional pillow under the wrist.

Procedure Using Nerve Stimulation Technique
At the elbow:
- Anesthetizing the ulnar nerve at the elbow may be uncomfortable for the patient. NS is not routinely used for localizing the ulnar nerve at the elbow, since the nerve is easily located (and palpated) in the cubital tunnel (ulnar groove) between the medial epicondyle of the humerus and the olecranon process of the ulna. Only a small volume (1 to 4 mL) of local anesthetic should be injected if performing the block at this location.

In the forearm:
- Similar to the median nerve, it may be difficult to blindly locate this nerve in the forearm using NS. Transcutaneous electrical stimulation[17] or percutaneous electrode guidance[18,19] can be used to locate the nerve. Once the nerve has been localized, an insulated needle attached to a nerve stimulator is inserted perpendicular to the plane of the forearm, and appropriate motor responses are sought. The appropriate responses for ulnar nerve block at this location are flexion of the ring (fourth) and little (fifth) fingers and ulnar deviation of the wrist. Injection of 5 mL local anesthetic is sufficient to block the nerve at the forearm. Combined US- and NS-guided technique provides good localization and accuracy with local anesthetic spread.

Procedure Using Ultrasound Imaging (Forearm, Fig. 36-25)
- Scanning: A high-frequency (10 to 15 MHz) linear probe is often used for this block. The probe is placed transversely just above the mid-forearm level to view the ulnar nerve in short axis as it approaches the ulnar artery. The nerve is positioned above the ulna and the belly of the flexor carpi ulnaris, on the anterior surface of the arm, rather than medially to contact the bone. The operator should scan downward slowly until the nerve and pulsatile artery are viewed adjacent to each other (Doppler may be valuable here) and retract the scanhead slightly so the artery and nerve appear clearly as separate structures (Fig. 36-25).
- Appearance: The nerve in short axis is seen as a honeycomb-like, oval-shaped structure, including hypoechoic fascicular structures surrounded by hyperechoic tissue. The adjacent ulnar artery appears anechoic and roughly similar in size to the nerve and lateral to it. The median nerve may be seen at the lateral edge of the image and appears similar to the ulnar nerve in size and shape.
- Needling: During IP needling, the image should be adjusted so that the nerve is toward the most lateral edge of the screen for good visibility of the needle shaft (not shown in Fig. 36-25). A short (20 to 30 mm) needle can be used in a medial-to-lateral direction to reduce the risk of vascular puncture.
- Local anesthetic spread: The aim is to spread approximately 5 mL of local anesthetic around the nerve in a circular fashion in order to obtain a complete block while avoiding nerve contact. The local anesthetic injection will appear as an expansion of hypoechogenicity surrounding the nerve, which may separate the nerve from the artery.

Clinical Pearls
- When performing regional anesthesia in the elbow, direct injection after eliciting a paresthesia or direct injection into the groove under pressure is not advised because of the risk of damage to the nerve. Small volumes (3 to 5 mL) of local anesthetic should be used.
- During nerve block in the forearm, blood withdrawal into the tubing suggests ulnar artery puncture, and the needle should be reinserted after holding pressure. Contact with the ulna indicates that the needle is too deep.
- US imaging facilitates the unique approach of blocking the ulnar nerve in the forearm. This technique may reduce complications such as ulnar nerve neuritis or neurapraxia compared to blocks at the cubital tunnel behind the medial epicondyle.
- A linear or curved array US probe with a small footprint (26 mm; e.g., a "hockey stick" probe) may be used. This size of probe is helpful for easy manipulation on the forearm and for good alignment of the needle using IP technique.
- At the wrist, the ulnar nerve lies between the ulnar artery and the tendon of the flexor carpi ulnaris muscle. A skin wheal is raised at the level of the styloid process on the palmar side of the forearm between these two landmarks, a small-gauge needle is inserted, and 3 mL of solution is injected into the area, with or without paresthesias.

Intravenous Regional Anesthesia (Bier Block)

Without using NS or US, arm anesthesia can be provided by the injection of local anesthetic into the venous system distal to an occluding tourniquet.

Procedure
- A small-gauge (20 or 22) intravenous catheter is inserted and taped on the dorsum of the hand in the arm to be blocked. A heparin lock or small syringe is attached, and saline is injected to maintain patency. A pneumatic tourniquet is applied over the upper arm. The tourniquet pressure should be set to 2.5 times the systolic blood pressure. The tourniquet should be inflated to confirm that the pressure is sufficient to occlude distal arterial blood flow and should be deflated before starting the block.

- The arm is elevated to promote venous drainage. An Esmarch bandage is then wrapped tightly around the limb from distal to proximal to produce further exsanguination. After exsanguination, the tourniquet is inflated to 300 mmHg or 2.5 times the patient's systolic blood pressure and is again tested for adequate occlusion of the distal radial pulse.
- The arm is returned to the horizontal position, a 50-mL syringe with 0.5% lidocaine (without preservative) is attached to the previously inserted cannula, and the contents are injected slowly. The forearm discolors, and the patient perceives a transient "pins and needles" sensation and warmth as anesthesia ensues over the following 5 minutes. Epinephrine should not be added to the local anesthetic solution.
- For short procedures, the cannula can be removed at this point. If surgery extends beyond 1 hour, the cannula can be left in place and used for reinjection after 90 minutes.
- Beyond 45 minutes of surgery, many patients experience discomfort at the level of the tourniquet. Special "double-cuff" tourniquets are available for this block to alleviate this problem. The distal cuff is inflated first followed by the proximal cuff. The distal cuff is then deflated, allowing anesthesia to be induced in the area under the distal cuff. If discomfort ensues, the distal cuff is inflated over the anesthetized area of skin, and the uncomfortable proximal cuff is released. This step is critical because the major risk of this procedure is premature release of the local anesthetic solution into the circulation. If a double cuff is used, both cuffs should be tested before starting, and the proper sequence for inflation and deflation followed meticulously. The potential for leakage of anesthetic into the circulation is greater with the narrower cuffs used in the double setup. Because the shifting process also increases the potential for unintentional release of anesthetic, the use of a single, wider cuff may be better for short procedures.
- If surgery is completed in less than 20 minutes, the tourniquet is left inflated for at least that total period of time. If 40 minutes has elapsed, the tourniquet can be deflated as a single maneuver. Between 20 and 40 minutes, the cuff can be deflated, reinflated immediately, and finally deflated after 1 minute to delay the sudden absorption of anesthetic into the systemic circulation, although this may not truly lower the eventual peak plasma local anesthetic levels achieved.
- Duration of anesthesia is minimal beyond the time of tourniquet release. The cardiotoxicity of systemic levels of bupivacaine makes this drug contraindicated for Bier block.

Clinical Pearls

- The simplicity of this technique is offset by the potentially significant risk of systemic local anesthetic toxicity if the tourniquet fails or is released prematurely. Complications related to systemic toxicity include seizures, cardiac arrest, and death; other noted complications include nerve damage, compartment syndrome, and thrombophlebitis.[137] Careful testing of the tourniquet and slow injection of solution into a peripheral (not antecubital) vein will reduce the chance of leakage under the tourniquet. Systemic blood levels are time-dependent, and careful attention should be paid to the sequence of tourniquet release and to patient monitoring during this period. A separate intravenous site for injection of resuscitation drugs is needed, as is ready availability of all appropriate resuscitative equipment. With careful attention to these details, this is one of the most effective and reliable technique available to the anesthesiologist.

Trunk Nerve Blocks

Anesthesia of the abdomen and chest is often obtained most simply with spinal and epidural injections of local anesthetics, but peripheral block of the spinal nerves in the paravertebral space or the intercostal or inguinal nerves is suitable for many uses. This is particularly relevant when either a narrow band of anesthesia (intercostal or paravertebral) or reduced motor block is preferable. In addition, epidural injection may be hazardous because of infection or coagulopathy. Epidural anesthesia also carries concerns of systemic hypotension and epidural hematoma, which can limit its use for some patients.[138] In many clinical situations, it may be desirable to use intercostal blocks to overcome the combined anesthesia of the somatic and sympathetic fibers that occurs with neuraxial blocks. The sympathetic nerves separate from their somatic counterparts early in their course, which makes independent somatic and sympathetic blockade a practical consideration. Likewise, although paravertebral blocks may result in both somatic and sympathetic blocks, hemodynamic responses are often less than those encountered during epidural block. Sympathetic blocks are performed commonly at the major ganglia, particularly the stellate, celiac, and lumbar plexus. These blocks may require multiple injections and are technically more difficult than axial anesthesia, but they offer advantages in certain clinical situations. The reader is referred to Chapter 56 for discussion of these blocks.

Ilioinguinal and iliohypogastric nerve blocks are used for procedures in the inguinal area, including hernia repair and orchidopexy. A lumbar plexus block is not optimal in these cases since these nerves exit the plexus more cranially (L1–L2) than those nerves targeted by the lumbar plexus block (L3–L5). Transversus abdominis plane (TAP) block[139,140] and rectus sheath blocks[141,142] can be performed for abdominal, umbilical, or other midline surgical procedures and are often performed bilaterally. Approaches to the rectus sheath block targets the terminal branches of the 9th, 10th, and 11th intercostal nerves within the rectus sheath; ideally, injection is between the posterior rectus sheath and the rectus abdominis muscle. The TAP block aims to impede innervation of the abdominal wall up to the level of T8 by injecting local anesthetic between the transversus abdominis and internal oblique muscles. The initial technique of multiple injections of local anesthetic in the abdominal wall was modified to a single injection using the landmark technique by locating the "lumbar triangle of Petit."[143] US-guided regional techniques allow the layers of musculature to be identified, and needle insertion and local anesthetic deposition between the fascial layers can be visualized in real time. Thus, the approach to the TAP block has evolved yet again and has become more common.

Intercostal Nerve Block

Anesthesia of the intercostal nerves provides both motor and sensory anesthesia of the abdominal wall from the xiphoid to the pubis. Intercostal nerve blockade is used for various conditions of acute and chronic pain affecting the thorax and upper abdomen (e.g., postoperative analgesia after thoracotomies, various cardiac surgeries, and both open and laparoscopic cholecystectomies). It can be performed through several means, including continuous infusions into the subpleural space, through interpleural catheters, and by direct intercostal nerve block. The surgical site (i.e., intraoperative anatomic access) determines the available options.

These nerve blocks involve injections along the easily palpated sharp posterior angulation of the ribs, which occurs between 5 and 7 cm from the midline in the back. The blocks may be performed more laterally (8 to 10 cm from the midline)[144] or more medially (immediately beyond the transverse processes). The levels of T1–T5 may be most amenable to paravertebral block due to the overlying scapula and bulky paraspinal musculature at this region. Establishing blockade of five or six levels of intercostal nerves is a useful anesthetic procedure for providing analgesia and motor relaxation for upper abdominal procedures such as cholecystectomy and gastric surgery. Unilateral blockade of these nerves is a useful treatment for the pain of rib fracture and also serves to reduce postoperative analgesia requirements in patients with subcostal incisions. Several segments must be blocked in each of these applications because of the overlap in supply of the intercostal nerves. This technique is also useful in reducing the pain associated with the insertion of chest tubes or percutaneous biliary drainage procedures.

For intercostal blocks, the patient may be in the lateral, sitting, or prone position. For operative anesthesia, the prone position is most practical. A pillow is placed under the abdomen to provide slight flexion of the thoracic spine. The arms are draped over the edge of the stretcher or operating table so that the scapula falls away laterally from the midline. The anesthesiologist stands at the patient's side. Most anesthesiologists prefer to stand on the side that allows their dominant hand to hold the syringe at the caudad end of the patient.

Procedure Using Landmark-based Technique

Landmarks. The reader is referred to the Clinical Anatomy section (see earlier) for descriptions of the locations of the relevant landmarks. The spinous processes in the midline from T6 to T12 are marked. The ribs are then identified along the line of their most extreme posterior angulation. The 6th and 12th ribs are marked first at their inferior borders, and a line is drawn between these two points. The rest of the ribs between them are identified, and a mark is placed on the inferior border of each rib along the angled parasagittal plane identified by the first line between the 6th and 12th ribs.

Needling. After aseptic preparation, light sedation is provided for the patient, and a skin wheal is raised at each mark on the inferior border of each respective rib. Starting with the lowest rib, the index finger of the cephalad hand retracts the skin above the identifying mark in a cephalad direction. Using the other hand, the anesthesiologist inserts a needle (22 gauge, 3.75 cm) directly onto the rib, maintaining a constant 10 degree cephalad angulation. After contact is made with the rib, the cephalad traction is slowly released, the cephalad hand takes over the needle and syringe, and the needle is allowed to "walk" down to below the rib at the same angle. The needle is then advanced approximately 4 mm under the rib.

Age influences the point of needle insertion in children. The needle is inserted at the intersection of the lower border of the rib and the mid-axillary line or posterior axillary line in children below 10 years old and above 10 years old, respectively. Anterior approaches are used rarely and will not be described here.

Injection. Once in the groove, aspiration is performed, and 3 to 5 mL of local anesthetic solution (lower volumes for children <3 years old) is injected. The needling and injection procedure is repeated for each segmental level and for both sides if applicable. Since the intercostal space is highly vascularized, local anesthetics are absorbed rapidly, and toxic levels of local anesthetic may be encountered when using large volumes, which can quickly lead to neurologic or cardiovascular sequelae. Maximum doses should be calculated and followed carefully for these blocks.

Procedure Using Ultrasound Imaging

The ribs can be visualized easily with the use of US. A high-frequency (5 to 15 MHz) probe is placed in a longitudinal axis. The rib will appear as a hyperechoic line casting a hypoechoic bony shadow underneath (Fig. 36-26). The pleurae can also be seen to "glitter" as they slide with respiration. The remainder of the procedure will be similar to that of the blind technique. If a more medial (proximal) intercostal nerve block is desired, such as to relieve the pain of herpes zoster or of proximal rib fractures, US imaging of the costotransverse joint and ribs may be helpful. The section on paravertebral block describes and illustrates this imaging.

Clinical Pearls

- Intercostal nerve blocks can be supplemented by a number of somatic paravertebral nerve blocks or sympathetic block of the celiac plexus. Care should be taken to adjust

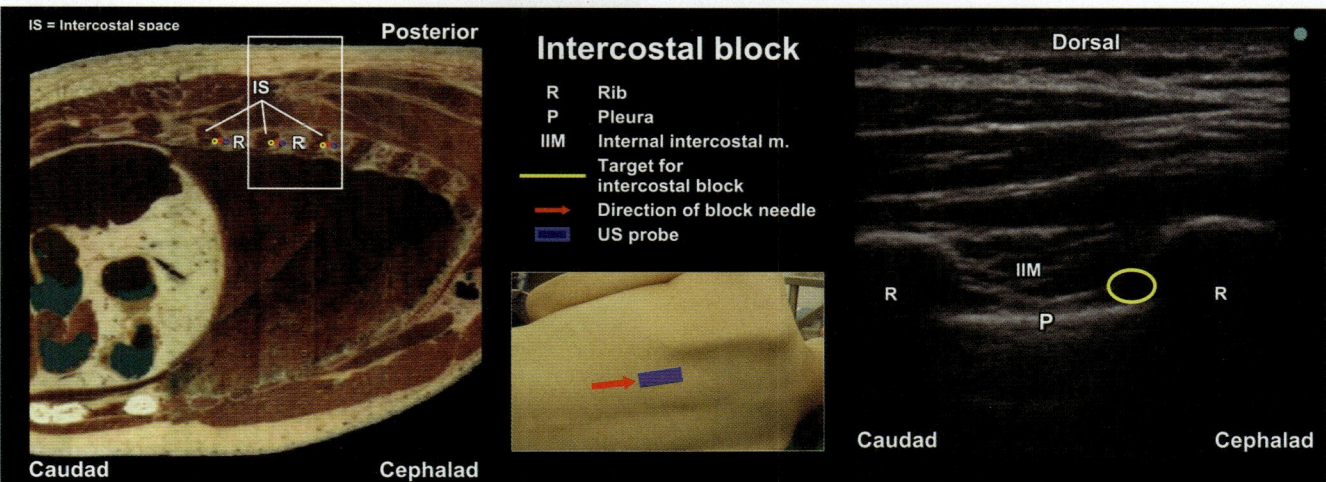

Figure 36-26 Arrangement of relevant anatomy for ultrasound-guided intercostal nerve block. The ultrasound image shows the hyperechoic lines of the ribs casting a hypoechoic bony shadow. The pleura is the hyperechoic line deep to that of the ribs and has a glittery appearance, especially on respiration.

the total dose of drug in these combined techniques so that the maximal recommended amounts are not exceeded.

- The advantages of intercostal block over sole intravenous opioid use include superior analgesia, opioid sparing, improved pulmonary mechanics (including earlier extubation), and reduced central nervous system depression.[144] Intercostal blocks are often used in addition to systemic analgesia (e.g., intravenous, patient-controlled analgesia).
- Despite frequent concern about the incidence of pneumothorax with intercostal blocks, this complication is rare, especially when US is used in experienced hands. This depends primarily on maintaining strict safety features of the described technique. Emphasis should be placed on absolute control of the syringe and needle at all times, particularly during injection.
- A common complication is related to the sedation required to perform this block in the prone position. Overdose can lead to airway obstruction and respiratory depression in the prone position. Attention must be paid to the patient's mental status because this block produces the highest blood levels of local anesthetics compared to any other regional anesthetic technique. When the block is performed for postoperative pain relief, the dose should be reduced to 0.25% bupivacaine or ropivacaine to minimize the risk of toxicity.
- It is possible to produce partial spinal or epidural anesthesia if the injection is made close to the midline and the local anesthetic tracks along a dural sleeve to the epidural or subarachnoid space. Respiratory insufficiency can also be seen if the intercostal muscles are blocked in a patient who depends on them for ventilation. Patients with chronic obstructive disease with ineffective diaphragm motion are not good candidates for this technique.

Paravertebral Block

Techniques

Paravertebral block is useful for segmental anesthesia, particularly of the upper thoracic segments. It is also useful if blockade more proximal (central) than that of the intercostal nerves is needed, such as to relieve the pain of herpes zoster or a proximal rib fracture. Thoracic paravertebral block is used for breast surgery and perioperatively for thoracic surgery. Thoracolumbar paravertebral anesthesia is used commonly for inguinal herniorrhaphy and postoperative analgesia following hip surgery. Lumbar paravertebral blockade has been used successfully for outpatient hernia operations, providing significant postoperative analgesia.

Single-injection paravertebral block used for surgical anesthesia has been shown to surpass general anesthesia with respect to postoperative pain relief, incidence of vomiting, and pain upon mobilization.[145] Paravertebral blocks are considered "unilateral epidurals" since they block spinal nerves selectively on the side of anesthetic application, although they also have the potential for epidural spread (i.e., they can be bilateral if desired). The anesthesia includes both somatic and sympathetic effects, with a reduced hemodynamic response (e.g., hypotension) compared to epidural anesthesia. This nerve block requires excellent knowledge of paravertebral anatomy but can be performed easily with experience.

The upper five ribs are more difficult to palpate laterally, and blockade of their associated intercostal nerves is best performed with a paravertebral injection. This approach is technically more difficult and has slightly greater potential for complications because of the proximity of the lung and intervertebral foramina.

The paravertebral block can be used at any level. At the lumbar spine, some prefer to perform lumbar plexus block to reduce the number of injections and avoid sympathetic block. The injection is made into the triangular paravertebral space where the spinal nerve has just left the intervertebral foramen. The nerve may be difficult to localize using bony landmarks in a blind fashion, and larger volumes of local anesthetic are often required. NS has been used to locate the nerve. US can be performed prior to the block to improve bony landmark identification, particularly for obese patients or those with a spinal deformity. However, real-time US guidance can be challenging and may offer limited additional value from preprocedural landmark identification since the overriding bone tissue reflects the US beam and provides dorsal shadowing, which obscures imaging (especially of the needle) to the depth of the paravertebral space.

Paravertebral block is performed with the patient in the lateral, sitting, or prone position, the latter using a pillow placed under the patient's abdomen to produce flexion of the thoracic and lumbar spine.

Procedure Using Nerve Stimulation or Loss-of-Resistance Technique

Landmarks. The paravertebral approach varies depending on the spinal level and the respective orientation of the vertebral spinous and transverse processes (see Clinical Anatomy section). Thus, paravertebral blocks in the upper thoracic region are performed at each level by identifying the spinous process of the vertebra above the level to be blocked; in the lumbar region, the spinous process of the level to be blocked is used to locate the transverse process. The appropriate spinous processes for the region to be blocked are marked, and transverse lines are drawn across the cephalad border and extended laterally to overlie the transverse process (approximately 2.5 cm) (Fig. 36-27). Finally, the transverse processes are marked individually or by drawing a vertical line parallel to the spine joining the ends of the transverse lines. For a diagnostic block, a single nerve may need to be anesthetized. For pain control, several levels must be identified. The injection of at least three segments (as in intercostal blockade) is required to

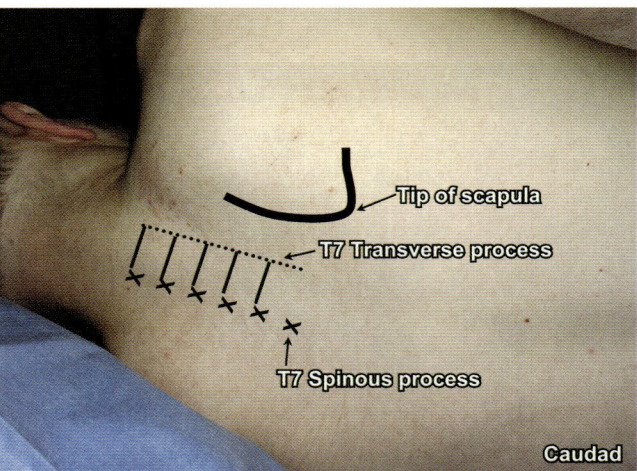

Figure 36-27 Landmarks for paravertebral block at the thoracic spine. The spinous process of the level below the block (e.g., spinous process of T7 for block at T6) is identified, and a line is drawn horizontally from the cranial aspect of the spinous process to mark the transverse process. The needle is inserted at appropriate spinal levels at the lateral line marking the transverse processes.

produce reliable segmental block because of sensory overlap from multiple nerves.

Needling. After aseptic skin preparation and patient sedation, skin wheals are raised at the marked transverse processes. A 22-gauge, 70-mm insulated needle is introduced through the skin wheal in the sagittal plane and directed slightly cephalad to contact the transverse process (usually at a depth of 2 to 4 cm in the thoracic region and 5 to 8 cm in the lumbar region) or—oftentimes likely—the costotransverse ligament. Gentle cephalad or caudad exploration may be required to identify the bone. The depth of the transverse process should be noted on the needle shaft. The needle is then withdrawn from the transverse process to the skin level and reinserted 10 degrees superiorly (to target the spinal nerve corresponding to the spinous process) or inferiorly (corresponding to the vertebral level below the spinous process) and 1 cm deeper than the point of bone contact. The needle should be angled slightly medially to avoid causing pneumothorax. There will be a subtle "give" at the midpoint between these landmarks (spinous and transverse processes), indicating entrance into the paravertebral space.

Nerve Localization. For NS, an initial current of 2.5 to 5 mA is used, and the needle is advanced until contractions of the appropriate muscles (e.g., abdominal muscles with lumbar paravertebral block) are observed, after which the current intensity is reduced to localize the nerves at 0.5 to 0.6 mA. A test dose of local anesthetic will confirm nerve localization upon elimination of the nerve response, resulting from the current dissipation at the needle tip from the conducting solution.[26] For loss of resistance, a 22-gauge Tuohy needle is used. After walking off the transverse processes, a "pop" or loss of resistance may be felt when entering the paravertebral space.

Injection. When the needle has entered the paravertebral space, 3 to 7 mL of local anesthetic, depending on the number of sites and patient size, is injected at each site following careful aspiration. Attention must be paid to the total milligram dose injected; the volume required to block each level limits the concentration that can be used and the total number of levels that can be blocked. If lumbar paravertebral injections are combined with intercostal blocks, the concentration and total volume for both blocks may have to be reduced.

Procedure Using Ultrasound Imaging

Imaging for these blocks is often used before block performance (i.e., "preprocedural," "supported," or "off-line" imaging) rather than during (i.e., "real-time" or "on-line" imaging) to identify the deep bony landmarks, including the articular and transverse processes. Real-time US-guided paravertebral block is an advanced block and should only be performed by experienced personnel.

Scanning. Placing the probe transversely at the midline will provide an overview of the vertebral lamina and processes, as well as costal structures if viewing the thoracic spine (Fig. 36-28, top). A medial-to-lateral scan using a longitudinally placed probe can then be used to locate and mark important bony landmarks (Fig. 36-28, bottom). For this, a 5 to 7 MHz curved-array US probe (lower frequency for obese patients and higher frequency linear probes for thin adult or pediatric patients) is positioned in the sagittal plane on top of the spinous processes of the target thoracic or lumbar region. Subsequent lateral scanning will allow consecutive identification of the lamina, articular, and transverse processes, and, in the thoracic spine, the ribs.

Appearance. The initial transverse scan will show a hyperechoic outline of the vertebral spinous and transverse processes, the lamina, and (in the thoracic spine) the associated rib. During the lateral scan with the probe placed longitudinally to the spine, the laminae will appear first as largely overlapping linear structures. The articular processes in long axis appear as "multiple lumps," just lateral to the spinous processes and are short rectangular structures with hyperechoic lines and underlying hypoechoic bony shadowing. Moving laterally, the transverse processes appear and will look similar to the articular processes; they will disappear from view when the probe is moved beyond their tips, which can help distinguish them from the articular processes and mark the lateral block location. Beyond the transverse processes, the rib heads appear as long shadows within hyperechoic borders, deep to the linear hyperechoic muscle fibers of the paravertebral muscles. The paravertebral space lies deep to the transverse processes, and the pleura can often be identified between and deep to the transverse process, as well as deep to the ribs.

Needling. Since multiple injections are generally needed to completely cover all the dermatomes of the surgical area in clinical practice, US imaging is more suitable for a preblock assessment ("supported" US) to visualize and measure the depth of needle penetration required for the needle to contact the transverse processes. Needling will be identical to that for the blind technique, with the exception that the depth to the transverse process will be known more accurately. It is possible to perform real-time US guidance, using either IP or OOP needle alignment. The reader is referred to the Clinical Pearls for advice related to important precautions when using US guidance.

Local Anesthetic Spread. In adults, visualization of local anesthetic spread will be difficult if using real-time US guidance. The overlying bones largely reflect the US beam and obstruct visibility beyond into the paravertebral space. However, local anesthetic spread may be seen with US in young children (<2 to 3 years old) since fusion of the neural arches and vertebral bodies has not yet occurred, allowing good visibility into the paravertebral space.

Clinical Pearls

- Since the paravertebral space is well vascularized, inadvertent vascular puncture will often occur, highlighting the need for frequent aspiration and injection in small aliquots.[146]
- Pneumothorax is more likely with a paravertebral technique than with intercostal block. The needle should be directed medially as it passes below the transverse process and never more than 2 cm beyond the transverse process. If cough or chest pain occurs, a chest radiograph should be performed to rule out pneumothorax.
- Subarachnoid injection is also more likely in the thoracic area because of the extension of the dural sleeves to the level of the intervertebral foramina. Careful aspiration is important but may not prevent unintentional injection of local anesthetic into the subdural space. Total spinal anesthesia can result with a 5- to 10-mL injection. Systemic toxicity is also a possibility because of the need for relatively large volumes of local anesthetic.
- If attempting real-time US guidance of paravertebral block, it is important to observe the angulation of the needle, and use of IP needle alignment with respect to a longitudinal probe position may be most prudent. The needle should not be inserted with a significant medial direction as there is a risk of spinal cord injury from intraforaminal insertion and injection. Likewise, a lateral direction increases the risk of pneumothorax. If choosing to use real-time US guidance during block procedure, note that: (1) with the

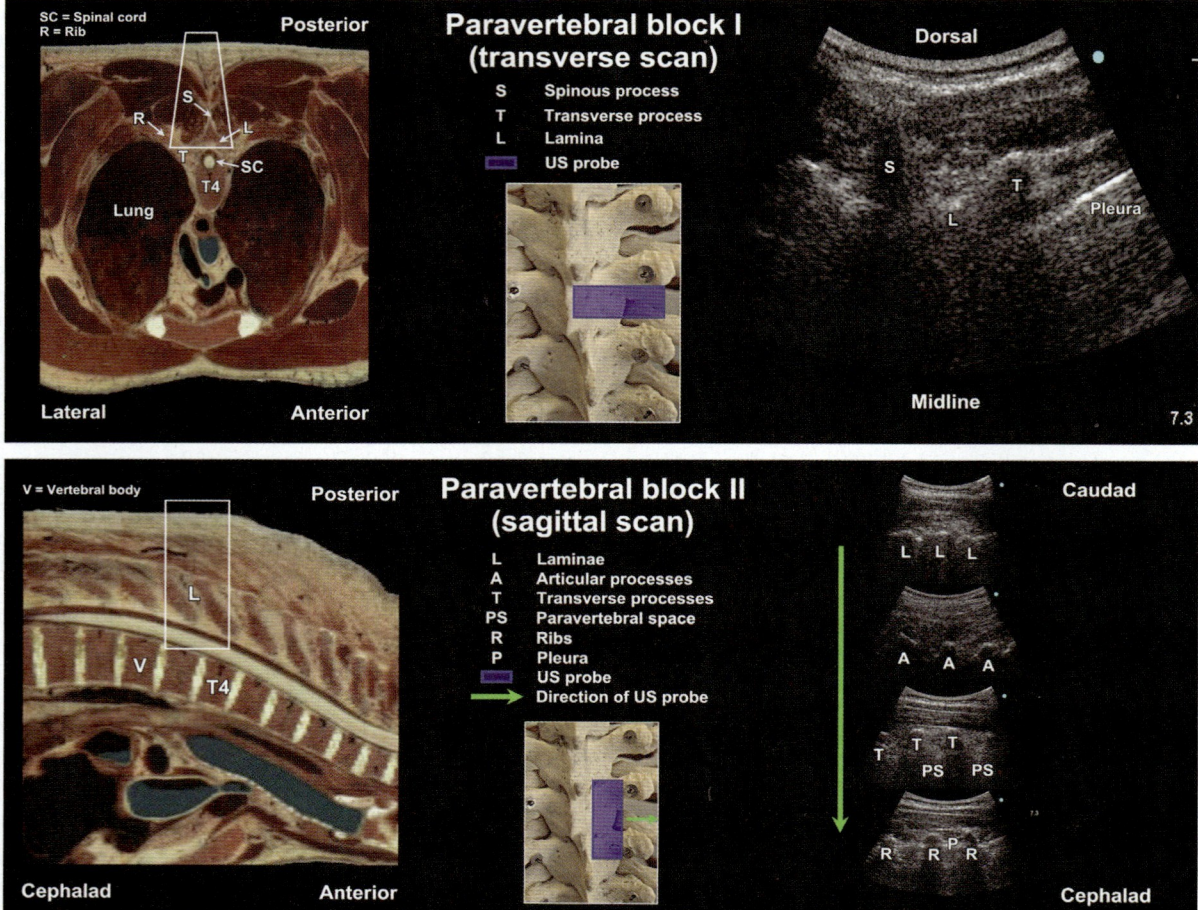

Figure 36-28 Arrangement of relevant anatomy and transverse probe placement for thoracic paravertebral block. **Top:** The probe is first placed in the midline of the spine to capture a transverse view of the vertebral and costal (if thoracic spine) elements. **Bottom:** The probe is then rotated longitudinally and moved laterally to view the laminae, articular processes, and transverse processes; the paravertebral space can be found deep to and between the latter.

probe placed in the sagittal/longitudinal plane, OOP needling may be more risky, as it often requires the medial or lateral angulations described earlier, and (2) an IP needling approach can be more risky when the probe is placed in the coronal/transverse plane.

- Traditionally, paravertebral blocks and other trunk blocks are performed blindly, with either sole use of landmarks, including a loss of resistance to needle penetration of the costotransverse ligament for paravertebral block, or combined landmark and NS technique. US imaging may be beneficial for these blocks, particularly paravertebral block, in order to facilitate landmark localization. For example, preprocedural scanning can identify the tips of the transverse processes, which will help to identify correct needle insertion site. US may be particularly useful for performing blocks in obese patients (where the depth of needle insertion will be modified) or those with anatomic variation (e.g., scoliosis). This section provides a detailed description of the technique using NS guidance but will also provide illustrations in the sections on paravertebral and inguinal blocks of US imaging prior to block performance.

Transversus Abdominis Plane Block

Procedure Using Landmark Technique

- The patient is positioned supine, and the "Triangle of Petit" is identified with the inferior margin the iliac crest, the posterior margin the latissimus dorsi muscle, and the external oblique muscle lying anterior.
- A blunted 22-gauge, 50- to 100-mm needle (depending on body habitus) is inserted perpendicularly, immediately posterior to the mid-axillary line and above the iliac crest.
- The first and second "pops" will be felt as the needle traverses through the fascial layer of the external and internal oblique muscles, respectively. The needle tip should be within the plane between the internal oblique and the transversus abdominis.

Procedure Using Ultrasound Imaging

- Scanning: A high-frequency (10 to 15 MHz) linear probe is often used for this block. With the patient lying supine, the probe is placed transversely in the midline to identify the rectus muscles. The probe is then moved laterally, and the three layers of muscles—the external oblique, the

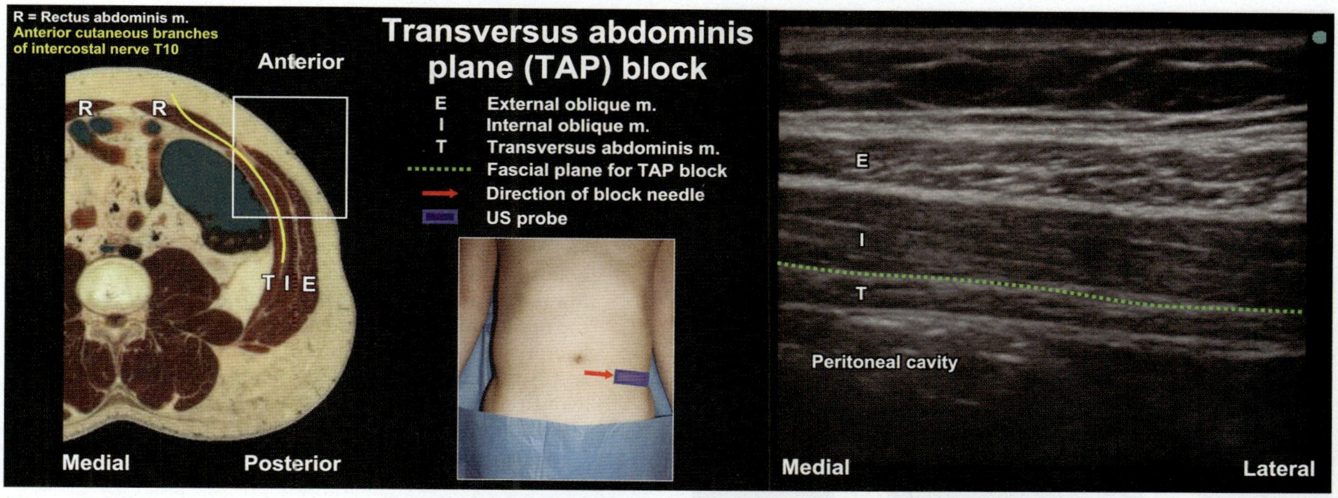

Figure 36-29 Arrangement of relevant anatomy for ultrasound-guided TAP block. A high frequency linear probe is placed transversely above the iliac crest on the anterior axillary line, revealing the three layers of abdominal muscles, the peritoneum, and the peritoneal cavity. The needle is at an IP alignment to the probe, inserted in a medial-to-lateral direction.

internal oblique, and the transversus abdominis—can be identified (Fig. 36-29). The probe should then be positioned above the iliac crest in the anterior axillary line.
- Appearance: The intercostal nerves can be too small and scattered to be identified under US imaging; therefore, the TAP block is predominantly a muscular plane block. The three layers of the abdominal muscles can be identified clearly since they are separated by the hyperechoic fascia. Beneath the abdominal muscles is the peritoneum, which is the hyperechoic line seen on US underneath the transversus abdominis. Below this lies the peritoneal cavity, in which bowel peristalsis can be seen in real time.
- Needling: During IP needling, the image should be adjusted so that the three layers of the abdominal muscles and a small portion of the peritoneal cavity are in view. A 22-gauge, 100-mm needle can be used in a medial-to-lateral direction to reduce the risk of peritoneal puncture, and it should aim toward the muscle plane between the internal oblique and transversus abdominis muscles.
- Local anesthetic spread: The aim is to spread 20 to 30 mL of local anesthetic, without exceeding the toxic dose (e.g., 2 mg/kg of bupivacaine or 3 mg/kg of ropivacaine; one-tenth of these volumes for children), on either side of the abdomen for transverse incision across the midline. The local anesthetic injection will appear as an expansion of hypoechogenicity deep to the fascial plane of the internal oblique and above that of the transversus abdominis muscle.

Clinical Pearls

- It is important to ensure local anesthetic spread in the correct fascial plane, rather than injecting local anesthetic intramuscularly.
- Color Doppler should be employed to ensure the needle trajectory is clear of blood vessels within the abdominal muscles.
- For midline incisions of the abdomen, rectus sheath block (described later) can be performed by targeting the local anesthetic injection between the rectus abdominis muscle and the posterior rectus sheath, which is formed by the aponeurosis of the three layers of abdominal muscles.

- TAP blocks have been demonstrated to provide effective analgesia in the obstetric and general surgery populations.[147–149]
- TAP catheters can be placed under direct vision by the surgeon to provide effective continuous postoperative analgesia. Following closure of the abdominal muscle layers, a catheter is inserted percutaneously above the incision, with the tip located at the most lateral point of the incision.
- TAP blocks can be modified into transversalis fascial plane (TFP) block by targeting the local anesthetic injection into the layer between the transversus abdominis muscle aponeurosis and the transversalis fascia. Local anesthetic will spread proximally over the inner surface of the quadratus lumborum muscle to anesthetize the proximal portions of the T12 and L1 nerves. The TFP block has been demonstrated to provide analgesia for anterior iliac bone graft harvesting.[150,151]

Other variations of abdominal field blocks have been described. Each block differs in the location where the injection is made (Fig. 36-30), but all use the transversus abdominis muscle as the primary landmark. The most well-studied of these blocks, including the rectus sheath block and ilioinguinal/iliohypogastric nerve block are described next.

Rectus Sheath Block

Procedure Using Landmark Technique

- The patient is positioned supine, and the umbilicus and linea semilunaris are identified. The external layer of the rectus sheath is marked on both sides, and a short-beveled needle is inserted at a point where the border of the rectus sheath intersects an imaginary horizontal line at the level of the umbilicus.
- The needle is advanced 60 degrees to the skin toward the umbilicus until a "pop" is felt as the needle penetrates the anterior rectus sheath. Local anesthetic is injected, and the same steps are repeated for the other side.

Procedure Using Ultrasound Imaging

- Scanning: A linear probe (6 to 15 MHz) is placed transversely on the anterior abdominal wall lateral to the intended site of

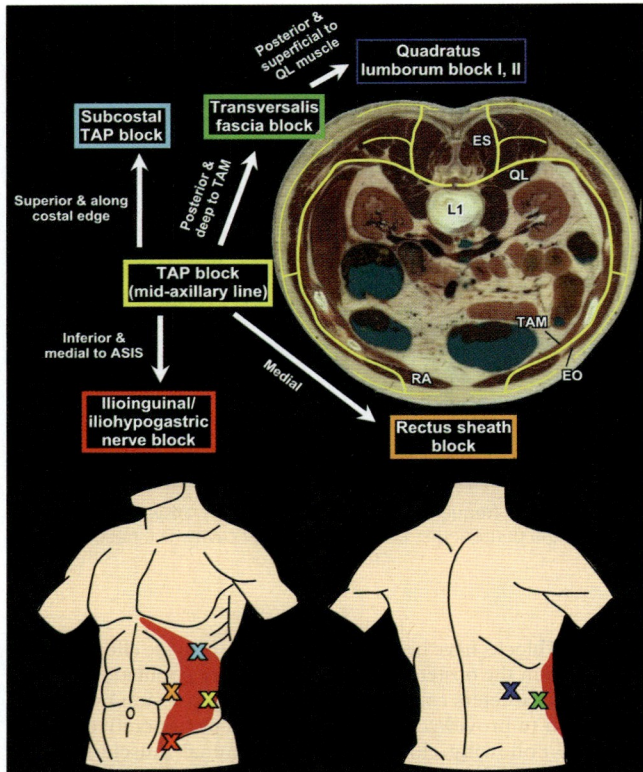

incision. Penetration depth varies with the thickness of the subcutaneous layer.

- **Appearance:** At the midline, the linea alba can be seen between the bellies of the rectus muscle, whereas the peritoneum can be visualized behind the posterior rectus sheath (Fig. 36-31). The external oblique, internal oblique, and transversus abdominis muscles can be seen lateral to the rectus muscle; the internal oblique muscle is on the same plane as the rectus muscle. Target nerves, which are not visible with US, are located between the internal oblique and transversus abdominis muscles before piercing the posterior rectus sheath and traversing the belly of the rectus muscle. The intended position of injection is the lateral space between the posterior rectus sheath and the rectus muscle. Color Doppler may be used to identify and avoid the inferior epigastric vessels that run through the rectus muscle.
- **Needling:** A 22-gauge, 50 to 100 mm needle (depending on subcutaneous fat depth) is inserted IP in a lateral-to-medial direction. A lateral insertion point will help to avoid inferior epigastric vessels. The needle is aimed through the external and internal oblique muscles toward the lateral gutter of the rectus muscle directly superior to the posterior rectus sheath. With this approach, the needle does not penetrate the belly of the rectus muscle and avoids the inferior epigastric vessels.
- **Local anesthetic spread:** Injection of 1 to 2 mL D5W can confirm needle tip position. A volume of 10 mL (0.2 mL/kg for children) local anesthetic (e.g., 0.5% ropivacaine) is injected on each side. The hypoechoic spread will be seen between the posterior rectus sheath and the rectus muscle.

Ilioinguinal and Iliohypogastric Nerve Blocks

These blocks are performed easily with a blind technique, although US imaging may be used to help improve the success rate of nerve localization and deposition of local anesthetic in the correct fascial plane proximal to the nerves.

Figure 36-30 Variations of abdominal field blocks. **Top:** The TAP block is performed at the mid-axillary line; moving the block site medially allows rectus sheath block, while moving the block site posteriorly allows transversalis fascia and quadratus lumborum block. Moving the insertion site superiorly or inferiorly from the TAP insertion site allows subcostal TAP and ilioinguinal/iliohypogastric block, respectively. **Bottom:** Needle insertion sites (X) for abdominal field blocks, color-coded according to the top figure. The approximate location of the transversus abdominis muscle is indicated in red.

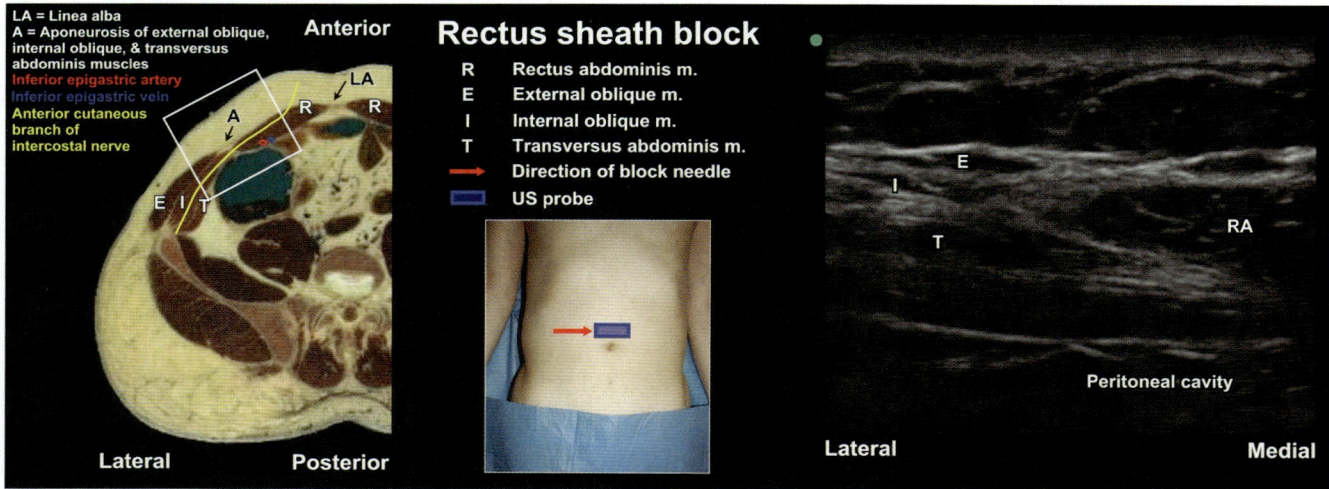

Figure 36-31 Arrangement of relevant anatomy for ultrasound-guided rectus sheath block. Placement of a transverse probe over the midline reveals the rectus abdominis and layers of the abdominal wall. Below these can be seen the peritoneum and peritoneal cavity. The needle is advanced in an IP alignment to the probe.

Procedure Using Blind Technique (Single-injection Fascial Click)

Landmarks. The injection site is located at about 1 to 2 cm medial and 1 to 2 cm inferior to the anterior superior iliac spine.

Needling and Injection. A 25-gauge, 36- to 50-mm blunted hypodermic needle can be used. The needle is inserted from the anterior abdomen (vertically) until a fascial click is detected, presumably at the junction of the internal oblique and transverse abdominis muscles. About 10- to 15-mL (0.3 to 0.5 mL/kg for children) local anesthetic can be injected. An additional 0.5 to 1 mL local anesthetic can be injected subcutaneously to block the iliohypogastric nerve.

Procedure Using Ultrasound Imaging

Scanning. Two different approaches have been used for US scanning of the ilioinguinal and iliohypogastric nerves.[61,152] In their clinical study, Willschke et al.[61] used a small footprint ("hockey stick"), 5 to 10 MHz probe, placed in transverse axis, just medial and superior to the anterior superior iliac spine. The cross-sectional view of the ilioinguinal nerve can be captured lying between the internal oblique and transverse abdominis muscles. In their cadaveric study, Eichenberger et al.[152] found that a 7.5 MHz probe was superior to one with a 10 MHz frequency. They used a position about 5 cm cranial and slightly posterior to the anterior superior iliac spine, where both nerves have been shown to be present between the above-mentioned muscles with a 90% probability. These authors visualized both nerves as distinct entities.

Appearance. The nerves appear hypoechoic with many hyperechoic dots and a distinct hyperechoic rim (Fig. 36-32). They have an oval, somewhat "boomerang" shape and appear embedded between the fascicular hypoechoic-appearing muscles. In the more cranial position, the iliac bone, with its hyperechoic border and dorsal shadowing, may be captured on the medial aspect of the screen. The thin external oblique muscle lies superficial at the cranial position, but it may not be visible more inferiorly.

Needling. An OOP alignment, with the needle placed caudad to the probe in its center, is preferred, although an IP approach is also feasible.

Local Anesthetic Spread. Either one or two injections can be made, depending on the number of distinct nerves localized. The dose of local anesthetic may be lower when using US imaging since the nerves are well localized. In children, 0.075 mL/kg has been shown to be effective for a single injection.[153] A hypoechoic area of solution should be visualized adjacent to the nerve(s).

Clinical Pearls

- The ilioinguinal and iliohypogastric nerves may exist as a common trunk at the level of the anterior superior iliac spine, which further supports the use of US guidance for localizing the individual nerve.[152]
- Since there is high variability in skin innervation from these nerves, it is impossible to confirm with clinical tests which nerve is blocked. Injecting lateral to the most laterally positioned ilioinguinal nerve, or medial to the iliohypogastric nerve, has been reported as one method to block these nerves individually.[152]
- Complications of this block are generally volume-related and include systemic toxicity and transient femoral nerve palsy. A recent assessment of the accuracy of the blind technique using US demonstrated that, even in experienced hands, needles were inserted deep to the transversus abdominis muscle over 40% of the time,[154] reinforcing the value of US in helping to prevent inaccurate needle placement or inappropriate anesthetic spread.

Penile Block

Penile block is used in children and adults for surgical procedures of the glans and shaft of the penis. The dorsal nerves (terminal branches of pudendal nerve; S2–S4) lie bilaterally on the outer aspect of the dorsal arteries of the penis. From the base of the penis, the nerves divide several times and encircle the shaft of the penis before reaching the glans. This block is often performed as a circumferential infiltration of the root of the penis (ring block). Two skin wheals are raised at the dorsal base of the penis, one on each side just below and medial to the pubic spine. A 25-gauge, 37.5-mm needle is introduced on each side, and

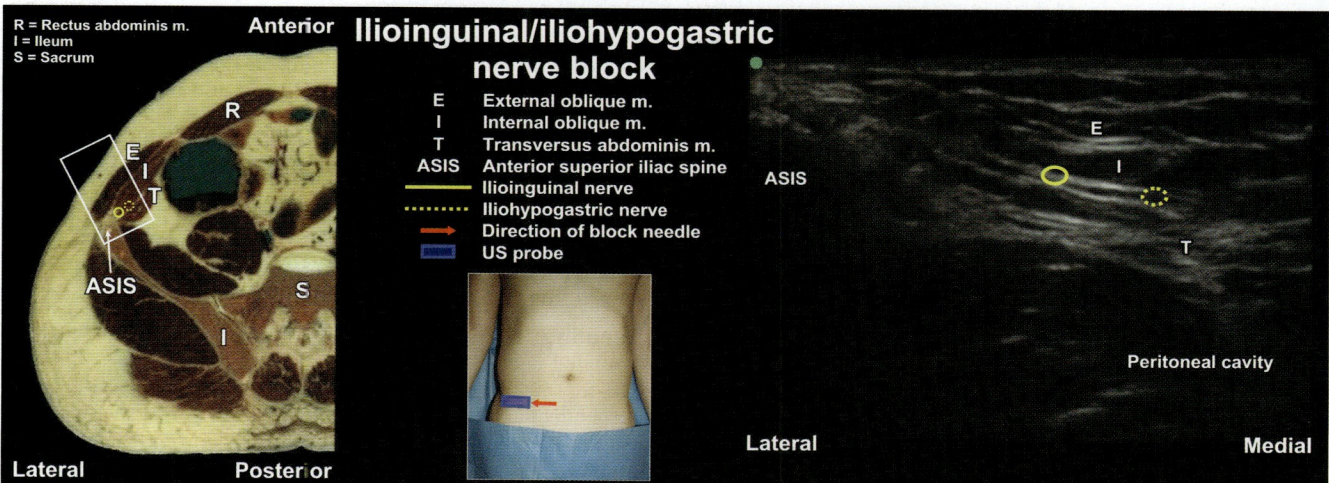

Figure 36-32 Arrangement of relevant anatomy for ultrasound-guided ilioinguinal/iliohypogastric nerve block. Transverse scanning on the abdomen just medial to the anterior superior iliac spine (ASIS) shows the nerves lying between the internal oblique and transversus abdominis muscles, just medial to the ASIS. These nerves can be blocked using an IP alignment and medial-to-lateral needle insertion to avoid puncturing through the peritoneum.

5 mL of anesthetic (0.5 to 1 mL for infants) is injected superficially and deep along the lower border of the pubic ramus to anesthetize the dorsal nerve. For a complete ring of infiltration, an additional 5 mL (adults) is infiltrated in the subcutaneous tissue around the underside of the shaft. A larger needle or a second injection site may be needed to complete the ring. Twenty to twenty-five milliliters of 0.75% lidocaine or 0.25% bupivacaine usually suffices in adults. Epinephrine-containing solutions should not be used to avoid compromising penile circulation. US can be used to improve the efficacy of penile blocks and, in one study, was found to decrease postoperative pain and delay the administration of postoperative analgesics,[155] although procedures using US were, on average, 10 minutes longer in duration compared to those performed blindly.

Lower Extremity

Combined blocks of the lumbar and sacral plexuses provide effective surgical anesthesia to the entire lower extremity. Prior to the 1990's, an "anterior lumbar block" approach (also referred to as the "femoral three-in-one" approach), which was first described by Winnie et al in 1973, had been commonly performed. This block was based on the assumption that a large volume local anesthetic injection into the femoral nerve sheath would produce spread of the solution proximally to anesthetize the obturator and lateral femoral cutaneous nerves as well. Later reports of failures to obtain obturator nerve block with this approach[157,158] led to the femoral block being considered as an individual nerve block and advocated the posterior lumbar block approach for accessing the whole lumbar plexus.

PNB is indicated when spinal or epidural techniques are contraindicated or when selective anesthesia of one leg or foot is needed. Because the anatomic landmarks identifying the fascial sheaths or compartments of the plexuses are not as clearly defined as those in the upper extremity, lower extremity blocks are often performed more distally, where the nerves have already separated into terminal branches. Thus, in addition to the fascial compartment approach (psoas block), there are peripheral approaches described at the anterior and posterior hip, knee, and ankle.

Techniques

Lumbar Plexus Block (Psoas Compartment Block)

Several techniques for blocking the lumbar plexus using a posterior approach have been described; however, the one at the psoas compartment, described first by Chayen et al.[159] in 1976, remains popular. This block is often performed with a single injection at a point some distance lateral to the spinous process of L4 since the nerves of the lumbar plexus are in proximity between the transverse processes of L4 and L5. Continuous psoas compartment blocks have also been shown to be effective for anesthesia (with sciatic nerve block) and perioperative analgesia in patients with hip fractures[160] and after hip arthroplasty.[161] A more cephalad approach, near L3, as described by Parkinson et al.,[158] may be used, although there have been reports of renal subcapsular hematomas with blocks performed at this level.[162] This block has the advantage of anesthetizing the entire lumbar plexus and therefore provides anesthesia/analgesia of the anterolateral and medial thigh, the knee, and the cutaneous distribution of the saphenous nerve below the knee. Although the sacral nerve roots may be anesthetized, this block will likely not provide complete

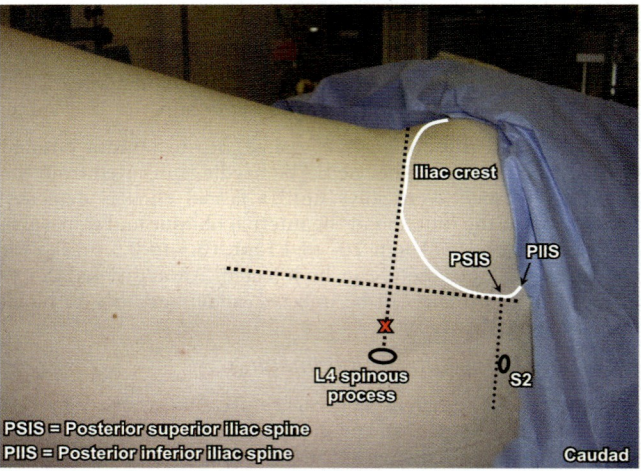

Figure 36-33 Surface landmarking for the lumbar plexus (psoas compartment) block. The needle insertion site (X) is one-third the distance along a horizontal line extending from the L4 transverse process to where it crosses a vertical line dissecting the posterior superior iliac spine.

anesthesia/analgesia for the entire upper leg, and sciatic nerve block will usually need to be performed as well. The patient is placed in the lateral position, with the operative side up. Adequate sedation should be provided since the plexus lies deep and the needle must penetrate several muscles.

Procedure Using Nerve Stimulation Technique

Landmarks. The landmarks developed by Capdevila et al.[161] using computed tomography are illustrated in Figure 36-33. Compared to the depth of the lumbar plexus or transverse processes, the distance between the L4 spinous process and the lumbar plexus is not affected by body mass index. The spinous process of L4 is estimated to lie approximately 1 cm cephalad to a line between the tops of the iliac crests (intercristal line); a horizontal line is drawn laterally from the L4 spinous processes to the far side of the body. A vertical line, running parallel to the spine, is then drawn at the point of the posterior superior iliac spine to intersect the horizontal line. The lumbar plexus is then located with an "X," below a point on the horizontal line and at the junction between the lateral third and medial two-thirds between the spine and posterior superior iliac spine. The mean skin-to-lumbar plexus depth at the level of L4 is 8.4 cm in adult men and 7.1 cm in adult women based on computed tomography assessment. The distance between the posterior edges of the transverse processes of the lumbar vertebrae and the lumbar plexus is about 1.8 cm. A strong correlation exists between weight and plexus depth in children; in one study, plexus depth ranged from 1.24 to 1.74 mm/kg in children aged 3 to 12.[163]

Needling. A skin wheal is raised at the marked block site. An insulated needle (17 to 20 gauge [22 to 25 gauge for children], 110 to 150 mm long, depending on body habitus) is inserted perpendicular to all planes at the "X" until contact with the L4 transverse process is made (approximately 5 to 6 cm deep). After contact, the needle is withdrawn and redirected caudad below the process to a maximum depth of 2 cm to the transverse process.

Nerve Localization. With the nerve stimulator set to deliver an output current of 1 to 1.5 mA, contraction of the quadriceps muscle (patellar twitch) is sought. The plexus is localized when the motor response is maintained at 0.3 to 0.5 mA. If a motor response is not obtained at first, moving the needle cautiously in a slight medial direction, without aiming toward the spinal cord, or in a direction 15 degree-caudad or cephalad, may help.

Injection. After the plexus is localized, 30 to 40 mL of local anesthetic is injected, using careful aspiration and administration of a test dose to rule out intravascular, epidural, or subarachnoid placement. Fifteen to twenty minutes may be required for spread of the anesthetic to all the roots of the lumbar plexus. It will take longer to produce anesthesia of the caudad branches (the lower sacral fibers that form the tibial nerve), and they may not become anesthetized at all.

Procedure Using Ultrasound Imaging

The lumbar plexus is difficult to view adequately since the target structures are deep. Similar to paravertebral block, US imaging may be best for identifying the exact location and depth of the transverse processes prior to the block procedure. If there is desire to perform the block at L3–L4, viewing the kidneys prior to and/or during the block may help prevent renal injury and hematoma. This is especially important in young children since the lower pole of the kidney can reach as low as L4–L5. The combined use of NS technique with US is still recommended to confirm correct needle placement.

Scanning. A curved array probe (5 to 8 MHz) is placed in the transverse plane in the midline at the level of the L4 spinous process to provide an overview of the L4 vertebra. The probe should be rotated to the longitudinal axis, parallel to the spine, which will allow a lateral scan to be performed to identify the tips of the transverse processes. The absence of associated ribs means that the tips of the transverse processes are fairly easily delineated. A 6 to 13 MHz "hockey stick" transducer may be used for young children and infants.

Appearance. For adults and older children, the deep location of this block precludes clear visibility of the lumbar plexus. Indeed, the transverse processes (which are the primary landmarks) are often only vaguely delineated. Therefore, it is important to switch between transverse and longitudinal scanning between the spinous processes and the tip of the transverse processes to survey the area. In the transverse scan, the spinous processes appear hypoechoic (likely due to dorsal shadowing effect) and extend superficially, whereas the transverse processes are hyperechoic masses/lines at the lateral edge of the vertebra. The fascicular-appearing musculature is evident surrounding the vertebra yet poorly delineated by most compact US machines. In the longitudinal scan, the lateral tips of the transverse processes will be identified at the most lateral point where a hyperechoic nodule is viewed.

Needling. Needling will be identical to that for the blind technique, with the exception that the depth to the transverse process will be more accurately known. If choosing to perform a more cephalad approach above L4, real-time imaging may be helpful to view the kidneys (especially during inspiration when they fall toward L3–L4) (Fig. 36-34). An IP needle alignment to a longitudinal probe may be most suitable to avoid excessive medial or lateral needle angulation (see Paravertebral Blockade Clinical Pearls).

Local Anesthetic Spread. In all patients except young children, it will be difficult to view local anesthetic spread when using US guidance. If seen, a hypoechoic mass will spread within the muscle mass lateral and deep to the transverse process.

Clinical Pearls

- The psoas compartment block can be beneficial for placing a catheter to provide long-lasting analgesia; the catheter is held securely by the psoas muscles and kept away from any active joint region. After obtaining good localization with the stimulating needle (bevel facing caudad and lateral), a stimulating catheter is advanced 3 to 5 cm. In some cases, injecting a nonconducting solution such as D5W to expand the perineural space, while maintaining the electrical characteristics, is helpful.[27] Quadriceps muscle contraction should be maintained during catheter advancement with a stimulating catheter.
- Prepuncture US may be beneficial prior to needle insertion and catheter placement. Using a higher frequency (6 to 13 MHz) linear array transducer, Ilfeld et al.[164] showed that

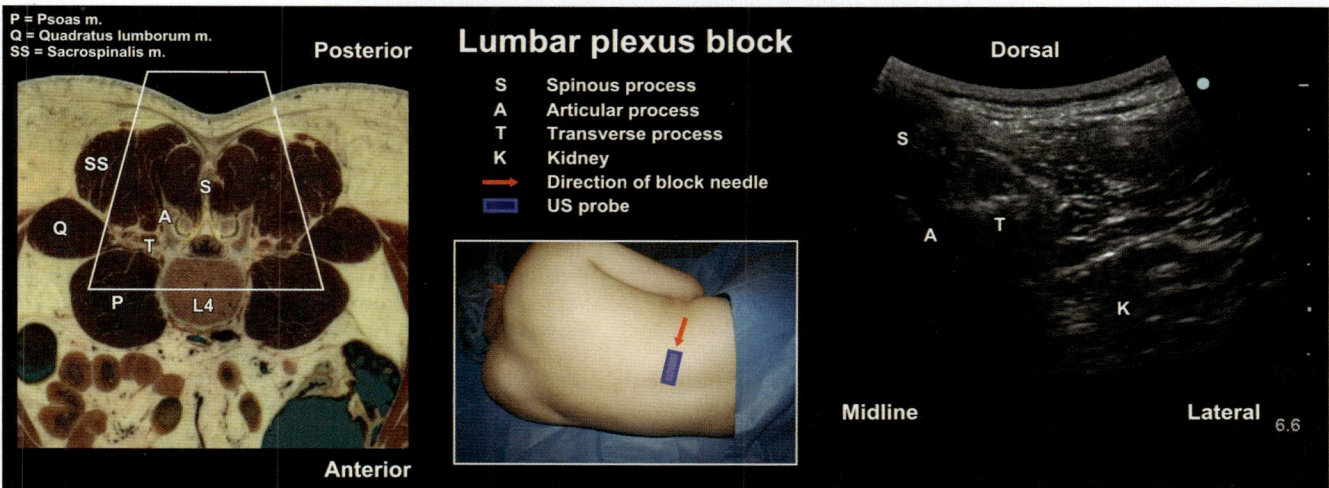

Figure 36-34 Arrangement of relevant anatomy for ultrasound-assisted lumbar plexus block. A curved array probe can be placed transversely to capture an overview of the spinous, articular, and transverse processes, with the psoas muscle just deep and lateral to the latter. Puncture of the kidney can be a potential complication of lumbar plexus block; if attempting real-time needle insertion, the safest needle alignment will be IP to a longitudinally placed probe over the L3–L5 transverse processes since the kidney may come to view at a more cephalad position.

the depth and location of each transverse process could be estimated accurately, allowing the user to minimize risks associated with needle/catheter insertion into the lumbar plexus.
- Complications of this technique include hematoma in the muscle sheath, retroperitoneal space, or kidney (hence, this block is contraindicated in patients with coagulopathy or bleeding diathesis); infection; and catheter placement within the peritoneum. Neuropathy is possible, and unintended spread to the epidural or even subarachnoid space has also been reported.

Separate Blocks of the Terminal Nerves of the Lumbar Plexus

Anesthesia can be performed for four terminal nerves of the lumbar plexus (lateral femoral cutaneous, femoral, obturator, and saphenous), although a psoas compartment block (described earlier) is preferable if anesthesia of all these nerves are required. Anesthesia of the lateral femoral cutaneous nerve is used occasionally to provide sensory anesthesia for obtaining a skin graft from the lateral thigh. It can also be blocked as a diagnostic/therapeutic tool to identify cases of meralgia paresthetica (a neurologic disorder of the lateral femoral cutaneous nerve). It has been shown that the obturator nerve provides variable sensory supply to the medial aspect of the thigh and knee joint and also gives off branches to the hip joint.[165] Obturator nerve block can be effective to prevent obturator reflex during transurethral bladder tumor resections, for treatment of pain in the hip area, for adductor spasm (as seen in multiple sclerosis patients), or as a diagnostic tool when studying hip mobility.[166] Saphenous nerve block often complements sciatic nerve block when anesthesia of the medial aspect of the ankle and foot are required. Procedures on the knee require anesthesia of the femoral and the obturator nerves, although postoperative analgesia of the knee can usually be provided by femoral nerve block alone. Single-injection femoral nerve block provides suitable postoperative analgesia after total knee arthroplasty while sparing the side effects of intrathecal morphine.[167] The use of a continuous technique can also reduce side effects as compared to continuous epidurals[168] and can facilitate rehabilitation.[169] A US-guided infrapatellar nerve block has been described for use for postoperative analgesia after outpatient arthroscopic surgery[170] but will not be discussed further here. Separate femoral nerve block is used extensively for analgesia, and US guidance has been described for this block; therefore, this chapter will provide a comprehensive description of this block. US guidance for obturator nerve block has been described and will be examined here. The other two nerve blocks will only be discussed briefly. The block sites for the femoral, lateral femoral cutaneous, and obturator nerves are illustrated in Figure 36-15.

Femoral Nerve/Fascia Iliaca Block

Procedure Using Nerve Stimulation
- Landmarks: The patient is placed in the supine position, with slight external rotation of the femur. A pillow can be placed under the patient's hip to facilitate palpation of the femoral pulse and accentuate other pertinent landmarks for ease of palpation. Vloka et al.[171] studied cadavers using four common needle insertion sites for femoral nerve block and found that the point where the nerve lies beneath the inguinal crease, immediately lateral to the femoral artery, was optimal for localizing the nerve. The femoral artery descends at the "mid-inguinal point," at the junction between the medial third and lateral two-thirds of the inguinal ligament, although it is most superficial at the femoral crease. It lies approximately 1 to 1.5 cm medial to the nerve. The inguinal crease is the skin fold located approximately 2.5 cm caudad and parallel to the inguinal ligament (Clinical Anatomy of lower extremity).
- Needling: A skin wheal is raised lateral to the area where the femoral artery pulsation is felt, and a 50-mm, 22-gauge insulated needle is inserted perpendicular to the skin or using a cephalad angle of approximately 30 degrees. Aspiration is performed frequently since the femoral artery is situated close to the nerve.
- Nerve localization: Using NS, a quadriceps muscle response (patellar twitch preferably) is sought, with an end point of 0.5 mA used for accurate localization. Branches to the sartorius muscle arise just inferior to the inguinal ligament and leave the femoral nerve proximal to the main block location site; a response of this muscle to stimulation often indicates that the needle is too superficial and medial to the main femoral nerve. For a fascia iliaca block, loss-of-resistance technique is used instead of NS. The needle is placed vertically 5 cm lateral to the artery at the inguinal crease. Two pops are felt when the needle traverses the fascia lata and fascia iliaca and enters the iliopsoas muscle.
- Injection: Injection of 20 mL (or less) of local anesthetic should suffice for sole femoral nerve anesthesia. Twenty to thirty milliliters of local anesthetic may be required for the fascia iliaca block. Intermittent injection with interval aspiration should be performed.

Procedure Using Ultrasound Imaging (Fig. 36-35)
- Scanning: A 10 MHz or higher transducer can be used for both blocks if the neurovascular structures are not located too deep (i.e., thin individuals), as this will show good distinction between the nerve and the surrounding structures (vessels and muscles). A midrange 5- to 8-MHz linear transducer is recommended if the nerve and artery are deep (>4 cm). Position the probe transverse to the nerve axis at the level of the inguinal crease. The nerve should appear approximately 1 cm deep and 1.5 cm lateral to the femoral artery, depending on body habitus (color Doppler may be used to identify the femoral artery and vein). A 5 to 10 MHz "hockey stick" transducer can be used for most children.
- Appearance: The nerve lies about 1 cm lateral and deep to the large, circular, anechoic, and pulsatile femoral artery. The nerve often appears triangular in shape and of variable size due to its irregular course; early branching above the inguinal ligament can increase the transverse diameter of the nerve. The fascia lata (most superficial) and fascia iliaca (immediately adjacent to the nerve and in fact separating the nerve from the artery) may be seen superficial to the femoral nerve and often appear bright and longitudinally angled.
- Needling: Place the nerve at the medial edge of the screen, with the probe capturing a transverse view of the neurovascular structures. A 50-mm, 22-gauge needle (for single-injection) can be inserted using either IP or OOP (Fig. 36-35) needle alignment. The needle should be inserted using an acute (30 to 45 degrees) angle to maximize viewing. IP blocks may be made easier by angling the needle tip slightly away from the nerve, whereas accuracy of catheter placement may be improved by tilting the needle hub in a caudad direction once the needle tip is positioned appropriately.[172] Inserting the catheter perpendicular or parallel to the nerve does not affect quality of analgesia, although the former technique may facilitate faster catheter insertion.[173]

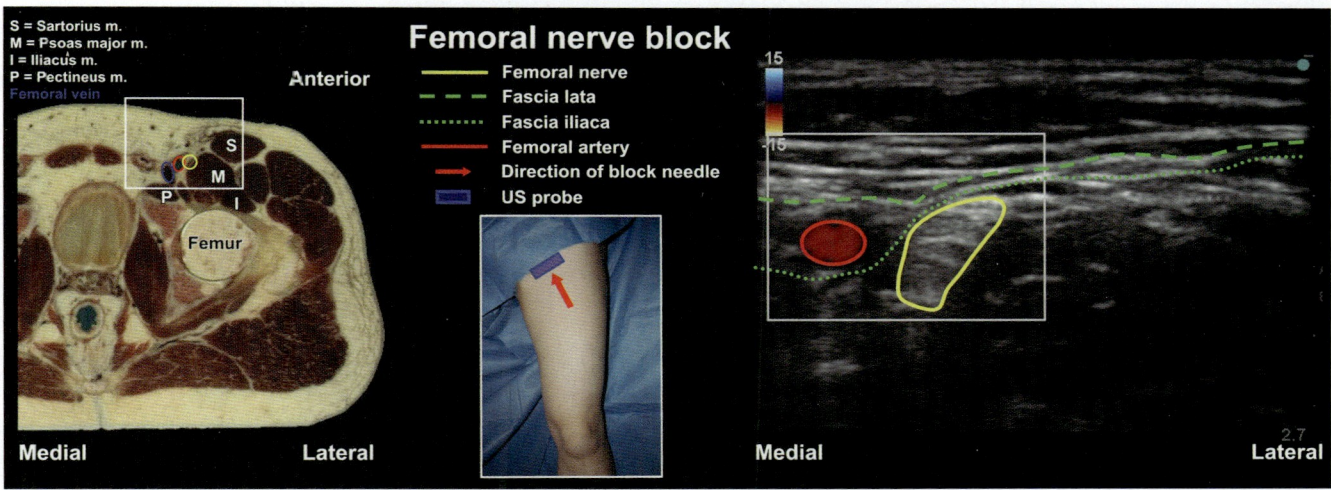

Figure 36-35 Arrangement of relevant anatomy for ultrasound-guided femoral nerve block. The probe is placed in a slightly oblique plane (at the level of and parallel to the inguinal crease) to capture the nerve in short axis lateral to the femoral artery. The needle (not shown) can be visualized as it transects the fascia lata and fascia iliaca. If IP needling is used, it should occur in a lateral-to-medial direction.

- For fascia iliaca block, the needle is generally placed more laterally than with conventional femoral nerve block.
- Local anesthetic spread: Performing a test dose with D5W is recommended prior to local anesthetic application to visualize the spread and confirm nerve localization. Local anesthetic spread should occur within the fascial space surrounding the nerve. The solution may displace the nerve medially toward or laterally away from the artery.

Clinical Pearls

- When inserting a catheter, it is debatable whether a stimulating catheter improves placement,[174,175] but using a solution to expand the perineural space has been shown to be beneficial in some cases.[176,177] If a stimulating catheter is used, injection of D5W for tissue expansion will maintain motor responses to NS.[26,27]
- With an IP needle alignment, lateral-to-medial needle insertion will ensure that the nerve is reached before encountering the femoral vessels.
- It is important to ensure that the US beam is perpendicular to the nerve's transverse axis to minimize the chance of anisotropic effects changing the echogenic properties of the structure. It has been shown that an approximate 10 degree cephalad or caudad tilt of the transducer can make the nerve isoechoic (similar-appearing) to the underlying iliopsoas muscle.[178]

Lateral Femoral Cutaneous Nerve

Using NS technique, Shannon et al.[179] found that the lateral femoral cutaneous nerve can be localized at the inguinal crease, approximately 0 to 1 cm medial to the anterior superior iliac spine (Fig. 36-15), although this mark may be highly variable[180] and should be confirmed with NS. An insulated needle (22 gauge, 50 mm; 35 mm for children) is inserted using a perpendicular approach if the puncture is close to the anterior superior iliac spine or in a lateral direction if it is at a distance. A "pop" may be felt as the needle penetrates the fascia lata. The primary end point for NS with this nerve is paresthesia over the lateral thigh (Fig. 36-14) with a current of approximately 0.5 to 0.6 mA. The sensory distribution may not extend proximal to the greater trochanter. Five to ten milliliters of a local anesthetic is usually sufficient to obtain a block.

A recent study demonstrated that nerve targeting may not be necessary in some cases; in patients undergoing knee surgery, injection of local anesthetic immediately under the inguinal ligament provided sufficient blockade without having to inject directly around the nerve.[181]

Obturator Nerve

Since the obturator nerve branches early after its descent from the obturator foramen, blocking the nerve within the foramen near the superior pubic ramus (i.e., before it branches) is often described for blind techniques. The patient is placed supine with their hip slightly externally rotated; the hip may also be slightly flexed and abducted. If using US imaging, a straight leg has been shown to be the best position. The pubic tubercle is located, and a mark is placed 1.5 cm both inferior and lateral to it (this mark should resemble that in Fig. 36-15). An inguinal approach is another option and may result in higher block success rates and fewer needle attempts in certain circumstances.[182]

Procedure Using Nerve Stimulation Technique

- An insulated needle (18 to 22 gauge, 90 to 100 mm for adults; 22 to 25 gauge, 35 to 50 mm for children) is inserted perpendicularly until contact with the inferior pubic ramus is obtained. The needle is then redirected laterally and caudally to enter the obturator foramen and is advanced 2 to 3 cm. NS using 0.5 mA for a current end point, with adductor muscle contraction, has been shown to greatly improve nerve localization.[166]

Procedure Using Ultrasound Imaging (Fig. 36-36).

Scanning: The use of US-guided obturator block at the proximal thigh is based predominantly on the identification of three muscle layers, namely, the adductor longus, adductor brevis, and adductor magnus muscles (from superficial to deep). The anterior branch of the obturator nerve usually lies on the lateral edge between the adductor longus and brevis muscles, whereas the posterior branch of the obturator nerve lies between the adductor brevis and magnus muscles; however, the obturator nerve shows a considerable degree of variability at this level.[183,184] Soong et al.[185] found that the anterior and posterior branches may be most easily visualized with the probe placed 2 cm laterally and

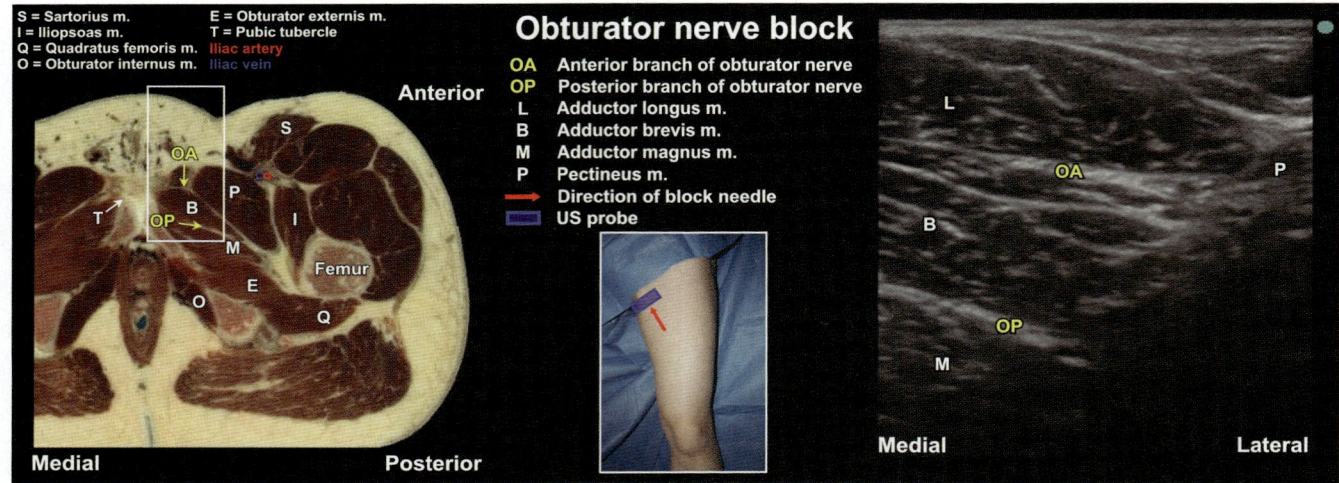

Figure 36-36 Arrangement of relevant anatomy for ultrasound-guided obturator nerve block (anterior and posterior branches) in the proximal thigh using an OOP approach. It is important to identify the three adductor muscles—the adductor longus, adductor brevis, and adductor magnus (from superficial to deep). The pectineus muscle should also be in view on the lateral side since the anterior branch of the obturator nerve is sandwiched between the adductor longus and adductor brevis deep to the pectineus muscle.

distally to the pubic tubercle. The branches may be localized on either side of the adductor brevis muscle if the fascial planes of the muscles are highly visible (hyperechoic). The depths of the anterior and posterior branches as measured during US guidance were 15.5 and 29.3 mm, respectively; tissue compression by the probe may influence this depth. The main (common) obturator nerve may be hard to view with US imaging. An IP needling technique and color Doppler can be used to help avoid adjacent blood vessels.

- Appearance: Using a high frequency probe, US visualization of the three layers of muscle—adductor longus, adductor brevis, and adductor magus—should be seen. The anterior branches of the nerve usually appear as hypoechoic circles in between a hyperechoic layer formed by the adductor longus and brevis, whereas the posterior branches are located between the layers of the adductor brevis and magnus muscles at this level. The nerve can also be blocked more distally at the knee.
- Needling: To anesthetize the anterior branch of the obturator nerve, a 22-gauge needle is inserted in either an IP or OOP fashion deep to the adductor longus muscle to deposit local anesthetic immediately beneath the muscle. Similarly, the needle can be inserted deeper to adductor brevis to reach the posterior branch. Five to ten milliliters of local anesthetic should suffice.
- Local anesthetic spread: A homogeneous, hypoechoic spread pattern between the muscle layers should appear during injection. It is important to avoid intramuscular injection.

Clinical Pearls

- Using cadavers and live subjects, Akkaya et al.[186] demonstrated that a hyperechoic triangle bordered by the superior pubic ramus, posterior edge of the pectineus muscle, and anterior aspect of the external obturator muscle is an ideal landmark to locate the obturator nerve, which lies just medial to the obturator vein.
- A report using US guidance suggested that a single injection of local anesthetic into the interfascial space (i.e., between the adductor longus and adductor brevis muscles) containing the anterior branch of the obturator nerve results in upward (cranial) spreading of anesthetic to block the posterior branch[187]; further spreading was encouraged by applying pressure distal to the needle insertion site.
- Aspiration is essential when injecting near the unbranched obturator nerve since the obturator artery lies adjacent to the nerve, and hemorrhage involving this artery can be life-threatening.[188]

Saphenous Nerve

Many approaches to saphenous nerve blockade have been described, with needle placement at various locations, including the mid-thigh, surrounding the knee, or at the ankle (as discussed in Ankle Block). A transsartorial block using a blind technique, first described by van der Wal et al.,[189] has been shown to be more effective compared to blockade at the medial femoral condyle (paracondylar block) or tibial tuberosity (below-knee field block) for producing anesthesia to the medial aspect of the foot.[190] US guidance has been used successfully with a transsartorius perifemoral,[191] subsartorial,[192] or perivenous (saphenous vein)[193,194] approach; the perifemoral approach will be discussed later. An effective approach using the sartorius and gracilis tendons as landmarks has also been described.[195] Using the more proximally located larger femoral artery (rather than the more distal saphenous branch of the descending genicular artery) as a highly visible landmark seems to help to identify the sartorius muscle and nerve.

Procedure Using Nerve Stimulation Technique (Transsartorial)

- Landmarks: The sartorius muscle is palpated at the medial aspect of the knee joint by asking the patient to raise their extended leg 5 to 10 cm off the table. The block location is marked by the end of a 4 cm vertical line drawn from this point in a proximal direction (Benzon et al.[190] used a slightly more cephalad point 3 to 4 cm superior and 6 to 8 cm posterior to the superomedial border of the patella).
- Needling: An insulated 22-gauge needle is inserted caudally using an angle of 45 degrees with a slight posterior angle advanced from the medial aspect of the knee, in a

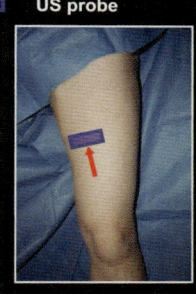

Figure 36-37 Arrangement of relevant anatomy for ultrasound-guided saphenous nerve block using a transsartorius perifemoral approach. The probe is placed in the coronal plane at the location where the femoral artery has yet to become the popliteal artery, approximately 10 to 12 cm proximal and 3 to 4 cm medial to the midpoint of the patella. Using the large femoral artery as a landmark may be beneficial to more distal approaches where the nerve lies adjacent to the smaller saphenous branch of the descending genicular artery (see text).

slight posterior and caudad angle, to penetrate the sartorius muscle at a depth of approximately 2 to 3 cm.
- **Nerve localization:** Since the saphenous nerve is purely sensory, paresthesia at the medial malleolus should be felt with the nerve stimulator at 0.6 mA or less at a depth of 3 to 5 cm. Elicitation of paresthesia is not usually performed in children, as it can be uncomfortable or painful.
- **Injection:** Following careful aspiration, 10 mL of local anesthetic (e.g., 1.5% to 2% lidocaine) is injected.

Procedure Using Ultrasound Imaging (Fig. 36-37)
- Using US, the sartorius muscle can be identified easily as being a superficial roof to the relatively large landmark of the femoral artery before the artery travels deep and becomes the popliteal artery via the adductor hiatus.[191] The nerve is located between the sartorius muscle and the artery in the thigh.
- **Scanning:** A high-frequency linear US transducer (e.g., L38, MicroMaxx, Sonosite, Bothell, WA, USA) is placed transversely to the longitudinal axis of the extremity at the mid-thigh, approximately 10 to 12 cm proximal and 3 to 4 cm medial to the midpoint of the patella. The femoral artery can be identified here with certainty by power Doppler, which in turn confirms the identity of the overlying sartorius muscle. The probe is then used to scan distally until it captures the point just prior to where the femoral artery becomes the popliteal artery.
- **Appearance:** Using color Doppler is important to visualize the femoral artery as a large hypoechoic (beneath the color) structure at a depth of approximately 2 to 3 cm in average-sized individuals. The sartorius muscle can then be identified as a highly delineated, lip-shaped muscle with hyperechoic borders immediately superficial to the artery. The nerve can be blocked as it lies sandwiched between the artery and the muscle at this level, or it can be blocked more distally at the knee.
- **Needling:** A 22-gauge needle is inserted in either an IP or OOP fashion to penetrate the sartorius muscle to deposit local anesthetic immediately beneath the muscle and medial to the artery. Five to ten milliliters of local anesthetic should suffice.

- **Local anesthetic spread:** A small hypoechoic mass on the medial surface of the femoral artery should appear during injection.

Sciatic Nerve Block Using Gluteal, Subgluteal, Posterior Popliteal, and Anterior Approaches

A sciatic nerve block can be used with lumbar plexus block for anesthesia of the lower extremity. Together with saphenous nerve block, the block produces adequate anesthesia of the sole of the foot and the lower leg. The large sciatic nerve is deep within the gluteal region and may be difficult to locate blindly or with US. Of benefit during US-guided blockade of the sciatic nerve and its terminal branches (tibial and common peroneal nerves) are the numerous bony and vascular landmarks that can be used for ease of identification. Knowledge of anatomy is paramount with these blocks, and the block location and approach will ultimately depend on the surgical requirement.

Posterior Sciatic Nerve Block: Classical Gluteal (Labat) Approach

Position the patient semiprone (Sims' position) with the hip and knee flexed and the operative side uppermost.

Procedure Using Nerve Stimulation
- **Landmarks (Fig. 36-38):** An oblique line is drawn joining the posterior superior iliac spine to the midpoint of the greater trochanter (on its medial aspect). Next, a horizontal line is drawn joining the greater trochanter (at above location) to the sacral hiatus. A perpendicular line drawn at the midpoint of the oblique line and reaching the parahorizontal line is the traditional puncture site (this intersection should be approximately 5 cm caudad along the perpendicular line).
- **Needling:** Raise a local anesthetic skin wheal after aseptic preparation. A 100-mm (shorter for pediatric patients), 22-gauge needle (insulated if NS is desired) is inserted perpendicular to the skin. For children, the depth to the nerve can be approximated as ~1 mm/kg weight, with less and more depth for younger and older individuals, respectively.

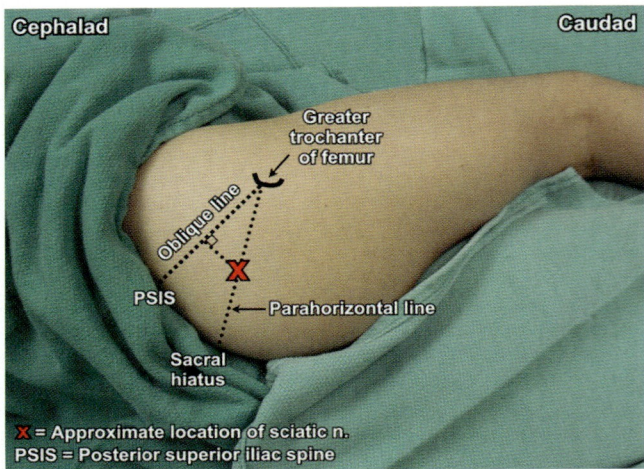

Figure 36-38 Landmarks for sciatic nerve block using a posterior gluteal (Labat) approach when using nerve stimulation procedure. This location will also serve as a reference point when applying ultrasound imaging.

- Nerve localization: Nerve responses of the lower leg and foot are sought. If they are not obtained at the full depth of the needle, the needle is withdrawn to the skin and reintroduced at a location perpendicular to the course of the nerve. Bone contact typically requires lateral needle adjustment.
- Injection: Injection of 20 to 30 mL of local anesthetic (e.g., 0.75% ropivacaine, 1% mepivacaine, 0.5% bupivacaine) is performed. If several blocks are required (i.e., lumbar plexus and/or saphenous nerve), a reduced concentration of local anesthetic may be necessary to prevent exceeding the toxic dose.

Procedure Using Ultrasound Imaging (Fig. 36-39)

- Scanning: A curved, lower frequency 2 to 5 MHz probe (higher frequency for young children) is generally used for scanning the gluteal region. Moving the probe cephalad and caudad in the gluteal region will help examine the ischial bone (a hyperechoic line with bony shadowing underneath); the widest portion of this bone, with the ischial spine medial, should be located. The bulky gluteus maximus muscle will be seen superficial and posterior to the sciatic nerve. The internal pudendal vessels (artery and vein), which may be identified using color Doppler, are adjacent to the ischial spine, which is medial to the sciatic nerve and adjacent inferior gluteal artery. Alternatively, the nerve can be first located at the subgluteal region, at about the midpoint between the greater trochanter and the ischial tuberosity, and traced proximally. Bony landmarks (e.g., medial aspect of greater trochanter, femoral condyles) are less visible in children, especially those under 7 years old.
- Appearance: The sciatic nerve in the gluteal region is found lateral to the ischial spine and superficial to the ischial bone. The nerve appears predominantly hyperechoic (bright) and is often wide and flat in short axis on US. Overlying the sciatic nerve is the large gluteus maximus, which is quite distinct with the usual "starry night" appearance. The inner muscle layers (superior and inferior gemellus muscles, obturator internus muscle, and quadratus femoris muscle) are often indistinct.
- Needling: Both IP and OOP approaches are appropriate for US-guided sciatic nerve block in the gluteal region. For an OOP approach, the needle is inserted inferior to the probe in a cephaloanterior direction. A fairly steep angle of insertion will be required, but placing the needle slightly inferior to the probe will reduce the angle somewhat for better visibility of the needle. With the IP approach, the needle may be moved in a lateral-to-medial direction to penetrate the gluteus maximus muscle before reaching the sciatic nerve above the ischial bone (Fig. 36-39).
- Local anesthetic spread: Performing a test dose with D5W is recommended prior to local anesthetic application to visualize the spread and confirm nerve localization. It is generally recommended to deposit the local anesthetic solution so that it spreads completely around the sciatic nerve.

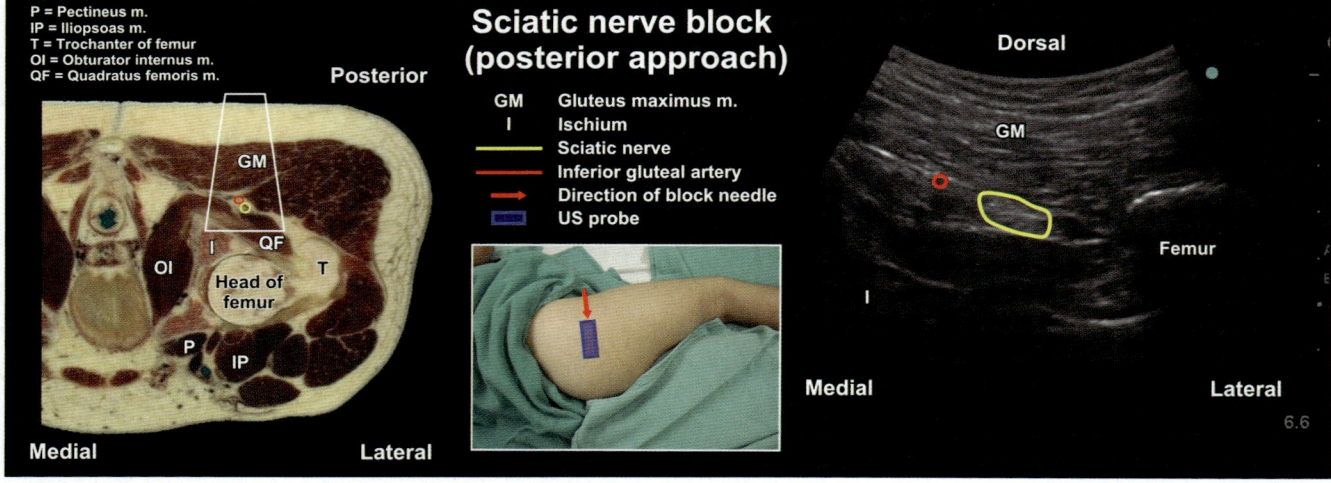

Figure 36-39 Arrangement of relevant anatomy for ultrasound-guided sciatic nerve block using a posterior gluteal (Labat) approach. An IP needle alignment to a curved low frequency probe is used. A lateral-to-medial needle direction may help avoid puncture of the inferior gluteal or internal pudendal vessels.

Clinical Pearls
- For both IP and OOP needling approaches, scanning before needling will determine the angle, distance, and depth of needle penetration.
- The OOP approach is often used for catheter insertion, and it is important to line up the site of needle insertion with the target nerve.

Posterior Sciatic Nerve Block: Subgluteal Approach

The patient is positioned semiprone (Sims position) with the hip and knee flexed and the foot resting on the dependent knee. In some patients, the supine position with the hip flexed and knee bent is either most comfortable or necessitated due to fracture or pain at the hip. The latter position requires an assistant to support the bent leg.

Procedure Using Nerve Stimulation Technique
- **Landmarks:** A horizontal line is drawn joining the medial aspect of the greater trochanter to the ischial tuberosity. The traditional puncture site is located on this line just medial to its midpoint.
- **Needling:** An insulated needle, 100 to 150 mm, depending on patient habitus, is used. The needle is inserted perpendicular to the skin. Shorter needles are recommended for use in children.
- **Nerve localization:** Confirming sciatic nerve localization with NS is important prior to local anesthetic application. Similar responses as those for the classic gluteal approach are sought, with ankle responses preferable. It is important to distinguish the tibial (inversion or plantar flexion) and common peroneal (eversion or dorsiflexion) components of the nerve and obtain both responses or, at minimum, the tibial response.
- **Injection:** Injection of 20 to 30 mL of local anesthetic is sufficient. If additional blocks of the lower extremity are performed, a solution with lower concentration should be considered to prevent exceeding the toxic dose of local anesthetic.

Procedure Using Ultrasound Imaging (Fig. 36-40)
- **Scanning:** A curved lower frequency 2 to 5 MHz probe or linear 4 to 7 MHz probe is suitable for scanning the subgluteal region; high frequency probes are recommended for scanning young children. The center of the probe should be aligned with the midpoint of a line between the ischial tuberosity and the greater trochanter. If the sciatic nerve is hard to localize at the subgluteal region, it can be traced proximally from the bifurcation point at or near the apex of the popliteal fossa.
- **Appearance:** On the lateral side of the screen, the medial aspect of the greater trochanter appears almost pear-shaped and hypoechoic when using a curved array probe. The sciatic nerve in the subgluteal region appears predominantly hyperechoic (bright) and is often elliptical in a short-axis view using US.
- **Needling:** Similar to the classic gluteal approach, both IP and OOP plane needling can be performed, with the needle directed from lateral to medial for the IP technique. Using an angle of insertion of approximately 45 degrees to the skin will provide the best view of the needle and will reach the nerve, although 60 to 70 degrees may be required in certain obese individuals.
- **Local anesthetic spread:** The goal is to deposit local anesthetic (20 to 30 mL) next to, but not directly within, the sciatic nerve structure in the subgluteal region. A hypoechoic local anesthetic fluid collection is often seen around the hyperechoic nerve within the sheath compartment during injection.

Clinical Pearls
- Since a low frequency curved array probe is necessary in many cases, the needle tip as viewed with an OOP approach will be even harder to identify than when using higher resolution linear probes. Nevertheless, this approach is used often since indwelling catheters are commonly placed in the subgluteal area. It will be important to use NS in addition to US-guided technique to confirm placement of the needle and local anesthetic.

Posterior Popliteal Sciatic Block

The sciatic nerve can be blocked below the hip at the lateral mid-femoral or lateral popliteal locations in addition to the posterior popliteal location,[196,197] but when using US guidance, the

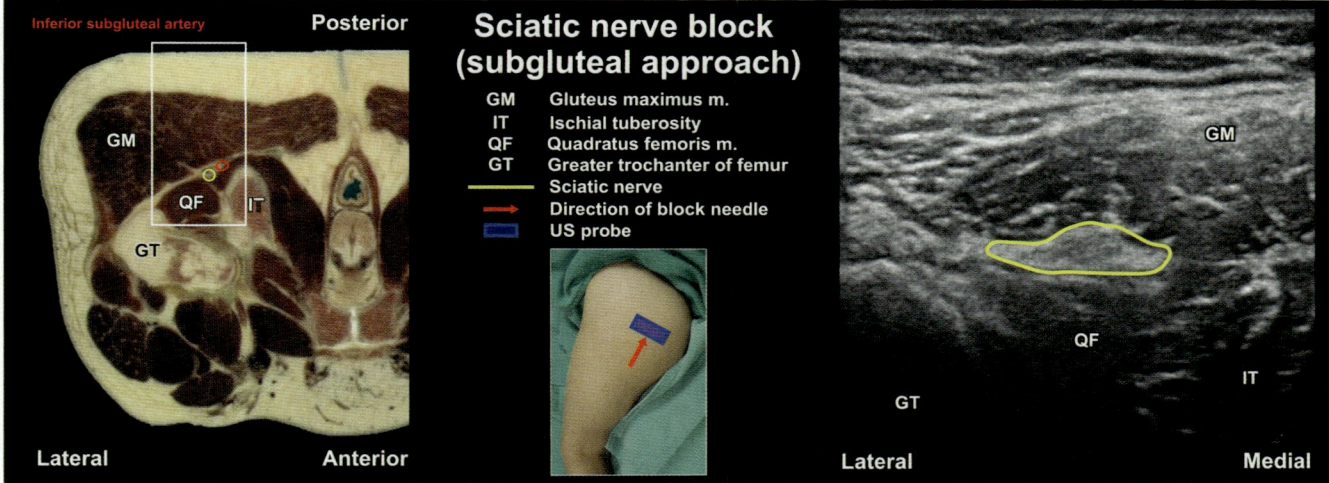

Figure 36-40 Arrangement of relevant anatomy for ultrasound-guided sciatic nerve block with a subgluteal approach. Out-of-plane approaches are preferred since this approach is used often for indwelling catheter placement, especially in children. The medially positioned ischial tuberosity is not captured in this image but will serve as a good bony landmark in most circumstances.

posterior approach allows the needle to be placed closely to the probe and thus may improve needle tracking and visibility. Furthermore, the posterior popliteal approach is most amenable to inserting indwelling catheters. The patient is positioned laterally or prone with the operative leg slightly flexed. Ideally, the ankles should be positioned beyond the end of the table so that motor responses to NS can be readily observed in the prone position. The landmarks become more visible when the knee is flexed against resistance.

Procedure Using Nerve Stimulation Technique

- **Landmarks:** The puncture site is often located at the tip of a triangle formed by the popliteal crease at the base, the biceps femoris tendon laterally, and the semimembranosus tendon medially (which generally lies medial to the tendon of the semitendinosus at this location). Alternatively, drawing lines 8 cm long in a cephalad direction from the insertion site of the medial and lateral tendons (above), the puncture point is at the midpoint of a line attaching the two (almost parallel) lines. It may be best to insert the needle at approximately 10 cm above the popliteal fossa in order to ensure that the sciatic nerve is blocked before its bifurcation. For children, the distance between the popliteal fold and the needle insertion point can be calculated based on patient weight: less than 10 kg = 1 cm, 10 to 20 kg = 2 cm, 20 to 30 kg = 3 cm, and so forth.
- **Needling:** Depending on the patient, a 50-mm insulated 22-gauge needle can be inserted using an angle of 45 degrees cephalad to the skin. A fan-wise search is conducted perpendicular to this line until the nerve is contacted. If the femur is contacted by the needle, the depth is noted; the nerve should lie midway between the skin and the femur.
- **Nerve localization:** NS is used to elicit motor responses at the ankle or foot. The aim should be to localize the sciatic nerve before its bifurcation into its tibial and common peroneal nerve components. If only ankle inversion and/or plantar flexion (tibial nerve) or eversion and/or dorsiflexion (common peroneal) is seen, adjust the needle insertion site a few centimeters cephalad to obtain complete ankle and foot movements. Otherwise, injecting after obtaining a sole tibial nerve response has been shown to provide similar success to that after both tibial and common peroneal responses (with two injections).[198] Maintaining a motor response with currents less than 0.5 mA will help ensure the nerve–needle distance is appropriate for a successful block.[199]
- **Injection:** Twenty to thirty milliliters of local anesthetic should be deposited at the final needle location.

Procedure Using Ultrasound Guidance (Fig. 36-41)

- **Scanning:** A linear, higher frequency 10 to 15 MHz probe is commonly used for scanning the sciatic nerve transversely in the popliteal fossa. A "hockey stick" probe is suitable for most children. A distal-to-proximal scan can effectively locate the sciatic nerve in the posterior popliteal fossa prior to its bifurcation (Fig. 36-41). At the popliteal crease, the transverse probe captures the tibial and common peroneal nerves, with the former being adjacent and lateral to the popliteal vessels (Doppler is valuable here). During a proximal scan, the tibial and common peroneal nerves approach each other and join to form the sciatic nerve.
- **Appearance:** At the level of the popliteal crease, the tibial and common peroneal nerves lie superficial and lateral to the popliteal vessels (the common peroneal nerve is the most lateral). Both nerves appear round-to-oval and hyperechoic compared to the surrounding musculature. The hyperechoic border of the femur (condyles) may be apparent. During the proximal scan, the tibial nerve moves away from the vessels and approaches the common peroneal nerve. More cephalad in the posterior thigh, the biceps femoris muscle lies superficial to the joining nerves and appears as a larger, oval-shaped structure with less internal punctate areas (hypoechoic spots) than the nerves. The sciatic nerve appears as a large, oval hyperechoic structure. The high fat and muscle content of the area may impair visualization of the nerve itself. Furthermore, the probe often needs to be tilted for optimal imaging since the nerve becomes more superficial as it descends distally.
- **Needling:** An OOP approach is performed commonly, especially if placing indwelling catheters. The probe is positioned directly above the sciatic nerve at or slightly cephalad to its bifurcation point and so that the nerve is in

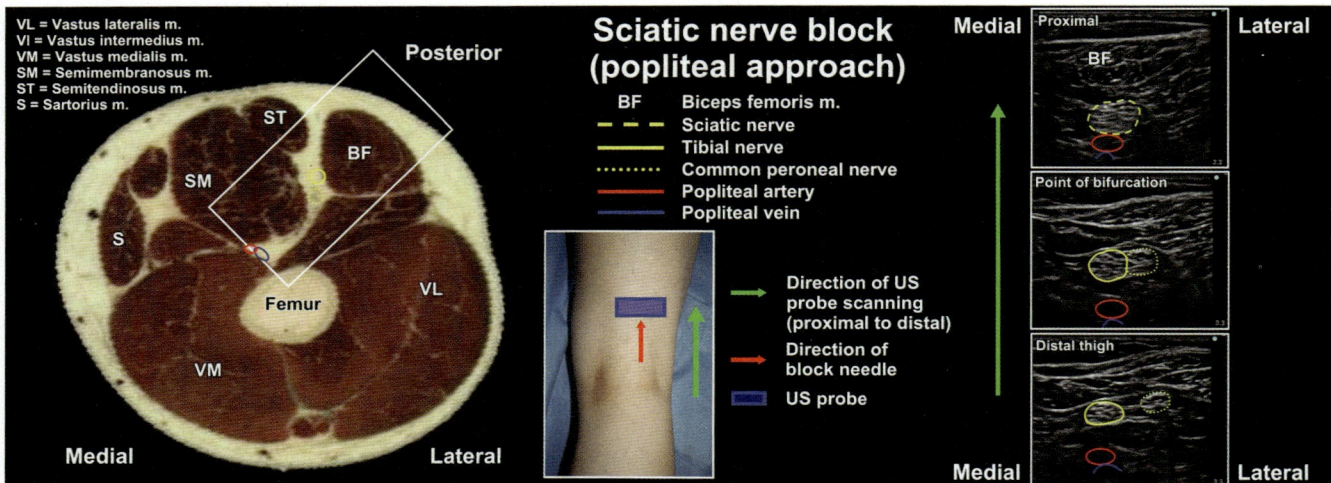

Figure 36-41 Arrangement of relevant anatomy for ultrasound-guided sciatic nerve block with a popliteal approach. The probe is placed initially at the popliteal crease and is used to scan proximally to capture the sciatic nerve just proximal to its bifurcation (i.e., the ideal block site), approximately 6 to 10 cm above the crease.

the center of the image. The needle should be inserted at the caudal surface of probe (especially if a catheter is to be inserted), with the needle tip contacting the skin approximately 3 to 4 cm caudal to the probe surface.
- Local anesthetic spread: For local anesthetic injection at the bifurcation, hypoechoic injectate will be seen to expand within the common epineural sheath. For injections above or below the bifurcation, a circumferential spread producing a "donut" shape surrounding the hyperechoic nerve structure is preferable. Several separate injections (medial and lateral) may be required for complete circumferential spread.

Clinical Pearls
- The ideal needle insertion point for sciatic nerve block using the popliteal approach remains debatable. The tibial and common peroneal branches may be blocked separately[200] or injection may occur between these nerves at the bifurcation.[201]
- Several groups have provided evidence that injection distal (caudad), rather than proximal, to the bifurcation point results in faster block onset and improved sensory block.[200–203] Recently, a randomized comparison between a single subepineural injection at the neural bifurcation and separate injections around the tibial and peroneal divisions demonstrated a higher success rate and shorter performance, onset, and total anesthesia-related times with the former approach.[204]
- Compared to NS guidance alone, US guidance, either alone or in conjunction with NS, was shown to improve the success of both single-injection and catheter-delivered local anesthetic as well as patient outcome with respect to postoperative pain.[205–207]
- The US probe may be rotated 90 degrees to show the sciatic nerve in the long axis. This is helpful to differentiate the sciatic nerve from other nonneural structures.
- During needle insertion using an OOP approach, it may be helpful to use incremental needle angulations. The needle may be best tracked within the tissue if an initial shallow angle is used to identify the needle tip clearly as a hyperechoic dot, which can then be followed with subsequent steeper needle angulations (see the description of the "walk-down" technique under Practical Approaches for US guidance).

Anterior Sciatic Nerve Block

This block is most suitable for patients who cannot be positioned laterally. The block is indicated for surgery below the knee, with the only sensory deficiency being the medial strip of skin supplied by the saphenous nerve. The anterior block is performed on a short portion of the sciatic nerve close to the lesser trochanter of the femur. This block may cause more discomfort since the needle traverses through more muscle layers than other approaches of sciatic nerve block. The patient is positioned supine, with the leg to be blocked externally rotated slightly.

Procedure Using Nerve Stimulation Technique
- Landmarks: A line is drawn connecting the anterior superior iliac spine with the pubic tubercle (inguinal ligament). A second line, parallel to the first, is drawn across the thigh from the greater trochanter. A line is then drawn downward from a point at the medial third of the upper line; the nerve is usually located at the intersection of the perpendicular line and the lower of the two parallel lines. Alternatively, the nerve is located lateral to the femoral artery pulse at the level of the inguinal crease.
- Needling: A 22-gauge, 100- to 150-mm insulated needle will be required for this deep block.
- The needle is inserted perpendicular to the skin and advanced until contact with the femur occurs. The needle is then withdrawn slightly, angulated slightly medial and cephalad, and introduced 5 cm further.
- Nerve localization: Motor responses of the ankle joint or foot are sought.
- Injection: Twenty to thirty milliliters of local anesthetic are injected after careful aspiration and administration of a test dose.

Procedure Using Ultrasound Imaging (Fig. 36-42)
- Scanning: It is most common to use a curved, lower frequency 2 to 5 MHz probe to scan the sciatic nerve in the proximal thigh. Place the probe over the proximal thigh approximately 8 cm distal to the femoral crease. A

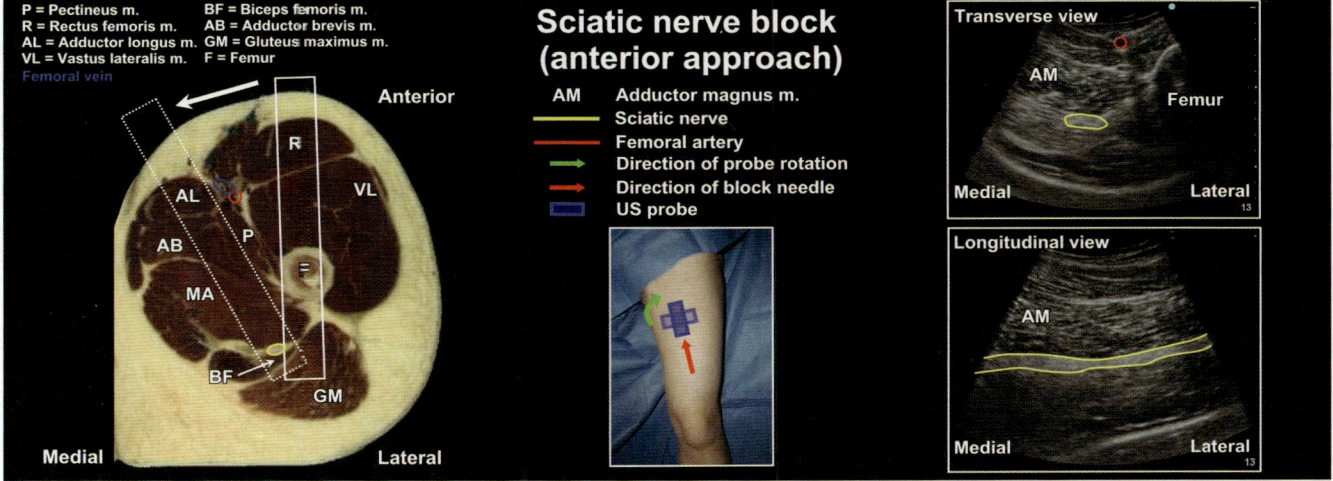

Figure 36-42 Arrangement of relevant anatomy for ultrasound-guided sciatic block using an anterior approach. Transverse probe positioning allows a short-axis view of the nerve (upper US image). A longitudinally placed probe captures the long axis of the nerve (lower US image), which may be beneficial if the transverse view is difficult to capture due to bony shadowing from the lesser trochanter.

transversely placed probe is commonly used, although the nerve may be best visualized by placing the probe axis longitudinally along the course of the nerve, since capturing a longitudinal axis of the nerve may improve its identification since it has a distinctive cable-like appearance. Moving in a medial-to-lateral direction may be helpful to capture an image of the nerve.
- Appearance: In transverse axis, the sciatic nerve often appears oval or round, predominantly hyperechoic, medial, and posterior to the lesser trochanter, and deep to the adductor magus muscle. If using Doppler, the femoral neurovascular structures are seen superficial below the hyperechoic fascial tissue and lateral to the sciatic nerve in this projection when the leg is externally rotated. A longitudinal view captures a broad, linear, and hyperechoic cable of fibers and may allow easier identification of the nerve.[208]
- Needling: When using a probe positioned in transverse axis to the nerve, an IP approach involves advancing the needle in a medial-to-lateral and anterior-to-posterior direction, whereas an OOP approach involves inserting the needle along the midline of the probe at a location 2 to 3 cm inferior and perpendicular to the probe. If the probe is placed longitudinally, the needle direction for OOP alignment will be similar to that for the IP approach described earlier. Using an IP approach with the probe placed longitudinally, the needle will be placed in a cephalad-to-caudad direction, allowing it to be aimed easily toward a relatively larger target (i.e., the cable-like sciatic nerve). It is highly recommended to use combined US and NS guidance for this procedure.
- Local anesthetic spread: After careful aspiration and injection of a small amount of D5W to visualize the anesthetic spread, inject the local anesthetic while ensuring that it spreads circumferentially around the nerve.

Clinical Pearls
- Although depositing the local anesthetic around the nerve is desirable, it is technically challenging to reposition the needle on both sides of the nerve because of the nerve's depth within the muscle layers.
- As with other sciatic nerve blocks, if this block is being combined with others, the local anesthetic may need to be diluted to reduce the risk of toxicity.
- Complications are rare but can include intravascular injection (e.g., femoral artery), infection in the injection area, hematoma formation, nerve injury, and potential CNS toxicity.

Other Approaches to Sciatic Block
- A supine approach developed by Raj et al.,[209] in which the patient's leg is maximally flexed, stretches the nerve within the space between the greater trochanter and the ischial tuberosity; needle insertion occurs at the midpoint between these two structures. In this approach, landmarks are easy to find, and the position offers an alternative to patients who cannot accommodate prone or lateral positioning. This approach has also been shown to be amenable to catheter-delivered continuous anesthesia of the sciatic nerve.[210]
- Several novel approaches to sciatic nerve blockade have been described that may be useful when the patient cannot be positioned for traditional approaches:
  a. Le Corroller et al.[211] have described a lateral approach in which the patient is positioned supine, and injection occurs on the midpoint of a vertical line drawn cephalad from the greater trochanter to the anterior superior iliac spine.
  b. Osaka et al.[212] have described a medial approach at the mid-thigh, where the patient is positioned supine and the hip and knee flexed and externally rotated. The sciatic nerve is beneath the adductor magnus muscle, 1.5 to 2 cm posterior to the femur at the upper mid-thigh.

Ankle Block

All five nerves of the foot can be blocked at the level of the ankle. The superficial nerves—sural, superficial peroneal, and saphenous nerves—can be blocked by simple infiltration techniques. US guidance can be useful for blocking the posterior tibial and deep peroneal (fibular) nerves, as their locations can be easily identified next to reliable landmarks (i.e., bones and vessels) that are clearly visible with US.

Posterior Tibial Nerve
Procedure Using Landmark Technique
- Landmarks: The posterior tibial nerve is the major nerve to the sole of the foot. It can be approached with the patient either in the prone position or lying supine with the hip and knee flexed so that the foot rests on the bed. The medial malleolus is identified, along with the pulsation of the posterior tibial artery behind it. The nerve is located posterior to the artery.
- Needling: A needle is introduced through the skin just behind the posterior tibial artery and directed 45 degrees anteriorly, seeking a paresthesia in the sole of the foot. Motor responses that may be seen with NS include twitches of the first (medial plantar branch) and fifth (lateral plantar branch) toes.
- Injection: Five milliliters of local anesthetic produces anesthesia if a paresthesia is identified. If not, a fan-shaped injection of 10 mL can be performed in the triangle formed by the artery, the Achilles tendon, and the tibia itself.

Procedure Using Ultrasound Imaging (Fig. 36-43)
- Scanning: A linear ("hockey stick"), 10 MHz probe with a small footprint is positioned in transverse (short) axis to the nerve just posterior and inferior to the medial malleolus. Alternatively, the nerve can be identified 3 to 5 cm above the malleolus. The use of color Doppler may be helpful, since the nerve lies posterior and deep to the posterior tibial artery at both of these locations. The nerve should be localized before it branches into the medial and lateral plantar nerves.
- Appearance: Immediately anterior to the artery lies the hypoechoic circular posterior tibial vein, although it may be compressed and not apparent on the screen. Posterior to the artery, the nerve appears slightly more hyperechoic than the surrounding tissues and has a condensed, honeycomb-like structure.
- Needling: A 36- to 50-mm needle is inserted using an OOP approach with the needle caudal or an IP approach with the needle anterior to the transversely positioned probe.

Sural Nerve
The patient is placed either in the prone position or supine with the hip and knee flexed so that the foot rests on the bed. The posteriorly located sural nerve can be blocked by injection on the lateral side. Subcutaneous injection of 5 mL of local anesthetic behind the lateral malleolus, filling the groove between it and the calcaneus, produces anesthesia of the sural nerve. The effectiveness of a sural nerve block was found to be improved using a perivascular approach (i.e., identifying the lesser saphenous vein

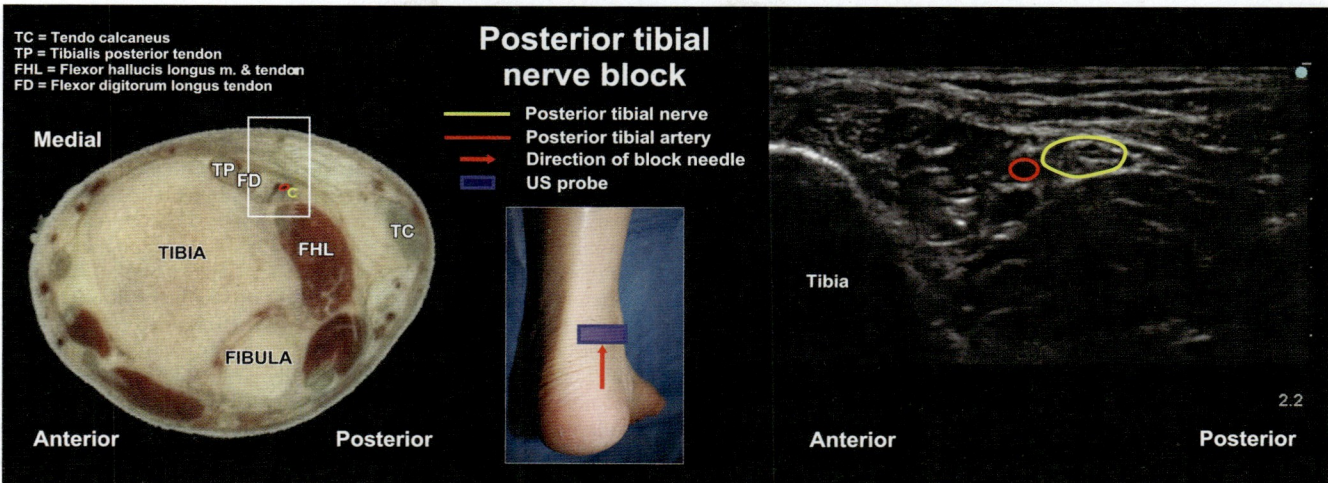

Figure 36-43 Arrangement of relevant anatomy for ultrasound-guided posterior tibial nerve block at the ankle using an IP approach. The nerve is imaged adjacent to the posterior tibial artery before the nerve divides into the medial and lateral plantar nerves.

1 cm proximal to the lateral malleolus), rather than a traditional, surface landmark-based approach, under US guidance.[213]

Deep Peroneal Nerve

Procedure Using Landmark Technique
- Landmarks: This is the major nerve to the dorsum of the foot and lies in the deep plane of the anterior tibial artery. The patient is positioned supine, generally with the leg extended. Pulsation of the artery is sought at the level of the skin crease on the anterior midline surface of the ankle. If the artery is not palpable, the tendon of the extensor hallucis longus can be identified (the nerve lies immediately lateral to this) by asking the patient to extend the big toe.
- Needling and Injection: If the artery pulse can be felt, 5 mL of local anesthetic is injected just lateral to it. If the artery is not palpable, the tendon of the extensor hallucis longus can be identified (see earlier). If using NS, toe extension is sought for this nerve. Injection can be made into the deep planes below the fascia using either one of these landmarks.

Procedure Using Ultrasound Imaging (Fig. 36-44)
- Scanning: A small footprint linear ("hockey stick") 10 MHz probe is placed in transverse (short) axis to the nerve at the anterior surface of the ankle joint. Alternatively, the nerve can also be found 3 to 5 cm above the ankle joint. However, the nerve itself can be difficult to see, and only the artery can be located consistently. Color Doppler can be used at both locations to identify the anterior tibial artery lying medial to the nerve.
- Appearance: If seen, the nerve appears as a small cluster of hyperechoic, fascicular-appearing fibers immediately lateral to the artery, with both the nerve and the artery adjacent to the well-demarcated distal end of the tibia.
- Needling: An OOP approach will be most suitable here since the tendons lie on either side of the nerve. A 36- to 50-mm needle is inserted OOP and caudal to the transversely positioned small footprint probe.

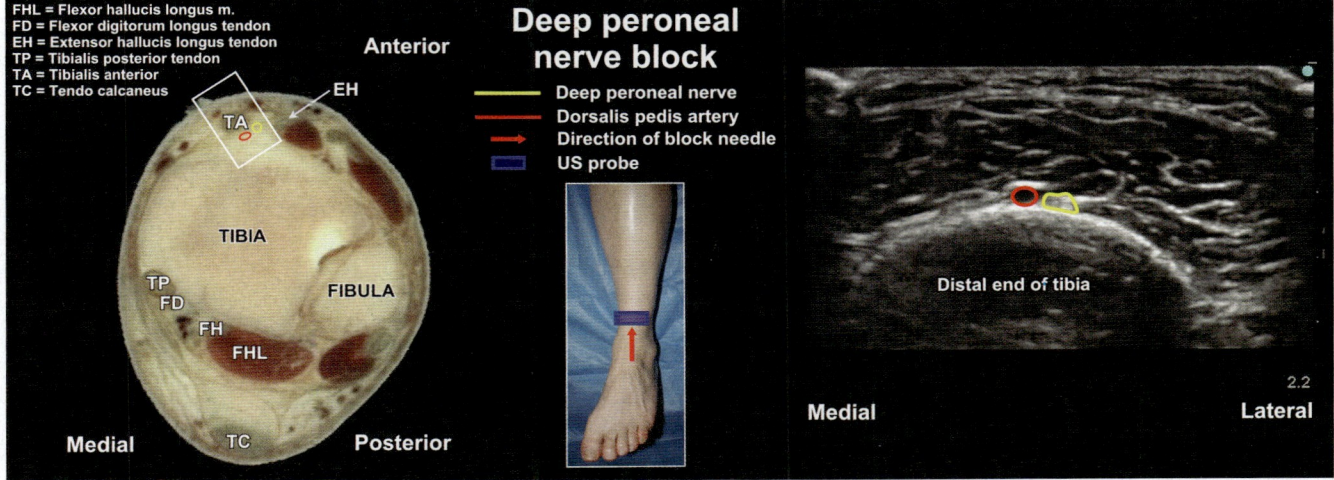

Figure 36-44 Arrangement of relevant anatomy for ultrasound-guided deep peroneal nerve block at the anterior ankle. If possible, the medially located anterior tibial artery should be localized with Doppler to differentiate between the nerve and surrounding tendons.

- Local anesthetic spread: Injection of 4 to 5 mL of local anesthetic lateral to the nerve will help to avoid the anterior tibial artery, which lies medial to the nerve. It is important to perform aspiration prior to injection.

Saphenous Nerve

The patient is placed supine with the leg extended. The saphenous nerve is anesthetized by infiltrating 5 mL of local anesthetic around the saphenous vein at the level where it passes anterior to the medial malleolus. A wall of anesthesia between the skin and the bone itself suffices to block the nerve. Alternatively, this nerve can be blocked at a more proximal site in the thigh. See the section on Separate Blocks of the Terminal Nerves of the Lumbar Plexus for blockade of this nerve more proximally in the thigh.

Superficial Peroneal Branches

A subcutaneous ridge of local anesthetic solution is injected along the skin crease between the anterior tibial artery and the lateral malleolus. This subcutaneous ridge overlies the subfascial injection used for the deep peroneal nerve. Another 5 to 10 mL of local anesthetic may be required to cover this area. The superficial peroneal nerve may be visualized using US, which may aid in more accurate injection of local anesthetic.[214]

Clinical Pearls

- Anesthesia of the foot usually ensues within 15 minutes of these five injections.
- Complications of ankle block are rare, although neuropathy can be produced. Care should be taken not to pin any of the deep nerves against the bone at the time of injection, and intraneural injection should be avoided. Epinephrine should not be added to local anesthetics used for this block in order to avoid compromising the distal circulation.
- US imaging for the deep nerves may help to avoid bone contact and multiple injections with the infiltration technique.

Continuous Catheter Technique

Continuous catheter regional anesthesia has been well documented to provide effective pain relief with reduced incidence of side effects and an improved quality of life.[215,216] Traditionally, catheters have been introduced blindly once neural structures are identified using a peripheral nerve stimulator and often after the initial local anesthetic dose has been injected via the needle. Although continuous delivery of local anesthetic has been used successfully at a number of block sites following blind catheter insertion,[217] the method is associated with at least 10% to 40% secondary block failure due to the catheters being in a suboptimal location.[218,219] This high failure rate resulted in the development of stimulating catheters to aid in their positioning close to the nerve,[220] which improved success rates. However, insertion and precise positioning of stimulating catheters requires technical expertise and can be a time-consuming process. Moreover, needle insertion with stimulating catheters remains a blind procedure since neurostimulation and anatomic landmarks are still required to locate the nerve.

In recent years, ultrasonography has been used extensively to initiate regional blocks,[221,222] and several large-scale studies have shown its efficacy in guiding the placement of perineural catheters.[223,224] However, catheter insertion for continuous regional anesthesia, whether guided by NS or US, suffers from several fundamental problems owing to the design of current needle-catheter assemblies, including dislodgement or movement of the catheter, leakage at the insertion site, and imprecise catheter placement.[217] The increasing popularity of US technology in regional anesthesia has facilitated increased use of catheter-over-needle approaches to continuous catheter placement. Several commercially available catheter-over-needle kits are marketed throughout the world. The primary benefit of this approach is that the catheter is held tightly by the surrounding skin since the needle—which enables initial skin puncture—is housed within the catheter and is removed once the needle tip is located appropriately. This overcomes the common problems described earlier for the traditional catheter-though-needle approach.[225,226] Another benefit over traditional catheter assemblies is that the catheter tip can be positioned with a high degree of accuracy proximal to the intended target nerve. Indeed, a catheter-over-needle approach has been used successfully for supraclavicular,[225] infraclavicular,[227] interscalene,[228] femoral nerve,[229] TAP,[230] and rectus sheath block.[231] Moreover, the stable indwelling catheter provides a means to deliver intermittent boluses[122,232] and, if desired, to reverse a nerve block with saline injection through the catheter.[233] A drawback of the catheter-over-needle approach is that needle/catheter assemblies are fixed length, limiting their use for neuraxial anesthesia and targeting of deeper nerves unless one is able to estimate accurately the length required prior to placement.

Continuous peripheral nerve catheter techniques, provided by the catheter-over-needle approach, are a reliable and practical option to facilitate intermittent bolusing of local anesthetic as a means of delivering continuous analgesia. Since the catheter tip can be targeted next to the nerve with relative accuracy and is stable once placed, multiple boluses can be injected through the catheter, avoiding the need for an infusion pump. This method potentially reduces the total dose delivered, minimizing the associated risk of local anesthetic toxicity.[232,234,235] Recently, remote control of local anesthetic infusion was described,[236] enabling pain management according to patient need and allowing the anesthesiologist to access pump information remotely. The main advantage of this technology is that there is no need for a nurse or physician to be physically present to manage the pump.

Acknowledgments

The authors thank Drs. Gareth Corry and Saadat Ali and the Department of Anesthesiology and Pain Medicine, University of Alberta, for their contributions to the text. The authors acknowledge the Ecole Polytechnique Federale de Lausanne, Switzerland, Visible Human Web Server (http://visiblehuman.epfl.ch) as the data source for the anatomic sections used in some of the figures. Most of the material was adapted from one of the author's (B.T.) textbooks, *Atlas of Ultrasound and Nerve Stimulation-Guided Regional Anesthesia*, 2nd edition (in press)[237] and *Pediatric Atlas of Ultrasound and Nerve Stimulation-Guided Regional Anesthesia*.[86] B.T. also has a patent licensing agreement with Pajunk.

REFERENCES

1. Tziavrangos E, Schug SA. Regional anaesthesia and perioperative outcome. *Curr Opin Anaesthesiol.* 2006;19:521–525.
2. Brown DL, Ransom DM, Hall JA, et al. Regional anesthesia and local anesthetic-induced systemic toxicity: Seizure frequency and accompanying cardiovascular changes. *Anesth Analg.* 1995;81:321–328.
3. Borgeat A, Schappi B, Biasca N, et al. Patient-controlled analgesia after major shoulder surgery: Patient-controlled interscalene analgesia versus patient-controlled analgesia. *Anesthesiology.* 1997;87:1343–1347.
4. Greengrass RA. Regional anesthesia for ambulatory surgery. *Anesthesiol Clin North Am.* 2000;18:341–353.
5. Singelyn FJ, Gouverneur JM. Postoperative analgesia after total hip arthroplasty: i.v. PCA with morphine, patient-controlled epidural analgesia, or

continuous "3-in-1" block? A prospective evaluation by our acute pain service in more than 1,300 patients. *J Clin Anesth.* 1999;11:550–554.
6. Nielsen KC, Steele SM. Outcome after regional anaesthesia in the ambulatory setting: Is it really worth it? *Best Pract Res Clin Anaesthesiol.* 2002;16:145–157.
7. Auroy Y, Narchi P, Messiah A, et al. Serious complications related to regional anesthesia: Results of a prospective survey in France. *Anesthesiology.* 1997;87:479–486.
8. Tsui B. Ultrasound-guidance and nerve stimulation: Implications for the future practice of regional anesthesia. *Can J Anaesth.* 2007;54:165–170.
9. Greenblatt GM, Denson JS. Needle nerve stimulator locator: Nerve blocks with a new instrument for locating nerves. *Anesth Analg.* 1962;41:599–602.
10. Sarnoff S. Functional localization of interspinal catheters. *Anesthesiology.* 1950;11:360.
11. Boezaart AP, De Beer JF, du Toit C, et al. A new technique of continuous interscalene nerve block. *Can J Anaesth.* 1999;46:275–281.
12. Copeland SJ, Laxton MA. A new stimulating catheter for continuous peripheral nerve blocks. *Reg Anesth Pain Med.* 2001;26:589–590.
13. Perlas A, Niazi A, McCartney C, et al. The sensitivity of motor response to nerve stimulation and paresthesia for nerve localization as evaluated by ultrasound. *Reg Anesth Pain Med.* 2006;31:445–450.
14. Urmey WF, Stanton J. Inability to consistently elicit a motor response following sensory paresthesia during interscalene block administration. *Anesthesiology.* 2002;96:552–554.
15. Hadzic A, Vloka J, Hadzic N, et al. Nerve stimulators used for peripheral nerve blocks vary in their electrical characteristics. *Anesthesiology.* 2003;98:969–974.
16. Urmey WF. Using the nerve stimulator for peripheral or plexus nerve blocks. *Minerva Anestesiol.* 2006;72:467–471.
17. Ganta R, Cajee RA, Henthorn RW. Use of transcutaneous nerve stimulation to assist interscalene block. *Anesth Analg.* 1993;76:914–915.
18. Urmey WF, Grossi P. Percutaneous electrode guidance: A noninvasive technique for prelocation of peripheral nerves to facilitate peripheral plexus or nerve block. *Reg Anesth Pain Med.* 2002;27:261–267.
19. Bosenberg AT, Raw R, Boezaart AP. Surface mapping of peripheral nerves in children with a nerve stimulator. *Pediatr Anesthiol.* 2002;12:398–403.
20. Tsui BC, Gupta S, Finucane B. Confirmation of epidural catheter placement using nerve stimulation. *Can J Anaesth.* 1998;45:640–644.
21. Tsui BC, Finucane B. Epidural stimulator catheter. *Tech Reg Anesth Pain Manage.* 2002;6:150–154.
22. Koscielniak-Nielsen ZJ, Rassmussen H, Jepsen K. Effect of impulse duration on patients' perception of electrical stimulation and block effectiveness during axillary block in unsedated ambulatory patients. *Reg Anesth Pain Med.* 2001;26:428–433.
23. Hadzic A, Vloka JD, Claudio RE, et al. Electrical nerve localization: Effects of cutaneous electrode placement and duration of the stimulus on motor response. *Anesthesiology.* 2004;100:1526–1530.
24. Borgeat A. Regional anesthesia, intraneural injection, and nerve injury: Beyond the epineurium. *Anesthesiology.* 2006;105:647–648.
25. Raj PP, Rosenblatt R, Montgomery SJ. Use of the nerve stimulator for peripheral blocks. *Reg Anesth.* 1980;5:14–21.
26. Tsui BC, Wagner A, Finucane B. Electrophysiologic effect of injectates on peripheral nerve stimulation. *Reg Anesth Pain Med.* 2004;29:189–193.
27. Tsui BC, Kropelin B, Ganapathy S, et al. Dextrose 5% in water: fluid medium for maintaining electrical stimulation of peripheral nerves during stimulating catheter placement. *Acta Anaesthesiol Scand.* 2005;49:1562–1565.
28. Sites BD, Beach ML, Spence BC, et al. Ultrasound guidance improves the success rate of a perivascular axillary plexus block. *Acta Anaesthesiol Scand.* 2006;50:678–684.
29. Williams SR, Chouinard P, Arcand G, et al. Ultrasound guidance speeds execution and improves the quality of supraclavicular block. *Anesth Analg.* 2003;97:1518–1523.
30. Marhofer P, Sitzwohl C, Greher M, et al. Ultrasound guidance for infraclavicular brachial plexus anaesthesia in children. *Anaesthesia.* 2004;59:642–646.
31. Soeding PE, Sha S, Royse CE, et al. A randomized trial of ultrasound-guided brachial plexus anaesthesia in upper limb surgery. *Anaesth Intensive Care.* 2005;33:719–725.
32. Liu FC, Liou JT, Tsai YF, et al. Efficacy of ultrasound-guided axillary brachial plexus block: A comparative study with nerve stimulator-guided method. *Chang Gung Med J.* 2005;28:396–402.
33. Marhofer P, Harrop-Griffiths W, Willschke H, et al. Fifteen years of ultrasound guidance in regional anaesthesia. Part 2. Recent developments in block techniques. *Br J Anaesth.* 2010;104:673–683.
34. Marhofer P, Harrop-Griffiths W, Kettner SC, et al. Fifteen years of ultrasound guidance in regional anaesthesia: Part 1. *Br J Anaesth.* 2010;104:538–546.
35. Tsui BC, Twomey C, Finucane BT. Visualization of the brachial plexus in the supraclavicular region using a curved ultrasound probe with a sterile transparent dressing. *Reg Anesth Pain Med.* 2006;31:182–184.
36. Tsui BC, Finucane BT. The importance of ultrasound landmarks: A "traceback" approach using the popliteal blood vessels for identification of the sciatic nerve. *Reg Anesth Pain Med.* 2006;31:481–482.
37. Tsui BC, Dillane D. Needle puncture site and a "walkdown" approach for short-axis alignment during ultrasound-guided blocks. *Reg Anesth Pain Med.* 2006;31:586–587.
38. Tsui BC. Facilitating needle alignment in-plane to an ultrasound beam using a portable laser unit. *Reg Anesth Pain Med.* 2007;32:84–88.
39. Selander D, Dhuner KG, Lundborg G. Peripheral nerve injury due to injection needles used for regional anesthesia. An experimental study of the acute effects of needle point trauma. *Acta Anaesthesiol Scand.* 1977;21:182–188.
40. Steele SM, Klein SM, D'Ercole FJ, et al. A new continuous catheter delivery system. *Anesth Analg.* 1998;87:228.
41. Claudio R, Hadzic A, Shih H, et al. Injection pressures by anesthesiologists during simulated peripheral nerve block. *Reg Anesth Pain Med.* 2004;29:201–205.
42. Hadzic A, Dilberovic F, Shah S, et al. Combination of intraneural injection and high injection pressure leads to fascicular injury and neurologic deficits in dogs. *Reg Anesth Pain Med.* 2004;29:417–423.
43. Selander D, Sjostrand J. Longitudinal spread of intraneurally injected local anesthetics. An experimental study of the initial neural distribution following intraneural injections. *Acta Anaesthesiol Scand.* 1978;22:622–634.
44. Tsui BC, Li LX, Pillay JJ. Compressed air injection technique to standardize block injection pressures. *Can J Anaesth.* 2006;53:1098–1102.
45. Asghar S, Bjerregaard LS, Lundstrom LH, et al. Distal infrared thermography and skin temperature after ultrasound-guided interscalene brachial plexus block: A prospective observational study. *Eur J Anaesthesiol.* 2014;31:626–634.
46. Asghar S, Lundstrom LH, Bjerregaard LS, et al. Ultrasound-guided lateral infraclavicular block evaluated by infrared thermography and distal skin temperature. *Acta Anaesthesiol Scand.* 2014;58:867–874.
47. Tsui BC, Shakespeare TJ, Leung DH, et al. Reproducibility of current perception threshold with the Neurometer((R)) vs the Stimpod NMS450 peripheral nerve stimulator in healthy volunteers: An observational study. *Can J Anaesth.* 2013;60:753–760.
48. Gaudreault F, Drolet P, Fallaha M, et al. The reliability of the current perception threshold in volunteers and its applicability in a clinical setting. *Anesth Analg.* 2015;120:678–683.
49. Bromage PR. *Epidural Analgesia.* Philadelphia, PA: WB Saunders; 1978: 301–320.
50. Borgeat A, Blumenthal S. Nerve injury and regional anaesthesia. *Curr Opin Anaesthesiol.* 2004;17:417–421.
51. Kaufman BR, Nystrom E, Nath S, et al. Debilitating chronic pain syndromes after presumed intraneural injections. *Pain.* 2000;85:283–286.
52. Selander D. Neurotoxicity of local anesthetics: Animal data. *Reg Anesth.* 1993;18:461–468.
53. Ben-David B. Complications of peripheral blockade. *Anesthesiol Clin North America.* 2002;20:695–707.
54. Graf BM, Abraham I, Eberbach N, et al. Differences in cardiotoxicity of bupivacaine and ropivacaine are the result of physicochemical and stereoselective properties. *Anesthesiology.* 2002;96:1427–1434.
55. Knudsen K, Beckman SM, Blomberg S, et al. Central nervous and cardiovascular effects of i.v. infusions of ropivacaine, bupivacaine and placebo in volunteers. *Br J Anaesth.* 1997;78:507–514.
56. Muller M, Litz RJ, Huler M, et al. Grand mal convulsion and plasma concentrations after intravascular injection of ropivacaine for axillary brachial plexus blockade. *Br J Anaesth.* 2001;87:784–787.
57. Petitjeans F, Mion G, Puidupin M, et al. Tachycardia and convulsions induced by accidental intravascular ropivacaine injection during sciatic block. *Acta Anaesthesiol Scand.* 2002;46:616–617.
58. Reinikainen M, Hedman A, Pelkonen O, et al. Cardiac arrest after interscalene brachial plexus block with ropivacaine and lidocaine. *Acta Anaesthesiol Scand.* 2003;47:904–906.
59. Ruetsch YA, Fattinger KE, Borgeat A. Ropivacaine-induced convulsions and severe cardiac dysrhythmia after sciatic block. *Anesthesiology.* 1999;90:1784–1786.
60. Marhofer P, Schrogendorfer K, Wallner T, et al. Ultrasonographic guidance reduces the amount of local anesthetic for 3-in-1 blocks. *Reg Anesth Pain Med.* 1998;23:584–588.
61. Willschke H, Marhofer P, Bosenberg A, et al. Ultrasonography for ilioinguinal/iliohypogastric nerve blocks in children. *Br J Anaesth.* 2005;95:226–230.
62. Weinberg GL, VadeBoncouer T, Ramaraju GA, et al. Pretreatment or resuscitation with a lipid infusion shifts the dose-response to bupivacaine-induced asystole in rats. *Anesthesiology.* 1998;88:1071–1075.
63. Litz RJ, Popp M, Stehr SN, et al. Successful resuscitation of a patient with ropivacaine–induced asystole after axillary plexus block using lipid infusion. *Anaesthesia.* 2006;61:800–801.
64. Rosenblatt MA, Abel M, Fischer GW, et al. Successful use of a 20% lipid emulsion to resuscitate a patient after a presumed bupivacaine–related cardiac arrest. *Anesthesiology.* 2006;105:217–218.
65. Fremling MA, Mackinnon SE. Injection injury to the median nerve. *Ann Plast Surg.* 1996;37:561–567.
66. Shah S, Hadzic A, Vloka JD, et al. Neurologic complication after anterior sciatic nerve block. *Anesth Analg.* 2005;100:1515–1517.
67. Selander D, Edshage S, Wolff T. Paresthesiae or no paresthesiae? Nerve lesions after axillary blocks. *Acta Anaesthesiol Scand.* 1979;23:27–33.

68. Winchell SW, Wolfe R. The incidence of neuropathy following upper extremity nerve blocks. *Reg Anesth.* 1985;10:12–15.
69. Enneking FK, Chan V, Greger J, et al. Lower–extremity peripheral nerve blockade: Essentials of our current understanding. *Reg Anesth Pain Med.* 2005;30:4–35.
70. Gentili F, Hudson AR, Hunter D, et al. Nerve injection injury with local anesthetic agents: A light and electron microscopic, fluorescent microscopic, and horseradish peroxidase study. *Neurosurgery.* 1980;6:263–272.
71. Selander D. *Peripheral Nerve Injury After Regional Anesthesia, Complications of Regional Anesthesia.* Edited by Finucane BT. Philadelphia, PA: Churchhill Livingstone; 1999:105–115.
72. Sauter AR, Smith HJ, Stubhaug A, et al. Use of magnetic resonance imaging to define the anatomical location closest to all three cords of the infraclavicular brachial plexus. *Anesth Analg.* 2006;103:1574–1576.
73. Retzl G, Kapral S, Greher M, et al. Ultrasonographic findings of the axillary part of the brachial plexus. *Anesth Analg.* 2001;92:1271–1275.
74. Chan VWS, Perlas A, McCartney CJL, et al. Ultrasound guidance improves success rate of axillary brachial plexus block. *Can J Anaesth.* 2007;54:176–182.
75. Bonnel F. Microscopic anatomy of the adult human brachial plexus: An anatomical and histological basis for microsurgery. *Microsurgery.* 1984;5:107–118.
76. Klaastad O, Smedby O, Thompson GE, et al. Distribution of local anesthetic in axillary brachial plexus block: A clinical and magnetic resonance imaging study. *Anesthesiology.* 2002;96:1315–1324.
77. Kessler J, Gray AT. Sonography of scalene muscle anomalies for brachial plexus block. *Reg Anesth Pain Med.* 2007;32:172–173.
78. Uysal II, Seker M, Karabulut AK, et al. Brachial plexus variations in human fetuses. *Neurosurgery.* 2003;53:676–684.
79. Orebaugh SL, Pennington S. Variant location of the musculocutaneous nerve during axillary nerve block. *J Clin Anesth.* 2006;18:541–544.
80. Venieratos D, Anagnostopoulou S. Classification of communications between the musculocutaneous and median nerves. *Clin Anat.* 1998;11:327–331.
81. Amoiridis G. Median–ulnar nerve communications and anomalous innervation of the intrinsic hand muscles: An electrophysiological study. *Muscle Nerve.* 1992;15:576–579.
82. Bigeleisen PE. The bifid axillary artery. *J Clin Anesth.* 2004;16:224–225.
83. Kutiyanawala MA, Stotter A, Windle R. Anatomical variants during axillary dissection. *Br J Surg.* 1998;85:393–394.
84. Uglietta JP, Kadir S. Arteriographic study of variant arterial anatomy of the upper extremities. *Cardiovasc Intervent Radiol.* 1989;12:145–148.
85. Tsui BC. *Atlas of Ultrasound- and Nerve Stimulation-Guided Regional Anesthesia.* New York, NY: Springer; 2007.
86. Tsui BC, Suresh S. *Pediatric Atlas of Ultrasound- and Nerve Stimulation-Guided Regional Anesthesia.* New York, NY: Springer; 2015.
87. Tsui BC. Ultrasound imaging to localize foramina for superficial trigeminal nerve block. *Can J Anaesth.* 2009;56:704–706.
88. Pascal J, Charier D, Perret D, et al. Peripheral blocks of trigeminal nerve for facial soft–tissue surgery: Learning from failures. *Eur J Anaesthesiol.* 2005;22:480–482.
89. Nguyen A, Girard F, Boudreault D, et al. Scalp nerve blocks decrease the severity of pain after craniotomy. *Anesth Analg.* 2001;93:1272–1276.
90. Knize DM. A study of the supraorbital nerve. *Plast Reconstr Surg.* 1995;96:564–569.
91. Naja MZ, Al-Tannir M, Naja H, et al. Repeated nerve blocks with clonidine, fentanyl and bupivacaine for trigeminal neuralgia. *Anaesthesia.* 2006;61:70–71.
92. Haas DA. Alternative mandibular nerve block techniques: A review of the Gow-Gates and Akinosi-Vazirani closed-mouth mandibular nerve block techniques. *J Am Dent Assoc.* 2011;142:8S–12S.
93. Winnie AP, Ramamurthy S, Durrani Z, et al. Interscalene cervical plexus block: A single-injection technic. *Anesth Analg.* 1975;54:370–375.
94. Usui Y, Kobayashi T, Kakinuma H, et al. An anatomical basis for blocking of the deep cervical plexus and cervical sympathetic tract using an ultrasound-guided technique. *Anesth Analg.* 2010;110:964–968.
95. Stoneham MD, Doyle AR, Knighton JD, et al. Prospective, randomized comparison of deep or superficial cervical plexus block for carotid endarterectomy surgery. *Anesthesiology.* 1998;89:907–912.
96. de Sousa AA, Filho MA, Faglione W, Jr., et al. Superficial vs combined cervical plexus block for carotid endarterectomy: A prospective, randomized study. *Surg. Neurol.* 2005;63(Suppl 1):S22–S25.
97. Pandit JJ, Bree S, Dillon P, et al. A comparison of superficial versus combined (superficial and deep) cervical plexus block for carotid endarterectomy: A prospective, randomized study. *Anesth Analg.* 2000;91:781–786.
98. Castresana MR, Masters RD, Castresana EJ, et al. Incidence and clinical significance of hemidiaphragmatic paresis in patients undergoing carotid endarterectomy during cervical plexus block anesthesia. *J Neurosurg Anesthesiol.* 1994;6:21–23.
99. Masters RD, Castresana EJ, Castresana MR. Superficial and deep cervical plexus block: Technical considerations. *AANA J.* 1995;63:236–243.
100. Stoneham MD, Knighton JD. Regional anaesthesia for carotid endarterectomy. *Br J Anaesth.* 1999;82:910–919.
101. Chen H, Sokoll LJ, Udelsman R. Outpatient minimally invasive parathyroidectomy: A combination of sestamibi-SPECT localization, cervical block anesthesia, and intraoperative parathyroid hormone assay. *Surgery.* 1999;126:1016–1021.
102. Miccoli P, Barellini L, Monchik JM, et al. Randomized clinical trial comparing regional and general anaesthesia in minimally invasive video-assisted parathyroidectomy. *Br J Surg.* 2005;92:814–818.
103. Tran DQ, Dugani S, Finlayson RJ. A randomized comparison between ultrasound-guided and landmark-based superficial cervical plexus block. *Reg Anesth Pain Med.* 2010;35:539–543.
104. Herring AA, Stone MB, Frenkel O, et al. The ultrasound-guided superficial cervical plexus block for anesthesia and analgesia in emergency care settings. *Am J Emerg Med.* 2012;30:1263–1267.
105. Spanknebel K, Chabot JA, DiGiorgi M, et al. Thyroidectomy using local anesthesia: A report of 1,025 cases over 16 years. *J Am Coll Surg.* 2005;201:375–385.
106. Specht MC, Romero M, Barden CB, et al. Characteristics of patients having thyroid surgery under regional anesthesia. *J Am Coll Surg.* 2001;193:367–372.
107. Tobias JD. Cervical plexus block in adolescents. *J Clin Anesth.* 1999;11:606–608.
108. Burtles R. Analgesia for 'bat ear' surgery. *Ann R Coll Surg Engl.* 1989;71:332.
109. Afridi SK, Shields KG, Bhola R, et al. Greater occipital nerve injection in primary headache syndromes—prolonged effects from a single injection. *Pain.* 2006;122:126–129.
110. Anthony M. Cervicogenic headache: Prevalence and response to local steroid therapy. *Clin Exp Rheumatol.* 2000;18:S59–S64.
111. Winnie AP. Interscalene brachial plexus block. *Anesth Analg.* 1970;49:455–466.
112. Gadsden JC, Tsai I, Iwata T, et al. Low intescalene block provides reliable anesthesia for surgery at or about the elbow. *J Clin Anesth.* 2009;21:98–102.
113. Kim JH, Chen J, Bennett H, et al. A low approach to interscalene brachial plexus block results in more distal spread of sensory-motor coverage compared to the conventional approach. *Anesth Analg.* 2011;112:987–989.
114. Benumof JL. Permanent loss of cervical spinal cord function associated with interscalene block performed under general anesthesia. *Anesthesiology.* 2000;93:1541–1544.
115. Yang WT, Chui PT, Metreweli C. Anatomy of the normal brachial plexus revealed by sonography and the role of sonographic guidance in anesthesia of the brachial plexus. *AJR Am J Roentgenol.* 1998;171:1631–1636.
116. Demondion X, Herbinet P, Boutry N, et al. Sonographic mapping of the normal brachial plexus. *AJNR Am J Neuroradiol.* 2003;24:1303–1309.
117. Sheppard DG, Iyer RB, Fenstermacher MJ. Brachial plexus: Demonstration at US. *Radiology.* 1998;208:402–406.
118. Ip VH, Tsui BC. Continuous interscalene block: The good, the bad and the refined spread. *Acta Anaesthesiol Scand.* 2012;56:526–530.
119. Boezaart AP, Koorn R, Rosenquist RW. Paravertebral approach to the brachial plexus: An anatomic improvement in technique. *Reg Anesth Pain Med.* 2003;28:241–244.
120. Klaastad O, VadeBoncouer TR, Tillung T, et al. An evaluation of the supraclavicular plumb-bob technique for brachial plexus block by magnetic resonance imaging. *Anesth Analg.* 2003;96:862–867.
121. Apan A, Baydar S, Yilmaz S, et al. Surface landmarks of brachial plexus: Ultrasound and magnetic resonance imaging for supraclavicular approach with anatomical correlation. *Eur J Ultrasound.* 2001;13:191–196.
122. Ip VH, Tsui BC. The catheter-over-needle assembly facilitates delivery of a second local anesthetic bolus to prolong supraclavicular brachial plexus block without time-consuming catheterization steps: A randomized controlled study. *Can J Anaesth.* 2013;60:692–699.
123. Kapral S, Jandrasits O, Schabernig C, et al. Lateral infraclavicular plexus block vs. axillary block for hand and forearm surgery. *Acta Anaesthesiol Scand.* 1999;43:1047–1052.
124. Klaastad O, Smith HJ, Smedby O, et al. A novel infraclavicular brachial plexus block: The lateral and sagittal technique, developed by magnetic resonance imaging studies. *Anesth Analg.* 2004;98:252–256.
125. Raj PP, Montgomery SJ, Nettles D, et al. Infraclavicular brachial plexus block—a new approach. *Anesth Analg.* 1973;52:897–904.
126. Rettig HC, Gielen MJ, Boersma E, et al. A comparison of the vertical infraclavicular and axillary approaches for brachial plexus anaesthesia. *Acta Anaesthesiol Scand.* 2005;49:1501–1508.
127. Whiffler K. Coracoid block—a safe and easy technique. *Br J Anaesth.* 1981;53:845–848.
128. Wilson JL, Brown DL, Wong GY, et al. Infraclavicular brachial plexus block: Parasagittal anatomy important to the coracoid technique. *Anesth Analg.* 1998;87:870–873.
129. Klaastad O, Lilleas FG, Rotnes JS, et al. Magnetic resonance imaging demonstrates lack of precision in needle placement by the infraclavicular brachial plexus block described by Raj et al. *Anesth Analg.* 1999;88:593–598.
130. Koscielniak-Nielsen ZJ, Rasmussen H, Hesselbjerg L, et al. Clinical evaluation of the lateral sagittal infraclavicular block developed by MRI studies. *Reg Anesth Pain Med.* 2005;30:329–334.
131. Groen GJ, Gielen MJ, Jack NT, et al. At the cords, the pinkie towards: Interpreting infraclavicular motor responses to neurostimulation. *Reg Anesth Pain Med.* 2004;29:505–507.

132. Borene SC, Edwards JN, Boezaart AP. At the cords, the pinkie towards: Interpreting infraclavicular motor responses to neurostimulation. Reg Anesth Pain Med. 2004;29:125–129.
133. Borene SC, Edwards JN, Boezaart A. Response to: At the cords, the pinkie towards: Interpreting infraclavicular motor responses to neurostimulation. Reg Anesth Pain Med. 2004;29:505–507.
134. Brull R, McCartney CJ, Chan VW. A novel approach to infraclavicular brachial plexus block: The ultrasound experience. Anesth Analg. 2004;99:950–951.
135. Imasogie N, Ganapathy S, Singh S, et al. A prospective, randomized, double-blind comparison of ultrasound-guided axillary brachial plexus blocks using 2 versus 4 injections. Anesth Analg. 2010;110:1222–1226.
136. Urmey WF, Grossi P. Percutaneous electrode guidance and subcutaneous stimulating electrode guidance Modifications of the original technique. Reg Anesth Pain Med. 2003;28:253–255.
137. Guay J. Adverse events associated with intravenous regional anesthesia (Bier block): A systematic review of complications. J Clin Anesth. 2009;21:585–594.
138. Horlocker TT. Peripheral nerve blocks-regional anesthesia for the new millennium. Reg Anesth Pain Med. 1998;23:237–240.
139. McDonnell JG, O'Donnell B, Curley G, et al. The analgesic efficacy of transversus abdominis plane block after abdominal surgery: A prospective randomized controlled trial. Anesth Analg. 2007;104:193–197.
140. O'Donnell BD, McDonnell JG, McShane AJ. The transversus abdominis plane (TAP) block in open retropubic prostatectomy. Reg Anesth Pain Med. 2006;31:91.
141. Courreges P, Poddevin F, Lecoutre D. Para-umbilical block: A new concept for regional anaesthesia in children. Ped Anesth. 1997;7:211–214.
142. Ferguson S, Thomas V, Lewis I. The rectus sheath block in paediatric anaesthesia: New indications for an old technique? Ped Anesth. 1996;6:463–466.
143. Rafi AN. Abdominal field block: A new approach via the lumbar triangle. Anaesthesia. 2001;56:1024–1026.
144. Pourseidi B, Khorram-Manesh A. Effect of intercostals neural blockade with Marcaine (bupivacaine) on postoperative pain after laparoscopic cholecystectomy. Surgical Endoscopy. 2007;21:1557–1559.
145. Pusch F, Freitag H, Weinstabl C, et al. Single-injection paravertebral block compared to general anaesthesia in breast surgery. Acta Anaesthesiol Scand. 1999;43:770–774.
146. Naja Z, Lonnqvist PA. Somatic paravertebral nerve blockade: incidence of failed block and complications. Anaesthesia. 2001;56:1184–1188.
147. Belavy D, Cowlishaw PJ, Howes M, et al. Ultrasound-guided transversus abdominis plane block for analgesia after Caesarean delivery. Br J Anaesth. 2009;103:726–730.
148. El-Dawlatly AA, Turkistani A, Kettner SC, et al. Ultrasound-guided transversus abdominis plane block: Description of a new technique and comparison with conventional systemic analgesia during laparoscopic cholecystectomy. Br J Anaesth. 2009;102:763–767.
149. Niraj G, Searle A, Mathews M, et al. Analgesic efficacy of ultrasound-guided transversus abdominis plane block in patients undergoing open appendicectomy. Br J Anaesth. 2009;103:601–605.
150. Chin KJ, Chan V, Hebbard P, et al. Ultrasound-guided transversalis fascia plane block provides analgesia for anterior iliac crest bone graft harvesting. Can J Anaesth. 2012;59:122–123
151. Hebbard PD. Transversalis fascia plane block, a novel ultrasound-guided abdominal wall nerve block. Can J Anaesth. 2009;56:618–620.
152. Eichenberger U, Greher M, Kirchmair L, et al. Ultrasound-guided blocks of the ilioinguinal and iliohypogastric nerve: Accuracy of a selective new technique confirmed by anatomical dissection. Br J Anaesth. 2006;97:238–243.
153. Willschke H, Bosenberg A, Marhofer P, et al. Ultrasonographic-guided ilioinguinal/iliohypogastric nerve block in pediatric anesthesia: What is the optimal volume? Anesth Analg. 2006;102:1680–1684.
154. Randhawa K, Soumian S, Kyi M, et al. Sonographic assessment of the conventional 'blind' ilioinguinal block. Can J Anaesth. 2010;57:94–95.
155. Faraoni D, Gilbeau A, Lingier P, et al. Does ultrasound guidance improve the efficacy of dorsal penile nerve block in children? Pediatr Anesth. 2010;20:931–936.
156. Winnie AP, Ramamurthy S, Durrani Z. The inguinal paravascular technic of lumbar plexus anesthesia: The "3-in-1 block." Anesth Analg. 1973;52:989–996.
157. Marhofer P, Nasel C, Sitzwohl C, et al. Magnetic resonance imaging of the distribution of local anesthetic during the three-in-one block. Anesth Analg. 2000;90:119–124.
158. Parkinson SK, Mueller JB, Little WL, et al. Extent of blockade with various approaches to the lumbar plexus Anesth Analg. 1989;68:243–248.
159. Chayen D, Nathan H, Chayen M. The psoas compartment block. Anesthesiology. 1976;45:95–99.
160. Chudinov A, Berkenstadt H, Salai M, et al. Continuous psoas compartment block for anesthesia and perioperative analgesia in patients with hip fractures. Reg Anesth Pain Med. 1999;24:563–568.
161. Capdevila X, Macaire P, Dadure C, et al. Continuous psoas compartment block for postoperative analgesia after total hip arthroplasty: New landmarks, technical guidelines, and clinical evaluation. Anesth Analg. 2002;94:1606–1613.
162. Aida S, Takahashi H, Shimoji K. Renal subcapsular hematoma after lumbar plexus block. Anesthesiology. 1996;84:452–455.
163. Kirchmair L, Enna B, Mitterschiffthaler G, et al. Lumbar plexus in children: A sonographic study and its relevance to pediatric regional anesthesia. Anesthesiology. 2004;101:445–450.
164. Ilfeld BM, Loland VJ, Mariano ER. Prepuncture ultrasound imaging to predict transverse process and lumbar plexus depth for psoas compartment block and perineural catheter insertion: A prospective, observational study. Anesth Analg. 2010;110:1725–1728.
165. Capdevila X, Coimbra C, Choquet O. Approaches to the lumbar plexus: Success, risks, and outcome. Reg Anesth Pain Med. 2005;30:150–162.
166. Magora F, Rozin R, Ben-Menachem Y, et al. Obturator nerve block: An evaluation of technique. Br J Anaesth. 1969;41:695–698.
167. Sites BD, Beach M, Gallagher JD, et al. A single injection ultrasound-assisted femoral nerve block provides side effect-sparing analgesia when compared with intrathecal morphine in patients undergoing total knee arthroplasty. Anesth Analg. 2004;99:1539–1543.
168. Barrington MJ, Olive D, Low K, et al. Continuous femoral nerve blockade or epidural analgesia after total knee replacement: A prospective randomized controlled trial. Anesth Analg. 2005;101:1824–1829.
169. Singelyn FJ, Deyaert M, Joris D, et al. Effects of intravenous patient-controlled analgesia with morphine, continuous epidural analgesia, and continuous three-in-one block on postoperative pain and knee rehabilitation after unilateral total knee arthroplasty. Anesth Analg. 1998;87:88–92.
170. Lundblad M, Kapral S, Marhofer P, et al. Ultrasound-guided infrapatellar nerve block in human volunteers: Description of a novel technique. Br J Anaesth. 2006;97:710–714.
171. Vloka JD, Hadzic A, Drobnik L, et al. Anatomical landmarks for femoral nerve block: A comparison of four needle insertion sites. Anesth Analg. 1999;89:1467–1470.
172. Niazi AU, Prasad A, Ramlogan R, et al. Methods to ease placement of stimulating catheters during in-plane ultrasound-guided femoral nerve block. Reg Anesth Pain Med. 2009;34:380–381.
173. Wang A-Z, Gu L, Zhou Q-H, et al. Ultrasound-guided continuous femoral nerve block for analgesia after total knee arthroplasty: Catheter perpendicular to the nerve versus catheter parallel to the nerve. Reg Anesth Pain Med. 2010;35:127–131.
174. Hayek SM, Ritchey RM, Sessler D, et al. Continuous femoral nerve analgesia after unilateral total knee arthroplasty: Stimulating versus nonstimulating catheters. Anesth Analg. 2006;103:1565–1570.
175. Morin AM, Eberhart LH, Behnke HK, et al. Does femoral nerve catheter placement with stimulating catheters improve effective placement? A randomized, controlled, and observer-blinded trial. Anesth Analg. 2005;100:1503–1510.
176. Ip VH, Tsui BC. Injection of injectates is more than just for "opening the perineural space." Reg Anesth Pain Med. 2011;36:89–90.
177. Pham Dang C., Guilley J, Dernis L, et al. Is there any need for expanding the perineural space before catheter placement in continuous femoral nerve blocks? Reg Anesth Pain Med. 2006;31:393–400.
178. Soong J, Schafhalter-Zoppoth I, Gray AT. The importance of transducer angle to ultrasound visibility of the femoral nerve. Reg Anesth Pain Med. 2005;30:505.
179. Shannon J, Lang SA, Yip RW, et al. Lateral femoral cutaneous nerve block revisited. A nerve stimulator study. Reg Anesth. 1995;20:100–104.
180. Murata Y, Takahashi K, Yamagata M, et al. The anatomy of the lateral femoral cutaneous nerve, with special reference to the harvesting of iliac bone graft. J Bone Joint Surg Am. 2000;82:746–747.
181. Hara K, Sakura S, Shido A. Ultrasound-guided lateral femoral cutaneous nerve block: Comparison of two techniques. Anaesth Intensive Care. 2011;39:69–72.
182. Jo YY, Choi E, Kil HK. Comparison of the success rate of inguinal approach with classical pubic approach for obturator nerve block in patients undergoing TURB. Korean J Anesthesiol. 2011;61:143–147.
183. Anagnostopoulou S, Kostopanagiotou G, Paraskeuopoulos T, et al. Obturator nerve block: From anatomy to ultrasound guidance. Anesth Analg. 2008;106:350–351.
184. Saranteas T, Anagnostopoulou S, Chantzi C. Obturator nerve anatomy and ultrasound imaging. Reg Anesth Pain Med. 2007;32:539–540.
185. Soong J, Schafhalter-Zoppoth I, Gray AT. Sonographic imaging of the obturator nerve for regional block. Reg Anesth Pain Med. 2007;32:146–151.
186. Akkaya T, Ozturk E, Comert A, et al. Ultrasound-guided obturator nerve block: A sonoanatomic study of a new methodologic approach. Anesth Analg. 2009;108:1037–1041.
187. Lee SH, Jeong CW, Lee HJ, et al. Ultrasound guided obturator nerve block: A single interfascial injection technique. J Anesth. 2011;25:923–926.
188. Akata T, Murakami J, Yoshinaga A. Life-threatening haemorrhage following obturator artery injury during transurethral bladder surgery: A sequel of an unsuccessful obturator nerve block. Acta Anaesthesiol Scand. 1999;43:784–788.
189. van der Wal M, Lang SA, Yip RW. Transsartorial approach for saphenous nerve block. Can J Anesth. 1993;40:542–546.
190. Benzon HT, Sharma S, Calimaran A. Comparison of the different approaches to saphenous nerve block. Anesthesiology. 2005;102:633–638.
191. Tsui BC, Ozelsel T. Ultrasound-guided transsartorial perifemoral artery approach for a saphenous nerve block. Reg Anesth Pain Med. 2009;34:177–178.

192. Horn JL, Pitsch T, Salinas F, et al. Anatomic basis to the ultrasound-guided approach for saphenous nerve blockade. *Reg Anesth Pain Med.* 2009;34:486–489.
193. de Mey JC, Deruyck LJ, Cammu G, et al. A paravenous approach for the saphenous nerve block. *Reg Anesth Pain Med.* 2001;26:504–506.
194. Gray AT, Collins AB. Ultrasound-guided saphenous nerve block. *Reg Anesth Pain Med.* 2003;28:148.
195. Sahin L, Sahin M, Isikay N. A different approach to an ultrasound-guided saphenous nerve block. *Acta Anaesthesiol Scand.* 2011;55:1030–1031.
196. Pham Dang C. Midfemoral block: A new lateral approach to the sciatic nerve. *Anesth Analg.* 1999;88:1426.
197. Zetlaoui PJ, Bouaziz H. Lateral approach to the sciatic nerve in the popliteal fossa. *Anesth Analg.* 1998;87:79–82.
198. March X, Pineda O, Garcia MM, et al. The posterior approach to the sciatic nerve in the popliteal fossa: A comparison of single- versus double-injection technique. *Anesth Analg.* 2006;103:1571–1573.
199. Vloka JD, Hadzic A. The intensity of the current at which sciatic nerve stimulation is achieved is a more important factor in determining the quality of nerve block than the type of motor response obtained. *Anesthesiology.* 1998;88:1408–1411.
200. Buys MJ, Arndt CD, Vagh F, et al. Ultrasound-guided sciatic nerve block in the popliteal fossa using a lateral approach: Onset time comparing separate tibial and common peroneal nerve injections versus injecting proximal to the bifurcation. *Anesth Analg.* 2010;110:636–637.
201. Ip VH, Tsui BC. Kill 2 birds with 1 stone: injection at the bifurcation during popliteal sciatic nerve block. *Reg Anesth Pain Med.* 2011;36:633–634.
202. Germain G, Levesque S, Dion N, et al. A comparison of an injection cephalad or caudad to the division of the sciatic nerve for ultrasound-guided popliteal block: A prospective randomized study. *Anesth Analg.* 2012;114:233–235.
203. Prasad A, Perlas A, Ramlogan R, et al. Ultrasound-guided popliteal block distal to sciatic nerve bifurcation shortens onset time: A prospective randomized double-blind study. *Reg Anesth Pain Med.* 2010;35:267–271.
204. Tran DQ, Dugani S, Pham K, et al. A randomized comparison between subepineural and conventional ultrasound-guided popliteal sciatic nerve block. *Reg Anesth Pain Med.* 2011;36:548–552.
205. Bendtsen TF, Nielsen TD, Rohde CV, et al. Ultrasound guidance improves a continuous popliteal sciatic nerve block when compared with nerve stimulation. *Reg Anesth Pain Med.* 2011;36:181–184.
206. Mariano ER, Cheng GS, Choy LP, et al. Electrical stimulation versus ultrasound guidance for popliteal-sciatic perineural catheter insertion: A randomized controlled trial. *Reg Anesth Pain Med.* 2009;34:480–485.
207. Perlas A, Brull R, Chan VW, et al. Ultrasound guidance improves the success of sciatic nerve lock at the popliteal fossa. *Reg Anesth Pain Med.* 2008;33:259–265.
208. Tsui BC, Ozelsel TJ. Ultrasound-guided anterior sciatic nerve block using a longitudinal approach: "Expanding the view." *Reg Anesth Pain Med.* 2008;33:275–276.
209. Raj PP, Parks RI, Watson TD, et al. A new single-position supine approach to sciatic-femoral nerve block. *Anesth Analg.* 1975;54:489–493.
210. Robards C, Wang RD, Clendenen S, et al. Sciatic nerve catheter placement: Success with using the Raj approach. *Anesth Analg.* 2009;109:972–975.
211. Le Corroller T, Wittenberg R, Pauly V, et al. A new lateral approach to the parasacral sciatic nerve block: An anatomical study. *Surg Radiol Anat.* 2011;33:91–95.
212. Osaka Y, Kashiwagi M, Nagatsuka Y, et al. Ultrasound-guided medial mid-thigh approach to sciatic nerve block with a patient in a supine position. *J Anesth.* 2011;25:621–624.
213. Redborg KE, Sites BD, Chinn CD, et al. Ultrasound improves the success rate of a sural nerve block at the ankle. *Reg Anesth Pain Med.* 2009;34:24–28.
214. Canella C, Demondion X, Guillin R, et al. Anatomic study of the superficial peroneal nerve using sonography. *Am J Roentgenol.* 2009;193:174–179.
215. Capdevila X, Ponrouch M, Choquet O. Continuous peripheral nerve blocks in clinical practice. *Curr Opin Anaesthesiol.* 2008;21:619–623.
216. Chelly JE, Ghisi D, Fanelli A. Continuous peripheral nerve blocks in acute pain management. *Br J Anaesth.* 2010;105:i86–i96.
217. Ilfeld BM. Continuous peripheral nerve blocks: A review of the published evidence. *Anesth Analg.* 2011;113:904–925.
218. Ilfeld BM, Morey TE, Wright TW, et al. Continuous interscalene brachial plexus block for postoperative pain control at home: A randomized, double-blinded, placebo-controlled study. *Anesth Analg.* 2003;96:1089–1095.
219. Salinas FV. Location, location, location: Continuous peripheral nerve blocks and stimulating catheters. *Reg Anesth Pain Med.* 2003;28:79–82.
220. Kick O, Blanche E, Pham-Dang C, et al. A new stimulating stylet for immediate control of catheter tip position in continuous peripheral nerve blocks. *Anesth Analg.* 1999;89:533–534.
221. Chin KJ, Chan V. Ultrasound-guided peripheral nerve blockade. *Curr Opin Anaesthesiol.* 2008;21:624–631.
222. Marhofer P, Chan VW. Ultrasound-guided regional anesthesia: Current concepts and future trends. *Anesth Analg.* 2007;104:1265–1269.
223. Bryan NA, Swenson JD, Greis PE, et al. Indwelling interscalene catheter use in an outpatient setting for shoulder surgery: Technique, efficacy, and complications. *J Shoulder Elbow Surg.* 2007;16:388–395.
224. Davis JJ, Swenson JD, Greis PE, et al. Interscalene block for postoperative analgesia using only ultrasound guidance: The outcome in 200 patients. *J Clin Anesth.* 2009;21:272–277.
225. Ip V, Bouliane M, Tsui B. Potential contamination of the surgical site caused by leakage from an interscalene catheter with the patient in a seated position: A case report. *Can J Anesth.* 2012;59:1125–1129.
226. Tsui BC, Tsui J. Less leakage and dislodgement with a catheter-over-needle versus a catheter-through-needle approach for peripheral nerve block: An ex vivo study. *Can J Anesth.* 2012;59:655–661.
227. Shakespeare TJ, Tsui BC. Catheter-over-needle method facilitates effective continuous infraclavicular block. *Can J Anesth.* 2013;60:948–949.
228. Ip VH, Rockley MC, Tsui BC. The catheter-over-needle assembly offers greater stability and less leakage compared with the traditional counterpart in continuous interscalene nerve blocks: A randomized patient-blinded study. *Can J Anaesth.* 2013;60:1272–1273.
229. Herring AA, Liu B, Kiefer MV, et al. ED placement of perineural catheters for femoral fracture pain management. *Am J Emerg Med.* 2014;32:287.e1–e3.
230. Gomez-Rios MA. Postoperative analgesia with transversus abdominis plane catheter infusions of levobupivacaine after major gynecological and obstetrical surgery. A case series. *Rev Esp Anestesiol Reanim.* 2015;62:165–169.
231. Tsui BC, Green JS, Ip VH. Ultrasound-guided rectus sheath catheter placement. *Anaesthesia.* 2014;69:1174–1175.
232. Spencer AO, Tsui BC. Intermittent bolus via infraclavicular nerve catheter using a catheter-over-needle technique in a pediatric patient. *Can J Anaesth.* 2014;61:684–685.
233. Tsui BC, Dillane D. Reducing and washing off local anesthetic for continuous interscalene block. *Reg Anesth Pain Med.* 2014;39:175–176.
234. Byeon GJ, Shin SW, Yoon JU, et al. Infusion methods for continuous interscalene brachial plexus block for postoperative pain control after arthroscopic rotator cuff repair. *Korean J Pain.* 2015;28:210–216.
235. Patkar CS, Vora K, Patel H, et al. A comparison of continuous infusion and intermittent bolus administration of 0. 1% ropivacaine with 0. 0002% fentanyl for epidural labor analgesia. *J Anaesthesiol Clin Pharmacol.* 2015;31:234–238.
236. Macaire P, Nadhari M, Greiss H, et al. Internet remote control of pump settings for postoperative continuous peripheral nerve blocks: A feasibility study in 59 patients. *Ann Fr Anesth Reanim.* 2014;33:e1–e7.
237. Tsui BC. *Atlas of Ultrasound- and Nerve Stimulation-Guided Regional Anesthesia.* 2nd ed. New York, NY: Springer; 2016.

Section 7
ANESTHESIA SUBSPECIALITY CARE

37 Anesthesia for Neurosurgery

JOHN F. BEBAWY • JEFFREY J. PASTERNAK

Introduction
Neuroanatomy
Neurophysiology
Pathophysiology
Monitoring
   Central Nervous System Function
   Influence of Anesthetic Technique on Evoked Potentials
Cerebral Perfusion
   Transcranial Doppler Ultrasonography
   Laser Doppler Flowmetry
   Intracranial Pressure Monitoring
   Cerebral Oxygenation and Metabolism Monitors
Cerebral Protection
   Ischemic and Reperfusion
   Hypothermia
   Pharmacologic Therapy for Cerebral Protection
   Glucose and Cerebral Ischemia
   A Practical Approach
Anesthetic Management
   Preoperative Evaluation
   Induction of Anesthesia and Airway Management
   Maintenance of Anesthesia
   Ventilation Management
   Fluids and Electrolytes
   Transfusion Therapy
   Glucose Management
   Emergence
Common Surgical Procedures
   Surgery for Tumors
   Pituitary Surgery
   Cerebral Aneurysm Surgery and Endovascular Treatment
   Arteriovenous Malformations
   Carotid Surgery
   Epilepsy Surgery
   Awake Craniotomy
Anesthesia and Traumatic Brain Injury
   Anesthetic Management
Anesthesia for Spine Trauma and Complex Spine Surgery
   Spinal Cord Injury
   Comorbid Injuries
   Initial Management
   Intraoperative Management
   Complications of Anesthesia for Spine Surgery
Conclusion

KEY POINTS

1. The brain receives approximately 70% of its blood supply from two internal carotid arteries anteriorly and 30% from two vertebral arteries posteriorly forming the basilar artery, that subsequently converge to form the Circle of Willis, an anastomotic ring at the base of the skull.

2. The spinal cord receives its blood supply from one anterior spinal artery and two posterior spinal arteries. The anterior spinal artery originates from 6 to 8 major radicular arteries derived from the aorta, with the largest one being the artery of Adamkiewicz (usually occurring at T11 or T12 and generally supplying T8 to the conus medullaris terminus).

3. Cerebral blood flow (CBF) is regulated by "flow-metabolism coupling," whereby increases in regional neuronal electrical activity require corresponding increases in regional blood flow. Such coupling occurs on the order of seconds, with very little variation in the amount of oxygen extraction by the brain tissue (i.e., CBF matches cerebral metabolic rate of oxygen consumption very quickly and efficiently in the healthy brain).

4. Moderate changes in mean arterial pressure (MAP) (or cerebral perfusion pressure) will yield a consistent CBF of 50 mL/100 g/min, due to the normal brain's ability to autoregulate its blood flow. Cerebral autoregulation of blood flow is thought to remain intact between a MAP of approximately 60 and 160 mmHg and functions by altering cerebrovascular resistance (CVR) on the order of 5 to 60 seconds. The alteration in CVR is accomplished in both a rapid phase ("dynamic autoregulation") and a slow phase ("static autoregulation").

5. CBF is linearly associated with arterial carbon dioxide tension between 20 and 80 mmHg. Hyper- and hypoventilation, both patient-determined and iatrogenic, play critical roles in decreasing or increasing CBF, respectively. A change in arterial carbon dioxide tension of 1 mmHg roughly correlates to a similar change in CBF of 1 to 2 mL/100 g/min. Below the lower limit of this linear effect (i.e., with arterial carbon dioxide tension below 20 mmHg), maximal cerebral vasoconstriction leads to tissue hypoxia and a reflex vasodilation.

6. Intravenous drugs, such as propofol, etomidate, benzodiazepines, and thiopental, decrease CBF by virtue of a drug-induced decrease in cerebral metabolic rate of oxygen consumption and subsequent flow-metabolism coupling. Autoregulation and arterial carbon dioxide tension responsiveness remain intact with these agents.

7. Potent volatile anesthetics, such as isoflurane, sevoflurane, and desflurane, are direct cerebral vasodilators. However, this direct vasodilation is offset by a drug-induced decrease in cerebral metabolic rate of oxygen consumption, and via flow-metabolism coupling, an attenuation of the direct effect on CBF. This leads to minimal, if any, increase in CBF at lower doses. However, at high doses where maximal suppression of cerebral metabolic rate of oxygen consumption has occurred are direct vasodilatory effects observed leading to a dose-dependent increase in CBF. Furthermore, autoregulation is inhibited with potent volatile anesthetic drugs in a dose-dependent fashion, although the cerebral vasculature remains responsive to changes in arterial carbon dioxide tension.

8. The Monro–Kellie doctrine states that "an increase in the volume of one intracranial compartment will lead to a rise in intracranial pressure unless it is matched by an equal reduction in the volume of another compartment." Since the brain parenchyma is relatively incompressible, cerebrospinal fluid and cerebral blood volume play an integral role in accommodating increases in intracranial pressure (ICP).

9. The most commonly used modalities of evoked potential monitoring are somatosensory evoked potentials, motor evoked potentials, and electromyography, with brainstem auditory evoked potentials and visual evoked potentials being less commonly used. Anesthetic drugs play a major role in facilitating the success of intraoperative evoked potential monitoring.

10. Reliable pharmacologic and nonpharmacologic therapies to prevent neuronal ischemic injury are currently not readily available for use in the perioperative period. At the present time, one can only hope to attenuate injury by preventing secondary insults to surrounding neuronal tissue (e.g., ensuring adequate oxygen and substrate delivery).

11. The preoperative evaluation of the neurosurgical patient is of paramount importance to ensure a safe and successful anesthetic. Specific problems must be identified so as to formulate appropriate plans for intraoperative and postoperative management. For patients with intracranial mass lesions, the most important fact to ascertain is the presence and extent of intracranial hypertension and this should be assumed until information proves otherwise. Choice of drugs for maintenance of general anesthesia depends to a great extent on the ICP and whether neuromonitoring is being employed.

Introduction

Neuroanesthesia is the practice of perioperative medicine related to the treatment of diseases or injury to the central nervous system (CNS) or peripheral nervous system (PNS). The CNS encompasses the brain and spinal cord, whereas the PNS includes all of the peripheral nerves of the body emanating from the brain and spinal cord. As such, neuroanesthesia is the provision of anesthesia and analgesia for a multitude of procedures, including invasive, minimally invasive, neurodiagnostic, and neurointerventional procedures, and involving the brain, spinal cord, and peripheral nerves.

Neuroanatomy

The CNS is composed of the brain and the spinal cord. The brain is enclosed by the cranium, a fixed bony cavity, and is physically and functionally divided into two compartments: the supratentorium and the infratentorium (Fig. 37-1). The supratentorium contains the paired cerebral hemispheres and the diencephalon that is composed of the thalamus and hypothalamus. Each cerebral hemisphere is divided into four lobes (frontal, temporal, parietal, and occipital). Eloquent cortical areas are generally considered to be regions responsible for gross motor function and language. The primary somatosensory and motor cortex strips lie adjacent to the central sulcus in the parietal and frontal lobes, respectively, and extend inferiorly to the Sylvian fissure. Cortical regions that are responsible for language are located in the left hemisphere in almost all right-handed people as well as in the majority of left-handed people. The two primary regions responsible for language are Broca area, located in the premotor frontal cortex and responsible for language formation,[1] and Wernicke area, located in the posterior superior temporal cortex and responsible for language acquisition. Lesions in Broca area lead to expressive aphasia whereas those in Wernicke area cause receptive aphasia.

The extrapyramidal system consists of a group of brain structures that modify motor function but are not components of the corticospinal tract and primary motor cortex. These structures include the basal ganglia (comprised of the caudate nucleus, globus pallidus, putamen, substantia nigra, and red nucleus), cerebellum, and components of the auditory and vestibular pathways. Dysfunction of structures in the extrapyramidal system results in difficulty with motor control without frank weakness. This includes Parkinson disease, essential tremor, and ataxia.

The diencephalon lies cephalad to the midbrain and is composed of the thalamus and hypothalamus. The thalamus acts as a sensory and motor "relay station," functionally and physically connecting the cortex with the rest of the nervous system. The hypothalamus, lying below the thalamus, has autonomic and endocrine functions and is connected to the pituitary gland via the infundibulum.

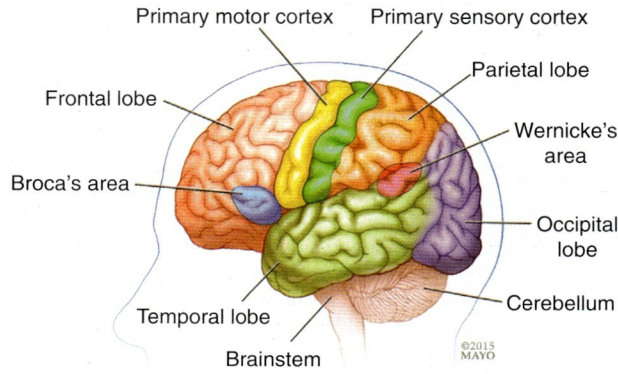

Figure 37-1 Gross anatomy of the brain. (Used with permission of Mayo Foundation for Medical Education and Research. All rights reserved.)

The limbic system consists of a group of structures that play a role in cognitive function, memory consolidation, and emotional responses. Components of the limbic system include, but are not limited to, the hippocampus, amygdala, part of the hypothalamus, and some regions of the cortex (e.g., insular region). The hypothalamus, although generally considered a component of the diencephalon, also functions in the limbic system due to its role in the regulation of autonomic and endocrine function in addition to modulation of behavior and sexual function.

The infratentorium encompasses the brainstem and the cerebellum. The brainstem is comprised of the midbrain, pons, and medulla and is responsible for consciousness via the reticular activating system, a variety of autonomic functions including respiratory and cardiovascular control, and many reflexes (e.g., cough/gag, pupillary reflexes). The brainstem contains nuclei for cranial nerves III to XII. The cerebellum, among the most rudimentary parts of the brain, lies in the posterior fossa and is responsible for such actions as processing proprioceptive input and establishing axial posture and gait.[2]

The brain receives approximately 70% of its blood supply from two internal carotid arteries anteriorly and 30% from two vertebral arteries posteriorly forming the basilar artery, that subsequently converge to form the Circle of Willis, an anastomotic ring at the base of the skull (Fig. 37-2). The common carotid artery, originating from the aortic arch, divides at the level of the thyroid cartilage into the internal and external carotid arteries. The internal carotid artery traverses the skull base through the foramen lacerum and subsequently travels through the cavernous sinus and into the carotid groove. Thereafter, the artery divides into the posterior communicating artery (PCOM), the anterior cerebral artery (ACA), and the middle cerebral artery (MCA).

The bilateral vertebral arteries originate from the subclavian arteries and converge to form the basilar artery at the pontomedullary junction. When reaching the midbrain (along the ventral surface of the brainstem), the basilar artery divides into the posterior cerebral arteries (PCAs) and also anastomoses with the PCOMs, thus completing the circle of Willis. Interestingly, less than 50% of people demonstrate a "complete" circle of Willis.[3]

The venous system of the brain consists of both deep and superficial veins that ultimately drain into the dural venous sinuses (Fig. 37-3). These sinuses are valveless endothelialized channels lying between the dura mater and skull periosteum. All of the sinuses eventually drain into the sigmoid sinus and thereafter into the internal jugular veins.

The entire CNS is insulated from its bony encasement by cerebrospinal fluid (CSF) that is produced mostly by the choroid plexus of the lateral and third ventricles (Fig. 37-4). The average volume of CSF in an adult is approximately 150 mL. CSF is created at a rate of 15 to 20 mL/hr and moves from these ventricles via the aqueduct of Sylvius to the fourth ventricle. From there, CSF flows out of the fourth ventricle via the foramen of Magendie and the lateral foramina of Luschka to the subarachnoid space in the cranium. It does so via a series of interconnected cisterns at the base of the brain, to be subsequently reabsorbed into the dural venous sinuses, primarily the superior sagittal sinus, via arachnoid villi and granulations.[4] Some CSF traverses the foramen magnum, entering the subarachnoid space within the

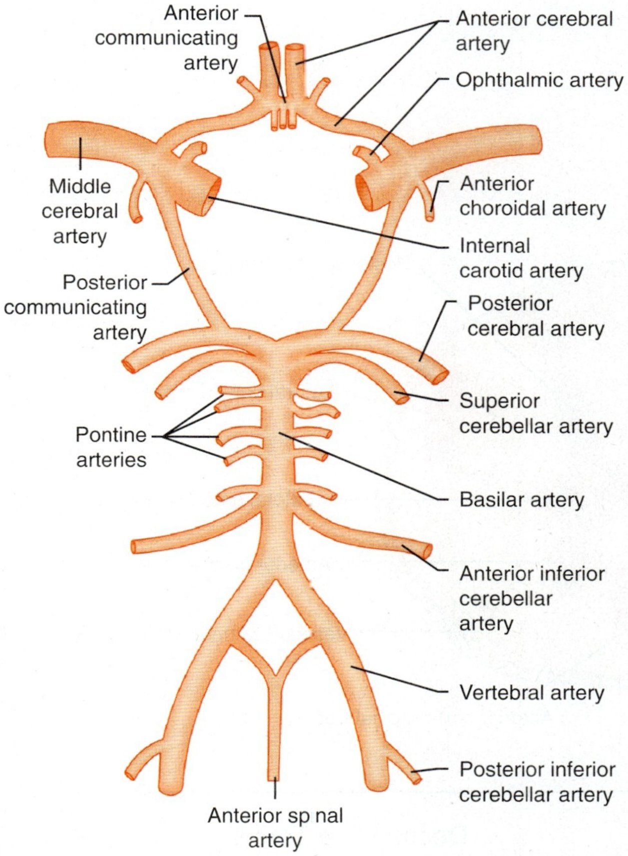

Figure 37-2 The circle of Willis, demonstrating the anterior and posterior blood supply to the brain.

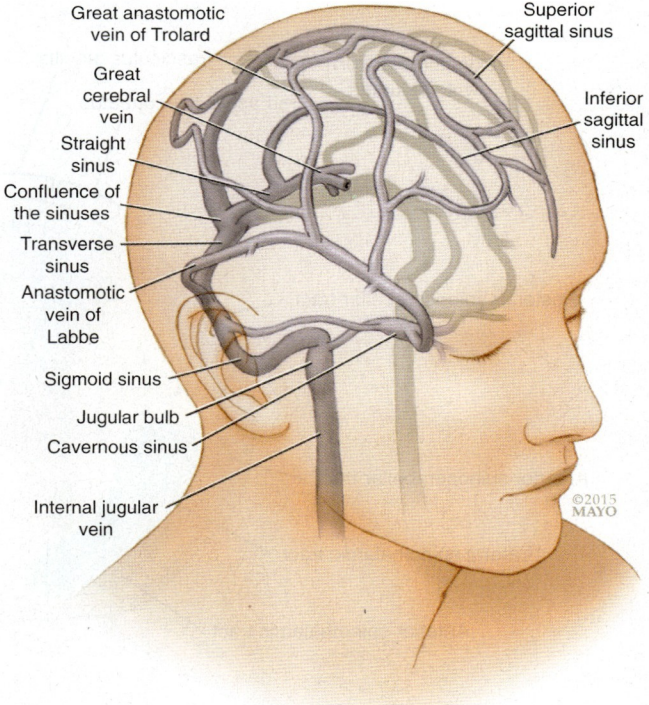

Figure 37-3 Gross anatomy of the venous drainage system of the brain, including the major venous sinuses. (Used with permission of Mayo Foundation for Medical Education and Research. All rights reserved.)

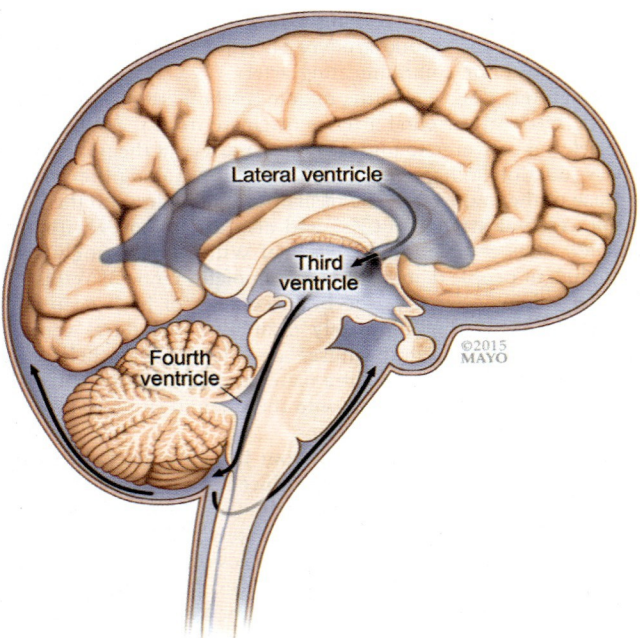

Figure 37-4 Cerebrospinal fluid compartments within and around the brain. This includes the ventricular system and gross cerebral spinal fluid flow patterns. (Used with permission of Mayo Foundation for Medical Education and Research. All rights reserved.)

spinal column. This movement of CSF is important for acute and chronic compensation in elevated ICP states.

The spinal column is composed of 33 vertebrae (7 cervical, 12 thoracic, 5 lumbar, and 9 fused sacral and coccygeal), with nerve roots leaving the enclosed spinal cord and exiting through corresponding intervertebral foramina. The spinal cord itself is composed of central gray matter, the dorsal columns containing tracts responsible for proprioception and light touch, lateral spinothalamic tracts responsible for pain and temperature, and outer white matter containing the lateral corticospinal tracts (Fig. 37-5). The lateral gray columns contain the cell bodies of the preganglionic neurons that eventually enter the sympathetic chain (running on either side of the vertebral bodies), arising from T1 to L2 or L3. The spinal cord itself terminates at L1 or L2 in adults, ending in structures known as the conus medullaris terminus and filum terminale.

The spinal cord receives its blood supply from one anterior spinal artery and two posterior spinal arteries (Fig. 37-6). The anterior spinal artery originates from six to eight major radicular arteries derived from the aorta, with the largest one being the artery of Adamkiewicz (usually occurring at T11 or T12 and generally supplying T8 to the conus medullaris terminus). Thus, the artery of Adamkiewicz is responsible for supplying arterial blood to the anterior two-thirds of the spinal cord. The posterior spinal arteries originate from the posterior cerebral circulation and supply the dorsal horns and white matter (posterior third of the spinal cord).[5]

Various regions of the brain and spinal cord responsible for distinct functions are shown in Table 37-1.

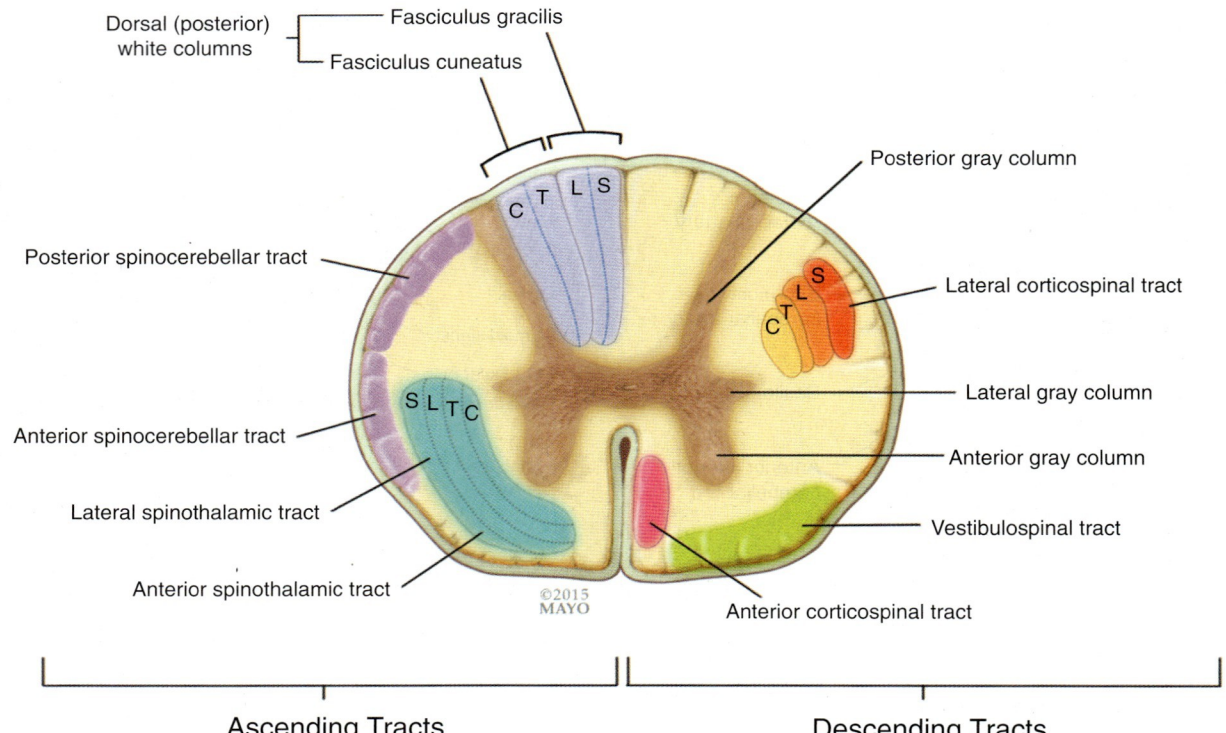

Figure 37-5 Major ascending and descending spinal cord tracts (cross-section). C, cervical; T, thoracic; L, lumbar; and S, sacral. (Used with permission of Mayo Foundation for Medical Education and Research. All rights reserved.)

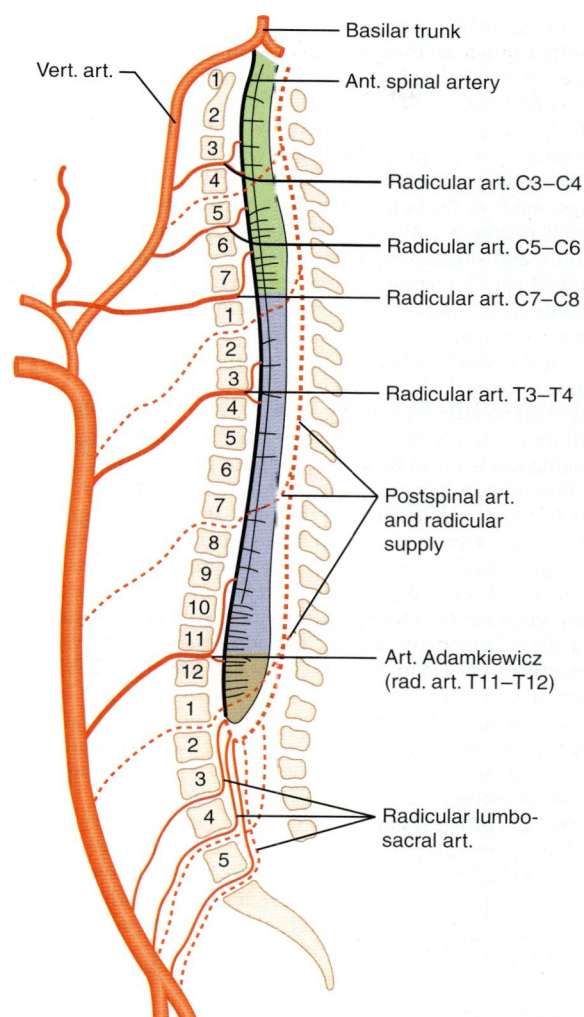

Figure 37-6 The spinal cord blood supply. Note that the cervical spine is served by the posterior circulation emanating from the circle of Willis.

Neurophysiology

Although the adult brain accounts for only 2% of total body weight, it is responsible for 20% of total body oxygen consumption and 25% of total body glucose consumption. The cerebral metabolic rate of oxygen consumption ($CMRO_2$) is normally 3 to 3.8 mL/100 g/min and brain glucose consumption is approximately 5 mg/100 g/min. Normal cerebral blood flow (CBF) is 50 mL/100 g/min or 750 mL/min. Therefore, the brain receives about 15% of the cardiac output to meet these high metabolic requirements. The brain depends on a continuous supply of oxygen and glucose, with irreversible injury potentially occurring after only 4 to 5 minutes of global ischemia.[6]

CBF is regulated by "flow-metabolism coupling," whereby increases in regional neuronal electrical activity require corresponding increases in regional blood flow. Such coupling occurs on the order of seconds, with very little variation in the amount of oxygen extraction by the brain tissue (i.e., CBF matches $CMRO_2$ very quickly and efficiently in the healthy brain).[7,8]

CPP is the difference between mean arterial pressure (MAP) and either intracranial pressure (ICP) or central venous pressure (CVP), depending on which is higher. CBF itself is equal to CPP/cerebrovascular resistance (CVR). Fortunately, even moderate changes in MAP (or CPP) will yield a consistent CBF of 50 mL/100 g/min, due to the normal brain's ability to autoregulate its blood flow. Cerebral autoregulation of blood flow is thought to remain intact between a MAP of approximately 60 to 160 mmHg and functions by altering CVR on the order of 5 to 60 seconds (Fig. 37-7). However, the lower limit of autoregulation (LLA) is likely to be not only higher than an MAP of 60 mmHg but also dynamic throughout the day and differs among individuals. In those with otherwise healthy brains, the LLA may be as high as a MAP of 80 mmHg in some individuals.[9] The alteration in CVR is accomplished in both a rapid phase ("dynamic autoregulation") and a slow phase ("static autoregulation").[10] Dynamic autoregulation is thought to respond to pulsatility changes more closely linked to the systolic systemic blood pressure,[11] whereas static autoregulation is a phenomenon that accommodates to changes in MAP over longer time intervals.[12] Above the upper limit of autoregulation and below the LLA, CBF is pressure-dependent. Below the LLA maximal cerebral vasodilation occurs and cerebral ischemia can

Table 37-1 Functionality of CNS Structures

Anatomic Location	Structure	Function
Postcentral gyrus	Primary somatosensory cortex	Sensation
Precentral gyrus	Primary motor cortex	Movement
Occipital lobe	Primary visual cortex	Vision
Temporal lobe	Primary auditory cortex	Hearing
Wernicke area (angular gyrus of dominant hemisphere)	Primary language association cortex	Language
Broca area (frontal lobe of dominant hemisphere)	Primary language expression cortex	Language
Frontal lobe	Primary personality cortex	Personality/Intellect
Temporal lobe	Limbic cortex	Emotion
Temporal lobe	Hippocampus	Memory
Diencephalon	Hypothalamus	Vegetative regulation
Brain stem	Reticular activating system	Consciousness
Brain stem	Vasomotor center	Circulatory/respiratory control
Spinal cord	Dorsal horn (sensory)/ventral horn (motor)	Movement/sensation/reflexes

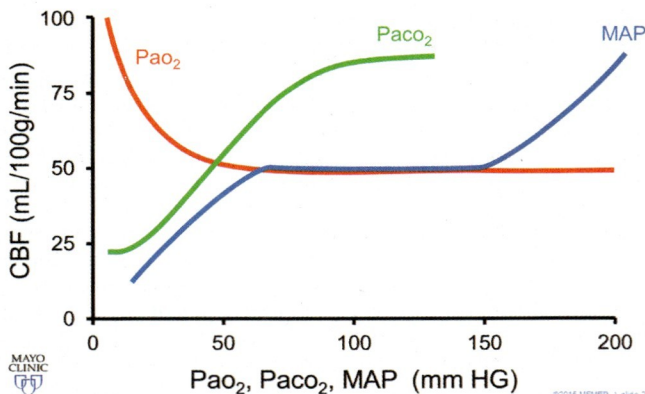

Figure 37-7 Autoregulation in the central nervous system: cerebral blood flow (CBF) remains constant between mean arterial pressures (MAP) of approximately 60 to 160 mmHg (*blue*). CBF varies linearly between arterial carbon dioxide partial pressures ($PaCO_2$) of 20 to 80 mmHg (*green*). Cerebral blood flow remains constant above an arterial oxygen partial pressure (PaO_2) of 50 mmHg (*red*). (Used with permission of Mayo Foundation for Medical Education and Research. All rights reserved.)

result. Above the upper limit of autoregulation, cerebral vessels are maximally vasoconstricted and increases in perfusion pressure may lead to disruption of the blood–brain barrier (BBB), cerebral edema, or cerebral hemorrhage.[13]

CVR changes responsible for autoregulation are the result of both myogenic responses in cerebral resistance vessels and neurogenic forces (e.g., sympathetic activation due to chronic hypertension). The autoregulatory curve is shifted rightward in cases of chronic hypertension. Anesthetics, especially the potent volatile anesthetics, have a dose-dependent effect of decreasing the extent of autoregulation.[14]

Besides MAP, other physiologic parameters play an important role in regulating CBF. Arterial carbon dioxide tension ($PaCO_2$) is the most important of these variables. CBF is linearly associated with $PaCO_2$ between 20 and 80 mmHg (Fig. 37-7). Hyper- and hypoventilation, both patient-determined and iatrogenic, play critical roles in decreasing or increasing CBF, respectively. A change in $PaCO_2$ of 1 mmHg roughly correlates to a similar change in CBF of 1 to 2 mL/100 g/min. Below the lower limit of this linear effect (i.e., with $PaCO_2$ below 20 mmHg), maximal cerebral vasoconstriction leads to tissue hypoxia and a reflex vasodilation. This phenomenon is the basis for spontaneous hyperventilation that develops in response to acutely elevated ICP.[15] This beneficial reflex, however, can be detrimental as low regional CBF and ischemia can occur.[16] Furthermore, the effect of hyperventilation on CBF and ICP is only sustainable for approximately 6 hours, as the pH of the CSF will renormalize.

Oxygen tension in the arterial blood (PaO_2) has minimal effect on CBF unless marked hypoxemia ($PaO_2 < 50$ mmHg) occurs, below which CBF increases dramatically (Fig. 37-7). When PaO_2 is greater than 350 mmHg, slight cerebral vasoconstriction can occur. It is unclear why this reflex occurs, but it may be a method by which the brain protects itself from "oxygen toxicity" (i.e., oxygen free radical formation).[17] Temperature is also an important determinant of CBF, with a 6% to 7% decrease in CBF per 1°C decrease in core temperature.

Regional CBF is more complex than global CBF (as described earlier) and is governed by both humoral and neurogenic factors. Certain circulating catecholamines and other mediators such as α_1-adrenergic agonists, ionic calcium, endothelin, and thromboxane A_2 may have cerebral vasoconstrictive effects, whereas other factors such as β_2-adrenergic agonists, nitric oxide, adenosine, and prostaglandins play a role in regional cerebral vasodilation.[18] Neurogenic influences over local regulation of CBF include effects mediated by the release of acetylcholine, dopamine, serotonin, and substance P.[19]

Anesthetics can have profound effects on CBF. Intravenous drugs, such as propofol, etomidate, benzodiazepines, and thiopental, decrease CBF by virtue of a drug-induced decrease in $CMRO_2$ and subsequent flow-metabolism coupling. Autoregulation and $PaCO_2$ responsiveness remain intact with these agents.[20] Opioids have very little effect on $CMRO_2$, CBF, autoregulation, or $PaCO_2$ responsiveness. Ketamine is unique in that it increases CBF and $CMRO_2$, with little effect on autoregulation or $PaCO_2$ responsiveness.[21]

Potent volatile anesthetics, such as isoflurane, sevoflurane, and desflurane are direct cerebral vasodilators. However, this direct vasodilation is offset by a drug-induced decrease in $CMRO_2$, and via flow-metabolism coupling, an attenuation of the direct effect on CBF. These effects lead to minimal, if any, increase in CBF at lower doses. However, at high doses where maximal suppression of $CMRO_2$ has occurred are direct vasodilatory effects observed leading to a dose-dependent increase in CBF.[22] Furthermore, autoregulation is inhibited with potent volatile anesthetic drugs in a dose-dependent fashion, although the cerebral vasculature remains responsive to changes in $PaCO_2$. Nitrous oxide is a direct cerebral vasodilator and causes minimal effect on $CMRO_2$.[23,24] Nitrous oxide may have a variable effect on cerebral autoregulatory capacity leading to preserved autoregulation during propofol anesthesia but further impairment of autoregulation during sevoflurane anesthesia.[25,26]

Spinal cord physiology is very similar to brain physiology in that autoregulation is maintained and spinal cord perfusion pressure (SCPP) = MAP − SSSP (spinal subarachnoid space pressure). The specific effects of different anesthetic drugs on spinal cord physiology are not as well characterized as the effects of these drugs on the brain.

Pathophysiology

ICP is the pressure within the intracranial cavity, which is a closed vault containing the brain parenchyma (1,400 mL), CSF (150 mL), and the cerebral blood volume (CBV) (150 mL). The Monro–Kellie doctrine states that "an increase in the volume of one intracranial compartment will lead to a rise in ICP unless it is matched by an equal reduction in the volume of another compartment."[27] Since the brain parenchyma is relatively incompressible, CSF and CBV play an integral role in accommodating increases in ICP. CSF will tend to egress out of the cranial cavity and into the spinal subarachnoid space, whereas CBV will be decreased by both a reflex arterial vasoconstriction and increased venous efflux from the brain and venous sinuses. Since these compartments are relatively low in volume, their ability to compensate for large increases in ICP is greatly limited. When these compensatory effects are exhausted, a small increase in volume can lead to a dramatic increase in the pressure within the cranium (Fig. 37-8). The results can be neurologically devastating with impaired perfusion and possible herniation of the brain. This can cause irreversible brain injury or even death. Hence, meticulous care in those patients in whom elevated ICP is suspected is critical. This includes avoiding hypoventilation, maintaining adequate CPP, implementing techniques to reduce intracranial volume (i.e., mannitol, CSF diversion, cerebral vasoconstricting anesthetics), and considering decompressive craniectomy.

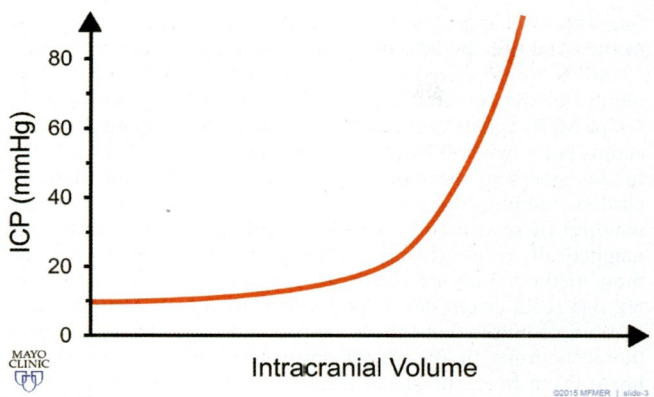

Figure 37-8 Intracranial elastance curve. The intracranial elastance curve is composed of three sections. Intracranial pressure (ICP) remains low and relatively constant at low volumes until the "elbow" of the curve is reached. At this point, small changes in volume lead to moderate changes in pressure. When a critical intracranial volume is reached, the pressure increases precipitously. (Used with permission of Mayo Foundation for Medical Education and Research. All rights reserved.)

Normal ICP is 7 to 15 mmHg. Poor neurologic outcome is associated with prolonged ICP above 20 to 25 mmHg.[28] Normal ICP is subject to fluctuation with such activities as the Valsalva maneuver or patient position. Kety and Schmidt demonstrated in 1948 that increases in ICP can lead to CBF reduction, which led many investigators to question the safe management of elevated ICP in terms of its effects on cerebral ischemia.[29]

The intracranial elastance curve is quite useful in visualizing the ICP–volume relationship. The initial "flat part of the curve," where intracranial elastance is low, demonstrates that in non-pathologic brain states, changes in intracranial volume are compensated for quite easily by CSF and CBV buffering. When this compensation is exhausted ("elbow of the curve") and elastance increases, small increases in volume lead to rapid rises in ICP. Cerebral elastance ($E = dP/dV$) can be estimated with invasive cerebral and spinal monitoring devices (e.g., lumbar drain, extraventricular drain).

Elevated ICP may be caused by a variety of pathophysiologic mechanisms. The most common contributing factor to increased ICP is cerebral edema. Edema in the brain is generally classified into three major types: cytotoxic, vasogenic, and interstitial.[30,31] Cytotoxic edema is characterized by increased *intracellular* water. This commonly occurs in the setting of cerebral ischemia, where failure of membrane ionic pumps leads to accumulation of ions, and thus water, within cells. Vasogenic edema occurs when there is loss of integrity of the BBB, leading to accumulation of extracellular water. Vasogenic edema commonly occurs in regions of brain surrounding tumors, abscesses, or contusions. Dexamethasone is effective at decreasing only vasogenic edema, due in part to its effect at upregulating expression of proteins responsible for the integrity of the tight junctions between endothelial cells in the brain.[32] Interstitial edema is characterized by increased extracellular fluid in the setting of an intact BBB. Interstitial edema occurs in patients with hydrocephalus due to permeation of CSF into the interstitial space and in those with a significant osmotic difference between the brain interstitial space and the intravascular space as occurs in acute hyponatremia. In many circumstances, cerebral edema may be due to a combination of cytotoxic, vasogenic, and interstitial edema.

In addition to edema, there are a variety of other causes that can contribute to intracranial hypertension. Increased CBV, because of either increased arterial inflow or decreased venous efflux, can lead to increases in ICP. Increased arterial inflow is due to cerebral arterial vasodilation from factors such as use of vasodilatory drugs, hypercapnia, severe hypoxemia, or acidosis and decreased venous efflux can be caused by jugular venous obstruction, or elevated pressures within the airways. Likewise, inadequate CSF absorption, due to diminished absorption at the arachnoid villi as may occur with subarachnoid hemorrhage (SAH) or obstructive hydrocephalus as may occur with tumor, can cause hydrocephalus and elevated ICP. Lastly, mass effect from tumors, hematomas, or abscesses can elevate ICP by a direct space-occupying effect.

Clinical symptoms of intracranial hypertension include headache, nausea, vomiting, and papilledema. As ICP continues to increase, Cushing triad, consisting of hypertension, bradycardia, irregular respiration, may appear. Patients risk brain herniation and death with very severe intracranial hypertension. The signs of herniation will depend on the structures that are herniating and may include pupillary dilation, oculomotor weakness, absent pupillary light reflex, and cardiorespiratory arrest. Radiologically, computed tomography (CT) is most commonly used, and ICP elevation may manifest itself as effacement of sulci, compression of the ventricles, midline shift, or even ventriculomegaly, depending on the etiology.

Acute spinal cord injury is distinctly different from chronic spinal cord injury. Although both may involve loss of sensory, motor, and possibly autonomic function below the level of injury, flaccid paralysis and hypotension are evident in the acute phase whereas spastic paralysis, pain, and possible risk for autonomic hyperreflexia are observed in the chronic phase. Acute spinal cord compression, due to trauma or tumor, is usually a surgical emergency, as time to decompression has been correlated with functional outcome in some populations.[33] The role of steroids in preventing secondary injury is much more controversial.[34] Cervical injuries necessitate extremely careful management of the airway, and these injuries are associated with more physiologic perturbations than lower injuries, including diaphragmatic paralysis, cardiac disturbances, and death.

Monitoring

Central Nervous System Function

The most important monitor of CNS function is the neurologic examination of an awake and responsive patient. Although some neurosurgical procedures are specifically performed with mild sedation, most are performed in patients who receive general anesthesia. In this latter circumstance, other modes to monitor the integrity of the nervous system may be necessary. Electrophysiologic monitoring techniques are commonly used in the operating room to assess the functional integrity of the nervous system during surgeries that might put neurologic structures at risk. There is some consensus that these monitoring techniques can detect reversible changes in neurologic function in the patient during general anesthesia, allowing a surgical or physiologic change of plan that may avert permanent neurologic injury. However, there is a paucity of definitive data proving that such monitoring will prevent neurologic injury and improve outcomes.

The most commonly used modalities of evoked potential monitoring are somatosensory evoked potentials (SSEPs), motor evoked potentials (MEPs), and electromyography (EMG), with brainstem auditory evoked potentials (BAEPs) and visual evoked potentials (VEPs) being less commonly used (Fig. 37-9). The peaks and troughs of evoked potential waveforms can be

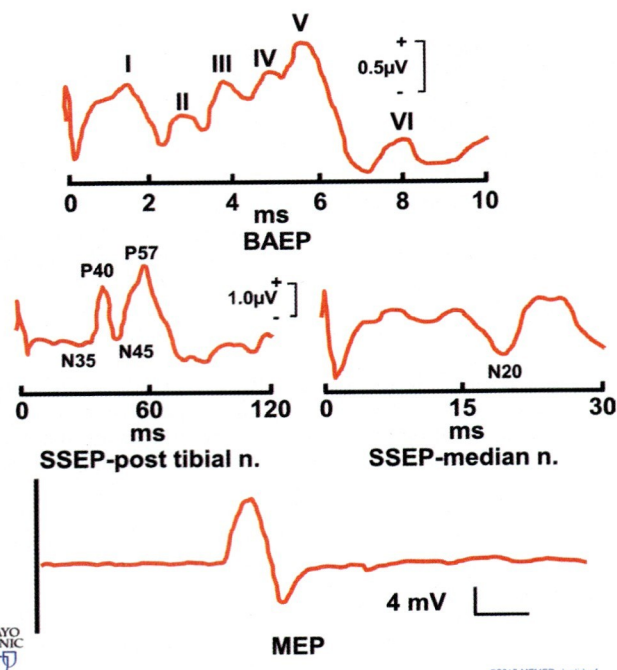

Figure 37-9 Representative brainstem auditory evoked potential (BAEP), somatosensory evoked potential (SSEP), and motor evoked potential (MEP) tracings. (Used with permission of Mayo Foundation for Medical Education and Research. All rights reserved.)

characterized by two parameters: amplitude and latency. Amplitude, measured in microvolts (for SSEPs and BAEPs) or millivolts (for MEPs), refers to the measured signal voltage of a peak relative to a baseline voltage or an adjacent peak. Latency, usually measured in milliseconds, refers to the delay in peak signal following stimulation and reflects transit time along the neural pathway.

SSEPs are elicited in a cyclical, repetitive manner from a peripheral nerve (e.g., median, ulnar, posterior tibial) and usually measured at the level of the subcortex (upper cervical spine, inion) and cortex (scalp). Stimuli predominantly travel via the posterior column/medial lemniscus pathway in the CNS. This modality is especially useful for monitoring the integrity of the peripheral nerves, dorsal columns of the spinal cord, the brainstem, the subcortex, and the sensory cortex of the brain. Any insult to this pathway may alter the SSEP response. Since sensory tracts decussate at the brainstem before proceeding through the thalamus and up to the sensory cortex, stimuli are recorded on the contralateral scalp. Notably, SSEPs are inherently small in amplitude, requiring a prolonged stimulation time, signal averaging, conversion from analog to digital format, and signal filtration to achieve a stable waveform. Therefore, it may take minutes to obtain a waveform. Muscle relaxants may be helpful as they tend to remove artifact caused by spontaneous EMG activity. SSEPs are commonly used during spine surgery, especially when posterolateral sensory elements are at risk of ischemia from surgical distraction.[35] They may also be useful during neurovascular brain surgery to ensure sufficient perfusion to the somatosensory cortex during procedures that may put this cortex at risk, such as cerebral aneurysm clipping.[36] Lower extremity SSEPs tend to correlate with the integrity of cortex supplied by the ACA whereas upper extremity SSEPs tend to correlate with the cortex supplied by the MCA distribution. The commonly used definitions of "significant changes" to the SSEP waveform include a decrease in the amplitude by 50% or an increase in the latency by 10%.[37]

MEPs are produced at the level of the cortex by direct stimulation of the cerebral cortex or by indirect stimulation of the scalp. MEP signals are usually measured as compound muscle action potentials (CMAPs) at the muscular level. MEPs are useful for assessing the motor cortex and the anterolateral spinal cord (containing the corticospinal tracts) during surgeries that may put these structures at risk. Stimulation may be performed magnetically or electrically, with the latter being the more common method. Indirect electrical stimulation of the motor cortex, via scalp electrodes, is performed, usually in a single pulse or train of pulses that travels caudad and depolarizes the upper motor neurons in the spinal cord, summating in the ventral horn. From here, the signal travels to the α-motor neurons via the internuncial pathways, descending to the motor endplates, where muscle movement related to an action potential can be measured.[38] Unlike SSEPs, MEPs do not require signal averaging or filtration and are produced by a single pulse or train of a few pulses requiring only seconds. Measurement of a response in muscles is severely inhibited by muscle relaxants. MEPs are useful during spine surgery, especially when anterior elements are at risk, and during intracranial surgery during procedures where the motor cortex or descending motor pathway are at risk for injury or ischemia. Although there is no formal definition of "significant changes" that warrant concern for altered neural pathway function, a decrease in amplitude of 50% is considered "significant" as is a need to increase the stimulation intensity required to maintain a reproducible signal. Latency of MEPs has much less of a role in defining a worrisome change than with SSEPs.[39]

EMG is a monitoring modality that is used to continually assess the integrity of distinct peripheral or cranial nerves or nerve roots. Spontaneous neural electrical activity can be monitored or, in stimulated EMG, electrical current can be induced in a nerve and then that signal can be detected as a means to monitor nerve integrity or identify a nerve.[40] EMG is sensitive to both mechanical and thermal injury. EMG, unlike SSEPs and MEPs, is not a monitor of ischemia. Needle electrodes are placed in a muscle known to be innervated by a particular nerve root, and if that nerve root is disturbed, EMG activity is recorded from that muscle. For example, EMG can be monitored in muscles innervated by spinal nerves during spine surgery or in muscles innervated by cranial nerves during various intracranial procedures that may put cranial nerves at risk, such as during acoustic neuroma resection. In addition, a surgeon may use stimulated EMG to identify cranial nerves during surgery.[41] "Triggered EMG," as is commonly performed with pedicle screw testing during spine surgery, relies on direct stimulation of the screws being placed within the bony pedicle. If there is disruption of the bony pedicle, and hence contact or near-contact between the screw and neural elements, the amount of current necessary to stimulate the corresponding nerve root will be much less than if the pedicle were intact.[42] Like MEPs, EMG is particularly sensitive to the effects of muscle relaxants.[43]

BAEPs are used to assess the integrity of the auditory canal, tympanic membrane, hair cells, spiral ganglion, vestibulocochlear nerve (cranial nerve VIII), cochlear nuclei, superior olivary complex, lateral lemniscus, inferior colliculus, and medial geniculate thalamic nuclei. A device that produces auditory stimuli (i.e., clicking sounds) is placed in the external auditory canal and responses are recorded from the scalp. Thousands of signals are averaged, yielding a typical waveform consisting of six waves. In general, any injury to CN VIII will affect all of the waves after wave I, decreasing their amplitude and prolonging their latency.[44] Retraction on the cerebellum may prolong the latency of the tracing between waves I and V. BAEPs are often performed during surgery at or near the brainstem such as microvascular decompression of cranial nerves V or VII or for acoustic neuroma resection. Fortunately, BAEPs are extremely robust with little effect from any anesthetic regimen.[45]

VEPs are used to assess the integrity of the visual pathway, including the eye, optic nerve, optic chiasm, and visual cortex in the occipital lobe. A bright stimulus is applied to the eyes using special goggles or contact lenses, and responses are recorded from scalp electrodes. VEPs may be useful during surgery at or near the optic chiasm or the occipital cortex. Unfortunately, VEPs are exquisitely sensitive to almost any anesthetic regimen and the difficulty in the ability to obtain and interpret the signals make them very infrequently used.[46]

Influence of Anesthetic Technique on Evoked Potentials

Anesthetic drugs play a major role in facilitating the success of intraoperative evoked potential monitoring. With regard to cortical SSEPs, potent volatile anesthetics and nitrous oxide have the greatest inhibitory effect causing a decrease in amplitude and an increase in wave latency. These drugs may limit the acquisition of robust SSEP signals, doing so in a nearly linear dose-dependent fashion. Robust signals can, however, usually be obtained in neurologically intact patients with up to 0.5 MAC of inhaled agent.[47] In neurologically impaired patients, such as those with peripheral neuropathy, total intravenous anesthesia (TIVA) might be required and is commonly performed with a hypnotic (e.g., propofol) and an opioid infusion. Nitrous oxide has more of a depressant effect on signal amplitude rather than latency. Intravenous anesthetics such as propofol tend to have a very limited effect on SSEPs, unless administered in very high doses. Likewise, opioids tend to have a very minimal effect on SSEPs, except with bolus administration, which may decrease amplitudes transiently. Etomidate and ketamine are exceptions in that they actually can increase cortical amplitudes at clinical doses and have been used to enhance SSEP waveforms. Muscle relaxants are generally beneficial for SSEP monitoring as they eliminate myogenic interference. Lastly, it is important to note that these anesthetic effects are much less prominent with regard to subcortical, cervical, and peripheral signal acquisition, as these areas are much more resistant to the inhibitory effects of anesthesia.

MEPs elicited from the scalp are exquisitely sensitive to the effects of anesthesia. Potent volatile anesthetics are greatly inhibitory to the acquisition of MEPs, though doses of 0.5 MAC can still be used. Above this concentration, a nonlinear and greatly accelerated suppression of MEP amplitudes occurs. As with SSEPs, nitrous oxide depresses MEP amplitudes. Intravenous anesthetics are generally conducive to MEP acquisition, except at very high doses. As such, TIVA is commonly employed when MEPs are being monitored. Like SSEPs, ketamine and etomidate may improve MEP amplitudes and lower the electrical threshold required to obtain a response.[48,49] Muscle relaxants must be given very judiciously or avoided completely so as not to abolish the MEP response or prohibitively increase its variability, rendering it difficult to follow over time.[50]

Muscle relaxants can impair or, with deep neuromuscular blockade, abolish, EMG signals. Inhaled and intravenous anesthetics have very little effect on the acquisition of spontaneous or "triggered" EMG. Hence, it is wise to avoid muscle relaxation or reverse the effects of muscle relaxants prior to pedicle screw testing or cranial nerve identification.

BAEPs, as mentioned earlier, are quite robust regardless of the anesthetic regimen being used. Small increases in latency can be seen with deep inhalational or intravenous anesthesia. Notably, cold irrigation fluids at the brainstem will also cause some increases in interwave latencies.

VEPs are the most sensitive neuromonitoring modality with regards to anesthesia. Inhalational-based anesthetics, with and without nitrous oxide, are more inhibitory to VEPs than TIVA techniques in general. One proposed anesthetic technique for facilitating VEP monitoring might involve an opioid-based TIVA with muscle relaxants and BIS monitoring, although other techniques may be used.[51]

Cerebral Perfusion

Transcranial Doppler Ultrasonography

Transcranial Doppler Ultrasonography (TCD) is a tool used in neurology, neurosurgery, and neurocritical care. An ultrasound probe is placed over a "window" that is a thinner region of the cranium, such as the temporal bone above the zygomatic arch, to measure blood flow velocities in major cerebral vessels, including the MCA, PCA, and ACA and the basilar artery. The ultrasound probe emits a high-frequency sound wave that reflects off red blood cells and returns to the probe at a different frequency determined by the Doppler Effect. Specifically, the velocity of blood cells relative to the ultrasound probe will cause a change in the frequency of ultrasound waves that are reflected back to the probe. This "Doppler shift" is proportional to the velocity of blood and the sign (positive or negative) of the Doppler shift is determined by direction of blood flow. Positive (increase in frequency) occurs when blood is moving toward the probe and negative (decrease in frequency) occurs when blood is moving away from the probe. Flow velocity that is greater than expected can indicate stenosis, emboli, or vasospasm. It is important to note that TCD cannot determine actual CBF (reported as flow; that is unit volume per unit time). Rather, TCD measure blood flow velocity (in units of m/s). This distinction is significant as decreased arterial diameter will lead to an increased blood flow velocity but a decrease in blood flow volume. However, in other circumstances, such as cerebral autoregulatory failure, increases in CBF velocity occur with increases in CBF. Therefore, thoughtful interpretation of TCD data is required.[52,53] Also, other parameters that can influence CBF and blood flow velocity must be held constant to minimize their effect on the data. These variables include $PaCO_2$, systemic blood pressure, angle of insonation, and doses of drugs that can impact cerebral hemodynamics including anesthetics. Most TCD monitors are capable of deriving a variety of parameters in addition to mean flow velocity, including pulsatility of the waveform, which reflects distal CVR—commonly called the *pulsatility index*. TCD is also useful in quantifying the status of both static and dynamic autoregulation, using parameters known as the *index of autoregulation* and the *rate of restoration of flow velocity*, respectively.[54]

Laser Doppler Flowmetry

Laser Doppler Flowmetry (LDF) is a relatively new monitoring technology used to quantify blood flow in human tissue such as the brain. LDF employs a very small fiberoptic laser that is 0.5 to 1 mm in diameter and is implanted into the brain. LDF measures the Doppler shift caused by passing red blood cells in microscopic vessels in real-time. Unlike ultrasound that uses sound waves, LDF is based on the Doppler shift in the frequency of light. This signal is then processed to yield the regional CBF. Such measurements are useful in detecting the effects of various physiologic changes, such as anemia and hyperventilation, on CBF. LDF yields measurements of CBF similar to the Xenon (^{133}Xe) washout technique, one of the established gold standard techniques used to determine CBF.[55]

Intracranial Pressure Monitoring

ICP monitoring is a useful tool for patients suffering from any cause of elevated ICP. ICP monitoring is probably most studied in patients with traumatic brain injury (TBI) at risk for intracranial hemorrhage, worsening cerebral edema, and diminished CPP. Normal ICP is 7 to 15 mmHg, and monitoring is generally initiated when ICP is thought to be above 20 mmHg or one is unable to assess for increased ICP by clinical means. ICP greater than 40 mmHg represents severe, life-threatening intracranial hypertension. Knowledge of the ICP alone can be useful but further information about cerebral well-being can be obtained from observing changes in ICP over time. Specifically, the presence of characteristic Lundberg waves can provide valuable information about the state of the brain. There are three, classically described Lundberg waves: A, B, and C (Fig. 37-10). "A waves," also called plateau waves, occur in the setting of severely exhausted compensatory mechanisms for elevated ICP. ICP increases to 50 to 100 mmHg and remains elevated for minutes. "A waves" occur due to intense vasodilation in response to decreased cerebral perfusion and are always pathologic. "B waves" are elevations in ICP of 20 to 30 mmHg above baseline, occurring once or twice a minute and reflecting changes in vascular tone when CPP is at the LLA. "C waves" are small oscillations occurring four to eight times per minute, where ICP is in the normal range, and reflect systemic changes in vasomotor tone, with little pathologic significance.[56]

Monitoring can be accomplished using a variety of devices, most of which are invasive at this time, with a few notable exceptions (e.g., CT scan, optic nerve sheath diameter).[57] Although invasive modalities allow for actual pressure measurement, they have associated risks (described later). Noninvasive modalities, although associated with fewer risks, rely on surrogate variables to estimate ICP and therefore are prone to inaccuracy. The most commonly used device is a ventriculostomy or external ventricular drain (EVD) that measures ICP by way of a transducer (zeroed at the external auditory meatus) connected via tubing placed in the lateral ventricle. Currently, this is the gold standard of ICP monitoring. In addition to pressure transduction, a ventriculostomy also allows for drainage of CSF to attenuate elevated ICP and to provide CSF samples for laboratory diagnostic purposes. Also, a ventriculostomy can be used to deliver drugs, such as antibiotics and thrombolytic agents. There are certain disadvantages with EVD monitoring, including difficulty in placement, fluid leaks, clots, and air bubbles, all of which can lead to inaccurate recording. Most notably, infection is a great risk, since the intraventricular drain pierces the meninges and brain parenchyma. CSF sepsis can lead to increased morbidity and mortality in these patients, and aseptic technique in placement of EVDs is of prime importance.[58]

Intraparenchymal devices are also used to measure ICP, though much less frequently. Two such systems currently exist. The first is a microtransducer system attached to a flexible wire, and the second is a fiberoptic system with a pressure transducer at its tip. Both systems require a hollow screw to be inserted in the skull, whereby the wire or fiberoptic cables can traverse the brain parenchyma. These systems are highly accurate (second only to EVDs), are more easily placed than a ventriculostomy, and are associated with fewer infectious and hemorrhagic risks. Unfortunately, these devices are incapable of removing CSF or allowing drugs to be administered into the CSF.

Subarachnoid "bolts" are not commonly used anymore, but remain an alternative to EVDs. These systems rely on a small bolt that is threaded through a burr hole in the skull, with the tip placed 1 mm beneath the dura. The bolt is then attached to a stopcock assembly and transducer. Subarachnoid bolts are capable of diverting CSF, with lower infectious and hemorrhagic risks than EVDs, but are notoriously inaccurate in measuring ICP; therefore, they are rarely used.[59] Epidural sensor/transducer systems have lower infectious and hemorrhagic risks than EVDs. They are unacceptably inaccurate, however, reflecting only the epidural space and not the entire intracranial compartment.

Cerebral Oxygenation and Metabolism Monitors

Other devices used to monitor the homeostasis of the brain, including its oxygenation and metabolism, are available but may not be commonly employed in the clinical setting. Jugular bulb venous oximetry is the most common of these techniques and involves a fiberoptic catheter placed in a retrograde fashion into the internal jugular vein. The catheter is advanced cephalad beyond the common facial vein and into the jugular bulb that lies at the skull base. Proper placement entails x-ray confirmation of the catheter tip at the level of the mastoid process. This catheter is capable of measuring the mixed cerebral venous oxygen tension ($SjVO_2$) that is indicative of the brain's global oxygen consumption/extraction. Other metabolites that can be measured from this source include lactate and glucose concentrations. Measurement can be accomplished by serial sampling but this method only gives information about the status of the brain at single points in time. Furthermore, extracranial blood may contaminate the sample. More useful perhaps is the continuous fiberoptic measurement of $SjVO_2$. High $SjVO_2$ (80% to 85%) may reflect high oxygen delivery or low $CMRO_2$ whereas low $SjVO_2$ usually indicates low oxygen delivery (e.g., low CBF or hypoxemia) or high $CMRO_2$. $SjVO_2$ below 55%, commonly used to

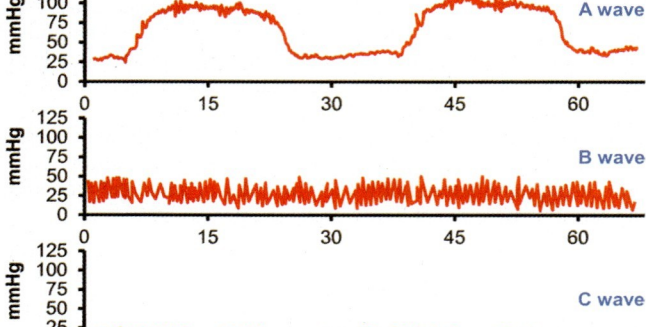

Figure 37-10 Lundberg A, B, and C wave morphologies. (Used with permission of Mayo Foundation for Medical Education and Research. All rights reserved.)

define critical jugular bulb desaturation, may be caused by cerebral ischemia in the setting of systemic hypotension or markedly elevated ICP.[60] SjVO$_2$ may be useful in guiding hyperventilation that results in a reduction in SjVO$_2$ due to vasoconstriction, with the goal of maintaining the saturation above 55%.[61]

Other monitors used to measure cerebral metabolism include brain tissue oxygen monitors and microdialysis catheters. Brain tissue oxygen monitors measure the partial pressure of oxygen (PbtO$_2$) in a portion of brain interstitium 15 to 20 mm wide, directly and invasively, via a Clark-type electrode. PbtO$_2$ is normally 25 to 48 mmHg. PbtO$_2$ values reflect the balance between oxygen supply and demand in the region of brain surrounding the electrode. Factors that affect PbtO$_2$ include local oxygen delivery, predicted by the fraction of inspired oxygen, cardiac output, hemoglobin concentration, local oxygen extraction, PaO$_2$, and CBF. Generally, values below 20 mmHg in pathologic brain states are considered significant and may portend secondary injury to otherwise healthy brain tissue.[62] Indications for brain tissue oxygen monitoring are most commonly TBI and SAH, and experience is growing with this type of monitoring.

Cerebral microdialysis is becoming more popular in neurocritical care units. A filamentous catheter is placed into the brain parenchyma, consisting of outer and inner tubes and a semipermeable membrane at its tip. A pump is used to perfuse the inner catheter with a crystalloid solution that is iso-osmolar with CSF. At the tip of the catheter, metabolites in the extracellular fluid are driven by a concentration gradient into the outer tubing and are eventually collected into a microvial. This solution is then analyzed for its metabolite contents and their concentrations, including glucose, pyruvate, lactate, glutamate, and glycerol. Clinical correlation with attention to the location of the catheter tip and comparison of values over time, is required. Although glucose, pyruvate, and lactate concentrations are measures of adequate aerobic metabolism, glutamate and glycerol levels represent ischemic neuronal stress and cell membrane degradation, respectively.[63] Indeed, one of the major limitations of cerebral microdialysis as well as brain tissue oxygen monitors is that findings will depend on the location of measurement. For example, measurement of values obtained from regions of brain remote from the site of brain injury might indicate minimal, if any, abnormality. Therefore, microdialysis and measurement of oxygen partial pressure is best obtained from locations where "at risk" brain exists.

Lastly, cerebral oximetry has become more prevalent in the clinical setting recently. This technology involves a noninvasive, transcutaneous, measurement of regional cerebral blood oxygenation (rSO$_2$) over the frontal cortices bilaterally. Oxygenation is given as a percentage of maximum hemoglobin saturation. This reflects the contribution of both arterial and venous blood. A decrease of at least 20% from baseline values is considered significant hypoxia, though definitive data in this regard do not exist.[64] Mechanistically, light from the probe placed on the forehead is transmitted through the skull. Hemoglobin oxygen saturation is determined by the ratio of the absorbances of two or more different wavelengths of light allowing for the determination of oxyhemoglobin and deoxyhemoglobin. This technology differs from pulse oximetry in that it uses two photodetectors, thereby allowing for subtraction of the absorbance from hemoglobin in the scalp and skull. Specifically, near-field photodetection is subtracted from far-field photodetection, yielding a value of brain tissue oxygenation. Cerebral oximetry also differs from pulse oximetry in that it does not rely on pulsatile blood flow. Regional estimates of cerebral oxygenation in the frontal cerebral cortices provide a sensitive method of detecting changes in oxygen delivery due to the very limited oxygen reserve of this highly metabolic area. Factors that may play a role in averting long-term injury based on low cerebral oximetry values include increasing systemic blood pressure, increasing cardiac output, increasing oxygen delivery (FiO$_2$), increasing PaCO$_2$ to ameliorate cerebral vasoconstriction, or red blood cell transfusion to increase oxygen-carrying capacity and delivery.[65]

Cerebral Protection

Ischemic and Reperfusion

Because of its high rate of oxygen and glucose consumption, inability to store substrate, and inability to dispose of toxic metabolites quickly, the brain is especially susceptible to rapid ischemic injury. With the accumulation of intracellular calcium (Ca^{2+}) under ischemic conditions, neuronal damage quickly occurs and is compounded by the accumulation of lactic acid.[66] Global ischemia, as can occur during severe hypotension and severe anemia, may be responsive to interventions that restore total cerebral perfusion and oxygen-carrying capacity, such as cardiopulmonary resuscitation (CPR) or red blood cell transfusion. Focal ischemia occurs due to a regional insult such as an embolus or arterial disruption. Treatment of focal ischemia must be focused on restoring perfusion to the region in question. In cases of focal ischemia, a penumbra of salvageable tissue usually surrounds a necrotic core of dead parenchyma. Efforts must also be directed at restoring oxygen and substrate delivery to the ischemic penumbra that is being supplied by some collateral circulation. Much of the research being performed in cerebral protection today deals with this concept of "saving the penumbra," and practical methods include augmentation of CPP and reducing brain edema in the acute setting (see later).[67] Another area under study is that of reperfusion and "reperfusion injury." Specifically, reperfusion of previously ischemic brain tissue can actually worsen neurologic outcome largely due to the production of free radicals derived from oxygen and mediators of inflammation and exacerbation of injury of the microvasculature upon restoration of flow.[68,69]

Hypothermia

Induced systemic hypothermia has been regarded as a potentially beneficial intervention in certain subgroups of the neurologically injured population, though definitive human studies regarding its consistent efficacy have been lacking. Theoretically, hypothermia should be extremely protective to the brain and spinal cord from a metabolic standpoint, as it lowers the CMRO$_2$ of the CNS to a much greater extent than anesthetics are capable of doing. Although anesthetics can cause an isoelectric EEG, reducing the brain's metabolic activity by up to 60%, hypothermia can do far more by reducing even the brain's homeostatic need for oxygen, required for basic neuronal survival. Animal models have shown that cerebral protection is possible with even a decrease of 1°C in core temperature, demonstrating that the possible protective effects of hypothermia on the CNS are not simply a result of decreased metabolism, but rather may involve other mechanisms as well.[70]

The use of hypothermia in patients with global ischemia may be promising. Profound hypothermia in humans (27°C), as is currently used for cold-cardiopulmonary bypass, and deep hypothermia (12°C to 18°C) used during circulatory arrest, have been shown to provide cerebral protection.[71] When adults who have sustained an out-of-hospital cardiac arrest and return of spontaneous circulation, are cooled to 32°C to 34°C for

12 to 24 hours, neurologic outcome may be improved.[72] Clinical improvement has also been seen in neonates with hypoxic-ischemic encephalopathy treated with mild hypothermia within 6 hours of delivery.[73]

The use of hypothermia in those with focal ischemia is less promising. The Intraoperative Hypothermia for Aneurysm Surgery Trial (IHAST) demonstrated no improvement in neurologic outcome but higher rates of infectious complications in patients who had cerebral aneurysm clipping with mild total-body hypothermia compared to those that had normothermic management.[74] Data involving TBI patients and mild hypothermia have yielded mixed results, with "short-term" cooling (24 to 48 hours) showing little benefit, whereas "long-term" cooling for up to 5 days showing some promise.[75]

What is clearly known in both humans and animals is that cerebral hyperthermia is detrimental, with focal cerebral ischemic infarct size in animals tripling for each 1°C rise in core temperature.[76] Hyperthermia must be avoided in the setting of cerebral ischemia.

Pharmacologic Therapy for Cerebral Protection

As with induced hypothermia, there is promise for cerebral protection in the setting of neuronal ischemia by both anesthetic and nonanesthetic drugs. However, most of this data comes from animal stroke models and not definitive human studies. Anesthetics may mitigate the effects of CNS ischemia both by their reduction on $CMRO_2$ as well as by other molecular mechanisms. Volatile anesthetics may reduce ischemia-induced glutamate release, increase the availability of antiapoptotic mediators, activate ATP-dependent potassium channels, reduce excitotoxic stressors, and augment CBF.[77,78] Likewise, barbiturates (of proven benefit in focal ischemia in animal studies),[79] nitrous oxide, propofol, etomidate, ketamine, and lidocaine have been associated with beneficial effects on cerebral ischemia in animal and preclinical studies.[80,81]

Nonanesthetic agents, too, have been the focus of many studies for their possible neuroprotective effects. Calcium-channel blockers, by inhibiting the effects of voltage-gated calcium channels, have been investigated, although they do not seem clinically useful for this indication.[82] Likewise, magnesium has been investigated as a possible neuroprotective agent, by virtue of its antagonistic effect on various voltage-gated and transmitter-activated channels, though so far human clinical studies are disappointing.[83]

Other agents, such as free radical scavengers (e.g., tirilazad, α-tocopherol, NXY-059),[84] amino acid modulators (e.g., gavestinel),[85] erythropoietin (activates antiapoptotic pathways and decreases inflammation),[86] and most recently statins for their upregulation of nitric oxide synthase and both anti-inflammatory and antioxidative effects are currently under investigation. Interestingly, patients treated with statins for 1 to 6 months, without cardiac disease, showed a 16% reduction in stroke risk in a recent human study, though other human data demonstrate no protective effect, or even a deleterious effect, on patients having already suffered a hemorrhagic stroke.[87] Despite ongoing, and often promising, work in this field, it is important to note that a single and definitive neuroprotective agent in human clinical studies has never been identified.

Glucose and Cerebral Ischemia

As mentioned earlier, ischemia is rapidly detrimental to the nervous system not only because of oxygen starvation but also because glucose is the only substrate that can be aerobically metabolized by the brain under normal conditions. Glucose is not stored in the nervous system, so when glucose is reduced or absent due to limited cerebral circulation, adenosine triphosphate (ATP) is no longer produced at a rate that supplies the energy requirement of neurons and cellular injury quickly ensues. Cerebral glucose consumption (5 mg/100 g/min) parallels $CMRO_2$, so hypoxemia and hypoglycemia are roughly equally detrimental to the brain. With cerebral ischemia and hypoglycemia, lactate is metabolized to some extent in the brain, but with much less efficacy than glucose.[88] Hyperglycemia (serum blood glucose over 180 mg/dL) in the setting of cerebral ischemia has also been shown to worsen neurologic outcomes, presumably by worsening cerebral acidosis in an anaerobic setting, in which glucose is converted to lactic acid.[89,90]

A Practical Approach

Reliable pharmacologic and nonpharmacologic therapies to prevent neuronal ischemic injury are currently not readily available for use in the perioperative period. One can only hope to attenuate injury. With some exceptions, inhaled and intravenous anesthetics may protect the brain from ischemic injury. For surgeries in which there is planned regional ischemia, such as temporary clipping of cerebral vessels during aneurysm surgery, propofol given in a large bolus (1 to 2 mg/kg) followed by a high-dose infusion (150 μg/kg/min) is often used and titrated to induce burst-suppression *prior* to the planned ischemia. In cardiac or neurologic surgeries in which circulatory and pulmonary arrest is planned, such as aortic arch repair or giant basilar aneurysm clipping, deep hypothermia (12°C to 18°C) can be instituted to protect the nervous system. Another example of practical neurologic protection involves the placement of a lumbar CSF drain prior to thoracoabdominal aortic aneurysm repair. This technique is used to lower CSF pressure and ostensibly maintain spinal cord perfusion when radicular arteries originating from the aorta are at surgical risk.

Anesthetic Management

Preoperative Evaluation

The preoperative evaluation of the neurosurgical patient is of paramount importance to ensure a safe and successful anesthetic. Specific problems must be identified so as to formulate appropriate plans for intraoperative and postoperative management. For patients with intracranial mass lesions, the most important fact to ascertain is the presence and extent of intracranial hypertension and this should be assumed until information proves otherwise. This information can be obtained most readily from the history and physical examination, CT and magnetic resonance imaging (MRI) scans, and ICP measurements, if available. Patients with elevated ICP may complain of headaches, dizziness, visual or gait disturbances, nausea or vomiting, and seizures. On physical examination, such patients may exhibit abnormalities such as altered level of consciousness, confusion, papilledema, loss of strength or sensation, and cranial nerve dysfunction. Radiologic studies are generally most helpful in quantifying the degree of ICP derangement with "slit ventricles," or a shift of midline brain structure of more than 5 mm indicating advanced pathology.[91] As part of a preoperative evaluation of the neurosurgical patient, findings on routine blood tests can also prove useful. A careful evaluation of laboratory values may demonstrate electrolyte disturbances, which can be due to pituitary pathology (e.g., syndrome of inappropriate antidiuretic hormone secretion [SIADH]), diuretics, steroids, or anticonvulsants being taken by the patient.

In patients with elevated ICP, premedication must be carefully titrated, or avoided completely. Benzodiazepines and opioids, even in small doses, can depress respiration, leading to elevated PaCO$_2$ and subsequent exacerbation of intracranial hypertension. Corticosteroids, such as dexamethasone, and anticonvulsants should be continued preoperatively.[92]

Preoperative evaluation of patients presenting for spine surgery, especially in the acute setting, should focus on the airway examination, current hemodynamic conditions, the level of injury, the degree of injury (complete versus incomplete), the timing of injury (i.e., less than 8 hours or 8 hours or more), and the complete neurologic examination. Carefully planning for endotracheal intubation and subsequent hemodynamic management of these patients is vital, as advanced airway techniques and critical fluid management with concomitant vasopressor use may be required.

Induction of Anesthesia and Airway Management

Induction of general anesthesia and airway management are critically important periods, especially in those patients who have elevated ICP, an unsecured aneurysm, or cervical spinal cord injury. Constant attention to hemodynamics is critical in patients with elevated ICP in order to maintain CPP. To that end, the induction of general anesthesia in patients with elevated ICP should be "slow and controlled," with constant attention to the blood pressure throughout the process.[93] In many cases, preinduction arterial catheterization, osmotic diuresis, or CSF drainage may be helpful. Hypotension must be avoided. Patients with elevated ICP may receive a short-acting opioid and lidocaine (1.5 mg/kg) intravenously to blunt the sympathetic response to laryngoscopy. Also, hypoventilation and hypercapnia should be avoided. Following induction of anesthesia, a muscle relaxant should be administered. Succinylcholine should be used with caution in patients with pre-existing motor deficits as upregulation of nicotinic receptors at the neuromuscular junction can lead to increased risk of hyperkalemia. Also, succinylcholine can increase ICP but this effect is of short duration.[94] During intubation, strict control of blood pressure is important, as a rapid increase in arterial blood pressure will worsen ICP, especially in patients with autoregulatory failure, or put an unsecured aneurysm at risk of rupture. Hypotension and decreased CPP can also be detrimental. In the case of a cervical spinal cord injury, maintenance of MAP is very important during induction of anesthesia, whereas the actual performance of intubation may require more complex techniques (e.g., awake fiberoptic intubation, midline and sagittal stabilization) to ensure that the spinal cord is not further compromised.

Maintenance of Anesthesia

The maintenance of general anesthesia in neurosurgical patients requires regimens that vary depending on the hemodynamic and monitoring goals for that procedure. For intracranial surgeries, ICP control is paramount until the dura mater is opened. To this end, once Mayfield fixation of the head and positioning are safely completed, mannitol (0.5 to 1.5 g/kg) may be administered if ICP control is needed, as are steroids (e.g., dexamethasone 10 mg) and, in some cases, a prophylactic anticonvulsant. Choice of drugs for maintenance of general anesthesia depends to a great extent on the ICP and whether neuromonitoring is being employed. For patients with elevated ICP, volatile anesthetics are often limited to 0.5 MAC, if used at all, to minimize the degree of cerebral vasodilation and inhibition of autoregulation that can result. Anesthesia is either maintained or supplemented with intravenous drug infusions such as propofol with or without a short-acting opioid such as remifentanil or sufentanil. This regimen works well in neuromonitoring cases as well, where more than 0.5 MAC of volatile agent may interfere with SSEP and MEP monitoring. Muscle relaxants are generally used, unless limited by MEP or EMG monitoring, and nitrous oxide may be considered in select neurosurgical cases. Because of its mild vasodilating effects, potential for expanding pneumocephalus, and unfavorable effects on neuromonitoring, N$_2$O should be avoided in cases where the patient has significantly increased ICP, the potential for intradural air, or where it will interfere with monitoring modalities. In the absence of muscle relaxant, immobility can be achieved with remifentanil infusions approaching 0.2 μg/kg/min.[95] Throughout the procedure, CPP must be maintained, possibly requiring a vasopressor. If autoregulation is greatly inhibited due to the disease process or the anesthetic drugs, CBF will be directly dependent on MAP, thus hypertension should be avoided. In cases of acute spinal cord injury, many of the same principles apply in regards to maintenance of anesthesia, as spinal cord perfusion (especially in cervical spine surgery) and the ability to perform neuromonitoring are of great concern.

Ventilation Management

Ventilatory management of patients undergoing neurosurgery is also a key consideration. For patients undergoing an intracranial procedure, tidal volume should be maintained at 6 to 8 mL/kg to minimize potential inflammatory injury to the lungs, with peak pressures kept at less than 40 cmH$_2$O.[96] These principles hold especially true for patients with SAH or TBI, who may already exhibit acute lung injury (ALI) or adult respiratory distress syndrome (ARDS). Positive end-expiratory pressure (PEEP) should be avoided unless needed to improve oxygenation, as it increases intrathoracic pressure and may impede cerebral venous drainage.[97] Positive pressure ventilation (PPV) is generally used for neurosurgical procedures, as it allows direct control of PaCO$_2$, and is especially beneficial during sitting craniotomies, where negative intrathoracic pressure may contribute to the development of venous air embolism (VAE).

Fluids and Electrolytes

For many years, the teaching of fluid maintenance during craniotomy was to keep the patient "dry," so as to minimize the amount of reactive cerebral edema both during the surgery and postoperatively. This strategy is generally not considered optimal, as the primary goal of fluid management in neurosurgical cases should be to maintain cerebral perfusion, which is a more important consideration and will actually lessen the amount of cerebral edema produced.[98] Hence, the goal of fluid management should be to keep the patient euvolemic. Isotonic or slightly hypertonic solutions (e.g., 0.9% sodium chloride) should be used if large amounts of fluid are to be administered. Hypotonic solutions, such as Ringer lactate, when administered in large amounts, can contribute to cerebral edema. Glucose-containing solutions are avoided, as hyperglycemia is detrimental to cerebral metabolism (see section Glucose and Cerebral Ischemia), and because glucose is quickly metabolized and not osmotically active, leaving free water that can worsen brain edema.

Depending on patient comorbidities and length of the surgery, electrolyte derangements may be common and require close monitoring. Certainly, patients with SIADH, diabetes insipidus (DI), or cerebral salt wasting syndrome, will require careful monitoring of electrolytes. Hypertonic saline (3%) supplementation (given slowly at a rate of 50 to 100 mL/hr, and with the serum sodium level checked hourly) may be required in moderate to severe hyponatremic states.[99] Rapid rises in serum sodium (more than 3 to 4 mEq/L/hr) must be avoided as this poses a risk for central pontine myelinolysis.[100] In patients with DI, hypotonic solutions such as Ringer lactate or 0.45% sodium chloride might be required and their administration should be carefully titrated based on volume status and serum electrolyte concentrations. Mannitol, especially at large doses, can cause mild electrolyte derangements which are generally short-lived (e.g., hyponatremia, hyperkalemia), and these should be monitored and possibly corrected. Also, diuresis from mannitol can result in dehydration that can impair cerebral perfusion.[101] Sodium chloride solution (0.9%), given in large amounts, can cause hyperchloremic metabolic acidosis and subsequent acute kidney injury due to renal tubular acidosis.[102]

Transfusion Therapy

The transfusion of blood products may be required perioperatively in patients having neurosurgical procedures. Preoperatively, coagulation studies, if available, should be carefully noted and are required in patients receiving anticoagulants.[103] Preoperative coagulopathies should be corrected as intraoperative or postoperative bleeding can have a significantly adverse impact on outcome. Neurosurgical patients having nonurgent surgery should have a platelet count over 100,000/mm³. For patients having craniotomy for indications that would that would be at low risk for intraoperative bleeding, a "type and screen" with a negative antibody screen may be adequate. Red blood cells that are "typed and crossed" should be available for procedures with high risk for bleeding such as neurovascular procedures (e.g., aneurysm clipping, arteriovenous malformation [AVM] resection) or tumor craniotomies that invade the cranial sinuses. For coagulopathies that may develop with the release of brain tissue thromboplastin, fresh frozen plasma, platelets, and cryoprecipitate may be needed. Complex spine surgery (especially with planned osteotomies or due to tumor) is usually associated with more profound blood loss, volume shifts, and the need for transfusion therapy. In these cases, multiple units of blood products should be immediately available and close, repetitive monitoring of the complete blood count (CBC) and coagulation studies should be performed.[104]

Glucose Management

As discussed earlier, glucose management is very important in neurosurgical cases for the prevention of both hypo- and hyperglycemia. In 2001, van den Berghe et al.[105] showed that strict glycemic control (i.e., target serum glucose concentration of 80 to 110 mg/dL) in critically ill surgical patients was associated with improved outcome. In recent years, however, strict glycemic control has been associated with increased risk for hypoglycemia that can be detrimental to the brain.[106,107] To reduce the risk of both hypoglycemia and excessive hyperglycemia, most authors agree that serum glucose during neurosurgical procedures should be maintained in the 90- to 180-mg/dL range. For hyperglycemia exceeding this range, short-acting insulin should be readily available and can be given intravenously as a bolus with or without an infusion. In these cases, monitoring of serum glucose must be frequent enough to capture episodes of hypoglycemia.[108] In cases of hypoglycemia, 50% dextrose should be available, and 20 to 50 mL of this solution is administered with further titration based on continued close monitoring of serum glucose concentration.

Emergence

Emergence from general anesthesia following neurosurgical procedures requires meticulous attention to hemodynamic and ventilatory parameters, while also ensuring a prompt neurologic examination. Postcraniotomy hypertension is a well-described, albeit poorly understood, phenomenon, but can certainly be detrimental as it may increase bleeding from the surgical site and worsen cerebral edema.[109,110] Careful analgesia (so as not to obtund the patient postoperatively) is helpful to minimize risk for hypertension, but usually antihypertensive medications are required. These can include labetalol, esmolol, nicardipine, or clevidipine. Control of hypertension is especially important for patients emerging from cerebral AVM resection, as bleeding from the resection bed may be very significant. In patients having undergone posterior fossa surgery, and those in whom a pre-existing ventilatory disturbance was present due to brainstem compromise, emergence may be much slower and the time to safe extubation much more prolonged.[111] Coughing on emergence for all patients should be avoided due to the risk of bleeding and elevation in ICP, and a low-dose remifentanil infusion or either intravenous or intratracheal lidocaine may be helpful in this regard. Likewise, postoperative nausea and vomiting should be prophylactically treated in these cases for the same reasons.[112] Dexamethasone used for this indication should be avoided in patients in whom the diagnosis of lymphoma is being considered (or at least delayed until an adequate pathology specimen is obtained), as steroids can causes tumor lysis of lymphoma and potentially interfere with diagnosis. Also, dexamethasone should also be avoided following pituitary surgery as it can suppress the hypothalamic–pituitary–adrenal axis and significantly increase the false positive rate for diagnosis of postoperative hypopituitarism.[113]

Common Surgical Procedures

Surgery for Tumors

One of the most common indications for neurosurgery is the removal of both benign and malignant tumors that emanate from or spread to the CNS or PNS. In adults, supratentorial lesions are more common and include tumors derived from support cells in the CNS (e.g., gliomas, astrocytomas, oligodendrogliomas), meningiomas, or metastases. The most common metastatic tumors to the brain include melanoma or those that originate in the lung, breast, or kidney. Infratentorial tumors in the posterior fossa are more common in children and include medulloblastoma, pilocytic astrocytoma, ependymoma, and brainstem glioma.[114]

Independent of their histology, the morbidity of brain tumors is associated with their size, rate of growth, and proximity to and invasion of nearby structures. Furthermore, glial disruption of the BBB may cause significant vasogenic edema, which may persist even after tumor resection, and autoregulation is usually impaired in parenchyma surrounding tumors.[115] Fortunately, most brain tumors grow slowly, allowing adaptive and compensatory mechanisms to accommodate increases in ICP due to edema or mass effect. Unfortunately, this same fact often leads to delayed diagnosis.

The anesthetic management of these patients must take all of these factors into account, as patients with dangerously elevated ICP preoperatively must be treated with great caution, sometimes requiring preoperative CSF diversion and dexamethasone. Surgery for intracranial tumors can be safely accomplished with a careful preoperative evaluation and a smooth induction, maintenance, and emergence regimen. Preoperative assessment should include an understanding of the lesion site and dimensions, plan for surgical approach, neurologic symptomatology, ICP concerns, and medical comorbidities. Anxiolysis with benzodiazepines must be carefully considered, as even small increases in $PaCO_2$ in otherwise asymptomatic patients can quickly lead to dangerously elevated ICP due to increased intracranial elastance. Steroids and anticonvulsants should be continued, and in many cases supplemented, prior to and during craniotomy. Hemodynamic instability during any part of the anesthetic should be minimized due to the possibility of impaired autoregulation in peritumoral brain parenchyma. Hypertension can increase the risk of bleeding and exacerbate brain edema. Generally, propofol is administered for induction of general anesthesia. Lidocaine (1 to 1.5 mg/kg) and fentanyl (1 to 2 µg/kg) may be given intravenously to blunt the hemodynamic and ICP response to laryngoscopy. Adequate vascular access (usually two large-bore peripheral intravenous catheters, and arterial catheter, and possibly a central venous catheter) is mandatory for brain tumor resection. ICP and CPP are of great concern throughout these procedures, and an arterial catheter is very helpful to monitor CPP closely while also allowing the titration of $PaCO_2$ by revealing its gradient with end-expired CO_2 via arterial blood gas measurement.[116] After vascular access is established and any neuromonitoring modalities are applied, the Mayfield pins are usually applied to the skull. The hemodynamic response is similar to laryngoscopy, and optimal control of blood pressure must again be sought, often by using propofol, opioids, or short-acting β-adrenergic antagonists such as esmolol.

Excessive flexion, extension, or rotation of the neck may impair cerebral venous drainage via compression of the internal jugular veins. A head-up position is also favorable to promote venous drainage. PEEP should be avoided, or used cautiously, as this may also impair venous drainage, although if oxygenation is impaired, a PEEP up to 10 cm H_2O can be considered. In patients with large tumors or known significant intracranial hypertension, efforts should be made to decrease brain volume for optimal surgical exposure and to minimize retractor-related edema. This can include mild hyperventilation and use of mannitol (0.5 to 1.5 g/kg) or hypertonic saline (3% starting at 50 to 100 mL/hr with hourly sodium surveillance).[117] Mannitol should be given as a bolus to achieve its full effect, although great care should be taken in patients with congestive heart failure, pulmonary edema, or renal failure as the initial elevation in central circulatory volume may be detrimental in these patients prior to the diuretic phase.[118] For maintenance of general anesthesia, the choice of anesthetics is heavily dictated by avoiding increases in ICP (at least until the dura is open), maintaining CPP, neuromonitoring requirements, and ensuring a rapid emergence. Short-acting and easily titratable drugs are generally preferred. These include propofol, remifentanil, sevoflurane, desflurane, and possibly nitrous oxide unless otherwise contraindicated. Muscle relaxants are beneficial if not precluded by neuromonitoring. Fluid maintenance should be accomplished with dextrose-free iso-osmolar crystalloids or colloids, with the goal of euvolemia (see earlier).

Patients who demonstrated a normal level of consciousness (Glasgow Coma Score [GCS] of 13 to 15) preoperatively are generally extubated at the conclusion of the case, and as with induction, hemodynamic stability is paramount during this period. Aberrations in blood pressure, usually systemic hypertension, can lead to worsening cerebral edema or tumor resection bed bleeding postoperatively, and short-acting and easily titratable drugs, such as labetalol, nicardipine, or esmolol should be immediately available. Coughing at extubation, and vomiting after extubation, which may both worsen ICP, can be minimized with careful opioid titration and a prophylactic antiemetic. Adequate analgesia must be ensured as well, as craniotomy is painful and inadequate analgesia can worsen systemic hypertension. At the same time, avoiding analgesic doses which may obtund the patient and preclude a careful neurologic assessment is vitally important. In this regard, the use of short-acting opioids (i.e., remifentanil, fentanyl), local anesthetic infiltration, intravenous acetaminophen, or dexmedetomidine can be considered.[119-122]

Infratentorial tumors and tumors of the posterior fossa, due to their proximity to the brainstem, may be associated with more hemodynamic perturbations intraoperatively and postoperatively, as well as changes in respiratory control and arousal levels postoperatively. These patients may more frequently require postoperative intubation and mechanical ventilation, due to altered levels of consciousness and delayed emergence.

In adults, tumors of the posterior fossa include acoustic neuromas, metastases, meningiomas, and hemangioblastomas. These tumors, because of their proximity to the brainstem and cranial nerves, can cause altered respiratory patterns, cardiac dysrhythmias, or cranial nerve dysfunction. Surgery for these tumors can be performed in the prone, lateral, or sitting positions, and may require specific cranial nerve monitoring, such as EMG or BAERs of cranial nerves. The sitting position requires special attention, as the risk of VAE is increased. VAE occurs when the operative site is above the level of the right atrium in the presence of open, noncollapsible venous channels. VAE occurs in 30% to 75% of all sitting posterior fossa surgery, but is usually hemodynamically insignificant. It is estimated that 8% to 15% of episodes of VAE cause significant hemodynamic change.[123,124] When air is entrained into the heart and pulmonary circulation, it can lead to impaired gas exchange, intrapulmonary shunting, hypoxemia, and a concomitant decrease in end-expired CO_2. If air entrainment becomes severe, arrhythmias, decreased cardiac output, severe pulmonary hypertension, and hemodynamic collapse can result. Monitoring for VAE in the sitting position may include precordial Doppler ultrasonography, which can detect 0.25 mL of air in the heart. A more sensitive monitor is transesophageal echocardiography, which is much more cumbersome, invasive, and requires an observer familiar with this technique. Also, transesophageal echocardiography may not allow for continuous monitoring for air as the device will cease working when probe temperature rises from normal use to a preset value. However, transesophageal echocardiography allows for a quantitative assessment of intracardiac air whereas precordial Doppler sonography is a qualitative monitor for VAE (i.e., indicates only if air is present in the heart).

Prevention of VAE entails decreasing the height difference between the operative site and the heart as much as possible, maintaining euvolemia, and the use of bone wax by the surgeon to occlude visibly open dural venous sinuses or larger veins. Treatment of VAE includes notifying the surgeon to flood the surgical field, administering 100% oxygen, aspirating air through a multiorifice central venous catheter positioned at the junction of the superior vena cava and right atrium, and supportive hemodynamic care. Depending on the degree of hemodynamic perturbation, treatment may include vasopressors, fluids, inotropes, and adjusting the OR table position so that the head is at the level of the heart. This final maneuver is saved for severe or unremitting manifestations of VAE as it likely will disrupt the surgical field. If nitrous oxide was being used, it should be stopped not only to deliver 100% oxygen but also because nitrous oxide may increase air bubble volume, potentially exacerbating the clinical effects of VAE. The application of PEEP, although theoretically favorable, is generally not helpful.[125]

Pituitary Surgery

Pituitary surgery is usually performed endoscopically and transnasally. Anesthetic concerns for pituitary surgery include systemic manifestations of any associated endocrinopathy, electrolyte and fluid disturbances caused by endocrine disease, SIADH, or DI, and inadvertent surgical trespass into the cavernous sinus or internal carotid artery. Patients with a sellar mass may exhibit visual field defects, and a careful history and physical examination preoperatively is important to differentiate between organic and anesthetic causes of visual problems after surgery.

Growth hormone (GH) secreting tumors cause acromegaly. A large mandible and hypertrophy of tissue leads to decreased airway aperture and predisposes to obstructive sleep apnea and difficulty with mask ventilation and intubation. Also, a smaller sized endotracheal tube and additional tools and strategies to secure the airway, such as awake fiberoptic intubation or a video laryngoscope–based intubation may be considered. Furthermore, longstanding acromegalics are prone to cardiac rhythm disturbances and hypertrophic cardiomyopathy, and caution with cardiac depressant medications is warranted.

Adrenocorticotropic hormone (ACTH) secreting tumors cause Cushing syndrome by causing hypercortisolism. Cushing syndrome is associated with glucose intolerance or diabetes mellitus, increased skin fragility (potentially making peripheral intravenous access difficult), impaired wound healing, and secondary hypertension. There is some data to suggest, however, that Cushing syndrome are not significantly associated with airway difficulty.[126]

Patients with thyroid-stimulating hormone (TSH) secreting pituitary adenomas should be rendered euthyroid before surgery unless vision is threatened. Such patients may have inadvertently been treated for Grave disease preoperatively, thereby decreasing the production of free T4 and T3 hormones and reducing the amount of negative feedback to the pituitary adenoma, which may predispose to rapid tumor growth.[127]

SIADH is common with sellar tumors, due to compression of the posterior pituitary and an excess of circulating antidiuretic hormone (ADH), which may lead to intravascular volume overload and hyponatremia. Extracellular body water is usually normal, and edema or hypertension is usually not characteristic. Treatment of perioperative SIADH involves water restriction (to the extent that it is safe to do so), treating the underlying cause, and demeclocycline which is a tetracycline antibiotic that inhibits ADH action in the renal tubules. The hallmark of DI is polyuria with dilute urine output. Fluid replacement is required and desmopressin may be needed for persistent or severe cases.[128]

Because accidental surgical entry into the cavernous sinus or internal carotid artery is a known, albeit infrequent, complication of pituitary surgery, adequate vascular access and an arterial catheter are recommended. A lumbar subarachnoid catheter is sometimes placed before or after pituitary surgery.

Intraoperatively, injection of air or sterile saline or withdrawal of CSF can facilitate exposure of the tumor as increases or decreases in intracranial volume can serve to move the sellar structures inferiorly or superiorly, respectively. Postoperatively, a lumbar CSF drainage catheter can be used to drain CSF that will decrease CSF volume where a dural sealant or fat graft has been used and reduce the risk for chronic CSF leakage.[129]

Cerebral Aneurysm Surgery and Endovascular Treatment

The development of cerebral aneurysms, and their likeliness to rupture causing SAH, is associated with age over 40 years, female sex, cigarette smoking, systemic hypertension, or connective tissue disorders.[130] Ruptured aneurysms are the most common cause of spontaneous SAH, accounting for 80% of nontraumatic SAH. Aneurysms are thought to arise from turbulent blood flow at arterial branching points, causing "sac-like" or "fusiform" dilatations to occur. Cerebral aneurysms most commonly occur at the anterior communicating arteries (40%), PCOMs (25%), and MCA (25%), with only 10% arising from the vertebrobasilar system.[131]

Following SAH, an acute increase in ICP is accompanied by a decrease in CPP. These changes result in an increase in systemic blood pressure to maintain CBF. Patients may present with severe headache (classically, the "worst headache of my life"), nausea and vomiting, photophobia, seizures, focal neurologic deficits, and altered consciousness. A noncontrast head CT scan is usually sufficient to diagnose SAH, but more sophisticated imaging, such as digital-subtraction angiography, CT angiography, or MRI angiography, is required to identify the location and morphology of the aneurysm.

Cerebral aneurysms, and their neurologic sequelae, are categorized by a variety of ways for both treatment and prognostication. The Hunt and Hess Grading Scale (based on clinical symptoms) (Table 37-2),[132] the World Federation of Neurological Surgeons Grading Scale (based on GCS and motor deficits) (Table 37-3),[133] and the Fisher Grade System (based on radiologic bleeding) (Table 37-4)[134] are commonly used. Aneurysm size is an important factor when considering management. "Small" aneurysms are less than 10 mm in diameter, "large" aneurysms are 10 to 24 mm in diameter, and "giant" aneurysms are more than 24 mm in diameter. Rupture risk increases with aneurysm diameter, with those larger than 6 mm generally requiring treatment.[135]

Preoperative assessment must include knowledge of the aneurysm size and location and whether it is intact or ruptured. Caring for patients with ruptured aneurysms must take into account the presence and possibility of rebleeding, vasospasm of cerebral arteries, hydrocephalus, cardiac dysfunction, neurogenic pulmonary

Table 37-2	Hunt and Hess Grading System
Hunt and Hess Grade	Clinical Symptoms
0	Unruptured aneurysm/asymptomatic
1	Minimal headache, slight nuchal rigidity
2	Moderate to severe headache, nuchal rigidity, cranial nerve palsy
3	Mildly obtunded, confused, focal deficits
4	Severely obtunded, hemiparesis, early decerebrate posturing
5	Coma, decerebrate posturing

Table 37-3 World Federation of Neurological Surgeons (WFNS) Grading Scale

WFNS Grade	Glasgow Coma Scale Score	Motor Deficit
1	15	No
2	14–13	No
3	14–13	Yes
4	12–7	Yes or no
5	6–3	Yes or no

edema, and seizures. Cerebral vasospasm rarely occurs within 72 hours of rupture. Surgical or endovascular treatment of ruptured aneurysms is generally undertaken within the first 48 hours after presentation of SAH, to minimize the risk of rebleeding but prior to increased risk for cerebral vasospasm. Cardiac and pulmonary conditions should be optimized to the greatest extent possible, which may require inotropes, antiarrhythmics, hypertonic saline supplementation if SIADH or cerebral salt wasting syndrome are present, maintenance of euvolemia, and maintenance of tissue oxygenation, all without delay of surgical treatment. Furthermore, enteral nimodipine and a statin drug should be administered per ICU protocol. Nimodipine is the only intervention that decreases risk for cerebral vasospasm. Statins, via their pleotropic effects, may also decrease risk of vasospasm.

Aneurysms amenable to surgical clipping are usually saccular as opposed to fusiform in morphology. Great caution must be taken to minimize risk for rupture by avoiding hypertension during intubation, Mayfield head fixation, and during the surgical procedure. Also, in patients with prior rupture, adequate CPP must be maintained as ICP may be elevated. If the rupture was more than 3 days prior, patients may have cerebral arterial vasospasm. In any case, a plan must be in place in the event of intraoperative aneurysm rupture. Anesthetic induction is controlled with the above-mentioned ICP considerations in mind. In those with prior rupture, CPP is maintained, sometimes requiring careful vasopressor use in an effort to also prevent hypertension that can increase risk for rerupture.

In patients without prior rupture and a normal ICP, excessive hypertension should be avoided. A maintenance anesthetic technique similar to the one described earlier for brain tumors is used, not necessarily because of ICP concerns, but because neuromonitoring may be employed to detect regional ischemia. During exposure of the aneurysm, burst-suppression on the EEG may be desired to decrease the impending ischemic burden on the brain from temporary occlusion of large cerebral vessels. Burst-suppression can be accomplished with propofol

Table 37-4 Fisher Grade System

Fisher Grade	Blood on Computed Tomography Scan
1	No subarachnoid blood seen
2	Diffuse vertical layers of blood <1 mm thick
3	Localized clot and/or vertical layer of blood ≥1 mm thick
4	Intracerebral or intraventricular clot with diffuse or absent subarachnoid hemorrhage

administered as a 1- to 2-mg/kg bolus followed by infusion of 100 to 150 μg/kg/min. Additional vasopressor may be required during this time to maintain CPP.

Prior to direct clipping of the aneurysmal neck, the surgeon may place one or more temporary clips on parent or feeding arteries to "soften" the neck and make it more amenable to direct clipping while minimizing the chances of rupture. Alternatively, when temporary clips are anatomically difficult to place, adenosine 0.3 to 0.4 mg/kg may be safely given as a bolus to cause a transient circulatory arrest and profound hypotension, allowing safe permanent clip application.[136,137] Other techniques, such as deep hypothermic circulatory arrest (DHCA), retrograde suction decompression, or rapid ventricular pacing achieve the same end point but are logistically more difficult to perform. During temporary and permanent clipping, SSEP and MEP monitoring may be performed as this is the period of time during which the brain is at greatest ischemic risk.

Inadvertent rupture is possible during dissection around the aneurysm. A plan must be in place to contend with this potentially devastating complication, including the availability of blood products and adenosine (0.3 to 0.4 mg/kg), or another rapidly acting antihypertensive medication (e.g., sodium nitroprusside), for rescue. In this regard, large-bore intravenous access is required, especially for large aneurysms over 10 mm and ruptured aneurysms; and, central venous access is recommended. Arterial catheters are routinely used for aneurysm surgery.

Endovascular treatment of aneurysms involves groin arterial access and the deployment of coils into the aneurysmal sac or another means to occlude blood flow into the sac. An example of the latter technique is the pipeline treatment or the deployment of a stent into the parent artery to prevent blood from entering the aneurysmal sac. The International Subarachnoid Aneurysm Trial (ISAT) demonstrated that, despite a greater occurrence of rebleeding, there was a 25% decrease in poor neurologic outcomes at 1 year in patients undergoing coiling versus surgical clipping of aneurysms.[138] Other data, however, do not suggest a significant benefit of coiling *versus* clipping of aneurysms. Furthermore, certain aneurysms may not be amenable to coiling, due to their morphology. The major disadvantage of coiling is incomplete obliteration of the aneurysm, requiring recoiling that may be necessary in up to 30% of cases. General anesthesia is used, with adequate muscle relaxation, as movement should be prevented. An arterial catheter is needed to monitor the blood pressure closely and to obtain blood samples for coagulation measurements at repeated intervals, as heparin is given periodically. The anesthesiologist should communicate very closely with the interventionalist throughout the procedure, as any extravasation of dye into the brain parenchyma may be indicative of aneurysmal or feeding vessel rupture. In this circumstance, protamine must be immediately available; to reverse the effects of heparin, and hyperventilation, mannitol, burst-suppression, and placement of an EVD should be available on an emergency basis, with the possibility of emergency craniotomy as a strong possibility. Embolism of coils to unintended locations in the brain is also possible throughout the procedure; thus, a prompt neurologic examination at the conclusion of the procedure is very important.

Arteriovenous Malformations

Cerebral AVMs are congenital abnormalities in which a plexus of arteries and "arterialized" veins form a nidus that may lead to cerebral hemorrhage, headaches, seizures, or signs of cerebral ischemia due to a "steal" effect. AVMs are usually detected

Table 37-5 Spetzler–Martin Grading System	
Feature of Arteriovenous Malformation	**Score**
Size	
Small (<3 cm)	1
Medium (3–6 cm)	2
Large (>6 cm)	3
Adjacent brain	
Noneloquent	0
Eloquent	1
Venous drainage pattern	
Superficial	0
Deep	1

between the ages of 10 and 40 years, with approximately 70% being supratentorial.[139] Morphologically, these structures have a nidus of dysplastic vessels of varying size, and are drained by one or more superficial or deep veins. Characteristically, there is no capillary bed between arteries and veins within AVMs. These lesions can be diagnosed by MRI or cerebral angiography, and treatment modalities include embolization in the interventional radiology suite preoperatively to minimize intraoperative burden or improve curativity. In addition, stereotactic radiosurgery or surgical removal can be considered. The Spetzler–Martin Grading System is used to predict surgical outcome, and is based on size, eloquence of adjacent brain, and pattern of venous drainage (i.e., superficial versus deep) of the AVM (Table 37-5).[140] Notably, about 7% of cerebral AVMs include a flow-related cerebral aneurysm as well, and this information should be sought and accounted for in the anesthetic plan.[141]

Vascular access, more than in any other intracranial neurosurgical procedure, is of great importance, and a central venous catheter is highly recommended. The greatest risk of AVM resection is bleeding, both intraoperatively as surgical hemostasis can be challenging due to poor visualization of arterial and especially venous vessels and postoperatively. Strict control of blood pressure is required to maintain CPP without worsening blood loss from the resection bed due to ongoing systemic hypertension. At the same time, avoidance of hypotension is crucial as these patients often present with seizures or focal neurologic deficits due to an ischemic "steal" phenomenon. Because most AVMs are high-flow and low-resistance shunts, the incidence of sudden rupture with *acute* rises in systemic blood pressure (as with direct laryngoscopy) is low unless there is an accompanying aneurysm. Blood products should be immediately available, and antihypertensives are very often needed, especially during emergence from anesthesia. The phenomenon of "normal perfusion pressure breakthrough," or NPPB, is controversial in terms of its mechanism, but very much clinically relevant to the anesthesiologist. NPPB is thought to be a type of autoregulatory inhibition caused by the AVM and affecting the surrounding "normal" brain, in which previously normal cerebral vessels are maximally vasodilated due to longstanding "steal" caused by the AVM. When the AVM has been resected, these "vasoparalyzed" vessels are unable to vasoconstrict, leading to cerebral hyperemia, cerebral edema, headache, and possibly increased risk for postoperative bleeding.[142,143] Another phenomenon that may lead to perioperative hyperemia and postoperative morbidity is "occlusive hyperemia."[144] This phenomenon is primarily related to arterial and venous obstruction occurring in normal brain tissue that surrounded the AVM due to surgical disruption of these vessels. This obstruction can impact flow in brain parenchyma that surrounded the AVM leading to ischemia from poor arterial flow and edema and increased risk for hemorrhage from impaired venous outflow.[145] Postoperatively, up to 50% of patients may experience seizures, thus prophylactic anticonvulsants are typically administered.[146] Neuromonitoring is increasingly being used to facilitate cerebral AVM resections, and a maintenance anesthetic regimen that allows neuromonitoring may be required. Arterial catheterization and careful induction and intubation, as described with cerebral aneurysms, are standard.

Carotid Surgery

Surgery to remove carotid plaque that may be causing symptomatic cerebral ischemia is generally indicated when the plaque burden is over 70% occlusive in the ipsilateral ICA. Up to 20% of strokes may be due to cerebral ischemia caused by intimal narrowing of the ICA, either unilaterally or bilaterally. Carotid revascularization has proven to be a useful procedure for reducing the risk of stroke in cases of severe occlusion of the ICA (i.e., 70% to 99% occlusion) in the presence of symptoms of ischemia. However, benefit in less severe occlusive states or in asymptomatic patients may not outweigh risks and medical management may be preferred.[147] Currently, procedural treatments of carotid artery stenosis include carotid endarterectomy or carotid artery stenting. The most significant advantage of carotid endarterectomy over stenting is that it has an overall lower incidence of postoperative stroke and restenosis, whereas potential disadvantages of this surgery include the need for a general or regional anesthetic technique, a possible increased risk for cardiac events, and a higher incidence of cranial nerve dysfunction.[148] However, carotid artery stenting may be accomplished with very minimal sedation and carries a lower incidence of cranial nerve injury, although it has been associated with a higher risk of restenosis and stroke in the postprocedural period.[149]

Carotid endarterectomy is performed either "awake" with regional anesthesia or "asleep" with general anesthesia. Neither technique has been found to be superior at improving neurologic outcome.[150] "Awake" carotid surgery usually involves a superficial and sometimes deep cervical plexus block to provide anesthesia within the C2 to C4 dermatomes.[151] Low-dose analgesia and sedation with remifentanil or propofol may be considered. It is important to ensure that the patient is responsive to commands and able to perform manual tasks on the contralateral side. This technique requires a cooperative patient who is able to tolerate lying flat for a prolonged period of time, and patients with chronic obstructive pulmonary disease or uncompensated congestive heart failure may be unsuitable candidates. Advantages of an "awake" technique include a direct monitor of the patient's neurologic status, better hemodynamic stability, shorter hospital length of stay, and decreased bleeding complications. If the patient becomes agitated, confused, or unresponsive following carotid occlusion, the anesthesiologist should assume that cerebral ischemia has ensued and assure adequate perfusion and oxygenation by increasing systemic blood pressure to up to 20% greater than preoperative values.

"Asleep" carotid surgery employs general endotracheal anesthesia, and frequently some form of monitoring for cerebral ischemia is used. EEG is probably the most common and ischemia presents as ipsilateral slowing of oscillations. SSEPs and MEPs can also be used with ischemia appearing as a decrease in waveform amplitude or an increase in waveform latency. Carotid stump pressure is the pressure measured in the internal carotid artery distal to the cross-clamp and is thought to reflect adequate collateral blood flow via the circle of Willis. A stump pressure greater than 50 mmHg is desirable. Cerebral oximetry or TCD are other, less commonly employed techniques used to monitor for cerebral ischemia. To date, no modality of neuromonitoring has been shown to ensure adequate collateral blood flow or definitively decrease the incidence of neurologic complications perioperatively.

General anesthesia provides the advantages of a motionless patient, the ability to ensure eucapnia, and control of the airway at all times. Eucapnia is preferred, as hyperventilation will cause cerebral vasoconstriction and decreased CBF, whereas hypoventilation and hypercapnia may lead to a "steal" phenomenon from watershed areas of cerebral perfusion.

Regardless of the type of anesthesia performed, invasive arterial blood pressure monitoring is preferred as operative morbidity is generally due to neurologic complications whereas mortality is usually due to cardiac complications. Therefore, blood pressure control is critical. Patients are generally chronically hypertensive preoperatively and may have cardiovascular disease and other significant comorbidities. Blood pressure should be maintained at baseline levels prior to cross-clamping. Patients having regional anesthesia often maintain baseline blood pressure but those having general anesthesia may require pharmacologic manipulation of blood pressure. Cross-clamping occurs above and below the area of plaque, usually at the levels of the common carotid artery below and the ICA above and heparinization is commonly performed prior to cross-clamping. Upon cross-clamp occlusion of the common carotid artery, blood pressure should be augmented to improve collateral flow from the contralateral side, often requiring a vasopressor. During manipulation of the carotid baroreceptor, bradycardia and possibly hypotension are not uncommon, and the surgeon may infiltrate the carotid sinus with lidocaine to prevent this response. Following restoration of flow in the carotid artery, hypertension may persist, probably due to surgical denervation of the carotid baroreceptor.[152] Since cerebral vessels distal to the stenotic carotid artery have been maximally vasodilated, autoregulation may not be intact. Hypertension with cerebral vasomotor paralysis can lead to cerebral edema and increased risk for cerebral hemorrhage. Any neurologic compromise postoperatively may also be indicative of cerebral emboli or ICA thrombosis, and patients must be monitored extremely closely in the recovery room or intensive care unit for these complications. Lastly, the anesthesiologist must be keenly aware of the potential for a postoperative neck hematoma, which may quickly compromise the airway. Immediate intubation, which may be more difficult and surgical exploration of the wound is required.[153]

Other modalities of treating ICA stenosis, including carotid angioplasty, have gained popularity in the last few years, with some evidence supporting their safety and efficacy over traditional endarterectomy.

Epilepsy Surgery

Epilepsy affects about 1% of the general population and is characterized by recurrent seizure activity of both the generalized and partial varieties. Complex partial seizures, including temporal lobe epilepsy, are most common, involving an initial focus of abnormal neuronal discharge that spreads with a subsequent loss of consciousness. Epilepsy may occur idiopathically, or as part of a constellation of symptoms related to head injury, tumors, neurovascular disease, metabolic derangement, or infection. Approximately 30% of patients with drug resistant epilepsy undergo surgical treatment for their disease.[154] Perioperative management of patients having surgery for epilepsy requires a keen understanding of the pharmacologic effects of both anesthetics and antiepileptic drugs. Surgery for epilepsy is generally indicated when there is a discrete epileptic focus, most often identified in the temporal lobe. Thus, temporal lobectomy with amygdalohippocampectomy is a very common surgical procedure performed for the treatment of epilepsy.

Preoperative evaluation is critical, with particular attention paid to the patient's preoperative antiepileptic regimen, their known side effects, and in some cases plasma concentrations of drugs with known therapeutic windows. Antiepileptic drugs are generally continued throughout the perioperative period unless seizure focus mapping is intended. Antiepileptics taken by the patient can induce liver enzymes and increase the metabolism of muscle relaxants, opioids, and dexmedetomidine, leading to a need for higher dosages.[155] Anesthetics have mixed and variable excitatory and inhibitory effects on seizure activity. Thus, if used improperly, can be detrimental to seizure focus mapping, which is often necessary to perform this surgery. Benzodiazepines should be avoided when electrocorticography (ECoG) is planned. Induction of anesthesia with propofol, a muscle relaxant, and an opioid is acceptable. During maintenance of anesthesia and prior to ECoG, any anesthetic regimen conducive for craniotomy can be used, but 30 minutes prior to ECoG initiation, propofol infusion should be stopped and potent volatile anesthetic held to a minimum (0.5 MAC) or stopped as well. To prevent awareness, scopolamine, nitrous oxide, and high-dose opioid infusion can be used with very little adverse effect on ECoG. Dexmedetomidine is also thought to be useful in this regard. In any case, the patient should be counseled about the possibility of intraoperative awareness during the procedure. In some cases, methohexital, etomidate, or alfentanil (50 μg/kg) can be used to enhance epileptiform activity and assist in mapping.[156] Once ECoG is complete, the general anesthetic technique used prior to ECoG can be resumed during the resection. Postoperatively, patients should be monitored closely for seizure activity, and any seizures, which might signify postoperative bleeding, metabolic derangements, hypercapnia, or hypoxemia, should be treated aggressively so as to avoid cerebral damage or status epilepticus.

Awake Craniotomy

Craniotomy performed with monitored anesthesia care, also known as "awake craniotomy," has gained popularity in some institutions and is used in cases in which a lesion lies adjacent to primary cortex that controls motor function, speech, or sensory function. Awake craniotomy allows for speech, motor, or sensory cortical mapping in real-time, hence facilitating a more aggressive resection of the tumor and minimizing risk to motor, sensory, or speech function. A motivated patient is critical to the success of the procedure, and the preoperative assessment should include a detailed explanation of the anesthetic so as to ensure cooperation and allay anxiety. Awake craniotomy can be performed with the patient sedated for the duration of the procedure, or with an "asleep–awake–asleep" technique employing a supraglottic airway device or nasopharyngeal tubes for general anesthesia prior to and following the awake mapping.[157,158] During awake mapping, the airway device is removed so that the patient can communicate and then replaced following mapping (or alternately the patient kept sedated for surgical closure). For a fully "awake" craniotomy, an arterial catheter is placed and sedation prior to and following awake mapping may be facilitated with propofol, remifentanil, or dexmedetomidine infusions.

A selective scalp nerve block may be performed preoperatively, either unilaterally or bilaterally, blocking the six nerves on each side which innervate the scalp and dura mater. These include the supratrochlear, supraorbital, zygomaticotemporal, auriculotemporal, lesser occipital, and great occipital nerves.[159] Otherwise, the surgeon may choose to perform a field block. Care must be taken to avoid local anesthetic toxicity, particularly as the surgeon infiltrates the dura mater with additional local anesthetic. During cortical mapping, electrical stimulation is used by the surgeon *via* a probe stimulator, in conjunction with neuropsychologic testing, to map critical cortical regions. This allows the surgeon to determine safe resection margins and is of particular significance if the tumor is located near major language areas in cortex (usually located in the left hemisphere).

Regardless of the anesthetic technique used, close attention to the airway is critical, as hypoventilation and hypercapnia are detrimental to surgical exposure and apnea requiring emergent intubation may be very difficult in a patient in whom the head is turned and fixed in a Mayfield head-holder. In this regard, the surgical drape should be positioned in a manner allowing direct and constant access to the patient's face. Patient positioning is very important, and careful padding and positioning should be accomplished before any sedation is administered. Lastly, and often overlooked in these cases, is the importance of constant communication with the patient, not only to facilitate speech or motor testing but also to comfort the patient who may be very anxious.

Complications of awake craniotomy intraoperatively may include a disinhibited or uncooperative patient, oversedation prohibitive to neuropsychologic testing, respiratory depression, airway obstruction, intractable brain edema, seizures, or uncontrollable pain. Emergency airway equipment allowing for mask ventilation, placement of a supraglottic airway device, or fiberoptic intubation must be immediately available. Seizures should be treated with cold saline applied to the brain surface by the surgeon and a small bolus of propofol (20 mg) intravenously. Postoperatively, patients may be observed in the PACU or the ICU with similar considerations as for general anesthesia craniotomies, including adequate analgesia.

Anesthesia and Traumatic Brain Injury

TBI is a significant public health problem in the developed and underdeveloped world, accounting for 15% to 20% of mortality in people 5 to 35 years old.[160] TBI is often associated with other trauma such as thoracic, abdominal, and orthopedic injuries. It is important to note that the primary insult to the brain is often irreversible. Death following TBI is often associated with secondary insults from hypotension, hypoxemia, and malignantly increased ICP due to hematoma or edema.[161] Emergency and anesthetic management of patients with TBI should focus on minimizing these secondary insults to optimize perfusion of the injured brain. Patients presenting with TBI are stratified according to the GCS on presentation (3 to 15). GCS 13 to 15 corresponds to mild head injury, GCS 9 to 12 corresponds to moderate head injury, and GCS below 9 represents severe head injury. Patients with TBI are often intubated when GCS is 8 or less owing to high risk for impaired airway protection. A GCS of 8 or less also corresponds to 35% mortality.[162] Noncontrast CT scan that shows midline shift of more than 5 mm or absent ventricles should also lead to immediate intubation, as ICP may be significantly elevated potentially impairing ventilation.

ICP monitoring is frequently used in patients with acute TBI, and can be instituted in the emergency department by an EVD, where mannitol, hyperventilation, and propofol can be used to control elevated ICP. Operative management, such as decompressive craniectomy, is normally indicated for depressed skull fractures, dural breech, midline shift more than 5 mm, basal cistern compression, refractory ICP elevation, and acutely expanding intracranial hemorrhage, including subdural and epidural hematomas.[163,164]

Anesthetic Management

Patients presenting with TBI are assumed to have concomitant cervical spine injury, and intubation, if not already performed, must take this into account. Furthermore, 40% of patients will have an associated life-threatening injury.[165,166] A detailed but rapid primary survey, along with a focused neurologic examination is critical. Hypoxemia is common, which may be further exacerbated by pulmonary injury. Doses of anesthetic drugs must be tailored so as to avoid worsening systemic hypotension as patients may have hypovolemia from an associated injury. Succinylcholine is controversial following an acute closed head injury, as it may raise ICP very transiently but can be considered if there is a need to rapidly secure an airway and no other contraindications to its use exist. Nasal intubation is contraindicated if a basilar skull fracture is present or presumed. Once the airway is secured, attention must be paid to hemodynamics, as systolic blood pressure less than 80 mmHg is associated with a worse neurologic outcome. Fluid resuscitation and vasopressors are often needed to assure an adequate systemic and cerebral perfusion pressure. There is some evidence that achieving euvolemia with hypertonic saline may be beneficial in TBI patients, especially pediatric patients, as intravascular volume is repleted and CPP is maintained with less cerebral edema.[167] Euglycemia should be maintained. Intravascular access should include an arterial catheter and large-bore intravenous cannulae, and possibly a central venous line. Cross-matched red blood cells and other blood products should be available, and any available results relating to red blood cell counts and clotting function should be reviewed.

Choice of an anesthetic maintenance technique depends on an understanding of ICP management (see earlier), with inhalational drugs in higher doses used with caution to avoid excessive cerebral vasodilation. Additional mannitol or hypertonic saline may be required to control edema. Hyperventilation should not continue beyond 2 to 6 hours, as its effect to decrease ICP may not be durable after this time.[168] After this acute phase of hyperventilation, a $PaCO_2$ of 30 to 35 mmHg is desirable. Of particular importance for TBI management, CPP should always be kept above 60 mmHg to maintain cerebral perfusion but excessive hypertension should be avoided to reduce risk of exacerbating edema or increasing risk for hemorrhage.[169] The release of brain tissue thromboplastin into the systemic circulation may lead to disseminated intravascular coagulation and coagulopathy must be aggressively sought and treated. Likewise, ARDS or neurogenic pulmonary edema may be present, and a lung-protective ventilation strategy using PEEP and low tidal volumes may be needed to maintain oxygenation.

Complications that may occur during and immediately following operative management of TBI include seizures, intracranial hemorrhage, sudden and profound hypotension following decompression of large hematomas, and cerebral edema. The latter can be treated with propofol, mannitol, or hypertonic saline, temporary hyperventilation, CSF diversion, and possibly avoiding replacement of the bone flap at the conclusion of surgery.

Extubation at the conclusion of surgery depends on the degree of ICP elevation, the severity of injury, and concomitant injuries. Most patients are admitted to the neurointensive care unit after surgery and require continued intubation, mechanical ventilation, and sedation.

Anesthesia for Spine Trauma and Complex Spine Surgery

Spinal Cord Injury

Acute spinal cord injury often necessitates emergency surgery to stabilize the spinal column and prevent secondary injury. Cervical spine injuries are most common, as this is the most mobile part of the spine.[170] Cervical injuries are also the most devastating injuries from a neurologic perspective. Cervical cord injuries cause more functional motor, sensory, and autonomic deficits than lower cord injuries. Also, higher cord injuries can impact respiratory muscle function to a greater extent with intercostal function being impacted by thoracic and cervical injuries and phrenic function being impaired by lesions at C5 or higher. Although voluntary respiratory effort remains with injury at the C4 level, vital capacity may be diminished by up to 25%.[171] Sympathetic nervous system function is usually impaired following higher thoracic and cervical cord injuries and cardiac accelerator nerve function (derived from the T1 to T5 segments), may lead to profound hypotension and bradycardia. Likewise, temperature control is lost with SCI because of a loss of sweating function and cutaneous vasodilation due to loss of sympathetic function. The American Spinal Injury Association (ASIA) score is used to stratify spinal cord injury based on sensory, motor, and reflex function (Table 37-6).[172]

Following acute spinal cord injury, spinal cord autoregulation is impaired and the phenomena of spinal shock may be present. Spinal shock is characterized by sensory–motor deficits below the level of the injury and flaccid paralysis, usually lasting up to 6 weeks.[173] After this initial period, spasticity of the affected muscles tends to occur. Hypotension can result from autonomic impairment and hypovolemia associated with other injuries (e.g., long bone fractures, intra-abdominal bleeding). During this time, it is critical to prevent secondary injury by providing aggressive hemodynamic support. Although primary injury may be due to stretching, compression, or transection of the spinal cord or its blood supply due to hyperflexion, hyperextension, or impingement of the fractured spinal column, secondary injury is a more complicated biochemical phenomenon involving the release of inflammatory mediators, cytokines, and amino acids leading to cellular edema, apoptosis, and free radical formation.[174] As with TBI, mitigating these secondary insults, by avoiding hypoxemia, hypotension, and worsening cord edema, is of paramount importance in ensuring the best outcome possible.

Comorbid Injuries

Many patients presenting with acute spinal cord injury may also have comorbid injuries. These include TBI, nonvertebral fractures, facial injuries, chest or abdominal injuries (including pneumothorax and pulmonary contusion), and traumatic amputations. Obviously during this time, life-threatening injuries must be addressed, all the while ensuring that spinal alignment is maintained to avoid adding secondary injury to the spinal cord. Comorbid injuries pose a significant problem in the SCI population, as they may be the cause or contribute to hypotension and hypoxemia. They may also be more difficult to diagnose and treat in a patient for whom manipulation may be difficult or dangerous.

Initial Management

Patients presenting with acute spinal cord injury, depending on the level and extent of injury, may be compromised from a ventilatory and hemodynamic standpoint, and immediate control of these parameters is crucial. A detailed neurologic examination is critical to establish the operative plan and subsequent prognostication. Airway management in cervical spinal injury focuses on maintaining in-line stabilization throughout, and may require the use of fiberoptic intubation or other adjuncts to secure the airway. In a stable patient, radiographic studies are helpful in assessing the degree of cervical injury and options for intubation.[175] However, plain x-ray imaging of the cervical spine is not sensitive for ligamentous injury thus underestimating risk. Succinylcholine is safe in the initial 24 hours following spinal cord injury as new junctional and extrajunctional nicotinic receptors have not yet been fully expressed. In addition to intravenous fluids and blood products, vasopressors and inotropes are often required to support the blood pressure as hypotension and anemia can contribute to secondary injury of the spinal cord. Arterial blood pressure monitoring and large-bore intravenous access (preferably central venous access) are required. MAP should be maintained above 85 mmHg to ensure adequate spinal cord perfusion for at least 7 days from the date of injury.[176]

Other strategies to protect the spinal cord, such as corticosteroids, naloxone, or hypothermia, may be instituted at this time, but convincing human data for these therapies is lacking. Corticosteroids have received particular attention in this regard, both in animal and human studies. The mechanism to account for their potential neuroprotective effect is largely unknown, but thought to include reduction of vasogenic edema, improvement of spinal cord perfusion, anti-inflammatory effects, and free radical scavenging. The most comprehensive human trials were the National Acute Spinal Cord Injury Studies (NASCIS) I to III, which

Table 37-6 American Spinal Cord Association (ASIA) Impairment Scale

ASIA Impairment Class	Deficit	Deficit Description
A	Complete	No motor or sensory function
B	Incomplete	Sensory but no motor function below neurologic level including S4–5
C	Incomplete	Motor function preserved below neurologic level + ≥50% key muscles have severe weakness
D	Incomplete	Motor function preserved below neurologic level + ≥50% key muscles have mild weakness
E	None	Normal motor and sensory function

demonstrated that early steroid intervention may improve neurologic outcome in SCI patients. These studies were highly suspect, however, in that their results were not reproducible, their populations were skewed, and survival or quality of life did not improve with the intervention (methylprednisolone).[177] Furthermore, corticosteroids are known to have untoward effects, including the predisposition to infection and glucose dysregulation that must be weighed against their potential benefits. Currently, both the American Association of Neurological Surgeons and Congress of Neurological Surgeons do not recommend the use of high-dose steroids in patients with acute spinal cord injury.[178]

Intraoperative Management

The choice of technique for maintenance of anesthesia in patients with spinal cord injury should focus on two key considerations: maintaining blood pressure and allowing for intraoperative neuromonitoring. Again, MAP should be maintained above 85 mmHg. Complex spine surgery, which often involves multiple level fusions and osteotomies, should also take into account the real possibility of significant, and sometimes profound, surgical bleeding and the need for postoperative mechanical ventilation following massive transfusion.[179] Depending on the spinal levels requiring intervention and the extent of the planned surgery, the patient may be placed in Mayfield head-fixation. Clearly, adequate intravascular access is vitally important. Measurements of arterial blood gas, coagulation parameters, hemoglobin concentration, and platelet counts should be undertaken very frequently, as coagulopathy and anemia are quite common and need to be corrected rapidly as they can contribute to secondary injury. Close communication with the surgeon is very important, as these large operations often may benefit from early closure and staging of the procedure. Use of antifibrinolytics, such as tranexamic acid or aminocaproic acid, can decrease risk of bleeding with minimal, if any, increased risk for thrombotic complications.[180] In noninfectious, nontumor cases, intraoperative cell salvage can be quite helpful in reducing the total amount of allogeneic blood transfused.[181] Other blood-sparing techniques, such as acute normovolemic hemodilution and deliberate hypotension, have largely fallen out of favor, due to the known harmful effects of anemia and hypotension on the neurologic and cardiovascular systems.

Complications of Anesthesia for Spine Surgery

Fortunately, complications specifically related to anesthesia for spine surgery are rare, but they are often devastating when they occur. Postoperative visual loss is one such complication, with an incidence of 0.088 to 1.2 per 1000 after spine surgery.[182–184] Most cases are due to posterior ischemic optic neuropathy, with central retinal artery occlusion and cortical blindness being much less common. Risk factors include male sex, obesity, use of the Wilson frame, longer surgery and anesthesia duration, and high estimated blood loss, whereas use of colloid may be protective.[185] Ophthalmologic consultation should be immediately undertaken if this complication is suspected.

Another complication of spine surgery is anterior spinal artery syndrome. This syndrome is caused by sustained hypoperfusion of the anterior spinal artery, owing to either surgical distraction or hypotension, and leads to motor weakness.[186,187] MEPs may be helpful in detecting and averting this devastating complication.

Deliberate hypotension, hypothermia, and hypovolemia may predispose spine surgery patients to the formation of deep venous thromboses (DVT) and subsequent pulmonary emboli (PE). Lumbar fusion is associated with an incidence of symptomatic DVT of up to 4%, with a 2% incidence of PE.[188,189] Because prophylaxis with an anticoagulant is often impossible prior to spine surgery for fear of worsening blood loss and formation of epidural hematoma, an inferior vena cava filter is often placed prior to surgery in high risk patients.

Autonomic dysreflexia (AD) is an important physiologic phenomenon that is not a complication of spine surgery, but rather a late complication of complete SCI. AD occurs weeks to months after such injury, in 60% to 80% of such SCI patients, and is characterized by a profound hypertensive response to any stimulus below the level of injury, such as distention of a hollow organ such as the bladder, pain, or surgery.[190] The most common manifestation of AD is profound systemic hypertension, accompanied by headache, profuse sweating, and flushing above the level of injury and oftentimes bradycardia, cardiac arrhythmias, or cardiac dysfunction. The pathophysiology of this phenomenon is thought to be due to a disruption of descending inhibitory tracts with intact sympathetic reflex arcs below the level of injury. The primary goal in patients at risk for AD is prevention. Triggers should be minimized (i.e., appropriate bowel and bladder care) and anesthesia should still be used for painful or stimulating procedures in insensate regions. Treatment of an acute episode of AD involves removing the inciting stimulus and deepening the level of anesthesia along with the administration of potent vasodilators. Recommended vasodilators include calcium-channel blockers, nitrates, or hydralazine.[191] There is some controversy regarding the preferred anesthetic technique for these patients, although general and spinal anesthesia are usually preferred to epidural anesthesia or mild-to-moderate sedation. Spinal anesthesia had the advantage over epidural anesthesia as it is generally a denser block and does not risk sparing of sacral segments that may occur with epidural anesthesia. If general anesthesia is used, succinylcholine should generally be avoided as it may trigger a profound hyperkalemic response. As with all neurosurgical patients, careful monitoring for these patients in the postoperative period is critical, as AD may manifest itself at this time.

Conclusion

The perioperative care of neurosurgical patients requires a sound understanding of neurophysiologic and neuropharmacologic principles, the timely application of these principles, and vigilance to often rapidly changing clinical conditions. At the core of neuroanesthesia practice are the ideas of maintaining cerebral oxygen and substrate delivery, facilitating intraoperative neuromonitoring, and assuring for a rapid emergence to facilitate neurologic examination in appropriate patients. Expert application of the requisite knowledge to achieve these goals, along with efficient resource utilization, will provide the safest neurologic outcome possible for this vulnerable patient population.

REFERENCES

1. Tate MC, Herbet G, Moritz-Gasser S, et al. Probabilistic map of critical functional regions of the human cerebral cortex: Broca's area revisited. *Brain.* 2014;137:2773–2782.
2. Gilman S, Newman S. *Manter and Gatz's Essentials of Clinical Neuroanatomy and Neurophysiology.* Philadelphia, PA: FA Davis; 2002.
3. Kapoor K, Singh B, Dewan LI. Variations in the configuration of the circle of Willis. *Anat Sci Int.* 2008;83:96–106.

4. Johanson CE, Duncan JA, 3rd, Klinge PM, et al. Multiplicity of cerebrospinal fluid functions: new challenges in health and disease. *Cerebrospinal Fluid Res.* 2008;5:10.
5. Melissano G, Bertoglio L, Rinaldi E, et al. An anatomical review of spinal cord blood supply. *J Cardiovasc Surg (Torino).* 2015;56:699–706.
6. Xu F, Liu P, Pascual JM, et al. Effect of hypoxia and hyperoxia on cerebral blood flow, blood oxygenation, and oxidative metabolism. *J Cereb Blood Flow Metab.* 2012;32:1909–1918.
7. Hill RA, Tong L, Yuan P, et al. Regional blood flow in the normal and ischemic brain is controlled by arteriolar smooth muscle cell contractility and not by capillary pericytes. *Neuron.* 2015;87:95–110.
8. Lebrun-Grandie P, Baron JC, Scussaline F, et al. Coupling between regional blood flow and oxygen utilization in the normal human brain: a study with positron tomography and oxygen 15. *Arch Neurol.* 1983;40:230–236.
9. Sanders RD, Degos V, Young WL. Cerebral perfusion under pressure: is the autoregulatory 'plateau' a level playing field for all? *Anaesthesia.* 2011;66:968–972.
10. Menon DK. Cerebral circulation. In: Priebe HJ, Skarvan K, eds. *Cardiovascular Physiology.* London: BMJ Publishing; 2000:240–277.
11. Deegan BM, Devine ER, Geraghty MC, et al. The relationship between cardiac output and dynamic cerebral autoregulation in humans. *J Appl Physiol (1985).* 2010;109:1424–1431.
12. Strebel S, Lam AM, Matta B, et al. Dynamic and static cerebral autoregulation during isoflurane, desflurane, and propofol anesthesia. *Anesthesiology.* 1995;83:66–76.
13. Hori D, Brown C, Ono M, et al. Arterial pressure above the upper cerebral autoregulation limit during cardiopulmonary bypass is associated with postoperative delirium. *Br J Anaesth.* 2014;113:1009–1017.
14. Werner C, Lu H, Engelhard K, et al. Sevoflurane impairs cerebral blood flow autoregulation in rats: reversal by nonselective nitric oxide synthase inhibition. *Anesth Analg.* 2005;101:509–516.
15. Brothers RM, Lucas RA, Zhu YS, et al. Cerebral vasomotor reactivity: steady-state versus transient changes in carbon dioxide tension. *Exp Physiol.* 2014;99:1499–1510.
16. Meng L, Gelb AW. Regulation of cerebral autoregulation by carbon dioxide. *Anesthesiology.* 2015;122:196–205.
17. Sjoberg F, Singer M. The medical use of oxygen: a time for critical reappraisal. *J Intern Med.* 2013;274:505–528.
18. Zauner A, Daugherty WP, Bullock MR, et al. Brain oxygenation and energy metabolism: Part I-biological function and pathophysiology. *Neurosurgery.* 2002;51:289–301.
19. Wilson TD, Shoemaker JK, Kozak R, et al. Reflex-mediated reduction in human cerebral blood volume. *J Cereb Blood Flow Metab.* 2005;25:136–143.
20. Fox J, Gelb AW, Enns J, et al. The responsiveness of cerebral blood flow to changes in arterial carbon dioxide is maintained during propofol-nitrous oxide anesthesia in humans. *Anesthesiology.* 1992;77:453–456.
21. Schmidt A, Ryding E, Akeson J. Racemic ketamine does not abolish cerebrovascular autoregulation in the pig. *Acta Anaesthesiol Scand.* 2003;47:569–575.
22. Kuroda Y, Murakami M, Tsuruta J, et al. Preservation of the ration of cerebral blood flow/metabolic rate for oxygen during prolonged anesthesia with isoflurane, sevoflurane, and halothane in humans. *Anesthesiology.* 1996;84:555–561.
23. Dashdorj N, Corrie K, Napolitano A, et al. Effects of subanesthetic dose of nitrous oxide on cerebral blood flow and metabolism: a multimodal magnetic resonance imaging study in healthy volunteers. *Anesthesiology.* 2013;118:577–586.
24. Pasternak JJ, Lanier WL. Is nitrous oxide use appropriate in neurosurgical and neurologically at-risk patients? *Curr Opin Anaesthesiol.* 2010;23:544–550.
25. Harrison JM, Girling KJ, Mahajan RP. Effects of propofol and nitrous oxide on middle cerebral artery flow velocity and cerebral autoregulation. *Anaesthesia.* 2002;57:27–32.
26. Iacopino DG, Conti A, Battaglia C, et al. Transcranial Doppler ultrasound study of the effects of nitrous oxide on cerebral autoregulation during neurosurgical anesthesia: A randomized controlled trial. *J Neurosurg.* 2003;99:58–64.
27. Macintyre I. A hotbed of medical innovation: George Kellie (1770-1829), his colleagues at Leith and the Monro-Kellie doctrine. *J Med Biogr.* 2013;22:93–100.
28. Majdan M, Mauritz W, Wilbacher I, et al. Timing and duration of intracranial hypertension versus outcomes after severe traumatic brain injury. *Minerva Anestesiol.* 2014;80:1261–1272.
29. Kety SS, Skenkin HA, Schmidt CF. The effects of increased intracranial pressure on cerebral circulatory functions in man. *J Clin Invest.* 1948;27:493–499.
30. Ho ML, Rojas R, Eisenberg RL. Cerebral edema. *AJR Am J Roentgenol.* 2012;199:W258–W273.
31. Michinaga S, Koyama Y. Pathogenesis of brain edema and investigation into anti-edema drugs. *Int J Mol Sci.* 2015;16:9949–9975.
32. Dietrich J, Rao K, Pastorino S, et al. Corticosteroids in brain cancer patients: benefits and pitfalls. *Expert Rev Clin Pharmacol.* 2011;4:233–242.
33. La Rosa G, Conti A, Cardali S, et al. Does early decompression improve neurological outcome of spinal cord injured patients? Appraisal of the literature using a meta-analytical approach. *Spinal Cord.* 2004;42:503–512.
34. Hurlbert RJ. Methylprednisolone for acute spinal cord injury: an inappropriate standard of care. *J Neurosurg.* 2000;93:1–7.
35. Pajewski TN, Arlet V, Phillips LH. Current approach on spinal cord monitoring: the point of view of the neurologist, the anesthesiologist and the spine surgeon. *Eur Spine J.* 2007;16(Suppl. 2): S115–S129.
36. Wicks RT, Pradilla G, Raza SM, et al. Impact of changes in intraoperative somatosensory evoked potentials on stroke rates after clipping of intracranial aneurysms. *Neurosurgery.* 2012;70:1114–1124; discussion 1124.
37. Koht A, Sloan T, Toleikis JR. *Neuromonitoring for the Anesthesiologist.* New York, NY: Springer-Verlag; 2012:20.
38. Sloan TB, Heyer EJ. Anesthesia for intraoperative neurophysiologic monitoring of the spinal cord. *J Clin Neurophysiol.* 2002;19:430–443.
39. Pankowski R, Dziegiel K, Roclawski M, et al. Intraoperative Neurophysiologic Monitoring (INM) in scoliosis surgery. *Stud Health Technol Inform.* 2012;176:319–321.
40. Yingling CD, Gardi JN. Intraoperative monitoring of facial and cochlear nerves during acoustic neuroma surgery. *Otolaryngol Clin North Am.* 1992;25:413–448.
41. Prell J, Strauss C, Rachinger J, et al. Facial nerve palsy after vestibular schwannoma surgery: Dynamic risk-stratification based on continuous EMG-monitoring. *Clin Neurophysiol.* 2014;125:415–421.
42. Holdefer RN, Heffez DS, Cohen BA. Utility of evoked EMG monitoring to improve bone screw placements in the cervical spine. *J Spinal Disord Tech.* 2013;26: E163–E169.
43. Rattenni RN, Cheriyan T, Lee A, et al. Intraoperative spinal cord and nerve root monitoring a hospital survey and review. *Bull Hosp Jt Dis (2013).* 2015;73:25–36.
44. Thirumala PD, Ilangovan P, Habeych M, et al. Analysis of interpeak latencies of brainstem auditory evoked potential waveforms during microvascular decompression of cranial nerve VII for hemifacial spasm. *Neurosurg Focus.* 2013;34:E6.
45. Nakatomi H, Miyazaki H, Tanaka M, et al. Improved preservation of function during acoustic neuroma surgery. *J Neurosurg.* 2015;122:24–33.
46. Kamio Y, Sakai N, Sameshima T, et al. Usefulness of intraoperative monitoring of visual evoked potentials in transsphenoidal surgery. *Neurol Med Chir (Tokyo).* 2014;54:606–611.
47. Sloan TB, Toleikis JR, Toleikis SC, et al. Intraoperative neurophysiological monitoring during spine surgery with total intravenous anesthesia or balanced anesthesia with 3% desflurane. *J Clin Monit Comput.* 2015;29:77–85.
48. Sloan T, Rogers J. Dose and timing effect of etomidate on motor evoked potentials elicited by transcranial electric or magnetic stimulation in the monkey and baboon. *J Clin Monit Comput.* 2009;23:253–261.
49. Yang LH, Lin SM, Lee WY, et al. Intraoperative transcranial electrical motor evoked potential monitoring during spinal surgery under intravenous ketamine or etomidate anaesthesia. *Acta Neurochir (Wien).* 1994;127:191–198.
50. Kim WH, Lee JJ, Lee SM, et al. Comparison of motor-evoked potentials monitoring in response to transcranial electrical stimulation in subjects undergoing neurosurgery with partial vs no neuromuscular block. *Br J Anaesth.* 2013;110:567–576.
51. Rozet I, Metzner J, Brown M, et al. Dexmedetomidine does not affect evoked potentials during spine surgery. *Anesth Analg.* 2015;121:492–501.
52. Czosnyka M, Brady K, Reinhard M, et al. Monitoring of cerebrovascular autoregulation: Facts, myths, and missing links. *Neurocrit Care.* 2009;10:373–386.
53. Wakerley BR, Kusuma Y, Yeo LL, et al. Usefulness of transcranial Doppler-derived cerebral hemodynamic parameters in the noninvasive assessment of intracranial pressure. *J Neuroimaging.* 2015;25:111–116.
54. Rasulo FA, De Peri E, Lavinio A. Transcranial doppler ultrasonography in intensive care. *Eur J Anaesthesiol Suppl.* 2008;42:167–173.
55. Rejmstad P, Akesson G, Hillman J, et al. A laser Doppler system for monitoring of intracerebral microcirculation. *Conf Proc IEEE Eng Med Biol Soc.* 2012;2012:1988–1991.
56. Kim DJ, Czosnyka Z, Kasprowicz M, et al. Continuous monitoring of the Monro-Kellie doctrine: is it possible? *J Neurotrauma.* 2012;29:1354–1363.
57. Mehrpour M, Oliaee Torshizi F, Esmaeeli N, et al. Optic nerve sonography in the diagnostic evaluation of pseudopapilledema and raised intracranial pressure: a cross-sectional study. *Neurol Res Int.* 2015;2015:146059.
58. Fargen KM, Hoh BL, Neal D, et al. The burden and risk factors of ventriculostomy occlusion in a high-volume cerebrovascular practice: results of an ongoing prospective database. *J Neurosurg.* 2015:1–8.
59. Hutchinson PJ, Hutchinson DB, Barr RH, et al. A new cranial access device for cerebral monitoring. *Br J Neurosurg.* 2000;14:46–48.
60. Chieregato A, Calzolari F, Trasforini G, et al. Normal jugular bulb oxygen saturation. *J Neurol Neurosurg Psychiatry.* 2003;74:784–786.
61. Verweij BH, Amelink GJ, Muizelaar JP. Current concepts of cerebral oxygen transport and energy metabolism after severe traumatic brain injury. *Prog Brain Res.* 2007;161:111–124.
62. Zweifel C, Dias C, Smielewski P, et al. Continuous time-domain monitoring of cerebral autoregulation in neurocritical care. *Med Eng Phys.* 2014;36:638–645.
63. Reis C, Wang Y, Akyol O, et al. What's new in traumatic brain injury: Update on tracking, monitoring and treatment. *Int J Mol Sci.* 2015;16:11903–11965.

64. Colak Z, Borojevic M, Bogovic A, et al. Influence of intraoperative cerebral oximetry monitoring on neurocognitive function after coronary artery bypass surgery: a randomized, prospective study. *Eur J Cardiothorac Surg.* 2015;47:447–454.
65. Moerman A, De Hert S. Cerebral oximetry: the standard monitor of the future? *Curr Opin Anaesthesiol.* 2015;28:703–709.
66. Han L, Tian R, Yan H, et al. Hydrogen-rich water protects against ischemic brain injury in rats by regulating calcium buffering proteins. *Brain Res.* 2015;1615:129–138.
67. Bonova P, Danielisova V, Nemethova M, et al. Scheme of ischaemia-triggered agents during brain infarct evolution in a rat model of permanent focal ischaemia. *J Mol Neurosci.* 2015;57:73–82.
68. Bai J, Lyden PD. Revisiting cerebral postischemic reperfusion injury: new insights in understanding reperfusion failure, hemorrhage, and edema. *Int J Stroke.* 2015;10:143–152.
69. Granger DN, Kvietys PR. Reperfusion injury and reactive oxygen species: The evolution of a concept. *Redox Biol.* 2015;6:524–551.
70. Wass CT, Lanier WL, Hofer RE, et al. Temperature changes of >or =. 1 degree C alter functional neurologic outcome and histopathology in a canine model of complete cerebral ischemia. *Anesthesiology.* 1995;83:325–335.
71. Alam HB, Duggan M, Li Y, et al. Putting life on hold-for how long? Profound hypothermic cardiopulmonary bypass in a Swine model of complex vascular injuries. *J Trauma.* 2008;64:912–922.
72. Bernard SA, Smith K, Cameron P, et al. Induction of prehospital therapeutic hypothermia after resuscitation from nonventricular fibrillation cardiac arrest. *Crit Care Med.* 2012;40:747–753.
73. Shankaran S. Therapeutic hypothermia for neonatal encephalopathy. *Curr Opin Pediatr.* 2015;27:152–157.
74. Todd MM, Hindman BJ, Clarke WR, et al. Mild intraoperative hypothermia during surgery for intracranial aneurysm. *N Engl J Med.* 2005;352:135–145.
75. Clifton GL, Miller ER, Choi SC, et al. Lack of effect of induction of hypothermia after acute brain injury. *N Engl J Med.* 2001;344:556–563.
76. Favero-Filho LA, Borges AA, Grassl C, et al. Hyperthermia induced after recirculation triggers chronic neurodegeneration in the penumbra zone of focal ischemia in the rat brain. *Braz J Med Biol Res.* 2008;41:1029–1036.
77. Codaccioni JL, Velly LJ, Moubarik C, et al. Sevoflurane preconditioning against focal cerebral ischemia: Inhibition of apoptosis in the face of transient improvement of neurological outcome. *Anesthesiology.* 2009;110:1271–1278.
78. Inoue S, Davis DP, Drummond JC, et al. The combination of isoflurane and caspase 8 inhibition results in sustained neuroprotection in rats subject to focal cerebral ischemia. *Anesth Analg.* 2006;102:1548–1555.
79. Warner DS, Takaoka S, Wu B, et al. Electroencephalographic burst suppression is not required to elicit maximal neuroprotection from pentobarbital in a rat model of focal cerebral ischemia. *Anesthesiology.* 1996;84:1475–1484.
80. Zaidan JR, Klochany A, Martin WM, et al. Effect of thiopental on neurologic outcome following coronary artery bypass grafting. *Anesthesiology.* 1991;74:406–411.
81. Bilotta F, Stazi E, Zlotnik A, et al. Neuroprotective effects of intravenous anesthetics: a new critical perspective. *Curr Pharm Des.* 2014;20:5469–5475.
82. D'Souza S. Aneurysmal subarachnoid hemorrhage. *J Neurosurg Anesthesiol.* 2015;27:222–240.
83. Saver JL, Starkman S, Eckstein M, et al. Prehospital use of magnesium sulfate as neuroprotection in acute stroke. *N Engl J Med.* 2015;372:528–536.
84. Sutherland BA, Minnerup J, Balami JS, et al. Neuroprotection for ischaemic stroke: translation from the bench to the bedside. *Int J Stroke.* 2012;7:407–418.
85. Haley EC Jr., Thompson JL, Levin B, et al. Gavestinel does not improve outcome after acute intracerebral hemorrhage: an analysis from the GAIN International and GAIN Americas studies. *Stroke.* 2005;36:1006–1010.
86. Larpthaveesarp A, Ferriero DM, Gonzalez FF. Growth factors for the treatment of ischemic brain injury (growth factor treatment). *Brain Sci.* 2015;5:165–177.
87. O'Regan C, Wu P, Arora P, et al. Statin therapy in stroke prevention: a meta-analysis involving. 121,000 patients. *Am J Med.* 2008;121:24–33.
88. Dienel GA. Brain lactate metabolism: The discoveries and the controversies. *J Cereb Blood Flow Metab.* 2012;32:1107–1138.
89. Pasternak JJ, McGregor DG, Schroeder DR, et al. Hyperglycemia in patients undergoing cerebral aneurysm surgery: Its association with long-term gross neurologic and neuropsychological function. *Mayo Clin Proc.* 2008;83:406–417.
90. Wass CT, Lanier WL. Glucose modulation of ischemic brain injury: review and clinical recommendations. *Mayo Clin Proc.* 1996;71:801–812.
91. Wolfe TJ, Torbey MT. Management of intracranial pressure. *Curr Neurol Neurosci Rep.* 2009;9:477–485.
92. Weston J, Greenhalgh J, Marson AG. Antiepileptic drugs as prophylaxis for post-craniotomy seizures. *Cochrane Database Syst Rev.* 2015;3:CD007286.
93. Kandasamy R, Tharakan J, Idris Z, et al. Intracranial bleeding following induction of anesthesia in a patient undergoing elective surgery for refractory epilepsy. *Surg Neurol Int.* 2013;4:124.
94. Kovarik WD, Mayberg TS, Lam AM, et al. Succinylcholine does not change intracranial pressure, cerebral blood flow velocity, or the electroencephalogram in patients with neurologic injury. *Anesth Analg.* 1994;78:469–473.
95. Maurtua MA, Deogaonkar A, Bakri MH, et al. Dosing of remifentanil to prevent movement during craniotomy in the absence of neuromuscular blockade. *J Neurosurg Anesthesiol.* 2008;20:221–225.
96. Zhang Z, Hu X, Zhang X, et al. Lung protective ventilation in patients undergoing major surgery: a systematic review incorporating a Bayesian approach. *BMJ Open.* 2015;5:e007473.
97. de Jong MA, Ladha KS, Melo MF, et al. Differential Effects of Intraoperative Positive End-expiratory Pressure (PEEP) on respiratory outcome in major abdominal surgery versus craniotomy. *Ann Surg.* 2015.
98. Tommasino C. Fluids and the neurosurgical patient. *Anesthesiol Clin North America.* 2002;20:329–346, vi.
99. Shao L, Hong F, Zou Y, et al. Hypertonic saline for brain relaxation and intracranial pressure in patients undergoing neurosurgical procedures: A meta-analysis of randomized controlled trials. *PLoS One.* 2015;10:e0117314.
100. Rafat C, Flamant M, Gaudry S, et al. Hyponatremia in the intensive care unit: How to avoid a Zugzwang situation? *Ann Intensive Care.* 2015;5:39.
101. Tommasino C, Picozzi V. Volume and electrolyte management. *Best Pract Res Clin Anaesthesiol.* 2007;21:497–516.
102. Lira A, Pinsky MR. Choices in fluid type and volume during resuscitation: impact on patient outcomes. *Ann Intensive Care.* 2014;4:38.
103. Bachelani AM, Bautz JT, Sperry JL, et al. Assessment of platelet transfusion for reversal of aspirin after traumatic brain injury. *Surgery.* 2011;150:836–843.
104. Zeeni C, Carabini LM, Gould RW, et al. The implementation and efficacy of the Northwestern High Risk Spine Protocol. *World Neurosurg.* 2014;82:e815–e823.
105. van den Berghe G, Wouters P, Weekers F, et al. Intensive insulin therapy in critically ill patients. *N Engl J Med.* 2001;345:1359–1367.
106. Bilotta F, Caramia R, Paoloni FP, et al. Safety and efficacy of intensive insulin therapy in critical neurosurgical patients. *Anesthesiology.* 2009;110:611–619.
107. Thiele RH, Pouratian N, Zuo Z, et al. Strict glucose control does not affect mortality after aneurysmal subarachnoid hemorrhage. *Anesthesiology.* 2009;110:603–610.
108. Bebawy JF, Ramaiah VK, Hemmer LB, et al. Clinical pharmacology of insulin confounds stroke trials. *Ann Neurol.* 2012;71:148.
109. Jian M, Li X, Wang A, et al. Flurbiprofen and hypertension but not hydroxyethyl starch are associated with post-craniotomy intracranial haematoma requiring surgery. *Br J Anaesth.* 2014;113:832–839.
110. Bebawy JF, Houston CC, Kosky JL, et al. Nicardipine is superior to esmolol for the management of postcraniotomy emergence hypertension: a randomized open-label study. *Anesth Analg.* 2015;120:186–192.
111. Flexman AM, Merriman B, Griesdale DE, et al. Infratentorial neurosurgery is an independent risk factor for respiratory failure and death in patients undergoing intracranial tumor resection. *J Neurosurg Anesthesiol.* 2014;26:198–204.
112. Bergese SD, Antor MA, Uribe AA, et al. Triple therapy with scopolamine, ondansetron, and dexamethasone for prevention of postoperative nausea and vomiting in moderate to high-risk patients undergoing craniotomy under general anesthesia: A pilot study. *Front Med (Lausanne).* 2015;2:40.
113. Burkhardt T, Rotermund R, Schmidt NO, et al. Dexamethasone PONV prophylaxis alters the hypothalamic-pituitary-adrenal axis after transsphenoidal pituitary surgery. *J Neurosurg Anesthesiol.* 2014;26:216–219.
114. Nabors LB, Portnow J, Ammirati M, et al. Central nervous system cancers, Version. 1.2015. *J Natl Compr Canc Netw.* 2015;13:1191–1202.
115. Bebawy JF. Perioperative steroids for peritumoral intracranial edema: A review of mechanisms, efficacy, and side effects. *J Neurosurg Anesthesiol.* 2012;24:173–177.
116. Luostarinen T, Dilmen OK, Niiya T, et al. Effect of arterial blood pressure on the arterial to end-tidal carbon dioxide difference during anesthesia induction in patients scheduled for craniotomy. *J Neurosurg Anesthesiol.* 2010;22:303–308.
117. Gelb AW, Craen RA, Rao GS, et al. Does hyperventilation improve operating condition during supratentorial craniotomy? A multicenter randomized crossover trial. *Anesth Analg.* 2008;106:585–594, table of contents.
118. Stiff JL, Munch DF, Bromberger-Barnea B. Hypotension and respiratory distress caused by rapid infusion of mannitol or hypertonic saline. *Anesth Analg.* 1979;58:42–48.
119. Garavaglia MM, Das S, Cusimano MD, et al. Anesthetic approach to high-risk patients and prolonged awake craniotomy using dexmedetomidine and scalp block. *J Neurosurg Anesthesiol.* 2014;26:226–233.
120. Guilfoyle MR, Helmy A, Duane D, et al. Regional scalp block for postcraniotomy analgesia: a systematic review and meta-analysis. *Anesth Analg.* 2013;116:1093–1102.
121. Rajan S, Hutcherson MT, Sessler DI, et al. The effects of dexmedetomidine and remifentanil on hemodynamic stability and analgesic requirement after craniotomy: A randomized controlled trial. *J Neurosurg Anesthesiol.* 2015.
122. Song J, Ji Q, Sun Q, et al. The opioid-sparing effect of intraoperative dexmedetomidine infusion after craniotomy. *J Neurosurg Anesthesiol.* 2015.
123. Mammoto T, Hayashi Y, Ohnishi Y, et al. Incidence of venous and paradoxical air embolism in neurosurgical patients in the sitting position: Detection by transesophageal echocardiography. *Acta Anaesthesiol Scand.* 1998;42:643–647.

124. Young ML, Smith DS, Murtagh F, et al. Comparison of surgical and anesthetic complications in neurosurgical patients experiencing venous air embolism in the sitting position. *Neurosurgery*. 1986;18:157–161.
125. Giebler R, Kollenberg B, Pohlen G, et al. Effect of positive end-expiratory pressure on the incidence of venous air embolism and on the cardiovascular response to the sitting position during neurosurgery. *Br J Anaesth*. 1998;80:30–35.
126. Nemergut EC, Zuo Z. Airway management in patients with pituitary disease: A review of 746 patients. *J Neurosurg Anesthesiol*. 2006;18:73–77.
127. Clarke MJ, Erickson D, Castro MR, et al. Thyroid-stimulating hormone pituitary adenomas. *J Neurosurg*. 2008;109:17–22.
128. Dunn LK, Nemergut EC. Anesthesia for transsphenoidal pituitary surgery. *Curr Opin Anaesthesiol*. 2013;26:549–554.
129. Lam G, Mehta V, Zada G. Spontaneous and medically induced cerebrospinal fluid leakage in the setting of pituitary adenomas: review of the literature. *Neurosurg Focus*. 2012;32:E2.
130. Kang HG, Kim BJ, Lee J, et al. Risk factors associated with the presence of unruptured intracranial aneurysms. *Stroke*. 2015;46:3093–3098.
131. Rinkel GJ, Djibuti M, Algra A, et al. Prevalence and risk of rupture of intracranial aneurysms: a systematic review. *Stroke*. 1998;29:251–256.
132. Hunt WE, Hess RM. Surgical risk as related to time of intervention in the repair of intracranial aneurysms. *J Neurosurg*. 1968;28:14–20.
133. Teasdale GM, Drake CG, Hunt W, et al. A universal subarachnoid hemorrhage scale: report of a committee of the World Federation of Neurosurgical Societies. *J Neurol Neurosurg Psychiatry*. 1988;51:1457.
134. Fisher CM, Kistler JP, Davis JM. Relation of cerebral vasospasm to subarachnoid hemorrhage visualized by computerized tomographic scanning. *Neurosurgery*. 1980;6:1–9.
135. Ramachandran M, Retarekar R, Raghavan ML, et al. Assessment of image-derived risk factors for natural course of unruptured cerebral aneurysms. *J Neurosurg*. 2015;124:1–8.
136. Bebawy JF, Gupta DK, Bendok BR, et al. Adenosine-induced flow arrest to facilitate intracranial aneurysm clip ligation: Dose-response data and safety profile. *Anesth Analg*. 2010;110:1406–1411.
137. Bebawy JF, Zeeni C, Sharma S, et al. Adenosine-induced flow arrest to facilitate intracranial aneurysm clip ligation does not worsen neurologic outcome. *Anesth Analg*. 2013;117:1205–1210.
138. Molyneux A, Kerr R, Stratton I, et al. International Subarachnoid Aneurysm Trial (ISAT) of neurosurgical clipping versus endovascular coiling in. 2143 patients with ruptured intracranial aneurysms: A randomised trial. *Lancet*. 2002;360:1267–1274.
139. Rutledge WC, Ko NU, Lawton MT, et al. Hemorrhage rates and risk factors in the natural history course of brain arteriovenous malformations. *Transl Stroke Res*. 2014;5:538–542.
140. Spetzler RF, Martin NA. A proposed grading system for arteriovenous malformations. *J Neurosurg*. 1986;65:476–483.
141. Flores BC, Klinger DR, Rickert KL, et al. Management of intracranial aneurysms associated with arteriovenous malformations. *Neurosurg Focus*. 2014;37:E11.
142. Rangel-Castilla L, Spetzler RF, Nakaji P. Normal perfusion pressure breakthrough theory: A reappraisal after 35 years. *Neurosurg Rev*. 2015;38:399–404; discussion 404–405.
143. Gutierrez-Gonzalez R, Gil A, Serna C, et al. Normal perfusion pressure breakthrough phenomenon: What still remains unknown. *Br J Neurosurg*. 2012;26:403–405.
144. Zacharia BE, Bruce S, Appelboom G, et al. Occlusive hyperemia versus normal perfusion pressure breakthrough after treatment of cranial arteriovenous malformations. *Neurosurg Clin N Am*. 2012;23:147–151.
145. al-Rodhan NR, Sundt TM Jr., Piepgras DG, et al. Occlusive hyperemia: a theory for the hemodynamic complications following resection of intracerebral arteriovenous malformations. *J Neurosurg*. 1993;78:167–175.
146. von der Brelie C, Simon M, Esche J, et al. Seizure outcomes in patients with surgically treated cerebral arteriovenous malformations. *Neurosurgery*. 2015;77:762–768.
147. Kolos I, Troitskiy A, Balakhonova T, et al. Modern medical treatment with or without carotid endarterectomy for severe asymptomatic carotid atherosclerosis. *J Vasc Surg*. 2015;62:914–922.
148. Hye RJ, Mackey A, Hill MD, et al. Incidence, outcomes, and effect on quality of life of cranial nerve injury in the Carotid Revascularization Endarterectomy versus Stenting Trial. *J Vasc Surg*. 2015;61:1208–1214.
149. Zhang L, Zhao Z, Ouyang Y, et al. Systematic review and meta-analysis of carotid artery stenting versus endarterectomy for carotid stenosis: A chronological and worldwide study. *Medicine (Baltimore)*. 2015;94:e1060.
150. Lewis SC, Warlow CP, Bodenham AR, et al. General anaesthesia versus local anaesthesia for carotid surgery (GALA): A multicentre, randomised controlled trial. *Lancet*. 2008;372:2132–2142.
151. Pasin L, Nardelli P, Landoni G, et al. Examination of regional anesthesia for carotid endarterectomy. *J Vasc Surg*. 2015;62:631–644 e1.
152. Marrocco-Trischitta MM, Cremona G, Lucini D, et al. Peripheral baroreflex and chemoreflex function after eversion carotid endarterectomy. *J Vasc Surg*. 2013;58:136–144 e1.
153. Shakespeare WA, Lanier WL, Perkins WJ, et al. Airway management in patients who develop neck hematomas after carotid endarterectomy. *Anesth Analg*. 2010;110:588–593.
154. Perry MS, Duchowny M. Surgical versus medical treatment for refractory epilepsy: Outcomes beyond seizure control. *Epilepsia*. 2013;54:2060–2070.
155. Flexman AM, Wong H, Riggs KW, et al. Enzyme-inducing anticonvulsants increase plasma clearance of dexmedetomidine: A pharmacokinetic and pharmacodynamic study. *Anesthesiology*. 2014;120:1118–1125.
156. Chui J, Manninen P, Valiante T, et al. The anesthetic considerations of intraoperative electrocorticography during epilepsy surgery. *Anesth Analg*. 2013;117:479–486.
157. Cai T, Gao P, Shen Q, et al. Oesophageal naso-pharyngeal catheter use for airway management in patients for awake craniotomy. *Br J Neurosurg*. 2013;27:396–397.
158. Rajan S, Cata JP, Nada E, et al. Asleep-awake-asleep craniotomy: A comparison with general anesthesia for resection of supratentorial tumors. *J Clin Neurosci*. 2013;20:1068–1073.
159. Pinosky ML, Fishman RL, Reeves ST, et al. The effect of bupivacaine skull block on the hemodynamic response to craniotomy. *Anesth Analg*. 1996;83:1256–1261.
160. Gomez PA, de-la-Cruz J, Lora D, et al. Validation of a prognostic score for early mortality in severe head injury cases. *J Neurosurg*. 2014;121:1314–1322.
161. Corral L, Javierre CF, Ventura JL, et al. Impact of non-neurological complications in severe traumatic brain injury outcome. *Crit Care*. 2012;16:R44.
162. Rudehill A, Bellander BM, Weitzberg E, et al. Outcome of traumatic brain injuries in. 1,508 patients: Impact of prehospital care. *J Neurotrauma*. 2002;19:855–868.
163. Wang R, Li M, Gao WW, et al. Outcomes of early decompressive craniectomy versus conventional medical management after severe traumatic brain injury: A systematic review and meta-analysis. *Medicine (Baltimore)*. 2015;94:e1733.
164. Sauvigny T, Gottsche J, Vettorazzi E, et al. New radiological parameters predict clinical outcome after decompressive craniectomy. *World Neurosurg*. 2015;88:519–525.
165. Budisin B, Bradbury CC, Sharma B, et al. Traumatic brain injury in spinal cord injury: Frequency and risk factors. *J Head Trauma Rehabil*. 2015;31:E33–E42.
166. Korley FK, Kelen GD, Jones CM, et al. Emergency department evaluation of traumatic brain injury in the United States,. 2009–2010. *J Head Trauma Rehabil*. 2015.
167. Piper BJ, Harrigan PW. Hypertonic saline in paediatric traumatic brain injury: a review of nine years' experience with. 23.4% hypertonic saline as standard hyperosmolar therapy. *Anaesth Intensive Care*. 2015;43:204–210.
168. Carrera E, Steiner LA, Castellani G, et al. Changes in cerebral compartmental compliances during mild hypocapnia in patients with traumatic brain injury. *J Neurotrauma*. 2011;28:889–896.
169. Griesdale DE, Ortenwall V, Norena M, et al. Adherence to guidelines for management of cerebral perfusion pressure and outcome in patients who have severe traumatic brain injury. *J Crit Care*. 2015;30:111–115.
170. Kanna RM, Gaike CV, Mahesh A, et al. Multilevel non-contiguous spinal injuries: incidence and patterns based on whole spine MRI. *Eur Spine J*. 2015;25:1163–1169.
171. Ledsome JR, Sharp JM. Pulmonary function in acute cervical cord injury. *Am Rev Respir Dis*. 1981;124:41–44.
172. El Masry WS, Tsubo M, Katoh S, et al. Validation of the American Spinal Injury Association (ASIA) motor score and the National Acute Spinal Cord Injury Study (NASCIS) motor score. *Spine (Phila Pa. 1976)*. 1996;21:614–619.
173. Phillips AA, Krassioukov AV. Contemporary cardiovascular concerns after spinal cord injury: Mechanisms, maladaptations, and management. *J Neurotrauma*. 2015;32:1927–1942.
174. Bank M, Stein A, Sison C, et al. Elevated circulating levels of the pro-inflammatory cytokine macrophage migration inhibitory factor in individuals with acute spinal cord injury. *Arch Phys Med Rehabil*. 2015;96:633–644.
175. Chew BG, Swartz C, Quigley MR, et al. Cervical spine clearance in the traumatically injured patient: Is multidetector CT scanning sufficient alone? Clinical article. *J Neurosurg Spine*. 2013;19:576–581.
176. Ryken TC, Hurlbert RJ, Hadley MN, et al. The acute cardiopulmonary management of patients with cervical spinal cord injuries. *Neurosurgery*. 2013;72(Suppl. 2):84–92.
177. Evaniew N, Noonan VK, Fallah N, et al. Methylprednisolone for the treatment of patients with acute spinal cord injuries: A propensity score-matched cohort study from a Canadian multi-center spinal cord injury registry. *J Neurotrauma*. 2015;32:1674–1683.
178. Hurlbert RJ, Hadley MN, Walters BC, et al. Pharmacological therapy for acute spinal cord injury. *Neurosurgery*. 2013;72(Suppl. 2):93–105.
179. Carabini LM, Zeeni C, Moreland NC, et al. Development and validation of a generalizable model for predicting major transfusion during spine fusion surgery. *J Neurosurg Anesthesiol*. 2014;26:205–215.
180. Yang B, Li H, Wang D, et al. Systematic review and meta-analysis of perioperative intravenous tranexamic acid use in spinal surgery. *PLoS One*. 2013;8:e55436.

181. Liang J, Shen J, Chua S, et al. Does intraoperative cell salvage system effectively decrease the need for allogeneic transfusions in scoliotic patients undergoing posterior spinal fusion? A prospective randomized study. *Eur Spine J.* 2015;24:270–275.
182. Stevens WR, Glazer PA, Kelley SD, et al. Ophthalmic complications after spinal surgery. *Spine (Phila Pa. 1976).* 1997;22:1319–1324.
183. Shen Y, Drum M, Roth S. The prevalence of perioperative visual loss in the United States: A 10-year study from. 1996 to. 2005 of spinal, orthopedic, cardiac, and general surgery. *Anesth Analg.* 2009;109:1534–1545.
184. Chang SH, Miller NR. The incidence of vision loss due to perioperative ischemic optic neuropathy associated with spine surgery: The Johns Hopkins Hospital Experience. *Spine (Phila Pa. 1976).* 2005;30:1299–1302.
185. Postoperative Visual Loss Study Group. Risk factors associated with ischemic optic neuropathy after spinal fusion surgery. *Anesthesiology.* 2012;116:15–24.
186. Rigney L, Cappelen-Smith C, Sebire D, et al. Nontraumatic spinal cord ischaemic syndrome. *J Clin Neurosci.* 2015;22:1544–1549.
187. Stockl B, Wimmer C, Innerhofer P, et al. Delayed anterior spinal artery syndrome following posterior scoliosis correction. *Eur Spine J.* 2005;14:906–909.
188. McClendon J Jr., Smith TR, O'Shaughnessy BA, et al. Time to event analysis for the development of venous thromboembolism after spinal fusion >/= 5 levels. *World Neurosurg.* 2015;84:826–833.
189. Yang SD, Liu H, Sun YP, et al. Prevalence and risk factors of deep vein thrombosis in patients after spine surgery: A retrospective case-cohort study. *Sci Rep.* 2015;5:11834.
190. Hou S, Rabchevsky AG. Autonomic consequences of spinal cord injury. *Compr Physiol.* 2014;4:1419–1453.
191. Caruso D, Gater D, Harnish C. Prevention of recurrent autonomic dysreflexia: a survey of current practice. *Clin Auton Res.* 2015;25:293–300.

38 Anesthesia for Thoracic Surgery

JAMES B. EISENKRAFT • EDMOND COHEN • STEVEN M. NEUSTEIN

Preoperative Evaluation
  History
  Physical Examination
  Evaluation of the Cardiovascular System
  Pulmonary Function Testing and Evaluation for Lung Resectability

Preoperative Preparation
  Smoking
  Infection
  Hydration and Removal of Bronchial Secretions
  Wheezing and Bronchodilation
  Pulmonary Rehabilitation

Intraoperative Monitoring
  Direct Arterial Catheterization
  Central Venous Pressure Monitoring
  Pulmonary Artery Catheterization
  Transesophageal Echocardiography
  Monitoring of Oxygenation and Ventilation

One-lung Ventilation
  Absolute Indications for One-lung Ventilation
  Relative Indications for One-lung Ventilation
  Methods of Lung Separation
  Lung Separation in the Patient with a Tracheostomy
  Lung Separation in the Patient with a Difficult Airway

Management of One-lung Ventilation
  Confirmation of Correct Position of DLT or Endobronchial Blocker
  Inspired Oxygen Fraction
  Tidal Volume and Respiratory Rate
  Positive End-expiratory Pressure to the Dependent Lung
  Continuous Positive Airway Pressure to the Nondependent Lung
  Clinical Approach to Management of One-lung Ventilation

Choice of Anesthesia for Thoracic Surgery

Hypoxic Pulmonary Vasoconstriction
  Effects of Anesthetics on Hypoxic Pulmonary Vasoconstriction
  Other Determinants of Hypoxic Pulmonary Vasoconstriction
  Potentiators of Hypoxic Pulmonary Vasoconstriction
  Nitric Oxide and One-lung Ventilation

Anesthesia for Diagnostic Procedures
  Bronchoscopy

Diagnostic Procedures for Mediastinal Mass
  Mediastinoscopy
  Thoracoscopy
  Video-assisted (Minimally Invasive) Thoracoscopic Surgery

Anesthesia for Special Situations
  High-frequency Ventilation
  Bronchopleural Fistula and Empyema
  Lung Cysts and Bullae
  Anesthesia for Resection of the Trachea
  Bronchopulmonary Lavage
  Myasthenia Gravis
  Myasthenic Syndrome (Eaton–Lambert Syndrome)

Postoperative Management and Complications
  Postoperative Pain Control
  Complications Following Thoracic Surgery

KEY POINTS

1. It is important to determine prior to the onset of anesthesia and surgery whether the patient will be able to tolerate the planned lung resection.
2. Preoperative assessment of vital capacity is critical because at least three times the tidal volume (V_T) is necessary for an effective cough.
3. Smoking increases airway irritability, decreases mucociliary transport, and increases secretions. It also decreases forced vital capacity and forced expiratory flow 25% to 75%, thereby increasing the incidence of postoperative pulmonary complications.
4. The absolute indications for lung separation using a double-lumen tube have been for protection against spillage of blood, infectious material, or lavage fluid from one lung, or for ventilation in the case of bronchopleural fistula or bullae. A lobectomy or pneumonectomy is a relative indication.
5. The most important advance in checking the proper position of a double-lumen tube is the introduction of the pediatric flexible fiberoptic bronchoscope.
6. During one-lung ventilation (OLV), the dependent lung should be ventilated using a V_T that results in a plateau airway pressure less than 25 cm H_2O at a rate adjusted to maintain $Paco_2$ at 35 ± 3 mmHg.
7. The choice of anesthetic technique for OLV must take into consideration the effects on oxygenation and therefore on hypoxic pulmonary vasoconstriction.
8. The need for OLV is much greater with video-assisted thoracoscopic surgery than with open thoracotomy because it is not possible to retract the lung during video-assisted thoracoscopic surgery as it is during an open thoracotomy.
9. The potential advantages offered by high-frequency positive-pressure ventilation during thoracic anesthesia are that lower V_T and inspiratory pressures result in a quiet lung field for the surgeon, with minimal movements of airway, lung tissue, and mediastinum.
10. Myasthenia gravis is a disorder of the neuromuscular junction, characterized by weakness and fatigability of voluntary muscles with improvement following rest. Surgical thymectomy is a commonly performed therapy.
11. In addition to a more comfortable patient, important benefits of adequate pain relief are avoidance of postoperative atelectasis and limited inspiratory thoracic cage expansion.

Lung cancer is the most common cause of cancer mortality in the United States in men, and surpassed breast cancer as the leading cause of cancer deaths in women in 1987 (Fig. 38-1).[1] It is currently estimated to be responsible for 1.59 million deaths annually worldwide. Each year there are more deaths from lung cancer than from colon, breast, and prostate cancers combined. The most recent statistics from the American Cancer Society indicated that approximately 221,200 new cases of lung cancer would be diagnosed in 2015 (115,610 among men and 105,590 among women). The Society also estimated that there would be 158,040 deaths from lung cancer, which represents 27% of all cancer deaths.[2] The increased incidence of lung cancer has led to an increase in the amount of noncardiac thoracic surgery performed in the United States. The overall risk of developing lung cancer is greater in women than in men (1 in 13 vs. 1 in 16). Most lung cancers are found in the older population, the average age at time of diagnosis is about 70 years. Less than 2% of all cases occur in those age 45 years or less.[2]

In this chapter, the physiologic, pharmacologic, and clinical considerations for the patient undergoing pulmonary surgery are reviewed, followed by sections on anesthesia for diagnostic and therapeutic procedures, high-frequency ventilation, and special situations, including bronchopleural fistula (BPF) and tracheal reconstruction. A discussion of myasthenia gravis (MG) is included because of its relationship to the thymus gland and because thymectomy is one of the most commonly performed surgical procedures in these patients. The chapter concludes with a review of the postoperative management of the patient who has undergone noncardiac thoracic surgery.

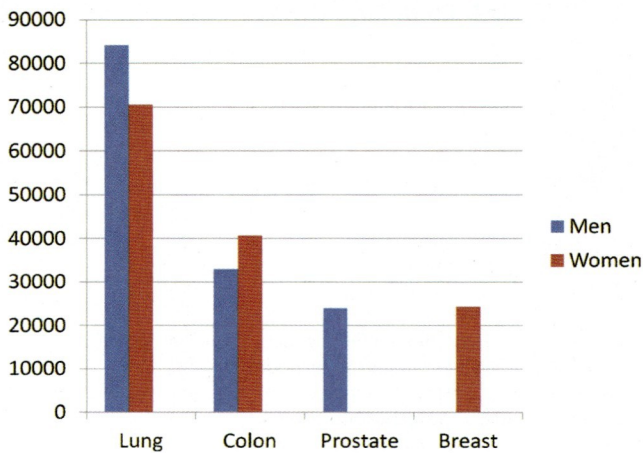

Figure 38-1 Estimated 2011 deaths from cancer in the United States. Lung cancer is the leading cause of cancer-related mortality. (Based on data from The American Cancer Society, Cancer Statistics, 2010. A presentation from the American Cancer Society. 2011 Estimated U.S. Cancer Deaths. Available at: http://www.cancer.org/acs/groups/content/@epidemiologysurveillance/documents/document/acspc-029997.pptx. Accessed November 26, 2012.)

Preoperative Evaluation

The preoperative evaluation of the patient for thoracic surgery should focus on the extent and severity of pulmonary disease and cardiovascular involvement (see Chapter 22). It is important to determine whether the patient will be able to tolerate the planned lung resection. To discover postoperatively that the patient cannot tolerate the resection would be catastrophic.

The most common complications following thoracic surgery are pulmonary in nature, the most frequent being pneumonia and atelectasis.[3] It is more difficult to predict postoperative pulmonary complications following elective cardiothoracic, compared with noncardiothoracic surgery.[4] Thoracic surgery is known to be high risk, and patient factors that have been associated with increased risk include advanced age, poor general health status, chronic obstructive pulmonary disease (COPD), body mass index higher than 30 kg/m^2, low FEV_1 and low predicted postoperative FEV_1.[5,6]

History

Dyspnea

Dyspnea occurs when the requirement for ventilation is greater than the patient's ability to respond appropriately (see Chapter 11). Dyspnea is quantified by the degree of physical activity required to produce it, the level of activity possible (e.g., ability to walk on level ground or climb stairs), and management of daily activities. Severe exertional dyspnea usually implies a significantly diminished ventilatory reserve and a forced expiratory volume in 1 second (FEV_1) later 1,500 mL, with possible need for postoperative ventilatory support.

Cough

Recurrent productive cough for 3 months of the year for two consecutive years is necessary to make the diagnosis of chronic bronchitis. Cough indirectly increases airway irritability. If the cough is productive, the volume, consistency, and color of the sputum should be assessed. Sputum should be cultured to rule out infection and to establish whether there is a need for preoperative antibiotic therapy. Blood-stained sputum or episodes of gross hemoptysis should alert the anesthesiologist to the possibility of a tumor invading the respiratory tract (e.g., the main stem bronchus), which might interfere with endobronchial intubation.

Cigarette Smoking

Cigarette smoking is the main risk factor for developing lung cancer and in the United States, is linked to about 90% of lung cancers. Using other tobacco products such as cigars or pipes also increases the risk for lung cancer. Tobacco smoke is a toxic mix of more than 7,000 chemicals. Cigarette smokers have a 15 to 30 times greater likelihood of developing and/or dying from lung cancer than nonsmokers. Former smokers have a lower risk of lung cancer than if they had continued to smoke, but their risk is still greater than the risk for people who never smoked. Stopping smoking at any age decreases the risk of lung cancer.[7]

Cigarette smoking increases the risk of chronic lung disease and other malignancies (mouth, nose, throat, voicebox [larynx], esophagus, liver, bladder, kidney, pancreas, colon, rectum, cervix, stomach, blood, and bone marrow [acute myeloid leukemia]), as well as the incidence of postoperative pulmonary complications. The number of pack-years (packs smoked per day multiplied by the number of years) is directly related to measurable changes in respiratory gas flow and closing capacity, making these patients prone to postoperative atelectasis and arterial hypoxemia.

Exercise Tolerance

Patients who can walk up three or more flights of stairs are at reduced risk, and those unable to climb two flights are generally at increased risk.[8] The best evaluation is actually the history of the patient's quality of life. An otherwise healthy patient, with good exercise tolerance, generally does not require additional screening tests. Quality of life measures alone have been shown to correlate poorly with such measures as FEV_1, diffusion capacity for carbon monoxide (DLCO), and exercise testing, and should not substitute for actual testing.

Risk Factors for Acute Lung Injury

In some cases, thoracic surgery may lead to acute lung injury (ALI) postoperatively. Perioperative risk factors that have been identified include preoperative alcohol abuse and patients undergoing pneumonectomy. Intraoperative risk factors include high ventilatory pressures and administration of excessive amounts of fluid.[9] Poor preoperative pulmonary function and positive fluid balance on postoperative day 1 have been identified as independent risk factors for lung injury in patients undergoing open thoracotomy.[10]

Physical Examination

The physical examination of the patient should address the following aspects.

Respiratory Pattern

The presence of cyanosis and clubbing, the breathing pattern, and the type of breath sounds should be noted.

Cyanosis. The presence of peripheral cyanosis (in the fingers, toes, or ears) should be distinguished from causes of poor circulation (acrocyanosis). The presence of central cyanosis (in the buccal mucosa) is usually secondary to arterial hypoxemia. If cyanosis is present, the arterial hemoglobin saturation with oxygen is 80% or less (Pao_2 <50 to 52 mmHg), which indicates a limited margin of respiratory reserve.

Clubbing. Clubbing of fingers and toes is often seen in patients with chronic lung disease, malignancies, or congenital heart disease associated with right-to-left shunt.

Respiratory Rate and Pattern. A patient's inability to complete a normal sentence without pausing for breath is an indication of severe dyspnea. Inspiratory paradox, the abdomen moving in while the chest moves out, suggests diaphragmatic fatigue and respiratory dysfunction. The patient should be assessed for paroxysmal retraction (Hoover sign), limited diaphragmatic movement because of hyperinflation, asymmetry of chest movement secondary to phrenic nerve involvement, hemothorax, pleural effusion, and pneumothorax. The pattern and rate of breathing have important roles in distinguishing between obstructive and restrictive lung diseases. For constant minute ventilation, the work done against airflow resistance decreases when breathing is slow and deep. Work done against elastic resistance decreases when breathing is rapid and shallow (e.g., as in pulmonary infarct or pulmonary fibrosis).

Breath Sounds. Wet sounds (crackles) are usually caused by excessive fluid in the airways and indicate sputum retention or edema. Dry sounds (wheezes) are produced by high-velocity gas flow through bronchi and are a sign of airways obstruction. Distant sounds are an indication of emphysema and possibly bullae. The trachea should be in the midline. Displacement of the trachea may be secondary to a number of causes, including mediastinal mass, and should alert the anesthesiologist to a potentially difficult intubation of the trachea or airway obstruction on induction of anesthesia.

Evaluation of the Cardiovascular System

One of the most important factors in the evaluation of a patient scheduled for thoracic surgery is the presence of an increase in pulmonary vascular resistance secondary to a fixed reduction in the cross-sectional area of the pulmonary vascular bed. The pulmonary circulation is normally a low-pressure, high-compliance system capable of handling an increase in blood flow by recruitment of normally underperfused vessels. This acts as a compensatory mechanism that normally prevents an increase in pulmonary arterial pressure. In COPD, there is distention of the pulmonary capillary bed with decreased ability to tolerate an increase in blood flow (decreased compliance). Such patients demonstrate an increase in pulmonary vascular resistance when cardiac output increases because of a decreased ability to compensate for an increase in pulmonary blood flow. This results in pulmonary hypertension, signs of which include a narrowly split second heart sound, increased intensity of the pulmonary component of the second heart sound, and right ventricular and atrial hypertrophy. An increase in pulmonary vascular resistance is of significance in the management of the patient during anesthesia because several factors, such as acidosis, sepsis, hypoxia, and application of positive end-expiratory pressure (PEEP), all further increase the pulmonary vascular resistance and increase the likelihood of right ventricular failure.

In patients with ischemic or valvular heart disease, the function of the left side of the heart should also be carefully evaluated.

Electrocardiogram

A patient with COPD may present with electrocardiographic features of right atrial and ventricular hypertrophy and strain. These include a low-voltage QRS complex due to lung hyperinflation and poor R-wave progression across the precordial leads. An enlarged P wave ("P pulmonale") in standard lead II is diagnostic of right atrial hypertrophy. The electrocardiographic changes of right ventricular hypertrophy are an R/S ratio of greater than 1 in lead V_1 (i.e., R-wave voltage exceeds S-wave voltage).

Chest Radiography

Hyperinflation and increased vascular markings are usually present with COPD. Prominent lung markings often occur in bronchitis, while they are decreased in emphysema, particularly at the bases, where actual bullae may be present in severe cases. Hyperinflation, with an increased anteroposterior chest diameter, may be present, together with an enlarged retrosternal air space of greater than 2 cm in diameter seen in a lateral chest radiograph.

The location of the lung lesion should be assessed by posteroanterior and lateral projections on chest radiography. In addition to tracheal or carinal shift, a mediastinal mass may indicate difficulty with ventilation, a difficult and bloody dissection, difficulty in placing a double-lumen tube (DLT; because of deviation of the main stem bronchus), or a collapsed lobe owing to bronchial obstruction with possible sepsis. Review of a computed tomography (CT) study is also useful, and often provides more information about tumor size and location than the chest radiograph.

Arterial Blood Gas Analysis

A common finding in arterial blood gas analysis of patients with COPD is hypoventilation and CO_2 retention. The "blue bloaters" (chronic bronchitis) are cyanotic, hypercarbic, hypoxemic, and usually overweight. They are in a state of chronic respiratory failure and have a decreased ventilatory response to CO_2. In these patients, the high Pa_{CO_2} increases cerebrospinal fluid bicarbonate concentration, the medullary chemoreceptors become reset to a higher level of CO_2, and sensitivity to CO_2 is decreased. Such patients hypoventilate when given high concentrations of oxygen to breathe because of a decreased hypoxic drive.

The "pink puffers" (patients with emphysema) are typically thin, dyspneic, and pink, with essentially normal arterial blood gas values. They present with an increase in minute ventilation to maintain their normal Pa_{CO_2}, which explains the increase in work of breathing and dyspnea. The preoperative Pa_{O_2} correlates with the intraoperative Pa_{O_2} during one-lung ventilation (OLV), but the intraoperative Pa_{O_2} during two-lung ventilation correlates more closely.[11]

Pulmonary Function Testing and Evaluation for Lung Resectability

There are three goals in performing pulmonary function tests in a patient scheduled for lung resection. The first goal is to identify the patient at risk of increased postoperative morbidity and mortality. In thoracic surgery for lung cancer, the specific question is: How much lung tissue may be safely removed without making the patient a pulmonary cripple? This should be weighed against the 1-year mean survival rate of the patient with surgically untreated lung carcinoma. The second goal is to identify the patient who will need short-term or long-term postoperative ventilatory support. The third goal is to evaluate the beneficial effect and reversibility of airway obstruction with the use of bronchodilators.

Effects of Anesthesia and Surgery on Lung Volumes

Anesthesia and postoperative medications can cause changes in lung volumes and ventilatory pattern. Total lung capacity (TLC) decreases after abdominal surgery but not after surgery on an extremity. Vital capacity is decreased by 25% to 50% within 1 to 2 days after surgery and generally returns to normal after 1 to 2 weeks. Residual volume (RV) increases by 13%, whereas expiratory reserve volume decreases by 25% after lower abdominal surgery and 60% after upper abdominal and thoracic surgery. Tidal volume (V_T) decreases by 20% within 24 hours after surgery and gradually returns to normal after 2 weeks. Pulmonary compliance decreases by 33% with similar reductions in functional residual capacity (FRC) secondary to small airway closure. Most of the patients who undergo lung resection are smokers with a certain degree of COPD. They are prone to postoperative complications in direct relation to the amount of lung to be resected (lobectomy or pneumonectomy) and to the severity of the preoperative lung disease.

Spirometry

Forced vital capacity (FVC), forced expired volume in 1 second (FEV_1), maximum voluntary ventilation (MVV), and RV/TLC correlate with outcome following thoracic surgery (see Chapter 11).[12] An abnormal preoperative vital capacity can be identified in 30% to 40% of postoperative deaths. A patient with an abnormal vital capacity has a 33% likelihood of complications and a 10% risk of postoperative mortality.

FEV_1 is a more direct indication of airway obstruction. In the past, an FEV_1 of less than 800 mL in a 70-kg man had been considered an absolute contraindication to lung resection. However, with the advent of thoracoscopic surgery and improved postoperative pain management, patients with smaller lung volumes are now successfully undergoing surgery. It is preferable to indicate the percentage of predicted value, rather than just using the actual results in liters. The percentage of predicted value takes into account the age and size of the patient, and the same number may have a different implication in another patient. The ratio FEV_1/FVC is useful in differentiating between restrictive and obstructive pulmonary diseases. It is normal in restrictive disease because both FEV_1 and FVC decrease, whereas in obstructive disease the ratio is usually low because the FEV_1 is markedly decreased. MVV is a nonspecific test and is an indicator of both restriction and obstruction. Although MVV has not been systematically evaluated as a predictor of morbidity, it is generally accepted that an MVV less than 50% of predicted value is an indication of high risk. A ratio of RV to TLC (RV/TLC) of greater than 50% is generally indicative of a high-risk patient for pulmonary resection. By multiplying the preoperative FEV_1 by the percentage of lung tissue expected to remain following resection, a predicted postoperative FEV_1 can be calculated. Patients with a predicted postoperative FEV_1 value above 40% are at reduced risk and those with predicted postoperative FEV_1 below 30% are at increased risk.[13] Those patients who fall into the latter category are more likely to need postoperative ventilation.

Flow–Volume Loops

The flow–volume loop displays essentially the same information as a spirometer but is more convenient for measurement of specific flow rates (Fig. 38-2). The shape and peak airflow rates during expiration at high lung volumes are effort dependent, but indicate the patency of the larger airways. Effort-independent expiration occurs at low lung volumes and usually reflects small airway resistance, best measured by forced expiratory flow (FEF) during the middle half of the FVC ($FEF_{25\%-75\%}$).

In general, patients with obstructive airway disease (Fig. 38-3), such as asthma, bronchitis, and emphysema, have grossly decreased FEV_1/FVC ratios because of increased airway resistance and a decrease in FEV_1. Peak expiratory flow rate and MVV are usually decreased, whereas TLC increases secondary to increases in RV. In these patients, the effort-independent portion of the flow–volume curve is markedly depressed inward, with reduction of the flow rate at 25% to 75% of FVC.

In patients with restrictive disease (Fig. 38-3), such as pulmonary fibrosis and scoliosis, there is a decrease in FVC with a relatively normal FEV_1. Because the airway resistance is normal, FEV_1/FVC is also normal. TLC is markedly decreased, whereas MVV and $FEF_{25\%-75\%}$ are usually normal. The flow–volume curves of these patients are normal in shape, but the lung volumes and peak flow rates are decreased.

Significance of Bronchodilator Therapy. Pulmonary function tests are usually performed before and after bronchodilator therapy to assess the reversibility of the airway obstruction. This is useful in the assessment of the degree of airway obstruction and the patient's effort ability. After treatment with bronchodilators, increases in peak expiratory flow compared with a baseline indicate reversibility of airway obstruction (often seen in asthmatic patients). A 15% improvement in pulmonary function tests may be considered a positive response to bronchodilator therapy and indicates that this therapy should be initiated before surgery.

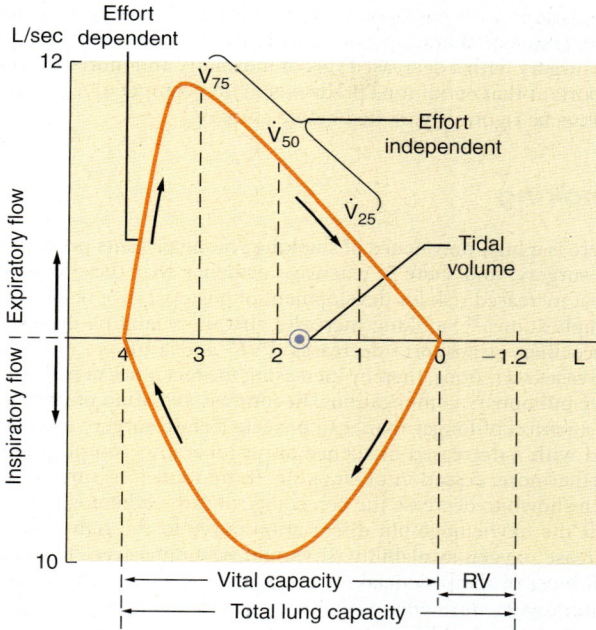

Figure 38-2 Flow–volume loop in a normal subject. $\dot{V}_{75}$, $\dot{V}_{50}$, and $\dot{V}_{25}$ represent flow at 75%, 50%, and 25% of vital capacity, respectively. RV, residual volume. (Adapted from Goudsouzian N, Karamanian A. *Physiology for the Anesthesiologist*. 2nd ed. Norwalk, CT: Appleton-Century-Crofts; 1984.)

The overall prognosis of COPD is better related to the level of spirometric function after bronchodilator therapy than to a baseline function.

Split-Lung Function Tests

Regional lung function studies serve to predict the function of the lung tissue that would remain after lung resection. A whole (two)-lung test may fail to estimate whether the amount of postresection lung tissue will allow the patient to function at a reasonable level of activity without disabling dyspnea or cor pulmonale.

Regional Perfusion Test. This involves the intravenous injection of insoluble radioactive xenon (^{133}Xe). The peak radioactivity of each lung is proportional to the degree of perfusion of each lung.

Regional Ventilation Test. Using an inhaled, insoluble radioactive gas, the peak radioactivity over each lung is proportional to the degree of ventilation. Combining radiospirometry with whole-lung testing (FEV$_1$, FVC, maximal breathing capacity) has resulted in a fair degree of correlation between predicted volumes and pulmonary function tests measured after pneumonectomy.

Computed Tomography and Positron Emission Tomography Scans. Patients normally undergo CT scanning. The CT scan provides anatomic sections through the chest and can delineate the size of the tumor. It can also reveal if there is airway or cardiovascular compression.

Positron emission tomography (PET) scans use a glucose analog that is labeled with a radionuclide positron emitter. This scan can detect tumor based on the metabolic activity. Because malignant tumors are growing at such a fast rate compared with healthy tissue, the tumor cells will use up more of the sugar that has the radionuclide attached to it. There is greater uptake by malignant mediastinal lymph nodes than benign nodes. PET may be more accurate than CT for mediastinal staging.[14] Currently, PET scans can be used to further evaluate lesions that are seen on a CT scan. The PET scan can also be used to follow the results of lung cancer treatments.[15]

The CT and PET scans can be done at the same time to produce a PET–CT scan. A mass that is seen on the CT scan is more likely to be malignant if it also demonstrates enhanced glucose uptake on the PET scan.

Diffusing Capacity for Carbon Monoxide

The ability of the lung to perform gas exchange is reflected by the diffusing capacity for carbon monoxide (DL$_{CO}$). It is impaired in such disorders as interstitial lung disease, which affects the alveolar-capillary site. A predicted postoperative DL$_{CO}$ below 40% is associated with increased risk. Predicted postoperative diffusing capacity percent is the strongest single predictor of risk of complications and mortality after lung resection. There is little interrelationship of predicted postoperative diffusing capacity percent and predicted postoperative FEV$_1$, indicating that these values should be assessed independently when estimating operative risk.[13] In a study of 956 patients, a lower DL$_{CO}$PPO (diffusing capacity for carbon monoxide, predicted postoperative) and the preoperative administration of chemotherapy, were found to be predictive of postoperative complications. In that study, FEV$_1$ was not found to be predictive of complications.[16] In another study, the DL$_{CO}$PPO was the most predictive factor for postoperative morbidity and mortality.[17] It has been demonstrated that PPO FEV$_1$ and DL$_{CO}$ are predictive for postoperative pulmonary complications in both minimally invasive and open lobectomies.[18] If the PPO FEV$_1$ and DL$_{CO}$ are greater than 60%, the patient is at low risk, and no further testing is needed.[19]

Maximal Oxygen Consumption. The maximal oxygen consumption (VO$_2$ max) is a predictor of postoperative complications. Patients with a VO$_2$ max over 15 to 20 mL/kg/min are at reduced risk.[20] A VO$_2$ max below 10 mL/kg/min indicates very high risk for lung resection.[21] A simpler test that can be performed is exercise oximetry—a decrease of 4% during exercise is associated with increased risk.[22] A 6-minute walk test of less than 2,000 feet has been correlated both with a VO$_2$ max below 15 mL/kg/min and with a decrease in oximetry reading during exercise.

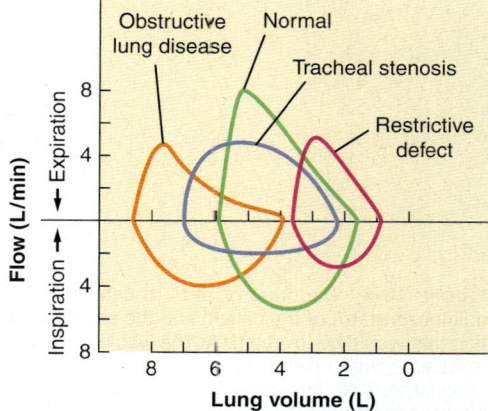

Figure 38-3 Flow–volume loops relative to lung volumes in a normal subject, in a patient with COPD, in a patient with fixed obstruction (tracheal stenosis), and in a patient with pulmonary fibrosis (restrictive defect). Note the concave expiratory form in the patient with COPD and the flat inspiratory curve in the patient with a fixed obstruction. (Adapted from Goudsouzian N, Karamanian A. *Physiology for the Anesthesiologist*. 2nd ed. Norwalk, CT: Appleton-Century-Crofts; 1984.)

It has been suggested that the percentage of predicted VO_2 max may be a better indicator for risk, and a threshold of 50% to 60% could be established without an increase in surgical mortality.[23] Brunelli and Fianchini[24] had patients climb the maximum number of stairs possible. On the basis of the results of this study, these authors recommended that patients who were able to climb more than 14 m can safely undergo surgery, and those who were able to climb less than 12 m, with predicted postoperative function FEV_1 below 35% not be considered for major lung resection. The inability to do a maximal stair climbing has been correlated with an increased mortality following major lung resection.[25] In a recent study, climbing to 20 m with a speed of at least 15 m/min, correlated with meeting qualifying criteria for pneumonectomy. The results for stair climbing correlated with VO_2 consumption during treadmill exercise.[26] Climbing 22 m has been correlated with at least VO_2 of 15 mL/kg/min, although the stair climbing is not standardized.[27] Evaluation of lung function with spirometry and DLCO, and estimating peak oxygen consumption helps to predict risk of postoperative complications.[28] An 11-point scoring scale has been developed for predicting postoperative pulmonary complications.[29] ASA physical status of 3 or higher, emergency or high risk surgery, and history of CHF or chronic lung disease were independent predictors for reintubation following extubation. The preoperative evaluation of the patient for lung resection is summarized in Figure 38-4.

Preoperative Preparation

The wide spectrum of physiologic changes that occur during thoracic surgery puts patients at great risk of developing postoperative complications. Morbidity and mortality increase when these changes are superimposed on an acutely or chronically compromised patient. Several conditions, including infection, dehydration, electrolyte imbalance, wheezing, obesity, cigarette smoking, cor pulmonale, and malnutrition, show particular correlations with postoperative complications. Proper, vigorous preoperative preparation can improve the patient's ability to face the surgery with a decreased risk of morbidity and mortality. It is important that conditions predisposing to postoperative complications be rigorously treated before surgery.

Smoking

There is a high prevalence of smoking among patients presenting for surgery, and there is extensive evidence that these patients are at increased risk for development of postoperative respiratory complications.[30] Smoking increases airway irritability, decreases mucociliary transport, decreases FVC and $FEF_{25\% \text{ to } 75\%}$, and increases secretions, thereby increasing the incidence of postoperative pulmonary complications. In contrast, cessation of smoking for a period of longer than 4 to 6 weeks before surgery is associated with a decreased incidence of postoperative complications. Furthermore, cessation of smoking 48 hours before surgery has been shown to decrease the percentage of carboxyhemoglobin, to shift the oxyhemoglobin dissociation curve to the right, and to increase oxygen availability. It should be emphasized, however, that most of the beneficial effects of cessation of smoking, such as improvement in ciliary function, improvement in closing volume, increase in $FEF_{25\% \text{ to } 75\%}$, and reduction in sputum production, usually occur 2 to 3 months after smoking has ceased. In one study, there was no evidence of a paradoxical increase in postoperative complications in patients who stopped smoking within 2 months before undergoing thoracic resection for lung tumor.[31] Smoking is associated with increased mortality and pulmonary complications, but these can be decreased by preoperative cessation; the risk decreases with a longer cessation.[32] A recent study indicated that the discontinuation of smoking for more than 8 weeks prior to surgery can help improve postoperative pulmonary function.[33] One meta-analysis indicated that there was no improvement with cessation of smoking for less than 8 weeks[34]

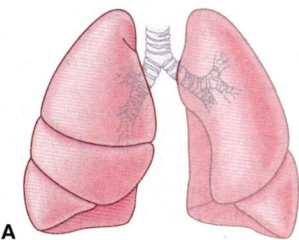

Whole-lung function

ABG (FiO_2 = 0.21) $PaCO_2$ >46 mmHg
                      PaO_2 <60 mmHg
FVC   <50% or 1.5 mL/kg
FEV_1 <50%
VC   <2 L
MVV   <50% or <50 L/min
Lung Volume   RV/TLC >50%
DL_{CO} <50%

A

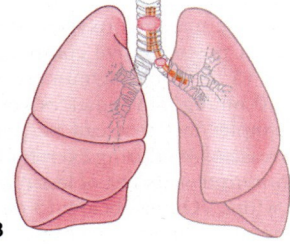

Split-lung function

1. Split-lung spirometry with DLT
2. Regional lung radiospirometry
   Regional perfusion (^{133}Xe, ^{131}I-MAA)
   Regional ventilation ^{133}Xe

Predicted postresection FEV_1 <800 mL

Blood flow to the resected lung >70%

B

Figure 38-4 The order of tests to determine the cardiopulmonary status of the patient and the extent of lung resection that would be tolerated. **A:** The whole-lung function test is a basic screening test. **B:** The split-lung function tests are regional tests to determine the involvement of the diseased lung to be removed. ABG, arterial blood gas; FVC, forced vital capacity; FEV_1, forced expiratory volume in 1 second; VC, vital capacity; MVV, maximum voluntary ventilation; RV/TLC, residual volume/total lung capacity; DLT, double-lumen tube, D_{LCO}, diffusing capacity for carbon monoxide. (Adapted from Neustein SM, Cohen E. Preoperative evaluation of thoracic surgical patients. In: Cohen E, ed. *The Practice of Thoracic Anesthesia*. Philadelphia: JB Lippincott; 1995:187.)

but another meta-analysis indicated a progressive improvement with each week of abstinence from smoking.[35]

Infection

Acute or chronic infection should be vigorously treated before surgery. Broad-spectrum antibiotics are commonly used. Treatment of the acutely ill patient depends on the results of the Gram stain of the sputum and blood cultures. Unless there are other modifying circumstances such as allergic history or patients are already receiving antibiotics, cefazolin is routinely administered perioperatively. To be most effective, it needs to be given prior to skin incision.[36] In one prospective study, the incidence of mortality was lower in the group treated with prophylactic antibiotics compared with the untreated group (9% vs. 17%), and a lower incidence of postoperative pulmonary infection was also found.[37] Although not all surgeons routinely administer antibiotics prophylactically to their patients, any infection present before surgery should be vigorously treated.

Hydration and Removal of Bronchial Secretions

Correction of hypovolemia and electrolyte imbalance should be accomplished before surgery because adequate hydration decreases the viscosity of bronchial secretions and facilitates their removal from the bronchial tree. Humidification of inspired gas is extremely useful. The use of mucolytic drugs, such as acetylcysteine (Mucomyst), or oral expectorants (potassium iodide) can be beneficial to patients with viscous secretions. Commonly used methods for removing secretions from the bronchial tree include postural drainage, vigorous coughing, chest percussion, deep breathing, and the use of an incentive spirometer. These modalities often require patient cooperation and frequent verbal encouragement to maximize the benefit.

Wheezing and Bronchodilation

The presence of acute wheezing represents a medical emergency, and elective surgery should be postponed until effective treatment has been instituted. Chronic wheezing is often seen in patients with COPD and is attributable to the presence of gas flow obstruction secondary to smooth muscle contraction, accumulation of secretions, and mucosal edema. Smooth muscle contraction may occur in small airways only (detectable by changes in $FEF_{25\% \text{ to } 75\%}$) or may be widespread, with a large reduction of FEV_1 and FVC. The efficacy of bronchodilators in reversing the bronchospastic component is extremely important. A trial of bronchodilators and measurement of their effects on pulmonary function should be performed in any patient who shows evidence of airflow obstruction. Several classes of bronchodilators are available.

Sympathomimetic Drugs

Sympathomimetic drugs increase the formation of 3′,5′-cyclic adenosine monophosphate (cAMP). The balance between cAMP, which produces bronchodilation, and cyclic guanosine monophosphate, which produces bronchoconstriction, determines the state of contraction of the bronchial smooth muscle. Increasing cAMP production therefore causes relaxation of the bronchial tree. Sympathomimetic drugs, such as epinephrine, isoproterenol, isoetharine, and ephedrine, all have mixed β_1 and β_2 sympathetic agonist effects. The β_1 (cardiac effects) of these drugs are often undesirable in patients with COPD. Selective β_2 sympathomimetic drugs, such as albuterol, terbutaline, and metaproterenol, given as inhaled aerosols, are the preferred drugs for the treatment of bronchospasm, particularly in patients with cardiac disease.

Phosphodiesterase Inhibitors

Phosphodiesterase inhibitors inhibit the breakdown of cAMP by cytoplasmic phosphodiesterase. The methylxanthines, such as aminophylline, increase the level of cAMP, resulting in bronchodilation. In addition, aminophylline improves diaphragmatic contractility and increases the patient's resistance to fatigue. Therapeutic blood levels of aminophylline are 5 to 20 μg/mL and can be achieved by infusing a loading dose of 5 to 7 mg/kg over 20 minutes, followed by a continuous intravenous infusion of 0.5 to 0.7 mg/kg/hr. Aminophylline may cause ventricular dysrhythmias, and this side effect should be borne in mind when treating patients who have myocardial ischemia. Because newer medications have fewer side effects, aminophylline is now rarely used.

Steroids

Although not true bronchodilators, steroids are traditionally considered to decrease mucosal edema and may prevent the release of bronchoconstricting substances. They are of questionable benefit in acute bronchospasm. Steroids may be administered orally, parenterally, or in aerosol form, such as beclomethasone by inhaler.

Cromolyn Sodium

Cromolyn sodium stabilizes mast cells and inhibits degranulation and histamine release. It is useful in the prevention of bronchospastic attacks but is of little value in the treatment of the acute situation (see Chapter 8).

Parasympatholytic Drugs

Parasympatholytics include atropine and ipratropium (see Chapter 14). In the past, atropine has been avoided in patients with COPD and bronchitis because of the concern regarding increases in the viscosity of mucus produced by this agent. However, atropine blocks the formation of cyclic guanosine monophosphate and therefore has a bronchodilator effect.

Pulmonary Rehabilitation

Sekine et al. reported that pulmonary rehabilitation led to reduced hospital stay and improved postoperative FEV_1, compared with a historical control group.[37] The pulmonary rehabilitation included education in a variety of areas such as breathing, exercise, and nutrition. Preoperative physical therapy in patients undergoing surgery for lung cancer led to better oxygenation and shortened hospital stay in the treatment group.[38]

Intraoperative Monitoring

All patients undergoing anesthesia for thoracic surgical procedures require adherence to the Standards of Basic Anesthetic Monitoring American Society of Anesthesiologists (ASA) (see

Chapter 26). In particular, these include an electrocardiogram (lead II and, if possible, V_5), chest or esophageal stethoscopes for heart and breath sound auscultation, and a temperature probe. A chest stethoscope may be placed over the dependent hemithorax to assess dependent lung ventilation. Pulse oximetry, which is a standard of care, is especially valuable during thoracic surgery because hypoxemia may occur during OLV.

Dysrhythmias occur commonly both during and after thoracic surgery, making the usual need for continuous electrocardiographic monitoring even more important. Intraoperative supraventricular tachyarrhythmias may be caused by cardiac manipulation. Dysrhythmias that occur during OLV may be a sign of inadequate oxygenation or ventilation. Postoperative dysrhythmias may be related to sympathetic nervous system stimulation from pain or to a decreased pulmonary vascular bed following lung resection. Patients who present for lung resection often have COPD due to cigarette smoking, have right-sided heart strain, and are prone to multifocal atrial tachyarrhythmias.

The axis of electrocardiogram lead II parallels that of the P wave, making this lead useful for dysrhythmia detection. The simultaneous monitoring of lead V_5 also allows for monitoring of anterolateral wall myocardial ischemia. The use of multiple leads increases the sensitivity for ischemia detection.[39] The following invasive monitors are also indicated and have led to marked improvements in patient care.

Direct Arterial Catheterization

Peripheral arterial catheterization has become an essential tool for the anesthesiologist in the management of patients undergoing major thoracic surgical procedures (see Chapter 26). It allows for continuous beat-to-beat measurement of blood pressure and frequent sampling for the determination of arterial blood gases. Continuous blood pressure readings are critical during thoracic surgery because surgical manipulations may result in cardiac compression and there may be sudden bleeding. Immediate recognition of these changes allows time for proper identification of the etiology and the institution of appropriate treatment.

Serial arterial blood gas analyses are performed as needed in the management of patients undergoing one-lung anesthesia or during cases in which a part of the lung may be "packed away" for a period. Arterial hypoxemia may occur because of shunting of mixed venous through the collapsed lung and an inadequate hypoxic pulmonary vasoconstriction (HPV) response. Significant changes in acid–base status and hyperventilation or hypoventilation can also be identified.

A radial artery catheter (see Chapter 26) can be placed in either extremity during thoracic surgery. For a mediastinoscopic examination, one approach is to place the catheter in the right arm and to use it to monitor for possible compression of the innominate artery by the mediastinoscope. This can help avoid central nervous system complications that might result from inadequate cerebral blood flow via the right carotid artery (see "Mediastinoscopy"). The other approach would be to place the arterial catheter in the left radial artery, allowing for continuous blood pressure measurements, uninterrupted by innominate artery compression. If this is done, a pulse oximeter probe should be placed on the right upper extremity to monitor for innominate artery compression. During thoracotomy, placement of the arterial catheter in the dependent arm can be used to monitor for possible axillary artery compression, which may occur if the patient is not properly positioned. For a brief thoracoscopy case in a relatively healthy patient, it would be acceptable to proceed without an arterial catheter, as long as the pulse oximeter is functioning reliably. Such an example might be a healthy patient presenting for bilateral VAT sympathectomy for hyperhidrosis.

The patient undergoing a pulmonary resection, and especially a right pneumonectomy, is at risk for postoperative pulmonary edema. It is especially important to not fluid overload such a patient, as the likelihood of postoperative edema is greater with increased intraoperative fluid administration. Prior to its administration it would be preferable to be able to identify which patients would be likely to respond favorably to a fluid bolus. The central venous pressure (CVP) may not accurately reflect intravascular volume status, and is no longer recommended as a guide for fluid responsiveness.[40] Systolic pressure variation (SPV) and pulse pressure variation (PPV) have been reported as being able to predict fluid responsiveness.[41] In a recent paper, a PPV greater than 13% predicted fluid responsiveness, less than 9% predicted that the patient would not be responsive, and 9% to 13% reflected a gray zone.[42] Stroke volume variation has been reported to predict fluid responsiveness, specifically in patients undergoing thoracic surgery, during OLV.[43]

Central Venous Pressure Monitoring

The CVP may reflect the patient's blood volume, venous tone, and right ventricular performance; however, it is also affected by central venous obstructions and alterations of intrathoracic pressure such as PEEP (see Chapter 26). The CVP reflects right-sided heart function, not left ventricular performance. Catheters for measuring CVP may be placed for thoracotomies, and in particular, patients undergoing pneumonectomy. Uses of CVP catheters or large-bore introducers include (1) insertion of a transvenous pacemaker where necessary, (2) infusion of vasoactive drugs, and (3) insertion of a pulmonary artery (PA) catheter, which may subsequently be required during surgery or in the postoperative period. A recent study in healthy subjects indicated that, contrary to common belief, the CVP did not reflect intravascular volume status.[44]

The CVP catheter can be placed centrally from either the external or the internal jugular vein, from the subclavian veins, or from one of the arm veins. The success rate is highest using the right internal jugular vein, and a pacemaker or PA catheter can be inserted most easily from this vein. The major disadvantage of using the external jugular vein during thoracotomy is that the catheter often kinks when the patient is turned to the lateral decubitus position. The subclavian technique leads to a higher incidence of pneumothorax, which can be disastrous if it occurs in the dependent lung during OLV. If necessary and if possible, a subclavian catheter should be placed ipsilateral to the surgery. As discussed earlier, the CVP is no longer considered an accurate guide for fluid responsiveness. However, it is a common practice among thoracic anesthesiologists to place a CVP catheter for certain thoracic cases such as esophagectomy and pneumonectomy.

Pulmonary Artery Catheterization

The PA catheter is most reliably inserted through the right internal jugular vein using a modified Seldinger technique (see Chapter 26). Insertion of the PA catheter through either the external jugular vein or the subclavian vein often leads to obstruction of the catheter when the patient is placed in the lateral decubitus position. Misinterpretation of data from a PA catheter is a real risk in a patient with cardiac and pulmonary diseases undergoing thoracic surgery with OLV. These errors can be produced by altered ventilatory modes, the location of the PA catheter tip, ventricular compliance changes, or ventricular interdependence.[45] A major limitation of the PA catheter is the assumption that the pulmonary capillary wedge pressure (PCWP) provides a good approximation of left ventricular end-diastolic volume. The use of PCWP directly to assess preload assumes a linear relationship between ventricular end-diastolic volume and ventricular end-diastolic pressure. However, alterations in ventricular compliance affect this pressure–volume relationship during surgery. Decreases in ventricular compliance can occur with myocardial ischemia, shock, right ventricular overload, or pericardial effusion. Numerous investigators have demonstrated a poor correlation between PCWP and left ventricular end-diastolic volume in acutely ill patients.[46] This correlation is further worsened by the application of PEEP. In addition, ventricular interdependence can cause misdiagnosis when the interventricular septum encroaches on the left ventricular cavity, leading to increased values of PCWP. A PCWP associated with a decreased cardiac output can be interpreted as left ventricular failure, when in fact, left ventricular end-diastolic volume may not be increased but decreased because of compression of the left ventricle by a distended right ventricle. This situation can occur with acute respiratory failure and high levels of PEEP. Techniques such as echocardiography, which directly measure ventricular dimensions, may facilitate resolution of this complex situation.

Because most of the pulmonary blood flow is to the right lower lobe, the tip of a flow-directed PA catheter is usually located in the right lower lobe. During a left thoracotomy with OLV, the catheter tip would then be in the dependent lung and should provide accurate hemodynamic measurements. However, during a right thoracotomy with OLV, the catheter tip would most likely be in the nondependent lung, and may not be accurate. The use of intraoperative mean pulmonary artery pressure has been reported to be an indicator of safety for lung resection under thoracotomy.[47] The authors concluded that following occlusion of the main PA, upper safety limits of 33 mmHg for right, and 35 mmHg for left thoracotomy could be used. The authors noted that the difference between sides was minimal, and less than expected. The monitoring of $S\bar{v}O_2$ has been evaluated in patients undergoing one-lung anesthesia.[48] Changes in $S\bar{v}O_2$ were mainly dependent on changes in Sao_2. Currently, the use of the PA catheter for monitoring during thoracic surgery is generally unnecessary, and may be reserved for patients with pulmonary hypertension.

Transesophageal Echocardiography

Transesophageal echocardiography (TEE) is a useful intraoperative monitor for ventricular function, valvular function, and wall motion changes that might reflect ischemia (see Chapter 27). Its use in thoracic surgical patients has been limited, but it is widely used in patients undergoing lung transplant. The use of TEE requires special training, and may not be available at all centers. A recent review concluded that although the intraoperative use of TEE is not routinely indicated, it may be useful for diagnosing right ventricular dysfunction, in the setting of hypotension or arrhythmias following lung resection.[49] Right ventricular dysfunction may occur during OLV, clamping of the pulmonary artery for pneumonectomy, or lung transplantation. TEE may be used to help determine if it is necessary to utilize cardiopulmonary bypass during lung transplantation.[50]

TEE may be useful in visualizing hilar lung tumors, and evaluating possible extension into the heart. In one study, central lung tumors were seen with TEE in nine of the nine patients, peripheral lung tumors in one of the three patients, and an anterior mediastinal mass in one of one patient.[51] In this study, TEE revealed PA compression in five patients and PA infiltration in two patients. In another study investigating echocardiographic recognition of mediastinal tumors, TEE revealed that the tumors were often adjacent to the heart and identified those patients in whom there was compression of the innominate vein or PA, or infiltration of the heart.[52]

Intraoperative TEE has also revealed tumor invasion of the heart, indicating that a resection by thoracotomy without cardiopulmonary bypass was not feasible.[53] In one case report, TEE monitoring during an attempted resection of a tumor invading the left atrium showed embolization of the tumor.[54] Fragments of the tumor were seen to pass through the aortic valve. This patient subsequently died of disseminated metastases. In an exploratory thoracotomy for hemothorax, intraoperative TEE revealed the presence of a subacute aortic dissection, which was believed to be the cause of the hemothorax.[55] TEE was used intraoperatively to evaluate a large anterior mediastinal mass, providing data on right ventricular outflow compression, and ventricular contractility and filling status.[56] In another recent report, a mediastinal mass was diagnosed intraoperatively using TEE; in that case, the mass had been misdiagnosed preoperatively with transthoracic echocardiography as a pericardial effusion.[57]

Additional Noninvasive Monitoring

Although data are presently limited, it has been reported that decreased cerebral oximetry values by absolute cerebral oximetry during OLV have been correlated with postoperative complications.[58] In a subsequent study, the larger decreases in cerebral oxygen saturation occurred in patients with better preoperative lung function.[59] At this time, the data are still too limited to recommend cerebral oximetry as a routine monitor during thoracic surgery.

A meta-analysis of the use of noninvasive cardiac output measurements during surgery revealed poor agreement with thermodilution. Noninvasive cardiac output measurements are not commonly utilized during thoracic surgery and thus are recommended at this time.[60]

Monitoring of Oxygenation and Ventilation

Oxygenation

During the administration of all thoracic surgical anesthetics, the concentration of inspired oxygen in the breathing system must be measured using an oxygen analyzer with a low oxygen concentration limit alarm (see Chapter 25). Such analyzers vary in sophistication from fuel cells to rapidly responding paramagnetic analyzers that monitor oxygen breath-by-breath and display an oxygram (analogous to, and a mirror image of, the capnogram). Adequacy of blood oxygenation must also be ensured, and adequate illumination and exposure of the patient are helpful to assess the color of shed blood or the presence of cyanosis of the lips, nail beds, or mucous membranes. Most patients undergoing thoracic surgical or diagnostic procedures have an arterial catheter in place for continuous monitoring of blood pressure and sampling of arterial blood for blood gas analyses.

Pulse oximetry is a standard of care for noninvasive assessment of blood oxygenation. The use of pulse oximetry is especially important during OLV, when rapid assessment of oxygenation is critical. A low Spo_2 reading provides the clinician with an indication for blood gas sampling and laboratory analysis of arterial blood. The traditional two-wavelength pulse oximeter may display spurious readings of Sp_{O_2} in the presence of dyshemoglobins, methemoglobin, and carboxyhemoglobin. Multiwavelength (8 or 12 wavelengths) pulse oximeters are available that can measure carboxyhemoglobin, methemoglobin, deoxygenated hemoglobin, and oxygenated hemoglobin (HbO_2%).[61,62] Continuous noninvasive monitoring of total hemoglobin concentration is also available.[63–65]

Ventilation

All patients must be continually monitored to ensure adequacy of ventilation. Monitoring includes qualitative signs such as chest excursion (visual observation of the lungs when the chest is open) and auscultation of breath sounds. In addition, during OLV, a stethoscope can be placed on the chest wall under the ventilated dependent lung. During controlled ventilation, circuit low-pressure and high-pressure alarms with an audible signal must be used. The respiratory rate, V_T, minute volume, and inflation pressures should be monitored.

Adequacy of ventilation is confirmed by monitoring arterial blood gas analyses and Pa_{CO_2}, in particular. This may be estimated continuously and noninvasively by capnography (see Chapter 26). The end-tidal CO_2 concentration represents alveolar CO_2 (PA_{CO_2}), which approximates Pa_{CO_2}. There is normally a small arterial-to-alveolar CO_2 difference (4 to 6 mmHg), depending on alveolar dead space. The capnogram waveform is also helpful in diagnosing airway obstruction, incomplete relaxation, and even malposition of the DLT.[66,67] During OLV, systemic hypoxemia is usually a greater problem than hypercarbia.[68] This is because CO_2 is approximately 20 times more diffusible than oxygen and Pa_{CO_2} is more dependent on ventilation, compared with Pa_{O_2}, which is more dependent on perfusion.

Physiology of One-lung Ventilation

Physiology of the Lateral Decubitus Position. Ventilation and blood flow in the upright position are discussed in Chapters 15 and 29. These variables will now be considered as they pertain to the lateral decubitus position under six circumstances that are encountered during thoracic surgery.

Lateral Position, Awake, Breathing Spontaneously, Chest Closed. In the lateral decubitus position, the distribution of blood flow and ventilation is similar to that in the upright position, but turned by 90 degrees (Fig. 38-5). Blood flow and ventilation to the dependent lung are significantly greater than that to the nondependent lung. Good V̇/Q̇ matching at the level of the dependent lung results in adequate oxygenation in the awake patient who is breathing spontaneously. There are two important concepts in this situation. First, because perfusion is gravity-dependent, the vertical hydrostatic pressure gradient is smaller in the lateral than in the upright position; therefore, zone 1 is usually less extended. Second, in regard to ventilation, the dependent hemidiaphragm is pushed higher into the chest by the abdominal contents compared with the nondependent lung hemidiaphragm. During spontaneous ventilation, the conserved ability of the dependent diaphragm to contract results in an adequate distribution of V_T to the dependent lung. Because most of the perfusion is to the dependent lung, the V̇/Q̇ matching in this position is maintained similar to that in the upright position.

Lateral Position, Awake, Breathing Spontaneously, Chest Open. Controlled positive-pressure ventilation is the most common way to provide adequate ventilation and ensure gas exchange in an open-chest situation. Frequently, thoracoscopy is performed

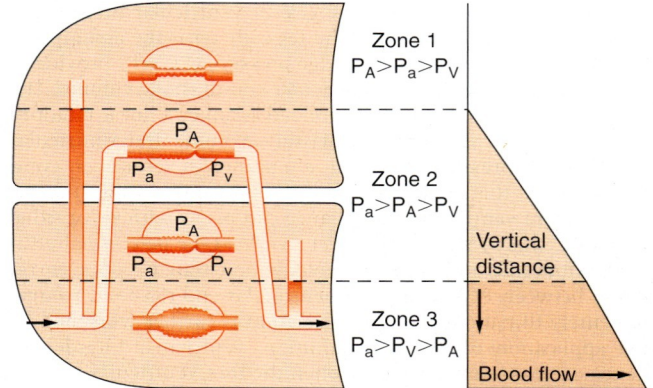

Figure 38-5 Schematic representation of the effects of gravity on the distribution of pulmonary blood flow in the lateral decubitus position. Vertical gradients in the lateral decubitus position are similar to those in the upright position and cause the creation of West zones 1, 2, and 3. Consequently, pulmonary blood flow increases with lung dependency, and is largest in the dependent lung and least in the nondependent lung. P_a, pulmonary artery pressure; P_A, alveolar pressure; P_v, pulmonary venous pressure. (Adapted from Benumof JL. Physiology of the open-chest and one lung ventilation. In: *Thoracic Anesthesia*. New York, NY: Churchill Livingstone; 1983:288.)

using intercostal blocks with the patient breathing spontaneously to allow proper lung examination. The thoracoscope provides an adequate seal of the open chest to prevent a "free" open-chest situation. Two complications can arise from the patient breathing spontaneously with an open chest. The first is mediastinal shift, usually occurring during inspiration (Fig. 38-6). The negative pressure in the intact hemithorax, compared with the less negative pressure of the open hemithorax, can cause the mediastinum to move vertically downward and push into the dependent hemithorax. The mediastinal shift can create circulatory and reflex changes that may result in a clinical picture similar to that of shock and respiratory distress. Sometimes, depending on the severity of the distress, the patient needs to be tracheally intubated immediately, with initiation of positive-pressure ventilation, and the anesthesiologist must be prepared to intubate in this position without disturbing the surgical field.

The second phenomenon is paradoxical breathing (Fig. 38-7). During inspiration, the relatively negative pressure in the intact hemithorax compared with atmospheric pressure in the open hemithorax can cause movement of air from the nondependent lung into the dependent lung. The opposite occurs during expiration. This gas movement reversal from one lung to the other represents wasted ventilation and can compromise the adequacy of gas exchange. Paradoxical breathing is increased by a large thoracotomy or by an increase in airway resistance in the dependent lung. Positive-pressure ventilation or adequate sealing of the open chest eliminates paradoxical breathing.

Lateral Position, Anesthetized, Breathing Spontaneously, Chest Closed. The induction of general anesthesia does not cause significant change in the distribution of blood flow, but it has an important impact on the distribution of ventilation. Most of the V_T enters the nondependent lung, and this results in a significant V̇/Q̇ mismatch. Induction of general anesthesia causes a reduction in the volumes of both lungs secondary to a reduction in FRC. Any reduction in volume in the dependent lung is of a greater magnitude than that in the nondependent lung for several reasons. First, the cephalad displacement of the dependent diaphragm by the abdominal contents is more pronounced and is

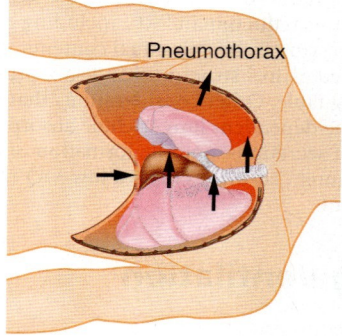
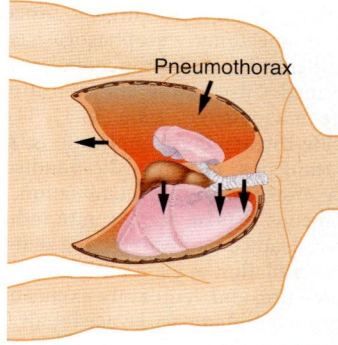

Figure 38-6 Schematic representation of mediastinal shift in the spontaneously breathing, open-chested patient in the lateral decubitus position. During inspiration, negative pressure in the intact hemithorax causes the mediastinum to move downward. During expiration, relative positive pressure in the intact hemithorax causes the mediastinum to move upward. (Adapted from Tarhan S, Moffitt EA. Principles of thoracic anesthesia. *Surg Clin North Am.* 1973;53:813.)

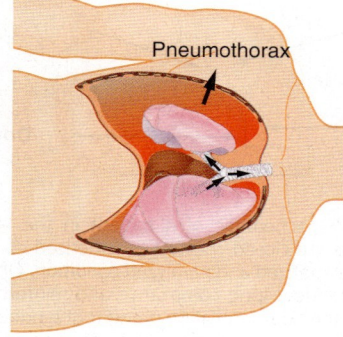
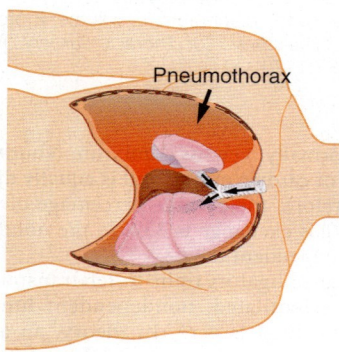

Figure 38-7 Schematic representation of paradoxical respiration in the spontaneously breathing, open-chested patient in the lateral decubitus position. During inspiration, movement of gas from the exposed lung into the intact lung and movement of air from the environment into the open hemithorax cause collapse of the exposed lung. During expiration, the reverse occurs, and the exposed lung expands. (Adapted from Tarhan S, Moffitt EA. Principles of thoracic anesthesia. *Surg Clin North Am.* 1973;53:813.)

increased by paralysis. Second, the mediastinal structures pressing on the dependent lung or poor positioning of the dependent side on the operating table prevents the lung from expanding properly. The aforementioned factors will move lungs to a lower volume on the S-shaped volume–pressure curve (Fig. 38-8). The nondependent lung moves to a steeper position on the compliance curve and receives most of the V_T, whereas the dependent lung is on the flat (noncompliant) part of the curve.

Lateral Position, Anesthetized, Breathing Spontaneously, Chest Open. Opening the chest has little impact on the distribution of perfusion. However, the upper lung is now no longer restricted by the chest wall and is free to expand, resulting in a further increase in $\dot{V}/\dot{Q}$ mismatch as the nondependent lung is preferentially ventilated, owing to a now increased compliance.

Lateral Position, Anesthetized, Paralyzed, Chest Open. During paralysis and positive-pressure ventilation, diaphragmatic displacement is maximal over the nondependent lung, where there is the least amount of resistance to diaphragmatic movement caused by the abdominal contents (Fig. 38-9). This further compromises the ventilation to the dependent lung and increases the $\dot{V}/\dot{Q}$ mismatch.

OLV, Anesthetized, Paralyzed, Chest Open. During two-lung ventilation in the lateral position, the mean blood flow to the nondependent lung is assumed to be 40% of cardiac output, whereas 60% of cardiac output goes to the dependent lung

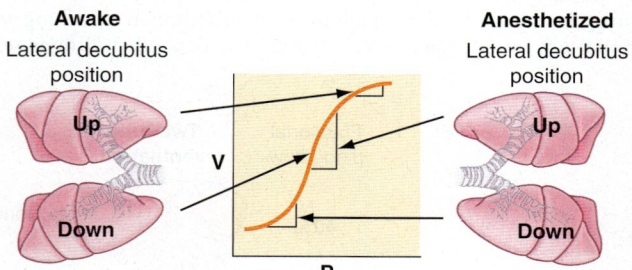

Figure 38-8 The left side of the schematic shows the distribution of ventilation in the awake patient (closed chest) in the lateral decubitus position, and the right side shows the distribution of ventilation in the anesthetized patient (closed chest) in the lateral decubitus position. The induction of anesthesia has caused a loss in lung volume in both lungs, with the nondependent (up) lung moving from a flat, noncompliant portion to a steep, compliant portion of the pressure–volume curve, and the dependent (down) lung moving from a steep, compliant part to a flat, noncompliant part of the pressure–volume curve. Thus, the anesthetized patient in the lateral decubitus position has most tidal ventilation in the nondependent lung (where there is the least perfusion) and less tidal ventilation in the dependent lung (where there is the most perfusion). V, volume; P, pressure. (Adapted from Benumof JL. *Anesthesia for Thoracic Surgery.* Philadelphia, PA: WB Saunders; 1987:112.)

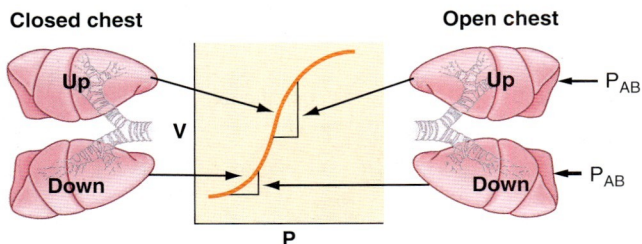

Figure 38-9 This schematic of a patient in the lateral decubitus position compares the closed-chested anesthetized condition with the open-chested anesthetized and paralyzed condition. Opening the chest increases nondependent lung compliance and reinforces or maintains the larger part of the tidal ventilation going to the nondependent lung. Paralysis also reinforces or maintains the larger part of tidal ventilation going to the nondependent lung because the pressure of the abdominal contents (P_{AB}) pressing against the upper diaphragm is minimal, and it is therefore easier for positive-pressure ventilation to displace this less resisting dome of the diaphragm. V, volume; P, pressure. (Adapted from Benumof JL. *Anesthesia for Thoracic Surgery*. Philadelphia, PA: WB Saunders; 1987:112.)

(Fig. 38-10). Normally, venous admixture (shunt) in the lateral position is 10% of cardiac output and is equally divided as 5% in each lung. Therefore, the average percentage of cardiac output participating in gas exchange is 35% in the nondependent lung and 55% in the dependent lung.

OLV creates an obligatory right-to-left transpulmonary shunt through the nonventilated, nondependent lung because the $\dot{V}/\dot{Q}$ ratio of that lung is zero. In theory, an additional 35% should be added to the total shunt during OLV. However, assuming active HPV, blood flow to the nondependent hypoxic lung will be decreased by 50% and therefore is (35/2) = 17.5%. To this, 5% must be added, which is the obligatory shunt through the nondependent lung. The shunt through the nondependent lung is therefore 22.5% (Fig. 38-10). Together with the 5% shunt in the dependent lung, total shunt during OLV is 22.5% + 5% = 27.5%. This results in a Pa_{O_2} of approximately 150 mmHg ($FI_{O_2} = 1$).[69]

Because 72.5% of the perfusion is directed to the dependent lung during OLV, the matching of ventilation in this lung is important for adequate gas exchange. The dependent lung is no longer on the steep (compliant) portion of the volume–pressure curve because of reduced lung volume and FRC. There are several reasons for this reduction in FRC, including general anesthesia, paralysis, pressure from abdominal contents, compression by the weight of mediastinal structures, and suboptimal positioning on the operating table. Other considerations that impair optimal ventilation to the dependent lung include absorption atelectasis, accumulation of secretions, and the formation of a transudate in the dependent lung. All these create a low $\dot{V}/\dot{Q}$ ratio and a large $P(A–a)_{O_2}$ gradient.

One-lung Ventilation

Absolute Indications for One-lung Ventilation

Currently, a variety of thoracic surgical procedures such as lobectomy, pneumonectomy, esophagogastrectomy, pleural decortication, bullectomy, and bronchopulmonary lavage are commonly performed. Customarily, the indications are classified either as absolute or as relative (Table 38-1). The absolute indications include life-threatening complications, such as massive bleeding, sepsis, and pus, in which the nondiseased contralateral lung must be protected from contamination. Bronchopleural and bronchocutaneous fistulae are absolute indications because they offer a low-resistance pathway for the delivered V_T during positive-pressure ventilation. A giant unilateral bulla may rupture under positive pressure, and ventilatory exclusion is mandatory. Finally, during bronchopulmonary lavage for alveolar proteinosis or cystic fibrosis, prevention of drowning the contralateral lung is necessary.

Video-assisted thoracoscopy (VAT) is now widely used in clinical practice. Unlike conventional thoracoscopy, VAT allows for an extensive variety of diagnostic and therapeutic procedures. Improvements in video-endoscopic surgical equipment and a growing enthusiasm for minimally invasive surgical approaches have contributed to its use. In most cases general anesthesia with OLV is required. The lung should be well collapsed to provide the surgeon with an optimal view of the surgical field, and to facilitate palpation of the lesion in the lung parenchyma. In addition, it is difficult to place the stapler on a lung that is not completely collapsed, and there is an increase in incidence of

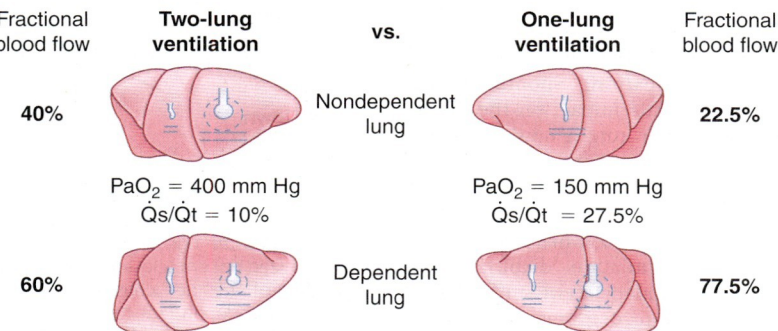

Figure 38-10 Schematic representation of two-lung ventilation versus one-lung ventilation (OLV). Typical values for fractional blood flow to the nondependent and dependent lungs, as well as Pa_{O_2} and $\dot{Q}S/\dot{Q}t$ for the two conditions, are shown. The $\dot{Q}S/\dot{Q}t$ during two-lung ventilation is assumed to be distributed equally between the two lungs (5% to each lung). The essential difference between two-lung ventilation and OLV is that, during OLV, the nonventilated lung has some blood flow and therefore an obligatory shunt, which is not present during two-lung ventilation. The 35% of total flow perfusing the nondependent lung, which was not shunt flow, was assumed to be able to reduce its blood flow by 50% by hypoxic pulmonary vasoconstriction. The increase in $\dot{Q}S/\dot{Q}t$ from two-lung to OLV is assumed to be due solely to the increase in blood flow through the nonventilated, nondependent lung during OLV. (Adapted from Benumof JL. *Anesthesia for Thoracic Surgery*. Philadelphia, PA: WB Saunders; 1987:112.)

Table 38-1 Indications for One-lung Ventilation

Absolute
1. Isolation of each lung to prevent contamination of a healthy lung
   a. Infection (abscess, infected cyst)
   b. Massive hemorrhage
2. Control of distribution of ventilation to only one lung
   a. Bronchopleural fistula
   b. Bronchopleural cutaneous fistula
   c. Unilateral cyst or bullae
   d. Major bronchial disruption or trauma
3. Unilateral lung lavage
4. Video-assisted thoracoscopic surgery

Relative
1. Surgical exposure—high priority
   a. Thoracic aortic aneurysm
   b. Pneumonectomy
   c. Lung volume reduction
   d. Minimally invasive cardiac surgery
   e. Upper lobectomy
2. Surgical exposure—low priority
   a. Esophageal surgery
   b. Middle and lower lobectomies
   c. Mediastinal mass resection, thymectomy
   d. Bilateral sympathectomies

Modified from Benumof JL. Physiology of the open-chest and one lung ventilation. In: Kaplan JA, ed. *Thoracic Anesthesia*. New York, NY: Churchill Livingstone; 1983:299.

postoperative air leak in these circumstances. The increased use of VAT has significantly increased the number of procedures that require lung separation. In some institutions, 80% to 90% of the procedures are now performed using the thoracoscopic approach. In contemporary anesthesia practice, VAT is an absolute indication for lung separation.

Relative Indications for One-lung Ventilation

In clinical practice, a DLT is commonly used for a lobectomy or pneumonectomy; these represent relative indications for lung separation when performed through an open thoracotomy. Upper lobectomy, pneumonectomy, and thoracic aortic aneurysm repair are high-priority indications. These procedures are technically difficult, and optimal surgical exposure and a quiet operative field are highly desirable. Lower or middle lobectomy and esophageal resection are of lower priority. There are a number of additional procedures that have not been traditionally included as indications for OLV. Nevertheless, many surgeons are accustomed to operating with the lung collapsed for these cases. OLV minimizes lung trauma from retractors and manipulation, improves visualization of the lung anatomy, and facilitates identification and separation of anatomic structures and lung fissures. These procedures include minimally invasive cardiac surgery, lung volume reduction, thoracic aneurysm repair, thoracic spinal procedures, mediastinal mass resection, thymectomies, and mediastinal lymph node dissection.

It is important to distinguish between the need for lung isolation versus lung separation.

Lung Isolation. Whenever the nondiseased lung is threatened with contamination by blood or pus from the diseased lung, the lungs must be isolated to prevent potentially life-threatening complications. Other indications are bronchopleural and bronchocutaneous fistulas because they offer a low-resistance pathway for the delivered V_T during positive-pressure ventilation. Finally, during bronchopulmonary lavage for alveolar proteinosis or cystic fibrosis, protection of the contralateral lung from drowning is necessary. These situations, however, are relatively uncommon and in modern anesthesia practice constitute less than 10% of all thoracic procedures.

Lung Separation. All other indications for OLV can be considered as lung separations, in which there is no risk of contamination of the dependent lung. This includes all the relative indications that are primarily for surgical exposure. VAT for diagnostic and therapeutic procedures, which requires a well-collapsed lung, should also be included in this category. The majority of procedures where OLV is used are for lung separation; only a minority require lung isolation.[70,71]

Methods of Lung Separation

Double-Lumen Endobronchial Tubes

Double-lumen endobronchial tubes are currently the most widely used means of achieving lung separation and OLV. There are several different types of DLT, but all are essentially similar in design in that two endotracheal tubes are "bonded" together. One lumen is long enough to reach a main stem bronchus, and the second lumen ends with an opening in the distal trachea. Lung separation is achieved by inflation of two cuffs: A proximal tracheal cuff and a distal bronchial cuff located in the main stem bronchus (see "Positioning Double-lumen Tubes"). The endobronchial cuff of a right-sided tube is slotted or otherwise designed to allow ventilation of the right upper lobe because the right main stem bronchus is too short to accommodate both the right lumen tip and a right bronchial cuff.

Robertshaw Tube. The Carlens tube (which had a carinal hook) was the first clinically available DLT and was used by pulmonologists for split function spirometry testing (Fig. 38-11A). Subsequently, the Robertshaw-design DLT (which lacked a carinal hook) was developed to facilitate thoracic surgery (Fig. 38-11B). This DLT is available in left-sided and right-sided forms. The absence of a carinal hook facilitates insertion. This tube design has the advantages of having D-shaped, large-diameter lumens that allow easy passage of a suction catheter, offer low resistance to gas flow, and have a fixed curvature to facilitate proper positioning and reduce the possibility of kinking. The original red rubber Robertshaw tubes were available in three sizes: small, medium, and large. Red rubber tubes are rarely used now and have been replaced by clear, polyvinyl chloride (PVC) disposable Robertshaw-design DLTs. These are available in both right-sided and left-sided versions and in 35 French (Fr), 37 Fr, 39 Fr, and 41 Fr sizes. A 32-Fr left-sided DLT is available for small adults, and a 28 Fr for use in pediatric cases. The advantages of the disposable tubes include the relative ease of insertion and proper positioning as well as easy recognition of the blue color of the endobronchial cuff when fiberoptic bronchoscopy is used. Other advantages are the confirmation of the position on a chest radiograph using the radiopaque lines in the wall of the tube and the continuous observation of tidal gas exchange and respiratory moisture through the clear plastic. The right-sided endobronchial tube is designed to minimize occlusion of the opening of the right upper lobe bronchus. The right endobronchial cuff is doughnut-shaped and

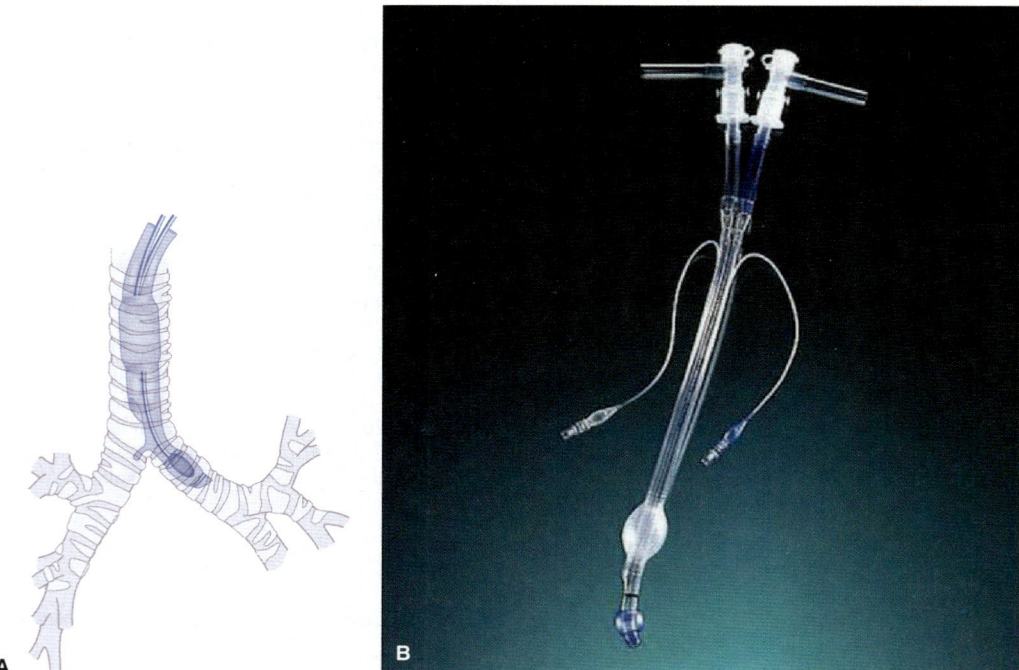

Figure 38-11 **A:** Left main stem endobronchial intubation using a Carlens tube. Note carinal "hook" used for correct positioning. (Reprinted with permission from Hillard EK, Thompson PW. Instruments used in thoracic anaesthesia. In: Mushin WW, ed. *Thoracic Anaesthesia*. Oxford: Blackwell Scientific; 1963:315.) **B:** A left-sided Robertshaw type double-lumen tube constructed from polyvinyl chloride. (Courtesy of Nellcor Puritan Bennett, Inc., Pleasanton, California.)

allows the right upper lobe ventilation slot to ride over the opening of the right upper lobe bronchus. The tube is also suitable for use in long-term ventilation in the intensive care unit (ICU) because it has a high-volume, low-pressure cuff. These disposable PVC tubes are generally considered the tubes of choice for achieving lung separation and OLV.

A rubber–silicone left-sided DLT, Silbronco (Silbronco DLT, Fuji Systems, Tokyo, Japan), is also available. This tube has a D-shaped wire-reinforced lumen to maintain the tip at a 45-degree angle. The reinforced wall tends to prevent obstruction or kinking of the bronchial lumen, yet at the same time maintains flexibility. It is especially useful if the left main stem bronchus is angled at 90 degrees from the trachea, making it almost impossible to position a PVC DLT. This clinical scenario can be seen in patients who have previously undergone a left upper lobectomy and the expansion of the left lower lobe displaces the left main bronchus upward.[72] As the left main bronchus is considerably longer than the right bronchus, there is a narrow margin of safety on the right main bronchus, with potentially a greater risk of upper lobe obstruction whenever a right-sided DLT is used. A left-sided DLT is preferred for both right- and left-sided procedures. A left-sided DLT was selected for 1,166 of the 1,170 patients in one report, and was used successfully in over 98% of those patients.[73] The authors recommended selecting the largest DLT that will safely fit the bronchus. This will provide less resistance to ventilation and is less likely to dislocate.

Some authors have suggested using the patient height as a basis for selecting a DLT. However, the correlation between airway size and height is extremely poor. Tracheal and bronchial dimensions can be also directly measured from the chest radiograph or chest CT scan. It is possible to measure the diameter of the left bronchus from the chest radiograph in almost 75% of patients.

In patients in whom the left main bronchus cannot be directly measured, the left bronchial diameter can be accurately estimated by measuring tracheal width. The width of the left bronchus is directly proportional to tracheal width. The left bronchial width is estimated by multiplying the tracheal width by 0.68.[74] Typically, most women will need a 37-Fr DLT and most men will be adequately managed with a 39-Fr DLT. In the past it was a more common practice to use the largest size DLT possible to avoid distal migration of the tube, and so that the pressure in the bronchial cuff could be minimized by needing less air for a seal. The common practice of fiberoptic bronchoscopy has decreased the risk of undetected distal placement or migration of the bronchial tip. A study showed that the routine use of a 35-Fr DLT in adults regardless of height was not associated with an increase in hypoxemia or any other adverse clinical outcomes.[75]

The depth required for insertion of the DLT correlates with the height of the patient. For any adult 170 to 180 cm tall, the average depth for a left-sided DLT is 29 cm. For every 10 cm increase or decrease in height, the DLT is advanced or withdrawn 1 cm.[76]

Recently introduced to clinical practice is the VivaSight-DL disposable DLT (ET View Ltd., Misgav, Israel) which consists of a high-resolution camera embedded on the DLT between the tracheal cuff and the bronchial cuff.[77,78] This device allows continuous real-time viewing of the DLT position, which can be important in cases where the patient's head is away from the anesthesiologist, such as during robotic thoracic surgery. The VivaSight tube is also available as a single-lumen tube (VivaSight-SL) through which an independent blocker may be inserted without the need of a FB. A prospective study of 71 adult patients, compared intubation times using either the VivaSight-DL or a conventional DLT.[79] The duration of intubation with visual confirmation of tube position was significantly reduced using the VivaSight-DL compared with the conventional DLT (51 vs. 264 seconds). None of the patients allocated to the VivaSight-DL required fiberoptic bronchoscopy during intubation or surgery. One limitation of the VivaSight compared with a FB is that its position of the camera is set at the distal part of the tracheal lumen of the tube and therefore it cannot be used to inspect either main stem bronchus if this is deemed necessary. The VivaSight DLT will not allow complete elimination of the use of a FB in lung isolation procedures, but may instead lead to a significant reduction.

Placement of Double-lumen Tubes. This section concentrates on the insertion of disposable Robertshaw-design DLTs because they are the most widely used. Before insertion, the DLT should be prepared and checked. The tracheal cuff (high volume, low pressure) can accommodate up to 20 mL of air, and the bronchial cuff can be checked using a 3-mL syringe. The tube should be coated liberally with water-soluble lubricant and the stylet should be withdrawn, lubricated, and gently placed back into the bronchial lumen without disturbing the tube's preformed curvature. A Macintosh laryngoscope blade is preferred for intubation of the trachea because it provides the largest area through which to pass the tube. The insertion of the tube is performed with the distal concave curvature facing anteriorly. After the tip of the tube is past the vocal cords, the stylet is removed and the tube is rotated through 90 degrees. A left-sided tube is rotated 90 degrees to the left, and a right-sided tube is rotated to the right. Advancement of the tube ceases when moderate resistance to further passage is encountered, indicating that the tube tip has been firmly seated in the main stem bronchus. It is important to remove the stylet before rotating and advancing the tube to avoid tracheal or bronchial laceration. Rotation and advancement of the tube should be performed gently and under continuous direct laryngoscopy to prevent hypopharyngeal structures from interfering with proper positioning. Once the tube is believed to be in the proper position, a sequence of steps should be performed to check its location.

First the tracheal cuff should be inflated, and equal ventilation of both lungs established. If breath sounds are not equal, the tube is probably too far down, and the tracheal lumen opening is in a main stem bronchus or is lying at the carina. Withdrawal of the tube by 2 to 3 cm usually restores equal breath sounds. The second step is to clamp the right side (in the case of the left-sided tube) and remove the right cap from the connector. Then the bronchial cuff is slowly inflated to prevent an air leak from the bronchial lumen around the bronchial cuff into the tracheal lumen. This ensures that excessive pressure is not applied to the bronchus and helps avoid laceration. Inflation of the bronchial cuff rarely requires greater than 2 mL of air. The third step is to remove the clamp and check that both lungs are ventilated with both cuffs inflated. This ensures that the bronchial cuff is not obstructing the contralateral hemithorax, either totally or partially. The final step is to clamp each side selectively and watch for absence of movement and breath sounds on the ipsilateral (clamped) side; the ventilated side should have clear breath sounds, chest movement that feels compliant, respiratory gas moisture with each tidal ventilation, and no gas leak. If peak airway pressure during two-lung ventilation is 20 cm H_2O, it should not exceed 40 cm H_2O for the same V_T during OLV.

Other methods that have been used for ensuring the correct placement of a DLT include fluoroscopy, chest radiography, selective capnography, and use of an underwater seal. Determination of the presence of gas leaks when positive pressure is applied to one lumen of a DLT is easily done in the operating room (OR). If the bronchial cuff is not inflated and positive pressure is applied to the bronchial lumen of the DLT, gas leaks past the bronchial cuff and returns through the tracheal lumen. If the tracheal lumen is connected to an underwater seal system, gas will be seen to bubble up through the water. The bronchial cuff can then be gradually inflated until no gas bubbles are seen and the desired cuff seal pressure can be attained. This test is of extreme importance when absolute lung separation is needed, such as during bronchopulmonary lavage.

The most important advance in checking for proper position of a DLT is the introduction of the pediatric flexible fiberoptic bronchoscope (Fig. 38-12). Smith et al.[80] showed that when the disposable DLT was believed to be in correct position by auscultation and physical examination, subsequent fiberoptic bronchoscopy showed that 48% of tubes were, in fact, malpositioned. Such malpositions, however, are usually of no clinical significance.[81] When using a left-sided DLT, the bronchoscope is usually first introduced through the tracheal lumen. The carina is visualized, but no bronchial cuff herniation should be seen. The upper surface of the blue endobronchial cuff should be just below the tracheal carina. The bronchial cuff of the disposable DLT is easily visualized because of its blue color. The bronchoscope should then be passed through the bronchial lumen, and the left upper lobe bronchial orifice should be identified. When a right-sided DLT is used, the carina should be visualized through the tracheal lumen but, more importantly, the orifice of the right upper lobe bronchus should be identified when the bronchoscope is passed through the right upper lobe ventilating slot of the DLT. Pediatric fiberoptic bronchoscopes are available in several sizes: 5.6, 4.9, and 3.6 mm in external diameter. The 4.9-mm diameter bronchoscope can be passed through DLTs of 37 Fr and larger. The 3.6-mm diameter bronchoscope is easily passed through all sizes of DLT. In general, it is recommended that the largest size that can pass through the lumen of a DLT be used because it provides better visualization and facilitates identification of the bronchial anatomy. Excellent fiberoptic images of the tracheobronchial tree can be seen by accessing the website thoracicanesthesia.com.

Problems of Malposition of the Double-Lumen Tube. The use of a DLT is associated with a number of potential problems, the most important of which is malposition. There are several possibilities for tube malposition. The DLT may be accidentally directed to the side opposite the desired main stem bronchus. In this case, the lung opposite the side of the connector clamp will collapse. Inadequate separation, increased airway pressures, and instability of the DLT usually occur. In addition, because of the morphology of the DLT curvatures, tracheal or bronchial lacerations may result. If a left-sided DLT is inserted into the right main stem bronchus, it obstructs ventilation to the right upper lobe. It is therefore essential to recognize and correct such a malposition as soon as possible.

Second, the DLT may be passed too far down into either the right or the left main stem bronchus (Fig. 38-13). In this case, breath sounds are very diminished or not audible over the contralateral side. This situation is corrected when the tube is withdrawn and the opening of the tracheal lumen is above the carina.

Third, the DLT may not be inserted far enough, leaving the bronchial lumen opening above the carina. In this position, good breath sounds are heard bilaterally when ventilating through the bronchial lumen. No breath sounds are audible when ventilating through the tracheal lumen because the inflated bronchial cuff obstructs gas flow arising from the tracheal lumen. The cuff should be deflated and the DLT rotated and advanced into the desired main stem bronchus.

Fourth, a right-sided DLT may occlude the right upper lobe orifice. The mean distance from the carina to the right upper lobe orifice is 2.3 ± 0.7 cm in men and 2.1 ± 0.7 cm in women.[82] With right-sided DLTs, the ventilatory slot in the side of the bronchial

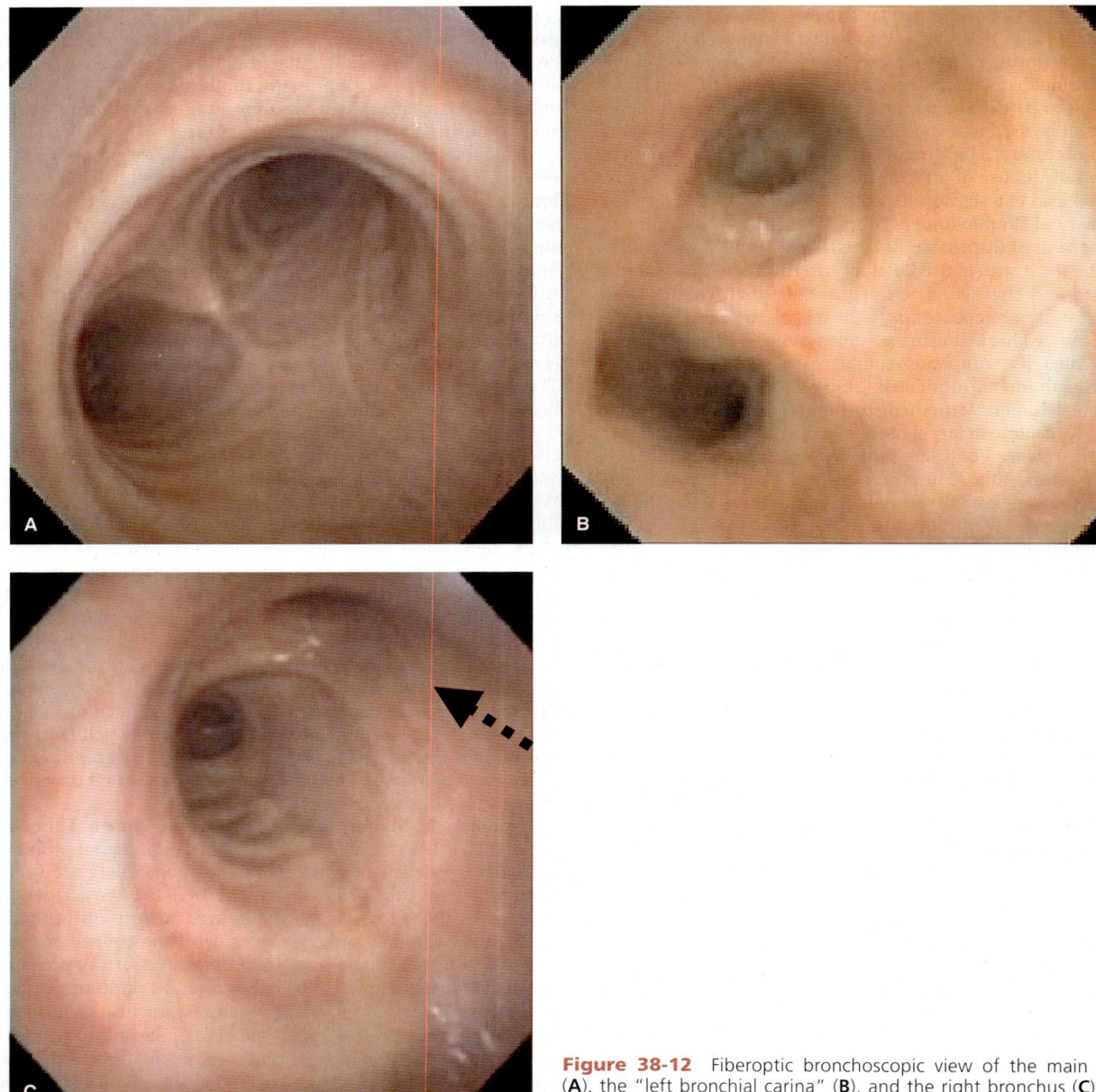

Figure 38-12 Fiberoptic bronchoscopic view of the main carina (**A**), the "left bronchial carina" (**B**), and the right bronchus (**C**). Note the right upper lobe orifice (*arrow*).

catheter must overlie the right upper lobe orifice to permit ventilation of this lobe. However, the margin of safety is extremely small, and varies from 1 to 8 mm.[82] It is therefore difficult to ensure proper ventilation to the right upper lobe and avoid dislocation of the DLT during surgical manipulation. When right endobronchial intubation is required, a disposable right-sided DLT is perhaps the best choice because of the slanted doughnut shape of the bronchial cuff, which allows the ventilation slot to ride off the right upper lobe ventilation orifice and increases the margin of safety.

Fifth, the left upper lobe orifice may be obstructed by a left-sided DLT. Traditionally, it was believed that the take-off of the left upper lobe bronchus was at a safe distance from the carina and that it would not be obstructed by a left-sided DLT. However, the mean distance between the left upper lobe orifice and the carina is 5.4 ± 0.7 cm in men and 5 ± 0.7 cm in women.[82] The average distance between the openings of the right and left lumens on the left-sided disposable tubes is 6.9 cm. Therefore, an obstruction of the left upper lobe bronchus is possible while the tracheal lumen is still above the carina. There is also a 20% variation in the location of the blue endobronchial cuff on the disposable tubes because this cuff is attached to the tube at the end of the manufacturing process.

Bronchial cuff herniation may occur and obstruct the bronchial lumen if excessive volumes are used to inflate the cuff. The bronchial cuff has also been known to herniate over the tracheal carina, and in the case of a left-sided DLT, to obstruct ventilation to the right main stem bronchus.

Another rare complication with DLTs is tracheal laceration or rupture (Fig. 38-14). Overinflation of the bronchial cuff,

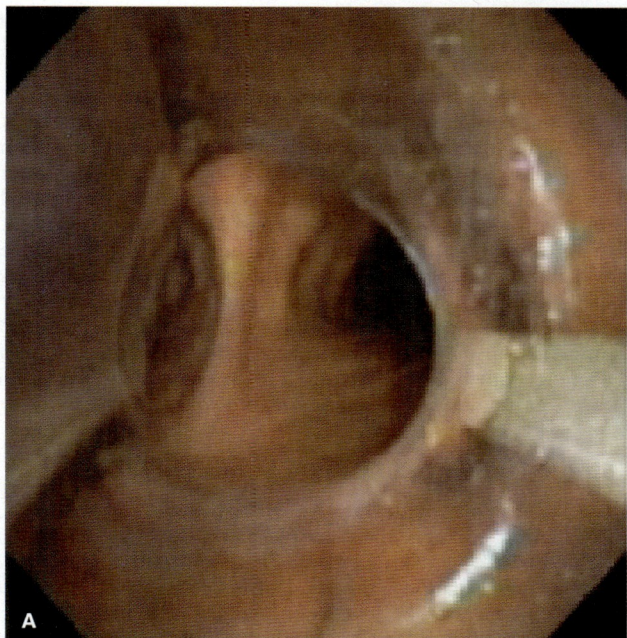
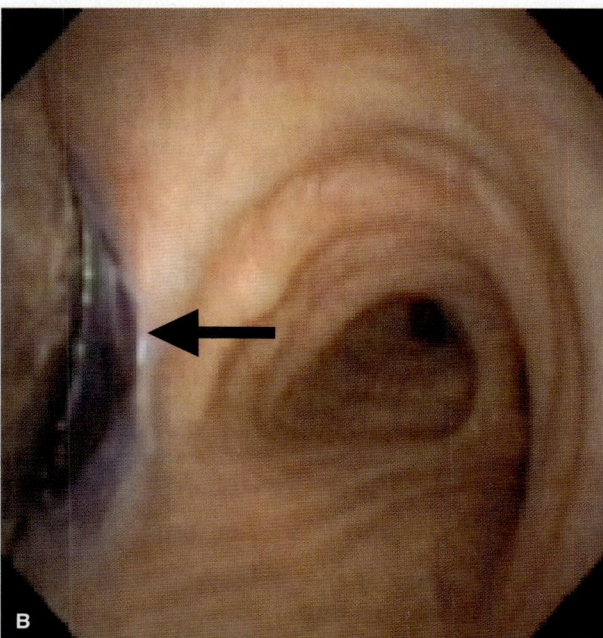

Figure 38-13 Malposition of the left bronchial limb of the double-lumen tube (DLT). **A:** The limb is too far into the left bronchus because the cuff is not evident. **B:** DLT is withdrawn and the balloon is now in view, indicating appropriate position of the DLT (*arrow*).

inappropriate positioning, and trauma owing to intraoperative dislocation that resulted in bronchial rupture have been described in association with the Robertshaw tube and the disposable DLT.[83,84] Therefore, the pressure in the bronchial cuff should be assessed and decreased if the cuff is found to be overinflated. If absolute separation of the lungs is not needed, the bronchial cuff should be deflated and then reinflated slowly to avoid excessive pressure on the bronchial walls. The bronchial cuff should also be deflated during any repositioning of the patient unless lung separation is absolutely required during this time.

In a prospective trial, 60 patients were randomly assigned to two groups.[85] OLV was achieved with either an endobronchial blocker (blocker group) or a DLT (double-lumen group). Postoperative hoarseness and sore throat were assessed at 24, 48, and 72 hours following surgery. Bronchial injuries and vocal cord lesions were examined by bronchoscopy immediately after surgery. Postoperative hoarseness occurred significantly more frequently in the double-lumen group compared with the blocker group (44% vs. 17%, respectively). Similar findings were observed for vocal cord lesions (44% vs. 17%). The incidence of bronchial injuries was comparable between groups. Clayton-Smith et al.[86] performed a review and meta-analysis of 39 randomized controlled trials comparing bronchial blockers with DLTs. They concluded that while bronchial blockers are associated with a lower incidence of airway injury, DLTs can be placed more rapidly and reliably.

Lung Separation in the Patient with a Tracheostomy

Occasionally, a patient with a permanent tracheostomy is scheduled for surgery on the lung that requires isolation. Examples of such patients include those who have undergone resection of a tumor in the floor of the mouth or on the base of the tongue, followed by extensive reconstructive surgery with the creation of a permanent tracheal stoma. Routine follow-up may reveal a lung lesion that requires a diagnostic procedure. Conventional double-lumen endobronchial tubes are designed to be inserted through the mouth, not through a tracheal stoma. The standard

Figure 38-14 Bronchoscopic view showing laceration in left mainstem bronchus.

DLTs are usually too stiff to negotiate the curve required for insertion through a tracheal stoma and are difficult to position.[87] A separately inserted bronchial blocker may permit adequate lung separation.[88]

Saito et al.[89] described a spiral, wire-reinforced, double-lumen endobronchial tube made of silicone (Koken Medical, Tokyo, Japan) that is designed for placement through a tracheostomy. The middle section of the tube consists of two thin-walled silicone catheters with an internal diameter of 5 mm, glued together and reinforced with a stainless steel spiral wire and covered with a silicone coating with two pilot balloons. The distal section, which contains the bronchial lumen and the bronchial cuff, is made of wire-reinforced silicone to avoid excessive flexibility. The dimensions are based on the Mallinckrodt DLT (Hazelwood, MD). The bronchial cuff is located 1.2 cm from the tip, and the distance between the tip orifice and the tracheal orifice is 4.9 cm. In a clinical trial in patients with permanent tracheal stomas, the tubes functioned well in achieving lung separation, with no sign of kinking or movement, and permitted easy passage of a suction catheter.

Lung Separation in the Patient with a Difficult Airway

An airway may be recognized initially as difficult when conventional laryngoscopy reveals a grade III or IV view (see Chapter 28, Airway Management). When separation of the lungs is required and the patient has a clearly recognized difficult airway, then awake intubation using a flexible fiberoptic bronchoscope can be used to place a DLT, Univent tube, or single-lumen tube (SLT) (Fig. 38-15). The SLT may then be exchanged for a DLT or Univent tube using a tube exchanger. Furthermore, depending on the extent and duration of the surgical procedure, and the amount of fluid shift, an airway that was not initially classified as difficult may become difficult secondary to facial edema, secretions, and laryngeal trauma from the initial intubation.[90,91]

A logical approach to lung separation is shown in Figure 38-15. The same approach may be used for the patient with an unrecognized difficult airway and a failure to intubate with conventional laryngoscopy. When using a DLT over a fiberoptic bronchoscope, the anesthesiologist should keep in mind that it is a bulky tube with a large external diameter and because of the length of the DLT, only a limited part of the fiberoptic bronchoscope is available for manipulation. In addition, the mismatch between the flexibility of the fiberoptic bronchoscope and the rigidity of the DLT makes it more difficult to advance over the fiberoptic bronchoscope. The Univent tube has the same bulky external diameter and is also often difficult to pass between the vocal cords, particularly in a patient who is awake.

Single-Lumen Tube Can Be Successfully Placed

If a failure to provide lung separation could result in a life-threatening situation, there are two possibilities to provide OLV when an SLT is already in place. First, depending on the indication for lung isolation, a tube exchanger can be used to switch to a DLT or a Univent tube. The second possibility is to direct a bronchial blocker through the SLT into the selected main stem bronchus. These two methods, however, offer limited protection or an inadequate seal in cases such as lung lavage, pulmonary abscess, or hemoptysis, where a DLT would be the tube of choice.

Use of a Tube Exchanger

Several tube exchangers are commercially available (Cook Critical Care, Bloomington, IN; Sheridan Catheter Corporation, Argyle, NY). On these tube exchangers, the depth is marked in centimeters; they are available in a wide range of external diameters

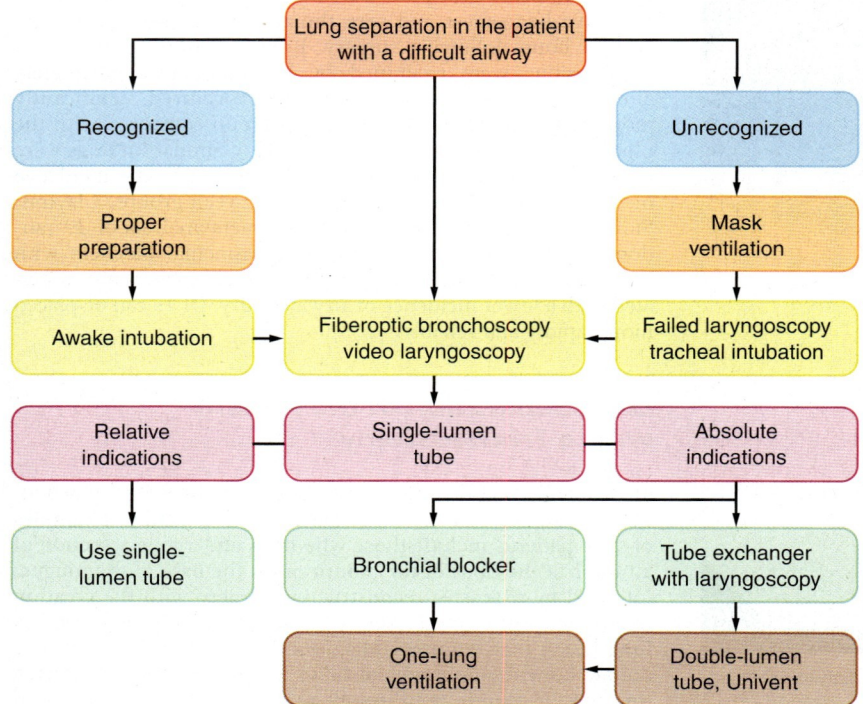

Figure 38-15 Lung separation in the patient with a difficult airway. (Adapted with permission from Cohen E, Benumof JL. Lung separation in the patient with a difficult airway. *Curr Opin Anesthesiol.* 1999;12:29.)

and easily adapted for either oxygen insufflation or jet ventilation. The size of the tube exchanger and the size of the tube to be inserted should be tested before use in a patient. The 11-Fr tube changer will pass through a 35- to 41-Fr DLT, whereas the 14-Fr tube exchanger does not pass through a 35 Fr. To prevent lung laceration, the tube exchanger should never be inserted against resistance. Because the first generation of tube exchangers was very stiff, there was a risk for tracheal or bronchial laceration. Tube exchangers that have a soft flexible tip are now available and should be safer to use and is less likely to cause airway laceration. Finally, when passing any tube over an airway guide, a laryngoscope should be used to facilitate passage of the tube over the airway guide past supraglottic tissues.

Use of Modern Bronchial Blockers

Bronchial Blocker (BB). Lung separation can be achieved with a reusable bronchial blocker.[92] Magill described an endobronchial blocker that is placed using a bronchoscope and directed to the nonventilated lung. Inflation of the cuff at the distal end of the blocker serves to block ventilation to that lung. The lumen of the blocker permits suctioning of the airway distal to the catheter tip. Depending on the clinical circumstance, oxygen can be insufflated through the catheter lumen. A conventional tracheal tube is then placed in the trachea. This technique can be useful in achieving selective ventilation in children younger than 12 years of age. However, because the blocker balloon requires a high distending pressure, it may easily slip out of the bronchus into the trachea, obstructing ventilation and losing the seal between the two lungs. This displacement can be secondary to changes in position or to surgical manipulation. The loss of lung separation can be a life-threatening situation if it was performed to prevent spillage of pus, blood, or fluid from bronchopulmonary lavage. For this reason, bronchial blockers are rarely used for these types of cases.

Indications for the use of a bronchial blocker are shown in Table 38-2. An independently passed bronchial blocker may be used with an SLT to obtain lung isolation, thereby avoiding the use of a DLT in a patient with a difficult airway. The use of a bronchial blocker also eliminates the potential risk of needing to change a DLT to an SLT at the conclusion of the procedure. The individual blockers are discussed later, in the chronologic order in which they were developed, and introduced into practice. In the past, Fogarty vascular embolectomy catheters were used for

Table 38-2 Indications for the Use of Endobronchial Blockers

The Difficult Airway
Avoids the need for tube exchange (DLT to SLT)
Following laryngeal surgery
Patient with a tracheostomy
Distorted bronchial anatomy due to compression by aneurysm or tumor
Patient who requires nasotracheal intubation

Management
Makes possible segmental blockade in a patient who cannot tolerate OLV
Morbid obesity
Small size and pediatric patients
Patients from the ICU who arrive to the OR tracheally intubated

Surgical Procedures Not Involving the Lung
Esophageal surgery
Spine surgery that requires a transthoracic approach
Minimally invasive cardiac surgery

ICU, Intensive care unit; OLV, one-lung ventilation; SLT, single-lumen tube; DLT, double-lumen tube; OR, operating room.

lung separation, but there is no indication for their use in the current practice of thoracic anesthesia. The balloon of the Fogarty is high pressure, low volume, and there is no lumen to allow egress of gas from the lung to facilitate deflation.

Univent Tube. The Univent (Fuji Systems Corp., Tokyo, Japan) is a single-lumen tracheal tube with a movable endobronchial blocker (Fig. 38-16). In the Univent tube, the bronchial blocker is housed in a small channel bored in the wall of the tube. The blocker contains a high-volume, low-pressure balloon, and is angled to permit external direction into the desired bronchus under direct fiberoptic bronchoscopic (FB) vision. After intubation of the trachea, the movable blocker is manipulated into the desired main stem bronchus with the aid of a fiberoptic bronchoscope. The Univent tube may be ideal for cases in which a tube change (e.g., from single to double lumen) may be difficult (e.g., mediastinoscopy followed by thoracotomy), or in cases of bilateral lung transplantation. The Univent tube has

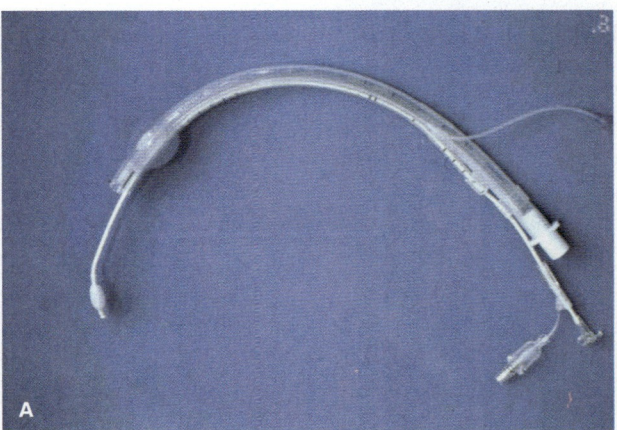
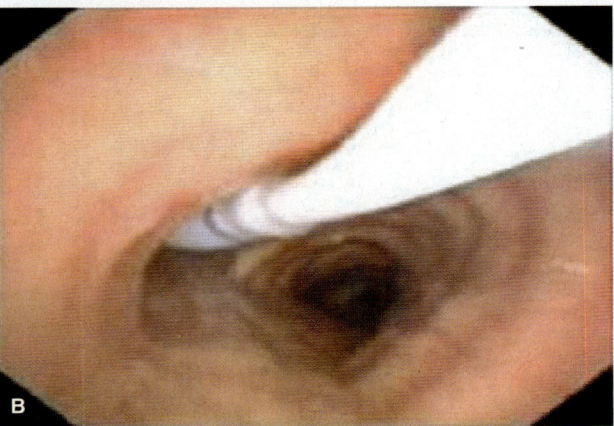

Figure 38-16 A: The Univent tube also allows lung separation using a single-lumen endotracheal tube. **B:** The Univent bronchial blocker positioned in left main stem bronchus.

the advantage common to all bronchial blockers: It is an SLT, and there is no need to change the tube at the end of the procedure if postoperative ventilatory support is required. This is particularly important in cases of difficult intubation, prolonged surgery with airway edema, such as thoracic aortic aneurysm surgery or extensive neurosurgical procedures on the spine with massive fluid replacement, and altered anatomy of the airway. It is also possible to suction through the blocker lumen or to apply continuous positive airway pressure (CPAP) to improve oxygenation in cases of hypoxemia.

The disadvantages of the Univent tubes are that correct positioning of the blocker may be difficult to achieve or maintain and that the external diameter of the tube is relatively large. Many anesthesiologists prefer to avoid postoperative ventilation with such a large-diameter tube, and in that case, change it to a standard tube at the conclusion of the surgery. The blocker can dislocate during surgical manipulation, and satisfactory bronchial seal and lung separation are sometimes difficult to achieve. The bronchial blocker is somewhat stiff and sometimes will not easily be directed into the main bronchus. This is particularly true for the left side. The bulky external diameter can also make it difficult to pass the tube between the vocal cords.

The first-generation Univent tube's bronchial blocker was difficult to direct into the selected main bronchus. The blocker would spin (torque) on its long axis, which made it difficult to control. The second generation, the Torque Control Blocker Univent, was introduced more recently. It consists of a silicon endotracheal tube that has a high friction coefficient. The Torque Control Blocker provides better control, which facilitates direction of the blocker into the target main stem bronchus.

Arndt Blocker. In an attempt to overcome the potential problems described previously, a snare-guided bronchial blocker was introduced (Cook Critical Care) (Fig. 38-17A). It is a wire-guided catheter with a loop snare. A fiberscope is passed through the loop of the bronchial blocker and then guided into the desired bronchus. The blocker is then slid distally over the fiberscope and into the selected bronchus. Bronchoscopic visualization confirms blocker placement and bronchial occlusion. This balloon-tipped catheter has a hollow lumen of 1.6 mm, which allows suction to facilitate the collapse of the lung and insufflation of oxygen to the nondependent lung. The balloon is available in spherical or elliptic shape. The set contains a multiport adapter, which allows uninterrupted ventilation during the positioning of the blocker. The wire may then be removed, and a 1.6-mm lumen may be used as a suction port or for oxygen insufflation. With the first generation of this device it was not possible to reinsert the string once it had been pulled out, losing the ability to redirect the bronchial blocker if necessary. External reinforcement of the wire now allows for its reintroduction through the lumen. Finally, the external diameter necessitates a large size

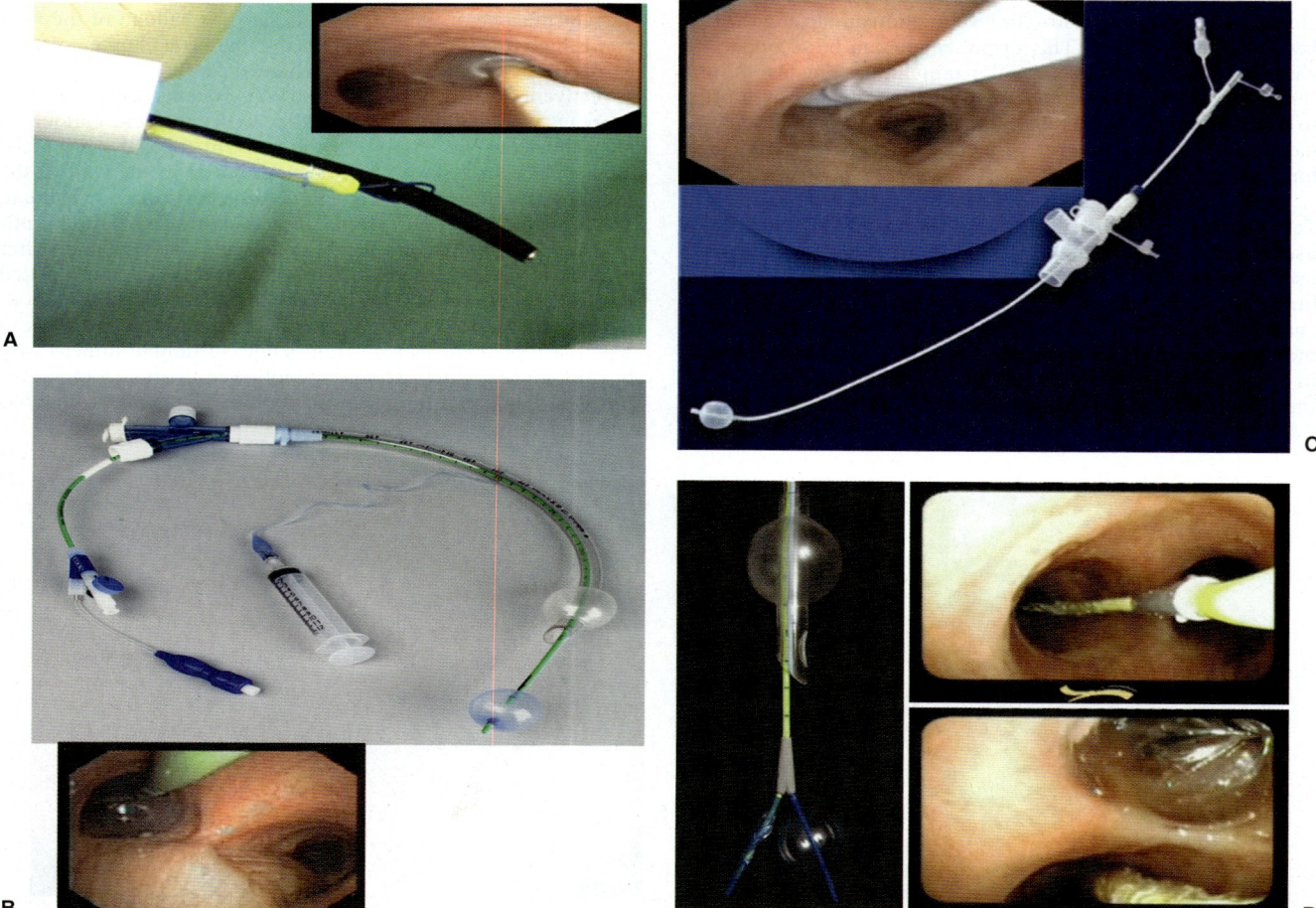

Figure 38-17 **A:** Arndt blocker. **B:** Cohen blocker. **C:** Uniblocker. **D:** EZ blocker.

SLT (at least 8 mm) to be able to accommodate the bronchial blocker. The Arndt blocker is available in a 7-Fr and in a 5-Fr pediatric size. One disadvantage of the Arndt Blocker is that it is advanced blindly over the FB into the desired main bronchus. In some occasions the tip of the blocker may get caught at the main carina or at the Murphy eye of the SLT.

Cohen Blocker. The Cohen Flexitip endobronchial blocker (Cook Critical Care) is designed for use as an independent bronchial blocker. It is inserted through a single-lumen endotracheal tube with the aid of a small-diameter (4-mm) fiberoptic bronchoscope (Fig. 38-17B).[93] The blocker has a rotating wheel that deflects the soft tip by more than 90 degrees and easily directs it into the desired bronchus. The blocker cuff is a high-volume, low-pressure balloon inflated via 0.4-mm lumen inside the wall of the blocker. It has a pear shape that provides adequate seal of the bronchus. Generally, it takes between 6 and 8 mL of air to seal the bronchus with the cuff. The cuff is a distinctive blue color that is easily recognizable by fiberoptic bronchoscopy. It is best to inflate the cuff under "direct vision" via the fiberoptic bronchoscope. The blocker size is 9 Fr. It has a central main lumen (1.6 mm) that allows limited suctioning of secretions and insufflation of oxygen to the collapsed lung in case of hypoxemia. This blocker and the FB do not have to pass through the tracheal tube at the same time for placement; the blocker can be passed ahead of the FB beyond the tracheal tube tip. Therefore, it can be used with a 7-mm tracheal tube.

Uniblocker. Fuji Systems introduced a 9-Fr balloon-tipped, angled blocker with a multiple port adapter that is essentially the same design as the Univent tube blocker, but can be used as an independent blocker passed via a special connector through a standard tracheal tube (Fig. 38-17C).

EZ-Blocker. The most recent addition to the endobronchial blocker design is the EZ Blocker (Teleflex, Morrisville, NC). This is a 7-Fr, 4-lumen, 75-cm, disposable endobronchial blocker to facilitate selective lung ventilation (Fig. 38-17D). It has a symmetric Y-shaped bifurcation and both branches have an inflatable cuff and a central lumen. The bifurcation resembles the bifurcation of the trachea. During insertion via a standard tracheal tube, each of the two distal ends is placed into a main stem bronchus. The selected lung is isolated by inflating the blocker's balloon to the least volume necessary to occlude the main stem bronchus under bronchoscopic visualization. This blocker should offer an advantage during bilateral procedures because each lung can be deflated without the need for repositioning the blocker.[94] The characteristics of the various bronchial blockers are summarized in Table 38-3.

The effectiveness of lung isolation among three devices—the left-sided DLT Broncho-Cath, the Torque Control Blocker Univent, and the wire-guided Arndt—has been compared in a prospective randomized trial. There was no significant difference in tube malpositions among the three groups: It took longer to position the Arndt blocker (3 minutes) compared with the left-sided DLT (2 minutes) and the Univent (2 minutes). Excluding the time for tube placement, the Arndt group also took longer for the lung to collapse (26 minutes), compared with the DLT group (17 minutes) or Univent group (19 minutes). Furthermore, unlike the other two groups, the majority of the Arndt patients required suction to achieve lung collapse. Once lung isolation was achieved, overall surgical exposure was rated excellent for the three groups. One minute longer to position a bronchial blocker or 6 minutes longer to collapse the lung with the bronchial blocker is insignificant when considering the duration of the thoracic procedure. The risk benefit and the patient safety of each individual patient should be considered when choosing the methods for lung isolation.[95,96]

A study evaluated the use of the Cohen blocker, the Arndt blocker, the Uniblocker, and DLT in 4 groups of 26 patients in each group. They found no differences among the groups in the time taken to insert these lung isolation devices or in the quality of the lung collapse.[97] The grading was done by the operating surgeons who were blinded as to which device was used. The number of cuff dislocations was higher among the bronchial blocker (BB) groups. Regardless of the type of BB or DLT selected to provide OLV, the decision as to which technique to use depends on the clinical circumstances and the physician's experience and comfort with a particular device. It is important, however, that the clinician does not limit his/her practice to the use of only one device but rather be versatile and comfortable in the use of several.

A recent comprehensive meta-analysis and randomized controlled trials analysis was performed for a comparison of the efficacy and adverse effects of DLTs and EBB in thoracic Surgery.[86] The authors performed a systematic literature search for RCTs comparing BBs and DLTs using databases up to October 2013. The search produced 39 RCTs published between 1996 and 2013. The authors concluded that DLTs were quicker to place and less likely to be incorrectly positioned than EBB. The EBB was associated with fewer patients having a postoperative sore throat, less hoarseness, and fewer airway injuries than DLTs. Most importantly, the time taken for adequate lung collapse as well as the quality of the lung collapse showed no significant difference between the EBB and the DLT.

DLTs have been used to achieve lung separation for more than 50 years and will remain the "gold standard" lung separation. However, there are many clinical situations where DLT may not be the method of choice or may be impossible to use. The anesthesiologist should become familiar with the various devices used to achieve lung separation. Bronchial blockers can be safely and

Table 38-3 Comparison of Bronchial Blockers (BBs)

	Arndt Blocker	Cohen Blocker	Uniblocker	EZ Blocker
Size	5 Fr, 7 Fr, 9 Fr	9 Fr	9 Fr	7 Fr
Guidance Feature	Wire loop to snare FOB	Deflecting tip	Prefixed bend	Double-lumen bifurcated tip
Recommended Tracheal Tube Size	9 Fr 8 mm 7 Fr 7 mm 5 Fr 4.5 mm	8 mm	8 mm	8 mm
Central Lumen	1.8 mm	1.8 mm	2 mm	
Murphy Eye	Present in 9 Fr	Present	None	None
Disadvantages	BB not visualized during insertion	Expensive	No steering mechanism. Prefixed bend	Lumen too small. Impossible to suction

effectively used either for simple procedures such as a brief wedge resections or for more complexes extended procedure such as lobectomy or pneumonectomy. The fact that there are several EBBs available for clinical use may be a reflection of the search for the ideal blocker. It is of benefit to the patient if the need to change tubes (DLT to SLT) during the case or at case-end can be avoided because the change may expose the patient to a period during which his/her airway is unprotected.[98]

Conclusion of the Surgical Procedure

Depending on the extent and the duration of the surgical procedure and the degree of fluid shift, an airway that was initially not classified as difficult may become difficult secondary to facial edema, secretions, and laryngeal trauma from the original intubation. In these cases, when planning to provide lung separation, the postoperative period should be considered and the appropriate tube placed. Many procedures that are not considered to represent absolute indications for lung separation are lengthy and complex. Complex lung resection, with or without chest wall resection, thoracoabdominal esophagogastrectomy, thoracic aortic aneurysm resection with or without total circulatory arrest, or an extensive vertebral tumor resection, may result in facial edema, secretion, and hemoptysis, requiring postoperative ventilatory support. Other indications for postoperative ventilatory support are marginal respiratory reserve, unexpected blood loss or fluid shift, hypothermia, and inadequate reversal of residual neuromuscular blockade.

If a Univent tube was used to provide OLV, the blocker may be fully retracted and the Univent tube can be used as an SLT. If an independent bronchial blocker was used, then the blocker is removed, leaving the SLT in place. The problem arises when a DLT was inserted for lung separation. In a patient with a difficult airway and subsequent facial edema, the DLT may be left in place after surgery.

If the decision to leave the DLT in place is made, it is important to keep in mind that the ICU staff is usually less experienced in managing such a tube, which may easily become dislocated. In addition, it is more difficult to suction through the lumens, and a longer, narrower suction catheter is needed to reach the tip of the endobronchial lumen. Another possibility is to withdraw the DLT to place the 19- to 20-cm mark at the teeth so that the endobronchial lumen is above the carina and both lungs can be ventilated via the bronchial lumen. Tracheal extubation from the DLT should be considered after diuresis and steroid therapy to allow reduction of the facial and airway edema.

If it is necessary to change the DLT to an SLT, a tube exchanger should be used to maintain access to the airway, as previously discussed. The tube exchanger can be passed through the bronchial limb of the DLT. Alternatively, the tube exchange may be performed under direct vision using one of several commercially available video laryngoscopes, such as the GlideScope (Verathon Medical), C-Mac (Karl Storz), or the Mc Grath (Aircraft Medical) (see Chapter 28). With these video laryngoscopes, the tube exchanger can be placed under direct vision between the vocal cords alongside the existing tube to permit passage of an SLT (Fig. 38-18). The Airtraq DL (King Systems) is a disposable video blade that is manufactured with a large channel that is large enough to accommodate a DLT.

In summary, the clinician should be able to master different methods of lung separation and make himself/herself familiar with the devices available to provide OLV. In addition, one should always plan in advance for the postoperative period when selecting the method of lung separation. Finally, in these cases, a close dialog with the surgical team is of vital importance.

Management of One-lung Ventilation

This section discusses the management of OLV in a paralyzed patient in the lateral decubitus position with an open chest. Inspired oxygen fraction (F_{IO_2}), V_T and respiratory rate, dependent lung, PEEP, and nondependent lung CPAP are reviewed, and an approach to the management of OLV is presented.

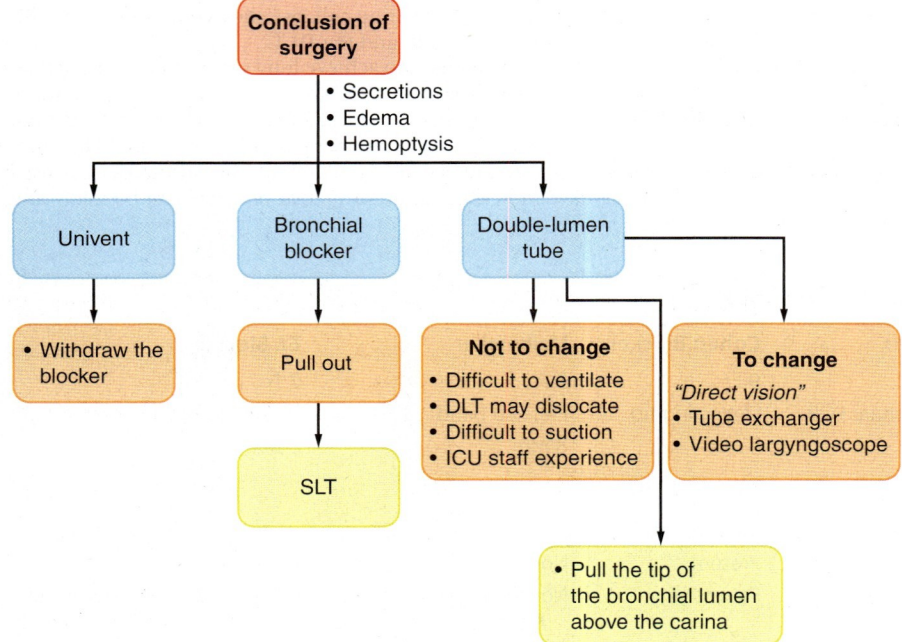

Figure 38-18 Conclusion of the surgical procedure. See text for discussion. SLT, single-lumen tube; DLT, double-lumen tube; ICU, intensive care unit.

Confirmation of Correct Position of DLT or Endobronchial Blocker

Following intubation with a DLT or placement of an endobronchial blocker, the correct position should be checked by clinical assessment, visualization of chest movement, auscultation, and pressure/volume flow profile. In modern anesthesia practice, a standard 4.0-mm fiberscope should be passed down the tracheal lumen to check for correct depth, or alongside the endobronchial blocker that was passed through the single lumen tracheal tube. It is a common practice to visualize the tip of the blue bronchial cuff at the level of the carina to ensure that the left upper lobe orifice is not obstructed. Once the patient is turned into the lateral position, the position of the DLT should be rechecked to exclude dislocation of the tube during positioning.[99]

Inspired Oxygen Fraction

An F_{IO_2} of 1 is generally recommended during OLV. High oxygen concentration serves to protect against hypoxemia during the procedure and provides a higher margin of safety. A high F_{IO_2} may, however, cause absorption atelectasis and potentially further increase the amount of shunt because of the collapsed alveoli. The use of an F_{IO_2} less than 1 during OLV has the potential benefits of decreasing the risk of absorption atelectasis and, if N_2O is used, may allow potent inhaled anesthetics to be used in lower concentrations. Some clinicians use an O_2 80%/N_2O 20% mixture as long that the SpO_2 is maintained in a safe range. The rate of the lung collapse during OLV was addressed by Ko et al.[100] They compared the effects of three different gas mixtures (air/oxygen, F_{IO_2} 0.4; N_2O/O_2, F_{IO_2} 0.4; and oxygen, F_{IO_2} 1) during OLV on lung collapse and oxygenation during subsequent OLV: They found that deflation of the nonventilated lung during thoracic surgery was delayed if air was used as part of the anesthetic gas mixture during the initial period of OLV. For thoracic procedures in which delayed collapse of the nonventilated lung will impede surgical exposure, the optimal anesthetic technique should include thorough denitrogenation of the lung by using F_{IO_2} of 1.

Tidal Volume and Respiratory Rate

It has been recommended that during OLV, the dependent lung be ventilated with a V_T of 10 to 12 mL/kg. Tidal volumes (V_T) ranging between 8 and 15 mL/kg produced no significant effect on transpulmonary shunt or PaO_2.[101] A V_T less than 8 mL/kg can result in a decrease in FRC and increased formation of atelectasis in the dependent lung. A V_T greater than 15 mL/kg may recruit the atelectatic alveoli in the dependent lung. It will increase the pulmonary vascular resistance of the dependent lung (similar to the application of PEEP) and divert blood flow into the nondependent lung. It has been common practice during OLV to maintain the same V_T as during two-lung ventilation.

Recently, more attention has been directed toward protection of the ventilated lung with the use of smaller V_T to avoid acute lung injury (ALI) (see Chapter 57).[102] This concept stimulated a debate over the optimal V_T that should be used during OLV. A pro and con editorial argued that a (large) V_T of 12 mL/kg during OLV may cause overdistention and stretching of the lung parenchyma and therefore would increase the risk of ALI.[103] However, a (small) V_T of 6 mL/kg could lead to atelectasis in the dependent lung. Furthermore, a small V_T with PEEP may cause dynamic hyperinflation secondary to the increase in respiratory rate necessary to maintain $PaCO_2$.[104]

Vegh et al.[105] evaluated the effect of low (5 mL/kg) and high (10 mL/kg) tidal volume on arterial oxygenation during OLV. For the first 30 minutes of OLV, 50 patients received a tidal volume of 10 mL/kg at a respiratory rate of 10/min, whereas another 50 patients received a tidal volume of 5 mL/kg with 5 cm H_2O of PEEP at a rate of 20 breaths/min. For the subsequent 30 minutes of OLV each patient received the alternative ventilatory parameters. These authors found that a tidal volume of 5 mL/kg with 5 cm H_2O PEEP resulted in comparable PaO_2 and shunt fractions during OLV as tidal volumes of 10 mL/kg without PEEP. The smaller TV significantly increased $PaCO_2$.

Mechanical ventilation practice has changed over the past few decades, with V_T decreasing significantly, especially in patients with ALI. The lungs of patients without ALI are still ventilated with large, and perhaps too large, V_T. Studies of ventilator-associated lung injury in subjects without ALI demonstrate inconsistent results. Retrospective clinical studies, however, suggest that the use of large V_T favors the development of lung injury in these patients.[106]

In a multicenter, prospective ARDS Network trial, the results unambiguously confirmed that mechanical ventilation with smaller V_T (6 mL/kg) rather than traditional V_T (12 mL/kg) resulted in a significant increase in the number of ventilator-free days and reduction of inhospital mortality.[107]

Although there is good evidence from studies in the ICU for a detrimental effect of high V_T and parenchymal overdistension, the data concerning lung injury during OLV is limited. Ventilation strategies during OLV have been compared to ARDS, because both involve ventilation of a decreased lung capacity due to unrecruited alveoli, otherwise known as the concept of "baby lung."[108] There is no evidence that these findings in patients with acute respiratory distress syndrome are applicable to patients undergoing a thoracic procedure requiring a relatively short period of controlled ventilation.

In one study, patients undergoing elective thoracotomy or laparotomy were randomly assigned to receive either mechanical ventilation with V_T of 12 or 15 mL/kg, respectively, and without PEEP, or V_T of 6 mL/kg with PEEP of 10 cm H_2O. In this study, neither time course nor concentrations of pulmonary or systemic inflammatory mediators (cytokines) differed between the two ventilatory settings within 3 hours.[109]

There are data indicating damaging effects of large V_T in patients who were ventilated for only several hours. In one study of patients undergoing pneumonectomy, 18% developed postoperative respiratory failure. The patients who developed respiratory failure had been ventilated with larger intraoperative V_T than those who did not (median, 8.3 vs. 6.7 mL/kg predicted body weight).[110] However, the authors recommended that protective lung ventilation (PV) with low V_T 6 to 7 mL/kg, PEEP to the dependent lung, frequent recruitment maneuvers, and limited administration of fluid be used during OLV.

In patients undergoing general anesthesia, lung recruitment maneuvers proved to be easy to perform and effective in reversing alveolar collapse, hypoxemia, and decreased compliance. The beneficial effect of an alveolar recruitment strategy on arterial oxygenation and respiratory compliance in anesthetized patients undergoing nonthoracic surgery in the supine position has been demonstrated by Tusman et al.,[111] who studied 10 patients undergoing open lobectomy and who received lung recruitment maneuvers. This was done by increasing peak inspiratory pressure to 40 cm H_2O, together with a PEEP of 20 cm H_2O for 10 respiratory cycles. They found that alveolar recruitment in the dependent lung augments PaO_2 values during OLV. It is important to apply the maneuvers over several minutes with a pressure of at least 20 cm H_2O and a peak of 40 cm H_2O.

Pressure-controlled ventilation (PCV) was also compared with volume-controlled ventilation (VCV) during OLV. The authors suggested that PCV may be preferred for management of OLV because the lower peak airway pressure was associated with greater perfusion of the dependent lung and smaller transpulmonary shunt.[112] A study has investigated whether PCV results in improved arterial oxygenation compared with VCV during OLV.[113] Fifty-eight patients with good preoperative pulmonary function scheduled for thoracic surgery were prospectively randomized into two groups. Those in group A underwent OLV initially with VCV for 30 minutes followed by PCV for a similar period of time. Those in group B underwent OLV initially with PCV for 30 minutes followed by VCV for a similar duration. Airway pressures and arterial blood gases were obtained during OLV at the end of each ventilatory mode period. The authors found no differences in arterial oxygenation during OLV between VCV (Pa_{O_2}, 206.1 ± 62.4 mmHg) and PCV (Pa_{O_2}, 202.1 ± 56.4 mmHg; $p = 0.534$).[113]

Cruz Pardons et al.[114] studied 110 patients scheduled for thoracic surgery requiring a minimum of 1 hour of OLV. The patients were randomized into two groups: VCV or PCV, both providing a V_T of 8 mL/kg. Measurements were taken intraoperatively and up to 24 hours postoperatively. There were no differences in the intra- or early postoperative arterial oxygenation, airway plateau pressure, and mean arterial pressure between groups, except for higher peak airway pressures in the VCV group. The respiratory rate should be adjusted to maintain a Pa_{CO_2} of 35 ± 3 mmHg. Elimination of CO_2 is usually not a problem during OLV if the DLT is positioned correctly. The shunt during OLV has little influence on Pa_{CO_2} values because the arteriovenous PCO_2 difference is normally only 6 mmHg. Furthermore, CO_2 is 20 times more diffusible than O_2 and will be eliminated faster. It is also important not to hyperventilate the patient's lungs because hypocapnia increases vascular resistance in the dependent lung, inhibits nondependent lung HPV, increases shunt, and decreases Pa_{O_2}. Hypocarbia is believed to inhibit HPV secondary to a vasodilator effect. Because hypocapnia can only be achieved by hyperventilating the dependent lung, it raises the mean intra-alveolar pressure and therefore increases the vascular resistance in that lung.

OLV is known to cause an inflammatory response and ALI.[115] Hypercapnia has been shown to have beneficial effects in patients with lung injuries such as ARDS. Gao et al.[116] therefore studied the effect of deliberate hypercapnia on the inflammatory responses to OLV in patients undergoing lobectomy. Fifty patients having lobectomy under intravenous anesthesia were randomly assigned to ventilation with either air (PCO_2 35 to 45 mmHg) or CO_2 (60 to 70 mmHg) from a CO_2 tank connected to the anesthesia machine. FIO_2 was maintained at greater than 0.8 during OLV. Duration of OLV was not significantly different between the two groups (means ~ 180 minutes). Alveolar lavage fluid was collected and assayed for inflammatory factors. The authors found that induced hypercapnia during the OLV period inhibited the local inflammatory response, decreased airway pressure as well as increased lung compliance and PaO_2/FIO_2 following surgery. No severe adverse effects were reported in relation to the therapeutic hypercarbia. The potential beneficial effect of inhalation of CO_2 (60 to 70 mmHg) during OLV merits further investigation in patients receiving potent inhaled anesthetics, which have already been shown to inhibit the inflammatory response during lung surgery.

Positive End-expiratory Pressure to the Dependent Lung

The beneficial effect of selective PEEP 10 cm H_2O ($PEEP_{10}$) to the dependent lung is caused by an increased lung volume at end expiration (FRC), which improves the ventilation/perfusion ($\dot{V}/\dot{Q}$) relationship in the dependent lung. The increase in FRC prevents airway and alveolar closure at end-expiration. However, PEEP may lead to an increase in lung volume that could cause compression of the small interalveolar vessels and increase pulmonary vascular resistance. If this increase in resistance is limited to the dependent lung, blood flow can be diverted only to the nondependent (nonventilated) lung, increasing shunt fraction and further decreasing Pa_{O_2}.

The possibility that the application of PEEP can improve Pa_{O_2} in a diseased dependent lung (low lung volume and low $\dot{V}/\dot{Q}$ ratio) with a low Pa_{O_2} (<80 mmHg) during OLV was studied by Cohen et al.[117] They found that the application of $PEEP_{10}$ during OLV in patients with a low Pa_{O_2} may increase FRC to normal values, resulting in a lower pulmonary vascular resistance and in an improved $\dot{V}/\dot{Q}$ ratio and Pa_{O_2}. Presumably, patients with a higher Pa_{O_2} had a dependent lung with an adequate FRC, and the application of PEEP had the negative effect of redistributing blood flow away from the dependent ventilated lung (Fig. 38-19).

In summary, in most circumstances PEEP alone would not improve arterial oxygenation, unless it could increase FRC to normal values. Since PV with low V_T is the recommended mode of ventilation during OLV, it most likely would lead to formation of atelectasis. Therefore, combining low V_T with a small amount of PEEP (5 cm H_2O) to protect from development of atelectasis is the currently recommended ventilatory strategy.

Continuous Positive Airway Pressure to the Nondependent Lung

The single most effective maneuver to increase Pa_{O_2} during OLV is the application of CPAP to the nondependent lung.[118,119] A lower level of CPAP (5 to 10 cm H_2O) maintains the patency of the nondependent lung alveoli, allowing some oxygen uptake

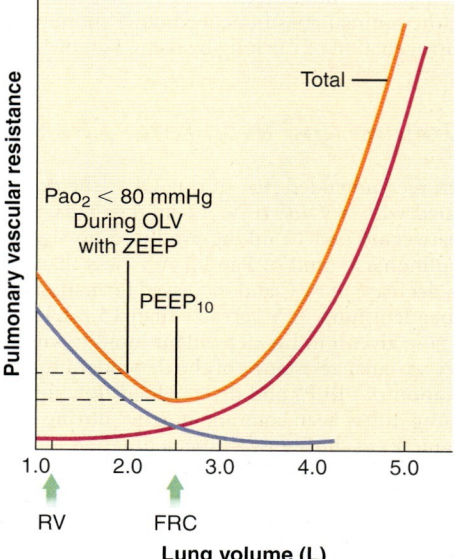

Figure 38-19 Effect of 10 cm H_2O positive end-expiratory pressure (PEEP) on functional residual capacity (FRC). It is postulated that, in patients having Pa_{O_2} below 80 mmHg with zero end-expiratory pressure (ZEEP), FRC is low. $PEEP_{10}$ increases FRC and thereby increases Pa_{O_2}. OLV, one-lung ventilation; $PEEP_{10}$, positive end-expiratory pressure (10 cm H_2O); RV, residual volume.

to occur in the distended alveoli. CPAP should be applied after delivering an inspiratory V_T to the nondependent lung to keep it slightly expanded. CPAP, applied by insufflation of oxygen under positive pressure, keeps this lung "quiet" and prevents it from collapsing completely. Insufflation of oxygen without maintaining a positive pressure failed to improve Pao_2. Intermittent reinflation of the collapsed (nondependent) lung with oxygen also resulted in a significant improvement in Pao_2.[120]

Unfortunately, most thoracic procedures are initiated thoracoscopically, and the application of CPAP to the nondependent lung is generally not acceptable to most surgeons. During VAT, the lung should be well collapsed to allow the surgeon an optimal view of the surgical field and to palpate the lesion in the lung parenchyma. In addition, it is difficult to place the stapler on a lung that is not completely collapsed, and there is an increase in incidence of postoperative air leak.

The beneficial effects of CPAP 10 cm H_2O ($CPAP_{10}$) are not attributable solely to the effect of positive pressure in diverting blood flow away from the collapsed lung because (in dogs) the hyperinflation of nitrogen into the nondependent lung under 10 cm H_2O failed to improve Pao_2.

The application of high-level CPAP (15 cm H_2O) is not beneficial. At this pressure, the lung becomes overdistended, which interferes with surgical exposure. Also, this level of CPAP might have hemodynamic consequences, whereas $CPAP_{10}$ has been shown to have no significant hemodynamic effects.[121]

CPAP can be applied to the nondependent lung using a number of simple systems, all of which have essentially the same features: an oxygen source, tubing to connect the oxygen source to the nonventilated lung, a pressure relief valve, and a pressure gauge. The catheter to the nondependent lung is usually insufflated with 5 L/min of oxygen using a modified Ayre's T-piece (pediatric) circuit, and the valve on the expiratory limb is adjusted to the desired pressure as read on the attached gauge. Instead of a pressure gauge or manometer inserted into the circuit, a spring-loaded adjustable PEEP valve can be used. The amount of CPAP applied should be titrated to the clinical circumstances. In most cases, even low levels of CPAP may be sufficient to increase the Pao_2 to an accepted safe level. CPAP greater than 10 cm H_2O is not beneficial because it creates an overdistention that interferes with surgical exposure and may have undesirable hemodynamic consequences.

High-frequency ventilation with oxygen to the nondependent lung and conventional ventilation (CV) to the dependent lung have also been used to improve Pao_2 during OLV (see "High-frequency Ventilation.").

Clinical Approach to Management of One-lung Ventilation

Once the patient is in the lateral decubitus position, the placement of the DLT should be rechecked. Two-lung ventilation should be maintained for as long as possible, and when OLV needs to be instituted, it is generally recommended that an Fio_2 of 1 be used (Table 38-4). The lung should be ventilated using a V_T that results in a plateau airway pressure greater than 25 cm H_2O at a rate adjusted to maintain $Paco_2$ at 35 ± 3 mmHg. This is usually monitored indirectly with the use of a capnometer or other multigas analyzer. The following measures are recommended during OLV: use of PV with low V_T 6 to 7 mL/kg, application of PEEP to the dependent lung, frequent recruitment maneuvers, and limiting the volume of fluid administered.

After initiation of OLV, depending on the lung pathology and the intensity of HPV, Pao_2 can continue to decrease for up to

Table 38-4 Clinical Approach to One-lung Ventilation (OLV) Management

1. Use Fio_2 of 1
2. Ventilate with a V_T of 6–8 mL/kg with PEEP 5 cm H_2O
3. Respiratory rate to maintain $Paco_2$ between 35 and 40 mmHg
4. Check the DLT/endobronchial blocker position subsequent to the lateral decubitus positioning
5. If peak airway pressure exceeds 40 cm H_2O during OLV, DLT/endobronchial blocker malposition should be excluded
6. For hypoxemia, apply CPAP 10 cm H_2O to the nondependent lung (not during VAT)
7. If additional correction of hypoxemia is necessary, add PEEP 5–10 cm H_2O to the ventilated lung
8. Frequent recruiting maneuvers
9. Avoid fluid overload
10. TIVA may be preferable to inhalation anesthetics
11. If necessary, intermittently inflate and deflate the operated lung

V_T, tidal volume; PEEP, positive end-expiratory pressure; DLT, double-lumen tube; CPAP, continuous positive airway pressure; VAT, video-assisted thoracoscopy; TIVA, total intravenous anesthetic.

45 minutes. Frequent monitoring of arterial blood gases and use of a pulse oximeter continue throughout the operative period. It is also essential to work closely with the surgeon in case reinsufflation of the lung is necessary. If hypoxemia occurs during OLV, the position of the DLT should be rechecked using a fiberoptic bronchoscope. If the dependent lung is not severely diseased, a satisfactory Pao_2 on two-lung ventilation should not decrease to dangerously hypoxic levels on OLV. If a left thoracotomy is being performed using a right-sided DLT, ventilation to the right upper lobe should be ensured. After the tube position has been confirmed as correct, $CPAP_{10}$ should be applied to the nondependent lung after a V_T that expands the lung. In most cases, the Pao_2 increases to a safe level. During thoracoscopy, application of CPAP is usually not possible because it impedes the surgeon. This is especially so during video-assisted thoracoscopic surgery (VATS) procedures. In this case, PEEP to the ventilated lung may be tried.

In the very rare case in which the Pao_2 remains low despite these maneuvers, intermittent two-lung ventilation can be reinstituted with the surgeon's cooperation. Also, depending on the stage of surgical dissection, if a pneumonectomy is being performed, ligation of the pulmonary artery eliminates the shunt.

During OLV, the peak airway pressure, the actual V_T delivered (measured by a spirometer), the shape of the capnogram, and, if available, the pressure–volume loop, should be checked continuously. A sudden increase in peak airway pressure may be secondary to tube dislocation because of surgical manipulation, resulting in impaired ventilation. In addition, the ability to auscultate by a stethoscope over the dependent lung is extremely important.

If there is any doubt about the stability of the patient, or if the patient becomes hypotensive, dusky, or tachycardic, two-lung ventilation should be resumed until the problem has been resolved. Because of pericardial manipulation (during left thoracotomy in particular) and pulling on the great vessels, cardiac dysrhythmias and hypotension are not uncommon. Cardiotonic drugs should be prepared and kept available for use during any thoracic surgical procedure. Most thoracic surgical procedures represent only relative indications for OLV, and the benefits of OLV should always be weighed against the risks to the patient.

Attention should be directed toward the protection of the ventilated lung. PV should be used with low V_T and the lowest peak airway pressure, an I:E ratio of 1:1, with high respiratory rate or using pressure control ventilation. Patients with COPD are of particular concern because the application of PEEP may cause dynamic hyperinflation secondary to the increase in respiratory rate to maintain $Paco_2$.

Frequent recruiting maneuvers should be applied to reduce the amount of atelectasis in the dependent lung. They should be applied with a sustained peak pressure of 40 cm H_2O to be effective. Fluid administration during the procedure must be limited to avoid fluid overload that could increase pulmonary capillary permeability. The risk of ALI and fluid overload increases in proportion to the amount of lung parenchyma resected.[122-124]

A balanced anesthetic technique using inhalational agents with low rates of propofol infusion alone or in combination with remifentanil is the technique of choice during OLV. It should have the least inhibitory effect on HPV and decrease the transpulmonary shunt through the nonventilated lung. Karzai et al.[125] published an excellent review on the prediction, prevention, and treatment of hypoxemia during OLV.

Yang et al.[126] compared PV with CV in two groups of 50 patients each undergoing OLV. Conventional strategy consisted of Fio_2 1, V_T 10 mL/kg, zero end-expiratory pressure (ZEEP), and VCV; the protective strategy (PV) consisted of Fio_2 0.5, V_T 6 mL/kg, PEEP 5 cm H_2O, and PCV. During OLV, although 58% of the PV group needed an increased Fio_2 to maintain an Spo_2 greater than 95%, peak airway pressure was significantly lower than in the CV group, whereas the mean $Paco_2$ values remained at 35 to 40 mmHg in both groups. Importantly, in the PV group, the incidence of the primary end point of pulmonary dysfunction was significantly lower than in the CV group (incidence of Pao_2/Fio_2 <300 mmHg, lung infiltration, or atelectasis: 4% vs. 22%). The mechanical ventilation strategies used during OLV are discussed in a recent comprehensive review by Şentürk et al.[127]

Choice of Anesthesia for Thoracic Surgery

The choice of anesthesia technique for a thoracic surgical procedure must take into account the patient's cardiovascular and respiratory status and the particular effects of anesthetic drugs on these and other organ systems. Thoracic surgical patients are more likely than others to have increased airway reactivity and a propensity to develop bronchoconstriction. This is because many of these patients are cigarette smokers and have chronic bronchitis or COPD. In addition, surgical manipulation of the airways and bronchial tree by instruments, a DLT, or the surgeon, makes bronchoconstriction more likely to occur. The potent inhaled anesthetic agents have all been shown to decrease airway reactivity and bronchoconstriction provoked by hypocapnia or inhaled or irritant aerosols. Their mechanism of action is probably a direct one on the airway musculature itself, and potent inhaled anesthetic agents are therefore the drugs of choice in patients with reactive airways. For an inhalation induction, halothane or sevoflurane might be preferable because they are the least pungent of the three drugs, although once the patient is asleep, isoflurane may be the preferred drug because it raises the cardiac dysrhythmia threshold and provides greater cardiovascular stability than halothane (see Chapter 18). Fentanyl does not appear to influence bronchomotor tone, but morphine may increase tone by a central vagotonic effect and by releasing histamine.

In most patients, anesthesia is safely induced with propofol or etomidate (since thiopental is no longer available in the United States). In patients with reactive airways, ketamine may be the drug of choice for induction because it has a bronchodilator effect and has been successfully used in the treatment of asthma. Shimizu et al.[128] compared the effects of isoflurane and sevoflurane on Pao_2 during OLV in 20 patients undergoing thoracotomy and found no significant difference between the groups in Pao_2, concluding that both agents can be used safely. In an in vitro study, Loer et al.[129] showed that desflurane inhibits HPV, with an ED_{50} of 1.6 minimum alveolar concentration (MAC). Propofol infused in doses of 6 to 12 mg/kg/hr does not abolish HPV during OLV in humans.[130] Propofol infusion in combination with remifentanil is probably the technique of choice for producing a stable OLV with no effect on HPV. Propofol is widely used during OLV and has been investigated in terms of its effect on oxygenation. Kellow et al.[131] compared the effects of propofol and isoflurane anesthesia on right ventricular function and shunt fraction during thoracic surgery and found that isoflurane, but not propofol, was associated with an increase in shunt fraction due to HPV inhibition. However, propofol was associated with a reduction in cardiac index and right ventricular ejection fraction.

In deciding between intravenous versus potent inhaled agent for anesthesia during OLV, consideration should be given to their effects on inflammatory alterations in the deflated lung. Studies have shown that ventilation with increased V_T and pressures can produce a proinflammatory reaction (e.g., tumor necrosis factor, interleukins) in the nondeflated, ventilated lung.[132] De Conno et al.[133] studied the effect on the pulmonary inflammatory response in the nonventilated lung before and after OLV in 54 adult patients undergoing thoracic surgery, and assessed if there were any immunomodulatory effects of propofol and sevoflurane. The results suggested an immunomodulatory role for sevoflurane. Compared with propofol there was a significant reduction in inflammatory mediators and a significantly better clinical outcome defined by postoperative adverse events with sevoflurane.[128] A subsequent study compared the effects of desflurane, sevoflurane, and propofol on pulmonary and systemic inflammation in 63 patients undergoing open thoracic surgery. The investigators found that OLV increases the alveolar concentrations of proinflammatory mediators in the ventilated lung and that desflurane and sevoflurane suppress the local alveolar, but not the systemic, inflammatory responses to OLV and thoracic surgery.[134] In murine models isoflurane has also been shown to have a protective effect against acute and ventilator-induced lung injury.[135,136]

The neuromuscular blocking drugs of choice for thoracic procedures are those that lack a histamine-releasing or vagotonic effect and that have some sympathomimetic effect (see Chapter 21). In this respect, pancuronium, vecuronium, rocuronium, and cisatracurium probably represent the drugs of choice. Succinylcholine is useful to provide rapid profound relaxation for intubation of the trachea and is not associated with an increase in airway reactivity.

Atropine or glycopyrrolate may be used to block the muscarinic effects of acetylcholine and thereby protect against cholinergically induced bronchoconstriction. It may be administered intravenously or in nebulized form (see Chapter 14).

Hypoxic Pulmonary Vasoconstriction

HPV was first described by Von Euler and Liljestrand in 1946.[137] They were studying changes in the pulmonary circulation of the cat in response to changes in inspired gas mixtures and found that 10.5% inspired O_2 (in N_2) mixtures caused an increase in pulmonary artery pressure. Breathing 100% O_2 caused a decrease in pulmonary artery pressure. They concluded that the increased pressure during hypoxia was caused by a direct effect on the pulmonary vessels. Whereas they delivered hypoxic gas mixtures to both lungs, others have studied the effects of the size of the hypoxic segment and the size of the hypoxic stimulus on perfusion pressure and on flow diversion.[138] Pulmonary perfusion pressure (in dogs) increased with the size of the hypoxic segment from zero (smallest hypoxic segment) to approximately 2.2 times baseline for the hypoxic whole lung. Flow diversion, as a percentage of flow to the test segment under normoxic conditions, decreased with increasing size of the hypoxic test segment from a maximum of 75% for very small segments to zero when the whole lung was made hypoxic. Flow diversion increased linearly as Pa_{O_2} was decreased over the range of 128 to 28 mmHg. In both flow diversion and changes in perfusion pressure, the response to HPV was predictable, continuous, and maximal at a predicted Pa_{O_2} of 30 mmHg (4% oxygen). Thus, HPV causes an increase in both perfusion (pulmonary artery) pressure and flow diversion.

The choice of anesthetic technique for OLV must take into consideration the effects on oxygenation and therefore on HPV. Normally, collapse of the nonventilated, nondependent lung results in activation of reflex HPV in this lung. This causes local increases in pulmonary vascular resistance and diversion of blood flow to other, better oxygenated parts of the pulmonary vascular bed (i.e., the dependent oxygenated and ventilated lung).

The relationship between Pa_{O_2} and the size of the hypoxic segment (Fig. 38-20) shows that, when not much of the lung is hypoxic, HPV has little effect on Pa_{O_2} because shunt is small in this situation. When most of the lung is hypoxic, there is no significant normoxic region to which the hypoxic region can divert flow, and then it does not matter, in terms of Pa_{O_2}, whether the hypoxic region has active HPV. When the amount of lung made hypoxic is 30% to 70%, such as occurs during OLV, there may be a large difference between the Pa_{O_2} to be expected with normal HPV compared with that expected in its absence. HPV can raise Pa_{O_2} from potentially dangerous levels to higher and safer ones. Conversely, inhibition of HPV may cause or contribute to hypoxemia during anesthesia.

The response is believed to be accounted for by each smooth muscle cell in the pulmonary arterial wall responding to the oxygen tension in its vicinity. The mechanism of HPV has been the subject of many studies that have been recently summarized in an excellent review.[139]

Effects of Anesthetics on Hypoxic Pulmonary Vasoconstriction

The inhalation anesthetics and many of the intravenous drugs used in anesthesia have been studied for their effects on HPV. The results have not always been consistent. Benumof[140] classified the preparations used to study these effects as in vitro, in vivo nonintact, in vivo intact, and human studies. On the basis of the results of these three types of preparation, it is generally believed that inhaled agents inhibit HPV, whereas intravenous drugs do not have this effect.[141] The effects of anesthetics and other drugs in HPV in humans is difficult since during a surgical procedure there are many confounding variables, in particular the effects of inhaled agents on hemodynamics, for which to account.[142-144] Clinical studies therefore often fail to show a difference between inhaled and intravenous agents. For example, studies have shown no clinical difference in Pa_{O_2} and shunt between OLV patients anesthetized using propofol or sevoflurane,[145] or propofol versus isoflurane.[146] Another study[131] reported finding a larger shunt with isoflurane. A study comparing sevoflurane with propofol, both titrated to a BIS reading of 40 to 60, found no difference in effect on oxygenation.[147]

Beck et al.[145] studied 40 patients requiring OLV randomized to receive propofol (4 to 6 mg/kg/hr) or sevoflurane (1 MAC) for anesthesia maintenance. During OLV shunt fraction increased in both groups, but there was no significant difference between groups. It was concluded that inhibition of HPV by sevoflurane may only account for small increases in shunt fractions and that much of the overall shunt fraction during OLV has other causes.

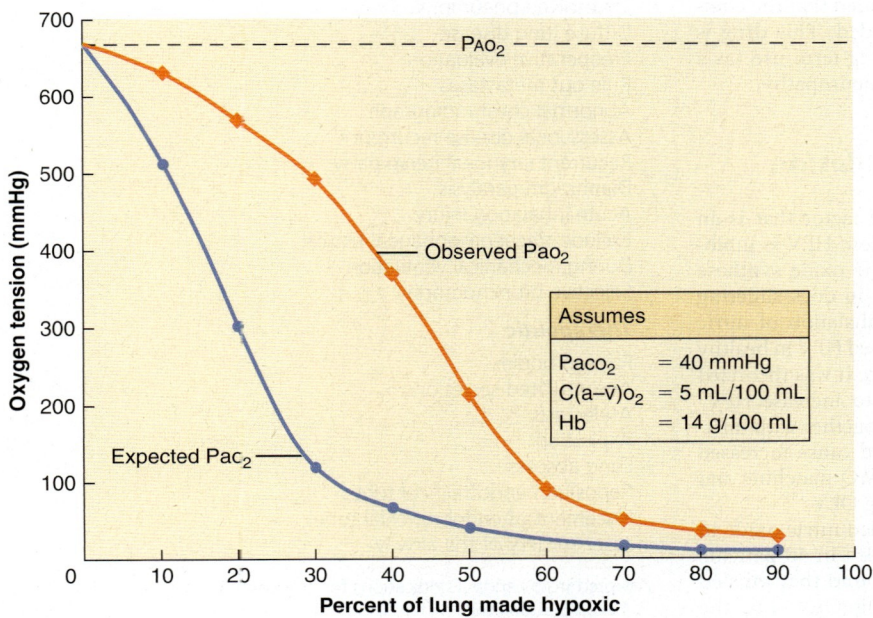

Figure 38-20 Role of hypoxic pulmonary vasoconstriction (HPV) in preserving Pa_{O_2} (in dogs). Assumptions are shown in inset. Lung is ventilated with $Fi_{O_2} = 1$, while increasing portions of lung are subjected to hypoxia or atelectasis. In the absence of HPV, the expected Pa_{O_2} would follow the *blue line*, whereas in the presence of an active HPV response, observed Pa_{O_2} is maintained close to the *red line*. PA_{O_2}, alveolar P_{O_2}; Pa_{O_2}, arterial P_{O_2}. (Adapted from Marshall BE, Marshall C, Benumof JL, et al. Hypoxic pulmonary vasoconstriction in dogs: Effects of lung segment size and alveolar oxygen tension. *J Appl Physiol.* 1981;51:1543.)

Overall, the potent inhaled anesthetics are the drugs of choice during thoracic surgery. However, the technique chosen should always be dictated by the needs of the particular patient, so in the presence of cardiovascular instability or poor oxygenation when depression of HPV is a possibility, a balanced technique may be chosen.

Other Determinants of Hypoxic Pulmonary Vasoconstriction

Aside from potent inhaled agents, other drugs and maneuvers used during anesthesia may also have an inhibitory effect on regional or whole-lung HPV. Factors associated with an increase in pulmonary artery pressure antagonize the effect of increased resistance caused by HPV and result in increased flow to the hypoxic region. Such indirect inhibitors of HPV include mitral stenosis, volume overload, thromboembolism, hypothermia, vasoconstrictor drugs, and a large hypoxic lung segment. Direct inhibitors of HPV include infection, vasodilator drugs such as nitroglycerin and nitroprusside, nitric oxide, acetazolamide, phosphodiesterase inhibitors, prostacyclin, angiotensin-converting enzyme inhibitors, hypocarbia, and metabolic alkalemia. All these potential inhibitors should be considered when evaluating a patient for hypoxemia during thoracic surgery.[148]

Potentiators of Hypoxic Pulmonary Vasoconstriction

Almitrine, a respiratory stimulant drug, in low dose has been reported to improve Pa_{O_2} in patients with COPD and to have this effect in the absence of ventilatory stimulation.[149] In large doses it causes vasoconstriction in normoxic lung.[150] Its mechanism of action is not known. Since almitrine potentiates HPV and potent inhaled anesthetics inhibit HPV, Bermejo et al.[151] studied the effect of almitrine versus placebo in patients who were receiving sevoflurane-remifentanil anesthesia for open chest procedures. The results showed that almitrine failed to improve PaO_2 or shunt fraction during OLV and sevoflurane anesthesia and increased pulmonary artery pressure. The authors concluded that the combination of almitrine and sevoflurane be avoided. This drug is not approved for use in the United States. Long-term use (as a respiratory stimulant) may cause a peripheral neuropathy.

Nitric Oxide and One-lung Ventilation

Nitric oxide is an endothelial-derived relaxing factor that is an important mediator for smooth muscle relaxation. HPV is inhibited by inhaled nitric oxide. Inhibition of nitric oxide synthase improved, but did not completely restore HPV in dogs suffering from sepsis.[152] Frostell et al.[153] showed that inhalation of nitric oxide selectively induced vasodilation and reversed HPV in healthy humans without causing systemic vasodilatation. It was theorized that intravenous administration of almitrine (to increase HPV) causing vasoconstriction throughout the lung, together with inhalation of nitric oxide to inhibit HPV locally and cause increased flow in the ventilated regions, would improve $\dot{V}/\dot{Q}$ matching and Pa_{O_2} in patients with $\dot{V}/\dot{Q}$ mismatching or during OLV.[154]

Moutafis et al.[155] studied the effects of inhaled nitric oxide in combination with almitrine infusion during OLV in 40 patients undergoing thoracoscopic procedures. They found that inhaled nitric oxide alone did not affect Pa_{O_2} during OLV, but the additional infusion of almitrine 16 mg/kg/min caused a marked increase in Pa_{O_2}. These authors suggested that this nonventilatory technique should be of value during special thoracic procedures, such as thoracoscopy, where there is a need to manipulate the pulmonary circulation to improve Pa_{O_2} but measures such as PEEP and CPAP cannot be used. Moutafis et al.[155] also reported the use of almitrine infusion/nitric oxide inhalation to improve Pa_{O_2} during OLV for bronchopulmonary lavage.

Although the use of almitrine appears to be attractive, this drug is not without side effects.[156] Also, the manufacturer has not made it available outside France. Phenylephrine could be a possible alternative to almitrine.[157]

Anesthesia for Diagnostic Procedures

Bronchoscopy

Early bronchoscopes were rigid tubes, but in 1966 the Machida and Olympus Companies introduced the first practical bronchofiberscopes. Since then, they have been improved dramatically and have simplified many otherwise complicated bronchoscopies. The indications for bronchoscopy are shown in Table 38-5 and the instruments of choice in Table 38-6. Operator preferences and experience may play a major role in the choice of instrument.

Before bronchoscopy is performed, the patient must be evaluated for chronic lung disease, respiratory obstruction, bronchospasm, coughing, hemoptysis, and infectivity of secretions. Medications should be reviewed, and the need for a more major

Table 38-5 Indications for Bronchoscopy

Diagnostic
Cough
Hemoptysis
Wheeze
Atelectasis
Unresolved pneumonia
Diffuse lung disease
Preoperative evaluation
Rule out metastases
Abnormal chest radiograph
Assess local disease recurrence
Recurrent laryngeal nerve palsy
Diaphragm paralysis
Acute inhalation injury
Exclude tracheoesophageal fistula
During mechanical ventilation
Selective bronchography

Therapeutic
Foreign bodies
Accumulated secretions
Atelectasis
Aspiration
Lung abscess
Reposition endotracheal tubes
Placement of endobronchial tubes
Laser surgery of the airway

Adapted from Landa JF. Indications for bronchoscopy. *Chest.* 1978;73(Suppl):686.

Table 38-6 Instruments of Choice for Bronchoscopy

Rigid
Foreign bodies
Massive hemoptysis
Vascular tumors
Small children
Endobronchial resections

Fiberoptic/Flexible
Mechanical problems of neck
Upper lobe and peripheral lesions
Limited hemoptysis
During mechanical ventilation
Pneumonia, for selective cultures
Positioning of double-lumen tubes
Difficult intubation
Checking position of endotracheal tube
Bronchial blockade

Adapted from Landa JF. Indication for bronchoscopy. *Chest.* 1978; 73(suppl):686.

procedure should always be anticipated. Thus bronchoscopy may lead to thoracotomy or sternotomy. The planned technique for bronchoscopy should be discussed with the surgeon before the operation, and all equipment and connectors should be checked for compatibility. Monitoring during bronchoscopy should include an electrocardiogram, a blood pressure cuff, a precordial stethoscope, and a pulse oximeter. If thoracotomy is planned, an arterial cannula should also be placed, as well as other monitors (e.g., PA or CVP catheters) that may be indicated by the patient's condition. Many anesthetic techniques are useful for bronchoscopy.

Local Anesthesia

The patient should first be pretreated with a drying agent such as glycopyrrolate. The local anesthetics most commonly used are lidocaine and tetracaine. In all cases, the total dose of anesthetic must be considered and the potential for toxicity recognized. A nebulizer can be used to spray the oropharynx and base of the tongue, or the patient may gargle with viscous (2%) lidocaine. Alternatively, the tongue may be held forward, and pledgets soaked in local anesthetic held in each piriform fossa using Krause forceps to achieve block of the internal branch of the superior laryngeal nerve (see Chapter 28). Tracheal anesthesia is achieved by a transtracheal injection of local anesthetic, or by spraying the vocal cords and trachea under direct vision using a laryngoscope or through the suction channel of the bronchofiberscope. Alternatively, a superior laryngeal nerve block can be performed by an external approach, and a glossopharyngeal block can be used to depress the gag reflex. These blocks cause depression of airway reflexes, so patients must be kept on nothing by mouth status for several hours after the examination. If fiberoptic bronchoscopy is to be performed transnasally, the nasal mucosa should be pretreated topically with 4% cocaine, or viscous lidocaine may be administered through the nares. Local anesthesia for bronchoscopy has the advantages of a patient who is awake, cooperative, and breathing spontaneously. Sedatives may be added to make the patient more comfortable. Disadvantages of local anesthesia include poor tolerance of any bleeding by the patient and the occasional lack of patient cooperation.

General Anesthesia

General anesthesia for bronchoscopy is often combined with topical laryngeal anesthesia so less general anesthesia is needed. A balanced technique uses N_2O/O_2, incremental doses of an intravenous drug such as propofol, an opioid, and a neuromuscular blocking drug. A potent inhalational anesthesia technique is also satisfactory. Alternatively, an intravenous-based technique may be used to avoid contamination of the OR atmosphere by potent inhaled agents. If desired, limited scavenging of waste gases may be achieved by placing a suction catheter in the patient's oropharynx. Unless there is some contraindication, ventilation of the lungs is usually controlled. In any patient undergoing a thoracic diagnostic procedure for a suspected malignancy, the possibility of the myasthenic syndrome with sensitivity to nondepolarizing muscle relaxants must always be considered. The doses of neuromuscular blocking drugs should be titrated to effect using a neuromuscular monitoring system.

Rigid Bronchoscopy

A modern rigid ventilating bronchoscope is essentially a hollow tube with a blunted, beveled tip. Various sizes and designs are available; however, in all of them, a side arm is provided for connection to an anesthetic gas source. A number of techniques have been described for maintaining ventilation and oxygenation during rigid bronchoscopic examination.[158]

Apneic Oxygenation. After preoxygenation and induction of general anesthesia, skeletal muscle paralysis and cessation of intermittent positive-pressure ventilation, the Pa_{CO_2} increases. During the first minute, the increase is approximately 6 mmHg. Subsequently, the average rate of increase is 3 mmHg/min.[159] Oxygen is insufflated at 10 to 15 L/min through a small catheter placed above the carina. The apneic period should be kept to the minimum necessary, particularly in high-risk patients, because the technique is limited by buildup of CO_2, respiratory acidosis, and cardiac dysrhythmias.

Apnea and Intermittent Ventilation. Oxygen and anesthesia gases are delivered to the bronchoscope via the anesthesia circuit. Ventilation is possible only when the eyepiece is in place, which limits the period for instrumentation by the surgeon. Intermittent ventilation of the lungs is achieved by squeezing the reservoir bag. In this way, assuming a good bronchoscope fit in the airway, compliance is constantly monitored, the risk of barotrauma is reduced, and V_T may be estimated. The disadvantage of this technique is that there may be a leak around the bronchoscope, which could lead to hypoventilation and hypercarbia. Packing of the oropharynx can reduce the leak, and improve ventilation in the case of such a gas leak.

Sanders Injection System. Oxygen from a high-pressure source (50 psig) is delivered, using a controllable pressure-reducing valve and toggle switch, to a 2.5- to 3.5-cm 18- or 16-gauge needle inside and parallel to the long axis of the bronchoscope.[160] When the toggle switch is depressed, the jet of oxygen entering the bronchoscope entrains room air, and the air–oxygen mixture resulting at the distal tip of the bronchoscope emerges at a pressure to provide adequate ventilation and oxygenation. The intraluminal tracheal pressure depends on the driving pressure from the reducing valve, the size of the needle jet, the length, internal diameter, and design of the bronchoscope. Increasing the size of the needle jet increases the total gas flow for any given driving pressure. For each combination of gas-driving pressure, jet orifice, and bronchoscope diameter, only one inflation pressure can be attained, regardless of the volume or compliance of the lung. As long as the proximal end of the bronchoscope is open, the system is strictly pressure limited, and the pressure does not increase because of obstruction at the distal end. Pressure varies inversely with the cross-sectional area of the bronchoscope, so insertion of a suction catheter or biopsy forceps into the lumen causes the intratracheal pressure to increase. Provided there is not a tight fit between the bronchoscope and the airway, the risk of barotrauma is low. If the fit is tight, driving pressure should be decreased.

The advantages of the Sanders system are that because continuous ventilation is possible (because the presence of an eyepiece is not necessary for ventilation of the lungs), the duration of the bronchoscopy procedure is minimized, but the efficiency also permits extended bronchoscopy. A disadvantage is that entrainment of air by the oxygen jet results in a variable F_{IO_2} at the distal end of the bronchoscope, ventilation of the lungs may be inadequate if compliance is poor, and adequacy of ventilation may be difficult to assess.

Mechanical Ventilator. Ventilation of the lungs may be achieved by connecting a mechanical ventilator to an anesthesia circuit that is connected to the bronchoscope side arm. One disadvantage of this ventilation technique is the presence of a leak of anesthesia gases, and consequentially, light anesthesia.

High-Frequency Positive-Pressure Ventilation. HFPPV has been used in conjunction with rigid bronchoscopy and has been compared with the Sanders injector in patients with tracheobronchial stenosis. With HFPPV of up to 150 breaths/min, blood gases were identical with both techniques. At a frequency of 500 breaths/min, oxygenation deteriorated and CO_2 was not removed effectively. HFPPV has the advantage that the tracheobronchial wall remains immobilized during ventilation.

Fiberoptic Bronchoscopy

New generations of fiberscopes, with their improved optics and smaller diameters, have revolutionized bronchoscopy. The flexibility has also been applied in preoperative assessment of the airway, management of difficult tracheal intubations, endotracheal tube positioning and change, bronchial toilet, correct positioning of DLTs, bronchial blockade, and evaluation of the larynx and trachea. Nasal fiberoptic bronchoscopy under topical anesthesia is well tolerated by most awake patients. The administration of an antisialagogue such as glycopyrrolate is useful in reducing secretions. Oral insertion is also possible in both awake and asleep patients and should be performed with a bite block in place to prevent damage to the bronchoscope.

Physiologic Changes Associated with Fiberoptic Bronchoscopy. In all patients, insertion of the fiberoptic bronchoscope is associated with hypoxemia. The average decline in Pa_{O_2} is 20 mmHg and lasts for 1 to 4 hours after the procedure. By 24 hours, the blood gas tensions are usually back to normal. It is therefore recommended that if the initial Pa_{O_2} is 70 mmHg ($F_{IO_2} = 0.21$), bronchoscopy should be performed only with the administration of supplemental oxygen. This can be provided using mouth-held nasal prongs, a special face mask with a diaphragm through which the fiberscope can be passed, or an endotracheal tube with a T-piece diaphragm adapter.

During and after fiberoptic bronchoscopy, patients experience increased airway obstruction. Thus in 35 patients, insertion of the bronchoscope was associated with an increase in FRC (17% to 30%) and decreases in Pa_{O_2}, vital capacity, FEV_1, and forced inspiratory flow.[161] All returned to baseline by 24 hours. These changes are believed to be secondary to direct mechanical activation of irritative reflexes in the airway and, possibly, to mucosal edema. They may be avoided if atropine, either intramuscular or aerosolized into the airway, is administered before the procedure.

The standard adult fiberoptic bronchoscope has an external diameter of 5.7 mm and a 2-mm diameter suction channel. If suction at 1 atm is applied to the fiberscope, air is removed at a rate of 14 L/min. If the fiberscope is in the airway, this causes decreases in F_{IO_2}, Pa_{O_2}, and FRC, leading to decreased Pa_{O_2}. Suctioning should therefore be kept brief. The adult fiberscope can be passed through endotracheal tubes of 7 mm or greater internal diameter. Clearly, passage through an endotracheal tube decreases the cross-sectional area available for ventilating the patient, so if fibroscopy is planned, an endotracheal tube of the largest possible diameter should be used.

Insertion of the bronchoscope also causes a significant PEEP effect that may result in barotrauma in ventilated patients. If PEEP is already being used, it should be discontinued before passage of the fiberscope. A postendoscopy chest radiograph is advisable to exclude the presence of mediastinal emphysema or pneumothorax. In patients whose tracheas are intubated with endotracheal tubes of less than 7 mm internal diameter, use of pediatric fiberscopes, which have smaller diameters, would be more appropriate.

The suction channel of the adult fiberoptic bronchoscope has been used to oxygenate and ventilate the lungs of patients. By attaching a jet ventilation system (similar to that used to drive the Sanders injector for rigid bronchoscopy) to the suction connection at the head of a fiberoptic bronchoscope, successful ventilation of the lungs of patients undergoing gynecologic procedures was achieved.[160] A driving pressure of 50 psig of oxygen was used with a ventilatory rate of 18 to 20 breaths/min. This technique permitted adequate ventilation of patients with normally compliant lungs and chest walls. Ventilation of the lungs should be performed only with the tip of the instrument in the trachea because a more peripheral location may produce barotrauma.

Neodymium-yttrium-aluminum garnet (Nd-YAG) lasers are used for the resection of obstructing and endobronchial lesions (see Chapter 48). This procedure is performed under general anesthesia. The lasers may be introduced into the bronchial tree through a fiberoptic bundle passed via the suction port of the fiberoptic bronchoscope. During laser resection, F_{IO_2} should be kept to a minimum and titrated to oxygen saturation (as continuously monitored by pulse oximeter) to make endotracheal fire less likely (see Chapter 5). Laser therapy of bronchial tumors is also possible using a rigid bronchoscope. HFPPV through a rigid bronchoscope provides satisfactory operating conditions for laser resection of tracheal tumors and has the advantage of producing airway immobility.

Complications of Bronchoscopy

Complications of rigid bronchoscopy include mechanical trauma to the teeth, hemorrhage, bronchospasm, loss of a sponge, bronchial or tracheal perforation, subglottic edema, and barotrauma. The incidence of complications is much lower with fiberoptic bronchoscopy. Nevertheless, complications may arise owing to overdose with topical anesthetic, insertion trauma, local trauma, hemorrhage, upper airway obstruction related to passage of the instrument through an area of tracheal stenosis, hypoxemia, and bronchospasm. In most cases, it is best to intubate the trachea with an endotracheal tube after bronchoscopy under general anesthesia. This permits avoidance or treatment of some of these problems, particularly the increased airway irritability. Intubation also facilitates effective suctioning of the trachea and bronchi, and allows the patient to recover more gradually from general anesthesia.

8 ▸ Diagnostic Procedures for Mediastinal Mass

Patients with an anterior mediastinal mass may present a special problem for the anesthesiologist. Although such masses may cause obvious superior vena cava obstruction, they may also cause obstruction of major airways and cardiac compression, which are less obvious and may become apparent only on induction of anesthesia. Many cases of anesthetic-related airway compression from anterior mediastinal mass have been reported. In one case, total occlusion of the trachea starting 2 to 3 cm above the carina and extending to both main stem bronchi was observed, and a bronchoscope was passed through the obstruction.[162] In the second case of this report, extrinsic compression of the left main stem bronchus occurred on inspiration during recovery from anesthesia. In the third case, flow–volume studies were performed with the patient in the upright and supine positions, with marked reductions in FEV_1 and peak expiratory flow in the latter position. These findings suggested potential obstruction with onset of anesthesia; radiation therapy to the mediastinum was commenced, after which the flow–volume studies showed improved function. The planned surgical procedure was then performed under local anesthesia. In a subsequent series of 105 patients with mediastinal masses, the incidence of intraoperative cardiorespiratory complications was 38%, and the incidence of postoperative respiratory complications was 11%.[163] No cases of airway collapse were reported during anesthesia. In this series, patients were at increased risk of complications if there were preoperative cardiorespiratory signs and symptoms, obstructive and restrictive dysfunction on pulmonary function tests, and greater than 50% tracheal compression on CT scan. In another series of patients with mediastinal mass, four patients had abnormal spirometry but underwent general anesthesia without sequelae.[164] In severe cases of airway compression, the femoral vessels should be cannulated prior to induction of anesthesia so that if the airway is lost completely cardiopulmonary bypass can be instituted immediately.[165]

The mass may be sensitive to radiation therapy, which could shrink the tumor and make an induction of general anesthesia less hazardous. However, a serious potential disadvantage of preoperative radiation therapy is that it may affect tissue histologic appearance, thereby preventing an accurate diagnosis. Furthermore, if the patient is a child, it may be difficult to obtain tissue samples under local anesthesia. No fatalities occurred in a series of 44 patients aged 18 years of age or younger with anterior mediastinal masses who underwent general anesthesia before radiation or chemotherapy. However, seven patients did have airway compromise.[166] In another report in a series of children, it was found to be safe to induce general anesthesia if the CT scan revealed that the tracheal cross-sectional area and peak expiratory flow rates were at least 50% of predicted.[167] Airway obstruction caused by an anterior mediastinal mass has been attributed to changes in lung and chest wall mechanics associated with changes in position or to onset of paralysis in muscles that previously maintained airway patency. Preoperative evaluation of a patient with an anterior mediastinal mass to avoid life-threatening total airway obstruction is shown in Figure 38-21. It is important to determine in the history if the patient has dyspnea in the supine position and to examine the CT scan to determine the extent of the tumor and its effect on surrounding structures. If such obstruction occurs, it may be relieved by passage of a rigid bronchoscope or anode tube past the obstruction, by direct laryngoscopy,[168] or by changing the position of the patient.

Airway collapse and inability to ventilate has been reported in a previously asymptomatic patient with a mediastinal mass

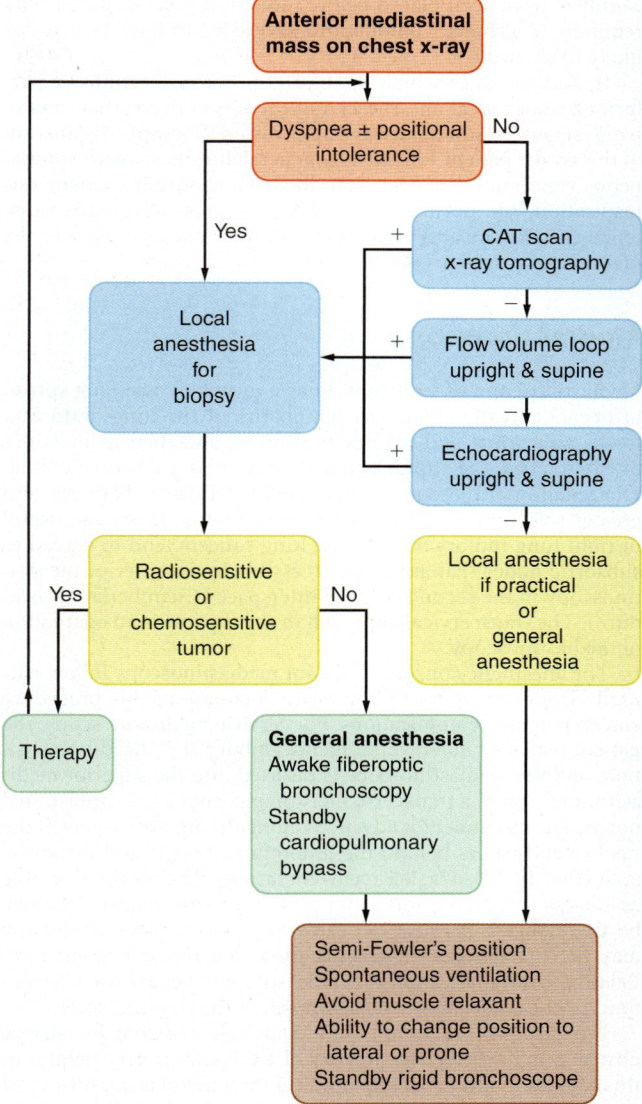

Figure 38-21 Flow chart describing the preoperative evaluation of the patient with an anterior mediastinal mass. + indicates positive finding; − indicates negative workup. (Reprinted with permission from Neuman GG, Weingarten AE, Abramowitz RM, et al. Anesthetic management of the patient with an anterior mediastinal mass. *Anesthesiology.* 1984;60:144.)

despite spontaneous ventilation with an inhaled anesthetic and an endotracheal tube.[169] This resulted in sudden cardiopulmonary collapse. Positive-pressure ventilation was impossible, a rigid bronchoscopy was requested and the surgeons began to prepare femoral vessel access for emergent cardiopulmonary bypass. Fortunately, the airway patency was re-established when the patient's spontaneous respiratory efforts improved as he awoke from general anesthesia. The authors emphasize the need for immediate availability of a rigid bronchoscope and that if a patient is at high risk, then serious consideration should be given to insertion of the femoral cannulas with cardiopulmonary bypass standing by before general anesthesia is induced. Cardiopulmonary bypass is not a suitable rescue modality unless the cannulae have been placed before induction because in the time required to achieve cannulation, severe neurologic damage is likely to occur.[170]

In a situation in which the biopsy procedure cannot be performed under local anesthesia and there is concern that muscle paralysis may result in airway compression, fiberoptic intubation of the awake patient followed by general anesthesia with spontaneous ventilation has been described. Thus during spontaneous inspiration, the normal transpulmonary pressure gradient distends the airways and helps maintain their patency, even in the presence of extrinsic compression.

9 Mediastinoscopy

Mediastinoscopy was introduced as a means of assessing spread of bronchial carcinoma. The lymphatics of the lung drain first to the subcarinal and paratracheal areas, and then to the sides of the trachea, the supraclavicular areas, and the thoracic duct. Examination of these nodes has provided a tissue diagnosis and greater selectivity of patients for thoracotomy. It is most useful in right lung tumors because left lung cancers tend to spread to subaortic nodes that are more accessible by an anterior mediastinoscopy in the second or third interspace (Chamberlain procedure). The transcervical approach to the thymus is an adaptation of mediastinoscopy.

The anesthetic considerations for mediastinoscopy follow naturally from an understanding of the anatomy of this procedure and its potential complications. For cervical mediastinoscopy, the patient is placed in a reverse Trendelenburg (i.e., head-up) position, and the mediastinoscope is inserted into the superior mediastinum through a transverse incision just above the suprasternal notch. The instrument is advanced along the anterior aspect of the trachea and passes behind the innominate vessels and the aortic arch (Fig. 38-22). The left recurrent laryngeal nerve is vulnerable as it loops around the aortic arch, and any of these structures may be traumatized. Because of scarring, previous mediastinoscopy may be considered a contraindication to a repeat examination. Relative contraindications include superior vena cava obstruction, tracheal deviation, and aneurysm of the thoracic aorta.

Preoperative evaluation should include a search for airway obstruction or distortion. Review of a CT scan is very helpful in this regard. Evidence of impaired cerebral circulation, history of stroke, or signs of the Eaton–Lambert syndrome resulting from oat cell carcinoma should be sought. Blood must be available for the procedure because hemorrhage is a real risk and may be life-threatening.

Most surgeons and anesthesiologists prefer general anesthesia using an endotracheal tube and continuous ventilation because this offers a more controlled situation and greater flexibility in terms of surgical manipulation. The anesthetic technique should include a muscle relaxant to prevent the patient from coughing because this may produce venous engorgement in the chest or trauma by the mediastinoscope to surrounding structures.

The incidence of morbidity with mediastinoscopy has been reported as 1.5% to 3.0%, and that of mortality as 0.09%. The most common complication is hemorrhage (0.73%) because of the proximity of major vessels and the vascularity of certain tumors. Tamponade may be the only recourse, and thoracotomy or median sternotomy may be required to achieve hemostasis. Needle aspiration of any structure is essential before any biopsy is taken. If severe bleeding occurs, induced arterial hypotension may be helpful in reducing the size of the tear in a vessel. If bleeding is venous, fluids given via an upper limb vein may enter the mediastinum, in which case a large-bore catheter should be

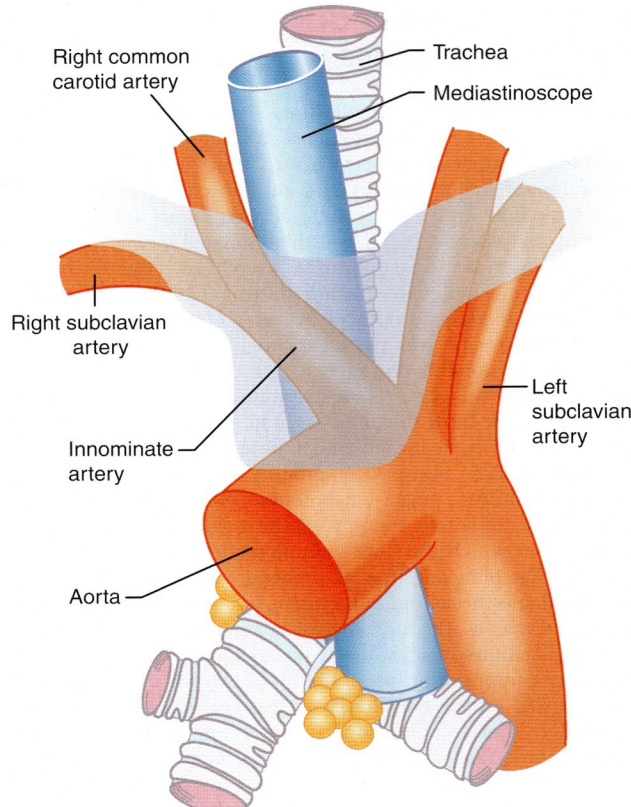

Figure 38-22 Anatomic relationships during mediastinoscopy. Note the position of the mediastinoscope behind the right innominate artery and aortic arch and anterior to the trachea. (Adapted from Carlens E. Mediastinoscopy: A method for inspection and tissue biopsy in the superior mediastinum. *Dis Chest.* 1959;36:343.)

placed in a lower limb vein. A venous laceration may also result in air embolism, particularly if the patient is breathing spontaneously. Some recommend the use of a precordial Doppler probe if the risk of air embolism is likely.

Pneumothorax is the second most common complication (0.66%). It is usually right-sided, often recognized at the time of the occurrence, and is treated according to the size. A symptomatic pneumothorax should be treated by chest tube decompression.

Recurrent laryngeal nerve injury occurred in 0.34% of cases and was permanent in 50% of these cases. The nerve may be damaged by the mediastinoscope or be involved in tumor. Such injury is not a problem unless both nerves are damaged, in which case upper airway obstruction may result. Autonomic reflexes may be triggered by manipulation of the trachea or the aorta, the latter having pressor receptors located in the arch. Vagally mediated reflexes may be blocked by atropine.

"Factitious" cardiac arrest has been reported when the right radial pulse was monitored using a plethysmograph, and the tracing suddenly disappeared in the presence of a normal electrocardiogram. A normal pulse returned after the mediastinoscope was removed, and the cause of the apparent arrest was pressure on the innominate artery by the instrument. Decreases in right arm as compared with left arm blood pressure have been reported in cases undergoing mediastinoscopy. Duration was 15 to 360 seconds. This is of particular significance if there is a history of impaired cerebral circulation or transient ischemic attacks, or if a carotid bruit is present, because transient left hemiparesis may occur after mediastinoscopy. It is therefore recommended that blood pressure be monitored in the left arm and that the right radial pulse be monitored continuously during mediastinoscopy. A decrease in the right radial pulse amplitude is an indication for repositioning the mediastinoscope, especially in a patient with a history of cerebrovascular disease.

Other reported complications include acute tracheal collapse, tension pneumomediastinum, mediastinitis, hemothorax, and chylothorax. A chest radiograph taken in the immediate postoperative period is a useful precaution in all patients after mediastinoscopy.

Thoracoscopy

Thoracoscopy (medical thoracoscopy) involves the insertion of an endoscope into the thoracic cavity and pleural space. It is used for the diagnosis of pleural disease, effusions, and infectious disease (especially in immunosuppressed patients and those with acquired immunodeficiency syndrome) and for staging procedures, chemical pleurodesis, and lung biopsy. It is usually performed by the pulmonary physician in the clinic, under local anesthesia. It is also used in therapeutic procedures such as CO_2 laser treatment of spontaneous pneumothorax or bullous emphysema[171] and Nd-YAG laser vaporization of malignant pleural tumors. A small incision is made in the lateral chest wall, and with the insertion of the instrument, fluid and biopsy specimens are easily obtained.

This procedure may be performed using local, regional, or general anesthesia; the choice depending on the expected duration of the procedure and the physical status of the patient. Pneumothorax is a potential complication of an intercostal block, but it would not have clinical sequelae during a thoracoscopy because it is created as part of the surgical procedure. The collapse of the lung provides the surgeon with a working space, and a chest tube is placed at the conclusion of the surgery. The addition of a stellate ganglion block helps suppress the cough reflex that is sometimes provoked during manipulation of the hilum of the lung.

When air enters the pleural cavity under inspection, a partial pneumothorax occurs, permitting good surgical visualization. Changes in Pao_2, $Paco_2$, and cardiac rhythm are usually minimal when the procedure is performed using local or regional anesthesia.

With local anesthesia, the spontaneous pneumothorax is usually well tolerated because the skin and chest wall form a seal around the thoracoscope and limit the degree of lung collapse. Occasionally, however, the procedure is poorly tolerated, and general anesthesia must be induced. The insertion of a DLT with the patient in the lateral position may be difficult, in which case the patient may be temporarily placed in the supine position for the intubation.

If general anesthesia is required, a DLT is preferable to an SLT because positive-pressure ventilation via an SLT would interfere with endoscopic visualization. In addition, if pleurodesis is being performed, general anesthesia through a DLT allows for re-expansion of the lung and avoids the pain associated with instillation of talc for recurrent pneumothorax.

Video-assisted (Minimally Invasive) Thoracoscopic Surgery

VATS entails making small incisions in the chest wall, which allows the introduction of a video camera and surgical instruments into the thoracic cavity.[172] Generally, it is performed by a thoracic surgeon in the operating room under general anesthesia. Although the first thoracoscopy was performed by Jacobeus in 1910, using what was at that time a cystoscope, in more recent years the surgical techniques, instruments, and video technology have been improved to permit a wide variety of procedures to be performed using VATS. These now include diagnostic procedures for evaluation of pleural disease and effusions, staging of lung cancer, and the identification of parenchymal disease, including nodules, mediastinal tumors, and pericardial disease. They also include therapeutic procedures such as operations for pleural disease, including pleurodesis, decortication and drainage of empyema, resection of lung tissue or bullae, pericardial window or stripping, and esophageal surgery. Lung lobectomies are now usually performed by VATS, and an increasing number are being performed robotically.[173-175]

Anesthesia Considerations

As with a traditional thoracotomy, the patient needs to be in the lateral decubitus position, and lung collapse is needed for adequate surgical exposure. This generally mandates the use of a lung-separation technique. VATS is most commonly performed under general anesthesia with OLV. The need for OLV is much greater in VATS procedures than in open thoracotomy procedures. This is because during VATS, it is not possible to retract the lung, whereas during open thoracotomy lung retraction is possible. Deflation of the non-dependent (operated) lung should begin as soon as possible following tracheal intubation and patient positioning because it can take more than 30 minutes to achieve complete collapse of the lung. Also, the surgeon enters the thoracic cavity much sooner during VATS than with open thoracotomy. Suction applied to the airway can help facilitate a more rapid deflation of the lung. In some cases, carbon dioxide is insufflated into the pleural cavity to facilitate visualization. Insufflation pressures should be maintained as low as possible and the CO_2 inflow rate kept less than 2 L/min. Higher pressures can cause mediastinal shift, hemodynamic compromise, increases in airway pressure, and increases in end-tidal CO_2. Hemodynamic compromise presents a picture similar to that because of tension pneumothorax. Significant hemodynamic changes can be produced when pressures as little as 5 mmHg are used to insufflate CO_2 into the chest cavity.[176]

CPAP is commonly used for the treatment of hypoxemia during OLV for thoracotomy and is usually very effective. However, during VATS, CPAP interferes with the surgical exposure and is therefore best avoided. It would be preferable to use PEEP to the nonoperated (dependent lung). In addition, a lower Pao_2 may have to be tolerated during VATS compared with a thoracotomy.[177]

Postoperative Concerns

There is less pain after VATS than open thoracotomy, and an epidural catheter is usually placed before surgery only if there is a likelihood that a thoracotomy may need to be performed. Although a lobectomy can be performed by VAT, sometimes conversion to an open thoracotomy may be required. The patient's respiratory function is better preserved after VATS, and their recovery is faster. However, postoperative dysrhythmias, which commonly occur after thoracotomy, have also been reported after VATS.[178] Other complications that may occur include bleeding, pulmonary edema, and pneumonia.

Anesthesia for Special Situations

Management of patients with BPF, empyema, cysts, and bullae, as well as those requiring tracheal reconstruction, is considered here. Many of these patients are appropriately managed using high-frequency ventilatory techniques; therefore, these techniques are described first (see Chapter 28).

High-Frequency Ventilation

With conventional positive-pressure ventilation, V_T and rates usually exceed or approach those in the normal, spontaneously breathing patient. Gas transport to the alveoli occurs by convection in the larger airways, and then by convection and molecular diffusion in the more distal airways and alveoli. High-frequency ventilation differs from conventional positive-pressure ventilation in that smaller V_T and more rapid rates are used. Gas transport may depend more on molecular diffusion, high-velocity flow, and coaxial gas flow in the airways, with gas in the center moving distally and that in the periphery moving proximally.

There are several different types of high-frequency ventilation.[179] HFPPV uses small V_T at rates of 60 to 120 breaths/min (1 to 2 Hz). The ventilator used has a negligible internal compliance so the V_T generated, which usually approximates the dead space volume, equals the volume set on the ventilator and represents all fresh gas. The high instantaneous gas flows generated facilitate gas exchange and movement in the conducting airways.

HFPPV may be delivered by an open or a closed system. An example of the former is the percutaneous placement of a transtracheal catheter or placement of a catheter through the nose or mouth with its distal end above the carina. Inflow is intraluminal and outflow is extraluminal. This technique has been used during bronchoscopy, tracheal resection, and reconstructive surgery. When open systems are used, the gas outflow pathway is not established mechanically and depends on natural airway patency. It is therefore subject to compromise. Also, aspiration is a potential complication with open systems.

The closed system is superior because it integrates both airway patency and outflow protection. A closed system is represented by a catheter placed in a short segment of an endotracheal tube for delivery of the HFPPV, whereas the remainder of the tube lumen represents the exit pathway for gas. A quadruple-lumen endotracheal tube (Hi-Lo Jet Tracheal Tube, Mallinckrodt, Inc.) has been designed specifically for delivery of HFPPV. One lumen is for the HFPPV delivery, one for gas outflow, one for cuff inflation, and one for measuring airway pressures at the distal end of the tube. The use of a closed system also permits application of PEEP, a situation not possible with an open arrangement.

High-frequency jet ventilation (HFJV) uses a pulse of a small jet of fresh gas introduced from a high-pressure source (50 psig) into the airway through a small catheter or additional lumen in an endotracheal tube. Rates used are usually 100 to 400 breaths/min. The fresh gas jet entrains gas from an injection cannula side-port reservoir. This system is somewhat analogous to the Sanders injector system described in the "Bronchoscopy" section, and F_{IO_2} is similarly variable. The jet and entrained gas flows cause forward motion of the mass of gas in the airways. HFJV can be used with an open system or with a closed arrangement, as described earlier. In the latter, PEEP may be added to enhance oxygenation. Also, with use of high fresh gas flows from an anesthesia circuit, inhaled anesthetics may be delivered as an entrained gas mixture.

High-frequency oscillation ventilation uses a mechanism that oscillates gas at rates of 400 to 2,400 breaths/min. It has not been described in association with thoracic surgical procedures. In this system, V_T is small (50 to 80 mL), and gas exchange occurs through enhanced molecular diffusion and coaxial airway flow.

The potential advantages offered by HFPPV during thoracic anesthesia are that lower V_T and inspiratory pressures result in a quiet lung field for the surgeon, with minimal movements of airway, lung tissue, and mediastinum. Thus, HFPPV has been used to ventilate both the nondependent and the dependent lung during thoracic surgical procedures, with adequate arterial blood gas measurements obtained throughout. At high frequencies (>6 Hz), however, CO_2 retention may become a problem.

HFJV has been used to ventilate the nondependent lung to improve Pa_{O_2} during one-lung anesthesia, whereas the dependent lung is ventilated with conventional intermittent positive-pressure ventilation. Pa_{O_2} increased compared with that obtained during simple collapse of the nondependent lung. A study comparing HFJV with CPAP to the nondependent lung during conventional intermittent positive-pressure ventilation to the dependent lung found that both improved Pa_{O_2} significantly during closed and open stages of the surgery. When the chest was open, HFJV maintained satisfactory cardiac output, whereas CPAP usually decreased cardiac output; however, there were no significant differences in Pa_{CO_2} between HFJV and CPAP. Because similar increases in Pa_{O_2} may be obtained using selective CPAP to the nondependent lung and much simpler equipment than that necessary to deliver high-frequency ventilation, the use of CPAP would seem preferable to high-frequency ventilation to increase Pa_{O_2} during most one-lung anesthesia situations.

The lower pressures and V_T associated with high-frequency ventilation result in a small leak through BPFs, and HFJV is now generally considered the conservative treatment of choice in this condition. Another advantage of high-frequency ventilation is that the rapid-rate small V_T can be delivered through small tubes or catheters so if an airway has to be divided, the passage of a small tube across the surgical field permits ventilation of the distal airway and lung tissue. This use has been applied during sleeve resection of the lung, tracheal reconstruction, and surgery for tracheal stenosis. In all three situations, the surgeon is able to work easily around the small catheter used to provide the high-frequency ventilation.

Bronchopleural Fistula and Empyema

A BPF is an abnormal communication between the bronchial tree and the pleural cavity. Occasionally, there is an additional communication to the surface of the chest, a cutaneous BPF. BPF occurs most commonly after pulmonary resection for carcinoma. Other causes include traumatic rupture of a bronchus or bulla (sometimes caused by barotrauma or PEEP), penetrating chest wound, or spontaneous drainage into the bronchial tree of an empyema cavity or lung cyst. The incidence of BPF is higher after pneumonectomy than following other types of lung resection. The problems associated with BPF and empyema are that positive-pressure ventilation may result in contamination of healthy lung, loss of air, decreased alveolar ventilation leading to CO_2 retention, and the development of a tension pneumothorax.

If an empyema is present, it should be drained under local anesthesia before any surgery to close the BPF. Drainage is performed with the patient sitting up and leaning toward the affected side. Empyemas are often loculated, and complete drainage is not always possible. A drain to an underwater seal system is left in the cavity before administration of anesthesia for surgery of the BPF, and after drainage of an empyema, a chest radiograph should be obtained to determine the efficacy of the procedure.

The priorities in the anesthetic management of BPF are the isolation of the affected side in terms of contamination and ventilation. The ideal approach is intubation of the trachea while the patient is awake using a DLT with the patient breathing spontaneously. Supplemental oxygen should be administered, and the patient should be constantly reassured. Neuroleptanalgesia is satisfactory in providing a suitably cooperative patient, and the airway is then pretreated with topical anesthesia. The endobronchial tube selected should be such that the bronchial lumen is on the side opposite the BPF. Selection of the largest possible tube provides a close fit in the trachea, which helps stabilize the tube. Once the tube is adequately positioned in the trachea, there may be a considerable outpouring of pus from the tracheal lumen if an empyema is present; therefore, this lumen should be immediately suctioned using a large-bore suction catheter. The healthy and possibly the affected lung may then be ventilated; adequacy of oxygenation and ventilation is assessed by pulse oximetry and arterial blood gas analysis.

An alternative technique is to insert the DLT under general anesthesia, with the patient breathing spontaneously to avoid a tension pneumothorax. With either technique, the chest drainage tube must be left unclamped to avoid any bouts of coughing and to prevent the buildup of a tension pneumothorax in the event that a predisposing valvular mechanism exists. In patients who do not have an empyema, use of an SLT has been described and may be satisfactory if the BPF and air leak are small. A rapid-sequence induction with ketamine or propofol followed by a relaxant has also been described, but is associated with considerable risk of contamination and tension pneumothorax.

BPF may also be treated conservatively using various ventilatory techniques. Thus, the bronchus of the normal lung may be intubated and ventilated, allowing the BPF to rest and heal. This approach may result in an intolerable shunt, however, and PEEP may be necessary to maintain Pa_{O_2}. Differential lung ventilation using a DLT has also been described, the healthy lung being ventilated with normal V_T, while the affected lung is exposed to a smaller V_T or to CPAP with oxygen at pressures just below the critical opening pressure of the fistula. The critical opening pressure of the BPF can be assessed by determining the lowest level of CPAP that must be applied to the bronchus on the affected side to produce continuous bubbling through the underwater seal chest drain.

For a large BPF, HFJV may be the nonsurgical treatment of choice. The use of small V_T results in minimal gas loss through the fistula, which may heal more quickly. In addition, hemodynamic effects are usually minimal and spontaneous efforts at ventilation are usually abolished, thereby decreasing the work of breathing and eliminating the need for relaxants or excessive sedation.

Lung Cysts and Bullae

Air-filled cysts of the lung are usually bronchogenic, postinfective, infantile, or emphysematous. They may be associated with COPD or be an isolated finding. A bulla is a thin-walled space filled with air that results from the destruction of alveolar tissue. The walls are, therefore, composed of visceral pleura, connective tissue septa, or compressed lung tissue. In general, bullae represent an area of end-stage emphysematous destruction of the lung.

Patients may be considered for surgical bullectomy when dyspnea is incapacitating, when the bullae are expanding, when there are repeated pneumothoraces owing to rupture of bullae, or if the bullae compress a large area of normal lung. Most of these patients have severe COPD and CO_2 retention, and little functional respiratory reserve. The first consideration in management is maintenance of a high F_{IO_2}. If the bulla or cyst communicates with the bronchial tree, positive-pressure ventilation may cause it to expand or even to rupture, if it is compliant, producing a situation analogous to tension pneumothorax. If the bulla is very compliant, most of the applied V_T may be wasted in this additional dead space. Nitrous oxide should be avoided because it causes expansion of any air spaces in the body, including bullae. Once the chest is open, even more of the V_T may enter the compliant bulla, which is no longer limited by chest wall integrity, and an increase in ventilation is needed until the bulla is controlled.

The anesthetic management of these patients is challenging, particularly if the disease is bilateral. Ideally, a DLT is inserted with the patient awake or under general anesthesia but breathing spontaneously. The avoidance of positive-pressure ventilation (when possible) helps decrease the likelihood of the potential problems described previously, although oxygenation may be precarious with spontaneous ventilation. Once the endotracheal tube is in place, each lung may be controlled separately, and adequate ventilation can be applied to the healthy lung if bilateral disease is not present. Gentle positive-pressure ventilation with rapid, small V_T and pressures not to exceed 10 cm H_2O may be used during the induction and maintenance of anesthesia, especially if the bullae have been shown to have no or only poor bronchial communication by preoperative ventilation scanning. While the surgery is being performed, as each bulla is resected, the operated lung can be separately ventilated to check for air leaks and the presence of additional bullae.

If positive-pressure ventilation is to be applied before the chest is opened, the possibility of a tension pneumothorax must be kept in mind, and treatment should be readily available. The diagnosis of pneumothorax may be made by a unilateral decrease in breath sounds (this may be difficult to distinguish in a patient with bullous disease), increase in ventilatory pressure, progressive tracheal deviation, wheezing, or cardiovascular changes. Treatment of a pneumothorax involves the rapid placement of a chest tube. An added risk of chest tube placement is the creation of a cutaneous BPF, which causes problems for ventilation. Alternatively, general anesthesia is induced only after the surgeon has prepared the operative field and draped the patient. In the event of sudden deterioration in the patient's condition during induction, the surgeon may perform an immediate median sternotomy. In any event, the time from induction of anesthesia to sternotomy must be kept to a minimum.

To avoid these problems in a patient with known bullae, HFJV has been used in a patient with a large bulla undergoing coronary artery bypass graft and in another patient undergoing bilateral bullectomy. If bilateral bullectomy is to be performed, a median sternotomy is usually used. Benumof[180] described the use of sequential OLV using a DLT in the management of a patient needing bilateral bullectomy. The side with the largest bulla and least lung function, as assessed before surgery by ventilation and perfusion scans, should be operated on first. In this way, the lung with the better function should support gas exchange first. If hypoxemia develops during this one-lung situation, application of CPAP to the nonventilated lung during the deflation phase of a tidal breath should increase Pa_{O_2}.

Unlike most cases of pulmonary resection, patients after bullectomy are left with a greater amount of functional lung tissue than was previously available to them, and the mechanics of respiration are improved. At the end of the procedure, the DLT is replaced by an SLT, and the patients generally require several days to be weaned from the ventilator. During this time, the positive airway pressure used should be minimized to avoid causing a pneumothorax owing to rupture of suture or staple lines or of residual bullae.

Anesthesia for Resection of the Trachea

Tracheal resection and reconstruction are technically difficult for the surgeon and challenging for the anesthesiologist. Indications for this type of procedure include congenital lesions (agenesis, stenosis), neoplasia (primary or secondary), injuries (direct or indirect), infections, and postintubation injuries (caused by an endotracheal tube or tracheotomy). For the surgical team, the major problems are maintenance of ventilation to the lungs while the airway is being operated on and postoperative integrity of the anastomoses. In this respect, the presence of lung disease sufficiently severe to require postoperative ventilatory support is a relative contraindication to tracheal resection or reconstruction.

Monitoring of these patients should include placement of an arterial cannula in the left radial artery to permit continuous measurement of blood pressure during periods of innominate artery compression. Steroids should be administered to help reduce any tracheal edema, and a high F_{IO_2} should be used throughout the procedure to ensure an adequate oxygen reserve at all times in the FRC so that temporary interruptions of ventilation are less likely to produce hypoxemia.

Numerous methods have been reported to provide oxygenation and ventilation of the lungs during these procedures. A small-bore anode tube may be placed through and distal to an upper tracheal lesion so resection may occur around the tube. This technique is useful only in mild stenoses. Alternatively, an endotracheal tube may be passed through the glottis to above the stenosis, and a sterile endotracheal or bronchial tube may later be inserted into the trachea opened distal to the site of stenosis, with the sterile anesthesia tubing being led across the surgical field. After resection of the lesion, the sterile and distally placed endotracheal tube is withdrawn, and the upper tube (originally passed through the glottis) is advanced across the anastomosis. With low tracheal or bronchial lesions, resection and reconstruction may be performed around an endobronchial or DLT. During these procedures, the patient is kept in a head-down position to minimize aspiration of blood and debris into the alveoli, and ventilation must be carefully monitored throughout the procedure.

Clearly, the presence of a large-bore tube in the airway may make these resections technically difficult, and the use of high-frequency ventilation techniques may improve surgical access. Thus, a small-diameter catheter or catheters may be placed across or through the stenotic lesion or transected airway(s) and ventilation to the distal airways and lungs maintained using HFPPV or HFJV. Potential disadvantages of these high-frequency ventilation techniques are that, by necessity, the system is "open" (see "High-frequency Ventilation"), and egress of gas during exhalation may be compromised if the stenosis is tight. Also, the catheter may become occluded by blood and become displaced, and distal aspiration of debris or blood may occur. With complex resections, two anesthesia teams with two machines and anesthesia circuits or sets of ventilating equipment may be necessary to ensure adequate ventilation of the two distal airway segments. Although during carinal resections, HFPPV to the left lung alone usually provides adequate oxygenation and ventilation.

After tracheal resection or reconstructive surgery, patients should be kept with the neck and head flexed to reduce tension on the anastomotic suture lines. In some cases, this is maintained by using sutures between the chin and the anterior chest wall. Extubation of the trachea is performed as early as possible to minimize tracheal trauma due to the endotracheal tube and cuff.

Bronchopulmonary Lavage

This procedure involves irrigation of the lung and bronchial tree, and is used as a treatment for alveolar proteinosis, radioactive dust inhalation, cystic fibrosis, bronchiectasis, and asthmatic bronchitis. Lung lavage is performed under general anesthesia using a DLT so one lung may be ventilated while the other is being treated with lavage fluid.[181]

The preoperative assessment of these patients should include ventilation–perfusion scans so lavage can be performed first on the more severely affected lung (i.e., the one with the least ventilation). If involvement is equal, the left lung is generally lavaged first because gas exchange should be better through the larger, right lung. Patients are premedicated and supplied with supplemental oxygen en route to the operating room.

Anesthesia is induced with an intravenous drug and maintained with an inhaled agent in oxygen to maintain the highest possible F_{IO_2}. Muscle relaxation facilitates placement of the DLT, and the cuff seal should be checked to maintain perfect separation at a pressure of 50 cm H_2O to prevent leakage of lavage fluid around the cuff. A fiberoptic bronchoscope is useful to check the position of the bronchial cuff of the DLT. Monitoring should include an arterial catheter, and a stethoscope should be placed over the ventilated lung to check for rales, the presence of which may indicate leakage of lavage fluid into this lung.

The patient is maintained on an F_{IO_2} of 1 throughout the procedure. Before lavage, this serves to denitrogenate the lungs so only oxygen and carbon dioxide remain. Instillation of fluid then allows these gases to be absorbed, resulting in greater access by the fluid to the alveolar spaces than if the more insoluble nitrogen bubbles remained.

Once the trachea is intubated, the patient is turned so the side to be lavaged is lowermost, and the DLT position and seal are checked once again. With the patient in a head-up position, warmed heparinized isotonic saline is infused by gravity from a reservoir 30 cm above the midaxillary line into the catheter to the dependent lung, while the nondependent lung is ventilated. When fluid ceases to flow in (usually after 700 to 1,000 mL in an adult), the patient is placed in a head-down position and fluid is allowed to drain out. The lavage is continued until the effluent is clear (as opposed to the milky fluid that drains initially when lavage is being performed for alveolar proteinosis), at which point the lung is suctioned and ventilation is re-established with large V_T (and pressures) because compliance is decreased owing to loss of surfactant. With each lavage, inflow and outflow volumes are monitored so the patient is not "drowned" in fluid, and there is no excessive absorption or leakage to the ventilated side. At least 90% of the saline volume should be recovered with each lavage. Two-lung ventilation is re-established and, as compliance improves, an air–oxygen mixture (addition of nitrogen) may be introduced to help maintain alveolar patency. After a further period of ventilation, in most patients, the trachea can be extubated in the operating room. In the posttreatment period, patients are encouraged to cough and engage in breathing exercises to fully re-expand the treated lung. From 3 days to 1 week after lavage of the first lung, the patient may return to the operating room for lavage of the other lung.

Problems sometimes encountered with this procedure include spillage of lavage fluid from the treated to the ventilated lung. This must be managed by stopping the lavage and ensuring functional separation of the lungs before continuing. DLT positioning is critical. Spillage may cause profound decreases in oxygenation, which may necessitate terminating the procedure and maintaining two-lung ventilation with oxygen and PEEP.

During periods when lavage fluid is being instilled into the dependent lung, oxygenation usually improves because the increased intra-alveolar pressure caused by the fluid produces diversion of the pulmonary blood flow to the nondependent, ventilated lung. Conversely, when the fluid is drained out of the dependent lung, hypoxemia may occur. In some cases in which severe hypoxemia was anticipated during right lung lavage, the risk has been reduced by passing a balloon-tipped catheter into the right main pulmonary artery (checked by radiography) and inflating the balloon during periods of right lung drainage. In this way, blood flow to the dependent, right, nonventilated lung is minimized during periods of drainage. This technique is not without risk (e.g., pulmonary artery rupture) and is reserved for those patients considered to be at greatest risk for hypoxemia during lavage. If the patient has recently had a diagnostic open lung biopsy, a BPF may be present. If this is a possibility, a chest tube should be inserted on the side of the BPF, and this side should be lavaged first. The chest drain is removed several days later.

Limitations in the sizes of available DLTs preclude their use for lavage in patients weighing less than 40 kg. In such cases, cardiopulmonary bypass may be required to provide oxygenation during lavage.

Myasthenia Gravis

10 The thoracic anesthesiologist will most likely have to manage patients with MG for thymectomy, which is now considered the treatment of choice in most cases of MG. MG is a disorder of the neuromuscular junction, the function of which is altered routinely in the modern practice of anesthesia. The incidence of MG appears to be increasing. The most accurate estimate of incidence of MG was around 30/1,000,000 per year. The incidence in children and adolescents aged 0 to 19 years was found to be between 1 and 5/1 000,000 per year. These rates may well be an underestimate of the true incidence rates, as mild cases will have been missed and cases in the elderly will have been misdiagnosed.[182] People of any age may be affected, but peaks of incidence occur in the third decade for women and the fifth decade for men. MG is a chronic disorder characterized by a clinical course of fluctuating painless weakness and fatigability of voluntary muscles with improvement following rest.[183,184] Onset is usually slow and insidious, any skeletal muscle or group of muscles may be affected, and the condition is associated with relapses and remissions. The most common onset is ocular; if the disease remains localized to the eyes for 2 years, the likelihood of progression to generalized MG is low. In some cases, the disease is generalized and may involve the bulbar musculature, causing problems with breathing and swallowing. Peripheral muscle involvement may cause weakness, clumsiness, and difficulty in holding up the head or in walking. A commonly used clinical classification of MG[185] is shown in Table 38-7.

In MG, there is a decrease in the number of postsynaptic acetylcholine receptors (AChRs) at the endplates of affected muscles. This causes a decrease in the margin of safety of neuromuscular transmission. MG is an autoimmune disorder, and about 80% of the affected patients have detectable circulating antibodies to the nicotinic AChR. These anti-AChR antibodies may cause complement-mediated lysis of the postsynaptic membrane or direct blockade of the receptors, or may modulate the receptor turnover such that the degradation rate exceeds the resynthesis rate. Studies of the endplate area show loss of synaptic folds and a widening of the synaptic cleft. A variable proportion of the patients who do not have anti-AChR antibodies have antibodies to muscle-specific tyrosine kinase (MuSK).[186]

The diagnosis of MG is suspected from the patient's history and confirmed by clinical, pharmacologic, electrophysiologic, or immunologic testing. Patients cannot sustain or repeat muscular contraction. The electrical counterpart of this is a decrement in the compound muscle action potentials evoked by repetitive stimulation of a motor nerve. This is the most specific of the nerve tests for MG but it can be performed only on certain muscles, which may not be the ones affected in an individual patient. Mechanical and electrical (electromyography) decrements improve with 2 to 10 mg of intravenous edrophonium (Tensilon test). MG patients characteristically are sensitive to nondepolarizing muscle relaxants. When the routine electromyographic results are equivocal, a regional nondepolarizing muscle relaxant test may be performed using a tourniquet to isolate the limb and limit the action of the drug. In the regional nondepolarizer muscle relaxant test, electromyograms are performed before and after the administration of 0.2 mg of curare. In equivocal cases, a positive result of a test for anti-AChR antibodies is considered diagnostic.

Medical Therapy

Anticholinesterases are used to prolong the action of acetylcholine at the postsynaptic membrane and may also exert their own agonist effect at the AChRs. Anticholinesterases are the most

Table 38-7 Clinical Classification of Myasthenia Gravis (MG)

Class	Description
I	Ocular myasthenia—involvement of ocular muscles only. Mild with ptosis and diplopia. Electrophysiologic testing of other musculature is negative for MG.
IA	Ocular myasthenia with peripheral muscles showing no clinical symptoms but showing a positive electromyogram for MG.
II	Generalized myasthenia
IIA	Mild—slow onset, usually ocular, spreading to skeletal and bulbar muscles. No respiratory involvement. Good response to drug therapy. Low mortality rate.
IIB	Moderate—as IIA but progressing to more severe involvement of skeletal and bulbar muscles. Dysarthria, dysphagia, difficulty chewing. No respiratory involvement. Patient's activities limited. Fair response to drug therapy.
III	Acute fulminating myasthenia—rapid onset of severe bulbar and skeletal weakness with involvement of muscles of respiration. Progression usually within 6 mos. Poor response to therapy. Patient's activities limited. Low mortality rate.
IV	Late severe myasthenia—severe MG developing at least 2 yrs after onset of group I or group II symptoms. Progression of disease may be gradual or rapid. Poor response to therapy and poor prognosis.

Adapted from Osserman KE, Genkins G. Studies in myasthenia gravis: a review of a 20-year experience in over 1200 patients. *Mt Sinai J Med.* 1971;38:497.

Table 38-8 Anticholinesterase Drugs Used to Treat Myasthenia Gravis

Drug	Oral	IV	IM	Efficacy
	Dose (mg)			
Pyridostigmine (Mestinon)	60	2	2–4	1
Neostigmine (Prostigmine)	15	0.5	0.7–1	1

IV, intravenous; IM, intramuscular.

Table 38-9 Disorders Associated with Myasthenia Gravis

Thymoma
Thyroid disease
Hyperthyroidism
Hypothyroidism
Thyroiditis
Idiopathic thrombocytopenic purpura
Rheumatoid arthritis
Systemic lupus erythematosus
Anemias
Pernicious
Hemolytic
Multiple sclerosis
Ulcerative colitis
Leukemia
Lymphoma
Convulsive disorders
Extrathymic neoplasia
Sjögren syndrome
Scleroderma

commonly used medical therapy in MG (Table 38-8). Interestingly, no randomized controlled trial has been conducted on the use of acetylcholinesterase inhibitors in patients with MG because the response in observational studies is so obvious that a placebo group could not be justified.[187,188] Myasthenic patients learn to regulate their medication and titrate the dose against optimum effect. Overdosage causes the muscarinic effects of acetylcholine and may cause a cholinergic crisis. Underdosage causes weakness or a myasthenic crisis. In a patient with weakness, distinction between the two types of crisis may be made by performing a Tensilon test or by examining pupillary size, which will be large (mydriatic) in a myasthenic crisis but small (miotic) in a cholinergic crisis. Muscarinic side effects are treatable with atropine (see Chapter 14).

The immunologic basis of MG has led to the use of short- and long-term immunosuppressive drugs. Steroids are used for short-term immunosuppression, whereas for long-term effect azathioprine, cyclophosphamide, cyclosporine, methotrexate, mycophenolate mofetil, rituximab, and tacrolimus have been used.[184] Steroids often produce initial deterioration before an improvement. The usual regimen is prednisone 1 mg/kg on alternate days. Rapid short-term immunomodulation has been achieved in acute exacerbations or to improve muscle strength prior to surgery. Plasma exchange or plasmapheresis may produce dramatic but transient improvements in muscle strength with decreases in anti-AChR and anti-MuSK titers, as well as other inflammatory mediators. Usually reserved for severe MG, plasma exchange has been shown to improve respiratory function in both operated and nonoperated patients with MG. Plasmapheresis causes a decrease in plasma cholinesterase levels that may prolong the effect of drugs such as succinylcholine that are normally broken down by this enzyme system.

Long-term immunomodulation is achieved by surgical thymectomy.[189] Abnormalities are found in 75% of thymus glands removed from patients with MG (85% show hyperplasia, 15% show thymoma). After thymectomy, approximately 75% of patients either go into remission or show some improvement. Thymectomy is always indicated in those patients with thymoma, and now considered the treatment of choice in most patients with MG, except for those in Osserman class I (Table 38-7). Response to thymectomy is best if it is performed within the first 3 years following diagnosis. Clinical outcome from thymectomy is equivalent whether performed via a transsternal or video-assisted thoracoscopic approach.[190] A report describing anesthesia concerns in 17 patients who underwent robotic-assisted thoracoscopic thymectomy suggested that refinement of the surgical technique and positioning are required.[191]

Management of General Anesthesia

When possible, patients with MG should be admitted for elective surgery while in remission.[192] On admission, the patient's physical and emotional states should be optimized. Other diseases occasionally associated with MG should be excluded (Table 38-9).[193] The patient's current drug therapy should be reviewed and possible drug interactions considered. Because patients are less active while in the hospital, their anticholinesterase dosage may need to be decreased. If the patient has a history of respiratory disease or bulbar involvement, preoperative evaluation should include respiratory function studies. Breathing exercises and instruction in the use of incentive spirometers may be indicated. Patients should be told of the possible need for postoperative intubation of the trachea and ventilation of the lungs. Ideally, patients with MG should be scheduled to be the first case of the day in the operating room. Patients receiving steroid therapy should receive perioperative coverage. Interactions with other immunosuppressant drugs must be considered and if the patient is in crisis, preoperative plasmaphereses may be necessary.

Because the trachea is to be intubated and the lungs ventilated for the planned procedure in the patient with MG, traditional practice is to withhold anticholinesterase therapy on the morning of surgery so that the patient is weak on arrival at the operating room.[194] This avoids interactions with other drugs used in the operating room. Anticholinesterase therapy may be continued if the patient is physically or psychologically dependent on it. Others recommend continuing pyridostigmine, including an oral dose just before induction.[195] Premedication is satisfactorily achieved with a benzodiazepine or barbiturate. Opioids are usually avoided because of the risk of producing respiratory depression.

Monitoring should be dictated by the patient's state and planned surgical procedure, but should include an assessment of neuromuscular transmission (by means of a mechanomyogram/twitch monitor, an integrated electromyographic monitor, a kinemyograph, or an accelograph monitor)[196] if agents affecting neuromuscular transmission are to be used.

Induction of anesthesia is readily achieved with a short-acting barbiturate (if available) or propofol. In elective cases, intubation of the trachea, maintenance, and relaxation are readily achieved using potent inhaled anesthetics. Anesthesia may be deepened using a potent inhaled agent and the trachea intubated under its effect. Myasthenic patients are more sensitive than normal patients to the neuromuscular depressant effects of the potent inhaled agents. In patients with MG, isoflurane at 1.9 MAC end-tidal concentration induced a neuromuscular block of 30% to 50%, whereas halothane at 1.8 MAC induced a block of 10% to 20%. Both agents produced fade in the train-of-four ratio of 41% and 28%, respectively.[197] The less-soluble inhaled agents, sevoflurane and desflurane, are even more easily administered and withdrawn; they are now the most commonly used anesthetic drugs for patients with MG. Nitahara et al.[198] studied the neuromuscular effects of sevoflurane in 16 myasthenic patients and 12 normal patients. As expected, they found a concentration-dependent decrease in T1 and T4/T1 values. The depressant effects of sevoflurane were more prominent in those myasthenic patients with baseline T4/T1 less than 0.90. Whichever agent is used, at the end of the procedure, the inhaled agent is discontinued and recovery of neuromuscular function begins. Experience with desflurane in MG patients undergoing video-assisted thoracoscopic thymectomy was similar.[199]

Nondepolarizing Relaxants. In some cases, patients with MG cannot tolerate the cardiovascular depressant effects of the potent inhaled anesthetics, in which case neuromuscular blocking drugs may be used, titrating dose against monitored effect. Patients with MG are sensitive (i.e., show a decrease in ED_{50} and ED_{95} when compared with non-MG patients) to the nondepolarizing neuromuscular blocking drugs.[200] All nondepolarizing relaxants have been successfully and uneventfully used with careful monitoring in patients with MG (see Chapter 21). Since the sensitivity of any individual MG patient is unknown, these drugs should be titrated in 1/10 of the usual dose. Cisatracurium may be preferred because of its short elimination half-life, small volume of distribution, lack of cumulative effect, and high clearance.[201] Sensitivity to nondepolarizing relaxants is increased during the coadministration of a potent inhaled anesthetic.[201]

Other intermediate-duration nondepolarizing agents such as vecuronium and rocuronium may be used; long-acting relaxants are best avoided in patients with MG. If necessary, the residual relaxation produced by nondepolarizers may be reversed by increments of anticholinesterase drugs, whereas neuromuscular transmission is carefully monitored to obtain maximum antagonism yet avoid a cholinergic crisis. All anticholinesterases have been safely used. Edrophonium may be the drug of choice because its onset of action is rapid and higher doses have a prolonged duration of action. The sensitivity of patients with MG to nondepolarizing relaxants is very variable depending on the individual patient, the severity of MG, and the treatment. Mann et al.[202] showed that MG patients who have a T4/T1 ratio less than 0.9 in the preanesthetic period show increased sensitivity to atracurium. They suggest that neuromuscular monitoring using train-of-four stimulation should begin in the preinduction period following administration of adequate analgesia (fentanyl, 2 µg/kg). Itoh et al.[203] found that patients with ocular MG were less sensitive to vecuronium than were those with generalized MG. They also found that in patients with clinical MG, sensitivity to vecuronium was unrelated to the presence or absence of antibodies to the AChR. Seronegative patients were as sensitive to vecuronium as seropositive patients.[204] There are conflicting reports as to the sensitivity of patients with MG in remission. All such patients should be considered sensitive to nondepolarizers until proven otherwise.[205]

Sugammadex is a novel cyclodextrin drug that is designed to bind rocuronium with a great affinity. Before the introduction of sugammadex, anticholinesterase drugs were the only options for antagonism of residual neuromuscular blockade, and in MG patients anticholinesterases must be administered with caution so as to avoid myasthenic or cholinergic crises. Sugammadex has been reported to provide very rapid, complete, and lasting recovery from deep levels of rocuronium-induced neuromuscular blockade in normal patients.[206,207]

Sugammadex has since been reported to safely reverse deep rocuronium-induced neuromuscular blockade within 210 seconds in a patient with MG.[208] Sugammadex offers significant advantages in the management of the MG patient.[209] At the time of writing, this drug has been approved by the Food and Drug Administration for clinical use in the United States.

Succinylcholine. Myasthenic patients are resistant to the neuromuscular blocking effects of succinylcholine. The ED_{95} is 2.6 times normal in these patients.[210] Clinically, however, the use of succinylcholine has been without incident, with the usual clinical doses producing adequate relaxation for endotracheal intubation and a normal recovery time, despite the occasionally reported early onset of phase II block. Doses of 0.2 to 1 mg/kg have been used in a number of patients with MG, and most did not show fasciculation before becoming paralyzed. Fade in response to train-of-four stimulation was observed in some patients during recovery, but recovery was not delayed. Prior administration of an anticholinesterase may complicate the response to succinylcholine by delaying its metabolism.

When a rapid-sequence intubation of the trachea is required, rapid onset of muscle relaxation may be achieved with succinylcholine or with moderate doses of a nondepolarizer in the latter case, with an associated prolongation of effect. A succinylcholine (1.5 mg/kg)–vecuronium (0.01 mg/kg) sequence has been safely used in three patients with MG for thymectomy. The authors suggested that this technique may be particularly advantageous when rapid-sequence induction of anesthesia is indicated.[211] In the future, a combination technique of intubating dose rocuronium–sugammadex may replace succinylcholine for the MG patient who requires rapid-sequence induction.

Nonrelaxant Techniques. Because of concerns over the use of muscle relaxants in MG patients, there are many reports of successful use of nonrelaxant techniques. Della Rocca et al.[212] studied 68 consecutive MG patients undergoing transsternal thymectomy randomized to receive propofol/O_2/N_2O/fentanyl or sevoflurane/N_2O/O_2/fentanyl. All were tracheally extubated in the operating room, and none required intubation for postoperative respiratory depression. Madi-Jebara et al.[213] described the use of sevoflurane as the sole anesthetic combined with intrathecal sufentanil–morphine for analgesia in an adult patient who underwent transsternal thymectomy. Abe et al.[214] described propofol anesthesia combined with thoracic epidural anesthesia for thymectomy in 11 patients with MG. Chevalley et al.[215] reported use of propofol combined with epidural bupivacaine and sufentanil in 12 MG patients undergoing similar procedures. They commented that the shift away from use of muscle relaxants provided optimal operating condition and improved patient comfort. Lorimar and Hall[216] used a total intravenous anesthetic technique with propofol and remifentanil for transsternal thymectomy in an MG patient. Politis and Tobias[217] describe rapid-sequence intubation in a myasthenic patient with a full stomach using propofol, lidocaine, and remifentanil.

Baraka et al.[218] described a 19-year-old myasthenic patient with a thymoma who received remifentanil and sevoflurane anesthesia for a 2-hour thymectomy. Although the trachea was extubated 10 minutes after discontinuation of remifentanil, the patient was unresponsive to verbal stimuli and remained somnolent for 12 hours. Because the patient had been receiving pyridostigmine for the months prior to surgery, they suggest that the delayed arousal may have been the result of possible inhibition by pyridostigmine of the nonspecific esterases that normally hydrolyze remifentanil. Ingersoll-Weng et al.[219] reported use of a dexmedetomidine infusion/isoflurane technique for transsternal thymectomy in a

52-year-old woman. The patient was stable at the start of surgery but became asystolic on sternal retraction and received open cardiac massage. Resuscitation was successful, the dexmedetomidine infusion was discontinued, and surgery was completed uneventfully. Several factors may have contributed to the asystolic arrest, including a centrally mediated increase in parasympathetic activity resulting from dexmedetomidine in a patient who was also being treated with pyridostigmine, which also increases vagal tone. Thus, pyridostigmine may have interacted with dexmedetomidine in an additive or synergistic manner.

Other Drug Interactions. Medications with neuromuscular blocking properties should be used with caution in patients with MG, particularly if relaxants are being used concurrently. Such drugs include antiarrhythmics (quinidine, procainamide, calcium-channel blockers), diuretics (by causing hypokalemia), nitrogen mustards, quinine, and aminoglycoside antibiotics. Dantrolene has been used safely in a patient with MG.

Recovery from Anesthesia. Recovery from anesthesia must be carefully monitored in these patients. Extubation of the trachea should be performed when the patients are responsive and able to generate negative inspiratory pressures of greater than -20 cm H_2O. After extubation of the trachea, patients are carefully observed in the recovery area or the ICU. As soon as possible, patients should resume their usual pyridostigmine regimen. Cases of mild respiratory depression may be treatable with parenteral anticholinesterase; more severe cases may require reintubation of the trachea and mechanical ventilation of the lungs. In the immediate postoperative period, postthymectomy patients often show a marked improvement in their condition and a decreased need for anticholinesterase therapy.

Postoperative Respiratory Failure

Myasthenic patients are at increased risk for development of postoperative respiratory failure. There have been several attempts to predict before surgery which patients with MG will require prolonged postoperative ventilation of the lungs.[220] For patients who underwent transsternal thymectomy, positive predictors were a duration of MG more than 6 years, history of chronic respiratory disease other than that directly caused by MG, pyridostigmine dosage more than 750 mg/day, and a preoperative vital capacity less than 2.9 L. This predictive system was not found useful when applied in patients with MG undergoing transsternal thymectomy at other centers, and of no value in patients with MG undergoing other types of surgical procedures.[221] In a study of 52 MG patients following thymectomy, Mori et al.[222] concluded that those patients who received more than 250 mg of pyridostigmine were at greater risk for respiratory failure requiring reintubation. A more recent scoring system to predict postoperative myasthenic crisis and need for ventilatory support has been proposed which cites as its chief risk factors advanced staging of the patient's MG (bulbar involvement and rapid progression conferring greater risk), BMI greater than 28, history of prior myasthenic crisis, duration of symptoms more than 2 years, and association with a pulmonary resection.[223] Each patient should therefore be treated on his or her own merits.

A study of patients undergoing transsternal thymectomy suggested that the need for postoperative mechanical ventilation correlated best with preoperative maximum static expiratory pressure. It was concluded that expiratory weakness, by reducing cough efficacy and ability to clear secretions, was the main predictive determinant. Adequate clearance of secretions is essential in these patients and may occasionally necessitate bronchoscopy.

In general, the postoperative morbidity in terms of respiratory failure is lower after transcervical rather than transsternal thymectomy.[224] Techniques described that may be useful in reducing postoperative ventilatory failure include preoperative plasma exchange and high-dose perioperative steroid therapy. If the anticipated duration of the surgical procedure is 1 to 2 hours, preoperative oral anticholinesterase therapy may be of value because the peak effect of the drug coincides with the conclusion of the surgical procedure and attempts at tracheal extubation.

Postoperative Care

In the immediate postoperative period, pain relief for patients with MG is usually provided by opioid analgesics, such as meperidine, but in reduced doses. The analgesic effect of morphine and other opioid analgesics has been reported to be increased by anticholinesterases, which has led to the recommendation that the dose of opioid analgesics be reduced by one-third in patients receiving anticholinesterase therapy. Combined regional and general anesthesia techniques have also been used to provide good surgical conditions and improved postoperative analgesia in patients with MG undergoing thymectomy. Combined epidural–general anesthesia has been reported to provide excellent intraoperative and postoperative conditions for both surgeon and patient.[225,226]

Myasthenic Syndrome (Eaton–Lambert Syndrome)

The myasthenic syndrome is a very rare immune-mediated disorder of neuromuscular transmission, associated with antibodies to the presynaptic voltage-gated calcium channel. The prevalence is estimated to be about 1/100,000.[227] It is associated with small cell carcinoma of the lung in 50% to 60% of cases. Complaints of weakness may be mistaken for MG, but in Eaton–Lambert syndrome, symptoms do not respond to administration of anticholinesterases or steroids, and activity improves strength. The defect in this condition is prejunctional, is associated with diminished release of acetylcholine from nerve terminals, and improved by agents such as 4-aminopyridine,[228] guanidine, and germine that increase repetitive firing. Affected patients are particularly sensitive to the effects of all muscle relaxants, which should be used with great caution or avoided entirely.[229] Other therapies have included immunosuppression, immune globulins, and plasmapheresis.[230]

The possibility of Eaton–Lambert syndrome should be considered in all patients with known malignant disease and those patients undergoing diagnostic procedures for suspected carcinoma of the lung. Anesthesia considerations in these patients are essentially the same as in those with MG.[231,232]

Postoperative Management and Complications

Postoperative Pain Control

After extubation of the trachea, respiratory therapy and pain management become critical components of postoperative care. Adequate postoperative pain control is necessary to ensure a good respiratory effort.[233] Administration of intravenous opioids has been the standard form of pain management for years. The administration of sufficient opioid to treat pain adequately may cause sedation and respiratory depression. Patient-controlled analgesia (PCA) has been reported to decrease the amount of postoperative pain, drug use, sedation, and pulmonary complications.[234] PCA also eliminates the delays associated with personnel-administered medications and in general is very well accepted by patients.

There are other intravenous medications that can be used for pain management in addition to opioids. Low-dose ketamine infusion at 0.05 mg/kg/hr was reported to be a useful adjunct to epidural analgesia for postthoracotomy pain management.[235] Small doses of ketamine added to morphine for PCA administration have been shown to reduce the amount of morphine administered and improve respiratory parameters.[236] It reduced the incidence of oxygen desaturation below 90% during the first three postoperative nights. Ketamine may provide an anti-inflammatory effect. A meta-analysis indicated a reduction of interleukin 6,[237] and a subsequent prospective study did not corroborate that finding.[238] Ketamine can also be administered via the epidural route to relieve post thoracotomy pain.[239]

Gabapentin has also been successful in reducing pain following thoracic surgery.[240] Gabapentin may also reduce the incidence of postoperative delirium, and one approach could be to administer 900 mg 1 to 2 hours preoperatively.[241] Gabapentin has been reported to be not effective in reducing ipsilateral shoulder pain.[242] The injection of the periphrenic fat pad has been shown to reduce the ipsilateral shoulder pain that may occur following thoracic surgery.[243]

Intercostal nerve blocks can decrease pain and improve postoperative respiratory function. The intercostal blocks can be performed internally or externally before or after surgery using a standard technique. However, the easiest method during thoracic surgery is to have the surgeon perform the blocks under direct vision from inside the thorax while the chest is open. Bupivacaine 0.25% to 0.5%, in doses of 2 to 5 mL, can be placed in the five intercostal spaces around the incision and in intercostal spaces where chest tubes will be placed. This provides 6 to 24 hours of moderate pain relief, but patients still complain of diaphragmatic and shoulder discomfort caused by the chest tubes. Larger volumes of local anesthetics should not be used in the intercostal space because of the high absorption rate and attendant systemic toxicity that can be produced, as well as the possibility of pushing the drug centrally and producing a paravertebral sympathetic or epidural block with central sympatholysis and severe hypotension. The intraoperative placement of catheters in intercostal grooves allows for a continuous postoperative intercostal nerve block. The technique reduces pain and improves pulmonary function. Placement of a catheter in the paravertebral space allows for blockade of multiple levels of intercostal nerves. This technique has been reported to provide good analgesia, and with fewer side effects than epidural analgesia.[244] Paravertebral block may be as effective as epidural analgesia for pain relief following thoracic surgery, and is a good alternative.[245,246] Another approach to postoperative pain control after thoracic surgery is the use of epidural or subarachnoid opioids (see Chapter 20). Epidural morphine produces profound analgesia lasting from 16 to 24 hours after thoracotomy and does not cause a sympathetic block or sensory or motor loss. These are significant advantages over systemic opioids or infiltration of local anesthetics. Epidural opioids are most effective at alleviating pain when administered at the thoracic level. Epidural morphine has been shown to decrease pain and improve respiratory function in postthoracotomy patients.

On the basis of a meta-analysis of 100 studies in the National Library of Medicine's PubMed database from 1966 to 2002, Block et al.[247] concluded that epidural analgesia was superior to parenteral medication; this was true regardless of agent used in the epidural catheter or the level of catheter placement. There may be a reduction in both morbidity and mortality with epidural or spinal analgesia.[248] The technique most commonly employed in academic medical centers in the United States is an infusion of bupivacaine together with a narcotic such as fentanyl administered via a thoracic epidural catheter.[249] Data in the pediatric population are limited; in one study of adolescent patients, the use of thoracic epidural analgesia provided better postoperative pain relief following minimally invasive pectus excavatum repair.[250] Acetaminophen may be a useful adjunct to thoracic epidural analgesia for treatment of ipsilateral shoulder pain following thoracotomy.[251] Ketorolac may be given postoperatively, but carries a risk of bleeding if given intraoperatively.

Subarachnoid (intrathecal) morphine, in a dose of 10 to 12 µg/kg, has been successfully used after thoracic surgery.[252,253] With this technique, the drug acts directly on the spinal cord, and analgesia can be produced with a smaller dose than by the epidural or intravenous routes. When morphine is given intrathecally before the induction of anesthesia, a decrease in the dose of anesthetic drugs required may occur. All patients who have received subarachnoid or epidural opioids must be closely observed for potential side effects, including delayed respiratory depression, urine retention, pruritus, nausea, and vomiting. These effects appear to be dose-related and may be reversed with naloxone. Despite over 30 years of usage, it is still not clear what dosage is optimal for this type of surgery.[254]

Noxious stimuli, including surgical incision, may lead to changes in the central nervous system that exacerbate postoperative pain. The administration of analgesic agents before surgery is termed preemptive analgesia and may prevent these neuroplastic changes, thereby decreasing postoperative pain. This has more recently been termed preventive analgesia. In an early study of preemptive analgesia, the administration of lumbar epidural fentanyl before thoracotomy incision reduced postoperative pain scores and use of PCA morphine by a small but significant amount, compared with administration of lumbar epidural fentanyl after skin incision.[255] On the basis of a meta-analysis of randomized controlled studies published between 1966 and 2004, Bong et al.[256] concluded that thoracic epidural preemptive analgesia did not provide a statistically significant reduction in postoperative pain, but was associated with a trend toward a reduction in the incidence of such pain. A subsequent study investigating the preemptive analgesic effect of infiltration of the surgical incisions with lidocaine prior to bilateral VAT incisions did help relieve pain for 24 hours, but not thereafter.[257] In that study, since there was a bilateral incision, the infiltration was only done on one side, and each patient served as his or her own control.

Interpleural analgesia is another technique for postoperative pain treatment. The injection of local anesthetic between the pleural layers can block multiple thoracic intercostal nerves and/or pain fibers traveling with the thoracic sympathetic chain. The surgeon can place the catheter under direct vision while the chest is open. The chest tubes should not be suctioned for approximately 15 minutes after injection of local anesthetic to avoid loss of the anesthetic into the drainage. The surgeon can also place in the wound a soaker catheter, through which local anesthetics can be administered postoperatively. The On-Q PainBuster (I-Flow Corporation, Lake Forrest, CA) can be used for this purpose, and is an effective adjunct in alleviating pain following thoracic surgery.[258] There may be chronic pain following thoracotomy, and also following VAT, even though the incisions are smaller with this approach.[259,260] In one report, women were more likely than men to suffer from both perioperative pain and chronic pain.[261] If it occurs, it is important to treat this chronic postoperative pain early and aggressively.[262]

There is a high incidence of chronic pain following thoracotomy.[263,264] Approximately one-third of these have a neuropathic component.[265] Chronic post thoracotomy pain has been reported to occur with an incidence of approximately 30% to 50%.[266,267] Successful prevention and management of post thoracotomy chronic pain is hindered by an inadequate understanding of the pathophysiology. Thoracic epidural analgesia may reduce development of this chronic pain syndrome.

Peripheral nerve stimulation may provide relief in some cases.[268] Preventive analgesia has replaced the term preemptive analgesia, and involves treatment from before incision continuously until after wound healing is complete. Although ketamine reduces pain acutely, it does not have a long-term effect, either intravenously or by the epidural route. Although celecoxib has been shown to improve acute postoperative pain following thoracic surgery as an adjunct to epidural analgesia (Senard), there is no data on an impact on post thoracotomy pain syndrome. Once developed, post-thoracotomy chronic pain is difficult to treat, as it is a form of neuropathic pain.

In recent years, the use of VAT has become more common, and is often the initial approach for thoracic surgery. Although there can be expected to be less pain and respiratory impairment following VAT compared with thoracotomy, it is still important to have a pain management strategy as there can be a significant amount of postoperative pain. Acute postoperative pain may be either myofascial or neuropathic in origin. These can cause neuroplastic changes, which may result in chronic pain. In one study, there was a 47% incidence of chronic pain reported following VAT.[269] The incidence of chronic pain after VAT may be comparable with that following thoracotomy. The pain that occurs may be related to trauma to intercostal nerves by insertion of the surgical trocars or by compression during the surgery. In addition, an incision will be required to extract a lobe in the case of a lobectomy, which may exacerbate pain further.

If there is a relatively high likelihood of the surgeon converting the VAT to a thoracotomy, it may be preferable to place a thoracic epidural. If the preoperative lung function is poor, such that the patient may have difficulty breathing adequately postoperatively or may not tolerate systemic opioids, it also may be more prudent to place an epidural for that situation also. In contrast, for patients with good lung function who are scheduled to undergo a VAT in which a thoracotomy is unlikely, an epidural is probably unnecessary. The use of intercostal or paravertebral block combined with systemic opioids via PCA should be sufficient. In the United Kingdom, that approach has been reported to be more common for VATS lobectomy than the use of epidural analgesia.[270] In that survey, only 46% of patients undergoing VATS had a thoracic epidural placed. In contrast with an epidural, the paravertebral block is unilateral, and does not cause a sympathectomy. The administration of local anesthetic via the chest tubes is another approach which can successfully treat postoperative pain.[271] In a recent update in which the literature was reviewed regarding pain management for VAT, it was concluded that an epidural is not necessary.[272] The use of a single shot, multilevel, paravertebral block has been recommended for VATS in a recent update on the use of paravertebral blocks for thoracic surgery. The placement of a paravertebral catheter for VAT was shown to be effective for postoperative pain management in a recent prospective randomized trial.[273]

Complications Following Thoracic Surgery

Atelectasis

Patients who require thoracotomy often have pre-existing pulmonary disease that, when combined with the operative procedure, is likely to result in significant pulmonary dysfunction and possibly pneumonia. There is a reduction in respiratory complications with epidural analgesia including atelectasis and pneumonia.[274] Atelectasis, the most significant cause of postoperative morbidity, has been reported to occur in up to 100% of patients undergoing thoracotomy for pulmonary resection. It occurs more commonly in the basal lobes than in the middle or upper lung regions. It may be secondary to reduction of normal respiratory effort due to splinting from pain, obesity, intrathoracic blood and fluid accumulation, and decreased compliance, all of which lead to rapid, shallow, constant V_T. Such a respiratory pattern produces small airway closure and obstruction with inspissated secretions, resulting ultimately in alveolar air resorption and terminal airway collapse. A poor cough and limited clearance of secretions add to the problem. Other sources of atelectasis include mucus plugging, which can obstruct a lobe or even an entire lung, and incomplete re-expansion of the remaining lung tissue after one-lung anesthesia.

The diagnosis of atelectasis can be made by clinical findings, chest radiography, or arterial blood gas analysis. This problem is best resolved by increasing resting lung volume or FRC. The latter can be increased by an increase in transpulmonary pressure (difference between airway pressure and interpleural pressure) or in lung compliance.

The tracheas of many patients can be extubated shortly after thoracic surgical procedures. These patients should be observed in the operating room for at least 5 minutes following extubation, and many will require a high F_{IO_2} by face mask. Some patients with COPD undergoing extensive thoracic surgical procedures require postoperative ventilation to avoid atelectasis and other pulmonary complications. Mechanical ventilation increases airway pressure and, to a lesser extent, interpleural pressure; therefore, transpulmonary pressure increases.

The use of incentive spirometry and CPAP has been shown to reduce postoperative complications. Additional modalities that may be helpful in preventing atelectasis include bronchodilator treatment, coughing and clearance of secretions, chest physiotherapy, mobilizing the patient, and providing adequate analgesia. Atelectasis caused by collapse of lung tissue distal to a mucus plug can be treated by positioning the patient in the lateral decubitus position with the fully expanded lung in the dependent position. This improves $\dot{V}/\dot{Q}$ matching and facilitates clearance of mucus from the nondependent obstructed lung. However, the patient should not be placed with the operative side in the dependent position after a pneumonectomy because of the risk of cardiac herniation.

The other major complications after thoracic surgery can be grouped into cardiovascular, pulmonary, and related problems.

Cardiovascular Complications

Cardiovascular complications are often the most difficult to manage in patients with associated respiratory insufficiency. The low cardiac output syndrome and postoperative cardiac dysrhythmias may be life-threatening. Invasive hemodynamic monitoring may be needed to assist in diagnosis and fluid management therapy. Other diagnostic modalities, such as echocardiography, may be required to rule out the presence of pericardial effusions or tamponade after opening the pericardium during certain types of thoracic surgical procedures. The low cardiac output syndrome must be differentiated from hypovolemia resulting from intrathoracic hemorrhage, tamponade, pulmonary emboli, or the effects of mechanical ventilation with PEEP. Postoperative fluid administration can lead to pulmonary edema resulting from the resection of lung tissue and the concomitant reduction of the pulmonary vascular bed. Re-expansion of a chronically collapsed lung may in some cases lead to re-expansion pulmonary edema (RPE); rapid re-expansion and drainage of large amounts of pleural fluid increase the risk for RPE.[275] A postoperative pulmonary embolism can originate from the remaining pulmonary artery stump. Therapeutic interventions for postoperative myocardial dysfunction include inotropic drugs, vasodilators, and combinations of these drugs, as needed, to improve ventricular function. The goal is to shift the Starling function curve up and to the left by reducing preload of either the left or right side of the heart and increasing cardiac output. Vasodilators are very effective at decreasing right ventricular afterload and improving right ventricular function because this side of the heart is especially afterload-dependent. Combinations of inotropes and vasodilators, such as dopamine and nitroglycerin, or combined drugs, such as milrinone, can be especially useful in the treatment of right-sided heart failure.

Postoperative cardiac dysrhythmias are common after thoracic surgery. Patients following pulmonary resection have postoperative supraventricular tachycardias with a frequency and severity proportional to both their age and the magnitude of the surgical procedure. Many factors contribute to these dysrhythmias, including underlying cardiac disease, degree of surgical trauma, intraoperative cardiac manipulation, stimulation of the sympathetic nervous system by pain, a reduced pulmonary vascular bed, effects of anesthetics and cardioactive drugs, and metabolic abnormalities.

In a series of 300 thoracotomies for lung resection, atrial fibrillation occurred in 20% of patients with malignant disease but in only 3% with benign disease.[276] A similar incidence of dysrhythmias is observed after pneumonectomies. Multifocal atrial tachycardia often occurs in patients with COPD and concomitant right-sided cardiac dysfunction. The right side of the heart may be further strained by the reduction in the size of the pulmonary vasculature from the lung resection, especially after right pneumonectomy. Historically, the primary antidysrhythmic drug was used to treat atrial tachycardias in thoracic surgical patients. The prophylactic use of digitalis in thoracic surgical patients is controversial, particularly in patients with signs of congestive heart failure. Arguments against its use include the potential toxic effects of the drug and the difficulty in assessing adequacy of digitalization in the absence of heart failure. A prospective, placebo-controlled, randomized study demonstrated no advantage to prophylactic digitalization of patients undergoing thoracic surgery.[277] Part of the argument for its use is the drug's efficacy in reducing the incidence of potentially fatal complications in older patients. In some studies, it has been reported to reduce the incidence of perioperative dysrhythmias. If digitalis therapy is to be instituted, normokalemia should be ensured to reduce the likelihood of digitalis toxicity.

More recently, newer drugs have replaced digitalis for dysrhythmia control. Supraventricular tachycardias can also be treated with other agents such as β-blockers or calcium-channel–blocking drugs, after ruling out underlying reversible physiologic abnormalities, such as hypoxia. Verapamil has been the standard treatment for these problems until the introduction of the ultrashort-acting β-blocker, esmolol. Esmolol has been shown to be equally effective in controlling the ventricular rate in patients with postoperative atrial fibrillation or flutter and in increasing the conversion rate to regular sinus rhythm from 8% to 34%. Owing to its short duration of action (β elimination half-life of 9 minutes) and $β_1$-cardioselectivity, it is the drug of choice in the postoperative period to control these dysrhythmias. Esmolol, in an intravenous loading dose of 500 μg/kg given over 1 minute followed by an infusion of 50 to 200 μg/kg/min, has been shown to be effective in the control of supraventricular tachycardias. Amiodarone has been reported to be effective in restoring and maintaining sinus rhythm.[278]

Bleeding and Respiratory Complications

Hemorrhage and pneumothorax are always major concerns after intrathoracic surgery. Although there is less pain following VAT compared with thoracotomy, the risk of bleeding and intraoperative complications may be higher.[279]

Because of these problems, interpleural thoracostomy tubes with an underwater seal system are routinely used after thoracic surgery. Slippage of a suture on any major vessel or airway in the chest can lead to the slow or rapid development of hypovolemic shock or a tension pneumothorax. Drainage of more than 200 mL/hr of blood is an indication for surgical re-exploration for hemorrhage. Management of the pleural drainage system is fraught with confusion. The chest bottles must be kept below the level of the chest, and the tubes should not be clamped during patient transport. These tubes can be lifesaving, but errors in technique can lead to serious complications. The creation of a pneumothorax in the nonoperative chest by central venous catheter placement is very hazardous because this lung is essential both intraoperatively during one-lung anesthesia and postoperatively after contralateral lung resection. Dehiscence of the bronchial stump may lead to the formation of a BPF, which carries a mortality rate of 20%. Surgical treatment may be needed, in which case ventilation of the patient's lungs may be difficult because of loss of V_T through the fistula. A double-lumen endobronchial tube positioned in the contralateral main stem bronchus or the use of HFJV may be required for safe management. HFJV allows ventilation with lowered peak airway pressures. However, there have been reports in which ventilation by HFJV was difficult. If a double-lumen endobronchial tube is placed, the lung with the fistula can be ventilated independently with either CPAP or HFJV.

Neurologic Complications

Central and peripheral neurologic injuries can occur during intrathoracic procedures. Such injuries often result in serious and disabling loss of function. Peripheral nerves can also be injured, either in the chest or in other parts of the body, by pressure or stretching. The nerve injury may be apparent immediately after surgery or may not become obvious until several days later. These patients often complain of a variety of unpleasant sensations, including paresthesias, cold, pain, or anesthesia in the area supplied by the affected nerves. The brachial plexus is especially vulnerable to trauma during thoracic surgery, owing to its long superficial course in the axilla between two points of fixation, the vertebrae above, and the axillary fascia below. Stretching may be the primary cause of damage to the brachial plexus, with compression playing only a secondary role. Branches of the brachial plexus may also be injured lower in the arm by compression against objects such as an ether screen or other parts of the operating table. Intrathoracic nerves can be directly injured during a surgical procedure by being transected, crushed, stretched, or cauterized. The recurrent laryngeal nerve can become involved in lymph node tissue and injured at the time of a node biopsy, especially when the biopsy is performed through a mediastinoscope. This nerve can also be injured during tracheostomy or radical pulmonary dissections. The phrenic nerve may be injured during pericardiectomy, radical pulmonary hilar dissections, division of the diaphragm during esophageal surgery, or dissection of mediastinal tumors.

Prevention is the treatment of choice for these intraoperative nerve injuries. Analgesics may be necessary to control postoperative pain in the distribution of the nerve injury and to aid in maintaining joint mobility during the healing phase.

REFERENCES

1. Cancer: fact sheet no. 297. World Health Organization website. http://www.who.int/mediacentre/factsheets/fs297/en/. Updated February 2015; accessed January 10, 2016.
2. American Cancer Society. What are the key statistics about lung cancer. http://www.cancer.org/cancer/lungcancer-non-smallcell/detailedguide/non-small-cell-lung-cancer-key-statistics. Revised March 2015; accessed January 10, 2016.
3. Agostini P, Cieslik H, Rathinam S, et al. Postoperative pulmonary complications following thoracic surgery: Are there any modifiable risk factors? Thorax. 2010;65:815–818.
4. Bapoje SR, Whitaker JF, Schulz T, et al. Preoperative evaluation of the patient with pulmonary disease. Chest. 2007;132:1637–1645.
5. Smetanta GW. Preoperative pulmonary evaluation: Identifying and reducing risks for pulmonary complications. Cleve Clin J Med. 2006;73(Suppl 1):S36–S41.
6. Slinger P. Update on anesthetic management for pneumonectomy. Curr Opin Anesthesiol. 2009;22:31–37.
7. Centers for Disease Control and Prevention. What are the risk factors for lung cancer? Centers for Disease Control website. http://www.cdc.gov/cancer/lung/basic_info/risk_factors.htm. Accessed January 10, 2016.
8. Brunelli A, Socci L, Refai M. Quality of life before and after major lung resection for lung cancer: A prospective follow-up analysis. Ann Thorac Surg. 2007;84:410–416.
9. Licker M, Perrot M, Spiliopulos A. Risk factors for acute lung injury after thoracic surgery for lung cancer. Anesth Analg. 2003;97:1558–1565.
10. Yao S, Mao T, Fang W. Incidence and risk factors for acute lung injury after open thoracoctomy for thoracic diseases. J Thorac Dis. 2013;5:455–460.
11. Slinger PD, Susssa S, Triolet W. Predicting arterial oxygenation during one-lung anaesthesia. Can J Anaesth. 1992;39:1030–1035.
12. Slinger P, Johnston M. Preoperative evaluation of the thoracic surgery patient. Semin Anesth. 2002;21:168.
13. Nakahara K, Ohno K, Hashimoto J, et al. Prediction of postoperative respiratory failure in patients undergoing lung resection for cancer. Ann Thorac Surg. 1988;46:549–552.
14. Vansteenkiste J, Fischer BM, Dooms C, et al. Positron-emission tomography in prognostic and therapeutic assessment of lung cancer: Systematic review. Lancet Oncol. 2004;5:531–540.
15. Gould MK, Kuschner WG, Rydzak CE, et al. Test performance of positron emission tomography and computer tomography for mediastinal staging in patients with non-small-cell lung cancer: A meta-analysis. Ann Intern Med. 2003;139:879–892.
16. Amar D, Munoz D, Shi W. A clinical prediction rule for pulmonary complications after thoracic surgery for primary lung cancer. Anesth Analg. 2010;110:1343–1348.
17. Ferguson MK, Vigneswaran WT. Diffusing capacity predicts morbidity after lung resection in patients without chronic obstructive pulmonary disease. Ann Thorac Surg. 2008;85:1158–1165.
18. Zhang R, Lee SM, Wigfield C, et al. Lung function predicts pulmonary complication regardless of the surgical approach. Ann Thorac Surg. 2015;99:1761–1767.
19. Brunelli A, Kim AW, Berger KI, et al. Physiologic evaluation of the patient with lung cancer being considered for resectional surgery: Diagnosis and management of lung caner, 3rd ed. American College of Chest Physicians evidence-based clinical practice guidelines. Chest. 2013;143(5 Suppl):e166S–90S.
20. Walsh GL, Morice RC, Putnam JB. Resection of lung cancer is justified in high-risk patients selected by oxygen consumption. Ann Thorac Surg. 1994;58:704–710.
21. Bollinger CT, Wyser C, Roser H, et al. Lung scanning and exercise testing for the prediction of postoperative performance in lung resection candidates at increased risk for complications. Chest. 1995;108:341–348.
22. Ninan M, Sommers KE, Landranau RJ, et al. Standardized exercise oximetry predicts post pneumonectomy outcome. Ann Thorac Surg. 1997;64:328–332.
23. Win T, Jackson A, Sharples L, et al. Cardiopulmonary exercise tests and lung cancer surgical outcome. Chest. 2005;127:1159–1165.
24. Brunelli A, Fianchini A. Stair climbing test predicts cardiopulmonary complications after lung resection. Chest. 2002;121:1106–1110.
25. Brunelli A, Sabbatini A, Xiume F, et al. Inability to perform maximal stair climbing test before lung resection: A propensity score analysis on early outcome. Eur J Cardiothorac Surg. 2005;27:367–372.
26. Bernasconi M, Koegelenberg CF, von Groote-Bidingmaier F, et al. Speed of ascent during stair climbing identifies operable lung resection candidates. Respiration. 2012;84:117–122.
27. Spyratos D, Zarogoulidis P, Porpodis K. Preoperative evaluation for lung cancer resection. J Thorac Dis. 2014;6:S162–S166.
28. Mazzone P. Preoperative evaluation of the lung resection candidate. Cleve Clin J Med. 2012;79:eS17–eS22.
29. Brueckmann B, Villa-Uribe JL, Bateman BT, et al. Development and validation of a score for prediction of postoperative respiratory complications. Anesthesiology. 2013;118:1276–1285.
30. Nakagawa M, Tanaka H, Tsukuma H. Relationship between the duration of the preoperative smoke-free period and the incidence of postoperative pulmonary complications after pulmonary surgery. Chest. 2001;120:705–710.
31. Barrera R, Shi W, Amar D, et al. Smoking and cessation: impact on pulmonary complications after thoracotomy. Chest. 2005;127:1927–1983.
32. Mason DP, Subramanian S, Nowicki ER, et al. Impact of smoking cessation before resection of lung cancer: A society of thoracic surgeons general thoracic surgery database study. Ann Thorac Surg. 2009;88:362–371.
33. Mastracci TM, Carli F, Finley RJ, et al. Effect of preoperative smoking cessation interventions on postoperative complications. J Am Coll Surg. 2011;212:1094–1096.
34. Myers K, Hajek P, Hinds C, et al. Stopping smoking shortly before surgery and postoperative complications: A systematic review and meta-analysis. Arch Intern Med. 2011;171:983–989.
35. Mills E, Eyawo O, Lockhart I, et al. Smoking cessation reduces postoperative complications: A systematic review and meta-analysis. Am J Med. 2011;124:144–154.
36. Mauermann WJ, Nemergut EC. The anesthesiologist's role in the prevention of surgical infections. Anesthesiology. 2006;105:413–421.
37. Sekine Y, Chiyo M, Iwata T, et al. Perioperative rehabilitation and physiotherapy for lung cancer patients with chronic obstructive pulmonary disease. Jpn J Thorac Cardiovasc Surg. 2005;53:237–243.
38. Pehlivan E, Turna A, Gurses A. The effects of preoperative short-term intense physical therapy in lung cancer patients: A randomized controlled trial. Ann Thorac Cardiovasc Surg. 2011;17:461–468.
39. Landesberg G, Mosseri M, Wolf Y, et al. The probability of detecting perioperative myocardial ischemia in vascular surgery by continuous 12-lead ECG. Anesthesiology. 2002;96:264–270.
40. Marik P. Does central venous pressure predict fluid responsiveness? A systematic review of literature and tale of seven mares. Chest. 2008;134:172–178.
41. Marik P. Techniques for assessment of intravascular volume in critically ill patients. J Intensive Care Med. 2009;24:329–337.
42. Cannesson M, Le Manach YL, Hofer CK, et al. Assessing the diagnostic accuracy of pulse pressure variations for the prediction of fluid responsiveness. Anesthesiology. 2011;115:231–241.
43. Suehiro K, Okutani R. Stroke volume variation as a predictor of fluid responsiveness in patients undergoing one-lung ventilation. J Cardiothorac Vasc Anesth. 2010;24:772–775.
44. Kumar A, Anel R, Bunnell E, et al. Pulmonary artery occlusion pressure and central venous pressure fail to predict ventricular filling volume, cardiac performance, or the response to volume infusion in normal subjects. Crit Care Med. 2004;32:691–699.
45. Iberti TJ, Fischer EP, Leibowitz AB, et al. A multicenter study of physician's knowledge of the pulmonary artery catheter. JAMA. 1990;264:2928–2932.
46. Raper R, Sibbald WJ. Misled by the wedge. Chest. 1986;89:427–434.
47. Koji A. Mean pulmonary artery pressure under thoracotomy as an indicator of safety for lung resection. J Jpn Assoc Chest Surg. 2001;15:561.
48. Thys DM, Cohen E, Eisenkraft JB. Mixed venous oxygen saturation during thoracic anesthesia. Anesthesiology. 1988;69:1005–1009.
49. Pedotos A, Amar D. Right heart function in thoracic surgery: role of echocardiography. Curr Opin Anaesthesiol. 2009;22:44–49.
50. Serra E, Feltracco P, Barbieri S, et al. Transesophageal echocardiography during lung transplantation. Transplant Proc. 2007;39:1981–1982.
51. Pothoft G, Curtius JM, Wassermann K, et al. Transesophageal echography in staging of bronchial cancers. Pneumologie. 1992;446:111–117.
52. Manguso L, Pitrolo F, Bond F, et al. Echocardiographic recognition of mediastinal masses. Chest. 1988;93:144–148.
53. Neustein SM, Cohen E, Reich DL, et al. Transesophageal echocardiography and the intraoperative diagnosis of left atrial invasion by carcinoid tumor. Can J Anaesth. 1993;40:664–666.
54. Suriani RJ, Konstadt SN, Camunas J, et al. Transesophageal echocardiographic detection of left atrial involvement in a lung tumor. J Cardiothorac Vasc Anesth. 1993;7:73–75.
55. Neustein SM, Narang J. Spontaneous hemothorax due to subacute aortic dissection. J Cardiothorac Vasc Anesth. 1993;7:79–80.
56. Redford D, Kim A, Barber B. Transesophageal echocardiography for the intraoperative evaluation of a large anterior mediastinal mass. Anesth Analg. 2006;103:578–579.
57. Brooker RF, Zvara DA. Mediastinal mass diagnosed with intraoperative transesophageal echocardiography. J Cardiothorac Vasc Anesth. 2007;21:257–258.
58. Kazan R, Bracco D, Hemmerling TM. Reduced cerebral oxygen saturation measured by absolute cerebral oximetry during thoracic surgery correlates with postoperative complications. Br J Anaesth. 2009;103:811–816.

59. Suehero K, Okutai R. Cerebral desaturation during single-lung ventilation is negatively correlated with preoperative respiratory functions. *J Cardiothorac Vasc Anesth*. 2011;25:127–130.
60. Peyton P, Chong S. Minimally invasive measurement of cardiac output during surgery and critical care: a meta-analysis of accuracy and precision. *Anesthesiology*. 2010;113:1220–1235.
61. Zaouter C, Zavorsky GS. The measurement of carboxyhemoglobin and methemoglobin using a non-invasive pulse CO-oximeter. *Respir Physiol Neurobiol*. 2012;182(2-3):88–92.
62. Barker SJ, Badal JJ. The measurement of dyshemoglobins and total hemoglobin by pulse oximetry. *Curr Opin Anaesthesiol*. 2008;21:805–810.
63. Miller RD, Ward TA, Shiboski SC, et al. A comparison of three methods of hemoglobin monitoring in patients undergoing spine surgery. *Anesth Analg*. 2011;112:858–863.
64. Miller RD, Ward TA, McCulloch CE, et al. A comparison of lidocaine and bupivacaine digital nerve blocks on noninvasive continuous hemoglobin monitoring in a randomized trial in volunteers. *Anesth Analg*. 2014;118:766–771.
65. Berkow L, Rotolo S, Mirski E. Continuous noninvasive hemoglobin monitoring during complex spine surgery. *Anesth Analg*. 2011;113(6):1396–1402.
66. Giordano CR, Gravenstein N. Capnography. In: Ehrenwerth J, Eisenkraft JB, Berry JM, eds. *Anesthesia Equipment: Principles and Applications*. 2nd ed. New York, NY: Elsevier; 2013:245–255.
67. Shafieha MA, Sit J, Kartha R, et al. End-tidal CO_2 analyzers in proper positioning of double-lumen tubes. *Anesthesiology*. 1986;64:844–845.
68. Yam PCI, Innes PA, Jackson M, et al. Variation in the arterial to end-tidal Pco_2 difference during one-lung thoracic anaesthesia. *Br J Anaesth*. 1994;72:21–24.
69. Benumof JL. Isoflurane anesthesia and arterial oxygenation during one-lung ventilation. *Anesthesiology*. 1986;64:419–422.
70. Cohen E. Recommendations for airway control and difficult management in thoracic anesthesia: Are we ready for the challenge? *Minerva Anestesiol*. 2009;75:3–5.
71. Fischer GW, Cohen E. Update of anesthesia for thoracoscopic surgery. *Curr Opin Anaesthesiol*. 2010;23:7–11.
72. Lohser J, Brodsky J. Silibronco double-lumen tube. *J Cardiothorac Vasc Anesth*. 2006;20:129–131.
73. Brodsky JB, Lemmens HJM. Left double-lumen tubes: clinical experience with 1,170 patients. *J Cardiothorac Vasc Anesth*. 2003;17:289–298.
74. Brodsky JB, Lemmens HJ. Tracheal width and left double-lumen tube size: a formula to estimate left-bronchial width. *J Clin Anesth*. 2005;17:267–270.
75. Amar D, Desiderio D, Heerdt PM, et al. Practice patterns in choice of left double-lumen tube size for thoracic surgery. *Anesth Analg*. 2008;106:379–383.
76. Chow MY, Go MH, Ti LK. Predicting the depth of insertion of left-sided double-lumen endobronchial tubes. *J Cardiothorac Vasc Anesth*. 2002;16:456–458.
77. Massot J, Dumand-Nizard V, Fischler M, et al. Evaluation of the double-lumen tube Vivasight-DL (DLT-ETView): a prospective single-center study. *J Cardiothorac Vasc Anesth*. 2015;29:1544–1549.
78. Koopman EM, Barak M, Weber E, et al. Evaluation of a new double-lumen endobronchial tube with an integrated camera (VivaSight-DL™): A prospective multicentre observational study. *Anaesthesia*. 2015;70:962–968.
79. Levy-Faber D, Malyanker Y, Nir RR, et al. Comparison of VivaSight double-lumen tube with a conventional double-lumen tube in adult patients undergoing video-assisted thoracoscopic surgery. *Anaesthesia*. 2015;70:1259–1263.
80. Smith G, Hirsch N, Ehrenwerth J. Sight and sound: Can double-lumen endotracheal tubes be placed accurately without fiberoptic bronchoscopy? *Br J Anaesth*. 1987;58:1317.
81. Cohen E, Neustein SM, Goldofsky S, et al. Incidence of malposition of PVC and red rubber left-sided double lumen tubes and clinical sequelae. *J Cardiothorac Vasc Anesth*. 1995;9:122–127.
82. Benumof JL, Partridge BL, Salvatierra C, et al. Margin of safety in positioning modern double-lumen endotracheal tubes. *Anesthesiology*. 1987;67:729–738.
83. Sakuragi T, Kumano K, Yasumoto M, et al. Rupture of the left main-stem bronchus by the tracheal portion of a double-lumen endobronchial tube. *Acta Anaesthesiol Scand*. 1997;41:1218–1220.
84. Wagner DL, Gammage GW, Wong ML. Tracheal rupture following the insertion of a disposable double-lumen endotracheal tube. *Anesthesiology*. 1985;63:698–700.
85. Heike Knoll H, Stephan Ziegeler S, Jan-Uwe Schreiber JU, et al. Airway injuries after one-lung ventilation: A comparison between double-lumen tube and endobronchial blocker: a randomized, prospective, controlled trial. *Anesthesiology*. 2006;105:471–477.
86. Clayton-Smith A, Bennett K, Alston RP, et al. A comparison of the efficacy and adverse effects of double-lumen endobronchial tubes and bronchial blockers in thoracic surgery: a systematic review and meta-analysis of randomized controlled trials. *J Cardiothorac Vasc Anesth*. 2015;29:955–966.
87. Andros TG, Lennon PF. One-lung ventilation in a patient with a tracheostomy and severe tracheobronchial disease. *Anesthesiology*. 1993;79:1127–1128.
88. Bellver J, Garcia-Aguado A, Andres JD, et al. Selective bronchial intubation with the Univent system in patients with a tracheostomy. *Anesthesiology*. 1993;79:1453–1454.
89. Saito T, Naruke T, Carney E, et al. New double-lumen intrabronchial tube (Naruke tube) for tracheostomized patients. *Anesthesiology*. 1998;89:1038–1039.
90. Cohen E, Benumof JL. Lung separation in the patient with a difficult airway. *Curr Opin Anesthesiol*. 1999;12:29–35.
91. Benumof JL. Difficult tubes and difficult airways. *J Cardiothorac Vasc Anesth*. 1998;12:131–132.
92. Neustein SM. The use of bronchial blockers for providing one-lung ventilation. *J Cardiothorac Vasc Anesth*. 2009;23:860–868.
93. Cohen E. The Cohen flexitip endobronchial blocker: an alternative to a double lumen tube. *Anesth Analg*. 2005;101:1877–1879.
94. Mourisse J, Liesveld J, Verhagen A, et al. Efficiency, efficacy, and safety of EZ-blocker compared with left-sided double-lumen tube for one-lung ventilation. *Anesthesiology*. 2013;118:550–561.
95. Campos JH, Kernstine KH. A comparison of a left-sided Broncho-Cath with the torque control blocker Univent and the wire-guided blocker. *Anesth Analg*. 2003;96:283–289.
96. Campos JH. Progress in lung separation. *Thorac Surg Clin*. 2005;15:71–83.
97. Narayanaswamy M, McRae K, Slinger P, et al. Choosing a lung isolation device for thoracic surgery: A randomized trial of three bronchial blockers versus double-lumen tubes. *Anesth Analg*. 2009;108:1097–1101.
98. Cohen E. Strategies in lung isolation: To block or not to block? *Can J Anaesth*. 2016 April 29. Epub ahead of print.
99. Desiderio DP, Burt M, Kolker AC, et al. The effects of endobronchial cuff inflation on double-lumen endobronchial tube movement after lateral decubitus positioning. *J Cardiothorac Vasc Anesth*. 1997;11:595–598.
100. Ko R, McRae K, Darling G, et al. The use of air in the inspired gas mixture during two-lung ventilation delays lung collapse during one-lung ventilation. *Anesth Analg*. 2009;108:1092–1096.
101. Katz JA, Larlane RG, Fairly HB, et al. Pulmonary oxygen exchange during endobronchial anesthesia: Effect of tidal volume and PEEP. *Anesthesiology*. 1982;56:164–171.
102. Eichenbaum KD, Neustein SM. Acute lung injury following thoracic surgery. *J Cardiothorac Vasc Anesth*. 2010;24:681–690.
103. Slinger P. Low tidal volume is indicated during one-lung ventilation. *Anesth Analg*. 2006;103:268–270.
104. Gal T. Low tidal volume is not indicated during one-lung ventilation. *Anesth Analg*. 2006;103:271–273.
105. Vegh T, Juhasz M, Szatmari S, et al. Effects of different tidal volumes for one-lung ventilation on oxygenation with open chest condition and surgical manipulation: A randomised cross-over trial. *Minerva Anesthesiol*. 2013;79:24–32.
106. Schultz MJ, Jack J, Haitsma JJ, et al. What tidal volumes should be used in patients without acute lung injury? *Anesthesiology*. 2007;106:1226–1231.
107. Wrigge H, Uhlig U, Zinserling J, et al. The effects of different ventilatory settings on pulmonary and systemic inflammatory responses during major surgery. *Anesth Analg*. 2004;98:775–781.
108. Senturk M. New concepts of the management of one-lung ventilation. *Curr Opin Anesthesiol*. 2006;19:1–4.
109. Wrigge H, Zinserling J, Stuber F, et al. Effects of mechanical ventilation on release of cytokines into systemic circulation in patients with normal pulmonary function. *Anesthesiology*. 2000;93:1413–1417.
110. Fernandez-Perez ER, Keegan MT, Brown DR, et al. Intraoperative tidal volume as a risk factor for respiratory failure after pneumonectomy. *Anesthesiology*. 2006;105:14–18.
111. Tusman G, Böhm SH, Vazquez da Anda G, et al. "Alveolar recruitment strategy" improves arterial oxygenation during general anaesthesia. *Br J Anaesth*. 1999;82:8–13.
112. Tugrul M, Camici E, Karadeniz H, et al. Comparison of volume control with pressure control ventilation during one-lung anaesthesia. *Br J Anaesth*. 1997;79:306–310.
113. Carmen MU, Casas J, Moral I, et al. Pressure-controlled versus volume-controlled ventilation during one-lung ventilation for thoracic surgery. *Anesth Analg*. 2007;104:1029–1033.
114. Cruz Pardons P, Garutti I, Piñeiro P, et al. Effects of ventilatory mode during one-lung ventilation on intraoperative and postoperative arterial oxygenation in thoracic surgery. *J Cardiothorac Vasc Anesth*. 2009;23:770–774.
115. Sugasawa Y, Yamaguchi K, Kumakura S, et al. The effect of one-lung ventilation upon pulmonary inflammatory responses during lung resection. *J Anesth*. 2011;25:170-177.
116. Gao W, Dong-Dong L, Li D. Effect of therapeutic hypercapnia on inflammatory responses to one-lung ventilation in lobectomy patients. *Anesthesiology*. 2015;122:1235–1252.
117. Cohen E, Thys DM, Eisenkraft JB, et al. PEEP during one-lung anesthesia improves oxygenation in patients with low Pao2. *Anesth Analg*. 1985;64:200.
118. Capan LM, Turndorf H, Patel K, et al. Optimization of arterial oxygenation during one-lung anesthesia. *Anesth Analg*. 1980;59:847–851.
119. Hogue CW. Effectiveness of low levels of nonventilated lung continuous positive airway pressure in improving arterial oxygenation during one-lung ventilation. *Anesth Analg*. 1994;79:364–367.
120. Malmkvist G. Maintenance of oxygenation during one-lung ventilation: effect of intermittent reinflation of the collapsed lung with oxygen. *Anesth Analg*. 1989;68:763–766.
121. Cohen E, Eisenkraft JB, Thys DM, et al. Oxygenation and hemodynamic changes during one-lung ventilation. *J Cardiothorac Vasc Anesth*. 1988;2:34–40.

122. Wiedemann HP. A perspective on the fluids and catheters treatment trial (FACTT). Fluid restriction is superior in acute lung injury and ARDS. *Cleve Clin J Med*. 2008;75:42–48.
123. Wiedemann HP, Wheeler AP, Bernard GR, et al. Comparison of two fluid-management strategies in acute lung injury. *N Engl J Med*. 2006;354:2564–2575.
124. Rivers EP. Fluid-management strategies in acute lung injury: liberal, conservative, or both? *N Engl J Med*. 2006;354(24):2598–2600.
125. Karzai W, Schwarzkopf K. Hypoxemia during OLV: prediction, prevention and treatment. *Anesthesiology*. 2009;110:1402–1411.
126. Yang M, Joo H, Kim K, et al. Does a protective ventilation strategy reduce the risk of pulmonary complications after lung cancer surgery? A randomized controlled trial. *Chest*. 2011;139:530–537.
127. Şentürk M, Slinger P, Cohen E. Intraoperative mechanical ventilation strategies for one-lung ventilation. *Best Pract Res Clin Anaesthesiol*. 2015;29:357–369.
128. Shimizu T, Abe K, Kinovchik K, et al. Arterial oxygenation during one-lung ventilation. *Can J Anaesth*. 1997;44:1162–1166.
129. Loer SA, Scheeren TWL, Tarnow J. Desflurane inhibits HPV in isolated rabbit lungs. *Anesthesiology*. 1995;83:552–556.
130. Van Keer L, Van Aken H, Vandermeersch E, et al. Propofol does not inhibit HPV in humans. *J Clin Anesth*. 1989;1:284–288.
131. Kellow NH, Scott AD, White SA, et al. Comparison of the effects of propofol and isoflurane anaesthesia on right ventricular function and shunt fraction during thoracic surgery. *Br J Anesth*. 1995;75:578–582.
132. Schilling T, Kozian A, Huth C, et al. The pulmonary immune effects of mechanical ventilation in patients undergoing thoracic surgery. *Anesth Analg*. 2005;101:957–965.
133. De Conno E, Steurer MP, Wittlinge M, et al. Anesthetic-induced improvement of the inflammatory response to one-lung ventilation. *Anesthesiology*. 2009;110:1316–1326.
134. Schilling T, Kozian A, Senturk M, et al. Anesthetic-induced improvement of the inflammatory response to one-lung ventilation. *Anesthesiology*. 2011;115:65–74.
135. Faller S, Strosing KM, Ryter SW, et al. The volatile anesthetic isoflurane prevents ventilator-induced lung injury via phosphoinositide 3-kinase/Akt signaling in mice. *Anesth Analg*. 2012;114:747–756.
136. Englert JA, Macias AA, Amador-Munoz D, et al. Isoflurane ameliorates acute lung injury by preserving epithelial tight junction integrity. *Anesthesiology*. 2015;123:377–388.
137. Von Euler US, Liljestrand G. Observations on the pulmonary arterial blood pressure in the cat. *Acta Physiol Scand*. 1946;12:301.
138. Marshall BE, Marshall C, Benumof JL, et al. Hypoxic pulmonary vasoconstriction in dogs: Effects of lung segment size and alveolar oxygen tensions. *J Appl Physiol*. 1981;51:1543–1551.
139. Lumb AB, Slinger P. Hypoxic pulmonary vasoconstriction: physiology and anesthetic implications. *Anesthesiology*. 2015;122:932–946.
140. Benumof JL. One-lung ventilation and hypoxic pulmonary vasoconstriction: Implications for anesthetic management. *Anesth Analg*. 1985;64:821–833.
141. Eisenkraft JB. Effects of anesthetics on the pulmonary circulation. *Br J Anaesth*. 1990;65:63–78.
142. Rogers SM, Benumof JL. Halothane and isoflurane do not decrease PaO_2 during one-lung ventilation in intravenously anesthetized patients. *Anesth Analg*. 1985;64:946–954.
143. Benumof JL, Augustine SD, Gibbons JA. Halothane and isoflurane only slightly impair arterial oxygenation during one-lung ventilation in patients undergoing thoracotomy. *Anesthesiology*. 1987;67:910–915.
144. Slinger P, Scott WAC. Arterial oxygenation during one-lung ventilation: a comparison of enflurane and isoflurane. *Anesthesiology*. 1995;82:940–946.
145. Beck DH, Doepfmer UR, Sinemus C, et al. Effects of sevoflurane and propofol on pulmonary shunt fraction during one-lung ventilation. *Br J Anaesth*. 2001;86:38–43.
146. Reid CW, Slinger PD, Lenis S. A comparison of the effects of propofol-alfentanil vs. isoflurane on arterial oxygenation during one lung ventilation. *J Cardiovasc Thorac Anesth*. 1996;10:860–863.
147. Pruszkowski O, Dalibon N, Moutafis M, et al. Effects of propofol vs sevoflurane on arterial oxygenation during one-lung ventilation. *Br J Anaesth*. 2007;98:539–544.
148. Ng A, Swanevelder J. Hypoxaemia associated with one-lung anaesthesia: new discoveries in ventilation and perfusion. *Br J Anaesth*. 2011;106:761–763.
149. Moutafis M, Dalibon N, Liu N, et al. The effects of almitrine on oxygenation and hemodynamics during one-lung ventilation. *Anesth Analg*. 2002;94:830–834.
150. Dalibon N, Moutafis M, Liu N, et al. Treatment of hypoxemia during one-lung ventilation using intravenous almitrine. *Anesth Analg*. 2004;98:590–594.
151. Bermejo S, Gallart L, Silva-Costa-Gomes T, et al. Almitrine fails to improve oxygenation during one-lung ventilation with sevoflurane anesthesia. *J Cardiothorac Vasc Anesth*. 2014;28:919–924.
152. Fischer SR, Deyo DJ, Bone HG, et al. Nitric oxide synthase inhibition restores HPV in sepsis. *Am J Respir Crit Care Med*. 1997;156:833–839.
153. Frostell CG, Blomqvist H, Hedenstierna G, et al. Inhaled nitric oxide selectively reverses human HPV without causing systemic vasodilation. *Anesthesiology*. 1993;78:427–435.
154. Troncy E, Francoeur M, Blaise G. Inhaled nitric oxide: clinical applications, indications and toxicology. *Can J Anaesth*. 1997;44:973–988.
155. Moutafis M, Dalibon N, Colchen A, et al. Improving oxygenation during bronchopulmonary lavage using nitric oxide inhalation and almitrine infusion. *Anesth Analg*. 1999;89:32–36.
156. B'chir A, Mebassa A, Losserm MR, et al. Intravenous almitrine bimesylate reversibly inhibits lactic acidosis and hepatic dysfunction in patients with lung injury. *Anesthesiology*. 1998;89:823–830.
157. Doering EB, Hanson CW, Reily D, et al. Improvement in oxygenation by phenylephrine and nitric oxide in patients with adult respiratory distress syndrome. *Anesthesiology*. 1997;87:18–25.
158. Pathak V, Welsby I, Mahmood K, et al. Ventilation and anesthetic approaches for rigid bronchoscopy. *Ann Am Thorac Surg*. 2014;11:628–634.
159. Frumin MJ, Epstein RM, Cohen G. Apneic oxygenation in man. *Anesthesiology*. 1959;20:789–798.
160. Satyanarayana T, Capan L, Ramanathan S, et al. Bronchofiberscopic jet ventilation. *Anesth Analg*. 1980;59:350–354.
161. Matsushima Y, Jones RL, King EG, et al. Alterations in pulmonary mechanics and gas exchange during routine fiberoptic bronchoscopy. *Chest*. 1984;86:184–188.
162. Neuman GG, Weingarten AE, Abramowitz RM, et al. The anesthetic management of the patient with an anterior mediastinal mass. *Anesthesiology*. 1984;60:144–147.
163. Bechard P, Letourneau L, Lacasse Y. Perioperative cardiorespiratory complications in adults with mediastinal mass: incidence and risk factors. *Anesthesiology*. 2004;100:826–834.
164. Oley LTC, Hnatiuk MC, Corcoran MC, et al. Spirometry in surgery for anterior mediastinal masses. *Chest*. 2001;120:1152–1156.
165. Tempe DK, Arya R, Dubey S, et al. Mediastinal mass resection: femorofemoral cardiopulmonary bypass before induction of anesthesia in the management of airway obstruction. *J Cardiothorac Vasc Anesth*. 2001;15:233–236.
166. Ferrari LR, Bedford RF. General anesthesia prior to treatment of anterior mediastinal masses in pediatric cancer patients. *Anesthesiology*. 1990;72:991–995.
167. Shamberger RC. Preanesthetic evaluation of children with anterior mediastinal masses. *Semin Pediatr Surg*. 1999;8:61–68.
168. DeSoto H. Direct laryngoscopy as an aid to relieve airway obstruction in a patient with a mediastinal mass. *Anesthesiology*. 1987;67:116–117.
169. Gardner JC, Royster RL. Airway collapse with an anterior mediastinal mass despite spontaneous ventilation in an adult. *Anesth Analg*. 2011;113:239–242.
170. Slinger PD, Karsli C. Management of a patient with a large anterior mediastinal mass: recurring myths. *Curr Opin Anaesthesiol*. 2007;20:1–3.
171. Barker SJ, Clarke C, Trivedi N, et al. Anesthesia for thoracoscopic laser ablation of bullous emphysema. *Anesthesiology*. 1993;78:44–50.
172. Brodsky JB, Cohen E. Video-assisted thoracoscopic surgery. *Curr Opin Anaesthesiol*. 2000;13:41–45.
173. Kent M, Wang T, Whyte R, et al. Open, video-assisted thoracic surgery, and robotic lobectomy: Review of a national database. *Ann Thorac Surg*. 2014;97:236–242.
174. Steenwyk B, Lyerly R III. Advancements in robotic-assisted thoracic surgery. *Anesthesiol Clin*. 2012;30(4):699–708.
175. Velez-Cubian FO, Ng EP, Fontaine JP, et al. Robotic-assisted videothoracoscopic surgery of the lung. *Cancer Control*. 2015;22:314–325.
176. Plummer S, Hartley M, Vaughan RS. Anaesthesia for telescopic procedures in the thorax. *Br J Anaesth*. 1998;80:223–234.
177. Lohser J. Managing hypoxemia during minimally invasive thoracic surgery. *Anesthesiol Clin*. 2012;30:683–697.
178. Neustein SM, Kahn P, Krellenstein DJ, et al. Incidence of arrhythmias and predisposing factors after thoracic surgery: Thoracotomy versus video-assisted thoracoscopy. *J Cardiothorac Vasc Anesth*. 1998;12:659–661.
179. Courey AJ, Hyzy RC. High frequency ventilation in adults. UpToDate website. http://www.uptodate.com/contents/high-frequency-ventilation-in-adults. Updated May 2015.
180. Benumof JL. Sequential one-lung ventilation for bilateral bullectomy. *Anesthesiology*. 1987;67:268–272.
181. Cohen E, Eisenkraft JB. Bronchopulmonary lavage: effects on oxygenation and hemodynamics. *J Cardiothorac Anesth*. 1990;4:119–129.
182. McGrogan A, Sneddon S, de Vries CS. The incidence of myasthenia gravis: A systematic literature review. *Neuroepidemiology*. 2010;34:171–183.
183. Drachman DB. Myasthenia gravis. Review article. *N Engl J Med*. 1994;330:1797–1810.
184. Sathasivam S. Current and emerging treatments for the management of myasthenia gravis. *Ther Clin Risk Manag*. 2011;7:313–323.
185. Osserman KE, Genkins G. Studies in myasthenia gravis: review of a twenty-year experience in over 1200 patients. *Mt Sinai J Med*. 1971;38:497–537.
186. McConville J, Farrugia ME, Beeson D, et al. Detection and characterization of MuSK antibodies in seronegative myasthenia gravis. *Ann Neurol*. 2004;55:580–584.
187. Mehndiratta MM, Pandey S, Kuntzer T. Acetylcholinesterase inhibitor treatment for myasthenia gravis. *Cochrane Database Syst Rev*. 2011;16:CD006986.
188. Kumar V, Kaminski HJ. Treatment of myasthenia gravis. *Curr Neurol Neuroscience Rep*. 2011;11:89–96.

189. Maurizi G, D'Andrilli A, Sommella L, et al. Transsternal thymectomy. *Thorac Cardiovasc Surg.* 2015;63(3):178–186.
190. Meyer DM, Herbert MA, Sobhani NC, et al. Comparative clinical outcomes of thymectomy for myasthenia gravis performed by extended transsternal and minimally invasive approaches. *Ann Thorac Surg.* 2009;87:385–390.
191. Pandey R, Garg R, Chandralekha, et al. Robot-assisted thoracoscopic thymectomy: perianaesthetic concerns. *Eur J Anaesthesiol.* 2010;27:473–477.
192. Blichfeldt-Lauridsen L, Hansen BD. Anesthesia and myasthenia gravis. *Acta Anaesthesiol Scand.* 2012;56:17–22.
193. Gilhus NE, Nacu A, Andersen JB, et al. Myasthenia gravis and risks for comorbidity. *Eur J Neurol.* 2015; 22:17–23.
194. Tripathi M, Kaushik S, Dubey P. The effect of use of pyridostigmine and requirement for vecuronium with myasthenia gravis. *J Postgrad Med.* 2003; 49:311–314.
195. Dillon FX. Anesthesia issues in the perioperative management of myasthenia gravis. *J Postgrad Med.* 2003;49:311.
196. Kopman AF. The Datex-Ohmeda M-NMT module: a potentially confusing user interface. *Anesthesiology.* 2006;104:1110–1111.
197. Nilsson E, Muller K. Neuromuscular effects of isoflurane in patients with myasthenia gravis. *Acta Anaesthesiol Scand.* 1990;34:126–131.
198. Nitahara K, Sugi Y, Higa K, et al. Neuromuscular effects of sevoflurane in myasthenia gravis patients. *Br J Anaesth.* 2007;98:337–341.
199. Gritti P, Carrara A, Khotcholava M, et al. The use of desflurane or propofol in combination with remifentanil in myasthenic patients undergoing a video-assisted thoracoscopic-extended thymectomy. *Acta Anaesthesiol Scand.* 2009;53:380–389.
200. Eisenkraft JB, Book WJ, Papatestas AE. Sensitivity to vecuronium in myasthenia gravis: a dose-response study. *Can J Anaesth.* 1990;37:301–306.
201. Baraka A, Siddik S, Kawkabani N. Cisatracurium in a myasthenic patient undergoing thymectomy. *Can J Anaesth.* 1999;46:779–782.
202. Mann R, Blobner M, Jelen-Esselborn S, et al. Preanesthetic train-of-four fade predicts the atracurium requirement of myasthenia gravis patients. *Anesthesiology.* 2000;93:346–350.
203. Itoh H, Shibata K, Nitta S. Difference in sensitivity to vecuronium between patients with ocular and generalized myasthenia gravis. *Br J Anaesth.* 2001;87: 885–889.
204. Itoh H, Shibata K, Nitta S. Sensitivity to vecuronium in seropositive and seronegative patients with myasthenia gravis. *Anesth Analg.* 2003;96:1842.
205. Basaranoglu G, Erden V, Delatioglu H. Anesthesia of a patient with cured myasthenia gravis. *Anesth Analg.* 2003;96:1842–1843.
206. Naguib M. Sugammadex: Another milestone in clinical neuromuscular pharmacology. *Anesth Analg.* 2007;104:575–581.
207. Kopman AF. Sugammadex: A revolutionary approach to neuromuscular antagonism. *Anesthesiology.* 2006;104(4):631–633.
208. Unterbuchner C, Fink H, Blobner M. The use of sugammadex in a patient with myasthenia gravis. *Anaesthesia.* 2010;65:302–305.
209. de Boer HD, Shields MO, Booij LH. Reversal of neuromuscular blockade with sugammadex in patients with myasthenia gravis: A case series of 21 patients and review of the literature. *Eur J Anaesth.* 2014;31:715–721.
210. Eisenkraft JB, Book WJ, Papatestas AE, et al. Resistance to succinylcholine in myasthenia gravis: A dose-response study. *Anesthesiology.* 1988;69:760–763.
211. Baraka A, Tabboush Z. Neuromuscular response to succinylcholine-vecuronium sequence in three myasthenic patients undergoing thymectomy. *Anesth Analg.* 1991;72:827–830.
212. Della Rocca G, Coccia C, Diana L, et al. Propofol or sevoflurane anesthesia without muscle relaxants allow the early extubation of myasthenic patients. *Can J Anaesth.* 2003;50:547–552.
213. Madi-Jebara S, Yazigi A, Hayek M, et al. Sevoflurane anesthesia and intrathecal sufentanil-morphine for thymectomy in myasthenia gravis. *J Clin Anesth.* 2002;14:558–559.
214. Abe S, Takeuchi C, Kaneko T, et al. Propofol anesthesia combined with thoracic epidural anesthesia for thymectomy for myasthenia gravis: A report of eleven cases. *Masui.* 2001;50:1217.
215. Chevalley C, Spiliopoulos A, de Perrot M, et al. Perioperative medical management and outcome following thymectomy for myasthenia gravis. *Can J Anesth.* 2001;48:446–451.
216. Lorimer M, Hall R. Remifentanil and propofol total intravenous anaesthesia for thymectomy in myasthenia gravis. *Anaesth Intensive Care.* 1998;26:210–212.
217. Politis GD, Tobias JD. Rapid sequence intubation without a neuromuscular blocking agent in a 14 year old female patient with myasthenia gravis. *Paediatr Anaesth.* 2007;17:285–288.
218. Baraka AS, Haroun-Bizri ST, Georges FJ. Delayed postoperative arousal following remifentanil-based anesthesia in a myasthenic patient undergoing thymectomy. *Anesthesiology.* 2004;100:460–461.
219. Ingersoll-Weng E, Manecke GR, Thistlethwaite PA. Dexmedetomidine and cardiac arrest. *Anesthesiology.* 2004;100:738–739.
220. Eisenkraft JB, Papatestas AE, Kahn CH, et al. Predicting the need for postoperative mechanical ventilation in myasthenia gravis. *Anesthesiology.* 1986;65:79–82.
221. Grant RP, Jenkins LC. Prediction of the need for postoperative mechanical ventilation in myasthenia gravis: Thymectomy compared to other surgical procedures. *Can Anaesth Soc J.* 1982;29:112–116.
222. Mori T, Yoshioka M, Watanabe K, et al. Changes in respiratory condition after thymectomy for patients with myasthenia gravis. *Ann Thorac Cardiovasc Surg.* 2003;9:93–97.
223. Leuzzi G, Meacci E, Cusumano G, et al. Thymectomy in myasthenia gravis: proposal for a predictive score of postoperative myasthenic crisis. *Eur J Cardiothorac Surg.* 2014;45:e76–e88.
224. Zahid I, Sharif S, Routledge T, et al. Video-assisted thoracoscopic surgery or transsternal thymectomy in the treatment of myasthenia gravis? *Interact Cardiovasc Thorac Surg.* 2011;12:40–46.
225. Burgess FW, Wilcosky B. Thoracic epidural anesthesia for transsternal thymectomy in myasthenia gravis. *Anesth Analg.* 1989;69:529–531.
226. Gorback MS. Analgesic management after thymectomy. *Anesthesiol Rep.* 1990;2:262–266.
227. Petty R. Lambert Eaton myasthenic syndrome. *Pract Neurol.* 2007;7:265–267.
228. Keogh M, Sedehizadeh S, Maddison P. Treatment for Lambert-Eaton myasthenic syndrome. *Cochrane Database Syst Rev.* 2011:CD003279.
229. Itoh H, Shibata K, Nitta S. Neuromuscular monitoring in myasthenic syndrome. *Anesthesia.* 2001;56:562–567.
230. Verschuuren JJ, Wirtz PW, Titulaer MJ, et al. Available treatment options for the management of Lambert-Eaton myasthenic syndrome. *Expert Opin Pharmacother.* 2006;7:1323–1336.
231. Telford RJ, Hollway TE. The myasthenic syndrome: anesthesia in a patient treated with 3,4 diaminopyridine. *Br J Anaesth.* 1990;64:363–366.
232. Weingarten TN, Araka CN, Mogensen ME, et al. Lambert-Eaton myasthenic syndrome during anesthesia: a report of 37 patients. *J Clin Anesth.* 2014;28: 648-653.
233. Kavanagh BP, Katz J, Sandler AN. Pain control after thoracic surgery: A review of current techniques. *Anesthesiology.* 1994;81:737–759.
234. Whiting WG, Sandler AN, Lau LC, et al. Analgesic and respiratory effects of epidural sufentanil in post-thoracotomy patients. *Anesthesiology.* 1988;69: 36–43.
235. Suzuki M, Haraguti S, Sugimoto K, et al. Low-dose intravenous ketamine potentiates epidural analgesia after thoracotomy. *Anesthesiology.* 2006;105: 111–119.
236. Michelet P, Guervilly C, Helaine A. Adding ketamine to morphine for patient-controlled analgesia after thoracic surgery: Influence on morphine consumption, respiratory function, and nocturnal desaturation. *Br J Anaesth.* 2007;99:396–403.
237. Dale O, Somogyi AA, Li Y, et al. Does intraoperative ketamine attenuate inflammatory reactivity following surgery? A systematic review and meta-analysis. *Anesth Analg.* 2012;115:934–943.
238. D'Alonzo RC, Bennet-Guerrero E, Podgoreanu M, et al. A randomized, double blind, placebo controlled clinical trial of the preoperative use of ketamine for reducing inflammation and pain after thoracic surgery. *J Anesth.* 2011; 25:672–678
239. Ryu HG, Lee CJ, Kim YT, et al. Preemptive low-dose epidural ketamine for preventing chronic postthoracotomy pain: A prospective, double-blinded, randomized, clinical trial. *Clin J Pain.* 2011;27:304–308.
240. Kinney MA, Mantilla CB, Carns PE, et al. Preoperative gabapentin for acute post-thoracotomy analgesia: A randomized, double-blinded, active placebo-controlled study. *Pain Pract.* 2012;12:175–183.
241. Kong VK, Irwin MG. Gabapentin: A multimodal perioperative drug? *Br J Anaesth.* 2007;99:775–786.
242. Hout HP, Chouinard P, Girard, et al. Gabapentin does not reduce post thoracotomy shoulder pain: A randomized, double-blind placebo controlled study. *Can J Anaesth.* 2008;55:337–343.
243. Martinez-Barenys C, Busquets J, Lopez de Castro PE, et al. Randomized double-blind comparison of phrenic nerve infiltration and suprascapular nerve block for ipsilateral shoulder pain after thoracic surgery. *Eur J Cardiothorac Surg.* 2011;40(1):106–112.
244. Davies RG, Myles PS, Graham JM. A comparison of the analgesic efficacy and side-effects of paravertebral vs epidural blockade for thoracotomy: A systematic review and meta-analysis of randomized controlled trials. *Br J Anaesth.* 2006;96:418–426.
245. Scarci M, Joshi A, Attia R. In patients undergoing thoracic surgery is paravertebral block as effective as epidural analgesia for pain management? *Interact Cardiovasc Thorac Surg.* 2010;10:92–96.
246. Wenk M, Schug. Perioperative pain management after thoracotomy. *Curr Opin Anaesthesiol.* 2011;24:8–12.
247. Block BM, Spencer SL, Rowlingson BA, et al. Efficacy of postoperative epidural analgesia: A meta-analysis. *JAMA.* 2003;290:2455–2463.
248. Rodgers A, Walker N, Schug S, et al. Reduction of postoperative mortality and morbidity with epidural or spinal anesthesia: Results from an overview of randomized trials. *Br Med J.* 2000;321:1493.
249. Minzler B, Grimm BJ, Johnson RF, et al. The practice of thoracic epidural analgesia: A survey of academic centers in the United States. *Anesth Analg.* 2002;95:472–475.
250. Weber T, Matzl J, Rokitansky A, et al. Superior postoperative pain relief with thoracic epidural analgesia versus intravenous patient-controlled analgesia after minimally invasive pectus excavatum repair. *J Thorac Cardiovasc Surg.* 2007;132:865–870.

251. Mac TB, Girard F, Chouinard P, et al. Acetaminophen decreases early post-thoracotomy ipsilateral shoulder pain in paients with thoracic epidural analgesia. *J Cardiothorac Vasc Anesth.* 2005;19:475–478.
252. Cohen E, Neustein SM. Intrathecal morphine during thoracotomy. *J Thorac Cardiovasc Anesth.* 1993;7:154–156.
253. Askar FZ, Kocabas S, Yucel S, et al. The efficacy of intrathecal morphine in post-thoracotomy pain. management. *J Int Med Res.* 2007;35:314–322.
254. Meylan N, Elia N, Lysakowski C, et al. Benefit and risk of intrathecal morphine without local anaesthetic in patients undergoing major surgery: Meta-analysis of randomized trials. *BJA.* 2009;102:156–162.
255. Katz J, Kavanagh BP, Sandler AN, et al. Preemptive analgesia. *Anesthesiology.* 1992;77:439–446.
256. Bong CL, Samuel M, Ng JM, et al. Effects of preemptive epidural analgesia on post-thoracotomy pain. *J Cardiothorac Vasc Anesth.* 2005;19:786–793.
257. Fiorelli A, Vicidomini G, Laperuta P, et al. Pre-emptive local analgesia in video assisted thoracosic surgery sympathectomy. *Eur J Cardiothorac Surg.* 2010;37:588–593.
258. Detterbeck FC. Subpleural catheter placement for pain relief after thoracoscopic resection. *Ann Thorac Surg.* 2006;81:1552–1553.
259. Gotoda Y, Kambara N, Sakai T, et al. The morbidity, time course and predictive factors for persistent post-thoracotomy pain. *Eur J Pain.* 2001;5:89–96.
260. Hutter J, Miller K, Moritz E. Chronic sequels after thoracoscopic procedures for benign diseases. *Eur J Cardiothoracic Surg.* 2000;17:687–690.
261. Ochroch EA, Gottschalk A, Troxel AB, et al. Women suffer more short and long-term pain than men after major thoracotomy. *Clin J Pain.* 2006;22:491–498.
262. Gottschalk A, Cohen S, Yang S, et al. Preventing and treating pain after thoracic surgery. *Anesthesiology.* 2006;104:594–600.
263. Wildgaard K, Ravn J, Kehlet H. Chronic post-thoracotomy pain: a critical review of pathogenic mechanisms and strategies for prevention. *Eur J Cardiothorac Surg.* 2009;36:170–180.
264. Wildgard K, Ravn J, Nikolajsen L, et al. Consequences of persistent pain after lung cancer surgery: a nationwide questionnaire study. *Acta Anaesthesiol Scand.* 2011;55:60–68.
265. Guastella V, Mick G, Soriano C, et al. A prospective study of neuropathic pain induced by thoracotomy: incidence, clinical description, and diagnosis. *Pain.* 2011;152:74–81.
266. Khelemsky Y, Noto C. Preventing post-thoracotomy pain syndrome. *Mt Sinai J Med.* 2012;79:133–139.
267. Mongardon N, Pinton-Connet C, Szekely B, et al. Assessment of chronic pain after thoracotomy: a 1 year prevalence study. *Clin J Pain.* 2011;27:677–681.
268. Goyal GN, Gupta D, Jain R, et al. Peripheral nerve field stimulation for intractable post-thoracotomy scar pain not relieved by conventional treatment. *Pain Pract.* 2010;10:366–369.
269. Steegers MA, Snik DM, Verhagen AF, et al. Only half of the chronic pain after thoracic surgery shows a neuropathic component. *J Pain.* 2008;9:955–961.
270. Kotemane NC, Gapinath N, Vaja R. Analgesic techniques following thoracic surgery: a survey of United Kingdom practice. *Eur J Anaesthesiol.* 2010;27:897–899.
271. Demmy TL, Nwagu C, Solan P, et al. Chest-tube delivered bupivacaine improves pain and decreases opioid use after thoracoscopy. *Ann Thorac Surg.* 2009;87:1040–1046.
272. Kaplowitz J, Papadakos PJ. Acute pain management for video-assisted thoracoscopic surgery: An update. *J Cardiothorac Vasc Anesth.* 2012;26(2):312–321.
273. Fibla JJ, Molis L, Mier JM, et al. The efficacy of paravertebral block using a catheter technique for postoperative analgesia in thoracoscopic surgery: A randomized trial. *Eur J Cardiothorac Surg.* 2011;40(4):907–911.
274. Manion SC, Brennan TJ. Thoracic epidural analgesia and acute pain management. *Anesthesiology.* 2011;115:181–188.
275. Neustein SM. Reexpansion pulmonary edema. *J Cardiothorac Vasc Anesth.* 2007;21:887–891.
276. Beck-Nielsen J, Sorensen HR, Alstrup P. Atrial fibrillation following thoracotomy for non-cardiac cases, in particular, cancer of the lung. *Acta Med Scand.* 1973;193:425–429.
277. Ritchie J, Bowe P, Gibbons JRP. Prophylactic digitalization for thoracotomy: a reassessment. *Ann Thorac Surg.* 1990;50:86–88.
278. Ciriaco P, Mazzone P, Canneto B, et al. Supraventricular arrhythmia following lung resection for non-small-cell lung cancer and its treatment with amiodarone. *Eur J Cardiothorac Surg.* 2000;18:12–16.
279. Gopaldas RR, Bakaeen FG, Dao TK, et al. Video-assisted thoracoscopic versus open thoracotomy lobectomy in a cohort of 13,619 patients. *Ann Thorac Surg.* 2010;89:1563–1570.

39 Anesthesia for Cardiac Surgery

NIKOLAOS J. SKUBAS • ADAM D. LICHTMAN • CINDY J. WANG • AARTI SHARMA • STEPHEN J. THOMAS

Introduction
Coronary Artery Disease
   Myocardial Oxygen Demand
   Myocardial Oxygen Supply
   Coronary Blood Flow
   Hemodynamic Goals
   Monitoring for Ischemia
   Selection of Anesthetic
   Opioids
   Inhalation Anesthetics
   Intravenous Sedative Hypnotics
   Treatment of Ischemia
Valvular Heart Disease
   Aortic Stenosis
   Hypertrophic Cardiomyopathy
   Aortic Insufficiency
   Mitral Stenosis
   Mitral Regurgitation
Aortic Diseases
   Aortic Dissection
   Aortic Aneurysm
Cardiopulmonary Bypass
   Circuits
   Oxygenators
   Pumps
   Heat Exchanger
   Prime
   Anticoagulation
   Blood Conservation in Cardiac Surgery
   Myocardial Protection
Preoperative and Intraoperative Management
   Current Drug Therapy
   Physical Examination
   Premedication
   Monitoring
   Selection of Anesthetic Drugs
   Intraoperative Management
Minimally Invasive Cardiac Surgery
Postoperative Considerations
   Bring Backs
   Tamponade
   Pain Management
Anesthesia for Children with Congenital Heart Disease
   Preoperative Evaluation
   Premedication
   Monitoring
   Anesthetic and Intraoperative Management
   Tracheal Extubation and Postoperative Ventilation
   Hybrid Procedures in Pediatric Cardiac Surgery

KEY POINTS

1. When treating myocardial ischemia, decreasing O_2 demand is more important than modifying O_2 supply.
2. The critical factors that modify coronary blood flow are the perfusion pressure and vascular tone of the coronary circulation, the time available for perfusion (determined mainly by heart rate), the severity of intraluminal obstructions, and the presence of (any) collateral circulation.
3. Slow rate, small chamber size, and adequate perfusion pressure are the goals in patients with coronary artery disease.
4. The pulmonary artery catheter is not a reliably monitor for detection of myocardial ischemia.
5. There is no "ideal" anesthetic in cardiac surgery.
6. In aortic stenosis, a preload-dependent, hypertrophic ventricle requires adequate diastolic time and perfusion pressure.
7. In chronic aortic insufficiency, a dilated ventricle requires increased preload and decreased afterload.
8. In mitral stenosis, the left ventricle is "lazy" and "underused" and requires a slow heart rate to fill.
9. In mitral regurgitation, a preload-dependent and dilated left ventricle benefits from afterload reduction and fast heart rate.
10. The most critical factor governing the selection and dose of the anesthetics and adjuvants is the degree of ventricular dysfunction.
11. Fast-track anesthetic techniques depend on higher concentration of inspired volatile agents, use of vasoactive medications (β-blockers), and smaller doses of benzodiazepines and opioids.
12. The combination of systolic systemic and diastolic pulmonary pressures characterizes the performance of the left ventricle, and the combination of systolic pulmonary and central venous pressures characterizes the performance of the right ventricle.

Introduction

Anesthetizing patients who undergo cardiac surgery is exciting, intellectually challenging, and emotionally rewarding. The cardiac anesthesiologist should have a thorough understanding of normal and altered cardiac physiology, cardiovascular and anesthetic medications pharmacology, and be familiar with the physiologic alterations associated with cardiopulmonary bypass (CPB) and the surgical procedures. This chapter presents a brief overview of the critical physiologic and technical considerations during cardiac surgical procedures.

Coronary Artery Disease

The prevention or treatment of myocardial ischemia during coronary artery bypass graft (CABG) surgery decreases the incidence of perioperative myocardial infarction. The hemodynamic management should avoid factors that increase myocardial oxygen demand ($M\dot{V}O_2$), particularly during the vulnerable pre-CPB period, while optimizing oxygen delivery to the myocardium, since it is well recognized that most ischemic events occur with minimal or no change in $M\dot{V}O_2$.[1,2] The determinants of myocardial oxygen supply and demand are shown in Figure 39-1 and are also discussed in Chapter 12, Cardiac Anatomy and Physiology.

Myocardial Oxygen Demand

The principal determinants of $M\dot{V}O_2$ are wall tension and contractility.[3] According to Laplace law, wall tension is directly proportional to intracavitary pressure and radius and inversely proportional to wall thickness. Therefore, $M\dot{V}O_2$ can be reduced by interventions that decrease intraventricular pressure and prevent or promptly treat ventricular distention.

Myocardial Oxygen Supply

1 Increases in myocardial oxygen requirements can be met only by increasing the coronary blood flow. Arterial blood oxygen content and myocardial oxygen extraction are infrequent reasons for intraoperative myocardial ischemia because oxygenation and blood volume are usually well controlled during anesthesia. In addition, since the coronary sinus blood is desaturated (P_{O_2} in the range of 15 to 20 mmHg), further oxygen extraction is inadequate to meet a significantly increased $M\dot{V}O_2$. Therefore, the principal mechanism for matching oxygen supply to alterations in $M\dot{V}O_2$ is exquisite regulation and control of coronary blood flow.

Coronary Blood Flow

2 The critical factors that modify coronary blood flow are the perfusion pressure and vascular tone of the coronary circulation, the time available for perfusion (determined mainly by heart rate), the severity of intraluminal obstructions, and the presence of (any) collateral circulation. The area most vulnerable to ischemia

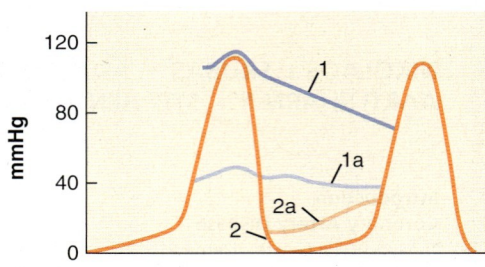

Figure 39-2 The pressure relationships between the aorta (1) and the left ventricle (2) determine coronary perfusion pressure. In coronary artery disease, myocardial perfusion may be compromised by decreased pressure distal to a significant stenosis (1a) (not quantifiable clinically) and/or by an increase in left ventricular end-diastolic pressure (2a). (Adapted from Gorlin R. *Coronary Artery Disease*. Philadelphia, PA: WB Saunders; 1976:75, with permission.)

is the subendocardium of the left ventricle (LV), because it is directly exposed to the intracavitary pressure and because it has the greatest metabolic requirements due to its greater systolic shortening than other areas of the myocardium.[4]

Perfusion of the LV subendocardium takes place almost entirely during diastole, whereas the right ventricular subendocardium is perfused in diastole and systole, assuming pulmonary hypertension is not present. This temporal disparity is explained by the different intraventricular pressures developing during systole.

The LV coronary perfusion pressure is often defined as the gradient between aortic diastolic (or mean) pressure and LV diastolic pressure (LVDP; usually approximated by the pulmonary artery occlusion pressure). In the presence of intraluminal obstruction or increased myocardial vascular tone, this pressure gradient is reduced (Fig. 39-2). A low LVDP is ideal for improving perfusion (higher pressure gradient) and reducing $M\dot{V}O_2$ (decreased LV volume and wall tension). On the other hand, increasing perfusion pressure by raising the aortic pressure will increase $M\dot{V}O_2$. However, this is not as important, when one considers that tachycardia is the most important cause of intraoperative and perioperative ischemia.

Alterations in the tone of the small intramyocardial arterioles regulate diastolic vascular resistance, allowing the matching of oxygen supply with $M\dot{V}O_2$ over a wide range of perfusion pressures.[5] The difference between auto regulated (basal) flow, and blood flow available under conditions of maximal vasodilation is termed *coronary vascular reserve* and is normally three to five times higher than basal flow. As epicardial coronary stenosis becomes more pronounced, progressive vasodilation of these resistance vessels allows preservation of basal flow, but at the cost of reduced reserve. Once perfusion pressure decreases to below 40 mmHg, autoregulation of subendocardial coronary flow is lost. Whenever $M\dot{V}O_2$ increases above available reserve, signs, symptoms, and metabolic evidence of ischemia develop.

Reversible ischemia may be caused by an inadequate supply of oxygen to the myocardium and/or the inability to respond to increased $M\dot{V}O_2$. Irreversible injury to the myocardium can occur if coronary blood flow is occluded for longer than 20 minutes, leading to myocardial cell death and necrosis. Supply-induced ischemia results from a transient coronary occlusion from vasospasm or temporary thrombus that leads to transmural ischemia and decreased LV compliance. Demand-induced ischemia results from the inability to increase coronary blood flow and oxygen delivery to the myocardium in response to increases in $M\dot{V}O_2$. In either case, the result is subendocardial ischemia and decreased LV compliance.[6]

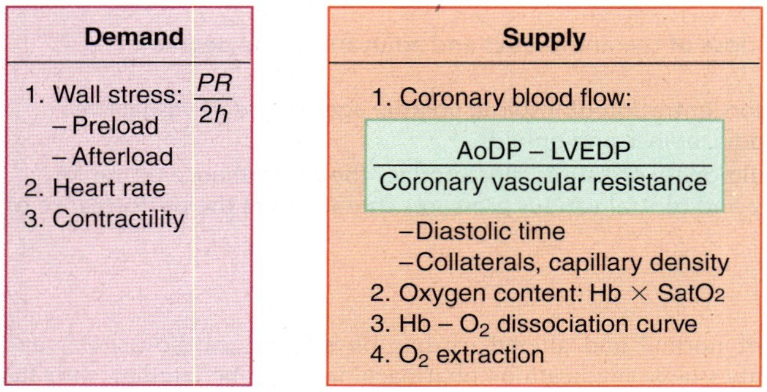

Demand	Supply

1. Wall stress: $\frac{PR}{2h}$
  – Preload
  – Afterload
2. Heart rate
3. Contractility
	1. Coronary blood flow:
	  $\frac{AoDP - LVEDP}{Coronary\ vascular\ resistance}$
	  – Diastolic time
	  – Collaterals, capillary density
	2. Oxygen content: $Hb \times SatO_2$
	3. $Hb - O_2$ dissociation curve
	4. O_2 extraction

Figure 39-1 Determinants of myocardial oxygen balance. P, intracavitary pressure; R, ventricular radius; h, wall thickness; AoDP, diastolic arterial pressure; LVEDP, left ventricular end-diastolic pressure; Hb, hemoglobin; $SatO_2$, arterial oxygen saturation.

In reversible ischemia, the myocardium remains viable and can be differentiated into stunned or hibernating myocardium. Stunning refers to a state of abnormal function that occurs after an acute, discrete episode of ischemia. No cell death occurs in stunning, but it may take several days or longer for the myocardium to recover, even though adequate blood flow has been restored. Hibernating myocardium refers to a chronic state of reduced coronary blood flow and abnormal function usually secondary to a fixed stenosis. In response to decreased oxygen supply, hibernating myocardial cells downregulate their metabolism and oxygen demand to maintain viability.[7]

Dead myocardium and viable myocardium (stunned or hibernating) may both appear hypokinetic on echocardiography making the two difficult to distinguish. Studies such as single photon emission CT (SPECT) or low-dose dobutamine echocardiography can help to differentiate viable myocardium that may benefit from revascularization. The current data for revascularization in patients with CAD and LV systolic dysfunction remains inconclusive with the most recent guidelines for CABG surgery published in 2011 recommending that the choice of revascularization in these patients should be based on clinical variables such as coronary anatomy, presence of diabetes mellitus or chronic kidney disease, magnitude of LV systolic dysfunction, patient preferences, clinical judgment, and consultation between the interventional cardiologist and the cardiac surgeon.[8]

Hemodynamic Goals

The primary goal of any successful cardiac anesthetic is prevention of myocardial ischemia and prompt identification and treatment of new ischemic episodes. The anesthetic interventions are geared at reducing and controlling the factors (Table 39-1) that increase $M\dot{V}O_2$ (heart rate, contractility, and wall tension). The first intervention is to optimize coronary blood flow, that is, maintain coronary perfusion pressure, while keeping in mind that the peripheral arterial systolic pressure is different (usually higher) than the aortic root pressure, and to increase diastolic time. Thus, the cardiac goals for patients with coronary artery disease are slow (heart rate), small (ventricular size), and well perfused (adequate blood pressure). Preoperative medications that may benefit coronary patients include statins[9] and angiotensin-converting enzyme inhibitors (to stabilize the atherosclerotic plaque) as well as β-blockers (to control heart rate).[10] Volatile anesthetics offer cardioprotection when applied prior to or even after the ischemic insult. A reduction in mortality and morbidity has been shown in patients undergoing CABG and aortic valve (AV) surgery. However, it is very difficult to associate these beneficial effects to pre- or postconditioning mechanisms.[11]

Monitoring for Ischemia

The continuous analysis and display of the ST segment in multiple leads (most commonly leads II and V_4 or V_5) is considered standard and recommended by the 2011 AHA/ACCF practice guidelines.[8] Patients likely to develop right ventricular ischemia or those with disease of the right coronary artery might benefit from monitoring of leads V_{4R} or V_{5R}.

Favorable conditions for $M\dot{V}O_2$ are those of lower heart rate and higher blood pressure rather than tachycardia and hypotension. Neither the ratio of mean arterial pressure over heart rate nor the diastolic to systolic pressure–time index is any more predictive or reliable than the product of heart rate and pressure (RPP),[12] which was once, but no longer, considered a reliable correlate of $M\dot{V}O_2$.

Certain changes of the invasively monitored hemodynamic waveforms with a pulmonary artery catheter (PAC) are suggestive of adverse hemodynamics. A sudden elevation in mean pulmonary artery occlusion pressure indicates LV dysfunction, which may be differentiated further into (i) primarily systolic dysfunction if there is an increase in the height of v wave indicating left atrial pressure hypertension that is associated with ischemia-induced papillary muscle dysfunction and/or mitral regurgitation (MR), or (ii) primarily diastolic dysfunction if there is a large a wave indicating decreased LV compliance. PAC-based monitoring of pressures, saturation of mixed venous blood in oxygen, and thermodilution cardiac output are common perioperative practices in cardiac surgery centers.[13,14] The 2011 AHA/ACCF CABG practice guidelines recommend the insertion of a PAC in a hemodynamically compromised patient, while recognizing that center-specific practices vary.[8] The PAC may be of little value as a monitor of myocardial ischemia[15] or indicate abnormal regional myocardial wall function,[16] whereas high-risk cardiac surgical patients may be safely managed without routine use of a PAC.[17] Compared with transesophageal echocardiography (TEE), PAC predicted normal left ventricular function well, but performed poorly in judging preload and ventricular dysfunction in the management of critically ill patients in the intensive care unit (ICU).[18] Other studies showed no benefit from PACs in high-risk surgical patients,[19,20] but these studies may not reflect the current era of perioperative management of such patients. It is difficult to determine the value of PAC in diagnosis and treatment when the physician's ability for correct interpretation of PAC information is still in doubt.[21] The most recent American Society of Anesthesiologists Practice Guidelines concluded that the evidence regarding the benefit that cardiac surgery patients receive from PAC is conflicting.[22]

Since its introduction in the 1980s, TEE has become an invaluable diagnostic and monitoring tool during cardiac surgery. TEE permits assessment of ventricular volume, global and regional function, estimation and quantitation of valvular pathology, measurement of valve gradients and calculation of filling pressures, visualization of the thoracic aorta, and detection of intracardiac air. The recent introduction of real-time three-dimensional TEE

Table 39-1 Coronary Artery Disease: Hemodynamic Goals

Preload	↓	A smaller heart size (TEE dimensions) decreases wall tension and PADP (LVEDP) and increases perfusion pressure gradient
Afterload	Maintain	Hypertension is better than hypotension
Contractility	↓	If LV function is normal
Rate	↓	
Rhythm	Sinus	Correct arrhythmias
$M\dot{V}O_2$		Monitor for and treat "supply"-related disturbances
Post-CPB		No need for increased PADP (LVEDP)

↑, increase; ↓, decrease; PADP, pulmonary artery diastolic pressure; LVEDP, left ventricular end-diastolic pressure; $M\dot{V}O_2$, myocardial oxygen consumption; CPB, cardiopulmonary bypass; TEE, transesophageal echocardiography.

introduced a real revolution in perioperative imaging. Practice guidelines for perioperative TEE have been recently published by the ASA.[23] Experienced cardiac anesthesiologists who are supported by continuous quality programs perform comprehensive TEE studies[24] and interpret TEE examinations at a level comparable with physicians whose primary practice is echocardiography.[25]

The American Society of Echocardiography/Society of Cardiovascular Anesthesiologists task force for intraoperative echocardiography has published guidelines for performing a comprehensive intraoperative echocardiographic examination.[26] These recommendations describe a series of standard tomographic views of the heart and great vessels that should be included in a complete intraoperative echocardiographic examination. With experience, a thorough examination can be performed in less than 10 minutes.

Selection of Anesthetic

[5] There is no one "ideal" anesthetic for patients with coronary artery disease. The choice of anesthetic should be based on known hemodynamic, pharmacologic, and pharmacokinetic effects of each drug as they apply to the particular patient, the experience of the anesthesiologist, and the relative cost–benefit of each agent, and should depend primarily on the extent of pre-existing myocardial dysfunction. If drugs are titrated to the desired effect, cardiovascular changes are minimized in healthy, as well as in patients with severe myocardial depression to facilitate a safe anesthetic. Most patients with mild or even moderate dysfunction may benefit from some degree of myocardial depression, which leads to decreased oxygen demand, and may alleviate or at least reduce episodes of ischemia.

Early extubation is common practice and is achieved by multiple approaches.[27,28] Volatile anesthetics with low-dose narcotics or total intravenous anesthesia with short-acting drugs (e.g., midazolam, alfentanil, remifentanil, propofol) have been used to achieve early extubation. The increased use of benzodiazepines and volatile agents has been associated with low incidence of awareness.[29] Intraoperative clinical variables, such as inotropic requirements or transfusion for bleeding, should be considered in the timing of postoperative extubation after fast-track cardiac surgery.[30] In general, the use of low-dose opioid based general anesthesia and time-directed protocols for fast-track interventions have similar risks of mortality and major postoperative complications to conventional (not fast-track) care, and appear to be safe in patients considered to be at low to moderate risk. However, despite a reduced time to extubation and shortened length of stay in the ICU, fast-track extubation protocols have not been shown to reduce the hospital length of stay.[31]

Opioids

The primary advantages of opioids are lack of myocardial depression, maintenance of a stable hemodynamic state, and reduction of heart rate. The current practice is to supplement the opioid with benzodiazepines and volatile agents. The planned time of extubation is now one of the major factors determining the selection and dosage of opioid. Shorter-acting opioids (sufentanil and remifentanil) produce equally rapid extubation, similar ICU stay, and similar costs to fentanyl. Thus, any of these opioids can be used for fast-track cardiac surgery.[32] The beneficial cardioprotective and anti-inflammatory effects of morphine have been reconsidered recently,[33,34] bringing back into the foray the opioid that reinvigorated the practice of cardiac anesthesia.[35]

Inhalation Anesthetics

The desirable features of volatile anesthetics include dose-dependent hemodynamic changes, easy reversibility, titratable myocardial depression, amnesia, and suppression of sympathetic responses to surgical stress and CPB. Volatile anesthetics protect the myocardium from ischemia and reperfusion injury and reduce myocardial infarct size.[36] This beneficial effect has been shown when volatile anesthetics are administered before a period of prolonged ischemia ("anesthetic preconditioning") as well as during reperfusion ("anesthetic postconditioning").[37] However, it is difficult to ascertain whether these laboratory-proven benefits have contributed to improved myocardial protection in clinical practice.[38] An anesthetic based primarily on volatile agents may cause systemic hypotension (whether induced by decreased contractility or vasodilation), which may compromise the oxygen supply and lack of postoperative analgesia. Instead, balanced techniques based on combinations of opioids and any of the volatile anesthetics are advantageous with minimal untoward effects.

Isoflurane is a coronary vasodilator, as are the other volatile anesthetics (although to a lesser degree). This dose-related effect is clinically insignificant in doses less than 1 MAC. Clinical studies using isoflurane to clinical rather than pharmacologic end points have not shown increased episodes of ischemia or a worsened outcome.[39] Desflurane and sevoflurane have the fastest recovery of all volatile anesthetics. Desflurane has a rapid uptake and distribution, allowing it to be useful in cases in which hemodynamic changes mandate rapid changes in anesthetic depth. It has a cardiac profile similar to that of isoflurane. When studying sympathetic nervous system activity, Helman et al.[40] found an increase in sympathetic activity and myocardial ischemia in patients anesthetized with desflurane as the sole anesthetic agent for coronary artery bypass surgery compared with patients anesthetized with sufentanil. Compared with isoflurane, in a technique combining fentanyl with the inhalational anesthetic, sevoflurane had an acceptable cardiovascular profile prior to CPB and similar outcome data.[41]

Intravenous Sedative Hypnotics

An alternative adjuvant anesthetic to a low-dose opioid technique is a titratable intravenous infusion of a short-acting sedative, such as midazolam,[42] propofol, or dexmedetomidine.[43] These can be continued postoperatively in the ICU and afford a predictable and fairly rapid awakening after discontinuation.[44] When compared with volatile anesthetics, propofol was associated with less favorable cardiac function, higher need for inotropic support, and elevated plasma troponins after cardiac surgery in elderly patients.[45,46]

Treatment of Ischemia

The use of anesthetics or vasoactive drugs is aimed at decreasing heart size, decreasing heart rate, and improving myocardial perfusion pressure. The principal vasoactive drugs are nitrates, β-blockers, peripheral vasoconstrictors, and calcium entry blockers. Clinical scenarios for their use are given in Table 39-2. Volatile anesthetics can also be used to control blood pressure and reduce contractility.

Nitrates

Nitroglycerin (TNG) is the drug of choice for the treatment of acute myocardial ischemia. Its action is via systemic venodilation

Table 39-2 Treatment of Intraoperative Ischemia	
Clinical Manifestation	**Suggested Intervention**
Increased Demand	
↑ Heart rate	Treat usual reasons including inadequate anesthesia, administer β-blocker
↑ Blood pressure	↑ Anesthetic depth
↑ PCWP	Nitroglycerin
Decreased Supply	
↓ Heart rate	Atropine, pacing
↓ Blood pressure	↓ Anesthetic depth, administer vasoconstrictor
↑ PCWP	Nitroglycerin, inotrope
No Changes	
	Nitroglycerin, calcium channel blockers, consider heparin

↑, increase(d); ↓, decrease(d); PCWP, pulmonary capillary wedge pressure.

that decreases LV preload, wall tension, $M\dot{V}O_2$, and coronary arterial dilation, which is operative in both stenosed coronaries and collateral beds.[47] There is no evidence for the prophylactic use of TNG for prevention of either intraoperative ischemic episodes or postoperative cardiac complications.[48] At higher doses, TNG dilates systemic arteries and may cause systemic hypotension, which is counterproductive for treatment of myocardial ischemia, as is compensatory tachycardia that may increase $M\dot{V}O_2$. The recommended TNG dose is 0.5 to 3 µg/kg/min and is reduced in the presence of hepatic and/or renal disease. TNG may cause methemoglobinemia especially in patients with methemoglobin reductase deficiency; this complication is more likely when large doses are administered over a prolonged time.[49]

Sodium Nitroprusside

Sodium nitroprusside (SNP) decreases peripheral vascular resistance via its metabolic or spontaneous reduction to nitric oxide. Similar to TNG, SNP improves ventricular compliance in the ischemic myocardium. The recommended SNP dose is 0.5 to 3 µg/kg/min and should be reduced in the presence of hepatic and/or renal disease. Adverse effects include cyanide and thiocyanate toxicity, rebound hypertension, intracranial hypertension, blood coagulation abnormalities, increased pulmonary shunting, and hypothyroidism. In vitro findings suggest that cardiac surgical patients may be at increased risk of cyanide toxicity in response to the perioperative administration of SNP.[50] Cyanide is a metabolite of SNP; toxic blood levels (>100 µg/dL) occur when more than 1.0 mg/kg SNP is administered within 2 hours or when more than 0.5 mg/kg/hr is administered within 24 hours. The presenting signs of cyanide toxicity include the triad of elevated mixed venous O_2 ($S\bar{v}O_2$), increasing requirements for SNP (tachyphylaxis), and metabolic acidosis.[51] In addition, the patient may appear flushed. Greater risk of cyanide toxicity exists in patients who are nutritionally deficient in cobalamine (vitamin B_{12} compounds) or in dietary substances containing sulfur. Measurement of blood cyanide and pH will enable detection of abnormalities in high-risk patients for whom larger than recommended amounts of SNP have been used (8 to 10 µg/kg/min). Treatment should consist of discontinuing infusion, administering 100% O_2, administering amyl nitrate (inhaler) or intravenous sodium nitrite and intravenous thiosulfate, except in those patients with abnormal renal function, for whom hydroxocobalamin is recommended. Circulating levels of thiocyanate increase when renal function is compromised, and central nervous system abnormalities result when thiocyanate levels reach 5 to 10 µg/dL. Lowering the SNP dose requirement or, better, replacing SNP with nicardipine, metoprolol, or esmolol reduces or eliminates the consequent accumulation of cyanide. SNP deteriorates in the presence of light and the solution container should be wrapped in nontransparent material. Other drugs should not be infused in the same solution as SNP.

Vasoconstrictors

Vasoconstrictors (phenylephrine, norepinephrine, vasopressin) are useful adjuncts in the prevention and treatment of ischemia because they increase systemic blood pressure, thereby improving coronary perfusion pressure, albeit at the expense of increasing afterload and perhaps $M\dot{V}O_2$. In addition, concomitant venoconstriction increases venous return and LV preload. TNG is sometimes added to counteract any increase in preload. In most situations, the increase in coronary perfusion pressure more than offsets any increase in wall tension. Peripheral vasoconstriction is needed during episodes of systemic hypotension, especially those caused by reduced surgical stimulation or drug-induced vasodilation. No one vasoconstrictor is superior to all others. Occasionally, a combination of vasoconstrictors (e.g., norepinephrine and vasopressin) may be needed to achieve the desired blood pressure.[52]

β-Blockers

β-Adrenergic blockade improves myocardial oxygen balance by decreasing the chronotropic and inotropic state. Indications for β-blockers include treatment of sinus tachycardia not caused by light anesthesia or hypovolemia, prophylaxis of, and slowing the ventricular response to, supraventricular dysrhythmias, hyperdynamic states, and control of ventricular dysrhythmias.[53,54] The use of β-blockers should aim at reducing the heart rate and increasing the diastolic filling time without, at the same time, decreasing the perfusion pressure and cardiac output. These therapy targets are even more important, since the POISE study revealed that death and stroke were side effects of β-blockers.[55,56] Nowadays intravenous preparations include, metoprolol, labetalol, esmolol and rarely propranolol. Propranolol is a nonselective β-blocker with an elimination half-life of 4 to 6 hours. Metoprolol is similar to propranolol but has the purported advantage of $β_1$-selectivity and is less likely to trigger bronchospasm in patients with reactive airway disease. Labetalol combines β-blocking properties with those of α-blockade and is useful in treating hyperdynamic and hypertensive situations. Esmolol is a short-acting $β_1$-blocker that is cardioselective, with a half-life of only 9.5 minutes. It is particularly useful in treating transient increases in heart rate owing to episodic sympathetic stimulation.

Calcium Channel Blockers

Calcium channel blockers depress contractility, reduce coronary and systemic vascular tone, decrease sinoatrial node firing rate, and impede atrioventricular conduction[57,58] at a remarkably variable degree. The negative inotropic effect is greatest with verapamil and less with nifedipine, diltiazem, and nicardipine (in decreasing order). Verapamil is particularly useful in the treatment of supraventricular tachycardia for slowing the ventricular response in atrial fibrillation and/or flutter, but its myocardial depressant effects limit its usefulness. In patients with reduced myocardial function, intravenous diltiazem is preferred. Calcium channel blockers have been found to have cardioprotective effects during reperfusion. Nicardipine in particular has coronary antispasmodic and vasodilatory effects more than systemic arterial vasodilatory effects.[59]

Nifedipine, and nicardipine are prominent systemic arterial dilators and are used in the treatment of postoperative hypertension in cardiac surgical patients.[60] The newer agent clevidipine was a better antihypertensive agent than SNP or TNG and was equivalent to nicardipine.[61] Magnesium has coronary arterial dilating properties, reduces the size of myocardial infarction in the setting of acute ischemia, and decreases mortality associated with infarction.[62] In addition, it is an antiarrhythmic and minimizes myocardial reperfusion injury. Although magnesium was found to prevent atrial fibrillation in coronary artery surgery,[63] in patients treated with β-blockers, the addition of prophylactic IV magnesium did not reduce the incidence of atrial arrhythmias.[64]

The most recent guidelines for CABG surgery were published in 2011.[65] They recommend:
- Volatile agent–based anesthetic aimed at early tracheal extubation
- Adequate perioperative analgesia
- Anesthetic care by a fellowship-trained or experienced, board-certified, TEE-trained anesthesiologist
- Utilization of intraoperative TEE for evaluation of acute, persistent, and life-threatening hemodynamic changes, for monitoring of ventricular function and regional wall motion abnormalities, and for concomitant valvular surgery
- Augmentation of the coronary arterial perfusion pressure to reduce the risk of perioperative myocardial ischemia and infarction
- Administration of β-blockers to reduce the incidence (or complications) of atrial fibrillation and cardiac mortality (particularly in patients with LVEF >30%)
- Administration of angiotensin-converting enzyme (ACE) inhibitors or angiotensin receptor blockers perioperatively
- Selective use of PAC
- Multimodal approach for management of perioperative bleeding and transfusion, based on use of lysine analogues, point-of-care testing, discontinuation of antiplatelet medications for at least 5 days preoperatively, among others.

The reader is encouraged to consult the full document at http://circ.ahajournals.org/content/124/23/e652.

Valvular Heart Disease

Alterations in loading conditions are the initial physiologic burdens imposed by valvular heart lesions, both stenotic and regurgitant: LV afterload is increased in aortic stenosis (AS), LV preload is increased in aortic insufficiency and MR, and both are decreased in mitral stenosis, whereas the right ventricle (RV) faces progressively increasing left atrial and pulmonary artery pressure. Compensatory mechanisms consist of chamber enlargement, myocardial hypertrophy, and variations in vascular tone and level of sympathetic activity. These mechanisms in turn induce secondary alterations, including altered ventricular compliance, development of myocardial ischemia, cardiac dysrhythmias, and progressive myocardial dysfunction.

Myocardial contractility in patients with MR is often transiently depressed but may progress to irreversible impairment even in the absence of clinical symptoms. Conversely, the patient with AS may complain of dyspnea, not because of impaired systolic function, but because the reduced ventricular compliance causes left atrial hypertension and pulmonary vascular congestion.

The patient presenting for valve repair or replacement may have pulmonary hypertension, significant ventricular dysfunction, and chronic arrhythmias. For a safe anesthetic, understanding the altered loading conditions, preserving the compensatory mechanisms, maintaining circulatory homeostasis, and anticipating problems that may arise during and after valve surgery are important. In this section, we briefly describe the pathophysiology, desirable hemodynamic profile, and other pertinent anesthetic considerations for each valvular lesion.

TEE has become the standard of care in the perioperative management of patients undergoing valve surgery. TEE can further refine the preoperative diagnosis, identify valvular pathology and the mechanism of disease, and quantify the degree of stenosis and/or regurgitation. A detailed review of the perioperative role of TEE is presented in Chapter 27.

Aortic Stenosis

AS is the most common valvular disease in the United States. In a normal adult, the AV is composed of three semilunar cusps attached to the wall of the aorta. The normal AV area is 2 to 4 cm^2. The AV cusps are suspended from the sinuses of Valsalva. The AV cusps and the corresponding sinuses are named according to their relation to the coronary ostia: left, right, and noncoronary (opposite the interatrial septum). On the ventricular side of the AV is the oval-shaped LV outflow tract (LVOT). Its borders are the inferior surface of the anterior leaflet of the mitral valve, the interventricular septum, and the LV wall. The normal diameter of the LVOT is 2.2 ± 0.2 cm.

Calcific AV disease has many similar features with coronary artery disease. What in the past was thought to be "degenerative" is a disease continuum, similar to atherosclerosis. The mechanism is the increased mechanical stress (higher on the aortic side of AV cusps, in the flexion area) that causes endothelial disruption and leads to lipoprotein deposition, chronic inflammation, and cusp calcification.[66] Increased calcification eventually leads to cusp immobility and outflow obstruction. Clinical factors associated with AS include older age, male gender, smoking, hypertension, and hyperlipidemia. Patients with bicuspid AV (increased mechanical stress) or with altered mineral metabolism (Paget disease, renal failure) have a higher prevalence of calcific AS disease. Rheumatic disease (an autoimmune disease, rarely seen in developed countries, leading to calcification and fusion along the commissures) causes mixed AS and AV regurgitation and usually coexists with mitral valve disease.

Pathophysiology

The classic symptoms of AS are angina (35%), syncope (15%), and dyspnea (50%) and are harbingers of poor outcome (death) within 5, 3, and 2 years, respectively, unless the AV is replaced. The progressive narrowing of the AV area results in chronic obstruction to LV ejection. As LV systolic pressure increases to preserve forward flow, concentric LV hypertrophy, in which the LV wall gradually thickens but the cavity size remains unchanged, is the compensatory response that normalizes the concomitant increase in LV wall tension. Contractility is preserved and ejection fraction is maintained at a normal range until late in the disease process (Fig. 39-3). Signs and symptoms of AS usually occur when the AV orifice is reduced to less than 0.8 to 1.0 cm^2.[67]

The relaxation of the thickened LV walls is slow ("stiff" LV), early diastolic LV filling is delayed, and LA contraction becomes

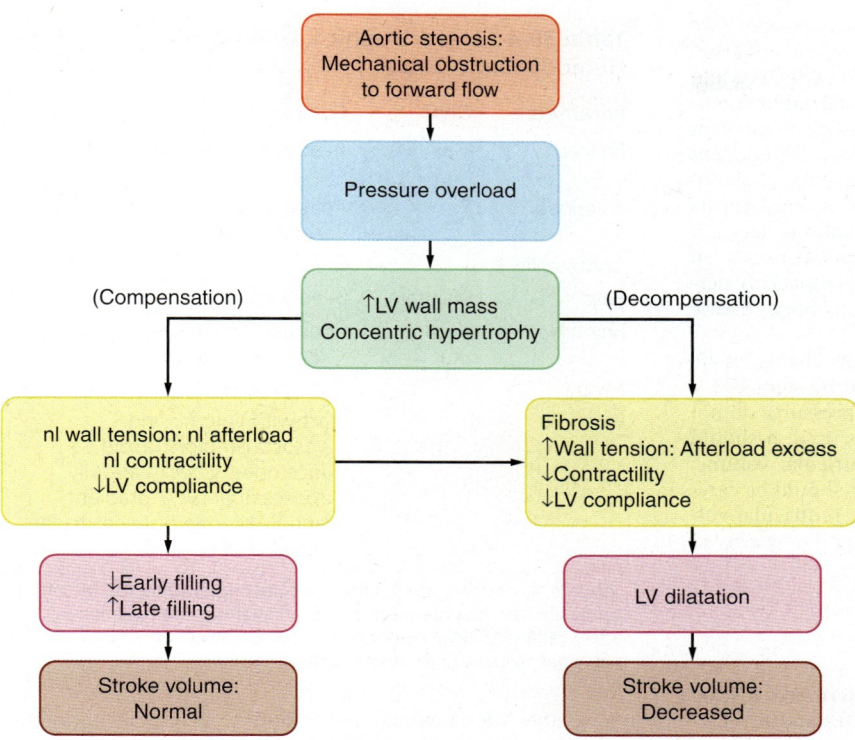

Figure 39-3 Pathophysiology of aortic stenosis. LV, left ventricle; nl, normal.

critical for maintaining adequate stroke volume. In AS, the "atrial kick" may account for up to 30% to 40% of LV end-diastolic volume. The ventricular filling pressure, as reflected by pulmonary capillary wedge pressure, may vary widely with only small changes in ventricular volume (reduced compliance). Additionally, the hypertrophic LV myocardium has increased basal $M\dot{V}O_2$, and demand further increases because of the elevated LV systolic pressure. As the capillary density is often inadequate for the hypertrophic muscle, any reduction in the coronary perfusion pressure (as when the aortic diastolic pressure is decreased and/or the LV filling pressure is increased) may compromise supply and vasodilatory reserve. These are more critical in the presence of coronary artery obstruction. Such AS patients often present with heart failure.

There is an inverse relationship between systolic wall stress (afterload) and LV ejection fraction. In patients with a substantial transvalvular pressure gradient (mean >40 mmHg), AV replacement corrects the afterload excess and improves outcome. In an LV with reduced contractility or decreased stroke volume the transvalvular pressure gradient is less than critical (<40 mmHg: "pseudo" or "low-gradient" AS) despite an echocardiographically stenosed AV. Although the response to pharmacologic intervention with dobutamine may clarify the diagnosis (increased SV and AS: true AS vs. increased AV area: less than severe AS vs. lack of SV increase: LV dysfunction and implications for increased surgical risk), surgical intervention has better long term than medical management alone.[68] In the high surgical risk AS patient, the option of a percutaneous transcatheter AV replacement (TAVR) is accepted as an alternative to surgical AVR.[69]

Anesthetic Considerations

The ideal hemodynamic environment for the patient with AS is summarized in Table 39-3. Noncardiac surgery in patients with asymptomatic severe AS may not be associated with complications, provided that their hemodynamics are appropriately monitored.[70,71] Although some studies report a marked increase in perioperative death and infarction rates, others do not.[72,73] The reasons for these differences are not clear, but

Table 39-3 Aortic Stenosis: Hemodynamic Goals

Parameter	Goal	Comment
Preload	Maintain or ↑	
Afterload	Maintain or ↑	To maintain coronary perfusion gradient
Contractility		Usually not a problem, may require inotropic support if hypotension persists
Rate		Avoid bradycardia (↓ CO) and tachycardia (ischemia)
Rhythm	Sinus	May need cardioversion or β-blockers in non-sinus or fast rhythms
$M\dot{V}O_2$		Treat tachycardia and hypotension (ischemia is an ever-present risk)
Post-CPB ↑ Blood pressure	↑ Contractility ↑ Contractility (suspected myocardial stunning); ↑ blood pressure	

↑, increase(d); ↓, decrease(d); CO, cardiac output; CPB, cardiopulmonary bypass; $M\dot{V}O_2$, myocardial oxygen consumption.

appropriate monitoring and perioperative management are considered essential for safe outcomes in noncardiac surgery.[74]

The perioperative management should aim at (a) avoidance and immediate detection and treatment of systemic arterial hypotension, (b) maintaining coronary perfusion pressure to prevent the vicious cycle of hypotension-induced ischemia, subsequent ventricular dysfunction, and worsening hypotension, (c) avoiding extremes of heart rate, tachycardia as well as, bradycardia (despite an increase in diastolic time the stroke volume does not increase in an LV with concentric hypertrophy, and causes a fall in cardiac output and further hypotension; this is especially pertinent in the elderly or diabetic patient with sinus node disease and reduced sympathetic responses).

Ischemia may be difficult to detect because the characteristic electrocardiographic changes are often obscured by signs of LV hypertrophy and strain, and elevated LV filling pressures do not necessarily reflect increased volume.[68] If TNG is used, it should be titrated to effect with minimal effects on ventricular volume. In the presence of LV dysfunction, nicardipine[75] should be carefully titrated to lower afterload without affecting ventricular volume. The utility of TEE in diagnosing and grading the severity of AS is described in Chapter 27.

Hypertrophic Cardiomyopathy

Hypertrophic cardiomyopathy is a genetically determined disease characterized by histologically abnormal myocytes and myocardial hypertrophy developing a priori, in the absence of a pressure or volume overload. The LV has a relatively small cavity relative to the wall thickness and a hyperdynamic function.[76,77]

Pathophysiology

The physiologic consequences of hypertrophic cardiomyopathy are similar to those detailed for AS and are depicted in Figure 39-4. A subset of patients (20% to 30%) have some degree of subvalvular obstruction (hypertrophic obstructive cardiomyopathy), which may result in an LVOT gradient from a combination of anatomic (systolic septal bulging into the LVOT, malposition of the anterior papillary muscle) and functional (drag forces, and hyperdynamic LV contraction causing a Venturi effect) factors. The LVOT gradient is dynamic in nature and increases when the LV cavity decreases (increased contractility and heart rate or decreased preload or afterload). The rapid blood ejection through the narrowed LVOT area pulls the anterior mitral valve leaflet closer to the septum (systolic anterior motion) and results in a variable MR jet, which, in the absence of organic mitral disease, is directed posteriorly.[78]

In hypertrophic cardiomyopathy the myocardial oxygen balance is tenuous, and angina during exercise occurs even in the absence of coronary artery disease, if the coronary blood flow is unable to meet the demands of the hypertrophied myocardium.

Anesthetic Considerations

Treatment options for hypertrophic cardiomyopathy include pharmacologic "thinning" of the proximal interventricular septum with intracoronary alcohol injection (provided that the diastolic septal thickness at the site of injection is <15 mm), cardiac pacing, and surgical septal myectomy that is aimed to decrease the flow gradient (target is <30 mmHg at rest or <50 mmHg during exercise). The anesthetic management of patients with hypertrophic cardiomyopathy is similar to that for AS and focuses on (a) avoiding bradycardia and tachycardia, (b) maintaining LV filling and avoiding the factors predisposing to outflow tract obstruction or ischemia (Table 39-4), (c) avoiding

Table 39-4 Hypertrophic Cardiomyopathy: Hemodynamic Goals

Parameter	Goal	Comment
Preload	Maintain or ↑	Treat as in aortic stenosis
Afterload	↑	Treat hypotension aggressively with α-adrenergic agonists
Contractility	↓	
Rate	Maintain	β-Blockers
Rhythm	Sinus	Consider atrial pacing modalities (PAC, esophageal)
MVO₂		Not a problem
Post-CPB		Start with volume and vasoconstrictors; avoid inotropes. Check carefully for residual LVOT gradient and SAM; rule out ventricular septal defect

↑, increase; ↓, decrease; LVOT, left ventricular outflow tract; LVEDP, left ventricular end-diastolic pressure; LV, left ventricle; PAC, pulmonary artery catheter; MVO₂, myocardial oxygen consumption; CPB, cardiopulmonary bypass; SAM, systolic anterior motion.

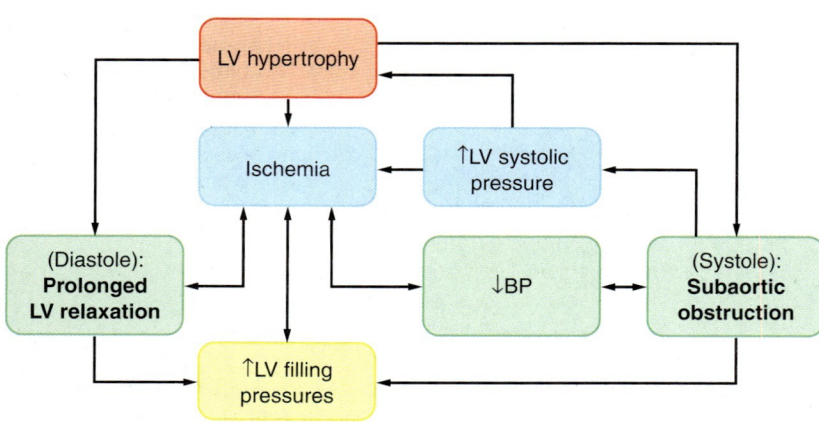

Figure 39-4 Pathophysiology of primary left ventricular (LV) hypertrophy in hypertrophic cardiomyopathy. BP, blood pressure.

increases in myocardial contractility for which the volatile anesthetics are useful, and (d) maintaining sinus rhythm since LV preload is dependent on atrial contraction; if junctional rhythm occurs, these patients may need atrial pacing with a transesophageal pacing probe or a PAC with pacing capability.

Although infrequent, valvular AS may occasionally coexist with hypertrophic cardiomyopathy and may explain unanticipated difficulties in separating from bypass or unexpected increased pressure gradient following a seemingly uncomplicated AV replacement. Nowadays, a comprehensive TEE examination of the LVOT area proximal to the AV should resolve such dilemmas. A dynamic LVOT obstruction may also result following MV repair, if an elongated anterior mitral leaflet is brought closer to the interventricular septum (anterior septal motion observed echocardiographically), and should be similarly treated.[79]

Aortic Insufficiency

Aortic valve insufficiency (AI) is the result of annular dilatation or structural AV cusp lesions. Chronic annular dilatation occurs with aneurysms (Marfan syndrome). Structural AV cusps lesions from calcific degeneration, rheumatic disease, or in bicuspid AV result in abnormal cusp motion and loss of coaptation and eventually AI. Acute AI is caused by bacterial endocarditis, aortic dissection, or trauma.

Pathophysiology

In AI, blood flows retrograde during diastole into the LV from the aorta and leads to volume and pressure overload (Fig. 39-5). In chronic AI, the LV cavity increases gradually and out of proportion to the LV wall thickness (eccentric LV hypertrophy), thus increasing the LV wall stress. The LV end-diastolic pressures are usually within the normal range, evidence of a significant increase in chamber compliance. As a result, and in contrast to AS, considerable fluctuations in LV volume can occur with only minimal changes in LV filling pressure. Although the LV may eject more than twice the normal cardiac output, $M\dot{V}O_2$ does not increase extraordinarily because the cost for muscle shortening (volume work) is low. The diastolic runoff and the moderate vasodilation reduce the LV afterload and increase the arterial pulse pressure. Thus, patients may be relatively symptom-free even when contractility is reduced. This is important in terms of planning the anesthetic, but perhaps even more so with respect to the timing of AV replacement. Ideally, the valve should be replaced just prior to the onset of irreversible myocardial damage. These patients should undergo AV replacement before LV ejection fraction decreases (<50%) or the LV dilates (LV end-diastolic diameter <65 mm).[80,81] Therefore, continued echocardiographic follow-up of these patients is paramount to detect decreased LV contractility.

In acute AI, the previously normal in size and compliance LV is faced with a rapidly increased end-diastolic volume and pressure whereas the diastolic aortic to LV pressure gradient is acutely decreased.[82] These will decrease the myocardial contractility and perfusion gradient with severe congestive heart failure as the cardinal clinical sign. The compensatory mechanisms of tachycardia and peripheral vasoconstriction further increase the $M\dot{V}O_2$. In such acutely ill patients, emergent AV replacement is required, whereas in less severe circumstances, mild systemic vasodilation and inotropic support may return hemodynamics toward normal.

Anesthetic Considerations

The main goal is to avoid further increases in LV wall stress (Table 39-5). Arterial vasodilation (nicardipine or SNP) promotes forward flow, although additional intravascular volume may be necessary to maintain adequate preload. The ideal heart rate is somewhat controversial; tachycardia reduces the diastolic runoff from the aorta to the LV, thereby reducing LV volume and wall tension, and increases the diastolic blood pressure

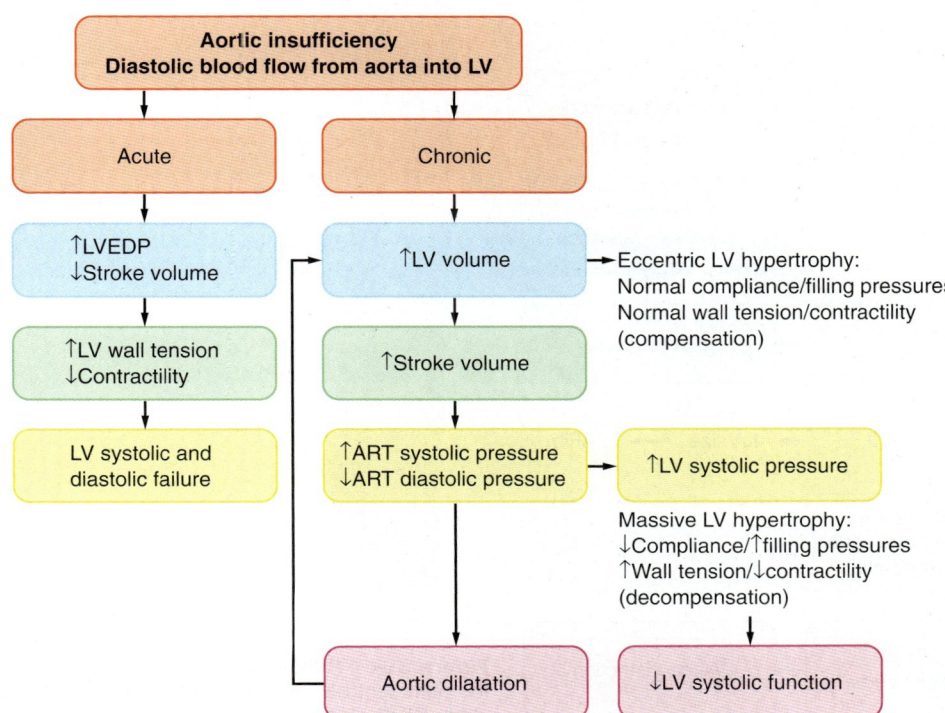

Figure 39-5 Pathophysiology of aortic insufficiency. LVEDP, left ventricular end-diastolic pressure; LV, left ventricle; ART, arterial.

Table 39-5 Aortic Insufficiency: Hemodynamic Goals

Parameter	Goal	Comment
Preload	↑ Slightly	↑ Slightly
Afterload	↓	Anesthetic depth ↑ or vasodilators (to decrease regurgitant fraction)
Contractility		Usually adequate
Rate	↑	Reduces ventricular volume and increases diastolic aortic pressure
Rhythm		Usually sinus; not a problem
$M\dot{V}O_2$		Usually not a problem
CPB		Beware (and observe) for ventricular distention pre- and post-AXC: regurgitant flow increases if ↓ HR and in non-beating heart

↑, increase; ↓, decrease; $M\dot{V}O_2$, myocardial oxygen consumption; CPB, cardiopulmonary bypass; AXC, aortic cross-clamp; HR, heart rate.

and coronary perfusion gradient, thus offsetting any increase in $M\dot{V}O_2$ secondary to increased heart rate. Bradycardia should be avoided as it results in ventricular distention, elevations in left atrial pressure, and pulmonary congestion.

Ventricular distention may occur with the onset of CPB in the setting of bradycardia or unexpected ventricular fibrillation (ineffective systolic ejection). Contextual monitoring with TEE, invasive pressure lines, and visual inspection of the heart is especially important. If LV distention occurs, insertion of an LV vent or immediate cross-clamping of the aorta should alleviate the problem. The approach to CPB is equally important: after application of the aortic cross-clamp, the incompetent AV prevents the cardioplegia delivered to the aortic root from reaching the coronary system. Instead, cardioplegia will fill and distend the LV, causing ischemia since the diastolic arrest of the heart is not achieved. In the presence of AI, the heart is arrested by injecting cardioplegia directly into the coronary ostia (after aortotomy) or retrograde, into the coronary sinus. The utility of TEE in diagnosing and grading the severity of AI is described in Chapter 27.

Mitral Stenosis

Mitral valve stenosis (MS) develops from leaflet thickening, commissural fusion, and chordal shortening and fusion due to chronic inflammation. The most frequent cause of MS is atherosclerosis-associated mitral annular calcification and endocarditis; rheumatic fever is a rare etiology in the United States.[83]

Pathophysiology

The spectrum of physiologic disruption in patients with MS is presented in Figure 39-6. Progressive decrease of the mitral valve area (MVA) impedes the blood flow from the left atrium (LA) to the LV, resulting in a pressure gradient across the MV during diastole. With worsening MS, the LV stroke volume is limited. The LV dysfunction is caused by the combination of decreased preload and increased afterload (from reflex vasoconstriction). Proximal to the decreased MVA, the LA pressure (LAP) is elevated. According to the formula by Gorlin and Gorlin[84]:

$$\text{Valve area} = \text{flow}/(K \cdot \sqrt{\text{Pressure gradient}}) \quad \text{or}$$
$$\text{Pressure gradient} = [\text{flow}/(K \cdot \text{MVA})]^2$$

where flow is cardiac output/diastolic filling time; pressure gradient is the difference between LAP and LVDP; and K is a hydraulic

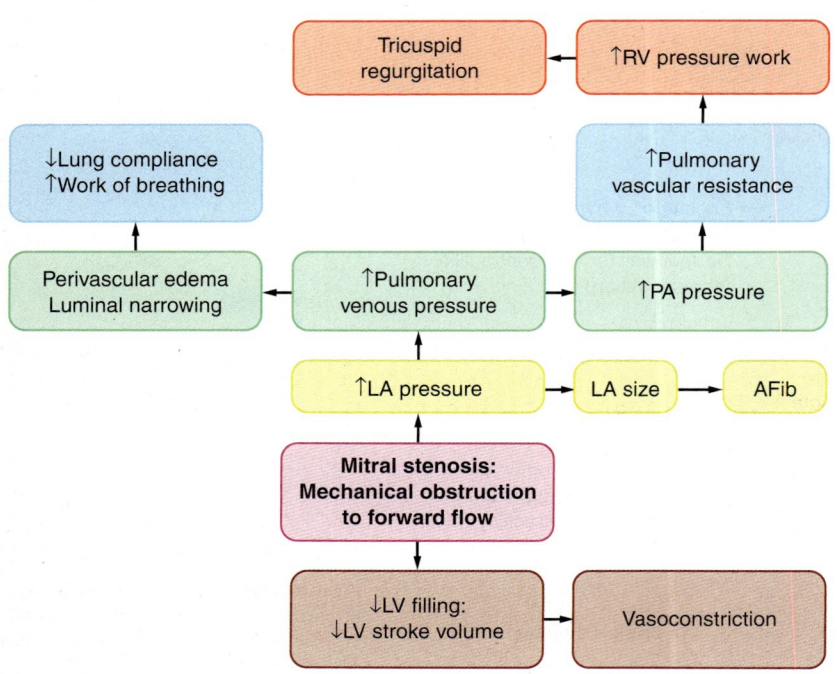

Figure 39-6 Pathophysiology of mitral stenosis. RV, right ventricle; PA, pulmonary artery; LA, left atrium; AFib, atrial fibrillation; LV, left ventricle.

pressure constant (this calculation assumes no regurgitant flow). At a constant MVA, rearrangement of the Gorlin formula reveals the clinical variables determining the elevated LAP in MS:

$$LAP - LVDP = [(cardiac\ output)/(diastolic\ time)/(K \cdot MVA)]^2$$

$$or\quad LAP = LVDP + [flow/(K \cdot MVA)]^2$$

Therefore, increased cardiac output or decreased diastolic filling period results in a geometric elevation of LAP. This explains why tachycardia or increased forward flow, seen classically with pregnancy, thyrotoxicosis, or infection, can precipitate pulmonary edema in a patient with MS. Similarly, atrial fibrillation causes hemodynamic deterioration because the rapid ventricular rate decreases the diastolic filling time, thereby increasing the LAP pressure. Upstream from the LA, a persistently elevated LAP eventually leads to LA dilatation and is reflected through the pulmonary circulation increasing the work of breathing. This causes right ventricular pressure overload with compensatory right ventricular hypertrophy. The progression and severity of pulmonary hypertension is variable and at some point irreversible reactive changes in the pulmonary vasculature (rales on auscultation, hemoptysis) occur. Once pulmonary vascular hypertension has developed, the operative risk is increased (12% vs. 3% to 8%).[85] Right ventricular dysfunction, tricuspid annular dilatation, and insufficiency (engorged neck veins) may develop once the right heart function worsens.

MS is not an LV problem, but mimics left heart failure, with pulmonary congestion and decreased systemic flow. The only definitive treatment is relief of obstruction with MV replacement; balloon valvuloplasty and open commissurotomy are palliative interventions. The medical therapy should aim at decreasing the heart rate (with β- or calcium channel blockers) or treating the cause(s) responsible for the increased diastolic transmitral flow. The measured pulmonary capillary wedge pressure is higher than the true LVDP at least by the amount of the transmittal diastolic pressure gradient.

Anesthetic Considerations

8 The hemodynamic goals listed in Table 39-6 are the cornerstones of prebypass anesthetic management (Table 39-6). Avoiding tachycardia helps prevent episodes of LA and pulmonary hypertension, potential right ventricular dysfunction, as well as inadequate LV filling with concomitant systemic hypotension. Preoperative maintenance of rate-control with β-blocking drugs, selection of anesthetics that minimize the risk of tachycardia, and attainment of anesthetic levels deep enough to suppress autonomic responses are methods to achieve these goals. Factors inducing pulmonary vasoconstriction, such as hypoxia, hypercarbia, and acidosis must be prevented to avoid the potential for right heart failure.

Treatment of hypotension in patients with MS can present a challenging dilemma, because hypovolemia is not usually the cause. The response to volume administration is often disappointing; instead, a vasoconstrictor is used to offset mild peripheral vasodilation, bearing in mind the effect of pulmonary vasoconstriction on right ventricular function. A drug with some inotropic effect, such as ephedrine or epinephrine, is preferred instead of relying on a pure vasoconstrictor, such as phenylephrine. In separating from CPB, attention is on avoiding right ventricular failure (discussed subsequently); more commonly, however, there is LV dysfunction. This may be because of intraoperative injury or sudden increase in flow to, and distention of, the chronically underloaded LV. After bypass, prominent v waves may be present in the pulmonary capillary wedge pressure

Table 39-6	Mitral Stenosis: Hemodynamic Goals	
Parameter	**Goal**	**Comment**
Preload	Maintain	Maintain, avoid hypovolemia
Afterload		Prevent ↑ RV afterload (due to pulmonary vasoconstriction hypoxia, hypercarbia); treat systemic hypotension with vasopressors
Contractility	↑ RV	May be decreased in long-standing pulmonary hypertension; (LV: usually intact)
Rate	Maintain	At low end of normal; avoid and treat tachycardia
Rhythm		Control ventricular response in atrial fibrillation
MVO$_2$		Not a problem
Post-CPB		LV preload and filling pressures may be elevated; cardiac function does not improve immediately

↑, increase(d); RV, right ventricle; MVO$_2$, myocardial oxygen consumption; CPB, cardiopulmonary bypass; MV, mitral valve; LV, left ventricle.

waveform, reflecting the increased LV filling, assuming a cardiac output increased from preinduction values. The echocardiographic evaluation of MS is described in Chapter 27.

Mitral Regurgitation

In MR, the valve is incompetent during systole and blood regurgitates from the LV to the LA. Etiologies of MR include excessive motion of one or both leaflets (prolapse or flail due to degenerative disease, or ruptured chordae tendineae following acute myocardial infarction), restricted leaflet motion due to rheumatic heart disease or myocardial ischemia (functional MR), or leaflet perforation from endocarditis. In functional MR the leaflet structure is normal, but the valve is incompetent due to either decreased LV systolic pressure (ischemic cardiomyopathy) that fails to "close" the leaflets or a dilated annulus (the fiber ring from where the leaflets are suspended) that decreases the coaptation surface of the leaflets (Table 39-7).

Pathophysiology

Volume overload similar to that described with AI is the cardinal feature of MR (Fig. 39-7). The LA acts as a low-pressure outlet during LV ejection; with the onset of ventricular systole blood is ejected retrograde (there is no isovolumetric contraction period) and the total LV output consists of forward (systemic, via the aorta) and retrograde (into the LA) blood volumes. The aftermaths of MR are atrial and ventricular chamber enlargement (due to "back-and-from" blood flow), LV wall hypertrophy (to compensate for the increased wall tension from chamber enlargement), and increased blood volume. The LV compliance is increased so that the large LV end-diastolic volume does not cause striking increase in LVDP. Initially, there is no concomitant increase in oxygen requirements because the systolic work is not increased. As a result, patients may have minimal symptoms

Table 39-7 Mechanisms of Mitral Regurgitation

Cause	Characteristics	Location
Degeneration	Excessive motion due to prolapse or flail Redundant tissue Ruptured chordae	Leaflet
Rheumatic	Thickened, calcified, restricted leaflets Commissural fusion	Leaflet
Congenital	Cleft mitral valve, double orifice mitral valve	Leaflet
Miscellaneous	Drug-related (fenfluramine)	Leaflet
Endocarditis	Perforation(s) Vegetations	Leaflet
Myocardial infarction	Papillary muscle rupture	Tensor apparatus
Dilated cardiomyopathy	Annular dilatation	Annulus
Ischemic heart disease	Papillary muscle dysfunction	Tensor apparatus

Table 39-8 Mitral Regurgitation: Hemodynamic Goals

Parameter	Goal	Comment
Preload	↑ Slightly	
Afterload	↓	With anesthetics, arterial vasodilators
Contractility		(May be ↑) titrate myocardial depressants carefully
Rate	↑ Slightly	↑ Avoid bradycardia
Rhythm		Control ventricular response if atrial fibrillation present
$M\dot{V}O_2$		Compromised if MR coexists with ischemic heart disease
Post-CPB		↑ Inotropy (afterload is increased with competent valve)

↑, increase(d); ↓, decrease(d); $M\dot{V}O_2$, myocardial oxygen consumption; MR, mitral regurgitation; CPB, cardiopulmonary bypass.

as well as normal or slightly reduced ejection fraction, despite progressive myocardial dysfunction and decreased contractility. The regurgitant blood volume is related to the size of the regurgitant MV orifice, the systolic ejection time, the pressure gradient across the MV, and the LA compliance. The regurgitant MV orifice size, in turn, depends on the type of MR mechanism and LV size. Therefore, increases in heart rate, reduction of preload, and arterial dilators are effective in reducing the regurgitation of blood volume from the LV to LA.

Repairing or replacing the MV increases the LV afterload and unmasks any underlying myocardial dysfunction. Administration of inotropes and/or vasodilators, as well as judicious increase in preload, may be necessary to successfully separate from bypass.

Acute-onset MR has a different hemodynamic picture; acute LA and LV volume overload occurs in the absence of compensatory LV enlargement. The acutely increased LV filling pressure is transmitted to the pulmonary vasculature, and concomitant to the decrease in cardiac output pulmonary edema develops. In the setting of acute myocardial infarction, contractility may be inadequate despite pharmacologic support, and intra-aortic balloon assistance and emergency surgery may be lifesaving.

Anesthetic Considerations

Selection of anesthetics that promote vasodilation and tachycardia is ideal in the patient with MR (Table 39-8). In chronic MR, vasoactive medications are usually not necessary because of LV compensatory mechanisms. However, patients with acute MR

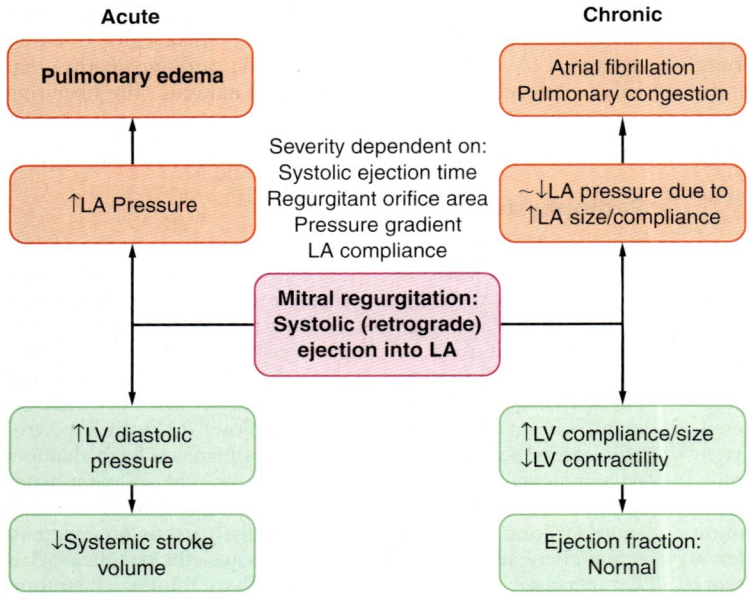

Figure 39-7 Pathophysiology of mitral regurgitation. LA, left atrial; LV, left ventricular.

may need aggressive pharmacologic management. In the absence of acute deterioration, pharmacologic intervention is not needed usually until the postbypass period. However, vasodilators and inotropes may lead to reoccurrence or worsening of MR if, following MV repair surgery, the anterior mitral leaflet is "sucked in" towards the intraventricular septum and results in LVOT obstruction. This pathophysiologic and clinical picture is similar to that of hypertrophic cardiomyopathy. The risk of systolic anterior motion after MV repair is increased when the anterior leaflet is longer than the posterior leaflet or when there is a narrow angle between the mitral and aortic annuli. If this scenario is suspected, a trial of volume expansion and vasoconstrictors is indicated. The echocardiographic evaluation of MR and its surgical treatment is described in Chapter 27.

Aortic Diseases

Acquired (hypertension, inflammation, deceleration trauma, or iatrogenic trauma) and genetic (connective tissue disorders, bicuspid AV) conditions are the cause of aortic diseases: aortic dissection, intramural hematoma, and aortic aneurysm. Weakening of the media layers of the aorta (the term *cystic medial degeneration* denotes the disappearance of smooth muscle cells and the degeneration of elastic fibers) leads to increased wall stress, which induces dilatation of the aortic lumen and formation of aneurysm, which may coexist with intramural hemorrhage or aortic dissection, or even lead to rupture.

Aortic Dissection

Aortic dissection[86] is one of the features of the acute aortic syndromes, which also include intramural hematoma and penetrating ulcer. Connective tissue disorders, such as Marfan syndrome and Ehlers–Danlos syndrome affect mostly the young (age <40 years), whereas hypertension is the most common risk factor in older patients. Aortic dissection is caused by a tear in the aortic intima and media, which propagates proximal and distally, creating a false lumen within the aortic media. When the false lumen involves aortic vessels, it causes malperfusion of vital organs (brain, spinal cord, abdominal organs). Rupture of the false lumen into the pericardium can cause cardiac tamponade, whereas interference with the AV may cause AI. Acute aortic dissection of the ascending aorta (type A) has a mortality rate of 1% to 2% per hour after onset of symptomatology and is a true surgical emergency. An aortic dissection distal to the left subclavian artery is called type B, has a 30-day mortality of 10%, and may be managed medically or with insertion of a scaffold (stent). Intramural hematoma originates from ruptured vasa vasorum in the media and is considered a precursor to classic dissection. Intramural hematoma has the same prognosis as aortic dissection and is treated similarly.

Severe neck or chest pain (type A) or back or abdominal pain (type B) is the most common symptom, although many patients have atypical symptoms mimicking stroke, myocardial infarction, vascular embolization, and abdominal pathology. Some diabetics may be totally asymptomatic. Syncope may indicate cardiac tamponade or cerebral hypoperfusion. Pulse deficits in extremities and/or differences in blood pressure are a significant sign and are related to impaired blood flow to a limb. It is important to diagnose correctly the type of dissection as this determines the proper treatment. A variety of diagnostic techniques are accurate (contrast-enhanced spiral computed tomography scanning or magnetic resonance imaging are slightly more sensitive and specific than TEE, which is more portable and available at bedside).[87]

Patients with a high clinical suspicion of acute aortic dissection may be sent directly to the operating room for TEE-based diagnostic workup and preparation for surgery, thus expediting surgical intervention.[88] Two-dimensional TEE identifies the intimal tear in 61% of the patients.[89] Apart from direct visualization of intimal tear and flap (the aortic wall separating the two lumens), the site of injury, thrombosis of the false lumen, coronary involvement, intramural hematoma, pericardial effusion, and AI can be diagnosed with high sensitivity and specificity.[90] However, dissections in the distal ascending aorta and proximal arch are difficult to visualize because of interposition of the left main stem bronchus between the esophagus (TEE) and aorta. Surgery is the definitive treatment for patients with type A acute aortic dissection to decrease mortality associated with aortic rupture, pericardial tamponade, and AI. It involves implantation of a composite graft in the ascending aorta with or without reimplantation of the coronary arteries. Type B aortic dissections can be managed medically if chronic or with implantation of a graft via an open or closed (percutaneous) approach if complicated (malperfusion symptomatology).

Anesthetic Considerations

Acute aortic dissection is a surgical emergency. Adequate intravenous access and invasive hemodynamic monitoring, including TEE, are mandatory. The hemodynamic goals are shown in Table 39-9.

Table 39-9 Acute Aortic Dissection: Hemodynamic Goals

Parameter	Goal	Comment
Preload	↓	If acute AI; (must ↑ further in tamponade)
Afterload	↓	With anesthetics, analgesics, arterial dilators (nitroprusside, nicardipine): keep systolic BP <100–120 mmHg
Contractility	Maintain or ↑	Titrate myocardial depressants carefully
Rate	↓ to <60–80 bpm	Use β-blocker; ensure contractility is adequate
Rhythm		Control ventricular response (If atrial fibrillation present)
MVO$_2$		Compromised if aortic dissection involves coronary vessels
CPB		Alternate site of inflow (arterial) cannulation, deep hypothermic circulatory arrest possible if cerebral vessels are involved

↑, increase(d); ↓, decrease(d); AI, aortic insufficiency; BP, blood pressure; bpm, beats per minute; MVO$_2$, myocardial oxygen consumption; CPB, cardiopulmonary bypass.

Aortic Aneurysm

Aortic aneurysms may involve one or more aortic segments (aortic root, ascending aorta, arch, descending aorta). Most patients are asymptomatic at the time of diagnosis. Aortic root aneurysms may cause AI (diastolic murmur or heart failure). When large, aortic aneurysms may cause local mass effect such as compression of the trachea (cough), esophagus (dysphagia), and/or recurrent laryngeal nerve (hoarseness). Detection and sizing can be done with contrast-enhanced computed tomography scanning and magnetic resonance angiography. The risk for rupture increases abruptly as aortic aneurysms reach a diameter of 6 cm.[91] Surgery is indicated for ascending aorta aneurysms greater than 5.5 cm or descending aortic aneurysms greater than 6 cm.[92] Composite aortic repair (Bentall procedure) using a tube graft with a prosthetic AV sewn into one end is performed for aortic root aneurysm associated with AI.[93] Alternatively, if AI is due to aortic root dilation, a valve-sparing procedure (preservation of the native AV cusps) is performed.[94]

The surgical replacement of aortic arch aneurysm requires circulatory arrest during the construction of distal anastomosis and carries a risk of neurologic damage from global ischemic injury or embolization of atherosclerotic debris. Cerebral protection methods during replacement of the aortic arch include use of deep hypothermic circulatory arrest with or without arrest of cerebral circulation. Retrograde (via a superior vena cava cannula) or selective antegrade (direct cannulation of cerebral vessels) cerebral perfusion is employed to improve outcomes by providing perfusion to the brain and flush out particulate matter from the cerebral and carotid arteries, with, so far, disputed results.[95]

Surgical replacement of the descending aorta is associated with postoperative paraplegia secondary to interruption of spinal cord blood supply (13% to 17%). A variety of methods (cerebrospinal fluid drainage, reimplantation of critical spinal arteries, maintenance of distal aortic perfusion with the use of an LA–left femoral artery bypass circuit, intraoperative epidural cooling, or use of somatosensory evoked potentials) are being used to avoid this complication, although outcome is heavily influenced by hospital and surgeon volume.[96] Alternatively, a transluminally placed endovascular stent-graft can be inserted.[97] Chapter 40 reviews recent advances in vascular stenting.

Anesthetic Considerations

The anesthetic technique is centered around two major organ systems: (1) preservation of cardiac function (most crucial in surgery of descending aortic aneurysms, where the "clamp-and-go" surgical technique imposes great fluctuations in systemic afterload and hemodynamic instability), and (2) neurologic integrity (in arch or descending aortic operations). Drainage of cerebrospinal fluid will augment the spinal cord perfusion pressure. Usually, increments of 10 mL are drained at a time and the cerebrospinal fluid pressure is monitored continuously, keeping a cerebrospinal fluid pressure below 15 mmHg at all times.[98,99] Left heart bypass (LA to femoral artery) provides nonpulsatile retrograde aortic perfusion and supplements blood flow during aortic flow interruption, but does not perfuse the excluded aortic segment. Blood is actively removed via a cannula inserted inside the LA and advanced distal to the aortic interruption site. This technique ameliorates LV stress by reducing LV preload and afterload. The bypass flow depends on adequate preload (as assessed by the pulmonary arterial diastolic pressure or LV size via TEE) and low-normal afterload distal to the aortic cross-clamp. Too high flow of the bypass system will lead to hypotension, whereas increased pump flow will help decrease systemic hypertension proximal to the aortic interruption.

Cardiopulmonary Bypass

Circuits

A CPB circuit consists of tubing (cannulae) that drain venous and return arterial blood; an oxygenator, where gas exchange occurs; and a mechanical pump that provides systemic perfusion (Fig. 39-8). The initiation of CPB involves the drainage of venous blood to the CPB machine. This is accomplished by placing a large-bore cannula(e) into the right atrium from which blood is drained to the venous reservoir of the CPB machine. For nonintracardiac procedures, a multi-orifice "dual-stage" cannula that drains blood from the right atrium, coronary sinus, and inferior vena cava is often used. However, where a bloodless field is required single cannula drainage may be suboptimal. In this case individual "single-stage" cannulae are placed into the superior and inferior venae cavae and then snared, thus preventing systemic venous blood from entering the heart. During CPB, venous drainage is passive and depends on several factors: proper placement of appropriately sized cannulae, intravascular volume status, and a hydrostatic pressure gradient (the difference in height between the right atrium and the venous reservoir). In the event of poor venous drainage, adjustment of the venous cannulae, raising the height of the operating table, or application of suction usually corrects the problem.

From the venous reservoir, blood enters the oxygenator/heat exchanger, which acts an artificial lung, and the blood is oxygenated and carbon dioxide is removed. Blood may then be warmed/cooled and returned to the arterial circulation via a large "arterial" cannula placed in the ascending aorta, femoral, or axillary arteries. This cycle of venous blood returning to the CPB machine where it is then oxygenated and retuned to arterial circulation continues for the duration of CPB.

Other ancillary functions of the CPB machine include delivery of cardioplegia, cardiotomy suction (scavenging shed blood from the surgical field), and venting (to decompress the LV and aspirate air from the heart during de-airing procedures). Venting prevents ventricular distention that may lead to myocardial ischemia and is particularly important in patients with aortic insufficiency. Common LV vent sites include a cannula placed

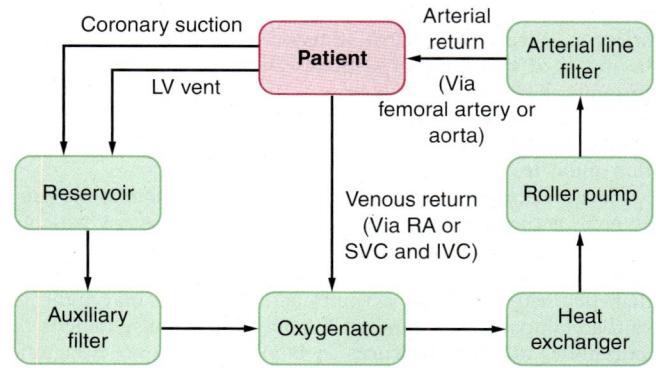

Figure 39-8 The basic circuit for cardiopulmonary bypass. LV, left ventricle; RA, right atrium; SVC, superior vena cava; IVC, inferior vena cava. (Adapted from Thomson IR. Technical aspects of cardiopulmonary bypass. In: Thomas SJ, ed. *Manual of Cardiac Anesthesia.* 2nd ed. New York: Churchill Livingstone; 1993:480, with permission.)

in the pulmonary artery, left atrium or LV via the left superior pulmonary vein or the aortic root.

In addition to providing cardiopulmonary support, CPB circuits contain filters for the removal of bubbles and debris, in-line blood gas monitors, and volatile agent vaporizers. Warning monitors are placed in key locations of the CPB circuit. These monitors are used to detect low blood levels in the venous reservoir/oxygenator (to prevent entrainment of air to the arterial side of the circuit), high systemic line pressure (to diagnose possible arterial cannula obstruction/aortic dissection; both cause elevated line pressure), and bubbles.

Oxygenators

The use of membrane oxygenators in modern CPB machines eliminates the destructive blood–gas interface seen with older bubble oxygenators. Membrane oxygenators use bundles of hollow microporous fibers contained in a plastic housing. Within this housing, blood flows around the fibers while fresh gas is passed though the fibers. The micropores act as channels allowing the diffusion of both oxygen and carbon dioxide. With this arrangement PO_2 on CPB is controlled by changes in FIO_2 and carbon dioxide elimination by changes in total gas flow or "sweep rate."

Pumps

7 During CPB, a mechanical pump is required to provide systemic perfusion and circulatory support. Centrifugal and roller pumps are used in clinical practice. Roller pumps are the simplest and earliest type of pump. A length of tubing is placed in the periphery of a rigid curved housing. At the center of this housing are two metal arms set 180 degrees apart with rollers at each end. When the arm rotates, the tubing is alternately compressed and released against the housing. Alternately compressing and releasing the tubing generates forward flow without the possibility of retrograde flow. This permits constant flow over a range of arterial resistance.

Roller pumps are simple and easy to use. The disadvantages include destruction of blood elements, spallation (development of plastic microemboli due to tubing compression), and complications from inflow and outflow occlusion of the pump. If pump inflow is occluded, negative pressure will develop in the roller head causing cavitation or the development of microscopic bubbles. If pump outflow becomes occluded, excessive pressure may develop proximal to the occlusion, causing the tubing connections to separate or the tubing to burst.

Centrifugal (CPs) or constrained vortex pumps have supplanted roller pumps for providing systemic support but they are still used for delivering cardioplegia and providing vent/cardiotomy suction.

CPs use magnetically controlled impellers placed within a rigid plastic housing. The impeller rotates to provide kinetic energy, that is then transferred to blood that becomes flow. The impeller is magnetically coupled to an electric motor located in the CPB machine and by rotating rapidly, a pressure drop across the impeller is generated, which creates a constrained vortex causing the displacement of blood. One major difference between roller head and centrifugal pumps is that flow from centrifugal pumps will vary with changes in pump preload and afterload. It is for this reason that a flow meter must be placed on the arterial side of the bypass circuit. Advantages of centrifugal pumps include less blood trauma, lower line pressures, lower risk of massive air emboli, and elimination of tubing wear and spallation.

Some potential complications of CPB include aortic dissection due to aortic cannulation (manifests as low blood pressure on CBP with high line pressure), catastrophic CPB machine failure (a hand crank may be used to mechanically operate the biohead of a centrifugal pump to develop adequate pump flow), and massive air emboli.

Heat Exchanger

A heat exchanger is a counter current device where either heated or cooled water is circulated around a conducting material with good thermal properties that is in contact with the patient's blood. In this way blood is subsequently warmed or cooled and maintained at a desired temperature.

Prime

The fluid contained within the CPB tubing is called prime. Using crystalloid solutions, such as lactated Ringer solution, allows the CPB prime to achieve similar osmolarity and electrolyte composition as blood. Other solutions such as albumin (to decrease postoperative edema), mannitol (to promote diuresis), additional electrolytes (calcium to prevent hypocalcemia due to citrate in transfused blood), and heparin (to ensure a safe level of anticoagulation) may be added to the prime. Many institutions use a standard volume prime for all adult patients, and others use a minimum volume based on body weight or body surface area (the average prime volume is about 1,500 mL). To prevent excessive dilutional anemia and decrease in oxygen-carrying capacity, blood may be added to the pump prime prior to initiating CPB in children, small adults, and patients with preoperative anemia. The lowest safe hematocrit on CPB is debated, but hematocrits of 22% are well tolerated.[100] Despite limited data the trend currently favors higher levels to avoid renal and neurologic consequences. Dilutional anemia on CPB is useful to the degree that it offsets changes in blood viscosity due to hypothermia. Thus, dilutional anemia may improve systemic flow. The use of cerebral oximetry on CPB may help identify patients at risk neurologic injury due to low intraoperative hematocrit or low flow. In an attempt to reduce the systemic inflammatory reaction, hemodilution, and coagulopathy associated with standard CPB circuits, miniaturized circuits have been developed. These miniaturized CPB circuits have a decreased surface area and consist of a smaller arterial venous loop/venous reservoir, pump, oxygenator, and filter. This reduction in surface area, and to a lesser extent a reduction in pump prime, may reduce blood usage.

Anticoagulation

Contact between patient's blood and components of the CPB circuit initiates activation of the coagulation cascade. To prevent thrombosis of the CPB circuit (and the patient's death), systemic anticoagulation is required prior to insertion of cannulae and initiation of CPB. The anticoagulant of choice is heparin, a polyionic mucopolysaccharide. Following intravenous injection, the peak onset of heparin is less than 5 minutes with a half-life of approximately 90 minutes in normothermic patients. In hypothermic patients, there is a progressive and proportional increase in the half-life of heparin. The anticoagulant effect of heparin is derived from its ability to potentiate the activity of antithrombin III (AT).

Heparin's binding to AT alters its structural configuration and increases its thrombin inhibitory potency more than 1,000-fold. By inhibiting thrombin, AT prevents formation of fibrin clot via both the intrinsic and extrinsic pathways, in addition to inhibiting factors IX, Xa, XIa, XIIa, kallikrein, and plasmin. In patients receiving heparin preoperatively and those with congenital AT deficiencies, higher than expected doses of heparin are required to achieve adequate anticoagulation.

In the event of inadequate anticoagulation due to a relative or absolute deficiency of AT, exogenous AT can be administered in the form of a commercially available concentrate. Postoperative heparin rebound and subsequent bleeding may be a concern following the administration of exogenous AT.

Currently, the two methods for determining adequate heparinization are measurement of the activated clotting time (ACT) or blood–heparin concentrations. The ACT test consists of adding blood to tubes containing either diatomaceous earth (celite) or kaolin, warming and rotating the tube, and then recording the time required for clot formation. Generally, ACTs above 480 seconds are considered acceptable for the initiation of CPB. Measuring heparin levels intraoperatively is an alternative method for determination of anticoagulation levels. In this method, known doses of protamine are added to a heparinized sample of blood sequentially, until the optimum dose of protamine that produces a clot in the shortest amount of time is determined. By knowing the neutralization ratio of heparin and protamine (usually 1 mg of protamine to 100 U of heparin), the heparin concentration in the sample can be determined. This method will correctly diagnose inadequate anticoagulation despite a therapeutic ACT.

Partial thromboplastin time is not used in cardiac surgery to measure heparin action. This is due to the fact that modern partial thromboplastin time assays are so sensitive that heparin levels far lower than those used for safe initiation of CPB cause the sample blood to become almost unclottable within the time frame of the test.

Allergies to heparin are rare; more commonly, patients may present with a history of heparin-induced thrombocytopenia (HIT). There are two subtypes of HIT. The first is generally mild and consists of a transient decrease in platelet count following the administration of heparin a few days following surgery. The second type is more severe, characterized by autoimmune-mediated decrease in the platelet count due to the formation of antigenic heparin compounds (anti-PF4) that activate platelets in the face of endothelial injury. This predisposes to platelet clumping and microvascular thrombosis. This thrombosis may occur anywhere in the body and cause bowel or limb ischemia to name a few. In patients with HIT who require systemic anticoagulation, heparin alternatives should be used instead. These include defibrinogenating agents (ancrod obtained from pit viper venom), hirudin, bivalirudin, and factor X inhibitors. Hirudin, which is isolated from the salivary gland of the medicinal leech (*Hirudo medicinalis*), and bivalirudin (hirulog) are both direct inhibitors of thrombin. Their action is independent of AT. The use of these agents is uncommon and the reader is advised to consult one of the several reviews on this subject.[101]

Blood Conservation in Cardiac Surgery

Blood and blood components are finite resources that are increasingly difficult to replace because of declining donation and restrictions on those that may donate. In addition, patients are increasingly demanding "bloodless" surgeries to lessen the risks of blood transfusion (infection, incompatibility reactions, transfusion error). However, because of the nature of cardiac surgery, the risk of blood and blood product transfusion is high. Bleeding as a result of reoperation, use of anticoagulants/platelet function inhibitors, and residual surgical bleeding contribute to this risk. Furthermore, the inherent risk of platelet dysfunction and coagulopathy due to CPB cannot be eliminated. The use of a multimodal approach to blood conservation including intraoperative autologous blood donation, the scavenging and reinfusion of shed blood, the use of antifibrinolytics (ε-aminocaproic acid, tranexamic acid), and other conservation techniques may all help to reduce the need for transfusion.[102,103]

Intraoperative autologous hemodilution is a well-described method of removing whole blood from a patient prior to systemic heparinization and CPB. Returning this blood following the separation from CPB returns red blood cells, active platelets, and functional coagulation factors that may mitigate surgical bleeding. Contraindications to intraoperative autologous blood donation include preoperative anemia, unstable angina/high-grade left main coronary artery disease, and aortic stenosis. Blood salvage (cell saver) is another key method of intraoperative blood conservation in cardiac surgery. Following processing, units of shed blood may have hematocrits of 70%. Unfortunately, as platelets and coagulation factors are removed in the washing process, reinfusion of shed blood may worsen the CPB-associated coagulopathy by promoting a dilutional thrombocytopenia and reduction of clotting factors. Contraindications to the use of intraoperative cell salvage include infection, malignancy, and the use of topical hemostatic agents.

Antifibrinolytic use in cardiac surgery is the standard in most cardiac centers, with ε-aminocaproic acid being the primary agent used in the United States. The lysine analogues ε-aminocaproic and tranexamic acid bind to plasminogen and block its ability to bind at lysine residues of fibrinogen. This prevents the lysis of fibrin clots. Administration of these antifibrinolytics decreases bleeding after CPB and reduces the risk of blood transfusion.[104]

Hemodilution due to the CPB prime is one undesired by-product of extracorporeal circulation. One method that has been used with success to avoid excess hemodilution and reduce the need for blood transfusion is retrograde autologous priming (RAP). In RAP, the crystalloid prime contained within the CPB circuit is displaced prior to the initiation of CPB and replaced by blood drained retrograde via the arterial and venous cannulae. RAP reduces hemodilution and diminishes the drop in systemic vascular resistance (SVR) associated with the initiation of CPB. When using this technique, care must be taken to avoid acute hypovolemic hypotension. Reported benefits of RAP include reduced extravascular lung water and weight gain.[105]

Ultrafiltration is another technique used in conjunction with CPB to reduce postoperative bleeding and transfusion needs. During ultrafiltration (hemoconcentration), plasma water is separated from low–molecular-weight solutes, intravascular cell components, and plasma proteins with a semipermeable membrane, using a hydrostatic pressure differential created by external suction. Conventional ultrafiltration is initiated during rewarming and is practiced more often in pediatric cardiac surgery. Advantages of hemoconcentration include a reduction in free water, increase in hemoglobin and hematocrit, preservation of hemostasis, and a decrease in levels of circulating inflammatory mediators.[106]

Myocardial Protection

The most common method of myocardial protection used today is that of intermittent hyperkalemic cold cardioplegia and systemic hypothermia. Systemic hypothermia is beneficial for both myocardial and neurologic protection during cardiac surgery. The benefits of hypothermia are a reduction in metabolic rate and oxygen consumption, preservation of high-energy phosphate substrates, and a reduction in excitatory neurotransmitter release. For each degree centigrade reduction in temperature, there is an 8% reduction in metabolic rate, so that at 28°C there is an approximate reduction in metabolic rate of 50%. Moderate systemic hypothermia can be achieved with either passive or active cooling. Using passive cooling, or "drifting" the patient's core temperature is allowed to equalize with the ambient temperature. This may be a slow or rapid process depending on variables such as patient's body surface area exposed and ambient temperature. Most patients undergoing cardiac surgery are actively cooled and then rewarmed using a heat exchanger.

The fundamental concept of cold cardioplegia is that a cold solution (10° to 15°C) of either blood or crystalloid with a supranormal concentration of potassium is injected into the coronary arteries or veins to induce diastolic electrical arrest. Cardioplegia may be employed via an anterograde, retrograde, or a combination of the two routes. Anterograde cardioplegia solution is injected via the aortic root following aortic cross-clamp which then follows the normal anatomic flow of blood into the native coronaries. In patients with severe coronary artery disease or AI, anterograde cardioplegia may provide inadequate myocardial protection due to an incompetent AV allowing cardioplegia to flow into the LV, bypassing the coronary ostia causing left ventricular distention and ischemia. In cases of significant AI, following aortic cross-clamping, an aortotomy is made and cardioplegia is delivered anterograde via handheld cannulae placed in the individual coronary ostia under direct vision. During coronary artery bypass surgery, individual grafts may be used to deliver cardioplegia once distal anastomoses have been completed. This will ensure the delivery of anterograde cardioplagia distal to any obstructive coronary artery disease. Retrograde cardioplegia is employed for myocardial protection by placing a catheter inside the coronary sinus. Retrograde cardioplegia is then injected via the cardiac venous system, bypassing obstructed coronaries and achieving greater myocardial protection. To maximize myocardial protection, both anterograde and retrograde are often used in combination. Depending on the time required for surgical repair, multiple injections of cardioplegia may be necessary to wash out metabolic by-products, add new high-energy and oxygen-carrying substrates, and maintain hypothermic diastolic arrest. There is gaining interest in single-dose cardioplegia solutions such as del Nido cardioplegia. This agent is administered once and is has been reported to protect aged cardiomyocytes during cardioplegic arrest and reperfusion.[107]

For the anesthesiologist monitoring a patient on CPB, the sentinel events of cardioplegic electrical arrest and resumption of electrical activity must be observed closely. LV distention and lack of rapid electrical arrest may be evidence of poor myocardial protection and the possibility of difficulty in separation from CPB. TEE is particularly helpful in diagnosing ventricular distention and its relief by venting or manual decompression of the LV.

Preoperative and Intraoperative Management

The preoperative visit should focus on the cardiovascular system but should not disregard the assessment of pulmonary, renal, hepatic, neurologic, endocrine, and hematologic functions. The depth and detail of the explanation should be custom-tailored to each patient and the anticipated events from transport to the operating room until emergence should be discussed with the patient.

Pertinent findings suggestive angina or ischemia-induced left and/or right ventricular dysfunction (Table 39-10), should be integrated to plan for monitoring and anesthetic techniques.

It is important to evaluate for conditions commonly associated with heart disease, such as hypertension, diabetes mellitus, and cigarette smoking, as well as the presence of pulmonary hypertension. Higher systemic arterial pressures may be desirable throughout surgery in patients with a history hypertension or evidence of carotid artery disease. Renal function must also be evaluated, since it is commonly affected postoperative.

Table 39-10 Preoperative Findings Suggestive of Ventricular Dysfunction

History
CAD: previous MI, chest pain/pressure
CHF (intermittent or chronic): fatigue, DOE, orthopnea, PND, ankle swelling

Physical Examination
Vital signs: hypotension, tachycardia (severe CHF)
Engorged neck veins, apical impulse displaced laterally, S_3, S_4, rales, pitting edema, pulsatile liver, ascites

Electrocardiogram
Ischemia/infarct, rhythm, conduction abnormalities

Chest Radiography
Cardiomegaly, pulmonary vascular congestion/pulmonary edema, pleural effusion, Kerley B lines

Cardiovascular Testing
Catheterization data: LVEDP >18 mmHg, EF <0.4, CI <2.0 L/min/m²

CAD, coronary artery disease; MI, myocardial infarction; CHF, congestive heart failure; DOE, dyspnea on exertion; PND, paroxysmal nocturnal dyspnea; LVEDP, left ventricular end-diastolic pressure; EF, ejection fraction; CI, cardiac index.

Current Drug Therapy

Almost without exception all cardiovascular drugs are continued until the time of surgery.[108] Interactions between these drugs and anesthetics are more often beneficial than harmful in maintaining hemodynamic control during periods of surgical stress and reducing morbidity and mortality. Contrary to common belief, there is a potential long-term benefit of ACE inhibitors provided that dosing is adjusted so that hypotension is avoided.[109] On the other hand, the protracted hypotension encountered on bypass and associated with poor outcome has been associated with preoperative β-blockers or calcium channel blockers.[110] Most cardiac antidysrhythmics should also be continued to the time of surgery.

Physical Examination

Physical examination should be part of the preoperative evaluation; signs of cardiac decompensation such as an S_3 gallop, rales, jugular venous distention, or pulsatile liver should be sought. Routes for vascular access should be assessed, and the pulse

Table 39-11	Preoperative Physical Examination
Parameter	Scope
Vital signs	Current values and range
Height, weight	For calculations of drug dosages, pump flow, cardiac index
Airway	Evaluate, identify difficulties for ventilation, intubation
Neck	Landmarks for jugular vein cannulation Vein engorgement (CHF) Bruits (carotid artery disease)
Heart	Murmurs: Characteristic of valve lesions, S_3 (elevated LVEDP), S_4 (decreased compliance), click (MVP prolapse) Lateral PMI displacement (cardiomegaly) Precordial heave, lift (hypertrophy, wall motion abnormality)
Lungs	Rales (CHF) Rhonchi, wheezes (COPD, asthma)
Vasculature	Peripheral pulses Sites for venous and arterial access
Abdomen	Pulsatile liver (CHF, tricuspid regurgitation)
Extremities	Peripheral edema (CHF)
Nervous system	Motor or sensory deficits

CHF, congestive heart failure; LVEDP, left ventricular end-diastolic pressure; MVP, mitral valve prolapse; PMI, point of maximal impulse; COPD, chronic obstructive pulmonary disease.

of peripheral arteries should be evaluated. As always, the airway should be carefully evaluated with respect to ease of mask ventilation and tracheal intubation. Other pertinent points are described in Table 39-11.

Premedication

These days, sedation is almost always given in the operating room after completion of regulatory paperwork. Premedication will assist in providing a calm, anxiety-free, arousable, and hemodynamically stable patient who is prepared for surgery. Selection of drug and dosage depends on the patient's age, cardiovascular state, level of anxiety, and location. Although heavy premedication is ideal there is inadequate time for premedication for the same-day-admit patient. Inadequate sedation may predispose to hypertension, tachycardia, or coronary vasospasm, and precipitate myocardial ischemia.

Monitoring

We emphasize only those aspects of monitoring particularly relevant to cardiac surgery because other monitoring techniques used commonly in cardiac surgery and other procedures are discussed extensively in Chapters 26 and 37.

Pulse Oximeter

Vascular cannulations may be challenging and the preinduction period may be prolonged. The pulse oximeter should be the first monitor placed to detect clinically unsuspected episodes of hypoxemia and tachycardia during the preinduction period.

Electrocardiogram

Regional ischemia may be diagnosed by appropriate lead monitoring: Lead II (and/or leads III, aVF) for the inferior myocardium (right coronary artery distribution), leads V_4 or V_5 for the anterior myocardium (left anterior descending [LAD] artery), and leads I and aVL for the lateral LV myocardial walls (circumflex artery). A strip-chart recorder or the "freeze pane" function of the hemodynamic monitor is useful for analysis and documentation of ST segment alterations and complex dysrhythmias.

Temperature

Central temperature can be measured with urinary bladder catheter or with a thermistor from a PAC.[111] Depending upon the case, nasopharyngeal or tympanic temperature probes may be used (as in cases of deep hypothermic circulatory arrest). Rectal and skin probes record peripheral temperatures, which lag behind central measurements during both cooling and rewarming periods.

Arterial Blood Pressure

Systemic arterial pressure should always be monitored invasively. The radial artery is usually cannulated,[112] although the femoral, brachial, and axillary arteries may also be used. The exact site is often a matter of personal or institutional preference. Criteria include convenience, selection of the arterial site with the "fullest" or most bounding pulse, and avoidance of the dominant hand. Occasionally, the site of surgery dictates appropriate placement; for example, the right radial artery should be used for procedures involving the descending thoracic aorta because the left subclavian artery may be included in the proximal aortic clamp. Following CPB, radial artery pressure is often misleading and may be as much as 30 mmHg lower than central aortic pressure. The mechanism may be due to peripheral vasodilation during rewarming or marked vasoconstriction.[113] Whenever a pressure discrepancy is suspected, the central aortic pressure should be estimated (by palpation by the surgeon) or directly measured (via femoral artery catheterization or with a needle placed directly into the aorta). Timely recognition will avoid unnecessary treatment of presumed hypotension. The gradient usually disappears within 45 minutes of separation from bypass. The optimal management of blood pressure during and immediately after CPB remains undefined.[114]

Central Venous Pressure and Pulmonary Artery Catheter

Access to the central circulation is mandatory for infusion of cardioactive drugs. In addition, right atrial (RAP) or central venous pressure (CVP) reflect right ventricular filling pressure and is of critical importance whenever right ventricular dysfunction is suspected. The relationship between the transduced RAP and the LV filling pressure is less predictable, more so in the presence of severe LV failure, pulmonary hypertension, or reduced LV compliance. The insertion of a PAC provides a better estimation of LV filling via measurement of the pulmonary capillary wedge pressure, although TEE data are far more accurate, because the actual volume can be better estimated. The PAC-facilitated calculation of stroke volume, cardiac output, PVR, and SVR offer additional information to guide hemodynamic and anesthetic management.

Indications for PAC insertion vary greatly among institutions.[22] In some, PAC are used routinely, whereas in others they are limited to patients with severe cardiac dysfunction or pulmonary hypertension. Insertion of a pacing PAC can be helpful whenever exact control of rate and rhythm is desirable before access to the epicardium is possible, for example, in patients with hypertrophic cardiomyopathy or those with significant bradycardia secondary to β-blockade. Before preinduction insertion of the PAC, in order to determine the baseline hemodynamics prior to the anesthetic induction, one should consider the anxiety and discomfort it may cause the patient.

The PAC often migrates distally with cardiac manipulation, as well as with acute preload changes. Therefore, it is prudent to pull the PAC back a few centimeters prior to the initiation of CPB to prevent permanent wedging or possible pulmonary artery rupture.[115] Despite the controversy concerning the routine use of these catheters, there is no disagreement that the capability to estimate or measure cardiac output and ventricular filling pressures must be available in any institution performing cardiac surgery.[65] Whether this is done with a PAC or TEE is immaterial. At any time, the ability of the practitioner to interpret correctly the PAC or TEE data cannot be overemphasized.

Echocardiography

The detection of ischemia by real-time evaluation of new regional wall motion abnormalities and the assessment of valvular function (before and after intervention) and of the ascending aorta with TEE have been mentioned. It is well known that, following CPB, the LV filling pressure, irrespective of the site of measurement (LV end-diastolic pressure, LA, pulmonary capillary wedge pressure), is a poor and often misleading indicator of LV volume status.[116] The estimation of LV volume with TEE should direct fluid infusion and selection of vasoactive drugs, particularly in patients who are difficult to wean from CPB. In addition, residual valve lesions, intracardiac air, or new areas of ischemia or global dysfunction (due to prolonged CPB, inadequate cardioplegia or reperfusion injury) can be detected with TEE. Please see Chapter 27 for a review of TEE applications.

Central Nervous System Function and Complications

Monitoring of the brain during CPB is difficult because of lack of standardized equipment or criteria. Neurologic complications after cardiac surgery can be devastating. The 1- and 5-year survival rates after stroke are about 65% and 45%, respectively, compared with more than 90% and 80% to 85% for patients not having stroke.[117] Many investigators have focused on methods to determine the etiology and improve the detection, prevention, and treatment of postoperative neurologic complications in patients undergoing cardiac surgery. The incidence of stroke after CABG surgery ranges from less than 1% (for patients <64 years) to more than 5% to 9% (for patients >65 years).[118] The incidence of subtle cognitive deficits that can be elicited by detailed neuropsychometric testing is much higher (60% to 70%). It is known that the neuropsychiatric deficits do improve over the initial 2 to 6 months after cardiac surgery; however, a significant percentage of patients (13% to 39%) have residual impairment. The etiology of perioperative neurologic complications is believed to be predominantly due to emboli (air, atheroma, other particulate matter) and not to hypoperfusion in susceptible patients (e.g., preexisting cerebrovascular disease). Most overt strokes after cardiac surgery are focal and likely due to macroemboli, whereas the cognitive changes are subtle and probably result from microemboli.

Risk factors for neurologic complications include advanced age (>70 years), pre-existing cerebrovascular disease (e.g., carotid artery stenosis >80%), history of prior stroke, peripheral vascular disease, ascending aortic atheroma, and diabetes. Operative factors include the duration of CPB, intracardiac procedure (e.g., valve replacement), excessive warming during and following CPB, and perhaps perfusion pressure on CPB.[119,120] Intraoperative hyperglycemia, which could theoretically result in worsened neurologic damage, has not been associated with poorer neurologic outcome.

The role of TEE in evaluating the ascending and descending aorta has been described previously. Management options for patients with severely diseased aortas, especially those with mobile atheromas who are at increased risk of stroke, include hypothermic fibrillatory arrest with LV vent and no aortic cross-clamp, single cross-clamp (i.e., distal and proximal grafts performed during same cross-clamp), relocation of proximal grafts to area of nondiseased aorta, no proximal grafts (internal mammary arteries only) either on CPB or using off-pump coronary artery bypass, or hypothermic circulatory arrest with resection and graft replacement of the diseased aortic segment. The technical means for cerebral protection such as the use of 20- to 40-μm arterial line filters and membrane oxygenators, newer modifications of the basic CPB apparatus, or the use of specialized equipment or procedures (including hypothermia and "tight" glucose control) have unproven benefit on neurologic outcomes.[121] Hypothermia is excellent in that it decreases cerebral metabolic rate and prolongs ischemic tolerance. However, during routine CPB the patient is normothermic when the risk of embolization is highest: during rewarming and unclamping of the aorta and with initial ventricular ejection.

Selection of Anesthetic Drugs

The choice of anesthetic has no effect on the outcome in CABG patients, as shown by Tuman[122] and Slogoff.[123] The most critical factor governing the selection and dose of the anesthetics and adjuvants is the degree of ventricular dysfunction. Any anticipated difficulties during tracheal intubation, the expected duration of surgery, and the anticipated time of tracheal extubation should be considered as well. The anesthetic depth should be rapidly adjustable, so as to counteract the varying intensity of surgical stress. The most intense stimulation and sympathetic response is expected during tracheal intubation, incision, sternotomy, pericardiotomy, and manipulation of the aorta. On the other hand, the period of preparing and draping following intubation of the trachea requires minimal levels of anesthetic, as does the period of hypothermic bypass.

Nowadays, volatile anesthetics are used as primary anesthetics and as adjuvants to prevent or treat "breakthrough" hypertension. They favorably balance the myocardial oxygen supply and demand by reducing contractility and afterload. At the same time, any unwanted declines in coronary perfusion pressure must be prevented or treated. Volatile agents have been used successfully in all types of valve surgery without untoward effects, although they are sometimes associated with more hemodynamic variability than is seen with opioids. Volatile anesthetics have been associated with cardioprotective effects from ischemia and reperfusion and allow for more rapid recovery of contractile function on reperfusion.[11] The ability to rapidly increase and decrease the alveolar concentration allows easy adjustment to the variable levels of surgical stimulation. Volatile anesthetics are also administered during CPB through a vaporizer mounted on the pump; they are also appropriate in the postbypass period,

Opioids

Opioids lack negative inotropic effects in the doses used clinically and have thus found widespread use as the primary agents for cardiac surgery. This era began in 1969, when high doses of morphine were used to anesthetize patients for AV replacement.[35] However, hypotension, histamine release, increased fluid requirements, and, often, inadequate anesthesia resulted in a decline in the use of morphine in favor of the more potent fentanyl and its analogues. Aside from bradycardia, fentanyl and its analogues are relatively devoid of cardiovascular effects and have proved to be effective anesthetics. As a primary anesthetic agent, fentanyl (50 to 100 μg/kg) or sufentanil (10 to 20 μg/kg) and oxygen provide hemodynamic stability, although they do not consistently prevent a hypertensive response to periods of increased surgical stimulation. The use of high-dose opioids prolongs the time until emergence and extubation when compared with techniques primarily based on volatile anesthetics and is no longer in fashion. In addition, although high doses of opioids produce unconsciousness and characteristic electrocardiographic slowing, recall of intraoperative events is not eliminated. Therefore, a current-era cardiac anesthetic includes benzodiazepines to provide amnesia and volatile anesthetics or vasodilators to control hypertension. Superiority of any one opioid has not been demonstrated for either coronary or valvular surgery. Remifentanil, an ultrashort-acting opioid, undergoes hydrolysis by nonspecific esterases in minutes. Its predictable and rapid elimination is unaffected by hepatic or renal disease, making it an optimal drug for infusion techniques. Combinations of the fentanyl-type drugs and benzodiazepines, whether given concomitantly or as premedication, result in hypotension secondary to a fall in SVR. Any opioid in high doses can produce excessive bradycardia. Abdominal and chest wall rigidity commonly occur with rapid injection of high doses of opioids and can be severe enough to render ventilation impossible. A low dose (priming) of nondepolarizing muscle relaxant should be given prior to a high-dose opioid administration.

Induction Drugs

Benzodiazepines, barbiturates, propofol, and etomidate can be used as supplements to either inhalation or opioid anesthetics, or as sole induction drugs in patients with cardiac disease depending on the adequacy of ventricular function and baseline sympathetic tone. All dosages must be altered to fit the clinical situation. Etomidate is favored for induction in patients with limited cardiac reserve, but rarely administered repeatedly or for prolonged periods because of the risk of adrenal dysfunction associated with prolonged use.

Neuromuscular Blocking Drugs

Muscle relaxants are components of a balanced anesthetic for cardiac surgery. Although they are not essential to surgical exposure of the heart, muscle paralysis facilitates intubation of the trachea and attenuates skeletal muscle contraction during defibrillation. They are necessary to prevent or treat opioid-induced truncal rigidity. The chief criteria for selection are the hemodynamic and pharmacokinetic properties associated with each relaxant, the patient's myocardial function, the presence of coexisting disease, current pharmacologic regimen, and anesthetic technique.[124]

Intraoperative Management

In this section we describe the anesthetic management of a patient undergoing a cardiac surgical procedure from the time of arrival in the operating room until his/her care is transferred to ICU personnel. Anticipation of needs specific to each stage of the procedure and immediate availability of necessary equipment and medications prevent untoward hemodynamic aberrations and last-minute rushed decisions.

Preparation

The operating room must be readied prior to arrival of the patient. Heparin may be drawn up prior to induction of anesthesia in the unlikely event of the need to "crash" onto CPB. Typed and cross-matched blood should be available in the operating suite. Table 39-12 provides a checklist to aid in proper preoperative preparation of the operating room.

Table 39-12 Anesthetic Preparation for Cardiac Surgery

Anesthesia Machine
Routine check

Airway
Nasal cannula for O_2
Ventilation/intubation equipment, including difficult airway devices
Suction
Inspired gas humidifier

Circulatory Access
Catheters (peripheral and central venous and arterial access)
Intravenous fluids and infusion tubing and pumps
Fluids warmer

Monitors
Standard ASA: ECG leads, blood pressure cuff, pulse oximeter, neuromuscular blockade monitor
Temperature probes (nasal, tympanic, bladder, rectal)
Transducers (arterial, pulmonary, and central venous pressure) zeroed and functioning
Cardiac output computer: Proper constant inserted
Awareness monitor (BIS)
Anticoagulation (ACT) monitor(s)
Recorder/printer

Medications
General anesthetic: hypnotic/induction, amnestic/benzodiazepine, volatile, opioid, muscle relaxant
Heparin (predrawn)
Cardioactive
- Predrawn: nitroglycerin/nicardipine, $CaCl_2$, phenylephrine/ephedrine, epinephrine
- Infusions: nitroglycerin, inotrope
Antibiotics*

Miscellaneous
Pacemaker with battery
Defibrillator/cardioverter with external paddles and ECG cables
Ultrasound system for central venous line insertion
Compatible blood in operating room

ASA, American Society of Anesthesiologists; ECG, electrocardiogram; BIS, bispectral index; ACT, activated clotting time.

Preinduction Period

The patient's general status and level of anxiety and the effectiveness of premedication (if ordered) should be assessed prior to entry to the operating room. Peripheral oxygen saturation monitor, ECG leads, and noninvasive blood pressure cuff are placed, and a set of baseline vital signs are recorded. Any angina should be promptly treated with supplemental oxygen, additional sedation, intravenous nitroglycerin, or, if related to anxiety-induced hypertension or tachycardia, with β-blocker and prompt induction of general anesthesia if possible.

Peripheral intravenous cannulae are inserted after site infiltration with local anesthetic (additional routes for infusion are desirable in patients undergoing repeat cardiac surgery). Although some anesthesiologists induce anesthesia and insert arterial and central venous cannulas following tracheal intubation, others prefer to have one or both of these cannulae inserted prior to induction of anesthesia. Preinduction or postinduction insertion of central venous or PAC has been discussed previously. Surface ultrasound for central venous access should be the standard practice, and at all times sterile barrier technique should be adhered to.[125,126] Once hemodynamic monitoring is established, baseline values for all pressures and cardiac output should be recorded, and baseline determinations of arterial blood gases, hematocrit, blood glucose, and activated coagulation time should be obtained.

Throughout the preinduction period, the anesthesiologist must never divert his or her attention from the patient. Continuous monitoring of the vital signs, careful observation of the patient, and periodic verbal contact facilitate detection of hemodynamic or ECG abnormalities, increased anxiety, or excessive response to intravenous sedation.

Induction and Intubation

The exact choice and sequence of drugs are a subtle—sometimes not so subtle—combination of art and science. The choice of specific agents (e.g., sedative, opioid, volatile drug, muscle relaxant), dose, and speed of administration depends primarily on the patient's cardiovascular reserve and desired cardiovascular profile. A smooth transition from consciousness to blissful sleep is desired without untoward airway difficulties (e.g., coughing, laryngospasm, truncal rigidity) or hemodynamic responses (e.g., hypotension from relative overdose, loss of sympathetic tone, or myocardial depression; hypertension caused by airway insertion; or jaw thrust). A "slow cardiac induction" sometimes causes, rather than alleviates, these potential problems. However, awake tracheal intubation, after proper sedation, may be appropriate in an obese patient with a wide neck if ventilation and intubation appear to be difficult. The necessity for individual approach to each patient cannot be overemphasized.

Deep planes of anesthesia, brief duration of laryngoscopy, and innumerable pharmacologic regimens have been proposed for eliminating the hypertension and tachycardia associated with intubation of the trachea. None is uniformly successful, and all drug interventions carry some degree of risk, even though they may be small. In patients with a slow heart rate prior to induction of anesthesia, the reflex response to tracheal intubation is primarily vagal, and severe bradycardia and rarely sinus arrest can occur. Identification of persistently abnormal hemodynamics or ischemia should be sought and treated.

Preincision Period

The period of time from tracheal intubation until skin incision is one of minimal stimulation as the surgical team attends to insertion of a urinary bladder catheter, temperature probe, positioning, preparing, and draping. As a result, hypotension often develops, regardless of the anesthetic used. It may be necessary to reduce the anesthetic depth or alternatively support the systemic pressure with a vasoconstrictor. The potential risks of vasoconstriction in patients with poor left or right ventricular performance must be kept in mind. The anesthetic depth should be increased immediately prior to incision and sternotomy.

Incision to Bypass

As previously emphasized, the prebypass period is characterized by periods of intense surgical stimulation that may cause hypertension and tachycardia, or induce ischemia. Anticipating these events and deepening the anesthetic may be effective, but a vasodilator or other adjuvant is often required. Hypotension can occur during the less stressful moments before CPB, but it is more commonly associated with cardiac manipulation in preparation for, and during, atrial cannulation. This may interfere with venous return or produce episodic ectopic beats or sustained supraventricular dysrhythmias, and atrial fibrillation is not uncommon. Depending on the blood pressure and heart rate response, appropriate treatment may range from observation to vasoconstrictors, cardioversion, or rapid cannulation and institution of bypass. Maintaining adequate intravascular volume may attenuate the extent of hypotension. This is a critical period, and continuous observation of the surgical field is essential.

It is important to identify any new ischemia pre bypass with ST segment analysis and frequent TEE examination. If it occurs, it should be treated appropriately and the surgeon notified. Communication between the anesthesiologist and the surgeon is necessary to keep both apprised of the situation and to ensure the heart gets a periodic "rest during periods of manipulation." In rare cases of inadvertent injury of a cardiac chamber and uncontrollable bleeding, heparin is administered and CPB commences via femoral vessel cannulation, using field suction as the major means of venous return.

Cardiopulmonary Bypass

After heparin administration, the cannulae are inserted, and adequate levels of anticoagulation are checked to ensure the patient is ready for the institution of CPB (Table 39-13). Attention is focused on adequacy of venous drainage (no pulsatility on CVP or PA waveforms), unobstructed arterial return (appropriate systemic arterial pressure), sufficient gas exchange, and provision of necessary anesthetics and muscle relaxants. The anesthetic requirements are decreased if systemic hypothermia is used.

Once full CPB is established, it is no longer necessary to ventilate the lungs. During the initial minutes of CPB, systemic arterial pressure initially drops to 30 to 40 mmHg as pulsatile flow ceases and the hemodilution effect of the CPB prime becomes apparent. Once adequate mixing is obtained, blood pressure increases to levels determined primarily by flow rate, and secondarily by total vascular resistance (Table 39-14). There is no consensus as to what constitutes the ideal blood pressure or flow rate for adequate vital organ perfusion, especially of the brain, during bypass.[114] Commonly, flow rates are maintained at approximately 50 to 60 mL/kg/min, with systemic blood pressures in the 50 to 60 mmHg range, whereas some believe that older patients benefit from a higher blood pressure (>70 mmHg).[127]

Monitoring and Management during Bypass

The common causes of blood pressure changes during CPB are listed in Table 39-14. Of primary importance is continuous

Table 39-13 Checklist before Initiating Cardiopulmonary Bypass

Laboratory Values
Heparinization adequate (ACT or other method)
Hematocrit

Anesthetic
Maintenance: amnestics, opioids, muscle relaxants are supplemented

Monitors
Arterial pressure: initial hypotension (followed by recovery)
CVP: if low, indicates adequate venous drainage
PCWP: if elevated, indicated LV distention (inadequate drainage, AI)
Pull back PAC 1–2 cm

Patient/field
Cannulae in place
- No kinks or clamps or air locks
- Arterial cannula is free of bubbles

Face
- Suffusion? Inadequate SVC drainage
- Unilateral blanching? Innominate artery cannulation

Heart
- Signs of distension (AI, ischemia)

Support
Usually not required

ACT, activated clotting time; CVP, central venous pressure; PCWP, pulmonary capillary wedge pressure; LV, left ventricle; AI, aortic insufficiency; PAC, pulmonary artery catheter; SVC, superior vena cava.

---

observation of the surgical field and cannulae to exclude mechanical obstruction to flow. Attention can then be directed to other causes of hypotension or hypertension and their treatment. Additional areas that require periodic monitoring and occasional intervention during CPB are also described in Table 39-14. Maintenance of adequate depths of anesthesia is obviously important during CPB, although clinical signs are few. Anesthetic requirements are decreased during the period of hypothermia but return toward normal when the patient is rewarmed.

Arterial pH and mixed venous oxygen saturation, often measured online, are used to assess the adequacy of perfusion. Urine output is monitored, but it is influenced by so many variables

---

Table 39-14 Checklist during Cardiopulmonary Bypass

Laboratory values	Heparinization adequate	ACT or other method
	ABGs	Is there acidosis?
	Hematocrit, Na$^+$, K$^+$, ionized Ca^{2+}, glucose	
Anesthetic	Discontinue ventilation	
Monitors		
Arterial hypotension	Inadequate venous return	Venous cannula malposition, clamp, kink, air lock
		Bleeding, hypovolemia, IVC obstruction, table too low
	Pump	Poor occlusion, low flow
	Arterial cannula	Misdirected, kinked, partially clamped, aortic dissection
	Decreased vascular tone	Anesthetics, hemodilution, idiopathic
	Transducer/monitor malfunction	Radial artery cannula malpositioned, dampened waveform
Arterial hypertension	Pump	High flow
	Arterial cannula	Misdirected
	Vasoconstriction	Light anesthetic plane, response to hypothermia
	Transducer/monitor malfunction:	Radial artery cannula malpositioned/kinked
Venous pressure	Decreased	Transducer higher than atrial level?
	Increased	True obstruction of chamber drainage (CVP: Right, PCWP/LA: left heart)
Adequate body perfusion	Flow and pressure?	
	Acidosis	
	Mixed venous blood oxygen saturation	
Temperature		
Urine output		
Patient/field	Heart	Distention, fibrillation
	Cyanosis, venous engorgement, skin temperature	
	Movement	
	Signs of light anesthesia/hypercapnia	Breathing/diaphragmatic movement
Support	Assist/adequacy of pump flow	Anesthetics/vasodilators for hypertension
		Constrictors for hypotension

ACT, activated clotting time; ABGs, arterial blood gases; IVC, inferior vena cava; CVP, central venous pressure; PCWP, pulmonary capillary wedge pressure; LA, left atrium; EEG, electroencephalogram.

(e.g., arterial and venous pressure, flow rate, temperature, diuretic history) that it is difficult to draw meaningful conclusions from this measurement.[128] In addition, postoperative renal failure develops from either aggravation of pre-existing renal dysfunction or persistent low cardiac output following bypass. Although many institutions administer diuretics routinely, they are just as assiduously avoided elsewhere.

Rewarming

When surgical repair is nearly complete, gradual rewarming of the patient begins. A gradient of 4° to 6°C is maintained between the patient and the perfusate to prevent formation of gas bubbles, and blood temperature should be less than 37°C. A slower rate of rewarming has been associated with better cognitive function 6 weeks post CABG surgery.[129] Patient awareness becomes a possibility as the potentiation of anesthetic effects due to hypothermia dissipates. If adequate doses of anesthetics have not been given, administration during rewarming should be considered to prevent recall of intraoperative events. Targeting an end-tidal concentration of the inhaled agent between 0.7 and 1.3 MAC is as effective as maintaining a BIS value between 40 and 60.[130] Use of volatile anesthetics is helpful if a smooth CPB course is anticipated and early weaning from mechanical ventilation and tracheal extubation are planned. On completion of the surgical repair any residual intracardiac air is removed as the anesthesiologist is vigorously ventilating the lungs to remove air from the pulmonary veins and aid in filling the cardiac chambers. TEE is particularly useful in assessing the effectiveness of the de-airing process. The heart is defibrillated (if needed) and externally paced or allowed to beat (if native rhythm is present) in preparation to separate from CPB.

Discontinuation of Cardiopulmonary Bypass

Prior to discontinuing CPB, the patient should be normothermic, no frank surgical bleeding must be present, the appropriate ABG values must be checked, the pulmonary compliance must be evaluated, and ventilation of the lungs must begun (Table 39-15). If necessary, heart rate and rhythm are regulated either pharmacologically or electrically (appropriate pacing, defibrillation, cardioversion), and vasoactive infusions started. The venous cannula(e) are then occluded incrementally and sufficient pump volume is transfused into the patient, while the bypass flow is slowly decreased (Fig. 39-9). During this time, the cardiac function is constantly evaluated from hemodynamic and TEE data and direct inspection of the heart, and the need for vasoactive or cardioactive drugs is re-assessed. The potential disparity between radial artery and aortic pressures must be kept in mind. Contractility, rhythm, and ventricular filling are continuously evaluated by careful observation of the beating heart and TEE. For example, a low blood pressure and a vigorously contracting, relatively empty ventricle suggest that volume and perhaps a vasoconstrictor are all that is needed to wean the patient from CPB, whereas adequate blood pressure in the presence of a sluggish and overdistended heart may be treated with a vasodilator and/or a small dose of an inotrope. Figure 39-10 presents a general approach to termination of CPB.

Inadequate cardiac performance must prompt a search for possible causes (Table 39-16); structural defects require more than mere regulation of inotropes or vasodilators. If the clinical picture is suggestive of coronary air emboli with diffuse ST segment elevation and a hypocontractile heart, continuous support on CPB with a high perfusion pressure and an unloaded ventricle is indicated to expel the air bubbles from the coronary circulation.

Table 39-15 Checklist before Separation from Cardiopulmonary Bypass

Laboratory Values
Hematocrit, ABGs
K^+: possibly elevated (cardioplegia)
Ionized Ca^{2+}

Anesthetic/machine
Lung compliance: Evaluate (hand ventilation)
Lungs are expanded, no atelectasis, both are ventilated (manual or mechanical)
Vaporizers: Off
Alarms: On

Monitors
Normothermia (37°C nasopharyngeal, 35.5°C bladder, 35°C rectal)
ECG: Rate, rhythm, ST
Transducers re-zeroed and leveled
Arterial and filling pressures
Recorder (if available)

Patient/field
Look at the heart!
De-aired: Check lead II, TEE
Eyeball contractility, size, rhythm
LV vent clamped/removed, caval snares released
Bleeding: No major sites (grafts, suture lines, LV vent site)
Vascular resistance: CPB flow ∝ MAP ÷ resistance

Support
As needed

ABGs, arterial blood gases; ECG, electrocardiogram; TEE, transesophageal echocardiography; LV, left ventricle; CPB, cardiopulmonary bypass; MAP, mean arterial pressure.

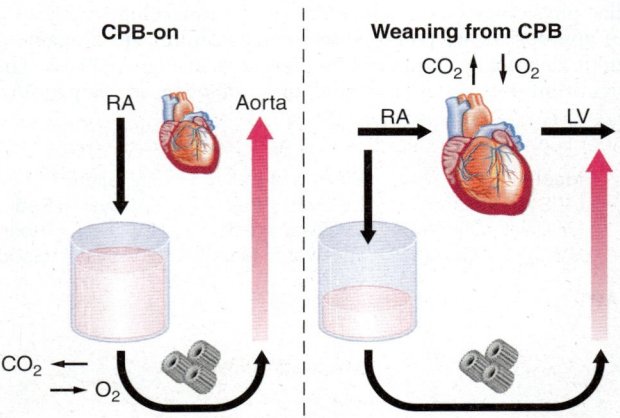

Figure 39-9 Weaning from cardiopulmonary bypass. While on cardiopulmonary bypass (CPB), the venous return to the heart is diverted from the right atrium (RA) to the CPB reservoir. The drainage is passive (by gravity). From the venous reservoir, the blood is "ventilated," CO_2 is removed, and O_2 is added, and then returned to the patient, usually into the aorta but occasionally via the femoral or axillary arteries. During weaning from CPB, the venous return to the CPB is reduced by gradually occluding the venous cannula, directing more of its contents to the right heart and lungs. LV, left ventricle.

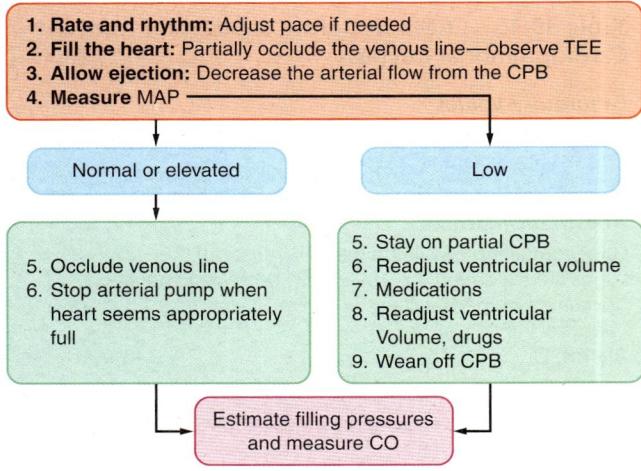

Figure 39-10 General approach to termination of cardiopulmonary bypass (CPB). TEE, transesophageal echocardiographic; MAP, mean arterial pressure; CO, cardiac output.

Table 39-16	Etiology of Right or Left Ventricular Dysfunction after Cardiopulmonary Bypass

Ischemia
Inadequate myocardial protection
Intraoperative infarction
Reperfusion injury
Coronary spasm
Coronary embolism (air, thrombus, calcium)
Technical difficulties (kinked or clotted grafts)

Uncorrected Structural Defects
Nongraftable vessels, diffuse coronary artery disease
Residual or new valve pathology
Hypertrophic cardiomyopathy
Shunts
Preexisting cardiac dysfunction

CPB-related Factors
Excessive cardioplegia
Unrecognized cardiac distention

An approach to patients with inadequate cardiac output is summarized in Table 39-17. The heart rate is adjusted first. Following that, ventricular filling is optimized by transfusing blood from the CPB pump. It is important not to overdistend the heart by transfusing to an arbitrary level of filling pressure because this may result in further myocardial dysfunction. It is important to image the cardiac chambers by TEE and directly look at the heart when evaluating the response to small incremental volume infusions. The ratio of systemic to pulmonary artery pressure is also helpful[131]; if increasing, the pulmonary artery pressure should increase at the same degree/rate as the systemic pressure (Fig. 39-11A). Change in opposite directions (e.g., pulmonary pressure increases and systemic pressure decreases; see Fig. 39-11C) is suggestive of LV failure, whereas an increasing CVP and decreasing pulmonary artery pressure indicate right ventricular failure.

If pharmacologic support is required, an integration of cardiac physiology (see Chapter 12) and pharmacology will lead to an appropriate selection. Numerous algorithms are available to guide decision making; one is presented in Figure 39-12. This algorithm uses systemic arterial and pulmonary artery pressures and cardiac output. If TEE is available, myocardial contractility and valvular function can be more readily assessed. After integrating available data, a diagnosis is made and appropriate treatment is begun. Continual reassessment of the situation is necessary to document the efficacy of treatment or to suggest new diagnoses and therapeutic approaches. If cardiac output is low and systemic pressure is adequate (Fig. 39-12A), an arteriolar dilator may improve forward flow by decreasing afterload. If systemic pressure is too low (Fig. 32-12C and D), thus prohibiting the use of vasodilators, an inotrope should be selected instead. Each inotropic drug has a distinct profile with respect to its effects on rate, contractility, SVR and PVR, and cardiac dysrhythmogenic potential (Table 39-18). If these initial therapies are insufficient to promote adequate forward flow, various combinations of drugs may be tested. If systemic perfusion is still inadequate, mechanical circulatory support (MCS) is required.

A therapeutic approach to right ventricular failure (Fig. 39-12D) is outlined in Table 39-19. When pulmonary arterial pressure is normal or decreased, the cause is usually severe right ventricular ischemia secondary to intraoperative events or air. The initial response is to return to full CPB, improve perfusion,

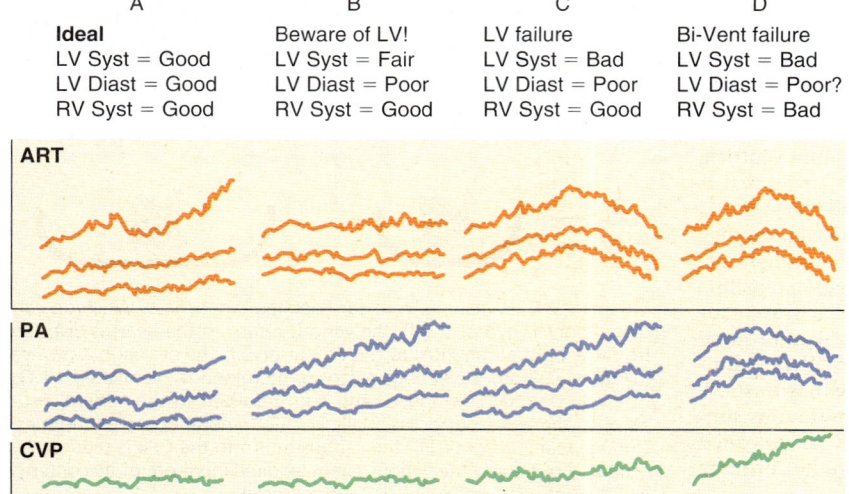

Figure 39-11 Hemodynamic abnormalities on termination of cardiopulmonary bypass. LV, left ventricle; syst, systolic; diast, diastolic; RV, right ventricle; ART, arterial pressure; PA, pulmonary artery; CVP, central venous pressure.

Table 39-17	Steps for Improving Systemic Flow
1	Heart rate (A-, V-, A/V-pacing) and rhythm
2	Preload: Optimize (beware of altered compliance postbypass)
3–4	Afterload reduction if blood pressure is high and/or contractility augmentation (inotrope if low CO)
5	Preload: Recheck and adjust
6	Combine therapies
7	IABP
8	VAD

A, atrial; V, ventricular; CO, cardiac output; IABP, intra-aortic balloon pump; VAD, ventricular assist device.

and await recovery and improvement of contractility. If this does not occur, inotropic and vasodilator therapy is established. In patients who have right ventricular failure secondary to high PVR, the mainstay of therapy is reduction of PVR with vasodilators, such as inhaled prostaglandin I_2 (PGE_2) or nitric oxide, and inotropic support. The phosphodiesterase III inhibitors, amrinone and milrinone, are particularly useful because they significantly decrease PVR and increase contractility. Overdistention of the ventricle must be assiduously avoided. Combination therapy with differential infusions refers to infusion of inotropes with vasoconstrictive properties into the left side of the circulation to maintain systemic perfusion, while avoiding an increase of the pulmonary circulation resistance. Persistent right ventricular failure precluding separation from CPB may require the insertion of a right ventricular assist device (RVAD).

Retrospective studies of patients undergoing CABG either alone or in combination with valve surgery showed that wall motion score index, combined CABG and mitral valve surgery, LV ejection fraction more than 35%, reoperation, moderate-to-severe MR, and aortic cross-clamp time were independent predictors for use of inotropes (39% of patients).[132] The use of

Table 39-18 Medications Given by Continuous Infusion

Drugs	Usual Initial Dose (µg/kg/min)	Usual Dose Range (µg/kg/min)
Amrinone[a]	2–5	2–20
Dopamine	2–5	2–20
Dobutamine	2–5	2–20
Epinephrine	0.01	0.01–0.1
Isoproterenol[b]	0.05–1	0.1–1
Lidocaine	20	20–50
Milrinone	50 µg/kg over 3 min	0.3–0.7
Nitroglycerin	0.5	0.5–5
Nitroprusside	0.5	0.5–5
Norepinephrine	0.1	0.1–1
Phenylephrine	1	1–3
Prostaglandin E_1	0.05–0.1	0.05–0.2
Vasopressin		0.0004

[a]Requires initial bolus of 750 µg/kg over 3 min before start of infusion.
[b]For chronotropic effect following cardiac transplantation, doses of 0.005–0.010 µg/kg/min are used.

more than one vasoactive drug or the need for mechanical support were found to be independent predictors of mortality and adverse outcome postoperatively.[133]

Intra-aortic Balloon Pump

The simplest and most readily available mechanical support device is the intra-aortic balloon pump.[132] It consists of a 25-cm long, sausage-shaped balloon composed of nonthrombogenic polyurethane mounted on a 90-cm vascular catheter. It is usually

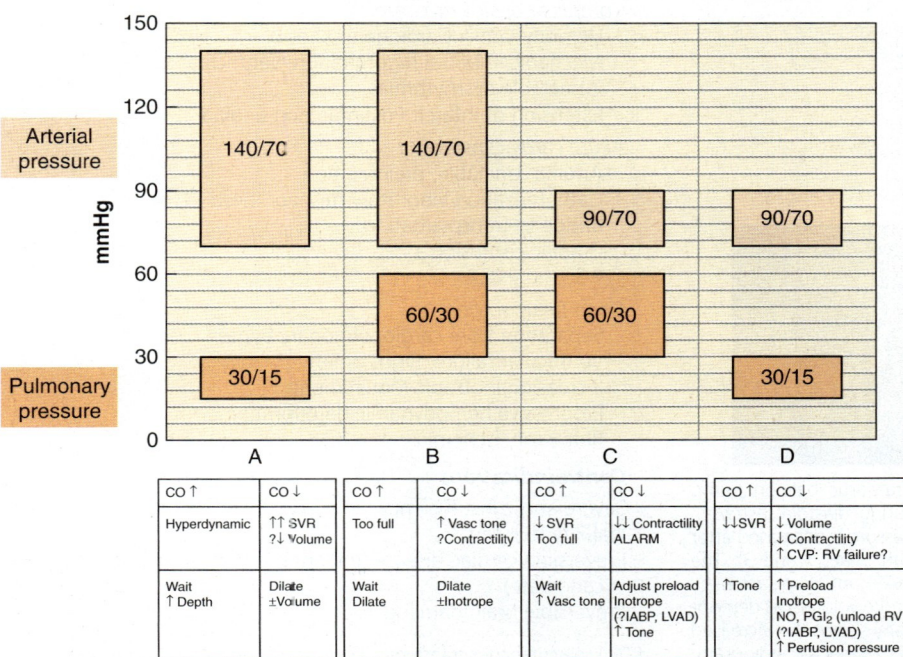

Figure 39-12 Algorithm for the diagnosis and treatment of hemodynamic abnormalities on termination of cardiopulmonary bypass. CO, cardiac output; SVR, systemic vascular resistance; vasc, vascular; IABP, intra-aortic balloon pump; LVAD, left ventricular assist device; CVP, central venous pressure; RV, right ventricle; NO, nitric oxide; PGI_2, prostacyclin; ?, possibly.

Table 39-19 Right Ventricular Failure

	Pulmonary Artery Pressure			
	Increased		Normal or Decreased	
	CVP Increased	CVP Decreased	CVP Increased	CVP Decreased
Diagnosis	RV and LV failure	LV failure	RV failure	Hypovolemia
Management	Inhaled NO or PGI$_2$, PDE-III Inotropes Differential infusions RVAD	Support on CPB	High perfusion pressure ?CABG	Volume

CVP, central venous pressure; RV, right ventricle; LV, left ventricle; NO, nitric oxide; PGI$_2$, prostaglandin I$_2$; PDE-III, phosphodiesterase III inhibitor; CPB, cardiopulmonary bypass; RVAD, right ventricular assist device; CABG, coronary artery bypass graft.

inserted into the femoral artery, either percutaneously or after surgical exposure, and advanced so the distal tip is below the left subclavian artery (to prevent emboli to the head vessels) and the proximal above the renal arteries.[134] Occasionally, when peripheral vascular disease prohibits passage of the balloon via the femoral artery, it is inserted via the ascending aorta.

The intra-aortic balloon pump decreases M$\dot{V}$O$_2$ and increases oxygen supply to the myocardium. It uses synchronized counterpulsation to assist a beating, ejecting heart: blood volume is moved in a direction "counter" to normal flow. The balloon is inflated during diastole and deflated during systole. The balloon inflation elevates aortic diastolic blood pressure (diastolic augmentation), thus increasing the coronary perfusion gradient proximally, and enhances forward flow distally. During the subsequent systole and balloon deflation, the LV ejects facing a lower systemic diastolic pressure (systolic unloading, reduced M$\dot{V}$O$_2$) (Fig. 39-13). Proper timing of balloon deflation is necessary to reduce end-diastolic pressure as much as possible to maximally off-load the ventricle. The indications and contraindications for intra-aortic balloon pump placement are listed in Table 39-20. Myocardial function often improves with the use of the intra-aortic balloon pump, and systemic perfusion and vital organ function are preserved.[135] It is crucial to control heart rate and suppress atrial and ventricular dysrhythmias to ensure proper balloon timing. As cardiac function returns, the assist ratio is gradually weaned from every beat to every other beat and so on and, assuming no further cardiac deterioration, until it is removed.

Complications associated with the intra-aortic balloon pump are primarily related to ischemia distal to the site of balloon insertion. Direct trauma to the vessel, arterial obstruction, and thrombosis are most common, although aortic perforation and balloon rupture occur rarely. Platelet destruction and thrombocytopenia may also occur.

Ventricular Assist Device

Infrequently (1%), the heart is unable to meet systemic metabolic demands despite revascularization, maximal pharmacologic

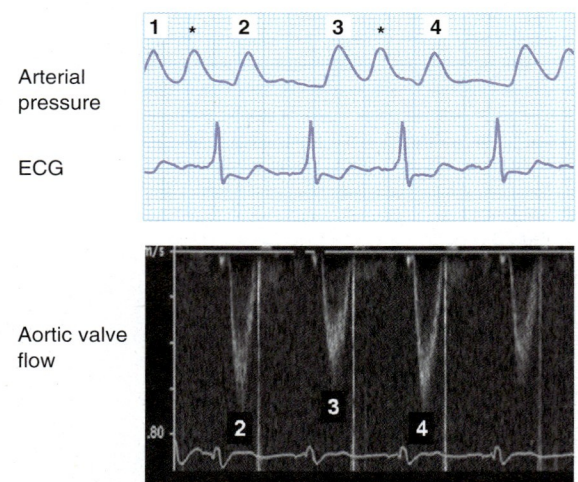

Figure 39-13 The physiologic effects of intra-aortic balloon pump (IABP) counterpulsation. The IABP is inflated during diastole (*asterisk*), every other beat (rate 1:2). The arterial systolic pressure is decreased after IABP augmentation (compare beats *2* and *4* with beats *1* and *3*). The diastolic arterial pressure is augmented during IABP inflation (*asterisk*). The flow through the aortic valve (approximate stroke volume) as demonstrated with pulsed wave Doppler echocardiography shows the increased forward flow after augmentation (beats *2* and *4*). ECG, electrocardiogram.

Table 39-20 Intra-aortic Balloon Pump Indications and Contraindications

Indications

Complications of myocardial ischemia
   Hemodynamic: Cardiogenic shock
   Mechanical: Mitral regurgitation, ventricular septal defect
   Intractable dysrhythmias
   Extension of infarct: Postinfarction angina

Acute cardiac instability
   Angina: Unstable, preinfarction
   Catheterization laboratory mishap: failed PTCA
   Bridge to transplantation
   Cardiac contusion
   ? Septic shock

Open heart surgery
   Separation from cardiopulmonary bypass
   Ventricular failure: Right or left
   Increasing inotropic requirement
   Progressive hemodynamic deterioration
   Refractory ischemia

Contraindications

Severe aortic insufficiency
Inability to insert
Irreversible cardiac disease (patient is not a transplant candidate)
Irreversible brain damage

PTCA, percutaneous transluminal coronary angioplasty; ?, possibly.

therapy, and insertion of the intra-aortic balloon pump. Under these circumstances, devices that provide cardiac output and/or bypass either the LV or RV are required. MCS is increasingly an option for patients suffering from either an acute or chronic myocardial insult. Maintenance of systemic perfusion, correction of metabolic acidosis, ventricular decompression, and reduced myocardial oxygen consumption by MCS may aid in myocardial recovery.[136] Where myocardial recovery is not possible, MCS can act as a bridge to allow for cardiac transplantation and has now become a destination therapy in its own right.

MCS can provide short or long-term support to a single failing ventricle or provide biventricular support to both ventricles. Ventricular assist devices (VAD) are named for the ventricles that is supported, that is, left ventricular assist device (LVAD), RVAD, or in biventricular support (BiVAD). The length of MCS support anticipated will often dictate the type of device that is used to provide MCS.

In an LVAD, the blood is drained to the device (which assumes the function of the failing ventricle) via a cannula placed in either the LA or the LV apex and is ejected into the systemic circulation via a cannula or graft placed in the aorta. In an RVAD, a cannula is placed in the right atrium to divert blood from the RV, which is then ejected into the pulmonary artery.

The types of MCS devices that are available include extracorporeal and fully implantable devices.[137] Extracorporeal devices use cannulae that divert the patient's blood to a pump or biohead that is outside the body and deliver it back to the systemic circulation. By adding an oxygenator to these extracorporeal devices extracorporeal membrane oxygenation (ECMO) can be provided. Once MCS is no longer required the device can be explanted. If there is no meaningful cardiac recovery long-term options are utilized. Long-term options include fully implantable devices that are placed in the patient's abdominal cavity with only the control lines exiting the body and can allow patients to return of the activities of daily living.

For acute short-term MCS of the LV, RV, or BiV the Thoratec CentriMag is often used. This device is composed of a single-use centrifugal pump, a motor, and a primary drive console. Using a bearingless magnetically levitated impeller, it provides continuous flow via a centrifugal-type rotary blood pump. The pump can rotate at speeds of 1,500 to 5,500 rpm and can provide flow rates of up to 9.9 L/min. Other short-term devices include the Abiomed AB5000 (Abiomed, Danvers, MA) and Thoratec PVAD (Thoratec Laboratories, Pleasanton, CA). Another short-term VAD that is inserted intravascularly and be used during high-risk coronary intervention or as a bridge to recovery is the Abiomed Impella (Abiomed).[138] This device is a catheter-based intravascular microaxial blood pump. This axial flow pump is capable of delivering either 2.5 or 5 L/min of flow (depending on the device used). It can be placed either percutaneously or via a cut down in either the femoral or axillary artery. The device is placed within the aorta with the distal/inflow portion crossing the AV and resting in the LV. LV blood is diverted to the outflow portion of the device via an impeller pump to the distal aorta providing improved systemic perfusion.

Long-term VADs include the Thoratec Heartmate II which uses nonpulsatile axial flow (Thoratec Laboratories, Pleasanton, CA).

Anesthetic Considerations for MCS

When considering an anesthetic plan for a patient requiring MCS one must take into account the degree of myocardial dysfunction. This may involve one or both ventricles. In addition to standard monitoring, preinduction arterial blood pressure monitoring is essential. The ablation of high sympathetic tone that heart failure patients possess may be catastrophic and cause cardiac arrest on the induction of anesthesia. As such, agents that maintain hemodynamic stability are chosen for these patients. These include the use of etomidate as an induction agent (due to its lack of vasodilatation and myocardial depression) and a careful "balanced technique." Incremental doses of midazolam and etomidate followed by a potent opioid (such as fentanyl or sufentanil) and neuromuscular blockade if titrated carefully are usually tolerated. One caveat is that, due to the slow circulation times in heart failure patients, care must be taken to allow medications time to circulate and reach the desired effect. Overzealous dosing may cause cardiovascular collapse. A good rule of thumb is that a 20% decrease in blood pressure should be treated using a direct acting agent such as phenylephrine or norepinephrine. This allows for a margin of safety and may prevent profound hypotension due to the long circulation time if the blood pressure is treated only as the patient becomes hypotensive. Volatile anesthetic agents are generally well tolerated in low doses. Following the induction of anesthesia a PAC and TEE are routinely placed. The PAC provides important information such as CVP (indication of RV function), pulmonary artery pressures, mixed venous oxygen saturation, and cardiac output. TEE is used in both the pre- and post-implant period.

Important information that needs to be determined by TEE prior to the initiation of CPB include anything that would restrict or impair LVAD filling (mitral stenosis, tricuspid regurgitation, severe RV dysfunction), the presence of aortic insufficiency (causing LV dilatation), and other anatomic issues that impact LVAD placement (PFO/ASD, intracardiac thrombus, severe atherosclerosis of the ascending aorta). Post-implant TEE is used to assess the adequacy of de-airing maneuvers, proper cannula position, and RV size and function.[139]

Considerations for VAD Patients

An in-depth discussion of the considerations for VAD patients is beyond the scope of this chapter and the reader is advised to consult one of the excellent review articles on the subject.[140]

Whether RVAD or LVAD support is required, several issues exist in common for both. In each case, maintenance of adequate preload is essential for proper device function. Once the failing ventricle is mechanically supported, the "cardiac output" of that chamber(s) is dependent upon adequate preload to fill the device and normal to low vascular resistance to promote forward flow and provide adequate systemic perfusion. Low to normal PVR is especially important in patients with an LVAD. The RV is exquisitely sensitive to changes in afterload and a failing RV will not "fill" the left side of the heart and therefore limit LVAD output. Despite extreme care, severe RV failure requiring biventricular support still occurs in approximately 30% of patients requiring an LVAD. Inotropic agents such as epinephrine, dobutamine, and milrinone as well as inhaled agents such as nitric oxide and iloprost are often used to support the RV and help maintain low PVR. Unfortunately, agents that lower PVR also tend to lower SVR. In addition, patients undergoing LVAD implantation tend to manifest profound vasodilatation following CPB. Vasopressin by virtue of not increasing PVR is preferred over norepinephrine as a vasopressor especially in patients with pulmonary hypertension.[141]

For patients on MCS that require noncardiac surgery the maintenance of adequate volume status and careful safeguarding of low to normal vascular resistance is important. The use of a PAC or TEE should be tailored to the specific patient and procedure. However, TEE is recommended in the case of patients with impaired RV function or in procedures with the potential for large volume shifts/transfusion requirements. No specific anesthetic technique is recommended in patients with MCS; however, abrupt changes in SVR due to neuraxial techniques such as spinal anesthesia make them less desirable. Patients with fully implantable devices should be considered at risk for pulmonary aspiration and treated accordingly.[142,143] Of note, in the event of cardiac arrest, chest compression is contraindicated due to the possible disruption or displacement of the VAD cannulae.

Postcardiopulmonary Bypass

Continued vigilance is mandatory during decannulation, protamine administration, "drying up," and chest closure. Anesthetics are administered as clinically indicated. Transient atrial or junctional dysrhythmias may be caused by removal of the atrial cannulae. Heparin is reversed with protamine following removal of the venous cannulae, whereas the arterial return cannula remains in place for transfusion of blood to the systemic circulation as needed. When this is completed and bleeding is controlled the arterial cannula is removed, and if bleeding is considered to be under control the chest is closed. During decannulation, the possibility exists for unexpected bleeding from the atrial or aortic suture lines, and this sometimes requires rapid transfusion. Continued vigilance for new ischemia (manifested by ST segment changes, ectopy, atrial dysrhythmia, regional wall motion abnormalities by TEE) is important because it may indicate a correctable problem with the grafts. All valve procedures are assessed by TEE for adequacy of the repair or replacement (i.e., perivalvular leak, residual stenosis).

Reversal of Anticoagulation

Protamine, a polycationic protein derived from salmon sperm, is used to neutralize heparin. The initial and total doses administered vary widely. Some use a fixed ratio of protamine to heparin, others use 1-mg protamine to 100-U heparin, and still others look to automated protamine titrations to suggest the initial dose. Regardless of the method selected, further requirements are assessed by repeated measures of the activated coagulation time or other clotting assay(s), as well as by the appearance of the surgical field.[144]

Protamine administration is associated with a broad spectrum of hemodynamic effects.[145] Idiosyncratic responses include type I anaphylactic reactions and both immediate and delayed anaphylactoid responses. True anaphylaxis is rare and characterized by increased airway pressure, vasodilation with systemic hypotension, and skin flushing. Increased incidence of reactions has been reported in patients sensitized to protamine from previous cardiac catheterization, hemodialysis, cardiac surgery, or exposure to neutral protamine Hagedorn insulin. Perhaps the most devastating complication associated with protamine is sudden and profound pulmonary hypertension accompanied by an elevated CVP, RV failure, and systemic hypotension. This complication, which may occur in approximately 1% of patients, is mediated by release of thromboxane and C5a anaphylatoxin. The reaction is extremely short-lived, and although reinstitution of CPB is required on rare occasions, it is usually not necessary. Whether protamine is administered via the RA, LA, or aorta, or peripherally, probably makes no difference to the occurrence of this rare reaction. Because systemic hypotension is more likely with rapid injection of protamine, slow administration into a peripheral venous site is advisable.

Postbypass Bleeding

Persistent oozing following heparin reversal is not uncommon. The usual causes include inadequate surgical hemostasis or reduced platelet count or function, and neither is identified by a prolonged activated coagulation time. Insufficient doses of protamine, dilution of coagulation factors, thrombocytopenia, and platelet dysfunction, and rarely "heparin rebound," belong in the differential diagnosis. Blood product transfusion based on point of care testing has been proven effective in treating nonsurgical bleeding.[146]

After adequate hemostasis is obtained, the chest is closed. This is occasionally associated with transient decreases in blood pressure, which usually respond to volume infusion. If hypotension persists, the chest should be reopened to rule out cardiac tamponade, a kinked coronary bypass graft, or other problems.

As the surgeon completes skin closure, the anesthesiologist prepares for an orderly transfer of the patient from the operating room to the recovery room or ICU. Medicated infusions must be maintained, as clinically indicated, with portable infusion pumps. Additional syringes with emergency cardiac medications and necessary equipment for airway management should be carried, and blood pressure(s) and ECG constantly monitored.

Minimally Invasive Cardiac Surgery

Despite advantages in cardiac surgery and perfusion technology, the deleterious effects of CPB and aortic cross-clamping are well documented. The desire to avoid these complications, as well as complications associated with sternotomy, was a factor leading to the development of minimally invasive techniques not requiring CPB.[147] As the population ages, older patients with multiple comorbid medical conditions requiring surgery are increasingly common. Avoidance of aortic manipulation and cross-clamping especially in elderly patients is associated with lower stroke rates.[148]

Newer procedures include minimally invasive direct coronary artery bypass (MIDCAB), off-pump coronary artery bypass (OPCAB), robotic surgery,[149] and percutaneous valve repair/replacement performed in the catheterization laboratory or a hybrid operating room,[69,150] MIDCAB is considered as an alternative to angioplasty for single-vessel LAD coronary artery disease. It is performed via a left thoracotomy using one-lung ventilation. In OPCAB surgery the exposure is via a sternotomy and CPB is not used. The development of retractors and stabilization devices allows the surgeon to operate on the beating heart without causing arrhythmia or hypotension. Other advances include the use of intracoronary shunts and sutureless anastomotic devices. OPCAB can provide complete multivessel coronary revascularization. Alternate incisions tutored as "minimally invasive" provide limited exposure and increase surgical difficulty. A type of minimally invasive cardiac surgery uses port access technology, with the assistance of a robotic system. A period of single-lung ventilation may be required under capnothorax for insertion of surgical access ports. Catheters are placed percutaneously in the femoral artery and internal jugular vein to facilitate CPB. These catheters include an endovascular aortic balloon that acts as cross-clamp, a modified PAC to act as an LV vent, and a coronary sinus catheter placed for retrograde cardioplegia administration.[151]

Changes in surgical technique have forced changes in anesthetic technique.[152] Shorter-acting agents are used to facilitate early extubation. The hemodynamics are monitored constantly and rapid intervention is needed in the face of changing hemodynamics. One major problem associated with OPCAB is that exposure of the diseased coronaries and subsequent graft placement requires positioning of the heart that is often associated with hypotension and ischemia. In such cases, standard monitors used in cardiac surgery may not be useful in detecting ST-T wave changes, because the positioning and retraction of the heart often results in a low-amplitude ECG with axis deviation. The placement of laparotomy pads in the pericardial well or lifting the heart out of the chest, makes TEE unreliable in detecting regional wall motion changes signifying ischemia. In addition, displacement of the heart may cause falsely elevated central venous and pulmonary pressures despite the presence of hypovolemia. Sudden changes in pulmonary artery pressure may be related to acute MR due to surgical positioning. Direct observation of the heart and communication with the surgeon are critical in managing hemodynamic swings.[153,154]

The coronary artery to be anastomosed is isolated proximally and distally using either an occluder clip or a snare. Following such an occlusion there is usually a period of myocardial ischemia. Pre-existing high-grade lesions might have caused formation of collateral circulation, which may ameliorate potential ischemia. Right coronary lesions will predispose to bradycardia, atrial dysrhythmias, and heart block. For these reasons, immediate access to cardiac pacing and cardioversion are essential. Left-sided coronary lesions may cause malignant ventricular dysrhythmias and hemodynamic collapse.

Several techniques are used to avoid rapid hemodynamic changes. These include optimizing preload prior to positioning, judicious use of inotropes and α-agonists, and placing the patient in Trendelenburg position, which allows redistribution of intravascular volume to support the heart in the vertical position.

Normothermia contributes to early extubation as well as prevention of coagulopathy. Aggressive pain control improves patient satisfaction and contributes to early extubation. Techniques for pain control in OPCAB and minimally invasive surgery include systemic opioids and nonsteroidal agents such as ketorolac (in patients without renal insufficiency), local infiltration of the surgical incision, and regional anesthesia. Regional techniques including thoracic epidurals and neuraxial narcotics are used with great success, although anticoagulation is a concern in patients with central regional anesthetics.[155] Anticoagulant protocols are controversial. Both heparin and protamine doses vary between centers. Some do not routinely reverse heparin or administer reduced doses of protamine because of the suspicion that OPCAB may cause hypercoagulability.[156]

Despite great interest in OPCAB as a way to decrease the complications associated with CPB, many remain skeptical as to the benefits. Several studies have shown the superiority of OPCAB in regard to improved neurologic outcome, whereas others have not.[157,158] Despite disappointing results in regard to neurocognitive and overall outcome, several short-term outcomes are improved following OPCABG. These include shorter ICU stays, decreased utilization of hospital resources, and decreased incidence of atrial fibrillation.[159]

Many have argued that the advantages of traditional CABG over OPCAB include a still bloodless field allowing for a better anastomosis and long-term graft patency.[160] Other studies have refuted this to prove equal long-term graft patency rates.[161] The proponents of OPCAB tend to be very familiar with the technique and perform off-pump surgery frequently. This frequency seems to make them technically facile in the peculiarities unique to OPCAB surgery. As such, this may account for varying results from center to center. Currently, there is no consensus as to the superiority of standard CABG versus OPCAB.

Postoperative Considerations

Bring Backs

Postoperative re-exploration is needed in 4% to 5% of cases. The indications are persistent bleeding, cardiac tamponade, and, infrequently, unexplained poor cardiac performance. Surgery is usually required within the first 24 hours but also later in cases of delayed tamponade. The possibility of cardiac tamponade must always be included in the differential diagnosis of the postoperative "dwindles" because the classic symptoms and signs are often absent.

Tamponade

In tamponade, the intracardiac pressures are deceptively elevated and do not reflect the actual intracardiac pressure or volume. Because the surrounding (intrapericardial) pressure is increased, the distending (transmural) pressure (intracavitary pressure–extracavitary pressure) is actually decreased. Cardiac chamber collapse is a critical feature of cardiac tamponade, and the chambers with the lowest intracardiac pressure (atria in systole and RV in diastole) are most likely to be compressed. The stroke volume is limited, and tachycardia maintains the cardiac output. Peripheral vasoconstriction to preserve venous return and systemic blood pressure is another compensatory mechanism. Myocardial ischemia may occur because of the tachycardia and reduced coronary perfusion pressure.

Clinically, awake patients present with dyspnea, orthopnea, tachycardia, paradoxical pulse, and hypotension, but the intubated, sedated, and mechanically ventilated patient in the postoperative care unit following cardiac surgery may have varied clinical and hemodynamic presentations. In the cardiac surgical patient the diagnosis of tamponade should be considered whenever hemodynamic deterioration or signs of low cardiac output occur. In postoperative cardiac patients, the pericardium is no longer intact, and loculated areas of clot may compress only one chamber, causing isolated increases in filling pressure (i.e., mimicking right and/or left ventricular dysfunction). Urine output is usually diminished. Serial chest films typically show progressive mediastinal widening. Diastolic collapse of the RA and right ventricular and/or LV diastolic collapse are the most sensitive and specific echocardiographic signs of cardiac tamponade.[162] In addition, there is excessive respiratory variation of the Doppler flow velocities across the tricuspid and mitral valves. The existing extracardiac compression augments the respiration-induced ventricular interdependence and affects the diastolic filling of the two ventricles differently. During mechanical inspiration the increased intrathoracic pressure will impede the RV and augment the LV filling. As a result, the diastolic tricuspid flow will show marked decrease as the filling gradient between the extrathoracic veins and the intrathoracic RV is further reduced. At the same time, the diastolic mitral flow will increase as the increased intrathoracic pressure, which is transmitted to the intrathoracic pulmonary veins, increases the filling gradient of the LV. The opposite effects take place during mechanical exhalation when the effects of positive ventilation dissipate. A TTE approach to document these reciprocal changes may be limited, as a retrosternal collection may be difficult to visualize in the postoperative patient, whereas subcostal views are rarely feasible early in the postoperative period because of the presence of chest tubes, pacemaker wires, and/or local tenderness in the subxiphoid area. TEE is a better diagnostic tool in the immediate postoperative period.

The treatment for cardiac tamponade is surgical. The selected anesthetics drugs should preserve the compensatory mechanisms that sustain forward flow. Drugs with vasodilator (either venous or arteriolar) or myocardial depressant properties should be avoided in patients with serious hemodynamic compromise and dosages of any induction agent should be appropriately reduced. Ketamine, because of its sympathomimetic effects, may be helpful in preserving heart rate and blood pressure response. It is not, however, a panacea and can induce hypotension in patients under maximal sympathetic stress. If on reopening the chest there is minimal fluid or if the patient shows little improvement, a thorough search for other causes of inadequate cardiac performance, such as clotted or kinked grafts, myocardial ischemia, or valve malfunction, is indicated.

Pain Management

Early awakening and extubation have brought the problem of postoperative pain management in cardiac surgery into focus. The standard practice has been intravenous opioids given as needed followed by conversion to oral pain medications. However, the quest is on to find an ideal postoperative pain management technique to complement the goal of early extubation and maximize patient satisfaction.[163] Several studies have shown the benefits of intrathecal administration of opioids.[164] The addition of nonsteroidal anti-inflammatory agents may play an increasing role. In cardiac patients with severe pain associated with sternal fractures due to the sternal retraction device during internal mammary harvest, epidural analgesia has been shown to be safe and effective and results in improved postoperative pulmonary function.

Anesthesia for Children with Congenital Heart Disease

Because "anatomy dictates the physiology," the anesthetic management of children with congenital heart disease (CHD) requires knowledge of anatomic defects, planned surgical procedures, and comprehensive understanding of the altered physiology. The overall incidence of CHD varies between 4 and 12 per 1,000 live births. CHD can be cyanotic or acyanotic. The best way to understand the impact of a congenital defect and how anesthetic agents will interact with this defect is to envision the path blood must follow to maintain flow to the pulmonary arteries and aorta. Table 39-21 classifies various types of lesions by their physiologic impact; however, it must be remembered that there is often more than one defect present.

Preoperative Evaluation

History

In infancy, heart failure usually becomes manifest through feeding difficulties, easy fatigability, vomiting, lethargy, and labored breathing. In the older child, heart failure causes easy fatigability, shortness of breath, and dyspnea on exertion. Child's age and weight, presence of an upper respiratory tract infection, baseline arterial saturation, and anticipated durations of surgery and CPB must be taken into consideration.[165]

In addition, a detailed medication and surgical history should be obtained. The previous surgical procedures may be key to understanding the patient's anatomy.

Physical Examination

The physical examination of a child should seek signs and symptoms of poorly compensated congenital cardiac lesions. These children most often present with failure to thrive, which could be due to pulmonary hypertension and/or poor peripheral

Table 39-21 Physiologic Effects of Congenital Cardiac Lesions

Volume overload (ventricle or atrium) resulting in increased pulmonary blood flow
- Atrial septal defect: ↑ flow, ↓ pressure
- Ventricular septal defect: ↑ flow, ↑ pressure
- Patent ductus arteriosus: ↑ flow, ↑ pressure
- Endocardial cushion defect: ↑ flow, ↑ pressure

Cyanosis resulting from obstruction to pulmonary blood flow
- Tetralogy of Fallot
- Tricuspid atresia
- Pulmonary atresia

Pressure overload to the ventricle
- Aortic stenosis
- Coarctation of the aorta
- Pulmonary stenosis

Cyanosis due to a common mixing chamber
- Total anomalous venous return
- Truncus arteriosus
- Double outlet right ventricle
- Single ventricle

Cyanosis due to separation of the systemic and pulmonary circulation
- Transposition of the great vessels

↑, increase; ↓, decrease.

oxygenation and organ perfusion. The physical examination should seek to discover other signs of congestive heart failure, such as irritability, diaphoresis, tachycardia, rales, jugular venous distention, and hepatomegaly. Clinical examination of extremities should include evaluation of cyanosis, clubbing, edema, pulse volume, and blood pressure. In children with Blalock–Taussig shunts (subclavian artery to pulmonary artery), upper extremity pulses may be absent or reduced on the side of the shunt. It is important to measure blood pressure in the arms as well as in the legs in all patients in whom CHD is suspected; thus, coarctation of aorta will not be missed. Auscultation of the heart in these patients can reveal different types of murmurs depending on the lesions (Table 39-22).

The possibility of associated congenital anomalies should be considered. The overall incidence of extracardiac anomalies among children with CHD may be as high as 20%.[166]

Laboratory Evaluations

The presence of anemia in these patients may require priming of the extracorporeal circuit with red blood cells. Children with cyanotic lesions manifest with polycythemia. Polycythemia results as a consequence of bone marrow stimulation (via release of erythropoietin from the kidneys) from arterial desaturation. Increased red cell mass can lead to hyperviscosity, peripheral sludging, and reduced oxygen delivery. Sludging is augmented by dehydration from preoperative fasting and by hypothermia from low ambient operating room temperatures. In patients with hematocrit above 70%, consideration should be given to preoperative electrophoresis if symptomatic hyperviscosity is present. Cyanotic children with low hematocrit may exhibit hypoxic spells more readily than if the hematocrit were normal. Polycythemia can induce a low-grade disseminated intravascular coagulation with activation of fibrinolysis, degranulation of platelets, and consumption of coagulation factors. Newborns often have

Table 39-22 Classification of Cardiac Murmurs

Systolic
Stenotic semilunar valves
Regurgitant atrioventricular valves
Atrial septal defect
Ventricular septal defect
Coarctation of the aorta

Diastolic
Regurgitant semilunar valves
Stenotic atrioventricular valves
Mitral flow rumble
Tricuspid flow rumble

Continuous
Patent ductus arteriosus
Arteriovenous fistula
Excessive bronchial collaterals
Aortopulmonary window
Venous hum
Surgical shunt
Severe peripheral pulmonic stenosis

inadequate liver-dependent coagulation factors because of immaturity of hepatic function. Platelet count, prothrombin time, and partial thromboplastin time should be evaluated.

Children on diuretic therapy are at risk for hypokalemia, particularly if they are receiving digitalis. Infants, particularly those with congestive heart failure, are also at risk for both hypoglycemia and hypocalcemia. Children who have undergone major cardiac procedures earlier in their lives may have been exposed to blood or blood products and are at increased risk of having abnormal serum antibodies to various blood antigens. Hence, samples of a child's blood should be sent to the blood bank for possible cross-matching.

Cardiac Evaluations

Echocardiography delineates most of the cardiac anatomy and permits noninvasive measurement of ventricular size and function, cardiac output, and severity of valve dysfunction. Cardiac catheterization is reserved for patients with poor echocardiographic windows and when there is intervening bone or air-filled lung (e.g., scoliosis or abnormalities of the peripheral pulmonary arteries). The chest radiograph of a child with CHD should be evaluated for cardiac position, size, shape, abnormal vessels, right aortic arch, scimitar syndrome (hypoplasia/aplasia of one or more lobes of right lung and hypoplasia of right pulmonary artery), aberrant pulmonary vessels, abnormal position of bronchi, vascular rings, or associated pulmonary abnormalities (e.g., pneumonia, atelectasis, or emphysema). The ECG should be reviewed for rate and rhythm abnormalities.

Premedication

The purpose of the premedication is to have a calm child without oversedation, loss of protective airway reflexes, or hemodynamic compromise. This will facilitate the separation of the child from the parents and ease the fear and anxiety associated with the perioperative period. Details on this topic are provided in Chapters 42 and 43.

Monitoring

In addition to standard monitors, additional monitors used during open heart procedures include peripheral and central temperature monitoring, invasive blood pressure monitoring, CVP monitoring (which can include right atrial or left atrial pressure line placement by the surgeon intraoperatively), and TEE.

Anesthetic and Intraoperative Management

Inhalational agents hold a prominent place as induction as well as maintenance agents in pediatric cardiac anesthesia. However, patients with poor ventricular function and those with critical dependence on SVR and/or PVR will need intravenous access pre-induction and avoidance or limitation of anesthetic agents that can further compromise hemodynamic function. The choice of anesthetic agents following induction is governed by ventricular function (presence or absence of congestive failure), anticipated use of CPB, and the possibility of mechanical ventilation or tracheal extubation at the end of the case. Opioids are used routinely to limit the stress response in the prebypass phase of pediatric cardiac surgery. Neonates and infants undergoing cardiac surgery and deep hypothermic CPB can generate a significant hormonal stress response. No specific relationship between opioid dose and stress response has been established. Details of dose and side effects are provided in Chapters 42 and 43. Of special note is the marked reduction in neuromuscular blocking requirements during hypothermic bypass.

The many advances in the CPB and surgical and anesthetic techniques have significantly improved the survival of children with CHD.[167] However, CPB produces marked hemostatic derangements including:
- Dilution of blood clotting factors
- Activation of the clotting cascade and consumption of clotting factors and platelets
- Reduction in coagulation enzymatic activity
- Activation of the fibrinolytic pathway.
- Aminocaproic acid or tranexamic acid has been used to attenuate coagulopathy during pediatric cardiac surgery associated with CPB.

Hemodilution is a prominent problem in CPB in pediatric and neonatal populations. Modified ultrafiltration during pediatric CPB reduces total body water and serum levels of inflammatory mediators. In neonates, modified ultrafiltration results in an elevated hematocrit, improved pulmonary compliance in the immediate postbypass period, and probably improved cerebral metabolic recovery after deep hypothermic circulatory arrest, although the long-term benefit on outcome is unclear.[168] Separation from CPB will require pharmacologic and/or pacing support in some patients. In lesions in which the presence of increased PVR is known or suspected, addition of nitric oxide may be of benefit. Inhaled nitric oxide works via cGMP, causing pulmonary vasodilatation. It is truly selective for the pulmonary vascular bed and, in addition, should improve the ventilation/perfusion matching in the lungs.

Drugs that are useful in the postbypass period are given in Table 39-18.

Tracheal Extubation and Postoperative Ventilation

Children with simple lesions who have undergone CPB for procedures that do not involve ventricular incisions (atrial septal defect, ventricular septal defect without failure repaired across the tricuspid valve) can often have the endotracheal tubes removed at the conclusion of surgery or shortly thereafter in the ICU.[169,170]

Children most at risk for ventilatory failure following cardiac surgery include:

- Patients with complex surgeries requiring long bypass time and circulatory arrest time
- Patients less than a year of age and those well under their predicted weight
- Patients with Down syndrome
- Patients with pulmonary hypertension requiring preoperative ventilatory support
- Patients with postoperative cardiovascular and pulmonary complications

In some cases, nasal continuous positive airway pressure can be employed instead of mechanical ventilation. In patients with Fontan physiology (passive pulmonary circulatory), decreasing PVR is paramount and is very much dependent on adequate ventilation, usually through mechanical means. The potentially detrimental effects of endotracheal intubation and positive pressure ventilation offset this advantage. Positive pressure ventilation is known to have a deleterious effect on pulmonary blood flow in patients with Fontan physiology. Resumption of pain-free spontaneous respiration does enhance hemodynamic performance in these patients.[169]

Regional anesthetic techniques can be used to supplement intraoperative anesthesia and provide postoperative analgesia. For example, caudal (epidural) opioids can be used in repair of coarctation of the aorta in the older child or ligation of a patent ductus arteriosus. Some physicians have used caudal or intrathecal morphine for cases involving CPB (and concomitant heparin administration), although this is not a common practice. The recommendation has been made that one allow 60 minutes to elapse between placement of a neuraxial block and administration of heparin, although there is no evidence to support this time interval.[171] Reported benefits of regional techniques include decreased stress response, improved pulmonary and gastrointestinal function, and resultant potential for cost reduction.[172] However, it is difficult to establish the superiority of a regional technique compared with intravenous analgesia.[173]

Hybrid Procedures in Pediatric Cardiac Surgery

Hybrid pediatric cardiac surgery is an emerging field that reaches across interdisciplinary lines and combines skills and techniques traditionally used by pediatric cardiac surgeons and interventional pediatric cardiologists. Advantages of hybrid procedure are real-time feedback obtained by continuous transesophageal echocardiographic monitoring, avoidance of CPB, ventricular incisions, or muscle transections.[174]

REFERENCES

1. Landesberg G. The pathophysiology of perioperative myocardial infarction: Facts and perspectives. *J Cardiothorac Vasc Anesth.* 2003;17:90–100.
2. Biccrd BM, Rodseth RN. The pathophysiology of peri-operative myocardial infarction. *Anaesthesia.* 2010;65:733–741.
3. Weber KT, Janicki JS. The metabolic demand and oxygen supply of the heart: physiologic and clinical considerations. *Am J Cardiol.* 1979;44:722–729.
4. Hoffman JI. Transmural myocardial perfusion. *Prog Cardiovasc Dis.* 1987;29:429–464.
5. Bassenge E, Heusch G. Endothelial and neuro-humoral control of coronary blood flow in health and disease. *Rev Physiol Biochem Pharmacol.* 1990;116:77–165.
6. Canty JM, Duncker DJ. Coronary blood flow and myocardial ischemia. In: Mann DL, Zipes DP, Libby P, et al., eds. *Braunwald's Heart Disease: A Textbook of Cardiovascular Medicine.* 10th ed. Philadelphia, PA: Saunders, 2015;49:1029–1056.
7. Kloner RA, Jennings RB. Consequences of brief ischemia: stunning, preconditioning, and their clinical implications: part 2. *Circulation.* 2001;104:3158–3167.
8. Hillis LD, Smith PK, Anderson JL, et al. 2011 ACCF/AHA guideline for coronary artery bypass graft surgery: a report of the American College of Cardiology Foundation/American Heart Association Task Force on Practice Guidelines. *Circulation.* 2011;124:e652–e735.
9. Hindler K, Eltzschig HK, Fox AA, et al. Influence of statins on perioperative outcomes. *J Cardiothorac Vasc Anesth.* 2006;20:251–258.
10. Ferrari R, Guardigli G, Ceconi C. Secondary prevention of CAD with ACE inhibitors: A struggle between life and death of the endothelium. *Cardiovasc Drugs Ther.* 2010;24:331–339.
11. De Hert SG, Turani F, Mathur S, et al. Cardioprotection with volatile anesthetics: Mechanisms and clinical implications. *Anesth Analg.* 2005;100:1584–1593.
12. Brazier J, Cooper N, Buckberg GD. The adequacy of subendocardial oxygen delivery: The interaction of determinants of flow, arterial oxygen content and myocardial oxygen need. *Circulation.* 1974;49:968–977.
13. Ramsay SD, Saint S, Sullivan SD, et al. Clinical and economic effects of pulmonary artery catheterization in nonemergent coronary artery bypass graft surgery. *J Cardiothorac Vasc Anesth.* 2000;14:113–118.
14. London MJ, Moritz TE, Henderson WG, et al. Standard versus fiberoptic pulmonary artery catheterization for cardiac surgery in the Department of Veteran Affairs: A prospective, observational, multicenter analysis. *Anesthesiology.* 2002;96:860–870.
15. Haggmark S, Hohner P, Ostman M, et al. Comparison of hemodynamic, electrocardiographic, mechanical, and metabolic indicators of intraoperative myocardial ischemia in vascular surgical patients with coronary artery disease. *Anesthesiology.* 1989;70:19–25.
16. Leung JM, O'Kelly B, Browner WS, et al. Prognostic importance of postbypass regional wall-motion abnormalities in patients undergoing coronary artery bypass graft surgery. *Anesthesiology.* 1989;71:16–25.
17. Tuman KJ, McCarthy RJ, Spiess BD, et al. Effect of pulmonary artery catheterization on outcome in patients undergoing coronary artery surgery. *Anesthesiology.* 1989;70:199–206.
18. Fontes ML, Bellows W, Ngo L, et al. Assessment of ventricular function in critically ill patients: Limitations of pulmonary artery catheterization. *J Cardiothorac Vasc Anesth.* 1999;13:521–527.
19. Sandham JD, Hull RD, Brant RF, et al. A randomized, controlled trial of the use of pulmonary-artery catheters in high-risk surgical patients. *N Engl J Med.* 2003;348:5–14.
20. Schwann NM, Hillel Z, Hoeft A, et al. Lack of effectiveness of the pulmonary artery catheter in cardiac surgery. *Anesth Analg.* 2011;113:994–1002.
21. Squara P, Bennett D, Perret C. Pulmonary artery catheter: Does the problem lie in the users? *Chest.* 2002;121:2009–2015.
22. Practice guidelines for pulmonary artery catheterization: an updated report by the American Society of Anesthesiologists Task Force on Pulmonary Artery Catheterization. *Anesthesiology.* 2003;99:988–1014.
23. Thys DM, Abel MD, Brooker RF, et al. Practice guidelines for perioperative transesophageal echocardiography. *Anesthesiology.* 2010;112:1084.
24. Miller JP, Lambert AS, Shapiro WA, et al. The adequacy of basic intraoperative transesophageal echocardiography performed by experienced anesthesiologists. *Anesth Analg.* 2001;92:1103–1110.
25. Mathew JP, Fontes ML, Garwood S, et al. Transesophageal echocardiography interpretation: a comparative analysis between cardiac anesthesiologists and primary echocardiographers. *Anesth Analg.* 2002;94:302–309.
26. Hahn RT, Abraham T, Adams MS, et al. Guidelines for performing a comprehensive transesophageal echocardiographic examination: recommendations from the American Society of Echocardiography and the Society of Cardiovascular Anesthesiologists. *J Am Soc Echocardiogr.* 2013;26:921–964.
27. Cheng DC. Fast track cardiac surgery pathways: early extubation, process of care, and cost containment. *Anesthesiology.* 1998;88:1429–1433.
28. Myles PS, Daly DJ, Djaiani G, et al. A systematic review of the safety and effectiveness of fast-track cardiac anesthesia. *Anesthesiology.* 2003;99:982–987.
29. Ranta SO, Herranen P, Hynynen M. Patients' conscious recollections from cardiac anesthesia. *J Cardiothorac Vasc Anesth.* 2002;16:426–430.
30. London MJ, Shroyer AL, Coll JR, et al. Early extubation following cardiac surgery in a veterans population. *Anesthesiology.* 1998;88:1447–1458.
31. Zhu F, Lee a, Chee YE. Fast-track cardiac care for adult cardiac surgical patients. *Cochrane Database Syst Rev.* 2012;10:CD003587.
32. Engoren M, Luther G, Fenn-Buderer N. A comparison of fentanyl, sufentanil, and remifentanil for fast-track cardiac anesthesia. *Anesth Analg.* 2001;93:859–864.
33. Murphy GS, Szokol JW, Marymont JH, et al. The effects of morphine and fentanyl on the inflammatory response to cardiopulmonary bypass in patients undergoing elective coronary bypass graft surgery. *Anesth Analg.* 2007;104:1334–1342.

34. Murphy GS, Szokol JW, Marymont JH, et al. Morphine-based cardiac anesthesia provides superior early recovery compared with fentanyl in elective cardiac surgery patients. *Anesth Analg.* 2009;109:311–319.
35. Lowenstein E, Hallowell P, Levine FH, et al. Cardiovascular response to large doses of intravenous morphine in man. *N Engl J Med.* 1969;281:1389–1393.
36. Jenkins DP, Pugsley WB, Alkhulaifi AM, et al. Ischemic preconditioning reduces troponin T release in patients undergoing coronary artery bypass surgery. *Heart.* 1997;77:314–318.
37. Tanaka K, Ludwig L, Kersten J, et al. Mechanisms of cardioprotection by volatile anesthetics. *Anesthesiology.* 2004;100:707–721.
38. Fraessdorf J, De Hert S, Schlack W. Anaesthesia and myocardial ischaemia/reperfusion injury. *Br J Anaesth.* 2009;103:89–98.
39. Belhomme D, Peynet J, Louzy M, et al. Evidence for preconditioning by isoflurane in coronary artery bypass graft surgery. *Circulation.* 1999;100(19 Suppl):II340–II344.
40. Helman JD, Leung JM, Bellows WH, et al. The risk of myocardial ischemia in patients receiving desflurane versus sufentanil anesthesia for coronary artery bypass graft surgery. *Anesthesiology.* 1992;77:47.
41. Searle N, Martineau RJ, Conzen P, et al. Comparison of sevoflurane/fentanyl and isoflurane/fentanyl during elective coronary artery bypass surgery. *Can J Anaesth.* 1996;43:890–899.
42. Smith FJ, Bartel PR, Hugo JM, et al. Anesthetic technique (sufentanil versus ketamine plus midazolam) and quantitative electroencephalographic changes after cardiac surgery. *J Cardiothorac Vasc Anesth.* 2006;20:520–525.
43. Dasta JF, Jacobi J, Sesti AM, et al. Addition of dexmedetomidine to standard sedation regimens after cardiac surgery: an outcomes analysis. *Pharmacotherapy.* 2006;26:798–805.
44. Muellejans B, Matthey T, Scholpp J, et al. Sedation in the intensive care unit with remifentanil/propofol versus midazolam/fentanyl: a randomised, open-label, pharmacoeconomic trial. *Crit Care.* 2006;10:R91.
45. De Hert SG, Cromheecke S, ten Broecke PW, et al. Effects of propofol, desflurane and sevoflurane on recovery of myocardial function after coronary surgery in elderly high-risk patients. *Anesthesiology.* 2003;99:314–323.
46. Cromheecke S, Pepermans V, Hendrickx E, et al. Cardioprotective properties of sevoflurane in patients undergoing aortic valve replacement with cardiopulmonary bypass. *Anesth Analg.* 2006;103:289–296.
47. Smulyan H. Nitrates, arterial function, wave reflections and coronary heart disease. *Adv Cardiol.* 2007;44:302–314.
48. Ali I, Buth K, Maitland A. Impact of preoperative intravenous nitroglycerin on in-hospital outcomes after coronary artery bypass grafting for unstable angina. *Am Heart J.* 2004;148:727–732.
49. Kaplan KJ, Taber M, Teagarden JR, et al. Association of methemoglobinemia and intravenous nitroglycerine administration. *Am J Cardiol.* 1985;55:181–183.
50. Cheung AT, Cruz-Shiavone GE, Meng QC, et al. Cardiopulmonary bypass, hemolysis, and nitroprusside-induced cyanide production. *Anesth Analg.* 2007;105:29–33.
51. Zerbe NF, Wagner BKJ. Use of vitamin B₁₂ in the treatment and prevention of nitroprusside-induced cyanide toxicity. *Crit Care Med.* 1993;21:465–467.
52. Egi M, Bellomo R, Langenberg C, et al. Selecting a vasopressor drug for vasoplegic shock after adult cardiac surgery: a systematic literature review. *Ann Thorac Surg.* 2007;83:715–723
53. Halonen J, Hakala T, Auvinen T, et al. Intravenous administration of metoprolol is more effective than oral administration in the prevention of atrial fibrillation after cardiac surgery. *Circulation.* 2006;114(1 Suppl):I1.
54. Booth JV, Ward EE, Colgan KC, et al. Metoprolol and coronary artery bypass grafting surgery: does intraoperative metoprolol attenuate acute beta-adrenergic receptor desensitization during cardiac surgery? *Anesth Analg.* 2004;98:1224–1231.
55. Longon MJ. Quo vadis, perioperative beta blockade? Are you "POISE'd" on the brink? *Anesth Analg.* 2008;106:1025–1030.
56. Warltier DC. β-Adrenergic-blocking drugs: incredibly useful, incredibly underutilized. *Anesthesiology.* 1998;88:2–5.
57. Opie L. Anti-ischemic properties of calcium-channel blockers: lessons from cardiac surgery. *J Am Coll Cardiol.* 2003;41:1506–1509.
58. Wijeysundera DN, Beattie WS, Rao V, et al. Calcium antagonists reduce cardiovascular complications after cardiac surgery: a meta-analysis. *J Am Coll Cardiol.* 2003;41:1496–1505.
59. Apostolidou IA, Despotis GJ, Hogue CW Jr, et al. Antiischemic effects of nicardipine and nitroglycerin after coronary artery bypass grafting. *Ann Thorac Surg.* 1999;67:417–422.
60. Kaplan J. Clinical considerations for the use of intravenous nicardipine in the treatment of postoperative hypertension. *Am Heart J.* 1990;119:443–446.
61. Aronson S, Dyke CM, Stierer KA, et al. The ECLIPSE trials: comparative studies of clevidipine to nitroglycerin, sodium nitroprusside, and nicardipine for acute hypertension treatment in cardiac surgery patients. *Anesth Analg.* 2008;107:1110–1121.
62. Garcia LA, Dejong SC, Martin SM, et al. Magnesium reduces free radicals in an in vivo coronary occlusion-reperfusion model. *J Am Coll Cardiol.* 1998;32:536–539.
63. Shepherd J, Jones J, Frampton GK, et al. Intravenous magnesium sulphate and sotalol for prevention of atrial fibrillation after coronary artery bypass surgery: a systematic review and economic evaluation. *Health Technol Assess.* 2008;12:iii.
64. Cook RC, Humphries KH, Gin K, et al. Prophylactic intravenous magnesium sulphate in addition to oral β-blockade does not prevent atrial arrhythmias after coronary artery or valvular heart surgery: a randomized, controlled trial. *Circulation.* 2009;120(Suppl II):S163.
65. Hillis LD, Smith PK, Anderson JL, et al. 2011 ACCF/AHA guidelines for coronary artery bypass graft surgery: executive summary. *Anesth Analg.* 2011;114:11–45.
66. Freeman RV, Otto CM. Spectrum of calcific aortic valve disease: pathogenesis, disease progression, and treatment strategies. *Circulation.* 2005;111:3316–3326.
67. Carabello BA. Clinical practice: aortic stenosis. *N Engl J Med.* 2002;346:677–682.
68. Zile MR, Gaasch WH. Heart failure in aortic stenosis: improving diagnosis and treatment. *N Engl J Med.* 2003;348:1735–1736.
69. Klein AA, Skubas NJ, Ender J. Controversies and complications in the perioperative management of transcatheter aortic valve replacement. *Anesth Analg.* 2014;119:784–798.
70. O'Keefe JH Jr, Shub C, Rettke SR. Risk of noncardiac surgical procedures in patients with aortic stenosis. *Mayo Clin Proc.* 1989;64:400–405.
71. Calleja AM, Dommaraju S, Gaddam R, et al. Cardiac risk in patients aged >75 years with asymptomatic, severe aortic stenosis undergoing noncardiac surgery. *Am J Cardiol.* 2010;105:1159–1163.
72. Kertai MD, Bountioukos M, Boersma E, et al. Aortic stenosis: an underestimated risk factor for perioperative complications in patients undergoing non-cardiac surgery. *Am J Med.* 2004;116:8–13.
73. Zahid M, Sonel AF, Saba S, et al. Perioperative risk of noncardiac surgery associated with aortic stenosis. *Am J Cardiol.* 2005;96:436–438.
74. Skubas NJ, Shernan SK, Bollen B. An overview of the American College of Cardiology/American Heart Association 2014 Valve Heart Disease Practice Guidelines: What is its relevance for the anesthesiologist and perioperative medicine physician? *Anesth Analg.* 2015;121:1132–1138.
75. Khot UN, Novato GM, Popović ZB, et al. Nitroprusside in critically ill patients with left ventricular dysfunction and aortic stenosis. *N Engl J Med.* 2003;348:1756–1763.
76. Ommen SR, Nishimura RA. Hypertrophic cardiomyopathy. *Curr Probl Cardiol.* 2004;29:239–291.
77. Ommen SR. Hypertrophic cardiomyopathy. *Curr Probl Cardiol.* 2011;36:409–453.
78. Fifer MA, Vlahakes GJ. Management of symptoms in hypertrophic cardiomyopathy. *Circulation.* 2008;117:429–439.
79. Hensley N, Dietrich J, Nyhan D, et al. Hypertrophic cardiomyopathy: a review. *Anesth Analg.* 2015;120:554–569.
80. Borer JS, Bonow RO. Contemporary approach to aortic and mitral regurgitation. *Circulation.* 2003;108:2432–2438.
81. Nishimura RA, Otto CM, Bonow RO, et al. 2014 AHA/ACC guideline for the management of patients with valvular heart disease: a report of the American College of Cardiology/American Heart Association Task Force on Practice Guidelines. *J Thorac Cardiovas Surg.* 2014;148:e1–132.
82. Bekeredjian R, Grayburn PA. Valvular heart disease: aortic regurgitation. *Circulation.* 2005;112:125–134.
83. Carabello BA. Modern management of mitral stenosis. *Circulation.* 2005;112:432–437.
84. Gorlin R, Gorlin SG. Hydraulic formula for calculation of area of the stenotic mitral valve, other cardiac valves, and central circulatory shunts. *Am Heart J.* 1951;41:1–29.
85. Cardoso LF, Grinberg M, Rati MA, et al. Comparison between percutaneous balloon valvuloplasty and open commissurotomy for mitral stenosis: a prospective and randomized study. *Cardiology.* 2002;98:186–190.
86. Thrumurthy SG, Karthikesalingam A, Patterson BO, et al. The diagnosis and management of aortic dissection. *BMJ.* 2011;344:d8290.
87. Bosner RS, Ranasinghe AM, Loubani M, et al. Evidence, lack of evidence, controversy and debate in the provision and performance of the surgery of acute type A aortic dissection. *J Am Coll Cardiol.* 2011;58:2455–2474.
88. Eltzschig HK, Rosenberger P, Lekowski RW Jr, et al. Role of transesophageal echocardiography in patients with suspected aortic dissection. *J Am Soc Echocardiogr.* 2005;18:1221.
89. Mohr-Kahaly S, Erbel R, Rennollet H, et al. Ambulatory follow-up of aortic dissection by transesophageal two-dimensional and color-coded Doppler echocardiography. *Circulation.* 1989;80:24.
90. Penco M, Paparoni S, Dagianti A, et al. Usefulness of transesophageal echocardiography in the assessment of aortic dissection. *Am J Cardiol.* 2000;86:53G–56G.
91. Davies RR, Goldstein LJ, Coady MA, et al. Yearly rupture or dissection rates for thoracic aortic aneurysms: simple prediction based on size. *Ann Thorac Surg.* 2002;73:17–27.
92. Hiratzka LF, Bakris GL, Beckman JA, et al. ACCF/AHA/AATS/ACR/ASA/SCA/SCAI/SIR/STS/SVM guidelines for the diagnosis and management of patients with thoracic aortic disease: executive summary. *Anesth Analg.* 2010;111:279.
93. Isselbacher EM. Thoracic and abdominal aortic aneurysms. *Circulation.* 2005;111:816–828.

94. David TE, Ivanov J, Armstrong S, et al. Aortic valve-sparing operations in patients with aneurysms of the aortic root or ascending aorta. *Ann Thorac Surg.* 2002;74:S1758.
95. Hagl C, Ergin MA, Galla JD, et al. Neurologic outcome after ascending aorta-aortic arch operations: effect of brain protection technique in high-risk patients. *J Thorac Cardiovasc Surg.* 2001;121:1107–1121.
96. Cowan JA Jr, Dimick JB, Henke PK, et al. Surgical treatment of intact thoracoabdominal aortic aneurysms in the United States: hospital and surgeon volume-related outcomes. *J Vasc Surg.* 2003;37:1169.
97. Conrad MF, Cambria RP. Contemporary management of descending thoracic and thoracoabdominal aortic aneurysms: endovascular versus open. *Circulation.* 2008;117:841–852.
98. Vaughn SB, LeMaire SA, Collard CD. Case scenario: anesthetic considerations for thoracoabdominal aortic aneurysm repair. *Anesthesiology.* 2011;115:1093–1102.
99. Federow CA, Moon MC, Mutch WA, et al. Lumbar cerebrospinal fluid drainage for thoracoabdominal aortic surgery: rationale and practical considerations for management. *Anesth Analg.* 2010;111:46–58.
100. Habib RH, Zacharias A, Schwann TA, et al. Adverse effects of low hematocrit during cardiopulmonary bypass in the adult: should current practice be changed? *J Thorac Cardiovasc Surg.* 2003;125:1438–1450.
101. Bouraghda A, Gillois P, Albaladejo P. Alternatives to heparin and protamine anticoagulation for cardiopulmonary bypass in cardiac surgery. *Can J Anaesth.* 2015;62:518–528.
102. Avgerinos DV, DeBois W, Salemi A. Blood conservation strategies in cardiac surgery: more is better. *Eur J Cardiothorac Surg.* 2014;46:865–870.
103. Ferraris VA, Brown JR, Despotis GJ, et al; The Society of Thoracic Surgeons Blood Conservation Guideline Task Force. 2011 update to the Society of Thoracic Surgeons and the Society of Cardiovascular Anesthesiologists blood conservation clinical practice guidelines. *Ann Thorac Surg.* 2011;91(3):944–982.
104. Koster A, Faraoni D, Levy JH. Antifibrinolytic therapy for cardiac surgery: an update. *Anesthesiology.* 2015;123:214–221.
105. Trapp C, Schiller W, Mellert F. Retrograde autologous priming as a safe and easy method to reduce hemodilution and transfusion requirements during cardiac surgery. *Thorac Cardiovasc Surg.* 2015;63:628–634.
106. Papadopoulos N, Bakhtiary F, Grün V. The effect of normovolemic modified ultrafiltration on inflammatory mediators, endotoxins, terminal complement complexes and clinical outcome in high-risk cardiac surgery patients. *Perfusion.* 2013;28:306–314.
107. O'Blenes SB, Friesen CH, Ali A, et al. Protecting the aged heart during cardiac surgery: the potential benefits of del Nido cardioplegia. *J Thorac Cardiovasc Surg.* 2011;141:762–770.
108. Filion KB, Pilote L, Rahme E, et al. Perioperative use of cardiac medical therapy among patients undergoing coronary artery bypass graft surgery: a systematic review. *Am Heart J.* 2007;154:407–414.
109. Lazar HL. All coronary artery bypass graft surgery patients will benefit from angiotensin-converting enzyme inhibitors. *Circulation.* 2008;117:6.
110. Levin MA, Lin HM, Castillo JG, et al. Early on-cardiopulmonary bypass hypotension and other factors associated with vasoplegic syndrome. *Circulation.* 2009;120:1664–1671.
111. Grocott HP. Perioperative temperature and cardiac surgery. *J Extra Corpor Technol.* 2006;38:77–80.
112. Brzezinski M, Luisetti T, London MJ. Radial artery cannulation: a comprehensive review of recent anatomic and physiologic investigations. *Anesth Analg.* 2009;109:1763–1781.
113. Baba T, Goto T, Yoshitake A, et al. Radial artery diameter decreases with increased femoral to radial artery pressure gradient during cardiopulmonary bypass. *Anesth Analg.* 1997;85:252–258.
114. Murphy GS, Hessel EA II, Groom RC. Optimal perfusion during cardiopulmonary bypass: an evidence-based approach. *Anesth Analg.* 2009;108:1394–1417.
115. Bussières JS. Iatrogenic pulmonary artery rupture. *Curr Opin Anaesthesiol.* 2007;20:48–52.
116. Hansen RM, Viquerat CE, Matthy MA, et al. Poor correlation between pulmonary arterial wedge pressure and left ventricular end-diastolic volume after coronary artery bypass graft surgery. *Anesthesiology.* 1986;64:764–770.
117. Puskas JD, Winston D, Wright CE, et al. Stroke after coronary artery operation. Incidence, correlates, outcome, and cost. *Ann Thorac Surg.* 2000;69:1053–1056.
118. Ahonen J, Salmenperä M. Brain injury after adult cardiac surgery. *Acta Anaesthesiol Scand.* 2004;48:4–19.
119. Newman MF, Kirchner JL, Phillips-Bute B, et al. Longitudinal assessment of neurocognitive function after coronary-artery bypass surgery. *N Engl J Med.* 2001;344:395–402.
120. Grocott HP, Mackensen GB, Grigore AM, et al. Postoperative hyperthermia is associated with cognitive dysfunction after coronary artery bypass graft surgery. *Stroke.* 2002;33:537–541.
121. Hogue CW Jr, Palin CA, Arrowsmith JE. Cardiopulmonary bypass management and neurologic outcomes: an evidence-based appraisal of current practices. *Anesth Analg.* 2006;103:21–37.
122. Tuman KJ, McCarthy RJ, Spiess BD, et al. Does choice of anesthetic agent significantly affect outcome after coronary artery surgery? *Anesthesiology.* 1989;70(2):189–198.
123. Slogoff S, Keats AS, Dear WS, et al. Steal-prone coronary anatomy and myocardial ischemia associated with four primary anesthetic agents in humans. *Anesth Analg.* 1991;72:22–27.
124. Murphy GS, Szokol JW, Marymont JH, et al. Recovery of neuromuscular function after cardiac surgery: pancuronium versus rocuronium. *Anesth Analg.* 2003;96:1301–1307.
125. Troianos CA, Hartman GS, Glas KE, et al. Guidelines for performing ultrasound guided vascular cannulation: recommendations of the American Society of Echocardiography and the Society of Cardiovascular Anesthesiologists. *Anesth Analg.* 2012;114:46–72.
126. American Society of Anesthesiologists Task Force on Central Venous Access, Rupp SM, Apfelbaum JL, Blitt C, et al. Practice guidelines for central venous access: a report by the American Society of Anesthesiologists task force on central venous access. *Anesthesiology.* 2012;116:539–573.
127. Barry AE, Chaney MA, London MJ. Anesthetic management during cardiopulmonary bypass: a systematic review. *Anesth Analg.* 2015;120:749–769.
128. Garwood S. Renal insufficiency after cardiac surgery. *Semin Cardiothorac Vasc Anesth.* 2004;8:227–241.
129. Grigore AM, Grocott HP, Mathew JP, et al. The rewarming rate and increased peak temperature alter neurocognitive outcome after cardiac surgery. *Anesth Analg.* 2002;94:4–10.
130. Avidan MS, Zhang L, Burnside BA, et al. Anesthesia awareness and bispectral index. *N Engl J Med.* 2008;358:1097–1108.
131. Robitaille A, Denault AY, Couture P, et al. Importance of relative pulmonary hypertension in cardiac surgery: the mean systemic-to-pulmonary artery pressure ratio. *J Cardiothorac Vasc Anesth.* 2006;20:331–339.
132. McKinlay KH, Schinderle DB, Swaminathan M, et al. Predictors of inotrope use during separation from cardiopulmonary bypass. *J Cardiothorac Vasc Anesth.* 2004;18:404–408.
133. Denault AY, Tardif JC, Mazer CD, et al. Difficult and complex separation from cardiopulmonary bypass in high-risk cardiac surgical patients: a multicenter study. *J Cardiothorac Vasc Anesth.* 2012;26:608–616.
134. Klopman MA, Chen EP, Sniecinski RM. Positioning an intraaortic balloon pump using intraoperative transesophageal echocardiographic guidance. *Anesth Analg.* 2011;113:40–43.
135. Field ML, Rengarajan A, Khan O, et al. Preoperative intra aortic balloon pumps in patients undergoing coronary artery bypass grafting. *Cochrane Database Syst Rev.* 2007;24:CD004472.
136. Rihal CS, Naidu SS, Givertz MM, et al. 2015 SCAI/ACC/HFSA/STS clinical expert consensus statement on the use of percutaneous mechanical circulatory support devices in cardiovascular care. *J Card Fail.* 2015;21:499–518.
137. Schumer EM, Black MC, Monreal G, et al. Left ventricular assist devices: current controversies and future directions. *Eur Heart J.* 2015; Epub ahead of print.
138. Anderson MB, Goldstein J, Milano C, et al. Benefits of a novel percutaneous ventricular assist device for right heart failure: the prospective RECOVER RIGHT study of the Impella RP device. *J Heart Lung Transplant.* 2015;34:1549–1560.
139. Chumnanvej S, Wood MJ, MacGillivray TE, et al. Perioperative echocardiographic examination for ventricular assist device implantation. *Anesth Analg.* 2007;105:583–601.
140. Nicolosi AC, Pagel PS. Perioperative considerations in the patient with a left ventricular assist device. *Anesthesiology.* 2003;98:565–70.
141. Currigan DA, Hughes RJ, Wright CE. Vasoconstrictor responses to vasopressor agents in human pulmonary and radial arteries: an in vitro study. *Anesthesiology.* 2014;121:930–936.
142. Stone M, Hinchey J, Sattler C, et al. Trends in the management of patients with left ventricular assist devices presenting for noncardiac surgery: a 10-year institutional experience. *Semin Cardiothorac Vasc Anesth.* 2016;20:197–204.
143. Slininger KA, Haddadin AS, Mangi AA. Perioperative management of patients with left ventricular assist devices undergoing noncardiac surgery. *J Cardiothorac Vasc Anesth.* 2013;27:752–759.
144. Schulman S, Bijsterveld NR. Anticoagulants and their reversal. *Transfus Med Rev.* 2007;21:37–48.
145. Levy JH, Adkinson NF Jr. Anaphylaxis during cardiac surgery: implications for clinicians. *Anesth Analg.* 2008;106:392–403.
146. Weber CF, Görlinger K, Meininger D, et al. Point-of-care testing: a prospective, randomized clinical trial of efficacy in coagulopathic cardiac surgery patients. *Anesthesiology.* 2012;117:531–547.
147. Ejiofor JI, Leacche M, Byrne JG. Robotic CABG and hybrid approaches: the current landscape. *Prog Cardiovasc Dis.* 2015;58:356–364.
148. Houlind K, Kjeldsen BJ, Madsen SN. On-pump versus off-pump coronary artery bypass surgery in elderly patients: results from the Danish on-pump versus off-pump randomization study. *Circulation.* 2012;125:2431–2439.
149. Leff JD, Enriquez LJ. Robotic-assisted cardiac surgery. *Int Anesthesiol Clin.* 2012;50:78–89.
150. Neely RC, Leacche M, Byrne CR, et al. New approaches to cardiovascular surgery. *Curr Probl Cardiol.* 2014;39:427–466.

151. Rehfeldt KH, Mauermann W, Burkhart HM, et al. Robot-assisted mitral valve repair. *J Cardiothorac Vasc Anesth.* 2011;25:721–730.
152. Chassot PG, van der Linden P, Zaugg M, et al. Off-pump coronary artery bypass surgery: physiology and anaesthetic management. *Br J Anaesth.* 2004;92:400–413.
153. Bainbridge D, Cheng DC. Minimally invasive direct coronary artery bypass and off-pump coronary artery bypass surgery: anesthetic considerations. *Anesthesiol Clin.* 2008;26:437–452.
154. Huffmyer J, Raphael J. The current status of off-pump coronary bypass surgery. *Curr Opin Anaesthesiol.* 2011;24(1):64–69.
155. Fillinger MP, Yeager MP, Dodds TM, et al. Epidural anesthesia and analgesia: effects on recovery from cardiac surgery. *J Cardiothorac Vasc Anesth.* 2002;16:15–20.
156. Kurlansky PA. Is there a hypercoagulable state after off-pump coronary artery bypass surgery? What do we know and what can we do? *J Thorac Cardiovasc Surg.* 2003;126:7–10.
157. Lev-Ran O, Ben-Gal Y, Matsa M, et al. 'No touch' techniques for porcelain ascending aorta: comparison between cardiopulmonary bypass with femoral artery cannulation and off-pump myocardial revascularization. *J Card Surg.* 2002;17:370.
158. Sharony R, Bizekis CS, Kanchuger M, et al. Off-pump coronary artery bypass grafting reduces mortality and stroke in patients with atheromatous aortas: a case control study. *Circulation.* 2003;108(Suppl 1):II15.
159. Cheng DC, Bainbridge D, Martin JE, et al. Does off-pump coronary artery bypass reduce mortality, morbidity, and resource utilization when compared with conventional coronary artery bypass? A meta-analysis of randomized trials. *Anesthesiology.* 2005;102:188.
160. Kim KB, Lim C, Lee C, et al. Off-pump coronary artery bypass may decrease the patency of saphenous vein grafts. *Ann Thorac Surg.* 2001;72:S1033–S1037.
161. Lamy A, Devereaux PJ, Prabhakaran D, et al. Off-pump or on-pump coronary-artery bypass grafting at 30 days. *N Engl J Med.* 2012;366:1489.
162. Little WC, Freeman GL. Pericardial disease. *Circulation.* 2006;113:1622–1632.
163. Roediger L, Larbuisson R, Lamy M. New approaches and old controversies to postoperative pain control following cardiac surgery. *Eur J Anaesthesiol.* 2006;23:539–550.
164. Chaney MA. Intrathecal and epidural anesthesia and analgesia for cardiac surgery. *Anesth Analg.* 2006;102:45–64.
165. Malviya S, Voepel-Lewis T, Siewert M, et al. Risk factors for adverse postoperative outcomes in children presenting for cardiac surgery with upper respiratory tract infections. *Anesthesiology.* 2003;98:628–632.
166. Greenwood RD, Rosenthal LA, Parisi L, et al. Extracardiac abnormalities in infants with congenital heart disease. *Pediatrics.* 1975;55:485–492.
167. Karamlou T, Hickey E, Silliman CC, et al. Reducing risk in infant cardiopulmonary bypass: the use of a miniaturized circuit and a crystalloid prime improves cardiopulmonary function and increases cerebral blood flow. *Semin Thorac Cardiovasc Surg Pediatr Card Surg Annu.* 2005;8:3–11.
168. Raja SG, Yousufuddin S, Rasool F, et al. Impact of modified ultrafiltration on morbidity after pediatric cardiac surgery. *Asian Cardiovasc Thorac Ann.* 2006;14:341–350.
169. Alghamdi AA, Singh SK, Hamilton BC, et al. Early extubation after pediatric cardiac surgery: systematic review, meta analysis and evidence-based recommendations. *J Card Surg.* 2010;25:586–595.
170. Mittnacht AJ, Hollinger I. Fast-tracking in pediatric cardiac surgery-the current standing. *Ann Card Anaesth.* 2010;13:92–101.
171. Ip P, Chiu CS, Cheung YF. Risk factors prolonging ventilation in young children after cardiac surgery: impact of noninfectious pulmonary complications. *Pediatr Crit Care Med.* 2002;3:269–274.
172. Lofland GK. The enhancement of hemodynamic performance in Fontan circulation using pain free spontaneous ventilation. *Eur J Cardiothorac Surg.* 2001;20:114–119.
173. Peterson KL, DeCampli WM, Pike NA, et al. A report of two hundred twenty cases of regional anesthesia in pediatric cardiac surgery. *Anesth Analg.* 2000;90:1014–1019.
174. Bacha EA, Hijazi ZM. Hybrid procedures in pediatric cardiac surgery. *Semin Thorac Cardiovasc Surg Pediatr Card Surg Annu.* 2005:78–85.

40 Anesthesia for Vascular and Endovascular Surgery

ELIZABETH A. VALENTINE • E. ANDREW OCHROCH

Introduction and Overview
Vascular Disease
   Pathophysiology of Atherosclerosis
   Concurrent Vascular Disease in Vascular Surgery Patients
   Medical Optimization Prior to Vascular Surgery
   Preoperative Anesthesia Evaluation for Vascular Surgery

Open Vascular Surgery
   Cerebrovascular Disease
   Aortic Reconstruction
   Peripheral Artery Disease
Endovascular Surgery
   Carotid Artery Stenting
   Endovascular Aortic Repair
   Endovascular Management of Peripheral Artery Disease
Conclusion

KEY POINTS

1. Atherosclerosis is the most common underlying pathophysiologic mechanism for the development of cardiovascular disease.
2. The same risk factors that lead to coronary artery disease also lead to vascular disease in other major vascular beds, including the cerebral, aortic, and peripheral circulation.
3. Improvements in the medical management of patients with atherosclerotic risk factors with antiplatelet agents, β-blockers, angiotensin-converting enzyme inhibitors, statins, and strict glucose control have revolutionized the management of vascular surgery patients. Meticulous optimization of comorbid conditions plays a critical role in the reduction of perioperative morbidity and mortality in this patient population.
4. Most vascular surgery patients are at elevated perioperative risk of major adverse cardiac events, which remain the single most important cause of both short- and long-term morbidity and mortality following vascular surgery.
5. The pathophysiology of aneurysmal aortic disease is a clinically distinct degenerative process, although many of the risk factors are shared between degenerative and atherosclerotic vascular disease.
6. Endovascular procedures have transformed the field of vascular surgery with an increasing number of procedures being performed via a minimally invasive approach. Perioperative improvements in morbidity and mortality must be weighed against the long-term risks of decreased durability and increased need for repeat intervention.

Introduction and Overview

Atherosclerotic cardiovascular disease (ASCVD) is the most important cause of morbidity and mortality in both the United States and throughout the world. More than 80 million adults in the United States carry a diagnosis related to ASCVD. Globally, ASCVD has overtaken communicable diseases as the leading cause of death worldwide. ASCVD currently accounts for more than 17.3 million deaths worldwide per year, and this number is expected to increase to greater than 23.6 million deaths by 2030 due to an aging population.[1,2] Advances in medical management have led to an overall decrease in the total number of deaths attributable to ASCVD over recent years, although nearly one out of every three deaths in the United States is related to ASCVD.[3,4]

Emphasis on increased screening and the increasing age of the population in Western societies will likely increase the number of vascular procedures performed on a yearly basis. It has been estimated that 1 to 2 million vascular procedures will be performed annually in the United States by the year 2030.[5] Improvements in optimal medical management may delay the need for surgical interventions until severe systemic ASCVD disease is present. As a result of recent advances in endovascular techniques, many patients who previously would be deemed too high risk for the operating room are increasingly considered surgical candidates. This combination of a high-risk patient population and complex, high-risk surgical procedures makes vascular anesthesia challenging even for the experienced clinician. Despite both the medical and surgical issues that this patient population presents, surgical mortality has fallen from greater than 25% for major aortic reconstruction in the 1960s to as low as 3% today. This is largely due to improved perioperative optimization and management. The anesthesiologist may have greater influence in reducing morbidity and mortality in vascular surgery than in any other area of anesthesia.

This chapter begins with a discussion of the pathophysiology of ASCVD and a suggested approach to the preoperative evaluation and perioperative optimization of vascular surgery patients. Coronary artery disease (CAD) will be discussed in particular detail, given the high incidence of concomitant CAD in vascular surgery patients and the increased morbidity and mortality in this patient population. The specific surgical goals, anatomic considerations, and perioperative concerns for cerebrovascular, aortic, and lower extremity revascularization will be discussed in the context of optimal anesthetic management and accounting for surgical technique (open versus endovascular repair).

Vascular Disease

Pathophysiology of Atherosclerosis

1 Atherosclerosis is the most common pathophysiologic mechanism underlying cardiovascular disease. At its simplest definition, atherosclerosis is a generalized inflammatory disorder of the arterial tree. Putative mechanisms include endothelial damage, hemodynamic shear stress, inflammation from chronic infections, hypercoagulability with resultant thrombosis, and the destructive effect of low-density lipoproteins (LDLs). Atherosclerotic plaque formation is a complex process involving endothelial dysfunction, lipid deposition, smooth muscle proliferation, and the proliferation of inflammatory and immunogenic mediators.[6]

The development of atherosclerosis occurs in two stages: injury and response to injury. An intact vascular endothelium serves as a barrier between the blood and the more thrombogenic subendothelial tissues. Injured epithelial cells express leukocyte adhesion molecules that increase the adherence of macrophages and other leukocytes. Increased permeability of the damaged endothelium permits entry of leukocytes and LDL particles into the subendothelial space, and modified LDL particles induce leukocyte adhesion. The earliest recognizable lesion of atherosclerosis is this "fatty steak" which is comprised of lipid-rich macrophages and T lymphocytes that accumulate within the intima of the vessel wall. Monocyte-derived macrophages act as scavenging and antigen-presenting cells and produce further proinflammatory mediators. A variety of cytokines and growth factors (including monocyte chemotactic protein-1, macrophage and granulocyte-macrophage colony stimulating factors, intercellular adhesion molecule-1, tumor necrosis factor α, and interleukins 1, 3, 6, 8, and 18) further recruit activated immune and smooth muscle cells.[7,8] In this enriched environment, macrophages transform into foam cells. Foam cells and extracellular lipid form the core of the plaque, which is surrounded by smooth-muscle cells and a collagen-rich matrix.[6] The progression of atherosclerotic plaque ultimately narrows the intravascular lumen and contributes to an imbalance between oxygen supply and demand. Depending on location of the atherosclerotic plaque, the end result is ischemia of the coronary, cerebral, mesenteric, or peripheral circulation.

The traditional teaching is that of the "vulnerable plaque" model. That is, over time, inflammatory mediators and proteolytic enzymes may weaken the thin fibrous cap overlying the atheromatous plaque, making it particularly prone to ulceration and rupture. Exposure of blood to the necrotic, lipid-rich central core can result in acute thrombosis. Plaque rupture has been detected in up to 60% to 70% of cases of acute coronary syndromes,[9] making treatment of presumed high-risk lesions the focus of great effort. More recent evidence, however, suggests that although such high-risk features may be valuable as a surrogate for overall disease burden, no conclusive evidence exists to support that high-risk plaque characteristics are an independent risk factor for a clinical event.[10,11] Focus on overall atherosclerotic disease burden rather than individual plaque features may be as, if not more, important (Fig. 40-1). When plaque rupture is the culprit event, platelets play a pivotal role. Platelet polymorphisms have been found to be an independent risk factor following vascular surgery.[12]

Concurrent Vascular Disease in Vascular Surgery Patients

2 The underlying risk factors for atherosclerotic disease are similar regardless of plaque location, though individual risk factors may be more strongly associated with disease in one vascular bed than another. Some risk factors, such as a strong family history, nonwhite ethnicity, male gender, and increasing age, are outside a patient's control. Modifiable risk factors include smoking, atherogenic dyslipidemia (hypertriglyceridemia, elevated LDL, and decreased high-density lipoprotein [HDL]), abdominal obesity, hypertension, insulin resistance, renal insufficiency, and proinflammatory states.[13,14] With aggressive lifestyle and pharmacologic interventions, atherosclerotic disease progression can be significantly slowed.

ASCVD in one vascular bed often predicts significant disease in other areas of the body (Fig. 40-2).[13] The presence of

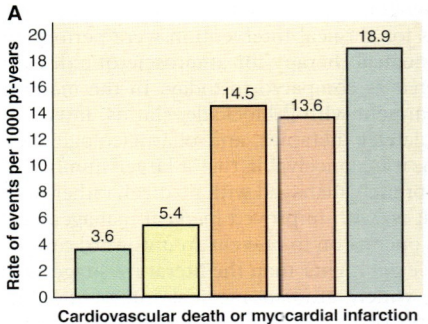
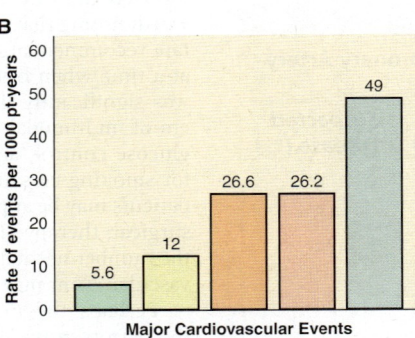
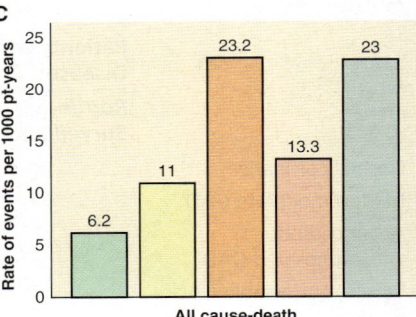

Figure 40-1 Rate of cardiovascular death, myocardial infarction, or major adverse cardiac event by presence, severity, and extent of coronary artery disease (CAD). Both obstructive and nonobstructive atherosclerotic plaque may result in significant cardiovascular morbidity and mortality. Overall disease burden may be as important a contributor as individual plaque characteristics to adverse events. (Reprinted with permission from Bittencourt MS, Hulten E, Ghoshhajra B, et al. Prognostic value of nonobstructive and obstructive coronary artery disease detected by coronary computed tomography angiography to identify cardiovascular events. CAD is coronary artery score, SIS is coronary segment involvement score. *Circ Cardiovasc Imaging*. 2014;7:282–291.)

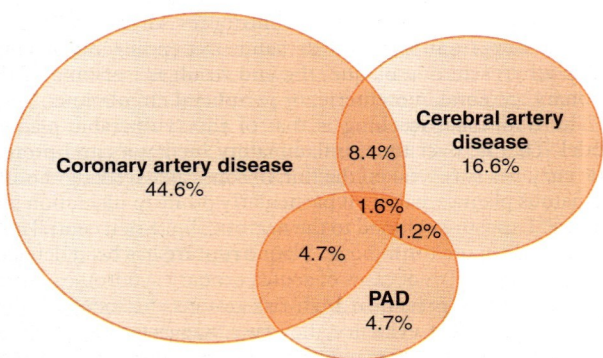

Figure 40-2 Typical overlap of atherosclerotic cardiovascular disease by vascular bed. Atherosclerotic disease in one vascular bed often predicts disease in other areas. (Reprinted with permission from Norgren L, Hiatt WR, Dormandy JA, et al. Inter-Society Consensus for the Management of Peripheral Arterial Disease [TASC II]. J Vasc Surg. 2007;45[Suppl S]:S5–S67. Copyright © 2007 The Society for Vascular Surgery. Published by Mosby, Inc. All rights reserved.)

cerebrovascular disease (CVD) has long been used as a surrogate marker for CAD. Multiple studies have demonstrated an association between carotid intima-media thickness (CIMT) and CAD and cardiovascular death. A meta-analysis of the literature demonstrated that for each 0.1-mm increase in CIMT, the future risk of myocardial infarction (MI) was increased by 10% to 15%.[15] Conversely, every 0.01 mm/yr decrease in the progression of CIMT has been associated with a nearly 20% reduction of the risk of nonfatal MI.[15] The overall presence of carotid atherosclerotic plaque, independent of CIMT, also predicts an increase in incidence of MI and cardiovascular death.[16]

Hertzer et al.[17] performed coronary angiography on 1,000 consecutive patients presenting for elective vascular surgery and identified an overall prevalence of CAD of approximately 50% in this patient population. Severe, correctable CAD was noted in 25% of the entire series (Table 40-1). Surgically correctable

Table 40-1 Coronary Artery Disease (CAD) Severity for Vascular Surgery Patients Who Underwent Routine or Selective Coronary Angiography[a]

	Patients with Coronary Artery Disease	
	Routine Surveillance (%)	Suspected Disease (%)
Normal coronaries	14	4
Mild to moderate CAD	49	18
Advanced but compensated CAD	22	34
Severe, correctable CAD	14	34
Severe, inoperable CAD	1	10

[a]A significant portion of patients who underwent coronary artery angiography prior to vascular surgery were found to have advanced disease. This held true even for patients without a high clinical suspicion for significant coronary artery disease.
Adapted with permission from Hertzer NR, Beven EG, Young JR, et al. Coronary artery disease in peripheral vascular patients: a classification of 1000 coronary angiograms and results of surgical management. Ann Surg. 1984;199:223–233.

disease was more frequent in patients with known risk factors for coronary disease than those without (34% vs. 14%). Subsequent analysis demonstrated that the severity of CAD could be accurately predicted by clinical risk factors.[18] The absence of: (1) diabetes mellitus, (2) prior angina, (3) previous MI, or (4) history of congestive heart failure (CHF) predicted the absence of severe CAD with a positive predictive value of 96%. The absence of critical CAD (greater than or equal to 70% stenosis of left main or triple vessel disease) could be predicted with a positive predictive value of 94% in patients without (1) prior angina, (2) previous MI, or (3) history of CHF.

The clinical prevalence of CAD or CVD in patients with diagnosed peripheral artery disease (PAD) ranges from 40% to 60%. The extent of CAD, measured by either computed tomography (CT) detection of coronary artery calcium or coronary angiography, correlates with the ankle–brachial index.[13] Approximately 10% to 30% of patients with documented CAD have concurrent PAD. Concurrent carotid and peripheral arterial disease occurs in approximately 25% to 50% of patients. Autopsy studies have demonstrated that patients with fatal MI are twice as likely to have a significant disease in the cerebral and peripheral arterial beds.

Medical Optimization Prior to Vascular Surgery

Cardiovascular complications are a major source of morbidity and mortality following vascular surgery. Nearly 10% of patients demonstrate evidence of significant myocardial injury in the perioperative period, and 2% of patients suffer a major adverse cardiac event (MACE).[19–21] Patient who experience an MI following noncardiac surgery have an elevated in-hospital mortality rate of 15% to 25%, and nonfatal perioperative MI is an independent predictor for cardiovascular death in the 6 months following surgery.[20,22,23] Thus, medical optimization of ASCVD in the perioperative period has been a focus of significant study.

Lifestyle modifications such as regular exercise, weight loss, diet modification, and smoking cessation may forestall the progression of atherosclerotic disease and improve fitness for surgery. Patients undergoing vascular surgery should also be aggressively treated for underlying medical conditions that predispose to ASCVD such as hypertension, dyslipidemia, and diabetes. Improvements in pharmacologic therapy have revolutionized the care of patients with atherosclerotic disease. It is worth noting that many of the landmark trials that currently dictate recommendations for surgical intervention were performed at a time when best medical therapy for atherosclerotic disease was significantly limited as compared to today. In the modern era of multimodal treatment with β-blockade, statins, intensive glucose control, antiplatelet therapies, and pharmacologic aids for smoking cessation, it is conceivable that a larger number of patients may be appropriately managed with medical, rather than surgical, therapy. That is, with improved medical management, the number needed to operate on to prevent an untoward cardiovascular event may be even higher than the literature suggests.

Perhaps the most widely studied medical intervention in the perioperative period is the use of β-blockade. A significant proportion of postoperative ischemic events are thought to be secondary to a persistently exaggerated sympathetic response. Substantial elevations in heart rate increase myocardial oxygen demand while simultaneously decreasing oxygen supply, with resultant demand ischemia. It has been proposed that modulating this heart rate response may decrease both the incidence and severity of the ischemia (Fig. 40-3).[24,25] Several randomized controlled studies demonstrated a significant benefit to β-blockade

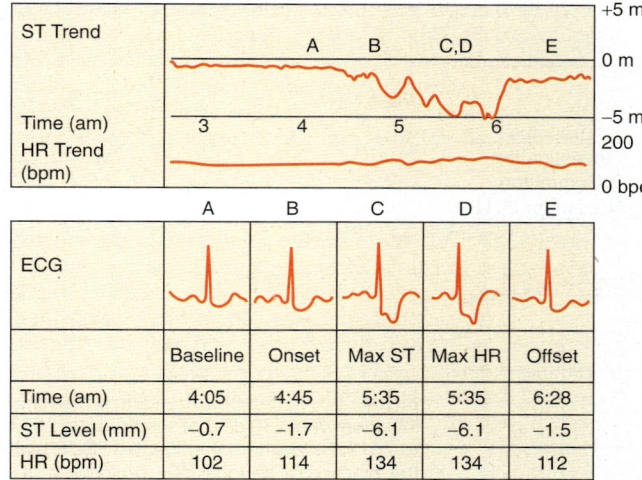

Figure 40-3 ST segment changes with heart rate (HR) during an ischemic episode. Tachycardia can increase the myocardial oxygen demand (due to increased work) while decreasing supply (due to decreased diastolic filling time), culminating in demand ischemia. (Reprinted with permission from Mangano DT, Hollenberg M, Fegert G, et al. Perioperative myocardial ischemia in patients undergoing noncardiac surgery–I: Incidence and severity during the 4 day perioperative period. The Study of Perioperative Ischemia [SPI] Research Group. *J Am Coll Cardiol.* 1991;17:843–850.)

as a means to reduce the risk of MACE,[25–27] although other studies have failed to validate these findings.[28–30] Some of the most compelling evidence in support of perioperative β-blockade came from the Dutch Echocardiographic Cardiac Risk Evaluation Applying Stress Echocardiography Study Group (DECREASE-1 and DECREASE-IV),[26,31] the validity of which has been called into question in light of allegations of scientific misconduct. The PeriOperative Ischemic Evaluation (POISE-1) trial, a large randomized controlled trial of more than 8,000 patients, found that perioperative β-blockade was associated with a decrease in perioperative MI, at the expense of an even greater increased risk of death or stroke.[32] In light of these new findings, updated recommendations for the role of perioperative β-blockade in noncardiac surgery were released by the American College of Cardiology (ACC) and American Heart Association (AHA).[19] This systemic review examined 17 large (>100 patients) randomized controlled or cohort studies comparing perioperative β-blockade against placebo in adult patients undergoing noncardiac surgery. For patients started on β-blockade 1 day or less before surgery, this review demonstrated an overall moderate reduction in nonfatal MI, even with the exclusion of the DECREASE studies. There was, however, an overall increased risk of all-cause death and trend toward increased risk of cardiovascular death. There was also a significant increase in the risk of nonfatal stroke, as well the risk for significant hypotension and bradycardia, in the group receiving β-blockade. For patients in whom β-blockade was initiated 2 or more days prior to surgery, current data were deemed insufficient to recommend for or against β-blockade therapy in the perioperative period. Further multicenter, randomized controlled trials are needed to address this gap in knowledge.

The 2014 update to the ACC/AHA clinical practice guideline for perioperative cardiovascular evaluation and management of patients undergoing noncardiac surgery also made specific recommendations regarding the management of perioperative β-blockade.[33] This task force recommended that β-blockers should be continued in the perioperative period in patients who are chronically on β-blocker therapy (Class I, Level of Evidence B) and that it may be reasonable to begin β-blockers in the perioperative period on those patients with intermediate- to high-risk myocardial ischemia noted on preoperative testing (Class IIb, LOE C) or in patients with three or more cardiac risk factors (Class IIb, LOE B). It is reasonable to start such therapy in advance of surgery to establish safety and tolerability (Class IIb, Level of Evidence: B). They further recommend that β-blockers should not be started on the day of surgery (Class III, LOE B).

Studies of perioperative β-blockade specific to the vascular surgery population have found similar conclusions to those in the general surgical population. A recent retrospective cohort analysis of the Society for Vascular Surgery Vascular Quality Initiative (SVS-VQI) found that, exclusive of high-risk open abdominal aortic aneurysm repair (OAR), preoperative institution of β-blockade did not decrease mortality or rate of MACE, but did increase the rates of other adverse events following major vascular surgery.[34] The Perioperative Beta Blockade (POBBLE)[30] trial evaluated more than 100 patients undergoing infrarenal vascular surgery and the Metoprolol after Vascular Surgery (MaVS)[28] included nearly 500 patients undergoing abdominal aortic surgery, axillofemoral revascularization, or infrainguinal revascularization. Both studies failed to find a significant difference in MACE between patients who received β-blockers in the perioperative period and placebo. A recent Cochrane Review concluded that there is no evidence that perioperative β-blockade reduces all-cause mortality, cardiovascular mortality, nonfatal MI, arrhythmia, heart failure, stroke, or composite cardiovascular events in patients undergoing vascular surgery.[35] It further concluded that strong evidence suggests that β-blockade increases the risk of perioperative bradycardia and hypotension.

As a result of a shift in both the strength and direction of evidence, the practice of β-blocker initiation in the immediate perioperative period has precipitously declined over recent years (Fig. 40-4), although the practice remains relatively common in patients with higher cardiac risk and those undergoing vascular surgery.[36] The choice of β-blocker in the perioperative period has also been studied. An epidemiologic analysis of nearly 40,000 high-risk patients found a decreased mortality at both 30 days and 1 year in patients who received atenolol as compared to metoprolol.[37] A retrospective analysis of nearly 60,000 patients found that both preoperative metoprolol (compared to atenolol) and intraoperative metoprolol (compared to esmolol or labetalol) was associated with an increased risk of stroke after noncardiac surgery.[38]

The marked sympathetic stimulation that occurs in the perioperative period has led to significant interest in α_2-adrenergic agonists to blunt the surgical stress response and reduce cardiovascular morbidity and mortality. Evidence for the utility of α_2-agonists in the perioperative period is conflicting. Several studies have suggested that the perioperative use of α_2-agonists reduces intraoperative myocardial ischemia, postoperative catecholamine levels, and mortality in high-risk noncardiac surgery.[39,40] A recent meta-analysis[41] found data to be encouraging, but insufficient, to suggest that this class of medication can reduce the risk of cardiac morbidity and mortality, and a second specific to the vascular surgery population found a decreased risk of mortality and perioperative MI.[42] Despite these encouraging results, other evidence calls the perioperative benefit of α_2-agonists into question. The PeriOperative Ischemic Evaluation-2 (POISE-2) trial was a multicenter, international, randomized, blinded trial that evaluated over 10,000 patients with, or at risk for, ASCVD undergoing noncardiac surgery.[43] In this study, α_2-agonists did not reduce the incidence of perioperative MI or the composite outcome of death or nonfatal MI. Patients receiving α_2-agonists

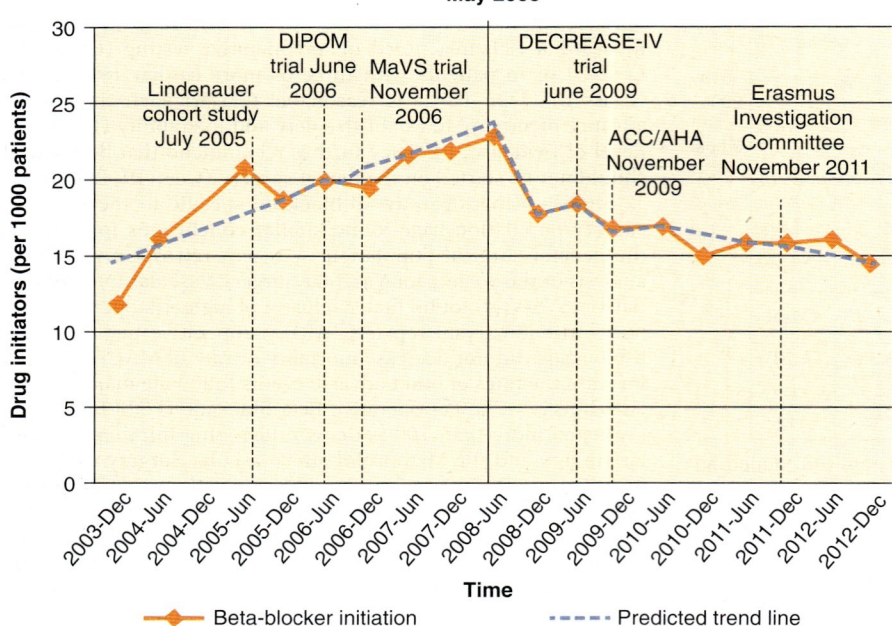

Figure 40-4 Temporal trends in β-blockade initiation within 30 days of surgery from 2003 to 2012. Following the influential POISE trial, the practice of perioperative β-blockade initiation within 30 days of surgery decreased significantly. ACC/AHA, American College of Cardiology/American Heart Association. (Reprinted with permission from Patorno E, Wang SV, Schneeweiss S, et al. Patterns of beta-blocker initiation in patients undergoing intermediate- to high-risk noncardiac surgery. *Am Heart J.* 2015;170:812–820.e6.)

had more clinically significant hypotension and an increase incidence of nonfatal cardiac arrest. In light of these recent findings, the most recent ACC/AHA guidelines state that α_2-agonists are not recommended for prevention of MACE in patients undergoing noncardiac surgery (Class III; LOE B).[33] Although evidence to support the initiation of α_2-agonists is lacking, it is important to recognize that the abrupt discontinuation of this class of medication in patients who are chronic users can result in a rebound sympathetic surge including profound hypertension and tachycardia, diaphoresis, and pulmonary edema. Thus, the relative risks and benefits of continuing versus withdrawing this class of medication must be considered in patients who chronically receive α_2-agonists.

Renin–angiotensin system (RAS) blockers (including angiotensin-converting enzyme inhibitors and angiotensin-receptor blockers) are a commonly used class of antihypertensive agents that have several benefits in regard to prevention of acute cardiovascular events independent of their antihypertensive effects. The RAS has been shown to influence the progression of ASCVD via effects on inflammation, endothelial function, and overall plaque stability.[44] RAS blocking agents have demonstrated beneficial effects on ventricular remodeling following acute MI,[45] ischemia–reperfusion injury,[46] and perioperative acute kidney injury.[47] Despite beneficial long-term effects, a recent large, retrospective study in the cardiac surgery population found an increased risk of perioperative morbidity (including significant vasoplegia, need for inotropic support, dysrhythmia, and renal dysfunction) and mortality when ACE inhibitors were continued in the perioperative period.[48] A similar association was found between perioperative RAS blockade and 30-day mortality following major vascular surgery.[49] To date, no studies provide definitive evidence for the independent ability of RAS blockers to reduce perioperative cardiovascular risk, and further randomized controlled trials are warranted. The most recent ACC/AHA guidelines suggest that continuation of RAS blocking agents is reasonable in the perioperative period (Class IIa; LOE B), and that if they stopped preoperatively, it is reasonable to restart as soon as clinically feasible (Class IIa; LOE C).[33] However, many choose to hold this class of medication in the preoperative period due to a well-recognized association between RAS blocking medications and refractory vasoplegia.

Statins are widely utilized for both primary and secondary prevention of ASCVD for their beneficial effects on lipid profile. More recent evidence also suggests more pleiotropic effects on events critical to the surgical stress response. Statins have been shown to inhibit the inflammatory response, reduce ischemia–reperfusion injury, reduce thrombosis, enhance fibrinolysis, decrease platelet reactivity, and restore endothelial function.[50,51] Use of preoperative statins has been associated with reduced cardiac morbidity and mortality following both cardiac and vascular surgery.[52–57] The abrupt discontinuation of statins interferes with endothelial functioning and increases markers of inflammation and oxidative stress in acute coronary syndromes,[58] and the discontinuation of statins in the postoperative period is similarly associated with increased in-hospital death and myonecrosis.[52,54] A recent meta-analysis demonstrated a reduction in all-cause mortality, combined fatal and nonfatal cardiovascular disease, combined fatal and nonfatal coronary events, and combined fatal and nonfatal stroke in patients treated with statins for primary prevention of ASCVD.[59] Meta-analyses specific to the vascular surgery population have had conflicting results. One analysis found no difference in 30-day mortality or MACE in patients not already receiving a statin medication following noncardiac vascular surgery,[60] whereas another found no significant difference in cardiovascular mortality but a lower risk of all-cause mortality, MI, stroke, and the composite outcome of MI, stroke, and death.[61] The ACC/AHA recommendations propose that patients who take a statin should be continued on this medication during the perioperative period (Class I; LOE B). They further suggest that it is reasonable to initiate treatment in patients undergoing vascular surgery if statin naïve (Class IIa; LOE B).[33]

Antiplatelet agents are commonly employed for secondary prevention of MACE. Multiple studies have found that antiplatelet agents, and particularly dual antiplatelet therapy (DAPT), can reduce the rate of ischemic events. A recent retrospective review found that aspirin withdrawal precedes more than 10% of acute cardiovascular events.[62] Patients who have suffered previous ischemic stroke should be continued on mono or dual antiplatelet therapy,[63] and evidence suggests that patients undergoing carotid endarterectomy (CEA) have a lower rate of perioperative stroke when antiplatelet agents are continued in the perioperative period.[64,65] Similarly, DAPT is essential following coronary stent implantation.[33] Despite the purported benefits of antiplatelet agents, however, a recent review from the Vascular Quality Initiative found no difference in the rate of in-hospital MI or death in patients who did and did not receive antiplatelet agents before major vascular surgery.[66] There was, however, an increased rate of blood loss for all procedures and increased transfusion rate for infrainguinal bypass. Similarly, the POISE-2 trial found no difference in the primary outcome of composite of death or nonfatal MI at 30 days between those who did and did not receive aspirin, or in the secondary outcome which also included nonfatal stroke.[67] A greater risk of major bleeding was observed in the aspirin group. In contrast to these two trials, a recent prospective review from the Vascular Study Group of New England evaluated the use of clopidogrel, aspirin, or DAPT for more than 10,000 patients at 15 centers undergoing nonemergent CEA, lower extremity bypass, endovascular aortic repair (EVAR), and OAR and found no difference in major bleeding complications between the three groups.[68] Thus, although the use of antiplatelet agents is important for long-term management of ASCVD, the purported risks and benefits of antiplatelet therapy in the perioperative period must be carefully weighed in noncardiac, noncarotid vascular surgery.

The lack of perceived benefit of aspirin on perioperative MI observed in the Vascular Quality Initiative and POISE-2 studies may be related to a difference in the causative mechanism of MI in the perioperative period compared to the nonoperative setting. Specifically, type I MI (characterized by morphologically complex coronary plaque prone to rupture and thrombus) may not be the dominant mechanism in the perioperative setting. A recent study demonstrated that this "classic" lesion occurs in only 45% of perioperative MI.[69] Rather, the increase in major bleeding caused by antiplatelet agents may lead to a demand ischemia related to anemia, tachycardia, and hypotension (type II MI).[67,69] The most recent ACC/AHA guidelines suggest that the management of perioperative antiplatelet therapy should be determined by consensus of the treating clinicians (Class I; LOE C). It may be reasonable to continue aspirin in patients undergoing nonemergent/nonurgent noncardiac surgery who have not had previous coronary stenting when the perceived risk of MACE outweighs the risk of increased bleeding (Class IIb; LOE B). These guidelines recommend against the initiation or continuation of aspirin in patients undergoing elective noncardiac, noncarotid surgery who have not had previous coronary stenting (Class III; LOE B), unless the risk of ischemic event is greater than the risk of surgical bleeding (Class III; LOE C).[33]

Hyperglycemia has been associated with increased morbidity and mortality in critically ill patients. Of the oral hypoglycemic agents, it is reasonable to hold sulfonylureas due to the risk of hypoglycemia in the setting of preoperative fasting. Metformin is associated with lactic acidosis and should also be held preoperatively due the increased risk of lactic acidosis with hypovolemia and renal dysfunction (which may be comorbid or provoked by iodinated contrast agents used during endovascular procedures). Patients on these medications can be managed with insulin, which is the treatment modality most intensively studied in the perioperative period. Initial work suggested that tight glucose control (glucose 80 to 110 mg/dL) in critically ill patients led to significant decrease in mortality and multiorgan system failure, resulting in a call for stringent control of hyperglycemia in hospitalized patients.[70] Subsequent studies, however, have failed to replicate these results and instead have found an increase in unrecognized hypoglycemia and an increased risk of death in patients in the intensive glucose control group.[71,72] Hyperglycemia may exacerbate neurologic injury and thus may be especially important for carotid and thoracic aortic procedures with elevated risk of perioperative stroke. In the intraoperative period, both hyperglycemia (glucose >200 mg/dL) and tight glucose control (glucose <140 mg/dL) have been associated with an increased risk of adverse outcomes.[73] Thus, although severe hyperglycemia should be avoided, it is likely prudent to maintain glucose levels in the 140 to 180 mg/dL range rather than attempt normoglycemia.

It has been suggested that anemia (hematocrit <28%) may increase the incidence of postoperative myocardial ischemia and MACE in high-risk patients undergoing noncardiac surgery,[74] and a traditional practice is to transfuse patients deemed high risk for adverse cardiac events to a hematocrit of 30%. More recently, two studies have suggested no benefit to liberal (hemoglobin goal 10 to 12 mg/dL) rather than restrictive (hemoglobin goal 7 to 8 mg/dL) transfusion practices.[75,76] The Functional Outcomes in Cardiovascular Patients Undergoing Surgical Hip Fracture Repair (FOCUS) trial,[80] in specific, found no outcomes differences between patients transfused intraoperatively with a restrictive versus liberal strategy, even in a perceived high-risk population. In vascular surgery, specifically, perioperative transfusion has been independently associated with increased 30-day morbidity and mortality.[77] Decision for perioperative transfusion should be based on evidence of compromised end organ perfusion, rate and cause of blood loss, and likelihood of obtaining control of ongoing hemorrhage. Hypothermia is also associated with increased adrenergic tone and postoperative myocardial ischemia and events in vascular surgery patients.[78] In addition, maintaining perioperative normothermia reduces blood loss and transfusion requirement by clinically important amounts.[79] Therefore, aggressive heat conservation and warming measures are appropriate perioperatively. Shivering should be avoided in the perioperative period to prevent increased myocardial demand, and extubation should be postponed in hypothermic patients.

Cardiac morbidity and mortality is higher following vascular surgery than after other types of noncardiac surgery, and the presence of uncorrected CAD appears to double the 5-year mortality following vascular surgery. Given the high likelihood of concurrent CAD in patients presenting for vascular surgery, and given that myocardial revascularization may have long-term benefits in patients with triple vessel CAD, left main disease, or poor left ventricular (LV) function, the question of preoperative coronary revascularization prior to elective vascular surgery has been a subject of study. Initial observational studies suggested that preoperative cardiac revascularization improves patient outcomes prior to high-risk noncardiac surgery.[80,81] Whether preoperative coronary revascularization actually protects against perioperative MACE is controversial in prospective studies. Monaco and colleagues[82] randomized more than 200 patients undergoing vascular surgery to routine preoperative coronary angiography versus selective angiography based on the results of noninvasive testing and risk stratification. Myocardial revascularization was more common in the routine surveillance group, although there was no significant different in-hospital MACE rate between groups. Notably, however, long-term survival and freedom from death/cardiovascular events was improved in the group who underwent routine preoperative coronary angiography (Fig. 40-5). The multicenter Coronary Artery Revascularization Prophylaxis (CARP) trial evaluated more than 500 patients who underwent prophylactic cardiac revascularization prior to major vascular surgery based on the presence of ischemia on a noninvasive stress imaging study.[83] Patients were randomized to either percutaneous coronary intervention (PCI) or coronary artery bypass (CABG). With aggressive medical therapy (>80% of patients on β-blockers, >70% on aspirin, and >50% on statins in both groups), no long-term benefit was noted with preoperative revascularization. A subsequent subgroup analysis examined the value of CABG versus PCI and found that patients who underwent CABG had fewer MIs and shorter hospital stays than their counterparts in the PCI group.[84] This difference may be due to more complete revascularization in the CABG group. It is worth noting that the CARP study randomized patients on the basis of abnormal stress testing, whereas the Monaco study performed coronary angiography on all patients in the routine group. Thus, in the CARP study, patients with CAD but limited or no ischemia at stress testing may have missed on a benefit to revascularization prior to the procedure. Furthermore, most patients in the CARP trial had single-vessel or two-vessel disease with normal LV ejection fraction. Exclusion criteria in this study included left main disease or ejection fraction less than 20%, thus limiting patients with more severe disease. A subsequent analysis of the CARP data found that patients with unprotected left main disease may be the only subset of patients who benefits from prophylactic revascularization.[85] In large part due to the CARP trial, preoperative coronary revascularization (either surgical or interventional) is not recommended prior to even high-risk surgery, unless revascularization is independently indicated according to current practice guidelines.[86,87]

For patients who have suffered recent MI who need noncardiac surgery, evidence suggests that the risk of postoperative MI decreases significantly with time. Furthermore, the risk of postoperative MI may be modified by the occurrence and type of revascularization performed (CABG vs. PCI) prior to elective

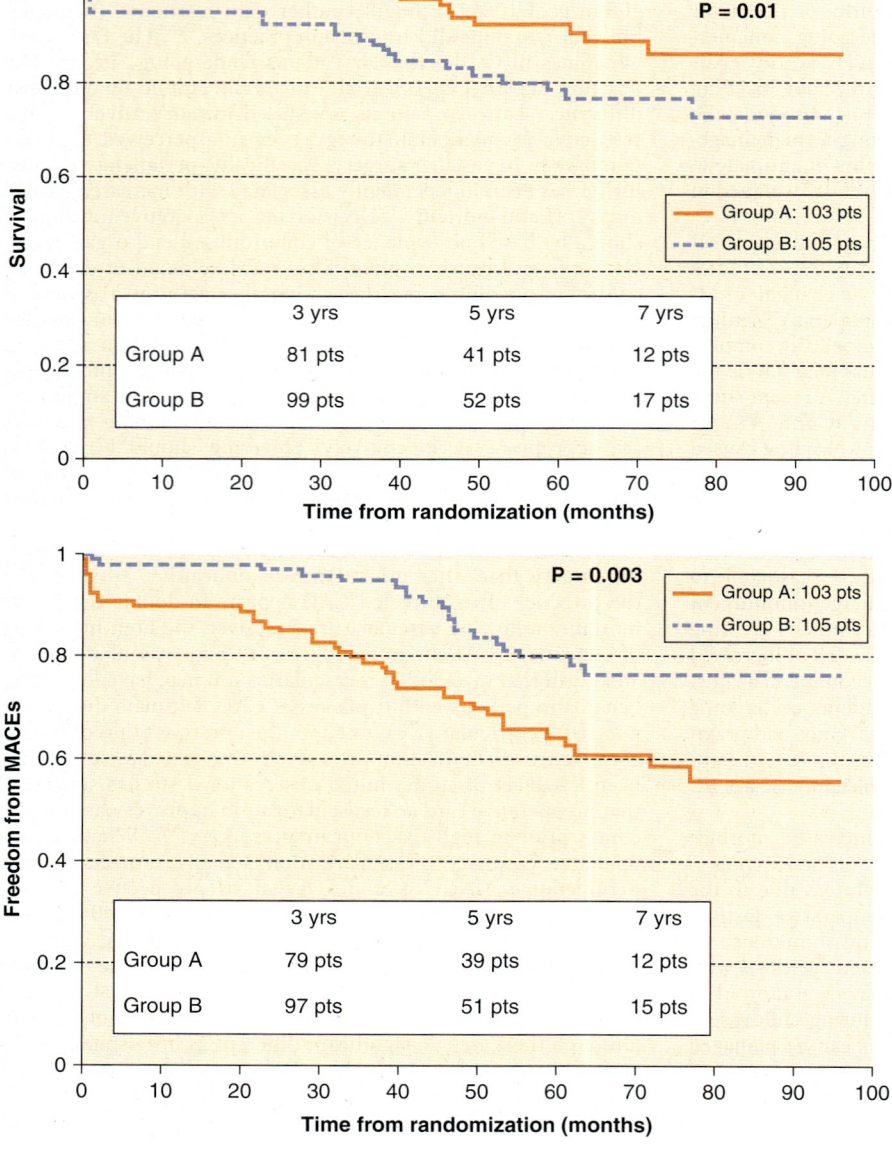

Figure 40-5 Cumulative survival and freedom from major adverse cardiac event for routine versus selective coronary angiography prior to major vascular surgery in intermediate- to high-risk patients. Long-term survival, and survival free from MACE, were greater in the group who underwent routine preoperative coronary angiography. (Reprinted with permission from Monaco M, Stassano P, Di Tommaso L, et al. Systematic strategy of prophylactic coronary angiography improves long-term outcome after major vascular surgery in medium- to high-risk patients: a prospective, randomized study. J Am Col Cardio. 2009;54:989–996.)

surgery.[88,89] Current guidelines recommend waiting at least 60 days following MI before elective noncardiac surgery in the absence of intervention.[33] For patients for whom preoperative coronary revascularization is deemed necessary prior to elective surgery, the timing of originally proposed procedure depends on the type of coronary intervention performed. The most recent ACC/AHA guidelines make no specific recommendation on appropriate timing on noncardiac surgery following CABG. In this case, the clinical urgency of the procedure, medical optimization, and overall fitness of surgery must all be taken into consideration. Specific recommendations are made following PCI, and the ACC/AHA released a focused update on duration of dual antiplatelet therapy (DAPT) for patients with CAD in 2016.[90] The updated guidelines suggest delaying elective noncardiac surgery 30 days following bare metal stent (BMS) placement and ideally 6 months following drug eluting stent (DES) placement (Class I; LOE B-NR). For patients treated with DAPT following coronary stent placement who must undergo surgical procedures that mandate discontinuation of their platelet receptor inhibitor (P2Y12) therapy, it is recommended that aspirin be continued when possible and the P2Y12 inhibitor be restarted as soon as possible following surgery (Class 1; LOE C-EO). A consensus decision among treating clinicians as to the relative risk of surgery and the discontinuation or continuation of antiplatelet agents can be useful (Class IIa; LOE C-EO). Elective noncardiac surgery after DES placement for whom P2Y12 inhibitor must be discontinued may be considered after 3 months if the risk of further delaying surgery outweighs the expected risk of stent thrombosis (Class IIb; LOE C-EO). Elective noncardiac surgery should not be performed within 30 days following BMS placement or within 3 months for DES implantation in patients in whom DAPT will need to be discontinued perioperatively (Class III; LOE B-NR).

Preoperative Anesthesia Evaluation for Vascular Surgery

The purpose of the preoperative anesthesia evaluation is to delineate the extent of any underlying comorbid pathology and medically optimize the patient for surgery. In vascular surgery, the preoperative assessment predominantly focuses on the presence of, or risk factors for, coronary or noncoronary ASCVD. A careful history must be taken to define the extent of any diagnosed ASCVD and to screen for any undiagnosed concurrent disease (e.g., angina or equivalent, symptoms of transient ischemic attack (TIA), or mesenteric or peripheral ischemia). Physical examination should evaluate for any evidence of end organ involvement (e.g., diminished pulses, S_4 gallop, or residual deficit from previous stroke) or cardiovascular decompensation (e.g., new or worsened murmur, jugular venous distention, third heart sound on cardiac auscultation, rales, shortness of breath, or peripheral edema). It is important to evaluate the control of any comorbid conditions such as diabetes or hypertension. The strong association between smoking and vascular disease mandates a thorough assessment of any underlying pulmonary disease. Medications should be optimized as discussed earlier.

For any major vascular surgery, it is prudent to obtain baseline laboratory studies. A complete blood count should be obtained due to the risk of major blood loss and possibility of concurrent medical diseases that may predispose to anemia. Coagulation studies should be considered if the patient is on anticoagulant medications or if regional anesthesia is anticipated. A metabolic panel should be obtained due to an increased likelihood of underlying renal insufficiency with resultant electrolyte abnormalities. It is also useful to have a baseline given an elevated risk of postoperative renal dysfunction. Cardiac biomarkers (e.g., troponin I, N-terminal pro-brain natriuretic peptide, cystatin C, and C-reactive protein) and risk factors identified on advanced imaging modalities (coronary artery calcium scores or CIMT) have long been studied for their ability to predict long-term cardiovascular outcomes; their utility in the perioperative setting to predict high-risk patients, however, is a relatively new area of interest.[91] A preoperative 12-lead electrocardiogram (ECG) is reasonable as a baseline because of the increased risk of perioperative MACE. A preoperative echocardiogram to assess LV function is reasonable for patients with previously documented LV dysfunction, worsening clinical status or if not assessed within the previous year, or for patients with dyspnea of unknown origin.[33] Routine echocardiography in asymptomatic patients cannot be recommended.

Determining which patients require additional preoperative cardiac testing is a source of frequent debate. Vascular surgery patients are known to be at elevated risk of perioperative MACE. It has been predicted that postoperative troponin elevation and MI predict a 26% and 55% lower survival rate, respectively, in the 5 years following vascular surgery compared with patients who do not experience an event (Fig. 40-6).[92] Thus, significant effort has focused on identifying patients at elevated cardiac risk. Conversely, over utilization of advanced testing modalities can put undue stress on the health-care system, result in false positive tests, delay necessary surgery, and ultimately cause patient harm in further invasive workup and treatment. The most well-recognized clinical practice guidelines for perioperative cardiovascular evaluation for patients undergoing noncardiac surgery are jointly developed by the ACC/AHA and were most recently revised in 2014 (Fig. 40-7).[33] The first step in evaluation for fitness for surgery is to determine the urgency of surgery. Clinical emergencies (e.g., ruptured abdominal aortic aneurysm [AAA]) should proceed to the operating room without delay and with best medication optimization, recognizing that the risk or perioperative MACE is elevated in this situation. Situations that are urgent, but not emergent (e.g., critical limb ischemia [CLI]) may allow for an abbreviated cardiac workup, if such workup will impact clinical management. The second step is to evaluate whether the patient has an acute coronary syndrome (new, crescendo, or unstable angina; MI within the last 60 days) or other major cardiac pathophysiology (symptomatic heart failure; new or worsening valvular heart disease; or unstable arrhythmia or conduction disease). If present, these conditions should be evaluated and optimized per clinical practice guidelines prior to elective surgery. The third step involves estimation of perioperative risk of MACE based on combined clinical and surgical risk factors. Commonly used estimations include the American College of Surgeons National Surgical Quality Improvement Program risk calculator[93] or the revised cardiac risk index (RCRI)[94] with an estimation of surgical risk; however, The Vascular Study Group of New England developed a vascular surgery-specific model for the prediction of cardiac events that more accurately predicted the risk of cardiac complications in vascular surgery patients than the RCRI, which was found to underestimate the risk of MACE by 1.7- to 7.4-fold in vascular surgery patients.[95] Independent predictors of MACE in this study included: increasing age, smoking, insulin-dependent diabetes, CAD, CHF, abnormal cardiac stress test, long-term β-blocker therapy, chronic obstructive pulmonary disease, and elevated creatinine. Regardless of the risk calculator used, functional status dictates the necessity for further cardiac workup prior to surgery for any patient deemed at elevated (>1%) risk of perioperative MACE. Patients

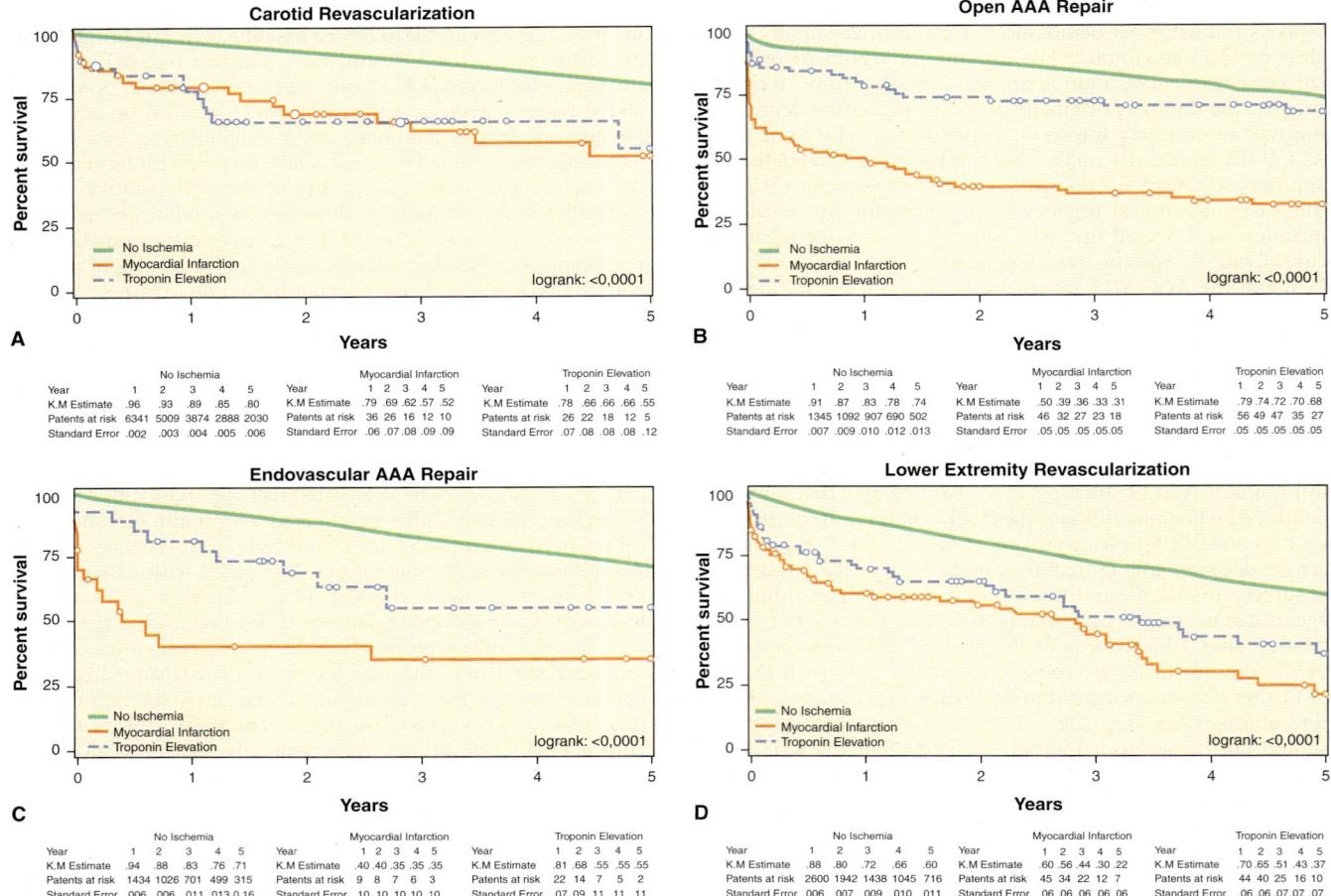

Figure 40-6 Univariate Kaplan–Meier (K-M) survival curves, stratified according to postoperative myocardial ischemia, for different major vascular surgical procedures. Vascular surgery patients who suffer from perioperative myocardial ischemia have significantly worse outcomes with decreased survival at 5 years for (**A**) carotid, (**B**) open aortic, (**C**) endovascular aortic, and (**D**) peripheral interventions. AAA, abdominal aortic aneurysm. (Reprinted with permission from Simons JP, Baril DT, Goodney PP, et al. The effect of postoperative myocardial ischemia on long-term survival after vascular surgery. *J Vasc Surg*. 2013;58:1600–1608.)

with moderate (4 metabolic equivalents [METs]) to excellent (>10 METs) exercise capacity may proceed to surgery with no further cardiac testing. For patients with poor or unknown functional capacity, a collaborative decision must be made between the patient and treating clinicians to determine the next step. Further cardiac testing (in the form of stress testing or cardiac catheterization) is reasonable if the results of the additional testing will change management decisions (e.g., coronary revascularization prior planned surgery or alternate plan for palliative care). Since most vascular surgery patients will fall in the elevated risk category and many will have poor to unknown functional status due to comorbid conditions, additional cardiac testing is not unreasonable prior to major vascular procedures.

Open Vascular Surgery

Cerebrovascular Disease

An imbalance between cerebral oxygen supply and demand leads to cerebral ischemia, which can be temporary or permanent. Nearly 800,000 patients per year suffer a stroke in the United States, and nearly 6.6 million patients in total have suffered a stroke for an overall prevalence of almost 3%.[3] From 2001 to 2011, the number of stroke deaths declined by more than 20%, primarily due to intensive efforts to control cardiovascular risk factors. Efforts to control hypertension appear to have had the greatest influence on the decline in stroke mortality, although improved management of diabetes mellitus and hyperlipidemia, as well as smoking cessation campaigns, have also contributed. The use of DAPT (aspirin plus clopidogrel) has been proven effective for both primary and secondary prevention of stroke in patients with cardiovascular risk factors.[96] Despite an overall decrease in stroke-related mortality, it is still the fourth leading cause of death in the United States.[3] Equally importantly, the combination of a significant psychological consequences and new disability may lead to profound impact on quality of life. Stroke has been called the most burdensome chronic condition.

Most strokes are ischemic, rather than hemorrhagic, in origin. Carotid atherosclerotic disease accounts for approximately 20% of all ischemic strokes, although the mechanism of pathophysiology is typically embolic rather than occlusive. Stroke symptomatology depends on the distribution of ischemia. Carotid disease may manifest as transient attacks of monocular blindness (amaurosis fugax), paresthesia, weakness or clumsiness, facial drooping, or speech problems. These symptoms may

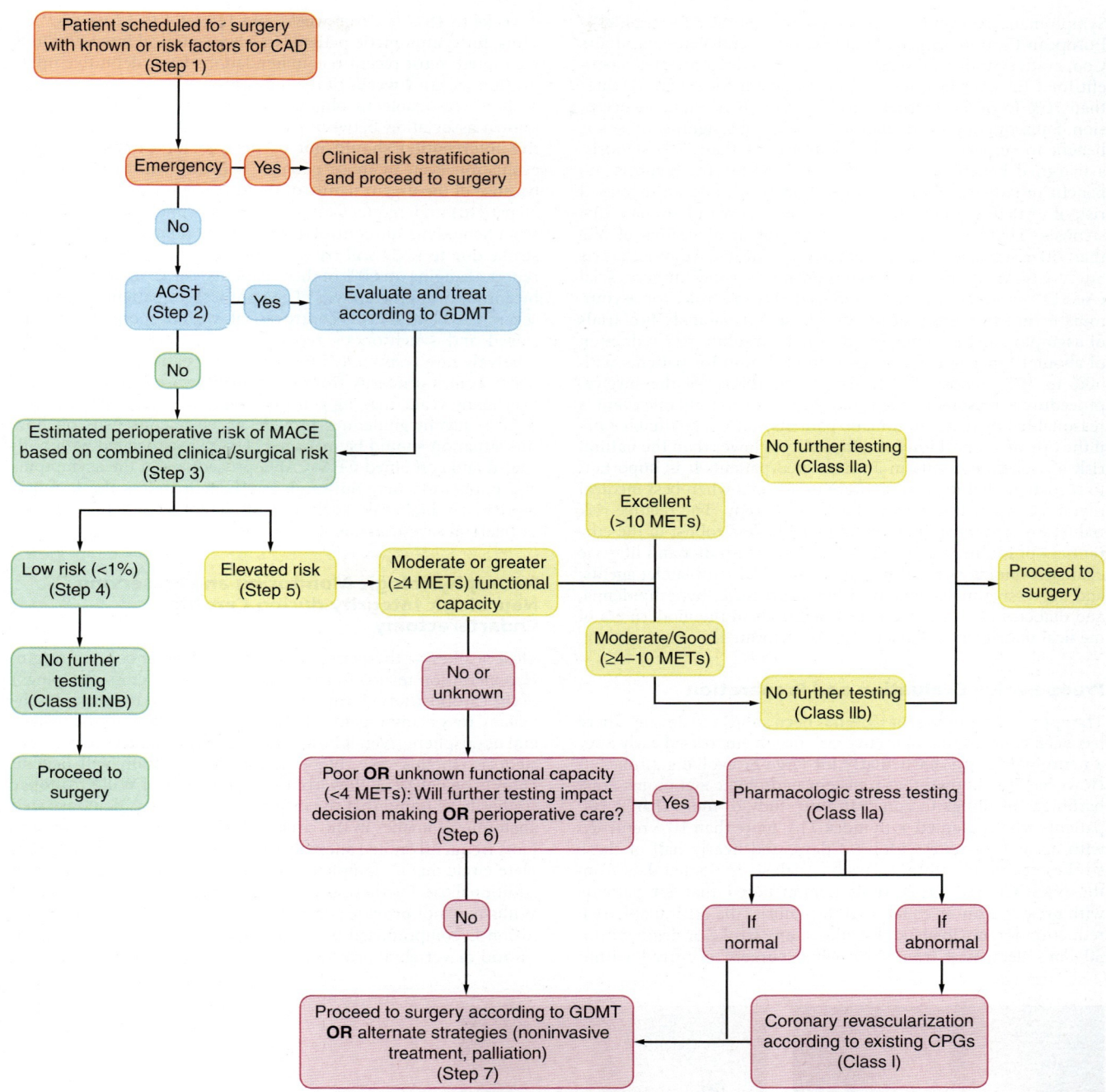

Figure 40-7 Proposed algorithm for cardiovascular evaluation and management of patients undergoing noncardiac surgery. In this most recent iteration of the ACC/AHA clinical practice guidelines, individual consideration of patient medical versus surgical risk has been combined into overall perioperative risk. A combination of clinical urgency, patient risk of major adverse cardiac event, and patient functional status helps to guide the necessity of further preoperative cardiac work up. CAD, coronary artery disease; ACS, acute coronary syndrome; GDMT, guideline directed medical therapy; MACE, major adverse cardiac event; MET, metabolic equivalent; NB, no benefit; CPG, clinical practice guideline. (Reprinted with permission from Fleisher LA, Fleischmann KE, Auerbach AD, et al. 2014 ACC/AHA guideline on perioperative cardiovascular evaluation and management of patients undergoing noncardiac surgery: executive summary: a report of the American College of Cardiology/American Heart Association Task Force on Practice Guidelines. *Circulation*. 2014;130:2215–2245.)

resolve spontaneously after a short period. Any focalized neurologic deficit lasting less than 24 hours' duration with no evidence of permanent infarction is known as a TIA. It has been estimated that up to 15% of strokes are heralded by TIA,[97] and the most important risk factor for future stroke is the presence of recent TIA symptoms. The risk of stroke following TIA is elevated in the initial days to weeks following the initial event.[98,99] Thus, TIA symptoms should prompt an immediate workup and referral for definitive intervention.

Several high profile randomized controlled trials have demonstrated clinical benefit for CEA for both symptomatic and asymptomatic carotid atherosclerosis. The North American

Symptomatic Carotid Endarterectomy (NASCET) trial,[100,101] European Carotid Surgery Trial (ECST),[102] and Veterans Affairs Cooperative Studies (VACS) Program,[103] all demonstrated a benefit for CEA over best medical management for severe (greater than 70% to 80%) internal carotid artery (ICA) stenosis occlusion. Subsequent pooled analyses[104,105] found a significant 5-year benefit to surgery for patients with greater than 70% stenosis, a marginal benefit for patients with 50% to 70% stenosis, no benefit in patients with 30% to 49% stenosis, and an increased risk of ipsilateral ischemic stroke in patients with less than 30% stenosis. There was no benefit to treatment of lesions of less than 50% stenosis. The Asymptomatic Carotid Atherosclerosis Study (ACAS)[106] and the Asymptomatic Carotid Surgery Trial (ACST)[107,108] demonstrated a reduced risk of stroke for asymptomatic carotid disease, albeit less robust. A meta-analysis of trials of asymptomatic patients found a small absolute risk reduction of about 1% per year for surgical intervention for patients with 50% to 70% stenosis.[109] Because the morbidity of the surgical procedure is reasonably high, and the risk of an ischemic event is reasonably low in asymptomatic patients, CEA is justifiable only if the operative morbidity and mortality is lower than the natural risk of ischemic events in an untreated patient. It is important to recognize that these trials were performed when best medical therapy consisted primarily of aspirin therapy. The relative risk reduction of surgical intervention may be less robust in the current era of multimodal medical treatment with diet and lifestyle changes; smoking cessation campaigns; dual antiplatelet agents; and aggressive management of blood pressure, hyperlipidemia, and diabetes. Randomized controlled trials in the modern era of medical management have not been performed.

Preoperative Evaluation and Preparation

The appropriate timing for CEA has been subject to debate. There has been concern that operative risk may be increased early after a neurologic event, particularly for large or evolving strokes.[110] However, it is known that transient neurologic symptoms are a harbinger of things to come. In one study of more than 1,700 patients who presented with index TIA, more than 10% returned with an acute stroke within 90 days, and nearly half of these strokes occurred within 2 days.[111] Analysis of pooled data from the NASCET and ECST trials demonstrated that for patients with greater than or equal to 70% stenosis, the attributable risk reduction for any ipsilateral stroke or any stroke or death within 30 days decreased from 30% when surgery occurred within 2 weeks to 18% at 2 to 4 weeks and 11% at 4 to 12 weeks.[110,112] Thus, for symptomatic patients in whom surgical intervention is warranted, most recent recommendations favor definitive intervention within 2 weeks of the index event.[113]

It is reasonable to obtain a cardiac evaluation due to the known association between carotid and CAD; however, definitive intervention should not be delayed for extensive cardiac evaluation even in those patients with known cardiac disease because of the urgent nature of the surgery. It is prudent to treat all patients undergoing CEA as if they have underlying CAD with strict hemodynamic control. Fifty percent of patients with TIA or stroke due to CVD will have an abnormal stress test despite no report of angina; in 60% of these patients, the CAD will be severe by coronary angiography.[114] The approach to patients with both severe CAD and CVD is controversial, with proponents for both staged and synchronous repair. Because these operations are relatively rare (especially in symptomatic patients), current evidence comes primarily from poor-quality case series performed over many years, making generalizability to current practice difficult. Current guidelines provide no clear consensus on how this situation should be managed. The risk associated with both staged and combined CEA–CABG procedures in the asymptomatic population may outweigh any benefit unless the lesion is particularly high risk, such as contralateral complete occlusion or bilateral severe stenosis.[115]

Neurophysiologic Monitoring and Preserving Neurologic Integrity during Carotid Endarterectomy

Most strokes in the perioperative period are embolic in origin. Hypoperfusion related to temporary occlusion ("cross-clamping") of the carotid artery during surgery can also lead to cerebral ischemia. Cross-clamping acutely disrupts blood flow to the ipsilateral hemisphere, even if flow was markedly diminished by severe stenosis. In this case, blood supply to the brain will depend entirely on collateral flow from an intact circle of Willis. Autopsy studies have found that the majority of specimens demonstrated anatomic anomalies in the circle of Willis.[116] Hypoplasia was the most frequently noted anomaly (24%) (Fig. 40-8), and an incomplete circle due to complete absence of a vessel was noted in an additional 6%. Furthermore, even an anatomically intact circle of Willis may not provide adequate cerebral blood if collateral perfusion is compromised by occlusive disease of the contralateral carotid or vertebral arteries, or if the patient becomes relatively

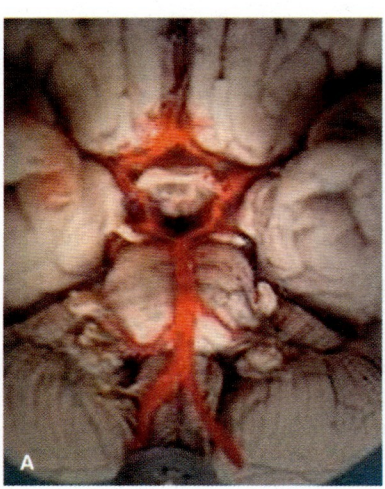
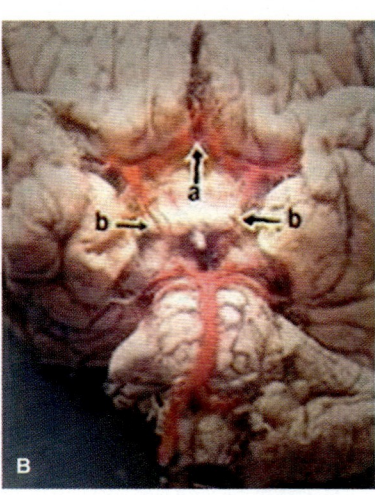

Figure 40-8 Intact and hypoplastic circle of Willis. (**A**) demonstrates an anatomically normal circle of Willis. (**B**) demonstrates hypoplastic (*a*) anterior and (*b*) posterior communicating arteries. (Reprinted with permission from Iqbal S. A comprehensive study of the anatomical variations of the circle of Willis in adult human brains. *J Clin Diagn Res.* 2013;7:2423–2427.)

hypotensive compared to baseline. Phenylephrine infusions are commonly used to augment cerebral blood flow but the practice has been associated with an increase in postoperative MI following CEA.[117] However, the short-term use of phenylephrine to augment cerebral collateral perfusion pressure, particularly in instances of electroencephalogram (EEG)-detected reversible cerebral ischemia, seems to be without significant long-term detriment to the heart.

A temporary carotid shunt can be employed to bypass the cross-clamp and restore cerebral blood flow. Significant practice variation exists among surgeons regarding the use of carotid shunts in CEA. Some surgeons never use shunts and rely on expedient surgery and meticulous hemodynamic control (including permissive hypertension) to maintain adequate collateral cerebral perfusion pressures. Others may shunt selectively based on changes in neurophysiologic monitoring, and still others shunt routinely. Shunt placement is not an entirely benign undertaking, with morbidity including atheromatous or air emboli, arterial dissection, nerve injury, hematoma, infection, and long-term restenosis. Perhaps most compellingly, shunting has been demonstrated to be unnecessary in approximately 85% of patients.[118] Furthermore, a shunt is only beneficial if the cause of neurologic dysfunction is inadequate blood flow. However, the majority of studies suggest that as many as 65% to 95% of all neurologic deficits during CEA are caused by thromboembolic events. A recent review of the literature found no difference in outcomes including rate of all stroke, ipsilateral stroke, or death up to 30 days after surgery between selective and routine shunting.[119]

Neurophysiologic monitoring is commonly employed to assess overall cerebral perfusion and to help determine which patients may benefit from carotid shunting. Some monitoring techniques, such as electroencephalography (EEG), somatosensory evoked potentials (SSEP), and motor evoked potentials (MEP), assess the overall integrity of cerebral function. Others, including transcranial Doppler (TCD) or carotid stump pressure, assess the blood flow in the large cerebral vessels. A third group, including near-infrared spectroscopy (NIRS) and jugular venous bulb saturation, estimate cerebral metabolism.[120] The gold standard for cerebral monitoring remains serial neurologic examination on an awake patient. No matter the modality employed, the goal of neurophysiologic monitoring is to identify patients who may benefit from selective shunting and to avoid shunting in patients where it is unnecessary.

EEG monitoring is perhaps the most commonly employed neurophysiologic monitor for carotid surgery. EEG records the electrical activity of the brain, and changes in cerebral blood flow can be reflected in the EEG waveform. Normal cerebral blood flow is approximately 50 mL/min/100 g brain tissue. In the perioperative period, decreases in cerebral blood flow as low as approximately 22 mL/min/100 g brain tissue may be well tolerated with no EEG changes.[121] EEG deterioration usually begins below a threshold of approximately 15 to 18 mL/min/100 g brain tissue, and frank cellular failure appears to occur below 10 to 12 mL/min/100 g brain tissue (Fig. 40-9).[122] The most common manifestations of cerebral ischemia on EEG are ipsilateral slowing and/or attenuation. Deterioration in EEG can be noted within seconds of carotid cross-clamping, and these changes are typically reversible with appropriate augmentation of hemodynamics and/or temporary shunt placement.

EEG monitoring is not without limitations. The sensitivity of EEG for predicting cerebral ischemia is poor; in one series of more than 300 patients, EEG identified cerebral ischemia in fewer than 60% of patients with a false positive rate of 1%.[123] In patients with pre-existing or fluctuating neurologic deficits, the EEG may be falsely negative. In these patients, there may be areas of brain parenchyma that are electrically silent or immediately adjacent to regions of infarction, and therefore not reliably monitored by EEG. These still-viable regions may progress to irreversible injury over the length of the procedure. EEG monitors cortical structures and not deep brain structures, and strokes in this distribution will be missed. Interpretation of EEG may be complicated by other intraoperative parameters such as hypothermia or rapid or sudden changes in anesthetic depth. This may be particularly relevant when propofol-based anesthetics are

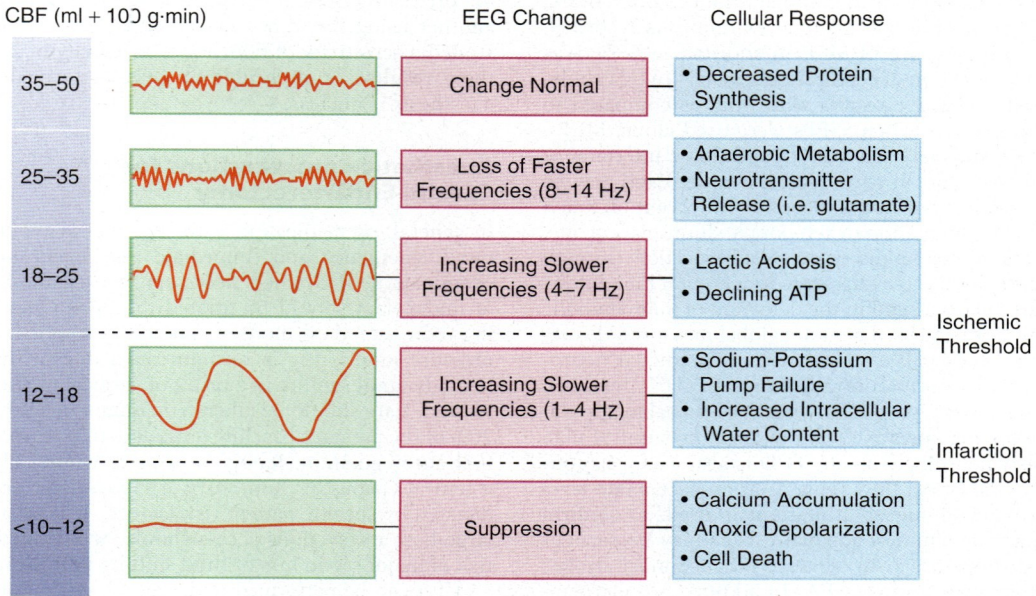

Figure 40-9 Characteristic electroencephalogram (EEG) changes with reduction in cerebral blood flow. Decreases in cerebral blood flow are associated with characteristic changes in the EEG and predictable cellular response. CBF, coronary blood flow; EEG, electroencephalogram; ATP, adenosine triphosphate. (Reprinted with permission from Foreman B, Claassen J. Quantitative EEG for the detection of brain ischemia. *Crit Care*. 2012;16[2]:216.)

used, although in general EEG changes secondary to anesthetic agents are more likely to be bilateral, whereas changes due to cross-clamping or hypoperfusion tend to involve the ipsilateral hemisphere. Finally, it is important to recognize that EEG is a global monitor of cerebral activity. It is unable to reliably detect strokes related to smaller thromboembolic phenomena, which is the most likely etiology of perioperative stroke.

SSEP monitoring employs electrical stimuli to peripheral nerves and evaluates the amplitude and latency of the signal over the cerebral cortex. In contrast to EEG, which only evaluates cortical functioning, SSEP monitoring also reflects the deep brain structures. Most commonly, the median and/or tibial nerves are assessed. A decrease in signaling for the median nerve suggests hypoperfusion in the watershed of the middle cerebral artery, whereas deterioration of tibial nerve signaling may reflect ischemia of the parenchyma supplied by the anterior cerebral artery.[120] A decrease in signal amplitude of greater than 50% is typically accepted as indicative of ischemia, which may occur when cerebral blood flow is critically low (i.e., at 15 mL/min/100 g brain tissue). SSEP monitoring may be particularly useful in patients with baseline cerebral ischemia in whom EEG interpretation is more difficult. Although some studies have been optimistic about the value of SSEP monitoring in the detection of cerebral ischemia, others have questioned both the sensitivity and specificity of SSEP for the detection of cerebral ischemia. A recent comparison of different neurophysiologic monitoring demonstrated a sensitivity of approximately 80% and a specificity of 57% for the detection of cerebral ischemia.[124] Furthermore, SSEPs are sensitive to virtually all commonly used anesthetic agents which may complicate intraoperative interpretation and lead to a high false positive rate. A light plane of anesthesia must be maintained if increased latencies and decreased amplitude of SSEP are to be ascribed to inadequate cerebral perfusion. False negatives with intraoperative SSEP monitoring has also been described; focal ischemia of the internal capsule has been suggested as a potential mechanism in this circumstance. Monitoring motor, rather than sensory, evoked potentials is one mechanism to overcome this problem. To monitor MEP, transcranial electrodes are utilized to stimulate the cerebral cortex, and motor response in the contralateral extremity is recorded. In one recent study, the use of MEP in addition to SSEP was more sensitive for detection of cerebral ischemia.[125] In this study, there were no false negative results with MEP as compared to a 1.5% false negative rate when SSEPs were used alone. MEPs, however, can be exquisitely sensitive to anesthetic interference (neuromuscular blockade, in particular, is avoided) and may be more prone to false positives and unnecessary intervention (such as blood pressure augmentation or temporary shunt placement).

TCD measures the maximum velocity of blood flow through the middle cerebral artery as a surrogate for cerebral blood flow. TCD may be particularly useful in the detection of microembolic phenomena that may be missed by more global measures of cerebral functioning. In a small case series, TCD predicted neurologic events despite a normal intraoperative EEG.[126] Detection of microembolic showers, particularly during surgical manipulation, may allow for the operative team to alter the surgical plan to prevent further neurologic insult. TCD is also useful in confirming that cerebral blood flow remains at an acceptable level after carotid cross-clamping or, if a shunt is used, to confirm that flow through the shunt is adequate. TCD may be particularly useful in postoperative surveillance because most strokes occur after, rather than during, CEA. In addition to microembolic showers, TCD can also identify patients with acute postoperative thrombosis or those at risk for cerebral hyperperfusion syndrome.[127] TCD has the benefit of being quick, easy to apply, is more easily interpretable without expertise (as compared to EEG or evoked potentials), and allows for serial evaluation. Disadvantages to TCD include operator dependence and technical limitation. In approximately 10% to 20% of patients, adequate temporal windows (a prerequisite for accurate monitoring) cannot be obtained.

Carotid stump pressure estimates ipsilateral hemispheric blood flow by directly measuring the pressure in the carotid stump distal to the clamp. Purported advantages of this technique are that it is a direct gauge of collateral cerebral perfusion, quick to obtain, cost effective, and does not require sophisticated equipment or expert interpretation. Stump pressures greater than 40 to 50 mmHg are generally considered adequate to avoid temporary shunt placement, although a critical value for stump pressure is not known.[121] Some patients may have adequate perfusion below values of 40 to 50 mmHg, whereas others may not have sufficient collateral flow despite maintaining stump pressure above this range. A retrospective series of more than 400 patients performed under regional anesthesia found that a stump pressure cutoff of 40 mmHg was as reliable as EEG monitoring in predicting cerebral ischemia on cross-clamp application during CEA.[128] The generalizability to patients undergoing CEA under general anesthesia is unclear.

NIRS uses the relative absorption of specific wavelengths of light by oxyhemoglobin and deoxyhemoglobin to estimate frontal lobe cerebral perfusion (rSO_2) and estimate cerebral oxygen balance. A decrease in rSO_2, theoretically, reflects a decrease in cerebral blood flow below a critical level. NIRS is easily portable, inexpensive, and simple to interpret without special training.[121] Limitations include potential inaccuracy over areas of previous infarction, as well as in the fact that NIRS is a global assessment of cerebral oxygenation only in the frontal grey matter. Thus, ischemia in other areas of the brain may be missed. Data on the sensitivity and specificity of NIRS for predicting cerebral ischemia during CEA are conflicting. One study performed under regional anesthesia demonstrated that a drop in rSO_2 more than 19% following carotid cross-clamping has sensitivity of 100% and a specificity of 98% (yielding PPV of 82% and NPV of 100%) for predicting need for temporary shunt placement,[129] whereas another using the same device and ischemic threshold demonstrated a sensitivity of 60% and a specificity of 25%.[130] Whether these results are applicable to CEA performed under general anesthesia is unclear.

Anesthetic Considerations for Carotid Endarterectomy

In general, premedication with sedatives is avoided to facilitate rapid emergence and immediate assessment of a neurologic examination. If deemed necessary, the smallest effective dose of midazolam should be titrated to effect. Once in the operating room, standard monitors should be applied. Invasive blood pressure monitoring is recommended due to the potential for hemodynamic lability as a result of surgical or anesthetic manipulation. Care should be taken to maintain hemodynamics within 20% of the patient's baseline range due to potential shifts in cerebral autoregulation. Rarely is invasive central monitoring with a central venous or pulmonary artery catheter necessary, unless dictated by specific patient risk factors. At least one medium- to large-bore intravenous access should be obtained, although the risk of major blood loss or fluid shifting in this procedure is low.

CEA can be performed under either general or regional anesthesia. A regional anesthetic allows for continuous monitoring of a patient's neurologic status, which is the ultimate monitor for cerebral ischemia. An abrupt change in mental status will alert the operative team sooner and more definitely than indirect neuromonitoring methods and will also avoid morbidity associated with unnecessary interventions. Regional anesthesia avoids hemodynamically labile periods such as induction and emergence of general anesthesia as well as the need to administer negative inotropic anesthetic agents to patients with underlying cardiovascular disease. Superficial cervical plexus blockade has been found to be as efficacious as deep or combined block while avoiding the known complications of a deep cervical plexus block.[131] Complications associated with deep cervical plexus block include accidental subarachnoid injection with resultant brainstem anesthesia; intravascular injection with potential seizure; or accidental blockade of the phrenic, vagus, or recurrent laryngeal nerves with respiratory complications. Patient cooperation is vital as the patient will have to lie still for the duration of the operation (inability to communicate, orthopnea, and painful arthritis are relative contraindications) and patients cannot be claustrophobic as the surgical drapes will be in close proximity to the patient's face.

General anesthesia affords improved patient comfort, particularly for highly anxious patients, and may allow for more frank intraoperative communication amongst the operative team. Perhaps most compellingly, it avoids an urgent conversion to general anesthesia should complications arise such as deterioration of neurologic status or oversedation. It is not uncommon for the operating room table to be positioned with the head away from the anesthesia provider to allow the surgical team adequate room to work. Thus, emergent conversion to general anesthesia, with an ongoing operation in the neck, is not a trivial task. Overall conversion rates to general anesthesia are generally less than 5%[132]; nevertheless, the ability to rapidly convert to general anesthesia in case of surgical or anesthetic misadventure must be ensured.

Whether one anesthetic technique is superior to the other has been the subject of extensive debate. The most well-known study in this patient population is the General Anesthesia versus Local Anesthesia for carotid surgery (GALA) trial,[132] an international, multicenter, randomized controlled trial of more than 3,500 patients. There was no difference in the primary end point of proportion of patients with stroke, MI, or death between randomization and 30 days after surgery between the two groups. A recent meta-analysis of 14 randomized trials involving more than 4,500 operations (the largest trial included being the GALA trial) similarly demonstrated no difference in death, stroke, or MI rates between the general and local anesthesia groups (Fig. 40-10).[133] There were also no difference in major morbidity, postoperative cardiovascular or pulmonary complications, hospital length of stay, or patient satisfaction between the two groups. Currently available literature does not suggest a benefit of one anesthetic approach over another. Rather, a mutually agreeable decision should be made between the surgeon and anesthesiologist, bearing in mind patient preference and potential limitations. Regardless of technique chosen, the anesthetic goals are the same: mitigate perioperative cerebral insult, ensure hemodynamic stability, and allow for a smooth and rapid emergence for anesthesia to allow for early neurologic assessment.

General anesthesia for CEA is typically performed with an endotracheal tube (ETT), although the use of laryngeal mask airway (LMA) has been described. ETT offers a more secure airway, potential better control of gas exchange, and may distort the anatomy of the neck less than an LMA. LMA may cause less hemodynamic lability during periods of induction and emergence since direct laryngoscopy is avoided. General anesthesia is maintained at a "light" level that ensures amnesia but minimally interferes with neurophysiologic monitoring. Typically, a balanced technique is employed and a variety of agents have been successfully employed. General anesthesia is typically induced with a short-acting hypnotic agent, titrated to effect. Both etomidate and propofol decrease cerebral metabolic rate and thus cerebral oxygen requirements. Etomidate may preserve cardiovascular stability and thus be beneficial for patients in whom cardiac reserve is limited. The addition of a short-acting opioid such as fentanyl or remifentanil is frequently employed to blunt the hemodynamic stimulation of intubation. The trachea may be sprayed with atomized lidocaine prior to intubation in an attempt to minimize stimulation by the ETT during surgery and to prevent coughing upon emergence. Small amounts of short-acting opioid can be titrated intraoperatively as needed; however, large doses or long-acting opioids are typically avoided so as to not confound the neurologic examination at the end of surgery. The combined use of a cervical plexus block and/or surgeon-administered local anesthetic can significantly reduce or eliminate the need for perioperative opioids. Muscle relaxation is not mandated for this surgery, but often allows for the "lighter" plane of anesthesia and reduces muscular interference with the EEG.

General anesthesia can be maintained with either volatile or intravenous agents. No evidence has reliably demonstrated a benefit for one technique over another.[134,135] All of the commonly used volatile agents decrease cerebral metabolic rate and oxygen requirements to a comparable degree.[136] No differences in intraoperative hemodynamics have been described between inhalational and intravenous anesthetic techniques. Patients undergoing a propofol-based anesthetic have been noted to have fewer intraoperative regional wall motion abnormalities suggestive of ischemia than those undergoing isoflurane-based anesthetics; however, no postoperative differences in troponin levels, EKG changes, or clinical outcomes were noted in study.[135] The transient intraoperative regional wall motion abnormalities were attributed to isoflurane-induced ventricular loading changes as a result of arterial and venous dilation and unrelated to myocardial oxygen balance. Intravenous anesthesia with propofol and remifentanil may be associated with less hemodynamic lability upon emergence of anesthesia,[134] at the expense of longer recovery room stays and medical intervention for hypertension.[135] The authors attribute this difference not to the ultrashort duration of action of analgesia, but rather the more rapid awakening from propofol/remifentanil than isoflurane/fentanyl-based regimens. This assertion is supported by comparable pain scores and analgesic requirements. The more rapid recovery from intravenous-based anesthetic techniques and ability to obtain a postoperative neurologic examination makes intravenous-based anesthetics attractive to many providers. Intravenous regimens had the added benefit of lower rates of postoperative nausea and vomiting, which prevents retching on a fresh neck incision and may decrease the risk of postoperative hematoma, a feared complication. Intravenous techniques, at approximately nine times the cost of inhalational based anesthetics, were less cost effective in comparison. Regardless of whether an inhalation or intravenous based technique is chosen, short-acting agents are preferable to allow for rapid awakening. Desflurane or sevoflurane may be preferable to isoflurane due to their rapid offset and salutary effects, on cognitive recovery and cerebral ischemia.[136]

Normocapnia should be maintained during CEA. Hyperventilation may lead to cerebral vasoconstriction and decrease cerebral blood flow during critical periods of carotid cross-clamping. Hypercapnia may be equally detrimental if it leads to dilation of the cerebral vasculature in normal areas of the brain, whereas vessels in ischemic areas are already maximally dilated and are unable to further respond. The net effect is a "steal" phenomenon with diversion of blood flow from hypoperfused to normal areas of the brain. Hypothermia can depress cerebral activity and

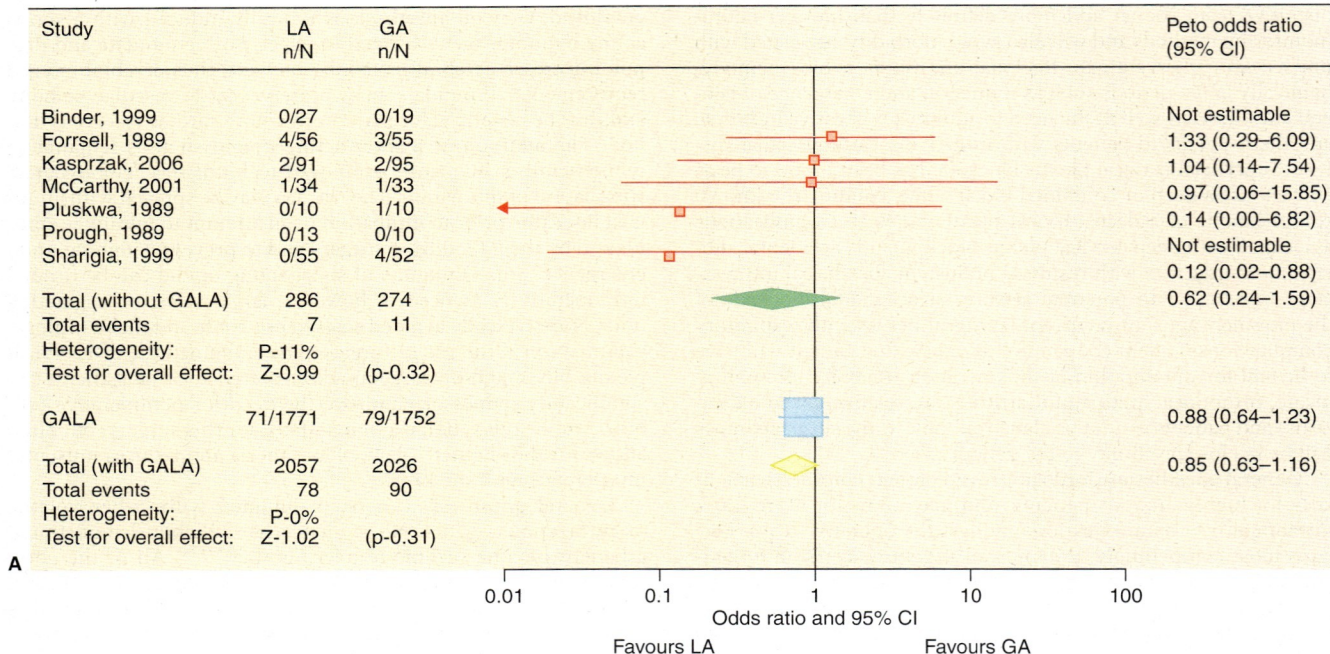

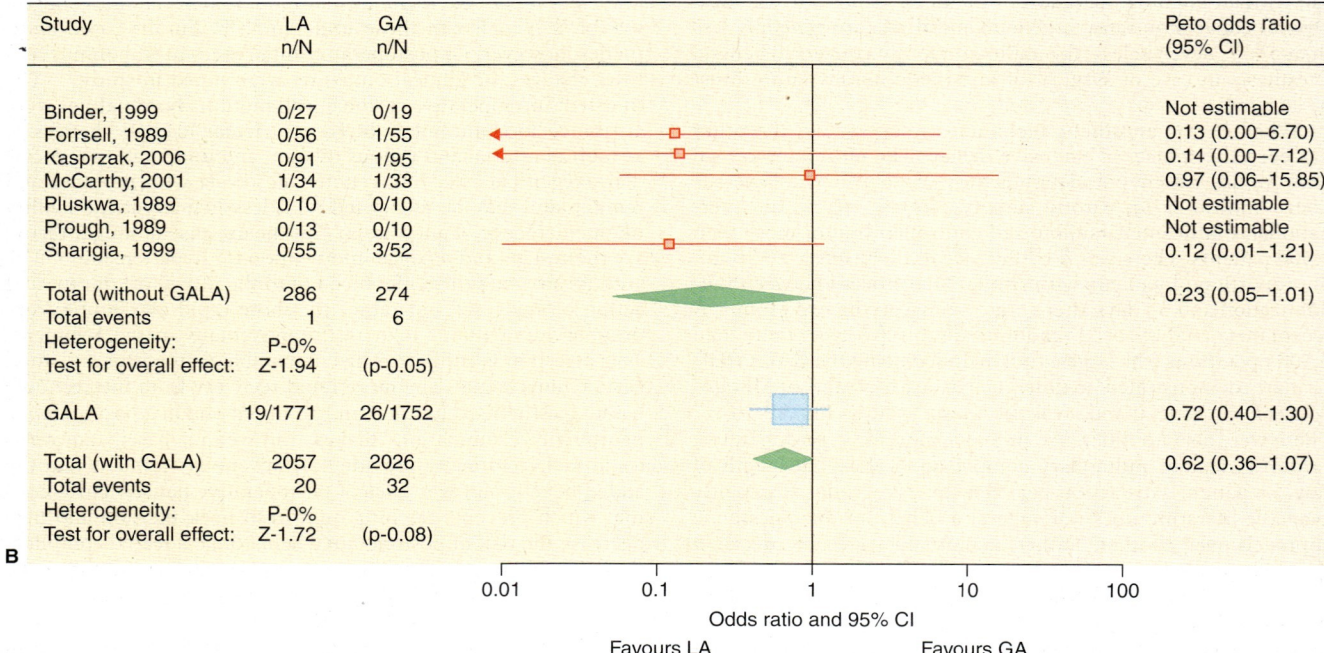

Figure 40-10 Odds ratio for outcome of (**A**) stroke or death, or (**B**) death for carotid endarterectomy performed under general versus local anesthesia. Plots show odds ratios and 95% confidence interval for the specified outcomes. No difference in any of the primary outcomes was noted in either the GALA trial or a meta-analysis of the literature. GA, general anesthesia; LA, local anesthesia. (Reprinted with permission from Lewis SC, Warlow CP, Bodenham AR, et al. General anaesthesia versus local anaesthesia for carotid surgery [GALA]: a multicentre, randomised controlled trial. Lancet. 2008;372:2132–2142.)

decrease cellular oxygen requirements below the minimum levels normally required to maintain cellular viability. In theory, hypothermia represents the most effective method of cerebral protection; even a mild decrease in temperature may reduce ischemic damage to the brain. However, even mild hypothermia can induce shivering that significantly increases myocardial oxygen consumption and work.[137] Currently, the literature provides no definitive evidence to support the hypothesis that hypothermia protects that brain sufficiently to justify the myocardial risks imposed by hypothermia and shivering.

Patients are nearly always extubated at the end of the surgical procedure. A deep extubation may be considered in those patients who were easy to ventilate, intubate, and are at minimal risk for aspiration. The rationale for deep extubation is to mitigate the hemodynamic lability that may accompany emergence and to prevent coughing or straining against an ETT with a fresh vascular anastomosis in the neck. Tight blood pressure control must continue through extubation and into the postoperative period. Whether performed before or after extubation, neurologic integrity must be confirmed prior to leaving the operating room. New neurologic deficits may lead to noninvasive imaging, cerebral angiography, or surgical re-exploration. It is rare to require postoperative intensive care unit (ICU) monitoring, and this is typically limited to particularly high-risk patients. In one study, postoperative ICU surveillance was necessary only for patients with four or more of the following risk factors: stroke, CHF, chronic kidney failure, hypertension, dysrhythmia, and MI.[138]

Postoperative Considerations

The paradox of carotid surgery is that, though the goal is to reduce the long-term patient risk of stroke, the patient is put at small but real risk of perioperative stroke. The incidence of postoperative stroke following CEA has been estimated to be approximately 6%.[101,102] Three interventions in the modern era, however, have decreased the incidence of perioperative stroke to approximately 1%: improved perioperative medication management (namely, DAPT), perioperative neurophysiologic monitoring (primarily intraoperative TCD and completion angiography), and perioperative hemodynamic control (preventing cerebral hyperperfusion and hemorrhage).[139] Cerebral hyperperfusion syndrome (CHS) is a rare but devastating complication of CEA, reported in 0% to 3% of cases.[140] CHS occurs as a consequence of impaired cerebral autoregulation following relief of high grade stenosis, which may result in ipsilateral cerebral edema, headache, seizures, focal neurologic deficit, or intracerebral hemorrhage. Management of CHS consists of pharmacologic control of hypertension and limitation of rises in cerebral perfusion. Early recognition and treatment is paramount, and complete recovery is possible.

Hemodynamic lability is common in the perioperative period; hypertension is more common than hypotension. Both acute tachycardia and hypertension may precipitate acute myocardial ischemia and failure, and hypertension is associated with CHS as discussed earlier. Post-CEA hypertension is significantly associated with adverse events such as stroke, death, and a trend toward cardiac complications, whereas postoperative hypotension and bradycardia do not appear to correlate with adverse primary or secondary outcomes. A large review of more than 60,000 patients suggests the risk of perioperative MI is below 1%.[141] Despite the low incidence, MI remains a leading cause of death following CEA. Appropriate perioperative medication management as discussed earlier is critical to decrease the risk of MACE. Uncontrolled pain may contribute to hemodynamic lability, although it is important to balance pain control with the need to follow neurologic status. Total perioperative fluid should be limited in this case due to relatively small intraoperative losses (either blood or evaporative). a short surgical time with limited exposure, and frequent diastolic dysfunction. Fluid overload is relatively common cause of demand ischemia, congestion, and respiratory or cardiovascular morbidity following CEA. Other common causes of hypertension should also be ruled out such as full bladder, hypoxemia, or hypercarbia. Once secondary causes of hypertension are ruled out, pharmacologic treatment should be initiated with goal hemodynamics typically within 20% of the patient's baseline values. In some centers, a postoperative ECG is to be obtained in the recovery room to evaluate for new ischemia.

Postoperative respiratory insufficiency following CEA may result from underlying pulmonary pathophysiology, recurrent laryngeal nerve or hypoglossal nerve injury, neck hematoma, or altered carotid body chemoreceptor response to hypercapnia or hypoxia. Surgical manipulation may damage the nerve supply to the carotid body, resulting in impaired chemo- and baroreceptor responses. Although unilateral loss of carotid body chemoreceptor function is unlikely to be significant, a bilateral loss may prevent the patient from appropriately increasing ventilation in response to hypercapnia or hypoxemia. This may be particularly important for a patient undergoing CEA who has had previous contralateral surgery. Supplemental oxygen should be utilized in the postoperative period. Similarly, drugs that depress respiratory drive (e.g., narcotics) should be limited and avoided whenever possible. Cranial nerve injury is usually temporary.

Wound hematomas develop in up to 2% of patients following CEA. Small hematomas which are likely caused by venous oozing may be managed conservatively with reversal of residual heparin or with compression. A rapidly expanding hematoma is a clinical emergency and must be evaluated immediately due to the risk of tracheal compression and impending loss of airway. Impaired lymphatic drainage can produce sudden and severe pharyngolaryngeal edema; it is prudent to have difficult airway equipment (including videolaryngoscopy, small ETT, and surgical airway equipment) available prior to reinstrumentation of the airway. A high index of suspicion for arterial bleeding may preclude the ability to open and evacuate the hematoma at bedside. Management of a rapid enlarging or symptomatic hematoma is best undertaken in the operative room, both for airway management and surgical re-exploration.

Aortic Reconstruction

Surgical manipulation of the aorta can result in significant and potentially catastrophic effects on patient hemodynamics. The anesthetic management of aortic reconstruction is perhaps the most technically challenging for the vascular anesthesiologist. Aortic surgery typically comes in two flavors: reconstruction for aneurysmal disease or reconstruction for aortic dissection.

An aneurysm is defined as a greater than 50% dilation of normal expected arterial diameter; for most patients, this corresponds to an abdominal aortic diameter greater than 3.0 cm. The abdominal aorta is the most frequent location of arterial aneurysm and is approximately nine times more common than a thoracic aortic aneurysm.[142] Thoracic aortic aneurysms may involve the ascending (40%), descending (35%), or aortic arch (15%).[143] Approximately 15% involve both the thoracic and abdominal aorta. Thoracic aortic aneurysms are discussed in more detail in Chapter 39 (Anesthesia for Cardiac Surgery). AAAs are classified as infrarenal, juxtarenal, or suprarenal. Approximately 85% of AAAs are infrarenal, with a minority involving the suprarenal aorta.[144] It is vital to understand the location of the aneurysm because it will dictate the level of aortic cross-clamp applied, which has significant implications to the anesthetic management.

Though many of the risk factors are shared between the two processes, the pathophysiology of aortic aneurysm formation is distinct from atherosclerotic disease. Aortic aneurysm formation is a degenerative process involving the degradation of aortic wall connective tissue (primarily, the medial and adventitial layers), inflammation and immune responses, and biomechanical wall stress.[145] The size of the aortic aneurysm is the single most important predictor of subsequent rupture and mortality.

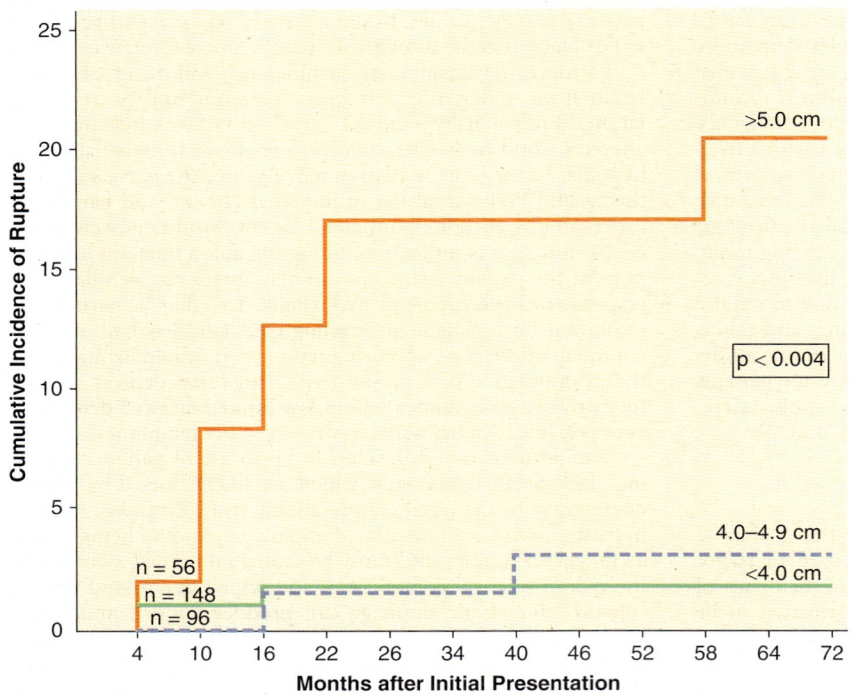

Figure 40-11 Cumulative incidence of abdominal aortic aneurysm rupture, according to aneurysm diameter at diagnosis. The incidence of rupture is significantly higher for aneurysms greater than 5.0 cm in diameter. (Reprinted with permission from Guirguis EM, Barber GG. The natural history of abdominal aortic aneurysms. *Am J Surg.* 1991;162:481–483.)

A prospective study followed 300 consecutive patients who were initially managed nonoperatively.[146] The median increase in aneurysm diameter was 0.3 cm per year. The 6-year cumulative incidence of rupture was 1% in patients among patients with aneurysms less than 4.0 cm, 2% for patients with aneurysms 4.0 to 4.9 cm, but 20% among patients with aneurysms more than 5.0 cm in diameter (Fig. 40-11). Current recommendations are for serial monitoring of known aneurysms and surgical repair when AAAs exceed 5.5 cm or descending thoracic aortic aneurysms exceed 6.5 cm.[147,148] Other risk factors for rupture include rapid growth, symptomatology (e.g., abdominal or back pain), aneurysm shape (saccular vs. fusiform), sex, family history, and degree of control of other comorbidities. Aneurysm rupture is nearly always lethal with mortality rates of 85% to 90%.[149] Thus, close follow-up for known aneurysms is essential, particularly as they enlarge.

Acute aortic dissection is a life-threatening medical catastrophe that is associated with very high rates of morbidity and mortality. More than 20% of patients with aortic dissection die before hospital admission.[150] The hallmark lesion of aortic dissection is a tear in the intimal layer of the arterial wall that creates a false lumen, which is then propagated by pulsatile blood flow. Aortic dissections are classified anatomically and temporally. Acute dissections are those in which clinical symptomatology has lasted fewer than 14 days. Dissections with symptoms exceeding 2 weeks' duration are deemed chronic. Approximately half of aortic dissections originate from the ascending aorta; ascending aortic aneurysms are a surgical emergency. Death from an ascending aortic aneurysm is usually due to acute aortic regurgitation, pericardial tamponade, or myocardial ischemia secondary to coronary ostial compromise. The next most common site of origin is just distal to the left subclavian artery, in the vicinity of the ligamentum arteriosum. Isolated abdominal aortic dissections are rare, with a reported incidence of 1.3%.[151] Death from acute descending aortic dissection is typically secondary to end-organ compromise due to malperfusion of the visceral vessels.

Uncomplicated descending aneurysms may be managed medically, whereas complicated (i.e., visceral or limb compromise) require surgical intervention.

Pathophysiology of Aortic Occlusion and Reperfusion

The pathophysiologic response to aortic cross-clamping depends on the level of the occlusion, the overall volume status of the patient, and overall cardiac function (Fig. 40-12).[152] Aortic cross-clamping has little to no effect on heart rate. The most dramatic and consistent effect of aortic cross-clamping is an increase in systemic vascular resistance and mean arterial pressure as a result of the sudden impedance to aortic flow. The extent to which afterload increases depends upon the level the cross-clamp applied. Infrarenal cross-clamping may increase arterial blood pressure 2% to 10%, where as a supraceliac clamp has a significantly greater effect and may increase the mean arterial pressure up to 50% (Table 40-2).

A complex interaction between splanchnic venous tone, blood volume redistribution, coronary blood flow, and myocardial contractility may result in an increase or decrease in cardiac preload, central filling pressures, and cardiac output (Fig. 40-13). Placement of the aortic cross-clamp results in blood volume redistribution proximal to the clamp placement. Infraceliac cross-clamping is relatively well tolerated compared with supraceliac cross-clamping. With lower clamping, blood volume can shift into the compliant splanchnic vasculature, thus limiting preload changes. With the placement of a supraceliac cross-clamp, the splanchnic circulation is unable to absorb this shift in blood volume. Instead, the decrease in splanchnic arterial flow is associated with a decrease in venous capacitance as a result of elastic recoil. The net result is an increase in venous return, central filling pressures, and cardiac output. The increase in preload and afterload increases myocardial work, which in turn leads to coronary vasodilation to maximize coronary blood flow and

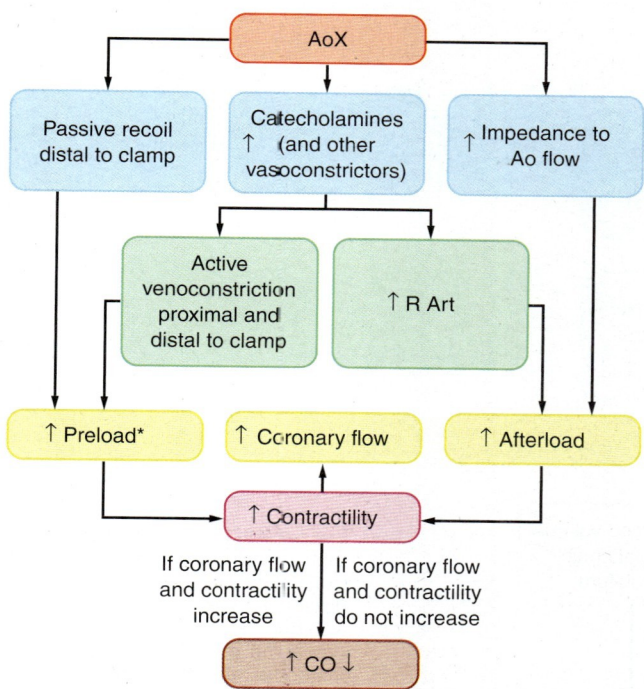

Figure 40-12 Systemic hemodynamic response to aortic cross-clamping (AoX). Preload does not necessarily increase. The most dramatic and consistent effect of aortic cross-clamping is an increase in systemic vascular resistance and mean arterial pressure as a result of the sudden impedance to aortic flow. Ao, aorta. (Adapted with permission from Gelman S. The pathophysiology of aortic cross-clamping and unclamping. *Anesthesiology.* 1995;82:1026–1060.)

placement. Despite a decrease in ejection fraction, cardiac output and stroke volume increased by expanding the cavity size of the left ventricle.

Anticipation of aortic cross-clamp placement should prompt hemodynamic manipulation. A pragmatic approach is to initially use esmolol to decrease heart rate to a target of around 60 to 65 beats per minute. This decreases the risk of myocardial oxygen imbalance. Direct vasodilators are then employed to control arterial pressure. This can be accomplished via bolus (+/− continuous infusion) of intravenous vasodilating agents (e.g., sodium nitroprusside, nitroglycerin, or nicardipine), local anesthetic administration via thoracic epidural, or deepening of anesthetic depth. The goal is to offset the increase in afterload and myocardial work with systemic vasodilation. It is important to recognize that attempts to normalize systemic vascular resistance above the level of the clamp can even further compromise blood flow distal to the clamp. The administration of sodium nitroprusside has been shown to decrease aortic pressure distal to the level of cross-clamp placement; this decrease was unresponsive to increases in preload via volume challenge or cardiac output.[154] It is critical to maintain a perfusion pressure below the level of the cross-clamp that will not potentiate visceral or spinal cord ischemia.

There are two distinct aortic unclamping events. Even if the initial aortic clamp was supraceliac, the anastomosis is most commonly infrarenal. Once the proximal anastomosis is made, the clamp is moved from native aorta to graft in order to allow reperfusion of the celiac and renal beds. This is usually hemodynamically insignificant due to the relatively short duration of ischemia and rapid reapplication of the cross-clamp distal to the visceral vessels until the distal anastomosis (or, in the case of bifurcated graft, anastomoses) are complete. The subsequent release of the distal clamp(s) results in the release of inflammatory mediators, decreased cardiac output, hypoxemia-mediated vasodilation, and a reactive hyperemia that ultimately culminates in profound vasodilation and arterial hypotension (Fig. 40-14). Systemic vascular resistance may decrease up to 80%, with similarly profound decrease in LV pressure. A relative central hypovolemia develops as blood pools in tissue distal to the cross-clamp. Various therapies have been employed to counteract this response, with no evidence to suggest superiority of one method over another. Most anesthesiologists employ some degree of volume loading during the period of cross-clamp application. Vasoconstrictors such as phenylephrine or norepinephrine, or inotropic agents such as epinephrine or calcium chloride are frequently employed in conjunction with volume loading. It may also be prudent to decrease anesthetic depth and/or discontinue

oxygen delivery. Patients with limited cardiac reserve, such as those with a decreased ejection fraction or significant CAD (in whom the coronary vasculature is already maximally dilated), may not tolerate this increase in myocardial work. In such cases, myocardial ischemia or failure may develop. New LV wall abnormalities have been demonstrated in up to one-third of patients with a suprarenal aortic cross-clamp placement, and more than 90% of patients with a supraceliac aortic cross-clamp.[153] Patients with an infrarenal cross-clamp, by comparison, did not have evidence of regional wall motion abnormalities during cross-clamp

Table 40-2 Effect of Level of Aortic Occlusion on Changes in Cardiovascular Variables[a]

Cardiovascular Variable	% Change in Variable, by Level of Aortic Occlusion		
	Supraceliac	Suprarenal	Infrarenal
Mean arterial blood pressure	54	5	2
Pulmonary capillary wedge pressure	38	10	0
End diastolic area	28	2	9
End systolic area	69	10	11
Ejection fraction	−38	−10	−3
Abnormal motion of wall, % of patients	92	33	0
New myocardial infarction, % of patients	8	0	0

[a]The degree of hemodynamic derangements with aortic cross clamping is dictated in large part by the level of aortic occlusion.
Adapted with permission from Roizen MF, Ellis JE, Foss JF, et al. Intraoperative management of the patient requiring supraceliac aortic occlusion. In: Veith FJ, Hobson RW, Williams RA, et al. New York, NY: McGraw-Hill; 1994:256.

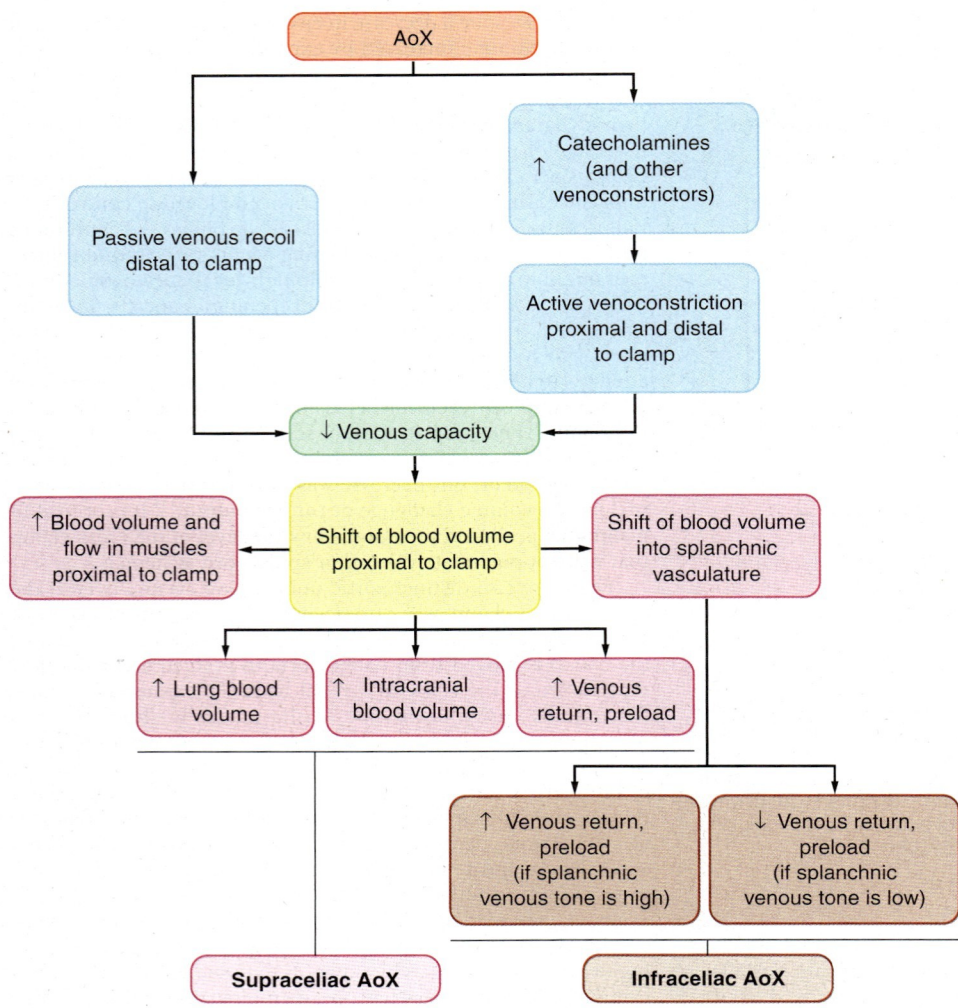

Figure 40-13 Blood volume redistribution following aortic cross-clamp (AoX) placement. Passive venous recoil distal the aortic cross-clamp results in a shift in blood volume from distal to the aortic occlusion to proximal to the occlusion. If the aorta is occluded above the level of the celiac axis, the splanchnic reserve is redistributed to the organs and tissues proximal to the clamp. If an infraceliac cross-clamp is placed, the blood volume may shift into the splanchnic system in addition to other organs proximal to the clamp. The ability to shift into or out of the splanchnic vasculature accounts for variability in preload augmentation. (Adapted with permission from Gelman S. The pathophysiology of aortic cross-clamping and unclamping. *Anesthesiology.* 1995;82:1026–1060.)

epidural infusions in anticipation of these predictable changes. Preferable to pharmacologic manipulation is a gradual release of the cross-clamp to allow for a slow, controlled release of vasoactive and cardiodepressant mediators. If bilateral iliac clamps are employed, the lower extremities can be reperfused sequentially to allow for a more controlled release and appropriate resuscitation. Clear communication with the vascular surgeon is vital to coordinate appropriate management. For example, bleeding at the anastomosis requires immediate reclamping; if vasopressors and inotropes are administered as boluses and then the clamp is reapplied, profound proximal hypertension can ensue.

Renal Hemodynamics and Renal Protection

Postoperative mortality is four- to fivefold higher in those who develop acute renal failure when compared with those who do not. Preoperative renal dysfunction is the most powerful predictor of postoperative renal dysfunction. There is no proven renal protective strategy other than minimizing the length of ischemia and avoidance of profound or prolonged hypotension.[155,156] Though the level of the cross-clamp can markedly impact renal blood flow, renal failure is a commonly encountered source of perioperative morbidity even with infrarenal cross-clamp placement. The incidence of acute renal failure is approximately 5% following infrarenal cross-clamping and approaches 13% after suprarenal cross-clamping. With suprarenal occlusion, renal blood flow decreases by up to 80%. Blood flow is not only reduced but also redistributed, favoring flow to the cortical and juxtamedullary layers over the hypoxia-prone renal medulla.[157] Even with an infrarenal occlusion, renal blood flow is decreased by nearly 50% compared to baseline, whereas renal vascular resistance increases by almost 70%. These alterations are predominantly a result of neurohumoral activation rather due to changes in hemodynamics or cardiac output. Physiologic fluctuations do not immediately revert after the release of cross-clamping and may persist for at least 30 minutes beyond systemic cardiovascular return to baseline. Thus, tincture of time may be the best management of decreased urine output in the immediate post–cross-clamping period.

Many different pharmacologic methods of renal protection have been advocated, most centering on improving renal blood flow or glomerular flow. Mannitol increases diuresis and functions as a free radical scavenger. No clinical trials to date have demonstrated any reduction in the incidence of postoperative renal failure in patients undergoing repair of an AAA who have been given mannitol.[158] Diuretics, and particularly loop diuretics, are often considered in the case of low urine output, despite the fact that no significant correlation has been demonstrated

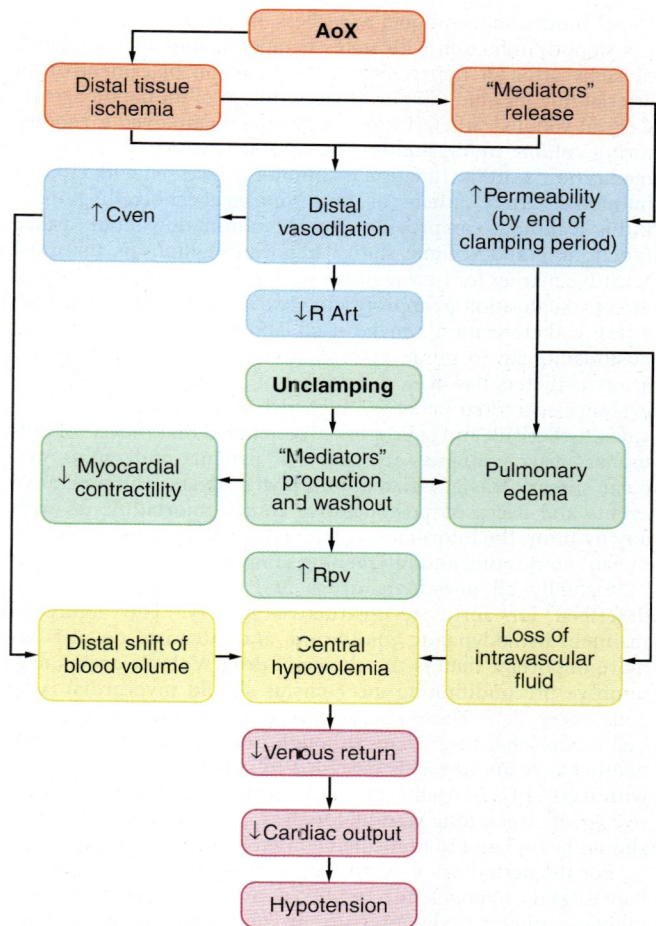

Figure 40-14 Hemodynamic response to aortic cross-clamp (AoX) release. A complex cascade of events, including release of inflammatory mediators, distal vasodilation, increased vascular permeability, and decreased myocardial contractility results in a relative central hypovolemia, decreased cardiac output, and systemic hypotension. (Adapted with permission from Gelman S. The pathophysiology of aortic cross-clamping and unclamping. *Anesthesiology*. 1995;82:1026–1060.)

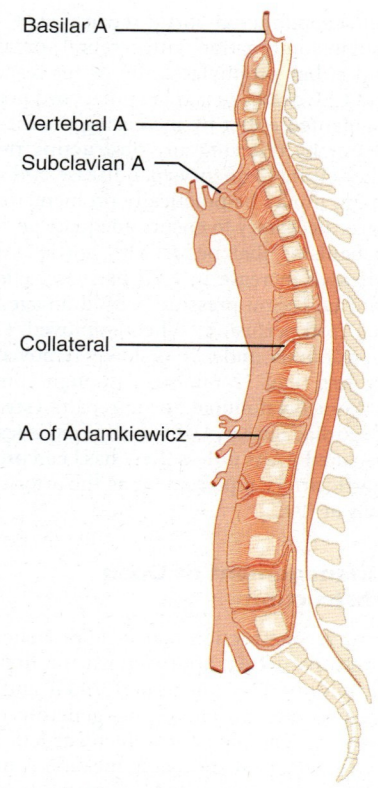

Figure 40-15 Vascular supply to the spinal cord. The singular anterior spinal artery and paired posterior spinal arteries arise from the posterior circulation and provide blood supply to the spinal cord. Radicular arteries arising from the aorta supplement this blood supply. The artery of Adamkiewicz is the most clinically significant contributor. Variability in collateral flow helps to explain, in part, the unpredictability of paraplegia following aortic surgery. (Adapted from Piccone W, DeLaria GA, Najafi H. Descending thoracic aneurysms. In: Bergan JJ, Yao JST, eds. *Aortic Surgery*. Philadelphia, PA: WB Saunders; 1989:249.)

between intraoperative mean urinary output or lowest hourly urinary output and the development of acute renal insufficiency.[159] The use of diuretic medications for the sole purpose of increasing urine output only converts an oliguric to polyuric renal failure. In the interim, significant fluid shifting may result in depletion of intravascular volume, adding further renal insult. Diuretics should be reserved only for patients who are demonstrably volume overloaded and then used judiciously to effect. Dopamine does not appear to improve postoperative renal dysfunction. Fenoldopam, a selective dopamine agonist, has shown promise in some clinical trials but results have been conflicting in cardiovascular surgery.[156,160,161] Ali and colleagues[162] investigated the role of ischemic preconditioning on renal and myocardial injury with aortic cross-clamping and found a beneficial effect on both. In this study, ischemic preconditioning was found to decrease the incidence of postoperative renal insufficiency by 23%.

Spinal Cord Ischemia and Protection

The spinal cord is supplied primarily by the single anterior and paired posterior spinal arteries, arising from the posterior circulation (Fig. 40-15). The posterior spinal arteries supply approximately 25% of spinal cord blood flow and supply the sensory tracts of the posterior columns. The anterior spinal artery supplies the anterolateral cord, including motor tracts, and supplies 75% of the spinal cord blood flow. The anterior spinal artery is fed by a series of radicular arteries arising from the aorta, although collateralization is variable. This leaves areas of the spinal cord vulnerable to watershed ischemia, particularly with aortic occlusion or prolonged hypotension. The single most important radicular artery supplying the thoracolumbar cord is derived from the artery of Adamkiewicz. The artery of Adamkiewicz originates between T8 and T12 in 75% of cases and at the level of L1 or L2 in an additional 10% of cases.

Spinal cord ischemia is a feared complication of aortic reconstruction and occurs in up to 10% of patients involving a distal aortic repair. Pertinent risks for spinal cord ischemia include previous aortic surgery (particularly with vascular exclusion of major thoracic radicular collaterals), open surgical repair, aortic cross-clamp location and duration, length of aortic replacement, and intraoperative hypotension/hypoperfusion. The definitive measures to prevent spinal cord ischemia are a short cross-clamp time, maintenance of normal cardiac function, and higher perfusion pressures. Segmental sequential surgical repair may minimize the duration of ischemia to any given vascular bed. A markedly reduced incidence of neurologic deficits has been reported in thoracoabdominal aortic repairs when distal aortic perfusion is used in combination with cerebral spinal fluid (CSF) drainage, placed either prophylactically or for rescue.[166,164] The rationale behind CSF drainage is that spinal cord perfusion pressure can be augmented either by increasing the forward driving pressure (MAP) or by relieving any obstructing pressure (CSF pressure). In the setting of aneurysmal disease and major vascular reconstruction, it may be practically problematic to augment MAP to the degree necessary to ensure adequate perfusion. Autoregulatory mechanisms that occur with aortic cross-clamping results in a reflexive increase in CSF pressure, effectively lowering spinal cord perfusion pressure. CSF drainage, then, favors improved spinal cord perfusion. When employed, CSF monitoring is usually continuous, and CSF is slowly removed to maintain a CSF pressure less than 12 mmHg. Although commonly used in thoracic or thoracoabdominal aortic repairs (see Chapter 39, Anesthesia for Cardiac Surgery), this technique is less commonly employed for isolated AAAs unless there has been previous extensive thoracic aortic artery replacement as the artery of Adamkiewicz is less likely at risk.

Anesthetic Management of Open Aortic Reconstruction

Abdominal aortic reconstruction may be approached via a transabdominal or retroperitoneal approach. In the first case, a thoracoabdominal midline incision is performed and the aorta is accessed via the peritoneum. This allows generous exposure and is usually favored for complex aortic reconstruction or replacement. In the retroperitoneal approach, incision is made over the lateral order of the left rectus muscle, from the level of the 12th rib to several centimeters below the umbilicus. This approach allows access to the aorta from the crux of the diaphragm to its bifurcation. Benefits of the retroperitoneal approach include comparable surgical exposure with decreased fluid shifting, fewer postoperative pulmonary complications, faster return of bowel function, shorter ICU stays, and decreased hospital costs with average savings of $4,000 to $5,000.[165] This technique may be favored in cases of significant truncal obesity, chronic obstructive pulmonary disease, intra-abdominal adhesions, and juxtarenal aneurysms. Regardless of the surgical technique employed, OAR requires a large vertical incision. Barring contraindication to neuraxial instrumentation, an epidural catheter should be considered. A functional epidural may be used intraoperatively to manage the hemodynamic lability of aortic cross-clamping, decrease postoperative sympathetic stimulation, aid in postoperative pain control, and potentially aid in weaning from mechanical ventilation. Although most ischemic complications are the result of dislodgment of atheromatous material off the disease aorta and not de novo clot formation, most surgeons administer intravenous heparin to reduce the risk of thromboembolic events before aortic cross-clamping. If neuraxial instrumentation is attempted, heparin dosing should be delayed per current guidelines.[166] In the case of traumatic placement or intravascular catheter, a frank consideration of the risks and benefits of proceed to surgery versus delaying the case must be undertaken by the operative team due to the small but catastrophic risk of epidural hematoma.

General anesthesia is typically employed for open repair of AAA. Induction of general anesthesia and intubation can be associated with dramatic hemodynamic lability and sympathetic stimulation, which may put the aneurysm at risk of rupture. It is prudent to ensure adequate blood product availability in the operating room and large-bore peripheral intravenous access prior to the induction of general anesthesia. There is no single "best" induction technique; regardless of agents chosen, the goal is a smooth induction with stable hemodynamics and avoidance of tachycardia or hypertension. Preinduction placement of an arterial line may aid in appropriate titration of induction agents. Central venous catheterization is generally employed for monitoring volume trends and for the reliable delivery of vasoactive medication. Cardiac function is commonly assessed with either a pulmonary artery catheter or transesophageal echocardiography. Either technique can provide valuable information about cardiac functioning and volume status. Echocardiography is the most sensitive marker for new regional wall motion abnormalities and direct visualization of appropriate ventricular filling. Pulmonary artery catheterization can be useful both intraoperatively and postoperatively to guide resuscitation. The use of pulmonary artery catheters has been the subject of debate, with conflicting evidence as to their benefit in high-risk surgical patients.[167,168] A study by Berlauk and colleagues[169] concluded that the use of pulmonary artery catheters to "tune up" patients undergoing vascular surgery was associated with fewer adverse intraoperative events and deceased postoperative cardiac morbidity. As with any monitor, the information obtained is only as good as the clinician interpreting and intervening upon the data.

Virtually all anesthetic drugs and techniques have been described for aortic reconstructive surgery. The ability to maintain hemodynamic equilibrium and attend to detail is far more important than is the choice of drug. Volatile agents may improve preconditioning mechanisms should myocardial ischemia occur.[162,170] These effects have been demonstrated in animal models and in cardiac, although not vascular surgery. The maintenance anesthetic is designed to maintain hemodynamics within 20% of the baseline range. An array of short-acting vasoactive agents (including vasodilators, vasopressors, and inotropes) should be on hand to immediately treat hemodynamic lability.

For the period prior to cross-clamp placement, the patient is kept slightly hypovolemic (typically, as assessed by CVP, pulmonary catheter wedge pressure or echocardiography) to limit hypertensive extremes with aortic occlusion. At the time of cross-clamp placement, vasodilating infusions may be required. Alternatively, deepening the anesthetic or injection of the epidural catheter with local anesthetic will increase vasodilation, although both of these approaches require careful attention to avoid unintended hypotension. When there is concern about spinal cord perfusion, it may be prudent to allow permissive hypertension, to the extent possible, above the level of the clamp to provide higher distal perfusion pressure and avoid distal ischemia. This choice may come at the expense of myocardial well-being.

After the vascular clamps are placed and the aneurysm sac is incised, blood loss is swift from any vessels arising from the aorta between the two clamps. Adequate peripheral and central venous access is imperative. Blood loss can be considerable without the onset of hypotension or tachycardia because a significant portion of the vascular tree is excluded from circulation during aortic occlusion. An autotransfusion device should be employed to reduce the amount of autologous blood needed. It is prudent to volume load during the period of aortic cross-clamping in anticipation for the vasoplegic washout and reactive hyperemia that will occur with the removal of aortic cross-clamp. It is the practice of the authors to resuscitate with a combination of crystalloid, colloid, and blood products as the clinical scenario dictates to a CVP or pulmonary capillary wedge pressure 2 to 3 mmHg higher than the initial wedge pressure, or according to echocardiographic estimates of volume. This augmentation of central volume will then fill the increased capacitance distal to the aortic clamp when it is subsequently released.

Immediately prior to the removal of the aortic clamp, vasodilating agents are discontinued. The surgeon opens the aortic clamp gradually to ensure that severe hypotension or bleeding does not develop. Ongoing fluid resuscitation and vasopressor and inotropic support is frequently necessary. Severe refractory hypotension can be temporarily abated with reapplication of the aortic cross-clamp until appropriate measures can be instituted. Over the course of the reconstruction, there may be frequent instances of cross-clamp application and release to limit the ischemic time to vital organs and to "test" the anastomoses. It is imperative for the anesthesiologist to be flexible and adaptable, and to have a variety of short-acting vasoactive agents available for hemodynamic manipulation. Each time the cross-clamp is removed, a "washout" of vasoactive agents occurs with the potential for hemodynamic instability. Central and pulmonary filling pressures may be elevated despite systemic hypotension because of the washout of lactic acid and other inflammatory mediators, which results in pulmonary vasoconstriction and cardiac stunning.

At the end of the procedure, the decision regarding emergence and extubation must take into account any ongoing hemodynamic instability, metabolic derangements, and ongoing need for resuscitation. β-Blocking agents are continued in the perioperative period, as tolerated. Reinstitution of the epidural catheter allows for adequate pain control and may help with weaning from mechanical ventilation, particularly in those with concomitant chronic obstructive pulmonary disease. For those patients who remain intubated, the use of the epidural catheter for pain control permits a reasonably light intravenous sedation, which allows for continued monitoring of neurologic status.

Peripheral Artery Disease

It has been estimated that up to 20% of the population is affected by PAD. Though the majority of patients are asymptomatic, PAD is a risk factor for adverse cardiovascular events, with an annual rate of 5% to 7%.[13,171] Risk factors include nonwhite race, male gender, age, smoking, diabetes, hypertension, dyslipidemia, chronic renal insufficiency, hyperviscous/hypercoagulable states, hyperhomocysteinemia, and patients with elevated inflammatory markers. There are three clinical indications for elective surgery for PAD: intermittent claudication (IC), ischemic rest pain or ulceration, or gangrene.

Most patients with PAD have either asymptomatic disease or IC, defined as reproducible discomfort in a defined muscle group that is induced by activity and relieved with rest. Approximately 10% to 35% of patients with PAD will present with symptoms of IC.[172] The clinical manifestations of IC depend on the location of the occlusion, its severity, and the presence (or absence) or collateral blood flow. Aortoiliac occlusive disease (AIOD), or "inflow" disease, tends to result in claudication in the buttock or hip. AIOD disease usually originates in the distal aorta or proximal common iliac arteries. "Outflow" disease, defined as femoropopliteal or infrapopliteal lesions, results in claudication of the thigh or leg.

IC is the first and most common symptom associated with PAD. The natural history of PAD is typically indolent with a slow, progressive decline in function. Aggressive management of risk factors with pharmacologic, exercise, and lifestyle modification prevents disease progression in the vast majority of cases.[13] Because of the relatively slow and benign progression of symptoms, the decision for surgical intervention for IC must be individualized. Decision making should consider response to therapy, loss of function, and effect on quality of life.[173] A very active person may be debilitated by relatively mild symptoms, whereas more severe symptoms may be well tolerated by a sedentary individual.

CLI occurs when the existing arterial blood flow is unable to meet even basal metabolic demands, resulting in rest pain, ulceration, and gangrene. CLI is an especially aggressive manifestation of PAD associated with more severe, multisegmental occlusion. Risk factors for accelerated disease progression include age, diabetes, smoking, and hyperlipidemia.[13] PAD progresses to CLI in approximately 1% to 2% of the population. Patients with CLI may have progressive ischemia and are at variable risk for imminent limb loss; thus, urgent surgical intervention is warranted. It is estimated that within 1 year, 25% of patients will progress to amputation, and an additional 25% will die from cardiovascular causes.[13,173] Not surprisingly, these patients also have more severe ASCVD in other vascular beds. Approximately 50% of patients with CLI will have concomitant CAD, with a higher mortality from MI or stroke amongst patients with CLI compared to less aggressive forms of PAD. These patients, then, are at elevated perioperative risk due to both medical and surgical factors related to disease severity.

AIOD may be repaired via direct reconstruction (aortoiliac or aortofemoral bypass), or with extra-anatomic reconstruction (axillary-femoral +/− femoral-femoral bypass). Direct reconstruction has better long-term patency rates (greater than 80%), at the expense of greater perioperative morbidity and mortality. Extra-anatomic bypass, although less morbid, has also proven less durable, with 5-year patency rates are reported between 55% and 80%.[171,174] As such, extra-anatomic bypass is typically reserved for patients deemed particularly high risk for direct surgical reconstruction such as previous graft or stent complication, infection, or previous intra-abdominal surgery with resultant abdominal adhesions. Open revascularization of infrainguinal disease depends on the level of the lesion(s), and may involve the femoral, popliteal, or infrapopliteal vessels.

Anesthetic Management of Lower Extremity Revascularization

The anesthetic management of AIOD depends on whether anatomic or extra-anatomic bypass is performed. Anesthetic considerations for aortofemoral bypass are similar to OAR. Barring contraindication, a preinduction epidural catheter should be considered for postoperative pain control. General anesthesia with an ETT is typically employed due to length of the case as well as the potential for hemodynamic lability. Large-bore peripheral IV access and an arterial line should be placed to help guide resuscitation and to allow instantaneous assessment of hemodynamic changes. Although aortic cross-clamping and uncross-clamping is required for aortofemoral bypass, it is typically better tolerated than for aneurysmal disease because the patient is already accustomed to high aortic resistance. Hemodynamics tend to be more stable both as a result of clamp location (typically, distal aortic) as well as the likelihood of extensive collateralization related to chronic atherosclerotic obstruction. This stands in stark contrast to aneurysmal disease, which has limited preexisting collateral flow. Central venous access is reasonable to ensure reliable delivery of necessary vasoactive medications. Additional cardiac monitoring, such as pulmonary artery catheter placement or transesophageal echocardiography, may be considered depending on patient and surgical factors.

By definition, extra-anatomic bypass does not involve aortic manipulation and thus avoids the need for aortic cross-clamping and uncross-clamping. Typically, extra-anatomic bypass is undertaken from the axillary artery to the ipsilateral femoral artery,

+/− subsequent femoral to femoral artery bypass. Typically, less hemodynamic lability is noted with axillary and femoral artery cross-clamping than with aortic cross-clamping. Thus, although large-bore peripheral IV and arterial line placement is still prudent, the need for extensive central or cardiac monitoring is less critical unless independently indicated due to medical comorbidities. Arterial line placement should be contralateral to the surgical bypass, as arterial cross-clamp placement will render an ipsilateral arterial line nonfunctional. The extra-anatomic bypass must be tunneled subcutaneously in the mid-axillary line to prevent kinking of the graft, which may be more sympathetically stimulating than cross-clamp placement. Close attention must be paid to prevent untoward hemodynamic swings or patient movement during this period.

The choice of anesthetic technique for infrainguinal revascularization is individualized for each patient. Lower extremity revascularization can be performed under general, neuraxial, or regional anesthesia. Purported benefits of regional anesthesia include avoidance of hyperdynamic responses to tracheal intubation and extubation, blunted perioperative catecholamine response, improved vascular blood flow, higher graft patency rates, and lower pulmonary complications. A recent review of the NSQIP database compared nearly 15,000 receiving neuraxial (spinal or epidural) versus general anesthesia for lower extremity revascularization.[175] In this study, neuraxial anesthesia was associated with a decreased likelihood of reintervention, decreased rates of graft failure, and decreased rates of postoperative respiratory and cardiovascular complications. In an analysis of patients in the NSQIP database with CLI, however, no differences in perioperative morbidity were noted between patients who underwent general versus neuraxial anesthesia.[176] A Cochrane review of general versus regional anesthesia for lower extremity revascularization concluded that there was insufficient evidence to rule out clinically important differences for most clinical outcomes (mortality, MI, or rate of lower-limb amputation).[177] Thus, anesthetic technique should be governed by clinical expertise, patient, and surgeon preferences.

Morbidity and mortality following lower extremity revascularization is typically cardiac in origin. Perioperative MI is reported to occur in 4% to 15% of patients undergoing peripheral vascular surgery and accounts for more than 50% of perioperative mortality.[178] A recent review of the NSQIP database suggests an overall cardiac mortality rate of 2.7% with 30-day combined mortality/major morbidity rate of nearly 20%.[179] Patients who undergo surgery for CLI as compared to IC are at increased risk, likely due to greater disease burden and more technically challenging repairs due to multilevel, extensive disease.

Endovascular Surgery

6 The advent of the endovascular era has revolutionized the field of vascular surgery. Endovascular procedures are minimally invasive and are generally associated with decreased perioperative mortality and major morbidity, shorter hospital and intensive care stays, and quicker return to baseline function, particularly for the elderly or frail. In addition to a lower level of surgical stress, endovascular techniques may obviate the need for general anesthesia. Despite overall improvements in short- and intermediate-term outcomes, long-term benefits to endovascular repairs have not been sustained. In addition, endovascular repairs have proven less durable and more prone to reintervention than traditional open repairs. In this section, we will consider the anesthetic implications for endovascular approaches to vascular disease.

Carotid Artery Stenting

Carotid artery angioplasty and stenting was first described in the late 1970s and early 1980s, but early complications related to distal plaque embolization during stent deployment limited initial enthusiasm for an endovascular approach to cerebral vascular disease. The development of embolic protection devices in the 1990s led to a renewed interest in an endovascular approach to carotid disease, especially in patients deemed high risk for open surgery. Five landmark randomized controlled trials have compared traditional open CEA to carotid artery stenting.[180–184] A recent meta-analysis of these data concluded that, for symptomatic patients, carotid artery stenting was associated with a decreased risk of perioperative MI at the expense of an increased risk of the primary composite outcome of death or any stroke as well as an increased risk of perioperative stroke.[185] There was no difference in rates of death or major disabling stroke. Recent work by Kuliha and colleagues[186] demonstrates an increase in silent ischemia in patients who undergo carotid artery stenting compared to CEA but no significant difference in postoperative cognitive function.

These findings stand in contrast to other head-to-head trials of endovascular versus open repairs (such as treatment of aortic and peripheral disease, discussed later), where short-term perioperative morbidity and mortality tend to be improved with endovascular treatment. Most of the differences in perioperative morbidity were limited to the elderly. Long-term outcomes beyond the perioperative period, including functional outcomes, are comparable between patients who undergo open versus endovascular intervention for carotid disease. Thus, a short-term increased risk of minor, nondisabling stroke must be weighed against a decreased risk of perioperative MI. At present, the contemporary literature fails to reach a consensus on the superiority of either open or endovascular technique for the treatment of carotid disease. Individual medical, surgical, and operator considerations must be weighed in the decision for open versus endovascular repair. Though CEA remains the gold standard for repair, continuous advances in endovascular techniques, and particularly in cerebral protection devices, is changing the trends in the management of carotid disease. Recent 30-day perioperative outcomes reported from the Safety and Efficacy Study for Reverse Flow Used During Carotid Artery Stenting Procedure (ROADSTER) trial, utilizing a novel transcarotid neuroprotection system, has reported the lowest perioperative stroke rates (1.4%) for endovascular techniques.[187] Current data suggests that the use of carotid artery stenting is increasing, from less than 3% of interventions in 1998 to more than 13% in 2008.[188] Carotid stenting is strongly preferred over open repair for reoperation, in patients who have had neck radiation, and very high lesions.

A major benefit of carotid artery stenting lies in the ability to continuously monitor neurologic integrity during the procedure. The minimally invasive vascular approach requires little, if any, sedation beyond local anesthetic to the access site. It is vital that the patient remains alert and cooperative with the proceduralist for serial neurologic examinations. A candid preoperative discussion to set appropriate patient expectations is perhaps the most critical anesthetic intervention. The lowest necessary doses of short-acting sedatives should be titrated to effect; patient disinhibition must be avoided. Standard intraoperative monitoring and a single medium- to large-bore peripheral intravenous line is typically sufficient for the procedure; invasive arterial access may be considered but is rarely warranted. In an emergency, arterial pressure may be monitored from the surgical access site. It is important to recognize that carotid angioplasty and stent deployment may trigger the carotid baroreceptor reflex, with resultant bradycardia and hypotension, similar to external carotid manipulation. If this occurs, cessation of manipulation should extinguish the response; prophylaxis with an anticholinergic agent may be considered. Altered postoperative carotid baroreceptor function is possible as with open repair; hemodynamic instability should be treated as for CEA.

Endovascular Aortic Repair

Prior to the endovascular era, options for AAA management were limited to OAR or medical management. Morbidity and mortality associated with OAR is significant. At the same time, risk of rupture increases significantly as aneurysms enlarge, with near 100% mortality rate for out-of-hospital rupture. The advent of the endovascular era revolutionized the management of AAAs. Parodi[189] pioneered an endovascular approach to aortic aneurysms in the early 1990s. Initially, this technique was reserved for high-risk patients with straightforward anatomy deemed unfit for open surgical repair. Recent advances in stent technology and surgical skill, including customized fenestrated stents and chimney techniques, have made endovascular repair an option for patients who previously would have been considered unfit due to anatomic considerations. In fact, the broad application of EVAR technology has rapidly overtaken the use of OAR as the primarily modality for AAA treatment over the last decade.[190,191] In 2000, EVAR accounted for 5.2% of AAA repairs. In 2004, EVAR surpassed OAR as the more commonly employed technique. By 2010, this percentage had risen dramatically to 74%. Endovascular repair has also become the treatment modality of choice for complicated acute type B dissections.[192]

Several rigorous, large, multicenter, randomized controlled trials have addressed the issue of open versus endovascular aneurysm repair.[193–196] The Dutch Randomized Endovascular Aneurysm Management (DREAM), EndoVascular Aneurysm Repair (EVAR), and Open Versus Endovascular Repair (OVER) trials all demonstrated significantly lower perioperative mortality with EVAR than with OAR, although this benefit was lost in intermediate- to long-term follow-up. The Aneurysme de l'aorte abdominale: Chirurgie versus Endoprothese (ACE) trial, in contrast, found no significant difference in perioperative or longer-term mortality between the EVAR and OAR groups, although it is worth noting that these patients were considered low- to intermediate-risk for surgery. Taken together, a pooled analysis of these results suggests a decrease in short-term mortality, but no significant difference in either intermediate- (up to 4 years) or long-term outcomes.[197] Major operative morbidity, including myocardial, neurologic, and renal complications, were similar in pooled analysis. Pulmonary complications were found to be significantly higher in the OAR compared to EVAR group, and a similar trend was noted in pulmonary-related deaths. The long-term reintervention rate was significantly higher in the EVAR than OAR group; the unique complication profile of endovascular repair necessitates a lifetime of surveillance. In general, the majority of reinterventions are also endovascular with low associated morbidity and mortality. Even so, repeated exposure to radiation and contrast exposure, and potentially surgery and anesthesia, should be considered when deciding between open- versus endovascular-based interventions. An otherwise young, fit patient with a lower perioperative risk profile may be a reasonable candidate for OAR to avoid the associated risks of lifetime surveillance and potential for reintervention; however, a recent review of the NSQIP database suggests that the perioperative reduction in mortality and major morbidity persists even in patients deemed low risk for infrarenal OAR.[198]

The EVAR-2 trial was designed to compare maximum medical therapy versus EVAR in patients deemed unfit for OAR.[199] Patient factors that were associated with ineligibility for OAR included major cardiac, pulmonary, or renal comorbidities. This trial concluded that EVAR reduces aneurysm-related, but not overall, mortality as compared to medical therapy. Presumably, the same factors that made patients too high risk for OAR likely contributed to a high subsequent rate of all-cause mortality. Thus, the authors suggest that patients with a poor life expectancy due to coexisting disease do not benefit from EVAR. The EVAR-2 study has been criticized both for methodologic flaws that may have biased against the EVAR group as well as unacceptably high mortality rates.[200] A more recent evaluation of patients considered unfit for surgery at single, high-volume center demonstrated a survival benefit, even in a presumed high-risk population.[201] Pertinently, patients in this study were more likely to be optimized with antiplatelet and statin agents than the patients enrolled in EVAR-2, which may also have made them better surgical candidates. In addition, endovascular repair was undertaken at a single, high volume center. This is in contrast to EVAR-2 in which multiple centers, with variable expertise, took part. As with most interventions, proceduralist experience and skill is likely associated with outcomes and success.

A question that persists after the EVAR-2 trial is which patients, in particular, should be considered high risk for endovascular repair. Egorova and colleagues[202] evaluated close to 67,000 patients who underwent EVAR in the inpatient Medicare database. A risk model for perioperative mortality was developed and validated. Table 40-3 lists the baseline risk factors that significantly predicted mortality with a corresponding score. The vast majority of patients (96.6%) had additive scores below ten, which correlated with a 30-day mortality of less than 5%, whereas less than 1% had a mortality rate greater than 10%. The authors conclude that although a high-risk cohort exists that should not be treated with EVAR due to prohibitively high 30-day mortality, that cohort is quite small. Giles et al.[203] also developed an aneurysm scoring system that was predictive of mortality for both open and endovascular repair. The EVAR Risk Assessment model[204] has been shown to predict not only perioperative mortality but also morbidity, mid-term survival, and reintervention rates. The eight variables included in this model were aneurysm

Table 40-3 Risk Scores for 30-day Mortality for EVAR Patients[a]

Risk Factor	Score
Renal failure with dialysis	7
Lower extremity ischemia	5
Age ≥85 yrs	4
Liver disease	3
Congestive heart failure	3
Age 80–84 yrs	2
Female	2
Neurologic comorbidity	2
Chronic pulmonary disease	1
Surgeon case experience <3	1
Hospital annual volume <7	1
Age 57–59 yrs	1

[a]A total score between 10 and 12 predicts a 5% mortality rate. A total score greater than 13 predicts a 10% operative rate.
EVAR, EndoVascular Aneurysm Repair. Adapted with permission from Egorova N, Giacovelli JK, Gelijns A, et al. Defining high-risk patients for endovascular aneurysm repair. *J Vasc Surg*. 2009;50(6):1271–1279.e1.

size, age, ASA, gender, creatinine, aortic neck angle, infrarenal neck diameter, and infrarenal neck length.

Evolution of Endovascular Repair for Complex Aneurysms

The field of endovascular surgery has rapidly expanded since Parodi[189] first described the use of a custom-made Dacron tube endograft, which limited its use to infrarenal aortic segments only. The development of bifurcated and modular grafts soon followed, allowing for the extension beyond the aortic bifurcation. Until recently, however, device design constraints excluded patients with more complicated anatomy from endovascular repair. For example, patients with juxta- or suprarenal aneurysms, in whom the visceral vasculature may arise from the aneurysmal aorta, were not candidates for endovascular repair because blood flow to critical organs would be interrupted. Similarly, up to 15% of infrarenal aneurysms have an inadequate length of normal infrarenal aorta to allow for an adequate proximal seal without compromising visceral blood flow. Recent advances in stent technology have revolutionized management of these more complicated repairs. The development of branched or fenestrated grafts (f-EVAR) allows for continued blood flow to visceral organs while still permitting proximal graft extension. These devices are custom made based on three-dimensional reconstructions (typically, CT angiography) so that the fenestrations or branches are appropriately positioned for the corresponding arterial orifices. Because they are custom designed, these devices are both costly and take significant time to manufacture. Thus, they are typically not an option for emergent repair. An alternative technique is that of a chimney graft (Ch-EVAR). With this approach, a distinct endograft is positioned in parallel to the body of the main aortic stent graft (between the aortic wall and the main stent) to allow for preserved flow to the visceral branch (Fig. 40-16). The "snorkel" technique allows for blood flow from above the level of the main stent while the "periscope" technique allows blood flow from below. The end result is preservation of visceral blood flow to vessels that otherwise would have been excluded by the main body of the graft. A "sandwich" technique has even been described, in which the visceral snorkels are sandwiched between two segments of aortic grafts. Chimney grafts

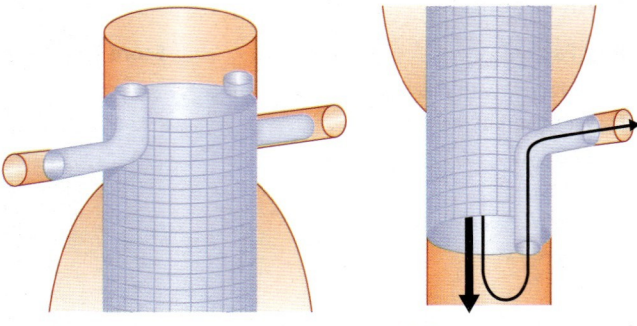

Figure 40-16 Snorkel and periscope stents. Coaxial placement of stents into vital mesenteric vessels allow for both adequate blood flow to visceral organs and exclusion of the aneurysm sac for supra- or juxtarenal aneurysms or aneurysms with insufficient proximal (**A**) or distal (**B**) landing zones. In the case of a periscope, blood exiting the body of the main stent flows back up into the coaxial periscope, providing blood flow to the visceral branch that would otherwise be excluded from the circulation. (Reprinted with permission from Wilson A, Zhou S, Bachoo P, et al. Systematic review of chimney and periscope grafts for endovascular aneurysm repair. *Br J Surg.* 2013;100:1557–1564.)

are available "off the shelf" and thus remain an option in urgent situations in which no time exists to manufacture a custom made fenestrated stent. They are also less prohibitively expensive than their custom made counterparts.

No randomized controlled trials exist to compare the use of open, fenestrated, or chimney techniques for complex aneurysm repairs. It is important to recognize the inherent bias in the published literature. Patient cohorts are likely not comparable based on pre-existing morbidity, complexity of anatomy, and urgency of procedure. A recent systematic review demonstrated a trend toward decreased perioperative mortality with f-EVAR compared to OAR, although this difference did not reach statistical significance.[205] Similar trends were appreciated in perioperative cardiovascular and pulmonary morbidity, blood loss, and hospital and ICU length of stay. A second systemic review and meta-analysis of the existing literature have found f-EVAR to have acceptable short- and mid-term outcomes in terms of mortality, technical success rate, target vessel patency rate, and need for reintervention.[206] As with any new technique, an early steep learning curve must be considered in the interpretation of these data. In addition, this technique was primarily reserved for high-risk patients who were not suitable candidates for open repair in the early years. Further study is warranted now that f-EVAR is a standard practice in major aortic centers to evaluate outcomes.

The perioperative mortality rate for Ch-EVAR has been demonstrated to be comparable to OAR (4% to 5%) but higher than for standard EVAR.[207] Both the medical complexity of the patient and surgical complexity of the aneurysm are likely to account for this difference. One concern for the Ch-EVAR approach is an increased risk of type I endoleak (discussed later) due the coaxial deployment of the main and chimney stents. A review of the literature concluded that Ch-EVAR clearly produced more endoleaks than f-EVAR, although many of these were successfully treated intraoperatively with additional balloon dilation or disappeared during subsequent follow-up.[205] Ch-EVAR was also associated with an increased risk of ischemic stroke compared to either OAR or f-EVAR. The chimney technique requires vascular access from the brachial or axillary artery in order to appropriately align and deploy the chimney graft. This upper extremity approach, particularly with an atherosclerotic or difficult arch anatomy, increases the risk for iatrogenic stroke.[205] An increasing amount of data suggests that this is a safe and valuable technique, particularly for complex patients with urgent need for surgical repair.[65] The technical success and patency rates in the short- and intermediate-term is promising for both f-EVAR and Ch-EVAR, although long-term results have yet to be determined.

Anesthetic Management of Endovascular Aneurysm Repair

EVAR can be successfully performed under almost any type of anesthesia including local, regional, neuraxial, and general techniques. Which technique is employed will depend on a variety of factors. Concurrent use of antiplatelet agents or therapeutic anticoagulation may preclude the use of neuraxial or regional anesthetics. Patient factors, such as inability to lie flat for an extended period or an inability to effectively communicate, may sway the provider toward general anesthesia. Finally, surgical considerations such as anticipated duration or difficulty of surgery must be considered. Many nonrandomized analyses address the question of local or regional versus general anesthesia for EVAR. A study of more than 5,500 patients who underwent EVAR repair in 164 centers under general, regional, or local anesthesia demonstrated that local or regional techniques resulted in reduced operative time, ICU admissions, duration of hospital stay, and a number of systemic complications.[208] A review of more than 5,500 patients in the NSQIP database demonstrated a decrease in pulmonary morbidity and a 10% to 20% decrease in hospital length of stay when local or regional anesthesia was utilized as compared to general anesthesia.[209] A meta-analysis of the current literature suggests a decrease in operative time, hospital stay, and postoperative complications with local compared to general anesthesia, in spite of the fact that patient receiving local anesthesia tended to be older with an increase burden of cardiovascular or respiratory disease.[210] However, there are no randomized controlled trials to suggest the superiority of one technique over another.

The minimally invasive nature of EVAR means that hemodynamic changes should be relatively insignificant during the case; however, the possible need for urgent conversion must always be considered. Perioperative conversion rates from EVAR to OAR is less than 1% and may occur in the setting of difficult arterial access, vessel dissection, poor anatomic parameters, stent malposition or migration, or aneurysm rupture. The ability to rapidly convert to general anesthesia is necessary if other techniques are primarily employed. Adequate resuscitative equipment such as cell saver and rapid infusion devices should be readily available. Two large-bore peripheral intravenous should be placed and adequate blood product availability should be ensured.

Short periods of hypertension and increased afterload should be anticipated if aortic ballooning is needed for stent deployment, analogous to external cross-clamping. Most stents self-deploy without ballooning. These episodes typically do not require intervention due to their brevity. Blood loss should be minimal in experienced hands. In case of rupture, emergent proximal control is first obtained via endoscopic balloon occlusion which is then replaced with cross-clamp upon open conversion. In this setting, proximal arterial access is indispensable due to the hemodynamic changes anticipated during OAR. Central venous access is not typically warranted for EVAR because hemodynamic changes are rare during routine surgery, vasoactive infusions are rarely warranted, and postoperative ICU stay is rare. Exceptions to this rule may include thoracic endovascular aneurysm repair (TEVAR) cases or complicated repairs including snorkel/periscope techniques. Central venous access may be considered for TEVAR for the ability to rapidly place a pulmonary artery catheter should that case convert to an open TAAA, which would require cardiopulmonary bypass (discussed in Chapter 39, Anesthesia for Cardiac Surgery). Central venous access may be considered for snorkel/chimney cases because each additional stent placed requires separate arterial sheaths. These cases can be longer, more complicated, and associated with greater blood loss. Thus, more aggressive resuscitation and/or vasoactive infusions may be necessary. Before device insertion, systemic anticoagulation with intravenous heparin will be requested with a goal activated clotting time of 200 seconds or longer. At the time of device deployment, the patient will be asked to hold their breath (or, for anesthetized patients, a request will be made to hold ventilation) to allow for accurate stent deployment. At the same time, a request for temporary lowering of the mean arterial pressure may be made to minimize distal migration of the stent. After device deployment, a completion angiogram is performed to evaluate for technical success and any complications related to the procedure, anticoagulation is reversed, and the patient is typically extubated in the operating room.

Complications of Endovascular Aneurysm Repair

The unique complication profile related to endovascular repair mandates a lifetime of surveillance and a higher rate for reintervention as compared to OAR (29.6% vs. 18.1%).[193] Most reinterventions are graft-related complications including endoleaks, stent graft occlusion, migration, kinking, or infection. The majority of reinterventions tend to be catheter-based with limited morbidity and mortality. Nevertheless, each iterative intervention exposes the patient to the risks of radiation, iodinated contrast dye, and potentially the risks of anesthesia.

The most common indication for reintervention following EVAR is for endoleak. An endoleak is characterized by persistent blood flow into the aneurysm sac outside of the stent graft. The failure to exclude the aneurysm from the circulation may cause an increase in sac pressure over time, expansion, and potential rupture. Endoleaks complicate approximately 10% to 25% of EVAR cases[211,212] and require reintervention in upward of 12%.[212] Five types of endoleaks exist (Fig. 40-17). Types I and III involve direct communication with the systemic arterial circulation and thus mandate reintervention. Type I endoleaks are typically treated with repeat balloon molding or proximal or distal stent extension, whereas stent relining is the treatment for Type III endoleaks. The treatment of Type II endoleaks, caused by retrograde filling of the aneurysm sac by branch vessels, is controversial. Though retrograde flow can lead to aneurysm enlargement and increase in sac pressure, the majority of these aneurysms remain stable or decrease in size due to low flow and spontaneous thrombosis.[211] The EUROSTAR registry found no significant difference in the rate of aneurysm rupture between patients with and without type II endoleak.[213] If treatment is warranted, endovascular embolization of the feeding vessel is typically employed. Type IV endoleaks are related to graft porosity and are typically self-limited once the patient's coagulation status returns to baseline. Type V endoleak, also called "endotension," refers to an enlarging aneurysm sac without demonstrable endoleak. The etiology of endotension has not been completely elucidated. Although there may be a role for conservative management or endovascular reintervention, open conversion is the mainstay of management for endotension. Endoleak remains the single leading cause of late (more than 30-day) conversion to open repair, accounting for more than 60% of late reinterventions.[214] The incidence of late conversions has been reported to be as low as 2% but more recent evidence suggests a rate as high as 4%. This may be related to the increased number of endovascular repairs, and particularly complex endovascular repairs, performed. Late conversion to open repair is a technically challenging procedure with a relatively high mortality rate, particularly if performed emergently. Mortality rates for nonelective repair have been reported to be as high as 30%.[214]

The pulsatile nature of blood flow results in an ongoing downward pressure on the stent graft and may result in stent migration. Over time, this may re-expose the aneurysm to systemic pressurization. Risk factors include aneurysm anatomy (e.g., hostile angulation of the aortic neck or short proximal landing zone) and graft properties (e.g., inadequate fixation and short overlaps).[212] Aortic stent graft infection occurs in up to 1% of cases and may be a result of direct primary contamination or occur later from a secondary source. Clinical findings may be nonspecific such as fever, back pain, or leukocytosis. Initial treatment involves broad spectrum antibiotics but may require explanation of the stent graft and open bypass. Stent graft kinking or infolding occurs in less than 5% of cases but may result in flow-restricting stenosis, graft thrombosis, and occlusion. Acute occlusion is frequently treated with catheter-directed thrombolysis or may be treated with mechanical thrombectomy if pharmacologic treatment is contraindicated.

Renal damage after EVAR is multifactorial. Preoperative renal insufficiency best predicts perioperative renal failure/dialysis

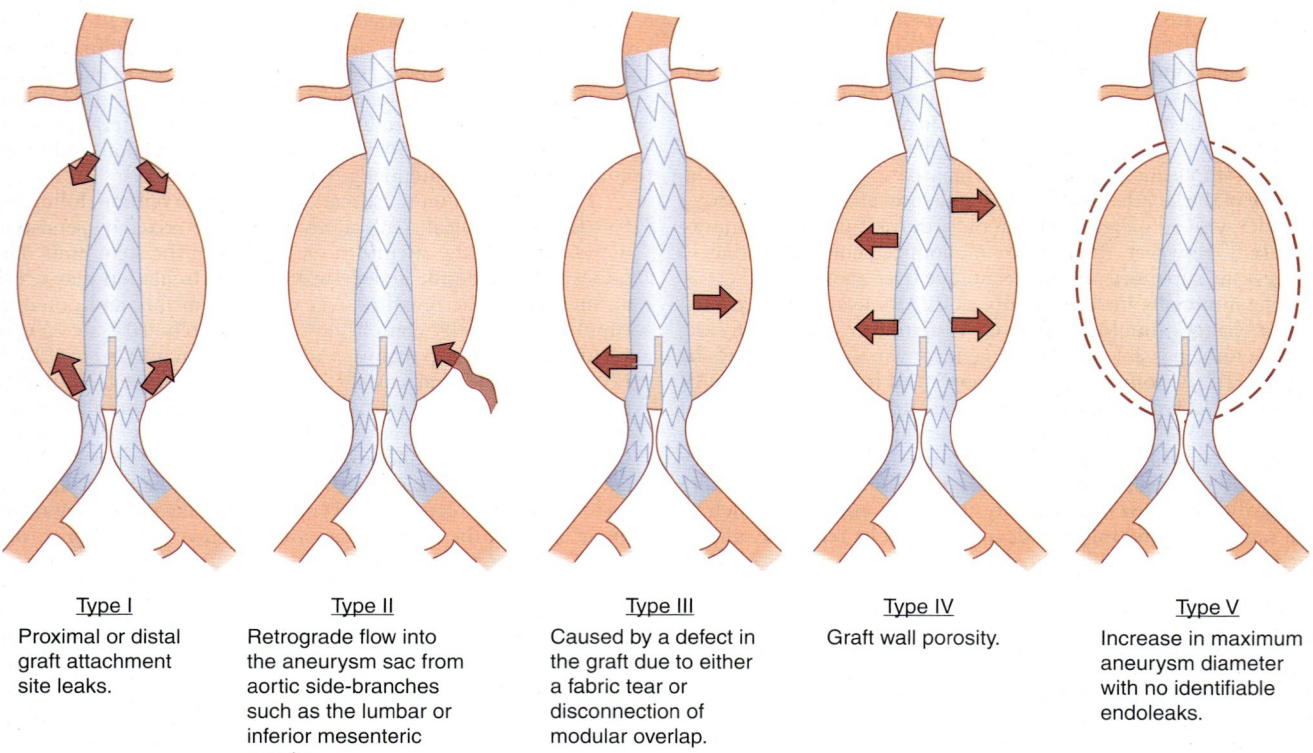

Figure 40-17 Types of endoleaks. Five types of endoleaks exist depending on the mechanism of persistent blood flow. Subsequent management depends on the type of endoleak present. The possibility of endoleak requires lifelong surveillance following EVAR, and endoleak remains the primary indication for late reintervention. (Reprinted with permission from England A, McWilliams R. Endovascular Aortic Aneurysm Repair [EVAR]. *Ulster Med J.* 2013;82[1]:3–10.)

need. Serial creatinine or GFR should be followed to ensure that the patient has sufficiently recovered from diagnostic angiography prior to surgery. The best way to limit renal damage is to limit contrast use. Gadolinium and CO_2 have been used. Better x-ray equipment and operator experience allows for lower contrast dosing. Preoperative fluid loading with 1 mL/kg/hr over 12 hours prior to surgery seems to be optimum management, but most patients are outpatients. Thus initial fluid loading seems prudent. Sodium bicarbonate infusions and N-acetyl cysteine infusions may play a small role in preventing renal damage.

Endovascular Management of Peripheral Artery Disease

The Inter-Society Consensus for the Management of PAD (TASC II) recommends endovascular revascularization for focal, discrete lesions and open surgical revascularization for severe disease.[13] Evidence suggests, however, that national trends in revascularization approach skew heavily toward endovascular repair even for more diffuse, complex disease. Endovascular interventions have increased more than threefold while open peripheral bypass surgery has decreased by more than 40% in recent years.[215] This trend is likely due, in large part, to continued improvement in technology available for endovascular repair (e.g., stents, imaging techniques, and drug–device combinations).[216] This paradigm shift is reflected in the most recent recommendations from the Society for Vascular Surgery practice guidelines, which endorses endovascular treatment as a reasonable first-line approach in most circumstances, even for complex disease.[171] In some cases, a hybrid approach to PAD may be employed. In one study, nearly 25% of complex AIOD repairs combined open femoral endarterectomy with endovascular iliac intervention due to disease severity.[217] In other cases, a percutaneous approach to femoropopliteal disease may be combined with traditional open surgery below the knee. The development of hybrid operating rooms, with a full array of imaging equipment, allows for real-time decision making and completion of multiple procedures (both endovascular and open) under one anesthetic. Ultimately, the decision making must take into account disease severity and location, patient risk factors, and proceduralist skill.

Few randomized controlled trials exist to guide management decisions for the surgical management of PAD; the majority of the evidence is based on observational data. No large randomized controlled trials have compared open versus endovascular repair for complex AIOD. A systematic review of more than 5,300 patients undergoing open versus endovascular repair demonstrated greater perioperative morbidity and mortality but better long-term durability with open repair.[218] A recent meta-analysis of endovascular revascularization of AIOD demonstrated 4- to 5-year primary patency rates from 60% to 86% and secondary patency rates from 80% to 98%.[219] The majority of reinterventions in this study were percutaneous or noninvasive in nature. The Bypass versus Angioplasty in Severe Ischaemia of the Leg (BASIL) trial was a multicenter, randomized controlled trial that demonstrated that endovascular therapy resulted in less short-term morbidity and similar amputation-free survival for femoropopliteal disease.[220] For patients who survived at least 2 years, however, open revascularization was associated with increased overall survival and a trend toward amputation-free survival.[221] A recent meta-analysis evaluating endovascular versus surgical revascularization for femoropopliteal disease endorses an endovascular approach as first-line therapy.[61] Endovascular repair of infrapopliteal disease has traditionally been reserved for patients with CLI due to limited success and unacceptable rates restenosis, dissection, and thrombosis early after the intervention. However, the advent of new technologies (namely, drug eluting stents) is changing the treatment paradigm for infrapopliteal disease. Several recent randomized controlled trials and meta-analyses support the use of drug eluting stents for symptomatic infrapopliteal disease that is anatomically suitable for intervention.[222]

Endovascular repair of PAD is typically performed under local anesthesia or monitored anesthesia care. Small doses of short-acting agents should be utilized to allow for patient cooperation throughout the procedure. The patient must be able to tolerate lying flat on the procedure table for several hours. Patients who are particularly anxious or who are unable to cooperate may require general anesthesia. Because the risk of blood loss is minimal and significant hemodynamic alterations are not anticipated intraoperatively, invasive hemodynamic monitoring is rarely indicated for these procedures. A single medium- to large-bore intravenous line is sufficient for vascular access.

Conclusion

Vascular surgery patients are generally elderly patients with significant cardiovascular disease in multiple vascular beds. They frequently have complex medical problems including CAD, COPD, diabetes mellitus, and renal insufficiency. A thorough preoperative evaluation for concurrent disease and pharmacologic optimization is paramount. The use of preoperative cardiac testing is controversial but current recommendations suggest it is reasonable to obtain preoperative cardiac testing for patients with poor or unknown exercise capacity if it will change perioperative management. Major morbidity in the perioperative setting is related to cardiovascular events; therefore, the heart should be the major focus of the anesthesiologist's attention. The skill of the anesthesiologist can greatly influence perioperative outcome. The field of vascular surgery is increasingly moving toward an endovascular focus. Improvements in imaging technique, equipment, and proceduralist skill are pushing the frontiers of what can be accomplished via minimally invasive techniques. Consequently, open repair is increasingly reserved for more severe or surgically complex disease. Endovascular surgery has its own unique complication profile that mandates a lifetime of surveillance. Long-term outcomes of many recent advances remain to be seen.

REFERENCES

1. Laslett LJ, Alagona P Jr, Clark BA III, et al. The worldwide environment of cardiovascular disease: prevalence, diagnosis, therapy, and policy issues: a report from the American College of Cardiology. *J Am Coll Cardiol.* 2012;60(25 Suppl): S1–S49.
2. Smith SC Jr, Collins A, Ferrari R, et al. Our time: a call to save preventable death from cardiovascular disease (heart disease and stroke). *J Am Coll Cardiol.* 2012;60(22):2343–2348.
3. Mozaffarian D, Benjamin EJ, Go AS, et al. Heart disease and stroke statistics–2015 update: a report from the American Heart Association. *Circulation.* 2015;131(4):e29–322.
4. Go AS, Mozaffarian D, Roger VL, et al. Heart disease and stroke statistics–2013 update: a report from the American Heart Association. *Circulation.* 2013;127(1):e6–e245.
5. Anderson PL, Gelijns A, Moskowitz A, et al. Understanding trends in inpatient surgical volume: vascular interventions, 1980–2000. *J Vasc Surg.* 2004;39(6):1200–1208.
6. Hansson GK. Inflammation, atherosclerosis, and coronary artery disease. *N Engl J Med.* 2005;352(16):1685–1695.
7. Li H, Freeman MW, Libby P. Regulation of smooth muscle cell scavenger receptor expression in vivo by atherogenic diets and in vitro by cytokines. *J Clin Invest.* 1995;95(1):122–133.
8. Tintut Y, Patel J, Parhami F, et al. Tumor necrosis factor-alpha promotes in vitro calcification of vascular cells via the cAMP pathway. *Circulation.* 2000; 102(21):2636–2642.
9. Falk E, Shah PK, Fuster V. Coronary plaque disruption. *Circulation.* 1995; 92(3):657–671.
10. Arbab-Zadeh A, Fuster V. The myth of the "vulnerable plaque": transitioning from a focus on individual lesions to atherosclerotic disease burden for coronary artery disease risk assessment. *J Am Coll Cardiol.* 2015;65(8):846–855.
11. Bittencourt MS, Hulten E, Ghoshhajra B, et al. Prognostic value of nonobstructive and obstructive coronary artery disease detected by coronary computed tomography angiography to identify cardiovascular events. *Circ Cardiovasc Imaging.* 2014;7(2):282–291.
12. Faraday N, Martinez EA, Scharpf RB, et al. Platelet gene polymorphisms and cardiac risk assessment in vascular surgical patients. *Anesthesiology.* 2004;101(6):1291–1297.
13. Norgren L, Hiatt WR, Dormandy JA, et al. Inter-society consensus for the management of peripheral arterial disease (TASC II). *J Vasc Surg.* 2007;45 Suppl S:S5–67.
14. Grundy SM, Cleeman JI, Daniels SR, et al. Diagnosis and management of the metabolic syndrome: an American Heart Association/National Heart, Lung, and Blood Institute Scientific Statement. *Circulation.* 2005;112(17):2735–2752.
15. Goldberger ZD, Valle JA, Dandekar VK, et al. Are changes in carotid intima-media thickness related to risk of nonfatal myocardial infarction? A critical review and meta-regression analysis. *Am Heart J.* 2010;160(4):701–714.
16. Wyman RA, Mays ME, McBride PE, et al. Ultrasound-detected carotid plaque as a predictor of cardiovascular events. *Vasc Med (Lond).* 2006;11(2):123–130.
17. Hertzer NR, Beven EG, Young JR, et al. Coronary artery disease in peripheral vascular patients: a classification of 1000 coronary angiograms and results of surgical management. *Ann Surg.* 1984;199(2):223–233.
18. Paul SD, Eagle KA, Kuntz KM, et al. Concordance of preoperative clinical risk with angiographic severity of coronary artery disease in patients undergoing vascular surgery. *Circulation.* 1996;94(7):1561–1566.
19. Wijeysundera DN, Duncan D, Nkonde-Price C, et al. Perioperative beta blockade in noncardiac surgery: a systematic review for the 2014 ACC/AHA guideline on perioperative cardiovascular evaluation and management of patients undergoing noncardiac surgery: a report of the American College of Cardiology/American Heart Association Task Force on Practice Guidelines. *Circulation.* 2014;130(24):2246–2264.
20. Devereaux PJ, Goldman L, Cook DJ, et al. Perioperative cardiac events in patients undergoing noncardiac surgery: a review of the magnitude of the problem, the pathophysiology of the events and methods to estimate and communicate risk. *CMAJ.* 2005;173(6):627–634.
21. Devereaux PJ, Chan MT, Alonso-Coello P, et al. Association between postoperative troponin levels and 30-day mortality among patients undergoing noncardiac surgery. *JAMA.* 2012;307(21):2295–2304.
22. Mangano DT, Browner WS, Hollenberg M, et al. Long-term cardiac prognosis following noncardiac surgery: the Study of Perioperative Ischemia Research Group. *JAMA.* 1992;268(2):233–239.
23. Badner NH, Knill RL, Brown JE, et al. Myocardial infarction after noncardiac surgery. *Anesthesiology.* 1998;88(3):572–578.
24. Mangano DT, Hollenberg M, Fegert G, et al. Perioperative myocardial ischemia in patients undergoing noncardiac surgery. I. Incidence and severity during the 4 day perioperative period. The Study of Perioperative Ischemia (SPI) Research Group. *J Am Coll Cardiol.* 1991;17(4):843–850.
25. Mangano DT, Layug EL, Wallace A, et al. Effect of atenolol on mortality and cardiovascular morbidity after noncardiac surgery: multicenter study of Perioperative Ischemia Research Group. *N Engl J Med.* 1996;335(23):1713–1720.
26. Poldermans D, Boersma E, Bax JJ, et al. The effect of bisoprolol on perioperative mortality and myocardial infarction in high-risk patients undergoing vascular surgery. Dutch Echocardiographic Cardiac Risk Evaluation Applying Stress Echocardiography Study Group. *N Engl J Med.* 1999;341(24):1789–1794.
27. Beattie WS, Wijeysundera DN, Karkouti K, et al. Does tight heart rate control improve beta-blocker efficacy? An updated analysis of the noncardiac surgical randomized trials. *Anesth Analg.* 2008;106(4):1039–1048.
28. Yang H, Raymer K, Butler R, et al. The effects of perioperative beta-blockade: results of the Metoprolol after Vascular Surgery (MaVS) study, a randomized controlled trial. *Am Heart J.* 2006;152(5):983–990.
29. Juul AB, Wetterslev J, Gluud C, et al. Effect of perioperative beta blockade in patients with diabetes undergoing major non-cardiac surgery: randomised placebo controlled, blinded multicentre trial. *BMJ (Clin Res).* 2006;332(7556):1482.
30. Brady AR, Gibbs JS, Greenhalgh RM, et al. Perioperative beta-blockade (POBBLE) for patients undergoing infrarenal vascular surgery: results of a randomized double-blind controlled trial. *J Vasc Surg.* 2005;41(4):602–609.
31. Dunkelgrun M, Boersma E, Schouten O, et al. Bisoprolol and fluvastatin for the reduction of perioperative cardiac mortality and myocardial infarction in

intermediate-risk patients undergoing noncardiovascular surgery: a randomized controlled trial (DECREASE-IV). *Ann Surg.* 2009;249(6):921–926.
32. Devereaux PJ, Yang H, Yusuf S, et al. Effects of extended-release metoprolol succinate in patients undergoing non-cardiac surgery (POISE trial): a randomised controlled trial. *Lancet.* 2008;371(9627):1839–1847.
33. Fleisher LA, Fleischmann KE, Auerbach AD, et al. 2014 ACC/AHA guideline on perioperative cardiovascular evaluation and management of patients undergoing noncardiac surgery: executive summary: a report of the American College of Cardiology/American Heart Association Task Force on Practice Guidelines. *Circulation.* 2014;130(24):2215–2245.
34. Scali S, Patel V, Neal D, et al. Preoperative beta-blockers do not improve cardiac outcomes after major elective vascular surgery and may be harmful. *J Vasc Surg.* 2015;62(1):166–176.e2.
35. Mostafaie K, Bedenis R, Harrington D. Beta-adrenergic blockers for perioperative cardiac risk reduction in people undergoing vascular surgery. *Cochrane Database Syst Rev.* 2015;1:Cd006342.
36. Patorno E, Wang SV, Schneeweiss S, et al. Patterns of beta-blocker initiation in patients undergoing intermediate to high-risk noncardiac surgery. *Am Heart J.* 2015;170(4):812–820.e6.
37. Wallace AW, Au S, Cason BA. Perioperative beta-blockade: atenolol is associated with reduced mortality when compared to metoprolol. *Anesthesiology.* 2011;114(4):824–836.
38. Mashour GA, Sharifpour M, Freundlich RE, et al. Perioperative metoprolol and risk of stroke after noncardiac surgery. *Anesthesiology.* 2013;119(6):1340–1346.
39. Ellis JE, Drijvers G, Pedlow S, et al. Premedication with oral and transdermal clonidine provides safe and efficacious postoperative sympatholysis. *Anesth Analg.* 1994;79(6):1133–1140.
40. Wallace AW, Galindez D, Salahieh A, et al. Effect of clonidine on cardiovascular morbidity and mortality after noncardiac surgery. *Anesthesiology.* 2004;101(2):284–293.
41. Wijeysundera DN, Bender JS, Beattie WS. Alpha-2 adrenergic agonists for the prevention of cardiac complications among patients undergoing surgery. *Cochrane Database Syst Rev.* 2009(4):Cd004126.
42. Wijeysundera DN, Naik JS, Beattie WS. Alpha-2 adrenergic agonists to prevent perioperative cardiovascular complications: a meta-analysis. *Am J Med.* 2003;114(9):742–752.
43. Devereaux PJ, Sessler DI, Leslie K, et al. Clonidine in patients undergoing noncardiac surgery. *N Engl J Med.* 2014;370(16):1504–1513.
44. Husain K, Hernandez W, Ansari RA, et al. Inflammation, oxidative stress and renin angiotensin system in atherosclerosis. *World J Biol Chem.* 2015;6(3):209–217.
45. Sayer G, Bhat G. The renin-angiotensin-aldosterone system and heart failure. *Cardiol Clin.* 2014;32(1):21–32.
46. Lazar HL. The use of angiotensin-converting enzyme inhibitors in patients undergoing coronary artery bypass graft surgery. *Vasc Pharmacol.* 2005;42(3):119–123.
47. Benedetto U, Sciarretta S, Roscitano A, et al. Preoperative angiotensin-converting enzyme inhibitors and acute kidney injury after coronary artery bypass grafting. *Ann Thorac Surg.* 2008;86(4):1160–1165.
48. Miceli A, Capoun R, Fino C, et al. Effects of angiotensin-converting enzyme inhibitor therapy on clinical outcome in patients undergoing coronary artery bypass grafting. *J Am Coll Cardiol.* 2009;54(19):1778–1784.
49. Railton CJ, Wolpin J, Lam-McCulloch J, Belo SE. Renin-angiotensin blockade is associated with increased mortality after vascular surgery. *Can J Anaesth.* 2010;57(8):736–744.
50. Halcox JP, Deanfield JE. Beyond the laboratory: clinical implications for statin pleiotropy. *Circulation.* 2004;109(21 Suppl 1):II42–48.
51. Le Manach Y, Coriat P, Collard CD, et al. Statin therapy within the perioperative period. *Anesthesiology.* 2008;108(6):1141–1146.
52. Collard CD, Body SC, Shernan SK, et al. Preoperative statin therapy is associated with reduced cardiac mortality after coronary artery bypass graft surgery. *J Thorac Cardiovasc Surg.* 2006;132(2):392–400.
53. Schouten O, Boersma E, Hoeks SE, et al. Fluvastatin and perioperative events in patients undergoing vascular surgery. *N Engl J Med.* 2009;361(10):980–989.
54. Le Manach Y, Godet G, Coriat P, et al. The impact of postoperative discontinuation or continuation of chronic statin therapy on cardiac outcome after major vascular surgery. *Anesth Analg.* 2007;104(6):1326–1333, table of contents.
55. Durazzo AE, Machado FS, Ikeoka DT, et al. Reduction in cardiovascular events after vascular surgery with atorvastatin: a randomized trial. *J Vasc Surg.* 2004;39(5):967–975.
56. Leurs LJ, Visser P, Laheij RJ, et al. Statin use is associated with reduced all-cause mortality after endovascular abdominal aortic aneurysm repair. *Vascular.* 2006;14(1):1–8.
57. Berwanger O, Le Manach Y, Suzumura EA, et al. Association between preoperative statin use and major cardiovascular complications among patients undergoing non-cardiac surgery: the VISION study. *Eur Heart J.* 2016; 37(2):177–185.
58. Heeschen C, Hamm CW, Laufs U, et al. Withdrawal of statins increases event rates in patients with acute coronary syndromes. *Circulation.* 2002;105(12):1446–1452.
59. Taylor F, Huffman MD, Macedo AF, et al. Statins for the primary prevention of cardiovascular disease. *Cochrane Database Syst Rev.* 2013;1:Cd004816.
60. Sanders RD, Nicholson A, Lewis SR, et al. Perioperative statin therapy for improving outcomes during and after noncardiac vascular surgery. *Cochrane Database Syst Rev.* 2013;7:Cd009971.
61. Antoniou GA, Hajibandeh S, Hajibandeh S, et al. Meta-analysis of the effects of statins on perioperative outcomes in vascular and endovascular surgery. *J Vasc Surg.* 2015;61(2):519–532.e1.
62. Burger W, Chemnitius JM, Kneissl GD, et al. Low-dose aspirin for secondary cardiovascular prevention: cardiovascular risks after its perioperative withdrawal versus bleeding risks with its continuation—review and meta-analysis. *J Intern Med.* 2005;257(5):399–414.
63. Smith SC Jr, Benjamin EJ, Bonow RO, et al. AHA/ACCF Secondary Prevention and Risk Reduction Therapy for Patients with Coronary and other Atherosclerotic Vascular Disease: 2011 update: a guideline from the American Heart Association and American College of Cardiology Foundation. *Circulation.* 2011;124(22):2458–2473.
64. Batchelder A, Hunter J, Cairns V, et al. Dual antiplatelet therapy prior to expedited carotid surgery reduces recurrent events prior to surgery without significantly increasing peri-operative bleeding complications. *Eur J Vasc Endovasc Surg.* 2015;50(4):412–419.
65. Lindblad B, Persson NH, Takolander R, et al. Does low-dose acetylsalicylic acid prevent stroke after carotid surgery? A double-blind, placebo-controlled randomized trial. *Stroke.* 1993;24(8):1125–1128.
66. De Martino RR, Beck AW, Hoel AW, et al. Preoperative antiplatelet and statin treatment was not associated with reduced myocardial infarction after high-risk vascular operations in the Vascular Quality Initiative. *J Vasc Surg.* 2016;63(1):182–189.e2.
67. Devereaux PJ, Mrkobrada M, Sessler DI, et al. Aspirin in patients undergoing noncardiac surgery. *N Engl J Med.* 2014;370(16):1494–1503.
68. Stone DH, Goodney PP, Schanzer A, et al. Clopidogrel is not associated with major bleeding complications during peripheral arterial surgery. *J Vasc Surg.* 2011;54(3):779–784.
69. Gualandro DM, Campos CA, Calderaro D, et al. Coronary plaque rupture in patients with myocardial infarction after noncardiac surgery: frequent and dangerous. *Atherosclerosis.* 2012;222(1):191–195.
70. Van den Berghe G, Wilmer A, Hermans G, et al. Intensive insulin therapy in the medical ICU. *N Engl J Med.* 2006;354(5):449–461.
71. Finfer S, Chittock DR, Su SY, et al. Intensive versus conventional glucose control in critically ill patients. *N Engl J Med.* 2009;360(13):1283–1297.
72. Griesdale DE, de Souza RJ, van Dam RM, et al. Intensive insulin therapy and mortality among critically ill patients: a meta-analysis including NICE-SUGAR study data. *CMAJ.* 2009;180(8):821–827.
73. Duncan AE, Abd-Elsayed A, Maheshwari A, et al. Role of intraoperative and postoperative blood glucose concentrations in predicting outcomes after cardiac surgery. *Anesthesiology.* 2010;112(4):860–871.
74. Nelson AH, Fleisher LA, Rosenbaum SH. Relationship between postoperative anemia and cardiac morbidity in high-risk vascular patients in the intensive care unit. *Crit Care Med.* 1993;21(6):860–866.
75. Hebert PC, Wells G, Blajchman MA, et al. A multicenter, randomized, controlled clinical trial of transfusion requirements in critical care. Transfusion Requirements in Critical Care Investigators, Canadian Critical Care Trials Group. *N Engl J Med.* 1999;340(6):409–417.
76. Carson JL, Terrin ML, Noveck H, et al. Liberal or restrictive transfusion in high-risk patients after hip surgery. *N Engl J Med.* 2011;365(26):2453–2462.
77. Obi AT, Park YJ, Bove P, et al. The association of perioperative transfusion with 30-day morbidity and mortality in patients undergoing major vascular surgery. *J Vasc Surg.* 2015;61(4):1000–1009.e1.
78. Frank SM, Fleisher LA, Breslow MJ, et al. Perioperative maintenance of normothermia reduces the incidence of morbid cardiac events: a randomized clinical trial. *JAMA.* 1997;277(14):1127–1134.
79. Rajagopalan S, Mascha E, Na J, et al. The effects of mild perioperative hypothermia on blood loss and transfusion requirement. *Anesthesiology.* 2008;108(1):71–77.
80. Foster ED, Davis KB, Carpenter JA, et al. Risk of noncardiac operation in patients with defined coronary disease: the Coronary Artery Surgery Study (CASS) registry experience. *Ann Thorac Surg.* 1986;41(1):42–50.
81. Eagle KA, Rihal CS, Mickel MC, et al. Cardiac risk of noncardiac surgery: influence of coronary disease and type of surgery in 3368 operations. CASS Investigators and University of Michigan Heart Care Program. Coronary Artery Surgery Study. *Circulation.* 1997;96(6):1882–1887.
82. Monaco M, Stassano P, Di Tommaso L, et al. Systematic strategy of prophylactic coronary angiography improves long-term outcome after major vascular surgery in medium- to high-risk patients: a prospective, randomized study. *J Am Coll Cardiol.* 2009;54(11):989–996.
83. McFalls EO, Ward HB, Moritz TE, et al. Coronary-artery revascularization before elective major vascular surgery. *N Engl J Med.* 2004;351(27):2795–2804.
84. Ward HB, Kelly RF, Thottapurathu L, et al. Coronary artery bypass grafting is superior to percutaneous coronary intervention in prevention of perioperative myocardial infarctions during subsequent vascular surgery. *Ann Thorac Surg.* 2006;82(3):795–800.

85. Garcia S, Moritz TE, Ward HB, et al. Usefulness of revascularization of patients with multivessel coronary artery disease before elective vascular surgery for abdominal aortic and peripheral occlusive disease. *Am J Cardiol*. 2008;102(7):809–813.
86. Hillis LD, Smith PK, Anderson JL, et al. 2011 ACCF/AHA Guideline for Coronary Artery Bypass Graft Surgery: a report of the American College of Cardiology Foundation/American Heart Association Task Force on Practice Guidelines. Developed in collaboration with the American Association for Thoracic Surgery, Society of Cardiovascular Anesthesiologists, and Society of Thoracic Surgeons. *J Am Coll Cardiol*. 2011;58(24):e123–e210.
87. Levine GN, Bates ER, Blankenship JC, et al. 2011 ACCF/AHA/SCAI Guideline for Percutaneous Coronary Intervention: executive summary: a report of the American College of Cardiology Foundation/American Heart Association Task Force on Practice Guidelines and the Society for Cardiovascular Angiography and Interventions. *Catheter Cardiovasc Interv*. 2012;79(3):453–495.
88. Livhits M, Ko CY, Leonardi MJ, et al. Risk of surgery following recent myocardial infarction. *Ann Surg*. 2011;253(5):857–864.
89. Livhits M, Gibbons MM, de Virgilio C, et al. Coronary revascularization after myocardial infarction can reduce risks of noncardiac surgery. *J Am Coll Surg*. 2011;212(6):1018–1026.
90. Levine GN, Bates ER, Bittl JA, et al. 2016 ACC/AHA Guideline Focused Update on Duration of Dual Antiplatelet Therapy in Patients With Coronary Artery Disease: A Report of the American College of Cardiology/American Heart Association Task Force on Clinical Practice Guidelines. *J Am Coll Cardiol*. 2016;68(10):1082–115.
91. Zarinsefat A, Henke P. Update in preoperative risk assessment in vascular surgery patients. *J Vasc Surg*. 2015;62(2):499–509.
92. Simons JP, Baril DT, Goodney PP, et al. The effect of postoperative myocardial ischemia on long-term survival after vascular surgery. *J Vasc Surg*. 2013;58(6):1600–1608.
93. Bilimoria KY, Liu Y, Paruch JL, et al. Development and evaluation of the universal ACS NSQIP surgical risk calculator: a decision aid and informed consent tool for patients and surgeons. *J Am Coll Surg*. 2013;217(5):833–842.e1–e3.
94. Ford MK, Beattie WS, Wijeysundera DN. Systematic review: prediction of perioperative cardiac complications and mortality by the revised cardiac risk index. *Ann Intern Med*. 2010;152(1):26–35.
95. Bertges DJ, Goodney PP, Zhao Y, et al. The Vascular Study Group of New England Cardiac Risk Index (VSG-CRI) predicts cardiac complications more accurately than the Revised Cardiac Risk Index in vascular surgery patients. *J Vasc Surg*. 2010;52(3):674–683, 83.e1–83.e3.
96. Gouya G, Arrich J, Wolzt M, et al. Antiplatelet treatment for prevention of cerebrovascular events in patients with vascular diseases: a systematic review and meta-analysis. *Stroke*. 2014;45(2):492–503.
97. Johnston SC, Fayad PB, Gorelick PB, et al. Prevalence and knowledge of transient ischemic attack among US adults. *Neurology*. 2003;60(9):1429–1434.
98. Tsantilas P, Kuhnl A, Kallmayer M, et al. Stroke risk in the early period after carotid related symptoms: a systematic review. *J Cardiovasc Surg*. 2015;56(6):845–852.
99. Wu CM, McLaughlin K, Lorenzetti DL, et al. Early risk of stroke after transient ischemic attack: a systematic review and meta-analysis. *Arch Intern Med*. 2007;167(22):2417–2422.
100. Beneficial effect of carotid endarterectomy in symptomatic patients with high-grade carotid stenosis. *N Engl J Med*. 1991;325(7):445–453.
101. Barnett HJ, Taylor DW, Eliasziw M, et al. Benefit of carotid endarterectomy in patients with symptomatic moderate or severe stenosis. North American Symptomatic Carotid Endarterectomy Trial Collaborators. *N Engl J Med*. 1998;339(20):1415–1425.
102. Randomised trial of endarterectomy for recently symptomatic carotid stenosis: final results of the MRC European Carotid Surgery Trial (ECST). *Lancet*. 1998;351(9113):1379–1387.
103. Hobson RW II, Weiss DG, Fields WS, et al. Efficacy of carotid endarterectomy for asymptomatic carotid stenosis. The Veterans Affairs Cooperative Study Group. *N Engl J Med*. 1993;328(4):221–227.
104. Rothwell PM, Eliasziw M, Gutnikov SA, et al. Analysis of pooled data from the randomised controlled trials of endarterectomy for symptomatic carotid stenosis. *Lancet*. 2003;361(9352):107–116.
105. Rerkasem K, Rothwell PM. Carotid endarterectomy for symptomatic carotid stenosis. *Cochrane Database Syst Rev*. 2011;(4):Cd001081.
106. Walker MD, Marler JR, Goldstein M, et al. Endarterectomy for Asymptomatic Carotid Artery Stenosis. *JAMA*. 1995;273(18):1421–1428.
107. Halliday A, Mansfield A, Marro J, et al. Prevention of disabling and fatal strokes by successful carotid endarterectomy in patients without recent neurological symptoms: randomised controlled trial. *Lancet*. 2004;363(9420):1491–1502.
108. Halliday A, Harrison M, Hayter E, et al. 10-year stroke prevention after successful carotid endarterectomy for asymptomatic stenosis (ACST-1): a multicentre randomised trial. *Lancet*. 2010;376(9746):1074–1084.
109. Chambers BR, Donnan GA. Carotid endarterectomy for asymptomatic carotid stenosis. *Cochrane Database Syst Rev*. 2005;(4):Cd001923.
110. Rothwell PM, Eliasziw M, Gutnikov SA, et al. Endarterectomy for symptomatic carotid stenosis in relation to clinical subgroups and timing of surgery. *Lancet*. 2004;363(9413):915–924.
111. Johnston SC, Gress DR, Browner WS, et al. Short-term prognosis after emergency department diagnosis of TIA. *JAMA*. 2000;284(22):2901–2906.
112. Kernan WN, Ovbiagele B, Black HR, et al. Guidelines for the prevention of stroke in patients with stroke and transient ischemic attack: a guideline for healthcare professionals from the American Heart Association/American Stroke Association. *Stroke*. 2014;45(7):2160–2236.
113. Brott TG, Halperin JL, Abbara S, et al. 2011 ASA/ACCF/AHA/AANN/AANS/ACR/ASNR/CNS/SAIP/SCAI/SIR/SNIS/SVM/SVS guideline on the management of patients with extracranial carotid and vertebral artery disease: executive summary: a report of the American College of Cardiology Foundation/American Heart Association Task Force on Practice Guidelines, and the American Stroke Association, American Association of Neuroscience Nurses, American Association of Neurological Surgeons, American College of Radiology, American Society of Neuroradiology, Congress of Neurological Surgeons, Society of Atherosclerosis Imaging and Prevention, Society for Cardiovascular Angiography and Interventions, Society of Interventional Radiology, Society of NeuroInterventional Surgery, Society for Vascular Medicine, and Society for Vascular Surgery. *J Am Coll Cardiol*. 2011;57(8):1002–1044.
114. Chimowitz MI, Poole RM, Starling MR, et al. Frequency and severity of asymptomatic coronary disease in patients with different causes of stroke. *Stroke*. 1997;28(5):941–945.
115. Venkatachalam S, Shishehbor MH. Management of carotid disease in patients undergoing coronary artery bypass surgery: is it time to change our approach? *Curr Opin Cardiol*. 2011;26(6):480–487.
116. Iqbal S. A comprehensive study of the anatomical variations of the circle of willis in adult human brains. *J Clin Diagnost Res*. 2013;7(11):2423–2427.
117. Modica PA, Tempelhoff R, Rich KM, et al. Computerized electroencephalographic monitoring and selective shunting: influence on intraoperative administration of phenylephrine and myocardial infarction after general anesthesia for carotid endarterectomy. *Neurosurgery*. 1992;30(6):842–846.
118. Aburahma AF, Mousa AY, Stone PA. Shunting during carotid endarterectomy. *J Vasc Surg*. 2011;54(5):1502–1510.
119. Chongruksut W, Vaniyapong T, Rerkasem K. Routine or selective carotid artery shunting for carotid endarterectomy (and different methods of monitoring in selective shunting). *Cochrane Database Syst Rev*. 2014;6:Cd000190.
120. Apinis A, Sehgal S, Leff J. Intraoperative management of carotid endarterectomy. *Anesthesiol Clin*. 2014;32(3):677–698.
121. Guarracino F. Cerebral monitoring during cardiovascular surgery. *Curr Opin Anaesthesiol*. 2008;21(1):50–54.
122. Foreman B, Claassen J. Quantitative EEG for the detection of brain ischemia. *Crit Care (Lond)*. 2012;16(2):216.
123. Hans SS, Jareunpoon O. Prospective evaluation of electroencephalography, carotid artery stump pressure, and neurologic changes during 314 consecutive carotid endarterectomies performed in awake patients. *J Vasc Surg*. 2007;45(3):511–515.
124. Moritz S, Kasprzak P, Arlt M, et al. Accuracy of cerebral monitoring in detecting cerebral ischemia during carotid endarterectomy: a comparison of transcranial Doppler sonography, near-infrared spectroscopy, stump pressure, and somatosensory evoked potentials. *Anesthesiology*. 2007;107(4):563–569.
125. Malcharek MJ, Ulkatan S, Marino V, et al. Intraoperative monitoring of carotid endarterectomy by transcranial motor evoked potential: a multicenter study of 600 patients. *Clin Neurophysiol*. 2013;124(5):1025–1030.
126. Costin M, Rampersad A, Solomon RA, et al. Cerebral injury predicted by transcranial Doppler ultrasonography but not electroencephalography during carotid endarterectomy. *J Neurosurg Anesthesiol*. 2002;14(4):287–292.
127. Pennekamp CW, Moll FL, De Borst GJ. Role of transcranial Doppler in cerebral hyperperfusion syndrome. *J Cardiovasc Surg*. 2012;53(6):765–771.
128. Calligaro KD, Dougherty MJ. Correlation of carotid artery stump pressure and neurologic changes during 474 carotid endarterectomies performed in awake patients. *J Vasc Surg*. 2005;42(4):684–689.
129. Ritter JC, Green D, Slim H, et al. The role of cerebral oximetry in combination with awake testing in patients undergoing carotid endarterectomy under local anaesthesia. *Eur J Vasc Endovasc Surg*. 2011;41(5):599–605.
130. Stilo F, Spinelli F, Martelli E, et al. The sensibility and specificity of cerebral oximetry, measured by INVOS - 4100, in patients undergoing carotid endarterectomy compared with awake testing. *Minerva Anestesiol*. 2012;78(10):1126–1135.
131. Pandit JJ, Satya-Krishna R, Gration P. Superficial or deep cervical plexus block for carotid endarterectomy: a systematic review of complications. *Br J Anesth*. 2007;99(2):159–169.
132. Lewis SC, Warlow CP, Bodenham AR, et al. General anaesthesia versus local anaesthesia for carotid surgery (GALA): a multicentre, randomised controlled trial. *Lancet*. 2008;372(9656):2132–2142.
133. Vaniyapong T, Chongruksut W, Rerkasem K. Local versus general anaesthesia for carotid endarterectomy. *Cochrane Database Syst Rev*. 2013;12:Cd000126.
134. Mutch WA, White IW, Donen N, et al. Haemodynamic instability and myocardial ischaemia during carotid endarterectomy: a comparison of propofol and isoflurane. *Can J Anaesth*. 1995;42(7):577–587.

135. Jellish WS, Sheikh T, Baker WH, et al. Hemodynamic stability, myocardial ischemia, and perioperative outcome after carotid surgery with remifentanil/propofol or isoflurane/fentanyl anesthesia. *J Neurosurg Anesthesiol.* 2003;15(3):176–184.
136. Umbrain V, Keeris J, D'Haese J, et al. Isoflurane, desflurane and sevoflurane for carotid endarterectomy. *Anaesthesia.* 2000;55(11):1052–1057.
137. Ralley FE, Wynands JE, Ramsay JG, et al. The effects of shivering on oxygen consumption and carbon dioxide production in patients rewarming from hypothermic cardiopulmonary bypass. *Can J Anaesth.* 1988;35(4):332–337.
138. Lipsett PA, Tierney S, Gordon TA, et al. Carotid endarterectomy: is intensive care unit care necessary? *J Vasc Surg.* 1994;20(3):403–409.
139. Naylor AR, Sayers RD, McCarthy MJ, et al. Closing the loop; a 21-year audit of strategies for preventing stroke and death following carotid endarterectomy. *Eur J Vasc Endovasc Surg.* 2013;46(2):161–170.
140. van Mook WN, Rennenberg RJ, Schurink GW, et al. Cerebral hyperperfusion syndrome. *Lancet Neurol.* 2005;4(12):877–888.
141. Boulanger M, Cameliere L, Felgueiras R, et al. Periprocedural myocardial infarction after carotid endarterectomy and stenting: systematic review and meta-analysis. *Stroke.* 2015;46(10):2843–2848.
142. Kuivaniemi H, Elmore JR. Opportunities in abdominal aortic aneurysm research: epidemiology, genetics, and pathophysiology. *Ann Vasc Surg.* 2012;26(6):862–870.
143. Bickerstaff LK, Pairolero PC, Hollier LH, et al. Thoracic aortic aneurysms: a population-based study. *Surgery.* 1982;92(6):1103–1108.
144. Olsen PS, Schroeder T, Agerskov K, et al. Surgery for abdominal aortic aneurysms: a survey of 656 patients. *J Cardiovasc Surg.* 1991;32(5):636–642.
145. Wassef M, Baxter BT, Chisholm RL, et al. Pathogenesis of abdominal aortic aneurysms: a multidisciplinary research program supported by the National Heart, Lung, and Blood Institute. *J Vasc Surg.* 2001;34(4):730–738.
146. Guirguis EM, Barber GG. The natural history of abdominal aortic aneurysms. *Am J Surg.* 1991;162(5):481–483.
147. Chaikof EL, Brewster DC, Dalman RL, et al. The care of patients with an abdominal aortic aneurysm: the Society for Vascular Surgery practice guidelines. *J Vasc Surg.* 2009;50(4 Suppl):S2–S49.
148. Elefteriades JA. Natural history of thoracic aortic aneurysms: indications for surgery, and surgical versus nonsurgical risks. *Ann Thorac Surg.* 2002;74(5):S1877–S1880.
149. Kent KC. Clinical practice. Abdominal aortic aneurysms. *N Engl J Med.* 2014;371(22):2101–2108.
150. Meszaros I, Morocz J, Szlavi J, et al. Epidemiology and clinicopathology of aortic dissection. *Chest.* 2000;117(5):1271–1278.
151. Trimarchi S, Tsai T, Eagle KA, et al. Acute abdominal aortic dissection: insight from the International Registry of Acute Aortic Dissection (IRAD). *J Vasc Surg.* 2007;46(5):913–919.
152. Gelman S. The pathophysiology of aortic cross-clamping and unclamping. *Anesthesiology.* 1995;82(4):1026–1060.
153. Roizen MF, Beaupre PN, Alpert RA, et al. Monitoring with two-dimensional transesophageal echocardiography: comparison of myocardial function in patients undergoing supraceliac, suprarenal-infraceliac, or infrarenal aortic occlusion. *J Vasc Surg.* 1984;1(2):300–305.
154. Gelman S, Reves JG, Fowler K, et al. Regional blood flow during cross-clamping of the thoracic aorta and infusion of sodium nitroprusside. *J Thorac Cardiovasc Surg.* 1983;85(2):287–291.
155. Brinkman R, HayGlass KT, Mutch WA, et al. Acute kidney injury in patients undergoing open abdominal aortic aneurysm repair: a pilot observational trial. *J Cardiothorac Vasc Anesth.* 2015;29(5):1212–1219.
156. Sheinbaum R, Ignacio C, Safi HJ, et al. Contemporary strategies to preserve renal function during cardiac and vascular surgery. *Rev Cardiovasc Med.* 2003;4(Suppl 1):S21–S28.
157. Wahlberg E, Dimuzio PJ, Stoney RJ. Aortic clamping during elective operations for infrarenal disease: The influence of clamping time on renal function. *J Vasc Surg.* 2002;36(1):13–18.
158. Hersey P, Poullis M. Does the administration of mannitol prevent renal failure in open abdominal aortic aneurysm surgery? *Interact Cardiovasc Thorac Surg.* 2008;7(5):906–909.
159. Alpert RA, Roizen MF, Hamilton WK, et al. Intraoperative urinary output does not predict postoperative renal function in patients undergoing abdominal aortic revascularization. *Surgery.* 1984;95(6):707–711.
160. Oliver WC Jr, Nuttall GA, Cherry KJ, et al. A comparison of fenoldopam with dopamine and sodium nitroprusside in patients undergoing cross-clamping of the abdominal aorta. *Anesth Analg.* 2006;103(4):833–840.
161. Bove T, Zangrillo A, Guarracino F, et al. Effect of fenoldopam on use of renal replacement therapy among patients with acute kidney injury after cardiac surgery: a randomized clinical trial. *JAMA.* 2014;312(21):2244–2253.
162. Ali ZA, Callaghan CJ, Lim E, et al. Remote ischemic preconditioning reduces myocardial and renal injury after elective abdominal aortic aneurysm repair: a randomized controlled trial. *Circulation.* 2007;116(11 Suppl):I98–105.
163. Sinha AC, Cheung AT. Spinal cord protection and thoracic aortic surgery. *Curr Opin Anaesthesiol.* 2010;23(1):95–102.
164. Robertazzi RR, Cunningham JN Jr. Intraoperative adjuncts of spinal cord protection. *Semin Thorac Cardiovasc Surg.* 1998;10(1):29–34.
165. Ballard JL, Yonemoto H, Killeen JD. Cost-effective aortic exposure: a retroperitoneal experience. *Ann Vasc Surg.* 2000;14(1):1–5.
166. Horlocker TT, Wedel DJ, Rowlingson JC, et al. Regional anesthesia in the patient receiving antithrombotic or thrombolytic therapy: American Society of Regional Anesthesia and Pain Medicine Evidence-Based Guidelines (Third Edition). *Reg Anesth Pain Med.* 2010;35(1):64–101.
167. Sandham JD, Hull RD, Brant RF, et al. A randomized, controlled trial of the use of pulmonary-artery catheters in high-risk surgical patients. *N Engl J Med.* 2003;348(1):5–14.
168. Heringlake M, Sondermund-Adib B, Grossherr M, et al. [The use of a pulmonary artery catheter does not increase mortality in critical cancer care and can reduce the mortality of high-risk surgical patients]. *Der Anaesthesist.* 2007;56(3):275–276.
169. Berlauk JF, Abrams JH, Gilmour IJ, et al. Preoperative optimization of cardiovascular hemodynamics improves outcome in peripheral vascular surgery: a prospective, randomized clinical trial. *Ann Surg.* 1991;214(3):289–297.
170. Tanaka K, Ludwig LM, Kersten JR, et al. Mechanisms of cardioprotection by volatile anesthetics. *Anesthesiology.* 2004;100(3):707–721.
171. Conte MS, Pomposelli FB, Clair DG, et al. Society for Vascular Surgery practice guidelines for atherosclerotic occlusive disease of the lower extremities: management of asymptomatic disease and claudication. *J Vasc Surg.* 2015;61(3 Suppl):2s–41s.
172. Rooke TW, Hirsch AT, Misra S, et al. Management of patients with peripheral artery disease (compilation of 2005 and 2011 ACCF/AHA Guideline Recommendations): a report of the American College of Cardiology Foundation/American Heart Association Task Force on Practice Guidelines. *J Am Coll Cardiol.* 2013;61(14):1555–1570.
173. Hirsch AT, Haskal ZJ, Hertzer NR, et al. ACC/AHA 2005 Practice Guidelines for the management of patients with peripheral arterial disease (lower extremity, renal, mesenteric, and abdominal aortic): a collaborative report from the American Association for Vascular Surgery/Society for Vascular Surgery, Society for Cardiovascular Angiography and Interventions, Society for Vascular Medicine and Biology, Society of Interventional Radiology, and the ACC/AHA Task Force on Practice Guidelines (Writing Committee to Develop Guidelines for the Management of Patients With Peripheral Arterial Disease): endorsed by the American Association of Cardiovascular and Pulmonary Rehabilitation; National Heart, Lung, and Blood Institute; Society for Vascular Nursing; TransAtlantic Inter-Society Consensus; and Vascular Disease Foundation. *Circulation.* 2006;113(11):e463–e654.
174. Passman MA, Taylor LM, Moneta GL, et al. Comparison of axillofemoral and aortofemoral bypass for aortoiliac occlusive disease. *J Vasc Surg.* 1996;23(2):263–269.
175. Singh N, Sidawy AN, Dezee K, et al. The effects of the type of anesthesia on outcomes of lower extremity infrainguinal bypass. *J Vasc Surg.* 2006;44(5):964–968.
176. Ghanami RJ, Hurie J, Andrews JS, et al. Anesthesia-based evaluation of outcomes of lower-extremity vascular bypass procedures. *Ann Vasc Surg.* 2013;27(2):199–207.
177. Barbosa FT, Juca MJ, Castro AA, Cavalcante JC. Neuraxial anaesthesia for lower-limb revascularization. *Cochrane Database Syst Rev.* 2013;7:Cd007083.
178. Bode RH Jr, Lewis KP, Zarich SW, et al. Cardiac outcome after peripheral vascular surgery. Comparison of general and regional anesthesia. *Anesthesiology.* 1996;84(1):3–13.
179. LaMuraglia GM, Conrad MF, Chung T, et al. Significant perioperative morbidity accompanies contemporary infrainguinal bypass surgery: an NSQIP report. *J Vasc Surg.* 2009;50(2):299–304.e1–e4.
180. Mas JL, Trinquart L, Leys D, et al. Endarterectomy Versus Angioplasty in Patients with Symptomatic Severe Carotid Stenosis (EVA-3S) trial: results up to 4 years from a randomised, multicentre trial. *Lancet Neurol.* 2008;7(10):885–892.
181. Gurm HS, Yadav JS, Fayad P, et al. Long-term results of carotid stenting versus endarterectomy in high-risk patients. *N Engl J Med.* 2008;358(15):1572–1579.
182. Eckstein HH, Ringleb P, Allenberg JR, et al. Results of the Stent-Protected Angioplasty versus Carotid Endarterectomy (SPACE) study to treat symptomatic stenoses at 2 years: a multinational, prospective, randomised trial. *Lancet Neurol.* 2008;7(10):893–902.
183. Bonati LH, Dobson J, Featherstone RL, et al. Long-term outcomes after stenting versus endarterectomy for treatment of symptomatic carotid stenosis: the International Carotid Stenting Study (ICSS) randomised trial. *Lancet.* 2015;385(9967):529–538.
184. Brott TG, Hobson RW II, Howard G, et al. Stenting versus endarterectomy for treatment of carotid-artery stenosis. *N Engl J Med.* 2010;363(1):11–23.
185. Bonati LH, Lyrer P, Ederle J, et al. Percutaneous transluminal balloon angioplasty and stenting for carotid artery stenosis. *Cochrane Database Syst Rev.* 2012;9:Cd000515.
186. Kuliha M, Roubec M, Prochazka V, et al. Randomized clinical trial comparing neurological outcomes after carotid endarterectomy or stenting. *Br J Surg.* 2015;102(3):194–201.
187. Kwolek CJ, Jaff MR, Leal JI, et al. Results of the ROADSTER multicenter trial of transcarotid stenting with dynamic flow reversal. *J Vasc Surg.* 2015;62(5):1227–1234.e1.

188. Dumont TM, Rughani AI. National trends in carotid artery revascularization surgery. *J Neurosurg.* 2012;115(6):1251–1257.
189. Parodi JC, Palmaz JC, Barone HD. Transfemoral intraluminal graft implantation for abdominal aortic aneurysms. *Ann Vasc Surg.* 1991;5(6):491–499.
190. Dua A, Kuy S, Lee CJ, et al. Epidemiology of aortic aneurysm repair in the United States from 2000 to 2010. *J Vasc Surg.* 2014;59(6):1512–1517.
191. Sethi RK, Henry AJ, Hevelone ND, et al. Impact of hospital market competition on endovascular aneurysm repair adoption and outcomes. *J Vasc Surg.* 2013;58(3):596–606.
192. Singh M, Hager E, Avgerinos E, et al. Choosing the correct treatment for acute aortic type B dissection. *J Cardiovasc Surg.* 2015;56(2):217–229.
193. De Bruin JL, Baas AF, Buth J, et al. Long-term outcome of open or endovascular repair of abdominal aortic aneurysm. *N Engl J Med.* 2010;362(20):1881–1889.
194. Greenhalgh RM, Brown LC, Powell JT, et al. Endovascular versus open repair of abdominal aortic aneurysm. *N Engl J Med.* 2010;362(20):1863–1871.
195. Becquemin JP, Pillet JC, Lescalie F, et al. A randomized controlled trial of endovascular aneurysm repair versus open surgery for abdominal aortic aneurysms in low- to moderate-risk patients. *J Vasc Surg.* 2011;53(5):1167–1173.e1.
196. Lederle FA, Freischlag JA, Kyriakides TC, et al. Long-term comparison of endovascular and open repair of abdominal aortic aneurysm. *N Engl J Med.* 2012;367(21):1988–1997.
197. Paravastu SC, Jayarajasingam R, Cottam R, et al. Endovascular repair of abdominal aortic aneurysm. *Cochrane Database Syst Rev.* 2014;1:Cd004178.
198. Siracuse JJ, Gill HL, Graham AR, et al. Comparative safety of endovascular and open surgical repair of abdominal aortic aneurysms in low-risk male patients. *J Vasc Surg.* 2014;60(5):1154–1158.
199. Greenhalgh RM, Brown LC, Powell JT, et al. Endovascular repair of aortic aneurysm in patients physically ineligible for open repair. *N Engl J Med.* 2010;362(20):1872–1880.
200. Bush RL, Mureebe L, Bohannon WT, et al. The impact of recent European trials on abdominal aortic aneurysm repair: is a paradigm shift warranted? *J Surg Res.* 2008;148(2):264–271.
201. Sobocinski J, Maurel B, Delsart P, et al. Should we modify our indications after the EVAR-2 trial conclusions? *Ann Vasc Surg.* 2011;25(5):590–597.
202. Egorova N, Giacovelli JK, Gelijns A, et al. Defining high-risk patients for endovascular aneurysm repair. *J Vasc Surg.* 2009;50(6):1271–1279.e1.
203. Giles KA, Schermerhorn ML, O'Malley AJ, et al. Risk prediction for perioperative mortality of endovascular vs open repair of abdominal aortic aneurysms using the Medicare population. *J Vasc Surg.* 2009;50(2):256–262.
204. Barnes M, Boult M, Maddern G, et al. A model to predict outcomes for endovascular aneurysm repair using preoperative variables. *Eur J Vasc Endovasc Surg.* 2008;35(5):571–579.
205. Katsargyris A, Oikonomou K, Klonaris C, et al. Comparison of outcomes with open, fenestrated, and chimney graft repair of juxtarenal aneurysms: are we ready for a paradigm shift? *J Endovasc Ther.* 2013;20(2):159–169.
206. Di X, Ye W, Liu CW, et al. Fenestrated endovascular repair for pararenal abdominal aortic aneurysms: a systematic review and meta-analysis. *Ann Vasc Surg.* 2013;27(8):1190–1200.
207. Wilson A, Zhou S, Bachoo P, et al. Systematic review of chimney and periscope grafts for endovascular aneurysm repair. *Br J Surg.* 2013;100(12):1557–1564.
208. Ruppert V, Leurs LJ, Steckmeier B, et al. Influence of anesthesia type on outcome after endovascular aortic aneurysm repair: an analysis based on EUROSTAR data. *J Vasc Surg.* 2006;44(1):16–21; discussion 21.
209. Edwards MS, Andrews JS, Edwards AF, et al. Results of endovascular aortic aneurysm repair with general, regional, and local/monitored anesthesia care in the American College of Surgeons National Surgical Quality Improvement Program database. *J Vasc Surg.* 2011;54(5):1273–1282.
210. Karthikesalingam A, Thrumurthy SG, Young EL, et al. Locoregional anesthesia for endovascular aneurysm repair. *J Vasc Surg.* 2012;56(2):510–519.
211. Chen J, Stavropoulos SW. Management of endoleaks. *Semin Interv Radiol.* 2015;32(3):259–264.
212. Ilyas S, Shaida N, Thakor AS, et al. Endovascular aneurysm repair (EVAR) follow-up imaging: the assessment and treatment of common postoperative complications. *Clinical radiology.* 2015;70(2):183–196.
213. van Marrewijk C, Buth J, Harris PL, et al. Significance of endoleaks after endovascular repair of abdominal aortic aneurysms: The EUROSTAR experience. *J Vasc Surg.* 2002;35(3):461–473.
214. Kouvelos G, Koutsoumpelis A, Lazaris A, et al. Late open conversion after endovascular abdominal aortic aneurysm repair. *J Vasc Surg.* 2015;61(5):1350–1356.
215. Goodney PP, Beck AW, Nagle J, et al. National trends in lower extremity bypass surgery, endovascular interventions, and major amputations. *J Vasc Surg.* 2009;50(1):54–60.
216. Jaff MR, White CJ, Hiatt WR, et al. An update on methods for revascularization and expansion of the tasc lesion classification to include below-the-knee arteries: a supplement to the Inter-Society Consensus for the Management of Peripheral Arterial Disease (TASC II). *J Endovasc Ther.* 2015;22(5):663–677.
217. Leville CD, Kashyap VS, Clair DG, et al. Endovascular management of iliac artery occlusions: extending treatment to TransAtlantic Inter-Society Consensus class C and D patients. *J Vasc Surg.* 2006;43(1):32–39.
218. Indes JE, Pfaff MJ, Farrokhyar F, et al. Clinical outcomes of 5358 patients undergoing direct open bypass or endovascular treatment for aortoiliac occlusive disease: a systematic review and meta-analysis. *J Endovasc Ther.* 2013;20(4):443–455.
219. Jongkind V, Akkersdijk GJ, Yeung KK, et al. A systematic review of endovascular treatment of extensive aortoiliac occlusive disease. *J Vasc Surg.* 2010;52(5):1376–1383.
220. Adam DJ, Beard JD, Cleveland T, et al. Bypass versus angioplasty in severe ischaemia of the leg (BASIL): multicentre, randomised controlled trial. *Lancet.* 2005;366(9501):1925–1934.
221. Bradbury AW, Adam DJ, Bell J, et al. Bypass versus Angioplasty in Severe Ischaemia of the Leg (BASIL) trial: an intention-to-treat analysis of amputation-free and overall survival in patients randomized to a bypass surgery-first or a balloon angioplasty-first revascularization strategy. *J Vasc Surg.* 2010;51(5 Suppl):5s–17s.
222. Antoniou GA, Chalmers N, Kanesalingham K, et al. Meta-analysis of outcomes of endovascular treatment of infrapopliteal occlusive disease with drug-eluting stents. *J Endovasc Ther.* 2013;20(2):131–144.

41 Obstetric Anesthesia

FERNE R. BRAVEMAN • BARBARA M. SCAVONE • MARCELLE E. BLESSING • CYNTHIA A. WONG

Physiologic Changes of Pregnancy
   Hematologic Alterations
   Cardiovascular Changes
   Respiratory Changes
   Metabolism
   Gastrointestinal Changes
   Altered Drug Responses

Placental Transfer and Fetal Exposure to Anesthetic Drugs
   Placenta
   Hemodynamic Factors
   Fetus and Newborn

Analgesia for Labor and Vaginal Delivery
   Nonpharmacologic Methods of Labor Analgesia
   Systemic Medication
   Regional Analgesia

Anesthesia for Cesarean Delivery
   Neuraxial Anesthesia
   General Anesthesia

Anesthetic Complications
   Maternal Mortality
   Pulmonary Aspiration
   Hypotension
   Total Spinal Anesthesia
   Local Anesthetic Systemic Toxicity
   Postdural Puncture Headache
   Nerve Injury

Management of High-risk Parturients
   Hypertensive Disorders of Pregnancy
   Obstetric Hemorrhage
   Heart Disease
   Diabetes Mellitus
   Obesity
   Advanced Maternal Age

Preterm Delivery

Substance Abuse
   Tobacco Abuse
   Alcohol
   Opioids
   Marijuana
   Cocaine
   Amphetamines

Fetal Monitoring
   Electronic Fetal Monitoring
   Ancillary Tests and Fetal Pulse Oximetry

Newborn Resuscitation in the Delivery Room
   Fetal Asphyxia
   Neonatal Adaptations at Birth
   Resuscitation
   The APGAR Score
   Diagnostic Procedures

Anesthesia for Nonobstetric Surgery in Pregnant Women
   Practical Suggestions

KEY POINTS

1. As oxygen consumption increases during pregnancy, the maternal cardiovascular system adapts to meet the metabolic demands of a growing fetus.
2. Airway edema may be particularly severe in women with preeclampsia, in patients placed in the Trendelenburg position for prolonged periods, in those who have pushed during the second stage of labor, or with concurrent use of tocolytic agents.
3. A rapid-sequence induction of anesthesia, application of cricoid pressure, and intubation with a cuffed endotracheal tube are recommended for all pregnant women receiving general anesthesia after 20 weeks of gestation.
4. The driving force for placental drug transfer is the concentration gradient of free drug between the maternal and fetal blood.
5. Labor analgesia may benefit mother and fetus and should not be withheld if requested.
6. Although the case-fatality rate (maternal mortality) with general anesthesia remains greater than that with neuraxial anesthesia, in recent years, mortality during general anesthesia has decreased while mortality during neuraxial anesthesia has increased.
7. By virtue of age and gender as well as reduced epidural pressure after delivery, pregnant women are at a higher risk for developing postdural puncture headache.
8. Pregnancy and parturition are considered "high risk" when accompanied by conditions unfavorable to the well-being of the mother, fetus, or both.
9. Preeclampsia is considered severe if it is associated with severe hypertension, significant thrombocytopenia, or end-organ damage.
10. Hemorrhage is the leading cause of maternal mortality worldwide.
11. Heart disease during pregnancy is a leading nonobstetric cause of maternal mortality.
12. Obese parturients are more likely to have antenatal comorbidities, which may adversely affect outcome.
13. When a mother requires surgery during pregnancy, there is no data to suggest that any one anesthetic technique is preferred over another, provided oxygenation and blood pressure are maintained and hyperventilation is avoided.

Physiologic Changes of Pregnancy

During pregnancy, there are major alterations in nearly every maternal organ system. These changes are initiated by hormones secreted by the corpus luteum and placenta. The mechanical effects of the enlarging uterus and compression of surrounding structures play an increasing role in the second and third trimesters. This altered physiologic state has relevant implications for the anesthesiologist caring for the pregnant patient. The most relevant changes involving hematologic, cardiovascular, ventilatory, metabolic, and gastrointestinal functions are considered in Table 41-1.

Hematologic Alterations

Increased mineralocorticoid activity during pregnancy produces sodium retention and increased body water content. Thus, plasma volume and total blood volume begin to increase in early gestation, resulting in a final increase of 40% to 50% and 25% to 40%, respectively, at term. The relatively smaller increase in red blood cell volume (20%) accounts for a reduction in hemoglobin concentration (from 12 g/dL to 11 g/dL) and hematocrit (to 35%).[1] Plasma expansion and the resultant relative anemia of pregnancy plateau at approximately 32 to 34 weeks of gestation. The leukocyte count ranges from 8,000 to 10,000/mm^3 throughout pregnancy. Several procoagulant factor levels increase during pregnancy, most notably fibrinogen, which doubles in mass. Anticoagulant activity decreases, as evidenced by decreased protein S concentrations and activated protein C resistance, and fibrinolysis is impaired. Increases in D-dimer and thrombin–antithrombin complexes indicate increased clotting and probable secondary fibrinolysis. Indeed, pregnancy has been referred to as a state of *chronic compensated disseminated intravascular coagulation*.[2,3] These coagulation changes peak at the time of parturition.[4] The platelet count is decreased in pregnant women, due to both dilution and increased consumption, and 6% to 15% of pregnant women at term have a platelet count below 150×10^9/L, compared with only 1% of age-matched nonpregnant controls. A further 1% of women at term have platelet counts below 100×10^9/L.[5]

Table 41-1 Summary of Physiologic Changes of Pregnancy at Term

Variable	Change	Amount
Plasma volume	↑	40–50%
Total blood volume	↑	25–40%
Hemoglobin	↓	11–12 g/dL
Fibrinogen	↑	100%
Serum cholinesterase activity	↓	20–30%
Systemic vascular resistance	↓	50%
Cardiac output	↑	30–50%
Systemic blood pressure	↓	Slight
Functional residual capacity	↓	20–30%
Minute ventilation	↑	50%
Alveolar ventilation	↑	70%
Oxygen consumption	↑	20%
Carbon dioxide production	↑	35%
Arterial carbon dioxide tension	↓	10 mmHg
Arterial oxygen tension	↑	10 mmHg
Minimum alveolar concentration	↓	32–40%

↑, increase; ↓, decrease.

Serum cholinesterase activity declines to a level of 20% below normal by term and reaches a nadir in the puerperium. However, it is doubtful that moderate succinylcholine doses lead to prolonged apnea in otherwise normal circumstances.[6] Although the total amount of protein in the circulation increases, plasma protein concentration declines to below 6 g/dL at term because of dilution from increased plasma volume.[7] The albumin–globulin ratio declines because of the relatively greater reduction in albumin concentration. A decrease in serum protein concentration may be clinically significant because the free fractions of protein-bound drugs can be expected to increase.

Cardiovascular Changes

As oxygen consumption increases during pregnancy, the maternal cardiovascular system adapts to meet the metabolic demands of a growing fetus. Systemic vascular resistance (SVR) declines as maternal vessels lose their responsiveness to angiotensin and other pressors.[8,9] As a result, cardiac output increases by 30% to 50% above that of the nonpregnant state due primarily to a 20% to 50% increase in stroke volume and also to mild elevations in heart rate. Arterial blood pressure decreases slightly because the decrease in peripheral resistance exceeds the increase in cardiac output. Additional increases in cardiac output occur during labor (when cardiac output may reach 12 to 14 L/min) and also in the immediate postpartum period because of added blood volume from the contracted uterus. These changes are exaggerated in multiple gestation pregnancies.[10]

Supine hypotensive syndrome, which affects some women, occurs because the supine position leads to vena cava occlusion and thus decreased preload to the heart, resulting in lowered cardiac output and blood pressure, tachycardia, maternal mental status changes, nausea, and presyncope. From the second trimester, vena cava compression by the enlarged uterus becomes progressively more important, reaching its maximum at 36 to 38 weeks of gestation, after which it may decrease as the fetal head descends into the pelvis.[11] Studies of cardiac output, measured with the patient in the supine position during the last weeks of pregnancy, have indicated a decrease to nonpregnant levels; however, this decrease was not observed when patients were in the lateral decubitus position.[12] Therefore, left uterine displacement by placing a wedge under the right hip or providing left lateral pelvic tilt should be applied routinely during the second and third trimesters of pregnancy; many women may remain susceptible to vena cava compression unless provided with 30 degrees of tilt.[11]

Changes in the electrocardiogram (ECG) may also occur. In addition to heart rate increases, left axis deviation is observed in the third trimester. There is also a tendency toward premature atrial contractions, paroxysmal supraventricular tachycardia, and ventricular dysrhythmias.[13,14]

Respiratory Changes

Respiratory adaptations are necessary for adaptation to increasing metabolic demands, mechanical effects of the enlarging uterus, and cardiovascular changes of pregnancy. Increased extracellular fluid and vascular engorgement and hormonal changes may lead to edema of the upper airway. Many pregnant women complain of difficulty with nasal breathing, and the friable nature of the mucous membranes during pregnancy can cause severe bleeding, especially on insertion of nasopharyngeal airways or nasogastric or endotracheal tubes. Airway edema may be particularly severe in women with preeclampsia, in patients placed in the Trendelenburg position for prolonged periods, or with concurrent use of tocolytic agents. It may also be difficult to perform laryngoscopy in obese or short-necked parturients or those with enlarged breasts. Use of a short-handled laryngoscope may prove helpful. Mallampati scores increase during pregnancy and worsen further throughout labor when oropharyngeal volume also decreases.[15,16]

The diaphragm is displaced cephalad as the uterus increases in size. This is accompanied by an increase in the anteroposterior and transverse diameters of the thoracic cage so that total lung capacity decreases only slightly. From the fifth month, functional residual capacity (FRC) decreases by 20% to 30%, as do its subcomponents, expiratory reserve volume (ERV; 15% to 20%) and residual volume (RV; 20% to 25%). Concomitantly, there is an increase in inspiratory reserve volume. In most pregnant women, a decreased FRC does not cause problems, but those with pre-existing alterations in closing volume as a result of smoking, obesity, or scoliosis may experience early airway closure with advancing pregnancy, leading to hypoxemia. The Trendelenburg and supine positions also exacerbate the abnormal relationship between the closing volume and FRC. The FRC returns to normal shortly after delivery.

Airway resistance usually remains unchanged due to the competing effects of progesterone-induced relaxation of bronchiolar smooth muscle versus factors associated with increased airway resistance such as upper airway edema. Progesterone induces increases in minute ventilation, which increases from the beginning of pregnancy to a maximum of 50% above nonpregnant values at term. This is accomplished by a 30% to 50% increase in tidal volume and a small increase in respiratory rate. Alveolar dead space increases such that the dead space to tidal volume ratio remains unchanged. After delivery, as blood progesterone levels decline, ventilation returns to normal within 1 to 3 weeks.

Metabolism

Basal oxygen consumption increases during early pregnancy, with an overall increase of 20% by term; CO_2 production increases. However, increased alveolar ventilation leads to a reduction in the partial pressure of carbon dioxide in arterial blood (Pa_{CO_2}) to 28 to 32 mmHg and an increase in the partial pressure of oxygen in arterial blood (Pa_{O_2}) to 106 mmHg. The plasma buffer base decreases from 47 to 42 mEq/L; therefore, the pH remains practically unchanged. The maternal uptake and elimination of inhalational anesthetics are enhanced because of increased alveolar ventilation and decreased FRC. Also, the decreased FRC and increased metabolic rate predispose the mother to development of hypoxemia during periods of apnea/hypoventilation, such as may occur during airway obstruction or prolonged attempts at tracheal intubation.[17]

Human placental lactogen and cortisol increase the tendency toward hyperglycemia and ketosis, which may exacerbate pre-existing diabetes mellitus. The patient's ability to handle a glucose load is decreased, and the transplacental passage of glucose may stimulate fetal secretion of insulin, in turn leading to neonatal hypoglycemia in the immediate postpartum period.[18]

Gastrointestinal Changes

Pregnant women are at increased risk for aspiration of gastric contents compared to the general population. Aspiration pneumonitis is estimated to occur in 0.1% of cesarean deliveries performed under general anesthesia. Airway difficulties present during pregnancy may contribute to this risk.[19] In addition, gastric secretions are more acidic. Gastric emptying time is not prolonged during pregnancy, but overall gastrointestinal transit time is prolonged. In two contemporary studies of obese and nonobese, nonlaboring parturients at term, gastric emptying did not differ after ingestion of a moderate amount (300 mL) of water versus after an overnight fast.[20,21] Recent obstetric anesthesia practice guidelines by the American Society of Anesthesiologists and the Society for Obstetric Anesthesia and Perinatology allow for oral intake of modest amounts of clear liquids in uncomplicated laboring patients and for similar intake in patients scheduled for uncomplicated cesarean delivery up to 2 hours prior to induction of anesthesia; they recommend against ingestion of solid food during labor.[22] However, the guidelines state that patients with additional risk factors for aspiration (e.g., morbid obesity, diabetes, difficult airway) or patients at increased risk for operative delivery (e.g., nonreassuring fetal heart rate [FHR] pattern) may have further restrictions of oral intake.

The lower esophageal sphincter (LES) may become distorted and incompetent and progesterone may decrease its tone. The risk of regurgitation depends, in part, on the gradient between the LES and intragastric pressures. The gravid uterus may increase intra-abdominal and intragastric pressures, decreasing the gradient. After succinylcholine administration in most patients, the gradient increases because the increase in LES pressure exceeds the increase in intragastric pressure. However, in parturients with "heartburn," the LES tone is greatly reduced.[23]

The efficacy of prophylactic nonparticulate antacids may be diminished by inadequate mixing with gastric contents, improper timing of administration, and the tendency for antacids to increase gastric volume. Administration of histamine (H_2) receptor antagonists, such as ranitidine, may be useful. A case can be made for the administration of intravenous metoclopramide before elective cesarean delivery. This dopamine antagonist hastens gastric emptying and increases resting LES tone in both nonpregnant and pregnant women.[24] The aforementioned American Society of Anesthesiologists and Society for Obstetric Anesthesia and Perinatology practice guidelines advise practitioners to consider the administration of nonparticulate antacids, H_2 receptor antagonists, and/or metoclopramide for aspiration prophylaxis before surgical procedures and to use neuraxial anesthesia whenever possible.[22] A rapid-sequence induction of anesthesia, application of cricoid pressure, and intubation with a cuffed endotracheal tube are recommended for pregnant women receiving general anesthesia from 20 weeks of gestation, or earlier, if symptoms of reflux are present. These recommendations also pertain to women in the immediate postpartum period because there is uncertainty as to when the risk for aspiration of gastric contents returns to normal.

Altered Drug Responses

The minimum alveolar concentration (MAC) for inhalation agents is decreased by 8 to 12 weeks of gestation and may be related to an increase in progesterone levels.[25] In addition, maximal cephalad block level after neuraxial administration of local anesthetics is higher in the second and third trimesters of pregnancy.[26] Epidural venous engorgement, which decreases intrathecal volume, may lead to increased local anesthetic spread. Pregnancy increases median nerve sensitivity to lidocaine block[27] and in vitro preparations from pregnant animals demonstrate increased susceptibility to local anesthetic blockade. This increased sensitivity may be due to progesterone or other hormonal mediators.

Placental Transfer and Fetal Exposure to Anesthetic Drugs

Most drugs, including many anesthetic agents, readily cross the placenta. Several factors influence the placental transfer of drugs, including physicochemical characteristics of the drug itself, maternal drug concentrations in the plasma, properties of the placenta, and hemodynamic events within the fetomaternal unit.

Drugs cross biologic membranes by simple diffusion, the rate of which is determined by the Fick principle, which states that:

$$Q/t = KA(C_m - C_f)/D$$

where Q/t is the rate of diffusion, K is the diffusion constant, A is the surface area available for exchange, C_m is the concentration of free drug in maternal blood, C_f is the concentration of free drug in fetal blood, and D is the thickness of the diffusion barrier.

The diffusion constant (K) of the drug depends on physicochemical characteristics such as molecular size, lipid solubility, and degree of ionization. Compounds with a molecular weight less than 500 Da are unimpeded in crossing the placenta, whereas those with molecular weights of 500 to 1,000 Da are more restricted. Most drugs commonly used by the anesthesiologist have molecular weights that permit easy transfer.

Drugs that are highly lipid soluble cross biologic membranes more readily. The degree of ionization is important because the nonionized moiety of a drug is more lipophilic than the ionized one. Local anesthetics and opioids are weak bases, with a relatively low degree of ionization and considerable lipid solubility. In contrast, muscle relaxants are more ionized and less lipophilic, and their rate of placental transfer is therefore more limited.

The relative concentrations of drug existing in the nonionized and ionized forms can be predicted from the Henderson–Hasselbalch equation:

$$pH = pKa + \log(base)/(cation).$$

The pKa is the pH at which the concentrations of free base and cation are equal. The ratio of base to cation becomes particularly important with local anesthetics because the nonionized form penetrates tissue barriers, such as the placenta. For the amide local anesthetics, the pKa values (7.7 to 8.1) are sufficiently close to physiologic pH so that changes in maternal or fetal acid–base status may significantly alter the proportion of ionized and nonionized drugs present. At equilibrium, the concentrations of nonionized drug in the fetal and maternal plasma are equal. In an acidotic fetus, local anesthetics may be relatively more ionized than in maternal blood, and "ion trapping" may occur, leading to fetal drug accumulation.[28]

The effects of maternal plasma protein binding on the rate and amount of drug transferred to the fetus are not so well understood. In sheep, the low fetomaternal ratio of bupivacaine plasma concentrations has been attributed to the difference between fetal and maternal plasma protein binding, rather than to extensive fetal tissue uptake.[29] However, if enough time is allowed for fetomaternal equilibrium to be approached, substantial accumulation of highly protein-bound drugs, such as bupivacaine, can occur in the fetus.[30]

As already stated, the driving force for placental drug transfer is the concentration gradient of free drug between the maternal and fetal blood. On the maternal side, the following factors interact: The dose administered, the mode and site of administration, and, in the case of local anesthetics, the use of vasoconstrictors. The rates of distribution, metabolism, and excretion of the drug, which may vary at different stages of pregnancy, are equally important. In general, higher doses result in higher maternal blood concentrations. The absorption rate varies with the site of drug injection. Compared with other forms of administration, an intravenous bolus results in the highest blood concentrations. Increased maternal blood concentrations after repeated administration of a drug greatly depend on the dose and frequency of reinjection, in addition to the kinetic characteristics of the drug. The elimination half-life of amide local anesthetic agents is relatively long, so repeated injections may lead to accumulation in the maternal plasma. In contrast, 2-chloroprocaine, an ester local anesthetic, undergoes rapid enzymatic hydrolysis in the presence of pseudocholinesterase. After epidural injection, the mean half-life in the mother is approximately 3 minutes. After reinjection, 2-chloroprocaine can be detected in the maternal plasma for only 5 to 10 minutes, and no accumulation of this drug is evident.[31]

Placenta

Maturation of the placenta can affect the rate of drug transfer to the fetus, as the thickness of the trophoblastic epithelium decreases from 25 to 2 mm at term. Uptake and biotransformation of anesthetic drugs by the placenta would decrease the amount transferred to the fetus. However, placental drug uptake is limited, and there is no evidence to suggest that this organ metabolizes any of the agents commonly used in obstetric anesthesia.

Hemodynamic Factors

Any factor decreasing placental blood flow (e.g., aortocaval compression, hypotension, or hemorrhage) can decrease drug delivery to the fetus. During labor, uterine contractions intermittently reduce perfusion of the placenta. If a uterine contraction coincides with a rapid decline in plasma drug concentration after an intravenous bolus injection, by the time perfusion has returned to normal, the concentration gradient across the placenta has been greatly reduced. Thus, an intravenous injection of diazepam, administered at the onset of contraction compared to during uterine diastole, results in less drug being delivered to the fetus.

Several characteristics of the fetal circulation delay equilibration between the umbilical arterial and venous blood, and thus delay the depressant effects of anesthetic drugs (Fig. 41-1). The liver is the first fetal organ perfused by the umbilical venous blood, which carries drug to the fetus. Substantial uptake by this organ has been demonstrated for a variety of drugs, including thiopental, lidocaine, and halothane. During its transit to the arterial side of the fetal circulation, the drug is progressively diluted as blood in the umbilical vein becomes admixed with fetal venous blood from the gastrointestinal tract, the lower extremities, the head and upper extremities, and finally, the lungs. Because of this unique pattern of fetal circulation, continuous administration of anesthetic concentrations of nitrous oxide during elective cesarean sections caused newborn depression only if the induction-to-delivery interval exceeded 5 to 10 minutes. Rapid transfer of inhalation agents, including halothane, enflurane, and isoflurane, results in detectable umbilical arterial and venous concentrations after 1 minute.[32] Because of the rapid decline in maternal plasma drug concentrations, administration of thiopental or thiamylal as a single-bolus injection not exceeding 4 mg/kg was followed by fetal arterial concentrations of barbiturate below a level that would result in neonatal depression.[33]

Fetal regional blood flow changes can also affect the amount of drug taken up by individual organs. For example, during

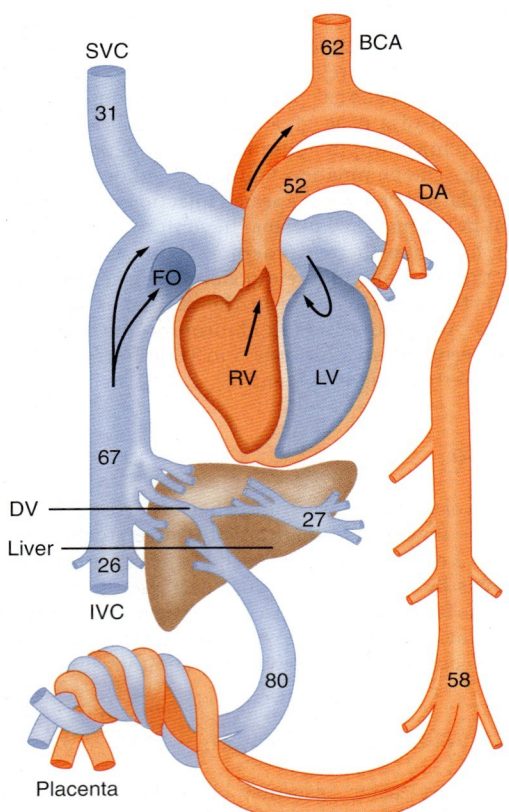

Figure 41-1 Diagram of the circulation in the mature fetal lamb. The numerals indicate the mean oxygen saturation (%) in the great vessels of six lambs: Right ventricle (RV), left ventricle (LV), superior vena cava (SVC), inferior vena cava (IVC), brachiocephalic artery (BCA), foramen ovale (FO), ductus arteriosus (DA), ductus venosus (DV). (Adapted from Born GVR, Dawes GS, Mott JC, et al. Changes in the heart and lungs at birth. *Cold Spring Harb Symp Quant Biol.* 1954;19:103.)

asphyxia and acidosis, a greater proportion of the fetal cardiac output perfuses the fetal brain, heart, and placenta. In asphyxiated baboon fetuses, infusion of lidocaine resulted in increased drug uptake in the heart, brain, and liver compared with control fetuses that were not asphyxiated.[34]

Fetus and Newborn

Any drug that reaches the fetus undergoes metabolism and excretion. In this respect, the fetus has an advantage over the newborn in that it can excrete the drug back to the mother once the concentration gradient of the free drug across the placenta has been reversed. With the use of local anesthetics, this may occur even though the total plasma drug concentration in the mother may exceed that in the fetus because there is lower protein binding in fetal plasma.[29] There is only one drug, 2-chloroprocaine, that is metabolized in the fetal blood so rapidly that even in acidosis, substantial accumulation in the fetus is avoided.[31]

In both the term and the preterm newborn, the liver contains enzymes essential for the biotransformation of amide local anesthetics. The metabolic clearance in the newborn is similar to, and renal clearance greater than, that in the adult. Elimination half-life is prolonged in the newborn due to a greater volume of distribution of the drug. Prolonged elimination half-lives in the newborn compared with the adult have been noted for other amide local anesthetics.[35]

It is not completely understood whether the fetus and the newborn are more sensitive than the adult to the depressant and toxic effects of local anesthetics. The relative central nervous system (CNS) and cardiorespiratory toxicity of lidocaine has been studied in adult ewes and lambs (fetal and neonatal).[36] The doses required to produce toxicity in the fetal and neonatal lambs were greater than those required in the adult, although serum concentrations at which toxicity occurred were not different. In the fetus, this was attributed to placental clearance of drug into the mother and better maintenance of blood gas tensions during convulsions. In the newborn, a larger volume of distribution was thought to be responsible for the higher doses needed to induce toxic effects.

Bupivacaine has been implicated as a possible cause of neonatal jaundice because its high affinity for fetal erythrocyte membranes may lead to a decrease in filterability and deformability, rendering them more prone to hemolysis (see Chapter 41). However, studies have failed to show increased bilirubin production in newborns whose mothers received bupivacaine for epidural anesthesia during labor and delivery.[37] Finally, observational neurobehavioral studies have revealed subtle changes in newborn neurologic and adaptive functions. In the case of most anesthetic agents, these changes are minor and transient, lasting for only 24 to 48 hours.

Analgesia for Labor and Vaginal Delivery

Most women experience moderate-to-severe pain during parturition. In the first stage of labor, pain is caused by uterine contractions, associated with dilation of the cervix and stretching of the lower uterine segment. Pain impulses are carried in visceral afferent type C fibers accompanying the sympathetic nerves. During the first stage of labor, pain is referred to the T10 to L1 spinal cord segments. In the late first and second stages of labor, additional pain impulses from distention of the vaginal vault and perineum are carried by the pudendal nerves, composed of sacral fibers (S2 to S4).

Well-conducted obstetric analgesia, in addition to relieving pain and anxiety, may have other benefits. Pain may result in maternal hypertension and reduced uterine blood flow. During the first and second stages of labor, epidural analgesia blunts the increases in maternal cardiac output, heart rate, and blood pressure that occur with painful uterine contractions and "bearing-down" efforts.[38] In reducing maternal secretion of catecholamines, epidural analgesia may convert a previously dysfunctional labor pattern to normal. Maternal analgesia may also benefit the fetus by eliminating maternal hyperventilation, which can result in reduced fetal arterial oxygen tension because of a leftward shift of the maternal oxygen–hemoglobin dissociation curve.

The most frequently chosen methods for relieving the pain of parturition are psychoprophylaxis, systemic medication, and regional analgesia. Inhalation analgesia, conventional spinal analgesia, and paracervical blockade are less commonly used. General anesthesia is rarely necessary but may be indicated for uterine relaxation in complicated deliveries. Labor varies in length and intensity, as do individual tolerance to pain and desire for pain relief. Women should be educated about the options for labor analgesia and supported in their choice for method of pain control. Analgesia should not be withheld if requested.[39]

Neonatal outcomes appear to be similar for healthy women who deliver without pharmacologic analgesia and for women who receive analgesia.

Nonpharmacologic Methods of Labor Analgesia

Nonpharmacologic methods to relieve the pain of childbirth include childbirth education, emotional support, massage, aromatherapy, audiotherapy, and therapeutic use of hot and cold. More advanced techniques that require specialized training or equipment include hydrotherapy, intradermal water injections, biofeedback, transcutaneous electrical nerve stimulation (TENS), acupuncture or acupressure, and hypnosis. Conclusions regarding the efficacy of most of these techniques are not possible, as the techniques have been inadequately studied.[40]

Prepared Childbirth and Psychoprophylaxis

The philosophy of prepared childbirth maintains that lack of knowledge, misinformation, fear, and anxiety can heighten a patient's response to pain and consequently increase the need for analgesics. The most popular method of prepared childbirth was introduced by Lamaze. It provides an educational program on the physiology of parturition and attempts to diminish cortical pain perception by encouraging responses such as specific patterns of breathing and focused attention on a fixed object.[41] Scientific data as to whether childbirth education and psychoprophylaxis are effective in reducing childbirth pain are inconsistent and lack scientific rigor. Education, intense motivation, and cultural influences can influence the affective and behavioral responses to pain, although their true effect on pain sensation is less clear.

Other Nonpharmacologic Methods

Continuous labor support refers to the presence during labor of nonmedical support by a trained person. Prospective, controlled trials and several systematic analyses have concluded that women who receive continuous labor support have shorter labors, fewer operative deliveries, fewer analgesic interventions, and better overall satisfaction.[42] Systematic reviews of randomized controlled trials of hydrotherapy (water baths) have concluded that women experience less pain and use less analgesia, without change in the duration of labor, rate of operative delivery, or neonatal outcome.[43] Intradermal water injection consists of the injection of 0.05 to 0.1 mL of sterile water at four sites on the lower back to treat back pain during labor. Although some randomized controlled trials have found that the technique is effective in reducing severe back pain during labor, a 2012 meta-analysis of seven studies concluded that there is little robust evidence that sterile water injections are effective for low back pain or other labor pain.[44] Hypnosis requires prenatal training of the mother by a trained hypnotherapist. A meta-analysis of seven randomized controlled trials concluded that the small number of trials precluded drawing conclusions about the usefulness of hypnotherapy for pain management during labor, although the technique shows some promise.[45] The results of studies using TENS are inconsistent, but in general, labor pain does not appear to be lessened by TENS, nor does it lower the use of other analgesic modalities.[46] In a meta-analysis including 13 trials, women who were randomized to receive acupuncture or acupressure versus control (no or "false" acupuncture) had modestly lower pain scores.[47] Similarly, relaxation techniques may also reduce pain intensity and improve satisfaction with pain relief compared to standard care.[48]

Systemic Medication

The advantages of systemic analgesics include ease of administration and patient acceptability. However, the drug, dose, time, and method of administration must be chosen carefully to avoid maternal or neonatal depression. Opioids are used most commonly, although tranquilizers and ketamine are used occasionally.

Opioids

Systemic opioids are commonly administered for labor analgesia, although existing data suggest that they provide little significant analgesia (see Chapter 20).[49-51] Meperidine has historically been the most commonly used systemic analgesic for the treatment of labor pain. Meperidine can be administered by intravenous injection (effective analgesia in 5 to 10 minutes) or intramuscularly (peak effect in 40 to 50 minutes). However, in the past decade, because of concerns of lack of efficacy and the presence of side effects, there has been a move away from its use for both labor pain and other pain conditions.[51] The major side effects are a high incidence of nausea and vomiting, maternal sedation, dose-related depression of ventilation, orthostatic hypotension, and the potential for neonatal depression. Meperidine may cause transient alterations of the FHR, such as decreased beat-to-beat variability and mild tachycardia. The risk of neonatal depression is related to the interval from the last drug injection to delivery. The placental transfer of an active metabolite, normeperidine, which has a long elimination half-life in the neonate (62 hours), has also been implicated in contributing to neonatal depression and subtle neonatal neurobehavioral dysfunction.

Synthetic opioids such as fentanyl, alfentanil, and remifentanil are more potent than meperidine; however, their use during labor is limited by their short duration of action. These drugs offer an advantage when analgesia of rapid onset but short duration is necessary (e.g., with forceps application). For more prolonged analgesia, fentanyl or remifentanil can be administered with patient-controlled delivery devices.[52] However, patient-controlled analgesia (PCA) administration of opioids does carry with it the potential for drug accumulation and the risk of neonatal depression. Remifentanil has the theoretical advantage of rapid onset and offset compared with the other opioids. Bolus doses ranging from 0.2 to 1 µg/kg with lockout intervals from 1 to 5 minutes and background infusion rates from 0 to 0.1 µg/kg/min[53] have been described. However, as with other systemic opioid techniques, it is unclear whether remifentanil PCA can provide satisfactory analgesia without an unacceptably high incidence of maternal, fetal, and neonatal side effects.[54]

Opioid agonists–antagonists, such as butorphanol and nalbuphine, have also been used for obstetric analgesia. These drugs have the proposed benefits of a lower incidence of nausea, vomiting, and dysphoria, as well as a "ceiling effect" on depression of ventilation. Butorphanol, 1 to 2 mg, or nalbuphine, 10 mg by intravenous or intramuscular injection, is probably the most popular. Unlike meperidine, these drugs are biotransformed into inactive metabolites and have a ceiling effect on depression of ventilation.

Naloxone, a pure opioid antagonist, should not be administered to the mother shortly before delivery to prevent neonatal ventilatory depression because it reverses maternal analgesia at a time when it is most needed. In addition, in some instances, it has caused maternal pulmonary edema and even cardiac arrest. If necessary to correct respiratory depression, the drug should be given directly to the newborn intramuscularly (0.1 mg/kg).

Ketamine

Ketamine is a potent analgesic. However, it may also induce unacceptable amnesia that may interfere with the mother's recollection of the birth. Nonetheless, ketamine is a useful adjuvant to inadequate regional analgesia during vaginal delivery or for obstetric manipulations. In low doses (0.2 to 0.4 mg/kg), ketamine provides adequate analgesia without causing neonatal depression. Constant communication is required with the patient to ensure that she is awake and able to protect her airway.

Regional Analgesia

Regional techniques provide excellent analgesia with minimal depressant effects on the mother and the fetus. The regional techniques most commonly used in obstetric anesthesia include central neuraxial blocks (spinal, epidural, and combined spinal/epidural [CSE]), paracervical and pudendal blocks, and, less frequently, lumbar sympathetic blocks (LSBs). Hypotension resulting from sympathectomy is the most frequent complication of central neuraxial blockade. Therefore, maternal blood pressure should be monitored at regular intervals, typically every 2 to 5 minutes for approximately 15 to 20 minutes after the initiation of the block and at routine intervals thereafter. The use of regional analgesia may be contraindicated in the presence of coagulopathy, acute hypovolemia, or infection at the site of needle insertion. Chorioamnionitis without frank sepsis is not a contraindication to central neuraxial blockade in obstetrics, provided antibiotics have been administered.

Because of ethical considerations and methodologic difficulties, it is difficult to design clinical studies to examine the effects of neuraxial analgesia on the progress of labor and mode of delivery. Randomized controlled trials have found no difference in the rate of cesarean delivery in women who received neuraxial compared with systemic opioid labor analgesia.[55] Meta-analyses suggest that neuraxial analgesia does not prolong the first stage of labor, although the data are heterogeneous.[55] There has been concern that early initiation of epidural analgesia during the latent phase of labor (<4 cm cervical dilation) in nulliparous women may result in a higher incidence of dystocia and cesarean delivery. However, large randomized trials and a meta-analysis of these trials found no difference in the rate of cesarean delivery in women randomized to early neuraxial compared with systemic opioid analgesia.[56] Neuraxial analgesia is, however, associated with prolongation of the second stage of labor in nulliparous women, possibly owing to a decrease in expulsive forces or malposition of the vertex.[55] Although the American College of Obstetricians and Gynecologists (ACOG) traditionally defined abnormally prolonged second stage of labor as more than 3 hours in nulliparous women with epidural analgesia and more than 2 hours in women without epidural analgesia, a 2014 consensus document developed jointly by the ACOG and the Society for Maternal-Fetal Medicine (SMFM) stated that "a specific absolute maximum length of the time spent in second stage labor beyond which all women should undergo operative delivery has not been identified." In addition, they suggested that longer durations (beyond the traditional 3 hours) may be appropriate on an individual basis.[57] Prolongation of the second stage in women with epidural analgesia may be minimized by the use of dilute local anesthetic solutions in combination with opioid.[58]

Epidural Analgesia

Epidural analgesia may be used for pain relief during labor and vaginal delivery, and if necessary, converted to anesthesia for cesarean delivery. Effective analgesia during the first stage of labor may be achieved by blocking the T10 to L1 dermatomes with low concentrations of local anesthetic, usually combined with lipid-soluble opioids. Combining drugs allows the use of lower doses of both drugs, thus minimizing side effects and complications of each. For the second stage of labor and delivery, the nerve block should be extended to include the S2 to S4 segments in order to block pain from vaginal and perineal distension and trauma.

Long-acting amides such as bupivacaine or ropivacaine are most frequently used because they produce excellent sensory analgesia while sparing motor function, particularly at low concentrations (<0.1%). Although some studies have found that ropivacaine is associated with less motor blockade than equipotent doses of bupivacaine, there was no difference in the rate of instrumental vaginal delivery among women randomized to receive epidural levobupivacaine, bupivacaine, or ropivacaine for maintenance of labor analgesia.[59]

Analgesia for the first stage of labor may be achieved with 5 to 10 mL of bupivacaine or ropivacaine (0.125%) combined with fentanyl (50 to 100 μg) or sufentanil (5 to 10 μg). There is controversy regarding the need for an epidural test dose when using dilute solutions of local anesthetic. Because catheter aspiration is not always diagnostic, particularly when using single-orifice epidural catheters, some experts believe that a test dose should be administered to improve detection of an intrathecally or intravascularly placed catheter.

Analgesia may be maintained with a continuous infusion (8 to 12 mL/hr) of bupivacaine (0.0625% to 0.1%) or ropivacaine (0.08% to 0.15%). The addition of fentanyl (1 to 2 μg/mL) or sufentanil (0.3 to 0.5 μg/mL) allows for more dilute local anesthetic solutions to be administered. Alternatively, analgesia may be maintained with patient-controlled epidural analgesia (PCEA) with similar solutions of local anesthetic and opioid. PCEA resulted in greater patient satisfaction, a lower average hourly dose of bupivacaine (and therefore less motor block), and less need for physician interventions[60,61] compared with a continuous epidural infusion. Protocols for PCEA vary widely. Data are conflicting as to whether a background infusion improves analgesia; however, a background infusion may be helpful in selected parturients (e.g., nulliparas with long labors).[61,62] Common PCEA parameters include a parturient-administered bolus dose of 5 to 10 mL, a lock-out interval of 10 to 20 minutes, and a background infusion of 0 to 10 mL/hr. Thirty percent to 50% of the hourly dose is often administered as a background infusion.

The timed, or programmed intermittent epidural bolus technique is a new method for maintaining epidural analgesia. In this technique, the pump is programmed to deliver a bolus dose at regular intervals. Presumably, the bolus administration of drugs into the epidural space results in better distribution of the drug solution. Randomized controlled trials comparing this technique with continuous epidural infusion or with PCEA have shown lower anesthetic dose, greater patient satisfaction, and a lower incidence of motor block and instrumental vaginal delivery.[63]

Women with hemodynamic stability and preserved motor function who do not require continuous fetal monitoring may ambulate with the assistance of a partner during the first stage of labor. Before ambulation, women should be observed for

30 minutes after initiation of neuraxial blockade to assess maternal and fetal well-being.

During delivery, the sacral dermatomes may be blocked with 10 mL of bupivacaine (0.25% to 0.5%), lidocaine (1.0%), or 2-chloroprocaine (2% to 3%). Many parturients have adequate analgesia for delivery without an additional bolus dose, particularly if epidural analgesia has been maintained for a long interval (hours). However, instrumental vaginal delivery may require a denser block than that obtained with dilute local anesthetic solutions.

Spinal Analgesia

A single subarachnoid injection for labor analgesia has the advantage of fast and reliable onset of neural blockade, and it is technically easier to initiate compared with epidural analgesia. However, repeated intrathecal injections may be required for a long labor, thus increasing the risk of postdural puncture headache (PDPH). Spinal analgesia with fentanyl (15 to 25 µg) or sufentanil (2 to 5 µg) in combination with plain bupivacaine (1.25 to 2.5 mg) may be appropriate in the multiparous patient whose anticipated course of labor does not warrant a catheter technique (duration, 1.5 hours). A potential disadvantage of single-shot spinal analgesia is that the duration of labor, even in a rapidly progressing multiparous woman, may be longer than anticipated. Furthermore, if the woman requires an urgent cesarean delivery, a new anesthetic will need to be initiated. However, spinal anesthesia (a "saddle block") is a safe and effective alternative to general anesthesia or pudendal nerve block for instrumental delivery in parturients without pre-existing epidural analgesia.

Combined Spinal/Epidural Analgesia

CSE analgesia is an ideal analgesic technique for use during labor. CSE analgesia combines the rapid, reliable onset of profound analgesia resulting from spinal injection with the flexibility and longer duration associated with a continuous epidural technique. After identification of the epidural space using a conventional (or specialized) epidural needle, a longer (127 mm), pencil-point spinal needle is advanced into the subarachnoid space through the epidural needle. After intrathecal injection, the spinal needle is removed and an epidural catheter is inserted. Intrathecal injection of fentanyl (10 to 25 µg) or sufentanil (2 to 5 µg) alone or more commonly in combination with bupivacaine (1.25 to 2.5 mg) produces profound analgesia lasting for 90 to 120 minutes with minimal motor block. Spinal opioid alone provides complete analgesia for the early latent phase of labor. However, the addition of bupivacaine is necessary for satisfactory analgesia during advanced labor. Continuous epidural analgesia, PCEA, or programmed intermittent epidural bolus may be initiated following the spinal injection to maintain analgesia.

The most common side effects of intrathecal opioids are pruritus, nausea, vomiting, and urinary retention. The incidence of pruritus is lower if opioid is coadministered with local anesthetic.[64] Rostral spread resulting in delayed respiratory depression may occur; the risk is highest in the first 30 minutes after injection. It is rare with the use of fentanyl or sufentanil. Transient nonreassuring FHR patterns may occur after initiation of either epidural or spinal analgesia, with or without opioids; however, the incidence may be higher after CSE compared to epidural analgesia. Presumably, uterine tachysystole and decreased uteroplacental perfusion occur as a result of rapid decrease in circulating maternal epinephrine levels after initiation of analgesia or as a result of hypotension after sympatholysis. The incidence of emergency cesarean delivery, however, is no greater after CSE than after conventional epidural analgesia.[65,66]

Mothers in early labor, or with preload-dependent medical conditions (e.g., aortic stenosis), may particularly benefit from opioid-only CSE analgesia. Spinal opioid provides complete analgesia without the need for local anesthetic in early labor, thus avoiding an acute decrease in preload, and almost always allowing motivated women to ambulate because there is no motor block. Multiparous women with advanced cervical dilation also benefit from CSE analgesia in which both intrathecal opioid and local anesthetic are injected. The onset of sacral analgesia is accomplished significantly faster with much less drug than initiation of lumbar epidural analgesia. Some experts advocate the cautious use of CSE analgesia in women who may require urgent cesarean delivery or are at increased risk from general anesthesia (e.g., morbidly obese or anticipated difficult airway) because the epidural component of a CSE is not initially tested. However, epidural catheters sited as part of a CSE technique fail less during labor and intrapartum cesarean delivery compared to catheters sited with a traditional epidural technique.[67,68]

Paracervical Block

Bilateral paracervical block interrupts transmission of nerve impulses from the uterus and cervix during the first stage of labor. Five to ten milliliters of dilute local anesthetic solution is injected submucosally via a needle guide in the vagina into the left and right lateral vaginal fornices. Although paracervical block effectively relieves pain during the first stage of labor, the technique has fallen out of favor during childbirth because it is associated with a high incidence of fetal asphyxia and poor neonatal outcome, particularly with the use of bupivacaine. Performing the block with dilute local anesthetic solutions, allowing 5 to 10 minutes to elapse between injections on the left and right sides, and limiting the block to women with less than 8 cm cervical dilation, may decrease the incidence of complications.

Paravertebral Lumbar Sympathetic Block

Paravertebral LSB is a reasonable alternative when contraindications exist to central neuraxial techniques. LSB interrupts the painful transmission of cervical and uterine impulses during the first stage of labor.[69] Although there is less risk of fetal bradycardia with LSB compared with paracervical blockade, unfamiliarity and technical difficulties associated with the performance of the block and risks of intravascular injection have decreased its use in standard practice.

Pudendal Nerve Block

The pudendal nerves, derived from the sacral nerve roots (S2 to S4), supply the vaginal vault, perineum, rectum, and parts of the bladder. The nerves are easily anesthetized transvaginally where they loop around the ischial spines. Ten milliliters of dilute local anesthetic solution deposited behind each sacrospinous ligament can provide adequate anesthesia for outlet forceps delivery and episiotomy repair.

Inhalation Analgesia and General Anesthesia

Inhalation labor analgesia is uncommon in the United States, although its use is more common in other parts of the world (see Chapter 18). Nitrous oxide, 50% by volume, is the most commonly used inhalation agent for analgesia during labor. The mother is trained to intermittently self-administer the gas at the onset of a contraction. Studies are conflicting as to whether nitrous oxide provides benefit to the parturient; its safety for the fetus and the neonate has also not been well studied.[70,71] A major disadvantage of inhalation analgesia is the need for a waste gas scavenging system.

General anesthesia is rarely used for vaginal delivery, and precautions against gastric aspiration must always be observed (see General Anesthesia in the section Anesthesia for Cesarean Delivery). General anesthesia may be required when time constraints prevent induction of regional anesthesia. Potent inhalation drugs (1.5 to 2 MAC for short periods) can provide uterine relaxation for obstetric maneuvers such as second twin delivery, breech presentation, or postpartum manual removal of a retained placenta. However, in current practice, intravenous nitroglycerin (50 to 250 µg) has largely replaced the need for general anesthesia for uterine relaxation.

Anesthesia for Cesarean Delivery

The most common indications for cesarean delivery include arrest of dilation, nonreassuring fetal status, cephalopelvic disproportion, malpresentation, prematurity, prior cesarean delivery, and prior uterine surgery involving the corpus. The choice of anesthesia depends on the urgency of the procedure, the condition of the mother and the fetus, and the mother's wishes.

A 2001 survey of obstetric anesthesia practices in the United States revealed that most patients undergoing cesarean delivery do so under spinal or epidural anesthesia.[72] Neuraxial techniques have several advantages, such as:
- Prevent airway manipulation
- Lessen the risk of gastric aspiration
- Avoid the use of depressant anesthetic drugs
- Allow the mother to remain awake during delivery
- May be associated with less operative blood loss

Compared with general anesthesia, there is also less immediate neonatal depression after neuraxial compared with general anesthesia.

Neuraxial Anesthesia

Blockade to the T4 dermatome is necessary to perform cesarean delivery without maternal discomfort. The most common complication of neuraxial anesthesia is hypotension and the attendant risk of decreased uteroplacental perfusion (see Hypotension in the section on Anesthetic Complications). Measures to decrease the incidence and severity of hypotension include left uterine displacement, intravenous fluid administration, and the liberal use of vasopressors to prevent and treat hypotension.

Most anesthesiologists administer a nonparticulate antacid before induction of anesthesia for pulmonary aspiration prophylaxis. Some practitioners also administer an H_2 receptor antagonist and metoclopramide. Sedative premedication is usually not necessary. Intraoperative monitoring mimics that for all anesthetics, although blood pressure should be measured frequently (every several minutes) for the first 20 minutes after initiation of anesthesia. Although supplemental oxygen is frequently administered, there is no evidence of benefit to the mother, the fetus, or the neonate.[73]

Multimodal analgesia, including systemic nonsteroidal antiinflammatory drugs and neuraxial opioids and/or local anesthetics, is optimal for postoperative pain management.

Although postcesarean delivery analgesia should take the nursing infant into account, very small amounts of drugs administered to the mother actually cross into breast milk, and even smaller amounts are absorbed from the neonatal gut. Prolonged (12 to 24 hours) postoperative pain relief in the postpartum patient can be provided by intrathecal morphine (100 to 150 µg)[74] or epidural morphine (3.5 to 4.0 mg).[75] PCEA with a dilute solution of local anesthetic and lipid-soluble opioid is another option after epidural anesthesia. Side effects of neuraxial morphine include nausea, vomiting, and pruritus. Delayed respiratory depression is a rare but potentially devastating complication; therefore, patients who receive neuraxial opioids must be monitored carefully in the postoperative period.[76] Morbidly obese women may be at higher risk for respiratory depression. Abdominal wall nerve block techniques (transversus abdominis plane [TAP] block) have also been described after cesarean delivery. Intrathecal morphine provides superior and longer-lasting analgesia compared to bilateral TAP block,[77] but TAP block is useful for women who do not or cannot receive neuraxial opioid analgesia.

Spinal Anesthesia

Subarachnoid block is probably the most commonly administered neuraxial anesthetic for cesarean delivery because of its simplicity, speed of onset, and reliability. It is an alternative to general anesthesia for almost all but the most emergent of cesarean deliveries. Hyperbaric 0.75% bupivacaine (12.5 to 13.5 mg [1.6 to 1.8 mL]) is the most commonly used local anesthetic in the United States. It reliably provides 90 to 120 minutes of surgical anesthesia.

Despite an adequate dermatomal level for surgery, women may experience varying degrees of visceral discomfort and nausea and vomiting, particularly during exteriorization of the uterus and traction on abdominal viscera. Improved perioperative anesthesia and analgesia can be provided with the addition of fentanyl (10 to 20 µg), sufentanil (2.5 to 5 µg), or morphine (0.1 to 0.15 mg) to the local anesthetic solution. Fentanyl has a rapid onset, but is short acting and provides little additional postoperative analgesia. In contrast, morphine has a longer latency than fentanyl, but will also provide anesthesia for 12 to 18 hours after delivery.

Lumbar Epidural Anesthesia

In contrast to spinal anesthesia, epidural anesthesia is associated with a slower onset of action and a larger drug requirement to establish adequate sensory block. The major advantages of epidural compared with single-shot spinal anesthesia are the ability to titrate the extent and duration of anesthesia. To avoid unintentional intrathecal or intravascular injection, correct placement of the epidural needle and catheter is essential. This is especially true because epidural anesthesia for cesarean delivery necessitates the administration of large doses of local anesthetic.

Aspiration of the epidural catheter for blood or cerebrospinal fluid is not reliable for detection of catheter misplacement, particularly with single-orifice catheters. Thus, most anesthesiologists administer a test dose before the initiation of surgical anesthesia. A small dose of local anesthetic (e.g., lidocaine, 45 mg, or bupivacaine, 5 mg) readily produces identifiable sensory and motor blocks if injected intrathecally. Addition of epinephrine (15 µg) with careful hemodynamic monitoring may signal intravascular injection if followed by a transient increase in heart rate and blood pressure. The use of an epinephrine test dose (15 µg) in obstetrics is controversial because false positive results do occur (10% increase in heart rate), especially in laboring women. In addition, epinephrine may reduce uteroplacental perfusion. Rapid injection of 1 mL of air with simultaneous precordial Doppler monitoring appears to be a reliable indicator of intravascular catheter placement.[78] It has also been suggested that fentanyl (100 μg) may be used to test epidural catheter placement.[79] A negative test, although reassuring, does not eliminate the need for incremental administration of local anesthetic.

The most commonly used agents for obstetric epidural anesthesia are 2% lidocaine with epinephrine, 5 μg/mL (1:200,000) and 3% 2-chloroprocaine. Adequate anesthesia is usually achieved with 15 to 25 mL of local anesthetic solution, administered in divided doses over 5 to 10 minutes. 2-Chloroprocaine provides rapid onset of a reliable block with minimal risk of systemic toxicity because of its extremely high rate of metabolism in maternal and fetal plasma. However, 2% lidocaine with epinephrine and sodium bicarbonate (1 mEq/10 mL lidocaine) and fentanyl may also be used when the rapid conversion of pre-existing epidural labor analgesia to surgical anesthesia is required for urgent cesarean delivery.[80] Lidocaine has an onset and duration intermediate to those of 2-chloroprocaine and bupivacaine. Lidocaine should be administered with epinephrine, as lidocaine without epinephrine does not consistently provide satisfactory surgical anesthesia. Bupivacaine is no longer commonly used for obstetric epidural anesthesia, as it is associated with a greater risk of local anesthetic systemic toxicity (LAST) compared with other amide local anesthetics. Unintentional intravascular injection of bupivacaine is associated with a high incidence of maternal mortality.[81] Ropivacaine 0.5% combined with fentanyl may be used for surgical anesthesia, as the risk of toxicity is less than that of bupivacaine. A meta-analysis of studies comparing different anesthetic solutions for extension of labor epidural analgesia for cesarean delivery concluded that ropivacaine provided denser anesthesia compared with bupivacaine or levobupivacaine.[80]

Combined Spinal/Epidural Anesthesia

Advantages of CSE anesthesia for cesarean delivery include the rapid onset of a dense block with a low anesthetic dose, and the ability to extend the duration of anesthesia, and perhaps to provide continuous postoperative analgesia. There is a lower incidence of breakthrough pain and intraoperative shivering, and maternal satisfaction was higher after CSE compared with epidural anesthesia for cesarean delivery.[82] Several variations of the CSE technique have been described. The standard technique uses the same spinal dose of local anesthetic as one would use for standard spinal anesthesia. In sequential CSE anesthesia, a smaller spinal dose is expected to result in inadequate anesthesia for some patients. After 15 minutes, if anesthesia is inadequate, the block is extended by injecting supplemental local anesthetic via the epidural catheter.[83] Although the incidence of hypotension is lower with this technique compared with full-dose spinal anesthesia, the induction to incision time is prolonged. A third technique is also associated with a lower incidence of hypotension without prolonging onset time. A small dose of spinal local anesthetic is followed by the routine injection of additional anesthetic through the epidural catheter approximately 5 minutes after the intrathecal dose.[84] Bupivacaine doses from 6 to 12 mg have been described for CSE anesthesia.

General Anesthesia

General anesthesia may be necessary when absolute or relative contraindications exist to neuraxial anesthesia (e.g., coagulopathy, or moderate or severe aortic stenosis), or when the need for emergency delivery precludes central neuraxial blockade. General anesthesia should be used cautiously in women with asthma, upper respiratory tract infection, obesity, or a history of difficult tracheal intubation. Preoperative airway evaluation is particularly important in pregnant women because the inability to intubate the trachea and provide effective ventilation is the leading cause of maternal death related to anesthesia.[85] Equipment to manage the difficult airway should be immediately available.[22] Mallampati classification scores worsen during labor in some parturients.[86] If airway difficulties are anticipated, a neuraxial anesthetic technique should be considered or an awake tracheal intubation performed. Pulmonary aspiration prophylaxis should be administered and the patient should be positioned with left lateral tilt to prevent aortocaval compression. Monitoring mimics that for all anesthetics.

To minimize the risk of hypoxemia during induction, denitrogenation for 3 to 5 minutes with a tight-fitting mask is essential. In an emergency, four deep breaths with 100% oxygen may suffice. A "defasciculating" dose of a nondepolarizing muscle relaxant is not necessary. Although somewhat controversial,[87] a rapid-sequence induction is usually performed. Induction with a sedative–hypnotic (e.g., propofol [2 mg/kg], ketamine [1 mg/kg], or etomidate [0.2 to 0.3 mg/kg]) is followed by succinylcholine (1 to 1.5 mg/kg) to facilitate tracheal intubation. A trained assistant applies cricoid pressure until the airway is properly secured with a cuffed endotracheal tube. Once correct placement of the endotracheal tube is confirmed with capnography and auscultation, the obstetrician may proceed with incision.

Historically, succinylcholine has been the preferred muscle relaxant. However, the availability of sugammadex may change this practice. High-dose rocuronium (1.0 mg/kg) may be a safe alternative if deep neuromuscular blockade can be rapidly reversed with sugammadex.[88]

If there is difficulty in securing the airway, the mother should be ventilated with 100% oxygen before a subsequent attempt at tracheal intubation is made. Although some experts advise attempting to maintain cricoid pressure throughout, this practice may actually make visualization of the glottis and mask ventilation more difficult in some patients.[89] The American Society of Anesthesiologists' Difficult Airway Algorithm should be modified to include assessment of fetal status and the need for immediate delivery (Fig. 41-2).[90] It may be safer for the mother to allow her to awaken and to reassess the method of induction and intubation, rather than to persist with traumatic efforts at tracheal intubation. However, if the fetus is in extremis, airway management with a mask or supraglottic airway device may be an acceptable alternative.[90]

In the interval between intubation and delivery, anesthesia is maintained with a 50:50 mixture of nitrous oxide in oxygen and a volatile anesthetic agent. In the past, it was common to limit the volatile agent concentration to 0.5 MAC to limit fetal exposure before delivery and to limit uterine relaxation after delivery. However, the incidence of intraoperative awareness appears to be unacceptably high with this technique.[91] Indeed, a significant number of women had bispectral index values greater than 60 during general anesthesia with sevoflurane 1% in nitrous oxide 50%.[92] Therefore, higher concentrations of volatile agent should be used before delivery. After delivery, the nitrous oxide concentration can be increased and/or an intravenous amnestic (e.g., midazolam) and opioids can be administered.

General anesthesia for cesarean delivery is associated with lower neonatal Apgar scores at 1 minute compared with neuraxial anesthesia[93]; however, the Apgar scores at 5 minutes are comparable. Therefore, an individual trained in neonatal resuscitation should be present at delivery of the infant. After delivery, prophylactic intravenous oxytocin is administered to decrease the risk of uterine atony and anesthesia may be deepened with an opioid and benzodiazepine, as necessary. At the end of the procedure, the mother's trachea is extubated once she is awake and extubation

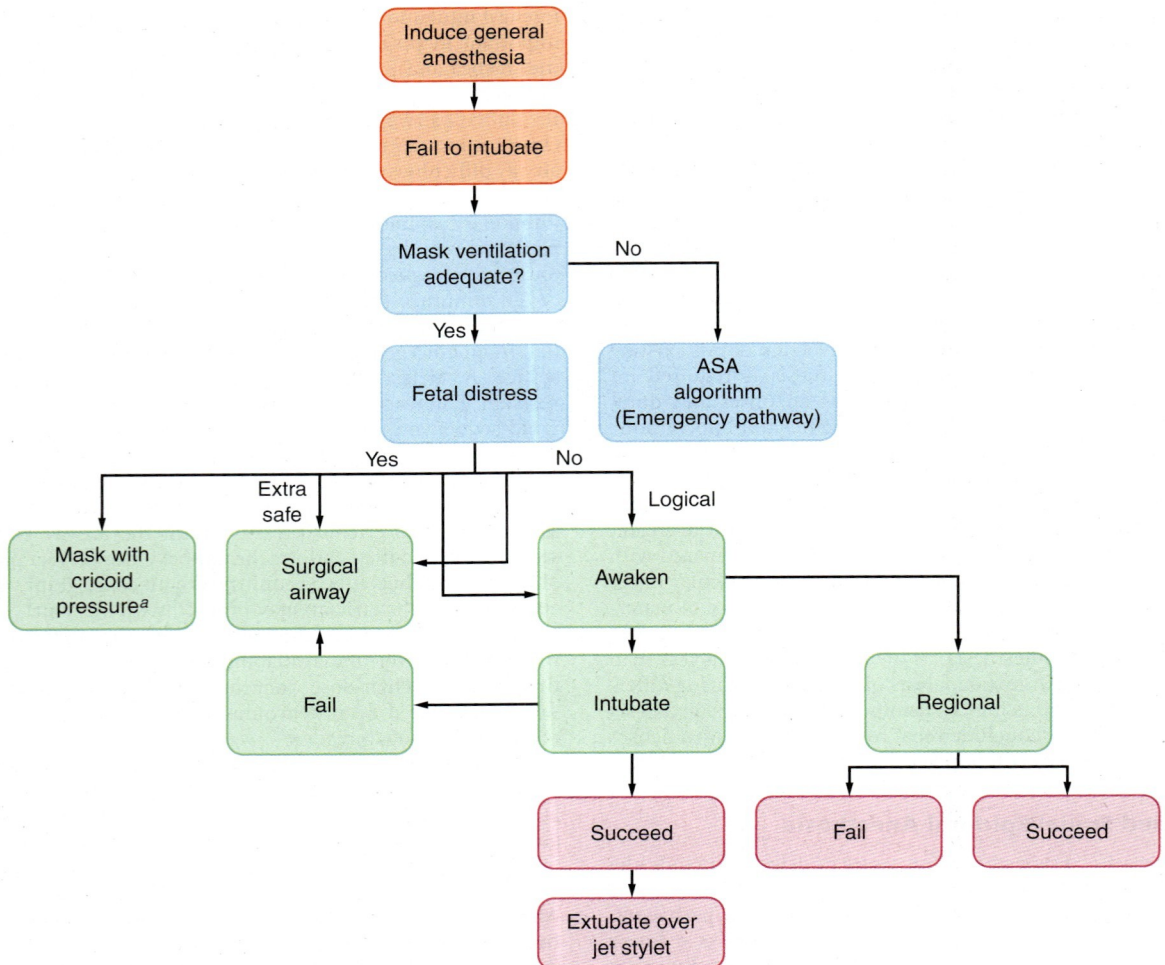

Figure 41-2 Management of the difficult airway in pregnancy with special reference to the presence or absence of fetal distress. When mask ventilation is not possible, the clinician is referred to the American Society of Anesthesiologists' (ASA) algorithm for emergency airway management found in Chapter 28. [a]Conventional face mask or laryngeal mask airway. (Reprinted with permission from Kuczkowski KM, Reisner LS, Benumof JL. The difficult airway: risk, prophylaxis, and management. In: Chestnut DH, ed. *Obstetric Anesthesia: Principles and Practice*. 3rd ed. St. Louis: Elsevier-Mosby; 2004:550.)

criteria have been met. The usual blood loss during cesarean delivery is 750 to 1,000 mL; transfusion is rarely necessary.

Anesthetic Complications

Maternal Mortality

A review of maternal mortality data from the US Centers for Disease Control and Prevention found that anesthesia-related maternal mortality decreased by nearly 60% from the dates 1979 to 1990 versus 1991 to 2002.[85] Historically, general anesthesia has been associated with a higher rate of anesthesia-related deaths than neuraxial anesthesia. During the most recent period, case-fatality rates from general anesthesia fell, whereas those for neuraxial anesthesia rose. The risk ratio for general to neuraxial was 1.7 (95% confidence interval 0.6 to 4.6). Anesthesia-related mortality was most often associated with cesarean delivery (86%). The leading causes of death were intubation failure or induction problems (23%), respiratory failure (20%), and high spinal or epidural block (16%).[85]

Pulmonary Aspiration

The risk of inhalation of gastric contents may be increased in pregnant women, particularly if difficulty occurs with airway management. Women who have recently eaten, are laboring, received systemic opioids, or have frequent heartburn are of greatest concern. Comprehensive airway evaluation, prophylactic administration of nonparticulate antacids, and use of regional anesthesia decrease the risk of aspiration. General anesthesia may be unavoidable occasionally; therefore, awake intubation may be indicated in women in whom airway difficulties are anticipated.

Hypotension

Neuraxial anesthesia is frequently associated with hypotension. Labor lowers the risk of hypotension in term pregnant women compared with nonlaboring women. Blood pressure should be monitored frequently (every 2 to 3 minutes) after the induction of neuraxial anesthesia. Techniques to reduce the incidence of hypotension during neuraxial anesthesia include left uterine displacement, intravenous fluid, and vasopressor administration. Maintaining the maternal blood pressure close to baseline reduces the incidence of maternal nausea and vomiting and is associated with higher umbilical artery pH values.[94] The administration of an intravenous bolus of crystalloid solution (1,000 to 1,500 mL) at the time of induction of neuraxial analgesia (co-load) is as effective as administration of the same volume of solution prior to the initiation of anesthesia (preload).[95] Colloid (500 mL) is superior to crystalloid solution in preventing hypotension[96] and may be considered in woman at high risk for hypotension or its consequences.

Phenylephrine is equally efficacious to ephedrine for treating maternal hypotension and results in less fetal acidosis.[97] Ephedrine crosses the placenta to a greater extent than phenylephrine and undergoes less early metabolism.[98] Stimulation of fetal β-adrenergic receptors by ephedrine increases the fetal metabolic rate; however, the clinical significance of this effect is not known. Phenylephrine may be administered as a bolus dose (100 to 150 μg) to treat hypotension[99] or as a continuous prophylactic infusion (starting rate, 25 to 50 μg/min).[100] Managing spinal anesthesia-induced hypotension using a prophylactic phenylephrine infusion results in fewer physician interventions and less patient nausea than treating hypotension with bolus-dose phenylephrine after it occurs.[101]

Total Spinal Anesthesia

High or total spinal anesthesia is a rare complication of intrathecal or epidural local anesthetic injection that occurs after excessive cephalad spread of local anesthetic in the subarachnoid or epidural space. Unintentional intrathecal administration of epidural medication as a result of dural puncture or catheter migration may also result in this complication. There is rapid ascent of sensory–motor blockade and patients may complain of dyspnea, inability to phonate, and difficulty swallowing. Profound hypotension may lead to brainstem and cerebral hypoperfusion and cause loss of consciousness. Immediate vasopressor administration, continued fluid administration, left uterine displacement, and leg elevation might be necessary to achieve hemodynamic stability. Reverse Trendelenburg position should not be used if hyperbaric anesthetic solution was used for spinal blockade, as there is a risk of cerebral hypoperfusion. Rapid control of the airway is essential, and endotracheal intubation may be necessary to ensure oxygenation without aspiration.

Local Anesthetic Systemic Toxicity

LAST may occur after unintended intravascular injection or drug accumulation (see Chapter 22). Resuscitation equipment (intravenous access, airway equipment, emergency drugs, and suction equipment) should always be available when using local anesthetics. To avoid systemic toxicity of local anesthetic agents, strict adherence to recommended dosages, methods to detect misplaced needles and catheters, and fractional administration of the induction dose are essential.

Despite these precautions, life-threatening convulsions and, rarely, cardiovascular collapse may occur. Seizure activity should be treated with an intravenous benzodiazepine, such as midazolam (1 to 5 mg), or other sedative–hypnotic. Hemodynamics, ventilation, and oxygenation must be maintained. Lipid emulsion (20%, 1.5 mL/kg over 1 minute, followed by 0.25 mL/kg/min for at least 10 minutes after attainment of hemodynamic stability) should be administered concurrent with basic and advanced cardiac life support protocols.[102] Vasopressin, along with calcium channel blockers and β-adrenergic blockers should be avoided. Amiodarone may be used to treat ventricular dysrhythmias, particularly those due to bupivacaine. Failure to respond to lipid emulsion and vasopressor therapy should prompt consideration of cardiopulmonary bypass. Perimortem cesarean delivery may be required to relieve aortocaval compression and to ensure the efficacy of cardiac massage.[103]

Postdural Puncture Headache

By virtue of age and gender, pregnant women are at a higher risk for developing PDPH (see Chapter 35). In addition, after delivery, reduced epidural pressure may increase the risk of cerebrospinal fluid leakage through the dural rent, and estrogen withdrawal after delivery may exacerbate vascular headaches.

The incidence of PDPH is related to the diameter of the dural puncture, ranging from in excess of 70% after the use of 16-gauge spinal needles to less than 1% with 25- or 26-gauge spinal needles. The incidence of cephalalgia is reduced with the use of pencil-point needles (Whitacre or Sprotte), compared with cutting bevel (Quincke) needles. Conservative treatment is indicated in the presence of mild-to-moderate discomfort, and includes bed rest, hydration, and simple analgesics. Caffeine (500 mg intravenously or 300 mg orally) has also been used in the treatment of PDPH, but the therapeutic effect is transient. Severe headache that does not respond to conservative measures for 24 hours is best treated with an autologous epidural blood patch. Using aseptic technique, approximately 20 mL of the patient's blood is injected into the epidural space close to the site of dural puncture.[104] Prophylactic administration of autologous blood (after delivery, before removal of the epidural catheter) does not influence the incidence and severity of PDPH, although the duration of headache is less, compared with expectant management.[105] Data supporting the use of intrathecal catheter placement for prevention of PDPH are inconsistent.[106]

Nerve Injury

Neurologic sequelae of central neuraxial blockade, although rare, have been reported. Pressure or trauma exerted by a needle or catheter on spinal nerve roots or the spinal cord produces immediate pain. Needle or catheter advancement should stop immediately on patient complaint of paresthesia or pain, and if the symptom does not resolve within seconds, the needle or catheter should be withdrawn and repositioned. Anesthetics should *not* be injected when there are paresthesias. Infections are rare; epidural abscess is usually caused by skin contaminants and meningitis by contamination of drugs or needles with clinicians' nasopharyngeal flora.[107] Epidural hematoma can also occur, usually in association with coagulation defects. Nerve root irritation may have a protracted recovery, lasting weeks or months. Postpartum peripheral nerve injury as a result of instrumentation, lithotomy position, or compression by the fetal head is not uncommon and is not related to neuraxial anesthesia.[108]

Management of High-risk Parturients

Pregnancy and parturition are considered "high risk" when accompanied by conditions unfavorable to the well-being of the mother, the fetus, or both. Maternal problems may be related to pregnancy, such as preeclampsia–eclampsia and other hypertensive disorders of pregnancy, or antepartum hemorrhage resulting from placenta previa or abruptio placentae. Diabetes mellitus, cardiac, chronic renal, neurologic, or sickle cell disease; and asthma, obesity, and drug abuse are not related to pregnancy but affect or are affected by it. Advanced maternal age (AMA)—usually defined as age 35 or more at the time of delivery—is associated with an increased risk of maternal and fetal complications. Prematurity (gestation of <37 weeks), postmaturity (≥42 weeks), intrauterine growth retardation (IUGR), and multiple gestation are fetal conditions associated with increased risk. During labor and delivery, fetal malpresentation (breech, transverse lie), placental abruption, compression of the umbilical cord (prolapse, nuchal cord), precipitous labor, or intrauterine infection (prolonged rupture of membranes) may increase the risk to the mother or the fetus.

In general, the anesthetic management of the high-risk parturient is based on the same maternal and fetal considerations as the management of healthy mothers and fetuses. These include maintenance of maternal cardiovascular function and oxygenation, maximization of uteroplacental blood flow, and creation of optimal conditions for a painless, atraumatic delivery of an infant without significant drug effects. However, there is less physiologic reserve because many of these functions may be compromised before the induction of anesthesia. For example, significant acidosis is prone to develop in fetuses of diabetic mothers when delivered by cesarean section with spinal anesthesia complicated by even brief maternal hypotension. Because the high-risk parturient may have received a variety of drugs, anesthesiologists must be familiar with potential interactions between these drugs and the anesthetic drugs they plan to administer.

Hypertensive Disorders of Pregnancy

3

Hypertensive disorders, which occur in up to 10% of pregnancies, are a major cause of maternal morbidity and mortality.[109] The ACOG[110] has modified the diagnosis and management of hypertensive disorders of pregnancy. The four categories are as follows. *Gestational hypertension* which describes the development of elevated blood pressure after 20 weeks of gestation without proteinuria or severe features of preeclampsia. *Chronic hypertension* is pre-existing hypertension or hypertension developing before 20 weeks of gestation. *Chronic hypertension with superimposed preeclampsia* includes elevated blood pressure with new onset of proteinuria or other signs/symptoms of preeclampsia. The ACOG task force[110] does not recommend treatment of hypertension unless the blood pressure is above 160 mmHg systolic or 110 mmHg diastolic to minimize fetal risk. Above these parameters, treatment is indicated to reduce maternal risk. *Preeclampsia/eclampsia* is the fourth category. *Preeclampsia* is defined by hypertension with proteinuria or any of the severe features of preeclampsia. Proteinuria is no longer necessary for the diagnosis of preeclampsia. Mild preeclampsia has been replaced by preeclampsia without severe features. *Eclampsia* is present if convulsions occur. Preeclampsia–eclampsia is a disease of unknown etiology but is unique to human pregnancy. Symptoms can appear before the 20th week, with a hydatidiform mole. The condition requires the presence of a trophoblast but not a fetus.[110]

Many of the symptoms associated with preeclampsia, including placental ischemia, systemic vasoconstriction, and increased platelet aggregation, may result from an imbalance in placental production of prostacyclin and thromboxane (Figs. 41-3 and 41-4). During normal pregnancy, the placenta produces equivalent quantities of these prostaglandins, whereas in preeclamptic

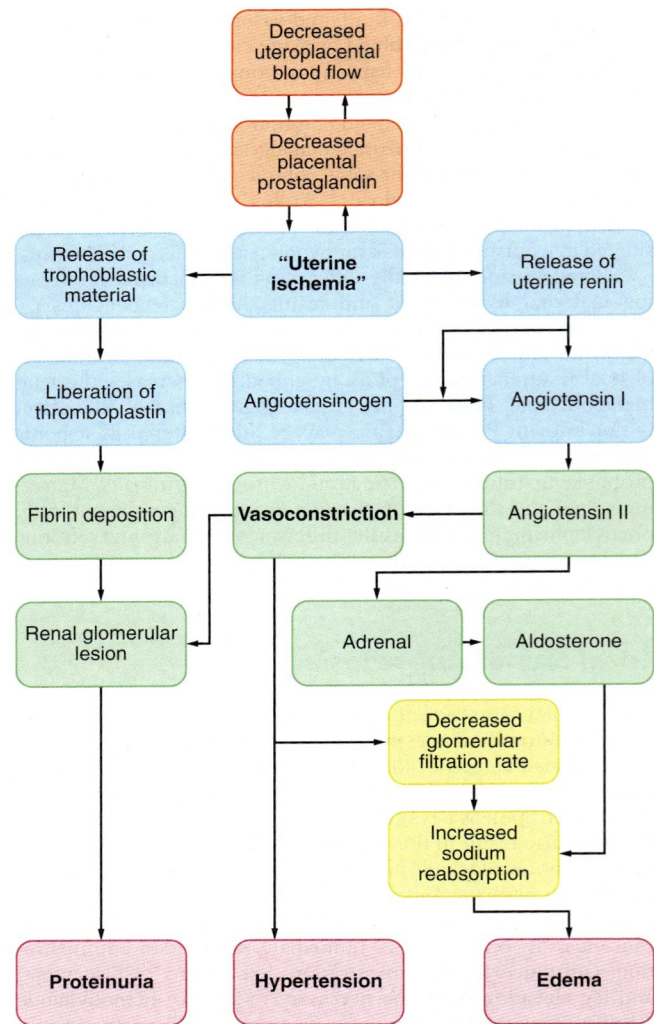

Figure 41-3 Proposed scheme of pathophysiologic changes in toxemia of pregnancy. (Reprinted with permission from Speroff L. Toxemia of pregnancy: mechanism and therapeutic management. *Am J Cardiol.* 1973;32:582.)

pregnancy, there is seven times more thromboxane than prostacyclin.[111] An alternative etiology may be related to an inhibition of the normal trophoblastic migration of placental arterioles during the second trimester, thus preventing a low-resistance, high-flow placental circulation from developing.[112] Endothelial dysfunction is central to the development of preeclampsia. In preeclamptic women, there appears to be an imbalance between proangiogenic factors (vascular endothelial growth factor [VEGF]) and antiangiogenic factors (soluble fms–like tyrosine kinase 1 [sFlt-1]). Increased sensitivity to angiotensin II has also been observed in patients with preeclampsia. This may be the result of the presence of autoantibodies to the angiotensin AT-1 receptor.

Placental ischemia results in a release of uterine renin and an increase in angiotensin (Fig. 41-3). Widespread arteriolar vasoconstriction occurs, causing hypertension, tissue hypoxia, and endothelial damage. Adherence of platelets at sites of endothelial damage results in coagulopathy. Enhanced angiotensin-mediated aldosterone secretion may lead to increased sodium

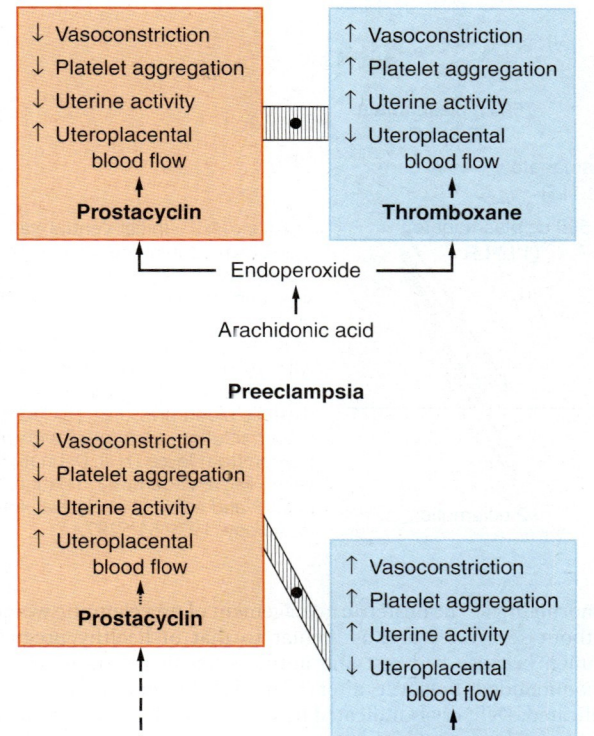

Figure 41-4 Comparison of the balance in the biologic actions of prostacyclin and thromboxane in normal pregnancy with the imbalance of increased thromboxane and decreased prostacyclin in preeclamptic pregnancy. (Reprinted with permission from Walsh SW. Preeclampsia: an imbalance in placental prostacyclin and thromboxane production. *Am J Obstet Gynecol.* 1985;152:335.)

reabsorption and edema. Proteinuria may also be attributed to placental ischemia, which would lead to local tissue degeneration and a release of thromboplastin with subsequent deposition of fibrin in constricted glomerular vessels, as well as increased permeability to albumin and other plasma proteins. Furthermore, there is believed to be a decreased production of prostaglandin E, a potent vasodilator secreted in the trophoblast, which normally would balance the hypertensive effects of the renin–angiotensin system. The HELLP syndrome is a particular form of severe preeclampsia characterized by hemolysis, elevated liver enzymes, and low platelet count (thrombocytopenia). In contrast to preeclampsia, elevations in blood pressure and proteinuria may be mild.

Severe features of preeclampsia include:
- Severe hypertension
  - Systolic blood pressure more than 160 mmHg
  - Diastolic blood pressure more than 110 mmHg
- Thrombocytopenia (platelet count < 100×10^9/L)
- Impaired liver function
- Renal insufficiency (either serum creatinine concentration >1.1 mg/dL, or doubling of the baseline serum creatinine concentration)
- Pulmonary edema
- New-onset cerebral or visual disturbances

Severe preeclampsia–eclampsia is a multisystem disease. Global cerebral blood flow is not diminished, but focal hypoperfusion may occur. Postmortem examination has revealed hemorrhagic necrosis in the proximity of thrombosed precapillaries, suggesting intense vasoconstriction. Cerebral edema and small foci of degeneration have been attributed to hypoxia. Petechial hemorrhages are common after the onset of convulsions. Symptoms related to these changes include headache, vertigo, cortical blindness, hyperreflexia, and convulsions. Blood pressure elevation correlates poorly with the incidence of seizures. Cerebral hemorrhage and edema account for 50% of deaths with preeclampsia–eclampsia. Intense ocular arteriolar constriction may cause blurred vision, even temporary blindness. In severe cases, heart failure may result due to peripheral vasoconstriction and increased blood viscosity secondary to hemoconcentration. Left ventricular hypertrophy, subendocardial hemorrhages, and fatty and hyaline degeneration may occur.

Decreased blood supply to the liver may lead to periportal necrosis. Subcapsular hemorrhage results in epigastric pain. Rarely, there is rupture of the overstretched liver capsule and massive hemorrhage into the abdominal cavity. There may be elevated aspartate aminotransferase, lactate dehydrogenase, and alkaline phosphatase, whereas bilirubin is unaltered.

In the kidneys, there is swelling of glomerular endothelial cells and deposition of fibrin, leading to a constriction of the capillary lumina. Renal blood flow and glomerular filtration rate decrease, resulting in reduced uric acid clearance and, in severe cases, reduced clearance of urea and creatinine. Oliguria and proteinuria are characteristic symptoms of severe preeclampsia. The severity of renal involvement is reflected in the degree of proteinuria, which may reach nephrotic levels of 10 to 15 g/24 hr.

A mild pulmonary ventilation–perfusion imbalance has been reported in severe cases. It is not believed to be clinically important because the arterial oxygen tension was within normal limits. In contrast, airway edema, which may also occur in severe preeclampsia, is of great concern because it may lead to difficulty in tracheal intubation. Pulmonary edema occurs in approximately 2% of severe preeclamptic patients as a result of heart failure, circulatory overload, or aspiration of gastric contents during convulsions.

A reduction in intervillous blood flow may result from vasoconstriction or the development of occlusive lesions in decidual arteries, despite the elevated maternal blood pressure. Reduced placental blood flow leads to chronic fetal hypoxia and malnutrition. The risks of IUGR, premature birth, and perinatal death are substantially higher than in normal pregnancies and correlate with the severity of preeclampsia.

Although preeclampsia is accompanied by exaggerated retention of water and sodium, a shift of fluid and proteins from the intravascular into the extravascular compartment may result in hypovolemia, hypoproteinemia, and hemoconcentration. This phenomenon may be further affected by proteinuria. The risk of uteroplacental hypoperfusion and poor fetal outcome correlates with the degree of maternal plasma and protein depletion. The mean plasma volume in women with preeclampsia was found to be 9% less than normal, and in those with severe disease, 30% to 40% below normal.[113] The inverse relationship between the intravascular volume and the severity of hypertension was confirmed with measurements of central venous pressure (CVP) (Fig. 41-5). Volume expansion may improve maternal tissue perfusion in patients with severe preeclampsia, but must be performed cautiously because of the risk of pulmonary edema.

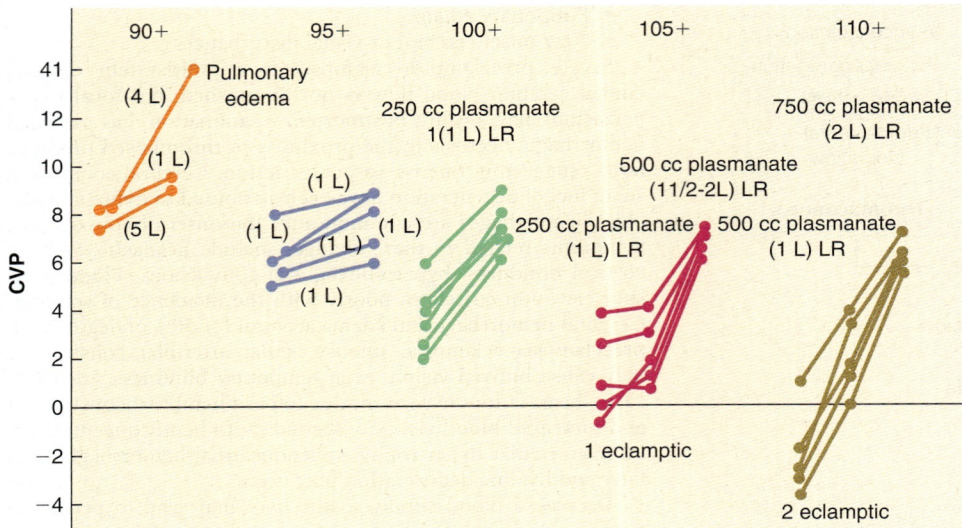

Figure 41-5 Initial central venous pressure measurements (three or more recordings of maternal diastolic pressure) and intravenous volume replacement required to attain the range of 6 to 8 cm H_2O in five groups of women with preeclampsia classified according to the severity of the disease (by diastolic blood pressure). LR, lactated Ringer solution. (Reprinted with permission from Joyce TH III, Debnath KS, Baker EA. Preeclampsia: relationship of CVP and epidural analgesia. *Anesthesiology*. 1979;51:S297.)

Adherence of platelets at sites of endothelial damage may result in consumptive coagulopathy and thrombocytopenia. It is usually mild, with the platelet count in the range of 100×10^9/L to 150×10^9/L. High-dose steroids (>24 mg of β- or dexamethasone in 24 hours) used to accelerate fetal lung maturity have been shown to prevent a worsening in platelet count or even increase platelet count in women with the HELLP syndrome (Fig. 41-6).[114] Elevated levels of fibrin degradation products are found less frequently, and plasma fibrinogen concentrations remain normal unless there is a placental abruption. Prolongation of prothrombin and partial thromboplastin times indicates consumption of procoagulant. Bleeding time is no longer considered a reliable test of clotting.

General Management

The definitive treatment of preeclampsia/eclampsia remains delivery of the fetus and placenta. Management is usually symptomatic until the obstetrician determines that delivery is appropriate. The goals are to prevent or control convulsions, improve organ perfusion, normalize blood pressure, and correct clotting abnormalities. The obstetric management of preeclamptic women without severe features is similar to that of healthy pregnant women because bed rest and antihypertensive therapy are not recommended; however, after 37 weeks of gestation, delivery is indicated. Delivery is indicated in severe cases if there is nonreassuring fetal status or if the pregnancy is beyond 34 weeks of gestation. In severe cases, aggressive management should continue for at least 24 to 48 hours after delivery.

The mainstay of anticonvulsant therapy is magnesium sulfate (see Chapter 16). Magnesium is only recommended for women with severe preeclampsia. The patient usually receives an intravenous loading dose of 4 g in a 20% solution over 5 minutes. Therapeutic blood levels are maintained by continuous infusion of 1 to 2 g/hr. Magnesium may cause mild peripheral arterial vasodilation. Magnesium ions cross the placenta readily and may lead to fetal and neonatal hypermagnesemia. There is poor correlation between magnesium concentrations in the umbilical cord blood and the incidence of low Apgar scores and depression of ventilation at birth, which are more likely due to fetal asphyxia and prematurity. In fact, there is evidence that magnesium therapy is neuroprotective for the fetus and reduces the risk of cerebral palsy.[115]

Magnesium potentiates the duration and intensity of action of depolarizing and nondepolarizing muscle relaxants by decreasing the amount of acetylcholine liberated from the motor nerve terminals, diminishing the sensitivity of the end plate to acetylcholine, and depressing the excitability of the skeletal muscle membrane. Magnesium may also increase the severity of hypotension under regional anesthesia and make it more difficult to treat. Judicious hydration with a balanced salt solution may be required to replace intravascular volume. In all cases, careful monitoring of arterial pressure and urine output should be started as soon as possible. Invasive arterial blood pressure monitoring may be useful for patients with severe preeclampsia, but CVP monitoring is infrequently used. Monitoring should be extended into the postpartum period.

Antihypertensive therapy in preeclampsia is used to lessen the risk of cerebral hemorrhage in the mother while maintaining, even improving, tissue perfusion. Hydralazine is the most commonly used vasodilator in preeclampsia because it increases uteroplacental and renal blood flow. Nitroprusside, a potent vasodilator of resistance and capacitance vessels, with an

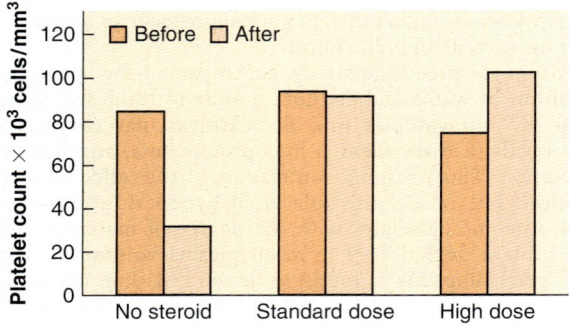

Figure 41-6 Mean platelet count in women with HELLP syndrome without steroids, and before and after standard steroid (<24 mg/day) and high steroid (>24 mg/day) therapy. (Adapted with permission from O'Brien JM, Milligan DA, Barton JR. Impact of high dose corticosteroid therapy for patients with HELLP [hemolysis, elevated liver function tests, and low platelets] syndrome. *Am J Obstet Gynecol*. 2000;183:921.)

immediate but evanescent action, is useful in preventing dangerous elevations in systemic and pulmonary artery blood pressure during laryngoscopy and intubation, and is ideal for treatment of hypertensive emergencies. Other agents used to control maternal blood pressure in preeclampsia include nitroglycerin and labetalol. Consumption coagulopathy may require infusion of fresh whole blood, platelet concentrates, fresh frozen plasma, and cryoprecipitate (see Chapter 17). Neuraxial anesthesia is contraindicated in patients with severe coagulopathy.

Anesthetic Management

Epidural, spinal, or CSE analgesia or anesthesia for labor and delivery should no longer be considered contraindicated in preeclamptic parturients, provided there is no severe clotting abnormality or plasma volume deficit.[116] In volume-repleted patients positioned with left uterine displacement, neuraxial analgesia does not cause an unacceptable reduction in blood pressure and leads to a significant improvement in placental perfusion.[117] With the use of radioactive xenon, it was shown that the intervillous blood flow increased by approximately 75% after the induction of epidural analgesia (10 mL of bupivacaine 0.25%).[118]

For cesarean delivery, the sensory level of anesthesia must extend to T3 to T4, making adequate fluid therapy and left uterine displacement even more critical. The use of spinal anesthesia in severely preeclamptic women has been discouraged in favor of the continuous epidural technique. The concern is related to the fact that severely preeclamptic women can have significant intravascular volume deficits related to widespread arteriolar vasoconstriction, which may result in catastrophic hypotension with the sudden onset of extensive sympathectomy associated with spinal anesthesia. In fact, women with severe preeclampsia appear to be at lower risk of hypotension than normotensive women having cesarean delivery.[119] Furthermore, studies to date have shown that the incidence and severity of hypotension is similar in women with severe preeclampsia having a cesarean delivery with spinal compared with epidural anesthesia.[120,121] Thus, spinal anesthesia is emerging as a suitable alternative to epidural anesthesia for cesarean delivery in severely preeclamptic women. It is important to note that severely preeclamptic women need to be adequately prepared prior to neuraxial anesthesia with judicious hydration and control of blood pressure.

General anesthesia in preeclamptic patients has its particular hazards. Rapid-sequence induction of anesthesia and intubation of the trachea are occasionally difficult because of a swollen tongue, epiglottis, or pharynx (see Chapter 28). In patients with impaired coagulation, laryngoscopy and intubation of the trachea may provoke profuse bleeding. Marked systemic and pulmonary hypertension occurring at intubation and extubation enhance the risk of cerebral hemorrhage and pulmonary edema (Fig. 41-7). However, these hemodynamic changes can be minimized with appropriate antihypertensive therapy, such as administration of labetalol or nitroprusside infusion. The use of ketamine and ergot alkaloids should be avoided. Magnesium may prolong the effects of all muscle relaxants through its actions on the myoneural junction. Therefore, relaxants should be administered with caution (using a nerve stimulator) to avoid overdosage. General anesthesia may be necessary in acute emergencies, such as abruptio placentae, and in patients who do not meet the criteria for neuraxial anesthesia.

Obstetric Hemorrhage

Worldwide, hemorrhage remains the leading cause of maternal mortality, causing 25% of peripartum deaths. The vast majority of these deaths occur in the developing world; however, there is evidence that the rate and severity of hemorrhage are increasing in developed nations, including the United States.[122,123] Obstetric hemorrhage can be defined in four "categories": Abnormal tissue (placentation), abnormal tone (atony), abnormal coagulation, and trauma (uterine rupture, cesarean delivery).

Antepartum hemorrhage occurs in association with placenta previa (abnormal placental implantation on the lower uterine segment and partial-to-total occlusion of the internal cervical

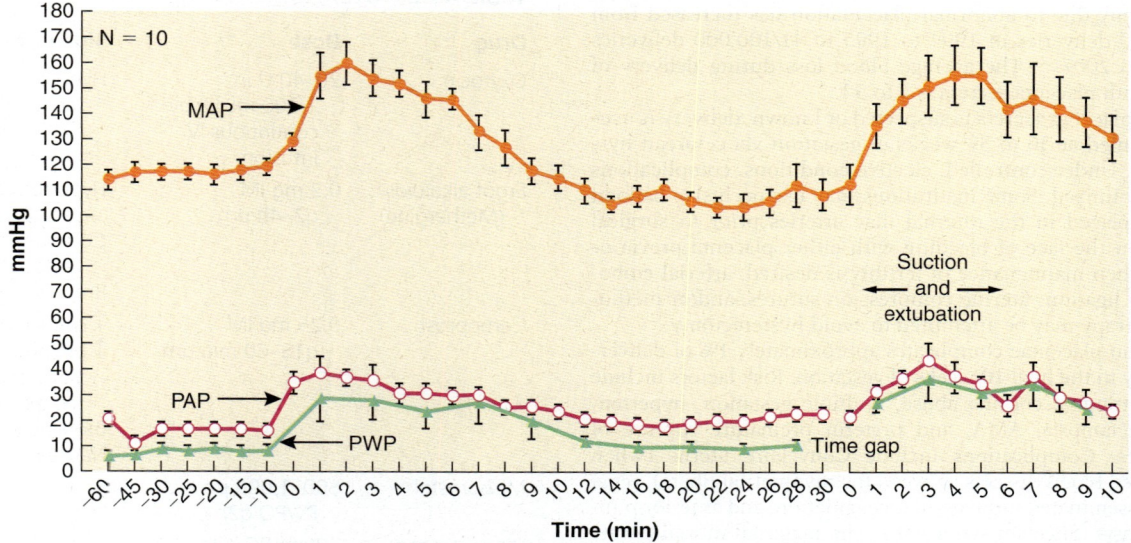

Figure 41-7 Mean and SE of mean arterial pressure (MAP), mean pulmonary artery pressure (PAP), and pulmonary wedge pressure (PWP) in patients with severe preeclampsia receiving thiopental and nitrous oxide (40%) with 0.5% halothane anesthesia for cesarean section. (Reprinted with permission from Hodgkinson R, Husain FJ, Hayashi RH. Systemic and pulmonary blood pressure during cesarean section in parturients with gestational hypertension. *Can Anaesth Soc J.* 1980;27:389.)

os) and abruptio placentae. Placenta previa complicates approximately 0.4% of pregnancies, resulting in up to 0.9% incidence of maternal mortality and a 17% to 26% incidence of perinatal mortality. Risk factors for placenta previa include previous cesarean delivery, uterine surgery, or pregnancy termination. Other risk factors include smoking, AMA, multiparity, multiple gestation, and cocaine abuse. The risk for placenta previa increases in a "dose-dependent" manner with the number of previous cesarean deliveries and greater parity. The relative risk is 4.5 (95% confidence interval, 3.6 to 5.5) with one previous cesarean delivery, and it increases to 44.9 (95% confidence interval, 13.5 to 139.5) with four prior cesarean deliveries.[124,125] The diagnosis should be suspected whenever a patient presents with painless, bright red vaginal bleeding, usually after the seventh month of pregnancy. Placenta previa may also be associated with an unstable or abnormal lie. The diagnosis is confirmed by ultrasonography. If bleeding is not profuse and the fetus is immature, obstetric management is conservative to prolong pregnancy. Admission to a high-risk unit is advisable if contractions or acute bleeding are present. Intravenous access and typed and cross-matched blood should be available at all times. In severe cases, or if the fetus is mature at the onset of symptoms, prompt delivery is indicated, usually by cesarean section.

Anesthesia for delivery of patients with placenta previa may be with neuraxial anesthesia, provided the mother is hemodynamically stable. Past recommendations for general anesthesia to provide "more control" are not supported by the literature, as there is no difference in complications between the two techniques, except that general anesthesia is associated with greater blood loss and greater need for transfusion. An emergency hysterectomy may be required if there is severe hemorrhage, even after delivery of the placenta, because of uterine atony. The risk of severe hemorrhage after attempted removal of the placenta is greatly increased in patients who have undergone prior uterine surgery, including cesarean delivery. This is related to a higher incidence of placenta accreta, which results from the penetration of myometrium by placental villi. The risk of placenta accreta in women with previa increases from 3% in primary cesarean section to 61% in quaternary section.[126] Indeed, placenta accreta is becoming the leading cause of cesarean hysterectomy, and the rate of cesarean hysterectomy due to abnormal placentation has increased from 33/100,000 deliveries in 1994 to 1995 to 41/100,000 deliveries in 2006 to 2007.[127] The average blood loss during delivery of patients with placenta accreta is 3 to 5 L.

When placenta accreta is suspected or known, delivery is usually scheduled at 36 to 37 weeks of gestation via cesarean hysterectomy. Under controlled, elective conditions, complications can be minimized. Some institutions may use occlusive balloon catheters placed in the internal iliac arteries prior to surgical delivery. In the face of bleeding with either placenta previa or accreta, when maintenance of fertility is desired, arterial embolization or ligation, uterine compression sutures, and/or methotrexate therapy may be attempted to avoid hysterectomy.[128]

Abruptio placentae complicates approximately 1% of deliveries, usually in the final 10 weeks of gestation. Risk factors include smoking, trauma, cocaine abuse, multiple gestation, hypertension, preeclampsia, AMA, and preterm premature rupture of membranes. Complications include Couvelaire uterus (when extravasated blood dissects between the myometrial fibers), renal failure, disseminated intravascular coagulation, and anterior pituitary necrosis (Sheehan syndrome). The maternal mortality rate is high (1.8% to 11.0%), and the perinatal mortality rate is even higher, in excess of 50%. The diagnosis of abruptio placentae is based on the presence of uterine tenderness and hypertonus as well as vaginal bleeding of dark, clotted blood. Bleeding may be concealed if the placental margins have remained attached to the uterine wall. If the blood loss is severe (>2 L), there may be changes in the maternal blood pressure and pulse rate, indicative of hypovolemia. Fetal movement may increase during acute hypoxia or decrease if hypoxia is gradual. Fetal bradycardia and death may ensue. When placental separation is more than 50%, stillbirth is the likeliest outcome. Management of abruption depends on presentation, gestational age, and the degree of compromise. Management of milder cases of abruption includes artificial rupture of amniotic membranes and oxytocin augmentation of labor, if required. Distant from term, expectant management with close observation is reasonable. In the presence of nonreassuring fetal status, an emergency cesarean delivery may be performed. If fetal death has occurred, usually with severe abruption, vaginal delivery is reasonable if the mother is stable.

Postpartum hemorrhage is usually defined as blood loss greater than 500 mL after vaginal delivery or greater than 1,000 mL after cesarean section. The incidence of postpartum hemorrhage is increasing in the United States, mainly due to an increase in uterine atony.[122,123] Predisposing factors to atony include multiple gestations, labor induction or augmentation, cesarean delivery, polyhydramnios, chorioamnionitis, hypertensive disorders of pregnancy, retained products of conception, and antepartum hemorrhage. Treatment of postpartum hemorrhage may require aggressive uterotonic therapy for atony, intrauterine balloon tamponade or evacuation of the uterus for retained products of conception (Table 41-2). If there is a need for dilation and curettage, the anesthesiologist may be asked to provide uterine relaxation. This can be accomplished with volatile agents if the patient is under general anesthesia or with intravenous nitroglycerin if regional anesthesia or general anesthesia is used.

The anesthesiologist's role in management of obstetric hemorrhage includes both maternal resuscitation and provision of anesthesia for cesarean delivery, cesarean hysterectomy, or dilation and curettage. The choice of anesthetic technique depends on the anticipated duration of surgery, maternal condition and volume status, the potential for coagulopathy, and

Table 41-2 Uterotonic Therapy

Drug	Dose	Side Effects
Oxytocin	20–40 U in 1,000 mL LR by continuous IV infusion	Hypotension, tachycardia
Ergot alkaloids (Methergine)	0.2 mg IM q2–4h prn	Hypertension, vasoconstriction Coronary vasospasm Bronchospasm
Carboprost	0.25 mg IM q15–60 min prn	↑ cardiac output ↑ pulmonary vascular resistance Bronchospasm Nausea
Misoprostol	800–1,000 μg PR/PV/PO q2h	Fever Nausea
Dinoprostone	20 mg PO q2h	Hypotension Nausea

LR, Lactated Ringer solution; IV, intravenous; IM, intramuscularly; prn, as needed; PR, rectally; PV, vaginally; PO, orally.

urgency of the procedure. General anesthesia is indicated in the presence of uncontrolled hemorrhage and/or severe coagulation abnormalities. Neuraxial anesthesia, usually continuous epidural anesthesia, has been successfully used for hysterectomy in planned, controlled situations. A saddle block is an option for anesthesia when dilation and curettage for treatment of postpartum hemorrhage is indicated and the patient is hemodynamically stable.

Maternal resuscitation in the setting of hemorrhage may require rapid securing of the airway if significant hemodynamic instability occurs, in addition to obtaining large-bore intravenous, arterial, and possibly central venous access. All of these tasks may be challenging in the parturient and consideration should be given to performing them in advance of hemorrhage when hemorrhage is anticipated. Prompt transfusion of blood component therapy is crucial for replacement of blood loss, maintenance of tissue oxygenation, and correction of coagulopathy. In recent years, transfusion rates for postpartum hemorrhage have increased 92% in the United States.[123,129,130]

The practice of transfusing packed red blood cells and fresh frozen plasma in a 1:1 ratio decreases mortality from hemorrhage in trauma patients. Early administration of platelets and cryoprecipitate has also become common in *hemostatic resuscitation protocols* for major traumatic hemorrhage, and crystalloid and colloid administration is minimized in favor of blood products (see Chapter 53). Hypothermia, metabolic acidosis, and coagulopathy commonly occur in traumatic and obstetric hemorrhage. Because of these commonalities, it has become common to extend these successful transfusion practices from the trauma literature to obstetric practice. Transfusion of cryoprecipitate or better, fibrinogen concentrate, should be incorporated early in obstetric hemorrhage because decreased fibrinogen levels strongly correlate with increased severity of postpartum hemorrhage.[129,131] Obstetric hemorrhage is associated with the rapid development of consumptive and dilutional coagulopathy and can be quickly assessed using point-of-care testing of clotting with thromboelastography (TEG) or rotational thromboelastometry (ROTEM) (see Chapter 17).

Other options are available to decrease transfusion requirements and reduce blood loss. Intraoperative cell salvage, formerly shunned because of concerns about the risk of amniotic fluid contamination of red cells, has been implemented safely during cesarean section in many centers.[132] There is also increasing interest in the use of prohemostatic agents for the treatment of obstetric hemorrhage. The antifibrinolytic drug tranexamic acid has been shown to decrease bleeding in both elective cesarean section and postpartum hemorrhage and is recommended for early use in resuscitation by a European task force[131]; however, further studies are needed to confirm its safety.[133] Case reports and series also describe the safe and effective use of activated recombinant factor VII for intractable hemorrhage.[134]

11 Heart Disease

Heart disease during pregnancy occurs in about 1.6% of patients and is a leading nonobstetric cause of maternal morbidity and mortality, with a mortality rate ranging from 0.4% among patients in class I or II of the New York Heart Association's functional classification to 6.8% among those in classes III and IV. Medical and surgical advancements have changed the types of cardiac problems seen in pregnancy. Patients with congenital heart disease are reaching childbearing age, and the number of patients with rheumatic heart disease has declined. Older parturients may present with aortic stenosis and insufficiency associated with a bicuspid aortic valve. AMA and obesity may be associated with coronary artery disease and myocardial ischemia. Deaths associated with congenital heart disease have decreased, but there appears to be an increase in deaths described as sudden arrhythmic death syndrome (SADS).[135] Peripartum cardiomyopathy continues to be associated with a high rate of maternal morbidity and mortality.[136,137]

Cardiac decompensation occurs most commonly at times of maximum hemodynamic stress—in the third trimester of pregnancy, during labor and delivery, and during the immediate postpartum period. The increase in maternal blood volume, which occurs at 20 to 24 weeks of gestation, may also precipitate cardiac decompensation. During labor, cardiac output increases progressively above antepartum levels; with each uterine contraction, approximately 200 mL of blood moves into the central circulation. Consequently, stroke volume, cardiac output, and left ventricular work increase, and each contraction consistently increases cardiac output by 10% to 25% above that of uterine diastole. The greatest change occurs immediately after delivery of the placenta, when cardiac output increases to an average of 80% above prepartum values; in some patients, it may increase by as much as 150%.

Evaluation of pre-existing heart disease is crucial and a multidisciplinary approach is necessary when managing patients with complicated cardiac disease during pregnancy and parturition.[138] Many symptoms of pregnancy can mimic those of cardiac disease, complicating new diagnoses of cardiac disease during pregnancy. Labored breathing and venous stasis from aortocaval compression may mimic pulmonary and peripheral edema associated with congestive heart failure. Flow murmurs may be difficult to distinguish from those due to organic lesions. Finally, elevation of the diaphragm causes the heart to rotate, signs of which may be mistaken for cardiac hypertrophy. For the anesthesiologist, it is particularly important to understand how the hemodynamic consequences of different anesthetic techniques might adversely affect mothers with specific cardiac lesions. Invasive monitoring during labor and delivery is rarely indicated. Exceptions are patients with pulmonary hypertension, right-to-left shunts, or coarctation of the aorta. Because hemodynamic changes observed during labor and delivery persist into the postpartum period, if used, invasive monitoring should continue for 24 to 48 hours postpartum.

Congenital Heart Disease

Many patients with successful surgical repair of congenital heart defects are asymptomatic with minimal cardiac findings. Patients with uncorrected or partially corrected lesions may have serious cardiac decompensation with pregnancy. This includes patients with corrected tetralogy of Fallot who may have recurrence of a small ventricular septal defect or develop outflow obstruction. Neuraxial labor analgesia is recommended to minimize hemodynamic changes associated with pain. Maintenance of SVR and venous return is necessary to prevent an increase in right-to-left shunt. Phenylephrine should be used to minimize and/or treat reduction in SVR associated with sympathetic blockade.

Patients with corrected ventricular septal defects or atrial septal defects require no special care, nor do those with small asymptomatic atrial septal defects or ventricular septal defects. In symptomatic patients, neuraxial analgesia will minimize the increase in SVR associated with elevated catecholamines due to pain and may slightly decrease SVR, thus minimizing left-to-right shunting through the defect. Large ventricular septal defects or atrial septal defects are associated with pulmonary hypertension. Patients with these lesions require invasive monitoring and an analgesic technique that maintains SVR, heart rate, and pulmonary vascular resistance.

Eisenmenger syndrome occurs when uncorrected left-to-right shunt results in pulmonary hypertension, which, when severe, reverses flow to a right-to-left shunt. Pregnancy is not well tolerated and mortality can approach 30%, most commonly from embolic phenomena. Management of these patients is challenging. Invasive monitoring of arterial and cardiac filling pressures is indicated. The right ventricle is at greater risk of dysfunction than the left ventricle. Thus, measuring the right atrial pressure is useful in this setting. Implementing labor analgesia that does not lead to deleterious hemodynamic changes is a challenge; opioid-based neuraxial techniques (e.g., CSE, continuous spinal) combined with a dilute local anesthetic may be the best option.

Cesarean delivery is most often accomplished under general anesthesia in women with Eisenmenger syndrome. It should be recognized that arm-to-brain circulation times are rapid owing to right-to-left intracardiac shunts; drugs given intravenously have a rapid onset of action. In contrast to parenteral drugs, the rate of rise of arterial concentrations of inhaled drugs is slow because of decreased pulmonary blood flow. The myocardial depressant and vasodilating actions of volatile drugs may be hazardous in patients with Eisenmenger syndrome, and nitrous oxide, which may increase pulmonary vascular resistance, should be avoided. Positive-pressure ventilation (PPV) of the lungs may also decrease pulmonary blood flow. Sympathetic blockade with CSE anesthesia may lead to cardiovascular decompensation. Thus, maintenance of preload using phenylephrine and fluids, guided by CVP measurements, is essential if regional anesthesia is selected. Hemodynamic monitoring for 48 hours postpartum is essential.

Valvular Heart Disease

The decrease in incidence of rheumatic heart disease in the developed world has resulted in fewer parturients with valvular heart disease. Aortic stenosis is now likely associated with a bicuspid valve in the patient with AMA. Table 41-3 summarizes the management goals of patients with valvular heart disease.

Patients with prosthetic heart valves present a different challenge in pregnancy. Bioprostheses avoid the risk of thrombosis and the need for anticoagulation. There is, however, concern that pregnancy hastens the rate of valve deterioration. Mechanical valves require anticoagulation. Compared to heparin, warfarin is associated with a lower incidence of thrombosis, but also an unacceptable fetal risk. Unfractionated heparin (UFH) and low-molecular-weight heparin (LMWH) do not cross the placenta but it is more difficult to ensure appropriate anticoagulation. The American College of Cardiology recommends any of the following options once pregnancy is confirmed[138]:
- Continue warfarin until 36 weeks, then convert to UFH or LMWH.
- Use UFH or LMWH from 6 to 12 weeks and after 36 weeks; use warfarin from 12 to 36 weeks.
- Use LMWH throughout pregnancy.

Primary Pulmonary Hypertension

Primary pulmonary hypertension (PPH) is seen predominantly in young women. Pulmonary hypertension is defined as mean pulmonary artery pressure over 25 mmHg at rest or 30 mmHg with exercise. The cause is unclear but is associated with endothelial dysfunction. Although uncommon in pregnancy, PPH is associated with a very high maternal mortality; pregnancy is discouraged and termination is advised should pregnancy occur.

The mode of delivery of these patients is contentious. Vaginal delivery is associated with smaller hemodynamic shifts and less risk for bleeding. However, emergency cesarean delivery for maternal or fetal deterioration may be needed. Planned cesarean delivery may offer the advantages of ensuring optimal conditions and the availability of experienced staff.

Pain during labor and vaginal delivery is especially detrimental because it may further increase pulmonary vascular resistance and decrease venous return. Neuraxial analgesia is useful for preventing pain-induced increases in pulmonary vascular resistance. Dilute local anesthetic solutions with the addition of opioids will minimize the decrease in SVR. General and epidural anesthesia have been used for cesarean delivery. Spinal anesthesia may result in a sudden decrease in SVR and is thus not recommended for cesarean delivery. Risks of general anesthesia include increased pulmonary artery pressures during laryngoscopy and tracheal intubation, the adverse effects of PPV on venous return, and the negative inotropic effects of volatile anesthetics. Nitrous oxide may further increase pulmonary vascular resistance and should not be used. In addition to oxygen, the administration of isoproterenol, inhaled nitric oxide, calcium channel blockers, or sildenafil may be useful for decreasing pulmonary vascular resistance. Hemodynamic monitoring, including systemic and pulmonary arterial pressures, remains controversial in these patients, with no evidence to support the use of pulmonary artery catheters. Pulmonary artery rupture and thrombosis are risks of pulmonary artery catheters in the presence of pulmonary hypertension, but some argue that the benefits in these critically ill patients offset these potential hazards. Maternal mortality is estimated between 30% and 55%, with most deaths due to right heart failure that occurs during labor and the early postpartum period.[138]

Cardiomyopathy of Pregnancy

Cardiomyopathy of pregnancy is left ventricular failure occurring late in pregnancy or in the first 6 weeks postpartum. It occurs in approximately 1 in 3,000 births and is associated with a maternal mortality of 25% to 50%. It is a diagnosis of exclusion, the etiology thought to be related to myocarditis or an abnormal immune response. Risk factors include AMA, multiparity, multiple gestation, obesity, hypertension, and preeclampsia.[137,139] Good long-term prognosis is related to recovery of left ventricular function within 6 months of delivery. A left ventricular ejection fraction of less than

Table 41-3 Hemodynamic Goals with Valvular Lesions	
Lesion	Goal
Aortic stenosis	Sinus rhythm Maintain HR Avoid ↓ SVR Maintain venous return
Aortic insufficiency	Mild ↑ HR Avoid ↑ SVR
Mitral stenosis	Sinus rhythm ↓ HR Maintain SVR Maintain venous return
Mitral insufficiency	Sinus rhythm Mild ↑ HR Avoid ↑ SVR Avoid ↑ venous return

SVR, systemic vascular resistance; HR, heart rate.

25% at diagnosis is associated with poor long-term outcome, even with recovery after pregnancy, and these patients should be counseled against future pregnancies. If the cardiomyopathy persists, the mortality may be as high as 50%; many patients with persistent cardiomyopathy become transplant candidates. Medical management includes preload optimization, afterload reduction, and therapy to improve myocardial contractility. Patients may require thromboprophylaxis. Intrapartum anesthetic management is directed at minimizing cardiac stress and thus decompensation, and may be aided by invasive hemodynamic monitoring.

Coronary Artery Disease and Myocardial Infarction

Acute myocardial infarction during pregnancy is rare, occurring in 1 in 10,000 to 30,000 women. It is associated with a maternal mortality as high as 37% as well as a high infant mortality rate (9%). As more women with risk factors become pregnant, this complication will increase in frequency. The left anterior descending artery is most commonly affected, with 47% of infarcts associated with coronary spasm (i.e., normal angiogram) and another 16% associated with coronary artery dissection. Risk factors include smoking, obesity, AMA, diabetes, hypertension, and hyperlipidemia. Women older than 35 years are at greatest risk; the risk is 30-fold higher in women older than 40 years, compared to women younger than 20 years. The ergot alkaloids should be avoided because they can lead to coronary vasospasm, as can cocaine use.[140]

Diagnosis may be difficult as symptoms of ischemia may mimic common nonspecific complaints during pregnancy. Thus the greatest obstacle to diagnosis is a low index of suspicion. Cardiac troponin I levels are increased if cardiac muscle injury occurs; however, preeclampsia and gestational hypertension may also increase troponin levels. Therefore, ECG is an important diagnostic tool.

Delivery within 2 weeks of the infarct is associated with a high rate of reinfarction and death. Thus, delaying delivery, if possible, should be considered. Vaginal delivery is associated with lower morbidity and mortality than cesarean delivery. Intrapartum monitoring should mimic intraoperative monitoring of the nonobstetric patient with a recent myocardial infarction.

In the event of cardiac arrest in late pregnancy, left lateral displacement of the uterus should be achieved, and if cardiopulmonary resuscitation is unsuccessful, the fetus should be delivered within 5 minutes to improve maternal and infant survival.[141]

Sudden Arrhythmic Death Syndrome

SADS is defined as sudden cardiac death where all other causes are eliminated. Under this diagnosis are those cases where the heart is normal on autopsy and all stimulant drugs ruled out as a cause of death. Some are identified as likely due to conduction defects by examination of relatives; the remainder are presumed to be related to arrhythmias.[135] An association between obesity and SADS has been suggested.

Diabetes Mellitus

Diabetes occurs in approximately 3% of pregnancies and 8% of gravidae of AMA. The incidence is increasing, in parallel with the increase in population obesity and type 2 diabetes.[142] Gestational diabetes mellitus is diabetes or glucose intolerance that is first diagnosed during pregnancy. Gestational diabetes mellitus is associated with increased adverse outcomes, including macrosomia, neonatal hypoglycemia, hyperbilirubinemia, and intrauterine fetal demise, as well as an increased risk of obesity and diabetes in offspring later in life. Women with gestational diabetes mellitus are at increased risk for development of type 2 diabetes later in life.

Pre-existing type 1 or 2 diabetes is also associated with adverse pregnancy outcomes, including congenital malformations. Vasculopathy, nephropathy, and retinopathy may be exacerbated by pregnancy. Tight glycemic control before and during pregnancy may decrease the risk of adverse outcomes. Although a rare occurrence, normal physiologic changes of pregnancy contribute to a propensity for diabetic women, especially type 1 diabetics, to develop diabetic ketoacidosis (DKA).[143] DKA occurs at lower glucose levels in pregnancy due to enhanced lipogenesis and ketogenesis. β-Adrenergic therapy and steroid administration may also increase the likelihood of developing DKA. Although maternal mortality from DKA is unusual, fetal mortality is high.

Guidelines for the management of pregnant diabetics focus on glycemic control. A blood sugar of 60 to 120 mg/dL is desirable and insulin therapy is needed if fasting blood sugar levels are above 100 mg/dL.[144] Maternal insulin requirements increase progressively during the second and third trimesters. Fetal surveillance is more intense in diabetic women. Antenatal surveillance with twice weekly nonstress tests often begins at 28 weeks. Delivery at 38 weeks of gestation may be considered if estimated fetal weight exceeds 4,500 g or fetal surveillance indicates the need for delivery.

There is no compelling evidence that one analgesic or anesthetic technique is superior to another when caring for diabetic parturients. Patients with pregestational diabetes should be assessed for comorbidities. Neuraxial labor analgesia does not appear to alter peripartum insulin and glucose requirements. Intrapartum blood glucose levels should be monitored frequently, and glucose administration and insulin therapy should be titrated to maintain maternal glucose concentration between 60 and 120 mg/dL. Insulin requirements decrease shortly after delivery.

Obesity

In the United States, over 60% of the adult population is overweight or obese; not surprising, obesity in pregnancy mimics this incidence. Obese women are more likely to have antenatal comorbidities, such as chronic hypertension, diabetes mellitus, and preeclampsia.[145] Obstetric outcome may also be affected by maternal obesity; there is a greater risk of fetal congenital cardiac anomalies, macrosomia, and shoulder dystocia. Abnormal labors and failed inductions of labor, are more likely to occur. Overall cesarean delivery rates, and specifically emergency cesarean delivery rates, increase with increasing body mass index. Preanesthetic evaluation of the obese parturient should be performed with anticipation of these complications and a multidisciplinary care plan should be generated. Careful airway evaluation is required, and alternative airway equipment must be readily available, especially as the use of general anesthesia for cesarean delivery is higher in the obese parturient than in her nonobese peers. In addition, the extent of comorbidities such as hypertension and diabetes mellitus should be assessed, as these occur more frequently in obese patients.[146] Continuous neuraxial analgesia is the preferred option for pain relief during labor because it provides excellent pain relief without sedation/obtundation and prevents additional demands on the cardiorespiratory system of the obese patient. Most importantly, a well-functioning neuraxial anesthetic for labor may also be used for anesthesia for instrumental vaginal or cesarean delivery, thus avoiding airway manipulation. For cesarean delivery, the choice of anesthetic depends on maternal and fetal conditions. The panniculus must be positioned carefully to prevent cardiorespiratory compromise. A continuous neuraxial anesthetic technique should be considered over a "single-shot" technique because there may be unpredictable spread of local anesthetic and because a prolonged surgical duration can be anticipated. Thus, the procedure itself may outlast the effective anesthesia from the latter. Obesity is associated with an increased risk for maternal death related to increased incidence of infection, diabetes, preeclampsia, and thromboembolism. Anesthesia-related maternal mortality is also increased, primarily related to airway difficulties.

Advanced Maternal Age

As reproductive technologies improve and more women are delaying childbearing, pregnancies in women of AMA will become more prevalent. In 2002, almost 14% of all births in the United States occurred in women aged 35 years or older.[147] In 2003, the percentage of primiparas 35 years and older was 10%.[148] In Canada in 2002, live births to women 30 to 34 years old accounted for 30.6% of all births; to women aged 35 to 39 years old, 14.1%; and to women 40 years and older, 2.6%. Some studies have reported higher maternal morbidity as well as perinatal morbidity and mortality in older gravidae,[149–151] suggesting that pregnancy in older women may be a "medical problem." As we care for these patients, we must remember that healthy women of AMA will likely have uncomplicated pregnancies and deliveries; the incidence of complications is largely related to comorbidities, which occur at a greater incidence in older women. In one study, almost half of the pregnant women older than 45 years of age had pre-existing medical problems.[150] Cleary-Goldman et al.[151] found that 38% of 36,000 patients older than 35 years of age took medication for pre-existing conditions. In addition, many older pregnant patients have been infertile or subfertile or had a previous poor obstetric outcome. Seven percent had prior preterm delivery and 26% had a previous miscarriage.[152] Obstetric management should be focused on the patient's comorbidities.

AMA is independently associated with gestational diabetes, preeclampsia, placental abruption, and cesarean delivery. Older gravidae are more likely to have a weight of more than 70 kg, hypertension, diabetes mellitus, and a bad obstetric history. These medical problems complicate the pregnancy and its management. Pregestational hypertension occurs more frequently in patients over 30 years of age.[153] Patients with chronic hypertension are more likely to develop superimposed preeclampsia (78%), deliver by cesarean section (71%), and deliver before 37 weeks of gestation than normotensive patients. Hypertensive parturients are at greater risk for placental abruption, congestive heart failure, pulmonary edema, and hypertensive encephalopathy. Further, older parturients are more likely to require prolonged hospitalization and are more likely to be admitted to the intensive care unit than younger parturients.

Cesarean delivery is performed more frequently in those with AMA. In some patients, the need for cesarean delivery is related to coexisting problems such as hypertension, preeclampsia, placental abruption, or fetal macrosomia. AMA is also independently associated with an increased likelihood for cesarean delivery. Lin et al.[154] reported that over a 5-year period, "request cesarean delivery" rates rose steadily in all patients but rose disproportionately in patients with AMA. Women over the age of 34 years were twice as likely to request cesarean delivery compared with those aged 25 years or younger. The cesarean delivery rate for mothers of 30 to 34 years of age was 37%, and for mothers older than 34 years, it was 48%.[154] The complex sociodemographic explanation for the increased requests for cesarean delivery is yet to be fully ascertained and the long-term medical cost has yet to be defined.[155,156] Cesarean delivery is associated with increased maternal risks compared with uncomplicated vaginal delivery. These include short-term risks of cesarean delivery such as hemorrhage, infection, ileus, and aspiration pneumonitis. In addition, hysterectomy occurs 10 times more frequently following cesarean delivery compared with vaginal delivery. The risk of maternal death is 16 times greater. Long-term morbidity includes adhesions, bowel obstruction, bladder injury, and increased risk for placenta previa or ectopic pregnancy in subsequent pregnancies.[157]

Older women may believe that their age makes their infant more vulnerable and, as such, that a controlled cesarean delivery is safer than a vaginal delivery. Other explanations for increased requests for cesarean delivery include concerns about physical stamina, protection of the pelvic floor from damage, refusal to undergo labor pain, and social convenience. Patient beliefs run counter to the many studies that show that cesarean delivery in the absence of clinical indications increases maternal mortality and perinatal morbidity.[155,156]

Perinatal complications are also significant in patients with AMA; multiple gestations,[157] both iatrogenic and naturally occurring, are more common in older gravidae. The incidence of miscarriage, congenital anomalies, preterm delivery, low birth weight, and intrauterine and neonatal death also increase with age.

Preterm Delivery

Preterm labor and delivery (before 37 completed weeks of gestation) present a significant challenge to the anesthesiologist because both mother and infant may be at risk. Although preterm deliveries occur in 8% to 10% of all births, they account for approximately 80% of early neonatal deaths. In general, the mortality and morbidity rates are higher among preterm infants than among small-for-gestational-age infants of comparable weight. Severe problems that may develop in preterm infants are respiratory distress syndrome, intracranial hemorrhage, hypoglycemia, hypocalcemia, and hyperbilirubinemia. With improved neonatal intensive care, preterm infants who weigh over 1,500 g often survive without severe long-term impairment. The very low-birth-weight infant (<1,500 g) is still at greater risk for significant long-term impairment.[158]

Obstetricians will try to stop preterm labor to enhance fetal lung maturity. Delaying delivery by even 24 to 48 hours may be beneficial if glucocorticoids are administered to the mother. Various agents have been used to suppress uterine activity (tocolysis), including ethanol, magnesium sulfate, prostaglandin inhibitors, b-sympathomimetics, and calcium channel blockers (Table 41-2). Magnesium sulfate may also be used to improve neonatal outcomes; available evidence suggests that if given early (before 30 to 33 weeks), it may reduce the risk for cerebral palsy.[159]

It is thought that the premature infant is more vulnerable than the term newborn to the effects of drugs used in obstetric analgesia and anesthesia. However, there have been few systematic studies to determine the maternal and fetal pharmacokinetics and dynamics of drugs throughout gestation. There are several postulated causes of enhanced drug sensitivity in the preterm newborn, including:

- Less protein available for drug binding
- Higher levels of bilirubin, which may compete with the drug for protein binding
- Greater drug access to the CNS because of a poorly developed blood–brain barrier
- Greater total body water and lower fat content
- A decreased ability to metabolize and excrete drugs

However, these deficiencies of the preterm infant may not be as serious as we have been led to believe. Serum albumin and α_1-acid glycoprotein concentrations are lower in the preterm fetus; however, this would primarily affect drugs that are highly bound to these proteins. Most drugs used in anesthesia exhibit only low-to-moderate degrees of protein binding in the fetal serum.

In selection of the anesthetic drugs and techniques for delivery of a preterm infant, concerns regarding drug effects on the newborn are far less important than prevention of asphyxia and trauma to the fetus. For labor and vaginal delivery, well-conducted neuraxial anesthesia is advantageous in providing good perineal relaxation. Preterm infants with breech presentation are usually delivered by cesarean as are very low-birth-weight infants (<1,500 g). If neuraxial anesthesia is used, nitroglycerin should be available for uterine relaxation. If vaginal delivery occurs with a breech infant and there is head entrapment, general anesthesia or nitroglycerin may be needed for uterine relaxation.

Substance Abuse

Nearly 90% of women who abuse tobacco, drugs, or alcohol are of childbearing age. The most commonly abused substances in society as well as in pregnancy are alcohol, tobacco, cocaine, marijuana, opioids, caffeine, amphetamines, and to a lesser extent, hallucinogens and solvents. Substance abuse may significantly impact intrapartum anesthetic management and may result in obstetric crises that require the intervention or assistance of an obstetric anesthesiologist. Diagnosis of the patient who is not under the effect of a substance at admission may be made when she, or her infant, develops withdrawal symptoms or the newborn is diagnosed with a syndrome related to in utero exposure. Women often abuse more than one drug, so the newborn's problems may reflect the impact of multiple drug exposures.

Tobacco Abuse

Smoking is the most commonly abused substance in pregnancy. Smoking during pregnancy has been associated with miscarriages, IUGR, and increased risk of premature rupture of membranes, placental previa, abruptio placentae, preterm delivery, impaired respiratory function in newborns, and sudden infant death syndrome. The pregnant patient is at greater risk for bronchitis, pneumonia, and asthma. Nicotine causes vasoconstriction and thus may decrease placental blood flow and oxygen delivery to the fetus; of interest, smoking appears to be protective for the development of preeclampsia.

Alcohol

In a pregnant female, heavy alcohol consumption may be associated with liver disease, coagulopathy, cardiomyopathy, and esophageal varies; it can also alter drug metabolism. In the fetus, alcohol has been linked to fetal alcohol syndrome. The prevalence of fetal alcohol syndrome is approximately one-third of infants of heavy maternal drinkers (>28 g absolute alcohol or two drinks per day). Neurobehavioral deficit and IUGR have been demonstrated in infants of moderate drinkers (>14 g absolute alcohol or 1 drink per day). The parturient who abuses alcohol is at further increased risk for aspiration compared with the average pregnant individual. She may have hepatic dysfunction, cardiac failure, or coagulopathy. Acute alcohol withdrawal may present within 6 to 48 hours of abstinence; thus, it may occur intrapartum or postpartum. The signs and symptoms of alcohol withdrawal include nausea and vomiting, hypertension, tachycardia, dysrhythmias, seizures, and cardiac failure. These are easily mistaken for other disease entities.

Opioids

Opioid abuse has multiple implications for both mother and fetus. The intravenous opioid abuser may have septic thrombophlebitis, human immunodeficiency virus, endocarditis, or hepatitis. These patients are at an increased risk for developing preeclampsia and third-trimester bleeding. They will develop withdrawal symptoms should an agonist/antagonist be administered for pain relief in labor.

The anesthetic management of a chronic opioid user should include the continuation of opioids throughout labor and into the postpartum period to prevent acute opioid withdrawal. These patients are likely to have increased opioid requirements. Those patients with a history of opioid abuse who are on methadone maintenance should have a stable peripartum course. Neuraxial anesthesia is safe in these patients, but one must continue a maintenance dose of systemic opioid to prevent withdrawal symptoms, despite neuraxial labor analgesia. Neonates will have neonatal abstinence syndrome, which will require close observation and treatment.[160]

Marijuana

Marijuana is frequently abused by women of childbearing age. Delta-9-tetrahydrocannabinol (THC) readily crosses the placenta and may directly affect the fetus. It has been associated with preterm labor and IUGR. The parturient who chronically uses marijuana has an increased incidence of respiratory problems, including bronchitis and emphysema, and thus may be at risk for respiratory complications related to general anesthesia. Acute marijuana use may be associated with cardiovascular stimulation at moderate doses and myocardial depression at higher doses.

Cocaine

Women acutely ingesting cocaine generally display euphoria, tachycardia, and hypertension. More serious manifestations may include seizure and coma, myocardial infarction, pulmonary edema, or subarachnoid hemorrhage. Sudden death may occur from a lethal ventricular dysrhythmia. Cocaine use in the first trimester may cause congenital anomalies. Later in pregnancy, cocaine use may be associated with premature labor, IUGR, and nonreassuring fetal status because of uteroplacental insufficiency or placental abruption. Therapy is supportive, primarily aimed at controlling cardiovascular and CNS consequences of cocaine use. Hypertension related to acute cocaine ingestion may be the primary etiology of cerebral hemorrhage, or cocaine may cause vasospasm and cerebral infarction. Pure β-antagonist drugs should be avoided because of the potential for worsening hypertension related to unopposed α-receptor stimulation by cocaine. The choice of anesthetic depends on maternal and fetal conditions, the planned procedure (vaginal or cesarean delivery), and urgency. General anesthesia may be associated with uncontrolled hypertension/tachycardia and life-threatening dysrhythmias in women using cocaine. Neuraxial anesthesia may also be complicated by cocaine use. Cocaine is a local anesthetic, and systemic toxicity may be additive when using amide local anesthetics for epidural

> **Table 41-4** Anesthetic Considerations Associated with Cocaine and/or Amphetamine Abuse
>
> - Uncontrolled hypertension
> - Cardiac dysrhythmias (ventricular tachycardia/fibrillation)
> - Myocardial ischemia
> - Ephedrine-resistant hypotension with neuraxial blockade (use direct-acting agent)
> - Acute intake may increase MAC of volatile agents
> - Chronic use may decrease dosage of anesthetic agents
> - May have increased sensitivity to arrhythmogenic effects of volatile agents

MAC, minimum alveolar concentration.

anesthesia. Esters compete with cocaine for metabolism, resulting in decreased metabolism of both drugs. Chronic cocaine use may be associated with thrombocytopenia. The incidence and severity of hypotension related to neuraxial anesthesia may be greater in chronic cocaine-abusing parturients compared with controls, and hypotension may be more difficult to treat. Direct-acting agents are more effective and predictable in chronic cocaine abusers. Fetal exposure to cocaine may alter the developing brain, contributing to an increased susceptibility to addiction.[161]

Amphetamines

Amphetamines are noncatecholamine sympathomimetic drugs. They are often abused in conjunction with other CNS stimulants such as cocaine. They can be taken orally or intravenously (methamphetamine) or smoked, as crystal methamphetamine. Ecstasy is an analog of methamphetamine that has become tremendously popular in young adults. Amphetamine use leads to an increased release of norepinephrine, leading to hypertension, tachycardia, dysrhythmias, dilated pupils, hyperpyrexia, proteinuria, agitation, confusion, and seizures. These signs and symptoms closely resemble those of cocaine abuse. Methamphetamine abuse has been associated with stroke in pregnant women as well as fetal and infant deaths. Amphetamines taken early in pregnancy can result in fetal anomalies and low birth weight infants. Later in pregnancy, placental abruption may lead to fetal death. The anesthetic management of patients who abuse amphetamines is similar to that of cocaine abusers (Table 41-4).

Fetal Monitoring

The development of biophysical monitoring of the fetus during labor and delivery has had a tremendous impact on obstetric practice since the early 1970s. Monitoring procedures are now performed routinely, and it is important that the anesthesiologist understand the basic principles of the technology as well as the interpretation of results. With the growing sophistication of electronic devices, and specifically the science of telemetry, surveillance of both mother and fetus may take place without the loss of maternal freedom and activity that monitoring entailed in the past.

Electronic Fetal Monitoring

Intrapartum electronic fetal heart rate (FHR) monitoring is the most common obstetric procedure performed.[162] An electronic fetal monitor is a two-channel recorder of FHR and uterine activity. In the internal system, the fetal ECG is obtained from an electrode attached to the presenting part. Intrauterine pressure is measured continuously with a transducer connected to a saline-filled catheter that is inserted transcervically. Internal monitoring is quantitative but requires rupture of the membranes and a cervical dilation of at least 1.5 cm. In addition, the presenting part must be in the true pelvis. External fetal monitoring uses data obtained indirectly from transducers secured to the mother's abdomen with adjustable straps. Ultrasound cardiography is the most commonly used method of obtaining FHR signals. Uterine activity is monitored with a tocodynamometer triggered by the changing shape of the uterus during the contraction. Indirect monitoring is mostly qualitative. Its advantage is that it can be applied without rupture of membranes, even before the onset of labor.

The following variables are considered when fetal well-being is being assessed: Uterine activity, baseline heart rate and variability, presence of accelerations, and periodic decelerations. Cervical dilation and descent of the presenting part during the first stage of labor result primarily from uterine contractions. During the active phase, contractions should occur every 2 to 3 minutes, with peak intrauterine pressures of 50 to 80 mmHg and resting pressures of 5 to 20 mmHg. When more than five contractions occur in 10 minutes, it is termed tachysystole. Tachysystole is sometimes seen after neuraxial labor analgesia and may result from a sudden drop in serum catecholamines, which normally serve to relax the uterus.[163] Poor uterine contractility may result from overdistention (polyhydramnios, multiple gestation) or aortocaval compression. The addition of epinephrine to a local anesthetic solution may have a dose-related inhibitory effect on uterine activity.

The baseline FHR is the mean rate during a 10-minute segment and ranges between 110 and 160 beats per minute in the normal fetus.[162] Persistently elevated rates may be associated with chronic fetal distress, maternal fever, or administration of drugs such as ephedrine and atropine. Abnormally low rates may be encountered in fetuses with congenital heart block or as a late occurrence during the course of fetal hypoxia and acidosis.

Baseline FHR variability refers to fluctuations in baseline FHR that are irregular in amplitude and frequency; baseline variability is quantified as the amplitude of the peak to the trough heart rate and normally ranges between 6 and 25 beats per minute.[162] Baseline variability reflects the beat-to-beat adjustments of the parasympathetic and sympathetic nervous systems to a variety of internal and external stimuli and is mediated by the CNS, the peripheral nervous system, and the cardiac conduction system itself. Presence of normal variability is a reassuring sign of normal fetal acid–base status. Fetal CNS depression by asphyxia may decrease baseline variability. Therefore, a smooth FHR tracing may be an ominous finding. However, drugs that depress the CNS (sedatives, opioids, barbiturates, anesthetics) can also decrease FHR variability. Atropine may decrease variability by blocking the transmission of control impulses to the cardiac pacemaker.

An acceleration of FHR is an abrupt increase over baseline and is a reassuring sign that the fetus is not acidemic.[162] Periodic FHR decelerations occur in association with uterine contractions (Fig. 41-8). There are three patterns observed: Early, late, and variable. Early decelerations are characterized by a symmetrical gradual decrease in FHR. The fetal heart usually begins to slow with the onset of the contraction, nadirs with the peak of the contraction, and returns to the baseline as the uterus relaxes. Early decelerations reach a nadir 30 seconds or more after the onset of the deceleration.[162] This type of deceleration has been attributed to fetal head compression, leading to increased vagal

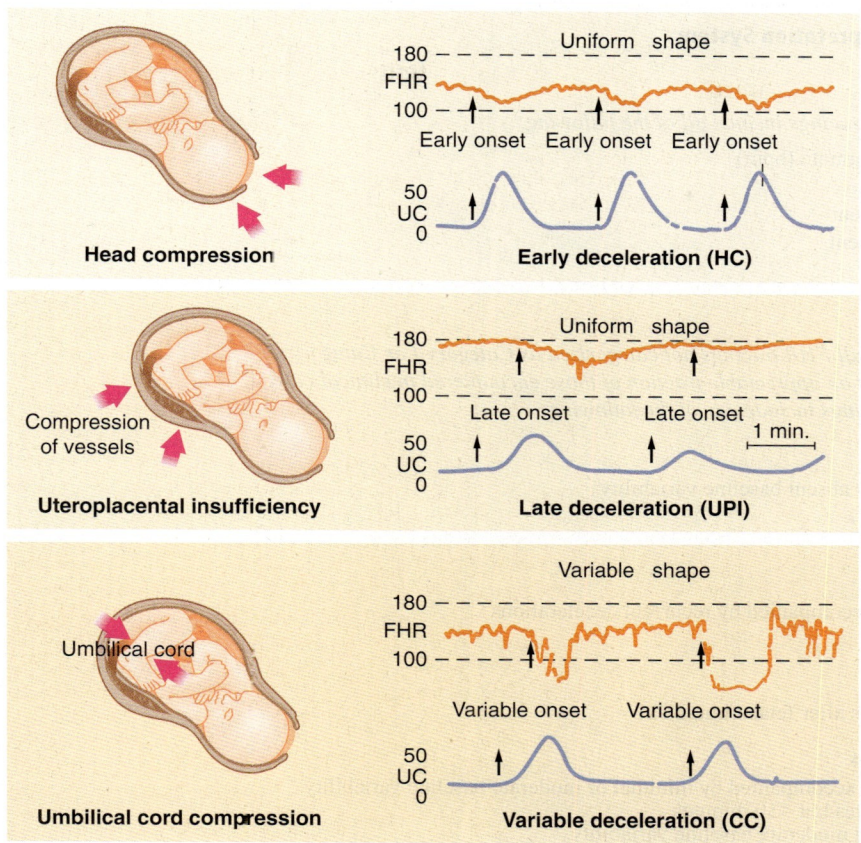

Figure 41-8 Classification and mechanism of fetal heart rate patterns. HC, head compression; UPI, uteroplacental insufficiency; CC, cord compression. (Adapted from Hon EH. *An Introduction to Fetal Heart Rate Monitoring*. New Haven, CT: Harty Press; 1969:29.)

tone. It is not ameliorated by increasing fetal oxygenation but is blocked by atropine administration. Early decelerations are transient and well tolerated by the fetus; there is no systemic hypoxemia or acidosis.

Late decelerations are also symmetric and gradual in onset. However, they begin after the onset of uterine contraction and the low point of the deceleration occurs well after its peak, at least 30 seconds after the onset of the deceleration.[162] CNS or myocardial ischemia resulting from uteroplacental insufficiency and fetal hypoxemia may cause late decelerations.

Variable decelerations are the most common periodic pattern observed in the intrapartum period. They are variable in shape and abrupt in onset, with the heart rate nadir occurring within 30 seconds of the onset.[162] Variable decelerations occur due to umbilical cord compression that results in activation of the carotid baroreceptor reflex. Although the initial FHR changes are of reflex origin, if the cord compressions are frequent or prolonged, fetal asphyxia may result in fetal hypoxemia and CNS insult or direct myocardial depression. If late or variable decelerations are recurrent (occur with at least one-half of contractions) or prolonged (≥15 beats per minute below baseline lasting ≥2 minutes but <10 minutes), there is a significant correlation with fetal acidosis and delivery may be undertaken.[164]

The ACOG currently recommends a three-tiered system for the evaluation of FHR tracings.[162] Category I tracings are those with normal baseline and variability, and no late or variable decelerations. They correlate strongly with normal fetus acid–base status at the time of observation. Category II tracings include all those that are not classified as either category I or III. They are predictive of neither normal nor abnormal acid–base status, and require continued observation and assessment. Category III tracings are abnormal. They are characterized by absent variability with any one of the following: Recurrent late decelerations, recurrent variable decelerations, or bradycardia (FHR <100 beats per minute). Sinusoidal patterns (a sine-wave like pattern) also fall into category III. Category III tracings may be corrected by improving fetal oxygenation, which may be accomplished with oxygen administration to the mother, correction of maternal hypotension or aortocaval compression, or by taking measures that reduce uterine activity. If the heart rate pattern does not respond to these conservative measures, imminent delivery may be required (Fig. 41-9).

Currently, experts agree regarding the reassuring value of a normal category I FHR tracing. There is also consensus regarding the potentially ominous nature of category III tracings. However, FHR patterns between these extremes present a clinical dilemma. The high false positive rate of FHR monitoring may lead to unnecessary cesarean deliveries. Recent recommendations regarding the approach to a category II tracing emphasize that clinicians should consider time spent with a category II tracing and progress of labor when determining delivery plans.[164] A recent ACOG Practice Bulletin opines not only the high false positive rate of nonreassuring FHR tracings for predicting adverse neonatal outcomes but also the excessive inter- and intraobserver variabilities in interpretation. It also notes that the practice is associated with an increase in both instrumental vaginal and cesarean deliveries, without decreasing the incidence of cerebral palsy. The bulletin recommends continuous FHR analysis for high-risk conditions, although it allows for intermittent auscultation in an uncomplicated patient.[162]

Three-Tier Fetal Heart Rate Interpretation System

Category I

Category I fetal heart rate (FHR) tracings include all of the following:

- Baseline rate: 110–160 beats per minute (bpm)
- Baseline FHR variability: moderate
- Late or variable decelerations: absent
- Early decelerations: present or absent
- Accelerations: present or absent

Category II

Category II FHR tracings include all FHR tracings not categorized as Category I or Category III. Category II tracings may represent an appreciable fraction of those encountered in clinical care. Examples of Category II FHR tracings include any of the following:

Baseline rate
- Bradycardia not accompanied by absent baseline variability
- Tachycardia

Baseline FHR variability
- Minimal baseline variability
- Absent baseline variability not accompanied by recurrent decelerations
- Marked baseline variability

Accelerations
- Absence of induced accelerations after fetal stimulation

Periodic or episodic decelerations
- Recurrent variable decelerations accompanied by minimal or moderate baseline variability
- Prolonged deceleration ≥2 minutes but <10 minutes
- Recurrent late decelerations with moderate baseline variability
- Variable decelerations with other characteristics, such as slow return to baseline, "overshoots," or "shoulders"

Category III

Category III FHR tracings include either:

- Absent baseline FHR variability and any of the following:
  - Recurrent late decelerations
  - Recurrent variable decelerations
  - Bradycardia
- Sinusoidal pattern

Figure 41-9 Three-tiered fetal heart rate interpretation system. (Reprinted with permission from The 2008 National Institute of Child Health and Human Development Workshop on Electronic Fetal Monitoring: Updates on Definitions, Interpretations, and Research Guidelines. *Obstet Gynecol.* 2008;112:661.)

Ancillary Tests and Fetal Pulse Oximetry

Fetal scalp pH testing has been used in the past to determine the presence of acidemia in fetuses with indeterminate FHR tracings; however, its use is decreasing, and less invasive ancillary tests such as vibroacoustic stimulation and digital scalp stimulation are more commonly employed. The elicitation of accelerations with such stimuli indicates acidemia is unlikely.

Fetal pulse oximetry is a technique in which a sensor is placed through the cervix in contact with fetal skin that evaluates intrapartum fetal oxygenation. Fetal O_2 saturation between 30% and 70% is considered normal, and saturation readings consistently below 30% for a prolonged period of time may be associated with fetal acidemia. The technique was initially touted as an adjunct to FHR monitoring in the hope that it could reduce the incidence of unnecessary cesarean delivery associated with that methodology. Unfortunately, two large studies failed to demonstrate a reduction in the incidence of cesarean delivery with the use of fetal pulse oximetry. Moreover, neonatal outcomes did not differ between subjects managed with versus without fetal pulse oximetry.[165,166] Similarly disappointing results have been seen with the addition of fetal ECG ST analysis to cardiotocography.[167] The ACOG does not currently endorse the routine use of fetal pulse oximetry or fetal ECG ST analysis.[167]

Newborn Resuscitation in the Delivery Room

Of the approximately 3.5 million infants newly born in the United States each year, 10% require resuscitation in the delivery room.[168] The following factors may contribute to depression of the newborn: Medications used during labor and delivery, including anesthetic agents, birth trauma, and birth asphyxia (i.e., hypoxia and hypercapnia with metabolic acidosis).

Fetal Asphyxia

Fetal asphyxia, the best-studied cause of neonatal depression, usually develops as a result of interference with maternal or fetal perfusion of the placenta. As stated previously, the normal fetus is neither hypoxic nor acidotic before labor. Experimental data have revealed that transplacental gradients for pH and PCO_2 are approximately 0.05 pH units and 5 mmHg, respectively. Although oxygen tension is low, oxygen saturation is relatively high (80% to 85%) by virtue of the leftward shift of the fetal oxyhemoglobin dissociation curve.

During labor, uterine contractions decrease or even eliminate the blood flow through the intervillous space of the placenta. On the fetal side, cord compression occurs during the final stages of approximately one-third of vaginal deliveries. Thus, mild degrees of hypoxia and acidosis occur even during normal labor and delivery and play an important role in initiation of ventilation immediately after birth. On average, healthy, vigorous infants have an oxygen saturation of 21%, a pH of 7.24, and a PCO_2 of 56 mmHg at birth.

Severe fetal asphyxia occasionally develops as a result of maternal or fetal complications, such as uterine hyperactivity, premature separation of the placenta, maternal hypotension, a tight nuchal cord, or a prolapsed cord. During asphyxia, changes in acid–base status are rapid. The decrease in pH results from accumulation of carbon dioxide (respiratory acidosis) and end products of anaerobic metabolism (metabolic acidosis). After oxygen stores are exhausted, the ability of fetal brain and myocardium to derive energy from anaerobic metabolism is essential for survival. However, anaerobic glycolysis is pH dependent, and its rate is greatly diminished when the pH decreases below 7. Other untoward effects of severe hypoxia and acidosis include depression of the myocardium, resulting from a decrease in its responsiveness to catecholamines; a shift to the right of the fetal oxyhemoglobin dissociation curve, resulting in reduced oxygen delivery; and an increase in pulmonary vascular resistance, which plays an important role during circulatory readjustment at birth.

Neonatal Adaptations at Birth

During birth and through the early hours and days of life, many morphologic and functional changes take place, with the cardiovascular and ventilatory systems undergoing the most dramatic alterations. In the normal newborn, two events occur almost simultaneously and within seconds of delivery: The end of umbilical circulation through the placenta and expansion of the lungs. These events change the fetal circulation toward the adult type.

Survival of the neonate depends primarily on prompt establishment of effective ventilation and expansion of the lungs, which dilates the pulmonary vascular bed, resulting in decreased resistance and a significant increase in pulmonary blood flow. Pulmonary vascular resistance further decreases as oxygen tension increases and carbon dioxide levels decrease. As soon as pulmonary resistance decreases, the foramen ovale, which is a communication between the right and the left atrium, undergoes functional closure because of relative pressure changes across the valve of the foramen (Fig. 41-1). Cessation of the umbilical circulation reduces pressure in the inferior vena cava and right atrium, whereas the increase in pulmonary blood flow increases venous return and pressure in the left atrium. The ductus arteriosus does not constrict abruptly or completely after birth; functional closure may take hours, even days. Thus, shunting may still occur in the neonatal period, its direction depending on relative resistances in the pulmonary and systemic vascular beds. The smooth muscle of the ductus arteriosus constricts in response to increased oxygen tension in the newborn's blood. Catecholamines, which exist in increased concentrations in the newborn, particularly during the first 3 hours of life, also constrict the ductus arteriosus. In contrast, prostaglandins I_2 and E_2, produced by the wall of the ductus arteriosus, relax the ductal smooth muscle. Administration of prostaglandin synthesis inhibitors to fetal animals promotes closure of the ductus arteriosus.

Cardiac output and its distribution also increase; left ventricular output increases approximately 150 to 400 mL/kg/min. Cardiac output changes closely parallel the increase in oxygen consumption. The redistribution of cardiac output also leads to increases in myocardial, renal, and gastrointestinal blood flow, and decreases in cerebral, adrenal, and carotid flow.

During fetal life, respiratory gas exchange takes place through the placenta. Delivery of the infant's trunk relieves the thoracic compression that occurs as the infant passes through the birth canal, and the thorax and the lungs expand. Most infants initiate respiratory efforts a few seconds after birth. Negative pressures in excess of 40 cm H_2O bring about the initial entry of air into fluid-filled alveoli. In the mature, normal neonate, the lungs expand almost completely after the first few breaths, and the pressure–volume changes achieved with each respiration resemble those of the adult. After lung expansion, the FRC approximates 70 mL in the term newborn and changes little over the first 6 days of life. The tidal volume varies between 10 and 30 mL, the breathing frequency ranges from 30 to 60 breaths per minute, and minute ventilation exceeds 500 mL. After delivery and prompt lung expansion, reoxygenation is rapid, but it takes 2 to 3 hours to achieve a relatively normal acid–base balance, primarily by pulmonary excretion of carbon dioxide. By 24 hours, the healthy neonate has reached the same acid–base state as that of the mother before labor.

Resuscitation

The delivery room must be prepared for adequate and prompt treatment of severe neonatal depression at birth. Members of the delivery room team should be trained in resuscitation methods because both mother and infant may encounter difficulty simultaneously. One person should be designated specifically to care for the newborn during every delivery. When continued resuscitation is anticipated, a team of skilled personnel should be present. Every piece of apparatus necessary for emergency resuscitation should be checked carefully before delivery (Table 41-5). An overview of resuscitation in the delivery room is provided in Figure 41-10.

Evaluation and Treatment

The American Heart Association has released guidelines to advise the practitioner providing neonatal resuscitation.[168] Immediately after delivery, the infant should be held head-down while the cord is clamped and cut. The initial appraisal of the newborn should start from the moment of birth, with particular attention paid to determining the answer to three questions:

- Is the newborn the result of a term gestation?
- Is the newborn crying or breathing vigorously?
- Does the newborn have good muscle tone?

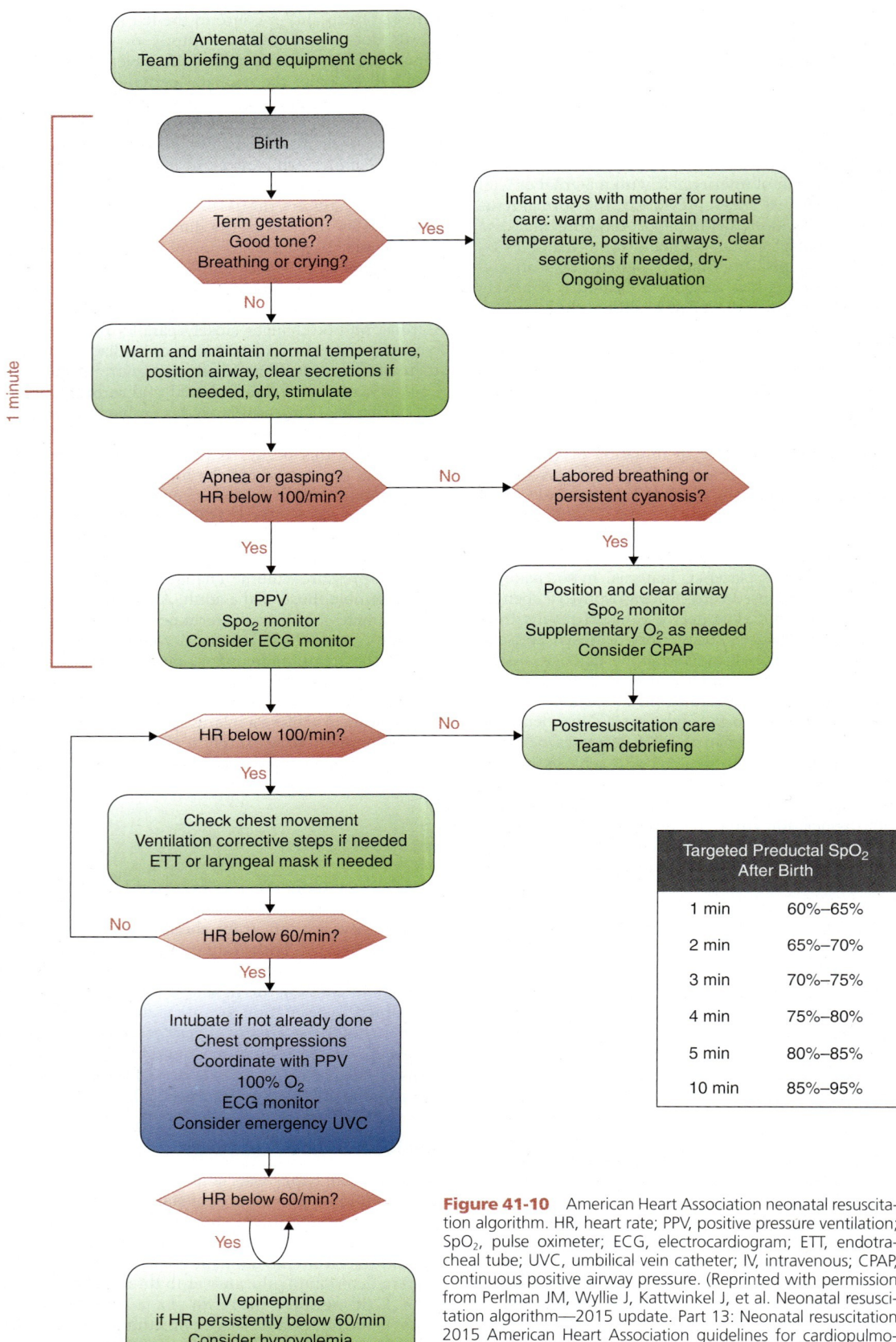

Figure 41-10 American Heart Association neonatal resuscitation algorithm. HR, heart rate; PPV, positive pressure ventilation; SpO₂, pulse oximeter; ECG, electrocardiogram; ETT, endotracheal tube; UVC, umbilical vein catheter; IV, intravenous; CPAP, continuous positive airway pressure. (Reprinted with permission from Perlman JM, Wyllie J, Kattwinkel J, et al. Neonatal resuscitation algorithm—2015 update. Part 13: Neonatal resuscitation 2015 American Heart Association guidelines for cardiopulmonary resuscitation and emergency cardiovascular care. *Circulation*. 2015;132(Suppl 2):S543.)

Table 41-5 Resuscitation Equipment in the Delivery Room

Radiant warmer
Suction with manometer and suction trap
Suction catheters
Wall oxygen with flow meter
Resuscitation bag (≤750 mL)
Infant face masks
Infant oropharyngeal airways
Endotracheal tubes—2.5, 3, 3.5, and 4 mm
Endotracheal tube stylets
Laryngoscope(s) and blade(s)
Sterile umbilical artery catheterization tray
Needles, syringes, three-way stopcocks
Medications and solutions
1:10,000 Epinephrine
Volume expanders

If the answer to all three questions is "yes," then the baby does not require further resuscitation and should be placed skin to skin with its mother if practical. If the answer to any of the above questions is "no," then further resuscitation should be provided, with the following steps taken in the order listed.

Initial Stabilization

One should place the infant supine under a radiant heat source, with the head kept low in the sniffing position. Breathing should be stimulating by slapping the infant's soles lightly or rubbing the back. Suctioning is only needed in the presence of obvious secretions, as it may provoke vagally-induced bradycaria.

Assessment of Respirations and Heart Rate

Presence of respiration versus apnea is assessed, and respiratory efforts are judged as unlabored versus gasping or labored.

An assistant should listen to the heartbeat immediately, indicating the rate by finger movement, or the rate can be detected from pulsation of the umbilical cord. Normally, the newborn's heart rate is above 100 beats per minute.

Ventilation

If the newborn is apneic or gasping, or if the heart rate is below 100 beats per minute after initial stabilization, then positive pressure ventilation (PPV) should begin. PPV via bag and mask should be instituted at a rate of 40 to 60 breaths per minute. The initial breath may require pressures of 30 to 40 cm H_2O. Subsequent inflation pressures should be reduced to 15 to 20 cm H_2O in an infant with normal lungs. A small plastic oropharyngeal airway may help maintain patency of the upper airway. Endotracheal intubation may be required if bag–mask ventilation is ineffective or prolonged. The administration of oxygen is controversial because studies demonstrate that both hypoxemia and excessive oxygen administration may be harmful to babies, and two recent meta-analyses suggest that room air resuscitation is associated with lower mortality than that with 100% oxygen.[169,170] Therefore, it is recommended that preductal pulse oximetry guides oxygen therapy with attention to target saturations listed in the box in Figure 41-10, and that oxygen therapy be titrated to positive heart rate response.

Chest Compressions

After adequate ventilation with oxygen for 30 seconds, if the heart rate is below 60 beats per minute, then chest compressions should be initiated. It is recommended that the operator encircle the chest with both hands, supporting the back with his hands and compressing the chest with his thumbs; alternatively, one may compress with two fingers. Compressions should take place on the lower third of the sternum, to a depth that is one-third of the anterior–posterior diameter of the chest. Care must be taken not to interfere with ventilation. Recommendations call for a 3:1 compression to ventilation ratio, with 90 compressions and 30 breaths delivered per minute.

Cardiac massage and ventilation should be maintained until the heart rate exceeds 60 beats per minute.

Medications and Volume Expansion

Persistent neonatal bradycardia is most often a result of hypoxemia, and usually responds to ventilatory efforts. If the heart rate continues at less than 60 beats per minute despite adequate ventilation with 100% oxygen, then the newborn may need epinephrine, volume expansion, or both. It is recommended that epinephrine be administered intravenously as soon as access is established, at a dose of 0.01 to 0.03 mg/kg. In the absence of intravenous access, one may consider endotracheal administration of 0.05 to 0.1 mg/kg.

The use of naloxone or other medications in the delivery room is no longer recommended.

Hypovolemia frequently follows severe birth asphyxia because a greater-than-normal portion of fetal blood remains in the placenta. The infant may appear pale and have low arterial pressure, tachycardia, and tachypnea. If heart rate does not respond to other measures, then acute blood volume expansion may be accomplished with the intravenous administration of normal saline or Lactated Ringer solution, 10 mL/kg over 5 to 10 minutes, or, when blood loss is suspected, a similar volume of O-negative blood. Albumin is not recommended (Table 41-6).

The APGAR Score

The scoring system introduced by Apgar is a useful method of clinically evaluating the infant, particularly at 1 and 5 minutes after delivery (Table 41-7).

Table 41-6 Therapeutic Guidelines for Neonatal Resuscitation

Drug or Volume Expander	Concentration	Dosage	Route/Rate
Epinephrine	1:10,000	0.01–0.03 mg/kg (IV) 0.05–0.1 mg (IT)	IV or IT Give rapidly
Volume expanders	PRBCs Normal saline Lactated Ringer	10 mL/kg	Give over 5–10 min

IV, intravenously; IT, intratracheally; PRBCs, packed red blood cells.

Table 41-7 APGAR Scores

Sign	0	1	2
Heart rate	Absent	<100 beats/min	>100 beats/min
Respiratory effort	Absent	Slow, irregular	Good, crying
Muscle tone	Limp	Some flexion of extremities	Active motion
Reflex irritability	No response	Grimace	Cough, sneeze, or cry
Color	Pale, blue	Body pink, extremities blue	Completely pink

Diagnostic Procedures

After the neonate is successfully resuscitated and stabilized, several diagnostic procedures may be indicated. To rule out choanal atresia, each nostril should be obstructed. Because newborns must breathe through their noses, occlusion of the nostril on the patent side causes respiratory obstruction. To rule out esophageal atresia, a suction catheter is inserted into the stomach. Gastric contents are aspirated; volume in excess of 12 mL after vaginal delivery and 20 mL after cesarean delivery may result from an abnormality of the upper gastrointestinal tract.

Exit Procedure

The EXIT (ex utero intrapartum treatment) procedure, which maintains uteroplacental support for a period of time after partial delivery of the fetus, is employed for certain fetal conditions that pose an immediate threat to neonatal life on separation from the placental circulation. The most common indications are treatment of large fetal neck masses and reversal of tracheal occlusion from clips placed for congenital diaphragmatic hernia.[171] The usual procedure involves partial delivery of the fetus, surgical treatment of fetal pathology (e.g., attainment of a patent fetal airway), and, finally, delivery of the fetus and clamping of the umbilical cord.

Anesthetic considerations include maintenance of uterine relaxation during the phase of fetal manipulation, administration of fetal anesthesia, ensuring adequate fetal oxygenation, fetal monitoring, and rapid reversal of uterine relaxation after cord clamping to minimize maternal blood loss. Most often the mother is anesthetized with deep inhalation general anesthesia following a standard rapid-sequence induction. Maintenance of anesthesia with high concentrations of volatile anesthetic agents provides for uterine relaxation during the procedure, although a report highlighted the use of intravenous nitroglycerin for this purpose.[172] The use of high inspired inhalational anesthesia or nitroglycerin may be associated with maternal hypotension. Therefore, intravenous vasopressors may be required in order to ensure adequate uteroplacental blood flow. Use of volatile anesthetic concentrations less than 2 MAC is recommended to minimize untoward effects on uterine blood flow.[173] An F_{IO_2} of 1 helps maximize oxygen delivery to the placental unit.

Inhalational anesthetics rapidly cross the placenta and contribute to fetal anesthesia; intravenous opioids may be used to provide additional fetal anesthesia.[173] Intramuscular anesthetic agents, neuromuscular blocking agents, and atropine are administered to the fetus as needed after partial delivery. During the period of fetal manipulation, FHR and oxygenation can be monitored by sterile ultrasound and pulse oximetry sensors. A retrospective review of 31 EXIT procedures reported a mean FHR of 153 beats per minute and a mean fetal oxygen saturation of 71%.[171] After cord clamping, uterine relaxation must be reversed rapidly by decreasing the inspired concentration of inhalation agent and administering uterotonic agents such as oxytocin, so as to minimize maternal blood loss. The retrospective study previously referenced reported a mean maternal estimated blood loss of 848 mL and a mean duration of uteroplacental support of 30 minutes.[171]

Usually, two anesthetic teams are employed: One to tend to the mother and the other to care for the fetus/newborn. Communication and coordination between surgical, pediatric, anesthesia, and nursing teams is mandatory for successful outcomes.

Anesthesia for Nonobstetric Surgery in the Pregnant Woman

In the United States, approximately 1% of pregnant women require nonobstetric surgical interventions during pregnancy.[174] The most frequent nonobstetric procedures are excision of ovarian cysts, appendectomy, cholesyectomy, breast biopsy, and surgery related to trauma. Serious conditions such as intracranial aneurysms, cardiac valvular disease, and pheochromocytoma present rarely during pregnancy and may not require surgical intervention until postpartum. Treatment of an incompetent cervix (cervical cerclage) typically occurs in early pregnancy or midpregnancy.

The goal for treating patients undergoing nonobstetric operative procedures is the same as with any patient; safe perioperative care. This goal is complicated by the need to consider the well-being of both mother and fetus. That said, surgical outcomes in pregnant patients are similar to nonpregnant patients. Miscarriage and rate of birth defects are not significantly different when compared to the general obstetric population.[175] One does need to recognize the effects of the patient's altered physiology. Induction and emergence from anesthesia is more rapid than in the nonpregnant state because of increased minute ventilation, decreased FRC, and the decreased MAC of volatile agents, which may be seen as early as 8 to 10 weeks of gestation. Supine hypotensive syndrome can occur as early as the second trimester. Gastric emptying is essentially normal in the first two trimesters, but is prolonged in the third. Gastroesophageal sphincter tone is decreased after 20 weeks, thus caution regarding the unprotected airway is essential.[23] The effects of altered physiology during pregnancy are not limited to general anesthesia. There is an increased effect of local anesthetics during pregnancy; thus, the amount of local anesthetic administered should be reduced by 25% to 30% during any stage of pregnancy.

Teratogenicity may be induced at any stage of gestation. However, most of the critical organogenesis occurs in the first trimester (days 13 to 60). Although many commonly used anesthetics are teratogenic at high doses in animals, few, if any, studies support teratogenic effects of anesthetic or sedative medications in the doses used for human anesthesia care. Medicinal doses of benzodiazepines are safe when needed to treat perioperative anxiety.

Nitrous oxide has also been suggested to be teratogenic in animals when administered for prolonged periods (1 to 2 days).[176] Its effect on DNA synthesis is of concern for its use in humans. Although teratogenesis has been seen only in animals under extreme conditions, not likely to be reproduced in clinical care, some believe that nitrous oxide use is contraindicated in the first two trimesters.

One of the largest studies regarding reproductive outcome after surgery during pregnancy is a Swedish registry review covering the years 1973 to 1981.[177] During this period, there were a total of 720,000 births, 5,405 of them after anesthesia and surgery during pregnancy. The results of this study are reassuring in that there was no increased incidence of congenital anomalies or stillbirths among infants exposed in utero to maternal surgery and anesthesia. However, in this group, there was an increased frequency of very low and low birth weights, and of deaths within 168 hours after delivery. The reasons for this are unclear and are not related to any specific type of operation. The authors postulated that the maternal illness itself might have been a major contributor to adverse neonatal outcome.

Recent studies showing accelerated neuronal cell death in immature rat brain exposed to anesthetics raise concerns regarding use of general anesthetics.[178] It is premature to suggest that impairment seen in the developing rat brain with general anesthesia can be extrapolated to humans. Further human studies are also inconclusive regarding anesthesia exposure in utero or in early childhood.[179]

Intrauterine fetal asphyxia is avoided by maintaining maternal Pa_{O_2}, Pa_{CO_2}, and uterine blood flow. Pa_{CO_2} can affect uterine blood flow as maternal alkalosis may cause direct vasoconstriction. Alkalosis also shifts the oxyhemoglobin dissociation curve, resulting in the release of less oxygen to the fetus at the placenta. Maternal hypotension leads to a reduction in uterine blood flow and thus fetal hypoxia. Uterine hypertension, as occurs with increased uterine irritability, will also decrease uterine blood flow.

To summarize, elective surgery should be delayed until the patient is no longer pregnant and she has returned to her nonpregnant physiologic state (approximately 2 to 6 weeks postpartum). Procedures that can be scheduled with some flexibility but cannot be delayed until postpartum are best scheduled in the second trimester. This lessens the risk for teratogenicity (first-trimester medication administration) or preterm labor (greater risk in the third trimester) (Fig. 41-11).

If emergency surgery is required, there is no data to suggest that any well-conducted anesthetic is preferred over another, provided oxygenation and blood pressure are maintained and hyperventilation is avoided. Despite this statement, regional anesthesia should be considered as it minimizes fetal exposure to medications. Left uterine displacement should be used during the second and third trimesters, and aspiration prophylaxis should be administered to all pregnant patients after approximately 20 weeks of gestation. At a minimum, pre- and postoperative FHR and uterine activity should be assessed.[180]

Practical Suggestions

It is generally agreed that only surgical procedures that cannot be delayed for months, including emergency surgery, should be performed during pregnancy, particularly in the first trimester. The possibility of pregnancy should be considered in all female surgical patients of reproductive age. On the basis of the maternal and fetal hazards already described, the following approach to anesthesia is suggested (Fig. 41-11):

1. Anesthesiologists and surgeons should obtain consultation from an obstetrician before performing nonobstetric surgery in pregnancy.
2. The patient's apprehension should be allayed as much as possible by personal reassurance during the preanesthetic visit and by adequate sedation and premedication.
3. Pain should be relieved whenever present.

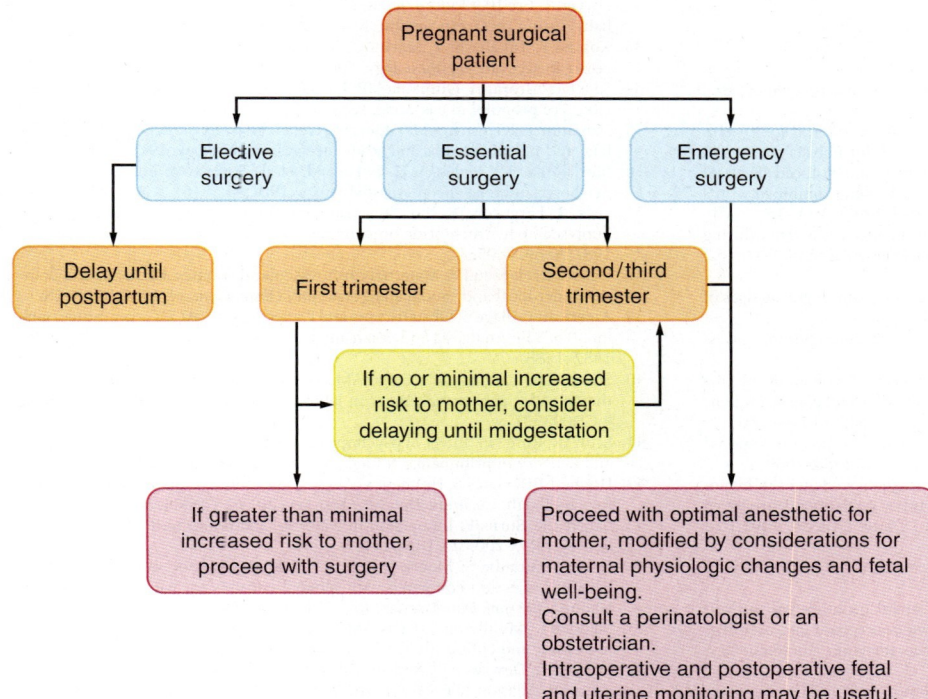

Figure 41-11 Recommendations for management of parturients and surgical procedures. (Adapted from Rosen MA. Management of anesthesia for the pregnant surgical patient. *Anesthesiology*. 1999;91:1159.)

4. A nonparticulate antacid (15 to 30 mL), should be administered within half an hour before induction of anesthesia. Ranitidine and metoclopramide may be useful.
5. Beginning in the second trimester, uterine displacement must be maintained at all times.
6. Hypotension related to spinal or epidural anesthesia should be prevented as much as possible by rapid intravenous infusion of crystalloid solution during induction of anesthesia. If the mother becomes hypotensive, ephedrine or phenylephrine should be promptly administered intravenously.
7. General anesthesia should be preceded by careful denitrogenation.
8. The risk of aspiration should be minimized by application of cricoid pressure and rapid tracheal intubation with a cuffed tube.
9. To reduce fetal hazard, particularly during the first trimester, it appears preferable to choose drugs with a long history of safety. These drugs include thiopental, morphine, meperidine, muscle relaxants, and low concentrations of nitrous oxide.
10. Avoid maternal hyperventilation and monitor end-expiratory Pa_{CO_2} or arterial blood gases.
11. FHR may be monitored continuously or intermittently throughout surgery and anesthesia, provided that placement of the transducer does not encroach on the surgical field (this becomes technically feasible from the 16th week of pregnancy). The decision to monitor the fetus should be made in conjunction with the obstetrician based on the severity of maternal disease, the potential for fetal jeopardy, whether the fetus is viable, and whether a physician able to perform a cesarean delivery plans to be immediately available. Uterine tone may also be monitored with an external tocodynamometer if the uterus reaches the umbilicus or above.
12. Monitoring uterine activity should be continued after the operation, and tocolytic agents may be required.

REFERENCES

1. Taylor DJ, Lind T. Red cell mass during and after normal pregnancy. *Br J Obstet Gynaecol.* 1979;86:364–370.
2. Brenner B. Haemostatic changes in pregnancy. *Thromb Res.* 2004;114:409–414.
3. Cerneca F, Ricci G, Simeone R, et al. Coagulation and fibrinolysis changes in normal pregnancy. Increased levels of procoagulants and reduced levels of inhibitors during pregnancy induce a hypercoagulable state, combined with a reactive fibrinolysis. *Eur J Obstet Gynecol Reprod Biol.* 1997;73:31–36.
4. Gerbasi FR, Bottoms S, Faraq A, et al. Changes in hemostasis activity during delivery and the immediate postpartum period. *Am J Obstet Gynecol.* 1990;162:1158.
5. Valera M, Varant O, Vayssiere C, et al. Physiologic and pathologic changes of platelets in pregnancy. *Platelets.* 2010;21:587–595.
6. Wildsmith JA. Serum cholinesterase, pregnancy and suxamethonium. *Anaesthesia.* 1972;27:90–91.
7. Coryell MN, Beach EF, Robinson AR, et al. Metabolism of women during the reproductive cycle. XVII. Changes in electrophoretic patterns of plasma proteins through the cycle and following delivery. *J Clin Invest.* 1950;29:1559–1567.
8. Gant NF, Daley GL, Chand S, et al. A study of angiotensin II pressor response throughout primigravid pregnancy. *J Clin Invest.* 1973;52:2682–2689.
9. Duvekot JJ, Cheriex EC, Pieters FA, et al. Early pregnancy changes in hemodynamics and volume homeostasis are consecutive adjustments triggered by a primary fall in systemic vascular tone. *Am J Obstet Gynecol.* 1993;169:1382–1392.
10. Kametas NA, McAuliffe F, Krampl E, et al. Maternal cardiac function in twin pregnancy. *Obstet Gynecol.* 2003;102:806–815.
11. Higuchi H, Takagi S, Zhang K, et al. Effect of lateral tilt angle on the volume of the abdominal aorta and inferior vena cava in pregnant and nonpregnant women determined by magnetic resonance imaging. *Anesthesiology.* 2015;122:286–293.
12. Kerr MG, Scott DB, Samuel E. Studies of the inferior vena cava in late pregnancy. *Br Med J.* 1964;1:532–533.
13. Carruth JE, Mivis SB, Brogan DR, et al. The electrocardiogram in normal pregnancy. *Am Heart J.* 1981;102:1075–1078.
14. Nakagawa M, Katou S, Ichinose M, et al. Characteristics of new-onset ventricular arrhythmias in pregnancy. *J Electrocardiol.* 2004;37:47–53.
15. Pilkington S, Carli F, Dakin MJ, et al. Increase in Mallampati score during pregnancy. *Br J Anaesth.* 1995;74:638–642.
16. Kodali B, Chandrasekhar S, Bulich LN, et al. Airway changes during labor and delivery. *Anesthesiology.* 2008;108:357–362.
17. Archer GW Jr, Marx GF. Arterial oxygen tension during apnoea in parturient women. *Br J Anaesth.* 1974;46:358–360.
18. Datta S, Kitzmiller JL, Naulty JS, et al. Acid-base status of diabetic mothers and their infants following spinal anesthesia for cesarean section. *Anesth Analg.* 1982;61:662–665.
19. McDonnell NJ, Peach MJ, Clavisi OM, et al. Difficult and failed intubation in obstetric anaesthesia: an observational study of airway management and complications associated with general anesthesia for caesarean section. *Int J Obstet Anesth.* 2009;17:292.
20. Wong CA, Loffredi M, Ganchiff JN, et al. Gastric emptying of water in term pregnancy. *Anesthesiology.* 2002;96:1395–1400.
21. Wong CA, McCarthy RJ, Fitzgerald PC, et al. Gastric emptying of water in obese pregnant women at term. *Anesth Analg.* 2007;105:751–755.
22. American Society of Anesthesiologists. Practice guidelines for obstetric anesthesia: An updated report by the American Society of Anesthesiologists Task Force on obstetric anesthesia and the Society for Obstetric Anesthesia and Perinatology. *Anesthesiology.* 2016;124:270–300.
23. Brock-Utne JG, Dow TG, Dimopoulos GE, et al. Gastric and lower oesophageal sphincter (LOS) pressures in early pregnancy. *Br J Anaesth.* 1981;53:381–384.
24. Wyner J, Cohen SE. Gastric volume in early pregnancy: effect of metoclopramide. *Anesthesiology.* 1982;57:209–212.
25. Gin T, Chan MT. Decreased minimum alveolar concentration of isoflurane in pregnant humans. *Anesthesiology.* 1994;81:829–832.
26. Hirabayashi Y, Shimizu R, Saitoh K, et al. Spread of subarachnoid hyperbaric amethocaine in pregnant women. *Br J Anaesth.* 1995;74:384–386.
27. Butterworth JF IV, Walker FO, Lysak SZ. Pregnancy increases median nerve susceptibility of lidocaine. *Anesthesiology.* 1990;72:962–965.
28. Brown WU Jr, Bell GC, Alper MH. Acidosis, local anesthetics, and the newborn. *Obstet Gynecol.* 1976;48:27–30.
29. Kennedy RL, Miller RP, Bell JU, et al. Uptake and distribution of bupivacaine in fetal lambs. *Anesthesiology.* 1986;65:247–253.
30. Kuhnert PM, Kuhnert BR, Stitts JM, et al. The use of a selected ion monitoring technique to study the disposition of bupivacaine in mother, fetus, and neonate following epidural anesthesia for cesarean section. *Anesthesiology.* 1981;55:611–617.
31. Kuhnert BR, Kuhnert PM, Prochaska AL, et al. Plasma levels of 2-chloroprocaine in obstetric patients and their neonates after epidural anesthesia. *Anesthesiology.* 1980;53:21–25.
32. Dwyer R, Fee JP, Moore J. Uptake of halothane and isoflurane by mother and baby during caesarean section. *Br J Anaesth.* 1995;74:379–383.
33. Kosaka Y, Takahashi T, Mark LC. Intravenous thiobarbiturate anesthesia for cesarean section. *Anesthesiology.* 1969;31:489–506.
34. Sanchez-Alcaraz A, Quintana MB, Laguarda M. Placenta transfer and neonatal effects of propofol in caesarean section. *J Clin Pharm Ther.* 1998;23:19–23.
35. Morishima HO, Finster M, Pedersen H, et al. Pharmacokinetics of lidocaine in fetal and neonatal lambs and adult sheep. *Anesthesiology.* 1979;50:431–436.
36. Morishima HO, Pedersen H, Finster M, et al. Toxicity of lidocaine in adult, newborn, and fetal sheep. *Anesthesiology.* 1981;55:57–61.
37. Gale R, Ferguson JE 2nd, Stevenson DK. Effect of epidural analgesia with bupivacaine hydrochloride on neonatal bilirubin production. *Obstet Gynecol.* 1987;70:692–695.
38. Ueland K, Hansen JM. Maternal cardiovascular dynamics. III. Labor and delivery under local and caudal analgesia. *Am J Obstet Gynecol.* 1969;103:8–18.
39. American College of Obstetricians and Gynecologists. ACOG committee opinion. No. 339: Analgesia and cesarean delivery rates. *Obstet Gynecol.* 2006;107:1487–1488.
40. Smith CA, Collins CT, Cyna AM, et al. Complementary and alternative therapies for pain management in labour. *Cochrane Database Syst Rev.* 2006;4:CD003521.
41. Scott JR, Rose NB. Effect of psychoprophylaxis (Lamaze preparation) on labor and delivery in primiparas. *N Engl J Med.* 1976;294:1205–1207.
42. Hodnett ED, Gates S, Hofmeyr GJ, et al. Continuous support for women during childbirth. *Cochrane Database Syst Rev.* 2013;7:CD003766.
43. Cluett ER, Burns E. Immersion in water in labour and birth. *Cochrane Database Syst Rev.* 2009;2:CD000111.
44. Derry S, Straube S, Moore RA, et al. Intracutaneous or subcutaneous sterile water injection compared with blinded controls for pain management in labour. *Cochrane Database Syst Rev.* 2012;1:CD009107.
45. Madden K, Middleton P, Cyna AM, et al. Hypnosis for pain management during labour and childbirth. *Cochrane Database Syst Rev.* 2012;11:CD009356.
46. Bedwell C, Dowswell T, Neilson JP, et al. The use of transcutaneous electrical nerve stimulation (TENS) for pain relief in labour: a review of the evidence. *Midwifery.* 2011;27:e141.

47. Smith CA, Collins CT, Crowther CA, et al. Acupuncture or acupressure for pain management in labour. Cochrane Database Syst Rev. 2011;7:CD009232.
48. Smith CA, Levett KM, Collins CT, et al. Relaxation techniques for pain management in labour. Cochrane Database Syst Rev. 2011;12:CD009514.
49. Nelson KE, Eisenach JC. Intravenous butorphanol, meperidine, and their combination relieve pain and distress in women in labor. Anesthesiology. 2005;102:1008–1013.
50. Ullman R, Smith LA, Burns E, et al. Parenteral opioids for maternal pain relief in labour. Cochrane Database Syst Rev. 2010;9:CD007396.
51. Anderson D. A review of systemic opioids commonly used for labor pain relief. J Midwifery Womens Health. 2011;56:222–239.
52. Leong WL, Sng BL, Sia AT. A comparison between remifentanil and meperidine for labor analgesia: a systematic review. Anesth Analg. 2011;113:818–825.
53. Hinova A, Fernando R. Systemic remifentanil for labor analgesia. Anesth Analg. 2009;109:1925–1929.
54. Kranke P, Girard T, Lavand homme P, et al. Must we press on until a young mother dies? Remifentanil patient controlled analgesia in labour may not be suited as a "poor man's epidural". BMC pregnancy and childbirth. 2013;13:139.
55. Anim-Somuah M, Smyth RM, Jones L. Epidural versus non-epidural or no analgesia in labour. Cochrane Database Syst Rev. 2011;12:CD000331.
56. Sng BL, Leong WL, Zeng Y, et al. Early versus late initiation of epidural analgesia for labour. Cochrane Database Syst Rev. 2014;10:CD007238.
57. Caughey AB, Cahill AG, Guise JM, et al. Safe prevention of the primary cesarean delivery. Am J Obstet Gynecol. 2014;210:179–193.
58. Sultan P, Murphy C, Halpern S, et al. The effect of low concentrations versus high concentrations of local anesthetics for labour analgesia on obstetric and anesthetic outcomes: a meta-analysis. Can J Anaesth. 2013;60:840–854.
59. Beilin Y, Guinn NR, Bernstein HH, et al. Local anesthetics and mode of delivery: bupivacaine versus ropivacaine versus levobupivacaine. Anesth Analg. 2007;105:756–763.
60. van der Vyver M, Halpern S, Joseph G. Patient-controlled epidural analgesia versus continuous infusion for labour analgesia: a meta-analysis. Br J Anaesth. 2002;89:459–465.
61. Halpern SH, Carvalho B. Patient-controlled epidural analgesia for labor. Anesth Analg. 2009;108:921–928.
62. Heesen M, Bohmer J, Klohr S, et al. The effect of adding a background infusion to patient-controlled epidural labor analgesia on labor, maternal, and neonatal outcomes: a systematic review and meta-analysis. Anesth Analg. 2015;121:149–158.
63. George RB, Allen TK, Habib AS. Intermittent epidural bolus compared with continuous epidural infusions for labor analgesia: a systematic review and meta-analysis. Anesth Analg. 2013;116:133–144.
64. Asokumar B, Newman LM, McCarthy RJ, et al. Intrathecal bupivacaine reduces pruritus and prolongs duration of fentanyl analgesia during labor: a prospective, randomized controlled trial. Anesth Analg. 1998;87:1309–1315.
65. Albright GA, Forster RM. Does combined spinal-epidural analgesia with subarachnoid sufentanil increase the incidence of emergency cesarean delivery? Reg Anesth. 1997;22:400–405.
66. Abrao KC, Francisco RP, Miyadahira S, et al. Elevation of uterine basal tone and fetal heart rate abnormalities after labor analgesia: a randomized controlled trial. Obstet Gynecol. 2009;113:41–47.
67. Pan PH, Bogard TD, Owen MD. Incidence and characteristics of failures in obstetric neuraxial analgesia and anesthesia: a retrospective analysis of 19,259 deliveries. Int J Obstet Anesth. 2004;13:227–233.
68. Lee S, Lew E, Lim Y, et al. Failure of augmentation of labor epidural analgesia for intrapartum cesarean delivery: a retrospective review. Anesth Analg. 2009;108:252–254.
69. Leighton BL, Halpern SH, Wilson DB. Lumbar sympathetic blocks speed early and second stage induced labor in nulliparous women. Anesthesiology. 1999;90:1039–1046.
70. Likis FE, Andrews JC, Collins JC et al. Nitrous oxide for the management of labor pain: A systemic review. Anesth Analg. 2014;118:153–167.
71. King TL, Wong CA. Nitrous oxide for labor pain: is it a laughing matter? Anesth Analg. 2014;118:12–14.
72. Bucklin BA, Hawkins JL, Anderson JR, et al. Obstetric anesthesia workforce survey: twenty-year update. Anesthesiology. 2005;103:645–653.
73. Chatmongkolchart S, Prathep S. Supplemental oxygen for caesarean section during regional anaesthesia. Cochrane Database Syst Rev. 2013;6:CD006161.
74. Palmer CM, Emerson S, Volgoropolous D, et al. Dose-response relationship of intrathecal morphine for postcesarean analgesia. Anesthesiology. 1999;90:437–444.
75. Palmer CM, Nogami WM, Van Maren G, et al. Postcesarean epidural morphine: a dose-response study. Anesth Analg. 2000;90:887–891.
76. American Society of Anesthesiologists. Practice guidelines for the prevention, detection, and management of respiratory depression associated with neuraxial opioid administration: an updated report by the American Society of Anesthesiologists Task Force on Neuraxial Opioids and the American Society of Regional Anesthesia and Pain Medicine. Anesthesiology. 2016;124:535–552.
77. Abdallah FW, Halpern SH, Margarido CB. Transversus abdominis plane block for postoperative analgesia after caesarean delivery performed under spinal anaesthesia? A systematic review and meta-analysis. Br J Anaesth. 2012;109:679–687.
78. Leighton BL, Norris MC, DeSimone CA, et al. The air test as a clinically useful indicator of intravenously placed epidural catheters. Anesthesiology. 1990;73:610–613.
79. Morris GF, Gore-Hickman W, Lang SA, et al. Can parturients distinguish between intravenous and epidural fentanyl? Can J Anaesth. 1994;41:667–672.
80. Hillyard SG, Bate TE, Corcoran TB, et al. Extending epidural analgesia for emergency caesarean section: a meta-analysis. Br J Anaesth. 2011;107:668–678.
81. Albright GA. Cardiac arrest following regional anesthesia with etidocaine or bupivacaine. Anesthesiology. 1979;51:285–287.
82. Choi DH, Kim JA, Chung IS. Comparison of combined spinal epidural anesthesia and epidural anesthesia for cesarean section. Acta Anaesthesiol Scand. 2000;44:214–219.
83. Thoren T, Holmstrom B, Rawal N, et al. Sequential combined spinal epidural block versus spinal block for cesarean section: effects on maternal hypotension and neurobehavioral function of the newborn. Anesth Analg. 1994;78:1087–1092.
84. Choi DH, Ahn HJ, Kim JA. Combined low-dose spinal-epidural anesthesia versus single-shot spinal anesthesia for elective cesarean delivery. Int J Obstet Anesth. 2006;15:13–17.
85. Hawkins JL, Chang J, Palmer SK, et al. Anesthesia-related maternal mortality in the United States: 1979–2002. Obstet Gynecol. 2011;117:69–74.
86. Kodali BS, Chandrasekhar S, Bulich LN, et al. Airway changes during labor and delivery. Anesthesiology. 2008;108:357–362.
87. de Souza DG, Doar LH, Mehta SH, et al. Aspiration prophylaxis and rapid sequence induction for elective cesarean delivery: time to reassess old dogma? Anesth Analg. 2010;110:1503–1505.
88. McGuigan PJ, Shields MO, McCourt KC. Role of rocuronium and sugammadex in rapid sequence induction in pregnancy. Br J Anaesth. 2011;106:418–419.
89. Apfelbaum JL, Hagberg CA, Caplan RA, et al. Practice guidelines for management of the difficult airway: an updated report by the American Society of Anesthesiologists Task Force on Management of the Difficult Airway. Anesthesiology. 2013;118:251–270.
90. Mushambi MC, Kinsella SM, Popat M, et al. Obstetric Anaesthetists' Association and Difficult Airway Society guidelines for the management of difficult and failed tracheal intubation in obstetrics. Anaesthesia. 2015;70:1286–1306.
91. Pandit JJ, Andrade J, Bogod DG, et al. 5th National Audit Project (NAP5) on accidental awareness during general anaesthesia: summary of main findings and risk factors. Br J Anaesth. 2014;113:549–559.
92. Chin KJ, Yeo SW. Bispectral index values at sevoflurane concentrations of 1% and 1.5% in lower segment cesarean delivery. Anesth Analg. 2004;98:1140–1144.
93. Ong BY, Cohen MM, Palahniuk RJ. Anesthesia for cesarean section: effects on neonates. Anesth Analg. 1989;68:270–275.
94. Ngan Kee WD, Khaw KS, Ng FF. Comparison of phenylephrine infusion regimens for maintaining maternal blood pressure during spinal anaesthesia for Caesarean section. Br J Anaesth. 2004;92:469–474.
95. Banerjee A, Stocche RM, Angle P, et al. Preload or coload for spinal anesthesia for elective Cesarean delivery: a meta-analysis. Can J Anaesth. 2010;57:24–31.
96. Morgan PJ, Halpern SH, Tarshis J. The effects of an increase of central blood volume before spinal anesthesia for cesarean delivery: a qualitative systematic review. Anesth Analg. 2001;92:997–1005.
97. Lee A, Ngan Kee WD, Gin T. A quantitative, systematic review of randomized controlled trials of ephedrine versus phenylephrine for the management of hypotension during spinal anesthesia for cesarean delivery. Anesth Analg. 2002;94:920–926.
98. Ngan Kee WD, Khaw KS, Tan PE, et al. Placental transfer and fetal metabolic effects of phenylephrine and ephedrine during spinal anesthesia for cesarean delivery. Anesthesiology. 2009;111:506–512.
99. George RB, McKeen D, Columb MO, et al. Up-down determination of the 90% effective dose of phenylephrine for the treatment of spinal anesthesia-induced hypotension in parturients undergoing cesarean delivery. Anesth Analg. 2010;110:154–158.
100. Allen TK, George RB, White WD, et al. A double-blind, placebo-controlled trial of four fixed rate infusion regimens of phenylephrine for hemodynamic support during spinal anesthesia for cesarean delivery. Anesth Analg. 2010;111:1221–1229.
101. Siddik-Sayyid SM, Taha SK, Kanazi GE, et al. A randomized controlled trial of variable rate phenylephrine infusion with rescue phenylephrine boluses versus rescue boluses alone on physician interventions during spinal anesthesia for elective cesarean delivery. Anesth Analg. 2014;118:611–618.
102. Neal JM, Mulroy MF, Weinberg GL. American Society of Regional Anesthesia and Pain Medicine checklist for managing local anesthetic systemic toxicity: 2012 version. Reg Anesth Pain Med. 2012;37:16–18.
103. Lipman S, Cohen S, Einav S, et al. The Society for Obstetric Anesthesia and Perinatology consensus statement on the management of cardiac arrest in pregnancy. Anesth Analg. 2014;118:1003–1016.

104. Paech MJ, Doherty DA, Christmas T, et al. The volume of blood for epidural blood patch in obstetrics: a randomized, blinded clinical trial. Anesth Analg. 2011;113:126–133.
105. Scavone BM, Wong CA, Sullivan JT, et al. Efficacy of a prophylactic epidural blood patch in preventing post dural puncture headache in parturients after inadvertent dural puncture. Anesthesiology. 2004;101:1422–1427.
106. Apfel CC, Saxena A, Cakmakkaya OS, et al. Prevention of postdural puncture headache after accidental dural puncture: a quantitative systematic review. Br J Anaesth. 2010;105:255–263.
107. Centers for Disease Control and Prevention (CDC). Bacterial meningitis after intrapartum spinal anesthesia: New York and Ohio, 2008–2009. MMWR Morb Mortal Wkly Rep. 2010;59:65–69.
108. Wong CA, Scavone BM, Dugan S, et al. Incidence of postpartum lumbosacral spine and lower extremity nerve injuries. Obstet Gynecol. 2003;101:279–288.
109. Ananth CV, Keyes KM, Wapner RJ. Pre-eclampsia rates in the United States 1980–2010: age-period-cohort analysis. BMJ. 2013;347:f6564.
110. American College of Obstetricians and Gynecologists; Task Force on Hypertension in Pregnancy. Hypertension in pregnancy. Report of the American College of Obstetricians and Gynecologists' Task Force on hypertension in pregnancy. Obstet Gynecol. 2013;122:1122–1131.
111. Wang Y, Walsh SW, Kay HH. Placental lipid peroxides and thromboxane are increased and prostacyclin is decreased in women with preeclampsia. Am J Obstet Gynecol. 1992;167:946–949.
112. Meekins JW, Pijnenborg R, Hanssens M, et al. A study of placental bed spiral arteries and trophoblast invasion in normal and severe pre-eclamptic pregnancies. Br J Obstet Gynaecol. 1994;101:669–674.
113. Chesley LC. Plasma and red cell volumes during pregnancy. Am J Obstet Gynecol. 1972;112:440–450.
114. O'Brien JM, Milligan DA, Barton JR. Impact of high dose corticosteroid therapy for patients with HELLP (hemolysis, elevated liver enzymes, and low platelet count) syndrome. Am J Obstet Gynecol. 2000;183:921–924.
115. Doyle LW, Crowther CA, Middleton P, et al. Magnesium sulphate for women at risk of preterm birth for neuroprotection of the fetus. Cochrane Database Syst Rev. 2009;2:CD004661.
116. Hogg B, Hauth JC, Caritis SN, et al. Safety of labor epidural anesthesia for women with severe hypertensive disease. National Institute of Child Health and Human Development Maternal Fetal Medicine Units Network. Am J Obstet Gynecol. 1999;181:1096–1101.
117. Newsome LR, Bramwell RS, Curling PE. Severe preeclampsia: hemodynamic effects of lumbar epidural anesthesia. Anesth Analg. 1986;65:31–36.
118. Jouppila P, Jouppila R, Hollmen A, et al. Lumbar epidural analgesia to improve intervillous blood flow during labor in severe preeclampsia. Obstet Gynecol. 1982;59:158–161.
119. Aya AG, Mangin R, Vialles N, et al. Patients with severe preeclampsia experience less hypotension during spinal anesthesia for elective cesarean delivery than healthy parturients: a prospective cohort comparison. Anesth Analg. 2003;97:867–872.
120. Wallace DH, Leveno KJ, Cunningham FG, et al. Randomized comparison of general and regional anesthesia for cesarean delivery in pregnancies complicated by severe preeclampsia. Obstet Gynecol. 1995;86:193–199.
121. Hood DD, Curry R. Spinal versus epidural anesthesia for cesarean section in severely preeclamptic patients: a retrospective survey. Anesthesiology. 1999;90:1276–1282.
122. Bateman BT, Berman MF, Riley LE, et al. The epidemiology of postpartum hemorrhage in a large, nationwide sample of deliveries. Anesth Analg. 2010;110:1368–1373.
123. Callaghan WM, Kuklina EV, Berg CJ. Trends in postpartum hemorrhage: United States, 1994–2006. Am J Obstet Gynecol. 2010;202:353.e1–353.e6.
124. Ananth CV, Smulian JC, Vintzileos AM. The association of placenta previa with history of cesarean delivery and abortion: a meta-analysis. Am J Obstet Gynecol. 1997;177:1071–1078.
125. Miller DA, Chollet JA, Goodwin TM. Clinical risk factors for placenta previa-placenta accreta. Am J Obstet Gynecol. 1997;177:210–214.
126. Silver RM, Landon MB, Rouse DJ, et al. Maternal morbidity associated with multiple repeat cesarean deliveries. Obstet Gynecol. 2006;107:1226–1232.
127. Bateman BT, Mhyre JM, Callaghan WM, et al. Peripartum hysterectomy in the United States: nationwide 14 year experience. Am J Obstet Gynecol. 2012;206:63.e1–63.e8.
128. ACOG Committee opinion. Number 266, January 2002: placenta accreta. Obstet Gynecol. 2002;99:169–170.
129. Charbit B, Mandelbrot L, Samain E, et al. The decrease of fibrinogen is an early predictor of the severity of postpartum hemorrhage. J Thromb Haemost. 2007;5:266–273.
130. Kuklina EV, Meikle SF, Jamieson DJ, et al. Severe obstetric morbidity in the United States: 1998–2005. Obstet Gynecol. 2009;113:293–299.
131. Girard T, Mörtl M, Schlembach D. New approaches to obstetric hemorrhage: the postpartum hemorrhage consensus algorithm. Curr Opin Anaesth. 2014;27:267–274.
132. Liumbruno GM, Liumbruno C, Rafenelli D. Intraoperative cell salvage in obstetrics: is it a real therapeutic option? Transfusion. 2011;10:2244–2256.
133. Gungorduk K, Yildirim G, Asicioglu O, et al. Efficacy of intravenous tranexamic acid in reducing blood loss after elective cesarean section: a prospective, randomized, double-blind, placebo-controlled study. Am J Perinatol. 2011;28:233–240.
134. Franchini M, Franchi M, Bergamini V, et al. The use of recombinant activated FVII in postpartum hemorrhage. Clin Obstet Gynecol. 2010;53:219–227.
135. Lucas S. (on behalf of the Centre for Maternal and Child Enquiries). Annex 9.1. Pathologic overview of cardiac deaths including sudden adult/arrhythmic death syndrome (SADS). BGOG. 2011;116:118(suppl 1).
136. Arafeh JM, Baird SM. Cardiac disease in pregnancy. Crit Care Nurs Q. 2006;29:32–52.
137. Ro A, Frishman WH. Peripartum cardiomyopathy. Cardiol Rev. 2006;14:35–42.
138. Curry R, Swan L, Steer P. Cardiac disease in pregnancy. Curr Opin Obstet Gynecol. 2009;21:508–513.
139. Palmer DG. Peripartum cardiomyopathy. J Perinat Neonatal Nurs. 2006;20:324–332.
140. Baird SM, Kennedy B. Myocardial infarction in pregnancy. J Perinat Neonatal Nurs. 2006;20:311–321; quiz 322.
141. Mallampalli A, Guy E. Cardiac arrest in pregnancy and somatic support after brain death. Crit Care Med. 2005;33:S325–S331.
142. Hunt KJ, Schuller KL. The increasing prevalence of diabetes in pregnancy. Obstet Gynecol Clin North Am. 2007;34:173–199, vii.
143. Parker JA, Conway DL. Diabetic ketoacidosis in pregnancy. Obstet Gynecol Clin North Am. 2007;34:533–543, xii.
144. Mulholland C, Njoroge T, Mersereau P, et al. Comparison of guidelines available in the United States for diagnosis and management of diabetes before, during, and after pregnancy. J Womens Health (Larchmt). 2007;16:790–801.
145. Perlow JH, Morgan MA, Montgomery D, et al. Perinatal outcome in pregnancy complicated by massive obesity. Am J Obstet Gynecol. 1992;167:958–962.
146. Centre for Maternal and Child Enquires (CMACE). Improving the health of mothers, babies and children. Maternal obesity in the UK: findings from a National Project. United Kingdom, 2010.
147. Hamilton BE, Martin JA, Sutton PD. Births: preliminary data for 2002. Natl Vital Stat Rep. 2003;51:1.
148. Montan S. Increased risk in the elderly parturient. Curr Opin Obstet Gynecol. 2007;19:110–112.
149. Joseph KS, Allen AC, Dodds L, et al. The perinatal effects of delayed childbearing. Obstet Gynecol. 2005;105:1410–1418.
150. Simchen MJ, Yinon Y, Moran O, et al. Pregnancy outcome after age 50. Obstet Gynecol. 2006;108:1084–1088.
151. Cleary-Goldman J, Malone FD, Vidaver J, et al. Impact of maternal age on obstetric outcome. Obstet Gynecol. 2005;105:983–990.
152. Callaway LK, Lust K, McIntyre HD. Pregnancy outcomes in women of very advanced maternal age. Aust N Z J Obstet Gynaecol. 2005;45:12–16.
153. Vigil-De Gracia P, Montufar-Rueda C, Smith A. Pregnancy and severe chronic hypertension: maternal outcome. Hypertens Pregnancy. 2004;23:285–293.
154. Lin HC, Sheen TC, Tang CH, et al. Association between maternal age and the likelihood of a cesarean section: a population-based multivariate logistic regression analysis. Acta Obstet Gynecol Scand. 2004;83:1178–1183.
155. Amu O, Rajendran S, Bolaji II. Should doctors perform an elective caesarean section on request? Maternal choice alone should not determine method of delivery. BMJ. 1998;317:463.
156. Bell JS, Campbell DM, Graham WJ, et al. Do obstetric complications explain high caesarean section rates among women over 30? A retrospective analysis. BMJ. 2001;322:894–895.
157. Oleszczuk JJ, Keith LG, Oleszczuk AK. The paradox of old maternal age in multiple pregnancies. Obstet Gynecol Clin North Am. 2005;32:69–80, ix.
158. Holcroft CJ, Blakemore KJ, Allen M, et al. Association of prematurity and neonatal infection with neurologic morbidity in very low birth weight infants. Obstet Gynecol. 2003;101:1249–1253.
159. Committee on Obstetric Practice. Number 455 March 2010: magnesium sulfate before anticipated preterm birth for neuroprotection. Obstet Gynecol. 2010;115:669–671.
160. Bagley SM, Wachman EM, Holland E, et al. Review of the assessment and management of neonatal abstinence syndrome. Addict Sci Clin Pract. 2014;9:19.
161. Estelles J, Rodriguez-Arias M, Maldonado C, et al. Gestational exposure to cocaine alters cocaine reward. Behav Pharmacol. 2006;17:509–515.
162. ACOG practice bulletin No. 106. Intrapartum fetal heart rate monitoring: Nomenclature, interpretation, and general management principles. Obstet Gynecol. 2009;114:192–202.
163. VandeVeld M, Vercauterren M, Vandermeersch E. Fetal heart rate abnormalities after regional analgesia for labor pain: the effect of intrathecal opioids. Reg Anesth Pain Med. 2001;26:257–262.
164. Timmins AE, Clark SL. How to approach intrapartum category II tracings. Obstet Gynecol Clin N Am. 2015;42:363–375.
165. Bloom SL, Spong CY, Thom E, et al. Fetal pulse oximetry and cesarean delivery. N Engl J Med. 2006;355:2195–2202.

166. Garite TJ, Dildy GA, McNamara H, et al. A multicenter controlled trial of fetal pulse oximetry in the intrapartum management of nonreassuring fetal heart rate patterns. *Am J Obstet Gynecol*. 2000;183:1049–1058.
167. Saccone G, Schuit E, Am-Wahlin I, et al. Electrocardiogram ST analysis during labor: a systemic review and meta-analysis of randomized controlled trials. *Obstet Gynecol*. 2016;127:127–135.
168. Kattwinkel J, Perlman JM, Aziz K, et al. Special Report—Neonatal Resuscitation: 2010 American Heart Association guidelines for cardiopulmonary resuscitation and emergency cardicvascular care. *Circulation*. 2010;122:S9.
169. Davis PG, Tan A, O'Donnell CPF, et al. Resuscitation of newborn infants with 100% oxygen or air: a systematic review and meta-analysis. *Lancet*. 2004;364:1329–1333.
170. Rabi Y, Rabi D, Yee W. Room air resuscitation of the depressed newborn: a systematic review and meta-analysis. *Resuscitation*. 2007;72:353–363.
171. Bouchard S, Johnson MP, Flake AW, et al. The EXIT procedure: experience and outcome in 31 cases. *J Pediatr Surg*. 2002;37:418–426.
172. Clark KD, Viscomi CM, Lowell J, et al. Nitroglycerin for relaxation to establish a fetal airway (EXIT procedure). *Obstet Gynecol*. 2004;103:1113–1115.
173. Gaiser RR, Cheek TG, Kurth CD. Anesthetic management of cesarean delivery complicated by ex utero intrapartum treatment of the fetus. *Anesth Analg*. 1997;84:1150–1153.
174. Stewart MK, Terhune KP. Management of pregnant patients undergoing general surgical procedures. *Surg Clin North Am*. 2015;95:429–442.
175. Cohen-Kerem R, Railton C, Oren D, et al. Pregnancy outcome following nonobstetrical surgical intervention. *Am J Surg*. 2005;190:467–473.
176. Smith BE, Gaub ML, Moya F. Teratogenic effects of anesthetic agents: nitrous oxide. *Anesth Analg*. 1965;44:726–732.
177. Duncan PG, Pope WD, Cohen MM, et al. Fetal risk of anesthesia and surgery during pregnancy. *Anesthesiology*. 1986;64:790–794.
178. Sanchez V, Feinstein S, Lunardi N, et al. General anesthesia causes long-term impairment of mitochondrial morphogenesis and synaptic transmission in developing rat brain. *Anesthesiology*. 2011;115:992–1002.
179. Sun LS, Li G, Miller TL, et al. Association between a single general anesthesia exposure before age 36 months and nuerocognitive outcomes in later childhood. *JAMA*. 2016;315:2312–2320.
180. ACOG Committee on Obstetric Practice. ACOG Committee opinion number 284. August 2003: nonobstetric surgery in pregnancy. *Obstet Gynecol*. 2003;102:431.

42 Neonatal Anesthesia

JUSTIN B. LONG • SANTHANAM SURESH

Physiology of the Infant and the Transition Period
   The Cardiovascular System
   The Pulmonary System
   The Renal System
   Fluid and Electrolyte Therapy in the Neonate
   Blood Component Therapy in the Neonate
   The Hepatic System
   Anatomy of the Neonatal Airway
   Anesthetic Drugs in Neonates
Anesthetic Management of the Neonate
   Preoperative Considerations
   Intraoperative Considerations
   Impact of Surgical Requirements on Anesthetic Technique
   Uptake and Distribution of Anesthetics in Neonates
   Anesthetic Dose Requirements of Neonates
   Regional Anesthesia
   Postoperative Pain Management
   Postoperative Ventilation
Special Considerations
   Maternal Drug Use during Pregnancy
   Temperature Control and Thermogenesis
   Respiratory Distress Syndrome
   Postoperative Apnea
   Retinopathy of Prematurity
   Neurodevelopmental Effects of Anesthetic Agents
Surgical Procedures in Neonates
   Surgical Procedures in the First Week of Life
   Surgical Procedures in the First Month of Life
Summary
Acknowledgment

KEY POINTS

1. Understanding the physiologic changes that occur during the transition from fetal to neonatal life is crucial to the anesthetic management of the neonate. The circulatory, pulmonary, hepatic, and renal systems are all affected in this process.
2. Important physiologic and anatomic factors account for the rapid rate of desaturation observed in neonates. These include an increase in oxygen consumption, a higher closing volume, a high ratio of minute ventilation to functional residual capacity, and a pliable rib cage.
3. Persistent pulmonary hypertension of the newborn is a pathologic condition that can be primary but is often secondary to other conditions, including meconium aspiration, sepsis, congenital diaphragmatic hernia, or pneumonia. Understanding the pathophysiologic characteristics of this condition helps guide therapy.
4. Knowledge of the major anatomic differences between the infant and the adult airway helps one understand why the infant's airway is often described as "anterior" and why airway management may be challenging. These differences include a relatively large tongue, a cephalad glottis with anterior slanting vocal folds, a larger occiput, and a narrowing at the cricoid ring.
5. Careful attention must be given to the choice of anesthetic agents and dosing of such agents in the neonatal population. Ongoing maturational changes in the renal and hepatobiliary systems, which occur during the first 30 days of life, will affect the metabolism and elimination of many anesthetic agents.
6. Although a host of anesthetic techniques are available, including regional anesthesia, multiple factors are considered when choosing an anesthetic plan for the neonate. These include the surgical requirements, the need for postoperative ventilation, the cardiovascular stability of the neonate, and the anticipated method of postoperative pain control.
7. Special considerations must be addressed when planning an anesthetic for a neonate. Some of the controversial issues include the risk of postoperative apnea, the role of oxygen concentration in the development of retinopathy of prematurity, and the neurocognitive effects of anesthetic agents on the fetal and neonatal brain.
8. True surgical emergencies are uncommon in the neonatal period. Knowledge of conditions with comorbidities, such as tracheoesophageal fistula, omphalocele, and congenital diaphragmatic hernia, and a thorough preoperative evaluation and stabilization of such neonates cannot be overemphasized.

Physiology of the Infant and the Transition Period

An infant's first year of life is characterized by a miraculous growth in size and maturity. The body weight alone changes by a factor of three, and there is no other period in extrauterine life when changes occur so rapidly. Before birth, fetal growth and development depend on the genetic composition of the fetus, the mother's placental function, and potential exposure to chemicals or infectious agents that can affect the mother, fetus, or both.

After birth, the newborn must rapidly adjust to the extrauterine environment to survive. The dramatic changes in functions of several systems will determine the viability of the neonate, as well as its ability to grow and develop properly.

The newborn period has been defined as the first 24 hours of life, and the neonatal period as the first 28 days of life. There is significant change in many physiologic systems during both of these periods. The first 72 hours are especially significant for the cardiovascular, pulmonary, and renal systems. The changes in these systems are interrelated; inadequate progression of change or a disease state altering one of these systems can quickly alter the maturation of one or more of the other systems. Understanding the differences in these systems from the older child, as well as the changes that occur in the neonatal period, is important in developing a comprehensive anesthetic approach.

The Cardiovascular System

Fetal Circulation

The fetal circulation is characterized by a parallel system in which both ventricles pump most of their output into the systemic circulation. Less than 10% of the combined cardiac output goes through the fetal circulation as a result of the ductus arteriosus (Fig. 42-1A). The placenta provides oxygenated blood into the ductus venosus, the inferior vena cava, and then into the right atrium. In the right atrium, the majority of the oxygenated blood primarily flows through the foramen ovale into the left atrium, bypassing the right ventricle and the pulmonary vascular bed. This preferential flow across the foramen occurs because of the relatively low pressure in the left atrium compared with that of the right atrium. Some blood from the right atrium does flow through the right ventricle and into the main pulmonary artery.

The pulmonary vascular resistance is quite high in utero because of alveolar collapse and compression of blood vessels, inhibiting flow through the pulmonary circulation. The pulmonary vascular resistance is also high at this point because of the relatively low Pa_{O_2} and pH of the blood that does flow through the vessels. Some blood in the pulmonary artery does flow through the pulmonary circulation and then into the left atrium, but the majority of flow goes through the ductus arteriosus into the descending aorta.

Changes at Birth

After birth, all of these shunts are eliminated or start to close quickly.[1] The placental shunt is eliminated and the ductus venosus is closed. The newborn's left ventricle is now pumping blood into the higher pressure systemic circulation exclusively. Expansion of the lungs and initiation of breathing lead to dramatic changes in both the circulatory and pulmonary systems (Fig. 42-1B). As alveoli fill with air, the compression of the pulmonary alveolar capillaries is relieved, reducing pulmonary vascular resistance and promoting flow through the pulmonary circulation. This blood is now oxygenated, raising the arterial PO_2, and further reducing pulmonary vascular resistance. Although the change in the first minutes to hours is dramatic, it usually takes

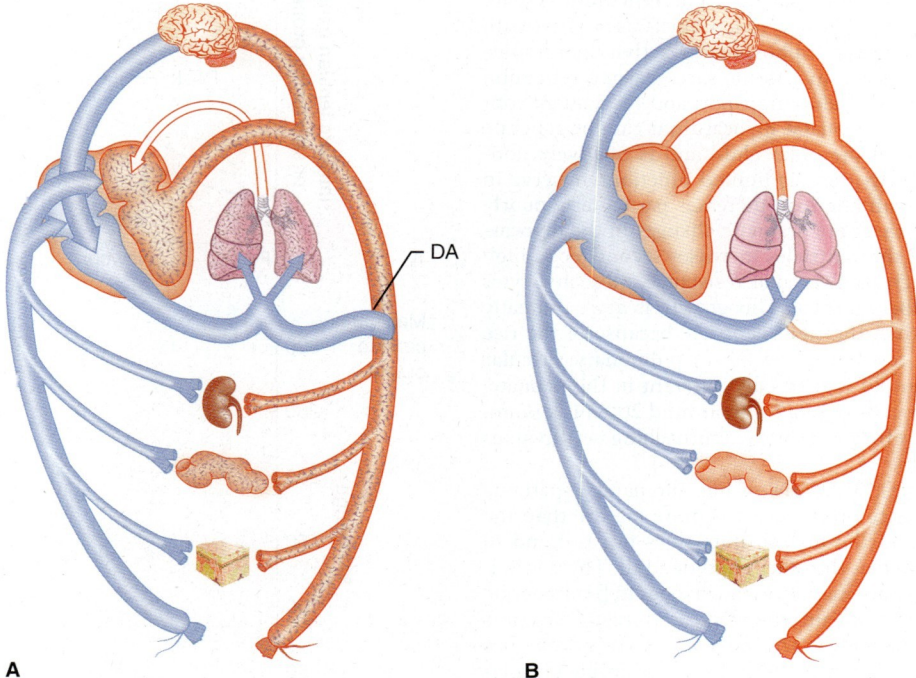

Figure 42-1 A: Schematic representation of the fetal circulation. Oxygenated blood leaves the placenta in the umbilical vein (*vessel without stippling*). Umbilical vein blood joins blood from the viscera (represented here by the kidney, gut, and skin) in the inferior vena cava. Approximately half of the inferior vena cava flow passes through the foramen ovale to the left atrium, where it mixes with a small amount of pulmonary venous blood, and this relatively well-oxygenated blood (denoted by *stippling*) supplies the heart and brain by way of the ascending aorta. The other half of the inferior vena cava stream mixes with superior vena cava blood and enters the right ventricle (blood in the right atrium and ventricle has little oxygen). Because the pulmonary arterioles are constricted, most of the blood in the main pulmonary artery flows through the ductus arteriosus (DA) so the descending aorta's blood has less oxygen (*heavy stippling*) than does blood in the ascending aorta (*light stippling*). **B:** Schematic representation of the circulation in the normal newborn. After expansion of the lungs and ligation of the umbilical cord, pulmonary blood flow and left atrial and systemic arterial pressures increase. When left atrial pressure exceeds right atrial pressure, the foramen ovale closes so all inferior and superior vena cava blood leaves the right atrium, enters the right ventricle, and is pumped through the pulmonary artery toward the lung. With the increase in systemic arterial pressure and decrease in pulmonary artery pressure, flow through the ductus arteriosus becomes left to right, and the ductus constricts and closes. The course of circulation is the same as in the adult. (Reprinted with permission from Phibbs R. Delivery room management of the newborn. In: Avery GB, ed. *Neonatology, Pathophysiology and Management of the Newborn*. 2nd ed. Philadelphia, PA: JB Lippincott; 1981:184.)

3 to 4 days for the pulmonary vascular resistance to decrease to normal levels. The foramen ovale will usually functionally close in the first hour of life as the increase in left atrial pressure from increased pulmonary circulation after the initiation of breathing exceeds right atrial pressure. The foramen is closed by a flap of tissue. This foramen can reopen if there is a relative increase in right atrial pressure such as is seen with elevated pulmonary vascular resistance or fluid overload. Anatomic closure usually occurs in the first year of life, but may remain probe-patent into adulthood in 10% to 20% of patients. The ductus arteriosus starts to close in the first day of life and is usually functionally closed in the second day of life. In utero, patency of the ductus was maintained by the combined relaxant effects of low oxygen tension and endogenously produced prostaglandins, especially prostaglandin E_2. In a full-term neonate, oxygen is the most important factor controlling ductal closure. When the Pa_{O_2} of blood in the ductus rises to about 50 mmHg, the muscle in the vessel constricts. It should be noted that the ductus of a preterm infant is less responsive to increased oxygen, even though its musculature is developed.

Myocardial function is different in the neonate. The neonatal cardiac myocyte has less organized contractile elements than the child or adult.[2] Not only are there fewer myofibril elements, but they are not organized in parallel roles, as seen in the child and adult heart, making them less efficient. The neonate myocyte also has a less mature sarcoplasmic reticulum system. The underdeveloped sarcoplasmic reticulum is associated with a decrease in Ca^{2+}-adenosine triphosphatase activity, an important component of contractility. As the sarcoplasmic reticulum matures, the efficiency of calcium transport and subsequent contractility increases.[3] The neonatal myocardium cannot generate as much force as that of the older child and is relatively noncompliant. Consequently, there is limited functional reserve in the neonatal period, with afterload increases particularly poorly tolerated. After birth, there are dramatic changes in the myocardium. As the work of the ventricles increases secondary to high stroke volume and increased vascular resistance, these myocytes grow quickly in number and size. This growth is more dramatic in the left ventricle than the right ventricle because of the rise in systemic vascular resistance and fall in pulmonary vascular resistance. Cardiac output is markedly different in the neonate, up to 400 mL/kg/min, falls in infancy to around 200 mL/kg/min, and is 100 mL/kg/min by adolescence approaching adult values of 70 to 80 mL/kg/min.

Especially in the first 3 months of life, the parasympathetic nervous system influence on the heart is more mature than the sympathetic system and the myocardium does not respond to inotropic support as well as the older child or adult. There is animal evidence that there are maturational changes in β-adrenergic receptor function that explain the decreased responsiveness to inotropes in the neonate.[4] The neonatal myocardium has increased glycogen stores and higher rates of anaerobic glycolysis, which may explain its relative resistance to hypoxia and better performance in the presence of an ischemic insult. Because the myocardium is relatively noncompliant in the newborn, preload changes can increase stroke volume and cardiac output, but not as effectively as in the older child.[5] In other words, the Frank–Starling relationship is present in the neonatal heart, but is not as effective as in the adult. Therefore, the clinical implication of a noncompliant ventricle is that, in the absence of significant increases in stroke volume, cardiac output is not well maintained in the presence of bradycardia. Finally, neonates have immature baroreceptors. The baroreceptor is responsible for reflex tachycardia that occurs in response to hypotension. Therefore, the immaturity of this reflex would limit the neonate's ability to compensate for hypotension by increasing heart rate. In addition, the baroresponse of the neonate is more depressed than that of the adult at the same level of anesthesia.

In summary, the neonatal heart has some significant differences when compared to the mature heart. Resting cardiac output is much higher relative to body weight than in the adult because of the higher O_2 consumption per kilogram of body weight. Stimulation of the myocardium produces a limited increase in contractility and cardiac output. The sympathetic nervous system, which usually provides the important chronotropic and inotropic support to the mature circulation during stress, is severely limited in the neonate because of relative lack of development when compared with the parasympathetic nervous system. Even in the absence of stress, the neonatal heart has limited ability to increase cardiac output compared with the mature heart (Fig. 42-2). The resting cardiac output of the immature heart is close to the maximal cardiac output, so there is limited reserve. The mature heart can increase cardiac output by 300%, whereas the immature heart can only increase cardiac output by 30% to 40%.

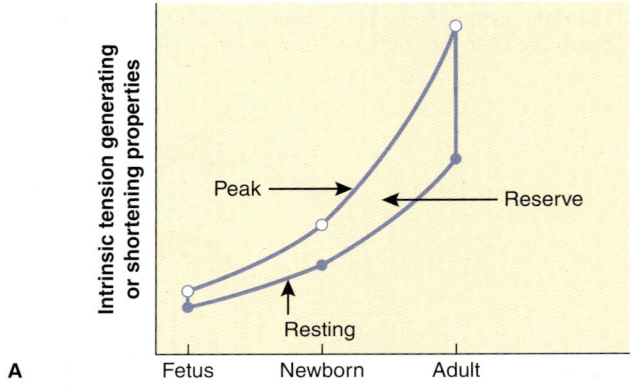

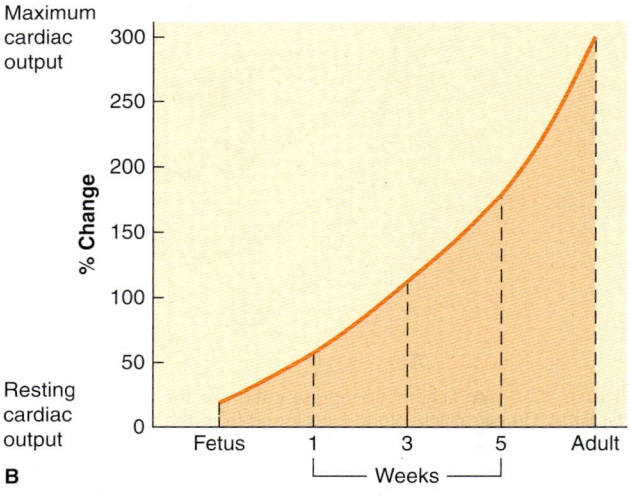

Figure 42-2 Schema of reduced cardiac reserve in fetal and newborn animal hearts compared with adult hearts. **A:** In the newborn infant, resting cardiac muscle performance is close to a peak of ventricular function because of limitations in diastolic, systolic, and heart rate reserve. **B:** Similarly, pump reserve early in life is limited by these factors and by much higher resting cardiac output relative to body weight, compared with that in adults. (Reprinted with permission from Friedman WF, George BL. Treatment of congestive heart failure by altering loading conditions of the heart. *J Pediatr.* 1985;106:700.)

Table 42-1 Normal Blood Gas Values in the Neonate

Subject	Age	PO$_2$ (mmHg)	PCO$_2$ (mmHg)	pH
Fetus (term)	Before labor	25	40	7.37
Fetus (term)	End of labor	10–20	55	7.25
Newborn (term)	10 min	50	48	7.2
Newborn (term)	1 h	70	35	7.35
Newborn (term)	1 wk	75	35	7.4
Newborn (preterm, 1,500 g)	1 wk	60	38	7.37

The Pulmonary System

The pulmonary system develops rapidly during the last trimester, with important changes in both the number of alveoli and the maturity of the pulmonary vascular system.[6] These systems have not matured enough to provide adequate gas exchange until about 24 to 26 weeks' gestation. The airways and alveoli continue to grow after birth, with alveoli increasing in number until about 8 years of age.[7] With the initiation of ventilation, the pulmonary system changes dramatically. The alveoli transition from a fluid-filled to an air-filled state and a normal ventilatory pattern with normal volumes develops in the first 5 to 10 minutes of life. In order to adequately expand the collapsed and fluid-filled alveoli, the newborn will generate an initial negative intrathoracic pressure in the range of 40 to 60 cm H$_2$O. By 10 to 20 minutes of life, the newborn has achieved its near-normal functional residual capacity (FRC), and the blood gases stabilize with the establishment of increased pulmonary blood flow. Table 42-1 lists the normal blood gases for the various periods of life. The initial breaths to expand the lungs and subsequently maintain FRC are necessary components of the stabilization of the ventilatory system, as well as the circulatory system. Failure to do so will quickly lead to deterioration of both systems.

Tidal volume is roughly the same in the neonate as the child or adult on a volume/kilogram body weight measure, but the respiratory rate is increased. Closing volumes are particularly high and may be within the range of the normal tidal volume (Fig. 42-3). This increased minute ventilation mirrors the higher oxygen consumption in neonates, which is about double that seen in an adult. Because the FRC in the newborn is comparable to that of the older child or adult, but the minute ventilation is much higher, the ratio of minute ventilation to FRC is two to three times higher in the newborn. The clinical significance of this ratio is twofold. First, anesthetic induction with a volatile anesthetic agent should be faster, as should emergence. Second, the decrease in FRC relative to minute ventilation and oxygen consumption means that there is less "oxygen reserve" in the FRC compared to that of older children and adults. There will be a more rapid drop in arterial oxygen levels in the newborn in the presence of apnea or hypoventilation. Table 42-2 compares normal respiratory parameters in the normal newborn and adult.

Lung compliance is relatively low, but chest wall compliance is relatively high, compared to that of older children. The pliable rib cage gives less mechanical support than in the older child, leading to significant retractions with less efficient gas exchange and functional airway closure, thus increasing the work of breathing. The intercostal muscles are poorly developed at birth, with the diaphragm providing most of the gas exchange. The diaphragm in the neonate has two types of fibers, the type 1, slow twitch, high-oxidative fibers that give sustained contraction with very little fatigue, and the type 2, fast twitch, low-oxidative fibers that give quick contractions but fatigue easily. The distribution of these fibers in the newborn shows only about 25% type 1 fibers, whereas 55% of the fibers are type 1 in the mature diaphragm at about 2 years of age. The preterm newborn has even fewer type 1 fibers at birth, in the 10% range. This relative lack of type 1 fibers means that the newborn, especially the preterm, is at risk for diaphragmatic fatigue in the presence of significant resistance to ventilation or periods of hyperventilation.

Finally, the continued presence of surfactant is necessary to maintain both the distensibility of the alveoli and the maintenance of an FRC at exhalation. Decreased surfactant production, due to prematurity or other conditions such as maternal diabetes, can cause respiratory distress syndrome (RDS). The decreased surfactant can cause alveolar collapse, decrease in lung compliance, hypoxia, increased work of breathing, and respiratory

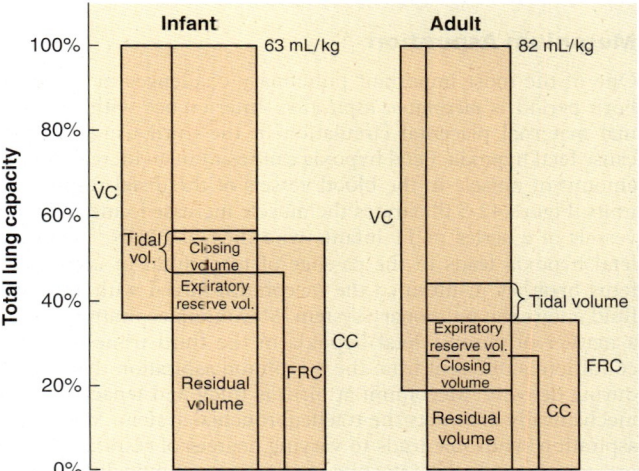

Figure 42-3 Static lung volumes of infants and adults. CC, closing capacity; FRC, functional residual capacity; VC, vital capacity. (Reprinted with permission from Smith CA, Nelson NM. *Physiology of the Newborn Infant*. 4th ed. Springfield, IL: Charles C Thomas; 1976:207.)

Table 42-2 Comparison of Normal Respiratory Values in Infants and Adults

Parameter	Infant	Adult
Respiratory frequency (breaths/min)	30–50	12–16
Tidal volume (mL/kg)	7	7
Dead space (mL/kg)	2–2.5	2.2
Alveolar ventilation (mL/kg/min)	100–150	60
Functional residual capacity (mL/kg)	27–30	30
Oxygen consumption (mL/kg/min)	7–9	3

failure. Commercially available surfactant is extraordinarily useful to both treat and prevent RDS in susceptible patients. In addition, surfactant can improve gas exchange in preterm neonates who may not have RDS, but are stressed by sepsis, heart failure, or other systemic problems.[8] Delivered through an endotracheal tube, it can be used prophylactically in the very preterm newborn to prevent RDS, as well as treat neonates who have developed RDS.

In addition to the mechanical aspects of the pulmonary system, control of breathing has unique aspects in the neonatal period, especially in the preterm neonate. Neonates respond less to hypercapnia than the older child. In addition, neonates respond to hypoxia with a brief period of hyperventilation, followed by hypoventilation. The initial hyperventilatory response is prevented by hypothermia, further increasing risk of hypoventilatory response to hypoxia. Finally, a periodic breathing pattern is common in neonates, especially in preterm newborns, and can persist up to a year of age.

Persistent Pulmonary Hypertension of the Newborn

The pulmonary circulation is extremely sensitive to oxygen, pH, and nitric oxide, a variety of mediators such as adenosine and prostaglandins, and mechanical factors such as lung inflation. Figure 42-4 illustrates the correlation of the mean pulmonary artery pressure with age during the first 3 days of life. Hypoxia and acidosis, along with inflammatory mediators, may cause pulmonary artery pressure either to persist at a high level or, after initially decreasing, to increase to pathologic levels. The result is termed *persistent pulmonary hypertension of the newborn* (PPHN), sometimes referred to as *persistent fetal circulation*. PPHN occurs in term and preterm infants, usually caused by precipitating conditions such as severe birth asphyxia, meconium aspiration, sepsis, congenital diaphragmatic hernia (CDH), and maternal use of nonsteroidal anti-inflammatory drugs with in utero constriction of the ductus arteriosus, although it is often idiopathic. Other risk factors include maternal diabetes, maternal asthma, and cesarean delivery.[9]

Elevated pulmonary vascular resistance causes both the ductus arteriosus and foramen ovale to remain open, with subsequent right-to-left shunting which bypasses the pulmonary circulation. These changes result in profound hypoxia from right-to-left shunting and a normal or elevated $PaCO_2$. The hypoxemia is often noted to be out of proportion to the other presenting signs of respiratory and cardiovascular compromise. Treatment starts with correcting any predisposing disease (hypoglycemia, polycythemia) and improving poor tissue oxygenation. The response to therapy is often unpredictable. However, the goals are to achieve a PaO_2 of 60 to 100 mmHg and maintain normocapnia.[10]

In addition to standard mechanical ventilation, high-frequency ventilation, exogenous surfactant, inhaled nitric oxide (iNO), alkalinization, and extracorporeal membrane oxygenation (ECMO) have been used with varying degrees of success. In particular, the use of iNO is becoming more common and is indicated when the newborn expresses an oxygen index of 15 or more. However, iNO has not been shown to reduce the need for ECMO in neonates with congenital diaphragmatic hernia.[11,12] iNO remains the only United States Food and Drug Administration (FDA) approved medication for treatment of PPHN. Additional vasodilator therapy with prostacyclin (epoprostenol), phosphodiesterase inhibitors (sildenafil), and endothelin receptor antagonists (bosentan) has enjoyed varying levels of success beyond the neonatal period, into infancy. Success in treatment, and survival, varies directly with correction the underlying cause. Significant prognostic factors for PPHN are the ability of therapy to reduce pulmonary vascular resistance and the occurrence of associated complications, such as ischemic encephalopathy.

Maintenance of right ventricular function is paramount to survival in PPHN. Use of dobutamine in a normotensive patient may provide inotropy and decreased systemic vascular resistance, which could increase right-to-left shunting and offload the right ventricle.[13] Therapy is now often guided with the use of point-of-care echocardiography as its availability continues to grow and technology improves.[14] Preoperative assessment of the echocardiogram by the pediatric anesthesiologist may help predict what problems may be encountered in the operative environment. Also, the availability of very small transesophageal echocardiogram (TEE) probes make the possibility of real-time monitoring of cardiac function in the operating room a reality. However, insertion of even the smallest TEE probes requires close attention to ventilator parameters in very small (<3 kg) neonates.[15]

Meconium Aspiration

One of the most important pulmonary challenges in the newborn period is *meconium aspiration*. Interference with the normal maternal placental circulation in the third trimester may cause fetal hypoxia. Fetal hypoxia can result in an increase in the amount of muscle in the blood vessels of the distal respiratory units. Figure 42-5 illustrates the muscle increase found in blood vessels of a series of 11 infants who died of PPHN.[16] Chronic fetal hypoxia leads to the passage of meconium in utero. The fetus breathes in utero so the meconium mixed with amniotic fluid enters the pulmonary system. Meconium aspiration can be a marker of chronic fetal hypoxia in the third trimester. This condition is different from the meconium aspiration that occurs during delivery. Meconium at birth is thick and tenacious, and mechanically obstructs the tracheobronchial system. Meconium aspiration syndrome leads to varying degrees of respiratory failure, which can be fatal in spite of all treatment modalities.

Current recommendations for intubation and suctioning for newborns at delivery with frank meconium aspiration or meconium staining (approximately 10% of newborns) emphasize a conservative approach.[17] Routine oropharyngeal suctioning of

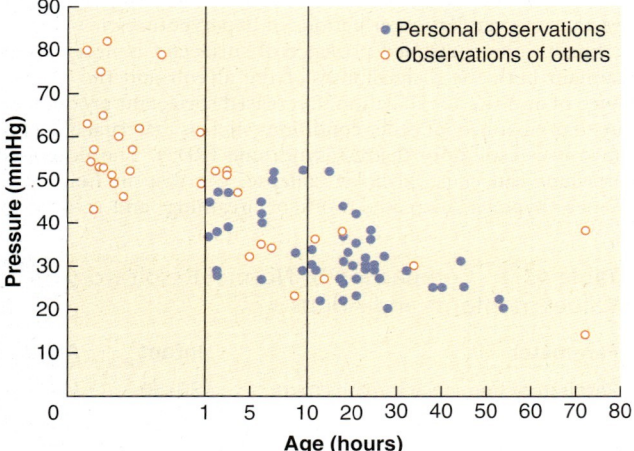

Figure 42-4 Correlation of mean pulmonary arterial pressure with age in 85 normal-term infants studied during the first 3 days of life. (Adapted from Emmanouilides GC, Moss AJ, Duffie ER, et al. Pulmonary arterial pressure changes in human newborn infants from birth to 3 days of age. *J Pediatr.* 1964;65:327.)

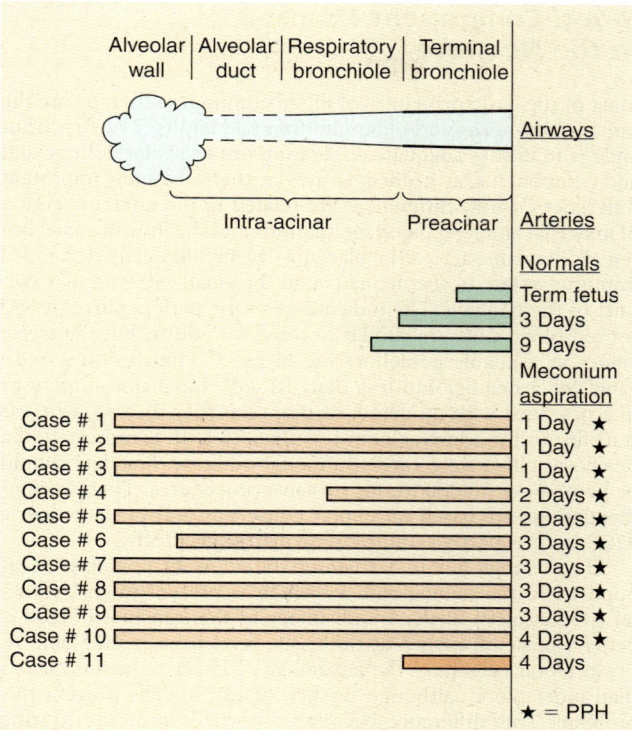

Figure 42-5 Diagram of muscle extension along pulmonary arterial branches (*shaded bars*). In the normal newborn, virtually no intra-acinar artery is muscular. In 9 of 10 infants with meconium aspiration and persistent pulmonary hypertension (PPH), muscle extended into the most peripheral arteries; the infant with meconium aspiration without PPH (case 11) had normal intra-acinar arteries. (Reprinted with permission from Murphy JD, Vawter GF, Reid LM. Pulmonary vascular disease in fetal meconium aspiration. *J Pediatr.* 1984;104:758.)

meconium is recommended immediately at the time of delivery, but tracheal intubation and suctioning should be performed selectively. If the newborn is vigorous and crying, no further suctioning is needed. If meconium is present and the newborn is depressed, the trachea should be intubated and meconium and other aspirated material suctioned from beneath the glottis. If meconium is retrieved and no bradycardia is present, reintubate and suction. If there is bradycardia, administer positive pressure ventilation and consider suctioning again later once the neonate is stabilized.

The Renal System

In utero, most of the fetal waste material is removed by the maternal placenta. In effect, the fetal kidneys are passive, receiving relatively little renal blood flow and having a low glomerular filtration rate (GFR).[8] There are four major reasons for the low renal blood flow and GFR: low systemic arterial pressure, high renal vascular resistance, low permeability of the glomerular capillaries, and the small size and number of glomeruli. In utero, the kidneys receive only about 3% of the cardiac output, whereas they will receive about 25% of cardiac output in adulthood. At birth, this changes dramatically. The systemic arterial pressure increases and the renal vascular resistance decreases, and the kidneys now receive a progressively increased part of the cardiac output. At birth, the GFR is low, but increases significantly in the first few days of life, doubles in the first 2 weeks, and reaches adult levels by about 2 years of age. The limited ability of the newborn's kidney to concentrate or dilute urine results from this low GFR and decreased tubular function. However, during the first 3 to 4 days, the circulatory changes increase renal blood flow and GFR, improving the neonate's ability to concentrate and dilute the urine. Part of the improvement in renal function is the establishment of gradients in the medullary interstitium that promotes resorption of sodium. This maturation continues in the normal, full-term neonate and the kidneys are approximately 60% mature by 1 month of age. Urine output is low in the first 24 hours, but increases to an expected level of at least 1 to 2 mL/kg/hr. Urine output, after the first day of life, of less than 1 mL/kg/hr should be considered indicative of either hypovolemia or decreased renal function from another cause.

Despite rapid maturation of renal function and increased capacity of the neonatal kidneys, they still have limitations. From an anesthetic standpoint, the half-life of medications excreted by means of glomerular filtration will be prolonged.[19] The relative inability to conserve water means that neonates, especially in the first week of life, tolerate fluid restriction poorly. In addition, the inability to excrete large amounts of water means the newborn tolerates fluid overload poorly. The newborn kidney is better able to conserve sodium than excrete sodium, making hypernatremia a risk if excess sodium is administered. However, because of the lack of tonicity in the medullary interstitium shortly after birth, there will be some obligate sodium loss in the first days of life. Sodium loss improves as the countercurrent multiplier is developed in the interstitium.

Fluid and Electrolyte Therapy in the Neonate

Total body water (TBW), which is usually described in terms of percent of body weight, varies by both age and gestational status. The highest TBW is found in the fetus, but decreases to about 80% of body weight for a term neonate at birth. Preterm neonates have a higher TBW than term infants, 85% of body weight, up to 90% of body weight in very low–birth-weight (VLBW) preterm neonates. TBW decreases during the first 6 months of life to about 60% of body weight, remaining this level through childhood.

TBW is distributed between two compartments, intracellular fluid (ICF) and extracellular fluid (ECF). The ECF volume is larger than the ICF volume in the fetus and newborn, usually in the 40% (ECF) and 20% (ICF) of body weight ranges. This ratio is the inverse of the ECF and ICF relationship observed in infants and children. There is a significant diuresis and natriuresis after birth that produces a decrease in the ECF volume. In addition, ICF volume increases because of the growth of cells in the body. The ECF and ICF volumes (20% and 40% of body weight) approach adult values per body weight by about 1 year of age. This dramatic shift is beneficial to the child, especially in increasing the mobility of reserves in the face of dehydration. Fluid can be easily mobilized from ICF volumes to replenish intravascular volume that is lost from fasting, fever, diarrhea, or other causes. Thus, an infant or child is better situated to maintain intravascular volume in these situations than a neonate.

The ECF is divided into the plasma and the interstitial fluid. The plasma water is usually about 5% of body weight and the related blood volume, assuming a hematocrit of 45%, is about 8% of body weight in infants and children. The water content is slightly higher in neonates and may approach 10% of body weight in preterm neonates. The interstitial fluid, usually about 15% of body weight, can demonstrate large increases in disease states such as liver failure, heart failure, renal failure, and other causes fluid retention, such as pleural effusions or ascites. Any condition that decreases oncotic pressure, such as loss of albumin in liver failure, promotes the loss of fluid into the interstitial fluid. On the other hand, raised hydrostatic pressures, such as seen in heart failure, can result in fluid leaving the plasma and accumulating in the interstitial space. Conditions that result in translocation of fluid from the plasma to the interstitial spaces, whether because of decreased oncotic pressure or increased hydrostatic pressure, are of significant consequence to the neonate. Loss of fluid from the plasma volume compromises the intravascular volume, potentially decreasing the perfusion of vital organs and systems.

The blood volume in the normal full-term newborn is approximately 90 mL/kg and approximately 100 mL/kg in preterm, VLBW, or critically ill newborns. However, these estimates of intravascular volumes are variable between studies. Approximately half of the intravascular volume in a newborn is plasma volume. For all practical purposes, electrolyte values in the neonatal period are the same as in the child and adult with the exception of potassium, which can be about 1 to 2 mmol/L higher than average for the first 2 days of life.[20]

Maintenance fluid requirements increase during the first days of life. They have been estimated to be 60, 75, 90, 105, 120, 135, and 150 mL/kg/24 hr for the first 7 days of life, respectively. For the rest of the neonatal period, a maintenance rate of 150 mL/kg/24 hr is appropriate.[21]

The appropriate type of maintenance fluid depends on several issues. Because of ongoing sodium loss secondary to the inability of the neonatal distal tubule to respond fully to aldosterone, intravenous fluids in the neonate must contain some sodium. Most operations on neonates involve loss of blood and ECF, which must be replaced with a fluid of similar electrolyte content (i.e., a near-isotonic solution such as lactated Ringer or Plasma-Lyte). Hypotonic solutions should not be used to replace these losses because they can cause significant hyponatremia. Thus, if the neonate is already stable on a maintenance solution, it is reasonable to continue this maintenance at a constant rate, adding balanced salt solution, colloid, or blood products as needed to offset ongoing surgical or insensible losses.

The other issues for fluid choice in the neonate center on appropriate glucose administration. In most cases, maintenance fluids containing 10% glucose and 0.2% saline with 20 mmol/L of potassium are reasonable in the first 48 hours of life. Beyond that time period, full-term infants may do well with 5% glucose instead of 10%, although preterm infants will often require the higher glucose load longer. Newborns of diabetic mothers, those who are small for gestational age, and those who have had continuous glucose infusions stopped have particular problems with hypoglycemia. These infants need to have their blood glucose values monitored. Neonates who are scheduled for surgery and have been receiving intravenous (parenteral) nutrition or supplementary glucose must continue to receive that fluid during surgery or must have their glucose levels monitored because of concerns of hypoglycemia. There is little consensus on the issue of what constitutes hypoglycemia.[22]

The concern about hypoglycemia must be balanced against the potential augmentation of ischemic injury from iatrogenic hyperglycemia. Interestingly, there are observational reports examining neonates undergoing cardiac surgery in which high glucose concentrations during or after the surgery were not associated with worse neurodevelopmental outcomes.[23] This finding supports the contention that avoiding hypoglycemia may be preferable to restricting glucose in newborns and risking hypoglycemia, at least in those having cardiac surgery.

Blood Component Therapy in the Neonate

Most of the basic principles of blood component therapy are the same in newborns and older children and adults. The first principle is to ensure adequate circulating intravascular volume and add components, as needed. However, there are a few important differences. These differences are related to the interconnection of maternal and fetal blood circulations and the flow of some, but not all elements, across the placenta, the incompletely developed immune system of the neonate, and the small intravascular volume of the neonate. The indications in the perioperative period for red blood cells are similar to those for adults, but the target values in available guidelines are higher.[24] Transfusion is indicated for a hemoglobin less than 10 g/dL for major surgery or in a newborn with moderate cardiopulmonary disease, whereas transfusion for a hemoglobin less than 13 g/dL is indicated in a newborn with severe cardiopulmonary disease. Platelets should be kept above 50,000/μL for invasive procedures. These recommendations are based on expert consensus and older pediatric data, not prospective studies in neonates specifically.

The hemoglobin in transfused blood is hemoglobin A, as opposed to the hemoglobin F, which is present in the neonatal circulation at birth. An advantage of the transfused blood is better release of oxygen at the tissue level from hemoglobin A. Fresh blood cells have the advantage of lower potassium levels than older blood, although washed or frozen cells prevent this problem. This difference becomes especially important during rapid, massive transfusion. Transfusion-associated graft-versus-host disease is a rare but potentially deadly complication of red blood cell transfusion. Transfused lymphocytes in the donor blood attack the recipient bone marrow and other tissues, causing fever, pancytopenia, diarrhea, and hepatitis. To prevent this, gamma irradiation of cellular blood components is used to destroy lymphocytes and prevent transfusion-associated graft-versus-host disease. Therefore, irradiated blood is routinely used for transfusion of preterm infants and, in many centers, for all neonates and infants under 6 months of age. Leukocyte reduction by filtration is also used to reduce cytomegalic virus transmission, decrease risk of alloimmunization, and decrease febrile hemolytic transfusion reactions. There is decrease in retinopathy of prematurity (ROP), bronchopulmonary dyplasia, and length of hospital stay when leukocyte reduction is used for transfusions in premature neonates.[25] Finally, because there is very weak expression of the ABO antigens at birth, ABO typing, Rh typing, and an initial antibody screen are commonly done prior to transfusion, although crossmatching is not always needed.

The Hepatic System

The functional capacity of the liver is immature in the newborn, especially synthetic and metabolic functions. Although most enzyme systems for both normal function and drug metabolism are present at birth, the systems have not yet been induced.[26] In utero, the maternal circulation and metabolism were responsible for the majority of drug elimination. As the newborn develops, the different hepatic metabolic pathways mature at different rates. Conjugation by sulfation and acetylation are relatively well developed in the newborn, with conjugation with glutathione and glucuronidation less well developed.[27] Some of these pathways do not achieve adult levels of activity until after 1 year of age.[28] Because of this immaturity, some drugs that undergo hepatic biotransformation, such as morphine, have prolonged elimination half-lives in newborns. Other drugs, such as lidocaine, do not undergo prolonged elimination in the newborn. In some drugs, such as caffeine, the lack of hepatic metabolism of the drug is balanced by excretion of an increased amount of unchanged drug through the kidney. Up to 85% of unmetabolized caffeine may be found in the urine in the newborn, compared with 1% in the adult.[29]

Finally, decreased metabolism of a drug may actually increase its safety profile. Acetaminophen undergoes less biotransformation by the cytochrome P450 system in the newborn, producing less reactive metabolites that are toxic. Paradoxically, neonates can tolerate dosages of acetaminophen that would be hepatotoxic in adults.[30] Synthetic function of the liver is also altered in the neonatal period. Levels of albumin and other proteins necessary for binding of drugs are low in term newborns (and are even lower in preterm infants) and impacts the ability to bind drugs, producing greater levels of free drug. This phenomenon is especially true for the binding of alkaline drugs that bind to α-1-acid glycoprotein, such as synthetic opioids and local anesthetics. The ability to bind to existing albumin may also be altered by hyperbilirubinemia for some medications. The need for exogenous vitamin K in the newborn is a consequence of this decreased ability. Because of decreased synthetic function, neonatal hepatic glycogen stores are low, especially in the preterm infant, increasing the risk of hypoglycemia in response to stress.

Anatomy of the Neonatal Airway

4 The anatomic and maturational factors unique to the neonatal airway are important to understand in order to effectively manage the airway (Fig. 42-6). Although traditional teaching is that all neonates, especially preterm infants, are *obligate* nasal breathers, the majority of neonates are actually *preferential* nose breathers.[31] Anything that obstructs the nares can compromise the neonate's ability to breathe.[32] For this reason, bilateral choanal atresia of the nasopharynx can be a life-threatening surgical condition for the neonate. The airway needs to be secured or the atresia opened to ensure adequate ventilation. The large tongue occupies relatively more space in the infant's oropharynx, promoting both soft tissue obstruction of the upper airway and increasing the difficulty of direct laryngoscopic examination and intubation of the infant's trachea. In the normal adult, the glottis is at the level of C5–C6. In the full-term infant, the glottis is at the level of C4, and in the premature infant, it is at the level of C3. The combination of a large tongue and a relatively cephalad glottis means that on laryngoscopic examination it is more difficult to establish a direct line of vision between the mouth and the larynx; there is relatively more tissue in a smaller distance. Therefore, the infant's larynx appears to be *anterior*, although the more anatomically accurate description is *cephalad*. The epiglottis is omega- or tubular-shaped, with a stubby base and thick, bulky aryepiglottic folds, making it difficult to elevate with a laryngoscope blade. Because the tip of the epiglottis lies at C1, its close apposition with the soft palate allows the newborn to simultaneously suckle and breathe, which contributes to the *preferential* nasal breathing found in the neonate. The vocal cords are anterior-slanting, making visualization more challenging. The slanting also occasionally provides some obstruction to the passage of the endotracheal tube, which is especially true with either nasal or "blind" intubation attempts because the bevel of the tube may hang up in the anterior commissure of the angulated vocal cords instead of easily passing into the subglottic larynx.

The neonatal subglottic area is funnel-shaped, unlike the infant, child, or adult airway (Fig. 42-7). In adults, the narrowest aspect of the upper airway is at the vocal cords, but in the neonate there is further narrowing ending at the level of the cricoid ring, the first complete cartilaginous ring. Although studies have challenged the funnel shape in infants and children, there has been no study further clarifying this relationship in neonates.[33,34] Because this narrowing is susceptible to trauma from intubation or too large an endotracheal tube, uncuffed tubes have traditionally been used in the neonatal period, although cuffed tubes are increasingly popular. The use of newer cuffed, small volume, high resistance endotracheal tubes have been demonstrated to provide an adequate airway with marginal changes to the diameter of the airway leading most practitioners to now use a cuffed tube, in even neonates and young infants.[35] Though cuffed endotracheal tubes may be gaining ground in use, it does not appear that they have supplanted the use of uncuffed endotracheal tubes in neonates.[36] Although the glottic opening may actually be the smallest measured point in the pediatric airway, it is more distensible than the cricoid ring, the first complete cartilaginous

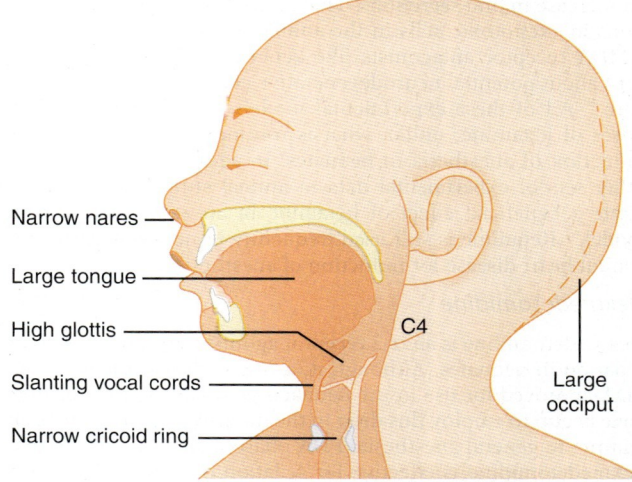

Figure 42-6 Complicating anatomic factors in infants. (Adapted from Smith RM. *Smith's Anesthesia for Infants and Children*. 4th ed. St Louis: Mosby; 1980:16.)

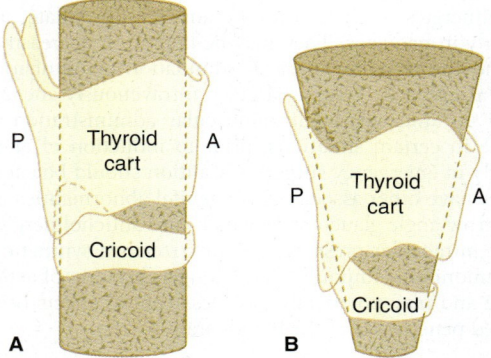

Figure 42-7 Configuration of the adult (**A**) versus the infant (**B**) larynx. The adult larynx has a cylindrical shape. The infant larynx is funnel-shaped because of the narrow, undeveloped cricoid cartilage. A, Anterior; P, Posterior. (Adapted from The pediatric airway, In: Ryan JF, Coté CJ, Todres ID, eds. *A Practice of Anesthesia for Infants and Children*. 2nd ed. Orlando, FL: Grune & Stratton; 1992:61.)

ring in the airway, thus, the cricoid ring is funtionally the smallest cross-sectional area in the airway. An endotracheal tube that passes easily through the glottic opening may not advance beyond the less distensible cricoid ring.

Finally, the infant has a large occiput so the head flexes forward onto the chest when the infant is lying supine with his or her head in the midline. Further flexion of the neck can cause obstruction. Extreme extension can also obstruct the airway, so a midposition of the head with slight extension is preferred for airway maintenance. Rarely, this may require placing a small roll at the base of the neck and shoulders.

Anesthetic Drugs in Neonates

[5] The pharmacokinetics of drugs in neonates are different than in older children and adults. Factors affecting the metabolism of drugs in neonates include a larger volume of distribution, decreased protein binding, decreased body fat percentage, and immature renal and hepatic function. The following physiologic changes alter pharmacokinetics and pharmacodynamics in neonates:

- Volume of distribution. Total body water represents a greater proportion of body weight in premature and full-term neonates, which increases the necessary dose for medications that are water-soluble.
- Protein binding. Neonates have decreased protein and hence have a decrease in protein binding of most drugs. This leads to increased free drug levels, which leads to increased activity and toxicity of drugs that are predominantly protein bound.
- Fat content. Neonates have a decreased amount of fat and muscle mass, which leads to greater levels of drugs that are primarily redistributed to muscle and fat. Decreased renal and hepatic function predisposes neonates to increased blood levels from normal doses that are used for induction and maintenance of anesthesia.

Neurotoxicity of anesthetic agents is a topic that has received much attention in the literature as well as in popular media. However, most surgical procedures in the neonatal period are not elective. There is a detailed discussion of neurotoxicity of anesthetic agents presented in Chapter 43.

Intravenous Agents

Anticholinergics

Anticholinergics, such as atropine and glycopyrrolate, are used frequently in neonates. They may be helpful in decreasing secretions and the response to vagal stimulation on intubation. The dose of atropine is 10 μg/kg if given intravenously and 20 μg/kg if given intramuscularly. Intramuscular administration may be desirable in certain situations, prior to induction of anesthesia, especially in emergency surgeries. Caution should be exercised if neonates have other associated congenital abnormalities, particularly narrow angle glaucoma in which case anticholinergics could increase intraocular pressure. Glycopyrrolate, a synthetic quaternary ammonium compound, has a longer duration of action than atropine and may potentially have less central effects because of decreased penetration of the blood–brain barrier.

Midazolam

Midazolam is a water-soluble benzodiazepine that can be used for premedication in infants prior to surgery. Clearance of midazolam is lower in neonates and premature infants, and hence caution has to be exercised with the amount of midazolam used. If combined with opioids, intravenous midazolam can cause severe hypotension. A common modality for midazolam administration in neonatal intensive care units is by continuous infusion. If a patient is receiving midazolam infusion, care should be taken to avoid large doses of opioids to prevent hypotension.

Sedative/Hypnotics

The common sedative/hypnotics used in neonates include propofol, thiopental, and ketamine.

Thiopental

Because of an ongoing shortage of thiopental in North America, it is now rarely used there. Because of the large volume of distribution in neonates, it may be necessary to use large doses of thiopental for induction of anesthesia. However, because of its reduced clearance, the effect may last longer than anticipated. Thiopental can cause hypotension in neonates who are volume depleted, especially in infants presenting for emergency surgery. It should be avoided in neonates with congenital heart disease because of its effect on myocardial function, leading to hypotension. A dose of 2 to 4 mg/kg is usually well tolerated by most neonates for induction of anesthesia. When compared with intubation without any hypnotic, the use of intravenous thiopental demonstrated adequate maintenance of heart rate and blood pressure.[37]

Propofol

Propofol, a phenol derivative sedative/hypnotic, is a commonly used induction agent in infants and children. In a randomized trial comparing intravenous propofol with atropine, succinylcholine, and morphine, it was noted that propofol maintained adequate hemodynamics in neonates.[38] There is variability in elimination of propofol in neonates and preterm infants with longer elimination times.[39] Hence, while using propofol, it is important to reduce the dose to ensure early wake up and extubation. Propofol is the most commonly used intravenous induction agent in the United States.

Ketamine

Ketamine, an N-methyl-D-aspartic acid (NMDA) antagonist, is used for induction of anesthesia in neonates who may have cardiovascular instability. An induction dose of 2 mg/kg intravenously with a higher dose of 4 to 7 mg/kg is used intramuscularly. Although it produces hemodynamic stability, it can cause an increase in oral secretions. There have been significant alterations in excitotoxic cells in the animal model when exposed to NMDA receptor antagonists like ketamine with resultant concern about potential neurodegenerative changes with their exposure.[40] All of these experimental models were using very high doses of ketamine, unlike what is routinely recommended for induction of anesthesia in neonates. In addition, there are also other sets of experimental data in animal studies that demonstrate a beneficial effect of ketamine in an experimental pain model.[41] Ketamine is still used frequently in neonates with congenital heart disease for induction of anesthesia.

Dexmedetomidine

Dexmedetomidine is an α-2 receptor agonist that can be used for sedation in neonates. Although it, as many drugs, has not been FDA-approved for use in the neonatal population, some centers have begun to employ this drug in the intensive care unit or as an adjunct to general anesthesia. FDA phase 2/3 trials indicate that dexmedetomidine is effective for sedation of term and preterm neonates undergoing mechanical ventilation, but preterm neonates exhibited decreased plasma clearance and increased elimination half-life of the drug. A study of 127 infants and neonates revealed that dexmedetomidine is likely to be safe in this patient population at doses similar to those used in adult intensive care for sedation, 0.2 to 0.6 μg/kg/hr.[42] Blood pressure and heart rate should be monitored as drop in systolic blood pressure and episodes of bradycardia may be noted. Dexmedetomidine may reduce required doses of midazolam and fentanyl needed to achieve the same level of sedation. Animal studies suggest that dexmedetomidine may be less neurotoxic than other traditionally used agents, such as midazolam.[43] Although much work remains to be done with this drug in the neonatal population, it is emerging as a viable sedative in neonates.

Opioids

Opioids are used extensively in the management of anesthesia in neonates. The advantage of using opioids is their ability to maintain cardiovascular stability during major surgery. The common opioids used in neonates include fentanyl, morphine, and remifentanil. Infants who are on long-term doses of opioids may develop dependence and have to be placed on methadone, a longer-acting opioid.[44]

Fentanyl

This synthetic opioid is commonly used for sedation in the neonate in the intensive care unit as well as in the operating room. A dose of 2 to 4 μg/kg/hr can maintain hemodynamic stability in these infants during surgery. The pharmacokinetics of fentanyl have been well studied in newborns.[45] The use of fentanyl in association with benzodiazepines may lead to hypotension and hemodynamic instability. Caution must be exercised when the combination is administered during the perioperative period. Fentanyl may result in respiratory depression even with small doses. Continuous infusions may predispose to respiratory depression more frequently than bolus doses.[46] Chest wall rigidity and glottic rigidity have been described with fentanyl.[47] Small doses, as little as 1 to 2 μg/kg, can result in significant chest wall rigidity, leading to desaturation and need for mechanical ventilation. There is no significant maturational change in the brain associated with fentanyl, compared with morphine. Hence, the sensitivity to fentanyl will not significantly change as the infant matures significantly. Fentanyl still continues to be the mainstay in newborns for sedation and analgesia.

Morphine

The kinetics of morphine have been studied in newborns. Premature babies have been shown to have decreased clearance. Morphine clearance (range, 0.8 to 6.5 mL/min/kg) directly correlates with gestational age ($r = 0.60$; $p < 0.01$) and birth weight ($r = 0.55$; $p < 0.01$).[48] Because of decreased clearance, dosing in neonates, especially premature infants, should occur on a 4- to 6-hour basis to allow for more predictable clearance of the drug.[49] Morphine is used frequently in the intensive care unit for postoperative pain control. Morphine infusions in the perioperative period have resulted in minor prolongation of postoperative ventilation. However, increased incidence of apnea or hypotension was not observed in neonates despite prolonged morphine infusions after successful extubation.[50]

Morphine is metabolized to morphine-3-glucuronide and morphine-6-glucuronide. Morphine-6-glucuronide predisposes to respiratory depression. The sensitivity to morphine-6-glucuronide increases with age because of increased maturation of the neuronal receptors.[51] A minority of infants who are scheduled for surgery may have been on ECMO. Kinetics of morphine have been carefully studied in neonates undergoing ECMO and do not show significant variability.[52]

Remifentanil

Remifentanil is an ultra short-acting opioid that is metabolized by nonspecific esterases in plasma and tissues and has a half-life of less than 10 minutes. The pharmacokinetics of remifentanil in neonates are similar to that of older children.[53] Remifentanil can be used for maintenance of anesthesia with avoidance of volatile anesthetic agents. The use of remifentanil infusion facilitated tracheal extubation in infants in a randomized trial when compared with volatile agents.[54]

Methadone

Methadone is a long-acting opioid that is used in neonates and infants in neonatal intensive care units, particularly when withdrawal from opioids is suspected. The pharmacokinetics of methadone are being studied in neonates; however, published data is not available. The FDA "black box" warning against the use of methadone in patients with prolonged QT intervals on their electrocardiogram is a valid concern and infants on long-term methadone use should be carefully monitored with serial ECGs. However, it is used frequently in managing opioid tolerance without significant complication.[44]

Neuromuscular Blocking Agents

Neuromuscular blocking agents (NMBAs) are frequently used during neonatal anesthesia to facilitate tracheal intubation, assist with controlled ventilation, relax abdominal musculature, and ensure immobility. Factors that influence the choice of agent include the time of onset, duration of action, cardiovascular effects, drug availability, and mechanism of clearance/elimination.

Succinylcholine

Succinylcholine, the only depolarizing muscle relaxant available, has the most rapid onset time of all the NMBAs. Neonates and infants have a larger ECF volume, leading to a larger volume of distribution and an increased dose requirement compared with children and adults. Thus, the recommended intravenous dose of succinylcholine for neonates and infants is 3 mg/kg, compared with 2 mg/kg in children, with an onset time of 30 to 45 seconds and duration of 5 to 10 minutes. The recommended intramuscular dose of succinylcholine is 4 mg/kg, with an onset time of 3 to 4 minutes and duration of approximately 20 minutes. Caution should be exercised when administering a second dose of succinylcholine because this can lead to vagally mediated bradycardia or sinus arrest. Pretreatment with atropine is recommended.[55]

The more recent succinylcholine controversy has called into question the use of succinylcholine in boys younger than 8 years. The reports of hyperkalemia with cardiac arrest in such children with unrecognized muscular dystrophy have led some clinicians to take the position that succinylcholine should not be used routinely for this group of patients. The occurrence of this problem is somewhere in the range of 1 in 250,000 anesthetics, with a mortality rate of 50%. Although a concern in young children, it is not a problem in the neonatal period. Succinylcholine is still recommended in rapid-sequence situations, potential difficult airway, or if there are airway emergencies with progressive desaturation. When it is evident that a neonatal airway is obstructed by laryngospasm or other reason and no progress is made in ventilation, intramuscular or intravenous succinylcholine should be administered. Hyperkalemia can be recognized by peaked T waves. However, the clinician may not see this particular electrocardiographic change because it occurs 2 to 3 minutes after drug administration, when the anesthesiologist is tending to the airway. The hyperkalemia interferes with cardiac conduction, leading to a bradycardia and, if severe enough, cardiac arrest. The drug of first choice is intravenous calcium chloride, 10 mg/kg. The use of sodium bicarbonate, 1 mEq/kg, to treat any metabolic acidosis that may occur with arrest is also believed to be useful because alkalosis decreases hyperkalemia. At the same time, the patient should be hyperventilated to reduce $PaCO_2$, thereby inducing respiratory alkalosis. If there is refractory hypotension, one option is to administer epinephrine 5 to 10 μg/kg. One of the actions of epinephrine is to stimulate the sodium–potassium pump and cause potassium to re-enter the cell, thereby reducing the serum level. If there is no response at this dose level, it should be increased incrementally until there is a response. Finally, magnesium has been described as a treatment for hyperkalemia, because it also antagonizes the effects of hyperkalemia, as does calcium. However, it is typically only employed for this purpose in the setting of digoxin toxicity.

Nondepolarizing Agents

The neonate's neuromuscular junction is more sensitive to nondepolarizing muscle relaxants, and the neonate has a larger volume of distribution because of a large ECF volume. These two effects tend to balance each other; therefore, the dose of a nondepolarizing muscle relaxant for an infant is similar to that for a child on an mg/kg basis. Ongoing organ maturation has a tremendous impact on the metabolism and clearance of the nondepolarizing agents. As a result, there is considerable variability and unpredictability in the duration of action of these agents in the neonatal period. Dosing should be titrated to effect and, when possible, guided by monitoring neuromuscular function with a nerve stimulator. However, reliable twitch monitoring may be challenging in this age group.

Intermediate Nondepolarizing Agents

Rocuronium

Rocuronium appears to be the drug of choice among the intermediate-acting, nondepolarizing muscle relaxants for neonates. The intubating dose of rocuronium is 0.6 mg/kg. The length of action of rocuronium in the neonate is similar to that in the older infant or child following an equipotent dose.[56] Smaller doses (0.45 mg/kg) have been demonstrated to provide adequate relaxation and predictable recovery in newborn infants. However, if a larger dose of rocuronium, 1 to 1.2 mg/kg, is administered to avoid using succinylcholine during a rapid-sequence induction, then rocuronium will be a relatively long-acting muscle relaxant. Rocuronium is metabolized by the liver; however, there are no active metabolites of rocuronium which is unlike vecuronium. Rocuronium has mild vagolytic properties and may slightly increase heart rate.

Vecuronium

Although vecuronium is considered an intermediate-acting muscle relaxant in children and adults, in infants younger than 1 year it is considered to be a long-acting muscle relaxant. The duration of action of vecuronium is approximately twice that observed in children because of liver immaturity. Vecuronium undergoes primarily hepatic metabolism with production of active metabolites that are dependent on renal excretion. The recommended dose of vecuronium is 0.1 to 0.15 mg/kg, with an onset time of 90 seconds and duration of action of 60 to 90 minutes in the neonate. Even with increased doses, vecuronium has no effect on the cardiovascular system.

Pancuronium

Pancuronium is a long-acting NMBA with a pharmacokinetic profile similar to vecuronium. The recommended dose of 0.1 to 0.15 mg/kg has an onset time of 120 seconds and duration of 60 to 75 minutes. Unlike vecuronium, however, pancuronium primarily undergoes renal excretion. Pancuronium has vagolytic and sympathomimetic actions that cause tachycardia and an increase in blood pressure.[57] In a relatively normal neonate with a normal blood pressure and normal blood volume, the use of pancuronium may result in hypertension, which has the potential to increase blood loss and increase the risk of hemorrhage in the extremely premature neonate. The risk for prolonged neuromuscular blockade in neonates, especially with altered renal function, makes pancuronium less desirable in neonates and infants undergoing minor outpatient surgical procedures. The use of pancuronium for prolonged durations especially in the intensive care units can lead to muscle weakness. Prolonged use has also been associated with sensorineural hearing loss in infants.[58]

Cis-atracurium

Cis-atracurium is an intermediate-acting NMBA of the bisbenzyltetrahydroisoquinolinium class. The unique aspect of this agent within its class is a lack of histamine release. The most important fact about this drug is its degradation through Hoffman elimination, which is an organ-independent chemodegradative mechanism. Because its elimination is not kidney or liver dependent, it offers a reliable recovery time even in neonates. In fact, when used for prolonged infusion in infants and neonates in intensive care, it offers a more reliable recovery time than vecuronium.[59] One theoretical concern with administration of cis-atracurium is the accumulation of one metabolite, laudanosine, which can decrease the seizure threshold. However, this does not seem to be relevant at clinical doses of cis-atracurium.[60] The typical dose is 0.15 to 0.2 mg/kg, has an onset time of 150 seconds, and a half-life of approximately 25 minutes.

Reversal Agents

The unpredictable nature of the NMBAs in the neonatal population, as well as the inability to accurately assess neuromuscular function in many situations, necessitates reversal of all nondepolarizing NMBA in neonates. The two commonly used reversal agents are edrophonium and neostigmine. Edrophonium in a dose of 1 mg/kg achieves a 90% reversal of a neuromuscular block in 2 minutes, whereas neostigmine in a dose of 0.07 mg/kg requires 10 minutes for a 90% reversal of neuromuscular block. This difference in time to peak effect allows the anesthesiologist to decide which agent is needed. Anticholinergic drugs like atropine or glycopyrrolate are coadministered to decrease the incidence of bradycardia. Neostigmine is the most common agent used for reversal of nondepolarizing muscle relaxants in neonates. The advantages of edrophonium over neostigmine are a more rapid reversal and fewer muscarinic side effects, but edrophonium is still less commonly used in clinical practice due to its shorter duration of action. Neostigmine administered without an anticholinergic is the most common drug error leading to perioperative cardiac arrest in the pediatric population.[61]

Volatile Agents

Volatile agents are used for maintenance of anesthesia in the neonatal period. Although halothane was the most commonly used volatile agent for many years and had a reasonable safety profile, the introduction of sevoflurane has clearly made a difference to the use of volatile agents in neonates. Isoflurane is used for maintenance of anesthesia for longer surgical procedures and desflurane may be desirable for rapid awakening in certain cases. Each of these agents will be discussed here.

Halothane

Halothane is still commonly used in developing countries and in veterinary medicine, although it is not currently used in the United States nor is it frequently used in other developed countries. Its long history for induction of anesthesia and its ease of use still make it a desirable agent in children. Halothane has a weak muscle relaxant property, facilitating induction and intubation without the use of a muscle relaxant. Halothane is a potent bronchodilator and may reduce the airway reflexes associated with intubation. The use of high doses of halothane for procedures including bronchoscopic evaluation of the airway may lead to significant myocardial depression. Infants less than 8 weeks old and with a history of RDS with longer period of preoperative fasting are prone to hypotension. Halothane also sensitizes the myocardium to cardiac dysrhythmias. Animal experiments demonstrate the increased sensitivity to epinephrine with halothane when compared with isoflurane or sevoflurane. Hence, when concurrent exogenous catecholamines are administered (including epinephrine in local anesthetic solution), careful attention to the maximum dose should be carefully monitored.

Isoflurane

Isoflurane has become a common maintenance volatile agent in neonates and infants. Its pungent odor does not allow its use for mask induction. Isoflurane has a greater effect in potentiation of muscle relaxation and hence plays an important role as a maintenance anesthetic. It is important to remember that the dose of muscle relaxants should be reduced when isoflurane anesthesia is used because of potentiation. The dose of rocuronium bromide may have to be reduced to 0.45 mg/kg compared with a normal maintenance dose of 0.6 mg/kg.[56] Isoflurane has less myocardial depression when compared with halothane in neonates.[62]

Sevoflurane

This volatile agent offers an advantage for rapid induction and rapid awakening. It has a less pungent smell than isoflurane, making it ideal for mask induction. Its pharmacodynamics have been studied in neonates and children with a reasonable safety profile.[63] In children with congenital cardiac disease, it has been shown to produce fewer hemodynamic changes when compared with isoflurane.[64] Although it produces less myocardial depression, it has a greater effect on respiratory depression compared with halothane. Minute ventilation and respiratory frequency were significantly lower during sevoflurane than halothane anesthesia (4.5 compared with 5.4 L/m^2/min, and 37.5 compared with 46.7 breaths per minute, respectively, $p < 0.05$). There was also significantly less thoracoabdominal asynchrony during sevoflurane anesthesia.[65]

Desflurane

Desflurane was touted to be the best volatile agent in children because of its partition coefficient being close to that of nitrous oxide, thereby allowing a rapid uptake. However, the pungent nature of the drug has made it nearly impossible to use for inhalation induction of anesthesia. When compared with sevoflurane, infants who were preterm were noted to wake up sooner with desflurane, but there were no reductions in postoperative respiratory events.[66] 1 MAC of desflurane in a neonate is estimated to be 9.2% end-tidal.[67] Pungency increasing the risk of laryngospasm and bronchospasm make this volatile agent less attractive in neonates, but its rapid elimination and awakening have secured its place in regular clinical use. In an animal model using neonatal mice, mice exposed to desflurane had greater neuroapoptosis than mice exposed to equipotent doses of isoflurane or sevoflurane.[68]

Local Anesthetics

Local anesthetic solutions are represented by two main classes, the amino-amides (amides) and the amino-esters (esters). The main difference between the two classes is that the amides undergo enzymatic degradation by the liver and the esters are hydrolyzed by plasma cholinesterases.

Amides

These are commonly used local anesthetic solutions in neonates and infants. Local anesthetics used in common clinical practice belonging to this class include lidocaine, bupivacaine, ropivacaine, and levobupivacaine. The main characteristics differentiating these drugs are their speed of onset, duration of action, and potential for cardiac toxicity. The ability of neonatal liver enzymes to metabolize and their ability to oxidize and reduce these drugs are decreased when compared with adults.[69] At approximately 3 months of age, the conjugation of these drugs in the liver reaches adult levels. Older children can also achieve higher levels of local anesthetic solution than adults because of alteration in pharmacokinetics of the drugs.

Local anesthetic solution levels have been shown to be higher in children undergoing intercostal nerve blocks compared with adults.[70] After caudal administration of local anesthetics, peak plasma level is obtained in children and adults in approximately 30 minutes.[71] The steady-state volume of distribution (Vd_{ss}) for amides is increased in children compared with adults, although clearance (CL) is similar.[71] Elimination half-life ($t_{1/2}$) is related to the volume of distribution and clearance as follows: $t_{1/2} = (0.693 \times Vd_{ss})/CL$. This results in a larger Vd_{ss} and prolongation of the elimination half-life, especially if a continuous infusion is used. Also, due to decreased circulating α-1-acid glycoprotein levels in neonates, more free (active) local anesthetic circulates in the bloodstream.

The systemic absorption of local anesthetics is often based on the site of injection. On a decreasing scale, the incidence of complications with local anesthetic solution injections decreases, with the highest concentrations seen in the intercostal area followed by the caudal space, the epidural space, and peripheral nerve blocks. With newer techniques in regional anesthesia, including ultrasound guidance, the volume and dose of local anesthetic solution can be significantly reduced.[72]

Bupivacaine. Bupivacaine is one of the most commonly used local anesthetic solutions in infants and children. The pharmacokinetics and the pharmacodynamics have been well studied in infants and children. The concentration of the local anesthetic solution used depends on the site of injection, the desired density of blockade (motor and sensory), and the potential for cardiovascular and neurotoxicity. The concomitant use of other local anesthetics including infiltration anesthesia must be taken into account before a total volume of local anesthetic solution is determined. This is especially true in neonatal surgery in which large quantities of local anesthetic solution can sometimes be injected for skin infiltration. If upper safe limits are likely to be approached, it is reasonable to avoid local anesthetic solution for infiltration and use a dilute epinephrine solution instead for vasoconstriction. The preferred concentration for peripheral nerve blockade is 0.25% bupivacaine or 0.2% ropivacaine, and the preferred concentration for single dose caudal is 0.25% or 0.125% solution of bupivacaine or 0.2% ropivacaine. When a continuous infusion is desired, a 0.1% or 0.125% solution of bupivacaine is preferred. In premature infants and in infants weighing under 1 kg, we prefer using 0.0625% bupivacaine, or intermittent bolus dosing every 12 hours. Although clear guidelines do not exist for local anesthetic solutions, a rough rule of thumb is to use 0.2 mg/kg/hr for continuous infusions of bupivacaine and 2 mg/kg for bolus doses.[73]

Metabolism and Toxicity. Bupivacaine in the circulation is heavily bound to α-1-acid glycoprotein. Levels of this circulating protein are lower in the neonatal period.[74] Bupivacaine is a racemic mixture of the levo and dextro enantiomers. Although the levo enantiomer is the active form that provides the clinical effect of the local anesthetic solution, the dextro enantiomer is responsible for the adverse effects related to local anesthesia, including cardiac toxicity and neurotoxicity.

The major adverse effect of bupivacaine is toxicity related to the cardiovascular and the CNS systems. Local anesthetics have the ability to cross the blood–brain barrier and can cause alterations in the CNS functions. Continuous infusions in neonates can predispose them to CNS toxicity sooner than older infants.[75] In pediatric patients, the incidence of cardiac toxicity occurs sooner than neurotoxicity,[75] which may be partly because children may be anesthetized and devastating neurotoxicity may not be noticed until significant cardiac toxicity is seen. Manifestation of bupivacaine toxicity may also be affected by the concomitant use of volatile agents for general anesthesia.

Dosage. Bupivacaine can be used for most peripheral nerve blocks as well as for epidural and caudal infusions in infants and children. The maximum dosage suggested for bolus injections in the caudal space or epidural space for older children is 4 mg/kg and 2 mg/kg for neonates and infants.[73] Dosage recommendations for continuous infusions is 0.4 mg/kg/hr in older children and 0.2 mg/kg/hr in neonates and infants.[26] The concentration of the solution used for peripheral nerve blocks is usually 0.25%, bearing in mind the ceiling limit for maximum dosage. Higher concentration such as 0.375% may be necessary for surgical blockade without sedation. An example of a continuous infusion in a 4-kg neonate will be 0.2 mg/kg/hr; this will be equivalent to 0.8 mL/hr of a 0.1% solution of bupivacaine (1 mg/mL of bupivacaine).

Ropivacaine. Ropivacaine is an amide local anesthetic. It is a levo enantiomer with relatively less cardiovascular and CNS side effects compared with bupivacaine.[76] The pharmacokinetics of ropivacaine are such that caudal blocks with ropivacaine (2 mg/kg) in children (aged 1 to 8 years) result in plasma concentrations of ropivacaine well below toxic levels in adults.[76] This dose was also noted to produce less motor block, but provide adequate analgesia. Mean maximum plasma concentration of total ropivacaine at 2 mg/kg was 0.47 mg/L. A threshold of CNS toxicity was noted at a plasma concentration of 0.6 mg/L. Body weight–adjusted clearance was the same as in adults (5 mL/min/kg). Ropivacaine clearance depends on the unbound fraction of ropivacaine rather than the liver blood flow.

Toxicity. Although the safety of ropivacaine has been demonstrated in animal experiments, there have been reports of CNS toxicity and cardiac toxicity associated with the use of epidural ropivacaine. It is important to understand that an overdose of ropivacaine can cause toxicity, making close attention to dosage as important with ropivacaine as with other local anesthetics. Our recommended dose is bolus dose of 2 mg/kg and an infusion rate of 0.2 mg/kg/hr in neonates.

Levobupivacaine. Levobupivacaine is a newer levo enantiomer that has fewer adverse effects than bupivacaine.[77] There are fewer pediatric trials available in literature. Because of the common use of bupivacaine in children and its low incidence of complications, levobupivacaine is not used abundantly in general pediatric anesthesiology practice. It is currently not available for use in the United States, although it is widely used in other parts of the world.

Toxicity. Levobupivacaine, in the animal model, has been shown to have less cardiac toxicity with lower degree of myocardial depression than bupivacaine. Although it is less toxic, the recommended doses remain the same for levobupivacaine as bupivacaine.

Lidocaine. Lidocaine is a frequently-utilized amide local anesthetic with an intermediate duration of action. It is a frequently used local anesthetic for postoperative catheter infusions because its level can be measured in most hospital laboratories in a time-efficient manner. A variety of concentrations are readily available on the market. A concentration of 1.5% in the epidural space is generally considered to be adequate for surgical blockade, whereas peripheral nerve blocks are typically done with 2% for surgical block. Lidocaine has a high hepatic extraction ratio, so its clearance is based on hepatic blood flow. Lidocaine has a longer half-life and volume of distribution in the neonate. Furthermore, the relatively low level of α-1-acid glycoprotein in neonates increases the proportion that is not protein-bound in the serum. When utilized for spinal blockade, the possibility of transient neurological symptoms is significant, so other local anesthetics have supplanted much of its use in spinal anesthesia.

Toxicity. Lidocaine has been an attractive local anesthetic for postoperative continuous infusion in the neonatal population. Because lidocaine has other uses in the intensive care setting, most hospital laboratories can measure its level reasonably quickly. Thus, serum levels of lidocaine may be monitored in the setting of continuous infusions for safety. Furthermore, convulsions are typically noted before the onset of cardiac toxicity, which also confers a greater safety level over bupivacaine.

Esters

Ester local anesthetics are metabolized by plasma cholinesterases. As a result, in populations with lower circulating pseudocholinesterase levels, there is a modestly increased serum half-life of these drugs. This includes infants and neonates particularly. The duration of action of the drug is short; hence, a continuous infusion of chloroprocaine is recommended even when used for only intraoperative anesthesia.

2-Chloroprocaine. This drug is experiencing a resurgence within the neonatal population as interest in its safety profile has reinvigorated its use. Even though neonates have a lower level of circulating pseudocholinesterase, the plasma half-life of chloroprocaine remains short. The plasma half-life of chloroprocaine in adults is 23 seconds, whereas in neonates it is 43 seconds. The plasma half-life of lidocaine, an intermediate-acting amide local anesthetic, is 90 to 120 minutes. Thus, the toxicity profile of chloroprocaine is expected to be much better across a range of doses, though studies in neonates have not been specifically designed to answer this clinical question.

Dosing. After a bolus dose of 1.5 mL/kg, a continuous infusion of chloroprocaine at 1.5 mL/kg/hr of 3% 2-chloroprocaine has been used to achieve a level of T4 to T2 through an intravenous catheter placed in the sacral canal.[78] This level will be effective in producing complete surgical anesthesia for neonates' major abdominal surgery. Lower doses such as 1 mL/kg bolus and an infusion of 1 mL/kg/hr have been used successfully for inguinal and penoscrotal surgery.[79] Given the high concentrations of local that can be used, motor block is easy to achieve with this local anesthetic. Postoperative infusion of chloroprocaine through an epidural catheter is a relatively common practice in neonates as observed in the Pediatric Regional Anesthesia Network (PRAN) database.

Management of Local Anesthetic Systemic Toxicity

Lipid emulsion therapy has been demonstrated to reverse the effects of LAST in experimental animal models.[80] Its effect on human models was parlayed in a case report where lipid was used as a last resort to reverse the effects of bupivacaine following a regional anesthesia technique.[81] Lipid should be readily available if local anesthetics are being used in neonates. There is a report where an infant received a caudal block which resulted in cardiac toxicity which was treated successfully with lipid rescue.[82] Although guidelines for neonatal administration of lipid rescue do not exist, lipid administration across a wide range of doses appears to be safe in neonates.[83] The present recommended dose of lipid rescue for LAST is 1.5 mL/kg bolus, which may be repeated for continued instability, followed by continuous infusion of 0.25 mL/kg/min, which may be increased for continued hypotension.[84]

Topical Anesthesia

Several local anesthetic preparations are now available for topical use. The most common local anesthetic preparations for topical use include lidocaine, tetracaine, benzocaine, and prilocaine. When these are applied to skin they produce effective but relatively short duration of analgesia. One topical anesthetic formulation, eutectic mixture of local anesthetic (EMLA), is a mixture of lidocaine 2.5% and prilocaine 2.5% and is used extensively for topical anesthesia in neonates, particularly for circumcision and venipunctures. The preparation has to be applied under an occlusive bandage for 45 to 60 minutes to obtain effective cutaneous analgesia. Although the incidence of methemoglobinemia from prilocaine is not very common in neonates, caution should be exercised when applying large doses of EMLA for procedures.[85]

Newer topical anesthetic solutions are now available that may offer a faster rate of onset. LMX-4, a 4% liposomal lidocaine solution can be used as topical anesthesia. There is no need for an occlusive dressing when LMX-4 is used, and it has the same efficacy as EMLA.[86] Liposome-encapsulated lidocaine or tetracaine has been shown to remain in the epidermis after topical application, affording a fast and lasting anesthetic effect.

Anesthetic Management of the Neonate

Effective evaluation, preparation, and anesthetic management of the neonate depend on appropriate knowledge, clinical skills, and vigilance on the part of the anesthesiologist. For safe and effective care, the anesthesiologist must take extraordinary caution to understand the current status of the patient, the nature of the planned surgery, and the potential need for stabilization and preparation before surgery. After ensuring that the patient has been adequately prepared, the anesthesiologist needs to develop a detailed plan that encompasses the issues of anesthetic equipment and monitoring, airway management, drug choice, fluid management, temperature control, anticipated surgical needs, pain management, and postoperative care.

Studies have shown that morbidity and mortality related to anesthesia is higher in infants, especially neonates, compared with infants, older children, and adults.[61,87,88] The rate of major complications may be as high as 23% in neonates undergoing surgical procedures and are more frequent in reoperations, surgery for congenital diaphragmatic hernia, prematurity of less than 32 weeks at birth, and abdominal surgery.[89] There are probably several causes for the higher complication rate observed with neonatal surgery, including the emergent nature of most surgical procedures that are performed at this age, the physiologic instability of the neonate, the relative lack of experience most clinicians have with patients in this age range, and the technical challenges of monitoring and treating a very small patient. Because of the specialized nature of neonatal surgery and care, it is important that each institution that provides care to these patients has the resources of equipment, critical care facilities, nursing, laboratory, blood bank, and social work necessary to meet the needs of these patients and their families, as well as systems in place to guarantee a robust quality assurance emphasis on the provision of care. Both the American Academy of Pediatrics and the American Society of Anesthesiologists have provided guidance to many of the systems issues that should be addressed in institutions caring for these patients.[90] Physicians who agree to participate in this care need to have the preparation and ongoing experience needed to provide a consistent, expert level of care.

In the distant past, concerns about physiologic instability and other challenges of caring for neonates led some practitioners to use minimal or no anesthesia for both minor and major procedures. It is now widely recognized that neonates have stress responses similar to those of older patients, and the lack of adequate anesthetic care is as inhumane in the neonate as it is in the older child or adult.[91] The neurologic system in neonates is sufficiently developed to transmit painful stimuli and lack of pain control may result in a higher morbidity rate, increased pain to subsequent events, and increased neuroendocrine response to painful stimuli.[92] Consequently, the same attention to adequate analgesia and anesthesia needs to be paid to the neonate as to other patients.

Preoperative Considerations

Preanesthetic Evaluation—History

The preanesthetic planning process starts with an evaluation of the course of intrauterine growth, events of labor and delivery, and the immediate postpartum course of the patient. The amount of history available to the anesthesiologist may vary widely. If the mother had received prepartum and postpartum care in the same institution where the neonate is admitted, a significant amount of detail may be available. If the neonate is transferred from another institution, there may be limited information available. Best efforts should be made to get as much relevant information as possible, with an emphasis on maternal factors that may have affected fetal growth as well as the current status of the neonate. Additional history of the child's course since birth is important, with a particular focus on the signs that identifies the surgical condition that is to be treated. Important factors include the history of feeding and hydration, need for oxygenation or ventilatory support, cardiovascular abnormalities, and any evidence of CNS problems such as seizures or intraventricular hemorrhage. Finally, an estimation of the gestational status is made, with an emphasis on the issues of prematurity and intrauterine growth retardation with subsequent small-for-gestational age status and VLBW neonates.

The World Health Organization's definition of prematurity is less than 37 weeks' gestation at birth. The determination of gestational age is based on the estimated date of full-term delivery, as well as physical examination of the newborn. Although these indicators are generally widely agreed on, they are subject to some degree of variation in interpretation. The greater the degree of prematurity, the more physiologic abnormalities will be expected. The implications for anesthesiologist are that the more preterm a newborn is, the greater the variability of responsiveness to anesthetic agents, fluids, vasoactive medications, and the stress of the surgical procedure.

In addition to prematurity, there is a second, related classification system. Low birth weight, defined as a birth weight of less than 2,500 g, can be due to prematurity, poor intrauterine growth, or both. Prematurity and intrauterine growth retardation are associated with increased neonatal morbidity and mortality, and it is difficult to completely separate factors associated with prematurity from those associated with intrauterine growth retardation. For discussion purposes, preterm infants are often divided into subgroups. Newborns born at 35 to 37 weeks' gestation are considered near term. These newborns have a lower incidence of major physiologic abnormalities typical of the more preterm newborn. Although they usually do not have significant pulmonary abnormalities, they may have some feeding problems or hyperbilirubinemia. This degree of prematurity does not usually have a significant impact on anesthetic management. However, infants born between 30 and 34 weeks' gestation are much more likely to show some abnormalities related to prematurity that can complicate anesthetic management.[93]

Although RDS had previously been a significant source of morbidity in this population, the widespread use of exogenous surfactant has decreased the incidence dramatically, as well as the later complications of chronic lung disease. This group does have more problems with inadequate feeding, persistent patency of the ductus arteriosus, apnea in response to stress, and temperature instability. However, infants born more prematurely than 30 to 34 weeks' gestation begin to demonstrate significant physiologic abnormalities related to prematurity.

For infants with VLBW, defined as less than 1,500 g, the presence of complicating problems and morbidity and mortality are inversely related to birth weight. Major surgery in VLBW infants is associated with a 50% greater risk of mortality or neurodevelopmental impairment at 18 to 22 months of age versus normal birth weight. RDS is found in approximately 80% of infants weighing 501 to 750 g, in 65% of those 751 to 1,000 g, in 45% between 1,001 and 1,250 g, and in 25% between 1,251 and 1,500 g. In addition, symptomatic intraventricular hemorrhage is found in about 25% of infants weighing 501 to 750 g, in 12% between 751 and 1,000 g, in 8% between 1,001 and 1,250 g, and in 3% between 1,251 and 1,500 g. Other complications, such as sepsis, necrotizing enterocolitis (NEC), and bronchopulmonary dysplasia (BPD) are very high in infants with VLBW. Table 42-3 lists some of the most common abnormalities found in the preterm population that have implications for anesthetic evaluation, preparation, and management.

Preanesthetic Evaluation—Physical Examination

Physical examination of the newborn is focused by the condition requiring surgical intervention. Hydration is often an important issue because of both fasting and losses related to the surgical lesion. Clinical signs of dehydration include a sunken fontanel, poor skin turgor, dry mucous membranes, sunken eyes, poor skin perfusion, delayed capillary refill, hypothermia, tachycardia, or absent urine output. If there are clinical signs of dehydration,

Table 42-3 Abnormalities Associated with the Preterm Infant: Common Anesthetic Concerns

Respiratory	Respiratory distress syndrome Apnea Pneumothorax, pneumomediastinum Pneumonia Pulmonary hemorrhage Bronchopulmonary dysplasia
Cardiovascular	Patent ductus arteriosus Hypotension Bradycardia Pulmonary hypertension Persistent transitional circulation Congenital heart disease
Central nervous system	Intraventricular hemorrhage Hypoxic–ischemic encephalopathy Seizures Kernicterus Drug withdrawal
Metabolic	Hypoglycemia Hyperglycemia Hypocalcemia Hypothermia Metabolic acidosis
Renal	Hyponatremia Hypernatremia Hyperkalemia Poor urine output
Gastrointestinal	Poor feeding Necrotizing enterocolitis Intestinal obstruction
Hematologic	Anemia Hyperbilirubinemia Vitamin K deficiency
Other	Retinopathy of prematurity Sepsis and infections

efforts should be made to correct the deficits before surgery, except in extreme, life-threatening situations. Physical examination also focuses on the respiratory and cardiovascular systems. The presence of any cardiovascular abnormalities should be noted, including poor perfusion or pulses, abnormal rhythm or rate, a murmur or gallop, hepatomegaly, or other signs of either heart failure or poor perfusion. The presence of a murmur is of concern in the neonatal period and warrants further evaluation, which is best done by a pediatric cardiologist. An electrocardiogram and echocardiogram will help define whether there is significant cardiovascular disease present that will affect the anesthetic management. Although this evaluation may take some effort and time, it is worthwhile to ensure that the anesthesiologist can plan the child's care with full knowledge of the limitations cardiovascular disease can impose.

The respiratory system also must be examined in some detail. The presence of stridor or other evidence of airway obstruction, such as sternal or chest wall retractions, should be identified and investigated. Although upper airway obstruction is relatively rare in the newborn, laryngeal webs, cysts of the tongue or supraglottic region, vocal cord paralysis after a traumatic delivery, and hemangiomas of the airway can cause obstruction and need to be identified. In addition, newborns that have been previously intubated may have some degree of subglottic edema related to previous intubation. More likely are signs of lower airway disease such as tachypnea, grunting, rhonchi, retractions, and cyanosis. This may be related to the early development of RDS, but may also represent meconium aspiration, pneumonia, pneumothorax, or heart failure. The cause of any respiratory distress needs to be evaluated expeditiously prior to anesthesia to identify treatable causes and begin therapy.

Preanesthetic Evaluation—Laboratory

Most laboratory investigations are related to the underlying surgical condition such as radiography, computed tomography, magnetic resonance imaging, and echocardiography. However, most newborns will have, at a minimum, a blood count and glucose level drawn. The hemoglobin in a newborn is primarily fetal hemoglobin, which has a higher affinity for oxygen than adult hemoglobin. Because of this higher affinity, the hemoglobin dissociation curve is shifted to the left, releasing less oxygen to the tissues than adult hemoglobin. Newborns have a higher hemoglobin than the infant or child, often in the 15 to 18 g/dL range.[94] Rarely, a newborn will have significant polycythemia, with hemoglobin levels above 20 g/dL. If symptomatic, these patients may benefit from therapeutic phlebotomy and volume replacement.

Glucose levels obtained close to the time of the proposed surgery are important. The stressed newborn, especially the stressed preterm or small-for-gestational age newborn, are at particular risk for hypoglycemia.[95] A glucose level between 60 and 80 mg/dL is expected in a full-term newborn, with a preterm often 10 mg/dL below that. Although there is some controversy about what actually constitutes hypoglycemia in these populations, most agree that levels less than 45 mg/dL warrant therapy with additional dextrose. Patients with diabetic mothers, those who have not been receiving either enteral or parenteral feeds, those who are VLBW, and those who have been septic are especially susceptible to hypoglycemia and require frequent monitoring and modification of parenteral fluids.

Other laboratory studies, such as electrolyte determinations and coagulation profiles, are indicated in specific patients. Hypocalcemia, in particular, can be troubling because signs of hypocalcemia are nonspecific. Unexplained hypotension, irritability, or even seizures can be presenting signs. Hypocalcemia is a problem with preterm newborns, but can also be seen in full-term newborns who have a delay in starting enteral feedings. Hyponatremia is not uncommon in newborns who have been receiving solutions with little or no salt in the first days of life, although hypernatremia may occur if there is inadequate resuscitation of the dehydrated patient when water loss is greater than salt loss. The longer a newborn has received parenteral fluids, the greater the chance of electrolyte abnormalities because of the difficulty in matching ongoing losses with replacement in the presence of an immature kidney.

Coagulation parameters are different in newborns compared with adults.[96] Although platelet counts in term newborns are usually similar to adult values, lower values are frequently seen in the preterm. Unexplained thrombocytopenia can be an early sign of sepsis, and a falling count should be an impetus to look for other signs of sepsis. Other coagulation tests are different in both the full-term and preterm newborn. The prothrombin time and partial thromboplastin time levels are about 10% longer in the newborn, but prothrombin time values approach adult levels in the first week of life and partial thromboplastin time levels within the first month of life. Prevention of early vitamin K deficiency bleeding (VKDB) of the newborn is the purpose of intramuscular vitamin K administration after birth and is standard of care in the United States.[97]

Preanesthetic Plan

The anesthesiologist has a host of anesthetic techniques from which to choose and can tailor the anesthetic to the requirements of the surgery and the condition of the neonate. Major factors that should be considered in planning the anesthetic include (1) anticipated blood loss and necessity for blood products to be available before beginning the case, (2) monitoring requirements, including invasive monitoring techniques, (3) additional equipment needs for airway and vascular access, (4) transport requirements, (5) postoperative recovery location risk of postoperative ventilation requirements, and (6) plan for postoperative pain relief. Both the medical status of the patient and the planned surgical procedure will impact this planning. The anesthesiologist has the responsibility of clarifying any medical issues with the neonatologist before finalizing the plan, as well as clarifying any issues related to the planned procedure with the surgeon. Occasionally, as planning progresses, it becomes obvious that the patient needs further medical resuscitation or evaluation before it is prudent to proceed with the procedure.

Once the anesthetic plan is clear, it should be discussed with the available parent or caregiver who has legal custody of the child. Informed consent is a process by which the anesthesiologist explains his/her understanding of the patient's status, the planned procedure, the plan for anesthetic management, alternatives to the plan, and some discussion of risks and benefits. Although there may be rare circumstances in which the legal guardian is not available to provide consent, efforts should be made in all except the most emergent of situations to have this discussion. It should be stressed that informed consent is a process, not a document. The goal of informed consent is to help the parent understand what care is being proposed, the risks and benefits involved, and reasonable alternatives. It is the discussion, in terms understandable to the parent, that is the basis of true informed consent.

Premedication

Premedication is not commonly used for neonatal anesthetics. Sedation is not usually necessary and analgesics are rarely indicated before taking the patient to the operating room. Atropine or glycopyrrolate may be used for vagolytic effect before induction. Because of the dominance of the parasympathetic nervous system, bradycardia on induction or in response to inhalation agents is of concern. Manipulation of the airway or administration of succinylcholine may cause bradycardia in neonates without administration of atropine or glycopyrrolate. Although it is not requisite to administer a vagolytic, it should be among the drugs immediately available and additional vigilance from the anesthesiologist is necessary to quickly respond to bradycardia. Although a dose of 20 µg/kg of atropine is most frequently used to prevent bradycardia, the question of a minimum dose of 100 to 200 µg has been a source of controversy. However, it appears that prior concerns over paradoxical bradycardia with small doses of atropine have not been evident in clinical trials, leading to a practice reversal where the minimum dose of atropine is no longer commonly used.[98]

Intraoperative Considerations

Monitoring

Neonatal patients are at a disadvantage when it comes to perioperative monitoring because of their small size. Many of the monitoring modalities that are easily employed in older children and adults are very difficult in the neonate. Other monitors that are used may occasionally not provide reliable information for technical reasons. Examples of this include neuromuscular blockade monitoring and automated blood pressure monitoring. Invasive monitoring such as arterial line and central venous line catheters may be technically difficult to insert, especially in the preterm. However, improvements in ultrasound guidance have made line placement much more efficient and the development of small transesophageal echocardiography (TEE) probes has extended this useful monitoring technique into the neonatal population, including premature newborns.[15] The overarching goal of monitoring should be to establish American Society of Anesthesiologists standard monitors at the beginning of the case and add invasive monitoring, as appropriate.

Although physical observation of the patient is important in preanesthetic evaluation, it is difficult to use this monitor effectively during a surgical procedure. Observation of the patient's color, capillary refill, warmth of skin, muscle tone, fullness of fontanelle, and chest expansion are useful monitors, but they are difficult to reliably observe once the patient is covered with surgical drapes. There is a large dependence on electronic monitors during the majority of the procedure. However, it should be remembered that heart and breath sounds heard through a precordial or esophageal stethoscope, the compliance determined during hand ventilation, the appearance of bleeding in the surgical field, and trends noted in the anesthetic record are all important observations that the anesthesiologist can use as part of the overall assessment of the patient.

Pulse oximetry is one of the most important monitors in neonatal anesthesia. Flexible probes designed for pediatric patients should be used. Placement is sometimes difficult because of the small fingers of the neonate. It may be necessary to place the probe across the web space between the thumb and the first finger, around the lateral aspect of the hand, or on the foot. Many anesthesiologists will place and check two pulse oximeter probes at the beginning of the case because of the clinical experience of having one probe malfunctioning secondary to changes in perfusion during the case. Because there may be differences in preductal and postductal saturations, probes on the left hand or either leg may give lower values than a probe on the right hand in the setting of high pulmonary pressures or low systemic pressures. Especially in the first 2 weeks of life, there is a preponderance of fetal hemoglobin. The pulse oximeter does not compensate for the left shift of the hemoglobin desaturation curve, and pulse oximeter values read about 2% higher than arterial blood saturations.[99]

The hallmark of the pediatric anesthesiologist had been the precordial stethoscope. Precordial stethoscopes have the advantage of being simple and effective in allowing continuous monitoring of heart rate, heart rhythm, strength of heart sounds, and breath sounds. A softening of heart sounds often is indicative of a drop in blood pressure. The esophageal stethoscope is more secure and less susceptible to external noise compared to the precordial stethoscope, while also providing the ability to measure core temperature. However, there has been recent skepticism about the usefulness of the stethoscope,[100] and a survey of pediatric anesthesiologists in the United Kingdom and Ireland revealed relatively little use of the precordial or esophageal stethoscope.[101]

The electrocardiograph is useful primarily to assess heart rate and rhythm. It is sometimes difficult to get the leads to adhere properly, but wiping the skin with alcohol before placement is often helpful. These leads, once applied, can bind tightly to skin, and care must be taken when removing them to avoid removal of skin, especially in the preterm newborn. ST–T wave abnormalities may be an indicator of significant electrolyte disturbances, but abnormalities related to myocardial ischemia are not common in the perioperative period unless coronary perfusion pressures are compromised.

Blood pressure measurements are important in the management of all newborns. Noninvasive automated machines are commonly used, but it is important that a proper-sized cuff—one-half to two-thirds of the length of the upper arm—be used, and that the arterial indicator, adjacent to the exit of the hoses, be placed over the artery. The cuff should not be routinely cycled excessively, more than every 3 minutes, because of the danger of venous stasis, especially in preterm neonates. In some cases, it is not possible to get reliable readings from an automated machine. An effective alternative is to use a manual cuff and place a Doppler probe over the brachial or radial artery. This system gives reliable systolic blood pressures over a very wide range; the Doppler probe can detect flow, even at very low blood pressures when the automated cuff may fail.

Direct arterial blood pressure monitoring offers the double advantage of accurate blood pressure readings and the ability to withdraw blood samples. A 22-gauge catheter is often used in full-term neonates and a 24-gauge catheter in preterm neonates. A variety of sites can be used, including the radial, dorsalis pedis, and posterior tibial arteries. Less commonly, the brachial or femoral arteries are used. Ultrasound guidance is a valuable tool in the placement of arterial access, even in neonates. It is imperative that ultrasound guidance be attempted before resorting to a cutdown for vascular access. Some patients may come to the operating room with an umbilical arterial line in place. Although these can be used for monitoring, umbilical lines have both infectious and embolic risks, and may be in the way of the surgical field. All arterial lines should be flushed, either continuously or intermittently, with small amounts of heparinized saline, but caution should be used because even small amounts of flush can transmit significant pressure retrograde and cause embolic damage to the brain.

Central venous monitoring is occasionally used in neonatal surgery. Access to blood samples and central venous pressures can be especially useful in procedures, such as gastroschisis repair, in which there are anticipated large changes in both blood loss and third-space losses. Central catheters can also be used for the administration of blood, total parenteral nutrition, and cardioactive drug infusion. Insertion of these lines can be in a variety of sites, including the subclavian, internal jugular, femoral, or external jugular veins using special precautions to maintain sterile technique. The umbilical vein is not recommended as a site for central monitoring because of the risk of portal vein thrombosis.

Percutaneous insertion may be assisted by ultrasound guidance. Central lines can be both challenging to insert, but also associated with significant complications related to infection, thrombosis, and emboli. Meticulous technique with insertion and maintenance of the line will help minimize these complications. The use of ultrasound guidance is now routine in many US children's hospitals to provide a presumably safe and consistent method for gaining central venous access; however, a meta-analysis did not demonstrate any significant decrease in complications when ultrasound was used to place internal jugular access versus placement by landmark techniques.[102] The rate of complications with central line placement appears to be lowest when the right internal jugular vein is used for central access in infants.[103] Peripherally inserted central catheter (PICC), are now common in neonatal practice and associated with a relatively low rate of complications, especially when the axillary vein site is used for access.[104]

Although there may be some differential between capnography and arterial PCO_2 readings, the trend data are accurate and the shape of the waveform can give significant information about changes in ventilation, obstruction, and rebreathing. Airway pressure measurements are particularly useful in assessing changes in resistance or compliance. Although it has been traditional that hand ventilation was important in determining changes in airway and chest compliance, there is controversy about the reliability of the "feel of the hand on the bag."[105,106] Airway pressure measurements are also useful in adapting adult anesthesia ventilators for use in neonatal and pediatric patients, using peak airway pressures as a guide for setting tidal volume.[107]

Anesthetic Systems

There is a long tradition in pediatric anesthesia of using semi-open, nonrebreathing systems for general anesthesia in newborns. Circuits such as the Jackson-Rees adaptation of the Ayre's T-piece and the Bain circuit have been the most commonly used. These, and related circuits, have the advantages of light weight, easy-to-open valves or lack of valves, rapid response to changes in anesthetic concentration, minimal work of breathing, and high circuit compliance. On the other hand, they require relatively high gas flows and require some modification for mechanical ventilation. These circuits were especially popular when spontaneous ventilation was more commonly used than it is now in neonatal patients. As the use of these circuits has diminished, familiarity with their use and application has dropped in favor of the semi-closed, rebreathing circle systems used in adult patients. There will be slower change in anesthetic concentration, less circuit compliance, and larger compression volume with these circuits, but they give the advantage of using the same circuit on patients of all ages, less environmental pollution with anesthetic gases, and allow accurate tidal volume delivery with modern anesthesia machines.

Because the loss of both heat and humidity through the endotracheal tube is of concern in the neonate, the anesthetic circuit should incorporate features to minimize water and heat loss. In the past, heated vaporizers were added to the circuit for this purpose. However, there is a danger of patient absorption of water and fluid overload with their use, as well as concerns about overheating the patient or an airway burn. It is now common to use a combination of low gas flows[108] and a disposable, neonatal humidity and heat exchanger to the circuit, with warming of the gases and retention of some of the exhaled humidity.[109]

Finally, the anesthesia machine used for anesthetizing neonates should have the capacity to administer medical air. There are two reasons for this. First, if nitrous oxide is contraindicated, such as in the newborn with bowel obstruction, air is mixed with oxygen to prevent the administration of only 100% oxygen. This is also used to minimize the risk of ROP by avoiding prolonged administration of 100% oxygen in preterm neonates. Second, some patients, such as those with hypoplastic left heart syndrome, may benefit from the administration of air with additional oxygen. Without an air flowmeter in the system, this will not be possible.

Induction of Anesthesia

There is no one method of induction and maintenance of anesthesia that is best for all patients. The current medical status of the patient, the surgical condition, the presence of ongoing fluid or blood losses, the gestational age of the patient, recent fasting, and the experience of the anesthesiologist are all important considerations. Most neonates who come to the operating room will have vascular access already established; if not, the first task before induction is to establish adequate vascular access after applying monitors. Although it may rarely be appropriate to use an inhalational induction if vascular access is difficult in the older newborn, near a month of age, it is mandatory to establish access first in the newborn who is preterm, medically unstable, has a full stomach, has a potentially difficult airway, or has ongoing fluid losses.

Airway Management

Establishing the airway in the neonate requires an appreciation of the differences between the newborn and the adult airway, as discussed earlier. It is rare to administer anesthesia in the newborn period without establishing an artificial airway. Although, with meticulous technique, a mask airway can successfully be used for short periods of time, the tolerances of mask fit, adequate airway pressure, and avoidance of gastric distention are small, making this a poor choice for any but the briefest of operations. In addition, controlled ventilation is used more commonly today than spontaneous ventilation for surgical procedures, making an artificial airway necessary.

Awake intubation has been used to secure the airway without the danger of loss of airway during the procedure, but it can be a traumatic experience for both the patient and the anesthesiologist, accompanied by pain, bradycardia, breath holding, desaturation, and tissue trauma.[110] The desaturation associated with this technique can be ameliorated by using an oxyscope, a Miller laryngoscope blade that has a side channel to allow insufflation of oxygen during the procedure. However, this technique is usually reserved for patients with severe hemodynamic compromise, an extraordinarily distended and tense abdomen, or a presumed difficult airway, especially the newborn with micrognathia. In the latter situation, the addition of sedation with an opioid or topical application of local anesthetic can help decrease some of the trauma of the procedure. It has also been suggested that an awake intubation may be best for the anesthesiologist who is not very experienced in intubating newborns. It may be better to have a more experienced clinician, if available, attend to the airway in that situation.

Most newborns are intubated after a rapid-sequence induction. Preoxygenation is useful in adding additional safety to the procedure. Although there may be a minor concern about a period of hyperoxia in the preterm, there is no evidence that a short exposure such as preoxygenation will increase the risk of ROP. Agents for induction and muscle relaxation are discussed elsewhere. If there is concern about the difficulty of intubation, it may be prudent to induce anesthesia, ensure adequacy of mask ventilation, and then give the muscle relaxant.

Positioning for intubation is based on the known differences in the neonatal airway. Because of the large occiput, the newborn already has a flexed neck. No changes in position are usually needed, although additional extension of the head may be accomplished by a shoulder roll. A Miller no. 1 blade is commonly used for the full-term newborn and a Miller no. 0 in the preterm, although there are other available blades that individual practitioners may prefer. Sliding the blade down the right side of the mouth allows the blade to be seated with minimal overlap by the tongue (Fig. 42-8). The tip of the blade is advanced to lift the epiglottis directly instead of placing it in the vallecula, as is commonly done with older patients. Every patient's anatomy is different, but if the laryngoscope is advanced in the direction parallel to the handle, one will get the best visualization. If the glottis is not easily seen, cricoid pressure can be applied with the little finger of the hand holding the handle or by an assistant, often improving the view (Fig. 42-9).

Uncuffed tubes have traditionally been used in newborns to minimize cuff pressure on the subglottic larynx, especially at

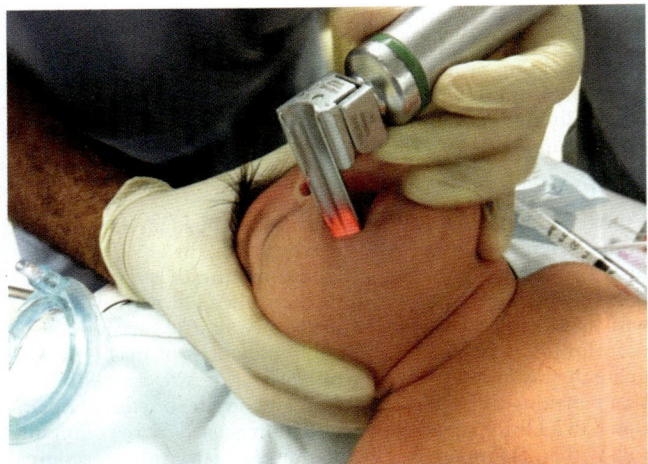

Figure 42-8 Insertion of Miller blade down the right side of the tongue. The blade is then turned and pressure is applied in the direction of the handle.

the level of the cricoid cartilage. Although there has been interest in the use of cuffed tubes in newborns and infants,[111] most clinicians continue to use uncuffed tubes in newborns to maximize the internal diameter (ID) and gas flow characteristics for a given external diameter of tube. Modern cuffed endotracheal tubes make minimal sacrifice in tube diameter to allow for the presence of a cuff, which has renewed interest in cuffed endotracheal tubes. Although various formulas have been proposed for how far to advance an uncuffed tube, it is prudent to use the depth markers at the end of the tube to ensure under direct vision that the tip is advanced 2 or 3 cm past the vocal cords. A 3- or 3.5-mm ID uncuffed tube is usually appropriate for a full-term newborn and a 2.5-mm ID tube is used in preterms, especially those under 1,500 g body weight. Once inserted, the presence of a positive capnograph tracing, bilateral expansion of the thorax, and bilateral breath sounds are used to ensure proper placement. Although some anesthesiologists prefer to advance the endotracheal tube past the carina and then withdraw until bilateral breath sounds are heard, there are two major disadvantages to the technique: trauma to the airway and lack of a guarantee that the tip of the tube is not sitting right at the carina, increasing the chance of migration into a bronchus with head movement. Finally, listen for an air leak at an airway pressure of about 20 cm H_2O to ensure that the tube is not too large for the airway, increasing the chances of subglottic edema and damage.

If intubation proves difficult, there are a variety of options. A supraglottic airway (SGA) can be used to provide ventilation in newborns as small as 1-kg body weight as preparations are made to use other intubating techniques.[112] The SGA has also successfully been used as the primary airway device in very small patients, but has not been extensively studied.[113] It is possible to use the SGA as a guide for blind intubations in newborns with the use of a stylletted tube.[114] The light wand can also be used in newborns,[115] and can be particularly useful in the newborn with micrognathia or retrognathia because of the ability to mold the wand to a "hockey stick" configuration with a sharp angle. Fiberoptic laryngoscopy, the most flexible of intubating tools routinely used in older children and adults, can also be used in the newborn. Fiberscopes are currently available that accept endotracheal tubes as small as 2.5-mm ID, although these scopes do not currently have the ability to change direction and are useful more for confirmation of tube placement. Fiberscopes that can actively change direction accept a 3.5-mm ID tube at the smallest. Insertion of the fiberscope can be done directly or through an SGA. A SGA as a conduit has been particularly useful in directly intubating newborns that could not be visualized by routine approaches.[116]

Finally, an old technique that is used infrequently is digital intubation in which two fingers are advanced along the midline of the tongue and onto the epiglottis, with a stylletted tube then advanced between the two fingers.[117] Once the airway is secured, ventilation is usually controlled during neonatal surgical procedures with hand ventilation or, more commonly, mechanical ventilation. After establishing a baseline of acceptable ventilation, it is important to continuously monitor the peak airway pressures, chest expansion, return volume, pulse oximetry, and capnograph tracings for changes. Initial tidal volumes of 6 to 7 mL/kg and rates of 20 to 25 breaths per minute are a reasonable starting point for most patients. With this rate and volume setting, it would be expected that peak airway pressures be approximately 20 cm H_2O. A level of positive end-expiratory pressure (PEEP) of 3 to 5 cm H_2O can be useful in preventing atelectasis. Lung protective strategies applied in the Neonatal Intensive Care Unit (NICU) may be appropriate to continue in the operating room,[118] which is facilitated by the modern anesthesia ventilator. Of course, this strategy must be modified for some patients with severe coexisting disease.

Mechanical ventilation of the neonate can be challenging for the anesthesiologist. Many of the patients presenting for surgery during the neonatal period will have complicating factors such as BPD or frequent mucous plugging that make ventilation continuously challenging during the case. Modern anesthetic systems make ventilation much easier than in the past, even in the smallest patients. Although the standard has been to use pressure control ventilation in this population, all modes of ventilation are now readily available on modern anesthesia machines. In the NICU, volume control ventilation has started to replace pressure control ventilation due to its more predictable and consistent delivery of a set minute ventilation. Table 42-4 shows the modes of ventilation and breath synchronization most commonly used in neonates. Use of high frequency ventilation in the operative setting will require use of a specialized ventilator and close consultation with a critical care physician and respiratory therapist. Table 42-5 lists some of the advantages and disadvantages to use of pressure control, volume targeted, and high frequency ventilation.

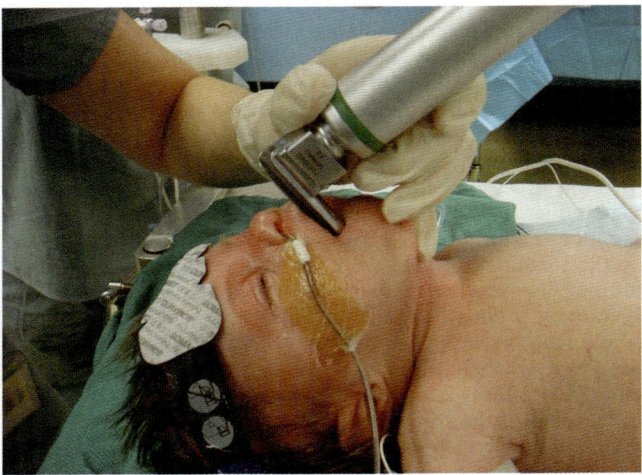

Figure 42-9 Cricoid pressure applied with little finger.

Table 42-4 Common Ventilator Strategies in Neonates

Conventional ventilation
    Breath initiation
        Intermittent mandatory ventilation
        Synchronized intermittent mandatory ventilation
        Pressure support ventilation
        Neurally adjusted ventilatory assist
    Pressure-limited ventilation
        Pressure-control
    Volume-targeted ventilation
        Volume-control
        Volume-guarantee
        Pressure-regulated volume control
High-frequency ventilation
    High-frequency oscillator ventilation
    High-frequency jet ventilation
    High-frequency flow interrupter

Impact of Surgical Requirements on Anesthetic Technique

6 Every procedure has its own unique challenges. With any surgery, issues related to presurgical resuscitation, perioperative fluid and blood loss, heat loss from the surgical field, likely perioperative complications, and the likely need for postoperative intubation and ventilation should be anticipated, both on the basis of experience and communication about the unique needs of the upcoming procedure. There is a dramatic increase in the use of laparoscopic and thoracoscopic approaches to lesions, even in the smallest neonates. The considerations for these approaches are different from open procedures. There may be less blood, fluid, and heat loss, but there are additional issues related to positioning, insufflation pressures in the chest and abdomen, and prolonged surgical time. As new techniques evolve, close communication between the anesthesiologist and the surgeon is necessary to ensure adequate preparation, monitoring, and resolution of problems or complications.

Uptake and Distribution of Anesthetics in Neonates

Various reasons for the faster uptake of anesthetics in infants have been proposed: (1) the ratio of alveolar ventilation to FRC is 5:1 in the infant and 1.5:1 in the adult; (2) in the neonate, more of the cardiac output goes to the vessel-rich group of organs, which includes the heart and the brain; (3) the neonate has a greater cardiac output per kilogram of body mass; and (4) the infant has a lower blood gas partition coefficient for volatile anesthetics. One not well-recognized factor that may result in higher concentrations of volatile anesthetics being administered to infants has to do with the use of nonrebreathing systems such as the Bain or a Mapleson "D" circuit. When an adult circle system is used with infant tubes and bag, the clinician experienced with this equipment is used to reading the inspired, end-tidal, and dialed concentrations of the volatile anesthetic. In the circle system, the inspired concentration is a result of the combination of the end-tidal concentration that is rebreathed through the soda lime absorber and the dialed concentration. The inspired concentration is always lower than the dialed concentration, unless the flow rates are so high that a nonrebreathing system has been created. In the nonrebreathing system, the dialed concentration is the inspired concentration. Clinicians who use both systems are accustomed to these subtle differences. However, if the clinician switches back and forth between the circle system and a nonrebreathing circuit, but does so infrequently, there is a

Table 42-5 Advantages of Particular Ventilator Strategies in Neonates

Mode	Advantages	Disadvantages
Pressure control ventilation	• Easy to use due to long-standing widespread use worldwide • Supported by almost all ventilators • Less affected by large leaks around endotracheal tube	• Constant variation in tidal volume and minute ventilation • Rapid changes in lung compliance may lead to volutrauma, hyperventilation, desaturation, or hypoventilation • Increased work of breathing during spontaneous breaths
Volume-targeted ventilation	• Standard, targeted tidal volume, resulting in a predictable minute ventilation • Associated with lower rate of death or bronchopulmonary dysplasia in NICU management of acute respiratory failure[119] • Reduces rates of pneumothorax, hypocarbia, days of ventilation, and significant neurologic injury over pressure control ventilation[120]	• Requires ventilators with capability of measuring very small tidal volumes • Relies on pressure limits set in ventilator (risk of single point of failure) • More difficult to implement than PCV due to complexity of the ventilators • Large leaks around endotracheal tube may significantly affect reliability of ventilation
High-frequency ventilation	• May provide better ventilation and oxygenation in neonates with severe respiratory disease • Allows for small tidal volumes that are less than total dead space but allow for oxygenation and ventilation • Minimizes barotrauma and volutrauma	• No significant morbidity or mortality advantage over conventional ventilation • Additional cost and difficulty of operation over conventional ventilation • Anesthesia providers are not very familiar with optimization of these devices • Difficult for use during transport or non-ICU locations

danger of not recognizing the possibility of excessive overpressure of volatile anesthetics with the nonrebreathing systems.

Anesthetic Dose Requirements of Neonates

Neonates and premature infants have lower anesthetic requirements than older infants and children.[69] The easiest way to remember the minimum alveolar concentration (MAC) values is that the MAC value in the mature state (i.e., late teenager or adult) is the same as for a full-term infant. By 6 months of age, the MAC value has increased by 50%. In the premature infant, the MAC value decreases by 20% to 30%. However, for sevoflurane anesthesia the highest MAC requirement may be the full-term neonate, decreasing throughout life to adult values (Fig. 42-10).

The reasons for the lower MAC requirements are believed to be an immature nervous system, progesterone from the mother, and elevated blood levels of endorphins, coupled with an immature blood–brain barrier. Progesterone has been shown to reduce the MAC of the pregnant mother. The newborn infant has elevated progesterone levels, similar to those of the mother. Elevated levels of β-endorphin and β-lipotropin have been demonstrated in infants in the first few days of postnatal life. Endorphins do not cross the blood–brain barrier in adults; however, it is believed that the neonate's blood–brain barrier is more permeable and that endorphins may pass into the CNS, thus elevating the pain threshold and reducing the MAC requirement.

Regional Anesthesia

There has been a tremendous increase in the use of regional anesthesia in infants and children. In general, regional techniques are combined with general anesthesia to permit early extubation

Table 42-6 Regional Anesthesia Techniques Useful in Neonates
Central neuraxial
Epidural (lumbar, thoracic, caudal)
Spinal
Peripheral nerve blocks
Infraorbital block
Brachial plexus block (supraclavicular, infraclavicular, axillary)
Lateral femoral cutaneous block
Penile block
Ilioinguinal block
TAP block (transversus abdominis plane block)
Scalp blocks

and provide postoperative pain relief. Useful regional anesthesia techniques include spinal anesthesia, caudal anesthesia, epidural analgesia, penile block, and other peripheral nerve blocks (Table 42-6). Regional anesthesia may even have other applications outside surgery, including management of neonatal limb ischemia.[121] Combined regional and general anesthesia is commonly provided for neonates for multiple procedures. The use of ultrasonography has revolutionized the use of regional anesthesia as vascular structures can be easily avoided while still providing a regional blockade.[122] It is important to remember that the dosage of local anesthetic solution used is limited and lipid emulsion is available to potentially treat any intravascular injections.[123] A dose of 1.5 mL/kg of intralipid has been suggested as a rescue dose for toxicity in children.

Spinal Anesthesia

Regional anesthesia can be provided as a sole anesthetic or in combination with general anesthesia. The use of sole regional anesthesia in neonates and infants is for avoidance of general anesthetics, for either theoretical decreased risk of apnea or decreased risk of neurotoxicity. Although neurotoxicity trials are still ongoing, it has been shown that spinal anesthesia decreases early apnea following surgery in premature neonates, but does not decrease the risk of overall apnea following surgery in premature neonates.[124] For patients receiving combined general and regional anesthesia, early extubation is possible because the addition of regional anesthetic techniques eliminates the need for intraoperative narcotics in neonates, reduces or eliminates the need for muscle relaxants, and reduces the concentration of volatile agents needed for relaxation.[125] Spinal anesthesia has been reported to be effective when used as the sole anesthetic technique in premature and high-risk infants, but this technique requires excellent cooperation between the anesthesiologist and an experienced surgeon.[126] Although this is technically feasible, because of increasing advancements in general anesthesia techniques, we may be able to provide safer anesthesia with fewer complications by using general anesthesia.[127] Even high doses of spinal anesthetic provide a relatively short time of surgical anesthesia.

Some patients may benefit from providing a caudal block in addition to the spinal anesthetic. This technique seems to provide a longer duration of surgical anesthesia. Total spinal anesthesia, produced either with a primary spinal technique or secondary to an attempted epidural puncture, will present as apnea, rather than as hypotension, because of the lack of sympathetic tone in infants. The exact mechanism for the lack of cardiovascular change with spinal anesthesia in infants and young children is not clear. Consequently, the first indication of a high spinal is

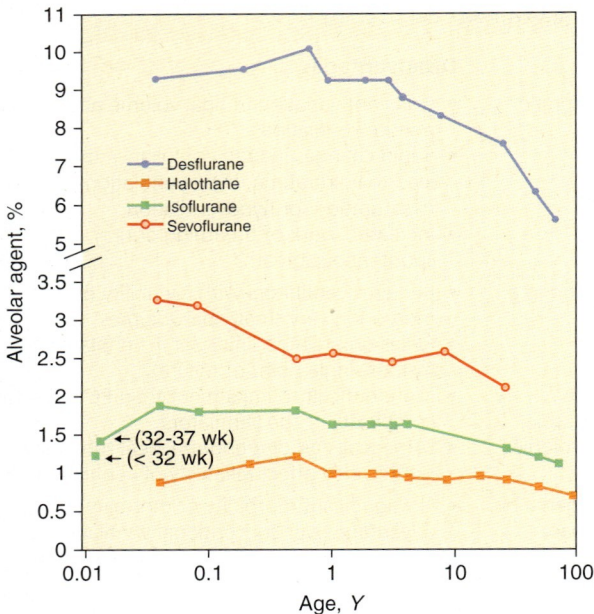

Figure 42-10 Effect of age on minimum alveolar concentration (MAC) of anesthetic gases. (Adapted from Greeley WJ. Pediatric anesthesia. In: Miller RD, ed. *Atlas of Anesthesia*. vol 7. Philadelphia, PA: Churchill Livingstone; 1999.)

falling oxygen saturation rather than a falling blood pressure. Sedation can be added to regional anesthesia but may cause problems with apnea in ex-premature infants.[128]

Caudal Block

Caudal epidural block is frequently used for abdominal surgery in neonates and is the most commonly used regional anesthetic technique in neonates and infants. There are several different techniques described for performing a caudal block. The landmarks are the coccyx, the two sacral cornua, and the posterior superior iliac spines (Fig. 42-11). Several needle types may be used, but the "pop" through the sacrococcygeal ligament is best observed with a blunt-tipped needle, whereas an intravenous catheter advanced over a needle may provide additional confirmation of sacral canal entry. The caudal space is identified by "pop" through the sacrococcygeal ligament, ease of local anesthetic injection, and absence of subcutaneous swelling upon dose delivery. Once the sacrococcygeal ligament is penetrated and there is a loss of resistance, gentle aspiration is applied to the needle to determine if there is blood or cerebrospinal fluid. Injection of the anesthetic is then attempted. If there is difficulty in injecting the solution, and the tip of the needle is not in the caudal space and it needs to be repositioned. The needle is not advanced up the sacral canal after proper placement in the caudal epidural space has been accomplished, this avoids dural puncture and accidental intrathecal injection. Other methods to identify the caudal space have been described, including stimulating technique[129] and ultrasound guidance.[130] Epinephrine is added to local anesthetic solutions for the purposes of determining if there is an intravascular injection of the anesthetic. Evidence of an intravascular injection include (1) peaked T waves (which may be of relatively short duration), (2) increase in heart rate, and (3) increase in blood pressure. Another technique to minimize the potential difficulties of an intravascular injection is to fractionate the dose by dividing the total dose into three aliquots and waiting approximately 20 to 30 seconds between each aliquot before continuing the injection. Caudal blocks are safe procedures as demonstrated in a large prospective database (PRAN) with very minimal risk overall so long as appropriate precautions are taken during performance.[131]

Caudal anesthesia is particularly effective at reducing the concentrations of volatile anesthetics needed, as well as relaxants and opioids. In addition, a single-injection caudal anesthetic can provide analgesia for 6 to 8 hours. The most common local anesthetics currently in use are 0.125% bupivacaine, 0.25% bupivacaine, or 0.2% ropivacaine. Epinephrine, 1:200,000, is added to local anesthetics to assist in determining if there has been an intravenous injection. Ropivacaine has been reported to be less cardiodepressant than equipotent doses of bupivacaine. If a caudal catheter is placed, an infusion of ropivacaine, bupivacaine, lidocaine, or chloroprocaine can be administered and provide analgesia for several days postoperatively. Current recommendations for infusions in neonates and young infants are for an initial loading dose of 0.2 to 0.25 mg/kg of bupivacaine; after 1 to 2 hours, an infusion can be begun in a dose of 0.2 mg/kg/hr.[73] The addition of clonidine, 1 to 2 µg/kg, to local anesthetic for caudal block has been used, but may not enhance analgesia.[132] Opioids can also be used for epidural infusions. However, caution must be exercised in neonates and infants who may be prone to apnea with even moderate doses of opioids in the epidural space. Ultrasonography can be used for localization of the caudal space in infants whose anatomy may not be apparent.[130]

Epidural Analgesia

With the introduction of newer and smaller needles and epidural catheters, we are able to provide epidural analgesia in neonates and infants. Although some practitioners prefer using a caudal route to place catheters in the epidural space, lumbar and thoracic epidural catheters can be easily placed in neonates.[133] Ultrasound or fluoroscopy can be used to provide additional reassurance of successful placement into the epidural space. It is imperative to limit the dose of local anesthetic solution in neonates and children to avoid toxicity.

Peripheral Nerve Blocks

Common peripheral nerve blocks in neonates include penile blocks, ilioinguinal nerve blocks, lateral femoral cutaneous blocks, transversus abdominis plane (TAP) blocks, brachial plexus blocks, and head and neck blocks for neurosurgical procedures.

Penile Block

This is a relatively simple block that can be performed easily. The dorsal nerves of the penis are located on either side of the shaft of the penis. A ring block using local anesthetic without epinephrine can be used to provide analgesia following circumcision.[134] The dorsal penile nerves may also be approached more proximally, using the pubic symphysis as the primary landmark and injecting the nerves at approximately the 2 o'clock position and 10 o'clock position if the pubic symphysis is at the 12 o'clock position. Because the penis is innervated by the two dorsal penile nerves which are branches of the bilateral pudendal nerves and also inntervated by the perineal nerves which are also branches of the pudendal nerves, the ventral surface of the penis may need a ring block with care to avoid the urethra for complete block of the penis. All of these techniques have also been described with ultrasound.[135]

Ilioinguinal Nerve Block

The ilioinguinal and iliohypogastric nerves supply sensory innervation to the inguinal area. These nerves can be easily visualized

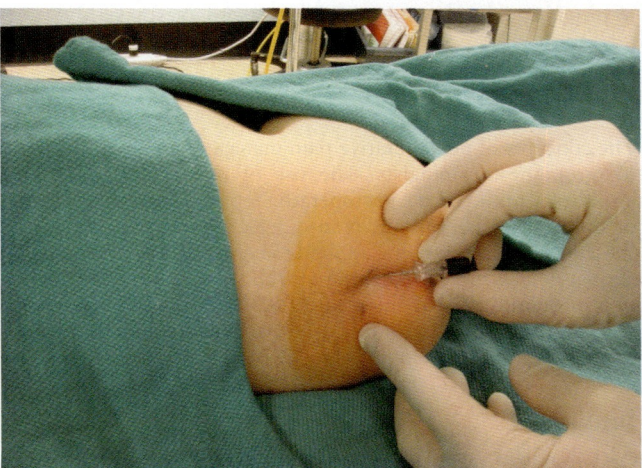

Figure 42-11 Caudal block. The sacral cornua are identified. A stylletted needle is introduced into the caudal space through the sacral hiatus. A "pop" is felt as the sacrococcygeal ligament is accessed. After aspiration, 0.8 to 1 mL/kg of local anesthetic solution is injected. This provides analgesia for hernia repair, circumcisions, and lower abdominal surgeries.

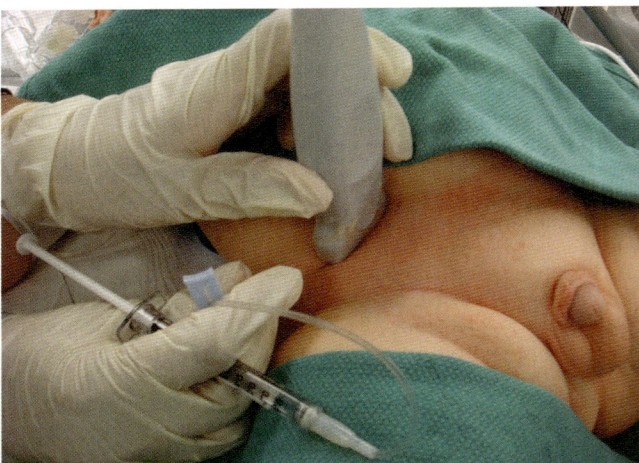

Figure 42-12 Ilioinguinal nerve block. Using a linear ultrasound probe, the anterior superior iliac spine is identified. The layers of the abdomen including the external oblique, transversus abdominis, and iliacus muscles are identified. The ilioinguinal and iliohypogastric nerves are located under the internal oblique muscle and in the plane between the internal oblique and the transversus abdominis muscle. A 27-gauge needle is inserted under ultrasound guidance in this plane. After aspiration, 0.075 to 0.1 mL/kg of local anesthetic solution is injected. This block can be used for pain relief following hernia surgery.

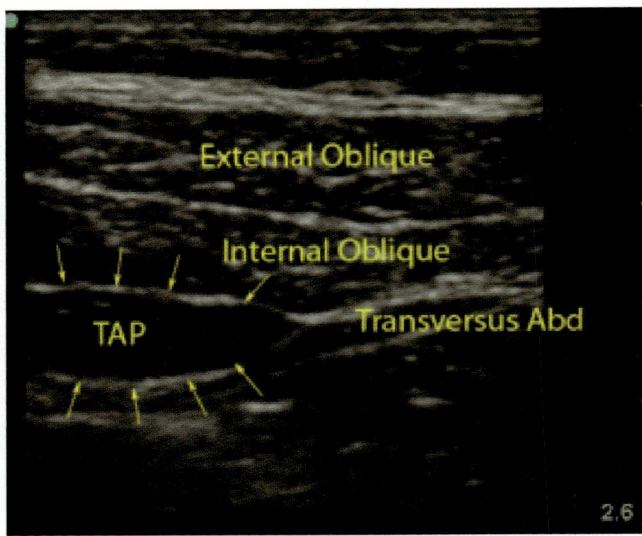

Figure 42-13 TAP (transversus abdominis plane) block using a linear ultrasound probe with a small footprint (25 mm), the abdominal wall is scanned from medial to lateral, the three layers of the abdominal muscles are recognized, a needle is inserted into the space between the internal oblique and the transversus abdominis muscle while hydro-dissecting to find the plane, 0.5 mL/kg of 0.125% bupivacaine is injected into each side to provide analgesia for the abdominal wall.

while operating. However, we find that blockade of these nerves can provide adequate postoperative analgesia (Fig. 42-12). The anterior superior iliac spine is identified. Immediately medial to the anterior superior iliac spine, a needle is inserted toward the umbilicus and local anesthesia is fanned into the area. The advantage with the use of ultrasonography is the ability to significantly reduce the dose of local anesthesia.[72] In fact, that study found the volume for ilioinguinal nerve block can be effectively reduced to 0.075 mL/kg of local anesthetic solution.

TAP Block

The TAP is a virtual space that exists between the internal oblique and the transversus abdominis muscle. This plane carries the thoracolumbar fibers from T8 to L1 (Fig. 42-13). This block has successfully been used to provide analgesia for infants and neonates undergoing major abdominal surgery, including colostomy placement.[136] This block provides cutaneous pain relief following abdominal procedures but does not provide visceral pain relief. It is a safe block in neonates with no evidence of toxicity.[137]

Lateral Femoral Cutaneous Nerve Block

The lateral femoral cutaneous nerve is a sensory branch of the lumbar plexus that supplies cutaneous innervation over the lateral aspect of the thigh. This block is particularly useful in neonates who undergo muscle biopsies of the lateral thigh.[125]

Brachial Plexus Block

This is performed for major limb surgery including major hand and arm surgical procedures. Using ultrasonography during the axillary approach to identify each branch of the brachial plexus allows selective block of each nerve,[138] thus reducing the total dose of local anesthetic. A single shot supraclavicular approach to the brachial plexus can also be used for providing analgesia for upper extremity surgery. It is important to visualize using ultrasonography because the pleura is relatively close to the area of interest and injection. For sustained pain relief, an infraclavicular catheter may be used and is easily held in place by additional muscle and fascial layers which make this a preferable approach to catheter placement for upper extremity surgery.[139]

Neurosurgical Blocks

Peripheral nerve blocks of the head and neck are useful for many surgical procedures. These may be useful in the sick neonate who requires a neurosurgical procedure. Peripheral nerve blocks of the trigeminal nerve and occipital nerve branches may be used to provide analgesia while avoiding general anesthesia.[140]

Postoperative Pain Management

The concepts of postoperative pain management are well known to most anesthesiologists. The use of intraoperative epidural anesthesia followed by postoperative epidural local anesthetics or opioids has been popular in older children and adults, and these techniques are being applied to neonates. In addition, most neonatologists are experienced with the intravenous administration of opioids for patient comfort. Each technique has its own risks and benefits. Commonly used systemic treatments for postoperative pain are listed in Table 42-7.

Oral Routes

Oral routes of medications have been used for decades in neonates and children for managing pain. The commonly used oral analgesics include nonsteroidal analgesics including acetaminophen (10 to 15 mg/kg) and ibuprofen (5 to 10 mg/kg), and opioids, including hydrocodone (0.1 mg/kg). There may be some pharmacogenetic changes associated with the use of codeine in infants; thus, it is falling out of favor in use across all ages.[141]

Table 42-7 Postoperative Pain Control for Neonates and Infants

Intravenous
  Opioids: morphine, fentanyl, methadone
  NSAIDs: ketorolac, ibuprofen
  Acetaminophen
Oral
  Acetaminophen
  Ibuprofen
  Hydrocodone
  Oxycodone
  Codeine
Rectal
  Acetaminophen
  Diclofenac
Regional and local anesthesia

NSAIDs, nonsteroidal anti-inflammatory drugs.

Rectal Routes

Rectal suppositories are used frequently in neonates and infants for managing pyrexia. Rectal acetaminophen is commonly used for postoperative analgesia. A larger dose than is usually given orally is needed in infants to achieve good blood levels, because of unreliable absorption. A dose of 20 to 30 mg/kg of rectal acetaminophen is generally recommended for postoperative pain control. Diclofenac, a commonly available rectal suppository in Europe, is frequently used in infants for postoperative pain control.

Intravenous Analgesia

Opioids are the mainstay of analgesia in neonates and infants in the postoperative period. Morphine and fentanyl are frequently used in the neonatal intensive care unit for analgesia. However, the potential for opioid tolerance after prolonged infusion of opioids is somewhat common. To decrease the likelihood of opioid tolerance,[44] one can rotate opioids or add other medications including continuous intravenous naloxone[142] and intravenous methadone. Other intravenous nonsteroidal anti-inflammatory medications and intravenous acetaminophen, have been introduced. Although not FDA approved for use in neonates, it has been gaining great interest in children for analgesia.[143] It is common to use decreased doses in neonates, 10 mg/kg, whereas the usual dose in older children is 15 mg/kg. Intravenous ketorolac, a nonsteroidal anti-inflammatory drug, has been used successfully in neonates and infants for pain control at a dose of 0.5 mg/kg.[144]

Postoperative Ventilation

The choice of an anesthetic drug should be guided by the need for postoperative management of ventilation, as well as the drug's effects on the circulation and other organs. If the surgical procedure or the neonate's condition is such that postoperative ventilation is likely, the prolonged respiratory effects of opioids or any other drug are of little concern. However, if the surgical procedure is relatively short and by itself does not require postoperative ventilation, the clinician should carefully select drugs, as well as doses of anesthetic drugs and relaxants, that will not necessitate prolonged postoperative ventilation or intubation. Postoperative ventilation places the neonate at added risk because of the problems associated with mechanical ventilation, the trauma to the subglottic area, and the potential development of postoperative subglottic stenosis or edema. However, if there is any question about the neonate's ability to maintain protective airway reflexes or normal ventilation after anesthesia, the neonate should be returned to the recovery room or neonatal intensive care unit with the trachea intubated, with controlled mechanical ventilation.

Special Considerations

Maternal Drug Use during Pregnancy

Many drugs taken during pregnancy can affect the fetus and neonate. One area of special concern is substance abuse. During pregnancy, maternal drug use of cocaine, marijuana, and others leads to a host of problems for the neonate. Cocaine use, for instance, results in a reduced catecholamine reuptake, which may result in the accumulation of catecholamines. This accumulation has circulatory effects on the uterus, the umbilical blood vessels, and the fetal cardiovascular system. Three major problems affecting the infant are premature birth, intrauterine growth retardation, and cardiovascular abnormalities, including low cardiac output.[145] The cardiac output and stroke volume are reduced on the first day of life but return to normal by the second day. The clinical implication of this finding is that these neonates may be unstable enough in the first day of life that it may be advantageous to postpone surgery, if possible, until the second or third day of life. There is also an increase in structural cardiovascular malformations and electrocardiographic abnormalities. The most frequent lesions are peripheral pulmonary stenosis, right ventricular conduction delay, right ventricular hypertrophy, and ST segment and T-wave changes.[146] Preanesthetic history should elicit the use of drugs, including illicit use, if possible, to evaluate potential alteration of the anesthetic approach.

Temperature Control and Thermogenesis

The newborn is at risk for significant metabolic derangements caused by hypothermia. Newborns, and especially preterms, do not have the normal compensatory mechanisms that infants and children have when exposed to a cold environment. The newborn does not shiver, increase activity, or effectively vasoconstrict like older children or adults do in response to cold. In addition, the newborn has a larger body surface area-to-weight ratio that promotes heat loss, as well as low levels of subcutaneous fat for insulation. The primary mechanism the newborn has to respond to heat loss is nonshivering thermogenesis.[147] When there is a 2-degree centigrade gradient between core and skin, there is a release of norepinephrine into the bloodstream. Norepinephrine stimulates increased metabolism in a specialized tissue, brown fat, which contains a high concentration of mitochondria and has abundant vascular supply. Stimulated lipolysis results in heat production, with side effects of increased oxygen consumption and production of ketone bodies and water. Ketone production causes both a metabolic acidosis and osmotic diuresis. The aerobic activity results in diversion of cardiac output to the deposits of brown fat around the kidneys, under the sternum, and between the scapulae. Because the diuresis, diversion of cardiac output away from the core circulation, and metabolic acidosis are maladaptive, every effort should be made to prevent nonshivering thermogenesis in the newborn.

Efforts to minimize nonshivering thermogenesis in the newborn are based on minimizing heat loss, both during transport to and from the neonatal intensive care unit and in the operating room. Transport should be done with the newborn in an incubator or in an open bed with overhead heaters. This will prevent heat loss from conduction and radiation. In the operating room, the room temperature is raised to its maximal level to minimize loss by conduction. Placing the patient on a forced-air warming blanket can reduce conductive heat loss. Using plastic wrap or commercially available covers and hats to minimize heat loss from the head and all other areas not in the surgical field is also beneficial. The goal of all these activities is to maintain a neutral thermal environment, minimizing the stress that hypothermia can induce in the perioperative period. A complicating factor is that anesthetic agents can reduce or eliminate thermogenesis, removing any ability to compensate for cold stress.[148]

Respiratory Distress Syndrome

Because of the enormous technical ability of the neonatologist and the resources of neonatal intensive care units, many small infants survive and some will require surgery. One of the frequent problems of preterm infants is the occurrence of the RDS secondary to a deficiency of surfactant. As discussed earlier, the use of exogenous surfactant has been widely used in premature infants of low birth weight either to prevent or to treat RDS. As a result, fewer infants now die of this entity, and the incidence of complications related to RDS has dropped. One of the long-term consequences of RDS is BPD. BPD refers to a continuum of chronic disease of the lung parenchyma and airways, as well as neurodevelopment that occurs in preterm infants, especially those born under 32 weeks' gestation, who have survived RDS.[149] The theories of the cause of this condition include toxicity from oxygen administration, infection, inflammation, and barotrauma. Characteristics include airway smooth muscle hyperplasia, peribronchiolar fibrosis, enlarged alveoli, and disorganized pulmonary vasculature. Many patients improve as they age, but reactive airways, recurrent pulmonary infections, and a prolonged oxygen requirement are seen in some patients. Anesthetic concerns in these patients include evaluation of baseline oxygenation and potential presence of active bronchoconstriction. These patients often benefit from prophylactic bronchodilator therapy before induction. The baseline measure of oxygenation is important because these patients have less pulmonary oxygen reserve and may desaturate quickly with induction of anesthesia and hypoventilation. In patients with severe BPD, ventilatory management may be complicated by poor lung compliance and hyperinflation, as well as reactive airway disease. Although postanesthetic ventilation is not usually required, a high index of suspicion should be used if there is significant clinical evidence of poor lung function preoperatively.

Postoperative Apnea

Apnea and bradycardia are well-recognized, major complications during and after surgery in neonates. The infants at highest risk are those born prematurely, those with multiple congenital anomalies, those with a history of apnea and bradycardia, and those with chronic lung disease. The etiology of neonatal apnea is multifactorial. Decreased ventilatory control and decreased responsiveness to hypoxia and hypercarbia may be potentiated by anesthetic agents. Respiratory muscle fatigue may also play a role because neonates have a smaller percentage of type I fibers in their diaphragm and intercostal muscles. In addition, hypothermia and anemia also contribute to the development of postoperative apnea.[150] The treatment of postoperative apnea or bradycardia may be as simple as tactile stimulation. However, some infants require mask ventilation or even prolonged intubation and ventilatory support. Infants with life-threatening apnea and bradycardia before surgery may be receiving CNS stimulants. Caffeine and theophylline (metabolized to caffeine) act by increasing central respiratory drive and lowering the threshold of response to hypercarbia, as well as stimulating contractility in the diaphragm. Caffeine is favored because of its wider therapeutic margin and decreased propensity for toxicity. Administering caffeine prophylactically to infants at risk of postoperative apnea to ensure adequate serum levels may prevent the need for prolonged periods of postoperative ventilatory support. The recommended loading dose is 10 mg/kg caffeine.[151] Spinal anesthesia may reduce the risk of early postoperative apnea, but does not reliably decrease the overall risk of postoperative apnea in premature infants.

The question remains as to which infant should be admitted and monitored after outpatient surgery and for how long. The most conservative approach is to monitor all infants younger than 60 weeks' postconceptual age overnight after surgery. Although the incidence of significant apnea and bradycardia is highest in the first 4 to 6 hours after surgery, it can occur up to 12 hours after surgery. In addition, the incidence of apnea directly correlates to postconceptual age. The risk of apnea goes up the younger the gestational age at birth. An insightful approach to interpreting the various small studies is to stratify the risk of apnea, as done by Cote et al.[150] Using a meta-analysis, the study determined that the risk of apnea could be correlated with a combination of gestational age and postconceptual age. Using 95% confidence limits, the authors found that the probability of apnea in nonanemic infants free of recovery room apnea was not less than 5% until postconceptual age was 48 weeks with gestational age of 35 weeks. This risk was not less than 1%, until a postconceptual age of 56 weeks with a gestational age of 32 weeks or a postconceptual age of 54 weeks and gestational age of 35 weeks. This type of analysis allows the clinician to determine which patients should be admitted on not only the criteria of gestational and postconceptual ages but also the amount of risk they are willing to assume.

Retinopathy of Prematurity

As the survival rate of increasingly preterm infants has grown, there is increasing concern about the development of ROP. The very preterm infant, especially those under 1,200 g of weight, are at highest risk, with an incidence of significant disease about 2%. Acute retinal changes are seen in about 45% of susceptible preterm neonates, but there is spontaneous regression in most, permitting development of normal vision. Other infants will progress to a severe form of ROP and potentially permanent blindness. Several complex factors may be responsible for the development of ROP. In the fetus, developing blood vessels grow gradually from the macula toward the edges of the developing retina. In full-term newborns, this process is complete at birth or in the first few weeks, but continues for a longer period in the preterm infant. These growing vessels are at risk for vasoconstriction and subsequent hemorrhage, followed by disorganized neovascularization or scarring. This scarring and lack of normal growth can eventually cause the retinal network to peel away resulting in retinal detachment. The spectrum or stages of disease is classified as follows:

Stage I. Mildly abnormal blood vessel growth. Many children who develop stage I improve with no treatment and eventually develop normal vision.

Stage II. Moderately abnormal blood vessel growth. Many children who develop stage II improve with no treatment and eventually develop normal vision. The disease resolves on its own without further progression.

Stage III. Severely abnormal blood vessel growth. The abnormal blood vessels grow toward the center of the eye instead of following their normal growth pattern along the surface of the retina. Some infants who develop stage III disease improve with no treatment and eventually develop normal vision. However, when infants have a certain degree of stage III and "plus disease" develops, treatment is considered. Plus disease means that the blood vessels of the retina have become enlarged and twisted, indicating a worsening of the disease. Treatment at this point provides a good chance of preventing retinal detachment.

Stage IV. Partially detached retina.

Stage V. Completely detached retina.

The most common cited cause of ROP is hyperoxia from administered oxygen, but hypoxemia, hypotension, sepsis, intraventricular hemorrhage, and other stresses have been implicated. At one time, there was concern that exposure to bright ambient light could cause ROP, but this has been disproven.[152] Although there may be spontaneous regression in early stages, there may also be progression to advanced stages and retinal detachment. The most common therapies involve using cryotherapy or laser therapy to destroy peripheral areas of the retina, slowing or reversing the abnormal growth of blood vessels. This is done to preserve the central vision from continuing distortion of the abnormal vessels in the periphery, although there is some loss of peripheral vision with this therapy.[153] In advanced stages, partial retinal detachment can be treated with a scleral buckle or vitrectomy.

Cryotherapy and laser therapies, as well as advanced procedures, are usually performed under general anesthesia in the operating room, although it is occasionally done at bedside with sedation in ventilated patients. These surgical procedures do not involve blood loss or significant surgical stress, but they do depend on a still surgical field for periods ranging from 30 to 90 minutes. The primary anesthetic challenge in these patients is related to the extreme prematurity and small size of the patients. Adequate monitoring, vascular access, and thermal stability are common challenges to management.

The risks of the development of ROP from hyperoxia have been of concern to anesthesiologists who anesthetize preterm infants for any type of surgery. Whether supplemental oxygen during anesthesia contributes to development of ROP has been a long-standing question in neonatal anesthesia. There is no direct answer to this question, but some evidence from a large collaborative study helps provide some guidance. Premature infants with confirmed early stages of ROP and a median pulse oximetry below 94% saturation were randomized to a conventional oxygen arm with pulse oximetry targeted at 89% to 94% saturation or a supplemental arm with pulse oximetry targeted at 96% to 99% saturation for at least 2 weeks.[154] The patients were then re-examined for progression of disease. Use of supplemental oxygen at pulse oximetry saturations of 96% to 99% did not cause additional progression of pre-threshold ROP. This study demonstrates that the use of supplemental oxygen for a prolonged period of time, not just for the short duration of a general anesthetic, was not deleterious as long as the pulse oximetry readings were kept in the 96% to 99% range. Consequently, keeping pulse oximetry readings in this range during an anesthetic should not be responsible for causing a progression of ROP in susceptible patients.

Neurodevelopmental Effects of Anesthetic Agents

There has been recent concern about the potential deleterious impact of anesthetic drugs on the developing brain. A variety of studies have shown that prolonged exposure of animal models to anesthetic agents can lead to neurodegenerative changes in the developing brain of neonatal rats.[155] However, these exposures to volatile agents and ketamine were for prolonged periods, the equivalent of several weeks of continuous exposure in the human. Nonetheless, this is an area of great concern for anesthesiologists.[156] Animal experiments have demonstrated neurocognitive changes in animals exposed to NMDA receptor antagonists like ketamine, volatile agents like isoflurane, as well as other agents including midazolam. The collective data that are currently available in literature do not support the withdrawal of these drugs from the practice of neonatal anesthesia. There has been a general recommendation to delay nonurgent surgery in children under 3 years of age made by the FDA/IARS public/private partnership SmartTots[157]; however, neonatal surgical problems cannot usually be delayed safely for years.

The neurotoxicity data seem to be reproducible in rodents but not in other species. Future prospective trials with prospective neurocognitive testing of infants exposed to anesthesia are needed. There currently exists no conclusive evidence to demonstrate the deleterious effect of inhaled or intravenous anesthetics on neurocognitive function in neonates and infants. Prospective studies, including a current study randomizing infants to getting a spinal anesthesia versus general anesthesia should be able to provide better information on this very complex problem that may face pediatric anesthesiologists. Early results from a prospective randomized general anesthesia and spinal study (GAS) has demonstrated no significant differences in neurocognitive outcomes in infants undergoing short procedures like hernia repair.[158] Several retrospective studies including data about children from a particular county in Minnesota has some data to lead to believe that there may be an association with the development of learning disability especially when exposed to multiple anesthetics before 2 years of age.[159] Although the data generated a lot of interest, it is important to understand that we need more concrete data and prospective studies to demonstrate that there are indeed clinically apparent neurocognitive changes associated with exposure to anesthesia in neonates and infants.

Surgical Procedures in Neonates

Surgical procedures in neonates are functionally divided into two periods: those performed in the first week and those performed in the first month. There has been a strong trend in recent years to put an emphasis of presurgical stabilization before taking the newborn to the operating room. This has reduced the emergent nature of newborn surgeries. Many procedures that used to be done on an emergent basis, even in the middle of the night, such as repair of CDH or omphalocele, are now done days later, after initial therapy has been instituted. Exceptions to this include gastroschisis, which is usually corrected within 12 to 24 hours, airway lesions such as webs that are causing significant airway obstruction, and acute subdural/epidural hematomas from traumatic delivery. In most cases, however, a period of 1 to 3 days can be allowed for stabilization of the newborn or transport to an appropriate pediatric center for treatment. There is more to neonatal emergency surgery than just the immediate anesthetic and surgical procedures. Many of these infants require the support services of specialized nursing units, pediatric radiologists, pediatric intensive care physicians, specialized laboratory facilities, and they must have their complete care be the main consideration of where their surgery should be done. Many procedures are now performed using laparoscopic techniques which decreases postoperative morbidity and pain and facilitates early extubation.

Surgical Procedures in the First Week of Life

The most frequent major surgical procedures performed in the first week of life are for CDH, omphalocele and gastroschisis, tracheoesophageal fistula (TEF), intestinal obstruction, and myelomeningocele. Some of these conditions, such as CDH, omphalocele and gastroschisis, and myelomeningocele, are obvious at birth. It may take hours or days for a TEF or intestinal obstruction to manifest. Because of the lack of expertise many hospitals have in the care of these patients, the transfer of these neonates to hospitals with greater expertise is often prudent after initial stabilization of the patient. Most hospitals that have expertise in these patients have a transport team that is well-qualified to help with stabilization and transport. Those centers that do not have transport teams often have extensive protocols and procedures to work with the sending institution to help ensure the safe transfer of the patient.

Two confounding factors in neonatal surgery are prematurity and associated congenital anomalies. The presence of one congenital anomaly increases the likelihood of another one. In conditions such as TEF, the mortality rate from an associated congenital heart defect is higher than that from the surgical correction of the TEF. Prematurity, particularly when associated with RDS, may adversely affect surgical outcome. The use of surfactant in the treatment of the RDS has greatly increased the number of survivors and has decreased the complexity of the issues of the infant with a combination of TEF and RDS. A neonatologist should be consulted in the case of any neonate with a congenital defect who is considered for surgery. The most serious associated congenital lesion is that of the cardiovascular system. More than 10% of infants with CDH have a cardiac anomaly,[160] with a higher incidence in newborns with associated syndromes, and approximately 15% to 25% of infants with TEF have an associated congenital cardiac anomaly.[161]

Congenital Diaphragmatic Hernia

CDH occurs with an incidence of approximately 1 in 4,000 live births. Traditionally, the mortality rate from CDH was in the range of 40% to 50%. The new strategy of permissive hypercapnia and delayed surgical repair has resulted in survival rates of more than 75% in some centers.[162] However, the morbidity remains high in survivors. A brief discussion of the embryologic characteristics of CDH will help the clinician understand the potentially enormous postoperative problems that may be encountered.

Embryology

Early in fetal development, the pleuroperitoneal cavity is a single compartment. The gut is herniated or extruded to the extraembryonic coelom during the ninth to tenth weeks of fetal life. During this period, the diaphragm develops to separate the thoracic and abdominal cavities (Fig. 42-14). The development of the diaphragm is usually completed by the seventh fetal week. In the ninth to tenth weeks, the developing gut returns to the peritoneal cavity. If there is delay or incomplete closure of the diaphragm, or if the gut returns early and prevents normal closure of the diaphragm, a diaphragmatic hernia will develop, producing varying degrees of herniation of the abdominal contents into the chest. The left side of the diaphragm closes later than the right side, which results in the higher incidence of left-sided diaphragmatic hernias (foramen of Bochdalek). Approximately, 90% of hernias detected in the first week of life are on the left side.

Clinical Presentation

The clinical presentation and the outcome from a diaphragmatic hernia are varied. The bowel contents may compress the lung buds and prevent development, leading to bilateral hypoplastic lungs with very little chance for survival. In most instances, however, a moderately small diaphragmatic hernia may develop later in fetal life so the lung is normal but compressed by the abdominal viscera. At the mild end of the scale, the infant might have a relatively normal pulmonary vascular bed with varying degrees of persistent pulmonary hypertension that may rapidly revert to normal. In more severe defects, significant pulmonary hypoplasia and abnormal pulmonary vasculature lead to greater mortality, largely a result of ongoing pulmonary hypertension.

After closure of the pleuroperitoneal membrane, muscular development of the diaphragm occurs. Incomplete muscularization of the diaphragm results in the development of a hernia sac because of intra-abdominal pressure. The condition is known as eventration of the diaphragm, and the diaphragm may extend well up into the thoracic cavity. The other possibility is that the innervation of the diaphragm is incomplete and the muscle is atonic. Eventration of the diaphragm is usually not symptomatic in the first week of life.

Antenatal Diagnosis

The diagnosis of CDH can be made prenatally by fetal ultrasonography or fetal magnetic resonance imaging. Antenatal diagnosis has led to the identification of a "hidden mortality" in CDH, fetuses who did not survive gestation and neonates who died before diagnosis. Various factors have been proposed to identify

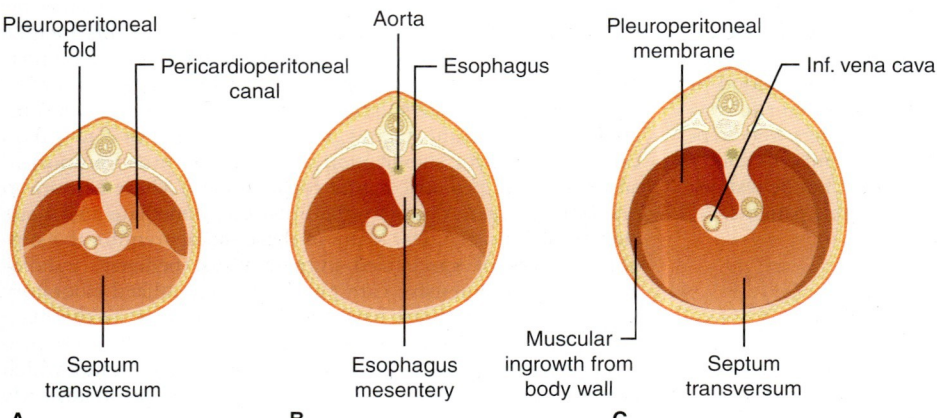

Figure 42-14 Schematic drawings illustrating the development of the diaphragm. **A:** The pleuroperitoneal folds appear at the beginning of the sixth week. **B:** The pleuroperitoneal folds have fused with the septum transversum and the mesentery of the esophagus in the seventh week, thus separating the thoracic cavity from the abdominal cavity. **C:** In a transverse section at the fourth month of development, an additional rim derived from the body wall forms the most peripheral part of the diaphragm. (Adapted from Langman J. Body cavities and serous membranes. In: Sadler TW, ed. *Langman's Medical Embryology*. 5th ed. Baltimore, MD: Williams & Wilkins; 1985:147.)

predictability of survival, including early gestation diagnosis, severe mediastinal shift, polyhydramnios, a small lung-to-thorax transverse area ratio, and the herniation of liver or stomach. New techniques in fetal surgery, such as temporary endoscopic fetal tracheal occlusion, may prove beneficial to fetuses with CDH who are identified to be at risk for not surviving to term.[163] The other obvious advantage of prenatal diagnosis is that plans can be made for maternal or neonatal transport to a center with advanced neonatal critical care with availability of ECMO. Early repair, on ECMO, or delayed repair with treatment of pulmonary hypertension on ECMO prior to repair remains an area of controversy, with literature in support of both approaches.[164,165] However, it is clear that introduction of ECMO has improved survival compared to historical data.[166]

Clinical Presentation

The occurrence of symptoms depends on the degree of herniation and interference with pulmonary function. At times, the degree of interference is so great that the neonate's clinical condition begins to deteriorate immediately and, in other situations, it may be several hours before the infant's condition is fully appreciated. In the severely affected newborn, the initial clinical findings are usually classic and readily discerned. The infant has a scaphoid abdomen secondary to the absence of intra-abdominal contents, which have herniated into the chest. Breath sounds on the affected side are reduced or absent. The diagnosis can be confirmed with a radiograph (Fig. 42-15). Immediate supportive care entails tracheal intubation and control of the airway along with decompression of the stomach. Excessive airway pressure carries a high risk for pneumothorax before and after the repair.

Preoperative Care

CDH was traditionally treated as a surgical emergency. The infants were taken immediately to surgery for decompression and repair. The thought was that removing the abdominal viscera from the thorax would allow for re-expansion of the atelectatic lung and improved oxygenation. However, as the pathophysiology of CDH was more clearly defined—pulmonary hypoplasia associated with a hyperreactive and hypoplastic pulmonary vasculature—a strategy of preoperative stabilization with delayed surgical repair was adopted.

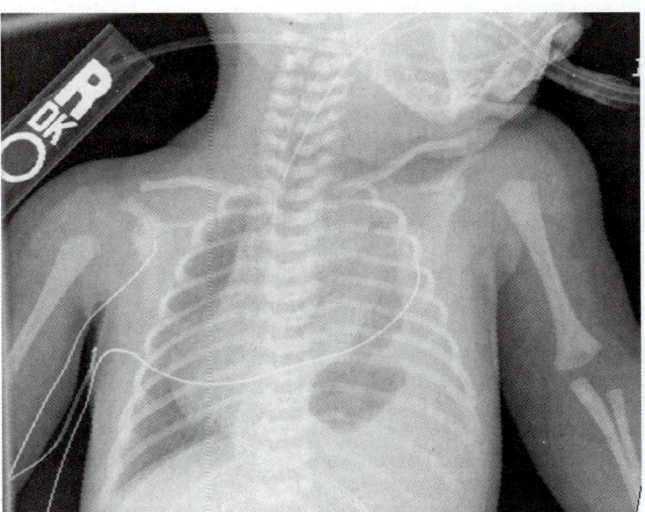

Figure 42-15 Infant with left-sided congenital diaphragmatic hernia. Note the loop of bowel gas in left hemithorax.

The stabilization of an infant with CDH may require multiple treatment modalities. The use of aggressive ventilation strategies to induce respiratory alkalosis has been abandoned secondary to the high incidence of iatrogenic lung injury. Conventional ventilation with permissive hypercapnia is now favored. The goal is to maintain preductal arterial saturation above 85% using peak inspiratory pressures below 25 cm H_2O and allowing the PCO_2 to rise to 45 to 55 mmHg.[162] High-frequency oscillatory ventilation, in addition to nitric oxide, has been used in place of conventional ventilation in an attempt to reduce barotrauma and has been demonstrated to be beneficial.[167] Neonates born with CDH may also have a component of surfactant deficiency, and studies have shown improvement in oxygenation in those infants given surfactant prophylactically. These have been well demonstrated in animal experiments when compared with tracheal ligation.[168]

The use of ECMO in infants with CDH was initiated in the mid-1980s. Despite extensive literature on the subject, there remains an ongoing debate as to whether ECMO improves survival in neonates with CDH. The Congenital Diaphragmatic Hernia Study Group analyzed data from the multicenter CDH Registry and determined that ECMO improves the survival rate in CDH neonates with a predicted high risk of mortality (≥80%) based on birth weight and 5-minute Apgar score. A right-sided CDH may carry a higher mortality and morbidity compared with a left-sided defect, despite the use of ECMO.[169] Repair of a right-sided CDH can be seen in Figure 42-16.

Perioperative Care

Because delayed surgical repair of CDH is now the norm, neonates with CDH frequently present to the operating room already intubated and on some form of ventilatory support. Despite a period of preoperative stabilization, some infants still have a component of reactive pulmonary hypertension. The goals of ventilatory management are to ensure adequate oxygenation and avoid barotrauma. Any sudden deterioration in oxygen saturation with or without associated hypotension should raise suspicion of pneumothorax. It is important to avoid hypothermia because this increases the oxygen requirement and could precipitate pulmonary hypertension. Blood loss and fluid shifts are usually not a problem, although maintenance of intravascular volume is essential to avoid acidosis, which could also precipitate pulmonary hypertension. Preoperative preparation may include multimodal treatment of pulmonary hypertension with nitric oxide, sildenafil (PDE-5 inhibitor), milrinone (PDE-3 inhibitor), epoprostenol or iloprost (PGI_2 inhibitor), bosentan (endothelin inhibitor), and imatinib (platelet derived growth factor inhibitor) which have all been attempted with varying degrees of success.[170]

Anesthetic Technique

The anesthetic technique chosen depends on the size of the defect and the anticipated postoperative respiratory status. In those infants who will remain intubated after surgery, inhalation agents and narcotics may be used as tolerated. In those infants with a small defect, who present to the operating room with little or no respiratory distress, it may be beneficial to avoid intraoperative narcotics and provide regional or neuraxial analgesia in anticipation of extubation. The use of nitrous oxide should be avoided, particularly in those situations in which abdominal closure could be difficult. Muscle relaxation is often needed to facilitate abdominal closure.

Postoperative Care

Most infants with CDH require intensive postoperative care. Recovery depends on the degree of pulmonary hypertension and pulmonary hypoplasia. It was previously believed that pulmonary

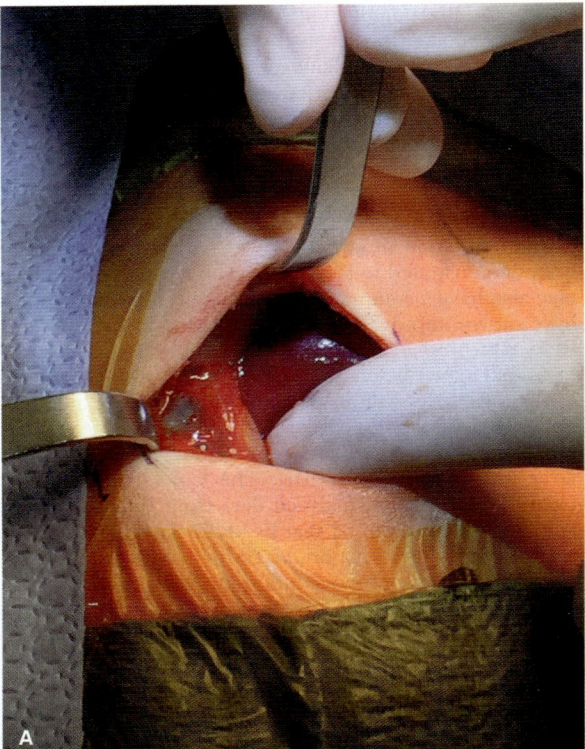 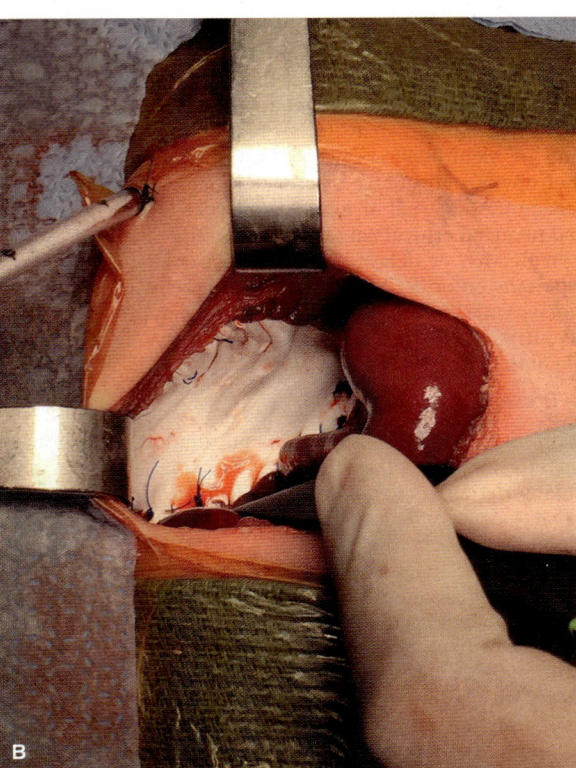

Figure 42-16 Another infant with congenital diaphragmatic hernia. In this patient, the defect is in the right diaphragm. **A:** The liver herniated into the right chest cavity. **B:** The complete repair with Gore-Tex graft material and the liver appropriately located in the abdominal cavity. (Photographs courtesy of Rashmi Kabre, MD.)

hypoplasia was responsible for most deaths; however, it is now believed that potentially reversible pulmonary hypertension may be responsible for as much as 25% of reported deaths.

There is evidence to suggest that cardiac development is impaired in infants with CDH. Relative left ventricular hypoplasia with an attenuated muscle mass and cavity size have been described.

Omphalocele and Gastroschisis

Although omphalocele and gastroschisis sometimes appear similar and may be confused, they have entirely different origins and associated congenital anomalies.[171] During the fifth to tenth weeks of fetal life, the abdominal contents are extruded into the extraembryonic coelom, and the gut returns to the abdominal cavity at approximately the tenth week. Failure of part of or all the intestinal contents to return to the abdominal cavity results in an omphalocele that is covered with a membrane called the amnion (Fig. 42-17). The amnion protects the abdominal contents from infection and the loss of ECF. The umbilical cord is found at approximately the apex of the sac. Gastroschisis, in contrast, develops later in fetal life, after the intestinal contents have returned to the abdominal cavity. It results from interruption of the omphalomesenteric artery, which results in ischemia and atrophy of the various layers of the abdominal wall at the base of the umbilical cord. The gut then herniates through this tissue defect. The degree of herniation may be slight, or major amounts of the abdominal viscera may be found outside the peritoneal cavity. The umbilical cord is found to one side of the intestinal contents (Fig. 42-18).

The intestines and viscera are not covered by any membrane and therefore are highly susceptible to infection and loss of ECF. There is a very high incidence of associated congenital anomalies with omphalocele, but much lower with gastroschisis.[172] The Beckwith–Wiedemann syndrome consists of mental retardation, hypoglycemia, congenital heart disease, a large tongue, and an

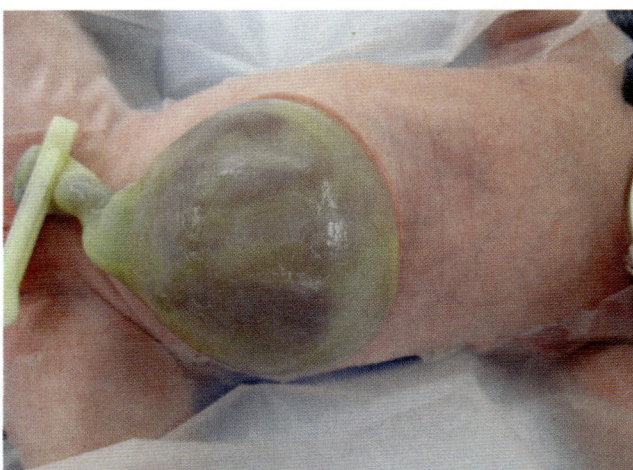

Figure 42-17 Omphalocele on day 1 of life. Note the abdominal contents covered in amnion and umbilical cord protruding from the apex of the sac. (Photograph courtesy of Matthew S. Clifton, MD, FACS, FAAP.)

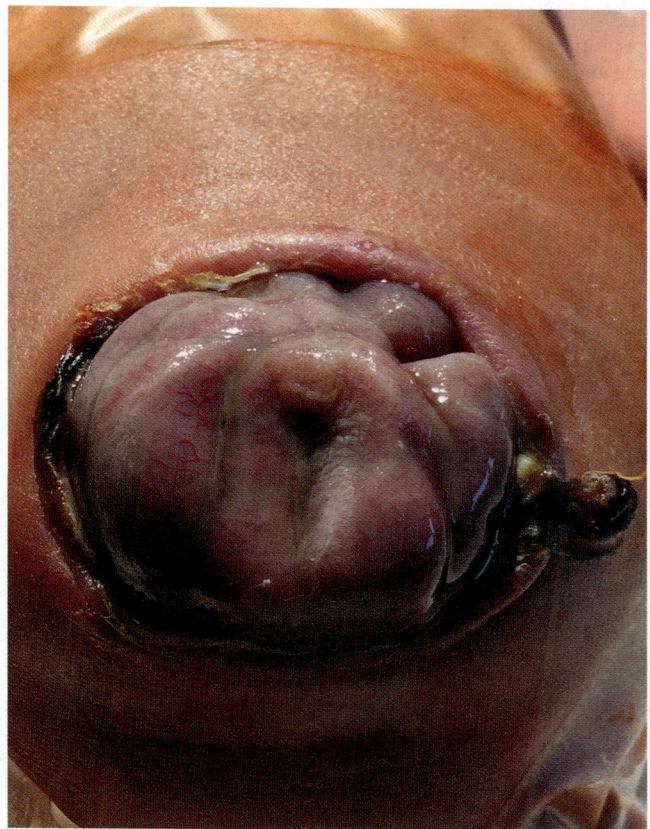

Figure 42-18 Gastroschisis. Note the umbilical cord is found to the side of the abdominal contents which are not covered in a sac. (Photograph courtesy of Linda Zekas, MSN, APN.)

omphalocele. Congenital heart lesions are found in approximately 20% of infants with omphalocele. Other associated congenital defects are found with gastroschisis and omphalocele; most involve the gastrointestinal tract and consist primarily of intestinal atresia, stenosis, or malrotation. Because of the uncovered gut irritating the uterine lining, premature delivery is more common in gastroschisis patients.

Antenatal Diagnosis

The overall incidence of these defects is about 1:5,000 live births. Screening for abdominal wall defects is accomplished through the use of maternal serum α-fetoprotein (AFP). AFP is a normal protein present in fetal tissues during fetal development. Closure of the abdominal wall and the neural tube (see "Myelomeningocele") prevents release of large quantities of this protein into the amniotic fluid. High levels of AFP in the amniotic fluid can cross the placenta and be detected in maternal blood. Thus, abnormal levels of maternal serum AFP in the mother raise concerns over the possibility of either an abdominal wall defect or a neural tube defect in the fetus, as do high levels of AFP in fluid obtained during amniocentesis. Levels tend to be higher when the defect is gastroschisis instead of omphalocele. The primary method of definitive fetal diagnosis of gastroschisis and omphalocele is ultrasonography. In a recent study, 88% of patients with gastroschisis and 69% with omphalocele were diagnosed prenatally with ultrasound.[173] An advantage of ultrasound is the ability to diagnose other complicating abnormalities, such as cardiac defects.

Preoperative Care

Most neonates with gastroschisis or omphalocele diagnosed prenatally are delivered by cesarean section. The advantages of this are the ability to prevent trauma to the exposed bowel and to allow better coordination of the various medical specialties needed for immediate surgical management of the defect. Priorities in the delivery room care unique to an infant with gastroschisis are the need to protect the exposed bowel and minimize fluid and temperature loss. An effective way to achieve these goals involves placing the defect and lower body in a sterile, clear plastic bag to protect the defect and minimize heat and fluid loss. The bag can be filled with warm saline and a drawstring can be used to tighten the bag against the infant's body.

Preoperative stabilization of the neonate with an abdominal wall defect includes management of respiratory insufficiency, establishment of adequate intravenous access, and an assessment for associated congenital anomalies. It is expected that a significantly higher incidence of congenital anomalies will be found in omphalocele patients. Respiratory failure at birth in infants with omphalocele is a significant predictor of mortality. Lung hypoplasia and abnormal thoracic development may be significant in infants with large omphaloceles. A difficult airway can be present in the patient with Beckwith–Wiedemann syndrome because of the large tongue.

Surgery is not urgent in the neonate with an omphalocele and can be delayed for several days until the infant is assessed and stabilized. In those infants with severe respiratory distress or congenital heart disease who are too unstable for surgery, nonsurgical treatment with topical antiseptics and delayed closure is an option.[174] Although there has been some interest in nonoperative, bedside-staged closure of gastroschisis defects, primary operative closure continues to be the most common approach.[175]

Perioperative Care

The two major perioperative concerns are fluid loss and ventilation. The fluid volume management of the infant often entails administration of large amounts of full-strength, balanced salt solution. The adequacy of the peripheral circulation and urine output is an indicator of the adequacy of the intravascular volume resuscitation. Both conditions may present an intraoperative challenge to the anesthesiologist because with an omphalocele, after the amniotic membrane is removed, large volumes of fluid may transude or exude from the exposed abdominal viscera. The fluid that is lost is ECF, which should be replaced with a balanced salt solution even in neonates. An arterial line is often used for blood pressure monitoring and frequent blood gas monitoring to assess acid–base status.

If the defect in the abdominal wall is small, a primary repair of the deficit can be accomplished. However, with a large defect, it may be difficult to return the abdominal viscera to the peritoneal cavity because the muscle and peritoneum are underdeveloped. Because of concern for the increase in the volume of gas in the intestine, nitrous oxide should not be used. Muscle relaxation is necessary to allow closure of the abdomen. With moderate size abdominal wall defects, it may not be possible to close the peritoneum, but there may be sufficient skin to close the defect. With large defects, the peritoneal cavity may be too small to contain the viscera, and attempted closure can impair circulation to the bowel, kidneys, and lower extremities, as well as compromise respiration. A pulse oximeter probe on the foot can be helpful in monitoring circulation to the lower extremities during abdominal wall closure.

Attempts have been made to find objective criteria by which to determine whether the infant will tolerate primary closure of the defect, and to avoid or minimize the circulatory and ventilatory problems. One method has been to measure intragastric pressure in infants who undergo primary closure. Intragastric pressure is measured by placing a nasogastric tube in the stomach and using a column of saline to measure the pressure.[176] Studies have used the criteria that if the intragastric pressure was less than 20 mmHg, primary closure can proceed. Above 20 mmHg pressures during closure, delayed closure and placement of a Dacron silo were used. With this approach, primary closure has been successful when used, with faster return to full feeds and shorter hospital length of stay compared with patients treated by delayed closure. Complications have been less with primary closure using this approach. Another method to predict successful closure of abdominal wall defects is to use central venous pressure, an increase with closure of the fascia of greater than 4 mmHg is predictive of unsuccessful primary closure.[177]

If primary closure is impossible, a silo (Fig. 42-19) is incorporated into the abdominal wall to contain and cover the abdominal viscera. The repair is then staged from this point onward. Every 2 or 3 days, the size of the silo is reduced, in much the same fashion that a tube of toothpaste is squeezed. The infant may feel some degree of discomfort as the peritoneum and skin are stretched. Institutions vary in how they accomplish the delay closure, with some surgeons bringing the patient to the operating room for each stage and others doing this at bedside, often with the assistance of small doses of ketamine or other analgesics. Some of these patients remain on mechanical ventilation during this period, and others are extubated. In either case, both blood pressure and oxygen saturation should be closely monitored during and immediately after each stage of closure to ensure that the increase in abdominal and intrathoracic pressure does not significantly impede ventilation, oxygenation, and venous return. In some cases, further reduction must be delayed until there is more abdominal growth. This is a situation that requires clinical judgment. After several stages of silo reduction, the final operation is complete closure of the abdominal wall defect under full anesthesia with complete muscle relaxation.

Postoperative Care

The postoperative care of infants with omphalocele or gastroschisis is critical. Some need tracheal intubation and assisted ventilation of the lungs for days to weeks. The ventilatory status of the patient is especially critical in omphalocele patients because up to half of these patients are born with pulmonary hypoplasia, making the balance of increased abdominal pressures and adequate ventilation and oxygenation especially challenging. Additional complications include postoperative hypertension and edema of the extremities. The increased abdominal pressure can reduce the circulation to the kidneys, which results in a release of renin. Renin activates the renin–angiotensin–aldosterone system, which is believed to cause the hypertension.

Tracheoesophageal Fistula

The treatment of esophageal atresia and TEF can be both challenging and satisfying for the anesthesiologist. Death in the perioperative period typically results from prematurity or from an associated congenital heart defect. TEF occurs in approximately 1 in 3,000 live births. Approximately 85% consist of a fistula from the distal trachea to the esophagus and a blind proximal esophageal pouch. In 10% of cases, there is a blind proximal esophageal pouch with no TEF (Fig. 42-20). The embryologic defect results from imperfect division of the foregut into the anteriorly positioned larynx and trachea and the posteriorly positioned esophagus; the division should occur between the fourth and fifth weeks of intrauterine life. Fifty percent of affected infants have associated congenital anomalies, of which approximately 15% to 25% involve the cardiovascular system.

Clinical Presentation

Atresia of the esophagus leads to inability of the fetus to swallow amniotic fluid and the subsequent development of polyhydramnios. Ultrasound may well raise the possibility of a congenital anomaly. For that reason, if polyhydramnios is present, attempts should be made to pass a nasogastric tube shortly after delivery. Passing a nasogastric tube is not routine in the delivery room;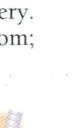

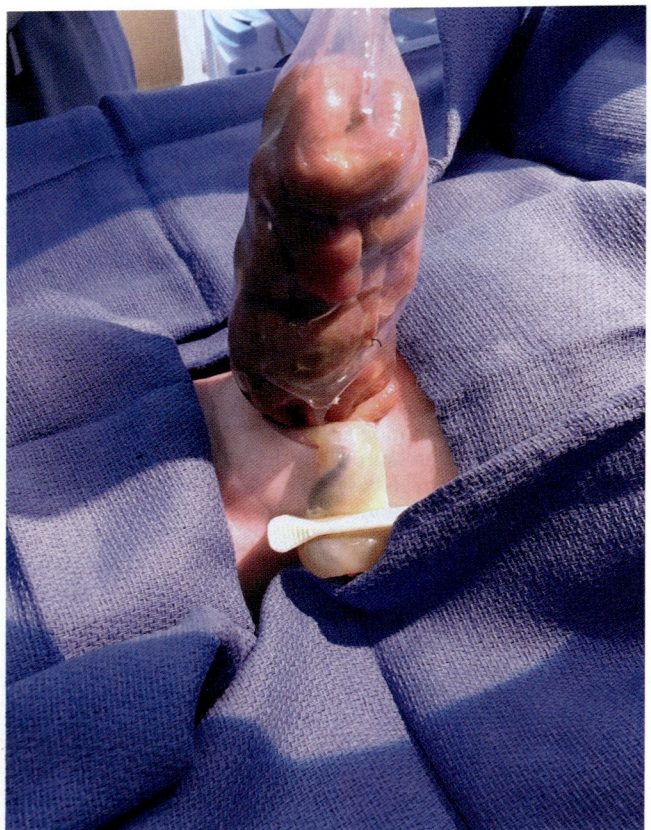

Figure 42-19 Silo placement on neonate with gastroschisis. The abdominal contents are now within a large silo, suspended above the neonate, with the umbilical cord observed protruding from one side of the defect. (Photograph courtesy of Linda Zekas, MSN, APN.)

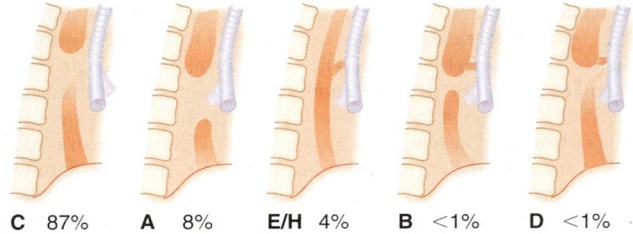

Figure 42-20 Diagrams of the five most commonly encountered forms of esophageal atresia and tracheoesophageal fistula, shown in order of frequency. (Adapted from Herbst JJ. Gastrointestinal tract. In: Behrman RE, Kleigman RM, Nelson WE, et al., eds. *Nelson's Textbook of Pediatrics*. 14th ed. Philadelphia, PA: WB Saunders; 1992:942.)

therefore, the diagnosis may not become apparent until the infant is fed. Cyanosis and choking with oral feedings should raise suspicion.

There are two major complications of esophageal atresia with a distal tracheal fistula: aspiration pneumonia and dehydration. The presence of a distal TEF increases the likelihood of reflux of gastric juice up the esophagus and into the pulmonary system. Dehydration results from the fact that the proximal esophagus does not communicate with the stomach. Therefore, preoperative preparation of these infants is aimed at evaluation and treatment of the pulmonary system, as well as at ensuring adequate hydration and electrolyte balance. Rarely, the degree of reflux and pneumonia is so great that a gastrostomy must be performed to protect the pulmonary system, and a period of several days is needed to improve the general condition of the infant. However, if the infant is in good condition, primary repair can be performed at 24 to 48 hours. This consists of ligation of the fistula and a primary repair with approximation of the two ends of the esophagus.

Anesthetic Considerations

The repair of TEF can be done in the conventional method or by using video-assisted thoracoscopic surgery (VATS) method. Both methods and the anesthetic implications for each technique will be described here. The presence of a gastrostomy reduces the potential for reflux of gastric juice during the surgical procedure. If a gastrostomy is present, the gastrostomy tube should be open to air and left at the head of the table under the anesthesiologist's observation to avoid kinking and obstruction.

Conventional Open TEF Closure. There are three approaches to tracheal intubation after induction of anesthesia. One is to use an inhalation induction, followed by topical spray of lidocaine and intubation while the infant is breathing spontaneously. Another technique is to use an intravenous or inhalation induction and intubate the trachea after muscle paralysis. This technique may lead to distention of the fistula and stomach with excessive positive-pressure ventilation. When controlled ventilation of the lungs is used, attempts must be made to minimize the distention of the stomach and the potential for reflux. If a gastrostomy tube is in place, the point is moot. A third technique is to intubate the neonates awake with mild sedation. This can protect the airway while reducing the chances of aspiration. Alternatively, because the fistula is usually located just above the carina on the posterior wall of the membranous trachea, the endotracheal tube can be placed just distal to the TEF. To do this, the endotracheal tube is inserted until it enters a main-stem bronchus. This is judged by unilateral expansion of the chest and unilateral breath sounds. The endotracheal tube is then slowly withdrawn until bilateral chest movement and breath sounds are confirmed.

The endotracheal tube might inadvertently enter the fistula when the infant is turned or during surgical manipulation. Intubation of the fistula should be suspected if there is increased difficulty in ventilation of the lungs, as well as decreased oxygen saturation and end-tidal CO_2. Because these findings may also be present when the lung is packed away to perform the surgery and because there are other explanations for these findings, intubation of the fistula should always be included in the differential diagnosis. At any time ventilation is difficult and desaturation is occurring, the surgeon must stop the procedure while the situation is clarified. The surgeon will be able to palpate the tip of the tube in the fistula if this is the problem.

The localization and isolation of H-type fistulas can be difficult. In this situation, direct laryngoscopy and bronchoscopy is performed by the surgeon, the fistula is identified, and a guidewire is fed through the fistula tract into the esophagus. The infant is then intubated, with care taken not to dislodge the guidewire. Once intubated, esophagoscopy is performed, the guidewire is visualized and brought out through the mouth. In this way, the surgeon can use fluoroscopy to determine the level of the fistula and decide whether a cervical or thoracic approach is necessary. During surgery, the anesthesiologist can apply traction to the wire loop to facilitate the localization of the fistula by the surgeon.

Endoscopic TEF Repair. The use of endoscopic methods for repair of TEF is now popular in pediatric surgery.[178] The infant should be kept spontaneously breathing until the fistula is ligated. Maintenance of spontaneous ventilation can be challenging considering that these infants may not tolerate the use of potent inhalation agents while spontaneous ventilation is established. This approach may shorten the duration of surgical operating time while providing a minimally invasive method. The anesthetic management is challenging.

Postoperative Care

Although there have been great advances in the treatment of TEF and esophageal atresia, postoperative care can be complicated by associated congenital heart disease, RDS, and a need for continued postoperative ventilation. The compression of the lung for several hours, along with pre-existing aspiration pneumonia in some of these infants, suggest the need, in the more difficult cases, for a short period of postoperative ventilation, or at least intubation with PEEP, as the most conservative technique for postoperative airway management. Some infants are in excellent condition at the time of surgery with no complicating factors and, therefore, should be considered for extubation immediately at the end of surgery or shortly thereafter. If extubation of the trachea is planned for the end of surgery, the anesthetic technique must be tailored accordingly. Neuraxial anesthesia as part of the technique is useful in these situations, reducing the concentration of maintenance volatile anesthetics, the amount of muscle relaxants, and the need for intraoperative narcotics. These catheters may remain in place after the procedure to allow for postoperative pain control with local anesthetic by continuous infusion or intermittent bolus. Another option is to place a unilateral, ultrasound-guided paravertebral block which can again provide analgesia for the hemithorax that is the operative site.[179]

A high percentage of infants with esophageal atresia have residual defects of the tracheobronchial tree and esophagus for many years. These defects include tracheomalacia, gastroesophageal reflux, esophageal stricture, and recurrent fistulas.

Intestinal Obstruction

A useful way of classifying gastrointestinal obstruction is to group lesions proximal and distal to the pylorus. Obstruction of the upper gastrointestinal tract is manifested by vomiting, especially after feeds, whereas obstruction of the lower gastrointestinal tract may present with abdominal distention, little or no stool passed, hematochezia, signs of pain, and vomiting.

Upper Gastrointestinal Tract Obstruction

The most common cause of upper gastrointestinal obstruction in the newborn is pyloric stenosis, but pyloric stenosis does not usually present in the first week of life. Other rare causes of obstruction, such as congenital webs, may occur. If there has been persistent vomiting, this usually means that a deficit of fluids or electrolytes will develop in the infant. Persistent vomiting results in the greatest deficit of sodium. Another major concern in the infant with upper gastrointestinal tract obstruction is aspiration of gastric contents.

The anesthetic management of these patients is directed toward ensuring adequate relaxation for abdominal exploration, repair of the congenital defect, and closure of the abdomen. Nitrous oxide can be used in high intestinal obstruction because there is essentially no gas in the upper gastrointestinal tract. The next concern is whether the infant's trachea should be extubated at the end of surgery. If the infant is robust, extubation of the trachea at the end of surgery can be anticipated. The preferred technique is for general anesthesia combined with neuraxial anesthesia. This allows light levels of volatile agent and minimal muscle relaxant use, and results in early extubation. Opioids may be administered, although the impact on the ability to ventilate at the end of the procedure should be considered. If the infant is moderately debilitated or if the surgical incision is extensive, a period of postoperative ventilation may well be indicated, particularly if moderate doses of opioids have been used.

Lower Gastrointestinal Tract Obstruction

Intestinal obstruction in the newborn can result from a variety of lesions. These include imperforate anus, duodenal atresia, jejunoileal atresia (Fig. 42-21), intussusception, malrotation, volvulus, choledochal cyst, or meconium ileus. Although these are all different in etiology, their presentation is similar. The problems associated with lower gastrointestinal tract obstruction usually develop within 1 to 7 days after birth. It may take this long for the lesion to become evident because it is low in the gastrointestinal tract. An imperforate anus should be recognizable shortly after birth. However, once intestinal obstruction is diagnosed in the newborn, it becomes a surgical emergency as these patients may deteriorate rapidly. Some of these infants may have vomiting secondary to the obstruction, which poses a problem for fluid and electrolyte management. An enormous amount of fluid can be sequestered within the intestinal tract. This fluid is essentially ECF and has high sodium content. Therefore, these infants should be prepared expeditiously for surgery and have a serum sodium level of at least 130 mEq/L as well as a urine output of 1 to 2 mL/kg/hr. In addition to fluid and electrolyte disturbances, delayed diagnosis or treatment of these patients can result in increased abdominal pressure, leading to respiratory embarrassment from pressure on the diaphragm and aspiration pneumonitis, as well as sepsis. Finally, some of these conditions are associated with other congenital anomalies that complicate preanesthetic evaluation and anesthetic management.[180] Duodenal atresia, for instance, can be associated with trisomy 21, cystic fibrosis, imperforate anus, or renal abnormalities.

The preanesthetic evaluation and perioperative management is similar for all these lesions. Preanesthetic evaluation is focused on the stabilization of fluid and electrolyte status, ensuring adequate oxygenation and ventilation, hemodynamic support if the patient is septic, and identification of complicating issues such as other congenital abnormalities.

In the operating room, the need for invasive arterial and central venous monitoring is determined by the current status of the patient and the urgency of the procedure. The primary anesthetic considerations are the same as those in the preoperative period, including ongoing fluid and electrolyte resuscitation. Because these cases are usually emergent and there may be associated vomiting and abdominal distention, either an awake intubation or rapid-sequence induction and intubation is indicated. Although awake intubation may be the best approach if the patient has a probable difficult airway or has hemodynamic decompensation, a rapid-sequence induction and intubation after preoxygenation is the approach normally taken. Any induction agent can be used if judicious doses are chosen, but ketamine or etomidate are often chosen because of a concern about cardiovascular instability.

Anesthetic agents for maintenance during these cases are chosen on the basis of the patient's status and the likely surgical course. Nitrous oxide should not be used in any infant who has gaseous distention of the intestine, which is easily determined from the preoperative radiograph. Providing adequate muscle relaxation for surgery can be accomplished with various anesthetic techniques such as volatile anesthesia, muscle relaxants, and caudal or epidural block.[181] There is increasing interest in the use of remifentanil in newborns and infants because of its titratability and short duration of action, potentially increasing the options for extubation at the end of the case for some patients.[182]

The criteria for tracheal extubation at the end of surgery are the same as those described for upper gastrointestinal tract obstruction. When in doubt, it is prudent to leave the tracheal tube in place and provide a period of postoperative ventilation during which the patient's status can be re-evaluated before deciding that extubation is safe.

Myelomeningocele

Clinical Presentation

Myelomeningocele is the most common congenital primary neural tube defect. Despite the known ability of folic acid supplementation during pregnancy to largely prevent this defect, the lesion still occurs in approximately 0.5 to 1 of every 1,000 live births.[183] It results from failure of neural tube closure during the fourth week of gestation. Neural tube defects can be identified on prenatal ultrasound. Elevated maternal serum AFP detects 50% to 90% of open neural tube defects but has a false-positive rate of 5%. Amniotic fluid AFP is more reliable and typically used for confirmation after elevated serum levels.

By definition, the lesion involves both the meninges and neural components, as compared with a meningocele, which does not contain neural elements. The infant is born with a cystic mass on the back comprising a neural placode, arachnoid, dura, nerve tissue and roots, and cerebrospinal fluid. The lesion most commonly occurs in the lumbosacral or sacral region, although

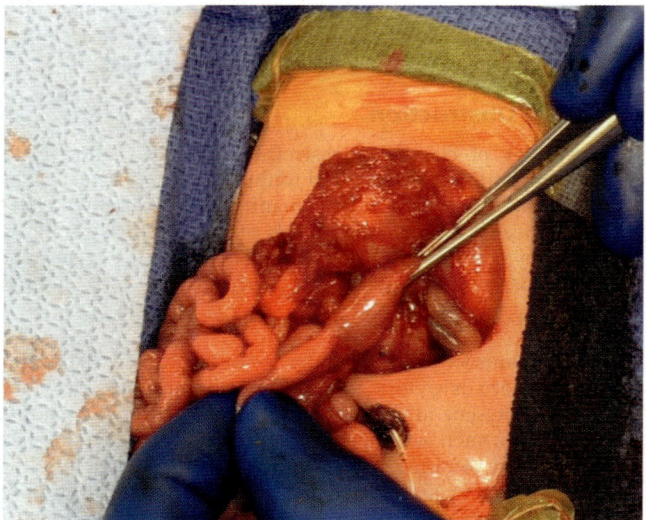

Figure 42-21 Jejunal atresia. (Photograph courtesy of Kurt Heiss, MD.)

it can extend to the thoracic region. The bony canal is also malformed, leading to multiple orthopedic problems as the child matures. Urologic complications correlate with the level of the spinal lesion.

Newborns born with myelomeningocele have an associated anomaly of the brainstem known as the Arnold–Chiari II (Chiari II) malformation. The Chiari II malformation is characterized by caudal displacement of the cerebellar vermis through the foramen magnum, caudal displacement of the medulla oblongata and the cervical spine, kinking of the medulla, and obliteration of the cisterna magna.[184] The cause of Chiari II malformation rests in the small size of the skull housing the posterior fossa, forcing CNS contents out during development. Hydrocephalus requiring shunting develops in approximately 80% to 90% of infants with myelomeningocele. In contrast, only 20% of patients have symptoms of brainstem dysfunction as a result of the Chiari II malformation, but the mortality rate among those symptomatic patients is high. Complications of brainstem dysfunction include stridor, apnea and bradycardia, aspiration pneumonia, sleep-disordered breathing patterns, vocal cord paralysis, lack of coordination, and spasticity. If the symptoms are not improved by shunting, posterior fossa decompression is necessary.[185]

The infant with a myelomeningocele is usually operated on within the first 24 to 48 hours of life. This reduces the risk for development of ventriculitis or progressive neurologic deficits. Most centers close the defect and place a shunt at the same time. However, some centers may delay placement of a shunt until the infant shows symptoms of hydrocephalus. There is ongoing work to determine the benefits of intrauterine repair of myelomeningocele, hopefully with the benefits of decreased development of a Chiari II malformation, decreased hydrocephalus, and increased lower limb function. As these studies continue, the role of intrauterine repair will become clearer.[186]

Preoperative Care

The preoperative stabilization period focuses on the prevention of infection, maintenance of ECF volume, avoidance of hypothermia, and assessment for other congenital anomalies. The exposed neural placode is susceptible to trauma, leakage, and infection. The infant is usually placed in the prone position, and the placode is covered with warm saline-soaked gauze to prevent desiccation. Because of the high risk of infection, antibiotic therapy is initiated in the preoperative period. Rupture of the cyst on the back can lead to ongoing cerebrospinal fluid leakage. This fluid is replaced with a full-strength, balanced salt solution. The infant is also assessed for any potentially life-threatening congenital anomalies.

Perioperative Care

The high prevalence of clinical latex allergy and latex sensitization in children with myelomeningocele has drawn much attention and led many individuals to believe that these patients have an impaired immune system that makes them more susceptible to latex allergy. The likely cause of the increased incidence of latex sensitization is repeated exposure to latex products through frequent hospitalizations and surgical procedures, as well as a program of daily bladder catheterization for those with neurogenic bladders.[187]

Positioning is critical in the infant with myelomeningocele. For induction of anesthesia, the infant may be placed supine with the defect resting in a "doughnut" to minimize trauma. Alternatively, the induction can be performed with the infant in the lateral position, although this makes intubation more challenging. The infant is turned prone for surgery. Rolls are positioned to ensure the abdomen and chest are free, avoiding pressure on the epidural venous plexus to minimize bleeding and allow adequate ventilation.

In most instances, the infant has an intravenous line placed before surgery and an intravenous induction is performed. Succinylcholine may be used to facilitate intubation without risking hyperkalemia.[188] Because increased intracranial pressure is rarely present before closure of the defect, inhalational induction is an alternative in the infant with difficult intravenous access. The anesthetic management of these newborns is rarely complicated unless there are other congenital anomalies that warrant special attention. There is no particular advantage of one technique over another because of the surgical lesion. Because these patients are usually extubated at the end of the case, a technique that allows this is usually chosen. Regional anesthesia has been reported as a safe adjunct or alternative to general anesthesia in the neonate with myelomeningocele. One small series has been published in which tetracaine spinals were used as the anesthetic for 14 infants undergoing repair of myelomeningocele.[189] In this series, there was no evidence of anesthetic-induced neurologic damage. Of note, 2 of the 14 infants had a postoperative respiratory event (1 transient apnea/bradycardia and 1 brief desaturation with bradycardia). Both of these infants had received intraoperative midazolam for sedation.

Postoperative Care

These infants must be monitored closely in the postoperative period. Respiratory complications, including stridor, apnea and bradycardia, cyanosis, and respiratory arrest, may develop after surgery in these infants with known brainstem abnormalities and potential disorders of central respiratory control. In addition, infants who were not shunted during repair may show signs of hydrocephalus, including lethargy, vomiting, seizures, apnea and bradycardia, or cardiovascular instability. These infants need to return to the operating room for insertion of a shunt. Although the majority of these patients will eventually require a shunt, a recent survey has shown that only about one-third of the patients receive one during the initial hospitalization.[190]

Hydrocephalus

Hydrocephalus in the first month of life may have several causes. It may occur after closure of a meningomyelocele because of the Chiari II malformation, it may be congenital in origin, or it may be related to intraventricular hemorrhage, especially in the very preterm newborn. The incidence of hydrocephalus has been stable in recent years, with a decrease related to Chiari II malformations, but an increase secondary to hemorrhage in the preterm.[191] The cranial sutures in the neonate are open, so intracranial pressure increases are blunted or minimized. However, infants with hydrocephalus eventually have an increase in head size and sometimes in intracranial pressure, resulting in lethargy, vomiting, and cardiorespiratory problems.

The anesthetic approach and the technique for tracheal intubation depend on the infant's condition. The major concern is protection of the airway and control of intracranial pressure. Awake tracheal intubation, crying, struggling, and straining can increase intracranial pressure. A rapid-sequence induction of anesthesia to control the airway and intracranial pressure is preferred. Volatile drugs, nitrous oxide, and opioids are all reasonable choices for maintenance of anesthesia, with no evidence that one technique is superior. Noninvasive intracranial pressure measurements in neurologically normal preterm infants have shown a decrease in intracranial pressure with all drugs, including ketamine, fentanyl, and isoflurane. The failure of volatile anesthetics and ketamine to increase intracranial pressure as in adults is attributed to the compliance of the neonate's open-sutured cranium. After surgery, the trachea of these infants may remain intubated if they were experiencing periods of apnea or bradycardia before surgery because of the intracranial abnormalities. If not, the trachea can be extubated as soon as the protective reflexes of the airway have recovered.

Surgical Procedures in the First Month of Life

Surgical procedures in the first month also are considered emergent, or at least urgent, surgery. The most frequent surgical procedures in the first month are exploratory laparotomy for NEC, inguinal hernia repair, correction of pyloric stenosis, patent ductus arteriosus (PDA) ligation, a shunt procedure for hydrocephalus, and placement of a central venous catheter.

Necrotizing Enterocolitis

NEC is a disease that primarily affects premature infants who have survived the first days of life, although it can be seen in full-term newborns. One of the theories about NEC is that earlier, more rapid feeding places infants at greater risk for development of NEC. The incidence of NEC among VLBW infants varies between 5% and 15%.[192] The exact pathophysiology of NEC has been the source of much study and some controversy, although it is likely multifactorial.[193] The condition is characterized by a cascade of pathologic events, beginning with an immature distal small and sometimes large intestine that has a decreased ability to absorb substrate, leading to stasis. The most common site is the ileocolic region, but can be seen in other areas and can be discontinuous, giving a patchy appearance. Stasis encourages bacterial proliferation, which leads to local infection. The picture is complicated by further pooling of fluid. The ischemia and infection may lead to necrosis of the intestinal mucosa, followed by perforation. The perforation leads to gangrene of the gut wall, fluid loss, peritonitis, septicemia, and disseminated intravascular coagulation. The first signs that NEC may be abdominal distention, irritability, and the development of metabolic acidosis. This may be followed by radiologic evidence of pneumatosis intestinalis, portal venous air, or free abdominal air. NEC is primarily a medical disease and is treated by cessation of oral intake, administration of antibiotics, fluid and electrolyte therapy, insertion of an orogastric tube, hemodynamic support, and in some cases, the insertion of a peritoneal drain.[194] In nonresponsive cases, the infant becomes more septic with severe peritonitis, and the only solution is to perform an exploratory laparotomy to remove the gangrenous bowel and create an ileostomy.

The preoperative problems are an acute abdomen with severe peritonitis, necrosis, and gangrene of the intestine, septicemia, metabolic acidosis, and hypovolemia. These neonates may also have disseminated intravascular coagulation. Preparation of the patient is directed toward stabilization of these problems. By the time the newborn becomes a surgical candidate, the septicemia, coupled with the distended abdomen and the overall clinical deterioration of the infant, often has necessitated the use of intubation and ventilation in the neonatal intensive care unit. Appropriate laboratory investigations include an arterial blood gas, hemoglobin, glucose, electrolytes, and coagulation profile. The deteriorating status of the patient may compromise both resuscitation efforts and the desire to establish adequate vascular access and monitoring, but focused efforts should be made to provide multiple vascular access lines, an arterial line, and central venous access.

The anesthetic requirements are continuation of resuscitation, provision of abdominal relaxation for the surgery, and careful titration of anesthetic drugs. These infants are often so critically ill that they are very sensitive to the depressant effects of anesthesia. If the patient is not already intubated and ventilated, a rapid-sequence induction with ketamine and succinylcholine is often used. The only caution with this technique is that some patients with NEC have significant hyperkalemia secondary to dead bowel, making the use of succinylcholine problematic. High-dose rocuronium is a reasonable alternative in that situation. Maintenance of anesthesia is usually based on an opioid technique, supplemented with additional doses of ketamine or, if the patient's condition improves, low-dose inhalation agent. The use of nitrous oxide should be avoided because of the gas pockets in the abdomen.

These infants are among the most challenging cases in pediatric anesthesia. The fluid loss can be enormous, both because of surgical losses and third-space losses. Fluid management starts with full-strength, balanced salt solution for maintenance of blood pressure and urine output. Blood products are often needed during these cases. If the hematocrit is below 30% to 35%, red blood cells should be administered. On the basis of both preoperative and intraoperative laboratory work, fresh frozen plasma, platelets, and cryoprecipitate may be needed. Due to bleeding, activated factor 7 or other prothrombotic agents may be needed. Inotropic support may also be needed. The surgical technique and length of surgery is variable, depending on the findings at laparotomy. A combination of bowel resection, primary anastomoses, and enterostomies may be used. At the end of the procedure, these infants are returned intubated and ventilated to the intensive care unit, where resuscitation is continued.[195] Long-term survival is based on several factors, including the degree of prematurity, associated congenital abnormalities, the degree of surviving bowel, the total length of affected bowel, and subsequent complications. Mortality rates, especially in newborns weighing less than 1,500 g, are poor with recent studies demonstrating 25% to 50% mortality before discharge.[196,197]

Inguinal Hernia Repair in the Neonate

The development of a hernia in the premature infant or neonate is a different clinical problem from the development of a hernia in an infant older than 1 year. In infants younger than 2 months who need inguinal hernia repair, there is a higher incidence of prematurity, history of RDS, history of incarceration, and congenital heart disease.[198] In preterms, the incidence of hernia may approach 20% to 30%. There is a concern about new or recurring incarceration in these patients, making hernia repair less an elective procedure than in older infants. Consequently, once identified, these patients usually are repaired within a relatively short time. If the patient is currently hospitalized, it is common to repair the hernia before discharge. Otherwise, the surgery should be scheduled within days to weeks of diagnosis.

Anesthetic Techniques for Hernia Repair

Surgical procedures below the umbilicus can be performed with either general or regional anesthesia. The choice of whether to use general or regional anesthesia depends on the preference of the surgeon and/or the anesthesiologist and expected length of procedure. However, the choice is influenced by the underlying status of the patient, previous complications, and the known risk of preterm patients to develop apnea and bradycardia during and after these procedures. There is a risk in any preterm for apnea and bradycardia after stressful procedures, but this has been most widely studied in association with inguinal hernia repair. Analysis of the many small studies have shown certain common elements.[150] Apneic events are inversely related to both gestational age and postconceptual age. The incidence of apnea is less in small-for-gestational age infants. Anemia increases the incidence of apneic events. Apneic events at home are associated with a higher incidence in the perioperative period. There have been multiple studies that were recently analyzed to determine if the choice of regional or general anesthetic techniques decreased the incidence of apnea and bradycardia.[199] Use of spinal anesthesia without sedatives does not decrease the risk of late apnea in preterm neonates in the best evidence to date. Consequently, the choice of anesthetic should not be based solely on the risk of preventing apneic spells. An adjunct that has some evidence in support of its use to minimize apneic spells is caffeine. The use of preservative-free caffeine in a single dose of 10 mg/kg has been suggested to decrease the incidence of apneic spells.[151]

Regional anesthesia can be used entirely for the surgery or as an adjunct to reduce general anesthetic requirements and provide postoperative analgesia. Other methods of providing intraoperative anesthesia and postoperative analgesia include the ilioinguinal–iliohypogastric nerve block or local infiltration. Ilioinguinal–iliohypogastric nerve block with 0.25% bupivacaine or 0.2% ropivacaine, with epinephrine, can be administered shortly after the induction of general anesthesia and affords excellent postoperative analgesia.

Discharge after inguinal hernia repair to home is an area of some controversy. There is significant institutional variation on the issue of monitoring for postoperative apnea, with the decision to admit overnight usually based on the postconceptual age in preterm neonates. Some centers use 46 weeks postconceptual age as the lower limit for admission, but other centers will use up to 60 weeks postconceptual age as the limit. In our institution, we have used a different approach. In order to make the limit easily understandable and also understanding that the basis of determining gestational age is not precise, we have all preterm infants admitted until they are 6 months of age. This ensures 26 weeks added to gestational age and is a compromise between the 46-week and 60-week limits, but is easy to administer. However, it may be overly conservative in the 36-week premature infant now 5 months of age. No matter what limits are used, if the infant has apneic or bradycardic spells during the perioperative period, he or she should be monitored in-house until the infant has been apnea-free for at least 12 hours.

Pyloric Stenosis

Pyloric stenosis is a relatively frequent surgical disease of the neonate and infant. It most commonly appears between weeks 2 and 6 of life. The pathologic characteristics include hypertrophy of the pyloric smooth muscle with edema of the pyloric mucosa and submucosa. This process, which develops over a period of days to weeks, leads to progressive obstruction of the pyloric valve, causing persistent vomiting. The vomiting leads to varying losses of fluids and electrolytes. The diagnosis is usually made at an early stage in the development of symptoms, especially with the help of ultrasound, so it is rare to find an infant with severe fluid and electrolyte derangements. However, an infant is occasionally seen whose problem has developed slowly over a period of weeks, resulting in severe fluid and electrolyte derangements. The stomach contents contain sodium, potassium, chloride, hydrogen ions, and water. The classic electrolyte pattern in infants with severe vomiting is hyponatremic, hypokalemic, and hypochloremic metabolic alkalosis with a compensatory respiratory acidosis. The anesthesiologist, pediatrician, and surgeon are all responsible for preparing these infants for surgery. Pyloric stenosis is a medical emergency, not a surgical emergency. The patient should not be operated on until there has been adequate fluid and electrolyte resuscitation. The infant should have normal skin turgor, and the correction of the electrolyte imbalance should produce a sodium level that is greater than 130 mEq/L, a potassium level that is at least 3 mEq/L, a chloride level that is greater than 85 mEq/L (trending upward), and a urine output of at least 1 to 2 mL/kg/hr. These patients need a resuscitation fluid of balanced salt solution and, after the infant begins to urinate, the addition of potassium.

Anesthetic Management

It is prudent to pass a large orogastric tube and aspirate the stomach contents because of the significant volume that may be present.[200] This procedure greatly reduces the quantity of gastric fluid. A rapid-sequence induction is advisable because of the potential for additional volume in the stomach. Although awake intubation had been popular with some clinicians in the past, it is associated with a higher incidence of complications and is traumatic to the child.[110] These patients have been fully resuscitated before coming to surgery, so there is little reason for an awake intubation. Anesthesia can be maintained by almost any technique the clinician prefers. There has been a need for muscle relaxation only for a short period during pyloromyotomy. Some surgeons may require muscle relaxation because most of these are now performed using minimally invasive laparasocpic procedures (Fig. 42-22). Careful attention has to be paid to ventilation and blood pressure as the abdominal pressure is increased during insufflation for laparoscopy. Controlled ventilation reduces or eliminates the need for muscle relaxants for this surgery. At the end of the case, the patient should be wide awake before extubation. A TAP block can be provided using ultrasound guidance for postoperative pain relief with good analgesia or local infiltration at laparoscopic port sites. Intravenous or rectal acetaminophen is commonly administered for pain relief as well.

Ligation of a Patent Ductus Arteriosus

As the number of small premature infants who survive has increased, so also has the number of infants who have a PDA

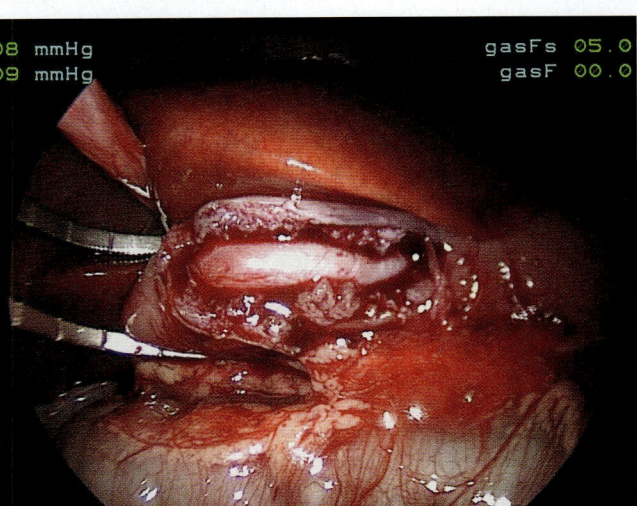

Figure 42-22 Laparoscopic repair of pyloric stenosis. In this image, the surgical cleft created in the hypertrophic muscles of the pylorus can be seen. This surgical intervention is curative of pyloric stenosis. (Photograph courtesy of Timothy Lautz, MD.)

with heart failure and respiratory failure. Prostaglandins relax the smooth muscle of the ductus so it cannot constrict. Indomethacin, a prostaglandin synthetase inhibitor, can be administered to encourage closure of the ductus. However, indomethacin is often unsuccessful in the small premature infant because of the lack of muscle within the ductus. Infants with a PDA and heart failure need maximal medical management with fluid restriction, diuretics, and inotropes. These infants are at special risk because of the reduced blood volume and precarious cardiopulmonary system. If the surgery is performed in the operating room, special attention is taken to maintain normothermia, ventilation, and oxygenation during transport. If the surgery is performed at bedside in the neonatal intensive care unit, the anesthesiologist must take time before the procedure to establish where he or she will be situated, where all venous access is, and that all drugs and fluids are already prepared. An opioid-based technique with muscle relaxant is a frequent choice for anesthesia. Probably the biggest challenge during these cases is the diagnosis and management of hypotension. There can be sudden, catastrophic blood loss if the ductus arteriosus ruptures during the procedure. Consequently, syringes of a balanced salt solution, albumin, and blood should be immediately available. The other common cause of hypotension is compression of the lungs, heart, and great vessels by the surgeon as they are gaining exposure. This must be a balance between stopping the procedure to allow the heart and blood pressure to recover versus the need to proceed with the operation. The answer comes in close communication between the anesthesiologist and the surgeon. These patients usually remain intubated after procedure, without a need to reverse the muscle relaxant. Residual opioid will provide good analgesia for the immediate postoperative period.

There are two newer techniques for closing the PDA in infants that are increasing in popularity.[201] Video-assisted thoracoscopic surgery (VATS) uses small endoscopes inserted through a series of small thoracotomy incisions to guide instruments to ligate the ductus. VATS can be done either in the operating room or, rarely, at bedside. The other approach is used by cardiologists in the cardiac catheterization to occlude the ductus arteriosus with a coil. A test clamp is often used to demonstrate continued aortic flow to the lower extremities and an improvement in diastolic blood pressure from decrease of diastolic run-off to the ductus arteriosus.

Placement of a Central Venous Catheter

The use of a central venous catheter for monitoring serum electrolytes, for parenteral nutrition, and for administering medications is a well-established part of modern perioperative care. It can be placed either as part of the surgical procedure or at some other time as a separate procedure. The three major concerns in central venous catheter placement are airway management, pneumothorax, and bleeding. The anesthetic technique depends on the infant's condition. If general anesthesia is selected, then intubation or laryngeal mask airway have each been successfully used. A pneumothorax may occur with attempts at subclavian vein puncture. The first indication of pneumothorax may be a decreasing oxygen saturation, hypotension, or difficulty with ventilation of the lungs. Because imaging using fluoroscopy is often used for central venous catheter placement, it can be used rapidly to diagnose a pneumothorax. If not, the chest should be rapidly aspirated for both diagnostic and therapeutic reasons. Bleeding is an unusual but serious complication of central venous catheter placement. It usually manifests in the perioperative period as hemothorax or as hypovolemia with a decreasing hematocrit or blood pressure. The establishment of intravenous access placed before proceeding with a central line is problematic for some patients. The reason for the central line may very well be the inability to obtain peripheral access, and the clinician is left with a trade-off between prolonged attempts at starting an intravenous catheter versus proceeding directly to obtain central venous line placement.

PICCs, placed in either the upper extremity or the femoral vein, are now common in practice. Often, these lines may be placed with local anesthetic only or with mild sedation, with ketamine for example. Strict attention to skin preparation, sterile glove and drape use, and minimizing access to the central line are components important to diminish catheter-related sepsis. Subclavian approach has a higher incidence of problems during line placement than internal jugular or femoral approaches, but may have fewer associated infections and fewer overall problems with the line once it is in use. PICCs have not been well-studied in the neonatal population, but continue to grow in their popularity.

Summary

The anesthetic management of the newborn is among the most challenging to anesthesiologists. A strong knowledge of neonatal anatomy, physiology, and pharmacology is needed, as well as an appreciation of the disease states and surgical procedures that are unique to this population. A thorough preanesthetic evaluation and preparation, a concise plan, and meticulous technique are the basis of an effective approach. The patient's neonatologist or pediatrician and the surgeon are strong allies in providing the best care, and close communication with them is necessary. Finally, the clinical status of a newborn can change remarkably quickly. Strict attention to detail and prospective management are the hallmarks of the anesthesiologist skilled in providing care in these difficult cases. Use of current technology including ultrasound guidance is suggested for facilitating vascular access as well as regional anesthesia for pain management in these fragile infants.

Acknowledgment

The authors of this edition would like to thank Dr. Steve Hall for his contributions to previous versions of this chapter as well as his career-long dedication to the field of pediatric anesthesiology.

REFERENCES

1. Friedman AH, Fahey JT. The transition from fetal to neonatal circulation: normal responses and implications for infants with heart disease. *Semin Perinatol.* 1993;17(2):106–121.
2. Baum VC, Palmisano BW. The immature heart and anesthesia. *Anesthesiology.* 1997;87(6):1529–1548.
3. Fu JD, Li J, Tweedie D, et al. Crucial role of the sarcoplasmic reticulum in the developmental regulation of Ca2+ transients and contraction in cardiomyocytes derived from embryonic stem cells. *FASEB J.* 2006;20(1):181–183.
4. Auman JT, Seidler FJ, Tate CA, et al. Are developing beta-adrenoceptors able to desensitize? Acute and chronic effects of beta-agonists in neonatal heart and liver. *Am J Physiol Regul Integr Comp Physiol.* 2002;283(1):R205–217.
5. Kishkurno S, Takahashi Y, Harada K, et al. Postnatal changes in left ventricular volume and contractility in healthy term infants. *Pediatr Cardiol.* 1997;18(2):91–95.
6. Hislop A. Developmental biology of the pulmonary circulation. *Paediatr Respir Rev.* 2005;6(1):35–43.
7. Mansell AL, Collins MH, Johnson E Jr, et al. Postnatal growth of lung parenchyma in the piglet: morphometry correlated with mechanics. *Anat Rec.* 1995;241(1):99–104.
8. Engle WA, American Academy of Pediatrics Committee on Fetus and Newborn. Surfactant-replacement therapy for respiratory distress in the preterm and term neonate. *Pediatrics.* 2008;121(2):419–432.

9. Hernandez-Diaz S, Van Marter LJ, Werler MM, et al. Risk factors for persistent pulmonary hypertension of the newborn. *Pediatrics.* 2007;120(2): e272–e282.
10. Jain A, McNamara PJ. Persistent pulmonary hypertension of the newborn: Advances in diagnosis and treatment. *Semin Fetal Neonatal Med.* 2015; 20(4):262–271.
11. Konduri GG, Solimano A, Sokol GM, et al. A randomized trial of early versus standard inhaled nitric oxide therapy in term and near-term newborn infants with hypoxic respiratory failure. *Pediatrics.* 2004;113(3 Pt 1):559–564.
12. Steinhorn RH. Nitric oxide and beyond: new insights and therapies for pulmonary hypertension. *J Perinatol.* 2008;28 Suppl 3:S67–S71.
13. Noori S, Seri I. Neonatal blood pressure support: the use of inotropes, lusitropes, and other vasopressor agents. *Clin Perinatol.* 2012;39(1):221–238.
14. El-Khuffash A, Herbozo C, Jain A, et al. Targeted neonatal echocardiography (TnECHO) service in a Canadian neonatal intensive care unit: a 4-year experience. *J Perinatol.* 2013;33(9):687–690.
15. Scohy TV, Gommers D, Jan ten Harkel AD, et al. Intraoperative evaluation of micromultiplane transesophageal echocardiographic probe in surgery for congenital heart disease. *Eur J Echocardiogr.* 2007;8(4):241–246.
16. Murphy JD, Vawter GF, Reid LM. Pulmonary vascular disease in fatal meconium aspiration. *J Pediatr.* 1984;104(5):758–762.
17. Velaphi S, Vidyasagar D. Intrapartum and postdelivery management of infants born to mothers with meconium-stained amniotic fluid: evidence-based recommendations. *Clin Perinatol.* 2006;33(1):29–42, v-vi.
18. Drukker A, Guignard JP. Renal aspects of the term and preterm infant: a selective update. *Curr Opin Pediatr.* 2002;14(2):175–182.
19. Alcorn J, McNamara PJ. Ontogeny of hepatic and renal systemic clearance pathways in infants: part 1. *Clin Pharmacokinet.* 2002;41(12):959–998.
20. Nash PL. Potassium and sodium homeostasis in the neonate. *Neonatal Netw.* 2007;26(2):125–128.
21. Chawla D, Agarwal R, Deorari AK, Paul VK. Fluid and electrolyte management in term and preterm neonates. *Indian J Pediatr.* 2008;75(3):255–259.
22. Cornblath M, Ichord R. Hypoglycemia in the neonate. *Semin Perinatol.* 2000;24(2):136–149.
23. Ballweg JA, Wernovsky G, Ittenbach RF, et al. Hyperglycemia after infant cardiac surgery does not adversely impact neurodevelopmental outcome. *Ann Thorac Surg.* 2007;84(6):2052–2058.
24. Wu Y, Stack G. Blood product replacement in the perinatal period. *Semin Perinatol.* 2007;31(4):262–271.
25. Fergusson D, Hebert PC, Lee SK, et al. Clinical outcomes following institution of universal leukoreduction of blood transfusions for premature infants. *JAMA.* 2003;289(15):1950–1956.
26. Alcorn J, McNamara PJ Pharmacokinetics in the newborn. *Adv Drug Deliv Rev.* 2003;55(5):667–686.
27. Strassburg CP, Strassburg A, Kneip S, et al. Developmental aspects of human hepatic drug glucuronidation in young children and adults. *Gut.* 2002;50(2):259–265.
28. Leeder JS, Kearns GL. Pharmacogenetics in pediatrics. Implications for practice. *Pediatr Clin North Am.* 1997;44(1):55–77.
29. Bory C, Baltassat P, Porthault M, et al. Metabolism of theophylline to caffeine in premature newborn infants. *J Pediatr.* 1979;94(6):988–993.
30. Green MD, Shires TK, Fischer LJ. Hepatotoxicity of acetaminophen in neonatal and young rats. I Age-related changes in susceptibility. *Toxicol Appl Pharmacol.* 1984;74(1):116–124.
31. deAlmeida VL, Alvaro RA, Haider Z, et al. The effect of nasal occlusion on the initiation of oral breathing in preterm infants. *Pediatr Pulmonol.* 1994;18(6):374–378.
32. Miller MJ, Carlo WA, Strohl KP, et al. Effect of maturation on oral breathing in sleeping premature infants. *J Pediatr.* 1986;109(3):515–519.
33. Dalal PG, Murray D, Messner AH, et al. Pediatric laryngeal dimensions: an age-based analysis. *Anesth Analg.* 2009;108(5):1475–1479.
34. Litman RS, Weissend EE, Shibata D, et al. Developmental changes of laryngeal dimensions in unparalyzed, sedated children. *Anesthesiology.* 2003;98(1):41–45.
35. Weiss M, Dullenkopf A, Fischer JE, et al. European Paediatric Endotracheal Intubation Study Group. Prospective randomized controlled multi-centre trial of cuffed or uncuffed endotracheal tubes in small children. *Br J Anaesth.* 2009;103(6):867–873.
36. Flynn PE, Black AE, Mitchell V. The use of cuffed tracheal tubes for paediatric tracheal intubation, a survey of specialist practice in the United Kingdom. *Eur J Anaesthesiol.* 2008;25(8):685–688.
37. Bhutada A, Sahni R, Rastogi S, et al. Randomised controlled trial of thiopental for intubation in neonates. *Arch Dis Child Fetal Neonatal Ed.* 2000; 82(1):F34–F37.
38. Ghanta S, Abdel-Latif ME, Lui K, et al. Propofol compared with the morphine, atropine, and suxamethonium regimen as induction agents for neonatal endotracheal intubation: a randomized, controlled trial. *Pediatrics.* 2007; 119(6):e1248–e1255.
39. Allegaert K, Peeters MY, Verbesselt R, et al. Inter-individual variability in propofol pharmacokinetics in preterm and term neonates. *Br J Anaesth.* 2007; 99(6):864–870.
40. Bhutta AT. Ketamine: a controversial drug for neonates. *Semin Perinatol.* 2007;31(5):303–308.
41. Anand KJ, Garg S, Rovnaghi CR, et al. Ketamine reduces the cell death following inflammatory pain in newborn rat brain. *Pediatr Res.* 2007;62(3):283–290.
42. Estkowski LM, Morris JL, Sinclair EA. Characterization of dexmedetomidine dosing and safety in neonates and infants. *J Pediatr Pharmacol Ther.* 2015;20(2):112–118.
43. Luo J, Guo J, Han D, et al. [Comparison of dexmedetomidine and midazolam on neurotoxicity in neonatal mice]. *Sheng Wu Yi Xue Gong Cheng Xue Za Zhi.* 2013;30(3):607–610.
44. Suresh S, Anand KJ. Opioid tolerance in neonates: a state-of-the-art review. *Paediatr Anaesth* 2001;11(5):511–521.
45. Santeiro ML, Christie J, Stromquist C, et al. Pharmacokinetics of continuous infusion fentanyl in newborns. *J Perinatol.* 1997;17(2):135–139.
46. Vaughn PR, Townsend SF, Thilo EH, et al. Comparison of continuous infusion of fentanyl to bolus dosing in neonates after surgery. *J Pediatr Surg.* 1996;31(12):1616–1623.
47. Fahnenstich H, Steffan J, Kau N, et al. Fentanyl-induced chest wall rigidity and laryngospasm in preterm and term infants. *Crit care Med.* 2000;28(3):836–839.
48. Saarenmaa E, Neuvonen PJ, Rosenberg P, et al. Morphine clearance and effects in newborn infants in relation to gestational age. *Clin Pharmacol Ther.* 2000;68(2):160–166.
49. Bhat R, Chari G, Gulati A, et al. Pharmacokinetics of a single dose of morphine in preterm infants during the first week of life. *J Pediatr.* 1990;117(3):477–481.
50. El Sayed MF, Taddio A, Fallah S, et al. Safety profile of morphine following surgery in neonates. *J Perinatol.* 2007;27(7):444–447.
51. Murphey LJ, Olsen GD. Morphine-6-beta-D-glucuronide respiratory pharmacodynamics in the neonatal guinea pig. *J Pharmacol Exp Ther.* 1994;268(1):110–116.
52. Peters JW, Anderson BJ, Simons SH, et al. Morphine metabolite pharmacokinetics during venoarterial extra corporeal membrane oxygenation in neonates. *Clin Pharmacokinet.* 2006;45(7):705–714.
53. Davis PJ, Cladis FP. The use of ultra-short-acting opioids in paediatric anaesthesia: the role of remifentanil. *Clin Pharmacokinet.* 2005;44(8):787–796.
54. Davis PJ, Galinkin J, McGowan FX, et al. A randomized multicenter study of remifentanil compared with halothane in neonates and infants undergoing pyloromyotomy. I. Emergence and recovery profiles. *Anesth Analg.* 2001;93(6):1380–1386, table of contents.
55. Hannallah RS, Oh TH, McGill WA, Epstein BS. Changes in heart rate and rhythm after intramuscular succinylcholine with or without atropine in anesthetized children. *Anesth Analg.* 1986;65(12):1329–1332.
56. Rapp HJ, Altenmueller CA, Waschke C. Neuromuscular recovery following rocuronium bromide single dose in infants. *Paediatr Anaesth.* 2004;14(4): 329–335.
57. Gronert BJ, Brandom BW. Neuromuscular blocking drugs in infants and children. *Pediatr Clin North Am.* 1994;41(1):73–91.
58. Cheung PY, Tyebkhan JM, Peliowski A, et al. Prolonged use of pancuronium bromide and sensorineural hearing loss in childhood survivors of congenital diaphragmatic hernia. *J Pediatr.* 1999;135(2 Pt 1):233–239.
59. Reich DL, Hollinger I, Harrington DJ, et al. Comparison of cisatracurium and vecuronium by infusion in neonates and small infants after congenital heart surgery. *Anesthesiology.* 2004;101(5):1122–1127.
60. Fodale V, Santamaria LB. Laudanosine, an atracurium and cisatracurium metabolite. *Eur J Anaesthesiol.* 2002;19(7):466–473.
61. Bhananker SM, Ramamoorthy C, Geiduschek JM, et al. Anesthesia-related cardiac arrest in children: update from the Pediatric Perioperative Cardiac Arrest Registry. *Anesth Analg.* 2007;105(2):344–350.
62. Murray DJ, Forbes RB, Mahoney LT. Comparative hemodynamic depression of halothane versus isoflurane in neonates and infants: an echocardiographic study. *Anesth Analg.* 1992;74(3):329–337.
63. Lerman J, Sikich N, Kleinman S, et al. The pharmacology of sevoflurane in infants and children. *Anesthesiology.* 1994;80(4):814–824.
64. Russell IA, Miller Hance WC, Gregory G, et al. The safety and efficacy of sevoflurane anesthesia in infants and children with congenital heart disease. *Anesth Analg.* 2001;92(5):1152–1158.
65. Brown K, Aun C, Stocks J, et al. A comparison of the respiratory effects of sevoflurane and halothane in infants and young children. *Anesthesiology.* 1998;89(1):86–92.
66. Sale SM, Read JA, Stoddart PA, et al. Prospective comparison of sevoflurane and desflurane in formerly premature infants undergoing inguinal herniotomy. *Br J Anaesth.* 2006;96(5):774–778.
67. Taylor RH, Lerman J. Minimum alveolar concentration of desflurane and hemodynamic responses in neonates, infants, and children. *Anesthesiology.* 1991;75(6):975–979.
68. Kodama M, Satoh Y, Otsubo Y, et al. Neonatal desflurane exposure induces more robust neuroapoptosis than do isoflurane and sevoflurane and impairs working memory. *Anesthesiology.* 2011;115(5):979–991.
69. Mazoit JX. Pharmacokinetic/pharmacodynamic modeling of anesthetics in children. therapeutic implications. *Paediatr Drugs.* 2006;8(3):139–150.
70. Rothstein P, Arthur GR, Feldman HS, et al. Bupivacaine for intercostal nerve blocks in children: blood concentrations and pharmacokinetics. *Anesth Analg.* 1986;65(6):625–632.

71. Ecoffey C, Desparmet J, Maury M, et al. Bupivacaine in children: pharmacokinetics following caudal anesthesia. *Anesthesiology*. 1985;63(4):447–448.
72. Willschke H, Bosenberg A, Marhofer P, et al. Ultrasonographic-guided ilioinguinal/iliohypogastric nerve block in pediatric anesthesia: what is the optimal volume? *Anesth Analg*. 2006;102(6):1680–1684.
73. Berde CB. Convulsions associated with pediatric regional anesthesia. *Anesth Analg* 1992;75(2):164–166.
74. Rapp HJ, Molnar V, Austin S, et al. Ropivacaine in neonates and infants: a population pharmacokinetic evaluation following single caudal block. *Paediatr Anaesth*. 2004;14(9):724–732.
75. McCloskey JJ, Haun SE, Deshpande JK. Bupivacaine toxicity secondary to continuous caudal epidural infusion in children. *Anesth Analg*. 1992;75(2):287–290.
76. Hansen TG, Ilett KF, Reid C, et al. Caudal ropivacaine in infants: population pharmacokinetics and plasma concentrations. *Anesthesiology*. 2001;94(4):579–584.
77. Chalkiadis GA, Eyres RL, Cranswick N, et al. Pharmacokinetics of levobupivacaine 0.25% following caudal administration in children under 2 years of age. *Br J Anaesth*. 2004;92(2):218–222.
78. Tobias JD, O'Dell N. Chloroprocaine for epidural anesthesia in infants and children. *AANA J*. 1995;63(2):131–135.
79. Henderson K, Sethna NF, Berde CB. Continuous caudal anesthesia for inguinal hernia repair in former preterm infants. *J Clin Anesth*. 1993;5(2):129–133.
80. Weinberg G, Ripper R, Feinstein DL, et al. Lipid emulsion infusion rescues dogs from bupivacaine-induced cardiac toxicity. *Reg Anesth Pain Med*. 2003;28(3):198–202.
81. Rosenblatt MA, Abel M, Fischer GW, et al. Successful use of a 20% lipid emulsion to resuscitate a patient after a presumed bupivacaine-related cardiac arrest. *Anesthesiology*. 2006;105(1):217–218.
82. Shah S, Gopalakrishnan S, Apuya J, et al. Use of Intralipid in an infant with impending cardiovascular collapse due to local anesthetic toxicity. *J Anesth*. 2009;23(3):439–441.
83. Mirtallo JM, Dasta JF, Kleinschmidt KC, et al. State of the art review: Intravenous fat emulsions: Current applications, safety profile, and clinical implications. *Ann Pharmacother*. 2010;44(4):688–700.
84. Neal JM, Mulroy MF, Weinberg GL, American Society of Regional Anesthesia and Pain Medicine. American Society of Regional Anesthesia and Pain Medicine checklist for managing local anesthetic systemic toxicity: 2012 version. *Reg Anesth Pain Med*. 2012;37(1):16–18.
85. Couper RT. Methaemoglobinaemia secondary to topical lignocaine/prilocaine in a circumcised neonate. *J Paediatr Child Health*. 2000;36(4):406–407.
86. Lehr VT, Taddio A. Topical anesthesia in neonates: clinical practices and practical considerations. *Semin Perinatol*. 2007;31(5):323–329.
87. Braz LG, Modolo NS, do Nascimento P Jr, et al. Perioperative cardiac arrest: a study of 53,718 anaesthetics over 9 yr from a Brazilian teaching hospital. *Br J Anaesth*. 2006;96(5):569–575.
88. Murat I, Constant I, Maud'huy H. Perioperative anaesthetic morbidity in children: a database of 24,165 anaesthetics over a 30-month period. *Paediatr Anaesth*. 2004;14(2):158–166.
89. Catre D, Lopes MF, Madrigal A, et al. Predictors of major postoperative complications in neonatal surgery. *Rev Col Bras Cir*. 2013;40(5):363–369.
90. Section on Anesthesiology and Pain Medicine, Polaner DM, Houck CS; American Academy of Pediatrics. Critical Elements for the Pediatric Perioperative Anesthesia Environment. *Pediatrics*. 2015;136(6):1200–1205.
91. Anand KJ, Carr DB. The neuroanatomy, neurophysiology, and neurochemistry of pain, stress, and analgesia in newborns and children. *Pediatr Clin North Am*. 1989;36(4):795–822.
92. Prevention and management of pain and stress in the neonate. American Academy of Pediatrics. Committee on Fetus and Newborn. Committee on Drugs. Section on Anesthesiology. Section on Surgery. Canadian Paediatric Society. Fetus and Newborn Committee. *Pediatrics*. 2000;105(2):454–461.
93. Tomashek KM, Shapiro-Mendoza CK, Davidoff MJ, et al. Differences in mortality between late-preterm and term singleton infants in the United States, 1995–2002. *J Pediatr*. 2007;151(5):450–456, 456 e451.
94. Ozyurek E, Cetintas S, Ceylan T, et al. Complete blood count parameters for healthy, small-for-gestational-age, full-term newborns. *Clin Lab Haematol*. 2006;28(2):97–104.
95. Deshpande S, Ward Platt M. The investigation and management of neonatal hypoglycaemia. *Semin Fetal Neonatal Med*. 2005;10(4):351–361.
96. Lippi G, Salvagno GL, Rugolotto S, et al. Routine coagulation tests in newborn and young infants. *J Thromb Thrombolysis*. 2007;24(2):153–155.
97. American Academy of Pediatrics Committee on Fetus and Newborn. Controversies concerning vitamin K and the newborn. American Academy of Pediatrics Committee on Fetus and Newborn. *Pediatrics*. 2003;112(1 Pt 1):191–192.
98. Barrington KJ. The myth of a minimum dose for atropine. *Pediatrics*. 2011;127(4):783–784.
99. Shiao SY. Effects of fetal hemoglobin on accurate measurements of oxygen saturation in neonates. *J Perinat Neonatal Nurs*. 2005;19(4):348–361.
100. Hubmayr RD. The times are a-changin': should we hang up the stethoscope? *Anesthesiology*. 2004;100(1):1–2.
101. Watson A, Visram A. Survey of the use of oesophageal and precordial stethoscopes in current paediatric anaesthetic practice. *Paediatr Anaesth*. 2001;11(4):437–442.
102. Sigaut S, Skhiri A, Stany I, et al. Ultrasound guided internal jugular vein access in children and infant: a meta-analysis of published studies. *Paediatr Anaesth*. 2009;19(12):1199–1206.
103. Han SH, Kim SD, Kim CS, et al. Comparison of central venous catheterization sites in infants. *J Int Med Res*. 2004;32(6):563–569.
104. Panagiotounakou P, Antonogeorgos G, Gounari E, et al. Peripherally inserted central venous catheters: frequency of complications in premature newborn depends on the insertion site. *J Perinatol*. 2014;34(6):461–463.
105. Schily M, Koumoukelis H, Lerman J, et al. Can pediatric anesthesiologists detect an occluded tracheal tube in neonates? *Anesth Analg*. 2001;93(1):66–70.
106. Spears RS Jr, Yeh A, Fisher DM, et al. The "educated hand". Can anesthesiologists assess changes in neonatal pulmonary compliance manually? *Anesthesiology*. 1991;75(4):693–696.
107. Tobin MJ, Stevenson GW, Horn BJ, et al. A comparison of three modes of ventilation with the use of an adult circle system in an infant lung model. *Anesth Analg*. 1998;87(4):766–771.
108. Hunter T, Lerman J, Bissonnette B. The temperature and humidity of inspired gases in infants using a pediatric circle system: effects of high and low-flow anesthesia. *Paediatr Anaesth*. 2005;15(9):750–754.
109. Luchetti M, Pigna A, Gentili A, et al. Evaluation of the efficiency of heat and moisture exchangers during paediatric anaesthesia. *Paediatr Anaesth*. 1999;9(1):39–45.
110. Cook-Sather SD, Tulloch HV, Cnaan A, et al. A comparison of awake versus paralyzed tracheal intubation for infants with pyloric stenosis. *Anesth Analg*. 1998;86(5):945–951.
111. Salgo B, Schmitz A, Henze G, et al. Evaluation of a new recommendation for improved cuffed tracheal tube size selection in infants and small children. *Acta Anaesthesiol Scand*. 2006;50(5):557–561.
112. Lonnqvist PA. Successful use of laryngeal mask airway in low-weight expremature infants with bronchopulmonary dysplasia undergoing cryotherapy for retinopathy of the premature. *Anesthesiology*. 1995;83(2):422–424.
113. Jagannathan N, Ramsey MA, White MC, et al. An update on newer pediatric supraglottic airways with recommendations for clinical use. *Paediatr Anaesth*. 2015;25(4):334–345.
114. Hansen TG, Joensen H, Henneberg SW, et al. Laryngeal mask airway guided tracheal intubation in a neonate with the Pierre Robin syndrome. *Acta Anaesthesiol Scand*. 1995;39(1):129–131.
115. Fisher QA, Tunkel DE. Lightwand intubation of infants and children. *J Clin Anesth*. 1997;9(4):275–279.
116. Cain JM, Mason LJ, Martin RD. Airway management in two of newborns with Pierre Robin Sequence: the use of disposable vs multiple use LMA for fiberoptic intubation. *Paediatr Anaesth*. 2006;16(12):1274–1276.
117. Moura JH, da Silva GA. Neonatal laryngoscope intubation and the digital method: a randomized controlled trial. *J Pediatr*. 2006;148(6):840–841.
118. Feldman JM. Optimal ventilation of the anesthetized pediatric patient. *Anesth Analg*. 2015;120(1):165–175.
119. Wheeler K, Klingenberg C, McCallion N, et al. Volume-targeted versus pressure-limited ventilation in the neonate. *Cochrane Database Syst Rev*. 2010(11):CD003666.
120. Wheeler KI, Klingenberg C, Morley CJ, et al. Volume-targeted versus pressure-limited ventilation for preterm infants: a systematic review and meta-analysis. *Neonatology*. 2011;100(3):219–227.
121. Piersigilli F, Bersani I, Giliberti P, et al. Neonatal limb ischemia: caudal blockade and NIRS monitoring. *Eur J Pediatr*. 2014;173(12):1599–1601.
122. Marhofer P, Willschke H, Kettner S. Imaging techniques for regional nerve blockade and vascular cannulation in children. *Curr Opin Anaesthesiol*. 2006;19(3):293–300.
123. Weinberg GL, Ripper R, Murphy P, et al. Lipid infusion accelerates removal of bupivacaine and recovery from bupivacaine toxicity in the isolated rat heart. *Reg Anesth Pain Med*. 2006;31(4):296–303.
124. Davidson AJ, Morton NS, Arnup SJ, et al. Apnea after Awake Regional and General Anesthesia in Infants: The General Anesthesia Compared to Spinal Anesthesia Study—Comparing Apnea and Neurodevelopmental Outcomes, a Randomized Controlled Trial. *Anesthesiology*. 2015;123(1):38–54.
125. Suresh S, Wheeler M. Practical pediatric regional anesthesia. *Anesthesiol Clin North America*. 2002;20(1):83–113.
126. Williams RK, Adams DC, Aladjem EV, et al. The safety and efficacy of spinal anesthesia for surgery in infants: the Vermont Infant Spinal Registry. *Anesth Analg*. 2006;102(1):67–71.
127. Suresh S, Hall SC. Spinal anesthesia in infants: is the impractical practical? *Anesth Analg*. 2006;102(1):65–66.
128. Welborn LG, Rice LJ, Hannallah RS, et al. Postoperative apnea in former preterm infants: prospective comparison of spinal and general anesthesia. *Anesthesiology*. 1990;72(5):838–842.
129. Tsui BC, Tarkkila P, Gupta S, et al. Confirmation of caudal needle placement using nerve stimulation. *Anesthesiology*. 1999;91(2):374–378.
130. Marhofer P, Bosenberg A, Sitzwohl C, et al. Pilot study of neuraxial imaging by ultrasound in infants and children. *Paediatr Anaesth*. 2005;15(8):671–676.

131. Suresh S, Long J, Birmingham PK, et al. Are caudal blocks for pain control safe in children? An analysis of 18,650 caudal blocks from the Pediatric Regional Anesthesia Network (PRAN) database. *Anesth Analg.* 2015;120(1):151–156.
132. Wheeler M, Patel A, Suresh S, et al. The addition of clonidine 2 microg.kg-1 does not enhance the postoperative analgesia of a caudal block using 0.125% bupivacaine and epinephrine 1:200,000 in children: a prospective, double-blind, randomized study *Paediatr Anaesth.* 2005;15(6):476–483.
133. Willschke H, Bosenberg A, Marhofer P, et al. Epidural catheter placement in neonates: sonoanatomy and feasibility of ultrasonographic guidance in term and preterm neonates. *Reg Anesth Pain Med.* 2007;32(1):34–40.
134. Brady-Fryer B, Wiebe N, Lander JA. Pain relief for neonatal circumcision. *Cochrane Database Syst Rev.* 2004(4):CD004217.
135. Sandeman DJ, Dilley AV. Ultrasound guided dorsal penile nerve block in children. *Anaesth Intensive Care.* 2007;35(2):266–269.
136. Bielsky A, Efrat R, Suresh S. Postoperative analgesia in neonates after major abdominal surgery: 'TAP' our way to success! *Paediatr Anaesth.* 2009;19(5):541–542.
137. Suresh S, De Oliveira GS Jr. Blood Bupivacaine Concentrations After Transversus Abdominis Plane Block in Neonates: A Prospective Observational Study. *Anesth Analg.* 2016;122(3):814–817.
138. Marhofer P, Greher M, Kapral S. Ultrasound guidance in regional anaesthesia. *Br J Anaesth.* 2005;94(1):7–17.
139. Marhofer P, Sitzwohl C, Greher M, et al. Ultrasound guidance for infraclavicular brachial plexus anaesthesia in children. *Anaesthesia.* 2004;59(7):642–646.
140. Suresh S, Voronov P. Head and neck blocks in children: an anatomical and procedural review. *Paediatr Anaesth.* 2006;16(9):910–918.
141. Williams DG, Patel A, Howard RF. Pharmacogenetics of codeine metabolism in an urban population of children and its implications for analgesic reliability. *Br J Anaesth.* 2002;89(6):839–845.
142. Cheung CL, van Dijk M, Green JW, et al. Effects of low-dose naloxone on opioid therapy in pediatric patients: a retrospective case-control study. *Int Care Med.* 2007;33(1):190–194.
143. Pacifici GM, Allegaert K. Clinical pharmacology of paracetamol in neonates: a review. *Curr Ther Res Clin Exp.* 2015;77:24–30.
144. Papacci P, De Francisci G, Iacobucci T, et al. Use of intravenous ketorolac in the neonate and premature babies. *Paediatr Anaesth.* 2004;14(6):487–492.
145. Rayburn WF. Maternal and fetal effects from substance use. *Clin Perinatol.* 2007;34(4):559–571, vi.
146. Lipshultz SE, Frassica JJ, Orav EJ. Cardiovascular abnormalities in infants prenatally exposed to cocaine. *J Pediatr.* 1991;118(1):44–51.
147. Hackman PS. Recognizing and understanding the cold-stressed term infant. *Neonatal Netw.* 2001;20(8):35–41.
148. Plattner O, Semsroth M, Sessler DI, et al. Lack of nonshivering thermogenesis in infants anesthetized with fentanyl and propofol. *Anesthesiology.* 1997;86(4):772–777.
149. Ehrenkranz RA, Walsh MC, Vohr BR, et al.; National Institutes of Child Health and Human Development Neonatal Research Network. Validation of the National Institutes of Health consensus definition of bronchopulmonary dysplasia. *Pediatrics.* 2005;116(6):1353–1360.
150. Cote CJ, Zaslavsky A, Downes JJ, et al. Postoperative apnea in former preterm infants after inguinal herniorrhaphy. A combined analysis. *Anesthesiology.* 1995;82(4):809–822.
151. Walther-Larsen S, Rasmussen LS. The former preterm infant and risk of post-operative apnoea: recommendations for management. *Acta Anaesthesiol Scand.* 2006;50(7):888–893.
152. Kennedy KA, Fielder AR, Hardy RJ, et al. Reduced lighting does not improve medical outcomes in very low birth weight infants. *J Pediatr.* 2001;139(4):527–531.
153. Reynolds JD, Dobson V, Quinn GE, et al. Evidence-based screening criteria for retinopathy of prematurity: natural history data from the CRYO-ROP and LIGHT-ROP studies. *Arch Ophthalmol.* 2002;120(11):1470–1476.
154. Lloyd J, Askie L, Smith J, et al. Supplemental oxygen for the treatment of prethreshold retinopathy of prematurity. *Cochrane Database Syst Rev.* 2003(2):CD003482.
155. Fredriksson A, Ponten E, Gordh T, et al. Neonatal exposure to a combination of N-methyl-D-aspartate and gamma-aminobutyric acid type A receptor anesthetic agents potentiates apoptotic neurodegeneration and persistent behavioral deficits. *Anesthesiology.* 2007;107(3):427–436.
156. Soriano SG, Anand KJ. Anesthetics and brain toxicity. *Curr Opin Anaesthesiol.* 2005;18(3):293–297.
157. Rappaport BA, Suresh S, Hertz S, et al. Anesthetic neurotoxicity–clinical implications of animal models. *N Engl J Med.* 2015;372(9):796–797.
158. Davidson AJ, Disma N, de Graaff JC, et al. Neurodevelopmental outcome at 2 years of age after general anaesthesia and awake-regional anaesthesia in infancy (GAS): an international multicentre, randomised controlled trial. *Lancet.* 2016;387(10015):239–50.
159. Flick RP, Katusic SK, Colligan RC, et al. Cognitive and behavioral outcomes after early exposure to anesthesia and surgery. *Pediatrics.* 2011;128(5):e1053–1061.
160. Lin AE, Pober BR, Adatia I. Congenital diaphragmatic hernia and associated cardiovascular malformations: type, frequency, and impact on management. *Am J Med Genet C Semin Med Genet.* 2007;145C(2):201–216.
161. Greenwood RD, Rosenthal A. Cardiovascular malformations associated with tracheoesophageal fistula and esophageal atresia. *Pediatrics.* 1976;57(1):87–91.
162. Harting MT, Lally KP. Surgical management of neonates with congenital diaphragmatic hernia. *Semin Pediatr Surg.* 2007;16(2):109–114.
163. Peralta CF, Jani JC, Van Schoubroeck D, et al. Fetal lung volume after endoscopic tracheal occlusion in the prediction of postnatal outcome. *Am J Obstet Gynecol.* 2008;198(1):60.e61–65.
164. Fallon SC, Cass DL, Olutoye OO, et al. Repair of congenital diaphragmatic hernias on Extracorporeal Membrane Oxygenation (ECMO): does early repair improve patient survival? *J Pediatr Surg.* 2013;48(6):1172–1176.
165. West KW, Bengston K, Rescorla FJ, et al. Delayed surgical repair and ECMO improves survival in congenital diaphragmatic hernia. *Ann Surg.* 1992;216(4):454–460; discussion 460–452.
166. Ssemakula N, Stewart DL, Goldsmith LJ, et al. Survival of patients with congenital diaphragmatic hernia during the ECMO era: an 11-year experience. *J Pediatr Surg.* 1997;32(12):1683–1689.
167. Ng GY, Derry C, Marston L, et al. Reduction in ventilator-induced lung injury improves outcome in congenital diaphragmatic hernia? *Pediatr Surg Int.* 2008;24(2):145–150.
168. Rodrigues CJ, Tannuri U, Tannuri AC, et al. Prenatal tracheal ligation or intra-amniotic administration of surfactant or dexamethasone prevents some structural changes in the pulmonary arteries of surgically created diaphragmatic hernia in rabbits. *Rev Hosp Clin Fac Med Sao Paulo.* 2002;57(1):1–8.
169. Fisher JC, Jefferson RA, Arkovitz MS, et al. Redefining outcomes in right congenital diaphragmatic hernia. *J Pediatr Surg.* 2008;43(2):373–379.
170. van den Hout L, Sluiter I, Gischler S, et al. Can we improve outcome of congenital diaphragmatic hernia? *Pediatr Surg Int.* 2009;25(9):733–743.
171. Hwang PJ, Kousseff BG. Omphalocele and gastroschisis: an 18-year review study. *Genet Med.* 2004;6(4):232–236.
172. Ledbetter DJ. Gastroschisis and omphalocele. *Surg Clin North Am.* 2006;86(2):249–260, vii.
173. Henrich K, Huemmer HP, Reingruber B, et al. Gastroschisis and omphalocele: treatments and long-term outcomes. *Pediatr Surg Int.* 2008;24(2):167–173.
174. Lee SL, Beyer TD, Kim SS, et al. Initial nonoperative management and delayed closure for treatment of giant omphaloceles. *J Pediatr Surg.* 2006;41(11):1846–1849.
175. Owen A, Marven S, Jackson L, et al. Experience of bedside preformed silo staged reduction and closure for gastroschisis. *J Pediatr Surg.* 2006;41(11):1830–1835.
176. Olesevich M, Alexander F, Khan M, et al. Gastroschisis revisited: role of intraoperative measurement of abdominal pressure. *J Pediatr Surg.* 2005;40(5):789–792.
177. Yaster M, Buck JR, Dudgeon DL, et al. Hemodynamic effects of primary closure of omphalocele/gastroschisis in human newborns. *Anesthesiology.* 1988;69(1):84–88.
178. Nguyen T, Zainabadi K, Bui T, et al. Thoracoscopic repair of esophageal atresia and tracheoesophageal fistula: lessons learned. *J Laparoendosc Adv Surg Tech A.* 2006;16(2):174–178.
179. Thompson ME, Haynes B. Ultrasound-guided thoracic paravertebral block catheter experience in 2 neonates. *J Clin Anesth.* 2015;27(6):514–516.
180. Dalla Vecchia LK, Grosfeld JL, West KW, et al. Intestinal atresia and stenosis: a 25-year experience with 277 cases. *Arch Surg.* 1998;133(5):490–496; discussion 496–497.
181. Cucchiaro G, De Lagausie P, El-Ghonemi A, et al. Single-dose caudal anesthesia for major intraabdominal operations in high-risk infants. *Anesth Analg.* 2001;92(6):1439–1441.
182. Welzing L, Roth B. Experience with remifentanil in neonates and infants. *Drugs.* 2006;66(10):1339–1350.
183. Shaer CM, Chescheir N, Schulkin J. Myelomeningocele: a review of the epidemiology, genetics, risk factors for conception, prenatal diagnosis, and prognosis for affected individuals. *Obstetr Gynecol sur.* 2007;62(7):471–479.
184. McLone DG, Dias MS. The Chiari II malformation: cause and impact. *Child's Nerv Syst.* 2003;19(7–8):540–550.
185. McLone DG. Care of the neonate with a myelomeningocele. *Neurosurg Clin N Am.* 1998;9(1):111–120.
186. Sutton LN. Fetal surgery for neural tube defects. *Best Pract Res Clin Obstet Gynaecol.* 2008;22(1):175–188.
187. Shah S, Cawley M, Gleeson R, et al. Latex allergy and latex sensitization in children and adolescents with meningomyelocele. *J Allergy Clin Immunol.* 1998;101(6 Pt 1):741–746.
188. Dierdorf SF, McNiece WL, Rao CC, et al. Failure of succinylcholine to alter plasma potassium in children with myelomeningocoele. *Anesthesiology.* 1986;64(2):272–273.
189. Viscomi CM, Abajian JC, Wald SL, et al. Spinal anesthesia for repair of meningomyelocele in neonates. *Anesth Analg.* 1995;81(3):492–495.
190. Sin AH, Rashidi M, Caldito G, et al. Surgical treatment of myelomeningocele: year 2000 hospitalization, outcome, and cost analysis in the US. *Child's Nerv Syst.* 2007;23(10):1125–1127.

191. Persson EK, Anderson S, Wiklund LM, et al. Hydrocephalus in children born in 1999–2002: epidemiology, outcome and ophthalmological findings. *Child's Nerv Syst*. 2007;23(10):1111–1118.
192. Lee JS, Polin RA. Treatment and prevention of necrotizing enterocolitis. *Semin Neonatol*. 2003;8(6):449–459.
193. Srinivasan PS, Brandler MD, D'Souza A. Necrotizing enterocolitis. *Clin Perinatol*. 2008;35(1):251–272, x.
194. Alfaleh K, Bassler D. Probiotics for prevention of necrotizing enterocolitis in preterm infants. *Cochrane Database Syst Rev*. 2008;23(1):CD005496.
195. Ehrlich PF, Sato TT, Short BL, et al. Outcome of perforated necrotizing enterocolitis in the very low-birth weight neonate may be independent of the type of surgical treatment. *Am Surg*. 2001;67(8):752–756.
196. Catre D, Lopes MF, Madrigal A, et al. Early mortality after neonatal surgery: analysis of risk factors in an optimized health care system for the surgical newborn. *Rev Bras Epidemiol*. 2013;16(4):943–952.
197. Blakely ML, Lally KP, McDonald S, et al. Postoperative outcomes of extremely low birth-weight infants with necrotizing enterocolitis or isolated intestinal perforation: a prospective cohort study by the NICHD Neonatal Research Network. *Ann Surg*. 2005;241(6):984–989; discussion 989–994.
198. Lau ST, Lee YH, Caty MG. Current management of hernias and hydroceles. *Sem Pediatr Surg*. 2007;16(1):50–57.
199. Craven PD, Badawi N, Henderson-Smart DJ, et al. Regional (spinal, epidural, caudal) versus general anaesthesia in preterm infants undergoing inguinal herniorrhaphy in early infancy. *Cochrane Database Syst Rev*. 2003;(3):CD003669.
200. Cook-Sather SD, Tulloch HV, Liacouras CA, et al. Gastric fluid volume in infants for pyloromyotomy. *Can J Anaesth*. 1997;44(3):278–283.
201. Jacobs JP, Giroud JM, Quintessenza JA, et al. The modern approach to patent ductus arteriosus treatment: complementary roles of video-assisted thoracoscopic surgery and interventional cardiology coil occlusion. *Ann Thorac Surg*. 2003;76(5):1421–1427; discussion 1427–1428.

43 Pediatric Anesthesia

JERROLD LERMAN

Anatomy and Physiology
  Airway
  Cardiovascular
  Central Nervous System
Pharmacology
  Developmental Pharmacology
  Inhalational Anesthetics
  Intravenous
Preoperative Assessment
  Fasting Guidelines
  Laboratory Testing
  Medical Conditions
  Preoperative History
  Allergies
  Preoperative Physical Examination
  Anesthetic Risks; Consent/Assent
Induction of Anesthesia
  Equipment
  Monitors
  Emergency Drugs
  Full Stomach and Rapid Sequence Induction

Preoperative Preparation
  Anxiolysis
  Induction Techniques
Problems during Induction of Anesthesia
  Hemoglobin Oxygen Desaturation
  Laryngospasm
  Bradycardia
Maintenance of Anesthesia
  Techniques
  Fluid Management
  Prophylaxis for Postoperative Vomiting
  Regional Anesthesia and Pain Management
Emergence and Recovery from Anesthesia
Transport to PACU
PACU Complications
  Laryngospasm, Postoperative Stridor, and Negative Pressure Pulmonary Edema
  Oxygen Desaturation
  Emergence Delirium
  Vomiting
  Postoperative Pain

KEY POINTS

1. The airway in infants and children presents unique features that require a clear understanding of the anatomy and physiology of the airway structures. Laryngospasm and airway obstruction increase perioperative morbidity and mortality. Treatment of laryngospasm includes continuous positive airway pressure with 100% oxygen, jaw thrust applied at the condyles of the mandible, and early administration of atropine and propofol and/or succinylcholine to prevent profound desaturation and bradycardia and to relax the vocal cords.

2. Evidence in young animals has raised concerns regarding the neurocognitive sequelae after general anesthetics. Recent laboratory evidence however, suggests that exercising and socializing the animals after an anesthetic mitigates the neurocognitive dysfunction. Neurocognitive function in young children assessed 2 years after a simple but brief sevoflurane anesthetic indicates similar neurocognitive function as after spinal anesthesia.

3. Drug dosing in children is complex. Several factors influence drug doses including organ homeostasis (cardiopulmonary, renal, and hepatic functions), coexisting diseases, obesity, and developmental maturation of the cytochrome enzyme system. Unusual drug responses may result from single nucleotide polymorphisms (SNFs).

4. Understanding the pharmacokinetics and pharmacodynamics of inhaled anesthetics, the most commonly used anesthetics in children, helps to anticipate unexpected responses such as an anesthetic overdose during controlled ventilation or awareness after sub-MAC dosing during stimulation.

5. Upper respiratory tract infections (URTIs) are the most common comorbidity in children who present for surgery. Caution should be exercised when anesthetizing infants (<1 year of age) with recent URTIs (i.e., respiratory syncytial and other viruses may be latent) and children with colds in the preceding 2 weeks as the rate of perioperative complications is increased. Surgery should be rescheduled if any one of the following signs complicates a URTI: fever (>38.5°C); the child is not behaving normally (e.g., lack of appetite); purulent, green secretions; or lower respiratory tract signs (e.g., wheezing that does not clear with a deep cough).

6. Obstructive sleep apnea (OSA) in children differs from adults in that large tonsils and adenoids are the primary causes of OSA. Perioperative respiratory complications in these children are linked to the severity of intermittent nocturnal desaturation (threshold is oxygen saturation [SaO_2] <85%) as hypoxemia upregulates the genes responsible for opioid sensitivity. Emerging evidence suggests that OSA in obese children is complicated by a systemic inflammatory response, resulting in less favorable improvement after adenotonsillar surgery.

7. Obesity is the most rapidly growing challenge in pediatric anesthesia. Although laryngoscopy and tracheal intubation has been considered challenging in these patients, a 25-degree head-up position and exaggerated sniffing position such that the tragus lies above a horizontal line through the sternal notch facilitates tracheal intubation. Drug dosing must be adjusted to the appropriate weight scalar for the drug. Perioperative respiratory complications and postoperative admission after surgery are more common in these children.

8 Allergies and anaphylaxis during anesthesia in children in North America are most commonly due to latex sensitivity. Antibiotics, particularly the penicillin analogues, constitute a distant second cause. Epinephrine is the definitive treatment. Propofol allergy is extraordinarily rare in children, occurring only in those with documented egg anaphylaxis (not allergy). Although more common in Europe, anaphylaxis to muscle relaxants in children in North America is rare we suspect because of the absence of sensitizing agents (such as pholcodine).

9 The philosophical shift in fluid management strategy for most children 6 months of age or older in perioperative volumes has been from hypotonic glucose-containing solutions in 4–2–1 mL/kg/hr to use balanced salt solutions of 10 to 40 mL/kg over 1–4 h. The underlying strategy is to downregulate antidiuretic hormone secretion to avoid perioperative hyponatremia. In neonates and young infants (<6 months), the 4–2–1 mL/kg/hr hypotonic glucose-containing fluid strategy remains appropriate for maintenance.

10 Efficient ambulatory surgery in children requires effective preventative pain and vomiting strategies. Pain should be prophylactically managed with local anesthetics and/or systemic analgesics during anesthesia to limit the need for postoperative analgesics. Continuous regional blocks are most effective in appropriate surgery. Prophylactic strategies to prevent postoperative vomiting are most effectively managed with a combination of aggressive perioperative IV fluid hydration, intravenous (IV) dexamethasone, and serotonin-receptor antagonists and avoiding forcing postoperative fluids. Ex-premature infants and full-term neonates should be monitored postoperatively in hospital until the risk of a perioperative apnea has waned (≥12 hours apnea-free).

Anatomy and Physiology

1 Airway

Understanding the anatomic differences between the infant and adult upper airways is key to managing the infant's airway safely. Table 43-1 summarizes these differences. With a large brain and occiput, the child's head is naturally in the "sniffing" or flexed position. The large tongue/mouth volume ratio presents difficulty if the mouth is closed during mask ventilation, particularly with the narrowed nares. Hence, mask ventilation requires particular skill to avoid airway obstruction. Ensuring safe mask anesthesia and a patent airway requires proper application of the "jaw thrust" as described later while avoiding pressure on the soft tissues in the submental triangle.

The most common airway problem in infants and young children is upper airway obstruction due to laryngomalacia. In this condition, the supraglottic structures converge on the glottic opening during inspiration preventing most, if not all, air entry through the glottis. The net effect is upper airway obstruction. This is characterized by suprasternal and supraclavicular retractions, paradoxical collapse of the chest wall and/or sternum, and exaggerated diaphragmatic excursions. The treatment is constant positive airway pressure. Laryngomalacia usually resolves with age and without treatment.

A number of congenital airway anomalies pose challenges during anesthesia. Pierre Robin sequence (defined as micrognathia, airway distress in the first 24 to 48 hours after birth, and glossoptosis) is a common airway anomaly in which direct laryngoscopy is often difficult. This airway anomaly improves with age, usually resolving by 2 years. In contrast, other airway anomalies become progressively more difficult to manage with age. Treacher Collins syndrome is one such anomaly in which the airway becomes increasingly difficult with age. Several other disorders present primarily as difficult mask ventilation (e.g., Crouzon and Apert diseases and Down syndrome), but tracheal intubation is not a problem. In children, it is uncommon to face a "cannot ventilate, cannot intubate" airway in a child. Nonetheless, it is essential to identify a child's syndrome and the airway issue if it exists and to design an appropriate treatment strategy.

Covered with pseudostratified, columnar epithelium, the cricoid ring is the only solid cartilaginous and ringed structure within the upper airway. This loosely adherent, columnar epithelium is subject to swelling if irritated, reducing the radius of the lumen. Because airflow in the upper airway is turbulent (Reynolds number >4,000), as the lumen of the ring narrows, the pressure drop increases in proportion to radius to the fifth power. Hence, a 50% reduction in the radius of the cricoid ring increases the pressure drop by 32-fold. This increases the work of breathing, which if sustained, may result in respiratory failure.

The short trachea in the infant and child facilitates inadvertent endobronchial intubation. Careful assessment of the position of the tracheal tube in the airway is crucial to avoid this problem. Persistent hemoglobin desaturation (SaO_2 <85%) may be the first sign of an endobronchial intubation.

The greater alveolar ventilation to functional residual capacity (FRC) ratio in the child (5:1) compared with the adult (1.5:1) increases the risk of hemoglobin desaturation. The increased

Table 43-1	Anatomic Features of the Upper Airway in Infants Compared with Adults
Head	Larger occiput in the infant naturally positions the head in the "sniffing" position Stabilize the head against lateral rotation Obligate nose breathers for the first few months
Mouth	Relative large tongue volume in the mouth in the infant reduces the available space for instrumentation Edentulous
Neck	Larynx is more cephalad in the neck (C3–C4) in the infant Epiglottis is omega shaped and longer Vocal cords slant caudally at their insertion in the arytenoids Narrowest part of the upper airway is the cricoid ring (a solid circumferential, cartilaginous structure) covered by pseudostratified columnar epithelium Trachea is short (4–5 cm)
Tracheobronchial tree	Acute angle of the right mainstem bronchus at the carina Turbulent gas flow until the fifth bronchial division (resistance is inversely related to the radius to the fifth power)

alveolar ventilation reflects the increased oxygen consumption per kilogram in the child. This oxygen requirement, combined with the increased compliance of the rib cage (due to both anatomic and physiologic features), reduced compliance of the lungs (due to the relative lack of elastin in the infant), and reduced percent of type 1 fibers (slow-twitch, high oxidative muscle fibers) in the diaphragm predisposes the basal segments of the lungs to atelectasis under the weight of the abdomen. Together, these factors predispose the infant to rapid desaturation and respiratory failure when faced with respiratory difficulties. Additional details of the physiology of the pulmonary system in the neonate may be found in Chapter 42.

Cardiovascular

Once the neonatal heart completes the transition to postnatal life, the changes in the cardiovascular system are less dramatic. In the early years, the heart has reduced ability to increase stroke volume, rendering cardiac output more dependent on heart rate than in the adult. In the infant, atropine increases cardiac output not only by increasing the heart rate but also by augmenting a calcium-dependent force-frequency response.[1] A corollary of this relationship is that hypotension in the child with a normal or increased heart rate is due to hypovolemia and is ideally managed with fluids rather than vasopressors (except possibly in those with congenital heart disease). Systemic vascular tone is poor in children up to 8 years of age, as evidenced by the lack of change in blood pressure when caudal/epidural blocks are administered.

Both heart rate and blood pressure increase with increasing age in childhood (Table 43-2)[2] and these provide a framework from which the definitions of bradycardia and hypotension were developed.

Central Nervous System

Physiology

Oxygen consumption in the brain of children (5.5 mL/100 g/min) is 50% greater than that in adults (3.5 mL/100 g/min).[3] As a result, cerebral blood flow (CBF) differs substantially from adults. In children, overall CBF is 50% to 70% greater than in adults (70 to 110 mL/min/100 g vs. 50 mL/min/100 g). More CBF is directed to gray matter in children, reaching a distribution similar to that in adults by adolescence. Autoregulation is intact in full-term and nonstressed infants. The details of autoregulation in children are not well defined, although evidence indicates there are no age-related changes in autoregulation throughout childhood.

Neuroapoptosis

That alcohol and NMDA receptor antagonists caused apoptosis (programmed cell death) in newborn rodents led investigators to discover that most general anesthetics and sedatives, which also act on NMDA and $GABA_A$ receptors, cause apoptosis in newborn rodents and nonhuman primates. Most anesthetics, with the exception of the α_2 agonists, opioids, muscle relaxants, and possibly xenon cause apoptosis and neurocognitive dysfunction in newborn animals. These effects are exacerbated when multiple anesthetics are coadministered and administered for more prolonged periods.[4] If the affected newborns are raised to adulthood, the neurocognitive changes remain. Interestingly, several drugs and interventions dramatically attenuate these effects including melatonin, lithium, hypothermia, and exercise.[5,6]

Whether these effects in newborn animals are translatable to humans remains contentious. First, the positive predictive value of animal effects in humans is less than 10%. Second, the doses of IV anesthetics and sedatives in rodents and primates are up to 10-fold greater than in humans[7]; such large doses may explain, in part, the neurocognitive dysfunction observed after IV anesthetics but do not explain the effects of inhalational anesthetics whose dosing is constant across species. Third, studies in humans who received anesthesia at a young age indicated that neurocognitive dysfunction in those who received anesthesia before the age of 3 years and who received multiple anesthetics was more severe than in those who did not.[4] However, most of those studies were seriously flawed in terms of their design (retrospective), limited external validity (no pulse oximetry or capnography), different anesthetics (halothane), nonstandardized metrics (learning disability tests were not applied equally to all children), and confounding variables (complex pregnancy, drugs such as magnesium) that were not standardized. A large cohort of identical twins who were discordant for general anesthesia at less than 3 years of age tested identically for intellectual aptitude 10 years later.[8] The 2-year follow-up of children in the prospective, randomized, and blinded GAS (sevoflurane anesthesia vs. spinal anesthesia) study demonstrated identical neurocognitive function in the two groups.[9]

Pharmacology

Developmental Pharmacology

Understanding the pharmacology of drugs in children is a complex subject that is briefly addressed later. Drugs must reach their effect site if they are to be effective. The steps involved in that process include absorption of the drug into the blood, transfer from the blood to the effect site, and termination of its action by redistribution, metabolism, and/or excretion.

The bioavailability of drugs depends on several factors including the route of administration, pK_a, the solubility of the drug and local perfusion. Some drugs such as midazolam are poorly absorbed from the stomach (15% bioavailability)[10] but are well absorbed from the nares,[11] whereas others such as acetaminophen are well absorbed from the stomach but are poorly and erratically absorbed from the rectum.[12] Age is another factor that may substantially affect drug absorption. For example, gastric juice is closer to neutral pH (pH ~6 to 8) at birth, only

Table 43-2 Normal Range of Resting Heart Rates and Blood Pressure in Children

Age	Heart Rate (beats/min)	Blood Pressure (mmHg)
0–3 mos	100–150	65–85/45–55
3–6 mos	90–120	70–90/50–65
6–12 mos	80–120	80–100/55–65
1–3 yrs	70–110	90–105/55–70
3–6 yrs	65–110	95–110/60–75
6–12 yrs	60–95	100–120/60–75
>12 yrs	55–85	110–135/65–85

Adapted with permission from Bernstein D. History and physical examination. In: Kliegman RM, Stanton BF, Geme JW, et al, eds. *Nelson Textbook of Pediatrics*. 19th ed. Philadelphia, PA: Saunders Elsevier; 2011:1529–1536.

reaching adult levels of acidity by ~3 years of age, thus affecting the absorption of lipophilic drugs at neutral pH values.[13] The route of administration also affects whether the drug undergoes first-pass metabolism through the liver. Rectal venous drainage from the superior hemorrhoidal veins drains into the portal venous system, whereas drainage from the middle and inferior hemorrhoidal veins bypasses the liver and flows directly into the iliac veins and into the heart. Hence, drugs that are administered rectally may undergo first-pass hepatic metabolism if they are absorbed via the superior rectal veins. Because drugs may be administered by any of these routes, it is critical to evaluate the bioavailability of the drug via each route and at each age to determine the appropriate dose to achieve a therapeutic blood concentration.

Once in the bloodstream, drugs partition between the protein and lipid-bound fractions and the free or active fraction. Two major proteins that bind drugs are synthesized in the liver: albumin and α_1-acid glycoprotein. The concentration of albumin, which is reduced at birth and in children with liver disease, cancer, nephropathy, and malnutrition, binds acidic drugs. The concentration of α_1-acid glycoprotein, which is also reduced at birth but increases with increasing age as well as during periods of stress and inflammation,[14] binds basic compounds such as lidocaine. Hence, the free fraction of lidocaine in young infants will be greater than in older children.[14] With reduced plasma concentrations of both albumin and α_1-acid glycoprotein in neonates and infants, the free fraction of drugs increases leading to a greater dose reaching the effect site and exerting physiologic as well as possible toxic effects.

Termination of the action of most IV drugs depends on their metabolism through phase 1 reactions (e.g., hydroxylation and oxidation) and/or phase 2 reactions (e.g., glucuronidation) in the liver. The rates at which these enzyme systems mature vary widely among and within individuals depending on a host of factors. Apart from a few enzyme systems that hold importance in fetal life (e.g., CYP450 3A7),[15] the activities of the vast majority of CYP450 enzyme systems (e.g., CYP450 3A4, 2E1, and 2D6) involved in phase 1 reactions increase from birth, but at varying rates (Fig. 43-1).[15] Moreover, genetic polymorphisms of several families of enzymes (e.g., 2D6) may dramatically affect the activity of the enzyme, resulting in a wide range of activity from zero to rapid and excessive (see Codeine).[16]

Phase 1 reactions are responsible for the majority of drug metabolism in the liver acting via the cytochrome P450 enzyme system: 3A4 metabolizes 50% of our drugs, 2D6 10% to 20%,[16] and 1A2, 2E1, and 2C9 the remainder. These isozyme systems mature from birth reaching adult activity levels by 1 to 5 years of age (Fig. 43-1). Phase 2 enzymes, which conjugate drugs and metabolites for excretion, are also immature at birth, giving rise to concerns about bilirubin toxicity. However, these systems also mature quickly with age.

Termination of the action of many drugs in anesthesia depends on either redistribution of the active compound away from the effect site to other vessel-rich organs (see Inhalational Anesthetics section) or muscle, or metabolism in the liver and excretion or direct excretion by the kidneys. Elimination of the metabolic by-products and residual active parent compounds depends on renal perfusion and elimination. The glomerular filtration rate is markedly reduced in the neonate and young infant but matures throughout childhood reaching adult rates by 5 to 15 years of age.[17]

Inhalational Anesthetics

The widespread appeal of the current inhalational anesthetics may be attributed to their physicochemical properties (Table 43-3), which provide a rapid onset and offset of action, cardiorespiratory homeostasis, and limited metabolism and toxicity. Halothane has all but disappeared from North American anesthetic practice, having been replaced by sevoflurane as the induction agent of choice in infants and children. Enflurane has been supplanted by its optical isomer, isoflurane, and more recently by desflurane. Desflurane offers the most favorable pharmacokinetic and in vivo metabolic characteristics in terms of its minimal blood and tissue solubilities and resistance to metabolism, although its use as an induction agent in children is proscribed because it is very irritating to the upper airway. Most recently, the noble gas xenon has generated much interest as an anesthetic because it is safe for the environment, lacks cardiovascular

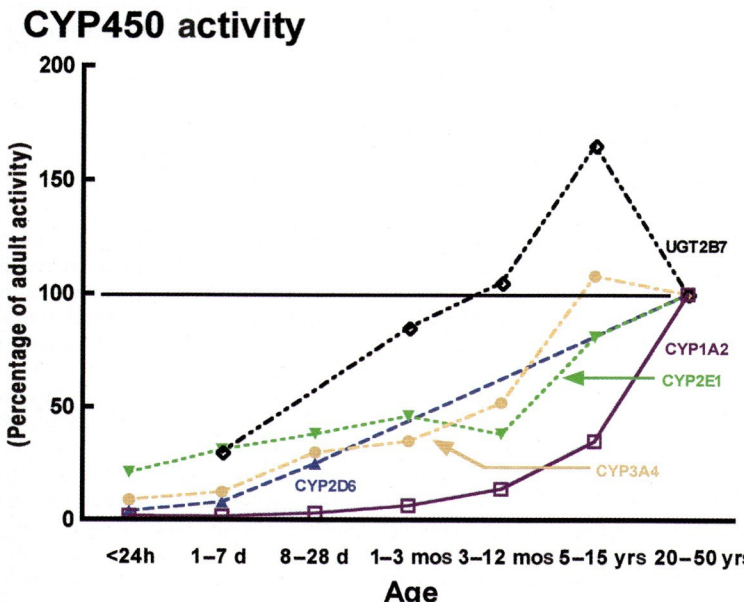

Figure 43-1 Developmental changes in common cytochromes of interest in pediatric anesthesia. (Adapted from Kearns GL, Abdel-Rahman SM, Alander SW, et al. Developmental pharmacology—drug disposition, action, and therapy in infants and children. *N Engl J Med*. 2003;349:1157–1167; and Alcorn J, McNamara PJ. Pharmacokinetics in the newborn. *Adv Drug Deliv Rev*. 2003;55:675.)

Table 43-3 Pharmacology of Inhaled Anesthetics

	Halothane	Enflurane	Isoflurane	Sevoflurane	Desflurane
Odor	Mild, pleasant	Etheric	Etheric	Pleasant, tolerated	Etheric
Solubility					
$\lambda_{b/g}$ adults	2.4	1.9	1.4	0.66	0.42
$\lambda_{b/g}$ neonates[a]	2.14	1.78	1.19	0.66	–
$\lambda_{brain/b}$ adults[b]	1.9	1.3	1.6	1.7	1.2
$\lambda_{brain/b}$ neonates[c]	1.5	0.9	1.3	–	–
$\lambda_{fat/b}$ adults[b]	51.1	–	45	48	27
MAC					
MAC_{adults}	0.75	1.7	1.2	2.05	7
$MAC_{neonates}$	0.87	–	1.60	3.2	9.2
Metabolism					
In vivo (%)	15–20	2.4	1.4	<5	0.2

λ is the partition coefficient; b/g is blood/gas; brain/b is brain/blood; fat/b is fat/blood; MAC is the minimum alveolar concentration (%).
[a]Data from Lerman J, Schmitt-Bantel BI, Gregory GA, et al. Effect of age on the solubility of volatile anesthetics in human tissues. *Anesthesiology*. 1986;65:307–311; and Malviya S, Lerman J. The blood/gas solubilities of sevoflurane, isoflurane, halothane, and serum constituent concentrations in neonates and adults. *Anesthesiology*. 1990;72:793–796.
[b]Data from Yasuda N, Targ AG, Eger EI II. Solubility of I-653, sevoflurane, isoflurane, and halothane in human tissues. *Anesth Analg*. 1989;69:370–373.
[c]Data from Lerman J, Gregory GA, Willis MM, et al. Age and solubility of volatile anesthetics in blood. *Anesthesiology*. 1984;61:139–143.

toxicity, and has no serious toxicity either in vivo or in vitro. However, xenon is not widely available (because it must be extracted from the atmosphere), is very expensive, has a minimum alveolar concentration (MAC) of 70%, and causes nausea and vomiting. There are no published data regarding the pharmacology of xenon in children.

All of the currently used inhalational anesthetics are methyl ethyl ether compounds with the exception of sevoflurane, which is a methyl isopropyl ether. Their physicochemical and pharmacodynamic effects are summarized in Table 43-3.

Pharmacokinetics

The rate of increase in alveolar to inspired anesthetic partial pressures—that is, fraction in the alveolus (F_A) to fraction in the inspired gas (F_I), known as the washin ratio (F_A/F_I)—depends on six factors (Table 43-4). The first three determine the delivery of anesthetic to the lungs and the second three determine the removal of anesthetic from the lung. The washin ratio increases from 0 toward 1 in the shape of an exponential curve for all inhalational anesthetics. The order of washin of the anesthetics is inversely related to the solubility of the anesthetics in blood; that is, the smaller the solubility in blood, the more rapid the washin (Table 43-3).[18,19]

The washin curve for inhalational anesthetics is characterized by the simple exponential equation

$$F_A/F_I = 1 - e^{-kt} \qquad (43\text{-}1)$$

where k is a constant (k = 1/time constant (τ)) and t is time in minutes. τ is the ratio of the volume of the organ to the blood flow to that organ. The smaller the time constant, the more rapidly F_A/F_I equilibrates. The time constants for most organs in children are less than those in adults, explaining in part the rapid equilibration of halothane in children compared with adults (Fig. 43-2).

In the case of infants and children, four factors explain the more rapid washin of halothane compared with adults. These

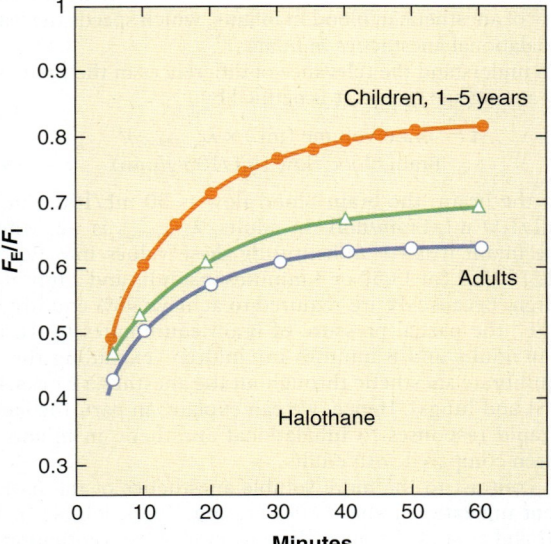

Figure 43-2 The more rapid washin of halothane in children compared with adults. The fractional end-tidal to inspired ratio (F_E/F_I) of halothane (Y-axis) over time (X-axis). The two *lower* curves (with *open symbols*) are from adults. (Adapted from Salanitre E, Rackow H. The pulmonary exchange of nitrous oxide and halothane in infants and children. *Anesthesiology*. 1969;30:391.)

Table 43-4 Determinants of the Washin and Washout of Inhalational Anesthetics

1. Inspired concentration
2. Alveolar ventilation
3. Functional residual capacity
4. Cardiac output
5. Solubility
6. Alveolar to venous anesthetic partial pressure gradient

Table 43-5 Factors That Explain the More Rapid Washin of Inhalational Anesthetics in Children Compared with Adults

- Alveolar ventilation:FRC ratio (5:1 in infants vs. 1.5:1 in adults)
- Greater distribution of cardiac output to the vessel-rich group in infants (vessel-rich group comprises 18% of the body weight in infants compared with 8% in adults)
- Reduced tissue solubility in infants[18]
- Reduced blood solubility in infants[20,21]

factors are listed in order of importance from the greatest to the least in Table 43-5.

The greater alveolar ventilation (VA):functional residual capacity (FRC) ratio in infants and children compared with adults may be attributed to the greater metabolic rate and oxygen demand in children. Increases in alveolar ventilation speed the equilibration of inspired to alveolar anesthetic partial pressures.[22] The net effect of a greater VA:FRC ratio is a reduction in the time constant, from 0.7 in adults to 0.2 in infants, which explains the speed of equilibration. Although a greater cardiac output should slow the rate of increase in F_A/F_I, it actually speeds the equilibration in neonates and infants. This paradoxical effect may be attributed to the greater cardiac output perfusing the vessel-rich group (VRG) (comprised of the heart, brain, gastrointestinal organs, kidneys, and endocrine glands) which comprises 18% of the body's weight in infants compared with only 8% in adults. Hence, the greater cardiac output in infants speeds the equilibration of F_A/F_I in the VRG, which takes up most of the anesthetic during the first couple of hours of anesthesia. The third factor is the reduced tissue solubility in infants compared with that in adults.[18] The solubility of all inhalational anesthetics is reduced in tissues in infants compared with adults including the brain, muscle, and heart. The fourth factor is the reduced solubility of anesthetic in blood in infants, which speeds the washin of inhalational anesthetics in infants.[21]

To understand the relevance of differences in the tissue solubility among age groups, τ is defined by

$$\tau = (\text{Brain volume (mL)} \times \lambda_{brain/blood})/\text{Brain blood flow (mL/100 g/min)} \quad (43\text{-}2)$$

In the brain, the brain blood flow is 50 mL/100 g/min or 50 mL/100 mL brain/min. In adults, $\lambda_{brain/blood}$ is ~2, whereas in the infant it is ~1. Substituting these values into Eq. 43-2 yields 100 × 2 (or 1)/50 or 4 minutes in adults and 2 minutes in children. Because 4τ are required to achieve 98% equilibration of F_A/F_I, the partial pressure of brain equilibrates by 16 minutes in adults and 8 minutes in children (excluding the time to equilibrate anesthetic throughout the anesthesia workstation [AWS] and lungs). Hence, we can explain, in part, the sudden and rapid responses to inhalational anesthetic in infants and children compared with adults.

In contrast to the more soluble anesthetics of the past, the current inhalational anesthetics are much less soluble in both blood and tissues. Because changes in alveolar ventilation and cardiac output affect the washin of less soluble anesthetics to a lesser extent than more soluble anesthetics, the effects of the first two factors in Table 43-5 on the washin of sevoflurane and desflurane in young children are attenuated. Therefore, the washin of these anesthetics in this age group may be similar in infants and adults. Furthermore, the solubilities of these agents in blood in infants are similar to those in adults[20]; however, the tissue solubilities in infants compared with adults have not been reported. Hence, we may expect the washin of sevoflurane and desflurane in infants to be, at the most, only marginally more rapid than in adults.

Estimates of the effect site equilibration half-life ($t_{1/2keo}$) for sevoflurane in children and adults have been reported using the bispectral index (BIS) to be 1.2 and 3.2 minutes, respectively.[23,24]

Two additional aspects of the pharmacokinetics of inhalational anesthetics in infants and children merit consideration. The first is the mode of ventilation. The washin of inhalational anesthetics increases rapidly during induction of anesthesia. In dogs, the washin of halothane was well tolerated during spontaneous respiration whether the inspired concentration was 0.4% or 4%.[25] The F_A/F_I plateaued in all instances at 0.6 to 0.7. As the anesthetic depth increased, ventilation was reduced, decreasing the uptake of anesthetic. As anesthetic was redistributed from the brain and the depth of anesthesia reduced, ventilation increased and the uptake and depth of anesthesia resumed. This process is known as a negative feedback control loop. However, when ventilation was controlled, 85% and 100% of the dogs that received 4% or 6% inspired halothane, respectively, died.[25] Controlled ventilation is a positive feedback control loop in which the delivery of inhalational anesthesia to the lungs continues unabated, deepening the level of anesthesia and thus cardiac output. The decreased cardiac output attenuates the pulmonary blood flow and thus the uptake of and removal of anesthetic from the lung. Thus, the partial pressure of anesthetic within the lungs increases steadily. These greater partial pressures in the lungs equilibrate with the reduced cardiac output, to further depress the VRG, ultimately resulting in a cardiac arrest. This study illustrates the inherent safety of the spontaneous compared with controlled ventilation during inhalational anesthesia in that the former protects against an overdose of an inhalational anesthetic; whether the same benefit holds true for sevoflurane remains unknown. In the past, multiple vaporizers could be used simultaneously, posing a hazard if ventilation were controlled. Interlocking devices were developed to prevent such an anesthetic overdose.

The second issue relates to shunts and their effects on the uptake and distribution of anesthetics. Left-to-right shunts have limited effects on the uptake and distribution of inhalational anesthetics provided the cardiac output is maintained.[5] However, right-to-left shunts present an entirely different and far more complex clinical situation. Irrespective of the source of these shunts (intrapulmonary or intracardiac or both), the washin of less soluble anesthetics are affected to a much greater extent by the presence of these shunts than more soluble anesthetics.[5] That is, it is much more difficult to maintain an adequate depth of anesthesia with sevoflurane in infants with significant right-to-left shunts whether it is an intrapulmonary or intracardiac shunt. To maintain anesthesia in infants with these shunts, supplemental IV anesthesia is often required. Understanding the differential effect of shunts on the washin of inhalational anesthetics is beyond the scope of this chapter, but the basis may be summarized by the differential effect of ventilation on the washin of less and more soluble anesthetics.[5]

The speed of washout of inhalational anesthetics follows an exponential decay, with the speed inversely related to the solubility of the anesthetics in blood (Table 43-3). That is, the washout is more rapid for anesthetics that are less soluble in blood: desflurane > sevoflurane > isoflurane ≥ halothane.[19,21] The only exception to this rule is the washout of halothane, which overlaps that of isoflurane in part, because the former is extensively metabolized in vivo, 15% to 25% (Table 43-3). Computer simulations demonstrated greater differences in recovery and greater than 90% decrement in the anesthetic concentration among the anesthetics after prolonged anesthesia.[26]

Substituting a less soluble anesthetic for a more soluble one during maintenance of anesthesia has been proposed to accelerate the washout of anesthetics and recovery from anesthesia. However, switching from isoflurane to desflurane 30 minutes before the end of surgery did not speed the recovery compared with a 2 h anesthetic with 1.25 MAC isoflurane in adult volunteers.[27] More recently, charcoal filters have been used to adsorb anesthetics and, when combined with hypercapnic hyperventilation, were shown to rapidly remove anesthetics and speed recovery in adults.[28,29] Comparable washout data in children are lacking.

Pharmacodynamics

The MAC is that concentration of inhalational anesthetic at which 50% of patients move in response to a skin incision. In children, the MAC is known to vary substantively with age. That is, as the fetus matures and reaches term, the MAC increases peaking in infants 1 to 6 months of age for halothane[30,31] and isoflurane[32,33] and then decreases steadily thereafter with increasing age (Fig. 43-3). In the case of sevoflurane, the MAC is 3.3% in neonates and 3.2% in infants 1 to 6 months of age.[34] For children 6 months to 12 years, the MAC is constant at 2.4%.[34] In the case of desflurane, the MAC increases throughout infancy peaking in infants 6 to 12 months of age and decreases thereafter with increasing age.[35] The reasons for the peak of MAC in infancy and the age-dependent changes in the MAC remain unclear.

The MAC values of inhalational anesthetics in children have shown several other peculiarities. The MAC of halothane is 25% less in children with cognitive dysfunction, especially those taking anti-seizure drugs.[36] The MAC of desflurane in adult homozygote redheads is 20% greater than in nonredheads[37]; the same response would be expected in children of similar genetic predisposition. The MAC values for halothane and isoflurane show simple additivity with N_2O in adults and children; however, 60% N_2O only contributes 25% to the MAC values for sevoflurane and desflurane in children.[34,38] The reason for this diminished effect of N_2O on the MAC values of sevoflurane and desflurane is unknown. The MAC also varies with the child's temperature. In children 4 to 10 years of age, the MAC of isoflurane decreases 5%/°C decrease in temperature.[39]

In addition to determining the MAC responses to skin incision, the ED_{50} to a number of other maneuvers including insertion and removal of laryngeal mask airways (LMAs), tracheal extubation, and others have been determined in children.[5]

Respiration

When administered in the absence of surgical stimulation, all anesthetics depress respiration and minute ventilation in a dose-dependent manner, by decreasing tidal volume and increasing respiratory rate.[40,41] Inhalational anesthetics relax intercostal muscles before the diaphragm, resulting primarily in diaphragmatic respiration. Respiratory rate increases during anesthesia, which offsets in part the reduced tidal volume. These effects are most pronounced with halothane; at concentrations 1.4 MAC or higher, sevoflurane depresses respiration to a greater extent than halothane in adults,[42] although the evidence is less clear in children.[41] As the concentration of sevoflurane increases, respiratory rate also diminishes ultimately resulting in apnea. This effect is augmented in the presence of a midazolam premedication. This central effect is offset by manually assisting ventilation. In the case of desflurane, concentrations greater than 1 MAC depress respiration in infants and children, an effect that exceeds the depression by other inhalational anesthetics.[43]

Inhalational anesthetics also depress the response to carbon dioxide and hypoxia in a dose-dependent manner.

Airway resistance increases during desflurane,[44] and decreases during sevoflurane anesthesia in children.[44,45] Hence, in children with asthma, sevoflurane is preferable. In both children and adults with refractory status asthmaticus, inhalational anesthetics have been effective to break the bronchospasm in the intensive care unit.[46,47]

Upper airway responses to inhalational anesthesia (by mask) depend on both the concentration and the particular anesthetic administered. Halothane and sevoflurane infrequently trigger these reflex responses[40,48] whereas isoflurane and desflurane are quite irritating to the airway, particularly at concentrations exceeding 1 MAC.[49,50] The package insert for desflurane cautions against using it for inhalational inductions in children. The mechanism by which inhalational anesthetics trigger upper airway reflex responses remains unclear.

When a tracheal tube is used, neither desflurane nor isoflurane triggers airway reflexes during maintenance or emergence from anesthesia.[50] When an LMA is used, extubation during deep desflurane anesthesia may increase the incidence of airway reflex responses when compared with extubation awake after desflurane or isoflurane.[51]

Cardiovascular

Inhalational anesthetics depress the heart in a dose-dependent manner. Direct effects of these anesthetics depress the heart rate, contractility, and peripheral vascular tone. Among the inhalational anesthetics, halothane slows the heart rate the most, often sensitizing the myocardium to catecholamines and inducing ventricular dysrhythmias. In the past, anticholinergics were commonly used to prevent bradycardia and arrhythmias in children given halothane; however, this practice is no longer necessary with the newer ether anesthetics that infrequently cause arrhythmias. Sevoflurane and the remaining ether anesthetics exert limited effects on the cardiac conduction system. Sevoflurane maintains or increases heart rate during induction of anesthesia in most instances likely due to withdrawal

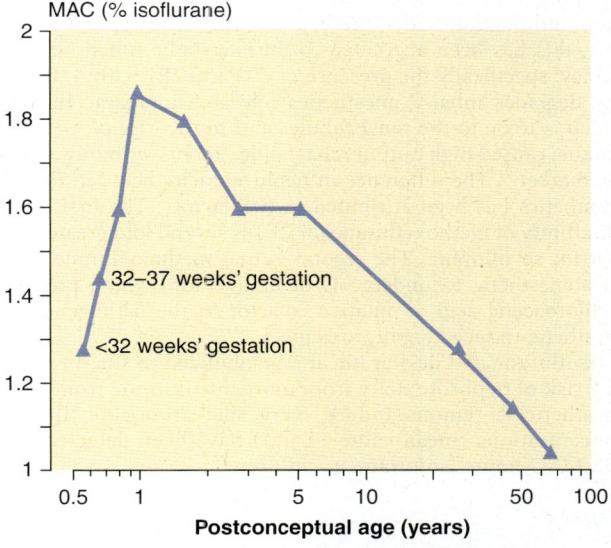

Figure 43-3 Age and the MAC of isoflurane from premature infants to adults. (Adapted from LeDez KM, Lerman J. The minimum alveolar concentration [MAC] of isoflurane in preterm neonates. *Anesthesiology*. 1987;67:301–307.)

of vagal tone,[52] although on occasion, nodal bradycardia may occur. This is usually a self-limited effect. Desflurane and isoflurane also tend to increase the heart rate. Desflurane, to a greater extent than isoflurane, causes a sympathetic discharge when the inspired concentration is increased substantively and in a stepwise manner, without pretreatment with opioids[53]; similar responses in children have not been forthcoming. This effect is mediated through the right and left lungs.[54] Sevoflurane and the other inhalational anesthetics prolong the QT interval, but do not increase the dispersion of repolarization, thus precluding torsades de pointes and other potentially fatal arrhythmias (see later).[55] However, arrhythmias have been reported in children with congenital long QT interval particularly during emergence from anesthesia.[56]

Halothane depresses myocardial contractility to the greatest extent; sevoflurane and the remaining ether anesthetics exert a much more attenuated effect in children. Sevoflurane and halothane decrease cardiac index in children similarly, ~10% at 1 × MAC and 20% to 30% at 2 × MAC, although sevoflurane may depress cardiac index in infants less than after halothane.[57,58] Compared with awake values, systolic blood pressure decreases ~20% to 30% at 1 × MAC of ether anesthetics, an effect that is usually reversed with surgical stimulation.[32,34,35]

Early studies showed that cardiac output depended on heart rate in young children; the calcium-dependent force contraction-rate effect is pronounced in infants and young children.[1] Furthermore, increasing the heart rate reversed the halothane-dependent decreases in cardiac output.[59] More recent evidence suggests that children can increase their stroke volume if needed to augment their cardiac output. Peripheral vascular resistance is reduced in children as evidenced by the absence of a change in blood pressure when a caudal/epidural block is administered.

Sevoflurane is preferred over halothane in children with congenital heart disease as it causes fewer arrhythmias and less hypotension than halothane.[60]

Most anesthetic drugs prolonged the QT interval, which is prolonged when it exceeds 500 milliseconds.[61] When the QT interval is prolonged in the presence of an increased dispersion of repolarization, there is a substantial risk for torsades de pointes. The risk of torsades de pointes is increased when anesthetics that prolong the QT interval are administered to children in the presence of congenital long QT interval (Romano–Ward and Jervell and Lange-Nielsen syndrome), nonanesthetic drugs that prolong the QT interval, several medical conditions (hypomagnesemia, hypokalemia, hypocalcemia, cardiac disease, hypothyroidism), bradycardia, and the female gender.[61,62]

Central Nervous System

All inhalational anesthetics decrease cerebral vascular resistance and cerebral metabolic rate for oxygen. The decrease in vascular resistance increases CBF in the following order: halothane > desflurane > isoflurane > sevoflurane.[3] Sevoflurane and isoflurane decrease oxygen consumption to greater extents than halothane. Hence, the most favorable ratio of CBF to oxygen consumption follows the reverse order: sevoflurane > isoflurane > desflurane > halothane.

The effects of changes in blood pressure as well as carbon dioxide and oxygen tensions on CBF during anesthesia in children have not been fully elucidated. Autoregulation of CBF in children of all ages is similar to that in adults, although it occurs at greater blood flow rates.[3] The lower limit of autoregulation in children of all ages appears to be similar, that is, the MAP of the 50th percentile for height or ~60 mmHg mean arterial pressure (MAP). However, in infants under 6 months, this limit may be as low as 38 mmHg or at 20% below the baseline MAP. All inhalational anesthetics impair autoregulation, although sevoflurane does not impair autoregulation in children 1.5 MAC or lower.[3] As in adults, hyperventilation restores autoregulation with isoflurane and sevoflurane. Cerebrovasodilatation and CBF increase as carbon dioxide tension increases in children up to ~50 mmHg, but beyond that level, maximum vasodilatation prevents any further response. Changes in CBF in response to changes in PCO_2 during isoflurane anesthesia are greater than during sevoflurane. Hence, hyperventilation may be more effective in attenuating increased intracranial pressure during isoflurane anesthesia than during sevoflurane.

The electroencephalogram during sevoflurane is characterized by sharp, slow waves in the lower frequency range. This pattern differs substantially from that of the isoflurane, the latter comprising the algorithm for the BIS. As a result, the BIS readings in children under 5 years are imprecise, readings decrease 10% to 20% as the child ages from 1 to 12 years, and the BIS values paradoxically increase as the sevoflurane concentration increases from 3% to 4% (see BIS Measurements).[63–67]

Myoclonic movement as well as EEG spike and wave activity (epileptiform) have been reported in a very small number of children during inhalational inductions with sevoflurane, at concentrations between 5% and 8%.[68] In patients with seizures, epileptiform EEG activity has been reported in 58% of those anesthetized with 1 to 2 MAC sevoflurane and in 25% of those with 1 to 2 MAC isoflurane, with hyperventilation and nitrous oxide curiously reducing the epileptiform activity.[69] With sevoflurane, these occurred not only in several patients with a history of seizures but also in the presence of hyperventilation. Indeed, at sevoflurane concentrations approaching 8% during induction of anesthesia, ventilation should be assisted, but not controlled with hyperventilation, if apnea occurs.

Renal

Inhalational anesthetics do not exert substantive effects on the kidneys in children except through their metabolism: the kidney is a site of degradation of inhalational anesthetics. Ether anesthetics, most notably methoxyflurane (no longer in use) and to a lesser extent sevoflurane, are degraded by CYP450 2E1[70] releasing inorganic fluoride into the circulation in similar concentrations, although only the former is known to be nephrotoxic. In part, this has been attributed to the metabolic function of the kidney: specifically the presence of CYP450 2E1 within the kidney degrades inhaled anesthetics releasing inorganic fluoride, which is toxic to the renal tubules and in the case of methoxyflurane, caused high output renal failure and its withdrawal from the market.[71] The difference in nephrotoxicity between the two anesthetics has been attributed to two factors: The first is that the affinity of methoxyflurane for 2E1 is several fold greater than that for sevoflurane. The second is that methoxyflurane is the only anesthetic to undergo O-demethylation, which produces dichloroacetic acid, a putative cofactor in the pathogenesis of anesthetic-induced nephrotoxicity.[72]

Isoflurane and desflurane are metabolized to small extents. The risk of nephrotoxicity from inorganic fluoride from either anesthetic is remote. Indeed, very small inorganic fluoride concentrations (mean value 11 μM) have been detected after 131 MAC-hours isoflurane in children.[73]

Hepatic

There are few data regarding the effects of inhalational anesthetics on hepatic function in children. However, isolated cases of hepatic dysfunction in children have been reported after uses of every inhalational anesthetic.[74,75] Most children who develop hepatic dysfunction recover without further treatment. In the case of halothane hepatitis, serologic markers in the form of antibodies to hepatic cell membrane antigens have been detected.[76] Similar immunologic markers have been detected after isoflurane and desflurane, although none have been identified for sevoflurane to date. Although it has been suggested that repeated anesthetics with halothane cause hepatitis, this author asserts there is insufficient evidence to avoid repeated inhalational anesthetics in children.

In Vitro Metabolism

Degradation of inhalational anesthetics in the presence of carbon dioxide absorbents has been the subject of intense research and concern in both adults and children.

Sevoflurane may be degraded via the Cannizzaro reaction in carbon dioxide absorbents. The reaction is accelerated in the presence of increased temperature and barium hydroxide, strong bases (potassium hydroxide), very low fresh gas flow, large sevoflurane concentrations, and dessicated absorbent. The reaction releases five compounds, of which compound A, fluoromethyl-2,2-difluoro-1-(trifluoromethyl) vinyl ether, is the most common.[77] Nephrotoxic concentrations of compound A are more than 100 ppm; in children 1 MAC sevoflurane produces 16 ppm after 5.6 MAC-hours in a circle circuit with a 2 L/min fresh gas flow.[77] To date, there have been no instances of compound A–induced nephrotoxicity in children.

Inhalational anesthetics may also be degraded in the presence of desiccated carbon dioxide absorbent yielding carbon monoxide. Desiccation may occur when a large fresh gas flows through a carbon dioxide absorber for an extended period (>48 hours) without a reservoir bag attached. Subsequently, when a potent inhalational anesthetic encounters the desiccated absorbent, carbon monoxide is produced. The rate of production of carbon monoxide follows the order: desflurane ≥ enflurane > isoflurane > halothane = sevoflurane.[78] This problem can be avoided if the AWS is turned off or the fresh gas is discontinued after each day or if the reservoir bag remains attached. Recently, carbon monoxide (≤18 ppm) was detected in the anesthesia breathing circuit in children although the source was unclear.[79]

Intravenous

IV drugs are distributed first to the VRG, just as inhalational anesthetics are, and then to the muscle, vessel-poor, and fat groups. The primary anesthetic effect occurs when an adequate brain concentration is achieved; thereafter, the anesthetic is redistributed to other tissues and metabolized to terminate its action. The pharmacokinetics of IV anesthetics depends on the dose and rate of drug administered, the binding of the drug in blood, the cardiac output and the distribution of cardiac output, metabolism, and excretion pathways.

Propofol

Diisopropylphenol is the most commonly used IV induction agent in children. This highly lipophilic drug distributes rapidly to the VRG to affect its anesthetic action. The effect site equilibration half-life ($t_{1/2keo}$) has been estimated at 0.8 or 1.2 minutes, depending on the model.[80] Its action is terminated by redistribution as well as hepatic and extrahepatic metabolism. Volume of distribution and clearance (to a lesser extent) decrease progressively during early childhood.[81] However, clearance increases throughout gestation and the neonatal period, reaching 90% of adult values by 3 months of age.[82] To maintain the 3 μg/mL blood concentration for anesthesia, a 50% greater induction and infusion dosing schedule is required in young children.[83] The net effect is a context-sensitive half-life that increases with time in children more rapidly than in adults.[83]

The ED_{50} for loss of the eyelash reflex in children varies with the child's age: 3 ± 0.2 mg/kg in infants 1 to 6 months; 1.3 to 1.6 mg/kg in children 1 to 12 years; 2.4 ± 0.1 mg/kg in children 10 to 16 years.[84] The ED_{50} and ED_{90} of propofol to insert an LMA in children is 3.5 and 5.4 mg/kg (4.7 to 6.8 mg/kg 95% CI), respectively.[85,86] The dose of propofol to facilitate tracheal intubation in children during sevoflurane anesthesia is 1 to 2 mg/kg.[87,88]

Propofol is an integral part of total IV anesthesia (TIVA) for maintenance of anesthesia in children undergoing medical/radiologic evaluations and surgery. For painless medical or radiologic (e.g., MRI) procedures in young children 2 to 6 years of age, an initial infusion rate of 15 mg/kg/hr (250 μg/kg/min) of propofol is recommended after either an inhalational induction or an IV induction.[83,89,90] This dose may have to be increased to stop spontaneous movement, particularly if the children have neurocognitive impairment or are younger.[91] Conversely, the infusion rate may be reduced in older children. Infusion rates in obese children are far more complex and are discussed under Obesity.

Based on pharmacokinetic modeling to maintain a blood concentration of 3 μg/mL, the infusion rate is decreased during prolonged surgery to facilitate rapid emergence. One recommended stepwise reduction in the infusion rate in children 3 to 11 years of age after an IV induction with 2.5 mg/kg propofol is 15 mg/kg/hr (250 μg/kg/min) for 15 minutes followed by 13 mg/kg/hr (215 μg/kg/min) for 15 minutes, followed by 11 mg/kg/hr (180 μg/kg/min) for 30 minutes, followed by 10 mg/kg/hr (166 μg/kg/min) for 60 minutes, followed by 9 mg/kg/hr (150 μg/kg/min) for the next 2 hours.[83] Target-controlled infusions (TCI) in children are available in Europe, but not in North America.[92,93] These devices use preset algorithms based on the pharmacokinetics that use similar dosing algorithms with modest success.

Propofol causes pain in 70% or more of patients during IV induction of anesthesia[94]; the pain is greater when it is injected into a small vein (as in the hand) than in the arm.[95] This pain is most reliably prevented by administering 70% nitrous oxide before propofol or by applying a mini-Bier block with 0.5 to 1 mg/kg IV lidocaine for 60 seconds.[94-96]

Propofol has profound effects on the airway. After a rapid induction dose, a transient apnea is followed by a return of spontaneous respiration. Propofol reduces the hypopharyngeal dimensions, although upper airway patency is maintained.[97] A jaw thrust maneuver reestablishes a patent airway, should obstruction occur.[98] An important and unique property of propofol is the ease by which an LMA can be inserted. Propofol relaxes the upper pharyngeal muscles to facilitate acceptance of the LMA. Although propofol induces apnea, atelectasis during spontaneous respiration occurs less frequently than with tracheal intubation.[99]

Propofol is the only anesthetic with effective antiemetic properties that may be used for children with a history of postoperative nausea and vomiting (PONV) and in emetogenic surgery.[100]

Although propofol is used for both sedation and general anesthesia, long-term sedation with propofol in infants and children is not recommended, after reports of unexpected death during propofol sedation with greater than 4 mg/kg/hr for more than 48 hours.[101] In the United States, 21 children and 68 adults died in association with propofol administration over a 10-year period.[102] Whether these deaths were the result of the long-chain triglycerides or propofol or both has not been clarified or were less commonly due to other rare disorders such as neonatal adrenoleukodystrophy. Partial exchange transfusions have been effective in preventing death.[103] At least three reports of incipient propofol infusion syndrome (PRIS) have been reported in children after only a few hours of anesthesia.[104] The smallest infusion rate reported to trigger PRIS was 1.9 to 2.6 mg/kg/hr. Currently, long-term sedation with propofol is avoided in infants and children, especially in those with suspected inflammatory responses including sepsis.

Although the original package insert recommended caution when propofol is administered to children with egg and soy allergies this author only avoids propofol in those with documented egg anaphylaxis (see section on Allergies).

Ketamine

Ketamine is a phencyclidine derivative that offers enormous flexibility in the clinical care of children. This anesthetic can be used as a premedication (orally, nasally, rectally, or intramuscularly [IM]), general anesthetic induction agent (IV or IM), and maintenance agent as an infusion, as a sedative (IV or IM), or as a neuroaxial analgesic (caudal/epidural).

Ketamine is available as a racemic mixture, in which the S enantiomer is four times more potent than the R enantiomer. Ketamine is extremely lipophilic with a rapid onset of action, within 30 seconds, and maximum effect by 1 minute; the half-time to equilibrate in the effect site (brain) is 11 seconds.[105] Effective blood concentration of ketamine for anesthesia is 3 μg/mL.[106] Clearance of ketamine is reduced in neonates, but reaches adult levels by 6 months of age.[107] Context-sensitive half-life for ketamine in a 10-kg child increases from 30 minutes after 1 hour to 55 minutes after 5 hours of infusion. Emergence after a prolonged infusion of ketamine, especially when combined with opioids and benzodiazepines, may be delayed. Ketamine is primarily metabolized via CYP450 3A4 to norketamine.

Oral ketamine may be used for premedication in a dose of 5 to 6 mg/kg.[108] It may cause nausea and vomiting postoperatively; nightmares are not common by this route. Ketamine may also be given intranasally, although the porous nature of the cribriform plate raises concern regarding the potential neurotoxicity of ketamine if it reaches the brain directly via this route. The dose of intranasal (IN) ketamine (racemic mixture) is 3 to 6 mg/kg and for S-ketamine 2 mg/kg.[109] The rectal ketamine dose for premedication is 5 to 10 mg/kg, with recovery increasing substantially in duration with larger doses of ketamine. For IM use, 2 to 5 mg/kg ketamine sedates an uncooperative child in 3 to 5 minutes with a duration of action of 30 to 40 minutes.

General anesthesia may be induced with 1 to 2 mg/kg IV, a technique that is useful in children with cyanotic heart disease, septic shock, and conditions in which spontaneous respiration should be preserved (as in a child with an anterior mediastinal mass [AMM]). Ketamine may also be given as a continuous infusion after a single bolus loading dose of 2 mg/kg IV[92]: consisting of 11 mg/kg/hr for 20 minutes followed by 7 and 5 mg/kg/hr for the same periods, then 4 mg/kg/hr for the next hour, and 3.5 mg/kg/hr thereafter. If midazolam and nitrous oxide were added, the same regimen starting at 7 mg/kg/hr would provide adequate sedation.[92]

Ketamine is used occasionally for perioperative analgesia and has made a small resurgence for this indication in children with obstructive sleep apnea (OSA).[110] It is also used for neuroaxial analgesia. S-ketamine is the more potent and preferred enantiomer to administer. If ketamine is administered in a neuroaxial block, a preservative-free formulation should be used. *Caution: The neurotoxic risk of the racemic mixture of ketamine in the epidural space has not been established.*[111]

Side effects associated with ketamine include increased secretions, nystagmus, and nausea and vomiting. The last effect may occur in up to 33% of children. Nightmares and hallucinations have been reported after ketamine but appear to be very infrequent. Coadministration of midazolam and awakening in a dark, quiet environment may reduce the risk of nightmares postoperatively.[112]

Ketamine has been contraindicated in children with increased intracranial pressure and in those at risk for seizures although the evidence for both is weak.[113]

Etomidate

This hypnotic anesthetic is infrequently used in children as its pharmacology has not been understood until recently. It is reserved for those who are hemodynamically unstable (e.g., septic shock). The dose of etomidate is 0.3 mg/kg IV in children. The pharmacokinetics have only recently been estimated: With greater clearance and volume of distribution in young children, larger doses are required in this age group than older children.[114] Although the elimination half-life or context-sensitive half-life of etomidate has not been reported in children, repeated doses or infusions have delayed emergence which limits the use of this drug. Because etomidate causes pain at the site of injection, pretreatment with IV lidocaine and mini-Bier block is advised.

The major impediment to the use of etomidate and to its approval in many countries has been the suppression of adrenal glands, particularly in critically ill patients.[115]

Recent molecular engineering has yielded changes to the compound that attenuate the adrenal suppression and facilitate emergence even after prolonged infusions although these compounds remain under investigation.[116]

Neuromuscular Blocking Agents

With standard twitch devices readily available, every child who receives a muscle relaxant should be assessed for their twitch response before attempting to antagonize the neuromuscular blockade. The role of neuromuscular agents in children has diminished in the past decade or more with the demise in routine use of succinylcholine and the adoption of propofol as the adjunctive drug to facilitate tracheal intubation after induction of anesthesia with sevoflurane.

In the USA, anaphylaxis to muscle relaxants is quite rare. In contrast, the most common cause of anaphylaxis during anesthesia in adults in Europe is muscle relaxants, with succinylcholine and rocuronium being the most common causes,[117] although in children, latex was the most common cause (42%) followed by muscle relaxants (32%) and antibiotics (9%).[117] The explanation for the frequency of anaphylaxis to relaxants in Europe remained elusive, although regional differences in the use of pholcodine, an over-the-counter cough medicine, suggested that epitopes in pholcodine (and certain cosmetics), which are structurally similar to those in the aminosteroidal relaxants, caused a cross-sensitivity with and anaphylactic reactions to relaxants, even upon first exposure.[118] Indeed, after pholcodine was banned in Norway, the incidence of anaphylactic reactions to muscle relaxants in that country decreased dramatically suggesting that this over-the-counter cough medicine sensitized the population to the relaxants.

Succinylcholine

As the only depolarizing muscle relaxant in clinical practice, succinylcholine remains the agent that provides the most rapid onset and offset of paralysis, without additional drugs to recover the normal twitch response. Succinylcholine comprises two acetylcholine molecules fused together; it acts by depolarizing the acetylcholine receptors of the neuromuscular endplate.

The IV dose of succinylcholine is 3 to 4 mg/kg in neonates and infants, 2 mg/kg in children, and 1 mg/kg in adolescents.[119] The larger dose requirement with decreasing age has been attributed to the larger volume of distribution in younger infants. Paralysis usually occurs within 30 to 60 seconds and lasts approximately 5 minutes.[119] In contrast, an IM dose of 4 mg/kg paralyzes 100% of children within 1 to 2 minutes, although the duration may be as great as 20 minutes.[120] Rarely is it necessary to administer succinylcholine intra- or sublingually, but this approach may be optimized with digital massage of the injection site.[121] The speed of onset of paralysis when 1.1 mg/kg is administered intralingually is intermediate between IV and IM rates, ~75 seconds.[122] It is imperative to avoid midline sublingual blood vessels to avoid a sublingual hematoma. To administer succinylcholine either IM or sublingually, a 25-gauge needle should be used to minimize vascular trauma. This author routinely administers atropine 20 μg/kg before succinylcholine given via any route to prevent bradycardia and asystole after a single dose in infants and children.

The action of succinylcholine is terminated by pseudocholinesterase (or plasma cholinesterase) which is located on 3q26.1 and 3q26.2.[123] The residual products of metabolism have no neuromuscular activity. Pseudocholinesterase activity may be modified by a number of factors, inherited or acquired (Table 43-6). The inheritance pattern for pseudocholinesterase is autosomal recessive, which yields a host of phenotypes. Four alleles code for most of the genetic variants of pseudocholinesterase (see later): "Usual" (U); "Atypical" (A); "Fluoride resistant" (F); and "Silent gene" (S).[123] Several minor variants (H, J, and K) have also been reported in specific populations. A second gene locus that codes for pseudocholinesterase in only 10% of Caucasians has been identified. It produces a C5 band on electrophoresis that yields 30% more pseudocholinesterase enzyme than normal (Neitlich variant) and rapidly metabolizes succinylcholine.[124] Another gene variant named E Cynthiana has been shown to have increased activity.[125]

The genetics of the pseudocholinesterase activity variant follows simple Mendelian inheritance. The vast majority of the population responds normally to succinylcholine; that is, they are homozygous "Usual" pseudocholinesterase, U/U. The most common allele that prolongs the action of succinylcholine is the "Atypical," which occurs as heterozygous atypical (U/A) with minimal (~15 minutes) prolongation of action and as 1:3,000 to 1:10,000 in homozygous atypical (A/A) with a prolongation of 1 hour. In the case of fluoride-resistant, the frequency of homozygous F/F is 1:150,000 with a duration of activity of 1 to 2 hours whereas with the homozygous silent gene variant, S/S, the frequency is 1:10,000 patients with a clinical duration of 6 to 8 hours. The other variants H, J, and K (Kalow) are associated with a 90%, 66%, and 30% reduction in pseudocholinesterase activity, respectively. The homozygous H variant yields the greatest duration of action of succinylcholine among these three at 1 to 2 hours. The K variant is thought to occur in 13% of the population and the homozygous K variant occurs in 1.5%, extending the duration of succinylcholine to less than 1 hour. Interestingly, the K variant was present in 89% of A variants suggesting that more than one mutation is often present, for example, U/AK. The C5 and E Cynthiana variants destroy succinylcholine at an ultrarapid speed that may provide such a brief period of paralysis that the child recovers before laryngoscopy is attempted. Management of delayed recovery from succinylcholine includes sedation/anesthesia and ventilation. Blood should be sent for identification of the specific gene defect and a MedicAlert bracelet ordered.

Identification of the specific gene defect depends on the laboratory analysis of pseudocholinesterase activity and gene identification. When benzoylcholine is added to the blood, dibucaine suppresses the degradation of benzoylcholine by normal pseudocholinesterase by more than 71% (hence a dibucaine number of 71 is normal) whereas the degradation by A/A is only suppressed by 20% (hence the dibucaine number is 20). Intermediate inhibition is a dibucaine number of 60. When fluoride is added to blood, it inhibits normal pseudocholinesterase but the atypical variant to a much smaller extent.

Side Effects. The salient side effects associated with succinylcholine include arrhythmias (most notably bradycardia), rhabdomyolysis (with hyperkalemia and myoglobinuria), raised intraocular pressure (IOP), fasciculations, and malignant hyperthermia (MH).

Succinylcholine causes bradycardia via acetylcholine-associated activation of the vagal nerves. Sinus bradycardia is the most common arrhythmia, which may progress to transient asystole after a single IV dose of succinylcholine in a child.[126] Bradycardia can be

Table 43-6 Pseudocholinesterase Variants			
Decreased Activity		Increased Activity	
Congenital Causes	Acquired Causes	Congenital Causes	Acquired Causes
Gene defects	Hepatic insufficiency	Gene defect	Thyroid disease
Usual or E^u	Renal failure	Cynthiana (C$_5$) or Neitlich	Obesity
Atypical or E^a	Malnutrition		Nephrotic syndrome
Fluoride resistant or E^f	Severe burns		Cognitively challenged children
Silent gene or E^s	Chronic infections		
Rare defects	Pregnancy		
H variant	Neonate		
J variant	Plasmapheresis		
K variant	Drug-induced: organophosphates, cyclophosphamide, echothiophate iodide, oral contraceptives, metoclopramide, glucocorticoids, smolol, chlorpromazine		

prevented by pretreatment with an anticholinergic such as atropine (10 to 20 µg/kg) or glycopyrrolate (5 to 10 µg/kg).

Rhabdomyolysis may occur when succinylcholine is administered to children with MH or a myopathy.[127,128] The muscle breakdown releases massive concentrations of potassium as well as myoglobin, both resulting in potentially fatal consequences.

Hyperkalemia may occur in children with myopathies, upper and lower motor neuron disorders, burns, severe sepsis, and chronic immobilization (e.g., drug-induced, trauma-induced) (usually for weeks).[127] There is no evidence that succinylcholine presents additional risks when administered to patients with renal failure or cerebral palsy.[129] Hyperkalemia causes multifocal premature ventricular contractions that may progress to ventricular tachycardia and fibrillation. This occurs because the potassium concentration increases the resting membrane potential such that it approaches the threshold potential, triggering depolarization of myocardial cells. IV calcium (calcium chloride 10 mg/kg) raises the threshold potential, thus restoring the gap between the resting membrane and threshold potentials to prevent arrhythmias.

Succinylcholine increases IOP 7 to 10 mmHg reaching a peak pressure 1 to 2 minutes after IV administration and returns to the baseline in 5 to 7 minutes.[130] This increase may be attenuated by pretreatment with anesthetics, although none completely eliminates the increase in IOP. In the presence of a lacerated globe, this increase in IOP may increase the extrusion of intraocular contents although greater increases in IOP may occur during crying and coughing.[130]

Fasciculations occur immediately after administration of IV succinylcholine. Adolescents with muscular builds are at an increased risk of developing postoperative muscle pain after succinylcholine. To prevent this problem, pretreat with small doses of a nondepolarizing relaxant or simply avoid succinylcholine in this age group. Some assert that fasciculations increase the risk of regurgitation by increasing the abdominal muscle tone. However, the crura of the diaphragm comprise skeletal muscle, also fasciculates, thus preventing any decrease in gastric barrier pressure.

MH is a pharmacogenetic disorder of calcium metabolism in skeletal muscle.[128] The triggers (succinylcholine and/or potent inhalational anesthetics) induce an exaggerated release of intracellular calcium, which causes sustained muscle contractions. These sustained contractions generate heat and muscle breakdown with the release of intracellular potassium, myoglobin, and CPK. The earliest sign of an MH reaction is an increase in end-tidal PCO_2 that is accompanied by an increase in respiratory rate and hemoglobin desaturation. Late signs include increases in core body temperature, disseminated intravascular coagulopathy, and sepsis. Preparation of the anesthetic workstation is discussed later. The definitive treatment for MH is IV dantrolene 2.5 mg/kg, repeated as needed until the reaction abates (Fig. 43-4).[131] (See later and Chapter 24 for further details on MH.)

Rocuronium

Rocuronium is a steroidal muscle relaxant that is an analogue of vecuronium but differs from the latter by a more rapid onset of action and reduced potency. It is eliminated almost exclusively by the liver; hence liver failure may prolong the duration of action.[132] In contrast, renal failure should have minimal effect on its elimination.

The potency of rocuronium is greatest in infants, least in children, and intermediate in adults. The dose should be adjusted according to the child's age: the ED_{95} in infants is 0.25 mg/kg and in children is 0.4 mg/kg.[133,134] In healthy children during sevoflurane anesthesia, 0.3 to 0.4 mg/kg rocuronium provides suitable intubating conditions in 2 to 3 minutes and permits antagonism within 20 minutes. Twice the ED_{95} or 0.6 mg/kg IV rocuronium

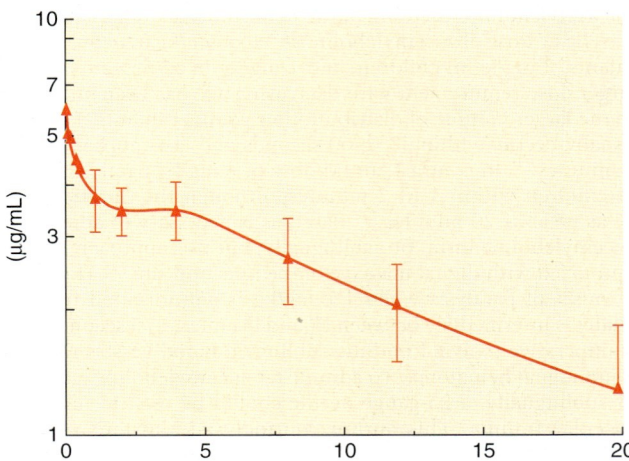

Figure 43-4 Pharmacokinetics of dantrolene in children 2 to 7 years of age. Blood concentrations after 2.4 mg/kg IV dantrolene decreased, leveling off at a therapeutic blood concentration of approximately 3.0 µg/mL between 1 and 4 hours and then decreased after 6.5 hours with an elimination half-life of 10 ± 2.6 hours. (Adapted with permission from Lerman J, McLeod E, Strong HA. Pharmacokinetics of intravenous dantrolene in children. *Anesthesiology*. 1989;70:625–629.)

provides relaxation in 1 to 1.5 minutes. Sevoflurane potentiates the effect of rocuronium compared with balanced anesthesia, a pharmacodynamic, not pharmacokinetic effect.[135] The time to 90% recovery of the twitch response after 0.6 mg/kg IV is 46 minutes in children. Recovery after rocuronium in infants is prolonged compared with that in children as a result of the reduced clearance and increased volume of distribution in the former.[134] At 3 to 4 × ED_{95}, 0.9 to 1.2 mg/kg IV rocuronium yields similar intubating conditions to succinylcholine within 60 seconds and may be used for rapid sequence induction (RSI), although recovery may be markedly prolonged.[136,137]

IM rocuronium (1.8 mg/kg) has been recommended in emergencies when an IV is not available. However, this dose and route provide poor intubating conditions after 4 minutes and a duration of 80 minutes. The author does not recommend this route and dose of administration.

Atracurium

Atracurium is a benzylisoquinolinium muscle relaxant that undergoes spontaneous degradation in blood primarily by Hofmann elimination yielding the major metabolite, laudanosine, which is devoid of neuromuscular blocking properties.[132] It is comprised of 10 isomers. A typical intubating dose in infants and children is 0.5 mg/kg IV (2 to 3 × ED_{95}) with an onset of 2 minutes and duration of 15 to 30 minutes. Complete recovery is usually achieved within 45 to 60 minutes. With its brief half-life, atracurium is suited for use as a continuous infusion in a dose of 6 µg/kg/min during isoflurane anesthesia and 9 µg/kg/min during a balanced IV anesthetic.[138] Neither renal nor hepatic failure affects the duration of action of atracurium. Side effects associated with atracurium include cutaneous erythema, bronchospasm, and wheezing after a rapid large bolus administration; rarely has anaphylaxis been reported.

Cis-atracurium

Cis-atracurium is one of the 10 isomers of atracurium that has supplanted atracurium. Its potency is threefold greater than that of atracurium resulting in more specificity for the receptor and fewer side effects such as histamine release.[132] It too is degraded by Hofmann elimination with a typical duration of action of 30 to 50 minutes. Suitable intubating conditions are achieved with 150 μg/kg (3 × ED$_{95}$) by 2 minutes after the dose.[139] Neither renal nor hepatic failure affect the duration of action of cis-atracurium. Side effects associated with the administration of cis-atracurium are minimal.

Neostigmine

This author strongly recommends antagonizing all neuromuscular blocking agents in infants and children when extubation is planned,[140] provided the time interval from the last dose has not exceeded 2 hours. The train-of-four should be 0.9 or greater before the trachea is extubated.[140] Any child who appears weak, as a "fish out of water," requires antagonism or a repeat dose of antagonism of the neuromuscular blockade. In order to successfully antagonize the relaxant, vital signs including temperature must be normal.

Neostigmine is an anticholinesterase compound that antagonizes neuromuscular blockade by preventing the degradation of acetylcholine. The acetylcholine competitively displaces the muscle relaxant from the neuromuscular junction. The dose of neostigmine in infants and children is 30% to 40% less than that in adults, or 20 to 40 μg/kg, which should be administered when at least one twitch is present in the train-of-four. If the recovery of neuromuscular blockade is incomplete, repeat doses of neostigmine may be administered up to 70 μg/kg. Care must be taken to avoid exceeding 100 μg/kg as acetylcholine-associated weakness may occur.

Neostigmine should be preceded by an anticholinergic, atropine 20 μg/kg or glycopyrrolate 10 μg/kg, to minimize the effect of neostigmine on the nicotinic receptors. Atropine causes a greater increase in heart rate but has a shorter duration of action than glycopyrrolate.

Sugammadex

This γ-cyclodextrin compound is a cylindrical oligosaccharide that uniquely binds rocuronium (and to a lesser extent vecuronium) to eliminate its activity.[141] When administered in the presence of moderate to profound rocuronium-induced neuromuscular blockade, sugammadex restored the twitch response thereby providing a direct intervention for a cannot ventilate, cannot intubate situation. The rocuronium/sugammadex complex is excreted unchanged in the kidney. Sugammadex has been used extensively in Europe but only recently in the United States. In children and adolescents, a single dose of 2 mg/kg or more sugammadex after partial recovery (two twitches of the train-of-four) from rocuronium yielded a train-of-four of 0.9 in approximately 2 minutes.[142] Dose response studies in children have not been forthcoming. In adults, 16 mg/kg can reverse rocuronium 3 minutes after administration for RSI. Most recently, two reports of sugammadex reversal of rocuronium-induced anaphylaxis refractory to vasopressors suggest another possible clinical role for sugammadex.[143]

Opioids

Morphine

Perioperative analgesia is usually accomplished with an intraoperative IV dose of 50 to 100 μg/kg and postoperative doses of 50 μg/kg morphine.[144] Perioperative infusions of morphine may also be administered by diluting morphine (1 mg/kg of the child's weight) in 100 mL of a balanced salt solution and infusing at 1 to 4 mL/hr. This provides analgesic blood concentrations of morphine, 10 to 40 ng/mL.[145] Morphine, 33 μg/kg, may also be administered via the caudal/epidural route with a prolonged duration of action and a small incidence of side effects (vomiting, pruritus).[145] Oral morphine has also been administered, although its bioavailability is 35% due to the first-pass effect.

Side effects after morphine include dose-dependent respiratory depression and incidence of vomiting (particularly at >100 μg/kg). Histamine release and urticaria at the site of injection are local, nonimmunologic reactions.

Fentanyl

This semi-synthetic opioid is the most widely used intraoperative analgesic in children. This very lipid-soluble opioid, which is bound primarily to α$_1$-acid glycoprotein in blood, has a very rapid onset of action, hemodynamic stability, and brief duration of action after a single dose.[146] It may be used via the IV, IM, oral, IN, and caudal/epidural routes. It is 50 to 100 times more potent than morphine, with doses 1 to 3 μg/kg IV attenuating the sympathetic responses to minor surgical procedures, up to doses of 12 to 50 μg/kg for neonatal surgery.[146] Fentanyl is infrequently administered IM; oral fentanyl, 10 to 20 μg/kg, is used in breakthrough cancer pain. IN fentanyl (1 to 2 μg/kg) has been used as a premedication and to reduce agitation in children undergoing myringotomy and tube surgery.[109,145] Epidural fentanyl has been administered to children via the epidural space in a dose of 1 to 2 μg/mL to supplement local anesthetics. There is very little evidence that fentanyl augments the analgesia provided by a lumbar epidural block in a child with an effective local anesthetic concentration (e.g., 0.125% bupivacaine or 0.0625% levobupivacaine)[147]; its addition to these local anesthetics causes pruritus, nausea/vomiting, and urinary retention.

The action of clinical doses of parenteral fentanyl is terminated by redistribution and, secondarily, by clearance in the liver. The initial redistribution is rapid; however, once tissue binding sites become saturated, the elimination half-life of fentanyl increases.[148] Fentanyl is metabolized extensively by CYP450 3A4 to inactive metabolites. The context-sensitive half-life of fentanyl in adults after a brief infusion for 1 hour, 20 minutes, increases dramatically to 4 hours after an 8-hour infusion.[148] Elimination half-life may exceed 20 hours after a prolonged chronic infusion or in some neonates. To offset the increasing context-sensitive half-life with time, the dose of fentanyl must be gradually reduced over time. After a prolonged infusion of fentanyl, it is necessary to slowly taper the dose and monitor for opioid withdrawal.

Meperidine

Meperidine is no longer recommended as an analgesic because of the risk of seizures (from normeperidine) and the accumulation of normeperidine after repeated doses of meperidine. It is currently recommended only for shivering.[145] The dose of meperidine for analgesia is 1 to 2 mg/kg and for shivering 25% to 50% of that dose. The elimination half-life of meperidine in children is 3 hours.[145]

Remifentanil

Remifentanil is a unique μ-receptor opioid that undergoes spontaneous degradation in blood by tissue esterases, with an elimination half-life of approximately 5 minutes that is independent of the duration of infusion.[149] With this brief half-life, remifentanil is usually administered as a continuous infusion. The context-sensitive half-life (the time to decrease the blood concentration by 50%) of remifentanil is 3 to 8 minutes. Metabolites of remifentanil do not effect analgesia.

Remifentanil is 10- to 60-fold more potent than alfentanil.[149,150] The infusion rate for remifentanil ranges from 0.05 to 0.25 μg/kg/

min (although larger doses have been administered), with the dose adjusted according to the presence of concomitant drugs (e.g., inhalational anesthetics). A loading dose (0.1 to 0.2 μg/kg) is usually not required as the infusion rapidly establishes an effective target organ concentration and hypotension is possible.

When administered in large doses, remifentanil may cause hypotension, bradycardia, and chest wall rigidity.[150] Prolonged administration has resulted in tachyphylaxis. Recent evidence suggests that nitrous oxide may attenuate the risk of tachyphylaxis.[151]

Hydromorphone

Hydromorphone (or Dilaudid) is a long-acting opioid analgesic. This μ-opioid receptor agonist is 5- to 10-fold more potent than morphine. Bolus dosing is 10 to 20 μg/kg IV or IM, followed by 1 μg/kg/hr IV or epidural continuous infusions.[145,152] Hydromorphone has an elimination half-life of 2.5 hours, similar to that of morphine. Metabolism is extensive (95%) via a single pathway to hydromorphone-3-glucuronide.

Codeine

Codeine has been the mainstay of postoperative analgesia in children for decades. However, it is a prodrug and its analgesic effect depends on its conversion to morphine (10%) and possibly to hydrocodone (11%) via CYP450 2D6.[153,154] Codeine received a blackbox warning from the US FDA for respiratory depression and deaths after tonsillectomy, particularly in children with OSA. This has led to codeine no longer being prescribed for postoperative pain in children in many jurisdictions.

Codeine may be administered IM, PO, and rectal.[145,154] IV codeine is not used as it causes cardiovascular depression and seizures. The dosing range for IM, PO, and rectal routes is similar, 0.5 to 1.5 mg/kg. Oral codeine reaches a peak blood level after 1 hour and an elimination half-life of 3 hours. When administered by the IM and rectal routes, the onset of action is more rapid than orally and the elimination half-life is less.

CYP450 2D6 is a noninducible enzyme that increases in activity from birth, reaching 20% of adult activity by 1 month of age (Fig. 43-1). It is mapped onto chromosome 22. 2D6 metabolizes 25% of the drugs in clinical use. More than 50 polymorphisms of 2D6 have been identified to date resulting in variability in the analgesia conferred from no analgesia (poor metabolizer) to an opioid overdose (an ultrarapid metabolizer), the latter being implicated in postoperative brain damage in one case and death in a second.[155,156] These polymorphisms vary along ethnic lines (e.g., 10% of Caucasians and 30% of Hong Kong Chinese are poor metabolizers whereas 29% of Ethiopians are ultra-extensive metabolizers) resulting in an unpredictable and varied response in children.[157,158] This has prompted some to substitute alternative analgesics postoperatively although few have been investigated in children. Care must be taken to prescribe the appropriate dose based on lean body weight (LBW) and whether the child's opioid receptors have been upregulated as a result of intermittent nocturnal desaturation.[159]

Acetaminophen

This nonsteroidal analgesic/antipyretic has been an effective analgesic for mild to moderate pain in children. Acetaminophen has no anti-inflammatory properties and is also free of platelet-inhibiting properties. Although its mechanism of action is not completely understood, it is believed to act on the peroxidase receptors of prostaglandin H_2 or via p-aminophenol.[160]

Oral doses of 10 to 15 mg/kg or rectal doses of 30 to 40 mg/kg yield adequate blood concentrations. Postoperative rectal dosing 20 mg/kg every 6 hours maintains blood concentrations after a rectal loading dose. Absorption after oral administration is rapid (~10 to 15 minutes) whereas after rectal administration it is slow and variable (1 to 2 hours).[161] Rectal suppositories should be lubricated to avoid mucosal tears. With an elimination half-life of 2 to 4 hours after any route, repeat doses may be administered every 4 to 6 hours, while maintaining the maximum 24-hour dose at less than 100 mg/kg confer both analgesia and antipyresis.

The most widely used IV formulations of acetaminophen is paracetamol.[162] An IV dose of 15 mg/kg may be administered every 6 hours.[162,163] Careful attention must be paid to the dosing as three overdoses involved 10- and 20-fold overdoses have been reported in infants, with one requiring treatment with IV N-acetylcysteine.[164,165] Furthermore, excessive dosing has occurred when clinicians failed to note previously administered doses on the electronic record. Acetaminophen dosing must be highlighted on the electronic record.

Paracetamol is metabolized via several pathways: the majority is eliminated by conjugation to either the glucuronide (55%) or sulfate (25%), less than 10% is oxidized (by CYP2E1, 3A4, and 2 other isozymes) to N-acetyl-p-benzoquinone (NAPQI) (toxic metabolite), and 1% to 4% is excreted unchanged by the kidney.

Ketorolac

Ketorolac is a parenteral nonsteroidal anti-inflammatory drug (NSAID) available for use in children. It possesses anti-inflammatory and analgesic properties for mild to moderate perioperative pain[166] and, like other NSAIDs, it also inhibits platelet adhesion by reducing the synthesis of thromboxane.

Ketorolac may be administered in doses of 0.5 to 2 mg/kg, with 0.5 mg/kg being the common dose administered to children.[167,168] The elimination half-life in infants and children is quite variable, 2 to 6 hours, and varies with whether the racemate (standard preparation) or stereoisomers are administered.[167,168]

The side effects of ketorolac have raised concerns limiting its use in the perioperative period. Some surgeons avoid ketorolac during tonsillectomy and adenoidectomy because of the risk of bleeding from COX-2 inhibition of platelet aggregation. Current evidence indicates that ketorolac increases the incidence of bleeding after adenotonsillectomy in adults but not children.[169] There is evidence that ketorolac inhibits bone healing in animals, but not in humans; a decision regarding its use during orthopedic surgery depends on the surgeon. All NSAIDs may trigger severe bronchoconstriction in asthmatics, and ketorolac is relatively contraindicated in this population, although some prescribe ketorolac in children with mild asthma.[170] Rarely, idiosyncratic renal failure has been reported after a single dose, which in most instances resolves spontaneously.

Diclofenac

This NSAID is also a cyclooxygenase inhibitor but with a 20-fold greater affinity for COX-2 rather than COX-1 receptors. Diclofenac may be administered IV, IM, PO, and rectally although in the United States only oral formulation is available. It is a potent analgesic, almost twice as effective for acute pain than acetaminophen during and after surgery.[171] The IV dose in children is 0.3 mg/kg and the oral dose is 1 mg/kg.[172,173] Its bioavailability after rectal administration is twice that of the oral route, hence the rectal dose is half the oral dose, 0.5 mg/kg. It is 99% bound to albumin, eliminated by CYP2C9, 3A4, and 3A5 phase 1 isozymes. Side effects are infrequent, 0.24% of children, with postoperative bleeding being the most frequent. Because of its limited affinity for COX-1 receptors, it is not a potent platelet inhibitor and causes far less risk of bleeding than the other NSAIDs. As with other NSAIDs, it is relatively contraindicated in children with asthma.

Ibuprofen

Ibuprofen is a widely used analgesic, antipyretic, and anti-inflammatory agent in the perioperative period in children. However, its use has been limited as it is only available in the oral form. A dose of 10 to 15 mg/kg oral q4–6h is widely prescribed for mild to moderate pain postoperatively, although some limit its use when postoperative bleeding may occur.

Recently, an IV formulation has been introduced and is undergoing clinical trials for use in children in the perioperative period.[174] A dose of 10 mg/kg up to max of 400 mg IV q4-6h or a maximum of 2400 mg/d is recommended.

Sedatives

Midazolam

This benzodiazepine is the most widely used anxiolytic in children in North America. It is water soluble, with a rapid onset of action when administered orally and a brief elimination half-life.[175] Unlike diazepam, it does not cause pain upon parenteral administration. Midazolam may be administered orally, sublingually, nasally, IV, IM, and rectally.[11,175] The oral and nasal doses are discussed under Anxiety, later. The dose for sublingual midazolam is the same dose as for the nasal route, 0.2 to 0.3 mg/kg.[11] Empirical IV dosing of 0.1 to 0.2 mg/kg should be administered, with larger doses being required in adolescence. IM midazolam is infrequently used in children because of the risk of sterile abscess and pain. Rectal dose of midazolam is 0.5 mg/kg, although this route is limited to children under 5 years of age.[11]

Midazolam is metabolized by CYP450 3A4 enzyme system; this enzyme reaches 30% to 40% of adult levels by 1 month and adult levels by 1 year (Fig. 43-1).[176] Approximately 50% of glucuronidated metabolite of midazolam is excreted via the kidneys.[176] Metabolism of midazolam is affected by renal and hepatic failures as well as enzyme systems that interfere with 3A4. The effects of midazolam may be antagonized by IV flumazenil in a dose of 0.01 mg/kg, which may be repeated to a maximum dose of 0.2 mg.

Dexmedetomidine

Dexmedetomidine is an α_2-agonist sedative whose relative affinity for $\alpha_2:\alpha_1$ receptors is eightfold greater than clonidine. It may be administered via the oral, nasal, IV, IM, and rectal routes.[177]

The oral dose, which requires 30 to 60 minutes to provide sedation, is 2 to 4 µg/kg, with increasing doses being more effective but with delayed recovery.[177] The IN dose is 1 to 2 µg/kg with 1 µg/kg sedating ~60% of children within 1 hour. The dose of IV dexmedetomidine may include a loading dose of 1 µg/kg infused over 10 minutes and followed by an IV infusion of 0.3 to 0.7 µg/kg/hr. *This infusion rate must be carefully transcribed because unlike other drugs, the infusion rate is in µg/kg/hr, not µg/kg/min.* When a loading dose is administered before the infusion, the risk of hypotension in the peri-induction period increases.

The pharmacokinetics of dexmedetomidine show a rapid early redistribution phase (half-life of 7 minutes) but a slow terminal elimination half-life, approximately 2 hours in children.[178,179] It is metabolized in the liver primarily via uridine glucuronyltransferase to inactive metabolites.

Unlike other sedative/anxiolytics, dexmedetomidine exerts its clinical effects via α_2 receptors with sedation in the locus coeruleus, hemodynamic manifestations via direct and indirect action on the sympathetic nervous system, and a host of miscellaneous side effects.[177] The unique feature of this sedative/anxiolytic is the *absence* of substantial respiratory depression.[180]

Dexmedetomidine is not a complete anesthetic. It decreases the MAC of inhalational anesthetics approximately 30%, provides suitable sedation for radiologic investigations (although a dose of 0.1 mg/kg IV midazolam is required to prevent movement unless large doses of dexmedetomidine are used),[89,181] facilitates awake fiberoptic intubation and awake craniotomy, provides sedation that is closest to natural sleep, provides analgesia, reduces emergence delirium (ED),[177] and facilitates motor- and sensory-evoked monitoring for spine surgery.[182]

Side effects of dexmedetomidine relate primarily to its hemodynamic effects. Bradycardia has been reported after larger infusion rates (up to 2 to 3 µg/kg/hr) and in younger age infants, with an incidence as great as 16%.[181] Do not treat the bradycardia (heart rates may reach 30 beats/min) with glycopyrrolate as profound hypertension may occur.[183]

Rapid administration of dexmedetomidine has been reported to cause transient hypertension, although this is uncommon in children. Hypotension (>20% decrease from baseline) has occurred during dexmedetomidine infusions.[181] The frequency of hypotension increases with an increasing dose and younger age: The greatest incidence occurs in infants, 8%. IV fluid loading may attenuate the hypotension but awaits additional studies.

Preoperative Assessment

Fasting Guidelines

The American Society of Anesthesiologists framed the fasting guidelines for infants and children in 2006.[184] The guidelines, which were based on a consensus panel and a review of the literature, concluded that the fasting intervals before elective anesthesia could be summarized as 2, 4, 6, and 8 hours as delineated in Table 43-7.[184] These guidelines are not age-adjusted. Gastric emptying times after breast milk and formula have only been evaluated in infants[185]; there are no data for comparable emptying times in children (≥1 year of age).

The child who presents chewing gum must expectorate the gum or surgery will be cancelled as aspirated gum will be very difficult to extricate from the airway. Gastric fluid volume after chewing sugar or sugarless gum is doubled, with approximately 50% showing a gastric fluid volume more than 0.8 mL/kg, but without a substantive change in the gastric fluid pH.[186] Hence, the gastric fluid characteristics in the child who is chewing gum are similar to those in the fasted child. Thus, induction of anesthesia does not need to be delayed in the child who has been chewing gum.

Obesity does not increase the risk of pneumonitis should aspiration occur.[187] Gastric fluid volume is increased slightly, but pH is unchanged. Thus, the risk of pneumonitis is unchanged in these children.

The risk of regurgitation and aspiration in children who present for emergency surgery is far more difficult to assess. Several factors relate to this risk including the severity and nature of the trauma, existing medical conditions, drugs that were

Table 43-7 Fasting Guidelines for Children Requiring Elective Anesthesia[184]

Clear fluids[a]	2 h
Breast milk	4 h
Infant formula and cow's milk	6 h
Solids	8 h

[a]Includes clear tea. If milk is added, we recommend a 6-hour fast. Gum should be expectorated, fasting need not be prolonged.

administered, and the timing and nature of the foods ingested. The only evidence upon which to assess the risk of a full stomach relates to the interval between the last food ingested and the trauma or injury.[188] Because gastroparesis and intestinal stasis occur after acute pain, an inflammatory response, and opioid drugs, it is likely that gastrointestinal peristalsis stops after a trauma. There is no evidence in children that administration of a prokinetic drug empties the stomach after trauma. Auscultation of bowel sounds in the abdomen does not ensure gastric emptying, although passing gas does imply peristalsis of the small and large bowels is present but does not ensure return of gastric motility. We consider children who ingested solid foods within 8 hours of a trauma to be at risk for regurgitation and aspiration and take appropriate precautions for managing the airway.

Certain medical conditions delay gastric emptying. Although diabetes mellitus delays gastric emptying, this may require years before the gastroparesis develops. Recent evidence suggests that gastroparesis may be multifactorial.[189,190] Indeed, hyperglycemia alone can delay gastric emptying in both diabetics and nondiabetics.

Laboratory Testing

Preoperative laboratory testing is infrequently ordered in healthy children without a pre-existing medical condition. A preoperative hemoglobin is indicated in those who are at risk for massive bleeding, those with pre-existing anemia in whom bleeding is highly probable, those with chronic nutritional deficiency, and those with sickle cell disease (see later).

A preoperative pregnancy test is required before anesthesia and sedation in most children of childbearing years in most jurisdictions. The reason for this test is the risk that some drugs that are administered in the perioperative period may cause a miscarriage or, less likely, teratogenicity of an unborn fetus. The incidence of unexpected and unknown pregnancies is approximately 0.3%.[191] Evidence suggests that history alone does not reliably predict pregnancy. Two pregnancy tests are available: urine and blood. The former test yields more rapid results, is cheaper but has a false-negative rate early after conception. Both tests have a known false-positive rate. There is debate regarding the threshold age to begin pregnancy testing. Many institutions and states require preoperative pregnancy testing in females who have reached menarche; some require testing in all females who are older than a specific age. If the pregnancy test is positive and the surgery is elective, the results must be conveyed to the patient. Due consideration should be given to the risk that anesthesia and surgery might pose to the unborn fetus if surgery proceeds. If, however, the surgery is emergent, then the risk benefit ratio of proceeding must be carefully assessed.

Medical Conditions

Upper Respiratory Tract Infection

Approximately 65% of children with upper respiratory tract infections (URTIs) have viruses as the cause of their infection; the remaining 34% have bacterial infections. Children who have had a recent URTI should not undergo elective anesthesia for 4 weeks after the infection to ensure resolution of the pathologic effects in the small airways. Because young children have 6 to 7 URTIs per year, most clinicians proceed with anesthesia 2 to 4 weeks after the original infection.[192]

When children present for elective surgery with a URTI, the author recommends canceling the anesthetic if any one of the four criteria listed in Table 43-8 is present.[193] The presence of each of these increases the risk of perioperative airway events. Additional factors that increase the risk of adverse airway events include cigarette smoking in the house, atopy, asthma, prematurity, young age, and secretions.[192,194] If an infant (<1 year of age) presents for surgery with a URTI, the chest should be examined very carefully and a low threshold maintained for cancellation as perioperative respiratory complications are substantive in this age group[195] including respiratory syncytial virus that may rapidly lead to pneumonia and a protracted recovery possibly involving prolonged tracheal intubation in the intensive care unit.[196]

Children who present with clear rhinorrhea, whether due to a mild URTI or allergic rhinitis, should be treated with 1 to 2 drops of oxymetazoline or neosynephrine (0.25%) nose drops per nostril to dry up the nasopharyngeal secretions during anesthesia. Care must be taken to use a dilute solution of neosynephrine, as concentrated solutions may cause a hypertensive crisis. We prefer to manage these children with a face mask if possible in order to minimize the risk of triggering airway reflex responses. However, if the airway must be manipulated, a supraglottic airway is less likely to trigger airway reflex responses than a tracheal tube.

Asthma

Up to 20% of children have asthma or an asthmatic history, but many fewer present with severe asthma that may complicate anesthesia.[197]

Children with a history of asthma should have their pulmonary condition optimized before surgery and be stable from their chest perspective, without a recent exacerbation or recent hospitalization. In the preoperative assessment, the age of onset of asthma, number and date of the most recent hospital admissions for asthma, treatment (β_2-agonists or steroids by inhalation), and current state of asthma should be recorded. Most children with asthma have never been admitted to hospital because of their asthma. However, if they have, the asthma should be considered severe. If oral steroids have been prescribed recently for an acute exacerbation of asthma, careful preoperative examination of the chest must be performed to ensure that there is no lingering reactive airway component. On the morning of the surgery, the child's lungs should be examined to check for wheezing. If wheezing is present, the child should be instructed to cough deeply to clear any airway secretions present, and bronchodilator therapy should be initiated. Preoperative bronchodilator therapy should be administered to children with mild to moderate asthma even if they are not wheezing, as this reduces airway resistance by approximately 25% during sevoflurane anesthesia and tracheal intubation.[198] If wheezing persists, the child should be referred to their pulmonologist for reassessment and the anesthetic deferred.

Preoperative bronchodilator therapy should be administered to children who are wheezing and present for emergency or

Table 43-8 Criteria to Cancel Anesthesia with an Upper Respiratory Tract Infection[194]

- Fever >38.5°C
- Altered behavior (not playing as usual) and habits (not feeding as usual)
- Purulent, productive discharge from the upper airway
- Lower respiratory tract signs (wheezing, rhonchi) that do not clear with coughing

urgent nonairway surgery. If tracheal intubation can be avoided, a face mask or LMA should be used. Equipment should be prepared to administer intraoperative bronchodilator therapy should the need arise.

6 Obstructive Sleep Apnea

OSA is the most serious form of sleep-disordered breathing in children.[199] Children have obstructed airways during sleep that are associated commonly with hypercapnia and intermittent hypoxia. The gold standard for the diagnosis is a polysomnogram, although many children present for surgery with a diagnosis of OSA but without a polysomnogram. In these cases, the diagnosis is made "clinically" by the presence of loud snoring, witnessed apneas, nocturnal enuresis, attention deficit disorder and behavioral problems, and inability to concentrate in school or poor school performance. OSA occurs equally in boys and girls and in asthenic and obese children. Daytime somnolence is not a common feature in children with OSA.

Two important decisions must be made when planning to anesthetize a child with OSA: (1) whether the child requires admission and overnight monitoring postoperatively[159] and (2) whether they are at risk for increased opioid sensitivity, that is those whose minimum nocturnal SaO_2 is less than 85%.[200,201] Although children with OSA may be premedicated with very small risk, those with persistent minimum nocturnal SaO_2 less than 85% are at increased risk for perioperative desaturation and airway events when the usual doses of opioids are administered. Alternative analgesic strategies including local anesthetic, NSAID agents, ketamine, and α_2-agonists should be considered.[202]

Ex-premature Infants

Infants who were born prematurely (<37 weeks gestational age) and are under 60 weeks postconceptional age (defined as the sum of the gestational and postnatal ages) require 12 to 24 hours of postanesthesia monitoring for apnea and hemoglobin oxygen desaturation, irrespective of the type of surgery (see Chapter 42).[203] Factors that increase the risk of perioperative apnea in ex-premature infants include age (<60 weeks postconceptual age), anemia (<12 g% Hb), and secondary diagnoses (e.g., intraventricular hemorrhage).[203,204] Opioids are best avoided in these infants; local anesthetic blocks are preferred. Caffeine 10 mg/kg IV may be administered intraoperatively to reduce the frequency of perioperative apneas, but it will not completely eliminate the risk of apnea.[205] Once the infant has been 12 hours apnea-free, he/she may be discharged home.

In contrast to general anesthesia, regional anesthesia does not increase the risk of perioperative apnea and does not require perioperative monitoring, unless the infant also received sedation, has multisystem disease, or has a history of perioperative apneas.[206] Spinal or caudal anesthesia will provide sufficient anesthesia to perform hernia surgery, the most common surgery in ex-premature infants. If the parents have an apnea monitor at home and have been trained to manage apnea, the child may be discharged home in the parents' care.

Malignant Hyperthermia

Most children who present with an MH diagnosis are offspring of a blood relative with an MH reaction or positive muscle biopsy.[128] The first task in such a case is to verify, as best as possible, the credibility of the past MH reaction from history or records. These children should be scheduled as the first case of the day to minimize their exposure to inhaled anesthetics in both the operating room and the postanesthetic care unit (PACU). If the child is anxious, he/she should be premedicated with oral midazolam (see later) in a dose appropriate for the child's age.

To prepare the AWS for an MH-susceptible child, either a designated inhaled anesthetic-free AWS should be used or a contaminated AWS should be flushed to reduce the anesthetic concentration to less than 10 ppm. In the latter situation, after removing the vaporizers from the AWS, the anesthetic breathing circuit and carbon dioxide canisters should be replaced with new equipment. The fresh gas flow should be set to 10 L/min oxygen/air mixture while the ventilator ventilates an artificial lung or reservoir bag to reduce the concentration of anesthetics in the machine to 10 ppm or less, considered to be the anesthetic threshold to trigger MH reactions. The time required to achieve 10 ppm or less varies amongst the current AWSs (Table 43-9), although there is no way of verifying that the threshold gas concentration was achieved by flushing a particular AWS.[207,208] Some recommend replacing components of the AWS to expedite the washout process whereas others recommend using charcoal absorbent in the inspiratory limb of the breathing circuit.[208] Once the breathing circuit has been flushed, the fresh gas flow should NOT be reduced to less than the flow rate used during flushing (if a charcoal filter is not used), lest a rebound in the anesthetic concentration occurs.[208] Interestingly, MH reactions have not been reported after reducing the fresh gas flow in a flushed AWS.

A trigger-free anesthetic includes propofol, opioids, benzodiazepines, nondepolarizing muscle relaxants, nitrous oxide, and regional anesthesia.[128] Of the standard monitors, end-tidal CO_2 (the earliest indicator of an MH reaction) and temperature (preferably axillary temperature because it will reflect temperature in the largest muscle bulk in the chest) are essential. IV dantrolene should be available in the facility in sufficient quantity to treat a reaction should it occur (2.4 mg/kg IV as an initial dose, and repeated until the reaction abates). The initial dose should maintain blood concentrations of dantrolene (>3 μg/mL) for 6 hours, after which its elimination half-life is 10 hours (Fig. 43-4).[131]

Ryanodex is a new formulation of dantrolene, which contains 250 mg of dantrolene per vial, only 125 mg of mannitol, and requires only 5 mL of sterile water for dissolution. This is sufficient dantrolene in a single vial for a loading dose in a 100 kg patient, far more dantrolene than is needed to treat the initial reaction in a child. If dantrolene is administered, a urinary catheter may be indicated depending on the dantrolene formulation used.

There is a host of additional strategies that may be used to stabilize the child including cooling strategies, and antiarrhythmics. Refer to Chapter 24 for more on MH.[128]

Table 43-9 Washout Times for Inhalational Anesthetics from Current Anesthesia Workstations

Ohmeda Machines (min)		Other Machines (min)	
Modulus 1	5–15	Narkomed GS	20
Excel 210	7	Drager Primus	70
AS/3	30	Drager Fabius GS	104
Aestiva (sevo)	22	Kion	>25
Aisys (sevo)	25		

Data from Kim TW, Nemergut ME. Preparation of modern anesthesia workstations for malignant hyperthermia-susceptible patients; a review of past and present practice. *Anesthesiology*. 2011;114:205–212; and Sabouri S, Lerman J, Heard C. Effects of fresh gas flow, tidal volume, and charcoal filters on the washout of sevoflurane from the Datex Ohmeda® (GE) Aisys®, Aestiva®/5, and Excel 210 SE Anesthesia Workstations. *Can J Anesth* 2014;61,935–42.

Children who are MH susceptible may undergo surgery as outpatients provided an MH reaction does not occur and the parents receive detailed instructions regarding how to monitor for possible MH reactions after discharge, as well as who to call and where to go if such a reaction occurs. Discharge times after a trigger-free anesthetic in an MH susceptible child may be similar to that after any other child undergoing similar elective surgery provided signs of an MH reaction do not occur.

Myopathies

The anesthetic for children with common myopathies, including Duchenne muscular dystrophy (DMD), Becker muscular dystrophy, and Emery–Dreifuss syndrome, should avoid drugs that are known to disrupt skeletal muscle membranes in children under 8 years of age and excessive cardiac depressants in children 10 years or older with cardiomyopathy.[128] DMD is an X-linked recessive gene in which the underlying defect is the lack of dystrophin (<3% of normal) in skeletal and cardiac muscles. The onset of the disease is 2 to 6 years of age. Becker dystrophy is a milder form of the disease with an onset in the second decade of life. Emery–Dreifuss syndrome is also a milder form of the disease often presenting with cardiac conduction defects, with syncope as the presenting finding.

The dystrophin protein complex is essential for the stability of the cytoskeleton of muscles. Muscle contractions, whether natural or drug induced, may tear the muscle membrane and release intracellular contents including high concentrations of potassium, myoglobin, and CPK. The administration of an inhalational anesthetic (halothane > sevoflurane > isoflurane) as well as succinylcholine may cause skeletal muscle contractions, damaging membranes and releasing intracellular contents.[209] In DMD, most muscle degradation occurs before the age of 10 years during which time this author would prefer propofol.[128] However, by adolescence muscle wasting abates and the predominant anesthetic concern is a progressive cardiomyopathy, which may be managed with careful titration by any anesthetic. In the case of Emery–Dreifuss, heart block may be a complicating finding. Hence, preoperative echocardiogram and electrocardiogram are warranted before anesthetizing adolescents with DMD or Emery–Dreifuss syndrome.

Mitochondrial myopathies are a complex group of disorders that result from defects in the protein complexes of the respiratory chain in mitochondria.[128,210] The protein complexes in the chain are under bigenomic control: 85% arise from nuclear DNA and 15% from mitochondrial DNA. In children, most mitochondrial myopathies result from defects in the nuclear DNA. The distribution of defective DNA in tissues in utero determines the spectrum of the disease.[128] Children with a history of lactic acidosis during infancy should be fasted for brief periods, not receive a lactate-containing solution, and receive an infusion of glucose intraoperatively. Both IV and inhalational anesthetics have been administered to children with mitochondrial myopathies without untoward events.[210]

Sickle Cell Disease

Sickle cell disease (SCD) or sickle cell anemia occurs primarily in children of sub-Saharan descent, with a frequency of sickle cell trait in African Americans of 8% and a form of SCD of 1:600.[211] A point genetic mutation results in the replacement of the Hb AA (where A is the normal hemoglobin) with Hb SS (S is the sickle hemoglobin) in every red blood cell. Thus, 100% of the cells in children with Hb SS are at risk for sickling; these children chronically have low hemoglobin concentrations (6 to 8 g%), may have had acute vaso-occlusive crises, and may have received multiple red cell transfusions in the past. Vaso-occlusive crises may involve a number of areas including bone, chest, and brain. Some children suffer from repeated vaso-occlusive crises whereas others never experience them. These crises are not related to hypoxia, hypovolemia, or hypothermia, but rather to a systemic inflammatory response, the nature of which remains unclear. Evidence suggests that those with SCD and vaso-occlusive crises have markers of a systemic inflammatory response to the disease that upregulates endogenous factors, including an adhesive factor that traps sickle red cells in arterioles and precipitates occlusive crises.[212] Whether the traditional factors of hypoxia, hypovolemia, and hypothermia exacerbate the initial process or compound the underlying inflammatory process has not been clearly established.

Two other forms of SCD, Hb SC and Hb SD, occur much less frequently than Hb SS and have an equal risk of sickling as Hb SS but have hemoglobin concentrations that are closer to normal values, approximately 10 to 11 g%. These children should be managed in a manner similar to those with Hb SS disease.[211]

Sickle cell may also present in a heterozygote form known as sickle trait, Hb AS. This disorder presents few problems during routine general and regional anesthesia and surgery provided extreme conditions, such as hypothermia and cardiopulmonary bypass, are not employed. Children with Hb AS have normal hemoglobin concentrations.

Preoperatively, a history of the frequency, severity, and precipitating triggers of sickle and vaso-occlusive crises in the child should be elicited. Consultation with the treating hematologist should provide insight into the current local strategies for managing this patient. However, if the child's sickle status has not been clearly established, a sickledex test may be used to diagnose SCD in infants above 6 months of age and in children. This test can be performed rapidly, inexpensively, and reliably. The sickledex test is unreliable in infants under 6 months of age because Hb F interferes with the sickling process and renders the test nonconfirmatory. Infants under 6 months of age rarely sickle because of the presence of Hb F, which gradually wanes in concentration beyond 3 months of age. If the test is negative, the child may still have sickle trait. If the test is positive or if the child is suspected of having sickle hemoglobin from history, then a hemoglobin electrophoresis should be performed to identify the particular hemoglobinopathy that is present. The definitive diagnostic test for SCD is the hemoglobin electrophoresis or high-performance liquid chromatography.

To attenuate the risk of a sickle cell crisis in children with SCD in the perioperative period, many hematologists transfuse the children with packed red cells to a total hemoglobin of 10 g%.[213] Others believe that both prophylactic blood transfusions and the need for transfusions in all children undergoing *minor* surgery are without merit.[214] The disadvantages of frequent transfusions in children who are at risk for sickle crises include sensitizing the recipient to minor antibodies (i.e., Kell and Duffy), iron overload, and transfusion reactions. It is important to consult local hematologists regarding the institutional management of children with SCD before the day of surgery to avoid surgical delays and document that discussion and management plan preoperatively with the parents and in the patient record. Optimal management of these children includes maintaining neutral thermoregulation and adequate hydration and oxygenation throughout the perioperative period.

Anterior Mediastinal Mass

Children with AMM require general anesthesia and/or sedation for a tissue (lymph node) biopsy, CT scan or MRI for diagnosis, or indwelling central line for chemotherapy.[215] Children with these tumors present a significant risk for anesthesia, because cardiac arrest has been reported in the past. Understanding the pathophysiology of the disease enables the clinician to anticipate complications and prepare the anesthetic to avoid them.

Four tissues can be found in AMMs in children: lymphomas, teratomas, thymomas, and thyroid.[215] The most rapidly growing tumor in the anterior mediastinum is the lymphoblastic T cell lymphoma, a non-Hodgkin's lymphoma, which has a doubling time of only 12 to 24 hours. These children may present with minor findings (e.g., night sweats) that rapidly progress over 1 to 2 days to life-threatening problems (e.g., orthopnea, superior vena cava syndrome). In children, anesthesia is usually required to delimit the extent of and tumor effects on mediastinal structures in radiology as well as for tissue biopsy and chronic chemotherapy access in the operating room.

The decision to proceed with local, regional, or general anesthesia depends on the age and level of cooperation of the child, the extent of mediastinal organ compromise, and the accessibility of the node or tumor being biopsied. A multidisciplinary team that includes the surgeon, anesthesiologist, and oncologist should review all radiologic and preoperative data before embarking on the surgery.

Older children often can tolerate the surgery under local anesthesia and sedation. Younger children and those whose tumor severely compromises the airway and/or pulmonary artery may require general anesthesia. In the latter conditions, attempts to shrink the tumor using a 12- to 24-hour course of IV steroids or a round of radiation should be considered to reduce the perioperative risk of cardiorespiratory complications. However, these alternatives should not be used without first a multidisciplinary discussion with the oncologists[216] because there is a risk of widespread tumor necrosis that may both render the diagnosis of the cell type difficult and/or induce tumor lysis syndrome.[217]

For most children who require a radiologic investigation, tumor biopsy, or chemotherapy access, general anesthesia with spontaneous respiration is preferred. If the child cannot lie flat, anesthesia can be induced and the trachea intubated with the child positioned in the left lateral decubitus or less desirably, in the sitting position. The trachea should be intubated at induction of anesthesia to ensure a patent airway should it become necessary to turn the child prone to reverse circulatory collapse. Tracheal intubation is performed without muscle relaxation to preserve spontaneous respiration. Spontaneous respiration best preserves the negative intrathoracic pressure gradient to suspend the tumor above the mediastinal structures and avoid pressure on the pulmonary artery and right atrium as well as the tracheobronchial tree. It is important to remember that the capnogram may be a very useful monitor to confirm the adequacy of the pulmonary circulation (and cardiac output); the sudden loss of or reduction in the capnogram may herald compression of the pulmonary artery before systemic cardiovascular sequelae occur.

Subacute Endocarditis (SBE) Prophylaxis

In 2007, the American Heart Association significantly revised the indications for SBE prophylaxis.[218] The new recommendations were crafted for dental procedures and adopted by the American Dental Association. The American Heart Association no longer recommends SBE prophylaxis for children undergoing gastrointestinal, urologic, and genitourinary surgeries, although many specialists in these areas continue to request SBE prophylaxis. Accordingly, it is incumbent upon the anesthesiologist to inquire of the specific specialist whether SBE prophylaxis should be administered.

Table 43-10 Subacute Bacterial Endocarditis Prophylaxis Recommendations by American Heart Association[218]

1. Prosthetic cardiac valve or material used to repair the cardiac valve
2. Previous infectious endocarditis
3. Congenital heart disease:
    a. Unrepaired cyanotic congenital heart disease, including palliative shunts and conduits
    b. Completely repaired congenital heart defect with prosthetic material or device, whether placed by surgery or by catheter intervention, during the first 6 mos after the procedure
    c. Repaired congenital heart disease with residual defects at the site or adjacent to the site of a prosthetic patch or prosthetic device (which inhibits endothelialization)
4. Cardiac transplantation recipients who develop cardiac valvulopathy

For dental procedures, the indications for SBE prophylaxis are listed in Table 43-10.[218] The antibiotic regimen for SBE prophylaxis has not changed since previously published.

Obesity

Obesity in children is an epidemic worldwide. In children, definitions are based on growth curves, not BMI, because height and weight change with age.[219] The definitions in children are as follows: Overweight is a BMI above the 85th percentile, obesity is a BMI above the 95th percentile, and super (morbid) obesity is a BMI above the 99th percentile for age and sex where BMI is defined as weight (kg)/[height (cm)/100]^2. In order to refine drug dosing in obese children, additional scalars should be defined. First, an easy, quick, and simple approach to estimate the IBW based on a child's age is

For children <8 years: Wt (kg) = 2 × Age (year) + 9

For children ≥8 years: Wt (kg) = 3 × Age (year)

Second, LBW, which accounts for the excess body muscle and bone masses that results from carrying the excess body fat is estimated to be IBW + 1/3(TBW − IBW).

Ninety-five percent of cases of obesity is attributable to environmental and lifestyle factors. Fewer than 5% of cases of obesity are attributable to diseases and genes such as Prader–Willi syndrome (Laurence–Moon–Biedl syndrome), inborn errors of metabolism, Cushing disease, and immobility (DMD). The underlying mechanisms for these disorders include leptin mutations (receptor and prohormone convertase 1), proopiomelanocortin mutation, and MCR4 (melanocortin receptor).

Thirty percent of overweight children have restrictive pulmonary pattern results from body fat encasing the pliable chest with decreased chest wall compliance, FRC, and vital capacity. The increased work of breathing compounds the reduced lung volumes as the closing volume approaches the tidal volume and V/Q mismatch occurs. Nocturnal hypoxemia from the above factors combined with large tonsils (see later) sets the stage for the development of pulmonary hypertension and right heart failure. Sleep-disordered breathing occurs in 17% (up to 33% if BMI >150%) of obese children.

Cardiovascular effects of obesity include systemic hypertension, left ventricular hypertrophy, and premature atherosclerosis.

Table 43-11 Drug Dosing for Obese Children

Drug	Induction Dose Based on	Maintenance Dose Based on
Thiopental	LBW	
Propofol	LBW	TBW
Synthetic opioids (fentanyl, alfentanil, and sufentanil)	TBW	LBW
Morphine	IBW	IBW
Remifentanil	LBW	LBW
Nondepolarizing neuromuscular blockers	IBW	IBW
Succinylcholine	TBW	
Sugammadex	TBW	

TBW, total body weight; LBW, lean body weight; IBW, ideal body weight.

Intermittent hypoxia during sleep apnea may lead to pulmonary hypertension. Both blood volume and cardiac output are increased.

Insulin resistance and metabolic syndrome are present in 40% of moderately obese children and 50% of severely obese adolescents. Increased abdominal weight predisposes to gastroesophageal reflux, which occurs in approximately 20% of children with severe obesity. Gastric emptying rates and the risk of pneumonitis from aspiration (based on gastric fluid pH and volume) in obese children do not differ from those in normal children. NPO times are the same in obese and nonobese children. Glomerular filtration rate is increased. Fatty infiltration of the liver leads to nonalcoholic fatty liver disease, which leads to abnormal liver function tests and possibly hepatic fibrosis.

Drug dosing in obese children is complex, varying with several factors including lipid solubility, volume of distribution, and the route of elimination, hepatic or renal.[219] The drug dosing for several commonly used drugs in obese children may be estimated on the basis of their weight (Table 43-11).

These children should be positioned 25-degree head-up during preoxygenation to reduce V/Q mismatch and to facilitate tracheal intubation. The tragus should be positioned above the level of the sternal notch to ensure that tracheal intubation will be successful.[220] IV access may be difficult. Desflurane is preferred for maintenance of anesthesia because it is the least fat soluble of the inhalational anesthetics and has the smallest context-sensitive half-life. However, if the child has asthma or is exposed to smoking, sevoflurane may be preferrable. Compression devices should be applied to the legs to prevent stasis and deep vein thrombosis.

Perioperative respiratory events including difficult mask ventilation, greater Mallampati airway class, bronchospasm, rapid hemoglobin desaturation, and prolonged PACU times are more common in obese children.[219]

Preoperative History

Medical, surgical, and family histories including complications should be recorded. The details of all allergies should be carefully elicited in terms of the clinical manifestations and severity. A systems approach should review each organ system including recent URTIs recorded.

Allergies

Most allergies that are reported in hospital records are of little relevance to the conduct of anesthesia. All allergies reported by patients and families are dutifully transcribed into the hospital record with neither censure nor regard for their relevance or authenticity. Examples of recognized side effects that do not constitute allergies include headaches after epinephrine, vomiting after opioids, and diarrhea or rash after amoxicillin. Only true allergies should be recorded on the anesthetic record: these include anaphylactic reactions and allergic reactions diagnosed and confirmed by an allergist/immunologist. The remainder should be identified as hypersensitivity or idiosyncratic reactions, although this is not the current practice. Cross-sensitivity between penicillin allergy and first-generation cephalosporins is possible; however, there is no cross-reactivity with second or later generation of cephalosporins.[226] If the parents report a possible penicillin allergy or sensitivity to cephalosporin in their child that occurred more than 5 years ago and not confirmed by an immunologist, then this author offers to test the child using a small test dose of the IV antibiotic while monitoring the child and informs the parent of the outcome.

Few, if any, allergies have been reported to propofol. Although the package insert for propofol cautions against the use of propofol in children with egg allergy, the only egg allergy that precludes the use of propofol is possibly egg anaphylaxis.[227] Egg lecithin, a phospholipid in propofol, is not a protein and therefore cannot induce anaphylaxis. However, it may carry trace concentrations of yolk proteins with it into the formulation. The manufacturer states that no soy protein is present in their North American formulation of propofol. Hence, children with soy allergy (usually <5 years of age) may receive propofol.

Latex allergy should be documented when preparing the operating room for children although its significance is waning.[228] In the past, numerous children with spina bifida, congenital urologic surgery, and multiple surgeries (>5 exposures) were exposed to latex products by repeated bladder catheterizations or latex gloves multiple times and developed IgE-mediated latex anaphylaxis. Children who are latex allergic and who touch toy balloons to their lips or in whom dentists insert a rubber dam, will react with lip or tongue swelling, respectively. Because latex products both in and out of hospital have been replaced with nonlatex substitutes, the prevalence of latex allergy in the children is decreasing; this is an acquired, not a congenital condition. It is imperative to avoid contaminating the surgical (and anesthetic) setup with latex in order to prevent latex anaphylaxis. Removing all latex products from the operating room has eliminated latex anaphylactic reactions and should be adopted worldwide.[229] If the child has latex anaphylaxis, each operating room door should have signage indicating that a latex-allergic patient is present. Epinephrine, in a dose of 1 to 10 μg/kg, is the drug of choice to reverse latex anaphylaxis; 1 to 2 μg/kg reverses isolated bronchospasm (but may need to be repeated), whereas 10 μg/kg is reserved for cardiac arrests.

Preoperative Physical Examination

The airway, respiratory, and cardiovascular systems should be examined preoperatively in every child. The airway examination should include visual inspection of the face in the anterior and profile views to detect any disproportions in facial features that might suggest a congenital facial or airway anomaly. The child should open their mouth fully, stick out their tongue, and extend their neck. Loose teeth should be identified and any removable dental appliances stored. Piercings in and around the mouth should be removed as these may become dislodged and aspirated if they are intraoral. The respiratory examination includes auscultation of the chest (front and back) with full inspiration and expiration through the mouth. If rales or rhonchi do not clear with deep coughing, then a chest x-ray and pulmonary consultation should be ordered. Cardiovascular examination includes auscultation of the heart. If a murmur is detected, then further inquiry regarding the presence of cardiac symptoms (syncope, arrhythmias, tachycardia, heart failure, shortness of breath) should be solicited. If the murmur is heard during diastole, has not been diagnosed previously, or is associated with any cardiac symptomatology, then a cardiology consultation should be sought. If the child has a history of cardiac surgery, then a recent cardiology note together with an electrocardiogram and echocardiogram should be reviewed.

Anesthetic Risks; Consent/Assent

The mortality associated with anesthesia in healthy children is 1:10,000 or less.[221] Perioperative cardiac arrest rate is greater in children who are young (under 1 year of age), with congenital heart disease, and undergoing emergency surgery. This author does not give a number for the risk of cardiac arrest to parents of healthy children undergoing elective anesthesia (unless specifically requested to do so) but rather uses an analogy that the risk is greater that they would be hit by a car crossing the busy street outside the hospital than to have a serious adverse outcome during general anesthesia. Perioperative morbidity may be greater than the incidence of cardiac arrest, but depends on the child's comorbidities and the severity of the current diseases.

Specific risks discussed preoperatively include the most common complications, pain, nausea, and vomiting. In addition, the author reviews the small risk of unforeseen complications that may result from as yet latent diseases, dental damage, corneal abrasion, aspiration, awareness, allergic reactions, and cardiac arrest.

If asked about awareness, this author informs the parents/guardians that the incidence of awareness in children is extremely rare (1:60,000),[222] although some have reported an ~1% incidence of awareness in their center.[223] The latter may be attributed, for the most part, to inadvertent light anesthesia during periods of stimulation.

If asked about cognitive dysfunction after anesthesia, the author informs the parents/guardians that neuroapoptosis has been reported after almost every anesthetic in neonatal animals and some nonhuman primates.[224] Several studies in children investigated the risk of anesthesia on the maturing human brain; in a sibling cohort study of a single anesthetic before 3 yr, IQ scores in later childhood were similar.[225] In a prospective randomized controlled study of sevoflurane versus spinal anesthesia, neurodevelopmental outcome at the 2-year (preliminary) follow-up was similar.[9] Accordingly, this author advises parents that there is insufficient evidence to suggest that anesthesia causes cognitive dysfunction in young children, but urges parents to consider all of the risks and benefits of anesthesia and surgery for their child when considering whether to proceed with surgery.

Induction of Anesthesia

Equipment

To ensure that the anesthetizing location is properly and completely prepared, it is useful to use a checklist. Appropriately sized equipment should be available for each child. A range of face mask sizes, oral airways, laryngoscope blades, tracheal tubes, and LMAs should be present. The author prefers cushioned clear face masks that fit the contour of the child's face and permit rapid identification of either fluid or solid material within the mask. Reliance on oral airways in establishing a patent upper airway in children has been supplanted, in part, by an appropriately applied jaw thrust maneuver.[98] The Miller and Wisconsin straight blades are preferred for tracheal intubation in infants and children, although we recently demonstrated that the Macintosh blade provides a similar view to that of the Miller blade in children 1 month to 2 years of age.[230] A range of sizes of laryngoscope blades should be available in every anesthetizing location. For laryngoscopy the child should be positioned flat on the table, with the head stabilized to prevent lateral movement. The large occiput of the child puts the head in the sniffing position naturally. In infants and children with limited oxygen reserve, or when performing tracheal intubation during sedation, the Oxyscope, a straight blade fitted with a source of oxygen at the tip of the blade, may prevent oxygen desaturation.

The classic laryngeal mask airway (cLMA) was introduced to replace face masks in adults and has subsequently proven to be a versatile and useful airway device in some circumstances in children.[231] To fit pediatric airways, the dimensions of the adult cLMA were simply scaled down in size from the adult and unmodified otherwise for infants and children. The cLMA has also proven to be effective in circumstances other than elective anesthesia, including neonatal resuscitation and fiberoptic intubation. A range of sizes of the cLMA should be available.

Although effective, the cLMA does not "protect" the airway from regurgitation and laryngospasm. Because the tone of the gastroesophageal sphincter is reduced in children, compared with adults, children may be at greater risk for regurgitation in the presence of a full stomach or positive pressure ventilation. Hence, it is best to avoid LMAs in these clinical situations. Modifications of the cLMA to include a vent for regurgitant gas or liquid from the esophagus, as in the ProSeal supraglottic airway, may better protect the airway against aspiration.

Complications associated with the cLMA in children are infrequent but may include gastric inflation, aspiration, airway obstruction, and laryngospasm.[232] When compared with tracheal tubes, supraglottic airway devices are associated with fewer postanesthetic complications.[233] The frequency of complications with cLMA in infants under 1 year of age is greater than that in older children and in infants managed with a face mask. Studies suggested that the epiglottis folds down into the bowl of the cLMA in a majority of children although the LMA is otherwise functioning properly; this finding may simply be moot.

A range of diameters of tracheal tubes appropriate for the child's age, as well as tubes 0.5 mm ID (internal diameter in mm) smaller and larger, should always be available. The appropriate size of the uncuffed tracheal tube is based on the ID of the tube. Guidelines for uncuffed tracheal tube sizes in infants and children are as follows: infant's weight (<1,500 g, 2.5 mm ID; 1,500 g to full-term gestation, 3 mm ID); neonate to 6 months postnatal age, 3.5 mm ID; and 0.5 to 1.5 years, 4 mm ID. For children above 2 years of age, the size of uncuffed tubes may be estimated using the formula: Age (in years)/4 + 4 (or 4.5) mm ID. The size of cuffed tubes (mm ID) may be estimated using the formula: Age (in years)/4 + 3 (for children <2 years) or +3.5 (for those >2 years).

The length of a tube from the lips to mid-trachea in infants less than 1,000 g in weight is 6 cm, 1,000 to 3,000 g is 7 to 9 cm, in term neonates 10 cm, and for infants and children, 10 + age (years) mm.

In the past, uncuffed tracheal tubes were commonly used to secure the airway of children under 8 years of age. The circular shape of the tracheal tube was suited to the round shape of the lumen within the cricoid ring,[234] which allowed for a good seal without the need for a cuff on the tube. Cuffs were avoided in children out of the concern that compression of the loosely adherent pseudostratified columnar epithelium that lines the cricoid ring would swell and encroach on this narrowest portion of the upper airway and cause stridor. To preclude this potentially serious airway complication, the tracheal tube was carefully selected so that it either passed through the cricoid ring without resistance or did so with an audible leak at a peak inspiratory pressure 10 to 20 cm H_2O.

Recently, there has been a shift from uncuffed to cuffed tracheal tubes in infants and children. Cuffed tubes contaminate the environment less with anesthetic gases, are associated with fewer laryngoscopies and reintubations, and deliver more consistent tidal volumes (as chest wall and abdominal compliance change during surgery) and positive end-expiratory pressure than uncuffed tubes. This shift in practice has been accelerated by the introduction of the soft, high-compliance cuffed Microcuff tube (Microcuff GMbH, Weinheim, Germany).[235] The latter tubes are uniquely designed as they have no Murphy eye, and the cuff is positioned closer to the tip of the tube (than standard cuffed tubes), is made of polyurethane, and shaped as a cylinder (rather than a sphere), thus mimicking the shape of the larynx. Microcuff tubes seal the airway at much lower cuff pressures (~11 cm H_2O) than other cuffed tubes.[236] The cost of the Microcuff tube is several fold greater than that of the uncuffed tube. All cuffs expand when nitrous oxide is used, although the time interval until the cuff pressure in the Microcuff tube reaches 25 cm H_2O exceeds that with other tubes because the former seals the airway at lower pressures. The cuff pressure should be monitored during surgery to preclude excessive cuff pressures. In a retrospective study, the incidence of post-extubation stridor in neonates whose airways were intubated with these tubes was almost threefold greater than that after uncuffed tubes, suggesting that caution be exercised when using Microcuff tubes in neonates.[237]

Optimizing ventilation during anesthesia and surgery in infants and children has been the subject of much interest.[238] Traditional strategies held that volume-controlled pressure-limited ventilators were effective for most infants and children. However, these ventilators accounted for neither the compliance of the breathing circuit nor the variable leak around the tracheal tube. Further concerns focused on the shape of the pressure tracing during inspiration and the risk of delivering excessive peak airway pressures. In the neonatal intensive care units, pressure-controlled ventilation has been used successfully, in part because the peak inspiratory pressure is restricted and the risk of barotrauma is decreased with the constant inspiratory pressure pattern. The inspiratory pressure pattern also more evenly distributes the inspiratory gas throughout the lungs, reducing the risk of ventilation/perfusion (V/Q) mismatch. Despite the advantages of the pressure-controlled ventilators, many anesthesia ventilators were simply unable to compensate for decreases in abdominal and chest wall compliance that occurred during surgery. The new generation of anesthetic machines offers markedly improved ventilators and ventilation strategies that are hybrids of the best aspects of both volume- and pressure-regulated ventilation. These new ventilators may prove to be ideal for both preterm and term neonates. Ventilation strategies, such as the hybrid pressure-regulated volume-controlled mode, maintain a fixed tidal volume by taking into account the compressible volume of the breathing circuit. This mode is used during controlled ventilation, and a pressure support mode is used once spontaneous respiration commences. For most children, the ventilation strategy will not impact on the outcome, but for those with lung disease, a poor ventilation strategy could result in a panoply of irreversible pulmonary problems. Whichever ventilation mode or strategy is planned for a particular child, it is crucial that the limits on ventilation including peak inspiratory pressure, rate, and positive end-expiratory pressure are set before the child is connected to the ventilator.

Monitors

The ASA recommends basic patient monitoring during all anesthetics including electrocardiogram, arterial blood pressure, SaO_2, capnogram, and temperature, as well as additional monitors specific for the child's medical or anesthetic condition, for example, depth of anesthesia monitor. Many infants and preschool-age children fight the application of monitors while awake. Although induction of anesthesia is usually well-tolerated and safe in expert hands, every effort should be made to apply at least a pulse oximeter before inducing anesthesia. The remaining monitors should be applied as soon as the child loses consciousness. Understanding the role of these monitors in pediatric anesthesia requires a basic understanding of these instruments, although three specific monitors merit further consideration: capnography, temperature, and depth of anesthesia monitoring.

Capnography

Respiratory rate and apnea may be detected by measuring the carbon dioxide tension in the anesthesia breathing circuit. The most commonly used technique is infrared analysis using one of two approaches: sidestream or mainstream capnography. The former requires aspiration of gas into an analyzer whereas the latter detects carbon dioxide with a detector inserted into the breathing circuit.

The accuracy of sidestream capnometry improved dramatically when circle system breathing circuits replaced T-piece circuits because there is less dilution of expiratory gas. Sidestream capnometry using gas obtained from the elbow of the circle breathing circuit provides accurate data, even in neonates who have small tidal volumes. On the other hand, mainstream capnography is infrequently used and is unpopular among pediatric anesthesiologists, particularly for use in infants and neonates, because it increases the dead space of the breathing circuit, must be fitted at the tracheal tube/elbow and is heavy, increasing the risk of kinking or obstructing the tracheal tube.

The end-tidal PCO_2 may also be accurately monitored while the child is sedated and breathing spontaneously through a face mask or through baffled nasal prongs. This noninvasive but accurate measure of capnometry allows continuous assessment of ventilation in remote sites such as the MRI and CT scanners amongst other locations.

Temperature

Thermoregulatory homeostasis requires an understanding of the physiology of heat transfer in the child as well as the effects of anesthesia. Children have large surface areas to body weight and as such are at risk for rapid and extensive heat loss to the environment. In children, heat loss follows the order: radiation (39%) > convection (34%) > evaporation (24%) > conduction (3%).[242] When anesthesia is induced, heat is redistributed from the central core to the periphery, and from there, it is lost to the environment. There is little that can be done to prevent the redistribution of heat with induction of anesthesia but there are a number of strategies that may attenuate the net loss of heat from the child.

The temperature of the operating room should be increased to about 28°C (80°F) before nonfebrile neonates and infants arrive. Because there may be a substantial (up to 1 hour) lag time between setting the operating room temperature and achieving it, the room temperature should be adjusted as the previous child leaves. The increased temperature warms the walls and the air within the room, thereby reducing both radiation and convection heat losses, respectively.

Several other modalities have been used to maintain thermoneutrality in infants and children during anesthesia including water mattresses, radiant overhead heaters, and forced air warmers. Water mattresses address heat loss primarily through conductive paths and because this accounts for an insignificant fraction of the heat loss, they are unnecessary. Radiant overhead heaters are used primarily in neonates and infants. Feedback control to avoid skin burns is best served using an accurate measure of the distance of the heater from the infant's skin surface as well as continuous surface temperature monitoring on the infant's skin. However, for the majority of infants and children who require temperature control in the operating room, the most important modality is the forced air warmer. These warmers are the single most effective strategy available to minimize heat loss in children who undergo surgery lasting 1 hour or more.[243] Although it is comforting to the child to preheat the air mattress before the child enters the operating room, this practice does not affect the child's temperature at the end of anesthesia. These warmers may predispose to airborne contamination and possible surgical infection, although evidence is conflicting. It remains this author's recommendation to turn the forced air warmer off when the skin is prepped and resume heating after the surgical drapes are in place.

A heat and moisture exchanger may be used to add humidity to the circuit although its efficiency is poor, particularly for surgery less than 1 hour and in infants.

Temperature should be monitored continuously throughout the anesthetic and in the PACU of all children who receive anesthesia or sedation. Core temperature is ideally measured at the level of the mid-esophagus using an esophageal temperature probe. Although alternative sites to measure the core temperature include the rectum, nasopharynx, and axilla, each site has its limitations. Rectal temperature probes may yield inaccurate temperatures if the probe falls out of the rectum or is buried in stool. Nasopharyngeal temperature may detect brain temperature but more likely underestimates the core temperature by cooler gas passing through the breathing circuit. Axillary temperature may under- or overestimate the core temperature if it is positioned on the ipsilateral arm where the IV fluid is infusing or if the probe is either in the airspace behind the axilla being bathed by cool room air or in the heat from the forced air warmer. The author prefers proper positioning of the axillary temperature probe in the arm without the IV and with the shoulder completely adducted. In this position, an increase in temperature may be detected as an early sign of an MH reaction given the proximity of the large deltopectoral muscle group. Although some use a forehead skin temperature to track temperature, 10 MH reactions occurred in which these devices failed to reflect an increase in temperature.[244]

Temperature monitoring is important not only in MH but also to detect hypothermia. Hypothermia delays emergence from inhalational anesthesia, reduces the rate of degradation of drugs, and increases infectious risks.

Depth of Anesthetic Monitoring

Recent reports of awareness in up to 1% of children who received general anesthesia for elective surgery have attracted considerable attention.[223] Careful review of the studies suggests that many of these episodes may be attributed to local practices that expose the children to concentrations of anesthesia that were insufficient for the level of stimulation. To reduce the risk of awareness, the anesthetic concentration of sevoflurane should be neither interrupted nor dramatically decreased early in anesthesia or during surgical stimulation; at least 0.7 MAC of the inhaled anesthetic should be maintained.

The most widely studied anesthetic depth monitor in children in North America is the BIS, although other monitors such as the cerebral state index and spectral entropy monitor are available. BIS readings are affected by a number of variables that raise questions regarding their validity in children. First, the determinations vary with the anesthetic administered. For example, at equi-MAC values, the BIS measurements during halothane anesthesia are 50% greater than those during sevoflurane.[245] This likely reflects the substantial differences in the EEGs between the two anesthetics. Second, the variability in the BIS measurements during sevoflurane among children precludes precise interpretation of the BIS measurement.[64] Third, age directly affects the BIS readings, because BIS measurements in children under 5 years of age are less reliable than those in children above 5 years of age.[63-65] This likely stems from maturational differences in the EEG from birth to school age, which was not incorporated in the BIS algorithm. Fourth, the BIS readings decrease as the sevoflurane concentration increases but beyond 3%, BIS paradoxically increases.[64] Additional curiosities with the BIS that are not pediatric specific include the changes in the BIS readings in the presence of nitrous oxide and ketamine and with the onset of paralysis,[246] and finally, the effect of position on the BIS reading with Trendelenburg position (30-degree head-down) increasing the BIS by 20%.[247]

This author's indications for the use of the BIS monitor in children include those who cannot tolerate general anesthesia because of hemodynamic instability, those in whom nitrous oxide is not used, and those who require TIVA.

Emergency Drugs

Emergency drugs should always be available before inducing anesthesia. Syringes with a small gauge (23G or 25G) needle that contain weight-appropriate doses of atropine and succinylcholine should be immediately available to facilitate IM or sublingual drug injection in an emergency. A syringe of propofol (1 to 2 mg/kg) should also be available to facilitate tracheal intubation or insert an LMA, as well as to break laryngospasm and increase the depth of anesthesia quickly.[241] Inotropic drugs are not routinely prepared for children undergoing elective surgery, unless the child has congenital heart disease or is critically ill. In the latter situations, preloaded syringes of phenylephrine (10 µg/mL) and epinephrine (10 µg/mL) should also be available.

Full Stomach and Rapid Sequence Induction

The term full stomach refers to the presence of residual solid or liquid foods in the stomach at induction of anesthesia, a condition that places the child at risk for regurgitation and aspiration.

A full stomach is assumed to be present in children who require emergency surgery, in those with gastric dysmotility syndromes, and in those with diabetes. A full stomach may be caused by the trauma, pain, and stress of the injury as well as by the administration of opioids, which increase gastric and intestinal paresis and further delay emptying of food from the stomach. In emergency surgery, the only time interval that correlates with the risk of food remaining in the stomach is the interval between ingestion of food and the trauma or opioid administration.[188]

There are three important principles to remember in such cases: (1) there is no safe time interval after an injury that guarantees the stomach is empty of food; (2) there is no safe time interval after an injury that guarantees that there is no risk of regurgitation of gastric contents; and (3) all children (even those treated with prokinetic motility drugs) are at risk for regurgitation and aspiration during induction of, maintenance of, and emergence from anesthesia.

To protect the airways of children who are at risk for regurgitation and aspiration during induction of anesthesia, an RSI is widely practiced. Although there is no evidence that an RSI is the best strategy, it seems reasonable to induce anesthesia as quickly as possible and to insert a tracheal tube into the larynx as quickly as possible and inflate the cuff, if a cuffed tube is used. To perform an RSI, a tracheal tube with a stylet as well as tubes 0.5 mm ID greater or less, a functioning laryngoscope, active suction, IV access, and predetermined doses of anesthetic agents should be prepared. Induction of anesthesia may include propofol (2 to 4 mg/kg), ketamine (1 to 2 mg/kg), or etomidate (0.2 to 0.3 mg/kg), with the latter two favored in hemodynamically unstable conditions. We recommend succinylcholine 2 mg/kg (preceded by atropine 0.02 mg/kg) for paralysis, although rocuronium 0.8 to 1 mg/kg has also been used. (Note: *Recent concern regarding unexpected hyperkalemia and ventricular tachycardia in male children with undiagnosed muscle (wasting) diseases who received succinylcholine requires the immediate availability of IV calcium chloride (10 mg/kg IV) or calcium gluconate (30 mg/kg IV) (repeated as necessary to restore normal sinus rhythm).*) If the child has a muscle wasting disorder, succinylcholine should be avoided and rocuronium used to secure the airway. However, if the airway appears to be difficult or precarious, then alternative strategies to secure the airway should be considered, including an inhalational anesthetic or topical local anesthetic and TIVA sedation. If an inhalational induction is performed, unexpected regurgitation may necessitate rotating the child quickly into the left lateral decubitus position and pharyngeal suctioning to prevent aspiration.

There is much debate regarding the importance and relevance of cricoid pressure in an RSI in children.[239] Currently, there is no evidence to support or refute the use of cricoid pressure during RSI. However, there are some concerns regarding the application of cricoid pressure in infants. In both infants and children, the cricoid ring and trachea are mobile and deformable, and as little as 5 N force can compress the infant's airway by 50%.[240] This is one-fourth to one-sixth the force recommended for cricoid pressure in adults.

Cricoid pressure may also increase the level of difficulty of tracheal intubation by distorting tracheal anatomy or compressing the cricoid ring. Very few assistants are trained properly in locating the cricoid ring and in how much force is required to occlude the esophagus. *It remains this author's view that cricoid pressure has not been shown to reduce regurgitation in children at risk for aspiration and is not required for RSI. The practitioner should understand the advantages and disadvantages of cricoid pressure in infants and children in order to make an informed decision regarding its use.*

Preoperative Preparation

Anxiolysis

It is important to reduce anxiety in children undergoing anesthesia and surgery. Anxiety is greater when preschool age and withdrawn children are separated from their parents, when anxious parents accompany their children, and when multiple personnel, bright lights, and loud noises are present at induction of anesthesia. Each of these factors should be addressed on an institutional basis to reduce the overall anxiety in young children scheduled for surgery. Goal-directed therapy for the child should primarily attenuate the child's anxiety preoperatively and anticipate more anxiety at induction of anesthesia and, secondarily, address the parental anxiety.[248]

Parental Presence at Induction of Anesthesia

Two systematic reviews established that parental presence at induction of anesthesia (PPIA) reduced the anxiety of parents but not the children.[249,250] Children 1 to 6 years of age are those for whom PPIA may be most beneficial. Parents who are most insistent on being present at induction of anesthesia are often the most disruptive, least likely to calm their child, and actually promote further noncompliant behavior in their child. Parents should never be invited to accompany their child for induction, lest both the hospital and the medical personnel find themselves responsible for any untoward sequelae that occur. The entire OR team must be like-minded regarding PPIA including detailed plans for escorting the parents out of the OR at the appropriate time. Before entering the OR, the parents must be instructed on the normal behavior of children during induction of anesthesia. If the parent is unable to cope with the OR environment or the child's loss of consciousness, he/she should not be present at their child's induction of anesthesia.

Some cognitively challenged adolescents and children may resist the transfer to the operating room. In such cases, the parents may have to be enlisted to accompany the child to the OR. Those children who resist attempts to bring them to the OR and are physically abusive despite enlisting the parent's assistance may require IM ketamine (see later).

Distraction Techniques

Preoperative coloring books, stories, videos, and websites may be used to help children of all ages learn about surgery and anesthesia and the equipment that will be used for induction of anesthesia.[250] Some children's hospitals conduct operating room tours during which time the children become familiar and touch the face masks and breathing circuits. Child-life providers may help children defuse anxiety on the day of surgery by having the children play with the mask and flavor the inside using lip balm. Other distraction techniques including video games, earphones, and portable Internet devices as well as music and clowns all reduce children's anxiety. Once the child enters the operating room, the anesthesiologist should establish rapport (distract) with the child by telling a story, engaging them in conversation about a recent birthday, holiday, or vacation, or by singing as they prepare for induction of anesthesia.

Pharmacologic Sedation

For some, a premedication may be required to facilitate smooth separation from their parents. In North America, midazolam is the most widely used premedication for children because it can be given orally, nasally, rectally, IM, or IV to provide anxiolysis before induction of anesthesia. It should be noted that most premedications do not delay recovery and/or hospital discharge for surgeries at least 30 minutes in duration.

The dose of oral midazolam increases with decreasing age, although few bother to consider this very important factor.[251] Failure to adequately premedicate the child may lead to parents questioning the practitioner's abilities, but more importantly, may fail to provide adequate anxiolysis for separation from the parents and induction of anesthesia. The bioavailability of oral midazolam is poor, with 27% at 0.15 mg/kg and 15% at 0.45 and 1 mg/kg.[10] This author administers 0.75 to 1 mg/kg (maximum dose 15 to 20 mg) to children 18 months to 3 years of age, 0.6 to 0.75 mg/kg to children 3 to 6 years of age, 0.5 mg/kg to children 6 to 10 years of age, and 0.3 mg/kg to children above 10 years to a maximum of 15 to 20 mg to ensure a 98% success rate of sedating children within 10 to 15 minutes.[252] Because oral midazolam leaves a bitter aftertaste, the current formulation is dissolved in a thick, strawberry flavored-syrup. To minimize the aftertaste, the dose should be swallowed in a single bolus and then followed with a small volume of water. For children too young to swallow midazolam from a cup, it should be instilled into the lateral gutters of the mouth using a needleless syringe to prevent the child from spitting it out. Judgment should be exercised when considering oral midazolam premedication for a child who is crying continuously as few strategies, including parental presence at induction, may provide anxiolysis.

Alternative oral premedications include ketamine (5 to 6 mg/kg),[108] clonidine (2 μg/kg),[253] and dexmedetomidine (2 μg/kg).[254] Ketamine is prepared by suspending it in a thick, flavored syrup. It offers few advantages over midazolam and may cause more postoperative vomiting (POV).[108] Postoperative hallucinations and nightmares are uncommon after oral premedication. Some have combined oral midazolam and ketamine in a 50:50 mixture with good success. Both clonidine and dexmedetomidine take 60 to 90 minutes to effect sedation and anxiolysis. They may produce bradycardia and sedation that persist beyond the duration of the anesthetic.

The IN route is effective in the crying child, although nasal administration of drugs is unpleasant for most.[248] A volume of 0.5 mL is well tolerated and covers adequate mucosal surface for rapid absorption. IN midazolam 0.1 to 0.2 mg/kg causes effective premedication, but older children complain of the bitter burning aftertaste.[255] IN sufentanil 1 to 2 μg/kg is also an effective premedication, although in one study, 23% of patients desaturated to less than 90% after 2 μg/kg of IN sufentanil and 45% developed chest wall rigidity after 4.5 μg/kg.[256] Succinylcholine may be required to resolve chest wall rigidity after IN sufentanil. IN dexmedetomidine (0.5 to 1 μg/kg) also provides anxiolysis and sedation,[257] although it may require up to 1 hour to affect sedation and the sedation may extend into the recovery period.

For older children and adolescents who are cognitively challenged, uncooperative, and/or behaviorally problematic despite their parents' presence, IM ketamine 2 to 5 mg/kg (concentration 100 mg/mL) administered via a small gauge, long needle (large enough to not break off if the encounter became combative) into the deltoid muscle of an arm may be the only means to ensure safe delivery of the child to the OR.[258] These children should be seated on a gurney before administering the ketamine, as they quickly lose consciousness and motor tone, becoming difficult to lift or move on to a gurney. By this route, ketamine has an onset of action of 3 to 5 minutes and a duration of 30 to 40 minutes.

Induction Techniques

Inhalational Induction

In North America, the most common technique for inducing anesthesia in children undergoing elective surgery is an inhalational induction. Infants and children of all ages, including those who are crying and upset, can be successfully anesthetized using this approach. Distracting upset and crying children using a warm, reassuring, and calm manner often permits a successful induction of anesthesia by face mask. The notion that distraught children should be treated with "brutane" by holding children down and forcing a mask on their face with 8% sevoflurane flowing has no place in pediatric anesthesia and may psychologically scar the child for life. If the child had a poor previous experience with anesthesia, it is important to understand the nature of the past experience and design an anesthetic to minimize their anxiety.

In preschool-age children, distraction techniques and premedication are key strategies to minimize the anxiety associated with separating from their parents and undergoing induction of anesthesia. The author offers children (>3 years of age) a choice of several flavored lip balms to mark inside the mask. For younger children (<3 years of age), the author flavors the face mask for them. The smell obscures the plastic smell of the mask but more importantly it distracts the child and offers a topic for discussion. Troposmia, which means a distorted perception of an odor, is an interesting strategy in which the child is told that the flavor that was applied to the mask will transform into his/her favorite flavor as anesthesia is induced. Using this approach, 80% of children interviewed postoperatively confirmed that they smelled their favorite flavor as they were anesthetized.[259] Other distraction techniques include music, story and joke telling, magic, video and handheld games, and clowns (see earlier).

With the child seated on the operating table with his/her back to the anesthesiologist's chest (or on your lap if a diaper is worn) and at least a pulse oximeter (with more monitors as tolerated), a flavored face mask is applied over the mouth and nose with 5 to 7 L/min of a mixture of 70% nitrous oxide and 30% oxygen. The adjustable pressure-limiting valve should be completely open to avoid resistance to exhalation. During this time, the child should be distracted by singing a song or telling a joke or story until the end-tidal N_2O concentration exceeds ~50% or the child ceases to respond to verbal stimulation. At this point, the inspired concentration of sevoflurane is increased in one step from 0% to 8%. If the sevoflurane concentration is increased in smaller increments, then a protracted period of excitement may ensue. If sevoflurane is introduced at the same time as the nitrous oxide, unpremedicated children will reject the mask because of the strong odor of sevoflurane, potentially resulting in an aversion to or fear of face masks, which almost certainly will present difficulties for future anesthetics.

As the child loses consciousness, he/she is placed supine. If apneic or hypopnea occurs (as is common after premedication), ventilation may be assisted manually and gently. To reduce the risk of awareness, this author recommends maintaining 8% sevoflurane and 70% nitrous oxide until IV access has been established. At that time, 1 to 2 mg/kg IV propofol is administered, the nitrous oxide may be discontinued, and an LMA or tracheal tube is inserted.[87] Bilateral air entry in the chest, the presence of a capnogram, and no air entry audible over the upper epigastrium confirm proper placement of the tube. After inflation of the cuff of the LMA, absence of excessive air leak at 20 cm H_2O confirms proper LMA placement. The inspired concentration of sevoflurane may be reduced to 2% to 3% inspired and nitrous oxide reintroduced.

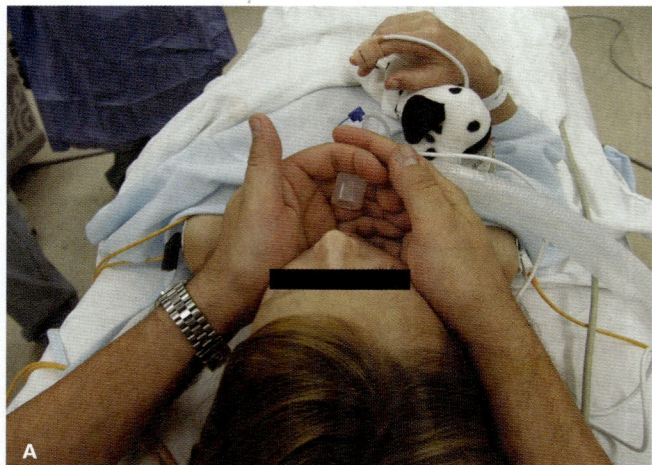 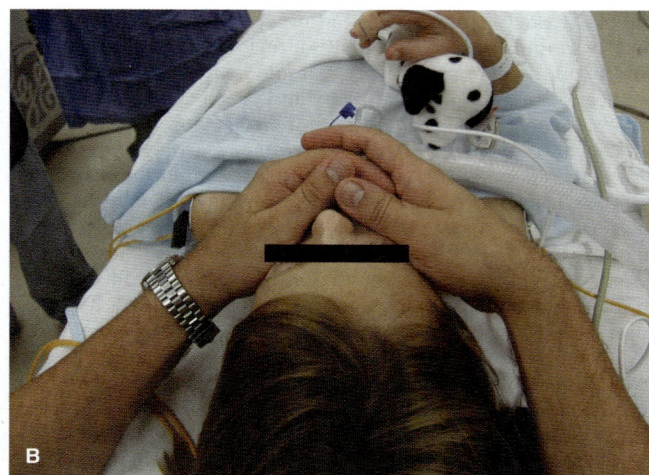

Figure 43-5 For the child who fears the face mask, the mask is removed and the elbow of the breathing circuit is inserted between interlaced fingers in the hand. **A:** At this time, the fresh gas comprises 70% nitrous oxide in oxygen. The hands are gradually brought closer to the child's mouth from below the chin (nitrous oxide is heavier than air), until they completely cover the mouth. **B:** At that point, either sevoflurane may be added to the fresh gas or a face mask applied to the face, or both.

The child with mask phobia poses a real challenge for those attempting to induce anesthesia by mask.[248,260] Besides refusing a mask, these frightened children often steadfastly refuse needles, leaving few options for induction of anesthesia. There are many reasons why children may be fearful of face masks, including the unappealing odor of 8% sevoflurane administered to an unpremedicated child previously, a partially closed APL valve that prevented the child from exhaling, and claustrophobia. Irrespective of the reason for the mask phobia, if the mask is the focal point of the fear, it should be eliminated. In these cases, anesthesia may be induced without a face mask by inserting the elbow of the breathing circuit between two fingers and interlacing the fingers of his/her two hands (with flavor applied to the gloves) (Fig. 43-5A and B). With the hands cupped under the child's chin and 70% nitrous oxide in oxygen flowing, the hands slowly close in over the child's mouth. Because nitrous oxide is heavier than air, the cupped hands act as a reservoir for the nitrous oxide. Suction tubing may be held in close proximity to minimize spread of anesthetic to those nearby. Although this technique causes OR pollution, this author believes it is the optimal approach for managing children with mask and IV phobias. Once the hands are tight over the mouth, 8% sevoflurane may be introduced. As soon as the child stops responding, the elbow of the circuit is inserted into the mask and the mask is applied to the face to seal the airway.

If the child is not mask-phobic, the anesthesiologist may deliver sevoflurane from the outset of the anesthetic without the child smelling the sevoflurane by rotating the face mask 90 degrees so the cuff on the mask occludes the nares. This eliminates/decreases the smell of sevoflurane and allows anesthesia to be induced smoothly.

For older children (usually >6 years of age) who understand how to hold their breath, a single-breath induction of anesthesia may be employed.[261] With this technique, the eyelash reflex is lost within 20 seconds of the breath-hold. However, to be successful, the child should practice inhaling maximally through the mouth and exhaling to residual volume (e.g., until there is no air left in their lungs) before the induction. The anesthesia breathing circuit should be primed with 8% sevoflurane (with or without 70% nitrous oxide) as evidenced by the agent analyzer. This is achieved by flushing the circle circuit and a 2- to 3-L reservoir bag three to four times with 8% sevoflurane in 70% nitrous oxide, exhausting the contents of the circuit each time through the scavenging system. Once the child has mastered the breathing maneuver, the child exhales to residual volume, at which point the face mask and the primed breathing circuit is applied and held tightly to the face. The child is instructed to take a single deep breath through the mouth and hold it for as long as he/she can. While the child is holding his/her breath, the anesthesiologist counts aloud slowly to distract the child. The child may be supine or sitting for this induction, but if the child is sitting, an assistant stand behind the child to support him/her when he/she loses consciousness. In general, the child loses consciousness before the count reaches 15 seconds. As discussed earlier, a gradual introduction of the inhaled anesthetics may proceed smoothly in cooperative patients and one variation on that approach is demonstrated in the video.

IV Induction

For children without IV access, there are several approaches to establishing access. First, a topical local anesthetic cream can be applied to the skin to prevent the pain of the needle puncture. Topical local anesthetic creams that are available include the eutectic mixture of local anesthetics (EMLA) cream (AstraZeneca, Wilmington, DE), which requires a 45- to 60-minute application time to produce topical anesthesia and may cause skin blanching and venoconstriction; Ametop (4% tetracaine) (Smith and New, Canada); ELA-Max (liposomal 4% lidocaine); and Synera (Zars Pharma Inc., Salt Lake City, UT).[262] Ametop, ELA-Max, and Synera require a 30-minute application time and do not cause skin blanching or venoconstriction. A meta-analysis of EMLA and amethocaine reported that amethocaine was more effective than EMLA in children.[263] The J-tip injector of powder lidocaine anesthetizes the skin, although it itself causes moderate pain in 20% of children. Investigation of the factors that predispose to painful response to IV placement include young age, more numerous previous painful procedures, greater state and trait anxiety, more active, and the presence of polymorphisms to endothelin receptor A (EDNRA rs5333) compared with those with less pain.[264] Second, 50% to 70% nitrous oxide may be administered for 1 to 2 minutes by a tight mask fit to permit IV insertion, yielding better results than with EMLA.[265] Third, IN sufentanil may be useful for IV placement. These approaches may be particularly useful for children with MH and myopathies in whom a potent inhalational anesthetic must be avoided.

Once IV access has been established, IV anesthesia with propofol, ketamine, or etomidate may be used for induction of anesthesia; sodium thiopental is only available outside of the US.

Propofol is the most widely available induction agent. It is available as Diprivan in a 1% solution that includes Intralipid (long-chain triglycerides derived from soybean oil), ethylenediaminetetraacetic acid (EDTA, a bacteriostatic agent), egg lecithin (a phospholipid membrane stabilizer), and propofol (2,6-diisopropylphenol). Because propofol is a phenol derivative, it causes pain when injected into the small peripheral veins of children. Several strategies have been investigated to attenuate or prevent pain, but only two techniques reliably prevent pain associated with IV propofol in small veins: 70% nitrous oxide in oxygen by inhalation or a modified Bier block using 0.5 to 1 mg/kg of 1% lidocaine injected into a vein while the arm is occluded for 45 to 60 seconds.[94-96] Propofol is a very safe induction agent for children. A bolus injection of propofol causes transient hypopnea or apnea with a minor decrease in heart rate and blood pressure.

Ketamine is also used for induction of anesthesia, although it is a second-tier induction agent because of concerns for postoperative nightmares. It is often used in the presence of circulatory instability (shock) or cyanotic heart disease.

Etomidate is only approved for children over 10 years of age in the United States. A recent population pharmacokinetic study of etomidate in children concluded that the dose of etomidate should increase as age decreases because both clearance and volume of distribution increase with decreasing age.[114] However, dosing recommendations have not been forthcoming. In adults, 0.2 to 0.3 mg/kg IV etomidate is effective for induction of anesthesia. Like ketamine, it maintains blood pressure even in the presence of circulatory instability. It decreases CBF by 20% to 30%. Minor side effects include pain on injection and myoclonic jerking. However, a far more serious side effect is suppression of adrenal function for up to 24 hours after both a single dose and a brief infusion of etomidate.

Sodium thiopental has been used for almost half a century as the IV induction agent of choice, but in the past two decades, it was gradually supplanted by propofol as the induction agent of choice and more recently supply was cutoff to the United States out of ethical concerns regarding its use for lethal injection. Thiopental remains available in Europe and Asia. Dosing for induction of anesthesia is 3 to 5 mg/kg IV. It causes no serious side effects when administered as an IV bolus. However, because it is only metabolized at 10%/hr, emergence is delayed if it is administered as a continuous infusion.

IM Induction

The IM route is infrequently used for induction of anesthesia in children because it is painful, induction is slow, and there is a risk of sterile abscess formation. The only anesthetic currently used for IM injections in children is ketamine.[258] This approach is usually reserved for adolescent children who are cognitively impaired, extremely uncooperative, and large in size. For further details, see IM premedication, earlier.

Rarely do children who require emergent securing of their airways present without IV access. When it does occur, one of several approaches may be undertaken. IV access may be established before induction of anesthesia, after anesthesia is induced with an inhalational agent, or after IM injection of ketamine (3 to 5 mg/kg), atropine (0.02 mg/kg), and succinylcholine (4 mg/kg).

Rectal Induction

Rectal induction of anesthesia has been popular in young children (<5 years of age) in the past, particularly for those who were unwilling to take oral premedication or who were very frightened. Several regimens have been used for rectal induction: methohexital 15 to 25 mg/kg, midazolam 1 mg/kg, ketamine 5 mg/kg, or thiopental 30 to 40 mg/kg.[266] A number of problems were identified with rectal anesthesia inductions, including poor bioavailability of the induction agent (due to unpredictable rectal venous absorption or evacuation of the drug from the rectum), laryngospasm (with methohexital), and delayed recovery from anesthesia. In immune-compromised patients, rectal administration of drugs may lead to sepsis. Today, rectal inductions are rarely employed. Most anesthetists prefer to involve the parents in managing the child's behavior at induction of anesthesia rather than administer a rectal medication.

Problems during Induction of Anesthesia

Hemoglobin Oxygen Desaturation

Pulse oximetry may be the only monitor that remains functional during induction of anesthesia in the restless young child. All current oximeters include motion-artifact compensating software to ensure fairly accurate measurements even when the child is moving. As the child becomes anesthetized, respiration is reduced resulting in hypoventilation. Despite the use of oxygen-enriched inspired gases, many children, particularly those with a history of a mild URTI or who become deeply anesthetized, hypoventilate or become apneic. This immediately leads to oxygen desaturation, which may be exacerbated if nitrous oxide was coadministered. The primary diagnosis at this time is segmental atelectasis and intrapulmonary shunting, providing upper airway obstruction (often referred to as mild laryngospasm) has been ruled out. To restore the SaO_2, 10 to 20 cm H_2O of positive end-expiratory pressure should be applied using the adjustable pressure limit valve. The peak pressure that is delivered should be carefully adjusted to avoid inflation of the stomach. If, however, the lungs are not being ventilated, then laryngospasm should be suspected quickly and the management followed as described later.

Laryngospasm

Laryngospasm is an infrequent, but potentially life-threatening complication that occurs in children during induction and emergence from anesthesia. The frequency ranges from 0.4% to 10% among studies.[267,268] Several factors are known to increase the risk of laryngospasm in children (Table 43-12).[268]

Laryngospasm is defined as the reflex closure of the false and true vocal cords, although the precise pathogenesis of this reflex remains debated. Complete laryngospasm is defined as closure of the false vocal cords and apposition of the laryngeal surface of the epiglottis and interarytenoids. The net effect is complete cessation of air movement and noisy respiration, absence of movement of the reservoir bag, and an absent capnogram. In contrast, incomplete (or partial) laryngospasm is defined as incomplete apposition of the vocal cords with a residual small gap between the cords posteriorly that permits a persistent inspiratory stridor,

Table 43-12 Factors Associated with Laryngospasm[267]

Age: greater in infants than older children and adults; the risk decreases with increasing age
Recent URTI (<2 weeks)
History of reactive airway disease
Exposure to second-hand smoke
Airway anomalies
Airway surgery
Airway devices (tracheal tubes, LMA)
Stimulating the glottis during a light plane of anesthesia
Secretions in the oropharynx (e.g., blood, excess saliva, gastric juice)
Inhaled anesthesia (desflurane and isoflurane)
Inexperienced anesthesiologist

URTI, upper respiratory tract infection; LMA, laryngeal mask airway.

limited movement of the reservoir bag, and progressively increasing respiratory effort. Some assert that incomplete laryngospasm is not laryngospasm at all, but for treatment purposes this is a moot point.

The clinical findings in laryngospasm begin with faint inspiratory stridor, suprasternal and supraclavicular in-drawing due to increased inspiratory effort, increased diaphragmatic excursions, and flailing of the lower ribs. As greater inspiratory effort is expended, the intensity and volume of the stridor increases, and the chest wall movement resembles that of a rocking horse. As laryngospasm progresses, air movement through the almost closed glottis ceases and the inspiratory effort becomes completely silent. This is an ominous sign. If the progression of the laryngospasm is not interrupted, oxygen desaturation will quickly ensue. This may be followed by a decrease in heart rate. This downward spiral must be interrupted as described later.

Management of laryngospasm requires a multifaceted and immediate response (Fig. 43-6).[267] As soon as the diagnosis is

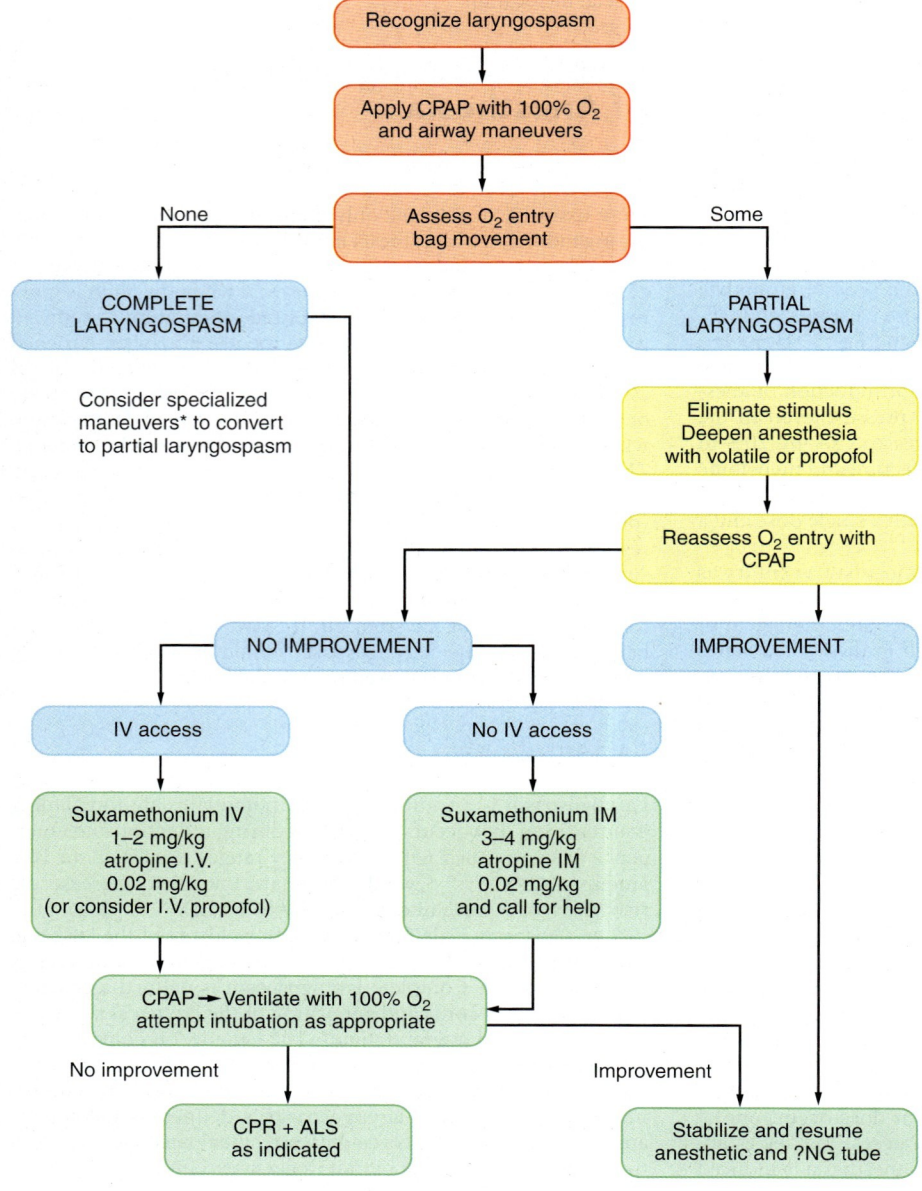

Figure 43-6 Algorithm to diagnose and manage laryngospasm in children. *Apply the jaw thrust maneuver as described on p. 1247. CPAP, continuous positive airway presure; CPR, cardiopulmonary resuscitation; ALS, advanced life support; NG, nasogastric tube. (Adapted with permission from Hampson-Evans D, Morgan P, Farrar M. Pediatric laryngospasm. *Paediatr Anaesth*. 2008;18:303–307.)

suspected, a tight-fitting face mask should be applied to the child's face and 100% oxygen delivered with continuous positive airway pressure (15 to 20 cm H_2O dialed into the adjustable pressure limiting valve). Pressures in excess of 20 cm H_2O may cause gastric inflation. Note that the reservoir bag should not be squeezed except during the child's inspiratory efforts, lest gas be driven into the stomach. If the triggering event is blood, secretions, or foreign material in the airway, these should be removed immediately. As soon as the offending agent has been expunged, the jaw thrust maneuver should be applied. This maneuver requires familiarity with the anatomy of the retromandibular notch, an area subtended by the condylar process of the ascending ramus of the mandible anteriorly, the mastoid process posteriorly, and the external auditory canal superiorly.[98] Bilateral digital pressure is applied to the most cephalad point on the posterior edge of the condylar process of the ascending ramus of the mandible, and the force directed toward the frontal hairline. The force should be applied for 3 to 5 seconds at a time and then released for 5 to 10 seconds, while maintaining a tight seal with the face mask against the child's face. By applying and releasing pressure on the condylar processes, the repeated painful stimuli may cause sufficient pain to induce the child to cry, which opens the vocal cords terminating the laryngospasm. In addition to causing pain, the jaw thrust maneuver serves to relieve upper airway obstruction in the anesthetized child by both translocating the ramus of the mandible anteriorly and rotating the temporomandibular joint so the mouth opens. Together, these maneuvers lift the tongue off the posterior pharyngeal wall establishing a patent upper airway.

The jaw thrust maneuver is not as effective when applied at the angle of the mandible as this region contains many fewer pain fibers and does not rotate the temporomandibular joint. Hence, the ability of the maneuver to establish a clear upper airway is not nearly as effective. Remember, laryngospasm cannot develop or persist if the vocal cords are moving and the child is vocalizing or crying. If positive pressure ventilation, 100% oxygen, and jaw thrust maneuver fail to break the laryngospasm, further intervention should be undertaken before desaturation and bradycardia develop. Appropriate treatment would include in the following order: IV or IM atropine (0.02 mg/kg), IV propofol (1 mg/kg), and IV or IM succinylcholine (1 to 2 mg/kg IV or 4 to 5 mg/kg IM).[267-269]

Some suggest that gentle chest compressions effectively break laryngospasm in children. To add chest compressions to the management of laryngospasm requires a pair of free hands. If no free hands are available, do not abandon the maneuvers described earlier to perform chest compressions unless there is a cardiac arrest. The risk associated with this maneuver includes sternal or rib fractures. Currently, the author believes there is excellent alternative treatment for laryngospasm and insufficient evidence to recommend chest compressions to relieve laryngospasm in children.

Bradycardia

Bradycardia is a slowing of the heart rate below age-defined limits. For infants (<1 year of age) this is 100 beats/minute (bpm); for young children 1 to 5 years of age, 80 bpm; and for children above 5 years of age, 60 bpm. Because cardiac output of infants and children is heart rate dependent, a slow heart rate means a reduced cardiac output. If the heart rate decreases below these limits, corrective action should be taken to restore the heart rate, and if necessary cardiopulmonary resuscitation should be initiated.

Although hypoxia is the foremost cause of bradycardia in children, drug-associated causes include halothane and succinylcholine. Because sevoflurane has replaced halothane in developed countries, this cause of bradycardia has all but disappeared.[48] This is not the case in many developing countries. A single dose of succinylcholine remains a cause of bradycardia in children but is a much less common cause today because succinylcholine is not routinely used in children for tracheal intubation. The incidence of bradycardia during the first 6 minutes of sevoflurane anesthesia in children with Down syndrome is fivefold greater than that in matched controls.[270] Children who are rate dependent for cardiac output and develop bradycardia may require treatment with atropine or isoproterenol. Atropine increases the cardiac output not only by increasing the heart rate, but also by increasing contractility through the force frequency response.[1]

The causes of bradycardia in healthy children are listed in Table 43-13. To stop progressive slowing of the heart rate, the underlying cause of bradycardia should be corrected (e.g., correct hypoxia when present and administer atropine 0.02 mg/kg). Atropine is only effective when myocardial electrical activity is present and the bradycardia is of vagal origin. If asystole occurs, however, atropine cannot restore the heart rhythm, and the only definitive treatment is IV epinephrine (10 μg/kg). Secondary treatment may include isoproterenol.

Table 43-13 Causes of Bradycardia in Infants and Children

1. Hypoxia (e.g., laryngospasm, obstructed airway, atelectasis)
2. Vagal reflex response (e.g., laryngoscopy, prolonged stretch on the extraocular muscles)
3. Increased intracranial pressure
4. Medications (e.g., clonidine, β-blockers, α-adrenergic eye drops, succinylcholine without pretreatment with atropine, sevoflurane [more common with Down syndrome], propofol infusion syndrome)
5. Electrolyte disturbance (e.g., hyperkalemia, hypocalcemia)
6. Congenital heart disease, congenital or acquired rhythm disturbance
7. Hypothermia
8. Air embolism
9. Tension pneumothorax

Maintenance of Anesthesia

Techniques

Inhalational anesthetics, supplemented with IV analgesics and antiemetics, have been the mainstay of anesthesia although, of late, TIVA has emerged as a reasonable alternative. One key advantage that distinguishes inhalational anesthetics from IV anesthesia is the ability to continuously measure the end-tidal (alveolar) anesthetic concentrations of inhaled agents. This measurement provides invaluable information regarding the accuracy of our delivery system and the anesthetic partial pressures in the VRG of tissues. Currently, isoflurane, sevoflurane, and desflurane are used to maintain anesthesia in children.

TIVA has become the primary anesthetic technique for children with MH, for those undergoing spine surgery with motor-evoked potential monitoring, for those with a history of severe perioperative nausea and vomiting, and, in some institutions, for all children. Propofol and ketamine are the primary general anesthetics used with TIVA, although, unlike propofol, ketamine is emetogenic and associated with prolonged emergence when infused for prolonged periods. Propofol has been proscribed as a continuous sedative for children in ICU because of the risk of PRIS but not in anesthesia. Dosing for bolus and infusions of propofol is described earlier.

Supplemental analgesics are also used during both inhalational and IV anesthesia to prevent physiologic responses and movement to pain. Remifentanil (with a 5-minute context-sensitive half-life) 0.05 to 0.1 µg/kg/min can be administered as an infusion, whereas other opioids (fentanyl and morphine) are more often administered by IV boluses. Fentanyl (1 to 2 µg/kg) or morphine (0.05 to 0.1 mg/kg) can be administered IV; the dose is adjusted up or down depending on the child's exposure to opioids, the severity of the pain, and concomitantly administered analgesics.

9 Fluid Management

General Principles

IV fluid administration sets should be prepared before the child arrives in the operating room. For young children, a 500-mL bag of LR solution with a graduated buretrol is appropriate; for infants (<1 year), a 250-mL bag with a buretrol is preferable. *These recommendations for the use of a buretrol and IV fluid bag are intended to limit the risk of adverse events should the entire bag inadvertently be infused in the child.* All pediatric IV sets should include a manual controller, a one-way valve (to prevent medications from passing retrograde up the IV tubing), and needleless ports and/or three-way stopcocks for medication administration. For children above 8 years of age, the IV infusion set may be prepared with a macro or micro-drip without a buretrol and a 1,000-mL bag of balanced salt solution.

Intralipid infusions from total parenteral nutrition should be discontinued before transfer to the OR to reduce the risk of contaminating the Intralipid and central venous access line by repeated line accessing, although concentrated sugar solutions should be continued.

Most IV fluids administered to healthy children during elective surgery consist of a nonglucose-containing isotonic salt solution, commonly LR solution in North America. These solutions replaced glucose-containing hypotonic solutions that were associated with perioperative seizures, aspiration, and brain damage after large volumes were administered during surgery. LR solution is slightly hypotonic (280 mOm/L) and contains small concentrations of potassium and lactate. Normal saline (0.9% NaCl) is isotonic (308 mOsm/L), acidic (pH 5), and contains no ionic moieties. Normal saline is not routinely used as the primary maintenance solution because large volumes may lead to a hyperchloremic metabolic acidosis (nonanion gap type). We advocate glucose-containing solutions, such as 1% or 2.5% glucose in LR solution, as a maintenance solution in infants under 6 months of age and for young children who are cachectic, chronically malnourished, tolerate fasting poorly (maple sugar disease), and suffer from debilitating disease who may be at risk for hypoglycemia.[271] These solutions should not lead to intraoperative hyperglycemia or hyponatremia. Although the shift to isotonic salt solutions dramatically decreased the incidence of perioperative hyponatremia, some specific surgeries (e.g., craniofacial surgery) may warrant perioperative monitoring of serum electrolytes.[272]

Children with specific medical conditions should have tailored IV solutions. For children with renal failure or renal insufficiency, normal saline has been the preferred balanced salt solution because it contains no potassium although evidence suggests it may lead to greater serum potassium concentrations than LR.[273] Children with a mitochondrial myopathy who had lactic acidosis in infancy should be fasted briefly preoperatively (to avoid acidosis and hypoglycemia) and should receive only nonlactate-containing solutions with glucose supplementation as needed.

Infants and children under 2 years of age who may be hypovolemic should be assessed preoperatively to determine the magnitude of their fluid deficit: mild, moderate, or severe. The signs of mild dehydration (5% body weight loss: approximately 50 mL/kg deficit) include poor skin turgor and dry mouth. The signs of moderate fluid dehydration (10% of body weight loss: 100 mL/kg deficit) include sunken fontanel (if present), tachycardia, and oliguria in addition to the signs of mild dehydration. The signs of severe fluid dehydration (15% of body weight loss: 150 mL/kg deficit) include sunken eyeballs, hypotension, and anuria plus the signs of moderate dehydration.

Correction of hypovolemia requires staged infusion of iso-osmolar fluid administration. Approximately 50% of the deficit should be replaced in the first hour, 25% in the second, and 25% in the third. A balanced salt solution should be used to restore euvolemia.

Elective Surgery

For elective surgery, the traditional calculation for the hourly fluid infusion rate has been based on replacing the triad of fluid deficit during fasting, ongoing maintenance, and blood and third-space losses. In children, a hypotonic glucose-containing solution was used as the maintenance solution at the rate of 4–2–1 mL/kg/hr rule where 4 mL/kg is for the first 10 kg, 2 mL/kg is for the second 10 kg, and 1 mL/kg is for the third 10 kg and any additional body weight thereafter.[274] However in the past 25 years, the maintenance solution has shifted to a balanced salt solution to prevent intraoperative hyponatremia. Holliday and Segar reappraised their 1957 recommendation recently,[274] seeking to address the risks associated with both administering hyponatremic solutions to children who were hypovolemic and applying their 4–2–1 fluid infusion rule to isotonic solutions. They reasoned that the antidiuretic hormone is upregulated in all children who are fasted for elective surgery, presenting with sepsis or an acute inflammatory response, or receiving medications such as opioids and this is the cause of perioperative hyponatremia and water intoxication. To address this problem, they recommended infusing 10 mL/kg/h isotonic solution for each hour for 2–4 h (except for those with cardiac or renal failure) after induction of anesthesia to re-establish euvolemia and downregulate the antidiuretic hormone.[275]

Blood Transfusion Therapy

Initial blood loss may be replaced with balanced salt solution at a rate of 3 mL of solution for every 1 mL of blood loss. For third-space losses, the replacement volume is based on the severity of the losses: 1 to 2 mL/kg/hr for minor surgery, 2 to 5 mL/kg/hr for moderate surgery, and 6 to 10 mL/kg/hr for major surgery and large third-space losses.

Although most pediatric surgeons are careful to minimize bleeding during surgery, it is important to remain vigilant regarding all blood loss during surgery. For procedures that are likely to result in significant tissue trauma or blood loss, appropriate size IV access must be provided for transfusion of the blood and blood products needed for volume replacement. Packed red cells cannot be rapidly infused through either 24-gauge IV catheters or most peripherally inserted central catheters. A 22-gauge catheter is the smallest IV cannula through which blood can be infused rapidly. Every effort should be expended to insert the largest IV catheter that the child's veins will accommodate. This replacement, together with the maintenance requirement, should be logged on the anesthetic record. As the combined volume of balanced salt solution approaches 75 to 100 mL/kg, it is important to consider the possibility of dilutional thrombocytopenia and dilution of coagulation factors; coagulation indices should be measured at this time.

The threshold for initiating packed RBC transfusions in children has undergone a renaissance in the past decade as evidence that the outcome and complications associated with a transfusion threshold of 7 g% hemoglobin is similar to that of 9 g%.[276]

The estimated blood volume in children decreases with increasing age from 95 to 100 mL/kg in premature infants to 70 mL/kg in adults.[276] Note that the estimated blood volume of obese children is reduced 10% from that of nonobese children of similar age. To estimate the allowable blood loss during surgery, the following equation is used[277]:

$$\text{Maximum allowable blood loss} = \frac{(\text{starting Hct} - \text{target Hct})}{(\text{starting Hct})} \quad (43\text{-}3)$$

Some modify Eq. 3 and replace the "starting Hct" in the denominator with the "average Hct." This increases the allowable blood loss before transfusion. Irrespective of which equation is used, the actual Hct should be determined before initiating blood transfusion to ensure that the Hct has actually decreased to the desired level. When initiating a blood transfusion in a child, two formulae provide rough estimates of the amount of blood required to increase the hemoglobin concentration by 1 g%: 4 to 5 mL/kg packed cells and 6 mL/kg whole blood.[276] Massive transfusion protocols have also been developed for children and may be accessed at http://pediatrictraumasociety.org/multimedia/files/clinical-resources/MTP-3.pdf (accessed January 15, 2017).

10 Prophylaxis for Postoperative Vomiting

The incidence of POV in children depends on a number of factors that relate to the child (motion sickness history, age), the anesthetic (inhalational anesthetics, nitrous oxide [in specific instances], opioids), perioperative oral fluid ingestion, and the type of surgery (inguinal/orchidopexy, tonsillectomy and adenoidectomy, strabismus, and middle ear surgery).[278]

To reduce PONV after elective surgery, children should be fasted for brief periods and not forced to drink oral fluids postoperatively until they request them (to reduce the risk of vomiting).[279] Intraoperatively, IV fluids should be aggressively administered 20 to 30 mL/kg to reduce PONV.[280] Pain should be controlled using regional anesthesia and NSAIDs or ketamine; opioids should be used only if necessary. If the child is scheduled for emetogenic surgery or has a history of POV, the optimal anesthetic regimen recommended is propofol oxygen/air and two antiemetics, although conflicting evidence exists regarding the role of substituting propofol and nitrous oxide in PONV.[281,282]

The optimal prophylactic antiemetic strategy to administer to children during anesthesia is dexamethasone and a 5-HT$_3$ receptor antagonist, such as ondansetron.[283] There is no dose–response relationship for dexamethasone: doses between 0.0625 and 1 mg/kg are equally effective, although this author limits the maximum dose to 10 mg.[284] The dose of ondansetron for prophylaxis in children is 0.05 to 0.15 mg/kg.

Although a single study suggested that dexamethasone increases the incidence of postoperative tonsil bleeding, their results are inconsistent with the author's experience and the subsequent literature.[285,286] A single dose of glucocorticoids has been associated with several reports of tumor lysis syndrome in patients with undiagnosed acute lymphoblastic lymphoma, a very rare but potentially fatal outcome if unrecognized.[217] A single dose of dexamethasone has also been associated with a transient increase in serum glucose concentration that peaked at 2 hours postoperatively, in obese adults with poorly controlled type 2 diabetes. Data in children have not been forthcoming.

Regional Anesthesia and Pain Management

There are numerous regional blocks that may be performed to reduce nociception during and after surgery. Three common neuroaxial blocks performed in children today are caudal, epidural, and spinal blocks and these are described later. There has been a shift from neuroaxial to peripheral nerve blocks, both single-dose and continuous local anesthetic administration for perioperative pain management facilitated by the introduction of ultrasound guidance. Morbidity and mortality associated with regional anesthesia in children is exceedingly small and is not considered a substantive argument against its routine use in skilled hands.

Caudal Blockade

This block is useful for both lower abdominal and lower extremity surgeries in infants and children (<5 to 6 years) who are undergoing ambulatory surgery. It is usually performed under general anesthesia although in neonates, awake caudal and spinal blocks have been performed using local anesthetic infiltration and/or sedation. Single-shot caudal blocks with local anesthetic alone are commonly performed in ambulatory surgery. These blocks may last 4 to 6 hours, but if adjuvant medications are added, they may last even longer.

After induction of anesthesia and once that airway is secured, the child is turned onto the lateral decubitus (the side is determined by the anesthesiologist; left-handed anesthesiologists generally prefer the right lateral decubitus position for the child), and the key anatomic sites on the sacrum are palpated: posterior superior iliac spines and the sacral hiatus subtended by the two sacral cornua (see also Chapter 42, Caudal Block section). The sacrococcygeal ligament traverses the space between the two cornua and the coccyx. The skin is then prepared with antiseptic solution and allowed to dry while local anesthetic is prepared. Once the drug has been prepared, the skin site is cut with a blunt needle (to prevent the transfer of epidermis to the caudal space) and the IV catheter (22 gauge for those ≤2 years or 20 gauge for >2 years) is passed through the subcutaneous tissue and between or just caudal to the level of the two cornua at a 45-degree angle to the skin. Once the sacrococcygeal ligament has been pierced, the cannula is laid almost flat against the skin (forming a 10-degree angle of the skin) and advanced 2 to 3 mm through the ligament. At that point, the catheter is slipped off the needle and advanced 2 to 3 mm. If any resistance is felt as the catheter is inserted, it is not within the caudal space and the entire cannula should be removed and the process repeated. If you are not certain the catheter is in the caudal canal, hold your thumb over the sacral hiatus and inject no more than 0.5 mL. If resistance or a bulge is felt, desist from injecting fluid; subcutaneous fluid will obscure the anatomy and preclude a successful caudal block. If the catheter is properly positioned, then remove the needle and examine for blood or cerebrospinal fluid leaking out the catheter. Do not apply negative pressure to the catheter as veins collapse easily. Connect the syringe with local anesthetic and inject slowly 2 to 3 mL every 2 minutes, while observing the electrocardiogram. Peak T waves and an increased ST segment are sensitive indicators of an inadvertent intravascular injection during inhalational anesthesia, although blood pressure increases are more sensitive during TIVA.[287] Once the injection is complete, remove the catheter, clean the caudal skin area, and position the child for surgery.

This author prefers to administer 1 mL/kg bupivacaine 0.175% with epinephrine (1:250,000) for all surgical procedures as a single-shot caudal block. This concentration may be prepared by combining 7 mL of 0.25% bupivacaine with 3 mL of saline to give a total volume of 10 mL. This concentration permits excellent analgesic with motor blockade that resolves within 1 hour of placement. Others use ropivacaine 1 mL/kg of 0.2% or levobupivacaine 1 mL/kg of 0.15%, although a comparative study of 0.2% ropivacaine, levobupivacaine, or bupivacaine concluded that the latter two local anesthetics were more effective than the first. Adjunctive medications have been used to prolong the duration of the caudal block for several hours at best.[111,288]

If a continuous caudal block is planned for the child remaining in hospital for a period, then an 18-ga IV catheter should be used to facilitate passage of a 21-ga epidural catheter. The catheter is inserted exactly as described above for caudal blocks and the catheter threaded to the spinal level necessary for perioperative analgesia. The catheter should be taped away from the anus or, alternately, tunneled under the skin to the side opposite the surgery. This reduces the risk of superficial infections at the catheter insertion site. Catheters that are smaller than 21 ga may not thread to the desired dermatome level. Alternative strategies that may be used to achieve the desired level of block include the Tsui approach[289] and inserting the catheter at an intervertebral space closer to the level of surgery.

Local anesthetics may be infused continuously epidurally for up to 3 days. In infants and young children, 0.2 to 0.4 mg/kg/hr bupivacaine may be administered using 0.3 mL/kg/hr of a 0.1% bupivacaine solution.[290] In older children, 0.4 to 0.5 mg/kg/hr may be administered using 0.3 mL/kg/hr of a 0.1% or 0.125% bupivacaine solution. In neonates 0.2 mg/kg/hr bupivacaine solution may be infused for 3 days as 0.2 mL/kg/hr of a 0.1% solution. To reduce absorption of local anesthetic, epinephrine is routinely added to the bupivacaine. Fentanyl (1 to 2 μg/mL) is often added to the caudal/epidural solution, although there is no evidence that this improves the quality of the block in children provided the tip of the catheter is properly positioned, 0.2 to 0.3 mL/kg/hr volume of local anesthetic is administered, and at least 0.1% bupivacaine or its equivalent concentration of local anesthetic is used.[147] The addition of fentanyl to the epidural solution yields side effects that include urinary retention, pruritus, nausea, and vomiting. In the case of levobupivacaine, a large study demonstrated no demonstrable benefit from the addition of fentanyl to epidural levobupivacaine in concentrations as small as 0.0625%.[147] Ropivacaine is also suited for continuous epidural infusion for perioperative analgesia using a 0.2% concentration at 0.1 mL/kg/hr for infants under 6 months of age and 0.2 mL/kg/hr for infants above 6 months of age and children, for up to 72 hours.[291]

Careful attention must be paid to the dose of the local anesthetic (although ropivacaine and levobupivacaine are several fold less cardiotoxic than bupivacaine) in infants and children as toxic blood concentrations may cause ventricular fibrillation and cardiac arrest, which, in the case of bupivacaine, is very difficult to successfully resuscitate. The most effective treatment for ventricular arrhythmias from local anesthetics is 1.5 mL/kg (LBW) IV of 20% Intralipid,[292] repeating the bolus up to twice or by continuous infusion of 0.25 to 0.5 mL/kg/min for up to 10 minutes while monitoring vital signs. [NB. Propofol cannot substitute for Intralipid if the latter is unavailable.] The incidence of complications after caudal/epidural block is small, approximately 1.5:1,000.[293] Postoperatively, each child and parents/guardian should be interviewed daily for the efficacy of the block, side effects, and complications from the caudal/epidural block. Side effects of the block include nausea, vomiting, pruritus, urinary retention if opioids were included, and excessive motor blockade or twitching from local anesthetics. Local infection, fluid leakage, and bleeding at the catheter site are important to recognize and treat as indicated.

Local skin infection at the catheter skin site may appear as red and swollen. These superficial infections do not migrate internally causing epidural abscesses; rather abscesses are due to a bacteremia. In any case, the catheter should be removed and the skin cleansed and dressed.

Epidural Block

Epidural anesthesia is performed in the same manner as in adults except that a shorter 5-cm Tuohy 18G needle is more manageable. The distances from the skin to the dura in infants and children, for example, are much smaller as are the doses.

Spinal Block

This block is useful in preterm infants and neonates who require lower abdominal superficial surgery (see Chapter 42, Spinal Anesthesia section).

Emergence and Recovery from Anesthesia

As surgery concludes, recovery of neuromuscular function should be assured by monitoring the twitch response and antagonizing the blockade, and the child should be normothermic before contemplating removing the tracheal tube. Equipment including active suction, a face mask, and a source of oxygen should be immediately available to manage the airway and any complications that may ensue. The trachea may be extubated when the child is either fully awake or deeply anesthetized. Evidence suggests that the advantages and disadvantages of the two techniques are similar, notwithstanding confounding effects by comorbidities and concomitant drugs.[294]

The optimal time to extubate the trachea "awake" requires that the child has sufficiently recovered from anesthesia to support his/her own airway, thus minimizing the risk of adverse airway events. For an awake extubation, the practitioner can follow one of two strategies: either the no-touch technique or direct stimulation. With the no touch technique, emergence from inhalational anesthesia follows three distinct phases: early, middle, and late. The early phase may last for several minutes depending on the anesthetic drugs present and the age of the child. During this phase, the child coughs intermittently, gags, struggles, and moves nonpurposefully. This phase passes relatively quickly as the child continues to emerge from anesthesia. During the second or quiescent phase, the child remains generally unresponsive, becoming apneic, agitated, or even breath-holding, straining, and/or desaturating. Desaturation should be treated immediately with continuous positive pressure airway pressure by dialing the adjustable pressure relief valve close until the SaO_2 is more than 95%. As the child enters the third and final phase of emergence, respiration resumes at a regular rate, purposeful movement begins and the child flexes the hips. As these intensify, the child begins to cough and gag on the tracheal tube, and then grimaces and opens his/her eyes spontaneously. Removing the tracheal tube during either the early or middle phase markedly increases the risk of triggering an adverse airway event (e.g., laryngospasm). It is only once the child is in this third phase of emergence that the practitioners should consider extubating the trachea. As I often say: "if you think it is time to remove the tube, don't! Leave the tube in situ for another minute (or two) until the child is definitely in the late or third phase of emergence. Complications do not occur from leaving a tube in for an extra minute, they only occur when the tube is removed prematurely."

With the no touch technique, the child breathes 100% oxygen undisturbed and remains unstimulated until the third and final phase of emergence (as described later). The MAC-awake for tidal sevoflurane concentration in children 2 to 5 years is 0.66% and in 5 to 12 years, 0.45%.[295] This author finds that emergence only begins when the anesthetic concentration is empirically less than 0.3% sevoflurane or less than 0.25% isoflurane, depending on the presence of concomitant medications. As the inhaled concentration decreases below these values, the child opens his/her eyes spontaneously and reaches for the tracheal tube, gags, and grimaces, all of which are consistent with a successful extubation. In the case of infants, flexion of the hips indicates good muscle tone. In contrast, with the direct stimulating technique, the anesthetic concentration decreases toward the same concentrations (sevoflurane <0.3% and isoflurane <0.25%) at which time digital pressure may be applied to the most cephalad portion of the ascending ramus of the mandible, to the condylar process (as described earlier in the jaw thrust maneuver), for 3 to 5 seconds while directing the force toward the frontal hairline.[98] The child becomes highly aroused and gags on the tracheal tube for several seconds, but then falls back to a semiconscious state when the stimulation abates. During this quiescent period, the child may breathe shallowly or breath-hold, but if desaturation occurs, positive pressure ventilation with 100% oxygen must be instituted. When the child resumes coughing and gagging, opens their eyes, their respirations are sustained and regular, and they make purposeful movement (e.g., reaches for the tube), then the trachea may be extubated. Both the no-touch and the direct stimulation strategies provide similar outcomes with safe and protected airways in children in experienced hands.

If the tube has been removed prematurely, breath-holding, upper airway obstruction, and laryngospasm may ensue. The child's face mask should be immediately available in order to deliver 100% oxygen through a tight fit to the face with 100% oxygen and dial 10- to 20-cm H_2O continuous positive airway pressure on the adjustable pressure limiting valve. To force the child through this "light" phase of anesthesia, pressure should be applied to the condyle of the mandible (see jaw thrust) in 3- to 5-second intermittent applications until the child begins to breathe. If laryngospasm develops, see earlier for treatment.

Deep tracheal extubation requires an organized plan. In order to extubate the trachea deep, the depth of inhalational anesthesia must be at least 1.5 to 2 × MAC. In the case of sevoflurane, this means between 3.6% and 5% end-tidal concentration for at least 10 minutes. Some prefer to inspect the larynx at that time for foreign substances and fluids by performing laryngoscopy. Others gently stimulate the airway by moving the tube slightly up and down. The absence of a response and the continuation of regular respirations indicate an adequate depth of anesthesia is present to remove the tube. If, however, the child coughs or breath-holds, then either a further period of anesthesia is required before a trial laryngoscopy is attempted or the deep extubation approach is abandoned and the child is awakened.

Appropriate airway equipment should be available to transfer the child once the trachea has been extubated. Either a self-inflating Laerdal bag or a T-piece should be available with a source of oxygen. The nurses who manage these children in PACU must have the skills to manage an intubated airway, emergence from anesthesia, and the airway after tracheal extubation.

In children, the primary focus during emergence from anesthesia is the airway, the child's ability to breathe, and whether the child can protect his/her airway should bleeding or regurgitation occur during or after extubation. It is this author's practice to remove the tracheal tube or LMA when the child has fully recovered airway reflexes and is responsive. There are very few surgical or medical indications to remove the airway during a deep level of anesthesia, although opinion varies on this matter. The concern regarding a deep extubation of the trachea is that a child who is deeply anesthetized and transported with an unsecured airway depends on the expertise of the caregiver in the PACU to manage the airway until that child awakens. If the anesthesiologist must return to the operating room and if there is no physician assigned to PACU, then the caregivers may have inadequate backup should an airway emergency arise.

The timing of removing the LMA, either awake or during deep anesthesia, in general, does not affect the incidence of upper airway adverse events. However, the presence of a URTI, specific anesthetics (e.g., desflurane, isoflurane ~ halothane, sevoflurane), and specific surgeries (e.g., airway surgery) increase the risk of perioperative airway events. When the LMA has been removed during deep anesthesia, upper airway reflex responses may only develop when the child begins to emerge from anesthesia, in the PACU. To avoid this potential problem, this author recommends that all LMAs be removed when the children are awake and only then should they be transferred to PACU.

In the vast majority of children, emergence from anesthesia progresses smoothly as described earlier. However, children who do not emerge from anesthesia in a timely fashion must be assessed for possible causes for delayed emergence from anesthesia (Table 43-14). The most common causes of delayed emergence include drug overdoses, increased sensitivity to drugs (e.g., OSA and opioid sensitivity), failure to taper or reduce the dose of inhalational or IV anesthetic, or the presence of hypothermia. Other, less frequent but potentially catastrophic events should also be considered including hypoglycemia, increased intracranial pressure, and metabolic causes including hyponatremia.

A rare but potentially fatal arrhythmia may develop during emergence in a child with an undiagnosed congenital long QT syndrome.[56] Administering medications (such as 5-HT_3 receptor antagonists) that are known to prolong the QT interval and in the presence of factors known to trigger torsades de pointes may suddenly trigger the arrhythmia.[296] Treatment with IV lidocaine (1 to 2 mg/kg), magnesium (15 to 30 mg/kg), and/or shock may be necessary to convert to sinus rhythm.

Transport to PACU

Transferring children from the operating room to the PACU requires a stable airway, adequate oxygenation and ventilation, stable heart rate and blood pressure, and adequate pain control. The child must be accompanied by an expert who has been trained to diagnose and manage postoperative problems, most notably airway obstruction.

Most children are transported to PACU without an artificial airway, breathing spontaneously. The optimal position for transfer

Table 43-14 Causes of Delayed Emergence from Anesthesia in Children

Cause	Investigation/Intervention
Anesthetic-related	
Residual anesthetic effects: Inhalational anesthetics, opioids, propofol	• End-tidal concentration • Evaluate total drug dose
Non-anesthesia medications: Recreational drug use (cocaine, crack), herbal medicines (valerian, St. John's wort)	• History; drug toxicology screen
Depressed neuromuscular junction, residual neuromuscular blockade, or pseudocholinesterase deficiency	• Assess train-of-four
Hypothermia	• Measure the child's temperature. • Introduce heating modalities as indicated (e.g., forced air warmer, heat operating room)
Severe hypercapnia (minimum alveolar concentration CO_2 ~200–245 mmHg)	• Blood gas and end-tidal PCO_2
Metabolic/other	
Hypo or hyperglycemia; diabetic ketoacidosis	• Measure blood glucose, urinary glucose, and ketones • Arterial blood gas and electrolytes for pH and anion gap
Electrolyte and metabolic disorder	• Serum electrolytes (e.g., hyponatremia, hypomagnesemia)
Acid–base disturbance	• Blood gas analysis (anion gap or nonanion gap acidosis)
Encephalopathy	• Hepatic, renal, endocrinopathy (e.g., hypothyroidism, Addison disease), or sepsis • Blood gas analysis, electrolytes, and blood cultures if indicated
Cerebrovascular accident/hypoxic-insult	• Check bilateral pupil size • Check responsiveness to light and pain stimulus bilaterally • Assess the presence of a gag reflex, symmetrical limb reflexes • Assess the fontanelle pressure in infants

of a child after surgery is the lateral decubitus position, known as the "recovery position."[297] In this position, the upper leg is flexed at the hip and resting on the bed in front of the lower leg. The child's upper hand should be placed under his lower cheek (Fig. 43-7). This position facilitates drainage of secretions, blood, or vomitus out of the mouth rather than onto the larynx, and the tongue falls to the lower cheek or out of the mouth rather than posteriorly onto the larynx. This position permits direct airway monitoring and intervention should the need arise.

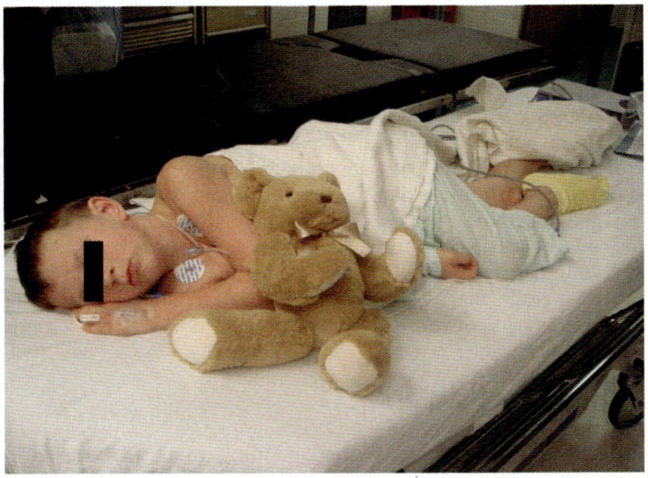

Supplemental oxygen may be administered by nasal prongs or face mask during transport to the PACU to prevent desaturation during the transport. However, in the absence of nitrous oxide and in children whose lungs are normal, the most common reason for desaturation during transport is upper airway obstruction, an emergency that is difficult to detect by pulse oximetry when supplemental oxygen is administered. The reason for this difficulty is that the large reserve of oxygen maintains the oxygen desaturation several minutes even in the presence of complete airway obstruction or hypopnea. Therefore, this author places the child in the recovery position, extends the child's neck with the base of his hand (thenar and hypothenar eminences) and positions his fingertips over the mouth/nose to feel the warm temperature in the exhaled gases to monitor respiration (but never closes the child's mouth).

Transporting the recovering child in the supine position predisposes to airway obstruction from posterior displacement of the tongue and facilitates the accumulation of secretions or other fluids in the supraglottic region. Furthermore, opioids depress the hypoglossal motor nuclei centrally, which relaxes the genioglossus muscle allowing the tongue to fall back and potentially obstruct the airway in the supine position.[298]

Figure 43-7 Position of the child after tracheal extubation in preparation for transfer to PACU and the pediatric ICU. This is known as the "recovery position" with the child lying in the lateral decubitus position, neck extended and mouth opened. In this position, oropharyngeal secretions, blood, or vomitus will drain onto the gurney rather than collect in the parapharyngeal region and trigger upper airway reflex responses.

PACU Complications

Approximately 5% of children have complications in the PACU,[299] with 77% from vomiting, 22% from respiratory causes, and 1% or less from cardiac causes. The age distribution of the complications showed that children above 8 years of age vomited more than twice as frequently as those under 8 years, whereas respiratory complications in infants under 1 year of age occurred twice as frequently as in those above 1 year of age.

Laryngospasm, Postoperative Stridor, and Negative Pressure Pulmonary Edema

Laryngospasm, postoperative stridor, and negative pressure pulmonary edema occur both during induction of anesthesia and during or after emergence from anesthesia. Factors that increase the risk of laryngospasm are enumerated in Table 43-12.

Postextubation stridor may also occur after tracheal extubation. Stridor usually results from the epithelium within the cricoid ring swelling after the tracheal tube is removed. The swelling reduces the internal cross-sectional diameter of the cricoid ring and increases the pressure gradient (and therefore work of breathing) across the ring. Because airflow in the upper airway is turbulent, the resistance to air flow increases as the fifth power of the radius of the cricoid ring decreases. That is, if the radius of the airway within the cricoid ring decreases by 50%, the resistance to airflow increases 32-fold (based on the Fanning equation). In infants with increased oxygen requirements and metabolic rates, residual opioids, muscle weakness, and anesthesia may further compromise their ability to maintain an increased work of breathing during stridor, which could hasten fatigue and respiratory failure. Postextubation stridor is more common in Down syndrome and children with recent URTIs. Treatment for stridor includes humidified oxygen, sitting the child upright, reassurance, light sedation, IV dexamethasone (0.6 mg/kg IV), and nebulized racemic epinephrine (0.5 mL epinephrine in 2 mL saline). Heliox has been effective in reducing the work of breathing, oxygen consumption, and distress although it limits the inspired oxygen fraction. If hypoxemia or respiratory failure occurs, the trachea should be reintubated with a smaller size tube than the one originally used. To avoid further irritating the epithelium, an audible leak should be present after intubation. If a racemic epinephrine treatment is repeated more than twice, the child should be observed for rebound edema in either the PACU or a monitored unit.

Negative pressure pulmonary edema or postextubation pulmonary edema is an infrequent complication that usually occurs immediately or within several minutes after tracheal extubation in healthy, muscular adolescents and young adults, although it has been reported in infants.[300] Shortly after the trachea is extubated, the airway may become increasingly obstructed while the child appears somnolent and unresponsive. The presumptive diagnosis is laryngospasm, which may range in severity from very mild (i.e., hiccups) to severe. Ventilation by mask with 100% oxygen may be ineffective in restoring vital signs, necessitating tracheal reintubation using propofol and a muscle relaxant. As soon as the tube passes the vocal cords, pink frothy pulmonary edema fluid may appear in the tube or appear upon suctioning the tube. SaO_2 can be restored to more than 94% using positive pressure ventilation with positive end-expiratory pressure and 100% oxygen. Tracheal intubation and positive pressure ventilation are usually sufficient to resolve the pulmonary edema although in some instances, IV furosemide may be required. In a dose of 0.5 to 1 mg/kg, furosemide venodilates the vasculature rapidly resolving the pulmonary congestion and improving oxygenation. Although some may recover from the pulmonary edema very rapidly, others require sedation and tracheal intubation for 12 to 24 hours or more, until the pulmonary edema resolves.

Oxygen Desaturation

Failure to maintain adequate SaO_2 in the recovery room is a common problem. Unrecognized hypoxia may lead to deterioration in the child's clinical status and lead to sudden bradycardia and cardiac arrest. Continuous monitoring of the child's SaO_2 in the PACU is essential to provide an early warning sign of respiratory distress. The minimum acceptable SaO_2 in PACU is 94%. Administration of oxygen by face mask may be required to maintain the SaO_2, particularly if residual anesthesia or opioids and/or a craniofacial or muscular abnormality is present, or the child is obese or fluid overloaded. In healthy children, oxygen desaturation in PACU is generally indicative of hypoventilation and/or airway obstruction. Because there is no means of assessing ventilation in children in the PACU who do not have artificial airways, we must rely on clinical signs to quickly diagnose and treat airway obstruction and hypoventilation before complications develop.

Children should be weaned from oxygen dependency (assuming they did not require supplemental oxygen preoperatively) before they are discharged to the floor or the step-down unit. Some children remove their face masks themselves when they awake from anesthesia; if their SaO_2 is 94% or more while breathing room air, then no additional oxygen is required. If the SaO_2 is maintained with a face mask, then the oxygen supply can be weaned to nasal prongs and then to room air provided the SaO_2 is maintained at each stage. If the child cannot maintain his/her SaO_2 despite weaning attempts, further investigation may be required (such as a chest x-ray) to rule out aspiration, pneumonia, or pneumothorax.

Emergence Delirium

The introduction of sevoflurane and desflurane anesthesia in children has caused a recrudescence of emergence agitation (also known as emergence delirium) during recovery from anesthesia. ED, with a prevalence of 20% to 80%, has a peak incidence in children (of both sexes) at 2 to 6 years of age, is more common after certain anesthetics (sevoflurane ~ desflurane ~ isoflurane > halothane ~ TIVA), lasts 10 to 15 minutes, and is terminated either spontaneously or after an IV dose of propofol, midazolam, clonidine, dexmedetomidine, ketamine, opioids, or a host of other medications.[301]

The diagnosis of ED in children has proven difficult for several reasons. First, the presence of pain has proved to be a significant confounding variable in establishing the diagnosis. When ED was assessed in children undergoing MRI with either sevoflurane or halothane, the incidence of ED after sevoflurane was fivefold greater than it was after halothane.[302] Second, the diagnosis of ED has been a challenge without a validated scale. To address this difficulty, we developed the pediatric anesthesia emergence delirium (PAED) score and validated it as an objective measure of ED; a score above 10 or, more recently, above 12 is considered strongly indicative of ED.[303]

Vomiting

The frequency of vomiting in the PACU and after hospital discharge has decreased dramatically with the introduction of prophylactic antiemetics for children at risk for PONV. Prophylaxis for PONV is recommended for surgeries with the greatest incidence of vomiting: hernia, orchidopexy, tonsillectomy and adenoidectomy, ear surgery, strabismus surgery, and laparoscopic surgery. The incidence of vomiting increases with increasing age, peaking in females 10 to 16 years.[278] IV dexamethasone (0.0625 to 0.15 mg/kg (maximum 10 mg) and ondansetron (0.05 to 0.15 mg/kg) reduce the perioperative incidence of PONV by up to 80% or more.[283] In fact, few children vomit in the PACU; most children who vomit do so after ingesting their first fluids on the ward, in the car on the way home, or at home. Hence, we administer large volumes of IV fluids intraoperatively and in PACU (total 10 to 40 mL/kg over 1–4 h) and recommend oral fluids only when the child requests to drink.[279,280] If the child continues to vomit, there is no magic solution. First, oral fluids should be withheld and IV access should be maintained or restarted and IV balanced salt solution administered. Second, if the child has either the ultrarapid polymorphism of CYP450 2D6 or a polymorphism of adenosine triphosphate–binding cassette subfamily B member 1 (ABCB1) non-TT type (e.g., 2677 or 3435 non-TT type) or both, then ondansetron may be ineffective.[304] Rapid assays are not available for these polymorphisms so we can only speculate as to the reasons for the vomiting. A second dose of ondansetron (0.1 mg/kg) may be given if at least 2 hours have passed since the first dose or IV metoclopramide (0.15 mg/kg) may be given.

Postoperative Pain

Management of pain in the PACU and on the ward depends on the origin of the pain, its severity, the medications already administered, and the status of the child. Regional anesthesia with neuroaxial or local blocks (penile, iliohypogastric/ilioinguinal or popliteal nerve blocks) may be used. Regional anesthesia is usually performed during general anesthesia in children (except in older adolescents) using either a direct nerve block or nerve stimulation or more recently ultrasound guidance.[305] When regional block is unsuitable, impractical, contraindicated, or refused by the parents, opioids, NSAID agents (diclofenac, tramadol, ibuprofen, and acetaminophen), and ketamine may be employed (see earlier).[306]

Continuous morphine infusions have been used to manage pain in children.[145] Morphine infusions may be prepared by dissolving the child's weight as milligram of morphine in 100 mL of saline and infused at 1 to 3 mL/hr. These children are best monitored continuously using pulse oximetry.

To tailor the morphine dose to the severity of the pain, patient-controlled analgesia (PCA) was developed for which the patient received morphine upon demand as well continuously for background pain, if needed. PCA has been shown to be effective in children as young as 5 years. For those under 5 years of age and those who are cognitively impaired, caregivers and parents who were educated regarding the use of PCAs have been very effective in controlling the children's pain.[307] A typical morphine PCA may be programmed for a child as follows: PCA bolus 10 to 30 µg/kg; continuous rate of 10 to 40 µg/kg/hr (or in children at risk of apnea, 0 µg/kg/hr); lockout interval 6 to 10 minutes; and a 4-hour limit of 0.25 to 0.4 mg/kg.[145] Smaller doses and background infusions of PCA morphine are used in infants.[145,308] Dilaudid (hydromorphone), which is three- to fivefold more potent than morphine, may be used in place of morphine. The attending nurse should routinely monitor the child's pain and if the pain is not adequately controlled, the pump settings should be reviewed and adjusted accordingly.

REFERENCES

1. Wiegerinck RF, Cojoc A, Zweidenweber CM, et al. Force frequency relationship of the human ventricle increases during early postnatal development. *Pediatric Res.* 2009;65:414–419.
2. Bernstein D. History and physical examination. In: Kliegman RM, Stanton BF, Geme JW et al., eds. *Nelson Textbook of Pediatrics.* 19th ed. Philadelphia, PA: Saunders Elsevier; 2011:1529–1536.
3. Szabó EZ, Luginbuehl I, Bissonnette B. Impact of anesthetic agents on cerebrovascular physiology in children. *Paediatr Anaesth.* 2009;19:108–118.
4. Stratmann G. Neurotoxicity of anesthetic drugs in the developing brain. *Anesth Analg.* 2011;113:1170–1179.
5. Coté CJ, Lerman J, Ward RM, et al. A practice of anesthesia for infants and children. In: Cote CJ, Lerman J, Todres ID, eds. *Pharmacokinetics and Pharmacology of Drugs Used in Children.* Philadelphia, PA: Saunders Elsevier; 2009:108.
6. Liu J, Rossaint R, Sanders RD, Coburn M. Toxic and protective effects of inhaled anaesthetics on the developing animal brain. Systematic review and update of recent experimental work. *Eur J Anaesthesiol.* 2014;31:669–677.
7. Slikker W Jr, Zou X, Hotchkiss CE. Ketamine-induced neuronal cell death in the perinatal rhesus monkey. *Toxicol Sci.* 2007;98:145–158.
8. Bartels M, Althoff RR, Boomsma DI. Anesthesia and cognitive performance in children: No evidence for a causal relationship. *Twin Res Hum Genet.* 2009;12:246–253.
9. Davidson AJ, Disma N, de Graaff JC, et al. Neurodevelopmental outcome at 2 years of age after general anaesthesia and awake-regional anaesthesia in infancy (GAS): an international multicenter, randomized controlled trial. *Lancet.* 2016;387(10015);239–259.
10. Payne K, Mattheyse FJ, Liebenberg D, et al. The pharmacokinetics of midazolam in paediatric patients. *Eur J Clin Pharmacol.* 1989;37:267–272.
11. Kogan A, Katz J, Efrat R, et al. Premedication with midazolam in young children: A comparison of four routes of administration. *Paediatr Anaesth.* 2002;12:685–689.
12. Anderson BJ, Holford NH, Woollard GA, et al. Perioperative pharmacodynamics of acetaminophen analgesia in children. *Anesthesiology.* 1999;90:411–421.
13. Koren G. Therapeutic drug monitoring principles in the neonate. *Clin Chem.* 1997;43:221–227.
14. Lerman J, Strong HA, LeDez KM, et al. Effects of age on the serum concentration of α1-acid glycoprotein and the binding of lidocaine in pediatric patients. *Clin Pharmacol Ther.* 1989;46:219–225.
15. Hines RN. Ontogeny of human hepatic cytochromes P450. *J Biochem Mol Toxicol.* 2007;21:169–175.
16. Ingelman-Sundberg M. Genetic polymorphisms of cytochrome P4502D6 (CYP2D6): Clinical consequences, evolutionary aspects and functional diversity. *Pharmacogenomics J.* 2005;5:6–13.
17. Hines RN. The ontogeny of drug metabolism enzymes and implications for adverse drug events. *Pharmacol Ther.* 2008;118:250–267.
18. Lerman J, Schmitt-Bantel BI, Gregory GA, et al. Effect of age on the solubility of volatile anesthetics in human tissues. *Anesthesiology.* 1986;65:307–311.
19. Yasuda N, Lockhart SH, Eger EI II, et al. Comparison of kinetics of sevoflurane and isoflurane in humans. *Anesth Analg.* 1991;72:316–324.
20. Malviya S, Lerman J. The blood/gas solubilities of sevoflurane, isoflurane, halothane, and serum constituent concentrations in neonates and adults. *Anesthesiology.* 1990;72:793–796.
21. Lerman J, Gregory GA, Willis MM, et al. Age and solubility of volatile anesthetics in blood. *Anesthesiology.* 1984;61:139–143.
22. Eger EI II. *Anesthetic Uptake and Action.* Baltimore, MD: Williams & Wilkins; 1974.
23. Olofsen E, Dahan A. The dynamic relationship between end-tidal sevoflurane and isoflurane concentrations and bispectral index and spectral edge frequency of the electroencephalogram. *Anesthesiology.* 1999;90:1345–1353.
24. Fuentes R, Cortínez LI, Struys MM, et al. The dynamic relationship between end-tidal sevoflurane concentrations, bispectral index, and cerebral state index in children. *Anesth Analg.* 2008;107:1573–1578.
25. Gibbons RT, Steffey EP, Eger EI II. The effect of spontaneous versus controlled ventilation on the rate of rise of alveolar halothane concentration in dogs. *Anesth Analg.* 1977;56:32–34.
26. Eger EI II, Shafer SL. Tutorial: Context-sensitive decrement times for inhaled anesthetics. *Anesth Analg.* 2005;101:688–696.
27. Neumann MA, Weiskopf RB, Gong DH, et al. Changing from isoflurane to desflurane toward the end of anesthesia does not accelerate recovery in humans. *Anesthesiology.* 1998;88:914–921.
28. Sakata DJ, Gopalakrishnan NA, Orr JA, et al. Hypercapnic hyperventilation shorten emergence time from isoflurane anesthesia. *Anesth Analg.* 2007;104:587–591.
29. Sakata DJ, Gopalakrishnan NA, Orr JA, et al. Rapid recovery from sevoflurane and desflurane with hypercapnia and hyperventilation. *Anesth Analg.* 2007;105:79–82.
30. Lerman J, Robinson S, Willis MM, et al. Anesthetic requirements for halothane in young children 0–1 month and 1–6 months of age. *Anesthesiology.* 1983;59:421–424.
31. Gregory GA, Eger EI II, Munson ES. The relationship between age and halothane requirements in man. *Anesthesiology.* 1969;30:488–491.
32. LeDez KM, Lerman J. The minimum alveolar concentration (MAC) of isoflurane in preterm neonates. *Anesthesiology.* 1987;67:301–307.
33. Cameron CB, Robinson S, Gregory GA. The minimum anesthetic concentration of isoflurane in children. *Anesth Analg.* 1984;63:418–420.

34. Lerman J, Sikich N, Kleinman S, et al. The pharmacology of sevoflurane in infants and children. *Anesthesiology.* 1994;80:814–824.
35. Taylor RH, Lerman J. Minimum alveolar concentration of desflurane and hemodynamic responses in neonates, infants, and children. *Anesthesiology.* 1991; 75:975–979.
36. Frei FJ, Haemmerle MH, Brunner R, et al. Minimum alveolar concentration for halothane in children with cerebral palsy and severe mental retardation. *Anaesthesia.* 1997;52:1056–1060.
37. Liem EB, Lin CM, Suleman MI, et al. Anesthetic requirement is increased in redheads. *Anesthesiology.* 2004;101:279–283.
38. Fisher DM, Zwass MS. MAC of desflurane in 60% nitrous oxide in infants and children. *Anesthesiology.* 1992;76:354–356.
39. Liu M, Hu X, Liu J. The effect of hypothermia on isoflurane MAC in children. *Anesthesiology.* 2001;94:429–432.
40. Hatch DJ. New inhalation agents in paediatric anaesthesia. *Br J Anaesth.* 1999;83:42–49.
41. Walpole R, Olday J, Haetzman M, et al. A comparison of the respiratory effects of high concentrations of halothane and sevoflurane. *Paediatr Anaesth.* 2001;11:157–160.
42. Doi M, Ikeda K. Respiratory effects of sevoflurane. *Anesth Analg.* 1987;66: 241–244.
43. Behforouz N, Dubousset AM, Jamali S, et al. Respiratory effects of desflurane anesthesia on spontaneous ventilation in infants and children. *Anesth Analg.* 1998;87:1052–1055.
44. von Ungern-Sternberg BS, Saudan S, Petak F, et al. Desflurane but not sevoflurane impairs airway and respiratory mechanics in children with susceptible airways. *Anesthesiology.* 2008;108:216–224.
45. Dikmen Y, Eminoglu E, Salihoglu Z, et al. Pulmonary mechanics during isoflurane, sevoflurane and desflurane anaesthesia. *Anaesthesia.* 2003;58: 745–748.
46. Tobias JD. Inhalational anesthesia: Basic pharmacology, end organ effects, and applications in the treatment of status asthmaticus. *J Intensive Care Med.* 2009;24:361–371.
47. Vaschetto R, Bellotti E, Turucz E, et al. Inhalational anesthetics in acute severe asthma. *Curr Drug Targets.* 2009;10:826–832.
48. Lerman J, Davis PJ, Welborn LG, et al. Induction, recovery, and safety characteristics of sevoflurane in children undergoing ambulatory surgery: A comparison with halothane. *Anesthesiology.* 1996;84:1332–1340.
49. Lindgren L, Randell T, Saarnivaara L. Comparison of inhalation induction with isoflurane or halothane in children. *Eur J Anaesthesiol.* 1991;8:33–37.
50. Taylor RH, Lerman J. Induction, maintenance and recovery characteristics of desflurane in inhalants and children. *Can J Anaesth.* 1992;39:6–13.
51. Lerman J, Hammer GB, Verghese S, et al. Airway responses to desflurane during maintenance of anesthesia and recovery in children with laryngeal mask airways. *Paediatr Anaesth.* 2010;20:495–505.
52. Wodey E, Senhadji L, Pladys P, et al. The relationship between expired concentration of sevoflurane and sympathovagal tone in children. *Anesth Analg.* 2003; 97:377–382.
53. Ebert TJ, Muzi M. Sympathetic hyperactivity during desflurane anesthesia in healthy volunteers. A comparison with isoflurane. *Anesthesiology.* 1993;79: 444–453.
54. Muzi, M, Ebert TJ, Hope WG, et al. Site(s) mediating sympathetic activation with desflurane. *Anesthesiology.* 1996;85:737–747.
55. Whyte SD, Sanatani S, Lim J, et al. A comparison of the effect on dispersion of repolarization of age-adjusted MAC values of sevoflurane in children. *Anesth Analg.* 2007;104:277–282.
56. Nathan AT, Berkowitz DH, Montenegro LM, et al. Implications of anesthesia in children with long QT syndrome. *Anesth Analg.* 2011;112:1163–1168.
57. Kawana S, Wachi J, Nakayama M, et al. Comparison of haemodynamic changes induced by sevoflurane and halothane in paediatric patients. *Can J Anaesth.* 1995;42:603–607.
58. Wodey E, Pladys P, Copin C, et al. Comparative hemodynamic depression of sevoflurane versus halothane in infants: An echocardiographic study. *Anesthesiology.* 1997;87:795–800.
59. Barash PG, Glanz S, Katz JD, et al. Ventricular function in children during halothane anesthesia: An echocardiographic evaluation. *Anesthesiology.* 1978;49:79–85.
60. Russell IA, Miller Hance WC, Gregory G, et al. The safety and efficacy of sevoflurane anesthesia in infants and children with congenital heart disease. *Anesth Analg.* 2001;92:1152–1158.
61. Cubeddu L. QT prolongation and fatal arrhythmias: A review of clinical implications and effects of drugs. *Am J Ther.* 2003;10:452–457.
62. Abriel H, Schlpafer J, Keller DI, et al. Molecular and clinical determinants of drug-induced long QT syndrome: An iatrogenic channelopathy. *Swiss Med Wkly.* 2004;134:685–694.
63. Wallenborn J, Kluba K, Olthoff D. Comparative evaluation of bispectral index and narcotrend index in children below 5 years of age. *Paediatr Anaesth.* 2007;17:140–147.
64. Kim HS, Oh AY, Kim CS, et al. Correlation of bispectral index with end-tidal sevoflurane concentration and age in infants and children. *Br J Anaesth.* 2005;95:362–366.
65. Tirel O, Wodey E, Harris R, et al. The impact of age on bispectral index values and EEG bispectrum during anaesthesia with desflurane and halothane in children. *Br J Anaesth.* 2006;96:480–485.
66. Davidson AJ, Huang GH, Rebmann CS, et al. Performance of entropy and bispectral index as measures of anaesthesia effect in children of different ages. *Br J Anaesth.* 2005;95:674–679.
67. Valkenburg AJ, de Leeuw TG, Tibboel D, et al. Lower bispectral index values in children who are intellectually disabled. *Anesth Analg.* 2009;109:1428–1433.
68. Wappler F, Bischoff P. Is fast induction with sevoflurane associated with an increased anesthetic risk in pediatric patients? *Anesth Analg.* 2003;96: 1239–1240.
69. Iijima T, Nakamura Z, Iwao Y, et al. The epileptogenic properties of the volatile anesthetics sevoflurane and isoflurane in patients with epilepsy. *Anesth Analg.* 2000;91:989–995.
70. Kharasch ED, Thummel KE. Identification of cytochrome P450 2E1 as the predominant enzyme catalyzing human liver microsomal defluorination of sevoflurane, isoflurane, and methoxyflurane. *Anesthesiology.* 1993;79:795–807.
71. Kharasch ED, Hankins DC, Thummel KE. Human kidney methoxyflurane and sevoflurane metabolism. Intrarenal fluoride production as a possible mechanism of methoxyflurane nephrotoxicity. *Anesthesiology.* 1995;82:689–699.
72. Kharasch ED, Schroeder JL, Liggitt D, et al. New insights into the mechanism of methoxyflurane nephrotoxicity and implications for anesthetic development (part 2). *Anesthesiology.* 2006;105:737–745.
73. Arnold JH, Truog RD, Rice SA. Prolonged administration of isoflurane to pediatric patients during mechanical ventilation. *Anesth Analg.* 1993;76:520–526.
74. Jang Y, Kim AI. Severe hepatotoxicity after sevoflurane anesthesia in a child with mild renal dysfunction. *Paediatr Anaesth.* 2005;15:1140–1144.
75. Coté G, Bouchard S. Hepatotoxicity after desflurane anesthesia in a 15-month-old child with Mobius syndrome after previous exposure to isoflurane. *Anesthesiology.* 2007;107:843–845.
76. Reichle FM, Conzen PF. Halogenated inhalational anaesthetics. *Best Pract Res Clin Anaesthesiol.* 2003;17:29–46.
77. Frink EJ Jr, Green WB Jr, Brown EA, et al. Compound A concentrations during sevoflurane anesthesia in children. *Anesthesiology.* 1996;84:566–571.
78. Fang ZC, Eger EI II, Laster MJ, et al. Carbon monoxide production from degradation of desflurane, enflurane, isoflurane, halothane, and sevoflurane by sodalime and Baralyme®. *Anesth Analg.* 1995;80:1187–1193.
79. Levy RJ, Nasr VG, Rivera O, et al. Detection of carbon monoxide during routine anesthetics in infants and children. *Anesth Analg.* 2010;110:747–753.
80. Munoz HR, Cortínez LI, Ibacache ME, et al. Estimation of the plasma effect site equilibration rate constant (k_{eo}) of propofol in children using the time to peak effect. *Anesthesiology.* 2004;101:1269–1274.
81. Murat I, Billard V, Vernois J, et al. Pharmacokinetics of propofol after a single dose in children aged 1–3 years with minor burns. *Anesthesiology.* 1996;84: 526–532.
82. Allegaert K, De Hoon J, Verbesselt R, et al. Maturational pharmacokinetics of single intravenous bolus of propofol. *Paediatr Anaesth.* 2007;17:1028–1034.
83. McFarlan CS, Anderson BJ, Short TG. The use of propofol infusions in paediatric anaesthesia: A practical guide. *Paediatr Anaesth.* 1999;9:209–216.
84. Westrin P. The induction dose of propofol in infants 1–6 months of age and in children 10–16 years of age. *Anesthesiology.* 1991;74:455–458.
85. Allsop E, Innes P, Jackson M, et al. Dose of propofol required to insert the laryngeal mask airway in children. *Paediatr Anaesth.* 1995;5:47–51.
86. Martlew RA, Meakin G, Wadsworth R, et al. Dose of propofol for laryngeal mask airway insertion in children: Effect premedication with midazolam. *Br J Anaesth.* 1996;76:308–309.
87. Lerman J, Houle TT, Matthews BT, et al. Propofol for tracheal intubation in children anesthetized with sevoflurane: A dose-response study. *Paediatr Anaesth.* 2009;19:218–222.
88. Kim H, Hong JY, Suk EH, et al. Optimum bolus dose of propofol for tracheal intubation during sevoflurane induction without neuromuscular blockade in children. *Anaesth Intensive Care.* 2011;39:899–903.
89. Heard C, Burrows F, Johnson K, et al. A comparison of dexmedetomidine-midazolam with propofol for maintenance of anesthesia in children undergoing magnetic resonance imaging. *Anesth Analg.* 2008;107:1832–1839.
90. Usher AG, Kearney RA, Tsui BCH. Propofol total intravenous anesthesia for MRI in children. *Paediatr Anaesth.* 2005;15:23–28.
91. Asahi Y, Kubota K, Omichi S. Dose requirements for propofol anaesthesia for dental treatment for autistic patients compared with intellectually impaired patients. *Anaesth Intensive Care.* 2009;37:70–73.
92. Mani V, Morton NS. Overview of total intravenous anesthesia in children. *Paediatr Anaesth.* 2010;20:211–222.
93. Sepúlveda P, Cortínez LI, Sáez C, et al. Performance evaluation of paediatric propofol pharmacokinetic models in healthy young children. *Br J Anaesth.* 2011;107:593–600.
94. Picard P, Tramer MR. Prevention of pain on injection with propofol: A quantitative systematic review. *Anesth Analg.* 2000;90:963–995.
95. Jalota L, Kalira V, George E, et al. Prevention of pain on injection of propofol: Systematic review and meta-analysis. *BMJ.* 2011;342:d1110.
96. Beh T, Splinter W, Kim J. In children, nitrous oxide decreases pain on injection of propofol mixed with lidocaine. *Can J Anaesth.* 2002;49:1061–1063.

97. Evans RG, Crawford MW, Noseworthy MD, et al. Effect of increasing depth of propofol anesthesia on upper airway configuration in children. *Anesthesiology.* 2003;99:596–602.
98. Larson PC Jr. Laryngospasm—the best treatment. *Anesthesiology.* 1998;89:1293–1294.
99. Lutterbey G, Wattjes MP, Doerr D, et al. Atelectasis in children undergoing either propofol infusion or positive pressure ventilation anesthesia for magnetic resonance imaging. *Paediatr Anaesth.* 2007;17:121–125.
100. Gan TJ, Diemunsch P, Habib AS, et al. Consensus guidelines for management of postoperative nausea and vomiting. *Anesth Analg.* 2014;118:85–113.
101. Fodale V, La Monaca E. Propofol infusion syndrome. An overview of a perplexing disease. *Drug Saf.* 2008;31:293–303.
102. Wysowski DK, Pollock ML. Reports of death with use of propofol (Diprivan) for nonprocedural (long-term) sedation and literature review. *Anesthesiology.* 2006;105:1047–1051.
103. Da-Silva SS, Wong R, Coquillon P, Gavrilita C, Asuncion A. Partial-exchange blood transfusion: An effective method for preventing mortality in a child with propofol infusion syndrome. *Pediatric.* 2010;125:e1493–e1499.
104. Westhout FD, Muhonen MG, Nwagwu CI. Early propofol infusion syndrome following cerebral angiographic embolization for giant aneurysm repair. *J Neurosurg.* 2007;106:139–142.
105. Herd DW, Anderson BJ, Keene NA, et al. Investigating the pharmacodynamics of ketamine in children. *Paediatr Anaesth.* 2008;18:36–42.
106. Dallimore D, Anderson BJ, Short TG, et al. Ketamine anesthesia in children–exploring infusion regimens. *Paediatr Anaesth.* 2008;18:708–714.
107. Anderson BJ, McKee AD, Holford NH. Size, myths and the clinical pharmacokinetics of analgesia in paediatric patients. *Clin Pharmacokinet.* 1997;33:313–327.
108. Gutstein HB, Johnson KL, Heard MB, et al. Oral ketamine preanesthetic medication in children. *Anesthesiology.* 1992;76:28–33.
109. Wolfe TR, Braude DA. Intranasal medication delivery for children: A brief review and update. *Pediatrics.* 2010;126:532–537.
110. Aspinall RL, Mayor A. A prospective randomized controlled study of the efficacy of ketamine for postoperative pain relief in children after adenotonsillectomy. *Paediatr Anaesth.* 2001;11:333–336.
111. Ansermino M, Basu R, Vandebeek C, et al. Nonopioid additives to local anaesthetics for caudal blockade in children: A systematic review. *Paediatr Anaesth.* 2003;13:561–573.
112. Funk W, Jakob W, Riedl T, et al. Oral preanesthetic medication for children: Double-blind randomized study of a combination of midazolam and ketamine vs midazolam or ketamine alone. *Br J Anaesth.* 2000;84:335–340.
113. Zeiler FA, Teitelbaum J, West M, Gillman LM. The ketamine effect on intracranial pressure in nontraumatic neurological illness. *J Crit Care.* 2014;29:1096–1106.
114. Lin L, Zhang JW, Huang Y, et al. Population pharmacokinetics of intravenous bolus etomidate in children over 6 months of age. *Paediatr Anaesth.* 2011;22:318–326.
115. Forman SA. Clinical and molecular pharmacology of etomidate. *Anesthesiology.* 2011;114:695–707.
116. Raines DE. The pharmacology of etomidate and etomidate derivatives. *Intl Anesth Clin.* 2015;53:63–75.
117. Mertes PM, Alla F, Tréchot P, et al. Anaphylaxis during anesthesia in France: An 8-year national survey. *J Allergy Clin Immunol.* 2011;128:366–373.
118. Florvaag E, Johansson SGO, Irgens A, et al. IgE-sensitization to the cough suppressant pholcodine and the effects of its withdrawal from the Norwegian market. *Allergy.* 2011;66:955–960.
119. Meakin G, Walker RW, Dearlove OR. Myotonic and neuromuscular blocking effects of increased doses of suxamethonium in infants and children. *Br J Anaesth.* 1990;65:816–818.
120. Liu LMP, DeCook TH, Goudsouzian NG, et al. Dose response to intramuscular succinylcholine in children. *Anesthesiology.* 1981;55:599–602.
121. Redden RJ, Miller M, Campbell RL. Submental administration of succinylcholine in children. *Anesth Prog.* 1990;37:296–300.
122. Mazze RI, Dunbar RW. Intralingual succinylcholine administration in children: An alternative to intravenous and intramuscular routes? *Anesth Analg.* 1968;47:605–615.
123. Davis L, Britten JJ, Morgan M. Cholinesterase. Its significance in anaesthetic practice. *Anaesthesia.* 1997;52:244–260.
124. Neitlich HW. Increased plasma cholinesterase activity and succinylcholine resistance: A genetic variant. *J Clin Invest.* 1966;45:380–387.
125. Yoshida A, Motulsky AG. A pseudocholinesterase variant (E Cynthiana) associated with elevated plasma enzyme activity. *Am J Hum Genet.* 1969;21:486–498.
126. Leigh MD, McCoy DD, Belton MK, et al. Bradycardia following intravenous administration of succinylcholine chloride to infants and children. *Anesthesiology.* 1957;18:698–702.
127. Martyn JA, Richtsfeld M. Succinylcholine-induced hyperkalemia in acquired pathologic states. *Anesthesiology.* 2006;104:58–69.
128. Lerman J. Perioperative management of the paediatric patient with coexisting neuromuscular disease. *Br J Anaesth.* 2011;107(S1):i79–i89.
129. Thapa S, Brull SJ. Succinylcholine-induced hyperkalemia in patients with renal failure: An old question revisited. *Anesth Analg.* 2000;91:237–241.
130. Chidiac EJ, Rasikin AO. Succinylcholine and the open eye. *Ophthalmol Clin North Am.* 2006;19:279–285.
131. Lerman J, McLeod ME, Strong HA. Pharmacokinetics of intravenous dantrolene in children. *Anesthesiology.* 1989;70:625–629.
132. Meakin GH. Muscle relaxants in children. *Curr Opin Anaesthesiol.* 2007;20:227–231.
133. Taivainen T, Meretoja OA, Erkola O, et al. Rocuronium in infants, children and adults during a balanced anaesthesia. *Paediatr Anaesth.* 1996;6:271–275.
134. Wierda JM, Meretoja OA, Taivainen T, et al. Pharmacokinetics and pharmacokinetic-dynamic modelling of rocuronium in infants and children. *Br J Anaesth.* 1997;78:690–695.
135. Woloszczuk-Gebicka B, Wyska E, Grabowski T, et al. Pharmacokinetic–pharmacodynamic relationship of rocuronium under stable nitrous oxide-fentanyl or nitrous–sevoflurane anesthesia in children. *Paediatr Anaesth.* 2006;16:761–768.
136. Fuchs-Buder T, Tassonyi E. Intubating conditions and time course of rocuronium-induced neuromuscular block in children. *Br J Anaesth.* 1996;77:335–338.
137. Cheng CA, Aun CS, Gin T. Comparison of rocuronium and suxamethonium for rapid tracheal intubation in children. *Paediatr Anaesth.* 2002;12:140–145.
138. Brandom BW, Cook DR, Woelfel SK, et al. Atracurium infusion requirements in children during halothane, isoflurane, and narcotic anesthesia. *Anesth Analg.* 1985;64:471–476.
139. Meakin G, Meretoja OA, Perkins R, et al. Tracheal intubating conditions and pharmacodynamics following cisatracurium in infants and children undergoing halothane and thiopental-fentanyl anesthesia. *Paediatr Anaesth.* 2007;17:113–120.
140. Meretoja OA. Neuromuscular block and current treatment strategies for its reversal in children. *Paediatr Anaesth.* 2010;20:591–604.
141. Fields AM, Vadivelu N. Sugammadex: A novel neuromuscular blocker binding agent. *Curr Opin Anaesthesiol.* 2007;20:307–310.
142. Plaud B, Meretoja O, Hofmockel R, et al. Reversal of rocuronium-induced neuromuscular blockade with sugammadex in pediatric and adult surgical patients. *Anesthesiology.* 2009;110:284–294.
143. McDonnell NJ, Pavy TJG, Green LK, et al. Sugammadex in the management of rocuronium-induced anaphylaxis. *Br J Anaesth.* 2011;106:199–201.
144. Kart T, Christrup LL, Rasmussen M. Recommended use of morphine in neonates, infants and children based on a literature review: Part 2—clinical use. *Paediatr Anaesth.* 1997;7:93–101.
145. Brislin RP, Rose JB. Pediatric acute pain management. *Anesthesiol Clin North America.* 2005;23:789–814.
146. Robinson S, Gregory GA. Fentanyl-air-oxygen anesthesia for ligation of patent ductus arteriosus in preterm infants. *Anesth Analg.* 1981;60:331–334.
147. Lerman J, Nolan J, Eyres R, et al. Efficacy, safety and pharmacokinetics of levobupivacaine with and without fentanyl after continuous epidural infusion in children: A multicenter study. *Anesthesiology.* 2003;99:1166–1174.
148. Hughes MA, Glass PS, Jacobs JR. Content-sensitive half-time in multicompartment pharmacokinetic models for intravenous anesthetic drugs. *Anesthesiology.* 1992;76:334–341.
149. Davis PJ, Cladis FP. The use of ultra-short-acting opioids in paediatric anaesthesia: The role of remifentanil. *Clin Pharmacokinet.* 2005;44:787–796.
150. Marsh DF, Hodkinson B. Remifentanil in paediatric anaesthetic practice. *Anaesthesia.* 2009;64:301–308.
151. Echevarria G, Elgueta F, Fierro C, et al. Nitrous oxide (N_2O) reduces postoperative opioid-induced hyperalgesia after remifentanil-propofol anaesthesia in humans. *Br J Anaesth.* 2011;107:959–965.
152. Berde CB, Sethna NF. Analgesics for the treatment of pain in children. *N Engl J Med.* 2002;347:1094–1103.
153. Williams DG, Hatch DJ, Howard RF. Codeine phosphate in paediatric medicine. *Br J Anaesth.* 2001;86:413–421.
154. Oyler JM, Cone EJ, Joseph RE, et al. Identification of hydrocodone in human urine following controlled codeine administration. *J Anal Toxicol.* 2000;24:530–536.
155. Voronov P, Przybylo HJ, Jagannathan N. Apnea in a child after oral codeine: A genetic variant—an ultra-rapid metabolizer. *Paediatr Anaesth.* 2007;17:684–687.
156. Ciszkowski C, Madadi P, Phillips MS, et al. Codeine, ultrarapid-metabolism genotype, and postoperative death. *N Engl J Med.* 2009;361:827–828.
157. Williams DG, Patel A, Howard RF. Pharmacogenetics of codeine metabolism in an urban population of children and its implications for analgesic reliability. *Br J Anaesth.* 2002;89:839–845.
158. Palmer SN, Giesecke NM, Body SC, et al. Pharmacokinetics of anesthetic and analgesic agents. *Anesthesiology.* 2005;102:663–671.
159. Lerman J. A disquisition on sleep-disordered breathing in children. *Paediatr Anaesth.* 2009;19(suppl 1):100–108.
160. Jahr JS, Lee VK. Intravenous acetaminophen. *Anesthesiol Clin.* 2010;28:619–645.

161. Birmingham PK, Tobin MJ, Fisher DM, et al. Initial and subsequent dosing of rectal acetaminophen in children: A 24-hour pharmacokinetic study of new dose recommendations. *Anesthesiology*. 2001;94:385–389.
162. Anderson BJ, Pons G, Autret-Leca E, et al. Pediatric intravenous paracetamol (propacetamol) pharmacokinetics: A population analysis. *Paediatr Anaesth*. 2005;15:282–292.
163. Prins SA, Van Dijk M, Van Leeuwen P, et al. Pharmacokinetics and analgesic effects of intravenous propacetamol vs rectal paracetamol in children after major craniofacial surgery. *Paediatr Anaesth*. 2008;18:582–592.
164. Nevin DG, Shung J. Intravenous paracetamol overdose in a preterm infant during anesthesia. *Paediatr Anaesth*. 2010;20:105–107.
165. Beringer RM, Thompson JP, Parry S, et al. Intravenous paracetamol overdose: Two case reports and a change to national treatment guidelines. *Arch Dis Child*. 2011;96:307–308.
166. Shende D, Das K. Comparative effect of intravenous ketorolac and pethidine on perioperative analgesia and postoperative nausea and vomiting (PONV) for paediatric strabismus surgery. *Acta Anaesthesiol Scand*. 1999;43:265–269.
167. Lynn AM, Bradford H, Kantor ED. Postoperative ketorolac tromethamine use in infants aged 6–18 months: The effect on morphine usage, safety assessment, and stereo-specific pharmacokinetics. *Anesth Analg*. 2007;104:1040–1051.
168. Cohen MN, Christians U, Henthorn T, et al. Pharmacokinetics of single-dose intravenous ketorolac in infants aged 2–11 months. *Anesth Analg*. 2011;112:655–660.
169. Chan DK, Parikh SR. Perioperative ketorolac increases post-tonsillectomy hemorrhage in adults but not children. *Laryngoscope*. 2014;124:1789–1793.
170. Campobasso CP, Procacci R, Caligara M. Fatal adverse reaction to ketorolac tromethamine in asthmatic patient. *Am J Forensic Med Pathol*. 2008;29:358–363.
171. Standing JF, Savage I, Pritchard D, et al. Diclofenac for acute pain in children. *Cochrane Database Syst Rev*. 2009;4:CD005538.
172. Standing JF, Tibboel D, Korpela R, et al. Diclofenac pharmacokinetic meta-analysis and dose recommendations for surgical pain in children aged 1–12 years. *Paediatr Anaesth*. 2011;21:316–324.
173. Standing JF, Howard RF, Johnson A, et al. Population pharmacokinetics of oral diclofenac for acute pain in children. *Br J Clin Pharmacol*. 2008;66:846–853.
174. Moss JR, Watcha MF, Bendel LP, et al. A multicenter, randomized, double-blind placebo-controlled, single dose trial of the safety and efficacy of intravenous ibuprofen for treatment of pain in pediatric patients undergoing tonsillectomy. *Pediatr Anesth*. 2014;24:483–489.
175. Reed MD, Rodarte A, Blumer JL, et al. The single-dose pharmacokinetics of midazolam and its primary metabolite in pediatric patients after oral and intravenous administration. *J Clin Pharmacol*. 2001;41:1359–1369.
176. Alcorn J, McNamara PJ. Ontogeny of hepatic and renal systemic clearance pathways in infants. Part I. *Clin Pharmacokinet*. 2002;41:959–998.
177. Mason KP, Lerman J. Dexmedetomidine in children: Current knowledge and future applications. *Anesth Analg*. 2011;113:1129–1142.
178. Petroz GC, Sikich N, James M, et al. A phase I, two-center study of the pharmacokinetics and pharmacodynamics of dexmedetomidine in children. *Anesthesiology*. 2006;105:1098–1110.
179. Vilo S, Rautiainen P, Kaisti K, et al. Pharmacokinetics of intravenous dexmedetomidine in children under 11 yr of age. *Br J Anaesth*. 2008;100:697–700.
180. Belleville JP, Ward DS, Bloor BC, et al. Effects of intravenous dexmedetomidine in humans. I. Sedation ventilation and metabolic rate. *Anesthesiology*. 1992;77:1125–1133.
181. Mason DP, Zurakowski D, Zgleszewski SE, et al. High dose dexmedetomidine as the sole sedative for pediatric MRI. *Paediatr Anaesth*. 2008;18:403–411.
182. Tobias JD, Goble TJ, Bates G, et al. Effects of dexmedetomidine on intraoperative motor and somatosensory evoked potential monitoring during spinal surgery in adolescents. *Paediatr Anaesth*. 2008;18:1082–1088.
183. Mason KP, Zgleszewski S, Forman RE, et al. An exaggerated hypertensive response to glycopyrrolate therapy for bradycardia associated with high-dose dexmedetomidine. *Anesth Analg*. 2009;108:906–908.
184. Apfelbaum JL, Caplan RA, Connis RT, et al. Updated by the American Society of Anesthesiologists (ASA) Committee on standards and practice parameters. Practice guidelines for preoperative fasting and the use of pharmacologic agents to reduce the risk of pulmonary aspiration: Application to healthy patients undergoing elective procedures. *Anesthesiology*. 2011;114:495–511.
185. Cavell B. Gastric emptying in infants. *Acta Paediatr Scand*. 1971;60:370–371.
186. Poulton TJ, Gum chewing during pre-anesthetic fasting. *Pediatr Anesth*. 2012;22:288–296.
187. Cook-Sather SD, Gallagher PR, Kruge LE, et al. Overweight/obesity and gastric fluid characteristics in pediatric day surgery: Implications for fasting guidelines and pulmonary aspiration risk. *Anesth Analg*. 2009;109:727–736.
188. Bricker SR, McLuckie A, Nightingale DA. Gastric aspirates after trauma in children. *Anaesthesia*. 1989;44:721–724.
189. Samsom M, Bharucha A, Gerich JE, et al. Diabetes mellitus and gastric emptying: Questions and issues in clinical practice. *Diabetes Metab Res Rev*. 2009;25:502–514.
190. Ma J, Rayner CK, Jones KL, et al. Diabetic gastroparesis. Diagnosis and management. *Drugs*. 2009;69:971–986.
191. Manley S, de Kelaita G, Joseph NJ, et al. Preoperative pregnancy testing in ambulatory surgery. Incidence and impact of positive results. *Anesthesiology*. 1995;83:690–693.
192. von Ungern-Sternberg BS, Boda K, Chambers NA, et al. Risk assessment for respiratory complications in paediatric anaesthesia: A prospective cohort study. *Lancet*. 2010;376:773–783.
193. Tait AR, Malviya S. Anesthesia for the child with an upper respiratory tract infection: Still a dilemma? *Anesth Analg*. 2005;100:59–65.
194. Tait AR, Malviya S, Voepel-Lewis T, et al. Risk factors for perioperative adverse respiratory events in children with upper respiratory tract infections. *Anesthesiology*. 2001;95:299–306.
195. Cohen MM, Cameron CB. Should you cancel the operation when a child has an upper respiratory tract infection? *Anesth Analg*. 1991;72:282–288.
196. Pavia AT. Viral infections of the lower respiratory tract: Old viruses, new viruses, and the role of diagnosis. *Clin Infect Dis*. 2011;52(suppl 4):S284–S289.
197. Netuveli G, Hurwitz B, Levy M, et al. Ethnic variations in UK asthma frequency, morbidity, and health-service use; a systematic review and meta-analysis. *Lancet*. 2005;365(9456):312–317.
198. Scalfaro P, Sly PD, Sims C, et al. Salbutamol prevents the increase of respiratory resistance caused by tracheal intubation during sevoflurane anesthesia in asthmatic children. *Anesth Analg*. 2001;93:898–902.
199. Carroll JL. Obstructive sleep-disordered breathing in children: New controversies, new directions. *Clin Chest Med*. 2003;24:261–282.
200. Brown KA, Laferriere A, Lakheeram I, et al. Recurrent hypoxemia in children is associated with increased analgesic sensitivity to opiates. *Anesthesiology*. 2006;105:665–669.
201. Raghavendran S, Bagry H, Detheux G, et al. An anesthetic management protocol to decrease respiratory complications after adenotonsillectomy in children with severe sleep apnea. *Anesth Analg*. 2010;110:1093–1101.
202. Aydin ON, Ugur B, Ozgun S, et al. Pain prevention with intraoperative ketamine in outpatient children undergoing tonsillectomy or tonsillectomy and adenotomy. *J Clin Anesth*. 2007;19:115–119.
203. Cote CJ, Zaslavsky A, Downes JJ, et al. Postoperative apnea in former preterm infants after inguinal herniorrhaphy: A combined analysis. *Anesthesiology*. 1995;82:809–822.
204. Murphy JJ, Swanson T, Ansermino M, et al. The frequency of apneas in premature infants after inguinal hernia repair: Do they need overnight monitoring in the intensive care unit? *J Pediatr Surg*. 2008;43:865–868.
205. Henderson-Smart DJ, Steer P. Postoperative caffeine for preventing apnea in preterm infants. *Cochrane Database Syst Rev*. 2001;4:CD000048.
206. Frawley G, Ingelmo P. Spinal anaesthesia in the neonate. *Best Pract Res Clin Anaesthesiol*. 2010;24:337–351.
207. Kim TW, Nemergut ME. Preparation of modern anesthesia workstations for malignant hyperthermia-susceptible patients; a review of past and present practice. *Anesthesiology*. 2011;114:205–212.
208. Sabouri AS, Lerman J, Heard C. Effects of fresh gas flow, tidal volume, and charcoal filters on the washout of sevoflurane from the Datex Ohmeda (GE) Aisys, Aestiva/5, and Excel 210SE anesthesia workstations. *Can J Anaesth*. 2014;61:935–942.
209. Gurnaney H, Brown A, Litman RS. Malignant hyperthermia and muscular dystrophies. *Anesth Analg*. 2009;109:1043–1048.
210. Footitt EJ, Sinha MD, Raiman JAJ, et al. Mitochondrial disorders and general anaesthesia: A case series and review. *Br J Anaesth*. 2008;100:436–441.
211. Firth PG. Anesthesia and hemoglobinopathies. *Anesthesiol Clin*. 2009;27:321–327.
212. Firth PG. Anaesthesia for peculiar cells—a century of sickle cell disease. *Br J Anaesth*. 2005;95:287–299.
213. Yawn BP, Buchanan GR, Afenyi-Annan AN, et al. Management of sickle cell disease. Summary of the 2014 evidence-based report by expert panel members. *JAMA*. 2014;312:1033–1048.
214. Fu T, Corrigan NJ, Quinn CT, et al. Minor elective surgical procedures using general anesthesia in children with sickle cell anemia without pre-operative blood transfusion. *Pediatr Blood Cancer*. 2005;45:43–47.
215. Lerman J. Anterior mediastinal masses in children. *Semin Anesth Perioper Med Pain*. 2007;26:133–140.
216. Borenstein SH, Gerstle T, Malkin D, et al. The effects of pre-biopsy corticosteroid treatment on the diagnosis of mediastinal lymphoma. *J Pediatr Surg*. 2000;35:973–976.
217. McDonnell C, Barlow R, Campisi P, et al. Fatal peri-operative acute tumour lysis syndrome precipitated by dexamethasone. *Anaesthesia*. 2008;63:652–655.
218. Wilson W, Taubert KA, Gewitz M, et al. Prevention of infection endocarditis. Guidelines from the American Heart Association. A guideline from the American Heart Association Rheumatic Fever, Endocarditis, and Kawasaki Disease Committee, Council on Cardiovascular Disease in the Young, and the Council on Clinical Cardiology, Council on Cardiovascular Surgery and Anesthesia, and the Quality of Care and Outcomes Research Interdisciplinary Working Group. *Circulation*. 2007;116:1736–1754, e376–e377.
219. Mortensen A, Lenz K, Abildstrom H, et al. Anesthetizing the obese child. *Paediatr Anaesth*. 2011;21:623–629.

220. Greenland KB, Edwards MJ, Hutton NJ. External auditory meatus-sternal notch relationship in adults in the sniffing position: A magnetic resonance imaging study. *Br J Anaesth.* 2010;104:268–269.
221. van der Griend BF, Lister NA, McKenzyie IM, et al. Postoperative mortality in children after 101,885 anesthetics at a tertiary pediatric hospital. *Anesth Analg.* 2011;112:1440–1447.
222. Pandit JJ, Andrade J, Bogod DG, et al. 5th National audit project (NAP5) on accidental awareness during general anaesthesia: summary of main findings and risk factors. *Br J Anaesth.* 2014;113:549–559.
223. Davidson AJ, Huang GH, Czarnecki C, et al. Awareness during anesthesia in children: A prospective cohort study. *Anesth Analg.* 2005;100:653–661.
224. Hansen TG. Anesthesia-related neurotoxicity and the developing animal brain is not a significant problem for children. *Pediatr Anesth.* 2015;25:66–72.
225. Sun LS, Li G, Miller TLK, et al. Association between a single general anesthesia exposure before age 36 months and neurocognitive outcomes in later childhood. *JAMA.* 2016:315(21)2312–2320.
226. Pichichero ME. A review of evidence supporting the American Academy of Pediatrics recommendation for prescribing cephalosporin antibiotics for penicillin-allergic patients. *Pediatrics.* 2005;115:1048–1057.
227. Murphy A, Campbell DE, Baines D, et al. Allergic reactions to propofol in egg-allergic children. *Anesth Analg.* 2011;113:140–144.
228. Sampathi V, Lerman J. Perioperative latex allergy in children. *Anesth Analg.* 2011;114:673–680.
229. de Queiroz M, Combet S, Bérard J, et al. Latex allergy in children: Modalities and prevention. *Paediatr Anaesth.* 2009;19:313–319.
230. Passi Y, Sathyamoorthy M, Lerman J, et al. Comparison of the laryngoscopy views with the size 1 Miller and Macintosh laryngoscope blades lifting the epiglottis or the base of the tongue in infants and children <2 years of age. *Br J Anaesth.* 2014;113(5):869–874.
231. White MC, Cook TM, Stoddart PA. A critique of elective pediatric supraglottic airway devices. *Paediatr Anaesth.* 2009;19(suppl 1):55–65.
232. Park C, Bahk JH, Ahn WS, et al. The laryngeal mask airway in infants and children. *Can J Anaesth.* 2001;48:413–417.
233. Luce V, Harkouk H, Michelet D, et al. Supraglottic airway devices vs tracheal intubation in children: A quantitative meta-analysis of respiratory complications. *Pediatr Anesth.* 2014;24:1088–1098.
234. Dalal PG, Murray D, Messner AH, et al. Pediatric laryngeal dimensions: an age-based analysis. *Anesth Analg.* 2009;108:1475–1479.
235. Dullenkopf A, Gerber A, Weiss M. The Microcuff™ tube allows a longer time interval until unsafe cuff pressures are reached in children. *Can J Anaesth.* 2004;51:997–1001.
236. Dullenkopf A, Schmitz A, Gerber AC, et al. Tracheal sealing characteristics of pediatric cuffed tracheal tubes. *Pediatr Anesth.* 2004;14:825–830.
237. Sathyamoorthy M, Lerman J, Asariparamil R, Penman AD, Lakshminrusimha S. Stridor in neonates after using the Microcuff and uncuffed tracheal tubes: A retrospective review. *Anesth Analg.* 2015;121:1321–1324.
238. Habre W. Neonatal ventilation. In: *Neonatal Anesthesia.* Lerman J (Ed), New York: Springer; 2015:213–224.
239. Lerman J. On cricoid pressure: "May the force be with you." *Anesth Analg.* 2009;109:1363–1366.
240. Walker RWM, Ravi R, Haylett K. Effect of cricoid force on airway calibre in children: A bronchoscopic assessment. *Br J Anaesth.* 2010;104:71–74.
241. Batra YK, Ivanova M, Ali SS, et al. The efficacy of a subhypnotic dose of propofol in preventing laryngospasm following tonsillectomy and adenoidectomy in children. *Paediatr Anaesth.* 2005;15:1094–1097.
242. Luginbuehl I, Bissonnette B. Thermal regulation. In: Coté CJ, Lerman J, Todres ID, eds. *A Practice of Anesthesia for Infants and Children.* 4th ed. Philadelphia, PA: Elsevier Inc; 2009:557–567.
243. Murat I, Berniere J, Constant I. Evaluation of the efficacy of a forced-air warmer (Bair Hugger) during spinal surgery in children. *J Clin Anesth.* 1994;6:425–429.
244. Larach MG, Gronert GA, Allen GC, et al. Clinical presentation, treatment, and complications of malignant hyperthermia. *Anesth Analg.* 2010;110:498–507.
245. Edwards JJ, Soto RG, Bedford RF. Bispectral Index™ values are higher during halothane vs. sevoflurane anesthesia in children, but not in infants. *Acta Anaesthesiol Scand.* 2005;49:1084–1087.
246. Schuller PJ, Newell S, Strickland PA, Barry JJ. Response of bispectral index to neuromuscular block in awake volunteers. *Br J Anaesth.* 2015;i95–i103.
247. Kaki AM, Almarakbi WA. Does patient position influence the reading of the bispectral index monitor? *Anesth Analg.* 2009;109:1843–1846.
248. Banchs RJ, Lerman J. Preoperative anxiety management, emergence delirium, and postoperative behavior. *Anesthesiol Clin* 2014;32:1–23.
249. Chundamala J, Wright JG, Kemp SM. An evidence-based review of parental presence during anaesthesia induction and parent/child anxiety. *Can J Anaesth.* 2009;56:57–70.
250. Yip P, Middleton P, Cyna AM, et al. Non-pharmacological interventions for assisting the induction of anaesthesia in children. *Cochrane Database Syst Rev.* 2009;8:CD006447.
251. Kain ZN, MacLaren J, McClain BC, et al. Effects of age and emotionality on the effectiveness of midazolam administered preoperatively to children. *Anesthesiology.* 2007;107:545–552.
252. Coté CJ, Cohen IT, Suresh S, et al. A comparison of three doses of a commercially prepared oral midazolam syrup in children. *Anesth Analg.* 2002;94:37–43.
253. Bergendahl H, Lonnqvist PA, Eksborg S. Clonidine in paediatric anaesthesia: Review of the literature and comparison with benzodiazepines for premedication. *Acta Anaesthesiol Scand.* 2006;50:135–143.
254. Zub D, Berkenbosch JW, Tobias JD. Preliminary experience with oral dexmedetomidine for procedural and anesthetic premedication. *Paediatr Anaesth.* 2005;15:932–938.
255. Karl HW, Rosenberger JL, Larach MG, et al. Transmucosal administration of midazolam for premedication in pediatric patients; comparison of the nasal and sublingual routes. *Anesthesiology.* 1993;78:885–891.
256. Karl HW, Keifer AT, Rosenberger JL, et al. Comparison of the safety and efficacy of intranasal midazolam or sufentanil for preinduction of anesthesia in pediatric patients. *Anesthesiology.* 1992;76:209–215.
257. Yuen VM, Hui TW, Irwin MG, et al. Optimal timing for the administration of intranasal dexmedetomidine for premedication in children. *Anaesthesia.* 2010;65:922–929.
258. Hannallah RS, Patel RI. Low-dose intramuscular ketamine for anesthesia preinduction in young children undergoing brief outpatient procedures. *Anesthesiology.* 1989;70:598–600.
259. Fukumoto M, Arima H, Ito S, et al. Distorted perception of smell by volatile agents facilitated inhalational induction of anesthesia. *Paediatr Anaesth.* 2005;15:98–101.
260. Przybylo HJ, Tarbell SE, Stevenson GW. Mask fear in children presenting for anesthesia: Aversion, phobia, or both? *Paediatr Anaesth.* 2005;15:366–370.
261. Agnor R, Sikich N, Lerman J. Single-breath vital capacity rapid inhalation induction in children: 8% sevoflurane versus 5% halothane. *Anesthesiology.* 1998;89:379–384.
262. Kumar M, Chawla R, Goyal M. Topical anesthesia. *J Anaesthesiol Clin Pharm.* 2015;31:450–456.
263. Lander JA, Weltman BJ, So SS. EMLA and amethocaine for reduction of children's pain associated with needle insertion. *Cochrane Database Syst Rev.* 2009;3:CD004236.
264. Kleiber C, Schutte DL, McCarthy AM, et al. Predictors of topical anesthetic effectiveness in children. *J Pain.* 2007;8:168–174.
265. Vetter T. A comparison of EMLA cream versus nitrous oxide for pediatric venous cannulation. *J Clin Anesth.* 1995;7:486–490.
266. Tanaka M, Sato M, Saito A, et al. Reevaluation of rectal ketamine premedication in children: Comparison with rectal midazolam. *Anesthesiology.* 2000;93:1217–1224.
267. Hampson-Evans D, Morgan P, Farrar M. Pediatric laryngospasm. *Paediatr Anaesth.* 2008;18:303–307.
268. Al-alami AA, Markakis Zestos M, Baraka AS. Pediatric laryngospasm: Prevention and treatment. *Curr Opin Anaesthesiol.* 2009;22:388–295.
269. Afshan G, Chohan U, Qamar-Ul-Hoda M, et al. Is there a role of a small dose of propofol in the treatment of laryngeal spasm? *Paediatr Anaesth.* 2002;12:625–628.
270. Kraemer FW, Stricker PA, Gurnaney HGG, et al. Bradycardia during induction of anesthesia with sevoflurane in children with Down syndrome. *Anesth Analg.* 2010;111:1259–1263.
271. Dubois MC, Gouyet L, Murat I, et al. Lactated Ringer with 1% dextrose: An appropriate solution for peri-operative fluid therapy in children. *Paediatr Anaesth.* 1992;2:99–104.
272. Rando K, Zunini G, Negroto A. Intraoperative hyponatremia during craniofacial surgery. *Paediatr Anaesth.* 2009;19:358–363.
273. O'Malley CMN, Frumento RJ, Hardy MA, et al. A randomized, double-blind comparison of Lactated Ringer's solution and 0.9% NaCl during renal transplantation. *Anesth Analg.* 2005;100:1518–1524.
274. Holliday MA, Segar WE. The maintenance need for water in parenteral fluid therapy. *Pediatrics.* 1957;19:823–832.
275. Holliday MA, Friedman AL, Segar WE, et al. Acute hospital-induced hyponatremia in children: A physiologic approach. *J Pediatr.* 2004;145:584–587.
276. Morley SL. Red blood cell transfusions in acute paediatrics. *Arch Dis Child Educ Pract Ed.* 2009;94:65–73.
277. Barcelona SL, Thompson AA, Coté CJ. Intraoperative pediatric blood transfusion therapy: A review of common issues. Part II: Transfusion therapy, special considerations, and reduction of allogenic blood transfusions. *Paediatr Anaesth.* 2005;15:814–830.
278. Lerman J. Surgical and patient factors involved in postoperative nausea and vomiting. *Br J Anaesth.* 1992;69 (Suppl 1): 24S-32S.
279. Schreiner MS, Nicolson SC, Martin I, et al. Should children drink before discharge from day surgery? *Anesthesiology.* 1992;76:528–533.
280. Goodarzi M, Matar MM, Shafa M, et al. A prospective randomized blinded study of the effect of intravenous fluid therapy on postoperative nausea and vomiting in children undergoing strabismus surgery. *Paediatr Anaesth.* 2006;16:49–53.
281. Apfel CC, Kortilla K, Abdalla M, et al. A factorial trial of six interventions for the prevention of postoperative nausea and vomiting. *NEJM.* 2004;350:2441–2451.
282. Peyton PJ, Wu CY. Nitrous oxide-related postoperative nausea and vomiting depends on duration of exposure. *Anesthesiology.* 2014;120:1137–1145.

283. Engelman E, Salengros JC, Barvais L. How much does pharmacologic prophylaxis reduce postoperative vomiting in children? Calculation of prophylaxis effectiveness and expected incidence of vomiting under treatment using Bayesian meta-analysis. *Anesthesiology.* 2008;109:1023–1035.
284. Kim MS, Coté CJ, Cristoloveanu C, et al. There is no dose-escalation response to dexamethasone (0.0625–1.0 mg/kg) in pediatric tonsillectomy or adenotonsillectomy patients for preventing vomiting, reducing pain, shortening time to first liquid intake, or the incidence of voice change. *Anesth Analg.* 2007;104:1052–1058.
285. Mahant S, Keren R, Localio R, et al. Dexamethasone and risk of bleeding in children undergoing tonsillectomy. *Otolarynol Head Neck Surg.* 2014;150:872–879.
286. Bellis JR, Pirmohamed M, Nunn AJ, et al. Dexamethasone and haemorrhage risk in paediatric tonsillectomy: A systematic review and meta-analysis. *Br J Anaesth.* 2014;113:23–42.
287. Polaner DM, Zuk J, Luong K, et al. Positive intravascular test dose criteria in children during total intravenous anesthesia with propofol and remifentanil are different than during inhaled anesthesia. *Anesth Analg.* 2010;110:41–44.
288. Kumar P, Rudra A, Pan AK, et al. Caudal additives in pediatrics: A comparison among midazolam, ketamine, and neostigmine coadministered with bupivacaine. *Anesth Analg.* 2005;101:69–73.
289. Tsui BC, Wagner A, Cave D, et al. Thoracic and lumbar epidural analgesia via the caudal approach using electrical stimulation guidance in pediatric patients: A review of 289 patients. *Anesthesiology.* 2004;100:683–689.
290. Berde CB. Convulsions associated with pediatric regional anesthesia. *Anesth Analg.* 1992;175:164–166.
291. Bosenberg AT, Thomas J, Cronje L, et al. Pharmacokinetics and efficacy of ropivacaine for continuous epidural infusion in neonates and infants. *Paediatr Anaesth.* 2005;15:739–749.
292. Ciechanowicz S, Patil V. Lipid emulsion for local anesthetic systemic toxicity. *Anesth Res Pract.* 2012;2012:131784.
293. Ecoffey C. Safety in pediatric regional anesthesia. *Paediatr Anaesth.* 2012;22:25–30.
294. Pounder DR, Blackstock D, Steward DJ. Tracheal extubation in children: Halothane versus isoflurane, anesthetized versus awake. *Anesthesiology.* 1991;74:653–655.
295. Davidson AJ, Wong A, Knottenbelt G, et al. MAC-awake of sevoflurane in children. *Pediatr Anesth.* 2008;18:702–707.
296. Zeltser D, Justo D, Halkin A, et al. Torsade de Pointes due to noncardiac drugs: Most patients have easily identifiable risk factors. *Medicine.* 2003;82:282–290.
297. Arai YCP, Fukunaga K, Hirota S, et al. The effect of chin lift and jaw thrust while in the lateral position on stridor score in anesthetized children adenotonsillar hypertrophy. *Anesth Analg.* 2004;99:1638–1641.
298. Hajiha M, DuBord MA, Liu H, et al. Opioid receptor mechanisms at the hypoglossal motor pool and effects on tongue muscle activity in vivo. *J Physiol.* 2009;587:2677–2692.
299. Murat I, Constant I, Maud'huy H. Perioperative anaesthetic morbidity in children: A database of 24,165 anaesthetics over a 30-month period. *Paediatr Anaesth.* 2004;14:158–166.
300. Holmes JR, Hensinger RN, Wojtys EW. Postoperative pulmonary edema in young, athletic adults. *Am J Sports Med.* 1992;19:365–371.
301. Dahmani S, Stany I, Brasher C, et al. Pharmacological prevention of sevoflurane- and desflurane-related emergence agitation in children: A meta-analysis of published studies. *Br J Anaesth.* 2010;104:216–223.
302. Cravero J, Surgenor S, Whalen K. Emergence agitation in paediatric patients after sevoflurane anaesthesia and no surgery: A comparison with halothane. *Paediatr Anaesth.* 2000;10:419–424.
303. Sikich N, Lerman J. Development and psychometric evaluation of the pediatric anesthesia emergence delirium scale. *Anesthesiology.* 2004;100:1138–1145.
304. Ho KY, Gan TJ. Pharmacology, pharmacogenetics, and clinical efficacy of 5-hydroxytryptamine type 3 receptor antagonists for postoperative nausea and vomiting. *Curr Opin Anaesth.* 2006;19:606–611.
305. Ecoffey C. Pediatric regional anesthesia—update. *Curr Opin Anaesthesiol.* 2007; 20:232–235.
306. Anderson BJ, Palmer GM. Recent developments in the pharmacological management of pain in children. *Curr Opin Anaesthesiol.* 2006;19:285–292.
307. Birmingham PK, Suresh S, Ambrosy A, et al. Parent-assisted or nurse-assisted epidural analgesia: Is this feasible in pediatric patients? *Paediatr Anaesth.* 2009; 19:1084–1089.
308. Kart T, Christrup LL, Rasmussen M. Recommended use of morphine in neonates, infants and children based on a literature review: Part 1—pharmacokinetics. *Paediatr Anaesth.* 1997;7:5–11.

Section 8
ANESTHESIA FOR SELECTED SURGICAL SERVICES

44 Anesthesia for Laparoscopic and Robotic Surgeries

GERARDO RODRIGUEZ • SHARMA E. JOSEPH

Introduction
Laparoscopic Surgery
   Surgical Approach and Positioning
   Ambulatory Laparoscopic Surgery
   Robotic Laparoscopic Surgery
Physiologic Impact of Laparoscopy
   Cardiovascular System
   Respiratory System
   Regional Perfusion Effects
Intraoperative Management
   Monitoring
   Anesthesia Maintenance
   Mechanical Ventilation
   Body Temperature
   Fluid Management

Complications Related to Surgery
   Intraoperative
   Patient Shifting and Falls
   Ocular Injuries
   Peripheral Nerve and Brachial Plexus Injuries
   Airway Edema
Postoperative Complications
   Respiratory Dysfunction
   Venous Thrombosis
Postoperative Management
   Acute Pain Management
   Postoperative Nausea and Vomiting
Conclusion

KEY POINTS

1. Small incisions, decreased postoperative pain, and lower surgical complication rates are some of the benefits of laparoscopy over laparotomy.
2. Pneumoperitoneum- and position-related physiologic changes are a significant disadvantage, to the anesthesiologist.
3. Risk of perioperative complications may be significant in patients with body mass index > 40 kg/m^2 and obesity-related comorbidities.
4. Advances in robotic-assisted laparoscopic surgery have expanded its application to multiple subspecialties.
5. Access to the patient during robotic-assisted surgery may be seriously limited during an intraoperative cardiopulmonary or airway emergency.
6. Severe hypercarbia and acidosis from absorbed carbon dioxide can lead to reduced inotropy, dysrhythmias, and arterial vasodilation.
7. High intra-abdominal pressures during hypovolemia can severely impair venous return and cardiac filling.
8. Endobronchial intubation can occur during diaphragmatic displacement into the thorax and Trendelenburg positioning.
9. Renal blood flow, glomerular filtration, and urine output are reduced during pneumoperitoneum.
10. The assessment of neuromuscular blockade during laparoscopic surgery remains highly subjective.
11. Major vascular injuries occur rarely during abdominal entry and are associated with significant morbidity and mortality.
12. Severe hypotension during pneumoperitoneum should be treated with deinsufflation, and possible conversion to an open procedure.
13. Risk factors for complications of subcutaneous emphysema include operative times more than 200 minutes, lower BMI, high intra-abdominal pressure, and Nissen fundoplication surgery.
14. Tension capnothorax is a life-threatening condition that requires a high index of suspicion and immediate action from the operating room team.
15. Perioperative use of preemptive multimodal strategies and postoperative nausea and vomiting prophylaxis are integral components for optimal patient recovery after laparoscopic surgery.

Introduction

Over a century ago, laparoscopy was first introduced as a therapeutic alternative to laparotomy. Since then, the field of laparoscopic surgery has evolved and grown tremendously, to the extent that it has now become a conventional approach for many surgical diseases traditionally treated with open procedures. In fact, laparoscopy is now the gold standard approach for cholecystectomy and bariatric surgery. The growth of the specialty has been fueled, in large part, by the benefits of "minimally invasive" surgery (Table 44-1). Improved surgical cosmesis, reduced postoperative pain, faster return to work, and lower surgical-related complications continue to make laparoscopy, in many cases, preferable to open surgery.[1-4] Advances in anesthesia have also facilitated the expansion of laparoscopy into noninpatient facilities. Today, a large number of surgeries that once required prolonged hospital stays are now performed in outpatient surgery centers and short-stay facilities.[5-9] The creation of protocolized, fast-track programs that maximize the benefits of minimally invasive surgery has improved surgical outcomes and reduced health-care costs.[10]

Despite its outcome advantages, the practice of traditional laparoscopic surgery has been fraught with technical challenges for the surgeon, derived from the act of operating through small access ports, using long rigid surgical instruments—all while having a limited sense of pressure and depth. Technological advances have now introduced robotics to laparoscopic surgery to address many of its technical issues that affect all laparoscopic surgeons. Robotic-assisted laparoscopic surgery provides surgeons with a close approximation of the fine motor skills and depth of vision used in traditional open surgery, all while positioned comfortably away from the patient's bedside.

Disadvantages exist in laparoscopy for patients and medical providers alike (Table 44-2). A significant source of intraoperative and postoperative issues during laparoscopy stems from the creation of pneumoperitoneum. Physiologic derangements, particularly affecting the cardiopulmonary system, are common during pneumoperitoneum, and are further aggravated by steep positioning changes common in laparoscopy. A patient's age and comorbidities can greatly affect the severity of pneumoperitoneum-related changes observed by clinicians. In robotic surgery, long operative time and limited access to the patient, due to prominent robotic equipment, can further complicate management of urgent conditions. As the application of laparoscopy and robotic-assisted surgery continues to expand to more complex patients and diseases, the anesthetist must be increasingly attentive to avoid or minimize serious patient harm.

In this chapter, a general overview is provided regarding the anesthetic management of laparoscopic and robotic-assisted surgery for the adult patient undergoing abdominal and pelvic exploration. For additional discussion on their application in other areas of surgery, we refer the reader to other relevant chapters within this textbook.

Laparoscopic Surgery

Surgical Approach and Positioning

Laparoscopic surgery is a minimally invasive surgical technique where specialized tubes are inserted for surgical access. Small skin incisions are made, approximately 1 cm in length, to facilitate insertion of rigid tubes, called trocars. Trocars are sharp, multiport, one-way conduits used to insufflate gas and to guide various specialized surgical instruments. Intraperitoneal viewing is conducted using a video-capable telescopic camera, called a laparoscope.

Exposure of the intraperitoneal space can be achieved either by intraperitoneal pressurization, called pneumoperitoneum, or by external abdominal wall retraction.

Conventional laparoscopy uses carbon dioxide (CO_2) for intraperitoneal (e.g., bariatric and cholecystectomy surgery) and extraperitoneal insufflation (e.g., adrenal and inguinal hernia repair surgery). In contrast to other insufflation gases, such as helium and nitrous oxide, CO_2 has a desirable safety profile. CO_2 is highly soluble in blood, facilitating rapid pulmonary removal and minimizing the consequences of inadvertent extraperitoneal or intravascular insufflation. CO_2 is nonflammable, nonoxidizing, and safe to use during electrocautery. Despite its safety profile, CO_2 insufflation has known side effects discussed in subsequent sections of this chapter.

Intraperitoneal insufflation is generally established by creating a small subumbilical incision, through which a stainless steel, spring-loaded, blunt needle, called a Veress needle, is inserted. An automated, self-regulating insufflator with adjustable preset parameters is connected to the Veress stopcock to deliver low-flow rates of CO_2 until adequate abdominal distention is achieved. Maximal preset intra-abdominal pressures (IAP) above 15 mmHg should be avoided as to minimize CO_2-related complications and significant cardiopulmonary instability. The Veress needle is replaced with a trocar for laparoscope insertion. Several other incisions are then made through which trocars are sequentially inserted under direct laparoscope visualization and transillumination to avoid inadvertent intra-abdominal injury. The surgery is conducted using a laparoscope for video monitoring, and various long, handheld surgical instruments. If the surgeon's hand is needed for intra-abdominal tissue manipulation or large specimen extraction during laparoscopic surgery, a larger surgical access can be provided for a laparoscopic hand-assisted approach. A single 5- to 7.5-cm abdominal wall opening is made for insertion of a flexible, self-retaining, circular sleeve used for intra-abdominal hand insertion.

Table 44-1	Benefits of Laparoscopic Surgery	
Patient-specific	**Surgeon-specific**	**Anesthesiologist-specific**
Improved cosmetic results	↓Medical risk	↓Incisional stress response
Shorter recovery time	Better clinical outcomes	↓Opioid requirements
Earlier return to work	Earlier return of bowel function	↓Postoperative pain
Faster return to normal activities	↓Postoperative complications	↓Fluid shifts
↓Costs		↓Postoperative respiratory dysfunction

Table 44-2	Disadvantages of Laparoscopy Surgery	
Patient-specific	**Surgeon-specific**	**Anesthesiologist-specific**
↑Risk of PONV Referred pain from CO_2 insufflation	Highly-specialized training Ergonomics Limited tactile sense Longer operating times Complex equipment and setup Use in reoperation or scar tissue more challenging	Pneumoperitoneum-induced stress response Positioning Mechanical ventilatory challenges Extraperitoneal CO_2-related complications Limited access to patient (robotic surgery)

As an alternative to CO_2 pneumoperitoneum, exposure of the intraperitoneal space can be achieved by external abdominal wall retraction, called abdominal wall lift. This technique requires a specialized horizontal lifting apparatus inserted into the abdominal wall for suspension of the anterior abdominal wall away from the abdominal viscera. Gas insufflation is, usually not necessary. Despite the benefits of avoiding gas insufflation and its side effects, abdominal wall lift is generally believed to be inferior to pneumoperitoneum laparoscopy due to longer operative times and an unclear safety profile.[11,12]

Patient positioning during laparoscopic surgery is uniquely affected by several aspects. Long, rigid laparoscopic instruments facilitate minimal access, but limit the ease of tissue manipulation. Bed tilting is usually needed to passively optimize surgical exposure with minimal surgical retraction. Steep, reverse Trendelenburg position (i.e., "head up") exposes upper abdominal structures, such as in gastric bypass surgery. Steep Trendelenburg position (i.e., "head down") is used to expose lower abdominal structures, such as in uterine or prostate surgery. The lateral jackknife position is used to expose the retroperitoneal space during radical nephrectomy surgery. Leftward tilting exposes the appendix, whereas rightward tilting exposes the left colon. The addition of lithotomy is dependent on the need for genital, urologic access. An in-depth discussion on patient positioning and potential injuries is discussed elsewhere (see Chapter 29).

Ambulatory Laparoscopic Surgery

Laparoscopic surgery performed as day or outpatient surgery has a long history that continues to grow. The earliest reports of outpatient laparoscopy date back to the 1970s, when it was first used in gynecological surgeries.[13] Female sterilization entailed some of the first outpatient surgeries performed with minimal reported complications and low readmission rates.[14,15] Since then, general surgical procedures have surpassed all other outpatient laparoscopic surgery performed worldwide. Laparoscopic cholecystectomy for symptomatic cholelithiasis is now the most commonly performed outpatient laparoscopic surgery. Its safety and dependability has been well established.[5,6] When comparing outpatient versus overnight admission for laparoscopic cholecystectomy, day surgery has been shown to be equally safe with similar pain scores and recovery times.[16]

Ambulatory laparoscopic surgery is also being performed in the bariatric population with increasing frequency. Common laparoscopic weight loss procedures include gastric bypass, sleeve gastrectomy, and adjustable gastric band. Due to its low rates of complications, and readmissions, and predictably short operative time, gastric banding is the most commonly performed outpatient bariatric surgery.[8,17]

The expansion of sleeve gastrectomy and, particularly, gastric bypass into the ambulatory setting, is in large part due to advancements in minimally invasive surgery, patient screening and anesthetic management. Nonetheless, postoperative complications, unanticipated admissions, and readmission rates for these procedures remain concerns for suitability and safety. Based on a comprehensive retrospective review of ambulatory laparoscopic gastric bypass surgery, unplanned admission and readmission rates were 16% and 1.82%, respectively.[9] Causes for unanticipated readmission in both gastric bypass and sleeve gastrectomy surgery include dysphagia, nausea, and uncontrolled pain. More serious complications include unexpected gastric leaks after sleeve gastrectomy, gastrointestinal bleeding, and pulmonary embolism.[9,18,19]

Appropriate patient presurgical screening is ideal for optimizing good surgical results and avoiding unexpected complications. Assessing the body mass index (BMI) and severity of obesity-related comorbidities is important for preoperative risk stratification. Patients with a BMI of less than 40 kg/m^2 and well-optimized comorbid conditions, such as type II diabetes, heart disease, and obstructive sleep apnea, may have acceptable risk for ambulatory surgery. Concerns for greater risk of perioperative complications exist for patients with BMI greater than 40 kg/m^2 and poorly managed obesity-related comorbidities. Ultimately, well-supported recommendations for weight limits in obese patients being screened for ambulatory surgery are lacking, and may only be based on expert opinion.[19]

Other laparoscopic surgeries routinely performed in an outpatient setting include several general surgical and gynecological procedures, such as inguinal or ventral hernia repair, diagnostic laparoscopy, ovarian cystectomy, and endometrial laser ablation. An in-depth review on the practice of ambulatory anesthesia (see Chapter 31) and anesthesia in obesity are presented elsewhere (see Chapter 45).

Robotic Laparoscopic Surgery

Robotic laparoscopic surgery is a highly sophisticated, technologic variation on conventional laparoscopic surgery, requiring modification of both surgical and anesthetic management.[1,3,4] The approach was developed to address several limitations of conventional laparoscopy, including reduced range of motion and instrument dexterity, and a two-dimensional view of the operative field. The advanced technology has transformed technically challenging procedures into feasible ones via a minimally invasive approach. Although it was first popularized in urology for radical prostatectomies, robotic-assisted surgery has since gained ground in other fields, in part, due to reports of improved surgical outcomes, lower complication rates, shortened lengths of hospital stay, and improved surgeon ergonomics. It currently has applications and FDA approval in other types of urological surgeries, general laparoscopic surgeries, general noncardiovascular thoracoscopic surgeries, thoracoscopically-assisted cardiotomy

Table 44-3 Examples of Robotic-assisted Laparoscopic Surgery

Cardiac
Coronary artery bypass, valvuloplasty
Thoracic
Lung resection, esophagectomy
Gastrointestinal
Fundoplication, colectomy, gastrectomy, hepatectomy
Urologic
Radical cystectomy, pyeloplasty, prostectomy
Gynecologic, Oncologic
Hysterectomy, lymph node dissection, oophorectomy

procedures, and may be used with adjunctive mediastinotomy to perform coronary anastomosis during cardiac revascularization (Table 44-3).

Robotic surgery is performed most commonly employing the Da Vinci Surgical System (Intuitive Surgical Inc., Sunnyvale, CA) that uses a surgeon control console, a robot cart with interactive surgical arms, and a high-definition (HD) 3D video tower (Fig. 44-1). Similar to conventional laparoscopy, robotic laparoscopic surgery entails the creation of a pneumoperitoneum, insertion of a video laparoscope, and insertion of trocars for surgical access. From there, the differences in approach far outweigh their similarities. The surgical robot is positioned near the patient with robotic arms inserted into the insufflated cavity. The robotic arms are controlled remotely by a surgeon seated at an ergonomically designed control console. Remote handling of instruments via a specialized control allows for movements that mimic natural maneuvers, improved degrees of freedom, and optimal surgical instrument rotation and pivoting. Surgical visualization is achieved via a goggle viewfinder with an HD, magnified, 3D video display. An assistant near the surgical field provides surgical support, such as robotic arm adjustments, tissue retraction, and suctioning. Other clinicians in the operating room suite visualize the laparoscopic surgical field using 2D HD video screens.

Anesthetic management during laparoscopic robotic surgery requires preparing for patient accessibility limitations and adjusting for patient positioning challenges. Prominent surgical robotic equipment near the patient can greatly limit anesthesia provider access to the patient in case of an emergency. Though newer surgical robotic systems are becoming more compact, with thinner robotic arms, and improved motorized maneuverability functions for steering and engaging, the robotic systems in use today have a large footprint near and above the operating room bed. In the rare event of an airway or cardiopulmonary emergency, the robotic surgical arms must first be carefully disengaged from the trocars, before the robot can be removed safely and the patient positioned in a manner consistent with that needed for airway management or cardiopulmonary resuscitation, respectively.

Steep Trendelenburg positioning used in many robotic surgeries requires greater vigilance of the patient. Ocular injury risk in steep Trendelenburg during robotic surgery may be greater than in conventional laparoscopic surgery (see Complications Related to Surgery). Robotic arms often extend above the patient's face in this position, increasing the potential risk of both accidental endotracheal tube dislodgement and facial injury. Careful endotracheal tube taping and protective foam padding can be placed on the patient's face for extra security.

Physiologic Impact of Laparoscopy

Laparoscopic surgery induces complex physiologic changes that impact multiple organ systems. Direct mechanical stress placed on the patient, as well as neuroendocrine stimulation during laparoscopy are the primary forces responsible for much of the physiologic derangement observed. The degree of observed effect is modified by a patient's pre-existing comorbidities, positioning, surgical factors, and anesthetic approach.[20,21] Although physiologic changes during minimally invasive surgery are well tolerated in healthy patients, minimizing complications and optimizing conditions for a successful surgical result, require an understanding of the interplay between physiology and laparoscopic surgery.

Cardiovascular System

The cardiovascular system is exquisitely challenged during laparoscopy by multiple stressors on preload, inotropy, rhythm, and afterload (Table 44-4). In patients, the cumulative effect is an increase in mean arterial pressure (MAP), myocardial oxygen demand, and systemic vascular resistance (SVR). Modifiable factors that affect hemodynamics during laparoscopy include the intravascular volume status of the patient, positioning, baseline comorbidities, and surgical technique.

Carbon dioxide gas is highly soluble and, during insufflation, rapidly moves from the peritoneal cavity into the circulation. Prolonged surgeries and high insufflation pressures can lead to increased CO_2 gas absorption. Systemic CO_2 gas then exerts both direct and indirect effects on the cardiovascular system via adrenergic pathways. Mild hypercarbia ($PaCO_2$ of 45 to 50 mmHg) alters hemodynamics very little, whereas severe hypercarbia ($PaCO_2$ 55 to 70 mmHg) and acidosis can lead to myocardial depression, dysrhythmias from catecholamine-induced myocardial sensitization, and peripheral vasodilation. Further complicating the response of the myocardium to transient hypercarbia is the potential for acute elevations in right ventricular afterload from hypercarbia-induced pulmonary vasoconstriction. The potential hemodynamic effects of severe hypercarbia are counteracted by sympathetic nervous system stimulation during laparoscopy, that concurrently produces tachycardia, an increase in MAP, and vasoconstriction from an increase in SVR.[21,22]

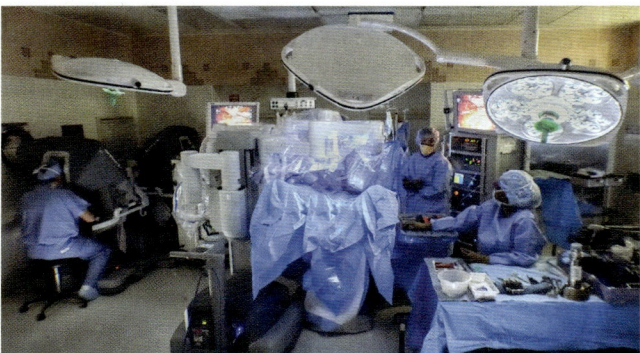

Figure 44-1 Robotic surgery room setup. Surgeon at the console (*left*), robot and patient (*center*), and video tower (*right*).

Table 44-4 Causes of Hemodynamic Changes during Laparoscopy

Determinants of Blood Pressure in Laparoscopy[a]	Effect on Blood Pressure
Preload (venous return)	
IVC compression	↑ or no change
Intra-abdominal organ compression	↑ or no change
Trendelenburg position	↑
Cardiac output or inotropy[a]	
Venous return	↑ or no change
Peripheral Vasoconstriction	↑ or no change
Rhythm (brady- or tachyarrhythmia)[a]	
Hypercapnia/acidosis	↑ or no change
Hypoxia	↓ or no change
Peritoneal irritation	↑,↓ or no change
Afterload and MAP[a]	
Hypercapnia/acidosis	↑,↓ or no change

[a]Autonomic nervous system stimulation and neurohumoral factors, such as catecholamines, vasopressin, and cortisol, released during laparoscopy contribute to physiologic changes. IVC, inferior vena cava; MAP, mean arterial pressure.

The peritoneum and abdominal viscera are highly innervated by autonomic nerve fibers. Stimulation of these autonomic pathways during pneumoperitoneum, typically results in sympathetic nervous system activation, catecholamine release, activation of the renin–angiotensin system, and release of the neurohypophysial hormone vasopressin.[23] This potent endogenous hormone can cause intense vasoconstriction, an increase in MAP, and increases in left ventricular afterload. Left ventricular wall tension and myocardial work needed to maintain intraventricular pressure and cardiac index (CI), respectively, are raised with significant increases in SVR. Mechanical stretch on the peritoneum and abdominal viscera can result in parasympathetic stimulation through the vagus nerve, but sympathetic tone usually predominates.

Intravascular volume status is an important modifier of the mechanical effects of pneumoperitoneum.[22] In instances where low right atrial pressures reflect low cardiac filling volumes, an increase IAP can result in compression of the inferior vena cava (IVC), causing a decrease in venous return and cardiac filling. However, where high right atrial pressures reflect hypervolemia, and not increased intrathoracic pressures from pneumoperitoneum, the IVC can resist collapse resulting in a rapid but transient increase in venous return[2,3] from splanchnic compression.

Patient positioning can further modify the effects of IAP. Steep Trendelenburg positioning during pneumoperitoneum may augment venous return and cardiac filling.[24] In contrast, reverse Trendelenburg position during pneumoperitoneum can result in an increase in SVR and minor reductions in CI that are soon reversed.[25] Initiating insufflation while supine and maintaining IAP within the recommended range (12 to 15 mmHg) can minimize any reduction in preload.[20] Nonetheless, extremely high IAP, in addition to hypovolemia, can result in severe compression of the venous system, as well as a perilous reduction in venous return and cardiac filling.

Preoperative comorbidities have varying effects on hemodynamics. Morbidly obese patients undergoing laparoscopic gastric bypass surgery show similar hemodynamic changes as nonbariatric patients. It is hypothesized that the morbidly obese better tolerate insufflation because of an intrinsically elevated IAP at 9 to 10 mmHg compared with nonobese patients.[26] Geriatric patients[21] can generally tolerate minimally invasive surgery. However, complex hemodynamic changes in elderly patients with cardiovascular disease may be significant during pneumoperitoneum, despite a lack of observable myocardial ischemia by electrocardiogram.[27] In geriatric patients with at least 1 cardiac risk factor (i.e., history of hypertension, coronary artery disease, heart failure, or myocardial ischemia), the initiation of pneumoperitoneum in the supine position results in an increase in SVR, a reduction in ejection fraction (EF), and CI. Preload and left ventricular stroke work index (LVSWI) remain unchanged. Trendelenburg positioning increases preload, EF, and CI. Return to supine positioning with deinsufflation decreases SVR below baseline and increases EF, CI, and LVSWI—all above baseline.[27] In patients with significant pulmonary hypertension or right ventricular failure, ventricular function may be strained in the setting of changing preload and pulmonary vascular resistance (PVR). Acute increases in preload can strain an already stressed right ventricle. Hypercarbia and acidosis can lead to increased pulmonary vasoconstriction and increased right ventricular afterload, in addition to impaired inotropy. Significant volume loading of a dilated right ventricle can in turn compress the left ventricle through the mechanism of ventricular interdependence leading to reduced global ventricular function.[28]

The type of surgical procedure may also influence the degree of hemodynamic derangement. Surgical disruption of the esophageal hiatus during laparoscopic fundoplication may increase mediastinal and pleural pressures, resulting in a significant reduction in CI.[29] Laparoscopic robotic prostatectomy results in hemodynamics similar to conventional laparoscopic surgery.[30,31] In healthy patients placed in steep Trendelenburg position during robotic prostatectomies, ventricular filling pressure is increased, whereas cardiac markers of ventricular performance remain unchanged.

Respiratory System

Laparoscopic abdominal surgery exerts changes on the pulmonary system by mechanically displacing thoracic structures, altering lung mechanics (i.e., volumes, compliance, resistance) and disrupting gas exchange through ventilation–perfusion mismatch (Table 44-5). An early effect of insufflation on the pulmonary system is the displacement of the diaphragm into the

Table 44-5 Causes of Pulmonary Changes during Laparoscopy

Anatomic Displacement	VQ Mismatch	Altered Lung Mechanics
Carinal cephalad displacement	Lung volume reduction/ uneven gas distribution	Lung compliance decrease and resistance increase
Diaphragm elevation	↑Alveolar-arterial oxygen gradient	↑Pleural pressure
Endobronchial intubation		↑Airway pressure

Table 44-6 Causes of Severe Hypercarbia during Laparoscopy

Excessive CO$_2$ Absorption	Excessive CO$_2$ Production	Inadequate CO$_2$ Removal
CO$_2$ venous embolism	Hypermetabolic conditions (e.g., fever, malignant hyperthermia)	Hypoventilation
Subcutaneous emphysema	Morbid obesity	Endobronchial intubation
Capnothorax (CO$_2$ pneumothorax)		Atelectasis
Capnomediastinum		Cardiogenic shock
Capnopericardium		Exhausted CO$_2$ absorber

thorax, which can be further aggravated by Trendelenburg positioning.[20,21] This shifts the carina cephalad, increasing the risk of endobronchial intubation. Elevated IAP and diaphragmatic displacement also lead to compression of the lung bases, atelectasis, ventilation–perfusion mismatch, and hypoxemia. However, abnormally low levels of oxygen are rarely observed in patients with normal preoperative pulmonary function. The change in pulmonary compliance can be observed as an increase in peak inspiratory pressure (PIP) during positive pressure ventilation. Ventilator adjustments may be needed to minimize peak airway pressure, while maintaining acceptable minute ventilation. Hypercarbia from CO$_2$ pneumoperitoneum frequently requires adjustments in mechanical ventilation.

Hypercarbia routinely develops in all patients from the absorption of intraperitoneal CO$_2$ into the circulatory system (Table 44-6). The concentration gradient that develops preferentially drives CO$_2$ from the pulmonary capillaries into the alveolar network, where it is removed during exhalation and measured by capnography as end-tidal CO$_2$ (EtCO$_2$.) Exhaled CO$_2$ and the degree of gas absorption vary based on the route of insufflation, preoperative comorbidities, and acute intraoperative pathology. In lieu of CO$_2$ absorption, calculated CO$_2$ elimination during intraperitoneal and extraperitoneal laparoscopy could increase rapidly then reach a steady state within 30 minutes, regardless of surgery duration.[32] Extraperitoneal insufflation may result in a higher CO$_2$ elimination than during intraperitoneal insufflation, due to a greater likelihood of tissue gas accumulation.[32]

In healthy patients undergoing intraperitoneal laparoscopy, hypercarbia and changes in pulmonary mechanics may have limited clinical significance. Compensatory hyperventilation can readily normalize hypercapnia. Despite speculation that a ventilation–perfusion mismatching contributes to hypercapnia during laparoscopy, minimal changes occur in alveolar dead space and pulmonary shunting during prolonged and steep Trendelenburg positioning with pneumoperitoneum used in robotic-assisted hysterectomy and prostatectomy.[33] Elevated EtCO$_2$ levels with a stable PaCO$_2$ in these types of surgeries is likely due to insufflated CO$_2$ absorption and not impaired alveolar ventilation. Furthermore, steep Trendelenburg positioning with pneumoperitoneum can produce close to a 50% reduction in lung compliance while simultaneously producing in an unexpected improvement in oxygenation by mechanisms that remain unclear.[31]

Hypoxia during laparoscopy is usually due to a transient ventilation–perfusion mismatch that is commonly attributed to pulmonary shunting (Table 44-7). Physiologic changes induced during pneumoperitoneum and extreme positioning can reduce the number of ventilated alveolar units being perfused. Nonetheless, this ventilation–perfusion relationship during laparoscopy is still unclear, given the observation in the porcine animal model of hypoxic pulmonary vasoconstriction–mediated improvements in arterial oxygenation (PaO$_2$) after pneumoperitoneum, possibly due to perfusion redistribution away from atelectatic areas.[34,35]

Morbid obesity and chronic obstructive pulmonary disease (COPD) are common pre-existing conditions that may complicate ventilation and gas exchange during laparoscopy. Compensating for hypercarbia, managing inspiratory resistance, and maintaining normoxia in morbidly obese patients are common intraoperative dilemmas. The degree of instituted compensatory hyperventilation is a balance between the detrimental effects of extreme hypercarbia and the potential benefits of mild hypercapnia, which can improve tissue oxygenation, vasodilatation, and rightward shift of the oxyhemoglobin dissociation curve.[36,37] Before the induction of pneumoperitoneum under general anesthesia, morbidly obese patients can have an inspiratory resistance about 70% higher than nonobese patients. After Trendelenburg positioning, inspiratory resistance increases significantly. A sizable reduction in functional residual capacity (FRC) from pneumoperitoneum and Trendelenburg positioning in morbid obesity may greatly impair PaO$_2$.[38] High BMI alone may also be a stronger predictor of impaired PaO$_2$, despite compensatory ventilatory maneuvers.[39] Termination of pneumoperitoneum in morbidly obese patients can result in a

Table 44-7 Causes of Hypoxia during Laparoscopy

Pre-existing Comorbidities	Inadequate O$_2$ Supply or Gas Exchange	Low Cardiac Output State
Morbid obesity	Hypoventilation	Vena cava compression
Cardiopulmonary disease (e.g., congestive heart failure, chronic obstructive pulmonary disease)	Atelectasis	CO$_2$ venous embolism
	Endobronchial intubation	Capnothorax (CO$_2$ pneumothorax)
	Low inspired oxygen concentration	Capnomediastinum
		Capnopericardium
		Acute dysrhythmias
		Severe hemorrhage

prolonged return to baseline exhaled CO_2 compared to healthy patients,[40] potentially extending the need for ventilatory support. In patients with advanced COPD, severe hypercarbia and limited correlation with standard capnography is expected. A reduced number of intact pulmonary units and decreased effective alveolar ventilation can lead to a rapid and severe rise in $PaCO_2$ during pneumoperitoneum, that may be refractory to hyperventilation maneuvers. Increased alveolar physiologic space in these patients leads to a wide $PaCO_2$–$EtCO_2$ difference. As a result, $EtCO_2$ monitoring in COPD may underestimate the actual $PaCO_2$. Eventually, $PaCO_2$ levels return to a baseline values after deinsufflation.[41]

Regional Perfusion Effects

In healthy patients undergoing laparoscopy the splanchnic, renal, cerebral, and ocular organ systems undergo physiologic changes that are transient and of limited clinical significance (Table 44-8). Nonetheless, the magnitude of physiologic derangement and likelihood of iatrogenic injury are modified by the patients' underlying pathophysiology.

Splanchnic blood flow during laparoscopy may decrease both from external compression during pneumoperitoneum, and systemic vasoconstriction from released neuroendogenous hormones. IAP produced during pneumoperitoneum is known to reduce hepatic vein flow.[42] This physiologic occurrence may be advantageous during laparoscopic hepatic transection surgery, such that CO_2 peritoneum between 10 and 14 mmHg may be used to minimize bleeding.[43] Diminished mesenteric flow during pneumoperitoneum has been implicated in unusual cases of intraoperative mesenteric ischemia in cardiovascularly compromised patients.[44] Although splanchnic vasodilatation from absorbed CO_2 during pneumoperitoneum may offset any potential reductions in mesenteric blood flow in healthy patients, caution should be used in patients with known gastrointestinal coexisting diseases.

Renal function is reduced during pneumoperitoneum. IAP and neurohumoral effects of pneumoperitoneum may partly account for the reductions in renal blood flow, glomerular filtration, and urine output. Prolonged insufflation times at 15 mmHg IAP have been shown to correlate with reduced urine output without permanent renal sequelae.[45,46] Vasopressin release is induced partially by reduced renal perfusion, resulting in increased renal water reabsorption in the collecting ducts, and oliguria.[47,48] Preoperative risk factors for renal dysfunction may increase the risk of acute kidney injury (AKI) postoperatively. In bariatric surgery, increasing BMI and both insulin- and noninsulin-dependent diabetes mellitus was associated with acute kidney injury within 72 hours of surgery.[49] Though the use of intermittent sequential pneumatic compression devices during bariatric surgery has been shown to improve renal blood flow and urine output,[50] the mechanisms of action remain unclear, as well as its potential future role in AKI prevention.

Both intracranial pressure and cerebral perfusion increase during Trendelenburg positioning and pneumoperitoneum,[51] likely due to diminished cerebral venous outflow and hypercarbia-induced cerebral hyperperfusion. Although the cerebral venous blood fraction is increased from a reduction in cerebral venous drainage, regional cerebral tissue oxygen saturation appears to increase in this setting, possibly due to an increase in cerebral oxygen delivery from an elevated cerebral perfusion pressure and cerebral hyperperfusion.[52] Though these cerebral physiologic changes are usually well tolerated in healthy patients, prolonged steep Trendelenburg positioning with pneumoperitoneum has been associated with acute postoperative cerebral edema.[53] Cerebral physiologic changes during laparoscopy and extreme positioning carry serious theoretical implications for patients with known or occult cerebral vascular disease and intracranial tumors.

Intraocular pressure (IOP) increases during robotic prostatectomy surgery in steep Trendelenburg positioning.[54,55] The determinants of elevated IOP in this setting are theorized to be elevations in CVP from Trendelenburg positioning and increases in choroidal blood volume from absorbed CO_2 during insufflation.[54] Though IOP increases time-dependently and remains elevated during Trendelenburg positioning, postoperative visual function appears to remain unchanged.[54] Nonetheless, the role of IOP and other contributing factors in the development of postoperative ischemic optic neuropathy remains controversial. Rare cases of postoperative blindness after prolonged steep Trendelenburg positioning in laparoscopic prostatectomy[56] and colorectal surgery[57] have been reported. Pre-existing diseases, such as atherosclerotic disease, diabetes, and glaucoma, may lower the threshold of physiologic tolerance to acute intraocular derangements during laparoscopic surgery.

Intraoperative Management

General anesthesia with endotracheal intubation (GETA), muscle relaxation, and controlled mechanical ventilation remains the preferred anesthetic technique for laparoscopic surgery. Some factors that make laparoscopic surgery best suited for general anesthesia versus other anesthetic techniques include extreme patient positioning, discomfort from pneumoperitoneum, prolonged operative times, and induced cardiopulmonary derangements. Regional anesthesia, if considered, may be suited for brief laparoscopy procedures with minimal positioning changes.[22,58]

Table 44-8 Causes of Regional Perfusion Changes during Laparoscopy		
Cerebral	**Splanchnic**	**Systemic Vasculature**
↑Cerebral blood flow	↓ or, unchanged, intestinal flow Hypercapnic mesenteric vasodilatation Pneumoperitoneum bowel compression	↓Femoral vein flow IVC compression
↑Intracranial pressure	↓Hepatic flow Pneumoperitoneum hepatic compression ↓Renal flow Pneumoperitoneum renal compression	

Monitoring

Electrocardiography, noninvasive blood pressure, capnography, pulse oximetry, and body temperature monitors are mandatory for all laparoscopic procedures. Mechanical ventilation settings and pulmonary mechanics should be modified and measured via the anesthesia machine. Invasive or advanced noninvasive monitoring, such as arterial catheter, pulse contour analysis, pulmonary artery catheter, or echocardiography, may be considered if significant pre-existing cardiopulmonary disease is present. Reliability of CVP monitoring may be misleading, especially during steep Trendelenburg positioning. The role of additional monitors in laparoscopic procedures continue to evolve. Transcutaneous CO_2 monitoring, for example, may provide a close approximation to $PaCO_2$ in bariatric surgery,[59] and, in the future, may become a complementary device to $EtCO_2$ monitoring.

Anesthesia Maintenance

Inhaled Anesthetics and Propofol

The induction agent of choice in laparoscopy is propofol given its predictable pharmacokinetic profile, and its antiemetic properties.

Anesthesia maintenance with inhaled volatile anesthetics remains the standard anesthetic approach in laparoscopic surgery. Desflurane and sevoflurane are inhaled anesthetics with short-acting and easily titratable properties, ideally suited for ambulatory surgery.[44] Propofol-based total intravenous anesthesia (propofol-TIVA) has become a common anesthetic approach. Recent popularity of propofol-TIVA has been driven primarily by its associated lower incidence of postoperative nausea and vomiting (PONV), compared to inhaled anesthetics.[60] However, its cost, limited titratability, and infusion equipment set up have limited its broad appeal among anesthesia providers.[25,29] Choice of propofol as a maintenance anesthetic, compared to inhaled anesthetics, remains controversial. The incidence of PONV among patients with low PONV risk factors has been shown to be similar among patients receiving either a propofol-TIVA or an inhaled anesthetic combined with prophylactic antiemetics.[29] On the other hand, compared to balanced anesthesia with desflurane, propofol-TIVA during robotic laparoscopic prostatectomy may reduce the incidence and severity of PONV during the early postoperative recovery period.[61]

Nitrous Oxide

The use of nitrous oxide (N_2O) during laparoscopic surgery remains controversial. N_2O during anesthesia is believed to diffuse into air spaces, such as intestinal lumina, leading to adverse pressurization. However, detectable intestinal distension and disruption of laparoscopic surgical conditions does not appear to occur during an N_2O-based anesthetic.[62] N_2O is avoided by some practitioners due to a potentially greater risk of PONV. Although the risk of PONV with N_2O-based anesthetics seems to be greater than non-N_2O based anesthetics, particularly in young female patients, the overall risk in laparoscopy appears to be equivocal.[63] Additionally, the PONV risk associated with N_2O appears to be counterbalanced by antiemetic prophylaxis and propofol-based anesthetics. N_2O is known to support combustion during a spark ignition. During an N_2O-based anesthetic, N_2O has been shown to accumulate in the peritoneal cavity to combustion levels as early as 30 minutes[64] to as late as 2 hours.[64] Nonetheless, the incidence of spontaneous intra-abdominal laparoscopic surgical fire with N_2O is exceedingly rare. This may be explained by the mechanical circulation of peritoneal gases during pneumoperitoneum.

Pharmacologic Adjuncts

Lower postoperative pain is a benefit of laparoscopic surgery over conventional open surgery. A number of pharmacologic adjuncts are available for use during a balanced anesthetic to minimize intraoperative sympathetic stimulation, while optimizing postoperative recovery. Remifentanil significantly suppresses sympathetic stimulation and the neuroendocrine stress response during pneumoperitoneum[65] without the prolonged respiratory effects of longer-acting opioids. Dexmedetomidine infusion during bariatric surgery reduces fentanyl use, PONV, and PACU length of stay.[66] Lidocaine infusion administered during laparoscopic abdominal surgery has been associated with significant early postoperative pain reduction, as well as earlier return of gastrointestinal motility.[67–70] Wound infiltration or intraperitoneal instillation with a local anesthetic is routinely performed as part of a preemptive analgesia strategy.[71–73] Improvements in early postoperative pain scores have been shown in both wound infiltration[75,76] and intraperitoneal installation[77,78] of a long-acting local anesthetic. Continuous local anesthetic wound infiltration may have a role in laparoscopic-assisted surgical procedures with longer incisions.[74] Ultimately, controversy remains regarding medication safety, due to unclear concentration and dosing parameters for administered local anesthetics.

Neuromuscular Blockade

Neuromuscular blocking agents are routinely used to improve surgical exposure during pneumoperitoneum. Still, controversy remains about how to best define the role of neuromuscular blockade (NMB) in laparoscopic surgery,[79] while minimizing the potential respiratory complications associated with residual paralysis. Surrounding these concerns remains the topic of how surgeons and anesthetists define "optimal surgical working conditions." Subjective assessments of surgical working conditions during laparoscopy continue to vary between surgeons and anesthetists, as well as between surgeons.[82,83] Satisfaction scores from surgeons during laparoscopy are consistently higher during deep NMB than other levels of NMB.[82–84] Small trials show a correlation between deep NMB and improved surgical exposure during laparoscopic cholecystectomy at an IAP less than 15 mmHg,[80,81] thereby supporting the view that more muscle relaxation is invariably better for optimal surgical exposure. A more nuanced view of NMB in laparoscopy, however, might be preferable given that multiple factors, such as BMI, gender, and older age, may play a role in determining expected abdominal wall compliance changes.[81] Ultimately, until more effective reversal agents are widely available, such as Sugammadex, anesthetists must continue to balance the task of optimizing perceived operating conditions using NMB while minimizing risks to patients that may be more susceptible to postoperative respiratory complications from residual NMB.[85–87]

Mechanical Ventilation

Volume control (VC) and pressure control (PC) ventilation with positive end-expiratory pressure (PEEP) are the conventional modes of ventilation available during general endotracheal anesthesia (GETA). Both modes of ventilation are suitable to handle the transient effects of laparoscopy on lung mechanics and to control minute ventilation during pneumoperitoneum.[88]

Extreme positioning during pneumoperitoneum creates unique challenges to each mode. During VC in steep Trendelenburg, tidal volume remains constant while peak airway pressure increases and lung compliance decreases. In PC, peak airway pressure remains constant while tidal volume typically decreases. Conversely, reverse Trendelenburg typically induces the opposite ventilatory effects, that is, lower peak airway pressure and increased compliance with VC, and increased tidal volume with PC. Though switching from VC to PC during Trendelenburg may result in dynamic lung mechanic improvements, the effects do not appear to result in significant static lung changes, oxygenation improvements, or any other short-term benefit.[89]

Compensatory hyperventilation and PEEP may be employed if either hypercarbia or hypoxia are suspected. Hypercapnia during laparoscopic cholecystectomies in healthy patients may be normalized by increasing the minute ventilation about 25% above baseline.[90] Ventilation strategies that utilize PEEP can significantly improve ventilation–perfusion matching and preserve oxygenation.[91,92] The use of PEEP during pneumoperitoneum for extended laparoscopy may improve oxygenation.[93] Furthermore, alveolar recruitment maneuvers (RM) with the application of PEEP may have a profound effect in preventing the development of ventilator-induced lung injury by keeping alveoli open, especially in obese subjects.

The role of PEEP as a cause for hypotension in laparoscopy remains controversial. High PEEP levels in the presence of elevated IAP can further increase intrathoracic pressure and can contribute to a decrease in cardiac index.[21] However, a recent meta-analysis concluded that adding RM to PEEP in obese patients improved oxygenation and lung compliance without increasing the risk of hypotension from decreased preload.[88] Furthermore, the postoperative impact of RM and PEEP in the obese population remains controversial. Beach chair position and PEEP improve ventilatory mechanics and oxygenation during pneumoperitoneum.[94,95] Unfortunately, the beneficial effects of PEEP and recruitment maneuvers may only be short term and may induce hemodynamic instability in the hypovolemic patient. Ultimately, caution should be used when using compensatory ventilatory maneuvers because increased peak airway pressure may occur, especially during steep Trendelenburg positioning in morbidly obese patients.

The ideal inspired oxygen fraction (FiO_2) continues to be debated.[96] Oxygen delivery intraoperatively is speculated to have secondary effects in antiemesis, wound healing, and ventilation–perfusion mismatching. Yet, to date, data appear only to support the role of high FiO_2 in reducing surgical site infection with only a modest effect on PONV. Its role in inducing absorption atelectasis is not well supported. Therefore, judicious use of oxygen to assure adequate oxygenation, especially in obese populations and those with significant lung pathology, is prudent until more data are available.

Optimal ventilation strategies during GETA continue to be defined in light of limited trials convincingly showing harm with conventional ventilation strategies.[97,98] Nonetheless, rationale for using lung-protective ventilation strategies in the operating room borrows greatly from historical experience managing adult respiratory distress syndrome in the intensive care unit. Low tidal volumes (6 to 8 cc/kg IBW), optimized PEEP (5 to 10 cm H_2O, or greater), and RM continue to be the key components used to avoid ventilator-induced lung injury.

Body Temperature

Debate continues regarding the effects of CO_2 gas insufflation on heat loss during laparoscopic surgery. CO_2 gas used in laparoscopy is stored in pressurized cylinders in its cold, liquid phase. Phase transition from liquid to gas results in rapid heat extraction from the environment that is associated with release of a cold, desiccated gas. Convective heat losses during insufflation have been theorized to be worse when intraperitoneal contents are exposed to cold and dry CO_2 gas,[99] leading to the practice of actively warming and humidifying insufflated gas with an inline heating device.[100] To date, however, insufflation with heated and humidified CO_2 gas, compared to cold and dry CO_2 gas, for laparoscopic abdominal surgery has not been shown to be superior to conventional hypothermia preventive methods.[101] Temperature control and monitoring should follow standard ASA guidelines.

Fluid Management

Perioperative fluid management (see Chapter 16) is a controversial topic that in laparoscopy is further complicated by a unique interplay of surgical and physiologic alterations. Moreover, growing acceptance of enhanced recovery protocols in abdominal surgery,[102] which include clear, carbohydrate-rich fluid loading up to the morning of surgery, has changed perceptions of the classic intravascular "volume depleted" preoperative patient. Pneumoperitoneum may create volume shifts that can alter expected perioperative fluid therapy goals. In patients undergoing ambulatory laparoscopic cholecystectomy, intraoperative fluid loading with 40 mL/kg, compared with 15 mL/kg, of Ringer's lactate resulted in unexpected postoperative improvements in pulmonary function, exercise capacity, and overall well-being. Surgical stress markers were also reduced.[103] These findings suggest a benefit to high volume loading in the healthy patient undergoing elective ambulatory laparoscopy. In major abdominal laparoscopic surgery, however, perioperative fluid management approaches continue to be defined. In fluid therapy for robotic surgery, increasing age may impart a negative effect on the relationship between length of hospital stay and anastomosis integrity. Geriatric patients (age >70) who received more crystalloid or colloids showed higher rates of anastomotic leaks and longer hospital stays.[104]

Intraoperative fluid therapy based on classic hemodynamic and physiologic indicators may not be reliable. Pneumoperitoneum and steep Trendelenburg positioning, as previously discussed, alter the predictive value of heart rate, blood pressure, and central venous pressure. Pneumoperitoneum dramatically impacts the role of urine output as a surrogate for intravascular volume status. In laparoscopic bariatric surgery, high volume loading (10 mL/kg/h) compared to low volume loading (4 mL/kg/h) of Ringer's lactate resulted in similar rates of oliguria with no difference in renal dysfunction.[105,106] Though restricted fluid therapy approaches have gained momentum recently, insufficient evidence exists regarding the optimal total volume delivery, fluid timing, and role of intraoperative hemodynamic monitoring.[102,107] Intraoperative monitors for goal-directed fluid therapy, such as esophageal Doppler, pulse contour analysis, and bioreactance, are available for use at a clinician's discretion.

Positioning changes may alter fluid management. Steep Trendelenburg positioning may result in more craniofacial edema and airway compromise,[104] which might be ameliorated with intraoperative fluid restriction. A change to steep reverse Trendelenburg position during laparoscopic surgery for morbidly obese patients, compared to healthy normal weight patients, induces a significant change in pulse pressure variation, suggesting a low preload state and a need for rapid volume loading.[108]

Complications Related to Surgery

In properly selected patients and surgical procedures, laparoscopy continues to be as safe as open surgery worldwide.[109] Nonetheless, perioperative complications during laparoscopic surgery still occur with varying frequency and severity, including those attributable to surgical abdominal entry, pneumoperitoneum, and extreme patient positioning.[110] Greater risk of complications may exist in laparoscopy for upper abdominal procedures, robotic surgery, and in patients with significant preexisting diseases.[111–115] Any recognized life-threatening complication intraoperatively should result in immediate termination of laparoscopy and serious consideration to convert to an open laparotomy, if deemed appropriate.

Intraoperative

Intra-abdominal Injuries

Over 50% of complications related to laparoscopy are due to the abdominal entry techniques using the Veress needle and primary trocar insertion.[109] Major vascular injuries are infrequent, but are associated with high mortality rates when they do occur. Furthermore, they occur almost five times more often during blind abdominal entry than during the laparoscopic phase of the surgery. Major vessels at risk for injury during midline abdominal entry include the abdominal aorta, iliac vessels, and IVC. Abdominal entry away from the midline puts other vessels at risk, such as the superior and inferior mesenteric arteries, epigastric artery, and other small vessels of the abdominal wall. Vessels proximal to the site of surgical dissection are at increased risk of injury, such as the cystic and hepatic artery during laparoscopic cholecystectomy, and the dorsal vein complex during robotic prostatectomy. Though frank bleeding may be seen during a major vascular injury, most significant bleeding events during laparoscopy remain occult, requiring clinicians to have a high level of suspicion throughout the procedure. The anesthesiologist should be prepared for immediate surgical conversion to an open laparotomy to control severe bleeding, while managing possible hemodynamic instability due to hemorrhagic shock. Intraoperative testing and interpretation of hematocrit as an assessment of acute blood loss anemia should be performed cautiously, given the confounding effects of preoperative hematocrit collection, active bleeding, and intravascular dilution from crystalloid infusion. Transfusion triggers should be made on an individual basis, taking into account severity of bleeding, hemodynamics, and the patient's coexisting diseases. Preoperative requirement for type and screen testing for laparoscopy continues to be defined.[116] It has become less routine for ambulatory laparoscopy,[117] but continues to be determined by risk of more than minimal blood loss.

Gastrointestinal and urological structures can be injured during both the abdominal entry and the intra-abdominal portion of laparoscopic surgery.[109] Bowel injuries are infrequent but are a major cause of morbidity and mortality, resulting in high rates of laparotomy. Because most intestinal injuries go unrecognized, the risk of postoperative intra-abdominal sepsis is high, making it a common cause of death related to laparoscopy. Deflation of the stomach with an orogastric tube should be routinely performed to minimize the risk of gastric injury during left upper quadrant trocar insertion. Bladder perforation and ureter ligation or transection are also possible during laparoscopy and may present with low urine output, hematuria, and, rarely, pneumaturia. Postoperative hemodynamic instability or unexpected gross hematuria should trigger immediate suspicion of occult injury. Consultation with the surgeon and critical care specialist may be warranted postoperatively.

Cardiopulmonary

Acute cardiovascular complications associated with laparoscopy include hypertension, hypotension, dysrhythmias, and rarely cardiac arrest.[21] Hypertension is most common during the initial insufflation when an increase in IAP displaces blood from the splanchnic vasculature and leads to an increase in preload and cardiac output. Catecholamine release further aggravates hypertension by increasing afterload. Hypotension can sometimes be the result of a low cardiac output from vagal stimulation and impaired venous return during insufflation. Preload can be further reduced during positive pressure ventilation and steep reverse Trendelenburg positioning. Hypercapnia can increase PVR. This effect may further impact preload in patients with pulmonary hypertension or right ventricular failure. Tachyarrhythmias during intraperitoneal CO_2 insufflation are commonly due to catecholamine release and hypercapnia. A vagal-mediated cardiovascular reflex triggered by peritoneal stretching can induce bradyarrhythmias, which can range from sinus bradycardia to more life-threatening nodal rhythms. Profound vasovagal reaction to rapid peritoneal distention during insufflation has been implicated in acute cardiovascular collapse and cardiac arrest.[21,118] Treatment of acute cardiovascular disturbances should be based on the cardiophysiologic disturbance. Acute hypertension is often transient, and may be ameliorated by adjusting the depth of anesthesia. More severe cases may require short-acting vasoactive agents. Hypotension is usually responsive to decreasing depth of anesthesia, volume expansion, lower IAP insufflation, and short-acting vasopressors. If treatment of hypotension involves peritoneal deflation, slow re-insufflation with lower IAP should be attempted. Conversion to open laparotomy or termination of surgery may be indicated if there is recurrent hypotension. Refractory hypotension may require immediate abdominal decompression, return to neutral patient position, and exploration of occult life-threatening conditions, such as severe bleeding or capnothorax.

Pulmonary complications that develop during laparoscopy can present as acute hypercarbic (Table 44-6) and hypoxemic (Table 44-7) events. Treatment of refractory hypercarbia usually involves cessation of insufflation. If severe hypercarbia persists during emergence, particularly in the setting of significant pulmonary disease, such as severe OSA, or if airway compromise from subcutaneous emphysema is suspected, persistent ventilator support should be considered. Treatment of hypoxemia should be swift, focusing on confirming O_2 delivery and endotracheal tube positioning. Immediate pneumoperitoneum release, 100% O_2 ventilation, and neutral positioning should be instituted for refractory hypoxia.

CO_2 Extravasation

Subcutaneous Emphysema

The inadvertent introduction of CO_2 gas into subcutaneous, preperitoneal, or retroperitoneal tissue leads to trapped gas pockets called subcutaneous emphysema.[119,120] Extension of extraperitoneal CO_2 gas along fascial planes can lead to distant anatomic areas being affected, such as the upper and lower extremities, neck, and face, as well as large cavities, such as the thorax, mediastinum, and pericardium. Risk factors for the development of subcutaneous emphysema include longer operative times (i.e., more than 200 minutes), greater number of surgical ports, lower BMI, older patient age, higher IAP, higher insufflation flow rates, and Nissen fundoplication surgery.[119–122] Subcutaneous emphysema may present as crepitus on physical exam, but remains largely undetected unless a computed tomography or x-ray is performed postoperatively. Unexplained sudden or persistent hypercarbia or acute hypotension may be early signs of subcutaneous emphysema or capnothorax, respectively.[122] The treatment of subcutaneous emphysema is peritoneal deinsufflation; however, no intervention is required in most cases. Reinsufflation at a lower IAP is recommended if pneumoperitoneum must be resumed. Postoperative treatment is supportive. Extravasated CO_2 resolves within 24 hours due to its high rate of diffusion. If concerns for persistent or recurrent hypercarbia from subcutaneous emphysema exist during the postoperative recovery, clinicians should maintain oxygen therapy and monitor for somnolence and acute respiratory acidosis by arterial blood gas. Cervical emphysema should be evaluated with a chest x-ray and the airway should be evaluated for signs of obstruction.

Capnothorax

Carbon dioxide gas accumulation within the pleural space is called capnothorax. It is an unintentional complication of CO_2 insufflation that occurs when CO_2 travels outside the peritoneum, enters the mediastinum, and subsequently dissects along the pleura. Tension capnothorax may occur from uncontrolled pressurization of the thoracic cavity, leading to an increase in intrathoracic pressure, mediastinal shift, decreased venous return, and subsequent right ventricular compression—a potentially life-threatening condition.[110,119]

Insufflated CO_2 can pass from the abdomen and into the thorax through various routes.[123,124] There are several anatomic defects in the diaphragm that connect the abdominal and thoracic cavities, most notably the aortic hiatus, esophageal hiatus, and caval opening. These defects, in addition to other smaller openings, are believed to serve as channels through which CO_2 can exit out of the abdomen and into the pleural spaces. Risk factors for capnothorax are similar to those for subcutaneous emphysema; however, greater risk exists during procedures near the diaphragm.[111,125] Tension capnothorax can occur during dissection along the diaphragm (e.g., Nissen fundoplication), unrecognized mechanical injury of the diaphragm (e.g., unrecognized trocar injury), or, very rarely, through congenital pleuro-diaphragmatic channels.[119]

Early signs of capnothorax may include palpable subcutaneous emphysema in the upper torso, severe hypercarbia, and changes in electrical axis and reduced amplitude of the ECG. Physical exam findings may include reduced breath sounds bilaterally or unilaterally, as well as reduced chest excursion.[126] Tension capnothorax may present more acutely with high peak airway pressure, hypoxia, and severe hypotension.[124] Tension capnothorax can be a life-threatening condition that may be difficult to accurately diagnose intraoperatively, therefore, a high index of suspicion and quick communication with the surgical team is often necessary to rescue a patient from harm. Postoperative imaging may be useful to confirm diagnosis of capnothorax. Transthoracic echocardiography is increasingly being used to assess lung pathology, including intraoperative pneumothorax.[127] However, its role in diagnosing capnothorax has not been well defined.

Primary treatment of capnothorax is immediate peritoneal deinsufflation. Hyperventilation can be used to expedite CO_2 reabsorption. Also, the addition of PEEP can reduce the pressure gradient between the abdomen and the thorax during both inspiration and expiration. Close observation is usually adequate for healthy patients with minimal physiologic derangements.[123,124,128] Patients with baseline cardiac dysfunction may be more likely to require supportive therapy. The hemodynamic unstable patient should be supported with fluids or vasoactive agents while the capnothorax is reabsorbed. In severe cases, emergent needle decompression or chest tube insertion may be necessary intraoperatively. If tension capnothorax and hemodynamic instability recur after reinsufflation, termination of laparoscopy and conversion to an open surgical procedure may be indicated.

Other thoracic structures rarely at risk for CO_2 dissection and compression include the mediastinum and pericardium. Severe capnomediastinum and capnopericardium may be associated with severe hemodynamic instability due to excessive pressure of large mediastinal vascular structures and cardiac chambers. Treatment and postoperative management is similar to tension capnothorax.

Venous Gas Embolism

Venous CO_2 gas embolism is a potentially fatal complication of laparoscopy that occurs when large CO_2 gas bubbles enter the venous system, circulate to the heart, and result in right ventricular chamber gas lock and a subsequent venous outflow obstruction.[129] Although the consequence of CO_2 embolism can be severe, clinically significant occurrence is rare. Fatalities from suspected gas embolism occurred in seven patients in a retrospective review of 500,000 closed-entry laparoscopies, over three decades.[130] The reported incidence is varied. According to several case-series, the risk of gas embolism during laparoscopic major hepatectomy may be less than 1.5%, with an unclear correlation to morbidity and mortality.[131] Availability of ultrasound for intraoperative monitoring has allowed clinicians to detect previously undetected gas embolisms during laparoscopic surgery. Clinicians using intraoperative transesophageal echocardiography (TEE) have reported subclinical CO_2 gas embolisms in approximately 20% of laparoscopic radical prostatectomies to almost 100% of laparoscopic total hysterectomies.[132,133]

The etiology of a venous CO_2 gas embolism during laparoscopic surgery, and its degree of hemodynamic impact, is likely multifactorial. Direct Veress needle insertion into a vein or solid organ during insufflation could potentially result in CO_2 entry into the venous system. Open, transected vessels during laparoscopic surgical dissection may result in sudden gas venous ingress and a CO_2 gas embolism. Round ligament transection and broad ligament dissection during laparoscopic hysterectomy have resulted in gas embolisms.[133] The deep dorsal venous complex is a major source of bleeding during radical prostatectomies and a potential source of gas embolism during vessel transection.[134] Patient positioning may play a role in the degree of CO_2 gas entrainment into the right heart chambers. In the animal model, laparoscopic hepatectomies in the reverse Trendelenburg position preferentially resulted in venous gas embolisms.[135] Steep Trendelenburg positioning during robotic radical prostatectomies appears to protect against venous gas embolism compared to open radical retropubic prostatectomies.[134]

Vigilance is important for the early detection of a venous CO_2 gas embolism. Diagnosis is usually dependent on the constellation of clinical signs associated with gas emboli. The severity and presence of these signs vary widely. Acute tachycardia, cardiac arrhythmias, QRS complex widening, hypotension, hypoxemia, and low end-tidal CO_2 may be seen by monitoring. Physical exam findings may include cyanosis and a "mill wheel" murmur

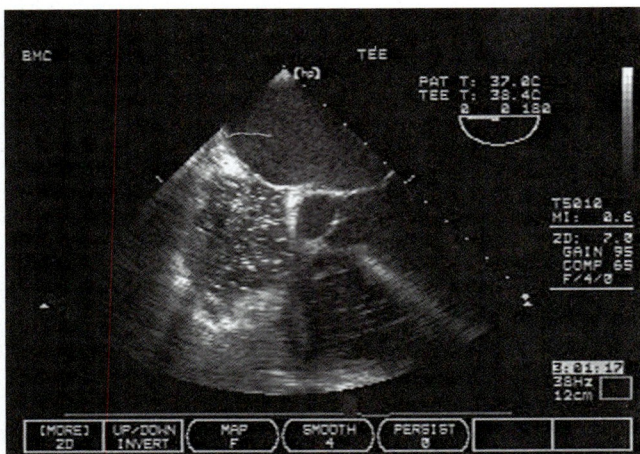

Figure 44-2 Venous air embolism of the right atrium visible with transesophageal echocardiographic monitoring.

by auscultation. TEE is considered the most sensitive method for detecting gas emboli in the heart.[136] A large bolus of CO_2 gas would appear as a near white-out of the right heart chambers, potentially leading to a right ventricular air lock (Fig. 44-2). Because micro air bubbles are present in most peripherally injected solutions, clinicians using TEE must be ready to distinguish CO_2 gas bubbles from peripherally injected bubbles. This can be facilitated by viewing the IVC during TEE monitoring.

Treatment of a massive CO_2 gas embolism requires immediate action. Pneumoperitoneum should be immediately terminated and the abdomen decompressed. Advanced cardiac life support should be initiated for cardiac arrest. Rapid intravenous fluid may be initiated for hypotension. CO_2 gas removal may be accelerated with hyperventilation and administration of 100% O_2. If deemed necessary, the patient may be placed in Trendelenburg with a left lateral decubitus position to help minimize the severity of right ventricular air lock.

Patient Shifting and Falls

Extreme positioning and potential for injury are common in laparoscopic procedures, particularly in robot-assisted laparoscopy. Patients undergoing laparoscopy in steep reverse Trendelenburg and steep Trendelenburg are at risk of unexpectedly shifting down or up on the operating room table. Operating rooms table falls are rare,[137] but potentially devastating. The anesthesiologists should actively take part in positioning and ensuring safe securement of the anesthetized patient. A patient in steep Trendelenburg may be secured from moving by using an operating table belt strap. Additional accessories may include an underbody gel pad for skid prevention, lithotomy stirrups with Velcro straps, and a surgical beanbag device. Careful attention should be paid to pressure points created by the securing devices. During steep reverse Trendelenburg positioning, a padded footrest can be attached to the operating room table to keep a patient from shifting down and off the table.

Ocular Injuries

Steep Trendelenburg positioning during laparoscopic robotic surgery alters ophthalmic physiology and may increase the risk of both corneal abrasion and ischemic optic neuropathy–associated blindness.[56,138] The theorized mechanisms of injury may be independent or an interplay between external and internal stressors.[139] The mechanism of corneal abrasion is proposed to be mediated predominantly by external risk factors, such as direct ocular trauma, corneal exposure, and corneal dehydration.[140] Eye patches, in addition to eye taping, may further reduce risk of corneal abrasions in robotic prostatectomies.[104] Prolonged steep Trendelenburg position and large volume fluid therapy may increase IOP and venous congestion acutely, thereby potentially leading to optic canal ischemia and subsequent blindness.

Peripheral Nerve and Brachial Plexus Injuries

A large number of nerve injuries acquired intraoperatively are due to patient positioning.[141] The mechanism of injury may involve excessive compression, stretch, and ischemia. Risk factors include prolonged operative times, high BMI, inadequate padding, arm tucking, steep Trendelenburg positioning, and improper beanbag use. The brachial plexopathy is highly associated with steep Trendelenburg and longer operative time in laparoscopic colorectal surgery,[142] and caudad shoulder displacement during robotic prostatectomy.[143] Recommendations for risk reduction continue to evolve. In the meantime careful attention to positioning throughout the operative course is imperative.

Airway Edema

Prolonged steep Trendelenburg position during robotic prostatectomy and large volume fluid resuscitation may induce facial and pharyngo-laryngeal edema,[104] which can result in airway compromise postoperatively. A recumbent sitting position may expedite reversal of any orofacial edema during emergence and postoperative recovery. A cuff leak test may be reasonable to perform prior to extubation; however, its role in ruling out significant laryngeal edema in the intraoperative, noncritically ill, patient is not well defined. If concerns for severe airway edema exist intraoperatively, a plan for continued intubation and ventilatory support should be made.[104]

Postoperative Complications

Respiratory Dysfunction

A significant benefit of laparoscopy over laparotomy is improved pulmonary function and reduced postoperative respiratory complications. Albeit rare, the potential for postoperative respiratory dysfunction after laparoscopy surgery still exists and may be modified by coexisting diseases, surgery specific factors, and any reported intraoperative pulmonary challenges. In bariatric surgery, patients with active reflux disease may be at risk for postoperative aspiration events and exacerbation of reactive airway disease.[144] Significant subcutaneous emphysema in the setting of coexisting lung disease may overwhelm a patient's ability to compensate for severe hypercarbia. Diaphragmatic dysfunction after laparoscopy has been reported[145,146] and can infrequently lead to respiratory dysfunction.[147]

Venous Thrombosis

Coagulation cascade activation and venous outflow obstruction during CO_2 pneumoperitoneum are suspected pathophysiologic factors for acute venous thromboembolism (VTE).[148,149] Prevalence of deep venous thrombosis and pulmonary embolism associated with laparoscopic surgery is low. Still, surgical disease, associated comorbidities, and age modify the patient's risk of VTE in laparoscopic surgery.[151] The prevalence of in-hospital VTE after laparoscopic cholecystectomy increases with age, but overall remains low.[150,151] Obesity is a known hypercoagulable risk factor with a greater negative impact on women than men.[152] Lymph node dissection during radical prostatectomy carries a significant risk of DVT and PE postoperatively, albeit lower if the surgery is performed robotically.[153]

Postoperative Management

Acute Pain Management

Postoperative pain has a significant impact on patient recovery, early mobilization, length of hospital stay, and a return to normal activity. Compared to open abdominal surgery, laparoscopic surgery results in less pain, shorter duration of pain, and less opioid consumption.[154] A number of surgical techniques can reduce the severity of postoperative pain after laparoscopy. These include the use of lower IAP,[11] shorter duration of pneumoperitoneum, and evacuation of subdiaphragmatic CO_2 gas prior to wound closure.[155] Parenteral analgesics and regional anesthesia are common options for postoperative pain management. However, a preferred approach is a preemptive multimodal strategy[71,156] that relies predominately on nonopioids, such as NSAIDS, COX-2 inhibitors,[157] and acetaminophen,[158-160] and minimal weak opioids.[71] These nonopioid analgesics may adequately control acute postoperative pain, while minimizing adverse effects of opioids. Although the role of transversus abdominis plane block remains unclear, this procedure remains a viable option for postoperative pain management after laparoscopic surgery.[161-164] Neuraxial analgesia is not a routine strategy employed in laparoscopic abdominal surgery,[154,165] unless potential exists for conversion to open laparotomy.

Postoperative Nausea and Vomiting

Evidence suggests that patients undergoing laparoscopic surgery are at greater risk of PONV than patients undergoing nonlaparoscopic surgery. Cholecystectomy has been reported to be the highest, independent predictor of PONV, followed by laparoscopic surgery.[166] In laparoscopic bariatric surgery, PONV is a common cause of prolonged anesthesia recovery.[167] Several additional PONV risk factors exist for patients undergoing laparoscopic surgery, including inhaled volatile anesthetics, perioperative opioids administration, younger age, female gender, and nonsmoking status. PONV management should be based on assessing level of PONV risk, baseline risk reduction of known PONV triggers, patient consideration, and cost effectiveness.[168] Optimal antiemetic prophylaxis is the key for minimizing prolonged postanesthesia recovery.

Conclusion

Laparoscopic surgery has been a revolutionary alternative to many open surgical procedures. Its ability to provide surgeons the means to operate with minimal surgical trauma while providing patients a shorter postoperative recovery has made it critical to the growth of ambulatory surgery. Advances in technology have introduced robotics as a common and growing feature of minimally invasive surgery. For the anesthetists, "minimally invasive" surgery requires maximally attentive anesthesia. Pneumoperitoneum in conjunction with extreme patient positioning induces transient, but significant, multiorgan derangements that require short-term manipulation of physiology to minimize complications. Because serious complications related to surgery can occur at any stage during the intraoperative and postoperative course, constant vigilance and action are critical to avoiding permanent injury or death. Preemptive multimodal analgesia and PONV prophylaxis strategies in laparoscopy are the keys to optimal postoperative recovery.

REFERENCES

1. Weinberg L, Rao S, Escobar PF. Robotic surgery in gynecology: an updated systematic review. *Obstet Gynecol Int.* 2011;2011:852061.
2. Finkelstein J, Eckersberger E, Sadri H, et al. Open versus laparoscopic versus robot-assisted laparoscopic prostatectomy: the European and US Experience. *Rev Urol.* 2010;12(1):35–43.
3. Hanly EJ, Talamini MA. Robotic abdominal surgery. *Am J Surg.* 2004;188 (4A Suppl):19S–26S.
4. Mack MJ. Minimally invasive and robotic surgery. *JAMA.* 2001;285(5):568–572.
5. Gurusamy K, Junnarkar S, Farouk M, Davidson BR. Meta-analysis of randomized controlled trials on the safety and effectiveness of day-case laparoscopic cholecystectomy. *Br J Surg.* 2008;95(2):161–168.
6. Gurusamy KS, Junnarkar S, Farouk M, et al. Day-case versus overnight stay in laparoscopic cholecystectomy. *Cochrane Database Syst Rev.* 2008;(1):CD006798.
7. Thomas H, Agrawal S. Systematic review of day-case laparoscopic fundoplication. *J Laparoendosc Adv Surg Tech A.* 2011;21(9):781–788.
8. Thomas H, Agrawal S. Systematic review of same-day laparoscopic adjustable gastric band surgery. *Obes Surg.* 2011;21(6):805–810.
9. Thomas H, Agrawal S. Systematic review of 23-hour (outpatient) stay laparoscopic gastric bypass surgery. *J Laparoendosc Adv Surg Tech A.* 2011;21(8):677–681.
10. Walter CJ, Collin J, Dumville JC, et al. Enhanced recovery in colorectal resections: a systematic review and meta-analysis. *Colorectal Dis.* 2009;11(4):344–353.
11. Gurusamy KS, Samraj K, Davidson BR. Low pressure versus standard pressure pneumoperitoneum in laparoscopic cholecystectomy. *Cochrane Database Syst Rev.* 2009;15(2):CD006930.
12. Gurusamy KS, Koti R, Davidson BR. Abdominal lift for laparoscopic cholecystectomy. *Cochrane Database Syst Rev.* 2013;8:CD006574.
13. Gunning JE RB. Evolution of endoscopic surgery. In: White RA, ed. *Endoscopic Surgery.* Boston, MA: Mosby Year Book; 1991:1–9.
14. Brash JH. Outpatient laparoscopic sterilization. *Br Med J.* 1976;1(6022):1376–1377.
15. Thompson B, Wheeless RC. Outpatient sterilization by laparoscopy: a report of 666 patients. *Obstet Gynecol.* 1971;38(6):912–915.
16. Vaughan J, Gurusamy KS, Davidson BR. Day-surgery versus overnight stay surgery for laparoscopic cholecystectomy. *Cochrane Database Syst Rev.* 2013;7: CD006798.
17. Hinojosa MW, Varela JE, Parikh D, et al. National trends in use and outcome of laparoscopic adjustable gastric banding. *Surg Obes Relat Dis.* 2009;5(2):150–155.
18. Abou Rached A, Basile M, El Masri H. Gastric leaks post sleeve gastrectomy: review of its prevention and management. *World J Gastroenterol.* 2014;20(38):13904–13910.
19. Joshi GP, Ahmad S, Riad W, et al. Selection of obese patients undergoing ambulatory surgery: a systematic review of the literature. *Anesth Analg.* 2013;117(5):1082–1091.
20. O'Malley C, Cunningham AJ. Physiologic changes during laparoscopy. *Anesthesiol Clin North Am.* 2001;19(1):1–19.
21. Gutt CN, Oniu T, Mehrabi A, et al. Circulatory and respiratory complications of carbon dioxide insufflation. *Dig Surg.* 2004;21(2):95–105.
22. Collins LM, Vaghadia H. Regional anesthesia for laparoscopy. *Anesthesiol Clin North Am.* 2001;19(1):43–55.
23. Sammour T, Mittal A, Loveday BPT, et al. Systematic review of oxidative stress associated with pneumoperitoneum. *Br J Surg.* 2009;96(8):836–850.
24. Gannedahl P, Odeberg S, Brodin LA, et al. Effects of posture and pneumoperitoneum during anaesthesia on the indices of left ventricular filling. *Acta Anaesthesiol Scand.* 1996;40(2):160–166.
25. Tonner PH, Scholz J. Total intravenous or balanced anaesthesia in ambulatory surgery? *Curr Opin Anaesthesiol.* 2000;13(6):631–636.

26. Nguyen NT, Wolfe BM. The physiologic effects of pneumoperitoneum in the morbidly obese. *Ann Surg.* 2005;241(2):219–226.
27. Harris SN, Ballantyne GH, Luther MA, Perrino AC. Alterations of cardiovascular performance during laparoscopic colectomy: a combined hemodynamic and echocardiographic analysis. *Anesth Analg.* 1996;83(3):482–487.
28. Chin KM, Kim NHS, Rubin LJ. The right ventricle in pulmonary hypertension. *Coron Artery Dis.* 2005;16(1):13–18.
29. Joshi GP. Inhalational techniques in ambulatory anesthesia. *Anesthesiol Clin North America.* 2003;21(2):263–272.
30. Falabella A, Moore-Jeffries E, Sullivan MJ, et al. Cardiac function during steep Trendelenburg position and CO_2 pneumoperitoneum for robotic-assisted prostatectomy: a trans-oesophageal Doppler probe study. *Int J Med Robot.* 2007; 3(4):312–315.
31. Lestar M, Gunnarsson L, Lagerstrand L, et al. Hemodynamic perturbations during robot-assisted laparoscopic radical prostatectomy in 45° Trendelenburg position. *Anesth Analg.* 2011;113(5):1069–1075.
32. Kadam PG, Marda M, Shah VR. Carbon dioxide absorption during laparoscopic donor nephrectomy: a comparison between retroperitoneal and transperitoneal approaches. *Transplant Proc.* 2008;40(4):1119–1121.
33. Schrijvers D, Mottrie A, Traen K, et al. Pulmonary gas exchange is well preserved during robot assisted surgery in steep Trendelenburg position. *Acta Anaesthesiol Belg.* 2009;60(4):229–233.
34. Strang CM, Fredén F, Maripuu E, et al. Ventilation-perfusion distributions and gas exchange during carbon dioxide pneumoperitoneum in a porcine model. *Br J Anaesth.* 2010;105(5):691–697.
35. Strang CM, Ebmeyer U, Maripuu E, et al. Improved ventilation-perfusion matching by abdominal insufflation (pneumoperitoneum) with CO_2 but not with air. *Minerva Anestesiol.* 2013;79(6):617–625.
36. Hager H, Reddy D, Mandadi G, et al. Hypercapnia improves tissue oxygenation in morbidly obese surgical patients. *Anesth Analg.* 2006;103(3): 677–681.
37. Fleischmann E, Herbst F, Kugener A, et al. Mild hypercapnia increases subcutaneous and colonic oxygen tension in patients given 80% inspired oxygen during abdominal surgery. *Anesthesiology.* 2006;104(5):944–949.
38. Pelosi P, Croci M, Ravagnan I, et al. The effects of body mass on lung volumes, respiratory mechanics, and gas exchange during general anesthesia. *Anesth Analg.* 1998;87(3):654–660.
39. Sprung J, Whalley DG, Falcone T, et al. The effects of tidal volume and respiratory rate on oxygenation and respiratory mechanics during laparoscopy in morbidly obese patients. *Anesth Analg.* 2003;97(1):268–274.
40. Perilli V, Vitale F, Modesti C, et al. Carbon dioxide elimination pattern in morbidly obese patients undergoing laparoscopic surgery. *Surg Obes Relat Dis.* 2012;8(5):590–594.
41. Kwak HJ, Jo YY, Lee KC, et al. Acid-base alterations during laparoscopic abdominal surgery: a comparison with laparotomy. *Br J Anaesth.* 2010; 105(4):442–447.
42. Takagi S. Hepatic and portal vein blood flow during carbon dioxide pneumoperitoneum for laparoscopic hepatectomy. *Surg Endosc.* 1998;12(5):427–431.
43. Tranchart H, O'Rourke N, Van Dam R, et al. Bleeding control during laparoscopic liver resection: a review of literature. *J Hepatobiliary Pancreat Sci.* 2015;22(5):371–378.
44. Leduc LJ, Mitchell A. Intestinal ischemia after laparoscopic cholecystectomy. *JSLS.* 2006;10(2):236–238.
45. McDougall EM, Monk TG, Wolf JS, et al. The effect of prolonged pneumoperitoneum on renal function in an animal model. *J Am Coll Surg.* 1996; 182(4):317–328.
46. Nguyen NT, Perez R V, Fleming N, et al. Effect of prolonged pneumoperitoneum on intraoperative urine output during laparoscopic gastric bypass. *J Am Coll Surg.* 2002;195(4):476–483.
47. Viinamki O, Punnonen R. Vasopressin release during laparoscopy: role of increased intra-abdominal pressure. *Lancet.* 1982;1(8264):175–176.
48. Melville RJ, Frizis HI, Forsling ML, et al. The stimulus for vasopressin release during laparoscopy. *Surg Gynecol Obstet.* 1985;161(3):253–256.
49. Weingarten TN, Gurrieri C, McCaffrey JM, et al. Acute kidney injury following bariatric surgery. *Obes Surg.* 2013;23(1):64–70.
50. Bickel A, Loberant N, Bersudsky M, et al. Overcoming reduced hepatic and renal perfusion caused by positive-pressure pneumoperitoneum. *Arch Surg.* 2007;142(2):119–124.
51. Halverson A, Buchanan R, Jacobs L, et al. Evaluation of mechanism of increased intracranial pressure with insufflation. *Surg Endosc.* 1998;12(3):266–269.
52. Kalmar AF, Foubert L, Hendrickx JF, et al. Influence of steep Trendelenburg position and CO_2 pneumoperitoneum on cardiovascular, cerebrovascular, and respiratory homeostasis during robotic prostatectomy. *Br J Anaesth.* 2010; 104(4):433–439.
53. Pandey R, Garg R, Darlong V, et al. Unpredicted neurological complications after robotic laparoscopic radical cystectomy and ileal conduit formation in steep Trendelenburg position: two case reports. *Acta Anaesthiol Belg.* 2010;61(3):163–166.
54. Hoshikawa Y, Tsutsumi N, Ohkoshi K, et al. The effect of steep Trendelenburg positioning on intraocular pressure and visual function during robotic-assisted radical prostatectomy. *Br J Ophthalmol.* 2014;98(3):305–308.
55. Awad H, Santilli S, Ohr M, et al. The effects of steep Trendelenburg positioning on intraocular pressure during robotic radical prostatectomy. *Anesth Analg.* 2009;109(2):473–478.
56. Weber ED, Colyer MH, Lesser RL, et al. Posterior ischemic optic neuropathy after minimally invasive prostatectomy. *J Neuroophthalmol.* 2007;27(4): 285–287.
57. Kumar G, Vyakarnam P. Postoperative vision loss after colorectal laparoscopic surgery. *Surg Laparosc Endosc Percutan Tech.* 2013;23(2):e87–e88.
58. Smith I. Anesthesia for laparoscopy with emphasis on outpatient laparoscopy. *Anesthesiol Clin North Am.* 2001;19(1):21–41.
59. Dion JM, McKee C, Tobias JD, et al. Carbon dioxide monitoring during laparoscopic-assisted bariatric surgery in severely obese patients: transcutaneous versus end-tidal techniques. *J Clin Monit Comput.* 2015;29(1):183–186.
60. Kumar G, Stendall C, Mistry R, et al. A comparison of total intravenous anaesthesia using propofol with sevoflurane or desflurane in ambulatory surgery: systematic review and meta-analysis. *Anaesthesia.* 2014;69(10):1138–1150.
61. Yoo Y-C, Bai S-J, Lee K-Y, et al. Total intravenous anesthesia with propofol reduces postoperative nausea and vomiting in patients undergoing robot-assisted laparoscopic radical prostatectomy: a prospective randomized trial. *Yonsei Med J.* 2012;53(6):1197–1202.
62. Taylor E, Feinstein R, White PF, et al. Anesthesia for laparoscopic cholecystectomy. Is nitrous oxide contraindicated? *Anesthesiology.* 1992;76(4):541–543.
63. Fernández-Guisasola J, Gómez-Arnau JI, Cabrera Y, et al. Association between nitrous oxide and the incidence of postoperative nausea and vomiting in adults: a systematic review and meta-analysis. *Anaesthesia.* 2010;65(4):379–387.
64. Neuman GG, Sidebotham G, Negoianu E, et al. Laparoscopic explosion hazards with nitrous oxide. *Anesthesiology.* 1993;78(5):875–879.
65. Watanabe K, Kashiwagi K, Kamiyama T, et al. High-dose remifentanil suppresses stress response associated with pneumoperitoneum during laparoscopic colectomy. *J Anesth.* 2014;28(3):334–340.
66. Tufanogullari B, White PF, Peixoto MP, et al. Dexmedetomidine infusion during laparoscopic bariatric surgery: the effect on recovery outcome variables. *Anesth Analg.* 2008;106(6):1741–1748.
67. Kranke P, Jokinen J, Pace NL, et al. Continuous intravenous perioperative lidocaine infusion for postoperative pain and recovery. *Cochrane Database Syst Rev.* 2015;7:CD009642.
68. Marret E, Rolin M, Beaussier M, et al. Meta-analysis of intravenous lidocaine and postoperative recovery after abdominal surgery. *Br J Surg.* 2008;95(11): 1331–1338.
69. McCarthy GC, Megalla SA, Habib AS. Impact of intravenous lidocaine infusion on postoperative analgesia and recovery from surgery: a systematic review of randomized controlled trials. *Drugs.* 2010;70(9):1149–1163.
70. Vigneault L, Turgeon AF, Côté D, et al. Perioperative intravenous lidocaine infusion for postoperative pain control: a meta-analysis of randomized controlled trials. *Can J Anaesth.* 2011;58(1):22–37.
71. Kehlet H, Gray AW, Bonnet F, et al. A procedure-specific systematic review and consensus recommendations for postoperative analgesia following laparoscopic cholecystectomy. *Surg Endosc.* 2005;19(10):1396–1415.
72. Møiniche S, Jørgensen H, Wetterslev J, et al. Local anesthetic infiltration for postoperative pain relief after laparoscopy: a qualitative and quantitative systematic review of intraperitoneal, port-site infiltration and mesosalpinx block. *Anesth Analg.* 2000;90(4):899–912.
73. Gupta A. Local anaesthesia for pain relief after laparoscopic cholecystectomy—a systematic review. *Best Pract Res Clin Anaesthesiol.* 2005;19(2):275–292.
74. Thornton PC, Buggy DJ. Local anaesthetic wound infusion for acute postoperative pain: a viable option? *Br J Anaesth.* 2011;107(5):656–658.
75. Loizides S, Gurusamy KS, Nagendran M, et al. Wound infiltration with local anaesthetic agents for laparoscopic cholecystectomy. *Cochrane Database Syst Rev.* 2014;3:CD007049.
76. Gurusamy KS, Nagendran M, Guerrini GP, et al. Intraperitoneal local anaesthetic instillation versus no intraperitoneal local anaesthetic instillation for laparoscopic cholecystectomy. *Cochrane Database Syst Rev.* 2014;3:CD007337.
77. Kahokehr A, Sammour T, Soop M, et al. Intraperitoneal use of local anesthetic in laparoscopic cholecystectomy: systematic review and meta-analysis of randomized controlled trials. *J Hepatobiliary Pancreat Sci.* 2010;17(5):637–656.
78. Kahokehr A, Sammour T, Srinivasa S, Hill AG. Systematic review and meta-analysis of intraperitoneal local anaesthetic for pain reduction after laparoscopic gastric procedures. *Br J Surg.* 2011;98(1):29–36.
79. Kopman AF, Naguib M. Laparoscopic surgery and muscle relaxants: is deep block helpful? *Anesth Analg.* 2015;120(1):51–58.
80. Staehr-Rye AK, Rasmussen LS, Rosenberg J, et al. Surgical space conditions during low-pressure laparoscopic cholecystectomy with deep versus moderate neuromuscular blockade: a randomized clinical study. *Anesth Analg.* 2014; 119(5):1084–1092.
81. Van Wijk RM, Watts RW, Ledowski T, et al. Deep neuromuscular block reduces intra-abdominal pressure requirements during laparoscopic cholecystectomy: a prospective observational study. *Acta Anaesthesiol Scand.* 2015; 59(4):434–440.
82. Martini CH, Boon M, Bevers RF, et al. Evaluation of surgical conditions during laparoscopic surgery in patients with moderate vs deep neuromuscular block. *Br J Anaesth.* 2014;112(3):498–505.

83. Blobner M, Frick CG, Stäuble RB, et al. Neuromuscular blockade improves surgical conditions (NISCO). Surg Endosc. 2015;29(3):627–636.
84. Dubois PE, Putz L, Jamart J, et al. Deep neuromuscular block improves surgical conditions during laparoscopic hysterectomy: a randomised controlled trial. Eur J Anaesthesiol. 2014;31(8):430–436.
85. Murphy GS, Brull SJ. Residual neuromuscular block: lessons unlearned. Part I: definitions, incidence, and adverse physiologic effects of residual neuromuscular block. Anesth Analg. 2010;111(1):120–128.
86. Brull SJ, Murphy GS. Residual neuromuscular block: lessons unlearned. Part II: methods to reduce the risk of residual weakness. Anesth Analg. 2010;111(1):129–140.
87. Plaud B, Debaene B, Donati F, et al. Residual paralysis after emergence from anesthesia. Anesthesiology. 2010;112(4):1013–1022.
88. Aldenkortt M, Lysakowski C, Elia N, et al. Ventilation strategies in obese patients undergoing surgery: a quantitative systematic review and meta-analysis. Br J Anaesth. 2012;109(4):493–502.
89. Balick-Weber C-C, Nicolas P, Hedreville-Montout M, et al. Respiratory and haemodynamic effects of volume-controlled vs pressure-controlled ventilation during laparoscopy: a cross-over study with echocardiographic assessment. Br J Anaesth. 2007;99(3):429–435.
90. Baraka A, Jabbour S, Hammoud R, et al. End-tidal carbon dioxide tension during laparoscopic cholecystectomy: correlation with the baseline value prior to carbon dioxide insufflation. Anaesthesia. 1994;49(4):304–306.
91. Loeckinger A, Kleinsasser A, Hoermann C, et al. Inert gas exchange during pneumoperitoneum at incremental values of positive end-expiratory pressure. Anesth Analg. 2000;90(2):466–471.
92. Hazebroek EJ, Haitsma JJ, Lachmann B, et al. Mechanical ventilation with positive end-expiratory pressure preserves arterial oxygenation during prolonged pneumoperitoneum. Surg Endosc. 2002;16(4):685–689.
93. Meininger D, Byhahn C, Mierdl S, et al. Positive end-expiratory pressure improves arterial oxygenation during prolonged pneumoperitoneum. Acta Anaesthesiol Scand. 2005;49(6):778–783.
94. Futier E, Constantin J-M, Pelosi P, et al. Intraoperative recruitment maneuver reverses detrimental pneumoperitoneum-induced respiratory effects in healthy weight and obese patients undergoing laparoscopy. Anesthesiology. 2010;113(6):1310–1319.
95. Valenza F, Vagginelli F, Tiby A, et al. Effects of the beach chair position, positive end-expiratory pressure, and pneumoperitoneum on respiratory function in morbidly obese patients during anesthesia and paralysis. Anesthesiology. 2007;107(5):725–732.
96. Hovaguimian F, Lysakowski C, Elia N, et al. Effect of intraoperative high inspired oxygen fraction on surgical site infection, postoperative nausea and vomiting, and pulmonary function: systematic review and meta-analysis of randomized controlled trials. Anesthesiology. 2013;119(2):303–316.
97. Fernandez-Bustamante A, Hashimoto S, Serpa Neto A, et al. Perioperative lung protective ventilation in obese patients. BMC Anesthesiol. 2015;15:56.
98. Coppola S, Froio S, Chiumello D. Protective lung ventilation during general anesthesia: is there any evidence? Crit Care. 2014;18(2):210.
99. Gray RI, Ott DE, Henderson AC, et al. Severe local hypothermia from laparoscopic gas evaporative jet cooling: a mechanism to explain clinical observations. JSLS. 1999;3(3):171–177.
100. Davis SS, Mikami DJ, Newlin M, et al. Heating and humidifying of carbon dioxide during pneumoperitoneum is not indicated: a prospective randomized trial. Surg Endosc. 2006;20(1):153–158.
101. Birch DW, Manouchehri N, Shi X, et al. Heated CO_2 with or without humidification for minimally invasive abdominal surgery. Cochrane Database Syst Rev. 2011;(1):CD007821.
102. Lassen K, Soop M, Nygren J, et al. Consensus review of optimal perioperative care in colorectal surgery: Enhanced Recovery After Surgery (ERAS) Group recommendations. Arch Surg. 2009;144(10):961–969.
103. Holte K, Klarskov B, Christensen DS, et al. Liberal versus restrictive fluid administration to improve recovery after laparoscopic cholecystectomy: a randomized, double-blind study. Ann Surg. 2004;240(5):892–899.
104. Danic MJ, Chow M, Alexander G, et al. Anesthesia considerations for robotic-assisted laparoscopic prostatectomy: a review of 1,500 cases. J Robot Surg. 2007;1(2):119–123.
105. Matot I, Paskaleva R, Eid L, et al. Effect of the volume of fluids administered on intraoperative oliguria in laparoscopic bariatric surgery: a randomized controlled trial. Arch Surg. 2012;147(3):228–234.
106. Chakravartty S, Sarma DR, Patel AG. Rhabdomyolysis in bariatric surgery: a systematic review. Obes Surg. 2013;23(8):1333–1340.
107. Jacob M, Chappell D, Rehm M. Perioperative fluid administration: another form of "work-life balance." Anesthesiology. 2011;114(3):483–484.
108. Guenoun T, Aka EJ, Journois D, et al. Effects of laparoscopic pneumoperitoneum and changes in position on arterial pulse pressure wave-form: comparison between morbidly obese and normal-weight patients. Obes Surg. 2006;16(8):1075–1081.
109. Magrina JF. Complications of laparoscopic surgery. Clin Obstet Gynecol. 2002;45(2):469–480.
110. Joshi GP. Complications of laparoscopy. Anesthesiol Clin North Am. 2001;19(1):89–105.
111. Coelho JC, Campos AC, Costa MA, et al. Complications of laparoscopic fundoplication in the elderly. Surg Laparosc Endosc Percutan Tech. 2003;13(1):6–10.
112. Pareek G, Hedican SP, Gee JR, et al. Meta-analysis of the complications of laparoscopic renal surgery: comparison of procedures and techniques. J Urol. 2006;175(4):1208–1213.
113. Fischer B, Engel N, Fehr J-L, et al. Complications of robotic assisted radical prostatectomy. World J Urol. 2008;26(6):595–602.
114. Coelho RF, Palmer KJ, Rocco B, et al. Early complication rates in a single-surgeon series of 2500 robotic-assisted radical prostatectomies: report applying a standardized grading system. Eur Urol. 2010;57(6):945–952.
115. Lasser MS, Renzulli J, Turini GA, et al. An unbiased prospective report of perioperative complications of robot-assisted laparoscopic radical prostatectomy. Urology. 2010;75(5):1083–1089.
116. Dexter F, Ledolter J, Davis E, et al. Systematic criteria for type and screen based on procedure's probability of erythrocyte transfusion. Anesthesiology. 2012;116(4):768–778.
117. Usal H, Nabagiez J, Sayad P, et al. Cost effectiveness of routine type and screen testing before laparoscopic cholecystectomy. Surg Endosc. 1999;13(2):146–147.
118. Yong J, Hibbert P, Runciman WB, Coventry BJ. Bradycardia as an early warning sign for cardiac arrest during routine laparoscopic surgery. Int J Qual Health Care. 2015;27(6):472–477.
119. Ott DE. Subcutaneous emphysema—beyond the pneumoperitoneum. JSLS. 2014;18(1):1–7.
120. Siu W, Seifman BD, Wolf JS. Subcutaneous emphysema, pneumomediastinum and bilateral pneumothoraces after laparoscopic pyeloplasty. J Urol. 2003;170(5):1936–1937.
121. Murdock CM, Wolff AJ, Van Geem T. Risk factors for hypercarbia, subcutaneous emphysema, pneumothorax, and pneumomediastinum during laparoscopy. Obstet Gynecol. 2000;95(5):704–709.
122. Stern JA, Nadler RB. Pneumothorax masked by subcutaneous emphysema after laparoscopic nephrectomy. J Endourol. 2004;18(5):457–458.
123. Joris JL, Chiche JD, Lamy ML. Pneumothorax during laparoscopic fundoplication: diagnosis and treatment with positive end-expiratory pressure. Anesth Analg. 1995;81(5):993–1000.
124. Yee R, Hyde PR, Currie JS. Pneumothorax during laparoscopic Nissen fundoplication. Anaesth Intensive Care. 1996;24(1):93–96.
125. Phillips S, Falk GL. Surgical tension pneumothorax during laparoscopic repair of massive hiatus hernia: a different situation requiring different management. Anaesth Intensive Care. 2011;39(6):1120–1123.
126. Hawasli A. Spontaneous resolution of massive laparoscopy-associated pneumothorax: the case of the bulging diaphragm and review of the literature. J Laparoendosc Adv Surg Tech A. 2002;12(1):77–82.
127. Ueda K, Ahmed W, Ross AF. Intraoperative pneumothorax identified with transthoracic ultrasound. Anesthesiology. 2011;115(3):653–655.
128. Venkatesh R, Kibel AS, Lee D, et al. Rapid resolution of carbon dioxide pneumothorax (capno-thorax) resulting from diaphragmatic injury during laparoscopic nephrectomy. J Urol. 2002;167(3):1387–1388.
129. Cottin V, Delafosse B, Viale JP. Gas embolism during laparoscopy: a report of seven cases in patients with previous abdominal surgical history. Surg Endosc. 1996;10(2):166–169.
130. Bonjer HJ, Hazebroek EJ, Kazemier G, et al. Open versus closed establishment of pneumoperitoneum in laparoscopic surgery. Br J Surg. 1997;84(5):599–602.
131. Otsuka Y, Katagiri T, Ishii J, et al. Gas embolism in laparoscopic hepatectomy: what is the optimal pneumoperitoneal pressure for laparoscopic major hepatectomy? J Hepatobiliary Pancreat Sci. 2013;20(2):137–140.
132. Hong J-Y, Kim WO, Kil HK. Detection of subclinical CO_2 embolism by transesophageal echocardiography during laparoscopic radical prostatectomy. Urology. 2010;75(3):581–584.
133. Kim CS, Kim JY, Kwon J-Y, et al. Venous air embolism during total laparoscopic hysterectomy: comparison to total abdominal hysterectomy. Anesthesiology. 2009;111(1):50–54.
134. Hong JY, Kim JY, Choi YD, et al. Incidence of venous gas embolism during robotic-assisted laparoscopic radical prostatectomy is lower than that during radical retropubic prostatectomy. Br J Anaesth. 2010;105(6):777–781.
135. Fors D, Eiriksson K, Arvidsson D, et al. Gas embolism during laparoscopic liver resection in a pig model: frequency and severity. Br J Anaesth. 2010;105(3):282–288.
136. Couture P, Boudreault D, Derouin M, et al. Venous carbon dioxide embolism in pigs: an evaluation of end-tidal carbon dioxide, transesophageal echocardiography, pulmonary artery pressure, and precordial auscultation as monitoring modalities. Anesth Analg. 1994;79(5):867–873.
137. Dauber MH, Roth S. Operating table failure: another hazard of spine surgery. Anesth Analg. 2009;108(3):904–905.
138. Newman NJ. Perioperative visual loss after nonocular surgeries. Am J Ophthalmol. 2008;145(4):604–610.
139. American Society of Anesthesiologists Task Force on Perioperative Visual Loss. Practice advisory for perioperative visual loss associated with spine surgery: an updated report by the American Society of Anesthesiologists Task Force on Perioperative Visual Loss. Anesthesiology. 2012;116(2):274–285.

140. Roth S, Thisted RA, Erickson JP, et al. Eye injuries after nonocular surgery: a study of 60,965 anesthetics from 1988 to 1992. *Anesthesiology.* 1996;85(5):1020–1027.
141. Sukhu T, Krupski TL. Patient positioning and prevention of injuries in patients undergoing laparoscopic and robot-assisted urologic procedures. *Curr Urol Rep.* 2014;15(4):398.
142. Eteuati J, Hiscock R, Hastie I, et al. Brachial plexopathy in laparoscopic-assisted rectal surgery: a case series. *Tech Coloproctol.* 2013;17(3):293–297.
143. Phong SV, Koh LK. Anaesthesia for robotic-assisted radical prostatectomy: considerations for laparoscopy in the Trendelenburg position. *Anaesth Intensive Care.* 2007;35(2):281–285.
144. Avriel A, Warner E, Avinoach E, et al. Major respiratory adverse events after laparascopic gastric banding surgery for morbid obesity. *Respir Med.* 2012;106(8):1192–1198.
145. Sharma RR, Axelsson H, Oberg A, et al. Diaphragmatic activity after laparoscopic cholecystectomy. *Anesthesiology.* 1999;91(2):406–413.
146. Erice F, Fox GS, Salib YM, et al. Diaphragmatic function before and after laparoscopic cholecystectomy. *Anesthesiology.* 1993;79(5):966–975.
147. Sadovnikoff N, Maxwell LG. Respiratory failure after laparoscopic cholecystectomy in a patient with chronic hemidiaphragm paralysis. *Anesthesiology.* 1997;87(4):996–998.
148. Milic DJ, Pejcic VD, Zivic SS, et al. Coagulation status and the presence of postoperative deep vein thrombosis in patients undergoing laparoscopic cholecystectomy. *Surg Endosc.* 2007;21(9):1588–1592.
149. Schwenk W, Böhm B, Fügener A, et al. Intermittent pneumatic sequential compression (ISC) of the lower extremities prevents venous stasis during laparoscopic cholecystectomy. *Surg Endosc.* 2014;12(1):7–11.
150. Stein PD, Matta F, Sabra MJ. Pulmonary embolism and deep venous thrombosis following laparoscopic cholecystectomy. *Clin Appl Thromb Hemost.* 2014;20(3):233–237.
151. Stein PD, Matta F. Pulmonary embolism and deep venous thrombosis following bariatric surgery. *Obes Surg.* 2013;23(5):663–668.
152. Stein PD, Beemath A, Olson RE. Obesity as a risk factor in venous thromboembolism. *Am J Med.* 2005;118(9):978–980.
153. Tyritzis SI, Wallerstedt A, Steineck G, et al. Thromboembolic complications in 3,544 patients undergoing radical prostatectomy with or without lymph node dissection. *J Urol.* 2015;193(1):117–125.
154. Veldkamp R, Gholghesaei M, Bonjer HJ, et al. Laparoscopic resection of colon cancer: consensus of the European Association of Endoscopic Surgery (EAES). *Surg Endosc.* 2004;18(8):1163–1185.
155. Atak I, Ozbagriacik M, Akinci OF, et al. Active gas aspiration to reduce pain after laparoscopic cholecystectomy. *Surg Laparosc Endosc Percutan Tech.* 2011;21(2):98–100.
156. Joshi GP. Multimodal analgesia techniques and postoperative rehabilitation. *Anesthesiol Clin North Am.* 2005;23(1):185–202.
157. Gajraj NM, Joshi GP. Role of cyclooxygenase-2 inhibitors in postoperative pain management. *Anesthesiol Clin North Am.* 2005;23(1):49–72.
158. McNicol ED, Tzortzopoulou A, Cepeda MS, et al. Single-dose intravenous paracetamol or propacetamol for prevention or treatment of postoperative pain: a systematic review and meta-analysis. *Br J Anaesth.* 2011;106(6):764–775.
159. Ong CK, Seymour RA, Lirk P, et al. Combining paracetamol (acetaminophen) with nonsteroidal anti-inflammatory drugs: a qualitative systematic review of analgesic efficacy for acute postoperative pain. *Anesth Analg.* 2010;110(4):1170–1179.
160. Maund E, McDaid C, Rice S, et al. Paracetamol and selective and non-selective non-steroidal anti-inflammatory drugs for the reduction in morphine-related side-effects after major surgery: a systematic review. *Br J Anaesth.* 2011;106(3):292–297.
161. Baeriswyl M, Kirkham KR, Kern C, et al. The analgesic efficacy of ultrasound-guided transversus abdominis plane block in adult patients: a meta-analysis. *Anesth Analg.* 2015;121(6):1640–1654.
162. Fields AC, Gonzalez DO, Chin EH, et al. Laparoscopic-assisted transversus abdominis plane block for postoperative pain control in laparoscopic ventral hernia repair: a randomized controlled trial. *J Am Coll Surg.* 2015;221(2):462–469.
163. Elamin G, Waters PS, Hamid H, et al. Efficacy of a laparoscopically delivered transversus abdominis plane block technique during elective laparoscopic cholecystectomy: a prospective, double-blind randomized trial. *J Am Coll Surg.* 2015;221(2):335–344.
164. Petersen PL, Mathiesen O, Torup H, Dahl JB. The transversus abdominis plane block: a valuable option for postoperative analgesia? A topical review. *Acta Anaesthesiol Scand.* 2010;54(5):529–535.
165. Levy BF, Tilney HS, Dowson HMP, Rockall TA. A systematic review of postoperative analgesia following laparoscopic colorectal surgery. *Colorectal Dis.* 2010;12(1):5–15.
166. Apfel CC, Heidrich FM, Jukar-Rao S, et al. Evidence-based analysis of risk factors for postoperative nausea and vomiting. *Br J Anaesth.* 2012;109(5):742–753.
167. Weingarten TN, Hawkins NM, Beam WB, et al. Factors associated with prolonged anesthesia recovery following laparoscopic bariatric surgery: a retrospective analysis. *Obes Surg.* 2015;25(6):1024–1030.
168. Gan TJ, Diemunsch P, Habib AS, et al. Consensus guidelines for the management of postoperative nausea and vomiting. *Anesth Analg.* 2014;118(1):85–113.

45 Anesthesia and Obesity

ANA FERNANDEZ-BUSTAMANTE • BRENDA A. BUCKLIN

Definition and Epidemiology
  Introduction
  Management of Obesity
Pathophysiology
  Respiratory System
  Cardiovascular and Hematologic Systems
  Gastrointestinal System
  Renal and Endocrine Systems
Pharmacology
  Pharmacologic Principles
  Other Perioperative Agents
Preoperative Evaluation
Intraoperative Considerations
  Equipment and Monitoring
  Airway Management
  Induction and Maintenance
  Fluid Management
  Mechanical Ventilation
  Emergence
  Monitored Anesthesia Care and Sedation
  Regional Anesthesia
Postoperative Considerations
  Ventilatory Evaluation and Management
  Postoperative Analgesia
  Monitoring
Ambulatory Anesthesia
Critical Care and Resuscitation
Morbidity and Mortality

KEY POINTS

1. Obstructive sleep apnea (OSA) is common in obese patients and predisposes to airway difficulties during anesthesia.
2. Obese patients may appear asymptomatic even when they have significant cardiovascular disease because they often have limited exercise tolerance.
3. Neck circumference is the single best predictor of problematic intubation in morbidly obese patients. A larger neck circumference is associated with male sex, higher Mallampati score, grade 3 laryngoscopic views, and OSA.
4. Elevated liver function tests (mostly elevated alanine aminotransferase) are seen in many obese patients, but no clear correlation exists between abnormalities of routine liver function tests and the capacity of the liver to metabolize drugs.
5. Morbid obesity is a major independent risk factor for deep venous thrombosis and sudden death from acute postoperative pulmonary embolism. Mobilization in the morbidly obese is often difficult but critically important in the prevention of postoperative complications.
6. Positive end-expiratory pressure is the only ventilatory parameter that has consistently been shown to improve respiratory function in obese patients, but it decreases venous return, cardiac output, and subsequent oxygen delivery.
7. Forearm blood pressure is a fairly good predictor of upper arm blood pressure in most patients, but in obese patients, forearm measurements with a standard cuff may overestimate both systolic and diastolic blood pressures.
8. The head-elevated laryngoscopy position elevates the obese patient's head, upper body, and shoulders above the chest and can improve laryngoscopy and intubation.
9. Larger doses of induction agents may be required by obese patients because blood volume, muscle mass, and cardiac output increase linearly with the degree of obesity. An increased dose of succinylcholine is necessary because of an increase in pseudocholinesterase activity.
10. Prompt but safe extubation reduces the likelihood that the morbidly obese patient will become ventilator-dependent, especially in patients with cardiopulmonary disease.
11. Because of the risk of perioperative hypoxemia and apnea in obese patients, postoperative pain management should include opioid-sparing multimodal analgesic techniques. Regional anesthetic techniques reduce the risk of opioid-related complications.
12. Obese patients who have received either neuraxial or parenteral opioids require careful postoperative monitoring. Delayed respiratory depression with centrally administered neuraxial opioids, when coupled with a potentially difficult airway in the obese patient, suggests that close monitoring is prudent.

Definition and Epidemiology

Introduction

The World Health Organization defines obesity as a condition with excess body fat to the extent that health and well-being are adversely affected.[1] Over the past three decades, there has been a sharp increase in rates of obesity worldwide.[2] Estimates suggest that the number of obese individuals now exceeds the number of underweight individuals. More than one-third of Americans (33.8%) and 17% of youth are currently obese.[3] Prevalence of obesity in the United States is unevenly distributed geographically, by race and ethnicity, and by socioeconomic status. The Centers for Disease Control and Prevention (CDC) monitor the epidemiology of obesity and publish periodically updated data at http://www.cdc.gov/obesity/.

Obesity-related conditions including diabetes, cardiovascular disease, obstructive sleep apnea, nonalcoholic fatty liver disease (NAFLD), osteoarthritis, and some types of cancer are leading causes of morbidity and mortality in this population.[4,5] Although there has been an exponential increase in the number of bariatric procedures performed, obese and morbidly obese patients undergo all types of surgical procedures. Surgery in this patient population is considered high-risk; however, careful planning, preoperative risk assessment, adequate anesthetic management, strict venothrombotic event prevention, and effective postoperative pain control will all help to reduce the risk. With appropriate perioperative management, obese surgical patients can achieve safe and effective surgical outcomes.

The definition of obesity includes the presence of excessive body weight for the patient's age, gender, and height, and is based or estimated on calculation of the following concepts:

- Ideal Body Weight (IBW) is a concept derived by life insurance companies by referencing height-weight tables. It is the weight associated with the lowest mortality rate for a given height and gender and can be estimated using the Broca index: IBW (kg) = height (cm) − x, where x is 100 for adult males and 105 for adult females.
- Predicted Body Weight (PBW) is a similar concept as the IBW, and more commonly used in the medical literature. PBW is usually calculated with the following formulas in adults[6]:
  Males: PBW (kg) = 50 + 0.91 × (height (cm) − 152.4)
  Females: PBW (kg) = 45.5 + 0.91 × (height (cm) − 152.4)
- Lean Body Weight (LBW) is the total body weight (TBW) minus the adipose tissue. It is a combination of body cell mass, extracellular water, and nonfat connective tissue. It approximates 80% and 75% of TBW for males and females, respectively, although more accurate formulas like the following have been proposed[7]:
  Males: 1.10 × TBW − 0.0128 × BMI × TBW; Females: 1.07 × TBW − 0.0148 × BMI × TBW
  In morbidly obese patients, increasing the IBW by 20% to 30% gives an estimate of LBW. In nonobese and nonmuscular individuals, TBW approximates IBW.[8]
- Body Mass (Quetelet) Index (BMI) is used in clinical practice to estimate the degree of obesity:

$$BMI = \frac{body\ weight\ (kg)}{height^2\ (m)}$$

Obesity is defined as having a BMI 30 kg/m^2 or more. Obesity is further classified according to systemic disease risk (Table 45-1).

Morbid obesity, defined as a BMI 40 kg/m^2 or more, can also be further classified into super obesity (BMI ≥ 50 kg/m^2) and super-super obesity (BMI ≥ 60 kg/m^2).[9] BMI differentiates obese from nonobese adults and it estimates body fat because it adjusts for height while strongly correlating with body weight; however, it cannot distinguish between overweight and overfat, as heavily muscled individuals can be easily classified as overweight using BMI. Therefore, other factors such as age, fat content, and distribution (i.e., waist circumference and waist-to-hip ratio) should be taken into consideration, along with other health risk predictors that use the concept of BMI.

The anatomic distribution of body fat has associated pathophysiologic implications.[10,11] In android (central) obesity, adipose tissue is located predominantly in the upper body (truncal distribution) and is associated with increased oxygen consumption and increased incidence of cardiovascular disease. Visceral fat is particularly associated with cardiovascular disease and left ventricular dysfunction. In gynecoid (peripheral) obesity, adipose tissue is located predominantly in the hips, buttocks, and thighs. This fat is less metabolically active so it is less closely associated with cardiovascular disease. Body circumference indices such as waist circumference, waist-to-height ratio, and waist-to-hip ratio help to classify these patterns of obesity (e.g., android vs. gynecoid obesity) and correlate with mortality and the risk for developing obesity-related diseases. Waist circumference correlates with abdominal fat and is an independent risk predictor of disease (Table 45-1).

Management of Obesity

Medical Therapy

Indications for drug treatment include a BMI 30 kg/m^2 or more or a BMI between 27 and 29.9 kg/m^2 in conjunction with an obesity-related medical complication. Although conventional treatments of obesity including lifestyle changes and medications have demonstrated little success in long-term weight loss,[12–14] medications are often used to treat obesity because of their ability to reduce energy intake, increase energy utilization, or decrease absorption of nutrients. Phentermine, phentermine–topiramate, lorcaserin, bupropion–naltrexone, liraglutide, and orlistat are FDA-approved antiobesity medications.[15] Most pharmacologic therapies target appetite mechanisms with the exception of orlistat. Phentermine (Adipex-P) is primarily a noradrenergic and possibly dopaminergic sympathomimetic amine that decreases

Table 45-1 Classification of Obesity, and Systemic Disease Risk According to Waist Circumference

		Waist Circumference/Risk	
BMI (kg/m^2)	Description	Male: <102 cm Female: <88 cm	Male: ≥102 cm Female: ≥88 cm
<18.5	Underweight		
18.5–24.9	Normal		
25.0–29.9	Overweight		
30.0–34.9	Obesity (class I)	Average	Average
35.0–39.9	Obesity (class II)	Increased	High
≥40	Morbid obesity (class III)	High	Very high
≥50	Super obesity	Very high	Very high
≥60	Super-super obesity	Extremely high	Extremely high

BMI, body mass index.

appetite. Although it is only approved for 3 months' use, it can induce, tachycardia, palpitations, and hypertension, as well as dependence, abuse, and withdrawal symptoms. It is no longer combined with fenfluramine (Phen-Fen) due to concerns of pulmonary hypertension and valvular heart disease. It is now being combined with topiramate (Topamax).[16] However, this combination often causes dry mouth, paresthesias, constipation, insomnia, and dizziness. Lorcaserin is a serotonin receptor antagonist and stimulates the serotonin type 2c receptor. Bupropion is combined with naltrexone and is a dopamine and norepinephrine reuptake inhibitor[17] which stimulates pro-opiomelanocortin neurons. In combination with naltrexone, efficacy of bupropion is enhanced due to the release of feedback inhibition of pro-opiomelanocortin neurons that naltrexone potentiates. Liraglutide is associated with weight loss without an effect on appetite. It promotes weight loss by preventing resorption of glucose and water in the renal tubules.[18] Orlistat (over-the-counter Alli, prescribed Xenical) or tetrahydrolipstatin blocks the absorption of dietary fat by inhibiting lipases in the gastrointestinal tract. It leads to weight loss and improved blood pressure, fasting blood glucose levels, and lipid profile.[19] Fat malabsorption causes common complaints of oily spotting, liquid stools, fecal urgency, flatulence, and abdominal cramping. Chronic use of orlistat may result in fat-soluble vitamin deficiency. A prolonged prothrombin time with a normal partial thromboplastin time during orlistat treatment may reflect vitamin K deficiency, and this coagulopathy should be corrected 6 to 24 hours before elective surgery.[20]

Although over-the-counter preparations are widely used as a weight loss strategy, evidence to support their efficacy and safety is limited. Plant extracts or herbs are often used to combat obesity and include: pancreatic lipase inhibitors (e.g., caffeine, green or black tea), appetite suppressants (e.g., hoodia, Korean ginseng, ephedra, sunflower oil), stimulants of energy expenditure (e.g., acai berry, caffeine), and regulators of lipid metabolism (e.g., soybean, fish oil, oolong tea, caffeine).[21] The American Society of Anesthesiologists warns patients to tell their anesthesiologists about medications they are taking, including vitamins, herbs, and other supplements. Since these products can interfere with anesthesia, they can cause complications during surgery.[22]

Bariatric Surgery

Bariatric surgery is currently the most effective treatment for morbid (class III) obesity. Current guidelines recommend bariatric surgery for patients with BMI above 40 kg/m² or below 35 kg/m² with obesity-related comorbidities not controlled with medical therapy.[23] However recent calls suggest to alter the threshold for bariatric surgery to BMI 35 kg/m² or 30 kg/m² with comorbidities in order to reduce the lifetime cost associated with diabetes, hypertension, high cholesterol, colon cancer, and cardiovascular disease.[24] Procedures are classified into malabsorptive (e.g., jejunoileal bypass and biliopancreatic diversion, biliopancreatic diversion with duodenal switch), restrictive (vertical-banded gastroplasty, adjustable gastric banding, sleeve gastrectomy), or combined (Roux-en-Y gastric bypass [RYGB]). The RYGB combines gastric restriction with a minimal degree of malabsorption. RYGB adjustable gastric banding, sleeve gastrectomy, and vertical-banded gastroplasty can all be performed laparoscopically. Laparoscopic bariatric surgery is associated with less postoperative pain, lower morbidity, faster recovery, and less "third-spacing."[25] Several procedures (e.g., jejunoileal bypass) are no longer performed due to the risk for revisions and adverse health effects. RYGB is the most commonly performed bariatric procedure and produces safe short- and long-term weight loss in severely obese patients. With RYGB, patients lose an average of 50% to 60% excess body weight and show a BMI decrease of approximately 10 kg/m² during the first 12 to 24 postoperative months. Type II diabetes resolves in a majority of patients. Sleeve or partial gastrectomy is the second most commonly performed restrictive bariatric procedure. Laparoscopic adjustable gastric banding (LAGB) is a restrictive gastric operation that utilizes an adjustable inflatable band to alter stomach capacity for individual weight loss needs. Vertical-banded gastroplasty also restricts food intake.

Less invasive bariatric techniques are being developed. An implantable abdominal vagal nerve stimulator is placed laparoscopically and emits electrical impulses to control gastric emptying and signal the satiety center in the brain.[26] This device can be adversely affected by defibrillation, electrocautery, lithotripsy, magnetic resonance imaging, and therapeutic radiation. Intragastric balloons and prostheses, at different stages of development, are placed endoscopically as a temporary measure to increase satiety. They are often considered to be a bridge to more definitive bariatric procedures.[27] Adequate control of postoperative nausea and vomiting is critical to avoid possible stimulator lead or balloon dislodgement.

Pathophysiology

Obesity comes with adverse health implications of multiple organ systems. Table 45-2 provides a list of the most relevant organ systems with implications for clinical management. These systems will be discussed separately in this section.

Respiratory System

Fat accumulation on the thorax and abdomen decreases chest wall and lung compliance. Decreased lung compliance is partially explained by increased pulmonary blood volume because of an overall increase in blood volume. Increased elastic resistance and decreased compliance of the chest wall are further reduced while supine, leading to shallow and rapid breathing, increased work of breathing, and limited maximum ventilatory capacity. Respiratory muscle efficiency is below normal in obese individuals. Decreased pulmonary compliance leads to decreased functional residual capacity (FRC), vital capacity, and total lung capacity. Reduction in FRC is primarily a result of reduced expiratory reserve volume (ERV), but the relationship between FRC and closing capacity, the volume at which small airways begin to close, is adversely affected (Fig. 45-1). Decreases in FRC and ERV are the most commonly reported abnormalities of pulmonary function in obese patients.[28,29] Residual volume and closing capacity are unchanged. Reduced FRC (due to decreased ERV) can result in lung volumes below closing capacity in the course of normal tidal ventilation, leading to small airway closure, ventilation–perfusion mismatch, right-to-left shunting, and arterial hypoxemia. Anesthesia and supine positioning worsen this situation such that up to a 50% reduction in FRC occurs in the obese anesthetized patient compared with 20% in the nonobese individual. Forced expiratory volume in 1 second and forced vital capacity are usually within normal limits. ERV is the most sensitive indicator of the effect of obesity on pulmonary function.

Obesity increases oxygen consumption and carbon dioxide production even at rest. This is because of the metabolic activity of excess fat and the increased workload on supportive tissues. The body attempts to meet these metabolic demands by increasing both cardiac output and alveolar ventilation. Basal

Table 45-2 Implications of Medical Consequences of Obesity

System	Practical Anesthesia Key Points
Respiratory	Increased risk of perioperative hypoxemia Careful monitoring needed Use of supplemental oxygen CPAP (when indicated) Nonsupine positioning (if possible) Extreme caution when administering respiratory depressant drugs
Cardiovascular	Increased blood volume, cardiac output, left ventricular wall thickness Increased proinflammatory and prothrombotic mediators Higher perioperative complications related to hypertension, thromboembolic events, and left ventricular diastolic dysfunction
Gastrointestinal	Risk of regurgitation Higher gastric volume and lower pH increases risk of severe pneumonitis should aspiration occur Current preoperative fasting guidelines (6h for solids, 2h for clear liquids) are acceptable Careful assessment of preoperative liver function is recommended
Endocrine/metabolic	High prevalence of hyperglycemia, insulin resistance, and diabetes Careful perioperative glucose monitoring Metabolic syndrome (combination of central obesity, hypertension, dyslipidemia, and impaired glucose metabolism) is frequent and doubles the cardiovascular risk
Genitourinary	Increased risk of renal disease Higher incidence of preeclampsia and eclampsia
Neurologic	Careful positioning with extra padding needed
Hematology	Increased hypercoagulability and risk of perioperative thromboembolic events Preoperative polycythemia suggests prolonged history of apnea
Musculoskeletal	Increased prevalence of osteoarthritis
Psychology/psychiatry	Depression, reduced self-esteem, social stigma

CPAP, continuous positive airway pressure.

metabolic activity is usually within normal limits in relationship to body surface area and normocapnia is usually maintained by an increase in minute ventilation. This requires increased oxygen consumption because most obese patients retain their normal response to hypoxemia and hypercapnia. Arterial oxygen tension in morbidly obese patients breathing room air is lower than that predicted for similarly aged nonobese subjects in both sitting and supine positions. Chronic hypoxemia may lead to polycythemia, pulmonary hypertension, and cor pulmonale.

Obese patients often suffer from obstructive sleep apnea (OSA) characterized by periodic, partial, or complete obstruction of the upper airway during sleep. In obese patients, sleep apnea is more

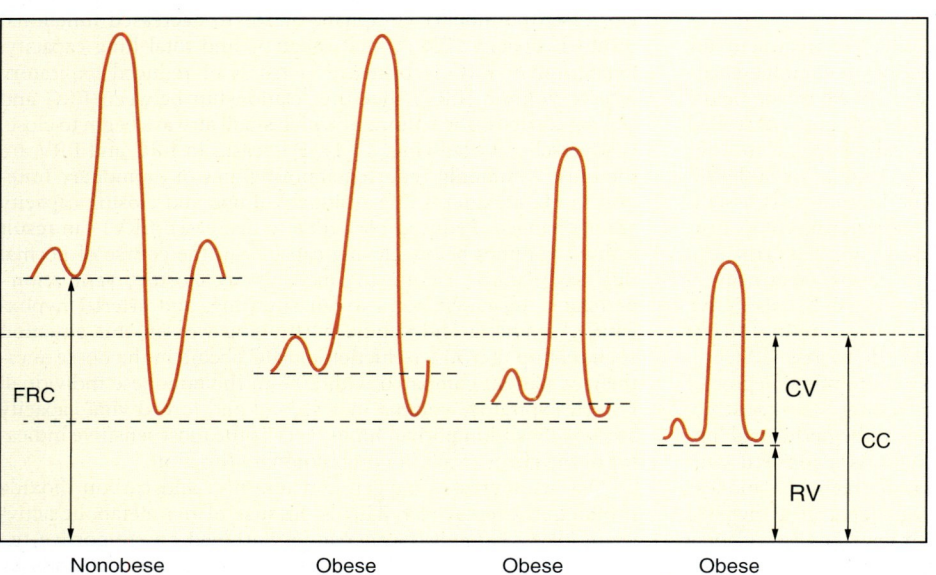

Figure 45-1 Effects of obesity, positioning, and anesthesia on lung volumes. FRC, functional residual capacity; CC, closing capacity; CV, closing volume; RV, residual volume.

likely to result from airway obstruction produced by excess soft tissue. However, centrally mediated forms of sleep apnea can also occur. Physiologic abnormalities resulting from OSA include hypoxemia, hypercapnia, pulmonary hypertension, systemic vasoconstriction, hypertension, and secondary polycythemia (from recurrent hypoxemia). These result in an increased risk of ischemic heart disease and cerebrovascular disease. Right ventricular failure can occur from hypoxic pulmonary vasoconstriction. Respiratory acidosis is usually limited only to periods of sleep.

The gold standard technique for diagnosing OSA is overnight polysomnography (OPS). The inconvenience, time, and expense of polysomnography lead to a significant fraction of obese patients presenting for surgery with suspicion for but no formal diagnosis of OSA.[30] Screening questionnaires such the STOP-BANG and others[31] are increasingly used for identifying patients at high risk for OSA. Suggestive signs of OSA include witnessed episodes of apnea during sleep, BMI 35 or more, neck circumference 16 in or more (women) or 17 in or more (men), hyperinsulinemia, and elevated glycosylated hemoglobin. Symptoms of snoring, frequent arousals during sleep and daytime sleepiness, impaired concentration, memory problems, and morning headaches are common but not predictive.[32] Ideally, a thorough preoperative evaluation for OSA should occur long enough before elective surgery to allow preparation of a perioperative management plan. Preoperative initiation of continuous positive airway pressure (CPAP), especially in severe OSA cases, should be considered.[33] A recent study found improvements in blood pressure, glucose, and lipid metabolism in obese OSA patients treated with CPAP in addition to a weight-loss intervention.[34] The frequent lack of compliance or intolerance to CPAP has spearheaded the development of alternative therapies. For example, the implantable hypoglossal nerve stimulator has shown promising results in a selected group of OSA patients. In general, patients with either confirmed or suspected OSA should be considered at high risk for a difficult airway and postoperative pulmonary complications, and managed accordingly.[35,36] To avoid postoperative hypoxemia and hypoventilation in patients either with or at high risk for OSA, experts recommend a semi-upright position, continuous pulse-oximetry monitoring, avoidance of opioid-based analgesia, and therapy with titrated oxygen and/or CPAP as needed.[37]

Obesity hypoventilation (Pickwickian) syndrome (OHS) may result from long-term OSA and is seen in 5% to 10% of morbidly obese patients. OHS is a combination of obesity and chronic hypoventilation that is frequently misdiagnosed and untreated,[38] resulting in pulmonary hypertension and cor pulmonale, increased risk of postoperative complications, and death.[39,40] The presence of both obesity (BMI >30 kg/m^2) and awake arterial hypercapnia (PaCO$_2$ >45 mmHg) in the absence of known causes of hypoventilation supports the diagnosis. Prolonged OSA also alters the control of breathing, leading to central nervous system (CNS)-mediated apneic events. This increases reliance on hypoxic drive for ventilation. The main ventilatory impairment of OHS is alveolar hypoventilation independent of intrinsic lung disease in a patient with obesity, daytime hypersomnolence, hypercapnia, hypoxemia, and polycythemia. Right ventricular failure eventually ensues. These patients also have an increased sensitivity to the respiratory depressant effects of general anesthetics.

Cardiovascular and Hematologic Systems

Total blood volume is increased in the obese individual, but on a volume-to-weight basis, it is less than in nonobese individuals (50 mL/kg compared with 70 mL/kg). Most of this extra volume is distributed in adipose tissue. Renal and splanchnic blood flows are increased. Cardiac output increases with increasing weight by as much as 20 to 30 mL/kg of excess body fat because of ventricular dilation and increases in stroke volume. The resulting increased left ventricular wall stress leads to hypertrophy, reduced compliance, and impairment of left ventricular filling (diastolic dysfunction) with elevated left ventricular diastolic pressure and pulmonary edema.[41] When left ventricular wall thickening fails to keep pace with dilation, systolic dysfunction ("obesity cardiomyopathy") and eventual biventricular failure result (Fig. 45-2).

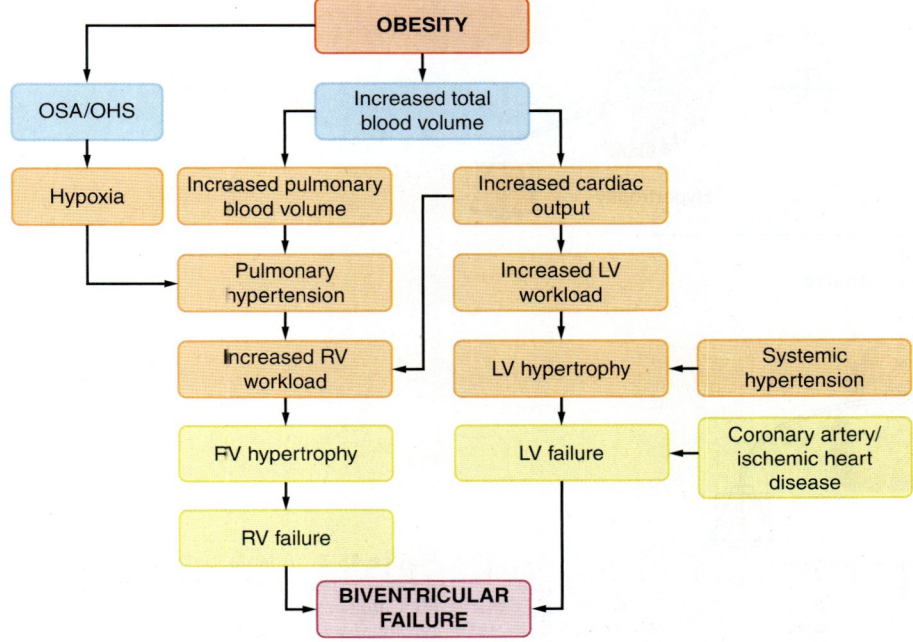

Figure 45-2 Interrelationship of cardiovascular and pulmonary sequelae of obesity. OSA, obstructive sleep apnea; OHS, obesity hypoventilation syndrome; LV, left ventricular; RV, right ventricular.

2 Obesity accelerates atherosclerosis. Symptoms such as angina or exertional dyspnea occur only occasionally because morbidly obese patients often have very limited mobility and may appear asymptomatic even when they have significant cardiovascular disease.

Blood flow to fat is 2 to 3 mL/100 g of tissue. Excess fat requires an increase in cardiac output, to parallel an increase in oxygen consumption. This leads to a systemic arteriovenous oxygen difference that remains normal or slightly above normal. Intraoperative ventricular failure may occur from rapid intravenous fluid administration (indicating left ventricular diastolic dysfunction), the negative inotropism of anesthetic agents, or pulmonary hypertension precipitated by hypoxia or hypercapnia. Cardiac dysrhythmias may be precipitated by fatty infiltration of the conduction system, hypoxia, hypercapnia, electrolyte imbalance, coronary artery disease, increased circulating catecholamines, OSA, and myocardial hypertrophy. Frequent electrocardiogram (ECG) findings seen in morbidly obese patients include low QRS voltage, multiple criteria for left ventricular hypertrophy (LVH), left atrial enlargement, and T-wave flattening in the inferior and lateral leads.[42] In addition, there is a leftward shift of the P-wave, QRS complex, and T-wave axes; lengthening of the corrected QT interval; and prolongation of the QT interval. Substantial weight reduction reverses many of these ECG abnormalities.[43]

Cardiac output rises faster in response to exercise in the morbidly obese and is often associated with a rise in left ventricular end-diastolic pressure and pulmonary capillary wedge pressure. Similar changes occur during the perioperative period, which should prompt a low threshold for performing detailed cardiac investigations. Many obese patients have mild-to-moderate hypertension, with a 3 to 4 mmHg increase in systolic and a 2 mmHg increase in diastolic arterial pressure for every 10 kg of weight gained. Normotensive obese patients have reduced systemic vascular resistance, which rises with the onset of hypertension. Their expanded blood volume causes increased cardiac output with a lower calculated systemic vascular resistance for the same level of arterial blood pressure. The renin–angiotensin system plays a major role in the hypertension of obesity by increased circulating levels of angiotensinogen, aldosterone, and angiotensin-converting enzyme. As little as 5% reduction in body weight leads to a significant reduction in renin–angiotensin activity in both plasma and adipose tissue, contributing to a reduction in blood pressure.[44]

Obese patients have normal-to-increased levels of sympathetic nervous system activity, which predispose to insulin resistance, dyslipidemia, and hypertension.[41] These obesity-induced comorbidities are responsible for the increased cardiovascular risk in obese patients.[45,46] Insulin resistance enhances the vasopressor activity of norepinephrine and angiotensin II. Hyperinsulinemia further activates the sympathetic nervous system, causing sodium retention and contributing to obesity-induced hypertension. Hypertension causes concentric hypertrophy of the ventricle in

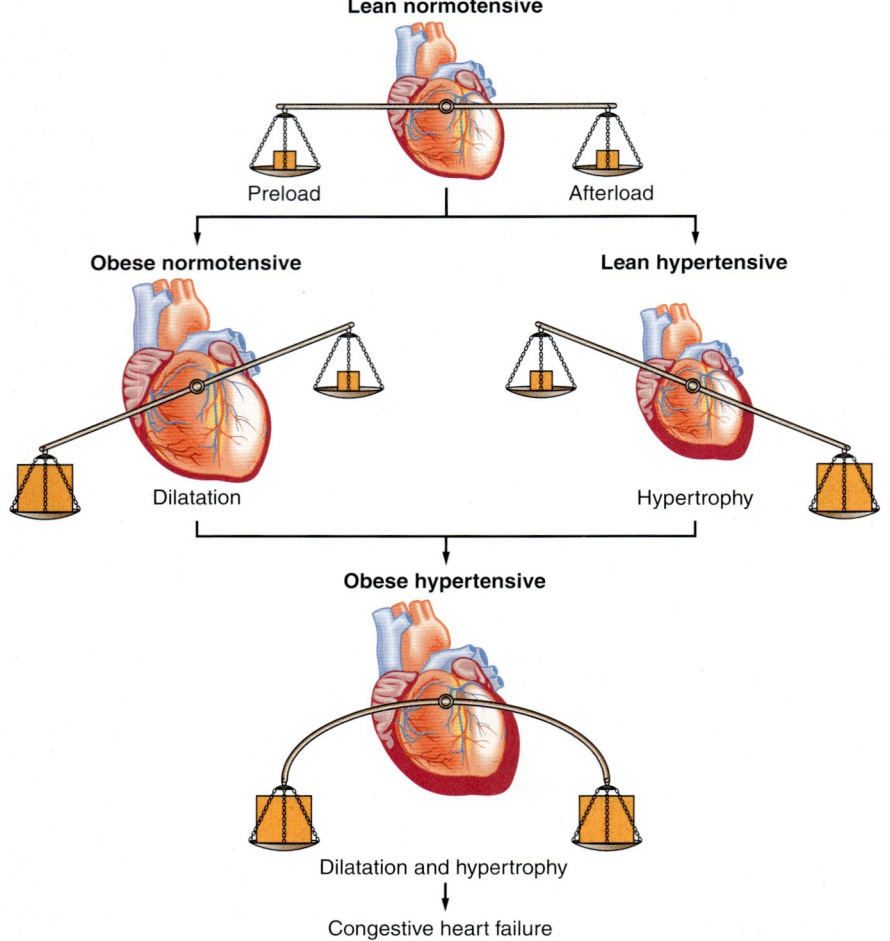

Figure 45-3 Adaptation of the heart to obesity and hypertension. (Adapted from Messerli FH. Cardiovascular effects of obesity and hypertension. *Lancet*. 1982;1:1165.)

normal-weight individuals but causes eccentric dilation in obese individuals. It is associated with increased preload and stroke work. The combination of obesity and hypertension causes left ventricular wall thickening and a larger heart volume; therefore, there is increased likelihood of cardiac failure (Fig. 45-3).

Obese individuals are also prone to cardiovascular disease because adipose tissue releases a large number of bioactive mediators. These can result in abnormal lipids, insulin resistance, inflammation, and coagulopathies.[45,46] Obese individuals have higher levels of fibrinogen (a marker for the inflammatory process of atherosclerosis), factor VII, factor VIII, von Willebrand factor, and plasminogen activator inhibitor-1 (PAI-1). Increased levels of fibrinogen, factor VII, factor VIII, and hypofibrinolysis are associated with hypercoagulability. High factor VIII levels are associated with increased cardiovascular mortality. Increased fasting triglyceride levels correlate with increased factor VII concentrations, and postprandial lipemia causes activation of factor VII. Endothelial dysfunction induced by insulin increases von Willebrand factor and factor VIII levels, predisposing to fibrin formation. Increased secretion of PAI-1 inhibits the fibrinolytic system and is associated with visceral obesity.[47]

Gastrointestinal System

Gastric volume and acidity are increased, hepatic function is altered, and drug metabolism is adversely affected by obesity. Many fasting morbidly obese patients who present for elective surgery have gastric volumes in excess of 25 mL and gastric fluid pH lower than 2.5 (the generally accepted volume and pH indicative of high risk for pneumonitis should regurgitation and aspiration occur). Delayed gastric emptying occurs because of increased abdominal mass that causes antral distention, gastrin release, and a decrease in pH with parietal cell secretion.[48,49] Abdominal obesity increases intragastric pressure, increasing the frequency of transient lower esophageal sphincter relaxation, and/or hiatal hernia formation. An increase of more than 3.5 kg/m^2 in BMI is associated with a 2.7-fold increase in risk for developing new reflux symptoms.[48] An increased incidence of hiatal hernia and gastroesophageal reflux further increases aspiration risk.

Gastric emptying is faster with high-energy content intake such as fat emulsions, but because of larger gastric volume (up to 75% larger), the residual volume is increased. The combination of hiatal hernia, gastroesophageal reflux, and delayed gastric emptying, coupled with increased intra-abdominal pressure and high-volume/low pH gastric content, puts the obese patient at risk for increased incidence of severe pneumonitis should aspiration occur. Unpremedicated, nondiabetic fasting obese surgical patients who are free from significant gastroesophageal pathology are unlikely to have high volume, low pH gastric contents after routine preoperative fasting.[50] They should follow the same fasting guidelines as nonobese patients and be allowed to drink clear liquids up until 2 hours before elective surgery.[51] Weight loss significantly improves gastroesophageal reflux symptoms.[52]

Peculiar morphologic and biochemical abnormalities of the liver are associated with obesity and include fatty infiltration (high prevalence of NAFLD), inflammation (nonalcoholic steatohepatitis [NASH]), focal necrosis, and cirrhosis. Fatty infiltration reflects the duration rather than the degree of obesity. Histologic and liver function test abnormalities are relatively common, but drug clearance usually is not reduced. Abnormal liver function tests are seen in up to one-third of obese patients who have no evidence of concomitant liver disease. The most common abnormality is an increased alanine aminotransferase (ALT). Despite these histologic and enzymatic changes, no clear correlation exists between liver function abnormalities and the capacity of the liver to metabolize drugs.[53] Morbidly obese patients who have undergone intestinal bypass surgery have a particularly high prevalence of hepatic dysfunction and cholelithiasis. This is also common in the general obese population due to abnormal cholesterol metabolism. The high prevalence of NAFLD, NASH, and cirrhosis necessitates careful assessment for pre-existing liver disease in obese patients scheduled for surgery. Features suggestive of NASH include hepatomegaly, elevated liver enzymes, and abnormal liver histology (steatosis, steatohepatitis, fibrosis, and cirrhosis).[45]

Renal and Endocrine Systems

Impaired glucose tolerance in the morbidly obese is reflected by a high prevalence of type II diabetes mellitus as a result of resistance of peripheral adipose tissue to insulin.[41] Many obese patients have an abnormal glucose tolerance test, and the relative risk of developing diabetes increases by 25% for every 1 kg/m^2 increase in BMI above 22 kg/m^2.[41] Hyperglycemia, insulin resistance, and diabetes predispose obese patients to wound infections and an increased risk of myocardial infarction. Exogenous insulin may be required perioperatively even in obese patients with type II diabetes mellitus to oppose the catabolic response to surgery.

In addition to these concerns, subclinical hypothyroidism occurs in about 25% of all morbidly obese patients. Thyroid-stimulating hormone levels are frequently elevated, suggesting the possibility that obesity leads to a state of thyroid hormone resistance in peripheral tissues. Hypothyroidism may be associated with hypoglycemia, hyponatremia, and impaired hepatic drug metabolism.

Obesity is associated with glomerular hyperfiltration as evidenced by increased renal blood flow and increased glomerular filtration rate. Excessive weight gain increases renal tubular resorption and impairs natriuresis through activation of the sympathetic and renin–angiotensin system, as well as physical compression of the kidney. With prolonged obesity, there may be a loss of nephron function, with further impairment of natriuresis and further increases in arterial pressure. However, the increased risk of acute kidney injury by obesity per se is unclear.[54] Obesity-related glomerular hyperfiltration decreases after weight loss, which decreases the incidence of overt glomerulopathy.[55]

Metabolic Syndrome. Metabolic syndrome, sometimes referred to as syndrome X and insulin resistance syndrome, is a cluster of metabolic abnormalities associated with an increased risk of diabetes and cardiovascular events. Individuals with this syndrome have up to a fivefold greater risk of developing type 2 diabetes mellitus (if not already present) and are also twice as likely to die from a myocardial infarction or stroke compared with those without the syndrome.[56] Furthermore, patients with metabolic syndrome are more likely to have perioperative adverse events including cardiovascular, pulmonary, and renal complications and wound infections.[57] Although there are several different definitions of metabolic syndrome, the National Cholesterol Education Program (NCEP) Adult Treatment Panel III (ATP III) definition is the most widely used.[58] It defines metabolic syndrome when three out of the following five conditions exist: (1) Central obesity: Waist circumference 102 cm or more (≥40 in) in males, 88 cm or more (≥35 in) in females; (2) Dyslipidemia: Triglycerides 150 mg/dL or more; (3) Dyslipidemia: HDL 40 mg/dL or less in males, 50 mg/dL or less in females; (4) Hypertension: at least 130/85 mmHg or use of antihypertensives; (5) Elevated fasting glucose: 100 mg/dL or more (≥5.6 mmol/L) or use of medication for hyperglycemia.

Weight loss and lifestyle changes can improve metabolic syndrome features.[56] However, bariatric surgery resolves metabolic syndrome in more that 95% of patients who achieve expected weight loss.[59] Because of the increased risk in the metabolic syndrome patient population, anesthesiologists should formulate perioperative management strategies to mitigate perianesthetic and surgical risk.

Pharmacology

Pharmacologic Principles

General pharmacokinetic principles dictate, with certain exceptions, that drug dosing should take into consideration the volume of distribution (VD) for administration of the loading dose, and the clearance for the maintenance dose.[60] A drug that is mainly distributed to lean tissues should have the loading dose calculated based on LBW. If the drug is equally distributed between adipose and lean tissues, dosing should be calculated based on TBW. For maintenance, a drug with similar clearance values in both obese and nonobese individuals should have the maintenance dose calculated based on LBW. However, a drug whose clearance increases with obesity should have the maintenance dose calculated according to TBW. Use of LBW and TBW in drug dosing for obese individuals is still under discussion.[61]

The relative volume of the central compartment in which drugs are first distributed remains unchanged in obese patients, but absolute body water content is decreased. Lean body and adipose tissue mass are increased, affecting lipophilic and polar drug distribution (Fig. 45-4). The VD in obese patients is affected by multiple factors including reduced total body water, increased total body fat, increased lean body mass, altered protein binding, increased blood volume, increased cardiac output, increased blood concentrations of free fatty acids, triglycerides, cholesterol, and α_1-acid glycoprotein, lipophilicity of the drug, and organomegaly.[7] Increased redistribution of a drug prolongs its elimination half-life even when clearance is unchanged or increased. Hyperlipidemia and an increased concentration of α_1-acid glycoprotein may affect protein binding, leading to a reduction in free drug concentration. Plasma albumin and total plasma protein concentrations and binding are not significantly changed by obesity, but when compared with normal-weight individuals, a relative increase in plasma protein binding may be evident. Splanchnic blood flow, blood volume, and cardiac output are all increased in obese patients. In contrast to the expected decrease in bioavailability of orally administered medications because of increased splanchnic blood flow, there is no significant difference in absorption and bioavailability when comparing obese and normal-weight subjects. Drugs that undergo phase I metabolism (oxidation, reduction, hydrolysis) are generally unaffected by changes induced by obesity, whereas phase II reactions (glucuronidation, sulfation) are enhanced.[7]

Histologic abnormalities of the liver are common in the obese, with concomitant deranged liver function tests, but drug clearance is not usually affected. Renal clearance of drugs is increased in obesity because of increased renal blood flow and glomerular filtration rate.[55,62] As a result of the increases in glomerular filtration rate and tubular secretion, drugs such as cimetidine and aminoglycoside antibiotics that depend on renal excretion may require increased dosing. Highly lipophilic substances such as barbiturates and benzodiazepines show significant increases in VD for obese individuals.[7] These drugs have a more selective distribution to fat stores and therefore a longer elimination half-life, but have comparable clearance values to normal individuals. Less lipophilic compounds have little or no change in VD with obesity. Exceptions to this rule include the highly lipophilic drugs digoxin, procainamide, and remifentanil.[63-65] Drugs with weak or moderate lipophilicity may be dosed on the basis of LBW. Adding 20% to the estimated IBW dose of hydrophilic medications is sufficient to include the obese patient's extra lean mass. Nondepolarizing muscle relaxants can be dosed in this manner. A recent study evaluated recovery times after reversal of neuromuscular blockade with sugammadex in obese (BMI >30 kg/m^2) and nonobese (BMI <30 kg/m^2) patients.[66] In the study, recovery time did not correlate with BMI. The authors recommend sugammadex dosing be based on actual body weight in both obese and nonobese patients.

Increased blood volume in the obese patient decreases plasma concentrations of rapidly injected intravenous drugs. Fat, however, has poor blood flow, and doses calculated on actual body weight could lead to excessive plasma concentrations. Calculating initial doses based on LBW with subsequent doses determined by pharmacologic response to the initial dose is a reasonable approach. Repeated injections may accumulate in fat, leading to a prolonged response because of subsequent release from this large depot. Table 45-3 presents dosing of intravenous agents used in obese patients.[67,68]

Other Perioperative Agents

Patients' usual medications should be continued until the time of surgery, with the possible exception of certain antihypertensives, insulin, and oral hypoglycemics. Antibiotic prophylaxis is usually indicated because of an increased incidence of wound infections in the obese. A recent prospective, cross-sectional study of 896 patients undergoing RYGB determined that the rate of surgical site infection was less in patients receiving a continuous infusion of cefazolin (1.55%) throughout the procedure compared to patients receiving either bolus dose ampicillin/sulbactam (4.16%) or ertapenem (1.98%).[69] Anxiolysis and prophylaxis against both aspiration pneumonitis and deep vein thrombosis (DVT) should

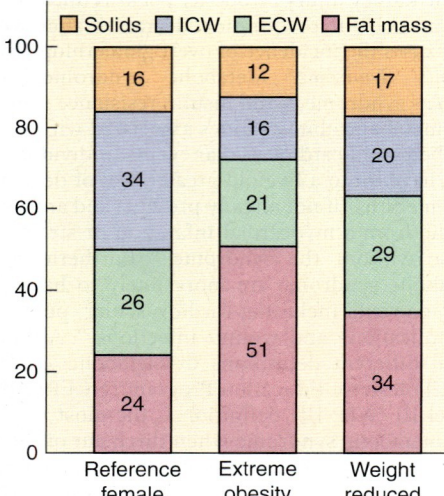

Figure 45-4 Body composition in extremely obese and weight-reduced states compared with reference female values. ICW, intracellular water; ECW, extracellular water. (Adapted from Das SK, Roberts SB, Kehayias JJ, et al. Body composition methods in extreme obesity. *Am J Physiol Endocrinol Metab*. 2003;284:E1080.)

Table 45-3 Intravenous Drug Dosing in Obesity[66–68]

Drug	Dosing	Practical Anesthesia Key Points
Thiopental	Induction: LBW (somewhat increased)	Increased initial dose due to increased blood volume, cardiac output, muscle mass Rapid distribution from plasma to periphery Increased absolute dose Prolonged duration of action due to high lipophilicity and increased VD Longer elimination half-life
Propofol	Induction: LBW (somewhat increased) Maintenance infusion: TBW	Short duration of action due to rapid redistribution Highly lipophilic Cardiac output is major determinant of peak plasma concentration Increased VD at steady state and increased clearance prevent increases in elimination half-life Total clearance and VD at steady state correlate with TBW during maintenance infusion Negative cardiovascular effects High affinity for fat and well-perfused organs High hepatic extraction and conjugation relate to TBW
Succinylcholine	TBW	Pseudocholinesterase activity increases linearly with increasing weight and large extracellular fluid compartment Dose of succinylcholine should be increased
Rocuronium	LBW	Dosing according to LBW to prevent delayed recovery due to increased VD Faster onset and longer duration when dosed according to TBW Pharmacokinetics and pharmacodynamics not altered in obese female patients
Vecuronium	LBW	Prolonged action when dosed according to TBW Dosing according to LBW to prevent delayed recovery due to increased VD and impaired hepatic clearance Obesity does not alter distribution or elimination of the drug
Atracurium	LBW	VD, absolute clearance, and elimination half-life unchanged by obesity Unchanged dose per unit body weight without prolongation of recovery because of organ function-independent elimination
Cis-atracurium	LBW	Pharmacokinetics similar to atracurium but prolonged duration of action when dosed according to TBW
Benzodiazepines		Highly lipophilic drugs with larger VD in obese patients result in longer duration of action Midazolam has potential for prolonged sedation because larger initial doses are required to achieve adequate serum concentrations
Fentanyl	LBW	Measured total body clearance has a nonlinear relationship to TBW and overestimates plasma concentration Fentanyl dosing based on a derived LBW or "pharmacokinetic mass" model correlates better with clearance than TBW dosing Dosing based on TBW overestimates dose requirements in the obese patient
Sufentanil	LBW	Highly lipid soluble Increased VD and prolonged elimination half-life, which correlates with degree of obesity Distributes extensively in excess body fat Similar pharmacokinetic parameters in obese and nonobese predict similar plasma concentrations Overestimation of plasma concentration occurs in the morbidly obese range (BMI >40 kg/m^2)
Remifentanil	LBW	Pharmacokinetics similar in obese and nonobese patients (i.e., more closely related to lean body mass than LBW) Systemic clearance and VD corrected per kilogram of TBW are significantly smaller in the obese patient; consider age and LBW for dosing
Dexmedetomidine	TBW	Highly selective α_2-adrenergic agonist Sedative-hypnotic, anesthetic-sparing analgesic, sympatholytic properties Lacks significant effects on respiration Ideal analgesic adjuvant in the morbidly obese patient As part of a balanced anesthetic, infusion rates of 0.2–0.7 µg/kg/hr produce clinically effective sedation with decreased analgesic and anesthetic requirements
Neostigmine	TBW	Prompt early reversal but delayed full recovery during neostigmine-induced reversal of vecuronium dosed according to TBW
Sugammadex	TBW	A modified γ-cyclodextrin compound that encapsulates rocuronium (and other steroid-based neuromuscular blockers to a lesser extent) May prove invaluable for more rapid and complete neuromuscular blockade reversal in obese patients

LBW, lean body weight; VD, volume of distribution; TBW, total body weight; BMI, body mass index.
Adapted with permission from Ogunnaike BO, Jones SB, Jones DB, et al. Anesthetic considerations for bariatric surgery. *Anesth Analg.* 2002;95:1793.

be addressed preoperatively. Oral benzodiazepines are reliable for anxiolysis and sedation. Intravenous midazolam can also be titrated in small doses for anxiolysis during the immediate preoperative period. Dexmedetomidine, because of its minimal respiratory depressant effects, should be considered. Pharmacologic intervention with H_2-receptor antagonists, nonparticulate antacids, or proton pump inhibitors will reduce gastric volume, acidity, or both, thereby reducing the risk and severity of aspiration pneumonitis.

Preoperative Evaluation

A comprehensive preoperative evaluation of the obese surgical patient is critical to identify and address possible multisystem comorbidities, and to allow the development of an individualized perioperative care plan.[70–72]

Airway—Preoperative airway assessment in obese patients is of paramount importance. Obesity played a significant role in US closed malpractice insurance claims related to airway management at induction.[73] Anatomic changes associated with obesity that contribute to a potentially difficult airway include limitation of movement of the atlantoaxial joint and cervical spine by upper thoracic and low cervical fat pads; excessive tissue folds in the mouth and pharynx; short, thick neck; thick submental fat pad; suprasternal, presternal, and posterior cervical fat; and large breasts in females. Excess pharyngeal tissue deposited in the lateral pharyngeal walls may not be noticed during routine airway examination. The history obtained from the patient and examination of previous records may help predict airway difficulties.

Obesity is an accepted risk factor for difficult mask ventilation and airway management. However, with adequate positioning and airway resources available, most obese patients can be adequately and safely managed. Overall, the magnitude of BMI does not significantly influence the difficulty of laryngoscopy.[74] Such difficulty in most studies correlates instead with increased age, male sex, temporomandibular joint pathology, Mallampati classes 3 and 4, OSA, and abnormal upper teeth.[75–77] The predictive role of OSA per se on difficult intubation has been recently disputed.[78] In a prospective study of bariatric patients by Neligan et al.[78] only a Mallampati score of 3 or more and male gender, but not BMI, OSA, or the apnea–hypopnea index (AHI), predicted the risk of difficult intubation. The patient's neck circumference has been identified as the single biggest predictor of problematic intubation in morbidly obese patients.[76] The probability of a problematic intubation is approximately 5% with a 40-cm (16-in) neck circumference compared with a 35% probability at 60-cm (24-in) neck circumference. In this study by Brodsky et al.[76] a larger neck circumference was associated with male gender, a higher Mallampati score, laryngoscopy grade 3 views, and OSA.

Cardiopulmonary—Attention should focus on issues peculiar to the obese patient including evaluation of the cardiopulmonary systems and the airway. Previous anesthetic experiences as detailed by the patient and previous anesthetic records are useful. Obese patients should be evaluated for systemic hypertension, pulmonary hypertension, signs of right and/or left ventricular failure, and ischemic heart disease. Signs of cardiac failure such as elevated jugular venous pressure, pathologic heart sounds, pulmonary crackles, hepatomegaly, and peripheral edema may all be difficult to detect because of excess adiposity. Pulmonary hypertension is fairly common in this patient population because of the chronic pulmonary impairment. The common features of pulmonary hypertension are exertional dyspnea, fatigue, and syncope (which reflect an inability to increase cardiac output during activity). Tricuspid regurgitation on echocardiography is the most useful confirmatory test of pulmonary hypertension but should be combined with clinical evaluation. An ECG may demonstrate signs of right ventricular hypertrophy such as tall precordial R waves, right axis deviation, and right ventricular strain. The higher the pulmonary artery pressure the more sensitive the ECG. Chest radiographs may show evidence of underlying lung disease and prominent pulmonary arteries.[79] Further cardiac testing may be individually required.[80]

Evidence of OSA and OHS should be obtained preoperatively because they are frequently associated with difficult airway management and increased perioperative pulmonary complications. A history of hypertension or a neck circumference greater than 40 cm (16 in) correlates with an increased probability of OSA. OSA is a legitimate reason to delay surgery for a proper evaluation.[33] OSA patients should generally be treated as inpatients; however, outpatient surgery can be considered under certain circumstances, including mild OSA, use of local or regional anesthesia with minimal sedation, availability of a 23-hour observation postanesthesia care unit (PACU), and when patients can resume oral medication at the time of discharge. OSA patients using a CPAP device at home should be instructed to bring it with them to the hospital, as it may be needed postoperatively. The possibility of invasive monitoring, prolonged intubation, and postoperative mechanical ventilation should be discussed with obese patients. Arterial blood gas measurements help evaluate ventilation, as well as the need for perioperative oxygen administration and postoperative ventilation. Routine pulmonary function tests and liver function tests are not cost-effective in asymptomatic obese patients.

Metabolic—Patients scheduled for repeat bariatric surgery should be screened preoperatively for long-term metabolic and nutritional abnormalities. The high prevalence of insulin resistance and diabetes in obese patients justifies the need of considering glycemia checks preoperatively, and correcting abnormalities if present. Preoperative evaluation should include assessment of therapies for glycemic control, last time and dose of preoperative administration, and usual glucose values for a specific patient. Electrolytes should be checked before surgery, particularly in patients with poor compliance to medications or acutely ill patients. Other nutritional deficiencies include vitamin B_{12}, iron, calcium, and folate. Vitamin and nutritional deficiencies can lead to a collective form of postoperative polyneuropathy, known as acute postgastric reduction surgery (APGARS) neuropathy, a polynutritional multisystem disorder characterized by protracted postoperative vomiting, hyporeflexia, and muscular weakness.[81] Differential diagnoses of this disorder include thiamine deficiency (Wernicke encephalopathy, beriberi), vitamin B_{12} deficiency, and Guillain–Barré syndrome. Close attention to dosing and monitoring of neuromuscular blocking agents is recommended in cases of suspected or diagnosed APGARS neuropathy. Chronic vitamin K deficiency may lead to coagulation abnormalities, requiring administration of vitamin K analog or fresh-frozen plasma.

Hematology—Morbid obesity is a known risk factor for perioperative thromboembolic events, including both DVT and sudden death from acute pulmonary embolism.[82] Several thrombo-prophylaxis protocols exist or are being developed,[83] but preoperative evaluation should confirm these plans. Guidelines from the American College of Chest Physicians recommend, in patients undergoing bariatric surgery, the combination of intermittent pneumatic compression devices with heparin (unfractionated or low molecular weight heparin), and warn that greater doses in obese patients may be needed than in non-obese ones.[84] Prolonged postoperative regimens (1 to 3 weeks) are being explored in bariatric patients.[83] Four important risk factors, namely venous stasis disease, BMI 60 or more, central obesity, and OHS and/or OSA, are significant in the development of postoperative DVT. If any of these factors are present, preoperative prophylactic placement of an inferior vena cava filter should be considered.[82] A combination of short duration of surgery, lower extremity pneumatic compression, and routine early ambulation may preclude mandatory heparin anticoagulation, except in patients with a history of previous DVT, a known hypercoagulable state, or a significant family history of DVT.[85]

Intraoperative Considerations

Equipment and Monitoring

Specially designed tables or two regularly sized operating room tables may be required for safe anesthesia and surgery in obese patients. Regular operating room tables have a maximum weight limit of approximately 200 kg, but operating room tables capable of holding up to 455 kg, with a greater width or side accessories to accommodate the extra girth, are available. Strapping obese patients to the operating room table in combination with a malleable beanbag helps keep them from falling off the operating room table.

Supine positioning causes ventilatory impairment and inferior vena cava and aortic compression in obese patients. FRC and oxygenation are decreased further with supine positioning (Fig. 45-1). Head-down positioning, often required during bariatric procedures, further worsens FRC and should be avoided if possible. Simply changing the obese patient from a sitting to supine position can cause a significant increase in oxygen consumption and cardiac output. The head-up position provides the longest safe apnea period during induction of anesthesia.[86] The extra time gained may help preclude hypoxemia if tracheal intubation is delayed. Both intraoperative positive end-expiratory pressure (PEEP) and the head-up position significantly decrease the alveolar–arterial oxygen tension difference and increase total respiratory compliance to a similar degree, but the head-up position results in lower airway pressures. Both, however, decrease cardiac output significantly, which partially counteracts the beneficial effects on oxygenation. Prone positioning, rarely required in the obese patient, should be correctly performed with freedom of abdominal movement to prevent detrimental effects on lung compliance, ventilation, and arterial oxygenation. Lateral decubitus positioning allows for better diaphragmatic excursion and should be favored over prone positioning whenever the surgical procedure permits. Particular care should be paid to protecting pressure areas, because pressure sores, neural injuries, and rhabdomyolysis may occur. Brachial plexus and lower extremity nerve injuries are frequent. Carpal tunnel syndrome is the most common mononeuropathy after bariatric surgery.[87] Other reported neurologic complications include encephalopathy (Wernicke), optic neuropathy, and myelopathy associated with vitamin B_{12} and copper deficiencies.[88]

Monitoring the surgical obese patient poses additional challenges. Careful selection of properly sized blood pressure cuff and its location are important. Blood pressure measurements can be falsely elevated if a cuff is too small. Cuffs with bladders that encircle a minimum of 75% of the upper arm circumference or, preferably, the entire arm, should be used. Forearm measurements with a standard cuff overestimate both systolic and diastolic blood pressures in obese patients.[89] Invasive arterial pressure monitoring may be indicated for the super morbidly obese patient, not only for those patients with cardiopulmonary disease but also for those patients in whom the noninvasive blood pressure cuff does not fit properly. Central venous catheterization, though not routinely needed, may be required for intravenous access in patients with inadequate peripheral access for perioperative fluid management.[90] Central venous catheters, pulmonary artery catheters, and/or transesophageal echocardiography can be used selectively in patients with significant cardiopulmonary disease or in patients undergoing extensive surgery.

Airway Management

Adequate preoxygenation is vital in obese patients because of rapid desaturation after loss of consciousness related to increased oxygen consumption and decreased FRC. Although 100% oxygen increases the formation of atelectasis, it extends the nonhypoxic apnea period after induction of anesthesia. Recent recommendations encourage the addition of a head-up position during preoxygenation for prolonging the nonhypoxic apneic period in the obese patient.[91–93] The extra time gained may help preclude hypoxemia if tracheal intubation is delayed. The head-up position can be achieved with reverse Trendelenburg or semi-sitting positions[86,94,95] and may also help to prevent aspiration and facilitate visualization during laryngoscopy. Preoperative use of noninvasive positive pressure ventilation (NIPPV) or application of CPAP during induction will also delay peri-induction hypoxemia.[96,97] Passive apneic oxygenation adjuvant techniques have been proposed to delay apneic hypoxemia, via oxygen supplementation by nasal cannula or laryngeal mask airway (LMA).[91]

Obese patients are more likely than nonobese patients to present with difficult mask ventilation and tracheal intubation, especially if they have a short thick neck and OSA.[73–75,98,99] If a difficult intubation is anticipated, awake fiberoptic intubation using topical or regional anesthesia is a prudent approach to maintain spontaneous ventilation. During awake intubation, sedative-hypnotic medications should be minimized. Sedation with dexmedetomidine during awake intubation provides adequate anxiolysis and analgesia without respiratory depression.[100] Hypoxia and aspiration of gastric contents should be prevented at all costs during tracheal intubation. An experienced colleague who is present or immediately available during induction and airway management can be helpful with mask ventilation or attempts at intubation. A surgeon capable of accessing the airway surgically should be readily available. The "ramped" position elevating the obese patient's upper body improves laryngoscopic view compared with the standard "sniffing" position.[101] Towels or folded blankets under the shoulders and head can compensate for the exaggerated flexed position of posterior cervical fat (Fig. 45-5). The objective of this maneuver, known as "stacking," is to position

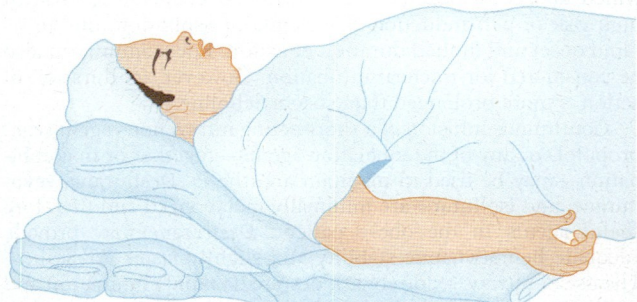

Figure 45-5 Ramped position with "stacking" of towels and blankets.

the patient so that the tip of the chin is at a higher level than the chest to facilitate laryngoscopy and tracheal intubation.

Although direct laryngoscopy is used successfully in many obese patients with optimal positioning, the immediate availability of other intubating tools is highly recommended. These include videolaryngoscopes, intubating stylettes (e.g., Eschmann stylet, tube exchanger), LMAs, and fiberoptic bronchoscopes. Videolaryngoscopes have proven to be efficient tools for intubating obese patients, reducing the duration and number of intubation attempts, with a similar or better glottic view than standard direct laryngoscopy.[99,102,103] Multiple laryngoscopic attempts and repeated attempts at intubation are associated with increased airway and hemodynamic complications.[104] Closed malpractice claims data also support the recommendations to limit conventional tracheal intubation attempts to three before using other strategies.[73] LMAs can be useful for temporarily achieving airway patency in patients with difficult mask ventilation and tracheal intubation[105] or for placing a definitive endotracheal tube (intubating LMA).[36,106]

Induction and Maintenance

Concerns of hypoxemia, gastric regurgitation, and aspiration during induction and tracheal intubation justify the common use of rapid sequence induction (RSI) strategies. Gastroesophageal reflux disease is relatively common in obese patients, and the incidence of regurgitation and severe pneumonitis in case of aspiration is increased in this population (as discussed earlier). Findings suggest that nonpremedicated nondiabetic fasting obese surgical patients with no significant gastroesophageal pathology are unlikely to have high volume, low pH gastric contents after routine preoperative fasting,[50] and that routine preoperative fasting guidelines (6 hours for solids, 2 hours for clear liquids) may be safe in obese patients.[107] In any case, the use of an RSI versus standard induction should be routinely and carefully evaluated in obese patients, and the final decision individualized based on the patient's risk of difficult mask ventilation, difficult tracheal intubation, hypoxemia, and gastric aspiration during induction.

No systematic comparison of anesthetic agents or techniques is available in obese patients. Larger doses of induction agents may be required because blood volume, muscle mass, and cardiac output increase linearly with the degree of obesity. Any of the commonly available intravenous induction agents may be employed after taking into consideration problems peculiar to individual patients. An increased dose of succinylcholine is necessary because of an increase in pseudocholinesterase activity. Myalgia is not frequently seen following succinylcholine use in morbidly obese patients.[108] Succinylcholine is highly recommended for tracheal intubation especially in obese patients in which airway management is considered challenging or with high risk of peri-induction hypoxemia or aspiration, due to its rapid onset and limited duration of action. Rocuronium can also be considered for tracheal intubation. However, its duration of action is more prolonged than succinylcholine.

Continuous infusion of a short-acting intravenous agent (e.g., propofol) or any of the inhalation agents—together or in combination—may be used to maintain anesthesia. Desflurane, sevoflurane, and isoflurane are minimally metabolized and therefore useful agents in the obese patient. Desflurane may provide adequate hemodynamic stability and slightly faster washout.[109] The use of nitrous oxide (N_2O), despite its rapid elimination and analgesic properties, is limited by the high oxygen demand in this patient population. Short-acting opioid analgesics are preferred in obese patients to minimize postoperative respiratory depression. Remifentanil and fentanyl, carefully titrated to clinical effect, are the most common choices.[70] Dexmedetomidine, an α_2-agonist with sedative and analgesic properties, has no clinically significant adverse effects on respiration and is an attractive anesthetic adjunct in obese patients.[110] Furthermore, it reduces postoperative opioid analgesic requirements.[110,111]

Profound muscle relaxation is important during laparoscopic bariatric procedures both to facilitate ventilation and to maintain an adequate working space for visualization and safe manipulation of laparoscopic instruments. It also facilitates extraction of excised tissues. Collapse of the pneumoperitoneum and tightening of the patient's musculature around port sites are early indications of inadequate muscle relaxation.[67] Vecuronium, rocuronium, and cis-atracurium are useful nondepolarizing muscle blocking agents for maintenance of muscle relaxation. Pneumoperitoneum should not be increased above 15 mmHg since intra-abdominal pressures of 20 mmHg or greater can cause caval compression and decrease cardiac output.[70] Cephalad displacement of the diaphragm and carina from a pneumoperitoneum during laparoscopy can cause a firmly secured endotracheal tube to displace into a main stem bronchus.[112]

Anesthesia personnel may be asked to facilitate the proper placement of an intragastric balloon to help the surgeon size the gastric pouch, and also to facilitate performance of leak tests with saline or methylene blue through a nasogastric tube. Care should be taken to ensure a tight seal of the endotracheal tube cuff, otherwise aspiration of saline or methylene blue can occur. All endogastric tubes should be completely removed (not just merely pulled back into the esophagus) before gastric division to avoid unplanned stapling and transection of these devices.

Fluid Management

Excess adipose tissue may mask peripheral perfusion, making fluid balance difficult to assess. Blood loss is usually greater in the obese than in the nonobese patient for the same type of surgery, because technical difficulties accessing the surgical site necessitate larger incisions and more extensive dissection. Because intravenous fluid requirements are generally greater than predicted, fluid management is particularly challenging in the obese patient. Normovolemia should be the goal, to avoid increased hemodynamic instability, postoperative nausea and vomiting, and acute tubular necrosis (ATN) from hypovolemia. ATN occurs in approximately 2% of patients undergoing bariatric surgery. Associated risk factors include BMI greater than 50 kg/m^2, prior history of renal disease, intraoperative hypotension, and prolonged surgical times.[113] Normovolemia also reduces the risk of hypervolemia resulting in decompensated congestive heart failure, peripheral tissue edema, and pulmonary complications. Rapid infusion of intravenous fluids should be avoided because pre-existing congestive cardiac failure is common in the obese patient. The use of IBW estimates and appropriate monitoring can help to avoid potential hyperhydration in morbidly obese patients.[114] Preliminary findings demonstrate that during laparoscopic bariatric surgery, urine output does not correlate with the rate of intraoperative fluid administration,[115] and the total volume of fluids infused does not seem to affect the incidence of postoperative rhabdomyolysis.[116]

Mechanical Ventilation

Obesity makes titration of ventilatory settings challenging, since increasing weight does not imply a proportional growth of the lung. Obese patients are more likely to be exposed to higher tidal volumes because of miscalculation of PBW or IBW,[117-119] and also to higher airway pressures due to the decreased respiratory system compliance. Although similar ventilatory parameters in nonobese patients can be used, it may be challenging to maintain end-expiratory (plateau) pressures of no more than 30 cm H_2O.[6] Greater inflation pressures may be tolerated in obese patients,[120] possibly because the extra adipose tissue partially attenuates lung overdistention.[121] In any case, 6 to 8 mL/kg PBW tidal volumes are often recommended for obese patients.[92,122] Larger tidal volumes offer no added advantages during ventilation of anesthetized morbidly obese patients.[123] Further increasing tidal volumes only increases the peak inspiratory airway pressure and plateau airway pressure without significantly improving arterial oxygen tension.[124] No specific ventilatory mode (volume vs. pressure control ventilation [PCV]) has been found significantly better for oxygenation and carbon dioxide clearance in obese patients, although pressure modes have in some studies correlated with increased oxygenation.[91,125-127]

PEEP is the only ventilatory parameter consistently shown to improve respiratory function in obese subjects, although the ideal PEEP value is still unknown.[128-130] Recruitment maneuvers in addition to the use of PEEP are the most effective ventilatory techniques to prevent postoperative atelectasis in obese patients and are increasingly recommended.[122,127] These techniques for alveolar recruitment are clearly beneficial in obese patients, compared to nonobese ones.[91,131] Different methods for performing recruitment maneuvers exist. A simple one proposed by Pelosi et al.[123] is a series of three short (6 seconds) inflations with PCV to administer a large tidal volume by reaching an inspiratory pressure of 40 to 55 cmH2O. Other recruitment techniques are summarized by Shah et al.[91] These higher-than-usual airway pressures may be needed to compensate for the decreased chest wall compliance, achieving an adequate transpulmonary pressure to avoid alveolar collapse. The combination of recruitment maneuvers and PEEP targets the opening and patency of small airway units, thereby improving ventilation–perfusion matching. This practice leads to less atelectasis and improved oxygenation,[130,132] shorter stay in the PACU, and decreased postoperative pulmonary complications[132] after laparoscopic bariatric surgery. Attention should be paid to avoid decreased venous return and cardiac output with PEEP or recruitment maneuvers, although they have been adequately tolerated in normovolemic morbidly obese patients.[124] Inspired oxygen fraction (FiO_2) should be titrated to the minimum level that assures acceptable oxygenation levels, but avoids reabsorption atelectasis. Some experts recommend the FiO_2 to be kept lower than 0.8 in obese patients.[123]

Emergence

Prompt but safe extubation reduces the likelihood that the morbidly obese patient will become ventilator-dependent. This is especially important in patients with underlying cardiopulmonary disease. The patient should be extubated in the semirecumbent position and recovered in the sitting position, which has less adverse effect on respiration.[123] In some institutions, policies have been developed for the mandatory presence of two anesthesia providers at emergence and extubation of morbidly obese patients.[133] Supplemental oxygen should be administered after extubation. Some authors recommend an observation period of at least 5 minutes after extubation before transporting the patient away from the operating room.[133] The risk of hypoventilation in the immediate postoperative period, with the consequent hypercapnia with or without hypoxemia, is leading to the development

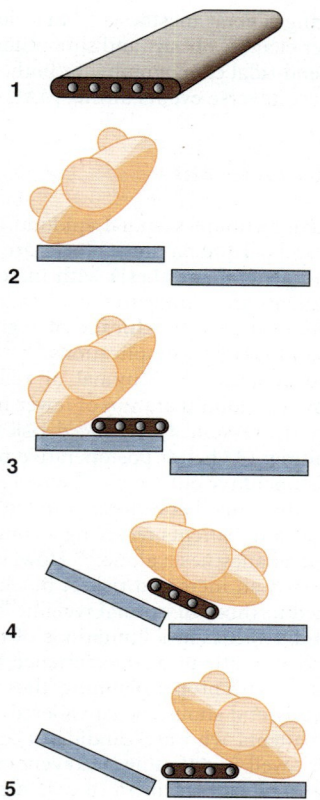

Figure 45-6 Illustration of the Walter Henderson maneuver. **1.** Patient transfer device (PTD, i.e., roller); **2.** patient tilted to slip roller underneath; **3.** roller slipped under patient; **4.** table tilted to roll patient "downhill" onto bed; **5.** patient rolled onto bed. (Reprinted with permission from Ogunnaike BO, Whitten CW. In response to Rosenblatt MA, Reich DL, Roth R, et al. [Letter]. *Anesth Analg.* 2004;98:1810.)

of noninvasive monitoring techniques and the increasing use of CPAP.[33]

Lifting devices such as the HoverMatt (Patient Handling Technologies, Allentown, PA), the patient transfer device (PTD; Alimed, Dedham, MA), and gantry-style, mechanical sling lifting devices are useful for transporting morbidly obese patients to and from the operating room table. The PTD can be combined with the Walter Henderson Maneuver (Fig. 45-6) to safely and gently transfer obese patients onto their postoperative beds.[133]

Monitored Anesthesia Care and Sedation

Monitoring of the adequacy of ventilation and oxygenation is extremely important in obese patients. Obese patients present a higher risk of sedation-induced respiratory depression, so careful titration of benzodiazepines, opioids, and propofol is mandatory to avoid hypercapnia and/or hypoxemia. Hypoxemia may require unplanned tracheal intubation, so a thorough airway examination and preparation for unintended airway management is critical even in monitored anesthesia care (MAC) or sedation cases. The prevalence of closed malpractice claims related to adverse respiratory events during monitored anesthesia cases is increasing, compared to respiratory complications or airway management complications encountered during general anesthesia.[134] In a closed claims analysis by Bhananker et al.,[135] obesity and suboptimal monitoring of pulse oximetry, end-tidal capnography, or both, were significant key factors in these adverse events during MAC.

Regional Anesthesia

Neuraxial anesthetic techniques (spinal, epidural, combined spinal-epidural [CSE]) and peripheral nerve blocks are used alone or in combination with general anesthesia with increasing frequency as more obese patients are coming to the operating room. Several studies have demonstrated the efficacy of regional techniques in reducing opioid-related complications,[136,137] but there are other distinct advantages: (1) Minimal or reduced manipulation of the airway; (2) administration of fewer medications with cardiopulmonary depression; (3) reduced risk of postoperative nausea and vomiting; (4) better postoperative pain control; and (5) improved postoperative outcomes.[138] When epidural anesthesia is combined with general anesthesia, time to tracheal extubation may be reduced in patients receiving a combined technique compared to general anesthesia alone.[139] However, studies demonstrate that there is an increased risk of block failure in obese patients compared to those of normal weight.[140] Failure is often due to technical difficulties and limitations of regional anesthesia. In addition, these patients also experience an increased risk of complications.[141] With proper planning, these techniques may be used successfully and should be considered in the anesthetic plan for obese patients who are candidates for regional anesthesia. However, well-functioning intravenous access should be secured prior to block placement in case high spinal or local anesthetic systemic toxicity occurs following regional anesthesia.

Neuraxial Anesthesia

Physiologic changes associated with neuraxial anesthesia. Neuraxial anesthesia can produce serious cardiopulmonary alterations in obese patients undergoing surgery. Because pulmonary mechanics, lung volumes, FRC, oxygenation, and ventilation are altered in these individuals, supine and Trendelenburg positioning during neuraxial anesthesia can lead to deterioration of lung volumes and further reductions in FRC. FRC may fall below closing capacity promoting small airway collapse, atelectasis, ventilation–perfusion mismatch, and hypoxia, especially during supine and Trendelenburg positioning (Fig. 45-1).[142] It is often helpful to measure the oxygen saturation in the sitting and supine positions to indicate the degree of pulmonary reserve prior to initiating neuraxial anesthesia. In addition to these pulmonary concerns, there are cardiovascular changes that warrant careful monitoring. The excess weight of the abdominal wall can compress the vena cava, causing decreased cardiac preload, reflex tachycardia, and decreased cardiac output. In a large series of obese patients undergoing nonobstetric surgery who had received spinal anesthesia, more than one-third developed hypotension.[143] Three of the 1,000 patients in this series also experienced cardiac arrest. There are other reports of cardiac arrest after supine positioning in morbidly obese patients.[144] Changes to the supine position likely contributed to the circulatory changes resulting in these arrests.

Despite these important considerations, use of neuraxial techniques can offer important advantages when compared to general anesthesia alone. Parenteral opioid administration can be hazardous in these patients because of increased sensitivity to opioids, risk of hypoxemia, a high incidence of OSA, and increased incidence of adverse respiratory events following surgery. The American Society of Anesthesiologists has published guidelines for the care of patients with OSA and recommends that regional anesthetic techniques should be considered to reduce or eliminate the requirements for systemic opioids in patients with sleep apnea.[33]

Positioning and placement. Positioning is an important step in placement of a successful neuraxial anesthetic. Spinal or epidural placement in the sitting position will assist with identification of the midline. The patient's back should be parallel to the edge of the bed to prevent lateral needle deviation away from the midline. Lateral deviation of the midline will increase the depth to the epidural or spinal spaces and can result in block failure and an increased risk for intraoperative conversion to general anesthesia in less-than-ideal circumstances. Anatomic landmarks are often obscured in these patients. If spinal processes cannot be appreciated with deep palpation, a line can be drawn from the cervical vertebral spinal process to the uppermost portion of the gluteal cleft. This line approximates the midline of the patient over the vertebral column. Ultrasound imaging can also be helpful to identify spinal processes and has been shown to significantly reduce the number of needle passes and decrease the time for spinal block placement in morbidly obese patients undergoing orthopedic surgery.[145] Since the iliac crests may also be difficult to appreciate, the patient's skin folds can be used to aid in drawing a line perpendicular to the vertical line so that the intersection point can serve as a reasonable spinal or epidural needle insertion guide.

Neuraxial anesthetic placement can be particularly difficult, especially when bony landmarks are nonpalpable, there is limited back flexion,[146] and there are false losses of resistance due to fat deposition. It is often difficult to predict the depth to the epidural space, although it generally correlates with BMI.[147] A recent study suggests that prepuncture ultrasonography may be useful to facilitate epidural placement in obese parturients to predict the depth to the epidural space.[148] However, ultrasound has limitations in this patient population because the image quality can be compromised due to fat overlying the epidural space and the distance to the epidural space may be inaccurate if the subcutaneous tissue is compressed. Future development of ultrasound technologies may incorporate the use of ultrasound-guided needle techniques to aid epidural placement in challenging patients.[149] In some cases, a long 25-gauge needle can be used for infiltration of local anesthetic, as well as to identify spinous processes. The patient is often helpful in determining whether needle placement is midline or lateral and directing the needle to the midline (e.g., Does it feel like I'm in the middle of your back?). A recent study demonstrated that obese women were less likely to identify the midline by pinprick compared to nonobese. However, both groups of women were correct 99% of the time in identifying whether a stimulus (fingertip or pinprick) was to the right or left of the midline.[150] In most cases, standard neuraxial needles (9 to 10 cm) are of sufficient length if placement is midline.[151] However, longer needles (16 cm) are sometimes needed in extremely obese parturients. These needles can cause serious injury so they should only be used after careful assessment of the midline when standard needles are inadequate.

Spinal anesthesia. Single injection spinal anesthesia is a popular neuraxial anesthetic technique but there are concerns about technical difficulties, exaggerated spread of local anesthetic, hypotension, and an inability to prolong the block, especially in the obese patient. Spinal anesthesia is reasonable if the airway examination is normal, there is no cardiopulmonary disease, and the surgery is expected to be less than 90 minutes. It is often easier to insert the spinal needle when a large gauge stiff epidural needle is used as a guide for the smaller flexible spinal needle.

Decreased cerebral spinal fluid (CSF) volumes have been confirmed in obese patients by magnetic resonance imaging[152] suggesting that the effective dose of spinal local anesthetic is reduced in obese patients compared to a nonobese patient. The decreased spinal fluid volume results from displacement of the CSF by soft tissue movement into the intervertebral foramen caused by an increase in abdominal pressure. This results in a direct positive correlation between the height of the block and the degree of obesity when patients receive the same volume and dose of spinal bupivacaine in the sitting position.[153] Others have demonstrated higher sensory levels of spinal anesthesia in obese patients[154] and the need for smaller volumes of bupivacaine in obese individuals to achieve similar sensory levels.[155] In addition to these factors, the large buttocks of obese patients may place the vertebral column in the Trendelenburg position, exaggerating the cephalad spread of spinal anesthesia. In order to avoid a high block when hyperbaric bupivacaine is used, a ramp can be placed under the patient's chest to elevate the cervical and thoracic spines to avoid the Trendelenburg position induced by a large buttocks. Although there are other studies that report no clinical differences in the height of sensory block after hypobaric[156] and hyperbaric[157] spinal anesthesia in obese compared to nonobese parturients, spinal anesthesia should be performed with caution because of the consequences of extensive blockade, prolonged surgery, and the hazards of intraoperative induction of general anesthesia.

Epidural anesthesia. Epidural anesthesia offers several advantages over single-injection spinal anesthesia including titratable dosing of local anesthetics, ability to prolong the block, decreased risk of excessive motor block, more controllable hemodynamic changes, and utilization for postoperative analgesia. However, in laboring patients, a multicenter prospective observational study found that epidural anesthesia failed more often than spinal or CSE techniques.[158] Increased maternal BMI was significantly related to failure of neuraxial techniques. Hood and Dewan[159] also demonstrated an increased initial failure rate of epidural catheters in obese laboring patients—42% compared to 6% in the nonobese control group. In addition, Hodgkinson and Hussain[160] demonstrated that the height of an epidural block for a given volume of local anesthetic is proportional to BMI and maternal weight but not height. Incremental dosing of epidural-administered local anesthetics will reduce the risk of hypotension and high block.

Catheter dislodgment is another potential problem in obese patients. Because the ligamentum flavum has a mild grip on the epidural catheter, body repositioning allows the epidural catheter to be pulled into or out of the subcutaneous fat. Therefore, before securing the epidural catheter, a patient should move from an upright sitting position to a lateral position. Hamilton et al.[161] evaluated changes in epidural catheter distance to skin with patient position modifications (sitting flexed to upright, upright to lateral, flexed to lateral). These changes were significantly increased with BMI, and averaged a maximum of 0.67 cm to 1.04 cm in parturients with BMIs lower than 25 and greater than 30, respectively. A more than 4 cm change was observed in one obese patient.[161] After repositioning, the catheter is subsequently taped in place without adjusting the catheter. This maneuver is helpful in reducing the incidence of catheter dislodgement and block failure.

In cases of inadvertent dural puncture, catheters may be threaded into the subarachnoid space for continuous spinal analgesia. Continuous spinal anesthesia offers the benefits of a single-injection spinal (i.e., reliability, density); however, converting to spinal anesthesia does not appear to affect the rate of postdural puncture headache or epidural blood patch.[162] Each case must be handled individually and if a continuous spinal catheter is placed, care must be used to avoid accidental administration of an epidural dose of local anesthetic through the spinal catheter that will increase risk of a high spinal, respiratory compromise, and loss of the airway patency. Higher levels of spinal anesthesia may result from reduced CSF volume[152] and large buttocks may increase cephalad spread. These catheters should be carefully marked so that they are not mistaken for an epidural catheter.

Combined spinal-epidural (CSE). CSE anesthesia is an alternative to conventional spinal or epidural anesthesia; however, there is concern that the technique is more complicated than either spinal or epidural alone, and the epidural catheter is "unproven" during the duration of spinal analgesia. Although CSE catheters fail at similar rates compared with conventional epidural catheters,[163] delayed recognition of a nonfunctional epidural catheter is a disadvantage of this technique, and is particularly problematic for prolonged surgical cases. This can increase the risk of intraoperative conversion to general anesthesia. However, even if the patient does not receive a "spinal dose" during CSE placement, the return of CSF in the spinal needle is confirmation of midline needle placement. This increases the likelihood of bilateral block, and improves sacral spread and onset of analgesia in laboring parturients.[164]

Peripheral Nerve Block

The use of peripheral nerve blocks with and without general anesthesia is increasingly common for surgical procedures. In obese patients, these blocks can be technically challenging and have an increased failure rate compared to techniques performed in patients of normal weight.[141,165] Although experience of the anesthesiologist with these blocks may influence their success, a large prospective study evaluating peripheral nerve blocks determined that the risk of block failure increased proportionately with BMI.[165] Continuous supraclavicular, paravertebral, superficial cervical plexus, and epidural blocks had the highest failure rates. Supplemental general anesthesia was also needed to supplement these blocks more often in obese patients. Another study compared success rates of supraclavicular blocks in obese and nonobese patients, and reported a lower success rate in obese patients.[166] However, the rate of successful blocks in the obese patients remained high (94.3%). Case reports have also described the use of oblique subcostal transversus abdominis plane (TAP) catheters as an alternative to epidural analgesia after upper abdominal surgery.[167,168]

Dosing of local anesthetics during regional anesthesia can be challenging in the obese. For instance, if a patient receives too large of a dose, hypotension, systemic toxicity, or respiratory compromise related to diaphragmatic hemiparesis may occur. If the dose is too small, there is a risk of block failure. Although absorption of local anesthetics is dependent on the site of injection (i.e., greatest with intercostal blocks, followed by epidural and spinal blocks), calculation of the maximum safe local anesthetic dose is important because this dose is often based on patient weight. However, basing the dose on the actual weight in this patient population will increase the risk for systemic toxicity. Therefore, local anesthetic dosing should be based on IBW rather than actual weight.

Although there are advantages of peripheral nerve blocks in these patients, placement is often difficult due to difficult positioning, obscure anatomic landmarks, and inadequate needle length. Since increased BMI is associated with increased number of attempts and risk of block failure,[141] the use of ultrasound in these patients may be a helpful tool to increase both block success[169,170] and safety. Unlike nerve stimulator or paresthesia techniques, ultrasound has the advantage of real-time identification of landmarks below the skin surface. Although real-time ultrasound has been shown to increase success rates,[169–171] decrease procedure time,[172] and decrease the minimum effective dose of local anesthetic solutions[173] in patients receiving peripheral nerve blocks who are of normal weight, reports of use of this technique in the obese are more limited. Because of greater soft tissue mass in the obese, the ultrasound must penetrate greater depths to visualize target structures.[174] Although low-frequency transducers increase depth of penetration, higher frequency transducers produce the best images.[174] Consequently, ultrasound images in the obese may be compromised, both due to an increased number of reflective surfaces as well as greater depth to the structures. Reports confirm increased success rates in the obese undergoing peripheral nerve blocks with ultrasound.[169,170] However, successful use of ultrasound for peripheral nerve blocks in patients of all sizes requires training and experience. The American Society of Regional Anesthesia and Pain Medicine and the European Society of Regional Anesthesia have recommended education and training guidelines for ultrasound-guided regional anesthesia.[175]

Postoperative Considerations

Ventilatory Evaluation and Management

There is an increased incidence of atelectasis in morbidly obese patients after general anesthesia, which persists into the postoperative period. Consequently, initiation of CPAP or bilevel positive airway pressure (BiPAP) has been advocated. Despite a theoretical risk, the use of NIPPV does not seem to increase the incidence of major anastomotic leakage after gastric bypass surgery. Postoperative CPAP may improve oxygenation, but does not facilitate CO_2 elimination.[176] Adequate analgesia, use of a properly fitted elastic binder for abdominal support, early ambulation, deep breathing exercises, and incentive spirometry are all useful adjuncts to avoid postoperative hypoventilation and atelectasis. Pulse oximetry and arterial blood gases should be monitored when they are indicated.

Postoperative Analgesia

Pain management is an important part of the postoperative care plan of obese patients. The goal of pain management in these individuals is not only to provide adequate analgesia but also to facilitate early mobilization and adequate respiratory function. Mobilization in these individuals is often difficult, yet critically important in the prevention of complications. Pressure ulcerations, pulmonary emboli, deep venous thrombosis, and pneumonia are some of the common complications that can be prevented by early mobilization. Plans for pain management should include: (1) Multimodal analgesics; (2) regional anesthesia/analgesia techniques; (3) early mobilization; (4) supplemental oxygen; and (5) elevation of the head of the bed. Besides delivery of a safe analgesic technique, adequate postoperative monitoring is required to ensure safety.

Obese patients with OSA have an increased likelihood of postoperative pulmonary complications.[30] Opioids increase the risk of central apnea in all patients, but those with OSA are at particular risk for opioid-induced apnea.[33] Because of the risk of hypoventilation and hypoxemia in obese patients with and without OSA, postoperative pain management should include opioid-sparing multimodal analgesic techniques, including regional anesthesia. These techniques are known to reduce the risk of opioid-related complications.[136,137] In patients with regional anesthesia contraindications, the use of multimodal analgesics (e.g., local anesthetics, NSAIDs) will reduce opioid consumption and the risk of respiratory depression. The American Society of Anesthesiologists practice guidelines encourage the use of regional analgesic techniques instead of systemic opioids in the postoperative pain management of patients with OSA, and are summarized in Table 45-4.

Monitoring

Obese patients who have received either neuraxial or parenteral opioids require careful postoperative monitoring for respiratory depression. However, routine admission to intensive care or high acuity care units is unnecessary since admission to these units has not been shown to reduce the risk of pulmonary complications or change perioperative outcome.[177] Patients with a history of OSA and being treated with CPAP should be encouraged to bring their own equipment to the hospital to reduce the risk of respiratory depression.[178] All patients receiving neuraxial opioids should be monitored for adequacy of ventilation (respiratory rate, depth of respiration), oxygenation (pulse oximetry when appropriate), and level of consciousness.[178]

Ambulatory Anesthesia

Identifying obese patients who are suitable candidates for ambulatory surgery depends upon early identification of patient comorbidities, invasiveness of the procedure, anesthetic technique, postoperative pain management, and skills of both the surgeon and anesthesiologist.[179] Although a number of studies have identified obesity as a risk factor for perioperative complications, a recent systematic review determined that BMI alone

---

Table 45-4 Summary of Practice Guidelines for the Perioperative Management of Patients with Obstructive Sleep Apnea (OSA): A Report by the American Society of Anesthesiologists Task Force on Perioperative Management of Patients with Obstructive Sleep Apnea

Regional anesthetic techniques should be considered to reduce or eliminate the requirements for systemic opioids in patients with OSA.
If neuraxial anesthesia is planned, the benefits and risks of using an opioid or opioid-local anesthetic mixture as compared to local anesthetic alone must be considered.
If patient-controlled systemic opioids are used, continuous background infusions should be avoided or used with extreme caution.
Nonsteroidal anti-inflammatory agents and other modalities should be considered to reduce opioid requirements.
Supplemental oxygen should be administered continuously to all patients who are at increased perioperative risk from OSA until they are able to maintain their baseline oxygen saturation while breathing room air.
Hospitalized patients at increased risk of respiratory compromise from OSA should be monitored with continuous pulse oximetry after discharge from the recovery room.

does not increase the risk for perioperative complications or unexpected admission after ambulatory surgery.[180] However, the authors caution that most super-obese patients (i.e., BMI ≥50 kg/m^2) are not candidates for ambulatory surgery.

Because many morbidly obese patients are diagnosed with sleep-disordered breathing, these patients may be considered for ambulatory procedures if their comorbid conditions are optimized and postoperative pain control is easily achieved with nonopioid techniques. The morbidly obese and those with OSA present unique and increasingly frequent challenges to ambulatory practices. Estimates suggest that 60% to 90% of all OSA patients have a BMI greater than or equal to 30 kg/m^2.[181] However, many patients with OSA do not carry the formal diagnosis, yet are more likely to experience major anesthetic problems throughout the perioperative period. A recent prospective cohort study of ambulatory surgical patients with propensity for OSA revealed an increase in number of laryngoscopy attempts, difficult laryngoscopic grade view, and the use of fiberoptic intubation.[182] These patients may also have respiratory insufficiency soon after extubation, as well as increased risks for emergent re-intubation, respiratory failure, mechanical ventilation, aspiration pneumonia, atrial fibrillation, and acute respiratory distress syndrome (ARDS).[35,183,184] These patients are also more likely to suffer from respiratory arrest with preoperative sedation or postoperative analgesia, because they are particularly sensitive to the respiratory depressant effects of even small dosages of sedatives or analgesics. Recent data suggest that patients who have a pre- or postoperative diagnosis of OSA are twice as likely to have respiratory complications compared to controls.[185] However, patients with a preoperative diagnosis of OSA who utilized CPAP were less likely to experience cardiovascular complications compared with patients who are diagnosed postoperatively.

Some recommend close postoperative monitoring of oxygen saturation in ambulatory OSA patients in an intensive care unit setting prior to discharge.[186] Use of local or regional anesthesia with minimal sedation and availability of a 23-hour observation PACU can facilitate such cases in the ambulatory setting. The possibility of invasive monitoring, prolonged tracheal intubation, and postoperative mechanical ventilation should also be discussed with obese patients. Although well-designed prospective trials are needed to assess the suitability of OSA patients for ambulatory surgery, patients receiving CPAP preoperatively should be advised to bring the CPAP device with them to the hospital and to use it for several days postoperatively.[187]

Recently, the American College of Surgeons National Surgical Quality Improvement Program (NSQIP) database identified risk factors for morbidity and mortality with 72 hours after ambulatory surgery.[188] Although the incidence of morbidity and mortality was only 0.1% in nearly 250,000 cases, independent risk factors for perioperative morbidity included: high BMI, chronic obstructive pulmonary disease, hypertension, history of transient ischemic attack or stroke, previous cardiac surgery, and longer surgical times. In the cohort, unplanned postoperative intubation, pneumonia, and wound disruption were the most commonly identified comorbidities. Others have determined that increased BMI, ASA 3 or more, age above 80 years, and length of surgery above 1 hour all increased the risk for unplanned hospital admission. Because increased BMI is a contributor for increased perioperative risk, exclusion criteria should be developed for patients undergoing ambulatory surgery.

Critical Care and Resuscitation

Caring for critically ill obese patients outside of the operating room poses the same challenges as during surgery, in terms of equipment, monitoring, and multiple comorbidities.[120] In addition, nutritional status of the critically ill obese patient is often paradoxical and difficult to address. Hyperglycemia from pre-existing or stress-induced diabetes is common and should be corrected because hyperglycemia is associated with a higher mortality rate. Obese patients are more likely to become ventilator-dependent than nonobese patients. The risks of obesity and commonly associated comorbidities (e.g., diabetes)[189] for the development acute lung injury (ALI) and/or ARDS is still unclear. Although BMI has been associated with an increased risk of developing ALI/ARDS,[119,190] its effect on clinical outcomes is still being explored.[119,191,192]

The possible need for cardiopulmonary resuscitation should be entertained when caring for the morbidly obese critically ill patient, including both equipment and technical concerns. Chest compressions may not be effective and mechanical compression devices may be required. The maximum 400 J of energy on regular defibrillators is usually sufficient for morbidly obese patients because their chest wall is usually not much thicker, but the higher transthoracic impedance from the fat may require a greater number of attempts. Airway management by conventional means may be very difficult. Tracheostomy, percutaneous cricothyrotomy, transtracheal jet ventilation, and retrograde wire intubation are time-consuming and technically difficult procedures in such emergency situations and should be reserved as final options and be performed by experienced practitioners.[193] Direct visualization of anatomic hallmarks during emergent cricothyroidotomy can also be extremely challenging in the obese patient. A novel technique has recently been proposed, in which palpation of the cricothyroid membrane can facilitate placement of an Eschmann stylette preloaded with a tracheal tube and inserted using a Seldinger-like technique.[194]

Morbidity and Mortality

Postoperative morbidity is increased in obese patients, but increased mortality is controversial.[192,195,196] The most common postoperative complications are respiratory (atelectasis, pneumonia), vascular (thrombophlebitis, DVT), and wound complications (infection, dehiscence). In addition, rhabdomyolysis is more common in morbidly obese patients undergoing laparoscopic procedures when compared with open procedures, especially with prolonged procedures. The incidence of perioperative adverse events is strongly associated with pre-existing disease more so than BMI alone.[197] For example, a patient with previously diagnosed metabolic syndrome has significantly greater risk of perioperative morbidity and mortality than an obese patient with no metabolic syndrome features.[198,199] Obese patients present a higher risk of perioperative pulmonary complications, especially if preoperative respiratory conditions (e.g., OSA) are present.[30,70] Obesity increases the risk of surgical site infections.[200,201] Some known contributing factors are hyperglycemia or diabetes,[201] longer duration of surgical procedures,[201] hypoperfusion or low tissue oxygen tension,[202,203] and low tissue antibiotic concentration. Morbid obesity significantly increases the risk of postoperative thromboembolic events.[82] Sequential compression devices (SCDs), routine early ambulation, and careful perioperative anticoagulation decrease the risk of thromboembolism.[85] Because of the higher risk of postoperative complications than in nonobese patients, outpatient surgery in this population should be individualized,[70,204] although it is becoming more accepted and safe in selected patients and procedures.[70,205]

REFERENCES

1. Obesity: preventing and managing the global epidemic. Report of a WHO consultation. *World Health Organ Tech Rep Ser.* 2000;894:i–xii, 1–253.
2. World Health Organization. Obesity and Overweight Fact Sheet #311. 2015. Accessed October 12, 2015.
3. Ogden CL, Carroll MD, Kit BK, et al. Prevalence of childhood and adult obesity in the United States, 2011–2012. *JAMA.* 2014;311:806–814.
4. Ng M, Fleming T, Robinson M, et al. Global, regional, and national prevalence of overweight and obesity in children and adults during 1980–2013: a systematic analysis for the Global Burden of Disease Study 2013. *Lancet.* 2014; 384:766–781.
5. Berrington de Gonzalez A, Hartge P, Cerhan JR, et al. Body-mass index and mortality among 1.46 million white adults. *N Engl J Med.* 2010;363:2211–2219.
6. ARDSNet. Ventilation with lower tidal volumes as compared with traditional tidal volumes for acute lung injury and the acute respiratory distress syndrome. The Acute Respiratory Distress Syndrome Network. *N Engl J Med.* 2000; 342:1301–1308.
7. Leykin Y, Miotto L, Pellis T. Pharmacokinetic considerations in the obese. *Best Pract Res Clin Anaesthesiol.* 2011;25:27–36.
8. Pai MP, Paloucek FP. The origin of the "ideal" body weight equations. *Ann Pharmacother.* 2000;34:1066–1069.
9. Leykin Y, Pellis T, Del Mestro E, et al. Anesthetic management of morbidly obese and super-morbidly obese patients undergoing bariatric operations: hospital course and outcomes. *Obes Surg.* 2006;16:1563–1569.
10. Menke A, Muntner P, Wildman RP, et al. Measures of adiposity and cardiovascular disease risk factors. *Obesity.* 2007;15:785–795.
11. Leitzmann MF, Moore SC, Koster A, et al. Waist circumference as compared with body-mass index in predicting mortality from specific causes. *PLoS One.* 2011;6:e18582.
12. Lagerros YT Rossner S. Obesity management: what brings success? *Therap Adv Gastroenterol.* 2013;6:77–88.
13. Tsai AG, Wadden TA. Systematic review: an evaluation of major commercial weight loss programs in the United States. *Ann Intern Med.* 2005;142:56–66.
14. Hemmingsson E, Johansson K, Eriksson J, et al. Weight loss and dropout during a commercial weight-loss program including a very-low-calorie diet, a low-calorie diet, or restricted normal food: observational cohort study. *Am J Clin Nutr.* 2012;96:953–961.
15. Apovian CM, Aronne LJ, Bessesen DH, et al. Pharmacological management of obesity: an Endocrine Society clinical practice guideline. *J Clin Endocrinol Metab.* 2015;100:342–362.
16. Aronne LJ, Wadden TA, Peterson C, et al. Evaluation of phentermine and topiramate versus phentermine/topiramate extended-release in obese adults. *Obesity (Silver Spring).* 2013;21:2163–2171.
17. Carroll FI, Blough BE, Mascarella SW, et al. Bupropion and bupropion analogs as treatments for CNS disorders. *Adv Pharmacol.* 2014;69:177–216.
18. Wadden TA, Hollander P, Klein S, et al. Weight maintenance and additional weight loss with liraglutide after low-calorie-diet-induced weight loss: the SCALE Maintenance randomized study. *Int J Obes (Lond).* 2013;37: 1443–1451.
19. Bray GA, Ryan DH. Drug treatment of the overweight patient. *Gastroenterology.* 2007;132:2239–2252.
20. MacWalter RS, Fraser HW, Armstrong KM. Orlistat enhances warfarin effect. *Ann Pharmacother.* 2003;37:510–512.
21. Yun JW. Possible anti-obesity therapeutics from nature—a review. *Phytochemistry.* 2010;71:1625–1641.
22. Abe A, Kaye AD, Gritsenko K, et al. Perioperative analgesia and the effects of dietary supplements. *Best Pract Res Clin Anaesthesiol.* 2014;28:183–189.
23. Arterburn D, Powers JD, Toh S, et al. Comparative effectiveness of laparoscopic adjustable gastric banding vs laparoscopic gastric bypass. *JAMA Surg.* 2014;149:1279–1287.
24. Sinha AC, Singh PM, Bhat S. Are we operating too late? Mortality analysis and stochastic simulation of costs associated with bariatric surgery: Reconsidering the BMI threshold. *Obes Surg.* 2016;26(1):219–228.
25. Nguyen NT. Open vs. laparoscopic procedures in bariatric surgery. *J Gastrointest Surg.* 2004;8:393–395.
26. U.S. Food and Drug Administration. Vagal nerve stimulator. 2015; http://www.fda.gov/NewsEvents/Newsroom/PressAnnouncements/ucm430223.htm. Accessed October 12, 2015.
27. Zerrweck C, Maunoury V, Caiazzo R, et al. Preoperative weight loss with intragastric balloon decreases the risk of significant adverse outcomes of laparoscopic gastric bypass in super-super obese patients. *Obes Surg.* 2012;22: 777–782.
28. Steier J, Lunt A, Hart N, et al. Observational study of the effect of obesity on lung volumes. *Thorax.* 2014;69:752–759.
29. Salome CM, King GG, Berend N. Physiology of obesity and effects on lung function. *J Appl Physiol.* 2010;108:206–211.
30. Memtsoudis SG, Besculides MC, Mazumdar M. A rude awakening—the perioperative sleep apnea epidemic. *N Engl J Med.* 2013;368:2352–2353.
31. Abrishami A, Khajehdehi A, Chung F. A systematic review of screening questionnaires for obstructive sleep apnea. *Can J Anaesth.* 2010;57:423–438.
32. Yeh PS, Lee YC, Lee WJ, et al. Clinical predictors of obstructive sleep apnea in Asian bariatric patients. *Obes Surg.* 2010;20:30–35.
33. American Society of Anesthesiologists Task Force on Perioperative Management of Patients with Obstructive Sleep Apnea. Practice guidelines for the perioperative management of patients with obstructive sleep apnea: an updated report by the American Society of Anesthesiologists Task Force on Perioperative Management of Patients with Obstructive Sleep Apnea. *Anesthesiology.* 2014;120:268–286.
34. Chirinos JA, Gurubhagavatula I, Teff K, et al. CPAP, weight loss, or both for obstructive sleep apnea. *N Engl J Med.* 2014;370:2265–2275.
35. Memtsoudis S, Liu SS, Ma Y, et al. Perioperative pulmonary outcomes in patients with sleep apnea after noncardiac surgery. *Anesth Analg.* 2011;112: 113–121.
36. Apfelbaum JL, Hagberg CA, Caplan RA, et al. Practice guidelines for management of the difficult airway: an updated report by the American Society of Anesthesiologists Task Force on management of the difficult airway. *Anesthesiology.* 2013;118:251–270.
37. Porhomayon J, Nader ND, Leissner KB, et al. Respiratory perioperative management of patients with obstructive sleep apnea. *J Intensive Care Med.* 2014;29:145–153.
38. Marik PE, Desai H. Characteristics of patients with the "malignant obesity hypoventilation syndrome" admitted to an ICU. *J Intensive Care Med.* 2013; 28:124–130.
39. Cullen A, Ferguson A. Perioperative management of the severely obese patient: a selective pathophysiological review. *Can J Anaesth.* 2012;59:974–996.
40. Chau EH, Lam D, Wong J, et al. Obesity hypoventilation syndrome: a review of epidemiology, pathophysiology, and perioperative considerations. *Anesthesiology.* 2012;117:188–205.
41. Finer N. Medical consequences of obesity. *Medicine.* 2011;39:18–23.
42. Fraley MA, Birchem JA, Senkottaiyan N, et al. Obesity and the electrocardiogram. *Obes Rev.* 2005;6:275–281.
43. Alpert MA, Terry BE, Hamm CR, et al. Effect of weight loss on the ECG of normotensive morbidly obese patients. *Chest.* 2001;119:507–510.
44. Engeli S, Bohnke J, Gorzelniak K, et al. Weight loss and the renin-angiotensin-aldosterone system. *Hypertension.* 2005;45:356–362.
45. Haslam DW, James WP. Obesity. *Lancet.* 2005;366:1197–1209.
46. Van Gaal LF, Mertens IL, De Block CE. Mechanisms linking obesity with cardiovascular disease. *Nature.* 2006;444:875–880.
47. Birgel M, Gottschling-Zeller H, Rohrig K, et al. Role of cytokines in the regulation of plasminogen activator inhibitor-1 expression and secretion in newly differentiated subcutaneous human adipocytes. *Arterioscler Thromb Vasc Biol.* 2000;20:1682–1687.
48. Nilsson M, Johnsen R, Ye W, et al. Obesity and estrogen as risk factors for gastroesophageal reflux symptoms. *JAMA.* 2003;290:66–72.
49. Ayazi S, Hagen JA, Chan LS, et al. Obesity and gastroesophageal reflux: quantifying the association between body mass index, esophageal acid exposure, and lower esophageal sphincter status in a large series of patients with reflux symptoms. *J Gastrointest Surg.* 2009;13:1440–1447.
50. Harter RL, Kelly WB, Kramer MG, et al. A comparison of the volume and pH of gastric contents of obese and lean surgical patients. *Anesth Analg.* 1998; 86:147–152.
51. American Society of Anesthesiologists Committee on Standards and Practice Parameters. Practice guidelines for preoperative fasting and the use of pharmacologic agents to reduce the risk of pulmonary aspiration: application to healthy patients undergoing elective procedures: an updated report by the American Society of Anesthesiologists Committee on Standards and Practice Parameters. *Anesthesiology.* 2011;114:495–511.
52. Frezza EE, Ikramuddin S, Gourash W, et al. Symptomatic improvement in gastroesophageal reflux disease (GERD) following laparoscopic Roux-en-Y gastric bypass. *Surg Endosc.* 2002;16:1027–1031.
53. Cheymol G. Effects of obesity on pharmacokinetics implications for drug therapy. *Clin Pharmacokinet.* 2000;39:215–231.
54. Suneja M, Kumar AB. Obesity and perioperative acute kidney injury: a focused review. *J Crit Care.* 2014;29:694.e1–696.e1.
55. Chagnac A, Weinstein T, Herman M, et al. The effects of weight loss on renal function in patients with severe obesity. *J Am Soc Nephrol.* 2003;14:1480–1486.
56. Kastorini CM, Milionis HJ, Esposito K, et al. The effect of Mediterranean diet on metabolic syndrome and its components: a meta-analysis of 50 studies and 534,906 individuals. *J Am Coll Cardiol.* 2011;57:1299–1313.
57. Tzimas P, Petrou A, Laou E, et al. Impact of metabolic syndrome in surgical patients: should we bother? *Br J Anaesth.* 2015;115:194–202.
58. Alberti KG, Eckel RH, Grundy SM, et al. Harmonizing the metabolic syndrome: a joint interim statement of the International Diabetes Federation Task Force on Epidemiology and Prevention; National Heart, Lung, and Blood Institute; American Heart Association; World Heart Federation; International Atherosclerosis Society; and International Association for the Study of Obesity. *Circulation.* 2009;120:1640–1645.
59. Frezza EE, Wachtel M. Metabolic syndrome: a new multidisciplinary service line. *Obes Surg.* 2011;21:379–385.
60. Casati A, Putzu M. Anesthesia in the obese patient: pharmacokinetic considerations. *J Clin Anesth.* 2005;17:134–145.

61. Friesen JH. Lean-scaled weight: a proposed weight scalar to calculate drug doses for obese patients. *Can J Anaesth.* 2013;60:214–215.
62. Hall JE. The kidney, hypertension, and obesity. *Hypertension.* 2003;41:625–633.
63. Christoff PB, Conti DR, Naylor C, et al. Procainamide disposition in obesity. *Drug Intell Clin Pharm.* 1983;17:516–522.
64. Egan TD, Huizinga B, Gupta SK, et al. Remifentanil pharmacokinetics in obese versus lean patients. *Anesthesiology.* 1998;89:562–573.
65. Abernethy DR, Greenblatt DJ, Smith TW. Digoxin disposition in obesity: clinical pharmacokinetic investigation. *Am Heart J.* 1981;102:740–744.
66. Monk TG, Rietbergen H, Woo T, et al. Use of Sugammadex in patients with obesity: A pooled analysis. *Am J Ther.* 2015;Sept 21 [e-pub ahead of print].
67. Ogunnaike BO, Jones SB, Jones DB, et al. Anesthetic considerations for bariatric surgery. *Anesth Analg.* 2002;95:1793–1805.
68. Suzuki T, Masaki G, Ogawa S. Neostigmine-induced reversal of vecuronium in normal weight, overweight and obese female patients. *Br J Anaesth.* 2006;97:160–163.
69. Ferraz AA, Siqueira LT, Campos JM, et al. Antibiotic prophylaxis in bariatric surgery: a continuous infusion of cefazolin versus ampicillin/sulbactam and ertapenem. *Arq Gastroenterol.* 2015;52:83–87.
70. Schumann R. Anaesthesia for bariatric surgery. *Best Pract Res Clin Anaesthesiol.* 2011;25:83–93.
71. Bein B, Scholz J. Anaesthesia for adults undergoing non-bariatric surgery. *Best Pract Res Clin Anaesthesiol.* 2011;25:37–51.
72. Schug SA, Raymann A. Postoperative pain management of the obese patient. *Best Pract Res Clin Anaesthesiol.* 2011;25:73–81.
73. Peterson GN, Domino KB, Caplan RA, et al. Management of the difficult airway: a closed claims analysis. *Anesthesiology.* 2005;103:33–39.
74. Ezri T, Medalion B, Weisenberg M, et al. Increased body mass index per se is not a predictor of difficult laryngoscopy. *Can J Anaesth.* 2003;50:179–183.
75. El-Orbany M, Woehlck HJ. Difficult mask ventilation. *Anesth Analg.* 2009;109:1870–1880.
76. Brodsky JB, Lemmens HJ, Brock-Utne JG, et al. Morbid obesity and tracheal intubation. *Anesth Analg.* 2002;94:732–736.
77. Juvin P, Lavaut E, Dupont H, et al. Difficult tracheal intubation is more common in obese than in lean patients. *Anesth Analg.* 2003;97:595–600.
78. Neligan PJ, Porter S, Max B, et al. Obstructive sleep apnea is not a risk factor for difficult intubation in morbidly obese patients. *Anesth Analg.* 2009;109:1182–1186.
79. McLaughlin VV, Archer SL, Badesch DB, et al. ACCF/AHA 2009 expert consensus document on pulmonary hypertension: a report of the American College of Cardiology Foundation Task Force on Expert Consensus Documents and the American Heart Association: developed in collaboration with the American College of Chest Physicians, American Thoracic Society, Inc., and the Pulmonary Hypertension Association. *Circulation.* 2009;119:2250–2294.
80. Katkhouda N, Mason RJ, Wu B, et al. Evaluation and treatment of patients with cardiac disease undergoing bariatric surgery. *Surg Obes Relat Dis.* 2012;8:634–640.
81. Chang CG, Adams-Huet B, Provost DA. Acute post-gastric reduction surgery (APGARS) neuropathy. *Obes Surg.* 2004;14:182–189.
82. Sapala JA, Wood MH, Schuhknecht MP, et al. Fatal pulmonary embolism after bariatric operations for morbid obesity: a 24-year retrospective analysis. *Obes Surg.* 2003;13:819–825.
83. Magee CJ, Barry J, Javed S, et al. Extended thromboprophylaxis reduces incidence of postoperative venous thromboembolism in laparoscopic bariatric surgery. *Surg Obes Relat Dis.* 2010;6:322–325.
84. Geerts WH, Bergqvist D, Pineo GF, et al. Prevention of venous thromboembolism: American College of Chest Physicians Evidence-Based Clinical Practice Guidelines (8th Edition). *Chest.* 2008;133:381S–453S.
85. Gonzalez QH, Tishler DS, Plata-Munoz JJ, et al. Incidence of clinically evident deep venous thrombosis after laparoscopic Roux-en-Y gastric bypass. *Surg Endosc.* 2004;18:1082–1084.
86. Boyce JR, Ness T, Castroman P, et al. A preliminary study of the optimal anesthesia positioning for the morbidly obese patient. *Obes Surg.* 2003;13:4–9.
87. Koffman BM, Greenfield LJ, Ali II, et al. Neurologic complications after surgery for obesity. *Muscle Nerve.* 2006;33:166–176.
88. Juhasz-Pocsine K, Rudnicki SA, Archer RL, et al. Neurologic complications of gastric bypass surgery for morbid obesity. *Neurology.* 2007;68:1843–1850.
89. Pierin AM, Alavarce DC, Gusmao JL, et al. Blood pressure measurement in obese patients: comparison between upper arm and forearm measurements. *Blood Press Monit.* 2004;9:101–105.
90. Juvin P, Blarel A, Bruno F, et al. Is peripheral line placement more difficult in obese than in lean patients? *Anesth Analg.* 2003;96:1218.
91. Shah U, Wong J, Wong DT, et al. Preoxygenation and intraoperative ventilation strategies in obese patients: a comprehensive review. *Curr Opin Anaesthesiol.* 2016;29(1):109–118.
92. Ortiz VE, Vidal-Melo MF, Walsh JL. Strategies for managing oxygenation in obese patients undergoing laparoscopic surgery. *Surg Obes Relat Dis.* 2015;11:721–728.
93. Murphy C, Wong DT. Airway management and oxygenation in obese patients. *Can J Anaesth.* 2013;60 929–945.
94. Dixon BJ, Dixon JB, Carden JR, et al. Preoxygenation is more effective in the 25 degrees head-up position than in the supine position in severely obese patients: a randomized controlled study. *Anesthesiology.* 2005;102:1110–1115.
95. Altermatt FR, Munoz HR, Delfino AE, et al. Pre-oxygenation in the obese patient: effects of position on tolerance to apnoea. *Br J Anaesth.* 2005;95:706–709.
96. Delay JM, Sebbane M, Jung B, et al. The effectiveness of noninvasive positive pressure ventilation to enhance preoxygenation in morbidly obese patients: a randomized controlled study. *Anesth Analg.* 2008;107:1707–1713.
97. Gander S, Frascarolo P, Suter M, et al. Positive end-expiratory pressure during induction of general anesthesia increases duration of nonhypoxic apnea in morbidly obese patients. *Anesth Analg.* 2005;100:580–584.
98. Corso RM, Piraccini E, Calli M, et al. Obstructive sleep apnea is a risk factor for difficult endotracheal intubation. *Minerva Anestesiol.* 2011;77:99–100.
99. Kheterpal S, Healy D, Aziz MF, et al. Incidence, predictors, and outcome of difficult mask ventilation combined with difficult laryngoscopy: a report from the multicenter perioperative outcomes group. *Anesthesiology.* 2013;119:1360–1369.
100. Abdelmalak B, Makary L, Hoban J, et al. Dexmedetomidine as sole sedative for awake intubation in management of the critical airway. *J Clin Anesth.* 2007;19:370–373.
101. Collins JS, Lemmens HJ, Brodsky JB, et al. Laryngoscopy and morbid obesity: a comparison of the "sniff" and "ramped" positions. *Obes Surg.* 2004;14:1171–1175.
102. Maassen R, Lee R, Hermans B, et al. A comparison of three videolaryngoscopes: the Macintosh laryngoscope blade reduces, but does not replace, routine stylet use for intubation in morbidly obese patients. *Anesth Analg.* 2009;109:1560–1565.
103. Marrel J, Blanc C, Frascarolo P, et al. Videolaryngoscopy improves intubation condition in morbidly obese patients. *Eur J Anaesthesiol.* 2007;24:1045–1049.
104. Mort TC. Emergency tracheal intubation: complications associated with repeated laryngoscopic attempts. *Anesth Analg.* 2004;99:607–613.
105. Keller C, Brimacombe J, Kleinsasser A, et al. The Laryngeal Mask Airway ProSeal(™) as a temporary ventilatory device in grossly and morbidly obese patients before laryngoscope-guided tracheal intubation. *Anesth Analg.* 2002;94:737–740.
106. Combes X, Sauvat S, Leroux B, et al. Intubating laryngeal mask airway in morbidly obese and lean patients: a comparative study. *Anesthesiology.* 2005;102:1106–1109.
107. Maltby JR, Pytka S, Watson NC, et al. Drinking 300 mL of clear fluid two hours before surgery has no effect on gastric fluid volume and pH in fasting and non-fasting obese patients. *Can J Anaesth.* 2004;51:111–115.
108. Lemmens HJ, Brodsky JB. The dose of succinylcholine in morbid obesity. *Anesth Analg.* 2006;102:438–442.
109. La Colla L, Albertin A, La Colla G, et al. Faster wash-out and recovery for desflurane vs sevoflurane in morbidly obese patients when no premedication is used. *Br J Anaesth.* 2007;99:353–358.
110. Feld JM, Hoffman WE, Stechert MM, et al. Fentanyl or dexmedetomidine combined with desflurane for bariatric surgery. *J Clin Anesth.* 2006;18:24–28.
111. Hofer RE, Sprung J, Sarr MG, et al. Anesthesia for a patient with morbid obesity using dexmedetomidine without narcotics. *Can J Anaesth.* 2005;52:176–180.
112. Ezri T, Hazin V, Warters D, et al. The endotracheal tube moves more often in obese patients undergoing laparoscopy compared with open abdominal surgery. *Anesth Analg.* 2003;96:278–282.
113. Ricciardi R, Town RJ, Kellogg TA, et al. Outcomes after open versus laparoscopic gastric bypass. *Surg Laparosc Endosc Percutan Tech.* 2006;16:317–320.
114. Poso T, Kesek D, Aroch R, et al. Morbid obesity and optimization of preoperative fluid therapy. *Obes Surg.* 2013;23:1799–1805.
115. Matot I, Paskaleva R, Eid L, et al. Effect of the volume of fluids administered on intraoperative oliguria in laparoscopic bariatric surgery: A randomized controlled trial. *Arch Surg.* 2011;147:228–234.
116. Wool DB, Lemmens HJ, Brodsky JB, et al. Intraoperative fluid replacement and postoperative creatine phosphokinase levels in laparoscopic bariatric patients. *Obes Surg.* 2010;20:698–701.
117. Bender SP, Paganelli WC, Gerety LP, et al. Intraoperative lung-protective ventilation trends and practice patterns: A report from the multicenter perioperative outcomes group. *Anesth Analg.* 2015;121:1231–1239.
118. Fernandez-Bustamante A, Wood CL, Tran ZV, et al. Intraoperative ventilation: Incidence and risk factors for receiving large tidal volumes during general anesthesia. *BMC Anesthesiol.* 2011;11:22.
119. Anzueto A, Frutos-Vivar F, Esteban A, et al. Influence of body mass index on outcome of the mechanically ventilated patients. *Thorax.* 2011;66:66–73.
120. Lewandowski K, Lewandowski M. Intensive care in the obese. *Best Pract Res Clin Anaesthesiol.* 2011;25:95–108.
121. Dreyfuss D, Soler P, Basset G, et al. High inflation pressure pulmonary edema. Respective effects of high airway pressure, high tidal volume, and positive end-expiratory pressure. *Am Rev Respir Dis.* 1988;137:1159–1164.
122. Fernandez-Bustamante A, Hashimoto S, Serpa Neto A, et al. Perioperative lung protective ventilation in obese patients. *BMC Anesthesiol.* 2015;15:56.
123. Pelosi P, Gregoretti C. Perioperative management of obese patients. *Best Pract Res Clin Anaesthesiol.* 2010;24:211–225.
124. Bohm SH, Thamm OC, von Sandersleben A, et al. Alveolar recruitment strategy and high positive end-expiratory pressure levels do not affect hemodynamics in morbidly obese intravascular volume-loaded patients. *Anesth Analg.* 2009;109:160–163.

125. Cadi P, Guenoun T, Journois D, et al. Pressure-controlled ventilation improves oxygenation during laparoscopic obesity surgery compared with volume-controlled ventilation. Br J Anaesth. 2008;100:709–716.
126. Zoremba M, Kalmus G, Dette F, et al. Effect of intra-operative pressure support vs pressure controlled ventilation on oxygenation and lung function in moderately obese adults. Anaesthesia. 2010;65:124–129.
127. Aldenkortt M, Lysakowski C, Elia N, et al. Ventilation strategies in obese patients undergoing surgery: a quantitative systematic review and meta-analysis. Br J Anaesth. 2012;109:493–502.
128. Bardoczky GI, Yernault JC, Houben JJ, et al. Large tidal volume ventilation does not improve oxygenation in morbidly obese patients during anesthesia. Anesth Analg. 1995;81:385–388.
129. Pelosi P, Ravagnan I, Giurati G, et al. Positive end-expiratory pressure improves respiratory function in obese but not in normal subjects during anesthesia and paralysis. Anesthesiology. 1999;91:1221–1231.
130. Reinius H, Jonsson L, Gustafsson S, et al. Prevention of atelectasis in morbidly obese patients during general anesthesia and paralysis: a computerized tomography study. Anesthesiology. 2009;111:979–987.
131. Prove Network Investigators for the Clinical Trial Network of the European Society of Anaesthesiology, Hemmes SN, Gama de Abreu M, et al. High versus low positive end-expiratory pressure during general anaesthesia for open abdominal surgery (PROVHILO trial): a multicentre randomised controlled trial. Lancet. 2014;384:495–503.
132. Talab HF, Zabani IA, Abdelrahman HS, et al. Intraoperative ventilatory strategies for prevention of pulmonary atelectasis in obese patients undergoing laparoscopic bariatric surgery. Anesth Analg. 2009;109:1511–1516.
133. Rosenblatt MA, Reich DL, Roth R. Bariatric surgery and the prevention of postoperative respiratory complications. Anesth Analg. 2004;98:1810.
134. Metzner J, Posner KL, Lam MS, et al. Closed claims' analysis. Best Pract Res Clin Anaesthesiol. 2011;25:263–276.
135. Bhananker SM, Posner KL, Cheney FW, et al. Injury and liability associated with monitored anesthesia care: a closed claims analysis. Anesthesiology. 2006;104:228–234.
136. von Ungern-Sternberg BS, Regli A, Reber A, et al. Effect of obesity and thoracic epidural analgesia on perioperative spirometry. Br J Anaesth. 2005;94:121–127.
137. Kehlet H, Holte K. Effect of postoperative analgesia on surgical outcome. Br J Anaesth. 2001;87:62–72.
138. Marret E, Remy C, Bonnet F, et al. Meta-analysis of epidural analgesia versus parenteral opioid analgesia after colorectal surgery. Br J Surg. 2007;94:665–673.
139. Gelman S, Laws HL, Potzick J, et al. Thoracic epidural vs balanced anesthesia in morbid obesity: an intraoperative and postoperative hemodynamic study. Anesth Analg. 1980;59:902–908.
140. Brodsky JB, Mariano ER. Regional anaesthesia in the obese patient: lost landmarks and evolving ultrasound guidance. Best Pract Res Clin Anaesthesiol. 2011;25:61–72.
141. Nielsen KC, Guller U, Steele SM, et al. Influence of obesity on surgical regional anesthesia in the ambulatory setting: an analysis of 9,038 blocks. Anesthesiology. 2005;102:181–187.
142. Damia G, Mascheroni D, Croci M, et al. Perioperative changes in functional residual capacity in morbidly obese patients. Br J Anaesth. 1988;60:574–578.
143. Catenacci AJ, Anderson JD, Boersma D. Anesthetic hazards of obesity. JAMA. 1961;175:657–665.
144. Tsueda K, Debrand M, Zeok SS, et al. Obesity supine death syndrome: reports of two morbidly obese patients. Anesth Analg. 1979;58:345–347.
145. Chin KJ, Perlas A, Chan V, et al. Ultrasound imaging facilitates spinal anesthesia in adults with difficult surface anatomic landmarks. Anesthesiology. 2011;115:94–101.
146. Ellinas EH, Eastwood DC, Patel SN, et al. The effect of obesity on neuraxial technique difficulty in pregnant patients: a prospective, observational study. Anesth Analg. 2009;109:1225–1231.
147. Clinkscales CP, Greenfield ML, Vanarase M, et al. An observational study of the relationship between lumbar epidural space depth and body mass index in Michigan parturients. Int J Obst Anesth. 2007;16:323–327.
148. Balki M, Lee Y, Halpern S, et al. Ultrasound imaging of the lumbar spine in the transverse plane: the correlation between estimated and actual depth to the epidural space in obese parturients. Anesth Analg. 2009;108:1876–1881.
149. Chiang HK, Zhou Q, Mandell MS, et al. Eyes in the needle: novel epidural needle with embedded high-frequency ultrasound transducer–epidural access in porcine model. Anesthesiology. 2011;114:1320–1324.
150. Butcher M, George RT, Ip J, et al. Identification of the midline by obese and non-obese women during late pregnancy. Anaesthesia. 2014;69:1351–1354.
151. Watts RW. The influence of obesity on the relationship between body mass index and the distance to the epidural space from the skin. Anaesth Intensive Care. 1993;21:309–310.
152. Hogan QH, Prost R, Kulier A, et al. Magnetic resonance imaging of cerebrospinal fluid volume and the influence of body habitus and abdominal pressure. Anesthesiology. 1996;84:1341–1349.
153. McCulloch WJ, Littlewood DG. Influence of obesity on spinal analgesia with isobaric 0.5% bupivacaine. Br J Anaesth. 1986;58:610–614.
154. Taivainen T, Tuominen M, Rosenberg PH. Influence of obesity on the spread of spinal analgesia after injection of plain 0.5% bupivacaine at the L3–4 or L4–5 interspace. Br J Anaesth. 1990;64:542–546.
155. Pitkanen MT. Body mass and spread of spinal anesthesia with bupivacaine. Anesth Analg. 1987;66:127–131.
156. Wong CA, Cariaso D, Johnson EC, et al. Body habitus does not influence spread of sensory blockade after the intrathecal injection of a hypobaric solution in term parturients. Can J Anaesth. 2003;50:689–693.
157. Norris MC. Patient variables and the subarachnoid spread of hyperbaric bupivacaine in the term parturient. Anesthesiology. 1990;72:478–482.
158. Bloom SL, Spong CY, Weiner SJ, et al. Complications of anesthesia for cesarean delivery. Obstet Gynecol. 2005;106:281–287.
159. Hood DD, Dewan DM. Anesthetic and obstetric outcome in morbidly obese parturients. Anesthesiology. 1993;79:1210–1218.
160. Hodgkinson R, Husain FJ. Obesity and the cephalad spread of analgesia following epidural administration of bupivacaine for Cesarean section. Anesth Analg. 1980;59:89–92.
161. Hamilton CL, Riley ET, Cohen SE. Changes in the position of epidural catheters associated with patient movement. Anesthesiology. 1997;86:778–784.
162. Russell IF. A prospective controlled study of continuous spinal analgesia versus repeat epidural analgesia after accidental dural puncture in labour. Int J Obstet Anesth. 2012;21:7–16.
163. Pan PH, Bogard TD, Owen MD. Incidence and characteristics of failures in obstetric neuraxial analgesia and anesthesia: a retrospective analysis of 19,259 deliveries. Int J Obstet Anesth. 2004;13:227–233.
164. Cappiello E, O'Rourke N, Segal S, et al. A randomized trial of dural puncture epidural technique compared with the standard epidural technique for labor analgesia. Anesth Analg. 2008;107:1646–1651.
165. Cotter JT, Nielsen KC, Guller U, et al. Increased body mass index and ASA physical status IV are risk factors for block failure in ambulatory surgery—an analysis of 9,342 blocks. Can J Anaesth. 2004;51:810–816.
166. Franco CD, Gloss FJ, Voronov G, et al. Supraclavicular block in the obese population: an analysis of 2020 blocks. Anesth Analg. 2006;102:1252–1254.
167. Bugada D, Guardia Nicola F, Carboni V, et al. TAP block for opioid-free postoperative analgesia in obese surgery. Minerva Anestesiol. 2013;79:1447–1448.
168. Niraj G, Kelkar A, Fox AJ. Oblique sub-costal transversus abdominis plane (TAP) catheters: an alternative to epidural analgesia after upper abdominal surgery. Anaesthesia. 2009;64:1137–1140.
169. Chantzi C, Saranteas T, Zogogiannis J, et al. Ultrasound examination of the sciatic nerve at the anterior thigh in obese patients. Acta Anaesthesiol Scand. 2007;51:132.
170. Schwemmer U, Papenfuss T, Greim C, et al. Ultrasound-guided interscalene brachial plexus anaesthesia: differences in success between patients of normal and excessive weight. Ultraschall in der Medizin. 2006;27:245–250.
171. Chan VW, Perlas A, McCartney CJ, et al. Ultrasound guidance improves success rate of axillary brachial plexus block. Can J Anaesth. 2007;54:176–182.
172. Brull R, Lupu M, Perlas A, et al. Compared with dual nerve stimulation, ultrasound guidance shortens the time for infraclavicular block performance. Can J Anaesth. 2009;56:812–818.
173. Casati A, Baciarello M, Di Cianni S, et al. Effects of ultrasound guidance on the minimum effective anaesthetic volume required to block the femoral nerve. Br J Anaesth. 2007;98:823–827.
174. Sites BD, Brull R, Chan VW, et al. Artifacts and pitfall errors associated with ultrasound-guided regional anesthesia. Part II: a pictorial approach to understanding and avoidance. Reg Anesth Pain Med. 2007;32:419–433.
175. Sites BD, Chan VW, Neal JM, et al. The American Society of Regional Anesthesia and Pain Medicine and the European Society of Regional Anaesthesia and Pain Therapy Joint Committee recommendations for education and training in ultrasound-guided regional anesthesia. Reg Anesth Pain Med. 2009;34:40–46.
176. Gaszynski T, Tokarz A, Piotrowski D, et al. Boussignac CPAP in the postoperative period in morbidly obese patients. Obes Surg. 2007;17:452–456.
177. Grover BT, Priem DM, Mathiason MA, et al. Intensive care unit stay not required for patients with obstructive sleep apnea after laparoscopic Roux-en-Y gastric bypass. Surg Obes Relat Dis. 2010;6:165–170.
178. American Society of Anesthesiologists Task Force on Neuraxial Opioids, Horlocker TT, Burton AW, et al. Practice guidelines for the prevention, detection, and management of respiratory depression associated with neuraxial opioid administration. Anesthesiology. 2009;110:218–230.
179. Abdullah HR, Chung F. Perioperative management for the obese outpatient. Curr Opin Anaesth. 2014;27:576–582.
180. Joshi GP, Ahmad S, Riad W, et al. Selection of obese patients undergoing ambulatory surgery: a systematic review of the literature. Anesth Analg. 2013;117:1082–1091.
181. Lopez PP, Stefan B, Schulman CI, et al. Prevalence of sleep apnea in morbidly obese patients who presented for weight loss surgery evaluation: more evidence for routine screening for obstructive sleep apnea before weight loss surgery. Amer Surg. 2008;74:834–838.
182. Stierer TL, Wright C, George A, et al. Risk assessment of obstructive sleep apnea in a population of patients undergoing ambulatory surgery. J Clin Sleep Med. 2010;6:467–472.

183. Mokhlesi B, Hovda MD, Vekhter B, et al. Sleep-disordered breathing and postoperative outcomes after elective surgery: analysis of the nationwide inpatient sample. *Chest*. 2013;144:903–914.
184. Memtsoudis SG, Stundner O, Rasul R, et al. The impact of sleep apnea on postoperative utilization of resources and adverse outcomes. *Anesth Analg*. 2014;118:407–418.
185. Mutter TC, Chateau D, Moffatt M, et al. A matched cohort study of postoperative outcomes in obstructive sleep apnea: could preoperative diagnosis and treatment prevent complications? *Anesthesiology*. 2014;121:707–718.
186. Seet E, Chung F. Management of sleep apnea in adults—functional algorithms for the perioperative period: continuing professional development. *Can J Anaesth*. 2010;57:849–864.
187. Joshi GP, Ankichetty SF, Gan TJ, et al. Society for Ambulatory Anesthesia consensus statement on preoperative selection of adult patients with obstructive sleep apnea scheduled for ambulatory surgery. *Anesth Analg*. 2012;115:1060–1068.
188. Mathis MR, Naughton NN, Shanks AM, et al. Patient selection for day case-eligible surgery: identifying those at high risk for major complications. *Anesthesiology*. 2013;119:1310–1321.
189. Honiden S, Gong MN. Diabetes, insulin, and development of acute lung injury. *Crit Care Med*. 2009;37:2455–2464.
190. Gong MN, Bajwa EK, Thompson BT, et al. Body mass index is associated with the development of acute respiratory distress syndrome. *Thorax*. 2010;65:44–50.
191. Hogue CW Jr., Stearns JD, Colantuoni E, et al. The impact of obesity on outcomes after critical illness: a meta-analysis. *Intensive Care Med*. 2009;35:1152–1170.
192. Nafiu OO, Kheterpal S, Moulding R, et al. The association of body mass index to postoperative outcomes in elderly vascular surgery patients: a reverse J-curve phenomenon. *Anesth Analg*. 2011;112:23–29.
193. Brunette DD. Resuscitation of the morbidly obese patient. *Am J Emerg Med*. 2004;22:40–47.
194. King DR. Emergent cricothyroidotomy in the morbidly obese: a safe, no-visualization technique. *J Trauma*. 2011;71:1873–1874.
195. Childers DK, Allison DB. The 'obesity paradox': a parsimonious explanation for relations among obesity, mortality rate and aging? *Int J Obes*. 2010;34:1231–1238.
196. Mullen JT, Davenport DL, Hutter MM, et al. Impact of body mass index on perioperative outcomes in patients undergoing major intra-abdominal cancer surgery. *Ann Surg Oncol*. 2008;15:2164–2172.
197. Mullen JT, Moorman DW, Davenport DL. The obesity paradox: body mass index and outcomes in patients undergoing nonbariatric general surgery. *Ann Surg*. 2009;250:166–172.
198. Tung A. Anaesthetic considerations with the metabolic syndrome. *Br J Anaesth*. 2010;105(Suppl 1):i24–i33.
199. Glance LG, Wissler R, Mukamel DB, et al. Perioperative outcomes among patients with the modified metabolic syndrome who are undergoing noncardiac surgery. *Anesthesiology*. 2010;113:859–872.
200. Anaya DA, Dellinger EP. The obese surgical patient: a susceptible host for infection. *Surg Infect*. 2006;7:473–480.
201. Cheadle WG. Risk factors for surgical site infection. *Surg Infect*. 2006;7(Suppl 1):S7–S11.
202. Kabon B, Nagele A, Reddy D, et al. Obesity decreases perioperative tissue oxygenation. *Anesthesiology*. 2004;100:274–280.
203. Kabon B, Rozum R, Marschalek C, et al. Supplemental postoperative oxygen and tissue oxygen tension in morbidly obese patients. *Obes Surg*. 2010;20:885–894.
204. Sabers C, Plevak DJ, Schroeder DR, et al. The diagnosis of obstructive sleep apnea as a risk factor for unanticipated admissions in outpatient surgery. *Anesth Analg*. 2003;96:1328–1335.
205. Thomas H, Agrawal S. Systematic review of same-day laparoscopic adjustable gastric band surgery. *Obes Surg*. 2011;21:805–810.

46 The Liver: Surgery and Anesthesia

RANDOLPH H. STEADMAN • MICHELLE Y. BRAUNFELD

Hepatic Function in Health
Assessment of Hepatic Function
Hepatobiliary Imaging
Liver Biopsy
Hepatic and Hepatobiliary Diseases
    Acute Liver Failure
    Acute Hepatitis
    Alcoholic Hepatitis
    Drug-induced Liver Injury
    Pregnancy-related Liver Diseases
Cirrhosis and Portal Hypertension
    Hemostasis
    Cardiac Manifestations
    Renal Dysfunction
    Pulmonary Complications
    Hepatic Encephalopathy
    Ascites
    Varices

Chronic Cholestatic Disease
Chronic Hepatocellular Disease
Hepatocellular Carcinoma
Nonalcoholic Fatty Liver Disease
Preoperative Management
    Hepatic Evaluation
    Perioperative Risk Associated with Liver Disease
Intraoperative Management
    Monitoring and Vascular Access
    Selection of Anesthetic Technique
    Pharmacokinetic and Pharmacodynamic Alterations
    Vasopressors
    Volume Resuscitation
    Transjugular Intrahepatic Portosystemic Shunt Procedure
    Hepatic Resection
Postoperative Liver Dysfunction
Conclusions
Acknowledgment

KEY POINTS

1. The liver is the largest internal organ, accounting for 2% of the total body mass of adults. It receives 25% of the cardiac output via a dual afferent blood supply. The portal vein supplies 75% of the hepatic blood flow, whereas the hepatic artery supplies the remainder. Because of the higher oxygen content in the hepatic artery, each vessel provides roughly 50% of the hepatic oxygen supply.

2. The liver plays a pre-eminent role in the intermediary metabolism of nutrients (glucose, nitrogen, and lipids) and the detoxification of chemicals, including lipophilic medications. Liver dysfunction affects the metabolism of nutrients and xenobiotics, and negatively impacts nearly every other organ system.

3. Portal hypertension, the end result of hepatic injury and fibrotic changes, results in portosystemic shunts that bypass the liver's metabolic and detoxification capabilities. When nitrogenous waste and other substances normally cleared by the liver enter the central circulation, hepatic encephalopathy ensues.

4. Additional complications of portal hypertension include variceal hemorrhage, ascites, and hepatorenal syndrome. Cardiac sequelae include hyperdynamic circulation due to decreased systemic vascular resistance, which results in an increase in cardiac output.

5. Perioperative complications encountered by cirrhotic patients include liver failure, postoperative bleeding, infection, and renal failure. Patients with a model for end-stage liver disease (MELD) score of less than 11 have a low postoperative mortality and represent an acceptable surgical risk. End-stage liver disease patients with a risk of postoperative liver failure should have elective abdominal surgery at institutions with a liver transplant program. In patients with a MELD score of 20 or higher, the high mortality risk contraindicates elective procedures until after liver transplantation.

6. Medical management undertaken to optimize cirrhotic patients undergoing surgery should be directed toward treating active infection, minimizing vasoactive infusions, optimizing central blood volume and renal status, minimizing ascites, and improving encephalopathy and coagulopathy.

7. The perioperative risk of patients with end-stage liver disease depends more on the operative site and the degree of liver impairment than the anesthetic technique.

Hepatic Function in Health

The liver is the largest internal organ and is the body's metabolic headquarters. It weighs 1.5 kg or about 2% of the total body weight in an adult. The functional unit of the liver is the lobule, a structure roughly 1×2 mm that consists of plates of hepatocytes located in a radial distribution about a central vein. The afferent blood supply from the portal vein and hepatic arteriole enters at the periphery of the lobule. Bile, formed in the hepatocytes, flows into canaliculi located between the plates of hepatocytes and drains into bile ducts located at the periphery of the lobule next to portal venules and hepatic arterioles. The large pores in the endothelium lining, the sinusoids, allow plasma and its proteins to move readily into the tissue spaces surrounding hepatocytes, an area known as the spaces of Disse. This fluid drains into the lymphatic system. The liver generates about half of the body's lymph (Fig. 46-1).

The liver receives approximately 25% of the cardiac output via a dual supply. The portal venules conduct blood from the portal vein, which drains the gastrointestinal tract. The portal vein supplies 75% of the liver inflow, or about 1 L/min. The hepatic arterioles supply the remaining 25% of the hepatic blood

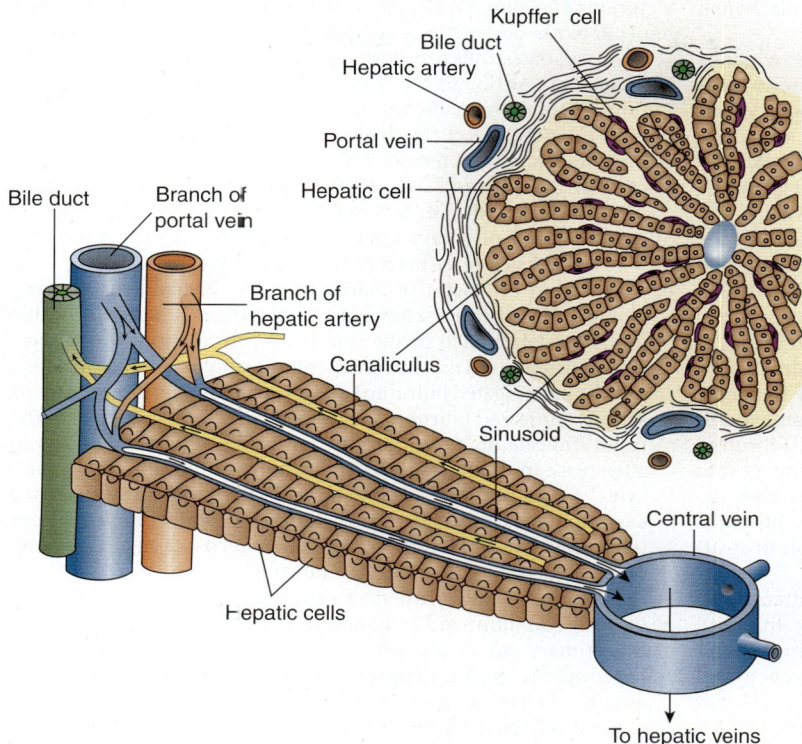

Figure 46-1 A magnified cross-section of a liver lobule **(right)** with its component cells and structures is juxtaposed to a 90-degree rotated view of a portion of this cross-section **(left)** showing the mixing of hepatic portal and arterial blood in the hepatic sinusoids. The sinusoids empty into the central vein, which sends blood to the hepatic vein and from there into the vena cava. (Adapted with permission from Porth CM. Disorders of hepatobiliary and exocrine pancreas function. *Essentials of Pathophysiology: Concepts of Altered Physical States*. 4th ed. Philadelphia, PA: Wolters Kluwer; 2015:726.)

flow. Due to the higher oxygen content of arterial blood, each vessel contributes about 50% of the hepatic oxygen supply.

The liver's high blood flow is due to low vascular resistance in the portal vein. The average portal vein pressure is 8 to 10 mmHg, which exceeds hepatic venous pressure by 4 to 5 mmHg. However, when injured hepatocytes are replaced by fibrous tissue, blood flow is impeded and portal hypertension ensues. A hepatic venous pressure gradient (HVPG) greater than 5 mmHg is abnormal and defines portal hypertension.[1] Sympathetic innervation from T3 to T11 controls resistance in the hepatic venules. Changes in compliance in the hepatic venous system contribute to the regulation of cardiac output and blood volume. In the presence of reduced portal venous flow, the hepatic artery can increase flow by as much as 100% to maintain hepatic oxygen delivery. The reciprocal relationship between flow in the two afferent vessels is termed the "hepatic arterial buffer response."[2]

The microcirculation of the liver lobule is divided into three zones that receive varying oxygen content.[3] Zone 1 receives oxygen-rich blood from the adjacent portal vein and hepatic artery. As blood moves through the sinusoid it passes from the intermediate zone 2 into zone 3, which surrounds the central vein. Blood entering zone 3 is oxygen poor. Pericentral hepatocytes have a greater quantity of cytochrome P450 enzymes and are the site of anaerobic metabolism. Hypoxia and reactive metabolic intermediates from biotransformation affect zone 3 more prominently than other zones.

Due to its ability to distend, the liver is capable of storing up to 1 L of blood. The liver serves as a reservoir capable of accepting blood, or releasing blood at times of low blood volume. The liver also stores vitamins, particularly vitamins B_{12} (1-year supply), D (3-month supply), and A (10-month supply). Excess body iron is transported via apoferritin to the liver for storage as ferritin, which is released when circulating iron levels are low. Thus, the liver apoferritin system serves as a blood iron buffer.

Reticuloendothelial cells called Kupffer cells line the venous sinusoids. These macrophages phagocytize bacteria that enter the sinusoids from the intestines. Less than 1% of bacteria that enter the liver pass through the systemic circulation.

The liver is involved in energy production and storage of nutrients absorbed from the intestines. The liver aids in blood glucose regulation through its glucose buffer function. This is accomplished by storing glucose as glycogen, converting other carbohydrates (principally fructose and galactose) to glucose, and synthesizing glucose from amino acids and triglyceride (gluconeogenesis).[4] In patients with altered liver function, blood glucose concentration can rise several fold higher than the postprandial levels found in patients with normal hepatic function.

The liver synthesizes fat, cholesterol, phospholipids, and lipoproteins. It also efficiently metabolizes fat, converting fatty acids to acetyl coenzyme A (CoA), an excellent source of energy, which can be diverted to the citric acid cycle to liberate energy for the liver. The liver generates more acetyl-CoA than it consumes. The excess is packaged as acetoacetic acid for use elsewhere in the body. The majority of cholesterol synthesized in the liver is converted to bile salts and secreted in the bile. The remainder is distributed to the rest of the body where it is used to form cellular membranes and other vital structures. Fat synthesis from protein and carbohydrates occurs almost exclusively in the liver, and the liver is responsible for most fat metabolism.

The liver also plays a key role in protein metabolism. The liver synthesizes all of the plasma proteins with the exception of γ-globulins, which are formed in plasma cells. The liver is capable of forming 15 to 50 g of protein per day, an amount sufficient to replace the body's entire supply of protein in several weeks. Albumin is the major protein synthesized by the liver and is the primary determinant of plasma oncotic pressure. The liver also synthesizes the nonessential amino acids from keto acids, which are also synthesized in the liver.

The liver is capable of deamination of amino acids, which is required for energy production or the conversion of amino acids to carbohydrates or fats. Deamination produces ammonia, which is toxic. Intestinal bacteria are an additional source of ammonia. The liver removes ammonia through the formation of urea.

All of the blood clotting factors, with the exception of factors III (tissue thromboplastin), IV (calcium), and VIII (von Willebrand factor), are synthesized in the liver. Vitamin K is required for the synthesis of prothrombin (factor II) and factors VII, IX, and X.

Hepatocytes produce roughly 500 mL of bile daily. Between meals, the high pressure in the sphincter of Oddi diverts bile to the gallbladder for storage. The gallbladder holds 35 to 50 mL of bile in concentrated form. The presence of fat in the duodenum causes release of the hormone cholecystokinin from duodenal mucosa, which reaches the gallbladder via circulation and stimulates gallbladder contraction. Bile contains bile salts, bilirubin, and cholesterol. Bile salts act as a detergent, solubilizing fat into micelles, which are absorbed. Bile salts return to the liver via the portal vein, completing the enterohepatic circulation. Bile salts are needed for fat absorption, and cholestasis can result in steatorrhea and vitamin K deficiency.

The liver has the unique ability to restore itself after injury or partial hepatectomy. As much as two-thirds of the liver can be removed with regeneration of the remaining liver in a matter of weeks.[5] Hepatocyte growth factor, produced by mesenchymal cells in the liver, and other growth factors, such as epidermal growth factor (EGF), cytokines, tumor necrosis factor (TNF), and interleukin-6, are involved in stimulating regeneration. Growth factor-β, a known inhibitor of hepatocyte proliferation, is involved in halting the regenerative process, which appears to be related to the ratio of liver-to-body weight.[5,6] Inflammation, such as with a viral infection of the liver, impairs regeneration.

Assessment of Hepatic Function

A number of laboratory tests are available to assess the liver. Collectively termed *liver function tests* (LFTs), many, including aspartate aminotransferase (AST) and alanine aminotransferase (ALT), do not assess function but rather cellular injury. Increased serum levels of these enzymes, AST (formerly serum glutamic oxaloacetic transaminase; SGOT) and ALT (formerly serum glutamic pyruvic transaminase; SGPT), occur in many types of hepatic disease. Because AST is also found in nonhepatic tissues (including the heart, skeletal muscle, kidney, and brain), elevations are not specific for hepatic disease. ALT is primarily localized to the liver.

Fatty liver and chronic infections are associated with mild (several fold) elevations of AST and ALT. Acute hepatitis produces larger increases, but the highest concentrations, which can exceed 50 times normal, are seen with acute hepatic necrosis. Absolute levels of these enzymes are not always helpful, as declining values may indicate recovery or conversely a lack of surviving hepatocytes. The AST/ALT ratio may be helpful in differentiating alcoholic liver disease, in which the ratio is typically greater than 2, from viral hepatitis, which is associated with a ratio lower than 1.

Indices of bile flow obstruction include serum levels of alkaline phosphatase (AP), 5′-nucleotidase (5′-NT), γ-glutamyl transferase (GGT), and bilirubin. AP isoenzymes are found in multiple organs including the liver, bone, kidney, intestines, placenta, and leukocytes. Normally, most circulating AP originates from liver and bone. Hepatic AP is concentrated in the microvilli of bile canaliculi and the sinusoidal surface of hepatocytes. Elevations of serum AP disproportionate to changes in AST and ALT occur with obstructions to bile flow. However, AP elevations may originate from other tissues, including the placenta during pregnancy. Although 5′-NT is also found in many tissues, elevations are highly specific for hepatobiliary obstruction. Elevations of 5′-NT may reflect the detergent action of bile salts on plasma membranes, a requirement for its release. Because 5′-NT is specific for liver diseases, it is useful to determine whether elevated AP is of hepatic origin. Serum GGT is the most sensitive laboratory indicator of biliary tract disease but it is less specific than 5′-NT and has largely been replaced by 5′-NT.

Bilirubin originates primarily from the breakdown of hemoglobin released from senescent red blood cells. Serum bilirubin levels are determined by the van den Bergh reaction, which separates bilirubin into two fractions: A lipid-soluble, indirect-reacting form (unconjugated bilirubin) and a water-soluble, direct-reacting form (conjugated bilirubin). Elevated levels of unconjugated bilirubin indicate an excess production of bilirubin (hemolysis) or a decrease in the uptake and conjugation of bilirubin by hepatocytes. Conjugated bilirubin is elevated by impaired intrahepatic excretion or extrahepatic obstruction. Even with complete biliary tract obstruction, the bilirubin rarely exceeds 35 mg/dL because of renal excretion of conjugated bilirubin.

Tests of hepatic synthetic function focus on the measurement of serum albumin and coagulation testing. Although the liver is the primary site of albumin synthesis, excessive protein losses (enteropathy, burns, nephrotic syndrome) can also result in low albumin levels. Because of its 3-week half-life, serum albumin is not a reliable indicator of acute liver disease. In contrast, the prothrombin time (PT) and international normalized ratio (INR) are sensitive indicators of hepatic disease because of the short half-life of factor VII. The PT depends upon sufficient intake of vitamin K, which in turn depends upon adequate biliary secretion of bile salts. In patients with biliary obstruction, the PT can be prolonged despite preserved hepatic function. Other conditions that can affect the PT in the absence of liver disease include congenital coagulation factor deficiencies, consumptive coagulopathies such as disseminated intravascular coagulation (DIC), and warfarin therapy.

A number of other tests exist to assess hepatic function, though their use in the United States is limited primarily to research applications. Indocyanine green (ICG) elimination estimates hepatic blood flow and hepatocellular function due to the high extraction ratio of ICG (>70%). The MEGX test measures the conversion of lidocaine to monoethylglycinexylidide (MEGX) via hepatic demethylation. Other metabolic tests include antipyrine clearance, aminopyrine breath test, caffeine breath test, galactose elimination capacity, and urea synthesis.

Ancillary tests to confirm specific diagnoses include serologic tests for the various hepatitis viruses, autoantibodies (for the diagnosis of primary biliary cirrhosis [PBC]), ceruloplasmin (Wilson disease), ferritin (hemochromatosis), α_1-antitrypsin (α_1-antitrypsin deficiency), and α-fetoprotein (hepatocellular carcinoma [HCC]). Serum ammonia is useful for following patients with hepatic encephalopathy (HE).

Hepatobiliary Imaging

Selection of the appropriate imaging technique depends on the differential diagnosis and whether a concurrent therapeutic intervention is planned. Plain radiography has a limited role in the evaluation of liver disease. Abdominal x-rays can be useful to detect calcified or gas-containing lesions. Examples include calcified gallstones, chronic calcific pancreatitis, gas-containing liver abscesses, portal venous gas, and emphysematous cholecystitis.

Ultrasonography is the primary screening test for hepatic parenchymal disease and extrahepatic biliary disease. It is the method of choice for detecting gallstones, the presence of ascites, and portal or hepatic vein thrombosis. Its major limitations are its dependence on the operator's skill and its inability to penetrate bone or air, including bowel gas.

Radioisotope scanning has largely been replaced by computed tomography (CT) scanning. However, it is still in use in patients with suspected acute cholecystitis. Radioisotopes visualized in the gallbladder rule out obstruction of the cystic duct, whereas visualization of the biliary tree and common bile duct without the gallbladder indicates cystic duct obstruction and the presence of cholecystitis.

CT scanning supplements ultrasonography, providing information on the liver texture, gallbladder disease, bile duct dilatation, and mass lesions of the liver and pancreas. CT provides more resolution than ultrasonography and is less operator-dependent. Lesions can be biopsied under CT guidance. The disadvantages of CT include radiation exposure and cost.

Magnetic resonance imaging (MRI) is increasingly used for the evaluation of hepatobiliary disease. MRI is superior to CT for the assessment of malignant focal liver lesions and diffuse liver disease.[7] MRI is also useful for the evaluation of biliary disease.[8] MRI also offers the advantages of avoidance of radiation and contrast nephropathy. The primary disadvantage is the need for breath-hold sequences, which can require sedation or anesthesia in young and/or uncooperative patients.

Percutaneous transhepatic cholangiography (THC) is the percutaneous injection of contrast into the bile ducts under fluoroscopic guidance. It can be used to determine the site and cause of biliary obstruction and to evaluate whether cholangiocarcinoma is surgically resectable. It can also be used for balloon dilatation of biliary strictures and/or placement of an internal stent or external drain. Endoscopic retrograde cholangiopancreatography (ERCP) uses endoscopy to visualize the ampulla of Vater and selectively inject contrast material into the pancreatic and common bile ducts. ERCP has the advantage over THC of not requiring a dilated biliary tree to achieve a high probability of success. ERCP permits sphincterotomy and stone extraction, biopsy, brushings, balloon dilatation, and stent insertion.

Liver Biopsy

Liver biopsy continues to have a role in the evaluation of patients with liver disease. It is the method of choice to determine whether liver damage is due to necrosis, inflammation, steatosis, or fibrosis. The presence of coagulopathy or thrombocytopenia may contraindicate percutaneous liver biopsy, although transjugular liver biopsy is often performed under these conditions.

Hepatic and Hepatobiliary Diseases

Liver disease may be the result of a variety of causes, which include developmental or genetic defects, metabolic abnormalities, autoimmune diseases, infectious diseases, neoplasm, alcohol, environmental toxins, and drug toxicity. A preliminary report from the National Vital Statistics System for the year 2013 lists liver disease as the 12th leading cause of death in the United States, being responsible for over 36,000 deaths in that year.[9] A minimum estimated 33.4 million people in the United States have chronic liver disease (CLD) and another 20 million have biliary disease, together affecting slightly more than a third of the adult population.[10–12]

Liver disease can be divided into two main groups on the basis of the primary anatomy affected. Processes may be considered primarily hepatocellular (parenchymal) or biliary. Progressive biliary disease may eventually lead to fibrotic changes and cirrhosis, but it is characteristic of the biliary diseases that cholestasis precedes hepatocellular dysfunction. In hepatocellular diseases evidence of cholestasis and synthetic dysfunction appear synchronously (Table 46-1). The fact that hepatocellular function is preserved until late in the course of cholestatic disease disadvantages patients with cholestatic liver disease awaiting liver transplantation.

Liver disease may also be described as acute or chronic. The most common causes for acute liver disease are drug toxicity and infection. Acute illnesses may resolve spontaneously, segue into chronic disease, or result in acute liver failure (ALF). Although the primary cause of ALF in the United States was once infectious (presumed acute hepatitis A and B), acetaminophen toxicity

Table 46-1 Blood Tests and the Differential Diagnosis of Hepatic Dysfunction

	Bilirubin Overload (Hemolysis)	Parenchymal Dysfunction	Cholestasis
Aminotransferases	Normal	Increased (may be normal or decreased in advanced stages)	Normal (may be increased in advanced stages)
Alkaline phosphatase	Normal	Normal	Increased
Bilirubin	Increased Unconjugated	Increased Conjugated	Increased Conjugated
Serum proteins	Normal	Decreased	Normal (may be decreased in advanced stages)
Prothrombin time	Normal	Decreased (may be normal in early stages)	Normal (may be prolonged in advanced stages)
Blood urea nitrogen	Normal	Normal (may be decreased in advanced stages)	Normal
Sulfobromophthalein/ indocyanine green	Normal	Retention	Normal or retention

From Gelman S. Anesthesia and the liver. In: Barash P, Cullen B, Stoelting R, eds. *Clinical Anesthesia*. 3rd ed. Philadelphia, PA: Lippincott-Raven; 1997:1011.

is currently the leading cause of this condition. Other causes of acute liver dysfunction include alcoholic hepatitis, nonacetaminophen drug toxicity, and pregnancy-related hepatic diseases. The most common causes for CLD are chronic viral hepatitis, alcoholic liver disease, and nonalcoholic fatty liver disease (NAFLD). Although the prevalence rates of chronic viral hepatitis and alcoholic liver disease have been relatively stable over the past 10 years, the prevalence of NAFLD has grown significantly and appears to be linked to the current epidemic of obesity.[13] The most important consequences of CLD are portal hypertension, cirrhosis, and malignancy.

Acute Liver Failure

ALF (previously termed fulminant hepatic failure) is defined as the appearance of encephalopathy together with coagulopathy, usually an INR 1.5 or more, in a patient who has no previous history of liver disease and who has had an illness of shorter than 26 weeks' duration. Although further distinctions in duration of disease, such as hyperacute and subacute, were once used, they are no longer considered useful for prognosis and have been abandoned. ALF is a rare entity with an incidence of about 2,000 cases per year in the United States. Drug-related toxicity accounts for over half of the cases of ALF in the United States. Of these drug-related cases, over 80% are the result of acetaminophen ingestion. In descending order the next most common causes are idiopathic, acute viral hepatitis, autoimmune, and ischemic.[14] The natural history of adult ALF in the United States is one of spontaneous recovery in approximately 45% of patients, liver transplantation in 25%, and death without transplantation in 30%.[15] Etiology has a significant bearing on outcome, with the most favorable prognosis for patients with acetaminophen overdose, ischemic injury, and hepatitis A and poor prognoses for those with nonacetaminophen drug-induced liver injury (DILI), acute hepatitis B, Wilson disease, and autoimmune hepatitis.[16]

Patients with no previous history of liver disease who present with signs or symptoms and laboratory evidence of a significant hepatitis should have an INR measured and undergo a careful mental status examination. An INR of 1.5 or more and any evidence of encephalopathy should lead to admission to the hospital for ALF. History should include questions about potential infectious or toxic exposures and a detailed history of recent medications or ingestions. Questions should include details about herbal and nutritional supplements, because these have been associated with ALF as well. Except for the finding of encephalopathy, physical examination may be unrevealing. In particular, evidence of CLD should not be present, as the patient should not have had adequate time to develop the stigmata of portal hypertension and cirrhosis. Acute decompensation of CLD or "acute on chronic" liver disease is a separate condition with different etiologies, therapy, and prognostic indicators.

Standard initial laboratory tests are indicated in Table 46-2.[16] Further laboratory and investigative studies are directed by the history, for example, radiologic imaging or ultrasound for suspected hepatic vein thrombosis. Although etiologies of ALF are heterogeneous, there are manifestations that are common to all patients who have massive hepatic necrosis, regardless of its provenance. The most serious, and often the proximate cause of death, is acute cerebral edema and intracranial hypertension. Effects on other organ systems include coagulopathy, circulatory dysfunction and hypotension, acute kidney injury, and metabolic derangements. Encephalopathy is a necessary finding to diagnose ALF. Encephalopathy is graded on a I to IV scale and is described in Table 46-3. The presence of cerebral edema is directly related to the depth of encephalopathy. The incidence of cerebral edema is almost negligible in stage I to stage II coma, but increases to 25% to 35% with stage III and 75% with stage IV.[17] As with the encephalopathy of cirrhosis, the underlying mechanism is not completely understood but hyperammonemia plays a significant role. Ammonia, which is toxic, is generally metabolized via the urea cycle in the liver. The brain has no cells capable of utilizing the urea cycle and thus must resort to

Table 46-2 Initial Laboratory Analysis of Suspected Acute Liver Failure

Prothrombin time/INR
Chemistries
  Sodium, potassium, chloride, bicarbonate, calcium, magnesium, phosphate glucose
  AST, ALT, alkaline phosphatase, GGT, total bilirubin, albumin creatinine, blood urea nitrogen
Arterial blood gas
Arterial lactate
Complete blood count
Blood type and screen
Acetaminophen level
Toxicology screen
Viral hepatitis serologies
  Anti-HAV IgM, HBSAg, anti-HBc IgM, anti-HEV,[a] anti-HCV[b]
Ceruloplasmin level[c]
Pregnancy test (females)
Ammonia (arterial if possible)
Autoimmune markers
  ANA, ASMA, immunoglobulin levels
HIV status[d]
Amylase and lipase

[a]If clinically indicated.
[b]Done to recognize potential underlying infection.
[c]Done only if Wilson disease is a consideration (e.g., in patients less than 40 yrs without another obvious explanation for ALF); in this case uric acid level and bilirubin to alkaline phosphatase ratio may be helpful as well.
[d]Implications for potential liver transplantation.
INR, international normalized ratio; AST, aspartate aminotransferase; ALT, alanine aminotransferase; GGT, gamma-glutamyl transferase; HAV, hepatitis A virus; IgM, immunoglobulin M; HBSAg, hepatitis B surface antigen; HEV, hepatitis E virus; HCV, hepatitis C virus; ANA, antinuclear antibody; ASMA, anti-smooth muscle antibody.
Adapted with permission from Polson J, Lee WM. AASLD position paper: the management of acute liver failure. *Hepatology.* 2005;41:1179.

Table 46-3 Grades of Encephalopathy

I.	Changes in behavior with minimal change in level of consciousness
II.	Gross disorientation, drowsiness, possibly asterixis, inappropriate behavior
III.	Marked confusion, incoherent speech, sleeping most of the time but arousable to vocal stimuli
IV.	Comatose, unresponsive to pain, decorticate or decerebrate posturing

Note: Some patients will overlap grades; clinical judgment is required.
Adapted from Conn HO, Leevy CM, Vhlahcevic ZR, et al. Comparison of lactulose and neomycin in the treatment of chronic portal-systemic encephalopathy: a double blind controlled trial. *Gastroenterology.* 1977;72:573.

detoxifying ammonia by synthesizing glutamine from ammonia and glutamate within astrocytes. Glutamine is osmotically active and results in osmotic astrocyte edema. Other contributors to the observed cerebral edema may include a systemic inflammatory response[18,19] and the loss of cerebral autoregulation, which leads to cerebral hyperemia.[20] Potential targets for therapy include osmotic and mechanical reduction of cerebral edema, elimination of ammonia, manipulation of cerebral blood flow and metabolism, and reduction of the inflammatory response.

General measures to reduce cerebral edema include maintaining the patient in a 30-degree head-up position and making sure the head is in neutral position so as not to impede venous return. Once a patient is intubated, muscle relaxants should be considered to minimize rises in intracranial pressure (ICP) from coughing, bucking, and shivering. Mannitol can be used to induce an osmotic diuresis, but may have limited utility in the patient with compromised renal function. Another option may be hypertonic saline, ideally targeting a serum sodium of 145 to 155 mEq/L.[21]

Although hyperventilation may acutely reduce the cerebral hyperemia associated with ALF, the response is short-lived. There is no evidence that chronic hyperventilation affords any decrease in episodes of intracranial hypertension or any survival benefit.[22] Current recommendations are to maintain normocarbia and to reserve hyperventilation for response to acute rises in ICP. Barbiturates can be used to decrease cerebral metabolism; however, their use may be limited by hypotension.

Ammonia can be eliminated by the administration of lactulose or nonabsorbable antibiotics such as rifaximin or neomycin; however, there is no evidence to support their use in the setting of ALF. Furthermore, neomycin is specifically contraindicated because of the risk of nephrotoxicity.

Corticosteroids have not been shown to be effective in ALF, but there may be a place for prophylactic antibiotics to prevent sepsis and minimize the inflammatory mediator burden. The US Acute Liver Failure Study Group has recommended empiric administration of antibiotics in the following settings: (a) when surveillance cultures reveal significant isolates; (b) progression to stage III or stage IV coma; (c) refractory hypotension; or (d) when the patient exhibits elements of the systemic inflammatory response syndrome, that is, temperature greater than 38°C or lower than 36°C, heart rate more than 90 bpm, white blood cell count more than 12,000 or less than 4,000.[23] Other potential modalities to decrease the inflammatory response include modest hypothermia to a target temperature of 32°C to 34°C and indomethacin.[24]

How to monitor the presence and progression of cerebral edema and intracranial hypertension is controversial. Serial head CTs are often obtained for patients who progress to stage III or stage IV coma, but they are not reliable for diagnosing or quantitating intracranial hypertension due to a lack of sensitivity. CT can, however, provide information on structural abnormalities such as intracranial hemorrhage.[25] Although many centers will place an ICP monitor to guide therapy in patients with stage III to stage IV coma, there are no randomized controlled studies to support this practice. Furthermore, ICP monitor placement is not a benign procedure, frequently entailing aggressive correction of coagulopathy and transport to and from the OR for a critically ill, fragile patient. Nonetheless, many believe that ICP monitors are invaluable for guiding acute therapy and for helping to determine who may no longer be a viable candidate for transplantation. In addition to measuring ICP, these monitors allow calculation of cerebral perfusion pressure (CPP = MAP − ICP), which should be kept between 50 and 80 mmHg. In one case series, a sustained CPP lower than 40 mmHg for greater than 2 hours was associated with a poor neurologic outcome.[26]

Table 46-4 ICP Management Protocol
Initiate in rapid stepwise fashion for ICP >20 mmHg for >5 min
Keep CPP >60 mmHg with norepinephrine or phenylephrine infusion
Mannitol 1 g/kg IV bolus, may repeat if serum osmolarity <320 mOsm/kg
Hyperventilation to target PCO_2 30–35 mmHg
Hypothermia using cooling blanket to core temperature of 33°–34°C
Initiate neuromuscular blockade if needed with cis-atracurium 0.2 mg/kg IV bolus, 3 µg/kg/min infusion—adjust to 2/4 on train of four
Pentobarbital 5 mg/kg bolus, repeated 3–5 mg/kg boluses as necessary—titrate to ICP effect
3% saline: Calculate dose to achieve serum sodium in 145–155 mEq/L range

ICP, intracranial pressure; CPP, cerebral perfusion pressure; IV, intravenous.
Adapted with permission from Raschke RA, Curry SC, Rempe S, et al. Results of a protocol for the management of patients with fulminant liver failure. *Crit Care Med.* 2008;36:2244.

An effective protocol for managing intracranial hypertension in patients with stage III or stage IV encephalopathy has been described (Table 46-4) and resulted in a 95% response to treatment of episodes of ICP greater than 20 mmHg. Furthermore, in this prospective series, ICP was monitored in all patients, and no patients died of isolated cerebral edema. The authors used a protocol that included activated recombinant factor VII (rFVIIa) to correct coagulopathy prior to ICP placement. Significant bleeding complications from ICP monitoring were not encountered.[27]

Deciding which patient should receive a transplant, which may recover spontaneously, and which are unlikely to benefit from transplantation is one of the most difficult decisions encountered during the management of patients with liver disease. Unfortunately there is no ideal guideline for making these decisions. The two most widely used prognostic models are the Clichy or Paul Brousse Hospital criteria and the King's College Hospital criteria. The Clichy criteria recommend transplantation for patients in stage III or stage IV coma on the basis of age and factor V levels. The transplantation threshold is 20% factor V activity for patients under 30 years or 30% factor V activity for patients above 30 years.[28] There is no distinction made for the etiology of ALF, which is felt to be a weakness of these criteria. The King's College Hospital (Table 46-5) criteria accounted for better spontaneous outcomes of patients who had ALF on the basis of acetaminophen toxicity and divided their criteria accordingly. Although the positive predictive value of King's College Hospital criteria has been shown to be clinically acceptable in ALF patients, the negative predictive value drops below 50% in nonacetaminophen patients.[29] Thus, patients who fail to fulfill these criteria include a number of patients who will die without being properly considered for transplantation. Modifications to the King's College Hospital criteria to improve performance and other prognostic scoring models for specific etiologies have been proposed, such as consideration of serum lactate levels[30] or the addition of an apoptosis marker.[31] However, these marginally improved specificity at the expense of sensitivity. It has been suggested that the Sequential Organ Failure Assessment (SOFA) or Acute Physiology and Chronic Health Evaluation II (APACHE II) scores may provide significantly more specificity with a minimal decrement in sensitivity compared to the King's College criteria and that the discriminative value of these indices deserve further investigation.[32]

Table 46-5 King's College Selection Criteria for Liver Transplantation According to the Etiology of Acute Liver Failure	
Etiology	**Selection Criteria for Transplantation**
Acetaminophen	Arterial pH <7.30 despite normal intravascular filling pressures (irrespective of grade of encephalopathy) OR Prothrombin time >100 s + serum creatinine >300 μmol/L in patients in grade III or IV encephalopathy
Nonacetaminophen	Prothrombin time >100 s (irrespective of grade of encephalopathy) OR Any three of the following (irrespective of grade of encephalopathy): Non-A, non-B hepatitis (cryptogenic), halothane hepatitis, or other drug toxicity Age <10 yrs or >40 yrs Jaundice to encephalopathy interval >7 d Prothrombin time >50 s Serum bilirubin >300 μmol/L

Adapted with permission from O'Grady JG, Alexander GJ, Hayllar KM, et al. Early indicators of prognosis in fulminant liver failure. *Gastroenterology*. 1989;97:439.

Coagulopathy is also a necessary finding for the diagnosis of ALF; however, clinically significant spontaneous bleeding is uncommon. Traditional standard of care recommends correction of thrombocytopenia to 50,000/mm³ or more and INR to 1.5 or less for the bleeding patient or the patient about to undergo an invasive procedure.[16,23] However, it has become clear that conventional coagulation studies such as INR and platelet count are poor predictors of bleeding complications of invasive procedures in liver disease.[33–35] Small studies suggest that whole blood viscoelastic studies are more accurate predictors of bleeding in both high- and low-risk invasive procedures[36,37]; however, they have not yet been fully validated for this purpose. Specific treatment thresholds for the nonbleeding patient are difficult to define, but it is suggested that prophylactic therapy not be undertaken except for severe abnormalities, for example, platelet count 10,000/mm³ or less, INR greater than 7, and fibrinogen less than 100 mg/dL.[16] Occasionally, the use of rFVIIa or prothrombin complex concentrate is used to correct a resistant INR abnormality or to avoid fluid overload. It should be kept in mind that these agents carry a thrombotic risk and are contraindicated when the etiology of ALF is associated with hypercoagulability, such as pregnancy or Budd–Chiari syndrome.

Hypotension in ALF may be the result of several days of gastrointestinal losses, poor intake, or myocardial dysfunction, but likely includes a component of decreased arterial tone as liver necrosis progresses. The hypotensive ALF patient should undergo volume status and cardiac function assessment prior to consideration of inotropes or vasopressors. Vasopressors may be used either to treat systemic hypotension or to maintain an adequate CPP. On the basis of recommendations for septic patients, either norepinephrine or dopamine may be used. The use of arginine vasopressin (AVP) or its analogues cannot be recommended as there is evidence that their use is associated with increases in ICP.[38]

Acute Hepatitis

The most common causes of acute viral hepatitis are, collectively, the five identified viral hepatitides: A (HAV), B (HBV), C (HCV), D (HDV or delta-virus), and E (HEV). HAV and HBV have been well characterized and vaccines have been developed to prevent their transmission. As a result of widespread vaccination, the incidence of new cases of HAV and HBV has decreased steadily worldwide. Unfortunately, the same cannot be said for HCV, for which there is no currently available vaccine. The number of reported new cases of HCV is decreasing but this is likely the result of better screening of transfused blood products and the adoption of universal precautions. HDV is a single-strand RNA genome that requires the helper function of HBV for virion assembly and so must occur either as a coinfection or as a superinfection with HBV. HEV is a small RNA virus that has been responsible for several epidemics of hepatitis, primarily in underdeveloped countries with poor sanitation.

The diagnosis of acute hepatitis is made on the basis of classic signs and symptoms, together with laboratory studies to assess liver damage and serologic assays. Symptoms can be nonspecific, such as fatigue, poor appetite, nausea, vomiting, and abdominal pain, and many infections are subclinical. Signs may include jaundice, or a serum-sickness–type presentation with fever, arthralgia or arthritis, and rash that results from circulating hepatitis antigen–antibody complexes. Incubation periods can be several weeks to even months and patients may undergo surgery without awareness of illness. For this reason viral hepatitis should be part of the differential diagnosis when there is any evidence of postoperative liver injury.

HAV is a picornavirus that is spread primarily by the fecal–oral route or via contaminated food or water. HAV has a wide range of manifestation from asymptomatic disease (particularly in children) to ALF. ALF is rare (<1%) and is more likely than other causes to result in spontaneous recovery (69%) in patients without underlying liver disease. There is no chronic disease state associated with HAV.

HBV is a DNA virus that is spread via parenteral, cutaneous, or mucosal exposure to infected blood or body fluids. HBV surface antigen (HBsAg) is the hallmark of active HBV infection and usually appears during the incubation period, 1 to 10 weeks after exposure. ALF caused by acute HBV infection occurs in less than 1% of cases, but has only a 20% rate of spontaneous recovery. Maintenance of seropositivity for HBsAg for more than 6 months after recovery suggests chronic infection and occurs in 2% to 5% of infected adults.

HDV infection occurs in conjunction with HBV infection and is estimated to be present in 5% of patients with chronic HBV. Two types of HDV infection are described: coinfection with acute HBV and superinfection on top of chronic HBV. Both types cause severe infection and may cause ALF.

HCV, once referred to as non-A, non-B hepatitis until its identification in 1989, is transmitted primarily parenterally. Because the identification of HCV, the ability to serologically screen blood products for its presence has all but eliminated it as a source of posttransfusion hepatitis. Causes of transmission are often not identifiable, but the most commonly known risk factor is parenteral drug use. HCV has a high rate of progression to chronic disease (50% to 85%) and a risk of developing cirrhosis ranging from 5% to 25% over 25 to 30 years.[32] HCV is currently the leading cause for liver transplantation in the United States, which is performed for cirrhosis and/or associated HCC. The therapy of chronic HCV infection has recently been revolutionized by the use of combination direct-acting antiviral agents that have achieved reported cure rates of 84% to 100% depending on patient population, drug combination, and viral genotype.[39–42]

Alcoholic Hepatitis

Alcoholic hepatitis is the syndrome marked by the development of jaundice and liver dysfunction in the setting of heavy alcohol use. Encephalopathy may be present in severe alcoholic hepatitis and, if so, portends a poorer prognosis. Laboratory studies show moderate serum aminotransferase elevations (<300 IU/mL), with AST being elevated more than ALT. The AST:ALT ratio is more than 2 in about 70% of patients with alcoholic hepatitis.[43] Elevations of serum creatinine are particularly ominous as they may indicate impeding hepatorenal syndrome (HRS).

A history of excessive alcohol use is supportive of the diagnosis of alcoholic hepatitis, but up to 20% of these patients may have a coexisting cause of liver disease.[44] Although liver biopsy is not required to make the diagnosis of alcoholic hepatitis, it is important to investigate other potential causes of acute liver disease.

The key component of therapy for alcoholic hepatitis is abstinence. For those patients with severe alcoholic hepatitis, medical therapy should also be considered. This consists of nutritional therapy that takes into account not only protein-calorie nutrition but vitamin and mineral deficiencies as well.

Drug-induced Liver Injury

Often considered as an afterthought when a patient presents with new abnormalities in liver-related laboratory studies, DILI is a significant cause of morbidity and mortality. Although the process of diagnosing DILI is not well defined and it is largely a diagnosis of exclusion, DILI should always be considered when formulating the differential diagnosis of patients presenting with liver abnormalities. Moreover, DILI is a serious problem for the pharmaceutical industry, as it is the most common reason for regulatory actions such as failure of approval, removal from market, or restrictions or indications for use. Nonacetaminophen drug-induced idiosyncratic liver injury accounts for 11% to 13% of cases of ALF and, with a 20% rate of survival with supportive care, has a poorer than average rate of spontaneous recovery.[14,45]

A recent report from the international DILI Expert Working Group has defined laboratory criteria for diagnosing DILI (Table 46-6). DILI can further be characterized as hepatocellular, cholestatic, or mixed, on the basis of the relative abnormalities of laboratory values. This is done by calculating the R value, such that $R = (ALT/ULN)/(ALP/ULN)$, where ALT is the alanine aminotransferase, ALP is the alkaline phosphatase, and ULN is the upper limit of normal value. The higher the R value, the more abnormal the ALT in comparison to the ALP. Thus R values 5 or more are used to define a hepatocellular pattern of damage. R values 2 or less define a cholestatic pattern, and R values between 2 and 5 define a mixed pattern. A prognostic rule of thumb is eponymously named "Hy law" after Hyman J. Zimmerman, a leader in DILI research. It was his observation that jaundice (defined as bilirubin >2 ULN) in patients with hepatocellular DILI carried a poor prognosis, with a mortality of more than 10%. This observation has been confirmed and recognized for many years by the FDA as a tool for identifying which drugs may be expected to cause significant hepatotoxicity.[46]

Table 46-6 Clinical Chemistry Criteria for Drug-Induced Liver Injury (DILI)

Any one of the following:
- ALT at least fivefold elevation above the ULN
- ALP at least twofold elevation above the ULN (particularly with accompanying elevations in concentrations of 5′-nucleotidase or γ-glutamyl transpeptidase in the absence of known bone pathology driving the rise in ALP level)
- ALT at least threefold elevation in concentration plus simultaneous elevation of bilirubin concentration exceeding twice the ULN

Level of evidence: 2b (exploratory/retrospective cohort studies)

ALT, alanine aminotransferase; ALP, alkaline phosphatase; ULN, upper limit of normal.
Adapted with permission from Aithal GP, Watkins PB, Andrade RJ, et al. Case definition and phenotype standardization in drug-induced liver injury. *Clin Pharmacol Ther.* 2011;89:806.

The liver is commonly involved in drug toxicity because of its central role in drug metabolism. Drugs may either be directly hepatotoxic or propagate toxic metabolites, most often as products of phase I drug metabolism and the cytochrome P450.[47] Cell injury follows via cell stress, mitochondrial injury, or immune-mediated injury. Cell stress may result from glutathione depletion or the binding of reactive metabolites to intracellular enzymes, proteins, or lipids. Mitochondrial injury may result from the uncoupling of mitochondrial respiration with the depletion of ATP and accumulation of reactive oxygen species (ROS). Immune-mediated injury may result from the binding of reactive metabolites to cell structures, creating antigenic entities that can invoke the formation of antibodies against the cell structures themselves.

In anesthesiology perhaps the best known potentially hepatotoxic drug is halothane. Halothane was introduced to patient care in 1956 and, because of its clinical advantages of lack of flammability, potency, and patient tolerance of administration, rapidly enjoyed widespread use. However, reports of postoperative liver injury began to appear shortly thereafter and, by 1963, over 300 cases of "halothane hepatitis" had been reported.[48] The National Academy of Sciences produced a retrospective epidemiologic study on the use of halothane from these reports. The National Halothane Study reviewed cases of fatal hepatic necrosis occurring within 6 weeks of the administration of a general anesthetic, from among 34 centers in the United States. Of the 856,000 anesthetics reviewed, about 255,000 involved halothane, and 82 cases of fatal hepatic necrosis were identified. Sixty-three of these cases could be ascribed to an identifiable clinical factor, leaving 19 with otherwise unexplained hepatic necrosis. Fourteen of the nineteen had received a halothane anesthetic, but did not have consistent histologic findings. Uncertainty over the direct association between halothane and the cases of fatal hepatic necrosis, together with the calculated incidence of 1 in 35,000 anesthetics even if such association did exist, led to the conclusion that halothane overall had a good safety record. The possible association with repeated exposure to halothane did not go unrecognized, and there was an editorial recommendation that halothane be avoided in patients with a history of unexplained fever and jaundice following a general anesthetic.[49]

It is generally agreed that halothane hepatitis is composed of two different manifestations. A relatively mild, self-limited form is characterized by elevations in liver-related laboratory studies without evidence of liver failure. This may occur in up to 20% of patients after halothane exposure.[50] A proposed mechanism for this hepatocellular damage is the combination of halothane degradation products and hypoxia caused by imbalance in the hepatic oxygen supply–demand relationship.[51] There is strong evidence that the severe, fulminant form of halothane hepatitis is an immune-mediated process. The association with repeated halothane exposure and the appearance of rash and eosinophilia support this hypothesis. Furthermore, circulating IgG antibodies against liver proteins, modified by the reactive trifluoroacetyl (TFA) metabolite of halothane, have been identified in the sera of patients with clinical halothane hepatitis.[52] Although other halogenated inhalational anesthetics that produce TFA metabolites such as enflurane, isoflurane, and desflurane have been associated with acute hepatic failure, the incidences of hepatitis attributed to them have been very small. Because halothane is by far the most extensively metabolized of these agents (20% halothane metabolized vs. 2% enflurane, 0.2% isoflurane, and 0.01% desflurane) the production of TFA metabolites would seem to correlate with the incidence of associated hepatitis. Indeed, an animal study examining the extent of hepatic tissue trifluoroacylation after exposure to halogenated anesthetics showed that halothane produced significantly more tissue acylation than enflurane, isoflurane, or desflurane.[53]

Pregnancy-related Liver Diseases

Abnormalities in liver studies occur in 3% to 5% of pregnancies. Although many causes reflect underlying hepatic or biliary disease, the most common causes are one of the five acute, pregnancy-related conditions: Hyperemesis gravidarum; intrahepatic cholestasis of pregnancy; preeclampsia; preeclampsia complicated by hemolysis, low platelet count, and elevated liver enzymes (HELLP syndrome); and acute fatty liver of pregnancy (AFLP; Table 46-7). Hyperemesis gravidarum is a feature of the first trimester of pregnancy and is characterized by vomiting of sufficient severity to warrant intravenous (IV) hydration. Risk factors include hyperthyroidism, molar pregnancy, and multiple pregnancies.[54] Liver enzymes may be elevated in 50% of patients, with up to 20-fold elevation, but little if any elevation of bilirubin.[55,56] It is important to distinguish hyperemesis from acute viral hepatitis or from drug toxicity with appropriate laboratory values and a careful medication history. Therapy is primarily supportive and the condition usually resolves by the second trimester.

Intrahepatic cholestasis of pregnancy usually presents in the second to third trimester of pregnancy. The proposed etiology is interference with bile acid transport across the canalicular membrane, resulting in elevated serum bile acid elevation and pruritus. In addition to modest increases in bilirubin (usually <5 mg/dL) aminotransferases may also be elevated up to 20-fold and serum bile acids may be elevated up to 100-fold.[56] As with hyperemesis gravidarum, treatment is primarily supportive, aimed at relieving pruritus. Unlike hyperemesis, intrahepatic cholestasis of pregnancy may be associated with chronic placental insufficiency, premature labor, and sudden fetal death. Therefore, pregnancies complicated by intrahepatic cholestasis of pregnancy are considered fetal high-risk pregnancies.

The three remaining uniquely pregnancy-related conditions all present in the third trimester. Preeclampsia is diagnosed by the triad of hypertension, edema, and proteinuria. Elevation of aminotransferases is indicative of severe preeclampsia. The appearance of microangiopathic hemolytic anemia (MAHA), elevated liver enzymes, and low platelet count in the preeclamptic patient comprises the HELLP syndrome and occurs in 20% of severely preeclamptic patients. MAHA is the result of

Table 46-7 Distinguishing Features of Intrahepatic Cholestasis of Pregnancy (ICP), the HELLP Syndrome, and Fatty Liver of Pregnancy (AFLP)

	ICP	HELLP	AFLP
Pregnancies	0.1% (United States)	0.2–0.6%	0.005–0.01%
Onset	25–32 wks	3rd trimester or postpartum	3rd trimester or postpartum
Family history	Often	No	Occasionally
Presence of preeclampsia	No	Yes	50%
Typical clinical features	Pruritus, mild jaundice, elevated bile acids, decreased vitamin K	Hemolysis, thrombocytopenia (<50,000 often)	Liver failure with coagulopathy, encephalopathy hypoglycemia, DIC
Aminotransferases	Mild to 10- to 20-fold elevation	Mild to 10- to 20-fold elevation	300–500 typical but variable elevation
Bilirubin	<5 mg/dL	<5 mg/dL unless massive necrosis	Often <5 mg/dL, higher if severe
Hepatic imaging	Normal	Hepatic infarcts, hematomas, rupture	Fatty infiltration
Histology	Normal–mild cholestasis, no necrosis	Patchy/extensive necrosis and hemorrhage	Microvesicular fat in zone 3
Maternal mortality	0%	1–25%	7–18%
Fetal/perinatal mortality	0.4–1.4%	11%	9–23%
Recurrence in subsequent pregnancies	45–70%	4–19%	α-Subunit, long-chain 3-hydroxyacyl-CoA dehydrogenase (LCHAD) defect—yes No fatty acid oxidation defect—rare

DIC, disseminated intravascular coagulation.
Adapted with permission from Hay JE. Liver disease in pregnancy. *Hepatology.* 2008;47:1067.

vascular endothelial injury with subsequent fibrin deposition and platelet consumption. This also leads to areas of hepatic infarction and subsequent hemorrhage, which may coalesce into large hematomas and lead to capsular rupture and intraperitoneal bleeding. Laboratory studies show elevated aminotransferases, up to 10- to 20-fold, and modest increases in bilirubin. A peripheral smear will show the characteristic schistocytes and burr cells of MAHA. Platelet count may be used to distinguish between mild, moderate, and severe HELLP, with platelet counts of 100,000 to 150,000/mm^3, 50,000 to 100,000/mm^3, and less than 50,000/mm^3, respectively.

Abdominal CT imaging is the preferred study to detect major hepatic complications of infarct, hematoma, or rupture. Contained hepatic hemorrhage can be managed conservatively with correction of volume deficit and coagulopathy. Capsular rupture or rapid extension of a hematoma is life-threatening and demands more aggressive treatment for control of bleeding, usually emergency laparotomy. Rarely, there may be an indication for transplantation for the patient in whom bleeding cannot be controlled. Delivery is definitive therapy for HELLP syndrome. Therapy remains the same regardless of timing of presentation and most patients will rapidly resolve abnormalities after delivery.

AFLP is the result of rapid microvesicular fatty infiltration of the liver resulting in acute portal hypertension and encephalopathy. Although the exact mechanism of AFLP is unknown, there is an association between it and abnormalities in the enzymes involved in β-oxidation of fatty acids. Symptoms are similar to severe preeclampsia and HELLP syndrome; however, the AFLP patient may additionally have laboratory and clinical findings more unique to liver failure, such as hypoglycemia, elevated ammonia, asterixis, and encephalopathy.

Arrangements for rapid delivery should follow diagnosis of AFLP, as recovery can only follow delivery. Recovery may be prolonged in patients who are severely ill upon presentation, and there is a role for transplantation in the patient who continues to deteriorate into ALF after delivery.

Cirrhosis and Portal Hypertension

Cirrhosis is the end product of the long course of CLD, during which there have been either steady or recurrent episodes of parenchymal inflammation and necrosis with resultant disruption of normal hepatic architecture. Areas of fibrosis and regenerative nodules replace the normal arrangement of hepatic lobules. Blood flow through the liver is disrupted as well, with the formation of shunts between afferent (portal venous and hepatic arterial) and efferent (hepatic venous) vessels.[57] Increased resistance to blood flow through the liver leads to portal hypertension. When portal hypertension becomes severe (generally defined as an HVPG of >10 to 12 mmHg), CLD becomes a systemic illness, affecting other organ systems as well.[58]

Hemostasis

Hemostasis is a dynamic process that is the product of interaction between coagulation, platelets, and fibrinolysis, resulting in the formation and revision of clot. Liver disease affects all three of these components, both quantitatively and qualitatively.

The liver is the site of synthesis for all procoagulant and anticoagulant factors, with the exception of tissue thromboplastin (III), calcium (IV), and von Willebrand factor (VIII). It is also the site for clearance of activated factors.

Cirrhotic patients are customarily considered to have a bleeding diathesis on the basis of abnormalities in conventional tests of coagulation such as PT and partial thromboplastin time (PTT). However, such tests reflect the activity of only a portion of the procoagulant factors and do not consider the concomitant decrease in anticoagulant factors, which are not customarily measured. It is the balance of procoagulant and anticoagulant forces, not the isolated measurement of either portion of the coagulation system, that indicates the effective generation of thrombin.[59,60] Not surprisingly, PT and PTT abnormalities correlate poorly with bleeding complications following invasive procedures, such as liver biopsy.[61–63] In fact there is evidence that, should one account for differences in the anticoagulant levels between normal and cirrhotic patients by adding thrombomodulin (an activator of the anticoagulant protein C) to the PT assay, normal and cirrhotic patients generate the same amounts of thrombin.[64] Thus, one may conclude that the decreased levels of protein C in cirrhotic patients balance the decreased levels of procoagulants, leaving thrombin generation in vivo unaltered.

Even more counterintuitive is the increasing evidence that cirrhotic patients not only have normal thrombin generation but may actually also have a procoagulant imbalance on the basis of reduced levels of anticoagulants protein C and antithrombin III, together with an increase in FVIII and von Willebrand factor.[59,60,65] Clinically, this is supported by studies reporting not only the lack of protection of liver disease against the formation of venous thromboembolism (VTE)[66,67] but also an increased risk of VTE formation associated with the presence of cirrhotic and noncirrhotic liver disease.[68]

The cholestatic diseases (e.g., PBC, sclerosing cholangitis) may eventually progress to cirrhosis, but until that happens the coagulopathy of these diseases has a different nature from that of hepatocellular dysfunction. The coagulopathy of biliary disease is characterized by functional deficiencies in the vitamin K–dependent procoagulants II, VII, IX, and X and anticoagulants protein C and protein S. Vitamin K is a fat-soluble cofactor necessary for the final step in the production of these factors: Carboxylation of the precursor produced by the liver. Bile salts are necessary for absorption of vitamin K, and impaired bile secretion in cholestasis results in vitamin K deficiency. Parenteral vitamin K can correct this deficiency and return coagulation to normal as long as the liver is still capable of manufacturing adequate amounts of factor precursors. It cannot, however, correct the coagulopathy of hepatocellular dysfunction.

Dysfibrinogenemia has been described in acute, chronic, and neoplastic liver disease and is the most common qualitative defect of coagulation factors, occurring in 70% to 80% of cirrhotics.[69] Its presence does not appear to be related to the severity of hepatic dysfunction, but instead to be associated with hepatic tissue regeneration. Excess sialic acid residues on the fibrinogen interfere with the enzymatic activity of thrombin and cause abnormal polymerization of fibrin monomers. Thus, although serum fibrinogen levels may be adequate, function is not accurately reflected.

Platelets provide primary hemostasis by interaction with the vessel wall at the site of injury and forming a physical plug. Thrombocytopenia is a well-known feature of cirrhosis. Estimates of incidence range from 30% to 64% of chronic cirrhotics, but platelet counts below 30,000/mm^3 are rare.[70] Because the liver is the primary site of thrombopoietin production, decreased levels of thrombopoietin contribute. Other factors include immunologic mechanisms, direct bone-marrow suppression, and consumptive processes such as DIC. However, the primary cause is splenic sequestration in the setting of portal hypertension. Up to 90% of the platelet population may be sequestered in the spleen.

Elevated levels of von Willebrand factor are felt to compensate for decreased platelet counts, augmenting the platelet–endothelial cell interaction on vessel walls.

A second function of platelets is to promote thrombin generation. Activated platelets provide negatively charged phospholipids on their surfaces, which act as receptors for the assembly of coagulation factors and thus promote coagulation. A series of assays measuring thrombin generation concluded that platelet counts below a threshold of 100,000/mm^3 negatively correlated with thrombin production. It was further estimated that the minimum platelet count necessary to support near-normal thrombin generation was 56,000/mm^3.[64] This information provides further support to the use of platelet transfusion in the bleeding patient with platelet counts in and below that range. Platelet transfusions are not indicated in the absence of bleeding.

The fibrinolytic system limits and revises clot formation. The initial step is activation of plasmin from plasminogen by enzymes such as tissue plasminogen activator (tPA). Plasmin consumes fibrin, producing fibrin degradation products such as D-dimer. The fibrinolytic system in cirrhotic patients has many abnormalities which may account for accelerated fibrinolysis, which has a reported incidence of 30% to 46% in patients with end-stage liver disease.[71,72] The liver is the site of tPA clearance, and elevated tPA levels have been noted in patients with cirrhosis.[73] Furthermore, the liver is the site of synthesis for plasmin inhibitors, such as plasmin activator inhibitor-1 (PAI-1) and thrombin-activatable fibrinolysis inhibitor (TAFI). However, as with the process of coagulation, what matters is the balance of these factors that promote and inhibit fibrinolysis and where their net forces lie. Commonly used studies for assessing the presence and severity of accelerated fibrinolysis include the euglobulin clot lysis time (ECLT) and thromboelastography (TEG). A clot lysis index in TEG has been defined as the ratio of the clot amplitude at 60 minutes post achievement of maximum amplitude (A60) to the clot maximum amplitude (MA). A ratio of less than 0.85 indicates the presence of accelerated fibrinolysis and suggests the need for an antifibrinolytic agent such as epsilon aminocaproic acid or tranexamic acid in the presence of otherwise unexplained bleeding.

DIC is primarily a thrombotic diathesis, followed by widespread secondary fibrinolysis. As factors are consumed, DIC becomes a bleeding diathesis of factor and platelet deficiencies. Whether or not DIC is a feature of stable CLD is controversial. Because cirrhosis shares common laboratory abnormalities with DIC, standard laboratory values cannot distinguish between consumption and decreased synthesis and so have little utility. More recent approaches to answer this question have utilized assays for substances that would be expected to be elevated as the result of excessive thrombin production, the sine qua non of DIC. These include the cleaved by-products of coagulation factor activation such as prothrombin fragment F1 + 2, fibrinopeptide A, and thrombin–antithrombin (TAT) complexes. Elevation of these would suggest that low levels of procoagulation factors are the result of consumption rather than underproduction.

It is generally agreed on the basis of examination of these special assays that overt DIC is probably not a feature of stable CLD.[74] However, an entity called "accelerated intravascular coagulation and fibrinolysis (AICF)" has been described. This may be considered a low-grade consumptive process that occurs in less than 30% of cirrhotics, primarily in those with severe, decompensated disease.[75] Although it may not have immediate clinical consequence, patients who exhibit this phenomenon are considered at increased risk to progress to DIC in the presence of a known stimulus, such as sepsis or spontaneous bacterial peritonitis (SBP).

Cardiac Manifestations

The cirrhotic patient typically has a hyperdynamic circulation, characterized by a high cardiac output, low arterial blood pressure, and low systemic vascular resistance. On examination the patient is warm and appears well perfused despite systolic arterial pressures in the 80s and 90s. Although pulmonary arterial pressures may be mildly elevated, the pulmonary vascular resistance (PVR) is usually within the normal range. Consideration of the formula for calculating PVR (mean pulmonary artery pressure, mPAP, minus pulmonary capillary wedge divided by cardiac output) reveals the explanation: The cardiac output is elevated proportionally to the transpulmonary gradient (the numerator in the equation). Although these patients have an elevated intravascular volume this is not usually reflected in an elevated wedge pressure. This is due to sequestration of this volume into the massively dilated and collateralized splanchnic vascular bed. Thus, the effective circulating volume is reduced, which has consequences on other organ systems as well.

At the heart of these circulatory changes is portal hypertension. Portal hypertension causes local production of vasodilators such as natriuretic peptides, vasoactive intestinal peptide, endotoxin, glucagon, and especially nitric oxide.[76] Elevated production of nitric oxide has been observed to precede the formation of the hyperdynamic circulation in cirrhosis, and inhibition of nitric oxide formation has been shown to increase arterial pressure in cirrhotic patients. Furthermore, there is reduced circulatory responsivity to sympathetic stimulation primarily due to overproduction of vasodilators.[77]

In addition to hyperdynamic circulation, the cirrhotic patient may have a combination of other cardiac functional abnormalities that are not immediately apparent in the baseline state. These abnormalities comprise four key components of a condition termed "cirrhotic cardiomyopathy." They include (1) the aforementioned increase in cardiac output and decrease in peripheral vascular resistance, (2) systolic and diastolic dysfunction, (3) cardiac resistance to β-adrenergic stimulation, and (4) electrophysiologic abnormalities.

Historically, cirrhosis has not been associated with cardiomyopathy because the hyperdynamic circulation was presumed to reflect cardiac vigor and the few patients who had overt dilated cardiomyopathy were thought to be manifesting alcoholic cardiomyopathy. However, elevated cardiac output is only a consequence of the profound decrease in afterload resulting from the dilated peripheral circulation. Systolic incompetence is revealed by physiologic or pharmacologic stress and is manifested by an inability to increase cardiac output in response to exercise and an inability to increase ejection fraction despite an increase in end-diastolic volume. Furthermore, the severity of cardiac dysfunction seems to be directly correlated with the severity of liver disease.[78]

Diastolic dysfunction has been described in cirrhotic patients as well, on the basis of diagnostic echocardiographic findings of abnormalities in transmitral flow during diastole. This consists of decrement or reversal of the E/A wave ratio and prolongation of E wave deceleration time, reflecting ventricular resistance to diastolic filling. Also supportive of the presence of diastolic dysfunction is the finding of septal and left ventricular hypertrophy on echo examination. Diastolic dysfunction renders cirrhotic patients very sensitive to changes in cardiac filling making them vulnerable to both heart failure and prerenal insufficiency.

Autonomic dysfunction is another characteristic of the altered cirrhotic cardiovascular system. Chronotropic and hemodynamic incompetence in response to various challenges such as sustained handgrip, ice water hand submersion, Valsalva maneuver, and tilt table testing has demonstrated autonomic neuropathy in 43% of cirrhotic patients. Although apparently unrelated to autonomic dysfunction, prolonged Q–Tc interval is also observed in cirrhotic patients with an incidence ranging from 30% in Child's A to 60% in Child's C patients (see later).[79] This should be kept in mind when treating these patients with drugs known to prolong Q–T interval.

Coronary artery disease (CAD) in cirrhotic patients has become an area of interest particularly as the application of liver transplantation has expanded to include older patients with comorbidities. Risk factors for coronary artery disease in cirrhotic patients are similar to those of other patient populations: hypertension, dyslipidemia, age, gender, and obesity. However, Nonalcoholic Steatohepatitis (NASH) has been recognized as an increasingly important cause for transplantation and carries with it both the cardiac disease risks of its attendant maladies, obesity and diabetes, and a chronic inflammatory state. The optimal test for identifying cirrhotic patients with significant CAD is unclear. Because many of these patients cannot exercise, pharmacologic stress testing is most commonly employed. Unfortunately, studies investigating the predictive value of noninvasive functional testing, particularly dobutamine stress echocardiography, have generally shown poor sensitivity and variable quality of negative predictive value (75% to 89%).[80] Thus, among liver transplantation candidates, consideration should be given to proceeding with coronary angiography if the patient is judged to have a high likelihood of CAD.[81] For less complex surgeries, however, this may not be warranted.

Renal Dysfunction

The hallmarks of renal dysfunction in cirrhosis are the seemingly inappropriate avid retention of sodium and free water, together with renal hypoperfusion and consequent decreased glomerular filtration. The extreme manifestation of this is the HRS, a prerenal functional abnormality that is the renal response to the circulatory abnormalities of advanced cirrhosis. Renal function is an important risk factor for mortality, a fact that is emphasized by its presence as one of only three variables used in calculating the MELD score, the primary predictor of 3-month mortality for patients on the liver transplantation waiting list.

Although the most dramatic and unique renal manifestation of CLD is the HRS, cirrhotic patients are also at high risk for more prosaic causes of renal dysfunction, such as parenchymal renal disease, sepsis, nephrotoxicity, and hypovolemia. It is important to remember that HRS is a diagnosis of exclusion and that other possible potentially treatable causes must be ruled out because therapies will differ.

Despite the fact that the cirrhotic patient's liver disease predominates, one should be mindful of any comorbidities that exist. Glomerulonephritis and diabetic nephropathy are not infrequent findings. NAFLD, the most common nonviral cause for adult CLD, is associated with type II diabetes. Immune complex nephropathies such as IgA nephropathy and membranous proliferative glomerulonephropathy are associated with chronic hepatitis C infection.[82] In addition, some underlying causes of liver failure are directly associated with renal dysfunction. These include such diseases as amyloidosis, systemic lupus erythematosus, autoimmune hepatitis, polycystic liver disease, and Alagille syndrome.

The cirrhotic circulatory system is characterized by marked sympathetic stimulation, and activation of the renin–angiotensin–aldosterone and vasopressin systems in response to the loss of effective circulating volume to the massively dilated splanchnic vasculature of portal hypertension. These systems combine to save salt and water and reduce renal perfusion. Elevated levels of renal prostaglandins help to maintain renal perfusion. Thus, cirrhotic patients are very sensitive to the prostaglandin inhibition of nonsteroidal anti-inflammatory medications. Aminoglycosides, angiotensin-converting enzyme inhibitors, and angiotensin receptor blockers are other drug groups associated with nephrotoxicity in cirrhotic patients. Despite the expectation that contrast administration would be nephrotoxic, there is no evidence to support that concern.[83]

Cirrhotic patients are at risk for hypovolemia from a number of causes, including gastrointestinal bleeding, diuretic use, and diarrhea resulting from lactulose or rifaximin administration. Unfortunately, it can be difficult to assess intravascular volume status in patients who are total-body volume overloaded, whose measured central filling pressures may reflect transmitted elevated intra-abdominal pressures because of ascites, and whose measured serum creatinine levels are poor estimates of GFR due to decreased muscle mass.[84,85] Nonetheless, pursuit of a diagnosis by discontinuing diuretics and providing volume expansion with albumin can help differentiate hypovolemia from the other prerenal etiology of interest, HRS. Failure to improve creatinine in response to such measures is strongly suggestive of HRS as the underlying cause.

HRS is the end-stage renal manifestation of the systemic circulatory derangement of cirrhosis. It is considered a functional derangement, primarily on the basis of successful transplantation of kidneys from HRS patients.[86] Although it is often invoked in the differential diagnosis of acute renal dysfunction in cirrhotic patients, it accounts for only about 23% of the cases of acute kidney injury in hospitalized cirrhotic patients.[87] Nonetheless, in cirrhotic patients with ascites, the incidence of HRS is 18% at 1 year and 39% at 5 years.[88]

The generally agreed-upon criteria for diagnosing HRS are those proposed by the International Ascites Club.[89,90] Two manifestations of HRS are recognized, called type I and type II. Although they were once considered variants of the same disorder, it has become increasingly clear that they must be treated as two different entities.

Type I HRS is characterized by rapidly progressive renal failure, typically represented by at least a doubling of serum creatinine over the course of 2 weeks in close proximity to a precipitating cause such as SBP, sepsis, gastrointestinal bleeding, or surgical stress. Patients with type I HRS have a median survival of 2 to 4 weeks without therapy.[88,91] Type I HRS is associated with failure of other organ systems, including adrenal insufficiency. Most notably, however, when type I HRS responds to medical therapy that response is usually sustained, even after withdrawal of therapy.[92]

Type II HRS is more indolent and may be considered the expected consequence of continuous and progressive activity of the circulatory homeostatic triad of the sympathetic renin–angiotensin–aldosterone and vasopressin systems in an attempt to compensate for the progressive loss of effective circulating blood volume to the increasingly dilated splanchnic vasculature. The most compelling clinical problem in these patients is refractory ascites. Patients with type II HRS have a median survival of about 6 months.[93]

Although profound renal vasoconstriction is the proximate cause of HRS, therapy aimed at directly increasing renal perfusion by the use of prostaglandins, dopamine agonists, or endothelin antagonists has not proved successful. More effective has been therapy targeting the underlying pathology that leads to the renal vasoconstrictive response, that is, reduction of portal hypertension and/or splanchnic vasodilation.

Vasoconstrictors such as AVP or its analogues, somatostatin or its analogues, and α-agonists such as norepinephrine and midodrine, combined with volume expansion, have shown efficacy in reversing type I HRS (typically defined as a reduction in creatinine to 1.5 mg/dL).[94] AVP and its analogues are particularly attractive, because they interact with V1 receptors, which mediate vasoconstriction and are particularly well represented in the splanchnic circulation. Choices among these therapies are to some extent dictated by drug availability because, for example, terlipressin is not available in the United States. Terlipressin is perhaps the most studied vasopressor for HRS and is effective in 40% to 60% of type I patients.[94,95] Predictive factors of successful treatment include a starting creatinine lower than 5 mg/dL and a sustained rise in MAP from baseline throughout the 1- to 2-week course of treatment.[96] More importantly, when therapy is withdrawn, recurrence is uncommon and occurs in lower than 15% of patients.[95] Although response to vasopressor plus volume expansion has been observed in type II HRS, recurrence after withdrawal of therapy is the rule.

Placement of a transjugular intrahepatic portal shunt (TIPS) lowers portal pressures and would be expected to decompress the splanchnic circulation, returning volume directly to the central circulation. Although pilot studies have shown TIPS capable of reversing both types of HRS, it has limited application primarily because of the exclusionary criteria used in these studies; for example, Child–Pugh score above 12, active infection, and serum bilirubin above 5 mg/dL, as well as risk of de novo development or worsening of HE.[97] Furthermore, even when initially successful there is a high rate of shunt stenosis and migration.

Liver transplantation is the definitive therapy for HRS. For patients with HRS who are transplant candidates, renal replacement therapy is the typical bridge to transplantation. In countries where terlipressin is available, terlipressin plus albumin volume expansion is also an option. In fact there is evidence that treatment of HRS I with terlipressin and albumin while awaiting liver transplantation may improve posttransplant outcome. Although renal recovery is anticipated, 35% of patients with pretransplant HRS will continue to require support in the immediate postoperative period, compared to 5% of patients without pretransplant HRS.[98] Gradual improvement in GFR occurs over the following 1 to 2 months, reaching 30 to 40 mL/min. There is some sense that, if allowed to continue, HRS that requires renal replacement therapy may not be reversible. In the First International Liver Transplantation Society Expert Panel Consensus on Renal Insufficiency in Liver Transplantation, it was recommended that patients who had received dialysis at least twice weekly for more than 6 weeks prior to transplantation be considered for combined liver–kidney transplantation.[99]

Pulmonary Complications

Pulmonary complications have long been associated with portal hypertension with or without intrinsic hepatic disease. Estimates of as high as 50% to 70% of patients with CLD complain of shortness of breath.[100] There are many commonplace mechanisms underlying pulmonary abnormalities observed in patients with liver disease. The differential diagnoses include ventilation–perfusion abnormalities associated with underlying obstructive airways disease, fluid retention, pleural effusion, and decreased lung capacities secondary to large volume ascites. $α_1$-Antitrypsin disease is a metabolic syndrome that has both lung and liver manifestations, as may cystic fibrosis. In addition, there are two types of vascular abnormalities unique to the setting of portal hypertension, which have significant morbidity and mortality.

These abnormalities have been termed hepatopulmonary syndrome (HPS) and portopulmonary hypertension (PPHTN). Their severity may even overshadow the underlying liver disease, so much so that their presence and severity influences candidacy for liver transplantation.

HPS consists of the triad of liver dysfunction, otherwise unexplained hypoxemia, and intrapulmonary vascular dilation (IPVD) that may be present in up to 20% of patients who present for liver transplantation. The diagnostic criteria for HPS are as follows[101]:

- Oxygenation defect: Partial pressure of oxygen below 80 mmHg or alveolar–arterial oxygen gradient of at least 15 mmHg while breathing ambient air
- Pulmonary vascular dilatation: Positive findings on contrast-enhanced echocardiography or abnormal uptake in the brain (>6%) with radioactive lung-perfusion scanning
- Liver disease: Portal hypertension (most common) with or without cirrhosis

Staging of HPS is given in Table 46-8.

IPVDs are of two types. Type I lesions are more common and are manifested as precapillary dilations at the alveolar level. Type II lesions are larger dilations that are more centrally located in the lungs and behave as anatomic shunts. Demonstration of IPVD may be made by agitated saline contrast-enhanced echocardiography or by technetium-labeled microaggregated albumin (TcMAA). In the absence of HPS, microbubbles and albumin microaggregates injected into the venous circulation are trapped by the pulmonary capillary bed. The delayed (>3 cardiac cycles) appearance of microbubbles in the left atrium or increased (>5%) extrapulmonary uptake of TcMAA suggests direct arteriovenous communication in the lungs and the presence of IPVDs. Type I IPVDs are functional, rather than true anatomic shunts. IPVDs result in a massive increase in pulmonary capillary diameter, from 8 to 15 μm to 50 to 500 μm. This, together with the usually hyperdynamic circulation of the cirrhotic patient, allows insufficient time for oxygen diffusion through the entire stream of capillary blood. This results in a central stream of poorly oxygenated blood that is functionally shunted. This lesion is easily correctable with the administration of oxygen, because increased FiO_2 increases oxygen diffusion through the dilated capillary. In fact, failure of 100% oxygen to correct the PaO_2 to greater

Table 46-8 Staging of the Hepatopulmonary Syndrome

Stage	Alveolar–Arterial Oxygen Gradient (mmHg)	Partial Pressure of Oxygen (mmHg)
Mild	≥15	≥80
Moderate	≥15	≥60–<80
Severe	≥15	≥50–<60
Very severe	≥15	<50 (<300 while the patient is breathing 100% oxygen)

The alveolar–arterial gradient is determined as follows:
$PAO_2 - PaO_2 = (FiO_2 - P_{atm} - PH_2O) - [PaCO_2/R]) - PaO_2$
where PAO_2 denotes partial pressure of alveolar oxygen, PaO_2 partial pressure of arterial oxygen, FiO_2 fraction of inspired oxygen, P_{atm} atmospheric pressure, PH_2O partial pressure of water vapor at body temperature, and $PaCO_2$ partial pressure of arterial carbon dioxide, and R the respiratory quotient.
Data from Rodriguez-Roisin R, Krowka MJ. Hepatopulmonary syndrome: a liver-induced lung vascular disorder. *N Engl J Med.* 2008;358:2378.

than 150 mmHg is suggestive of the presence of true anatomic or type II shunt.[102] Also of interest is the unique positional oxygenation change that occurs with this syndrome, called orthodeoxia. Because IPVDs predominate in the bases of the lungs, standing worsens hypoxemia and the supine position improves oxygenation as blood is redistributed from the bases to the apices.

The natural history of HPS is usually one of progressive hypoxemia. The pathogenesis of HPS is poorly understood, hampering the development of effective therapy. Suspected contributing factors include nitric oxide, splanchnic endotoxemia, decreased clearance of inflammatory mediators, and angiogenesis. Genetic factors are thought to contribute also. Post-liver-transplantation correction of hypoxemia is almost universal, although it may take up to a year to do so.[103,104] Mortality without transplantation is greater than in a matched cohort, with a median survival of 24 months and a 5-year survival of 23% versus a median survival of 87 months and a 5-year survival of 63% in transplant candidates without HPS.[105] A PaO_2 no more than 50 mmHg or a TcMAA-quantitated shunt fraction 20% or more are predictors of increased mortality regardless of whether the patient receives a transplant. However, in the largest single-center series of liver transplantation for HPS the overall 5-year survival was 76%, an outcome comparable to transplantation in non-HPS patients.[103,105,106] Taken together, these findings suggest that timely transplantation in patients with HPS results in good outcomes. The transplant community has recognized this by granting MELD exception points to patients with HPS and room air PaO_2 less than 60 mmHg.[107]

PPHTN is defined as pulmonary hypertension that exists in a patient who has portal hypertension with no other known cause. The specific diagnostic criteria put forth by the European Respiratory Society Task Force on Hepatopulmonary Diseases[108] follow:

1. Clinical evidence of portal hypertension with or without hepatic disease.
2. mPAP of 25 mmHg at rest or 30 mmHg during exercise.
3. Mean pulmonary artery occlusion pressure (mPAOP) less than 15 mmHg.
4. PVR more than 240 dynes/sec/cm^5 or 3 Wood units.

There is support for replacing the requirement that the mPAOP be less than 15 mmHg with one that requires the transpulmonary gradient (TPG = mPAP − mPAOP) to be more than 12 mmHg. Patients with pulmonary hypertension may be fluid overloaded as well, and such a measurement would help distinguish the contribution of volume status to an elevated mPAP. A TPG more than 12 mmHg would be consistent with increased PVR, suggesting a component of pulmonary hypertension in the increased mPAP. The requirement for calculation of the PVR is a reflection of the fact that many cirrhotic patients have mildly elevated mPAP simply on the basis of an elevated cardiac output. Calculated PVR in these hyperdynamic patients is often normal. Severity of PPHTN is graded by mPAP, with mild, moderate, and severe PPHTN defined as less than 35 mmHg, 35 to 50 mmHg, and more than 50 mmHg, respectively.

The occurrence of PPHTN is 2% in a population of patients with known portal hypertension,[109] as compared to 0.13% in an unselected population.[110] Among liver transplant candidates the prevalence is 4% to 6%.[111,112] The occurrence of PPHTN is unrelated to the severity of the underlying liver disease or portal hypertension, with one epidemiologic study documenting a distribution of 51% Child's class A, 38% Child's class B, and 11% Child's class C patients among a population of patients sent to a referral center with the diagnosis of PPHTN.[113] Female patients as well as patients with underlying autoimmune hepatitis are at increased risk for PPHTN, and patients with chronic hepatitis C are at decreased risk.[111,113]

Although a theory commonly put forth for the pathophysiology of PPHTN invokes a vascular proliferative reaction to the shear stress of a chronically elevated cardiac output, the increased incidence in women and in autoimmune hepatitis suggests hormonal and immunologic processes may also contribute. Furthermore, as with other types of pulmonary hypertension, increased levels of endothelin are also thought to play a role. Clinical improvement in PPHTN patients with the endothelin antagonist, bosentan, has been documented albeit in a small study.[114]

Similar to HPS patients, symptoms of PPHTN are nonspecific, commonly consisting of dyspnea, generalized weakness, and decreased exercise tolerance. Although HPS and PPHTN may coexist, such an occurrence is uncommon and PPHTN patients may have only a modest decrease in PaO_2 if at all. The single best screening study for PPHTN is the 2D transthoracic echocardiography (TTE). TTE allows estimation of RV systolic pressure (RVSP) via the velocity of the tricuspid regurgitant jet. TTE screening has a sensitivity of 97% and a specificity of 77% in diagnosing moderate to severe PPHTN in patients undergoing pretransplantation workup.[115] However, right-sided cardiac catheterization is necessary, both to confirm elevated pressures and to measure PVR.

Therapy includes conventional measures such as diuresis, as well as some specific vasodilator therapy. Calcium channel blockers, often used in other patients with pulmonary hypertension, are contraindicated in this population because they promote mesenteric vasodilation and worsen portal hypertension. Other drugs used include prostanoids, phosphodiesterase inhibitors, and endothelin antagonists. Reported success with these modalities is on the basis of case reports or case series, and no one therapy has emerged as definitive. Nonetheless, one goal of therapy is to make the patient transplant-eligible by reducing mPAP and PVR into an acceptable range.

Epoprostenol (PgI) has been shown to reduce pulmonary pressures in PPHTN and has been documented to have a survival benefit in pulmonary hypertension.[116] Epoprostenol also has an antiplatelet effect and promotes vascular remodeling. However, it must be administered as a continuous infusion via central access with little tolerance for interruption of the infusion. It has also been associated with splenomegaly and worsening thrombocytopenia, sufficient to limit its use.[117] The phosphodiesterase inhibitor sildenafil has also shown ability to reduce pulmonary pressures at 3 months, but without a sustained response at 12 months.[118] Nonetheless, it may be useful in combination therapy or it may provide a window for transplantation. Bosentan is the best studied of the endothelin antagonists. Although there are concerns for hepatic toxicity, published case reports and case series have not documented significant increases in liver enzymes with its use.[119]

The role of liver transplantation in the treatment of PPHTN is not well defined because outcomes of transplantation are not predictable. Some patients have resolution of PPHTN with transplant, some may have no or incomplete resolution and continue to require medical therapy, and some may experience worsening of their PPHTN. Nonetheless, it is an option for a select group of patients whose pulmonary hemodynamics and cardiac function suggest they will tolerate the procedure. Evaluation of the patient for potential transplantation must include a right-heart catheterization to measure mPAP and calculate PVR. Patients with mPAP less than 35 mmHg can be expected to tolerate transplant and do well postoperatively. Those with mPAP 35 mmHg or more and elevated PVR may be considered if they respond to therapy sufficiently to reduce their mPAP below 35 mmHg and PVR below 400 dynes/sec/cm^5.[120,121]

Hepatic Encephalopathy

HE is a serious, albeit reversible, neuropsychiatric complication that is a feature of both CLD and acute liver disease. The manifestations range from subtle, subclinical abnormalities that can only be discerned by formal psychometric tests (minimal HE) to clearly evident neurologic and behavioral derangements that are easily diagnosed at the bedside (overt HE). Although HE can appear as the result of portal–systemic shunting without intrinsic liver disease, the onset of HE is generally associated with advanced hepatocellular disease. Moreover, even minimal HE can affect the patient's ability to maintain employment, drive a car, perform quotidian activities, and interact with family. The fact that HE is frequently reversible emphasizes the importance of identifying and treating this condition.

The diagnosis of overt HE encompasses two sets of criteria: Neuropsychologic and neuromotor. Neuropsychologic assessment focuses on level of consciousness, attention and ability to follow commands, and effect. This is most often graded on a 0 to 4 scale using the West Haven criteria (Table 46-9).[122] Physical examination may elicit asterixis or other evidence of hyperreflexiveness such as clonus or Babinski sign. Other focal findings can include nystagmus or decerebrate posturing. However, focal neurologic findings should prompt appropriate imaging to rule out structural neurologic lesions, because these patients are at risk for intracranial bleeding and are not immune to other neurologic pathologies such as ischemic brain disease, abscess, and tumor.

It is generally agreed that HE is the result of the failure of the liver to adequately metabolize certain substances that when accumulated are neurotoxic, rather than failure to synthesize substances critical to normal neurotransmission. The proposed World Congress definitions support this by recognizing a type of HE that is associated with normal hepatocellular function but shunting of blood around the liver (type B). Historically, HE has been attributed to hyperammonemia resulting from inadequate hepatic metabolism of ammonia. Although ammonia continues to be considered an important contributor, severity of HE does not necessarily correlate with ammonia levels. This may be explained by recent investigations which have provided evidence for a multitude of other factors and mechanisms contributing to HE, including other gut-derived neurotoxins, γ-aminobutyric acid (GABA) and other endogenous GABA receptor agonists, oxidative stress, inflammatory mediators, hyponatremia, and abnormal serotonin and histamine neurotransmission.[123,124] Nonetheless, ammonia and its effect on astrocytes play a central role in the pathogenesis of HE. Ammonia is a by-product of nitrogen-containing compounds that is toxic and must be removed from the body. The liver is the primary site of ammonia metabolism and excretion via the urea cycle, but the brain, skeletal muscle, and possibly kidneys contribute as well. Unfortunately, neither the brain nor the skeletal muscle is capable of utilizing the urea cycle and instead use glutamine synthetase to synthesize glutamine from ammonia and glutamate. Astrocytes are major constituents of the blood–brain barrier and are the primary location for glutamine synthetase in the brain. Because these are the cells capable of metabolizing ammonia, as ammonia levels rise intracellular levels of glutamine rise in concert. There are two consequences to this: (1) Glutamine, which is osmotically active, pulls water intracellularly, causing astrocyte swelling and cerebral edema; and (2) glutamate, which is an important excitatory neurotransmitter, is first released and then consumed in producing glutamine. Experimental in vitro evidence has demonstrated a glutamate release from astrocytes in response to elevated levels of ammonia.[125] It is thought that this release may be related to the neuroexcitatory signs such as agitation and seizures observed in acute HE (type A). On the other hand, a neuroinhibitory state is characteristic of the HE associated with cirrhosis (type C) and may reflect chronic adaptive changes that include downregulation of glutamate receptors, inactivation of astrocyte glutamate transporters, and an increase in GABAergic tone (Table 46-10).[125] GABA is a major inhibitory neurotransmitter whose receptor complex can be activated by benzodiazepines and inhibited by flumazenil. Subsequent studies of plasma and CSF from HE patients were reported to demonstrate increased benzodiazepine-like substances. Improvement in mental status following flumazenil administration was observed in HE patients who had not received benzodiazepines, leading to the proposal that the production of endogenous benzodiazepine-like substances contributed to HE.[126,127] Unfortunately, the benefits of flumazenil appear to be limited by its short duration of action and lack of demonstrable survival or recovery advantage.[128,129]

Sepsis is a well-known precipitating factor for HE. Inflammatory mediators such as TNF-α, and cytokines IL-1 and IL-6 cause cytotoxic compromise of the blood–brain barrier, leading to or worsening cerebral edema. Astrocyte swelling is a trigger for production of ROS and RNOS, which can mediate local cell membrane damage and cause further blood–brain barrier permeability.[130]

The initial step in evaluating the patient with liver disease who presents with encephalopathy is to rule out causes other than HE. The differential diagnosis includes other metabolic encephalopathies such as uremia, sepsis, glucose and electrolyte abnormalities, and endocrinopathies. Structural and vascular CNS lesions or CNS infections should also be considered. Because cirrhotic patients are exquisitely sensitive to sedative medications and have impaired hepatic (and often renal) metabolism, careful search for possible drug-related encephalopathy should be undertaken. Once other potential causes have been eliminated, the next step should be a systematic search for an underlying cause or precipitating factor (Table 46-11). Once identified, treatment or elimination should commence as soon as possible and may be sufficient for clinical improvement.

If addressing the underlying cause does not produce improvement, the next step is to employ therapy designed to either reduce the production of or increase the excretion of ammonia.

Table 46-9 West Haven Criteria for Semiquantitative Grading of Mental State

Grade 1	Trivial lack of awareness Euphoria or anxiety Shortened attention span Impaired performance of addition
Grade 2	Lethargy or apathy Minimal disorientation for time or place Subtle personality change Inappropriate behavior Impaired performance of subtraction
Grade 3	Somnolence to semistupor, but responsive to verbal stimuli Confusion Gross disorientation
Grade 4	Coma (unresponsive to verbal or noxious stimuli)

Adapted with permission from Ferenci P, Lockwood A, Mullen K, et al. Hepatic encephalopathy—definition, nomenclature, diagnosis, and quantification: Final report of the working party at the 11th World Congresses of Gastroenterology, Vienna, 1998. *Hepatology*. 2002;35:716.

Table 46-10 Proposed Nomenclature of Hepatic Encephalopathy

HE Type	Nomenclature	Subcategory	Subdivisions
A	Encephalopathy associated with acute liver failure		
B	Encephalopathy associated with portal–systemic bypass and no intrinsic hepatocellular disease		
C	Encephalopathy associated with cirrhosis and portal hypertension/or portal–systemic shunts	Episodic HE	Precipitated Spontaneous[a] Recurrent
		Persistent HE	Mild Severe Treatment-dependent
		Minimal HE	

For definitions, see text.
[a]Without recognized precipitating factors.
Adapted with permission from Ferenci P, Lockwood A, Mullen K, et al. Hepatic encephalopathy—definition, nomenclature, diagnosis, and quantification: Final report of the working party at the 11th World Congresses of Gastroenterology, Vienna, 1998. *Hepatology*. 2002;35:716.

Historically, the nonabsorbable disaccharide lactulose has been the mainstay of therapy and remains the first-line drug for treating HE.[131] Although the basis for its benefit is unclear there are two proposed mechanisms for its salutary effect. First, anaerobic bacteria in the colon ferment lactulose to produce weak acids and acidify the colon. This acid milieu converts ammonia into ammonium, which is poorly absorbed. Secondly, it is proposed that this acid milieu is also cathartic, and that catharsis augments reduced absorption.

Although simple reduction in protein intake seems an intuitive solution, in fact protein restriction may be harmful for cirrhotic patients who tend to have little nutritional reserve due to poor intake and who have likely lost nutritional ground with every hospitalization. Practice guidelines for the treatment of HE patients recommend a normal protein intake (1 to 1.5 g/kg/day), preferably in the form of plant-based rather than animal protein because of its higher calorie to nitrogen ratio.[131]

Zinc is a cofactor in the urea cycle and may be a dietary deficiency in cirrhotic patients. Although it is unclear which patients might benefit, practice guidelines recommend consideration of chronic zinc supplementation to HE patients.

Table 46-11 Precipitating Factors in Hepatic Encephalopathy

Constipation
Dehydration
Gastrointestinal bleeding
Bowel obstruction or ileus
Infection—esp. spontaneous bacterial peritonitis, sepsis
Excessive dietary protein
Hypokalemia
Hypoglycemia
Hypothyroidism
Hypoxia
Metabolic alkalosis
Anemia
Azotemia/uremia
Hepatic malignancy
Transjugular intrahepatic portal shunt, surgical shunt
Vascular occlusion

Ascites

Ascites is the most common complication of cirrhosis leading to hospitalization.[132] The occurrence of ascites marks a threshold in the nature of the underlying liver disease and is associated with a 50% mortality rate within 3 years.[133] Thus, the current recommendation is that patients who present with ascites and who are potential candidates for liver transplantation should be referred for liver transplantation evaluation. Not all ascites is hepatic in nature; about 15% has a nonhepatic etiology. Nonhepatic causes include malignancy, cardiac failure, renal disease, pancreatitis, and tuberculosis. Perhaps the most expeditious study to define the nature of new-onset ascites is a paracentesis. In particular, the serum–ascites albumin gradient (SAAG) is extremely useful for delineating portal hypertensive ascites from other causes. It is calculated as the difference between simultaneously measured serum and ascites albumin levels. An SAAG 1.1 mg/dL or more indicates portal hypertension with 97% accuracy.[134] Standard initial therapy for portal hypertensive ascites is salt restriction (2 g/day) and diuretics. Hyponatremia is common among cirrhotic patients with ascites and generally does not warrant fluid restriction unless the serum sodium level is below 120 to 125 mEq/L.[132] Rapid correction of hyponatremia is undesirable because cirrhotic patients are particularly at risk for central pontine myelinolysis, a potentially devastating neurologic complication. Observations in liver transplant recipients suggest limiting correction to 16 mEq/L or less over an 8-day period.[135]

Refractory ascites, defined as ascites that is immutable to sodium restriction, maximum doses of diuretics, and paracentesis, heralds another change in the nature of the underlying cirrhosis. It is the hallmark complication of type II HRS and indicates increased disease severity. Once patients become refractory to maximum standard medical therapy, the 6-month mortality is 21%.[136] Therapeutic options for patients are limited and include serial paracentesis, liver transplantation, TIPS placement, and peritoneovenous shunt. Although current practice is to replace albumin when ascitic fluid is drained, this practice is not well supported by randomized prospective trials. The reasons for using albumin replacement include preventing paracentesis-induced circulatory dysfunction, minimizing electrolyte disturbances, minimizing the nutritional impact of albumin loss, and preventing renal impairment. Current recommendations are that patients with drainage volumes less than 5 L do not need albumin replacement, and for larger volume paracentesis 6 to 8 g albumin/L may be considered.[132] TIPS placement can generally be expected to improve quality of life by obviating the need for serial paracentesis, but this must be balanced against an increase in encephalopathy and the high incidence of shunt malfunction.[137,138] Peritoneovenous shunting is an older intervention that has generally fallen into disuse because of associated complications and lack of survival benefit. However, for patients who cannot easily travel for serial paracentesis and who are not candidates for TIPS or transplantation, this may be the only option.

Infections of ascitic fluid are sufficiently common that the American Association for the Study of Liver Diseases recommends paracentesis for all hospitalized patients with ascites. SBP is diagnosed when the PMN count in ascitic fluid is 250 cells/mm^3 or more in the absence of any other identifiable intra-abdominal source. Bacterial translocation from the bowel is the most common source of SBP, although nosocomial infection from bacteremia associated with invasive procedures occurs as well. Because cell counts are available more quickly than culture results, the decision to treat is made empirically on that basis. Patients should immediately be treated with a broad-spectrum antibiotic. Sepsis may develop rapidly in these patients and SBP is a recognized precipitating factor for type I HRS. Because of this, timely administration of antibiotics in this fragile population is so important that empiric antibiotics are warranted even for patients who do not meet the diagnostic ascitic fluid PMN cell count but who exhibit signs and symptoms suggesting infection such as fever, abdominal pain, evidence of worsening hepatic or renal function, and otherwise unexplained worsening encephalopathy.[132]

Varices

Varices, particularly esophageal varices, are one of the end results of portal hypertension. In cirrhosis, increases in portal pressure result from distorted hepatic architecture left in the wake of inflammatory insults. Fibrosis and regenerative nodules cause impedance to splanchnic flow through the liver and lead to formation of portosystemic collaterals, particularly with the gastric and esophageal venous systems. Progression of portal hypertension leads to increased local production of nitric oxide and, eventually, massive splanchnic vasodilation. Thus, portal hypertension becomes a problem not only of impedance to flow but also of a massive increase in flow to the liver. Rupture of the high-pressure collaterals that are formed is a highly lethal and feared complication of portal hypertension.

Portal hypertension is diagnosed by measurement of the wedged hepatic venous pressure (WHVP). Although this is not a direct measure of portal pressure WHVP has been demonstrated to correlate well with it.[139] This is done by advancement of a catheter into a hepatic vein to wedge position. To correct for the contribution of increased intra-abdominal pressure from ascites, a free hepatic venous pressure or an inferior vena caval pressure should be subtracted from the measured WHVP to give the HVPG. A normal HVPG is 3 to 5 mmHg. Patients with esophageal varices can be expected to have HVPGs of at least 10 to 12 mmHg.[140,141]

Esophagogastroduodenoscopy is the gold-standard procedure for diagnosing varices. Presence of varices correlates with the severity of the underlying liver disease, with incidence increasing from 40% in Child's A patients to 85% in Child's C patients.[142]

Nonselective β-blockers reduce portal pressure by two mechanisms: A decrease in cardiac output ($β_1$) and splanchnic vasoconstriction ($β_2$). There is no evidence that they prevent formation of varices; however, they are effective as primary prophylaxis for variceal bleeding. For those patients who cannot tolerate β-blockers or in whom they are contraindicated, another option for primary prophylaxis of variceal bleeding is endoscopic ligation. TIPS is associated with a higher incidence of encephalopathy and higher mortality and is not indicated for primary prophylaxis.[142]

Acute variceal bleed should be managed with a combination of volume resuscitation, correction of severe coagulopathy, pharmacologic manipulation of portal pressure, and endoscopic variceal ligation. Although the temptation to vigorously volume resuscitate and completely correct all coagulation abnormalities can be overwhelming in this setting, it should be resisted. Because bleeding is, to some extent, a pressure-related phenomenon, aggressive volume replacement may lead to resistant or recurrent bleeding.[143,144] The goal instead should be adequate resuscitation to maintain a hemoglobin level of 8 mg/dL and consideration of blood product transfusion to improve significant abnormalities in platelet count and INR.[142] Elective intubation for airway protection is often warranted in these patients as well. Medications to reduce portal pressure include vasopressin and its analogues and somatostatin and its analogues. Although β-blockers can reduce portal pressures, their effect on systemic pressures makes them undesirable in this setting. Early endoscopic variceal ligation in combination with pharmacotherapy is the preferred treatment for acute variceal bleed.

Resistant or early recurrent variceal bleeding occurs in about 10% to 20% of patients. A measured HVPG above 20 mmHg is a risk factor for failure of standard therapy, predicting greater length of ICU stay as well as greater transfusion requirements.[145] Balloon tamponade can be effective in this setting, but is associated with significant and potentially lethal complications such as esophageal rupture or necrosis and perforation, migration of the balloon components, and aspiration. If employed, it is recommended as a bridge to more definitive therapy such as surgical shunt or TIPS.[142]

Chronic Cholestatic Disease

Biliary obstruction increases pressures in the bile ducts, leading to reflux of bile into the liver sinusoids where it may also communicate with the vascular system. Serum levels of bilirubin, bile salts, and AP (which is synthesized by the biliary epithelium) rise. If bacteria are present in bile, the patient is at risk for infectious complications such as ascending cholangitis, hepatic abscess, and sepsis as well. Cholestasis and hyperbilirubinemia are associated with an increased incidence of acute kidney injury. This may be mediated by endotoxemia, as the result of both sepsis and loss of bile salts to the vascular space. Bile salts are normally secreted into the intestine where they prevent bacterial overgrowth and bind endotoxin, thereby preventing its absorption into the portal circulation. Loss of intestinal bile salts because of biliary obstruction may cause portal and systemic endotoxemia, leading to kidney injury. Kidney injury may additionally be exacerbated by the induced diuresis, as well as impairment of myocardial contractility, resulting from elevated serum levels of bile salts.[146,147] It has also been noted that patients who come to transplant for the chronic cholestatic diseases, PBC and primary sclerosing cholangitis (PSC), have evidence of preserved or hypercoagulability on the basis of increased incidence of portal venous thrombosis, elevated levels of TAT complexes, and thromboelastographic indices consistent with hypercoagulability.[148,149]

Chronic cholestatic disease in the adult population is primarily the result of immunologic mechanisms resulting in PBC or PSC. These diseases are frequently associated with other autoimmune pathology.

PBC is a disease characterized by the progressive destruction of small intrahepatic bile ducts, together with portal inflammation that eventually leads to cirrhosis. The laboratory hallmark of PBC is the antimitochondrial antibody, which is present in 95% of patients. Liver biopsy confirms diagnosis, as well as providing histologic disease staging. The typical disease course is one of steady progressive loss of small bile ducts together with increasing fibrosis, leading to cirrhosis over the course of 10 to 20 years. Ursodeoxycholic acid, which may have immunomodulatory effects, is the only drug demonstrated to retard progression of the disease and offer survival benefit. Liver transplantation is the most definitive therapy, but is associated with a recurrence rate of 10% to 35%.[150]

PSC is a progressive inflammatory disease of the medium and large intra- and extrahepatic bile ducts. The diagnostic studies of choice are ERCP and magnetic resonance cholangiopancreatography (MRCP), which reveal the characteristic beaded pattern of the biliary tree caused by multiple stenotic lesions. PSC has an extremely high association with inflammatory bowel disease (IBD), primarily ulcerative colitis but occasionally Crohn disease. It is also associated with other autoimmune diseases, such as insulin-dependent diabetes and psoriasis. Other contributors to the morbidity of PSC are recurrent bacterial cholangitis, cholangiocarcinoma, and, particularly in those patients with coexisting IBD, colon carcinoma. Over the average 15-year disease course of PSC, 15% to 30% of patients are likely to develop cholangiocarcinoma, which carries a very poor prognosis and may cause ineligibility for transplant.[151] Liver transplantation is the most definitive therapy for PSC, but is associated with disease recurrence.

Chronic Hepatocellular Disease

CLD is a major public health burden in the United States, with an increase in prevalence from 11.78% in the period 1988 to 1994 to 14.78% in the period 2005 to 2008. Chronic viral hepatitis, particularly hepatitis C, has historically been the most common cause of CLD, but recent data show that NAFLD has overtaken chronic hepatitis for this distinction. In the period 2005 to 2008, the prevalence of the most common causes of CLD was hepatitis B 0.3%, hepatitis C 1 7%, alcoholic liver disease 2.0%, and NAFLD 11.0%.[13] In 2013, NAFLD overtook alcoholic liver disease to become the second leading etiology for new registration on the liver transplantation waitlist.[152] Although chronic hepatitis C is still the leading cause of liver transplantation and is implicated in the increase in cases of HCC, the rise in prevalence of NAFLD together with the recognition that it can progress to cirrhosis and is a risk factor for HCC suggests that it is poised to become the next hepatic scourge.

Hepatocellular Carcinoma

Worldwide, HCC is the third leading cause of cancer-related death. Within the United States, it is the fifth most common cancer in men and the seventh in women.[153] Risk factors include chronic viral hepatitis infection, hemochromatosis, and cirrhosis of any provenance. The prevalence of underlying cirrhosis in patients with HCC is 80% to 90%. Even if the HCC patient does not have cirrhosis, there is almost always an underlying chronic hepatitis/chronic necroinflammatory state that seems to be key ingredient for HCC. Among patients with chronic viral hepatitis, the presence of cirrhosis or evidence of active inflammation (characterized by elevations in serum ALT) leads to increased HCC occurrence compared to patients without cirrhosis or those with persistently normal to near-normal ALT.[154] The American Association for the Study of Liver Diseases recommends surveillance of at-risk patients. Ideally this should be in the form of liver ultrasonography every 6 months, with the use of α-fetoprotein only if ultrasound is not available.[155] α-Fetoprotein lacks adequate sensitivity and specificity to be an effective screening tool, but may be valuable in diagnosis because a level above 200 ng/mL in a cirrhotic patient with a hepatic mass has a high positive predictive value for HCC.[155] Diagnosis of HCC can often be made with noninvasive studies, with biopsy reserved for lesions with atypical or discordant imaging.

Surgical resection is the optimal treatment for HCC for those patients who have sufficient hepatic reserve. Unfortunately many patients with HCC have cirrhosis and are unable to tolerate resection. In the United States, fewer than 5% of patients are candidates for resection.[153] Liver transplantation can be an option for those patients who are not resection candidates but whose disease can be expected to have transplant outcomes similar to that of other indications for transplant. The Milan criteria (one tumor <5 cm or three tumors all <3 cm) define those patients, and those patients who meet the criteria and are transplanted have 5-year survival rates of 65% to 78% compared to 5-year survival of 68% to 87% for nontumor indications.[156]

Patients who are neither surgical candidates nor transplant candidates may be managed by radiofrequency ablation or chemoembolization of their tumors. In addition, some centers use these therapies to maintain transplant eligibility for patients on the waiting list.

Nonalcoholic Fatty Liver Disease

NAFLD describes a range of conditions characterized by excessive fat deposition in the liver. NAFLD ranges in severity from simple fat deposition (steatosis) to fat deposition together with inflammation and hepatocellular necrosis (steatohepatitis or NASH). Primary NAFLD is associated with insulin resistance and its attendant manifestations, which are components of the metabolic syndrome: Obesity, central adiposity, type II diabetes, arterial hypertension, and hypertriglyceridemia. In fact it is often referred to as the hepatic manifestation of the metabolic syndrome. The prevalence of NAFLD increases with age, is greater in males, and differs by ethnicity. In the United States, the prevalence of NAFLD is 45% in Hispanics, 33% in Caucasians, and 24% in African-Americans,[157] with an estimated overall prevalence of 30%. Unsurprisingly, NAFLD is the most common cause of elevated liver enzymes in adults.[158] NAFLD may coexist with other hepatic pathologies and exacerbates damage when it appears together with chronic hepatitis C, hemochromatosis, or alcoholic liver disease.[159] Within the disease spectrum of NAFLD, only NASH is associated with the serious consequences of HCC and cirrhosis. The gold standard for distinguishing NASH from other NAFLD is liver biopsy with the key features of macrovesicular steatosis, lobular inflammation, hepatocyte ballooning, and often perisinusoidal fibrosis. The prevalence of NASH in the United States is estimated to be 3% to 5%.[158] There is evidence, although from small studies and with different end points, that lifestyle modifications that improve insulin sensitivity such as weight loss and exercise can reduce intrahepatic lipid content in NASH.[160] Medications that may augment weight loss, such as orlistat and rimonabant, have been shown to result in histologic improvement in NASH when associated with actual weight loss. For those patients who are unable to lose weight by more conservative means, bariatric surgery has been shown to result in dramatic histologic and chemical improvement, with decreased steatosis/inflammation on biopsy and decreases in serum aminotransferases. In a meta-analysis of morbidly obese patients who underwent bariatric surgery, the pooled patient incidence of biopsy-proven NASH was 53.87%. Of these patients, 81.3% showed improvement or resolution of steatohepatitis on follow-up biopsy, with 69.5% showing complete resolution.[161]

Preoperative Management

Hepatic Evaluation

The evaluation of hepatic function begins with a thorough history, starting with an inquiry into risk factors and the presence of symptoms attributable to CLD. Prior episodes of jaundice, particularly in relationship to surgical procedures and anesthesia, should be thoroughly investigated. Alcohol consumption, use of recreational or illicit drugs, medications (including herbal products), presence of tattoos, sexual promiscuity, consumption of raw seafood, and a history of travel to areas in which hepatitis is endemic should be sought. Symptoms of fatigue, anorexia, weight loss, nausea, vomiting, easy bruising, pruritus, dark-colored urine, biliary colic, abdominal distention, and gastrointestinal bleeding warrant further investigation for the presence of liver disease.

Physical examination findings suggestive of active liver disease include icterus, palmar erythema, spider angiomas, gynecomastia, hepatosplenomegaly, ascites, testicular atrophy, petechiae, ecchymoses, and asterixis.

In the absence of findings suggestive of liver disease, routine laboratory tests to assess hepatocellular integrity and hepatic synthetic function are not warranted. Routine laboratory testing may yield false-positive results, and true-positive results are infrequent in asymptomatic patients. Among over 19,000 Air Force trainees, 0.5% had liver-enzyme elevations; however, the cause was found in only 12 of the 99 with elevations.[162] In a study of over 7,600 surgical patients who underwent routine preoperative screening, liver-enzyme tests were abnormal in roughly 1 of 700 (0.1%) asymptomatic patients. Of the 11 patients with elevations, 3 (1 in 2,500 or 0.04%) developed jaundice.[163]

Because the normal range for laboratory tests is defined as the mean plus or minus two standard deviations, 5% of normal patients can be expected to fall outside the normal range, with 2.5% following above the upper limit of normal. As a result, minor elevations of liver-enzyme results—those less than twice the normal range—may be of no clinical importance.[164] The recommended approach is to avoid testing liver enzymes in asymptomatic patients. Nonetheless, in the presence of abnormal results (in an asymptomatic patient) the safest approach is to repeat the results; in the absence of elevations greater than twice the upper limits of normal it is reasonable to proceed with surgery.

In patients with more substantial elevations of liver enzymes, causes include alcohol abuse, medications, chronic hepatitis B and C, NASH, autoimmune hepatitis, hemochromatosis, Wilson disease, and α_1-antitrypsin deficiency. Nonhepatic causes include celiac sprue and muscle diseases. Medications include selected antibiotics, antiepileptic drugs, lipid-lowering agents, nonsteroidal anti-inflammatory agents, and sulfonylureas. Herbal medications and drugs of abuse are also associated with liver-enzyme abnormalities.[164]

Perioperative Risk Associated with Liver Disease

In patients with known liver disease, the etiology of hepatic dysfunction should be determined. Based on retrospective, small case series from the 1960s and 1970s, acute hepatitis confers a prohibitive risk for elective surgery. In a series of 36 patients with undiagnosed hepatitis who underwent laparotomy (for suspected biliary obstruction or hepatic malignancy) nearly one-third died. All patients with acute hepatitis, due to either virus or alcohol, died. The majority of patients suffered complications that included bacterial peritonitis, wound dehiscence, and hepatic failure.[165]

With improved diagnostic testing, which includes serologic testing for hepatitis C, ultrasound testing for gallstones, and improved imaging techniques for hepatic cancer, it is far more likely today that accurate diagnoses can be made preoperatively. As a result laparotomies are unlikely in patients with unsuspected hepatitis. In the absence of accumulating evidence, consensus opinion is that elective surgery should be postponed in patients with acute hepatitis.[166,167]

In patients with CLD it is not feasible to postpone surgery until recovery. A number of studies have investigated the risk of surgery in patients with cirrhosis.[168–171] Each of the studies identified various components of the Child–Turcotte–Pugh score, as well as the composite score, as important prognostic factors for perioperative mortality.

Child and Turcotte first described their classification system in 1964. They identified five factors—albumin, bilirubin, ascites, encephalopathy, and nutritional status—as important prognostic factors for patients with cirrhosis. Each of the factors was categorized according to three levels of severity and combined to generate a composite score leading to an assignment of one of three classes of severity (class A, B, or C, with C representing the most severe hepatic dysfunction). In 1972 Pugh modified the score, replacing nutritional status with PT (Table 46-12). The score was originally designed for patients undergoing portosystemic shunt procedures, but has subsequently been applied to patients with cirrhosis undergoing other surgeries. In studies conducted over multiple decades, the modified Child score performed similarly in predicting postoperative mortality: 10% in Child A, 17% to 30% in Child B, and 60% to 80% in Child C.[170–172] The 3-month mortality for hospitalized patients not undergoing surgery was 4% for Child A, 14% for Child B, and 51% for Child C.[171]

The MELD score was originally designed to predict mortality for patients undergoing transjugular intrahepatic portocaval

Table 46-12	Modified Child–Pugh Score		
	Points[a]		
Presentation	1	2	3
Albumin (g/dL)	>3.5	2.8–3.5	<2.8
Prothrombin time			
Seconds prolonged	<4	4–6	>6
International normalized ratio	<1.7	1.7–2.3	>2.3
Bilirubin (mg/dL)[b]	<2	2–3	>3
Ascites	Absent	Slight–moderate	Tense
Encephalopathy	None	Grade I–II	Grade III–IV

[a]Class A = 5 to 6 points; B = 7 to 9 points; C = 10 to 15 points.
[b]Cholestatic diseases (e.g., primary biliary cirrhosis) produce bilirubin elevations that are disproportionate to the hepatic dysfunction. Thus, the following adjustments should be made: Assign 1 point for a bilirubin level of 4 mg/dL; 2 points for bilirubin concentrations between 4 and 10 mg/dL; and 3 points for bilirubin >10 mg/dL.

shunt (TIPS) procedures.[173] Subsequently it was identified as an improvement to the Child score for the allocation of organs for liver transplant candidates due to its replacement of the subjective elements of the Child score (ascites, encephalopathy) with more objective ones, INR and creatinine. The MELD score is a useful predictor of 90-day wait list mortality in liver transplant candidates.[174] The MELD score weighs the continuous variables linearly or logarithmically instead of assigning arbitrary categories, as is the case with the Child score: MELD score = 9.57 × $\log_e$ (creatinine mg/dL) + 3.78 × $\log_e$ (bilirubin mg/dL) + 11.2 × $\log_e$ (INR) + 6.43.

The MELD score appears to predict perioperative mortality of cirrhotic patients. In a single-center study of 140 surgical procedures, the c-statistic for the MELD score's ability to predict 30-day mortality was 0.72. A c-statistic of 0.5 indicates predictive ability similar to chance (a 50:50 likelihood of predicting the outcome), whereas a c-statistic of 0.7 and higher is considered useful. In the cohort of patients undergoing abdominal surgery, the c-statistic improved to 0.80. In this study a MELD score between 25 and 30 was associated with a 30-day mortality of 50% after abdominal surgery.[175] Each point in the MELD score up to a score of 20 equated to an additional 1% mortality; each MELD point over 20 equated to an additional 2% mortality. A larger study of 772 cirrhotics found similar results. In this study, 75% of the patients underwent abdominal surgery. A MELD score of 25 was associated with 30-day mortality of 50%. Other than the MELD score, the other important predictors of perioperative mortality in cirrhotics were age (age >70 equated to 3 MELD points) and coexisting disease (ASA physical status > IV equated to 5 MELD points).[176] The perioperative complications encountered by cirrhotic patients include liver failure, postoperative bleeding, infection, and renal failure. These authors concluded that patients with a MELD score of less than 11 have a low postoperative mortality and represent an acceptable surgical risk. However, based on the list of complications, the authors recommend that these patients should preferably have surgery at institutions with a liver transplant center. In patients with a MELD score of 20 or higher, the high mortality risk contraindicates elective procedures until after liver transplantation.[176]

Medical management undertaken to optimize cirrhotic patients undergoing surgery should be directed toward treating active infection, optimizing central blood volume and renal status while minimizing ascites, and improving encephalopathy and coagulopathy. However, there is little evidence to support specific goal-directed targets for preoperative care. The perioperative risk depends more on the operative site and the degree of liver impairment than the anesthetic technique. Upper abdominal surgery (cholecystectomy), when compared to hysterectomy, was associated with liver-enzyme abnormalities, whereas the anesthetic technique (halothane, enflurane, or fentanyl) was not.[177] In a retrospective study of 733 cirrhotic patients mortality was associated with a number of factors in addition to the Child score: male gender, the presence of ascites, cryptogenic cirrhosis (vs. other etiologies), elevated creatinine, preoperative infection, higher ASA physical status, and surgery on the respiratory system.[178] The presence of each additional factor conferred additional risk. For instance, 1-year mortality in patients with six risk factors was over 80%; mortality with two risk factors was approximately 30%.

In addition to optimizing medical management, efforts should be made to minimize surgical risk through the consideration of less invasive surgery. Gallstones are twice as common in cirrhotic patients as in patients without cirrhosis.[168] Laparoscopic surgery appears safe in patients with Child–Pugh A and B cirrhosis. In uncontrolled retrospective studies the advantages included low mortality and shorter hospital stay.[179,180] However, Child's C patients may benefit from percutaneous drainage of the gallbladder rather than a laparoscopic approach.[180] In a series of over 4,200 laparoscopic cholecystectomies from Taiwan, the group with cirrhosis (n = 226) had a mortality of approximately 1:100, whereas mortality was 1:2,000 for those without cirrhosis.[181] Meta-analyses of randomized trials in cirrhotic patients showed the laparoscopic approach was associated with less blood loss, shorter operative time, and shorter hospitalization compared to an open approach.[182,183] Preoperative decompression of portal hypertension by TIPS may improve outcomes in patients with severe portal hypertension.[184] However, TIPS is associated with increases in pulmonary artery pressure and can worsen encephalopathy.[97,185]

Intraoperative Management

Monitoring and Vascular Access

In addition to routine noninvasive monitors, the need for arterial pressure monitoring should be considered for patients with end-stage liver disease. The decision is based on the presence of preoperative systemic hypotension due to vasodilation, anticipated blood loss, the need for intraoperative laboratory studies, coexisting disease, and age. Arterial cannulation should be considered in patients undergoing liver resection. The usefulness of CVP monitoring to predict fluid responsiveness has been questioned.[186] Some experts have abandoned CVP monitoring in the setting of liver resection.[187–189] In our practice we do not place a CVP catheter exclusively for monitoring. Pulmonary artery catheterization is used for patients with known or suspected pulmonary artery hypertension and for patients with a low cardiac ejection fraction. Transesophageal echocardiography (TEE) is a sensitive monitor for the assessment of preload, contractility, ejection fraction, regional wall motion abnormalities, and emboli. In a small series of patients with esophageal varices, TEE universally aided in diagnosis and was not associated with bleeding complications, although transgastric views were avoided to minimize esophageal manipulation.[190] Other authors have confirmed the safety of TEE in this population.[191,192] Viscoelastic coagulation testing using TEG or thromboelastometry, if available, may be a useful guide for coagulation management.[59] Viscoelastic tests reflect the overall effects of altered levels of endogenous pro- and anticoagulant factors, which may be in balance if both are reduced proportionally. Recently the clinical significance of an abnormal PT as a predictor of bleeding risk has been questioned because this test reflects only procoagulant factor levels rather than the rebalanced hemostatic system, which may be capable of normal thrombin generation.[60]

Selection of Anesthetic Technique

Neuraxial versus General Anesthesia

The effect of neuraxial anesthesia on hepatic blood flow appears related to alterations of systemic blood pressure.[193,194] More recent studies support the conclusion that hepatic blood flow is reduced by epidural anesthesia and, interestingly, further reduced by an infusion of norepinephrine.[195] However, other studies suggest that vasopressors (ephedrine and dopamine) restore hepatic blood flow.[196,197] Other data conflict with this, suggesting that dopamine does not improve splanchnic blood flow.[198] Despite this confusing picture high (T-5) neuraxial blocks appear to reduce hepatic blood flow, and this effect may not be reversed when block-related hypotension is corrected with catecholamines. Thus, avoidance of high neuraxial block and hypotension seems prudent in patients with advanced liver disease.

Standard contraindications to neuraxial blockade should be considered and weighed against the procedure's benefits on a case-by-case basis. Many patients with advanced hepatic disease may not warrant consideration for neuraxial techniques due to coagulopathy and/or thrombocytopenia. Nerve blockade may be appropriate even when neuraxial blockade is contraindicated. The transversus abdominal plane (TAP) block has been used successfully for abdominal surgery, including hepatobiliary procedures.[199,200] However, the efficacy has been questioned and complications, including abdominal wall hematoma, have been reported.

Volatile Anesthetics

Volatile anesthetics decrease hepatic blood flow, albeit to a variable degree.

Halothane is more likely than other inhaled anesthetics to cause cardiovascular depression and results in the greatest reduction of hepatic blood flow. Newer volatile agents, including isoflurane and sevoflurane, have less significant effects on hepatic blood flow.[201] At anesthetic concentrations of 1 MAC these agents produce very little reduction in hepatic blood flow. However, desflurane appears to more substantially decrease hepatic blood flow at 1 MAC, causing a 30% reduction at this anesthetic depth.[202] Animal studies suggest desflurane preserves total hepatic blood flow.[203] At higher anesthetic concentrations isoflurane results in a dose-dependent reduction in hepatic blood flow beyond that seen at 1 MAC. This dose-dependent reduction in hepatic blood flow does not occur with sevoflurane. In animal studies both sevoflurane and isoflurane maintain the hepatic arterial buffer response, which increases hepatic arterial blood flow in the presence of reductions of portal blood flow.[204,205]

In addition to variable effects on hepatic blood flow, concern exists regarding the production of reactive intermediates during the metabolism of volatile anesthetics. Halothane hepatitis, described earlier in this chapter, is largely responsible for these concerns. However, there is little evidence to suggest that other volatile anesthetics are responsible for hepatic complications. With the exception of sevoflurane, volatile anesthetics undergo metabolism that yields reactive TFA intermediates. These bind to hepatic proteins and produce an immunologic reaction. However, the incidence of liver injury correlates with the extent to which inhaled anesthetics undergo oxidative metabolism. Although 20% of halothane and 2.5% of enflurane are metabolized to TFA intermediates, the corresponding percentages for isoflurane and desflurane are 0.2% and 0.02%, respectively.[53]

Although there is a lack of evidence supporting a role for current volatile anesthetics in causing hepatic injury, several reports describe instances when repeated exposure to halogenated anesthetics is associated with hepatic dysfunction. Because there is no pathognomonic liver pathology, the diagnosis is based on the exclusion of other causes and a history of recent exposure. The potential for toxic metabolites seems related to the degree of in vivo biotransformation of the various halogenated anesthetics.[206] Nonetheless, desflurane, which undergoes the least biotransformation, has been implicated in a case of hepatotoxicity in a patient who may have been sensitized by previous halothane exposure.[207]

Sevoflurane undergoes more extensive metabolism than isoflurane or desflurane, rapidly producing detectable plasma concentrations of fluoride and hexafluoroisopropanol (HFIP), which are conjugated by the liver and excreted by the kidney. In distinction to the other agents, sevoflurane does not produce reactive TFA metabolites or fluoroacetylated liver proteins. This fact led to the suggestion that patients sensitized to other volatile anesthetics could be safely anesthetized with sevoflurane.[208] Indeed, despite the more extensive metabolism, there is no evidence that sevoflurane's metabolites, including compound A (produced in a reaction with carbon dioxide absorbents), produce hepatic injury.[209] In rodents there is evidence that sevoflurane protects against hepatic ischemia–reperfusion injury while isoflurane does not.[210] However, there is a single case report of ALF occurring 2 days after sevoflurane exposure for heart surgery.[211] Although the cause in this case is not certain, this report suggests that patients who are sensitized to one volatile anesthetic (i.e., evidence of hepatic injury following prior exposure) should not subsequently receive any other fluorinated anesthetic.

Nitrous Oxide

Nitrous oxide administration has not been shown to cause hepatocellular injury in the absence of hepatic hypoxemia.[212] In patients with mild alcoholic hepatitis, a nitrous oxide/narcotic technique was compared to nitrous oxide/enflurane and tetracaine spinal techniques for peripheral surgery. None of the techniques were associated with biochemical worsening.[213] Due to sympathomimetic effects, nitrous oxide can lead to decreased hepatic blood flow, and inhibition of methionine synthase can occur after even brief exposures. However, the clinical significance of these effects is unclear, although prolonged or repeated exposure could induce a vitamin B_{12} deficiency.[214]

Intravenous Anesthetics

IV anesthetics, such as propofol, etomidate, and midazolam, do not appear to alter hepatic function when given for a short duration during minor procedures. The effects of IV anesthetics after prolonged infusions and in patients with advanced liver disease are not well studied. A rare syndrome of lactic acidosis, lipemia, rhabdomyolysis, hyperkalemia, myocardial failure, and death has been reported after prolonged infusions of propofol. The initial reports were in children.[215] Liver dysfunction resulting in altered lipid metabolism may predispose to the propofol infusion syndrome, as may genetic defects.[216] Patients on prolonged propofol infusions should be monitored for worsening lactic acidosis and escalating vasopressor requirements. In the event of such findings, propofol should be discontinued.

There is no evidence that opioids have an effect on hepatic function that is independent of hepatic blood flow. All opioids increase sphincter of Oddi pressure. Some authors have suggested that morphine causes spasm in the sphincter of Oddi, but a review failed to show a differential effect, concluding that morphine may be preferred over meperidine for the treatment of patients with acute pancreatitis due to less risk of seizures.[217]

Pharmacokinetic and Pharmacodynamic Alterations

The decreased functional mass of hepatocytes and reduced hepatic blood flow due to portocaval shunts lead to reduced metabolism of drugs that rely on hepatic metabolism for clearance.

Factors that affect hepatic clearance include blood flow to the liver, the fraction of the drug unbound to plasma proteins, and intrinsic clearance. Drugs with low extraction ratios, less than 0.3, have restrictive hepatic clearance. Clearance of drugs in this class is affected by protein binding, the induction or inhibition of hepatic enzymes, age, and hepatic pathology, but clearance is not significantly affected by hepatic blood flow. Drugs with a high extraction ratio (greater than 0.7) undergo extensive first-pass metabolism, which alters their bioavailability after oral administration. Regardless of the route of administration, drugs with high extraction ratios are significantly affected by alteration in hepatic blood flow, which can occur with hemodynamic changes or hepatic inflow clamping during liver resection. High extraction ratio drugs tend to have short elimination half-lives (e.g., propranolol $t_{1/2}$ = 3.9 hours).

Benzodiazepines are an example of a drug with a low extraction ratio. As is commonly the case for drugs with low extraction ratios, the elimination half-life can be prolonged (diazepam $t_{1/2}$ = 43 hours). Studies have shown conflicting effects of cirrhosis on the metabolism of midazolam, possibly due to changes in protein binding.[218,219] As hepatic protein synthesis declines with advancing liver disease, the drug fraction bound to protein decreases. Because only the unbound drug is available for metabolism by hepatic enzymes, the elimination may be unaffected despite a reduction in intrinsic hepatic clearance.[220] Bilirubin and bile acids can increase the unbound drug fracture by displacing drugs from protein binding sites. An increase in the free fraction of a drug leads to enhanced effects. The volume of distribution can increase with an increase in the unbound drug. However, the volume of distribution of thiopental, another drug with a low extraction ratio, is not altered in cirrhotic patients.[221] This illustrates the complex interactions that affect pharmacokinetics in patients with end-stage liver disease. However, the altered pharmacodynamic effects that occur in patients with encephalopathy frequently lead to an increased sensitivity to sedatives and analgesics.

Opioid metabolism is reduced in patients with liver disease. Dosing intervals should be increased to avoid drug accumulation. Prolonged elimination is more prominent with morphine and meperidine than the shorter-duration synthetic opioids, although contradictory data exist that suggest pharmacokinetics is not significantly altered by liver disease. The clearance of the meperidine metabolite normeperidine is reduced in liver disease, which can lead to neurotoxicity.[222] The elimination of a single IV opioid bolus is less affected than a continuous infusion due to redistribution to storage sites. Remifentanil, rapidly hydrolyzed by blood and tissue esterases, is an exception among the opioids as its elimination is independent of both hepatic function and the duration of infusion. The pharmacodynamic effects of opioids are altered by liver disease, which argues for a dose reduction in patients with advanced disease because of the ability to precipitate or worsen encephalopathy.

Most induction agents, including ketamine, etomidate, propofol, and thiopental, are highly lipophilic and have high extraction ratios.[223] Although elimination should be prolonged in the presence of liver disease, clearance in cirrhotics is similar to normal patients. However, the pharmacodynamic effects are more pronounced, and in some cases, as with dexmedetomidine and the benzodiazepines, the duration of action can be prolonged.[224]

The intermediate-duration neuromuscular blocking agents metabolized by the liver, vecuronium and rocuronium, exhibit a prolonged duration of action in patients with liver disease.[225,226] Pancuronium's action is also prolonged. Despite this, a resistance to the initial dose of neuromuscular blocker typically occurs due to elevated γ-globulin concentrations and an increase in the volume of distribution (due to edema and/or ascites). Atracurium and cis-atracurium undergo organ-independent elimination. Their durations of action are not affected by liver disease. However, their metabolite, laudanosine, is eliminated by the liver but neurotoxicity has not been reported.[227] Succinylcholine metabolism is altered due to reduced plasma cholinesterase activity in cirrhotic patients; however, the clinical impact is rarely significant.

Vasopressors

In contrast to the increased response to sedatives, patients with liver disease exhibit a reduced response to endogenous vasoconstrictors, including angiotensin II, AVP, and norepinephrine.[228]

Hyporesponsiveness to catecholamines may be modulated by the release of nitric oxide, prostacyclin, and other endothelial-derived factors in response to humoral and mechanical stimuli.[229]

Volume Resuscitation

The selection of fluid and blood products for volume resuscitation is, in general, similar in patients with and without liver disease. However, in end-stage liver disease serum albumin function is quantitatively and qualitatively decreased.[230] Albumin has three major indications in the treatment of cirrhotic patients.[231] The first is after large volume (4 to 5 L) paracentesis.[232] The second is in the presence of SBP to prevent renal impairment, specifically in patients with bilirubin greater than 4 mg/dL or creatinine higher than 1 mg/dL.[232] The third situation is in the presence of type I HRS, where its use is beneficial in conjunction with splanchnic vasoconstrictors. In a randomized trial of terlipressin with and without concomitant albumin, a higher proportion (77%) of the group that received albumin showed a complete response (defined as a creatinine <1.5 mg/dL) compared to the terlipressin-only group (25%).[233]

Transjugular Intrahepatic Portosystemic Shunt Procedure

TIPS creates a connection between the portal and systemic circulations using a minimally invasive technique (Fig. 46-2). The indications are to decompress portal hypertension in the setting of esophageal varices and/or intractable ascites.

Sedation is commonly used to facilitate placement, though some proceduralists prefer general anesthesia, as it limits patient movement, controls diaphragmatic excursion, and reduces the

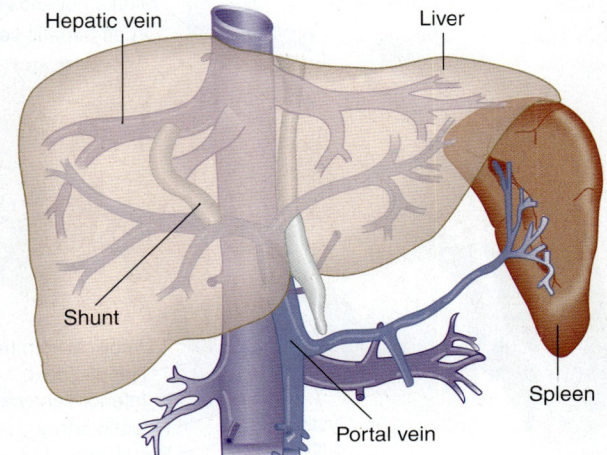

Figure 46-2 Transjugular intrahepatic portosystemic shunt procedure. A stent (or stents) is passed through the internal jugular vein over a wire into the hepatic vein. The wire and stent or stents are then advanced into the portal vein, after which blood can pass through the portal vein into the hepatic vein and bypass and decompress dilated esophageal veins.

risk of aspiration. In patients with recent variceal bleeding, volume resuscitation may be necessary. Due to coagulopathy, patients may require clotting factors and/or platelets before the procedure.[234] Complications include pneumothorax or vascular injury during access to the jugular vein. Dysrhythmias can occur during catheter insertion due to stimulation of the endocardium. Providers should be prepared for the possibility of hemorrhage, which can occur in the presence of extrahepatic artery or portal vein puncture.[235]

Hepatic Resection

In the late 1800s, the first gastrectomies and cholecystectomies were performed in Europe, but surgery on the liver was regarded as dangerous, if not impossible.[236] In 1908, Pringle described the technique of digital compression of the hepatic hilar vessels to control bleeding, which was a significant advance. Lortat-Jacob is credited with the first right hepatectomy in 1952. Another advance occurred in 1957 when segmental liver anatomy was described by Couinaud and others (Fig. 46-3).[237]

Despite these advances, hepatic surgery was associated with operative mortality rates of 20% or more as recently as the 1980s. Hemorrhage was a significant cause of morbidity and mortality. Persistence, along with further advances in surgery, anesthesia, and intensive care led to a reduction of mortality. Today hepatic resections are performed with mortality rates of 5% or less. Partial hepatectomy in normal, noncirrhotic livers is associated with mortality rates of 1% to 2%.[238] The percentage of patients requiring major hepatectomy (resection of three or more liver segments) for primary or secondary cancer appears to be decreasing; however, the perioperative mortality of major hepatectomy appears unchanged over time.[239] Further improvements in outcome are most likely to come from efforts to preserve parenchyma and prevent abdominal infection.

Improved surgical technique with avoidance of the thoracoabdominal approach, which was associated with high morbidity, contributes to improved outcomes. Smooth fracture of liver parenchyma accompanied by bipolar coagulation made parenchymal transection possible. New transection techniques using ultrasonic dissectors, high-pressure water jets, and/or harmonic scalpels may be helpful, but they have not been proven to be superior to conventional clamp crush techniques.[240–242] Preoperative imaging techniques delineate variations in portal, arterial, and bile duct anatomy. Transfusion is necessary in less than 20% of patients.[243,244]

Yet, bleeding remains a major complication, and the hepatic veins are a significant source of blood loss. Techniques to maintain CVP at normal or even low (<5 cm H_2O) levels has been suggested as a technique to limit blood loss.[245] Whether a low CVP is deleterious to renal function is uncertain. In a single-center, uncontrolled series of nearly 500 hepatic resection patients who were managed with low CVP, no cases of renal failure were attributed to the technique.[246] Others have suggested that peripheral venous pressure is an acceptable surrogate for CVP during hepatic resection and liver transplantation.[247,248]

A number of authors question the necessity of a low CVP technique given that blood loss is less significant in the current era.[187–189,240] Others question whether CVP is a reliable monitor of fluid responsiveness.[186] Lastly, two single-center series of living liver donors came to the same conclusion that CVP is not a predictor of blood loss during hepatic resection.[249,250] A recent meta-analysis concluded that optimal methods to lower CVP are uncertain, and that low CVP does not reduce morbidity.[251]

Vasopressors have a direct effect on splanchnic vessels, which reduces splanchnic pressure and decreases blood loss.[252] Portal triad clamping (of the afferent vessels) and total vascular occlusion

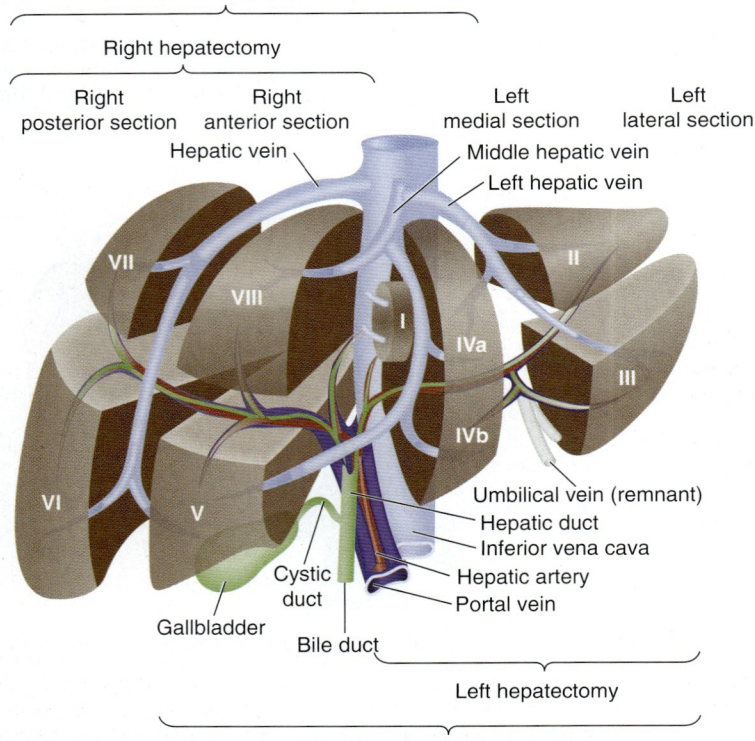

Figure 46-3 Schematic depiction of Couinaud segmental liver anatomy and the normal portal venous structures.

(of the afferent vessels plus the supra- and infrahepatic vena cava) are both effective in decreasing blood loss during hepatic resection. Portal triad clamping is better tolerated and as effective as total vascular occlusions.[253] Portal triad clamping is well tolerated hemodynamically and has little effect on liver function if intermittent.[254,255] Ischemic preconditioning (10-minute inflow occlusion, followed by a 10-minute reperfusion period) followed by continuous inflow clamping for up to 75 minutes was equally effective to intermittent inflow clamping (15-minute periods followed by 5-minute reperfusion) with regard to protection against postoperative liver injury in noncirrhotic patients undergoing hepatic resection. Ischemic preconditioning plus continuous clamping resulted in less blood loss than intermittent clamping.[256]

Air embolism, a known complication of hepatic resection, can be predicted on the basis of the need for a large hepatectomy (such as a right lobectomy) or when the tumor is near the vena cava or involves portal vessels. Low CVP may increase the risk of venous air embolism, though this has not been substantiated.[257]

Even in patients with normal preoperative coagulation profiles, the INR and platelet count can be abnormal after liver resection. The severity of the derangement correlates with the extent of the resection, peaks postoperative day 1 to 2, and takes up to 5 or more days to resolve.[258,259] This has implications in regards to postoperative continuous epidural analgesia. Some authors advise against preoperative epidural catheter placement, whereas others recommend correcting coagulation abnormalities prior to catheter removal.[260] Others, using viscoelastic testing, report brief hypercoagulability after liver resection despite prolonged PTs.[261] Nonetheless, alternatives that avoid epidural catheter placement have been sought. These include intrathecal opioid combined with IV analgesics, and local anesthesia infusion systems.[262]

Surgical techniques for hepatic resection continue to evolve, though indications for newer procedures are not always clearly defined. Examples include minimally invasive liver surgery, thermal ablation of hepatic tumors, and portal vein embolization to induce hypertrophy of the remnant liver. Despite this, complications are common after hemihepatectomy (52% of 144 patients); these include pleural effusions, biliary leakage, wound dehiscence, ascites and, intra-abdominal abscess.[263] In this series a higher preoperative MELD score was associated with the development of complications.

Postoperative Liver Dysfunction

Postoperative liver dysfunction is considered in the presence of asymptomatic elevation of hepatic transaminases, jaundice, and/or symptoms suggestive of liver failure, such as encephalopathy. Mild elevations of liver enzymes can occur after surgery, particularly upper abdominal procedures. Elevations that are less than two times the upper limit of normal are frequently transient and do not require investigation. More severe elevations suggest hepatocellular injury, which can result from a number of causes including hypoxemia, viral or bacterial insult, trauma, and chemical toxicity.

Asymptomatic, mild elevations of hepatic enzymes are not unusual within hours after surgery, but they do not usually persist for more than 2 days. Such elevations were more common after halothane than enflurane (incidence of 50% vs. 20%, respectively) but are uncommon in patients without hepatic dysfunction following currently used inhaled anesthetics.[264–268]

Jaundice, or more severe elevations of hepatic enzymes, requires investigation. Hepatic hypoxemia can result from a number of causes (Table 46-13) including cardiopulmonary etiologies (pneumonia, atelectasis, heart failure), hypoperfusion (secondary to shock), anemia, or fever. Surgery itself decreases hepatic blood flow.[269] Reabsorption of surgical or traumatic hematomas and transfusion of red blood cells are major causes of postoperative jaundice. Ten percent of transfused red cells hemolyze within 24 hours of transfusion. The bilirubin load per unit transfused is 250 mg. The liver may take time to clear the bilirubin load that results from significant hemolysis.

Unconjugated hyperbilirubinemia suggests hemolysis or an inherited disorder such as Gilbert syndrome, or the less common Crigler–Najjar syndrome. In both syndromes the absence or marked decrease of bilirubin glucuronyltransferase produces an unconjugated hyperbilirubinemia. Surgical and anesthetic problems are uncommon in patients with Gilbert and Crigler–Najjar syndromes. Hemoglobinopathies (e.g., sickle cell disease), erythrocyte metabolism defects (e.g., glucose-6-phosphate dehydrogenase deficiency), transfusion reactions, and prosthetic heart valves can also cause hemolysis.

If over 50% of bilirubin is conjugated cholestasis, hepatocellular dysfunction is likely. Hypoxemia, toxic reactions, unsuspected pre-existing liver disease, trauma, and congenital disorders should be considered (Table 46-14). Dubin–Johnson and Rotor syndromes are congenital disorders associated with a defect in bilirubin excretion, which causes a conjugated bilirubinemia. Surgery can worsen these syndromes.

The nature and site of the surgical procedure is an important risk factor for postoperative liver failure.[167] Abdominal surgery appears to reduce hepatic blood flow significantly. Abdominal traction can elevate prostaglandin levels, which may be responsible.[270] Not surprisingly, hepatic resection is a risk factor for postoperative liver failure. The indication for resection in many patients is HCC, which is associated with chronic hepatitis or cirrhosis.[167] The functional reserve of the remnant hepatic parenchyma is difficult to estimate in the cirrhotic liver. In a series of 747 hepatic resections, patients with obstructive jaundice due to malignancy had a higher postoperative mortality (21%) than those with cirrhosis (8.7%), whereas patients with a normal liver had a postresection mortality of 1%.[271] In a series of 373 patients undergoing surgery for obstructive jaundice, those with malignancy or markedly elevated bilirubin had a 1-month mortality higher than 20%.[272] When renal failure accompanies hyperbilirubinemia, the mortality exceeds 50%.[273] Low intestinal levels of bile salts appear to promote the absorption of endotoxin from the gastrointestinal tract, whereas vasoconstrictive inflammatory mediators can precipitate renal hypoperfusion.[274]

Table 46-13 Causes of Postoperative Liver Dysfunction

Hepatocellular
Drugs
Anesthetics
Ischemia
Shock, hypotension, iatrogenic injury
Viral hepatitis

Cholestasis
Benign postoperative cholestasis
Sepsis
Bile duct injury
Drugs
Antibiotics, antiemetics
Choledocholithiasis or pancreatitis
Cholecystitis
Gilbert syndrome

Table 46-14 Causes of Hyperbilirubinemia

Unconjugated (indirect)
Excessive bilirubin production (hemolysis)
Immaturity of enzyme systems
Physiologic jaundice of newborn
Jaundice of prematurity
Inherited defects
Gilbert syndrome
Crigler–Najjar syndrome
Drug effects

Conjugated (direct)
Hepatocellular disease (hepatitis, cirrhosis, drugs)
Intrahepatic cholestasis (drugs, pregnancy)
Benign postoperative jaundice, sepsis
Congenital conjugated hyperbilirubinemia
Dubin–Johnson syndrome
Rotor syndrome
Obstructive jaundice
Extrahepatic (calculus, stricture, neoplasm)
Intrahepatic (sclerosing cholangitis, neoplasm, primary biliary cirrhosis)

Adapted from Friedman L, Martin P, Munoz S. Liver function tests and the objective evaluation of the patient with liver disease. In: Zakim D, Boyer T, eds. *Hepatology: A Textbook of Liver Disease*. 3rd ed. Philadelphia, PA: WB Saunders; 1996:791.

Cardiac surgery in patients with cirrhosis is not well tolerated. Cardiopulmonary bypass exacerbates pre-existing hepatic disease by unknown mechanisms. The overall perioperative mortality in patients with cirrhosis was 31%, and 80% in patients with Child's class B cirrhosis.[275] Another series of cardiac patients reported 1-year mortality of 20%, 55%, and 84% in Child's class A, B, and C patients, respectively.[276] For comparison, the mortality in patients without cirrhosis is approximately 2%.[277] These authors concluded that cardiac surgery that involves cardiopulmonary bypass can be performed in cirrhotic patients with Child's class A cirrhosis and in selected patients with class B.

Conclusions

In patients with new-onset liver disease, elective surgery should be postponed until the course of the disease is known. In patients with pre-existing liver disease, the severity of the disease should be characterized in order to assess risk. Elective high-risk procedures (abdominal and cardiac surgery) in patients with Child's C cirrhosis should be deferred until after liver transplantation. Child's A and B patients should be medically optimized prior to surgery. Although no anesthetic technique is universally preferred, the presence of coagulopathy may contraindicate neuraxial regional techniques. The chosen technique should be designed to maintain splanchnic, hepatic, and renal perfusion. When surgery is unavoidable in patients with advanced liver disease, transfer to a liver transplant center should be considered in order to facilitate pretransplant evaluation and listing.

Acknowledgment

The authors are indebted to Brian S. Kaufman and J. David Roccaforte for their permission to use text, figures, and tables from their chapter in a prior version of *Clinical Anesthesia*.

REFERENCES

1. Merkel C, Montagnese S. Hepatic venous pressure gradient measurement in clinical hepatology. *Dig Liver Dis.* 2011;43(10):762–767.
2. Lautt WW. Mechanism and role of intrinsic regulation of hepatic arterial blood flow: hepatic arterial buffer response. *Am J Physiol.* 1985;249(5 Pt 1):G549–G556.
3. Jones, A. Anatomy of the normal liver. In: Zakim D, Boyer T.D, eds. *Hepatology: A Textbook of Liver Disease.* Philadelphia, PA: WB Saunders; 1996.
4. Nordlie RC, Foster JD, Lange AJ. Regulation of glucose production by the liver. *Annu Rev Nutr.* 1999;19:379–406.
5. Olthoff KM. Hepatic regeneration in living donor liver transplantation. *Liver Transpl.* 2003;9(10 Suppl 2):S35–S41.
6. Viebahn CS, Yeoh GC. What fires prometheus? The link between inflammation and regeneration following chronic liver injury. *Int J Biochem Cell Biol.* 2008;40(5):855–873.
7. Balci NC, Befeler AS, Leiva P, et al. Imaging of liver disease: comparison between quadruple-phase multidetector computed tomography and magnetic resonance imaging. *J Gastroenterol Hepatol.* 2008;23(10):1520–1527.
8. Weinreb JC, Cohen JM, Armstrong E, et al. Imaging the pediatric liver: MRI and CT. *AJR Am J Roentgenol.* 1986;147(4):785–790.
9. Xu J, Murphy SL, Kochanek KD, et al. Deaths: final data for 2013. *Natl Vital Stat Rep.* 2016;64(2):1–100.
10. Digestive diseases statistics for the United States. National Institute of Diabetes and Digestive and Kidney Diseases website. http://www.niddk.nih.gov/health-information/health-statistics/Pages/digestive-diseases-statistics-for-the-united-states.aspx. Published November 2014; Accessed December 22, 2015.
11. Hepatitis statistics: Surveillance for viral hepatitis—United States. 2013. Centers for Disease Control and Prevention website. http://www.cdc.gov/hepatitis/statistics/2013surveillance/commentary.htm. Updated October 19, 2015; Accessed December 22, 2015.
12. Lazo M, Hernaez R, Eberhardt MS, et al. Prevalence of nonalcoholic fatty liver disease in the United States: the Third National Health and Nutrition Examination Survey, 1988–1994. *Am J Epidemiol.* 2013;178(1):38–45.
13. Younossi ZM, Stepanova M, Afendy M, et al. Changes in the prevalence of the most common causes of chronic liver diseases in the United States from 1988 to 2008. *Clin Gastroenterol Hepatol.* 2011;9(6):524–530 e1; quiz e60.
14. Lee WM, Squires RH, Jr., Nyberg SL, et al. Acute liver failure: summary of a workshop. *Hepatology.* 2008;47(4):1401–1415.
15. Bernal W, Lee WM, Wendon, J, et al. Acute liver failure: a curable disease by 2024? *J Hepatol.* 2015;62(1 Suppl):S112–S120.
16. Polson J, Lee WM. AASLD position paper: the management of acute liver failure. *Hepatology.* 2005;41(5):1179–1197.
17. Munoz SJ. Difficult management problems in fulminant hepatic failure. *Semin Liver Dis.* 1993;13(4):395–413.
18. Blei AT. Infection, inflammation and hepatic encephalopathy, synergism redefined. *J Hepatol.* 2004;40(2):327–330.
19. Jalan R. Intracranial hypertension in acute liver failure: pathophysiological basis of rational management. *Semin Liver Dis.* 2003;23(3):271–282.
20. Larsen FS. Cerebral circulation in liver failure: Ohm's law in force. *Semin Liver Dis.* 1996;16(3):281–292.
21. Murphy N, Auzinger G, Bernel W, et al. The effect of hypertonic sodium chloride on intracranial pressure in patients with acute liver failure. *Hepatology.* 2004;39(2):464–470.
22. Ede RJ, Gimson AE, Bihari D, et al. Controlled hyperventilation in the prevention of cerebral oedema in fulminant hepatic failure. *J Hepatol.* 1986;2(1):43–51.
23. Stravitz RT, Kramer AH, Davern T, et al. Intensive care of patients with acute liver failure: recommendations from the U.S. Acute Liver Failure Study Group. *Crit Care Med.* 2007;35(11):2498–2508.
24. Frontera JA, Kalb T. Neurological management of fulminant hepatic failure. *Neurocrit care.* 2011;14(2):318–327.
25. Munoz SJ, Robinson M, Northrup B, et al. Elevated intracranial pressure and computed tomography of the brain in fulminant hepatocellular failure. *Hepatology.* 1991;13(2):209–212.
26. Lidofsky SD, Bass NM, Prager MC, et al. Intracranial pressure monitoring and liver transplantation for fulminant hepatic failure. *Hepatology.* 1992;16(1):1–7.
27. Raschke RA, Curry SC, Rempe S, et al. Results of a protocol for the management of patients with fulminant liver failure. *Crit Care Med.* 2008;36(8):2244–2248.
28. Bismuth H, Samuel D, Castaing D, et al. Orthotopic liver transplantation in fulminant and subfulminant hepatitis. The Paul Brousse experience. *Annals of Surgery.* 1995;222(2):109–119.
29. Riordan SM, Williams R. Mechanisms of hepatocyte injury, multiorgan failure, and prognostic criteria in acute liver failure. *Semin Liver Dis.* 2003;23(3):203–215.
30. Macquillan GC, Seyam MS, Nightingale P, et al. Blood lactate but not serum phosphate levels can predict patient outcome in fulminant hepatic failure. *Liver Transpl.* 2005;11(9):1073–1079.
31. Larson AM, Polson J, Fontana RJ, et al. Acetaminophen-induced acute liver failure: results of a United States multicenter, prospective study. *Hepatology.* 2005;42(6):1364–1372.

32. Cholongitas E, Theocharidou E, Vasianopoulou P, et al. Comparison of the sequential organ failure assessment score with the King's College Hospital criteria and the model for end-stage liver disease score for the prognosis of acetaminophen-induced acute liver failure. *Liver Transpl.* 2012;18(4):405–412.
33. Lisman T, Caldwell SH, Burroughs AK, et al. Hemostasis and thrombosis in patients with liver disease: the ups and downs. *J Hepatol.* 2010;53(2):362–371.
34. Tripodi A, Caldwell SH, Hoffman M, et al. Review article: the prothrombin time test as a measure of bleeding risk and prognosis in liver disease. *Aliment Pharmacol Ther.* 2007;26(2):141–148.
35. Townsend JC, Heard R, Powers ER, et al. Usefulness of international normalized ratio to predict bleeding complications in patients with end-stage liver disease who undergo cardiac catheterization. *Am J Cardiol.* 2012;110(7):1062–1065.
36. De Pietri L, Bianchini M, Montalti R, et al. Thrombelastography-guided blood product use before invasive procedures in cirrhosis with severe coagulopathy. A randomized controlled trial. *Hepatology.* 2016;63(2):566–573
37. Mallett, SV. Clinical utility of viscoelastic tests of coagulation (TEG/ROTEM) in patients with liver disease and during liver transplantation. *Semin Thromb Hemost.* 2015;41(5):527–537.
38. Shawcross DL, Davies NA, Williams R, et al. Systemic inflammatory response exacerbates the neuropsychological effects of induced hyperammonemia in cirrhosis. *J Hepatol.* 2004;40(2):247–254.
39. Feld JJ, Moreno C, Trinh R, et al. Sustained virologic response of 100% in HCV genotype 1b patients with cirrhosis receiving ombitasvir/paritaprevir/and dasabuvir for 12 weeks. *J Hepatol.* 2016;64(2):301–307
40. Sulkowski MS, Vargas HE, Di Bisceglie AM, et al. Effectiveness of Simeprevir plus Sofosbuvir, with or without Ribavirin, in real-world patients with HCV genotype 1 infection. *Gastroenterology.* 2016;150(2):419–429.
41. Kanda T, Nakamoto S, Nakamura M, et al. Direct-acting antiviral agents for the treatment of chronic hepatitis C virus infection. *J Clin Transl Hepatol.* 2014;2(1):1–6.
42. Nakamoto S, Kanda T, Shirasawa H, et al. Antiviral therapies for chronic hepatitis C virus infection with cirrhosis. *World J Hepatol.* 2015;7(8):1133–1141.
43. Cohen JA and Kaplan MM. The SGOT/SGPT ratio—an indicator of alcoholic liver disease. *Dig Dis Sci.* 1979;24(11):835–838.
44. Levin DM, Baker AL, Riddell RH, et al. Nonalcoholic liver disease. Overlooked causes of liver injury in patients with heavy alcohol consumption. *Am J Med.* 1979;66(3):429–434.
45. Ostapowicz G, Fontana RJ, Schiødt FV, et al. Results of a prospective study of acute liver failure at 17 tertiary care centers in the United States. *Ann Intern Med.* 2002;137:947–954.
46. U.S. Food and Drug Administration. Guidance for Industry on Drug-Induced Liver Injury: Premarketing Clinical Evaluation. 2009 December 20, 2015; Available from: http://www.fda.gov/downloads/Drugs/GdidanceCompliance RegulatoryInformation/Guidances/UCM174090.
47. Watkins PB, Seeff LB. Drug-induced liver injury: summary of a single topic clinical research conference. *Hepatology.* 2006;43(3):618–631.
48. Ray DC, Drummond GB. Halothane hepatitis. *Br J Anaesth.* 1991;67(1):84–99.
49. Bunker JP. Final report of the national halothane study. *Anesthesiology.* 1968;29(2):231–232.
50. Wright R, Eade OE, Chisholm M, et al. Controlled prospective study of the effect on liver function of multiple exposures to halothane. *Lancet.* 1975;1(7911):817–820.
51. Reichle FM, Conzen PF. Halogenated inhalational anaesthetics. *Best Pract Res Clin Anaesthesiol.* 2003;17(1):29–44.
52. Kenna JG, Satoh H, Christ DD, et al. Metabolic basis for a drug hypersensitivity: antibodies in sera from patients with halothane hepatitis recognize liver neoantigens that contain the trifluoroacetyl group derived from halothane. *J Pharmacol Exp Ther.* 1988;245(3):1103–1109.
53. Njoku D, Laster MJ, Gong DH, et al. Biotransformation of halothane, enflurane, isoflurane, and desflurane to trifluoroacetylated liver proteins: association between protein acylation and hepatic injury. *Anesth Analg.* 1997;84(1):173–178.
54. Fell DB, Dodds L, Joseph KS, et al. Risk factors for hyperemesis gravidarum requiring hospital admission during pregnancy. *Obstet Gynecol.* 2006;107(2 Pt 1):277–284.
55. Hay JE. Liver disease in pregnancy. *Hepatology.* 2008;47(3):1067–1076.
56. Bacq Y. Liver diseases unique to pregnancy: a 2010 update. *Clin Res Hepatol Gastroenterol.* 2011;35(3):182–193.
57. Pinzani M, Rosselli M, Zuckermann M. Liver cirrhosis. *Best Pract Res Clin Gastroenterol.* 2011;25(2):281–290.
58. Ripoll C, Groszmann R, Garcia-Tsao G, et al. Hepatic venous pressure gradient predicts clinical decompensation in patients with compensated cirrhosis. *Gastroenterology.* 2007;133(2):481–488.
59. Tripodi A, Primignani M, Chantarangkul V, et al. An imbalance of pro- vs anti-coagulation factors in plasma from patients with cirrhosis. *Gastroenterology.* 2009;137(6):2105–2111
60. Lisman T, Bakhtiari K, Pereboom IT, et al. Normal to increased thrombin generation in patients undergoing liver transplantation despite prolonged conventional coagulation tests. *J Hepatol.* 2010;52(3):355–361.
61. Diaz LK, Teruya J. Liver biopsy. *N Engl J Med.* 2001;344(26):2030.
62. Terjung B, Lemnitzer I, Dumoulin FL, et al. Bleeding complications after percutaneous liver biopsy. An analysis of risk factors. *Digestion.* 2003;67(3):138–145.
63. Segal JB, Dzik WH. Paucity of studies to support that abnormal coagulation test results predict bleeding in the setting of invasive procedures: an evidence-based review. *Transfusion.* 2005;45(9):1413–1425.
64. Tripodi A, Primignani M, Chantarangkul V, et al. Thrombin generation in patients with cirrhosis: the role of platelets. *Hepatology.* 2006;44(2):440–445.
65. Lisman T, Bongers TN, Adelmeijer J, et al. Elevated levels of von Willebrand factor in cirrhosis support platelet adhesion despite reduced functional capacity. *Hepatology.* 2006;44(1):53–61.
66. Dabbagh O, Oza A, Prakash S, et al. Coagulopathy does not protect against venous thromboembolism in hospitalized patients with chronic liver disease. *Chest.* 2010;137(5):1145–1149.
67. Northup PG, McMahon MM, Ruhl AP, et al. Coagulopathy does not fully protect hospitalized cirrhosis patients from peripheral venous thromboembolism. *Am J Gastroenterol.* 2006;101(7):1524–1528; quiz 1680.
68. Sogaard KK, Horvath-Puho E, Gronbaek H, et al. Risk of venous thromboembolism in patients with liver disease: a nationwide population-based case-control study. *Am J Gastroenterol.* 2009;104(1):96–101.
69. Francis JL, Armstrong DJ. Acquired dysfibrinogenaemia in liver disease. *J Clin Pathol.* 1982;35(6):667–672.
70. Amitrano L, Guardascione MA, Brancaccio V, et al. Coagulation disorders in liver disease. *Semin Liver Dis.* 2002;22(1):83–96.
71. Hu KQ, Yu AS, Tiyyagura L, et al. Hyperfibrinolytic activity in hospitalized cirrhotic patients in a referral liver unit. *Am J Gastroenterol.* 2001;96(5):1581–1586.
72. Kujovich JL. Hemostatic defects in end stage liver disease. *Crit Care Clin.* 2005;21(3):563–587.
73. Puoti C, Bellis L, Guarisco R, et al. Quantitation of tissue polypeptide antigen (TPA) in hepatic and systemic circulation in patients with chronic liver diseases. *J Gastroenterol Hepatol.* 2009;24(12):1847–1851.
74. Ben-Ari Z, Osman E, Hutton RA, et al. Disseminated intravascular coagulation in liver cirrhosis: fact or fiction? *Am J Gastroenterol.* 1999;94(10):2977–2982.
75. Joist JH. AICF and DIC in liver cirrhosis: expressions of a hypercoagulable state. *Am J Gastroenterol.* 1999;94(10):2801–2803.
76. Moller S, Henriksen JH. Cardiovascular complications of cirrhosis. *Gut.* 2008;57(2):268–278.
77. Schepke M, Heller J, Paschke S, et al. Contractile hyporesponsiveness of hepatic arteries in humans with cirrhosis: evidence for a receptor-specific mechanism. *Hepatology.* 2001;34(5):884–888.
78. Wong F, Girgrah N, Graba J, et al. The cardiac response to exercise in cirrhosis. *Gut.* 2001;49(2):268–275.
79. Puthumana L, Chaudhry V, Thuluvath PJ. Prolonged QTc interval and its relationship to autonomic cardiovascular reflexes in patients with cirrhosis. *J Hepatol.* 2001;35(6):733–738.
80. Raval Z, Harinstein ME, Skaro AI, et al. Cardiovascular risk assessment of the liver transplant candidate. *J Am Coll Cardiol.* 2011;58(3):223–231.
81. Ehtisham J, Altieri M, Salame E, et al. Coronary artery disease in orthotopic liver transplantation: pretransplant assessment and management. *Liver Transpl.* 2010;16(5):550–557.
82. McGuire BM, Julian BA, Bynon JS, Jr., et al. Brief communication: glomerulonephritis in patients with hepatitis C cirrhosis undergoing liver transplantation. *Ann Intern Med.* 2006;144(10):735–741.
83. Guevara M, Fernandez-Esparrach G, Alessandria C, et al. Effects of contrast media on renal function in patients with cirrhosis: a prospective study. *Hepatology.* 2004;40(3):646–651.
84. Takabatake T, Ohta H, Ishida Y, et al. Low serum creatinine levels in severe hepatic disease. *Arch Int Med.* 1988;148(6):1313–1315.
85. Papadakis MA, Arieff AI. Unpredictability of clinical evaluation of renal function in cirrhosis. Prospective study. *Am J Med.* 1987;82(5):945–952.
86. Koppel MH, Coburn JW, Mims MM, et al. Transplantation of cadaveric kidneys from patients with hepatorenal syndrome. Evidence for the functional nature of renal failure in advanced liver disease. *N Engl J Med.* 1969;280(25):1367–1371.
87. Garcia-Tsao G, Parikh CR, Viola A. Acute kidney injury in cirrhosis. *Hepatology.* 2008;48(6):2064–2077.
88. Gines A, Escorsell A, Gines P, et al. Incidence, predictive factors, and prognosis of the hepatorenal syndrome in cirrhosis with ascites. *Gastroenterology.* 1993;105(1):229–236.
89. Salerno F, Gerbes A, Gines P, et al. Diagnosis, prevention and treatment of hepatorenal syndrome in cirrhosis. *Gut.* 2007;56(9):1310–1318.
90. Salerno F, Guevara M, Bernardi M, et al. Refractory ascites: pathogenesis, definition and therapy of a severe complication in patients with cirrhosis. *Liver Int.* 2010;30(7):937–947.
91. Moreau R. Hepatorenal syndrome in patients with cirrhosis. *J Gastroenterol Hepatol.* 2002;17(7):739–747.
92. Arroyo V, Terra C, Gines P. Advances in the pathogenesis and treatment of type-1 and type-2 hepatorenal syndrome. *J Hepatol.* 2007;46(5):935–946.
93. Gines P, Guevara M, Arroyo V, et al. Hepatorenal syndrome. *Lancet.* 2003;362(9398):1819–1827.

94. Kiser TH, Maclaren R, Fish DN. Treatment of hepatorenal syndrome. *Pharmacotherapy*. 2009;29(10):1196–1211.
95. Sola E, Gines P. Renal and circulatory dysfunction in cirrhosis: current management and future perspectives. *J Hepatol*. 2010;53(6):1135–1145.
96. Boyer TD, Sanyal AJ, Garcia-Tsao G, et al. Predictors of response to terlipressin plus albumin in hepatorenal syndrome (HRS) type 1: relationship of serum creatinine to hemodynamics. *J Hepatol*. 2011;55(2):315–321.
97. Guevara M, Gines P, Bandi JC, et al. Transjugular intrahepatic portosystemic shunt in hepatorenal syndrome: effects on renal function and vasoactive systems. *Hepatology*. 1998;28(2):416–422.
98. Gonwa TA, Morris CA, Goldstein RM, et al. Long-term survival and renal function following liver transplantation in patients with and without hepatorenal syndrome—experience in 300 patients. *Transplantation*. 1991;51(2):428–430.
99. Charlton MR, Wall WJ, Ojo AO, et al. Report of the first International Liver Transplantation Society expert panel consensus conference on renal insufficiency in liver transplantation. *Liver Transpl*. 2009;15(11):S1–S34.
100. Palma DT, Fallon MB. The hepatopulmonary syndrome. *J Hepatol*. 2006;45(4):617–625.
101. Rodriguez-Roisin R, Krowka MJ. Hepatopulmonary syndrome—a liver-induced lung vascular disorder. *N Engl J Med*. 2008;358(22):2378–2387.
102. Krowka MJ. Hepatopulmonary syndrome: recent literature (1997 to 1999) and implications for liver transplantation. *Liver Transpl*. 2000;(4 Suppl 1):S31–S35.
103. Arguedas MR, Abrams GA, Krowka MJ, et al. Prospective evaluation of outcomes and predictors of mortality in patients with hepatopulmonary syndrome undergoing liver transplantation. *Hepatology*. 2003;37(1):192–197.
104. Iyer VN, Swanson KL, Cartin-Ceba R, et al. Hepatopulmonary syndrome: favorable outcomes in the MELD exception era. *Hepatology*. 2013;57(6):2427–2435.
105. Swanson KL, Wiesner RH, Krowka MJ. Natural history of hepatopulmonary syndrome: impact of liver transplantation. *Hepatology*. 2005;41(5):1122–1129.
106. Gupta S, Castel H, Rao RV, et al. Improved survival after liver transplantation in patients with hepatopulmonary syndrome. *Am J Transplant*. 2010;10(2):354–363.
107. Fallon MB, Mulligan DC, Gish RG, et al. Model for end-stage liver disease (MELD) exception for hepatopulmonary syndrome. *Liver Transpl*. 2006;12(12 Suppl 3):S105–S107.
108. Rodriguez-Roisin R, Krowka MJ, Herve P, et al. Pulmonary-hepatic vascular disorders (PHD). *Eur Respirat J*. 2004;24(5):861–880.
109. Hadengue A, Benhayoun MK, Lebrec D, et al. Pulmonary hypertension complicating portal hypertension: prevalence and relation to splanchnic hemodynamics. *Gastroenterology*. 1991;100(2):520–528.
110. McDonnell PJ, Toye PA, Hutchins GM. Primary pulmonary hypertension and cirrhosis: are they related? *Am Rev Respir Dis*. 1983;127(4):437–441.
111. Kawut SM, Krowka MJ, Trotter JF, et al. Clinical risk factors for portopulmonary hypertension. *Hepatology*. 2008;48(1):196–203.
112. Castro M, Krowka MJ, Schroeder DR, et al. Frequency and clinical implications of increased pulmonary artery pressures in liver transplant patients. *Mayo Clin Proc*. 1996;71(6):543–551.
113. Le Pavec J, Souza R, Herve P, et al. Portopulmonary hypertension: survival and prognostic factors. *Am J Resp Crit Care Med*. 2008;178(6):637–643.
114. Hoeper MM, Halank M, Marx C, et al. Bosentan therapy for portopulmonary hypertension. *Eur Resp J*. 2005;25(3):502–508.
115. Kim WR, Krowka MJ, Plevak DJ, et al. Accuracy of Doppler echocardiography in the assessment of pulmonary hypertension in liver transplant candidates. *Liver Transpl*. 2000;6(4):453–458.
116. McLaughlin VV, Archer SL, Badesch DB, et al. ACCF/AHA 2009 expert consensus document on pulmonary hypertension a report of the American College of Cardiology Foundation Task Force on Expert Consensus Documents and the American Heart Association developed in collaboration with the American College of Chest Physicians; American Thoracic Society, Inc.; and the Pulmonary Hypertension Association. *J Am Col Cardiol*. 2009;53(17):1573–1619.
117. Findlay JY, Plevak DJ, Krowka MJ, et al. Progressive splenomegaly after epoprostenol therapy in portopulmonary hypertension. *Liver Transplant Surg*. 1999;5(5):362–365.
118. Reichenberger F, Voswinckel R, Steveling E, et al. Sildenafil treatment for portopulmonary hypertension. *Eur Resp J*. 2006;28(3):563–567.
119. Porres-Aguilar M, Zuckerman MJ, Figueroa-Casas JB, et al. Portopulmonary hypertension: state of the art. *Ann Hepatol*. 2008;7(4):321–330.
120. Ramsay M. Portopulmonary hypertension and right heart failure in patients with cirrhosis. *Curr Opin Anaesthesiol*. 2010;23(2):145–150.
121. Krowka MJ, Mandell MS, Ramsay MA, et al. Hepatopulmonary syndrome and portopulmonary hypertension: a report of the multicenter liver transplant database. *Liver Transpl*. 2004;10(2):174–182.
122. Ferenci P, Lockwood A, Mullen K, et al. Hepatic encephalopathy—definition, nomenclature, diagnosis, and quantification: final report of the working party at the 11th World Congresses of Gastroenterology, Vienna, 1998. *Hepatology*. 2002;35(3):716–721.
123. Munoz SJ. Hepatic encephalopathy. *Med Clin North Am*. 2008;92(4):795–812, viii.
124. Bass NM, Mullen KD, Sanyal A, et al. Rifaximin treatment in hepatic encephalopathy. *New Eng J Med*. 2010;362(12):1071–1081.
125. Prakash R, Mullen KD. Mechanisms, diagnosis and management of hepatic encephalopathy. Nature reviews. *Gastroenterol Hepatol*. 2010;7(9):515–525.
126. Mullen KD, Szauter KM, Kaminsky-Russ K. "Endogenous" benzodiazepine activity in body fluids of patients with hepatic encephalopathy. *Lancet*. 1990. 336(8707):81–83.
127. Perney P, Butterworth RF, Mousseau DD, et al. Plasma and CSF benzodiazepine receptor ligand concentrations in cirrhotic patients with hepatic encephalopathy: relationship to severity of encephalopathy and to pharmaceutical benzodiazepine intake. *Metab Brain Dis*. 1998;13(3):201–210.
128. Lock BG, Pandit K. Evidence-based emergency medicine/systematic review abstract. Is flumazenil an effective treatment for hepatic encephalopathy? *Ann Emerg Med*. 2006;47(3):286–288.
129. Barbaro G, Di Lorenzo G, Soldini M, et al. Flumazenil for hepatic encephalopathy grade III and IVa in patients with cirrhosis: an Italian multicenter double-blind, placebo-controlled, cross-over study. *Hepatology*. 1998;28(2):374–378.
130. Haussinger D, Schliess F. Pathogenetic mechanisms of hepatic encephalopathy. *Gut*. 2008;57(8):1156–1165.
131. Blei AT, Cordoba J. Hepatic encephalopathy. *Am J Gastroenterol*. 2001;96(7):1968–1976.
132. Runyon BA. Management of adult patients with ascites due to cirrhosis: an update. *Hepatology*. 2009;49(6):2087–2107.
133. Arroyo V, Colmenero J. Ascites and hepatorenal syndrome in cirrhosis: pathophysiological basis of therapy and current management. *J Hepatol*. 2003;38(Suppl 1):S69–S89.
134. Runyon BA, Montano AA, Akriviadis EA, et al. The serum-ascites albumin gradient is superior to the exudate-transudate concept in the differential diagnosis of ascites. *Ann Int Med*. 1992;117(3):215–220.
135. Wszolek ZK, McComb RD, Pfeiffer RF, et al. Pontine and extrapontine myelinolysis following liver transplantation. Relationship to serum sodium. *Transplantation*. 1989;48(6):1006–1012.
136. Gines P, Cardenas A, Arroyo V, et al. Management of cirrhosis and ascites. *New Engl J Med*. 2004;350(16):1646–1654.
137. Albillos A, Banares R, Gonzalez M, et al. A meta-analysis of transjugular intrahepatic portosystemic shunt versus paracentesis for refractory ascites. *J Hepatol*. 2005;43(6):990–996.
138. D'Amico G, Luca A, Morabito A, et al. Uncovered transjugular intrahepatic portosystemic shunt for refractory ascites: a meta-analysis. *Gastroenterology*. 2005;129(4):1282–1293.
139. Perello A, Escorsell A, Bru C, et al. Wedged hepatic venous pressure adequately reflects portal pressure in hepatitis C virus–related cirrhosis. *Hepatology*. 1999;30(6):1393–1397.
140. Garcia-Tsao G, Groszmann RJ, Fisher RL, et al. Portal pressure, presence of gastroesophageal varices and variceal bleeding. *Hepatology*. 1985;5(3):419–424.
141. Lebrec D, De Fleury P, Rueff B, et al. Portal hypertension, size of esophageal varices, and risk of gastrointestinal bleeding in alcoholic cirrhosis. *Gastroenterology*. 1980;79(6):1139–1144.
142. Garcia-Tsao G, Sanyal AJ, Grace ND, et al. Prevention and management of gastroesophageal varices and variceal hemorrhage in cirrhosis. *Hepatology*. 2007;46(3):922–938.
143. Castaneda B, Morales J, Lionetti R, et al. Effects of blood volume restitution following a portal hypertensive-related bleeding in anesthetized cirrhotic rats. *Hepatology*. 2001;33(4):821–825.
144. Kravetz D, Sikuler E, Groszmann RJ. Splanchnic and systemic hemodynamics in portal hypertensive rats during hemorrhage and blood volume restitution. *Gastroenterology*. 1986;90(5 Pt 1):1232–1240.
145. Moitinho E, Escorsell A, Bandi JC, et al. Prognostic value of early measurements of portal pressure in acute variceal bleeding. *Gastroenterology*. 1999;117(3):626–631.
146. Green J, Beyar R, Bomzon L, et al. Jaundice, the circulation and the kidney. *Nephron*. 1984;37(3):145–152.
147. Green J, Beyar R, Sideman S, et al. The "jaundiced heart": a possible explanation for postoperative shock in obstructive jaundice. *Surgery*. 1986;100(1):14–20.
148. Ben-Ari Z, Panagou M, Patch D, et al. Hypercoagulability in patients with primary biliary cirrhosis and primary sclerosing cholangitis evaluated by thrombelastography. *J Hepatol*. 1997;26(3):554–559.
149. Segal H, Cottam S, Potter D, et al. Coagulation and fibrinolysis in primary biliary cirrhosis compared with other liver disease and during orthotopic liver transplantation. *Hepatology*. 1997;25(3):683–688.
150. El-Masry M, Puig CA, Saab S. Recurrence of non-viral liver disease after orthotopic liver transplantation. *Liver Intl*. 2011;31(3):291–302.
151. McGill JM, Kwiatkowski AP. Cholestatic liver diseases in adults. *Am J Gastroenterol*. 1998;93(5):684–691.
152. Wong RJ, Aguilar M, Cheung R, et al. Nonalcoholic steatohepatitis is the second leading etiology of liver disease among adults awaiting liver transplantation in the United States. *Gastroenterology*. 2015;148(3):547–555.
153. El-Serag HB. Hepatocellular carcinoma. *N Engl J Med*. 2011;365(12):1118–1127.
154. Benvegnu L, Fattovich G, Noventa F, et al. Concurrent hepatitis B and C virus infection and risk of hepatocellular carcinoma in cirrhosis. A prospective study. *Cancer*. 1994;74(9):2442–2448.
155. Bruix J, Sherman M. Management of hepatocellular carcinoma: an update. *Hepatology*. 2011;53(3):1020–1022.

156. Mazzaferro V, Bhoori S, Sposito C, et al. Milan criteria in liver transplantation for hepatocellular carcinoma: an evidence-based analysis of 15 years of experience. *Liver Transpl.* 2011;17(Suppl 2):S44–S57.
157. Browning JD, Szczepaniak LS, Dobbins R, et al. Prevalence of hepatic steatosis in an urban population in the United States: impact of ethnicity. *Hepatology.* 2004;40(6):1387–1395.
158. Vernon G, Baranova A, Younossi ZM. Systematic review: the epidemiology and natural history of non-alcoholic fatty liver disease and non-alcoholic steatohepatitis in adults. *Aliment Pharmacol Ther.* 2011;34(3):274–285.
159. Ratziu V, Bellentani S, Cortez-Pinto H, et al. A position statement on NAFLD/NASH based on the EASL 2009 special conference. *J Hepatol.* 2010;53(2):372–384.
160. Torres DM, Harrison SA. Diagnosis and therapy of nonalcoholic steatohepatitis. *Gastroenterology.* 2008;134(6):1682–1698.
161. Mummadi RR, Kasturi KS, Chennareddygari S, et al. Effect of bariatric surgery on nonalcoholic fatty liver disease: systematic review and meta-analysis. *Clin Gastroenterol Hepatol.* 2008;6(12):1396–1402.
162. Kundrotas LW, Clement DJ. Serum alanine aminotransferase (ALT) elevation in asymptomatic US Air Force basic trainee blood donors. *Dig Dis Sci.* 1993;38(12):2145–2150.
163. Schemel WH. Unexpected hepatic dysfunction found by multiple laboratory screening. *Anesth Analg.* 1976;55(6):810–812.
164. Pratt DS, Kaplan MM. Primary care: evaluation of abnormal liver-enzyme results in asymptomatic patients. *N Engl J Med.* 2000;342(17):1266–1271.
165. Powell-Jackson P, Greenway B, Williams R. Adverse effects of exploratory laparotomy in patients with unsuspected liver disease. *Br J Surg.* 1982;69(8):449–451.
166. Rizvon MK, Chou CL. Surgery in the patient with liver disease. *Med Clin North Am.* 2003;87(1):211–227.
167. Friedman LS. Surgery in the patient with liver disease. *Trans Am Clin Climatol Assoc.* 2010;121:192–204; discussion 205.
168. Aranha GV, Sontag SJ, Greenlee HB. Cholecystectomy in cirrhotic patients: a formidable operation. *Am J Surg.* 1982;143(1):55–60.
169. Doberneck RC, Sterling WA, Jr., Allison DC. Morbidity and mortality after operation in nonbleeding cirrhotic patients. *Am J Surg.* 1983;146(3):306–309.
170. Garrison RN, Cryer HM, Howard DA, et al. Clarification of risk factors for abdominal operations in patients with hepatic cirrhosis. *Ann Surg.* 1984;199(6):648–655.
171. Mansour A, Watson W, Shayani V, et al. Abdominal operations in patients with cirrhosis: still a major surgical challenge. *Surgery.* 1997;122(4):730–735; discussion 735–736.
172. Neeff H, Mariaskin D, Spangenberg H-C, et al. Perioperative mortality after non-hepatic general surgery in patients with liver cirrhosis: an analysis of 138 operations in the 2000s using Child and MELD scores. *J Gastrointest Surg.* 2011;15(1):1–11.
173. Malinchoc M, Kamath PS, Gordon FD, et al. A model to predict poor survival in patients undergoing transjugular intrahepatic portosystemic shunts. *Hepatology.* 2000;31(4):864–871.
174. Freeman RB, Wiesner RH, Harper A, et al. The new liver allocation system: Moving toward evidence-based transplantation policy. *Liver Transpl.* 2002;8(9):851–858.
175. Northup PG, Wanamaker RC, Lee VD, et al. Model for End-Stage Liver Disease (MELD) predicts nontransplant surgical mortality in patients with cirrhosis. *Ann Surg.* 2005;242(2):244–251.
176. Teh SH, Nagorney DM, Stevens SR, et al. Risk factors for mortality after surgery in patients with cirrhosis. *Gastroenterology.* 2007;132(4):1261–1269.
177. Viegas O, Stoelting RK. LDH changes after cholecystectomy or hysterectomy in patients receiving halothane, enflurane, or fentanyl. *Anesthesiology.* 1979;51(6):556–558.
178. Ziser A, Plevak DJ, Wiesner RH, et al. Morbidity and mortality in cirrhotic patients undergoing anesthesia and surgery. *Anesthesiology.* 1999;90(1):42–53.
179. Shaikh AR, Muneer A. Laparoscopic cholecystectomy in cirrhotic patients. *JSLS.* 2009;13(4):592–596.
180. Curro G, Iapichino G, Melita G, et al. Laparoscopic cholecystectomy in Child–Pugh class C cirrhotic patients. *JSLS.* 2005;9(3):311–315.
181. Yeh CN, Chen MF, Jan YY. Laparoscopic cholecystectomy in 226 cirrhotic patients. Experience of a single center in Taiwan. *Surg Endosc.* 2002;16(11):1583–1587.
182. Laurence JM, Tran PD, Richardson AJ, et al. Laparoscopic or open cholecystectomy in cirrhosis: a systematic review of outcomes and meta-analysis of randomized trials. *HPB (Oxford).* 2012;14(3):153–161.
183. Cheng Y, Xiong XZ, Wu SJ, et al. Laparoscopic vs. open cholecystectomy for cirrhotic patients: a systematic review and meta-analysis. *Hepatogastroenterology.* 2012;59(118):1727–1734.
184. Azoulay D, Buabse F, Damiano I, et al. Neoadjuvant transjugular intrahepatic portosystemic shunt: a solution for extrahepatic abdominal operation in cirrhotic patients with severe portal hypertension. *J Am Coll Surg.* 2001;193(1):46–51.
185. Van der Linden P, Le Moine O, Ghysels M, et al. Pulmonary hypertension after transjugular intrahepatic portosystemic shunt: effects on right ventricular function. *Hepatology.* 1996;23(5):982–987.
186. Marik PE, Baram M, Vahid B. Does central venous pressure predict fluid responsiveness? A systematic review of the literature and the tale of seven mares. *Chest.* 2008;134(1):172–178.
187. Mansour N, Lentschener C, Ozier Y. Do we really need a low central venous pressure in elective liver resection? *Acta Anaesthesiol Scand.* 2008;52(9):1306–1307.
188. Schroeder RA, Kuo PC. Pro: low central venous pressure during liver transplantation—not too low. *J Cardiothorac Vasc Anesth.* 2008;22(2):311–314.
189. Niemann CU, Feiner J, Behrends M, et al. Central venous pressure monitoring during living right donor hepatectomy. *Liver Transpl.* 2007;13(2):266–271.
190. Spier BJ, Larue SJ, Teelin TC, et al. Review of complications in a series of patients with known gastro-esophageal varices undergoing transesophageal echocardiography. *J Am Soc Echocardiogr.* 2009;22(4):396–400.
191. Myo Bui CC, Worapot A, Xia W, et al. Gastroesophageal and hemorrhagic complications associated with intraoperative transesophageal echocardiography in patients with model for end-stage liver disease score 25 or higher. *J Cardiothorac Vasc Anesth.* 2015;29(3):594–597.
192. Markin NW, Sharma A, Grant W, et al. The safety of transesophageal echocardiography in patients undergoing orthotopic liver transplantation. *J Cardiothorac Vasc Anesth.* 2015;29(3):588–593.
193. Kennedy WF, Everett GB, Cobb LA, et al. Simultaneous systemic and hepatic hemodynamic measurements during high spinal anesthesia in normal man. *Anesth Analg.* 1970;49(6):1016–1024.
194. Kennedy WF, Everett GB, Cobb LA, et al. Simultaneous systemic and hepatic hemodynamic measurements during high peridural anesthesia in normal man. *Anesth Analg.* 1971;50(6):1069–1077.
195. Meierhenrich R, Wagner F, Schutz W, et al. The effects of thoracic epidural anesthesia on hepatic blood flow in patients under general anesthesia. *Anesth Analg.* 2009;108(4):1331–1337.
196. Greitz T, Andreen M, Irestedt L. Effects of ephedrine on hemodynamics and oxygen-consumption in the dog during high epidural block with special reference to the splanchnic region. *Acta Anaesthesiol Scand.* 1984;28(5):557–562.
197. Tanaka N, Nagata N, Hamakawa T, et al. The effect of dopamine on hepatic blood flow in patients undergoing epidural anesthesia. *Anesth Analg.* 1997;85(2):286–290.
198. Hiltebrand LB, Krejci V, Sigurdsson GH. Effects of dopamine, dobutamine, and dopexamine on microcirculatory blood flow in the gastrointestinal tract during sepsis and anesthesia. *Anesthesiology.* 2004;100(5):1188–1197.
199. McDonnell JG, O'Donnell B, Curley G, et al. The analgesic efficacy of transversus abdominis plane block after abdominal surgery: A prospective randomized controlled trial. *Anesth Analg.* 2007;104(1):193–197.
200. Niraj G, Kelkar A, Jeyapalan I, et al. Comparison of analgesic efficacy of subcostal transversus abdominis plane blocks with epidural analgesia following upper abdominal surgery. *Anaesthesia.* 2011;66(6):465–471.
201. Frink EJ, Jr. The hepatic effects of sevoflurane. *Anesth Analg.* 1995;81(6 Suppl):S46–S50.
202. Schindler E, Muller M Zickmann B, et al. [Blood supply to the liver in the human after 1 MAC desflurane in comparison with isoflurane and halothane]. *Anasthesiol Intensivmed Notfallmed Schmerzther.* 1996;31(6):344–348.
203. Hartman JC, Pagel PS, Proctor LT, et al. Influence of desflurane, isoflurane and halothane on regional tissue perfusion in dogs. *Can J Anaesth.* 1992;39(8):877–887.
204. Matsumoto N, Koizumi M, Sugai M. Hepatolobectomy-induced depression of hepatic circulation and metabolism in the dog is counteracted by isoflurane, but not by halothane. *Acta Anaesthesiol Scand.* 1999;43(8):850–854.
205. Crawford MW, Lerman J, Saldivia V, et al. Hemodynamic and organ blood flow responses to halothane and sevoflurane anesthesia during spontaneous ventilation. *Anesth Analg.* 1992;75(6):1000–1006.
206. Lewis JH, Zimmerman HJ, Ishak KG, et al. Enflurane hepatotoxicity—a clinicopathological study of 24 cases. *Ann Int Med.* 1983;98(6):984–992.
207. Berghaus TM, Baron A, Geier A, et al. Hepatotoxicity following desflurane anesthesia. *Hepatology.* 1999;29(2):613–614.
208. Martin JL. [Volatile anesthetics and liver injury: a clinical update or what every anesthesiologist should know]. *Can J Anaesth.* 2005;52(2):125–129.
209. Obata R, Bito H, Ohmura M, et al. The effects of prolonged low-flow sevoflurane anesthesia on renal and hepatic function. *Anesth Analg.* 2000;91(5):1262–1268.
210. Bedirli N, Ofluoglu E, Kerem M, et al. Hepatic energy metabolism and the differential protective effects of sevoflurane and isoflurane anesthesia in a rat hepatic ischemia-reperfusion injury model. *Anesth Analg.* 2008;106(3):830–837.
211. Lehmann A, Neher M, Kiessling AH, et al. Case report: fatal hepatic failure after aortic valve replacement and sevoflurane exposure. *Can J Anaesth.* 2007;54(11):917–921.
212. Prys-Roberts C, Sear JW, Low JM, et al. Hemodynamic and hepatic effects of methohexital infusion during nitrous oxide anesthesia in humans. *Anesth Analg.* 1983;62(3):317–323.
213. Zinn SE, Fairley HB, Glenn JD. Liver function in patients with mild alcoholic hepatitis, after enflurane, nitrous oxide-narcotic, and spinal anesthesia. *Anesth Analg.* 1985;64(5):487–490.
214. Nunn JF. Clinical aspects of the interaction between nitrous oxide and vitamin B12. *Br J Anaesth.* 1987;59(1):3–13.

215. Parke TJ, Stevens JE, Rice AS, et al. Metabolic acidosis and fatal myocardial failure after propofol infusion in children: five case reports. *BMJ*. 1992;305(6854):613–616.
216. Otterspoor LC, Kalkman CJ, Cremer OL. Update on the propofol infusion syndrome in ICU management of patients with head injury. *Curr Opin Anaesthesiol*. 2008;21(5):544–551.
217. Thompson DR. Narcotic analgesic effects on the sphincter of Oddi: A review of the data and therapeutic implications in treating pancreatitis. *Am J Gastroenterol*. 2001;96(4):1266–1272.
218. Trouvin JH, Farinotti R, Haberer JP, et al. Pharmacokinetics of midazolam in anesthetized cirrhotic-patients. *Br J Anaesth*. 1988;60(7):762–767.
219. Macgilchrist AJ, Birnie GG, Cook A, et al. Pharmacokinetics and pharmacodynamics of intravenous midazolam in patients with severe alcoholic cirrhosis. *Gut*. 1986;27(2):190–195.
220. Susla GM. *AA. Principles of Clinical Pharmacology*. 2nd ed. Philadelphia, PA: Elsevier; 2007.
221. Pandele G, Chaux F, Salvadori C, et al. Thiopental pharmacokinetics in patients with cirrhosis. *Anesthesiology*. 1983;59(2):123–126.
222. Tegeder I, Lotsch J, Geisslinger G. Pharmacokinetics of opioids in liver disease. *Clin Pharmacokinet*. 1999;37(1):17–40.
223. Servin F, Desmonts JM, Haberer JP, et al. Pharmacokinetics and protein-binding of propofol in patients with cirrhosis. *Anesthesiology*. 1988;69(6):887–891.
224. Baughman VL, Cunningham FE, Layden T, et al. Pharmacokinetic/pharmacodynamic effects of dexmedetomidine in patients with hepatic failure. *Anesth Analg*. 2000;90(2):U231.
225. Hunter JM, Parker CJ, Bell CF, et al. The use of different doses of vecuronium in patients with liver dysfunction. *Br J Anaesth*. 1985;57(8):758–764.
226. Magorian T, Wood P, Caldwell J, et al. The pharmacokinetics and neuromuscular effects of rocuronium bromide in patients with liver disease. *Anesth Analg*. 1995;80(4):754–759.
227. Fodale V, Santamaria LB. Laudanosine, an atracurium and cisatracurium metabolite. *Eur J Anaesth*. 2002;19(7):466–473.
228. Cahill PA. Vasoconstrictor responsiveness of portal hypertensive vessels. *Clin Science*. 1999;96(1):3–4.
229. Cahill PA, Redmond EM, Sitzmann JV. Endothelial dysfunction in cirrhosis and portal hypertension. *Pharmacol Therap*. 2001;89(3):273–293.
230. Alves de Mattos A. Current indications for the use of albumin in the treatment of cirrhosis. *Ann Hepatol*. 2011;10(Suppl 1):S15–S20.
231. Bernardi M, Ricci CS, Zaccherini G. Role of human albumin in the management of complications of liver cirrhosis. *J Clin Exp Hepatol*. 2014;4(4):302–311.
232. Terg R, Gadano A, Cartier M, et al. Serum creatinine and bilirubin predict renal failure and mortality in patients with spontaneous bacterial peritonitis: a retrospective study. *Liver Int*. 2009;29(3):415–419.
233. Ortega R, Gines P, Uriz J, et al. Terlipressin therapy with and without albumin for patients with hepatorenal syndrome: results of a prospective, nonrandomized study. *Hepatology*. 2002;36(4 Pt 1):941–948.
234. Patel IJ, Davidson, JC, Nikolic B, et al. Consensus guidelines for periprocedural management of coagulation status and hemostasis risk in percutaneous image-guided interventions. *J Vasc Interv Radiol*. 2012;23(6):727–736.
235. Quiroga J, Sangro B, Nunez M, et al. Transjugular intrahepatic portal-systemic shunt in the treatment of refractory ascites: effect on clinical, renal, humoral, and hemodynamic parameters. *Hepatology*. 1995;21(4):986–994.
236. Sicklick JD, DAM Fong Y. The liver. In: J.C. Townsend, ed. *Sabiston Textbook of Surgery*. Philadelphia, PA: Elsevier Saunders; 2012:1411–1475.
237. Fortner JG, Blumgart LH. A historic perspective of liver surgery for tumors at the end of the millennium. *J Am Coll Surg*. 2001;193(2):210–222.
238. Jarnagin WR, Gonen M, Fong Y, et al. Improvement in perioperative outcome after hepatic resection: analysis of 1,803 consecutive cases over the past decade. *Ann Surg*. 2002;236(4):397–406; discussion 406–407.
239. Kingham TP, Correa-Gallego C, D'Angelica MI, et al. Hepatic parenchymal preservation surgery: decreasing morbidity and mortality rates in 4,152 resections for malignancy. *J Am Coll Surg*. 2015;220(4):471–479.
240. Franco D. Liver surgery has become simpler. *Eur J Anaesth*. 2002;19(11):777–779.
241. Lentschener C, Ozier Y. Anaesthesia for elective liver resection: some points should be revisited. *Eur J Anaesth*. 2002;19(11):780–788.
242. Clavien PA, Petrowsky H, DeOliveira ML, et al. Strategies for safer liver surgery and partial liver transplantation. *N Engl J Med*. 2007;356(15):1545–1559.
243. Lentschener C, Benhamou D, Mercier FJ, et al. Aprotinin reduces blood loss in patients undergoing elective liver resection. *Anesth Analg*. 1997;84(4):875–881.
244. Jones RM, Moulton CE, Hardy KJ. Central venous pressure and its effect on blood loss during liver resection. *Br J Surg*. 1998;85(8):1058–1060.
245. Wang WD, Liang LJ, Huang XQ, et al. Low central venous pressure reduces blood loss in hepatectomy. *World J Gastroenterol*. 2006;12(6):935–939.
246. Melendez JA, Arslan V, Fischer ME, et al. Perioperative outcomes of major hepatic resections under low central venous pressure anesthesia: blood loss, blood transfusion, and the risk of postoperative renal dysfunction. *J Am Coll Surg*. 1998;187(6):620–625.
247. Stephan F, Rezaiguia-Delclaux S. Usefulness of a central venous catheter during hepatic surgery. *Acta Anaesthesiol Scand*. 2008;52(3):388–396.
248. Hoftman N, Braunfeld M, Hoftman G, et al. Peripheral venous pressure as a predictor of central venous pressure during orthotopic liver transplantation. *J Clin Anesth*. 2006;18(4):251–255.
249. Kim YK, Chin JH, Kang SJ, et al. Association between central venous pressure and blood loss during hepatic resection in 984 living donors. *Acta Anaesthesiol Scand*. 2009;53(5):601–606.
250. Chhibber A, Dziak J, Kolano J, et al. Anesthesia care for adult live donor hepatectomy: Our experiences with 100 cases. *Liver Transpl*. 2007;13(4):537–542.
251. Hughes MJ, Ventham NT, Harrison EM, et al. Central venous pressure and liver resection: a systematic review and meta-analysis. *HPB (Oxford)*. 2015;17(10):863–871.
252. Massicotte L, Perrault MA, Denault AY, et al. Effects of phlebotomy and phenylephrine infusion on portal venous pressure and systemic hemodynamics during liver transplantation. *Transplantation*. 2010;89(8):920–927.
253. Belghiti J, Noun R, Zante E, et al. Portal triad clamping or hepatic vascular exclusion for major liver resection—a controlled study. *Ann Surg*. 1996;224(2):155–161.
254. Belghiti J, Noun R, Malafosse R, et al. Continuous versus intermittent portal triad clamping for liver resection: a controlled study. *Ann Surg*. 1999;229(3):369–375.
255. Torzilli G, Makuuchi M, Inoue K. The vascular control in liver resection: revisitation of a controversial issue. *Hepatogastroenterology*. 2002;49(43):28–31.
256. Petrowsky H, McCormack L, Trujillo M, et al. A prospective, randomized, controlled trial comparing intermittent portal triad clamping versus ischemic preconditioning with continuous clamping for major liver resection. *Ann Surg*. 2006;244(6):921–930.
257. Giordano C, Deitte LA, Gravenstein N, et al. What is the preferred central venous pressure zero reference for hepatic resection? *Anesth Analg*. 2010;111(3):660–664.
258. Matot I, Scheinin O, Eid A, et al. Epidural anesthesia and analgesia in liver resection. *Anesth Analg*. 2002;95(5):1179–1181, table of contents.
259. Borromeo CJ, Stix MS, Lally A, et al. Epidural catheter and increased prothrombin time after right lobe hepatectomy for living donor transplantation. *Anesth Analg*. 2000;91(5):1139–1141.
260. Elterman KG and Xiong, Z. Coagulation profile changes and safety of epidural analgesia after hepatectomy: a retrospective study. *J Anesth*. 2015;29(3):367–372.
261. Barton JS, Riha GM, Differding JA, et al. Coagulopathy after a liver resection: is it over diagnosed and over treated? *HPB (Oxford)*. 2013;15(11):865–871.
262. Lee SH, Gwak MS, Choi SJ, et al. Prospective, randomized study of ropivacaine wound infusion versus intrathecal morphine with intravenous fentanyl for analgesia in living donors for liver transplantation. *Liver Transpl*. 2013;19(9):1036–1045.
263. Alghamdi T, Abdel-Fattah M, Zautner A, et al. Preoperative model for end-stage liver disease score as a predictor for posthemihepatectomy complications. *Eur J Gastroenterol Hepatol*. 2014;26(6):668–675.
264. Evans C, Evans M, Pollock AV. The incidence and causes of postoperative jaundice. A prospective study. *Br J Anaesth*. 1974;46(7):520–525.
265. Ebert TJ, Frink EJ, Jr., Kharasch ED. Absence of biochemical evidence for renal and hepatic dysfunction after 8 hours of 1.25 minimum alveolar concentration sevoflurane anesthesia in volunteers. *Anesthesiology*. 1998;88(3):601–610.
266. Ebert TJ, Messana LD, Uhrich TD, et al. Absence of renal and hepatic toxicity after four hours of 1.25 minimum alveolar anesthetic concentration sevoflurane anesthesia in volunteers. *Anesth Analg*. 1998;86(3):662–667.
267. Bito H, Ikeda K. Renal and hepatic function in surgical patients after low-flow sevoflurane or isoflurane anesthesia. *Anesth Analg*. 1996;82(1):173–176.
268. Suttner SW, Schmidt CC, Boldt J, et al. Low-flow desflurane and sevoflurane anesthesia minimally affect hepatic integrity and function in elderly patients. *Anesth Analg*. 2000;91(1):206–212.
269. Gelman SI. Disturbances in hepatic blood flow during anesthesia and surgery. *Arch Surg*. 1976;111(8):881–883.
270. Seltzer JL, Goldberg ME, Larijani GE, et al. Prostacyclin mediation of vasodilation following mesenteric traction. *Anesthesiology*. 1988;68(4):514–518.
271. Belghiti J, Hiramatsu K, Benoist S, et al. Seven hundred forty-seven hepatectomies in the 1990s: An update to evaluate the actual risk of liver resection. *J Am Coll Surg*. 2000;191(1):38–46.
272. Dixon JM, Armstrong CP, Duffy SW, et al. Factors affecting morbidity and mortality after surgery for obstructive jaundice: a review of 373 patients. *Gut*. 1983;24(9):845–852.
273. Wait RB, Kahng KU. Renal failure complicating obstructive jaundice. *Am J Surg*. 1989;157(2):256–263.
274. Kramer HJ. Impaired renal function in obstructive jaundice: roles of the thromboxane and endothelin systems. *Nephron*. 1997;77(1):1–12.
275. Klemperer JD, Ko W, Krieger KH, et al. Cardiac operations in patients with cirrhosis. *Ann Thorac Surg*. 1998;65(1):85–87.
276. Filsoufi F, Salzberg SP, Rahmanian PB, et al. Early and late outcome of cardiac surgery in patients with liver cirrhosis. *Liver Transpl*. 2007;13(7):990–995.
277. Abramov D, Tamariz MG, Fremes SE, et al. Trends in coronary artery bypass surgery results: a recent, 9-year study. *Ann Thorac Surg*. 2000;70(1):84–90.

47 Endocrine Function

JEFFREY J. SCHWARTZ • SHAMSUDDIN AKHTAR • STANLEY H. ROSENBAUM

Thyroid Gland
   Thyroid Metabolism and Function
   Tests of Thyroid Function
   Hyperthyroidism
   Hypothyroidism
Parathyroid Glands
   Calcium Physiology
   Hyperparathyroidism
   Hypoparathyroidism
Adrenal Cortex
   Glucocorticoid Physiology
   Mineralocorticoid Physiology
   Glucocorticoid Excess (Cushing Syndrome)
   Mineralocorticoid Excess
   Adrenal Insufficiency (Addison Disease)
   Exogenous Glucocorticoid Therapy
   Mineralocorticoid Insufficiency

Adrenal Medulla
   Pheochromocytoma
Diabetes Mellitus
   Classification
   Physiology
   Diagnosis
   Treatment
   Anesthetic Management
   Hyperglycemia and Perioperative Outcomes
   Perioperative Glycemic Control
   Glycemic Goals
   Management of Perioperative Hyperglycemia
   Emergencies
Pituitary Gland
   Anterior Pituitary
   Posterior Pituitary
Endocrine Response to Surgical Stress

KEY POINTS

1. The major risk of anesthesia in the poorly controlled thyrotoxic patient is thyroid storm, which must be aggressively treated with β-blockers, iodide, and antithyroid drugs.
2. Asymptomatic or mild hypothyroidism does not appear to significantly increase anesthetic risk and is not a contraindication to surgery. Moderate to severe hypothyroidism should be corrected before surgery to prevent multisystem complications.
3. Patients who have received corticosteroids for more than 1 week in the past year may have adrenal suppression and should receive supplemental steroids in the perioperative period.
4. Preoperative preparation of the pheochromocytoma patient with α-blockers decreases intraoperative hemodynamic instability.
5. Pheochromocytoma manipulation is associated with severe hypertension that should be treated aggressively with nitroprusside, phentolamine, or other rapidly acting vasodilators.
6. The major perioperative risks to the diabetic patient come from coexisting disease, especially coronary artery disease. Coexisting disease must be aggressively sought and optimized.
7. Very tight control of perioperative blood glucose levels appears to increase the risk of hypoglycemic complications without clearly reducing the risk of hyperglycemic complications.
8. Endotracheal intubation may be unpredictably difficult in patients with acromegaly.

Thyroid Gland

The thyroid gland secretes thyroid hormones, thyroxine (T_4) and 3,3′,5-triiodothyronine (T_3), which are the major regulators of cellular metabolic activity. Thyroid hormones exert a variety of actions by regulating the synthesis and activity of various proteins. They are necessary for proper cardiac, pulmonary, and neurologic function during both health and illness.

Thyroid Metabolism and Function

The production of thyroid hormone is initiated by the active uptake and concentration of iodide in the thyroid gland (Fig. 47-1). Dietary iodine is reduced to iodide in the gastrointestinal (GI) tract. Circulating iodide is taken up by the thyroid gland, where it is then bound to tyrosine residues to form various iodotyrosines. After organification, monoiodotyrosine or diiodotyrosine is coupled enzymatically by thyroid peroxidase to form either T_3 or T_4. These hormones are attached to the thyroglobulin protein and stored as colloid in the gland. The release of T_3 and T_4 from the gland is accomplished through proteolysis from the thyroglobulin and diffusion into the circulation. Thyrotropin (thyroid-stimulating hormone [TSH]) is produced in the anterior pituitary gland, and its secretion is regulated by thyrotropin-releasing hormone produced in the hypothalamus. TSH is responsible for maintaining the uptake of iodide and proteolytic release of thyroid hormone. Excess iodide inhibits the synthesis and secretion of thyroid hormone. Circulating thyroid hormone inhibits thyrotropin-releasing hormone and TSH secretion in a negative-feedback loop. The thyroid gland is solely responsible for the daily secretion of T_4 (80 to 100 μg/day). The half-life of T_4 in the circulation is about 7 days.

Approximately 80% of T_3 is produced by the extrathyroidal deiodination of T_4 and 20% is produced by direct thyroid secretion. The half-life of T_3 is 24 to 30 hours. Most of the effects of thyroid hormones are mediated by the more potent and less protein-bound T_3. The degree to which these hormones are

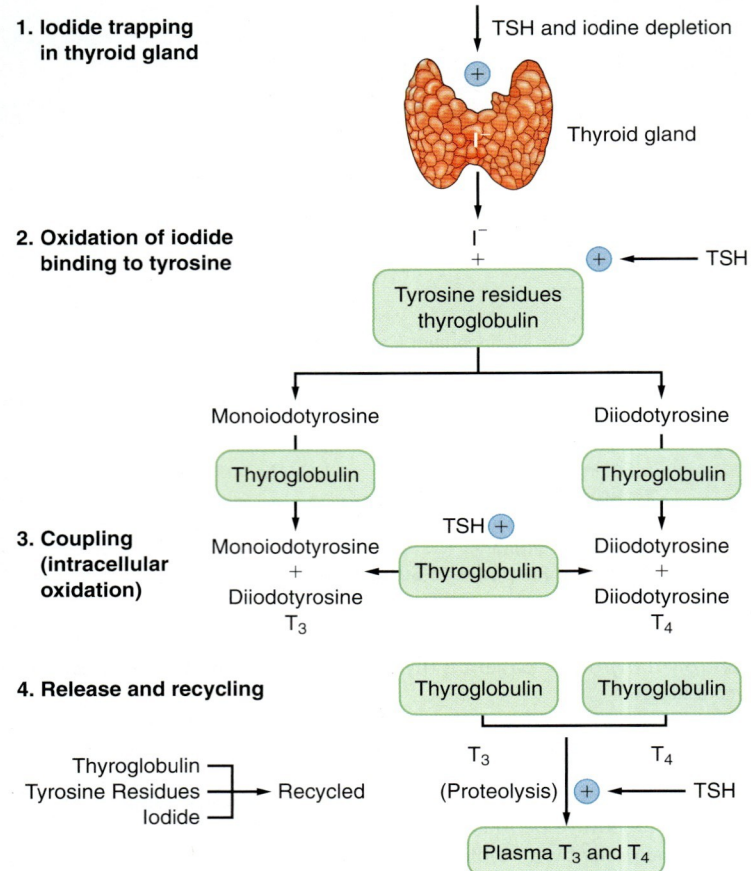

Figure 47-1 Thyroid hormone biosynthesis consists of four stages: (1) organification, (2) binding, (3) coupling, and (4) release. TSH, thyroid-stimulating hormone; T_3, triiodothyronine; T_4, thyroxine.

protein bound in the circulation is the major factor influencing their activity and degradation. T_4 is metabolized by monodeiodination to either T_3 or reverse T_3 (rT_3). T_3 is biologically active, whereas rT_3 is inactive. The major fraction of circulating hormone is bound to thyroxine-binding globulin (TBG), with a smaller fraction bound to albumin and transthyretin. Less than 0.1% is present as free, unbound hormone. Changes in serum-binding protein concentrations have a major effect on total T_3 and T_4 serum concentrations. The plasma normally contains 5 to 12 μg/dL of T_4 and 60 to 180 ng/dL of T_3. Many drugs can affect thyroid function, including amiodarone and dopamine.[1]

Although the thyroid hormone is important to many aspects of growth and function, the anesthesiologist is most often concerned with the cardiovascular manifestations of thyroid disease.[2] Thyroid hormones affect tissue responses to sympathetic stimuli and increase the intrinsic contractile state of cardiac muscle.

β-Adrenergic receptors are increased in number, and cardiac α-adrenergic receptors are decreased by thyroid hormone.[3]

Tests of Thyroid Function

Serum Thyroxine

The serum T_4 assay is a standard test for evaluation of thyroid gland function (Table 47-1). The total T_4 is elevated in approximately 90% of patients with hyperthyroidism, and it is low in 85% of those who are hypothyroid. The concentration of T_4 is measured by radioimmunoassay (RIA). The serum T_4 concentration is influenced by thyroid hormone protein–binding capacity. An increase or decrease in TBG levels or in protein binding may therefore alter the total T_4 but not the concentration of the free T_4. Because of the effect of TBG on circulating total T_4, the T_4 levels should never be used alone to evaluate thyroid disease. Elevations in the TBG concentration are the most common cause of hyperthyroxinemia in euthyroid patients. Increases in TBG due to acute liver disease, pregnancy, or drugs (oral contraceptives, exogenous estrogens, clofibrate, opioids) may be the causative factor. Because a total T_4 can be misleadingly high in euthyroidism or normal in hypothyroidism, some measure of free thyroid hormone activity (free T_4) must also be used.

Serum Triiodothyronine

The serum T_3 is also measured by RIA. Serum T_3 levels are often determined to detect disease in patients with clinical evidence of hyperthyroidism in the absence of elevations of T_4. T_3 may be the only thyroid hormone produced in excess. T_3 concentrations may be depressed by factors that impair the peripheral conversion of T_4 to T_3 (sick euthyroid syndrome). In 50% of hypothyroid patients, the serum T_3 concentration is low; in the remaining 50%, it is normal.

Tests for Assessing Thyroid Hormone Binding

Because conventional assays measure total hormone levels, which can be affected by protein binding without affecting free

Table 47-1 Tests of Thyroid Gland Function

	T$_4$	T$_3$	THBR	TSH
Hyperthyroidism	Elevated	Elevated	Elevated	Normal or low
Primary hypothyroidism	Low	Low or normal	Low	Elevated
Secondary hypothyroidism	Low	Low	Low	Low
Sick euthyroidism (decreased peripheral conversion of T$_4$ to T$_3$)	Normal	Low	Normal	Normal
Pregnancy	Elevated	Normal	Low	Normal

T$_4$, total serum thyroxine; T$_3$, serum triiodothyronine; THBR, thyroid hormone binding rate; TSH, thyroid-stimulating hormone.

hormone levels, it is necessary to correct for thyroid-binding proteins to correctly interpret total thyroxine levels. Most commonly, a direct measurement of unbound T$_3$ and T$_4$ can be performed by free immunoassays. The T$_3$ uptake test measures the ability of the patient's serum to bind exogenously introduced T$_3$ and reflects the amount of TBG and the extent of T$_3$ saturation on TBG. The T$_3$ uptake is inversely related to the degree of unsaturation of TBG. Indirect measurement of free hormone levels can be calculated by multiplying the total hormone level by the thyroid hormone binding ratio, which can be calculated from the T$_3$-resin uptake. This product is the free T$_3$ or T$_4$ index.

Thyroid-stimulating Hormone

The RIA for thyroid-stimulating hormone is sensitive and specific enough to become the first test in evaluating suspected thyroid dysfunction. It is often higher than 20 µIU/mL in primary hypothyroidism (normal 0.4 to 4.5 µIU/mL). Hyperthyroidism can be suspected from depressed TSH levels. A condition characterized by elevated TSH and normal T$_4$ may represent subclinical hypothyroidism. A low TSH level in a clinically hypothyroid patient indicates disease at the pituitary or hypothalamic level. The goal of thyroid replacement therapy is to normalize TSH levels.[3] Starvation, fever, stress, corticosteroids, and T$_3$ or T$_4$ can all depress TSH levels.

Radioactive Iodine Uptake

The thyroid gland has the ability to concentrate large amounts of inorganic iodide. The oral administration of radioactive iodine (^{131}I) can be used to indicate thyroid gland activity. Thyroid uptake is elevated in hyperthyroidism unless the hyperthyroidism is caused by thyroiditis, in which case the uptake is low or absent. Because of overlap in values, it is difficult to distinguish euthyroid from hypothyroid people. Radioactive iodine uptake may be increased by a variety of factors, including dietary iodine deficiency, renal failure, and congestive heart failure. Because uptake is under TSH control, elevated free T$_4$ levels and corticosteroids decrease radioactive iodide uptake. Functioning ("hot") thyroid tissue is rarely malignant. Nonfunctioning ("cold") tissue may be malignant or benign.

Hyperthyroidism

Hyperthyroidism results from the exposure of tissues to excessive amounts of thyroid hormone (Table 47-2). The most common cause is the multinodular diffuse goiter of Graves disease. This typically occurs between the ages of 20 and 40 years and is predominant in women. Most patients with this condition demonstrate a syndrome characterized by diffuse glandular enlargement, ophthalmopathy, dermopathy, and clubbing of the fingers. A thyroid-stimulating autoantibody may be present. Thyroid adenoma is the second most common cause. Another cause of increased thyroid hormone synthesis is thyroiditis. Subacute thyroiditis frequently follows a respiratory illness and is characterized by a viral-like illness with a firm, painful gland. This type of thyroiditis is frequently treated with anti-inflammatory agents alone. Rarely, subacute thyroiditis may occur in a patient with a normal-sized painless gland. Hashimoto thyroiditis is a chronic autoimmune disease that usually produces hypothyroidism but may occasionally produce hyperthyroidism. Hyperthyroidism may also be associated with pregnancy, ^{131}I therapy, thyroid carcinoma, trophoblastic tumors, or TSH-secreting pituitary adenomas. Iatrogenic hyperthyroidism may follow thyroid hormone replacement or may occur after iodide exposure (angiographic contrast media) in patients with chronically low iodide intake (Jod-Basedow phenomenon). The antiarrhythmic agent amiodarone is iodine rich and is another cause of iodine-induced thyrotoxicosis.[4]

The major manifestations of hyperthyroidism are weight loss, diarrhea, skeletal muscle weakness and stiffness, warm and moist skin, heat intolerance, and nervousness. Cardiovascular manifestations include increased left ventricular contractility and ejection fraction, tachycardia, elevated systolic blood pressure, and decreased diastolic blood pressure. Hypercalcemia, thrombocytopenia, and a mild anemia may be present. Elderly patients may present with heart failure, atrial fibrillation, or other cardiac dysrhythmias. They may also present with apathetic

Table 47-2 Causes of Hyperthyroidism

Intrinsic thyroid disease
- Hyperfunctioning thyroid adenoma
- Toxic multinodular goiter

Abnormal TSH stimulator
- Graves disease
- Trophoblastic tumor

Disorders of hormone storage or release
- Thyroiditis

Excess production of thyroid-stimulating hormone
- Pituitary thyrotropin (rare)

Extrathyroidal source of hormone
- Struma ovarii
- Functioning follicular carcinoma

Exogenous thyroid
- Iatrogenic
- Iodine induced

TSH, thyroid-stimulating hormone.

hyperthyroidism characterized by depression and withdrawal, without the usual systemic signs or symptoms.

Treatment and Anesthetic Considerations

The most important goal in managing the hyperthyroid patient is to make the patient euthyroid before any surgery, if possible. The drugs propylthiouracil and methimazole are thiourea derivatives that inhibit organification of iodide and the synthesis of thyroid hormone.[5] Propylthiouracil also decreases the peripheral conversion of T_4 to T_3. Normal thyroid glands usually contain a store of hormone that is large enough to maintain a euthyroid state for several months, even if synthesis is abolished. Therefore, hyperthyroid patients are unlikely to be regulated to a euthyroid state with antithyroid drugs alone in less than 6 to 8 weeks. Toxic reactions from these drugs are uncommon but include skin rash, nausea, fever, agranulocytosis, hepatitis, and arthralgias.

Inorganic iodide inhibits iodide organification and thyroid hormone release—the Wolff–Chaikoff effect. Iodide is also effective in reducing the size and vascularity of the hyperplastic gland and has a role in the preparation of the patient for emergency thyroid surgery. Antithyroid drugs should be started before iodide treatment because of the possibility of worsening the thyrotoxicosis.

β-Adrenergic antagonists are effective in attenuating the manifestations of excessive sympathetic activity and should be used in all hyperthyroid patients unless contraindicated. β-Adrenergic blockade alone does not inhibit hormone synthesis, but specifically propranolol does impair the peripheral conversion of T_4 to T_3 over 1 to 2 weeks. Propranolol given over 12 to 24 hours decreases tachycardia, heat intolerance, anxiety, and tremor. Any β-blocker may be used, and long-acting agents are more convenient. The combination of propranolol (in doses titrated to effect) plus potassium iodide (2 to 5 drops every 8 hours) is frequently used before surgery to ameliorate cardiovascular symptoms and reduce circulating concentrations of T_4 and T_3. Preoperative preparation usually requires 7 to 14 days.

Heart failure secondary to poorly controlled paroxysmal atrial fibrillation may improve with slowing of the ventricular rate, but abnormalities of left ventricular function secondary to hyperthyroidism may not be corrected with the use of β-antagonists. If a hyperthyroid patient with clinically apparent disease requires emergency surgery, β-adrenergic blockade should be administered to achieve a heart rate below 90 beats per minute. β-Blockers do not prevent thyroid storm. Glucocorticoids such as dexamethasone (8 to 12 mg/day) are used in the management of severe thyrotoxicosis because they reduce thyroid hormone secretion and the peripheral conversion of T_4 to T_3.

Radioactive iodine therapy is an effective treatment for some patients with thyrotoxicosis.[6] However, it should not be administered to patients who are pregnant because it crosses the placenta and may destroy the fetal thyroid. A side effect of radioiodine therapy is hypothyroidism; 10% to 60% of cases occur in the first year of therapy and an additional 2% occur per year thereafter.

A variety of anesthetic techniques and drugs have been used for hyperthyroid patients undergoing surgery. All antithyroid medications are continued through the morning of surgery. The goal of intraoperative management in the hyperthyroid patient is to achieve a depth of anesthesia that prevents an exaggerated sympathetic response to surgical stimulation while avoiding the administration of medication that stimulates the sympathetic nervous system. Pancuronium should be avoided. It is best to avoid using ketamine for induction, even when a patient is clinically euthyroid. Hypotension that occurs during surgery is best treated with direct-acting vasopressors rather than a medication

Table 47-3 Management of Thyroid Storm

Administer IV fluids
Administer sodium iodide, 250 mg PO or IV q6h
Administer propylthiouracil, 200–400 mg PO or via NGT q6h
Administer hydrocortisone, 50–100 mg IV q6h
Administer propranolol, 10–40 mg PO q4–6h, or esmolol infusion to treat hyperadrenergic signs
Cooling blankets and acetaminophen and meperidine (25–50 mg) IV q4–6h may be used to prevent shivering
Use digoxin for heart failure especially in the presence of atrial fibrillation with rapid ventricular response

NGT, nasogastric tube.

that provokes the release of catecholamines. The incidence of myasthenia gravis is increased in hyperthyroid patients; thus, the initial dose of muscle relaxant should be reduced and a twitch monitor should be used to titrate subsequent doses. Regional anesthesia is an excellent alternative when appropriate; however, epinephrine-containing solutions should be avoided.

Thyroid storm is a life-threatening exacerbation of hyperthyroidism that most commonly develops in the undiagnosed or untreated hyperthyroid patient because of the stress of surgery or nonthyroid illness.[7] Operating on an acutely hyperthyroid gland may provoke thyroid storm, although this is probably not due to mechanical release of hormone.[8] Its manifestations include hyperthermia, tachycardia, dysrhythmias, myocardial ischemia, congestive heart failure, agitation, and confusion. It must be distinguished from, or considered with, pheochromocytoma, malignant hyperthermia, and light anesthesia. Although free T_4 levels are often markedly elevated, no laboratory test is diagnostic. Treatment involves large doses of propylthiouracil and supportive measures to control fever and restore intravascular volume (Table 47-3). Invasive hemodynamic monitoring is especially useful in guiding the treatment of patients with significant left ventricular dysfunction (Table 47-3). Again, it is essential to remove or treat the precipitating event.

Anesthesia for Thyroid Surgery

Thyroidectomy as an alternative to prolonged medical therapy is used less frequently now than in the past. Indications include failed medical therapy, underlying cancer, and symptomatic goiter. It is usually performed under general endotracheal anesthesia, although the use of the laryngeal mask airway is increasing.[9] Use of a laryngeal mask airway allows real-time visualization of vocal cord function because the patient is allowed to breathe spontaneously. Limited thyroidectomy may also be performed under bilateral superficial cervical plexus block. The anesthesiologist must be prepared to manage an unexpected difficult intubation because the incidence of difficult intubation during goiter surgery is 5% to 8%.[10] Thyroid cancer increases the risk of difficult intubation, but the size of the goiter is not predictive. Large goiters, especially if associated with evidence of significant airway obstruction or tracheal deviation, may warrant securing the airway while the patient is awake. Large substernal goiters can behave as anterior mediastinal masses and cause intrathoracic airway obstruction after induction of general anesthesia. Computed tomography (CT) or magnetic resonance imaging (MRI) should be reviewed. Minimally invasive procedures such as robot-assisted transaxillary[11] and transoral thyroidectomies are beginning to occur. Nasal intubations are required for the transoral approach. The complications after thyroidectomy include recurrent laryngeal nerve (RLN) damage, tracheal compression secondary to hematoma or tracheomalacia, and hypoparathyroidism. Pneumothorax may occur during resection of substernal goiters. Hypoparathyroidism secondary to the inadvertent surgical removal of parathyroid glands is most frequently seen after total thyroidectomy. The symptoms of hypocalcemia develop within 24 to 96 hours after surgery (see Chapter 14).[12] Laryngeal stridor progressing to laryngospasm may be one of the first indications of hypocalcemic tetany. Intravenous (IV) administration of calcium chloride or calcium gluconate is warranted in this situation. Magnesium levels should also be monitored and corrected if low. Bilateral injury is an extremely rare injury and necessitates reintubation. Unilateral nerve injury is more common and is often transient.[13] Unilateral damage to the RLN is characterized by hoarseness and a paralyzed vocal cord, whereas bilateral injury causes aphonia (see Chapter 28). It is wise to evaluate vocal cord function before and after surgery by laryngoscopy or by asking the patient to phonate by saying the sound for "E." Routine postoperative visualization of the vocal cords is not warranted. Some surgeons elect to monitor RLN function intraoperatively. A nerve stimulator may be used by the surgeon to stimulate suspicious structures and contraction of the laryngeal muscles noted. Alternatively, the NIM (Nerve Integrity Monitor; Medtronic Xomed) endotracheal tube can be used. This endotracheal tube has two pairs of electrodes embedded in the shaft of the endotracheal tube just above the cuff. When properly positioned, the electrodes will be in contact with the vocal cords and an electromyographic signal can be monitored. Muscle relaxants and topical laryngeal anesthesia must be avoided to obtain appropriate signals during surgery. Succinylcholine or a small dose of rocuronium can be used to facilitate intubation. Care must be taken that the NIM tube is still positioned properly after the head and neck position have been optimized for surgery.[14] Postoperative extubation of the trachea should be performed under optimal conditions. Intraoperative laryngeal nerve injury or collapse of the tracheal rings from previous weakening may mandate emergency reintubation.

Hypothyroidism

Hypothyroidism is a relatively common disease (0.3% to 5% of the adult population) that results from inadequate circulating levels of T_4, T_3, or both.[15] The development of hypothyroidism is often slow and progressive, making the clinical diagnosis difficult, especially in more subtle cases. Hypofunctioning of the thyroid gland has many causes (Table 47-4). Primary failure of the thyroid gland refers to decreased production of thyroid hormone, despite adequate TSH production, and accounts for 95% of all cases of thyroid dysfunction. The remainder of the cases are caused by either hypothalamic or pituitary disease (secondary hypothyroidism) and are associated with other pituitary deficiencies.

A lack of thyroid hormone produces a variety of signs and symptoms. These early findings are often nonspecific and difficult to recognize. A history of radioiodine therapy, external neck irradiation, or the presence of a goiter is helpful in diagnosis. There is a generalized reduction in metabolic activity resulting in lethargy, slow mental functioning, cold intolerance, and slow movements. The cardiovascular manifestations of hypothyroidism reflect the importance of thyroid hormone for myocardial contractility and catecholamine function. These patients exhibit bradycardia, decreased cardiac output, and increased peripheral resistance.[16] The accumulation of a cholesterol-rich pericardial fluid produces low voltage on the electrocardiogram (ECG). Heart failure only rarely occurs in the absence of coexisting heart disease. Angina pectoris itself is unusual in hypothyroidism but can appear when thyroid hormone treatment is initiated. Ventilatory responsiveness to hypoxia and hypercapnia is depressed in hypothyroid patients. This depression is potentiated by sedatives, opioids, and general anesthesia. Postoperative ventilatory failure requiring prolonged ventilation is rarely seen in hypothyroid patients in the absence of coexisting lung disease, obesity, or myxedema coma. Other abnormalities found in hypothyroidism include anemia, coagulopathy, hypothermia, sleep apnea, and impaired renal free water clearance with hyponatremia. Decreased GI motility can compound the effect of postoperative ileus. In longstanding or severe disease, the stress response may be blunted and adrenal depression may occur.

Treatment and Anesthetic Considerations

Treatment of symptomatic hypothyroidism is with hormone replacement therapy.[17] Controversy remains regarding the preoperative anesthetic management of the hypothyroid patient. Although it seems logical, given the multisystem effects of thyroid hormone, to recommend that all hypothyroid surgical candidates be restored to a euthyroid state before surgery, such a recommendation is, in general, based on individual case reports. There have been few controlled studies to support the position that most hypothyroid patients are unusually sensitive to anesthetic drugs, have prolonged recovery times, or have a higher incidence of cardiovascular instability or collapse.

No increase in serious complications in patients with mild or moderate hypothyroidism undergoing general anesthesia has been noted.[18] One study noted a higher incidence of intraoperative hypotension and postoperative GI and neuropsychiatric complications in mild and moderately hypothyroid patients undergoing noncardiac surgery, but still noted there were no compelling clinical reasons to postpone surgery in these patients.[19] Surgery in severely hypothyroid patients should be postponed when possible until these patients are at least partially treated.

The management of hypothyroid patients with symptomatic coronary artery disease has been a subject of particular controversy.[20] The need for thyroid hormone replacement therapy must be weighed against the risk of precipitating myocardial ischemia. Several studies and a literature review found no differences in the frequency of intraoperative or postoperative complications when mild or moderately hypothyroid patients underwent cardiac surgery. In symptomatic patients or unstable patients with cardiac ischemia, thyroid replacement should probably be delayed until after coronary revascularization.

Table 47-4 Causes of Hypothyroidism

Primary hypothyroidism
- Autoimmune
- Irradiation to the neck
- Previous ^{131}I therapy
- Surgical removal
- Thyroiditis (Hashimoto disease)
- Severe iodine depletion
- Medications (iodines, propylthiouracil, methimazole)
- Hereditary defects in biosynthesis
- Congenital defects in gland development

Secondary or tertiary hypothyroidism
- Pituitary
- Hypothalamic

Adapted from Petersdorf RG, ed. *Harrison's Principles of Internal Medicine.* 10th ed. New York, NY: McGraw-Hill; 1983.

Table 47-5 Management of Myxedema
Tracheal intubation and controlled ventilation as needed
Levothyroxine, 200–300 µg IV over 5–10 min initially, and 100 µg IV q24h
Hydrocortisone, 100 mg IV, then 25 mg IV q6h
Fluid and electrolyte therapy as indicated by serum electrolytes
Cover to conserve body heat; no warming blankets

IV, intravenous(ly).

There appears to be little reason to postpone surgery in patients who have mild or moderate hypothyroidism. However, thyroid replacement therapy is indicated for patients with severe hypothyroidism or myxedema coma and for pregnant patients who are hypothyroid. Untreated hypothyroidism in pregnant patients is associated with an increased incidence of spontaneous abortion and mental and physical abnormalities in the offspring.

A number of anesthetic medications have been used without difficulty in hypothyroid patients. Although ketamine has been proposed as the ideal induction agents, all IV induction agents have been used in the hypothyroid patient. The maintenance of anesthesia may be safely achieved with either IV or inhaled anesthetics. There appears to be little, if any, decrease in the minimum alveolar concentration for volatile agents. Regional anesthesia is a good choice in the hypothyroid patient, provided the intravascular volume is well maintained. Monitoring is directed toward the early recognition of hypotension, congestive heart failure, or hypothermia. Scrupulous attention should be paid to maintaining normal body temperature.

Myxedema coma represents a severe form of hypothyroidism characterized by stupor or coma, hypoventilation, hypothermia, hypotension, and hyponatremia. This is a medical emergency with a high mortality rate (25% to 50%) and, as such, requires aggressive therapy (Table 47-5). Only lifesaving surgery should proceed in the face of myxedema coma. IV thyroid replacement is initiated as soon as the clinical diagnosis is made. An IV loading dose of T_4 (sodium levothyroxine, 200 to 300 µg) is given initially and followed by a maintenance dose of T_4, 50 to 200 µg/day intravenously.[21] Alternatively, T_3 may be used because it has a more rapid onset. Improvements in heart rate, blood pressure, and body temperature may occur within 24 hours. However, replacement therapy with either form of thyroid hormone may precipitate myocardial ischemia. There is also an increased likelihood of acute primary adrenal insufficiency in these patients, and they should receive stress doses of hydrocortisone. Steroid replacement continues until normal adrenal function can be confirmed.

Parathyroid Glands

Calcium Physiology

The normal adult body contains approximately 1 to 2 kg of calcium (Ca^{2+}), of which 99% is in the skeleton.[22] Plasma calcium is present in three forms: (a) a protein-bound fraction (50%), (b) an ionized fraction (45%), and (c) a diffusible but nonionized fraction (5%) that is complexed with phosphate, bicarbonate, and citrate (see Chapter 14). This division is interesting because it is the ionized fraction that is physiologically active and homeostatically regulated. The normal total serum calcium concentration is 8.8 to 10.4 mg/dL. Albumin binds approximately 90% of the protein-bound fraction of calcium, and total serum Ca^{2+} consequently depends on albumin levels. In general, an increase or decrease in albumin of 1 g/dL is associated with a parallel change in total serum Ca^{2+} of 0.8 mg/dL. The serum ionized Ca^{2+} concentration is affected by temperature and blood pH through alterations in Ca^{2+} protein binding to albumin. Acidosis decreases protein binding (increases ionized Ca^{2+}), and alkalosis increases protein binding (decreases ionized Ca^{2+}). The concentration of free Ca^{2+} ion is of critical importance in regulating skeletal muscle contraction, coagulation, neurotransmitter release, endocrine secretion, and a variety of other cellular functions. As a consequence, the maintenance of serum Ca^{2+} concentration is subject to tight hormonal control by parathyroid hormone (PTH) and vitamin D (Fig. 47-2).

PTH acts to maintain the extracellular fluid Ca^{2+} concentration through direct effects on bone resorption and renal Ca^{2+} resorption at the distal tubule and indirectly through its effects on the synthesis of 1,25-dihydroxyvitamin D. The renal effects of PTH include phosphaturia and bicarbonaturia, in addition to enhanced Ca^{2+} and magnesium resorption. Most evidence suggests that rapid changes in blood Ca^{2+} levels are primarily the result of hormonal effects on bone and, to a lesser extent, on renal Ca^{2+} clearance, whereas maintenance of overall Ca^{2+} balance depends more on the indirect effects of the hormone on intestinal calcium absorption.

PTH secretion is primarily regulated by the serum ionized Ca^{2+} concentration. This negative-feedback mechanism is exquisitely sensitive in maintaining calcium levels in a normal range. Release of PTH is also influenced by phosphate, magnesium, and catecholamine levels. Acute hypomagnesemia directly stimulates PTH release, whereas chronic magnesium depletion appears to inhibit proper functioning of the parathyroid gland. The plasma phosphate concentration has an indirect influence on PTH secretion by causing reciprocal changes in the serum ionized Ca^{2+} concentration.

Vitamin D is absorbed from the GI tract and can be produced enzymatically by ultraviolet irradiation of the skin. Vitamin D (cholecalciferol) is made from cholesterol metabolites and is inactive. Calciferol is hydroxylated in the liver to 25-hydroxycholecalciferol (25-OHD) and in the kidney is further hydroxylated to 1,25-dihydroxycholecalciferol [$1,25(OH)_2D$] or 24,25-dihydroxycholecalciferol [$24,25(OH)_2D$]. 25-OHD is the major circulating form of vitamin D. The synthesis of this form is not regulated by a hormone or by Ca^{2+} or phosphate levels. $1,25(OH)_2D$ and $24,25(OH)_2D$ are the major active metabolites of vitamin D, and their production is reciprocally regulated at the kidney. Hypocalcemia and hypophosphatemia cause an increased production of $1,25(OH)_2D$ and a decreased production of $24,25(OH)_2D$. $1,25(OH)_2D$ stimulates bone, kidney, and intestinal absorption of calcium and phosphate. Vitamin D deficiency can lead to decreased intestinal absorption of Ca^{2+} and secondary hyperparathyroidism.

Hyperparathyroidism

Primary hyperparathyroidism is most commonly due to a benign parathyroid adenoma (90% of cases) or hyperplasia (9%) and very rarely to a parathyroid carcinoma.[23] Primary hyperparathyroidism may also exist as part of a multiple endocrine neoplastic (MEN) syndrome. Hyperplasia usually involves all four glands. Although most patients with primary hyperparathyroidism are hypercalcemic, most are asymptomatic at the time of diagnosis. When symptoms occur, they usually result from the hypercalcemia that accompanies the disease. Primary hyperparathyroidism occurring during pregnancy is associated with a high maternal and fetal morbidity rate (50%). The placenta allows the fetus to concentrate

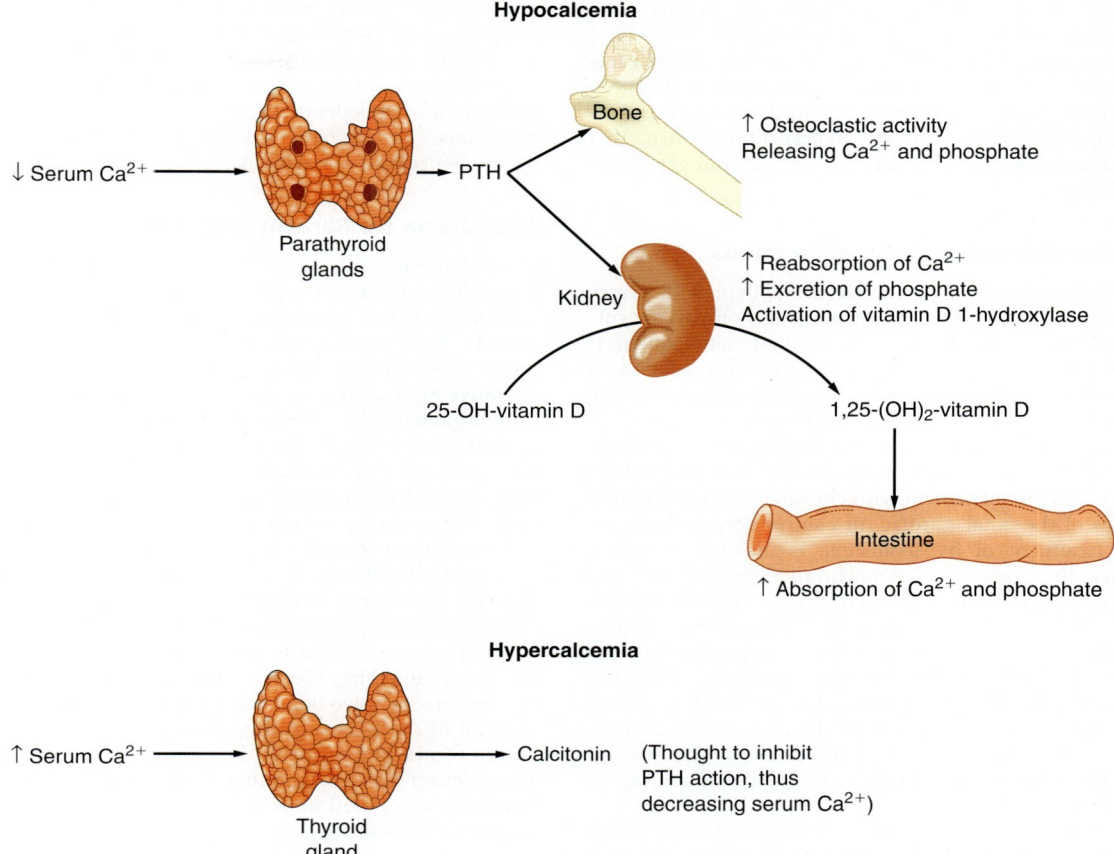

Figure 47-2 Parathyroid hormone (PTH) and vitamin D metabolism and action. 25-OH, 25-hydroxycholecalciferol; 1,25-(OH)$_2$, 1,25-dihydroxycholecalciferol. (Reprinted with permission from McClatchey KD. *Clinical Laboratory Medicine*. 2nd ed. Philadelphia, PA: Lippincott Williams & Wilkins; 2002.)

calcium, promoting fetal hypercalcemia and leading to hypoparathyroidism in the newborn. Pregnant women with primary hyperparathyroidism should generally be treated with surgery.

Hypercalcemia is responsible for a broad spectrum of signs and symptoms. Nephrolithiasis is the most common manifestation, occurring in 60% to 70% of patients. Polyuria and polydipsia are also common complaints. An increase in bone turnover may lead to generalized demineralization and subperiosteal bone resorption; however, only a small group of patients (10% to 15%) have clinically significant bone disease. Patients may experience generalized skeletal muscle weakness and fatigability, epigastric discomfort, peptic ulceration, or constipation. Psychiatric manifestations include depression, memory loss, confusion, or psychosis. Between 20% and 50% of patients are hypertensive, but this usually resolves with successful treatment of the disease. Cardiac function is enhanced in the early stages of hypercalcemia. Calcium flux into the cells is reflected in the plateau phase of the action potential (phase 2). As extracellular calcium increases, the inward flux is more rapid, and phase 2 is shortened (see Chapter 12). The corresponding ECG change is a shorter QT interval. Cardiac contractility may increase until a level between 15 and 20 mg/dL is reached. At this point, there is a prolongation of the PR segment and QRS complex that can result in heart block or bundle-branch block. Bradycardia also occurs.

An elevated serum Ca^{2+} concentration is a valuable diagnostic indicator of primary hyperparathyroidism. The serum phosphate concentration is nonspecific, with many patients having normal or near-normal levels. The reported incidence of hyperchloremic acidosis varies widely in primary hyperparathyroidism, but most patients usually have a serum chloride concentration in excess of 102 mEq/L. Rarely does a patient with hypercalcemia secondary to ectopic PTH production (malignancy) present with hyperchloremic acidosis. The definitive diagnosis of primary hyperparathyroidism is made by RIA demonstration of an elevation in PTH levels in the presence of hypercalcemia. An elevated nephrogenous cyclic adenosine monophosphate is noted in over 90% of patients with primary hyperparathyroidism.

Hypercalcemia may also result from the ectopic production of PTH or PTH-like substances from lung, genitourinary, breast, GI, or lymphoproliferative malignancies. Tumors may also produce hypercalcemia through direct bone resorption or the production of osteoclast-activating factor. In the absence of a clinically obvious neoplasm, there may be difficulty in differentiating between PTH-producing malignancies and primary hyperparathyroidism. PTH fragments from malignant tissue differ from native PTH, so precise laboratory identification may aid in distinguishing between ectopic PTH production and primary hyperparathyroidism.

Secondary hyperparathyroidism represents an increase in parathyroid function as a result of conditions that produce hypocalcemia or hyperphosphatemia. Chronic renal disease is a common cause of hyperphosphatemia (due to decreased phosphate excretion) and decreased vitamin D metabolism. The hypocalcemia that results leads to an increased production of PTH. GI disorders accompanied by malabsorption may also lead to a secondary increase in parathyroid activity. Tertiary hyperparathyroidism refers to the development of hypercalcemia in a patient who has had prolonged secondary hyperparathyroidism that has caused adenomatous changes in the parathyroid gland and unregulated PTH.

Treatment and Anesthetic Considerations

Surgery is the treatment of choice for the patient with symptomatic disease. However, there is considerable controversy surrounding the choice of treatment in the asymptomatic patient. It is not clear whether mild primary hyperparathyroidism decreases longevity. Surgery is often chosen over medical therapy because it offers definitive treatment and is generally safe.

Preoperative preparation focuses on the correction of intravascular volume and electrolyte irregularities. It is particularly important to evaluate the patient with chronic hypercalcemia for abnormalities of the renal, cardiac, or central nervous systems. Emergency treatment of hypercalcemia is undertaken before surgery when the serum Ca^{2+} concentration exceeds 15 mg/dL (7.5 mEq/L). Lowering of the serum Ca^{2+} concentration is initially accomplished by expanding the intravascular volume and establishing a sodium diuresis. This is achieved with the IV administration of normal saline and furosemide. Rehydration alone is capable of lowering the serum Ca^{2+} level by at least 2 mg/dL. Hydration dilutes the serum Ca^{2+}, and sodium diuresis promotes Ca^{2+} excretion through an inhibition of sodium and Ca^{2+} resorption in the proximal tubule. Hypokalemia and hypomagnesemia may result.

Another element in the treatment of hypercalcemia is the correction of hypophosphatemia. Hypophosphatemia increases GI absorption of Ca^{2+}, stimulates the breakdown of bone, and impairs the uptake of Ca^{2+} by bone. Low serum phosphate levels impair cardiac contractility and may contribute to congestive heart failure. Hypophosphatemia also causes skeletal muscle weakness, hemolysis, and platelet dysfunction.

Other medications that have a role in lowering the serum Ca^{2+} include bisphosphonates, mithramycin, calcitonin, and glucocorticoids. Bisphosphonates are pyrophosphate analogs that inhibit osteoclast action. They are the drugs of choice for severe hypercalcemia. Toxic effects include fever and hypophosphatemia. Mithramycin, a cytotoxic agent, inhibits PTH-induced osteoclast activity and can lower the serum Ca^{2+} levels by at least 2 mg/dL in 24 to 48 hours. Toxic effects include azotemia, hepatotoxicity, and thrombocytopenia. Calcitonin is useful in transiently lowering the serum Ca^{2+} level 2 to 4 mg/dL through direct inhibition of osteoclastic bone resorption. The advantages of calcitonin are the mild side effects (urticaria, nausea) and the rapid onset of activity. Calcitonin resistance usually develops within 24 to 48 hours. Glucocorticoids are effective in lowering the serum Ca^{2+} concentration in several conditions (sarcoidosis, some malignancies, hyperthyroidism, vitamin D intoxication) through their actions on osteoclast bone resorption, GI absorption of calcium, and the urinary excretion of calcium. Glucocorticoids are usually of no benefit in the treatment of primary hypercalcemia. Finally, hemodialysis or peritoneal dialysis can be used to lower the serum Ca^{2+} level when alternative regimens are ineffective or contraindicated.

There is no evidence that a specific anesthetic drug or technique has advantages over another. A thorough knowledge of the clinical manifestations attributable to hypercalcemia is of the greatest value in choosing an anesthetic technique. Special monitoring is usually not required. Because of the unpredictable response to neuromuscular-blocking drugs in the hypercalcemic patient, a conservative approach to muscle paralysis makes sense. There is an increased requirement for vecuronium, and probably all nondepolarizing muscle relaxants, during onset of neuromuscular blockade.[24] Careful positioning of the osteopenic patient is necessary to avoid pathologic bone fractures.

Anesthesia for Parathyroid Surgery

General anesthesia is most commonly used for parathyroid surgery. Minimally invasive parathyroidectomy is superior to conventional bilateral cervical exploration in patients with sporadic primary hyperparathyroidism[25] and can usually be performed under bilateral cervical plexus block.[26] Some centers use an intraoperative rapid PTH assay to help determine when a hyperfunctioning gland has been removed. A freely back-flowing IV catheter is needed for frequent sampling. There is in vitro, but no clinical,[27] evidence that propofol can interfere with the assay, so many surgeons prefer that propofol not be used within 15 minutes of an assay. Postoperative complications include RLN injury, bleeding, and transient or complete hypoparathyroidism. Unilateral RLN is characterized by hoarseness and usually requires no intervention. Bilateral RLN injury is a rare complication, producing aphonia and requiring immediate tracheal intubation.

After successful parathyroidectomy, a decrease in the serum Ca^{2+} level should be observed within 24 hours. Patients with significant preoperative bone disease may have hypocalcemia after removal of the PTH-secreting glands. This "hungry bone" syndrome comes as a result of the rapid remineralization of bone. Thus, serum Ca^{2+}, magnesium, and phosphorus levels should be closely monitored until stable. The serum Ca^{2+} nadir usually occurs within 3 to 7 days.

Hypoparathyroidism

An underproduction of PTH or resistance of the end-organ tissues to PTH results in hypocalcemia (<8 mg/dL).[28] The normal physiologic response to hypocalcemia is an increase in PTH secretion and $1,25(OH)_2D$ synthesis, with an increase in Ca^{2+} mobilization from bone, GI absorption, and renal tubule reclamation. The most common cause of acquired PTH deficiency is unintentional removal of the parathyroid glands during thyroid or parathyroid surgery. Other causes of acquired hypoparathyroidism include ^{131}I therapy for thyroid disease, neck trauma, granulomatous disease, or an infiltrating process (malignancy or amyloidosis). Severe hypomagnesemia (<0.8 mEq/L) from any cause can produce hypocalcemia by suppressing PTH secretion and interfering with PTH action. Renal insufficiency leads to phosphorus retention and impaired $1,25(OH)_2D$ synthesis, which results in hypocalcemia. These patients are commonly treated with vitamin D, which increases intestinal calcium absorption and suppresses secondary increases in PTH secretion. Hypocalcemia due to pancreatitis and burns results from the suppression of PTH and from the sequestration of calcium.

Clinical Features and Treatment

The clinical features of hypoparathyroidism are a manifestation of hypocalcemia. Neuronal irritability and skeletal muscle spasms, tetany, or seizures reflect a reduced threshold of excitation. Latent tetany may be demonstrated by eliciting the Chvostek or Trousseau sign. A Chvostek sign is a contracture of the facial muscle produced by tapping the facial nerve as it passes through the parotid gland. A Trousseau sign is a contraction of the fingers and wrist after application of a blood pressure cuff inflated above the systolic blood pressure for approximately 3 minutes. Other common complaints of hypocalcemia include fatigue, depression, paresthesias, and skeletal muscle cramps. The acute onset of hypocalcemia after thyroid or parathyroid surgery may manifest as stridor and apnea. Cardiovascular manifestations of hypocalcemia include congestive heart failure, hypotension, and a relative insensitivity to the effects of β-adrenergic agonists (see Chapter 12). Delayed ventricular repolarization results in a prolonged QT interval on the ECG. Although prolongation of the QT interval may be a reliable sign of hypocalcemia in an individual patient, the ECG is relatively insensitive for the detection of hypocalcemia.

The treatment of hypoparathyroidism consists of electrolyte replacement. The objective is to have the patient's clinical symptoms under control before anesthesia and surgery. Hypocalcemia caused by magnesium depletion is treated by correcting the magnesium deficit. Serum phosphate excess is corrected by the removal of phosphate from the diet and the oral administration of phosphate-binding resins (aluminum hydroxide). The urinary excretion of phosphate can be increased with a saline volume infusion. Ca^{2+} deficiencies are corrected with Ca^{2+} supplements or vitamin D analogs. Patients with severe symptomatic hypocalcemia are treated with IV calcium gluconate (10 to 20 mL of 10% solution) given over several minutes and followed by a continuous infusion (1 to 2 mg/kg/hr) of elemental Ca^{2+}. The correction of serum Ca^{2+} levels should be monitored by measuring serum Ca^{2+} concentrations and following clinical symptoms. When oral or IV calcium is inadequate to maintain a normal serum–ionized calcium level, vitamin D is added to the regimen.

Adrenal Cortex

The adrenal cortex functions to synthesize and secrete three types of hormones. Endogenous and dietary cholesterol is used in the adrenal biosynthesis of glucocorticoids (cortisol), mineralocorticoids (aldosterone and 11-deoxycorticosterone), and androgens (dehydroepiandrosterone). Cortisol and aldosterone are the two essential hormones, whereas adrenal androgens are of relatively minor physiologic significance in adults. The major biologic effects of adrenal cortical hyperfunction or hypofunction occur as a result of cortisol or aldosterone excess or deficiency. Abnormal function of the adrenal cortex may render a patient unable to respond appropriately during a period of surgical stress or critical illness.

Glucocorticoid Physiology

Cortisol (hydrocortisone) is the most potent endogenous glucocorticoid and is produced by the inner portions of the adrenal cortex. Cortisol is produced under the control of adrenocorticotropic hormone (ACTH; corticotropin), a polypeptide synthesized and released by the anterior pituitary gland. Glucocorticoids exert their biologic effects by diffusing into the cytoplasm of target cells and combining with specific high-affinity receptor proteins.

The daily production of endogenous cortisol is approximately 20 mg. The maximal output is 150 to 300 mg. Most of the circulating hormone is bound to the α-globulin cortisol-binding globulin. It is the relatively small amount of free hormone that exerts the biologic effects. Endogenous glucocorticoids are inactivated primarily by the liver and are excreted in the urine as 17-hydroxycorticosteroids. Cortisol is also filtered at the glomerulus and may be excreted unchanged in the urine. Although the rate of cortisol secretion is decreased by approximately 30% in the elderly patient, plasma cortisol levels remain in a normal range because of a corresponding decrease in hepatic and renal clearance.

Cortisol secretion is directly controlled by ACTH, which in turn is regulated by the corticotropin-releasing factor from the hypothalamus. ACTH is synthesized in the pituitary gland from a precursor molecule that also produces β-lipotropin and β-endorphin. The secretion of ACTH and corticotropin-releasing factor is governed chiefly by glucocorticoids, the sleep–wake cycle, and stress. Cortisol is the most potent regulator of ACTH secretion, acting by a negative-feedback mechanism to maintain cortisol levels in a physiologic range. ACTH release follows a diurnal pattern, with maximal activity occurring soon after awakening. This diurnal pattern of activity occurs in normal subjects and in those with adrenal insufficiency. Psychological or physical stress (trauma, surgery, intense exercise) also promotes ACTH release, regardless of the level of circulating cortisol or the time of day.

Cortisol has multiple effects on intermediate carbohydrate, protein, and fatty acid metabolism, as well as maintenance and regulation of immune and circulatory function. Glucocorticoids enhance gluconeogenesis, elevate blood glucose, and promote hepatic glycogen synthesis. The catabolic effect of glucocorticoids is partially blocked by insulin. The net effect on protein metabolism is enhanced degradation of muscle tissue and negative nitrogen balance. In supraphysiologic amounts, glucocorticoids suppress growth hormone secretion and impair somatic growth. The anti-inflammatory actions of cortisol relate to its effect in stabilizing lysosomes and promoting capillary integrity. Cortisol also antagonizes leukocyte migration inhibition factor, thus reducing white cell adherence to vascular endothelium and diminishing leukocyte response to local inflammation. Phagocytic activity does not decrease, although the killing potential of macrophages and monocytes is diminished. Other diverse actions include the facilitation of free water clearance, maintenance of blood pressure, a weak mineralocorticoid effect, promotion of appetite, stimulation of hematopoiesis, and induction of liver enzymes.

Mineralocorticoid Physiology

Aldosterone is the most potent mineralocorticoid produced by the adrenal gland. This hormone binds to receptors in sweat glands, the alimentary tract, and the distal convoluted tubule of the kidney. Aldosterone is a major regulator of extracellular volume and potassium homeostasis through the resorption of sodium and the secretion of potassium by these tissues. The major regulators of aldosterone release are the renin–angiotensin system and serum potassium levels (Fig. 47-3). The juxtaglomerular apparatus that surrounds the renal afferent arterioles produces renin in response to decreased perfusion pressures and sympathetic stimulation. Renin splits the hepatic precursor angiotensinogen to form the decapeptide angiotensin I, which is then altered enzymatically by converting enzyme (primarily in the lung) to form the octapeptide angiotensin II. Angiotensin II is the most potent vasopressor produced in the body. It directly stimulates the adrenal cortex to produce aldosterone. The renin–angiotensin system is the body's most important protector of volume status. Other stimuli that increase the production of aldosterone include hyperkalemia and, to a limited degree, hyponatremia, prostaglandin E, and ACTH.

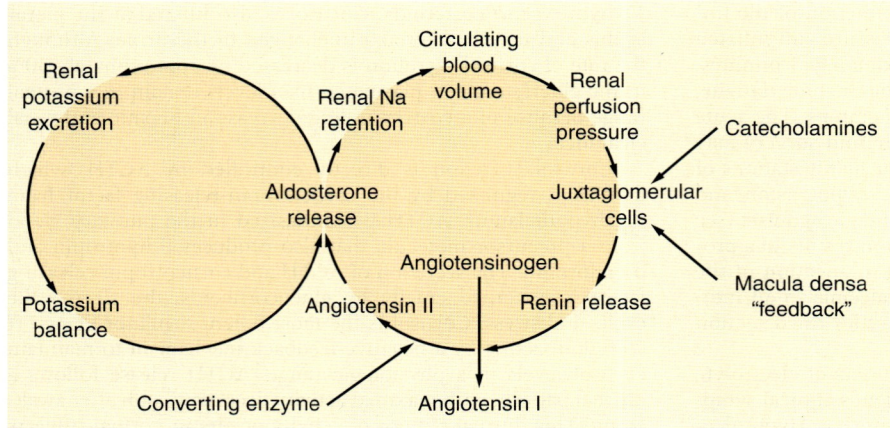

Figure 47-3 Interrelationship of the volume and potassium feedback loops on aldosterone secretion. (Adapted from Petersdorf RG, ed. *Harrison's Principles of Internal Medicine*. 10th ed. New York, NY: McGraw-Hill; 1983.)

Glucocorticoid Excess (Cushing Syndrome)

Cushing syndrome, caused by either overproduction of cortisol by the adrenal cortex or exogenous glucocorticoid therapy, is a syndrome characterized by truncal obesity, hypertension, hyperglycemia, increased intravascular fluid volume, hypokalemia, fatigability, abdominal striae, osteoporosis, and muscle weakness. Most cases of Cushing syndrome that occur spontaneously are due to bilateral adrenal hyperplasia secondary to ACTH produced by an anterior pituitary microadenoma or nonendocrine tumor (e.g., of the lung, kidney, or pancreas) (see Chapter 37). The primary overproduction of cortisol and other adrenal steroids is caused by an adrenal neoplasm in approximately 20% to 25% of patients with Cushing syndrome. These tumors are usually unilateral and approximately half are malignant. When Cushing syndrome occurs in patients older than 60 years of age, the most likely cause is an adrenal carcinoma or ectopic ACTH produced from a nonendocrine tumor. Finally, an increasingly common cause of Cushing syndrome is the prolonged administration of exogenous glucocorticoids to treat a variety of illnesses.

The signs and symptoms of Cushing syndrome follow from the known actions of glucocorticoids. Truncal obesity and thin extremities reflect increased muscle wasting and a redistribution of fat in facial, cervical, and truncal areas. Impaired calcium absorption and a decrease in bone formation may result in osteopenia. Sixty percent of patients have hyperglycemia, but overt diabetes mellitus (DM) occurs in less than 20%. Hypertension and fluid retention are seen in most patients. Profound emotional changes, ranging from emotional lability to frank psychosis, may be present. An increased susceptibility to infection reflects the immunosuppressive effects of corticosteroids. Hypokalemic alkalosis without distinctive physical findings is common when adrenal hyperplasia is caused by ectopic ACTH production from a nonendocrine tumor.

The laboratory diagnosis of hyperadrenocorticism is based on a variable elevation in plasma and urinary cortisol levels, urinary 17-hydroxycorticosteroids, and plasma ACTH. Once the diagnosis is established, simultaneous measurement of plasma ACTH and cortisol levels can determine whether the Cushing syndrome is due to primary pituitary or adrenal disease.[29]

Alternatively, a dexamethasone suppression test can be used. Patients with pituitary adenomas frequently show depression in cortisol and 17-hydroxycorticosteroid levels when a high dose of dexamethasone is administered because the tumor retains some negative-feedback control, and adrenal tumors do not.

Anesthetic Management

General considerations for the preoperative preparation of the patient include treating hypertension, diabetes, and normalizing intravascular fluid volume and electrolyte concentrations. Diuresis with the aldosterone antagonist spironolactone helps mobilize fluid and normalize potassium concentration. Careful positioning of the osteopenic patient is important to avoid fractures. Intraoperative monitoring is planned after evaluation of the patient's cardiac reserve and consideration of the site and extent of the proposed surgery. When either unilateral or bilateral adrenalectomy is planned, glucocorticoid replacement therapy is initiated at a dose equal to full replacement of adrenal output during periods of extreme stress (see Steroid Replacement during the Perioperative Period). The total dosage is reduced by approximately 50% per day until a daily maintenance dose of steroids is achieved (20 to 30 mg/day). Hydrocortisone given in doses of this magnitude exerts significant mineralocorticoid activity, and additional exogenous mineralocorticoid is usually not necessary during the perioperative period. After bilateral adrenalectomy, most patients require 0.05 to 0.1 mg/day of fludrocortisone (9-α-fluorohydrocortisone) starting around day 5 to provide mineralocorticoid activity. Slightly higher doses may be needed if prednisone is used for glucocorticoid maintenance because it has little intrinsic mineralocorticoid activity. The fludrocortisone dose is reduced if congestive heart failure, hypokalemia, or hypertension develops. For the patient with a solitary adrenal adenoma, unilateral adrenalectomy may be followed by normalization of function in the contralateral gland over time. Treatment plans should therefore be individualized and adjustments in dosage may be necessary. The production of glucocorticoids or ACTH by a neoplasm may not be eliminated if the tumor is unresectable. These patients often need continuous medical therapy with steroid inhibitors such as metyrapone to control their symptoms.

There are no specific recommendations regarding the use of a particular anesthetic technique or medication in patients with hyperadrenocorticism. When significant skeletal muscle weakness is present, a conservative approach to the use of muscle relaxants is warranted. Etomidate has been used for temporizing medical treatment of severe Cushing syndrome because of its inhibition of steroid synthesis.

Mineralocorticoid Excess

Hypersecretion of the major adrenal mineralocorticoid aldosterone increases the renal tubular exchange of sodium for potassium and hydrogen ions. This leads to hypertension, hypokalemic alkalosis, skeletal muscle weakness, and fatigue. Possibly as many as 1% of unselected hypertensive patients have primary hyperaldosteronism. The increase in renal sodium reabsorption and extracellular volume expansion is partly responsible for the high incidence of diastolic hypertension in these patients. Patients with primary hyperaldosteronism (Conn syndrome) characteristically do not have edema. Secondary aldosteronism results from an elevation in renin production. The diagnosis of primary or secondary hyperaldosteronism should be entertained in the nonedematous hypertensive patient with persistent hypokalemia who is not receiving potassium-wasting diuretics. Hyposecretion of renin that fails to increase appropriately during volume depletion or salt restriction is an important finding in primary aldosteronism. The measurement of plasma renin levels is useful in distinguishing primary from secondary hyperaldosteronism. It is of limited value in differentiating patients with primary aldosteronism from those with other causes of hypertension because renin activity is also suppressed in approximately 25% of patients with essential hypertension.

Anesthetic Considerations

Preoperative preparation for the patient with primary aldosteronism is directed toward restoring the intravascular volume and the electrolyte concentrations to normal. Hypertension and hypokalemia may be controlled by restricting sodium intake and administration of the aldosterone antagonist spironolactone. This diuretic works slowly to produce an increase in potassium levels, with dosages in the range of 25 to 100 mg every 8 hours. Total-body potassium deficits are difficult to estimate and may be in excess of 300 mEq. Whenever possible, potassium should be replaced slowly to allow equilibration between intracellular and extracellular potassium stores. The usual complications of chronic hypertension need to be assessed.

Adrenal Insufficiency (Addison Disease)

The undersecretion of adrenal steroid hormones may develop as the result of a primary inability of the adrenal gland to elaborate sufficient quantities of hormone or as the result of a deficiency in the production of ACTH.

Clinically, primary adrenal insufficiency is usually not apparent until at least 90% of the adrenal cortex has been destroyed. The predominant cause of primary adrenal insufficiency used to be tuberculosis; however, today, the most frequent cause of Addison disease is idiopathic adrenal insufficiency secondary to autoimmune destruction of the gland. Autoimmune destruction of the adrenal cortex causes both a glucocorticoid and a mineralocorticoid deficiency. A variety of other conditions presumed to have an autoimmune pathogenesis may also occur concomitantly with idiopathic Addison disease. Hashimoto thyroiditis in association with autoimmune adrenal insufficiency is termed Schmidt syndrome. Other possible causes of adrenal gland destruction include certain bacterial, fungal, and advanced human immunodeficiency virus infections; metastatic cancer; sepsis; and hemorrhage. Secondary adrenal insufficiency occurs when the anterior pituitary fails to secrete sufficient quantities of ACTH. Pituitary failure may result from tumor, infection, surgical ablation, or radiation therapy. Pituitary surgery may cause transient adrenal insufficiency requiring supplemental glucocorticoids.[30]

Patients receiving chronic corticosteroid therapy will not generally have frank adrenal insufficiency, but may have hypothalamic–pituitary–adrenal (HPA) suppression and may develop acute adrenal insufficiency during the stress of the perioperative period. Relative adrenal insufficiency is a common finding in critically ill surgical patients with hypotension requiring vasopressors.[31] Therefore, a patient with signs of chronic glucocorticoid excess can have findings of acute adrenal insufficiency.

Clinical Presentation

The cardinal symptoms of idiopathic Addison disease include chronic fatigue, muscle weakness, anorexia, weight loss, nausea, vomiting, and diarrhea. Hypotension is almost always encountered in the disease process. Female patients may exhibit decreased axillary and pubic hair growth because of the loss of adrenal androgen secretion. An acute crisis can present as abdominal pain, severe vomiting and diarrhea, hypotension, decreased consciousness, and shock. Diffuse hyperpigmentation occurs in most patients with primary adrenal insufficiency and is secondary to the compensatory increase in ACTH and β-lipotropin. These hormones stimulate an increase in melanocyte production. Mineralocorticoid deficiency is characteristically present in primary adrenal disease; as a result, there is a reduction in urine sodium conservation. Hyperkalemia may be a cause of life-threatening cardiac dysrhythmias. Adrenal insufficiency secondary to pituitary disease is not associated with cutaneous hyperpigmentation or mineralocorticoid deficiency. Salt and water balance is usually maintained unless severe fluid and electrolyte losses overwhelm the subnormal aldosterone secretory capacity. Organic lesions of pituitary origin require a diligent search for coexisting hormone deficiencies. Acute adrenal insufficiency from inadequate replacement of steroids on chronic steroid therapy is rare and can present as refractory, distributive shock. In critically ill patients, adrenal insufficiency may not present with classic symptoms. The clinical picture may resemble that of sepsis without a source of infection.[32] A high degree of suspicion must be maintained if the patient has cardiovascular instability without a defined cause.[33,34]

Diagnosis

The patient's pituitary–adrenal responsiveness should be determined when the diagnosis of primary or secondary adrenal insufficiency is first suspected. Biochemical evidence of impaired adrenal or pituitary secretory reserve unequivocally confirms the diagnosis. Patients who are clinically stable may undergo testing before treatment is initiated. Those believed to have acute adrenal insufficiency should receive immediate therapy.

Plasma cortisol levels are measured before and 30 and 60 minutes after the IV administration of 250 μg of synthetic ACTH. There are multiple determinants for adequate adrenal reserve; usually the plasma cortisol rises at least 500 nmol/L 60 minutes after the injection of the synthetic ACTH.[35] Patients with adrenal insufficiency usually demonstrate little or no adrenal response.

Treatment and Anesthetic Considerations

Normal adults secrete about 20 mg of cortisol (hydrocortisone) and 0.1 mg of aldosterone per day. Glucocorticoid therapy is usually given twice daily in sufficient dosage to meet physiologic requirements. A typical regimen in the unstressed patient may consist of prednisone, 5 mg in the morning and 2.5 mg in the

> **Table 47-6 Management of Acute Adrenal Insufficiency**
>
> Hydrocortisone, 100 mg IV bolus, followed by hydrocortisone, 100 mg q6h for 24 h
> Fluid and electrolyte replacement as indicated by vital signs, serum electrolytes, and serum glucose

> **Table 47-7 Management Options for Steroid Replacement in the Perioperative Period**
>
> Hydrocortisone, 25 mg IV, at the time of induction followed by hydrocortisone infusion, 100 mg over 24 h
> Hydrocortisone, 100 mg IV, before, during, and after surgery

evening, or hydrocortisone, 20 mg in the morning and 10 mg in the evening. The daily glucocorticoid dosage is typically 50% higher than basal adrenal output to cover the patient for mild stress. Replacement dosages are adjusted in response to the patient's clinical symptoms or the occurrence of intercurrent illnesses. Mineralocorticoid replacement is also administered on a daily basis; most patients require 0.05 to 0.1 mg/day of fludrocortisone. The mineralocorticoid dose may be reduced if severe hypokalemia, hypertension, or congestive heart failure develops, or it may be increased if postural hypotension is demonstrated.

Secondary adrenal insufficiency often occurs in the presence of multiple hormone deficiencies. A decrease in ACTH production results in the decreased secretion of cortisol and adrenal androgens, but aldosterone control by more dominant mechanisms remains intact. A liberal salt diet is encouraged. Glucocorticoid substitution follows the same guidelines previously outlined for primary adrenal insufficiency.

Immediate therapy of acute adrenal insufficiency is mandatory, regardless of the etiology, and consists of electrolyte resuscitation and steroid replacement (Table 47-6). Initial therapy begins with the rapid IV administration of an isotonic crystalloid solution. A dose of 100 mg of hydrocortisone is administered as an IV bolus over several minutes. Steroid replacement is continued during the first 24 hours with 100 mg of IV hydrocortisone given every 8 hours. If the patient is stable, the steroid dose is reduced starting on the second day. After adequate fluid resuscitation, if the patient continues to be hemodynamically unstable, inotropic support may be necessary. Invasive monitoring is extremely valuable as a guide to both diagnosis and therapy.

Steroid Replacement during the Perioperative Period

Perioperatively, patients with adrenal insufficiency and those with HPA suppression from chronic steroid use require additional corticosteroids to mimic the increased output of the normal adrenal gland during stress. The normal adrenal gland can secrete up to 100 mg/m^2 of cortisol per day or more during the perioperative period.[36] The pituitary–adrenal axis is usually considered to be intact if a plasma cortisol level higher than 19 μg/dL is measured during acute stress, but there is no precise threshold. The degree of adrenal responsiveness has been correlated with the duration of surgery and the extent of surgical trauma. The mean maximal plasma cortisol level measured during major surgery (colectomy, hip osteotomy) was 47 μg/dL. Minor surgical procedures (herniorrhaphy) resulted in mean maximal plasma cortisol levels of 28 μg/dL. Adrenal activity may also be affected by the anesthetic technique used. Regional anesthesia is effective in postponing the elevation in cortisol levels during surgery of the lower abdomen and extremities.[37] Deep general anesthesia may also suppress the elevation of stress hormones such as ACTH and cortisol during the surgical procedure.

Although symptoms indicative of clinically significant adrenal insufficiency have been reported during the perioperative period, these clinical findings have rarely been documented in direct association with glucocorticoid deficiency.[38] There is evidence in adrenally suppressed primates that subphysiologic steroid replacement causes perioperative hemodynamic instability and increased mortality.

Identifying which patients require steroid supplementation can be difficult. Though recommended by some, provocative testing with ACTH stimulation is too costly to justify compared with the risk of brief steroid supplementation. HPA suppression can occur after five daily doses of prednisone of at least 20 mg. Recovery of HPA function occurs gradually and can take up to 9 to 12 months. HPA suppression can occur with topical, regional, and inhaled steroids. Alternate-day therapy decreases the risk of HPA suppression.

The clinical problem is how much steroid to give. There is no proven optimal regimen for perioperative steroid replacement (Table 47-7). A low-dose cortisol replacement program using an IV infusion of 25 mg of cortisol before the induction of anesthesia, followed by a continuous infusion of cortisol (100 mg) in the next 24 hours, has been advocated (Fig. 47-4).[39] This low-dose cortisol replacement program was used in patients with proven adrenal insufficiency and resulted in plasma cortisol levels as high as those seen in healthy control subjects subjected to a similar operative stress. One study with a limited number of patients found no problems with cardiovascular instability if patients received their usual dose of steroids.[40] An extensive review concluded that the best evidence was that patients should receive their usual daily dose but no supplementation.[41] Although the low-dose approach appears logical, many clinicians are unwilling to adopt this regimen until further trials have been undertaken in patients receiving physiologic steroid replacement. A popular regimen calls for the administration of 200 to 300 mg of hydrocortisone per 70 kg body weight in divided doses on the day of surgery. The lower dose is adjusted upward for longer and more extensive surgical procedures. Patients who are using steroids at the time of surgery receive their usual dose on the morning of surgery and are supplemented at a level that is at least equivalent to the usual daily replacement. Glucocorticoid coverage is rapidly tapered to the patient's normal maintenance dosage during the postoperative period. Although no conclusive evidence supports an increased incidence of infection or abnormal wound healing when supraphysiologic doses of supplemental steroids are used acutely, the goal of therapy is to use the minimal drug dosage necessary to adequately protect the patient.

Exogenous Glucocorticoid Therapy

The therapeutic use of supraphysiologic doses of glucocorticoids has expanded, and the anesthesiologist should be familiar with the various preparations (Table 47-8). Dexamethasone, methylprednisolone, and prednisone have less mineralocorticoid effect than cortisone or hydrocortisone. Prednisone and methylprednisolone are precursors that must be metabolized by the liver before anti-inflammatory activity can occur and should be used cautiously in the presence of liver disease.

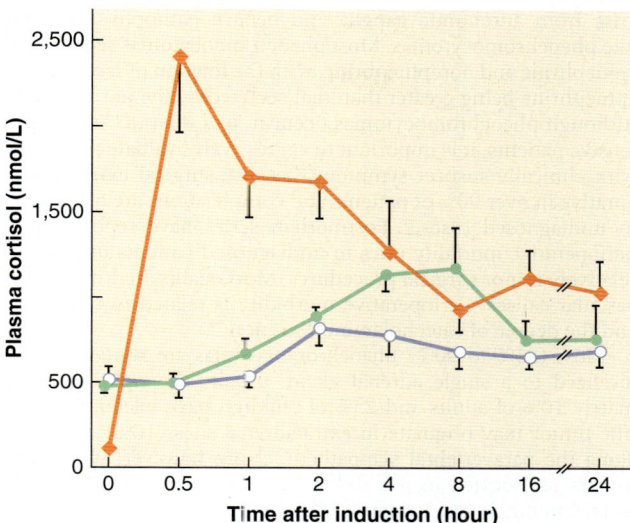

Figure 47-4 Plasma cortisol concentrations (mean ± SEM) were measured in three groups of patients undergoing elective surgery. Group I control patients, n = 8 (closed circles), had never received corticosteroids. Group II patients, n = 8 (open circles), received preoperative corticosteroids with a normal response to preoperative adrenocorticotropic hormone (ACTH; corticotropin) stimulation testing. These patients and control patients received no corticosteroid substitution during the perioperative period. Group III, n = 6 (closed diamonds), consisted of patients receiving long-term corticosteroid therapy with an abnormal response to ACTH stimulation testing during the perioperative period. These patients (group III) received intravenous (IV) cortisol, 25 mg, after the induction of anesthesia plus a continuous IV infusion of cortisol, 100 mg, during the next 24 hours. Plasma cortisol levels in group III were significantly lower than in the other two groups before the induction of anesthesia. After IV administration of cortisol to group III patients, plasma concentrations were significantly higher than in groups I and II for the next 2 hours ($p < 0.01$). Thereafter, the mean plasma concentrations were similar for all groups. There were no clinical signs of circulatory insufficiency in any group. (Reprinted with permission from Symreng T, Karlberg BE, Kagedol B, et al. Physiological cortisol substitution of long-term steroid-treated patients undergoing major surgery. Br J Anaesth. 1981;53:949.)

Mineralocorticoid Insufficiency

Isolated mineralocorticoid insufficiency has been reported as a congenital biosynthetic defect, after unilateral adrenalectomy for removal of an aldosterone-secreting adenoma, during protracted heparin therapy, and in patients with a deficiency in renin production. This syndrome is commonly seen in patients with mild renal failure and longstanding DM. A feature common to all patients with hypoaldosteronism is a failure to increase aldosterone production in response to salt restriction or volume contraction.

Most patients present with hypotension, hyperkalemia that may be life-threatening, and a metabolic acidosis that is out of proportion to the degree of coexisting renal impairment. Patients with low renin secretion, hypoaldosteronism, and renal dysfunction respond to ACTH stimulation. Nonsteroidal anti-inflammatory drugs, which inhibit prostaglandin synthesis, may further inhibit renin release and exacerbate the condition. Patients with isolated hypoaldosteronism are given fludrocortisone orally in a dose of 0.05 to 0.1 mg/day. Patients with low renin secretion usually require higher doses to correct the electrolyte abnormalities. Caution should be observed in patients with hypertension or congestive heart failure. An alternative approach in these patients is the administration of furosemide alone or in combination with mineralocorticoid.

Adrenal Medulla

The adrenal medulla is derived embryologically from neuroectodermal 3 cells. As a specialized part of the sympathetic nervous system, the adrenal medulla synthesizes and secretes the catecholamines epinephrine (80%) and norepinephrine (20%). Preganglionic fibers of the sympathetic nervous system bypass the paravertebral ganglia and pass directly from the spinal cord to the adrenal medulla. The adrenal medulla is analogous to a postganglionic neuron, although the catecholamines secreted by the medulla function as hormones, and not as neurotransmitters.

The synthesis of norepinephrine begins with hydroxylation of tyrosine to dopa (Fig. 47-5). This rate-limiting step in catecholamine biosynthesis is regulated so synthesis is coupled to release. In the adrenal medulla and in those rare central neurons using epinephrine as a neurotransmitter, most of the norepinephrine is converted to epinephrine by the enzyme phenylethanolamine-N-methyltransferase. It is likely that the capacity of the adrenal medulla to synthesize epinephrine is influenced by the flow of glucocorticoid-rich blood from the adrenal cortex through the intra-adrenal portal system because it is known that high concentrations of glucocorticoid are able to induce the enzyme phenylethanolamine-N-methyltransferase.

In the adrenal medulla, catecholamines are stored in chromaffin granules complexed with adenosine triphosphate and

Table 47-8	Glucocorticoid Preparations		
Generic Name	**Anti-inflammatory**	**Mineralocorticoid**	**Approximate Equivalent Dose (mg)**
Short-acting			
Hydrocortisone	1.0	1.0	20.0
Cortisone	0.8	0.8	25.0
Prednisone	4.0	0.25	5.0
Prednisolone	4.0	0.25	5.0
Methylprednisolone	5.0	—	4.0
Intermediate-acting			
Triamcinolone	5.0	—	4.0
Long-acting			
Dexamethasone	30.0	—	0.75

Relative milligram comparisons with cortisol. The glucocorticoid and mineralocorticoid properties of cortisol are set as 1.0.

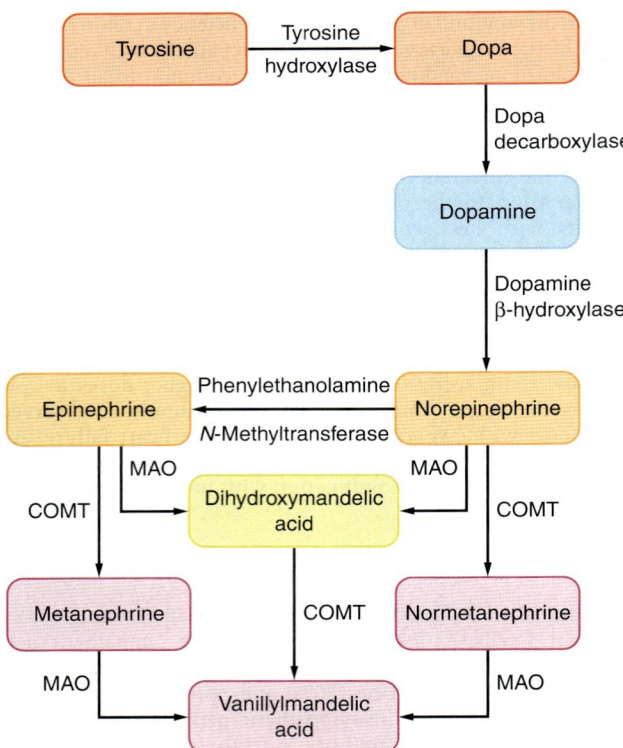

Figure 47-5 Synthesis and metabolism of endogenous catecholamines. COMT, catechol-*O*-methyltransferase; MAO, monoamine oxidase. (Adapted from Stoelting RK, Dierdorf SF, eds. *Anesthesia and Coexisting Disease*. New York, NY: Churchill-Livingstone; 1983.)

Ca^{2+}. The normal adrenal releases epinephrine and norepinephrine by exocytosis in response to stimulation by preganglionic sympathetic neurons. The circulatory half-life (10 to 30 seconds) of these catechols is considerably longer than the brief receptor activity of norepinephrine released as a neurotransmitter from postganglionic sympathetic nerve endings. Biotransformation of circulating norepinephrine and epinephrine is accomplished chiefly by the enzyme catechol-*O*-methyltransferase, located in the liver and kidney. Monoamine oxidase is of less importance in the metabolism of circulating catechols. Metanephrine and vanillylmandelic acid are the major end products of catecholamine metabolism. These metabolites and a small amount of unchanged catecholamine (1%) appear in the urine.

The outflow of postganglionic sympathetic neurotransmitters and circulating catecholamine from the adrenal medulla is coordinated by higher cortical centers connected to the brainstem. The intrinsic activity of the brainstem sympathetic areas is modulated by higher cortical functions, emotional reactions (anger, fear), and various physiologic stimuli, including changes in the physical and chemical properties of the extracellular fluid (hypoglycemia, hypotension). The adrenal medulla and sympathetic nervous system are often stimulated together in a generalized fashion, although many physiologic conditions exist in which they act independently.

Pheochromocytoma

The only important endocrine disease process associated with the adrenal medulla is pheochromocytoma. These tumors produce, store, and secrete catecholamines. Paragangliomas are tumors that arise from autonomic ganglia and behave pathophysiologically like pheochromocytomas. Most pheochromocytomas secrete both epinephrine and norepinephrine, with the fraction of secreted norepinephrine being greater than that secreted by the normal gland. Although pheochromocytomas occur in less than 0.2% of hypertensive patients, it is important to aggressively evaluate the patient with clinically suspect symptoms because surgical extirpation is curative in over 90% of patients and complications are often lethal in undiagnosed cases.[42] Postmortem series have reported high perioperative mortality rates in undiagnosed patients undergoing relatively minor surgical procedures. Most deaths are from cardiovascular causes. Perioperative morbidity is related to tumor size and the degree of catecholamine secretion.[43]

Most (85% to 90%) pheochromocytomas are solitary tumors localized to a single adrenal gland, usually the right. Approximately 10% of adults and 25% of children have bilateral tumors. The tumor may originate in extra-adrenal sites (10%), anywhere along the paravertebral sympathetic chain; however, 95% of the tumors are located in the abdomen, and a small percentage are located in the thorax, urinary bladder, or neck. Malignant spread of these highly vascular tumors occurs in approximately 10% of cases.

In approximately 5% of cases, this tumor is inherited as a familial autosomal dominant trait. It may be part of the polyglandular syndrome referred to as multiple endocrine neoplasia (MEN) IIA or IIB. Type IIA includes medullary carcinoma of the thyroid, parathyroid hyperplasia, and pheochromocytoma; type IIB consists of medullary carcinoma of the thyroid, pheochromocytoma, and neuromas of the oral mucosa. Pheochromocytomas may also arise in association with von Recklinghausen neurofibromatosis or von Hippel–Lindau disease (retinal and cerebellar angiomatosis). The pheochromocytoma of the familial syndromes is rarely extra-adrenal or malignant. Bilateral tumors occur in approximately 75% of cases. When these patients present with a single adrenal pheochromocytoma, the chances of subsequent development of a second adrenal pheochromocytoma are sufficiently high that bilateral adrenalectomy should be considered. Every member of a MEN family should be considered at risk for pheochromocytoma.

Clinical Presentation

Pheochromocytoma may occur at any age, but it is most common in young to middle adult life. The clinical manifestations are mainly due to the pharmacologic effects of the catecholamines released from the tumor. These tumors are not innervated, and catecholamine release is independent of neurogenic control. Most patients have sustained hypertension, although occasionally it is paroxysmal.[44] When true paroxysms occur, the blood pressure may rise to alarmingly high levels, placing the patient at risk for cerebrovascular hemorrhage, heart failure, dysrhythmias, or myocardial infarction. Headache, palpitations, tremor, profuse sweating, and either pallor or flushing may accompany an attack. Pheochromocytoma can masquerade as malignant hyperthermia. Physical examination of the patient with pheochromocytoma may be unrevealing during the period between attacks, unless the patient presents with symptoms and signs of sequelae related to longstanding hypertension. A catecholamine-induced cardiomyopathy may be accompanied by heart failure and cardiac dysrhythmias. Paroxysms are commonly not associated with clearly defined events, but may be precipitated by displacement of the abdominal contents or, in the case of a bladder tumor, by micturition.

Diagnosis

Biochemical determination of free catecholamine and catecholamine metabolites in the urine is the most common screening

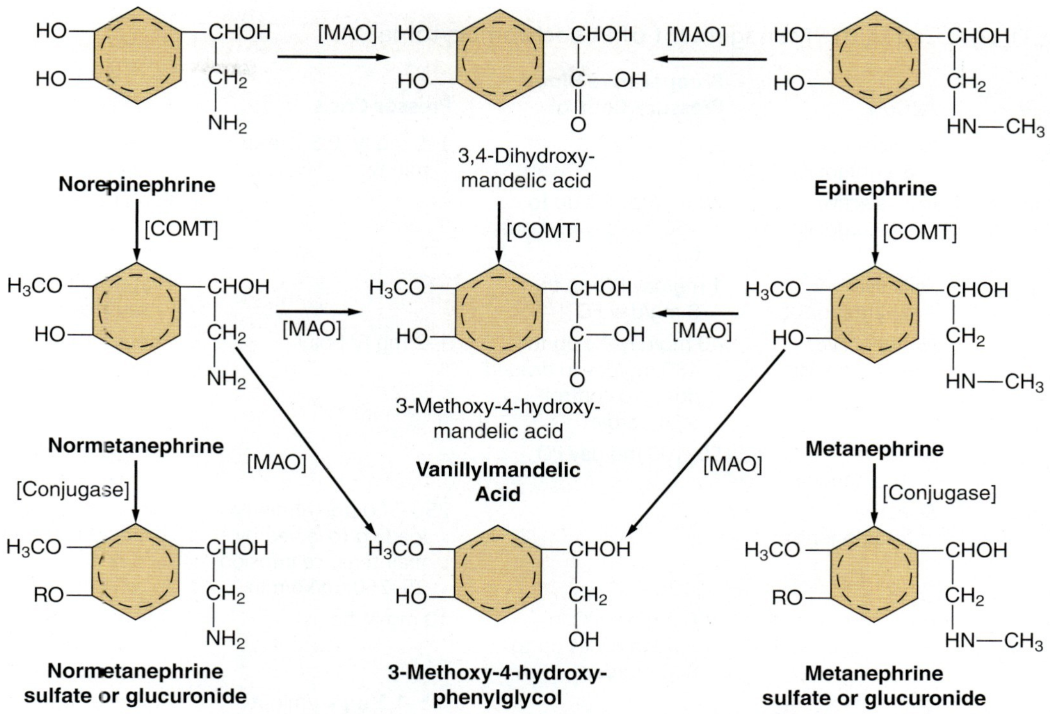

Figure 47-6 Catabolism of norepinephrine and epinephrine.

test used to establish the diagnosis of pheochromocytoma.[45] Urinary vanillylmandelic acid and unconjugated norepinephrine and epinephrine levels are measured in a 24-hour urine collection and are expressed as a function of the creatinine clearance (Fig. 47-6). Excess production of catecholamines is diagnostic for pheochromocytoma. Free catecholamines represent less than 1% of the originally released hormone, and urinary levels are not always elevated to a significant degree. Hence, differentiation from normal subjects may be difficult. A change in the ratio of unconjugated epinephrine to norepinephrine may be the only biochemical finding. Certain drugs interfere with urinary assays, and some patients with paroxysmal hypertension have normal values between attacks.

Although routine laboratory data are unlikely to provide specific diagnostic insight, ECG, chest radiograph, and complete blood cell count can provide valuable information about end-organ damage to the clinician who entertains the diagnosis. Left ventricular hypertrophy and nonspecific T-wave changes are two of the more common ECG findings. Evidence of acute myocardial infarction or tachyarrhythmia has also been reported. The chest radiograph may reveal cardiomegaly, and the blood count often shows an elevated hematocrit consistent with a reduced intravascular volume and hemoconcentration. Standardized imaging methods such as CT and MRI are used in the noninvasive localization of these tumors.[46] Ultrasound and MRI are especially useful in pregnant patients. ^{131}I-Metaiodobenzylguanidine scintigraphy is also effective in localizing recurrent or extra-adrenal masses.[47]

Anesthetic Considerations

Preoperative Preparation

4 Perioperative mortality rates have decreased from a high of 45% to between 0% and 3% for excision of pheochromocytoma followed by the introduction of α-antagonists for preoperative therapy. Perioperative blood pressure fluctuations, myocardial infarction, congestive heart failure, cardiac dysrhythmias, and cerebral hemorrhage all appear to be reduced in frequency when the patient has been treated before surgery with α-blockers and the intravascular fluid compartment has been re-expanded. Extended treatment with α-antagonists is also effective in treating the clinical manifestations of catecholamine myocarditis. However, α-blocker therapy has never been studied in a controlled way, and there are some groups that question its necessity in light of the availability of potent titratable vasodilators for intraoperative use.[48] A list of drugs frequently used in the management of pheochromocytoma is given in Table 47-9.

α-Adrenergic blockade is initiated once the diagnosis of pheochromocytoma is established (see Chapter 13). Phenoxybenzamine, a long-acting (24 to 48 hours), noncompetitive presynaptic (α_2) and postsynaptic (α_1) blocker, has traditionally been used at doses of 10 mg every 8 hours. Increments are added until the blood pressure is controlled and paroxysms disappear. Most patients need between 80 and 200 mg/day. The absorption after oral administration is variable, and side effects are common. Certain cardiovascular reflexes such as the baroreceptor reflex are blunted, and postural hypotension is common. Selective competitive α_1-blockers, such as doxazosin, terazosin, and prazosin, can also be used effectively with fewer side effects. Because postural hypotension can be pronounced with the commencement of therapy, the initial 1-mg dose is given at bedtime. Postural changes are also seen with maintenance therapy. A comparison of patients with pheochromocytoma receiving phenoxybenzamine or prazosin has shown both drugs to be equally effective in controlling blood pressure. Although the optimal period of preoperative treatment has not been established, most clinicians recommend beginning α-blockade therapy at least 10 to 14 days before the proposed surgery; however, periods as short as 3 to 5 days have been used.[49] During this time, the contracted intravascular volume

Table 47-9 Drugs Used in the Management of Pheochromocytoma

Drug	Action	Preoperative Blood Pressure Control	Pressor Crisis	Comment
Phentolamine	Nonselective α-antagonist	—	1–5 mg IV; 0.5–1 mg/min IV	Short duration of action ~5 min
Phenoxybenzamine	Nonselective α-antagonist	20 mg/day PO up to 160 mg/day in divided doses	—	Long half-life; may accumulate
Doxazosin (terazosin dosing similar)	Selective α_1-antagonist	1 mg/day PO up to 8 mg/day PO	—	First-dose phenomena; may cause syncope
Propranolol	Nonselective β-antagonist	40 mg/day PO up to 480 mg/day in divided doses to control tachycardia	1–2 mg IV bolus	Should never be given without first creating α-blockade
Atenolol	Selective β_1-antagonist	50–100 mg/day PO	—	Long-acting drug eliminated unchanged by kidney
Esmolol	Selective β_1-antagonist	—	250–500 µg/kg/min IV loading followed by maintenance infusion 25–250 µg/kg/min	Short acting; elimination half-life ~9 minute
Labetalol	α-antagonist and β-antagonist	200 mg/day PO in divided doses up to 800 mg/day	10 mg IV bolus	A much weaker α-blocker than β-blocker; may cause hypertensive response
Nitroprusside	Direct vasodilator	—	0.5–1.5 µg/kg/minute initially, increased to maximum of 8 µg/kg/min; titrate to effect	Powerful vasodilator; short acting
Magnesium sulfate	Direct vasodilator and membrane stabilizer	—	2–4 g IV bolus followed by 1–2 g/hour and additional 1–2 g boluses as needed	May potentiate neuromuscular blockade
Nicardipine	Calcium channel antagonist	—	1–2 µg/kg/min increased to 7.5 µg/kg/min; titrate to effect	—
α-Methyltyrosine	Inhibitor of biosynthesis of catecholamine	1–4 g/day PO in divided doses	—	Suitable for patients not amenable to surgery; may be nephrotoxic

and hematocrit return toward normal and the blood pressure is stabilized. Despite the real possibility of hypotension after vascular isolation of the tumor, most clinicians continue α-blockers until the morning of surgery. Calcium channel blockers can also be used alone or in combination with α-blockers.

β-Adrenergic blockade is occasionally added after α-blockade has been established. This addition is considered in patients with persistent tachycardia or cardiac dysrhythmias that may be caused by nonselective α-blockade or epinephrine-secreting tumors. β-Blockers should not be given until adequate α-blockade is ensured to avoid the possibility of unopposed α-mediated vasoconstriction. There is no clear preoperative advantage of one β-antagonist over another, although the short half-life of esmolol may allow better control of heart rate and arrhythmias in the perioperative setting. Labetalol, a β-adrenergic antagonist with α-blocking activity, is effective as a second-line medication, but can increase blood pressure when used alone.

α-Methyltyrosine is an agent that inhibits the enzyme tyrosine hydroxylase, the rate-limiting step in catecholamine biosynthesis. This medication is generally reserved for patients with metastatic disease or for situations in which surgery is contraindicated and long-term medical therapy is required though some institutions are including it as part of preoperative preparation. When α-methyltyrosine is used in combination with α-adrenergic–blocking agents, there is a significant reduction in catecholamine biosynthesis.

Unrecognized pheochromocytoma during pregnancy may be life-threatening to the mother and fetus. Although the safety of adrenergic-blocking agents during pregnancy has not been established, these agents probably improve fetal survival in pregnant patients with pheochromocytoma. The trend is to perform surgery during the first trimester or at the time of cesarean delivery. There is no reason to terminate an early pregnancy, but the patient should be aware of the risk of spontaneous abortion resulting from abdominal surgery to remove the tumor.[50]

Perioperative Anesthetic Management

Symptomatic patients continue to receive medical therapy until tachycardia, cardiac dysrhythmias, and paroxysmal elevations in blood pressure are well controlled. If it is not possible to initiate α-blocking therapy before surgery or if the patient has received less than 48 hours of intensive treatment, it may be necessary to infuse nitroprusside during the induction of anesthesia. A low-dose infusion is often initiated in anticipation of the marked blood pressure elevations that can occur with laryngoscopy and surgical stimulation.

Improvements in imaging now allow most patients with solitary tumors without evidence of metastases or local invasion to undergo a laparoscopic retroperitoneal approach. If the surgeon needs to assess for bilateral disease or the dissection is too difficult, then the procedure can be converted to an open one. During laparoscopic surgery, creation of the pneumoperitoneum may cause release of catecholamines and large changes in hemodynamics that can be controlled with a vasodilator.[51] Cortical sparing adrenalectomies are becoming more common to preserve adrenal function.

Continuous intra-arterial blood pressure monitoring is required for managing the patient with pheochromocytoma. Central venous access can be useful for secure administration of anticipated vasoactive medications. The presence of coexisting disease would dictate the need for more intensive monitoring.

Although there is no clear advantage to one anesthetic technique over another, drugs that are known to liberate histamine are avoided. Dopamine antagonists such as droperidol and metoclopramide can provoke catecholamine release and should not be used. A potent sedative hypnotic, in combination with an opioid analgesic, is used for induction. It is extremely important to achieve an adequate depth of anesthesia before proceeding with laryngoscopy to minimize the sympathetic nervous system response to this maneuver. Maintenance is provided with an opioid analgesic and a potent inhalation agent. Manipulation of the tumor may produce a marked elevation in blood pressure. Acute hypertensive crises are treated with IV infusions of nitroprusside or phentolamine or any vasodilator mentioned later. Phentolamine is a short-acting α-adrenergic antagonist that may be given as an IV bolus (2 to 5 mg) or by continuous infusion. Tachydysrhythmia is controlled with IV boluses of propranolol (1-mg increments) or by a continuous infusion of the ultrashort-acting selective β_1-adrenergic antagonist esmolol. The disadvantage of long-acting β-blockers may be persistence of bradycardia and hypotension after the tumor is removed. Even esmolol may be problematic because there are cases of cardiac arrest after clamping of the venous drainage in patients receiving large doses of esmolol. Almost every vasodilator has been tried and recommended as an adjuvant to control hypertension. Magnesium sulfate given as an infusion with intermittent boluses has successfully controlled blood pressure.[52] Nicardipine, clevidipine,[53] nitroglycerin, diltiazem, fenoldopam, and prostaglandin E_1 have all been used anecdotally. The reduction in blood pressure that may occur after ligation of the tumor's venous supply can be dangerously abrupt and should be anticipated through close communication with the surgical team. Restitution of any intravascular fluid deficit is the initial therapy in this situation. After replenishment of the intravascular volume, if the patient remains hypotensive, phenylephrine is administered. Norepinephrine or vasopressin may also be needed.[53] After surgery, catecholamine levels return to normal over several days. Approximately 75% of patients become normotensive within 10 days. Hypoglycemia must be watched for as insulin levels rise from loss of catecholamine-induced β-cell suppression.

Diabetes Mellitus

A fasting glucose level below 100 mg/dL is considered normal. Individuals with documented fasting glucose levels above 126 mg/dL (HbA1c ≥6.5%) are considered diabetics, whereas those with levels between 100 and 125 mg/dL (HbA1c 5.7 to 6.4) are considered prediabetics.[54] An estimated 29.1 million Americans (7% of the U.S. population) have DM and about 40 million Americans have prediabetes.[55] DM is the most commonly occurring endocrine disease found in surgical patients, and 25% to 50% of diabetics will require surgery at some point in their lives. Although the most serious complications of DM are related to its character as a chronic disease, it can cause difficulties in the short-term management of acute illness. DM can remain clinically unapparent until exacerbated by the stress of trauma or surgery.[56] Some observational studies report that hyperglycemia is present in 32% to 38% of patients in community hospitals, 41% of critically ill patients with acute coronary syndromes, and 80% of patients after cardiac surgery.[57] In these reports, approximately one-third of nonintensive care unit (non-ICU) patients and approximately 80% of ICU patients had no history of diabetes before admission.[57]

The principles of the treatment of DM will be easier to understand if one reviews the physiology of glucose metabolism and the stress response and then considers some of the specific pathologic entities that comprise the clinical picture of DM.

Classification

DM primarily manifests as a disease of glucose metabolism; however, it significantly affects lipid and protein metabolism and has an impact on a wide range of endocrinologic functions. Despite a variety of etiologic factors, its hallmark is a deficiency, either absolute or relative, in the amount of insulin effect to the tissues.

DM is classified into four broad types: type 1 diabetes, type 2 diabetes, gestational DM, and diabetes due to other causes.[54]

Type 1 is due to pancreatic β-cell destruction, usually leading to absolute insulin deficiency. It accounts for 5% to 10% of all DM cases and is distinguished from type 2, which accounts for the remaining 90% to 95% of all DM cases. Most patients with type 1 DM typically experience the onset of disease early in life. Consequently, this form was also referred to as juvenile-onset diabetes. However, type 1 diabetes and type 2 diabetes are heterogeneous diseases in which clinical presentation and disease progression may vary considerably. The traditional paradigms of type 2 diabetes presenting only in adults and type 1 diabetes only in children are no longer accurate, as both diseases occur in both cohorts.[58] Classification is important for determining therapy. Hyperglycemia in patients with type 1 diabetes cannot be controlled with diet or oral hypoglycemic agents; rather, it mandates treatment with insulin as there is an absolute deficiency of insulin. It is difficult to maintain an optimal glucose level in patients with type 1 DM. They are more likely to become ketotic and sustain progressive end-organ complications of diabetes.[54]

Patients with type 2 DM, also called adult-onset diabetes, typically experience a gradual onset of the disease later in life. It is due to a progressive loss of insulin secretion in the background of insulin resistance. However, type 2 form can occur in young people, and many older adults can acquire a severe and brittle form of type 1 diabetes. Because of the obesity epidemic, many adolescents and teenagers are presenting more frequently with this disorder.[54] Patients with type 2 DM are often obese, have resistance to the effects of insulin (commonly referred to as insulin resistance), and, hence, may have normal or even elevated levels of insulin, initially. In milder forms, this version of diabetes can often be treated with diet, lifestyle modifications, and oral hypoglycemic agents. Because these patients are relatively resistant to ketosis, their disease may not be clinically apparent until exacerbated by the stress of surgery or intercurrent illness.

Other types of DM can be a result of a disease that damages the pancreas and thus impairs insulin secretion. Pancreatic surgery, chronic pancreatitis, cystic fibrosis, and hemochromatosis can damage the pancreas and impair insulin secretion sufficiently to produce clinical DM. DM can also result from one of the endocrine diseases that produces a hormone that opposes the action of insulin. Hence, a patient with a glucagonoma, pheochromocytoma, or acromegaly may develop diabetes. An increased effect of glucocorticoids, from either Cushing disease or steroid or tacrolimus therapy (after organ transplantation), may also oppose the effect of insulin enough to elicit clinical diabetes and would certainly complicate the management of pre-existing diabetes. Thiazide diuretic and atypical antipsychotics (clozapine, olanzapine, risperidone, ziprasidone, quetiapine) increase the risk of diabetes.[59] Treatment of human immunodeficiency virus/acquired immunodeficiency syndrome, genetic defects in β-cell function, and genetic defects in insulin action can also induce diabetes (monogenic diabetes).[54] Gestational diabetes is typically diagnosed in the second or third trimester of pregnancy and may presage future type 2 DM. Different diagnostic criteria are used to diagnose gestational diabetes.[54]

Physiology

Insulin has multiple and complex interactions with lipid, protein, and glucose metabolism. It also has many nonmetabolic functions.[60] For our purposes, it is easiest to regard the effects of insulin on glucose metabolism as primary and to view its effects on other metabolic functions only as they relate to glucose.

Insulin is a small protein produced by the β cells of the islets of Langerhans in the pancreas. The basal rate of insulin secretion is about 1 unit/hr, which can increase by 5- to 10-fold after ingestion of food. Normal production in the adult human is approximately 40 to 50 units/day. Insulin acts through its specific receptor on cells. The half-life of insulin in the circulation is 5 minutes. However, it may clinically appear to have a longer duration of action, due to delays in binding and release from the cellular receptors.[61] These facts lead us to the important principle that once a high level of insulin saturates all the binding sites, insulin will not have a more potent effect, just a more long-lasting effect.

Insulin is metabolized in the liver and kidneys. In patients with hepatic dysfunction, the loss of gluconeogenesis and a prolongation of insulin effect increase the risk of hypoglycemia. Similarly, in patients with renal disease, the action of insulin is prolonged. They are more prone to hypoglycemia, and exogenous insulin should be administered judiciously in diabetic patients with renal disease.

Insulin release is related to a number of events. First is the direct effect of glucose and amino acids to stimulate insulin release. The mechanism involves interaction with hormones from the GI tract released during enteral feeding. The autonomic nervous system, also through vagal stimulation, increases insulin release, as does β-adrenergic stimulation and α-adrenergic blockade. Nitric oxide stimulates insulin secretion, and potassium depletion decreases insulin secretion.

The most fundamental action of insulin is to stimulate cellular uptake of glucose in skeletal muscle cells, adipose tissue, and cardiac cells. This is particularly important in skeletal muscle cells, where muscle activity also increases glucose uptake and is an important variable in the management of the physically active diabetic patient. The brain, liver, and immune cells are exceptions, where insulin does not affect glucose transport. Hence, the patient with diabetes has hyperglycemia because of inadequate cellular uptake of glucose in muscle and adipose tissue. Along with glucose, potassium enters the cells under the influence of insulin, so the diabetic patient is also likely to have an imbalance of potassium concentrations across cell membranes.

Other important metabolic functions of insulin include the stimulation of glycogen formation, as well as the suppression of gluconeogenesis and lipolysis. The patient with insulin deficiency has low glycogen stores and active gluconeogenesis. This implies that in the diabetic patient, because of an absence of glycogen, protein must be broken down to make glucose. Insulin also increases the uptake of amino acids into muscle cells. Hence, an insulin deficiency leads to catabolism and negative nitrogen balance.

Fat metabolism is also abnormal in the diabetic state, with acceleration of lipid catabolism and increased formation of ketone bodies. A deficiency of insulin leads to increased fatty acid liberation from adipose tissue. These fatty acids have multiple metabolic effects, including interference with carbohydrate phosphorylation in muscle, which leads to further hyperglycemia. Low concentrations of insulin, which may be inadequate to prevent hyperglycemia, are often sufficient to block lipolysis. This effect explains the common clinical situation in which a patient is hyperglycemic without being ketotic.

Glucagon is a polypeptide released from the α cells of the pancreas and acts both to stimulate the release of insulin and to oppose some of the effects of insulin. It has both a direct and an indirect ability to increase circulating glucose levels. In some patients, after total pancreatic resection, glucose balance is not as poor as might be expected because of the concomitant absence of glucagon. Glucagon release is stimulated by hypoglycemia, epinephrine, and cortisol and is suppressed by glucose ingestion.

The metabolic effects of stress are intricately involved with the same pathways as those involved in DM. During stress, elevations in the circulating levels of cortisol, glucagon, catecholamines, and growth hormone all act to stimulate gluconeogenesis and glycogenolysis and cause hyperglycemia. In addition, glucagon and adrenergic stimulation exert a suppressive effect on insulin release. Furthermore, inflammatory mediators released during stress enhance the release of the counter-regulatory hormones and directly affect the intracellular signaling pathways of insulin, culminating in significant insulin resistance.[62,63] Hence, mild hyperglycemia may occur in the stressed patient who does not have DM. In a patient with minimal or subclinical DM before the stressful episode, the hyperglycemia may become difficult to manage during the stress-related event and many patients require additional insulin to manage hyperglycemia.

Diagnosis

For decades, the diagnosis of diabetes was based on plasma glucose criteria, either the fasting plasma glucose (FPG) or the 2-hour value in the 75-g oral glucose tolerance test (OGTT). Starting in 2009, the criteria to diagnose DM was amended and now includes hemoglobin A1c (HbA1c) above 6.5%.[54] Correlation of HbA1c with average glucose levels is presented in Figure 47-7. Other criteria for diagnosing DM are listed in Table 47-10. As with most diagnostic tests, a test result diagnostic of diabetes should be repeated to rule out laboratory error, unless the diagnosis is clear on clinical grounds.[54,64]

Treatment

Patients with type 1 DM require exogenous insulin to survive. Further, the risk of microvascular complications can be decreased

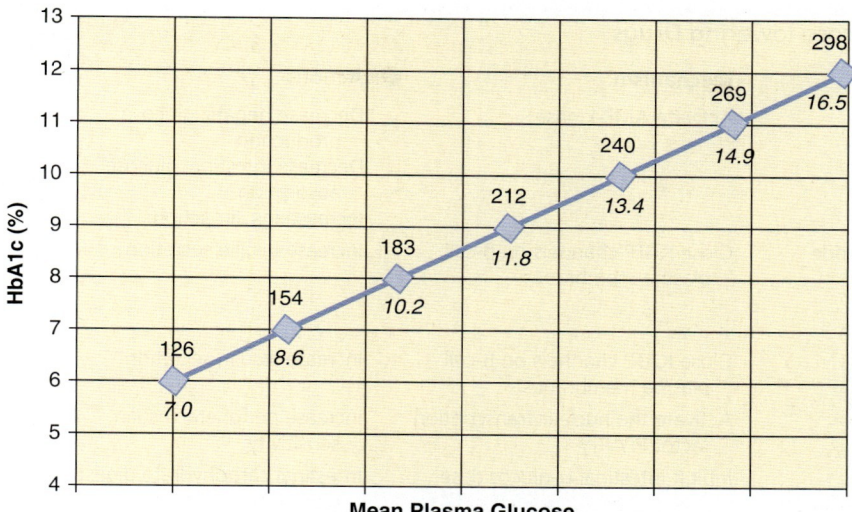

Figure 47-7 Correlation of hemoglobin A1c with average glucose. (Mean plasma glucose values above the line are in mg/dL and below the line and italic are in mmol/dL.) Estimates are based on 2,700 glucose measurements over 3 months per A1c measurement in 507 adults with type 1, type 2, and no diabetes. The correlation between A1c and average glucose was 0.92. (Data from Nathan DM, Kuenen J, Borg R, et al. A1c-derived average glucose study group: translating the A1c assay into estimated average glucose values. *Diabetes Care.* 2008;31:1473–1478.)

if glycemic control is maintained near normal levels of blood glucose (HbA1c <7%).[54,55] Patients may be on a range of doses of short-acting and long-acting insulin, with doses given three to four times per day, depending on the desire for tight control. In some clinical situations, an insulin pump may be used to administer a constant level of insulin. Intensive treatment of hyperglycemia in *newly* diagnosed patients may reduce long-term cardiovascular disease rates; however, intensive glycemic control (HbA1c <6.5% for 3.5 to 5.6 years) in patients with longstanding diabetes (8 to 11 years) showed no reduction in cardiovascular outcomes.[66]

Patients with type 2 DM may initially be treated with diet control, exercise, and metformin therapy.[67] Metformin is a biguanide that decreases hepatic glucose output and enhances the sensitivity of both hepatic and peripheral tissues to insulin.[68] If this fails to control glucose levels or the diabetes worsens, therapy with insulin and additional oral agents are indicated.[54] The goal is to decrease HbA1c levels below 7% safely, without causing hypoglycemia. Each new class of noninsulin agents added to initial therapy is expected to reduce HbA1c by 0.9% to 1.1%.[69] Selected properties of noninsulin glucose-lowering drugs are noted in Table 47-11. Sulfonylureas (glyburide, glipizide, glimepiride) and glinides (repaglinide, nateglinide) enhance β-cell insulin secretion. Rosiglitazone (Avandia) and pioglitazone (Actos) are thiazolidinediones that increase insulin sensitivity. α-Glucosidase inhibitors (acarbose, miglitol) decrease postprandial glucose absorption. Amylin analogs (pramlintide) suppress glucagon secretion and slow gastric emptying. Incretin mimetics (exenatide), as the name implies, emulate natural incretin hormones (glucagon-like peptide-1 [GLP-1], glucose-dependent insulinotropic polypeptide [GIP]) and increase insulin production, inhibit glucagon secretion, and decrease glucose absorption. Dipeptidyl-peptidase-4 inhibitors (sitagliptin) also slow degradation of incretin hormones, increase endogenous incretin hormone levels, and improve postprandial hyperglycemia. Sodium-glucose cotransporter 2 (SGLT2) inhibitors provide insulin-dependent glucose lowering by blocking glucose reabsorption in the proximal renal tubule by inhibiting SGLT2. There is an increased risk of ketoacidosis in patients with type 1 and type 2 diabetes who are treated with SGLT2 inhibitors.[70] Bariatric surgery may be considered for adults with a body mass index higher than 35 kg/m^2 and type 2 diabetes, especially if the diabetes or associated comorbidities are difficult to control with lifestyle and pharmacologic therapy.[54] Although small trials have shown a glycemic benefit of bariatric surgery in patients with type 2 diabetes with BMI 30 to 35 kg/m^2, there is currently insufficient evidence to generally recommend surgery in patients with BMI 35 kg/m^2 or lower.[71]

Anesthetic Management

Successful management of diabetic patients is as dependent on, or more dependent on, chronic complication management than acute hyperglycemia.

Preoperative

Preoperative evaluation and management has three important goals: One is determining end-organ complications of DM. This requires a thorough history and physical, a recent ECG, blood urea nitrogen, potassium, creatinine, glucose, and urinalysis. Second is determining the patient's glucose-lowering regimen. Patients may be on different types of insulin regimens and oral hypoglycemic agents. Preoperative counseling has to be specific to the patient's glucose-lowering regimen. The third goal is to

Table 47-10 Criteria for the Diagnosis of Diabetes

A1c ≥6.5%. The test should be performed in a laboratory using a method that is certified and standardized.[a]
Fasting plasma glucose ≥126 mg/dL (7 mmol/L). Fasting is defined as no caloric intake for at least 8 h.[a]
2-h plasma glucose ≥200 mg/dL (11.1 mmol/L) during an oral glucose tolerance test. The test should be performed as described by the World Health Organization, using a glucose load containing the equivalent of 75 g anhydrous glucose dissolved in water.[a]
In a patient with classic symptoms of hyperglycemia or hyperglycemic crisis, a random plasma glucose ≥200 mg/dL (11.1 mmol/L).

[a]In the absence of unequivocal hyperglycemia, result should be confirmed by repeat testing.
Adapted from Surks MI, Sievert R. Drugs and thyroid function. *N Engl J Med.* 1995;333:1688–1694.

Table 47-11 Properties of Selected Glucose-lowering Drugs

Class	Compounds	Mechanism	Actions
Biguanides	Metformin	Activate AMP-kinase	Decrease hepatic glucose production Decrease intestinal glucose absorption Increase insulin action
Sulfonylureas (second generation)	Glibenclamide/glyburide Glipizide Gliclazide Glimepiride	Close KATP channels on β-cell plasma membranes	Increase insulin secretion
Meglitinides (glinides)	Repaglinide Nateglinide	Close KATP channels on β-cell plasma membranes	Increase insulin secretion
Thiazolidinediones (glitazones)	Pioglitazone Rosiglitazone	Activate the nuclear transcription factor PPAR-γ	Increase peripheral insulin sensitivity
α-Glucosidase inhibitors	Acarbose Miglitol	Inhibit intestinal α-glucosidase	Intestinal carbohydrate digestion (consequently, absorption is slowed)
GLP-1 receptor agonists (incretin mimetics)	Exenatide Exenatide extended release Liraglutide Albiglutide Dulaglutide	Activate GLP-1 receptors (β-cells/endocrine pancreas; brain/autonomous nervous system)	Increase insulin secretion (glucose dependent) Decrease glucagon secretion (glucose dependent) Slow gastric emptying Increase satiety
DPP-4 inhibitors (incretin enhancers)	Sitagliptin Vildagliptin Saxagliptin Linagliptin Alogliptin	Inhibit DPP-4 activity, increasing postprandial, endogenously released, active incretin hormone concentration	Increase active GLP-1 concentration Increase active GIP concentration Increase insulin secretion Decrease glucagon secretion
Bile acid sequestrants	Colesevelam	Bind bile acids in the intestinal tract, increasing bile acid production	Decrease hepatic glucose production Increase incretin levels
Dopamine-2 agonists	Bromocriptine	Activate dopaminergic receptors	Alter hypothalamic regulation of metabolism Increase insulin sensitivity
SGLT2 inhibitors	Canagliflozin Dapagliflozin Empagliflozin	Inhibits SGLT2 in the proximal nephron	Block glucose reabsorption by the kidney, increasing glucosuria
Amylin mimetics	Pramlintide	Activates amylin receptors in the pancreas	Decrease glucagon secretion Slow gastric emptying Increase satiety

AMP, adenosine monophosphate; KATP, adenosine triphosphate potassium; PPAR, peroxisome proliferator-activated receptor; GLP, glucagon-like peptide; DPP, dipeptidyl peptidase; SGLT, sodium-glucose transport protein.
Adapted with permission from American Diabetes Association. Standards of medical care in diabetes–2016. *Diabetes Care.* 2016;39(Suppl 1):S1–S119.

determine patient glycemic control and the need for preoperative intervention to control glucose levels.

End-organ Complications of Diabetes

6 Atherosclerosis develops earlier and is more widespread in diabetic patients compared with nondiabetics. Manifestations include coronary artery disease, peripheral vascular disease, cerebrovascular disease, and renovascular disease. The incidence of postoperative myocardial infarction is increased in diabetic patients, and the complication rate is higher. Coronary artery disease can manifest at a young age or atypically in type 1 diabetics. Silent myocardial ischemia and infarction occur more commonly in diabetic patients, perhaps because of sensory neuropathy of the visceral afferents to the heart. DM may be associated with a cardiomyopathy in the face of angiographically normal coronary arteries, possibly with diffuse disease in arteries too small to be visualized. The American College of Cardiology (ACC)/American Heart Association guidelines recognize DM as a risk factor when evaluating patients for noncardiac surgery.[72] Preoperative hyperglycemia, as documented by increased HbA1c, has consistently been associated with poor perioperative outcomes in a variety of clinical situations.[61,73]

Diabetic nephropathy occurs in 20% to 40% of patients with diabetes and is the leading cause of end-stage renal disease (ESRD). Albuminuria usually precedes a steady decline in renal function. Microalbuminuria (30 to 299 mg/24 hrs) has been shown to be the earliest stage of diabetic nephropathy in type 1 diabetes and a marker for development of nephropathy in type 2 diabetes.[52,74]

Patients with diabetes can develop heterogeneous types of neuropathies with diverse clinical manifestations. Most common among the neuropathies are chronic sensorimotor distal symmetric polyneuropathy and autonomic neuropathy.[75] Cardiovascular autonomic neuropathy is clinically the most important. It presents as resting tachycardia, exercise intolerance, and orthostatic hypotension. Autonomic function may be tested by measuring the beat-to-beat variation in heart rate during breathing, heart rate response to a Valsalva maneuver, and orthostatic changes in diastolic blood pressure and heart rate. Diabetic patients with autonomic neuropathy are at increased risk for intraoperative hypotension, requiring vasopressor support, and perioperative cardiorespiratory arrest.[76-78] There may be an exaggerated pressor response to tracheal intubation.[79] Autonomic neuropathy predisposes to intraoperative hypothermia.[80]

Diabetic patients may also have GI neuropathies (e.g., esophageal enteropathy, gastroparesis, constipation, diarrhea, fecal incontinence). They may have delayed gastric emptying, and therefore they may be at increased risk of pulmonary aspiration of gastric contents. Autonomic function tests can predict the presence of solid food particles in gastric contents, but not increased gastric volume or acidity. Metoclopramide or erythromycin may be useful in emptying the stomach of solid food.[54]

In up to 40% of juvenile patients with DM presenting for renal transplantation, direct laryngoscopy can be difficult.[81] This may be due to diabetic stiff joint syndrome, a frequent complication of type 1 DM, leading to decreased mobility of the atlanto-occipital joint. The "prayer sign," an inability to approximate the palmar surfaces of the interphalangeal joints, is associated with stiff joint syndrome and may predict difficult laryngoscopy. Diabetic patients are at an increased risk of cognitive decline, dementia, fractures, cancer, obstructive sleep apnea, and hearing disorders.[54]

Determining Glucose-lowering Regimen and Preoperative Counseling

Though specific protocols vary from institution to institution, a typical protocol followed at our institution is as follows.[82] Patients who are on oral antihyperglycemic medications are advised to discontinue their medications the night before surgery. No oral hypoglycemic medications are administered or advised on the morning of surgery. Medications are reinstituted after the patient has resumed a normal diet. Patients who are on sulfonylureas are particularly at risk for developing hypoglycemia. Like other oral hypoglycemics, metformin should be discontinued preoperatively. Though it has been associated with severe lactic acidosis during episodes of hypotension, poor perfusion, or hypoxia, similar perioperative outcomes have been reported in patients who have undergone surgery without discontinuing metformin.[83]

For patients who are taking short- or long-acting insulin preparations, adjustment of the insulin should take into account the timing of their insulin regimen (Table 47-12). Patients who take both evening and morning doses of insulin should take their usual dose of evening short-acting insulin, but reduce their intermediate- or long-acting insulin dose by 20% the night before surgery. On the morning of surgery, they should omit their morning short-acting insulin and reduce the intermediate- or long-acting dose by 50% (and take this only if the fasting glucose is >120 mg/dL). If patients are using a premixed insulin, they are instructed to reduce their evening dose prior to surgery by 20% and hold insulin completely on the morning of the procedure.[82] Patients with type 1 diabetes need some basal insulin at all times. An estimated 400,000 patients with DM in the United States are receiving continuous subcutaneous insulin infusion (CSII) therapy (also called insulin pump therapy) to achieve optimal glucose control. Though insulin pumps have been safely utilized during surgery, there is no consensus regarding their management in the perioperative period. Specialized endocrinologic expertise may be needed in the care of patients with an insulin pump.[84] Blood glucose should be checked every hour if insulin infusion pump is continued during surgery.

Preoperative Glycemic Control

It is axiomatic that the patient should attain the best possible preoperative metabolic control; however, no randomized control study has documented that achieving a certain glycemic range preoperatively for a certain period of time will improve perioperative outcome.[85] Currently, no evidence-based guidelines exist regarding when to cancel a surgical procedure due to hyperglycemia. Given the multitude of patient factors involved as well as the variety of surgical procedures and procedure urgency, it is unlikely that recommendations based on outcomes will be forthcoming. Providers need to weigh several issues when considering this question. First, the urgency of surgery should be considered. Second, hyperglycemia could represent an unstable metabolic state, such as diabetic ketoacidosis (DKA), which should be rapidly assessed in the preoperative area. Elective surgery in an unstable metabolic state is not recommended (see "Emergencies"). Furthermore, the chronic glycemic state of the patient should be considered. If the patient has chronically elevated glucose values, this represents poor glucose control, as opposed to a new illness. In this situation, there are opportunities for providers to identify and address the problem prior to the patient arriving in the preoperative area. The value of canceling elective surgery in this situation is unclear. Another consideration is that the hyperglycemia may be caused by the illness for which the patient presented for surgery (e.g., wound infection, intra-abdominal sepsis, osteomyelitis), which would not be expected to improve until the patient undergoes surgery and source control is achieved. Providers must therefore assess the patient for stability, the need for the procedure, the risks of the procedure, and the ability of the patient to achieve glucose control if the surgery is postponed. Some institutions have used a cutoff value of 300 mg/dL as a trigger in the preoperative area for evaluation for ketoacidosis via either urine ketone dipstick or whole blood chemistry. In other institutions it is left to the discretion of the physician.[82] However, it is recommended to postpone nonurgent or elective surgery if there is an acute rise in glucose to above 400 mg/dL.[82]

Intraoperative

The details of the anesthetic plan depend intimately on the end-organ complications. Invasive monitoring may be indicated for

Table 47-12 Properties of Common Insulin Preparations

Insulin/Insulin Analogue Preparation	Onset	Peak	Duration
Lispro, Aspart, Glulisine (sc)	10–15 min	1–2 hr	3–5 hr
Regular (sc)	0.5–1 hr	2–4 hr	4–8 hr
Regular (iv)	15 min	15–30 min	0.5–1 hr
NPH (sc)	1–3 hr	4–10 hr	10–18 hr
Glargine (sc)	2–3 hr	none	24+ hr
Detemir (sc)	1 hr	none	Up to 24 hr

sc, subcutaneous; iv, intravenous.
Adapted from Inzucchi SE. The Yale Diabetes Center Diabetes Facts and Guidelines 2011–2012.

the patient with heart disease, awake intubation may be necessary if a difficult intubation is predicted, fluid management and drug choices may depend on renal function, and aspiration must be considered if there is gastroparesis.

Blood glucose levels should be measured before, during, and after surgery. Blood glucose should be monitored every 4 to 6 hours while the patient is NPO.[54] The need for additional measurements is determined by the duration and magnitude of surgery, as well as the brittleness of the diabetes. Hourly measurements are reasonable in high-risk patients, especially those receiving continuous insulin through either an insulin pump or infusion.

The standard glucose dosage for an adult patient is 5 to 10 g/hr (100 to 200 mL of 5% dextrose solution hourly). Intraoperative administration of glucose should be guided by the patient's glucose level with the goal of preventing hypoglycemia or hyperglycemia. Routine administration of additional glucose-containing IV fluids is not recommended. It is best to separately record dextrose administration and fluids given.

Monitoring of the patient who arrives in the operating room with significant metabolic impairment, such as DKA, is similar to management in the medical ICU, including hourly determinations of blood glucose, arterial pH, electrolytes, and fluid balance. Frequent reassessments with medical consultation as necessary guide the use of fluids and electrolytes, especially potassium, insulin, phosphate, and glucose.

Another area of monitoring that is extremely important in the diabetic patient is positioning on the operating table. Injuries to the limbs or nerves are more likely in the patient who arrives in the operating room already compromised by diabetic peripheral vascular disease or neuropathy. The peripheral nerves may already be partly ischemic and therefore particularly vulnerable to pressure or stretch injuries.[86]

Hyperglycemia and Perioperative Outcomes

Prior to the past decade, little attention was paid to the control of hyperglycemia in the perioperative period or in the acute phase of critical illness managed in the ICU. Permissive or stress-induced hyperglycemia was generally accepted as the norm. Stress-induced hyperglycemia is defined as a transient response to the stress of an acute injury or illness.[57] Observational studies have reported significant prevalence of hyperglycemia in hospitalized patients. Seventy percent of diabetic patients with acute coronary syndrome and 80% of cardiac surgery patients in the perioperative period may develop hyperglycemia.[67] Hyperglycemia in a hospital setting is defined as any blood glucose higher than 140 mg/dL.[87] Hyperglycemia significantly impairs chemotaxis, phagocytosis, generation of reactive oxygen species, and intracellular killing of bacteria.[88] Vascular reactivity is also decreased by hyperglycemia and is proposed to be related to decreased nitric oxide production. Acute hyperglycemia has also been shown to lead to poor outcomes in the setting of myocardial infarction and stroke.[88] There is evidence that hyperglycemia in hospitalized patients leads directly to adverse consequences.[88]

In surgical patients, *postoperative* hyperglycemia is associated with an increased risk of infection, renal and pulmonary complications, and also mortality (Fig. 47-8).[61,89–93] Many studies have addressed the effects of hyperglycemia *peri*operatively and confirmed similar associations.[85,94–96] One study demonstrated that for every 20 mg/dL increase in the mean intraoperative glucose, the risk of an adverse outcome increased by more than 30%.[94]

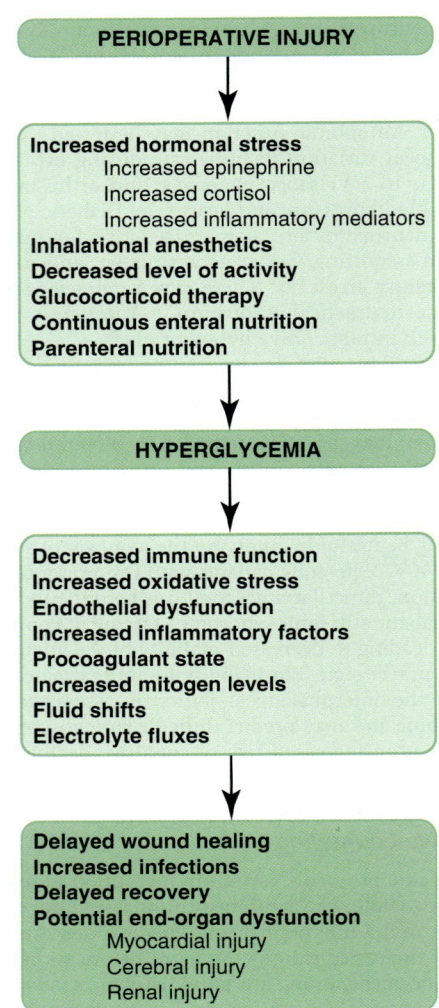

Figure 47-8 Relation among perioperative injury, hyperglycemia, and outcomes. (Reprinted with permission from Akhtar S, Barash PG, Inzucchi SE. Scientific principles and clinical implications of perioperative glucose regulation and control. *Anesth Analg*. 2010;110[2]: 478–497.)

Two other glycemic factors are also associated with poor perioperative outcomes. Hypoglycemia is a rare occurrence compared to hyperglycemia, but it is the principal factor limiting optimization of glycemic control and is associated with increased mortality.[97,98] Finally, glucose variability (changes in the measured level of blood glucose) is an independent predictor of mortality.[99] This indicates that measures of glycemia, other than glucose concentration, may be important in the pathophysiology of hyperglycemia. Three different methods of expression of glucose variability are utilized: standard deviation (SD) of glucose, the mean amplitude of glycemic excursions (MAGE), and the glycemic lability index (GLI). MAGE is the mean of absolute values of any change in glucose (consecutive values) that are more than 1 SD of the entire set of glucose values. GLI is the squared difference between consecutive glucose measures per unit of actual time between those samples. Of these three methods, the GLI may be the best discriminator for mortality.[100] However, no prospective trials have determined whether decreased glucose variability with insulin results in improved perioperative outcomes.

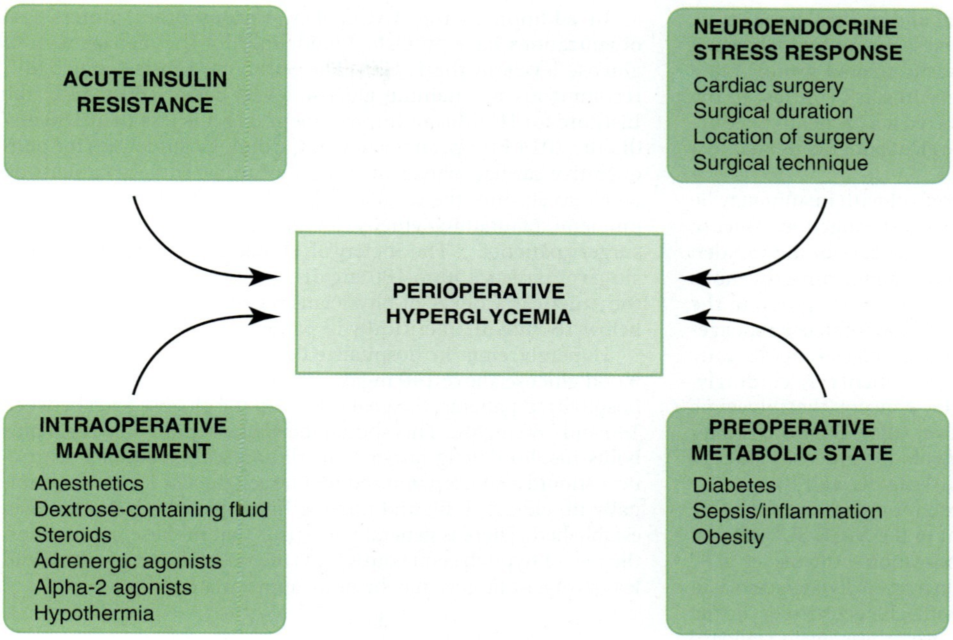

Figure 47-9 Modulators of perioperative hyperglycemia. (Reprinted with permission from Akhtar S, Barash PG, Inzucchi SE. Scientific principles and clinical implications of perioperative glucose regulation and control. *Anesth Analg.* 2010;110[2]:478–497.)

Perioperative Glycemic Control

Many factors influence the glucose levels in the perioperative period (Fig. 47-9). Endogenous insulin secretions, exogenous insulin administration, insulin resistance, endogenous glucose production, exogenous glucose administration, and overall glucose consumption are some of the key factors that determine glucose levels in a patient.

Insulin secretion can be decreased because of the direct effects of anesthetics, whereas significant insulin resistance develops postoperatively. Degree of insulin resistance is directly related to surgical trauma (Fig. 47-10). Insulin resistance not only can be modified by the stress of surgery and the inflammatory state but also may be affected by nutritional intake and level of activity. Postoperative ambulation and physical activity can alter glucose consumption acutely. Intraoperative and postoperative hyperglycemia are predicable in patients who present for cardiac and high-risk noncardiac surgery and/or have poor glycemic control preoperatively (e.g., diabetics, or patients who have an ongoing metabolic insult secondary to trauma or sepsis).[61]

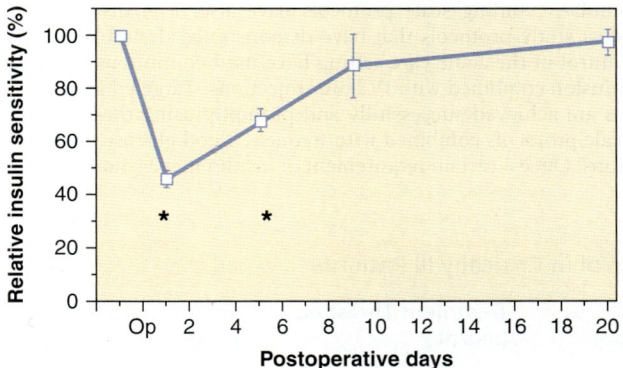

Figure 47-10 Time course for postoperative insulin resistance in patients undergoing open cholecystectomy. Relative insulin sensitivity represented as a percentage that is calculated as postoperative insulin sensitivity/perioperative insulin sensitivity × 100. Insulin sensitivity was determined within 5 days preoperatively and at days 1 (n = 9), 5, 9, and 20 (n = 5) postoperatively. *Statistically significant difference. Op, day of the operation. (Reprinted with permission from Thorell A, Efendic S, Gutnaik M, et al. Insulin resistance after abdominal surgery. *Br J Surg.* 1994;81:59–63.)

Glycemic Goals

In 2001, van den Berghe et al.[101] published a landmark paper that demonstrated a mortality benefit of tight glucose control in critically ill patients in the surgical ICU. From this study originated the concept of intensive insulin therapy (IIT) as a means of normalizing elevated glucose levels in critically ill patients. IIT was defined by a target glucose range of 80 to 110 mg/dL, and standard care implied a target glucose range of 180 to 200 mg/dL.[101] Although the study by van den Berghe et al. was a single-center, nonblinded trial, other retrospective studies also supported their findings and many centers adopted IIT protocols for management of hyperglycemia in the ICU. Furthermore, numerous studies documented clinical benefit of glycemic control in patients who underwent cardiac surgery.[61] However, most of the evidence was from prospective observational or retrospective studies. Over the course of the next few years, several studies comparing IIT to standard care failed to demonstrate a difference with respect to mortality. The IIT groups also demonstrated high incidences of hypoglycemia (8% to 28%), which was six times higher than the control group.[102–105]

The largest study to date, the NICE-SUGAR study, a multicenter, multinational randomized controlled trial, compared the effect of intensive glycemic control (target 81 to 108 mg/dL, mean blood glucose attained 115 mg/dL) to standard glycemic control (target 144 to 180 mg/dL, mean blood glucose attained 144 mg/dL) on outcomes among 6,104 critically ill participants, almost all of whom required mechanical ventilation.[106] Surprisingly, 90-day mortality was significantly higher in the intensive versus the conventional group in both surgical and medical patients, as was mortality from cardiovascular causes. Severe hypoglycemia was also more common in the intensively treated group (6.8% vs. 0.5%). The results of this study were in stark contrast to the van den Berghe et al. study, which reported a 42% relative reduction in ICU mortality in critically ill surgical patients treated to a target blood glucose of 80 to 110 mg/dL.

One situation where tight glucose control with insulin may be beneficial is in patients who are administered exogenous glucose via total parenteral nutrition.[107] This was the case in the van den Berghe et al. study, where patients received significant exogenous glucose early in the ICU. Furthermore, the control group in the NICE-SUGAR trial had reasonably good blood glucose management and was maintained at a mean glucose of 144 mg/dL, only 29 mg/dL above the intensively managed patients. Accordingly, this study's findings do not negate the concept that glycemic control in the ICU is important. However, they do strongly suggest that it may not be necessary to target blood glucose values to a highly stringent target of less than 110 mg/dL, and that it may actually be dangerous to control glucose too tightly.

Several studies published subsequent to the NICE-SUGAR trial underscored the findings of that investigation. Annane et al.[108] found no reduction in mortality and increased hypoglycemia in a randomized controlled trial of IIT with glucocorticoids in the treatment of septic shock. The control group was given standard insulin therapy plus glucocorticoids. Meta-analyses of randomized trials investigating IIT demonstrated no overall effect on mortality and increased hypoglycemia rates in the IIT groups compared with controls.[107,109-111] An observational cohort study published prior to the NICE-SUGAR trial compared outcomes before and after institution of an IIT policy. Hypoglycemia was increased and no survival benefit was noted with the institution of IIT.[112]

In summary, association between perioperative hyperglycemia and poor outcomes is strong. Though hyperglycemia develops frequently in patients who undergo cardiac or high-risk noncardiac surgery, the value of controlling glucose levels tightly *intraoperatively* has not been proven conclusively. Poor glycemic control is probably a marker of significant metabolic perturbation, which is beyond the regulatory capacity of the body. Given that in the NICE-SUGAR trial the standard insulin therapy control group (140 to 180 mg/dL range) had similar outcomes (if not better) than the IIT group, the 140 to 180 mg/dL range is now generally accepted as the new goal. In 2009, the American Association of Clinical Endocrinologists and the American Diabetes Association (AACE/ADA) released formal recommendations for the management of hyperglycemia in the ICU.[113] The recommended threshold to initiate an insulin infusion is no higher than 180 mg/dL. Once insulin therapy has been initiated, the 140 to 180 mg/dL goal range is targeted.

In addition to the AACE/ADA, various other professional organizations have published guidelines for the management of glucose levels in the ICU.[114] The Surviving Sepsis Campaign[115] recommends maintaining glucose levels below 180 mg/dL; the Institute for Healthcare Improvement target is less than 180 mg/dL; the 2014 European Society of Cardiology guidelines for perioperative cardiac management in noncardiac surgery patients do take into account the results of the NICE-SUGAR study and recommend maintaining glucose levels less than 180 mg/dL in postsurgery patients.[116] The Society of Thoracic Surgeons (for cardiac surgery) targets 150 to 180 mg/dL, whereas the guidelines from the American College of Physicians recommend keeping glucose below 180 mg/dL in critically ill patients (Table 47-13).[117]

Hyperglycemia in hospitalized patients has been defined as blood glucose above 140 mg/dL (7.8 mmol/L). In noncritically ill hospitalized patients, the goal is to keep the glucose level between 140 and 180 mg/dL. This should ideally be achieved by basal plus bolus insulin dosing rather than sliding scale insulin. Practitioners should also keep in mind that target glucose levels for terminally ill, elderly, frail, and nursing home patients have not been established. There is general consensus that in these populations, the risk of hypoglycemia outweighs the risk of hyperglycemia and less stringent targets may be more appropriate.[52,118]

Management of Perioperative Hyperglycemia

In view of the complex nature of glycemic control in the perioperative period, maintaining glucose levels within a specific range can be demanding. The narrower the desired glycemic range, the more resource intensive the protocol will be.

There are multiple insulin preparations, with varying duration of actions, which can be administered in many different ways.[119] The simplest way is to administer short-acting insulin subcutaneously. Only a few studies have adopted this route and have not been very successful in maintaining glucose in the desired range (40% to 60% of the time) and achieving it in a timely manner. In the perioperative setting, the state of peripheral perfusion is extremely variable and vasoconstriction is very common, often secondary to hypovolemia or hypothermia. Hence, absorption of any drug administered subcutaneously can be erratic and unreliable. Similarly, sliding scale protocols have also been disappointing. Most study protocols that have demonstrated desirable glycemic control in the acute care setting have used continuous IV insulin infusion combined with IV bolus injections. Targeted glucose levels are achieved successfully and promptly using these dynamic scale protocols combined with frequent blood glucose determinations. Once a certain requirement of insulin in a 24-hour period is

Table 47-13 Current Recommendations for Glycemic Control in Critically Ill Patients

Organization	Year	Patient Population	Treatment Threshold (mg/dL)	Target Glucose Level (mg/dL)
Society of Thoracic Surgeons	2009	Cardiac surgery in ICU	150	150–180
Institute for Healthcare Improvement	2009	ICU patients	180	<180
American College of Physicians	2011	ICU patients	180	140–180
Surviving Sepsis Campaign	2013	ICU patients	180	<180
European Society of Cardiology	2014	Patients after major noncardiac surgery	180	140–180
American Diabetes Association	2016	ICU patients	180	140–180

known, the patient can be transitioned to basal–bolus insulin protocol. This requires giving a certain amount of long-acting insulin (which provides a fraction of basal insulin requirement), supplemented by three or four doses of short-acting insulin bolus based on blood glucose measurements.[57] A randomized controlled trial has shown that basal–bolus treatment improved glycemic control and reduced hospital complications compared with sliding scale insulin in general surgery patients with type 2 diabetes.[120]

Blood glucose can be determined by central laboratory, blood–gas analysis machines, or various point-of-care testing devices that use capillary blood (fingerstick). Point-of-care devices are most commonly used in many acute care areas for glucose monitoring and management. Practitioners should keep in mind that the accuracy of these handheld meters can vary by 20%.[121] Glucose meter analysis (arterial and capillary blood) may provide higher glucose values, whereas blood–gas meter analysis of arterial blood may yield lower glucose values compared with central laboratory values. The hemodynamic state of the patient may also affect the accuracy of the blood glucose measurement by the point-of-care devices. Furthermore, whole blood glucose values and plasma glucose values are different, and the same is true for arterial and venous blood. Therefore, a real possibility exists of overdosing or underdosing a patient with insulin. Hence, aberrant glucose values should be verified by central laboratory measurements, and practitioners should be aware of the performance of the point-of-care devices used in their institutions.[122]

Type 1 Diabetes

Type 1 diabetics require exogenous insulin or they will rapidly develop ketoacidosis and its complications. This can be given by administering one-half to two-thirds of the patient's usual intermediate-acting insulin subcutaneously on the morning of surgery. In addition to this basal insulin, a regular insulin sliding scale (RISS) can be added and titrated to blood glucose measurement.[123] Alternatively, an insulin infusion of 0.5 to 2 units/hr (100 units of regular insulin in 1,000 mL normal saline at 5 to 20 mL/hr) can meet basal metabolic needs and be adjusted to maintain blood glucose at the desired level.[119] With either method, a slow glucose infusion (5% dextrose in water at 75 to 125 mL/hr) will prevent hypoglycemia while the patient is fasting.

Type 2 Diabetes

Patients who are on oral antihyperglycemic medications are advised to discontinue their medications the night before surgery. No oral hypoglycemic medications are administered or advised on the morning of surgery. Patients on chronic insulin are treated based on their insulin regimen. Perioperative glucose control can be achieved by insulin infusion titrated to blood glucose (typically in the ICUs) or basal long-acting insulin supplemented by an RISS. The use of an RISS as the sole method of control is to be discouraged, because it can predispose to wide glucose variations.[57]

Postoperatively, as the patient resumes oral intake, therapy can be transitioned to the patient's chronic regimen. Type 2 diabetics who have had a gastric bypass procedure can have rapid resolution of their glucose intolerance and will often need their oral agents and insulin reduced or even discontinued in the postoperative period. This effect appears to be due to changes in the incretin hormones such as GIP and GLP-1, rather than weight loss.[124]

Emergencies

Hyperglycemic hyperosmolar state (HHS) and DKA represent two extremes in the spectrum of decompensated DM. DKA is more common than HHS and accounts for 1% of diabetes-related emergencies. The mortality rate for HHS (10% to 20%) is greater than the mortality from DKA (5%).[125] Patients may present with a diabetic emergency, or it may develop perioperatively because stress, trauma, and infection may all lead to increased insulin requirements and insulin resistance.[126]

Hyperosmolar Nonketotic Coma

An occasional elderly patient with minimal or mild DM may present with remarkably high blood glucose levels (>600 mg/dL) and profound dehydration (9 to 12 L). Such patients usually have enough endogenous insulin activity to prevent lipolysis and ketosis; even with blood sugar concentrations of 1,000 mg/dL, they are not in ketoacidosis. It takes only *one-tenth* as much insulin to suppress lipolysis as it does to stimulate glucose utilization. Presumably, it is the combination of an impaired thirst response and mild renal insufficiency that allows the hyperglycemia to develop. The marked hyperosmolarity may lead to coma and seizures, with the increased plasma viscosity producing a tendency to intravascular thrombosis. It is characteristic of this syndrome that the metabolic disturbance responds quickly to rehydration and small doses of insulin. If there are no cardiovascular contraindications, 1 to 2 L (or 15 to 30 mL/kg) of normal saline should be infused over 1 hour. Insulin, by bolus or infusion, should be administered after initial volume has been administered.[127] Administering insulin before adequate fluid replacement can result in cardiovascular collapse. Insulin-mediated glucose uptake moves water out of the intravascular space and into cells causing severe hypovolemia. With rapid correction of the hyperosmolarity, cerebral edema is a risk, and recovery of mental acuity may be delayed after the blood glucose level and circulating volume have been normalized.[128]

Diabetic Ketoacidosis

DKA is defined by the biochemical triad of ketonemia, hyperglycemia, and acidemia.[129] If the diabetic patient has insufficient insulin effect to block lipolysis and the metabolism of free fatty acids, the metabolic by-products acetoacetate and β-hydroxybutyrate accumulate. These ketone bodies are organic acids and cause a metabolic acidosis with an increased unmeasured anion gap.[130] Clinically, the patient often presents because of intercurrent illness, trauma, or the untoward cessation of insulin therapy. Although hyperglycemia is almost always present, the degree of hyperglycemia does not correlate with the severity of acidosis. Blood sugar levels are often in the 250- to 500-mg/dL range. The patient is always dehydrated because of the combination of the hyperglycemia-induced osmotic diuresis and the nausea and vomiting typical of this syndrome. Because leukocytosis, abdominal pain, GI ileus, and mildly elevated amylase levels are all common in ketoacidosis, an occasional patient is misdiagnosed as having an intra-abdominal surgical problem.

Diagnostic criteria for DKA include ketonemia or significant ketonuria; blood glucose above 250 mg/dL or known DM; and serum bicarbonate below 18 mmol/L or arterial pH less than 7.3.[131] Treatment of DKA includes insulin administration and fluid and electrolyte replacement (Table 47-14). Route of administration of insulin is determined by the severity of DKA. Mild to moderate DKA can be treated with subcutaneously administered insulin analogs. However, severe DKA requires IV insulin administration. Typically, a continuous infusion is started at 0.1 unit/kg/hr as long as serum potassium is above 3.3 mEq/L. If the blood glucose does not fall by 10% in the first hour, a bolus of 0.1 unit/kg is administered. Another alternative is to administer 0.1 unit/kg as a bolus

Table 47-14 Management of Diabetic Ketoacidosis
Regular insulin, 10-unit IV bolus, followed by an insulin infusion nominally at (blood glucose/150) units/h
Isotonic IV fluids as guided by vital signs and urine output; anticipate 4–10 L deficit
When urine output is more than 0.5 mL/kg/h, give potassium chloride, 10–40 mEq/h (with continuous electrocardiographic monitoring when the rate is >10 mEq/h)
When serum glucose is decreased to 250 mg/dL, add dextrose 5% at 100 mL/h
Consider sodium bicarbonate to correct pH <6.9

followed by an infusion at 0.1 unit/kg/hr. When blood glucose levels decrease below 250 mg/dL, glucose should be added to the IV fluid while insulin therapy continues. Fluid requirements can be marked; 1 to 2 L of normal saline, or equivalent, should be given over 1 to 2 hours. After the first hour, they may need to be continued at 15 to 20 mL/kg/hr. Further deficits can be replaced more gradually. Potassium replacement is a key concern in patients with DKA. Because of the diuresis, the total-body potassium stores are reduced. However, acidosis by itself causes a shift of potassium ions out of the cell. Thus, the serum potassium concentration may be normal or even slightly elevated while the patient is acidotic. As soon as the metabolic acidosis is corrected, the potassium ions shift back into the cells. Consequently, the serum potassium concentration can decline acutely. Therefore, early and vigorous potassium replacement is required in these patients, with the exception of those patients in renal failure. Hypophosphatemia also occurs with the correction of the acidosis and, if severe, may cause impairment of ventilation, resulting from skeletal muscle weakness in the vulnerable patient. Instead of DKA, the diabetic patient with a metabolic acidosis may have lactic acidosis, which results from poor tissue perfusion or sepsis. It is diagnosed by the presence of an increased serum lactate concentration without an elevated ketone concentration. Several studies have shown that the use of bicarbonate in patients with DKA made no difference in resolution of acidosis or time to discharge.[132] Its use is not generally indicated unless the patient is hemodynamically unstable with pH below 7.1 or has pH below 6.9.

DKA must also be distinguished from the syndrome of alcoholic ketoacidosis. This typically occurs in the poorly nourished alcoholic patient after acute intoxication. Except for the presence of chemical ketoacidosis, alcoholic ketoacidosis is not clinically related in any way to DM. The alcoholic patient may be hypoglycemic or mildly hyperglycemic. The predominant ketone in this syndrome is β-hydroxybutyrate, which tends to react less sensitively in the standard laboratory nitroprusside reaction measurement of ketones. Hence, the diagnosis may be obscured. Administration of dextrose and parenteral fluids is the specific treatment for alcoholic ketoacidosis; insulin is not indicated (except in the rare circumstance in which the patient also has clear-cut DM).

Hypoglycemia

Hypoglycemia is the clinical occurrence most feared in the management of diabetic patients. The precise level at which symptomatic hypoglycemia occurs is variable. The normal, fasted patient may have blood sugar levels no higher than 50 mg/dL without symptoms. However, the diabetic patient who has a chronically elevated blood sugar level may be symptomatic at levels significantly above this glucose concentration. Hypoglycemia is almost impossible to diagnose clinically in the unconscious patient.

Clinically significant hypoglycemia is defined by Whipple triad: (a) Symptoms of neuroglycopenia, (b) simultaneous blood glucose concentration below 40 mg/dL, and (c) relief of symptoms with glucose administration. Although a subclinical stress response may be initiated at glucose levels below 70 mg/dL, a blood glucose level of approximately 55 mg/dL results in activation of the sympathetic nervous system and autonomic symptoms, which include sweating, palpitations, tremor, and hunger. Neuroglycopenic symptoms occur with blood glucose levels of approximately 45 mg/dL, and include behavioral and cognitive impairment, drowsiness, speech difficulty, blurred vision, seizures, coma, and death. Hypoglycemia in hospitalized patients has been defined as blood glucose below 70 mg/dL (3.9 mmol/L) and severe hypoglycemia as less than 40 mg/dL (2.2 mmol/L).[133] Many of the autonomic as well as the early neurologic symptoms are notably absent in the intubated, sedated, critically ill, or anesthetized patient. In the anesthetized patient, these signs of sympathetic hyperactivity can easily be misinterpreted as inadequate or "light" anesthesia. In the anesthetized, sedated, or seriously ill patient, the mental changes of hypoglycemia are also unrecognizable. Furthermore, in patients being treated with β-adrenergic–blocking agents or in patients with advanced diabetic autonomic neuropathy, the sympathetic hyperactivity of hypoglycemia may be obscured. Thus, the clinical diagnosis of hypoglycemia in the surgical patient may be difficult to make, and only a high degree of suspicion and frequent blood glucose checks can prevent this complication. Treatment is with 25 g of IV dextrose (50 mL of dextrose 50% in water) or 1 mg of intramuscular glucagon if the patient is not alert, and 8 ounces of juice if the patient is alert. The goal is to achieve a blood glucose level above 100 mg/dL.

Hypoglycemia is more likely to occur in the diabetic surgical patient if insulin or sulfonylureas are given without supplemental glucose. With renal insufficiency, the action of insulin and oral hypoglycemic agents is prolonged.

Pituitary Gland

The pituitary gland is located below the base of the brain in a bony structure called the sella turcica. The pituitary gland and the hypothalamus together form a central unit that regulates the release of various hormones. The pituitary gland is divided into two components. The *anterior pituitary* (adenohypophysis) secretes prolactin, growth hormone, gonadotropins (luteinizing hormone and follicle-stimulating hormone), TSH, and ACTH. The *posterior pituitary* (neurohypophysis) secretes the hormones vasopressin and oxytocin. Hormone release from the anterior and posterior pituitary is regulated by the hypothalamus. Regulatory peptides or preformed hormones from the hypothalamus are transported to the pituitary gland through vascular or tissue connections.

Anterior Pituitary

Hyposecretion of anterior pituitary hormones is usually due to compression of the gland by tumor. This may begin as an isolated deficiency, but it usually develops into multiglandular dysfunction. Male impotence or secondary amenorrhea in the woman is an early manifestation of panhypopituitarism. Panhypopituitarism after postpartum hemorrhagic shock (Sheehan syndrome) is due to necrosis of the anterior pituitary gland. Radiation therapy delivered to the sella turcica or nearby structures and surgical hypophysectomy are other causes of panhypopituitarism. Panhypopituitarism is treated with specific hormone replacement therapy, which should be continued in the perioperative period. Stress doses of corticosteroids are necessary for patients receiving steroid replacement because of inadequate ACTH.

The hypersecretion of various anterior pituitary hormones is usually caused by an adenoma. Excess prolactin secretion with galactorrhea is a common hormonal abnormality associated with pituitary adenoma. Cushing disease may occur secondary to excess ACTH production, and gigantism or acromegaly may occur as a consequence of excess growth hormone production in the child or adult, respectively. Excessive secretion of TSH is rare.

Acromegaly in the adult patient may pose several problems for the anesthesiologist.[134] Hypertrophy occurs in skeletal, connective, and soft tissues.[135] The tongue and epiglottis are enlarged, making the patient susceptible to upper airway obstruction. The incidence of difficult intubation is 20% to 30% and may be clinically unpredictable.[136] Hoarseness may reflect thickening of the vocal cords or paralysis of an RLN due to stretching. Dyspnea or stridor is associated with subglottic narrowing. Peripheral nerve or artery entrapment, hypertension, and DM are other common findings. The anesthetic management of these patients is complicated by distortion of the facial anatomy and upper airway. Induction of general anesthesia may put the patient at increased risk if mask fit is improper or vocal cord visualization is impaired. When the preoperative history suggests upper airway or vocal cord involvement, it is prudent to consider intubation of the trachea while the patient is awake.

Posterior Pituitary

The posterior pituitary, or neurohypophysis, is composed of terminal nerve endings that extend from the ventral hypothalamus. Vasopressin (antidiuretic hormone [ADH]) and oxytocin are the two principal hormones secreted by the posterior pituitary. Both hormones are synthesized in the supraoptic and paraventricular nuclei of the hypothalamus. They are bound to inactive carrier proteins, neurophysins, and transported by axons to membrane-bound storage vesicles located in the posterior pituitary. ADH is a nonapeptide that circulates as a free peptide after its release. The primary functions of ADH are maintenance of extracellular fluid volume and regulation of plasma osmolality. Oxytocin elicits contraction of the uterus and promotes milk secretion and ejection by the mammary glands.

Vasopressin

ADH promotes resorption of solute-free water by increasing cell membrane permeability to water alone. The target sites for ADH are the collecting tubules of the kidneys. A decrease in free water clearance causes a decrease in serum osmolality and a corresponding increase in circulating blood volume. Under normal conditions, the primary stimulus for the release of ADH is an increase in serum osmolality.

Osmoreceptors located in the hypothalamus are sensitive to changes in the normal serum osmolality of as little as 1% (normal osmolality is approximately 285 mOsm/L). Stretch receptors in the left atrium and perhaps pulmonary veins, which are sensitive to moderate reductions in the blood volume, are also capable of stimulating ADH secretion. The need to restore plasma volume may at times override osmotic inhibition of ADH release.

Various physiologic and pharmacologic stimuli also influence the secretion of ADH. Positive-pressure ventilation of the lungs, stress, anxiety, hyperthermia, β-adrenergic stimulation, and any histamine-releasing stimulus can promote the release of ADH.

ADH also has other actions. It can increase blood pressure by constricting vascular smooth muscle (see Chapter 39). This activity is most significant in the splanchnic, renal, and coronary vascular beds, and provides the rationale for administering exogenous vasopressin in the management of hemorrhage due to esophageal varices. Caution must be taken when this drug is used in patients with coronary artery disease. ADH (even in small doses) can precipitate myocardial ischemia through vasoconstriction of the coronary arteries. It is unclear whether selective arterial infusion is safer than systemic administration with regard to cardiac and vascular side effects. ADH is also often used in vasodilatory shock as an adjuvant to other pressor agents.

ADH also promotes hemostasis through an increase in the level of circulating von Willebrand factor and factor VIII. Desmopressin (DDAVP), an analogue of ADH, is commonly used to treat some types of von Willebrand disease (see Chapter 17). DDAVP is also frequently used to reverse the coagulopathy of renal failure.

Diabetes Insipidus

Diabetes insipidus results from inadequate secretion of ADH or resistance on the part of the renal tubules to ADH (nephrogenic diabetes insipidus). Failure to secrete adequate amounts of ADH results in polydipsia, hypernatremia, and a high output of poorly concentrated urine. Hypovolemia and hypernatremia may become so severe as to be life-threatening. This disorder usually occurs after destruction of the pituitary gland by intracranial trauma, infiltrating lesions, or surgery (see Chapter 37).[137] Patients in whom diabetes insipidus develops secondary to severe head trauma or subarachnoid hemorrhage often have impending brain death or are presenting for organ retrieval. Treatment of diabetes insipidus depends on the extent of the hormonal deficiency. During surgery, the patient with complete diabetes insipidus can be treated with DDAVP or vasopressin infusion combined with administration of an isotonic crystalloid solution.[138] The serum sodium and plasma osmolality are measured on a regular basis and therapeutic changes are made accordingly. If diabetes insipidus occurs postoperatively free access to water is often all that is needed. If persistent or severe, DDAVP administered intranasally has prolonged antidiuretic activity (12 to 24 hours). Nonhormonal agents that have efficacy in the treatment of incomplete diabetes insipidus include the oral hypoglycemic chlorpropamide (200 to 500 mg/day). This drug stimulates the release of ADH and sensitizes the renal tubules to the hormone. Hypoglycemia is a serious side effect that limits the usefulness of the drug. Carbamazepine and clofibrate are also capable of stimulating ADH release and have been used in the outpatient setting. None of these medications are effective in the patient with nephrogenic diabetes insipidus. Paradoxically, the thiazide diuretics exert an antidiuretic action in patients with this disorder.

Inappropriate Secretion of Antidiuretic Hormone

Inappropriate and excessive secretion of ADH may occur in association with a number of diverse pathologic processes, including head injuries, intracranial tumors, pulmonary infections, small cell carcinoma of the lung, and hypothyroidism (see Chapter 37). Surgery and trauma can cause transiently elevated ADH levels. The clinical manifestations occur as a result of a dilutional hyponatremia, decreased serum osmolality, and a reduced urine output with a high osmolality. Weight gain, skeletal muscle weakness, and mental confusion or convulsions are presenting symptoms. Peripheral edema and hypertension are rare. The diagnosis of the syndrome of inappropriate ADH secretion is one of exclusion, and other causes of hyponatremia must be ruled out first. The prognosis is related to the underlying cause of the syndrome.

The treatment for patients with mild or moderate water intoxication is restriction of fluid intake to 800 mL/day. Patients with severe water intoxication associated with hyponatremia (sodium <120 mEq/L) and central nervous system symptoms may require more aggressive therapy, with the IV administration of a hypertonic saline solution. This may be administered in conjunction with furosemide. Caution must be observed in patients with poor left ventricular function. Too-rapid correction of hyponatremia may induce osmotic demyelination and cause permanent brain damage. Serum sodium should not be raised by more than 9 mEq/L in 24 hours. Other drugs that may be used in the patient with syndrome of inappropriate ADH are demeclocycline and lithium. Demeclocycline interferes with the ability of the renal tubules to concentrate urine and is frequently used in outpatients. Lithium is usually not used because of the high incidence of toxicity. Vasopressin-2 receptor antagonists, such as conivaptan, may be useful in specific situations.

Endocrine Response to Surgical Stress

Anesthesia, surgery, and trauma elicit a generalized endocrine metabolic response characterized by an increase in the plasma levels of cortisol, ADH, renin, catecholamines, and endorphins and by metabolic changes such as hyperglycemia and a negative nitrogen balance.[139,140] There is also an increase in inflammatory markers such as C-reactive protein which would not be generally considered part of an endocrine response. Various neural and humoral factors (e.g., pain, anxiety, acidosis, local tissue factors, hypoxia) play a role in activating this stress response. There is an acute response to critical illness that is characterized by normal pituitary function, but targets organ insensitivity. During the chronic phase of critical illness, there is generalized endocrine hypofunction probably of a hypothalamic origin.[141]

The induction of anesthesia increases the levels of circulating catecholamines and is a form of metabolic stress. Regional anesthesia can block part, but not all, of the metabolic stress response during surgery, probably by blockade of the neural communication from the surgical area.[142] It is theorized that the persistently high levels of circulating catecholamines in trauma and critical illness lead to stress hyperglycemia through a direct inhibition of insulin release. Bypass of the gut hormonal actions in patients receiving IV glucose feedings, especially if given in large amounts, contributes to the impairment of insulin release during illness and can create a particularly difficult management problem for diabetic patients.

Endorphins are a group of endogenous peptides with opioid activity that have been isolated from the central nervous system. It is well documented that β-endorphin is released from the anterior pituitary, where it is contained as part of β-lipoprotein, a 91-chain amino acid, which is a cleavage product of the precursor peptide for ACTH. Large increases in the central nervous system and plasma concentrations of endorphins in response to emotional or surgical stimuli suggest that these substances play a role in the body's response to stress. These substances modulate painful stimuli by binding to opiate receptors located throughout the brain and spinal cord.

Numerous experiments have focused on the stress response and its relation to the depth of anesthesia. Regional anesthesia and general anesthesia appear to blunt the release of various stress hormones during the period of surgical stimulation in a dose-dependent fashion. Historically, anesthesiologists have relied on the indirect measurement of hemodynamic variables such as blood pressure and heart rate to evaluate the level of autonomic activity in response to anesthesia and surgery. It is assumed that the physiologic manifestations of stress are potentially harmful, especially in patients with limited functional reserve. As such, anesthetic techniques and pain management strategies are designed to limit this neurohormonal response in the hope of providing the patient with some benefit. Further investigations are needed to assess the impact of these efforts on perioperative morbidity and mortality.

REFERENCES

1. Surks MI, Sievert R. Drugs and thyroid function. *N Engl J Med*. 1995;333:1688–1694.
2. Deegan RJ, Furman WR. Cardiovascular manifestations of endocrine dysfunction. *J Cardiothorac Vasc Anesth*. 2011;25:705–720.
3. Klein I, Danzi S. Thyroid disease and the heart. *Circulation*. 2007;116:1725–1735.
4. Danzi S, Klein I. Amiodarone-induced thyroid dysfunction. *J Intensive Care Med*. 2015;30;179–185.
5. Cooper DS. Antithyroid drugs. *N Engl J Med*. 2005;352:905–917.
6. Cooper DS. Hyperthyroidism. *Lancet*. 2003;362:459–468.
7. Smallridge RC. Metabolic and anatomic thyroid emergencies: a review. *Crit Care Med*. 1992;20:276–291.
8. Chiha M, Samarasinghe S, Kabaker AS. Thyroid storm: an updated review. *J Intensive Care Med*. 2015;30(3):131–140.
9. Chun BJ, Bae JS, Lee SH, et al. A Prospective Randomized Controlled Trial of the Laryngeal Mask Airway Versus the Endotracheal Intubation in the Thyroid Surgery: Evaluation of Postoperative Voice, and Laryngopharyngeal Symptom. *World J Surg*. 2015;39:1713–1720.
10. Bouaggad A, Nejmi SE, Bouderka MA, et al. Prediction of difficult tracheal intubation in thyroid surgery. *Anesth Analg*. 2004;99:603–606.
11. Boccara G, Guenoun T, Aidan P. Anesthetic implications for robot-assisted transaxillary thyroid and parathyroid surgery: a report of twenty cases. *J Clin Anesth*. 2013;25:508–512.
12. Szubin L, Kacker A, Kakani R, et al. The management of post-thyroidectomy hypocalcemia. *Ear Nose Throat J*. 1996;75:612–614, 616.
13. Wagner HE, Seiler C. Recurrent laryngeal nerve palsy after thyroid gland surgery. *Br J Surg*. 1994;81:226–228.
14. Dionigi G, Chiang F, Dralle H, et al. Safety of neural monitoring in thyroid surgery. *Int J Surg*. 2013;11:S120–S126.
15. Lindsay RS, Toft AD. Hypothyroidism. *Lancet*. 1997;349:413–417.
16. Stathatos N, Wartofsky L. Perioperative management of patients with hypothyroidism. *Endocrinol Metab Clin North Am*. 2003;32:503–518.
17. Toft AD. Thyroxine therapy. *N Engl J Med*. 1994;331:174–180.
18. Bennett-Guerrero E, Kramer DC, Schwinn DA. Effect of chronic and acute thyroid hormone reduction on perioperative outcome. *Anesth Analg*. 1997;85:30–36.
19. Ladenson PW, Levin AA, Ridgway EC, et al. Complications of surgery in hypothyroid patients. *Am J Med*. 1984;77:261–266.
20. Whitten CW, Latson TW, Klein KW, et al. Anesthetic management of a hypothyroid cardiac surgical patient. *J Cardiothorac Vasc Anesth*. 1991;5:156–159.
21. Weinberg AD, Ehrenwerth J. Anesthetic considerations and perioperative management of patients with hypothyroidism. *Adv Anesth*. 1987;4:185–212.
22. Mihai R, Farndon JR. Parathyroid disease and calcium metabolism. *Br J Anaesth*. 2000;85:29–43.
23. Fraser WD. Hyperparathyroidism. *Lancet*. 2009;374:145–158.
24. Roland EJ, Wierda JM, Eurin BG, et al. Pharmacodynamic behaviour of vecuronium in primary hyperparathyroidism. *Can J Anaesth*. 1994;41:694–698.
25. Udelsman R, Lin Z, Donovan P. The superiority of minimally invasive parathyroidectomy based on 1650 consecutive patients with primary hyperparathyroidism. *Ann Surg*. 2011;253:585–591.
26. Shindo ML, Rosenthal JM, Lee T. Minimally invasive parathyroidectomy using local anesthesia with intravenous sedation and targeted approaches. *Otolaryngol Head Neck Surg*. 2008;138:381–387.
27. Kivela JE, Sprung J, Richards ML, et al. Effects of propofol on intraoperative parathyroid hormone monitoring in patients with primary hyperparathyroidism undergoing parathyroidectomy: a randomized control trial. *Can J Anaesth*. 2011;58:525–531.

28. Shoback D. Hypoparathyroidism. *N Engl J Med.* 2008;359:391–403.
29. Vaughan ED Jr. Diseases of the adrenal gland. *Med Clin North Am.* 2004;88:443–466.
30. Inder WJ, Hunt PJ. Glucocorticoid replacement in pituitary surgery: guidelines for perioperative assessment and management. *J Clin Endocrinol Metab.* 2002;87:2745–2750.
31. Rivers EP, Gaspari M, Abi Saad G, et al. Adrenal insufficiency in high-risk surgical ICU patients. *Chest.* 2001;119:889–896.
32. Lamberts SW, Bruining HA, DeJong FH. Corticosteroid therapy in severe illness. *N Engl J Med.* 1997;337:1285–1292.
33. Axelrod L. Perioperative management of patients treated with glucocorticoids. *Endocrinol Metab Clin North Am.* 2003;32:367–383.
34. Sutherland FW, Naik SK. Acute adrenal insufficiency after coronary artery bypass grafting. *Ann Thorac Surg.* 1996;62:1516–1517.
35. Charmandari E, Nicolaides NC, Chrousos GP. Adrenal insufficiency. *Lancet.* 2014;383:2152–2167.
36. Coursin DB, Wood KE. Corticosteroid supplementation for adrenal insufficiency. *JAMA.* 2002;287:236–240.
37. Engquist A, Brandt MR, Fernandes A, et al. The blocking effect of epidural analgesia on the adrenocortical and hyperglycemic responses to surgery. *Acta Anaesthesiol Scand.* 1977;21:330–335.
38. Salem M, Tainsh RE Jr, Bromberg J, et al. Perioperative glucocorticoid coverage: a reassessment 41 years after emergence of a problem. *Ann Surg.* 1994;219:416–425.
39. Symreng T, Karlberg BE, Kagedal B, et al. Physiological cortisol substitution of long-term steroid-treated patients undergoing major surgery. *Br J Anaesth.* 1981;53:949–954.
40. Glowniak JV, Loriaux DL. A double-blind study of perioperative steroid requirements in secondary adrenal insufficiency. *Surgery.* 1997;121:123–129.
41. Marik PE, Varon J. Requirement of perioperative stress doses of corticosteroids. *Arch Surg.* 2008;143(12):1222–1226.
42. Prys-Roberts C. Phaeochromocytoma: recent progress in its management. *Br J Anaesth.* 2000;85:44–57.
43. Kinney MA, Warner ME, van Heerden JA, et al. Perianesthetic risks and outcomes of pheochromocytoma and paraganglioma resection. *Anesth Analg.* 2000;91:1118–1123.
44. Kinney MA, Narr BJ, Warner MA. Perioperative management of pheochromocytoma. *J Cardiothorac Vasc Anesth.* 2002;16:359–369.
45. Chen H, Sippel RS, O'Dorisio MS, et al. The North American Neuroendocrine Tumor Society consensus guideline for the diagnosis and management of neuroendocrine tumors. *Pancreas.* 2010;39:775–783.
46. Witteles RM, Kaplan EL, Roizen MF. Sensitivity of diagnostic and localization tests for pheochromocytoma in clinical practice. *Arch Intern Med.* 2000;160:2521–2524.
47. Lenders JW, Duh QY, Eisenhofer G, et al. Pheochromocytoma and paraganglioma: an Endocrine Society clinical practice guideline. *J Clin Endocrinol Metab.* 2014;99:1915–1942.
48. Ulchaker JC, Goldfarb DA, Bravo EL, et al. Successful outcomes in pheochromocytoma surgery in the modern era. *J Urol.* 1999;161:764–767.
49. Pacak K. Preoperative management of the pheochromocytoma patient. *J Clin Endocrinol Metab.* 2007;92:4069–4079.
50. Hamilton A, Sirrs S, Schmidt N, et al. Anaesthesia for phaeochromocytoma in pregnancy. *Can J Anaesth.* 1997;44:654–657.
51. Joris JL, Hamoir EE, Hartstein GM, et al. Hemodynamic changes and catecholamine release during laparoscopic adrenalectomy for pheochromocytoma. *Anesth Analg.* 1999;88:16–21.
52. James MF, Cronje L. Pheochromocytoma crisis: the use of magnesium sulfate. *Anesth Analg.* 2004;99:680–686.
53. Lord MS, Augoustides JGT. Perioperative management of pheochromocytoma: Focus on magnesium, clevidipine, and vasopressin. *J Cardiothorac Vasc Anesth.* 2012;26:526–531.
54. Standards of medical care in diabetes—2016. *Diabetes Care.* 2016;39(Suppl 1):1–119.
55. Vijan S. In the clinic. Type 2 diabetes. *Ann Intern Med.* 2015:162:ITC 1–16.
56. Corathers SD, Falciglia M. The role of hyperglycemia in acute illness: supporting evidence and its limitations. *Nutrition.* 2011;27(3):276–281.
57. Smiley D, Umpierrez GE. Management of hyperglycemia in hospitalized patients. *Ann N Y Acad Sci.* 2010;1212:1–11.
58. Dabelea D, Rewers A, Stafford JM, et al. Trends in the prevalence of ketoacidosis at diabetes diagnosis: the SEARCH for diabetes in youth study. *Pediatrics.* 2014;133:e938–e945.
59. Erickson SC, Le L, Zakharyan A, et al. New-onset treatment-dependent diabetes mellitus and hyperlipidemia associated with atypical antipsychotic use in older adults without schizophrenia or bipolar disorder. *J Am Geriatr Soc.* 2012;60:474–479.
60. Kim JA, Montagnani M, Koh KK, et al. Reciprocal relationships between insulin resistance and endothelial dysfunction: molecular and pathophysiological mechanisms. *Circulation.* 2006;113(15):1888–1904.
61. Akhtar S, Barash PG, Inzucchi SE. Scientific principles and clinical implications of perioperative glucose regulation and control. *Anesth Analg.* 2010;110(2):478–497.
62. Bagry HS, Raghavendran S, Carli F. Metabolic syndrome and insulin resistance: perioperative considerations. *Anesthesiology.* 2008;108(3):506–523.
63. Biddinger SB, Kahn CR. From mice to men: insights into the insulin resistance syndromes. *Annu Rev Physiol.* 2006;68:123–158.
64. Sacks DB, Arnold M, Bakris GL, et al. Guidelines and recommendations for laboratory analysis in the diagnosis and management of diabetes mellitus. *Clin Chem.* 2011;57(6):e1–e47.
65. Nathan DM. Diabetes: advances in diagnosis and treatment. *JAMA.* 2015:314;1052–1062.
66. Skyler JS, Bergenstal R, Bonow RO, et al. Intensive glycemic control and the prevention of cardiovascular events: implications of the ACCORD, ADVANCE, and VA Diabetes Trials. *Diabetes Care.* 2009:32;187–192.
67. Qaseem A, Humphrey LL, Sweet DE, et al. Oral pharmacologic treatment of type 2 diabetes mellitus: a clinical practice guideline from the American College of Physicians. *Ann Intern Med.* 2012;156(3):218–231.
68. Bailey CJ, Turner RC. Metformin. *N Engl J Med.* 1996;334(9):574–579.
69. Bennett WL, Maruthur NM, Singh S, et al. Comparative effectiveness and safety of medications for type 2 diabetes: an update including new drugs and 2-drug combinations. *Ann Intern Med.* 2011;154(9):602–613.
70. FDA Drug Safety Communication: FDA revises labels of SGLT2 inhibitors for diabetes to include warnings about too much acid and serious urinary tract infections. FDA website. www.fda.gov/Drugs/DrugSafety/ucm475463.htm. Accessed March 4, 2016.
71. Brethauer SA, Aminian A, Rosenthal RJ, et al. Bariatric surgery improves the metabolic profile of morbidly obese patients with type 1 diabetes. *Diabetes Care.* 2014;37:e51–e52.
72. Fleisher LA, Fleischmann KA, Auerbach AD, et al. ACC/AHA guideline on perioperative cardiovascular evaluation and management of patients undergoing noncardiac surgery: A report of the American College of Cardiology Foundation/American Heart Association Task Force on practice guidelines. *J Am Coll Cardiol.* 2014;64:e77–e137.
73. Pichardo-Lowden A, Gabbay RA. Management of hyperglycemia during the perioperative period. *Curr Diab Rep.* 2012;12(1):108–118.
74. Garg JP, Bakris GL. Microalbuminuria: marker of vascular dysfunction, risk factor for cardiovascular disease. *Vasc Med.* 2002;7(1):35–43.
75. Freeman R. Not all neuropathy in diabetes is of diabetic etiology: differential diagnosis of diabetic neuropathy. *Curr Diab Rep.* 2009;9(6):423–431.
76. Charlson ME, MacKenzie CR, Gold JP. Preoperative autonomic function abnormalities in patients with diabetes mellitus and patients with hypertension. *J Am Coll Surg.* 1994;179(1):1–10.
77. Latson TW, Ashmore TH, Reinhart DJ, et al. Autonomic reflex dysfunction in patients presenting for elective surgery is associated with hypotension after anesthesia induction. *Anesthesiology.* 1994;80(2):326–337.
78. Page MM, Watkins PJ. Cardiorespiratory arrest and diabetic autonomic neuropathy. *Lancet.* 1978;1(8054):14–16.
79. Vohra A, Kumar S, Charlton AJ, et al. Effect of diabetes mellitus on the cardiovascular responses to induction of anaesthesia and tracheal intubation. *Br J Anaesth.* 1993;71(2):258–261.
80. Kitamura A, Hoshino T, Kon T, et al. Patients with diabetic neuropathy are at risk of a greater intraoperative reduction in core temperature. *Anesthesiology.* 2000;92(5):1311–1318.
81. Hogan K, Rusy D, Springman SR. Difficult laryngoscopy and diabetes mellitus. *Anesth Analg.* 1988;67(12):1162–1165.
82. Alexanian SM, McDonnell ME, Akhtar S. Creating a perioperative glycemic control program. *Anesthesiol Res Pract.* 2011;2011:465974.
83. Duncan AI, Koch CG, Xu M, et al. Recent metformin ingestion does not increase in-hospital morbidity or mortality after cardiac surgery. *Anesth Analg.* 2007;104(1):42–50.
84. Boyle ME, Seifert KM, Beer KA, et al. Guidelines for application of continuous subcutaneous insulin infusion (infusion pump) therapy in the perioperative period. *J Diabetes Sci Technol.* 2012:6;184–190.
85. King JT, Goulet JL, Perkal MF, et al. Glycemic control and infections in patients with diabetes undergoing noncardiac surgery. *Ann Surg.* 2011;253(1):158–165.
86. Harati Y. Diabetic peripheral neuropathies. *Ann Intern Med.* 1987;107(4):546–559.
87. Umpierrez GE, Hellman R, Korytkowski MT, et al. Management of hyperglycemia in hospitalized patients in non-critical care setting: an Endocrine Society clinical practice guideline. *J Clin Endocrinol Metab.* 2012;97(1):16–38.
88. Inzucchi SE. Clinical practice: management of hyperglycemia in the hospital setting. *N Engl J Med.* 2006;355(18):1903–1911.
89. Vriesendorp T, Morelis Q, Devries J, et al. Early post-operative glucose levels are an independent risk factor for infection after peripheral vascular surgery: a retrospective study. *Eur J Vasc Endovasc Surg.* 2004;28(5):520–525.
90. Pomposelli JJ, Baxter JK 3rd, Babineau TJ, et al. Early postoperative glucose control predicts nosocomial infection rate in diabetic patients. *JPEN J Parenter Enteral Nutr.* 1998;22(2):77–81.
91. Swenne CL, Lindholm C, Borowiec J, et al. Peri-operative glucose control and development of surgical wound infections in patients undergoing coronary artery bypass graft. *J Hosp Infect.* 2005;61(3):201–212.

92. Noordzij PG, Boersma E, Schreiner F, et al. Increased preoperative glucose levels are associated with perioperative mortality in patients undergoing noncardiac, nonvascular surgery. *Eur J Endocrinol.* 2007;156(1):137–142.
93. Schmeltz LR, DeSantis AJ, Thiyagarajan V, et al. Reduction of surgical mortality and morbidity in diabetic patients undergoing cardiac surgery with a combined intravenous and subcutaneous insulin glucose management strategy. *Diabetes Care.* 2007;30(4):823–828.
94. Gandhi GY, Nuttall GA, Abel MD, et al. Intraoperative hyperglycemia and perioperative outcomes in cardiac surgery patients. *Mayo Clin Proc.* 2005;80(7):862–866.
95. Frisch A, Chandra P, Smiley D, et al. Prevalence and clinical outcome of hyperglycemia in the perioperative period in noncardiac surgery. *Diabetes Care.* 2010;33(8):1783–1788.
96. Polito A, Thiagarajan RR, Laussen PC, et al. Association between intraoperative and early postoperative glucose levels and adverse outcomes after complex congenital heart surgery. *Circulation.* 2008;118(22):2235–2242.
97. Krinsley J, Preiser JC. Intensive insulin therapy to control hyperglycemia in the critically ill: a look back at the evidence shapes the challenges ahead. *Crit Care.* 2010;14(6):330.
98. Zoungas S, Patel A, Chalmers J, et al. Severe hypoglycemia and risks of vascular events and death. *N Engl J Med.* 2010;363(15):1410–1418.
99. Krinsley JS. Glycemic variability: a strong independent predictor of mortality in critically ill patients. *Crit Care Med.* 2008;36(11):3008–3013.
100. Mackenzie IM, Whitehouse T, Nightingale PG. The metrics of glycaemic control in critical care. *Intensive Care Med.* 2011;37(3):435–443.
101. van den Berghe G, Wouters P, Weekers F, et al. Intensive insulin therapy in critically ill patients. *N Engl J Med.* 2001;345(19):1359–1367.
102. van den Berghe G, Wilmer A, Hermans G, et al. Intensive insulin therapy in the medical ICU. *N Engl J Med.* 2006;354(5):449–461.
103. Arabi YM, Dabbagh OC, Tamim HM, et al. Intensive versus conventional insulin therapy: a randomized controlled trial in medical and surgical critically ill patients. *Crit Care Med.* 2008;36(12):3190–3197.
104. Brunkhorst FM, Engel C, Bloos F, et al. Intensive insulin therapy and pentastarch resuscitation in severe sepsis. *N Engl J Med.* 2008;358(2):125–139.
105. Preiser JC, Devos P, Ruiz-Santana S, et al. A prospective randomised multicentre controlled trial on tight glucose control by intensive insulin therapy in adult intensive care units: the Glucontrol study. *Intensive Care Med.* 2009;35(10):1738–1748.
106. Finfer S, Chittock DR, Su SY, et al. Intensive versus conventional glucose control in critically ill patients. *N Engl J Med.* 2009;360(13):1283–1297.
107. Marik PE, Preiser JC. Toward understanding tight glycemic control in the ICU: a systematic review and metaanalysis. *Chest.* 2010;137(3):544–551.
108. Annane D, Cariou A, Maxime V, et al. Corticosteroid treatment and intensive insulin therapy for septic shock in adults: a randomized controlled trial. *JAMA.* 2010;303(4):341–348.
109. Griesdale DE, de Souza RJ, van Dam RM, et al. Intensive insulin therapy and mortality among critically ill patients: a meta-analysis including NICE-SUGAR study data. *CMAJ.* 2009;180(8):821–827.
110. Kansagara D, Fu R, Freeman M, et al. Intensive insulin therapy in hospitalized patients: a systematic review. *Ann Intern Med.* 2011;154(4):268–282.
111. Buckleitner AM, Martinez-Alonso M, Hernandez M, et al. Perioperative glycaemic control for diabetic patients undergoing surgery (review). *Cochrane Database Syst Rev.* 2012;9:CD007315.
112. Treggiari MM, Karir V, Yanez ND, et al. Intensive insulin therapy and mortality in critically ill patients. *Crit Care.* 2008;12(1):R29.
113. Moghissi ES, Korytkowski MT, DiNardo M, et al. American Association of Clinical Endocrinologists and American Diabetes Association consensus statement on inpatient glycemic control. *Endocr Pract.* 2009;15(4):353–369.
114. Schricker T, Lattermann R. Perioperative catabolism. *Can J Anesth.* 2015;62:182–193.
115. Dellinger RP, Levy MM, Rhodes A. Surviving Sepsis Campaign: international guidelines for management of severe sepsis and septic shock: 2012. *Crit Care Med.* 2013;41:580–637.
116. Poldermans D, Bax JJ, Boersma E, et al. Guidelines for pre-operative cardiac risk assessment and perioperative cardiac management in non-cardiac surgery. *Eur Heart J.* 2009;30(22):2769–2812.
117. Qaseem A, Humphrey LL, Chou R, et al. Use of intensive insulin therapy for the management of glycemic control in hospitalized patients: a clinical practice guideline from the American College of Physicians. *Ann Intern Med.* 2011;154(4):260–267.
118. Sinclair AJ, Paolisso G, Castro M, et al. European Diabetes Working Party for Older People 2011 clinical guidelines for type 2 diabetes mellitus: executive summary. *Diabetes Metab.* 2011;37(Suppl 3):S27–S38.
119. Inzucchi SE. The Yale Diabetes Center Diabetes Facts and Guidelines 2011–2012. http://endocrinology.yale.edu/patient/50135_Yale%20National%20F.pdf. Accessed January 4, 2012.
120. Umpierrez GE, Smiley D, Jacobs S, et al. Randomized study of basal-bolus insulin therapy in the inpatient management of patients with type 2 diabetes undergoing general surgery (RABBIT 2 Surgery). *Diabetes Care.* 2011;334:256–261.
121. Rice MJ, Pitkin AD, Coursin DB. Review article: Glucose measurement in the operating room: more complicated than it seems. *Anesth Analg.* 2010;110(4):1056–1065.
122. Maerz LL, Akhtar S. Perioperative glycemic management in 2011: paradigm shifts. *Curr Opin Crit Care.* 2011;17(4):370–375.
123. Coursin DB, Connery LE, Ketzler JT. Perioperative diabetic and hyperglycemic management issues. *Crit Care Med.* 2004;32(4 Suppl):S116–S125.
124. Cummings DE, Overduin J, Foster-Schubert KE. Gastric bypass for obesity: mechanisms of weight loss and diabetes resolution. *J Clin Endocrinol Metab.* 2004;89(6):2608–2615.
125. Gosmanov AR, Gosmanova EO, Kitabchi AE. Hyperglycemic crises: diabetic ketoacidosis (DKA) and hyperglycemic hyperosmolar state (HHS). In: DeGroot LJ, Beck-Peccoz P, Chrousos G, et al., eds. *Endotext.* South Dartmouth, MA: MDText.com; 2015.
126. Nyenwe EA, Kitabchi AE. Evidence-based management of hyperglycemic emergencies in diabetes mellitus. *Diabetes Res Clin Pract.* 2011;94(3):340–351.
127. Scott AR. Management of hyperosmolar hyperglycaemic state in adults with diabetes. *Diabet Med.* 2015;32:714–724.
128. Pasquel FJ, Umpierrez GE. Hyperosmolar hyperglycemic state: a historic review of the clinical presentation, diagnosis, and treatment. *Diabetes Care.* 2014;37:3124–3131.
129. Savage MW, Dhatariya KK, Kilvert A, et al. Joint British Diabetes Societies guideline for the management of diabetic ketoacidosis. *Diabet Med.* 2011;28(5):508–515.
130. Kamel KS, Halperin ML. Acid-base problems in diabetic ketoacidosis. *N Engl J Med.* 2015;372:546–554.
131. Peterson C, Fox JA, Devallis P, et al. Starvation in the midst of cardiopulmonary bypass: diabetic ketoacidosis during cardiac surgery. *J Cardiothorac Vasc Anesth.* 2012;26:910–916.
132. Duhon B, Attridge RL, Franco-Martinez AC, et al. Intravenous sodium bicarbonate therapy in severely acidotic diabetic ketoacidosis. *Ann Pharmacother.* 2013;47:970–975.
133. Seaquist ER, Anderson J, Childs B, et al. Hypoglycemia and diabetes report of a workgroup of the American Diabetes Association and the Endocrine Society. *Diabetes Care.* 2013;36:1384–1395.
134. Melmed S. Acromegaly. *N Engl J Med.* 2006;355:2558–2573.
135. Smith M, Hirsch NP. Pituitary disease and anaesthesia. *Br J Anaesth.* 2000;85:3–14.
136. Schmitt H, Buchfelder M, Radespiel-Troger M, et al. Difficult intubation in acromegalic patients: incidence and predictability. *Anesthesiology.* 2000;93:110–114.
137. Nemergut EC, Dumont AS, Barry UT, et al. Perioperative management of patients undergoing transsphenoidal pituitary surgery. *Anesth Analg.* 2005;101:1170–1181.
138. Devin JK. Hypopituitarism and central diabetes insipidus perioperative diagnosis and management. *Neurosurg Clin North Am.* 2013;23:679–689.
139. Weissman C. The metabolic response to stress: an overview and update. *Anesthesiology.* 1990;73:308–327.
140. Desborough JP. The stress response to trauma and surgery. *Br J Anaesth.* 2000;85:109–117.
141. Langouche L, van den Berghe G. The dynamic neuroendocrine response to critical illness. *Endocrinol Metab Clin North Am.* 2006;35:777–791.
142. Fant F, Tina E, Sandblom D, et al. Thoracic epidural analgesia inhibits the neuro-hormonal but not the acute inflammatory stress response after radical retropubic prostatectomy. *Br J Anaesth.* 2013;110:747–757.

48 Anesthesia for Otolaryngologic Surgery

LYNNE R. FERRARI • RAYMOND S. PARK

Evaluating the Airway
Anesthesia for Pediatric Ear, Nose, and Throat Surgery
   Tonsillectomy and Adenoidectomy
   Preoperative Evaluation
   Sleep-disordered Breathing and Obstructive Sleep Apnea
   Anesthetic Management
   Complications
   Laryngology
   Ear Surgery
   Airway Surgery

Pediatric Airway Emergencies
   Epiglottitis
   Laryngotracheobronchitis
   Foreign Body Aspiration
Pediatric and Adult Surgery
   Laser Surgery of the Airway
   Nasal Surgery
   Skull Base Surgery
   Upper Airway Infections
   Maxillofacial Trauma
Acknowledgments

KEY POINTS

1. The restricted spaces in the airway require an understanding and cooperative relationship between surgeon and anesthesiologist, and the use of specially adapted equipment suitable to these cramped areas.
2. Despite only mild-to-moderate tonsillar enlargement on physical examination, children with obstructive sleep apnea have upper airway obstruction while awake and apnea during sleep. The clinician should not underestimate the severity of the problem based on tonsillar size alone.
3. Patients with obstructive sleep apnea have increased sensitivity to opioids and consequently the dose administered should be reduced by as much as 50%.
4. Post-tonsillectomy hemorrhage may result in unappreciated large volumes of swallowed blood originating from the tonsillar fossa. These patients must be considered to have a full stomach, and anesthetic precautions addressing this situation must be taken.
5. The middle ear and sinuses are air-filled, nondistensible cavities. During procedures in which the eardrum is replaced or perforation is patched, nitrous oxide should be discontinued or, if this is not possible, limited to a maximum of 50% during the application of the tympanic membrane graft to avoid pressure-related displacement.
6. Systemic absorption of vasoconstrictive agents during functional endoscopic sinus surgery may cause hypertension, bradycardia, tachycardia, and arrhythmias. Preoperative evaluation should include a thorough investigation of the patient's cardiovascular status. Rapid response by the anesthesiologist to these effects is necessary in preventing complications.
7. Patients with a history of head and neck cancer may have undergone prior chemotherapy, which can affect specific organ systems, or radiation, which can lead to fibrosis and ankylosis in the temporomandibular joint, rendering direct laryngoscopy difficult.
8. Facial trauma is commonly associated with other injuries such as cervical spine and head injuries, which can have implications for patient care beyond airway management.

Evaluating the Airway

Air flows through the upper respiratory passages into the trachea, bronchi, bronchioles, and alveoli in the healthy human. Airflow occurs seemingly without either thought or effort, and the actual work of respiration in the unobstructed airway is minimal. However, airway obstruction due to malformation, tumor, infection, or trauma may significantly alter the clinical presentation and make gas exchange a laborious, energy-consuming process. The increased work of breathing can leave the patient exhausted, incapable of maintaining adequate gas exchange, and finally succumbing to ventilatory failure. Significant obstruction and anatomic distortion may be present in a patient with minimal evidence of disease because clinically evident upper airway obstruction is a late sign. It is a most unwelcome experience for the anesthesiologist to unexpectedly discover an obstructed upper airway at the time of anesthetic induction or attempted tracheal intubation.

In the presence of tumor, other mass lesions, or infection in the airway, it may be useful to obtain radiologic evaluation of the airway with plain films of the tracheal and laryngeal air columns, computed tomography, or magnetic resonance imaging (MRI) studies of the airway. Significant anatomic distortion may be appreciated and help the anesthesiologist determine the most appropriate technique for securing the airway.

Anesthesia for Pediatric Ear, Nose, and Throat Surgery

The safe management of the pediatric patient undergoing surgery of the ear, nose, and throat is particularly challenging to the anesthesiologist. The restricted spaces in the airway of the child require an understanding and cooperative relationship between surgeon and anesthesiologist, and the use of specially adapted equipment suitable to these cramped areas.

Tonsillectomy and Adenoidectomy

Untreated adenoidal hyperplasia may lead to nasopharyngeal obstruction, causing failure to thrive, speech disorders, obligate mouth breathing, sleep disturbances, orofacial abnormalities with a narrowing of the upper airway, and dental abnormalities. Surgical removal of the adenoids is usually accompanied by tonsillectomy; however, purulent adenoiditis, despite adequate medical therapy, and recurrent otitis media with effusion secondary to adenoidal hyperplasia are improved with adenoidectomy alone.

Tonsillectomy is one of the more commonly performed pediatric surgical procedures.[1] Chronic or recurrent acute tonsillitis, peritonsillar abscess, tonsillar hyperplasia, and obstructive sleep apnea syndrome (OSAS) are the major indications for surgery. In addition, patients with cardiac valvar disease are at risk for endocarditis from recurrent streptococcal bacteremia secondary to infected tonsils. Tonsillar hyperplasia may lead to chronic airway obstruction resulting in sleep apnea, carbon dioxide (CO_2) retention, cor pulmonale, failure to thrive, swallowing disorders, and speech abnormalities. These risks are eliminated with removal of the tonsils.

Obstruction of the oropharyngeal airway by hypertrophied tonsils leading to apnea during sleep is an important clinical entity referred to as *obstructive sleep apnea syndrome*. Despite only mild-to-moderate tonsillar enlargement on physical examination, these patients have upper airway obstruction while awake and apnea during sleep. The goals of treatment are to relieve airway obstruction and increase the cross-sectional area of the pharynx.[2] Some patients require the use of nasal continuous positive airway pressure during sleep, whereas others may require a tracheostomy to bypass the chronic upper airway obstruction that is present. The two most frequent levels of obstruction during sleep are at the soft palate and the base of the tongue.[3,4] Most children have tremendous improvement in their symptoms after tonsillectomy.

In children with longstanding hypoxemia and hypercarbia, increased airway resistance can lead to cor pulmonale (Fig. 48-1). Patients may have electrocardiographic evidence of right ventricular hypertrophy and radiographic evidence consistent with cardiomegaly. Each apneic episode causes progressively increased pulmonary artery pressure with significant systemic and pulmonary artery hypertension, leading to ventricular dysfunction and cardiac dysrhythmias.[5] These patients often have dysfunction in the medulla or hypothalamic areas of the central nervous system causing persistently elevated CO_2, despite relief of airway obstruction as well as a hyperreactive pulmonary vascular bed. The increased pulmonary vascular resistance and myocardial depression in response to hypoxia, hypercarbia, and acidosis are far greater than what is expected for that degree of physiologic alteration in the normal population. Cardiac enlargement is frequently reversible with surgical removal of the tonsils and adenoids.

Preoperative Evaluation

A thorough history is the basis for the preoperative evaluation. A history of sleep-disordered breathing (SDB) should be sought. The physical examination should begin with observation of the patient. The presence of audible respirations, mouth breathing,

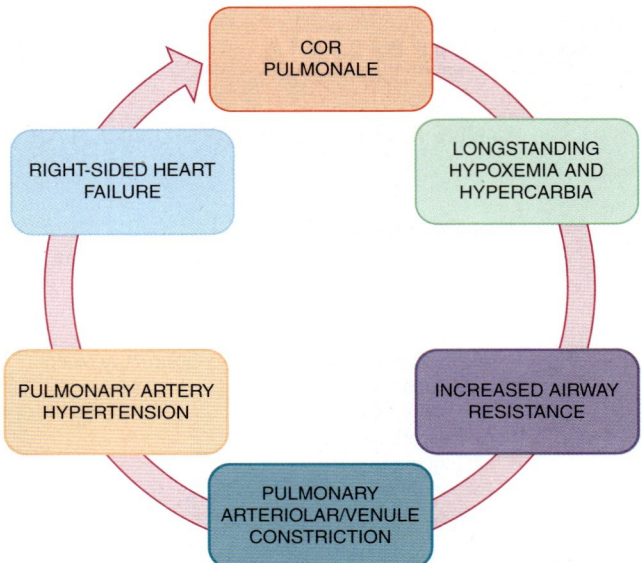

Figure 48-1 Events leading to cor pulmonale.

nasal quality of the speech, and chest retractions should be noted. Mouth breathing may be the result of chronic nasopharyngeal obstruction. An elongated face, a retrognathic mandible, and a high-arched palate may be present. The oropharynx should be inspected for evaluation of tonsillar size to determine the ease of mask ventilation and tracheal intubation (Fig. 48-2). The presence of wheezing or rales on auscultation of the chest may be a lower respiratory component of upper airway infection. The presence of inspiratory stridor or prolonged expiration may indicate partial airway obstruction from hypertrophied tonsils or adenoids.

Measurement of hematocrit and coagulation parameters is suggested. Because patients requiring tonsillectomy and adenoidectomy have frequent infections, the parent should be questioned for current use of antibiotics, antihistamines, or other medicines. Many nonprescription cold medications and antihistamines contain aspirin, which may affect platelet function, and this potential anticoagulation should be taken into consideration. Chest radiographs and electrocardiograms (ECGs) are not required unless specific abnormalities are elicited during the history, such as recent pneumonia, bronchitis, upper respiratory infection (URI), or history consistent with cor pulmonale, which is seen in children with OSAS. In those children with a history of cardiac abnormalities, an echocardiogram may be indicated.

Sleep-disordered Breathing and Obstructive Sleep Apnea

SDB is a spectrum of disorders ranging from primary snoring to OSAS. SDB affects 10% of the population, but only 1% to 4% will progress to OSAS. OSAS is characterized by periodic, partial, or complete obstruction of the upper airway during sleep.[6-9] Proper screening for and diagnosis of obstructive sleep apnea prior to surgery for both children and adults is essential in reducing the associated risks. The STOP-BANG questionnaire has been developed as a tool to screen adult patients for obstructive sleep apnea and includes information on *S*noring, daytime somnolence and *T*iredness, *O*bservation of apnea during sleep and elevations in

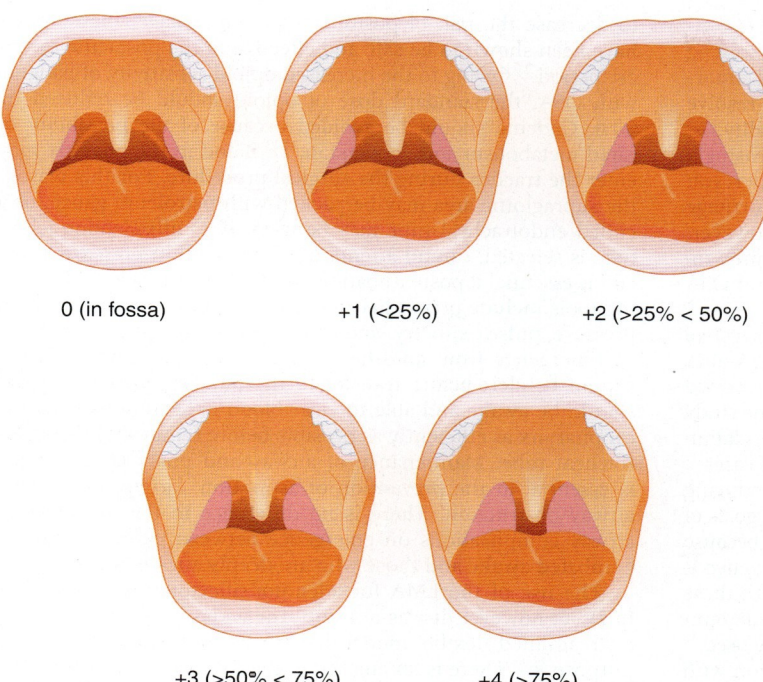

Figure 48-2 Classification of tonsil size, including percentage of oropharyngeal area occupied by hypertrophied tonsils.

blood Pressure. Predicting risk in children, however, is far more complicated.[10,11] The STBUR questionnaire has been proposed as an alternative for pediatric patients. It evaluates Snoring, Trouble Breathing, and Un-Refreshed after sleep and has the potential to be a reliable predictor of children at risk for perioperative respiratory events.[12]

Repetitive arousal from sleep to restore airway patency is a common feature, as are episodic sleep-associated oxygen desaturation, hypercarbia, and cardiac dysfunction as a result of airway obstruction. Individuals who experience obstruction during sleep may have snoring loud enough to be heard through closed doors or observed pauses in breathing during sleep. They may awaken from sleep with a choking sensation. Parents report restless sleep in affected children and frequent somnolence or fatigue while awake despite adequate sleep hours. These children fall asleep easily in nonstimulating environments and are difficult to arouse at usual awakening time. Type 1 OSAS is characterized by lymphoid hyperplasia without obesity, whereas type 2 OSAS patients are obese with minimal lymphoid hyperplasia. Approximately 10% of OSAS cases occur in preschool and school-aged children, and this number is thought to decline after 9 years of age.

Obesity changes craniofacial anthropometric characteristics. Therefore, a body mass index of 95% for age or greater is a predisposing physical characteristic that increases the risk of developing OSAS.[13,14] Children with craniofacial abnormalities including a small maxilla and mandible, a large tongue for a given mandibular size, and a thick neck have a similar increased risk. Many of these children have syndromes that are associated with additional comorbidities. Anatomic nasal obstruction and class 4 touching tonsils reduce oropharyngeal cross-sectional area, which constitutes an additional risk. Pharyngeal size is determined by the soft tissue volume inside the bony enclosure of the mandible; an anatomic imbalance between the upper airway soft tissue volume and craniofacial size will result in obstruction. The magnitude of pharyngeal muscle contraction is controlled by neural mechanisms, and the interaction between the anatomic balance and neural mechanisms determines pharyngeal airway size. Increased neural mechanisms can compensate for the anatomic imbalance in obstructive sleep apnea patients during wakefulness. When these neural mechanisms are suppressed during sleep or anesthesia, pharyngeal dilator muscles do not contract maximally, and therefore the pharyngeal airway severely narrows because of the anatomic imbalance. Increasing bony enclosure size will provide relief of airway obstruction. This is only accomplished surgically by mandibular advancement. Increasing the distance between the mentum and the cervical column by positioning will transiently relieve the obstruction so long as the sniffing position is maintained. Similarly, the sitting position displaces excessive soft tissue outside the bony enclosure through the submandibular space.

The long-term effects of OSAS are not limited to the airway. Increased body mass index and obesity may lead to increased cognitive vulnerability, as illustrated by the increased frequency of hyperactivity and increased levels of C-reactive protein. The duration of OSA has no relation to reversibility of neurobehavioral impairment, because many believe that episodic hypoxia alters the neurochemical substrate of the prefrontal cortex, causing neuronal cell loss. Metabolic syndrome consists of insulin resistance, dyslipidemia, and hypertension. It is thought that OSAS is a risk factor for metabolic syndrome in obese children but not in nonobese patients. Cardiovascular and hemodynamic comorbidities are more common in OSAS patients. These consist of altered regulation of blood pressure as well as alterations in sympathetic activity and reactivity. Also present are endothelial dysfunction and initiation and propagation of inflammatory response facilitated by increases in levels of C-reactive protein. Systemic inflammation with use of interleukins as a marker is a component of OSAS in both obese and nonobese children and is reversed after tonsillectomy. Systemic hypertension, changes in left ventricular geometry, and intermittent hypoxia leading to pulmonary artery hypertension are well-described comorbidities present in patients with OSAS.

The mainstay of the management is surgical removal of tonsils and adenoids, which carries an 85% success rate in resolving OSAS. Recurrence may occur in children with craniofacial abnormalities and in others. If surgical intervention does not resolve the problem, nocturnal CPAP is the next treatment modality.

Tonsillotomy, or partial tonsillectomy, is being increasingly utilized as an alternative therapy in patients with OSA as a result of evidence suggesting lower rates of postsurgical hemorrhage and decreased pain compared with tonsillectomy.[15,16] However, with tonsillotomy there remains concern for tonsillar regrowth, necessitating additional surgeries and inferior treatment of OSA because of subtotal removal of tonsillar tissue.[15]

For patients with severe or refractory OSA in whom corrective surgery is being considered or patients with persistent OSA after surgery, drug-induced sleep endoscopy (DISE) can be performed to better characterize the anatomic basis of obstruction. One study found that compared with clinical examination alone, information from DISE resulted in a change in surgical plan in 78% of cases.[17] During DISE, patients are sedated with the goal of reproducing obstructive symptoms that occur during sleep. One of the goals of sedation is maintenance of spontaneous respiration, and, because these patients are at high risk of obstruction, timely emergence is important for safe recovery and discharge. Coincident with these goals, agents with rapid offset such as propofol and dexmedetomidine infusion with or without ketamine bolus are typically used.[18] By nature, these patients are at increased risk of obstruction with sedation, and the anesthesiologist should have equipment immediately available (such as oral and nasal airways and laryngeal mask airways [LMAs]) to bypass and relieve obstruction. Once the patient is sedated, nasal endoscopic evaluation is performed to evaluate the upper airway for specific areas of obstruction that would be potentially corrected by surgical intervention.

Anesthetic Management

The goals of the anesthetic management for tonsillectomy and adenoidectomy are to render the child unconscious, to provide the surgeon with optimal operating conditions, to establish intravenous access to provide a route for volume expansion and medications when necessary, and to provide rapid emergence so that the patient is awake and able to protect the recently instrumented airway. Premedication may be used sparingly; sedative premedication should be avoided in children with obstructive sleep apnea, intermittent obstruction, or very large tonsils. Use of an antisialagogue will minimize secretions in the operative field.

Anesthesia is commonly induced with a volatile anesthetic agent, oxygen, and nitrous oxide (N_2O) by mask. Parental presence in the operating room (OR) during mask induction may be helpful in the anxious unpremedicated child. Tracheal intubation is best accomplished under deep inhalation anesthesia or aided by a short-acting nondepolarizing muscle relaxant. Many clinicians may choose to eliminate the neuromuscular blocking agent in favor of enhancing the depth of anesthesia with the use of propofol. Acetaminophen can be used as part of a multimodal pain regimen to reduce opioid consumption, particularly for patients having surgery for treatment of OSA. One study demonstrated that patients undergoing adenotonsillectomy who received fentanyl, 1 to 2 μg/kg, and acetaminophen, 15 mg/kg intravenously or 40 mg/kg rectally, had a median time to postoperative rescue analgesia of 7 and 10 hours, respectively.[19] The addition of 0.5 to 1 μg/kg of dexmedetomidine infused during the procedure may help to attenuate emergence delirium in toddlers at the conclusion of the anesthetic.[20] Although intraoperative nonsteroidal anti-inflammatory drugs should be avoided intraoperatively to decrease the risk of postoperative hemorrhage, these agents have been shown to be safe and effective in the postacute recovery period.[21] Owing to the increased opioid sensitivity of patients with OSA, the standard dose of opioid should be reduced by 50%. Codeine should be avoided because of the possibility of rapid metabolism and conversion.[22,23] Blood in the pharynx may enter the trachea during the surgical procedure. For this reason, the supraglottic area may be packed with petroleum gauze, or a cuffed endotracheal tube may be used. If a cuffed endotracheal tube is selected, careful attention to the inflation pressure of the cuff is essential if postextubation croup is to be avoided. Monitoring tools include precordial stethoscope, ECG, automated blood pressure, pulse oximetry, and end-tidal capnography.

Emergence from anesthesia should be rapid, and the child should be alert before transfer to the recovery area. The child should be awake and able to clear blood or secretions from the oropharynx as efficiently as possible before removal of the endotracheal tube. Maintenance of airway and pharyngeal reflexes is essential in the prevention of aspiration, laryngospasm, and airway obstruction. There is no difference in the incidence of airway complications on emergence between patients who are extubated awake and those who are deeply anesthetized.[24]

The use of the LMA for adenotonsillectomy was described in 1990; however, it was not until the widespread availability of a streamlined flexible model that it was routinely used for this purpose.[25,26] There is an emerging trend to use the flexible LMA for tonsillectomy, which protects the vocal cords from blood or secretions that may be present in the oropharynx.[27] The wide, rigid tube of the standard LMA model does not fit under the mouth gag and is easily compressed or dislodged during full mouth opening. The flexible model has a soft, reinforced shaft that easily fits under the mouth gag without becoming dislodged or compressed. Adequate surgical access can be achieved, and the lower airway is protected from exposure to blood during the procedure.[28,29] Because the cuff is larger and occupies a greater percentage of the posterior hypopharynx, there is a greater risk of airway fire if the electrocautery touches the LMA. Insertion is possible either after the intravenous administration of 3 mg/kg of propofol or when sufficient depth of anesthesia is achieved using a volatile agent administered by face mask. The same depth of anesthesia should be obtained during insertion of the LMA as would be required for performing laryngoscopy and endotracheal intubation. Positive-pressure ventilation should be avoided when the LMA is used during tonsillectomy, although gentle assisted ventilation is both safe and effective if peak inspiratory pressure is kept below 20 cm H_2O.

Tonsillar enlargement can make LMA insertion difficult; therefore, care in placement is essential. Maneuvers to overcome this include increased head extension, lateral insertion of the mask, anterior displacement of the tongue, pressure on the tip of the LMA using the index finger as it negotiates the pharyngeal curve, or use of the laryngoscope if all else fails. Dislodgment of the device does not occur during extreme head extension, assuming good position and ventilation were obtained before changes in head position.[30]

Advantages of the LMA over traditional endotracheal intubation are a decrease in the incidence of postoperative stridor and laryngospasm and an increase in immediate postoperative oxygen saturation. If the child is breathing spontaneously at a regular rate and depth, the LMA may be removed before emergence from anesthesia. The oropharynx should be gently suctioned with a soft flexible catheter, the LMA deflated and removed, an oral airway inserted, and the respirations assisted with 100% oxygen delivered by face mask. It is often distressing for young children to awaken with the LMA still in place. Although the device is an appropriate substitute for an oral airway in the adult population, this is not so in children. If the practitioner wants to remove the LMA when the child has emerged from anesthesia, it should be deflated and removed as soon as possible after the return to consciousness. In addition, because it is not possible to pass a nasogastric tube beyond the LMA cuff even when deflated, the stomach cannot be emptied at the conclusion of surgery.

Complications

The incidence of posttonsillectomy mortality within the first 48 hours in both children and adults has been reported to be increased in patients who are obese or have neurologic impairment or cardiopulmonary compromise.[31] The incidence of emesis after tonsillectomy ranges from 30% to 65%.[32] Whether emesis is due to irritant blood in the stomach or stimulation of the gag reflex by inflammation and edema at the surgical site remains unclear. Central nervous system stimulation from the gastrointestinal tract, as may be seen with gastric distention from the introduction of swallowed or insufflated air, may trigger the emetic center of the brain. Decompressing the stomach with an orogastric tube may be helpful in preventing this response. Treatment with ondansetron, 0.10 to 0.15 mg/kg, either with or without dexamethasone, 0.5 mg/kg, has been shown to be very effective in reducing posttonsillectomy nausea and vomiting.[33] Dehydration secondary to poor oral intake as a result of nausea, vomiting, or pain can occur after tonsillectomy in 1% of cases. Vigorous intravenous hydration during surgery can offset the physiologic effects of lower postoperative fluid intake.

The most serious complication of tonsillectomy is postoperative hemorrhage, which occurs at a frequency of 0.1% to 8.1%. The use of coblation tonsillectomy, which has recently increased in popularity, may result in an incidence of posttonsillectomy hemorrhage up to 11.1%.[34,35] Approximately 75% of postoperative tonsillar hemorrhage occurs within 6 hours of surgery. Most of the remaining 25% occurs within the first 24 hours of surgery, although bleeding may be noted until the sixth postoperative day (thus the "six hours or six days" guideline). Sixty-seven percent of postoperative bleeding originates from the tonsillar fossa, 26% in the nasopharynx, and 7% in both.[31] Initial attempts to control bleeding may be made using pharyngeal packs and cautery. If this fails, patients must return to the OR for exploration and surgical hemostasis.

Unappreciated large volumes of blood originating from the tonsillar bed may be swallowed. Patients must be considered to have a full stomach, and anesthetic precautions addressing this situation must be taken. A rapid-sequence induction accompanied by cricoid pressure and insertion of a styletted endotracheal tube is controversial but may be of benefit in some circumstances. Because the amount of blood swallowed can be considerable, blood pressure must be checked in both the erect and supine positions to exclude orthostatic changes resulting from decreases in vascular volume. Intravenous access and hydration must be established before the induction of anesthesia. A variety of laryngoscope blades and endotracheal tubes, as well as functioning suction apparatus, should be prepared in duplicate because blood in the airway may impair visualization of the vocal cords and cause plugging of the endotracheal tube.

Pain after adenoidectomy is usually minimal, but pain after tonsillectomy may be severe. This contributes to poor fluid intake and overall discomfort of patients. An increase in postoperative pain medication requirements has been noted in patients having laser or electrocautery as part of the operative tonsillectomy compared with those who have had sharp surgical dissection and ligation of blood vessels to achieve hemostasis. Intraoperative administration of corticosteroids may decrease edema formation and subsequent patient discomfort. Although infiltration of the peritonsillar space with local anesthetic and epinephrine has been shown to be effective in reducing intraoperative blood loss, it does not significantly decrease postoperative pain.[36]

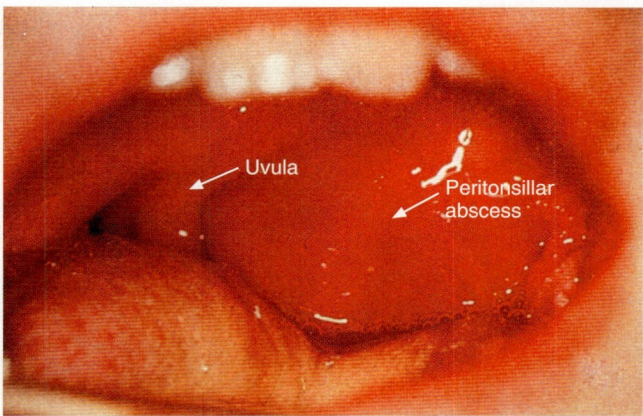

Figure 48-3 Patient with a peritonsillar abscess on the left side. Note the displacement of the uvula. (Courtesy of Michael Cunningham, MD, Boston, MA.)

Peritonsillar abscess, or quinsy tonsil, is a condition that may require immediate surgical intervention to relieve potential or existing airway obstruction. An acutely infected tonsil may undergo abscess formation, producing a large mass in the lateral pharynx that can interfere with swallowing and breathing (Figs. 48-3 to 48-5). Fever, pain, and trismus are frequent symptoms. Treatment consists of surgical drainage of the abscess, either with or without tonsillectomy, and intravenous antibiotic therapy. Although the airway seems compromised, the peritonsillar abscess is usually in a fixed location in the lateral pharynx and does not interfere with ventilation of the patient by face mask after induction of general anesthesia. Visualization of the vocal cords should not be impaired because the pathologic process is supraglottic and well above the laryngeal inlet. Laryngoscopy must be carefully performed, avoiding manipulation of the larynx and surrounding structures. Intubation should be gentle because the tonsillar area is tense and friable, and inadvertent rupture of the abscess can occur, leading to spillage of purulent material into the trachea. A head-down position may be useful during laryngoscopy to decrease risk of purulent aspiration in the event of abscess rupture.

Acute postoperative pulmonary edema is an infrequent but potentially life-threatening complication encountered when airway obstruction is suddenly relieved. One proposed mechanism is that during inspiration before adenotonsillectomy, the negative intrapleural pressure that is generated causes an increase in venous return, enhancing pulmonary blood volume. In the healthy child without airway obstruction, pleural pressure ranges from −2.5 cm to −10 cm H$_2$O during inspiration. Intrapleural pressure generated in the child with airway obstruction can be as much as −30 cm H$_2$O, which causes disruption of the capillary walls of the pulmonary microvasculature when transmitted to the interstitial peribronchial and perivascular spaces. Concurrent with a negative transpulmonary gradient is an increase in venous return to the right side of the heart, thus increasing preload, which in the setting of "leaky capillaries"

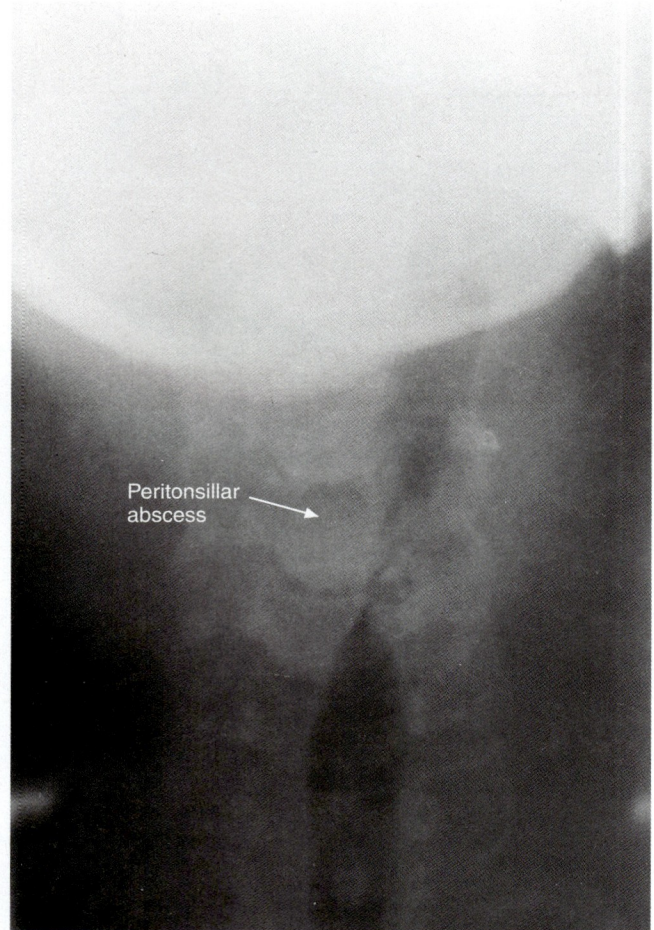

Figure 48-4 Neck radiograph of a patient with a peritonsillar abscess (*arrow*).

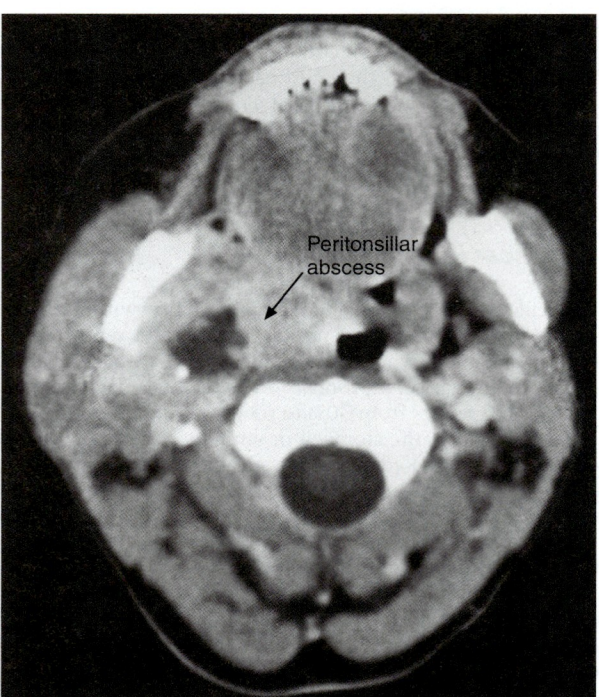

Figure 48-5 Computed tomography scan of a patient with a peritonsillar abscess (*arrow*).

facilitates transudation of fluid into the alveolar space. To counterbalance this negative gradient, positive intrapleural and alveolar pressures are generated during exhalation, which decreases pulmonary venous return and blood volume. This phenomenon is similar to an expiratory "grunt" mechanism, in which the transpleural pressures generated are similar to those present during a Valsalva maneuver.

The rapid relief of airway obstruction results in decreased airway pressure, an increase in venous return, an increase in pulmonary hydrostatic pressure, hyperemia, and finally pulmonary edema. The all-important counterbalance of the expiratory grunt in limiting pulmonary venous return is lost when the obstruction is relieved. Contributing factors are the increased volume load on both ventricles as well as the inability of the pulmonary lymphatic system to remove acutely large amounts of fluid. The anesthesiologist may attempt to prevent this situation during induction of anesthesia by applying moderate amounts of continuous positive pressure to the airway, thus allowing time for circulatory adaptation to take place. This physiologic sequence is similar to that seen in patients with severe acute airway obstruction secondary to epiglottitis or laryngospasm.

Negative-pressure pulmonary edema is signaled by the appearance of frothy pink fluid in the endotracheal tube of an intubated patient or the presence of decreased oxygen saturation, wheezing, dyspnea, and increased respiratory rate in the immediate postoperative period in a previously extubated patient. Mild cases may present with minimal symptoms. The differential diagnosis of negative-pressure pulmonary edema includes aspiration of gastric contents, adult respiratory distress syndrome, congestive heart failure, volume overload, and anaphylaxis. A chest radiograph illustrating diffuse, usually bilateral interstitial pulmonary infiltrates combined with an appropriate clinical history will confirm the diagnosis.[37,38] Treatment is usually supportive, with maintenance of a patent airway, oxygen administration, and diuretic therapy in some cases. Endotracheal intubation and mechanical ventilation with positive end-expiratory pressure may be necessary in severe cases. Resolution is usually rapid and may occur within hours of inception. Most cases resolve within 24 hours without treatment. There is currently no reliable method for predicting which children will experience this clinical syndrome after their airway obstruction has been resolved.

Adenoidectomy patients may be safely discharged on the same day after recovering from anesthesia. Although most tonsillectomy patients previously required postoperative admission to the hospital for observation, administration of analgesics, and hydration, many centers are discharging tonsillectomy patients on the day of surgery without adverse outcomes, and this trend will likely continue.[38] Patients should be observed for early hemorrhage for a minimum of 4 to 6 hours and be free from significant nausea, vomiting, and pain prior to discharge. The ability to take fluid by mouth is not a requirement for discharge home. However, intravenous hydration must be adequate to prevent dehydration. Excessive somnolence and severe vomiting are indications for hospital admission. There are patients for whom early discharge is not advised, and those patients should be admitted to the hospital after tonsillectomy. The characteristics of such patients are listed in Table 48-1. Recently, the American Academy of Pediatrics has recommended that children who exhibit oxygen saturation less than 80% in the posttonsillectomy recovery period be admitted

Table 48-1 Tonsillectomy and Adenoidectomy Inpatient Guidelines: Recommendation of the American Academy of Otolaryngology—Head and Neck Surgery

Admit patients to the hospital after adenotonsillectomy if they meet any of the following criteria:
- Age ≤3 yrs
- Severe OSA with an apnea–hypopnea index of 10 or more obstructive events/hr, oxygen saturation nadir <80%, or both
- Abnormal coagulation values with or without an identified bleeding disorder in the patient or family
- Systemic disorders that put the patient at increased preoperative cardiopulmonary, metabolic, or general medical risk
- Child with craniofacial or other airway abnormalities including, but not limited to, syndromic disorders such as Treacher Collins syndrome, Crouzon syndrome, Goldenhar syndrome, Pierre Robin anomalad, CHARGE syndrome, achondroplasia, and, most prominently, Down syndrome, as well as isolated airway abnormalities such as choanal atresia and laryngotracheal stenosis
- When extended travel time, weather conditions, and home social conditions are not consistent with close observation, cooperation, and ability to return to the hospital quickly at the discretion of the attending physician

CHARGE, coloboma of the eye, heart defects, atresia of the choanae, retardation of growth and/or development, genital and/or urinary abnormalities, and ear abnormalities.

to an inpatient unit and monitored for respiratory depression.[39] Despite removal of hypertrophied lymphoid tissue in the hypopharynx, there are some children who remain at risk for postoperative obstruction.[40] Admission to an intensive care unit (ICU) is controversial and reserved for those children with very severe OSA, comorbidities that cannot be managed on the floor, and children who have demonstrated significant airway obstruction and desaturation in the initial postoperative period that required intervention beyond repositioning and oxygen supplementation.[41]

Laryngology

There have been great advances in knowledge regarding voice disorders and strategies for managing them. This developed in adult practice, and the subspeciality of phoniatrics emerged. This expertise is now prevalent in surgeons for both pediatric and adult patient populations. The most common disorder is vocal nodules as a result of laryngeal hyperfunction, producing hoarseness. Papillomatosis of the vocal cords is another cause of voice disorder along with vocal fold paralysis.[42] Treatment of papillomatosis includes laser ablation, which is easily performed with a laser-reflective endotracheal tube in adults, and spontaneous ventilation with a natural airway in children. Medialization of the vocal cord or injection laryngoplasty is also accomplished during spontaneous ventilation with a natural airway. Although there are many different methods for providing general anesthesia with a natural airway, total intravenous anesthesia (TIVA) with topicalization of the vocal cords during spontaneous ventilation provides the best view of the surgical field for the surgeon.[43]

Ear Surgery

The ear and its associated structures are target organs for many pathologic conditions. General anesthesia for surgery of the ear has its own set of unique considerations that must be addressed.

Myringotomy and Tube Insertion

Chronic serous otitis in children can lead to hearing loss. Drainage of accumulated fluid in the middle ear is an effective treatment for this condition. Myringotomy, which creates an opening in the tympanic membrane for fluid drainage, may be performed alone. During healing, the drainage path may become occluded; therefore, ventilation tube placement is usually included. The insertion of a small plastic tube in the tympanic membrane serves as a vent for the ostium and allows for continued drainage of the middle ear until the tubes are naturally extruded in 6 months to 1 year or surgically removed at an appropriate time.

Myringotomy with tube insertion is a relatively short procedure, and anesthesia may be effectively accomplished with a potent inhalation agent, oxygen, and N_2O administered by face mask. Premedication is not recommended because most sedative drugs used for premedication will far outlast the duration of the surgical procedure. Patients with chronic otitis frequently have accompanying recurrent URI. It is often the eradication of middle ear fluid that resolves the concomitant URI. Because tracheal intubation is not required for routine patients, the criteria for cancellation of surgery and anesthesia may be different for this procedure. Insertion of myringotomy tubes may be undertaken in most children with a concomitant URI provided that this can be completed with face mask anesthesia and endotracheal intubation is avoided. No significant difference in perioperative morbidity between asymptomatic patients and those fulfilling URI criteria has been demonstrated.[44,45] It is recommended that patients with URI symptoms receive supplemental postoperative oxygen.

Middle Ear and Mastoid

Tympanoplasty and mastoidectomy are two of the most common procedures performed on the middle ear and accessory structures. To gain access to the surgical site, the head is positioned on a headrest, which may be lower than the operative table, and extreme degrees of lateral rotation may be required. Extreme tension on the heads of the sternocleidomastoid muscles must be avoided. The laxity of the ligaments of the cervical spine and the immaturity of odontoid process in children make them especially prone to C1 to C2 subluxation.

Ear surgery often involves surgical identification and preservation of the facial nerve, which requires isolation of the nerve by the surgeon and verification of its function by means of electrical stimulation (Fig. 48-6). This is accomplished by brainstem auditory evoked potential and electrocochleogram monitoring, which requires that complete muscle relaxation be avoided.[46] However, if an opioid-relaxant technique is chosen, at least 30% of the muscle response, as determined by a twitch monitor, should be preserved. This fact suggests that it is not mandatory to avoid skeletal muscle relaxants in the anesthetic management of patients undergoing surgical procedures when monitoring of facial nerve function is necessary.

Bleeding must be kept to a minimum during surgery of the small structures of the middle ear. Minimizing excessive increases in blood pressure and normotension can be helpful

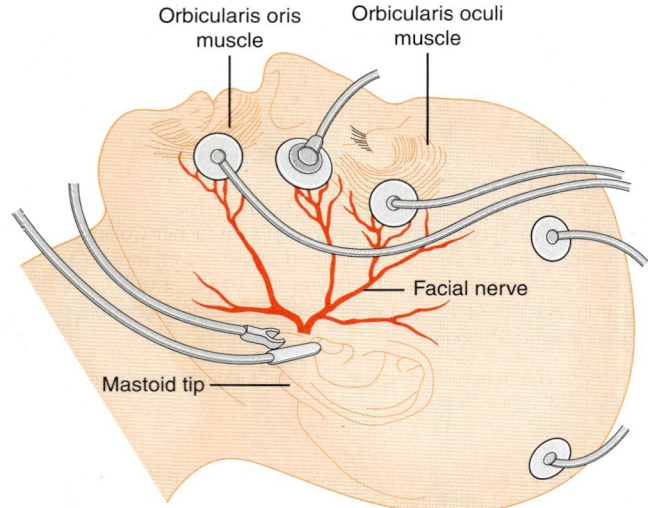

Figure 48-6 Illustration of facial nerve and monitoring electrodes. (Courtesy of Steve Ronner, PhD, Boston, MA.)

Table 48-2	Causes of Stridor	
Supraglottic Airway	**Larynx**	**Subglottic Airway**
Laryngomalacia	Laryngocele	Tracheomalacia
Vocal cord paralysis	Infection (tonsillitis, peritonsillar abscess)	Vascular ring
Subglottic stenosis	Foreign body	Foreign body
Hemangiomas	Choanal atresia	Infection (croup, epiglottitis)
Cysts	Cyst Mass Large tonsils Large adenoids Craniofacial abnormalities	

in improving the surgical field. Relative hypotension can also be effective, though careful consideration should be given to the risks of lowered blood pressure against the potential benefit of reduced surgical bleeding, because even short periods of hypotension may be associated with perioperative morbidity.[47] Additional specific contraindications to this technique include intracranial hypertension, hypovolemia, or history of vascular, cerebrovascular, or other end-organ disease.[48] Concentrated epinephrine solution, often 1:1,000, can be injected in the area of the tympanic vessels to produce vasoconstriction, though concentrations as low as 1:400,000 may give equivalent reductions in local blood flow with less potential for adverse effects from inadvertent intravascular injection.[49,50] Pay close attention to the volume of injected epinephrine so that dysrhythmias and wide swings in blood pressure may be avoided.

The middle ear and sinuses are air-filled, nondistensible cavities. An increase in the volume of gas in these structures results in an increase in pressure. N_2O diffuses along a concentration gradient into the air-filled middle ear spaces more rapidly than nitrogen moves out. Passive venting occurs at 20 to 30 cm H_2O pressure, and it has been shown that the use of N_2O results in pressures that exceed the ability of the eustachian tube to vent the middle ear within 5 minutes, leading to pressure buildup.[51] During procedures in which the eardrum is replaced or a perforation is patched, N_2O should be discontinued or, if this is not possible, limited to a maximum of 50% during the application of the tympanic membrane graft to avoid pressure-related displacement.

After N_2O is discontinued, it is quickly reabsorbed, creating a void in the middle ear with resulting negative pressure. This negative pressure may result in serous otitis, disarticulation of the ossicles in the middle ear (especially the stapes), and hearing impairment, which may last up to 6 weeks after surgery. The use of N_2O is related to a high incidence of postoperative nausea and vomiting, which is a direct result of negative middle ear pressure during recovery. The vestibular system is stimulated by traction placed on the round window by the negative pressure that is created. Although all patients have the potential for nausea and vomiting after surgery, children younger than 8 years of age seem to be most affected. If the use of N_2O cannot be avoided, vigorous use of antiemetics is warranted.

Airway Surgery

Stridor

Noisy breathing due to obstructed airflow is known as *stridor*. Inspiratory stridor results from upper airway obstruction; expiratory stridor results from lower airway obstruction; and biphasic stridor is present with midtracheal lesions. The evaluation of a patient with stridor begins with a thorough history. The age of onset suggests a cause: Laryngotracheomalacia is usually present at or shortly after birth, whereas cysts or mass lesions develop later in life (Table 48-2). Vocal cord paralysis may be congenital or acquired. Acquired vocal cord paralysis may be due to iatrogenic injury sustained during surgery, neurologic abnormalities such as Arnold–Chiari malformation, local invasion by tumors, and certain chemotherapy regimens. Information indicating positions that make the stridor better or worse should be obtained, and placing a patient in a position that allows gravity to aid in reducing obstruction can be of benefit during anesthetic induction.

Physical examination reveals the general condition of a patient and the degree of the airway compromise. Laboratory examination may include assessment of hemoglobin, a chest radiograph, and a barium swallow, which can aid in identifying lesions that may be compressing the trachea. Other radiologic examinations such as MRI and computed tomography may be indicated in isolated instances but are not routinely ordered. Specific note of the signs and symptoms listed in Table 48-3 should be made.

Laryngomalacia is the most common cause of stridor in infants. It is most often due to a long epiglottis that prolapses posteriorly and prominent arytenoid cartilages with redundant aryepiglottic folds that obstruct the glottic opening during inspiration.[52] Many times, laryngomalacia will improve as patients

Table 48-3 Clinical Component of the Evaluation of Patients with Stridor	
Respiratory rate	Chest retractions
Heart rate	Nasal flaring
Wheezing	Level of consciousness
Cyanosis	

grow older, though patients with severe obstructive symptoms may need surgical intervention.

Though the majority of patients with unilateral vocal cord paralysis (UVCP) are stridorous, they rarely have signs of overt airway obstruction, as would be the case with bilateral cord paralysis. Younger children with UVCP may have a weak cry and frequent aspiration from lack of ability to fully oppose their vocal cords and protect their airway, whereas older patients may have only symptoms of hoarseness and poor vocal projection.

The definitive diagnosis for both laryngomalacia and UVCP is obtained by direct laryngoscopy and rigid or flexible bronchoscopy. Preliminary examination is usually carried out in the surgeon's office. A small, flexible fiberoptic bronchoscope is inserted through the nares into the oropharynx, and the movement of the vocal cords is observed. Alternatively, it may be accomplished in the OR before anesthetic induction in an awake patient or in a lightly anesthetized patient during spontaneous respiration. Patients must be breathing spontaneously so that the vocal cords can move freely. After deepening of anesthesia and topicalization of the vocal cords is performed using 1% to 2% lidocaine, a rigid bronchoscope is inserted through the vocal cords, and the subglottic area is inspected; the lower trachea and bronchi are evaluated with a rigid or flexible fiberoptic bronchoscope. Treatment for laryngomalacia and UVCP can be performed in conjunction with direct laryngoscopy and bronchoscopy. During supraglottoplasty, redundant tissue is removed in a targeted manner to improve airflow mechanics. Interventional therapy for UVCP is aimed at medializing the paralyzed cord such that it can make contact with the contralateral functioning vocal cord and allow for airway protection. This can be accomplished with periodic injection laryngoplasty or with more permanent interventions such as medialization thyroplasty and reinnervation procedures. Reinnervation procedures do not return vocal cord mobility but restore tone such that the vocal cord assumes a more medial position.[53]

Bronchoscopy

Small infants may be brought into the OR unpremedicated. Older children and adults may experience respiratory depression and worsening of airway obstruction if heavy premedication is administered, so only light sedation is suggested. The airway must be protected from aspiration of gastric contents during prolonged airway manipulation; therefore, premedication with the full regimen of acid aspiration prophylaxis may be indicated.

The goals of the anesthetic are analgesia, an unconscious patient, and a "quiet" surgical field. Coughing, bucking, or straining during instrumentation with the rigid bronchoscope may cause difficulty for the surgeon and result in damage to the patient's airway. At the conclusion of the procedure, patients should be returned to consciousness quickly, with airway reflexes intact. For most patients, a pulse oximeter, blood pressure cuff, ECG leads, and precordial stethoscope are applied before induction of anesthesia. Inhalation induction by mask is accompanied by administration of oxygen and a volatile agent in increasing concentrations in children and intravenous drugs in adults. Patients should be placed in the position that produces the least adverse effect on airway symptoms (often the sitting position). An intravenously administered antisialagogue may help decrease secretions that might compromise the view through the bronchoscope.

The size of a bronchoscope refers to the internal diameter. Because the external diameter may be significantly greater than that of an endotracheal tube of similar size (Table 48-4), care must be taken to select a bronchoscope of proper external diameter to avoid damage to the laryngeal structures. A rigid bronchoscope

Table 48-4 Comparison of External Diameter of Standard Endotracheal Tubes versus Rigid Bronchoscope

Endotracheal Tube	Rigid Bronchoscope	
Internal Diameter (mm)	External Diameter (mm)	Internal Diameter (mm)
3.5	4.2	2.5
4.3	5	3
4.9	5.7	3.5
5.5	6.7	4
6.8	7.8	5
8.2	8.2	6

can be used for ventilation of the lungs during examination of the airway. It is inserted through the vocal cords, and ventilation is accomplished through a side port, which can be attached to the anesthesia circuit. During ventilation with the viewing telescope in place, high resistance may be encountered as a result of partial occlusion of the lumen. High fresh gas flow rates, large tidal volumes, and high inspired volatile anesthetic concentrations are often necessary to compensate for leaks around the ventilating bronchoscope and the high resistance encountered when the viewing telescope is in place. Manual ventilation at higher-than-normal rates is most effective in achieving adequate ventilation. Adequate time for exhalation must be provided for passive recoil of the chest.[54]

An alternative method of ventilation is the jet ventilation technique, which involves intermittent bursts of oxygen delivered under pressure.[55,56] Intermittent flow is accomplished by use of a programmed jet ventilator but can alternatively be accomplished with manual controls. The use of jet ventilation techniques is associated with the additional risks of pneumothorax or pneumomediastinum due to rupture of alveolar blebs or a bronchus.[57] Because ventilation may be intermittent and at times suboptimal, oxygen should be used as the carrier gas during bronchoscopic examination. Intravenous drugs that cause excessive respiratory depression should be avoided. It is wise to ask the surgeon if movement of the vocal cords will be required at the conclusion of the procedure or if tracheal or bronchial dynamics will be evaluated during the procedure so that the anesthetic may be planned accordingly (i.e., spontaneous respirations preserved during light levels of anesthesia vs. no respiratory efforts and the use of short-acting muscle relaxants).

Maintenance of anesthesia is usually accomplished with a volatile anesthetic augmented by propofol infusion (100 to 300 µg/kg/min). Intravenous anesthetics combined with muscle relaxation best maintain a constant level of anesthesia because the delivery of volatile anesthetics through the bronchoscope may be interrupted, and anesthetic depth can vary. At the conclusion of rigid bronchoscopy, an endotracheal tube is usually placed in the trachea to control the airway during recovery of anesthesia. Securing the airway is particularly important if muscle relaxants have been used because passive regurgitation of gastric contents may be more likely to occur in paralyzed patients. An additional advantage of placing an endotracheal tube is that if the surgeon should want to examine the distal airways, a small, flexible fiberoptic bronchoscope can be passed through the endotracheal tube.

Pediatric Airway Emergencies

Upper airway emergencies may be life-threatening and demand immediate treatment. Rapid respiratory failure can occur in patients with croup, epiglottitis, or foreign body aspiration, and few clinical situations are more challenging to the anesthesiologist.

Epiglottitis

Acute epiglottitis is one of the most feared infectious diseases in children and adults and is the result of *Haemophilus influenzae* type B. A conservative estimate of the incidence of epiglottitis is 10 to 40 cases per million people in the United States. Since 1985, with the widespread vaccination against *H. influenzae* type B (Hib), which was the most common organism related to epiglottitis, the overall incidence of the disease among children has dropped dramatically. It can progress with extreme rapidity from sore throat to airway obstruction to respiratory failure and ultimately to death if proper diagnosis and intervention are not rapidly implemented. Patients are usually between 2 and 7 years of age, although epiglottitis has been reported in younger children and in adults. Epiglottitis in the very young (younger than 1 year) is unusual and occurs in only about 4% of cases, and in adults it peaks between ages 20 to 40 years. Vaccination against *H. influenzae* type B polysaccharide is now recommended before 2 years of age to provide immunity before the greatest period of vulnerability in pediatric patients.

Characteristic signs and symptoms of acute epiglottitis include sudden onset of fever, dysphagia, drooling, thick muffled voice, and preference for the sitting position with the head extended and leaning forward. Retractions, labored breathing, and cyanosis may be observed in cases in which respiratory obstruction is present. However, in the early stages, the patient may be pale and toxic without respiratory distress. *Supraglottitis* may be a more appropriate designation because it is the tissues of the supraglottic structures—from the vallecula to the arytenoids—that are involved in the infectious process. At no time, especially in the emergency department or radiography suite, should direct visualization of the epiglottis be attempted in the unanesthetized patient. The differential resulting from negative pressure inside and atmospheric pressure outside the extrathoracic airway results in slight narrowing during normal inspiration. The pressure differential on inspiration is exaggerated in the patient with airway obstruction. This dynamic collapse of the airway may become life-threatening in the struggling, agitated patient, and every attempt should be made to keep the patient calm. Blood drawing, intravenous catheter insertion, and excessive manipulation of the patient, as well as sedation, should be avoided before securing the airway to avoid the possibility of total obstruction.

If the clinical situation allows, oxygen should be administered by mask, and lateral radiographs of the soft tissues in the neck may be obtained. Thickening of the aryepiglottic folds and swelling of the epiglottis may be noted (the "thumbprint" sign). Radiologic examination should be carried out only if skilled personnel and adequate equipment accompany the patient at all times. The patient with severe airway compromise should proceed from the emergency department directly to the operating suite accompanied by both the anesthesiologist and surgeon. Parental presence in this situation may calm an anxious and frightened child.

In all cases of epiglottitis, an artificial airway is established by means of tracheal intubation. In some centers in which personnel experienced in the management of the compromised airway are not available, tracheostomy is a less-favored alternative. In the OR, the child is kept in the sitting position while monitors are placed. A pulse oximeter and precordial stethoscope are essential. If it is believed to be helpful, one parent may accompany the child and remain in the OR during the induction of general anesthesia. The OR must be prepared with equipment and personnel for laryngoscopy, rigid bronchoscopy, and tracheostomy. Anesthetic induction is accomplished by inhalation of oxygen and increasing concentrations of sevoflurane. After loss of consciousness occurs, intravenous access should be secured and the child lowered into the supine position. Laryngoscopy followed by oral tracheal intubation is then accomplished without the use of muscle relaxants. The endotracheal tube chosen should be at least one size (0.5 mm) smaller than would normally be chosen, and a stylette is often useful. Once the surgeon has examined the larynx, noting the appearance of the epiglottis, aryepiglottic folds, and surrounding tissues, the endotracheal tube may be changed to a nasotracheal tube and secured. Tissue and blood cultures are taken, and antibiotic therapy is initiated. The child is then transferred to the ICU for continued observation and radiographic confirmation of tube placement. Sedation is appropriate at this time. Tracheal extubation is usually attempted 48 to 72 hours later in the OR, when a significant leak around the nasotracheal tube is present and visual inspection of the larynx by flexible fiberoptic bronchoscopy confirms reduction in swelling of the epiglottis and surrounding tissues.

Laryngotracheobronchitis

Laryngotracheobronchitis (LTB), or croup, occurs in children from 6 months to 6 years of age but is primarily seen in children younger than 3 years of age. It is usually viral in etiology, and its onset is more insidious than that of epiglottitis. The child presents with low-grade fever, inspiratory stridor, and a "barking" cough. Radiologic examination confirms the diagnosis, and subglottic narrowing of the airway column secondary to circumferential soft tissue edema produces the "steeple" sign characteristic of LTB. Approximately 6% of patients with LTB require admission to the hospital. Treatment includes cool, humidified mist and oxygen therapy, usually administered in a tent for mild-to-moderate cases. More severe cases of LTB are accompanied by tachypnea, tachycardia, and cyanosis. Racemic epinephrine administered by nebulizer is beneficial. The use of steroids has been surrounded by a great deal of controversy, but current opinion is that a short course of steroids may be beneficial. In rare circumstances, thick secretions are present in the airway, and the child requires intubation to allow pulmonary toilet and suctioning to be performed. Management in the ICU and extubation are carried out in the same fashion as for epiglottitis.

Foreign Body Aspiration

A major cause of morbidity and mortality in children and adults is aspiration of a foreign body. Any history of coughing, choking, or cyanosis while eating should suggest the possibility of foreign body aspiration. Peanuts, popcorn, jelly beans, and hot dogs are some of the ingested items most commonly associated with pulmonary aspiration. Any patient who presents to the emergency department with refractory wheezing should be suspected of this diagnosis. Physical findings include decreased breath sounds, tachypnea, stridor, wheezing, and fever. These signs indicate an obstructive process with inflammation present in the airway. Some foreign bodies are identifiable on radiologic examination;

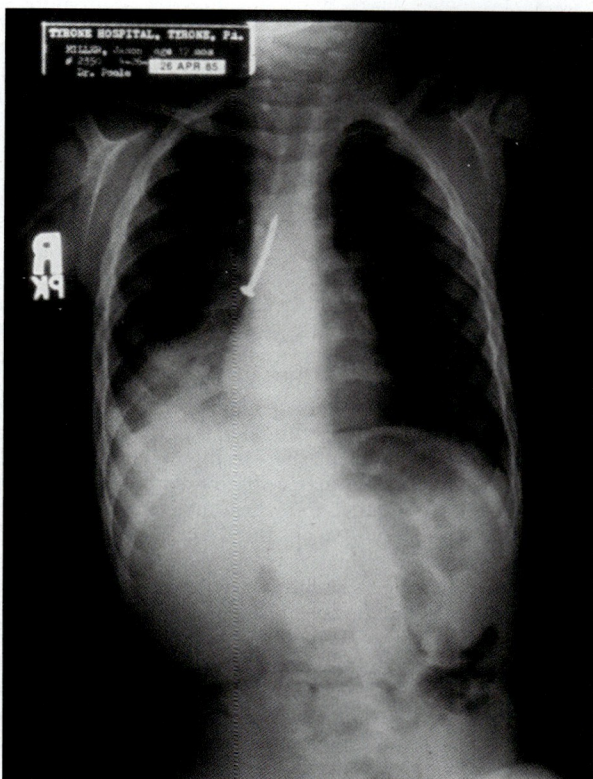

Figure 48-7 Aspirated foreign body in the right main stem bronchus.

however, 90% are radiolucent, and air trapping, infiltrate, and atelectasis are all that are noted.

The most common site of foreign body aspiration is the main stem bronchus, the right being more frequent than the left (Fig. 48-7). Food particles comprise the majority of aspirated items; however, beads, pins, and small toys are not unusual. Each type of aspirated item has potential complications associated with it. Vegetable items expand with moisture encountered in the respiratory tract and can fragment into multiple pieces, thus creating a situation in which the original foreign body is in one bronchus and, with coughing, a fragment is dislodged and transported to the other bronchus. Oil-containing objects, such as peanuts, cause a chemical inflammation, and sharp objects cause bleeding in addition to the obstruction.

All aspirated foreign bodies in the airway should be removed in the OR and considered to be emergency situations. No sedation should be administered to patients before removal of the foreign body. If the patient has recently eaten, full-stomach precautions must be taken, and anesthesia should be induced intravenously (topical anesthetic cream may be applied to the skin before intravenous catheter insertion in small children) by rapid sequence, with gentle cricoid pressure maintained during intubation of the trachea. If the child has not eaten recently, anesthesia may be induced by inhalation of sevoflurane in oxygen by mask. Inhalation induction can be prolonged secondary to obstruction of the airway, and N_2O should be avoided to prevent air trapping distal to the obstruction. After evacuation of the stomach by orogastric tube, the airway may be given over to the surgeon, who introduces a rigid bronchoscope and removes the aspirated object.

Spontaneous ventilation should be preserved until the location and nature of the foreign body have been determined.

Ventilation via the bronchoscope requires careful attention. Hypoxia and hypercarbia may occur because of inadequate ventilation caused by an excessively large leak around the bronchoscope or, more commonly, inability to provide adequate gas exchange through a narrow-lumen bronchoscope fitted with an internal telescope. These conditions are remedied by frequent removal of the telescope and withdrawal of the bronchoscope to the midtrachea, allowing effective ventilation. Bronchospasm may occur during examination of the respiratory tract and should be treated with increasing depths of anesthesia, nebulized albuterol, or intravenous bronchodilators. Although rare, pneumothorax should be suspected if acute deterioration occurs during the procedure.

Once the foreign body has been removed, examination of the entire tracheobronchial tree is carried out to detect any additional objects or fragments. Often, vigorous irrigation and suctioning distal to the obstruction are required to remove secretions and prevent the possibility of postobstructive pneumonia. Steroids are administered if inflammation of the airway mucosa is observed. Close postoperative observation of the patient is required so that early intervention may be instituted in the event of respiratory compromise secondary to airway edema or infection.

Pediatric and Adult Surgery

Certain surgical procedures are commonly performed in both adults and children, including nasal surgery and laser surgery of the airway.

Laser Surgery of the Airway

One of the greatest advances in airway surgery has been the use of the laser (light amplification by stimulated emission of radiation). For use in the airway, the laser provides precision in targeting lesions, minimal bleeding and edema, preservation of surrounding structures, and rapid healing. The laser consists of a tube with reflective mirrors at either end and an amplifying medium between them to generate electron activity, resulting in the production of light.[58] The CO_2 laser is the most widely used in medical practice, having particular application in the treatment of laryngeal or vocal cord papillomas, laryngeal webs, resection of redundant subglottic tissue, and coagulation of hemangiomas. The laser is an especially useful modality for the surgeon because the invisible beam of light affords an unobstructed view of the lesion during resection. The energy emitted by a CO_2 laser is absorbed by water contained in blood and tissues. Human tissue is approximately 80% water, and laser energy absorbed by tissue water rapidly increases the temperature, denaturing protein and vaporizing the target tissue. The thermal energy of the laser beam cauterizes capillaries as it vaporizes tissues; thus, bleeding and postoperative edema are minimized.

The properties that give the laser a high degree of specificity also supply the route by which a misdirected laser beam may cause injury to a patient or to unprotected OR personnel. The eyes are especially vulnerable, and all OR personnel should wear laser-specific eye goggles with side protectors to prevent injury. Because of the limited penetration (0.01 mm) of the CO_2 laser, it may cause injury only to the cornea. Other lasers such as the neodymium–yttrium-aluminum-garnet (Nd:YAG) have deeper penetration, and may cause retinal injury and scarring. The eyes of a patient undergoing laser treatment must be protected by taping them shut, followed by the application of wet gauze pads and a metal shield. Any stray laser beam is absorbed by the wet gauze, preventing penetration of the eyes. Laser radiation increases the temperature of the absorbent material, and flammable objects such as surgical drapes must be kept away from the path of the laser beam. To avoid cutaneous burns from deflected beams, wet towels should be applied to exposed skin of the face and neck when the laser is being used in the airway. Laser smoke plumes may cause damage to the lungs; interstitial pneumonia has been reported with long-term exposure. In addition, it has been postulated that cancer cells and virus particles, including human immunodeficiency virus, are vaporized during laser application, and the resultant smoke plume, if inhaled, may be a vehicle for spread. The use of specially designed surgical masks for filtering laser smoke is recommended.

Most anesthetic techniques are suitable for laser surgery, provided that patients are immobile and the laser beam can be directed at a target that is entirely still and in full view. Both N_2O and oxygen support combustion; therefore, the primary gas for anesthetic maintenance should consist of blended air and oxygen or helium and oxygen. A pulse oximeter should be used at all times to ensure adequate oxygenation at the lowest possible inspired concentration of oxygen. Anesthesia during laser surgery may be administered with or without an endotracheal tube. The choice of endotracheal tube used during laser surgery can affect the safety of the technique. All standard polyvinyl chloride endotracheal tubes are flammable and can ignite and vaporize producing hydrochloric acid when in contact with the laser beam. Cuffed endotracheal tubes should be inflated with sterile saline to which methylene blue has been added so that a cuff rupture from a misdirected laser spark is readily detected by the blue dye and extinguished by the saline.[59] Endotracheal tubes have been manufactured specifically for use during laser surgery. Some have a double cuff to ensure protection of the airway in the event of a cuff rupture, and some have a special matte finish that effectively prevents reflected laser beam scattering; some have both. Nonreflective flexible metal endotracheal tubes are also specifically manufactured for use during laser surgery. The outer diameter of each size of metal laser tube is considerably greater than the polyvinyl chloride counterpart, especially in the small sizes used for pediatric anesthesia (Table 48-5).

An apneic technique is preferred by some surgeons, especially when working on the airway of small infants and children. The advantage of this technique is an unobstructed surgical field owing to the absence of an endotracheal tube, which may obscure the surgical field. In this circumstance, a child is anesthetized and rendered immobile by the use of a muscle relaxant or deep inhalation of a volatile anesthetic. The patient's trachea is not intubated, and the airway is given over to the surgeon, who uses the laser for brief periods. Between laser applications, the patient's lungs are ventilated by mask. Because apnea is a component of this technique, it is prudent to ventilate the lungs with oxygen. Although this technique has been widely used with safety, there is a greater potential for debris and resected material to enter the trachea as well as the potential for airway trauma as a result of repeated endotracheal intubation.

The use of a jet ventilator is a modification of the apneic technique that does not require tracheal intubation but does provide for oxygenation; ventilation during laser surgery uses a jet ventilator. The operating laryngoscope is fitted with a catheter through which oxygen is delivered under pressure through a variable reducing valve. Additional room air is entrained, and the patient's lungs are ventilated with this combination of gases. This technique produces a quiet surgical field because large chest excursions of the diaphragm are eliminated and ventilation is uninterrupted. In morbidly obese patients and those with severe small airway disease, effective ventilation is difficult to impossible with this technique, and an alternate technique should be used.

The final technique that may be used is spontaneous ventilation without the aid of an endotracheal tube (Fig. 48-8). In this technique, a surgical laryngoscope fitted with an oxygen insufflation port is inserted into the larynx. Anesthesia may be induced with a volatile agent by mask but is maintained with total intravenous agents without muscle relaxant in the spontaneously breathing patient. Propofol may be infused with or without a short-acting narcotic, and the vocal cords may be sprayed with 4% lidocaine to decrease reactivity. This technique is advantageous in that longer periods of uninterrupted laser application may be provided. Disadvantages include the absence of complete control of the airway, limited protection from laryngospasm, limited protection from debris entering the airway, vocal cord motion, and difficult scavenging.

Nasal Surgery

Close communication between the anesthesiologist and the otorhinolaryngologist during nasal surgery is essential for a successful outcome and avoidance of major complications. Functional endoscopic sinus surgery (FESS) is the most common procedure performed in the nasal area. Historically, nasal procedures were completed under topical or local anesthesia with sedation so that the patient could signal the surgeon if problems arose.[60] As endoscopic nasal surgery grew larger in scope and duration, general anesthesia became preferred, and local anesthesia with sedation was reserved for the simpler cases.

To achieve optimal visualization of the surgical field, bleeding must be kept to a minimum. Current anesthetic practice includes the use of vasoconstrictors, elevation of the head, and avoiding excessive increases in blood pressure. Preoperative evaluation of the patient includes a focused cardiovascular history to document coronary artery disease, peripheral artery disease, and cardiac arrhythmias, which might be exacerbated by the use of sympathomimetic agents used for local vasoconstriction. Positive findings may alter the degree of head elevation, the use of topical constrictors, the anesthetic technique, and the lower limit of blood pressure that can be safely tolerated.

Intranasal vasoconstriction has been accomplished by the use of local anesthetics combined with cocaine, epinephrine, and phenylephrine. Systemic absorption of these agents can cause hypotension, hypertension, bradycardia, tachycardia, and arrhythmias.[61,62] For patients on β-blocker or calcium channel blocker therapy, α-agonist–induced hypertension may lead to pulmonary edema and cardiac failure. Prompt treatment is needed to prevent serious complications.

Table 48-5 Comparison of Standard Plastic versus Metal Endotracheal Tubes

Internal Diameter (mm)	External Diameter (mm)	
	Plastic	*Metal*
3 (uncuffed)	4.3	5.2
3.5 (uncuffed)	4.9	5.7
4 (uncuffed)	5.5	6.1
4.5 (cuffed)	6.2	7
5 (cuffed)	6.8	7.5
5.5 (cuffed)	7.5	7.9
6 (cuffed)	8.2	8.5

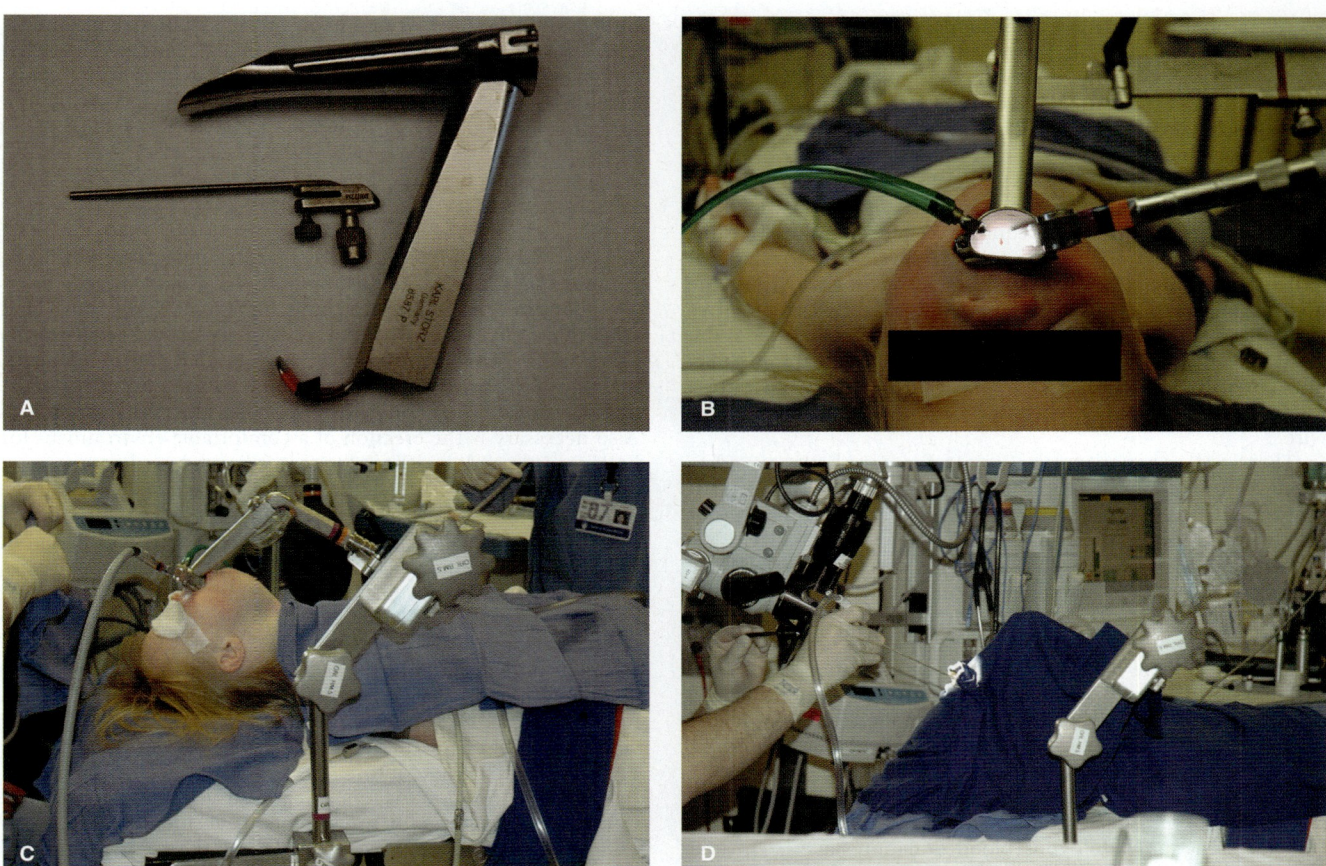

Figure 48-8 **A:** The surgical laryngoscope and the jet ventilator needle. **B:** The surgical view of the laryngoscope positioned in the patient's pharynx and connected to a continuous flow of oxygen through the jet ventilator needle. **C:** View of the anesthetized, spontaneously breathing patient. **D:** Laser-aided resection of vocal cord lesion.

The patient is positioned with the head elevated 15 degrees to facilitate venous drainage. This position may give some modest hypotension; however, there is the potential for venous pooling in the lower extremities. General anesthesia is maintained with either inhalation-based anesthesia or TIVA. Many surgeons now prefer TIVA because it has been shown to reduce blood loss and improve visualization of the surgical field. A comparison of isoflurane/fentanyl anesthesia to remifentanil/propofol TIVA resulted in better visualization and less blood loss for the TIVA group at equal reduction in blood pressure.[63,64] TIVA may also have the added benefit of reducing both coughing on emergence and postoperative nausea and vomiting.

Skull Base Surgery

Skull base surgery may be considered the logical extension of nasal surgery involving the practices of otorhinolaryngology, neurosurgery, and anesthesiology. The majority of adult patients undergoing skull base surgery have malignant tumors with a smaller group of patients having benign tumors, congenital malformations, or other abnormalities. These patients often require radiologic procedures to determine the location and extent of the lesion prior to surgery. Noninvasive tests include CAT scans and MRIs to ascertain the extent of bony and soft tissue abnormalities, whereas more invasive angiography may be needed to determine tumor location and blood supply. These studies may then be used to program intraoperative localizing systems to help guide the surgical dissection.[65] Finally, embolization of lesions may be performed a day or two prior to surgery to shrink the lesion and decrease blood loss during the operative procedure.[66]

Special attention during the preoperative assessment should be given to prior surgical procedures, which may affect the airway, chemotherapy, and radiation treatment. Prior surgical procedures may alter a previously easy airway, which subsequently may require advanced airway management techniques to intubate the trachea. Prior chemotherapy can have anesthetic implications depending on the agents used. Patients who have received cardiotoxic agents in which effects are dose dependent may require a cardiac evaluation including an echocardiogram. Decreased cardiac function may affect the type of anesthetic agents used and require invasive blood pressure monitoring with an arterial catheter. Prior treatment with neurotoxic agents may decrease the dose of muscle relaxants or cause their duration of action to be prolonged, requiring neuromuscular monitoring. Prior radiation therapy usually does not cause systemic problems unless the pituitary gland is damaged, which can give rise to the problems of panhypopituitarism leading to hypothyroidism, hypoadrenocorticism, and diabetes insipidus. Prior radiation therapy may lead to fibrosis and ankylosis in the temporomandibular joint, rendering direct laryngoscopy difficult. Previous radiation to the operative site may also increase blood loss and results in poor wound healing. Secondary radiation fibrosis may make the surgical dissection more difficult and time consuming. It may also necessitate the use of free or vascularized grafts to close the surgical site. In addition, the location of the donor site and potential anastomotic sites must be considered when positioning the patient.

Close attention must be paid to the evaluation of the head and neck during the physical examination. Usually these patients do not have a difficult airway or require special techniques for intubation. For lesions requiring a midline surgical approach, oral intubation is the preferred route. If the lesion does not cross the midline, an oral or nasal approach may be used. Nasal endotracheal tubes may be secured by use of a heavy suture through the nasal septum and around the tube. Oral endotracheal tubes may be secured by wiring the endotracheal tube to the teeth, suturing it to the gingival periosteum, or using a circummandibular wire.

There are two noteworthy points for anesthetic consideration: the use of muscle relaxation and blood conservation strategies. Similar to other procedures in which the facial nerve is at risk for injury or transection during dissection, it is necessary to avoid paralysis so that the facial nerve may be periodically stimulated to verify its integrity. Muscle relaxants may be given if nerve stimulation is no longer required. Minimizing blood loss and creating a plan for replacement with blood products must be considered. If there is anticipation for large-volume blood loss, various approaches can be utilized to potentially reduce the need for transfusion. Anemia identified preoperatively can be treated with iron and erythropoietin. Acute normovolemic hemodilution can be used to minimize blood loss during the procedure. Recently, antithrombolytic therapy has been used with success in craniofacial procedures and may be of benefit in these cases.[67,68] Directed donor or autologous blood donation have been used to minimize or decrease the exposure to allogenic blood products. Blood salvage techniques, such as cell saver, are usually not appropriate given that most surgical sites are not reached through sterile approaches, and they would also be relatively contraindicated in surgeries involving resection of tumors.

Upper Airway Infections

Infectious processes of the upper airway can occur in the adult and present the same problems of airway compression, distortion, and compromise. Inflammation of the upper airway caused mainly by gram-negative bacteria may present with the same symptoms as epiglottitis in the pediatric age group. Although these patients present with fever, chills, drooling, and difficulty in speaking and swallowing, they do not usually appear with critical airways from swelling. These same symptoms may occur with Ludwig angina, which is a generalized cellulitis of the submandibular region.[69] The infection is often the result of dental abscesses and extends into the submandibular, submental, and sublingual areas. Involvement of the sublingual spaces pushes the tongue upward and backward and can lead to asphyxiation due to obstruction of the airway. Should this occur, emergent surgical interventions may be required to drain the abscess and relieve the airway obstruction.

Airway management can be very difficult in these cases.[70] Awake tracheostomy with local anesthesia has been considered the safest in these patients. If awake tracheostomy is performed, positive-pressure ventilation should be avoided until confirmation of proper tracheal tube placement, because insufflation into a false or blind passage can lead to significant patient morbidity. Alternative techniques of intubation include fiberoptic nasal intubation and direct laryngoscopy after inhalational anesthesia. These patients require care in an ICU whether they have a tracheotomy or an endotracheal tube once the abscess has been drained because increased swelling may develop. The trachea should not be extubated until there is some resolution of the swelling.

Maxillofacial Trauma

Traumatic disruption of the bony, cartilaginous, and soft tissue components of the face and upper airway challenges the anesthesiologist to recognize the nature and extent of the injury and consequent anatomic alteration, create a plan for securing the airway safely, implement the plan without doing further damage, maintain the airway during the administration of an anesthetic, and determine when and how to extubate the patient's trachea. Also necessary is the creation of a comfortable environment for both surgeon and anesthesiologist in a limited workspace.

It is conventional to divide the facial skeleton into thirds. The lower third consists of the mandible, with its subdivisions of midline symphysis, body, angle, ramus, condyle, and coronoid process. The mandible has a unique, horseshoe shape that causes forces to gather at its points of vulnerability, often distant from the point of impact. Consequently, fractures of the mandible typically occur posteriorly where the cortex is also thinner—at the angle of the mandible, the ramus, and the condyle.[71,72] With a condylar fracture, there is potential for temporomandibular joint involvement and resulting limitations in jaw mobility. Another common point of fracture is in the body of the mandible at the level of the first or second molar. Clinical experience indicates that this distribution occurs after high-velocity, high-impact trauma, such as occurs in an automobile accident. After trauma inflicted by a fist, a blunt weapon, or a fall, there is a greater tendency for a fracture of the symphysis, parasymphysis, and body to occur.[73] Fractures of the mandible typically do not extend into the skull base. The middle third contains the zygomatic arch of the temporal bone, blending into the zygomaticomaxillary complex, the maxillae, nasal bones, and orbits. Force from a blow to the midface, especially from in front and above, does not follow a normal vector of force dispersion and redistribution. Rather, it tends to create an abnormal shearing force, which may tear the facial skeleton from the cranial skeleton and extend the fracture into the base of the skull. Therefore, in any patient with severe midfacial trauma, a fracture of the base of the skull must be considered. The superior third consists of the frontal bone.

In 1901, Rene Le Fort of Lille, France, determined the common lines of midface fracture, which are thus eponymous and called Le Fort I, Le Fort II, and Le Fort III fractures.

The Le Fort I fracture is a horizontal fracture of the maxilla, passing above the floor of the nose but involving the lower third of the septum, mobilizing the palate, maxillary alveolar process, and the lower third of the pterygoid plates and parts of the palatine bones. The fracture segment may be displaced posteriorly or laterally or rotated about a vertical axis. The Le Fort II fracture is pyramidal, beginning at the junction of the thick upper part of the nasal bone, with the thinner portion forming the upper margin of the anterior nasal aperture. The fracture crosses the medial wall of the orbit, including the lacrimal bone beneath the zygomaticomaxillary suture; crosses the lateral wall of the antrum; and passes posteriorly through the pterygoid plates. The fracture segment may be displaced posteriorly or rotated about an axis. In a Le Fort III fracture, the line of fracture parallels the base of the skull, separating the midfacial skeleton from the base of the cranium. The line of fracture passes through the base of the nose and the ethmoid bone in its depth and through the orbital plates. The cribriform plate of the ethmoid may or may not be fractured. The fracture line crosses the lesser wing of the sphenoid, then passes downward to the pterygomaxillary fissure and sphenopalatine fossa. From the base of the inferior orbital fissure, the fracture extends laterally and upward to the frontozygomatic suture and downward and backward to the root of the pterygoid plates. A Le Fort III fracture results from massive force applied to the midface. The zygomata are displaced, applying rotational force to the zygomatic arches. The arches are usually fractured as a result.

In a patient with a Le Fort III fracture, the midface is mobilized and often distracted posteriorly. The normal convexity of the face becomes concave, giving rise to the characteristic "dish face deformity" of a Le Fort III fracture. Even if this facial concavity is not clinically evident, the presence of a Le Fort III fracture should be suspected if the incisive edges of the maxillary and mandibular teeth are apposed instead of being in the normal position, in which the maxillary incisors shingle over the mandibular incisors. This apposition serves as a subtle clue to minimal posterior displacement of the midface.

Nasotracheal intubation is contraindicated in Le Fort II or III fractures when the cribriform plate of the ethmoid bone may be involved. Foreign material from the nasopharynx may result in meningitis or, even more devastating, the endotracheal tube can enter the cranial cavity. Even positive-pressure bag and mask ventilation can force foreign material or air into the skull.[74] Radiographic studies should be done prior to nasotracheal intubation whenever trauma to the skull base is suspected.

In the patient with facial trauma, concomitant injuries may not be apparent. One study revealed that in patients with maxillofacial injury due to low-velocity, low-impact blows, 4% had additional major life-threatening injuries and 10% had additional minor injuries. With high-velocity, high-impact accidents, 32% had major additional injuries and 31% had minor additional injuries.[75] Of great importance, cervical spine fractures occurred in 1.2% of high-velocity injuries. Multiple studies report cervical spine and significant head injury in patients with facial skeletal trauma, with incidence as high as 10.8% and 88.7%, respectively.[76,77] The area of cervical injury is frequently related to the site of maxillofacial trauma. Upper face injuries are associated with mid to lower cervical spine injuries, whereas unilateral mandibular injuries involve the upper cervical spine.[76]

To the extent that the patient's clinical situation allows, the degree of facial trauma and concomitant injuries should be assessed and incorporated into any plan for airway management. Patients with known or suspected cervical spine injuries should have appropriate protective precautions in place during airway management. Intubating patients with facial trauma can be potentially challenging owing to distorted or even disrupted anatomy, which can also be obscured by blood or emesis and displaced.[78] For cases in which there is concern about difficult airway management, intubation with a flexible fiberoptic bronchoscope should be considered, provided the patient is both cooperative and clinically stable. Fiberoptic bronchoscopy and videolaryngoscopy can also be used to assess the airway and as part of a rescue technique for failed direct laryngoscopy. Surgical airway placement may be required for patients with extensive airway injury that does not permit intubation, or for conditions such as laryngotracheal disruption that can be worsened with conventional intubation techniques such as direct laryngoscopy.[79]

If a patient cannot open the mouth during the preoperative evaluation, one must ascertain whether the restriction to mouth opening is the result of pain, trismus, or mechanical problem or some combination of the three. Simple fractures of the mandible can be very painful; however, once the patient is anesthetized, the mouth can be opened and tracheal intubation can proceed without difficulty. There may be mechanical interference with opening due to injury to the temporomandibular area either directly or indirectly. Direct trauma to the mandibular condyle or zygomatic arch may cause fractures that interfere with normal function of the temporomandibular joint. Indirect trauma is caused by transmittal of force up the body and ramus to the condyles. Compression fractures of condyles in the glenoid fossa and greenstick fractures of the condyles may result, impeding opening.

Trismus, spasm of the muscles of mastication, can result from trauma or infection and interfere with mouth opening. It too is usually overcome by general anesthesia and muscle relaxation. The caveat here is that should the trismus be of long standing, some degree of joint immobility will occur. If the trismus is caused by a facial infection, the affected muscles may become edematous and swell, causing a mechanical interference with opening.

Acknowledgments

The authors acknowledge Ms. Jessie Barnes Hurley for her tireless assistance in the preparation of this manuscript. They also would like to acknowledge the prior contributions of Drs. Alexander Gotta and Charles Nargozian to this chapter in previous editions.

REFERENCES

1. Cullen KA, Hall MJ, Golosinskiy A. Ambulatory surgery in the United States, 2006. *Natl Health Stat Rep.* 2009;11(11):1–25.
2. Schechter MS; Section on Pediatric Pulmonology, Subcommittee on Obstructive Sleep Apnea Syndrome. Clinical practice guideline: diagnosis and management of childhood obstructive sleep apnea syndrome. *Pediatrics.* 2002;109(4):704–712.
3. Myatt HM, Beckenham EJ. The use of diagnostic sleep nasendoscopy in the management of children with complex upper airway obstruction. *Clin Otolaryngol Allied Sci.* 2000;25(3):200–208.
4. Chaban R, Cole P, Hoffstein V. Site of upper airway obstruction in patients with idiopathic obstructive sleep apnea. *Laryngoscope.* 1988;98(6 Pt 1):641–647.
5. Blum RH, McGowan FX. Chronic upper airway obstruction and cardiac dysfunction: anatomy, pathophysiology and anesthetic implications. *Pediatr Anesth.* 2004;14(1):75–83.
6. Lerman J. Unraveling the mysteries of sleep-disordered breathing in children. *Anesthesiology.* 2006;105(4):645–647.
7. Gross JB, Bachenberg KL, Benumof JL, et al. Practice guidelines for the perioperative management of patients with obstructive sleep apnea: a report by the American Society of Anesthesiologists Task Force on Perioperative Management of patients with obstructive sleep apnea. *Anesthesiology.* 2006;104(5):1081–1093.
8. Brown KA. Outcome, risk, and error and the child with obstructive sleep apnea. *Pediatr Anesth.* 2011;21(7):771–780.
9. Patino M, Sadhasivam S, Mahmoud M. Obstructive sleep apnoea in children: perioperative considerations. *Br J Anaesth.* 2013;111(Suppl 1):i83–i95.
10. Chung F, Yegneswaran B, Liao P, et al. STOP questionnaire. *Anesthesiology.* 2008;108(5):812–821.
11. Chung SA, Yuan H, Chung F. A systemic review of obstructive sleep apnea and its implications for anesthesiologists. *Anesth Analg.* 2008;107(5):1543–1563.
12. Tait AR, Voepel-Lewis T, Christensen R, et al. The STBUR questionnaire for predicting perioperative respiratory adverse events in children at risk for sleep-disordered breathing. *Paediatr Anaesth.* 2013;23(6):510–516.
13. Tsuiki S, Isono S, Ishikawa T, et al. Anatomical balance of the upper airway and obstructive sleep apnea. *Anesthesiology.* 2008;108(6):1009–1015.
14. Coté CJ, Posner KL, Domino KB. Death or neurologic injury after tonsillectomy in children with a focus on obstructive sleep apnea: Houston, we have a problem! *Anesth Analg.* 2014;118(6):1276–1283.
15. Acevedo JL, Shah RK, Brietzke SE. Systematic review of complications of tonsillotomy versus tonsillectomy. *Otolaryngol Head Neck Surg.* 2012;146(6):871–879.
16. Windfuhr JP, Savva K, Dahm JD, et al. Tonsillotomy: facts and fiction. *Eur Arch Otorhinolaryngol.* 2015;272(4):949–969.
17. Eichler C, Sommer JU, Stuck BA, et al. Does drug-induced sleep endoscopy change the treatment concept of patients with snoring and obstructive sleep apnea? *Sleep Breath.* 2013;17(1):63–68.
18. Truong MT, Woo VG, Koltai PJ. Sleep endoscopy as a diagnostic tool in pediatric obstructive sleep apnea. *Int J Pediatr Otorhinolaryngol.* 2012;76(5):722–727.

19. Capici F, Ingelmo PM, Davidson A, et al. Randomized controlled trial of duration of analgesia following intravenous or rectal acetaminophen after adenotonsillectomy in children. *Br J Anaesth.* 2008;100(2):251–255.
20. Pestieau SR, Quezado ZM, Johnson YJ, et al. High-dose dexmedetomidine increases the opioid-free interval and decreases opioid requirement after tonsillectomy in children. *Can J Anesth.* 2011;58(6):540–550.
21. Kelly LE, Sommer DD, Ramakrishna J, et al. Morphine or Ibuprofen for post-tonsillectomy analgesia: a randomized trial. *Pediatrics.* 2015;135(2):307–313.
22. Brown KA, Laferriere A, Lakheeram I, et al. Recurrent hypoxemia in children is associated with increased analgesic sensitivity to opiates. *Anesthesiology.* 2006;105(4):665–669.
23. Voronov P, Przybylo HJ, Jagannathan N. Apnea in a child after oral codeine: a genetic variant—an ultra-rapid metabolizer. *Paediatr Anaesth.* 2007;17(7):684–687.
24. Patel RI1, Hannallah RS, Norden J, et al. Emergence airway complications in children: a comparison of tracheal extubation in awake and deeply anesthetized patients. *Anesth Analg.* 1991;73(3):266–270.
25. Alexander CA. A modified Intavent laryngeal mask for ENT and dental anaesthesia. *Anaesthesia.* 1990;45(10):892–893.
26. Haynes SR, Morton NS. The laryngeal mask airway: a review of its use in paediatric anaesthesia. *Pediatr Anaesth.* 1993;3(2):65–73.
27. Johr M. Anaesthesia for tonsillectomy. *Curr Opin Anaesthesiol.* 2006;19(3):260–261.
28. Williams PJ, Bailey PM. Comparison of the reinforced laryngeal mask airway and tracheal intubation for adenotonsillectomy. *Br J Anaesth.* 1993;70(1):30–33.
29. Nair I, Bailey PM. Review of uses of the laryngeal mask in ENT anaesthesia. *Anaesthesia.* 1995;50(10):898–900.
30. Goudsouzian NG, Cleveland R. Stability of the laryngeal mask airway during marked extension of the head. *Pediatr Anaesth.* 1993;3(2):117–119.
31. Goldman JL, Baugh RF, Davies L, et al. Mortality and major morbidity after tonsillectomy: etiologic factors and strategies for prevention. *Laryngoscope.* 2013;123(10):2544–2553.
32. Gunter JB, McAuliffe JJ, Beckman EC, et al. A factorial study of ondansetron, metoclopramide, and dexamethasone for emesis prophylaxis after adenotonsillectomy in children. *Paediatr Anaesth.* 2006;16(11):1153–1165.
33. Czarnetzki C. Dexamethasone and risk of nausea and vomiting and postoperative bleeding after tonsillectomy in children. *JAMA.* 2008;300(22):2621.
34. Windfuhr J, Chen Y, Remmert S. Hemorrhage following tonsillectomy and adenoidectomy in 15,218 patients. *Otolaryngology.* 2005;132(2):281–286.
35. Windfuhr JP, Deck JC, Remmert S. Hemorrhage following coblation tonsillectomy. *Ann Otol Rhinol Laryngol.* 2005;114(10):749–756.
36. Broadman LM, Patel RI, Feldman BA, et al. The effects of peritonsillar infiltration on the reduction of intraoperative blood loss and post-tonsillectomy pain in children. *Laryngoscope.* 1989;99(6):578–581.
37. Mehta VM, Har-El G, Goldstein NA. Postobstructive pulmonary edema after laryngospasm in the otolaryngology patient. *Laryngoscope.* 2006;116(9):1693–1696.
38. Brigger M, Brietzke S. Outpatient tonsillectomy in children: a systematic review. *Otolaryngol Head Neck Surg.* 2006;135(1):1–7.
39. Marcus CL, Brooks LJ, Draper KA, et al. Diagnosis and management of childhood obstructive sleep apnea syndrome. *Pediatrics.* 2012;130(3):576–584.
40. Brown KA, Brouillette RT. The elephant in the room: lethal apnea at home after adenotonsillectomy. *Anesth Analg.* 2014;118(6):1157–1159.
41. Statham MM, Elluru RG, Buncher R, et al. Adenotonsillectomy for obstructive sleep apnea syndrome in young children. *Arch Otolaryngol Head Neck Surg.* 2006;132(5):476–480.
42. Possamai V, Hartley B. Voice disorders in children. *Pediatr Clin North Am.* 2013;60(4):879–892.
43. Malherbe S, Whyte S, Singh P, et al. Total intravenous anesthesia and spontaneous respiration for airway endoscopy in children: a prospective evaluation. *Paediatr Anaesth.* 2010;20(5):434–438.
44. Tait AR. Malviya S. Anesthesia for the child with an upper respiratory tract infection: still a dilemma? *Anesth Analg.* 2005;100(1):59–65.
45. Tait AR, Malviya S, Voepel-Lewis T, et al. Risk factors for perioperative adverse respiratory events in children with upper respiratory tract infections. *Anesthesiology.* 2001;95(2):299–306.
46. Levine RA. Monitoring auditory evoked potentials during cerebellopontine angle tumor surgery: relative value of electrocochleography, brainstem auditory evoked potentials, and cerebellopontine angle recordings. *Intraoperative Neurophysiologic Monitoring in Neurosurgery.* New York, NY: Springer Science + Business Media; 1991:193–204.
47. Sun LY, Wijeysundera DN, Tait GA, et al. Association of intraoperative hypotension with acute kidney injury after elective noncardiac surgery. *Anesthesiology.* 2015;123(3):515–523.
48. Lavoie J. Blood transfusion risks and alternative strategies in pediatric patients. *Pediatr Anaesth.* 2011;21(1):14–24.
49. Gessler EM, Hart AK, Dunlevy TM, et al. Optimal concentration of epinephrine for vasoconstriction in ear surgery. *Laryngoscope.* 2001;111:1687–1690.
50. Dunlevy TM, O'Malley TP, Postma GN. Optimal concentration of epinephrine for vasoconstriction in neck surgery. *Laryngoscope.* 1996;106(11):1412–1414.
51. Casey WF, Drake-Lee AB. Nitrous oxide and middle ear pressure. *Anaesthesia.* 1982;37(9):896–900.
52. Zalzal GH. Stridor and airway compromise. *Pediatr Clin North Am.* 1989;36(6):1389–1402.
53. Butskiy O, Mistry B, Chadha NK. Surgical interventions for pediatric unilateral vocal cord paralysis: a systematic review. *JAMA Otolaryngol Head Neck Surg.* 2015;141(7):654–660.
54. Soriano SG, Kim C, Jones DT. Surgical airway, rigid bronchoscopy, and transtracheal jet ventilation in the pediatric patient. *Anesthesiol Clin North Am.* 1998;16(4):827–838.
55. Cook TM, Alexander R. Major complications during anaesthesia for elective laryngeal surgery in the UK: a national survey of the use of high-pressure source ventilation. *Br J Anaesth.* 2008;101(2):266–272.
56. Mausser G, Friedrich G, Schwarz G. Airway management and anesthesia in neonates, infants and children during endolaryngotracheal surgery. *Paediatr Anaesth.* 2007;17(10):942–947.
57. Jaquet Y, Monnier P, Van Melle G, et al. Complications of different ventilation strategies in endoscopic laryngeal surgery: a 10-year review. *Anesthesiology.* 2006;104(1):52–59.
58. Hermens JM, Bennett MJ, Hirshman CA. Anesthesia for laser surgery. *Anesth Analg.* 1983;62(2):218–229.
59. Apfelbaum JL, Caplan RA, Barker SJ, et al. Practice advisory for the prevention and management of operating room fires: an updated report by the American Society of Anesthesiologists Task Force on Operating Room Fires. *Anesthesiology.* 2013;118(2):271–290.
60. Lee WC, Kapur TR, Ramsden WN. Local and regional anesthesia for functional endoscopic sinus surgery. *Ann Otol Rhinol Laryngol.* 1997;106(9):767–769.
61. Groudine SB, Hollinger I, Jones J, et al. New York State guidelines on the topical use of phenylephrine in the operating room. The Phenylephrine Advisory Committee. *Anesthesiology.* 2000;92(3):859–864.
62. John G, Low JM, Tan PE, et al. Plasma catecholamine levels during functional endoscopic sinus surgery. *Clin Otolaryngol.* 1995;20(3):213–215.
63. Tirelli G, Bigarini S, Russolo M, et al. Total intravenous anaesthesia in endoscopic sinus-nasal surgery. *Acta Otorhinolaryngol Ital.* 2004;24(3):137–144.
64. Wormald PJ, van Renen G, Perks J, et al. The effect of the total intravenous anesthesia compared with inhalational anesthesia on the surgical field during endoscopic sinus surgery. *Am J Rhinol.* 2005;19(5):514–520.
65. Cartellieri M, Vorbeck F, Kremser J. Comparison of six three-dimensional navigation systems during sinus surgery. *Acta Otolaryngol.* 2001;121(4):500–504.
66. Gruber A, Bavinzski G, Killer M, et al. Preoperative embolization of hypervascular skull base tumors. *Minim Invasive Neurosurg.* 2000;43(2):62–71.
67. Goobie SM, Meier PM, Pereira LM, et al. Efficacy of tranexamic acid in pediatric craniosynostosis surgery. *Anesthesiology.* 2011;114(4):862–871.
68. Henry DA, Carless PA, Moxey AJ, et al. Anti-fibrinolytic use for minimising perioperative allogeneic blood transfusion. *Cochrane Database Syst Rev.* 2011;(3):CD001886.
69. Greenberg SL, Huang J, Chang RS, et al. Surgical management of Ludwig's angina. *ANZ J Surg.* 2007;77(5):540–543.
70. Kulkarni AH, Pai SD, Bhattarai B, et al. Ludwig's angina and airway considerations: a case report. *Cases J.* 2008;1(1):19.
71. Huelke DF, Patrick LM. Mechanics in the production of mandibular fractures: strain-gauge measurements of impacts to the chin. *J Dental Res.* 1964;43(3):437–446.
72. Nahum AM. The biomechanics of facial bone fracture. *Laryngoscope.* 1975;85(1):140–156.
73. Olson RA, Fonseca RJ, Zeitler DL, et al. Fractures of the mandible: a review of 580 cases. *J Oral Maxillofac Surg.* 1982;40(1):23–28.
74. Dacosta A, Billard JL, Gery P, et al. Posttraumatic intracerebral pneumatocele after ventilation with a mask: case report. *J Trauma.* 1994;36(2):255–257.
75. Luce EA, Tubb TD, Moore AM. Review of 1,000 major facial fractures and associated injuries. *Plast Reconstr Surg.* 1979;63(1):26–30.
76. Mithani SK, St-Hilaire H, Brooke BS, et al. Predictable patterns of intracranial and cervical spine injury in craniomaxillofacial trauma: analysis of 4786 patients. *Plast Reconstr Surg.* 2009;123(4):1293–1301.
77. Mulligan RP, Mahabir RC. The prevalence of cervical spine injury, head injury, or both with isolated and multiple craniomaxillofacial fractures. *Plast Reconstr Surg.* 2010;126(5):1647–1651.
78. Stephens CT, Kahntroff S, Dutton RP. The success of emergency endotracheal intubation in trauma patients: a 10-year experience at a major adult trauma referral center. *Anesth Analg.* 2009;109(3):866–872.
79. Jain U, McCunn M, Smith CE, et al. Management of the traumatized airway. *Anesthesiology.* 2016;124(1):199–206.

49 Anesthesia for Ophthalmologic Surgery

KATHRYN E. McGOLDRICK • STEVEN I. GAYER

Ocular Anatomy
Ocular Physiology
   Formation and Drainage of Aqueous Humor
   Maintenance of Intraocular Pressure
   Glaucoma
Effects of Anesthesia and Adjuvant Drugs on Intraocular Pressure
   Central Nervous System Depressants
   Ventilation and Temperature
   Adjuvant Drugs
Oculocardiac Reflex
Anesthetic Ramifications of Ophthalmic Drugs
   Anticholinesterase Agents
   Cocaine
   Cyclopentolate
   Epinephrine
   Phenylephrine
   Timolol and Betaxolol
   Intraocular Perfluorocarbons
   Systemic Ophthalmic Drugs
Preoperative Evaluation
   Establishing Rapport and Assessing Medical Condition
   Anesthesia Options

   Side of Anesthesia and Surgery
   Anesthesia Techniques
Anesthetic Management in Specific Situations
   "Open-Eye, Full-Stomach" Encounters
   Intraocular Surgery
   Retinal Detachment Surgery
   Strabismus Surgery
   Principles of Laser Therapy
Postoperative Ocular Complications
   Corneal Abrasion
   Chemical Injury
   Photic Injury
   Mild Visual Symptoms
   Hemorrhagic Retinopathy
   Retinal Ischemia
   Ischemic Optic Neuropathy
   Cortical Blindness
   Acute Glaucoma
   Postcataract Ptosis

KEY POINTS

1. Cataract surgery is one of the most frequently performed surgical procedures worldwide but represents just one aspect of the various ophthalmic subspecialties, which include cornea, retina, glaucoma, uveitis, strabismus, oculoplastic, and oncology surgeries.

2. Eye surgery patients are often at the extremes of age, ranging from premature babies with retinopathy of prematurity to nonagenarians with multiple coexisting diseases in which age-related anesthetic considerations are key.

3. With intraocular procedures, globe akinesia, patient movement, and control of intraocular pressure (IOP) are important variables; however, with extraocular surgery, the significance of IOP fades, whereas elicitation of the oculocardiac reflex becomes a concern.

4. Inhalation anesthetics cause dose-related reductions in IOP. The exact mechanisms are unknown, but postulated causes include depression of a control center in the diencephalon, reduction of aqueous humor production, enhancement of aqueous outflow, or relaxation of the extraocular muscles.

5. The oculocardiac reflex is triggered by pressure on the globe and by traction on the extraocular muscles as well as on the conjunctiva or on the orbital structures. This reflex, whose afferent limb is trigeminal and efferent limb is vagal, may also be elicited by performing a regional eye block, by ocular trauma, and by direct pressure on tissue remaining in the orbital apex after enucleation.

6. Ophthalmic drugs may significantly alter the patient's reaction to anesthesia. Similarly, anesthetic drugs and maneuvers may dramatically influence intraocular dynamics.

7. Several anesthetic options are available for many types of ocular procedures, including general anesthesia, retrobulbar (intraconal) block, peribulbar (extraconal) anesthesia, sub-Tenon block, topical analgesia, and intracameral injection.

8. The complications of ophthalmic anesthesia can be both vision- and life-threatening.

1 Cataract surgery is one of the most frequently performed surgical procedures worldwide but represents just one aspect of the ophthalmic subspecialties, which include cornea, retina, glaucoma, uveitis, strabismus, oculoplastic, and oncology surgeries. Anesthesia for ophthalmic surgery presents many unique challenges (Table 49-1). In addition to possessing technical expertise, the anesthesiologist must have detailed knowledge of ocular anatomy, physiology, and pharmacology. It is essential to appreciate that ophthalmic drugs may significantly alter the reaction to anesthesia and that concomitantly anesthetic drugs and maneuvers may dramatically influence intraocular dynamics. **2** Patients undergoing ophthalmic surgery may represent extremes

Table 49-1 Requirements of Ophthalmic Surgery
Safety
Akinesia
Analgesia
Minimal bleeding
Avoidance or obtundation of oculocardiac reflex
Control of intraocular pressure
Awareness of drug interactions
Smooth emergence

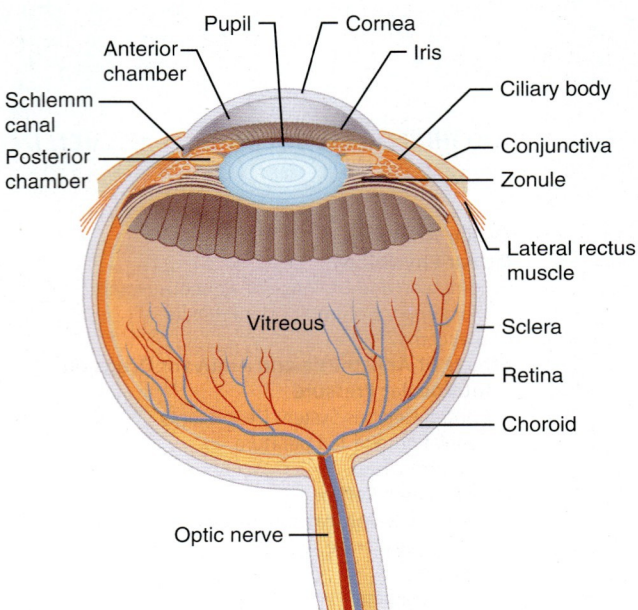

Figure 49-1 Diagram of ocular anatomy.

of age. They may have coexisting diseases (e.g., diabetes mellitus, coronary artery disease, essential hypertension, chronic lung disease), and they are likely to be elderly. Indeed, the elderly constitute the most rapidly growing subset of the U.S. population, with the census projecting that by 2030, one in five Americans will be age 65 or older. Furthermore, "the elderly" is a uniquely vulnerable group with reduced functional reserve and a myriad of age-related diseases. The economic implications are staggering. For example, age-related macular degeneration is the leading cause of blindness in individuals older than 65 years in the United States, affecting more than 1.75 million people. Because of the rapid aging of our population, this number will increase to almost 3 million by 2020.[1]

One must be knowledgeable about the numerous surgical procedures that are unique to the specialty of ophthalmology. Although the list of ocular surgical interventions is lengthy, these procedures may, in general, be classified as *extraocular* or *intraocular*. This distinction is important because anesthetic considerations are different for these two major surgical categories. For example, with intraocular procedures, globe akinesia, patient movement, and control of intraocular pressure (IOP) are important variables; however, with extraocular surgery, the significance of IOP fades, whereas elicitation of the oculocardiac reflex becomes a concern.

Ocular Anatomy

The anesthesiologist should be knowledgeable about ocular anatomy as a basis for learning ophthalmic regional anesthesia and to enhance understanding of surgical procedures (Fig. 49-1). Salient subdivisions of ocular anatomy include the orbit, the eye itself, the extraocular muscles, the eyelids, and the lacrimal system.

The orbit is a bony pyramidal cavity housing the globe and its associated structures in the skull. The walls of the orbit are composed of the following bones: frontal, zygomatic, greater wing of the sphenoid, maxilla, palatine, lacrimal, and ethmoid. A familiarity with the surface relationships of the orbital rim aids performance of regional blocks.

The optic foramen, located at the orbital apex, transmits the optic nerve and the ophthalmic artery as well as the sympathetic nerves from the carotid plexus. The superior orbital fissure transmits the superior and inferior branches of the oculomotor nerve; the lacrimal, frontal, and nasociliary branches of the trigeminal nerve; the trochlear and abducens nerves; and the superior and inferior ophthalmic veins. The inferior orbital or sphenomaxillary fissure contains the infraorbital and zygomatic nerves and communication between the inferior ophthalmic vein and the pterygoid plexus. The infraorbital foramen, located about 4 mm below the orbital rim in the maxilla, transmits the infraorbital nerve, artery, and vein. The lacrimal fossa contains the lacrimal gland in the superior temporal orbit. The supraorbital notch, located at the junction of the medial one-third and temporal two-thirds of the superior orbital rim, transmits the supraorbital nerve, artery, and vein. The supraorbital notch, the infraorbital foramen, and the lacrimal fossa are all clinically palpable.

The globe itself is actually one large sphere with part of a smaller sphere incorporated in the anterior surface, constituting a structure with two different radii of curvature. The coat of the eye is composed of three layers: sclera, uveal tract, and retina. The fibrous outer layer, or *sclera,* is protective, providing sufficient rigidity to maintain the shape of the eye. The anterior portion of the sclera, the cornea, is highly avascular and transparent, permitting light to pass into the internal ocular structures. The double-spherical shape of the eye exists because the corneal arc of curvature is steeper than the scleral arc of curvature. The focusing of rays of light to form a retinal image commences at the cornea.

The *uveal tract,* or middle layer of the globe, is vascular and in direct apposition to the sclera. A potential space, known as the *suprachoroidal space,* separates the sclera from the uveal tract. This potential space, however, may become filled with blood during an expulsive or suprachoroidal hemorrhage, often associated with surgical disaster. The iris, ciliary body, and choroid compose the uveal tract. The iris includes the pupil, which controls the amount of light entering the eye by contractions of three sets of muscles. The iris dilator is sympathetically innervated; the iris sphincter and the ciliary muscle have parasympathetic innervation. Posterior to the iris lays the ciliary body, which produces aqueous humor (see Formation and Drainage of Aqueous Humor, later). The ciliary muscles, situated in the ciliary body, adjust the shape of the lens to accommodate focusing at various distances. Large vessels and a network of small vessels and capillaries known as the *choriocapillaris* constitute the choroid, which supplies nutrition to the outer part of the retina.

The *retina* is a neurosensory membrane composed of 10 layers that convert light impulses into neural impulses. These neural impulses are then carried through the optic nerve to the brain. Located in the center of the globe is the vitreous cavity, filled with a gelatinous substance known as *vitreous humor*. This material is adherent to the most anterior 3 mm of the retina as well as to large blood vessels and the optic nerve. The vitreous humor may pull on the retina, causing retinal tears and retinal detachment.

The crystalline lens, located posterior to the pupil, refracts rays of light passing through the cornea and pupil to focus images on the retina. The ciliary muscle, whose contractile state causes tautness or relaxation of the lens zonules, regulates the thickness of the lens.

In addition, six extraocular muscles move the eye within the orbit to various positions. The bilobed lacrimal gland provides most of the tear film, which serves to maintain a moist anterior surface on the globe. The lacrimal drainage system—composed of the puncta, canaliculi, lacrimal sac, and lacrimal duct—drains into the nose below the inferior turbinate. Blockage of this system occurs frequently, necessitating procedures ranging from lacrimal duct probing to dacryocystorhinostomy, which involves anastomosis of the lacrimal sac to the nasal mucosa.

Covering the surface of the globe and lining the eyelids is a mucous membrane called the *conjunctiva*. Because drugs are absorbed across the membrane, it is a popular site for administration of ophthalmic drugs.

The eyelids consist of four layers: the conjunctiva, the cartilaginous tarsal plate, a muscle layer composed mainly of the orbicularis and the levator palpebrae, and the skin. The eyelids protect the eye from foreign objects; through blinking, the tear film produced by the lacrimal gland is spread across the surface of the eye, keeping the cornea moist.

Blood supply to the eye and orbit is by means of branches of both the internal and external carotid arteries. Venous drainage of the orbit is accomplished through the multiple anastomoses of the superior and inferior ophthalmic veins. Venous drainage of the eye is achieved mainly through the central retinal vein. All these veins empty directly into the cavernous sinus.

The sensory and motor innervations of the eye and its adnexa are very complex, with multiple cranial nerves supplying branches to various ocular structures. A branch of the oculomotor nerve supplies a motor root to the ciliary ganglion, which in turn supplies the sphincter of the pupil and the ciliary muscle. The trochlear nerve supplies the superior oblique muscle. The abducens nerve supplies the lateral rectus muscle. The trigeminal nerve constitutes the most complex ocular and adnexal innervation. In addition, the zygomatic branch of the facial nerve eventually divides into an upper branch, supplying the frontalis and the upper lid orbicularis, whereas the lower branch supplies the orbicularis of the lower lid.

Ocular Physiology

Despite its relatively diminutive size, the eye is a complex organ, concerned with many intricate physiologic processes. The formation and drainage of aqueous humor and their influence on IOP in both normal and glaucomatous eyes are among the most important functions, especially from the anesthesiologist's perspective. An appreciation of the effects of various anesthetic manipulations on IOP requires an understanding of the fundamental principles of ocular physiology.

Formation and Drainage of Aqueous Humor

Two-thirds of the aqueous humor is formed in the posterior chamber by the ciliary body in an active secretory process

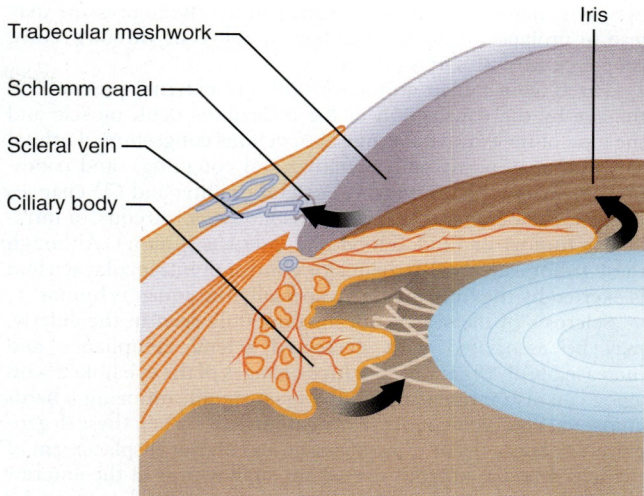

Figure 49-2 Ocular anatomy concerned with control of intraocular pressure.

involving both the carbonic anhydrase and the cytochrome oxidase systems (Fig. 49-2). The remaining third is formed by passive filtration of aqueous humor from the vessels on the anterior surface of the iris.

At the ciliary epithelium, sodium is actively transported into the aqueous humor in the posterior chamber. Bicarbonate and chloride ions passively follow the sodium ions. This active mechanism results in the osmotic pressure of the aqueous humor being many times greater than that of plasma. It is this disparity in osmotic pressure that leads to an average rate of aqueous humor production of 2 μL/min.

Aqueous humor flows from the posterior chamber through the pupillary aperture and into the anterior chamber, where it mixes with the aqueous formed by the iris. During its journey into the anterior chamber, the aqueous humor bathes the avascular lens and, once in the anterior chamber, it also bathes the corneal endothelium. Then the aqueous humor flows into the peripheral segment of the anterior chamber and exits the eye through the trabecular network, Schlemm canal, and episcleral venous system. A network of connecting venous channels eventually leads to the superior vena cava and the right atrium. Thus, obstruction of venous return at any point from the eye to the right side of the heart impedes aqueous drainage, elevating IOP accordingly.

Maintenance of Intraocular Pressure

IOP normally varies between 10 and 21.7 mmHg and is considered abnormal above 22 mmHg. This level varies from 1 to 2 mmHg with each cardiac contraction. Also, a diurnal variation of 2 to 5 mmHg is observed, with a higher value noted on awakening. This higher awakening pressure has been ascribed to vascular congestion, pressure on the globe from closed lids, and mydriasis—all of which occur during sleep. If IOP is too high, it may produce opacities by interfering with normal corneal metabolism.

During anesthesia, a rise in IOP can produce permanent visual loss. If the IOP is already elevated, a further increase can trigger acute glaucoma. If penetration of the globe occurs when the IOP is excessively high, rupture of a blood vessel with subsequent hemorrhage may transpire. IOP becomes atmospheric once the eye cavity has been entered, and any sudden rise in pressure may lead to prolapse of the iris and lens, and loss of vitreous. Thus, proper control of IOP is critical.

Three main factors influence IOP: (1) external pressure on the eye by the contraction of the orbicularis oculi muscle and the tone of the extraocular muscles, venous congestion of orbital veins (as may occur with vomiting and coughing), and conditions such as orbital tumor; (2) scleral rigidity; and (3) changes in intraocular contents that are semisolid (lens, vitreous, or intraocular tumor) or fluid (blood and aqueous humor). Although these factors affect IOP, the major control of intraocular tension is exerted by the fluid content, especially the aqueous humor.

Sclerosis of the sclera, not uncommonly seen in the elderly, may be associated with decreased scleral compliance and increased IOP. Other degenerative changes of the eye linked with aging can also influence IOP, the most significant being a hardening and enlargement of the crystalline lens. When these degenerative changes occur, they may lead to anterior displacement of the lens–iris diaphragm. A resultant shallowness of the anterior chamber angle may then occur, reducing access of the trabecular meshwork to the aqueous. This process is usually gradual, but if rapid lens engorgement occurs, angle-closure glaucoma may transpire.

Changes in the nature of the vitreous that affect the amount of unbound water also influence IOP. Myopia, trauma, and aging produce liquefaction of vitreous gel and a subsequent increase in unbound water, which may lower IOP by facilitating fluid removal. However, under different circumstances, the opposite may occur; that is, the hydration of more normal vitreous may be associated with elevation of IOP. Hence, it is often prudent to produce a slightly dehydrated state in the surgical patient with glaucoma.

Intraocular blood volume, determined primarily by vessel dilation or contraction in the spongy layers of the choroid, contributes importantly to IOP. Although changes in arterial or venous pressure may secondarily affect IOP, excursions in arterial pressure have much less importance than do venous fluctuations. In chronic arterial hypertension, ocular pressure returns to normal levels after a period of adaptation brought about by compression of vessels in the choroid as a result of increased IOP. Thus, a feedback mechanism reduces the total volume of blood, keeping IOP relatively constant in patients with systemic hypertension.

However, if venous return from the eye is disturbed at any point from Schlemm canal to the right atrium, IOP increases substantially. Trendelenburg position, a cervical collar, and even a tight necktie can produce increased intraocular blood volume and distention of orbital vessels as well as attenuated aqueous drainage.[2] Straining, vomiting, or coughing greatly increases venous pressure and raises IOP as much as 40 mmHg or more. The deleterious implications of these activities cannot be overemphasized. Laryngoscopy and tracheal intubation may also elevate IOP, even without any visible reaction to intubation, but especially when the patient coughs. Topical anesthesia of the larynx may attenuate the systemic hypertensive response to laryngoscopy but does not reliably prevent associated increases in IOP.[3] Ordinarily, the pressure elevation from such increases in blood volume or venous pressure dissipates rapidly. However, if the coughing or straining occurs during ocular surgery when the eye is open, as in penetrating keratoplasty, the result may be a disastrous expulsive hemorrhage, at worst, or a disconcerting loss of vitreous, at best.

Despite the notable role of venous pressure, scleral rigidity, and vitreous composition, maintenance of IOP is determined primarily by the rate of aqueous formation and the rate of aqueous humor outflow. The most important influence on formation of aqueous humor is the difference in osmotic pressure between aqueous humor and plasma. This fact is illustrated by the equation:

$$IOP = K[(OPaq - OPpl) + CP] \quad (49\text{-}1)$$

where K is the coefficient of outflow, OPaq is the osmotic pressure of aqueous humor, OPpl is the osmotic pressure of plasma, and CP is the capillary pressure. Hypertonic solutions such as mannitol are used to lower IOP because a small change in the solute concentration of plasma can markedly influence the formation of aqueous humor and hence IOP.

Fluctuations in aqueous humor outflow may also produce a dramatic alteration in IOP. The most significant factor controlling aqueous humor outflow is the diameter of Fontana spaces, as illustrated by the equation:

$$A = \frac{r^2(Piop - Pv)}{8\eta L} \quad (49\text{-}2)$$

where A is the volume of aqueous outflow per unit of time, r is the radius of Fontana spaces, Piop is the IOP, Pv is the venous pressure, η is the viscosity, and L is the length of Fontana spaces. When the pupil dilates, Fontana spaces narrow, resistance to outflow is increased, and IOP rises. Because mydriasis is undesirable in both closed-angle glaucoma and open-angle glaucoma, miotics are applied conjunctivally in patients with glaucoma.

Glaucoma

Glaucoma is a condition characterized by progressive optic nerve dysfunction and loss of vision. The terminology for glaucoma is complex because there are a number of variants, including acquired versus congenital, high-IOP versus normal pressure, acute versus chronic, and open-angle versus closed-angle. Angle-closure glaucoma may be either acute or chronic; notably, acute angle-closure glaucoma is an urgent condition, whereas chronic angle-closure disease is far more common and often asymptomatic.

With open-angle glaucoma, the elevated IOP exists within an anatomically open anterior chamber angle. It is believed that sclerosis of trabecular tissue results in impaired aqueous humor filtration and drainage. Treatment consists of medication to produce miosis and trabecular stretching. Commonly used eye drops are epinephrine, timolol, dipivefrin, and betaxolol. Closed-angle glaucoma is characterized by the peripheral iris moving into direct contact with the posterior corneal surface, mechanically obstructing aqueous humor outflow. People who have a narrow angle between the iris and the posterior cornea are predisposed to this condition. In these patients, mydriasis can produce such increased thickening of the peripheral iris that corneal touch occurs and the angle is closed. Another mechanism producing acute closed-angle glaucoma is swelling of the crystalline lens. In this case, pupillary block occurs, with the edematous lens blocking the flow of aqueous humor from the posterior to the anterior chamber. This situation can also develop if the lens is traumatically dislocated anteriorly, thus physically blocking the anterior chamber.

It was previously believed that intravenous atropine should not be administered to patients with glaucoma; however, atropine in the dose range used clinically has no effect on IOP in either open-angle or closed-angle glaucoma. When 0.4 mg of atropine is given parenterally to a 70-kg person, approximately 0.0001 mg is absorbed by the eye.[4] Garde et al.[5] reported, however, that scopolamine has a greater mydriatic effect than atropine and recommended not using scopolamine in patients with known or suspected closed-angle glaucoma.

Equation 49-2, describing the volume of aqueous outflow per unit of time, clearly demonstrates that outflow is exquisitely sensitive to fluctuations in venous pressure. Because a rise in venous pressure produces an increased volume of ocular blood and decreased aqueous outflow, it is obvious that considerable elevation of IOP occurs with any maneuver that increases venous pressure. Hence, in addition to preoperative instillation of miotics, consider avoiding IOP-elevating maneuvers such as overhydration, constriction around the patient's neck, prolonged Trendelenburg or prone position, and hypercapnia, which may induce choroidal vascular congestion. In some patients, such as those undergoing robotic-assisted laparoscopic prostatectomy with prolonged steep Trendelenburg position coupled with elevated CO_2, the optic nerve may be at risk due to narrow-angle glaucoma. In these situations, one may contemplate preoperative ophthalmology consultation and intraoperative prophylactic administration of acetazolamide and/or mannitol.[6]

A small percentage of glaucoma patients experience a marked decrement in vision following surgery, termed visual field "wipe out." Although no distinct etiology is known, several surgical, anesthetic, and postoperative reasons have been postulated. Proposed, but not validated, anesthesia mechanisms include pressure on the optic nerve or its circulation by local anesthetic, blood, or a compression device; direct optic nerve injury by a needle; and hypoperfusion of the optic nerve due to hypotension during general anesthesia or vasoconstrictors admixed with local anesthetic.

Primary congenital glaucoma is classified according to age of onset, with the infantile type presenting any time after birth until 3 years of age. The juvenile type presents between the ages of 37 months and 30 years. Moreover, childhood glaucoma may also occur in conjunction with various eye diseases or developmental anomalies such as aniridia, mesodermal dysgenesis syndrome, and retinopathy of prematurity.

Successful management of infantile glaucoma depends critically on early diagnosis. Presenting symptoms include epiphora, photophobia, blepharospasm, and irritability. Ocular enlargement, termed *buphthalmos*, or "ox eye," and corneal haziness secondary to edema are common. Buphthalmos is rare, however, if glaucoma develops after 3 years of age because by then the eye is much less elastic.

Because infantile glaucoma is frequently associated with obstructed aqueous humor outflow, management of it often requires surgical creation, by goniotomy or trabeculotomy, of a route for aqueous humor to flow into the canal of Schlemm. However, advanced disease may be unresponsive to even multiple goniotomies, and the more radical trabeculectomy or some other variety of filtering procedure may be necessary.

The juvenile form of glaucoma, in which the cornea and eye size are normal, is commonly associated with a family history of open-angle glaucoma and is treated similarly to primary open-angle glaucoma.

In cases of pediatric secondary glaucoma, goniotomy and filtering may be unsuccessful, whereas cyclocryotherapy may effect a reduction in IOP, pain, and corneal edema. The ciliary body is destroyed with a cryoprobe cooled to −70°C, thus dramatically decreasing aqueous formation.

It is essential to appreciate that the high IOP frequently encountered in infantile glaucoma can be significantly reduced when a surgical plane of general anesthesia is achieved. Some clinicians maintain that ketamine is a useful drug to use for examination under anesthesia when infantile glaucoma is part of the differential diagnosis because ketamine does not appear to give a spuriously low reading from drug-induced decreased IOP. Moreover, even normal infants sporadically have pressures in the mid-20s. Hence, diagnosis is not based exclusively on the numerical pressure recorded under anesthesia. Other factors such as corneal edema and increased corneal diameter, tears in Descemet membrane, and cupping of the optic nerve are considered in making the diagnosis. If these aberrations are noted, surgical intervention may be mandatory, even in the setting of a reputedly normal IOP.

Effects of Anesthesia and Adjuvant Drugs on Intraocular Pressure

Central Nervous System Depressants

Inhalation anesthetics purportedly cause dose-related decreases in IOP. The exact mechanisms are unknown, but postulated causes include depression of a central nervous system (CNS) control center in the diencephalon, reduction of aqueous humor production, enhancement of aqueous humor outflow, or relaxation of the extraocular muscles.[4] Moreover, virtually all CNS depressants—including barbiturates, neuroleptics, opioids, tranquilizers,[4] and hypnotics, such as etomidate and propofol—lower IOP in both normal and glaucomatous eyes. Etomidate, despite its proclivity to produce pain on intravenous injection and skeletal muscle movement, is associated with a significant reduction in IOP.[7] However, etomidate-induced myoclonus may be hazardous in the setting of a ruptured globe.

Controversy surrounds the issue of ketamine's effect on IOP. Administered intravenously or intramuscularly, ketamine initially was believed to increase IOP significantly, as measured by indentation tonometry.[8] Corssen and Hoy[9] also reported a slight but statistically significant increase in IOP that appeared unrelated to changes in blood pressure or depth of anesthesia. However, nystagmus made proper positioning of the tonometer difficult and may have resulted in less-than-accurate measurements.

Conflicting results arose from a study in which 2 mg/kg of ketamine given intravenously to adults failed to have a significant effect on IOP.[10] Furthermore, a pediatric study reported no increase in IOP after an intramuscular ketamine dose of 8 mg/kg. Indeed, values obtained were similar to those reported with halothane and isoflurane.[11,12]

Some of the confusion may arise from differences in premedication practices and from the use of different instruments to measure IOP. More recent studies have used applanation tonometry rather than indentation tonometry. However, even if future studies should confirm that ketamine has minimal or no effect on IOP, ketamine's proclivity to cause nystagmus and blepharospasm makes it a less-than-optimal agent for many types of ophthalmic surgery.

Ventilation and Temperature

Hyperventilation decreases IOP, whereas asphyxia, administration of carbon dioxide, and hypoventilation have been shown to elevate IOP.

Hypothermia lowers IOP. On initial consideration, hypothermia might be expected to raise IOP because of the associated increase in viscosity of aqueous humor. However, hypothermia is linked with decreased formation of aqueous humor and with vasoconstriction; hence, the net result is a reduction in IOP.

Adjuvant Drugs

Hypertonic Solutions and Acetazolamide

Intravenous administration of hypertonic solutions such as dextran, urea, mannitol, and sorbitol elevates plasma osmotic pressure, thereby decreasing aqueous humor formation and reducing IOP. As effective as urea is in reducing IOP, intravenous mannitol has the advantage of fewer side effects. Mannitol's onset, peak (30 to 45 minutes), and duration of action (5 to 6 hours) are similar to those of urea. Moreover, both drugs may produce acute intravascular volume overload. Sudden expansion of plasma volume secondary to efflux of intracellular water into the vascular compartment places a heavy workload on the kidneys and heart, often resulting in hypertension and dilution of plasma sodium. Furthermore, mannitol-associated diuresis, if protracted, may trigger hypotension in volume-depleted patients.

Intravenous administration of acetazolamide inactivates carbonic anhydrase and interferes with the sodium pump. The resultant decrease in aqueous humor formation lowers IOP. However, the action of acetazolamide is not limited to the eye, and systemic effects include loss of sodium, potassium, and water secondary to the drug's renal tubular effects. Such electrolyte imbalances may then be linked to cardiac dysrhythmias during general anesthesia.

An advantage of acetazolamide is its relative ease of administration. Whereas large volumes of hypertonic solutions must be infused to reduce IOP, acetazolamide is easily dispensed from a single small vial. Acetazolamide may also be given orally, and topical carbonic anhydrase inhibitors are commercially available.

Neuromuscular Blocking Drugs

Neuromuscular blocking drugs have both direct and indirect actions on IOP.

Equipotent paralyzing doses of all the nondepolarizing drugs directly lower IOP by relaxing the extraocular muscles (Fig. 49-3).[13] However, if paralysis of the respiratory muscles is accompanied by alveolar hypoventilation, the latter secondary effect may supervene to increase IOP.

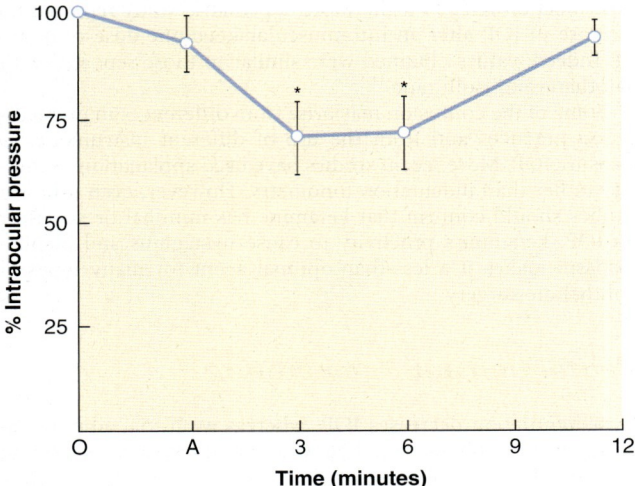

Figure 49-3 Mean intraocular pressure after administration of thiopental, 3 to 4 mg/kg, and pancuronium, 0.08 mg/kg at 0. *A*, loss of lid reflex; * = $p < 0.05$. (Adapted with permission from Litwiller RW, DiFazio CA, Rushia EF. Pancuronium and intraocular pressure. *Anesthesiology*. 1975;42:75.)

In contrast to nondepolarizing drugs, the depolarizing drug succinylcholine elevates IOP. Lincoff et al.[14] reported extrusion of vitreous after succinylcholine administration to a patient with a surgically open eye. An average peak IOP increase of about 9 mmHg is produced within 1 to 4 minutes of an intravenous dose. Within 7 minutes, return to baseline usually transpires.[15] The ocular hypertensive effect of succinylcholine has been attributed to several mechanisms, including tonic contraction of extraocular muscles,[4] choroidal vascular dilation, and relaxation of orbital smooth muscle. One study speculates that the succinylcholine-induced increase in IOP is multifactorial but primarily the result of the cycloplegic action of succinylcholine, producing a deepening of the anterior chamber and increased outflow resistance.[16] Because they studied eyes with the extraocular muscles detached and still observed an elevation in IOP, these investigators proposed that changes in extraocular muscle tone do not contribute substantially to the increase in IOP observed after succinylcholine administration.

A variety of methods have been advocated to prevent succinylcholine-induced elevations in IOP. However, although some attenuation of the increase results, none of these techniques consistently and completely block the ocular hypertensive response. Prior administration of such drugs as acetazolamide, narcotics, β-blockers, and nondepolarizing neuromuscular blocking drugs has been suggested. The efficacy of pretreatment with nondepolarizing drugs is controversial.

In 1968, using indentation tonometry, Miller et al.[17] reported that pretreatment with small amounts of gallamine or *d*-tubocurarine prevented succinylcholine-associated increases in IOP. However, in 1978, using the more sensitive applanation tonometer, Meyers et al.[18] were unable to consistently circumvent the ocular hypertensive response after similar pretreatment therapy (Table 49-2). In addition, Verma[19] claimed that a "self-taming" technique in which a small dose of succinylcholine is administered prior to induction was protective, but in a controlled study using applanation tonometry, Meyers et al.[20] challenged this claim. Although intravenous pretreatment with lidocaine, 1 to 2 mg/kg, may blunt the hemodynamic response to laryngoscopy,[3,21] such therapy does not reliably prevent the ocular hypertensive response associated with succinylcholine and intubation.[22] However, Grover et al.[23] claimed that pretreatment with lidocaine, 1.5 mg/kg intravenously, 1 minute before induction with thiopental and succinylcholine offered protection from IOP increases because of succinylcholine and may therefore be of value in rapid-sequence induction for open eye injuries.

In summary, succinylcholine is not the ideal agent for patients with penetrating ocular wounds, and one must carefully ponder giving it after the eye has been opened. Nonetheless, as explained in the later section, "Open-Eye, Full Stomach" Encounters, it is no longer valid to recommend that succinylcholine be used only with extreme reluctance in ocular surgery.

The forced duction test (FDT) is an intraoperative maneuver that helps the ophthalmologist to determine whether strabismus is due to muscle paresis versus a restrictive force. It is discussed in detail in the strabismus section of this chapter. Jampolsky[24] warned that succinylcholine should be avoided in patients undergoing repeat strabismus surgery because the FDT does not return to baseline for approximately 30 minutes after administration of the drug. Quantitatively sophisticated studies by Dell and Williams[25] supported this caveat, although the latter investigators suggest waiting only 20 minutes after administration of succinylcholine before performing the FDT. However, in light of the black box warning issued by the U.S. Food and Drug Administration stating that use of succinylcholine in children may

Table 49-2 Effects of Succinylcholine on Intraocular Pressure: Double-Blind d-Tubocurarine or Gallamine Pretreatment

Pretreatment[a]	Mean Age (yr)	Intraocular Pressure (mmHg, MEAN ± SE)		
		Baseline	3 min after Pretreatment	1 min after Succinylcholine[b]
d-Tubocurarine	13.4	13 ± 1	12.3 ± 1.2	24 ± 1.3
Gallamine	8.7	10.9 ± 1.1	10.6 ± 1	23.4 ± 2.3

[a]d-Tubocurarine, 0.09 mg/kg, or gallamine, 0.3 mg/kg.
[b]1 to 1.5 mg/kg intravenously.
Reprinted with permission from Meyers EF, Krupin T, Johnson M, et al. Failure of nondepolarizing neuromuscular blockers to inhibit succinylcholine-induced increased intraocular pressure: a controlled study. *Anesthesiology*. 1978;48:149.

rarely be associated with hyperkalemia and cardiac arrest, it should be reserved for emergency intubation or when immediate airway control is needed, so the drug is typically avoided in pediatric strabismus surgery.

Oculocardiac Reflex

Bernard Aschner and Giuseppe Dagnini first described the oculocardiac reflex in 1908. This reflex is triggered by pressure on the globe and by traction on the extraocular muscles as well as on the conjunctiva or the orbital structures. Moreover, the reflex may also be elicited by performance of an eye block, by ocular trauma, and by direct pressure on tissue remaining in the orbital apex after enucleation. The afferent limb is trigeminal and the efferent limb is vagal. Although the most common manifestation of the oculocardiac reflex is sinus bradycardia, a wide spectrum of cardiac dysrhythmias may occur, including junctional rhythm, ectopic atrial rhythm, atrioventricular blockade, ventricular bigeminy, multifocal premature ventricular contractions, wandering pacemaker, idioventricular rhythm, asystole, and ventricular tachycardia.[26] This reflex may appear during either local or general anesthesia; however, hypercarbia and hypoxemia are believed to augment the incidence and severity of the problem, as may inappropriate anesthetic depth.

Reports on the incidence of the oculocardiac reflex are remarkable in their striking variability. Berler[27] reported an incidence of 50%, but other sources quote rates ranging from 16% to 82%. Commonly, those articles disclosing a higher incidence included children, who tend to have more vagal tone, in the study population.

A variety of maneuvers to abolish or obtund the oculocardiac reflex have been promulgated. None of these methods have been consistently effective, safe, and reliable. Regional anesthesia can block the afferent limb of the reflex, but is not without other potential complications. Inclusion of intramuscular anticholinergic drugs such as atropine or glycopyrrolate in the usual premedication regimen for oculocardiac reflex prophylaxis is ineffective.[28] Atropine given intravenously within 30 minutes of surgery may reduce incidence of the reflex. For pediatric strabismus surgery, however, some anesthesiologists administer intravenous atropine, 0.02 mg/kg, before commencing surgery.[29] Alternatively, glycopyrrolate, 0.01 mg/kg administered intravenously, may be associated with less tachycardia than atropine in this setting. Moreover, some anesthesiologists claim that prior intravenous administration of atropine may yield more serious and refractory cardiac dysrhythmias than the reflex itself. Clearly, atropine may be considered a potential myocardial irritant. A variety of cardiac dysrhythmias[30] and several conduction abnormalities,[31] including ventricular fibrillation, ventricular tachycardia, and left bundle branch block, have been attributed to intravenous atropine.

It is generally believed that the aforementioned prophylactic measures, fraught with inherent hazards, are usually not indicated in adults. If a cardiac dysrhythmia appears, initially the surgeon should be asked to cease operative manipulation. Next, the patient's anesthetic depth and ventilatory status are evaluated. Commonly, heart rate and rhythm return to baseline within 20 seconds after institution of these measures. Moreover, Moonie et al.[32] noted that the reflex is attenuated with repeated manipulation. Bradycardia is less likely to recur, probably secondary to fatigue of the reflex arc at the level of the cardioinhibitory center. However, if the initial cardiac dysrhythmia is especially serious or if the reflex tenaciously recurs, atropine should be administered intravenously, but only after the surgeon stops ocular manipulation.

Delivery of chemotherapy via ophthalmic artery cannulation is a relatively new endovascular treatment modality for infants and children with retinoblastomas. This so-called superselective ophthalmic artery chemotherapy is performed under general anesthesia in a dedicated interventional radiology suite. The procedure involves insertion of a microcatheter into the ophthalmic artery with subsequent infusion of high-concentration chemotherapeutic agent, typically melphalan, directly to the eye. Serious adverse cardiopulmonary responses to cannulation of the ophthalmic artery or injection of the agent have been described.[33] These responses are characterized by *abrupt drop in end-tidal CO_2* followed by markedly reduced lung compliance akin to acute bronchospasm, profound hypoxia, systemic hypotension, and bradycardia. Harris reported an approximate 40% overall incidence,[34] whereas Phillips et al.,[33] who did not encounter the reaction during initial treatment, noted a 39% occurrence during the second or subsequent catheterization. Yamane et al.[35] confronted bradycardia with such frequency that they considered it to be an indicator of successful ophthalmic artery cannulation. Preoperative intravenous atropine did not alter the incidence or severity of the reaction. It has been postulated that superselective ophthalmic artery chemotherapy may trigger a trigeminal-afferent autonomic reflex response akin to the oculocardiac reflex. It has been referred to as a trigeminocardiac reflex (TCR) because the stimulus is decidedly posterior to the globe. Harris proposes that "trigeminal afferents, particularly in these young patients, act as exquisitely sensitive baroreceptors to the increased pressure during microcatheter insertion and infusion."[34] Analogous to the oculocardiac reflex, the TCR is often self-limited and is suppressed by removal of the stimulus, in this case, withdrawal of the catheter from the ophthalmic artery. Profound or refractory TCR can be treated with intravenous epinephrine.

Anesthetic Ramifications of Ophthalmic Drugs

[6] There is considerable potential for drug interactions during administration of anesthesia for ocular surgery. Topical ophthalmic drugs may produce undesirable systemic effects or may have deleterious anesthetic implications. Systemic absorption of topical ophthalmic drugs may occur from either the conjunctiva or the nasal mucosa after drainage through the nasolacrimal duct. In addition, from spillover, some percutaneous absorption through the immature epidermis of the premature infant may transpire. Occluding the nasolacrimal duct by pressing on the inner canthus of the eye for a few minutes after each instillation greatly decreases systemic absorption. Some of the potentially worrisome topical ocular drugs include anticholinesterases, cocaine, cyclopentolate, epinephrine, phenylephrine, and timolol. In addition, intraocular sulfur hexafluoride and other intraocular gases have important anesthetic ramifications. Furthermore, certain ophthalmic drugs given systemically may produce untoward sequelae germane to anesthetic management. Drugs in this category include glycerol, mannitol, and acetazolamide.

Anticholinesterase Agents

Echothiophate, also known as *phospholine iodide,* is a long-acting anticholinesterase miotic that lowers IOP by decreasing resistance to the outflow of aqueous humor. It is used to treat glaucoma that is refractory to other therapies and also to treat some children with accommodative esotropia. It is absorbed into the systemic circulation after instillation in the conjunctival sac. Any of the long-acting anticholinesterases may prolong the action of succinylcholine because, after at least 1 month of therapy, plasma pseudocholinesterase activity may be below 5% of normal. It is said, moreover, that normal enzyme activity does not return until 4 to 6 weeks after discontinuation of the drug.[36] Hence, the anesthesiologist should anticipate prolonged apnea after a usual dose of succinylcholine. In addition, a delay in metabolism of ester local anesthetics should be expected.

Cocaine

Cocaine, introduced to ophthalmology in 1884 by Koller, has limited topical ocular use because it can cause corneal pits and erosion. However, as the only local anesthetic that inherently produces vasoconstriction and shrinkage of mucous membranes, cocaine has been used in nasal packs during dacryocystorhinostomy. The drug is so well absorbed from mucosal surfaces that plasma concentrations are achieved that are comparable to those after direct intravenous injection. Because cocaine interferes with catecholamine uptake, it has a sympathetic nervous system potentiating effect.

The usual maximal dose of cocaine used in clinical practice is 200 mg for a 70-kg adult, or 3 mg/kg. Although 1 g is considered to be the usual lethal dose for an adult, considerable variation occurs. Furthermore, systemic reactions may appear with as little as 20 mg. Meyers[37] described two cases of cocaine toxicity during dacryocystorhinostomy, underscoring that cocaine is contraindicated in hypertensive patients or in patients receiving drugs such as tricyclic antidepressants or monoamine oxidase inhibitors. In addition, sympathomimetics, such as epinephrine or phenylephrine, should not be given with cocaine. The use of cocaine has largely been abandoned owing to its toxicity profile and potential for drug abuse. So-called pseudococaine solutions consisting of lidocaine 4%, oxymetazoline 0.05%, and peppermint oil are nearly as effective.

Obviously, before administering cocaine or another potent vasoconstrictor for dacryocystorhinostomy, doses of dilute solutions should be meticulously calculated and carefully administered. If serious cardiovascular effects occur, labetalol should be used to counteract them.[38] β-Blocking agents should not be administered in this situation owing to the potential to exacerbate hypertension as a result of unopposed α-adrenergic stimulation. Labetalol offers the advantages of combined α-blockade and β-blockade. In addition, labetalol is preferable to esmolol because of its longer duration of action. It is important to appreciate, however, that labetalol has not been shown to reverse coronary artery vasoconstriction in humans. In the setting of cocaine-associated chest pain and/or myocardial infarction, β-blockers should not be administered acutely. Rather, nitroglycerin should be given.

Cyclopentolate

Despite the popularity of cyclopentolate as a mydriatic, it is not without side effects, which include CNS toxicity. Manifestations include dysarthria, disorientation, and frank psychotic reactions. Purportedly, CNS dysfunction is more likely to follow use of the 2% solution as opposed to the 1% solution. Furthermore, cases of convulsions in children after ocular instillation of cyclopentolate have been reported. Hence, for pediatric use, 0.5% to 1% solutions are recommended. At higher concentrations, cyclopentolate also causes cycloplegia.

Epinephrine

Although topical epinephrine has proved useful in some patients with open-angle glaucoma, the 2% solution has been associated with such systemic effects as nervousness, hypertension, angina pectoris, tachycardia, and other dysrhythmias. Consequently, dipivefrin hydrochloride, a prodrug of epinephrine formed by the diesterification of epinephrine and pivalic acid, is often used instead. The addition of pivaloyl groups to the epinephrine molecule enhances its lipophilic character, greatly facilitating its penetration into the anterior chamber, where it reduces aqueous production and augments outflow. The prodrug delivery system is a more efficient way of delivering the therapeutic benefits of epinephrine, with less drug and with fewer side effects than conventional epinephrine therapy. Dipivefrin 0.1% is less irritating than 1% or 2% epinephrine, and, unlike cholinergic agents used to treat glaucoma, it does not produce miosis or accommodative spasm. Dipivefrin should not be used, however, in patients with narrow angles because any dilation of the pupil may trigger an attack of angle-closure glaucoma.

Phenylephrine

Pupillary dilation and capillary decongestion are reliably produced by topical phenylephrine. Although systemic effects secondary to topical application of prudent doses are rare,[39] severe hypertension, headache, tachycardia, and tremulousness have been reported.

In patients with coronary artery disease, severe myocardial ischemia, cardiac dysrhythmias, and even myocardial infarction may develop after topical 10% eye drops. Those with cerebral aneurysms may be susceptible to cerebral hemorrhage after phenylephrine in this concentration. In general, a safe systemic level follows absorption from either the conjunctiva or the nasal mucosa after drainage by the tear ducts. However, phenylephrine should not be given in the eye after surgery has begun and venous channels are patent.

Children are especially vulnerable to overdose and may respond in a dramatic and adverse fashion to phenylephrine drops. Hence, the use of only 2.5%, rather than 10%, phenylephrine is recommended in infants and the elderly, and the frequency of application should be strictly limited in these patient populations.

Timolol and Betaxolol

Timolol, a nonselective β-adrenergic blocking drug, historically has been a popular antiglaucoma drug. Because significant conjunctival absorption may occur, timolol should be administered with caution to patients with known obstructive airway disease, congestive heart failure, or greater than first-degree heart block. Life-threatening asthmatic crises have been reported after the administration of timolol drops to some patients with chronic, stable asthma.[40] The development of severe sinus bradycardia in a patient with cardiac conduction defects (left anterior hemiblock, first-degree atrioventricular block, and incomplete right bundle branch block) has been reported after timolol.[41] Moreover, timolol has been implicated in the exacerbation of myasthenia gravis[42] and in the production of postoperative apnea in neonates and young infants.[43]

In contrast to timolol, betaxolol, a $β_1$-blocker, is said to be more oculospecific and have minimal systemic effects.[44] However, patients receiving an oral β-blocker and betaxolol should be observed for potential additive effect on known systemic effects of β-blockade. Caution should be exercised in patients receiving catecholamine-depleting drugs. Although betaxolol has produced only minimal effects in patients with obstructive airway disease, caution should be exercised in the treatment of patients with excessive restriction of pulmonary function. Moreover, betaxolol is contraindicated in patients with sinus bradycardia, congestive heart failure, greater than first-degree heart block, cardiogenic shock, and overt myocardial failure.

Intraocular Perfluorocarbons

For a patient with a retinal detachment, a relatively insoluble expandable gas may be injected into the vitreous to mechanically tamponade reattachment. By varying the concentration, volume, and type of gas used, bubbles can be produced that last from 5 to 70 days before being completely absorbed. Nitrous oxide is manyfold more diffusible than perfluorocarbons, can readily expand the size of a gas bubble, and so should be discontinued 15 minutes prior to injection of a gas bubble.

Should the patient need another operation of any sort, it must be remembered that perfluorocarbons may linger in the eye for a protracted period.[45] If nitrous oxide is administered during this interval, the bubble can rapidly expand, risking retinal and optic nerve ischemia secondary to central retinal artery occlusion. Nitrous oxide should be avoided for 5 days after air injection, for 10 days after sulfur hexafluoride injection, and for 70 days following perfluoropropane (Table 49-3).[46] A MedicAlert bracelet is placed on the patient to warn against administration of nitrous oxide during the window of vulnerability (see section on Retinal Detachment Surgery).

Table 49-3 Differential Solubilities of Gases

Gas	Blood–Gas Partition Coefficients
Perfluoropropane	0.001
Sulfur hexafluoride	0.004
Nitrogen	0.015
Nitrous oxide	0.468

Systemic Ophthalmic Drugs

In addition to topical and intraocular therapies, various ophthalmic drugs given systemically may result in complications of concern to the anesthesiologist. These systemic drugs include glycerol, mannitol, and acetazolamide. For example, oral glycerol may be associated with nausea, vomiting, and risk of aspiration. Hyperglycemia or glycosuria, disorientation, and seizure activity may also occur after oral glycerol.

The recommended intravenous dose of mannitol is 1.5 g/kg given over a 30- to 60-minute interval. However, serious systemic problems may result from rapid infusion of large doses of mannitol. These complications include renal failure, congestive heart failure, pulmonary congestion, electrolyte imbalance, hypotension or hypertension, myocardial ischemia, and, rarely, allergic reactions. Clearly, the patient's renal and cardiovascular status must be thoroughly evaluated before mannitol therapy.

Acetazolamide, a carbonic anhydrase inhibitor with renal tubular effects, should be considered contraindicated in patients with marked hepatic or renal dysfunction or in those with low sodium levels or abnormal potassium values. As is well known, severe electrolyte imbalances can trigger serious cardiac dysrhythmias during general anesthesia. Furthermore, people with chronic lung disease may be vulnerable to the development of severe acidosis with long-term acetazolamide therapy. Topically active carbonic anhydrase inhibitors have been developed, are now commercially available, and appear to be relatively free of clinically important systemic effects.

Preoperative Evaluation

Establishing Rapport and Assessing Medical Condition

Preoperative preparation and evaluation of the patient begin with the establishment of rapport and communication among the anesthesiologist, the surgeon, and the patient. Most patients realize that surgery and anesthesia entail inherent risks, and they appreciate a candid explanation of potential complications, balanced with information concerning probability or frequency of permanent adverse sequelae. Such an approach also fulfills the medicolegal responsibilities of the physician to obtain informed consent.

A thorough history of the patient and physical examination are the foundation of safe patient care. Questionnaires in lieu of medical evaluation lack sensitivity to detect pertinent medical issues.[47] A complete list of medications that the patient is currently taking, both systemic and topical, must be obtained so potential drug interactions can be anticipated and essential medication will be administered during the hospital stay. Naturally, a history of any allergies to medicines, foods, or tape should be documented. Clearly, knowledge of any personal or family history of adverse reactions to anesthesia is mandatory.

The requisite laboratory data vary, depending on the medical history and physical status of the patient, as well as the nature of the surgical procedure. Indeed, the American Society of Anesthesiologists (ASA) task force on preoperative evaluation concluded that routine preoperative tests are commonly not useful in assessing and managing patients' perioperative experience. Schein et al.,[48] for example, demonstrated that "routine" testing does not improve cataract patient safety or outcome. Some physicians and laypersons misinterpreted the results and conclusions of this investigation, believing that patients having cataract surgery need no preoperative evaluation. It is vital to note that all patients in this trial received regular medical care and were evaluated by a physician preoperatively. Patients whose medical status indicated a need for preoperative laboratory tests were excluded from the study. Clearly, testing should be based on the results of the history and physical examination. The favorable economic impact of a "targeted" approach is obvious, because "routine" testing for the more than 1.5 million annual U.S. cataract operations neither decreases adverse events nor improves outcomes but is estimated to cost $150 million.[49]

The dilemma whether to continue or suspend antithrombotic therapy prior to surgery is not unique to the ophthalmic patient population. Many elderly eye surgery patients are on antiplatelet or anticoagulant therapy because of a history of coronary or vascular pathology. These individuals are at higher risk for perioperative hemorrhagic events, including retrobulbar hemorrhage, circumorbital hematoma, intravitreous bleeding, and hyphema. Although prior discontinuation of antithrombotic agents may diminish the potential for perioperative ocular bleeding, such strategy may increase the risk of adverse events like myocardial ischemia, infarction, cerebrovascular accident, and deep venous thrombosis.

The consensus of studies exploring this controversial issue suggest that cataract and other ophthalmic procedures can be safely performed under regional anesthesia without discontinuing antithrombotic agents.[50–52] A multicenter study of almost 20,000 elderly cataract patients attempted to establish the risks and benefits of continuing aspirin or warfarin therapy.[53] Despite the large population studied, the rate of complications was so low that absolute differences in risk were minimal. Patients who continued therapy did not have more ocular hemorrhage; those who discontinued treatment did not have a greater incidence of medical events. A meta-analysis of 11 studies revealed that continuing warfarin therapy for cataract patients was associated with an increased risk of bleeding, but almost all instances were self-limiting and not clinically relevant. No patient had bleeding-related compromise of visual acuity.[54]

Recent articles in the *Annals of Surgery*[55] and the *New England Journal of Medicine*[56] categorized retina surgery as being distinctly apart from other ophthalmic procedures owing to the high risk for intraoperative hemorrhage. However, contemporary ophthalmic literature suggests otherwise.[57,58] Retrospective studies of hemorrhagic complications in patients undergoing retina surgery taking antithrombotics demonstrate equivalent or higher rates of bleeding compared to controls. Nonetheless, in nearly all of these studies bleeding did not cause long-term visual sequelae; most were self-limited vitreous hemorrhages that rarely required returning to the operating room. Evolving surgical techniques including smaller gauge vitrectomy may further decrease the risk of perioperative hemorrhage.

Regional anesthesia for eye surgery also presents another bleeding risk. Traditionally, some physicians held that patients taking antithrombotic medications should not receive a regional eye block owing to increased hemorrhagic risk. Significantly, there are no data that conclusively substantiate this. In fact, the risks have been shown to be comparable regardless of antithrombotic continuation or interruption.[53,59]

The introduction of newer antithrombotic agents such as the anticoagulants dabigatran, rivaroxaban, and apixaban, as well as the antiplatelet medications prasugrel and ticagrelor, adds further complication because their efficacy cannot be monitored with conventional clotting assays.

The continuing evolution of this debate emphasizes the need to evaluate the systemic risk of stopping antithrombotics against the consequences associated with potential surgical/anesthetic hemorrhage. Currently, it is advocated to tailor guidelines such that most patients continue their antithrombotic medication regimens prior to ophthalmic surgery.

Another area of potential concern involves coronary artery disease patients with drug-eluting stents. Although bare-metal stents are susceptible to in-stent restenosis, drug-eluting stents are more vulnerable to stent thrombosis, a complication with a high mortality rate. Thus, patients with drug-eluting stents are typically on dual antiplatelet therapy with aspirin and clopidogrel, for example, for extended periods of time. A conclusion that is emerging is that the risk of thrombotic complications in patients with drug-eluting stents appears to outweigh the risk of bleeding complications. Therefore, given current information, a convincing case can be made for continuing dual antiplatelet therapy in the perioperative period and for delaying elective surgery for at least 4 to 6 weeks after placement of a bare metal stent and for 6 months after drug-eluting stent placement.[54,60,61]

Eye surgery patients are often at the extremes of age, ranging from premature babies with retinopathy of prematurity to nonagenarians. Hence, special age-related considerations such as altered pharmacokinetics and pharmacodynamics apply. In addition, elderly patients frequently have multiple comorbidities, including thyroid dysfunction, cardiopulmonary, and renal diseases. Hypertension is encountered in the majority of geriatric patients. Those with poorly controlled blood pressure should not receive dilating eye drops, such as phenylephrine, without consulting an anesthesiologist. Systemic absorption of high concentrations (e.g., >2.5% phenylephrine) or improperly instilled mydriatics can precipitate a hypertensive crisis with potentially devastating consequences.

As our society becomes increasingly geriatric, the number of ophthalmic surgery patients presenting with implanted cardiac defibrillators (ICDs) and pacemakers grows. The theoretical possibility of eye injury from patient movement in the event of ICD discharge during surgery exists. Although there is a broad spectrum of ophthalmic surgical procedures, the majority of cases use minimal bipolar cautery. For some, such as clear-corneal cataract surgery, no cautery is used. Thus, there is low risk of electromagnetic interference precipitating device discharge. Despite millions of procedures performed each year, there have not been any case reports of ICD activation during ophthalmic surgery and none of the device manufacturers have documented such an incident.[62,63] A retrospective survey of ophthalmic anesthesia providers found that over 80% did not use a magnet to reprogram or inactivate an ICD before surgery.[62]

Perioperative movement is a possible cause of patient eye injury and potential anesthesiologist liability. An analysis of ophthalmic monitored anesthesia care (MAC) closed claims cases that resulted in blindness or poor visual outcome found that more than 80% were associated with inadequate anesthesia and/or patient movement either during the block or intraoperatively.[64] Cough, orthopnea, and restlessness are the most common precipitators of excessive motion. Propofol sedation for eye block is associated with sneezing. Midazolam, fentanyl, and alfentanil given prior to propofol abate the sneeze reflex.[65] Intraoperative movement during general anesthesia may also induce dire visual consequences. Because most ophthalmic surgical procedures are elective, should an enhanced risk of perioperative movement be noted during the preoperative assessment, the prudent course may be to postpone surgery until the patient is in optimal condition to remain relatively still[66] or to perform the procedure under general anesthesia. Deliberate patient selection is requisite in order to prescribe the optimal anesthesia care plan.

The anesthesiologist must be aware of the anesthetic implications of congenital and metabolic diseases with ocular manifestations. Diabetic patients often present with ocular complications, and the anesthesiologist must be knowledgeable about the systemic disturbances of physiology that affect these patients. Indeed, the list of congenital and metabolic diseases associated with ocular pathologic effects that have important anesthetic implications is lengthy. A partial summary includes syndromes such as Crouzon, Apert, Goldenhar (oculoauriculovertebral dysplasia), Sturge–Weber, Marfan, Lowe (oculocerebrorenal syndrome), Down (trisomy 21), Wagner–Stickler, and Riley–Day (familial dysautonomia). Other diseases in this category are homocystinuria, myotonia dystrophica, and sickle cell disease.[67]

Anesthesia Options

The requirements of ophthalmic surgery include safety, akinesia, analgesia, minimal bleeding, avoidance or obtundation of the oculocardiac reflex, prevention of intraocular hypertension, awareness of drug interactions, and a smooth emergence devoid of vomiting, coughing, or retching (Table 49-1). Moreover, the exigencies of ophthalmic anesthesia mandate that the anesthesiologist be positioned remote from the patient's airway, sometimes creating certain logistic problems.

A number of anesthetic options exist, including general anesthesia, retrobulbar (intraconal) block, peribulbar (extraconal) anesthesia, sub-Tenon block, topical anesthesia, and intracameral injection. General anesthesia is typically administered for infants and children. Some adolescent and most adult patients can be cared for with regional or topical anesthesia and MAC, with or without sedation. The choice of anesthesia technique should be individualized on the basis of the patient's needs and preferences, the nature and duration of the procedure, and the preferences and skills of the anesthesiologist and the surgeon.

The retrobulbar block has traditionally been the most popular regional anesthetic technique for eye surgery. Since the mid-1990s, owing to a presumed superior safety profile, peribulbar injection has surpassed retrobulbar block in popularity. Recently, however, topical analgesia has prevailed for cataract surgery in the United States,[68] whereas use of sub-Tenon blocks has surged in the United Kingdom and New Zealand.[69] Although cataract surgery embodies the majority of eye procedures, there are a variety of other subspecialty operations, including corneal transplant and procedures for glaucoma, strabismus, and tumor, as well as oculoplastic, orbital, vitreoretinal, and eye trauma procedures. Most of these continue to be accomplished primarily with a regional eye block and sedation,[70] although some warrant general anesthesia. Anesthesiologists have had increasing interest in administering ocular anesthesia, so workshops in ophthalmic regional anesthesia are often conducted at major regional and national meetings. Many ophthalmologists and administrators encourage anesthesiologists to administer the blocks to facilitate operating room efficiency.

When a regional anesthetic of the orbit is administered, by either the anesthesiologist or the ophthalmologist, it is the responsibility of the anesthesiologist to monitor the patient's vital signs, electrocardiogram (ECG), and oxygen saturation. Sedation may be administered before performance of the block and/or initiation of surgery. The anesthesiologist must be vigilant for the oculocardiac reflex, signs of brainstem anesthesia, and the need for airway support or other interventions.

Side of Anesthesia and Surgery

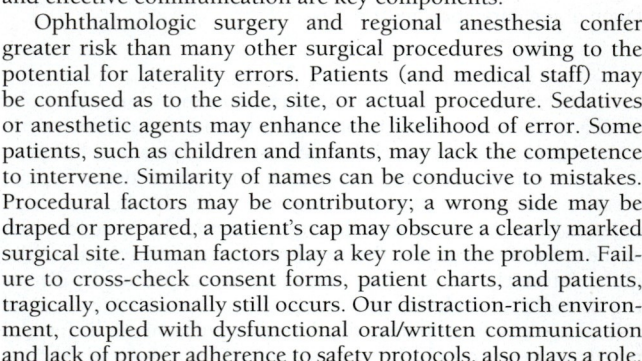

In an attempt to ensure proper patient, side, site, and procedure selection, The Joint Commission (formerly known as the Joint Commission on Accreditation of Healthcare Organizations) held a "Wrong Site Summit" in May 2003 in which they developed a universal protocol for preventing wrong site, wrong procedure, wrong person surgery. The policy is tripartite, involving preoperative verification, marking of the intended site, and a "time-out" immediately before the start of surgery.[71] Patient involvement and effective communication are key components.

Ophthalmologic surgery and regional anesthesia confer greater risk than many other surgical procedures owing to the potential for laterality errors. Patients (and medical staff) may be confused as to the side, site, or actual procedure. Sedatives or anesthetic agents may enhance the likelihood of error. Some patients, such as children and infants, may lack the competence to intervene. Similarity of names can be conducive to mistakes. Procedural factors may be contributory; a wrong side may be draped or prepared, a patient's cap may obscure a clearly marked surgical site. Human factors play a key role in the problem. Failure to cross-check consent forms, patient charts, and patients, tragically, occasionally still occurs. Our distraction-rich environment, coupled with dysfunctional oral/written communication and lack of proper adherence to safety protocols, also plays a role.

Anesthesia Techniques

In the past, ophthalmic procedures commonly involved large ocular incisions. General endotracheal anesthesia, with deep and sustained neuromuscular paralysis and placement of sandbags to surround the patient's head, were typical strategies to ensure perioperative immobility. Currently, general anesthesia typically is reserved for children and adults who are unable to communicate, cooperate, or remain suitably stationary. Supraglottic airways (SGAs) have been increasingly accepted as a means to secure the airway in patients with minimal risk for aspiration who are having eye surgery with general anesthesia.[72] The SGA is not only safe and effective in this setting but also offers the advantage of less increase in IOP on insertion and removal than is encountered with an endotracheal tube.[73] Similarly, less bucking and coughing on emergence and during the recovery phase have been noted.[74] Vigilance must be maintained, however, to detect initial misplacement or intraoperative displacement of the SGA. In addition, intraoperative laryngospasm in infants and neonates is not uncommon with an SGA.

Retrobulbar (Intraconal) and Peribulbar (Extraconal) Blocks

In 1844, Knapp described one of the first techniques for ophthalmic regional anesthesia.[75] In the early 20th century, Atkinson[76] introduced the retrobulbar block, a practical needle-based means to achieve analgesia and profound akinesia of the globe. For a retrobulbar block, the needle tip is situated behind (retro) the globe (bulbar). The peribulbar block, a more recently introduced needle-based technique, varies from the retrobulbar block in terms of the depth and angulation of needle placement within

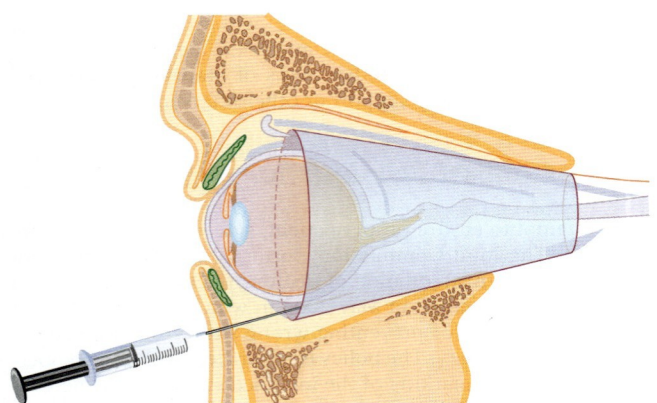

Figure 49-4 Intraconal (retrobulbar) block and schematic representation of the intraorbital muscle cone.

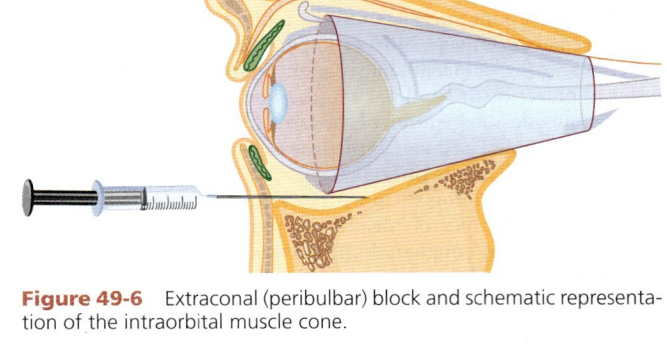

Figure 49-6 Extraconal (peribulbar) block and schematic representation of the intraorbital muscle cone.

the orbit. Here, the needle tip is placed around (peri) the globe (bulbar). The terminology is inadequate because "retro" and "peri" only vaguely describe the difference between the two techniques. The four rectus muscles, along with connective tissue septae, create a defined compartment known as the *orbital cone*, which extends from the rectus muscle origins around the optic foramen at the apex of the orbit to the attachment of the muscles onto the globe anteriorly. Retrobulbar blocks are accomplished by directing a needle through the eyelid or via the conjunctiva toward the orbital apex with sufficient depth and angulation such that the needle passes through the muscle cone (Figs. 49-4 and 49-5).[77] Local anesthetic is then instilled. The term intraconal injection is therefore a better, more descriptive name for the procedure than the older, retrobulbar block.[78]

Cadaveric dissections have shown that there is no complete intermuscular septum encircling the rectus muscles, linking them together to form an impermeable conal compartment behind the globe.[79] Ripart et al.[80] clearly demonstrated that extraconal injections of dye into cadaveric specimens diffused into the intraconal space, and solutions placed within the cone distributed to the extraconal space. Thus, the peribulbar or, more properly termed, extraconal block is executed by directing a needle through the eyelid or via the conjunctiva to less depth and with minimal angulation, parallel to the globe, toward the greater wing of the sphenoid bone (Figs. 49-6 and 49-7). Local anesthetic instilled in this extraconal space will eventually penetrate toward the optic nerve and other structures, establishing conduction anesthesia. The extraconal block may be theoretically safer because the needle tip is kept at a greater distance from vital intraorbital structures and brain.

The didactic classification of block nomenclature based on the relationship of the needle and the muscle cone is a useful means to conceptualize the differences between two types of needle-based eye blocks. It is important to emphasize, though, that needle path cannot always be predicted by clinical evaluation alone. Radiologic studies have shown that some percentage of intraconal blocks administered by experienced physicians is, in fact, extraconal, and vice versa.[81]

Again, a retrobulbar block is more precisely described as an intraconal injection. It positions local anesthetics deep within the orbit proximate to the nerves and muscle origins. Thus, it requires low volume, has rapid onset, and yields intense depth of anesthesia. The peribulbar or, more accurately labeled, extraconal block is placed further from the optic and other orbital nerves, requires larger volumes of local anesthetic, and has longer latency of onset. The needle entry point for both blocks is at the same inferotemporal location. The junction of the lateral third and medial two-thirds of the inferior orbital rim in line with the lateral limbal margin has been the conventional access point. However, locating the needle entry point more laterally

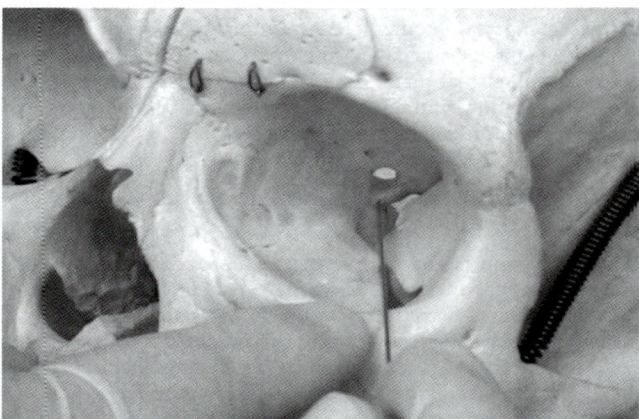

Figure 49-5 Needle placement for intraconal (retrobulbar) block.

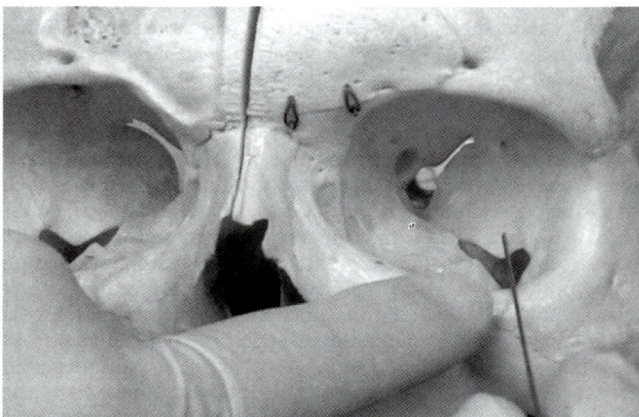

Figure 49-7 Needle placement for extraconal (peribulbar) block.

may serve to decrease the likelihood of injecting local anesthetics into the delicate inferior rectus or inferior oblique muscles. This is important because intramuscular injection of anesthetics has been postulated as a potential cause of postoperative strabismus.[82] Medial approaches at the caruncle have also been popularized.[83] Supplementation of anesthesia with an injection above the globe may not be prudent because the preponderance of vessels lie in the superior orbit. In addition, the belly of the superior oblique muscle and the trochlear muscle can be encountered superonasally.

Katsev et al.[84] demonstrated that the tips of commonly used 1.5-in (38-mm) needles can reach critical structures in the densely packed apex of the orbit in almost 20% of classic retrobulbar blocks. Consequently, needles 1.25 inches (31-mm) or shorter are appropriate. Controversy exists over the advantages of sharp versus dull needles. Dull needles may require more force to penetrate the globe. However, sharp needles are less painful to insert and may cause less damage in the face of inadvertent globe puncture.[85] In the past, patients were asked to gaze superonasally while a block was conducted. Unsold et al.[86] found that this maneuver caused the optic nerve to stretch directly in the path of the incoming needle during intraconal injection, exposing it to risk of needle trauma. Patients should be instructed to maintain gaze in the neutral position, leaving the optic nerve lax within the orbit in the course of needle insertion.[87] Elevations in IOP after an eye block can be minimized by application of gentle noncontinuous digital pressure or use of an ocular decompression device.[88]

Akinesia of the eyelids is obtained by blocking the branches of the facial nerve supplying the orbicularis muscle. Lid akinesia is often a direct consequence of the larger volume of local anesthetic used for extraconal blocks. Intraconal blocks, in contrast, often leave the orbicularis oculi fully functional. Thus, a facial nerve block is performed in conjunction with retrobulbar block to prevent squeezing of the eyelid, which could result in extrusion of intraocular contents during corneal transplantation, for example. Since facial nerve block was first used for ophthalmic surgery by Van Lint in 1914, numerous methods of facial nerve blockade have been described. These techniques block the facial nerve after its exit point from the skull in the stylomastoid foramen. Moving distally to proximally to the foramen, the techniques include the Van Lint, Atkinson, O'Brien, and Nadbath–Rehman methods. Although each has advantages and disadvantages, the Nadbath–Rehman approach can potentially produce the most serious systemic consequences. With this approach, a 27-gauge, 12-mm needle is inserted between the mastoid process and the posterior border of the mandibular ramus. Because of the proximity of the jugular foramen (10 mm medial to the stylomastoid foramen) to the injection site, ipsilateral paralysis of cranial nerves IX, X, and XI can occur, producing hoarseness, dysphagia, pooling of secretions, agitation, respiratory distress, or laryngospasm. Moreover, because the Nadbath–Rehman block produces complete hemifacial akinesia, which interferes with oral intake, this approach is not recommended for outpatients.

8 Complications associated with needle-based ophthalmic anesthetics may be local or systemic and may result in blindness or even death (Table 49-4). Bleeding may be superficial or deep, arterial or venous. Superficial hemorrhage may produce an unsightly circumorbital hematoma. Retrobulbar hemorrhage, when arterially based, may produce precipitous bleeding and a palpable, dramatic increase in IOP, as well as globe proptosis and entrapment of the upper lid. With the globe's vascular supply in jeopardy, the patient's long-term ultimate visual acuity may be quickly compromised. Consultation with an ophthalmologist should be immediately sought, and fundoscopic examination, tonometric measurement of IOP, ultrasound to assess presence/

Table 49-4 Complications of Needle-based Ophthalmic Anesthesia

Stimulation of oculocardiac reflex arc
Superficial hemorrhage → circumorbital hematoma
Retrobulbar hemorrhage ± retinal perfusion compromise → loss of vision
Globe penetration ± intraocular injection → retinal detachment, loss of vision
Trauma to optic nerve or orbital cranial nerves → loss of vision
Optic nerve sheath injection → orbital epidural anesthesia
Extraocular muscle injury, leading to postoperative strabismus, diplopia
Intra-arterial injection, producing immediate convulsions
Central retinal artery occlusion
Inadvertent brainstem anesthesia → contralateral amaurosis, mydriasis, muscle paresis
Neurocardiopulmonary compromise

location of blood, and even a lateral canthotomy may be warranted. Continuous ECG monitoring is indicated because the oculocardiac reflex may occur as blood extravasates from the muscle cone. The decision to proceed with surgery in the presence of a mild or moderate hemorrhage depends on numerous factors, including the degree of bleeding, the nature of the planned ophthalmologic surgery, and the patient's condition.

Penetration of the sclera is a distinct, although rare, possibility with needle-based anesthesia techniques. Mechanical trauma, with potential retinal detachment, and chemical injury to delicate retina tissue caused by local anesthetics can occur. Blindness or very poor vision may be the result. Globe puncture is defined as a single entry into the eye, whereas perforation is caused by two full-thickness wounds—an entry and a subsequent exit. The globe's posterior pole is the most commonly penetrated area. Risk factors for posterior pole needle injury include presence of an elongated globe, recessed orb, and/or atypical-shaped eye. The anteroposterior distance of an eye may be long because of myopia or presence of globe-enveloping intraorbital hardware such as a scleral buckle. Some patients have an abnormal outpouching of the eye, termed *staphyloma*. Most staphylomata are located at the posterior of the globe, surrounding the juncture of the eye with the optic nerve. By definition, an intraconal (retrobulbar) anesthetic is administered by purposefully angling the needle steeply and deeply within the orbit behind the globe. If the globe is longer than one assumes, it is at greater risk of penetration or puncture by the needle. In one study, ultrasound detection determined that the tip of the needle, placed in classic retrobulbar fashion, can be much closer to the posterior pole of the globe than presupposed by physicians.[89] Extraconal (peribulbar) anesthesia entails shallower placement of the needle without directing the needle inward toward the orbital apex; thus, it is associated with a lower incidence of globe needle injury. Be aware, however, that it is still possible to engage the needle with sclera laterally.

The risk of penetrating the sclera with a needle is also inversely proportional to the anesthesiologist's education and experience. This notion is affirmed by several reports of globe injuries rendered by inadequately educated or trained personnel in the early 1990s.[90] In a survey of 284 directors of anesthesiology and ophthalmology programs, no formal training or education in ophthalmic regional anesthesia techniques was provided to anesthesia residents in most academic programs.[91] This survey concluded that anesthesiologists who perform needle-based ophthalmic blocks should have knowledge of orbital anatomy and the ocular risk factors that were noted previously. Thus, appropriate preanesthesia history taking includes direct interrogation concerning myopia or previous scleral buckle surgery, because both imply increased globe length. Bayes et al.[92] showed that a history of correction for myopia as a child or young adult was both highly sensitive and highly specific for having an elongated axial length. Physical examination of surface anatomy should note the position of the globe within the orbit and whether enophthalmos is present. A recessed eye is at greater risk of needle-tip misadventure. The most important laboratory examination is the preoperative ultrasound. For patients undergoing cataract surgery, an ultrasound is *always* performed to calculate the appropriate intraocular lens to insert intraoperatively. In addition, it reveals the length and shape of the eye. An axial length greater than 26 mm confers greater risk of penetration or perforation. In the event that the ultrasound report is not found in the patient's chart, the anesthesiologist should inquire about the results before embarking on a needle-based block.

In the future, portable real-time ultrasonography may have a role in reducing the risk of penetrating injury (Fig. 49-8).[93] Needle-based eye blocks are "blind" techniques primarily dependent on surface anatomy landmarks to position the needle correctly. Ultrasound-guided direct visualization of both the needle and the spread of local anesthetic may improve the quality and safety of these blocks.

The eye is easily accessible, and its geometry and surrounding elements are relatively straightforward. Additionally, the tissue contents of the orbit lack gas-filled or osseous structures, making this a suitable area for ultrasonic imaging. Sonography of the eye, however, is not without risk. Owing to potential thermal and mechanical bioeffects, the U.S. Food and Drug Administration has imposed stricter physical parameters for ophthalmic ultrasound. In particular, limits on mechanical index and thermal index have been reduced to 0.23 and less than 1, respectively. Commercial ultrasound transducers marketed to anesthesiologists may not comply with these recommendations. A recent rabbit model study that compared thermal and mechanical changes induced by exposure to ophthalmic- and nonophthalmic-rated transducers showed significant changes in intraorbital temperature after moderate exposure to a nonophthalmic-rated device, emphasizing the need to ensure that proper eye-appropriate ultrasound equipment is employed for these blocks.[94]

Brainstem anesthesia and inadvertent intravascular injection of local anesthetics are two additional potentially devastating

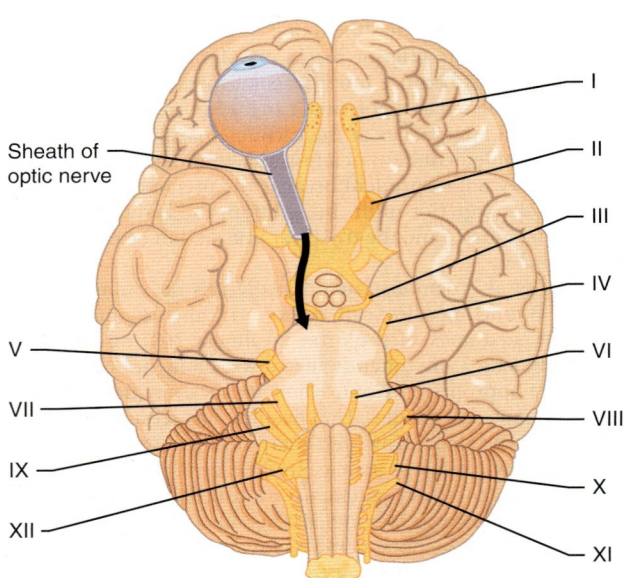

Figure 49-9 Base of the brain and the path that local anesthetic agents might follow if inadvertently injected into the subarachnoid space. This route includes the cranial nerves, pons, and midbrain. (Adapted with permission from Javitt JC, Addiego R, Friedberg HL, et al. Brain stem anesthesia after retrobulbar block. *Ophthalmology*. 1987;94:718.)

consequences of needle-based ocular anesthesia. In the course of accidental intravascular arterial injection, local anesthetics flow from the needle via a branch of the ophthalmic artery in retrograde fashion to the internal carotid artery and then to the circle of Willis. Rapid redistribution of local anesthetic to the brain results in immediate onset of convulsions. Cardiopulmonary instability may also occur.

Although the incidence of brainstem anesthesia is rare, it is even less common with extraconal versus intraconal blocks. Brainstem anesthesia is a consequence of the direct spread of local anesthetic agents to the brain along the meningeal sheath surrounding the optic nerve. In contradistinction to intra-arterial injection, symptoms are typically not immediate. There is a continuum of sequelae dependent on the concentration and volume of drug that gains access centrally, as well as the specific areas into which the anesthetic spreads (Fig. 49-9).[95] Nicoll et al.[96] reported 16 cases of apparently central spread of anesthetics in a series of 6,000 intraconal blocks. Eight patients developed respiratory arrest. Examination of the conscious patient's contralateral, non-blocked eye for amaurosis, mydriasis, and extraocular muscle paresis may confirm the diagnosis of brainstem anesthesia. The abducens and oculomotor nerves are more commonly affected than the superior oblique muscle's trochlear nerve. Other protean CNS signs may include violent shivering, eventual loss of consciousness, apnea, and hemiplegia, paraplegia, quadriplegia, or hyperreflexia. Blockade of cranial nerves VIII to XII results in deafness, vertigo, vagolysis, dysphagia, aphasia, and loss of neck muscle power. It is axiomatic that personnel skilled in airway maintenance and ventilatory and circulatory support should be immediately available whenever ophthalmic anesthetic blocks are administered.

Cannula-based Techniques

Cannula-based ophthalmic regional anesthesia was formally described by Swan[97] in 1956 and then rediscovered and popularized

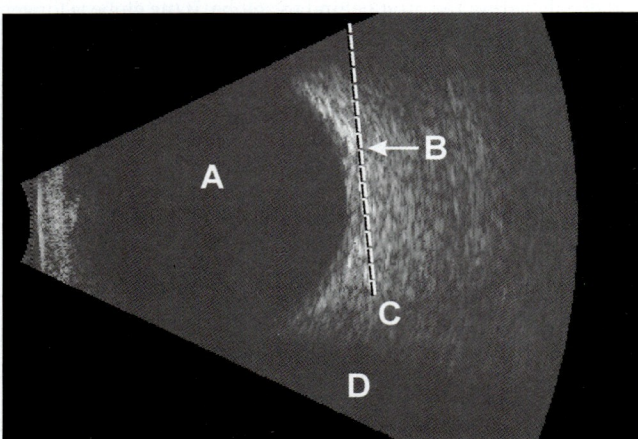

Figure 49-8 Ultrasound-guided block with overlay. **A:** Globe. **B:** Needleshaft. **C:** Needle tip. **D:** Optic nerve.

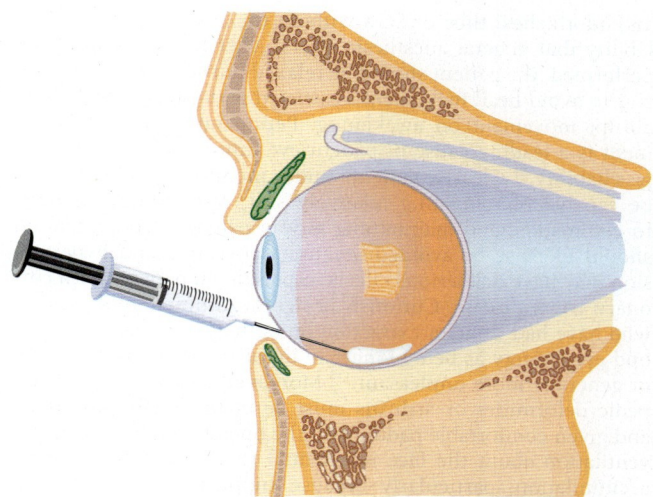

Figure 49-10 Sub-Tenon (episcleral) block with blunt cannula.

in the 1990s as another practical means to achieve analgesia and akinesia of the globe, while offering potential advantages in certain circumstances over needle-based blocks.[98] Imaging studies have shown that local anesthetics instilled beneath Tenon capsule spread into the posterior orbit.[99] The block is accomplished by inserting a blunt cannula through a small incision in the conjunctiva and Tenon capsule, also known as the *episcleral membrane*, with subsequent infusion of local anesthetics (Fig. 49-10). Onset of analgesia is rapid. The ultimate extent of globe akinesia is proportional to the volume of local anesthetic injected. One large prospective study by Guise[69] of 6,000 such blocks found this technique to be highly effective. Advantages, particularly for very myopic patients who have elongated axial lengths, include decreased risk of posterior pole penetration or perforation because needles are not placed into the posterior orbit.

After application of topical anesthetic, the episcleral space can be accessed from all quadrants with blunt-tipped scissors; however, the incision is most commonly made in the inferonasal quadrant. The cannula is guided through the opening with the aid of a toothless forceps. It is common for local anesthetics to leak retrogradely out of the incision site. Conjunctival bleeding, chemosis, and ballooning of the conjunctiva are also common. Fortunately, these are cosmetic issues that rarely affect outcome. Guise[69] estimated the incidence of minor hemorrhage to be below 10% and had to abandon only one case because of a large subconjunctival hemorrhage that was not sight threatening. Thus, the sub-Tenon block may be a prudent ocular anesthesia technique for the anticoagulated patient at risk for retrobulbar hemorrhage.

Major complications of sub-Tenon anesthesia include globe perforation,[100] hemorrhage, rectus muscle trauma, postoperative strabismus, orbital cellulitis, optic nerve neuritis, and brainstem anesthesia.[101] More complications are reported with longer (18 to 25 mm) rigid metallic cannulae. Shorter (12 mm), more flexible plastic cannulae may be preferable; however, they are associated with a higher incidence of conjunctival hemorrhage and chemosis. Variations of sub-Tenon blocks include use of ultrashort cannulae (6 mm) and needle-based episcleral block techniques.[102] A new technique of an incisionless sub-Tenon block has been pioneered by Allman et al.[103] There has been a report of a death associated with a sub-Tenon block, potentially secondary to central spread of local anesthetic.[104] However, the definitive pathogenesis remains an enigma.[105]

Topical Analgesia

Ophthalmologists have also been returning to a technique that was popularized during the early 1900s—the use of topical anesthetic agents, particularly when the surgical incision is made through clear cornea. Indeed, surface analgesia was the technique of choice for cataract surgery until the evolution of effective needle-based methods of regional anesthesia and improved safety of general anesthesia in the 1930s. Multiple advances in cataract surgery that have enabled faster operations with greater control and less trauma have allowed ophthalmologists to re-examine the use of topical anesthesia for this procedure.

Fully anticoagulated patients may be excellent candidates for topical analgesia, as are monocular patients who are spared the trauma of prolonged local anesthetic–induced postoperative amaurosis. Potential disadvantages of topical anesthesia include eye movement during surgery, patient anxiety or discomfort, and, rarely, allergic reactions. Patient selection is critical and should be restricted to individuals who are alert and able to follow instructions, and who can refrain from eye movement and lid squeezing. Patients who are demented or photophobic, or who cannot communicate, may be inappropriate candidates, as are those with active infection. Similarly, patients with dense cataracts or small pupils who may require significant iris manipulation or those who need large scleral incisions may be contraindicated for topical anesthesia.

Topical analgesia can be achieved with local anesthetic drops or gels. Anesthetic gels produce greater levels of drug in the anterior chamber than equal doses of drops and may afford superior surface analgesia.[106] Concerns about increased potential for postoperative endophthalmitis with gel-based topical analgesia exist because gels might theoretically form a barrier to bactericidal agents. Therefore, if administered, gels should be applied after antiseptic solutions, taking care to apply anesthetic drops before the use of caustic bactericidal preps.

Analgesia can be supplemented with intracameral injection of 0.1 to 0.2 mL of 1% preservative-free lidocaine into the anterior chamber. So-called shugarcaine, an intracameral admixture of 4% preservative-free lidocaine and 1:1000 bisulfite-free epinephrine in salt solution, provides analgesia, dilates the pupil, and stabilizes the iris.[107] It is employed for cataract surgery patients with benign prostatic hyperplasia who typically exhibit symptoms of floppy iris intraoperatively. This syndrome has strong association with oral α_1-selective adrenergic antagonists, particularly the α_{1a} class that includes tamsulosin and silodosin. It manifests as a triad of poor pupillary dilation, floppy iris tissue, and a tendency for the iris to prolapse during surgery, resulting in a higher rate of cataract surgical complications.[108] Of note, symptoms can persist for over a year after discontinuation of α_1 antagonists.

Choice of Local Anesthetics, Block Adjuvants, and Adjuncts

Anesthetics for ocular surgery are selected on the basis of onset and duration needed. Fast-onset, brief-duration local anesthetics are optimal for procedures such as cataract surgery or pterygium excision. Longer-acting agents are indicated for lengthier operations such as vitreoretinal surgery. Ophthalmic anesthesia has a tradition of mixing different local anesthetics to produce a block with shorter latency of onset yet longer duration of effect, although clinically there may not be true advantage to combining agents.[109] Bupivacaine 0.75% concentration has been shown to have potential to cause extraocular muscle toxicity. Lower concentrations do not have such a propensity.[110] Ropivacaine 0.75% or 1%, either alone or admixed with lidocaine, is an effective agent for eye block that has less cardiotoxic effects than 0.75% bupivacaine.[111,112]

Sodium bicarbonate, morphine sulfate, clonidine, and even vecuronium have been used as local anesthetic adjuvants in ophthalmic surgery. Vasoconstrictors may improve the quality of the block by delaying washout of drug from the orbit. There is concern, however, that epinephrine, the most common vasoconstrictor additive, may compromise retinal perfusion[113]; it is best avoided in patients with glaucomatous optic nerve damage.

Without question, however, hyaluronidase has been the most popular ancillary agent used to modify ocular local anesthetic actions since it was introduced by Atkinson in 1949. It acts by hydrolyzing hyaluronic acid, a natural substance that binds cells together, keeping them cohesive. Thus, hyaluronidase, in doses of 0.75 to 300 International Units per milliliter increases tissue permeability, serves to promote dispersion of local anesthetics through tissues within the orbit, reduces the increase in orbital pressure associated with the volume of injected anesthetics, and enhances the quality of orbital blockade.[114] Furthermore, hyaluronidase may reduce the risk of local anesthetic–induced extraocular muscle injury because clustered increases of postoperative diplopia were reported after national shortages of the drug in 1998 and 2000.[115] Studies since that time have supported these findings.[116] However, it is possible that technique was altered in response to the absence of hyaluronidase by placing needles deeper, using more injections, or depositing larger volumes of local anesthetics. Perhaps as a consequence of past national shortages, many facilities choose to obtain hyaluronidase from local compounding labs. In recent years, tainted medications from compounding facilities have led to multiple deaths due to fungal meningitis in chronic pain patients and permanent blindness in macular degeneration patients. Hyaluronidase is currently widely available in a human recombinant formulation, obviating the need for compounded formulations.

Digital pressure and mechanical devices have been used to soften the globe prior to surgery. Essentially, they are all variations on a ball, balloon, or bag theme. The Super Pinky ball and the Honan Intraocular Pressure Reducer (The Lebanon Corporation, Lebanon, Indiana) are examples.[88] Immediately after administration of regional orbital anesthesia, the compression device may be positioned on the eye for 5 to 20 minutes. Reduction of IOP to below baseline levels is not uncommon. However, excessive pressure on the globe by these devices may impede blood flow, causing ischemic optic neuropathy (ION) or central retinal artery occlusion, possibly leading to blindness.[117] The Honan device addresses this potentially catastrophic complication with a pneumatic bellows that maintains even compression of the globe coupled to a manometric gauge that indicates a numeric value of applied pressure. A safety valve limits the amount of inflation of the bellows. With the increasing popularity of smaller incisions, lower-profile prosthetic lenses, and topical analgesia for cataract surgery, there is less need for IOP-reducing devices.

General Principles of Monitored Anesthesia Care

Many advocate the intravenous administration of an appropriate agent immediately prior to ocular regional anesthesia to provide comfort and amnesia. Polypharmacy and deep sedation in the form of high doses of opioids, benzodiazepines, and hypnotics may be unwise because of the pharmacologic vagaries in the geriatric population and the attendant risks of respiratory depression, airway obstruction, hypotension, CNS aberrations, and prolonged recovery time. This undesirable technique has all the disadvantages of a general anesthetic in the absence of an endotracheal tube or SGA without the advantage of controllability that general anesthesia offers. After the block has been performed, the patient should be relaxed but sufficiently responsive to avoid head movement associated with snoring or sudden abrupt movement on awakening. Perioperative patient movement is a leading cause of patient eye injury and anesthesiologist liability.[64] Clearly, patients under monitored sedation must be capable of remaining relatively still, responding rationally to commands, and maintaining airway patency. Undersedation should likewise be avoided because tachycardia and hypertension may have deleterious effects, especially in patients with coronary artery disease. Curiously, a significant fraction of patients who have had cataract extraction on both eyes perceive the second eye surgery as being longer in duration, more painful, and/or generally more unpleasant.[118] Moreover, patients with orthopedic deformities or arthritis must be meticulously positioned and given comfortable padding on the operating table. Adequate ventilation about the face is essential to avoid carbon dioxide accumulation, particularly because supplemental oxygen can delay signs of desaturation and hypoventilation.[119] Use of exogenous oxygen can also contribute to surgical fire, particularly during oculoplastic surgery performed with electrocautery. Consider air or mixed air/oxygen instead of oxygen for these procedures. Tightly occluded drapes may also promote accumulation of oxygen. In fact, burn injuries during facial surgery with supplemental oxygen account for nearly one-third of MAC closed claims cases.[120] Patients must be comfortably warm because the hazards of shivering in patients having delicate eye surgery are well known. Further, shivering causes a risk for patients with coronary artery disease. Continuous ECG monitoring is vital, lest performance of the ophthalmic regional block, pressure on the orbit, or tugging on the extraocular muscles stimulates the oculocardiac reflex arc and produces dangerous cardiac dysrhythmias. Likewise, pulse oximetry is essential. The adequacy of the sedated patient's ventilation should be assessed by clinical signs as well as exhaled carbon dioxide. Unequivocally, MAC should reflect "maximum anesthesia caution, not minimal anesthesiology care."[121]

Studies have confirmed that most cataract operations performed in the United States are conducted with the patient under some form of local anesthesia (either retrobulbar, peribulbar, sub-Tenon, intracameral, or topical analgesia), with monitoring equipment used in 97% of cases and an anesthesiologist present in 78% of cases.[122] An international survey of ophthalmologists reported routine use of anesthesia-trained personnel in 96% and 97% of cases in the United States and Australia, respectively.[123] On the other side of the spectrum, ophthalmologists from Malaysia and Thailand had anesthesia monitoring 31% and 18% of the time, respectively. Indeed, many anesthesiologists fear that the Centers for Medicare and Medicaid Services will decide not to reimburse for MAC for "routine" cataract cases.

An important study by Rosenfeld et al.[124] assessed the need for MAC in cataract surgery. These investigators prospectively studied the incidence and nature of interventions required by anesthesia personnel in 1,006 consecutive cataract operations (both phacoemulsification and extracapsular techniques were included) performed under peribulbar block. They also analyzed germane information, including patient demographic data, medical history, and preoperative laboratory tests, for ability to predict those patients at greatest risk for intervention. They found that 37% of patients required some type of intervention and that in general the majority of those interventions could not have been predicted before surgery. Patients younger than 60 years required intervention in over 60% of cases. The interventions ranged from minor forms, such as verbal reassurance and hand holding, to administering such intravenous medications as supplemental sedation or antihypertensive, pressor, or antiarrhythmic agents, or to providing respiratory assistance. Although hypertension, lung disease, renal disease, and a diagnosis of cancer were related to interventions, these four conditions combined accounted for only a small portion of the needed interventions. Moreover, although many of the interventions were relatively minor, several were more serious, and 30% of the interventions were considered (by the involved anesthesia personnel) to be critical to the success of the operation. The investigators concluded that MAC by qualified anesthesia personnel is reasonable and justified and contributes to the quality of patient care when cataract surgery is performed with local anesthesia. Fung et al.[125] examined satisfaction scores for community-based cataract surgery via topical anesthesia and discovered that patients' value and regard for the anesthesiologist's role actually increased from the preoperative to the postoperative interview. In view of the fact that topical anesthesia produces analgesia that is less profound and provides operating conditions that are less ideal than regional or general anesthesia, it seems likely that anesthesia care is equally appropriate to provide comfort, support, and indicated drugs for these patients as well. For both ethical and surgical reasons, the ophthalmologist's attention must not be distracted from the microsurgical field.

Anesthetic Management in Specific Situations

"Open-Eye, Full-Stomach" Encounters

The anesthesiologist involved in caring for a patient with a penetrating eye injury and a full stomach confronts special challenges. He or she must weigh the risk of aspiration against the risk of blindness in the injured eye that could result from elevated IOP and extrusion of ocular contents.

As in all cases of trauma, attention should be given to the exclusion of other injuries, such as skull and orbital fractures, intracranial trauma associated with subdural hematoma formation, and the possibility of thoracic or abdominal bleeding.

Although regional anesthesia is often a valuable alternative for the management of nonfasted trauma patients, this option had traditionally been considered contraindicated with penetrating eye injuries because of the potential to extrude intraocular contents via pressure generated by injection of local anesthetics. Needle instrumentation of the orbit, squeezing of the eyelids, and pressure due to bleeding are additional reasons that regional anesthesia was typically avoided in open-globe scenarios. Nonetheless, some anecdotal case reports of successful use of ophthalmic blocks in this setting have been published.[126] Recognizing that there are several distinct permutations of eye injuries, Scott et al.[127] developed techniques to safely block patients with *select* open-globe injuries. In a 4-year period, 220 disrupted eyes were repaired via regional anesthesia. A significant number of injuries were caused by intraocular foreign bodies and dehiscence of cataract or corneal transplant incisions. Blocked eyes tended to have more anterior, smaller wounds than those repaired via general anesthesia. There was no outcome difference—that is, change of visual acuity from initial evaluation until final examination—between the eyes repaired via regional versus general anesthesia. Moreover, combined topical anesthesia and sedation for *selected* patients with open-globe injuries has also been reported.[128] Ophthalmologists' shift from the hospital operating room suite to ambulatory surgery facilities and specialty eye-care surgery centers has unbound their ties to hospitals. Many no longer maintain hospital privileges, creating impetus to operate on eye injury patients on an ambulatory surgical basis in their own facilities. For some patients, general anesthesia in an ambulatory surgery center may confer an unacceptable level of systemic risk. In those scenarios, selection of regional or topical anesthesia for repair of traumatic eye injuries may be a prudent alternative.

Nonetheless, general anesthesia remains the accepted modality for many traumatic eye injury patients. Preoperative prophylaxis against aspiration may involve administering H_2 receptor antagonists to elevate gastric fluid pH and to reduce gastric acid production. Metoclopramide may be given to induce peristalsis and enhance gastric emptying.

Traditionally, an induction agent with nondepolarizing neuromuscular blocking drug technique was described as the method of choice for the emergency repair of an open eye injury; however, this method has its disadvantages, including risk of aspiration and difficult airway. Performance of the Sellick maneuver may afford some protection. Furthermore, a premature attempt at intubation of the trachea produces coughing, straining, and a dramatic rise in IOP, emphasizing the need to confirm the onset of drug effect with a peripheral nerve stimulator while appreciating, nonetheless, that muscle groups vary in their response to muscle relaxants. Several studies have explored the use of large doses of nondepolarizing muscle relaxants to accelerate the onset of adequate relaxation for endotracheal intubation. Moreover, the cardiovascular side effects of tachycardia and hypertension may prove worrisome in patients with coronary artery disease.

Succinylcholine offers the distinct advantages of swift onset, superb intubating conditions, and brief duration of action. Although the advisability of this technique has been debated vociferously, McGoldrick[129] pointed out that the 1957 watershed article of Lincoff et al.[14] states: "Various communications have been received from ophthalmologists who have used succinylcholine in surgery. This includes several reports of cases in which succinylcholine was given to forestall impending vitreous prolapse only to have a prompt expulsion of vitreous occur." Under such desperate circumstances, it is extremely difficult to attribute the expulsion of vitreous directly to succinylcholine.[129]

Rocuronium, with its rapid onset, is a useful drug in these circumstances, provided adequate doses (1.2 mg/kg intravenously) are administered. Unfortunately, it has an intermediate duration of action that could be disadvantageous, compared with succinylcholine, in a patient with an unrecognized difficult airway. Sugammadex may provide a solution. It is an oligosaccharide chelating agent that rapidly reverses the effects of aminosteroid neuromuscular blocking agents, particularly rocuronium. Recovery of over 90% train-of-four responses may be accomplished in less than 120 seconds.[130] Thus, a new paradigm for the "open-globe, full-stomach" scenario may entail rapid-sequence induction with high-dose rocuronium to achieve swift onset of superb intubating conditions, followed by quick termination of neuromuscular blocking effect by sugammadex if one cannot intubate or cannot ventilate.[131] Sugammadex was approved for use in the United States in December 2015.

It was hoped that rapacuronium, with its swift onset, would emerge as a viable alternative to succinylcholine. However, rapacuronium is no longer available in the United States because of its role in triggering intractable bronchospasm in some patients. New ultrashort-acting nondepolarizing alternatives to succinylcholine are currently undergoing clinical investigation in human volunteers.

When confronted with a patient whose airway anatomy or anesthetic history suggests potential difficulties, the anesthesiologist should consult with the ophthalmologist concerning the probability of saving the injured eye. In selected instances, general anesthesia may be avoided by using topical or regional anesthesia. If this approach is not feasible, awake fiberoptic laryngoscopy and intubation may be the safest option, realizing that substantial increases in IOP may occur if the patient gags or coughs. These risks, which can be minimized by thorough topical anesthesia of the airway, assume relative unimportance when balanced against the risk of being unable to ventilate and oxygenate the patient.

Intraocular Surgery

Advances in both anesthesia and in technology now permit a level of controlled intraocular manipulation that was previously not possible (Table 49-5).

Proper control of IOP is crucial for intraocular procedures such as glaucoma drainage surgery, open sky vitrectomy, penetrating keratoplasty (corneal transplantation), and traditional intracapsular cataract extraction. Before scleral incision (when IOP becomes equal to atmospheric pressure), a low-normal IOP is essential because abrupt decompression of a hypertensive eye could result in iris or lens prolapse, vitreous loss, or expulsive choroidal hemorrhage. Available data have not demonstrated a major difference in the rate of complications such as vitreous loss and iris prolapse between local anesthesia and general anesthesia.

Vitrectomy is generally considered to be a low-risk procedure; however, in recent years, both the anesthesiology and ophthalmology literature have reported cases of sudden death during retina surgery. The presumed etiology is venous air embolism from air introduced into the choroid blood flow via a malpositioned infusion cannula.[132] An in vitro study of pars plana vitrectomy has confirmed the capacity for air infusion into the choroidal space, through the vortex veins, and on to the central circulation.[133] The majority of retina surgery has migrated to ambulatory facilities that are not typically capable of effective resuscitation from profound venous air embolism. It is important for anesthesiologists to confirm that vitreoretinal surgeons are aware of this rare phenomenon such that they ascertain the proper position of the infusion cannula prior to and during air infusion throughout vitrectomy.

Maximal pupillary dilation is important for many types of intraocular surgery and can be induced by continuous infusion of epinephrine 1:200,000 in a balanced salt solution, delivered through a small-gauge needle placed in the anterior chamber. Almost simultaneous with its administration, the drug is removed by aspirating it from the anterior chamber. The iris usually dilates immediately on contact with the epinephrine infusion, and drug uptake is presumably limited by the associated intense vasoconstriction of the iris and ciliary body. However, epinephrine may also be potentially absorbed by drainage through the canal of Schlemm into the venous system or by spillover of the infusion into the conjunctival vessels or drainage to the nasal mucosa.

Retinal Detachment Surgery

Surgery to repair retinal detachments involves procedures affecting intraocular volume, frequently using a synthetic silicone band or sponge to produce a localized or encircling scleral indentation (Table 49-5). Furthermore, internal tamponade of the retinal break may be accomplished by injecting an expandable gas such as sulfur hexafluoride into the vitreous. Because of blood gas partition coefficient differences, the administration of nitrous oxide may enhance the internal tamponade effect of the perfluorocarbon intraoperatively, only to be followed by a dramatic drop in IOP and volume on discontinuation of nitrous oxide. The injected bubble, in the presence of concomitant administration of nitrous oxide, can cause a rapid and dramatic rise in IOP, reaching a peak within 20 minutes[46,134] (see earlier section on Intraocular Perfluorocarbons). Because the resultant rise in IOP may compromise retinal circulation, Stinson and Donlon[134] recommended cessation of nitrous oxide administration 15 minutes before gas injection to prevent significant changes in the volume of the intravitreous gas bubble. Furthermore, Wolf et al.[46] stated that if a patient requires anesthesia after intravitreous gas injection, nitrous oxide should be omitted for 5 days after an air injection and for 10 days after sulfur hexafluoride injection. In cases in which perfluoropropane has been injected, the nitrous oxide proscription should be in effect for longer than 70 days. Alternatively, silicone oil, a vitreous substitute, may be injected to achieve internal tamponade of a retinal break. Moreover, it should be pointed out that cervicofacial subcutaneous emphysema and pneumomediastinum have been reported after the injection of pressurized gas during retinal detachment surgery.[135] Although the precise mechanism of injury remains speculative, it was hypothesized that the pressure indicator for the perfluorocarbon gas injection may have malfunctioned.

It should be emphasized that resorption time is not always uniform or predictable. For example, a diabetic 19-year-old woman was injected with sulfur hexafluoride 25 days before subsequent surgery and a diabetic 37-year-old man was injected with perfluoropropane gas 41 days before subsequent surgery. They were given nitrous oxide and developed central retinal artery occlusion and permanent blindness in the affected eye.[136] Because the pressure in the retinal arterial vessels is lower in patients with diabetes, the elderly, and those with atherosclerosis, these patients are likely at higher risk for this devastating complication.[137,138] The international distributors of medical-grade gases, in cooperation with the American distributors and the FDA, have begun to provide warning bracelets for patients who receive intraocular gas injection to alert health professionals to the presence of the bubble and the need to avoid nitrous oxide administration.

A scleral buckle procedure is basically an extraocular circumglobal placement of a band. During globe manipulation, rotation of the globe with traction on the extraocular muscles may elicit the oculocardiac reflex. The anesthesiologist must be vigilant

Table 49-5 Concerns with Various Ocular Procedures

Procedure	Concerns
Strabismus repair	Oculocardiac reflex
	Oculogastric reflex
	Forced duction testing
	Malignant hyperthermia
Intraocular surgery	Proper control of IOP
	Akinesia
	Drug interactions
	Associated systemic disease
Retinal detachment surgery	Nitrous oxide interaction with air, sulfur hexafluoride, or perfluorocarbon gas bubble
	Venous air embolism
	Oculocardiac reflex
	Proper control of IOP

IOP, intraocular pressure.

about potential cardiac dysrhythmias. Intravenous acetazolamide or mannitol to lower IOP may be requested to soften the globe during buckling.

Anesthesiologists are sometimes faced with the unpopular duty of triaging the order of unscheduled cases. Clearly salvage of life takes priority over salvage of limb, but where do nonelective eye operations fit in? A rhegmatogenous retinal detachment is the most common posterior segment emergency. It occurs when a break or tear in the retina allows vitreous fluid to dissect underneath the retina. There are two types: fovea-sparing and fovea-involving. For the former, the macula remains attached, preserving central vision and retaining high likelihood of ultimately achieving excellent visual acuity. In fovea-involving detachments, the macula is separated, so the prognosis for ultimate visual acuity of 20/40 or better is much lower. Although it seems logical that the sooner the retina is reattached, the better the prognosis, clinical evidence suggests that duration of macular detachment has little to no effect on visual outcome so long as the repair is accomplished within about 1 week.[139] It is generally considered safe to delay surgery to the next available elective surgical slot.[139] Fovea-sparing detachments, however, are more urgent, though still not emergent, and can likely be deferred for 1 to 3 days following the detachment without affecting ultimate visual acuity.[140]

There is debate regarding the urgency of removal of an intraocular foreign body. Studies have suggested that surgery within 72 hours reduces the incidence of vision-threatening endophthalmitis. Recent literature challenges this guiding principle, because not a single case of endophthalmitis or other deleterious side effects arose during Operation Iraqi Freedom and Operation Enduring Freedom despite a 21-day median time to foreign body removal.[141]

Strabismus Surgery

Approximately 3% of the population has malalignment of the visual axes, which may be accompanied by diplopia, amblyopia, and loss of stereopsis (Table 49-5). Indeed, strabismus surgery is the most common pediatric ocular operation performed in the United States, and it entails a variety of techniques to weaken an extraocular muscle by moving its insertion on the globe (recession) or to strengthen an extraocular muscle by eliminating a short strip of the tendon or muscle (resection).

Infantile strabismus occurs within the first 6 months of life and is often observed in the neonatal period. Although most patients with strabismus are healthy, normal children, the incidence of strabismus is increased in those with CNS dysfunction such as cerebral palsy and meningomyelocele with hydrocephalus. Moreover, strabismus may be acquired secondary to oculomotor nerve trauma or sensory abnormalities such as cataracts or refractive aberrations.

In addition to the well-known propensity of strabismus surgery to trigger the oculocardiac reflex (previously discussed), strabismus or ptosis patients are thought to have an increased incidence of malignant hyperthermia.[142] This observation is consistent with the impression that people susceptible to malignant hyperthermia often have localized areas of skeletal muscle weakness or other musculoskeletal abnormalities. Although recent studies have challenged this belief, anesthesiologists providing care for eye muscle surgery patients must be cognizant of the theoretically enhanced risk. Other aspects of strabismus surgery of interest to anesthesiologists include succinylcholine-induced interference with the FDT and an increased incidence of postoperative nausea and vomiting.

In formulating a surgical treatment plan for strabismus, ophthalmologists often find the FDT to be exquisitely helpful in differentiating between a paretic muscle and a restrictive force preventing ocular motion. To perform the FDT, the surgeon grasps the sclera of the anesthetized eye with a forceps near the corneal limbus and moves the eye into each field of gaze, concomitantly assessing tissue and elastic properties. This simple test provides valuable clues to the presence and site of mechanical restrictions of the extraocular muscles and is most valuable in patients who have previously undergone strabismus surgery, in those who may have paralysis of one of the extraocular muscles, and in those who have sustained orbital trauma.

France et al.[143] quantitated the magnitude and duration of change of the FDT after succinylcholine administration. They demonstrated that quantification of the force necessary to rotate the globe remained notably increased over control for 15 minutes, even though the rise in IOP and the skeletal muscle paralysis lasted less than 5 minutes. Because succinylcholine interferes with FDT, its use is contraindicated less than 20 minutes before testing. Hence, France et al.[143] suggested performing the FDT on the anesthetized patient while mask inhalation anesthesia is being administered, before intubation of the trachea; after intubation, facilitated by nondepolarizing neuromuscular blocking drugs; or after intubation under moderately deep inhalation anesthesia, unaided by succinylcholine. (As previously discussed, succinylcholine is widely avoided in elective pediatric surgical cases as a result of the FDA warning of rare reports of acute rhabdomyolysis, subsequent hyperkalemia, dysrhythmia, and potential cardiac arrest.)

During surgery, should bradycardia occur, the surgeon is asked to discontinue ocular manipulation, and the patient's ventilatory status and anesthetic depth are quickly assessed. If additional intravenous atropine is indicated, it is not given while the oculocardiac reflex is active in case even more dangerous cardiac dysrhythmias are triggered.

The SGA is gaining popularity for strabismus surgery in the United States, provided the patient is at minimal risk for aspiration. The laryngeal mask can be inserted without the use of muscle relaxants, causes less hemodynamic perturbation, and is associated with less straining and coughing on removal.

Vomiting after eye muscle surgery is common, giving credibility to the existence of the oculogastric reflex. The administration of droperidol, 0.075 mg/kg at induction of anesthesia before manipulation of the eye, has been shown to reduce the incidence of vomiting after strabismus surgery to a clinically acceptable level of approximately 10% without prolonging recovery time.[144] Moreover, a lower dose of droperidol, 0.02 mg/kg intravenously, administered immediately after anesthetic induction in patients with strabismus may decrease both the incidence and severity of nausea and vomiting.[145] Many physicians stopped using droperidol owing to the FDA's "black box" warning about QT-interval prolongation. However, the droperidol doses used for postoperative nausea and vomiting are extremely low and unlikely to be associated with notable cardiovascular events. Indeed, considerable concern has been expressed about the quality and quantity of evidence and the validity of the FDA conclusion.[146]

Prophylactic intravenous administration of a serotonin receptor antagonist such as ondansetron, dolasetron, or granisetron also appears to be efficacious. Combination therapy consisting of one or two antiemetics, each with a different mechanism of action, plus a glucocorticoid such as dexamethasone has been shown to be efficacious and safe in patients at high risk for postoperative nausea and vomiting.[146] Moreover, a total intravenous technique with propofol has also been associated with a low incidence of emesis after strabismus surgery.[147] In addition, avoiding narcotics may be helpful, although a recent paper found no difference in postoperative nausea or vomiting in children who received a remifentanil–sevoflurane mixture versus sevoflurane without the narcotic.[148] One study demonstrates that the nonopioid analgesic ketorolac, in a dose of 0.75 mg/kg intravenously, provides analgesia comparable with that of morphine in pediatric patients with strabismus, but with a much lower incidence of nausea and vomiting in the first 24 hours.[149]

Principles of Laser Therapy

In 1957, in a laboratory at Columbia University, the first design for the laser was born. The invention has revolutionized industry, refined scientific measurements, provided therapy for countless medical and surgical conditions, and inspired 13 Nobel Prizes. The principle is based on the consequences of a photon meeting an electron in an excited state. Sometimes the collision produces a second photon that has the same color and direction as the original. When repeated on a large scale, this process creates an orderly beam of light. The term *laser* was coined to describe this photon-cloning effect, and the acronym signifies light amplified by stimulated emission of radiation.

Laser radiation has many notable properties. Because it is monochromatic, all the photons have the same wavelength, energy, and frequency. It is coherent, with all the photons in phase. Moreover, laser radiation is collimated, so its beam is nondivergent. These properties allow the precision that is associated with laser surgery. The amount of radiant energy (joules) absorbed by tissues is the product of power (watts) multiplied by duration (seconds). Surgical lasers typically are used in either a continuous or a pulsed mode.

The effect that a particular laser beam exerts on tissue depends predominantly on its wavelength and power density. A specific laser's wavelength depends on its lasing medium, which also gives the laser its name. In general, the longer the wavelength, the more strongly absorbed the light. The converse is true; the shorter the wavelength, the more scattered the light. The power of the laser beam is converted to heat at a shallow depth. Coherent light of high-power density excels in cutting or vaporizing tissue. Lower-power densities are used to photocoagulate tissue and promote hemostasis. Of course, another variable that can be manipulated to produce a given effect is the duration of contact between laser beam and tissue. Additional uses of lasers of low-power density include the photoactivation of systemically administered dyes to precisely treat localized disease sites, such as with age-related macular degeneration.

Lasers are used to treat a wide spectrum of eye conditions, including three of the most common causes of visual loss in the United States: diabetic retinopathy, glaucoma, and age-related macular degeneration. The use of lasers expanded to include the rapidly growing field of refractive surgery. Argon, krypton, diode, dye-tuned, neodymium: yttrium-aluminum-garnet (Nd:YAG), and excimer lasers are among those commonly used for ophthalmic surgery. Owing to concerns that indirect exposure to laser energy could cause ocular damage to operating room personnel, staff working with or near the laser wear protective goggles designed to block the particular wavelength of light emitted by the laser in use.

The argon laser emits blue-green light with a wavelength of approximately 488 to 515 nm (approximately 0.5 µm). This laser has low maximum power and is easily transmitted by fiberoptic bundles. Light from the argon laser is strongly absorbed by hemoglobin, melanin, and other pigments, rendering it useful in retinal detachment surgery to photocoagulate or cauterize pigment epithelium and the adjacent neurosensory retina, thus creating an adhesion between the retina and the "wall of the eye" to keep the retina attached. This photocoagulative property of the argon and similar lasers achieves its therapeutic effect in the treatment of diabetic retinopathy by focal and controlled necrosis of a limited amount of ischemic retina. The argon laser is also used with some efficacy to treat the late complications that can develop in the natural history of retinal vein occlusion. Because emissions of the argon laser can penetrate the cornea and lens, causing severe retinal damage, personnel in the vicinity of the argon laser should wear orange protective goggles.

The Nd:YAG, commonly called the *YAG laser*, emits light in the infrared range (wavelength 1,064 nm [1.06 µm]) and is useful in posterior lens capsule surgery. The Nd:YAG laser has high-power density and is efficacious in creating an opening in opacified posterior capsule membranes that develop in approximately one-third of cases after phacoemulsification or other extracapsular cataract surgery. Personnel working in the vicinity of this laser should wear green goggles and realize that their ability to detect cyanosis will be impaired.

An excimer laser (sometimes, and more correctly, called an *exciplex laser*) is a form of high-power, ultraviolet chemical laser frequently used in the delicate refractive surgery commonly referred to as *laser corrective surgery* or *LASIK*. The term *excimer* is short for "excited dimer," and *exciplex* is short for "excited complex." An excimer laser generally uses a combination of inert gas (argon, krypton, or xenon) and a reactive gas (fluorine or chlorine). Under appropriate conditions of electrical stimulation, a pseudomolecule called a *dimer* is generated, which can exist only in an energized state and gives rise to laser light in the ultraviolet range, typically with wavelengths of 125 to 200 nm. The ultraviolet light from an excimer laser is well absorbed by biologic matter and organic compounds. Instead of burning or cutting material, the excimer laser supplies enough energy to disrupt the molecular bonds of surface tissue through ablation. This property allows removal of exceptionally fine layers of surface material with almost no heating or change to neighboring tissue. These lasers are usually operated with a pulse rate of around 100 Hz and a pulse duration of 10 ns, although some may operate as high as 8 kHz and 30 ns.

Age-related macular degeneration is the most common cause of blindness in the elderly and has become alarmingly prevalent. The treatment of the generally more severe wet form of age-related macular degeneration has interestingly progressed over the years from the initial photocoagulation of the neovascular membrane that develops in the central retina or macula. Cauterization obliterates this membrane but can also damage the adjacent healthy macular tissue. The next modality used to treat age-related macular degeneration was the cold laser to photoactivate an intravenously injected drug, verteporfin, which chemically changed on light exposure of 693 nm in the presence of oxygen. By precisely applying the cold laser light to the area of the neovascular membrane, the photoactivated verteporfin produced highly reactive oxygen radicals and "selectively" necrosed the diseased tissue. Because of ill effects on nearby healthy tissue, this approach has been superseded by a more effective, nonlaser treatment with intravitreous injection of monoclonal antibody drugs such as ranibizumab (FDA-approved) or bevacizumab (off-label).

Postoperative Ocular Complications

The incidence of eye injuries associated with nonocular surgery is low. In a study by Roth et al.[150] of 60,965 patients undergoing nonocular surgery from 1988 to 1992, the incidence of eye injury was 0.056% (34 patients). Twenty-one of these 34 patients sustained corneal abrasion, although other injuries included conjunctivitis, blurry vision, red eye, chemical injury, direct ocular trauma, and blindness. Independent risk factors for greater relative risk of ocular injury were protracted surgical procedures, lateral intraoperative positioning, head or neck surgery, general anesthesia, and (for some unknown reason) surgery on a Monday. A specific mechanism of injury could be identified in only 21% of cases. In the ASA Closed Claims Study published in 1992 (which analyzed only cases involving litigation), eye injuries represented merely 3% of all claims, but the serious nature of some of the injuries was reflected in large financial awards.[151] Similar to the findings of Roth et al., the specific mechanism of injury could be ascertained in only a minority of cases. Another Closed Claims Study, published in 2004, examining injuries associated with regional anesthesia, reported that the proportion of regional anesthesia claims linked to eye blocks increased from 2% in the 1980s to 7% in the 1990s.[152] These injuries were typically permanent and related to the anesthesiologist's block technique or patient movement. More than half of the claims resulted in blindness. As sub-Tenon and topical anesthesia for cataract removal became more common, it was thought that a reduction in claims would occur. This has not, in fact, been the case.[153]

Although infrequent and often transient, eye injuries occasionally can result in blindness or more limited but nonetheless permanent visual impairment. Postoperative complications after nonocular surgery include corneal abrasion and minor visual disturbances, chemical injuries, thermal or photic injury, and serious visual disturbances, including blindness. Serious injury may result from such diverse conditions as acute corneal epithelial edema, glycine toxicity and other visual disturbances associated with transurethral resection of the prostate, retinal ischemia, ION, cortical blindness, and acute glaucoma. It appears that certain types of surgery, including complex spinal surgery in the prone position, operations involving extracorporeal circulation, and neck, nasal, or sinus surgery may increase the risk of serious postoperative visual complications.

Corneal Abrasion

Although the most common ocular complication of general anesthesia is corneal abrasion,[154] the incidence varies widely, depending on the perioperative circumstances. In a prospective study, Cucchiara and Black[155] found a 0.17% incidence of corneal abrasion in 4,652 neurosurgical patients whose eyes were protected, whereas Batra and Bali[154] a decade earlier reported a 44% incidence of corneal abrasion when eyes were left unprotected and partly open. A more recent study of over 100,000 nonophthalmologic procedures found an incidence of 0.15%, which decreased to 0.079% following a teaching initiative.[156] A variety of mechanisms can result in corneal abrasion, including damage caused by the anesthetic mask, surgical drapes, and spillage of solutions. During intubation of the trachea, moreover, the end of plastic watch bands or hospital identification cards clipped to the laryngoscopist's vest pocket can injure the cornea. Ocular injury may also occur from loss of pain sensation, obtundation of protective corneal reflexes, and decreased tear production during anesthesia. Therefore, it may be prudent to tape the eyelids closed immediately after induction and during mask ventilation and laryngoscopy. In addition to taping the eyelids closed, applying protective goggles and instilling petroleum-based ointments into the conjunctival sac may provide protection. Disadvantages of ointments include occasional allergic reactions; flammability, which may make their use undesirable during surgery around the face and contraindicated during laser surgery; and blurred vision in the early postoperative period. The blurring and foreign body sensation associated with ointments may actually increase the incidence of postoperative corneal abrasions if they trigger excessive rubbing of the eyes while the patient is still emerging from anesthesia. Even water-based (methylcellulose) ointments may be irritating and cause scleral erythema. It would seem prudent, therefore, to close the eyelids with tape during general anesthesia for procedures away from the head and neck. For certain procedures on the face, ocular occluders or tarsorrhaphy may be indicated. Special attention should also be devoted to frequent checking of the eyes during procedures on a prone patient.

Patients with corneal abrasion usually complain of a foreign body sensation, pain, tearing, and photophobia. Pain is typically exacerbated by blinking and ocular movement. It is wise to consider early ophthalmologic consultation. Treatment typically consists of the prophylactic application of antibiotic ointment and patching the injured eye. Although permanent sequelae are possible, healing usually occurs within 24 hours.

Chemical Injury

Spillage of solutions during skin preparation may result in chemical damage to the eye. The FDA has reported serious corneal damage from eye contact with Hibiclens, a 4% chlorhexidine gluconate solution formulated with a detergent. Again, with meticulous attention to detail, this misadventure is preventable. Treatment consists of liberal bathing of the eye with balanced salt solution to remove the offending agent. After surgery, it may be desirable to have an ophthalmologist examine the eye to document any residual injury or lack thereof.

Photic Injury

Direct or reflected light beams may permanently damage the eye. For patients undergoing nonocular laser surgery, the potential for serious injury to the cornea or retina from certain laser beams requires that the patient's eyes be protected with moist gauze pads and metal shields and that operating room personnel wear protective glasses. These goggles must be appropriately tinted for the specific wavelength they are intended to block. Clear goggles may be worn when working with the carbon dioxide laser, whereas for work with the argon, Nd:YAG, or Nd:YAG-KTP (potassium titanyl phosphate) laser, the goggles must be tinted orange, green, or orange-red, respectively.

Mild Visual Symptoms

After anesthesia, transient mild visual disturbances such as photophobia or diplopia are common. Blurred vision in the early postoperative period may reflect residual effects of petroleum-based ophthalmic ointments or ocular effects of anticholinergic drugs administered in the perioperative period (see Corneal Abrasion).

In contrast, the complaint of postoperative visual loss is rare and is cause for alarm. Several of the following conditions may be associated with visual loss after anesthesia and surgery, and should be included in the differential diagnosis: hemorrhagic retinopathy, retinal ischemia, retinal artery occlusion, ION, cortical blindness, and acute glaucoma.

Hemorrhagic Retinopathy

Retinal hemorrhages that occur in otherwise healthy people secondary to hemodynamic changes associated with turbulent emergence from anesthesia or protracted vomiting are termed *Valsalva retinopathy*. Fortunately, these venous hemorrhages are usually self-limiting and resolve completely in a few days to a few months.

Because no visual changes occur unless the macula is involved, most cases are asymptomatic. However, if bleeding into the optic nerve occurs, resulting in optic atrophy, or if the hemorrhage is massive, permanent visual impairment may ensue. In some instances of massive hemorrhage, vitrectomy may offer some improvement.

Retinal venous hemorrhage has also been described after injections of local anesthetics, steroids, or saline into the lumbar epidural space, and these cases have been summarized by Purdy and Ajimal.[157] The patients all received large injections (≥40 mL) into the epidural space, and they subsequently developed blurry vision or headaches. On funduscopic examination, retinal hemorrhage was consistently observed. Eight of the nine patients described had complete recovery. It is believed that the hemorrhage is produced by rapid epidural injection, which causes a sudden increase in intracranial pressure. This increase in cerebrospinal fluid pressure causes an increase of retinal venous pressure, which may cause retinal hemorrhages. It is possible that obesity, hypertension, coagulopathies, pre-existing elevated cerebrospinal fluid pressure (as seen in pseudotumor cerebri), and such retinal vascular diseases as diabetic retinopathy may be risk factors. Caution is recommended when injecting drugs or fluid into the epidural space; a slow injection rate and using the minimal volume necessary to accomplish the desired objective are strongly recommended.

Retinal bleeding may also originate from the arterial circulation. This bleeding may be associated with extraocular trauma. Funduscopic examination shows cotton–wool exudates, and this condition is known as *Purtscher retinopathy*. Purtscher retinopathy should be ruled out when a trauma patient complains of postanesthetic visual loss. This condition is associated with a poor prognosis, and most patients sustain permanent visual impairment.

Retinal Ischemia

Retinal ischemia or infarction may also result from direct ocular trauma secondary to external pressure exerted by an ill-fitting anesthetic mask, especially in a hypotensive setting, from embolism during cardiac surgery, or from the intraocular injection of a large volume of sulfur hexafluoride or other gases in the presence of high concentrations of nitrous oxide. It may also result from increased ocular venous pressure associated with impaired venous drainage or elevated IOP.

The importance of carefully positioning patients and scrupulously monitoring external pressure on the eye cannot be overemphasized, especially when the patient is in the prone or jackknife position. When the head is dependently positioned, venous pressure may be elevated. If external pressure is applied to the globe from improper head support, perfusion pressure to the eye is likely to be reduced. An episode of systemic hypotension in this setting could further decrease perfusion pressure and thereby decrease intraocular blood flow, resulting in possible retinal ischemia.

It is imperative that a padded or foam headrest be used for procedures done with patients in the prone position. The patient's eyes must be in the opening of this headrest and they must be checked at frequent intervals for pressure. Alternatively, Mayfield tongs can be used. During some spine procedures, a steep head-down position may be used to decrease venous bleeding and enhance surgical exposure. This position, in combination with deliberate hypotension and infusion of large quantities of crystalloid, may increase the risk of compromising the ocular circulation. It seems prudent to avoid combining these three risk factors to any significant degree.

Central retinal arterial occlusion and branch retinal arterial occlusion are important, and frequently preventable, causes of postoperative visual loss. Most case reports follow spinal, nasal, sinus, or neck surgery, as well as coronary artery bypass graft (CABG) surgery. In addition to external pressure on the eye, causes can include emboli from carotid plaques or other sources as well as vasospasm or thrombosis after radical neck surgery complicated by hemorrhage and hypotension and after intranasal injection of α-adrenergic agonists. Several cases have followed intra-arterial injections of corticosteroids or local anesthetics in branches of the external carotid artery, with possible retrograde embolization to the ocular blood supply.[158] Mabry[159] suggested that the mechanism of injury involves positioning the needle intra-arterially to produce retrograde flow into the branches of the ophthalmic artery, as well as the perfusion pressure that must be overcome during the injection. Therefore, when injecting in the nasal and sinus areas, topical vasoconstrictors should be applied to decrease the size of the vascular bed, and a small (25-gauge) needle on a low-volume syringe should be used to minimize injection pressure. Moreover, because some cases have followed injections of corticosteroids combined with other drugs, it is believed that this practice may predispose to formation of drug crystals and therefore should be discouraged.

In cases of central retinal arterial occlusion, signs of eye injury including proptosis, chemosis, hyphema, corneal abrasion, and lid bruising are apparent. Pathognomonic findings on funduscopic examination reveal a pale, edematous retina and a cherry-red spot. Platelet-fibrin, cholesterol, calcific, or crystalloid emboli may be found in narrowed retinal arterioles. Embolic or arteritic causes may be discovered via echocardiogram, carotid ultrasound, and temporal artery biopsy. Computed tomography (CT) and magnetic resonance imaging (MRI) studies are usually negative.

Prevention is much more successful than treatment. It may be possible to apply ocular massage (contraindicated if glaucoma is a possibility) to dislodge an embolus to more peripheral sites, and intravenous acetazolamide and 5% carbon dioxide inhalation have been used to increase retinal blood flow. The prognosis, however, typically is poor, and approximately 50% of patients with central retinal arterial occlusion eventually have optic atrophy.

Ischemic Optic Neuropathy

Ischemic optic neuropathy in the nonsurgical setting is the most common cause of *sudden* visual loss in patients older than 50 years, and it may be either arteritic or nonarteritic. Our discussion is limited to postoperative ION and contrasts the similarities and differences between anterior ION and posterior ION. Because of a perceived increase in the incidence of postoperative visual loss since the mid-1990s, the Committee on Professional Liability of the ASA established the Postoperative Visual Loss Database on July 1, 1999, to better identify associated risk factors so these tragic complications might be prevented in the future.[160] Because the incidence of postoperative vision loss after spine surgery in the prone position is estimated to range from 0.017% to 0.1%, and the condition can occur in healthy individuals of all ages, it would seem prudent to discuss this potential complication preoperatively with the patient during the informed consent process.

Anterior Ischemic Optic Neuropathy

Although the multifactorial pathophysiology of anterior ION has not been completely established, it is believed to involve temporary hypoperfusion or nonperfusion of the vessels supplying the anterior portion of the optic nerve, although intra-axonal edema and disturbed autoregulation to the optic nerve head may also play a role.[161] Coexisting systemic disease, especially involving the cardiovascular system and (to a lesser extent) the endocrine system, is common in patients in whom anterior ION develops. Male gender also strongly predominates. Other risk factors for postoperative anterior ION include CABG and other thoracovascular operations, as well as spinal surgery. Although massive bleeding, anemia, and hypotension are commonly described intraoperative risk factors, a retrospective survey of surgeons who perform spinal fusion surgery disclosed that hypotension and anemia were equally prevalent in patients in whom ION developed and in those in whom it did not.[161] Other possible risk factors are increased IOP or orbital venous pressure. Although emboli may also play a role, anterior ION is not usually caused by emboli because emboli preferentially lodge in the central retinal artery rather than in the short posterior ciliary arteries that supply the anterior optic nerve.

Increased IOP caused by extrinsic compression of the eye decreases retinal blood flow, which can produce both retinal and optic nerve injuries. Moreover, increased IOP can result from large infusions of crystalloid when the head is steeply dependent, as during many spinal operations.[162] Increased orbital venous pressure results in a decreased perfusion pressure gradient to the optic nerve head. Interestingly, one patient who had ischemic optic neuropathy despite perioperative normotension had marked facial edema after surgery of protracted duration.[162] Similarly, a study in cardiac surgery patients revealed that increases in IOP correlated with the degree of hemodilution and the use of crystalloid priming solution.[163] Patients with anterior ION were more likely to have significant weight gain within 24 hours of open heart surgery, again suggesting the role of elevated ocular venous pressure in impeding blood flow to the optic nerve.

According to Roth and Gillesberg,[158] a complex interaction of factors such as ocular venous pressure, hemodilution, hypotension, release of endogenous vasoconstrictors, and individual risk factors such as atherosclerosis and aberrant optic nerve circulation may be implicated in the development of anterior ION. Therefore, specific recommendations for preventative strategies are elusive. Clearly, however, external pressure on the eyes must be meticulously avoided. It also seems prudent to minimize time in the prone position when the head is notably dependent. In patients with pre-existing cardiovascular disease, significant hypertension, or glaucoma, it seems advisable to maintain systemic blood pressure as close to baseline as possible.[158]

Patients with anterior ION typically have painless visual loss that may not be noted until the first postoperative day (or possibly later), an afferent pupillary defect, altitudinal field defects, and optic disc edema or pallor. MRI or CT initially shows enlargement of the optic nerve. However, optic atrophy is detected by MRI later.

The prognosis for anterior ION varies but is often grim. Although there is no recognized treatment for anterior ION Williams et al.[164] reviewed the various therapies that may be instituted. These include intravenous acetazolamide, furosemide, mannitol, and steroids. Maintaining the head-up position could be helpful if increased ocular venous pressure is operative. Surgical optic nerve sheath fenestration or decompression is not only ineffective but may actually be harmful.[165]

Posterior Ischemic Optic Neuropathy

The posterior optic nerve has a less luxuriant blood supply than the anterior optic nerve. Most perioperative ION cases associated with spine surgery occur in the posterior optic nerve where there is poor collateral flow, rendering the nerve vulnerable to prolonged pathophysiologic changes in blood flow. In contrast to anterior ION, relatively few cases have been reported after CABG, and posterior ION appears to be less related to coexisting cardiovascular disease. As with anterior ION, male patients outnumber female patients substantially. Many cases have been associated with surgery involving the neck, nose, sinuses, or spine. In approximately one-third of cases reported, facial edema has been noted.[158] Approximately 11% of cases were associated with cardiopulmonary bypass procedures.

Posterior ION is produced by reduced oxygen delivery to the retrolaminar part of the optic nerve. Compression of the pial vessels (supplied by small collaterals from the ophthalmic artery) or embolic phenomena have been postulated to produce ischemia.[158]

A hypoxic insult in this region results in a slower development of ischemic damage, so a symptom-free period often precedes the loss of vision. In some patients, the onset of symptoms may be delayed several days. Typical findings include an afferent pupillary defect or nonreactive pupil. Disc edema is not a feature of posterior ION because of its retro-orbital position. CT scan in the early postoperative period may reveal enlargement of the intraorbital portion of the optic nerve. Bilateral blindness is more common with posterior ION than with anterior ION, possibly indicating involvement of the optic chiasm. Concomitant disease of the eye or ocular blood supply may be related to posterior ION.[158] Some cases may show partial improvement spontaneously, but often no improvement is noted. Steroids may be considered for treatment. Preventive strategies are as outlined for anterior ION.

A review of the first 6 years of cases submitted to the ASA Postoperative Visual Loss Registry found that spinal surgery patients at greatest risk for ION and visual compromise include those with predisposing patient-specific factors, surgery exceeding 6 hours' duration, and blood loss of more than a liter.[166] In the 83 reported cases, there was no causative evidence of traumatic eye injury from edema or direct pressure on the globe. Mean blood pressures and hematocrits varied widely among those who developed postoperative blindness. However, 34% of cases had the lowest mean arterial blood pressure or systolic blood pressure at least 40% below baseline, and in only 6% of cases were the mean arterial or systolic pressures less than 20% below baseline. The ASA practice advisory for perioperative visual loss associated with spine surgery concludes that there is no established "transfusion threshold" and that deliberate intraoperative hypotension during surgery has not been proven as contributory to postoperative loss of vision.[167] The consultants and specialty society members, however, expressed concern about the use of deliberate hypotension in high-risk patients and recommended that the use of this technique be determined on a case-by-case basis. Further, they recommended that high-risk patients should be positioned so that their heads are level with or higher than the heart, if possible. Patients' heads should be maintained in a neutral forward position, avoiding neck flexion, extension, lateral flexion, or rotation, if at all possible. Finally, consideration should be given to using *staged* spine procedures to avoid excessively protracted periods in the prone position for high-risk patients.

In 2012, the first multicenter study to identify risk factors for ION patients compared with patients without ION after prone spinal fusion surgery using detailed perioperative data was published.[168] Cases with anterior and posterior ION were combined. After multivariate analysis, risk factors for ION after spinal fusion surgery included male sex, obesity, Wilson frame use, prolonged anesthesia duration, greater estimated blood loss, and lower-percent colloid administration. No statistically significant independent effect on ION of older age, hypertension, atherosclerosis, smoking, or diabetes was identified. These findings suggest that the etiology of ION may be more heavily influenced by intraoperative factors than by any known pre-existing comorbidities or vasculopathy. Fully half of the risk factors strongly support the speculation that acute venous congestion of the optic canal is a potential contributor to ION in this setting.[169] Perhaps over time, investigators will be able to determine what role, if any, an inflammatory response, either locally or systemically, plays in the genesis of ION.[169]

Cortical Blindness

Brain injury rostral to the optic nerve may cause cortical blindness. The impairment is produced by damage to the visual path beyond the lateral geniculate nucleus or the visual cortex in the occipital lobe. Similar to anterior ION, cortical blindness is a significant concern in patients undergoing CABG, and systemic disease is often present. Emboli and sustained profound hypotension are common causes. Other events implicated in the pathophysiology include cardiac arrest, hypoxemia, intracranial hypertension, exsanguinating hemorrhage, vascular occlusion, thrombosis, and vasospasm.

Differential diagnostic features include a normal optic disc on fundoscopy and normal pupillary responses. There is, however, loss of optokinetic nystagmus with normal eye motility. CT and MRI are helpful in delineating the extent of brain infarction associated with cortical blindness. Occipital lesions are frequently bilateral, and CT findings typically indicate posterior cerebral artery thrombosis, basilar artery occlusion, posterior cerebral artery branch occlusion, or watershed infarction. Lesions after CABG often include the parieto-occipital area.

Whereas most cases of ION do not improve significantly or completely, visual recovery from cortical blindness in previously healthy patients may be considerable but prolonged. Preventive strategies include maintenance of adequate systemic perfusion pressure and, in cardiac surgery, minimizing manipulation of the aorta, meticulous removal of air and particulate matter during valvular procedures, and use of an arterial line filter in selected patients during bypass.

Acute Glaucoma

Although topical application of mydriatic atropine and scopolamine is contraindicated in patients with known chronic glaucoma, the systemic use of anticholinergics in usual doses is safe for glaucomatous eyes. The atropine–neostigmine combination for reversal of neuromuscular blockade is also considered safe. Topical ophthalmic medications administered to control glaucoma should be continued through the perioperative period.

Acute angle-closure glaucoma typically occurs spontaneously but has been reported, albeit rarely, after both spinal and general anesthesia. Acute angle-closure glaucoma caused by pupillary block is a serious, multifactorial disease. Risk factors include genetic predisposition, shallow anterior chamber depth, increased lens thickness, small corneal diameter, female gender, and advanced age. One study[170] explored possible precipitating events in at-risk patients and found no evidence that the type of anesthetic agent, the duration of surgery, the volume of parenteral fluids, or the intraoperative blood pressure were related to the development of acute angle-closure glaucoma.

Despite its seriousness, acute angle-closure glaucoma may be difficult to recognize.[171] However, physicians should be knowledgeable about this potential complication because diagnostic delay may detrimentally affect visual outcome and cause permanent optic nerve damage. Those patients considered at risk should undergo a preoperative ophthalmic evaluation and perioperative miotic therapy. After surgery, these patients should be scrupulously watched for red eye or a fixed dilated pupil, as well as for complaints of pain and blurred vision. Acute glaucoma is a true emergency, and ophthalmologic consultation should be secured immediately to acutely decrease IOP with systemic and topical therapy. The intense periorbital pain typically described by these patients is an important aid in differential diagnosis.

Postcataract Ptosis

Ptosis after cataract surgery is not uncommon, and multiple factors have been implicated in its etiology.[172,173] These include the presence of a preexisting ptosis, injection of anesthetic solution into the upper lid when performing facial nerve block, injection of local anesthesia through the upper eyelid at the 12 o'clock position, ocular compression or massage, use of the eyelid speculum, placement of a superior rectus bridle suture with traction on the superior rectus–levator complex, creation of a large conjunctival flap, prolonged or tight patching in the postoperative period, and postoperative eyelid edema. Feibel et al.[172] believed that the development of postcataract ptosis is multifactorial and that no single aspect of cataract surgery is the sole contributor. Taylor et al.[173] used MRI immediately after diagnosis of diplopia in four patients who received extraconal block. They found peribulbar edema consistent with direct local anesthetic–induced myotoxicity after presumed inadvertent intramuscular injection. Although local anesthetics are clearly myotoxic, the local anesthetic injection cannot be isolated as the primary factor because postsurgical ptosis is also seen in patients undergoing surgery with general anesthesia.

REFERENCES

1. Eye Diseases Prevalence Research Group. Prevalence of age-related macular degeneration in the United States. *Arch Ophthalmol.* 2004;122:564–572.
2. Teng C, Gurses-Ozden R, Liebmann JM, et al. Effect of a tight necktie on intraocular pressure. *Br J Ophthalmol.* 2003;87:946–948.
3. Stoelting RK. Circulatory changes during direct laryngoscopy and tracheal intubation: influence of duration of laryngoscopy with or without prior lidocaine. *Anesthesiology.* 1977;47:381–384.
4. Duncalf D, Foldes FF. Effect of anesthetic drugs and muscle relaxants on intraocular pressure. In: Smith RB. eds. *Anesthesia in Ophthalmology.* Boston, MA: Little Brown; 1973:21.
5. Garde JF, Aston R, Endler GC, et al. Racial mydriatic response to belladonna preparations. *Anesth Analg.* 1978;57:572–576.
6. Awad H, Santilli S, Ohr M, et al. The effects of steep Trendelenburg positioning on intraocular pressure during robotic radical prostatectomy. *Anesth Analg.* 2009;109: 473–478.

7. Thompson MF, Brock-Utne JG, Bean P, et al. Anaesthesia and intraocular pressure: a comparison of total intravenous anaesthesia using etomidate with conventional inhalational anaesthesia. *Anaesthesia.* 1982;37:758.
8. Yoshikawa K, Murai Y. Effect of ketamine on intraocular pressure in children. *Anesth Analg.* 1971;50:199–202.
9. Corssen G, Hoy JE. A new parenteral anesthetic—CI581: its effect on intraocular pressure. *J Pediatr Ophthalmol.* 1967;4:20.
10. Peuler M, Glass DD, Arens JF. Ketamine and intraocular pressure. *Anesthesiology.* 1975;43:575–578.
11. Ausinsch B, Rayburn RL, Munson ES, et al. Ketamine and intraocular pressure in children. *Anesth Analg.* 1976;55:773–775.
12. Ausinsch B, Graves SA, Munson ES, et al. Intraocular pressure in children during isoflurane and halothane anaesthesia. *Anesthesiology.* 1975;42:167–172.
13. Litwiller RW, Difazio CA, Rushia EL. Pancuronium and intraocular pressure. *Anesthesiology.* 1975;42:750–752.
14. Lincoff HA, Breinin GM, DeVoe AG, et al. Effect of succinylcholine on the extraocular muscles. *Am J Ophthalmol.* 1957;44:440–444.
15. Pandey K, Badolas RP, Kumar S. Time course of intraocular hypertension produced by suxamethonium. *Br J Anaesth.* 1972;44:191–196.
16. Kelly RE, Dinner M, Turner LS, et al. Succinylcholine increases intraocular pressure in the human eye with the extraocular muscles detached. *Anesthesiology.* 1993;79:948–952.
17. Miller RD, Way WL, Hickey RF. Inhibition of succinylcholine-induced increased intraocular pressure by nondepolarizing muscle relaxants. *Anesthesiology.* 1968;29:123.
18. Meyers EF, Krupin T, Johnson M, et al. Failure of nondepolarizing neuromuscular blockers to inhibit succinylcholine-induced increased intraocular pressure: a controlled study. *Anesthesiology.* 1978;48:149–151.
19. Verma RS. "Self-taming" of succinylcholine-induced fasciculations and intraocular pressure. *Anesthesiology.* 1979;50:245–247.
20. Meyers EF, Singer P, Otto A. A controlled study of the effect of succinylcholine self-taming on IOP. *Anesthesiology.* 1980;53:72–74.
21. Stoelting RK. Blood pressure and heart rate changes during short duration laryngoscopy for tracheal intubation: influences of viscous or intravenous lidocaine. *Anesth Analg.* 1978;57:197–199.
22. Smith RB, Babinski M, Leano N. Effect of lidocaine on succinylcholine-induced rise in IOP. *Can Anaesth Soc J.* 1979;26:482–483.
23. Grover VK, Lata K, Sharma S, et al. Efficacy of lignocaine in the suppression of the intraocular pressure response to suxamethonium and tracheal intubation. *Anaesthesia.* 1989;44:22–25.
24. Jampolsky A. Strabismus: Surgical overcorrections. *Highlights Ophthalmol.* 1965;8:78.
25. Dell R, Williams B. Anaesthesia for strabismus surgery: a regional survey. *Br J Anaesth.* 1999;82:761–763.
26. Alexander JP. Reflex disturbances of cardiac rhythm during ophthalmic surgery. *Br J Ophthalmol.* 1975;59:518–524.
27. Berler DK. Oculocardiac reflex. *Am J Ophthalmol.* 1963;12(56):954–959.
28. Mirakur RK, Clarke RS, Dundee JW, et al. Anticholinergic drugs in anaesthesia: a survey of their present position. *Anaesthesia.* 1978;33:133–138.
29. Steward DJ. Anticholinergic premedication for infants and children. *Can Anaesth Soc J.* 1983;30:325–328.
30. Massumi RA, Mason DT, Amsterdam EA, et al. Ventricular fibrillation and tachycardia after intravenous atropine for treatment of bradycardias. *N Engl J Med.* 1972;287:336–338.
31. McGoldrick KE. Transient left bundle branch block during local anesthesia. *Anesthesiol Rev.* 1981;8(6):36.
32. Moonie GT, Rees DI, Elton D. Oculocardiac reflex during strabismus surgery. *Can Anaesth Soc J.* 1964;11:521–632.
33. Phillips TJ, McGuirk SP, Chahat HK, et al. Autonomic cardio-respiratory reflex reactions and super selective ophthalmic arterial chemotherapy for retinoblastoma. *Pediatric Anesth.* 2013;23:940–945.
34. Harris EA. Autonomic cardio-respiratory reflex reactions and super selective ophthalmic arterial chemotherapy for retinoblastoma (letter). *Pediatric Anesth.* 2014;24:230–231.
35. Yamane T, Kaneko A, Mohri M. The technique of ophthalmic arterial infusion therapy for patients with intraocular retinoblastoma. *Int J Clin Oncol.* 2004;9:69–73.
36. Ellis EP, Esterdahl M. Echothiophate iodide therapy in children: effect upon blood cholinesterase levels. *Arch Ophthalmol.* 1967;77:598–601.
37. Meyers EF. Cocaine toxicity during dacryocystorhinostomy. *Arch Ophthalmol.* 1980;98:842–843.
38. Gay GR, Loper KA. Control of cocaine-induced hypertension with labetalol (letter). *Anesth Analg.* 1988;67:92.
39. Brown MM, Brown GC, Spaeth GL. Lack of side effects from topically administered 10% phenylephrine eye drops: a controlled study. *Arch Ophthalmol.* 1980;98:487–489.
40. Jones FL, Eckberg NL. Exacerbation of asthma by timolol. *N Engl J Med.* 1979;301:170.
41. Kim JW, Smith PH. Timolol-induced bradycardia. *Anesth Analg.* 1980;59:301–303.
42. Shavitz SA. Timolol and myasthenia gravis. *JAMA.* 1979;242:1611–1612.
43. Bailey PL. Timolol and postoperative apnea in neonates and young infants. *Anesthesiology.* 1984;61:622.
44. Vinker S, Kaiserman I, Waitman DA, et al. Prescription of ocular beta-blockers in patients with obstructive pulmonary disease: does a central electronic medical record make a difference? *Clin Drug Investig.* 2006;26:495–500.
45. Lee EJK. Use of nitrous oxide causing severe visual loss 37 days after retinal surgery. *Br J Anaesth.* 2004;93:464–464.
46. Wolf GL, Capriano C, Hartung J. Effects of nitrous oxide on gas bubble volume in the anterior chamber. *Arch Ophthalmol.* 1985;103:418–419.
47. Marcus EN, Gayer S, Anderson DR. Medical evaluation of patients before ocular surgery (editorial). *Am J Ophthalmol.* 2003;136:338–339.
48. Schein OD, Katz J, Bass EB, et al. The value of routine preoperative medical testing before cataract surgery. *N Engl J Med.* 2000;342:168–175.
49. Chen CL, Lin GA, Bardash NT, et al. Preoperative medical testing in Medicare patients undergoing cataract surgery. *N Engl J Med.* 2015; 372;16:1530–1538.
50. Charles S, Rosenfeld PJ, Gayer S. Medical consequences of stopping anticoagulants prior to intraocular surgery or intravitreal injections. *Retina.* 2007; 27(7):813–815.
51. Feitl ME, Krupin T. Retrobulbar anesthesia. *Ophthalmol Clin North Am.* 1990;3:83.
52. Katz J, Feldman MA, Bass EB, et al. Risks and benefits of anticoagulant and antiplatelet medication use before cataract surgery. *Ophthalmology.* 2003;110: 1784–1788.
53. Jamula E, Anderson J, Douketis JD. Safety of continuing warfarin therapy during cataract surgery: a systematic review and meta-analysis. *Thomb Res.* 2009;124:292–299.
54. Douketis JD, Berger PB, Dunn AS, et al. The perioperative management of antithrombotic therapy: American College of Chest Physicians Evidence-Based Clinical Practice Guidelines (8th ed). *Chest.* 2008;133(6 suppl):299S–339S.
55. Gertein NS, Schulman WH, Petersen TR, et al. Should more patients continue aspirin therapy perioperatively? Clinical impact on aspirin withdrawal syndrome. *Ann Surg.* 2012;255:811–819.
56. Baron TH, Kamath PS, McBane RD. Management of antithrombotic therapy in patients undergoing invasive procedures. *N Engl J Med.* 2013;368:2113–2124.
57. McClellan AJ, Flynn HW, Smiddy, WE, Gayer S. The use of perioperative antithrombotic agents in posterior segment ocular surgery. *Am J Ophthalmol.* 2014;158:858–859.
58. McClellan AJ, Flynn HW, Gayer S. A novel issue for vitreoretinal surgeons. *Retina.* 2016;36:245–246.
59. Kallio H, Paloheimo M, Maunuksela E. Haemorrhage and risk factors associated with retrobulbar/peribulbar block: a prospective study in 1383 patients. *Br J Anaesth.* 2000; 85(5):708–711.
60. American Society of Anesthesiologists Committee on Standards and Practice Parameters. Practice alert for the perioperative management of patients with coronary artery stents: a report by the American Society of Anesthesiologists Committee on Standards and Practice Parameters. *Anesthesiology.* 2009;110: 22–23.
61. Hawn M, Graham L, Richman J, et al. Risk of major adverse cardiac events following noncardiac surgery in patients with coronary stents. *JAMA.* 2013; 310(14):1462–1472.
62. Bayes J. A survey of ophthalmic anesthetists on managing pacemakers and implanted cardiac defibrillators. *Anesth Analg.* 2006;103:1615–1616.
63. Stoller GL. Ophthalmic surgery and the implantable cardioverter defibrillator. *Arch Ophthalmol.* 2006;124:123–125.
64. Bhananker SM, Posner KL, Cheney FW, et al. Injury and liability associated with monitored anesthesia care: a closed claims analysis. *Anesthesiology.* 2006; 104:228–234.
65. Tao JP. Sneezing reflex associated with intravenous sedation and periocular anesthetic injection. *Am J Ophthalmol.* 2009;147(1):183–184.
66. Gayer S. Key components of risk associated with ophthalmic anesthesia. *Anesthesiology.* 2006;105:859.
67. McGoldrick KE. Ocular pathology and systemic diseases. In: McGoldrick KE, ed. *Anesthetic Implications: Anesthesia for Ophthalmic and Otolaryngologic Surgery.* Philadelphia, PA: WB Saunders; 1992:210.
68. Leaming DV. Practice styles and preferences of ASCRS members: 2002 survey. *J Cataract Refract Surg.* 2003;29:1412–1420.
69. Guise PA. Sub-Tenon anesthesia: a prospective study of 6000 blocks. *Anesthesiology.* 2003;98:964–968.
70. Gayer S, Flynn HW Jr. Sub-Tenon's injection for local anesthesia in posterior segment surgery (discussion). *Ophthalmology.* 2000;107:41–46.
71. Universal protocol for preventing wrong site, wrong procedure, wrong person surgery. Joint Commission on Accreditation of Healthcare Organizations website. http://www.jointcommission.org/standards_information/up.aspx. Accessed December 16, 2015.
72. Wainwright AC. Positive pressure ventilation and the laryngeal mask airway in ophthalmic anaesthesia. *Br J Anaesth.* 1995;75:249–250.
73. Lamb K, James MF, Janicki PK. The laryngeal mask airway for intraocular surgery: effects on intraocular pressure and stress responses. *Br J Anaesth.* 1992;69:143–147.
74. Thomson KD. The effect of the laryngeal mask airway on coughing after eye surgery under general anesthesia. *Ophthalmic Surg.* 1992;23:630–631.

75. Knapp H. On cocaine and its use in ophthalmic and general surgery. *Arch Ophthalmol.* 1884;13:402.
76. Atkinson WS. Retrobulbar injection of anesthetic within the muscular cone. *Arch Ophthalmol.* 1936;16:494.
77. Gayer S. Ophthalmic anesthesia: More than meets the eye. In: Schwartz AJ, ed. *American Society of Anesthesiologists Refresher Courses in Anesthesiology.* Philadelphia, PA: Lippincott Williams & Wilkins; 2006:55.
78. Gayer S, Kumar CM. Ophthalmic regional anesthesia techniques. *Minerva Anestesiol.* 2008;74:23–33.
79. Korneef L. The architecture of the musculofibrous apparatus in the human orbit. *Acta Morphol Neerl Scand.* 1977;15:35–64.
80. Ripart J, Lefrant J, de la Coussaye J, et al. Peribulbar versus retrobulbar anesthesia for ophthalmic surgery. *Anesthesiology.* 2001;94:56–62.
81. Carneiro HM, Tiexeira KI, de Avila MP, et al. Comparison of needle path, anesthetic dispersion, and quality of anesthesia in retrobulbar and peribulbar blocks. *Reg Anesth Pain Med.* 2016;41(1):37–42.
82. Capó H, Roth E, Johnson T, et al. Vertical strabismus after cataract surgery. *Ophthalmology.* 1996;103:918–921.
83. Ripart J, Lefrant J, Lalourcey L, et al. Medial canthus (caruncle) single injection periocular anesthesia. *Anesth Analg.* 1996;83:1234–1238.
84. Katsev DA, Drews RC, Rose BT. An anatomic study of retrobulbar needle path length. *Ophthalmology.* 1989;96:1221–1224.
85. Waller SG, Taboada J, O'Connor P. Retrobulbar anesthesia risk: do sharp needles really perforate the eye more easily than blunt needles? *Ophthalmology.* 1993;100:506–510.
86. Unsold R, Stanley JA, DeGroot J. The CT topography of retrobulbar anesthesia. *Graefes Arch Clin Exp Ophthalmol.* 1981;217:125–136.
87. Vohra SB. A review of the directions of gaze during intraocular anesthetic blocks. *Ophthal Surg Lasers Imag.* 2012;43:162–168.
88. Gayer S, Denham D, Alarakhia K, et al. Ocular decompression devices: liquid mercury balloon versus the tungsten powder balloon. *Am J Ophthalmol.* 2006;142:500–501.
89. Birch A, Evans M, Redembo E. The ultrasonic localization of retrobulbar needles during retrobulbar block. *Ophthalmology.* 1995;102:824–826.
90. Grizzard WS, Kirk NM, Pavan PR, et al. Perforating ocular injuries caused by anesthesia personnel. *Ophthalmology.* 1991;98:1011–1016.
91. Miller-Meeks MJ, Bergstrom T, Karp KO. Prevalent attitudes regarding residency training in ocular anesthesia. *Ophthalmology.* 1994;101:1353–1356.
92. Bayes J, Zheng H, Rosow CE. Early use of eyeglasses for myopia predicts long axial length of the eye. *Anesth Analg.* 2010;110:119–121.
93. Gayer S. Ocular ultrasound guided anesthesia. In: Singh AD, Hayden BC, eds. *Ophthalmic Ultrasonography.* Philadelphia, PA: Elsevier; 2012:195–200.
94. Palte HD, Gayer S, Arrieta E, et al. Are ultrasound-guided ophthalmic blocks injurious to the eye? A comparative rabbit model study of two ultrasound devices evaluating intraorbital thermal and structural changes. *Anesth Analg.* 2012;115(1):194–201.
95. Chin YC, Kumar CM. Brainstem anesthesia revisited: mechanism, presentation and management. *Trends Anesth Crit Care.* 2013;3:252–256.
96. Nicoll JM, Acharya PA, Ahlen K, et al. Central nervous system complications after 6000 retrobulbar blocks. *Anesth Analg.* 1987;66:1298–1302.
97. Swan KC. New drugs and techniques for ocular anesthesia. *Trans Am Acad Ophthalmol Otolaryngol.* 1956;60:368–375.
98. Gayer S, Cass GD. Sub-Tenon techniques should be one option among many. *Anesthesiology.* 2004;100:196.
99. Niemi-Murola L, Krootila K, Kivisaari R, et al. Localization of local anesthetic solution by magnetic resonance imaging. *Ophthalmology.* 2004;111:342–347.
100. Frieman BJ, Friedberg MA. Globe perforation associated with sub-Tenon's anesthesia. *J Ophthalmol.* 2001;131:520–521.
101. Ruschen H, Bremner FD, Carr C. Complications after sub-Tenon's eye block. *Anesth Analg.* 2003;96:273–277.
102. Ripart J, Metge L, Prat-Pradal D, et al. Medial canthus single-injection episcleral (sub-Tenon) anesthesia: computed tomography imaging. *Anesth Analg.* 1998;87:42.
103. Allman KG, Theron AD, Byles DB. A new technique of incisionless, minimally invasive sub-Tenon's anaesthesia. *Anaesthesia.* 2008;63(7):782–783.
104. Quantock C, Goswami T. Death potentially secondary to sub-Tenon's block. *Anaesthesia.* 2007;62:175–177.
105. Palte HD, Gayer S. Death after a sub-Tenon's block. *Anaesthesia.* 2007;62:531.
106. Bardocci A, Lofoco G, Perdicaro S, et al. Lidocaine 2% gel versus lidocaine 4% unpreserved drops for topical anesthesia in cataract surgery: a randomized controlled trial. *Ophthalmology.* 2003;110:144.
107. Shugar JK. Use of epinephrine for IFIS prophylaxis. *J Cataract Refract Surg.* 2006;32:1074–1075.
108. Bell CM, Hatch WV, Fischer HD, et al. Association between tamsulosin and serious ophthalmic adverse events in older man following cataract surgery. *JAMA.* 2009;301(19):1991–1996.
109. Jaichandran VV, Raman R, Laxmi G, et al. Local anesthetic agents for vitreoretinal surgery. *Ophthalmology.* 2015;120:1033.
110. Zhang C, Phamonvaechavan P, Rajan A, et al. Concentration-dependent bupivacaine myotoxicity in rabbit extraocular muscle. *J AAPOS.* 2010;14:323–327.
111. Borazan M, Karalezli A, Oto S, et al. Comparison of bupivacaine 0.5% and lidocaine 2% mixture with levobupivacaine 0.75% and ropivacaine 1% in peribulbar anaesthesia for cataract surgery with phacoemulsification. *Acta Ophthal Scand.* 2007;85:844–847.
112. Uy H, de Jesus AA, Paray AA, et al. Ropivacaine-lidocaine versus bupivacaine-lidocaine for retrobulbar anesthesia in cataract surgery. *J Cataract Refract Surg.* 2002;28:1023–1026.
113. Netland PA, Harris A. Color Doppler ultrasound measurements after topical and retrobulbar epinephrine in primate eyes. *Invest Ophthalmol Vis Sci.* 1997;38:2655–2661.
114. Adams L. Adjuvants to local anaesthesia in ophthalmic surgery. *Br J Ophthalmol.* 2011;95(10):1345–1349.
115. Brown SM, Coats DK, Collins ML, et al. Second cluster of strabismus cases after periocular anesthesia without hyaluronidase. *J Cataract Refract Surg.* 2001;27:1872–1875.
116. Hamada S, Devys JM, Xuan TH, et al. Role of hyaluronidase in diplopia after peribulbar anesthesia for cataract surgery. *Ophthalmology.* 2005;112(5):879–882.
117. Jay WM, Aziz MZ, Green K. Effect of intraocular pressure reducer on ocular and optic nerve blood flow in phakic rabbit eyes. *Acta Ophthalmol.* 1986;64:52–57.
118. Adatia FA, Munro M, Jivraj I, et al. Documenting the subjective patient experience of first versus second cataract surgery. *J Cataract Refract Surg.* 2015;41:116–121.
119. Downs JB. Has oxygen administration delayed appropriate respiratory care? Fallacies regarding oxygen therapy. *Respir Care.* 2003;48:611.
120. Mehta SP, Bhananker SM, Posner KL, et al. Operating room fires: a closed claims analysis. *Anesthesiology.* 2013;118:1133–1139.
121. Hug CC. MAC should stand for maximum anesthesia caution, not minimal anesthesiology care (editorial). *Anesthesiology.* 2006;104:221–223.
122. Norregaard JC, Schein OD, Bellan L, et al. International variation in anesthesia care during cataract surgery: results from the International Cataract Surgery Outcomes Study. *Arch Ophthalmol.* 1997;115:1304–1308.
123. Eichel R, Goldberg I. Anaesthesia techniques for cataract surgery: a survey of delegates to the Congress of the International Council of Ophthalmology, 2002. *Clin Experiment Ophthalmol.* 2005;33:469–472.
124. Rosenfeld SI, Litinsky SM, Snyder DA, et al. Effectiveness of monitored anesthesia care in cataract surgery. *Ophthalmology.* 1999;106:1256–1260.
125. Fung D, Cohen MM, Stewart S, et al. What determines patient satisfaction with cataract care under topical local anesthesia and monitored sedation in a community hospital setting? *Anesth Analg.* 2005;100:1644–1650.
126. Gayer S. Rethinking anesthesia strategies for patients with traumatic eye injuries: alternatives to general anesthesia. *Curr Anesth Crit Care.* 2006;17:191.
127. Scott IU, McCabe CM, Flynn HW Jr, et al. Local anesthesia with intravenous sedation for surgical repair of selected open globe injuries. *Am J Ophthalmol.* 2002;134:707–711.
128. Boscia F, La Tegola MG, Columbo G, et al. Combined topical anesthesia and sedation for open-globe injuries in selected patients. *Ophthalmology.* 2003;110:1555–1559.
129. McGoldrick KE. The open globe: Is an alternative to succinylcholine necessary? (editorial). *J Clin Anesth.* 1993;5:1–4.
130. de Boer H, Driessen JJ, Marcus MA, et al. Reversal of rocuronium-induced (1.2 mg/kg) neuromuscular block by sugammadex: a multicenter dose-finding and safety study. *Anesthesiology.* 2007;107:239–244.
131. Kopman AF. Sugammadex: A revolutionary approach to neuromuscular antagonism (editorial). *Anesthesiology.* 2006;104:631–633.
132. Ledowski T, Kiese F, Silke J, et al. Possible air embolism during eye surgery. *Anesth Analg.* 2005;100:1651–1652.
133. Morris R, Sapp M, Oltmanns M, et al. Presumed air by vitrectomy embolization (PAVE). *Br J Ophthalmol.* 2014;98:765–768.
134. Stinson TW, Donlon JV. Interaction of SF6 and air with nitrous oxide. *Anesthesiology.* 1979;51:S16.
135. Colson JD. Cervicofacial subcutaneous emphysema and pneumomediastinum after retinal detachment surgery: just another monitored anesthesia eye case. *J Clin Anesth.* 2011;23:410.
136. Seaberg RR, Freeman WR, Goldbaum MH, et al. Permanent postoperative vision loss associated with expansion of intraocular gas in the presence of a nitrous oxide-containing anesthetic. *Anesthesiology.* 2002;97:1309–1310.
137. Dallinger S, Findl O, Strenn K, et al. Age dependence of choroidal blood flow. *J Am Geriatr Soc.* 1998;46:484–487.
138. Recchia FM, Brown GC. Systemic disorders associated with retinal vascular occlusion. *Curr Opin Ophthalmol.* 2000;11:462–467.
139. Wykoff CC, Flynn HW, Scott IU. What is the optimal timing for rhegmatogenous retinal detachment repair? *JAMA Ophthalmol.* 2013;131(11):1399–1400.
140. Wykoff CC, Smiddy WE, Mathen T, et al. Fovea-sparing retinal detachments: time to surgery and visual outcomes. *Am J Ophthalmol.* 2010;150:205–210.
141. Colyer MH, Weber ED, Weichel ED, et al. Delayed intraocular foreign body removal without endophthalmitis during Operations Iraqi Freedom and Enduring Freedom. *Ophthalmology.* 2007;114(8):1439–1447.
142. Li G, Brady JE, Rosenberg H, et al. Excess comorbidities associated with malignant hyperthermia diagnosis in pediatric hospital discharge records. *Pediatr Anesth.* 2011;21:958–963.

143. France NK, France TD, Wordburn JD Jr, et al. Succinylcholine alteration of the forced duction test. *Ophthalmology*. 1980;87:1282–1287.
144. Lerman MD, Eustis S, Smith DR. Effect of droperidol pretreatment on postanesthetic vomiting in children undergoing strabismus surgery. *Anesthesiology*. 1986;65:322–325.
145. Brown RE, James DG, Weaver RG, et al. Low-dose droperidol versus standard-dose droperidol for prevention of postoperative vomiting after pediatric strabismus surgery. *J Clin Anesth*. 1991;3:306–309.
146. Gan TJ, Meyer TA, Apfel CC, et al. Society for Ambulatory Anesthesia guidelines for the management of postoperative nausea and vomiting. *Anesth Analg*. 2007;105:1615–1628.
147. Watcha MF, Simeon RM, White PF, et al. Effect of propofol on the incidence of postoperative vomiting after strabismus surgery in pediatric outpatients. *Anesthesiology*. 1991;75:204–209.
148. Oh AY, Kim JH, Hwang JW, et al. Incidence of postoperative nausea and vomiting after pediatric strabismus surgery with sevoflurane or remifentanil–sevoflurane. *Br J Anaesth*. 2010;104:756–760.
149. Munro HM, Riegger LQ, Reynolds PI, et al. Comparison of the analgesic and emetic properties of ketorolac and morphine for paediatric outpatient strabismus surgery. *Br J Anaesth*. 1994;72:624–628.
150. Roth S, Thisted RA, Erickson JP, et al. Eye injuries after nonocular surgery: a study of 60,965 anesthetics from 1988–1992. *Anesthesiology*. 1996;85:1020–1027.
151. Gild WA, Posner KL, Caplan RA, et al. Eye injuries associated with anesthesia. *Anesthesiology*. 1992;76:204–208.
152. Lee LA, Posner KL, Domino KB, et al. Injuries associated with regional anesthesia in the 1980s and 1990s: a closed claims analysis. *Anesthesiology*. 2004;101:143–152.
153. Szypula K, Ashpole KJ, Bogod D, et al. Litigation related to regional anesthesia: an analysis of claims against the NHS in England 1995–2007. *Anaesthesia*. 2010;65:443–452.
154. Batra YK, Bali M. Corneal abrasions during general anesthesia. *Anesth Analg*. 1977;56:363–365.
155. Cucchiara R, Black S. Corneal abrasion during anesthesia and surgery. *Anesthesiology*. 1988;69:978–979.
156. Martin DP, Weingarten TN, Gunn PW, et al. Performance improvement system and perioperative corneal injuries. *Anesthesiology*. 2009;111:320–326.
157. Purdy EP, Ajimal GS. Vision loss after lumbar epidural steroid injection. *Anesth Analg*. 1988;86:119–122.
158. Roth S, Gillesberg I. Injuries to the visual system and other sense organs. In: Benumof JL, Saidman LJ, eds. *Anesthesia and Perioperative Complications*. 2nd ed. St. Louis, MO: Mosby; 1999:377.
159. Mabry RL. Visual loss after intranasal corticosteroid injection. *Arch Otolaryngol*. 1981;107:484–486.
160. Lee LA. Postoperative visual loss data gathered and analyzed. *ASA Newsl*. 2000;64:25.
161. Myers MA, Hamilton SR, Bogosian AJ, et al. Visual loss as a complication of spinal surgery. *Spine*. 1997;22:1325–1329.
162. Dilger JA, Tetzlaff JE, Bell GR, et al. Ischemic optic neuropathy after spinal fusion. *Can J Anaesth*. 1998;45:63–66.
163. Shapira OM, Kimmel WA, Lindsey PS, et al. Anterior ischemic optic neuropathy after open heart operations. *Ann Thorac Surg*. 1996;61:660–666.
164. Williams EL, Hart WM, Tempelhoff R. Postoperative ischemic optic neuropathy. *Anesth Analg*. 1995;80:1018–1029.
165. The Ischemic Optic Neuropathy Decompression Trial Research Group. Optic nerve decompression surgery is not effective and may be harmful. *JAMA*. 1995;273:625.
166. Lee LA, Roth S, Posner KL, et al. The American Society of Anesthesiologists Postoperative Visual Loss Registry: analysis of 93 spine surgery cases with postoperative visual loss. *Anesthesiology*. 2006;105:652–659.
167. American Society of Anesthesiologists Task Force on Perioperative Visual Loss. Practice advisory for perioperative visual loss associated with spine surgery: an updated report by the American Society of Anesthesiologists Task Force on Perioperative Visual Loss. *Anesthesiology*. 2012;116:274–285.
168. The Postoperative Visual Loss Study Group. Risk factors associated with ischemic optic neuropathy after spinal fusion surgery. *Anesthesiology*. 2012;116:15–24.
169. Warner M. Cracking open the door on perioperative visual loss (editorial). *Anesthesiology*. 2012;116:1–2.
170. Drance SM. Angle-closure glaucoma among Canadian Eskimos. *Can J Ophthalmol*. 1973;8:252–254.
171. Gayer S. Prone to blindness: Answers to postoperative visual loss. *Anesth Analg*. 2010;112:11–12.
172. Feibel RM, Custer PL, Gordon MO. Postcataract ptosis: a randomized, double-masked comparison of peribulbar and retrobulbar anesthesia. *Ophthalmology*. 1993;100:660–665.
173. Taylor G, Devys JM, Heran F, et al. Early exploration of diplopia with magnetic resonance imaging after peribulbar anaesthesia. *Br J Anaesth*. 2004;92:899–901.

50 The Renal System and Anesthesia for Urologic Surgery

MARK STAFFORD-SMITH • AARON SANDLER • JAMIE R. PRIVRATSKY • CATHERINE KUHN

Introduction and Context
Renal Anatomy and Physiology
    Gross Anatomy
    Glomerular Filtration
    Clinical Assessment of the Kidney
Perioperative Nephrology
    Pathophysiology
    Electrolyte Disorders
    Acid–Base Disorders
    Acute Kidney Conditions
    Chronic Kidney Disease
    High Renal Risk Surgical Procedures
Nephrectomy
    Preoperative Considerations
    Intraoperative Considerations
    Postoperative Considerations
    Specific Procedures
Cystectomy and Other Major Bladder Surgeries
    Preoperative Considerations
    Intraoperative Considerations
    Postoperative Considerations
    Specific Procedures
Prostatectomy
    Preoperative Considerations
    Intraoperative Considerations
    Postoperative Considerations
    Specific Procedures
Transurethral Surveillance and Resection Procedures
    Preoperative Considerations
    Intraoperative Considerations
    Postoperative Considerations
    Specific Procedures
Therapies for Urolithiasis
    Preoperative Considerations
    Intraoperative Considerations
    Postoperative Considerations
    Specific Procedures
Urogynecology and Pregnancy-related Urologic Procedures
    Impotence Surgery and Medication
    Pediatric Surgical Urologic Disorders
    Nephrectomy and Adrenalectomy
    Reconstructive Urologic Procedures
Urologic Surgical Emergencies
    Testicular Torsion
    Fournier Gangrene
    Emergency Treatment of Nephrolithiasis

KEY POINTS

1. Renal filtration and reabsorption are susceptible to alterations by surgical illness and anesthesia. Autoregulation of renal blood flow (RBF) is effective over a wide range of mean arterial pressures (50 to 150 mmHg). Autoregulation of urine flow does not occur, but a linear relationship between mean arterial pressure above 50 mmHg and urine output is observed.
2. Renal medullary blood flow is low (2% of total RBF) but central to the kidneys' ability to concentrate urine. During periods of reduced renal perfusion, the metabolically active medullary thick ascending limb may be especially vulnerable to ischemic injury.
3. The physiologic response to surgical stress invokes intrinsic mechanisms for sodium and water conservation. Renal cortical vasoconstriction causes a shift in perfusion toward juxtamedullary nephrons, a decrease in glomerular filtration rate, and retention of salt and water result.
4. The stress response may induce a decrease in RBF and glomerular filtration rate, causing afferent arteriolar vasoconstriction. If this situation is not reversed, ischemic damage to the kidney may result in acute renal failure (ARF).
5. Anesthetic-induced reductions in RBF have been described for many agents but are usually clinically insignificant and reversible. Likewise, anesthetic agents have not been shown to interfere with the renal response to physiologic stress.
6. Isolated ARF carries a mortality of up to 80% in surgical patients, with acute tubular necrosis being the cause of ARF in most of these patients.
7. Surgical patients with non–dialysis-dependent chronic kidney disease are at higher risk of developing end-stage renal disease. The single most reliable predictor of new postoperative need for dialysis is preoperative renal insufficiency.
8. Overall, there are no conclusive comparative studies demonstrating superior renal protection or improved renal outcome with general versus regional anesthesia.
9. Maintaining adequate intravascular volume and hemodynamic stability with aggressive management of kidney hypoperfusion is a basic principle of anesthetic care to prevent acute kidney injury.
10. Urologic patients are often elderly, have numerous comorbidities, and require critical evaluation prior to any urologic procedure.

11. Combining epidural with general anesthetic techniques for some major urologic surgeries may offer advantages for accelerated recovery, improved analgesia, and even better outcomes, but these techniques must be conducted with respect for other perioperative issues, including thromboprophylaxis for prevention of deep venous thrombosis.
12. Watchful waiting, minimally invasive principles, and technologic innovation (e.g., laparoscopy, robotics) have changed the favored approach to many kidney, bladder, and prostate disorders, in some cases reducing the number of high-risk surgeries, in others creating other safer and less morbid alternate treatments.
13. Absorption of irrigating solution related most often to transurethral prostate or bladder tumor resections can cause "TUR syndrome," a condition that while becoming less common has the potential to be serious and even life-threatening during the several hours following surgery. Knowledge of specific concerns relevant to the different irrigating solutions, vigilance of the anesthesiologist to factors that minimize absorption, recognition of signs and symptoms, and appropriate treatment, are key to favorable outcomes with this condition.

Introduction and Context

The kidney plays a central role in implementing and controlling a variety of homeostatic functions; these include tight control of extracellular fluid volume and composition and efficient excretion of uremic toxins in the urine. Acute kidney injury (AKI) disturbs such functions and can occur as a result of systemic inflammation, nephrotoxin exposure, or prolonged reduction in renal oxygen delivery due to surgical or medical disease; practically speaking, several factors are often identified. The first part of this chapter reviews renal physiology and pathophysiologic states as they relate to anesthetic practice and then addresses strategies to recognize and manage patients at risk for AKI and renal failure. The second part describes current urologic procedures and their attendant anesthetic management issues.

Renal Anatomy and Physiology

Gross Anatomy

The two normal *kidneys* are reddish-brown organs and are ovoid in outline, but the medial margin is deeply indented and concave at its middle, where a wide, vertical cleft (the hilus) transmits items entering and leaving the kidney (Fig. 50-1). The *hilus* lies at approximately the level of the first lumbar vertebra. The kidneys lie in the paravertebral gutters, behind the peritoneum, with the right kidney resting slightly lower than the left one owing to the presence of the liver. At its upper end, the ureter is dilated to give rise to the *renal pelvis*, which passes through the hilus into the kidney proper. There it is continuous with several short funnel-like tubes (calyces) that unite it with the renal parenchyma. The renal blood vessels lie anterior to the pelvis of the kidney, but some branches may pass posteriorly. Renal pain sensation is conveyed back to spinal cord segments T10 through L1 by sympathetic fibers. Sympathetic innervation is supplied by preganglionic fibers from T8 to L1. The vagus nerve provides parasympathetic innervation to the kidney, and the S2 to S4 spinal segments supply the ureters.

Each kidney is enclosed in a thick, fibrous capsule, itself surrounded by a fatty capsule that fills the space inside a loosely applied renal (Gerota) fascia. The developing kidney is first formed in the pelvis and then ascends to its final position on the posterior abdominal wall. During its ascent, the kidney receives blood supply from several successive sources, such that an accessory renal artery from the aorta may be found entering the lower pole of the kidney. When first formed, the rudimentary kidneys are close together and may fuse to give rise to a horseshoe kidney. This organ is unable to ascend, "held in place" by the inferior mesenteric artery, and thus when present it remains forever a pelvic organ.

The *bladder* is located in the retropubic space and receives its innervation from sympathetic nerves originating from T11 to L2, which conduct pain, touch, and temperature sensations, whereas bladder stretch sensation is transmitted via parasympathetic fibers from segments S2 to S4. Parasympathetics also provide the bladder with most of its motor innervation.

The *prostate, penile urethra*, and *penis* also receive sympathetic and parasympathetic fibers from the T11 to L2 and S2 to S4 segments, respectively. The pudendal nerve provides pain sensation to the penis via the dorsal nerve of the penis. Sensory innervation of the *scrotum* is via cutaneous nerves, which project to lumbosacral segments, whereas testicular sensation is conducted to lower thoracic and upper lumbar segments.

Ultrastructure

Inspection of the cut surface of the kidney reveals the paler *cortex*, adjacent to the capsule, and the darker, conical pyramids of the renal *medulla* (Fig. 50-1). The pyramids are radially striated and are covered with cortex, extending into the kidney as the renal columns. *Collecting tubules* from each lobe of the kidney (pyramid and its covering of cortex) discharge urine into the calyceal system via renal papillae at the entrance of each pyramid into the calyx proper. These collecting tubules originate deep within the radial striations (medullary rays) of the kidney and convey urine formed in the structural units of the kidneys, the *nephrons*. The parenchyma of each kidney contains approximately 1×10^6 tightly packed nephrons, each one consisting of a tuft of capillaries (the *glomerulus*) invaginated into the blind, expanded end (glomerular corpuscle) of a long tubule that leaves the renal corpuscle to form the proximal convoluted tubule in the cortex. This leads into the straight tubule, which loops down into the medullary pyramid (*loop of Henle*) and hence back to the cortex to become continuous with the distal convoluted tubule. This then opens into a collecting duct that is common to a number of nephrons and passes through the pyramid to enter the lesser calyx at the papilla. It is in these parts of the nephron (proximal tubule, loop of Henle, distal tubule, and collecting duct) that urine is formed, concentrated, and conveyed to the ureters. The distal convoluted tubule comes into very close contact with the afferent glomerular arteriole, and the modified cells of each form the *juxtaglomerular apparatus*, a complex physiologic feedback control mechanism contributing in part to the precise control of intra- and extrarenal hemodynamics that is a hallmark feature of the normally functioning kidney.

As is the case for the renal tubules, the vasculature of the kidney is highly organized. The renal artery enters the kidney at the hilum and then divides many times before producing the

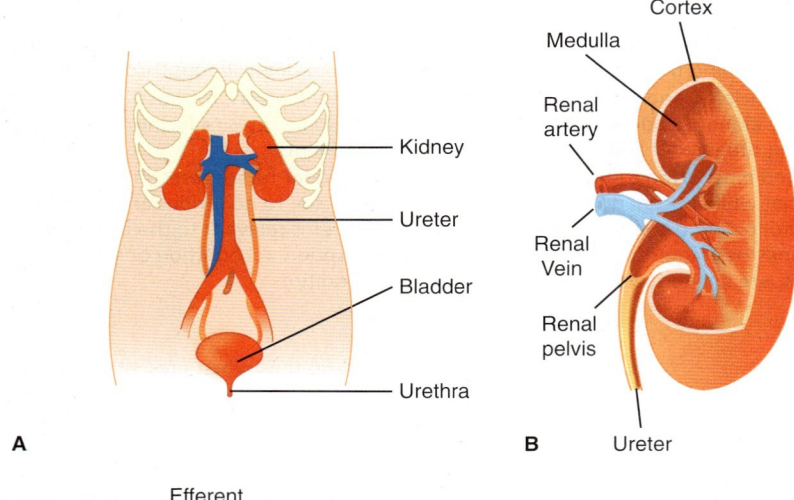
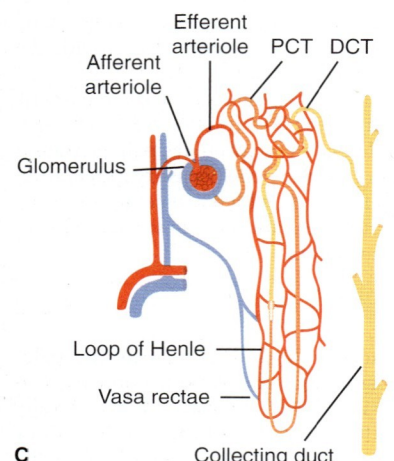
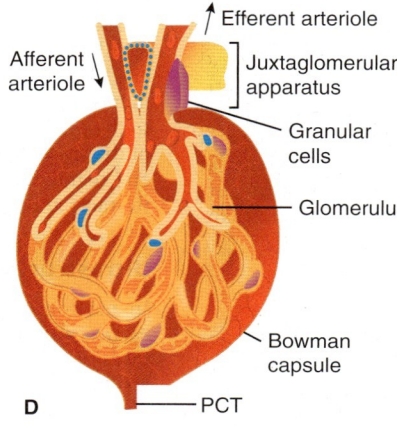

Figure 50-1 **A:** The gross anatomy and internal structure of the genitourinary system and kidney. **B:** Internal organization of the kidney includes cortex and medulla regions and the vasculature. **C:** The nephron is the functional unit of the kidney. **D:** Plasma filtration occurs in the glomerulus; 20% of plasma that enters the glomerulus passes through the specialized capillary wall into the Bowman capsule and enters the tubule to be processed and generate urine. PCT, proximal convoluted tubule; DCT, distal convoluted tubule.

arcuate arteries that run along the boundary between cortex and outer medulla. Interlobular arteries branch from arcuate arteries toward the outer kidney surface, giving rise as they pass through the cortex to numerous afferent arterioles, each leading to a single glomerular capillary tuft. The barrier where filtration from the vascular to tubular space within the glomerulus occurs is highly specialized and includes fenestrated negatively charged capillary endothelial cells and tubular epithelial cells (podocytes) separated by a basement membrane. Normally, selective permeability permits approximately 25% of the plasma elements to pass into the Bowman capsule; only cells and proteins more than 60 to 70 kDa cannot cross. However, abnormalities of this barrier can occur with disease, which may permit filtration of much larger proteins and even red blood cells; these changes manifest as the *nephrotic syndrome* (proteinuria >3.5 g/24 hr) or *glomerulonephritis* (hematuria and proteinuria). The glomerular capillaries exit Bowman capsule and merge to form the efferent arteriole and peritubular capillaries that nourish the tubules. The renal vasculature is unusual in having this arrangement of two capillary beds joined in series by arterioles. Blood supply to the entire tubular system comes from the glomerular efferent arteriole, which branches into an extensive capillary network. Some of these peritubular capillaries, the *vasa recta*, descend deep into the medulla to parallel the loops of Henle. The vasa recta then return in a cortical direction with the loops, join other peritubular capillaries, and empty into the cortical veins.

Correlation of Structure and Function

Because renal tissue makes up only 0.4% of body weight but receives 25% of cardiac output, the kidneys are by far the most highly perfused major organs in the body, and this facilitates plasma filtration at rates as high as 125 to 140 mL/min in young adults. The functions of the kidney are many and varied, including waste filtration, endocrine and exocrine activities, immune and metabolic functions, and maintenance of physiologic homeostasis. As well as tight regulation of extracellular solutes such as sodium, potassium, hydrogen, bicarbonate, and glucose, the kidney also generates ammonia and glucose and eliminates nitrogenous and other metabolic wastes including urea, creatinine, bilirubin, and other uremic toxins (i.e., substances that have toxic effects when they accumulate due to renal impairment). Finally, circulating hormones secreted by the kidney influence red blood cell generation, calcium homeostasis, and systemic blood pressure.

The kidney fulfills its dual roles of toxin excretion and body fluid management by filtering large amounts of fluid and solutes from the blood and secreting waste products into the tubular fluid. Effects on the normal filtration and reabsorption processes of comorbid disease, surgery, and anesthesia are the focus of the next section.

Glomerular Filtration

Production of urine begins with water and solute filtration from plasma flowing into the glomerulus via the afferent arteriole. The *glomerular filtration rate* (GFR) is a measure of glomerular function expressed as milliliters of plasma filtered per minute. The *ultrafiltration constant* (Kf) is directly related to glomerular capillary permeability and glomerular surface area. The two major determinants of filtration pressure are glomerular capillary pressure (P_{GC}) and glomerular oncotic pressure (p_{gc}). P_{GC} is directly related to renal artery pressure and is heavily influenced by arteriolar tone at points upstream (afferent) and downstream (efferent) from the glomerulus. An increase in afferent arteriolar tone, as occurs with intense sympathetic or angiotensin II stimulation, causes filtration pressure and GFR to fall. Milder degrees of sympathetic or angiotensin activity cause a selective increase in efferent arteriolar tone, which tends to increase filtration pressure and GFR. The p_{gc} is directly dependent on plasma oncotic pressure. Afferent arteriolar dilatation enhances GFR by increasing glomerular flow, which in turn elevates glomerular capillary pressure. Recent general revisions of Starling's original formula to incorporate the newly appreciated importance of the endothelial glycocalyx layer also appear to be relevant to glomerular filtration, particularly for pathologic states that involve proteinuria (e.g., diabetic nephropathy).[1-3]

Autoregulation of Renal Blood Flow and Glomerular Filtration Rate

Renal blood flow (RBF) *autoregulation* maintains relatively constant rates of RBF and glomerular filtration over a wide range of arterial blood pressure. Renal autoregulation of blood flow and filtration is accomplished primarily by local feedback signals that modulate glomerular arteriolar tone to protect the glomeruli from excessive perfusion pressure (Fig. 50-2).

In health, autoregulation of RBF is effective over a wide range of systemic arterial pressures. Several mechanisms for regulating blood flow to the glomerulus have been described, and all involve modulation of afferent glomerular arteriolar tone. The *myogenic reflex theory* holds that an increase in arterial pressure causes the afferent arteriolar wall to stretch and then constrict (by reflex); likewise, a decrease in arterial pressure causes reflex afferent arteriolar dilatation. The other proposed mechanism of RBF autoregulation is a phenomenon called *tubuloglomerular feedback*, which is also responsible for autoregulation of GFR.

Tubuloglomerular feedback allows the composition of distal tubular fluid to influence glomerular function through actions involving the juxtaglomerular apparatus. When RBF falls, the related decrease in GFR causes less chloride delivery to the juxtaglomerular apparatus, which in turn induces afferent arteriole dilation. As a result, glomerular flow and pressure then increase, and GFR returns to previous levels. Chloride also acts as the feedback signal for control of efferent arteriolar tone. When GFR falls, declining chloride delivery to the juxtaglomerular apparatus triggers release of *renin*, which ultimately causes the formation of *angiotensin II*. In response to angiotensin, efferent arteriolar constriction increases glomerular pressure, which increases glomerular filtration. It is important to realize that autoregulation of urine flow does not occur, and that above a mean arterial pressure of 50 mmHg there is a linear relationship between mean arterial pressure and urine output.

Tubular Reabsorption of Sodium and Water

Active, energy-dependent reabsorption of sodium begins almost immediately as the glomerular filtrate enters the proximal tubule. Here, an adenosine triphosphatase pump drives the sodium into tubular cells while chloride ions passively follow. Glucose, amino acid, and other organic compound reabsorption are strongly coupled to sodium in the proximal tubule. Normally, the proximal tubule reabsorbs two-thirds of the filtered sodium. Notably, no active sodium transport occurs in the loop of Henle until the medullary thick ascending limb is reached. Cells of the medullary thick ascending limb are metabolically active in their role of reabsorbing sodium and chloride and have a high oxygen consumption compared with the thin portions of the descending and ascending limbs.

Reabsorption of water is a passive, osmotically driven process tied to the reabsorption of sodium and other solutes. Water reabsorption also depends on peritubular capillary pressure; high capillary pressure opposes water reabsorption and tends to increase urine output. The proximal tubule reabsorbs approximately 65% of filtered water in an isosmotic fashion with sodium and chloride. The descending limb of the loop of Henle allows water to follow osmotic gradients into the renal interstitium. However, the thin ascending limb and medullary thick ascending limb are relatively impermeable to water and play a key role in the production of concentrated urine. Only 15% of filtered water is reabsorbed by the loop of Henle; the remaining filtrate volume flows into the distal tubule. There, and in the collecting duct, water reabsorption is controlled entirely by *antidiuretic hormone* (ADH) secreted by the pituitary gland. Conservation of water and excretion of excess solute by the kidneys would be impossible without the ability to produce concentrated urine. This is accomplished by establishing a hyperosmotic medullary interstitium and regulation of water permeability of the distal tubule and collecting duct via the action of ADH.

ADH increases the water permeability of the collecting ducts and allows for passive diffusion of water (under considerable osmotic pressure) back into the circulation. The posterior pituitary gland releases ADH in response to an increase in either extracellular sodium concentration or extracellular osmolality. In addition, ADH release can be triggered by an absolute or relative reduction in intravascular fluid volume. The arterial baroreceptors are activated when hypovolemia leads to a decrease

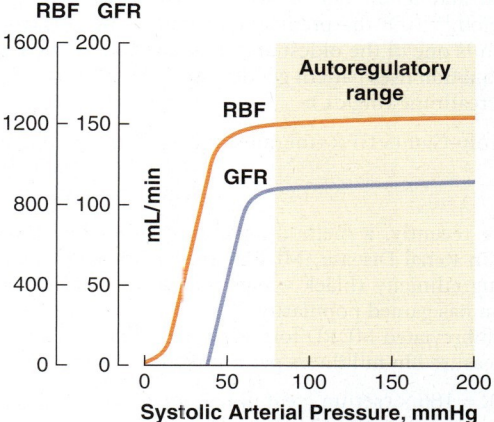

Figure 50-2 Renal blood flow (RBF) autoregulation maintains RBF and glomerular filtration rate (GFR) relatively constant with changes in systolic blood pressure from about 80 to 200 mmHg. (Adapted with permission from http://www2.kumc.edu/ki/physiology/course/two/2_8.htm.)

in blood pressure, whereas atrial receptors are stimulated by a decline in atrial filling pressure. Both of these circulatory reflex systems stimulate release of ADH from the pituitary and cause retention of water by the kidney in an effort to return the intravascular volume toward normal. ADH also causes renal cortical vasoconstriction when it is released in large amounts, such as during the physiologic stress response to trauma, surgery, or other critical illness. This induces a shift of RBF to the hypoxia-prone renal medulla.

The Renin–Angiotensin–Aldosterone System

Renin release by the afferent arteriole may be triggered by hypotension, decreased tubular chloride concentration, or sympathetic stimulation. Renin enhances *angiotensin II* production, which in turn induces renal efferent arteriolar vasoconstriction. Angiotensin II also promotes ADH release from the posterior pituitary, sodium reabsorption by the proximal tubule, and aldosterone release by the adrenal medulla. *Aldosterone* stimulates the distal tubule and collecting duct to reabsorb sodium (and water), resulting in intravascular volume expansion. Sympathetic nervous system stimulation may also directly cause release of aldosterone. This leads to renal cortical vasoconstriction, a decrease in GFR, and salt and water retention.

Renal Vasodilator Mechanisms

Opposing the saline retention and vasoconstriction observed in stress states are the actions of *atrial natriuretic peptide* (ANP), *nitric oxide*, and the renal *prostaglandin* system. ANP is released by the cardiac atria in response to increased stretch under conditions of volume expansion. Both natriuresis and aquaresis increase as ANP blocks reabsorption of sodium in the distal tubule and collecting duct. ANP also increases GFR, causes systemic vasodilatation, inhibits the release of renin, opposes production and action of angiotensin II, and decreases aldosterone secretion.[4] Likewise, nitric oxide produced in the kidney opposes the renal vasoconstrictor effects of angiotensin II and the adrenergic nervous system, promotes sodium and water excretion, and participates in tubuloglomerular feedback.

Prostaglandins are produced by the kidney as part of a complex system that modulates RBF and opposes the actions of ADH and the renin–angiotensin–aldosterone system. Stress states, renal ischemia, and hypotension stimulate the production of renal prostaglandins through the enzymes phospholipase A_2 and cyclooxygenase. Prostaglandins produced by cyclooxygenase activity cause dilatation of renal arterioles (antiangiotensin II), whereas their distal tubular effects result in an increase in sodium and water excretion (anti-ADH and aldosterone). The renal prostaglandin system is important in maintaining RBF and sodium and water excretion during times of high physiologic stress and poor renal perfusion.

Clinical Assessment of the Kidney

Most agree that immediate perioperative measures such as urine output correlate poorly with perioperative renal function[4]; however, much about the kidneys can be learned from knowing how effectively they clear circulating substances and inspection of the urine (i.e., urinalysis).

Renal Function Tests

Filtration is a useful method to clinically assess kidney function. As a key indicator of disease, knowledge of limited filtration capacity is important to guide drug dosing for agents cleared by the kidneys and helps with preoperative risk stratification. Also, acute declines in filtration capacity indicate kidney injury and predict a more complicated clinical course.[5] *GFR*, as previously mentioned, refers to the plasma volume filtered per unit time by the kidneys, and normal values range from 90 to 140 mL/min. Normal GFRs relate to the patient age, size, and gender. In general, GFR declines 10% per decade after age 30 and is approximately 10 mL/min higher in men than women. A GFR below 60 mL/min meets criteria for chronic kidney disease (CKD) and is considered impaired, whereas values lower than 15 mL/min are often associated with uremic symptoms and may require dialysis.

An "ideal" substance to assess GFR through its clearance from the circulation must have specific properties, including a steady supply, free filtration, and no tubular reabsorption or excretion; ideally, it is also cheap and easy to measure. Unfortunately, the perfect ideal substance is yet to be identified. The gold standard GFR tools involve expensive and cumbersome measurements (e.g., inulin, ^{51}Cr-EDTA, ^{99}Tc-DTPA clearance), whereas the most practical and inexpensive test involves an imperfect ideal substance, *creatinine*. However, despite creatinine's limitations, its relatively steady supply from muscle metabolism, modest tubular secretion, and proven usefulness in numerous clinical settings make it the most used renal filtration marker currently available. Although more ideal substances and other "early biomarkers" of AKI are being evaluated as clinical tools, current candidates (e.g., cystatin C) have yet to replace creatinine. The reader is referred to recent reviews on this subject.[9,10]

Estimates of GFR (eGFR) can be made by determining *creatinine clearance* (CrCl) from urine and blood creatinine tests. In stable, critically ill patients, 2-hour urine collections are sufficient to calculate CrCl,[11] using the following formula:

$$CrCl\ (mL/min) = (U_{cr}\ (mg/dl) \times V\ (ml))\ /\ (P_{cr}\ (mg/dl) \times time\ (min))$$

where U_{cr} = urine creatinine, V = total volume of urine collected, P_{cr} = plasma creatinine, and time = collection time.

However, if patient characteristics are known, GFR can also be estimated from a single steady-state serum creatinine value. Notably, predictive formulas are developed using data from stable (nonsurgical) populations, and factors such as fluid shifts, hemodilution, and hemorrhage add an "unsteadiness" to perioperative estimates of GFR using serum creatinine.

Nonetheless, serum creatinine remains, so far, an unsurpassed perioperative tool, particularly to reflect *trends* of change in renal filtration and to predict outcome, even during the perioperative period.[12-14] Of the predictive formulas, the Cockroft–Gault equation is one of the oldest and most durable.[15] The Cockroft–Gault equation uses patient gender, age (years), weight (kg), and serum creatinine (mg/dL):

$$Cockroft\text{–}Gault\ eGFR\ (mL/min) = (140 - age) \times weight\ (kg)/(Cr \times 72)(\times 0.85\ for\ female\ patients)$$

More recently, a method developed from the Modification of Diet in Renal Disease (MDRD) study that adds other factors including ethnicity (black versus nonblack) to Cockroft–Gault equation has gained popularity.[16]

An abbreviated MDRD formula is available that can estimate GFR measured in milliliters per minute per 1.73 m^2:

$$GFR = 186 \times (serum\ creatinine - mg/dL)^{-1.154} \times (age)^{-0.203}$$
$$(\times 0.742\ for\ female\ patients)$$
$$(\times 1.210\ for\ black\ patients)$$

However, even a detailed MDRD eGFR under ideal conditions sometimes correlates poorly with a gold standard–determined

GFR, with more than a 30% error in 10% of patients, and 2% deviating more than 50%.[16]

Some consensus definitions for significant perioperative renal dysfunction exist. The Society of Thoracic Surgeons defines postoperative AKI as either a new requirement for dialysis or a rise in serum creatinine to greater than 2 mg/dL involving at least a 50% increase in serum creatinine above baseline.[17] Another definition requires a creatinine rise of greater than 25% or 0.5 mg/dL (44 mmol/L) within 48 hours.[18] The Acute Dialysis Quality Initiative Group definition for critically ill patients grades AKI by an acute creatinine rise of 50% as "risk," 100% as "injury," or 200% as "failure" (the RIFLE criteria).[19] The Acute Kidney Injury Network definition, a 1.5-fold or 0.3 mg/dL (≥26.4 mmol/L) creatinine rise within a 48-hour period or more than 6 hours of oliguria (>0.5 mL/kg/hr), is a modification of its RIFLE predecessor.[19,20] The most recent consensus definition for AKI comes from Kidney Disease Improving Global Outcomes (KDIGO): an increase in serum creatinine by at least 0.3 mg/dL (≥26.5 µmol/L) within 48 hours; or increase in serum creatinine to at least 1.5 times baseline, which is known or presumed to have occurred within the prior 7 days; or urine volume below 0.5 mL/kg/h for 6 hours.[21] Notably, serum creatinine does not usually rise significantly until GFR rates fall below 50 mL/min, so preoperative serum creatinine may be normal in patients even with some degree of renal dysfunction (Fig. 50-3).

Blood urea nitrogen (BUN) is sometimes used to assess renal function but possesses few of the characteristics of an ideal substance for such a task. Tubular urea transport changes with some conditions (e.g., dehydration), and urea generation can be highly variable, particularly during the postoperative period (i.e., catabolic state). In addition, hemodilution (e.g., cardiopulmonary bypass [CPB]) may affect circulating BUN levels.

Urinalysis and Urine Characteristics

Urine inspection can reveal abnormal cloudiness or color and unexpected odors. Detailed descriptions of urine examination are available[22]; therefore, only a summary is provided here. Cloudy urine is due to suspended elements such as white or red blood cells and/or crystals. Lightly centrifuged urine sediment will normally contain 80 ± 20 mg of protein per day and up to two red blood cells per high-power field (400×); higher levels of red blood cells or protein reflect abnormal kidney function. Urine protein electrophoresis can differentiate proteinuria from a glomerular (filtering), tubular (reuptake), overflow (supply that saturates the reuptake system), or tissue (e.g., kidney inflammation) abnormality. In contrast, color changes reflect dissolved substances; this occurs most commonly with dehydration, but other causes include food colorings, drugs, and liver disease (e.g., bilirubin). Unusual odors are less common but can also be diagnostic (e.g., maple syrup urine disease). Chromogenic dipstick chemical tests can determine urine pH and provide a semiquantitative analysis of protein, blood, nitrites, leukocyte esterase, glucose, ketones, urobilinogen, and bilirubin. In addition, microscopy can identify crystals, cells, tubular casts, and bacteria.

Urine *specific gravity* (the weight of urine relative to distilled water) normally ranges between 1.001 and 1.035 and can be used as a surrogate for osmolarity (normal 50 to 1,000 mOsm/kg), with 1.010 reflecting a specific gravity similar to that of plasma. High specific gravity (>1.018) implies preserved renal concentrating ability, unless high levels of glucose, protein, or contrast dye injection have raised specific gravity without significantly changing osmolarity.

Although poor urine output (e.g., <400 mL urine/24 hr) may reflect hypovolemia or impending *prerenal* renal failure, a majority of perioperative AKI episodes develop in the absence of oliguria.[4] The normal response to hypovolemia is renal solute retention; fluid and electrolyte retention produces a concentrated urine with a low sodium content (<20 mEq/L). In contrast, impaired concentrating ability due to AKI causes urine to approach plasma osmolarity (isosthenuria) with a higher sodium content (>40 mEq/L). The kidneys' ability to retain electrolytes

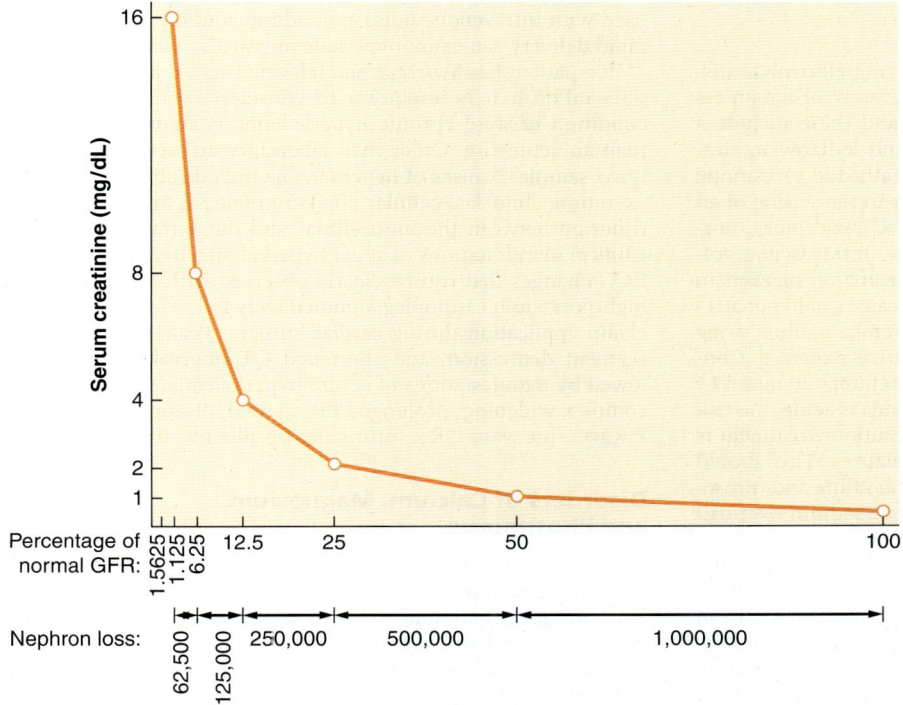

Figure 50-3 The nonlinear relationship between changes in renal filtration and serum creatinine level means that a large reduction (e.g., 75%, 120 to 30 mL/min) in glomerular filtration rate (GFR) may be associated with a modest rise in serum creatinine. Proportional reductions in GFR and (approximate) nephron loss (x axis) have an inverse logarithmic relationship with serum creatinine concentration (y axis). (Modified with permission from Faber MD, Kupin WL, Krishna G, et al. The differential diagnosis of ARF. In: Lazarus JM, Brenner BM, eds. *Acute Renal Failure.* 3rd ed. New York, NY: Churchill Livingstone; 1993:133.)

is also reflected in the *fractional excretion of sodium* (FE_{Na}), a test that uses a spot sample of urine and blood to compare sodium and creatinine excretion; this test can be useful to distinguish hypovolemia and renal injury:

$$FE_{Na} = U_{Na}/P_{Na} \times P_{Cr}/U_{Cr} \times 100$$

where U_{na} = urine sodium, P_{na} = plasma sodium, U_{cr} = urine creatinine, and P_{cr} = plasma creatinine.

FE_{Na} <1% implies that sodium is being normally conserved, whereas values above 1% are consistent with acute tubular necrosis (ATN).

Perioperative Nephrology

Pathophysiology

Altered renal function can be thought of as a clinical continuum ranging from the normal compensatory changes seen during stress to frank renal failure. Clinically, there is considerable overlap between compensated and decompensated renal dysfunctional states. The kidney under stress reacts in a predictable manner to help restore intravascular volume and maintain blood pressure. The sympathetic nervous system reacts to trauma, shock, or pain by releasing norepinephrine, which acts much like angiotensin II on the renal arterioles. Norepinephrine also activates the renin–angiotensin–aldosterone system and causes ADH release. The net result of modest activity of the stress response system is a shift of blood flow from the renal cortex to the medulla, avid sodium and water reabsorption, and decreased urine output. A more intense stress response may induce a decrease in RBF and GFR by causing afferent arteriolar constriction. If this extreme situation is not reversed, ischemic damage to the kidney may result, and AKI may become clinically manifest.

Electrolyte Disorders

Disorders of Sodium Balance

Hyponatremia is the most commonly occurring electrolyte disorder (see also Chapter 16).[24,25] Symptoms rarely occur unless sodium values are less than 125 mmol/L, and these include a spectrum ranging from anorexia, nausea, and lethargy to convulsions, dysrhythmias, coma, and even death due to osmotic brain swelling.[26–28] Hyponatremia may occur in the setting of an expanded (e.g., transurethral resection [TUR] syndrome), normal, or contracted extracellular fluid volume. Intravascular volume status and urinary sodium concentration are key markers in differentiating the large number of potential causes of hyponatremia. If water excess is a reason for hyponatremia, a dilute urine with a sodium concentration above 20 mmol/L is expected. Conversely, avid renal sodium retention (urine sodium <20 mmol/L) suggests sodium loss as a cause. If hyponatremia is acute, the risk of neurologic complications is higher, and cautious treatment is indicated to prevent cerebral edema and seizures. This should be accomplished with intravenous hypertonic saline and furosemide to enhance water excretion and prevent sodium overload (see transurethral resection syndrome section).

Hypernatremia (serum sodium >145 mmol/L) is generally the result of sodium gain or water loss, most commonly the latter. Dehydration of brain tissue can cause symptoms ranging from confusion to convulsions and coma. In cases of hypernatremia, laboratory studies often show evidence of hemoconcentration (increased hematocrit and serum protein concentrations). In addition, urine output is usually low (<500 mL/day) and hyperosmolar (>1,000 mOsm), with very low urinary sodium concentration and evidence of prerenal failure (elevations of BUN and serum creatinine). Occasionally, the urine is not maximally concentrated, suggesting an osmotic diuresis or an intrinsic renal disorder such as diabetes insipidus. The primary goal of treatment is restoration of serum tonicity, which can be achieved with isotonic or hypotonic parenteral fluids and/or diuretics unless irreversible renal injury is present, in which situation dialysis may be necessary.

Disorders of Potassium Balance

Even minor variations in serum potassium concentration can lead to symptoms such as skeletal muscle weakness, gastrointestinal ileus, myocardial depression, malignant ventricular dysrhythmias, and asystole. Nearly 98% of total body potassium is intracellular. Circulating potassium levels are tightly controlled via renal and gastrointestinal excretion and reabsorption, but potassium also moves between the intra- and extracellular compartments under the influence of insulin and β_2-adrenoceptors. In the kidney, 70% of potassium reabsorption occurs in the proximal tubule and another 15% to 20% in the loop of Henle. The collecting duct is responsible for potassium excretion under the influence of aldosterone.

Hypokalemia may be due to a net potassium deficiency or transfer of extracellular potassium to the intracellular space. Notably, total body depletion may exist even with normal extracellular potassium levels (e.g., diabetic ketoacidosis). Causes of hypokalemia include extrarenal loss (e.g., vomiting, diarrhea), renal loss (impaired processing due to drugs, hormones, or inherited renal abnormalities), potassium shifts between the extra- and intracellular spaces (e.g., insulin therapy), and, occasionally, inadequate intake. Clinical manifestations of hypokalemia include electrocardiography (ECG) changes (flattened T waves—"no pot, no T," U waves, prodysrhythmic state) and skeletal muscle weakness. Hypokalemia treatment involves supplementation by either intravenous or oral route; however, extreme caution should be used with intravenous potassium administration because overly rapid delivery can cause hyperkalemic cardiac arrest.

If a patient has *hyperkalemia* (elevated serum potassium level >5.5 mEq/L), it is important to consider the duration of the condition because chronic hyperkalemia is far better tolerated than an acute rise. Other than laboratory artifacts (e.g., hemolyzed sample), causes of hyperkalemia include abnormal kidney excretion, abnormal cellular potassium release, or abnormal distribution between the intracellular and the extracellular space. Clinical manifestations of acute hyperkalemia include a range of ECG changes that can be clearly observed with the infusion of high-potassium cardioplegia immediately following aortic cross-clamp application during cardiac surgery. Peaked T waves, ST segment depression, and shortened QT interval are soon followed by manifestations of severe hyperkalemia, including QRS complex widening, prolonged PR interval, disappearance of the P wave, sine wave QRS, ventricular fibrillation, and asystole.

Disorders of Calcium, Magnesium, and Phosphorus

Most of a grown adult's 1 to 2 kg of calcium is in bone (98%), with the remaining 2% in one of the three forms: ionized, chelated, or protein bound. Normal serum calcium values range between 8.5 and 10.2 mg/dL, but only the ionized fraction (50%) is biologically active and precisely regulated. Ionized extracellular calcium concentration (iCa^{++}) is controlled by the combined actions of parathyroid hormone (PTH), calcitonin, and vitamin D and further modulated by dietary and environmental factors. The clinical manifestations of *hypocalcemia* include cramping, digital numbness, laryngospasm, carpopedal spasm, bronchospasm, seizures, and respiratory arrest. A positive Chvostek sign (facial muscle twitching in response to tapping the facial nerve) or Trousseau sign (carpal spasm induced by brachial artery occlusion) are the classic hallmarks of hypocalcemia but in practice are often absent. Mental status changes, including irritability, depression, and impaired cognition may also occur. Cardiac manifestations include QT interval prolongation and dysrhythmias. Hypocalcemia may be due to several mechanisms, including a decrease in PTH secretion or action, reduced vitamin D synthesis or action, resistance of bone to PTH or vitamin D effects, or calcium sequestration. Acute hypocalcemia due to citrate toxicity can develop from rapid infusion of citrate-stored packed red blood cells, particularly with citrate accumulation during the anhepatic phase of liver transplant procedures. Parathyroidectomy, either selectively or as a complication of thyroidectomy during neck surgery, can acutely reduce PTH levels and precipitate hypocalcemia. Citrate used for regional anticoagulation with chronic dialysis can also cause hypocalcemia and may lead to hypomagnesemia from decreased PTH secretion. Hypocalcemia due to reduced serum protein levels is physiologically unimportant. Clinical symptoms of *hypercalcemia* correlate with its acuity and include constipation, nausea and vomiting, drowsiness, lethargy, weakness, stupor, and coma. Cardiovascular manifestations may include hypertension, shortened QT interval, heart block, and other dysrhythmias. The most frequent causes of hypercalcemia are primary hyperparathyroidism and malignancy. Other causes include thiazide (increases renal calcium reabsorption) or lithium (inhibits PTH release) therapy and rarer medical conditions including granulomatous disease, thyrotoxicosis, and multiple endocrine neoplasia types I and II.

Magnesium is a multifunctional cation that is found primarily in the intracellular space. Because extracellular magnesium represents only 0.3% of total (mainly intracellular) stores, normal serum levels (1.6 to 2.2 mg/dL) are a poor reflection of total body magnesium. *Hypomagnesemia* (<1.6 mg/dL) may sometimes be asymptomatic, but clinically important problems can and do manifest, including neuromuscular, cardiac, neurologic, and related electrolytic (hypokalemia and hypocalcemia) abnormalities. Causes of hypomagnesemia can be divided into four broad categories: decreased intake, gastrointestinal loss, renal loss, and redistribution. Nutritional hypomagnesemia can result from malabsorption syndromes in patients receiving parenteral nutrition, and it is also present in 25% of alcoholics. Redistribution occurs with acute pancreatitis, administration of catecholamines, and "hungry bone syndrome" after parathyroidectomy.[29] Magnesium can be supplemented orally or via the parenteral route. Clinical manifestations of *hypermagnesemia* (>4 to 6 mg/dL) are serious and potentially fatal. Minor symptoms include hypotension, nausea, vomiting, facial flushing, urinary retention, and ileus. In more extreme cases, flaccid skeletal muscular paralysis, hyporeflexia, bradycardia, bradydysrhythmias, respiratory depression, coma, and cardiac arrest may occur. Hypermagnesemia generally occurs in two clinical settings: compromised renal function (GFR < 20 mL/min) and excessive magnesium intake (e.g., excessive intravenous therapy in preeclampsia). Although mild hypermagnesemia in the setting of normal renal function can be treated with supportive care and withdrawal of the cause, in some cases dialysis is necessary.

Phosphorus is a major intracellular anion that plays a role in regulation of glycolysis, ammoniagenesis, and calcium homeostasis and is an essential component of adenosine triphosphate and red blood cell 2,3-diphosphoglyceric acid synthesis. *Hypophosphatemia* is clinically more important than hyperphosphatemia and can result in symptoms including muscle weakness, respiratory failure, and difficulty in weaning critically ill patients from mechanical ventilation when serum levels are less than 0.32 mmol/L. In addition, low phosphate levels may diminish oxygen delivery to tissues and rarely cause hemolysis. Hypophosphatemia can result from intracellular redistribution (from catecholamine therapy), from inadequate intake or absorption secondary to alcoholism or malnutrition, or from increased renal or gastrointestinal losses.[30] Intravenous and oral supplementation can be used to treat hypophosphatemia. *Hyperphosphatemia* (>5 mg/dL) is generally related to accompanying hypocalcemia although increased phosphate levels may also lead to calcium precipitation and decreased intestinal calcium absorption. Significantly elevated serum phosphate levels are most commonly due to reduced excretion from renal insufficiency but can also result from excess intake or redistribution of intracellular phosphorus. Treatment of chronic hyperphosphatemia includes dietary phosphate restriction and oral phosphate binders.

Acid–Base Disorders

The primary determinant of serum pH is the balance between plasma bicarbonate (HCO_3^-) concentration and the PCO_2 in the extracellular space. Acid–base homeostasis involves tight regulation of HCO_3^- and arterial PCO_2 ($PaCO_2$). Primary extracellular pH derangements due to abnormal bicarbonate reabsorption and proton (H^+) elimination by the kidney lead to metabolic acidosis or alkalosis, whereas factors that abnormally affect respiratory drive influence $PaCO_2$, leading to respiratory acidosis or alkalosis. Because combined problems are often seen in perioperative critically ill patients, an approach to both "pure" and "mixed" acid–base disorders is presented here.

Metabolic Acidosis

The *anion gap* (AG) represents the total serum concentration of unmeasured anions and can be calculated as $AG = (Na^+ + K^+) - (HCO_3^- + Cl^-)$. It allows differentiation of the causes of metabolic acidosis into normal AG (12 ± 4) and increased AG (>16 mmol/L) varieties. Conditions that cause an increase in negatively charged ions other than bicarbonate and chloride (e.g., lactate, salicylate) increase the AG. In contrast, non-AG metabolic acidosis results from renal or gastrointestinal HCO_3^- loss and is associated with high chloride levels (hyperchloremic metabolic acidosis). The usual compensatory response to all types of metabolic acidoses is hyperventilation, which leads to a partial pH correction toward normal. Winter's formula predicts expected $PaCO_2$ for a metabolic acidosis as follows: $PaCO_2 = (1.5 \times HCO_3^-) + 8$.

Metabolic Alkalosis

Metabolic alkalosis is a common primary acid–base disturbance associated with increased plasma HCO_3^-. Increased extracellular HCO_3^- is due to a net loss of H^+ and/or addition of HCO_3^-. The most common cause of metabolic alkalosis is gastrointestinal acid loss due to vomiting or nasogastric suctioning; the resulting hypovolemia leads to secretion of renin and aldosterone and enhanced absorption of HCO_3^-. Thiazides and loop diuretics both induce a net loss of chloride and free water and can cause a volume "contraction" alkalosis.

Respiratory Acidosis

If the lungs fail to eliminate CO_2, hypercapnia and respiratory acidosis result, characterized by increased $PaCO_2$ and decreased blood pH. Acute and chronic causes can be differentiated by examining arterial pH, $PaCO_2$, and HCO_3^- values. In the early phase of respiratory acidosis, increased $PaCO_2$ stimulates renal generation and secretion of H^+. The kidneys continue to adapt to the increased pH through greater titratable acid excretion (e.g., ammonium) and HCO_3^- generation. Therefore, acute respiratory acidosis is characterized by an elevated $PaCO_2$, acidemia, and a relatively normal HCO_3^-. In contrast, chronic respiratory acidosis is associated with an elevated HCO_3^- (often accompanied by a relatively normal pH) due to renal compensation.

Respiratory Alkalosis

Increased minute ventilation is the primary cause of respiratory alkalosis, characterized by decreased $PaCO_2$ and increased pH. Patients with acute, uncompensated respiratory alkalosis have normal plasma HCO_3^-. In chronic respiratory alkalosis, renal compensation leads to decreased plasma HCO_3^-. The causes of respiratory alkalosis relate to abnormal respiratory drive from stimulants or toxins (e.g., salicylate, caffeine, nicotine, progesterone), central nervous system abnormalities (e.g., anxiety, stroke, increased intracranial pressure), pulmonary abnormalities (e.g., pulmonary embolism, pneumonia), mechanical hyperventilation, or systemic conditions such as liver failure and sepsis.

Mixed Acid–Base Disorders

It is not uncommon for a metabolic derangement to coexist with a respiratory derangement, particularly in critically ill patients. A general approach to the diagnosis of mixed acid–base disorders requires a stepwise approach that begins with a focused history and physical examination. An arterial blood gas and a concurrent serum chemistry panel (including Na^+, K^+, Cl^-, and total CO_2 concentrations) should also be obtained, and the use of an acid–base map may help differentiate simple from mixed disorders (Fig. 50-4).

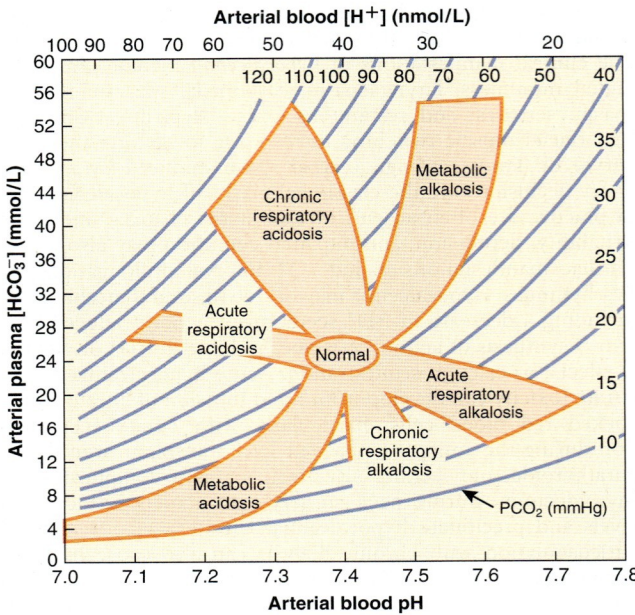

Figure 50-4 Acid–base map. Plotting the PCO_2 and H^+ (from the arterial blood gas) against plasma HCO_3^- (from the serum chemistry panel) for a patient can identify simple acid–base disorders. When mixed disorders exist, values may fall outside the shaded areas. (Adapted with permission from DuBose TD Jr. Acid-base disorders. In: Brenner BM, ed. *Brenner & Rector's The Kidney*. 7th ed. Philadelphia, PA: WB Saunders; 2004:938.)

Acute Kidney Conditions

Acute Kidney Injury

AKI is now the preferred term for an acute deterioration in renal function. It is associated with a decline in glomerular filtration and results in inability of the kidneys to excrete nitrogenous and other wastes. This manifests as an accumulation of creatinine and urea in the blood (uremia) and is often accompanied by reduced urine production, although nonoliguric forms of postoperative AKI are common.[31] In surgical patients, ATN is the most common cause of AKI. AKI frequently occurs in the setting of critical illness with multiple organ failure when the mortality is alarmingly high (up to 80%).[32] Notably, extracorporeal renal support appears to have little impact in altering the generally poor outcome associated with AKI in critically ill surgical patients.[32] Even studies that advocate the use of extracorporeal technology report mortality of between 50% and 70%.[33–35]

AKI can be caused by *prerenal* factors causing renal hypoperfusion, *intrinsic* renal causes, or *postrenal* causes (obstructive uropathy). There are many pathophysiologic similarities between the various causes of kidney injury.

Prerenal Azotemia

Prerenal azotemia is the increase in BUN associated with renal hypoperfusion or ischemia that has not yet caused renal parenchymal damage. The metabolically active cells of the medullary thick ascending limb of the loop of Henle are especially vulnerable to hypoxic damage because of their relatively high oxygen consumption. AKI ensues when necrosis of tubular cells releases debris into the tubules, causing flow obstruction, increased tubular back pressure, and leak of tubular fluid. Often, prerenal AKI is precipitated in patients with pre-existing renal vasoconstriction (e.g., volume depletion, heart failure, or sepsis) by nephrotoxin exposure or further reductions in cardiac output.

Intrinsic Acute Kidney Injury

The term *intrinsic* not only implies a primary renal cause of AKI but also includes AKI due to ischemia, nephrotoxins, and renal parenchymal diseases. ATN remains the most common ischemic lesion and represents an extension of prerenal azotemia, whereas cortical necrosis may follow a massive renovascular insult such as prolonged suprarenal aortic clamping or renal artery embolism. Nephrotoxins often act in concert with hypoperfusion or underlying renal vasoconstrictive states to damage renal tubules or the microvasculature. Several common nephrotoxins, some of which are difficult to avoid in a hospitalized patient population, are listed in Table 50-1.

Postrenal Acute Kidney Injury (Obstructive Uropathy)

Downstream obstruction of the urinary collecting system is the least common pathway to established AKI, accounting for less than 10% of cases.[37] Because it can generally be corrected, it is extremely important to exclude with a renal ultrasound

Table 50-1 Nephrotoxins Commonly Found in the Hospital Setting
Exogenous
Antibiotics (aminoglycosides, cephalosporins, amphotericin B, sulfonamide, tetracyclines, vancomycin)
Anesthetic agents (methoxyflurane, enflurane)
Nonsteroidal anti-inflammatory drugs (aspirin, ibuprofen, naproxen, indomethacin, ketorolac)
Chemotherapeutic–immunosuppressive agents (cisplatinum, cyclosporin A, methotrexate, mitomycin, nitrosoureas, tacrolimus)
Contrast media
Endogenous
Calcium (hypercalcemia)
Uric acid (hyperuricemia and hyperuricosuria)
Myoglobin (rhabdomyolysis)
Hemoglobin (hemolysis)
Bilirubin (obstructive jaundice)
Oxalate crystals
Paraproteins

examination as a source of AKI. The obstructing lesion may occur at any level of the collecting system, from the renal pelvis to the distal urethra. Intraluminal pressure rises and is eventually transmitted back to the glomerulus, thereby reducing glomerular filtration pressure and rate.

Nephrotoxins and Perioperative Acute Kidney Injury

Nephrotoxin exposure is a common occurrence in hospitalized patients and frequently plays a role in the cause of AKI in this population. Nephrotoxins may take the form of drugs, nontherapeutic chemicals, heavy metals, poisons, and endogenous compounds (Table 50-1). The nephrotoxins most likely to contribute to renal dysfunction/failure in the perioperative period are certain antimicrobial and chemotherapeutic–immunosuppressive agents, radiocontrast media, nonsteroidal anti-inflammatory drugs (NSAIDs), and the endogenous heme pigments myoglobin and hemoglobin. These diverse groups of renal toxins share a common pathophysiologic characteristic: They disturb either renal oxygen delivery or oxygen utilization and thereby promote renal ischemia.

Antimicrobial and chemotherapeutic–immunosuppressive agents are effective because they are cellular toxins. When these drugs are filtered, reabsorbed, secreted, and eventually excreted by the kidney, toxic concentrations in renal cells can be reached. The aminoglycoside antibiotics and amphotericin B are particularly difficult to avoid because they are effective antimicrobials, with few available alternatives. Their effect can be additive with other nephrotoxic factors causing impairment of kidney function. Hypovolemia, fever, renal vasoconstriction, and concomitant therapy with other nephrotoxic agents should be avoided wherever possible. Electrolyte disorders such as hypercalcemia, hypomagnesemia, hypokalemia, and metabolic acidosis can further enhance nephrotoxic damage to the kidney.

Cyclosporin A and tacrolimus are indispensable components of many immunosuppressive drug regimens, but in combination with other nephrotoxins and clinical factors, they can cause acute and exacerbate chronic kidney injuries in transplant recipients.[34]

Yacoub and colleagues[38] suggest that angiotensin-converting enzyme (ACE) inhibitors and angiotensin receptor blockers (ARBs) should not be given for 48 hours prior to routine cardiac surgery. In their meta-analysis of 29 retrospective studies (>50,000 procedures) these authors linked chronic ACE inhibitor or ARB use until the day of surgery with higher mortality risk (20%; $p = 0.005$) and AKI rates (17%; $p = 0.04$). ACE inhibitors and ARBs are also associated with increased AKI risk in patients receiving diuretic therapy; those with volume depletion, CHF, or diabetes; and the elderly.[39,40] Finally, although ACE inhibitors and ARBs are sometimes prescribed to slow the progression of CKD, their use with NSAIDs and other nephrotoxic agents such as cyclosporine, tacrolimus, and aprotinin is also associated with increased perioperative AKI risk.[39,41,42]

Discontinuing loop diuretic therapy on the day prior to surgery should also receive careful consideration. Two studies have linked chronic diuretic therapy with postoperative AKI,[43,44] with one differentiating loop (not thiazide) diuretics as having higher AKI and mortality risk.[44] Other retrospective studies report high furosemide dose as a risk factor for AKI following contrast exposure during coronary angiography and then subsequent off-pump cardiac surgery.[45] Short-term furosemide also worsened AKI in one randomized cardiac surgery trial and a retrospective study of noncardiac surgery patients.[46,47]

In contradistinction, patients taking statins prior to coronary artery bypass graft (but not isolated valve) surgery had lower dialysis and mortality rates in a meta-analysis of 17 studies (>47,000 patients) addressing this issue.[48]

Radiocontrast media pose a threat to the renal function of patients with diabetic nephropathy, pre-existing renal vasoconstriction (heart failure, hypovolemia), or renal insufficiency.[49] Radiocontrast dye has effects on renal function that develop 24 to 48 hours after exposure and peak at 3 to 5 days. Measures that may prevent AKI or lessen the severity of renal damage include prehydration, smaller contrast doses, and judicious withholding of other nephrotoxins, such as NSAIDs. Hu and colleagues[50] concluded that nonemergent cardiac procedures should be delayed for 24 hours after contrast administration to reduce the incidence of postoperative AKI in their meta-analysis of eight retrospective studies (>11,000 patients receiving dye within 3 days preoperatively).

NSAIDs produce reversible inhibition of prostaglandin synthesis and are well-known nephrotoxins.[51] Except in cases of massive overdose, NSAIDs produce renal dysfunction only in patients with coexisting renal hypoperfusion or vasoconstriction. Advanced age, hypovolemia, end-stage hepatic disease, heart failure, sepsis, chronic renal insufficiency, and major surgery are risk factors for development of NSAID-induced AKI.[52]

Myoglobin and hemoglobin are both capable of causing AKI in critically ill surgical patients. Myoglobin seems to be a more potent nephrotoxin than hemoglobin because it is more readily filtered at the glomerulus and can be reabsorbed by the renal tubules, where it chelates nitric oxide and thus induces medullary vasoconstriction and ischemia.[53] Hypovolemia and acidemia potentiate the toxicity of both pigments. Reduced intravascular volume causes a decrease in RBF and GFR, which results in a smaller volume of tubular fluid with a relatively higher concentration of pigment. There is also evidence suggesting that pigment precipitation inside the tubular lumen is enhanced under acidotic conditions and that tubular obstruction plays a role in the pathogenesis of AKI.[53,54]

Preventive treatment of pigment-induced AKI is directed at increasing RBF and tubular (urine) flow while correcting any existing acidosis. These goals may be accomplished by expanding the intravascular fluid volume with crystalloid infusion, stimulating an osmotic diuresis with mannitol, and increasing the urine pH with intravenous bicarbonate therapy.[55] Adequate systemic resuscitation from shock is a prerequisite if AKI is to be avoided, especially in massive crush injuries and electrical burns. Though high-quality evidence is lacking, forced mannitol-alkali diuresis is recommended as the second step in the preventive treatment of myoglobinuria, with urine flow rates of up to 300 mL/hour and a urine pH above 6.5 advocated for patients with massive crush injuries.[55]

The nephrotoxicity of volatile agents remains controversial. Inhalation anesthetics such as enflurane, isoflurane, and sevoflurane can generate free fluoride ions during their metabolism, which (when levels are >50 mm/L) may cause polyuric AKI by interfering with tubular concentrating ability. However, peak fluoride levels during administration of these agents seldom reach toxic levels, and there are few reports describing volatile agent–induced nephrotoxicity.[56] The potential of sevoflurane-induced nephrotoxicity has been related to the production of compound A during prolonged, low-fresh-gas-flow sevoflurane anesthesia.[57] Although there are insufficient data to conclude that sevoflurane-induced kidney injury occurs in the human population, even during low-gas-flow anesthesia, it is probably prudent to maintain a fresh gas flow of at least 2 L/min during sevoflurane anesthesia.[58]

Fluid resuscitation has also been associated with nephrotoxicity. Evidence of increased rates of renal replacement therapy in critically ill and septic patients receiving hydroxyethyl starches resulted in the elimination of these fluids from routine clinical practice.[59,60] In addition, excessive use of 0.9% "normal" saline (chloride liberal) was associated with higher risks of AKI and renal replacement therapy compared to a chloride-restrictive strategy in a prospective study of 1,543 critically ill patients.[61]

It appears that not only the type of fluid but also the amount of fluid can influence the development of AKI. It is well known that hypoperfusion of the kidney can lead to AKI; however, fluid overload can also worsen kidney injury through intra-abdominal hypertension and venous and interstitial congestion within the kidney.[62] In addition, a meta-analysis examining renal function in randomized controlled perioperative goal-directed therapy studies revealed a very modest role for fluid management in effective goal-directed therapy protocols, with the most effective reduction in AKI rates coming from significant inotropic intervention and less fluid resuscitation.[63] Thus, optimal fluid management in the perioperative period, in both the type and amount of fluid, has significant effects on renal function.

Chronic Kidney Disease

Patients with non–dialysis-dependent CKD are at increased risk of developing *end-stage renal disease* (ESRD). ESRD is the term used to describe a clinical syndrome characterized by renal dysfunction that would prove fatal without renal replacement therapy (i.e., dialysis). These patients have GFRs less than 25% of normal. Lesser degrees of renal dysfunction may be categorized as chronic renal insufficiency (25% to 40% of normal GFR) or decreased renal reserve (60% to 75% of normal GFR). Patients with decreased renal reserve are often asymptomatic and frequently do not have elevated blood levels of creatinine or urea. Established renal insufficiency results in patently abnormal serum creatinine and BUN values, but nocturia (due to reduced concentrating ability) may be the only symptom.

The *uremic syndrome* represents an extreme form of chronic renal failure, which occurs as the surviving nephron population and GFR decreases below 10% of normal. It results in inability of the kidney to perform its two major functions: regulation of the volume and composition of the extracellular fluid and excretion of waste products. Water balance in ESRD becomes difficult to manage because the number of functioning nephrons is too small either to concentrate or to fully dilute the urine. This results in failure both to conserve water and to excrete excess water. Patients with uremic syndrome often require frequent or continuous dialysis.

Life-threatening hyperkalemia may occur in CKD because of slower-than-normal potassium clearance. Situations predisposing patients with renal failure to hyperkalemia are presented in Table 50-2. Derangements in calcium, magnesium, and phosphorus metabolism are also commonly seen in CKD (Table 50-3).

Metabolic acidosis occurs in two forms in ESRD: a hyperchloremic, normal AG acidosis and a high AG acidosis from inability to excrete titratable acids. Both render patients susceptible to an endogenous acid load such as may occur in shock states, hypovolemia, or with an increase in catabolism.

Cardiovascular complications of the uremic syndrome are primarily due to volume overload, high renin–angiotensin activity, autonomic nervous system hyperactivity, acidosis, and electrolyte disturbances. Hypertension due to extracellular fluid volume expansion, autonomic factors, and hyperreninemia is an almost universal finding in ESRD. Together with volume overload, acidemia, anemia, and possibly the presence of high-flow arteriovenous fistulae created for dialysis access, hypertension may contribute to the development of myocardial dysfunction and heart failure. Pericarditis may occur secondary to uremia or dialysis, with pericardial tamponade developing in 20% of the latter group.[64] Pulmonary problems associated with CKD are limited to changes in lung water and control of ventilation. Pulmonary edema and restrictive pulmonary dysfunction are commonly seen in patients with renal failure and are usually responsive to dialysis. Hypervolemia, heart failure, reduced serum oncotic pressure, and increased pulmonary capillary permeability are relevant

Table 50-2 Factors Contributing to Hyperkalemia in Chronic Renal Failure

Potassium Intake
Increased dietary intake
Exogenous IV supplementation
Potassium salts of drugs
Sodium substitutes
Blood transfusion
Gastrointestinal hemorrhage

Potassium Release from Intracellular Stores
Increased catabolism, sepsis
Metabolic acidosis
β-Adrenergic blocking agents
Digitalis intoxication (Na–K-ATPase inhibition)
Insulin deficiency
Succinylcholine

Potassium Excretion
Acute decrease in GFR
Constipation
Potassium-sparing diuretics
Angiotensin-converting enzyme inhibitors (decreased aldosterone secretion)
Heparin (decreased aldosterone effect)

IV, intravenous; Na–K-ATPase, Na–K-adenosine triphosphatase; GFR, glomerular filtration rate.

Table 50-3   The Uremic Syndrome
Water Homeostasis
Extracellular fluid expansion
Electrolyte and Acid–Base
Hyponatremia
Hyperkalemia
Hypercalcemia or hypocalcemia
Hyperphosphatemia
Hypermagnesemia
Metabolic acidosis
Cardiovascular
Heart failure
Hypertension
Pericarditis
Myocardial dysfunction
Dysrhythmias
Respiratory
Pulmonary edema
Central hyperventilation
Hematologic
Anemia
Platelet hemostatic defect
Immunologic
Cell-mediated and humoral immunity defects
Gastrointestinal
Delayed gastric emptying, anorexia, nausea, vomiting, hiccups, upper gastrointestinal tract inflammation/hemorrhage
Neuromuscular
Encephalopathy, seizures, tremors, myoclonus
Sensory and motor polyneuropathy
Autonomic dysfunction, decreased baroreceptor responsiveness, dialysis-associated hypotension
Endocrine Metabolism
Renal osteodystrophy
↓ Glucose intolerance
Hypertriglyceridemia, ↑ atherosclerosis

factors in the development of pulmonary edema. Chronic metabolic acidosis may be responsible for the hyperventilation seen in patients with ESRD, but increased lung water and poor pulmonary compliance can also stimulate hyperventilation.

The anemia of CKD occurs as a result of reduced levels of erythropoietin, red cell damage, ongoing gastrointestinal blood loss, and iron or vitamin deficiencies. Platelet dysfunction may aggravate blood loss, but it is responsive to dialysis, cryoprecipitate administration, and desmopressin acetate (or 1-deamino-8-D-arginine vasopressin). Acquired defects in both cellular and humoral immunity probably account for the high prevalence of serious infections (60%) and high mortality from sepsis in CKD (30%).

Drug Prescribing in Renal Failure

If a drug depends solely on the kidney for clearance, then a simple approach to prescribing might involve a calculated percentage reduction in drug dosage that matches the reduction in GFR. Although GFR can be accurately measured, an estimated clearance derived from serum creatinine is usually adequate for these purposes. Unfortunately, clearance of most medications involves a more complex combination of both hepatic and renal functions, and drug level measurement or algorithms for specific drugs are often recommended.

AKI may affect absorption of a drug. For example, a reduced first-pass effect through the gastrointestinal tract and liver is associated with increased serum levels of oral β-blockers and opioids in patients with AKI. Also, an increase in the volume of distribution is seen in most patients with CKD owing to increased plasma volume and decreased plasma protein binding. However, plasma protein binding is highly variable, with acidic drugs having reduced binding and basic agents (e.g., amide local anesthetics) having increased binding. Importantly, for drugs with less binding, "normal" drug levels may reflect dangerously high active (unbound) drug levels. For example, therapeutic phenytoin levels are typically reported as being in the range of 10 to 20 mg/mL normally but 4 to 10 mg/mL in cases of renal failure. Finally, hepatic metabolism of drugs is difficult to predict in the setting of renal failure because some hepatic enzymes are inhibited whereas others are induced, and accompanying liver disorders may alter the relationship of drug clearance with GFR.

Anesthetic Agents in Renal Failure

With the exception of methoxyflurane and possibly enflurane, anesthetic agents do not directly cause renal dysfunction or interfere with the normal compensatory mechanisms activated by the stress response. The nephrotoxicity of methoxyflurane appears to be due to its metabolism, which results in release of the fluoride ions believed responsible for the renal injury.[65] It has been suggested that renal, not hepatic, metabolism of methoxyflurane may be responsible for generating fluoride ions locally that contribute to nephrotoxicity.[66] Enflurane nephrotoxicity may also occur[67] but is of minor clinical importance, even in patients with pre-existing renal dysfunction. Although direct anesthetic effects on the kidney are usually not harmful, indirect effects may combine with hypovolemia, shock, nephrotoxin exposure, or other renal vasoconstrictive states to produce renal dysfunction. If the chosen anesthetic technique causes a protracted reduction in cardiac output or sustained hypotension that coincides with a period of intense renal vasoconstriction, renal dysfunction or failure could result. This is true for either general or regional anesthesia. There are no comparative studies demonstrating superior renal protection or improved renal outcome with general versus regional anesthesia.

Significant renal impairment may affect the disposition, metabolism, and excretion of the commonly used anesthetic agents. Inhalation anesthetics are, of course, an exception to the rule that drugs with central nervous system activity (which generally are lipid soluble) must be converted to more hydrophilic compounds by the liver before being excreted by the kidney. The water-soluble metabolites of agents that are not inhaled may accumulate in renal failure and display prolonged pharmacodynamic effects if they possess even a small percentage of the pharmacologic activity of the parent drug. Drugs that are eliminated unchanged by the kidneys (e.g., certain nondepolarizing muscle relaxants, the cholinesterase inhibitors, many antibiotics, digoxin) have a prolonged elimination half-life when given to patients with kidney failure. Many drugs used in anesthesia are highly protein bound and may demonstrate exaggerated clinical effects when protein binding is reduced by uremia.

Induction Agents and Sedatives

Although now rarely used, sodium thiopental serves as a good illustrative example of how reduced protein binding in CKD may affect the clinical use of an anesthetic agent. Burch and Stanski[68] showed that the free fraction of an induction dose of thiopental is almost doubled in patients with renal failure. This accounts for the exaggerated clinical effects seen with thiopental in CKD patients and the substantial reduction in the necessary induction dose of this agent in uremic patients when compared with patients with normal renal function.

Ketamine is less extensively protein bound than thiopental, and renal failure appears to have less influence on its free fraction. Redistribution and hepatic metabolism are largely responsible for termination of the anesthetic effects, with less than 3% of the drug excreted unchanged in the urine. Norketamine, the major metabolite, has one-third the pharmacologic activity of the parent drug and is further metabolized before it is excreted by the kidney.[69]

Etomidate, although only 75% protein bound in normal patients, has a larger free fraction in patients with ESRD.[70] The decrease in protein binding does not seem to alter the clinical effects of etomidate anesthetic induction in patients with renal failure.

Propofol undergoes extensive rapid hepatic biotransformation to inactive metabolites that are renally excreted. Its pharmacokinetics appear to be unchanged in patients with renal failure,[71] and there are no reports of prolongation of its effects in ESRD.

The benzodiazepines, as a group, are extensively protein bound. CKD increases the free fraction of benzodiazepines in the plasma, and this potentiates their clinical effect. Certain benzodiazepine metabolites are pharmacologically active and have the potential to accumulate with repeated administration of the parent drug to anephric patients. For example, 60% to 80% of midazolam is excreted as its (active) α-hydroxy metabolite,[72] which accumulates during long-term infusions in patients with renal failure.[72] AKI appears to slow the plasma clearance of midazolam, whereas repeated diazepam or lorazepam administration in CKD may carry a risk of active metabolite-induced sedation. Alprazolam is one of the few drugs related to anesthesia practice that has undergone pharmacodynamic studies in patients with CKD. Schmith et al.[73] found that when decreased protein binding and increased free fraction of alprazolam are taken into account, patients with CKD are actually more sensitive to its sedative effects than healthy persons.

Dexmedetomidine is primarily metabolized in the liver. Volunteers with renal impairment receiving dexmedetomidine experienced a longer-lasting sedative effect than subjects with normal kidney function. The most likely explanation is that less protein binding of dexmedetomidine occurs in subjects with renal dysfunction.[74]

Opioids

Single-dose studies of the pharmacokinetics of morphine in renal failure demonstrate no alteration in its disposition. However, chronic administration results in accumulation of its 6-glucuronide metabolite, which has potent analgesic and sedative effects.[75] There is also a decrease in protein binding of morphine in ESRD, which mandates a reduction in its initial dose. Meperidine is remarkable for its neurotoxic, renally excreted metabolite (normeperidine) and is not recommended for use in patients with poor renal function. Hydromorphone is metabolized to hydromorphone-3-glucuronide, which is excreted by the kidneys. This active metabolite accumulates in patients with renal failure and may cause cognitive dysfunction and myoclonus.[76] Codeine also has the potential for causing prolonged narcosis in patients with renal failure and cannot be recommended for long-term use.[75]

Fentanyl appears to be a better choice of opioid for use in ESRD because of its lack of active metabolites, unchanged free fraction, and short redistribution phase.[77] Small-to-moderate doses, titrated to effect, are well tolerated by uremic patients.

Alfentanil has been shown to have reduced protein binding but no change in its elimination half-life or clearance in ESRD and is extensively metabolized to inactive compounds.[78] Therefore, caution should be exercised in administering a loading dose, but the total dose and infusion dose should be similar to those for patients with normal renal function. The free fraction of sufentanil is unchanged in ESRD; however, its pharmacokinetics are variable, and it has been reported to cause prolonged narcosis.[79]

Remifentanil is rapidly metabolized by blood and tissue esterases to a weakly active (about 4,600 times less potent) m-opioid agonist and renally excreted metabolite, remifentanil acid. Renal failure has no effect on the clearance of remifentanil, but elimination of the principal metabolite, remifentanil acid, is markedly reduced. However, the clinical implications of this metabolite are likely limited.[80]

Muscle Relaxants

Muscle relaxants are the most likely group of drugs used in anesthetic practice to produce prolonged effects in ESRD because of their dependence on renal excretion (Table 50-4). Only succinylcholine, atracurium, cis-atracurium, and mivacurium appear to have minimal renal excretion of the unchanged parent compound. Most nondepolarizing muscle relaxants must be either hepatically excreted or metabolized to inactive forms in order to terminate their activity. Some muscle relaxants have renally excreted active metabolites that may contribute to their prolonged duration of action in patients with ESRD. Although the following discussion focuses on the pharmacology of individual muscle relaxants, coexisting acidosis and electrolyte disturbances as well as drug therapy (e.g., aminoglycosides, diuretics, immunosuppressants, magnesium-containing antacids) may alter the pharmacodynamics of muscle relaxants in patients with renal failure.[81]

Succinylcholine has a long history of use in CKD that has been somewhat confused by conflicting reports of plasma cholinesterase activity in renal failure.[82,83] Provided the serum potassium concentration is not dangerously elevated, its use can be justified as part of a rapid-sequence anesthesia induction technique because its duration of action in ESRD is not significantly prolonged. However, use of a continuous succinylcholine infusion raises concerns because the major metabolite, succinylmonocholine, is weakly active and excreted by the kidney. The rise in serum potassium following succinylcholine administration (0.5 mEq/L in normal subjects) implies that levels of this electrolyte should be normalized to the best extent possible in patients with renal failure, but clinical experience suggests that the potassium rise following succinylcholine administration is usually well tolerated in patients with *chronically* elevated serum potassium levels. Use of the long-acting muscle relaxants doxacurium, pancuronium, and pipecuronium might also be questioned in patients with known renal insufficiency. In a single-dose study of doxacurium, Cook et al.[84] demonstrated an increased elimination half-life, reduced plasma clearance, and prolonged duration of effect in patients with renal failure. Similar findings have been reported for the pharmacokinetics of pipecuronium. Intermediate-acting muscle relaxants (atracurium, cis-atracurium, vecuronium, and

Table 50-4 Nondepolarizing Muscle Relaxants in Renal Failure

Drug	% Renal Excretion	Half-life (hr) Normal/ESRD	Renally Excreted Active Metabolite	Use in ESRD
D-Tubocurarine	60	1.4–2.2	–	Avoid
Metocurine	45–60	6/11.4	–	Avoid
Pancuronium	30	2.3/4–8	+	Avoid
Gallamine	>85	2.5/6–20	–	Avoid
Pipecuronium	37	1.8–2.3/4.4	+	Avoid
Doxacurium	30	1.7/3.7	–	Avoid
Vecuronium	30	0.9/1.4	+	Avoid infusion
Rocuronium	30	1.2–1.6/1.6–1.7	–	Variable duration
Atracurium/cis-atracurium	<5	0.3/0.4	–	Normal
Mivacurium	<7	2 min/2 min	–	Duration 1.5× normal
Rapacuronium	<12	0.5/0.5	++	Normal single dose

ESRD, end-stage renal disease.

rocuronium) have a distinct advantage in ESRD because of their shorter duration. The risk of a clinically significant prolonged block is much reduced. Atracurium and its derivative, cis-atracurium, undergo enzymatic ester hydrolysis and spontaneous nonenzymatic (Hoffman) degradation with minimal renal excretion of the parent compound. Their elimination half-life, clearance, and duration of action are not affected by renal failure,[85] nor have they been reported to cause prolonged clinical effects in ESRD. These characteristics strongly support their use in patients with renal disease. One potential concern is that an atracurium metabolite, laudanosine, may cause seizures in experimental animals and may accumulate with repeated dosing or continuous infusion.[86] However, this has not been realized in intensive care patients with renal failure receiving prolonged infusions of atracurium. Consistent with its greater potency and lower dosing requirements, cis-atracurium metabolism results in lower laudanosine blood levels than does atracurium in ESRD patients.

Initial reports suggested that the pharmacokinetics of vecuronium are unchanged in renal failure, but it has subsequently emerged that its duration of action is prolonged as a result of reduced plasma clearance and increased elimination half-life.[85] An intubating dose lasts approximately 50% longer in patients with ESRD.[87] In addition, the active metabolite, 3-desmethylvecuronium, accumulates in anephric patients receiving a continuous vecuronium infusion, producing a prolonged neuromuscular blockade.

Rocuronium has a pharmacokinetic profile in normal subjects similar to that of vecuronium.[88] Single-dose pharmacokinetic studies in patients with renal failure have reported conflicting results. Szenohradszky et al.[89] reported that renal failure increased the volume of distribution and elimination half-life of rocuronium but had no effect on its clearance. Cooper et al.[90] found that its clearance was reduced, and the duration of block was widely variable in patients with renal failure, although the mean duration of relaxation and spontaneous recovery was not statistically different from that in control subjects.

The short-acting muscle relaxant mivacurium is enzymatically eliminated by plasma pseudocholinesterase at a somewhat slower rate than succinylcholine. Low pseudocholinesterase activity correlates with slower recovery from a bolus dose of mivacurium in anephric patients.[83] The maintenance infusion dose has been reported to be both lower than[91] and similar[92] to that in normal control subjects.

The pharmacokinetics of the clinically available anticholinesterases are affected by renal failure.[93] They have a prolonged duration of action in ESRD because of their heavy reliance on renal excretion. The anticholinergic agents atropine and glycopyrrolate, used in conjunction with the anticholinesterases, are similarly excreted by the kidney. Therefore, no dosage alteration of the anticholinesterases is required when antagonizing neuromuscular blockade in patients with reduced renal function.

Sugammadex provides a novel approach to the reversal of muscle relaxants. This agent is a modified γ-cyclodextrin that encapsulates aminosteroidal neuromuscular blocking agents (e.g., rocuronium, vecuronium, pancuronium), which leads to a swift decline of free muscle relaxant in the plasma and rapid reversal.[94] A study has revealed that sugammadex-rocuronium complexes are cleared more slowly in patients with ESRD; however, reversal of neuromuscular blockade by sugammadex is still as timely and effective in these patients as in healthy controls.[95]

Diuretic Drugs: Effects and Mechanisms

When salt or water intake exceeds renal and extrarenal losses fluid overload results, leading to excess total body water and usually sodium. Fluid overload may be evenly distributed among the body compartments (e.g., congestive heart failure), or the interstitial space may be increased (i.e., edema) while the circulating blood volume may be normal or even decreased (e.g., posttraumatic or postoperative). Edema results when Starling forces favor passage of fluid into the interstitial space. Fluid overload due to a variety of chronic conditions (congestive heart failure, renal failure, or hepatic cirrhosis) may be first recognized during preoperative assessment and may require that elective surgery be delayed for treatment to reduce operative risk. The first line of therapy for fluid overload that includes all body compartments involves restriction of salt and water ingestion; however, diuretic therapy is often indicated.

The Physiologic Basis of Diuretic Action

Diuretics are typically grouped according to their site and mechanism of action (Fig. 50-5). Under normal conditions, kidney function assures that less than 1% of the filtered Na^+ load enters the urine (i.e., the FE_{Na} is <1%). The Na^+/K^+-ATPase pump on the basolateral surface (blood side) of renal tubular cells is primarily

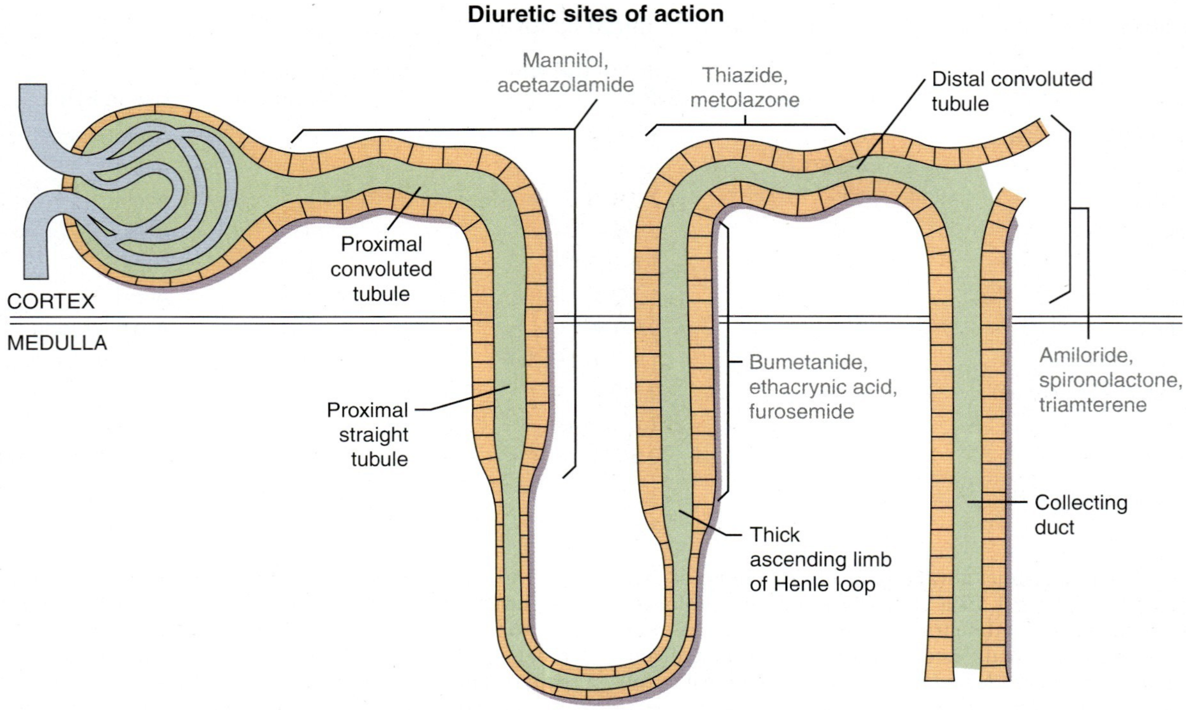

Figure 50-5 Site of action of commonly available diuretics. (Adapted with permission from Mende CW. Current issues in diuretic therapy. *Hosp Pract.* 1990;25[Suppl 1]:15.)

responsible for active pumping of Na^+ out of cells into blood in exchange for K^+. This pump causes a net movement of positive charge out of the cell (2 K^+ in, for every 3 Na^+ out) creating an electrochemical gradient that also causes Na^+ to enter the luminal (urine) side of the cell. Renal tubular cells in different portions of the nephron have different luminal "systems" to allow this Na^+ influx. These systems are the sites of action where the different diuretics work.

Proximal Tubule Diuretics

In the proximal tubule, a specialized luminal transporter exchanges protons (H^+) for sodium ions; the result is sodium reabsorption and acidification of the urine. The excreted H^+ combines with bicarbonate (HCO_3^-) in the tubule to form carbonic acid: $H^+ + HCO_3^- \rightarrow H_2CO_3$. Carbonic acid converts to water (H_2O) and carbon dioxide (CO_2) in a reaction catalyzed by carbonic anhydrase: $H_2CO_3 \rightarrow H_2O + CO_2$. The same enzyme, carbonic anhydrase, allows this reaction to occur in reverse within tubular cells, converting H_2CO_3 to HCO_3^- and H^+, generating more H^+ for countertransport with Na^+ and releasing bicarbonate, which passes into the circulation. Carbonic anhydrase inhibitors are drugs that inhibit this enzyme; the net effect of these agents is that sodium and bicarbonate, which would otherwise have been reabsorbed, remain in the urine and result in an alkaline diuresis.

Although patients may develop a metabolic acidosis when taking these agents, compensatory processes in the tubules accommodate the effects of carbonic anhydrase inhibitors so that their long-term use rarely causes this problem. However, these agents can be useful, for example, with contraction alkalosis from aggressive diuresis with loop diuretics (see later discussion); administration of these drugs can reduce $PaCO_2$ and improve PaO_2 for patients with little accompanying change in blood pH.

Specific uses for carbonic anhydrase inhibitors include treating mountain sickness and open-angle glaucoma and increasing respiratory drive in patients with central sleep apnea.[96,97]

Osmotic Diuretics

Substances such as mannitol that are freely filtered at the glomerulus but poorly reabsorbed by the renal tubule will cause an osmotic diuresis. In the water-permeable segments of the proximal tubule and loop of Henle, fluid reabsorption occurs, and filtered mannitol is concentrated. Eventually oncotic pressure in the tubular fluid resists further fluid reabsorption. Mannitol also draws water from cells into the plasma and effectively increases RBF.

Mannitol has been widely used for the treatment of increased intracranial pressure (see Chapter 35), but also as a strategy to prevent AKI. Although animal studies warranted hope, apart from AKI prophylaxis in kidney transplantation, there is no evidence to suggest mannitol is effective for either the prevention or treatment of AKI.[98,99] Even in cadaveric kidney transplant recipients, the data are modest to support a beneficial effect.[100] In a controlled trial of mannitol prophylaxis in patients with mild chronic renal failure, it was less effective than hydration alone for prevention of contrast-associated nephropathy.[99] Mannitol therapy is not without complications. As mannitol shifts water between fluid compartments, there can be effects on plasma and intracellular electrolyte concentrations, including hyponatremia and hypochloremia and intracellular increases in K^+ and H^+. Patients with normal renal function quickly correct these changes, but patients with renal impairment may develop significant circulatory overload with hemodilution and pulmonary edema, hyperkalemic metabolic acidosis, central nervous system depression, and even severe hyponatremia requiring urgent hemodialysis.[101]

Loop Diuretics

The electrochemical gradient established by the Na^+/K^+-ATPase in the loop of Henle drives the transport of one Na^+, one K^+, and two Cl^- ions into the tubule cells from the tubular fluid. Because the thick ascending limb segment of the loop of Henle is water impermeable, reabsorption of solute concentrates the interstitium and dilutes the tubular fluid. Loop diuretics, such as furosemide, bumetanide, and torsemide, directly inhibit the electroneutral transporter, preventing salt reabsorption from occurring. Because 25% of filtered NaCl is normally reabsorbed in the loop of Henle, loop diuretics cause a large salt load to pass to the distal convoluted tubule that is beyond the extra reserve of this tubular segment to reabsorb; consequently, large volumes of dilute urine ensue.

Loop diuretics are a first-line therapeutic modality for treatment of acute decompensated congestive heart failure. Although loop diuretics have no proven mortality benefit, they reduce left ventricular filling pressures and very effectively relieve the symptoms of congestion, pulmonary edema, extremity swelling, and hepatic congestion. Adverse effects of loop diuretics include hypokalemia, hyponatremia, and AKI. Heart failure patients with atrial fibrillation may also be prescribed digitalis, which in combination with furosemide can lead to hypokalemia-induced dysrhythmias. Loop diuretics, especially furosemide, may cause ototoxicity, particularly in patients with renal insufficiency.[102]

Distal Convoluted Tubule Diuretics

Distal convoluted tubule diuretics, such as thiazides (e.g., hydrochlorothiazide) and metolazone, act in the early part of this segment to block the NaCl cotransport mechanism across apical plasma membranes. Because the distal tubule is relatively water-impermeable, net NaCl absorption causes urinary dilution. Clinically, distal convoluted tubule diuretics are used for the treatment of hypertension (often as sole therapy) and volume overload disorders and to relieve the symptoms of edema in pregnancy.

Adverse reactions associated with distal tubule diuretics include electrolyte disturbances and volume depletion. Hydrochlorothiazide specifically has been associated with a number of other side effects including pancreatitis, jaundice, diarrhea, and aplastic anemia.

Distal (Collecting Duct) Acting Diuretics

Unlike in the more proximal nephron segments, NaCl absorption in the collecting duct cells is not electroneutral. That is, a net electrical gradient is maintained both by the Na^+/K^+-ATPase Na^+ ion channels and in the luminal membranes. As a result, the tubule lumen is negatively charged with respect to the blood. This normally causes K^+ secretion into the tubular lumen through K^+-specific ion channels. Distal K^+-sparing diuretics (e.g., amiloride and triamterene) directly inhibit luminal Na^+ entry, blocking this mechanism and resulting in a K^+-"sparing" effect. In addition, H^+ secretion is inhibited.

A second class of distal-acting, potassium-sparing diuretics is the competitive aldosterone antagonists (e.g., spironolactone and eplerenone). Ordinarily, the mineralocorticoid hormone aldosterone is released by the body in response to angiotensin II or hyperkalemia. Aldosterone normally stimulates Na^+ reabsorption and K^+ excretion by the collecting duct. Inhibition of the aldosterone effect by these drugs causes a mild natriuresis and K^+ retention. Distal K^+-sparing agents are used primarily for K^+-sparing diuresis (e.g., in patients with volume overload receiving digitalis or with hypokalemic alkalosis). In addition, these drugs are especially useful in treating disorders involving secondary hyperaldosteronism, such as cirrhosis with ascites.

Spironolactone treatment has been shown to improve survival with volume overload and left ventricular dysfunction or heart failure.[103] Hyperkalemia and hyperkalemic, hyperchloremic metabolic acidoses are significant complications of the injudicious use of spironolactone, triamterene, or amiloride.

Dopaminergic Agonists

Intravenous infusion of low-dose dopamine (1 to 3 mg/kg/min) is natriuretic owing primarily to a modest increase in the GFR and reduction in proximal Na^+ reabsorption mediated by dopamine type 1 (DA_1) receptors.[104] Fenoldopam is a selective DA_1 receptor agonist with little cardiac stimulation. At higher doses, the pressor response to dopamine is beneficial in patients with hypotension, but it has little or no renal effect in critically ill or septic patients.[104,105] The so-called "renal-dose" dopamine for the treatment of AKI, although widely used, has not been demonstrated to have significant renoprotective properties in numerous studies[106–108] and can cause worsened splanchnic oxygenation, impaired gastrointestinal function, impaired endocrine and immunologic system function, blunting of ventilatory drive, and increased risk of postcardiac surgery atrial fibrillation.[109–111]

High Renal Risk Surgical Procedures

Cardiac Surgery

Cardiac operations requiring CPB can be expected to result in AKI or renal failure in up to 7% of patients.[112,113] There are numerous risk factors associated with the development of postoperative AKI in this population (Fig. 50-6).[114] Interestingly, patients with preoperative CKD appear to tolerate surgery and CPB remarkably well.[115] Renal ischemia-reperfusion, inflammatory mediators, and toxin exposure are considered to be primary pathologic mechanisms involved in AKI. Renal risk factors contributing to each of these mechanisms include preoperative left ventricular dysfunction, duration of CPB, pulse pressure hypertension,[116] and aprotinin therapy.[117]

Although some retrospective studies suggest that "beating heart" off-pump coronary artery bypass grafting lowers renal risk compared with the traditional CPB techniques,[118] randomized studies have been inconclusive. However, despite the fact that pulsatile CPB suppresses plasma renin activity, postoperative renal function in patients with normal kidneys undergoing pulsatile or nonpulsatile CPB is equivalent.

Numerous agents have been used intraoperatively without success in attempts to protect the kidney during cardiac surgery. Mannitol use during CPB is partly aimed at avoiding hemoglobin-induced AKI by promoting urine flow and reducing renal cell swelling. Dopamine is infused at low doses (<5 mg/kg/min) as a renal vasodilator without benefit. Costa et al.[119] administered low-dose dopamine during CPB to patients with preoperative renal dysfunction and were able to induce a saluresis without affecting GFR or protecting the kidney from ischemic injury. Dopexamine improved CrCl and systemic oxygen delivery in one cardiac surgery study,[120] but a systemic review of 21 randomized controlled trials failed to confirm benefit.[121] Other studies examining the renal protective effects of fenoldapam, ANP, and insulin-like growth factor 1 in this population have not shown a consistently protective effect.

Noncardiac Surgery

Several common noncardiac surgical procedures can compromise previously normal renal function. Emergency surgery has been

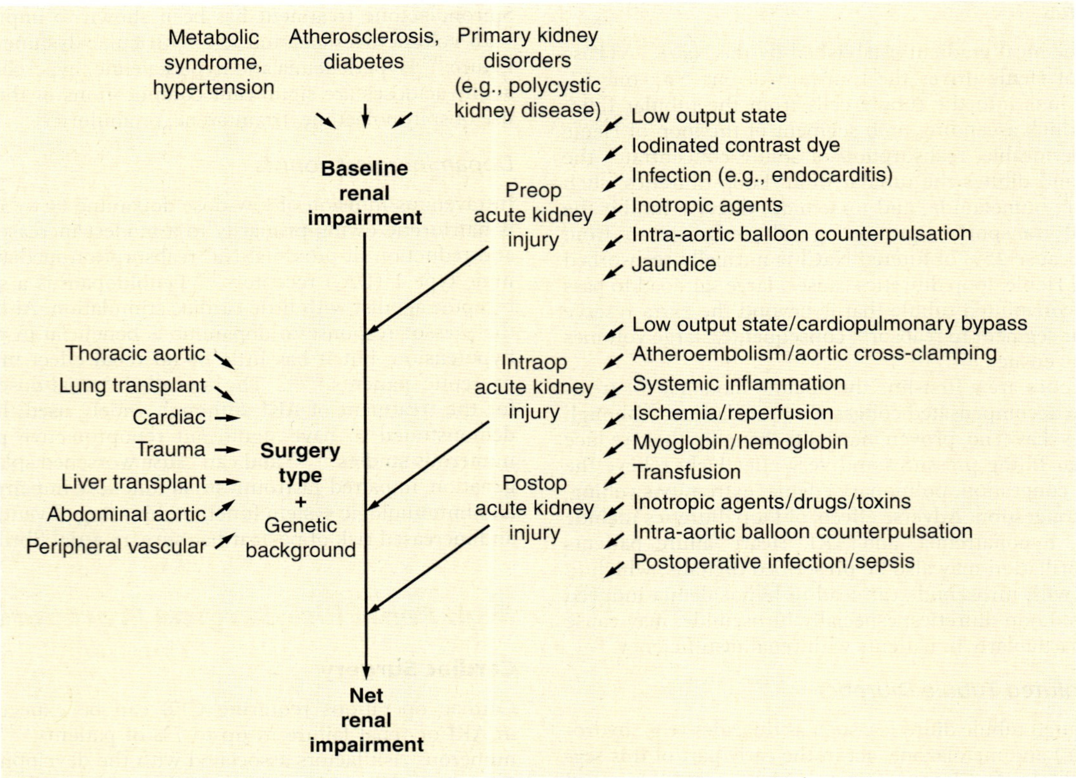

Figure 50-6 Clinical risk factors that predict perioperative acute kidney injury and renal dysfunction. Preop, preoperative; Intraop, intraoperative; Postop, postoperative. (Adapted with permission from Stafford-Smith M, Patel UD, Phillips-Bute BG, et al. Acute kidney injury and chronic kidney disease after cardiac surgery. *Adv Chronic Kidney Dis.* 2008;15:257–277.)

reported as a risk factor for AKI, with trauma surgery figuring as a prominent subgroup of emergency procedures.[122] ATN is the typical renal lesion associated with trauma, and it may be produced by a number of ischemic mechanisms. Most often, hypovolemic shock, pigmenturia, multiple organ failure, or exogenous nephrotoxins are responsible for sequential or simultaneous insults to the kidney. AKI that develops in the trauma patient may be characterized by an early oliguric picture related to inadequate volume resuscitation or by a later, sometimes nonoliguric syndrome associated with multiple organ failure, nephrotoxin exposure, or sepsis. The outcomes of these two posttraumatic AKI scenarios are dramatically different. The early form is associated with high mortality rates, whereas only 20% to 30% of patients will die in the case of nonoliguric AKI.[123] Not surprisingly, trauma victims with pre-existing renal insufficiency experience much higher mortality than previously healthy patients.[124]

Preventing AKI in patients presenting for emergency surgery begins with proper management of intravascular volume depletion and shock. Restoring euvolemia while maintaining cardiac output and systemic oxygen delivery is an important goal. Urine flow, once established, is maintained at 0.5 mL/kg/hr or more. Invasive hemodynamic monitoring may be required to guide intraoperative management of ongoing cardiovascular instability due to surgical manipulation, blood loss, fluid shifts, and anesthetic effects. Intraoperative transesophageal echocardiography provides excellent assessment of left and right ventricular functions as well as guidance of fluid resuscitation. Nephrotoxin exposure should be kept to a minimum in the unstable trauma victim. Radiocontrast media, NSAIDs, and myoglobin pose the greatest threat in this patient group. There is no place for either furosemide or mannitol therapy in the early, resuscitative phase of trauma management, except in the case of head injury with elevated intracranial pressure or when massive rhabdomyolysis is suspected.

Vascular surgery requiring aortic clamping has deleterious effects on renal function regardless of the level of clamp placement. Suprarenal clamping results in an attenuated ATN-like lesion.[125] Infrarenal clamping causes a smaller, short-lived reduction in GFR and is associated with a lower risk of AKI, whereas surgery involving the thoracic aorta has a 25% incidence of AKI.[126] Two major predictors of AKI following aortic surgery are pre-existing renal dysfunction and perioperative hemodynamic instability.[127] Olsen et al.[128] reported in a large series of patients undergoing abdominal aortic aneurysm repair that the overall incidence of AKI was 12%. Patients who had emergency surgery for ruptured aneurysm had a very high incidence of hemodynamic instability, and AKI developed in 26%; in contrast, elective aortic surgery was associated with good hemodynamic control and a 4% incidence of renal failure. Atheromatous renal artery emboli and prolonged aortic clamp time may contribute to ischemic renal injury in these patients.

The endovascular approach (endostent) to major aortic surgery has gained popularity.[129] The etiology of AKI after endovascular and open repair of aortic aneurysm is multifactorial (renal ischemia, atheroembolism, hemodynamic instability). Although hemodynamic changes during endovascular procedures on the aorta may be less dramatic than those accompanying open repair, the prevalence of renal complications appears to be similar. During endovascular procedures, patients may be exposed to substantial amounts of radiocontrast dye, which can exacerbate postoperative renal dysfunction, especially in those with pre-existing renal insufficiency. The long-term incidence of renal insufficiency/failure (followed up to 24 months postoperatively) is similar after endovascular and open repair of aortic aneurysm. It is thus important that before endovascular procedures, patients are adequately hydrated, and the total dose of radiocontrast dye is limited.

Most efforts to preserve renal function in aortic surgery have centered on diuretic and renal vasodilator therapies, although a large body of evidence no longer supports the use of either intravenous mannitol or dopamine to prevent AKI in this setting. Indeed, a clinical study of infrarenal aortic clamping found that combined mannitol and low-dose dopamine treatment was no more effective in preventing AKI than volume expansion with saline. Although increased urine flow rate is a consistent finding with low-dose infusion of dopamine, there is no evidence in collective analysis of numerous randomized studies that this is associated with preservation of renal function during aortic surgery. Other agents are being investigated for use as renoprotective drugs. Nifedipine attenuated a postoperative decrease in GFR in a small, placebo-controlled study of aortic surgery patients.[130] Insulin-like growth factor 1 has been shown to speed healing in experimental ischemic AKI[131] and to improve renal function in patients with ESRD[132] and in those undergoing aortic or renal artery surgery.[133] A synthetic form of ANP may be useful in managing established oliguric acute renal failure,[134] but it has not been used prophylactically in high-risk surgical patients. Fenoldopam, a selective dopamine-1 receptor agonist, showed some promise as a renal protective agent but has not been tested in large multicenter prevention trials in the perioperative setting. A new generation of early biomarker tests may soon be available, capable of recognizing AKI much earlier than possible with accumulation of serum creatinine. The hope is that earlier AKI recognition will improve the effectiveness of current interventions.

As previously discussed, patients with hepatic failure or cholestatic jaundice are particularly susceptible to AKI. When the serum conjugated bilirubin exceeds 8 mg/dL, endotoxins from the gastrointestinal tract are absorbed into the portal circulation, causing intense renal vasoconstriction. Intravenous mannitol and/or oral administration of bile salts in the preoperative period may limit renal dysfunction in patients with cholestatic jaundice. This phenomenon may contribute to the high incidence of AKI after liver transplantation and biliary surgery. AKI occurs in up to two-thirds of liver transplant recipients.[135] Many liver transplant candidates have overt hepatorenal syndrome, renal dysfunction, and presumably underlying renal vasoconstriction. When such patients are exposed to intraoperative hemodynamic instability, massive transfusion, and nephrotoxins, AKI frequently follows.[136]

Anesthetic Considerations for Urologic Procedures

A review of urologic surgical procedures follows, including sections on nephrectomy, cystectomy, prostatectomy, TUR procedures, and therapies for urolithiasis. For each section, general disease principles and treatment rationales are briefly discussed, perioperative management and potential complications reviewed, and then important aspects related to specific procedures within the section highlighted (e.g., simple versus radical nephrectomy). Selected additional topics are outlined at the end of the section. Notably, a deliberate approach has been taken to minimize repetition by referring the reader to other chapter sections whenever appropriate.

Nephrectomy

Nephrectomy procedures involve partial, radical, or simple resection of the kidney. Each year in the United States, there are approximately 46,000 nephrectomies for benign or malignant disease, and an additional 5,500 donor surgeries for renal transplant. Although radical nephrectomy is the standard for resectable kidney cancer, simple nephrectomy is typical for benign disease. Some kidney tumors invade the renal vein, extending as far as the inferior vena cava (IVC) or right atrium; these tumors require additional procedures to safely retrieve their intravascular component. Kidney transplant donor nephrectomy involves simple nephrectomy with measures to avoid organ trauma and optimize graft function. The so-called nephron-sparing or partial nephrectomy is indicated for limited benign disease but increasingly is being considered for wider indications, including selected cancerous lesions.

The approach and incision for nephrectomy are based on surgical priorities and surgeon preference. Retroperitoneal approaches require a flank incision and lateral decubitus positioning with flank extension (Fig. 50-7), allowing access to the kidney with avoidance of the peritoneal cavity. This approach has obvious advantages for treatment of infection but also simplifies procedures in those with prior abdominal surgery or obesity. Difficulties with the retroperitoneal approach include access to the vena cava, risk of unintentional pneumothorax, and the adverse effects of lateral decubitus position and flank extension on respiratory vital capacity, which can be reduced up to 20% (see Chapter 29).

Anterior approaches to nephrectomy involve supine positioning and breach of the peritoneal cavity through midline, subcostal, or thoracoabdominal incisions that provide direct access to both the kidney and major vascular structures. Although transperitoneal approaches add the risk of visceral injury and peritonitis, they improve access to the renal pedicle (e.g., trauma, hemorrhage) with best access to both kidneys being through midline incisions (e.g., bilateral nephrectomy for end-stage polycystic kidney disease). The thoracoabdominal approach enters both the peritoneal and pleural spaces and rarely may require single-lung ventilation.

In recent years, *laparoscopic* retro- and transperitoneal approaches to nephrectomy have surpassed their open equivalents in popularity, particularly for simple and donor procedures, but these techniques are even being used for nephron-sparing partial nephrectomy. Other recent innovations include robotic-assisted, single-port laparoscopic, and even transvaginal minimally invasive nephrectomies.

Preoperative Considerations

Recruits for donor nephrectomy surgery are typically healthy individuals; however, perioperative risk for other nephrectomy procedures often relates to the indication for surgery. Although smoking and obesity are the most important risk factors for renal cancer, many other cardiovascular risk factors are also strongly associated with renal cancer risk including advanced age, male gender, chronic renal disease or ESRD, and hypertension. Hence, protocols for assessment and management of perioperative cardiac risk are particularly relevant to nephrectomy surgery.[137]

Simple nephrectomy for infectious indications is uncommon but most often involves diabetic patients and can be grouped into two categories. Elective procedures involve irreversible kidney damage due to chronic pyelonephritis (e.g., xanthogranulomatous).[138] In contrast, emergent procedures are associated with very high mortality rates (up to 43%) and generally involve

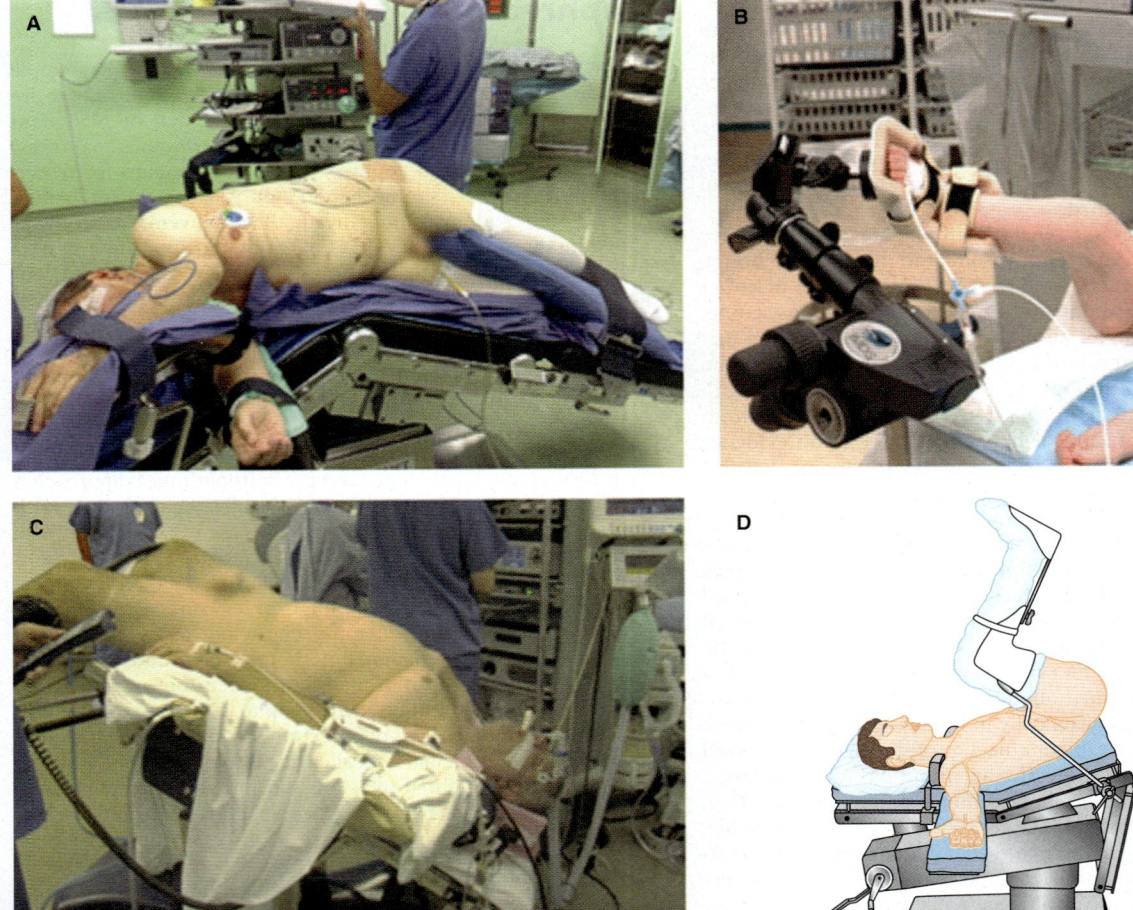

Figure 50-7 Common positioning options for urologic surgery include right lateral decubitus with waist extension (**A**), lithotomy (**B**), supine with steep (30 to 45 degrees) Trendelenburg (**C**), and exaggerated lithotomy (**D**). (**A**, reproduced with permission from http://www.opitek.dk/en/products/pedistirrup.)

critically ill patients with acute emphysematous pyelonephritis unresponsive to antibiotics.

Several hereditary conditions that are associated with kidney cancer also have attributes that must be considered in anesthetic planning;[139] for example, individuals with Birt–Hogg–Dubé syndrome have pulmonary cysts, which increase the risk of intraoperative spontaneous pneumothorax, whereas patients with von Hippel–Lindau syndrome, the commonest of these disorders, have high rates of pheochromocytoma and neuroendocrine tumors.

Ten to forty percent of patients presenting with renal cancer have associated paraneoplastic syndromes.[140] Beyond fever, cachexia, and weight loss, these subdivide into endocrine and nonendocrine categories. Tumor-related endocrine effects include hypercalcemia (PTH-like effects), hypertension (renin), anemia/polycythemia (erythropoietin), nonmetastatic hepatic dysfunction (Stauffer syndrome), galactorrhea, Cushing syndrome, and ectopic insulin and glucagon production, whereas nonendocrine effects include amyloidosis, neuromyopathies, vasculopathy, nephropathy, coagulopathy, and elevated prostaglandin levels. Of renal cancers presenting with hypercalcemia, 50% are paraneoplastic in origin. Renal tumors may also be associated with a hypercoagulable state; sudden intraoperative clot formation has been reported.[141]

As for most major urologic surgeries, other investigations for nephrectomy include routine ECG, chest x-ray, complete blood cell count, electrolyte profile with serum BUN and creatinine values, liver function tests, serum calcium assessment, coagulation testing, and urine analysis. Although normal serum creatinine level and evidence of contralateral function by means of intravenous pyelography are sometimes considered sufficient assessment to predict adequate postoperative renal function, a noninvasive differential renal scan (iodine-131 or technetium-99m computerized isotope renograph) is often performed for more precise prediction of postoperative GFR.

Urologic surgery patients often present with additional disease workup that can provide a wealth of information beyond routine studies and assessment of their urinary tract. Abdominal computed tomography (CT) scans detail tumor size and location and invasion of the renal collecting system or perirenal fat, whereas magnetic resonance imaging is most valuable to assess for vena caval and/or cardiac chamber involvement.

Standard recommended preoperative management of chronic drug therapies is all that is necessary for most nephrectomy procedures, although dose adjustment may be considered if significant changes in renal function are anticipated.

Intraoperative Considerations

Preparation for even the most straightforward nephrectomy surgery demands sufficient monitoring and vascular access to respond to complications, most notably significant hemorrhage, an uncommon but ever-present risk in such procedures. Beyond standard monitoring (e.g., American Society of Anesthesiologists guidelines) and two large-bore peripheral intravenous catheters, requirements for intravascular access and additional monitoring are dictated by patient condition and complexity of the procedure and may include a peripheral intra-arterial catheter for continuous blood pressure recording and repeated blood gas assessment and sometimes central venous access.

Although central venous line placement is not essential for most nephrectomy surgeries, patient and procedural factors such as comorbidities (e.g., cardiac history) and bleeding risk (e.g., tumor extension into venous structures) may warrant such access. If placement of a central venous catheter is deemed necessary, selection of the side *ipsilateral* to the nephrectomy surgery for subclavian or internal jugular central venous puncture should be considered to minimize the risk of bilateral pneumothorax.

Assessment of infection, bony metastases, and bleeding risk may influence the decision to include neuraxial procedures in the anesthesia plan. Sometimes spinal imaging from CT and magnetic resonance imaging scans can provide added detail useful when contemplating epidural catheter placement. If a lumbar or thoracic epidural catheter is placed, this is usually done prior to anesthesia induction to allow for a meaningful test dose sequence and to facilitate preincision administration of epidural opiates. Varied opinions regarding intraoperative local anesthetic dosing of the epidural catheter involve concerns over hemodynamic stability and the likelihood of significant blood loss during the procedure.

Neuraxial injection or catheter placement prior to anesthesia induction (e.g., epidural catheter insertion) can be followed by placement of intra-arterial and central venous access after anesthesia induction in most cases. Bladder catheter placement is essential for all nephrectomy procedures; urinary output monitoring provides information on intravascular volume status in the absence of central venous pressure monitoring, avoids the possibility of urinary retention, and also provides valuable information postoperatively regarding renal function, bleeding sources, and the possibility of clot-related urinary tract obstruction. Noninvasive cardiac output monitoring (e.g., esophageal Doppler, LiDCO [LiDCO Group plc, London, UK], noninvasive cardiac output) techniques may be useful in selected patients.

Standard preanesthesia induction considerations include postoperative planning (e.g., postanesthesia care unit versus stepdown versus intensive care unit disposition) and administration of intravenous antibiotic prophylaxis within 1 hour prior to surgical incision. Plans for postoperative analgesia strategy may dictate disposition particularly to involve a care team capable of recognizing and treating potential complications of the various analgesia strategies.

Anesthesia induction agent selection to achieve hypnosis, paralysis, and blunting of the hemodynamic intubation response should be matched to any use of regional anesthesia, the anticipated duration of the procedure, and the patient's renal function. Intraoperative and postoperative pain management can be accomplished by intravenous or other opioid therapies such as patient-controlled analgesia or neuraxial analgesia. Continuous epidural analgesia attenuates the neuroendocrine response but may also improve postoperative ventilatory mechanics and resolve ileus sooner, and has been associated with improved survival in intermediate- to high-risk noncardiac surgery.[142]

Potential intraoperative complications include injury to major blood vessels (e.g., IVC, aorta) or gastrointestinal organs (e.g., spleen, liver, pancreas) and unrecognized entry into the pleural space with resultant pneumothorax. Complications associated with hemorrhage during nephrectomy are uncommon but mandate preparatory steps beyond monitoring and generous intravenous access. Confirmation that blood products are present or readily available should occur immediately prior to surgery. Routine fluid and patient warming technology, availability of colloid volume expanders, and even a rapid transfusion device for selected cases should also be considered. Because unexplained changes in pulmonary mechanics or hypotension during a nephrectomy procedure may reflect diaphragmatic injury and pneumothorax, such changes should be discussed with the surgeon to facilitate prompt intervention. This may require direct repair of a rent in the diaphragm as well as needle decompression of a pneumothorax and chest tube insertion.

Particularly in the setting of limited renal reserve, in addition to consideration of transfusion triggers and strict avoidance of unjustifiable blood product administration, a note of caution is warranted regarding the potential for resuscitation "overshoot" in response to acute hemorrhage. Strict attention to appropriate monitors during fluid resuscitation and appropriate use of arterial blood gas assessment, assisted by good communication with the surgeon, will help avoid the risk of pulmonary edema from fluid overload.

Postoperative Considerations

Up to 20% of patients undergoing nephrectomy develop postoperative complications, and operative mortality rates following radical nephrectomy are as high as 2%. Added to standard concerns, such as hemorrhage and unrecognized visceral injury, are atelectasis, ileus, superficial and deep wound infections, temporary or permanent renal failure, and incisional hernia. The most common radical nephrectomy complications are adjacent organ (4% bowel, spleen, liver, diaphragm, or pancreas) and vascular injury (2%). Overall complication rates are similar whether an open or laparoscopic approach is used.[143-145] Bleeding requiring transfusion occurs in up to 5.7% of all cases.[146-148] Other less common major complications include myocardial infarction, congestive heart failure, pulmonary embolism, cerebrovascular accident, pneumonia, and thrombophlebitis.

A logical expectation of nephrectomy surgery would be the need to adjust postoperative dosing of drug therapies to accommodate the anticipated decrease in GFR associated with an approximate 50% loss of kidney tissue. Although a drop in GFR can be anticipated, interestingly, adaptation of the remaining kidney usually results in a modest 25% decline postoperatively.

The pain of nephrectomy, laparoscopic or open, is significant. Analgesia can be achieved with epidural or spinal analgesia strategies, systemic opioids, and nonopioid adjuncts. Recent findings of improved recovery using epidural analgesia for major abdominal surgeries[149] have not been assessed specifically for nephrectomy surgery.

Specific Procedures

Simple and Donor Nephrectomies

Simple nephrectomy is sufficient intervention for irreversible nonmalignant disease such as untreatable infection, unsalvageable kidney trauma, or a nonfunctioning kidney due to calculi or hypertensive disease. In up to 86% of patients with hypertension that is presumed to be renovascular in origin with noncorrectable unilateral renal artery disease, hypertension control improves after simple nephrectomy.

During donor procedures, several steps are added to simple nephrectomy, including administration of drugs intravenously just prior to explant to achieve low-level anticoagulation (e.g., 3,000-USP heparin units) and forced diuresis (e.g., mannitol, 12.5 g; furosemide, 40 mg), extension of (laparoscopic) incisions to ensure atraumatic organ extraction, and postharvest protamine administration. Procured organs are infused with cold preservative (e.g., University of Wisconsin or histidine–tryptophan–ketoglutarate solutions) and stored on ice and/or cold machine perfused. Just over one-third of renal transplants in the United States are from living donors, and, compared to cadavers, living kidney donation is associated with improved short- and long-term outcomes (i.e., recipient and graft survival).

Radical Nephrectomy

Renal cell carcinoma is the main indication for radical nephrectomy and accounts for 90% to 95% of kidney neoplasms and 3% of all malignancies in adults. With the exception of hereditary syndromes with high tumor rates (see earlier), a positive family history incurs a two- to threefold increased risk of kidney cancer, but such cases constitute only 2% of radical nephrectomies. Hematuria, a palpable mass, and flank pain compose the classic triad at presentation, but renal tumors are more often (approximately 72%) diagnosed incidentally during workup for other nonurologic problems. Occasionally, tumors are discovered owing to signs or symptoms of vena caval involvement such as dilated abdominal veins, (left) varicocele, lower extremity edema, or pulmonary embolism. Symptomatic tumors usually reflect more advanced disease and are more often associated with metastasis and a poor prognosis. Transitional cell cancers of the upper urothelial tract (ureters, renal pelvis) are also treated by radical nephrectomy with resection of the associated ureter, including a cuff of bladder tissue. Up to one-third of kidney cancer patients have metastases at diagnosis, but many are still candidates for surgery.

Radical nephrectomy involves renal artery and vein ligation with subsequent removal *en bloc* of the kidney, perinephric fat, Gerota fascia, proximal ureter, and often the adjacent adrenal gland. Lymph node dissection is then performed from the diaphragm to the aortic bifurcation. Most renal cancers stay within Gerota fascia and can be completely removed, but a disappointing 20% to 30% of patients with successful surgery still have their disease return. Although radical nephrectomy is standard for central and large tumors, the value of nephron-sparing partial nephrectomy for early-stage and small renal cell cancers is being evaluated. Although nonsurgical therapies are available, renal cell cancers are resistant to radiation and chemotherapy. Blood loss during radical nephrectomy is highly dependent on the location and extent of the tumor. Laparoscopic innovations have reduced bleeding for all types of nephrectomy surgeries.

Radical Nephrectomy with Inferior Vena Cava Tumor Thrombus

Between 4% and 10% of patients with renal cell carcinoma have the so-called tumor thrombus extension beyond the kidney, either limited to the renal vein or extending into the IVC. Although often restricted to the vessel lumen, the thrombus may become adherent to the vessel wall,[150] and right atrial involvement is present in 1% of cases. Radical nephrectomy procedures involving resection of tumor thrombus are particularly challenging owing to their risk of sudden major bleeding and potential for acute hemodynamic instability (e.g., inferior vena cava clamping or tumor pulmonary embolism).

Renal tumors with IVC thrombus are classified by the extent of tumor thrombus within the IVC and right atrium (levels I to IV; Fig. 50-8) and require different procedures in addition to radical nephrectomy.[151] In general, thrombus extraction can occur with simple proximal and distal caval control alone for tumors that go no further than the infrahepatic IVC. As thrombus extends into the intrahepatic IVC or higher, isolating the vessel to extract the thrombus becomes more challenging and ultimately can only be achieved safely using CPB with or without aortic cross-clamping and cardiac arrest. In addition to sternotomy incision, such procedures require standard heparin anticoagulation and employ an added circuit venous line filter to trap tumor fragments (Fig. 50-8). Other interventions used at some institutions in the treatment of renal tumor caval thrombus include venovenous bypass, inferior vena cava filter insertion, and even deep hypothermic circulatory arrest.

Appropriate considerations when monitoring these complex procedures include radial arterial catheterization, central venous or pulmonary artery catheter placement, and intraoperative transesophageal echocardiography (Fig. 50-8). In cases where supradiaphragmatic tumor thrombus is present, placement of a pulmonary artery catheter prior to thrombus resection is contraindicated owing to risk of embolization of tumor fragments. If the thrombus extends into the suprahepatic IVC, hepatic mobilization with the Pringle maneuver (clamping of the hepatoduodenal ligament to interrupt blood flow through the hepatic artery and portal vein) may be required, generally for less than 30 minutes.[152] Additional preparation includes all steps standard for procedures involving CPB (see Chapter 39), including large-bore peripheral intravenous access, vasoactive infusions, fluid, and blood products. Preoperative therapeutic embolization of the tumor is sometimes also used in cases of arterial thrombus or extensive parasitic vessel formation or when there is anticipated difficulty in isolating the renal artery. Despite the potential for significant blood loss, cell saver technology use is discouraged owing to the potential for returning tumor cells to the circulation.

Nephron-sparing Partial Nephrectomy

Minimizing unnecessary loss of healthy tissue is a logical part of surgical planning for any kidney resection. Partial nephrectomy is often sufficient for benign tumors, but this procedure is also becoming an alternate to radical nephrectomy for some cancerous renal cell tumors, particularly when renal parenchyma must be preserved; examples include bilateral tumors, CKD, tumors in a single remaining kidney, or when the contralateral kidney is at risk for future disease or tumor. Even when the contralateral kidney is normal, studies are now demonstrating comparable long-term results with nephron-sparing partial nephrectomy procedures as with radical nephrectomy for patients with a single, localized small tumor (<4 cm) or even medium-sized (<7 cm) peripherally located tumors. Limitations of partial nephrectomy include a higher perioperative risk of bleeding and urine leak, and a local tumor recurrence rate of 1% to 6%.

Laparoscopic and Robotic Nephrectomies

Laparoscopic and robotic techniques can be applied to retroperitoneal and transperitoneal approaches and all types of nephrectomies (i.e., radical, simple, or partial). Compared to open

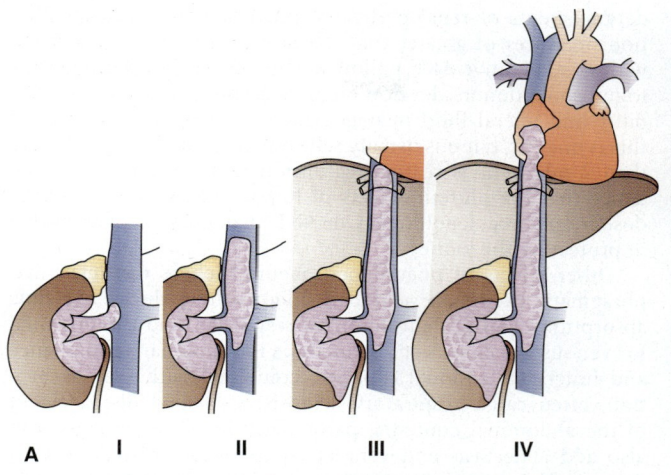
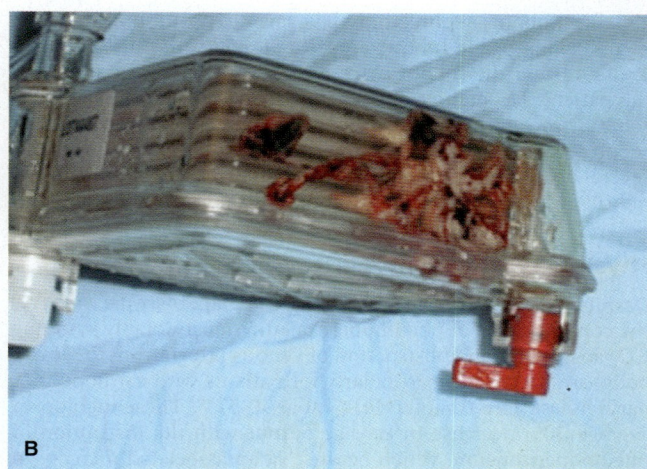
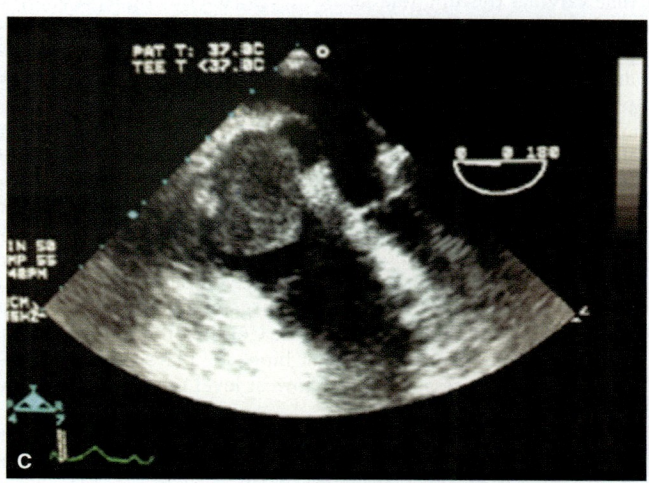

Figure 50-8 Radical nephrectomy with inferior vena cava thrombus removal for renal cell carcinoma is a major operative procedure. **A:** Surgical complexity is predicted by the extent of intravascular tumor thrombus, as classified by the most proximal level of tumor extension (levels I to IV). **B:** Evidence of thrombus emboli in the venous filter following cardiopulmonary bypass highlights the friability of intravascular renal cell carcinoma thrombus. **C:** Intraoperative transesophageal echocardiography demonstrates right atrial extension of a renal cell tumor. (**A,** Adapted with permission from Nesbitt JC, Soltero ER, Dinney CP, et al. Surgical management of renal cell carcinoma with inferior vena cava tumor thrombus. *Ann Thorac Surg.* 1997;63:1592–1600.)

approaches, these minimally invasive strategies employ access through small airtight ports. Insufflation of carbon dioxide into the peritoneal cavity or retroperitoneal space is used to separate structures and enhance visibility. In recent years, laparoscopic techniques have surpassed open nephrectomies in popularity, particularly for simple and radical procedures. Laparoscopic approaches to radical nephrectomy are even being successfully employed in the treatment of locally invasive kidney cancer. Laparoscopic partial nephrectomy is technically more demanding than its open counterpart and currently involves temporary clamping of the renal hilum to optimize visibility during excision and minimize blood loss. The warm ischemic time related to clamping can cause AKI, particularly if the duration exceeds 30 minutes.[153,154]

Some studies have reported comparisons of equivalent open and laparoscopic procedures. Laparoscopic radical nephrectomy for cancer involves smaller incisions, less blood loss, decreased postoperative analgesic requirement, shorter hospital stay and convalescent period, and similar long-term outcomes when compared with open radical nephrectomy.[155,156] Likewise, laparoscopic nephron-sparing partial nephrectomy results in less bleeding and a shorter hospital stay and for selected tumors has 5- and 10-year outcomes similar to those of open partial nephrectomy.[157,158] Laparoscopic donor nephrectomy has no adverse effects on the success of kidney transplant but is associated with less pain and analgesic requirement, faster hospital discharge, and better quality of life compared with open donor nephrectomy.[159] Institutional experience with laparoscopic and robotic assistance with nephrectomy procedures may influence anesthetic planning and the perceived need for invasive procedures (e.g., central venous cannulation).

Traditional open nephrectomy is associated with a significant incidence of chronic pain ranging from 5% to 26%.[160,161] The hope is that laparoscopic approaches will reduce the incidence of chronic pain syndromes. The perceived differences between laparoscopic and open nephrectomy procedures have influenced clinical practice, including anesthesia planning for postoperative pain management. Compared to open nephrectomy, the reduced pain and shorter recovery times have meant that epidural anesthesia is less likely to be selected for laparoscopic approaches, with postoperative pain control for these procedures provided by a multimodal strategy involving opiates and appropriate nonopioid adjuncts. NSAIDs are used rarely to avoid their potential nephrotoxic effects. Recent small studies have reported good success with continuous local anesthetic infusions via catheters placed in the rectus and retroperitoneal sheaths intraoperatively (across the intercostal, ilioinguinal, and iliohypogastric nerves). Benefits include reduction of the following: pain levels, opioid requirements, nausea, time to recovery and discharge, and cost.[162,163]

Robotic approaches to nephrectomy surgery are beginning to be employed but have very similar considerations to laparoscopic nephrectomy in terms of issues such as pneumoperitoneum.

Notably, robotic nephrectomy has specific positioning requirements owing to the robotic equipment, and care must be taken to assure that the robotic arms do not cause pressure injury to the patient. Depending on the experience of the surgical team, robotic procedures may also take more time. Notably, the role of robotic assistance is being similarly explored and developed for several other major urologic surgeries (e.g., partial nephrectomy, radical cystectomy, pyeloplasty, and radical cystectomy).[164]

Physiology of Pneumoperitoneum

Despite potential surgical advantages of laparoscopic surgery, the consequences of pneumoperitoneum, most notably systemic CO_2 absorption and obstruction of venous return from the lower body, are important, particularly for patients with cardiopulmonary disease (see Chapter 44) (Table 50-5).[165] These include an average 30% decrease in cardiac output with the institution of pneumoperitoneum, which because of an associated increase in systemic vascular resistance (afterload), is often accompanied by little change or even an increase (up to 16%) in mean arterial blood pressure. Systemic vascular resistance and cardiac output usually return to near-normal values over the 10 minutes following institution of pneumoperitoneum. Preoperative fluid loading with additional preinduction colloid boluses before institution of pneumoperitoneum results in higher stroke volume and urine output compared to standard intraoperative fluid regimens, but studies are lacking regarding any evidence of improved outcome using this strategy.[166]

A strategy involving hydration and limiting insufflation pressures to below 12 mmHg is advocated. Presumably related to derangements of renal perfusion, pneumoperitoneum insufflation pressures of greater than 15 mmHg have been associated with postoperative AKI. Following laparoscopic donor nephrectomy, some donors develop oliguria despite hemodynamic stability and liberal fluid management strategies. The etiology of this is unclear, but it is usually self-limited. Urine output of more than 2 mL/kg/hr is reassuring, although there is no clear evidence that the diuretic effects of furosemide, mannitol, "renal dose" dopamine, fenoldopam, or ANP analogues are of any value in protecting the kidney.[167]

Other effects of pneumoperitoneum include restricted diaphragmatic excursion, acid–base abnormalities due to systemic absorption of CO_2, neurohumoral responses, and the potential for venous gas embolism. Reductions in pulmonary compliance and functional residual capacity, combined with CO_2 absorption, often cause respiratory acidosis. Cephalad displacement of the abdominal contents, particularly in obese patients, can also add atelectasis and ventilation–perfusion mismatch. Cardiac valvular dysfunction has been reported during laparoscopic nephrectomy,[168] and cardiac ischemia can develop in at-risk patients with coronary artery disease. There is also an immediate increase in intracranial pressure with the institution of the pneumoperitoneum.

Hemodynamic instability or hypoxia that occurs with CO_2 insufflation owing to the abovementioned perturbations must be addressed, and a small number of patients will require conversion to an open surgical approach. However, despite the numerous disturbances, a majority of patients can be safely managed through episodes of pneumoperitoneum with appropriate circulatory support, thoughtful ventilator management, and good communication between surgeon and anesthesiologist that includes a willingness to adjust CO_2 insufflation pressures. Notably, adequate neuromuscular blockade plays a role in keeping insufflation pressures at the lowest level required to achieve optimal surgical exposure.

Offsetting advantages of laparoscopic approaches are risks also seen in settings other than nephrectomy, including trauma during trocar placement (~0.5%) and increased rates of postoperative deep venous thrombosis.

Cystectomy and Other Major Bladder Surgeries

Cystectomy involves removal of all or part of the urinary bladder. Although radical cystectomy is standard for most muscle-invasive malignant disease, simple cystectomy is primarily for benign bladder disease. Of the estimated 69,250 cases of bladder cancer in 2011 in the United States, approximately 90% were expected to undergo a surgical procedure for their disease. Radical cystectomy combines bladder removal with resection of other pelvic organs and lymph nodes. Partial or simple cystectomy and transurethral resection of bladder tumor (TURBT) (see transurethral resection procedures section) are other procedures used in the treatment of benign and malignant bladder diseases.

As a result of removal of the entire bladder, simple and radical cystectomy procedures require a companion surgery to allow for future urine collection. The so-called diversion procedures involve redirecting the ureters, most commonly to a pouch fashioned from ileum (ileal conduit) that passively drains urine into a bag through a stoma on the patient's abdominal wall. Alternate options include the so-called continent diversion reconstructive procedures, which are becoming more popular. Because diversion surgeries can make future diagnosis of appendicitis difficult,

Table 50-5 Physiology of CO_2 Pneumoperitoneum in the Trendelenburg Position

Organ System	Effect
Cardiovascular	↑ Systemic vascular resistance ↑ Mean arterial pressure ↑ Myocardial oxygen consumption ↓ Renal, portal, and splanchnic flow
Respiratory	↑ Ventilation–perfusion mismatch ↓ Functional residual capacity ↓ Vital capacity ↓ Compliance ↑ Peak airway pressure Pulmonary congestion and edema Hypercarbia, respiratory acidosis
Central nervous system	↑ Intracranial pressure ↑ Cerebral blood flow ↑ Intraocular pressure Catecholamine release
Endocrine	Activation of renin–angiotensin system
Others	Gastroesophageal regurgitation Venous air embolism Neuropraxia, especially brachial Tracheal tube displacement Facial and airway edema

Reprinted with permission from Irvine M, Patil V. Anaesthesia for robot-assisted laparoscopic surgery. *Contin Educ Anaesth Crit Care Pain*. 2009;9:125–129.

some surgeons routinely also perform an appendectomy as part of urinary diversion procedures.

Supine or modified lithotomy positioning (Fig. 50-7) and midline incision with avoidance of the umbilicus are standard for open cystectomy surgery; however, a transverse abdominal incision is occasionally used. Much like nephrectomy, both retroperitoneal and transperitoneal approaches are feasible for cystectomy, and laparoscopic and robotic-assisted techniques are becoming popular for both cystectomy and diversion procedures.

Preoperative Considerations

The most common patients presenting for cystectomy are those with bladder cancer. Approximately 90% have transitional cell tumors, and approximately 90% of these have already invaded muscle at diagnosis. Bladder tumors occasionally present with urinary retention but are generally diagnosed by hematuria (microscopic or macroscopic) with or without voiding symptoms such as urgency, frequency, and dysuria. Prior to cystectomy, patients have usually undergone one or several cystoscopies for tumor biopsy or resection, and many have already received radiation and chemotherapy.

Risk factors for bladder cancer and atherosclerosis overlap, and perioperative protocols for cardiac risk assessment and management are relevant to cystectomy surgery.[137] Smoking history is most important, doubling the risk of bladder cancer, and occupational exposures in the leather, dye, and rubber industry and drinking water with high arsenic levels also contribute. Men are about four times more likely than women to be diagnosed with bladder cancer, with white men twice as susceptible as African-American men. The average patient presenting with bladder cancer is 65 years old. Paraneoplastic syndromes similar to those seen with kidney cancer have been reported with bladder cancer but are relatively rare.

Intraoperative Considerations

Anesthetic management for cystectomy is similar to that for nephrectomy surgery (see earlier), including preparation for the potential for major bleeding. Although patients could strictly undergo cystectomy surgery with epidural anesthesia alone, this is rarely chosen because of the extended duration of surgery. Particular attention should be paid to the approach to assessment of intravascular volume during cystectomy given the considerable potential for bleeding and hypovolemia and the absence of meaningful urine output data. Combining intraoperative epidural analgesia with a general anesthetic for cystectomy may reduce bleeding and improve postoperative analgesia without otherwise affecting complication rates.[169]

A trend in radical cystectomy has been toward the use of fast-track protocols (e.g., Enhanced Recovery After Surgery [ERAS]). Made popular by their use in colorectal surgeries, such protocols include a variety of evidence-based preoperative, intraoperative, and postoperative management strategies aimed at achieving early return of gastrointestinal function and good pain control, thereby minimizing the surgical stress response, reducing end-organ dysfunction, and improving overall recovery following major surgery. The use of such pathways has been reported to significantly reduce time to discharge and incidence of postoperative complications, with the best supporting evidence coming from colorectal surgery outcomes.

For radical cystectomy, the ERAS Society recommendations start with preoperative counseling, education, and optimization. Avoidance of oral mechanical bowel preparation is recommended. Rather than prolonged fasting, the patient can consume a light meal 6 hours prior to surgery, a clear carbohydrate drink for preoperative hydration and glucose and insulin optimization up until 2 hours before surgery. After arrival in the preoperative area, a multimodal analgesic regimen (often involving insertion of a thoracic epidural catheter for regional analgesia and a minimal approach to systemic opioid administration) is started, along with venous thromboembolism prophylaxis using subcutaneous heparin injection. Intraoperatively, a minimally invasive surgical approach is employed whenever possible. End-organ function is optimized through a goal-directed fluid management strategy involving noninvasive cardiac output monitoring.[170] Postoperatively, return of gastrointestinal function is encouraged through early mobilization and oral diet and avoidance of nasogastric intubation.[171]

Notably, evidence of improved outcomes with implementation of ERAS protocols for cystectomy remains scant compared to that in colorectal surgery.[172] However, small studies point to improvements in return of bowel function and lower-readmission rates at 30 days,[173] as well as improved wound healing, decreased fever and thrombosis, lower analgesic requirement, improved gastrointestinal function, and decreased time in the intermediate care unit.[174]

Postoperative Considerations

Simple cystectomy with diversion procedure involves a more limited dissection of pelvic structures relative to radical cystectomy and is generally associated with considerably less blood loss and lower complication rates.[175] Following radical cystectomy with diversion, some patients will require admission to an intensive care unit. Average blood loss ranges between 560 and 3,000 mL, and transfusion is common. Hospital lengths of stay can be long but vary considerably among centers. The mortality rate for radical cystectomy with diversion is approximately 1%, and perioperative complications are common (27.3%).[176] Early problems include acute pyelonephritis following ureteral catheter removal, ileus, injury to local structures such as the obturator nerve (adductor palsy and gait disturbance), and impaired lymph drainage (lymphocele, leg edema).

Specific Procedures

Partial Cystectomy

Nonmalignant indications for partial bladder resection include bladder endometriosis and benign tumors (e.g., lymphangioma). Whenever partial cystectomy will suffice, the effects of added surgery and poorer quality of life associated with a urinary diversion procedure can be eliminated; hence the current interest in methods to identify bladder cancer patients for whom partial cystectomy with pelvic lymph node dissection may be as good a treatment as radical cystectomy. Selective bladder-sparing protocols that use responsiveness of a tumor to chemotherapy and radiation therapy as a guide to surgical decision making appear to successfully identify about one-third of the patients whose long-term outcome with partial cystectomy is equivalent to radical cystectomy, without the need for a diversion procedure.[164]

Simple and Radical Cystectomy

Simple cystectomy is indicated for benign disease such as neurogenic bladder, refractory bladder pain syndrome (interstitial cystitis), bladder damage from radiation, and refractory incontinence.

Radical cystectomy involves resection of the bladder and related pelvic structures, including pelvic lymphadenectomy of obturator and iliac nodes. In the male, the bladder is removed *en bloc* with pelvic peritoneum, prostate and seminal vesicles, ureteric remnants, and a small piece of membranous urethra. In the female, the uterus, ovaries, fallopian tubes, vaginal vault, and urethra are removed. Alternate terminology to radical cystectomy for these major procedures include radical cystoprostatectomy in men and radical cystectomy with pelvic exenteration in women.

Ileal Conduit and Other Diversion Procedures

The concept of ileal conduit surgery is relatively straightforward, involving creation of an ileal pouch that is attached to both ureters and the abdominal wall as a stoma. In contrast, continent diversion procedures are numerous and diverse in their approaches to urine collection and drainage. Continent urinary diversions can be categorized into (1) ureterosigmoidostomy, (2) continent cutaneous diversions, and (3) neobladder diversions to the native urethra.[177] Ureterosigmoidostomy is only occasionally used and involves tunneling the ureters to the sigmoid colon, with urine storage and elimination being through the rectum. Continent cutaneous reservoirs resemble ileal conduit surgery, but the stomal attachment to the abdominal wall is modified to produce a valve mechanism, with urine drainage achieved by intermittent catheter drainage. Many continent cutaneous variants exist that involve the use of different bowel segments as the source for the reservoir (e.g., ileum, ileocecum, ascending colon, sigmoid colon, or transverse colon). Finally, continent orthotopic diversions involve neobladder construction from terminal ileum, cecum, or sigmoid colon, which is attached to proximal urethra and its intact rhabdosphincter mechanism. Notably, all urinary diversion procedures involve extensive dissection and are considerably more challenging if the patient has received preoperative radiation therapy. Complications of urinary diversion surgery include bowel obstruction, urinary tract infection, deep venous thrombosis and pulmonary embolism, pneumonia, upper urinary tract damage, and skin breakdown around the stoma.

After recovery, patients with urinary diversions are vulnerable to conditions that require subsequent surgeries; these include problems at the stoma site (e.g., stricture, hernia, prolapse, retraction; 5% to 10%), fistulae between urinary tract and bowel (3%), bowel obstruction, reservoir or other genitourinary stone diseases (5%), impotence, primary tumor recurrence, and even bowel cancer in the bladder pouch. In addition, post–radical cystectomy bladder cancer victims are subjected to frequent surveillance procedures owing to their high risk for future upper urinary tract urothelial malignancies (3%) and may require radical nephroureterectomy.

Anesthetic considerations for patients who present with existing diversion procedures include metabolic and electrolyte abnormalities such as hyperchloremic metabolic acidosis (common), hypokalemia, hypocalcemia and hypomagnesemia, and high rates of urinary tract infection and pyelonephritis. In addition, these individuals frequently suffer from chronic diarrhea and may have problems related to malabsorption (e.g., vitamin B_{12} deficiency).

Prostatectomy

Almost all procedures involving complete resection of the prostate (i.e., prostatectomy) are for adenocarcinoma of the prostate, because nonmalignant surgical disease of the prostate is typically so amenable to TUR (see the next section). Although prostate cancer is a disease limited to men, it is the second most common

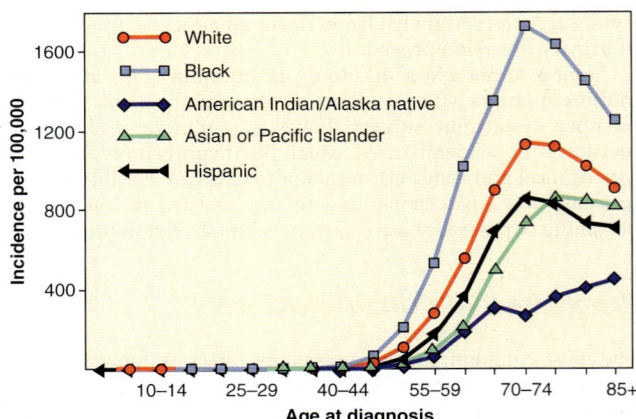

Figure 50-9 Crude incidence rates for prostate cancer, by race/ethnicity. (Adapted from www.seer.cancer.gov.)

cancer in most countries, with an incidence that increases significantly with age and is approximately 50% more common in African-American men than in Caucasian men (Fig. 50-9).[178]

Current evidence-based opinion on the optimal management of prostate cancer is rapidly evolving, including the relative value of intervention (i.e., hormonal, cryo-, chemo-, and internal and external radiation therapy; highly focused ultrasound ablation; and surgery) compared to an expanded role for watchful waiting in low-risk groups, as identified by measures such as tumor aggressiveness (e.g., Gleason score) and biomarkers (e.g., prostate-specific antigen levels). A second related concept is also emerging—that prostate cancer may exist in clinically significant (approximately 15%) and insignificant forms.[179] In general, surgical approaches are likely in younger men, whereas elderly patients who may die from disorders other than the prostate cancer are being more frequently advised to pursue nonsurgical therapy.

Prostatectomy can be performed using retropubic or perineal approaches and is amenable to endoscopic techniques with or without robotic assistance. The retropubic approach requires the patient to be supine with the bed extended and in Trendelenburg position (Fig. 50-7). This allows access to the prostate gland and related lymph nodes from behind the pubic symphysis (and the best chance of sparing the neurovascular bundle), using either a vertical midline or Pfannenstiel (horizontal low suprapubic) incision. In contrast, the perineal approach requires the patient to be in exaggerated lithotomy and steep Trendelenburg position (Fig. 50-7), with an incision between the scrotum and the anal sphincter that provides adequate access to the prostate (but not lymph nodes).

Preoperative Considerations

Beyond advanced age, relatively few factors predict likelihood of contracting prostate cancer. Family history more than doubles the chances of the disease, while African-American descent increases the risk by approximately 50% (Fig. 50-9). Otherwise, factors such as smoking, obesity, diet, history of vasectomy, prostatitis, or sexually transmitted diseases have little or no effect on prostate cancer risk. Owing to the advanced age of the population presenting for prostatectomy, an emphasis on comorbid disease in preoperative evaluation is particularly relevant. Paraneoplastic syndromes similar to those seen with kidney cancer are occasionally evident in prostate cancer patients.

Intraoperative Considerations

Anesthetic management for open prostatectomy is similar to that for cystectomy surgery (see earlier), including attentiveness to the potential for major bleeding. Epidural catheter placement is usually in the low thoracic spinal region, guided in part by the chosen option for anesthesia, including spinal/epidural alone, general alone, or combined spinal/epidural and general anesthesia. A surgical block to at least the T10 level is required for procedures performed using neuraxial block alone. In one study, patients experienced 33% less pain when preemptive epidural dosing occurred prior to incision.[180] Radical prostatectomy may take longer than the duration of a single-dose spinal anesthetic, so epidural or combined spinal–epidural is recommended. Notably, a neuraxial-alone strategy for perineal prostatectomy is likely to be poorly tolerated owing to the uncomfortable exaggerated lithotomy and head-down positioning requirements. Exaggerated lithotomy position for prostatectomy has also been associated in some studies with higher rates of neurologic injury (21% with transient sensory or motor deficit); patients appear to be at greater risk when surgery lasts longer than 180 minutes.[181,182] In addition, even with general anesthesia, some patients tolerate the exaggerated lithotomy–head-down position for perineal prostatectomy poorly owing to elevated ventilation pressures and impaired oxygenation.

As with cystectomy, the approach to intravascular volume assessment during prostatectomy must consider the potential for bleeding and hypovolemia and limited meaningful urine output data; the need for arterial and/or pressure central venous monitoring should be guided by patient comorbidities. Neuraxial anesthesia for prostatectomy has been associated with decreased blood loss in some studies.[183] However, any blood-sparing benefits of neuraxial anesthesia appear to be lost when it is combined with mechanical ventilation (and general anesthesia), possibly as a result of the effect of increased intrathoracic pressure on prostatic venous pressures.[184] Notably, breaching of the rich prostatic venous plexuses also creates the potential for acute hemodynamic instability from major venous air embolism, which has been reported during both retropubic and perineal prostatectomy approaches; suspicion of this complication warrants immediate steps to flood the surgical field and alter patient positioning to raise venous pressures above atmospheric, in addition to other standard resuscitation measures.[185]

Postoperative Considerations

Simple prostatectomy requires a limited dissection relative to radical prostatectomy and is generally associated with less blood loss and lower complication rates. Nonetheless, most radical prostatectomy patients are not admitted to an intensive care unit. Average blood loss for radical prostatectomy is between 500 and 1500 mL,[186] and approximately 10% of patients will require a perioperative blood transfusion.[187] In addition to vascular injury, the most common serious intraoperative complication is bowel or ureteral injuries. The mortality rate for radical prostatectomy is less than 1%. Impaired lymph drainage (lymphocele, leg edema) is associated in some studies with increased rates of postoperative deep venous thrombosis and pulmonary embolism.[187]

Transversus abdominis plane local anesthetic blocks are used at some institutions for pain management to facilitate retropubic prostatectomy fast-track recovery protocols[188]; ultrasound guidance for these procedures can minimize procedure-related risk of adjacent structure injury (e.g., bowel).

Specific Procedures

Simple Prostatectomy

Simple open prostatectomy is occasionally required for resection of very large prostate glands affected by benign prostatic hypertrophy (BPH),[189] but, in the era of medical therapies such as α-1 selective adrenergic receptor blockers and 5α-reductase inhibitors, this is an infrequent procedure. Currently, retropubic prostatectomy is the most common approach in the United States.

Radical Prostatectomy

Radical prostatectomy involves removal of the entire prostate gland, seminal vesicles, and generally the surrounding nerves and veins. The part of the urethra within the prostate gland's transition zone is also removed. Preservation of one or both cavernous nerves (part of the neurovascular bundle on each side of the prostate) can improve postsurgery quality of life (i.e., reduced urinary incontinence and erectile dysfunction) but limits the extent of possible resection. Notably, the incidence of positive margins with tumor resection during radical prostatectomy is significant (~30%). The value of more aggressive resection with sural nerve grafting to address erectile dysfunction remains unclear.[190] Controversial early data on the association of epidural anesthesia and analgesia with lower rates of cancer recurrence[191] have not been substantiated in more recent reports.

Laparoscopic and Robotic Prostatectomy

Minimally invasive laparoscopic and robotic-assisted approaches to prostatectomy are gaining popularity (see Chapter 44). Although these techniques are characterized by less pain, shorter hospital stays, faster recovery, and improved patient satisfaction,[192] they also present added challenge for the anesthesiologist, including prolonged procedure duration, the risk of hypothermia, occult blood loss, and the physiologic stresses of pneumoperitoneum and exaggerated Trendelenburg with or without lithotomy positioning.

Laparoscopic and robotic prostatectomy procedures require general anesthesia with endotracheal intubation. Standard monitoring and adequate intravenous access must be established prior to patient positioning because access after positioning is very difficult (Fig. 50-10). Pulse oximeter probe placement should avoid the earlobe to anticipate the potential for inaccurate readings in this location, presumably related to the venous engorgement with head-down positioning and pneumoperitoneum.[193] Intra-arterial and central venous monitoring are not routine but may be indicated based on patient comorbidities. As with all robotic surgeries, because of the fixed position of the robot arms, movements such as coughing can cause injury internally or at port sites, so care must be taken to maintain adequate depth of anesthesia and neuromuscular blockade. Exaggerated Trendelenburg positioning is required for the procedure, and some practitioners deliberately refrain from dosing epidural catheters to avoid cephalad spread of epidural drugs during the procedure.

Steep Trendelenburg positioning (30 to 45 degrees head-down) to facilitate pelvic access during laparoscopic and robotic prostatectomy increases the risk of several important complications (Fig. 50-7). To prevent sliding, patients must be well situated on the operating table (e.g., within a vacuum bean bag) then firmly secured (e.g., tape, safety belt). Arms should be placed on angled armboards *prior* to lowering the end table section during lithotomy positioning to minimize the risk of pinched or crushed fingers. The patient's arms are generally tucked at the side, and pressure points are carefully padded. Additional padding should distribute

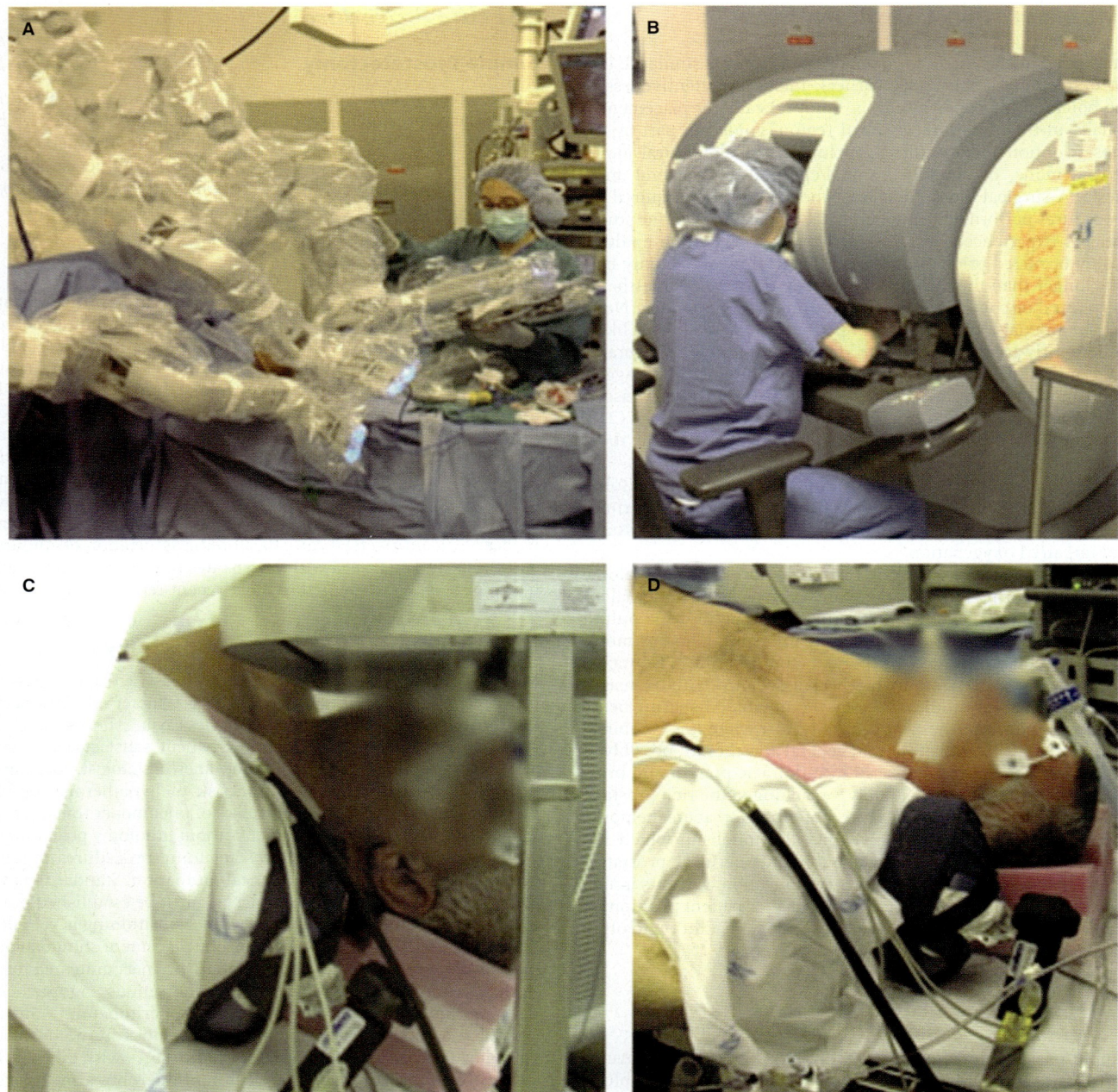

Figure 50-10 Images from a robotic radical prostatectomy procedure highlight the significant difficulty in accessing patients after the robot is docked (**A**), the remote location of the surgeon (**B**), the utility of a carefully placed Mayo stand to protect the patient's face and endotracheal tube (**C**), and the value of shoulder support padding to avoid pressure injuries (**D**).

localized pressure from shoulder braces, which sometimes support a significant fraction of the patient's body weight (Fig. 50-10). Beyond brachial plexus protection with shoulder padding, attention should be paid to radial (at the humerus), ulnar (at the elbow), and lateral femoral cutaneous (by the lithotomy leg holders) nerves to minimize axonal injuries. Finally, because oral ulceration and even conjunctival burns have been attributed to lithotomy-related reflux of gastric contents, steps such as preoperative antacid therapy, stomach drainage by orogastric tube, and waterproof eye taping should all be considered.[194]

Lack of easy access to the patient is a concern during robotic prostatectomy, primarily caused by the sheer size of current robot arms (Fig. 50-10). Hence, positioning preparation must be thorough and completed prior to robot docking. A Mayo instrument standing directly above the patient's head can help prevent robotic arms from causing pressure-related facial injuries and/or endotracheal tube displacement (Fig. 50-10).[195] Operating room staff must also be trained for robot emergencies, particularly timely removal of the device. Notably, although cardioversion and defibrillation are possible with the robot docked, cardiopulmonary resuscitation with chest compressions is nearly impossible.

The physiology of steep Trendelenburg positioning is well tolerated by healthy patients,[196] but this cannot be assumed for those with serious comorbidities. Adding to the stresses of head-down positioning during laparoscopic prostatectomy are the effects of CO_2 pneumoperitoneum (see nephrectomy section; Table 50-5). Although no formal guidelines exist, additional monitoring for patients with cardiac disease (e.g., compensated congestive heart failure) may be justified to assess responses to position-related intravascular volume shifts. Respiratory effects of robotic prostatectomy are numerous and often require considerable adjustments to mechanical ventilation parameters. Endotracheal tube cuff location should be just beyond the vocal cords to minimize the potential for developing a main stem intubation with the cephalad shift of the diaphragm and mediastinum from the combination of head-down positioning and pneumoperitoneum.[193] The related encroachment of abdominal contents onto the diaphragm also has significant effects on pulmonary function, particularly in obese patients, including reductions in functional residual capacity, vital capacity, and overall lung compliance, which translate into the need for higher peak airway pressures for equivalent tidal volumes. In addition, obese patients experience greater ventilation/perfusion mismatching. One study reported an average 8% lower tidal volumes, 22% higher respiratory rates, and 38% higher peak inspiratory pressures to maintain similar end-tidal carbon dioxide levels, but lower oxygen saturation during robotic compared to open retropubic radical prostatectomy.[197] Interestingly, CO_2 insufflation for retroperitoneal laparoscopic procedures requires greater increases in minute ventilation to compensate for absorbed CO_2 than equivalent transperitoneal procedures.[194] Tolerance of mildly elevated CO_2 levels (permissive hypercarbia) during some phases of the surgery may be a good strategy in some patients, but is potentially ill advised for patients with CKD, in which even mild respiratory acidosis can be associated with significant hyperkalemia.[198] Transcranial Doppler[199] and cerebral oximetry[196] to monitor intracranial perfusion have been suggested for patients with cerebrovascular disease. Potential adverse effects on intraocular pressure of head-down positioning in at-risk patients (e.g., poorly controlled glaucoma) have not been rigorously studied. Despite all these physiologic perturbations, the need to convert from laparoscopic/robotic assisted to open techniques for major urologic procedures is remarkably infrequent.[194]

During robotic prostatectomy, one of the major surgical steps involves reanastomosis of the severed urethral ends after prostate gland resection. This is often made more complicated by urine from the bladder neck's spilling directly into the operative field, obscuring the surgeon's view and impeding progress. Anticipation of this problem by the anesthesiologist can assist the surgeon through cautious fluid restriction, particularly prior to urethral anastomosis. A generally restrictive approach to fluid administration may also attenuate the development of mild facial, periorbital, and even occasionally laryngeal edema associated with prolonged steep lithotomy position.[193,194] However, edema accumulation is rarely sufficient to threaten airway patency after tracheal extubation.

Transurethral Surveillance and Resection Procedures

Transurethral endoscopy is a commonly used, relatively noninvasive surgical tool in the armamentarium of the urologist that can play an important role in the management and treatment of urothelial cancers (e.g., cystoscopy/ureteroscopy surveillance, TURBT), urolithiasis (e.g., ureteroscopic stent placement, basket stone retrieval), and BPH (e.g., transurethral resection of the prostate [TURP]). Despite the benign and noninvasive appearance of transurethral tissue resection surgeries (TURBT, TURP), these procedures are occasionally associated with significant morbidity and even mortality.

Cystoscopy and TURBT procedures are used in the surveillance, staging, and management of transitional cell bladder cancers (see cystectomy section). For patients with superficial cancers that do not invade the bladder muscle, bladder biopsy and subsequent TURBT may be curative, but such patients require ongoing cystoscopy surveillance and often receive biologic therapies (e.g., Bacillus Calmette–Guérin vaccine) that reduce the recurrence rate of bladder cancer, presumably by boosting the immune response. Nonetheless, about 50% of patients with a resected bladder cancer will develop another bladder or ureteral cancer in the future.

TURP is a mainstay and even gold standard therapy to alleviate urine obstructive symptoms related to BPH. BPH describes the smooth muscle and epithelial cell proliferation within the transition zone of the prostate that histologically characterizes this disorder. The symptoms of BPH reflect the combination of bladder outlet obstruction (static) and increased smooth muscle tone (dynamic). Although TURP surgery with electrocautery has been for many decades central to the treatment of BPH, a proliferation of other options explains the steady decrease in the use of TURP for BPH treatment, partly owing to the significant side effects that can occur with this procedure (e.g., incontinence, impotence). Medical therapy for BPH is common, directed at both static and dynamic components of the disease (α-1 adrenergic antagonists and α-1A reductase inhibitors), and is part of the current more conservative watchful waiting approach to surgical treatment of BPH. Numerous alternate procedures to TURP are now being used for BPH; in 2005, TURP represented only 39% of BPH procedures compared to 81% in 1999.[200] Description of these alternate procedures is beyond the scope of this text, but some of these include transurethral needle ablation, transurethral microwave thermal therapy, transurethral ablation prostatectomy, holmium laser ablation of the prostate, interstitial laser coagulation, high intensity focused ultrasound, and water intensity hyperthermia.

Positioning concerns for cystoscopy, TURBT, and TURP are the same as for other procedures in lithotomy position (Fig. 50-10) and in particular relate to adequate padding of pressure points and avoidance of peroneal nerve compression.

Preoperative Considerations

Patients presenting for TURP are likely to be elderly and may have other serious comorbidities. Cardiovascular and pulmonary status should be carefully assessed to evaluate the patient's ability to tolerate the intravascular volume changes associated with the procedure. Patients on anticoagulant therapy may not be candidates for spinal anesthesia, depending on the indication for anticoagulation. The risk of stopping the anticoagulant perioperatively may or may not be worth the advantages of spinal anesthesia for a particular patient. Decisions about this should be made in conjunction with the surgeon, because the risk of postoperative bleeding following TURP will likely dictate an interval of normal coagulation or bridging treatment with short-acting anticoagulants such as heparin.

Intraoperative Considerations

Choice of anesthetic technique for cystoscopy, TURBT, and TURP procedures should be tailored to the individual and can be performed safely with either general or regional anesthesia.[201] Neuraxial block allows the patient to remain awake and may hasten the diagnosis of bladder or prostatic capsule perforation and the TUR syndrome and may also decrease blood loss compared with general anesthesia.[202,203] For ambulatory surgery patients, care must be taken in the selection of spinal anesthetic medications so as to avoid prolonged anesthetic duration and delayed discharge from the facility. Combined spinal–epidural techniques or general anesthesia may have advantages if the length of surgery is unpredictable. Notably, the lower central venous pressure associated with regional anesthesia may actually increase the likelihood of significant irrigation fluid absorption.[204]

Hypothermia can complicate TURP procedures. Body temperature decreases approximately 1°C per hour of surgery, and shivering occurs in 16% of patients who receive room-temperature irrigation fluids. Hypothermia does not develop if irrigation solutions are warmed to body temperature.[205]

Approximately 2.5% of patients require transfusion during TURP surgery. Average blood loss is 2 to 4 mL/min,[206] but individual bleeding rates can be difficult to assess owing to mixing with irrigating fluid. The patient's vital signs may be useful to guide transfusion,[207] but, with prolonged resections, serial assessments of hemoglobin level are advisable.

Surgical perforation of the prostatic capsule occurs in 2% of TURP procedures, usually resulting in extraperitoneal fluid extravasation. Awake patients with a neuraxial anesthetic may complain during surgery of new-onset pain localized to the lower abdomen and back.[207,208] Bladder perforation during TURBT more commonly results in extravasation of fluid intraperitoneally and may produce abdominal distension and complaints of abdominal and shoulder pain in awake patients.[209] Notably, evidence of perforation often only becomes clear postoperatively.

Postoperative Considerations

Although abnormal bleeding after TURP occurs in fewer than 1% of resections,[206] 2% to 3% of patients will require transfusion perioperatively.[210,211] Blood loss following TURBT is usually less than 100 mL, although postoperative hemorrhage can rarely occur. Thromboplastin, a thrombogenic stimulant found in high concentrations in prostate cancer cells, can rarely trigger disseminated intravascular coagulation.[207] Another cause of post-TURP bleeding is release of prostatic tissue plasminogen activators. These factors convert plasminogen to plasmin, causing fibrinolysis. Treatment of these conditions is supportive and may include transfusion of coagulation factors and platelets.[212] Prophylactic administration of antifibrinolytics (e.g., tranexamic acid) demonstrated some success but has not gained widespread acceptance as standard practice.[213] Nevertheless, it may be considered in cases of refractory bleeding.

As outlined earlier, bladder, prostatic capsule, or urethral perforations are uncommon but serious complications that may manifest postoperatively with or without symptoms of TUR syndrome (see later). Fever related to TURP procedures may indicate bacteremia secondary to spread of bacteria through open prostatic venous sinuses, particularly with a history of infectious prostatitis.

The most common complications following TURP surgery are the need for urinary recatheterization (4%), prostatic capsule perforation (2%), and postoperative hemorrhage requiring transfusion (1%).[214] The 30-day mortality following TURP is 0.2%[208,215–218] and most commonly relates to serious cardiac and respiratory complications.[219]

Specific Procedures

Cystoscopy and Ureteroscopy

Although surveillance cystoscopy is often performed under local anesthesia outside the operating room with minimal monitoring or sedation and without the involvement of anesthesia personnel, some cystoscopy and most ureteroscopy procedures, particularly for those patients with comorbidities, occur in the operating room setting. Cystoscopy and ureteroscopy are rarely associated with significant complications, and perioperative considerations should generally parallel those for the disease being screened for or managed (see related sections).

Transurethral Bladder Tumor Resection

During any simple cystoscopy or ureteroscopy procedure, abnormal tissue may require one or more planned or unanticipated diagnostic biopsies or biopsy/resections. As outlined earlier (see cystectomy section), risk factors for bladder cancer and atherosclerosis overlap, and cardiac risk assessment is relevant to TURBT surgery.[220] A serious intraoperative complication of TURBT is bladder perforation by the rigid cystoscope during tissue resection, which occasionally occurs owing to unexpected patient movement. For this reason, muscle relaxation is preferred during general anesthesia, particularly in lateral wall resections, where the obturator nerve may be stimulated by electrocautery, producing a violent contraction of the ipsilateral thigh muscles. Neuraxial anesthesia to the T9 to T10 dermatomal level also provides adequate anesthesia for the procedure and prevents the obturator reflex. Regional anesthesia may facilitate detection of bladder perforation. Postoperative pain is usually minimal and responds well to nonopiate and opiate medications.

Transurethral Prostate Resection

Standard procedure during TURP surgery involves inserting a resectoscope, a specialized endoscopy instrument with an electrode capable of both coagulating and cutting tissue, into the urethra, then the bladder; the tissue protruding into the prostatic urethra is then resected.[221] There has been much recent interest in the use of lasers rather than electrocautery to resect excess prostate tissue. A variety of different lasers have been utilized. Laser techniques have advantages over traditional electrocautery approaches, particularly related to traditional irrigation fluid restrictions. Laser resection has no requirement for a nonconductive fluid, so 0.9% saline may be used, avoiding complications of absorption related to hypo-osmolarity and solute toxicity (see TUR syndrome). Furthermore, the potential for systemic absorption may be reduced owing to the lower irrigation infusion rates and pressures necessary for laser procedures.[222,223] Lasers also have coagulative properties, resulting in less blood loss and lower rates of transfusion.

Irrigating Solutions and Transurethral Resection Syndrome

Key to a surgeon's endoscopic view during transurethral procedures is a visually clear irrigating solution, infused with a pump or via gravity (and drained away) to flush out blood and resected

Table 50-6 Properties of Commonly Used Irrigating Solutions for Transurethral Resection Procedures

Solution	Osmolality (mOsm/L)	Advantages	Disadvantages
Distilled water	0	Improved visibility	Hemolysis Hemoglobinemia Hemoglobinuria Hyponatremia
Glycine (1.5%)	200	Less likelihood of TUR syndrome	Transient postoperative visual syndrome Hyperammonemia Hyperoxaluria
Sorbitol (3.3%)	165	Same as glycine	Hyperglycemia, possible lactic acidosis Osmotic diuresis
Mannitol (5%)	275	Isosmolar solution Not metabolized	Osmotic diuresis Possibility of acute intravascular volume expansion

TUR, transurethral resection.
Adapted with permission from Krongrad A, Droller MJ. Complications of transurethral resection of the prostate. In: Marshall FF, ed. Urologic Complications: Medical and Surgical, Adult and Pediatric. 2nd ed. St. Louis: Mosby-Year Book; 1990.

tissue and keep space between structures. Safety characteristics of the irrigating solution are important because with tissue resection or urinary tract injury, significant amounts of the fluid may inadvertently enter the circulation, for example, during TURP through openings in the venous plexus or retroperitoneal rents in the prostatic capsule or consequent to perforation of the urinary bladder into the peritoneal space during TURBT. Other procedures where inadvertent perforation can cause the TUR syndrome include cystoscopy, ureteroscopy, percutaneous nephrolithotomy (PNL), and laser vaporization of the prostate.

The spectrum of morbidities associated with irrigating solution absorption is termed the TUR syndrome. A variety of nonconductive *nonelectrolytic* solutions are in common use. The crystalloids have current-dispersing properties owing to their ionic characteristics that make them unsuitable for use with unipolar electrocautery. When absorbed in significant amounts, nonelectrolytic irrigation solutions combine electrolyte disturbances with hypervolemia. Notably, newer transurethral *bipolar* electrocautery and laser techniques now allow irrigation with isotonic crystalloid solutions (e.g., 0.9% saline), but until these technologies totally replace unipolar electrocautery, nonconducting osmotically active irrigating solutions will continue to be used, each variant having its own concerns (Table 50-6).[200]

It is therefore important for anesthesiologists to be aware of solutions used for transurethral procedures at their own institutions, because TUR syndrome for each irrigating solution has its own profile (Table 50-6). Nonetheless, *TUR syndrome* historically describes a common cluster of symptoms related to hypervolemic water intoxication; the principal components are (1) excessive volume expansion (respiratory distress, congestive heart failure, pulmonary edema, hypertension, bradycardia, hypotension, etc.), (2) hyponatremia (mental confusion, nausea, etc.; Table 50-7), and (3) other problems specific to each of the irrigating solutions.[224–226] Notably, any future trend toward limiting irrigation to physiologic solutions (e.g., 0.9% saline) should eliminate all but the hypervolemic component of the TUR syndrome.

Of available irrigating solutions, distilled water is rarely utilized owing to its hypotonicity. Water intoxication with distilled water rapidly causes severe hyponatremia leading to hemolysis, hemoglobinemia, and renal failure. Sorbitol and glucose solutions cause hyperglycemia when they are absorbed. Glycine, an amino acid normally metabolized to ammonia, may cause a depressed mental status and even coma (due to hyperammonemia) that can last 24 to 48 hours postoperatively.[227,228] Also reported with glycine are blurred vision, minimally or nonreactive pupils, and transient blindness.[229,230] Because glycine has structural similarities to aminobutyric acid, these visual disturbances are thought to reflect neurotransmitter-mediated brainstem or cranial nerve inhibition rather than cerebral edema.[230]

Absorption of very large amounts of irrigant (>2 L) is usually required to manifest the TUR syndrome. The incidence of symptomatic TUR syndrome is highest during TURP procedures, where it may be as high as 1.4%.[210] Typically, intraoperative irrigation infusion rates of 300 mL/min are used during TURP procedures for optimal surgical visualization.[219] Some intravascular absorption is to be expected; rates of 20 mL/min are typical, but these can reach as high as 200 mL/min.[231] Factors that predict increased irrigation fluid absorption during a TURP procedure include the number and size of open venous sinuses (i.e., greater blood loss implies greater potential for irrigation absorption), surgical disruption of the prostatic capsule, longer duration of resection, higher hydrostatic pressure of the irrigating fluid, and lower venous pressure at the irrigant–blood interface.[206]

To minimize fluid absorption, procedural guidelines include limiting resection time to less than 1 hour and suspending the irrigating fluid bag no more than 30 cm above the operating table at the beginning and 15 cm above in the final stages of resection.[206,232] In addition, avoidance of hypotonic intravenous

Table 50-7 Signs and Symptoms of Acute Hyponatremia

Serum Na+ (mEq/L)	CNS Changes	ECG Changes
120	Confusion Restlessness	Possible widening of QRS complex
115	Somnolence Nausea	Widened QRS complex Elevated ST segment
110	Seizures Coma	Ventricular tachycardia or fibrillation

CNS, central nervous system; ECG, electrocardiogram.
Adapted with permission from Jensen V. The TURP syndrome. Can J Anaesth. 1991;38:90.

fluids and treatment of regional anesthesia-induced hypotension with judicious use of intravenous vasopressor agents rather than intravenous fluids should be considered.

Symptomatic TUR syndrome is much less common following TURBT (and usually related to symptoms of bladder perforation), but it is important to be aware of the possibility of its occurrence because it may present somewhat differently owing to the slower rate of fluid absorption.[209] Most notably, the time course of symptoms following bladder perforation during TURBT reflects the slower absorption from the abdominal cavity compared to direct prostatic venous plexus entry with TURP. For example, nadir serum sodium values are generally reached between 1 and 6 hours following TURP, whereas TUR syndrome following TURBT occurs between 2 and 9 hours postoperatively.[209]

Clinical manifestations of the TUR syndrome range from mild (restlessness, nausea, shortness of breath, dizziness) to severe (seizures, coma, hypertension, bradycardia, cardiovascular collapse). In the awake patient with a regional block, a classic triad of symptoms has been described that consists of an increase in both systolic and diastolic pressures associated with an increase in pulse pressure, bradycardia, and mental status changes.[207,224]

Early symptoms associated with TUR syndrome are mostly related to acute intravascular volume expansion independent of changes in serum osmolality and sodium.[226] Initial hypertension and bradycardia from acute volume overload may evolve into left heart failure, pulmonary edema, and even cardiovascular collapse.[233] With the continued absorption of hypotonic irrigation fluid, cerebral edema as a consequence of dilutional hyponatremia may develop. Rapid change, as opposed to a specific low-threshold serum sodium concentration, is responsible for most of the signs and symptoms of TUR syndrome (Table 50-7).[224]

When neurologic or cardiovascular complications of TURP procedures are recognized intraoperatively, prompt intervention is necessary (Table 50-8). First, the surgeon should be informed of the patient's status change so that the procedure can be completed or terminated as quickly as possible. The hallmark of patient treatment is to restore extracellular tonicity. Although the traditional recommended rate of serum sodium correction is 0.5 mEq/L/hr, this is for chronic hyponatremia, and no established rate for correction of acute hyponatremia exists. Symptomatic patients with serum sodium concentrations less than 120 mEq/L should have their extracellular tonicity corrected with hypertonic saline. Sodium chloride in a 3% solution should be infused at a rate no greater than 100 mL/hr. Serum electrolytes should be followed closely and the hypertonic saline discontinued when the patient is asymptomatic or serum sodium concentration exceeds 120 mEq/L. Treatment with hypertonic saline has been associated with development of demyelinating central nervous system lesions (central pontine myelinolysis) owing to rapid increases in plasma osmolality, and this approach should be reserved for patients with severe, life-threatening symptoms.[234] The demyelination is the result of excessive shrinkage of brain cells after rapid hydration with hyperosmolar solution, because the brain cells have extruded important osmoles to compensate for the chronic hypotonicity. Notably, reports of demyelination after correction of acute symptomatic hyponatremia are rare, and there are no reports of demyelination after treatment of acute TUR syndrome.[226]

Therapies for Urolithiasis

Stone disease of the urinary tract, urolithiasis, can be subdivided on the basis of the location of the stone into nephrolithiasis (kidney), ureterolithiasis (ureter), or cystolithiasis (bladder). Nephrolithiasis is a common clinical problem, with an increasing incidence. The lifetime prevalence of nephrolithiasis is 10% in men and 5% in women. Up to 50% of patients with an initial stone episode will have a recurrence within 5 years.[235]

The composition of kidney stones varies (Table 50-9). The most common type of stones contains calcium and is radiopaque. Stones form when the concentration of stone-forming salts in the urine is elevated (e.g., oxalate) or when the level of stone inhibitors in the urine is low (e.g., citrate). This results in supersaturation of the urine with salts, allowing crystals to form and grow, particularly in situations where urine volume is low. This pathophysiology explains the principles of the medical management of kidney stones: increasing urine volume and maneuvers to restore urinary salt balance through dietary and medical treatment.[236,237]

The preferred diagnostic modality for urolithiasis is helical noncontrast CT scan, which can identify radiopaque and radiolucent stones in the entire urinary system and determine whether hydronephrosis is present. Ultrasound imaging is also informative for stones in the kidney and proximal ureter but cannot show the distal ureter and may miss smaller stones. Compared to helical CT and ultrasonography, plain radiographs (kidney–ureter–bladder [KUB]) provide no additional information about obstruction or hydronephrosis and can miss stones in the kidney or ureter. Intravenous pyelography is rarely used because it offers no added information compared to other diagnostic modalities and exposes the patient to radiation and contrast-related renal injury.[237]

Patients with kidney stones typically present with intermittent or continuous moderate to severe colicky pain in the ipsilateral flank and upper abdomen. Testicular or labial pain is more typical with distal ureteric stones. Occasionally, patients present with painless urinary infection or hematuria. Conservative nonsurgical therapy for smaller stones consists of analgesics (e.g., NSAIDs and/or opiates) and aggressive fluid administration to promote urine flow and passage of the stone. The so-called medical expulsive therapy to promote ureter relaxation and the spontaneous passage of small ureteral stones involves treatment with calcium channel blockers (e.g., nifedipine), α-blockers (e.g., tamsulosin), and sometimes corticosteroids.[237,238] The likelihood of stone passage without surgery relates to the size of the stone, its location, and the presence or absence of urinary system anatomic abnormalities such as strictures. If stones do not pass spontaneously or respond to medical expulsive therapy, various surgical options can be considered, as discussed earlier (Fig. 50-11).

Table 50-8 Treatment of the Transurethral Resection Syndrome

Ensure oxygenation and circulatory support
Notify surgeon and terminate procedure as soon as possible
Consider insertion of invasive monitors if cardiovascular instability occurs
Send blood to laboratory for evaluation of electrolytes, creatinine, glucose, and arterial blood gases
Obtain 12-lead electrocardiogram
Treat mild symptoms (with serum Na^+ concentration >120 mEq/L) with fluid restriction and loop diuretic (furosemide)
Treat severe symptoms (if serum Na^+ <120 mEq/L) with 3% sodium chloride intravenously at a rate <100 mL/hr
Discontinue 3% sodium chloride when serum Na^+ >120 mEq/L

Table 50-9 Spectrum of Kidney Stones Types: Composition, Frequency, and Causes

Stone Composition	Frequency	Mechanism
Calcium oxalate or calcium phosphate	70%–80%	Hypercalciuria • High sodium and protein diet • Hypercalcemia, e.g., hyperparathyroidism • Chronic metabolic acidosis Low urine output • Chronic dehydration Hyperuricosuria • High purine, high protein intake • Gout Hyperoxaluria • Low dietary calcium • High oxalate diet • Genetic Low urine citrate • Chronic metabolic acidosis • Renal tubular acidosis • Inflammatory bowel disease
Uric acid	10%–15%	Low urine pH Chronic metabolic acidosis Hyperuricosuria Obesity Lesch–Nyhan syndrome
Magnesium ammonium phosphate (struvite)	10%–15%	Urinary infections (urea-splitting bacteria), e.g., Proteus, Klebsiella, Staphylococcus, Pseudomonas, Providentia, and *Corynebacterium urealyticum*
Cystine	<1%	Cystinuria—autosomal recessive
Others: indinavir	<1%	Antiretroviral drug for HIV
Triamterene		Potassium-sparing diuretic
Xanthine		Xanthine oxidase inhibitor therapy, e.g., allopurinol

Data from Hall PM. Nephrolithiasis: treatment, causes, and prevention. *Cleve Clin J Med.* 2009;76:583–591; and Brown P. Management of urinary tract infections associated with nephrolithiasis. *Curr Infect Dis Rep.* 2010;12:450–454.

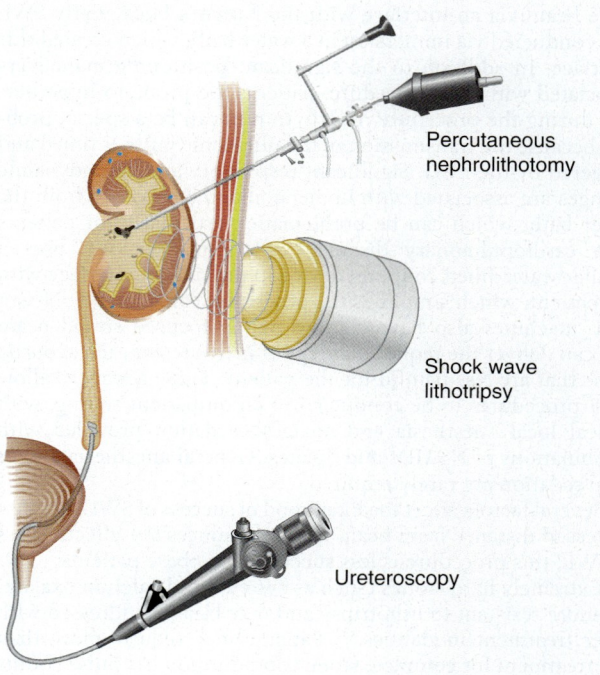

Figure 50-11 Intervention choices for urinary tract stones. (Adapted with permission from Samplaski MK, Irwin BH, Desai M. Less-invasive ways to remove stones from the kidneys and ureters. *Cleve Clin J Med*. 2009;76:592–598.)

Preoperative Considerations

Anesthetic planning for urolithiasis surgery should include standard considerations. Typical calcium salt stone disease presents in the third to fifth decades of life[237] and is commonly associated with comorbidities such as obesity, hypertension, and hyperparathyroidism. Patients with renal failure or CKD should be assessed for the sequelae of these conditions, including platelet dysfunction, anemia, and electrolyte abnormalities. Bladder stones are often diagnosed in patients with poor voiding capacity, for example, paraplegic patients, and the associated perioperative concerns for these patients should be addressed. Although paraplegic patients with sensory deficits below T6 lack pain perception for cystoscopy procedures, they are at risk for *autonomic hyperreflexia* and require anesthesia to block the afferent stimulation that can provoke this reaction (e.g., bladder distension). This can be achieved with deeper levels of general anesthesia or regional anesthesia.[239] Patients with idiopathic hypercalciuria are often treated with thiazide diuretics, and serum potassium should be assessed preoperatively.[237]

3

Perioperative opioid analgesic dosing for urolithiasis procedures can be challenging. Patients with recurrent nephrolithiasis may be receiving chronic opioid therapy and demonstrate tolerance intra- and postoperatively. In contrast, when severe colic is alleviated by surgery for an opioid-naive patient already treated with opiates, postoperative somnolence is quite common. Renal colic is often associated with nausea and vomiting, and preoperative aspiration prophylaxis should be considered.

Unless open surgery is planned, there is rarely a need for blood transfusion for stone surgery. Selection of appropriate monitors should be dictated by patient comorbidities, because significant blood loss or fluid shifts are unusual with these procedures. However, if difficulty achieving vascular access during a procedure is anticipated (e.g., percutaneous nephrolithotripsy), there should be a low threshold for establishing central access prior to the procedure. Antibiotic prophylaxis is important, particularly with infected stones or pyelonephritis. When lasers are required, appropriate eye protection should be provided for the perioperative team and patient.

Intraoperative Considerations

Compared with other more invasive urologic procedures, stone surgeries generally do not involve large amounts of blood loss or fluid shifts, with the possible exception of percutaneous nephrolithotripsy (see later). Information about anesthetic choice and potential intraoperative issues is discussed in the individual sections and in the sections on nephrectomy and transurethral surgery elsewhere in this chapter. Monitoring decisions and anesthetic choices should be made on the basis of patient comorbidity, and intraoperative care should focus on those as well.

Postoperative Considerations

Postoperative concerns for urolithiasis procedures are generally minor. Interestingly, patients with severe renal colic prior to less invasive surgeries (e.g., ureteroscopy) may have less or no pain postoperatively with relief of their urinary obstruction and stone retrieval. However, immediately following urinary tract instrumentation, many patients experience rather uncomfortable bladder and ureteral spasms. These spasms are typically more responsive to NSAIDs, oxybutynin, and belladonna and opium suppositories than to parenteral opioids.

Occasionally, open surgery is required for upper urinary tract stone removal, with postoperative concerns comparable to those for nephrectomy patients having similar incisions; these include pain, which may be sufficient to require epidural analgesia, and monitoring requirements to ensure that adequate resuscitation related to any blood loss has occurred.

Monitoring the adequacy of urine output and maintaining any urinary irrigation or drainage system (e.g., stents, three-way Foley catheters) to promote clearance of blood in the urinary system are important, because clots or stone fragments can cause acute urinary obstruction.

After extraction or lithotripsy of stones, particularly struvite stones or in the setting of pyelonephritis, patients may develop a pattern of rigors, hypotension, and fever, which can lead to shock. Urine culture results can be misleading in predicting which patients will develop sepsis because urine below the level of a stone may be clean, yet urine upstream of the stony obstruction may be infected. A sepsis picture can be noted during the procedure but is more likely to occur postoperatively. Indications of intravascular bacterial seeding from infected urine needs prompt attention with blood cultures, fluids and resuscitation, and institution of appropriate antibiotic therapy to prevent more serious sequelae of a sepsis syndrome. The potential acuity of this situation should not be underestimated, because even healthy ASA 1 to 2 patients can develop systemic inflammatory response syndrome and require aggressive resuscitation and intensive care.[240]

Specific Procedures

Shock Wave Lithotripsy

Shock wave lithotripsy (SWL) is best suited for intranephric stones that are small-to-moderate in size but can be used for proximal ureteral stones as well. The principle of SWL is to use focused sound waves to break the stone into pieces small enough to pass through the ureters, bladder, and urethra during normal urination. This requires transmission of the sound wave beam via an interface with the patient's body. Early SWL was conducted via immersion in a water bath, which created this interface. In addition to the significant positioning maneuvers associated with this procedure, patients are prone to hypothermia during the procedure. Dysrhythmias can be a special problem because the transmission of the ultrasonic pulse is timed and triggered by the ECG. Significant respiratory and hemodynamic changes are associated with immersion and emergence from the water bath, which can be problematic particularly for patients with cardiopulmonary disease.[241] Modern dry SWL uses a smaller water-filled coupling device to provide an interface with the patient, which simplifies the procedure considerably. Newer SWL machines also have a more tightly focused sound beam and can deliver the required energy at pressures in each acoustic pulse that are less painful for the patient. These advances allow most procedures to be conducted in an outpatient setting, with topical local anesthesia and analgesia/sedation provided with combinations of NSAIDs and opiates. General anesthesia and/or deep sedation are rarely required.

4

Several factors affect the likelihood of success of SWL. Because increased distance from beam to stone reduces the effectiveness of SWL, this procedure is less successful in obese patients.

Extremely hard stones (such as cysteine and calcium oxalate) are more resistant to lithotripsy and may best be addressed with other treatment modalities.[242] Patients may require more than one treatment for complete stone comminution. As pulse counts increase, so does the risk of kidney injury and even subcapsular

Table 50-10 Contraindications to Shock Wave Lithotripsy	
Absolute contraindications	Bleeding disorder or anticoagulation Pregnancy
Relative contraindications	Large calcified aortic or renal artery aneurysms Untreated urinary tract infection Obstruction distal to the renal calculi Pacemaker, ICD, or neurostimulation implant Morbid obesity

ICD, implantable cardioverter-defibrillator.

hematoma.[236] SWL is the least invasive and most commonly performed procedure for the management of stone disease; however, even for this approach, several relative and absolute contraindications exist (Table 50-10).

Percutaneous Nephrolithotomy

PNL is useful for the management of larger intranephric stones, especially those resistant to SWL, staghorn calculi, and some proximal ureteral stones. PNL requires initial placement of a ureteral stent via cystoureteroscopy performed in the lithotomy position. This stent will prevent ureteral obstruction as fragments of stone pass through the ureter following PNL. Following stent placement, the patient is repositioned to an oblique prone position for percutaneous puncture of the renal pelvis under fluoroscopic guidance, which is followed by placement of a nephrostomy tube to facilitate placement of a nephroscope for stone extraction with forceps or other instruments. Large stones may require use of an ultrasound or laser probe, also placed via the nephrostomy, to fragment them to facilitate removal. The combination of fluoroscopy and direct vision of the renal pelvis and ureters with nephro- and ureteroscopy is used to ensure that complete removal of the stone(s) has been achieved. Large volumes of irrigation are used to cool the ultrasound probe and wash away the debris, making TUR syndrome an occasional complication of PNL. Because of the large irrigant volume, blood loss can be underappreciated, and unexplained hemodynamic instability during these procedures is often a manifestation of blood loss. Published rates of transfusion during or after PNL range from 5% to 14%.[243] Pneumothorax, though rare, is a possible complication of the procedure depending on the approach used for insertion of the nephroscope.

General anesthesia with endotracheal intubation allows for a secure airway for positioning into the prone position and is most commonly used in many centers; however, spinal anesthesia can also be used.[244] For certain patients, local infiltration with sedation may even suffice.[245]

Ureteroscopy for Removal of Stones (URS)

URS is the procedure of choice for midureteral and distal ureteral stones that have failed conservative management. It is also indicated for treatment of bilateral ureteral stones and can be considered in patients for whom cessation of anticoagulation is not advisable. Morbidly obese patients for whom SWL is not advised are also candidates for this procedure.[236] Although more invasive than SWL, URS generally achieves a higher stone-free rate and can be used to remove stones in all portions of the ureter. Newer technology has allowed smaller, more flexible ureteroscopes, and lasers are now incorporated to facilitate stone disintegration. Various basket and other retrieval devices can be inserted through the ureteroscope. The postoperative complications from ureteroscopic stone retrieval include perforation of the ureter (5%) and stricture formation (<2%) and rarely TUR syndrome.[246] The procedure can be performed using urethral local anesthesia with intravenous sedation and monitored anesthesia care, spinal anesthesia, or general anesthesia. The previous section addresses anesthetic concerns related to cystoscopy and URS.

Open and Laparoscopic Pyelolithotomy or Nephrectomy

With the advent of the previously discussed modalities for the treatment of urolithiasis, the use of laparoscopic or open surgery for removal of stones has declined considerably, and they should not be considered first-line treatment for stone disease. Patients who have failed SWL or PNL or who require open surgery for other indications are candidates for open treatment of stone disease. This can be accomplished laparoscopically (retroperitoneal or transperitoneal) or open, depending on the capabilities of the surgeon. Compared with less-invasive approaches, both laparoscopic and open procedures result in more postoperative pain and longer hospital stays and recovery and are associated with higher complication rates.

Urogynecology and Pregnancy-related Urologic Procedures

A variety of urogynecologic procedures that treat pelvic floor prolapse are directed at symptomatic improvement of stress incontinence. These procedures are relatively noninvasive, often accomplished using a transvaginal approach with the patient in the lithotomy position, and frequently performed as outpatient procedures with same-day discharge home. Anesthesia can be accomplished with local infiltration accompanied by heavy sedation and monitored anesthesia care, neuraxial anesthesia using spinal or combined spinal/epidural local anesthetic injection, or general anesthesia. Local preferences may dictate anesthetic choice, as suggested by reports from some centers regarding the selection of spinal anesthesia that describe on the one hand improved patient and surgeon satisfaction[247] and on the other a fourfold higher urinary retention rate[248] and 1 hour longer postanesthesia care unit stay.

Renal colic is the most common nonobstetric cause of abdominal pain requiring hospitalization in pregnant women.[236] Medical management of these patients must consider the fetal gestational age in decisions about appropriate analgesics (e.g., NSAIDs in the third trimester may cause premature closure of the fetal ductus arteriosus and adverse renal effects). Diagnostic tests preferably avoid ionizing radiation and favor the use of ultrasound whenever possible. Interventions in pregnant patients with symptomatic nephrolithiasis have traditionally been limited to ureteral stents to relieve pain and prevent obstruction, with definitive therapy delayed post partum; however, the need for repeated stent exchanges is common. More recent data support the safety and efficacy of URS for stone removal during pregnancy. SWL is contraindicated in pregnancy.[249,250]

Surgical urologic issues related to the obstetric patient are uncommon, with the exception of inadvertent injury to the ureter or bladder during cesarean section, which, if recognized, should be repaired intraoperatively.[251] Ureteral stenting is also occasionally required to enable ureter identification during a cesarean/hysterectomy procedure for placenta accreta or percreta.[252]

Impotence Surgery and Medication

The impotence drugs sildenafil (Viagra), tadalafil (Cialis), and vardenafil (Levitra) all inhibit cyclic GMP–specific phosphodiesterase type 5 (PDE5) in vascular smooth muscle (Fig. 50-12). Blocking PDE5 impairs cyclic GMP breakdown, the mediator of nitric oxide effects that produce erectile responses to sexual stimulation through penile arterial vasodilation and corpus cavernosum smooth muscle relaxation. These agents have effects on other vessels and can be a useful treatment for pulmonary artery hypertension (trade names; sildenafil—Revatio, tadalfil—Adcirca).

Rational perioperative management of PDE5 inhibitor agents is important. Notably, although impotence therapies should be discontinued before surgery to minimize the risk of hypotension, pulmonary hypertension therapies must continue throughout the perioperative period. Although inhaled nitric oxide therapy can safely be used with PDE5 inhibitors, because its effects are limited to the pulmonary vasculature, whenever these agents are combined with systemic nitric oxide donors such as nitroglycerin or sodium nitroprusside exaggerated hypotensive responses are likely because of their dramatic potentiation of the peripheral vasodilator effects of nitric oxide.

Erectile dysfunction refractory to medical therapies can be treated by penile prosthesis implantation. Most prostheses are inflatable, with a secondary fluid reservoir and/or pump either behind the abdominal wall or inside the scrotum. Semirigid prostheses that do not involve pumps or reservoirs are also available, but these are less commonly used. Although penile implant procedures are relatively noninvasive, many recipients are elderly with multiple comorbidities, including vascular disease and diabetes. Traditionally, implantation has been performed under general or neuraxial anesthesia, but regional block (combined proximal dorsal nerve block and crural block) with sedation and monitored anesthesia care is also suitable if an abdominal incision is not required.[253]

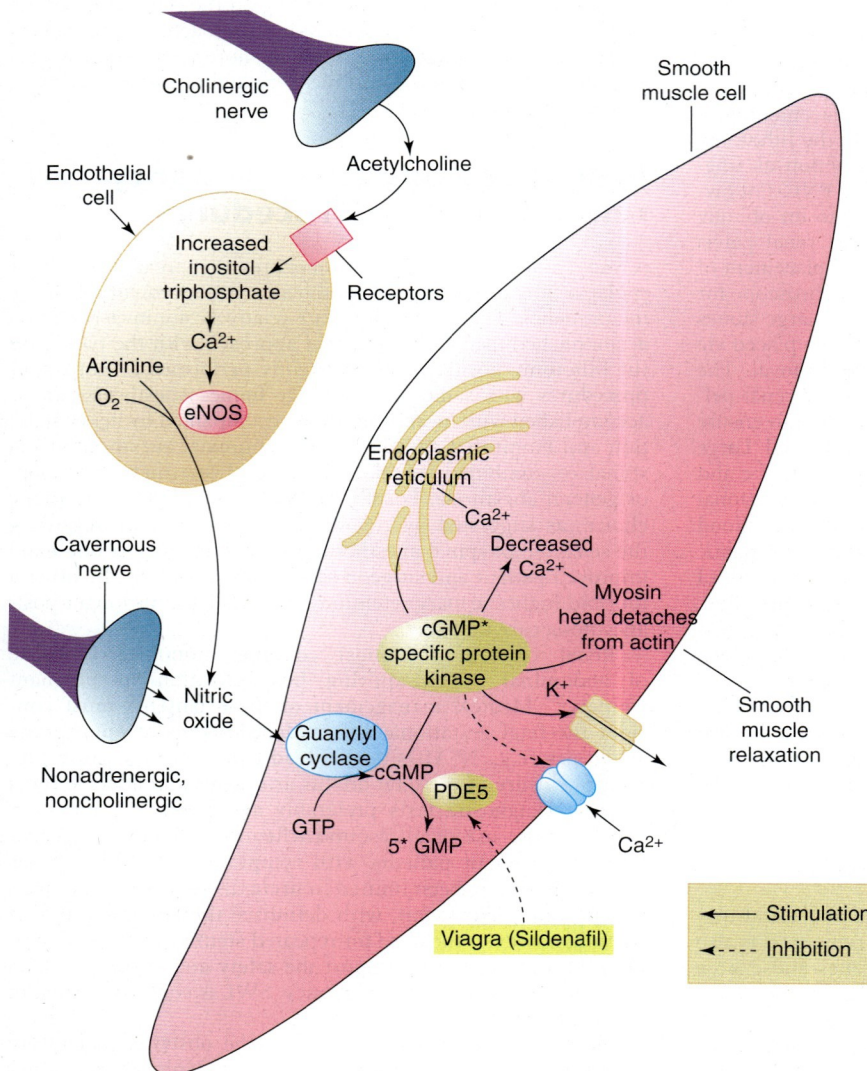

Figure 50-12 Nitric oxide–mediated vascular smooth muscle relaxation, including the inhibiting effects of sildenafil on cyclic GMP-specific phosphodiesterase type 5 (PDE5). (From www.wiley.com/college/boyer/0470003790/cutting_edge/viagra/viagra.htm. Reproduced with permission of John Wiley & Sons, Inc.)

Pediatric Surgical Urologic Disorders

The anesthesiologist caring for a pediatric patient undergoing a urologic procedure must first and foremost have a strong grasp of concepts of pediatric anesthesiology. General anesthesia is typical for these procedures, although a caudal block may provide good postoperative pain control (see Chapter 43).

Nephrectomy and Adrenalectomy

Many adult urologic procedures are also performed in children, although frequently for different indications. Nephrectomy, for example, is used to treat Wilms tumor and nonfunctioning kidney due to obstructive uropathy, stone disease, vesicoureteral reflux, or multicystic dysplastic kidney. Pediatric nephrectomy is amenable to open or laparoscopic approaches with general anesthesia.[254]

Adrenalectomy for neuroblastoma (28%), pheochromocytoma (21%), or adenoma (14%) can most often be achieved laparoscopically, although conversion to an open procedure, most often necessary owing to tumor adherence to surrounding organs, is more common than in adults (10%).[255]

As with adults, the preoperative workup and preparation of patients with pheochromocytoma should be thorough. Because inherited syndromes such as neurofibromatosis, von Hippel–Lindau disease, tuberous sclerosis, Sturge–Weber syndrome, and multiple endocrine neoplasia are commonly associated with pediatric pheochromocytoma, other related characteristics of these conditions should also be considered in preoperative preparation.[256] As with adult pheochromocytoma, preoperative therapy with α-1 adrenergic blocking agents (e.g., phenoxybenzamine) is recommended (see Chapter 46).[257]

Reconstructive Urologic Procedures

A number of urologic procedures related to congenital urologic deformities are performed almost exclusively on children. Many of these procedures are reconstructive in nature, intended to functionally repair a defect present at birth.

Bladder exstrophy, where part of the urinary bladder remains outside the body through a defect in the abdominal wall, occurs in 1 per 10,000 to 50,000 live births with a 2:1 male:female ratio.[258] Associated abnormalities are frequently present in the pelvic bones and external genitalia. Repair requires one or more of the following three procedures in a staged fashion: primary closure of the abdominal wall and osteotomy, usually occurring before 4 months of age; epispadias repair between 8 and 24 months of age; and bladder neck reconstruction at 40 to 60 months.[259]

Repair of ureteropelvic junction obstruction and ureterovesical reimplantation to treat vesicoureteral reflux requires general anesthesia and may be performed open or laparoscopically. Reconstruction of the lower urinary tract is more frequently achieved using an open approach, although laparoscopy is beginning to gain favor.

Posterior urethral valves (PUVs) are persistent embryonic membranes that cause bladder outlet obstruction and can lead to incomplete emptying, bladder hypertrophy, and even renal insufficiency or failure. PUVs occur exclusively in males, with an incidence of 1 to 2 per 10,000 male births, and may be diagnosed before or after birth by ultrasound. Although temporary treatment involves catheterization and antibiotics to prevent infection, definitive surgical repair is required, usually in the early postnatal period. Nonetheless, approximately one-third of the patients with PUV develop ESRD and require dialysis and/or renal transplantation.[260]

Undescended testis (cryptorchidism) affects 2% to 4% of male newborns. Cryptorchidism that persists at 1 year of age (1%) requires surgical repair (orchiopexy), normally as an outpatient procedure under general anesthesia.[261]

Hypospadias, an abnormal location of the urethral meatus on the ventral aspect of the penis resulting from incomplete embryologic development, occurs in 0.3% to 0.8% of male infants. Surgical repair is most commonly performed around 6 months of age as an outpatient procedure under general anesthesia, often supplemented with caudal analgesia. More complex repairs may require a second staged procedure around 12 months.

Circumcision of newborns is usually accomplished under ring block or local anesthetic infiltration without the presence of an anesthesiologist, although in older children general anesthesia with or without neuraxial anesthesia may be more appropriate.

Urologic Surgical Emergencies

Urologic emergencies are relatively rare, but three urologic emergency surgeries are worthy of mention. *Testicular torsion* requires emergency attention owing to the high risk, if otherwise untreated, for infarction or gangrene, which would require orchiectomy. In contrast, patients with *Fournier gangrene* or *sepsis* associated with nephrolithiasis are noteworthy because emergent definitive surgical therapy is the most effective way to reverse their infectious process and improve their prognosis. These latter patients are generally very seriously ill, and often the anesthesiologist provides ongoing resuscitation and applies critical care principles while delivering anesthetic care.

Testicular Torsion

Testicular torsion has a bimodal incidence, in the neonatal period and during early pubertal to teenage years. Testicular torsion affects approximately 1 in 4,000 young men, and 65% of cases occur in teenagers. When the spermatic cord twists, venous outflow from a testicle is obstructed, and eventually this compromises arterial flow, leading to ischemia and infarction.[262] Patients with testicular torsion present with acute scrotal pain and tenderness, most cases not involving a history of trauma. A predisposing anatomic bell-clapper deformity, which allows the testes to rotate freely in the tunica vaginalis, is the most common cause of this problem. Other risk factors include testicular tumors, a history of cryptorchidism, and an increase in testicular volume (e.g., puberty). Common misdiagnoses include epididymitis/orchitis, incarcerated hernia, and varicocele.[262] Absence of the cremasteric reflex is usually present on physical examination, and Doppler ultrasonography demonstrates decreased or absent blood flow. Equivocal physical examination findings dictate surgical exploration.

Apart from the considerable pain that torsion causes, the most important priority is the viability of the testicle. Testicular torsion requires immediate intervention, because viability decreases significantly with the duration of testicular ischemia. Success in saving the testicle relates to the timing from symptom onset to detorsion, with success rates of 90%, 50%, and 10% with delays of 6, 12, and greater than 24 hours, respectively.[263]

Anesthesia for testicular torsion surgery must respect its emergent nature, including the likelihood that the patient has not fasted. Regional or general anesthesia is appropriate, but spinal anesthesia is relatively contraindicated owing to the high risk of postdural puncture headache in the young population where the problem is most often manifested.

Fournier Gangrene

Fournier gangrene is a form of necrotizing fasciitis affecting the genitalia. It presents most commonly in older men, and frequently associated comorbidities include diabetes mellitus, morbid obesity, and immune suppression.[264] Minor genital trauma is often the inciting event, but rapid widespread inflammation, infection, and ultimately polymicrobial sepsis characterize the condition. Fournier gangrene patients often present with already established septic shock warranting the emergent status for surgery, but fluid resuscitation and institution of broad-spectrum antibiotic therapy (commonly staphylococci, streptococci, enterobacteriaceae, and anaerobes) are also priorities.[265] Surgical management consists of incision, drainage, and debridement of affected tissue. Hyperbaric oxygen therapy is also employed at some centers[266,267] but does not replace emergent surgical debridement. Morbidity and mortality are significant, with advanced age and presence of septic shock at presentation portending the highest risk.[268]

Anesthetic planning must incorporate assessment of the degree of sepsis and hemodynamic status of the patient. General anesthesia with endotracheal intubation and positive-pressure ventilation is standard. Intra-arterial and central venous access are often indicated to facilitate resuscitation of the patient. Transfusion may be necessary because the extensive tissue resection can involve significant blood loss. Patients often require postoperative intensive care admission to manage the sequelae of sepsis and often undergo repeated procedures for additional debridement, wound care, and eventually wound closure.[265]

Emergency Treatment of Nephrolithiasis

Most patients who require surgical or interventional treatment of nephrolithiasis can be managed electively, but patients with infection associated with urinary tract obstruction, AKI, bilateral obstructing stones, intractable pain or vomiting, or obstruction in a solitary (native or transplanted) kidney should be managed urgently to avoid sepsis and preserve renal function.[242] Procedures indicated for these conditions to alleviate obstruction include cystoscopy with stent insertion, percutaneous nephrostomy, and, very rarely, open pyelolithotomy or nephrectomy for definitive treatment related to stones unsuccessfully treated by less-invasive interventions. Identification of patients who have infected urine and obstruction is important because they are at high risk of developing sepsis, which can manifest preoperatively, intraoperatively, or postoperatively. As with any infection, the principles of drainage and institution of appropriate antibiotic therapy are paramount, and in the presence of complete urinary obstruction, antibiotic therapy alone is insufficient treatment. If the urinary tract can be decompressed with a stent or nephrostomy, definitive management can be postponed until the patient has responded to antibiotic therapy.[236] Patients with nephrolithiasis complicated by urinary tract infection are at higher risk for infection with antibiotic-resistant pathogens, which requires targeted antibiotic therapy.[269]

Another category of patients requiring urgent surgery are patients with declining renal function in the setting of urinary obstruction (e.g., ureteral obstruction from renal papillary necrosis, blood clots, or urethral obstruction due to blood clots or stricture).[235] Other situations (e.g., obstructed solitary or transplanted kidney, hemorrhage, and blood clots) may dictate urgent, rather than elective, surgery to relieve the urinary obstruction and preserve renal function, though in the absence of infection this group of patients may not be as acutely ill.

Anesthetic considerations for emergent nephrolithiasis surgery are similar to those for equivalent elective procedures (see earlier). Additional considerations include the potential need for more invasive monitoring, for example, direct arterial blood pressure monitoring in the setting of sepsis. Similarly, hemodynamically unstable septic patients often have ongoing needs for fluid resuscitation and pharmacologic support of the circulation and, in the setting of deteriorating renal function, may require alterations from standard anesthetic agent selections. Because evidence of sepsis may not manifest until the postoperative period, raised awareness for such concerns should continue into the postanesthetic recovery period.

REFERENCES

1. Woodcock TE, Woodcock TM. Revised starling equation and the glycocalyx model of transvascular fluid exchange: An improved paradigm for prescribing intravenous fluid therapy. *Br J Anaesth*. 2012;108(3):384–394.
2. Singh A, Satchell SC, Neal CR, et al. Glomerular endothelial glycocalyx constitutes a barrier to protein permeability. *J Am Soc Nephrol*. 2007;18(11):2885–2893.
3. Garsen M, Rops AL, Rabelink TJ, et al. The role of heparanase and the endothelial glycocalyx in the development of proteinuria. *Nephrol Dial Transplant*. 2014;29(1):49–55.
4. Alpert RA, Roizen MF, Hamilton WK, et al. Intraoperative urinary output does not predict postoperative renal function in patients undergoing abdominal aortic revascularization. *Surgery*. 1984;95(6):707–711.
5. Conlon PJ, Stafford-Smith M, White WD, et al. Acute renal failure following cardiac surgery. *Nephrol Dial Transplant*. 1999;14(5):1158–1162.
6. Levin A. Cystatin C, serum creatinine, and estimates of kidney function: Searching for better measures of kidney function and cardiovascular risk. *Ann Intern Med*. 2005;142(7):586–588.
7. Grubb A, Bjork J, Lindstrom V, et al. A cystatin C-based formula without anthropometric variables estimates glomerular filtration rate better than creatinine clearance using the Cockcroft-Gault formula. *Scand J Clin Lab Invest*. 2005;65(2):153–162.
8. Alpert MA, Govindarajan G, Del Rosario ML, et al. The role of the renin-angiotensin system in the pathophysiology, prevention, and treatment of renal impairment in patients with the cardiometabolic syndrome or its components. *J Cardiometab Syndr*. 2009;4(1):57–62.
9. Srisawat N, Murugan R, Kellum JA. Repair or progression after AKI: A role for biomarkers? *Nephron Clin Pract*. 2014;127(1-4):185–189.
10. Wasung ME, Chawla LS, Madero M. Biomarkers of renal function, which and when? *Clin Chim Acta*. 2015;438:350–357.
11. Sladen RN, Endo E, Harrison T. Two-hour versus 22-hour creatinine clearance in critically ill patients. *Anesthesiology*. 1987;67(6):1013–1016.
12. Bloor GK, Welsh KR, Goodall S, et al. Comparison of predicted with measured creatinine clearance in cardiac surgical patients. *J Cardiothorac Vasc Anesth*. 1996;10(7):899–902.
13. Gowans EM, Fraser CG. Biological variation of serum and urine creatinine and creatinine clearance: Ramifications for interpretation of results and patient care. *Ann Clin Biochem*. 1988;25(Pt 3):259–263.
14. Morgan DB, Dillon S, Payne RB. The assessment of glomerular function: Creatinine clearance or plasma creatinine? *Postgrad Med J*. 1978;54(631):302–310.
15. Cockcroft DW, Gault MH. Prediction of creatinine clearance from serum creatinine. *Nephron*. 1976;16(1):31–41.
16. Levey AS, Bosch JP, Lewis JB, et al. A more accurate method to estimate glomerular filtration rate from serum creatinine: A new prediction equation. Modification of Diet in Renal Disease Study Group. *Ann Intern Med*. 1999;130(6):461–470.
17. Ferguson TB Jr, Dziuban SW Jr, Edwards FH, et al. The STS national database: Current changes and challenges for the new millennium. Committee to establish a national database in cardiothoracic surgery, The Society of Thoracic Surgeons. *Ann Thorac Surg*. 2000;69(3):680–691.
18. Barrett BJ, Parfrey PS. Prevention of nephrotoxicity induced by radiocontrast agents. *N Engl J Med*. 1994;331(21):1449–1450.
19. Bellomo R, Ronco C, Kellum JA, et al. Acute renal failure – definition, outcome measures, animal models, fluid therapy and information technology needs: The second international consensus conference of the Acute Dialysis Quality Initiative (ADQI) group. *Crit Care*. 2004;8(4):R204–R212.
20. Mehta RL, Kellum JA, Shah SV, et al. Acute kidney injury network: Report of an initiative to improve outcomes in acute kidney injury. *Crit Care*. 2007;11(2):R31.
21. Kidney Disease: Improving Global Outcomes (KDIGO) Acute Kidney Injury Work Group. KDIGO clinical practice guideline for acute kidney injury. *Kidney Int Suppl*. 2012;2(1):1–138.

22. Greenberg A, ed. *Primer on Kidney Diseases*. 4th ed. Philadelphia, PA: Elsevier Saunders; 2005.
23. Stafford-Smith M. Antifibrinolytic agents make alpha1- and beta2-microglobulinuria poor markers of post cardiac surgery renal dysfunction. *Anesthesiology*. 1999;90:928–929.
24. Anderson RJ, Chung HM, Kluge R, et al. Hyponatremia: A prospective analysis of its epidemiology and the pathogenetic role of vasopressin. *Ann Intern Med*. 1985;102(2):164–163.
25. Verbalis JG. Hyponatremia: Epidemiology, pathophysiology, and therapy. *Curr Opin Nephrol Hypertens*. 1993;2(4):636–652.
26. Arieff AI. Hyponatremia, convulsions, respiratory arrest, and permanent brain damage after elective surgery in healthy women. *N Engl J Med*. 1986;314(24):1529–1535.
27. Arieff AI, Ayus JC, Fraser CL. Hyponatraemia and death or permanent brain damage in healthy children. *BMJ*. 1992;304(6836):1218–1222.
28. Ayus JC, Wheeler JM, Arieff AI. Postoperative hyponatremic encephalopathy in menstruant women. *Ann Intern Med*. 1992;117(11):891–897.
29. Witteveen JE, van Thiel S, Romijn JA, et al. Hungry bone syndrome: Still a challenge in the post-operative management of primary hyperparathyroidism: A systematic review of the literature. *Eur J Endocrinol*. 2013;168(3):R45–R53.
30. Amanzadeh J, Reilly RF Jr. Hypophosphatemia: An evidence-based approach to its clinical consequences and management. *Nat Clin Pract Nephrol*. 2006;2(3):136–148.
31. Anderson RJ, Linas SL, Berns AS, et al. Nonoliguric acute renal failure. *N Engl J Med*. 1977;296(20):1134–1138.
32. Doi K, Rabb H. Impact of acute kidney injury on distant organ function: Recent findings and potential therapeutic targets. *Kidney Int*. 2016;89(3):555–564.
33. Bagshaw SM, Laupland KB, Doig CJ, et al. Prognosis for long-term survival and renal recovery in critically ill patients with severe acute renal failure: A population-based study. *Crit Care*. 2005;9(6):R700–R709.
34. Wilkinson A, Cohen D. Renal failure in the recipients of nonrenal solid organ transplants. *J Am Soc Nephrol*. 1999;10(5):1136–1144.
35. Uchino S, Kellum JA, Bellomo R, et al. Acute renal failure in critically ill patients: A multinational, multicenter study. *JAMA*. 2005;294(7):813–818.
36. Alonso A, Lau J, Jaber B, et al. Prevention of radiocontrast nephropathy with N-acetylcysteine in patients with chronic kidney disease: A meta-analysis of randomized, controlled trials. *Am J Kidney Dis*. 2004;43(1):1–9.
37. Liano F, Pascual J. Epidemiology of acute renal failure: a prospective, multicenter, community-based study. Madrid Acute Renal Failure Study Group. *Kidney Int*. 1996;50(3):811–818.
38. Yacoub R, Patel N, Lohr JW, et al. Acute kidney injury and death associated with renin angiotensin system blockade in cardiothoracic surgery: A meta-analysis of observational studies. *Am J Kidney Dis*. 2013;62(6):1077–1086.
39. Knight EL, Glynn RJ, McIntyre KM, et al. Predictors of decreased renal function in patients with heart failure during angiotensin-converting enzyme inhibitor therapy: Results from the studies of left ventricular dysfunction (SOLVD). *Am Heart J*. 1999;138(5 Pt 1):849–855.
40. Schoolwerth AC, Sica DA, Ballermann BJ, et al. Council on the Kidney in Cardiovascular Disease, the Council for High Blood Pressure Research of the American Heart Association. Renal considerations in angiotensin converting enzyme inhibitor therapy: A statement for healthcare professionals from the Council on the Kidney in Cardiovascular Disease and the Council for High Blood Pressure Research of the American Heart Association. *Circulation*. 2001;104(16):1985–1991.
41. Adhiyaman V, Asghar M, Oke A, et al. Nephrotoxicity in the elderly due to co-prescription of angiotensin converting enzyme inhibitors and nonsteroidal anti-inflammatory drugs. *J R Soc Med*. 2001;94(10):512–514.
42. Kincaid EH, Ashburn DA, Hoyle JR, et al. Does the combination of aprotinin and angiotensin-converting enzyme inhibitor cause renal failure after cardiac surgery? *Ann Thorac Surg*. 2005;80(4):1388–1393.
43. Metz LI, Lebeau ME, Zlabek JA, et al. Acute renal failure in patients undergoing cardiothoracic surgery in a community hospital. *WMJ*. 2009;108(2):109–114.
44. Reynolds A, White W, Stafford-Smith M, et al. The relationship of loop diuretics with acute kidney injury and mortality after cardiac surgery. *Anesth Analg*. 2013;116(Suppl):SCA3.
45. Zhang Y, Ye N, Chen YP, et al. Relation between the interval from coronary angiography to selective off-pump coronary artery bypass grafting and postoperative acute kidney injury. *Am J Cardiol*. 2013;112(10):1571–1575.
46. Lassnigg A, Donner E, Grubhofer G, et al. Lack of renoprotective effects of dopamine and furosemide during cardiac surgery. *J Am Soc Nephrol*. 2000;11(1):97–104.
47. Kheterpal S, Tremper KK, Englesbe MJ, et al. Predictors of postoperative acute renal failure after noncardiac surgery in patients with previously normal renal function. *Anesthesiology*. 2007;107(6):892–902.
48. Singh I, Rajagopalan S, Srinivasan A, et al. Preoperative statin therapy is associated with lower requirement of renal replacement therapy in patients undergoing cardiac surgery: A meta-analysis of observational studies. *Interact Cardiovasc Thorac Surg*. 2013;17(2):345–352.
49. Rudnick M, Feldman H. Contrast-induced nephropathy: What are the true clinical consequences? *Clin J Am Soc Nephrol*. 2008;3(1):263–272.
50. Hu Y, Zhong Q. Contrast-induced nephropathy may constitute a marker of underlying limited renal reserve for cardiac surgical procedures? *Ann Thorac Surg*. 2013;95(5):1841.
51. Taber SS, Mueller BA. Drug-associated renal dysfunction. *Crit Care Clin*. 2006;22(2):357–374.
52. Huerta C, Castellsague J, Varas-Lorenzo C, et al. Nonsteroidal anti-inflammatory drugs and risk of ARF in the general population. *Am J Kidney Dis*. 2005;45(3):531–539.
53. Oh KJ, Lee HH, Lee JS, et al. Reversible renal vasoconstriction in a patient with acute renal failure after exercise. *Clin Nephrol*. 2006;66(4):297–301.
54. Melli G, Chaudhry V, Cornblath DR. Rhabdomyolysis: An evaluation of 475 hospitalized patients. *Medicine (Baltimore)*. 2005;84(6):377–385.
55. Singh D, Chander V, Chopra K. Rhabdomyolysis. *Methods Find Exp Clin Pharmacol*. 2005;27(1):39-48.
56. Eichhorn JH, Hedley-Whyte J, Steinman TI, et al. Renal failure following enflurane anesthesia. *Anesthesiology*. 1976;45(5):557–560.
57. Eger EI, Gong D, Koblin DD, et al. Dose-related biochemical markers of renal injury after sevoflurane versus desflurane anesthesia in volunteers. *Anesth Analg*. 1997;85(5):1154–1163.
58. Conzen PF, Kharasch ED, Czerner SF, et al. Low-flow sevoflurane compared with low-flow isoflurane anesthesia in patients with stable renal insufficiency. *Anesthesiology*. 2002;97(3):578–584.
59. Myburgh JA, Finfer S, Bellomo R, et al. Hydroxyethyl starch or saline for fluid resuscitation in intensive care. *N Engl J Med*. 2012;367(20):1901–1911.
60. Perner A, Haase N, Guttormsen AB, et al. Hydroxyethyl starch 130/0.42 versus Ringer's acetate in severe sepsis. *N Engl J Med*. 2012;367(2):124–134.
61. Yunos NM, Bellomo R, Hegarty C, et al. Association between a chloride-liberal vs chloride-restrictive intravenous fluid administration strategy and kidney injury in critically ill adults. *JAMA*. 2012;308(15):1566–1572.
62. Prowle JR, Kirwan CJ, Bellomo R. Fluid management for the prevention and attenuation of acute kidney injury. *Nature Rev Nephrol*. 2014;10(1):37–47.
63. Prowle JR, Chua HR, Bagshaw SM, et al. Clinical review: Volume of fluid resuscitation and the incidence of acute kidney injury: A systematic review. *Crit Care*. 2012;16(4):230.
64. Gunukula SR, Spodick DH. Pericardial disease in renal patients. *Semin Nephrol*. 2001;21(1):52–56.
65. Crandell WB, Pappas SG, Macdonald A. Nephrotoxicity associated with methoxyflurane anesthesia. *Anesthesiology*. 1966;27(5):591–607.
66. Kharasch ED, Hankins DC, Thummel KE. Human kidney methoxyflurane and sevoflurane metabolism: Intrarenal fluoride production as a possible mechanism of methoxyflurane nephrotoxicity. *Anesthesiology*. 1995;82(3):689–699.
67. Mazze RI, Calverley RK, Smith NT. Inorganic fluoride nephrotoxicity: Prolonged enflurane and halothane anesthesia in volunteers. *Anesthesiology*. 1977;46(4):265–271.
68. Burch PG, Stanski DR. Decreased protein binding and thiopental kinetics. *Clin Pharmacol Ther*. 1982;32(2):212–217.
69. Gan TJ. Pharmacokinetic and pharmacodynamic characteristics of medications used for moderate sedation. *Clin Pharmacokinet*. 2006;45(9):855–869.
70. Carlos R, Calvo R, Erill S. Plasma protein binding of etomidate in patients with renal failure or hepatic cirrhosis. *Clin Pharmacokinet*. 1979;4(2):144–148.
71. Kirvela M, Olkkola KT, Rosenberg PH, et al. Pharmacokinetics of propofol and haemodynamic changes during induction of anaesthesia in uraemic patients. *Br J Anaesth*. 1992;68(2):178–182.
72. Vinik HR, Reves JG, Greenblatt DJ, et al. The pharmacokinetics of midazolam in chronic renal failure patients. *Anesthesiology*. 1983;59(5):390–394.
73. Schmith VD, Piraino B, Smith RB, et al. Alprazolam in end-stage renal disease. II. Pharmacodynamics. *Clin Pharmacol Ther*. 1992;51(5):533–540.
74. De Wolf AM, Fragen RJ, Avram MJ, et al. The pharmacokinetics of dexmedetomidine in volunteers with severe renal impairment. *Anesth Analg*. 2001;93(5):1205–1209.
75. Chan GL, Matzke GR. Effects of renal insufficiency on the pharmacokinetics and pharmacodynamics of opioid analgesics. *Drug Intell Clin Pharm*. 1987;21(10):773–783.
76. Babul N, Darke AC, Hagen N. Hydromorphone metabolite accumulation in renal failure. *J Pain Symptom Manage*. 1995;10(3):184–186.
77. Murphy EJ. Acute pain management pharmacology for the patient with concurrent renal or hepatic disease. *Anaesth Intensive Care*. 2005;33(3):311–322.
78. Davis PJ, Stiller RL, Cook DR, et al. Effects of cholestatic hepatic disease and chronic renal failure on alfentanil pharmacokinetics in children. *Anesth Analg*. 1989;68(5):579–583.
79. Wiggum DC, Cork RC, Weldon ST, et al. Postoperative respiratory depression and elevated sufentanil levels in a patient with chronic renal failure. *Anesthesiology*. 1985;63(6):708–710.
80. Pitsiu M, Wilmer A, Bodenham A, et al. Pharmacokinetics of remifentanil and its major metabolite, remifentanil acid, in ICU patients with renal impairment. *Br J Anaesth*. 2004;92(4):493–503.
81. Szenohradszky J, Caldwell JE, Wright PM, et al. Influence of renal failure on the pharmacokinetics and neuromuscular effects of a single dose of rapacuronium bromide. *Anesthesiology*. 1999;90(1):24–35.

82. Ryan DW. Preoperative serum cholinesterase concentration in chronic renal failure. Clinical experience of suxamethonium in 81 patients undergoing renal transplant. Br J Anaesth. 1977;49(9):945–949.
83. Cook DR, Freeman JA, Lai AA, et al. Pharmacokinetics of mivacurium in normal patients and in those with hepatic or renal failure. Br J Anaesth. 1992;69(6):580–585.
84. Cook DR, Freeman JA, Lai AA, et al. Pharmacokinetics and pharmacodynamics of doxacurium in normal patients and in those with hepatic or renal failure. Anesth Analg. 1991;72(2):145–150.
85. Della Rocca G, Pompei L, Coccia C, et al. Atracurium, cisatracurium, vecuronium and rocuronium in patients with renal failure. Minerva Anestesiol. 2003;69(7-8):605–611.
86. Fahey MR, Rupp SM, Canfell C, et al. Effect of renal failure on laudanosine excretion in man. Br J Anaesth. 1985;57(11):1049–1051.
87. Lynam DP, Cronnelly R, Castagnoli KP, et al. The pharmacodynamics and pharmacokinetics of vecuronium in patients anesthetized with isoflurane with normal renal function or with renal failure. Anesthesiology. 1988;69(2):227–331.
88. Robertson EN, Driessen JJ, Booij LH. Pharmacokinetics and pharmacodynamics of rocuronium in patients with and without renal failure. Eur J Anaesthesiol. 2005;22(1):4–10.
89. Szenohradszky J, Fisher DM, Segredo V, et al. Pharmacokinetics of rocuronium bromide (ORG 9426) in patients with normal renal function or patients undergoing cadaver renal transplantation. Anesthesiology. 1992; 77(5):899–904.
90. Cooper RA, Maddineni VR, Mirakhur RK, et al. Time course of neuromuscular effects and pharmacokinetics of rocuronium bromide (Org 9426) during isoflurane anaesthesia in patients with and without renal failure. Br J Anaesth. 1993;71(2):222–226.
91. Phillips BJ, Hunter JM. Use of mivacurium chloride by constant infusion in the anephric patient. Br J Anaesth. 1992;68(5):492–498.
92. Blobner M, Jelen-Esselborn S, Schneider G, et al. Effect of renal function on neuromuscular block induced by continuous infusion of mivacurium. Br J Anaesth. 1995;74(4):452–454.
93. Morris RB, Cronnelly R, Miller RD, et al. Pharmacokinetics of edrophonium in anephric and renal transplant patients. Br J Anaesth. 1981;53(12):1311–1314.
94. Epemolu O, Bom A, Hope F, et al. Reversal of neuromuscular blockade and simultaneous increase in plasma rocuronium concentration after the intravenous infusion of the novel reversal agent Org 25969. Anesthesiology. 2003;99(3):632–637.
95. Staals LM, Snoeck MM, Driessen JJ, et al. Reduced clearance of rocuronium and sugammadex in patients with severe to end-stage renal failure: A pharmacokinetic study. Br J Anaesth. 2010;104(1):31–39.
96. Larson EB, Roach RC, Schoene RB, et al. Acute mountain sickness and acetazolamide: Clinical efficacy and effect on ventilation. JAMA. 1982;248(3):328–332.
97. White DP, Zwillich CW, Pickett CK, et al. Central sleep apnea. Improvement with acetazolamide therapy. Arch Intern Med. 1982;142(10):1816–1819.
98. Conger JD. Interventions in clinical acute renal failure: What are the data? Am J Kidney Dis. 1995;26(4):565–576.
99. Solomon R, Werner C, Mann D, et al. Effects of saline, mannitol, and furosemide to prevent acute decreases in renal function induced by radiocontrast agents. N Engl J Med. 1994;331(21):1416–1420.
100. Better OS, Rubinstein I, Winaver JM, et al. Mannitol therapy revisited (1940-1997). Kidney Int. 1997;52(4):886–894.
101. Borges HF, Hocks J, Kjellstrand CM. Mannitol intoxication in patients with renal failure. Arch Intern Med. 1982;142(1):63–66.
102. Gallagher KL, Jones JK. Furosemide-induced ototoxicity. Ann Intern Med. 1979;91(5):744–745.
103. Pitt B, Zannad F, Remme WJ, et al. The effect of spironolactone on morbidity and mortality in patients with severe heart failure. Randomized Aldactone Evaluation Study Investigators. N Engl J Med. 1999;341(10):709–717.
104. Jose PA, Felder RA. What we can learn from the selective manipulation of dopaminergic receptors about the pathogenesis and treatment of hypertension? Curr Opin Nephrol Hypertens. 1996;5(5):447–451.
105. Bellomo R, Cole L, Ronco C. Hemodynamic support and the role of dopamine. Kidney Int Suppl. 1998;66:S71–S74.
106. Marik PE. Low-dose dopamine: A systematic review. Intensive Care Med. 2002;28(7):877–883.
107. Kellum JA, Decker JM. Use of dopamine in acute renal failure: A meta-analysis. Crit Care Med. 2001;29(8):1526–1531.
108. Prins I, Plotz FB, Uiterwaal CS, et al. Low-dose dopamine in neonatal and pediatric intensive care: A systematic review. Intensive Care Med. 2001;27(1):206–210.
109. Holmes CL, Walley KR. Bad medicine: Low-dose dopamine in the ICU. Chest. 2003;123(4):1266–1275.
110. Argalious M, Motta P, Khandwala F, et al. "Renal dose" dopamine is associated with the risk of new-onset atrial fibrillation after cardiac surgery. Crit Care Med. 2005;33(6):1327–1332.
111. Denton MD, Chertow GM, Brady HR. "Renal-dose" dopamine for the treatment of acute renal failure: Scientific rationale, experimental studies and clinical trials. Kidney Int. 1996;50(1):4–14.
112. Abel RM, Buckley MJ, Austen WG, et al. Etiology, incidence, and prognosis of renal failure following cardiac operations. Results of a prospective analysis of 500 consecutive patients. J Thorac Cardiovasc Surg. 1976;71(3):323–333.
113. Swaminathan M, Shaw A, Phillips-Bute B, et al. Trends in acute renal failure associated with coronary artery bypass graft surgery in the United States. Crit Care Med. 2007;35(10):2286–2291.
114. Filsoufi F, Rahmanian PB, Castillo JG, et al. Early and late outcomes of cardiac surgery in patients with moderate to severe preoperative renal dysfunction without dialysis. Interact Cardiovasc Thorac Surg. 2008;7(1):90–95.
115. Bechtel JF, Detter C, Fischlein T, et al. Cardiac surgery in patients on dialysis: Decreased 30-day mortality, unchanged overall survival. Ann Thorac Surg. 2008;85(1):147–153.
116. Aronson S, Fontes ML, Miao Y, et al. Risk index for perioperative renal dysfunction/failure: Critical dependence on pulse pressure hypertension. Circulation. 2007;115(6):733–742.
117. Mangano DT, Tudor IC, Dietzel C. The risk associated with aprotinin in cardiac surgery. N Engl J Med. 2006;354(4):353–365.
118. Hix JK, Thakar CV, Katz EM, et al. Effect of off-pump coronary artery bypass graft surgery on postoperative acute kidney injury and mortality. Crit Care Med. 2006;34(12):2979–2983.
119. Costa P, Ottino GM, Matani A, et al. Low-dose dopamine during cardiopulmonary bypass in patients with renal dysfunction. J Cardiothorac Anesth. 1990;4(4):469–473.
120. Berendes E, Mollhoff T, Van Aken H, et al. Effects of dopexamine on creatinine clearance, systemic inflammation, and splanchnic oxygenation in patients undergoing coronary artery bypass grafting. Anesth Analg. 1997;84(5):950–957.
121. Renton MC, Snowden CP. Dopexamine and its role in the protection of hepatosplanchnic and renal perfusion in high-risk surgical and critically ill patients. Br J Anaesth. 2005;94(4):459–467.
122. Novis BK, Roizen MF, Aronson S, et al. Association of preoperative risk factors with postoperative acute renal failure. Anesth Analg. 1994;78(1):143–149.
123. Stene JK. Renal failure in the trauma patient. Crit Care Clin. 1990;6(1):111–119.
124. Cachecho R, Millham FH, Wedel SK. Management of the trauma patient with pre-existing renal disease. Crit Care Clin. 1994;10(3):523–536.
125. Myers BD, Miller DC, Mehigan JT, et al. Nature of the renal injury following total renal ischemia in man. J Clin Invest. 1984;73(2):329–341.
126. Godet G, Fleron MH, Vicaut E, et al. Risk factors for acute postoperative renal failure in thoracic or thoracoabdominal aortic surgery: A prospective study. Anesth Analg. 1997;85(6):1227–1232.
127. Svensson LG, Coselli JS, Safi HJ, et al. Appraisal of adjuncts to prevent acute renal failure after surgery on the thoracic or thoracoabdominal aorta. J Vasc Surg. 1989;10(3):230–239.
128. Olsen PS, Schroeder T, Perko M, et al. Renal failure after operation for abdominal aortic aneurysm. Ann Vasc Surg. 1990;4(6):580–583.
129. Svensson LG, Kouchoukos NT, Miller DC, et al. Expert consensus document on the treatment of descending thoracic aortic disease using endovascular stent-grafts. Ann Thorac Surg. 2008;85(1 Suppl):S1–S41.
130. Antonucci F, Calo L, Rizzolo M, et al. Nifedipine can preserve renal function in patients undergoing aortic surgery with infrarenal crossclamping. Nephron. 1996;74(4):668–673.
131. Ding H, Kopple JD, Cohen A, et al. Recombinant human insulin-like growth factor-I accelerates recovery and reduces catabolism in rats with ischemic acute renal failure. J Clin Invest. 1993;91(5):2281–2287.
132. Vijayan A, Franklin SC, Behrend T, et al. Insulin-like growth factor I improves renal function in patients with end-stage chronic renal failure. Am J Physiol. 1999;276(4 Pt 2):R929–R934.
133. Franklin SC, Moulton M, Sicard GA, et al. Insulin-like growth factor I preserves renal function postoperatively. Am J Physiol. 1997;272(2 Pt 2):F257–F259.
134. Allgren RL, Marbury TC, Rahman SN, et al. Anaritide in acute tubular necrosis. Auriculin Anaritide Acute Renal Failure Study Group. N Engl J Med. 1997;336(12):828–834.
135. Yalavarthy R, Edelstein CL, Teitelbaum I. Acute renal failure and chronic kidney disease following liver transplantation. Hemodial Int. 2007;11(Suppl 3):S7–S12.
136. Lopez Lago AM, Fernandez Villanueva J, Garcia Acuna JM, et al. Evolution of hepatorenal syndrome after orthotopic liver transplantation: Comparative analysis with patients who developed acute renal failure in the early postoperative period of liver transplantation. Transplant Proc. 2007;39(7):2318–2319.
137. Fleisher LA, Beckman JA, Brown KA, et al. ACC/AHA 2007 Guidelines on perioperative cardiovascular evaluation and care for noncardiac surgery: Executive summary: A report of the American College of Cardiology/American Heart Association Task Force on Practice Guidelines (Writing Committee to Revise the 2002 Guidelines on Perioperative Cardiovascular Evaluation for Noncardiac Surgery): Developed in Collaboration With the American Society of Echocardiography, American Society of Nuclear Cardiology, Heart Rhythm Society, Society of Cardiovascular Anesthesiologists, Society for Cardiovascular Angiography and Interventions, Society for Vascular Medicine and Biology, and Society for Vascular Surgery. Circulation. 2007;116(17):1971–1996.
138. Khaira HS, Shah RB, Wolf JS Jr. Laparoscopic and open surgical nephrectomy for xanthogranulomatous pyelonephritis. J Endourol. 2005;19(7):813–817.

139. Richard S, Lidereau R, Giraud S. The growing family of hereditary renal cell carcinoma. *Nephrol Dial Transplant.* 2004;19(12):2954–2958.
140. Palapattu GS, Kristo B, Rajfer J. Paraneoplastic syndromes in urologic malignancy: The many faces of renal cell carcinoma. *Rev Urol.* 2002;4(4):163–170.
141. Galvez JA, Clebone A, Garwood S, Popescu WM. Fatal intraoperative cardiac thrombosis in a patient with renal cell carcinoma. *Anesthesiology.* 2011;114(5):1212.
142. Wijeysundera DN, Beattie WS, Austin PC, et al. Epidural anaesthesia and survival after intermediate-to-high risk non-cardiac surgery: A population-based cohort study. *Lancet.* 2008;372(9638):562–569.
143. Dunn MD, Portis AJ, Shalhav AL, et al. Laparoscopic versus open radical nephrectomy: A 9-year experience. *J Urol.* 2000;164(4):1153–1159.
144. Permpongkosol S, Link RE, Su LM, et al. Complications of 2,775 urological laparoscopic procedures: 1993 to 2005. *J Urol.* 2007;177(2):580–585.
145. Pareek G, Hedican SP, Gee JR, et al. Meta-analysis of the complications of laparoscopic renal surgery Comparison of procedures and techniques. *J Urol.* 2006;175(4):1208–1213.
146. Gill IS, Matin SF, Desai MM, et al. Comparative analysis of laparoscopic versus open partial nephrectomy for renal tumors in 200 patients. *J Urol.* 2003;170(1):64–68.
147. Simmons MN, Gill IS. Decreased complications of contemporary laparoscopic partial nephrectomy: Use of a standardized reporting system. *J Urol.* 2007;177(6):2067–2073.
148. Turna B, Frota R, Kamoi K, et al. Risk factor analysis of postoperative complications in laparoscopic partial nephrectomy. *J Urol.* 2008;179(4):1289–1294.
149. Lassen K, Soop M, Nygren J, et al. Consensus review of optimal perioperative care in colorectal surgery: Enhanced Recovery After Surgery (ERAS) Group recommendations. *Arch Surg.* 2009;144(10):961–969.
150. Schefft P, Novick AC, Straffon RA, et al. Surgery for renal cell carcinoma extending into the inferior vena cava. *J Urol.* 1978;120(1):28–31.
151. Neves RJ, Zincke H. Surgical treatment of renal cancer with vena cava extension. *Br J Urol.* 1987;59(5) 390–395.
152. Nesbitt JC, Soltero ER, Linney CP, et al. Surgical management of renal cell carcinoma with inferior vena cava tumor thrombus. *Ann Thorac Surg.* 1997;63(6):1592–1600.
153. Porpiglia F, Renard J, Billia M, et al. Is renal warm ischemia over 30 minutes during laparoscopic partial nephrectomy possible? One-year results of a prospective study. *Eur Urol.* 2007;52(4):1170–1178.
154. Desai MM, Gill IS, Ramani AP, et al. The impact of warm ischaemia on renal function after laparoscopic partial nephrectomy. *BJU Int.* 2005;95(3):377–383.
155. Eskicorapci SY, Teber D, Schulze M, et al. Laparoscopic radical nephrectomy: The new gold standard surgical treatment for localized renal cell carcinoma. *Sci World J.* 2007;7:825–836.
156. Permpongkosol S, Chan DY, Link RE, et al. Long-term survival analysis after laparoscopic radical nephrectomy. *J Urol.* 2005;174(4 Pt 1):1222–1225.
157. Russo P. Is laparoscopic partial nephrectomy as effective as open partial nephrectomy in patients with renal cell carcinoma? *Nat Clin Pract Urol.* 2008;5(1):12–13.
158. Gill IS, Kavoussi LR, Lane BR, et al. Comparison of 1,800 laparoscopic and open partial nephrectomies for single renal tumors. *J Urol.* 2007;178(1):41–46.
159. Nicholson ML, Elwell R, Kaushik M, et al. Health-related quality of life after living donor nephrectomy: A randomized controlled trial of laparoscopic versus open nephrectomy. *Transplantation.* 2011;91(4):457–461.
160. Waller JR, Hiley AL, Mullin EJ, et al. Living kidney donation: A comparison of laparoscopic and conventional open operations. *Postgrad Med J.* 2002;78(917):153–157.
161. Owen M, Lorgelly P, Serpell M. Chronic pain following donor nephrectomy: A study of the incidence, nature and impact of chronic post-nephrectomy pain. *Eur J Pain.* 2010;14(7):732–734.
162. Biglarnia AR, Tufveson G, Lorant T, et al. Efficacy and safety of continuous local infusion of ropivacaine after retroperitoneoscopic live donor nephrectomy. *Am J Transplant.* 2011;11(1):93–100.
163. Panaro F, Gheza F, Piardi T, et al. Continuous infusion of local anesthesia after living donor nephrectomy: A comparative analysis. *Transplant Proc.* 2011;43(4):985–987.
164. Yates DR, Vaessen C, Roupret M. From Leonardo to da Vinci: The history of robot-assisted surgery in urology. *BJU Int.* 2011;108(11):1708–1713.
165. Branche PE, Duperret SL, Sagnard PE, et al. Left ventricular loading modifications induced by pneumoperitoneum: A time course echocardiographic study. *Anesth Analg.* 1998;85(3):482–487.
166. Mertens zur Borg IR, Di Biase M, et al. Comparison of three perioperative fluid regimes for laparoscopic donor nephrectomy: A prospective randomized dose-finding study. *Surg Endosc.* 2008;22(1):146–150.
167. Feltracco P, Ori C. Anesthetic management of living transplantation. *Minerva Anestesiol.* 2010;76(7):525–533.
168. Fahy BG, Barnas GM, Nagle SE, et al. Changes in lung and chest wall properties with abdominal insufflation of carbon dioxide are immediately reversible. *Anesth Analg.* 1996;82(3):501–505.
169. Ozyuvaci E, Altan A, Karaceniz T, et al. General anesthesia versus epidural and general anesthesia in radical cystectomy. *Urol Int.* 2005;74(1):62–67.
170. Gan TJ, Soppitt A, Maroof M, et al. Goal-directed intraoperative fluid administration reduces length of hospital stay after major surgery. *Anesthesiology.* 2002;97(4):820–826.
171. Cerantola Y, Valerio M, Persson B, et al. Guidelines for perioperative care after radical cystectomy for bladder cancer: Enhanced Recovery After Surgery (ERAS®) society recommendations. *Clin Nutr.* 2013;32(6):879–887.
172. Mir MC, Zargar H, Bolton DM, et al. Enhanced recovery after surgery protocols for radical cystectomy surgery: Review of current evidence and local protocols. *ANZ J Surg.* 2015;85(7-8):514–520.
173. Persson B, Carringer M, Andren O, et al. Initial experiences with the enhanced recovery after surgery (ERAS) protocol in open radical cystectomy. *Scand J Urol.* 2015;49(4):302–307.
174. Karl A, Buchner A, Becker A, et al. A new concept for early recovery after surgery for patients undergoing radical cystectomy for bladder cancer: Results of a prospective randomized study. *J Urol.* 2014;191(2):335–340.
175. Rowley MW, Clemens JQ, Latini JM, et al. Simple cystectomy: outcomes of a new operative technique. *Urology.* 2011;78(4):942–945.
176. Novotny V, Hakenberg OW, Wiessner D, et al. Perioperative complications of radical cystectomy in a contemporary series. *Eur Urol.* 2007;51(2):397–401.
177. Mullen R, Scollay JM, Hecht G, et al. Death within 48 h: Adverse events after general surgical procedures. *Surgeon.* 2012;10(1):1–5.
178. Www.seer.cancer.gov
179. Ploussard G, Epstein JI, Montironi R, et al. The contemporary concept of significant versus insignificant prostate cancer. *Eur Urol.* 2011;60(2):291–303.
180. Gottschalk A, Smith DS, Jobes DR, et al. Preemptive epidural analgesia and recovery from radical prostatectomy: A randomized controlled trial. *JAMA.* 1998;279(14):1076–1082.
181. Price DT, Vieweg J, Roland F, et al. Transient lower extremity neurapraxia associated with radical perineal prostatectomy: A complication of the exaggerated lithotomy position. *J Urol.* 1998;160(4):1376–1378.
182. Keller H. Re: Transient lower extremity neurapraxia associated with radical perineal prostatectomy: A complication of the exaggerated lithotomy position. *J Urol.* 1999;162(1):171.
183. Salonia A, Crescenti A, Suardi N, et al. General versus spinal anesthesia in patients undergoing radical retropubic prostatectomy: Results of a prospective, randomized study. *Urology.* 2004;64(1):95–100.
184. Malhotra V. Anesthesia considerations radical prostatectomy. *Rev Mex Anestesiol.* 2006;29(S1):89–92.
185. Memtsoudis SG, Malhotra V. Catastrophic venous air embolus during prostatectomy in the Trendelenburg position. *Can J Anaesth.* 2003;50(10):1084–1085.
186. Whalley DG, Berrigan MJ. Anesthesia for radical prostatectomy, cystectomy, nephrectomy, pheochromocytoma, and laparoscopic procedures. *Anesthesiol Clin North Am.* 2000;18(4):899–917.
187. Klevecka V, Burmester L, Musch M, et al. Intraoperative and early postoperative complications of radical retropubic prostatectomy. *Urol Int.* 2007;79(3):217–225.
188. Dudderidge T, Doyle P, Mayer E, et al. Evolution of care pathway for laparoscopic radical prostatectomy. *J Endourol.* 2012;26(6):660–665.
189. Sutherland DE, Perez DS, Weeks DC. Robot-assisted simple prostatectomy for severe benign prostatic hyperplasia. *J Endourol.* 2011;25(4):641–644.
190. White WM, Kim ED. Interposition nerve grafting during radical prostatectomy: cumulative review and critical appraisal of literature. *Urology.* 2009;74(2):245–250.
191. Biki B, Mascha E, Moriarty DC, et al. Anesthetic technique for radical prostatectomy surgery affects cancer recurrence: A retrospective analysis. *Anesthesiology.* 2008;109(2):180–187.
192. Fuchs KH. Minimally invasive surgery. *Endoscopy.* 2002;34(2):154–159.
193. Irvine M, Patil V. Anaesthesia for robot-assisted laparoscopic surgery. *Contin Educ Anaesth Crit Care Pain.* 2009;9(4):125–129.
194. Conacher ID, Soomro NA, Rix D. Anaesthesia for laparoscopic urological surgery. *Br J Anaesth.* 2004;93(6):859–864.
195. Pathan H, Gulati S. A case of airway occlusion in robotic surgery. *J Robotic Surg.* 2007;1:169–170.
196. Kalmar AF, Foubert L, Hendrickx JF, et al. Influence of steep Trendelenburg position and CO_2 pneumoperitoneum on cardiovascular, cerebrovascular, and respiratory homeostasis during robotic prostatectomy. *Br J Anaesth.* 2010;104(4):433–439.
197. Gainsburg DM, Wax D, Reich DL, et al. Intraoperative management of robotic-assisted versus open radical prostatectomy. *JSLS.* 2010;14(1):1–5.
198. Sladen RN. Anesthetic considerations for the patient with renal failure. *Anesthesiol Clin North Am.* 2000;18(4):863–882.
199. Colomina MJ, Godet C, Pellise F, et al. Transcranial Doppler monitoring during laparoscopic anterior lumbar interbody fusion. *Anesth Analg.* 2003;97(6):1675–1679.
200. Rocco B, Albo G, Ferreira RC, et al. Recent advances in the surgical treatment of benign prostatic hyperplasia. *Ther Adv Urol.* 2011;3(6):263–272.
201. Reeves MD, Myles PS. Does anaesthetic technique affect the outcome after transurethral resection of the prostate? *BJU Int.* 1999;84(9):982–986.
202. Mackenzie AR. Influence of anaesthesia on blood loss in transurethral prostatectomy. *Scott Med J.* 1990;35(1):14–16.

203. Mcgowan SW, Smith GF. Anaesthesia for transurethral prostatectomy: A comparison of spinal intradural analgesia with two methods of general anaesthesia. *Anaesthesia*. 1980;35(9):847–853.
204. Gehring H, Nahm W, Baerwald J, et al. Irrigation fluid absorption during transurethral resection of the prostate: Spinal vs. General anaesthesia. *Acta Anaesthesiol Scand*. 1999;43(4):458–463.
205. Allen TD. Body temperature changes during prostatic resection as related to the temperature of the irrigating solution. *J Urol*. 1973;110(4):433–435.
206. Hatch PD. Surgical and anaesthetic considerations in transurethral resection of the prostate. *Anaesth Intensive Care*. 1987;15(2):203–211.
207. Krongrad A, Droller M. Complications of transurethral resection of the prostate. In: Marshall F, ed. *Urologic Complications: Medical and Surgical, Adult and Pediatric*. 2nd ed. St. Louis, MO: Mosby-Year Book; 1990:305.
208. Mebust WK, Holtgrewe HL, Cockett AT, et al. Transurethral prostatectomy: Immediate and postoperative complications: A cooperative study of 13 participating institutions evaluating 3,885 patients. *J Urol*. 1989;141(2):243–247.
209. Dorotta I, Basali A, Ritchey H, et al. Transurethral resection syndrome after bladder perforation. *Anesth Analg*. 2003;97(5):1536–1538.
210. Reich O, Gratzke C, Bachmann A, et al. Morbidity, mortality and early outcome of transurethral resection of the prostate: A prospective multicenter evaluation of 10,654 patients. *J Urol*. 2008;180(1):246–249.
211. Ahyai SA, Gilling P, Kaplan SA, et al. Meta-analysis of functional outcomes and complications following transurethral procedures for lower urinary tract symptoms resulting from benign prostatic enlargement. *Eur Urol*. 2010;58(3):384-397.
212. Ansell J. Acquired bleeding disorders. In: Rippe J, Irwin R, Alpert J, Dalen J, eds. *Intensive Care Medicine*. 2nd ed. Boston, MA: Little, Brown; 1991:1013.
213. Rannikko A, Petas A, Taari K. Tranexamic acid in control of primary hemorrhage during transurethral prostatectomy. *Urology*. 2004;64(5):955–958.
214. Wasson JH, Reda DJ, Bruskewitz RC, et al. A comparison of transurethral surgery with watchful waiting for moderate symptoms of benign prostatic hyperplasia. The Veterans Affairs Cooperative Study Group on Transurethral Resection of the Prostate. *N Engl J Med*. 1995;332(2):75–79.
215. Melchior J, Valk WL, Foret JD, et al. Transurethral prostatectomy: Computerized analysis of 2,223 consecutive cases. *J Urol*. 1974;112(5):634-642.
216. Perrin P, Barnes R, Hadley H, et al. Forty years of transurethral prostatic resections. *J Urol*. 1976;116(6):757–758.
217. Fuglsig S, Aagaard J, Jonler M, et al. Survival after transurethral resection of the prostate: A 10-year followup. *J Urol*. 1994;151(3):637–639.
218. Matani Y, Mottrie AM, Stockle M, et al. Transurethral prostatectomy: a long-term follow-up study of 166 patients over 80 years of age. *Eur Urol*. 1996;30(4):414–417.
219. Fitzpatrick JM. Minimally invasive and endoscopic management of benign prostatic hyperplasia. In: Wein A, Kavoussi L, Novick A, et al, eds. *Campbell-Walsh Urology*. 9th ed. Philadelphia, PA: Saunders Elsevier; 2007:2803.
220. Gettman M, Segura J. Indications and outcomes of ureteroscopy for urinary stones. In: Stoller M, Meng M, eds. *Urinary Stone Disease*. Totowa, NJ: Humana Press; 2004.
221. Freiha F, Deem S, Pearl RG. Urology: Transurethral resection of the protate (TURP). In: Jaffe RA, Samuels SI, eds. *Anesthesiologist's Manual of Surgical Procedures*. New York, NY: Raven Press; 1994:553.
222. Shah HN, Kausik V, Hegde S, et al. Evaluation of fluid absorption during holmium laser enucleation of prostate by breath ethanol technique. *J Urol*. 2006;175(2):537–540.
223. Akata T, Yoshimura H, Matsumae Y, et al. [Changes in serum Na+ and blood hemoglobin levels during three types of transurethral procedures for the treatment of benign prostatic hypertrophy]. *Masui*. 2004;53(6):638–644.
224. Jensen V. The TURP syndrome. *Can J Anaesth*. 1991;38(1):90–96.
225. Agin C. Anesthesia for transurethral prostate surgery. In: Lebowitz P, ed. *Anesthesia for Urologic Surgery*. Boston, MA: Brown; 1993:25.
226. Gravenstein D. Transurethral resection of the prostate (TURP) syndrome: A review of the pathophysiology and management. *Anesth Analg*. 1997;84(2):438–446.
227. Roesch RP, Stoelting RK, Lingeman JE, et al. Ammonia toxicity resulting from glycine absorption during a transurethral resection of the prostate. *Anesthesiology*. 1983;58(6):577–579.
228. Hoekstra PT, Kahnoski R, Mccamish MA, et al. Transurethral prostatic resection syndrome: A new perspective: Encephalopathy with associated hyperammonemia. *J Urol*. 1983;130(4):704–707.
229. Ovassapian A, Joshi CW, Brunner EA. Visual disturbances: An unusual symptom of transurethral prostatic resection reaction. *Anesthesiology*. 1982;57(4):332–334.
230. Barletta JP, Fanous MM, Hamed LM. Temporary blindness in the TUR syndrome. *J Neuroophthalmol*. 1994;14(1):6–8.
231. Hahn RG, Ekengren JC. Patterns of irrigating fluid absorption during transurethral resection of the prostate as indicated by ethanol. *J Urol*. 1993;149(3):502–506.
232. Rippa A. Transurethral resection of the prostate: Aids and accessories. In: Smith A, ed. *Smith's Textbook of Endourology*. St. Louis, MO: Quality Medical; 1996:1190.
233. Hahn RG, Stalberg HP, Ekengren J, et al. Effects of 1.5% glycine solution with and without 1% ethanol on the fluid balance in elderly men. *Acta Anaesthesiol Scand*. 1991;35(8):725–730.
234. Black R. Disorders of plasma sodium and plasma potassium. In: Rippe J, Irwin R, Alpert J, Dalen J, eds. *Intensive Care Medicine*. 2nd ed. Boston, MA: Little, Brown; 1991:794.
235. Hall PM. Nephrolithiasis: Treatment, causes, and prevention. *Cleve Clin J Med*. 2009;76(10):583–591.
236. Preminger GM, Tiselius HG, Assimos DG, et al. 2007 Guideline for the management of ureteral calculi. *Eur Urol*. 2007;52(6):1610–1631.
237. Hollingsworth JM, Rogers MA, Kaufman SR, et al. Medical therapy to facilitate urinary stone passage: A meta-analysis. *Lancet*. 2006;368(9542):1171–1179.
238. Auge BK, Preminger GM. Update on shock wave lithotripsy technology. *Curr Opin Urol*. 2002;12(4):287–290.
239. Lambert DH, Deane RS, Mazuzan JE Jr. Anesthesia and the control of blood pressure in patients with spinal cord injury. *Anesth Analg*. 1982;61(4):344–348.
240. Mariappan P, Tolley DA. Endoscopic stone surgery: minimizing the risk of post-operative sepsis. *Curr Opin Urol*. 2005;15(2):101–105.
241. Abbott MA, Samuel JR, Webb DR. Anaesthesia for extracorporeal shock wave lithotripsy. *Anaesthesia*. 1985;40(11):1065–1072.
242. Samplaski MK, Irwin BH, Desai M. Less-invasive ways to remove stones from the kidneys and ureters. *Cleve Clin J Med*. 2009;76(10):592–598.
243. Stoller ML, Lee KL, Schwartz BF, et al. Autologous blood use in percutaneous nephrolithotomy. *Urology*. 1999;54(3):444–449.
244. Mehrabi S, Karimzadeh Shirazi K. Results and complications of spinal anesthesia in percutaneous nephrolithotomy. *Urol J*. 2010;7(1):22–25.
245. Aravantinos E, Karatzas A, Gravas S, et al. Feasibility of percutaneous nephrolithotomy under assisted local anaesthesia: A prospective study on selected patients with upper urinary tract obstruction. *Eur Urol*. 2007;51(1):224–227.
246. Johnson DB, Pearle MS. Complications of ureteroscopy. *Urol Clin North Am*. 2004;31(1):157–171.
247. Foon R, Toozs-Hobson P, Cooper G. Anaesthesia for incontinence surgery: Spinal anaesthesia or sedation? *J Obstet Gynaecol*. 2010;30(6):605–608.
248. Wohlrab KJ, Erekson EA, Korbly NB, et al. The association between regional anesthesia and acute postoperative urinary retention in women undergoing outpatient midurethral sling procedures. *Am J Obstet Gynecol*. 2009;200:571.e1–e5.
249. Lifshitz DA, Lingeman JE. Ureteroscopy as a first-line intervention for ureteral calculi in pregnancy. *J Endourol*. 2002;16(1):19–22.
250. Ulvik NM, Bakke A, Hoisaeter PA. Ureteroscopy in pregnancy. *J Urol*. 1995;154(5):1660–1663.
251. Yossepowitch O, Baniel J, Livne PM. Urological injuries during cesarean section: Intraoperative diagnosis and management. *J Urol*. 2004;172(1):196–199.
252. Belfort MA. Placenta accreta. *Am J Obstet Gynecol*. 2010;203(5):43043–43049.
253. Hsu GL, Hsieh CH, Chen HS, et al. The advancement of pure local anesthesia for penile surgeries: Can an outpatient basis be sustainable? *J Androl*. 2007;28(1):200–205.
254. Casale P, Kojima Y. Robotic-assisted laparoscopic surgery in pediatric urology: An update. *Scand J Surg*. 2009;98(2):110–119.
255. St Peter SD, Valusek PA, Hill S, et al. Laparoscopic adrenalectomy in children: A multicenter experience. *J Laparoendosc Adv Surg Tech A*. 2011;21(7):647–649.
256. Waguespack SG, Rich T, Grubbs E, et al. A current review of the etiology, diagnosis, and treatment of pediatric pheochromocytoma and paraganglioma. *J Clin Endocrinol Metab*. 2010;95(5):2023–2037.
257. Ein SH, Pullerits J, Creighton R, et al. Pediatric pheochromocytoma. A 36-year review. *Pediatr Surg Int*. 1997;12(8):595–598.
258. Meinhardt H. Computational modelling of epithelial patterning. *Curr Opin Genet Dev*. 2007;17(4):272–280.
259. Baird AD, Nelson CP, Gearhart JP. Modern staged repair of bladder exstrophy: A contemporary series. *J Pediatr Urol*. 2007;3(4):311–315.
260. Nasir AA, Ameh EA, Abdur-Rahman LO, et al. Posterior urethral valve. *World J Pediatr*. 2011;7(3):205–216.
261. Barthold JS, Gonzalez R. The epidemiology of congenital cryptorchidism, testicular ascent and orchiopexy. *J Urol*. 2003;170(6 Pt 1):2396–2401.
262. Ringdahl E, Teague L. Testicular torsion. *Am Fam Physician*. 2006;74(10):1739–1743.
263. Davenport M. ABC of general surgery in children: acute problems of the scrotum. *BMJ*. 1996;312(7028):435–437.
264. Paty R, Smith AD. Gangrene and Fournier's gangrene. *Urol Clin North Am*. 1992;19(1):149–162.
265. Norton KS, Johnson LW, Perry T, et al. Management of Fournier's gangrene: An eleven year retrospective analysis of early recognition, diagnosis, and treatment. *Am Surg*. 2002;68(8):709–713.
266. Korhonen K, Hirn M, Niinikoski J. Hyperbaric oxygen in the treatment of Fournier's gangrene. *Eur J Surg*. 1998;164(4):251–255.
267. Mindrup SR, Kealey GP, Fallon B. Hyperbaric oxygen for the treatment of fournier's gangrene. *J Urol*. 2005;173(6):1975–1977.
268. Corcoran AT, Smaldone MC, Gibbons EP, et al. Validation of the Fournier's gangrene severity index in a large contemporary series. *J Urol*. 2008;180(3):944–948.
269. Brown P. Management of urinary tract infections associated with nephrolithiasis. *Curr Infect Dis Rep*. 2010;12(6):450–454.

51 Anesthesia for Orthopedic Surgery

MEGHAN A. KIRKSEY • STEPHEN C. HASKINS • ELLEN M. SOFFIN • SPENCER S. LIU

Introduction to Orthopedic Anesthesia
Preoperative Assessment
Selection of Anesthetic Technique
Anesthesia for Spine Surgery
   Preoperative Assessment
   Positioning for Spine Surgery
   Blood Conservation
   Spinal Cord Monitoring
   Spinal Cord Injury
   Scoliosis
   Muscular Disorders
   Degenerative Vertebral Column Disease
   Postoperative Care of the Spine Patient
   Complications of Spine Surgery
Upper Extremity Surgery
   Surgery to the Shoulder and Upper Arm
   Surgical Approach and Positioning
   Anesthetic Management
   Surgery to the Elbow, Wrist, and Hand
   Postoperative Regional Analgesia
Lower Extremity Surgery
   Surgery to the Hip and Pelvis
   Surgery to the Knee
   Surgery to the Foot and Ankle
Pediatric Orthopedic Anesthesia
Special Considerations in Orthopedics
   Amputation
   Microvascular Surgery
   Acute Compartment Syndrome
   Tourniquets
   Fat Embolus Syndrome/Bone Cement Implantation Syndrome
   Venous Thromboembolism and Thromboprophylaxis

KEY POINTS

1. Optimal anesthetic management for orthopedic surgery requires expertise in regional anesthesia and analgesia techniques.
2. Regional anesthesia can provide physiologic benefits and facilitate recovery compared to general anesthesia.
3. General anesthesia is appropriate for surgeries not amenable to and/or patients with contraindications to regional techniques.
4. Orthopedic surgery patients may have limited mobility and may require special attention to avoid positioning-related injury.
5. Patients presenting for spine surgery should be evaluated carefully for potential airway challenges and/or impaired respiratory function.
6. Major spine surgery frequently involves significant bleeding, and blood conservation techniques should be considered.
7. Intraoperative monitoring of spinal cord function should be used for surgeries where the cord is at risk of injury.
8. Catastrophic venous air embolism during spine surgery may present as unexplained hypotension with high end-tidal nitrogen and low end-tidal carbon dioxide.
9. Nerve injury may result from surgical trauma and/or nerve blockade in the setting of pre-existing neurologic deficits.
10. In the sitting position, for every 20 cm of difference in height of the head from the heart, there is a 15-mmHg difference in mean arterial pressure.
11. Ephedrine, atropine, and glycopyrrolate should be available for management of hypotensive bradycardic events occurring during surgery in the beach chair position.
12. Interscalene blocks cause hemidiaphragmatic paresis and can cause respiratory compromise in patients with reduced pulmonary function.
13. Venous thromboembolism is a common complication of lower extremity orthopedic surgery performed with inadequate thromboprophylaxis.
14. The American Society of Regional Anesthesia has released guidelines for safe use of regional anesthesia in the setting of antithrombotic or thrombolytic therapy.

Introduction to Orthopedic Anesthesia

1 Perioperative management of the patient undergoing orthopedic surgery involves knowledge of orthopedic surgical techniques and associated complications, including nerve injury. Expertise in regional anesthetic techniques for both surgical anesthesia and postoperative analgesia is of paramount importance. Appropriate patient positioning produces optimal surgical conditions while avoiding complications related to stretch, pressure, and hemodynamic changes. Orthopedic procedures can be associated with major blood loss; therefore, one must be familiar with tourniquet use, controlled intraoperative hypotension, blood

salvage techniques, use of antifibrinolytics, fluid resuscitation (see Chapter 16), transfusions, and related complications (see Chapter 17).

Orthopedic surgical patients benefit greatly from early mobilization and rehabilitation, both of which can be expedited by specific anesthetic techniques and proactive postoperative analgesia. A multimodal approach, often utilizing neuraxial and/or peripheral nerve blocks, can enhance recovery and improve functional outcomes. Patients undergoing major orthopedic surgery are at high risk for venous thromboembolism. Knowledge of current pharmacologic and mechanical methods of thromboprophylaxis is required, and regional techniques must be managed so as to minimize associated bleeding risk.

Preoperative Assessment

All patients should undergo medical and laboratory testing appropriate to their medical history and planned procedure (see Chapter 23). Preoperative assessment of the orthopedic patient must include special attention to potential airway difficulties, considerations relating to mobility and intraoperative positioning, and medication history related to opioid dependence and anticoagulation status. Cardiopulmonary symptoms and exercise tolerance may be difficult to assess in this population because of limitations in mobility. As a result, pharmacologic functional cardiovascular testing and formal pulmonary function testing may be warranted in patients with concerning risk factors. Overall, patients undergoing orthopedic procedures are considered at intermediate risk for perioperative cardiac complications.

Patients with rheumatoid arthritis (RA) often require orthopedic surgery and merit special attention. RA can affect the pulmonary, cardiac, and musculoskeletal systems. Airway management can be challenging in these patients. Involvement of the cervical spine and temporomandibular joints results in limited neck range of motion and mouth opening. Atlantoaxial instability, with subluxation of the odontoid process, can lead to spinal cord injury during neck extension. Patients with RA on chronic steroid therapy may require perioperative steroid replacement.

All medications should be reviewed during a preoperative visit with detailed instructions as to which medications to hold and which to continue until surgery. Patients taking opioids for greater than 4 weeks often develop tolerance and opioid-induced hyperalgesia.[1] Although abrupt cessation of opioids is not advised, weaning of chronic opioids under the direction of a pain management specialist prior to elective surgery may be beneficial. Antihypertensives without a significant rebound effect may be held on the day of surgery if there is concern for excessive intraoperative hypotension or renal injury related to angiotensin-converting enzyme inhibitors or angiotensin receptor blockers. A plan for management of anticoagulants including heparins, warfarin, factor Xa inhibitors, and antiplatelet agents must be agreed upon by the medical and surgical teams and communicated clearly to the patient.[2] Anesthetic techniques must take into account the specifics of each patient's anticoagulation status and plan.

Preoperative evaluation should include a standard focused physical examination (see Chapter 23). Orthopedic patients may have coexisting disease or trauma requiring special attention to distorted airway anatomy or limited neck mobility. Proposed sites of needle placement for regional anesthesia and line placement should be assessed for evidence of infection and anatomic abnormalities. A brief neurologic examination with documentation of pre-existing deficits is crucial. Potential positioning difficulties related to body habitus, joint pain or instability, fractures, and/or fusions should be considered. Ideally, preoperative education regarding the surgical procedure, anesthetic/analgesic options, and postoperative rehabilitation plan should be provided.

Selection of Anesthetic Technique

Many orthopedic surgical procedures, because of their localized peripheral sites, lend themselves to regional anesthetic techniques. Neural structures may be blocked at the peripheral nerve, plexus, or neuraxial level (see Chapters 35 and 36). Regional anesthetics offer several advantages over general anesthetics including enhanced rehabilitation, accelerated hospital discharge, improved analgesia, decreased nausea and vomiting, less respiratory and cardiac depression, improved perfusion, reduced blood loss, and decreased risk of infection and thromboembolism. It is important to communicate potential benefits and encourage regional anesthesia when appropriate.

The optimal regional technique and local anesthetic depend on factors including surgery duration, indication for postoperative sympathectomy, and degree and duration of postoperative sensory/motor block needed for active and passive physical therapy. General anesthesia is appropriate for orthopedic surgery at sites not amenable to regional and in patients with contraindications to regional techniques owing to factors such as anticoagulation status, infection at the needle insertion site, pre-existing nerve injury or disease, and patient refusal. Of note, a contraindication to one regional technique may not preclude the use of another. For example, coagulopathy may prevent the use of neuraxial or deep plexus blocks, but a superficial peripheral nerve block may be appropriate. In contrast, a neuraxial block is likely to be safer in a patient with peripheral neuropathy.

Anesthesia for Spine Surgery

Preoperative Assessment

Preoperative evaluation for spine surgery should assess involvement of the respiratory, cardiovascular, and neurologic systems. Difficult airways are common in patients presenting for surgery involving the upper thoracic or cervical spine; therefore, airway evaluation should focus on restricted neck movement, cervical spine stability, and exacerbation of symptoms with movement or position. Both clinical and radiographic assessment of cervical spine stability should be discussed with the surgeon prior to neck manipulation. The decision to secure the airway awake, asleep, or with advance airway devices should be made prior to surgery and the patient counseled accordingly. Awake tracheal intubation is preferred when assessing for neurologic function prior to use of a traction device.

Patients presenting for spine surgery often have impaired respiratory function. Scoliosis can cause restrictive lung disease, neuromuscular diseases can be associated with recurrent chest infections, and patients with spinal cord injury may already be ventilator dependent. Physical exam and history should focus on functional impairment. Chest radiograph, arterial blood gas, and pulmonary function tests may be indicated in patients with restrictive pulmonary disease. A preoperative vital capacity less than 30% to 35% of predicted is associated with prolonged postoperative ventilation after scoliosis surgery.[3] Optimization of pulmonary function targets treatment of reversible causes with the use of preoperative physical therapy, antibiotics, and bronchodilators as indicated.

Cardiac dysfunction is often associated with spine pathology and may be a primary manifestation of the disease as seen in muscular dystrophies. Rarely, scoliosis can cause cor pulmonale secondary to chronic hypoxemia and pulmonary hypertension. An electrocardiogram (ECG) and echocardiogram should be obtained to assess left ventricular function and pulmonary arterial pressures. Dobutamine stress echocardiography may be necessary to assess cardiac function in patients with limited exercise tolerance or mobility.

Neurologic deficits of spine patients generally relate to the underlying disease and should be discussed in detail with the patient and surgeon and documented. With cervical spine surgery, extra care must be taken to avoid injury during tracheal intubation and positioning. Neuromuscular diseases increase risk of aspiration during airway manipulation. In patients with spinal cord injury, spinal shock and autonomic dysreflexia are of particular concern.

Positioning for Spine Surgery

Positioning for spine surgery depends on the level and approach of the procedure. Patients may be transitioned between supine, lateral, and prone positions intraoperatively. Overall goals of positioning are to (1) pad as needed to protect peripheral nerves, bony prominences, and the eyes, (2) avoid displacement of unstable fractures during surgery, and (3) ensure low venous pressures and thereby minimize blood loss at the surgical site. Low venous pressures can be facilitated by maintaining a free abdomen and reverse Trendelenburg position.

The posterior approach to spine surgery requires prone positioning (Fig. 51-1). Pressure on the abdomen causes inferior vena cava compression, increasing bleeding from valveless epidural veins, reducing cardiac output, and increasing the risk of lower limb thrombosis.[4] Therefore, adequate foam padding should be placed under the chest (below the axillae) and the anterior superior iliac spines. The arms should not be abducted to more than 90 degrees and should be positioned with slight internal rotation to reduce the risk of brachial plexus stretching. With the elbow flexed in the prone position, the ulnar nerve is at particular risk of pressure-related injury and should be protected. The eyes should be taped closed; appropriate positioning with a ProneView (Mizuho OSI, Union City, CA) or Mayfield fixator will avoid pressure on the eyes/orbits while maintaining a neutral neck position.

The anterior approach to the thoracolumbar spine is achieved in the lateral position. For scoliosis surgery, the convexity of the curve is usually uppermost, and removal of one or more ribs may be necessary for surgical exposure. Placement of a double-lumen endotracheal tube to collapse the lung on the operative side may be required for surgery above T8.

For cervical spine surgery, anterior approaches require the supine position and posterior approaches require prone positioning (Fig. 51-1). The patient may be positioned with the head 180 degrees away from the anesthetic machine to allow surgical access. Therefore, extensions may be needed for breathing circuits and intravascular lines, and it may be necessary to place venous access in the patient's foot. Endotracheal tubes must be carefully secured without disruption of the surgical field. The head may be supported on a padded head ring or the "horseshoe" of a Mayfield attachment. If neck traction is required, it is generally achieved by placing pins and weights onto the outer skull. Reverse Trendelenburg minimizes venous bleeding and provides

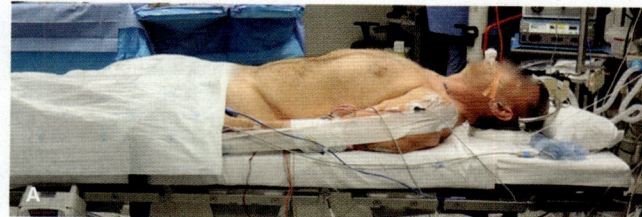
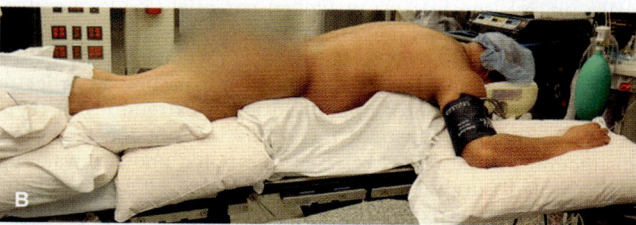

Figure 51-1 Positioning for spine surgery. **A:** Supine positioning for anterior approach. The neck is maintained in a neutral-flexed position and the head is supported with a round foam pillow or other supportive device. The shoulders are taped in caudal traction to aid exposure. In-line traction is applied via Gardner-Wells tongs. **B:** Prone positioning for posterior approach. The head and neck are neutral with the face supported on a head frame (ProneView) to avoid any direct pressure to the eyes. The shoulders are abducted to less than 90 degrees. The forearms are placed on padded supports at the level of the mattress to minimize direct pressure on the ulnar nerve at the elbow. The pelvis and chest are supported to minimize intra-abdominal pressure.

countertraction. Venous pooling in the lower limbs and carotid artery retraction can cause swift and significant hemodynamic changes; therefore, an arterial line is advisable. Because the arms will typically be tucked at the sides, the arterial line should be placed prior to positioning.

Blood Conservation

The frequency of transfusion in adult spine surgery ranges from 50% to 81%.[5] Most of the blood loss during spinal instrumentation and fusion occurs with decortication and is proportional to the number of vertebral levels involved.[6]

Patients may become coagulopathic perioperatively owing to fibrinolysis or dilution of coagulation factors and/or platelets. The detailed mechanisms of coagulopathy and the role of factor testing during spine surgery are poorly defined. However, it appears that a significant deviation from baseline of either the prothrombin time or activated partial thromboplastin time is predictive of bleeding and may be used to guide transfusion therapy.[7] A rare cause of bleeding during spine surgery is trauma to the aorta, vena cava, or iliac vessels. Unexplained rapidly evolving hypotension with signs of hypovolemia should alert the anesthesiologist to this possibility.

Measures to decrease blood loss and transfusion requirements during major spine surgery include preoperative autologous donation, proper positioning, the use of intraoperative blood salvage, and the administration of antifibrinolytics such as tranexamic acid (TXA) (see Chapter 17).[5,8] Recent data indicate that TXA not only reduces surgical bleeding and transfusion requirements but also does so without increased incidence of pulmonary embolism (PE), deep venous thrombosis (DVT), or myocardial infarction.[9,10]

Spinal Cord Monitoring

7 Intraoperative monitoring (IOM) of spinal cord function is now considered mandatory for all surgeries in which the cord is at risk of injury. Risk is incurred when corrective forces are applied to the spine, osteotomies are made, or the spinal canal is surgically invaded. Data suggest that IOM may reduce the incidence of motor deficits or paraplegia after scoliosis surgery from 3% to 7%[11,12] to 0.5%.[13] There are three main methods of IOM: the wake-up test, somatosensory evoked potential (SSEP) monitoring, and motor evoked potential (MEP) recording.

The wake-up test involves intraoperative awakening of the patient after completion of spinal instrumentation in order to assess motor function of upper and lower extremities. If there is satisfactory movement of the hands but not the feet, then distraction on the rod is released one notch and the wake-up test repeated. Surgical anesthesia can be achieved with a volatile anesthetic, nitrous oxide, and opioids, with or without propofol. Opioids are important for analgesia and tolerance of the endotracheal tube while the patient is awake. Although recall of the event occurs in only 0% to 20% of patients and is rarely viewed as unpleasant,[14] it is important to describe the wake-up test prior to surgery to minimize anxiety should the patient have recall.

The wake-up test has a number of disadvantages, including the risk that an uncooperative patient could move, dislodge the endotracheal tube, or even fall from the table. Additionally, the wake-up test assesses function only at the time it is performed and has the potential to provide false reassurance after instrumentation but prior to an unexpected neurologic injury. Thus, the wake-up test is most suitable if other monitoring techniques are not available or equivocal or if they fail.

SSEPs assess the dorsal column pathways of proprioception and vibration that are supplied by the posterior spinal artery. SSEPs are altered by neural injury, volatile anesthetics, hypercarbia, hypoxia, hypotension, and hypothermia.[15,16] Motor pathways are supplied by the anterior spinal artery and are monitored by MEPs. MEPs are considered technically more difficult to use, in part because they are impeded by use of muscle relaxants. If both SSEP and MEP are to be monitored during spine surgery, a suitable anesthetic regimen would include an ultrashort-acting opioid infusion with a low-dose inhaled anesthetic or total intravenous anesthesia with monitoring of the electroencephalogram or bispectral index to minimize the potential for intraoperative awareness (see Chapter 37).

Postoperative paraplegia has occurred despite preservation of intraoperative SSEPs; however, MEPs in combination with SSEPs may increase the early detection of spinal cord ischemia.[14,17] Acute alterations in signal amplitude or latency can signify spinal cord compromise and may be the result of direct trauma, ischemia, compression, or hematoma. If changes occur, it is recommended that surgery be discontinued, blood pressure returned to normal or 20% above normal, and volatile agents decreased or discontinued. Arterial blood gases can help rule out a metabolic derangement. If the signal does not return to normal, the surgeon should release distraction on the cord. A wake-up test can be performed at this time to definitely exclude neurologic deficits.

Spinal Cord Injury

Patients with a suspected spinal cord injury should be examined immediately to assess for signs of respiratory insufficiency, airway obstruction, rib fractures, and chest wall or facial trauma. Spinal cord function above the level of the injury should be determined. If the muscles controlled by the C5 nerve roots (deltoid, biceps, brachialis, and brachioradialis) are flaccid, partial diaphragmatic paralysis should also be expected.

Patients requiring spine stabilization surgery may present with spinal shock, which occurs immediately after the injury and lasts up to 3 weeks. Injuries at or above T5 are associated with hypotension due to a physiologic sympathectomy and loss of tone from the splanchnic vascular beds. Lesions above the cardiac accelerator fibers (T1 to T4) cause bradycardia. Hypotension due to spinal injury is poorly responsive to intravenous fluids and vasopressors, and excessive fluid administration may contribute to the development of pulmonary edema.

With complete cord transection above T5, following recovery from spinal shock, 85% of patients go on to exhibit autonomic hyperreflexia. The syndrome can also occur with injuries at lower levels and is characterized by severe paroxysmal hypertension with bradycardia from the baroreceptor reflex, dysrhythmias, and cutaneous vasoconstriction below and vasodilation above the level of the injury. Episodes are typically precipitated by distention of the bladder or rectum but can be induced by any noxious stimulus including surgery. Treatment involves removal of the stimulus, deepening of anesthesia, and administration of direct-acting vasodilators. Untreated, the hypertensive crisis may progress to seizures, intracranial hemorrhage, or myocardial infarction.

Ventilatory impairment increases with higher levels of spinal injury. A high cervical lesion that includes the diaphragmatic segments (C3 to C5) results in respiratory failure and death without mechanical ventilation. Lesions between C5 and T7 cause significant alterations in respiratory function due to loss of abdominal and intercostal support. Flaccid thoracic muscles can lead to paradoxic respirations and a vital capacity reduction of 60%. Inability to cough and effectively clear secretions causes atelectasis and increased risk of infection.

Succinylcholine can be administered safely for the first 48 hours after spinal cord injury. After that time, a proliferation of acetylcholine receptors in the muscle can cause hypersensitivity to depolarizing muscle relaxants leading to marked hyperkalemia.[18] Maximal hyperkalemia risk from succinylcholine occurs between 4 weeks and 5 months after spinal injury. Serum potassium levels may rise as high as 14 mEq/L, causing ventricular fibrillation and cardiac arrest. Although succinylcholine should be avoided in all patients with spinal cord injury after 48 hours, nondepolarizing paralytic agents can be used.

Patients with spinal cord injury are poikilothermic owing to disruption of sympathetic pathways carrying temperature sensation and subsequent loss of vasoconstriction below the level of injury. Normothermia can be achieved by applying exogenous heat to the skin, increasing ambient air temperature, warming intravenous fluids, and humidifying gases.

Scoliosis

Scoliosis involves a lateral and rotational deformity of the spine and occurs in up to 4% of the population. Most cases are idiopathic (70%), with a male to female ratio of 1:4. Surgery is considered when the Cobb angle, a measure of curvature, exceeds 50 degrees in the thoracic or 40 degrees in the lumbar spine. Surgery aims to halt progression of the condition and partially correct the deformity, preventing further respiratory and cardiovascular deterioration.

Scoliosis can cause chronic hypoxia, hypercapnia, and pulmonary vascular constriction resulting in irreversible pulmonary vascular changes, pulmonary hypertension, and eventually right ventricular hypertrophy and cor pulmonale. Thus, untreated idiopathic scoliosis can progress rapidly and is often fatal by the fourth or fifth decade of life. Scoliosis is also often associated with congenital heart conditions, including mitral valve prolapse, coarctation of the aorta, and cyanotic heart disease, suggesting a common embryonic insult or collagen defect.

Although the long-term effect of scoliosis repair is to halt the decline in respiratory function, pulmonary function acutely deteriorates for 7 to 10 days after surgery. Preoperative vital capacity is a reliable prognostic indicator of respiratory reserve, and postoperative ventilator support is likely to be required for patients with a vital capacity less than 40% of predicted.

Anesthetic considerations for surgical correction of scoliosis by spinal fusion and instrumentation include management in the prone position, hypothermia during long procedures with extensive exposure, and replacement of blood and fluid losses.[19] Adequate hemodynamic monitoring and venous access are essential. An arterial line allows for close hemodynamic monitoring and assessment of blood gases, whereas a central venous catheter may be helpful in evaluating blood and fluid management and can be used to aspirate air in the case of venous air embolism. Patients with evidence of pulmonary hypertension or severe coexistent cardiovascular or pulmonary disease may require a pulmonary artery catheter.

Muscular Disorders

Muscular dystrophy and cerebral palsy are important causes of scoliosis. Duchenne muscular dystrophy (DMD) has an incidence of 1:3,300 male births and is inherited as a sex-linked recessive condition affecting skeletal, cardiac, and smooth muscle. Patients with DMD lack a membrane cytoskeletal protein, dystrophin, and typically present between the ages of 2 and 6 years, with progressive weakness of proximal muscle groups. Up to one-third have intellectual impairment. DMD patients have a high incidence of cardiac abnormalities (50% to 70%). In the later stages of the disease, dilated cardiomyopathy may occur in association with mitral valve incompetence. Up to 50% of patients have cardiac conduction defects predisposing to dysrhythmias that can, in some cases, lead to cardiac arrest during spine surgery. Patients with DMD are sensitive to nondepolarizing neuromuscular blocking agents, and hyperkalemia may occur with use of succinylcholine. In general, the prognosis of scoliosis associated with neuromuscular disease is worse than that of idiopathic scoliosis, and these patients frequently require postoperative ventilatory support.

Degenerative Vertebral Column Disease

Spinal stenosis, spondylosis, and spondylolisthesis are all forms of degenerative vertebral column disease, causing pain and/or progressive neurologic symptoms requiring surgical intervention.

A preoperative assessment of C-spine symptoms and the airway should be performed, as described earlier. Intraoperatively, the anterior incision approximates the border of the sternocleidomastoid muscle, near critical anatomic structures. Lateral retraction of the carotid artery may endanger cerebral perfusion, particularly in the elderly patient. Retraction of the esophagus and trachea medially may cause pharyngeal laceration, laryngeal edema, and recurrent laryngeal nerve paralysis. Cerebrospinal fluid leaks and trauma to the vertebral artery have also been reported.

General anesthesia is preferred for nearly all thoracic and cervical procedures because of the high spinal level that would be required with a regional technique. General anesthesia ensures airway access, is associated with greater patient acceptance, and can be used for prolonged operations. For lower thoracic and lumbar spine surgery, either general or neuraxial anesthesia may be safely administered. A randomized trial in 2009 concluded that general anesthesia was associated with higher surgeon satisfaction and less nausea and vomiting.[20] Succinylcholine should be avoided if there are progressive neurologic deficits.

Postoperative Care of the Spine Patient

Most patients can be extubated immediately after spine surgery if the procedure was uncomplicated and preoperative vital capacity values were acceptable. Postoperative ventilation may be required in patients with neuromuscular disorders, severe restrictive pulmonary dysfunction with a preoperative vital capacity of less than 35% of predicted, right ventricular failure, obesity, or sleep apnea. Patients with prolonged procedures, thoracic cavity invasion, or blood loss greater than 30 mL/kg^{-1} may require postoperative ventilation.[21] In the event of significant blood loss requiring aggressive resuscitation, particularly in the prone position, facial and laryngeal edema may compromise an uncontrolled airway and extubation is not advisable. Residual opioid or muscle relaxant may lead to hypoventilation or apnea, especially in patients with neuromuscular disease. Neurologic status must also be monitored closely to determine appropriateness for extubation.

Postoperative mechanical ventilation may be maintained for a few hours, with the head of the bed elevated when possible, until hypothermia and metabolic derangements have been corrected and facial and airway edema have improved. Aggressive postoperative pulmonary therapy, including incentive spirometry, is necessary to avoid postextubation atelectasis and pneumonia. Careful monitoring of systemic pressures, urine output, and wound drainage is essential to ensure adequate resuscitation and absence of significant postoperative hemorrhage.

After spine surgery, analgesia is traditionally provided by systemic opioids. Adequate and safe opioid administration can often be accomplished using patient-controlled analgesia devices with or without background infusions. Side effects of opioids can include respiratory depression, sedation, and gastrointestinal ileus. These concerns are amplified after major spine surgery when breathing may be compromised. Neurologic status must be followed closely and bowel dysmotility is common. Wound infiltration with local anesthetic and injection of intrathecal morphine have been associated with improved pain scores and decreased side effects in the early postoperative period.[22] Multimodal analgesia has become the gold standard for postoperative pain relief and can be useful after spine surgery. The addition of nonopioid analgesics, including nonsteroidal anti-inflammatories, corticosteroids, acetaminophen, or anticonvulsant pain medications, can reduce opioid use, improve analgesia, and decrease opioid-related side effects (Table 51-1). The surgical team should be consulted prior to use of nonsteroidal anti-inflammatory drugs because they may cause delayed bone healing after spine fusion.

Complications of Spine Surgery

Venous air embolus (VAE) is a catastrophic event that is a particular risk during laminectomy because of the large amount of exposed bone and location of the surgical site above the level of the heart. VAE presents as unexplained hypotension with an increase in the end-tidal nitrogen concentration or a precipitous

Table 51-1 Multimodal Analgesia for Orthopedic Surgery

Drug Name	Mechanism of Action	Common Side Effects	Additional Considerations
Paracetamol/Acetaminophen			
Acetaminophen	COX inhibition (predominantly COX-2)	Hepatoxicity	Avoid in liver disease and alcoholism
NSAIDs			
Ketorolac, meloxicam, ibuprofen	COX-1/2 inhibition	Nephrotoxicity; Gastritis; May impair bone healing	Avoid in renal impairment and/or inflammatory bowel disease
Celecoxib	Selective COX-2 inhibition	Nephrotoxicity; Gastritis	Avoid in renal impairment and coronary artery disease; Avoid in patients with sulfa allergy
Anticonvulsants			
Gabapentin, Pregabalin	Binds to voltage-gated Ca^{2+} channels	Drowsiness, dizziness, peripheral edema	Adjust dose for renal impairment
Nontraditional Opioids			
Methadone	Opioid agonist, NMDA receptor antagonist, inhibits reuptake of NE	Drowsiness, sedation, constipation, dizziness, nausea/vomiting	Promotility bowel regimen required
Tramadol, Tapentadol	Weak μ-opioid agonist, inhibits reuptake of NE		Tramadol also blocks reuptake of 5-HT; opioid receptor binding affinity is 6000x lower than morphine.
Miscellaneous			
Ketamine	NMDA receptor antagonist	Tachycardia, dysphoria	Avoid with increased ICP, asthma; Transdermal patch or infusion
Lidocaine	Blocks Na^+ gated channels thereby blocking nerve conduction	Hepatic dysfunction	Transdermal patch or infusion
Dexmedetomidine	α-2 adenoreceptor agonist	Bradycardia; Hypotension	Infusion only

COX, cyclooxygenase; NSAIDs, nonsteroidal anti-inflammatory drugs; NMDA, *N*-methyl-D-aspartate; NE, norepinephrine; ICP, intracranial pressure.

---

fall in the end-tidal carbon dioxide concentration. Prompt diagnosis and treatment increase patient survival with VAE. Prevention and management measures include intravascular volume expansion, careful positioning, positive end-expiratory pressure, and jugular venous compression. Treatment includes flooding the surgical site with saline, controlling sites of air entry, repositioning the patient with the surgical site below the right atrium, aspiration of air from a multiorifice central venous catheter, cessation of inhaled nitrous oxide, and resuscitation with oxygen, intravenous fluids, and inotropic agents. Massive embolism may necessitate supine repositioning and cardiopulmonary resuscitation.

Vision loss is a rare, nonfatal yet catastrophic complication associated with spine surgery. A notable number of cases of unilateral and bilateral blindness have been reported after spine surgery.[23–25] The etiology of vision loss can be optic neuropathy, retinal artery occlusion, or cerebral ischemia. Most cases are associated with complex instrumented fusions,[26] significant sustained intraoperative hypotension, anemia, large intraoperative blood loss, and prolonged surgery.[25]

The American Society of Anesthesiologists (ASA) Postoperative Visual Loss Registry reported on 93 cases of visual loss after spine surgery submitted anonymously to the ASA Closed Claims Study. Ischemic optic neuropathy was the most common cause of visual loss and accounted for 83 of 93 cases.[26] Risk factors for ischemic optic neuropathy after spinal surgery include male sex, obesity, Wilson frame use, long anesthetic duration, large blood loss, and use of noncolloid fluids.[27]

Upper Extremity Surgery

Orthopedic surgical procedures to the upper extremity are well suited to regional anesthetic techniques. Peripheral nerve block adjuvants that prolong block duration can provide significant postoperative analgesia.[28] Continuous catheter techniques can also provide sustained analgesia and facilitate early limb mobilization.

The benefits of regional anesthesia for upper extremity surgery are well established. However, orthopedic patients may have concurrent cervical spine disease, and upper extremity surgical procedures may involve peripheral nerves with pre-existing deficits. Physicians must be cognizant of the risk of nerve injury resulting from the "second hit phenomenon" in the setting of surgical trauma and nerve blockade. The decision to perform regional anesthesia in a patient with pre-existing neurologic deficits or who is at risk for perioperative neurapraxia should be made on an individual basis after discussion with the patient and surgeon. Meticulous regional anesthetic technique with ultrasound guidance, appropriate use of local anesthetic solutions, careful patient positioning, and serial postoperative neurologic examinations may reduce the incidence of neurologic dysfunction.

Local anesthetic selection is based on the duration and degree of sensory or motor block required. The patient should be informed of the anticipated block duration prior to surgery and instructed to protect the extremity until block resolution. If there is a possibility of block resolution overnight, it is not unreasonable to recommend that patients commence oral pain medication at bedtime, even while numb, to minimize the risk of sudden and severe pain overnight. It should also be noted that supraclavicular and infraclavicular blocks can rarely be complicated by pneumothorax that may not manifest until 6 to 12 hours after surgery. Although these blocks are routinely performed safely for inpatient and ambulatory surgeries, each patient should be told to contact his or her surgeon immediately if any respiratory difficulties develop postoperatively.

Surgery to the Shoulder and Upper Arm

Reconstructive shoulder surgery, including total shoulder arthroplasty (TSA) and rotator cuff repair, presents unique management and positioning considerations to the anesthesiologist. For example, a recent institutional review of 1,569 patients who underwent TSA between 1993 and 2007 revealed a 2.2% rate of perioperative nerve injury.[29] It is notable that although a significant percentage of TSA-associated nerve injuries occur at the level of the brachial plexus, this study found a lower rate of perioperative nerve injury in patients who received interscalene blocks.[30] It is important to communicate both the risk of nerve injury after major shoulder surgery and the lack of evidence that brachial plexus nerve blocks contribute significantly to this risk.

Likewise, nerve injury can occur in association with trauma. For example, radial nerve palsy is identified in up to 17% of patients with humeral shaft fractures,[30] whereas axillary nerve and brachial plexus injury are often associated with proximal humerus fractures. This highlights the need for careful examination and documentation of deficits prior to use of a regional anesthetic and clear communication with patients regarding current evidence about associated risk and benefits.

Surgical Approach and Positioning

Surgical procedures to the upper arm and shoulder are typically performed with the patient sitting in the "beach chair" or lateral decubitus position (see Chapter 29). In either position, the patient's head, neck, and hips must be secured to prevent lateral movement during surgical manipulation, with frequent reassessment throughout the case. Excessive rotation or flexion of the head away from the operative side results in stretch injury to the brachial plexus. Care must be taken to avoid pressure on the eyes and ears. Access to the patient's face and airway is often limited, so any airway devices and connections must be carefully secured. In spontaneously breathing patients with unsecured airways, good airflow must be maintained to minimize carbon dioxide rebreathing and pockets of oxygen that present a fire safety risk.

Depending on the surgery and surgeon preference, the lateral position or the beach chair (sitting) position may be chosen. The lateral position has been associated with increased rates of neurapraxia from stretch injuries and is a challenging position from which to convert from an arthroscopic to an open procedure should this become necessary.[31] The beach chair position allows for easy conversion to open procedures but presents several hemodynamic challenges for the anesthesiologist. Blood pressure at the head will be lower than at the arm or leg, with every 20 cm of height difference equating to approximately 15-mmHg difference in mean arterial pressure (Fig. 51-2). Association between hypotension and cerebral desaturation has been reported, and there have been cases reports of strokes in the sitting position. However, The Anesthesia Patient Safety Foundation Beach Chair Study recently described decreased cerebral autoregulation and regional cerebral oxygenation in the sitting position with no associated increase in adverse neurologic outcomes or markers of neuronal injury.[32]

Up to 25% of patients undergoing surgery in the beach chair position under general or regional anesthesia can experience hemodynamically significant hypotensive bradycardic events thought to be caused by ventricular underfilling and the Bezold–Jarisch reflex. Studies have found that intraoperative epinephrine and fentanyl use are associated with increased risk of hypotensive bradycardic events.[33,34] In contrast, preincision administration of ondansetron or metoprolol may significantly decrease this risk.[35,36] Ephedrine, atropine, and glycopyrrolate have been used successfully to manage such events and should

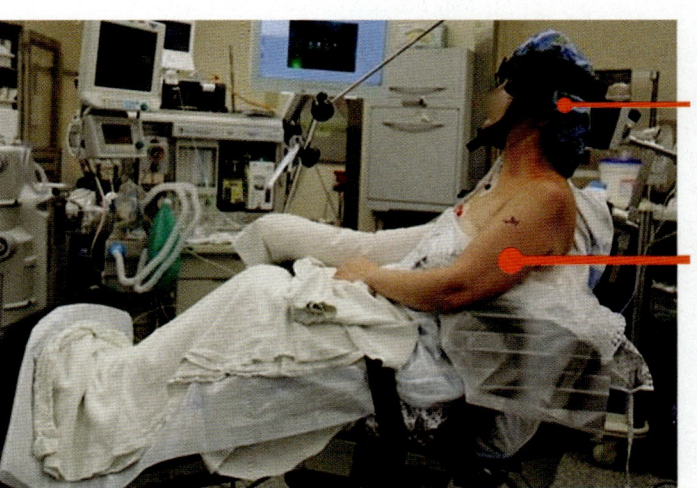

Figure 51-2 Positioning for upper extremity surgery: beach chair position. The patient is placed semi-recumbent with the head, neck, and torso supported in neutral position by a head harness and padding. Hips are flexed to 45 to 60 degrees and the knees to 30 degrees resting on a knee pillow. The chair is in 10 to 15 degrees of Trendelenburg. Pressure points are padded and the eyes are protected. The nonoperative arm is placed on an arm support. The major risk during surgery in the beach chair position is hypotension; for every 1-cm rise above the heart, there is a 0.75-mmHg drop in mean arterial pressure (MAP). Thus, a 20-cm rise in the head causes a 15-mmHg fall in cerebral MAP.

be immediately available when patients are undergoing surgery in the beach chair position.

A tourniquet cannot be used during proximal upper extremity procedures, and significant blood loss may occur. Moreover, patients are at risk of sudden hemodynamic instability from embolic syndromes caused by fat, air, and/or cement. Arterial cannulation for continuous direct blood pressure measurement and monitoring of hemoglobin concentration should be considered–particularly during TSA and humeral fracture reduction/fixation.

Anesthetic Management

Surgery to the shoulder and humerus may be performed under regional or general anesthesia. With careful positioning and appropriate sedation, interscalene or supraclavicular blockade alone can provide excellent surgical anesthesia (Table 51-2). However, a combination of regional and general anesthesia may be chosen because of limited access to the patient's airway, need for neuromuscular relaxation (i.e., during shoulder stabilization procedures), or a surgical field extending outside of the block dermatomes. General anesthesia without a nerve block should be considered in patients with a pre-existing brachial plexopathy or significant cervical spine disease because of the risk of perioperative exacerbation of neurologic deficits.

Historically, it was noted that interscalene blocks caused ipsilateral diaphragmatic paresis[37] in 100% of patients. With a functioning contralateral diaphragm, this leads to a 25% loss of pulmonary function. However, if the contralateral diaphragm is significantly impaired, complete respiratory failure will occur, and, therefore, bilateral interscalene blocks should be avoided. Recent studies have shown good analgesic efficacy of low-volume interscalene blocks in combination with general anesthesia for elective shoulder surgery with rates of hemidiaphragmatic paresis ranging from 13% to 93%.[38,39] In one study, rates of phrenic nerve blockade were 0% with ultrasound-guided supraclavicular blocks and 53% for those performed using a nerve stimulator.[38] Interscalene and superclavicular blocks should be used with caution in patients with severe pulmonary disease and should be performed using ultrasound guidance whenever possible. Care should also be taken when considering these blocks in obese patients and those with sleep apnea because they are also at increased risk of clinically significant reductions in pulmonary function.[40] Diaphragmatic paresis, when it occurs, is present for the duration of the block, so extra caution should be used when considering administration of adjuvants that will prolong these blocks.

Surgery to the Elbow, Wrist, and Hand

In patients without contraindications, surgery in the areas of the distal humerus, elbow, forearm, wrist, and hand can be performed with supraclavicular, infraclavicular, or axillary nerve blocks (Table 51-2). Infraclavicular and supraclavicular approaches to the brachial plexus are the most reliable and provide consistent anesthesia to the four major peripheral nerves of the brachial plexus. The medial aspect of the upper arm, supplied by the intercostobrachial nerve, is generally spared by infraclavicular and axillary blocks and may be blocked by a subcutaneous injection of local anesthetic immediately distal to the axilla for the prevention of tourniquet pain.

Minor hand procedures such as carpal tunnel release, reduction of phalanx fractures, and superficial wound debridements without a tourniquet may require only local infiltration or peripheral blockade at the midhumeral, elbow, or wrist level. Intravenous regional anesthesia (Bier block) using a double tourniquet permits more extensive surgery and longer tourniquet times than distal peripheral block but does not provide postoperative analgesia.

Postoperative Regional Analgesia

Peripheral nerve blocks are associated with earlier discharge and decreased risk of hospital admission following rotator cuff repair.[41,42] For TSA, peripheral nerve blocks improve pain management with no increase in complications or resource usage.[43] Indwelling perineural catheters may reduce hospital admission/readmission, decrease opioid-related side effects and sleep

Block	Nerves Blocked	Applications	Comments
Interscalene	Entire brachial	Shoulder Humerus Partial coverage of lateral clavicle	May not cover inferior trunk/ulnar nerve High rate of phrenic nerve block; inadequate for hand/forearm surgery
Supraclavicular	Entire brachial	Shoulder Humerus Elbow Forearm Wrist Hand	Moderate rate of phrenic nerve block
Infraclavicular	Radial, ulnar, median, and axillary nerves	Distal humerus Elbow Forearm Wrist Hand	Musculocutaneous nerve may be spared Intercostobrachial nerve not blocked; supplementation of medial arm may be required
Axillary	Radial, ulnar, median	Elbow Forearm Wrist Hand	Musculocutaneous nerve can be blocked reliably at this level with ultrasound guidance

Table 51-2 Regional Techniques for Upper Extremity Surgery

disturbance, and improve rehabilitation.[44,45] Brachial plexus catheters may be inserted using interscalene, infraclavicular, and axillary approaches. After surgery, catheters may be left indwelling for 4 to 7 days without adverse effects.

Lower Extremity Surgery

Orthopedic surgeries involving the lower extremity are among the most commonly performed operations in the United States. Demand for total joint arthroplasty of the hip and knee is rising due to increased life expectancy and an increasing emphasis on improving quality of life. General anesthesia and/or regional anesthesia can be utilized for surgery to the lower extremities. However, there is evidence that regional anesthesia improves mortality and morbidity, particularly in older fragile patients.[46]

When compared to general anesthesia, neuraxial techniques for total hip arthroplasty (THA) and total knee arthroplasty (TKA) are associated with lower 30-day mortality, decreased incidence of thromboembolic events, less blood loss, and lower transfusion requirements, along with decreased length of stay (LOS), cost, and in-hospital complications.[47] Regional anesthesia also provides superior postoperative pain control for painful procedures like TKA and foot reconstruction.

A major complication of orthopedic lower extremity surgery is perioperative DVT formation and venous thromboembolism. Knowledge of anticoagulant dose and timing is essential to prevent the rare yet devastating complication of an epidural hematoma as a result of neuraxial technique (Table 51-3) (see Venous Thromboembolism and Thromboprophylaxis).[48]

Surgery to the Hip and Pelvis

Primary partial or total hip arthroplasties are performed with increasing frequency, with almost 500,000 operations performed each year in the United States alone.[49] Including total hip revision and hip fracture surgery, there is significant associated anesthetic demand. The majority of hip fracture and arthroplasty patients are in the geriatric population and present with multiple comorbidities. Optimal perioperative conditions are essential for these patients.

Surgical Approach and Positioning

The anterior surgical approach for hip arthroplasty is gaining favor because it is tissue sparing, allowing for a smaller incision

Table 51-3 Summary of ASRA Practice Advisory Guidelines for Neuraxial Anesthesia and Antithrombotics

Agent	American Society of Regional Anesthesia Guidelines for Neuraxial Anesthesia
Warfarin	Stop 4–5 days prior to neuraxial block, confirm normalization of INR prior to needle insertion. Catheters should be removed with INR <1.5. Removal with INR between 1.5 and 3.0 merits close neuromonitoring. Warfarin dose should be held for INR >3.0.
Antiplatelets	
ASA	No contraindications
Clopidogrel	Stop for 7 days prior to neuraxial block. If neuraxial considered between 5 and 7 days, restoration of platelet function should be confirmed.
Prasugrel	Stop for 7–10 days prior to neuraxial block. Wait 9 hours after neuraxial block or catheter removal before administration of drug.
Ticagrelor	Stop for 5–7 days prior to neuraxial block. Wait 10 hours after neuraxial block or catheter removal before administration of drug.
Ticlopidine	Stop for 14 days prior to neuraxial block.
Heparins	
LMWH	Preoperatively: Wait 10–12 hours after prophylactic dose, 24 hours after treatment dose. Postoperatively: Catheters should be removed at least 2 hours prior to initiation of twice-daily dosing regimens. For single daily dosing of LMWH, catheters can be maintained but should only be removed 10–12 hours after last dose.
Subcutaneous	10,000 units per day or less: no contraindication; >10,000 units per day, use extra caution. Check platelet count if >4 days on heparin.
Intravenous	Stop for 2–4 hours prior to catheter removal. Wait 1 hour after neuraxial block or catheter removal before administration of drug.
Thrombin and Xa Inhibitors	
Dabigatran	Stop for 5 days prior to neuraxial block. Wait 6 hours after neuraxial block or catheter removal before administration of drug
Apixaban	Stop for 3 days prior to neuraxial block. Wait 7 hours after neuraxial block or catheter removal before administration of drug.
Rivaroxaban	Stop for 3 days prior to neuraxial block. Wait 8 hours after neuraxial block or catheter removal before administration of drug.
Thrombolytics/fibrinolytics/thrombin inhibitors	Neuraxial techniques contraindicated except in unusual circumstances.

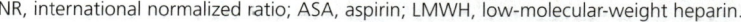
INR, international normalized ratio; ASA, aspirin; LMWH, low-molecular-weight heparin.

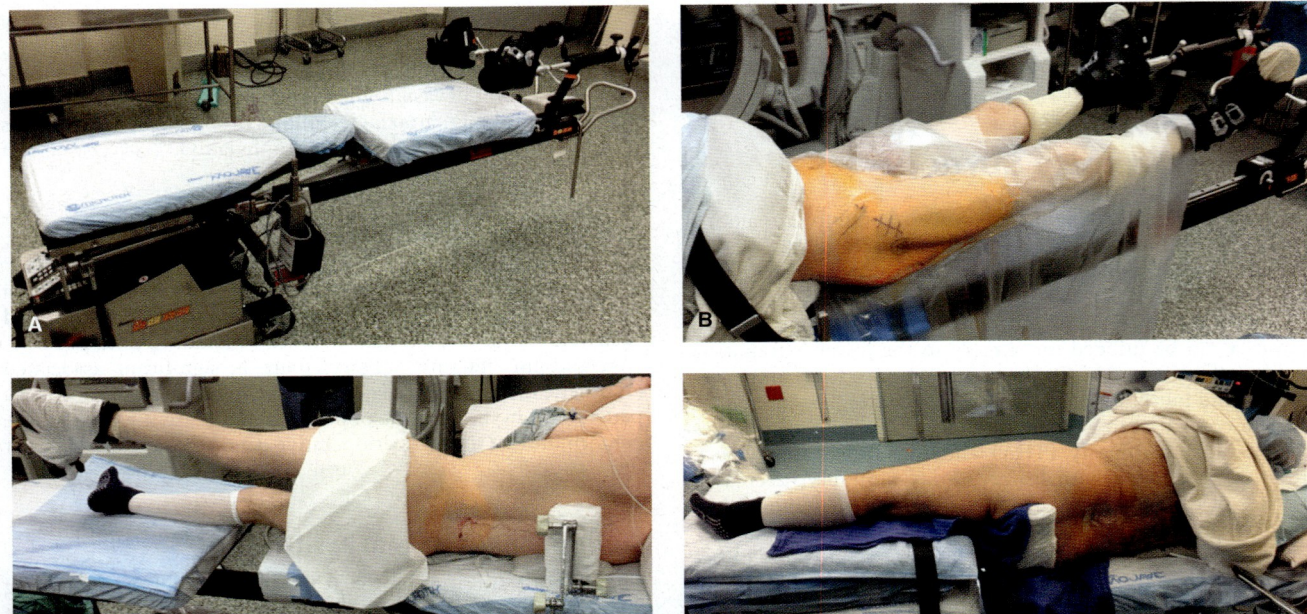

Figure 51-3 Positioning for hip surgery. **A:** The Mizuho OSI Hana trauma table utilized for anterior total hip arthroplasty. **B:** Patient positioned for anterior total hip arthroplasty on Mizuho OSI Hana trauma table. A padded post is placed between the legs to allow for traction, dislocation, and rotation of the femoral head. **C:** Lateral positioning for hip arthroscopy. The surgical leg is placed in a boot for traction, dislocation, and rotation of the femoral head from the acetabulum. **D:** Lateral positioning for total hip arthroplasty. An inflatable axillary roll prevents pressure on the axillary artery and brachial plexus.

and the potential for less pain, faster recovery, and improved mobility (Fig. 51-3).[50] However, most surgery to the hip and femur is performed using a posterior approach. For this approach, the patient is placed in the lateral decubitus position with the arms neutral and abducted/flexed less than 90 degrees, and an axillary roll is placed to prevent compression of the brachial plexus and axillary artery (Fig. 51-3). With general anesthesia, the airway should be accessed with the patient supine, prior to surgical positioning. A neuraxial anesthetic can be performed with the patient sitting or in the lateral position. The cervical spine and head must be kept neutral during positioning. Mild airway obstruction often improves in the lateral decubitus position; however, the airway should be secured prior to lateral positioning if there are any significant concerns.

Anesthesia Technique

General anesthesia is commonly used for hip and femur surgery as a result of institutional preference, perceived delays in surgical readiness, concern regarding lack of reliability, or prevention of urinary retention.[51] However, evidence supports the recommendation that neuraxial anesthesia should be utilized whenever possible for hip or femur surgery given the potential for improved mortality and morbidity.[52] Neuraxial anesthesia, when performed properly and with adherence to anticoagulation guidelines, is low risk. Epidural hematomas and neurologic complications are extremely rare (less than 0.04%).[53–55]

For hip fracture surgery, neuraxial techniques may decrease hospital LOS, but their overall mortality benefit is controversial.[56] Hip fracture patients are inherently fragile and difficult to optimize; however, surgery performed within 48 hours of admission will decrease inpatient mortality and development of pressure sores.[57] Therefore, surgery should be performed as soon as is safely possible.

Extra care should be taken when considering the impact of associated sympathectomy and hypotension in patients with major comorbidities, particularly severe aortic stenosis. Prior to epidural or spinal anesthesia, a fluid bolus will help avoid a precipitous drop in blood pressure. Slow and controlled dosing through an epidural catheter can also prevent rapid hypotension. Both hyperbaric and isobaric local anesthetics can be used for a spinal anesthetic.

A lumbar plexus block (LPB) or psoas compartment block is an anatomically deep block that provides a potent analgesic for hip surgery. The needle depth increases the risk of inadvertent intravascular injection; therefore, the LPB is avoided in anticoagulated patients. It should also be noted that performing an LPB can rarely result in inadvertent intrathecal injection. Femoral nerve block (FNB) is a useful alternative; however, quadriceps weakness may increase postoperative fall risk during rehabilitation.[58] For both LPB and FNB, continuous nerve catheters decrease postoperative opioid requirements.[58,59]

As THA surgical technique has evolved to include smaller implants, smaller incisions, and less cementing, recovery has become faster and less painful. As a result, some surgeons perform injections of a "cocktail" that may contain a local anesthetic, epinephrine, a nonsteroidal anti-inflammatory, a corticosteroid, and/or an antibiotic into the periarticular space. Some surgeons will place an epicapsular catheter for postoperative pain management. Utilization of these techniques can avoid urinary retention associated with epidural opioids and weakness associated with peripheral nerve blocks. Although superior to placebo,[60] further studies are needed to establish noninferiority of this technique for pain control compared to percutaneous regional anesthesia techniques.

Blood Loss and Transfusion

Deliberate hypotension using neuraxial anesthesia during hip surgery decreases blood loss and intraoperative transfusion needs when compared to general anesthesia.[61,62] This can be accomplished with either a lumbar spinal anesthetic utilizing a high dose of a short-acting local anesthetic such as mepivacaine, or a low thoracic epidural. In this setting, the inotropic effect of a low-dose epinephrine infusion prevents significant hypotension while maintaining cardiac output.[63] Maintaining normothermia improves intraoperative coagulation. Similar to spine surgery, TXA can be given intravenously or topically in the perioperative setting to decrease blood loss and transfusion requirements.[64]

Ambulatory Hip Surgery

Hip arthroscopy is a common procedure to repair labral tears and to treat hip dysplasia and femoroacetabular impingement. Patients are placed in either the supine or lateral position (Fig. 51-3). Maximal relaxation is necessary while the leg is placed in traction to facilitate dislocation of the femoral head from the acetabulum for access to the hip joint. Relaxation can be achieved by spinal, epidural, or general anesthesia.

A potentially life-threatening complication of hip arthroscopy is extravasation of the arthroscopy fluid from the hip joint into the peritoneal cavity. In extreme cases, intra-abdominal fluid extravasation (IAFE) can cause abdominal compartment syndrome resulting in hemodynamic instability, cardiovascular collapse, and, in tragic cases, death.[65] Iliopsoas tenotomy with concomitant high pump pressures is a risk factor for IAFE. Treatment ranges from clinical observation to diuresis and, in severe cases, abdominal laparotomy.[66] IAFE should be considered in a hemodynamically unstable patient experiencing severe abdominal or pelvic pain postoperatively. Diagnosis can be made with bedside ultrasound utilizing the focused assessment with sonography in trauma exam.[67] Hip arthroscopy is a painful procedure, and an LPB can improve postoperative analgesia[68] but may prolong recovery.[69]

Surgery to the Knee

Total Knee Arthroplasty

Nearly 700,000 TKAs are performed each year in the United States with a global projection of approximately 3.5 million in 2030.[70] Because TKA involves the cutting and cementing of two long bones, the femur and tibia, these procedures have a painful recovery with a high incidence of chronic pain following both primary and revision procedures.[71] It is important to create an appropriate postoperative analgesia plan to ensure mobility and range of motion.

Positioning and Anesthesia Technique

Knee arthroplasties and arthroscopies are performed in the supine position to allow for easy access to and evaluation of the knee joint in extension and flexion. For TKA, neuraxial anesthesia should be used whenever possible, as described earlier. A thigh tourniquet will minimize bleeding and improve surgical visualization. Tourniquets should be used with caution in patients with active infections or thromboses in the lower extremity, because the exsanguination prior to tourniquet inflation may cause systemic spread of infection or PE. In patients with severe atherosclerosis, the tourniquet may not optimally compress the arteries. If a tourniquet is not applied, consider deliberate hypotension as described earlier for hip surgery.

Analgesia for Total Knee Arthroplasty

The optimal analgesia for TKA is a complex and evolving topic (Table 51-4).[72] Regional anesthesia improves patient pain outcomes compared to traditional opioid regimens. Epidural catheters with a continuous infusion of dilute local anesthetic and low-dose opioid can provide excellent pain control, particularly when paired with patient-controlled epidural analgesia. Management of an epidural catheter for postoperative analgesia must account for pharmacologic venous thromboprophylaxis. Ultrasound-guided regional anesthesia has led to a significant increase

Table 51-4 Anesthetic Techniques and Nerve Blocks for Lower Extremity Surgery

Procedure	Anesthetic (*Optimal Anesthetic)	Nerve Block Options *(Preferred Blocks)
• Partial or total hip arthroplasty • Hip fracture surgery • Hip arthroscopy	• *Neuraxial • General anesthesia	• *Lumbar plexus (psoas compartment) block • Femoral nerve block • Fascia iliaca block
• Partial or total knee arthroplasty	• *Neuraxial • General anesthesia	• *Femoral nerve block (FNB) • *Saphenous (adductor canal) block • Lumbar plexus (psoas compartment) block • Sciatic nerve block (in combination with FNB) • Selective tibial nerve block (in combination with FNB) • Obturator nerve block (in combination with FNB)
• Anterior cruciate ligament reconstruction	• Neuraxial • General anesthesia	• *Saphenous (adductor canal) block • Femoral nerve block
• Bunionectomy • Hammer toe correction • Midfoot fusion • Ankle fracture • Achilles tendon repair	• Neuraxial • General anesthesia • Ankle block (surgery involving toes)	• *Popliteal fossa sciatic nerve block • Ankle block • Saphenous (adductor canal block) (in combination with popliteal fossa sciatic nerve block)

in use of peripheral nerve blocks and catheters as components of postoperative analgesic regimens. A balanced multimodal analgesic regimen can include pharmacologic treatment with anti-inflammatories, acetaminophen, opioids, and medications that manage neuropathic components of pain, such as pregabalin. Such a multimodal approach has the potential to maximize analgesic efficacy while minimizing side effects.

The femoral, sciatic, and obturator nerves provide sensation to the knee joint. The most commonly utilized peripheral nerve blocks are the LBP, fascia iliaca (3-in-1 block), FNB, and adductor canal (or saphenous) nerve blocks (see Chapter 36). These blocks can be performed in combination with a sciatic nerve block and/or an obturator nerve block. Literature and clinical practice continue to evolve regarding which blocks or combination of blocks best facilitate rehabilitation and postoperative mobilization, thereby reducing time to hospital discharge, enhancing cost effectiveness, and reducing the risk for complications such as ambulation-related falls.[73]

The FNB is currently considered the peripheral nerve block of choice for TKA analgesia because it has a low complication profile and is easy to perform with either nerve stimulation or ultrasound guidance owing to well-defined anatomic landmarks. FNBs can be performed in a single shot or via catheter; both techniques are associated with reduced morphine consumption after TKA.[74] A major drawback to FNB is quadriceps weakness (up to 80%)[75] and associated fall risk; however, the correlation between FNB and postoperative falls is disputed.[76]

The saphenous nerve block (or adductor canal block) is gaining popularity as a means to avoid quadriceps weakness from an FNB while providing similar pain control and minimizing opioid consumption.[77] Performing the block requires ultrasound guidance and a low local anesthetic volume placed distally within the adductor canal to avoid motor blockade to the vastus medialis.

The sciatic nerve provides sensation to the posterior compartment of the knee and, in combination with an FNB, can reduce opioid consumption after TKA.[73,78] Sciatic nerve blockade causes a "foot drop" that can increase postoperative fall risk and delay diagnosis of common peroneal nerve palsy, a complication seen with large valgus corrections of the knee.[79] A selective tibial nerve block is an alternative that provides similar analgesia without the corresponding foot drop.[80] Sole obturator nerve block is insufficient for TKA analgesia[81]; however, it may be beneficial in combination with FNB.[82]

Periarticular injections (local infiltration technique) with cocktails of medications (see Surgery to the Hip and Pelvis, Anesthesia Technique) performed by the surgeon can reduce LOS and improve resting pain scores[83]; however, its use with an FNB results in lower pain scores with ambulation and during continuous passive movement. Liposomal bupivacaine can be added to periarticular injections as a means to prolong the effect of the local anesthetic. The benefit of liposomal bupivacaine over standard local anesthetics is not conclusive, however, and both the safety profile[84] and cost[85] should be taken into consideration.

Ambulatory Knee Surgery

Ambulatory knee surgery has increased because health-care costs have encouraged outpatient management of less complex cases. An optimal anesthetic has a rapid onset and fast offset with minimal side effects so as to prevent prolonged postanesthesia care unit stays or unexpected overnight admissions. Neuraxial anesthesia results in a lower rate of nausea and vomiting than general anesthesia. However, in a practice with rapid turnover time and/or limited postanesthesia care unit capacity, the need to wait for block resolution may not be practical. In such settings, the use of general anesthesia with multimodal antinausea prophylaxis may be appropriate.

In performing a spinal anesthetic in an ambulatory setting, a short-to-intermediate–acting local anesthetic should be utilized. Intrathecal lidocaine causes a high rate of transient neurologic symptoms (TNSs) and is rarely used. The reported incidence of TNS with 1.5% mepivacaine is approximately 6%[86]; however, in our practice the observed rates are much lower. This may be due to concomitant use of the anti-inflammatory ketorolac and dexamethasone for nausea prophylaxis. TNS is rare with 2% chloroprocaine[87] and 0.5% bupivacaine; however, bupivacaine may not be appropriate for ambulatory cases owing to its longer duration. Short-acting narcotics (e.g., fentanyl) can be added to spinal blocks to increase anesthetic potency, but the resulting pruritus may not be tolerated. Evidence has not demonstrated a clinically significant difference in patient outcome with respect to anesthetic technique for ambulatory knee surgery.[88]

Anterior cruciate ligament (ACL) reconstruction is a common ambulatory procedure performed with a cadaveric allograft or an autograft from the patellar tendon or hamstring. In younger and more active patients the autograft is preferred, but patellar tendon and hamstring grafts cause significant postoperative pain. An epidural or spinal block can provide intraoperative anesthesia, in combination with an FNB or catheters for analgesia. However, recent data suggest that FNB is not superior to multimodal analgesia[89] and may prolong discharge. Additionally, quadriceps weakness can be a complication of ACL reconstructions owing to muscle atrophy and activation failure, and FNB may cloud the clinical picture.[90] An adductor canal block can provide similar analgesia to an FNB after ACL surgery without causing quadriceps weakness.[91]

Surgery to the Foot and Ankle

Innervation of the foot and ankle is provided by the femoral nerve (via the saphenous nerve) and the sciatic nerve (via the posterior tibial, sural, and deep and superficial peroneal nerves). Anesthesia for foot surgery can be performed with an ankle block or a sciatic nerve block in the popliteal fossa with a saphenous nerve block as needed for coverage of the medial foot and ankle (see Chapter 36). Some surgeons prefer ankle blocks in order to avoid the foot drop caused by a sciatic nerve block. A neuraxial or general anesthetic may be required to minimize patient movement and allow for thigh tourniquet inflation.

Surgery to the foot and ankle can cause severe postoperative pain, and regional anesthesia provides optimal postoperative analgesia, particularly in the outpatient setting. Long-acting local anesthetics such as bupivacaine and ropivacaine can provide up to 24 hours of analgesia, and the addition of adjuvants like preservative-free dexamethasone can consistently extend analgesia beyond 24 hours.[28,92] Local anesthetic infusion through an indwelling catheter is also common for major foot and ankle surgery and allows for prolonged analgesia with minimal opioid-related side effects, including in the outpatient setting.[93] Peripheral nerve catheters may be challenging for noncompliant patients or those with limited access to follow-up care. In the outpatient setting, care must be taken to prevent accidental trauma to an anesthetized extremity, and patients should be instructed on how to best protect the limb upon discharge.

Pediatric Orthopedic Anesthesia

Pediatric patients present with a variety of orthopedic conditions, including congenital deformities, trauma, infections, and malignancies (see Chapter 43). Orthopedic procedures may be performed under regional, general, or a combination of anesthetic techniques depending on patient age, operative site, positioning, and surgical duration.

The Pediatric Regional Anesthesia Network database has established the safety of regional anesthetic blocks and catheters in children.[94,95] Upper and lower extremity blocks may be performed with similar safety profiles in children who are awake as in those who are receiving sedation or general anesthesia.[96,97] The anatomic differences between the pediatric and adult spine and spinal cord must be appreciated, and caudal blocks should be considered for lower extremity surgery in very young children (see Chapter 35).

Special Considerations in Orthopedics

Amputation

Following amputation, many patients experience phantom limb pain, phantom limb sensations, and/or stump pain that can be chronic, debilitating, and difficult to manage. The incidence of persistent phantom limb pain is approximately 40% with upper extremity amputation[98] and up to 85% after lower limb amputation.[99] Prolonged outpatient local anesthetic administration (median 30 days) via perineural catheter may prevent phantom limb pain, with 84% of patients in one study reporting no pain at 12 months following lower limb amputation.[100] In contrast, a study of short-term (3 days) perioperative epidural and perineural analgesia found phantom limb pain rates of 38% and 50%, respectively, at 12 months.[101]

Microvascular Surgery

Microvascular surgery is often required for restoration of blood flow following orthopedic trauma. Microvascular surgery can take many hours to perform, often requiring general anesthesia to maintain patient comfort and prevent movement. Mechanical ventilation can help avoid vasoconstriction caused by hyperoxia and hypocarbia as well as by hypercarbia-induced catecholamine release. Moreover, optimal anesthetic management for microvascular surgery utilizes regional techniques that provide sympathectomy (maximizing vasodilation) and diminish the stress response (minimizing vasospasm and thrombotic risk).[102–104] Maintenance of normothermia is essential to minimize vasoconstriction,[104] and volume replacement is recommended at a rate of should read 3.5 to 6 mL/kg per hour.[105] Permissive hemodilution to a hematocrit of 30% can be considered for optimization of blood viscosity, and oxygen-carrying capacity. Surgeons generally discourage vasopressors except in emergency situations, so their use must be discussed with the surgical team prior to initiation. However, rather than supporting adverse effects of vasopressor use, evidence suggests they may be beneficial for maintenance of flap flow.[105,106] Postoperative local anesthetic neuraxial and/or perineural infusions are recommended to help maintain adequate perfusion postoperatively.[107–111] Antithrombotics, including unfractionated and low–molecular-weight heparins, are often used to prevent graft thrombosis and must be taken into consideration when managing catheter insertion and removal postoperatively.

Acute Compartment Syndrome

Acute compartment syndrome (ACS) occurs when soft tissue pressures in a closed extremity compartment exceed capillary perfusion pressure, resulting in ischemic tissue damage. This complication is most commonly seen following tibial and forearm fractures.[112] ACS is often first heralded by symptoms of pain out of proportion to injury; therefore, the benefits of regional analgesic techniques must be weighed against the risk of delayed diagnosis of compartment syndrome. The severity of ACS-related pain is reported to "break through" the analgesic effects of low-dose neuraxial or perineural local anesthetic infusions.[113–116] However, dense blocks have been reported to mask episodes of ACS.[117,118] Thus, the use of regional analgesic techniques requires careful clinical monitoring for ACS, and the decision for their use should be made in collaboration with the surgical team.[112]

Tourniquets

Tourniquets are often used to minimize blood loss and provide a bloodless operating field for extremity orthopedic surgery. The cuff should be large enough to comfortably encircle the limb, and the width should be more than half the limb diameter. Damage to underlying vessels, nerves, and muscles can be caused by excessively high tourniquet pressures and/or prolonged inflation times. In general, a cuff pressure 100 mmHg above a patient's measured systolic pressure is adequate for the thigh and 50 mmHg above systolic pressure is adequate for the arm. The duration of safe tourniquet inflation is generally considered to be 2 hours[119,120]; however, a perfusion break followed by repeat exsanguination may be considered if longer total tourniquet times are required. Breakthrough bleeding during tourniquet inflation is often due to intramedullary blood flow in long bones or small arterial vessels between the two bones of a distal extremity and cannot be resolved by tourniquet overinflation.

Tourniquet pain can become significant over time and can be mitigated with opioids and/or hypnotics or definitively managed by tourniquet deflation. Transient systemic metabolic acidosis, increased arterial carbon dioxide levels, and a drop in systemic blood pressure can be expected with tourniquet deflation and are generally well tolerated in healthy patients. Special care should be taken at the time of tourniquet deflation in patients with significant comorbidities who may be susceptible to such changes.

Fat Embolus Syndrome/Bone Cement Implantation Syndrome

Fat embolus syndrome (FES) is associated with multiple traumatic injuries, surgery involving long-bone fractures, and bilateral arthroplasty.[121–123] The incidence of FES in isolated long-bone fractures is 3% to 4%, and the associated mortality rate is significant, ranging from 10% to 20%. Early corticosteroid use in long-bone fracture patients may be beneficial in preventing the syndrome.[124] Symptoms of FES usually occur 12 to 40 hours after the injury and can range from mild dyspnea to frank coma; however, fulminant episodes can occur within hours of traumatic injury. Decreased arterial oxygen tension is the most consistent abnormal laboratory value. Major and minor clinical and laboratory criteria for FES diagnosis are listed in Table 51-5, as classified by Gurd and Schonfeld.[125,126] Management of FES is largely supportive and may require early mechanical ventilation.

Table 51-5 Criteria for Fat Embolism Syndrome[125,126]

Gurd's Criteria	Major	Minor	Laboratory
Requires 1 major and 4 minor/laboratory signs	Petechiae (axillary/subconjunctival)	Tachycardia	Microglobulinemia (required for diagnosis)
	Hypoxemia	Fever	Thrombocytopenia
	Depressed consciousness	Retina: fat emboli	Anemia
	Pulmonary edema	Sputum: fat globules	Elevated erythrocyte sedimentation rate
		Urine: fat globules	
Schonfeld fat embolism index	**Criteria**	**Points**	
Requires 5 or more points	Petechial rash	5	
	Diffuse alveolar infiltrates	4	
	Hypoxemia	3	
	Confusion	1	
	Fever	1	
	Tachycardia	1	
	Tachypnea	1	

Bone cement implantation syndrome (BCIS) is a poorly defined syndrome of hypoxemia, hypotension, and/or altered mental status observed in patients undergoing fracture repair or arthroplasty with cementation. The syndrome is defined as occurrence of these events in temporal proximity to cementation, prosthesis insertion, joint reduction, or tourniquet deflation, with its severity defined by degree of hypoxemia and hypotension.[127] Although BCIS has historically been attributed to circulation of methyl methacrylate cement monomers, it has since been shown that monomer levels are too low to account for the severity of observed signs and symptoms. It is likely that the syndrome overlaps extensively with FES and results from embolization of fat and other debris that is exacerbated by high-pressure intramedullary expansion of cement. Such embolization can trigger a cascade of endothelial damage, histamine release, and complement activation that contributes to the severity of FES and BCIS.[127] Invasive monitoring with an arterial line is recommended when cemented implants are being placed. Central venous pressure and possibly pulmonary artery catheter placement should be considered in medically fragile patients in whom cementation cannot be avoided.

Venous Thromboembolism and Thromboprophylaxis

Without prophylaxis, DVT develops in 40% to 80% of orthopedic patients. A range of 1% to 28% show clinical or laboratory evidence of PE, and fatal PE occurs in 0.1% to 8% of patients.[95] In the absence of prophylaxis, several studies report a lower incidence of DVT and PE in patients undergoing hip or knee surgery under epidural[46,128–131] and spinal[132–134] anesthesia. With appropriate mechanical and/or pharmacologic thromboprophylaxis, significant decreases in rates of DVT and PE have also been noted.

Given the significant risk of thromboembolism following orthopedic surgery, the American College of Chest Physicians (ACCP) has issued guidelines recommending a minimum of 14 days of pharmacologic thromboprophylaxis and/or use of portable mechanical compression devices.[135] However, given concerns regarding perioperative bleeding risks, the American Academy of Orthopedic Surgeons does not support the ACCP recommended target international normalized ratio of 2.0 to 3.0 for warfarin use, with most orthopedic surgeons preferring a target of 1.5 to 2.0.[136,137]

Following introduction of a multimodal prophylaxis protocol for THA (consisting of preoperative discontinuation of procoagulant medication, autologous blood donation, hypotensive epidural anesthesia, intravenous administration of heparin during surgery, aspiration of intramedullary contents, pneumatic compression, knee-high elastic stockings, and early mobilization and chemoprophylaxis), one study found rates of symptomatic DVT and PE to be 2.5% and 0.6%, respectively.[138] Similarly, two recent institutional reviews comprising over 36,000 orthopedic surgery patients found that 1.1% to 1.3% of patients developed symptomatic PE.[139,140] The mortality rate in the larger of the two studies was 0.02%, and risk factors for symptomatic PE included elevated body mass index, elevated Charlson comorbidity index, knee arthroplasty, chronic obstructive pulmonary disease, anemia, depression, and presence of DVT.[140]

The 2010 American Society of Regional Anesthesia practice advisory for the use of regional anesthesia in the setting of antithrombotic or thrombolytic therapy provides essential guidelines for minimizing the risk of clinically significant hematomas in at-risk patients.[48] A summary of recommendations for neuraxial blockade in the setting of anticoagulants and draft updates from the fourth American Society of Regional Anesthesia Practice Advisory for Regional Anesthesia in the Patient Receiving Antithrombotic or Thrombolytic Therapy is presented in Table 51-3.[141] It is generally recommended that the same guidelines be followed when deep plexus blocks are performed or peripheral nerve blocks are being placed near poorly compressible vessels.

REFERENCES

1. Buvanendran A, Thillainathan V. Preoperative and postoperative anesthetic and analgesic techniques for minimally invasive surgery of the spine. *Spine*. 2010;35(26 Suppl):S274–S280.

2. American Society of Anesthesiologists Committee on Standards and Practice Parameters. Practice alert for the perioperative management of patients with coronary artery stents: A report by the American Society of Anesthesiologists committee on standards and practice parameters. *Anesthesiology*. 2009;110(1):22–23.
3. Jenkins JG, Bohn D, Edmonds JF, et al. Evaluation of pulmonary function in muscular dystrophy patients requiring spinal surgery. *Crit Care Med*. 1982;18(9):645–649.
4. Edgcombe H, Carter K, Yarrow S. Anaesthesia in the prone position. *Br J Anaesth*. 2008; 100: 165–183.
5. Elgafy H, Bransford RJ, McGuire RA, et al. Blood loss in major spine surgery: Are there effective measures to decrease massive hemorrhage in major spine fusion surgery? *Spine*. 2010;35(9 Suppl):S47–S56.
6. Nuttall GA, Horlocker TT, Santrach PJ, et al. The predictors of blood transfusions in spinal instrumentation and fusion surgery. *Spine*. 2000;25:596–601.
7. Rajpal S, Gordon DB, Pellino TA, et al. Comparison of perioperative oral multimodal analgesia versus IV PCA for spine surgery. *J Spinal Disord Tech*. 2010;23:139–145.
8. Tse EY, Cheung WY, Ng KF, et al. Reducing perioperative blood loss and allogeneic blood transfusion in patients undergoing major spine surgery. *J Bone Joint Surg Am*. 2011;93:1268–1277.
9. Cheriyan T, Bianco K, Maier SP, et al. Efficacy of tranexamic acid and aminocaproic acid on bleeding in spine surgery: a meta-analysis. *Spine J*. 2013:13:S81.
10. Cheriyan T, Maier SP, Bianco K, et al. Efficacy of tranexamic acid on surgical bleeding in spine surgery: a meta-analysis. *Spine J*. 2015:15:752–761.
11. Epstein NE, Danto J, Nardi D. Evaluation of intraoperative somatosensory evoked potential monitoring during 100 cervical operations. *Spine*. 1993;18:737–747.
12. Meyer PR Jr, Cotler HB, Gireesan GT. Operative neurological complications resulting from thoracic and lumbar spine internal fixation. *Clin Orthop Relat Res*. 1988;237:125–131.
13. Nuwer MR, Dawson EG, Carlson LG, et al. Somatosensory evoked potential monitoring reduces neurological deficits after scoliosis surgery: results of a large multicenter study. *Electroencephalogr Clin Neurophysiol*. 1995; 96:6–11.
14. Pathak KS, Brown RH, Nash CL Jr, et al. Continuous opioid infusion for scoliosis fusion surgery. *Anesth Analg*. 1983;62:841–845.
15. Burke D, Hicks RG. Surgical monitoring of motor pathways. *J Clin Neurophysiol*. 1998;15:194–205.
16. Pathak KS, Ammadio M, Kalamchi A, et al. Effects of halothane, enflurane, and isoflurane on somatosensory evoked potentials during nitrous oxide anesthesia. *Anesthesiology*. 1987;66:753–757.
17. Schwartz DM, Auerbach JD, Dormans JP, et al. Neurophysiological detection of impending spinal cord injury during scoliosis surgery. *J Bone Joint Surg Am*. 2007;89:2440–2449.
18. Martyn JA, White DA, Gronert GA, et al. Up-and-down regulation of skeletal muscle acetylcholine receptors. Effects on neuromuscular blockers. *Anesthesiology*. 1992;76:822–843.
19. Fehlings MG, Brodke DS, Norvell DC, et al. The evidence for intraoperative neurophysiological monitoring in spine surgery: does it make a difference? *Spine*. 2010;35(9 Suppl):S37–S46.
20. Sadrolsadat SH, Mahdavi AR, Moharari RS, et al. A prospective randomized trial comparing the technique of spinal and general anesthesia for lumbar disk surgery: a study of 100 cases. *Surg Neurol*. 2009;71:60–65.
21. Vedantam R, Lenke LG, Eridwell KH, et al. A prospective evaluation of pulmonary function in patients with adolescent idiopathic scoliosis relative to the surgical approach used for spinal arthrodesis. *Spine*. 2000;25:82–90.
22. Steel T, Jones R, Crossman J, et al. Intraoperative wound infiltration with bupivacaine in patients undergoing lumbar spine surgery. *J Clin Neurosci*. 1998;5:298–303.
23. Dilger JA, Tetzlaff JE, Bell GR, et al. Ischaemic optic neuropathy after spinal fusion. *Can J Anaesth*. 1998;45:63–66.
24. Myers MA, Hamilton SR, Bogosian AJ, et al. Visual loss as a complication of spine surgery. A review of 37 cases. *Spine*. 1997;22:1325–1329.
25. Warner ME, Warner MA, Garrity JA, et al. The frequency of perioperative vision loss. *Anesth Analg*. 2001;93:1417–1421.
26. Lee LA, Roth S, Posner KL, et al. The American Society of Anesthesiologists Post-operative Visual Loss Registry: analysis of 93 spine surgery cases with postoperative visual loss. *Anesthesiology*. 2006;105:652–659.
27. Postoperative Visual Loss Study Group. Risk factors associated with ischemic optic neuropathy after spinal fusion surgery. *Anesthesiology*. 2012;116:15–24.
28. Kirksey MA, Haskins SC, Cheng J, et al. Local anesthetic peripheral nerve block adjuvants for prolongation of analgesia: a systematic qualitative review. *PLoS One*. 2015;10:e0137312.
29. Sviggum HP, Jacob AK, Mantilla CB, et al. Perioperative nerve injury after total shoulder arthroplasty: assessment of risk after regional anesthesia. *Reg Anesth Pain Med*. 2012;37:490–494.
30. Liu GY, Zhang CY, Wu HW. Comparison of initial nonoperative and operative management of radial nerve palsy associated with acute humeral shaft fractures. *Orthopedics*. 2012;35:702–708.
31. Li X, Eichinger JK, Hartshorn T, et al. A comparison of the lateral decubitus and beach-chair positions for shoulder surgery: advantages and complications. *J Am Acad Orthop Surg*. 2015;23:18–28.
32. Laflam A, Joshi B, Brady K, et al. Shoulder surgery in the beach chair position is associated with diminished cerebral autoregulation but no differences in postoperative cognition or brain injury biomarker levels compared with supine positioning: the anesthesia patient safety foundation beach chair study. *Anesth Analg*. 2015;120:176–185.
33. Sia S, Sarro F, Lepri A, et al. The effect of exogenous epinephrine on the incidence of hypotensive/bradycardic events during shoulder surgery in the sitting position during interscalene block. *Anesth Analg*. 2003;97:583–588.
34. Song SY, Son SH, Kim SO, et al. Intravenous fentanyl during shoulder arthroscopic surgery in the sitting position after interscalene block increases the incidence of episodes of bradycardia hypotension. *Korean J Anesthesiol*. 2011;60:344–350.
35. Liguori GA, Kahn RL, Gordon J, et al. The use of metoprolol and glycopyrrolate to prevent hypotensive/bradycardic events during shoulder arthroscopy in the sitting position under interscalene block. *Anesth Analg*. 1998;87:1320–1325.
36. Nallam SR, Dara S. Effect of intravenous ondansetron on reducing the incidence of hypotension and bradycardia events during shoulder arthroscopy in sitting position under interscalene brachial plexus block: a prospective randomized trial. *Indian J Anaesth*. 2015;59:353–358.
37. Urmey WF, Talts KH, Sharrock NE. One hundred percent incidence of hemidiaphragmatic paresis associated with interscalene brachial plexus anesthesia as diagnosed by ultrasonography. *Anesth Analg*. 1991;72:498–503.
38. Renes SH, Rettig HC, Gielen MJ, et al. Ultrasound-guided low-dose interscalene brachial plexus block reduces the incidence of hemidiaphragmatic paresis. *Reg Anesth Pain Med*. 2009;34:498–502.
39. Sinha SK, Abrams JH, Barnett JT, et al. Decreasing the local anesthetic volume from 20 to 10 mL for ultrasound-guided interscalene block at the cricoid level does not reduce the incidence of hemidiaphragmatic paresis. *Reg Anesth Pain Med*. 2011;36:17–20.
40. Erickson JM, Louis DS, Naughton NN. Symptomatic phrenic nerve palsy after supraclavicular block in an obese man. *Orthopedics*. 2009;32:368.
41. Hadzic A, Williams BA, Karaca PE, et al. For outpatient rotator cuff surgery, nerve block anesthesia provides superior same-day recovery over general anesthesia. *Anesthesiology*. 2005;102:1001–1007.
42. Danninger T, Stundner O, Rasul R, et al. Factors associated with hospital admission after rotator cuff repair: the role of peripheral nerve blockade. *J Clin Anesth*. 2015;27:566–573.
43. Stundner O, Rasul R, Chiu YL, et al. Peripheral nerve blocks in shoulder arthroplasty: how do they influence complications and length of stay? *Clin Orthop Relat Res*. 2014;472:1482–1488.
44. Ilfeld BM, Wright TW, Enneking FK, et al. Total elbow arthroplasty as an outpatient procedure using a continuous infraclavicular nerve block at home: a prospective case report. *Reg Anesth Pain Med*. 2006;31:172–176.
45. Ilfeld BM, Morey TE, Wright TW, et al. Interscalene perineural ropivacaine infusion: a comparison of two dosing regimens for postoperative analgesia. *Reg Anesth Pain Med*. 2004;29:9–16.
46. Sharrock NE, Haas SB, Hargett MJ, et al. Effects of epidural anesthesia on the incidence of deep-vein thrombosis after total knee arthroplasty. *J Bone Joint Surg Am*. 1991;73:502–506.
47. Memtsoudis SG, Sun X, Chiu Y-L, et al. Perioperative comparative effectiveness of anesthetic technique in orthopedic patients. *Anesthesiology*. 2013;118:1046–1058.
48. Horlocker TT, Wedel DJ, Rowlingson JC, et al. Regional anesthesia in the patient receiving antithrombotic or thrombolytic therapy: American Society of Regional Anesthesia and Pain Medicine Evidence-Based Guidelines (Third Edition). *Reg Anesth Pain Med*. 2010;35:64–101.
49. Fingar KR (Truven Health Analytics), Stocks C (AHRQ), Weiss AJ (Truven Health Analytics), Steiner CA (AHRQ). Most Frequent Operating Room Procedures Performed in U.S. Hospitals, 2003-2012. HCUP Statistical Brief #186. December 2014. Agency for Healthcare Research and Quality, Rockville, MD. http://www.hcup-us.ahrq.gov/reports/statbriefs/sb186-Operating-Room-Procedures-United-States-2012.pdf.
50. Moskal JT, Capps SG, Scanelli JA. Anterior muscle sparing approach for total hip arthroplasty. *World J Orthop*. 2013;4:12–18.
51. Miller AG, McKenzie J, Greenky M, et al. Spinal anesthesia: should everyone receive a urinary catheter?: a randomized, prospective study of patients undergoing total hip arthroplasty. *J Bone Joint Surg Am*. 2013;95:1498–1503.
52. Opperer M, Danninger T, Stundner O, et al. Perioperative outcomes and type of anesthesia in hip surgical patients: an evidence based review. *World J Orthop*. 2014;5:336–343.
53. Pumberger M, Memtsoudis SG, Stundner O, et al. An analysis of the safety of epidural and spinal neuraxial anesthesia in more than 100,000 consecutive major lower extremity joint replacements. *Reg Anesth Pain Med*. 2013;38:515–519.
54. Chelly JE, Schilling D. Thromboprophylaxis and peripheral nerve blocks in patients undergoing joint arthroplasty. *J Arthroplasty*. 2008;23:350–354.
55. Brull R, McCartney CJ, Chan VW, et al. Neurological complications after regional anesthesia: contemporary estimates of risk. *Anesth Analg*. 2007;104:965–974.

56. Neuman MD, Rosenbaum PR, Ludwig JM, et al. Anesthesia Technique, Mortality, and Length of Stay After Hip Fracture Surgery. *JAMA.* 2014;311: 2508–2517.
57. Moja L, Piatti A, Pecoraro V, et al. Timing matters in hip fracture surgery: patients operated within 48 hours have better outcomes. A meta-analysis and meta-regression of over 190,000 patients. *PLoS ONE.* 2012;7:e46175.
58. Johnson RL, Kopp SL, Hebl JR, et al. Falls and major orthopaedic surgery with peripheral nerve blockade: a systematic review and meta-analysis. *Br J Anaesth.* 2013;110:518–528.
59. Ilfeld BM, Mariano ER, Madison SJ, et al. Continuous femoral versus posterior lumbar plexus nerve blocks for analgesia after hip arthroplasty: a randomized, controlled study. *Anesth Analg.* 2011;113:897–903.
60. Aguirre J, Baulig B, Dora C, et al. Continuous epicapsular ropivacaine 0.3% infusion after minimally invasive hip arthroplasty: a prospective, randomized, double-blinded, placebo-controlled study comparing continuous wound infusion with morphine patient-controlled analgesia. *Anesth Analg.* 2012;114: 456–461.
61. Maurer SG, Chen AL, Hiebert R, et al. Comparison of outcomes of using spinal versus general anesthesia in total hip arthroplasty. *Am J Orthop.* 2007;36:E101–E106.
62. Guay J. The effect of neuraxial blocks on surgical blood loss and blood transfusion requirements: a meta-analysis. *J Clin Anesth.* 2006;18:124–128.
63. Sharrock NE, Bading B, Mineo R, et al. Deliberate hypotensive epidural anesthesia for patients with normal and low cardiac output. *Anesth Analg.* 1994;79:899–904.
64. Poeran J, Rasul R, Suzuki S, et al. Tranexamic acid use and postoperative outcomes in patients undergoing total hip or knee arthroplasty in the United States: retrospective analysis of effectiveness and safety. *BMJ.* 2014;349:g4829.
65. Kocher MS, Frank JS, Nasreddine AY, et al. Intra-abdominal fluid extravasation during hip arthroscopy: a survey of the MAHORN group. *Arthroscopy.* 2012;28:1654–1660.
66. Bardakos NV, Papavasiliou AV. Death after fluid extravasation in hip arthroscopy. *Arthroscopy.* 2012;28:1584.
67. Haskins S, Desai N, Fields K, et al. Diagnosis of Intra-Abdominal Fluid Extravasation Following Hip Arthroscopy With Point-of-Care Ultrasonography Can Identify Patients at an Increased Risk of Postoperative Pain. Abstract: American Society for Anesthesiology Annual Meeting 2015.
68. YaDeau JT, Tedore T, Goytizolo EA, et al. Lumbar plexus blockade reduces pain after hip arthroscopy: a prospective randomized controlled trial. *Anesth Analg.* 2012;115:968–972.
69. Schroeder KM, Donnelly MJ, Anderson BM, et al. The analgesic impact of preoperative lumbar plexus blocks for hip arthroscopy: a retrospective review. *Hip Int.* 2013;23:93–98.
70. Kurtz S, Ong K, Lau E, et al. Projections of primary and revision hip and knee arthroplasty in the United States from 2005 to 2030. *J Bone Joint Surg Am.* 2007;89:780–785.
71. Petersen KK, Simonsen O, Laursen MB, et al. Chronic postoperative pain after primary and revision total knee arthroplasty. *Clin J Pain.* 2015;31:1–6.
72. Danninger T, Opperer M, Memtsoudis SG. Perioperative pain control after total knee arthroplasty: an evidence based review of the role of peripheral nerve blocks. *World J Orthop.* 2014;5:225–232.
73. Abdallah FW, Brull R. Is sciatic nerve block advantageous when combined with femoral nerve block for postoperative analgesia following total knee arthroplasty? A systematic review. *Reg Anesth Pain Med.* 2011;36:493–498.
74. Paul JE, Arya A, Hurlburt L, et al. Femoral nerve block improves analgesia outcomes after total knee arthroplasty: a meta-analysis of randomized controlled trials. *Anesthesiology.* 2010;113:1144–1162.
75. Charous MT, Madison SJ, Suresh PJ, et al. Continuous femoral nerve blocks: varying local anesthetic delivery method (bolus versus basal) to minimize quadriceps motor block while maintaining sensory block. *Anesthesiology.* 2011;115:774–781.
76. Memtsoudis SG, Danninger T, Rasul R, et al. Inpatient falls after total knee arthroplasty: the role of anesthesia type and peripheral nerve blocks. *Anesthesiology.* 2014;120:551–563.
77. Kim DH, Lin Y, Goytizolo EA, et al. Adductor canal block versus femoral nerve block for total knee arthroplasty: a prospective, randomized, controlled trial. *Anesthesiology.* 2014;120:540–550.
78. Morin AM, Kratz CD, Eberhart LH, et al. Postoperative analgesia and functional recovery after total-knee replacement: comparison of a continuous posterior lumbar plexus (psoas compartment) block, a continuous femoral nerve block, and the combination of a continuous femoral and sciatic nerve block. *Reg Anesth Pain Med.* 2005;30:434–445.
79. Park JH, Restrepo C, Norton R, et al. Common peroneal nerve palsy following total knee arthroplasty: prognostic factors and course of recovery. *J Arthroplasty.* 2013;28:1538–1542.
80. Sinha SK, Abrams JH, Arumugam S, et al. Femoral nerve block with selective tibial nerve block provides effective analgesia without foot drop after total knee arthroplasty: a prospective, randomized, observer-blinded study. *Anesth Analg.* 2012;115:202–206.
81. Kardash K, Hickey D, Tessler MJ, et al. Obturator versus femoral nerve block for analgesia after total knee arthroplasty. *Anesth Analg.* 2007;105:853–858.
82. Macalou D, Trueck S, Meuret P, et al. Postoperative analgesia after total knee replacement: the effect of an obturator nerve block added to the femoral 3-in-1 nerve block. *Anesth Analg.* 2004;99:251–254.
83. YaDeau JT, Goytizolo EA, Padgett DE, et al. Analgesia after total knee replacement: local infiltration versus epidural combined with a femoral nerve blockade: a prospective, randomised pragmatic trial. *Bone Joint J.* 2013;95-B: 629–635.
84. Richard BM, Rickert DE, Newton PE, et al. Safety evaluation of EXPAREL (DepoFoam bupivacaine) administered by repeated subcutaneous injection in rabbits and dogs: species comparison. *J Drug Deliv.* 2011;2011:467429.
85. Lambrechts M, O'Brien MJ, Savoie FH, et al. Liposomal extended-release bupivacaine for postsurgical analgesia. *Patient Prefer Adherence.* 2013;7: 885–890.
86. YaDeau JT, Liguori GA, Zayas VM. The incidence of transient neurologic symptoms after spinal anesthesia with mepivacaine. *Anesth Analg.* 2005;101:661–665.
87. Goldblum E, Atchabahian A. The use of 2-chloroprocaine for spinal anaesthesia. *Acta Anaesthesiol Scand.* 2013;57:545–552.
88. Horlocker TT, Hebl JR. Evidence based report: outpatient knee arthroscopy–is there an optimal anesthetic technique? *Reg Anesth Pain Med.* 2003;28:58–63.
89. Mall NA, Wright RW. Femoral nerve block use in anterior cruciate ligament reconstruction surgery. *Arthroscopy.* 2010;26:404–416.
90. Thomas AC, Wojtys EM, Brandon C, et al. Muscle atrophy contributes to quadriceps weakness after anterior cruciate ligament reconstruction. *J Sci Med Sport.* 2016;19:7–11.
91. Chisholm MF, Bang H, Maalouf DB, et al. Postoperative analgesia with saphenous block appears equivalent to femoral nerve block in ACL reconstruction. *HSS J.* 2014;10:245–251.
92. YaDeau JT, Paroli L, Fields KG, et al. Addition of dexamethasone and buprenorphine to bupivacaine sciatic nerve block: a randomized controlled trial. *Reg Anesth Pain Med.* 2015;40:321.
93. Ilfeld BM, Morey TE, Wang RD, et al. Continuous popliteal sciatic nerve block for postoperative pain control at home: a randomized, double-blinded, placebo-controlled study. *Anesthesiology.* 2002;97:959–965.
94. Polaner DM, Taenzer AH, Walker BJ, et al. Pediatric regional anesthesia network (PRAN): a multi-institutional study of the use and incidence of complications of pediatric regional anesthesia. *Anesth Analg.* 2012;115:1353–1364.
95. Walker BJ, Long JB, De Oliveira GS, et al. Peripheral nerve catheters in children: an analysis of safety and practice patterns from the pediatric regional anesthesia network (PRAN). *Br J Anaesth.* 2015;115:457–462.
96. Taenzer AH, Walker BJ, Bosenberg AT, et al. Asleep versus awake: does it matter?: pediatric regional block complications by patient state: a report from the pediatric regional anesthesia network. *Reg Anesth Pain Med.* 2014;39: 279–283.
97. Taenzer A, Walker BJ, Bosenberg AT, et al. Interscalene brachial plexus blocks under general anesthesia in children: is this safe practice?: a report from the pediatric regional anesthesia network (PRAN). *Reg Anesth Pain Med.* 2014;39: 502–505.
98. Schley MT, Wilms P, Toepfner S, et al. Painful and nonpainful phantom and stump sensations in acute traumatic amputees. *J Trauma.* 2008;65:858–864.
99. Hsu E, Cohen SP. Postamputation pain: epidemiology, mechanisms, and treatment. *J Pain Res.* 2013;6:121–136.
100. Borghi B, D'Addabbo M, White PF, et al. The use of prolonged peripheral neural blockade after lower extremity amputation: the effect on symptoms associated with phantom limb syndrome. *Anesth Analg.* 2010;111:1308–1315.
101. Lambert A, Dashfield A, Cosgrove C, et al. Randomized prospective study comparing preoperative epidural and intraoperative perineural analgesia for the prevention of postoperative stump and phantom limb pain following major amputation. *Reg Anesth Pain Med.* 2001;26:316–321.
102. Shanahan PT. Replantation anesthesia. *Anesth Analg.* 1984;63:785–786.
103. Hahnenkamp K, Theilmeier G, Van Aken HK, et al. The effects of local anesthetics on perioperative coagulation, inflammation, and microcirculation. *Anesth Analg.* 2002;94:1441–1447.
104. Hagau N, Longrois D. Anesthesia for free vascularized tissue transfer. *Microsurgery.* 2009;29:161–167.
105. Motakef S, Mountziaris PM, Ismail IK, et al. Emerging paradigms in perioperative management for microsurgical free tissue transfer: review of the literature and evidence-based guidelines. *Plast Reconstr Surg.* 2015;135:290–299.
106. Motakef S, Mountziaris PM, Ismail IK, et al. Perioperative management for microsurgical free tissue transfer: survey of current practices with a comparison to the literature. *J Reconstr Microsurg.* 2015;31:355–363.
107. van den Berg B, Berger A, van den Berg E, et al. Continuous plexus anesthesia to improve circulation in peripheral microvascular interventions. *Handchir Mikrochir Plast Chir.* 1983;15:101–104.
108. Berger A, Tizian C, Zenz M. Continuous plexus blockade for improved circulation in microvascular surgery. *Ann Plast Surg.* 1985;14:16–19.
109. Kurt E, Ozturk S, Isik S, et al. Continuous brachial plexus blockade for digital replantations and toe-to-hand transfers. *Ann Plast Surg.* 2005;54:24–27.
110. Su HH, Lui PW, Yu CL, et al. The effects of continuous axillary brachial plexus block with ropivacaine infusion on skin temperature and survival of crushed fingers after microsurgical replantation. *Chang Gung Med J.* 2005;28:567–574.

111. Taras JS, Behrman MJ. Continuous peripheral nerve block in replantation and revascularization. *J Reconstr Microsurg.* 1998;14:17–21.
112. Gadsden J, Warlick A. Regional anesthesia for the trauma patient: improving patient outcomes. *Local Reg Anesth.* 2015;8:45–55.
113. Walker BJ, Noonan KJ, Bosenberg AT. Evolving compartment syndrome not masked by a continuous peripheral nerve block: evidence-based case management. *Reg Anesth Pain Med.* 2012;37:393–397.
114. Cometa MA, Esch AT, Boezaart AP. Did continuous femoral and sciatic nerve block obscure the diagnosis or delay the treatment of acute lower leg compartment syndrome? A case report. *Pain Med.* 2011;12:823–828.
115. Uzel AP, Steinmann G. Thigh compartment syndrome after intramedullary femoral nailing: possible femoral nerve block influence on diagnosis timing. *Orthop Traumatol Surg Res.* 2009;95:309–313.
116. Kucera TJ, Boezaart AP. Regional anesthesia does not consistently block ischemic pain: two further cases and a review of the literature. *Pain Med.* 2014; 15:316–319.
117. Noorpuri BS, Shahane SA, Getty CJ. Acute compartment syndrome following revisional arthroplasty of the forefoot: the dangers of ankle-block. *Foot Ankle Int.* 2000;21:680–682.
118. Hyder N, Kessler S, Jennings AG, et al. Compartment syndrome in tibial shaft fracture missed because of a local nerve block. *J Bone Joint Surg Br.* 1996;78:499–500.
119. Pedowitz RA. Tourniquet-induced neuromuscular injury. A recent review of rabbit and clinical experiments. *Acta Orthop Scand Suppl.* 1991;245:1–33.
120. Horlocker TT, Hebl JR, Gali B, et al. Anesthetic, patient, and surgical risk factors for neurologic complications after prolonged total tourniquet time during total knee arthroplasty. *Anesth Analg.* 2006;102:950–955.
121. Urban MK, Chisholm M, Wukovits B. Are postoperative complications more common with single-stage bilateral (SBTKR) than with unilateral knee arthroplasty: guidelines for patients scheduled for SBTKR. *HSS J.* 2006;2:78–82.
122. Swanson KC, Valle AG, Salvati EA, et al. Perioperative morbidity after single-stage bilateral total hip arthroplasty: a matched control study. *Clin Orthop Relat Res.* 2006;451:140–145.
123. Akhtar S. Fat embolism. *Anesthesiol Clin.* 2009;27:533–550, table of contents.
124. Bederman SS, Bhandari M, McKee MD, et al. Do corticosteroids reduce the risk of fat embolism syndrome in patients with long-bone fractures? A meta-analysis. *Can J Surg.* 2009 52:386–393.
125. Gurd AR. Fat embolism: an aid to diagnosis. *J Bone Joint Surg Br.* 1970;52: 732–737.
126. Schonfeld SA, Ploysongsang Y, DiLisio R, et al. Fat embolism prophylaxis with corticosteroids: a prospective study in high risk patients. *Ann Int Med.* 1983; 99:438–443.
127. Donaldson AJ, Thomson HE, Harper NJ, et al. Bone cement implantation syndrome. *Br J Anaesth.* 2009;102:12–22.
128. Sculco TP. Global blood management in orthopaedic surgery. *Clin Orthop Relat Res.* 1998;(357):43–49.
129. Modig J, Borg T, Bagge L, et al. Role of extradural and of general anaesthesia in fibrinolysis and coagulation after total hip replacement. *Br J Anaesth.* 1983;55:625–629.
130. Modig J, Borg T, Karlstrom G, et al. Thromboembolism after total hip replacement: role of epidural and general anesthesia. *Anesth Analg.* 1983;62:174–180.
131. Nielsen PT, Jorgensen LN, Albrecht-Beste E, et al. Lower thrombosis risk with epidural blockade in knee arthroplasty. *Acta Orthop Scand.* 1990;61:29–31.
132. Davis FM, Laurenson VG, Gillespie WJ, et al. Deep vein thrombosis after total hip replacement. A comparison between spinal and general anaesthesia. *J Bone Joint Surg Br.* 1989;71:181–185.
133. Donadoni R, Baele G, Devulder J, et al. Coagulation and fibrinolytic parameters in patients undergoing total hip replacement: influence of the anaesthesia technique. *Acta Anaesthesiol Scand.* 1989;33:588–592.
134. Thorburn J, Louden JR, Vallance R. Spinal and general anaesthesia in total hip replacement: frequency of deep vein thrombosis. *Br J Anaesth.* 1980;52:1117–1121.
135. Falck-Ytter Y, Francis CW, Johanson NA, et al. Prevention of VTE in orthopedic surgery patients: antithrombotic therapy and prevention of thrombosis, 9th ed: American College of Chest Physicians evidence-based clinical practice guidelines. *Chest.* 2012;141(2 Suppl):e278S-325S.
136. Lieberman JR. The new AAOS clinical practice guidelines on venous thromboembolic prophylaxis: how to adapt them to your practice. *J Am Acad Orthop Surg.* 2011;19:717–721.
137. Lieberman JR, Pensak MJ. Prevention of venous thromboembolic disease after total hip and knee arthroplasty. *J Bone Joint Surg Am.* 2013;95:1801–1811.
138. Gonzalez Della Valle A, Serota A, Go G, et al. Venous thromboembolism is rare with a multimodal prophylaxis protocol after total hip arthroplasty. *Clin Orthop Relat Res.* 2006;444:146–153.
139. Kim HJ, Walcott-Sapp S, Leggett K, et al. The use of spiral computed tomography scans for the detection of pulmonary embolism. *J Arthroplasty.* 2008;23 (6 Suppl 1):31–35.
140. Parvizi J, Huang R, Raphael IJ, et al. Symptomatic pulmonary embolus after joint arthroplasty: stratification of risk factors. *Clin Orthop Relat Res.* 2014;472:903–912.
141. Horlocker TT, Wedel DJ, Rowlingson JC, et al. Interim Update from the 4th ASRA Practice Advisory for Regional Anesthesia in the Patient Receiving Antithrombotic or Thrombolytic Therapy Web site. https://www.asra.com/advisory-guidelines/article/1/anticoagulation-3rd-edition. Accessed December 07, 2015.

52 Transplant Anesthesia

MARIE CSETE • GERARD MANECKE • DALIA BANKS

Anesthetic Management of Organ Donors
   Brain-dead Donors (Donation after Neurologic Death)
   Donation after Cardiac Death (Donation after Circulatory Determination of Death)
   Living Kidney Donors
   Living Liver Donors
Immunosuppressive Agents
   Calcineurin Inhibitors
   Corticosteroids
   Polyclonal and Monoclonal Antibodies
   Mammalian Target of Rapamycin Inhibitors
   Purine Antagonists
   Cell Therapies
Corneal Transplantation
Renal Transplantation
   Preoperative Considerations
   Intraoperative Procedures
Liver Transplantation
   Preoperative Considerations
   Intraoperative Procedures
   Pediatric Liver Transplantation
   Acute Liver Failure
Pancreas and Islet Transplantation
Small Bowel and Multivisceral Transplantation
Composite Tissue Allografts
Lung Transplantation
   Recipient Selection
   Intraoperative Management
   Primary Graft Dysfunction
   Inhaled Nitric Oxide
Heart–lung Transplant (Adult and Pediatric)
Heart Transplantation
   Left Ventricular Assist Devices
   Recipient Selection
   Preanesthetic Considerations
   Intraoperative Management
   Pediatric Heart Transplantation
Management of the Transplant Patient for Nontransplant Surgery

KEY POINTS

1. Brain death is declared when the clinical picture is consistent with irreversible cessation of all brain functions.
2. Anesthesiologists have a significant role to play in organ procurement and should consult with local organ procurement personnel for protocols to optimize healthy graft retrieval.
3. Extended criteria organs, including donation after cardiac death (DCD), are used because of ongoing organ shortage; cold ischemia times should be minimized for extended criteria donor organs.
4. Living kidney and liver donors must be healthy and without significant cardiopulmonary, neurologic, or psychiatric disease, diabetes, obesity, or hypertension.
5. Immune suppression is associated with severe infections, increased risk of malignancy, and progressive vascular disease.
6. Renal transplant recipients are often anemic, with hyperdynamic cardiac indices.
7. For renal transplantation, the major anesthetic consideration is maintenance of renal blood flow. Typical hemodynamic goals during transplant are systolic pressure above 90 mmHg, mean systemic pressure above 60 mmHg, and central venous pressure above 10 mmHg.
8. Patients with end-stage liver disease have multiorgan dysfunction with secondary cardiac, pulmonary, renal, and neurologic complications.
9. Liver transplantation is traditionally described in three phases: dissection, anhepatic phase, and neohepatic phase, with graft reperfusion marking the start of the neohepatic phase.
10. Intraoperative management of lung transplant patients should focus on fluid and ventilatory strategies designed to minimize acute lung injury and primary graft dysfunction.
11. Left ventricular assist devices are increasingly common in patients presenting for heart transplantation.
12. Nonischemic cardiomyopathy has replaced ischemic cardiomyopathy as the most common indication for heart transplantation.
13. For all transplant recipients, antibiotic, antiviral, antifungal, immunosuppressive, and disease-specific drug regimens should be disrupted minimally in the perioperative period.

Transplantation begins with the donor, and an anesthesiologist's exquisite attention to the details of organ donor management affects the life of multiple organ recipients. Most anesthesiologists will have little experience managing donors, and high-quality literature in this area is lacking, so that experienced personnel from local organ procurement organizations should be consulted. The United Network of Organ Sharing (UNOS; www.unos.org) was created by the 1984 National Organ Transplant Act to manage the organ procurement and transplant network for efficient and equitable distribution of donated organs. The system for organ placement received a technology upgrade in 2006 with the launch of DonorNet, an electronic resource for matching and distribution of organs around the United States. Speed of placement is important because brain-dead donors are unstable, and it is particularly important to transplant extended criteria donor (ECD) grafts with minimal cold ischemia times.

In general, maximum cold ischemia times are ideally less than 6 hours for heart or lung grafts, 12 to 24 hours for livers, and up to 72 hours for kidneys. The UNOS website data contain center- and region-specific transplant databases, regularly updated. The Scientific Registry of Transplant Recipients (www.ustransplant.org) is also a source of transplant data for clinicians, patients, and researchers.

About 122,000 patients were on solid-organ transplant waiting lists in the United States as of March 2016. Transplantation starts with the donor, and donation has not kept pace with demand, as seen by transplant numbers in 2015. A total of 30,973 transplants in the United States from 15,064 donors were reported in 2015. The ongoing gap between need for and availability of donor organs continues to push practice changes to increase the donor pool and more equitably distribute organs, including use of grafts from "donation after cardiac death" (DCD) donors as well as paired kidney donations (kidney swaps), and new modifications to the Model for End-Stage Liver Disease (MELD) scoring.

Anesthetic Management of Organ Donors

Brain-dead Donors (Donation after Neurologic Death)

Brain-dead, heart-beating donors deserve expert intensive care unit (ICU) and anesthetic management because they contribute life to many transplant recipients.[1] Particular attention should be paid to communication because anesthesiologists may be interacting with unfamiliar personnel from organ procurement organizations and surgical procurement teams.

Brain death is declared when the clinical picture is consistent with irreversible cessation of all brain functions.[2] Legal and medical brain death criteria differ from state to state, but all require cessation of both cerebral and brainstem functions. Brain-dead donors are unresponsive to sensory stimuli and have no brainstem reflexes, including ventilatory drive with apnea testing, but may have complex motor activity. Physicians involved in the transplant recipient process should not be involved in declaration of brain death of a donor. Potentially reversible causes of coma must be ruled out (hypothermia, hypotension, drugs, toxins) before declaration of brain death. A flat electroencephalogram is consistent with brain death. Transcranial Doppler and traditional or isotope angiography are used to confirm the clinical examination and lack of circulation to the brain.[3] Brain-dead patients may have intact spinal reflexes, so they may require neuromuscular blockade during organ procurement. Hospitals should incorporate the most recent recommendations of the Quality Standards Subcommittee of the American Academy of Neurology for brain death assessment.[1]

Brain death is associated with hemodynamic instability, wide swings in hormone levels, systemic inflammation, and oxidant stress, all of which negatively impact donor organ function.[4] Just after brain death, adrenergic surges can cause ischemia and ischemia–reperfusion injuries. Studies of head trauma patients suggest that the onset of brain death is associated with a transient period of hypotension with increased cardiac index and tissue perfusion. During this period, vasoactive drugs administered to increase blood pressure can cause rapid circulatory deterioration.[5] This period precedes the autonomic storm associated with herniation of the brain and emphasizes the wide dynamic swings in blood chemistries and hemodynamics after brain death. Of note, bradycardia after brain herniation is often unresponsive to atropine. The timing of therapies to support hemodynamics is difficult because catecholamine storm is often followed quickly by pituitary failure. Once pituitary failure ensues, hormone therapy may help stabilize donors hemodynamically and thereby extend the donor pool.[6] Hormone therapy regimens include triiodothyronine (4-μg intravenous [IV] bolus, then 3 μg/hr, though its use is not well supported by meta-analyses) and desmopressin, 1 unit, then 0.5 to 4 units/hr to maintain systemic vascular resistance (SVR) at 800 to 1,200 dyne/s/cm^5 (and reduce the polyuria of diabetes insipidus). Low-dose vasopressin is also commonly used to treat diabetes insipidus. Methylprednisolone is often used, though variably applied, despite insufficient study on its benefits, but a prospective trial of hydrocortisone in 259 brain-dead subjects showed that its use was associated with significantly less vasopressor need.[7]

High doses of catecholamines should be avoided. Evidence suggests that use of vasopressin (1 to 2 units/hr) reduces pressor requirement,[8] protects lung function,[9] and increases the rate of successful organ procurement.[10] Terlipressin also can reduce norepinephrine requirements in brain-dead donors.[11] Because there is little deep research on hormone replacement therapy, clinical practice varies widely. Insulin infusion to maintain blood glucose at 120 to 180 mg/dL is also recommended, and recent studies support glucose control for maintaining donor kidney graft quality.[12] Other medications that should be available for the donor operation are broad-spectrum antibiotics, mannitol and loop diuretics, and heparin (Table 52-1). Coagulopathies may require correction for active bleeding before and during organ recovery, but thromboprophylaxis is important because of the high incidence of pulmonary emboli found with organ retrieval.[13]

Table 52-1 Anesthesiology Setup for Organ Procurement

- **Equipment and supplies**

  Ventilator as in intensive care unit
  Bronchoscope
  Warming blankets
  Blood warmers
  Ice

- **Recheck items**

  Declaration of death
  Cause of death
  Consent
  Blood type

- **Fluids**

  Lactated Ringer's
  Albumin

- **Medications**

  Pressors (vasopressin, norepinephrine, dobutamine, phenylephrine, ephedrine, dopamine)
  Antibiotics
  Neuromuscular blocker
  Heparin
  Corticosteroids (per procurement team)
  Povidone-iodine (per nasogastric tube if pancreas procured)
  N-acetylcysteine (per organ procurement organization)
  Insulin
  Mannitol, furosemide
  Prostaglandin E_1

Lung-protective ventilatory strategies, with tidal volumes of 6 to 8 mL/kg and positive end-expiratory pressure (PEEP) adjusted to allow minimal fraction of inspired oxygen (FiO_2), are important in lung donors.[14] Pre-, post- and remote ischemic preconditioning in brain-dead and living donors has not been translated to clinical practice despite interesting preclinical studies.[15] In early trials ex vivo perfusion of beating donor hearts yielded similar results to traditional preservation methods.[16]

Donor heart history is very important in identifying heart donors, and electrocardiography and echocardiography are mandatory. The ideal heart donor is less than 50 years old and hemodynamically stable. Presence of major chest trauma, cardiac disease, active infection, prolonged cardiac arrest, malignancy, human immunodeficiency virus (HIV) or hepatitis, or intracardiac injections moves the donor from ideal to marginal status. Overall health status of the donor prior to determination of brain death can facilitate a directed laboratory evaluation, which may include cardiac catheterization. For recipients with pulmonary hypertension, younger donors, short ischemic time, low donor inotrope requirement, and oversized organs are preferred. Human leukocyte antigen typing and ABO blood group compatibility are determined. The donor heart size should be within 20% to 30% of the recipient's heart size.

Anesthetic management during organ procurement is guided by the needs of the procurement teams, who may come from several centers and have discrepant requests, depending on the organs procured. UNOS has created a resource for managing organ donors in an effort to improve donor care and, therefore, the function of donated organs.[1] Transport of ventilated donors to the operating room (OR) often requires PEEP valves; if more complex ventilator settings are used in the ICU, they should be continued during transport and in the OR.

The mainstay of donor management is maintenance of euvolemia and perfusion; therefore, central venous pressure (CVP) monitoring is standard. CVP is maintained at 6 to 12 mmHg, and when pulmonary artery (PA) catheters are used to assess cardiac function, pulmonary capillary wedge pressure is maintained at lower than 12 mmHg. Surgeons procuring the lungs will want to keep the CVP low, and diuretics may be requested just prior to collection of the lungs. Surgeons procuring kidneys usually want high filling pressures. Efforts should be made to maintain serum sodium levels below 155 mmol/L; higher levels are associated with poor liver graft function.[17]

Donor oxygenation, perfusion, and normothermia are all important anesthetic goals, and the precise end points of therapy require coordination and communication with the various surgical teams. Generally, arterial PCO_2 is maintained at 30 to 35 mmHg.

Prior to lung removal, surgeons will perform bronchoscopy. Glucocorticoids may be requested, and prostaglandin E_1 may be requested to improve circulation of the lung preservation solution.

Donor lungs are more susceptible to injury in brain-dead patients before procurement than are other organs, likely from contusion, aspiration, or edema with fluid resuscitation. Consequently, many multiorgan donors do not meet the idealized strict criteria for lung donors (Table 52-2). Extended criteria are used for donor lungs because of ongoing shortages. For example, a review of UNOS data showed that lung donors less than 64 years old show no major differences from those less than 55 years old.[19] Another example of working outside the strict criteria is acceptance of some lungs from donors with a smoking history. Sputum Gram stains and cultures are routinely obtained on all lung donors. Antibiotics for a donor with a positive Gram stain can lower the risk of posttransplant infection; however, organisms on bronchoalveolar lavage are associated with decreased survival.[20] One study suggested that evidence of aspiration seen on bronchoscopy, bilateral pulmonary infiltrates, or persistent purulent secretions are criteria for donor exclusion.[21] Ischemic times should still be less than 7 hours.[22] In addition to the usual immunologic criteria, donor–recipient compatibility is based on height and/or total lung capacity. DCD donors are still useful for lung transplantation, and ex vivo lung perfusion is emerging as a way to extend the lung donor pool.[23]

For heart retrieval, the surgeons perform a pericardiotomy, and the aortic root is cannulated for infusion of cardioplegia solutions. Following ligation of the great veins, the heart is compressed and exsanguinated, cardioplegia is given to induce cardiac arrest, and the aorta is cross clamped. After cardiectomy the donor heart is preserved in cold ice slush. For donors who provide both lungs and the heart to a single recipient, a combined cardiopulmonary surgical extraction is performed. Surgical techniques have been developed to allow three recipients from one thoracic donor: two single-lung transplants and a heart transplant.[18] The heart is removed first, leaving a small cuff of left atrium attached to the lungs. The harvesting team will ask for systemic heparinization just prior to exsanguination and excision. Cardioplegia is administered, the heart stops ejecting, and the heart is removed. The trachea is transected and the lungs are removed *en bloc* for later separation.

A shortage of available donors has led to increased use of marginal (extended criteria) donors and separate alternate transplant lists of recipients who consent to accept ECDs. Increased risk of primary graft dysfunction (PGD) is the main reason to avoid marginal donors. Marginal donors are typically used for patients who do not meet the standard recipient criteria, with advanced age a common reason for alternative listing. Common donor factors that lead to marginal status are abnormal hepatitis screening tests, left ventricular (LV) dysfunction or coronary artery disease, advanced age, and DCD.

Donation after Cardiac Death (Donation after Circulatory Determination of Death)

In 2007 US hospitals were mandated by The Joint Commission, in collaboration with organ procurement organizations, to develop DCD policies and protocols in response to organ donor shortages. DCD protocols have not been adopted uniformly. DCD donors accounted for 16.3% of donors in the United States in 2015 (per the Association of Organ Procurement Organizations).

Table 52-2 Ideal Deceased Lung Donor Characteristics

- Age <55 years
- ABO compatibility
- Clear chest radiograph
- Smoking history NONE; Tobacco history <20 pack years
- Ventilation <5 days
- PaO_2 >300 on FiO_2 1, positive end-expiratory pressure 5 cm H_2O
- Absence of chest trauma
- No evidence of aspiration or sepsis
- Negative sputum Gram stain
- Clear bronchoscopy

So DCD donors represent a fairly large portion of donors, but the number of organs used from DCD donors is less than from donation after brain death (DBD) donors, pointing to the need to optimize DCD protocols further. Pediatric DCD donors also provide quality organs for transplantation, and the American Academy of Pediatrics has endorsed their use.[24] Experience with DCD grafts suggests that DCD kidneys have an increased risk of delayed graft function, increasing costs, but long-term function is not reduced in DCD versus DBD grafts; DCD livers generally have worse survival than DBD livers.[1]

The protocols of planning for and managing DCD donors differ from center to center. Because any one center is unlikely to have considerable experience with these donors, an excellent quick reference was developed by UNOS, available at https://www.unos.org/wp-content/uploads/unos/Critical_Pathway_DCD_Donor.pdf. DCD donors typically have severe brain damage considered not recoverable but may have brain electrical activity. Death is defined by cessation of circulation (arterial monitoring showing pulse pressure is zero, or Doppler monitoring showing no flow) and respiration after withdrawal of futile treatment measures. Timing of withdrawal of support is to maximize the function of organs from these donors. Optimally, end-of-life care is provided by the same medical team responsible for the care of the patient in the ICU. Informed consent is required for organ donation and for any preorgan recovery procedures, such as drug administration or vascular cannulation.

Suitable DCD donors are those in whom death is anticipated within 1 to 2 hours of withdrawal of life support. A plan for the donor's care should be in place if the patient does not die within the anticipated time frame, and ideally care should be transferred back to the team that knows the patient and family. Predicting death within an hour of withdrawal of support is not an exact science, so evaluation tools to help predict which patients will die within this time frame are useful (Table 52-3). For death to be declared, circulation and respiration must be absent for a minimum of 2 minutes before the start of organ recovery. A scoring system for predicting death of pediatric DCD donors has also been developed and validated.[25]

Organ recovery started more than 5 minutes after respiratory and circulatory arrest may compromise donor organ quality, but this limit has been extended with reasonable transplant outcomes. The major goal of surgical management during procurement is to limit warm ischemia time (with rapid cooling techniques and minimal in situ dissection).[26]

No major differences in *intraoperative* events during the transplant procedure between DCD and DBD kidney grafts have been reported. A recent report suggests that withdrawal of support in the OR (after heparin administration) may lead to better function of the donor liver than withdrawal of support in the ICU.[27]

Living Kidney Donors

Safety and comfort are the primary considerations in the care of living donors. Living donors must be healthy and without significant cardiopulmonary, neurologic, or psychiatric disease; diabetes; obesity; or hypertension. Renal function must be normal, with no history of renal stones or proteinuria. The vast majority of living kidney grafts are retrieved laparoscopically with only a small number of these robotically assisted.[28] A recent national study suggests that robotically assisted surgeries are still associated with increased complications over hand-assisted laparoscopic kidney retrieval.[28] An estimated 2.4% of kidney donors experience anesthetic/surgical complications of donation,[28] pointing to the need for enhanced recovery protocols including preoperative carbohydrate loading, an opioid-free anesthetic, and transversus abdominis blocks.[29] Both anesthetics and insufflation of the peritoneum with carbon dioxide (CO_2), which are necessary for the laparoscopic procedure, decrease renal blood flow, so that a variety of fluid regimens have been suggested to blunt prerenal damage to the kidneys. Fluid loading overnight before surgery (versus fluid administration starting with surgery) is associated with better creatinine clearance acutely during the procedure,[30] and some suggest a colloid bolus just before pneumoperitoneum.[31] When a CVP end point is used for fluid goals, the CVP may not accurately reflect volume status with the patient in lateral decubitus position and with pneumoperitoneum.[32] Nitrous oxide is contraindicated for laparoscopic donor nephrectomy because distended bowel can get in the way of the surgeons.[33] For patient comfort, central venous lines (if used) are generally placed after induction of anesthesia.

Donor nephrectomy should be an uncomplicated procedure, and donor tracheas can be extubated in the OR. Deep venous thrombosis prophylaxis is warranted. For open nephrectomy, the patient is positioned in the lateral decubitus position with the bed flexed to expose and arch the flank. Donors are generally managed with general anesthesia, but epidural and combined epidural–spinal techniques (supplemented with intravenous propofol)[34] as well as general–epidural combined techniques are used. Postoperative pain following donor nephrectomy can be severe, and patient-controlled analgesia is often used. The pain can still be severe enough to limit respiratory effort and mobilization of the patient, however. Furthermore, a survey of 123 donors showed that one-third of them had chronic pain after the open procedure,[35] suggesting postoperative pain management is often not optimal. Early complications include pulmonary (atelectasis, pneumothorax, pneumonia), urinary tract infections, and wound problems; long-term complications include reduced renal function, hypertension, albuminuria, and psychiatric issues (anxiety, depression).[36] Some centers admit donors to a step-down or medical ICU for a day after surgery, but the total hospital stay is usually only 2 to 4 days. Bladder catheters are removed on postoperative day 1. Patients should be advised that full recovery (i.e., feeling normal) takes 4 to 6 weeks, especially after the open procedure. Fortunately, perioperative mortality is rare but cannot be denied as a possible outcome during preoperative patient discussions.

Table 52-3 UNOS Consensus Committee Criteria for Prediction of DCD Death within 60 Minutes of Withdrawal of Life-sustaining Treatment

- Apnea
- Respiratory rate <8 or >30 breaths/min
- Dopamine ≥15 µg/kg/min
- Left or right ventricular assist device
- Venoarterial or venovenous extracorporeal membrane oxygenation
- Positive end-expiratory pressure ≥10 and SaO_2 ≤92%
- FiO_2 ≥0.5 and SaO_2 ≤92%
- Norepinephrine or phenylephrine ≥0.2 µg/kg/min
- Pacemaker-unassisted heart rate <30
- IABP 1:1 or dobutamine or dopamine ≥10 µg/kg/min and CI ≤2.2 L/min/m²
- IABP 1:1 and CI ≤1.5 L/min/m²

UNOS, United Network of Organ Sharing; DCD, donation after cardiac death; SaO_2, arterial oxygen saturation; IABP, intra-aortic balloon pump; CI, cardiac index.

Living Liver Donors

Living liver donors have traditionally been employed in a stepwise manner to limit the chances of coercion, but increasingly living donors are being used for recipients with acute liver failure (ALF).[37] Left lobe liver donation (segments II and III) is usually done in the context of parent-to-child donation with recipients smaller than 15 kg. Although left lateral segmentectomy is a big operation, it is generally well tolerated (Fig. 52-1). Nonetheless, living left lobe donors must be healthy and without a history of or risk for thromboembolic disease. By comparison, donor right hepatectomy needed for adult-to-adult liver transplantation is a major procedure (Fig. 52-2) and carries significant risk. The residual liver volume of the donor must be greater than 35% of original volume to prevent "small for size" syndrome in the donor. Because risk for this syndrome is increased in older donors or in patients with cholestatic or hepatocellular disease, including steatosis,[38] adult-to-adult living donors should have no liver disease. Early death among live liver donors in the United States is estimated to be 1.7 per 1,000 donors[39] but is obviously devastating for both donor and recipient families. Serious complication rates are high for right liver donors (up to a third of donors depending on the center), including air embolism, atelectasis, pneumonia, respiratory depression, and biliary tract damage.[40–42] Nonetheless, experienced centers that report complication rates of 10% are developing enhanced recovery protocols for right liver donors.[43] Most centers do not perform living adult-to-adult liver transplants in very ill recipients.

Large liver resections may require virtually complete hepatic venous exclusion (cross-clamping of the hepatic pedicle usually without cava clamping). Not unexpectedly, venous return falls significantly. Without the collaterals developed by patients with chronic liver disease, normal donors may experience significant hypotension when the hepatic pedicle is cross clamped. Blood pressure is maintained largely through reflex increases in endogenous vasopressin and norepinephrine levels.[44] For these reasons, volume loading is reasonable prior to clamping, but some centers try to reduce blood loss by maintaining low CVP, whereas CVP monitoring is not routine in other centers. Sufficiently powered studies to prove that the benefits of low CVP

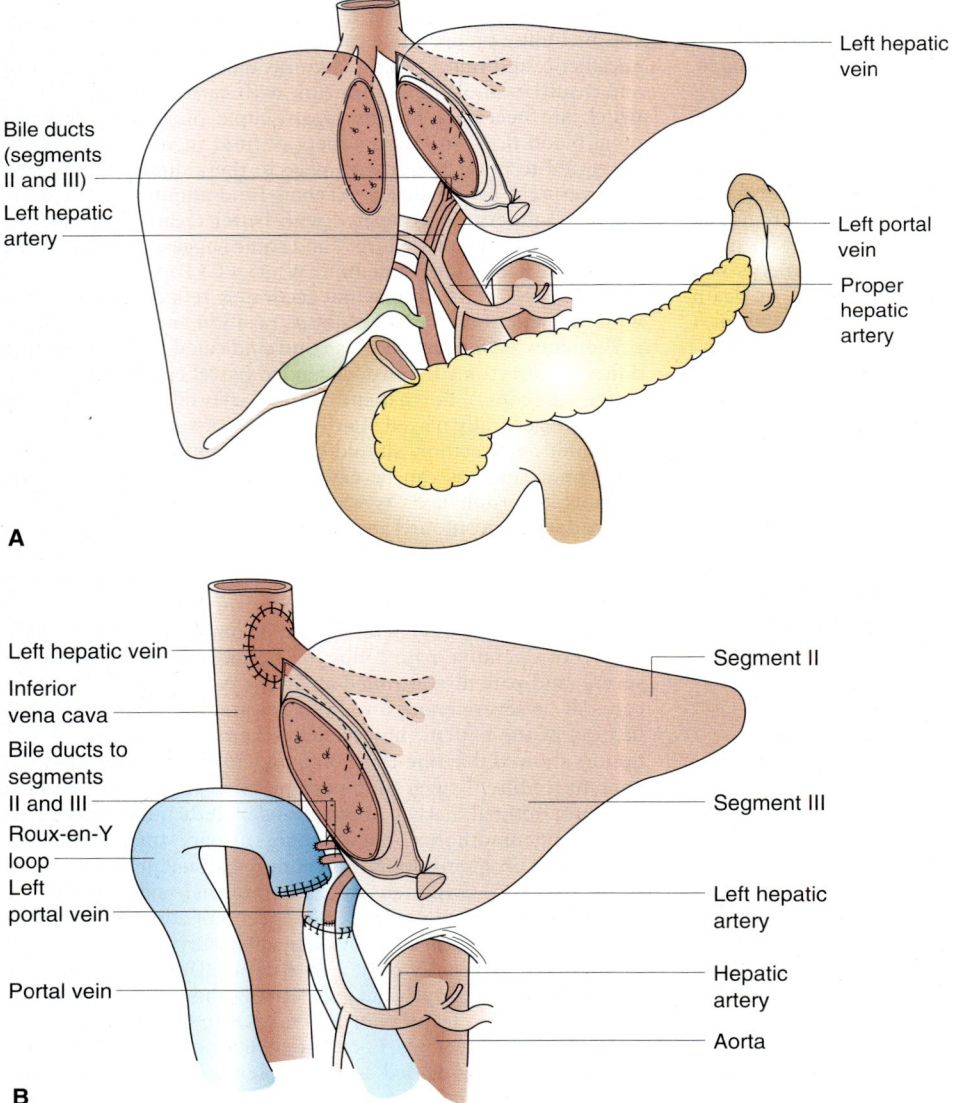

Figure 52-1 Left lateral segment (segments II and III) living donor transplantation. **A:** Donor operation. **B:** Recipient operation complete.

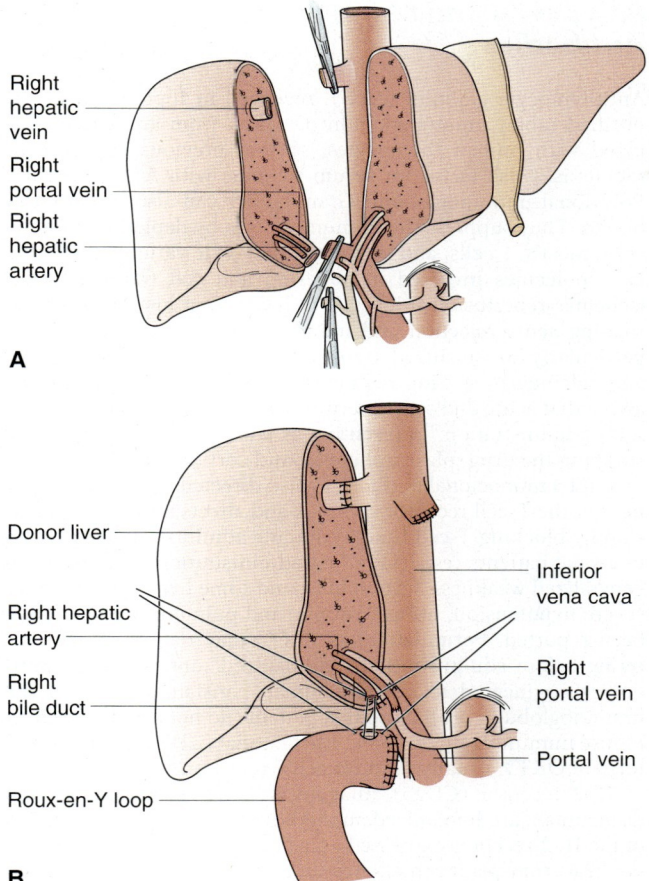

Figure 52-2 Right lobe (segments V to VIII) living donor transplantation. **A:** Donor operation. **B:** Recipient operation completed.

sodium phosphate infusions to maintain phosphate levels of 3.5 to 5.4 mg/dL, unless patients have significant renal compromise (creatinine clearance <50 mL/hr). Liver function tests including international normalized ratio (INR) are also abnormal in the postoperative period after liver resection and usually return to baseline levels within 3 months, although small changes in liver function tests can persist for up to a year after hepatectomy. Some living liver donors can experience chronic low platelet counts after hepatectomy.[50]

Immunosuppressive Agents

Pharmacologic suppression of the immune response to allografts is associated with major side effects. Considerable variability in intestinal absorption, genetic and induced differences in metabolism of these drugs, changing dosage requirements with aging, and idiosyncratic complications all mandate individualization of immunosuppressive regimens. Immunosuppressed patients who are undertreated risk rejection; overimmunosuppression can be toxic, especially to the kidneys. All immunosuppression regimens carry major risks, such as infection, malignancy, and progressive vascular disease. Immunosuppression regimens differ considerably from center to center, and anesthesiologists must communicate with the transplant team to obtain the schedule and dose of immunosuppressive agents for each patient, especially because immunosuppression drug options have expanded.[51] It is particularly important to review drug regimens with transplant coordinators when posttransplant patients are scheduled for surgery because the transplant team needs information about peak and trough drug levels that may not be accessible on the hospital record.

Immunosuppressed patients coming to the OR deserve special attention to sterile technique and maintenance of antibiotic, antifungal, and antiviral regimens during the perioperative period. Complications of chronic immunosuppression are summarized in Table 52-4.

(reduced transfusion requirements) outweigh the risks (renal compromise, air embolism) are unlikely to be performed, and institutional practices vary widely. If vasopressors are needed, vasopressin and norepinephrine are reasonable choices to enhance normal endogenous reflexes. Isovolemic hemodilution has been reported to reduce allogeneic red cell requirements in major hepatic resections.[45] At experienced centers, blood loss is usually less than 1 L, and transfusion requirements are usually not high. Blood salvage is useful, and some centers offer autologous donation programs for donors. Both can reduce the need for allogeneic blood transfusions. Transesophageal echocardiography (TEE), if expertise is available, is ideal and may obviate central line placement. Most donor tracheas can be extubated safely in the OR. Hypothermia is a preventable reason for not extubating in the OR. A wide variety of general anesthetics are used for liver donors, and epidural analgesia is useful for pain management,[46] though patient-controlled analgesia is preferred in some centers because of the potential for perioperative coagulopathy. Abdominal wall catheters placed by the surgeons may be useful for postoperative pain management.[47] Laparoscopic liver resection of left lobe (segments II and III) and right lobe is available in some centers, though concern has been raised about standardization for right lobe laparoscopic resections.[48]

Hypophosphatemia (with excessive loss of phosphate in the urine) is common after hepatectomy[49] and should be treated with

Table 52-4 Complications of Chronic Immune Suppression
Central Nervous System
Lowered seizure threshold
Cardiovascular
Diabetes
Hypertension
Hyperlipidemia
Atherosclerosis
Renal/Electrolyte
Decreased glomerular filtration rate
Hyperkalemia
Hypomagnesemia
Hematologic/Immune
Increased risk of infections
Increased risk of malignancy
Pancytopenia
Endocrine/Other
Osteoporosis
Poor wound healing

Calcineurin Inhibitors

The modern transplant era began with the introduction of the calcineurin inhibitor (CNI) cyclosporine into clinical practice. CNIs are still a mainstay of immunosuppression for solid-organ transplant recipients; tacrolimus is widely used. Inhibition of calcineurin, among other effects, modifies nuclear factor of activated T cells and frees nuclear factor-κB to translocate to the nucleus, where it enhances transcription of T-cell interleukin-2 (IL-2). Via these signal transduction pathways, CNI inhibits T-lymphocyte activation, differentiation, and cytokine production.[52]

Calcineurin is involved in diverse cellular processes, so its inhibition can cause many significant side effects. These include hypertension (often requiring therapy), hyperlipidemia, ischemic vascular disease (including in heart recipients), diabetes, and nephrotoxicity. Cyclosporine causes acute nephropathy, which is usually reversible with drug cessation. But chronic renal damage from cyclosporine is a more refractory problem. A variety of other drugs are used with CNI to reduce the amount of CNI required. Certain drugs, however, may cause renal dysfunction when coadministered with CNI, including amphotericin, cotrimoxazole, cimetidine, vancomycin, ranitidine, tobramycin, melphalan, gentamicin, and nonsteroidal anti-inflammatory drugs.[53]

Ischemic cardiac disease is the leading cause of death of kidney transplant recipients, in part because of underlying disease that preceded transplantation. But CNI can exacerbate risk factors for coronary artery disease. It is important to note that end-stage liver disease (ESLD) does not confer protection from coronary artery disease, and liver transplant patients are also at risk for progression of ischemic cardiac disease after transplantation. Neurologic side effects also complicate CNI therapy, including tacrolimus-induced polyneuropathy[54] and encephalopathy.[55] When immunosuppression is interrupted by surgery or when multiple potentially interacting drugs are used, tacrolimus trough levels should be reassessed.

Tacrolimus is metabolized by cytochrome P450 3A4 and causes its upregulation. Cyclosporine may rarely prolong the action of pancuronium.[56,57] To switch from oral to intravenous dosing of cyclosporine, usually about one-third the oral dose is used. Usual dosage of tacrolimus is 0.15 to 0.3 mg/kg/day given in two doses. To switch from oral to intravenous tacrolimus, a starting dose of about one-tenth the oral dose can be used. Statin–cyclosporine interactions deserve vigilance because rhabdomyolysis has been reported in a few patients taking simvastatin and cyclosporine.[58]

Corticosteroids

Corticosteroids disrupt expression of many cytokines in T cells, antigen-presenting cells, and macrophages. These drugs are used both for maintenance immunosuppression and in pulse dosing for acute rejection. Especially for growing children, corticosteroid-sparing regimens are increasingly popular. The well-known side effects are hypertension, diabetes, hyperlipidemia, weight gain (including cushingoid features), and gastrointestinal ulceration (see Chapter 47). Communication with the transplant service is important in determining timing and dose of steroid administration perioperatively in patients who are taking the drug chronically. Corticosteroids may be withheld during liver transplantation in recipients with hepatitis C because of concern that the drugs contribute to hepatitis C recurrence.[59]

Polyclonal and Monoclonal Antibodies

Antithymocyte globulin (ATG), reviewed in Ippoliti et al.,[60] is purified rabbit immunoglobulin G taken from animals immunized with human thymocytes, so that previous exposure to rabbits is a risk factor for serum sickness with ATG exposure. Polyclonal immunoglobulin G antibodies can also be raised in horses. They suppress the immune system by depleting immune cells, mostly T cells, and interact with a wide variety of cell surface molecules involved in adhesion and cell trafficking and ischemia–reperfusion injury. ATG has a long history of use in treating acute rejection and induction of immunosuppression, particularly in sensitized transplant recipients and in steroid- and calcineurin-sparing regimens. Anesthesiologists should be aware that acute and severe serum sickness is a rare side effect of ATG administration,[61] presenting as jaw pain, and is treated by stopping the drug, plasmapheresis, and corticosteroids.[62]

OKT3 monoclonal antibody is also directed against a component of the T-cell receptor complex and affects immunosuppression by blocking T-cell function. Acute administration of OKT3 in awake patients (especially first administration) may result in generalized weakness, fever, chills, and some hypotension. More severe hypotension, bronchospasm, and pulmonary edema have been reported. Formulations of OKT3 may require syringe filtering before administration. "Humanized" antibodies are antibodies engineered to contain human constant regions in the immunoglobulin protein, so that patients do not develop an antimouse immunologic response. Muromonab-CD3 is a humanized form of OKT3, usually used for acute rejection.[63]

IL-2 receptor (CD25) antagonists, such as basiliximab and daclizumab, are humanized antibodies directed against a portion of the IL-2 receptor expressed on activated T cells. About half of the heart transplant centers now use IL-2 receptor antagonists in their initial immunosuppression regimen to reduce the dose and cardiovascular side effects of CNIs. Gastrointestinal upset is the most commonly cited side effect of these drugs. However, basiliximab has been implicated in causing pulmonary edema in young renal transplant patients.[64] Generally these newer antibodies are associated with fewer side effects than other antibody therapies.[65]

Belatacept is directed against the CD80/CD86 ligands on antigen-presenting cells that activate T cells through the CD28 (costimulatory) pathway. It is approved for maintenance immunosuppression for kidney transplant recipients and is associated with fewer cardiovascular complications than CNI drugs.[64] Infusion reactions can include hypotension, but acute reactions are usually mild. New targets for immunosuppressive drugs include complement and B cells as well as drugs directed at molecules that exacerbate ischemia–reperfusion.[66] Coagulopathy has been reported as a side effect of alemtuzumab (Campath),[67] which recognizes CD52 on B cells. Rituximab is another anti–B-cell antibody that acts at CD20 and is used for humoral rejection.

Mammalian Target of Rapamycin Inhibitors

Mammalian target of rapamycin inhibitors are often used in combination with CNI to decrease the complications of dose-related side effects (calcineurin-sparing regimens) such as nephrotoxicity. Target of rapamycin is involved in complex signaling processes that promote synthesis of proteins, including several that regulate cellular proliferation. Thus, mammalian target of rapamycin inhibitors such as sirolimus (Rapamycin) are antiproliferative, used both in immunosuppression and increasingly in cancer therapies. Similar to cyclosporine and tacrolimus, sirolimus is metabolized in liver via P450 CYP3A isoenzymes, but coadministration of sirolimus and a CNI does not increase CNI drug requirements. In fact, the combination may be synergistic.[68] Diltiazem raises the plasma concentration of sirolimus.[69]

Purine Antagonists

Purine antagonists include mycophenolate mofetil and azathioprine. Azathioprine is hydrolyzed in blood to 6-mercaptopurine, a purine analogue and metabolite with the ability to incorporate into DNA during the S phase of the cell cycle. Because DNA synthesis is a necessary prerequisite to mitosis, azathioprine exerts an antiproliferative effect. Antiproliferative drugs rely on the fact that immune activation implies explosive proliferation of lymphocytes. Side effects occur because other proliferating cells (gastrointestinal tract, bone marrow) are also affected. Repression of bone marrow cell cycling can cause pancytopenia. Cardiac arrest and severe upper airway edema are rare complications.[70] The intravenous dose is about half the oral dose.

Mycophenolate mofetil is metabolized into a molecule that inhibits purine synthesis. It too can cause leukopenia and thrombocytopenia as side effects, as well as red cell aplasia[71]; it is considered teratogenic.[72] The usual oral dose is 1 to 1.5 g twice a day.

Cell Therapies

Tolerance of organ grafts without pharmacologic immunosuppression, the Holy Grail of transplantation, is possible using combined bone marrow and solid-organ transplants with marrow and the solid organ derived from the same donor.[73]

Mesenchymal stem cells (MSCs) are anti-inflammatory stem cells, currently in multiple clinical trials as adjuncts to transplant immunosuppression. MSCs are multipotent cells easily derived from marrow or fat (and other sources), and can be used autologously or from allogeneic sources without risk of cytotoxic T cell rejection. Their first use in the context of organ transplantation was for the treatment of grade IV graft versus host disease in marrow transplant recipients.[73] MSCs have pleiotropic effects on the immune response, including antiproliferative T-cell function. The goal of MSC trials for solid-organ transplantation is to reduce the amount of pharmacologic immunosuppression needed, and clinical trials are ongoing for liver, renal, heart, lung and islet transplantation. No adverse acute reactions to MSC infusion or injection have been reported after thousands of treatments.

Corneal Transplantation

Corneas are the most common organs transplanted in the United States, with ~46,000 transplants per year. Corneal transplants can be performed under local anesthesia (often with IV sedation), topical anesthesia, or general anesthesia depending on the details of surgery. The use of laryngeal masks versus endotracheal intubation may reduce the potential for ocular hypertension from coughing postoperatively.[74] Recipients of cornea grafts are often elderly. A major anesthetic goal is maintaining low intraocular pressure (see Chapter 49). Patient positioning (head-up angle of the bed) on transfer from the OR should be directed by the surgeon. For patients undergoing endothelial keratoplasty, less invasive than full cornea replacement, positioning in the prone or Trendelenburg position may rarely be requested. Rejection of corneal allografts is the most common cause of graft loss in the first year after transplantation.

Renal Transplantation

Preoperative Considerations

Allocation of kidneys in the United States changed in December 2014 with use of the Kidney Donor Risk Index (KDRI), and for deceased donors, the Kidney Donor Profile Index (KDPI), intended to provide the best grafts to patients with longest predicted posttransplant survival. Replacing extended donor criteria that were more limited, KDRI factors in age, height, weight, ethnicity, history of hypertension, history of diabetes, cause of death, creatinine, hepatitis C status, and DCD status. This system was intended to particularly benefit patients who were on dialysis for long periods of time, blood type B recipients, and highly sensitized patients. Systematic analysis of the impact of this change has not yet been reported. A living donor KDPI was recently proposed to compare the quality of liver donor kidneys.[75]

The prevalence of end-stage renal disease (ESRD) is about 0.17% in the United States, where 17,1017 kidney transplants were performed in 2014. Of these 11,570 came from deceased donors and 5,537 came from living donors. The most common recipient age group was 50 to 64 years (6,645 patients), and 3,325 recipients were over 65 years. In 2014, 4,761 patients died while waiting for a kidney transplant, and another 3,668 became too sick to undergo transplantation (http://optn.transplant.hrsa.gov).

Diseases treated with renal transplants are shown in Table 52-5. Many of these underlying diagnoses are also risk factors for coronary artery disease, so preoperative evaluation is focused on cardiovascular function, but a comprehensive medical workup is essential.

About half the mortality of patients on dialysis is due to heart failure. Cardiovascular disease is the leading cause of death (and therefore graft loss) after renal transplantation.[76] Therefore, cardiovascular risk factor modification is imperative before and after transplantation, including hypertension and hyperlipidemia. Renal transplant recipients are often anemic, with hyperdynamic cardiac indices. Patients above 50 years (with or without risk factors for coronary disease) are generally screened with dobutamine stress tests or myocardial scintigraphy. The interval at which these studies are repeated in patients listed for

Table 52-5 Diagnoses of Patients on Adult Renal Transplant Waiting List

Diagnosis	Patients on List (%)
Type 2 diabetes	29.1
Hypertension (and malignant hypertension)	21.7
Retransplant/failing transplant	6.8
Polycystic kidney disease	6.4
Focal glomerular sclerosis	5.1
Type 1 diabetes	3.7
IgA nephropathy	3.4
Systemic lupus erythematosus	2.6
Other/not reported	9.7

Data from optn.transplant.hrsa.gov.

transplantation varies from center to center. Peripheral vascular disease should also be assessed. Pulmonary function tests (PFTs) should be reviewed by anesthesiologists prior to transplantation (see Chapter 15). PFTs are particularly important in type 1 diabetics, who often present with reduced lung volumes and diffusing capacity. The precise cause of abnormal PFTs in these patients is not known, but clinical studies suggest that long-term normoglycemia after kidney or pancreas transplantation is associated with improved pulmonary function.[77] Hypercoagulable states are common in patients with renal disease and deserve detailed evaluation so that they can be managed perioperatively.[78]

All solid-organ transplant patients are screened for tumors (mammography, Papanicolaou test, colonoscopy, prostate-specific antigen) and infection (dental evaluation, viral serologies). Patients should have good control of their diabetes before transplantation and have an evaluation for psychiatric stability and social support. Severe heart, lung, or liver disease; most malignancies; and active or untreatable infections such as tuberculosis are exclusion criteria for renal transplantation.

Dialysis-dependent patients should be dialyzed before surgery. Cadaveric grafts can be safely transplanted after 24 hours of cold ischemia time, and potentially after 36 hours, allowing scheduling of preoperative dialysis. With preoperative dialysis, severe hyperkalemia during surgery is unusual. ECDs are often used for kidney transplantation. Factors used in designation of ECD kidneys are age (>60 yr), creatinine value, stroke as cause of death, and hypertension. DCD donors are also an ECD category. ECDs affect the scheduling of transplantation because minimization of cold ischemia times is essential and delayed graft function may complicate the intraoperative course of DCD graft recipients,[79] but recently the UK Transplant Registry reported that long-term outcomes after DCD and DBD donor kidney transplants were similar.[80]

Kidney allocation protocols were changed in late 2014 with the goal of improving longevity matching between donor and recipient, and better access to patients who have been historically difficult to match (highly sensitized patients) or those on long-term dialysis. Initial indications suggest that these goals have been met but at the cost of increased cold ischemia times associated with higher rates of delayed graft function.[81] Kidney allocation is much more complicated than liver allocation; updated rules for kidney allocation can be found at optn.transplant.hrsa.gov.

Intraoperative Procedures

Renal transplantation can be done using epidural or spinal anesthesia, and most renal transplantation is done under general anesthesia, though patients with epidurals reportedly have better postoperative pain relief.[82] Concerns over uremic platelet dysfunction and residual heparin from preoperative dialysis have limited the use of regional anesthesia for kidney transplantation. The patient's preoperative medication lists should be reviewed; antihypertensives are common in this population. Although recommendations vary and renal transplant patients have not been well studied, consideration should be given to maintaining β-blockers and withholding angiotensin II receptor blockers before transplantation.[83]

Rapid-sequence induction (preceded by oral sodium bicitrate) is indicated in diabetic patients with gastroparesis. Esmolol may be useful for blunting the hemodynamic response to intubation.[83] Anemic, hyperdynamic patients may have higher dose requirements for induction agents such as propofol.[84] Rocuronium is useful for patients in whom rapid-sequence induction is indicated, but the duration of block is variable in patients with ESRD.[85] Similarly, plasma clearance of rapacuronium is reduced with renal failure, but titration of dose to neuromuscular blockade monitoring end points prevents delayed recovery.[86] Generally, the long-acting nondepolarizing muscle relaxants are avoided and shorter-acting agents such as cisatracurium (cleared by Hoffman elimination) are used. Before incision, antibiotics are given. A central venous catheter (usually triple lumen) is often placed for CVP monitoring and drug administration in most centers, and a bladder catheter is placed.

Incision is usually in the lower right abdomen to facilitate placement of the graft in the iliac fossa. The recipient iliac artery and vein are used for graft vascularization, followed by connection of the ureter to the recipient bladder. If the kidney is too large for the iliac fossa, it can be positioned in the retroperitoneal space. Iliac vessels may be used for anastomoses, or the aorta and inferior vena cava may be required.

The major anesthetic consideration is maintenance of renal blood flow. No data are available to determine whether inhaled versus balanced intravenous techniques are better at preserving (graft) renal flow. Similarly, the choice of inhaled gas has not been shown to significantly affect posttransplant renal function. Isoflurane, sevoflurane, and desflurane are all used to manage renal transplant patients. Morphine effect is prolonged in the setting of ESRD, and high doses of meperidine can cause accumulation of its metabolite, normeperidine, in these patients. Similarly, remifentanil metabolite accumulation occurs in ESRD, whereas fentanyl, alfentanil, and sufentanil pharmacokinetics are clinically normal, though heterogeneity in pharmacokinetics in this population warrants increased vigilance for postoperative respiratory depression.[87]

Hypertensive renal transplant patients often require antihypertensive drugs perioperatively. Calcium channel blockers have been best studied for renal protection of cyclosporine-treated hypertensive transplant patients. But after surgery, angiotensin-converting enzyme inhibitors, increasingly used, and α-blockers may be as effective as calcium channel blockers.[88] Typical hemodynamic goals during transplant are systolic pressure greater than 90 mmHg, mean systemic pressure greater than 60 mmHg, and CVP greater than 10 mmHg. These goals are usually achievable without vasopressors, using isotonic fluids and adjustment of anesthetic doses. Hemodynamic management varies widely from center to center, so close communication between surgeon and anesthesiologist is imperative. Plasma Lyte is the crystalloid of choice for kidney transplantation, and it preserves acid–base balance and electrolytes when compared with Ringer's lactate or normal saline.[89]

Once the first anastomosis is started, diuresis is initiated (both mannitol and furosemide are often given). Heparin and verapamil should also be available in the OR. In some centers, anesthesiologists are asked to administer the first doses of immunosuppression. A kidney graft is defective in concentrating urine and reabsorbing sodium, so attention to electrolytes is important.

Glucose control is also important for patients undergoing transplantation.[90] A small, single-center prospective study of living kidney donor recipients identified glucose above 160 mg/dL as a risk factor for acute perioperative renal dysfunction, likely associated with more severe ischemia–reperfusion injury.[90] Tight glucose control after kidney transplant is associated with less rejection, and diabetics with poorly controlled glucose levels after transplantation have increased mortality.[91] For these reasons, tight blood glucose control (80 to 110 mg/dL) is a reasonable anesthetic management goal during renal transplantation. Dopamine does not reliably improve renal function in this setting. The selective DA1 agonist fenoldopam is used to preserve renal function during kidney transplantation in some centers and is a superior renal protectant compared to dopamine,[92] although not extensively studied.

Transfusion is rarely required in the OR, although renal transplant patients are often anemic coming to surgery (and may be receiving erythropoietin). Because of immunosuppression, if cytomegalovirus (CMV)-negative patients receiving a CMV-negative organ are transfused, CMV-negative blood is preferred. Leukocyte filters are also effective in preventing CMV transmission but are probably inferior to CMV-negative blood.[93] The entire surgery should take less than 3 hours.

Most surgical complications of renal transplantation are not recognized in the OR. The common postoperative complications are ureteral obstruction and fistulae, vascular thromboses, lymphoceles, wound complications,[94] and bleeding. Vascular complications can lead to early graft loss.[95]

Patient-controlled analgesia is a good choice for postoperative pain management, and despite prolonged action, morphine can be used safely if patients are well monitored. Nonsteroidal anti-inflammatory agents and cyclooxygenase-2 inhibitors are contraindicated. Pain can be severe, prompting some centers to explore combination blocks (ilioinguinal–iliohypogastric and intercostal nerve blocks)[96] or transversus abdominis plane blocks[97] for posttransplant pain control. Chronic pain after kidney transplantation is common,[98] suggesting that more attention should be given to early postoperative pain management.

In children, the most common causes of ESRD requiring transplantation are congenital (largely anatomic developmental) anomalies. Kidney size mismatch can complicate the surgery in small children. Adult donor kidneys may have to be placed in the retroperitoneum of small children. Although chronic peritoneal dialysis may help expand the abdominal volume,[99] attention to peak inspiratory pressures at closure is important, and increased pressures should be reported to the surgical team. Pediatric renal transplantation is associated with somewhat lower rates of success than adult transplantation, with vascular thromboses of the grafts more common in younger children as well as problems with adherence to immunosuppressive regimens.

Liver Transplantation

Preoperative Considerations

In June of 2013 Share 35 was initiated for liver transplantation to get donor livers to the sickest patients (with MELD scores >35), resulting overall in sicker patients transplanted since that time. The program mandated extended regional sharing of livers and intestines to liver–intestine candidates. Though overall mortality after liver transplantation did not change with Share 35, some regions experienced poorer outcomes.[100] Hyponatremia in liver transplant recipients is associated with increased mortality on the waiting list, especially in less sick patients.[101] For this reason, MELD score itself was modified in January 2016 to include sodium, the first score change since its implementation in 2002.[102]

MELD is calculated as follows:
$10 \times [(0.957 \times \ln(\text{creatinine})) + [(0.378 \times \ln(\text{bilirubin})) = 1.12 \times \ln(\text{INR})] + 6.43$.

MELD-Na is $\text{MELD} - \text{Na} - [0.025 \times \text{MELD} \times (140 - \text{Na})] + 140$.

Mathematical modeling suggests that this change will save about 60 lives per year.

Liver transplant programs vary considerably in the number of transplants performed; however, the number of transplants performed in a given center is only a percentage of patients evaluated for liver transplantation, for which anesthesiology expertise will be sought. The anesthesiologist's input into the workup of liver transplant recipients is essential for decisions regarding candidacy and optimal preparation of patients for transplantation. Patients with ESLD have multiorgan dysfunction with cardiac, pulmonary, and renal compromise because of their liver disease (Table 52-6). Furthermore, many liver transplant

Table 52-6 Multisystem Complications of End-stage Liver Disease

System	Consequence
Central Nervous System	
Encephalopathy (confusion to coma)	Fatigue
	Blood–brain barrier disruption and intracranial hypertension (acute liver failure)
Pulmonary	
Respiratory alkalosis	
Reduced diffusing capacity	Hypoxemia/hepatopulmonary syndrome
Pulmonary hypertension	Reduced right heart function
Cardiovascular	
Reduced systemic vascular resistance	Hyperdynamic circulation
Diastolic dysfunction	
Prolonged QT interval	
Blunted responses to inotropes	
Blunted responses to vasopressors	
Diabetes	
Gastrointestinal	
Gastrointestinal bleeding from varices	
Ascites	
Delayed gastric emptying	
Hematologic	
Decreased synthesis of clotting factors	Risk of massive surgical bleeding
Hypersplenism (pancytopenia)	
Impaired fibrinolytic mechanisms	
Renal	
Hepatorenal syndrome	Impaired renal excretion of drugs
Hyponatremia	
Endocrine	
Glucose intolerance	
Osteoporosis	Fracture susceptibility
Nutritional/metabolic	Muscle wasting and weakness
Other	
Poor skin integrity; pruritus	
Increased volume of distribution for drugs	
Decreased citrate metabolism	Calcium requirement with rapid fresh-frozen plasma infusion

> **Table 52-7 Diagnoses Leading to Liver Transplantation in Adults**
>
> ***Hepatocellular Disease***
> Hepatitis C
> Laennec cirrhosis (alcoholic)
> Combined hepatitis C virus/Laennec cirrhosis
> Autoimmune hepatitis
> Cryptogenic (idiopathic) cirrhosis
> Hepatitis B
> Small hepatocellular carcinoma (usually with other hepatocellular diseases)
> Nonalcoholic steatohepatitis
>
> ***Cholestatic Disease***
> Primary biliary cirrhosis
> Primary sclerosing cholangitis
>
> ***Acute Liver Failure***
> Viral (unknown)
> Acute hepatitis viruses (A, B, C)
> Drug-induced liver failure
> Wilson disease

recipients are more than 60 years old. Common liver diagnoses leading to liver transplantation are shown in Table 52-7. With the availability of pharmacologic cures for hepatitis C, the number of these patients requiring transplantation is expected to fall, and these drugs open new opportunities for treating posttransplant recurrence of hepatitis C virus.

Pediatric patients are prioritized for transplant using the pediatric (<12 years) ESLD score or pediatric end-stage liver disease (PELD) score, calculated as follows:

$10 \times [(0.48 \times Ln(\text{serum bilirubin})) + [1.857 \times Ln(INR)] - [0.687 \times Ln(\text{albumin})] = \text{Listing age factor} + \text{Growth}$.

For pediatric patients, exception diagnoses are urea cycle disorders, organic acidemia, and hepatoblastoma.

Patients with ALF are given priority for donor livers, then the patients with the highest MELD/PELD score and compatible blood group are next.

All liver transplant patients are screened for infectious diseases including HIV, CMV, and Epstein–Barr virus. As for other solid-organ transplants, major infection and malignancy may exclude patients from consideration for transplantation. Several centers have had good experience transplanting HIV-positive patients (kidney or liver), though these patients have somewhat increased mortality compared to HIV-negative controls. Nonetheless in HIV-positive patients with high MELD, transplantation confers a survival benefit.[103]

Renal dysfunction is common in patients undergoing liver transplantation and should be the focus of anesthetic regimens for patients with chronic liver disease undergoing transplantation. Serum creatinine levels are not extremely useful in capturing renal function in patients with liver disease. Even a small increase in serum creatinine in these patients suggests significant renal dysfunction; hence, creatinine is emphasized in MELD scoring.

Difficult decisions about patient candidacy are common in evaluating liver transplant candidates. Several are discussed here to highlight the need for regular involvement of a transplant anesthesiologist in the candidacy evaluation process. Patients with ESLD generally have very low SVR, high cardiac index, and increased mixed venous oxygen saturation. Liver disease is not protective against coronary artery disease. Because cardiovascular disease is the most common cause of 30-day mortality following liver transplantation,[104] a rigorous cardiac workup is warranted. Most patients are screened for cardiac disease using dobutamine stress echocardiography or myocardial stress scintigraphy, although the effectiveness of diagnosing coronary artery disease in these patients is not well established.[105] Patients with evidence of significant coronary lesions usually require cardiac catheterization to identify stenoses amenable to angioplasty preoperatively. These studies can be done safely even in patients with significant renal dysfunction.[106] Patients with severe coronary artery disease are generally not candidates for liver transplantation. Functional assessment of patients in addition to laboratory and imaging studies is important, and one study found that achieving a distance of less than 250 m on a 6-minute walk test is an independent predictor of death on the transplant waiting list.[107] A small retrospective study suggests that troponin I levels greater than 0.07 ng/mL may predict liver transplant patients at risk for cardiovascular complications.[108]

Every effort should be made to maximize therapy for coronary artery disease and other heart disease before transplantation. Patients with hypertrophic obstructive cardiomyopathy (HOCM) and LV outflow tract obstruction can be treated with alcohol ablation of the septum before surgery to improve cardiac function during transplantation.[109] HOCM patients can benefit particularly from TEE monitoring because PA capillary wedge pressure does not accurately reflect LV volume in this population. Patients with patent foramen ovales may be at risk for intraoperative stroke, and some centers work with cardiologists to close larger shunts noninvasively before surgery. Nonalcoholic steatohepatitis is increasingly an indication for liver transplantation and may be associated with increased major postoperative cardiac events.[110]

Portopulmonary hypertension (PPH) patients coming to transplantation are particularly challenging. Diagnosis of PPH is made in the setting of liver disease or a mean pulmonary artery (PA) pressure of 25 mmHg or higher, pulmonary vascular resistance (PVR) greater than 240 dyne/s/cm^5, and PA occlusion pressure 12 mmHg or lower.[111] Echocardiography is also used to screen patients for PPH and intracardiac shunts. Systolic PA pressure estimates are made by capturing the maximum velocity of regurgitant flow across the tricuspid valve, and this velocity is used in the Bernoulli equation for the pressure gradient between the right ventricle and the right atrium ($\Delta P = 4V^4$). If moderate-to-severe pulmonary hypertension (estimated systolic PA pressure >50 mmHg) is suggested, right heart catheterization is needed for direct pressure measurements. Multiple case reports and small retrospective reviews demonstrate that patients with PPH are at substantial risk of perioperative death. There is general agreement that a mean PA pressure greater than 50 mmHg is an absolute contraindication to liver transplantation. Patients with PA pressures between 35 and 50 mmHg and PVR greater than 250 dyne/s/cm^{-5} are also likely at increased risk. Efforts to lower PA pressure before transplantation pay off and considerably reduce the risk of transplantation.[111] Epoprostenol is the usual first-line therapy for PPH and is effective in lowering PA pressures significantly in many patients, but it requires home IV delivery. Inhaled iloprost has been used in Europe for PPH patients with good results.[112] Sildenafil is also useful for treatment of PPH[113] and can be given via nasogastric tube during surgery. Controlling PA pressures is critical in patients with the most severe PPH, and patients have been successfully managed with the mixed endothelin antagonist bosentan[114] or the selective endothelin-A receptor antagonist ambrisentan[115] or imatinib.[116] Right heart dysfunction that does not reverse after treatment of primary pulmonary hypertension is considered a contraindication to liver transplantation.[117] Inhaled nitric oxide (iNO) can be extremely useful for managing PA pressures during liver transplantation.

PFTs are often abnormal in ESLD, with most patients showing reduced diffusion capacity for carbon monoxide. Hepatopulmonary syndrome (HPS, a widened alveolar–arterial gradient in room air owing to liver disease) can lead to severe hypoxemia. Contrast echocardiography is used to diagnose intrapulmonary vasodilation using agitated saline. The microbubbles act as a contrast, and, if intracardiac shunts are present, they appear within three heartbeats after injection in the left ventricle. The later appearance of bubbles suggests intrapulmonary shunting. Once a contraindication to transplantation, HPS is now an indication for transplantation because it is the only therapy that can reverse the underlying physiology.[118] If HPS is severe and completely unresponsive to oxygen, transplantation is risky because the immediate perioperative period may be complicated by frank graft hypoxia and failure. Fortunately, most patients with HPS have some element of physiologic ventilation–perfusion mismatch, are oxygen responsive, and, with this "room to move," can be safely transplanted.

Some patients with refractory ascites and normal renal function can have relief from ascites with terlipressin treatment.[119] The FDA approved terlipressin in 2013 (orphan status) for treatment of ascites.

Recently, a large number of new drugs for the treatment of hepatitis C have entered the market,[120] including protease inhibitors, viral polymerase inhibitors, viral replication complex inhibitors, new interferon formulations, and new ribavirin formulations. Drug–drug interactions with the new anti–hepatitis C virus drugs are just being reported. Telaprevir inhibits CYP3A and induces a significant reduction in oral clearance of midazolam (and limits its oxidation) in liver microsomes.[121] Protease inhibitors used to treat HIV can interact with midazolam to cause prolonged sedation.[122]

Intraoperative Procedures

Uncomplicated liver transplants can take as few as 2 to 3 hours, and the trachea can be extubated at the end of the case, but predicting easy versus difficult cases is not an exact science. Consequently, intensive preparation for surgery is important. Rapid-sequence induction of general anesthesia is indicated because patients with ESLD often have gastroparesis[123] in addition to increased intra-abdominal pressure from ascites. For anticipated difficult cases, many centers place two arterial catheters; one can be in the femoral artery (left femoral if a kidney transplant is planned). PA catheters are still used in many centers to follow PVR, and TEE is increasingly used for monitoring volume status, particularly for patients with cardiac disease undergoing transplantation (see Chapter 27).[124] Major hemorrhagic complications of TEE use during liver transplantation in patients with esophageal varices are rare, but fear of these complications has limited TEE use in some centers.[125] For difficult cases, two large-bore (9 French) catheters are placed for rapid intravenous infusions. In many centers, anesthesiologists are capable of placing percutaneous lines specifically for use in venovenous bypass (VVB) if necessary, but most U.S. centers rarely use VVB with cava-sparing surgical techniques. Bladder catheters and nasogastric tubes are placed in all patients. A rapid infusion system with the ability to deliver at least 500 mL/min of warmed blood is primed and is in the room. Before surgical incision, blood product availability is confirmed. Normothermia, essential for optimal hemostasis, is maintained with fluid warmers and convective air blankets over the legs and over the upper body.

Liver transplantation is traditionally described in three phases: dissection, anhepatic phase, and neohepatic phase, with reperfusion of the graft marking the start of the neohepatic phase. The major issues during the first phase of transplantation are coagulation management and renal protection, so the major anesthetic goals of this phase are correction of coagulopathies and maintenance of intravascular volume for renal protection. Some centers advocate low CVP management of liver transplant patients to reduce blood loss,[126] but this technique may be not be tolerated by patients with higher MELD scores and marginal renal function. The incision in patients with massive ascites is a rapid paracentesis, and albumin infusion is warranted to prevent postparacentesis circulatory dysfunction, because cirrhotics often have very low albumin levels as well as poorly functioning albumin.[127]

Coagulation

Although standard laboratory coagulation studies do not predict bleeding well, they are still the gold standard for coagulation management. Though many transplants can be done with minimal transfusions, predicting bleeding is an inexact science, and anesthesiologists should be prepared for massive transfusion in these cases. Fresh frozen plasma (FFP) is used to maintain an INR of 1.5 or less in patients with anticipated or ongoing bleeding. Point-of-care INR is extremely useful in patients with massive blood loss, providing information in seconds. In the authors' experience, point-of-care INR and clinical laboratory INR values may be different, but once the offset is known, the two INR values track well. Rapid infusion of FFP can quickly lead to ionized hypocalcemia because of the citrate load that is not metabolized by a diseased liver. Infusion of calcium chloride ($CaCl_2$), adjusted to ionized Ca^{2+} levels, is better at maintaining constant calcium (Ca^{2+}) levels than are intermittent boluses. Use of calcium boluses will cause wide calcium swings and overuse of calcium. At this time, there is no sufficient U.S. experience with prothrombin complex concentrates[128] in liver transplant recipients to know the place for these factor concentrates. Platelet transfusion has traditionally been used to maintain platelet counts above 50,000/mm^3; however, platelet transfusion has been associated with worse graft and patient survival.[129,130] Importantly, we find that maintaining fibrinogen above 150 mg/dL with cryoprecipitate is critical for hemostasis and obviates the need for platelet transfusions in almost all patients. Cell-saver blood may also be used to limit allogeneic transfusions, although it is generally not used in patients with hepatocellular carcinoma.

Many other factors contribute to poor hemostasis in liver transplant patients besides poor clotting factor synthesis, including renal failure, infection, endothelial dysfunction, and high portal pressures.[131] This complexity in the etiology of underlying bleeding problems is likely a factor in the unpredictability of bleeding during liver transplantation.

In addition to complex coagulopathies of ESLD, many patients with liver disease have a superimposed hypercoagulable state (see Chapter 17). For example, patients with autoimmune liver diseases may have antiphospholipid antibodies. Many authors have suggested that the coagulation status of cirrhotics is "balanced" when procoagulant abnormalities are balanced by anticoagulant abnormalities.[132] But experienced transplant anesthesiologists recognize that both coagulopathy and hypercoagulability can cause simultaneous and serious problems—two diseases rather than a balanced system. In general, prohemostatic factors are also elevated in patients with liver disease, including von Willebrand factor and factor VIII, and low values of ADAMTS-13, antithrombin, protein C, and plasminogen disrupt the normal balance of hemostatic factors.[131] So in addition to monitoring discrete parts of the coagulation profile to guide transfusion therapies, it is important to look at a measure of whole-blood clotting to assess thrombotic potential. Most centers use thromboelastography (TEG) and increasingly thromboelastometry to help sort out complex coagulation disturbances and their evolution during liver transplantation, to help with interpretation of standard laboratory tests of coagulation, and to get a picture of overall clotting and fibrinolysis status. If TEG or thromboelastometry indicates normal or hypernormal whole clotting in the presence of high INR and low fibrinogen and platelets (and usually elevated D-dimers), this pattern is a caution that the patient may have a clinically significant hypercoagulable state. A formal hypercoagulability workup should be done as part of liver transplant evaluation. Under these circumstances, the authors' approach is to avoid pharmacologic procoagulant or antifibrinolytic drugs. For the majority of patients with coagulopathy dominated by synthetic dysfunction, thrombocytopenia, and hypofibrinogenemia, whole-blood clotting is delayed. If these patients have insufficient hemostasis, many centers supplement transfusion therapy with antifibrinolytic agents. Considerable center-dependent variation in use and dosing of antifibrinolytics makes generalizations difficult. In the authors' experience, ε-aminocaproic acid (EACA; 5-g load and 1 g/hr infusion) to support hemostasis during surgery is useful and safe[133] in most coagulopathic patients during liver transplantation, provided there is no evidence or history of hypercoagulability. Other centers use considerably less drug, less often. Fibrinolysis acutely worsens immediately after reperfusion to varying degrees, depending largely on the amount of tissue plasminogen activator released from the graft.[134] A (re)bolus of EACA is helpful to maintain hemostasis once this postreperfusion exacerbation of fibrinolysis is documented. Some centers use tranexamic acid instead of EACA, which is also a plasminogen inhibitor but has a longer half-life than EACA.

Activated factor VII can be used safely during liver transplantation but is usually reserved for rescue of refractory critical bleeding unresponsive to more standard management because of its expense and because the risk of thrombosis in liver disease patients is not known. Furthermore, its use may be associated with poor clinical outcomes.[135] When this drug is given, INR rapidly normalizes, although the amount of circulating clotting factors does not change, complicating interpretation of laboratory coagulation studies. NovoSeven administration is also useful for surgical hemostasis for placement of intracranial pressure (ICP) monitors in patients with ALF and for selected patients undergoing liver transplantation with difficult red cell crossmatches or in patients who refuse transfusion on religious grounds.

Pulmonary embolism is an unusual complication of liver transplantation, reflecting the complex coagulation imbalance of ESLD and liver transplantation. If diagnosed promptly, low-dose tissue plasminogen activator (0.5 to 4 mg) delivery into the CVP port of a pulmonary artery catheter (PAC) can lyse the clot quickly.[136]

Perioperative renal dysfunction is a major challenge in liver transplantation and can be exacerbated by hypovolemia and anesthetic-induced impairment of renal blood flow. Unsurprisingly a literature review showed that preoperative renal dysfunction and severity of liver disease as well as intraoperative hemodynamic instability and graft quality are associated with post–liver transplant renal dysfunction.[137] Creatinine levels can significantly underestimate the degree of renal dysfunction, especially in ESLD patients with significant muscle wasting.[138] Hepatorenal syndrome (HRS) is a functional renal disorder associated with liver disease, categorized as type 1 (acute severe decompensation), which is often fatal, and type 2 (chronic moderate renal failure with creatinine more than 1.5 and glomerular filtration rate less than 40 mL/min). Recently HRS type 1 was recategorized as a specific type of acute kidney injury, incorporating the idea that treatment should be based on relative changes in serum creatinine (>0.3 mg/dL over 48 hours) rather than an absolute threshold number for serum creatinine.[139] HRS in general is the diagnosis if the patient has ascites, is not in shock, has not been exposed to nephrotoxic drugs, has no parenchymal renal disease, has a creatinine level more than 1.5 mg/dL, and does not improve after 2 days of diuretic withdrawal and albumin therapy (1 g/kg/day up to 100 g/day).[140] HRS–acute kidney injury prevention best practices include SBP prophylaxis, intravenous albumin administration if SBP is present, and antibiotic prophylaxis for gastrointestinal bleeding.[139] In addition, large-volume (>5 L) drainage of ascites with incision is paracentesis and should be accompanied by albumin therapy to prevent renal decompensation, with recommended albumin doses of 6 to 8 g/L of ascites drained. Importantly, higher doses of albumin are associated with better survival in type 1 HRS.[141] Terlipressin and norepinephrine may be useful for HRS because they relieve splanchnic vasodilatation, though the data about these therapies are sparse.[142] The α_1-agonist midodrine in combination with octreotide is useful for improving renal function in some patients.[143] No prospective trials have been done to support use of one vasopressor over another during transplantation, and intraoperative pharmacologic renal support is largely guided by the hepatology literature. Dopamine is not useful for preserving renal function during liver transplantation. The most important consideration for patients with HRS is to ensure adequate volume replacement before instituting diuresis in the OR.

The *anhepatic phase* begins when the liver is functionally excluded from the circulation. Historically, the vena cava was clamped above (suprahepatic anastomosis) and below (infrahepatic anastomosis) the liver, and the portal vein and hepatic artery were clamped. With complete cava cross-clamping, venous return falls by 50% to 60%, often resulting in hypotension. VVB may be used to increase venous return and therefore blood pressure, to increase renal and gut perfusion pressures, and to decompress portal pressures for a better surgical field. VVB is rarely used in centers where surgeons use cava-sparing techniques, and hemodynamics during the anhepatic period can be managed with volume loading and vasopressors as needed. VVB carries potential complications, including arm lymphedema, air embolism, and vascular injury, and its benefit is limited when anhepatic times are short. Surgical techniques that preserve caval flow (e.g., piggyback technique) are standard in most U.S. centers and make intraoperative management significantly easier, but anesthesiologists should be familiar with managing both surgical situations.

Reperfusion of the graft is the most treacherous time of the liver transplant. Communication between the surgical and anesthesia teams is essential in precise preparation for reperfusion. Caval clamps are removed first, and the integrity of the caval anastomoses are ensured. Caval reperfusion is usually hemodynamically well tolerated. However, portal vein reperfusion often results in hemodynamic instability. The original descriptions of reperfusion syndrome emphasized (often severe) hypotension and bradycardia with portal reperfusion.[144] Now, with flushing techniques that precede reperfusion and changes in preservation solution, bradycardia is less common. Typically, reperfusion is associated with hypotension (further drop of already low SVR), which may or may not require treatment. The authors' preparation for reperfusion is to give sodium bicarbonate just before unclamping (25 to 50 mEq) to meet the acid load from the graft. For particularly prolonged acidosis, tris(hydroxymethyl) aminomethane infusion is useful.[145] Importantly, administration of 500 to 1,000 mg of $CaCl_2$ *precisely at the time of portal reperfusion* can counteract the effects of high potassium on the heart. If, despite these preparations, T waves on electrocardiogram (ECG) become elevated, the same treatment is repeated. Some anesthesiologists prefer to treat ECG changes only after they are diagnosed, but because the acid and potassium of reperfusion can be anticipated, the authors' practice is to counteract these prophylactically. Lidocaine, atropine, and norepinephrine are available at the time of reperfusion in case of ventricular dysrhythmias, bradyarrhythmias, and severe hypotension. Hepatic artery unclamping is usually hemodynamically uncomplicated.

Microemboli and right ventricular (RV) dysfunction are common at reperfusion, and intracardiac thromboemboli are not rare.[146] Intracardiac emboli and biventricular dysfunction are associated with adverse postoperative cardiac events.[146] Methylene blue is used by some to counteract the vasoplegic state of reperfusion, but its effects on outcome are unknown.[147] On the other hand, a study in which iNO was given during the entire transplant suggested significant acute benefits (decreased hepatocyte apoptosis) and earlier graft recovery, including faster coagulation factor synthesis.[148] Attempts to precondition the reperfused graft were analyzed in a well-designed trial, which showed no difference with propofol versus sevoflurane.[149]

In the *neohepatic phase*, calcium is not required after reperfusion; therefore one early indication of graft metabolic function is the lack of a calcium requirement, even when FFP is infused rapidly. Usually within 30 minutes, the base deficit improves with graft metabolism of citrate and lactate. Within the first hour, the CO decreases (after an acute increase after portal reperfusion) as SVR increases with graft metabolism of vasoactive substances unleashed at reperfusion. In addition, the graft appearance should be noted. It should have a smooth edge and no evidence of engorgement. Bile is made in the first half-hour after reperfusion in a well-functioning graft. Often, renal function improves after reperfusion, probably because of graft metabolism of renal vasoconstrictors. ECD grafts are often slow to function metabolically in the OR. (For these and other classes of ECD livers, cold ischemia times should be limited, which can significantly affect the OR schedule.) Fibrinolysis after reperfusion may require antifibrinolytic agents. Thromboelastometry may be more sensitive than thromboelastography in detecting fibrinolysis,[150] but decision to add or increase antifibrinolytics after reperfusion should be made by assessing surgical hemostasis as well as point-of-care tests.

During the neohepatic period, biliary anastomoses are completed and sources of surgical bleeding are corrected. Drains are placed and the abdomen is closed. Fast-tracking protocols for liver transplant patients are common in experienced centers.[151]

Pediatric Liver Transplantation

Indications for pediatric liver transplantation differ considerably from those of adults, with biliary atresia (44%) and inborn errors of metabolism (34%) being the most common indications.[152] PPH is rare in children, but biliary atresia is associated with cardiac defects and situs inversus.[153] Children younger than 1 year of age with inherited liver disease are often very small for age. In small children, a radial artery catheter and at least one large (18-g) peripheral intravenous line are placed after induction of anesthesia. Surgeons may place tunneled central lines before incision, which are useful for intraoperative transfusions, postoperative administration of drugs, and CVP monitoring. Children with previous Kasai operations for biliary atresia may have massive bleeding during dissection because of adhesions. Small children receiving large grafts may have respiratory compromise with abdominal closure. Because hepatic artery thrombosis (HAT) is a more common complication in children than adults, some centers choose to have the INR at the end of surgery in the 1.8 to 2 range; postoperative aspirin and alprostadil are often used to prevent HAT. If flow is inadequate (by poor Doppler signals) in the artery after anastomosis, intraoperative reanastomosis or a new anastomosis may be required acutely. Aortic cross-clamping may be required for these anastomoses. Biliary complications are also common in pediatric transplant recipients, especially those receiving adult left lateral segment grafts, with HAT a significant contributor to biliary complications. Use of split livers (one liver for two patients) puts a strain on transplant teams but is important for extending the donor pool.[154]

Acute Liver Failure

Anesthetic considerations for adults and children with ALF are focused on protection of the brain (see Chapter 37), so that in many ways management is opposite that of chronic liver failure, in which the kidneys are the most fragile organ requiring protection during liver transplantation. Patients with a diagnosis of ALF should be managed in the ICU, because they can have a rapidly progressive course of elevated ICP, leading to herniation and death. Because ALF is much less common than chronic liver disease, a single center gets little experience with ALF, so it is important to develop a detailed multidisciplinary protocol for managing these patients. ICP monitoring is useful in managing these patients but risks intracranial bleeding; nonetheless its use is advocated by the U.S. Acute Liver Failure Study Group in nonacetaminophen-induced ALF.[155] Some centers have gained expertise in transcranial Doppler monitoring in place of invasive ICP monitoring[156] thereby avoiding the risk of ICP monitoring in coagulopathic patients. In the authors' experience, bispectral index monitoring, especially in patients without ICP monitors, can help detect acute disruption of cerebral blood flow, such as with vascular clamping.

Anesthetic management of these patients starts in the ICU, with intubation as needed for airway protection in the setting of encephalopathy or for initiation of therapeutic hypothermia. Mild hypothermia (core temperature 34° to 35°C) is used in some centers for ALF, though recent retrospective analysis suggests no benefit.[157] The head is positioned midline and the head of the bed raised. Mild hyperventilation is also commonly used to manage ICP but is best used as a rescue therapy. Mannitol is used for osmotherapy to an end point of 310 to 315 mOsm/L. Hypertonic saline is also useful for lowering ICP in some patients, with a target serum Na of 145 to 155 mEq/L.[158] Liver-assist devices used to bridge patients with ALF to transplantation have not generally shown benefit, but cell-based assist devices are in active clinical trial.

Importantly, vasodilating anesthetics, including all inhaled agents, should be avoided, especially without ICP monitoring. In the authors' experience, pentothal is a good maintenance anesthetic, and acute rises in ICP can be managed with etomidate. With decreased availability of barbiturates, propofol is commonly used. Patients may come to the OR on *N*-acetylcysteine, a glutathione donor. When antihypertensive therapy is required, labetalol does not cause significant cerebral vasodilation in these patients.[159] Acute cerebral vasodilatation often accompanies reperfusion. Management of intracranial hypertension and cerebral edema is based on very small studies of patients with ALF and on adaptations of studies directed at control of intracranial hypertension in other settings (see Chapter 37).

Pancreas and Islet Transplantation

The majority of pancreas transplants (about 75%) are done as simultaneous pancreas and kidney transplants from a single deceased donor. Pancreata grafted in these procedures have historically had better long-term survival than grafts done after kidney transplantation or independent pancreas grafts. Independent pancreas grafts are usually performed for patients with type 1 diabetes, who have frequent metabolic complications (hypoglycemia) but preserved renal function. With proper donor selection and aggressive attention to targeted antibiotic coverage, better graft survival rates after isolated pancreas transplant have recently been reported.[160] Nonetheless, pancreas transplantation is becoming less frequent, and islet transplantation has increased,[161] likely because pancreas transplants are associated with higher rates of surgical and postoperative complications. Optimal immunosuppression for islet transplantation, to ward off both allo- and autoimmunity, remains a significant problem. Encapsulation of islets to create a barrier to immune cells has also been a surprisingly hard problem.[162]

The preoperative assessment of pancreas/islet transplant recipients focuses on the end-organ complications of type 1 diabetes (see Chapter 47). Monitoring will depend on cardiac status, but generally patients do not require PA catheters and have been evaluated for cardiac disease as part of the transplant workup. Nonetheless, cardiovascular disease is present in many patients undergoing pancreas transplantation, although they tend to be younger than liver transplant recipients.

The major difference between pancreas transplantation and other procedures is that strict attention to control of blood glucose is indicated to protect newly transplanted β cells from hyperglycemic damage. No formula for controlling blood glucose has emerged as a standard of intraoperative management. In general, if adult patients arrive with glucose above 250 mg/dL, 10 units of insulin can be given intravenously, followed by an infusion of insulin. The infusion starting rate varies, depending on the initial blood glucose level. Once blood glucose levels are controlled (<150 mg/dL), intravenous 5% dextrose (about 100 mL/hr) should also be infused as the insulin infusion is continued. The most important issue is to check the response to insulin frequently and adjust infusions as necessary. Little literature exists for a patient with an implanted insulin pump, though more than 400,000 have been implanted in the United States.[163] One center developed a protocol for patients undergoing surgery with insulin pumps, emphasizing preadmission contact with an endocrinologist and documentation of pump status from preoperative to postoperative settings.[163] A reasonable recommendation is to continue to use the pump at basal rates in these patients as long as its operation is reviewed and blood glucose levels are monitored regularly during surgery.

Islet transplants were revived by the Edmonton protocol, published in 2000.[164] The major changes introduced included a glucocorticoid-free immunosuppression regimen and immediate transplantation of islets after isolation. Since that time, islets have been cultured after isolation in many centers, which makes surgical scheduling easier. Islets are generally infused into the portal circulation; acute portal hypertension may result from the infusion. This surgery should not be complicated by significant blood loss.

Small Bowel and Multivisceral Transplantation

Indications for intestinal transplantation include impending liver failure in patients with intestinal failure (or short-gut syndromes requiring total parenteral nutrition [TPN]), frequent severe dehydration in patients with intestinal failure, and severe complications of central lines for TPN (sepsis, thrombosis of central veins). Patients who develop liver failure from TPN for intestinal failure are candidates for combined liver–intestine transplantation, and the presence of a liver in the graft may have a protective effect on the bowel graft.[165] In these cases, liver failure should be irreversible, and biopsy findings are often required to corroborate this conclusion in patients without overt ESLD. In general, intestinal transplantation is usually performed only in patients with life-threatening complications of intestinal failure, mostly in children, but increasingly in adult recipients.

A major hurdle for these transplants is line placement adequate for transfusion of blood products and fluids, need for which may be substantial during these long cases. Anesthesiologists should review angiographic studies to determine venous patency before attempting central line placement. Ultrasound devices are helpful in identifying the known patent vessels for cannulation, but surgical cutdowns for venous access may be necessary, including transhepatic or intraoperative renal vein catheterization. Superior vena cava or inferior vena cava obstruction may require preoperative intervention (surgical and/or lytic) for adequate vascular access for surgery.[166] Antibiotic regimens should be continued during the surgery. Nitrous oxide, as in liver transplantation, should be avoided.

Common complications of intestinal failure include dehydration and electrolyte abnormalities, gastric acid hypersecretion, pancreatic insufficiency, bone disease, and TPN-induced liver failure.[167] Because electrolyte abnormalities are common, they should be monitored continuously during surgery and appropriate replacement instituted. Because enteral feeding will not be possible until weeks after surgery, TPN should be continued in the perioperative period.

Like reperfusion of liver grafts, intestinal graft reperfusion is associated with an acute release of acid and potassium from the graft and a postreperfusion syndrome. Anticipatory bicarbonate and $CaCl_2$ administration is useful to counteract the effects of acid and potassium on the heart. After reperfusion, coagulopathy may worsen and is usually managed by reassessment of INR and fibrinogen and platelet counts and correction with blood products. Epidural anesthesia is useful for pain management in both intestine donors and recipients.[168]

Composite Tissue Allografts

Upper extremity and face transplants are extremely complex procedures performed only in a few centers. More than 85 patients have received hand or arm transplants, with the longest survivor 11 years posttransplant. More than 20 patients have received face transplants (hopkinsmedicine.org). For face donors, surgeons prefer to procure the face first, before other organs are procured. The graft recovery is complex, with isolation of motor and sensory nerves as well as venous and arterial vessels. Multiple surgeons are involved in both graft recovery and implantation. Recipient nose and mouth deformities will certainly require individualized airway care. Protocols for these patients are just being developed, but the choice of anesthetic and fluid management is directed at preventing microvasculature constriction and postoperative edema.

Anesthesiologists should be involved in perioperative protocol development for these new procedures from the initial planning stages of a program, especially because well-planned regional nerve blocks can be very useful for upper extremity transplants and other anesthesia-specific concerns can be addressed in advance.[169] Limb transplant recipients may be heparinized.[169] Bilateral limb allografts expose the recipient to two reperfusion events. The common feature of these grafts is that they contain multiple organs (blood vessels, nerves, muscle, skin). Multiple anastomoses imply a very long surgical procedure. Composite tissue recipients require intense immunosuppression, in part because the skin is highly antigenic, and some immunosuppressants that are unfamiliar to anesthesiologists may be administered intraoperatively. In addition to complex triple-drug immunosuppression, increasingly donor marrow infusions are used in an effort to induce tolerance to the allograft.[170] Preparation for massive blood loss in these cases is essential.

Face grafting also may require massive transfusion, and blood loss may be difficult to quantify because of bleeding into the drapes; the surgery can be very prolonged. Common complications include postoperative renal dysfunction, acute respiratory distress syndrome and jugular thrombosis. These cases are immunologically extremely complex.[171]

Lung Transplantation

Lung transplantation is accepted therapy for end-stage pulmonary and pulmonary vascular disease, based on documented improvement in longevity and quality of life.[172] The Department of Health and Human Services Organ Procurement and Transplantation Network reports more than 31,000 lung transplant procedures in the United States since 1988, and the 2015 Registry of the International Society for Heart and Lung Transplantation reports 51,400 lung transplants worldwide since 1989.[173] With median waiting time between 500 and 1,000 days, however, many patients die awaiting transplant because of the shortage of suitable organs. Over the past 20 years there has been a slow but steady improvement in overall outcome in lung transplantation. Data compiled from January 1990 to June 2013 reveal a median survival of 5.7 years and a 54% survival rate at 5 years. It has now become clear that long-term survival after bilateral lung transplantation is better than after single-lung transplantation (median 7.1 versus 4.5 years). The most common indications for lung transplantation are chronic obstructive pulmonary disease (32%), interstitial lung disease (24%), cystic fibrosis (CF) (16%), and α_1-antitrypsin deficiency (5%).[173]

Surgical options for lung transplantation are single-lung transplant, *en bloc* double, sequential double, and heart–lung transplantation. The International Society for Heart and Lung Transplantation registry for 2015 indicates a continued increase in double-lung transplants over the past two decades, with a relatively stable number of single-lung transplants, a trend likely related to reports of improved outcome after double-lung transplantation.[173] There has been a continued trend toward avoiding the use of cardiopulmonary bypass (CPB) in single and sequential double-lung transplantation, although CPB should always be available and is often used for patients with pulmonary hypertension. Double-lung transplantation is most commonly used in patients with pulmonary vascular disease and CF, although its use is increasing in chronic obstructive pulmonary disease and interstitial lung disease. Single-lung transplantation for emphysema has favor because of good short-term outcomes, with the added advantage of leaving a donor lung for another recipient. Lung transplant centers vary in applying single- or double-lung transplant to different diagnoses as well as in the application of CPB, and the procedure indications are still debated.[174] Double-lung transplantation, however, is indicated if a single-lung transplantation would allow a continuing pathologic process to jeopardize either the native or transplanted lung. For example, the presence of pulmonary infection, as in CF, in the native lung would likely spread to the transplanted lung. In pulmonary hypertension, remaining pulmonary vascular disease in the native lung would result in progressive pulmonary hypertension and thus hypertensive vasculopathy in a transplanted lung. Finally, a severely emphysematous lung, with its high compliance, would be at risk for air trapping and barotrauma when coexisting with a transplanted lung with normal compliance.

Recipient Selection

International Guidelines for the Selection of Lung Transplant Candidates were updated in 2006 by consensus agreement of several thoracic societies (summarized in Table 52-8).[175] In general, patients should be considered for lung transplantation if they exhibit poor pulmonary function despite maximal medical

Table 52-8 Lung Recipient Selection Guidelines

General Indications
End-stage lung disease
Failed maximal medical treatment of lung disease
Age within limits for planned transplant
Life expectancy <2–3 yr
Ability to walk and undergo rehabilitation
Sound nutritional status (70%–130% of ideal body weight)
Stable psychosocial profile
No significant comorbid disease

Disease-specific Indications

Chronic Obstructive Pulmonary Disease
FEV_1 <25% of predicted value after bronchodilators and/or $PaCO_2$ = 55 mmHg and/or pulmonary hypertension (especially with cor pulmonale)
Chronic O_2 therapy

Cystic Fibrosis
FEV_1 <30% predicted
Hypoxemia, hypercapnia, or rapidly declining lung function
Weight loss and hemoptysis
Frequent exacerbations, especially young females
Absence of antibiotic-resistant organisms

Idiopathic Pulmonary Fibrosis
Vital capacity <60%–65% of predicted
Resting hypoxemia
Progression of disease despite therapy (steroids)

Pulmonary Hypertension
NYHA functional status Class III or IV, despite prostacyclin therapy
Mean right atrial pressure <15 mmHg
Mean pulmonary artery pressure <55 mmHg
Cardiac index <2 L/min/m^2

Eisenmenger Syndrome
NYHA class III or IV, despite optimal therapy

Pediatric
NYHA class III or IV
Disease unresponsive to maximal therapy
Cor pulmonale, cyanosis, low cardiac output

FEV_1, forced expiratory volume in 1 second; NYHA, New York Heart Association.

therapy. Contraindications to lung transplantation are based on their impact on long-term survival. Patients with severe cardiac disease can be considered for heart–lung transplantation but are not candidates for isolated lung transplant. A Lung Allocation System, developed by the United Network for Organ Sharing, is used, with candidates given a lung allocation score to determine their wait-list status. This system weighs net benefit of transplant and clinical urgency.[176]

As for other transplants, patients are screened for malignancy (mammography, Papanicolaou test, and colonoscopy). PFT, left and right heart catheterization, and transthoracic echocardiography are used to evaluate potential recipients. Lung transplantation is not advocated for acute disease processes, such as acute respiratory distress syndrome. Specific age limits were recommended in the past; however, current guidelines list age more than 65 years as a relative contraindication only. CF is associated with complex pulmonary infections and colonization with microbial flora that can negatively affect transplant outcomes. However, with the exception of patients colonized with *Burkholderia cepacia*, most CF patients can be successfully transplanted despite chronic bacterial infections.[177]

Medical evaluation prior to listing a patient for transplantation requires many specialties. If the patient has been on the waiting list for an extended period, it is important to review recent laboratory and functional data; disease progression may have resulted in change in status since the original workup. It is critical to confirm ABO compatibility of donor and recipient prior to surgery. Lung transplant candidates have poor pulmonary status and are frequently receiving multiple therapies including oxygen, inhaled bronchodilators, steroids, and pulmonary vasodilators. These medications should be continued in the perioperative period. Although *ex vivo* lung perfusion is now used in many centers,[178,179] the transplant must still be done as soon as a lung becomes available. Because these procedures are done on an urgent or emergent basis, the patient often presents with a full stomach.

Although lung transplant patients are understandably anxious, they also have minimal pulmonary reserve, and sedation must be given carefully under monitored conditions. After determining oxygen saturation, slow incremental dosing of a short-acting benzodiazepine (0.25- to 1.0-mg of midazolam) may be used for anxiolysis. Premedication with narcotics such as fentanyl must be administered with extreme caution, if at all, because of their ventilatory depressant effect. Use of metoclopramide, histamine-2 antagonists, and a nonparticulate antacid are usually warranted because of "full stomach" status. Many patients are unable to rest in a supine or in Trendelenburg position for central venous catheterization. Placement of large-bore peripheral intravenous and arterial access is usually adequate for initiation of the anesthetic, with central access achieved after induction. Placement of a PAC is often warranted for monitoring cardiac output and PVR, with a catheter capable of continuous cardiac output and mixed venous oxygenation saturation (M_{VO_2}) preferable. Thoracic epidural catheters are placed preoperatively at some centers, especially in patients who are believed unlikely to require CPB with its associated anticoagulation. Another option is to place the epidural in the early postoperative period, after coagulopathies are corrected. The epidural can be placed using light sedation during weaning from mechanical ventilation, allowing better neurologic monitoring and pain control prior to tracheal extubation. Other options for postoperative pain relief include postoperative paravertebral blocks, and intercostal nerve blocks performed intraoperatively. Multimodal analgesic techniques, including dexmedetomidine infusion, intravenous acetaminophen, and nonsteroidal anti-inflammatory agents, are now standard components of enhanced recovery after surgery programs.[180] These will likely be useful after lung transplantation as well.

Intraoperative Management

Single-lung Transplantation

Lung transplant recipients are often chronically intravascularly volume depleted, and chronic pulmonary hypertension is common. These factors predispose the patients to hypotension and decreased cardiac output on anesthetic induction. Restriction of anesthetic doses because of this concern increases the risk of awareness in this patient population. Monitoring with processed electroencephalography may thus be useful; anesthetic management guided by bispectral index monitoring has been associated with a reduction of the incidence of intraoperative awareness in this population.[181] Because fluid restriction is beneficial for postoperative management,[182] small fluid boluses, particularly with colloid, and judicious induction with etomidate, benzodiazepine, and narcotics is prudent. A balanced technique combining narcotic and inhalation anesthetics or benzodiazepines is usually an effective approach to maintenance of the anesthetic. Possible plans for early extubation should be discussed with the surgeon, and minimizing narcotics while providing multimodal pain relief should be utilized if early extubation is planned. Muscle relaxation can be maintained with rocuronium or vecuronium and is associated with minimal hemodynamic side effects. Nitrous oxide is rarely used because it may exacerbate bullous emphysematous disease, pulmonary hypertension, or intraoperative hypoxemia.

Lung isolation, preferably with a double-lumen endobronchial tube, is necessary for single and bilateral sequential lung transplantation. The double-lumen tube, compared to bronchial blockade techniques, allows better suctioning of secretions, improved deflation of the operative lung during dissection, and application of continuous positive airway pressure to the operative lung if indicated. A bronchial blocker is more easily dislodged with surgical manipulation, may not provide isolation of the right upper lobe, and requires repositioning midsurgery in the case of a bilateral sequential procedure. A left-sided endobronchial tube is preferred, because a right-sided tube may be difficult to position relative to the right upper lobe bronchus.

Fluid restriction and lung ventilation strategies designed to protect the lung allograft are indicated, because these patients are at increased risk for acute lung injury and pulmonary edema. This implies use of small tidal volumes (6 mL/kg) and oxygenation techniques using PEEP and lowest acceptable F_{IO_2} settings.[182] Fluid restriction may decrease lung water in the newly transplanted lung, and there are data showing that elevated CVP is associated with increased mortality after lung transplantation.[183] Intermittent fluid boluses while keeping CVP less than 7 cm of H_2O and use of vasoactive drugs to maintain hemodynamics are recommended. Cardiac output monitoring using PAC, or minimally invasive techniques such as esophageal Doppler or pulse contour analysis, are useful for guiding fluid restriction while assuring adequate cardiac output. Lung recipients are susceptible to pulmonary hypertension and RV dysfunction or failure during single-lung ventilation. Optimizing oxygenation and ventilation does not always improve RV function, and vasodilator and/or inotropic support may be required. iNO is an option for improving respiratory and right heart function.

During single-lung ventilation, hypoxemia is common. Strategies to improve oxygenation and ventilation are discussed in detail in Chapter 38. They include application of PEEP to the dependent lung and CPAP to the nondependent lung and PA clamping of the nonventilated lung by the surgeon. Anesthesia machines with pressure-controlled ventilation and other advanced options have diminished the need for ICU ventilators during the operative procedure. CPB is indicated during lung transplantation if adequate oxygenation cannot be maintained despite ventilatory and pharmacologic maneuvers and PA clamping. Other indications for CPB include inability to provide adequate ventilation, or RV failure.

Single-lung transplantation can be performed via lateral thoracotomy. If the surgeon is concerned about possible need for CPB, then the patient must be positioned to allow rapid access to either the aorta and right atrium or the femoral artery and vein. This can be accomplished via either anterior thoracotomy with partial sternotomy or lateral thoracotomy with decreased angulation of the hips to allow access to the femoral vessels. Determination of operative side is based on preoperative ventilation–perfusion studies and prior thoracic surgeries. The lung with poorer function is typically the one replaced.

After pneumonectomy, the surgeon will size the donor vascular tissue to the recipient vessels and sequentially anastomose the atrial/pulmonary vein patch, bronchus, and PA. The lung is kept cold with ice in the surgical field until reperfusion. Circulation is restored to the donor lung, suture lines are checked for hemostasis, and then ventilation is begun. Systemic hypotension can occur during reperfusion but is usually not as significant as that with liver graft reperfusion. The anesthesiologist is often asked to assess the bronchial anastomosis using fiberoptic bronchoscopy and to perform bronchopulmonary toilet on the transplanted lung if necessary (removal of blood, secretions). TEE is useful to assess pulmonary venous drainage of the transplanted lung (see earlier). Along with *ex vivo* perfusion, Perfadex, a low–molecular-weight dextran solution, improves early graft function and is used widely for preservation during procurement.[184] There can nonetheless be reperfusion injury to the lung presenting as pulmonary edema. PEEP and lung protective strategies are particularly useful in this scenario.

Intraoperative TEE has become a valuable tool in the assessment of lung transplant patients. A comprehensive TEE examination should be performed after induction of anesthesia with attention focused on biventricular function, presence of valvular regurgitation, patent foramen ovale or atrial septal defect, and pulse wave Doppler flow patterns in the pulmonary veins. Significant RV dysfunction, valvular regurgitation, or intra-atrial shunt may lead to the decision to utilize CPB. TEE can be helpful in monitoring RV function during initial clamping of the PA; acute deterioration of RV function is an indication for the institution of CPB. After reperfusion, another TEE examination should be performed. Pulmonary vein anastomotic obstruction can be diagnosed with careful Doppler examination of the pulmonary venous inflow (see Chapter 27). Because this condition leads to acute graft failure, rapid diagnosis and treatment in the OR is essential.

At the completion of the procedure, the patient should be evaluated for exchange of the double-lumen endotracheal tube to a large (8-mm internal diameter or larger) single-lumen tube. The large diameter facilitates postoperative bronchopulmonary toilet and diagnostic bronchoscopy, as needed. Significant oropharyngeal edema, high PEEP requirement, or need for differential lung ventilation justifies leaving the double-lumen tube in place postoperatively to allow improvement in clinical status prior to endotracheal tube exchange.

Double-lung Transplantation

Bilateral lung transplant is performed in the supine position, using a "clamshell" incision. The arms can be suspended on a padded bar above the patient or tucked at the sides. If the arms are suspended, care must be taken to avoid stretching the brachial plexi. These cases can also be performed via midline sternotomy. *En bloc* double-lung transplantation requires CPB, and a single-lumen endotracheal tube is sufficient. Bilateral sequential transplantation requires lung isolation, preferably via a double-lumen endotracheal tube. Bilateral sequential transplantation is now the preferred procedure because a tracheal anastomosis is unnecessary, and there is less surgical bleeding. Most centers electively institute CPB for this procedure if preoperative pulmonary hypertension is present and urgent CPB if difficulties in oxygenation, ventilation, or RV function develop. Serial implantation implies longer ischemic time for the second lung, but this has not been shown to adversely affect outcome. In some institutions, sequential bilateral transplantation with CPB is performed using a double-lumen endobronchial tube, allowing immediate ventilation and oxygenation of the first transplanted lung while the second is being transplanted. In most institutions, the bronchial circulation is not re-established, so a transplanted lung on CPB does not receive oxygenated bronchial blood flow. Thus, ventilation of a newly transplanted lung with 50% oxygen, even during CPB, is advisable. The clamshell incision is extensive and can cause significant postoperative pain. Thoracic epidural may be very useful for managing postoperative pain.

Pediatric Lung Transplantation

The Registry of the International Society for Heart and Lung Transplantation Pediatric Report was last published in 2015.[185] Pediatric lung transplantation has increased over the past 15 years, with adolescents undergoing the majority of the procedures. One hundred and twenty-four pediatric lung transplants were reported worldwide in 2013, compared to only 73 in 1999. The most common diagnoses are CF, congenital heart disease, and idiopathic pulmonary hypertension. Overall survival is similar for pediatric and adult populations. There now appear to be age-related survival differences, with infants doing better than adolescents, but overall, survival is improving. An evaluation in 2007 of patients with CF listed for and/or receiving lung transplantation showed that only 1% of the patients showed a survival benefit from surgery.[186] However, a more recent study was more promising, with 5-year survival after transplant of 67%. Regardless of mortality outcome, quality of life still appears improved by lung transplantation in patients with CF. Efforts to quantify quality of life are ongoing.[174] The role of lung transplantation in treatment of CF deserves further study to determine optimal age, pretransplant diagnosis, status, and firm indications. Most pediatric patients receive double-lung transplantation with CPB, with a single-lumen endotracheal tube. The clamshell incision is used. Central and arterial access is necessary for perioperative monitoring.

Primary Graft Dysfunction (PGD)

The most common causes of acute transplanted lung failure are acute graft rejection, inadequate pulmonary venous drainage, and PGD. The etiology of PGD, a major cause of posttransplant morbidity and mortality, is multifactorial and complex.[187,188] PGD, defined as allograft dysfunction within 72 hours of transplantation, is graded on a scale of 0 to 3. Grade 3 is defined as Pa_{O_2}/F_{IO_2} less than 200 with radiographic infiltrates consistent with pulmonary edema. Grade 3 PGD is associated with statistically decreased 30-day mortality.[187] Grades 1 and 2 are also associated with infiltrates, but are less severe, with Pa_{O_2}/F_{IO_2} ratios greater than 300 and between 200 and 300, respectively. Grade 0 is essentially a normal lung, in which the PaO_2/FiO_2 ratio is greater than 300 and there are no pulmonary infiltrates. Possible contributing factors for PGD include prolonged organ ischemia time with ischemia/reperfusion injury, advanced donor age, recipient pulmonary hypertension, and the use of CPB. Specific anesthetic management factors have not emerged as a risk factor for PGD. To date there are no specific data to support a link between transfusion and PGD, although an association has been suspected. However, data are limited on transfusion during lung transplantation, in contradistinction to the data available on transfusion requirements during liver transplantation. Patients undergoing double-lung transplants or procedures with CPB or those with Eisenmenger syndrome or CF reportedly have increased transfusion requirements during lung transplantation. Further study is needed to determine whether transfusion negatively affects lung transplant outcomes. The transplant literature does not show a correlation between fluid management in the OR and outcome, although management of pulmonary transplant patients as if they have acute lung injury with a protective strategy as described earlier is recommended. Severe, life-threatening PGD has been successfully managed with extracorporeal membrane oxygenation (ECMO).[189]

Inhaled Nitric Oxide (iNO)

iNO therapy may be used to decrease PVR and improve oxygenation (see Chapter 38). iNO has an extremely short duration of action in vivo, rapidly inactivated by reacting with heme, resulting in methemoglobin. Because iNO is preferentially delivered to ventilated areas, vascular relaxation in these areas leads to improved blood flow and hence improvements in ventilation–perfusion matching and oxygenation. Rapid inactivation of iNO in the pulmonary vasculature prevents its systemic distribution and avoids systemic vasodilatation and hypotension.

Some anesthesiologists use iNO routinely for lung transplantation,[190] whereas others believe its potential adverse side effects should lead to restriction of its use.[191] Proponents argue that use of iNO in the recipient, and possibly even the donor, takes advantage of immunomodulatory and antimicrobial activities of NO that reduce recipient lung injury.[192] Opponents argue that iNO use should be limited to the population at risk for needing CPB during lung transplantation and to patients with reperfusion injury. They cite risks of methemoglobinemia, NO-metabolite–related lung injury, and decreased sensitivity of exhaled NO monitoring as a diagnostic tool for acute lung rejection. Some have suggested a prophylactic role for iNO, but the decision to use iNO should be based on specific clinical circumstances.[193] A randomized clinical trial of 30 patients undergoing double-lung transplant at an institution with high usage of CPB showed no benefit of prophylactic iNO in prevention of pulmonary edema.[194]

NO may mediate other clinically beneficial effects. NO activates guanylate cyclase in platelets to attenuate platelet aggregation and adhesion.[195] iNO can decrease PVR, improve oxygenation, decrease inflammatory response to surgery or trauma, impede microbial growth, and have a hemodynamic effect limited only to the pulmonary system. Its use in successful management of lung transplant patients is well documented.[196]

Heart–lung Transplant (Adult and Pediatric)

Heart–lung transplantation is the least common intrathoracic transplant procedure, with less than 40 per year currently being reported worldwide.[173] Bilateral sequential lung transplant has largely replaced heart–lung transplantation, and improved pharmacologic management of pulmonary hypertension and RV failure obviates the need for the heart–lung procedure. Because indications for lung transplantation have evolved to replace heart–lung transplant for diagnoses such as primary pulmonary hypertension and CF, congenital heart disease and idiopathic pulmonary hypertension are now the most common indications for heart–lung transplantation.[173] Pediatric heart–lung transplantation is now very infrequent, with only 11 performed in 2013.[185] Anesthetic management of heart–lung transplant patients is similar to that of isolated heart or lung transplant patients. Because a tracheal anastomosis is performed, a single-lumen endotracheal tube is sufficient. The endotracheal tube is either removed or withdrawn above the suture line during CPB to facilitate the tracheal anastomosis. Inotropes may be needed for RV dysfunction immediately after bypass. Pulmonary reperfusion injury can also occur, requiring management of acute lung injury as described for lung transplantation.

Heart Transplantation

Since Christian Barnard performed the first successful heart transplant in South Africa in 1967,[197] the procedure has become accepted practice for treatment of heart failure recalcitrant to medical therapy. Over 50,000 individuals have received heart transplants in the United States since 1988.[198] Unfortunately, more than 8,000 patients died while waiting for a donor during that time. Currently, more than 2,600 patients await heart transplants. Overall 1-year survival has improved from 74% in the early 1980s to 86% currently. The 5-year survival for primary transplantation is currently 72%. As our population ages and the use of cardiac transplantation and mechanical assist devices expands, increasing numbers of patients will present for transplantation, management of previous transplantation, or mechanical assist devices. In this section, anesthetic considerations for patients undergoing heart transplantation, as well as those with left ventricular assist devices (LVADs), are discussed.

Left Ventricular Assist Devices

Survival rates for patients with congestive heart failure (CHF) remain poor, despite improvements in medical therapy. One-year survival has been reported to be approximately 63%, with 5-year survival as low as 20%.[199] Patients with end-stage heart failure who have mechanical cardiac support experience better survival and quality of life than those receiving medical management alone.[200] Anesthesiologists often see heart failure patients for both initial device placement and perioperative management of LVADs. LVADs assist the heart by withdrawing blood from the failing left ventricle (inflow cannula in the left ventricle or left atrium) and pumping it into the aorta or femoral artery (outflow cannula) (Fig. 52-3). LVADs vary in significant ways, and it is important to understand the specifics of the LVAD being used. Variations include flow pattern (pulsatile or nonpulsatile), requirement for anticoagulation (none, aspirin, warfarin), filling pattern, power source (battery or alternating current), potential for electromagnetic interference, and impact of dysrhythmias and defibrillation on the device. Acetone-containing products and Betadine should be avoided near these devices because they can damage the cannula or drive lines.

LVAD pump flow is affected by intravascular volume and afterload. Failure to maintain adequate preload or afterload will result in decreased LVAD flow and hypotension because of low

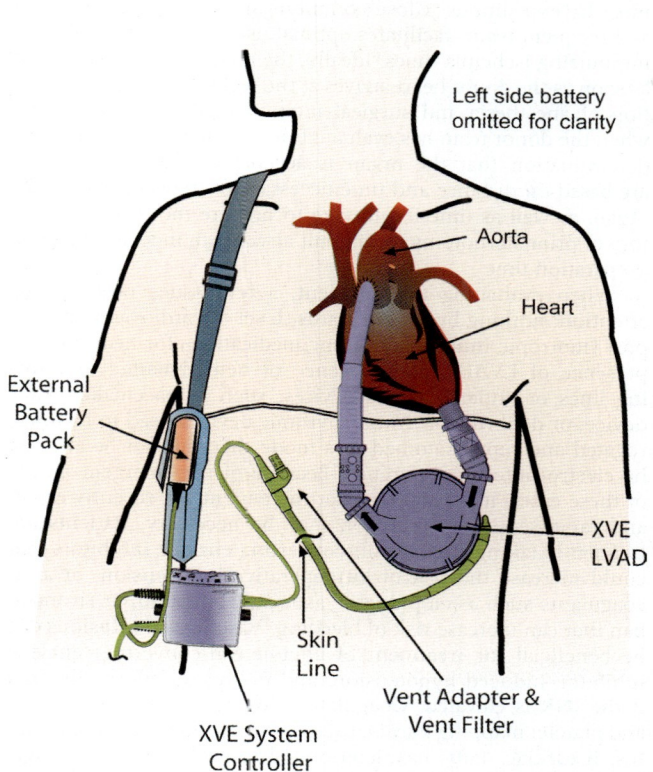

Figure 52-3 Implanted HeartMate XVE, an intracorporeal left ventricular assist device. An inflow cannula is in the left ventricle, and an outflow cannula is in the aorta. The prosthetic left ventricle (pump) propels blood from the left ventricle to the aorta, offloading some or all of the demand on the left ventricle. The cannulas and pump are within the patient, and the controller, drive line, and battery pack are external. (Courtesy of Thoratec Corp, Pleasanton, CA.)

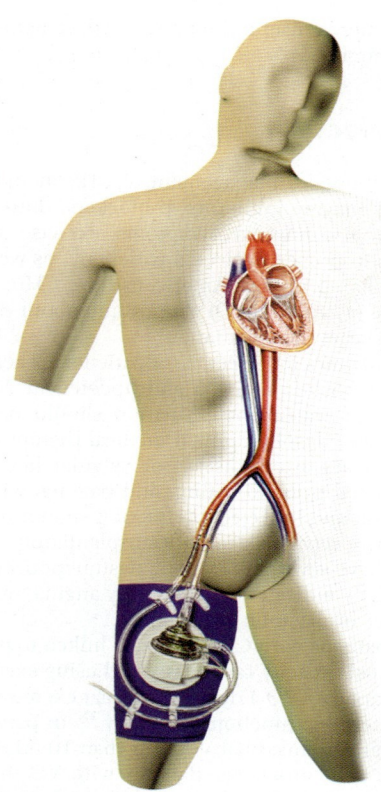

Figure 52-4 TandemHeart percutaneous ventricular assist device. Cannulas are placed percutaneously into the femoral vein and femoral artery, and the drive mechanism and power supply are external. The femoral venous line is placed across the atrial septum so as to drain the left atrium. Minimally invasive placement is a significant advantage of this system. (Courtesy TandemLife, Inc.)

functional cardiac output (LVAD flow plus native heart cardiac output). An individual familiar with the device should be present to assist with management and troubleshooting if the clinician does not have sufficient experience. Patients presenting for initial device placement are in various stages of decompensated heart failure and require advanced monitoring, often with an arterial line and either PA or central venous catheter. TEE is indicated to evaluate for valve pathologies and intracardiac shunts, which may complicate LVAD placement. TEE examination is repeated after device placement to confirm proper cannula placement and flow. These patients will likely need inotropic support until institution of CPB and device placement. Many clinicians advocate standard placement of TEE with central venous access. These facilitate perioperative management of volume status, assessment of forward flow, and administration of vasoactive medications.

LVADs are placed for rescue therapy, bridge to transplantation, and destination therapy. Most patients will show significant hemodynamic improvement with an LVAD, but some patients require support of the right ventricle via a right ventricular assist device or biventricular assist device. The TandemHeart (Cardiac Assist Inc., Pittsburgh, PA) is a percutaneous ventricular assist device usually placed in a cardiac catheterization laboratory. The indications are short-term hemodynamic support for patients in cardiogenic shock or temporary support of a patient undergoing high-risk percutaneous intervention. The left-sided cannula is advanced from the femoral vein into the left atrium by puncturing the interatrial septum (Fig. 52-4). The Abiomed options (Abiomed, Inc., Danvers, MA) are commonly used for postcardiotomy failure via direct cannulation. The chest is left open, and the cannulas can be left in place for up to 2 weeks. The Thoratec device (Thoratec Corporation, Pleasanton, CA) is an implanted device that can be used for long-term biventricular support. The HeartMate devices (Thoratec) are currently approved as therapy for patients with intractable heart failure who are not candidates for transplantation (destination therapy).

The most common conditions leading to transplantation are ischemic and idiopathic cardiomyopathies. Less common diagnoses include valvular heart disease, retransplant, and congenital heart disease.[198] Because of the limited availability of donor organs, technologies that can extend the life of patients awaiting donors have been developed. For transplants performed in 2009 to 2013, 40% of recipients were receiving intravenous inotropic support and 49% were receiving mechanical circulatory support.[198] In addition, cardiac resynchronization therapy (CRT) has been shown to reduce morbidity and mortality in patients with LV systolic dysfunction, prolonged QRS duration, and New York Heart Association Class III or IV heart failure despite optimal pharmacologic therapy.[201] Many patients presenting for heart transplantation have had a CRT device placed as part of their management, frequently with implantable cardioverter–defibrillator capability as well. Totally implantable artificial hearts are not currently in clinical use; however, their development is an active area of research.

Recipient Selection

Pharmacologic options for management of CHF include angiotensin-converting enzyme inhibitors, β-blockers, diuretics, and digoxin. CRT can also improve symptoms, exercise tolerance, and quality of life in properly selected patients,[202] as well as survival.[203,204] More than 5 million Americans have CHF, with the incidence increasing with age. Of these, only about 3,000 per year are listed for heart transplantation.

Consensus guidelines for selection of patients for heart transplantation were published in 2006 and updated in 2016.[205,206] Patients referred for transplant evaluation should have Class III or IV heart failure despite optimal medical therapy. Surgical correction of coronary artery disease or valvular heart disease should be considered prior to listing, and patients with severe mitral regurgitation and low ejection fraction should be considered for mitral valve repair instead of transplantation. Although most candidates have severe LV systolic dysfunction, transplantation is occasionally indicated for refractory angina, unmanageable dysrhythmias, or diastolic heart failure.

Prognosis in patients with CHF has been linked to functional capacity. Functional capacity can be assessed using exercise testing, and oxygen uptake (VO_2) during maximal exercise is a useful method to determine functional capacity.[207] In patients on a stable medical regimen, maximal VO_2 less than 10 mL/kg/min is associated with a poor prognosis. Patients with VO_2 more than 10 mL/kg/min have a better 1-year prognosis with medical therapy than transplantation.

Severe, irreversible pulmonary hypertension is a contraindication to transplant because of subsequent RV failure in the transplanted heart. Right heart catheterization is performed to determine transpulmonary gradient (the difference between mean PA pressure and pulmonary capillary wedge pressure) and pulmonary arteriolar resistance. Transpulmonary gradient above 12 mmHg indicates significant pathology. Pulmonary arteriolar resistance (the ratio of transpulmonary gradient to cardiac output, expressed as Wood units) greater than 2.5 also indicates a high risk of perioperative RV failure. Patients with elevated transpulmonary gradient or pulmonary arteriolar resistance require a trial with nitroprusside, prostacyclin, dobutamine, or milrinone in an attempt to decrease pulmonary resistance. Patients unresponsive to these therapies are often considered too high a risk for transplantation and may be candidates for LVAD or biventricular assist device insertion as definitive, destination therapy.

Contraindications to cardiac transplantation include some significant noncardiac diseases.[206] Because immunosuppressive agents have renal and hepatic side effects, the presence of intrinsic renal or hepatic disease increases perioperative risk of organ dysfunction or failure. Some patients with multiorgan disease can be considered for combined heart–kidney or heart–liver transplantation. Patients with forced expiratory volume in 1 second (FEV_1) less than 50% predicted despite optimal management of CHF are at increased risk for ventilatory failure and respiratory infections posttransplant. The presence of significant atherosclerosis is a contraindication because of the increased perioperative risk of atheroembolic complications.

Preanesthetic Considerations

Donor heart function worsens with donor cold ischemia times above 6 hours. For this reason, timing of transplantation depends on when the donor surgery can be done, frequently during night hours. Preoperative evaluation and preparation of the patient must be expeditious. Close communication between the donor and recipient teams facilitates optimal use of donor organs while minimizing ischemia times. Ideally, the recipient heart is excised as soon as the donor heart arrives at the recipient hospital. Induction of anesthesia and surgical incision of the recipient begin when the donor team has evaluated the donor and made the final determination that the organ is acceptable. Timing decisions are based on distance and time necessary to transport the donor organ, as well as time it will take to prepare the recipient. History of prior sternotomy or difficult airway can increase recipient preparation time.

When evaluating the recipient, a few issues need special attention: nothing by mouth status, level of cardiovascular support (inotropic infusions, chronic medications for heart failure, presence of LVAD), and presence of hemodynamic monitoring lines or antiarrhythmic devices, such as pacemaker, CRT device, or defibrillator. Antiarrhythmic devices need to be interrogated and reprogrammed to a mode that will not be affected by electrocautery interference. Because of the emergent nature of these cases, it is common that the patient has recently eaten, and rapid-sequence induction may be necessary. Patients are frequently taking angiotensin-converting enzyme inhibitors that could increase the risk of intraoperative hypotension, or anticoagulants such as clopidogrel, aspirin, Coumadin, or rivaraxaban that can increase risk of bleeding. Vasopressin infusions can be beneficial for treatment of angiotensin-converting enzyme inhibitor–induced hypotension, and plasma should be ordered if the INR is elevated. Coagulation function testing with TEG and platelet mapping may be useful in managing coagulation status. If cardiac status has deteriorated recently, the patient may be receiving infusions of inotropes, such as dobutamine or milrinone. On occasion, patients are receiving chronic dobutamine or milrinone therapy as outpatients. If patients have had multiple central lines, ultrasound evaluation of the central vessels may be helpful to determine vessel patency. Recent chest radiographs and laboratory studies must be reviewed to assess pulmonary, hepatic, and renal compromise associated with CHF.

Many anesthetic management issues related to the heart transplant patient are similar to those for open-heart surgeries (see Chapter 39). The notable differences are strictest attention to sterility and immunosuppression, poorer hemodynamic status of transplant candidates, and issues related to early donor heart function and denervation. The surgical team will request antibiotics specific to donor and recipient infection patterns, and immunosuppressive medications are often given prior to incision.

Placement of a PAC is favored by many centers. Invasive arterial pressure monitoring should be used during anesthetic induction. Large-bore intravenous access, central or peripheral, is necessary for administration of resuscitation medications and volume during induction. Inotropes should be readily available prior to induction. Dobutamine, epinephrine, milrinone, norepinephrine, dopamine, vasopressin, and phenylephrine have all been used effectively in the perioperative management of heart transplant patients.

Presence of an LVAD or prior sternotomy increases the length and the risks associated with the procedure. Where possible, old medical records should be reviewed to determine if the patient had prior aprotinin exposure. EACA or tranexamic acid can be used as an antifibrinolytic agent to decrease perioperative bleeding. Packed red blood cells should be immediately available prior to incision, particularly in repeat sternotomy. CMV status of the donor and recipient is needed to determine whether

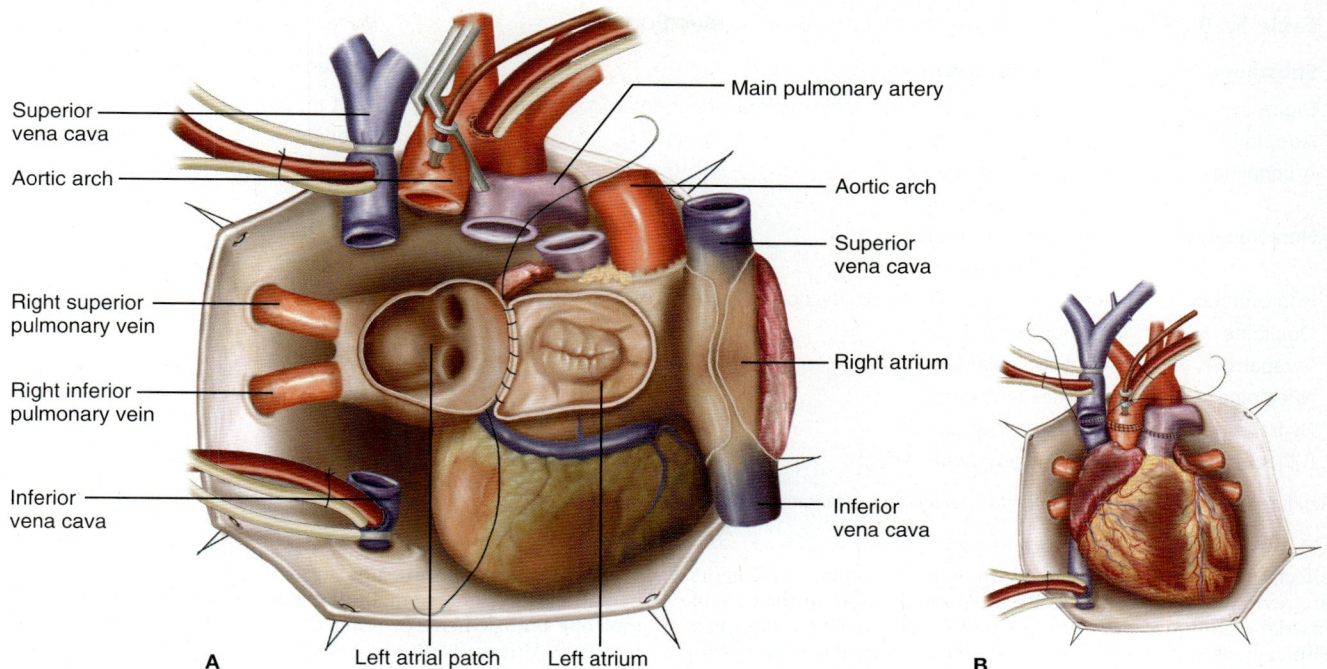

Figure 52-5 Anatomy of bicaval orthotopic heart transplant. **A:** A recipient left atrial patch including the four pulmonary veins remains in the recipient. Anastomoses are performed at the superior and inferior venae cavae, aorta, pulmonary artery, and left atrium. **B:** The completed transplantation. (Modified from Lima B, Gonzalez-Stawinski GV. Heart transplants: bicaval versus biatrial techniques. In: Grover FL, Mack MJ, eds. *Master Techniques in Surgery: Cardiac Surgery*. Philadelphia, PA: Wolters Kluwer; 2016:409–418.)

CMV-negative packed red blood cells should be ordered. Availability of plasma, platelets, and cryoprecipitate should be confirmed at the start of the procedure.

Intraoperative Management

Anesthetic induction in patients with poor ventricular function can be complicated by hemodynamic instability. Instituting or increasing inotrope infusions can be beneficial in these cases. Choice of anesthetic technique should be focused on minimizing cardiovascular instability and complications. High-dose narcotic techniques have been used for induction and management of cardiac transplant patients for many years with good results.[208] Balanced anesthetic techniques, using lower doses of narcotics, and inhalation anesthetics, can be used,[209] and early extubation using ultra fast-track protocols has been successful.[210] Neuromuscular blockade with a nondepolarizing agent is recommended. Hypotension may not respond to ephedrine or phenylephrine, and other inotropes and vasopressors such as epinephrine and vasopressin should be instituted rapidly in such cases.

A comprehensive TEE examination should be performed after induction of anesthesia and after weaning from CPB. The native heart can be monitored prior to CPB for changes in ventricular function or an increase in valvular regurgitation. Early diagnosis of deterioration can facilitate rapid therapy and hemodynamic stability. The risk of intracardiac thrombus is increased in the recipient heart. The left atrium and ventricle should be carefully examined. Surgical manipulation of the heart is minimized prior to aortic cross-clamping if thrombus is noted.

Median sternotomy is performed for orthotopic heart transplantation. After initiation of CPB, the recipient heart is excised, except for the left atrial tissue encompassing the pulmonary veins. In the classic biatrial approach, the atria are transected at the grooves, and there are right and left atrial anastomoses, along with PA and aortic anastomoses. The bicaval approach (Fig. 52-5), in which anastomoses are created in the superior and inferior vena cavae rather than the right atrium, is gaining popularity because it preserves tricuspid valve function and normal conduction in the right atrium.[211] A meta-analysis revealed benefits of the bicaval technique, so this technique is now performed frequently.[212]

Heparin dosing is similar to that for other CPB procedures. Cannulation of the aorta is performed high along the ascending aorta, near the aortic arch. The superior and inferior venae cavae are cannulated individually. By encircling the cavae with tourniquets, all blood flow is directed through the cannula in to the bypass circuit, and the surgical field is bloodless. Prior to resection of the native heart, the PAC should be withdrawn from the surgical field. The catheter can be readvanced after removal of the superior cava cannula. Maintenance of CPB and weaning from CPB are associated with the same issues as for other cardiac surgical procedures. Ischemic time for the donor heart starts with aortic cross-clamping during the harvest and ends with removal of the cross-clamp from the recipient aorta. Air should be evacuated prior to weaning from CPB.

Prior to weaning from CPB, the heart is reevaluated with TEE, with attention to ventricular and valvular function. Intracardiac shunts should be ruled out. Because the donor heart is denervated, normal physiologic feedback controlling inotropy and chronotropy are lost. Isoproterenol is used frequently for its direct effects on cardiac β-receptors to increase graft heart rate. Use of temporary epicardial pacing is sometimes needed until isoproterenol has had adequate time to reach maximal

Table 52-9 Effect of Denervation on Cardiac Pharmacology

Substance	Effect on Recipient	Mechanism
Digitalis	Normal increase of contractility, minimal effect on atrioventricular node	Direct myocardial effect, denervation
Atropine	None	Denervation
Adrenaline	Increased contractility Increased chronotropy	Denervation hypersensitivity
Noradrenaline	Increased contractility Increased chronotropy	Denervation No neuronal uptake
Isoproterenol	Normal increase in contractility, normal increase in chronotropy	
Quinidine	No vagolytic effect	Denervation
Verapamil	Atrioventricular block	Direct effect
Nifedipine	No reflex tachycardia	Denervation
Hydralazine	No reflex tachycardia	Denervation
β-Blocker	Increased antagonist effect	Denervation

Reprinted with permission from Deng MC. Cardiac transplantation. *Heart*. 2002;287:177.

effect. (Vasoactive drug effects in heart transplant recipients are reviewed in Table 52-9.) Residual atrial tissue, in the case of biatrial technique, may continue to have electrical activity, seen clinically as two P waves on ECG (one from native atrial tissue, one from donor). The native P wave has no physiologic effects on the donor heart.

Inotrope selection for weaning from CPB is similar to other cardiac surgical procedures (see Chapter 39). Special consideration should be given to recipients with preoperative pulmonary hypertension, donor hearts with long ischemic times, or donor hearts that are deemed marginal. The risk of donor right heart failure is increased in these cases. The donor right heart is not accustomed to high pulmonary resistance and may fail acutely. Therapy for graft right heart failure is similar to therapy for right heart failure in other cardiac cases. The goal is to improve contractility and decrease PVR. If intravenous agents do not facilitate weaning from CPB, iNO and inhaled prostacyclin (iloprost) have been shown to be beneficial in this population.[213–216]

Pediatric Heart Transplantation

UNOS reports over 5,000 pediatric heart transplants performed since 1988; 60% are performed in children less than 1 year or over 11 years old. The pretransplant diagnosis was congenital heart disease or idiopathic/viral cardiomyopathy in 75% of these patients, with retransplantation an increasing indication. The annual volume of pediatric cardiac transplantations reported to the International Society of Heart and Lung Transplantation is increasing, with a record 577 reported in 2013.[217] ECMO is used as a bridge to transplant at some centers, although it is acknowledged to be only a short-term option.[218] Even though ECMO is the therapeutic choice for circulatory support in most pediatric cardiac patients, some pediatric patients (mostly adolescents) benefit from placement of a ventricular assist device.[219]

Preoperative evaluation focuses on cardiopulmonary status and the particulars of the cardiac physiology in congenital heart disease patients (see Chapter 39). Palliative procedures may have been performed prior to transplant, and reoperation increases surgical risk. Central venous catheters and intra-arterial catheters are placed routinely, usually after induction. After an inhalation induction, anesthetic management frequently involves high-dose narcotics and intermittent benzodiazepines.

Marginal donors are, not surprisingly, also being used for pediatric heart grafts, including size mismatches, high donor inotrope requirement, prolonged ischemic time, and ABO mismatch.[220] Although ABO-incompatible transplantation is contraindicated in the adult population, it is more successful in infant recipients.[221,222] Hyperacute rejection does not occur because of the immaturity of the immune system and absence of antibodies to various antigens, including blood group antigens. For ABO mismatched grafts, recipient isohemagglutinin titers are obtained pretransplantation, then plasma exchange is performed during CPB. Four-year follow-up data show similar morbidity and mortality compared with ABO-compatible recipients. Furthermore, waiting list survival is improved because of expansion of the donor pool.

Management of the Transplant Patient for Nontransplant Surgery

As the population of transplant recipients increases, the incidence of elective or emergent nontransplant surgery becomes more commonplace. These patients cannot always return to the transplant center for surgery, so anesthesiologists outside transplant centers will encounter these patients. For solid-organ recipients, evaluation of patients is centered on the function of the grafted organ. In renal and liver transplant patients, the level of renal dysfunction will often determine the choice of drugs such as antibiotics, particularly neuromuscular blockers, and dose modification of drugs is dependent on renal excretion. Table 52-4 lists medications that can cause renal dysfunction when administered to a patient receiving immunosuppressive agents. A major consideration for renal transplant recipients is maintenance of renal perfusion with adequate volume replacement. Thus, CVP monitoring is useful for preventing prerenal damage to transplanted kidneys, but CVP lines must be placed using strict aseptic technique. It is important to note that signs of infection may be masked in transplant patients. Failing, rejecting, or reinfected liver grafts are often accompanied by deterioration of renal function. Protection of the kidneys is a central part of anesthesia plans, and CVP or TEE is useful to guide fluid replacement, especially in cases where large fluid shifts are anticipated.

13 For all transplant recipients, antibiotic, antiviral, antifungal, and immune suppression regimens should be disrupted as little as possible in the perioperative period. The types of infection to which transplant recipients are susceptible change over time, with donor-derived and hospital-acquired infections predominating in the first posttransplant month.[223] Infections acquired by transplant patients in months 2 to 6 versus later after transplantation are also distinct, and these patterns should guide surgical prophylaxis and perioperative diagnostic procedures. Infectious disease specialists are important consultants for preoperative transplant patients.

Complications of immune suppression are reviewed in Table 52-4. Significant intraoperative fluid shifts can cause an acute decrease in cyclosporine or tacrolimus blood levels. In these cases, consideration should be given to repeat testing of drug levels during the day of surgery. Nonsteroidal anti-inflammatory medications should be avoided for a number of reasons. First, many patients have underlying renal dysfunction related to immunosuppressive agents. Second, the risk of gastrointestinal hemorrhage is increased in patients already at risk for gastritis from chronic steroids.

Patients who present for surgery with signs of acute rejection or infection may benefit from delay of surgery to optimize their status. Both rejection and infection in the face of surgery are associated with increased risk of morbidity and mortality. Regional and general anesthetic techniques have been used successfully in posttransplant patients. In addition to the standard American Society of Anesthesiology monitors, invasive monitors should be used if warranted based on surgical procedure and general health status of the patient. Invasive monitoring is not indicated solely on the basis of prior transplantation. Nasal intubation should be avoided because of the potential risk for infection presented by nasal flora.

Virtually all liver diseases can recur in grafted livers, including autoimmune diseases, fatty liver, and hepatitis C. The degree of liver dysfunction from recurrent disease should be evaluated by hepatologists and by using standard laboratory tests.

For lung transplant recipients with a tracheal anastomosis, denervation has occurred below the level of the suture line, and the cough reflex is diminished or absent. These patients are at increased risk of retained secretions and pneumonia and have an increased airway hyperreactivity and bronchospasm. Because most lung transplants are now being done with bronchial instead of tracheal anastomoses, the risk of tracheal suture line stenosis or disruption with manipulation is markedly diminished. Advantages of regional anesthetic techniques in lung transplant patients include minimization of airway manipulation and decreased infectious risk. Comparison of preoperative PFT, arterial blood gas, and chest x-ray results with prior studies can help diagnose acute infection or rejection. Significant decreases in forced expiratory volume in 1 second, vital capacity, and total lung capacity and an obstructive pattern may indicate acute rejection. Arterial blood gas in the presence of rejection will show an increased alveolar–arterial gradient from stable baseline gases, along with perihilar infiltration on chest x-ray. However, rejection and infection can be difficult to distinguish clinically. If the patient is suspected of having an active pulmonary process, consultation with Pulmonary Medicine for a possible diagnostic bronchoscopy should be considered prior to surgery.

Transplanted hearts are denervated, affecting perioperative management significantly. The transplanted heart cannot respond to indirect acting agents, such as ephedrine and even dopamine, or to peripheral attempts to induce hemodynamic changes, such as carotid massage, Valsalva maneuver, or laryngoscopy. β-Receptor effects of epinephrine and norepinephrine are exaggerated in heart transplant recipients (versus α effects). Isoproterenol is the mainstay of chronotropic therapy in these patients. ECG analysis may show two P waves, one from the native atrium and one from the implanted atrium. The native P wave will not conduct to the implanted heart, and these nonconducted P waves should not be confused with complete heart block. Isoproterenol should be available as an inotrope and a chronotrope. Dobutamine can also be helpful; norepinephrine and epinephrine should be reserved for refractory cardiogenic shock. Because the denervated heart does not reflexively compensate for hemodynamic changes induced by regional anesthetics, general anesthesia is usually preferred.

Preoperative evaluation of heart transplant recipients should focus on cardiac functional status. Significant rejection will present with symptoms of heart failure. All heart transplant patients should be evaluated with ECG and transthoracic echocardiography prior to surgery. New findings should be discussed with the cardiology consultant to determine need for stress testing or myocardial biopsy. Invasive monitors should be placed only when warranted by the clinical status and surgical procedure. Use of TEE, CVP, or minimally invasive cardiac output monitoring such as esophageal Doppler or arterial pulse wave cardiac output can be helpful in managing fluids and inotropic support.

REFERENCES

1. Kotloff KM, Blosser S, Fulda GJ, et al. Management of the potential organ donor in the ICU: Society of Critical Care Medicine/American College of Chest Physicians/Association of Organ Procurement Organizations Consensus Statement. *Crit Care Med*. 2015;43:1291–1325.
2. A definition of irreversible coma. Report of the Ad Hoc Committee of the Harvard Medical School to Examine the Definition of Brain Death. *JAMA*. 1985;205:337–340.
3. Nijboer WN, Schuurs TA, van der Hoeven JA, et al. Effect of brain death and donor treatment on organ inflammatory response and donor organ viability. *Curr Opin Organ Transpl*. 2004;9:110.
4. Belzberg H, Shoemaker WC, Wo CC, et al. Hemodynamic and oxygen transport patterns after head trauma and brain death: implications for management of the organ donor. *J Trauma*. 2007;63:1032–1042.
5. Novitzky D, Cooper DK, Rosendale JD, et al. Hormonal therapy of the brain-dead organ donor: experimental and clinical studies. *Transplantation*. 2006;82:1396–1401.
6. Rosendale JD, Kauffman HM, McBride MA, et al. Aggressive pharmacologic donor management results in more transplanted organs. *Transplantation*. 2003;75:482–487.
7. Pinsard M, Ragot S, Mertes PM, et al. Interest of low-dose hydrocortisone therapy during brain-dead organ donor resuscitation: the CORTICOME study. *Crit Care*. 2014;18(4):R158.
8. Kim WR, Biggins SW, Kremers WK, et al. Hyponatremia and mortality among patients on the liver-transplant waiting list. *N Engl J Med*. 2008;359:1018–1026.
9. Callahan DS, Neville A, Bricker S, et al. The effect of arginine vasopressin on organ donor procurement and lung function. *J Surg Res*. 2014;186:452–457.
10. Plurad DS, Bricker S, Neville A, et al. Arginine vasopressin significantly increases the rate of successful organ procurement in potential donors. *Am J Surg*. 2012; 204:856–860.
11. Piazza O, Scarpati G, Rispoli F, et al. Terlipressin in brain-death donors. *Clin Transplant*. 2012;26:E571–E575.
12. Olmos A, Feiner J, Hirose R, et al. Impact of a quality improvement project on deceased organ donor management. *Prog Transplant*. 2015;25:351–360.
13. McKeown DW, Bonser RS, Kellum JA. Management of the heartbeating brain-dead organ donor. *Br J Anaesth*. 2012;108(S1):i96.
14. Mascia L, Pasero D, Slutsky AS, et al. Effect of a lung protective strategy for organ donors on eligibility and availability of lungs for transplantation: a randomized controlled trial. *JAMA*. 2010;304:2620–2627.
15. Selzner N, Boehnert M, Selzner M. Preconditioning, postconditioning, and remote conditioning in solid organ transplantation: basic mechanisms and translational applications. *Transplant Rev*. 2012;26:115.
16. Ardehali A, Hughes K, Sadeghi A, et al. Inhaled nitric oxide for pulmonary hypertension after heart transplantation. *Transplantation*. 2001;72:638–641.
17. Schnuelle P, Gottmann U, Hoeger S, et al. Effects of donor pretreatment with dopamine on graft function after kidney transplantation: a randomized controlled trial. *JAMA*. 2009;302:1067–1075.
18. Orens JB, Boehler A, Perrot M, et al. A review of lung transplant donor criteria. *J Heart Lung Transplant*. 2003;22:1183–1200.
19. Baldwin MR, Peterson ER, Easthausen I, et al. Donor age and early graft failure after lung transplantation: a cohort study. *Am J Transplant*. 2013;13:2685–2695.

20. Sekine Y, Waddell TK, Matte-Martyn A, et al. Risk quantification of early outcome after lung transplantation: donor, recipient, operative, and post-transplant parameters. *J Heart Lung Transpl.* 2004;23:96–104.
21. Klein AS, Messersmith EE, Ratner LE, et al. Organ donation and utilization in the United States, 1999–2008. *Am J Transplant.* 2010;10(Pt 2):973–986.
22. Meyer KC, Love RB, Zimmerman JJ. The therapeutic potential of nitric oxide in lung transplantation. *Chest.* 1998;113:1360–1371.
23. Chaney J, Suzuki Y, Cantu E III, et al. Lung donor selection criteria. *J Thorac Dis.* 2014;6:1032–1038.
24. Committee on Hospital Care, Section on Surgery, and Section on Critical Care, AAP. Policy statement: pediatric organ donation and transplantation. *Pediatrics.* 2010;125:822–828.
25. Das A, Anderson IM, Speicher DG, et al. Validation of a pediatric bedside tool to predict time of death after withdrawal of life support. *World J Clin Pediatr.* 2016;5:89–94.
26. LaMattina JC, Mezrich JD, Fernandez LA, et al. Simultaneous liver and kidney transplantation from donation after cardiac death donors: a brief report. *Liver Transpl.* 2011;17:591–595.
27. Cao Y, Shahrestani S, Chew HC, et al. Donation after circulatory death for liver transplantation: a meta-analysis on the location of life support withdrawal affecting outcomes. *Transplantation.* 2016;100:1513–1524.
28. Lentine KL, Lam NN, Axelrod D, et al. Perioperative complications after living kidney donation: a national study. *Am J Transpl.* 2015;16:1848–1857.
29. Waits SA, Hilliard P, Sheetz KH, et al. Building the case for enhanced recovery protocols in living kidney donors. *Transplantation.* 2015;99:405–408.
30. Biancofiore G, Amorese G, Lugli D, et al. Laparoscopic live donor nephrectomy: the anaesthesiologist's perspective. *Eur J Anaesthesiol.* 2004;21:74–76.
31. Mertens zur Borg IR, Di Biase M, Verbrugge S, et al. Comparison of three perioperative fluid regimes for laparoscopic donor nephrectomy: a prospective randomized dose-finding study. *Surg Endosc.* 2008;22:146–150.
32. Feldman LS, Anidiar M, Metrakos P, et al. Optimization of cardiac preload during laparoscopic donor nephrectomy: a preliminary study of central venous pressure versus esophageal Doppler monitoring. *Surg Endosc.* 2004;18:412–416.
33. El-Galley R, Hammontree L, Urban D, et al. Anesthesia for laparoscopic donor nephrectomy: Is nitrous oxide contraindicated? *J Urol.* 2007;178:225.
34. Haberal M, Emirolu R, Arslan G, et al. Living-donor nephrectomy under combined spinal-epidural anesthesia. *Transplant Proc.* 2002;34:2448–2449.
35. Owen M, Lorgelly P, Serpell M. Chronic pain following donor nephrectomy: a study of the incidence, nature and impact of chronic post-nephrectomy pain. *Eur J Pain.* 2010;14:732–734.
36. Fetracco P, Ori C. Anesthetic management of living transplantation. *Minerva Anestesiol.* 2010;76:525–533.
37. Goldaracena N, Spetzler VN, Marquez M, et al. Live donor liver transplantation: a valid alternative for critically ill patients suffering from acute liver failure. *Am J Transplant.* 2015;15:1591–1597.
38. Clavien PA, Petrowski H, DeOliveira ML, et al. Strategies for safer liver surgery and partial liver transplantation. *N Engl J Med.* 2007;356:1545–1559.
39. Muzaale AD, Dagher NN, Montgomery RA, et al. Estimates of early death, acute liver failure, and long-term mortality among live liver donors. *Gastroenterology.* 2012;142:273–280.
40. Azzam A, Uryuhara K, Taka I, et al. Analysis of complications in hepatic right lobe living donors. *Ann Saudi Med.* 2010;30:18–24.
41. Wadhawan M, Kumar A. Mangement issues in post living donor liver transplant biliary strictures. *World J Hepatol.* 2016;8:461–470.
42. Beebe D, Singh H, Jochan J, et al. Anesthetic complications including two cases of postoperative respiratory depression in living liver donor surgery. *J Anaesth Clin Pharmacol.* 2011;27:362.
43. Kim SH, Kim YK, Lee SD, et al. The impact of a surgical protocol for enhanced recovery on living donor right hepatectomy: a single-center cohort study. *Medicine (Balt)* 2016;95:e3227.
44. Eyraud D, Richard O, Borie DC, et al. Hemodynamic and hormonal responses to the sudden interruption of caval flow: insights from a prospective study of hepatic vascular exclusion during major liver resections. *Anesth Analg.* 2002;95:1173–1178.
45. Rhim CH, Johnson LB, Kitisin K, et al. Intra-operative isovolemic hemodilution is safe and effective in eliminating allogeneic blood transfusion during right hepatic lobectomy: comparison of living donor versus non-donors. *HPB (Oxf).* 2005;7:201.
46. Clarke H, Chandy T, Srinivas C, et al. Epidural analgesia provides better pain management after live liver donation: a retrospective study. *Liver Transpl.* 2011;17:315–323.
47. Khan J, Katz J, Montbriand J, et al. Surgically placed abdominal wall catheters on postoperative analgesia and outcomes after living liver donation. *Liver Transpl.* 2015;21:478–486.
48. Cauchy F, Schwarz L, Scatton O, et al. Laparoscopic liver resection for living donation: where do we stand? *World J Gastroenterol.* 2014;20:15590.
49. Nafidi O, Lepage R, Lapointe RW, et al. Hepatic resection-related hypophosphatemia is of renal origin as manifested by isolated hyperphosphaturia. *Ann Surg.* 2007;245:1000–1002.
50. Trotter JF, Gillespie BW, Terrault NA, et al. Adult-to-Adult Living Donor Transplantation Cohort Study Group: laboratory test results after living liver donation in the adult-to-adult living donor liver transplantation cohort study. *Liver Transpl.* 2011;17:409–417.
51. Axelrod D, Naik AS, Schnitzler MA, et al. National variation in use of immunosuppression for kidney transplantation: a call for evidence-based regimen selection. *Am J Transplant.* 2016;16:2453–2462.
52. Panther F, Strasen J, Czolbe M, et al. Inhibition of nuclear translocation of calcineurin suppresses T-cell activation and prevents acute rejection of donor hearts. *Transplantation.* 2011;91:597–604.
53. Kostopanagiotou G, Smyrniotis V, Arkadopoulos N, et al. Anesthetic and perioperative management of adult transplant recipients in nontransplant surgery. *Anesth Analg.* 1999;89:613.
54. De Weerdt A, Claeys KG, De Jonghe P, et al. Tacrolimus-related polyneuropathy: case report and review of the literature. *Clin Neurol Neurosurg.* 2008;110(3):291–294.
55. Wu Q, Marescaux C, Wolff V, et al. Tacrolimus-associated posterior reversible encephalopathy syndrome after solid organ transplantation. *Eur Neurol.* 2010;64:169–177.
56. Sidi A, Kaplan RF, Davis RF. Prolonged neuromuscular blockade and ventilatory failure after renal transplantation and cyclosporine. *Can J Anaesth.* 1990;37:543–548.
57. Crosby E, Robblee JA. Cyclosporine-pancuronium interaction in a patient with a renal allograft. *Can J Anaesth.* 1998;35:300–302.
58. Scarfia RV, Dlementi A, Granata A. Rhabdomyolysis and acute kidney injury secondary to interaction between simvastatin and cyclosporine. *Ren Fail.* 2013;35:1056–1057.
59. Kato T, Gaynor JJ, Yoshida H, et al. Randomization trial of steroid-free induction versus corticosteroid maintenance among orthotopic liver transplant recipients with hepatitis C virus: impact on hepatic fibrosis progression at one year. *Transplantation.* 2007;84:829.
60. Ippoliti G, Lucioni M, Leonardi G, et al. Immunomodulation with rabbit anti-thymocyte globulin in solid organ transplantation. *World J Transplant.* 2015;5:261–266.
61. Boothpur R, Hardinger KL, Skelton RM, et al. Serum sickness after treatment with rabbit anti-thymocyte globulin in kidney transplant recipients with previous rabbit exposure. *Am J Kidney Dis.* 2010;55:141–143.
62. Tanriover B, Chuang P, Fishback B, et al. Polyclonal antibody-induced serum sickness in renal transplant recipients: treatment with therapeutic plasma exchange. *Transplantation.* 2005;80:279–281.
63. ten Berge IJ, Parlevliet KJ, Raasveld MH, et al. Guidelines for the optimal use of muromonab CD3 in transplantation. *BioDrugs.* 1999;11:277–284.
64. Bamgbola FO, Del Rio M, Kaskel FJ, et al. Non-cardiogenic pulmonary edema during basiliximab induction in three adolescent renal transplant patients. *Pediatr Transplant.* 2003;7:31–37.
65. Webster AC, Ruster LP, McGee R, et al. Interleukin 2 receptor antagonists for kidney transplant recipients. *Cochrane Database Syst Rev.* 2010;20:CD003897.
66. Klipa D, Mahmud N, Ahsan N. Antibody immunosuppressive therapy in solid organ transplant: part II. *MAbs.* 2010;2:607–612.
67. Farid SG, Barwick J, Goldsmith PJ. Alemtuzumab (Campath-1H)-induced coagulopathy in renal transplantation. *Transplantation.* 2009;87:1751–1752.
68. Barten MJ, Streit F, Boeger M, et al. Synergistic effects of sirolimus with cyclosporine and tacrolimus: analysis of immunosuppression on lymphocyte proliferation and activation in rat whole blood. *Transplantation.* 2004;77:1154–1162.
69. Tsunoda SM, Aweeka FT. Drug concentration monitoring of immunosuppressive agents: focus on tacrolimus, mycophenolate mofetil and sirolimus. *BioDrugs.* 2000;14:355–369.
70. Jungling AS, Shangraw RE. Massive airway edema after azathioprine. *Anesthesiology.* 2000;92:888–890.
71. Engelen W, Verpooten GA, Van der Planken M, et al. Four cases of red blood cell aplasia in association with the use of mycophenolate mofetil in renal transplant patients. *Clin Nephrol.* 2003;60:119–124.
72. Perez-Aytes A, Ledo A, Boso V, et al. In utero exposure to mycophenolate mofetil: a characteristic phenotype? *Am J Med Genet A.* 2008;146:1–7.
73. Le Blanc K, Frassoni F, Ball L, et al. Mesenchymal stem cells for treatment of steroid-resistant, severe, acute graft-versus-host disease: a phase II study. *Lancet.* 2008;371:1579–1586.
74. Guerrier G, Boutboul D, Rondet S, et al. Comparison of a supraglottic gel device and an endotracheal tube in keratoplasty performed under general anesthesia: a randomized clinical trial. *Cornea.* 2016;35:37–40.
75. Massie AB, Leanza J, Fahmy LM, et al. A risk index for living donor kidney transplantation. *Am J Transpl.* 2016;16:2077–2084.
76. Stoumpos S, Jardine AG, Mark PB. Cardiovascular mobidity and mortality after kidney transplantation. *Transpl Int.* 2015;28:10–21.
77. Dieterle CD, Schmauss S, Arbogast H, et al. Pulmonary function in patients with type 1 diabetes before and after simultaneous pancreas and kidney transplantation. *Transplantation.* 2007;83:566–569.
78. Bunnapradist S, Danovitch GM. Evaluation of adult kidney transplant candidates. *Am J Kidney Dis.* 2007;7:2333.

79. Snoeijs MG, Winkens B, Heemskerk MB, et al. Kidney transplantation from donors after cardiac death: a 25-year experience. *Transplantation.* 2010;90:1106–1112.
80. Summers DM, Watson CJ, Pettigrew GJ, et al. Kidney donation after circulatory death (DCD): state of the art. *Kidney Int.* 2015;88:241–249.
81. Stewart DE, Kucheryavaya AY, Klassen DK, et al. Changes in deceased donor kidney transplantation one year after KAS allocation implementation. *Am J Transplant.* 2016;16:1834–1847.
82. Ricaurte L, Vargas J, Lozano E, et al. Anesthesia and kidney transplantation. *Transplant Proc.* 2013;45:1386–1391.
83. Spiro MD, Eilers H. Intraoperative care of the transplant patient. *Anesthesiol Clin.* 2013;31:705–721.
84. Goyal P, Puri GD, Pandey CK, et al. Evaluation of induction doses of propofol: comparison between end stage renal disease and normal renal function patients. *Anaesth Intensive Care.* 2002;30:584–587.
85. Robertson EN, Driessen JJ, Vogt M, et al. Pharmacodynamics of rocuronium 0.3 mg kg (−1) in adult patients with and without renal failure. *Eur J Anaesthesiol.* 2005;22:929–932.
86. Fisher DM, Dempsey GA, Atherton DP, et al. Effect of renal failure and cirrhosis on the pharmacokinetics and neuromuscular effects of rapacuronium administered by bolus followed by infusion. *Anesthesiology.* 2000;93:1384–1391.
87. Koehntop DE, Rodman JH. Fentanyl pharmacokinetics in patients undergoing kidney transplantation. *Pharmacotherapy.* 1997;17:746–752.
88. Olyaei AJ, deMattos AM, Bennett WM. A practical guide to the management of hypertension in renal transplant recipients. *Drugs.* 1999;58:1011–1027.
89. Hadimioglu N, Saadawy I, Saglam T, et al. The effect of different crystalloid solutions on acid-base balance and early kidney function after kidney transplantation. *Anesth Analg.* 2008;107:264–269.
90. Parekh J, Niemann CU, Dang K, et al. Intraoperative hyperglycemia augments ischemia reperfusion injury in renal transplantation: a prospective study. *J Transplant.* 2011;2011:652458.
91. Wiesbauer F, Heinze G, Regele H, et al. Glucose control is associated with patient survival in diabetic patients after renal transplantation. *Transplantation.* 2010;89:612–619.
92. Sorbello M, Morello G, Paratore A, et al. Fenoldopam vs dopamine as a nephroprotective strategy during living donor kidney transplantation: preliminary data. *Transplant Proc.* 2007;39:1794–1796.
93. Nichols WG, Price TH, Gooley T, et al. Transfusion-transmitted cytomegalovirus infection after receipt of leukoreduced blood products. *Blood.* 2003;101:4195–4200.
94. Parada B, Figueiredo A, Mota A et al. Surgical complications in 1000 renal transplants. *Transplant Proc.* 2003;35:1085–1086.
95. Ammi M, Daligault M, Sayegh J, et al. Evaluation of the vascular surgical complications of renal transplantation. *Ann Vasc Surg.* 2016;33:23–30.
96. Shoeibi G, Babakhani B, Mohammadi SS. The efficacy of ilioinguinal-iliohypogastric and intercostals nerve co-blockage for postoperative pain relief in kidney recipients. *Anesth Analg.* 2009;108:330–333.
97. Mukhtar K, Khattak I. Transversus abdominis plane block for renal transplant recipients. *Br J Anaesth.* 2010;104:663–664.
98. Masaitis-Zagaiewska A, Pietrasik P, Krawczyk J, et al. Similar prevalence but different characteristics of pain in kidney transplant recipients and chronic hemodialysis patients. *Clin Transplant.* 2011;25:E144–E151.
99. Healey PJ, McDonald R, Waldhausen JH, et al. Transplantation of adult living donor kidneys into infants and small children. *Arch Surg.* 2000;135:1035–1041.
100. Halazun KJ, Mathur AK, Rana AA, et al. One size does not fit all: regional variation in the impact of the Share 35 liver allocation policy. *Am J Transpl.* 2016;16:137–142.
101. Kim WR, Biggins SW, Kremers WK, et al. Hyponatremia and mortality among patients on the liver-transplant waiting list. *N Engl J Med.* 2008;359:1018–1026.
102. Freeman RB Jr, Wiesner RH, Harper A, et al; UNOS/OPTN Liver Disease Severity Score, UNOS/OPTN Liver and Intestine, and UNOS/OPTN Pediatric Transplantation Committees. The new liver allocation system: moving toward evidence-based transplantation policy. *Liver Transpl.* 2002;8:851–858.
103. Roland ME, Barin B, Huprikar S, et al. Survival in HIV-positive transplant recipients compared with transplant candidates and with HIV-negative controls. *AIDS.* 2016;30:435–444.
104. VanWagner LB, Lapin B, Levitsky J, et al. High early cardiovascular mortality following liver transplantation. *Liver Transpl.* 2014;20:1306–1316.
105. Ye C, Saincher M, Tandon P, et al. Cardiac work-up protocol for liver transplant candidates: experience from a single liver transplant centre. *Can J Gastroent.* 2012; 26:806–810.
106. Kumar N, Dahri L, Brown W, et al. Effect of elective coronary angiography on glomerular filtration rate in patients with advanced chronic kidney disease. *Clin J Am Soc Nephrol.* 2009;4:1907–1913.
107. Carey EJ, Steidley DE, Aqel BA, et al. Six-minute walk distance predicts mortality in liver transplant candidates. *Liver Transpl.* 2010;16:1373–1378.
108. Coss E, Watt KD, Pedersen R, et al. Predictors of cardiovascular events after liver transplantation: a role for pretransplant troponin levels. *Liver Transpl.* 2011;17:23–31.
109. Paramesh AS, Fairchild RB, Quinn TM, et al. Amelioration of hypertrophic cardiomyopathy using nonsurgical septal ablation in a cirrhotic patient prior to liver transplantation. *Liver Transpl.* 2005;11:236.
110. Van Wagner LB, Serper M, Kang R, et al. Factors associated with major adverse cardiovascular events after liver transplantation among a national sample. *Am J Transplant.* 2016;16:2684–2694.
111. Ashfaq M, Chinnakotla S, Rogers L, et al. The impact of treatment of portopulmonary hypertension on survival following liver transplantation. *Am J Transplant.* 2007;7:1258–1264.
112. Melgosa MT, Ricci GL, Garcia-Pagan JC, et al. Acute and long-term effects of inhaled iloprost in portopulmonary hypertension. *Liver Transpl.* 2010;16:348–356.
113. Makisalo H, Koivusalo A, Vakkuri A, et al. Sildenafil for portopulmonary hypertension in a patient undergoing liver transplantation. *Liver Transpl.* 2004;10:945–950.
114. Savale L, Magnier R, Le Pavec J, et al. Efficacy, safety and pharmacokinetics of bosentan in portopulmonary hypertension. *Eur Respir J.* 2013;41:96–103.
115. Cartin-Ceba R, Swanson K, Iyer V, et al. Safety and efficacy of ambrisentan for the treatment of portopulmonary hypertension. *Chest.* 2011;139:109–114.
116. Tapper EB, Knowles D, Heffron T, et al. Portopulmonary hypertension: imatinib as a novel treatment and the Emory experience with this condition. *Transplant Proc.* 2009;41:1969–1971.
117. Ramsay MA. Portopulmonary hypertension and hepatopulmonary syndrome, and liver transplantation. *Int Anesthesiol Clin.* 2006;44:69–82.
118. Pastor CM, Schiffer E. Therapy insight: hepatopulmonary syndrome and orthotopic liver transplantation. *Nat Clin Pract Gastroenterol Hepatol.* 2007;4:614–621.
119. Fimiani B, Guardia DD, Puoti C, et al. The use of terlipressin in cirrhotic patients with refractory ascites and normal renal function: a multicentric study. *Eur J Intern Med.* 2011;22:587–590.
120. Wang LS, D'Souza LS, Jacobson IM. Hepatitis C: a clinical review. *J Med Virol.* 2016;88:1844–1855.
121. Chapron B, Risler L, Phillips B, et al. Reversible, time-dependent inhibition of CYP3A-mediated metabolism of midazolam and tacrolimus by telaprevir in human liver microsomes. *J Pharm Pharm Sci.* 2015;18:101–111.
122. Hsu AJ, Carson KA, Yung R, et al. Severe prolonged sedation associated with coadministration of protease inhibitors and intravenous midazolam during bronchoscopy. *Pharmacotherapy.* 2012;32:538–545.
123. Verne GN, Soldevia-Pico C, Robinson ME, et al. Autonomic dysfunction and gastroparesis in cirrhosis. *J Clin Gastroenterol.* 2004;38:72–76.
124. De Pietri L, Mocchegiani F, Leuzzi C, et al. Transoesophageal echocardiography during liver transplantation. *World J Hepatol.* 2015;7:2432–2448.
125. Pai SL, Aniskevich S, Feinglass NG, et al. Complications related to intraoperative transesophageal echocardiography in liver transplantation. *Springerplus.* 2015;4:480.
126. Massicotte L, Lenis S, Thibeault L, et al. Effect of low central venous pressure and phlebotomy on blood product transfusion requirements during liver transplantations. *Liver Transpl.* 2006;12:117–123.
127. Bernardi M, Ricci CS, Zaccherini G. Role of albumin in the management of complications of cirrhosis. *J Clin Exp Hepatol.* 2014;4:302–311.
128. de Boer MT, Christensen MC, Asmussen M, et al. Impact of intraoperative transfusion of platelet and red blood cells on survival after liver transplantation. *Anesth Analg.* 2008;106:32–44.
129. Chin JL, Hisamuddin SH, O'Sullivan A, et al. Thrombocytopenia, platelet transfusion, and outcome following liver transplantation. *Clin Appl Thromb Hemost.* 2016;22:351–360.
130. Ghadimi K, Levy JH, Welsby IJ. Prothrombin complex concentrates for bleeding in the perioperative setting. *Anesth Analg.* 2016;122:1287–1300.
131. Tripoli A, Mannucci PM. The coagulopathy of chronic liver disease. *N Engl J Med.* 2011;365:147–156.
132. Northup PG, Caldwell SH. Coagulation in liver disease: a guide for the clinician. *Clin Gastroent Hepatol.* 2013;11:1064.
133. Nicolau-Raducu R, Ky TC, Ganier DR, et al. Epsilon-aminocaproic acid has no association with thromboembolic complications, renal failure, or mortality after liver transplantation. *J Cardiothorac Vasc Anesth.* 2016;30:917–923.
134. Porte RJ, Bontempo FA, Knot EA, et al. Systemic effects of tissue plasminogen activator-associated fibrinolysis and its relation to thrombin generation in orthotopic liver transplantation. *Transplantation.* 1989;47:978–984.
135. Scheffert JL, Taber DJ, Pilch NA, et al. Timing of factor VIIa in liver transplantation impacts cost and clinical outcomes. *Pharmacotherapy.* 2013;33: 483–488.
136. Boone JD, Sherwani SS, Herborn JC, et al. The successful use of low-dose recombinant tissue plasminogen activator for treatment of intracardiac/pulmonary thrombosis during liver transplantation. *Anesth Analg.* 2011;112: 319–321.
137. Caragata R, Wyssusek KH, Kruger P. Acute kidney injury following liver transplantation: a systematic review of published predictive models. *Anaesth Intensive Care.* 2016;44:251–261.
138. Sherman DS, Fish DN, Teitelbaum I. Assessing renal function in cirrhotic patients: problems and pitfalls. *Am J Kidney Dis.* 2003;41:269–278.

139. Levitsky J, O'Leary JG, Asrani S et al. Protecting the kidney in liver transplant recipients. *Am J Transplant.* 2016;16:2532–2544.
140. Guevara M, Arroyo V. Hepatorenal syndrome. *Expert Opin Pharmacother.* 2011;12:1405–1417.
141. Salerno F, Navickis RJ, Wilkes MM. Albumin treatment regimen for type 1 hepatorenal syndrome: a dose-response meta-analysis. *BMC Gastroenterol.* 2015;15:167.
142. Nassar Jr AP, Farias AQ, D'Albuquerque LA, et al. Terlipressin versus norepinephrine in the treatment of hepatorenal syndrome: a systematic review and meta-analysis. *PLos One.* 2014;9(9):e107466.
143. Angeli P, Volpin R, Gerunda G, et al. Reversal of type 1 hepatorenal syndrome with the administration of midodrine and octreotide. *Hepatology.* 1999;29:1690–1697.
144. Aggarwal S, Kang Y, Freeman JA, et al. Postreperfusion syndrome: hypotension after reperfusion of the transplanted liver. *J Crit Care.* 1993;8:154–160.
145. Nahas GG, Sutin KM, Fermon C, et al. Guidelines for the treatment of acidaemia with THAM. *Drugs.* 1998;55:191–224.
146. Shillicutt SK, Ringenberg KJ, Chacon MM, et al. Liver transplantation: intraoperative transesophageal echocardiography findings and relationship to major postoperative adverse cardiac events. *J Cardiothorac Vasc Anesth.* 2016;30:107.
147. Hosseinian L, Weiner M, Levin MA, et al. Methylene blue: magic bullet for vasoplegia? *Anesth Analg.* 2016;122:194–201.
148. Lang JD Jr, Teng X, Chumley P, et al. Inhaled NO accelerates restoration of liver function in adults following orthotopic liver transplantation. *J Clin Invest.* 2007;117:2583–2591.
149. Beck-Schimmer B, Bonvini JM, Schadde E, et al. Conditioning with sevoflurane in liver transplantation: results of a multicenter randomized controlled trial. *Transplantation.* 2015;99(8):1606–1612.
150. Abuelkasem E, Lu S, Tanaka K, et al. Comparison between thromboelastography and thromboelastometry in hyperfibrinolysis detection during adult liver transplantation. *Br J Anaesth.* 2016;116:507–512.
151. Taner CB, Willingham DL, Bulatao IG, et al. Is mandatory intensive care unit stay needed after liver transplantation? Feasibility of fast-tracking to the surgical ward after liver transplantation. *Liver Transpl.* 2012;18:361.
152. Wagenaar AE, Tashiro J, Sola JE, et al. Pediatric liver transplantation: predictors of survival and resource utilization. *Paediatr Surg Int.* 2016;32:439–449.
153. Guttman OR, Roberts EA, Schreiber RA, et al. Biliary atresia with associated structural malformations in Canadian infants. *Liver Int.* 2011;31:1485–1493.
154. Nemes B, Gaman G, Polak WG, et al. Extended-criteria donors in liver transplantation. Part II: reviewing the impact of extended-criteria donors on the complications and outcomes of liver transplantation. *Expert Rev Gastroenterol Hepatol.* 2016;10:841–859.
155. Karvellas CJ, Fix OK, Battenhouse H, et al. Outcomes and complications of intracranial pressure monitoring in acute liver failure: a retrospective cohort study. *Crit Care Med.* 2014;42:1157–1167.
156. Aggarwal S, Brooks DM, Kang Y, et al. Noninvasive monitoring of cerebral perfusion pressure in patients with acute liver failure using transcranial Doppler untrasonography. *Liver Transp.* 2008;14:1048.
157. Karvellas CJ, Stravitz RT, Battenhouse H, et al., for the US Acute liver Failure Study Group. Therapeutic hypothermia in acute liver failure: a multicenter retrospective cohort analysis. *Liver Transplant.* 2015;21:4.
158. Kandiah PA, Olson JC, Subramanian RM. Emerging strategies for the treatment of patients with acute hepatic failure. *Curr Opin Crit Care.* 2016;22:142–151.
159. Lidofsky SD, Bass NM, Prager MC, et al. Intracranial pressure monitoring and liver transplantation for fulminant hepatic failure. *Hepatology.* 1992;16:1–7.
160. Schnickel GT, Busuttil RW, Lipshutz GS. Improvement in short-term pancreas transplant outcome by targeted antimicrobial therapy and refined donor selection. *Am Surg.* 2011;77:1407–1411.
161. Markmann JF, Bartlett ST, Johnson P, et al. Executive summary of IPITS-TTS opinion leaders report on the future of B-cell replacement. *Transplantation.* 2016;100:e25–e31.
162. Farney AC, Sutherland DE, Opara EC. Evolution of islet transplantation for the last 30 years. *Pancreas.* 2016;45:8–20.
163. Boyle ME, Seifert KM, Beer KA, et al. Insulin pump therapy in the perioperative period: a review with careful implementation of institutional guidelines. *J Diabetes Sci Technol.* 2012;6:1016–1021.
164. Shapiro AM, Lakey JR, Ryan EA, et al. Islet transplantation in seven patients with type 1 diabetes mellitus using a glucocorticoid-free immunosuppressive regimen. *N Engl J Med.* 2000;343:230–238.
165. Boluda ER. Pediatric small bowel transplantation. *Curr Opin Organ Transplant.* 2015;20:550–556.
166. Mims TT, Fishbein TM, Feierman DE. Management of a small bowel transplant with complicated central venous access in a patient with asymptomatic superior and inferior vena cava obstruction. *Transplant Proc.* 2004;36:388–391.
167. Rege A, Sudan D. Intestinal transplantation. *Best Pract Res Clin Gastroenterol.* 2016;30:319–335.
168. Dalal A. Intestinal transplantation: the anesthesia perspective. *Transplant Rev (Orlando).* 2016;30:100–108.
169. Lang RS, Gorantla VS, Esper S, et al. Anesthetic management in upper extremity transplantation: the Pittsburgh experience. *Anesth Analg.* 2012;115:678–688.
170. Schneeberger S, Gorantla VS, Brandacher G, et al. Upper-extremity transplantation using a cell-based protocol to minimize immunosuppression. *Ann Surg.* 2013;257:345–351.
171. Chandraker A, Arscott R, Murphy GF, et al. The management of antibody-mediated rejection in the first presensitized recipient of a full-face allotransplant. *Am J Transplant.* 2014;14:1446–1452.
172. Reitz BA, Wallwork JL, Hunt SA, et al. Heart-lung transplantation: successful therapy for patients with pulmonary vascular disease. *N Engl J Med.* 1982;306:557–564.
173. Yusen RD, Edwards LB, Kucheryavaya AY, et al. The Registry of the International Society for Heart and Lung Transplantation: thirty-second Official Adult Lung and Heart-Lung Transplantation Report—2015. Focus theme: early graft failure. *J Heart Lung Transplant.* 2015;34:1264–1277.
174. Orens JB, Garrity ER Jr. General overview of lung transplantation and review of organ allocation. *Proc Am Thorac Soc.* 2009;6:13–19.
175. Orens JB, Estenne M, Arcasoy S, et al. International guidelines for the selection of lung transplant candidates: 2006 update. A consensus report from the Pulmonary Scientific Council of the International Society for Heart and Lung Transplantation. *J Heart Lung Transplant.* 2006;25:745.
176. Egan TM, Murray S, Bustami RT, et al. Development of the new lung allocation system in the United States. *Am J Transplant.* 2006;6:1212–1227.
177. Hadjiliadis D, Steele MP, Chaparro C, et al. Survival of lung transplant patients with cystic fibrosis harboring panresistant bacteria other than Burkholderia cepacia, compared with patients harboring sensitive bacteria. *J Heart Lung Transplant.* 2007;26:834–838.
178. Cypel M, Yeung JC, Liu M, et al. Normothermic ex vivo lung perfusion in clinical lung transplantation. *N Engl J Med.* 2011;364:1431–1440.
179. Tikkanen JM, Cypel M, Machuca TN, et al. Functional outcomes and quality of life after normothermic ex vivo lung perfusion lung transplantation. *J Heart Lung Transplant.* 2015;34:547–556.
180. Tan M, Law LS, Gan TJ. Optimizing pain management to facilitate Enhanced Recovery After Surgery pathways. *Can J Anaesth.* 2015;62:203–218.
181. Myles PS, Leslie K, McNeil J, et al. Bispectral index monitoring to prevent awareness during anaesthesia: the B-Aware randomised controlled trial. *Lancet.* 2004;363:1757–1763.
182. National Heart, Lung, and Blood Institute Acute Respiratory Distress Syndrome (ARDS) Clinical Trials Network, Wiedemann HP, Wheeler AP, et al. Comparison of two fluid-management strategies in acute lung injury. *N Engl J Med.* 2006;354:2564–2575.
183. Pilcher DV, Scheinkestel CD, Snell GI, et al. High central venous pressure is associated with prolonged mechanical ventilation and increased mortality after lung transplantation. *J Thorac Cardiovasc Surg.* 2005;129:912–918.
184. Oto T, Griffiths AP, Rosenfeldt F, et al. Early outcomes comparing Perfadex, Euro-Collins, and Papworth solutions in lung transplantation. *Ann Thorac Surg.* 2006;82:1842–1848.
185. Goldfarb SB, Benden C, Edwards LB, et al. The Registry of the International Society for Heart and Lung Transplantation: Eighteenth Official Pediatric Lung and Heart-Lung Transplantation Report—2015. Focus theme: early graft failure. *J Heart Lung Transplant.* 2015;34:1255–1263.
186. Liou TG, Adler FR, Cox DR, et al. Lung transplantation and survival in children with cystic fibrosis. *N Engl J Med.* 2007;357:2143–2152.
187. Barr ML, Kawut SM, Whelan TP, et al. Report of the ISHLT Working Group on Primary Lung Graft Dysfunction. Part IV: recipient-related risk factors and markers. *J Heart Lung Transplant.* 2005;24:1468–1482.
188. Christie JD, Van Raemdonck D, de Perrot M, et al. Report of the ISHLT Working Group on Primary Lung Graft Dysfunction. Part I: introduction and methods. *J Heart Lung Transplant.* 2005;24:1451–1453.
189. Oto T, Rosenfeldt F, Rowland M, et al. Extracorporeal membrane oxygenation after lung transplantation: evolving technique improves outcomes. *Ann Thorac Surg.* 2004;78:1230–1235.
190. Lang JD Jr, Lell W. Pro: inhaled nitric oxide should be used routinely in patients undergoing lung transplantation. *J Cardiothorac Vasc Anesth.* 2001;15:785–789.
191. McQuitty CK. Con: Inhaled nitric oxide should not be used routinely in patients undergoing lung transplantation. *J Cardiothorac Vasc Anesth.* 2001;15:790.
192. Meyer KC, Love RB, Zimmerman JJ. The therapeutic potential of nitric oxide in lung transplantation. *Chest.* 1998;113:1360–1371.
193. Griffiths MJ, Evans TW. Inhaled nitric oxide therapy in adults. *N Engl J Med.* 2005;353:2683–2695.
194. Perrin G, Roch A, Michelet P, et al. Inhaled nitric oxide does not prevent pulmonary edema after lung transplantation measured by lung water content: a randomized clinical study. *Chest.* 2006;129:1024.
195. Beghetti M, Sparling C, Cox PN, et al. Inhaled NO inhibits platelet aggregation and elevates plasma but not intraplatelet cGMP in healthy human volunteers. *Am J Physiol Heart Circ Physiol.* 2003;285:H637.
196. Cornfield DN, Milla CE, Haddad IY, et al. Safety of inhaled nitric oxide after lung transplantation. *J Heart Lung Transplant.* 2003;22:903.
197. Barnard CN. The operation. A human cardiac transplant: an interim report of a successful operation performed at Groote Schuur Hospital, Cape Town. *S Afr Med J.* 1967;41:1271.

198. Lund LH, Edwards LB, Kucheryavaya AY, et al. The Registry of the International Society for Heart and Lung Transplantation: Thirty-Second Official Adult Heart Transplantation Report—2015. Focus theme: early graft failure. *J Heart Lung Transplant.* 2015;34:1244–1254.
199. Goldberg RJ, Ciampa J, Lessard D, et al. Long-term survival after heart failure: a contemporary population-based perspective. *Arch Intern Med.* 2007;167:490.
200. Rose EA, Gelijns AC, Moskowitz AJ, et al. Long-term use of a left ventricular assist device for end-stage heart failure. *N Engl J Med.* 2001;345:1435–1443.
201. McAlister FA, Ezekowitz J, Hooton N, et al. Cardiac resynchronization therapy for patients with left ventricular systolic dysfunction: a systematic review. *JAMA.* 2007;297:2502–2514.
202. Seidl K, Rameken M, Vater M, et al. Cardiac resynchronization therapy in patients with chronic heart failure: pathophysiology and current experience. *Am J Cardiovasc Drugs.* 2002;2:219–226.
203. Goldenberg I, Kutyifa V, Klein HU, et al. Survival with cardiac-resynchronization therapy in mild heart failure. *N Engl J Med.* 2014;370:1694–1701.
204. Cleland JG, Freemantle N, Erdmann E, et al. Long-term mortality with cardiac resynchronization therapy in the Cardiac Resynchronization-Heart Failure (CARE-HF) trial. *Eur J Heart Fail.* 2012;14:628–634.
205. Mehra MR, Kobashigawa J, Starling R, et al. Listing criteria for heart transplantation: International Society for Heart and Lung Transplantation guidelines for the care of cardiac transplant candidates—2006. *J Heart Lung Transplant.* 2006;25:1024.
206. Mehra MR, Canter CE, Hannan MM, et al. The 2016 International Society for Heart Lung Transplantation listing criteria for heart transplantation: a 10-year update. *J Heart Lung Transplant.* 2016;35:1–23.
207. Fleg JL, Pina IL, Balady GJ, et al. Assessment of functional capacity in clinical and research applications: an advisory from the Committee on Exercise, Rehabilitation, and Prevention, Council on Clinical Cardiology, American Heart Association. *Circulation.* 2000;102:1591–1597.
208. Hensley FA Jr, Martin DE, Larach DR, et al. Anesthetic management for cardiac transplantation in North America—1986 survey. *J Cardiothorac Anesth.* 1987;1:429–437.
209. Demas K, Wyner J, Mihm FG, et al. Anaesthesia for heart transplantation: a retrospective study and review. *Br J Anaesth.* 1986;58:1357–1364.
210. Kianfar AA, Ahmadi ZH, Mirhossein SM, et al. Ultra fast-track extubation in heart transplant surgery patients. *Int J Crit Illn Inj Sci.* 2015;5:89–92.
211. Cheng A, Slaughter MS. Heart transplantation. *J Thorac Dis.* 2014;6:1105–1109.
212. Schnoor M, Schafer T, Luhmann D, et al. Bicaval versus standard technique in orthotopic heart transplantation: a systematic review and meta-analysis. *J Thorac Cardiovasc Surg.* 2007;134:1322–1331.
213. Ardehali A, Hughes K, Sadeghi A, et al. Inhaled nitric oxide for pulmonary hypertension after heart transplantation. *Transplantation.* 2001;72:638–641.
214. Mosquera I, Crespo-Leiro MG, Tabuyo T, et al. Pulmonary hypertension and right ventricular failure after heart transplantation: usefulness of nitric oxide. *Transplant Proc.* 2002;34:166–167.
215. Rajek A, Pernerstorfer T, Kastner J, et al. Inhaled nitric oxide reduces pulmonary vascular resistance more than prostaglandin E(1) during heart transplantation. *Anesth Analg.* 2000;90:523–530.
216. Sablotzki A, Czeslick E, Schubert S, et al. Iloprost improves hemodynamics in patients with severe chronic cardiac failure and secondary pulmonary hypertension. *Can J Anaesth.* 2002;49:1076–1080.
217. Dipchand AI, Rossano JW, Edwards LB, et al. The Registry of the International Society for Heart and Lung Transplantation: Eighteenth Official Pediatric Heart Transplantation Report—2015. Focus theme: early graft failure. *J Heart Lung Transplant.* 2015;34:1233–1243.
218. Burch M, Aurora P. Current status of paediatric heart, lung, and heart-lung transplantation. *Arch Dis Child.* 2004;89:386–389.
219. Fynn-Thompson F, Almond C. Pediatric ventricular assist devices. *Pediatr Cardiol.* 2007;28:149–155.
220. Conway J, Chin C, Kemna M, et al. Donors' characteristics and impact on outcomes in pediatric heart transplant recipients. *Pediatr Transplant.* 2013;17:774–781.
221. Kohler S, Engmann R, Birnbaum J, et al. ABO-compatible retransplantation after ABO-incompatible infant heart transplantation: absence of donor specific isohemagglutinins. *Am J Transplant.* 2014;14:2903–2905.
222. Irving CA, Gennery AR, Carter V, et al. ABO-incompatible cardiac transplantation in pediatric patients with high isohemagglutinin titers. *J Heart Lung Transplant.* 2015;34:1095–1102.
223. Fishman JA. Infection in solid-organ transplant recipients. *N Engl J Med.* 2007;357:2601–2614.

53 Trauma and Burns

LEVON M. CAPAN • SANFORD M. MILLER • COREY SCHER

Initial Evaluation and Resuscitation
  Airway Evaluation and Intervention
  Management of Breathing Abnormalities
  Management of Shock
Early Management of Specific Injuries
  Head Injury
  Spine and Spinal Cord Injury
  Neck Injury
  Chest Injury
  Abdominal and Pelvic Injuries
  Extremity Injuries

  Burns
Operative Management
  Monitoring
  Anesthetic and Adjunct Drugs
  Management of Intraoperative Complications
Early Postoperative Considerations
  Ventilatory Support
  Acute Kidney Injury
  Abdominal Compartment Syndrome
  Thromboembolism

KEY POINTS

1. Airway management is tailored to the type of injury, the nature and degree of airway compromise, and the patient's hemodynamic and oxygenation status.
2. Generally diagnosis of suspected cervical spine injury is reliably done for most patients by thin cut multidetector computed tomography scanning.
3. Generally it is reasonable to allow some relaxation of the manual inline stabilization of the cervical spine to improve the glottic view when visualization of the larynx is restricted.
4. A linear correlation exists between the rib score and development of pneumonia, acute respiratory failure, and need for tracheostomy.
5. A systolic blood pressure of 110 mmHg is accepted as a prehospital triage threshold for delivery to a Level I trauma center for trauma patients older than 65 years; systolic blood pressure of 90 mmHg remains a triage threshold for young patients.
6. The method of resuscitation of the hemorrhaging patient has changed since the Iraq and Afghanistan wars. The concept of damage control resuscitation has replaced the classic crystalloid resuscitation.
7. Damage control resuscitation consists of brief permissive hypotension; rapid control of any bleeding source; minimal crystalloid infusion; early administration of plasma and other blood products in a balanced ratio (preferably 1:1:1) of packed red blood cells, plasma, and platelets by activation of the massive transfusion protocol; early administration of tranexamic acid; and, if indicated, damage control surgery to control bleeding and sources of contamination. Definitive surgery is deferred until after normalization of the patient's physiologic condition.
8. Management strategies in the diagnosis and treatment of blunt aortic injuries have gone through major changes in the past 10 years with substantially improved early outcomes. In the area of diagnosis, computed tomography angiography replaced aortography, and, in the area of treatment, endovascular stenting practically replaced open repair, although in grade 3 or 4 blunt aortic injuries, open repair in the form of mostly "clamp and saw" technique is done.
9. Clinically, burn injury is manifested in two phases: burn shock, which is characterized by continued plasma loss from the intravascular space into burned, and often into intact, tissues for about the first day or two after injury, and the subsequent hypermetabolic or hyperdynamic phase, which may last for months.
10. In burn-injured patients, intravascular volume should be restored with utmost care to prevent excessive edema formation in both damaged and intact tissues which results from the generalized increase in capillary permeability caused by the injury. Edema from overaggressive resuscitation has many deleterious and potentially life-threatening effects.
11. Of the many resuscitation formulas available, the Parkland (Baxter) and modified Brooke formulas are tailored to the clinical condition of the patient and are accepted in most centers. Parkland formula uses crystalloid whereas Brooke formula uses combination of crystalloid and colloid during the first 24 hours. The addition of glucose is not necessary except in children, especially those weighing less than 20 kg. Albumin 5% may be administered after the first day following injury at a rate of 0.3, 0.4, or 0.5 mL/kg/24 hours for burns of 30% to 50%, 50% to 70%, or 70% to 100% of total body surface area, respectively. These formulas are guidelines only, and none can be expected to provide adequate restoration of intravascular volume in all burn victims, especially small children and patients with inhalation injuries.
12. Traditionally, monitoring of fluid therapy for burn injury is limited to hourly urine output, heart rate, systemic blood pressure, and base deficit. Indeed, there is some evidence to suggest that hourly monitoring of urine output as an end point of resuscitation compared to sophisticated hemodynamic monitoring provides similar outcomes in terms of mortality, organ function, length of hospital or intensive care stay, duration of mechanical ventilation, and burn-related complications such as pulmonary edema, compartment syndromes, or infection.

13. The transthoracic echocardiography (TTE) technique most commonly used in the trauma setting involves obtaining images through the subcostal long axis, subcostal inferior vena cava, parasternal long axis, parasternal short axis, and apical four-chamber windows. Placement of a phased-array, low-frequency (5 to 2 MHz) probe in these locations provides ideal views that are sufficient to inform the clinician of an underlying hemodynamic problem. TTE can be used in the emergency department, operating room, or intensive care unit and provides rapid information about the etiology of hypotension or other hemodynamic complications.

14. Unrecognized hypoperfusion may lead to splanchnic ischemia with resulting acidosis in the intestinal wall, permitting the passage of luminal microorganisms into the circulation and release of inflammatory mediators, causing sepsis and multiorgan failure. Base deficit and blood lactate level are considered acceptable markers of organ hypoperfusion in the *apparently* resuscitated patient and may be used intraoperatively to set the optimal end points of resuscitation.

15. Although trauma center laboratories cannot provide results of the standard coagulation tests rapidly, at least international normalized ratio can be monitored with a point-of-care device and provide some information. Thromboelastography and rotation transmission electron microscopy are point-of-care devices that provide a relatively rapid, comprehensive, and quantitative graphic evaluation of clotting function.

16. Anesthetic and adjunct drugs for general anesthesia need to be tailored to five major clinical conditions: airway compromise, hypovolemia, head or open eye injuries, cardiac injury, and burns. The varying contribution of these conditions to the clinical picture of a given patient necessitates priority-oriented planning.

17. Reducing or eliminating anesthesia to avoid abolishing the hemodynamic balance in hypovolemic patients is a natural and often utilized practice, especially when permissive hypotension, as part of damage control resuscitation, to limit bleeding is employed. This approach provides high pressure and low flow to the organs. Another concept, aggressive titrated administration of anesthetics and blood products to produce a high-flow and low-pressure hemodynamic state with vasodilation to improve organ flow and oxygenation and to reduce fibrinolytic activity and inflammation, has been proposed recently. Further research will determine the validity of these approaches.

18. Component transfusion therapy, used universally in civilian trauma, is inferior to the whole blood transfusion practiced by the military. During the preparation of platelets and fresh frozen plasma, 100 mL of nonhemostatic anticoagulants is put in each bag. This additional fluid lowers factor levels by 20%. Similarly 100 mL of solution is added to packed red blood cells for storage injury protection in addition to 100 mL of anticoagulant. During massive transfusion protocol, each blood product administered dilutes out the other two blood product components. Fresh frozen plasma will decrease the hematocrit and platelet count. Likewise, packed red blood cells lower coagulation factors and platelet counts. Thus a 1:1:1 ratio cannot be compared with whole blood in its hemostatic ability.

19. Death is a much greater threat during emergency trauma surgery than it is in any other operative procedure. Approximately 0.7% of patients admitted for acute trauma die in the OR, accounting for approximately 8% of postinjury deaths. Uncontrollable bleeding is the cause of approximately 80% of intraoperative mortality; brain herniation and air embolism are the most common causes of death in the remaining patients.

20. Recent advances in the management of acute trauma and critical care, such as limiting crystalloid infusion, hemostatic resuscitation, damage control, and open abdomen strategies, have substantially decreased the incidence of postinjury abdominal compartment syndrome.

Injury is responsible for 9% of the total annual mortality (more than 5 million people) in the world.[1] Traffic accidents alone killed 1.24 million people in 2010; almost half of the victims were pedestrians (22%), cyclists (5%), and motorcyclists (23%).[2] The death rate was higher in low- (18.3/100,000) and middle-income (20.1/100,000) countries than in high-income (8.7/100,000) countries. Homicide alone resulted in 475,000 deaths (6.7/100,000) in 2012, and violence, encompassing homicides, suicides, and war-related injuries, is estimated to kill about 1.5 million people every year in the world, of whom the vast majority reside in low- and middle-income countries.[3]

According to the National Trauma Institute, more than 192,000 people died as a result of trauma in the United States in 2014.[4] The National Safety Council[5] reported that intentional injuries (suicide, homicide, and assault) claimed 56,253 lives, unintentional (motor vehicle accidents, falls, drowning, poisoning, etc.) mortality claimed 126,438 lives, and additional undetermined injuries caused 4,773 deaths in 2011. Trauma especially afflicts young people; as of 2013 it was the leading cause of death for those aged between 1 and 46 years, and the third most common cause of death after cardiovascular diseases and cancer.[4] Unintentional injuries were the fifth, suicides the tenth, and assault the fifteenth leading causes of death overall.[5] Injuries account for 30% of life-years lost in the US, severely affecting productivity.[4] It has been estimated that worldwide for every trauma death there are dozens of cases of morbidity[1]; injury-related emergency department (ED) visits and hospital admissions reached 41 million and 2.3 million, respectively, in the US in 2014.[4] As such, the annual cost of trauma is estimated to be between $585 and $830 billion in the US. This includes the direct costs of fatal and nonfatal injuries, employer costs, vehicle damage, and fire losses.[4,5] As an interesting phenomenon, between 2000 and 2010 trauma deaths in the US increased out of proportion to population increase; population increased by 9.7%, whereas trauma-related deaths increased by 23%.[6] This has been attributed to the aging of the US baby boomer population, who, because of their age and pre-existing conditions, are more likely to die than younger patients. This trend may be more pronounced in the future with the increasing number of aging baby boomers.[6] Thus it is likely that the percentage of older trauma victims with pre-existing conditions coming to the operating room (OR) for surgery may increase.

Approximately 75% of hospital deaths from high-energy trauma such as motor vehicle accidents, falls, and gunshot or stab wounds occur within 48 hours after admission, most commonly from central nervous system (CNS), thoracic, abdominal, retroperitoneal, or vascular injuries.[7] CNS injury and hemorrhage are the most common causes of early trauma mortality.[8] Nearly one-third of these patients die within the first 4 hours after admission, representing the majority of OR trauma deaths. Of the hospital deaths, 5% to 10% occur between the third and seventh day of admission, usually from CNS injuries, and the rest in subsequent weeks, most commonly as a result of multiorgan failure.[7] Pulmonary thromboembolism and infectious complications may also contribute to mortality during this phase.[7] Interestingly, injuries caused by low-energy impacts, mainly from falls, usually in the elderly, also produce significant mortality from head injury and complications of skeletal injuries. Of these deaths, 20% occur within 48 hours, 32% after 3 to 7 days, and 48% after 7 days. Pre-existing conditions such as congestive heart failure, cirrhosis, warfarin intake, and/or β-blocker usage increase the mortality rate in trauma patients.[9]

Initial Evaluation and Resuscitation

Major trauma presents with a wide variety of clinical conditions in terms of the type and intensity of injury to individual organ systems, the combination of multiple injured locations, and the resulting physiologic disturbances. The strategy of initial management can be defined as a continuous, priority-driven process of patient assessment, resuscitation, and reassessment. After information has been obtained from paramedics about the mechanism of injury, possible injuries, vital signs at the field and during transport, prehospital treatment, and, if available, pre-existing medical disease(s), the general approach to evaluation of the acute trauma victim has three sequential components: rapid overview, primary survey, and secondary survey. Based on the findings of this evaluation, the patient is directed to an appropriate care unit for further management (Fig. 53-1). Resuscitation is initiated, if needed, at any time during this continuum. *Rapid overview* takes only a few seconds and is used to determine whether the patient is stable, unstable, dying, or dead. The *primary survey* involves rapid evaluation of functions that are crucial to survival. The ABCs of airway patency, breathing, and circulation are assessed. Then a brief neurologic examination is performed, and the patient is examined for any external injuries that might have been overlooked. A rapid limited transthoracic echocardiogram with parasternal long and short axis, apical, and subxiphoid views may give useful information about myocardial contractility, intravascular volume, and the presence of pericardial effusion at this point.[10]

The *secondary survey* involves a more elaborate systematic examination of the entire body to identify additional injuries. Radiography (focused assessment with sonography [FAST], computed tomography [CT], angiography, interventional radiologic procedures, magnetic resonance imaging [MRI]) and other diagnostic procedures may also be performed if the stability of the patient permits. With installation of multidetector CT scans

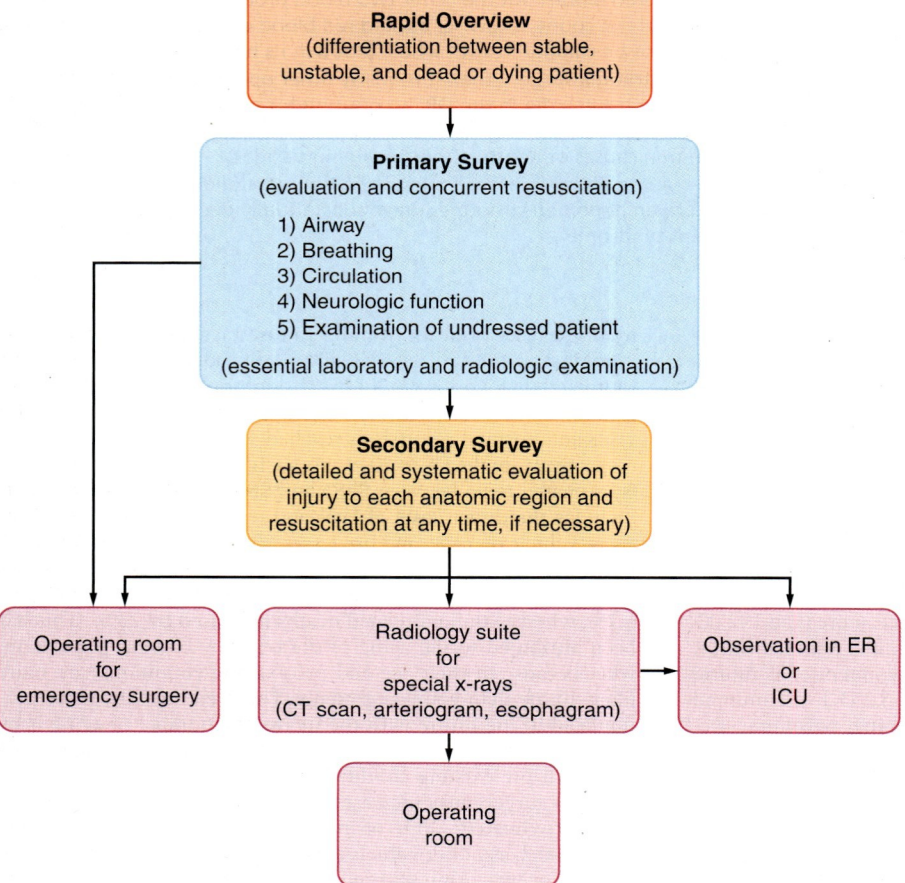

Figure 53-1 Clinical sequence for initial management of the major trauma patient. CT, computed tomography; ER, emergency room; ICU, intensive care unit.

(MDCT) in most Level 1 trauma centers, especially those in proximity to the ED, total body imaging is accomplished rapidly, helping substantially to direct subsequent surgical, interventional radiologic, or conservative management. In fact it has been emphasized that imaging by MDCT is most helpful in the unstable multiply injured patient.[11] Within this general framework the anesthesiologist, aside from managing the airway, contributes as part of the team for evaluation and resuscitation, while gathering information needed for possible future anesthetic management.

Injuries may be missed during initial evaluation and even during emergency surgery, resulting in significant pain, complications, residual disability, delay of treatment, or death.[12] Reported missed diagnoses include cervical spine, thoracoabdominal, pelvic, nerve, and external soft tissue injuries and extremity fractures. Some of these injuries may present during administration of anesthesia, such as spinal cord damage in a patient with unrecognized cervical spine injury, massive intraoperative bleeding from an unrecognized thoracoabdominal injury during extremity surgery, or sudden intraoperative hypoxemia in a patient with unrecognized pneumothorax.

A *tertiary survey* within the first 24 hours after admission (which may include a period of anesthesia) can potentially diagnose the majority of clinically significant injuries missed during initial evaluation by the care team's repeating the primary and secondary examinations and reviewing the results of radiologic and laboratory testing.[12]

Airway Evaluation and Intervention

Airway evaluation involves the diagnosis of any trauma to the airway or surrounding tissues, recognition and anticipation of the respiratory consequences of these injuries, and prediction of the potential for exacerbation of these or other injuries by any contemplated airway management maneuvers. Airway evaluation should be made for mask ventilation, tracheal intubation, and placement of a surgical airway. In obese patients with excessive pretracheal tissues, the cricothyroid membrane may be difficult to identify. Use of ultrasound can help to locate the trachea in these circumstances.[13] Although nontraumatic causes of airway difficulty, such as pre-existing factors, may be present, only the management of trauma-related problems is discussed in this section. Generally, the American Society of Anesthesiologists's (ASA) difficult airway algorithm can be applied with certain modifications to various trauma airway management scenarios. For instance, cancellation of airway management when difficulty arises may not be an option. Likewise, awake rather than anesthetized intubation or a surgical airway from the outset may be the preferred technique in some situations. The ASA's difficult airway algorithm as modified for various trauma conditions is available.[14] Airway management is tailored to the type of injury, the nature and degree of airway compromise, and the patient's hemodynamic and oxygenation status. Each of these conditions may present with great diversity, rendering trauma intubation difficult. Simultaneously performed resuscitation, time and environmental pressure, and possibly suboptimal equipment and assistance are additional factors increasing the difficulty. Continuous communication with members of the trauma team and obtaining information may help reduce the extent of the difficulty.

Airway Obstruction

Airway obstruction is probably the most frequent cause of asphyxia after trauma and may result from posteriorly displaced or lacerated pharyngeal soft tissues; cervical or mediastinal hematoma; bleeding, secretions, or foreign bodies within the airway; and/or displaced bone or cartilage fragments. Bleeding into the cervical region may produce airway obstruction not only because of compression by the hematoma but also from venous congestion and upper airway edema as a result of compression of neck veins. Signs of upper and lower airway obstruction include dyspnea, cyanosis, hoarseness, stridor, dysphonia, subcutaneous emphysema, and hemoptysis. Cervical deformity, edema, crepitation, tracheal tug and/or deviation, or jugular venous distention may be present before these symptoms appear and may help indicate that specialized techniques are required to secure the airway.

The initial steps in airway management are chin lift, jaw thrust, clearance of the oropharynx, placement of an oropharyngeal or nasopharyngeal airway, and, in inadequately breathing patients, ventilation with a self-inflating bag. Immobilization of the cervical spine and administration of oxygen should be applied simultaneously. Blind passage of a nasopharyngeal airway or a nasogastric or nasotracheal tube should be avoided if a basilar skull fracture is suspected because the airway may enter the anterior cranial fossa. A supraglottic airway may permit ventilation with a self-inflating bag, although these devices do not provide protection against aspiration of gastric contents. They may be used as temporary measures and can serve as a bridge for a brief period to re-establish the airway patency or to facilitate intubation aided by a flexible fiberoptic bronchoscope (FOB). If they do not provide adequate ventilation, the trachea must be secured immediately using direct laryngoscopy, video laryngoscopy, or cricothyroidotomy, depending on the results of airway assessment.

Maxillofacial, neck, and chest injuries, as well as cervicofacial burns, are some of the difficult trauma-related reasons for tracheal intubation. Airway assessment should include a rapid examination of the anterior neck for feasibility of access to the cricothyroid membrane. Tracheostomy is not desirable during initial management because it takes longer to perform than a cricothyroidotomy and requires neck extension, which may cause or exacerbate cord trauma in patients with cervical spine injuries. Conversion to a tracheostomy should be considered later to prevent laryngeal damage if a cricothyroidotomy will be in place for more than 2 to 3 days. Possible contraindications to cricothyroidotomy include age younger than 12 years and suspected laryngeal trauma. Permanent laryngeal damage may result in the former, and uncorrectable airway obstruction may occur in the latter situation.

Full Stomach

A full stomach is a background condition in acute trauma: The urgency of securing the airway often does not permit adequate time for pharmacologic measures to reduce gastric volume and acidity. Thus, rather than relying on these agents, the emphasis should be placed on selection of a safe technique for securing the airway when necessary: rapid-sequence induction with cricoid pressure for those patients without serious airway problems, and awake intubation with sedation and topical anesthesia, if possible, for those with anticipated serious airway difficulties.

In agitated and uncooperative patients, topical anesthesia of the airway may be impossible, whereas administration of sedative agents may result in apnea or airway obstruction, with an increased risk of aspiration of gastric contents and inadequate conditions for tracheal intubation. After locating the cricothyroid membrane and denitrogenating the lungs, a rapid-sequence induction may be used to allow securing of the airway with direct or video laryngoscopy or, if necessary, immediate cricothyroidotomy. Personnel and material necessary to perform translaryngeal ventilation or cricothyroidotomy must be in place before induction of general anesthesia.

Head, Open Eye, and Contained Major Vessel Injuries

The principles of tracheal intubation are similar for these injuries. Apart from the need to ensure adequate oxygenation and ventilation, these patients require deep anesthesia and profound muscle relaxation before airway manipulation. This helps prevent hypertension, coughing, and bucking, and thereby minimizes intracranial, intraocular, or intravascular pressure elevation, which can result in herniation of the brain, extrusion of eye contents, or dislodgment of a hemostatic clot from an injured vessel, respectively. The preferred anesthetic sequence to achieve this goal in patients who are not hemodynamically compromised includes preoxygenation and opioid loading, followed by relatively large doses of an intravenous anesthetic and muscle relaxant. Hemodynamic responses to this sequence should be carefully monitored and promptly corrected. Systemic hypotension, intracranial pressure (ICP) elevation, and decreased cerebral perfusion pressure (CPP; CPP equals mean arterial pressure minus ICP) may occur whether cerebral autoregulation is present or absent in patients with head injuries and if untreated can produce secondary ischemic insults. Ketamine, once thought to be contraindicated in patients with head and open eye injuries because it may potentially increase both intracranial and intraocular pressures (IOPs), is shown to be advantageous in this setting because it maintains the systemic blood pressure and does not cause an appreciable increase in ICP and IOP.[15,16] By increasing systemic blood pressure it can, however, cause dislodgment of a hemostatic plug, initiating bleeding in vascular injuries. Any muscle relaxant, including succinylcholine, may be used as long as the fasciculation produced by this agent is inhibited by prior administration of an adequate dose of a nondepolarizing muscle relaxant. Alternatively, rocuronium can provide intubating conditions within 60 seconds with a dose of 1.2 to 1.5 mg/kg; neuromuscular blockade produced by this dose lasts approximately 2 hours. Of course, neither muscle relaxants nor intravenous anesthetics are indicated when initial assessment suggests a difficult airway. As in any other trauma patient, hypotension, depending on its severity, dictates either reduced or no intravenous anesthetic administration. Tracheal intubation should be performed expeditiously, especially in head-injured patients, to prevent a decline in O_2 saturation, which may adversely influence outcome. Comparison of video laryngoscopy with direct laryngoscopy (Macintosh blade) in trauma patients showed longer intubation times with the video laryngoscope, resulting in a decline in O_2 saturation to 80% or less in more patients.[17] Although this finding should not discourage the use of a video laryngoscope in trauma patients, it should remind the clinician of the potential for the problem and that precautions such as applying appropriate preoxygenation are needed before attempting laryngoscopy and intubation.

Cervical Spine Injury

Overall, 2% to 4% of blunt trauma patients have cervical spine (C-spine) injuries, of which 7% to 15% are unstable.[18] The most common causes include high-speed motor vehicle accidents, falls, diving accidents, and gunshot wounds. Head injuries, especially those with a low Glasgow coma score (GCS) and focal neurologic deficits, are likely to be associated with C-spine injuries.

Approximately 2% to 10% of head trauma victims have C-spine injuries, whereas 25% to 50% of patients with C-spine injuries have an associated head injury.[18] The incidence of assault-related injuries depends on the mechanism, being highest after gunshot wounds (1.35%), lowest after stab wounds (0.12%), and intermediate after blunt trauma (0.4%) to the cervicothoracic region.

Initial Evaluation

Accurate and timely evaluation is important because 2% to 10% of blunt trauma–induced C-spine injury patients develop new or worsening neurologic deficits after admission, partly attributable to delayed diagnosis and improper C-spine protection and/or manipulation.[18] Often there is no time to evaluate the injury, and emergency airway management may have to be performed without ruling out C-spine injury while the patients are in a rigid collar and neck-stabilizing devices. Clearance of the neck at the earliest possible time after airway management should be performed to minimize the complications associated with the collar, such as pressure ulceration, ICP elevation in head-injured patients, compromised central venous access, and airway management challenges if reintubation is needed.

In the conscious patient with a suspected injury, diagnosis is relatively easy. According to the American National Emergency X-radiography Utilization Study (NEXUS), a clinical evaluation revealing no posterior midline neck tenderness and focal neurologic deficit, in an injured patient with a normal level of alertness, and no evidence of intoxication, and painful distracting injury indicates a low probability of a C-spine injury. There is thus no need for radiographic evaluation.[19] Recently, however, it has been shown that a significant number of major-trauma patients cleared by these criteria had clinically important unstable C-spine injuries requiring treatment. Therefore, routine CT in addition to clinical evaluation is recommended to rule out C-spine injury in major trauma victims.[20] Probably the reason for the lower reliability of the NEXUS criteria is the difficulty of evaluating distracting injuries.

The Canadian C-spine rule for radiography after trauma is another tool designed to identify low-risk patients.[18] With this diagnostic tool, proper answers to the following three questions eliminate the possibility of injury and the need for radiographic studies: Is there any high-risk factor mandating radiography? Are there low-risk factors that permit safe evaluation of the range of motion of the neck? Can the patient rotate the neck laterally for 45 degrees in each direction without pain (Fig. 53-2)? Comparison of these two sets of criteria showed that the Canadian rule is more reliable than NEXUS in diagnosing C-spine injury in responsive patients.[21] Generally patients without neck pain, tenderness, or upper extremity paresthesia are considered free of C-spine injury, especially in the absence of distracting pain from other anatomic locations. Absence of clinical findings is also shown to rule out C-spine injury in pre-elementary schoolchildren, eliminating the need for diagnostic studies and thus radiation exposure.[22] Children with persistent midline neck pain with no other clinical findings and negative initial imaging findings have also been shown to have very little possibility of an unstable C-spine.[23]

Currently in modern trauma centers radiographic evaluation of the C-spine is performed using thin-cut CT images with sagittal and coronal reconstruction. There is, however, a subset of patients with normal CT scans who are either comatose or obtunded or are awake but have neck pain. Given the fact that CT is not sensitive in diagnosing soft tissue and ligamentous injury, ruling out ligamentous C-spine injury in these patients is difficult, and the diagnostic strategy is somewhat controversial. Dynamic fluoroscopy to obtain flexion/extension series has limited value because it is extremely low yield, relatively dangerous,

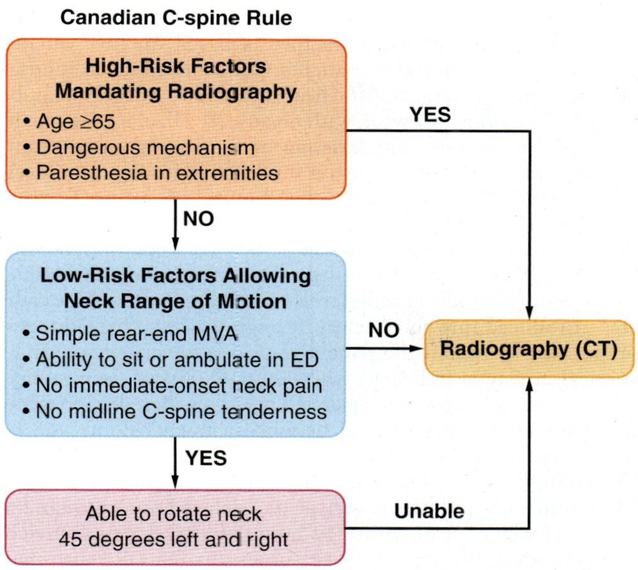

Canadian C-spine Rule

```
High-Risk Factors
Mandating Radiography
• Age ≥65
• Dangerous mechanism
• Paresthesia in extremities
         │ YES ──────────────┐
         │ NO                │
         ▼                   ▼
Low-Risk Factors Allowing    Radiography (CT)
Neck Range of Motion         ▲
• Simple rear-end MVA   NO   │
• Ability to sit or ambulate in ED
• No immediate-onset neck pain
• No midline C-spine tenderness
         │ YES               │
         ▼                   │
Able to rotate neck   Unable │
45 degrees left and right ───┘
```

Figure 53-2 Canadian cervical spine rule designed to diagnose cervical spine injury in conscious patients and identify patients who require further radiographic (computed tomography [CT]) evaluation. MVA, motor vehicle accident; ED, emergency department. (Adapted from Steill IG, Wells GA, Vandemheen K, et al. The Canadian C-Spine Rule for radiography in alert and stable trauma patients. *JAMA.* 2001;286:1841–1848; and Steill IG, Clement CM, McKnight RD, et al. The Canadian C-spine rule versus the NEXUS low-risk criteria in patients with trauma. *N Engl J Med* 2003;349:2510.)

and cost ineffective.[24] It requires repeat examinations, it is difficult to identify specific ligamentous injury, and often the lower cervical spine cannot be visualized. In many trauma centers it is no longer performed.

MRI is a reliable tool; a normal examination can conclusively exclude C-spine injury.[25] It is thus the gold standard for ruling C-spine injury in or out. However, it is so sensitive that it can detect subtle injuries that are clinically insignificant. It cannot be performed in multiple-trauma patients who have metallic skeletal fixators. It is expensive and requires patient transport. MRI may be useful in evaluating spinal cord–injured children without radiologic (CT) abnormalities. In this subgroup of patients, MRI can demonstrate the underlying pathology in some, but not all, patients.[26] A more recently proposed approach, which is practiced in many countries and in many, but not all, trauma centers in the US, is to rely on the MDCT study performed with less than 3-mm cuts. The diagnostic capability of this method is excellent, with the possibility of missing one unstable C-spine injury in about 5,000 patients not cleared by clinical examination.[27–29] Some clinicians advocate obtaining an MRI after CT as a definitive diagnostic measure to rule out C-spine injury, but the necessity for this strategy has not yet been shown.[30] In brain-injured children with suspected C-spine injury, this approach did not offer any yield.[31]

Interestingly, published series describe very few instances of neurologic deficits related to airway management in C-spine–injured patients. Recently, Hindman et al.[32] reviewed the closed claims data for perioperative cervical cord, nerve root, and spine injury between 1970 and 2007, which showed that overall airway management–related neurologic damage represented 11% of 48 claims. Nine patients in the series had unstable spines preoperatively and developed neurologic deficits. In two of these patients the injury was attributed to airway management following direct laryngoscopy and intubation without C-spine precautions. McLeod and Calder[33] reviewed nine allegedly intubation-related cervical spinal cord injuries. Of these, three patients in two reports developed increased neurologic deficit after laryngoscopy and intubation without stabilization of the neck. It is likely that two of these patients are the same patients described by Hindman et al.[32] Thus, it is possible that airway management–related cervical cord injury in C-spine–injured patients can occur, but, if it does, it is rare.

Airway Management

Almost all airway maneuvers, including jaw thrust, chin lift, head tilt, and oral airway placement, result in some degree of C-spine movement.[18] To secure the airway with direct laryngoscopy, manual inline stabilization (MILS) of the neck is the standard of care for these patients in the acute stage. A hard cervical collar alone, which is routinely placed, does not provide absolute protection, especially against rotational movements of the neck. MILS is best accomplished by having two operators in addition to the physician who is actually managing the airway. The first operator stabilizes and aligns the head in neutral position without applying cephalad traction. The second operator stabilizes both shoulders by holding them against the table or stretcher. The anterior portion of the hard collar, which limits mouth opening, may be removed after immobilization.

In the presence of MILS, the glottic view may be suboptimal during direct laryngoscopy in 10% to 15% of patients because of limitation of neck extension. Airway management may be further compromised in some patients because of enlargement of the prevertebral space by a hematoma from the vertebral fracture. Consequently, greater anterior pressure needs to be applied to the tongue by the laryngoscope blade in order to visualize the larynx. This increased anterior pressure is transmitted to the spine and can increase the movement of an unstable vertebral segment. Thus, the greater the restriction of the glottic view during direct laryngoscopy, the greater the pressure on the tongue, the spine, and the unstable segment with potential displacement of the unstable fragment. Santoni et al.[34] demonstrated that during various phases of direct laryngoscopy and intubation, the pressures exerted on the tongue and indirectly on the spine were greater with MILS than without MILS. This finding confirmed the results of a videofluoroscopic study by Lennarson et al.,[35] who demonstrated significant anteroposterior displacement when MILS was applied to cadavers with destabilized C-spines.

Although convincing, these data should not eliminate the current standard practice of applying MILS during airway management of these patients. Currently, there is no scientifically rigorous clinical trial to show conclusively that airway management without MILS is associated with a favorable spinal cord outcome. Based on the available data, it is, however, reasonable to allow some relaxation of the MILS to improve the glottic view when visualization of the larynx is restricted.[36]

Other measures such as videolaryngoscopy, use of a gum elastic bougie, translaryngeal (retrograde) intubation, and cricothyroidotomy can be used to secure the airway in the acute phase of cervical spine immobilization. Neck motion with modern videolaryngoscopes does not seem to be different from that produced by the Macintosh blade, although they do provide better glottic views. Cricoid pressure may optimize the view during laryngoscopy, but it should be applied with great care because it may produce undue motion of the unstable spine if excessive force is used. Supraglottic intubation of airways to facilitate intubation with or without the aid of FOB can be used, but neck movement with these devices appears to be comparable to that produced by conventional laryngoscopes. Flexible fiberoptic laryngoscopy, use of a lightwand, and possibly translaryngeal-guided intubation (see Maxillofacial Injuries) cause almost no neck movement, but blood or secretions in the airway, a long preparation time, and difficulty in their use in comatose, uncooperative, or anesthetized patients reduce their utility during initial management. Nasotracheal intubation carries the risks of epistaxis, failure of intubation, and possibility of entry of the endotracheal tube into the cranial vault or the orbit if there is damage to the cranial base or the maxillofacial complex. Absence of the usual signs of cranial base fracture (battle sign, raccoon eyes, or bleeding from the ear or the nose) cannot be relied on to exclude the possibility of its occurrence because with rapid prehospital transport, these signs may not be immediately apparent.

In the subacute phase of C-spine injury when time constraints, full stomach, and patient cooperation issues do not exist, the use of FOB in the awake sedated patient with appropriate topical anesthesia is preferred. Advantages of this technique are minimal movement of the neck, positioning of the patient awake, maintenance of protective reflexes, and ability to assess the neurologic status after intubation.

Direct Airway Injuries

Direct airway damage can occur anywhere between the nasopharynx and the bronchi. Sometimes more than one site may be involved, resulting in persistent airway dysfunction after one of the problems is corrected.[37] Head, face, and neck injuries are more common in military personnel in combat than in the civilian population; effective torso protection by body armor in combat leaves these regions unprotected.[38]

Maxillofacial Injuries

The mechanism of maxillofacial injuries can be divided into high-impact (motor vehicle accident, industrial explosion, free fall) and low-impact (altercation) trauma. Airway management is often challenging in patients with high-impact maxillofacial injuries. In addition to soft tissue edema of the pharynx and peripharyngeal hematoma, blood or debris in the oropharynx may be responsible for partial or complete airway obstruction in the acute stage of these injuries. Occasionally, teeth or foreign bodies in the pharynx may be aspirated into the airway, causing some degree of obstruction, which may occur or be recognized only during attempts at tracheal intubation. Another problem is the dynamic nature of soft tissue injuries in this region. A hematoma or edema of the face, tongue, or neck may expand during the first several hours after injury and ultimately occlude the airway. Serious airway compromise may develop within a few hours in up to 50% of patients with major penetrating facial injuries or multiple trauma, caused by progressive inflammation or edema resulting from liberal administration of fluids.

The face, head, and neck are vulnerable to missile and explosion injuries.[38] Although rare, massive hemorrhage, most frequently from the internal maxillary artery or its branches, and less frequently from the facial, external carotid, or sphenopalatine arteries and other small branches, may be life threatening, requiring anterior, posterior, or anteroposterior packing, intermaxillary fixation, and, when these measures are ineffective, angioembolization.[39,40] Tracheal intubation or a surgical airway is necessary as an initial measure to avert airway compromise in these circumstances.

Fracture-induced encroachment on the airway or limitation of mandibular movement, pain, and trismus may limit mouth opening. Fentanyl in titrated doses of up to 2 to 4 µg/kg over a period of 10 to 20 minutes may produce an improvement in the patient's ability to open the mouth if mechanical limitation is not present.

The selection of an airway management technique in the presence of a maxillofacial fracture is based on the patient's presenting condition. Most patients with isolated facial injuries do not require emergency tracheal intubation. Surgery may be delayed for as long as a week with no adverse effect on the repair. Patients who present with existing or impending airway compromise may be intubated using direct laryngoscopy; the decision about the use of anesthetics and muscle relaxants is based on the results of airway evaluation. When there is bleeding into the oropharynx, a flexible fiberoptic laryngoscope may be useless because of obstruction of the view. A retrograde technique, using a wire or epidural catheter passed through a 14-gauge catheter introduced into the trachea through the cricothyroid membrane, may be used if the patient can open his or her mouth. A surgical airway is indicated when there is airway compromise, when direct laryngoscopy has failed or is considered impossible, when the jaws will be wired, or when a tracheostomy will be performed anyway after definitive repair of the fracture.[41] Tracheostomy may be indicated as an emergency procedure in the ED within a few minutes of arrival, as a delayed procedure in the OR for airway control within 12 hours of arrival, or as an elective procedure during definitive surgery in the OR more than 12 hours following admission to the hospital.[38] Comminuted mandibular, midfacial bilateral Le Fort III, and panfacial fractures are likely to be managed with tracheostomy for definitive surgery.[41] To avoid the possible complications of tracheostomy, submental or submandibular intubation, which involves externalizing the proximal end of a flexible armored orotracheal tube through a small submental incision, has been performed. Thus, the trachea remains surgically intact and the endotracheal tube is not in the mouth, permitting comfortable surgical exposure and ability to apply intermaxillary fixation.[42] Nasogastric or nasotracheal intubation should be avoided when a basilar skull or maxillary fracture is suspected because of the possibility that the tube may enter the cranium or the orbit. Hemorrhagic shock and life-threatening cranial, laryngotracheal, thoracic, and cervical spine injuries may accompany major facial fractures, and airway management must be tailored accordingly. The likelihood of cranial injury increases in midface fractures involving the frontal sinus, as well as the orbitozygomatic and orbitoethmoid complexes.

Cervical Airway Injuries

Injury to the cervical air passages can result from blunt or penetrating trauma. The incidence of patients with blunt or penetrating laryngotracheal injuries admitted to major trauma centers is 0.34% and 4%, respectively.[43] Similar to maxillofacial injuries, wartime laryngotracheal trauma is more severe and more frequent (5% to 6%) than peacetime injuries (0.91%).[44] Although the pharynx and esophagus are close to the cervical air passages, their involvement in peacetime trauma is less likely than airway injuries (0.08% after blunt and 0.9% after penetrating trauma).[43] Clinical signs such as air escape, hemoptysis, and coughing are present in almost all patients with penetrating injuries, facilitating the diagnosis. In contrast, major blunt laryngotracheal damage may be missed, either because the patient is asymptomatic or unresponsive or because suggestive signs and symptoms are missed in the initial evaluation. The typical presentation includes hoarseness, muffled voice, dyspnea, stridor, dysphagia, odynophagia, cervical pain and tenderness, ecchymosis, subcutaneous emphysema, and flattening of the thyroid cartilage protuberance (Adam's apple). Whether the trauma is blunt or penetrating, attempts at blind tracheal intubation may produce further trauma to the larynx and complete airway obstruction if the endotracheal tube enters a false passage or disrupts the continuity of an already tenuous airway.[45] Thus, whenever possible,

Table 53-1 Classification of Laryngeal Injuries

Grade	Laryngeal Findings	Airway
1	No fractures Minor lacerations Minimal edema	Minimal airway symptoms
2	Undisplaced fractures Mucosal damage without cartilage exposure	Mild airway compromise
3	Displaced fractures Vocal fold immobility	Significant airway compromise
4	Multiple fractures with instability	Significant airway compromise
5	Laryngotracheal separation	Catastrophic airway obstruction

Data from Schaefer SD. Primary management of laryngeal trauma. *Ann Otol Rhinol Laryngol.* 1982;91:399; and Fuhrman GM, Stieg FH III, Buerk CA, et al. Blunt laryngeal trauma: classification and management protocol. *J Trauma.* 1990;30:87.

intubation of the trachea should be performed using an FOB, or the airway should be secured surgically. A CT scan of the neck provides valuable information and should be performed before any airway intervention in all stable patients without respiratory and hemodynamic compromise. Originally, the severity of laryngeal injury was classified based on endoscopic findings. With modern equipment, information similar to that provided by FOB can be obtained with CT scanning. A classification of laryngeal injuries is depicted in Table 53-1.[46,47]

The strategy for tracheal intubation depends on the clinical presentation.[45] The tracheas of some patients with penetrating airway injuries, especially stab wounds, may be intubated through the airway defect without the need for anesthetics or optical equipment. The presence of cartilaginous fractures or mucosal abnormalities necessitates awake intubation with an FOB or awake tracheostomy.[37] Laryngeal damage precludes cricothyroidotomy. Tracheostomy should be performed with extreme caution because up to 70% of patients with blunt laryngeal injuries may have an associated cervical spine injury.[45] Uncooperative or confused patients may not tolerate awake airway manipulation. It may be best to transport these patients to the OR, induce anesthesia with ketamine or inhalational agents, and intubate the trachea without muscle relaxants.[45] Episodes of airway obstruction during spontaneous breathing under an inhalational anesthetic can be managed by positioning the patient upright in addition to the usual maneuvers.

Complete transection of the trachea is rare, but when it occurs it is life threatening. The distal segment of the trachea retracts into the chest, causing airway obstruction either spontaneously or during airway manipulation. Surgery involves pulling up the distal end and performing an end-to-end anastomosis to the proximal segment or suturing it to the skin as a permanent tracheostomy. In extreme situations, such as complete or near-complete transection of the larynx and trachea, femorofemoral bypass or percutaneous cardiopulmonary support may be considered if time permits.[48]

Following repair, immediate or early extubation of the trachea is safe in patients with isolated cervical tracheal injuries. In patients who require prolonged airway control because of tracheal or extratracheal injuries, immediate tracheostomy and prolonged intubation are the two choices available. The former is associated with increased surgical site infection and the latter with pneumonia.[49] Thus every attempt should be made to aim for early extubation, and, if it is not possible, the risks and benefits of tracheostomy and prolonged intubation should be considered before final selection.

Thoracic Airway Injuries

Whereas penetrating trauma can cause damage to any segment of the intrathoracic airway, blunt injury usually involves the posterior membranous portion of the trachea and the main stem bronchi, usually within approximately 3 cm of the carina. A significant number of these injuries result from iatrogenic causes such as tracheal intubation.[50] Pneumothorax, pneumomediastinum, pneumopericardium, subcutaneous emphysema, and a continuous air leak from the chest tube are the usual signs of this injury. They occur frequently but are not specific for thoracic airway damage. In intubated patients without the suspicion of a tracheal injury, difficulty in obtaining a seal around the endotracheal tube or the presence on a chest radiograph of a large radiolucent area in the trachea corresponding to the cuff suggests a perforated airway. Other radiographic findings include a radiolucent line along the prevertebral fascia due to air tracking up from the mediastinum, peribronchial air or sudden obstruction along an air-filled bronchus, and the "dropped lung" sign when complete intrapleural bronchial transection causes the apex of the collapsed lung to descend to the level of the hilum. Occasionally, simultaneous esophageal injury with a tracheoesophageal fistula may be present.[51]

Airway management is similar to that for cervical airway injury. Anesthetics, and especially muscle relaxants, may produce irreversible obstruction, presumably because of relaxation of peritracheal or peribronchial structures that maintain airway patency in the awake patient. However, airway loss may also occur during attempts at awake intubation, often as a result of further distortion of the airway by the endotracheal tube, patient agitation, or rebleeding into the airway. After intubation of the trachea, the adequacy of airway intervention is evaluated mainly by auscultation and capnography. Pulmonary contusion, atelectasis, diaphragmatic rupture with thoracic migration of the abdominal contents, and pneumothorax may complicate the interpretation of chest auscultation. Likewise, carbon dioxide (CO_2) elimination may be decreased or absent in shock and cardiac arrest.

The outcome after surgical repair of these injuries is often suboptimal and complicated by stump leak and empyema, suture line stenosis, or the need for tracheostomy or pneumonectomy. The recent trend is selective conservative management with an endotracheal tube placed using bronchoscopic guidance distal to the tracheal injury.[52] Patients with lesions larger than 4 cm, cartilaginous rather than membranous injuries, concomitant esophageal trauma, progressive subcutaneous emphysema, severe dyspnea requiring intubation and ventilation, difficulty with mechanical ventilation, pneumothorax with an air leak through the chest drains, and mediastinitis are still managed surgically. Those without these problems may be treated nonoperatively with a reasonable outcome.[50,52] Following repair, early tracheal extubation should be the goal; it is likely that (as in cervical tracheal injuries) tracheostomy or prolonged intubation may be associated with infectious complications.[49]

Management of Breathing Abnormalities

Of the several causes that may alter respiration after trauma, tension pneumothorax, flail chest, and open pneumothorax are immediate threats to the patient's life and therefore require rapid diagnosis and treatment. Hemothorax, closed pneumothorax, pulmonary contusion, diaphragmatic rupture with herniation of abdominal contents into the thorax, and atelectasis from a mucous plug, aspiration, or chest wall splinting can also interfere with breathing and pulmonary gas exchange and deteriorate into life-threatening complications.

Although cyanosis, tachypnea, hypotension, neck vein distention, tracheal deviation, and diminished breath sounds on the affected side are the classic signs of tension pneumothorax, neck vein distention may be absent in hypovolemic patients and tracheal deviation may be difficult to appreciate. Inability to position most trauma patients upright and the likelihood of inadequate imaging decrease the diagnostic value of chest radiographs.[53] In the supine position the deep sulcus sign, which results from the tendency of pleural air to track in the lateral and caudal regions, is usually diagnostic of tension pneumothorax.[54] The definitive diagnosis is made by CT scanning.[55] However, in hypoxemic and hypotensive patients, immediate insertion of a 14-gauge angiocatheter through the fourth or fifth intercostal space in the midaxillary line or, at times, through the second intercostal space at the midclavicular line is essential. There is no time for radiologic confirmation in this setting.

A flail chest results from fractures at two or more sites of at least three adjacent ribs, or rib fractures associated with costochondral separation or sternal fracture. An underlying pulmonary contusion with increased elastic recoil of the lung and increased work of breathing is the main cause of respiratory insufficiency or failure and resulting hypoxemia.[56] It often develops over a 3- to 6-hour period, causing gradual worsening seen in the chest radiograph and deterioration of arterial blood gases (ABGs).[56] Coexisting hemopneumothorax, paradoxic chest wall movement, and/or pain-induced splinting may contribute to the gas exchange abnormalities. Repeat evaluation by physical examination, chest radiography, and ABG determinations is essential for early recognition of these complications. The fraction of lung volume contused, as determined by chest radiography or CT, may be predictive of the subsequent development of acute respiratory distress syndrome (ARDS). The likelihood increases abruptly once the contusion volume exceeds 20% of total lung volume.[57] There are other predictive signs of pulmonary complications after rib fractures. In the recently proposed *rib score* system, one point is assigned for each of the following types of rib fractures: six or more rib fractures, bilateral fractures, flail chest, three or more severely (bicortically) displaced fractures, first rib fracture, and at least one fracture in each of the anterior, lateral, and posterior regions of the ribs. A linear correlation exists between the rib score and development of pneumonia, acute respiratory failure and need for tracheostomy.[58] Vital capacity (VC) may be another predictive parameter. Patients with a VC greater than 50% of a nomogram-based normal VC had little likelihood of pulmonary complications, whereas the probability increased 2.5 times in those with VC below 30%.[59] Without significant gas-exchange abnormalities, chest wall instability alone is not an indication for respiratory support. There is evidence that liberal use of tracheal intubation and mechanical ventilation in the presence of a flail chest or pulmonary contusion increases the rate of pulmonary complications and mortality and prolongs the hospital stay.[56,60] Effective pain relief by itself can improve respiratory function and often avoids the need for mechanical ventilation. For this purpose, continuous epidural analgesia with local anesthetics and opioids, preferably directed to thoracic segments, and, if epidural access is not possible, thoracic paravertebral block with local anesthetics provide better pain relief and ventilatory function than parenteral opioids, reducing morbidity and mortality in elderly patients with chest wall trauma.[56] Other therapeutic measures include supplemental oxygen, continuous positive airway pressure of 10 to 15 cm water (H_2O) by face mask, airway humidification, chest physiotherapy, incentive spirometry, bronchodilators, airway suctioning (using FOB, if necessary), and nutritional support.[56] Overzealous infusion of fluids and transfusion of blood products may result in deterioration of oxygenation by worsening the underlying pulmonary injury.[56]

Severe pulmonary contusion, respiratory insufficiency or failure despite adequate analgesia, clinical evidence of severe shock, associated severe head injury or injury requiring surgery, airway obstruction, and significant pre-existing chronic pulmonary disease are indications for tracheal intubation and mechanical ventilation. The outcome in these patients may be dependent on the pattern of ventilation. Unless the clinical evidence suggests imminent cerebral herniation, hyperventilation must be avoided in head-injured patients because it increases cerebral vasoconstriction, thus decreasing perfusion, with accumulation of cerebral lactic acid immediately after its institution.[61] In hypovolemic patients, hyperventilation may interfere with venous return and cardiac output, leading to hypotension, further decrease in organ perfusion, and even cardiac arrest. Ventilation with low tidal volumes (6 to 8 mL/kg) and moderate positive end-expiratory pressure (PEEP), producing low inspiratory alveolar or plateau pressures, appears to be the best pattern to prevent hemodynamic deterioration and decrease the likelihood of ARDS.[62] In intubated, spontaneously breathing patients, airway pressure release ventilation, in which spontaneous breathing is superimposed on mechanical ventilation by an intermittent brief decrease of continuous positive airway pressure, provides improved ventilation/perfusion ($\dot{V}/\dot{Q}$) matching and systemic blood pressure, lower sedation requirements, greater oxygen (O_2) delivery, shorter periods of intubation, and a decreased incidence of ventilator-associated pneumonia, which occurs in up to 30% of ventilated patients with pulmonary contusion.[60,63,64] Severe unilateral pulmonary contusion unresponsive to these measures may be treated by differential lung ventilation via a double-lumen endobronchial tube. In bilateral severe contusions with life-threatening hypoxemia, high-frequency jet ventilation may enhance oxygenation and cardiac function, which may be compromised by concomitant myocardial contusion or ischemia.[65]

Systemic air embolism occurs mainly after penetrating lung trauma and blast injuries or, less frequently, after blunt thoracic trauma that produces lacerations of both distal air passages and pulmonary veins.[66] Positive-pressure ventilation after tracheal intubation may then result in entrainment of air into the systemic circulation. Hemoptysis, circulatory instability, and CNS dysfunction immediately after starting artificial ventilation, as well as detection of air in blood from the radial artery, establishes the diagnosis. Air bubbles may also be seen in the coronary arteries during thoracotomy. Surgical management involves immediate thoracotomy and clamping of the hilum of the lacerated lung. Respiratory maneuvers that minimize or prevent air entry into the systemic circulation include isolating and collapsing the lacerated lung by means of a double-lumen tube or ventilating with the lowest possible tidal volumes via a single-lumen tube.[66] Transesophageal echocardiography (TEE) of the left side of the heart may permit visualization of air bubbles and their disappearance with therapeutic maneuvers.

Management of Shock

Hemorrhage is the most common cause of traumatic hypotension and shock and is, after head injury, the second most common

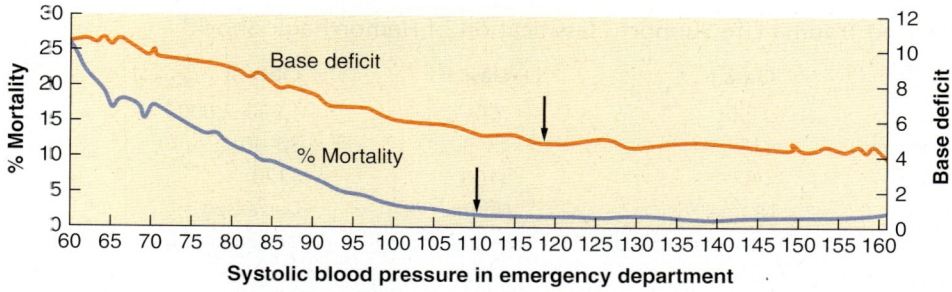

Figure 53-3 Relationship between emergency department systolic blood pressure, base deficit, and overall mortality rate of trauma patients; head injury patients are not included. Note that mortality and base deficit decrease as systolic blood pressure increases, stabilizing at 110 mmHg rather than at the generally accepted 90 mmHg. (Adapted from Eastridge BJ, Salinas J, Wade CE, et al. Hypotension begins at 110 mm Hg: redefining "hypotension" with data. J Trauma. 2007;63:291.)

cause of mortality after trauma. Other causes of hypotension are abnormal pump function (myocardial contusion, pericardial tamponade, pre-existing cardiac disease, or coronary artery or cardiac valve injury), pneumothorax or hemothorax, and spinal cord injury. Anaphylaxis occurs rarely in the acute stage, and sepsis, except in unrecognized bowel injury, is a cause of hypotension only several days after trauma.

In bleeding patients the primary goal is the urgent surgical control of the source. Certain types of bleeding, however, may be temporarily controlled with nonsurgical measures, such as finger compression of open neck injuries and tourniquet control of external bleeding from extremities. Tourniquets should be removed as soon as urgent surgical control is achieved to avoid pressure-induced nerve damage, skin necrosis, or limb ischemia.

Evaluation of the severity of hemorrhagic shock in the initial phase is based on the mechanism and anatomic pattern of injury, prehospital and ED hemodynamic data, and the response to fluid resuscitation. Free falls from heights over 6 meters, high-energy deceleration impact, and high-velocity gunshot wounds are very likely to produce major damage and bleeding. Noncompressible thoracoabdominal and pelvic injuries also are likely to be associated with major bleeding. Immediate evaluation of these anatomic sites clinically and with radiographs of the chest and pelvis, FAST, CT, or, rarely, diagnostic peritoneal lavage is necessary. Patients with significant intra-abdominal fluid recognized with these tests and hemodynamic instability require immediate surgical intervention. Those who are suspected to have occult abdominal bleeding based on a high-risk mechanism of injury but who are hemodynamically stable must undergo further evaluation with CT. The modern multislice CT devices available in most trauma centers can provide early whole-body scanning within a few minutes.[11,67]

Clinical assessment using hemodynamic data is based on a few relatively insensitive and nonspecific clinical signs. For example, tachycardia, which is traditionally used as an index of hypovolemia, may be absent in up to 30% of hypotensive trauma patients because of activated Bezold–Jarisch reflex, increased vagal tone, chronic cocaine use, or other reasons.[68] Inability of the patient to elevate the heart rate in the face of hypoperfusion is considered a predictor of increased mortality independent of severity of injury, systemic blood pressure, or presence of a head injury.[68] In contrast, by increasing catecholamine output, tissue injury and associated pain may result in maintenance of tachycardia and normal systemic blood pressure in the presence or absence of hypovolemia without necessarily increasing the cardiac index or tissue oxygen delivery. In fact, in this situation an increase in intestinal vascular resistance and a decrease in splanchnic blood flow may occur and, if prolonged, may allow entry of intestinal microorganisms into the circulation and increase the likelihood of subsequent sepsis and organ failure.[69,70] Thus, equating a normal heart rate and systemic blood pressure with normovolemia during initial resuscitation may lead to loss of valuable time for treating underlying occult hypovolemia or hypoperfusion. This is especially true in the elderly trauma population (age >65), in whom significant tissue hypoperfusion in the presence of normal blood pressure is more likely than in younger patients.[71] Traditionally, the normal systolic blood pressure (SBP) is defined as 90 mmHg. Recent findings suggest that trauma patients with ED SBP at this level or lower have higher mortality, higher blood lactate levels, and greater base deficits than civilian trauma patients with an SBP of 110 mmHg or injured soldiers with an SBP of 100 mmHg (Fig. 53-3).[72,73] Thus, the optimal SBP in the trauma patient appears to be 100 to 110 mmHg. Based on these findings, an SBP of 110 mmHg is accepted as a prehospital triage criterion for admission to a Level I trauma center for trauma patients over 65 years old[74]; 90 mmHg remains as a level for younger patients. Although traditional vital signs are relatively unreliable for recognizing life-threatening shock, heart rate, systemic blood pressure, pulse pressure, respiratory rate, urine output, and mental status are still used as early clinical indicators of the severity of hemorrhagic shock (Table 53-2).[69,75]

Efforts directed to early identification of uncontrolled hemorrhage led to several clinical diagnostic tools. Because of the immediate activation of transcapillary refill after hemorrhage, there is a decline in hematocrit (Hct) even in the absence of administration of fluids in both adults and children. Thus a low Hct on admission should elicit the suspicion of significant bleeding.[76,77] However, decision making based on a single Hct value may lead to erroneous management decisions. On the other hand, serial Hct measurements and consideration of the type and amount of fluid received may be useful in deciding the timing and amount of transfusion.[78] Among many scoring systems the most practical is the Assessment of Blood Consumption (ABC) score, which asks four yes/no questions: penetrating mechanism of injury, SBP of 90 mmHg or less, heart rate of 120/min or greater, and a positive FAST finding.[79] Shock index (SI), a value derived by dividing the heart rate by the SBP, appears to be another accurate indicator of early hemorrhagic shock and a predictor of mortality. In normal individuals, SI varies between 0.58 and 0.64 (mean 0.61), increasing from 0.70 to 0.80 (mean 0.75) after a moderate degree of blood loss. In the elderly, it has been demonstrated that age times SI identifies early shock and predicts mortality better than SI itself.[80] Additional predictive measures of major bleeding include blood lactate level greater than 2 mmol/L, low tissue O_2 saturation, and pulse oximeter–derived photoplethysmography analysis. Hypoperfusion of abdominal

Table 53-2 Advanced Trauma Life Support Classification of Hemorrhagic Shock[a]

	Class I	Class II	Class III	Class IV
Blood loss (mL)	≤750	750–1,500	1,500–2,000	≥2,000
Blood loss (% blood volume)	≤15	15–30	30–40	≥40
Pulse rate (per min)	<100	>100	>120	≥140
Blood pressure	Normal	Normal	Decreased	Decreased
Pulse pressure	Normal or increased	Decreased	Decreased	Decreased
Respiratory rate (breaths/min)	14–20	20–30	30–40	>35
Urine output (mL/h)	≥30	20–30	5–15	Negligible
Mental status	Slightly anxious	Mildly anxious	Anxious and confused	Confused, lethargic
Fluid replacement (3:1 rule)	Crystalloid[b]	Crystalloid	Crystalloid + blood	Crystalloid + blood

[a]For a 70-kg male patient, based on initial presentation.
[b]The 3:1 rule is based on empiric observation that most patients require 300 mL of balanced electrolyte solution for each 100-mL blood loss. Without other clinical and monitoring parameters, this guideline may result in excessive or inadequate fluid resuscitation.
Adapted from American College of Surgeons, Committee on Trauma. Shock. In: *Advanced Trauma Life Support Student Course Manual*. 8th ed. Chicago, IL: American College of Surgeons; 2008:55–71.

organs can also be detected by CT: Free peritoneal fluid, small bowel enhancement, and flattened inferior vena cava (IVC) and renal veins suggest hypoperfusion.[81]

One of the reasons scoring systems have been introduced for assessing the severity of hemorrhage is to determine the need for initiating the massive transfusion protocol (MTP). The ABC score represents the initially described basic form of these scoring systems. In this system, SBP lower or less than 90 mmHg, heart rate above 120 bpm, positive FAST, and presence of penetrating trauma each are given 1 point. In the US two more detailed scoring systems have been designed: the Cincinnati Individual Transfusion Trigger and the massive transfusion score, which has been recently revised.[82] In both these scoring systems additional parameters such as base deficit, international normalized ratio (INR), hemoglobin, and temperature are added to the simple ABC system to strengthen the predictive power for initiating MTP. Each criterion is given one point, and a minimum score of 1 or 2 suggests activation of the MTP. A sum of one point, although this may initiate MTP, may lead to some unnecessary activations. On the other hand, considering a sum of two points as indication for initiating MTP may result in omission of some patients who actually need activation of MTP. It has been realized that relying only on these scoring systems without using the clinical gestalt is likely to lead to under- or over use of MTP. Thus these scoring systems, preferably the revised massive transfusion score, should be relied upon only in conjunction with clinical judgment. Although the scoring systems are generally used for initial assessment in the ED, they also can be helpful in judging whether the MTP should be continued or stopped later during the process of management.[83] The method of resuscitation of the hemorrhaging patient has changed over the past several years since the Iraq and Afghanistan wars. The concept of damage control resuscitation has replaced the classic crystalloid resuscitation, which served to replenish depleted interstitial fluid and also to estimate the severity of intravascular volume depletion during the initial period. The response to initial fluid resuscitation with lactated Ringer's (LR) or normal saline solution of about 2 L, or 20 mL/kg in children, over a period of 15 to 30 minutes allowed estimation of the severity of hemorrhage.[64] Transient or no blood pressure response to this maneuver suggested major hemorrhage and dictated administration of blood products.

Damage control resuscitation is diametrically opposed to this principle. The severity of hemorrhage is estimated using the combination of clinical, laboratory, ultrasonographic, and radiologic diagnostic measures described earlier. After a major hemorrhage is identified, several components of the process are initiated. These consist of brief permissive hypotension; rapid control of any bleeding source; minimal crystalloid infusion; early administration of plasma and other blood products in a balanced ratio (preferably 1:1:1) of packed red blood cells (PRBCs), plasma, and platelets by activation of the MTP; and tranexamic acid. If indicated, damage control surgery may be required to control bleeding and sources of contamination. Definitive surgery is deferred until after normalization of the patient's physiologic condition. The purpose of damage control resuscitation is to prevent the pulmonary edema, ARDS, coagulopathy, multiple organ failure (MOF), and abdominal compartment syndrome attributed to administration of large volumes of resuscitative crystalloids. In addition, administration of large volumes of LR solution and normal saline are associated with elevated blood lactate levels and increasing base deficit, respectively.[84] An ever-increasing number of reports in the trauma literature indicate the deleterious effects of crystalloid resuscitation. Thus the amount of crystalloid administered during damage control resuscitation is limited to a carrier solution for blood products in most instances. Neil et al.[85] found that a cumulative crystalloid to PRBC ratio greater than 1.5:1 (liters to units) during the first 24 hours after admission was an independent cause of ARDS and abdominal compartment syndrome. Using ratios of less than 0.75:1 and more than 0.75:1 in two groups of trauma patients, another study found no statistical differences in oxygenation, ARDS and mortality between the low- and high-ratio groups, although fewer people in the low-ratio group died.[86] Thus, it is obvious that the crystalloid volume should be kept low during initial resuscitation.

Because management of the trauma patient is a continuum from the prehospital phase to the ED and then to the OR, the anesthesiologist should check the type and amount of resuscitation fluids administered before surgery and adjust the volume of crystalloids accordingly. The deleterious effects of crystalloid fluids are attributed to their effect on the glycocalyx and syndecan-1, a network of soluble plasma components on the endothelium stabilizing membrane integrity. Massive hemorrhage alters the integrity of the endothelial glycocalyx; damage to the cell membrane is thought to be the primary mechanism of shock in these patients. Although plasma is able to reconstitute syndecan-1, the main component of glycocalyx, crystalloids cause further destruction, worsening the endothelial dysfunction.[87]

Overinfusing fluids before control of the hemorrhage may lead to further bleeding by increasing arterial and venous pressures, displacing a hemostatic plug, diluting clotting factors and platelets, reducing body temperature, and decreasing blood viscosity.[88,89] Bickell et al.[90] showed that delaying fluid resuscitation until surgical control of bleeding in victims of penetrating trauma improved survival to hospital discharge and decreased the length of hospital stay. Although many experimental studies have confirmed the findings of Bickell et al.,[90] it has also become clear that withholding fluids completely can result in as much harm as vigorous resuscitation.[91] Feasibility of the time-sensitive permissive hypotension described by Bickell et al.[90] has been studied in a prospective randomized study comparing low-volume versus standard-volume (2L) crystalloid administration to hypotensive trauma patients during the prehospital phase.[92] Mortality was lower in patients who received low-volume crystalloids despite maintenance of hypotension.[92] Although controversial, this concept emphasizes the fact that fluid administration in excess of that needed to achieve normovolemia prior to control of hemorrhage may be deleterious. Permissive hypotension is also contraindicated in traumatic brain and spinal cord injuries and in elderly patients with chronic systemic hypertension in which adequate perfusion is crucial,[89] it emphasizes the fact that fluid administration in excess of that needed to achieve normovolemia prior to control of hemorrhage may be deleterious.[88] Early use of vasopressors to maintain hemodynamic stability also may be associated with deleterious effects. However judicious use of these drugs along with carefully titrated fluids may offer some advantages.

Some of the proven markers of organ perfusion can be used during early management to set the goals of resuscitation. Of these, the base deficit and blood lactate level are the most useful and practical tools during all phases of shock, including the earliest. The base deficit reflects the severity of shock, the oxygen debt, changes in O_2 delivery, the adequacy of fluid resuscitation, and the likelihood of MOF and survival with reasonable accuracy in *previously healthy* adult and pediatric trauma patients.[89] Base deficit is considered a better prognostic marker than the arterial pH. A base deficit between −2 and −5 mmol/L suggests mild shock, between −6 and −9 mmol/L indicates moderate shock, and more than 10 m/mol is a sign of severe shock.[89] An admission base deficit below −5 to −8 mmol/L correlates with increased mortality. Thus, normalization of the base deficit is one of the end points of resuscitation. Elevation of the blood lactate level is less specific than base deficit as a marker of tissue hypoxia because it can be generated in well-oxygenated tissues by increased epinephrine-induced skeletal muscle glycolysis, accelerated pyruvate oxidation, decreased hepatic clearance of lactate, and early mitochondrial dysfunction. All these conditions may be present in the trauma patient. Thus, blood lactate and base deficit may not closely correlate with each other. Nevertheless, in most trauma victims an elevated lactate level correlates with other signs of hypoperfusion, rendering it an important marker of dysoxia and an end point of resuscitation. The normal plasma lactate concentration is 0.5 to 1.5 mmol/L; levels over 5 mmol/L indicate significant lactic acidosis. The half-life of lactate is approximately 15 to 30 minutes in healthy individuals; thus, the level decreases rather rapidly after correction of the cause. Failure to clear lactate within 24 hours after reversal of circulatory shock is a predictor of increased mortality.[89,93]

The usefulness of hemoglobin (Hgb) or Hct as a PRBC transfusion threshold remains unclear, although the recommended target Hgb concentration in all phases of management is 7 to 9 g/dL, including in brain-injured patients in whom tissue oxygenation is most relevant.[89] Several studies demonstrated that increasing the Hgb level to 9 or 10 g/dL from lower levels with PRBCs of less than 19 days' storage increased brain oxygenation in 75% of head injured patients. However, data from other sources showed either increased morbidity and mortality with PRBC transfusion or improved neurologic outcome when the Hct was kept below 30 (Hgb <10 g/dL) for longer periods.[97] Transfusion of PRBCs has been shown to be an independent risk factor for mortality, lung injury, increased infection rate, renal failure, and intensive care unit (ICU) and hospital length of stay in trauma patients, especially when the transfused red cells are older than 14 days; this finding was independent of the severity of shock.[98,99] Nevertheless, this concern should not preclude timely and adequate administration of blood products.

Normally, type-specific crossmatched blood can be available in most centers in about 30 minutes, including transport time. Type-specific uncrossmatched blood can be available in even less time for patients with severe hemorrhage. However, if the situation dictates immediate transfusion, type O Rh-positive PRBCs and AB-negative fresh frozen plasma (FFP) are satisfactory in most situations. Controversy exists about the use of uncrossmatched type O PRBCs because of concern about the development of alloantibodies and allergic reactions. Dutton et al.,[100] reviewing their experience in 161 patients receiving 581 units of universal donor blood, demonstrated that only 1 of the 10 Rh-negative males receiving type O Rh-positive blood developed alloantibodies. All four females in the series received type O Rh-negative blood without apparent problem.

Most trauma patients are hypercoagulable when admitted to the ED and do not develop coagulopathy when administration of hemostatic agents is delayed. However, in the estimated 10% to 15% of patients with severe trauma and shock who enter the hospital in a hypocoagulable state[101] or rapidly develop hypocoagulation, resuscitative fluids and PRBCs may further worsen the coagulopathy and facilitate the vicious cycle. A computer simulation study by Hirshberg et al.[102] clearly demonstrated that with crystalloid resuscitation techniques, most major trauma patients are coagulopathic when they arrive at the OR. In their study, the prothrombin time (PT) increased to below hemostatic levels after replacement of 1 blood volume, fibrinogen function would become inadequate at replacement of 1.25 blood volumes, and platelets would become inadequate with replacement of 1.75 blood volumes. Experience gained in the Iraq and Afghanistan wars attests to the accuracy of the findings of Hirshberg et al.[102] Holcomb et al.[103] strongly recommend starting liquid plasma replacement along with fluids and PRBCs as soon as the patient arrives in the ED and continuing it throughout surgery. In a recent multicenter randomized clinical trial, Holcomb et al.[104] compared the effect of 2:1:1 with 1:1:1 ratios of PRBCs, FFP, and platelet resuscitation on mortality and continuation of hemorrhage during the initial 24-hour period after trauma and could not demonstrate a statistical difference in mortality, although patients treated with a 1:1:1 ratio had significantly decreased bleeding.

Liquid plasma differs from FFP in that it is never frozen and can be used up to 28 days after collection, but at a cost of containing a much lower level of hemostatic factors. Not all trauma center blood banks carry liquid plasma. Instead most centers keep thawed plasma stored in liquid form available to be used until FFP or PF 24 is thawed, which takes about 30 to 45 minutes. PF 24 is plasma frozen within 24 hours of collection, whereas FFP is frozen within 8 hours. It contains about 60% of the factors found in FFP except fibrinogen, which, because of its long half-life of 12 hours, is not affected. One unit of FFP contains approximately 7% of the coagulation factor activity of a 70-kg man. Available plasma preparations and their characteristics are shown in Table 53-3. Military data demonstrate that the death rate was 65% when the plasma to PRBC ratio was 1:8, 34% at 1:2.5, and 19% at 1:1.4.[105]

Table 53-3 Available Plasma Preparations and Their Features

	Collection to Freezing Interval (h)	Collection to Thawing Interval (h)	Factor Activity (%)	Time Taken to Thaw (min)	Comments
Fresh frozen plasma (FFP)	≤8	0–24	~100	45	Blood bank receives it frozen from the blood center
Plasma frozen 24 (PF24)	≤24	0–48	~60	45	All factors except fibrinogen are depleted
Liquid plasma	Never frozen	Never thawed	<30	—	Only few blood centers have it. It is good for 28 days.
Thawed plasma	8–24	0–48	20–30 Depending on the interval used after thawing	45	This product is kept thawed from 1 to 5 days and if not used discarded. It is released as the first group of plasma to be used until thawing of FFP or PF24 is completed

Currently many trauma centers use hemostatic resuscitation by activating MTPs during initial resuscitation of major traumatic hemorrhage in the ED and OR. These involve administering a relatively limited quantity of crystalloid solutions and volume replacement with FFP or PF 24 and PRBCs. In addition, platelets and cryoprecipitate are given regularly. One such protocol, used in Grady Memorial Hospital in Atlanta, Georgia, is shown in Table 53-4.[106]

Elderly (age >65 years) patients appear to tolerate MTP as well as their younger counterparts. Murray et al.[107] compared MTP in old (age >65 years) and young patients and found no difference in survival to discharge. For children the term *massive hemorrhage* is relatively new and is considered if transfusion volume exceeds 40 mL/kg.[108] A comparable definition is the administration of 50% of blood volume over 24 hours.[109] The adult definitions and treatments do not apply to the pediatric population because of the differences in size, physiology, nature of injury, and demographics. The circulating blood volume in the infant is 90 mL/kg and in children over 3 months, it is 70 mL/kg. Children have a greater hemodynamic reserve than adults, and vital signs deteriorate only if a significant quantity (about 35% to 40%) of blood is lost. A narrow pulse pressure is the most constant vital sign for early volume loss.[110] The high metabolic rate increases oxygen extraction, underscoring the importance of an adequate hemoglobin concentration. Above all, the procoagulant hemostatic proteins including the vitamin K-dependent factors are at subnormal levels until 6 months of age.[110] Neonatal platelet counts and function are normal, but fibrinogen is dysfunctional in the fetal form until 6 months to a year after birth. Plasmin generation and fibrinolysis are markedly reduced in infants. The PT and partial thromboplastin time (PTT) are mildly prolonged in infants and should not be used as a transfusion trigger. Thromboelastography, which looks at clot stability, is a better measure of coagulation status.

The 1:1:1 ratio that is often applied to adults translates to 20 mL/kg of PRBCs, 20 mL/kg of FFP, and 10 mL/kg of platelets in children.[111] This ratio has not been tested rigorously in pediatrics and serves as a guideline pending prospective investigation. Tranexamic acid and other procoagulants are given according to the comfort and experience of the clinician. This drug and many other procoagulants have also not been tested in pediatric trauma. In pediatric patients currently the actual trigger for activating the MTP is a high injury severity score. The decision to activate MTP is made by an experienced pediatric trauma surgeon or anesthesiologist. Bleeding into the retroperitoneal space and in the brain is more common in pediatric patients than in adults and should not be missed in the initial evaluation of the pediatric trauma patient. Although intracranial bleeding, if not accompanied by another injury, is not likely to cause hypotension in adults, it can cause significant hypotension in the pediatric age group. The

Table 53-4 Massive Transfusion Protocol Used in Grady Memorial Hospital in Atlanta

Package	PRBCs	Plasma	Platelets	Cryoprecipitate
Initiation	6 units (UD/TS)	6 U (UD)		
1 (0.5 hr)	6 units (UD/TS)	6 U (UD)	1 apheresis[a]	
2 (1 hr)	6 units (UD/TS)	6 U (TS)		10 U
3 (1.5 hr)	6 units (UD/TS)	6 U (TS)	1 apheresis[a]	
4 (2 hr)	6 units (UD/TS)	6 U (TS)		10 U
5 (2.5 hr)	6 units (UD/TS)	6 U (TS)	1 apheresis[a]	
6 (3 hr)	6 units (UD/TS)	6 U (TS)		10 U

UD, universal donor; TS, type specific.
[a]One apheresis unit of platelet is equal to 8 to 10 standard units.
Reprinted with permission from Dente CJ, Shaz BH, Nicholas JM, et al. Early predictors of massive transfusion in patients sustaining torso gunshot wounds in a civilian level 1 trauma center. *J Trauma.* 2010;68:298.

basic principles of administering blood components to promote both hemostatic and hemodynamic resuscitation in children are similar to the adult patient. Studies emphasize that a proper ratio of blood components (1:1:1) leads to better survival; presently evidence-based support for this is lacking in the pediatric population. There are several scoring systems that predict outcome for the massively transfused pediatric patient. The child who presents on admission with a base deficit above 6 or INR over 1.8 is predicted to have the highest mortality.[110]

One of the principal goals during early management of the hemorrhaging trauma victim is to avoid the development of the so-called vicious cycle or lethal triad, consisting of acidosis, hypothermia, and dilutional coagulopathy (Fig. 53-4). Both acidosis and hypothermia are major factors in the induction of coagulopathy. Resuscitation with crystalloids and PRBCs, which have no hemostatic activity, further adds to this effect by diluting platelets, already reduced in number and dysfunctional, and coagulation factors. Bleeding and intravascular coagulation further augment coagulopathy via loss or consumption of damaged or depleted platelets and coagulation factors. Augmented coagulopathy further increases the blood loss, necessitating additional fluid replacement and thus maintaining the vicious cycle, which ultimately results in MOF and death. More recent findings suggest that coagulopathy of the trauma patient has two components: acute traumatic coagulopathy (ATC) and resuscitation-associated coagulopathy (RAC). The former develops shortly after trauma and is caused by hyperfibrinolysis and severe tissue injury that releases tissue factor, which in turn activates the coagulation pathways. This type of coagulopathy appears to be independent of hypothermia or dilution of factors by crystalloids. The latter is caused by hypothermia, fluids, and possibly other resuscitation-related factors. In most severe trauma patients coagulopathy is caused by a combination of ATC and RAC. In fact patients presenting with ATC will require more intense resuscitation and likely develop hypothermia and dilutional coagulopathy. However, it appears that the presence of ATC has greater effect on the development of MOF and death than the components of the vicious cycle. Coagulopathy itself in one study was an independent predictor of MOF and mortality independent of shock, injury severity, and the vicious triad.[112] Thus initiating resuscitation with a high ratio of hemostatic fluids and PRBCs early enough, preferably in the prehospital phase, may improve outcome in this setting.

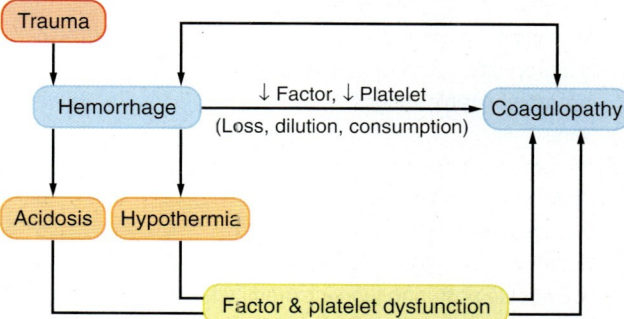

Figure 53-4 Schematic representation of bloody vicious cycle or lethal triad. Trauma-induced hemorrhage causes acidosis, hypothermia, and coagulopathy. Acidosis and hypothermia produce factor and platelet dysfunction, enhancing coagulopathy, which in turn causes increased bleeding. The cycle continues until death ensues, unless effective treatment by timely control of bleeding and correction of acidosis, hypothermia, and coagulopathy is instituted.

Rapid establishment of venous access with large-bore cannulae placed in peripheral veins that drain both above and below the diaphragm is essential for adequate fluid resuscitation in the patient who is severely injured. When vascular collapse and extremity injury impair access to arm or leg vessels, percutaneous cannulation of the internal jugular, subclavian, or femoral veins can be performed. Ultrasound guidance may facilitate cannulation of the internal jugular vein and prevent needle entry and infusion of fluids into the pleural space in patients with a large hemothorax. Ultrasound may also be used for infraclavicular access to the axillary vein, the cephalic or basilic veins at the midarm level, or the femoral vein. If necessary, a cutdown to a saphenous or arm vein can be rapidly performed in older children and adults. In children less than 5 years of age, intraosseous cannulation has a high success rate and a low incidence of complications. Infusion rates comparable with those obtained with intravenous lines are possible in small children, although a pressure infusion device may be necessary to achieve adequate flow.

Patients who arrive in the ED in cardiac arrest require advanced cardiac life support. However, the success rate of external cardiac massage in hypovolemic trauma victims is likely to be low.[113] ED thoracotomy not only permits performance of open cardiac massage but also aids resuscitation efforts by allowing drainage of pericardial blood, control of cardiac and great vessel bleeding, and application of a cross-clamp to the aorta. A small Foley catheter introduced into the right atrium or, in desperate situations, a large-bore catheter or introducer inserted in the descending aorta can be used for rapid administration of fluids. Not all patients who arrive in the ED in cardiac arrest benefit from ED thoracotomy. Countless reports attempted to identify predictors of survival to avoid fruitless ED thoracotomies and thereby decrease the risk of provider contamination with possibly infected patient blood. Some of the survival predictors include injury mechanism, anatomic injury location, extent of physiologic derangement, presenting signs of life, and presence of cardiac rhythm or vital signs. More recently, after review of available evidence-based studies, the survival rate with or without intact neurologic function after ED thoracotomy in different types of injuries in the presence and absence of signs of life has been reported.[114] Patients arriving with penetrating thoracic injury and signs of life have the greatest likelihood to survive (21.3%), and 11.7% have and a neurologically intact survival. In contrast patients arriving with pulseless blunt injury without signs of life have the least likelihood to survive (0.7%) and to have neurologically intact survival (0.1%). Signs of life include pupillary response, spontaneous ventilation, presence of carotid pulse, measurable or palpable blood pressure, extremity movement, and cardiac electrical activity. The highest survival with or without intact neurologic function occurred after penetrating thoracic trauma presented with signs of life. Those without signs of life on arrival had a lower rate of survival, but an ED thoracotomy could still be justified. Patients presenting pulseless after penetrating extrathoracic injury had more favorable outcome if they had some signs of life than those who did not. Those patients who had blunt injury with or without signs of life had a very poor survival rate, precluding ED thoracotomy.

Early Management of Specific Injuries

Head Injury

Approximately 40% of deaths from trauma are caused by head injury, and indeed even a moderate brain injury may increase the

Table 53-5 Effects on Outcome of Secondary Insults on the Brain Occurring from Time of Injury Through Resuscitation[a]

Secondary Insults	No. of Patients	Total Patients (%)	6-Month Outcome (%)		
			Good/Moderate	Severe/Vegetative	Dead
Total cases	717	100	43.0	20.2	36.8
Neither	308	43.0	63.9	10.2	26.9
Hypoxia	161	22.4	50.3	21.7	28.0
Hypotension	62	11.4	32.9	17.1	50.0
Both	166	23.2	20.5	22.3	57.2

[a]Data from hospital emergency departments enrolled in Traumatic Coma Data Bank.
Reprinted with permission from Prough DS, Lang J. Therapy of patients with head injuries: key parameters for management. *J Trauma.* 1997;42(Suppl):10S.

mortality rate of patients with other injuries. In nonsurvivors, progression of the damaged area beyond the directly injured region (secondary brain injury) can be demonstrated at autopsy.[115] The major factor in secondary injury is tissue hypoxia, which results in lactic acidosis; free radical generation; prostaglandin synthesis and release of excitatory amino acids (primarily glutamate); lipid peroxidation and breakdown of cell membranes; entry of large quantities of sodium, calcium, and water into the cells; and leakage of fluid from the blood vessels into the extracellular space.[116,117] This process results in brain edema and both regional and global disturbances of the cerebral circulation. Thus, of all the possible secondary insults to the injured brain, decreased oxygen delivery as a result of hypotension and hypoxia has the greatest detrimental impact (Table 53-5).[118,119]

Brain injury by itself does not cause hypotension in adults except as a preterminal event and in pediatric patients. However, more than half of the patients with severe head trauma have other injuries that render approximately 15% of them hypotensive. Approximately 30% are hypoxic on admission as a result of central respiratory depression or associated chest injuries. Furthermore, exposure to these insults is likely to occur during any phase of the continuum of hospital care: in the emergency room, the radiology unit, the OR, the postanesthesia care unit, the ICU, or elsewhere. The most common early complications of head trauma are intracranial hypertension, brain herniation, seizures, neurogenic pulmonary edema, cardiac dysrhythmias, bradycardia, systemic hypertension, and coagulopathy.

Diagnosis

Mental impairment after trauma may have any of several etiologies. However, the possibility of hypoxia and shock must always be considered first. If consciousness remains depressed despite ventilation and fluid replacement, a head injury is assumed to be present and the patient is managed accordingly. As noted, hypotension is the most important cause of death in the head-injured patient. Chesnut[119] demonstrated that a single episode of SBP less than 90 mmHg is associated with a 50% increase in mortality, and subsequent episodes or lower pressures increase mortality even further.[120] Therefore, every effort should be made to support the blood pressure with fluids and vasopressors (preferably phenylephrine, which does not constrict cerebral vessels) and ensure adequate oxygenation *before* the unconscious patient is evaluated. A baseline neurologic examination should be performed after initial resuscitation but before any sedative or muscle relaxant agents are administered, and this should be repeated at frequent intervals because the patient's condition may change rapidly.

Anesthetic and adjunct drugs may render an adequate neurologic examination impossible; thus, long-acting muscle relaxants, opioids, sedatives, or hypnotics should be given selectively.[118,121]

Consciousness can be initially assessed within a few seconds using the AVPU system (*a*lert; responds to *v*erbal stimuli; responds to *p*ain; *u*nresponsive) (Table 53-6). More precise information is provided by the GCS, which provides a standard means of

Table 53-6 Two-Level Initial Evaluation of Consciousness

Level 1. AVPU System
A = <u>A</u>lert
V = Responds to <u>v</u>erbal stimuli
P = Responds to <u>p</u>ainful stimuli
U = <u>U</u>nresponsive

Level 2. Glasgow Coma Scale (GCS)

Eye opening (E)	
Spontaneous, already open and blinking	4
To speech	3
To pain	2
None	1
Verbal response (V)	
Oriented	5
Answers but confused	4
Inappropriate but recognizable words	3
Incomprehensible sounds	2
None	1
Best motor response (M)	
Obeys verbal commands	6
Localizes painful stimulus	5
Withdraws from painful stimulus	4
Decorticate posturing (upper extremity flexion)	3
Decerebrate posturing (upper extremity extension)	2
No movement	1

GCS ≤8 = deep coma, severe head trauma, poor outcome
GCS 9–12 = conscious patient with moderate injury
GCS >12 = mild injury

evaluating the patient's neurologic status. In this test, the sum of the scores obtained for eye opening, verbal response, and motor activity correlates with the state of consciousness, the severity of the head injury, and the prognosis.[121] Assessment of motor function should be performed on the extremity that responds best. The limb affected by neurologic injury is examined, but the result is not considered in the GCS.

Dilatation and sluggish response of the pupil are signs of compression of the oculomotor nerve by the medial portion of the temporal lobe (uncus). A maximally dilated and unresponsive "blown" pupil suggests uncal herniation under the falx cerebri. The presence of similar findings in ocular injuries makes interpretation of pupillary findings difficult when eye and head injuries coexist. However, the pupillary reaction to light is usually more sluggish in the head-injured patient.

CT scanning is used for the diagnosis of most acute head injuries. Positive CT findings after acute head injury include midline shift, distortion of the ventricles and cisterns, effacement of the sulci in the uninjured hemisphere, and presence of a hematoma at any location in the cranial vault. Subdural hematomas usually have a concave border, whereas epidural hematomas present with a convex outline classically termed a *lenticular* configuration. Patients in severe coma (GCS <8) have a 40% likelihood of an intracranial hematoma. Those with higher GCS scores are less likely to have had intracranial bleeding although it is evident that the significant incidence of this complication even in these patients necessitates a CT study, preferably with contrast enhancement. Other benefits of CT scanning include detection of intracranial air and depressed skull fractures.

Management

The primary objective of the early management of brain trauma is to prevent or alleviate the secondary injury process that may follow any complication that decreases the oxygen supply to the brain, including systemic hypotension, hypoxemia, anemia, raised ICP, acidosis, and possibly hyperglycemia (serum glucose >200 mg/dL). These insults cause exacerbation of trauma-induced cerebral ischemia and metabolic derangements, worsening the outcome.[122,123] *The most important therapeutic maneuvers in these patients are aimed at normalizing ICP, CPP, and oxygen delivery.* The Brain Trauma Foundation and the American Association of Neurological Surgeons have published evidence-based guidelines for the treatment of head-injured patients.[118] Primary therapy includes normalization of the systemic blood pressure (mean blood pressure >80 mmHg) and maintaining the PaO$_2$ over 95, the ICP below 20 to 25 mmHg, and the CPP at 50 to 70 mmHg. Maintaining the CPP at levels above 70 mmHg, the former standard, is no longer advised because it may be associated with an increased incidence of ARDS.[118] The patient is kept at 30-degree head elevation, sedation and paralysis are employed as necessary, and cerebrospinal fluid is drained through a ventriculostomy catheter if available. Rapid and adequate restoration of the intravascular volume with isotonic crystalloid and, if necessary, with colloid solutions should be aimed at maintaining the CPP between 50 and 70 mmHg while attempting to minimize further brain swelling. LR solution, which is slightly hypotonic (Na$^+$ 130 mEq/L, osmolality ~255 mOsm/L), may promote swelling in uninjured areas of the brain if it is given in large quantities. Edema tends to occur in injured brain regions regardless of the type of solution administered because of increased permeability of the blood–brain barrier. To minimize edema formation, it is wise to monitor serum osmolality and to replace LR solution with isotonic normal saline. If serum osmolality cannot be measured, this change can be made empirically after 3 L of LR solution.

Much of the focus has been on in-hospital management of patients with brain trauma, but there is increasing interest in the impact of prehospital care on the outcome in these patients. Multiple studies have demonstrated an association between prehospital endotracheal intubation and mortality of patients with severe brain trauma.[124,125] In a large multicenter retrospective study, Davis et al.[126] found that patients with GCS no higher than 8, in whom endotracheal intubation was attempted at the accident site, had a higher mortality than those who were not intubated until arrival at the emergency room (adjusted odds ratio of 2.91; $p <0.01$). The authors speculated that this may result from physiologic insults during intubation (elevated ICP, oxygen desaturation, or inadvertent postintubation hyperventilation and cerebral hypoperfusion with ischemia) and concluded that there may be no benefit to prehospital endotracheal intubation.

Normalization of the ICP has been shown to reduce mortality.[127] Effective reduction in ICP can be provided, or at least aided, by administration of mannitol, an important part of the management of severe head injury. It is administered in boluses of 0.25 to 0.5 g/kg and repeated every 4 to 6 hours as needed to control the ICP.[118] Higher doses, up to 2 g/kg, are recommended by some authors.[128] In addition to its osmotic diuretic effect, this agent may improve cerebral blood flow (CBF) and O$_2$ delivery by reducing the Hct and thus the blood viscosity immediately after administration.[118] There is a risk of hypovolemia and resultant hypotension when therapeutic doses of mannitol are used. If the ICP elevation persists, additional doses of mannitol should be given cautiously. Acute mannitol toxicity, manifested by hyponatremia, high serum osmolality, and a gap between calculated and measured serum osmolality over 10 mOsm/L, may result when the drug is given in large doses (2 to 3 g/kg) or to patients with renal failure. Mannitol should be used with great care in the presence of hypotension, sepsis, nephrotoxic drugs, or pre-existing renal disease, because these may also precipitate renal failure.[118] Further, the effects of mannitol result from its activity in regions of the brain where the blood–brain barrier is intact. It may exacerbate edema in injured areas in which it may easily enter the tissues.

The addition of relatively small volumes of hypertonic saline in concentrations between 3% (6 to 8 mL/kg) and 7.5% (4 mL/kg) followed by infusion of LR may be beneficial in multiple-trauma patients with head injury.[129] In addition, hypertonic saline (15% solution), in bolus doses of 0.42 mL/kg, is as efficacious as mannitol for initial therapy of elevated ICP in this patient population.[128] Like mannitol, hypertonic saline draws fluid from the intracellular space, and thus in addition to restoring the blood volume, it reduces brain edema and prevents elevation of the ICP.[130] On the other hand, hypertonic saline may, also like mannitol, increase edema in the injured region of the brain.[131] However, administration of hypertonic saline cannot be maintained for long periods. It may cause hypernatremia, hyperosmolality, or hyperchloremic acidosis, probably from renal bicarbonate loss secondary to increased levels of chloride (Cl$^-$). Serum concentrations of sodium (Na$^+$) and Cl$^-$ and the patient's acid–base status should be followed, and the administration of hypertonic saline should be discontinued if plasma Na$^+$ reaches 160 mEq/L.

There have been several studies comparing hypertonic saline and mannitol for brain relaxation during craniotomy.[132] Although saline seems to be somewhat more effective in reducing brain swelling, the studies were all underpowered, and the clinical relevance of their results is questionable. Resuscitation with albumin 5% or 25% provides a sustained improvement in vital signs, but the increase in colloid osmotic pressure produced by these solutions may be associated with an increased risk of mortality.[133]

Hyponatremia in these patients results from intravascular volume expansion rather than sodium loss; thus treatment with saline solutions is not appropriate. Because of a synergistic action between mannitol and loop diuretics in improving the ICP, addition of furosemide may be a safer and more effective treatment than increasing the dose of mannitol when intracranial hypertension persists. Until about 1995, hyperventilation to a $PaCO_2$ of 25 to 30 mmHg was a mainstay of the therapy of head injury. However, brain ischemia, which is probably the most threatening consequence of head injury, is likely to occur during the first 6 hours after trauma even when the CPP is maintained above the generally recommended 50 to 70 mmHg.[134] Coles[134] has demonstrated by positron emission tomography scanning that a significant increase in the region of critical hypoperfusion may result from hyperventilation in these patients. This hypoperfusion seems to be caused largely by increased cerebral vascular resistance, which may be enhanced by hyperventilation. However, some degree of hyperventilation may be necessary for short periods of time in patients who have severe injuries and elevated ICP that does not respond to normal ventilation and diuretics, although this should not be used during the first 24 hours following injury.[118] Its use after the initial phase should be based on monitoring of the ICP. It should be noted that hyperventilation in the severely brain-injured patient may also be associated with acute lung injury.[135]

If the ICP remains elevated despite all of these measures, pentobarbital (3 to 10 mg/kg given over 0.5 to 2.5 hours, followed by a maintenance infusion of 0.5 to 3.0 mg/kg/hr, aimed at a serum concentration between 2.5 and 4.0 mg/dL) may be required. High-dose barbiturates are of no value in the routine therapy of head injury and should be used only for refractory ICP elevation. Of course, immediate surgical decompression, especially of epidural hematomas, is an important factor in reducing morbidity and mortality.

Over the past several years there has been much debate regarding optimal blood glucose level in critically ill patients. Brain-injured patients are unique members of this group because brain metabolism is altered by the injury and is heavily dependent on glucose. Hypoglycemia (<40 g/dL) may cause metabolic crisis, whereas hyperglycemia (>200 g/dL) can cause detrimental effects through excitotoxicity, oxidative stress, and inflammatory cytokine release. However, tight insulin control therapy (80 to 110 mg/dL) has been associated with episodes of hypoglycemia. As a result, the current recommendations are to maintain glucose levels of 110 to 180 mg/dL.[136]

Nearly 75% of severely brain-injured patients who die expire within the first 3 days following the initial trauma. Many of the survivors will later succumb to nonneurologic organ dysfunction involving pulmonary failure and cardiac impairment, which may be related to sympathetic hyperactivity. β-Blocker therapy has been proposed as a treatment that may be beneficial in these patients.[137] The optimal agent, the dose level, the timing, and the duration of treatment, however, remain to be determined.

If the patient is hemodynamically stable, a CT scan is performed. The strictest attention should be paid to ensure adequate oxygenation, ventilation, blood pressure, and ICP control during the procedure. If the patient is hemodynamically unstable or requires emergency surgery for associated injuries and has a history suggesting a head injury, even though a significant intracranial hematoma is unlikely on clinical grounds, intraoperative ICP monitoring is indicated to permit rapid detection of ICP elevation. Both intracranial hematomas and hemorrhage in other regions have a high surgical priority. In the multiple trauma victim, prioritization between the two is based on the severity of each injury. Because there is no time to obtain a CT scan of the head in patients with both profuse hemorrhage and brain herniation, the patient is brought directly to the OR for simultaneous control of the bleeding site and evacuation of the intracranial hematoma. The site of the craniotomy can be determined by a ventriculogram or an ultrasound examination with a pencil-tip probe; both tests may be performed under local anesthesia through a frontal burr hole.

Anesthetic Management

Intraoperative management is a continuation of the pre-existing intensive care.[138] Thus in addition to providing anesthesia, it is necessary to maintain the blood pressure, oxygenation, and CPP. It should be noted that there have been no studies comparing intravenous to inhalation techniques. It seems reasonable to assume that preserving the vital signs is more important than the specific means employed to accomplish this. Beyond the standard ASA monitors, an arterial line will permit beat-to-beat monitoring of the blood pressure, along with following blood gas levels and blood glucose. An ICP monitor will generally be placed by the neurosurgeons. Vital signs, PaO_2, and $PaCO_2$ should be maintained at the same levels as they are before the patient reaches the OR. Preoperative fluid management is also continued during surgery. Blood should be administered carefully, because overtransfusion may increase blood viscosity and thus decrease CBF.

It may be possible to improve the outlook for brain-injured patients, as outlined here:
1. The earlier definitive treatment is initiated, the better the outcome is likely to be. Rudehill et al.[139] have demonstrated improvement in outcomes in a large series of patients when care was initiated by anesthesiologists at the accident scene. On the other hand, Haltmeier et al.[140] found no difference between the outcomes for traumatic brain injury patients treated onsite by anesthesiologists in Bern or paramedics in US.
2. Meanwhile, the wide variety of types and severities of injury and of responses to treatment—both among different patients and in the same patient at different times—imply that therapeutic interventions must be individualized.[141,142] These aims may be met, at least partly, by carefully structured intensive care.[143,144] Therapeutic goals should be set explicitly and reviewed, and altered if necessary, at every change of shift.

   For instance, the traumatic brain injury pathway guideline of Bellevue Hospital Center, New York, generally follows the recommendations of the Brain Trauma Foundation guidelines, with adjustments depending on GCS and ICP.

Indeed, early intervention and controlled management may explain much of the improvement in outcomes that has been obtained over the past 20 years, including the results obtained by Patel et al.[145] and Palmer et al.[143] using strict protocol-driven therapies (in the latter case, the 1995 Brain Trauma Foundation guidelines) (Table 53-7).

Spine and Spinal Cord Injury

Initial Evaluation

The objective in the evaluation of spinal trauma is to diagnose instability of the spine and the extent of neurologic involvement. Not stabilizing the spine in the first hours after a major accident until a definitive diagnosis is established carries the risk of converting a neurologically intact patient into a paraplegic or quadriplegic. During transport to the hospital, the patient should be immobilized with a hard collar, a spine board, and tape. After

Table 53-7 6-Month Outcomes for Patients with Brain Injury In Various Studies

Name of Study	No. of Patients	Year Published	6-Month Outcome (%)			Comments
			Good/ Moderate	Severe/ Vegetative	Dead	
Three-country Jeanett and Teasdale[146]	700	1977	38	11	51	Various treatments, some untreated
Miller et al.[147]	158	1981	47	12	40	Vent, surgery, ICP monitoring, hyperventilation, and Rx
Traumatic Coma Data Bank (TCDB)[148]	717	1997	43	20	37	Total patients, standard therapy
TCDB[148]	308	1997	54	19	27	Patients without hypotension or hypoxia
Palmer et al.[143]	56	2000	70	14	16	1995 BTF Guidelines
Rudehill et al.[139]	1,508	2002	69	11	20	Standard protocol, early management
Patel et al.[149]	129	2002	63	13	20	NCCU Protocol

Results of various treatment protocols for brain injuries. The three-country study surveyed patients who had received a wide variety of treatment; some were untreated. Miller et al.[147] relied on hyperventilation and, when necessary, barbiturates. The TCBD patients were treated similarly; note the difference in outcome of the patients who did not experience hypotension or hypoxia. The final three studies are described in the text. ICP, intracranial pressure; BTF, Brain Trauma Foundation; Rx, other treatment; NCCU, neurosurgical critical care unit.

admission, patients should not be left on a rigid spine board for longer than 1 hour, especially when they are paralyzed, because of the risk of decubitus ulcers.

In the conscious patient, the diagnosis is relatively easy: a history of a motor vehicle, industrial, or athletic accident; an act of violence; a fall; penetrating trauma resulting in a neurologic deficit below a specific spinal level; or pain and tenderness over the involved vertebrae strongly suggest a spine injury. It should be noted, however, that spinal pain is not always localized to the level of injury.[150] Obviously, these symptoms are difficult to elicit in the comatose patient. In these circumstances, flaccid areflexia, loss of rectal sphincter tone, paradoxic respiration, and bradycardia in a hypovolemic patient suggest the diagnosis. In cervical spine trauma, an ability to flex but not to extend the elbow and response to painful stimuli above but not below the clavicle also indicate neurologic injury. Current guidelines consider absence of neck pain or paresthesia and a negative physical examination—lack of tenderness with palpation and during voluntary flexion and extension of the neck—in a neurologically intact, conscious patient as adequate indications for ruling out a cervical spine injury without further radiologic studies. Alcohol intoxication and distracting associated injuries do not seem to alter these criteria as long as the patient is alert, conscious, and able to concentrate. A large meta-analysis of obtunded trauma patients demonstrated that modern multislice helical CT imaging is sufficient to detect unstable cervical spine injuries. However, this approach may still miss some patients at risk for subsequent cervical cord insult.[151]

Depending on the degree of deficit, spinal cord injuries are categorized as *complete* or *incomplete*. Intact sensory perception over the sacral distribution and voluntary contraction of the anus (sacral sparing) are present in incomplete, but not in complete, injuries. There is practically no possibility of significant neurologic recovery in complete injury, whereas functional restoration may occur in up to 50% of patients after incomplete injuries. In some patients the development of *spinal shock*, which is manifested by absolute flaccidity and loss of reflexes, precludes distinguishing between complete and incomplete injuries during the initial phase of treatment. Therefore, even in the absence of sacral sparing, the possibility of neurologic recovery dictates that all possible efforts be made at this time to prevent further damage and to preserve cord function. A similar principle applies to the evaluation of the level of injury. After the first few days, spinal cord edema subsides, and the final injury level is commonly a few segments lower than on initial presentation. Thus, early therapeutic efforts should not be abandoned even in the patient with a high-level injury, which carries a grim functional prognosis.

Spinal shock is probably caused by direct trauma to the spinal cord and usually subsides within days to weeks. The term is frequently used as a misnomer for *neurogenic shock*, which is defined as hypotension and bradycardia caused by the loss of vasomotor tone and sympathetic innervation of the heart as a result of functional depression of the descending sympathetic pathways of the spinal cord. It is usually present after high thoracic and cervical spine injuries and improves within 3 to 5 days.[152]

Initial Management

The spinal cord, a microcosm of the brain, is also vulnerable to a secondary injury process that may be a product of hypotension, hypoxia, and probably other physiologic complications.[153] Prompt recognition and aggressive treatment of these insults, which may also result from associated trauma, may minimize exacerbation of spinal cord lesions and improve the long-term outlook of these patients.[122,154]

Immobilization and Intubation

Maintenance of immobilization of the injured spine is of paramount importance. If a cervical spine fracture is suspected, immobilization or MILS of the neck is necessary before the patient is moved. If the patient has a thoracic or lumbar injury, a careful logrolling maneuver should be used.[153,155]

About one-third of paraplegic patients require airway management, mostly within the first 24 hours after injury. Signs of respiratory distress or fatigue, or a rising respiratory rate or $PaCO_2$, are major indications for ventilatory assistance. Severe bradycardia or dysrhythmias may result from unopposed vagal activity during tracheal intubation or suctioning: The patient must be preoxygenated, and atropine (0.4 to 0.6 mg) should be given before any instrumentation. If bradycardia develops during airway management, treatment includes additional atropine, glycopyrrolate, isoproterenol, or, if necessary, cardiac pacing.

The techniques of intubation in spine-injured patients are discussed in the Airway Management section.

Respiratory Complications

Respiratory complications are common in all phases of the care of spinal cord–injured patients and are the most frequent cause of death in the acute stage.[156,157] In the initial period, these problems may be augmented by associated brain, neck, chest, or abdominal injury; alcohol intoxication; or the effects of self-administered or iatrogenic drugs. Injuries at C5 or lower are usually associated with normal tidal volumes because the function of the diaphragm is intact, whereas patients with injuries at C4 or above may require permanent ventilatory assistance. Nevertheless, accessory respiratory muscle paresis may cause a significant loss of expiratory reserve even when the injury involves the lower spinal segments.[158,159] Pulmonary edema is another significant cause of respiratory dysfunction. A severe catecholamine surge follows acute trauma to the spinal cord.[160] Although the resultant severe hypertension lasts for only a few minutes, its effects persist. It may produce both pulmonary capillary damage, as a result of shifting of a large portion of the blood volume into the pulmonary circulation, and left ventricular dysfunction. Overzealous fluid therapy to treat the patient's initial hypotension may lead to acute pulmonary edema when the sympathetic activity returns approximately 3 to 5 days after the injury.

Paradoxic respiration in the quadriplegic patient results from partial chest wall collapse during inspiration. It may produce limitation of the tidal volume and an increased risk of hypoventilation.[159] The situation is aggravated when the patient is in an upright position. The diaphragm cannot maintain its normal domed shape, the only way in which it can contract efficiently, because the weight of the thoracic contents is not opposed by the normal tone of the abdominal muscles. Thus, in contrast to other diseases that produce respiratory insufficiency, the supine position improves respiration in persons with quadriplegia (Fig. 53-5).[159] It should be noted that disordered breathing (probably mostly from obstructive sleep apnea) is common while the patient is asleep and may exacerbate the problems caused by other complications.[161]

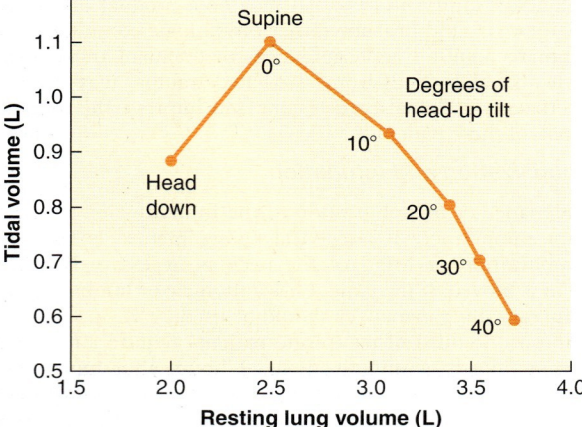

Figure 53-5 Effect of semi-Fowler's position on ventilation in quadriplegic patients. Adapted with permission from Winslow C, Rozovsky J: Effect of spinal cord injury on respiratory system. *Am J Phys Med Rehab*. 2003;82:803–14.

Other causes of inadequate respiration in the early phase of spinal cord injury are aspiration of gastric contents, atelectasis, pneumonia, and bronchoconstriction. Management includes careful observation of the patient's breathing and preparation to ventilate the lungs and intubate the trachea at the first sign of respiratory depression.[159]

Hemodynamic Management

Hemodynamic management of quadriplegic patients includes a complete assessment, with insertion of a central venous or pulmonary artery catheter (PAC) if necessary, as early as possible after injury. In as many as 25% of patients with cervical spinal cord injuries, left ventricular dysfunction may contribute to the hypotension.[162] There is evidence to support the maintenance of mean arterial pressure above 85 mmHg.[163] Decreased preload can be treated with fluid infusion using cardiac function curves as a guide. In general, volume may be safely replaced to a central venous or pulmonary capillary wedge pressure (PCWP) of 18 mmHg.[162] This avoids, or at least limits, the severity of the pulmonary edema described previously. Hypotension, despite adequate fluid infusion, acidosis, or low mixed venous PO_2, requires treatment with inotropes such as dopamine.

A review by Dhall et al.[164] indicates that these patients frequently experience deep vein thrombosis (DVT), which may adversely affect both hemodynamic and pulmonary function. The authors recommend the initiation of low–molecular-weight or low-dose unfractionated heparin therapy, combined with a rotating bed, compression stockings, or electrical stimulation, within 72 hours of the injury. This therapy should be held on the day of any surgical procedure.

Anesthetic Considerations

Any anesthetic technique compatible with the patient's general condition is satisfactory for the spinal cord–injured patient. Hypotension is very common during anesthesia in quadriplegics. Placement of a TEE or a central venous catheter or PAC may facilitate management of the patient's volume and blood pressure status.

Neck Injury

Both penetrating and blunt trauma may injure the major structures in the neck: vessels, respiratory and digestive tracts, and nervous system. Hemorrhage, asphyxia, mediastinitis, paralysis, stroke, or death may result if these injuries are not promptly recognized and treated.

Penetrating neck injuries usually present with obvious clinical manifestations; blunt cervical trauma may be more subtle. Airway compromise or obstruction, brisk bleeding from the wound site, an expanding pulsatile hematoma, and shock with or without external bleeding are obvious signs of cervical vascular injury and dictate immediate airway management and vascular control. Decreased or absent upper extremity or distal carotid pulses, as well as carotid bruit or thrill, are pathognomonic for cervical arterial injury. Hemothorax, pneumothorax, and signs of air embolism are also suggestive of cervical vascular injury. Respiratory distress, cyanosis, or stridor is an obvious sign of airway injury and requires immediate tracheal intubation. Other signs that strongly suggest airway injury are dysphonia, hoarseness, cough, hemoptysis, air bubbling from the wound, subcutaneous crepitus, and laryngeal tenderness. Because of their dynamic nature, cervical airway injuries may rapidly progress to obstruction. The patient, therefore, should be observed carefully and the trachea intubated at the first sign of problems.

Anatomic location of the penetrating neck injury is classified in to three zones. Zone I is the narrow area above the clavicles extending from the cricoid cartilage to the level of the sternal notch; zone II is the area between the cricoid cartilage and the angle of the mandible; and zone III comprises the area between the angle of the mandible and the cranial base. Penetrating injuries involving zones I and III are relatively infrequent and difficult to manage surgically because of availability of limited exposure. Neck injuries most commonly involve zone II. Physical examination as a screening tool for further overall management has utmost importance for these injuries. A prospective multicenter study showed that clinical signs and symptoms often reliably indicate the cervical structures injured and prevent unnecessary imaging, and, if imaging is needed, multidetector CT is a highly sensitive and specific screening tool.[165]

Patients present with hard and soft signs. Those with hard signs require urgent or emergent surgery, whereas those with soft signs can be evaluated further using CT angiography.[166] Hard signs include hypotension/shock, active bleeding, expanding hematoma, neurologic deficit, airway compromise, air bubbling through wound, massive subcutaneous emphysema, and hematemesis. Signs of airway compromise require management even before arrival at the OR.

Esophageal injuries, whether in the neck or in the chest, are insidious and difficult to diagnose. Dysphagia, odynophagia, hematemesis, subcutaneous crepitus, prevertebral air on a lateral cervical radiograph, and major concomitant injuries to other cervical structures suggest an esophageal injury and call for confirmation with an esophagram. A management algorithm for surgery of the esophageal injuries has been made available by the Western Trauma Association.[167]

The neurologic manifestations of a penetrating neck injury vary depending on the injured structure. Partial spinal cord transection produces Brown-Séquard syndrome with ipsilateral motor and contralateral sensory deficit below the injury. Complete spinal cord transection, depending on the level of injury, produces paraplegia or quadriplegia, usually with neurogenic shock. Occasionally, luminal occlusion of the carotid and vertebral arteries may lead to a hemispheric cerebrovascular accident; associated hypotension increases the likelihood of this event.

Blunt cervical vascular injuries usually present with a hematoma that may compress the cervical veins, displace the airway, and produce pharyngeal and laryngeal congestion. Injury to an artery may produce an intimal tear, pseudoaneurysm, fistula, or thrombosis. If a carotid or vertebral artery is involved, cerebral ischemia may occur. Often thrombosis develops gradually over minutes to a few hours; thus the appearance of neurologic symptoms is delayed in approximately 40% of patients. Symptomatic patients may present with a cervical bruit, altered mental status, or lateralizing neurologic deficits including hemiparesis, transient ischemic attacks, amaurosis fugax, or Horner syndrome. The mortality rate associated with blunt carotid injury varies between 15% and 28%, and 15% to 50% of survivors have neurologic deficits.[168] Identification of a blunt or penetrating carotid injury in an asymptomatic patient using ultrasound, CT, or CT angiography not only allows early institution of antiplatelet therapy, systemic anticoagulation, endovascular intervention, or surgical repair[168,169] but also occasionally prevents the neurologic deficits that may follow surgery for associated injuries in an unprotected patient.

Airway injuries after blunt trauma are rare but carry an overall mortality rate of 2%.[68] Their severity varies from a simple mucosal tear or hematoma to a comminuted laryngeal cartilage fracture or complete cricotracheal separation (Table 53-1). They frequently require primary laryngeal repair or tracheostomy. Anesthetic management is complicated not only by relatively complex airway management problems[45,48] (discussed in the airway evaluation and intervention section) but also by associated skull base, intracranial, open neck, cervical spine, esophageal, or pharyngeal injuries.[66,170]

Chest Injury

Although a high percentage of thoracic injuries can be treated conservatively, patients who need surgery may have major intraoperative physiologic disturbances.

Chest Wall Injury

Rib, scapula, and sternal fractures, in addition to interfering with adequate respiration, may be associated with severe underlying thoracic, abdominal, cranial, and skeletal injuries. The management principles for these injuries are similar to those previously described for flail chest, although the need for mechanical ventilation is less likely in single rib fractures treated with systemic analgesics than in a flail chest. Effective pain relief, preferably with continuous thoracic epidural anesthesia or paravertebral or intercostal block, is central to management.[66]

Pleural Injury

Occult pneumothorax is easy to miss in major trauma. The presence of subcutaneous emphysema, pulmonary contusion, and rib fractures should raise suspicion of coexisting pneumothorax.[54] Tension pneumothorax involving over 50% of a hemithorax presents with dyspnea, tachycardia, cyanosis, agitation, diaphoresis, neck vein distention, tracheal deviation, and displacement of the maximal cardiac impulse to the contralateral side.

Although an upright plain chest radiograph provides the best opportunity for detection of pneumothorax, this position may be impossible or contraindicated in patients who are experiencing major hemorrhage or those with suspected spine injury. Air in the pleural space tends to accumulate in the anteromedial sulcus first, and then in lateral and caudal regions, often producing hemodynamic alterations and the deep sulcus sign on the anteroposterior chest radiogram in supine or semirecumbent patients. Transthoracic ultrasound by positioning the ultrasound probe longitudinally over the intercostal space may be used for the emergency diagnosis of pneumothorax. Normally, movement of the lung beneath the chest wall, in addition to pleural sliding, produces vertical B lines, so-called comet tail artifacts from echo-dense areas on the lung surface. In addition, a two-dimensional ultrasound image of the normal lung shows echogenic horizontal lines (A lines), which appear at the same distances as the distance between the probe and the first A line. Comet tail B lines that appear during breathing erase A lines. In the presence of pneumothorax, neither lung motion, sliding, or comet tails can be seen. In the time–motion mode (M mode), lung tissue has a granular appearance. Pneumothorax in this mode appears in a horizontal line pattern. Often in the supine position pleural air moves anteriorly, compressing the lung posteriorly on the dependent side. The junction between the two appears as a vertical line called the lung point, which, if noted, is pathognomonic for pneumothorax.[171] A lung point may be seen when there is a relatively small volume of pneumothorax and during expiration, pleural air comes under one side of the ultrasound probe, producing a time–motion image that shows a granular pattern (normal lung) on one side and a horizontal line pattern (pneumothorax) on the other side of the screen. During inspiration with expansion of the lung, the entire lung tissue is under the probe, and a normal granular appearance may be obtained with time–motion image. It should be emphasized that diagnosis of pneumothorax with ultrasound relies primarily on the movement of the lung rather than frozen images. Thus lung sliding and comet tail artifacts, which are produced by the movement of the lung, are the most commonly utilized features. Ultrasound examination may also be helpful in detecting residual pleural air after placement of the thoracostomy tube and diagnosis of pulmonary embolism (PE), pneumonia, and hemothorax.[172] Chest CT is the definitive test for diagnosis of pneumothorax.[55] It has been suggested that a small closed pneumothorax can be safely managed by observation alone without a chest tube even in those patients who require positive-pressure ventilation as long as continuing vigilance is maintained.[173,174] Based on the most recent Advanced Trauma Life Support recommendation[174,175] and our own experience, we strongly believe that once diagnosed, a traumatic pneumothorax, no matter how small, should be treated with thoracostomy drainage before tracheal intubation and positive-pressure ventilation.

Bleeding intercostal vessels are responsible for most hemothoraces. Severe airway deviation with respiratory distress and shock may be produced by a hemothorax, although it is not as common as it is after a pneumothorax. Treatment consists of drainage with a #30- to #40-French catheter chest tube (#26- to #32-French catheter is used for pneumothorax). Initial drainage of 1,000 mL of blood or collection of over 200 mL/hr for several hours is an indication for thoracotomy. Retained clotted blood after tube thoracostomy may be treated conservatively with intrapleural fibrinolytic agents.[175] Additional indications for thoracotomy are a "white lung" appearance on the anteroposterior chest radiograph or a continuous major air leak from the chest tube, which may result from a direct airway injury or major lung laceration. Hemodynamically stable patients with persistent bleeding of less than 150 mL/hr are often managed with video-assisted thoracoscopic surgery (VATS) to control bleeding, which requires collapse of the lung on the involved side using a double-lumen tube or a bronchial blocker. VATS can also be useful in diagnosis of suspected diaphragmatic or mediastinal injuries, evaluation of some bronchopleural fistulas, and evacuation of clotted blood or an empyema that does not drain with a chest tube or respond to intrapleural fibrinolytic therapy.[175] Use of VATS decreases the need for open thoracotomy and the number of negative explorations in stable trauma patients.[176]

Pulmonary Contusion

Pulmonary contusion often accompanies chest wall injury but may also develop in isolation. Its management is discussed in the management of breathing abnormalities section.

Penetrating Cardiac Injury

Pericardial tamponade, cardiac chamber perforation, and fistula formation between the cardiac chambers and the great vessels are the consequences of a penetrating cardiac trauma. Any penetrating wound of the chest, especially one within the "cardiac window" (midclavicular lines laterally, clavicles superiorly, and costal margins inferiorly), can cause this injury. These injuries are often fatal at the scene, especially if they are gunshot rather than stab wounds and involve the right rather than the thicker-walled left ventricle. Because of the dynamic nature of cardiac injuries and the risk of sudden hemodynamic deterioration, these patients must be transported directly to the OR, and immediate sternotomy or left thoracotomy must be performed as soon as the injury is suspected. Emergency cardiopulmonary bypass may be needed. Pneumopericardium visible on a plain chest radiograph after penetrating chest trauma should increase the suspicion, although it is not seen in all patients. TTE can be used for screening stable patients, but it may be inconclusive in obese patients and in those with pneumothorax. The central venous pressure (CVP) is not always accurate. TEE provides an accurate diagnosis in these patients, but it is impractical during the initial evaluation phase of trauma.[177,178] A subxiphoid pericardial window created in the OR, often under general anesthesia, may not drain all the blood in the pericardium, but even partial drainage can improve hemodynamics temporarily in this setting. Two penetrating chest trauma surgical decision-making algorithms, one for damage control strategies in the unstable patient and the other for the management of definitive repair in the stable patient, are described by the Western Trauma Association.[179] Because of the high density of vital organs in the chest and their close proximity to each other, penetrating trauma often injures more than one organ, and as such the decision-making process requires consideration of the entire chest rather than a single organ such as the heart. These patients are often unstable, requiring immediate OR management, a damage-control surgical strategy with thoracic packing and vacuum-assisted closure of the open chest after control of life-threatening injuries, or intraoperative massive transfusion, and some may need postoperative renal replacement therapy for renal insufficiency and extracorporeal membrane oxygenation; mortality may be as high as 25%.[180]

Pericardial Tamponade

Both penetrating and blunt trauma can cause hemopericardium. The classic findings of pericardial tamponade—tachycardia, hypotension, distant heart sounds, distended neck veins, pulsus paradoxus, or pulsus alternans—are difficult to appreciate or may be absent in a hypovolemic trauma patient. A chest radiograph may reveal a globular heart, although this sign is often not appreciated. TTE with placement of the probe in the subxiphoid region, which is part of FAST, or intraoperative TEE can demonstrate blood in the pericardial sac and the presence of ventricular diastolic collapse, which indicates at least a 20% reduction in cardiac output.

Initial management consists of evacuation of the pericardial blood by ultrasound-guided pericardiocentesis or surgery as soon as possible. Even a small amount of blood drainage improves hemodynamics. Intracardiac volumes should be optimized with intravenous fluids. If anesthesia is contemplated for surgery, ketamine or etomidate, which produce relatively little myocardial depression, is preferred. Administration of anesthesia should be delayed until draping and preparation are completed. Patients in extremis with penetrating trauma-related pericardial tamponade may be candidates for ED thoracotomy. Rarely, laceration of the pericardium may permit complete or partial herniation of the heart through the defect with catastrophic consequences. Immediate thoracotomy and reduction of the heart are indicated.

Blunt Cardiac Injury

The term blunt cardiac injury (BCI) has replaced myocardial contusion and encompasses varying degrees of myocardial damage, coronary artery injury, and rupture of the cardiac free wall, septum, or a valve following blunt trauma.[181] Myocardial injury consists of myofibrillar disintegration, edema, bleeding, or necrosis that depending on its severity presents as minor

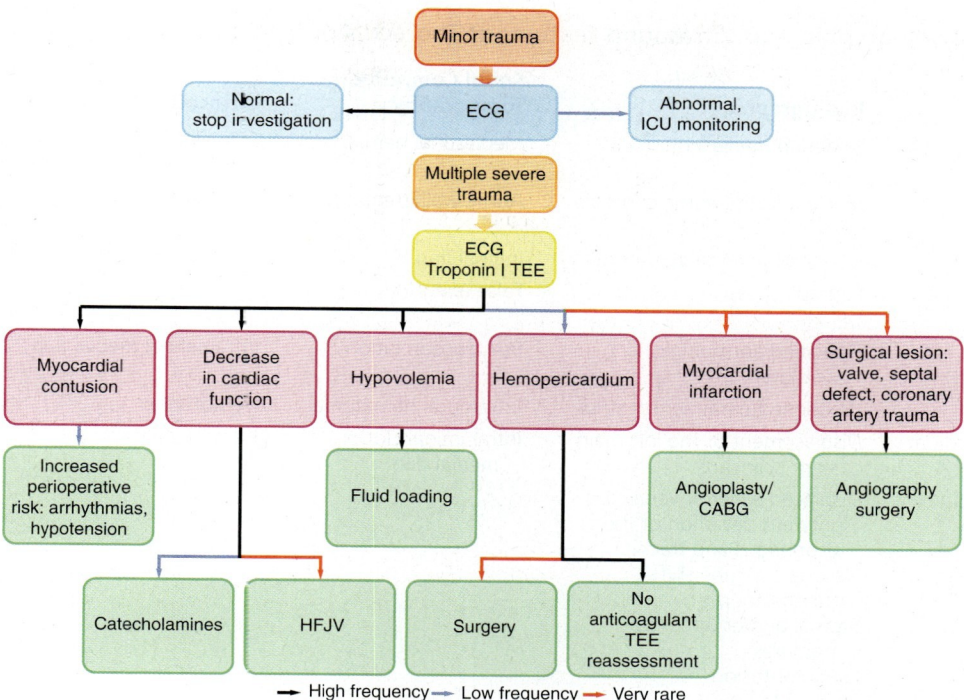

Figure 53-6 Algorithm for management of various clinical scenarios produced by severe blunt cardiac injury. Evaluation of severe multiple trauma-induced blunt cardiac injuries uses electrocardiogram (ECG), troponin I, and transesophageal echocardiography (TEE). *Colored lines* represent the frequency of occurrence of each scenario and the frequency of management measures. CABG, coronary artery bypass graft; HFJV, high-frequency jet ventilation. (Adapted from Orliaguet G, Ferjani M, Riou B. The heart in blunt trauma. *Anesthesiology.* 2001;95:544.)

electrocardiographic (ECG) or enzyme abnormalities, complex arrhythmias, or cardiac failure caused by direct mechanical impact or indirectly by coronary occlusion. Arrhythmias last no more than a few days, and ventricular wall motion abnormalities may persist longer. Pulmonary or systemic embolism may occur suddenly after a few days owing to development of clot in the hypokinetic cardiac chambers.

The prominent clinical findings are angina (sometimes responding to nitroglycerin), dyspnea, chest wall ecchymosis, and/or fractures; dysrhythmias of any type; and right-sided or left-sided congestive heart failure. Orliaguet et al.[181] proposed an algorithm for the diagnosis and treatment of several clinical scenarios caused by this injury (Fig. 53-6). The diagnosis is based on the 12-lead ECG, troponin I level, and echocardiography. The ECG is very sensitive, although not specific. A normal trace cannot rule out the diagnosis, but it is the best screening test. Common ECG abnormalities include almost any type of arrhythmia, ST- or T-wave changes, and conduction delays. Patients with a normal ECG undergoing minor surgery do not require any further testing. Patients with severe injuries need measurement of troponin I and TEE to diagnose any abnormalities caused by the cardiac injury. Echocardiography can demonstrate wall motion abnormalities, valve malfunction, hemopericardium, intracardiac thrombi, venous or systemic embolism, and fractional ventricular wall area changes. It thus aids not only in the diagnosis of BCI but also in hemodynamic management. Treatment options depend on the diagnosis. They include antiarrhythmic agents, inotropes, fluid loading, high-frequency jet ventilation to optimize cardiac function, and surgery for hemopericardium, valvular or septal lesions, or coronary artery injury or disease.

Valvular injuries present as insufficiency of the aortic, mitral, or tricuspid valves. Acute traumatic insufficiency of the aortic and mitral valves is poorly tolerated, increasing the ventricular wall stress and rapidly progressing to pulmonary edema. Ventricular septal defects can be recognized by increased pulmonary vascularity with a normal heart size on the chest radiograph. An atrial septal defect is usually missed in clinical examination but may be recognized by echocardiography.

Commotio cordis (agitated heart) is an entity characterized by the development of sudden ventricular tachyarrhythmias, cardiac arrest, and often death following a blow to the chest in young people, most often during competitive or recreational sports. The blow would have occurred during the 10- to 20-millisecond period of the T-wave upstroke. Commotio cordis differs from myocardial contusion because of the absence of any structural cardiac injury. Treatment involves immediate defibrillation.[182]

Thoracic Aortic Injury

Penetrating trauma can injure any part of the thoracic aorta, including its branches, to any extent. Blunt trauma, on the other hand, most commonly causes damage at the isthmus, the junction between the free and fixed portions of the descending aorta, which is just distal to the origin of the left subclavian artery. The ligamentum arteriosum and left main stem bronchus anchor the isthmus, fixing it in relation to the proximal aorta and making it vulnerable to traction forces and tearing. The thoracic aorta also may be injured at its root where it is fixed by the diaphragm, rendering it vulnerable to shearing forces of velocity changes. Blunt thoracic aortic injury is likely to be accompanied by various thoracic and abdominal visceral injuries.[183] The presenting symptoms, signs, and radiographic and ultrasound findings are shown in Table 53-8, although there may be no clinical findings or a constellation of symptoms or signs in the ED. Only 20% to 30% of patients with mediastinal widening actually have this injury.

Contrast-enhanced spiral CT with volume-rendered image reconstruction techniques permits a reliable noninvasive diagnosis of this injury. TEE is also capable of diagnosing subadventitial aortic injuries that require intervention.[184] Lesions of the intima and media and frequently encountered concomitant BCIs are also more likely to be detectable by TEE than CT.[184] However, CT, especially images obtained with multidetector devices,

Table 53-8 Common Clinical, Radiographic, and Ultrasound Features of Thoracic Aortic Injuries

Clinical	Radiographic	Spiral Computed Tomography	Ultrasound
Increased arterial pressure and pulse amplitude in upper extremities	Widened mediastinum	Mediastinal hematoma	Intimal flap
Decreased arterial pressure and pulse amplitude in lower extremities	Blurring of the aortic contours	Aortic wall irregularity	Turbulent flow
Absent or weak left radial artery pulse	Widened paraspinal interfaces	Intimal flap	Dilated aortic isthmus
Osler sign: discrepancy between left and right arm blood pressure	Left apical cap	False aneurysm	Acute false aneurysm
Retrosternal or interscapular pain	Opacified aortopulmonary window	Pseudocoarctation	Intraluminal medial flap
Hoarseness	Broadened paratracheal stripe	Intramural hematoma	Hemothorax
Systolic flow murmur over the precordium or medial to the left scapula	Displacement of the left main stem bronchus	Intraluminal clot or medial flap	Hemomediastinum
Neurologic deficits in the lower extremities	Displaced superior vena cava		
	Rightward deviation of the esophagus and trachea		
	Nasogastric tube shift		
	Left hemothorax		
	Sternal and/or upper rib fractures		
	Lung contusion		
	Pneumothorax		

is generally preferred for diagnosis because it provides an accurate diagnosis, and introducing a TEE probe under these circumstances is impractical and probably fraught with the danger of aortic rupture. Furthermore, many of these patients have suspected craniofacial or esophageal injuries, preventing introduction of the probe. TEE is especially useful for the anesthesiologist intraoperatively when associated injuries require immediate surgery without time for CT scanning of the chest.

Traumatic aortic injury can be classified into three categories: Grade 1 injury consists of an intramural hematoma, limited intimal flap, and/or mural thrombus; grade 2 injury consists of subadventitial rupture, injury to the media, altered aortic geometry, and/or small hemomediastinum; grade 3 injury consists of transsection with massive blood extravasation and intraluminal obstruction, causing pseudocoarctation and ischemia (Fig. 53-7).[185] Severity of the injury may also be judged by TEE measurement of maximum aortic diameter, the ratio between injured and normal aortic diameters, the size of pseudoaneurysm, the esophagus-to-aortic distance, aortic isthmus–to-left visceral–pleural distance, and the presence of hemothorax.[185] In another classification (Vancouver simplified classification), a fourth grade involving contrast extravasation is added.[186] Grade 1 injuries and some grade 2 injuries can be treated nonoperatively with serial observations using TEE or CT. Grade 2, 3, and 4 injuries require immediate or delayed surgery based on clinical findings.[185,186]

Management strategies in the diagnosis and treatment of blunt aortic injuries have gone through major changes during the past 10 years with substantially improved early outcomes (Table 53-9). In the area of diagnosis, contrast-enhanced CT angiography has practically replaced aortography and TEE, whereas endovascular thoracic aortic repair has replaced open surgery as the primary surgical treatment.[187] Intraoperatively, patients undergoing endovascular repair with a stent are monitored with contrast aortography and intravascular ultrasound. Thus, aortography has not been completely eliminated.

Although currently the vast majority of blunt thoracic aortic injuries are managed using endovascular stents, repairs via the traditional open left thoracotomy are still occasionally performed. This technique requires lung isolation with a double-lumen tube or a bronchial blocker, partial heparinization, and, at times, partial left heart bypass to decompress the left heart

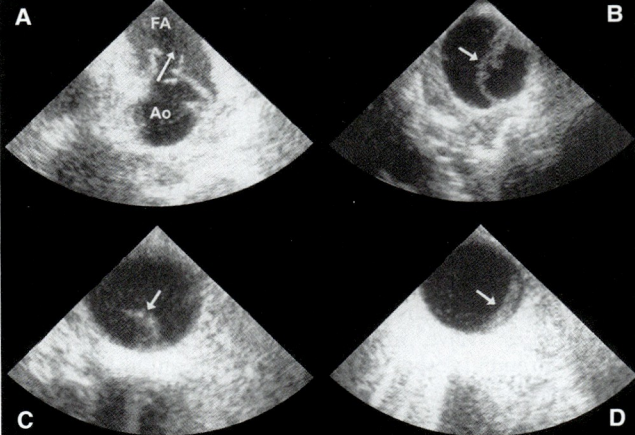

Figure 53-7 Typical transesophageal echocardiographic appearances of three grades of traumatic aortic injury. **A:** Grade 3 injury. Adventitia of the aortic wall is damaged and a false aneurysm (FA) is communicating (*arrow*) with the aortic lumen (Ao). **B:** Grade 2 injury. Large medial flap moves back and forth during each cardiac cycle. Adventitia is intact. **C, D:** Grade 1 injury. Intimal flap (**C**) and intramural hematoma (**D**) (shown with *arrows*) without hemomediastinum or alteration of aortic geometry. (Reprinted from Goarin J-P, Cluzel P, Gosgnach M, et al. Evaluation of transesophageal echocardiography for diagnosis of traumatic aortic injury. *Anesthesiology*. 2000;93:1373.)

Table 53-9 Change in the Management of Blunt Thoracic Aortic Injuries from 1997 to 2007

	AAST$_1$ N = 253	AAST$_2$ N = 193
Diagnosis		
Aortogram	220 (87%)	16 (8%)
CT scan	88 (35%)	180 (93%)
TEE	30 (12%)	2 (1%)
Repair		
Open	207 (100%)	68 (35%)
Endovascular	0	125 (65%)
Outcomes		
Mortality	53/241 (22%)	25/193 (13%)
Paraplegia		
All patients	18 (9%)	2 (2%)
Open repair	18 (9%)	2 (3%)
Endovascular	0	1/125 (1%)
Renal failure	18 (9%)	17 (9%)
Repair site complication	1/207 (1%)	25/125 (20%)

AAST$_1$, American Association for the Surgery of Trauma 1997 Study; AAST$_2$, American Association for the Surgery of Trauma 2007 Study; TEE, transesophageal echocardiogram; CT, computed tomography.
Reproduced with permission from Demetriades D, Velmahos GC, Scalea TM, et al. Diagnosis and treatment of blunt thoracic aortic injuries: changing perspectives. *J Trauma.* 2008;64:1415.

and perfuse the distal aorta during a "clamp and sew" technique. A clamp is placed just distal to the takeoff of the left subclavian artery. Although bleeding may be excessive, mortality and morbidity, especially paraplegia or renal dysfunction, are also frequent with this technique.[187,188] Lung isolation with a double-lumen endobronchial tube is necessary to prevent contamination of the contralateral lung from blood entering the airway during dissection of the aorta in proximity to the lung. It should be inserted under direct vision via FOB after ensuring that the left main stem bronchus lumen is not obliterated by the periaortic hematoma. Systemic blood pressure and potassium (K^+) should be monitored during aortic clamp release; a rise in K^+ should be treated with insulin and glucose.

Endovascular aortic repair is minimally invasive and is associated with fewer early complications such as paraplegia, stroke, bleeding, or death than are encountered after open thoracotomy (Table 53-9). An endoleak between the graft and the vascular wall is one of the early recognized complications. A radial artery cannula should be placed on the right side because sometimes the left subclavian artery is covered by the stent. A central venous catheter is placed for administration of vasoactive drugs. Embolization of aortic atheromas to the brain is one of the complications of this procedure. TEE may help to image the atheroma prior to stent deployment. During aortography and stent placement, ventilation may have to be stopped, and the systemic blood pressure may have to be lowered to a mean of 60 mmHg.

The incidence of long-term graft complications is not known, but it appears that the survival curves between open thoracotomy and endovascular techniques converge at 2 years, and the rates of aneurysm-related mortality converge at 6 years.[188]

Surgical prioritization when multiple injuries are present depends on the hemodynamic and neurologic status of the patient. Although the aorta should be repaired as early as possible, control of active hemorrhage from other sites and surgery for intracranial hematomas have a higher surgical priority, unless the aorta is leaking. Also heparinization needed for aortic repair may increase bleeding from associated injury sites. In most instances, a blood clot between the aorta and the mediastinal pleura occludes the vessel. Any disturbance of the tamponaded region may reinitiate bleeding. A rapid flow of blood in a large artery tends to pull its endothelium with it and thus may rupture an injured vessel that is sealed with a clot or a hematoma. Such an increase in the aortic blood flow is usually caused by increased myocardial contractility. Every effort should be made to prevent increased cardiac contractility and hypertension. The use of β-blocking agents should be considered.

Diaphragmatic Injury

Injury to the diaphragm may permit migration of abdominal contents into the chest, where they may compress the lung, producing abnormalities of gas exchange, or the heart, resulting in dysrhythmias and/or hypotension. Because the defect produced by blunt injury is usually larger than that resulting from a penetrating injury, migration of abdominal contents, which requires a defect of at least 6 cm in diameter, is also more common after blunt trauma. The liver protects the right side of the diaphragm; thus traumatic herniation is more common on the left side, but right-sided diaphragmatic injuries are more frequently missed.[189]

Clinically noting that the end of a nasogastric tube is above the diaphragm on the chest radiograph is a certain sign that the stomach is displaced into the chest. A chest radiograph that shows intestinal markings and lung compression or a contrast-enhanced abdominal CT scan that includes the lower third of the thorax can provide important information. A diaphragmatic tear alone may require laparoscopy for diagnosis and repair. In diagnosed patients anesthetic induction should be tailored to avoid aspiration of gastric contents. For those diaphragmatic injuries without thoracic migration of abdominal contents, some centers prefer to place a prophylactic chest tube before surgery to prevent pneumothorax during positive-pressure ventilation.

Abdominal and Pelvic Injuries

The abdomen, because of its lack of protection against external impacts, may be injured by blunt or penetrating trauma, producing solid organ, hollow viscus, and/or vascular injuries. Resulting intra- and retroperitoneal bleeding may cause hemorrhagic shock, which at times may be fatal. Spillage from intestines or another hollow viscus, if unrecognized, is responsible for the sepsis that may manifest hours or days after injury depending on the location of the injury; unrecognized left colonic injury may cause septic complications earliest. Table 53-10 summarizes the strengths and weaknesses of the currently available diagnostic tools used to diagnose and treat abdominal injuries.[190] Because of the unpredictable course of bullets in the body, exploratory laparotomy or, in selected cases, laparoscopy is required in most patients after a gunshot wound to the abdomen. Occasionally, in hemodynamically stable patients, abdominal and flank gunshot wounds may be evaluated with an initial CT scan. Stab wounds may be managed with tractotomy to determine whether the peritoneum is involved. Laparoscopy or laparotomy may be indicated after a positive tractotomy.

Overt abdominal signs such as evisceration in penetrating trauma, tenderness, guarding, and gross distension in blunt trauma during physical examination of the abdomen suggest

Table 53-10 Diagnostic Tools in Abdominal Trauma: Strengths and Weaknesses

Diagnostic Tool	Strength	Weakness
Physical examination	Expeditious, safe, and inexpensive; potential for serial examination	Diagnosis of specific injury (e.g., diaphragm)
Diagnostic peritoneal lavage	Expeditious, safe, and inexpensive	Diagnosis of diaphragmatic injury, hollow viscus injury, retroperitoneal injury; can be oversensitive and nonspecific
Computed tomography	Evaluation of peritoneum and retroperitoneum Staging of solid-organ injury	Diagnosis of diaphragmatic injury, hollow viscus injury Expensive; controversial need for contrast
Ultrasonography	Expeditious, safe, and inexpensive; accurate for free peritoneal fluid Potential for serial examinations	Diagnosis of diaphragmatic injury, hollow viscus injury, penetrating injury, good specificity, but moderate sensitivity Less accurate in the presence of large retroperitoneal hematomas
Laparoscopy	Diagnosis of peritoneal penetration, diaphragmatic injury Evaluation of bleeding or solid-organ injury Potential for therapy	Diagnosis of hollow viscus injury, retroperitoneal injury Expensive
Video-assisted thoracoscopic surgery	Evaluation of lung, diaphragm, mediastinum, chest wall, and pericardium; potential for treatment	Requires operating room; expensive Diagnosis of abdominal injuries

Reprinted with permission from Villavicencio RT, Aucar JA. Analysis of laparoscopy in trauma. *J Am Coll Surg.* 1999;189:11.

intra-abdominal pathology and necessitate further evaluation by CT scan unless the patient is hemodynamically unstable, in which case surgery without CT scan may be indicated. Absence of abdominal distention does not rule out intra-abdominal bleeding. At least 1 L of blood can accumulate before the smallest change in girth is apparent, and the diaphragm can also move cephalad, allowing further significant blood loss without any change in abdominal circumference. It is more likely for hemorrhagic shock to develop before perceptible distension.

Abdominal CT is capable of demonstrating solid-organ injuries and peritoneal bleeding. In fact CT is the best tool to grade the severity of solid-organ injuries. However, it is less likely to identify bowel and mesenteric injuries, unless relatively new 64-slice devices are used.[191]

The diagnostic ability of the FAST is inferior to CT scan evaluation, which has recently undergone significant technologic improvements. The FAST is operator dependent, has good specificity but only moderate sensitivity, can diagnose injuries associated with intraperitoneal fluid but not those without it, and cannot determine the severity of organ injury.[192] Nevertheless the FAST is most needed in hemodynamically unstable patients who may not be safely transported to the CT unit shortly after admission to the ED. Its sensitivity in those patients is found to be low, preventing the development of a reliable ultrasound-based clinical pathway to diagnose blunt abdominal injury and to decide between conservative and operative management.[192] Performing serial FAST examinations may decrease the false-negative results, but in the unstable patient there is often limited time for decision making. Known clinical conditions that decrease the sensitivity of the FAST include pelvic and spine injuries, subcutaneous emphysema, and obesity. On the other hand, the FAST requires one-third of the time, is less expensive to perform than CT, and is without the hazard of radiation. Screening with abdominal ultrasonography is performed by placing a 3.0- to 5.0-MHz probe on four distinct areas of the abdomen: subxiphoid, to detect pericardial blood; right upper quadrant, for blood in the hepatorenal pouch; left upper quadrant, to detect perisplenic blood; and just above the pubic symphysis, for blood in the rectovesical pouch.

Laparoscopy is an excellent screening tool in abdominal trauma patients.[193] An analysis showed that it avoided laparotomy in 63% of patients and missed only 1% of the injuries.[190] It is also possible to repair diaphragmatic, bladder, and solid-organ injuries with this technique. The complication rate of laparoscopy in trauma is approximately 1%, including pneumothorax, small bowel injury, intra-abdominal vascular injury, extraperitoneal CO_2 insufflation, and CO_2 embolization.[190]

"Selective surgical conservatism," which involves nonoperative management by careful evaluation and performance of surgery on a timely manner only for those who actually demonstrate signs of injuries that are not amenable to conservative treatment, replaced the old concept of mandatory laparotomy during the past few decades. Patient selection for nonoperative management is important. Penetrating trauma patients with a high injury severity score and profuse bleeding from liver, spleen, or major abdominal vessels requiring transfusion are unlikely to benefit from nonoperative management; in fact, they may succumb to death with this approach. Similarly, patients with blunt trauma with advanced age, low admission systolic pressure, high injury severity score, metabolic acidosis, lower GCS, and requirement for multiple units of transfusion cannot be managed nonoperatively.

Hypotension on opening the peritoneal cavity filled with blood is caused not only by hemorrhage but also by the sudden release of compression on the splanchnic vessels causing capacitance vessel dilation. Management includes fluid, preferably plasma, infusion but also vasopressor therapy to prevent overloading. After the repair, most patients develop bowel edema, which may potentially result in abdominal compartment syndrome if abdominal closure is demanded. Leaving the abdomen open with vacuum drainage may prevent this complication.

Fractures of the Pelvis

Pelvic fractures occur in widely varied anatomic forms and physiologic severity. Major hemorrhage, which is one of the major causes of mortality, occurs in about 25% of patients; exsanguination occurs in 1% of injuries. Other major causes of mortality include associated injuries, such as chest, brain, intra-abdominal, and long bone injuries, and postoperative complications, such as sepsis, PE, and renal failure. In most of these fractures, bleeding results from venous disruption by fragments of bone. Retroperitoneal pelvic bleeding is self-limited in most patients with venous injuries because of the tamponading effect, except in those with open fractures. Approximately 18% to 20% of patients have arterial bleeding that does not stop. The retroperitoneal space in these patients may serve as a distensible container that expands superiorly and anteriorly and may totally obliterate the lower part of the abdominal cavity. Component therapy with blood products is important in these patients until the bleeding is controlled.[194] Large retroperitoneal hematomas may also cause respiratory difficulty because of pressure on the diaphragm. An increase in ICP is also likely if there is a concomitant head injury.

Early detection and intervention to control bleeding are important. Pelvic ring disruption, arterial extravasation (CT blush), and elevated bladder pressure secondary to compression by hematoma volumes greater than 500 mL are important signs that can be detected on CT examination, making it a key diagnostic measure. In addition, continuing hemodynamic instability after adequate fracture stabilization is suggestive of pelvic hemorrhage. Following external pelvic ring stabilization using external fixators, a pelvic binder, or a C-clamp to decrease the mobility of the bone fragments and help control blood loss, angiography can indicate the type and location of bleeding. Arterial bleeding is treated with embolization. The angiography suite should be prepared in advance not only for anesthesia but also for invasive monitoring and resuscitation. In hemodynamically unstable patients, deciding whether to transport the patient to the OR to control bleeding from associated injuries or to proceed to interventional radiology for angiography and possible embolization is difficult, although surgery of abdominal, thoracic, and head injuries is given priority. In most centers, it takes at least 45 minutes to begin angiography, during which time a considerable amount of blood may be lost. Recent data suggest that after external stabilization of the pelvis, extraperitoneal (preperitoneal) packing in the OR under general anesthesia followed by angiography and, if arterial bleeding is noticed, embolization may be more beneficial than only external fixation and angiography.[195] In this manner, pelvic venous bleeding is managed expeditiously. Packing involves a 6- to 7-cm midline vertical incision starting from the pubic symphysis to access the hematoma with introduction of two or three abdominal lap pads deep into the pelvis. The incision for packing is not continuous with the abdominal incision. Although this concept contrasts with the traditional understanding that opening a retroperitoneal hematoma caused by a pelvic fracture must be avoided to prevent excessive bleeding, with the present approach hematoma is entered extraperitoneally instead of intraperitoneally, which indeed increases the bleeding. Laparotomy may be indicated, although it should be based on solid indications. Nontherapeutic laparotomy may worsen the outcome.[196] Pelvic fractures may also injure the bladder and the urethra. Thus, a urethrogram should be performed before insertion of a urinary catheter.

Extremity Injuries

Surgical repair of extremity fractures, whether open or closed, should be performed as soon as possible. Delayed fracture repair is associated with an increased risk of DVT, pneumonia, sepsis, and the pulmonary and cerebral complications of fat embolism. In open fractures, an additional important concern is infection. Wounds left unrepaired for more than 6 hours are likely to become septic.

Associated vascular trauma must be recognized early. Most vascular injuries exhibit at least some part of the classic syndrome of *pain, pulselessness, pallor, paresthesias,* and *paresis*. The definitive diagnosis is made with arteriography. In selected patients, a duplex ultrasound study may be used as a screening test. Patients with vascular trauma should be operated on expeditiously, often without preoperative angiography. The presence of a hybrid OR in the OR suite circumvents the need for an additional journey to the angiography unit. These patients may bleed slowly but substantially both pre- and intraoperatively; thus, delayed surgery and prolonged skeletal repair may lead to unrecognized hemorrhagic shock, which may at times become irreversible. Damage control, that is, controlling bleeding and external fixation of the fractures, may be the management of choice.

Compartment syndrome, which is characterized by severe pain in the affected extremity, should be recognized early so that emergency fasciotomy can be effective in preventing irreversible muscle and nerve damage. In unconscious patients, swelling and tenseness of the extremity indicate the presence of this complication. The definitive diagnosis is made by measuring compartment pressures using a transducer attached to a fluid-filled extension tube and a needle inserted into the various compartments of the extremity. A pressure exceeding 30 cm of H_2O is an indication for immediate surgery. Caution must be exercised when using epidural or nerve block analgesia for perioperative pain relief in the presence of extremity fractures. Absence of pain can delay the diagnosis of compartment syndrome.

Burns

Approximately 500,000 hospitalizations and 3,400 deaths resulted from burns and inhalation injuries in the US during 2013.[4] Significant improvement in outcome from burn injuries has been seen during recent decades because of effective resuscitation, modern nursing and critical care, early scar excision, infection control, and the ability to counteract the hypermetabolic response. Although during the 1950s, the lethal dose, 50%, of burn injury was about 40% to 50% of total body surface area (TBSA), the corresponding value is currently 90%, with a mortality of 4% in admitted patients.[197] Three risk factors determine the death rate: inhalation injury, burn size exceeding 40% of TBSA, and age greater than 60 years. Mortality has been shown to be 0.3%, 3%, 33%, and 90% in the presence of 0, 1, 2, and 3 risk factors, respectively.[198,199] Full-thickness burns involving over 10% of the TBSA; partial-thickness burns covering more than 25% of TBSA in adults or over 20% at the extremes of age; burns involving the face, hands, feet, or perineum; inhalation, chemical, and electrical burns; and burns in patients with severe pre-existing medical disorders are considered major burns.[200]

Clinically, burn injury is manifested in two phases: Burn shock is characterized by continued plasma loss from the intravascular space into burned and often into intact tissues for about the first day or two after injury, and the subsequent hypermetabolic or hyperdynamic phase, which may last for months.[198,200] Pathophysiologic changes in these two phases are somewhat different and often opposite to each other (Table 53-11).[96,194]

A severe burn is a systemic disease that stimulates the release of inflammatory mediators such as interleukins and tumor necrosis factor locally (producing wound edema) and into the circulation,

Table 53-11 Pathophysiologic Changes in the Early (First 2 Days) and Late Phases of the Burn Injury

	Early Phase	Late Phase
Cardiovascular system	↑ Heart rate ↓ Cardiac index ↓ Stroke volume ↓ Contractility ↑ PVR and SVR ↓ SvO$_2$	↑ Heart rate ↑ Cardiac index Normal or ↑ stroke volume ↓ Contractility ↓ SVR ↑ SvO$_2$
Blood	↑ Hematocrit	↓ Hematocrit
Lungs (inhalation injury)	Pulmonary edema Bronchospasm, bronchorrhea ARDS Atelectasis	Pulmonary edema Bronchospasm, bronchorrhea ARDS Atelectasis, pneumonia
Kidney	Oliguria Myoglobinuria FENa$^+$ < 1%	↑ GFR ↓ Tubular function
Brain	Altered mental status Possible cerebral edema ↑ Pain response	Altered mental status Possible cerebral edema ↑ Pain response
Endocrine and metabolic function	↑ Aldosterone ↑ Cortisol	↑ Insulin resistance ↑ O$_2$ consumption and CO$_2$ production Muscle catabolism

PVR, pulmonary vascular resistance; SVR, systemic vascular resistance; SvO$_2$, mixed venous O$_2$ saturation; ARDS, acute respiratory distress syndrome; FENa$^+$, fraction of excreted sodium; GFR, glomerular filtration rate.

resulting in immune suppression, hypermetabolism, protein catabolism, insulin resistance, sepsis, and multisystem organ failure. Patients with burns over 40% of TBSA consistently develop catabolism and weight loss, which may last up to 1 year. Prevention of sepsis, maintenance of normal body temperature, and pain management may decrease the extent of catabolism. Pharmacologically, recombinant human growth hormone, insulin-like growth factor 1, low-dose insulin infusion, β-blockade, and the synthetic testosterone analogue oxandrolone can decrease protein catabolism or improve anabolism.[201,202] Enteral and/or parenteral nutrition starting early after burn injury is effective in reducing the hypermetabolic response and replacing protein loss. Provided that the airway is secured, feeding via an ileostomy should continue during anesthesia for surgical procedures.[198] Enteral feeding should be stopped within a reasonable time before surgery if there is a chance that the airway will be unprotected intraoperatively for a period of time, as in tracheostomy.

Determination of the size and depth of a burn sets the guidelines for resuscitation as well as the indications for surgical intervention.[198,200] A partial-thickness burn is red, blanches to touch, and is sensitive to painful stimuli and heat. Superficial partial-thickness (first-degree) burns involve the epidermis and upper dermis and heal spontaneously. Deep partial-thickness (second-degree) burns involve the deep dermis and require excision and grafting to ensure rapid return of function. A full-thickness (third-degree) burn does not blanch, even with deep pressure, and is insensate. Complete destruction of the dermis requires wound excision and grafting to prevent a wound infection that may lead to local sepsis and systemic inflammation. Fourth-degree burns involve muscle, fascia, and bone, necessitating complete excision and leaving the patient with limited function. Laser Doppler imaging can be used as an aid to judge the burn depth.[203] The size of the burned area is estimated by the "rule of nines" to determine the TBSA involved. In an adult, the head contributes 9%; the upper extremities, 18%; the trunk, 36%; and the lower extremities, 36% of the TBSA.

These proportions are somewhat different in children, depending on the age and size. To estimate the size of a burn, the child's palmar surface (excluding the digits) represents about 0.5% of the TBSA over a wide range of ages. More accurate age-specific estimation of the TBSA can be obtained by using the Lund–Browder table (Table 53-12).[198]

Information about the mechanism of injury facilitates the diagnosis of associated clinical abnormalities. For example, thermal trauma caused by flames in a closed space is likely to be associated with airway damage. Burns resulting from motor vehicle, airplane, or industrial accidents may be complicated by other traumatic injuries. Finally, burns caused by electrocution may show little external evidence but may be associated with severe fractures, hematomas, visceral injury, and skeletal and cardiac muscle injury resulting in pain, myoglobinuria, and dysrhythmias or other ECG abnormalities.

Airway Complications

Injury to various parts of the airway occurs following inhalation of heated air, steam, or toxic substances. Airway and lung injury also may occur in the absence of inhalation via the inflammatory mediators released from the burned tissues, infection, and fluid resuscitation. Respiratory distress in the initial phase of a burn is usually caused by direct heat or steam injury to the pharynx or larynx. Singed facial hair, facial burns, dysphonia or hoarseness, cough, soot in the mouth or nose, and swallowing difficulties in patients with or without respiratory distress should increase the suspicion of upper (frequent) and lower (occasional) airway injury. In the upper airway, glottic and periglottic edema and copious thick secretions may produce respiratory obstruction. This may be aggravated by fluid resuscitation even in the absence of significant inhalation injury.[204] Injuries below the larynx are caused by smoke, hot particles, and aspiration involving the trachea and primary bronchi. Secondary bronchi also may

Table 53-12 Lund–Browder Body Surface Area Calculation Table Used during Admission of the Patient to Determine Percent Burn Size, Location, and Estimated Burn Depth

Area	Birth–1 yr	1–4 yr	5–9 yr	10–14 yr	15 yr	Adult	2°	3°	TOTAL
Head	9	17	13	11	9	7			
Neck	2	2	2	2	2	2			
Anterior trunk	13	13	13	13	13	13			
Posterior trunk	13	13	13	13	13	13			
Right buttock	2.5	2.5	2.5	2.5	2.5	2.5			
Left buttock	2.5	2.5	2.5	2.5	2.5	2.5			
Genitalia	1	1	1	1	1	1			
Right upper arm	4	4	4	4	4	4			
Left upper arm	4	4	4	4	4	4			
Right lower arm	3	3	3	3	3	3			
Left lower arm	3	3	3	3	3	3			
Right hand	2.5	2.5	2.5	2.5	2.5	2.5			
Left hand	2.5	2.5	2.5	2.5	2.5	2.5			
Right thigh	5.5	6.5	8	8.5	9	9.5			
Left thigh	5.5	6.5	8	8.5	9	9.5			
Right lower leg	5	5	5.5	6	6.5	7			
Left lower leg	5	5	5.5	6	6.5	7			
Right foot	3.5	3.5	3.5	3.5	3.5	3.5			
Left foot	3.5	3.5	3.5	3.5	3.5	3.5			
						TOTAL			

Only secondary and tertiary burns are included in the total burn percentage.
Adapted from Bittner E, Shank E, Woodson L et al. Acute and perioperative care of the burn-injured patient. *Anesthesiology* 2015;122: 448–464.

be involved if irritant gases are inhaled. In lower airway burns, decreased surfactant and mucociliary function, mucosal necrosis and ulceration, edema, tissue sloughing, and secretions produce bronchial obstruction, air trapping, and bronchopneumonia. The development of parenchymal lung injury takes approximately 1 to 5 days and presents with the clinical picture of ARDS. Pneumonia and PE are late complications that occur 5 or more days after burns. The presence of a lung injury markedly increases the fluid requirements (30% to 50%) and the mortality rate from thermal injuries.[198,205] Administration of the highest possible concentration of O_2 by face mask is the first priority in moderately to severely burned patients with a patent airway. In patients with massive burns, stridor, respiratory distress, hypoxemia, hypercarbia, loss of consciousness, or altered mentation, immediate tracheal intubation is indicated. The intubation technique selected depends on the operator's experience, the age of the patient, and the extent of airway compromise. In adults, awake fiberoptic intubation under adequate topical anesthesia, if feasible, is probably the safest approach, but other techniques using conventional blades or videolaryngoscopes with or without anesthetic induction or supraglottic airway–guided intubation may also be used. In most pediatric patients, awake intubation is not possible. An inhalation induction with O_2 and sevoflurane, followed by intubation using an FOB or conventional laryngoscope, is appropriate.[200] Alternatively, sedation with ketamine, which preserves pharyngeal tone, may provide good intubating conditions for FOB-guided intubation. The presence of full stomach may preclude the use of a supraglottic airway, except as a bridge to a secure airway. Methylnaltrexone, which antagonizes the peripheral but not the central effects of morphine, antagonizes gastric effect of morphine and facilitates its emptying without causing agitation.[198] A surgical airway entails a significant risk of pulmonary sepsis and late upper airway sequelae and should be reserved for those whose airway management cannot be handled in any other way, or in those who are likely to develop complications such as dysphagia or dysphonia following prolonged tracheal intubation.[198,200] Immediately after securing the airway, ventilation with low levels of PEEP will prevent the pulmonary edema that may develop secondary to loss of laryngeal auto-PEEP in patients with significant airway obstruction before intubation. Airway humidification, bronchial toilet, and bronchodilators if needed for bronchospasm are also indicated.

The pediatric airway is particularly challenging because its small diameter carries the risk of occlusion by minimal amounts of swelling. Prophylactic intubation may therefore be required in children who are suspected of having an inhalation injury, even though they are not yet in respiratory distress. Prophylactic tracheal intubation may also be indicated in adults when the resources for careful follow-up are insufficient. Information obtained from radiologic, ABG, and endoscopic examinations and pulmonary function testing may be useful for predicting which patient will need tracheal intubation and possibly decreasing the risks of airway manipulation. Prophylactic intubation carries the risk of dislodgment, especially during intra- or interhospital transport. It has been demonstrated that many patients who, according to the hospital policy, had indications for intubation did not need to have their airway secured as determined by serial airway examination with FOB. Thus tracheal intubation should be based on clear criteria such as large full-thickness burns, inability to protect the airway, or signs of airway obstruction.[198,206]

Serial fiberoptic laryngoscopy is easy to perform and can provide direct information about the glottic and periglottic structures. It may avoid tracheal intubation in patients who would otherwise be considered candidates for this procedure. Fiberoptic bronchoscopy has the additional advantage of providing information about the lower airway, although it is more uncomfortable for the patient and requires topical anesthesia of the tracheobronchial tree.

The chest radiograph, ABGs, and pulmonary function tests are usually normal in the immediate postburn period, even in patients with pulmonary complications.[198] However, these tests should be performed at this time for later comparison. The treatment of smoke inhalation in burns involves ventilatory management, intensive care, and treatment of carbon monoxide (CO) and cyanide (CN^-) toxicity.

Ventilation and Intensive Care

Hypoxemia may persist despite tracheal intubation, ventilation with PEEP, bronchodilators, and suction of airway secretions. In the first 36 hours, this is caused by acute pulmonary edema. From days 2 to 5, hypoxia may result from atelectasis, bronchopneumonia, and airway edema resulting from mucosal necrosis and sloughing, viscous secretions, and distal airway obstruction. Later there may be nosocomial pneumonia, hypermetabolism-induced respiratory failure, and ARDS. Treatment of these complications is individualized, using ventilatory maneuvers such as low tidal volume (5 to 6 mL/kg) with titrated PEEP, bronchoscopic lavage, antibiotics, chest physiotherapy, and other supportive measures. Lack of response to therapy because of severe ventilation–perfusion mismatching or shunt may be an indication for the use of nitric oxide, a potent, short-acting vasodilator, via the airway.[207] Patients with ARDS may benefit from high-frequency oscillatory ventilation, both intraoperatively and in the ICU.[208] Prophylactic measures against DVT, gastric ulcers, and hypothermia should be used routinely. Burns of at least 40% of TBSA and those necessitating ICU admission carry the risk of venous thromboembolism (VTE) requiring prophylaxis.[209] Further, pulmonary procoagulant activity with inhibited fibrinolysis in mechanically ventilated patients with burn and inhalation injuries results in alveolar fibrin deposition and pulmonary inflammation, which may decrease with anticoagulants.[210]

Carbon Monoxide Toxicity

In burn victims, CO inhalation is almost always associated with smoke inhalation, which increases morbidity and mortality compared with CO toxicity alone. CO produces tissue hypoxia by impairing O_2 unloading; it produces this effect by its 200-fold greater affinity for hemoglobin than oxygen and by its ability to shift the hemoglobin dissociation curve to the left and alter its shape. It also interferes with mitochondrial function, uncoupling oxidative phosphorylation and reducing adenosine triphosphate production, thus causing metabolic acidosis. Probably because of this effect on the mitochondria, CO can be a direct myocardial toxin, preventing survival in patients who suffer cardiac arrest even though they have been resuscitated and treated with a high concentration of O_2 or hyperbaric oxygen.

A normal oxygen saturation reading on most pulse oximeters does not exclude the possibility of CO toxicity, although low arterial O_2 saturation measured by a co-oximeter should raise the suspicion.[211] Portable devices such as the Masimo Rad-5 (Masimo Corp., East Irvine, CA) are capable of measuring carboxyhemoglobin and methemoglobin levels noninvasively via a finger sensor along with pulse oximetry, alerting the clinician about spuriously high O_2 saturation values. If CO toxicity is not accompanied by a lung injury and thus by decreased PaO_2, tachypnea

Table 53-13 Symptoms of Carbon Monoxide Toxicity as a Function of the Blood COHb Level

Blood COHb Level (%)	Symptoms
<15–20	Headache, dizziness, and occasional confusion
20–40	Nausea, vomiting, disorientation, and visual impairment
40–60	Agitation, combativeness, hallucinations, coma, and shock
>60	Death

COHb, carboxyhemoglobin.

is absent. The carotid bodies are sensitive to the arterial PO_2 and not to the O_2 content. The classic cherry-red color of the blood is also absent in most patients because it occurs only at carboxyhemoglobin (COHb) concentrations above 40%; it may also be obscured by coexistent hypoxia and cyanosis.

The greater the blood concentration of COHb, the more severe the presenting symptoms (Table 53-13). The patient's inspired oxygen should be maintained at the highest possible concentration, even when there is no evidence of significant smoke-induced lung injury, until CO toxicity is ruled out by measurement of blood COHb. A high fraction of inspired oxygen (FiO_2) not only improves oxygenation but also promotes elimination of CO; an FiO_2 of 1.0 decreases the blood half-life of COHb from 4 hours in room air to about 60 to 90 minutes, and to 20 to 30 minutes at 3 atm in a hyperbaric chamber.[198,200] The decision to institute this treatment should be based on comparing its risks and benefits; the risks include interhospital transport because most centers lack a hyperbaric chamber, decreased patient access during treatment, and delay in emergency treatment for the possible neurologic sequelae. Currently, hyperbaric O_2 is recommended for patients with COHb over 30% at admission if the treatment of life-threatening problems—shock, neurologic injury, metabolic acidosis, myocardial ischemia, infarction, or arrhythmias—will not be compromised.

Cyanide Toxicity

Another cause of tissue hypoxia in burned patients is CN^- toxicity. Cyanide or hydrocyanic acid is produced by incomplete combustion of synthetic materials and may be inhaled or absorbed through mucous membranes. The usual clinical presentation is unexplained metabolic acidosis in the absence of cyanosis. Nonspecific neurologic symptoms such as agitation, confusion, or coma are also common findings. Elevated plasma lactate levels in severe burns may result from hypovolemia or CO or CN^- toxicity. However, lactic acidosis after smoke inhalation in a patient without a major burn suggests CN^- toxicity.[212] The definitive diagnosis can be made only by determination of the blood cyanide level, which is toxic above 0.2 mg/L and lethal at levels beyond 1 mg/L. A spectrophotometric assay using methemoglobin as a colorimetric indicator provides timely and reliable determination of blood CN^-.[213] The pulse oximetry reading will be accurate in the absence of CO toxicity and nitrate therapy–induced methemoglobinemia.

Increased CN^- in the blood can cause generalized cardiovascular depression and cardiac rhythm disturbances, especially in patients with lactic acidosis. Fortunately, the half-life of CN^- is short (~1 hour),[212] and rapid improvement of hemodynamics should be expected after rescue of the victim from the toxic environment. Immediate administration of O_2, which is required for all burn victims, may be lifesaving for this complication. Although there are specific therapies for CN^- toxicity (e.g., amyl nitrate, sodium nitrite, thiosulfate), given the short half-life of the ion, it is not clear whether these measures offer significant help to the patient, whose blood CN^- usually decreases to low levels during transport from the field to the hospital.[214] Nevertheless exogenous thiosulfate combined with fast-acting hydroxycobalamin (vitamin B_{12}) can be administered to facilitate conversion to thiocyanate and cyanocobalamin, which are excreted in the urine.[198] Of course, if circumstances permit, hyperbaric O_2 treatment can be used for all the complications of thermal injury: CO and CN^- poisoning, smoke-induced lung damage, and cutaneous burns.

Fluid Replacement

Immediately after a serious burn microvascular permeability increases, causing the loss of a substantial amount of protein-rich fluid into the interstitial space. A major burn, a delay in initiation of resuscitation, or an inhalation injury increases the size of the leak.[198,200] Further, there seems to be a relation between inhalation injury and cutaneous burns in the production of edema: Pulmonary edema increases cutaneous edema and vice versa.[215] If resuscitation is successful, edema formation stops within 18 to 24 hours.[215] This fluid flux is enhanced by increased intravascular hydrostatic and interstitial osmotic pressures and decreased interstitial hydrostatic pressure. In addition, cardiac contractility may decrease because of circulating mediators, a diminished response to catecholamines, decreased coronary blood flow, and increased systemic vascular resistance.[200,216] This may result in shock, whose origin is primarily hypovolemic and, to a smaller extent, cardiogenic.[216] If the hypotension is treated appropriately with fluids, the hemodynamic picture is replaced within 24 to 48 hours by one resembling sepsis or septic shock, with increased heart rate, cardiac output, and diminished systemic vascular resistance caused by the release of inflammatory mediators.[216]

Fluid resuscitation is essential in the early care of the burned patient with an injury over 15% of TBSA. Smaller burns can be managed with oral or intravenous replacement at 150% of the calculated maintenance rate and careful monitoring of fluid status. Intravascular volume should be restored with utmost care to prevent excessive edema formation in both damaged and intact tissues resulting from the generalized increase in capillary permeability caused by the injury. Edema from overaggressive resuscitation has many deleterious and potentially life-threatening effects. Mention has already been made of the facilitation of upper airway edema after rapid fluid infusion in large cutaneous burns with or without smoke inhalation.[204] Likewise, chest wall edema may develop after administration of large quantities of fluid to patients with burns in this area, causing respiratory difficulties and necessitating excision of burned tissue from the anterior axillary line to improve breathing. Abdominal edema may also occur, and when resuscitation volume exceeds 300 mL/kg/24 hours, increased intra-abdominal pressure may produce *abdominal compartment syndrome* with impedance of venous return.[217,218] Edema formation may also increase the tissue pressure in the burned area, resulting in reduction of blood flow to distal sites. This, together with decreased tissue oxygen tension, may produce necrosis of damaged but viable cells, increasing the extent of injury and the risk of infection.

Crystalloid solutions are preferred for resuscitation during the first day following a burn injury; leakage of colloids during this phase may increase edema.[219] Nevertheless, crystalloid resuscitation, especially in children, may cause a rapid decline in plasma protein concentration and necessitate administration of 5% albumin in LR solution when the capillary leak stops after the first day following a burn greater than 30% of TBSA and/or significant inhalation injury.[220] It is believed that this will moderate the tendency to edema formation associated with the administration of large amounts of isotonic (0.9% saline or LR) solutions. Some centers use plasma with crystalloid routinely and partly attribute the good outcomes of their patients to this practice.[221] Administration of fluids in excess of the amount recommended by the Parkland formula appears to be relatively frequent in modern burn management and is termed *fluid creep*. Avoidance of early over-resuscitation, routine use of colloids, and adherence to protocols are recommended to prevent this problem.[222] Plasma exchange therapy may also remove inflammatory mediators and decrease capillary permeability, lowering fluid requirements and improving base deficit and blood lactate level in these patients.[223] Alternatively, hypertonic saline solutions draw intracellular water into the bloodstream and thus decrease the fluid volume needed to maintain perfusion and extracellular volume and limit the severity of edema in patients with burns occupying over 50% of TBSA, circumferential extremity burns, or inhalational injury.[200] Unfortunately, hypertonic solutions may cause hypernatremia and intracellular water depletion. Patients and experimental animals receiving these fluids for burn therapy often did not show an overall fluid-sparing effect and had an unacceptably high incidence of renal failure and death compared with those receiving LR solution.[219,224,225]

Of the many resuscitation formulas available, the Parkland (Baxter) and modified Brooke formulas are best tailored to the clinical condition of the patient and are accepted in most centers (Table 53-14).[220,226] The addition of glucose is not necessary except in children, especially those weighing less than 20 kg. Albumin 5% may be administered after the first day following

Table 53-14 Guidelines for Initial Fluid Resuscitation after Thermal Injury

Adults and Children >20 kg
Parkland Formula[a]
4.0 mL crystalloid/kg/% burn/first 24 h
20–60% of calculated plasma volume as colloid during second 24 h to maintain adequate urine output

Modified Brooke Formula[a]
2.0 mL lactated Ringer's/kg/% burn per first 24 h
0.3–0.5 mL/kg/% burn during second 24 h

Children <20 kg
Crystalloid 2–3 mL/kg/% burn per first 24 h[a]
Colloid 0.3–0.5 mL/kg/% burn + D_5W to maintain urine output
Crystalloid with 5% dextrose at maintenance rate
100 mL/kg for the first 10 kg and 50 mL/kg for the next 10 kg for 24 h

Clinical End Points of Burn Resuscitation
Urine output: 0.5–1 mL
Pulse: 80–140 beats per min (age dependent)
Systolic BP: 60 mmHg (infants); children 70–90 plus 2× age in years mmHg; adults MAP >60 mmHg
Base deficit: <2

BP, blood pressure; MAP, mean arterial pressure.
[a]50% of calculated volume is given during the first 8 hours, 25% is given during the second 8 hours, and the remaining 25% is given during the third 8 hours.

injury at a rate of 0.3, 0.4, or 0.5 mL/kg/24 hours for burns of 30% to 50%, 50% to 70%, or 70% to 100% of TBSA, respectively. These formulas are guidelines only, and none can be expected to provide adequate restoration of intravascular volume in all burn victims, especially small children and patients with inhalation injuries. Therefore, administration of fluids during the initial phase should be titrated to the specific goals described in Table 53-14, and, if a PAC is placed, to acceptable cardiac output, filling pressures, and a mixed venous oxygen tension (PvO_2) of 35 to 40 mmHg. Careful monitoring of the Hct may also guide fluid management. An increase in Hct during the first day suggests inadequate fluid resuscitation because hemolysis and sequestration are actually expected to cause a decrease in this parameter. Acute anemia, as may occur during excision and grafting of burns, is usually well tolerated. Blood replacement is usually not initiated until the Hct is decreased to 20% to 24% in healthy patients requiring limited operations, to approximately 25% in those who are healthy but need extensive procedures, and to 30% or more when there is a history of pre-existing cardiovascular disease.

When in rare instances fluid resuscitation fails despite administration of crystalloids in excess of 6 mL/kg per percentage of TBSA, and invasive or semi-invasive monitoring suggests adequate intravascular volume, vasopressor and/or inotropic agents may be indicated. Dopamine in small doses (5 μg/kg/min) and/or β-adrenergic agents may improve urine output without further need for fluids.[220] Electrolyte abnormalities may occur after the first day for several reasons but are primarily a result of topical agents applied to control pain, decrease vapor loss, prevent desiccation, and slow bacterial growth.[220] Nonaqueous topicals (silver sulfadiazine), if administered without providing free water such as 5% dextrose, may result in hypernatremia and its CNS consequences, including intracranial bleeding. In contrast, aqueous topical agents such as 5% silver nitrate solution may cause hyponatremia and its consequences of cerebral edema and seizure secondary to electrolyte leaching. Central pontine demyelination may occur if the hyponatremia is corrected rapidly with salt solutions. Serum ionized calcium and magnesium should also be monitored.

Traditionally, monitoring of fluid therapy for burn injury is limited to hourly urine output, heart rate, systemic blood pressure, and base deficit. The end points for these monitoring parameters are shown in Table 53-14. Indeed there is some evidence to suggest that hourly monitoring of urine output as an end point of resuscitation compared to sophisticated hemodynamic monitoring provides similar outcomes in terms of mortality, organ function, length of hospital or intensive care stay, duration of mechanical ventilation, and burn-related complications such as pulmonary edema, compartment syndromes, or infection.[227] On the other hand, there are criticisms about not using available sophisticated monitoring techniques during the initial 48 hours of burn injury.[226,228] The argument centers around the fact that in the presence of normal urine output, organ blood flow may still be compromised.[227,228] Some data suggest that using the minimally invasive lithium dilution cardiac output monitor (LiDCO Ltd., London, UK) or Pulsiocath thermistor-tipped catheter (Pulsion Medical Systems, Munich, Germany), which continuously measures systolic and pulse pressure variation (PPV) during positive-pressure ventilation and estimates preload dependence, resulted in administration of lower initial fluid volumes to burn patients than were administered with urine output and blood pressure measurement guidance.[229] Available monitoring tools that potentially can be used for this purpose are transthoracic echocardiography or TEE; hemodynamic parameters such as stroke volume variation (SVV), intrathoracic blood volume index, pulmonary artery occlusion pressure, cardiac index, and pulmonary capillary O_2 saturation; and markers of malperfusion such as base deficit, serum lactate level, near-infrared spectroscopy, or sidestream dark-field videomicroscopy.[227] Each of these monitoring tools provides distinct advantages but may also be difficult or not feasible to apply to burn patients. They may not be readily available in some burn units, may lack proof of accuracy, and may be invasive, presenting a risk to patients who are already in a critical clinical state.[227]

It seems that the initial fluid requirement of acute burn patients is often miscalculated for two reasons: erroneous estimation of burn size and computation of fluid volume to be administered. Not using the Lund–Browder chart is considered one of the reasons for wrong estimation of burn size. Several measures are suggested to improve the accuracy of computing fluid requirement, such as a nomogram or an electronic calculator.[230,231] Attributing part of the error to complicated initial resuscitation formulas, some authors have developed a simpler formula, the "Rule of Ten," which was designed and has been used by the US Army Institute of Surgical Research for the past several years.[228] With this method, the percentage of burned body surface area is multiplied by 10 to determine the estimated hourly fluid rate. For every 10 kg above 80 kg of body weight, 100 mL/hr is added to the calculated rate. The Rule of Ten appears accurate for patients weighing between 40 and 140 kg, overestimating the rate for patients below 40 kg and underestimating for those above 140 kg of body weight.[228] Generally, morbid obesity complicates initial fluid resuscitation. If actual body weight is used, the calculated fluid need is lower than that determined for normal-weight patients. If ideal body weight is used, which is rare in clinical practice, the patient may receive a higher resuscitation volume. Morbidly obese patients are likely to have higher acidosis, organ dysfunction, and mortality.[232]

Fluid management during the second 24-hour period after a burn is also important and involves the use of colloid, whether the Parkland or modified Brook formula is used as a guide. It has been shown that fluid intake in the second 24 hours correlates with that of the first 24-hour period; the higher the resuscitation volume during the first period, the higher the fluid intake during the second 24 hours.[233] Older victims, intubated patients, and those receiving high-dose narcotics require a larger volume of fluids during this period.[233] Although there are several formulae to calculate the hourly fluid volume needed, using 20% to 60% of the calculated plasma volume for colloid dose, or better the formula *(25+ %burn)(body surface area in m^2) mL for crystalloids + 0.3 to 0.5 mL/kg/% burn for colloids + maintenance fluid* provides a guideline for total fluid requirement. Generally the actual fluid volume administered exceeds the amount calculated by this formula by a factor of 1.5 to 1.9.[233] Maintenance fluid can be calculated by estimating 4 mL/kg/hr for the first 10 kg, 2 mL/kg/hr for the second 10 kg, and 1mL/kg/hr for additional weight thereafter.[233]

Operative Management

Monitoring

Hemodynamic Monitoring

Direct intra-arterial pressure monitoring, which permits beat-to-beat data acquisition and sampling for measurement of blood gases, should be in place before surgery. An ultrasound-guided technique or a surgical cutdown may be necessary to facilitate access. The radial artery is the vessel of choice in abdominal or chest trauma in which the aorta may be cross-clamped, making a femoral or dorsalis pedis cannula nonfunctional. The right radial artery is preferred in cases of chest trauma in which cross-clamping of the descending aorta might result in occlusion of the left subclavian artery. In mechanically ventilated patients, the magnitude of systolic pressure variation (the difference between the maximum and minimum systolic pressures over the respiratory cycle) and its delta down component (the difference between systolic pressures at end-expiration and the lowest value during the respiratory cycle) can provide reliable information about the intravascular volume status and predict responsiveness to fluid loading. A systolic pressure variation over 5 mmHg and a delta down over 2 mmHg suggest hypovolemia and responsiveness to fluid.[234]

The ability to predict fluid responsiveness is of crucial importance in preventing over- or underinfusion of fluids and its consequences. Interest has been centered on *automatically* obtaining systolic blood pressure variation, PPV, and SVV during the mechanical ventilation cycle to predict fluid responsiveness. Indeed several devices, such as the PiCCO (Pulsion Medical Systems, Munich, Germany), LiDCO (Lidco Ltd., London, UK), and FloTrac/Vigileo CO monitor (Edwards Lifesciences, Irvine, CA), are able to display systolic blood pressure variation, PPV, and SVV, which appear to predict responsiveness to fluid administration with greater accuracy than static markers of preload such as CVP, pulmonary artery occlusion pressure, and even global end-diastolic volume or left ventricular end-diastolic area.[235] Threshold values to discriminate responders from nonresponders to fluid infusion have been determined (PPV or SVV >12% for responders). These dynamic indices of preload can be obtained with an arterial line without central venous catheters or PACs. Limitations of this technology include ability to work only in intubated and mechanically ventilated patients with tidal volumes over 7 to 8 mL/kg, in a closed chest, and with normal cardiac rhythm; doubtful reliability in patients with stiff lungs or those receiving PEEP; and, most important, lack of information about accuracy in acutely injured patients.[236] An excellent review describing new methods of hemodynamic monitoring, including a pulse waveform analysis technique to determine fluid responsiveness and its possible application to trauma care, has recently become available.[237]

Delaying emergent surgery to place a central venous line is rarely indicated unless a large-bore catheter is needed for volume resuscitation. However, if the patient is elderly, if there is a likelihood of myocardial damage, or if there is multiple organ damage with a requirement for anticipated prolonged surgery, massive fluid replacement, and administration of vasoactive drugs, early placement of a CVP or PAC may be indicated before the development of coagulopathy renders it hazardous. If a PAC is placed, mixed venous O_2 and cardiac output measurement may convey information about organ perfusion. PACs with the capability of measuring right ventricular end-diastolic volume and ejection fraction (EF) provide better information about preload than regular PAC, but they are less accurate than TEE.[237]

The TEE provides valuable diagnostic information in BCI, cardiac septal or valvular damage, coronary artery injury, pericardial tamponade, and aortic rupture.[178] It also permits assessment of cardiac function, including right and left ventricular volume, EF, wall motion abnormalities, pulmonary hypertension, and cardiac output, and detects acute ischemia more accurately than either ECG or pulmonary artery pressure monitoring. Measuring the right ventricular volume alone can provide information about the adequacy of the intravascular volume. This technique also allows visualization of fat and air entry into the right heart, or into the left heart through a patent foramen ovale during internal fixation of lower extremity fractures.[238]

There is interest in using point-of-care TTE to qualitatively and quantitatively monitor preload and right and left cardiac function in trauma patients. Two excellent reviews have recently been published on this subject.[237,239] Obviously the purpose is not to perform a comprehensive TTE examination as practiced by cardiologists but to obtain goal-directed information about preload and cardiac function in symptomatic (hypotensive) trauma patients to select proper treatment. The TTE technique most commonly used in the trauma setting involves obtaining images through the subcostal long axis, subcostal inferior vena cava, parasternal long axis, parasternal short axis, and apical 4-chamber windows. Placement of a phased-array low-frequency (5 to 2 MHz) probe in these locations provides ideal views that are sufficient to inform the clinician of an underlying hemodynamic problem (Table 53-15 and Fig. 53-8).

Qualitatively, an empty heart and a flat IVC suggest hypovolemia. The patient is usually tachycardic and the ventricular walls contact each other (kissing) at the end of systole, producing a high EF. Likewise, the IVC collapses during the respiratory cycle. There are some pitfalls in interpretation of these findings. For example, in mechanically ventilated patients, the IVC may be large and may not collapse despite hypovolemia because of increased intrathoracic pressure. Also, patients in chronic heart failure may not show an empty hyperdynamic heart. Other qualitative findings to be looked for during evaluation of heart function with the parasternal short axis view at the level of the papillary muscles are inward motion of the endocardium, myocardial thickening, longitudinal motion of the mitral annulus, and geometry of the left ventricle. In addition, the presence of trauma-induced structural abnormalities such as pericardial effusion, or acute PE, which causes pulmonary hypertension and

Table 53-15 Transthoracic Echocardiographic Examination in the Trauma Setting

Window Used	Cardiac View	Probe Location	Direction of Probe Marker
Subcostal long axis	Four-chamber	Subcostal ~45-degree cephalad angle	Patient's left shoulder
Subcostal inferior vena cava	Inferior vena cava	Subcostal vertical	Patient's left shoulder
Parasternal long axis	Left atrium, left ventricle, left ventricular outflow tract, aortic root, right ventricle	Left parasternal third to fifth intercostal space	Patient's right shoulder
Parasternal short axis	Left ventricle and small portion of right ventricle	Left parasternal third to fifth intercostal space	Patient's left shoulder
Apical	All four chambers	Below the nipple	Patient's left back toward 2- and 3-o'clock position

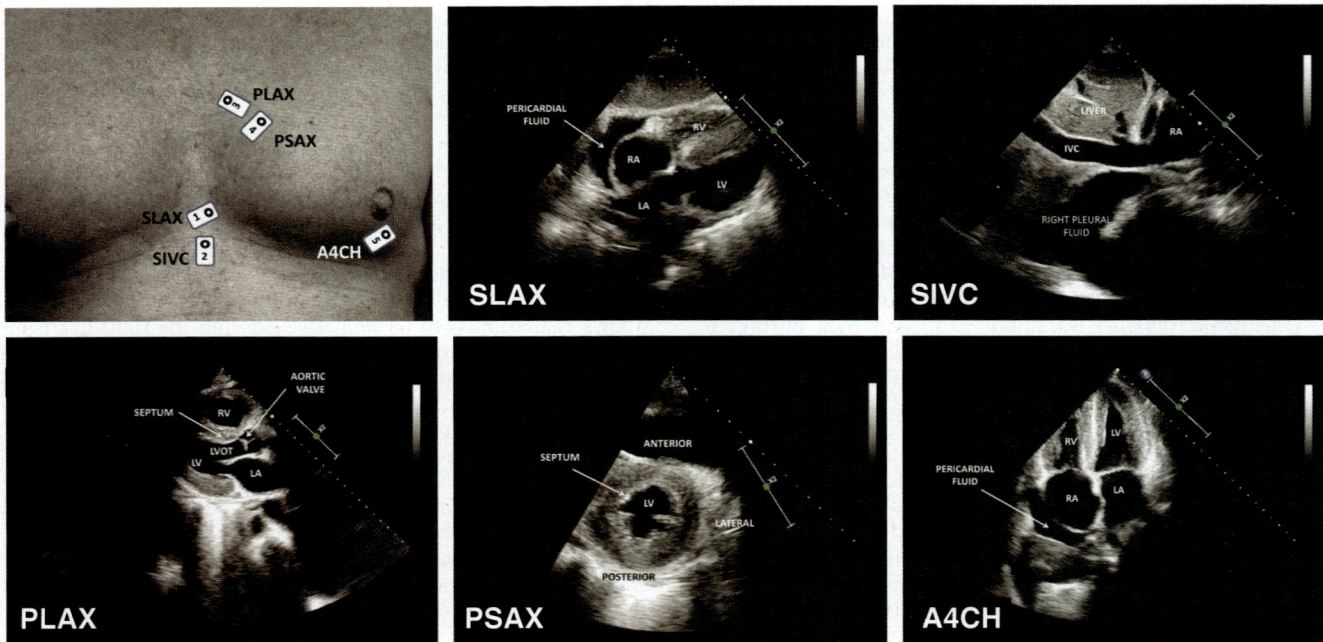

Figure 53-8 Transthoracic echocardiographic windows used in trauma patients and images obtained through each window. The photograph on the upper left shows location and position of the ultrasound probe and the direction of its marker (circle on the probe) for images of subxiphoid long axis (1, SLAX), subxiphoid inferior vena cava (2, SIVC), parasternal long axis (3, PLAX), parasternal short axis (4, PSAX) and apical four-chamber views (5, A4CH). Table 53-15 provides more detail about probe positioning. RA, right atrium; RV, right ventricle; LA, left atrium; LV, left ventricle; IVC, inferior vena cava; HV, heart valve; LVOT, left ventricular outflow tract. Right pleural fluid is shown on the SIVC and pericardial fluid in the A4CH views. (Courtesy of Drs. Ambika Nayar and Kenneth Sutin.)

right ventricular dilation with thinning of the walls, and tricuspid valve insufficiency can be detected.[239]

Quantitative evaluation of the TTE is more complex, but it permits calculation of stroke volume (SV), SVV after administration of fluids, EF, and cardiac output. These parameters can be determined from the two-dimensional image directly, or indirectly using the M mode, and by calculating fractional endocardial shortening during end-diastole and end-systole, which in turn provides end-diastolic and end-systolic volumes and thus permits calculation of SV, cardiac output, and EF.[239] The results of these measurements lead to four possibilities in the hypotensive trauma patient, each requiring different treatment: normal SV and EF requiring no treatment; low SV and high EF suggesting hypovolemia and necessitating fluids; low SV and low EF suggesting myocardial dysfunction and need for inotropic agents; or normal SV and high EF suggesting vasodilation, requiring vasopressor therapy.[237] With serial TTE determinations proper hemodynamic management is possible during the initial management of the trauma patient in shock whether in the ED or in the OR as long as access to the chest permits placement of the ultrasound probe. During ICU management, more detailed TTE examination is possible to guide therapy.

Urine Output

Urine output is routinely monitored as an indicator of organ perfusion, hemolysis, skeletal muscle destruction, and urinary tract integrity after trauma. Its reliability in monitoring perfusion is decreased by prolonged shock prior to surgery and osmotic diuresis caused by administration of mannitol or radiopaque dye. Dark, cola-colored urine in the trauma patient suggests either hemoglobinuria resulting from incompatible blood transfusion or myoglobinuria caused by massive skeletal muscle destruction after blunt or electrical trauma. Although the definitive diagnosis is made by serum electrophoresis, rapid differential diagnosis can be made by centrifugation of a blood specimen. Pink-stained serum suggests hemoglobinuria, whereas unstained serum indicates myoglobinuria. Both of these conditions may result in acute renal failure. Prevention involves inducing diuresis with fluids and mannitol and, in myoglobinuria, although controversial, additional alkalinization of the urine with sodium bicarbonate to pH greater than 5.6. Red-colored urine usually is caused by hematuria, which, in the traumatized patient, suggests urinary tract injury.

Oxygenation

Trauma patients frequently develop hypoxemia (O_2 saturation <90%), hypothermia, hypotension, and/or decreased peripheral perfusion. Of the available O_2 saturation (SpO_2) devices, finger or earlobe pulse oximeters are more affected by decreased perfusion than forehead probes, probably because the latter senses the pulsation of the supraorbital artery, a branch of the carotid artery, which is presumably less affected by shock or hypothermia. However, SpO_2 results with the forehead monitor may be affected by venous pulsation, especially in patients receiving positive-pressure ventilation or in any situation that distends the tributaries of the superior vena cava.[240] It has been suggested that using these sensors with a head band that exerts 10 to 20 mmHg of pressure may minimize the inaccuracy.[240]

With advances in technology, multi-wavelength pulse CO-oximeters are now capable of providing other physiologic data, including pulse rate, SpO_2, perfusion index, carboxyhemoglobin, and methemoglobin. They can also measure noninvasive continuous hemoglobin concentration with reasonable accuracy. The ability of these monitors (Masimo Rad-7 and Rad-57 Pulse CO-oximeters; Masimo, Irvine, CA) to measure methemoglobin and carboxyhemoglobin concentration noninvasively renders them useful in acute burn injury management. Although these devices are considered to provide more accurate information than conventional pulse oximeters, to the best of the authors' knowledge, they have not yet been systematically tested in major trauma victims.

Organ Perfusion and Oxygen Utilization

As discussed previously, unrecognized hypoperfusion may lead to splanchnic ischemia with resulting acidosis in the intestinal wall, permitting the passage of luminal microorganisms into the circulation and release of inflammatory mediators, causing sepsis and multiorgan failure.[69,70] Base deficit and blood lactate level, which have already been discussed in the section "Management of Shock," are considered acceptable markers of organ hypoperfusion in the *apparently* resuscitated patient and may be used intraoperatively to set the optimal end points of resuscitation.[70] Another parameter that may provide information about the global perfusion of the body is the arterial to end-tidal CO_2 difference. Values greater than 10 mmHg after resuscitation predict mortality.[241] It may be useful in the decision about when to perform damage control surgery and intraoperatively in guiding resuscitation with fluids, inotropes, and vasopressors. A large gap is usually due to decreased lung perfusion resulting in high $PaCO_2$ and low end-tidal CO_2. Severe chest trauma, hypotension, or metabolic acidosis also increases the likelihood of discordance between arterial and end-tidal CO_2.[242]

Oxygen transport variables, once routinely monitored as markers of organ perfusion, especially in the ICU setting, are used less frequently and in a limited number of centers primarily because they require pulmonary artery catheterization. They consist of oxygen delivery (DO_2), O_2 consumption (VO_2), and O_2 extraction ratio. The DO_2 index (DO_2I) is a particularly useful end point because it integrates three important variables: Hgb concentration, arterial oxygen saturation, and cardiac output. The minimum acceptable value for this marker is 500 mL/min/m^2,[243] which is as effective as the previously recommended DO_2I of at least 600 mL/min/m^2. A computerized ICU decision protocol developed to standardize shock resuscitation in some centers uses DO_2I above 500 mL/min/m^2 as a goal.[243] The oxygen consumption index (VO_2I) is also an important variable. Subsequent organ failure may occur if it decreases below a value of 170 mL/min/m^2, indicating a flow-dependent phase of O_2 utilization.[70] Increasing DO_2I until VO_2I attains flow independence may prevent organ failure; however, this approach is not practical clinically, mainly because there are also DO_2I-independent regulators of VO_2.[243]

Finally, a global O_2 extraction ratio below 0.25 to 0.3 suggests absence of dysoxia. However, it is possible that dysoxia may be present in an individual organ in the presence of a normal overall O_2 extraction ratio. Monitoring of O_2 transport variables, the most useful of which is DO_2I, is usually done in the ICU when invasive monitoring permits measurement of cardiac output and mixed venous O_2. These values can also be monitored in the OR whenever arterial and pulmonary artery lines are present.

It has recently been demonstrated that central venous, instead of pulmonary artery, monitoring with CVP above 10 mmHg, mean systemic blood pressure of 65 mmHg, and Hgb over 10 g/dL as threshold values also suggests adequate organ perfusion.[244] It should be emphasized that various pre-existing and trauma-related conditions may affect the interpretations of these perfusion markers. For example, the base deficit may reflect a nongap acidosis, elevated lactate may be secondary to impaired clearance owing to hepatic dysfunction, and arterial to end-tidal CO_2 gradient may be caused by chronic obstructive lung disease. Thus, management decisions must be individualized, taking into account the patient's general condition.

Coagulation

Conventional blood coagulation monitoring includes a baseline and subsequent serial measurements of INR, activated partial thromboplastin time (aPTT), platelet count, blood fibrinogen level, and fibrin degradation products (FDPs). Although trauma center laboratories cannot provide results of the standard coagulation tests rapidly, at least INR can be monitored with a point-of-care device and provide some information. Thromboelastography (TEG; Haemonetics, Boston, MA) and rotation transmission electron microscopy (ROTEM; Pentapharm, Munich, Germany) are point-of-care devices that provide a relatively rapid, comprehensive, and quantitative graphic evaluation of clotting function.[245,246] The TEG determines the time necessary for initial fibrin formation, the rapidity of fibrin deposition, the clot consistency, the rate of clot formation, and the times required for clot retraction and lysis (Fig. 53-9).[245] Basically, the R and K values are indices of formation, buildup, and crosslinking of fibrin and depend on the function of coagulation factors. The maximum amplitude is the widest portion of the curve and indicates the absolute strength of the fibrin clot. It represents platelet function. The α-angle is the slope of the external divergence of the tracing from the R-value point, indicating the speed of clot formation and fibrin crosslinking. The value of this parameter is determined by both coagulation factors and platelets. Hypothermia can cause coagulopathy by interfering with both platelets and coagulation factors.[247] When the blood of a cold and coagulopathic patient is placed in the TEG

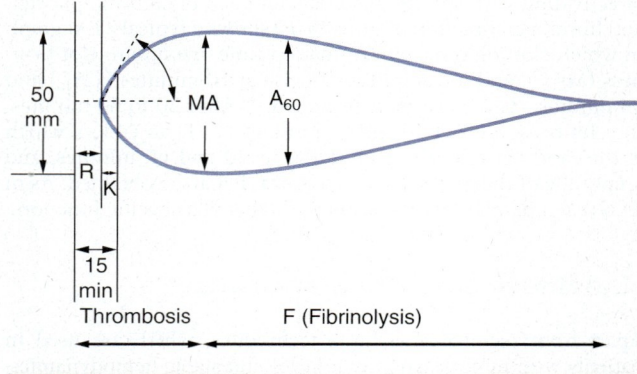

Figure 53-9 Thrombelastogram. R is the interval from blood deposition in the cuvette to an amplitude of 1 mm on the thrombelastogram; K is the time between the end of R and a point with an amplitude of 20 mm on the thrombelastogram; MA is the maximum amplitude of thrombelastogram; α angle is the slope of the external divergence of the tracing from the R value point; A_{60} is the amplitude of thromboelastogram 60 minutes after maximum amplitude; F is the time from MA to return to 0 amplitude (normal >300 minutes).

Normal Values:
- R = 6–8 min
- K = 3–7 min
- α angle = 50°–60°
- MA = 50–60 mm
- A_{60} = MA−5
- F = 300 min
- Clot lysis index (CLI) = A_{60}/MA × 100%
- CLI normal range >85%

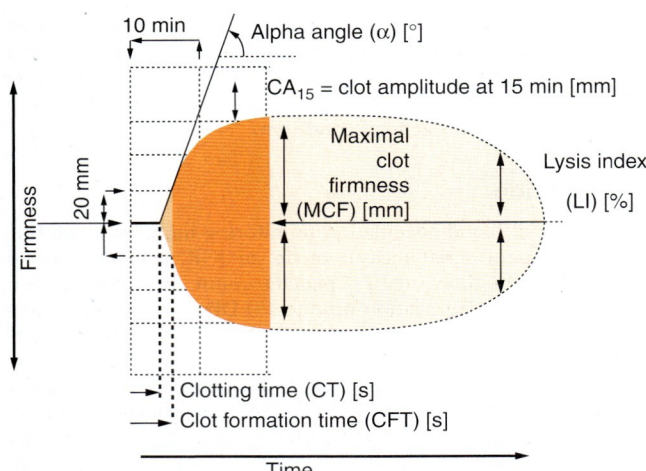

Figure 53-10 Rotation thromboelastometry graph depicting each clotting parameter. (Adapted with permission from Rugeri L, Levrat A, David JS, et al. Diagnosis of early coagulation abnormalities in trauma patients by rotation thromboelastography. *J Thromb Haemost.* 2007;5:289.)

cuvette, which is normally heated to 37°C, a near-normal trace may be obtained. Newer TEG devices are temperature adjustable. Thus, the temperature in the cuvette can be adjusted to that of the patient. Likewise, by using activators, rapid TEG (r-TEG) can be performed to obtain timely results.[248] ROTEM is a modified TEM that uses a ball-bearing system for power transduction and is less susceptible to movement or vibration that may affect the TEG.[246] It measures clot formation and fibrinolysis. Results of coagulation parameters are obtained within 10 to 15 minutes because of activation with specific materials for each of clotting, platelet, and fibrinogen function. Figure 53-10 shows a typical TEM graph in which clotting time, clot formation time, maximum clot firmness (MCF), and the amplitude of clot at 10 minutes (CA_{10}) and 15 minutes (CA_{15}) can be determined.[246] After 30 to 60 minutes, the clot lysis index at 30 and 60 minutes (CLI_{30} to CLI_{60}), which is the ratio between the amplitudes at 30 and 60 minutes, and amplitude of the graph at the point of CT may be obtained. As in TEG, each parameter represents the status of a specific function.

Anesthetic and Adjunct Drugs

Apart from regional anesthesia techniques, which are used in patients with minor extremity injuries and stable hemodynamics, anesthetic and adjunct drugs for general anesthesia need to be tailored to five major clinical conditions: airway compromise, hypovolemia, head or open eye injuries, cardiac injury, and burns. The varying contribution of these conditions to the clinical picture of a given patient necessitates priority-oriented planning.

Airway Compromise

Anesthetics and muscle relaxants should be avoided before the airway is secured if there is significant airway obstruction or if there is doubt as to whether the patient's trachea can be intubated because of anatomic limitations. If time permits, lateral neck radiographs, CT scanning, and endoscopy can be used to define the problems better. Topical anesthesia with mild sedation can be used to secure the airway with a conventional blade, videolaryngoscope, or FOB. If a rapid-sequence induction is contemplated, ketamine and etomidate may confer advantages over propofol. In equipotent doses in normovolemic patients, they produce less cardiovascular depression. Contrary to findings of increased mortality with prolonged etomidate infusion, a single induction dose (0.3 mg/kg) of etomidate did not affect organ function and outcome in acutely ill patients any more than ketamine, suggesting minimal effect on steroidogenesis.[249] Although succinylcholine, with its short onset time and duration, is still the muscle relaxant of choice for rapid-sequence induction, rocuronium (1.2 to 1.5 mg/kg) has almost the same onset time and does not have the undesirable side effects associated with succinylcholine (e.g., increased intragastric, intraocular, and intracranial pressures and potassium release in patients with burns and neurologic diseases). Its longer duration of action may be disadvantageous and may lead to hypoxia, if both ventilation and intubation prove to be impossible. Under these circumstances, one of the available videolaryngoscopes or other aids can be employed to overcome the problem. Sugammadex can also be utilized to encapsulate rocuronium or vecuronium and recover spontaneous breathing in a reasonably short period.[250,251] Surgical standby for cricothyroidotomy should be considered if failure of these techniques is anticipated. Bradycardia, dysrhythmias, and cardiac arrest may occur after succinylcholine in the presence of hypoxia and hypercarbia. Some of these complications may also follow an apparently uneventful intubation performed without succinylcholine.

Hypovolemia

In the absence of controlled human studies of anesthetic drug effects in hemorrhage and hemorrhagic shock, our current knowledge in this area is based on the results of experimental work, mostly in swine, and clinical experience from managing trauma victims. Our planning process for deciding how to use anesthetic agents is further complicated by the damage control resuscitation principle, specifically permissive hypotension. The facts that should drive decision making in this regard are as follows: First, anesthetic agents not only have direct cardiovascular depressant effects but also inhibit compensatory hemodynamic mechanisms such as central catecholamine output and baroreflex (neuroregulatory) mechanisms, which maintain systemic pressure in hypovolemia. Second, hemorrhage and hypovolemia alter the pharmacokinetics and pharmacodynamics of almost all anesthetic agents and often lead to a higher than normal blood concentration of intravenous agents and increased sensitivity of the brain and heart. Preferential distribution of the cardiac output to the brain and the heart, cerebral hypoxia, dilutional hypoproteinemia producing a larger free fraction of intravenous drugs, and acidosis all seem to be responsible for these effects. Third, hemorrhage and hypovolemia have different hemodynamic effects in the absence and presence of trauma. In the presence of trauma pain and a catecholamine surge, maintain blood pressure despite significant intravascular volume depletion and ischemia of vital organs such as the brain and the heart. Based on this knowledge, reducing or eliminating anesthesia to avoid abolishing the hemodynamic balance is a natural and often utilized practice, especially when permissive hypotension to limit bleeding is used. Dutton[252] recently suggested that proper management under these circumstances may be aggressive titrated administration of anesthetics and of blood products to produce a high-flow and low-pressure hemodynamic state with vasodilation to improve organ flow and oxygenation, which may reduce fibrinolytic activity and inflammation.[252] With serial blood lactate measurements the effect of either of these approaches can be monitored to aid further management. Further research is needed to help the clinician in selection of either of the approaches.

The pharmacokinetic and pharmacodynamic responses of intravenous agents to experimental hemorrhagic shock vary depending on the severity of the hemorrhage, the specific agent, and whether the effect analyzed is hypnosis or immobility to noxious stimuli. For example, in swine with compensated hemorrhage, when administered as a continuous infusion, blood propofol concentration increased by less than 20%, while during uncompensated shock (i.e., in hypotensive animals), it increased by almost four times.[253] On the other hand, under the same experimental conditions, plasma remifentanil concentration doubled during compensated shock but increased almost 27 times in uncompensated shock.[253] Remifentanil degradation relies on tissue and blood esterases. It is possible that hydrolysis by tissue esterases is more intense than by their blood counterparts because the decreased tissue blood flow in uncompensated shock is able to produce a major reduction in remifentanil metabolism. Another example is that hemorrhage has a similar potentiating effect on the production of hypnosis and immobility by propofol.[254] In contrast, the potentiating effect of hemorrhagic shock on isoflurane-induced hypnosis is much smaller than on its immobilizing effect.[254]

Because of the decrease in size of the central compartment and in systemic clearance, plasma concentrations of fentanyl and remifentanil are increased.[253,255] A decreased volume of distribution also increases the blood level of etomidate by 20% in shock,[256] and for propofol this effect is even greater. There is also variation in the extent of brain sensitivity to these agents. Although etomidate pharmacodynamics are unchanged,[257] a significant increase in the sensitivity of the brain and heart to propofol is noted in animals, even after fluid resuscitation.[256] Based on these experimental findings, Shafer[258] calculated that in patients with shock, the dose of propofol should be only 10% to 20% of that given to a healthy patient. Although he calculated that etomidate dose should not require adjustment for shock, the authors decrease the dose by at least 25% to 50% when hypovolemia is suspected. As to the opioids, the calculated dose for fentanyl and remifentanil is approximately one-half that for healthy patients (Fig. 53-11).[258] Of the remaining intravenous agents, midazolam is also known to have significant cardiovascular depressant activity, whereas ketamine has stimulatory effects when the autonomic nervous system is intact.

There are also differences among anesthetics in the direction and extent of their effects on compensatory mechanisms. For example, the baroreceptor depression produced by intravenous agents is usually milder than that of inhalational agents. Opioid agents have little direct cardiovascular or baroreflex depressant effect; however, these agents can cause hypotension by inhibiting central sympathetic activity, especially in the hypovolemic trauma patient whose apparent hemodynamic stability is maintained by hyperactive sympathetic tone.

Two important principles in the use of anesthetic agents are accurate estimation of the degree of hypovolemia and reduction of doses accordingly. The presence of hypotension suggests uncompensated hypovolemia, in which case anesthetics almost invariably produce further deterioration of systemic blood pressure and sometimes cardiac standstill. Intravascular volume, to the extent possible, must be restored before their use. When time constraints or continuing hemorrhage prevent restoration of blood volume, the airway may be secured without the benefit of anesthesia (perhaps using only rapidly acting muscle relaxants and small doses of opioids, etomidate, or ketamine), even though this approach may result in recall of induction and intraoperative events in up to 40% of patients, and, as mentioned before, vital organ ischemia.[259] Hypothermia, alcohol intoxication, illicit drug use before anesthesia, and metabolic disturbances in the acute trauma patient cannot reliably prevent recall. However, scopolamine (0.6 mg), and midazolam, if the patient can tolerate it, given before airway management may decrease the likelihood of this complication. Intraoperative use of the bispectral index monitor and, whenever possible, titrating anesthetics to bispectral index levels lower than 60 may prevent recall in trauma patients.

In normotensive but hypovolemic patients, restoration of volume and selection of an agent with the least cardiovascular depressant effect appears logical. Ketamine and etomidate are the preferred induction agents,[257] although at low doses other intravenous anesthetics are also unlikely to produce hypotension. Therefore, the use of any of these drugs in reduced doses is probably more important than the particular agent chosen.

Maintenance of anesthesia in the hypovolemic trauma patient raises concerns similar to those pertaining to induction. Experimental data have shown that depending on its severity, hemorrhagic shock decreases minimum alveolar concentration (MAC) by approximately 25%. Restoration of intravascular volume did not, but administration of naloxone did normalize MAC in these animals, suggesting that shock-induced release of endorphins is primarily responsible for this effect.[260]

Although nitrous oxide's (N_2O) myocardial depressant effect is normally somewhat counterbalanced by its ability to increase sympathetic outflow, in acute hemorrhage there is already a dramatic increase in sympathetic activity and stimulation of baroreceptors. Under these circumstances, patients are unlikely to respond to the sympathetic effect of N_2O, and the cardiovascular depressant properties of the gas are unmasked. These may be similar to those of other inhalation agents. In addition, by reducing FiO_2, use of N_2O incurs a risk of hypoxemia in patients with reduced cardiac output or pulmonary compromise. Despite causing little impairment of reflex tachycardia and having a vasodilatory activity that preserves organ blood flow in normovolemic patients, isoflurane can impair cardiac output and organ blood flow in hypovolemia—that is, it can cause cardiovascular depression. Desflurane and sevoflurane are not significantly better than isoflurane in this regard. However, because of their low solubility in blood, the severe hemodynamic depression produced by these

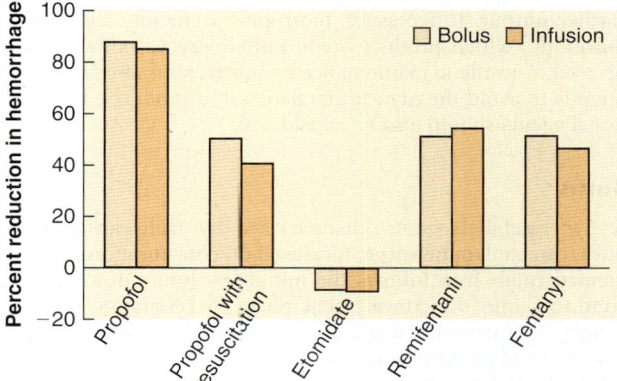

Figure 53-11 Calculated dose reduction of various anesthetics administered as bolus or infusion in moderate hemorrhagic shock. Calculation is based on pharmacokinetic and pharmacodynamic studies performed in experimental hemorrhagic shock. (Adapted from Shafer SL. Shock values. *Anesthesiology*. 2004;101:567.)

agents can be rapidly reversed, preventing suboptimal perfusion for a significant period of time. In summary, in the hypovolemic patient all inhalational agents may reduce both global and regional blood flows and therefore should be used only in low concentrations (<1 MAC). Opioid supplementation is usually well tolerated and often indicated.

Head and Open Eye Injuries

The importance of deep anesthesia and adequate muscle relaxation during airway management of patients with head or open eye injuries has already been discussed. Anesthetic agents selected for management of brain injury should produce the least increase in ICP, the least decrease in mean arterial pressure, and the greatest reduction in cerebral metabolic rate ($CMRO_2$). The most important factor causing cerebral ischemia is increased ICP from intracranial hematoma. Prompt decompression is the most crucial means of ensuring cerebral well-being. Hypotension caused by anesthetics or other factors contributes to the development or progression of cerebral ischemia. Utmost attention should be paid during anesthesia to avoidance of hypotension (mean arterial pressure <60 to 70 mmHg or SBP <90 to 100 mmHg). All intravenous anesthetics including ketamine cause comparable degrees of cerebrovascular constriction and ICP reduction.[261] $CMRO_2$ is also reduced by all of the available intravenous anesthetics. An important drawback to these agents, with the possible exception of ketamine, is that their cardiovascular depressant effects may reduce CPP. This problem can be ameliorated by administering pretreatment doses of opioids (fentanyl, 2 to 3 μg/kg), which permit reduction of the anesthetic dose. This may also prevent the myoclonic movements associated with etomidate and occasionally with propofol, and thus reduce the risks of ICP and IOP increase. Nevertheless, myoclonus is best prevented by careful timing of the dose of muscle relaxants. Another measure to preserve CPP during anesthesia is to administer vasopressors, being aware that hypovolemia may be masked by their use.

Ordinarily, administration of succinylcholine should follow pretreatment doses of nondepolarizing agents to prevent fasciculation-induced elevation of ICP and IOP.[262] Avoiding succinylcholine usually does not alleviate the problem because laryngoscopy and tracheal intubation produce a greater and longer-lasting increase in these pressures. Rocuronium, 1.2 to 1.5 mg/kg, has an onset time comparable with that of succinylcholine. None of the nondepolarizing muscle relaxants causes an elevation of ICP or IOP in the absence of associated tracheal intubation.

All inhalation anesthetics may increase CBF and cerebral blood volume, and thus the ICP. Cerebral autoregulation, CO_2 responsiveness, and $CMRO_2$ are reduced. Unlike intravenous anesthetics, which decrease both CBF and $CMRO_2$ in parallel, inhalational anesthetics decrease $CMRO_2$ while increasing the CBF. The extent of this uncoupling varies with the agent and the dose. Isoflurane has the least vasodilatory effect and thus is the most widely used inhalation anesthetic, although desflurane and sevoflurane have comparable effects on the cerebral circulation. In hyperventilated patients with cerebral tumors or mild edema, isoflurane does not raise the ICP if it is administered at an inspired concentration below 1 MAC. In the presence of severe head injury, when cerebral autoregulation and CO_2 responsiveness are impaired, isoflurane has the potential to increase CBF and ICP even at levels below 1 MAC and with hyperventilation. Therefore, it may be prudent not to use this agent in the presence of elevated ICP, at least until the skull is opened and the ICP is controlled. In these patients, anesthesia can be maintained initially with opioids plus propofol, midazolam, or etomidate.

Nitrous oxide may increase CBF, cerebral blood volume, and ICP when administered with inhalation anesthetics if the $PaCO_2$ is normal or increased. This effect may be eliminated when this agent is administered with adequate doses of barbiturates or hyperventilation. The effect on $CMRO_2$ is variable: Both increases and decreases have been observed. Thus, N_2O probably is not deleterious in patients with head injury with minimal ICP elevation if it is used after a bolus dose or during infusion of intravenous anesthetics.

A survey by Grathwohl et al.[16] compared the results of total intravenous anesthesia using ketamine with volatile agent anesthesia in a series of combat-related head injuries from Iraq. Although there are unavoidable shortcomings to the study, it nevertheless indicates that the specific anesthetic agents chosen probably do not affect the neurologic outcome as long as the vital signs are maintained.

Cardiac Injury

If there is pericardial tamponade, preload and myocardial contractility must be maintained. Any decrease in these parameters may exacerbate an already existing right ventricle (RV) inflow obstruction. A decrease in heart rate should also be treated promptly to maintain adequate cardiac output. Because all of the available anesthetics can depress myocardial contractility and cause vasodilation, it is preferable to administer these agents after evacuation of the pericardial blood under local anesthesia. If general anesthesia is required to relieve the tamponade, induction should be delayed until the patient is prepared and draped. Both anesthetics and controlled ventilation, particularly with PEEP, impair cardiac output. Deep anesthesia and high airway pressures should be avoided before evacuation of the hemopericardium. In chronic pericardial effusion, ketamine supports the cardiac index better than other intravenous agents. In acute pericardial tamponade, even minor insults can bring cardiac activity to a halt. Ketamine thus remains the agent of choice. It should be given in small doses after adequate fluid infusion. Similar principles apply to the use of maintenance agents, which should be given in the smallest possible doses until the heart is decompressed.

In blunt myocardial injury, the objective is not only to maintain cardiac contractility but also to lower the elevated pulmonary vascular resistance that may result from concomitant pulmonary contusion, atelectasis, or aspiration. All anesthetics should preferably be administered after restoration of intravascular volume and titrated to maintain adequate systemic blood pressure and cardiac output. If necessary, inotropes, preferably amrinone or milrinone, which produce some pulmonary vasodilation, may be used. Anesthetic maintenance by intravenous anesthetics and opioids to avoid the myocardial depression produced by inhalational agents should also be considered.

Burns

A hypermetabolic state characterized by tachycardia, tachypnea, catecholamine surge, increased O_2 consumption, and augmented catabolism follows the initial few hours of a burn and continues into the convalescent phase, necessitating increased oxygen, ventilation, and nutrition.[200,202,216,263] Early extensive and repeated escharotomies with coverage by skin grafts attenuate the postburn hypermetabolic response, decrease insulin resistance, decrease fluid loss, and improve survival.[264] They are usually performed between the second day and the second week, often necessitating massive transfusion, temperature control, and management of fluid, electrolyte, and coagulation abnormalities. Usually, an autograft harvested from either the patient, a cadaver, or both is used. An artificial skin substitute, INTEGRA (Integra Life Sciences, Plainsboro, NJ), consisting of a dermal inner layer made of bovine collagen and chondroitin-6-sulfate and a neoepidermal outer layer made of polysiloxane polymer, may also be used; it results in more favorable reduction of resting energy expenditure and elevation of serum proteins compared with that of cadaver skin.[265]

Anesthetic management of escharotomies presents several difficulties. Burned tissue may prevent access for ECG, pulse oximeter, neuromuscular function, and noninvasive blood pressure monitoring. Needle electrodes or surgical staples, a reflectance pulse oximeter, and an arterial catheter may be necessary. Large-bore intravenous catheters are essential. Hyperthermia occurs, but hypothermia is more likely in the OR and is to be avoided. Exposure and evaporative fluid loss necessitate maintenance of the OR temperature between 28°C and 32°C, use of fluid and blood warming devices, surface heating with forced dry warm air, and humidified inspired gases. Blood loss can be controlled by restricting the escharotomy to 15% to 20% of TBSA, using extremity tourniquets, applying topical thrombin and fibrin sealants to the excised area, using dilute epinephrine solution topically (1:10,000) or by injection (0.5 mg per 1,000 mL), and using compression bandages.[266] Epinephrine doses of up to 6.7 mg topically or 0.8 mg by injection into the surgical area are well tolerated. The affinity of β-adrenergic receptors to ligands is decreased after burns. The administration of a large amount of blood and blood products subjects the patient to complications of transfusion, such as hypocalcemia and coagulopathy, requiring monitoring of coagulation status and administration of adequate replacement therapy.[267]

Shock, hyperdynamic circulation, decreased serum albumin levels, increased α_1-acid glycoprotein concentration, and altered receptor sensitivity change the response to various drugs during the resuscitative and convalescent phases.[198,200] The doses of intravenous anesthetics should be reduced during the resuscitation phase to prevent excessive hemodynamic depression. During the hyperdynamic phase, blood flow to the liver and kidneys increases with increasing cardiac output. Thus drugs that rely on organ blood flow for elimination are cleared at a faster rate, requiring larger doses for effect, which may also be associated with hemodynamic depression.[198] Burn patients have excruciating pain and exceedingly high opioid requirements. Morphine may be the preferred opiate; in a preliminary study, patients receiving fentanyl experienced higher body temperatures than those who received morphine. This was attributed to the well-established anti-inflammatory properties of morphine.[268] A proven anesthetic regimen for excision and grafting of burns is volatile anesthetic agent plus large doses of opioid. Increased opioid requirement is related not only to the intense pain level but also to tolerance, which starts developing about 3 to 4 weeks after injury, reaching a maximum at 10 to 17 weeks and gradually declining to baseline about 6 months after injury. Similar tolerance to benzodiazepines may be noted.[198] Along with pharmacokinetic changes, pharmacodynamic alterations such as downregulation of the μ-opioid receptors and upregulation of the protein kinase C-γ and N-methyl-D-aspartate receptors appear to be responsible for opioid, benzodiazepine, and ketamine tolerance.[198] Clinically this problem can be overcome by supplementing opioids with clonidine, dexmedetomidine, ketamine, and, because of its long half-life, methadone.[198] A sedation analgesia guideline is proposed by Bittner et al.[198] for different burn-induced pain conditions.

For serial wound debridement, dressing or line changes, and insertion of urinary catheters in children, ketamine in intermittent doses provides a suitable alternative to inhalation anesthesia. Hemodynamic stability, preserved airway patency, bronchodilation, anti-inflammatory effect, counteraction of opioid hyperalgesia, and maintenance of hypoxic and hypercapnic responses are all advantages of this agent. Dysphoria and increased salivary output can be overcome by concomitant administration of benzodiazepines and anticholinergics. It should be kept in mind that in some catecholamine-depleted burn patients, hypotension may follow ketamine administration.

Regional anesthesia in its various forms can be effective to provide intraoperative anesthesia, postoperative analgesia, and assistance for rehabilitation. Pain in these patients originates from the burn site but also the area of skin harvesting, and often the latter is more intense. Tumescent infiltration in the form of continuous infusion of local anesthetic administered subcutaneously at the donor site may provide satisfactory analgesia. Lateral cutaneous nerve or transverse abdominis plane blocks provide analgesia to the lateral thigh, where skin harvesting is usually performed. These blocks may be combined with fascia iliaca blocks if the graft is taken from the anterior thigh. Paravertebral blocks with or without catheter placement can provide excellent analgesia to burnt areas at the torso. Brachial plexus and sciatic/femoral blocks can be useful for upper and lower extremity pain management. Finally, if the patient's back is free of burn injury, neuraxial blocks can be used.[198]

The response to depolarizing and nondepolarizing muscle relaxants remains unaltered during the first 24 hours after burn injury. After this period, succinylcholine should be avoided for at least 1 year because it can result in a potentially lethal increase of serum K^+ when the burn size exceeds 10% of TBSA. The mechanism of this response is related to upregulation (increase) of acetylcholine receptors, which ultimately occupy the entire muscle membrane, and the additional expression of two newly described isoforms of the acetylcholine receptor, and nicotinic (neural) α_7-acetylcholine receptors. The latter can be depolarized not only by acetylcholine and succinylcholine but also by choline, which thus plays an important role in the development of hyperkalemia.[269] Resistance develops to all nondepolarizing muscle relaxants including cisatracurium in patients with burns of more than 30% of TBSA starting at approximately 1 week and peaking 5 to 6 weeks after injury, probably from pharmacodynamic causes.[198,200,203] Increasing the dose can partly overcome this resistance. For instance, rocuronium, which is important for rapid-sequence induction and treatment of laryngospasm when succinylcholine is contraindicated, has an onset time delayed by about 50 seconds (30% longer than patients without burn) when a 0.9 mg/kg dose is used. Increasing the dose to 1.2 mg/kg decreases the delay by 30 seconds, but the onset time remains about 25 to 30 seconds longer than that observed in patients without burns. Intubating conditions also improve by increasing the dose. Recovery time from the block is shorter in burned patients than in normal individuals.[270]

Management of Intraoperative Complications

Persistent Hypotension

Persistent hypotension following trauma is usually the result of one of four mechanisms: bleeding, tension pneumothorax, neurogenic shock, or cardiac injury. Although many other causes, such as citrate intoxication (hypocalcemia), hypothermia, coronary artery disease, allergic reactions, or incompatible transfusion may be responsible for this complication, they occur infrequently.

Hypotension is most likely due to bleeding. The source may be obvious, such as external bleeding from the skull or an open vessel in the extremities, or occult. The thoracic and abdominal cavities and the pelvic retroperitoneal space are the most common sites of occult hemorrhage that results in hypotension. Management includes early diagnosis and control of the bleeding site plus effective fluid resuscitation with a rapid-infusion system, which should be connected to a 14-gauge or larger cannula, preferably inserted into veins both above and below the diaphragm. The Rapid Infuser systems (RI-2, Belmont Instrument Corp, Bellerica, MA; ThermaCor 1200, Smisson-Cartledge Biomedical, Macon, GA), which consist of a reservoir, heating system, roller pump, and large-diameter (5-mm) tubing, are capable of delivering up to 1,000 mL/min of warm fluids once the infusion rate is programmed.

Of the isotonic crystalloid solutions, LR is preferred over normal saline. Resuscitation with normal saline during uncontrolled hemorrhage is associated with greater urine output and thus greater fluid requirement compared with LR, hyperchloremic acidosis, and dilutional coagulopathy.[271] Acidosis does not occur with LR, but tissue edema may result from its slight hypotonicity (~255 mOsm/L), and neutralization of the citrate anticoagulant in PRBCs may occur because of its Ca^{2+} content. Human serum albumin (5% and 25%) is the most commonly used colloid, if the volume of hemostatic FFP exceeds the amount calculated by its ratio with transfused PRBC. Theoretically, the combined use of fluids and moderate doses of vasopressor may rapidly restore blood pressure to normal levels, limit the fluid volume infused, and improve short-term survival.

Neurogenic shock from spinal cord injury may be missed during initial evaluation, especially in unconscious patients. However, differentiation of neurogenic shock from hemorrhagic shock is important. Patients with spinal cord injury are often bradycardic and readily respond to catecholamine administration. Mistaking neurogenic shock for hemorrhagic shock may lead to excessive fluid infusion and pulmonary edema in the spinal cord–injured patient. The reverse error may also occur, depriving patients with hemorrhagic shock of fluids because of misdiagnosis of neurogenic shock. TTE or TEE may be helpful in differentiation. In some patients, of course, hemorrhagic shock and neurogenic shock may coexist.

Cardiac causes of persistent hypotension include BCI and pericardial tamponade. Intraoperative TEE can be useful in the differential diagnosis. The RV is most commonly involved in BCI. If there is a concomitant increase in pulmonary vascular resistance (e.g., from an associated pulmonary contusion), the RV pressure increases while its output decreases, resulting in an increased CVP. The raised RV pressure causes the interventricular septum to shift toward the left, decreasing left ventricular compliance, increasing its diastolic pressure, and decreasing cardiac output. These alterations in cardiac anatomy and ventricular dynamics can be displayed by TEE or TTE, information that can be useful during interpretation of elevated cardiac filling pressures.

In the absence of TEE, a PAC may be helpful. Equalization of pressures across the cardiac chambers during diastole suggests pericardial tamponade. A similar picture may also be seen in severe BCI, causing difficulty in differential diagnosis. This effect, however, is rare and is usually associated with critical hemodynamic instability. Differential diagnosis in these instances can be established by pericardiocentesis. Septal encroachment into the left ventricle from RV contusion results in an increase in pulmonary artery wedge pressure. Decreasing the rate of fluid infusion in these patients results in a further decrease in cardiac output. Treatment includes fluid infusion, pulmonary vasodilators if the systemic blood pressure is normal, and inotropic support if the systemic blood pressure is low. Absence of response to this treatment is an indication for placement of an intra-aortic balloon pump. Pulmonary artery catheterization may also help detect an oxygen step-up from a septal injury. During thoracotomy, a distended RV should also raise the suspicion of a septal defect.

Hypothermia

Shock, alcohol intoxication, exposure to cold, fluid resuscitation, and abnormalities in thermoregulatory mechanisms render the major trauma patient hypothermic during the initial phase of injury. A core body temperature below 35°C is often associated with acidosis, hypotension, and coagulopathy, which in turn may lead to an increased risk of severe bleeding, need for transfusion, and mortality.[89] Admission hypothermia, which is present in approximately 50% of patients, is an independent risk factor after major trauma,[272] and the mortality rate increases with decreasing temperature. Severe hypothermia, which in the trauma patient is defined as core temperature below 32°C,[273] was associated with a 100% mortality rate in one study,[274] although survival of a few patients with admission temperatures even lower than 32°C has been reported.[275] The intraoperative risk of hypothermia is also higher for trauma victims than for electively operated patients. Increased heat loss is seen most commonly in patients with spinal cord, extensive soft tissue, and burn injuries and in patients who consumed ethanol preoperatively or those undergoing body cavity surgery.

Other deleterious effects of hypothermia are cardiac depression, myocardial ischemia, arrhythmias, peripheral vasoconstriction, impaired tissue oxygen delivery, elevated oxygen consumption during rewarming, blunted response to catecholamines, increased blood viscosity, metabolic acidosis, abnormalities of K^+ and Ca^{2+} homeostasis, reduced drug clearance, and increased risk of infection.[272,276] Rewarming after hypothermia, especially at a rapid rate, may release accumulated metabolic products into the central circulation, causing further myocardial depression, hypotension, and increased acidosis.

Prevention of hypothermia and restoration of normal body temperature appear to decrease mortality rate, blood loss, fluid requirement, organ failure, and length of ICU stay.[277] Convective warming with forced dry air at 43°C can prevent a temperature drop in most trauma victims but cannot effectively treat severe hypothermia because the low specific heat of air has little heat content to transfer to the cold trauma patient, and often, owing to the nature of the surgical procedure, only a limited body surface area is exposed to warming.[277] Circulating-water warmers may produce faster rewarming even though they cover a relatively smaller body surface area than forced air warmers.[278] Airway warming can reduce the heat loss caused by the latent heat of vaporization, but this technique also transfers very little heat.[278] Administration of warm intravenous fluids may prevent and treat hypothermia in the trauma patient, provided they are administered at a relatively rapid rate. For each liter of fluid given at 40°C to a patient with a body temperature of 33°C, 29.33 kJ of heat energy are gained (the specific heat of water is 4.19 kJ/L/°C).

Coagulation Abnormalities

Multiple factors may be responsible for coagulopathy after trauma; they can be divided into two main categories. ATC develops shortly after trauma from tissue injury and hypoperfusion; this activates thrombomodulin from the endothelial cells and the thrombomodulin–thrombin complex, which in turn activates protein C inhibiting factors V and VIII.[279,280] RAC develops later and results from dilution of coagulation factors and platelets; tissue hypoperfusion; disturbance of fibrinogen/fibrin polymerization and platelet activity caused by decreased serum ionized Ca^{++} from infusion of colloids or binding to citrate in PRBCs, FFP, and platelet units[281]; hypoxia, hypothermia and acidosis; and disseminated intravascular coagulation (DIC). Primary fibrinolysis may develop early as a component of ATC or later as part of the RAC.[282,283] DIC results from acute release of thromboplastin from injured brain, fat, amniotic fluid, or other sources or subacutely from endothelial inflammation or failure interfering with clearance of activated coagulation factors, causing microthrombi and consumption coagulopathy.[284] Fibrinolysis may develop by depleted plasminogen activator inhibitor-1 (PA-1), which accelerates the formation of plasmin. Normally thrombin facilitates the conversion of fibrinogen to fibrin. In severe trauma, thrombin binds to thrombomodulin, which slows or reduces the activation of thrombin-activated fibrinolysis inhibitor, leading to hyperfibrinolysis.[285] More recently Johansson et al.[286] demonstrated elevated admission circulating syndecan-1 levels, a marker of degradation of the subendothelial glycocalyx, in trauma patients, suggesting that the precipitating event is vascular damage resulting from catecholamine release and increasing permeability, inflammation, and coagulopathy, probably implying that the interplay among these mechanisms is the pathogenesis of trauma-induced coagulopathy.[87,287]

Hypothermia affects platelet morphology, function, and sequestration; retards enzyme activity; and decreases coagulation factor function by about 10% for each 1°C drop in temperature, slowing the initiation and propagation of platelet plugs and fibrin clot as well as enhancing fibrinolytic activity.[101,282,288,289] The mechanism of hypothermia-induced coagulopathy is complex and depends on the extent of temperature decrease. Down to 33°C, there is little alteration in coagulation enzyme activity, explaining the practically unchanged values reported for aPTT.[290] Within this temperature range, coagulopathy results from altered platelet aggregation or adhesion.[290] Thus, the aPTT at temperatures from 33° to 37°C does not provide any meaningful information about coagulation status, even when the test is performed at the hypothermic patient's temperature, because it does not measure platelet adhesion. In contrast, TEG at the patient's temperature may be reflective of the degree of coagulopathy.[281] Both enzymatic activity and platelet aggregation are abnormal below 33°C.[290] Metabolic acidosis is probably a stronger coagulation enzyme inhibitor than hypothermia. It interferes with the generation of thrombin, a factor essential in activating cofactors, platelets, and enzymes, in addition to converting fibrinogen to fibrin. This effect of acidosis is potentiated by hypothermia.[291]

Diagnosis

The perioperative diagnosis of coagulopathy is often made by observing bleeding from wounds or puncture sites, rather than by interpretation of laboratory tests. However, the differential diagnosis between consumptive and dilutional coagulopathy requires laboratory testing. The availability of point-of-care coagulation testing (INR, TEG, and thromboelastometry) reduces the delay in obtaining the results of these tests.[248] In the absence of TEG or ROTEM, INR has been shown to be an acceptable alternative for this purpose.[292] In general, the inability to determine the type of coagulopathy does not present a problem because the initial treatment is similar for both conditions. Nevertheless, the diagnosis of DIC has prognostic significance because its treatment involves elimination of its cause(s). The presence of elevated circulating FDP, especially when above 40 mg/mL, is suggestive of DIC, but the result of this study will reach the clinician long after the completion of initial resuscitation. A fibrinogen level below 100 mg/dL is also suggestive of DIC, but reduction to this value often takes a long time, decreasing the diagnostic value of the test, although serial measurements may be useful. A diagnostic scoring system consisting of platelet count, PT or INR, fibrinogen level, and FDP measurements has been suggested to rule DIC in or out.[293]

Treatment

Red Blood Cell Transfusion and Hemostasis

Platelets function better in the presence of higher Hct, and a component therapy with 1:1:2 formula where 2 represents PRBCs.[294] Red blood cell administration should continue at least to a Hct of 30, at which point factors and platelets are active and can produce a solid clot. At lower Hct level, clot may develop but may not be strong enough to overcome bleeding. The optimal ratio of PRBCs:FFP:platelet during transfusion of the massively bleeding patient appears to be between 1:1:1 and 2:1:1.

Component transfusion therapy, used universally in civilian trauma, is inferior to the whole blood transfusion practiced by the military. During the preparation of platelets and FFP, 100 mL of nonhemostatic anticoagulants is put in each bag. This additional fluid lowers factor levels by 20%. Similarly 100 mL of solution is added to PRBCs for storage injury protection in addition to 100 mL of anticoagulant. During MTP, each blood product administered dilutes out the other two blood product components. FFP will decrease the Hct and platelet count. Likewise, PRBCs lower coagulation factors and platelet counts. Thus a 1:1:1 ratio cannot be compared with whole blood in its hemostatic ability.[252,294] Hemostatic capability of component therapy further decreases with storage injury of PRBCs. During storage, red cells undergo changes, including the loss of adenosine triphosphate, diphosphoglycerate, and potassium; oxidative injury to proteins, lipids, and carbohydrates; loss of shape and membrane; increased adhesiveness; decreased flexibility; reduced flow in capillaries; and decreased oxygen delivery. The success of a blood transfusion is defined as 75% of the red cells infused still being effective after 24 hours. The storage injury brings out the controversy about the safety and effectiveness of "new blood" versus "old blood."

New blood is generally defined as blood collected less than 14 days before administration, whereas old blood is considered blood that is 14 to 28 days past collection. Although banked blood can be stored for 42 days, the average age of blood units used in busy trauma centers is 16 days, essentially slightly older than "new blood." Blood at 42 days is rarely used. Of more than 15 studies on the effect of age of blood in trauma, all but one demonstrated that old blood transfusion had an increased risk of multiorgan failure, infection, vascular complications, greater ICU/hospital length of stay, and mortality.[295] From a clinical perspective, however, it is a challenge for the anesthesiologist to receive blood for massive transfusion that is always less than 14 days old.

Each unit of PRBCs as well as FFP has the additives of citrate, monobasic sodium phosphate, dextrose, and adenine.[296] Adenine extends red cell survival from 21 to 35 days and is intrinsic for the maintenance of red cell ATP levels. Dextrose and monobasic sodium monophosphate are nutritive. The significant complication of these additives is that citrate chelates calcium, which serves as a co-factor in the coagulation cascade, leading to hypocalcaemia. In addition to defective coagulation, signs and symptoms of hypocalcemia include hypotension, decreased pulse pressure, arrhythmias, change in mental status, and tetany. Citrate is in abundance in all component blood products.[296] Hypocalcemia is a rare event but must be considered after the goals of the MTP are met and the patient remains hypotensive. Citrate is metabolized by the liver, and in the condition of hypothermia, which is common in the trauma patient, liver metabolism is decreased and citrate intoxication may become the source of hypotension after administration of 6 units/hr or if a sustained rate of 35mL/min PRBC is transfused. Citrate metabolism is decreased by 50% at 31C°.

Fresh Frozen Plasma

FFP contains most of the components of the coagulation cascade and fibrinolytic and complement systems, proteins that enhance oncotic pressure and modulate immunity,[296] and fats, carbohydrates and minerals in similar concentrations to those in blood. In the trauma patient, FFP is used for hemostasis, intravascular volume restoration, reversal of coagulopathy in patients receiving vitamin K–antagonist oral anticoagulants (warfarin) who are actively bleeding or who require emergency surgery, and in patients who are anticoagulated with warfarin and are deficient in the functional vitamin K–dependent coagulation factors II, VII, IX, and X, as well as proteins C and S. The first-line treatment for warfarin reversal is prothrombin complex concentrate (PCC)[89,297]; if it is not available, FFP (or single-donor plasma) or factor IX concentrate can be used.

As discussed earlier, newer guidelines recommend administration of thawed AB Rh- FFP immediately after the arrival of severely traumatized, bleeding, coagulopathic patients.[89,298] The recommended dose is 10 to 15 mL/kg, but additional doses may be needed.[89,298] Following initial administration, FFP is indicated when the transfusion exceeds 10 units of PRBCs within a 6-hour period and when the PT and/or PTT values exceed 1.5 times normal.[89,298] Inspired by experience gained during recent wars, many trauma centers have changed their transfusion protocols and modified the PRBC to FFP ratio from 4:1 to 1:1 or 2:1. Many civilian studies indeed showed a benefit of early treatment with high FFP to PRBC ratios administered to bleeding trauma patients,[88,299,300] although others did not and suggested 2:1 or even 3:1 as a more optimal ratio.[298,301] Most recently, Holcomb et al.[104] in a multicenter study reported no difference in mortality between 1:1:1 and 1:1:2 ratios of FFP, platelet, and PRBC transfusion practices, but they noted less bleeding within the first 24 hours after trauma with a 1:1:1 ratio. It should be emphasized that large volumes of FFP may worsen traumatic intracerebral hematoma, increasing the mortality of head-injured patients.[302] The risks associated with FFP include circulatory overload, ABO incompatibility, transmission of infectious diseases, mild allergic reactions, and transfusion-related acute lung injury, in which platelet concentrates are also implicated.[89]

Platelets

Platelet transfusion is indicated when the platelet count falls below 50×10^9/L. It is possible that in patients with DIC or hyperfibrinolysis and in those with head injury and massive bleeding, higher levels (75 or 100×10^9/L) may be beneficial. High platelet to PRBC ratios (1:1 or 1:2) appear to decrease mortality in trauma patients.[299] Platelets can be administered either as pooled concentrates or single-donor apheresis units. From each unit of whole blood, platelet concentrates of 7.5×10^{10}/L can be prepared, which increase platelet count by 5 to 10×10^9/L; 4 to 8 U are usually sufficient. Apheresis platelet units contain 3 to 6×10^{11}/L of platelets, and a single unit is usually sufficient to provide hemostasis.[89] In the trauma patient who carries a high risk of infectious complications, is immunocompromised, and has tendency to develop ARDS, single-donor apheresis platelets are preferred over pooled concentrates.

Cryoprecipitate

Cryoprecipitate is produced by slowly thawing FFP at 4°C. This process causes the "cryoproteins" to precipitate out.[296] Cryoproteins include factor VIII, fibrinogen, von Willebrand factor, fibronectin, and factor XIII. After centrifuging and removing the supernatant, the remaining precipitate contains high concentrations of procoagulant factors in a small volume of plasma. Factor VIII and von Willebrand factors are now produced as purified recombinant concentrates, meaning that cryoprecipitate can be dedicated to the treatment of hypo- or dysfibrogenemia. Fibrinogen levels are commonly low upon arrival to the trauma emergency room and are effectively replaced with cryoprecipitate during the early phase of trauma management.

Fibrinogen

In the trauma patient, a plasma fibrinogen level below 1.5 g/L (normal 2 g/L) in the presence of nonsurgical bleeding indicates replacement with 3 to 4 g of fibrinogen concentrate or cryoprecipitate, 50 mg/kg (15 to 20 units).[89] However, obtaining a fibrinogen level from the laboratory not only may take about an hour but also may be erroneous; for example in patients receiving colloids, the fibrinogen level may be overestimated.[89] Repeated use of point-of-care devices, TEG, or thromboelastometry allows titration of fibrinogen or cryoprecipitate and other blood products (Fig. 53-10). For example, in normal individuals an MCF of 7 mm measured with thromboelastometry corresponds to a plasma fibrinogen concentration of 2 g/L; MCF values less than 7 mm require administration of fibrinogen or cryoprecipitate.[246]

Antifibrinolytic Agents

The synthetic lysin analogue antifibrinolytic agents, tranexamic acid and ε-aminocaproic acid, competitive inhibitors of plasmin and plasminogen, are effective in reducing bleeding in cardiac and elective surgery, even when a significant hyperfibrinolysis is absent.[89] The Clinical Randomization of Antifibrinolytics in Significant Hemorrhage (CRASH-2) study of 20,000 patients from 274 sites demonstrated that tranexamic acid given within 3 hours of injury (1 g in a 10-minute bolus and then 1 g infused over the next 8 hours) decreased mortality from hemorrhage; this reduction was 37% if the drug was given within 1 hour after injury. On the other hand, tranexamic acid given beyond 3 hours of injury increased bleeding-related mortality.[303] A survival benefit of tranexamic acid was also demonstrated by the military when used in soldiers early after injury.[304] Tranexamic acid may possibly be protective for the mucus membrane barrier of the gut, which is easily destroyed in shock, permitting development of severe inflammation.[305] Thus tranexamic acid may improve survival by simply preventing the inflammatory response to injury. Antifibrinolytics, especially tranexamic acid, should be considered in patients who demonstrate fibrinolysis during serial thromboelastographic or thromboelastometric monitoring. Currently most trauma centers are using tranexamic acid routinely during the initial resuscitation with continuation into the intraoperative phase. The usual dose of tranexamic acid is 10 to 15 mg/kg followed by 1 to 5 mg/kg/hr. The dose of ε-aminocaproic acid is 100 to 150 mg/kg followed by 15 mg/kg/hr.[89]

Factor VIIa

Once used frequently in coagulopathic trauma patients, factor VIIa is now used infrequently, and often without any benefit. It is also associated with thrombotic complications. By activating factor X, factor VIIa produces a thrombin burst, which in turn converts fibrinogen to fibrin. This thrombin release is augmented by platelet activation. Severe acidosis, hypothermia, and hemodilution block the effects of factor VIIa. Thus to obtain any benefit, it should be administered after platelet and fibrinogen levels are adequate and pH and hypothermia are corrected to at least

7.25 and 33°C, respectively. An initial dose of 100 to 140 μg/kg, with a similar dose repeated 1 and 3 hours later if needed, may provide adequate hemostatic plasma levels.[306]

Prothrombin Complex Concentrate (Factor IX Complex)

PCC comes in two forms: Bebulin—three factors (II, IX, and X) (factor IX complex) and Kcentra—four factors (II, VII, IX, and X). In the trauma setting, they are used for rapid reversal of vitamin K–antagonist oral anticoagulants (warfarin), especially in patients with intracranial bleeding.[307] The four-factor form is preferred over three factors. A similar effect can be obtained by administering FFP, but at a much slower rate and a larger infused volume.[308] PCC is not effective for reversing the novel oral anticoagulants, which are direct thrombin inhibitors (dabigatran [Pradaxa] and Eliquis [apixaban]). Recently a new agent Praxbind (idarucizumab) has been marketed, which reverses only dabigatran and none of the other novel oral anticoagulants. Whether PCC is effective in bleeding trauma patients who are not on warfarin is not clear. As with recombinant factor VIIa, thrombotic complications are increased with PCC.[308]

Transfusion-related Acute Lung Injury

Transfusion-related acute lung injury (TRALI) is responsible for 38% of deaths caused by transfusion, being the leading cause of mortality after blood product therapy.[309] All blood products have been associated with TRALI; however, the plasma-rich components, such as FFP and apheresis platelets, have been most frequently implicated. Although our understanding of TRALI is not yet comprehensive, we know that it occurs with transfusion of donor white blood cell antibodies (HLA class 1 or class 2 or human neutrophil antigen [HNA] antibodies).[310]

TRALI is a respiratory entity defined by pulmonary edema with subsequent hypoxia occurring within 6 hours of transfusion. Several other pulmonary disorders such as ARDS and aspiration pneumonia, which are seen in severe trauma, also may occur within 6 hours of transfusion but are unrelated to the transfusion itself. Thus the diagnosis remains clinical and is best determined by the unlikelihood of other trauma-related lung diseases following blood product administration.

TRALI occurs in the setting of the "two-hit model." The model refers to the concept that the cause may (HNA) or may not be from antibodies (HNA). If the patient has elevated interleukin-8 levels, the syndrome may become more severe. Other nonantibody contributions are from biologically activated lipids or neutrophil activation–stimulated cytokines. Nonantibody "granulocyte activation" causes capillary leakage leading to pulmonary edema.

In the antibody model, transfused anti–HNA-3 reacts with and activates neutrophils, causing agglutination and subsequent release of mediators of pulmonary injury. This model holds for platelet administration; thorough washing can mitigate antibody transfer. Prevention of antibody transfer, also known as "mitigation," is the first line of prevention. Treatment of TRALI is supportive, with mechanical ventilation, or extracorporeal membrane oxygenation in severe cases. Diuresis and steroids have not proven to be effective. The clinical course usually runs between 3 and 5 days.

Electrolyte and Acid–Base Disturbances

Intraoperative hyperkalemia may develop as a result of three mechanisms. First, in patients with irreversible shock, cell membrane permeability is altered; thus massive K^+ efflux results in severe hyperkalemia, and, in this situation, survival is unlikely. Second, after repair of a major vessel, subsequent reperfusion of the ischemic tissues results in a sudden release of K^+ into the general circulation. Third, transfusion at a rate faster than 1 unit every 4 minutes in an acidotic and hypovolemic patient may cause an increase in plasma K^+ levels. Frequent monitoring of serum K^+, gradual and intermittent unclamping of vascular shunts, and avoiding transfusion at higher rates than needed help reduce the rate of K^+ increase. If a rise in K^+ is detected, treatment with regular insulin, 10 units intravenously; 50% dextrose, 50 mL; and sodium bicarbonate, 8.4%, 50 mL is indicated. If there is a dysrhythmia, $CaCl_2$, 500 mg, should also be administered. Insulin and dextrose can be repeated two or three times at 30- to 45-minute intervals, if necessary. Hemodialysis may be indicated in desperate situations.

Metabolic acidosis is caused by shock in most trauma patients. Other rare causes of acidosis in this population are alcoholic lactic acidosis, alcoholic ketoacidosis, diabetic ketoacidosis, and CO or CN^- poisoning after inhalation injuries. The differential diagnosis between hypovolemic, diabetic, and alcoholic acidosis, all of which have anion gaps, requires measurement of blood lactate, urinary ketone bodies, and blood sugar and assessment of intravascular volume. Alcoholic ketoacidosis is treated with intravenous dextrose, whereas diabetic ketoacidosis is managed with insulin. No specific treatment except intravenous normal saline exists for alcoholic lactic acidosis.

Treatment of metabolic acidosis involves correction of the underlying cause: management of hypoxemia, restoration of intravascular volume, optimization of cardiac function, or treatment of CO or CN^- toxicity. Symptomatic treatment with sodium bicarbonate has serious disadvantages, including leftward shift of the oxyhemoglobin dissociation curve causing decreased O_2 unloading, a hyperosmolar state secondary to the excessive sodium load, hypokalemia, further hemodynamic depression, overshoot alkalosis a few hours after giving the drug, and intracellular acidosis if adequate ventilation or pulmonary blood flow cannot be provided. Nevertheless, because of the possibility that severe acidosis can cause dysrhythmias, myocardial depression, hypotension, and resistance to exogenous catecholamines, some clinicians administer bicarbonate to buy time if the pH is below 7.2.

Intraoperative Death

Death is a much greater threat during emergency trauma surgery than it is in any other operative procedure. Approximately 0.7% of patients admitted for acute trauma die in the OR, accounting for approximately 8% of postinjury deaths.[311] Uncontrollable bleeding is the cause of approximately 80% of intraoperative mortality; brain herniation and air embolism are the most common causes of death in the remaining patients.[311] A multicenter, retrospective study has defined certain features that increase the likelihood of OR death (Table 53-16).[311] Rapid transport to the OR, rapid stabilization of life-threatening injuries while deferring definitive surgery (damage control), simultaneous thoracotomy and laparotomy for thoracoabdominal injuries, appropriate management of retroperitoneal hematoma, and early correction of hypothermia and shock may reduce intraoperative mortality rates.[311]

Of these measures, the damage control principle has reduced not only the intraoperative but also the overall mortality from trauma surgery, although morbidity from sepsis, abscess formation, and gastrointestinal fistulas may increase.[312,313] Originally described in three stages, the current suggestion is that it should be managed in four phases. In the first phase, attention is directed in the ED to recognition of the pattern of injury, control of bleeding if possible, and rapid transport to the OR, as well as to the decision to initiate damage control resuscitation by

Table 53-16 Clinical Features Associated with Intraoperative Mortality

Category	Clinical Features
Mechanism of injury	Gunshot wound Pedestrian injuries
Injury severity	Mean injury severity score >41 Mean revised trauma score >3.0
Preoperative physiologic profile	Mean BP in the field <50 mmHg Mean BP on arrival to ED <60 mmHg Best systolic BP in the ED <90 mmHg Circulatory shock time >10 min Best mean pH <7.18 Mean preoperative crystalloid resuscitation >3,850 mL; mean red cell transfusion >834 mL
Type of injury	Significant head, chest, abdominal, and pelvic injuries individually or in combination after blunt trauma Significant chest and abdominal injuries individually or in combination after penetrating trauma
Organ injury	Brain Liver Aorta or other major vascular injury Cardiac injury
Operating room resuscitation and physiologic status	Systolic BP <90 mmHg during first h Systolic BP <90 mmHg for >30 min Deterioration of mean pH from 7.19 to 7.01 Mean intraoperative blood loss 5,172 mL; mean blood replacement 4,541 mL Mean platelet transfusion 784 mL Mean fresh frozen plasma 1,418 mL Mean intraoperative temperature 32.2°C Intraoperative cardiac arrest

BP, blood pressure; ED, emergency department.
Data from Hoyt DB, Bulger EM, Knudson MM, et al. Death in the operating room: an analysis of a multi-center experience. *J Trauma.* 1994;37:426

limiting crystalloid infusion, allowing permissive hypotension, activating rewarming, and initiating blood component replacement with early administration of FFP and platelets at high ratios with PRBCs.[313,314]

The second phase occurs in the OR where, in addition to efforts to maintain the patient's intravascular volume, temperature, acid–base status, and coagulation at near-normal levels with damage control resuscitation, the surgeons rapidly control bleeding and leave the abdominal cavity open without fascial closure but temporarily covered by a vacuum pack dressing, which allows an enlarged space for edematous organs and controlled egress of fluid.

The third phase takes place in the ICU where intravascular volume, hypothermia, acidosis, and coagulation abnormalities are corrected. In the fourth phase, the stabilized patient is returned to the OR for definitive surgery and abdominal closure. The fourth phase involves multiple returns to the OR at 24- to 48-hour intervals for organ repair, abdominal washout, and debridement before the final closure of the abdomen. The damage control principle, originally proposed for abdominal trauma, is now applied to injuries at other anatomic sites, including chest, pelvis, extremities, and soft tissues.[315]

Early Postoperative Considerations

To prevent multiple moves, major trauma patients should be admitted directly to the ICU. Postoperative care may involve obtaining a further medical history and description of the mechanism of injury from the patient, if he or she is awake, or from relatives, and performing tertiary survey to identify possible missed injuries. The concerns in the early postoperative period are similar to those of the intraoperative phase. Re-evaluation and optimization of the circulation, oxygenation, temperature, CNS function, coagulation, electrolyte and acid–base status, and renal function are the hallmarks of postoperative management. Pain control in this group of patients may have more than a humanitarian purpose; it can improve pulmonary function, ventilation, and oxygenation, especially in patients with chest and abdominal injury. A multidimensional pain control strategy may be used, including various combinations of regional analgesia, if coagulopathy is not a concern; intravenous opioids as patient-controlled analgesia or as bolus doses; nonsteroidal anti-inflammatory agents, if nephrotoxicity, gastric ulceration, or bleeding risks do not exist; acetaminophen; and low-dose (20 to 30 mg/hr) ketamine, particularly in patients with a known history of opioid. For sedation in mechanically ventilated patients, both propofol (25 to 75 μg/kg/min) and midazolam (0.1 to 20 μg/kg/min) infusions alone or in combination are equally effective and safe, although wake-up time in patients receiving midazolam is longer (660 ± 400 minutes) than in those receiving propofol alone (110 ± 50 minutes) or both agents combined (190 ± 200 minutes).[316] Morphine, 0.02 to 0.04 mg/kg/hr, or fentanyl, 1 to 3 μg/kg/hr, may be added for analgesia. Small boluses of midazolam (3 to 5 mg), propofol (50 mg), morphine (2 to 3 mg), or fentanyl (25 to 50 μg) may also be given as required.[316]

Ventilatory Support

Hypoxemia secondary to atelectasis due to bronchial plug, decreased breathing efforts, and pulmonary edema due to cardiac, neurologic, fluid overload, airway postobstructive, and various intrinsic pulmonary etiologies can occur, requiring chest physiotherapy, bronchoscopy, and artificial ventilatory maneuvers. PaO_2/FiO_2 ratio values of 300 or above, or 200 to 300, suggest the presence of ARDS or its less severe form, acute lung injury, respectively. Mechanical ventilation with VT no more than 6 mL/kg; an appropriate level of PEEP, allowing titration of FiO_2 to lowest possible level, plateau airway pressures below 35 cm H_2O, and avoidance of auto-PEEP with consideration of adjustment to hypo- or hypercapnia; and prevention of ventilator-induced pneumonia should be undertaken.

Acute Kidney Injury

Acute kidney injury (AKI), formerly called acute renal failure, is a possibility if prolonged shock or crush syndrome occurs during early management In a study aimed at finding the predictors of acute renal failure, trauma was one of the seven independent predictors of this complication.[317] Following an episode of shock in patients who have not received an osmotic load (radiopaque material, mannitol) or diuretic, determination of 2- or 6-hour creatinine and free water clearances may help predict the development of posttraumatic renal dysfunction.[318] Creatinine clearance below 25 mL/min and free water clearance of at least 15 mL/hr suggest the likelihood of acute renal failure. Decreased urine flow rate alone is not a good predictor, and the blood urea nitrogen does not rise until at least 24 hours after surgery or trauma.[318] In parallel with the reduction of glomerular filtration rate, AKI develops in varying intensities. Two diagnostic tools have been developed to predict and define each of these presentations: the RIFLE and AKIN classification schemes. They are comparable in their ability to differentiate the type and severity of kidney injury.[319,320] The RIFLE system is the most commonly used and defines the risk, injury, failure, loss and end-stage damage of kidney function based on increase in serum creatinine and duration of urine flow decrease (Table 53-17). Acute kidney injury network (AKIN) criteria also uses serum creatinine and urine flow parameters with somewhat different values than that used by RIFLE to define stages 1 to 3 of kidney dysfunction.

The cause of renal failure in crush syndrome is probably rhabdomyolysis-induced myoglobin release into the circulation. Serum creatinine kinase levels increase in these patients; levels above 5,000 units/L are associated with renal failure.[321] The differentiation of myoglobinuria from hemoglobinuria is described in the "Urine Output" section. A clear supernatant suggests myoglobin, whereas a rose color indicates hemoglobin. The traditional prophylaxis for renal failure after rhabdomyolysis includes fluids, mannitol, and bicarbonate. However, more recent data suggest that bicarbonate and mannitol are ineffective.[321] Additional causes of AKI after trauma are massive transfusion, sepsis, ureteral or urethral injury leading to obstruction, retroperitoneal hematoma compressing the kidney or ureters, and abdominal compartment syndrome. Often some of these etiologic factors coexist after trauma. Depending on the severity of kidney injury a nephrology consultation and renal replacement therapy is indicated.

Abdominal Compartment Syndrome

Abdominal compartment syndrome results from intra-abdominal hypertension with organ dysfunction after major abdominal trauma and surgery (primary syndrome), although other patients may develop the syndrome without surgery, for example, during massive fluid resuscitation following major trauma or burns (secondary syndrome).[322–324] The syndrome results from massive edema of abdominal organs produced by shock-induced inflammatory mediators, excessive fluid resuscitation, surgical manipulation, and closure of the abdominal fascia. The significant cardiac, pulmonary, renal, gastrointestinal, hepatic, and CNS dysfunctions caused by this syndrome result in a high mortality rate (Fig. 53-12).

Clinically, a tense severely distended abdomen, raised peak airway pressure, CO_2 retention, and oliguria should direct the clinician to measure the intravesical pressure, which reflects the

Table 53-17 Risk, Injury, Failure, Loss, and End-Stage Kidney Disease (RIFLE) Classification for Acute Kidney Injury

Class	Serum Creatinine Increase	GFR Decrease	Urine Output
Risk	×1.5	>25%	<0.5 mL/kg/h × 6 h
Injury	×2	>50%	<0.5 mL/kg/h × 12 h
Failure	×3	>75%	<0.3 mL/kg/h × 24 h or anuria × 12 h
Loss	Persistent ARF = complete loss of kidney function >4 wks		
ESKD	End-stage kidney disease (> 3 mos)		

GFR, glomerular filtration rate; ARF, acute renal failure; ESKD, end-stage kidney disease.

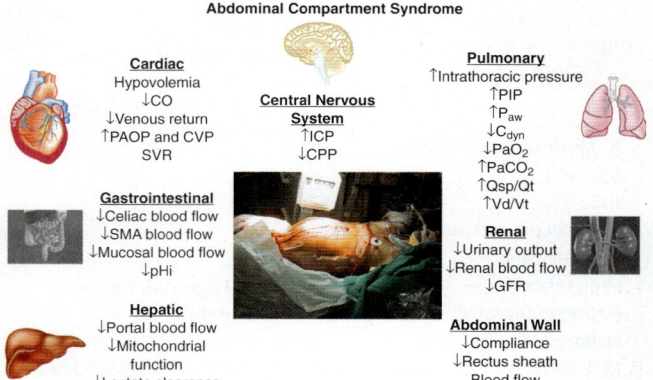

Figure 53-12 Physiologic effects of abdominal compartment syndrome. Image in the center is a patient whose abdomen was left open but covered with nonadhesive dressing. C_{dyn}, dynamic pulmonary compliance; CO, cardiac output; CPP, cerebral perfusion pressure; CVP, central venous pressure; GFR, glomerular filtration rate; ICP, intracranial pressure; PAOP, pulmonary artery occlusion pressure; P_{aw}, mean airway pressure; pHi, intramucosal pH; PIP, peak inspiratory pressure; Qsp/Qt, intrapulmonary shunt; SMA, superior mesenteric artery; SVR, systemic vascular resistance; Vd/Vt, dead space ventilation. (Adapted from Cheatham ML. Intra-abdominal hypertension and abdominal compartment syndrome. *N Horizons*. 1999;7:96.)

intra-abdominal pressure, via a Foley catheter. Values above 20 to 25 mmHg may indicate inadequate organ perfusion and necessitate abdominal decompression, which, if delayed, may result in progression to multiorgan failure and death.[322,323] Almost all of these patients require mechanical ventilation. If a PAC is in place, attributing a relatively high PCWP to the ventilator and continuing high-volume fluid infusion may further increase intra-abdominal edema and increase mortality.[325] Interestingly, patients who will develop abdominal compartment syndrome often do not respond to fluid administration with elevated cardiac output, despite an increasing PCWP.[325]

It should be emphasized that recent advances in the management of acute trauma and critical care, such as limiting crystalloid infusion, hemostatic resuscitation, damage control, and open abdomen strategies, have substantially decreased the incidence of postinjury abdominal compartment syndrome.[324] Postinjury intra-abdominal hypertension still occurs commonly in severely injured high-risk patients, but it is not associated with multiorgan failure in most instances. In other words, unlike in the past, intra-abdominal hypertension is seldom a harbinger of abdominal compartment syndrome or multiorgan failure. It is believed that limiting crystalloid infusion is the most important factor in this salutary evolution.[324]

Thromboembolism

The overall incidence of VTE involving DVT and PE is 3.2% in blunt trauma patients.[326] However, DVT occurs in 30% of major lower extremity injuries, 30% of spine injuries, 46% of major head injuries, 33% of major thoracic injuries, and 15% of serious injuries of the face or abdomen despite implementation of effective clinical management guidelines.[326] When injuries involve more than one of these high-risk regions, the likelihood of DVT is even higher.[326] Fortunately, only a relatively small fraction (0.3%) of severely injured patients have PE.[326] Statistically significant risk factors for VTE are mechanical ventilation for longer than 3 days, injury severity score above 15, spinal cord injury, major lower-extremity bony trauma, and pelvic ring injury.[326] In most instances, DVT is asymptomatic, and in many of those in whom leg swelling develops, concurrent lower-extremity injuries may be implicated. The diagnosis of proximal

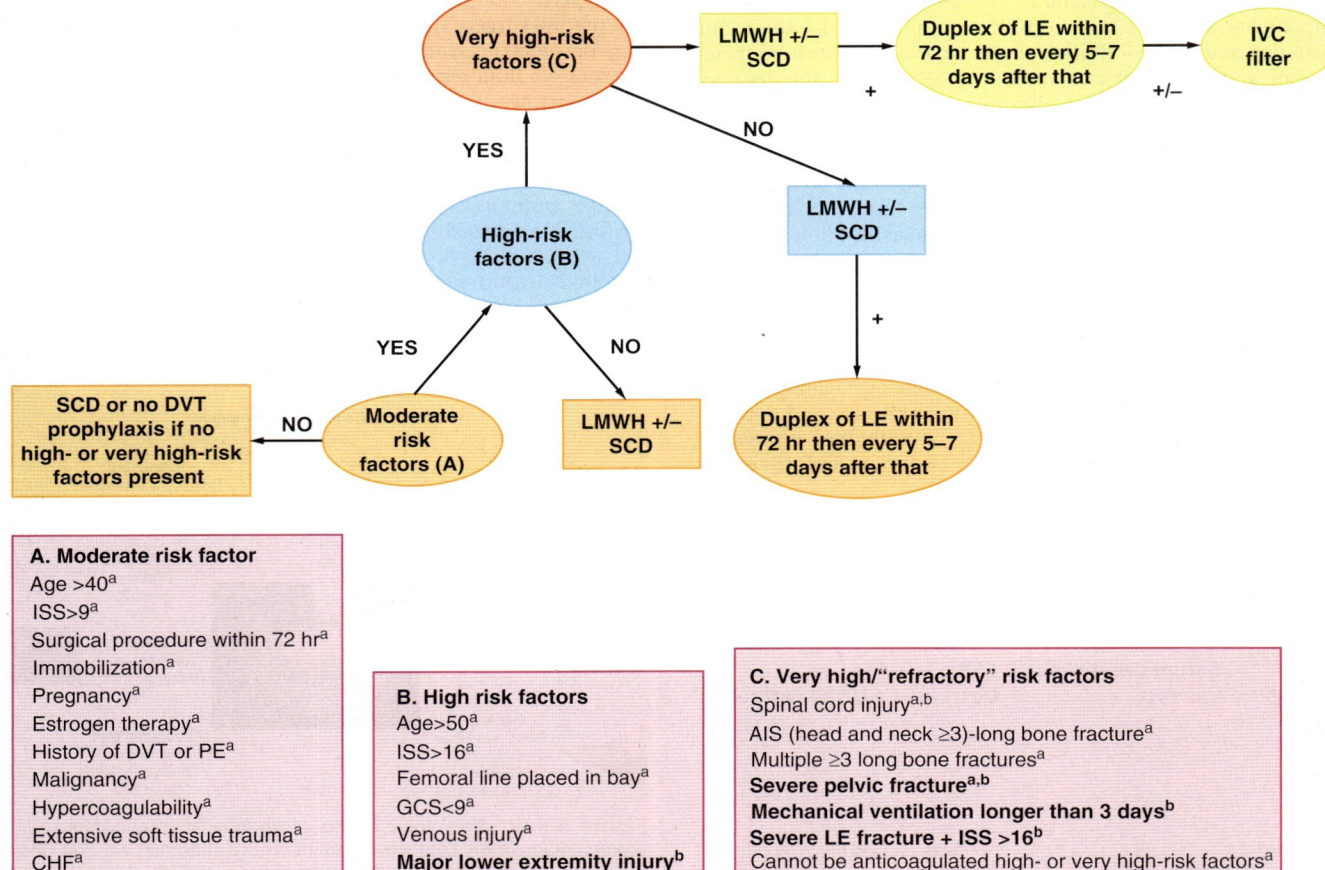

Figure 53-13 Prophylaxis model based on combination of Eastern Association for Surgery of Trauma (EAST) recommendations and the data from Baldwin et al. in blunt trauma patients. Venous thromboembolism risks are classified as moderate, high, and very high. Risk criteria in each of these groups are marked with a superscript of "a" (meaning based on EAST guidelines) or "b" (meaning based on Baldwin et al. data). Low–molecular-weight heparin (LMWH) is used unless contraindicated. AIS, abbreviated injury score; CHF, congestive heart failure; DVT, deep vein thrombosis; GCS, Glasgow coma score; IVC, inferior vena cava; ISS, injury severity score; LE, lower extremity; PE, pulmonary embolism; SCD, sequential compression device. (Adapted with permission from Baldwin K, Namdari S, Esterhai SL, et al. Venous thromboembolism in patients with blunt trauma: are comprehensive guidelines the answer? *Am J Orthop.* 2011;40:E83. Copyright © 2016, Frontline Medical Communications Inc.)

DVT in symptomatic patients can be made by duplex ultrasonography, but this method has low sensitivity in the absence of symptoms.[327] Venography, which is the gold standard, can be performed in equivocal cases, although it is associated with complications and inherent logistical problems. Hypoxemia, especially when sudden and associated with dyspnea and hemodynamic abnormalities, even very early after injury, is highly suggestive of PE. The definitive diagnosis is established by spiral CT and pulmonary angiography. In hemodynamically unstable patients, resuscitation takes precedence over radiologic diagnosis. Management is symptomatic and includes tracheal intubation, positive-pressure ventilation with FiO_2 of 1.0, administration of fluids and inotropes (amrinone or milrinone), and continuous arterial and CVP monitoring. TEE or TTE is helpful because it may demonstrate RV performance, tricuspid regurgitation, or, in some cases, the thrombus within the pulmonary artery, the right heart chambers, or in transit through a patent foramen ovale to the left atrium.

Baldwin et al.[326] reviewed their experience of VTE in more than 10,000 blunt trauma patients over a period of 10 years. These patients were managed using the clinical management guidelines recommended by the Eastern Association for the Surgery of Trauma.[328] Based on their experience, they proposed the management pathway shown in Figure 53-13, which combined their defined risks with their own for moderate, high, and higher risk factors; their modified pathway is based on this. Currently, prophylaxis involves application of sequential compression devices, even if one of the lower extremities is free of trauma, and low–molecular-weight heparin if bleeding is unlikely to exacerbate the injury. Low-dose unfractionated heparin appears to be ineffective in trauma patients.[329] Mechanical devices such as sequential compression boots should be applied as early as possible after injury. Late (>4 days) initiation of prophylaxis, whether because of massive transfusion, low anticipated risk owing to absence of comorbidity, or fear of intracranial bleeding after a severe head injury, has been shown to triple the risk of VTE.[330] Consideration should be given to placement of a vena cava filter if the risk of bleeding is unacceptably high. Removable vena cava filters are now available and are likely to be used prophylactically in high-risk patients more often than permanent filters, which are associated with long-term complications. In patients with severe hemodynamic depression or cardiac arrest unresponsive to resuscitative measures, thrombolytic agents may be considered despite the risk of hemorrhage.

REFERENCES

1. Injuries. World Health Organization. http://www.who.int/topics/en/injuries 2010. Accessed March 22, 2016.
2. World report on road traffic injury prevention. World Health Organization. http://www.who.int/topics/en/traffic injuries 2010. Accessed March 22, 2016.
3. World report on violence prevention. World Health Organization. http://www.who.int/topics/en/violence 2012. Accessed March 22, 2016.
4. Trauma Statistics. San Antonio, Texas: National Trauma Institute;2014. Accessed March 9, 2016.
5. Injury Facts: Annual Safety Report. Itasca, IL: National Safety Council; 2015.
6. Rhee P, Joseph B, Pandit V, et al. Increasing trauma deaths in the United States. Ann Surg. 2014;260:13–21.
7. Acosta J, Yang J, Winchell R, et al. Lethal injuries and time of death in a level 1 trauma center. J Am Coll Surg. 1998;186:528–531.
8. Sakellaridis N, Pavlou E, Karatzas S, et al. Comparison of mannitol and hypertonic saline in the treatment of severe brain injuries. J Neurosurg. 2011;114:545–548.
9. Ferraris V, Ferraris S, Saha SP. The relationship between mortality and preexisting cardiac disease in 5,971 trauma patients. J Trauma. 2010;69:645–652.
10. Ferrada P, Vanguri P, Anand R, et al. A,B,C,D, echo: limited transthoracic echocardiogram is a useful tool to guide therapy for hypotension in the trauma bay: A pilot study. J Trauma Acute Care Surg. 2012;74:220–223.
11. Chakraverty S, Zealley I, Kessel D. Damage control radiology in the severely injured patient: What the anesthetist need to know. Br J Anaesth. 2014;113:250–257.
12. Janjua K, Sugrue M, Deane S. Prospective evaluation of early missed injuries and the role of tertiary truama survey. J Trauma. 1998;44:1000–1005.
13. Chacko J, Nikahat J, Gagan B, et al. Real-time ultrasound-guided percutaneous dilatational tracheostomy. Intensive Care Med. 2012;38:920–921.
14. Wilson W. Trauma: Airway management. ASA difficult airway algorithm modified for trauma and five common intubation scenarios. ASA Newsl. 2005;69:9.
15. Himmelseher S, Durieux M. Revising a dogma: Ketamine for patients with neurological injury?. Anesth Analg. 2005;101:524–534.
16. Grathwohl K, Black I, Spinella P, et al. Total intravenous anesthesia including ketamine versus volatile gas anesthesia for combat-related operative traumatic brain injury. Anesthesiology. 2008;109:44–53.
17. Yeatts D, Dutton R, Hu P, et al. Effect of video laryngoscopy on trauma patient survival: A randomized controlled trial. J Trauma Acute Care Surg. 2013;75:212–219.
18. Crosby E. Airway management in adults after cervical spine trauma. Anesthesiology. 2006;104:1293–1318.
19. Hoffman J, Mower W, Wolfson A, et al. Validity of a set of clinical criteria to rule out injury to the cervical spine in patients with blunt trauma. National Emergency X-Radiography Utilization Study Group. N Engl J Med. 2000;343:94–99.
20. Duane T, Mayglothling J, Wilson S. National Emergency X-Radiography Utilization Study criteria is inadequate to rule out fracture after significant blunt trauma compared with computed tomography. J Trauma. 2011;70:829–831.
21. Stiell I, Clement C, McKnight R, et al. The Canadian C-spine rule versus the NEXUS low-risk criteria in patients with trauma. N Engl J Med. 2003;349:2510–2518.
22. Hale D, Fitzpatrick C, Doski J, et al. Absence of clinical findings reliably excludes unstable cervical spine injuries in children 5 years or younger. J Trauma Acute Care Surg. 2015;78:943–948.
23. Dorney K, Kimia A, Hannon M, et al. Outcomes of pediatric patients with persistent midline cervical spine tenderness and negative imaging result after trauma. J Trauma Acute Care Surg. 2015;79:822–827.
24. Anglen J, Metzler M, Bunn P. Flexion and extension views are not cost-effective in a cervical spine clearance protocol for obtunded trauma patients. J Trauma. 2002;52:54-59.
25. Muchow R, Resnick D, Abdel M, et al. Magnetic resonance imaging (MRI) in the clearance of the cervical spine in blunt trauma: A meta-analysis. J Trauma. 2008;64:179–189.
26. Boese C, Oppermann J, Siewe J, et al. Spinal cord injury without radiologic abnormality in children: A systematic review and meta-analysis. J Trauma Acute Care Surg. 2015;78:874–882.
27. Panczykowsky D, Tomycz N, Okonkwo D. Comparative effectiveness of using computed tomography alone to exclude cervical spine injuries in obtunded or intubated patients: Meta-analysis of 14,327 patients with blunt trauma. J Neurosurg. 2011;115:541–549.
28. Vanguri P, Young A, Weber W, et al. Computed tomographic scan: It's not just about the fracture. J Trauma Acute Care Surg. 2014;77:604–607.
29. Patel M, Humble S, Cullinane D, et al. Cervical spine collar clearance in the obtunded adult blunt trauma patient: A systemic review and practice management guideline from the Eastern Association for the surgery of trauma. J Trauma Acute Care Surg. 2015;78:430–441.
30. Schoenfeld A. Advocating policy with patient safety in the balance: The case of cervical spine clearance. J Trauma Acute Care Surg. 2015;78:639–640.
31. Qualls D, Leonard J, Keller M, et al. Utility of magnetic resonance imaging in diagnosing cervical spine in children with severe traumatic brain injury. J Trauma Acute Care Surg. 2015;78:1122–1128.
32. Hindman B, Palecek J, Posner K, et al. Cervical spinal cord, root, and bony spine injuries: A closed claims analysis. Anesthesiology. 2011;114:782–795.
33. McLeod A, Calder I. Spinal cord injury and direct laryngoscopy—the legend lives on. Br J Anaesth. 2000;84:705–709.
34. Santoni B, Hindman B, Puttlitz C, et al. Manual in-line stabilization increases pressures applied by the laryngoscope blade during direct laryngoscopy and orotracheal intubation. Anesthesiology. 2009;110:24–31.
35. Lennarson P, Smith D, Sawin P, et al. Cervical spinal motion during intubation: Efficacy of stabilization maneuvers in the setting of complete segmental instability. J Neurosurg. 2001;94:265–270.
36. Turner C, Block J, Shanks A, et al. Motion of cadaver model of cervical injury during endotracheal intubation with a Bullard laryngoscope or a Macintosh blade with and without in-line stabilization. J Trauma. 2009;67:61–66.
37. Verschueren D, Bell R, Begheri S, et al. Management of laryngo-tracheal injuries associated with craniomaxillofacial trauma. J Oral Maxillofac Surg. 2006;64:203–214.
38. Brennan J, Gibbons M, Lopez M, et al. Traumatic airway management in Operation Iraqi Freedom. Otolaryngol Head Neck Surg. 2011;144:376–380.
39. Cogbill T, Cothren C, Ahearn M, et al. Management of maxillofacial injuries with severe oronasal hemorrhage: A multicenter perspective. J Trauma. 2008;65:994–999.

40. Chen Y, Tzeng I, Li Y. Transcatheter arterial embolization in the treatment of maxillofacial trauma induced life-threatening hemmorrhages. *J Trauma.* 2009;66:1425–1430.
41. Holmgren E, Baghari S, Bell R. Utilization of tracheostomy in craniomaxillofacial trauma at a level-1 trauma center. *J Oral Maxillofac Surg.* 2007;65:2005–2010.
42. Gadre K, Waknis P. Transmylohyoid/submental intubation:review, analysis, and refinements. *J Craniofac Surg.* 2010;21:516–519.
43. Demetriades D, Velmahos G, Asensio J. Cervical pharyngoesophageal and laryngotracheal injuries. *World J Surg.* 2001;25:1044–1048.
44. Danic D, Prgomet D, Sekelj A, et al. External laryngotracheal trauma. *Eur Arch Otorhinolaryngol.* 2006;263:228–232.
45. O'Connor P, Russell J, Moriarty D. Anesthetic implications of laryngeal trauma. *Anesth Analg.* 1998;87:1283–1284.
46. Schaefer S. Primary management of laryngeal trauma. *Ann Otol Rhinol Laryngol.* 1982;91:399–402.
47. Fuhrman G, Stieg FR, Buerk C. Blunt laryngeal trauma: classification and management protocol. *J Trauma.* 1990;30:87–92.
48. Yamazaki M, Sasaki R, Masuda A. Anesthetic management of complete tracheal disruption using percutaneous cardiopulmonary support system. *Anesth Analg.* 1998;86:998–1000.
49. Harvin J, Taub E, Cotton B, et al. Airway management following repair of cervical tracheal injuries: A retrospective, multicenter study. *J Trauma Acute Care Surg.* 2016;80:366–371.
50. Gomez-Caro A, Ausin P, Moradiellos F, et al. Role of conservative medical management of tracheobronchial injuries. *J Trauma.* 2006;61:1426–1435.
51. Martel G, Al Sabti H, Mulder D. Acute tracheoesophageal burst injury afteer blunt chest trauma: Case report and review of the literature. *J Trauma.* 2007;62:236–242.
52. Beiderlinder M, Adamzik M, Peters J. Conservative treatment of tracheal injuries. *Anesth Analg.* 2005;100:210–214.
53. Ball G, Kirkpatrick A, Fox D, et al. Are occult pneumothoraces truly occult or simply missed? *J Trauma.* 2006;60:294–299.
54. Ball C, Kirkpatrick A, Laupland K. Incidence, risk factors, and outcomes for occult pneumpthoraces in victims of major trauma. *J Trauma.* 2005;59:917–925.
55. Kirkpatrick A, Sirois M, Laupland K. Handheld thoracic sonography for detecting post-traumatic pneumothoraces: The extended focused assessment with sonography for trauma (EFAST). *J Trauma.* 2004;57:288–295.
56. Cohn S, Dubose J. Pulmonary contusion: An update on recent advances in clinical management *World J Surg.* 2010;34:1959–1970.
57. Hamrick M, Duhn R, Ochsner M. Critical evaluation of pulmonary contusion in the early post-traumatic period: Risk of assisted ventilation. *Am Surg.* 2009;75:1054–1058.
58. Chapman B, Herbert B, Rodil M, et al. Rib score: A novel radiographic score based on fracture pattern that predicts pneumonia, respiratory failure, and tracheostomy. *J Trauma Acute Care Surg.* 2016;80:95–101.
59. Carver T, Milia D, Somberg C, et al. Vital capacity helps predict pulmonary complications after rib fractures. *J Trauma Acute Care Surg.* 2015;79:413–416.
60. Schweiger JW. The pathophysiology, diagnosis, and management strategies for flail chest injury and pulmonary contusion. *Anesth Analg.* 2001;92(Suppl):86–93.
61. Caufield E, Dutton R, Floccare D. Prehospital hypocapnia and poor outcome after severe traumatic brain injury. *J Trauma.* 2009;66:1577–1583.
62. Wolthuis E, Choi G, Dessing M. Mechanical ventilation with lower tidal volumes and positive end-expiratory pressure prevents pulmonary inflammation in patients without preexisting lung injury. *Anesthesiology.* 2008;108:46–54.
63. Walkey A, Nair S, Papadopulos S. Use of airway pressure release ventilation is associated witha reduced incidence of ventilator-associated pneumonia in patients with pulmonary contusion. *J Trauma.* 2011;70:E42–E47.
64. McCunn M, Habashi N. Airway pressure release ventilation in the acute respiratory distress syndrome following traumatic injury. *Int Anesthesiol Clin.* 2002;40:89–102.
65. Riou B, Zaier K, Kalfon P, et al. High frequency jet ventilation in life-threatening bilateral pulmonary contusion. *Anesthesiology.* 2001;94:927–930.
66. Ho A, Karmakar M, Critchley L. Acute pain management of patients with multipl fractured ribs: A focus on regional techniques. *Curr Opin Crit Care.* 2011;17:323–327.
67. Huber-Wagner S, Lefering R, Qvick LM, et al. Effect of whole-body CT during trauma resuscitation on survival: A retrospective study. *Lancet.* 2009;373:1455–1461.
68. Mizushima Y, Ueno M, Watanabe H. Discrepancy between heart rate and makers of hypoperfusion is a predictor of mortality in trauma patients. *J Trauma.* 2011;71:789–792.
69. American College of Surgeons, Committee on Trauma. Shock. In: *Advanced Trauma Life Support Student Course Manual.* 8th ed. Chicago, IL: American College of Surgeons; 2008:55–71.
70. Porter J, Ivatury R. In search of the optimal end points of resuscitation in trauma patients: A review. *J Trauma.* 1998;44:908–914.
71. Oyetunji T, Chang D, Crompton J. Redefining hypotension in the elderly: Normotension is not reassuring. *Arch Surg.* 2011;146:865–869.
72. Eastridge B, Salinas J, McManus J. Hypotension begins at 110 mm Hg: Redefining "hypotension" with data. *J Trauma.* 2007;63:291–299.
73. Eastridge B, Salinas J, Wade C. Hypotension is 100 mm Hg on the battlefield. *Am Surg.* 2011;202:404–408.
74. Brown J, Gestring M, Forsythe R, et al. Systolic blood pressure criteria in the national trauma triage protocol for geriatric trauma: 110 is the new 90. *J Trauma Acute Care Surg.* 2015;78:352–359.
75. Garrioch M. The body's response to blood loss. *Vox Sang.* 2004;87(Suppl):74–76.
76. Thorson C, Van Haren R, Ryan M, et al. Admission hematocrit and transfusion requirements after trauma. *J Am Coll Surg.* 2013;216:65–73.
77. Golden J, Dossa A, Goodhue C, et al. Admission hematocrit predicts the need for transfusion secondary to hemorrhage in pediatric blunt trauma patients. *J Trauma Acute Care Surg.* 2015;79:555–562.
78. Zehtabchi S, Sinert R, Goldman M, et al. Diagnostic performance of serial haematocrit measurements in identifying major injury in adult trauma patients. *Injury.* 2006;37:46–52.
79. Shackelford S, Colton K, Stansbury L, et al. Early identification of uncontrolled hemorrhage after trauma: Current status and future direction. *J Trauma Acute Care Surg.* 2014;77:S222–S227.
80. Zarzaur B, Croce M, Magnotti L, et al. Identifying life-threatening shock in the older injured patient: An analysis of the National Trauma Data Bank. *J Trauma.* 2010;68:1134–1138.
81. Smithson L, Morrell J, Kowalik U, et al. Correlation of computed tomographic signs of hypoperfusion and clinical hypoperfusion in adult blunt trauma patients. *J Trauma Acute Care Surg.* 2015;78:1162–1167.
82. Callcut R, Cripp M, Nelson M, et al. The massive transfusion score as a decision aid for resuscitation: Learning when to turn the massive transfusion protocol on and off. *J Trauma Acute Care Surg.* 2016;80:450–456.
83. Callcut R, Johannigman J, Kadon K. All massive transfusion criteria are not created equal: Defining the predictive value of individual transfusion triggers to better determine who benefits from blood. *J Trauma.* 2011;70:794–801.
84. Ross S, Christmas A, Fischer P, et al. Impact of common crystalloid solutions on resuscitation markers following Class 1 hemorrhage: A randomized control trial. *J Trauma Acute Care Surg.* 2015;79:732–740.
85. Neil M, Hoffman M, Cuschieri J. Crystalloid to packed red cell transfusion ratio in the massively transfused patient: When a little goes a long way. *J Trauma Acute Care Surg.* 2012;72:892–898.
86. Sharpe J, Magnotti L, Croce M, et al. Crystalloid administration during trauma resuscitation: Does less really equal more? *J Trauma Acute Care Surg.* 2014;77:828–832.
87. Kozar R, Pati S. Syndecan-1 restitution by plasma after hemorrhagic shock. *J Trauma Acute Care Surg.* 2015;78:S83–S86.
88. Maegele M, Lefering R, Yucel N, et al. Early coagulopathy in multiple injury: An analysis from the German Trauma Registry on 8724 patients. *Injury.* 2007;38:298–304.
89. Rossaint R, Bouillon B, Cerny V, et al. Management of bleeding following major trauma: An updated European guideline. *Crit Care.* 2010;14:R52.
90. Bickell W, Wall M, Pepe P, et al. Immediate versus delayed fluid resuscitation for hypotensive patients with penetrating torso injuries. *N Engl J Med.* 1994;331:1105–1113.
91. Stern S. Low-volume fluid resuscitation for presumed hemorrhagic shock: Helpful or harmful? *Curr Opin Crit Care.* 2001;7:422–430.
92. Schreiber M, Meier E, Tisherman S, et al. A controlled resuscitation strategy is feasible and safe in hypotensive trauma patients: Results of a prospective randomized pilot trial. *J Trauma Acute Care Surg.* 2015;78:687–697.
93. Dezman Z, Comer A, Smith G, et al. Failure to clear elevated lactate predicts 24-hour mortality in trauma patients. *J Trauma Acute Care Surg.* 2015;79:580–585.
94. Smith M, Stiefel M, Magge S, et al. Packed red blood cell transfusion increases local cerebral oxygenation. *Crit Care Med.* 2005;33:1104–1108.
95. Leal-Noval S, Munoz-Gomaz M, Arellano-Orden V, et al. Impact of age of transfused blood on cerebral oxygenation in male patients with severe traumatic brain injury. *Crit Care Med.* 2008;36:1290–1296.
96. Salim A, Hadjizacharia P, DuBose J. Role of anemia in traumati brain injury. *J Am Coll Surg.* 2008;207:398–406.
97. Carlson A, Schermer C, Lu S. Retrospective evaluation of anemia and transfusion in traumatic brain injury. *J Trauma.* 2006;61:567–571.
98. Malone D, Dunne J, Tracy J. Blood transfusion, independent of shock severity, is associated with worse outcome in trauma. *J Trauma.* 2003;54:898–907.
99. Weinberg J, McGwin GJ, Marques M. Does the age of transfused blood affect outcomes? *J Trauma.* 2008;65:794–798.
100. Dutton R, Shih D, Edelman B, et al. Safety of uncrossmatched type-O red cells for resuscitation from hemorrhagic shock. *J Trauma.* 2005;59:1445–1449.
101. Tieu B, Holcomb J, Schreiber M. Coagulopathy: Its pathophysiology and treament in the injured patient. *World J Surg.* 2007;31:1055–1064.
102. Hirshberg A, Dugas M, Banez E, et al. Minimizing dilutional coagulopathy in exsanguinating hemorrhage: A computer simulation. *J Trauma.* 2003;54:454–463.
103. Holcomb J, Jenkins D, Rhee P. Damage control resuscitation: Directly addressing the early coagulopathy of trauma. *J Trauma.* 2007;62:307–310.

104. Holcomb J, Tilley B, Baraniuk S, et al. Transfusion of plasma, platelets, and red blood cells in a 1:1:1 vs a1:1:2 ratio and mortality in patients with severe trauma: The PROPPR randomized clinical trial. *JAMA.* 2015;313:471–482.
105. Borgman M, Spinella P. Perkins J. Tha ratio of blood products transfused affects mortality in patients receiving massive transfusions at a combat support hospital. *J Trauma.* 2007;63:805–813.
106. Dente C, Shaz B, Nicholas J, et al. Early predictors of massive transfusion in patients sustaining torso gunshot wounds in a civilian level I trauma center. *J Trauma.* 2010;68:298–304.
107. Murray J, Saw A, Hoang D. Activation of massive transfusion for the elderly trauma patients. *Am Surg.* 2015;81:945–949.
108. Neff L, Cannon J, Morrison J, et al. Clearly defining pediatric massive transfusion: Cutting through the fog and the friction with combat data. *J Trauma Acute Care Surg.* 2015;78:22–29.
109. Stanworth S, Morris T, Gaarder C, et al. Reappraising the concept of massive transfusion in trauma. *Crit Care.* 2010;14(6):R239.
110. Nystrup K, Stensballe J, Bottger M, et al. Transfusion therapy in paediatric trauma patients: A review of the literature. *Scand J Trauma Resusc Emerg Med.* 2015;23:21.
111. Johansson P. Goal-directed hemostatic resuscitation for massively bleeding patients: The Copenhagen concept. *Transfus Apher Sci.* 2010;43(3):401–405.
112. Kutcher M, Howard B, Sperry J, et al. Evolving beyond the vicious triad: Differential mediation of traumatic coagulopathy by injury, shock, and resuscitation. *J Trauma Acute Care Surg.* 2015;78:516–523.
113. Luna G, Pavlin E, Kirkman T, et al. Hemodynamic effects of external cardiac massage in trauma shock. *J Trauma.* 1989;29:1430–1433.
114. Seamon M, Haut E, Arenconk K, et al. An evidence-based approach to patient selection for emergency department thoracotomy: A practice management guideline from the Eastern Association for the surgery of trauma. *J Trauma Acute Care Surg.* 2015;79:159–173.
115. Shackford S, Mackersie R. Davis J. Epidemiology and pathology of traumatic deaths occurring at a level I trauma center in a regionalized system: The importance of secondary brain injury. *J Trauma.* 1989;29:1392–1397.
116. Verweij B, Amelink G, Muizelaar J. Current concepts of cerebral oxygen transport and energy metabolism after severe traumatic brain injury. *Prog Brain Res.* 2007;161:111–124.
117. Werner C, Engelhard K. Pathophysiology of traumatic brain injury. *Br J Anaesth.* 2007;99:4–9.
118. Neurosurgeons BTFoAAo. Guidelines for the management of severe traumatic injury. *J Neurotrauma.* 2007;24(Suppl 1):S1–S106.
119. Chesnut R. Avoidance of hypotension: Conditio sine qua non of successful head injury management. *J Trauma.* 1997;42(Suppl):4S–9S.
120. McHugh G, Engel D, Butcher I, et al. Prognostic value of secondary insults in traumatic brain injury: results from the IMPACT study. *J Neurotrauma.* 2007;24:287–293.
121. American College of Surgeons, Committee on Trauma. Head trauma. In: *Advanced Trauma Life Support Student Course Manual.* 8th ed. Chicago, IL: American College of Surgeons; 2008:131–150.
122. Chesnut R. Management of brain and spine injuries. *Crit Care Clin.* 2004; 20:25–55.
123. Duncan T, Krost W, Mistovich J, et al. Beyond the basics: brain injuries. *Emerg Med Serv.* 2007;36:65–69; quiz 70–71.
124. Davis D, Peay J, Sise M, et al. The impact of prehospital endotracheal intubation on outcome in moderate to severe traumatic brain injury. *J Trauma.* 2005;58:933–939.
125. Wang H, Peitzman A, Cassidy L, et al. Out of hospital endotracheal intubation and outcome after traumatic brain injury. *Ann Emerg Med.* 2004;44:439–450.
126. Davis D, Koprowicz K, Newgard C. The relationship between out-of-hospital airway management and outcome among trauma patients with Glasgow Coma Scale Scores of 8 or less. *Prehosp Emerg Care.* 2011;15:184–192.
127. Farahvar A, Gerber L, Chiu Y. Response to intracranial hypertension treatment as apredictor of death in patients with severe traumatic injury. *J Neurosurg.* 2011;114:1471–1478.
128. Latorre J, Greer D. Management of acute intracranial hypertension: A review. *Neurologist.* 2009;15:193–207.
129. White H, Cook D, Venkatesh B. The use of hypertonic saline for treating intracranial hypertensionafter traumatic brain injury. *Anesth Analg.* 2006; 102:1836–1846.
130. Freshman S, Battistella F, Matteucci M, et al. Hypertonic saline (7.5%) versus mannitol: A comparison for treatment of acute head injuries. *J Trauma.* 1993; 35:344–348.
131. Lescot T, Degos V, Zouaoui A. Opposed effects of hypertonic saline on contusions and noncontused brain tissue in patients with severe traumatic brain injury. *Crit Care Med.* 2006;34:3029–3033.
132. Prabhakar H, Singh G, Anand V, et al. Mannitol versus hypertonic saline for brain relaation in patiente undergoing craniotomy. *Cochrane Database Syst Rev.* 2014;16(7):CD010026
133. Myburgh J, Cooper D, Finfer S, et al. Saline or albumin for fluid resuscitation in patients with traumatic brain injury. *N Engl J Med.* 2007;357:874–884.
134. Coles J. Regional ischemia after head injury. *Curr Opin Crit Care.* 2004;10: 120–125.
135. Mascia L, Zavala E, Bosma K. High tidal volume is associated with the development of acute lung injury after severe brain injury. *Crit Care Med.* 2007;35:1815–1820.
136. Jeremitsky E, Omert L, Dunham C, et al. The impact of hyperglycemia on patients with severe brain injury. *J Trauma.* 2005;58:47–50.
137. Heffernan D, Inaba K, Arbabi S. Sympathetic hyperactivity after traumatic brain injury and role of beta blocker therapy. *J Trauma.* 2010;69:1602–1609.
138. Sharma D, Vavilala M. Perioperative management of adult traumatic brain injury. *Anesthesiol Clin.* 2012;30:333–346.
139. Rudehill A, Bellander B, Weitzberg E, et al. Outcome of traumatic brain injuries in 1,508 patients: Impact of prehospital care. *J Neurotrauma.* 2002;19:855–868.
140. Haltmeier T, Schnurger B, Benjamin E, et al. Isolated blunt severe traumatic brain injury in Bern, Switzerland, and the United States: A matched cohort study. *J Trauma Acute Care Surg.* 2016;80:296–301.
141. Elf K, Nilsson P, Enblad P. Outcome after traumatic brain injury improved by an organized secondary insult program and standardized neurointensive care. *Crit Care Med.* 2002;30:2129–2134.
142. Warner D, Borel C. Tretment of traumatic brain injury: one size does not fit all. *Anesth Analg.* 2004;99:1208–1210.
143. Palmer S, Bader M, Qureshi A. The impact on outcomes in a community hospital setting of using the AANS traumatic brain injury guidelines. American Association for Neurologic Surgeons. *J Trauma.* 2001;50:657–664.
144. Watts D, Hanfling D, Waller M. An evaluation of the use of guidelines in prehospital management of brain injury. *Prehosp Emerg Care.* 2004;8:254–261.
145. Patel H, Menon D, Tebbs S, et al. Specialist neurocritical care and outcome from head injury. *Intensive Care Med.* 2002;28:547–553.
146. Jeanett B, Teasdale G, Galbraith S. Severe head injuries in three countries. *J Neurol Neurosurg Psychiatry.* 1977;40:291–298.
147. Miller J, Butterworth J, Gudeman S. Further experience in the management of severe head injury. *J Neurosurg.* 1981;54:289–299.
148. Prough D, Lang J. Therapy of patients with head injuries: Key parameters for management. *J Trauma.* 1997;42(Suppl):10S–18S.
149. Patel HC, Menon DK, Tebbs S, et al. Specialist neurocritical care and outcome from head injury. *Intensive Care Med.* 2002;28:547–553.
150. Domeier R, Evans R, Swor R, et al. Prehospital clinical findings associated with spinal injury. *Prehosp Emerg Care.* 1997;1:11–15.
151. Traynelis V, Kasliwal M. Cervical clearance. *J Neurosurg.* 2011;115:636–639.
152. Oh Y, Eun J. Cardiovascular dysfunction due to sympathetic hypoactivity after complete cervical spinal cord injury; a case report and literature review. *Medicine (Baltimore).* 2015;94:e686.
153. Stevens R, Bhardwaj A, Kirsch J, et al. Critical care and perioperative management in traumatic spinal cord injury. *J Neurosurg Anesthesiol.* 2003;15: 215–229.
154. Vale F, Burns J, Jackson A. Combined medical and surgical treatment after acute spinal cord injury: Results of a pilot study to assess the merits of sggressive medical resuscitation and blood pressure management. *J Neurosurg.* 1997; 87:239–246.
155. Bernhard M, Gries A, Kremer P, et al. Spinal cord injury (SCI): Prehospital management. *Resuscitation.* 2005;66:127–139.
156. Berlly M, Shem K. Respiratory management during the first five days after spinal cord injury. *J Spinal Cord Med.* 2007;30:309–318.
157. Brown R, DiMarco A, Hoit J. Respiratory dysfunctionand management in spinal cord injury. *Respir Care.* 2006;51:853–868.
158. Alexander M, Biering-Sorensen F, Bodner D, et al. International standards to document remaining autonomic function after spinal cord injury. *Spinal Cord.* 2009;47:36–43.
159. Winslow C, Rozovsky J. Effect of spinal cord injury on respiratory system. *Am J Phys Rehabil.* 2003:803–814.
160. Theodore J, Robin E. Pathogenesis of neurogenic pulmonary edema. *Lancet.* 1975;2:749–751.
161. Fuller D, Lee K, Tester N. The impact of spinal cord injury on breathing during sleep. *Respir Physiol Neurobiol.* 2013;188(3):344–354.
162. Mackenzie C, Shin B, Krishnaprasad D, et al. Assessment of cardiac and respiratory function during surgery on patients with acute quadriplegia. *J Neurosurg.* 1985;62:843–849.
163. Casha S, Christie S. A systematic review of intensive cardiopulmonary management after spinal cord injury. *J Neurotrauma.* 2011;28:1509–1514.
164. Dhall S, Hadley M, Aarabi B, et al. Deep venous thrombosis and thromboembolism in patients with cervical spinal cord injuries. *Neurosurgery.* 2013;72(Suppl 2):244–254.
165. Inaba K, Branco B, Menaker J, et al. Evaluation of multidetector computed tomography for penetrating neck injury: A prospective multicenter study. *J Trauma.* 2012;72:577–583.
166. Sperry J, Moore E, Coimbra R, et al. Western Trauma Association critical decisions in trauma: penetrating neck trauma. *J Trauma.* 2013;2013:936–940.
167. Biffl W, Moore E, Feliciano D, et al. Western trauma Association Critical Decisions in Trauma: Diagnosis and management of esophageal injuries. *J Trauma Acute Care Surg.* 2015;79:1089–1095.
168. Biffl W, Moore E, Ryu R, et al. The unrecognized epidemic of blunt carotid arterial injuries: Early diagnosis improves neurologic outcome. *Ann Surg.* 1998;228:462–469.

169. Jewett B, Shockley W, Rutledge R. External laryngeal trauma: Analysis of 392 patients. *Arch Otolaryngol Head Neck Surg.* 1999;125:877–880.
170. Demetriades D, Salim A, Brown C. Neck injuries. *Curr Probl Surg.* 2007; 44:13–85.
171. Lichtenstein D, Meziere G, Lascols N, et al. Ultrasound diagnosis of occult pneumothorax. *Crit Care Med.* 2005;33:1231–1238.
172. Reissig A, Copetti R, Kroegel C. Current role of emergency ultrasound of the chest. *Crit Care Med.* 2011;39:839–845.
173. Yadav K, Jalili M, Zehtabchi S. Management of traumatic occult pneumothorax. *Resuscitation.* 2010;81:1063–1068.
174. American College of Surgeons, Committee on Trauma. Thoracic trauma. In: *Advanced Trauma Life Support Student Course Manual.* 8th ed. Chicago, IL: American College of Surgeons; 2008:85.
175. Boersma R, Stigt J, Smit H. Treatment of haemothorax. *Respir Med.* 2010;104:1583–1587.
176. Mineo T, Ambrogi V, Cristino B. Changing indications for thoracotomy in blunt chest traum after the advent of videothoracoscopy. *J Trauma.* 1999;47: 1088–1091.
177. Porembka D, Johnson DN, Hoyt B, et al. Penetrating cardiac trauma: A perioperative role for transesophageal echocardiography. *Anesth Analg.* 1993;77: 1275–1277.
178. Porembka DT. Importance of transesophageal echocardiography in the critically ill and injured patient. *Crit Care Med.* 2007;35:S414–S430.
179. Karmy-Jones R, Namias N, Coimbra R, et al. Western Trauma Association critical decisions in trauma: Penetrating chest trauma. *J Trauma Acute Care Surg.* 2014;77:994–1001.
180. O'Connor J, DuBose J, Scalea T. Damage-control thoracic surgery: management and outcomes. *J Trauma Acute Care Surg.* 2014;77:660–665.
181. Orliaguet G, Ferjani M, Riou B. The heart in blunt trauma. *Anesthesiology.* 2001;95:544–548.
182. Maron B, Estes NR. Commotio cordis. *N Engl J Med.* 2010;362:917–927.
183. Teixeiera P, Inaba K, Barmparas G, et al. Blunt thoracic aortic injuries: An autopsy study. *J Trauma.* 2011;70:197–202.
184. Vignon P, Boncoeur M, Francois B. Comparison of multiplane transesophageal echocardiography and contrast-enhanced helical CT in the diagnosis of blunt traumatic cardiovascular injuries. *Anesthesiology.* 2001;94:615–622.
185. Goarin J, Cluzel P, Gosgnach M, et al. Evaluation of transesophageal echocardiography for diagnosis of traumatic aortic injury. *Anesthesiology.* 2000;93: 1373–1377.
186. Lamarche Y, Berger F, Nicolaou S, et al. Vancouver simplified grading system with computed tomographic angiography for blunt aortic injury. *J Thorac Cardiovasc Surg.* 2012;144:347–354.
187. Demetriades D, Velmahos G, Scalea T, et al. Diagnosis and treatment of blunt thoracic aortic injuries: Changing perspectives. *J Trauma.* 2008;64:1415–1419.
188. Singh K, Baum V. The anesthetic management of cardiovascular trauma. *Curr Opin Anaesthesiol.* 2011;24:98–103.
189. Morgan B, Watcyn-Jones J, Garner J. Traumatic diaphragmatic injury. *J R Army Med Corps.* 2010;156:139–144.
190. Villavicencio R, Aucar J. Analysis of laparoscopy in trauma. *J Am Coll Surg.* 1999;189:11–20.
191. Petrosoniak A, Engels P, Hamiltom P, et al. Detection of significant bowel and mesentericinjuries in blunt abdominal trauma with 64-slice computed sonograph. *J Trauma Acute Care Surg.* 2013;74:1081–1086.
192. Gaarder C, Kroepelien C, Loekke R. Ultrasound performed by radiologists: Confirming the truth about FAST in trauma. *J Trauma.* 2009;67:323–329.
193. Johnson J, Garwe T, Raines A, et al. The use of laparoscopy in the diagnosis and treatment of blunt and penetrating abdominal injuries: 10 year experience at a level 1 trauma center. *Am J Surg.* 2013;205:317–320.
194. White C, Hsu J, Holcomb J. Haemodynamically unstable pelvic fractures. *Injury.* 2009;40:1023–1030.
195. Cothren C, Osborn P, Moore E. Preperitoneal pelvic packing for hemodynamically unstable pelvic fractures: A paradigm shift. *J Trauma.* 2007;62: 834–839.
196. Verbeek D, Sugrue M, Balogh Z. Acute management of hemodynamically unstable pelvic trauma patients: Time for a change? Multicenter review of recent practice. *World J Surg.* 2008;32:1874–1882.
197. Fagan S, Bilodeau M, Goverman J. Burn intensive care. *Surg Clin North Am.* 2014;94:765–779.
198. Bittner E, Shank E, Woodson L, et al. Acute and perioperative care of the burn-injured patient. *Anesthesiology.* 2015;122:448–464.
199. Klein M, Goverman J, Hayden D, et al. Inflammation and host response to injury, and large-scale collaborative research program: Benchmarking outcomes in the critically injured burn patient. *Ann Surg.* 2014;259:833–841.
200. MacLennan N, Heimbach D, Cullen B. Anesthesia for major thermal injury. *Anesthesiology.* 1998;89:749–770.
201. Pereira C, Herndon D. The pharmacologic modulation of the hypermetabolic response to burns. *Adv Surg.* 2005;39:245–261.
202. Williams F, Branski L, Jeschke M. What, how, and how much should patients with burns be fed? *Surg Clin North Am.* 2011;91:609–629.
203. Hemmington-Gorse SJ. A comparison of laser Doppler imaging with other measurement techniques to assess burn depth. *J Wound Care.* 2005;14:151–153.
204. Haponik E, Meyers D, Munster A. Acute upper airway injury in burn patients: Serial changes of flow-volume curves and nasopharyngoscopy. *Am Rev Respir Dis.* 1997;1987:360–366.
205. Smith D, Cairns B, Ramadan F, et al. Effect of inhalation injury, burn size and age on mortality: A study of 1447 consecutive burn patients. *J Trauma.* 1994;37:655–659.
206. Muehlberger T, Kunar D, Munster A, et al. Efficacy of fiberoptic laryngoscopy in the diagnosis of inhalation injuries. *Arch Otolaryngol Head Neck Surg.* 1998;124:1003–1007.
207. Sheridan R, Hurford W, Kacmarek R, et al. Inhaled nitric oxide in burn patients with respiratory failure. *J Trauma.* 1997;42:629–634.
208. Walia G, Jada G, Cartotto R. Anesthesia and intraoperative high-frequency oscillatory ventilation during burn surgery. *J Burn Care Res.* 2011;32:118–123.
209. Pannucci C, Osborne N, Wahl W. Venous thromboembolism in thermally injured patients: analysis of the National Burn Repository. *J Burn Care Res.* 2011;32:6-12.
210. Hofstra J, Vlaar A, Knape P, et al. Pulmonary activation of coagulation and inhibition of fibrinolysis after burn injuries and inhalation trauma. *J Trauma.* 2011;70:1389–1397.
211. Vegfors M, Lennmarken C. Carboxyhemoglobinaemia and pulse oximetry. *Br J Anaesth.* 1991;66:625–626.
212. Baud F, Barriot P, Toffis V, et al. Elevated blood cyanide concentrations in victims of smoke inhalation. *N Engl J Med.* 1991;325:1761–1766.
213. Tung A, Lynch J, McDade W. A new biological assay for measuring cyanide in blood. *Anesth Analg.* 1997;85:1045–1051.
214. Breen P, Isserles S, Westley J, et al. Combined carbon monoxide and cyanide poisoning: A place for treatment? *Anesth Analg.* 1995;80:671–677.
215. Miller K, Chang A. Acute inhalation injury. *Emerg Med Clin North Am.* 2003;21:533–557.
216. Williams F, Herndon D, Suman O, et al. Changes in cardiac physiology after severe burn injury. *J Burn Care Res.* 2011;32:269–274.
217. Namias N. Advances in burn care. *Curr Opin Crit Care.* 2007;13:405–410.
218. Ivy M, Atweh N, Palmer J, et al. Intra-abdominal hypertension and abdominal compartment syndrome in burn patients. *J Trauma.* 2000;49:387–391.
219. Edgar D, Fish J, Gomez M, et al. Local and systemic treatments for acute edema after burn injury: A systematic review of the literature. *J Burn Care Res.* 2011;32:334–347.
220. Sheridan RL. Burns. *Crit Care Med.* 2002;30:S500–S514.
221. Fodor L, Fodor A, Ramon Y. Controversies in fluid resuscitation for burn management: Literature review and our experience. *Injury.* 2006;37:374–379.
222. Saffle J. The phenomenon of "fluid creep" in acute burn resuscitation. *J Burn Care Res.* 2007;28:382–395.
223. Klein M, Edwards J, Kramer C. The beneficial effects of plasma exchange after sever burn injury. *J Burn Care Res.* 2009;30:243–248.
224. Huang P, Stucky F, Dimick A. Hypertonic sodium resuscitation is associated with renal failure and death. *Ann Surg.* 1995;221:543–554.
225. Elgio G, Poli de Figueiredo L, Schenarts P. Hypertonic saline dextran produces early (8-12 hrs) fluid sparing in burn resuscitation: A 24-hr prospective, double-blind study in sheep. *Crit Care Ned.* 2000;28:163–171.
226. Rousseau AF, Massion P, Laungani A, et al. Toward targeted early burn care: Lessons from a European survey. *J Burn Care Res.* 2014;35:e234–e239.
227. Paratz J, Stockton K, Paratz E, et al. Burn resuscitation- hourly urine output versus alternative endpoints: A systematic review. *Shock.* 2014;42:295–306.
228. Alvarado R, Chung K, Cancio L, et al. Burn resuscitation. *Burns.* 2009;35:4–14.
229. Tokarik M, Sjoberg F, Balik M, et al. Fluid therapy LIDCO controlled trial: Optimization of volume resuscitation of extensively burne patients through noninvasive continuous real-time hemodynamic monitoring LIDCO. *J Burn Care Res.* 2013;34:537–542.
230. Dingley J, Cromey C, Bodger O, et al. Evaluation of 2 novel devices for calculation of fluid requirements in pediatric burns. *Ann Plast Surg.* 2015;74: 658–664.
231. Bodger O, Theron A, Williams D. Comparison of three techniques for calculation of the Parkland formula to aid fluid resuscitation in paediatric burns. *Eur J Anaesthesiol.* 2013;30:483–491.
232. Rae L, Pham T, Carrougher G, et al. Differences in rsuscitation in morbidly obese burn patients may contribute to high mortality. *J Burn Care Res.* 2013;34:507–514.
233. Mitchell K, Khalil E, Brennan A, et al. New management strategy for fluid resuscitation: Quantifying volume in the first 48 hours after burn injury. *J Burn Care Res.* 2013;34:196–202.
234. Rooke G, Schwid H, Shapira Y. The effect of graded hemorrhage and intravascular volume replacement on systolic pressure variation in humans during mechanical and spontaneous ventilation. *Anesth Analg.* 1995;80:925–932.
235. Marik P, Dellinger R. Is the cortrosyn test necessary in high basal corticoid patients with septic shock? *Crit Care Med.* 2009;37:386–387.
236. Michard F. Stroke volume variation: From applied physiology to improved outcomes. *Crit Care Med.* 2011;39:402–403.
237. Strumwasser A, Frankel H, Murthi S, et al. Hemodynamic monitoring of the injured patient: From central venous pressure to focused echocardiography. *J Trauma Acute Care Surg.* 2016;80:499–510.
238. Capan L, Miller S, Patel K. Fat embolism. *Anesth Clin North Am.* 1993;11:25–53.

239. Ferrada P. Image-based resuscitation of the hypotensive patient with cardiac ultrasound: An evidence-based review. *J Trauma Acute Care Surg*. 2016;80: 511–518.
240. Agashe G, Coakley J, Mannheimer P. Forehead pulse oximetry: Headband use helps alleviate false low readings likely related to venous pulsation artifact. *Anesthesiology*. 2006;105:1111–1116.
241. Tyburski J, Carlin A, Harvey E. End-tidal CO_2-arterial CO_2 differences: a useful intraoperative mortality marker in trauma surgery. *J Trauma*. 2003;55: 892–896.
242. Lee S, Hong Y, Han C. Concordance of end-tidal carbon dioxide and arterial carbon dioxide in severe traumatic brain injury. *J Trauma*. 2009;67:526–530.
243. McKinley B, Kozar R, Cocanour C. Normal versus supranormal oxygen delivery goals in shock resuscitation: The response is the same. *J Trauma*. 2002;53:825–832.
244. McKinley B, Sucher J, Todd S, et al. Central venous pressure versus pulmonary artery catheter-directed shock resuscitation. *Shock*. 2009;32:463–470.
245. Mallett S, Cox J. Thromboelastography. *Br J Anaesth*. 1992;69:307–313.
246. Rugeri L, Levrat A, David J. Diagnosis of early coagulation abnormalities in trauma patients by rotation thromboelastography. *J Thromb Haemost*. 2007;5:289–295.
247. Johnston T, Chen Y, Reed R. Functional equivalence of hypothermia to specific clotting factor deficiencies. *J Trauma*. 1994;37:413–417.
248. Cotton B, Faz G, Hatch Q. Rapid thromblastography delivers real-time results that predict transfusion within 1 hour of admission. *J Trauma*. 2011; 71:407–417.
249. Jabre P, Combes X, Lapostolle F, et al. Etomidate versus ketamine for rapid sequence intubation in acutely ill patients: A multicentre randomised controlled trial. *Lancet*. 2009;374:293–300.
250. Lemmens H, El-Orbany M, Berry J, et al. Reversal of profound vecuronium-induced neuromuscular block under sevoflurane anesthesia: Sugammadex versus neostigmine. *BMC Anesthesiol*. 2010;10:15.
251. Sacan O, White P, Tufanogullari B, et al. Sugammadex reversal of rocuronium-induced neuromuscular blockade: a comparison with neostigmine-glycopyrrolate and edrophonium-atropine. *Anesth Analg*. 2007;104:569–574.
252. Dutton R. Haemostatic resuscitation. *Br J Anaesth*. 2012;109(S1):i39–i46.
253. Kurita T, Uraoka M, Morita K. Influence of haemorrhage on the pseudo-steady-state remifentanil concentration in a swine model: A comparison with propofol and the effect of hemorrhagic shock stage. *Br J Anaesth*. 2011; 107:719–725.
254. Kurita T, Takata K, Morita K, et al. The influence of hemorrhagic shock on the electroencephalographic and immobilizing effects of propofol in a swine model. *Anesth Analg*. 2009;109:398–404.
255. Egar T, Kuramkote S, Gong G. Fentanyl pharmacokinetics in hemorrhagic shock: A porcine model. *Anesthesiology*. 1999;91:156–166.
256. Johnson K, Egan T, Kern S, et al. The influence of hemorrhagic shock on propofol: A pharmacokinetic and pharmacodynamic analysis. *Anesthesiology*. 2003;99:409–420.
257. Johnson K, Egan T, Layman J, et al. The influence of hemorrhagic shock on etomidate: A pharmacokinetic and pharmacodynamic analysis. *Anesth Analg*. 2003;96:1360–1368.
258. Shafer S. Shock values. *Anesthesiology*. 2004;101:567–568.
259. Weiskopf R, Bogetz M, Roizen M, et al. Cardiovascular and metabolic sequelae of inducing anesthesia with ketamine or thiopental in hypovolemic swine. *Anesthesiology*. 1984;60:214–221.
260. Kurita T, Takata K, Uraoka M, et al. The influence of hemorrhagic shock on the minimum alveolar anesthetic concentration of isoflurane in a swine model. *Anesth Analg*. 2007;105:1639–1643.
261. Zeiler F, Teitelbaum J, West M, et al. The ketamine effect on ICP in traumatic brain injury. *Neurocrit Care*. 2014;21:163–173.
262. Libonati M, Leahy M, Ellison N. The use of succinylcholine in open eye surgery. *Anesthesiology*. 1985;62:637–640.
263. Branski L, Herndon D, Byrd J, et al. Transpulmonary thermodilution for hemodynamic measurements in severely burned children. *Crit Care*. 2011;15:R118.
264. Chen X, Xia Z, Wei H. Eschaectomy and allografting during shock stage reduces insulin resistance induced by major burn. *J Burn Care Res*. 2011;32:e59–e66.
265. Branski L, Herndon D, Pereira C. Longitudinal assessment of Integra in primary burn management: A randomized pediatric clinical trial. *Crit Care Med*. 2007;35:2615–2623.
266. Sterling J, Heimbach D. Hemostasis in burn surgery: A review. *Burns*. 2011; 37:559–565.
267. Mitra B, Wasiak J, Cameron P, et al. Early coagulopathy of major burns. *Injury*. 2013;44:40–43.
268. Kahn S, Beers R, Lentz C. Do fentanyl and morphine influence body temperature after severe burn injury? *J Burn Care Res*. 2011;32:309–316.
269. Martyn J, Fukushima Y, Chon Y. Muscle relaxants in burns, trauma and critical illness. *Int Anesthesiol Clin*. 2006;44:123–143.
270. Han T, Kim H, Bae J, et al. Neuromuscular pharmacodynamics of rocuronium in patients with major burns. *Anesth Analg*. 2004;99:386–392.
271. Todd S, Malinoski D, Muller P. Lactated Ringer's is superior to normal saline in the resuscitation of uncontrolled hemorrhagic shock. *J Trauma*. 2007;62:636–639.
272. Wang H, Callaway C, Peitzman A, et al. Admission hypothermia and outcome after major trauma. *Crit Care Med*. 2005;33:1296–1301.
273. Tsuei B, Kearney P. Hypothermia in the trauma patient. *Injury*. 2004;35:7–15.
274. Jurkovich G, Greiser W, Luterman A, et al. Hypothermia in trauma victims: An ominous predictor of survival. *J Trauma*. 1987;27:1019–1025.
275. Ireland S, Endacott R, Cameron P, et al. The incidence and significance of accidental hypothermia in major trauma: A prospective observational study. *Resuscitation*. 2011;82:300–306.
276. Smith C, Soreide E. Hypothermia in trauma victims. *ASA Newslett*. 2005;69:17.
277. Gentilello L. Advances in the management of hypothermia. *Surg Clin North Am*. 1995;75:243–256.
278. Wadhwa A, Komatsu R, Orhan-Sungur M. New circulating-water devices warm more quickly than forced-air in volunteers. *Anesth Analg*. 2007;105: 1681–1687.
279. Brohi K, Cohen M, Ganter M. Acute traumatic coagulopathy initiated by hypoperfusion: Modulated through the protein C pathway? *Ann Surg*. 2007;245: 812–818.
280. Brohi K, Singh J, Heron M, et al. Acute trauma coagulopathy. *J Trauma*. 2003;54:1127–1130.
281. Mittermayr M, Streif W, Haas T, et al. Hemostatic changes after crystalloid or colloid fluid administration during major orthopedic surgery: The role of fibrinogen administration. *Anesth Analg*. 2007;105:905–917.
282. Kashuk J, Moore E, Sawyer M. Primary fibrinolysis is integral in the pathogenesis of the acute coagulopathy of trauma. *Ann Surg*. 2010;252:434–442.
283. Bolliger D, Gorlinger K, Tanaka K. Pathophysiology and treatment of coagulopathy in massive hemorrhage and hemodilution. *Anesthesiology*. 2010; 113:1205–1219.
284. Hess J, Lawson J. The coagulopathy of trauma versus disseminated intravascular coagulation. *J Trauma*. 2006;60:S12–S19.
285. Moore H, Moore E, Morton A, et al. Shock-induced systemic hyperfibrinolysis is attenuated by plasma first resuscitation. *J Trauma Acute Care Surg*. 2015;79:897–904.
286. Johansson P, Sternballe J, Rasmussen L. A high admission syndecan-1 level, a marker of endothelial glycocalyx degradation, is associated with inflammation, protein C depletion, fibrinolysis, and increased mortality in trauma patients. *Ann Surg*. 2011;254:194–200.
287. Holcomb JB. A novel and potentially unifying mechanism for shock induced early coagulopathy. *Ann Surg*. 2011;254:201–202.
288. Spahn D, Rossaint R. Coagulopathy and blood component transfusion in trauma. *Br J Anaesth*. 2005;95:130–139.
289. DeLoughery TG. Coagulation defects in trauma patients: Etiology, recognition, and therapy. *Crit Care Clin*. 2004;20:13–24.
290. Wolberg A, Meng Z, Monroe DR, et al. A systematic evaluation of the effect of temperature on coagulation enzyme activity and platelet function. *J Trauma*. 2004;56:1221–1228.
291. Martini W, Pusateri A, Uscilowicz J, et al. Independent contributions of hypothermia and acidosis to coagulopathy in swine. *J Trauma*. 2005;58:1002–1009.
292. Goodman M, Makley A, Hanseman D, et al. All the bang without the bucks: Defining essential point-of-care testing for traumatic coagulopathy. *J Trauma Acute Care Surg*. 2015;79:117–124.
293. Levi M. Disseminated intravascular coagulation. *Crit Care Med*. 2007;35: 2191–2195.
294. Gregory J, Huitron S, George A, et al. Optimizing transfusion ratios in massive transfusion protocols: An argument against the 1:1:1 dogma and approach to trauma resuscitation. *Lab Med*. 2015;46:e46–e52.
295. Sparrow R. Red blood cell storage and duration and trauma. *Transf Med Rev*. 2015;29:120–126.
296. Cardigan R, Macleenan S. Allogeneic blood components. *Transf Alter Transf Med*. 2008;10(3):92–101.
297. Milling TJ, Refaai M, Sarode R, et al. Safety of a 4-factor prothrombin complex concentrate versus plasma for vitamin K antagonist reversal: An integrated analysis of two phase IIIb clinical trials. *Acad Emerg Med*. 2016;23:466–475.
298. Kashuk J, Moore E, Sawyer M, et al. Postinjury coagulopathy management: Goal directed resuscitation via POC thrombelastography. *Ann Surg*. 2010;251:604–614.
299. Gunter OJ, Au B, Isbell J, et al. Optimizing outcomes in damage control resuscitation: Identifying blood product ratios associated with improved survival. *J Trauma*. 2008;65:527–534.
300. Duchesne J, Hunt J, Wahl G. Review of current blood transfusions strategies in a mature level I trauma center: Were we wrong for the last 60 years? *J Trauma*. 2008;65:272–278.
301. Snyder C, Weinberg J, McGwin GJ, et al. The relationship of blood product ratio to mortality: Survival benefit or survival bias? *J Trauma*. 2009;66:358–364.
302. Etemadrezaie H, Baharvahdat H, Shariati Z, et al. The effect of fresh frozen plasma in severe closed head injury. *Clin Neurol Neurosurg*. 2007;109:166–171.
303. Collaborators C-T. Effects of tranexamic acid on death, vascular occlusive events, and blood transfusion in trauma patients with significant haemorrhage (CRASH-2): A randomised, placebo-controlled trial. *Lancet*. 2010;376:23–32.
304. Morrison J, Dubose J, Rasmussen T, et al. Military application of tranexamic acid in trauma emergency resuscitation (MATTERs) study. *Arch Surg*. 2012; 147:113–119.

305. Diebel M, Diebel L, Manke C, et al. Early tranexamic acid administration: A protective effect on gut barrier function following ischemia/reperfusion injury. *J Trauma Acute Care Surg*. 2015;79:1015–1022.
306. Martinowitz U, Michaelson M. Guidelines for the use of recombinant activated factor VII (rFVIIa) in uncontrolled bleeding: A report by the Israeli Multidisciplinary rFVIIa Task Force. *J Thromb Haemost*. 2005;3:640–648.
307. Imberti D, Barillari G, Biasioli C. Emergency reversal of anticoagulation with a three-factor prothrombin complex concentrate in patients with intracranial hemorrhage. *Blood Transf*. 2011;9:148–155.
308. Sorensen B, Spahn D, Innerhofer P. Clinical review: Prothrombin complex concentrates-evaluation of safety and thrombogenicity. *Crit Care*. 2011;15:201.
309. US Food and Drug Administration. Transfusion related acute lung injury (TRALI). http://fda.gov/biologicsBloodVaccines/SafetyAvailability/BloodSafety/ucm095556.htm. Accessed March 28, 2016.
310. Storch E, Hillyer C, Shaz B. Spotlight on the pathogenesis of Trali:HNA-3a (CTL2) antibodies. *Blood*. 2014;124:1868–1871.
311. Hoyt D, Bulger E, Knudson M, et al. Death in the operating room: An analysis of a multi-center experience. *J Trauma*. 1994;37:426–432.
312. Nicholas J, Rix E, Easley K. Changing patterns in the management of penetrating abdominal trauma: the more things change, the more they stay the same. *J Trauma*. 2003;55:1095–1110.
313. Lamb C, MacGoey P, Navarro A, et al. Damage control surgery in the era of damage control resuscitation. *Br J Anaesth*. 2014;113:242–249.
314. Duchesne J, Kimonis K, Marr A, et al. Damage control resuscitation in combination with damage control laparotomy: A survival advantage. *J Trauma*. 2010;69:46–52.
315. Morshed S, Corrlaes L, Lin K, et al. Femoral nailing during serum bicarbonate-defined hypo-perfusion predicts pulmonary organ dysfunction in multisystem trauma patients. *Injury*. 2011;42:643–649.
316. Sanches-Izquierdo-Riera J, Caballero-Cubedo R, Perez-Vela J. Propofol versus midazolam: Safety and efficacy for sedating the severe trauma patient. *Anesth Analg*. 1998;86:1219–1224.
317. Kheterpal S, Tremper K, Englesbe M, et al. Predictors of postoperative acute renal failure after noncardiac surgery in patients with previously normal renal function. *Anesthesiology*. 2007;107:892–902.
318. Shin B, Mackenzie C, Helrich M. Creatinine clearance for early detection of posttraumatic renal dysfunction. *Anesthesiology*. 1986;64:605–609.
319. Chang CH, Lin CY, Tian YC, et al. Acute kidney injury classification: Comparison of AKIN and RIFLE criteria. *Shock*. 2010;33:247–252.
320. Lopes JA, Jorge S. The RIFLE and AKIN classifications for acute kidney injury: A critical and comprehensive review. *Clin Kidney J*. 2013;6:8–14.
321. Brown C, Rhee P, Chan L. Preventing renal failure in patience with rhabdomyolysis: do bicarbonate and mannitol make a difference? *J Trauma*. 2004;56:1191–1196.
322. Balogh Z, McKinley B, Cocanour C. Secondary abdominal compartment syndrome is an elusive early complication of traumatic shock resuscitation. *Am J Surg*. 2002;184:538–544.
323. Balogh Z, McKinley B, Holcomb J. Both primary and secondary abdominal compartment syndrome can be predicted early and are harbingers of multiple organ failure. *J Trauma*. 2003;54:848–859.
324. Balogh Z, Martin A, van Wessem KP, et al. Mission to eliminate postinjury abdominal compartment syndrome. *Arch Surg*. 2011;146:938–943.
325. Balogh Z, McKinley B, Cocanour C. Patients with impending abdominal compartment syndrome do not respond to early volume loading. *Am J Surg*. 2003;186:602–608.
326. Baldwin K, Namdari S, Esterhai J, et al. Venous thromboembolism in patients with blunt trauma: Are comprehensive guidelines the answer? *Am J Orthop*. 2011;40:E83–E87.
327. Jongbloets L, Lensing A, Koopman M. Limitations of compression ultrasound for the detection of syntomless postoperative deep vein thrombosis. *Lancet*. 1994;343:1142–1144.
328. Frankel H, FitzPatrick M, Gaskell S, et al. Strategies to improve compliance with evidence-based clinical management guidelines. *J Am Coll Surg*. 1999;189:533–538.
329. Geerts W, Jay R, Code K. A comparison of low-dose heparin with low-molecular-weight heparin as prophylaxis against venous thromboembolism after major trauma. *N Engl J Med*. 1996;335:701–707.
330. Nathens A, Mc Murray M, et al. The practice of venous thromboembolism prophylaxis in the major trauma patient. *J Trauma*. 2007;62:557–563.

Section 9

POSTANESTHETIC MANAGEMENT, CRITICAL CARE, AND PAIN MANAGEMENT

54 Postanesthesia Recovery

MICHAEL A. FOWLER • BRUCE D. SPIESS

Postanesthesia Recovery
   Standards for Postanesthesia Care
Value and Economics of Postanesthesia Care Unit
Levels of Postoperative/Postanesthesia Care
Postanesthesia Triage
Safety in the Postanesthesia Care Unit
Admission to the Postanesthesia Care Unit
Postoperative Pain Management
Discharge Criteria
Postoperative Evaluation
Cardiovascular Complications
Postoperative Pulmonary Dysfunction
   Inadequate Postoperative Ventilation
   Inadequate Respiratory Drive
   Increased Airway Resistance
   Decreased Compliance
   Neuromuscular and Skeletal Problems
   Increased Deadspace
   Increased Carbon Dioxide Production
   Inadequate Postoperative Oxygenation
   Distribution of Ventilation
   Distribution of Perfusion
   Inadequate Alveolar $P_{A}O_2$
   Reduced Mixed Venous PO_2
   Obstructive Sleep Apnea
   Anemia
   Supplemental Oxygenation
   Perioperative Aspiration
Postoperative Renal Complications
   Ability to Void
   Renal Tubular Function
   Oliguria
   Polyuria
Metabolic Complications
   Postoperative Acid–Base Disorders
   Glucose Disorders and Control
   Electrolyte Disorders
Miscellaneous Complications
   Incidental Trauma
   Skeletal Muscle Pain
   Hypothermia and Shivering
   Hyperthermia
   Persistent Sedation/Delayed Emergence
   Altered Mental Status
   Postoperative Nausea and Vomiting

KEY POINTS

1. The postoperative planning begins when a patient is scheduled for surgery. With emerging protocols for enhanced recovery after surgery (ERAS), specific evidence-based and best practice structure for patient care has the goal of providing care that is coordinated with the surgical team to provide the best outcomes and reduce unnecessary use of resources.

2. The level of postanesthesia care unit (PACU) care depends on the type/approach of surgery, type of anesthetic, intraoperative course of events, as well as patient pre-existing and evolving comorbidities. Typical recovery settings include inpatient recovery, ambulatory recovery (phase I for more intensive needs and phase II for less intensive needs), short stay (23-hour admit), and recovery from nonoperating room anesthesia (NORA) procedures (i.e., computed tomography, magnetic resonance imaging, invasive radiology, cardiac, pediatric, and radiation procedures).

3. The transfer of care to a PACU nurse includes assuring that the patient has had appropriate monitoring applied, admission vital signs were taken, and a direct and thorough report was received that allows for rapid evaluation should complications arise, as well as a nurse capable of handling the acuity of the patient's medical/surgical problems.

4. Postoperative analgesia should be individualized to requirements and expectations. A multimodal approach includes the appropriate use of nonsteroidal anti-inflammatory drugs, narcotics, adjuncts, regional and local anesthetics, as well as anxiety relief and appropriate emotional support.

5. Discharge criteria should be tailored to the individual patient's underlying disease, recovery course, and postdischarge level of care.

6. The cardiac risks during the postoperative stay include myocardial ischemia, which may be minimized with continued use of β-blockers, analgesia, nitrates, supplemental oxygen, adequate circulating volume, oxygen-carrying capacity, heart rate control, and an understanding of hypercoagulable states.

7. The respiratory risks of a patient must take into account the preoperative respiratory disease status. Residual anesthetics, muscle relaxants, opioids, and sedatives all impair responsiveness to increasing CO_2 and decreasing O_2 levels. Pain itself can decrease respiration/minute ventilation, leading to CO_2 retention and hypoxemia. Supplemental O_2 application alone does not guarantee hypoxemia will not occur.
8. The evaluation of a patient's ability to void may be affected by type of surgery (i.e., genitourinary surgery, hernia repairs) or type of anesthetic (i.e., regional, neuraxial, or opioids).
9. Relative hypovolemia should be evaluated and managed in PACU based on the patient's comorbidities, preoperative status (i.e., bowel preparation, postdialysis), type and duration of surgery, blood loss, and urine output.
10. Glycemic monitoring and control should persist as a continuum from intraoperative management. Good glycemic control may help with fighting infection and improve wound healing, which can result in better surgical outcomes. Hypoglycemia occurs because of nothing by mouth status, intraoperative administration of insulin, as well as the patient using programmable insulin pumps.
11. Hypothermia can lead to an increased length of stay in PACU, lethargy, decreased minute ventilation, decreased strength, and increased cardiac demand. It is important to assure that the patient is dry and insulated. The use of air warming blankets, warming mats, and intravenous fluid warmers all minimize hypothermia.
12. Many elderly patients experience a varied degree of postoperative confusion, delirium, or cognitive dysfunction in the PACU. Many pediatric patients also experience postemergence delirium leading to increased length of stay in the PACU.
13. Postoperative nausea and vomiting is a major cause of patient discomfort and dissatisfaction, as well as an aspiration risk and causes prolonged PACU stay.

Postanesthesia Recovery

Each patient recovering from an anesthetic has circumstances that require an individualized problem-oriented approach. Postanesthesia recovery must continue to adapt to meet the needs of the changing perioperative landscape, advances in technology, and changing surgical techniques, and to respond to improved evidence-based research. Dissemination of anesthesia services beyond the perisurgical arena has brought changes and greater demands on recovery units.

Standards for Postanesthesia Care

The American Society of Anesthesiologists (ASA) House of Delegates approved Standards for Postanesthesia Care on October 12, 1988. These standards were last amended on October 14, 2014.[28] These five standards of care are used to determine who needs managed recovery, types of recovery, who is responsible, and how the patient is monitored prior to discharge.

Value and Economics of Postanesthesia Care Unit

The quality of postanesthesia care is composed of many variables such as tracking of complications, time per patient spent in recovery, overall clinical outcomes, and patient satisfaction. The value of postanesthesia care is a measure of the quality of care provided compared with the amount of resources spent per patient outcome. The postanesthesia care unit (PACU) helps to use resources efficiently by having trained staff that routinely care for postsurgical patients, thereby recognizing/preventing complications, and by having physicians instituting appropriate and timely therapies.

The actual cost of PACU care incorporates costs of staffing, space, disposables, and hardware (resource utilization). Triage and discharge policies affect both how many admissions occur and what resources each admission consumes. Nurse staffing continues to be the largest direct cost in the PACU. The mix of nursing staff, experience of nurses, staffing ratios, and the complexity and duration of PACU stay affect the overall personnel cost per admission. The level of monitoring provided affects the capital expenditure for equipment, and disposable items account for operating expenditures. The patient acuity mix also determines needs for staffing and equipment such as ventilators, additional monitors, intravenous pumps, and patient-controlled analgesia pumps. The type of physician coverage—such as dedicated coverage versus on-demand coverage—can affect response time, efficiency of care, costs, and patient outcomes. The use of routine postoperative diagnostic testing and therapies without evidence-based need can lead to unnecessary treatments, increasing cost per patient and possible worse patient outcomes.

Cost comparisons between institutions are difficult because charges and cost factors vary widely across institutions, in different regions of the United States, and between countries. They constantly change over time. Regulatory requirements, standards of care, medical-legal climates, and institutional requirements vary greatly between regions and even between facilities in the same locale. It is difficult to establish cost-effectiveness goals of a single PACU because of the differing requirements of individual patients having the same procedures. This difference can be the result of levels of patient comorbidities, level of procedure complexity, surgeon, type of anesthetic, as well as patient perception and expectations. These are just some of the factors that can determine the type of care needed postoperatively. Continued pressures from many fronts to contain costs and maximize cost-effectiveness force each surgical facility to continually evaluate the value of its PACU care to each individual patient.

PACU directors are challenged to optimize clinical results while minimizing expenditures. Innovative PACU practices should guarantee safe care, minimize cost, and fulfill regulatory and institutional requirements. Medical professionals (physicians, nursing, and support staff) must work in concert to identify practices that are wasteful versus those that have proven yield/benefit. The impact of many PACU-proposed interventions on clinical outcomes are not easily substantiated by controlled scientific analysis. Useless testing, unnecessary or unjustifiable therapy, and inappropriate PACU admissions should be eliminated.

However, using a more expensive therapy may generate real savings by decreasing additional therapies, testing, admissions, or length of stay. Another important element essential for patient safety and efficiency in the PACU is communications with the intraoperative anesthesiology service. Communication is perhaps the least expensive tool in medicine and the one most universally proven to be involved in human error events. Utilization of PACU resources is directly related to anesthetic duration and technique. In one study, 22.1% of 37,000 patients had a minor anesthesia-related event or complication that prolonged PACU stays and consumed PACU resources.[1] Another study showed how postoperative adverse events increase the amount of nursing resources needed in the PACU.[2] Close coordination between the PACU and the anesthesiology service should reduce the frequency and impact of such events.

Continued collaboration with surgical teams and developing enhanced recovery after anesthesia (ERAS) protocols might create an opportunity to shorten the length of stay in the PACU. Providers in the recovery unit must be aware of these protocols and manage patients accordingly. Observed change is frequently seen by reducing transportation delays, persistence of pain or nausea, waiting for space, or surgeon discharge delays.[3] Cost-saving measures in other areas may also increase the cost of PACU care; for example, fast-tracking to discharge to home rather than to a hospital bed. The cost savings of not occupying a hospital bed is offset by an increase in PACU stay and therefore greater consumption of PACU resources.[4] The savings may be a cost savings for the patient and beneficial for the facility as a whole but at a greater expense to the PACU. True savings are only realized when operational changes yield a decrease in expenditures for staff, supplies, or equipment. For example, patients who are able to bypass the PACU create a savings opportunity only if paid nursing hours are reduced or if more surgical cases are covered with the same hours. With the use of less-invasive surgical techniques combined with innovative anesthetic techniques, such as regional anesthetics, shorter PACU stays can result in real savings opportunities. However, the areas of scheduling, clerical, or maintenance tasks must not consume excess staffing hours, without savings realized. Finally, trimming costs could entail an increase in unwanted risk to patients. Differentiating between cost-effective postanesthesia care and unsafe practice remains a matter of constant professional judgment and debate daily in most PACUs.

Levels of Postoperative/Postanesthesia Care

With continued demand to increase overall health-care efficiency, caution must be taken to provide the most appropriate care for each patient. As anesthesia services expand to cover a variety of patient types in ever-increasing areas outside the operating room, selecting the correct type of recovery is essential. For the many differing anesthesia areas ranging from inpatient surgery, ambulatory surgery, to off-site procedures, the level of postoperative care that a patient requires is determined by the degree of underlying illness, comorbidities, and the duration as well as the type of anesthesia and surgery. These factors are used to assess the risk of postoperative complications. Less-invasive surgeries or procedures combined with shorter-duration anesthetic regimens facilitate high levels of arousal and minimal cardiovascular or respiratory depression at the end of surgery.

Using a less intensive postanesthesia setting for selected patients can reduce costs for a surgical procedure and allow the facility to divert scarce PACU resources to patients with greater needs. Alert patients are more satisfied when spared the unnecessary assessments in interventions of PACU care. Amenities such as recliners, reading material, television, music, and food improve perceptions (emotional satisfaction) without affecting quality or safety. Earlier reunion with family or visitors in the low-intensity setting is desirable assuming that postoperative care is safe and appropriate. This notion is especially important in the pediatric population.

Creation of separate PACUs for inpatients, ambulatory, or off-site patients is one possible way to streamline PACU care for appropriately triaged patients. Phase I recovery would be reserved for more intense recovery and would require more one-on-one care for staff. Phase II recovery should be less intensive and is appropriate for patients after less invasive procedures requiring less attention from nursing while recovering. If separation of different phases of care is not possible, then providing the appropriate level of monitoring and coverage to the degree of postoperative impairment achieves similar results in a single PACU area. However, care equal to a full-intensity PACU must always be available, given the incidence of complications after anesthesia and surgery.[5] As the aging population generates an increase in the complexity of surgical care in the face of tighter control of resources, maintaining appropriate PACU capacity and safety by observing applicable PACU guidelines and standards will be increasingly important.[6,7]

Postanesthetic Triage

Patients must be carefully evaluated to determine which level of care is appropriate. Triage should be based on clinical condition, length/type of procedure and anesthetic, and the potential for complications that require intervention. Alternatives to PACU care must be used in a discriminatory fashion. Arbitrary criteria based on age, ASA classification, ambulatory versus inpatient versus off-site procedure status, or type of insurance should not be used for determining the level of recovery care. An individual patient undergoing a specific procedure or anesthetic should receive the same appropriate level of postoperative care whether the procedure is performed in a hospital operating room, an ambulatory surgical center, an endoscopy room, an invasive radiology suite, or an outpatient office. In accordance with the ASA Standards of Post Anesthesia Care, Standard I, an anesthesiologist familiar with the patient can determine which level of care is required or if time in a recovery area is needed. If doubt exists about a patient's safety in a lower intensity setting, the patient should be admitted to a higher level of care for recovery. Patient safety should always be favored regardless of the cost.

After superficial procedures using local infiltration, minor blocks, or sedation, patients can almost always recover with less intensive monitoring and coverage. Healthy patients undergoing more extensive procedures (e.g., hernia repairs, arthroscopic procedures, minor orthopedic procedures) under local, plexus, or peripheral nerve blockade might also bypass phase I recovery and go directly to phase II. The increasing use of continuous peripheral nerve catheters for surgery has shortened PACU times and can eliminate many hospital admissions.[8] Innovative anesthetic techniques, advanced surgical techniques, and use of bispectral index monitoring help facilitate fast-track postoperative care.[9]

For more intensive procedures and patients with greater acuity, bypassing the PACU and direct admission to intensive care units can reduce demands on the PACU as well as reduce errors with decreased number of hand offs. This transfer still requires proper postoperative reporting to the accepting unit including how to communicate with the surgical service and anesthesiologist. The intensive care units must be trained and prepared to receive immediate postoperative patients as well as meet the standards of the PACU.

Safety in the Postanesthesia Care Unit

Every PACU should have medical oversight in the form of a medical director. The PACU medical director must ensure the PACU environment is as safe as possible for both patients and staff. Beyond usual safety policies, maintain staffing and training to ensure that an appropriate coverage and skill mix is available to deal with unforeseen crises. Incidence of adverse events in the PACU correlates with nursing workload and staff availability.[2] Ideally, all staff should have PACU certification, and staffing ratios should never fall below acceptable standards.[7] Less-skilled or training staff must be appropriately supervised, and a sufficient number of certified personnel must always be available to handle worst-case scenarios.

The PACU staff protects patients who are temporarily incompetent and preserves patients' rights to observance of advanced directives, and to informed consent for additional procedures. The staff is obligated to optimize each patient's privacy and dignity, and to minimize the psychological impact of unpleasant or frightening events. Observance of procedures for handwashing, sterility, and infection control should be strictly enforced.[10] Medical directors must safeguard against potential for personal assault of patients during recovery such as unwarranted restraints and procedures without consent. Access to the PACU should be strictly controlled. With increasing acceptance of reuniting patients with family/friends, safety and privacy issues need to be continually addressed.

The PACU environment must also be safe for professionals. Air handling should guarantee that personnel are not exposed to unacceptable levels of trace anesthetic gases (although trace gas monitoring is not necessary), and ensure that staff members receive appropriate vaccinations, including those for hepatitis B, flu, and others required by their institution. Practitioners must adhere to policies for radiation safety, infection control, disposal of sharps, universal precautions for bloodborne diseases, and safeguarding against exposure to pathogens such as methicillin-resistant *Staphylococcus*, vancomycin-resistant *Enterococcus*, *Clostridium difficile*, or tuberculosis. Personal protective equipment (PPE) such as gloves and eye protection must be worn to protect both the patient and provider, and having masks, gowns, and appropriate particulate respiratory equipment easily accessible is needed for particular cases. Following current infection control policies and guidelines are essential for patient and staff safety. Ensure that sufficient help is available to avoid injury while lifting and positioning patients or while dealing with emergence situations. Precise documentation and clear delineation of responsibility is essential for proper care of patients and can protect staff against unnecessary medicolegal exposure.

Admission to the Postanesthesia Care Unit

Every patient admitted to a PACU should have vital signs, airway patency, peripheral oxygen saturation, ventilatory rate/character, and level of pain recorded and periodically monitored.[6] Assessment of the patient with periodic recording every 5 minutes for the first 15 minutes and every 15 minutes thereafter is a minimum. Document temperature, level of consciousness, mental status, neuromuscular function, hydration status, degree of nausea on admission/discharge, and more frequently if appropriate, are also minimum standards of care. Every patient should be continuously monitored with a pulse oximeter and at least a single-lead electrocardiogram (ECG). Extra leads, particularly precordial V3-6, are appropriate if left ventricular ischemia is likely. Capnography is necessary for patients receiving mechanical ventilation or those at risk for compromised ventilatory function. Transduction and recorded output from invasive monitors such as arterial, central venous, or pulmonary arterial catheters must be accomplished. Diagnostic (laboratory) testing should be ordered only for specific indications or part of a designed recovery protocol.

Anesthesiology personnel should manage the patient until a PACU nurse secures admission vital signs, attaches appropriate monitors, and care is transferred with a complete report to the nursing staff. A succinct but thorough report that includes sufficient information to allow rapid evaluation and intervention for postoperative complications must be legibly recorded using a standardized format printed on the PACU record or embedded in the PACU electronic medical record (Table 54-1). This report should be similar to the operating room (OR) timeout, providing patient identification, procedure performed, anesthetic type and continuing therapies. Documentation of the time and amount of all neuromuscular relaxants, respiratory depressant medications, and reversal agents should be standard. Outlined orders, specific therapeutic end points, and, most importantly, how to contact the responsible anesthesiologist all must be transmitted. The anesthesiologist should never transfer responsibility to PACU personnel until the patient's airway status, ventilation, and hemodynamics are appropriate for the caregivers to whom he or she entrusts the patient's care. Leaving a patient in the hands of someone unfamiliar or incapable of adequately handling the acuity of the medical situation in a rush to perform "the next case" may constitute abandonment of care. Check the function of indwelling cannulae, intravenous catheters, and monitors, and verify medication type and rates of any intravenous infusions before leaving.

Postoperative Pain Management

Relief of surgical pain with minimal side effects is a major goal during PACU care and a top priority for patients.[6,11-13] Level of pain should be assessed and documented periodically throughout recovery. The Joint Commission for Accreditation of Health Organizations mandated that a numerical pain scale be used with periodic recording and an acceptable score for discharge. Inadequate postoperative analgesia is a major source of preoperative fear and postoperative dissatisfaction for surgical patients. In addition to improving comfort, analgesia reduces sympathetic nervous system response, thereby avoiding hypertension, tachycardia, and dysrhythmias. In hypovolemic patients, the sympathetic nervous system activity may mask relative hypovolemia. Administration of analgesics can precipitate hypotension in an apparently stable patient, especially if direct or histamine-induced vasodilation occurs. It is important to carefully assess a tachycardic patient with low or normal blood pressure who complains of pain before giving analgesics that might precipitate or accentuate hypotension.

The actual degree of postoperative pain can be difficult to establish. Severity of pain varies among surgical procedures and anesthetic techniques. Staff members may be relatively ineffective

Table 54-1 Components of a Postanesthesia Care Unit Admission Report

Preoperative History/Procedures
- Medication allergies or reactions
- Pertinent earlier surgical procedures
- Underlying medical illness
- Chronic medications
- Acute problems (e.g., ischemia, acid–base status, dehydration)
- Premedications (e.g., antibiotics and time given, β-adrenergic blockers, antiemetics)
- Preoperative pain control (e.g., nerve blocks, adjunct medications, narcotics)
- Preoperative pain assessment (chronic and acute pain scores)
- NPO, *nil per os*, status

Intraoperative Factors
- Surgical procedure
- Type of anesthetic
- Type and difficulty of airway management
- Relaxant/reversal status
- Time and amount of opioids administered
- Type and amount of intravenous fluids administered
- Estimated blood loss
- Urine output
- Unexpected surgical or anesthetic events
- Intraoperative vital sign ranges
- Intraoperative laboratory findings
- Drugs given (e.g., steroids, diuretics, antibiotics, vasoactive medications, antiemetics)

Assessment and Report of Current Status
- Airway patency
- Ventilatory adequacy
- Level of consciousness
- Level of pain
- Heart rate and heart rhythm
- Endotracheal tube position
- Systemic pressure
- Intravascular volume status
- Function of invasive monitors
- Size and location of intravenous catheters
- Anesthetic equipment (e.g., epidural catheters, peripheral nerve catheters)
- Overall impression

Postoperative Instructions
- Expected airway and ventilatory status
- Acceptable vital sign ranges
- Acceptable urine output and blood loss
- Surgical instructions (e.g., positioning, wound care)
- Anticipated cardiovascular problems
- Orders for therapeutic interventions
- Diagnostic tests to be secured
- Therapeutic goals and end points before discharge
- Location of responsible physician

NPO, nothing by mouth.

at quantifying level of discomfort. Patients are often able to communicate despite having received sedative hypnotic drugs. Furthermore, patients may be impaired in their communication abilities coming into the hospital or may be affected by the entire medical experience, and thereby may be afraid to express their needs. Inexperienced nurses overestimate a patient's pain, whereas more experienced nurses tend to underestimate the pain.[14] Either error can lead to inappropriate treatment. Use of a numeric pain scale yields more reliable results but requires that a patient be willing to communicate. A wide divergence can exist between a patient's cognitive perception of pain and sympathetic nervous system response, and may be related to psychological, cultural, and cardiovascular differences among individuals. Some patients perceive severe pain with minimal sympathetic nervous system activity, whereas others exhibit hypertension and tachycardia with minimal complaint of discomfort. The best measure of analgesia is the patient's perception. Heart rate, respiratory rate and depth, sweating, nausea, and vomiting all may be signs of pain but their absence or presence is not in itself reliable as a measure of the presence of pain.

Careful identification of patient subgroups, assessment of individual analgesic requirements, and implementation of a planned, multimodal approach will provide seamless pain control through and beyond the PACU interval.[15] In a study of postoperative pain in 10,008 ambulatory patients, only 5.3% reported severe pain in the PACU and 1.7% in the discharge area (Fig. 54-1). However, a much higher percentage of patients report that moderate-to-severe pain recurs after discharge.[16,17] To avoid masking signs of an unrelated condition or a surgical complication, ascertain that the nature and intensity of pain are appropriate for the surgical procedure. The central nervous system (CNS) signs of hypoxemia, acidemia, or cerebral hypoperfusion often mimic those of pain, especially during emergence. Administration of parenteral analgesics or sedatives can acutely worsen hypoventilation, airway obstruction, or hypotension, causing sudden deterioration. Evaluating orientation, the level of arousal, and cardiovascular or pulmonary status usually identifies such patients.

Surgical pain can be effectively treated with a multimodal approach. Although usage of opioids continues, the use of regional and local anesthetic techniques and drugs such as acetaminophen, nonsteroidal anti-inflammatory drugs (NSAIDs), neurologics, and α agonists also have proven to be an effective in reducing pain. Sufficient analgesia is the end point, even if large doses of opioids are necessary in tolerant patients. Short-acting opioids are useful to expedite discharge and minimize nausea in ambulatory settings,[18] although duration of analgesia can be a problem. During intravenous titration of opioids, the patient should be assessed for incremental respiratory or cardiovascular depression. Oral and transdermal analgesics have a limited role in the PACU but are helpful for ambulatory patients transitioning to PACU discharge. Rectal analgesics are sometimes useful in small children. Interventions such as repositioning, reassurance, or extubation also help minimize discomfort.

Other analgesic modalities provide pain relief in and beyond the PACU.[19] Titration of intravenous opioids in the PACU is important for smooth transition to intravenous patient-controlled analgesia. Injection of opioids into the epidural or subarachnoid space during anesthesia or in the PACU yields prolonged postoperative analgesia in selected patients.[20,21] Nausea and pruritus are troubling side effects, and immediate or delayed ventilatory depression can occur related to vascular uptake and cephalad spread in cerebrospinal fluid. Nausea should resolve with antiemetics, whereas pruritus and ventilatory depression often respond to naloxone infusion. Addition of local anesthetic or clonidine to neuraxially administered drugs enhance analgesia and decrease the risk of side effects from epidural opioids, although local anesthetics add risk of hypotension and motor blockade. Epidural analgesia is effective after thoracic or abdominal procedures and helps wean obese patients or those with chronic obstructive pulmonary disease (COPD) from mechanical ventilation.

Continuous flow catheters with pressure delivery systems of local anesthetics have been used within the wound to reduce

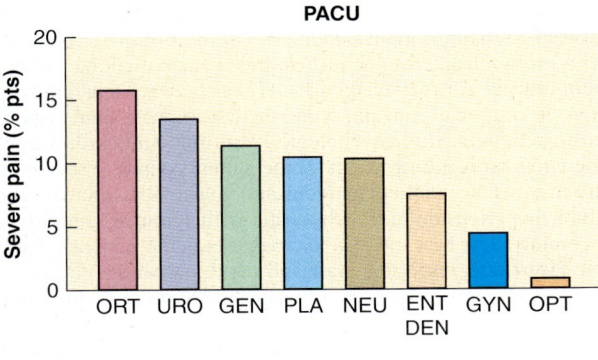
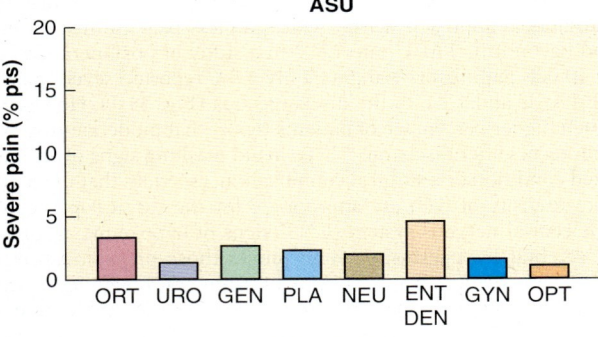
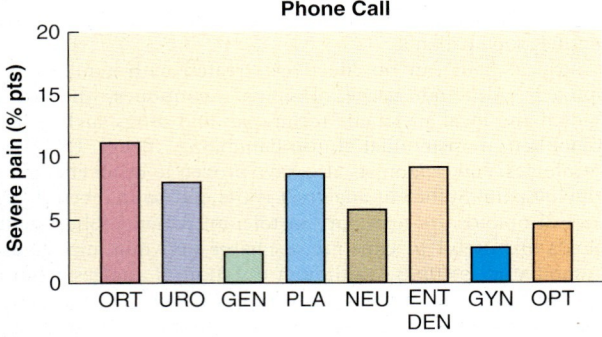

Figure 54-1 Percentage of patients experiencing severe pain in the postanesthesia care unit (PACU), the ambulatory surgery unit (ASU), and during phone call follow-up at 24 hours. ORT, orthopedics; URO, urology; GEN, general; PLA, plastics; NEU, neurology; ENT, ear, nose, throat; DEN, dental; GYN, gynecology; OPT, ophthalmology. (Reprinted with permission from Chung F, Ritchie E, Su J. Postoperative pain in ambulatory surgery. *Anesth Analg.* 1997;85:808.)

pain and opioid requirements, increase patient satisfaction, and reduce length of hospital stay.[22] These same delivery systems have been safely used with continuous peripheral nerve catheters for inpatient as well as outpatient use.[23,24] With the use of ultrasound-guided techniques for catheter placement, appropriately selected outpatients can safely receive the pain control benefits of regional anesthesia.[8] However, extensive written and oral postoperative instructions must be provided, with systems in place for 24-hour access by patients for catheter-related complications.

Placement of long-acting regional analgesic blocks reduces pain, controls sympathetic nervous system activity, and often improves ventilation.[19] After shoulder procedures, interscalene block yields almost complete pain relief with only moderate inconvenience from motor impairment. Paralysis of the ipsilateral diaphragm can impair postoperative ventilation in patients with marginal reserve, although the impact is small in most patients.[25] Suprascapular nerve block might be an alternative to avoid this potentially serious side effect. Percutaneous intercostal or paravertebral blocks reduce analgesic requirements after thoracic, breast, or high abdominal incision. Transversus abdominis plane (TAP) blocks are effective for lower abdominal surgeries as well as those innervated by the ilioinguinal and iliohypogastric nerves. Caudal analgesia or paravertebral blocks can also be effective in children after inguinal or genital procedures, whereas infiltration of local anesthetic into joints, soft tissues, or incisions decreases the intensity of pain. Other modalities, such as guided imagery, hypnosis, transcutaneous nerve stimulation, music, massage, or acupuncture, have limited utility for surgical pain but may provide a positive patient experience.

Use of patient-controlled analgesia, spinal opioids, or neural blockade mandates anticipation of risk beyond the PACU. The plan for extended postoperative analgesia should be established before induction of surgical anesthesia, and then the anesthetic and PACU care should be oriented toward that plan. These plans should be in agreement with the patient, surgeon, and anesthesiologist. If one analgesic modality proves inadequate, the team should take particular care when implementing a second technique.

Fear, anxiety, and confusion often accentuate postoperative pain during recovery, especially after general anesthesia. Titration of an intravenous sedative such as midazolam may attenuate this psychogenic component. It is important to distinguish between requirements for analgesia and anxiolysis. Opioids are poor sedatives and anxiolytics, whereas benzodiazepines are poor analgesics. However, when pain control modalities appear larger than what might be anticipated, one should consider the possibility that anxiety is playing a large role in the dysphoric event in the PACU.

Discharge Criteria

Before discharge from the postoperative unit to a lower level of care, each patient should be sufficiently oriented to assess his or her physical condition and be able to summon assistance. Airway reflexes and motor function must be adequate to maintain patency and prevent aspiration. One should ensure that ventilation and oxygenation are acceptable, with sufficient reserve to cover minor deterioration in unmonitored settings. Blood pressure, heart rate, and indices of peripheral perfusion should be relatively constant for at least 15 minutes and appropriately near baseline. Achieving normal body temperature is not an absolute requirement, but there should be resolution of shivering. Acceptable analgesia must be achieved and vomiting appropriately controlled. Patients should be observed for at least 15 minutes after the last intravenous opioid or sedative is administered to assess peak effects and side effects. If regional anesthetics have been administered, longer observation could be appropriate to assess effectiveness and rule out local toxicity. One should monitor oxygen saturation for 15 minutes after discontinuation of supplemental oxygen to detect hypoxemia. Ruling out likely complications of surgery (e.g., bleeding, vascular compromise, pneumothorax) or of underlying conditions (e.g., hypertension, myocardial ischemia, hyperglycemia, bronchospasm). One should also document a brief neurologic assessment to assure patient is at their baseline and review results of diagnostic tests. If these generic criteria cannot be met, postponement of discharge or transfer to a specialized unit is advisable. There is no demonstrable benefit from a mandatory minimum duration of PACU care.

Scoring systems such as the Modified Aldrete Score or Postanesthesia Discharge Scoring System (Table 54-2) are two commonly used systems for patient assessment and attempt to simplify and

Table 54-2 Two Most Commonly Used Postanesthesia Care Unit Discharge Criteria Systems

Modified Aldrete Scoring System	Postanesthetic Discharge Scoring System
Respiration	**Vital signs**
2 = Able to take deep breath and cough	2 = BP + pulse within 20% preop baseline
1 = Dyspnea/shallow breathing	1 = BP + pulse within 20%–40% preop baseline
0 = Apnea	0 = BP + pulse >40% preop baseline
O_2 saturation	**Activity**
2 = Maintains SpO_2 >92% on room air	2 = Steady gait, no dizziness or meets preop level
1 = Needs O_2 inhalation to maintain O_2 saturation >90%	1 = Requires assistance
0 = O_2 saturation <90% even with supplemental oxygen	0 = Unable to ambulate
Consciousness	**Nausea and vomiting**
2 = Fully awake	2 = Minimal/treated with PO medication
1 = Arousable on calling	1 = Moderate/treated with parenteral medication
0 = Not responding	0 = Severe/continues despite treatment
Circulation	**Pain**
2 = BP ± 20 mmHg preop	Controlled with oral analgesics and acceptable to patient:
1 = BP ± 20–50 mmHg preop	2 = Yes
0 = BP ± 50 mmHg preop	1 = No
Activity	**Surgical bleeding**
2 = Able to move four extremities voluntarily or on command	2 = Minimal/no dressing changes
1 = Able to move two extremities	1 = Moderate/up to two dressing changes required
0 = Unable to move extremities	0 = Severe/more than three dressing changes required
Score ≥9 for discharge	Score ≥9 for discharge

BP, blood pressure; PO, oral.

standardize patient discharge criteria. Fixed PACU discharge criteria must be used with caution because variability among patients is tremendous. Scoring systems that quantify physical status or establish thresholds for vital signs are useful for assessment but cannot replace individual evaluation.[26,27] Ideally, each patient should be evaluated for discharge by an anesthesiologist using a consistent set of criteria, considering the severity of underlying disease, the anesthetic and recovery course, and the level of care at the destination (Table 54-2). A plan for the continued management of likely postdischarge symptoms such as pain, nausea, headache, dizziness, drowsiness, and fatigue must be made prior to discharge.[17]

Postoperative Evaluation

The Centers for Medicare and Medicaid Services (CMS) have instituted compliance policies for those entities that participate in the Medicare and Medicaid programs. The policy for postanesthesia follow-up requires a written follow-up that is performed by an individual that is qualified to administer anesthesia no later than 48 hours post procedure. The time frame starts as soon as the patient arrives to the recovery area or intensive care unit (ICU). The evaluation should be performed only after the patient has sufficiently recovered from anesthesia to be able to participate, such as answer questions or perform simple tasks. The postanesthesia evaluation must contain the following elements:

- Respiratory function, including respiratory rate, airway patency, and oxygen saturation
- Cardiovascular function, including pulse rate and blood pressure
- Mental status
- Temperature
- Pain
- Nausea and vomiting
- Postoperative hydration

Cardiovascular Complications

The purpose of this section is not to entirely review all the possible cardiovascular events that might beset a patient in the PACU, rather it is to help the reader decide what events might be unique to the PACU. In the PACU, some reflexes previously blunted by general anesthetics, sedatives, and opioids return toward baseline revealing an unexpected cardiovascular compromise. Perhaps the two most common types of patients to encounter troubles will be the patient with coronary artery disease and the patient with congestive heart failure. Patients in the PACU may not complain of angina due to residual anesthetics and pain medications. The first sign of myocardial ischemia may well be hypotension, and the use of sedation techniques using drugs like dexmedetomidine can lead to hypotension postoperatively, which can cloud the picture of a patient's cardiac disease. The most common sign of myocardial ischemia is tachycardia. Tachycardia is very often a reaction to, not the cause of, myocardial ischemia. That does not mean that all tachycardia heralds myocardial ischemia, but in a patient who seems at risk for coronary artery disease, new-onset tachycardia that is not caused by pain should be taken seriously. The ECG may show classic ST-T wave elevation or depression depending on lead placement and area of ischemia. But the lack of ST-T wave elevation does not rule out coronary artery disease. Transmural myocardial infarctions outside the PACU show no

ECG diagnostic changes 10% to 30% of the time. So, the clinician must be especially suspicious of a series of hemodynamic changes in a person at risk for coronary artery disease. Early intervention with nitrates, opioids, β-blockers, and even anticoagulants may save a life. Cardiology should be involved to gain immediate and timely access to the cardiac catheterization laboratory or for anxiolytic drug therapy. With increasing use of bare metal and drug eluding stents (DES), recognition of those patients that have stopped antiplatelet therapy and are in postoperative hypercoagulable states can quickly occlude these stents. This requires quick recognition and response for intervention. Involvement and communication with the surgical service must be immediate and decisions, especially as to anticoagulation and lytic therapy, should be made among several services in consultation.

Congestive heart failure is epidemic in our ever-aging population. The outpatient cardiology services have an expanding armamentarium of new inotropic/vasodilator therapy, devices, and interventions that allow patients to compensate for their congestive heart failure. It is helpful to know not only the ejection fraction but also the activities of daily living, exercise tolerance, and other risk indices. The ejection fraction is only an estimate of the fractional shortening of the myocardial actin and myosin fibrils. Although it is a useful estimate of severity of impairment, one is struck by how stable some patients may be with a large dilated heart contracting at a 15% ejection fraction. They are compensated but have little reserve. The potential problems of bleeding, volume shifts, and respiratory compromise in the PACU could quickly cause decompensation. There are also no absolute numbers with regard to fluid restriction but precaution should be taken when giving fluid challenges. The usage of transesophageal echocardiography and transthoracic echo may be of great use in the PACU. Within a very few minutes a puzzling hypotensive situation might be explained by an echocardiogram. The echocardiogram allows rapid viewing of myocardial contractility, regional wall motion, volume status, and valvular dysfunction.

With evolving cardiac treatments and less invasive techniques, specialized PACU care can be safe and more cost effective than ICU admission. The natural extension is to establish some highly specialized PACUs that function as step-down or short-term ICUs. In a study of 85 prospective patients[29] undergoing "off-pump" coronary artery bypass graft procedures, the patients were extubated in 12 ± 2 minutes after the chest was closed. They were then taken to a special part of the PACU where they were monitored for a number of hours (up to 480 minutes in some situations). Patients were then either discharged to the cardiac floors or sent to an ICU. Of the 85 patients in this study, only 4 failed the PACU stay and had to be admitted to an ICU. Bradycardia was the cause for failure in three cases; the cause for the fourth failure was myocardial infarction. Two patients later returned to the ICU from the cardiac ward; there was one case of atrial fibrillation and another case of myocardial infarction. During the same time 304 patients who were not undergoing off-pump coronary artery bypass graft surgery were admitted to the cardiac ICU. The cost for PACU stay was $5,140.00 less than for an ICU-admitted patient. Although this study seems quite favorable, the two groups of patients were not comparable.

High-risk vascular and thoracic surgery patients have shown that they could each be adequately cared for in an adequately staffed and prepared PACU.[30] Hospitals can improve patient throughput by putting more resources into expanded PACU care and less into ICU services. Nursing reviews are available to give input as to how to structure such new units.[31,32]

Anesthesiology services are in increased demand throughout most hospitals. The PACU will likely need to prepare to care for those patients. Some facilities may elect to have separate recovery facilities and staff different from the traditional operating room PACU. Invasive cardiology suites are used for ablation techniques for dysrhythmias, and automated implantable defibrillators are placed in hybrid suites, operating rooms, or catheterization laboratories; these facilities may also be the sites of percutaneous valve replacements as well as some hybrid and percutaneous coronary revascularization procedures. If patients require deep sedation or general anesthesia, they will also require PACU care.

The cardiac patient is the common patient today. The new procedures and pressure to ever streamline operating room care is pressuring the PACU to become more and more a cardiac mini-ICU. The smart PACU medical director and hospital administrator will see that with targeted resources, patients may well be safely cared for in a more cost-effective manner with quicker throughput by using a PACU approach.

Postoperative Pulmonary Dysfunction

Mechanical, hemodynamic, and pharmacologic factors related to surgery and anesthesia impair ventilation, oxygenation, and airway maintenance.[33] Heavy smoking, obesity, sleep apnea, severe asthma, and COPD increase the risk of postoperative ventilatory events.[34] Preoperative pulmonary function testing has limited predictive value for postoperative complications,[35] perhaps with the exception of postoperative bronchospasm in smokers.[36]

Inadequate Postoperative Ventilation

In PACU patients, mild respiratory academia due to atelectasis and decreased minute ventilation is expected; thus, elevated Pa_{CO_2} does not necessarily indicate inadequate postoperative ventilation. Inadequate ventilation should be suspected when (1) respiratory acidemia occurs coincident with tachypnea, anxiety, dyspnea, labored ventilation, or increased sympathetic nervous system activity; (2) hypercarbia reduces the arterial pH below 7.30; or (3) $PaCO_2$ progressively increases with a progressive decrease in arterial pH.

Inadequate Respiratory Drive

During early recovery from anesthesia, residual effects of intravenous and inhalation anesthetics blunt the ventilatory responses to both hypercarbia and hypoxemia. Sedatives augment depression from opioids or anesthetics and reduce the conscious desire to ventilate (a significant component of ventilatory drive).

Hypoventilation and hypercarbia can evolve insidiously during transfer and admission to the PACU. Although effects of intraoperative medications are usually waning, the peak depressant effect of an intravenous opioid given just before transfer occurs in the PACU. Coincident depression of medullary centers that regulate the sympathetic nervous system can blunt signs of acidemia or hypoxemia such as hypertension, tachycardia, and agitation, concealing hypoventilation. Patients might communicate lucidly and even complain of pain while experiencing significant opioid-induced hypoventilation. A balance must be struck between an acceptable level of postoperative ventilatory depression and a tolerable level of pain or agitation. Patients with abnormal CO_2/pH responses from morbid obesity, chronic airway obstruction, or sleep apnea are more sensitive to respiratory depressants.[37] Risk for apnea after anesthesia in preterm infants depends on type of anesthetic, postconceptual age, and preoperative hematocrit. Preterm infants should be monitored for at least 12 hours. Children with active or recent upper respiratory infection are more prone to breath-holding, severe cough, and arterial desaturations below 90% during recovery, especially if they have a history of reactive airway disease or secondhand smoke exposure or have undergone intubation and/or airway surgery.[38] If hypoventilation from opioids is excessive, forced arousal and careful titration (20 to 40 µg at a time) of intravenous naloxone reverses respiratory depression without affecting analgesia. Flumazenil (0.1 mg titrated to effect up to 1.5 mg) directly reverses depressant effects of benzodiazepines on ventilatory drive but is usually unnecessary.

The abrupt diminution of a noxious stimulus (e.g., tracheal extubation, placement of a postoperative block) may promote hypoventilation or airway obstruction by altering the balance between arousal from discomfort and depression from medication. Intracranial hemorrhage or edema sometimes presents with hypoventilation, especially after posterior fossa craniotomy. Bilateral carotid body injury after endarterectomy can ablate peripheral hypoxic drive. Chronic respiratory acidemia from COPD alters CNS sensitivity to pH and makes hypoxic drive dominant, but hypoventilation from supplemental oxygen rarely occurs.

Increased Airway Resistance

High resistance to gas flow through airways increases work of breathing and CO_2 production. If inspiratory muscles cannot generate sufficient pressure gradients to overcome resistance, alveolar ventilation fails to match CO_2 production and progressive respiratory acidemia occurs.

In postoperative patients, increased upper airway resistance is caused by obstruction in the pharynx (posterior tongue displacement, change in anteroposterior and lateral dimensions from soft tissue collapse), in the larynx (laryngospasm, laryngeal edema), or in the large airways (extrinsic compression from hematoma, tumor, or tracheal stenosis). Weakness from residual neuromuscular relaxation,[39] myasthenia gravis or myasthenic syndromes can contribute, but it is seldom the primary cause of airway compromise. If the airway is clear of vomitus or foreign bodies, simple maneuvers such as improving the level of consciousness, lateral positioning, chin lift, mandible elevation, or placement of an oropharyngeal or nasopharyngeal airway may relieve obstruction. A nasopharyngeal airway may be better tolerated when the patient has functional gag reflexes. Acute extrinsic upper airway compression (e.g., an expanding neck hematoma) must be relieved.

During emergence, stimulation of the pharynx or vocal cords by secretions, blood, foreign matter, or extubation can generate laryngospasm.[40] Laryngeal constrictor muscles occlude the tracheal inlet and reduce gas flow. Patients who smoke or are chronically exposed to smoke have irritable airway conditions, have copious secretions, or have undergone upper airway surgery are at higher risk.[33,38] Laryngospasm usually can be overcome by providing gentle continuous positive pressure (10 to 20 mmHg) in the oropharynx by mask with 100% O_2. Prolonged laryngospasm is relieved with a small dose of succinylcholine (e.g., 0.1 mg/kg) or deepening sedation with propofol. An intubating dosage of succinylcholine should not be used to break postoperative laryngospasm, especially if the alveolar partial pressure of oxygen (P_AO_2) is decreased by hypoventilation. As little as 5 to 10 mg of succinylcholine can break the laryngospasm. Unless assisted ventilation is provided, declining P_AO_2 causes serious hypoxemia before spontaneous ventilation resumes (Fig. 54-2).[41]

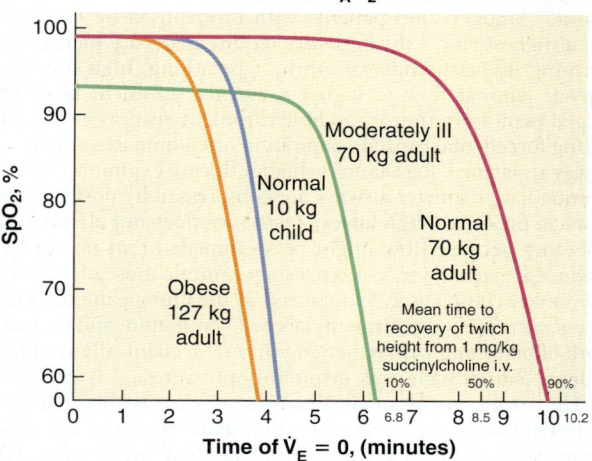

Figure 54-2 Rate of SpO_2 decline after onset of apnea. (Reprinted with permission from Benumof JL, Dagg R, Benumof R. Critical hemoglobin desaturation will occur before return to an unparalyzed state following 1 mg/kg intravenous succinylcholine. *Anesthesiology*. 1997;87:979.)

If the functional residual capacity (FRC) is abnormally reduced, the decreased volume of O_2 available in the lungs accelerates the development of hypoxemia. Severe laryngeal obstruction can occur secondarily because of acute hypocalcemia after parathyroid excision.

Soft-tissue edema worsens airway obstruction, especially in children and adults recovering from procedures on the neck. Nebulized vasoconstrictors like epinephrine help somewhat, but steroids have little effect acutely. Patients with C1 esterase inhibitor deficiency can develop severe angioneurotic edema after even slight trauma to the airway. Pathologic airway obstruction (e.g., severe edema, epiglottitis, retropharyngeal abscess, encroaching tumors) might require emergency tracheal intubation, but airway manipulation is dangerous because minor trauma from intubation attempts can convert a marginal airway into a total obstruction. Judgment by the individual anesthesiologist regarding timing, patient status, available equipment along with airway management skills all play a part of the decision as to where, when, and how to intubate. Sedatives or muscle relaxants used to facilitate intubation can worsen obstruction by compromising the patient's volitional efforts to maintain the airway and by eliminating spontaneous ventilation. Equipment and personnel necessary for emergency cricothyroidotomy or tracheostomy should be available. Needle cricothyroidotomy using a 14-gauge intravenous catheter or a commercially available kit permits oxygenation and marginal ventilation until the airway is secured, especially if jet ventilation with 100% oxygen is used.

Reduction of cross-sectional area in small airways increases overall airway resistance because resistance varies inversely with the fourth power of radius during turbulent flow. Pharyngeal or tracheal stimulation from secretions, suctioning, aspiration, or a tracheal tube can trigger a reflex constriction of bronchial smooth muscle in emerging patients with reactive airways. Histamine release precipitated by medication or allergic reactions also increases airway smooth muscle tone. Decreased radial traction on small airways reduces cross-sectional area in patients with COPD or with decreased lung volume secondary to obesity, surgical manipulation, excessive lung water, or splinting. Preoperative spirometric evidence of increased airway resistance predicts an increased risk of postoperative bronchospasm.[36] Smokers and patients with bronchospastic conditions are at highest risk.[42] If ventilatory requirements are increased by warming, hyperthermia, or work of breathing, high flow rates convert laminar flow to higher-resistance turbulent flow. Prolonged expiratory time or audible turbulent air flow (wheezing) during forced vital capacity expiration often unmasks subclinical airway resistance. Resistance is higher during expiration because intermediate-diameter airways are compressed by positive intrathoracic pressure. High airway resistance does not always cause wheezing because flow might be so impeded that no sound is produced. Signs of increased resistance mimic those of decreased pulmonary compliance. Spontaneously breathing patients exhibit accessory muscle recruitment, labored ventilation, and increased work of breathing with either condition. Mechanically ventilated patients exhibit high peak inspiratory pressures.

The treatment of small airway resistance is directed at an underlying etiology. One must eliminate laryngeal or airway stimulation. Patients often respond to their pre-existing regimen of their inhalers. Levalbuterol or metaproterenol nebulized in oxygen resolves postoperative bronchospasm with minimal tachycardia. Nebulized racemic epinephrine effectively relaxes smooth muscle, but side effects of tachycardia and flushing can be seen. Isoproterenol has also been nebulized with good results. Intramuscular or sublingual terbutaline can be added. Administration of steroid therapy offers little acute improvement, but may prevent later recurrence. Bronchospasm that is resistant to β_2-sympathomimetic medication may improve with an anticholinergic medication such as atropine or ipratropium. If bronchospasm is life-threatening, an intravenous epinephrine infusion yields profound bronchodilation. Increased small airway resistance caused by mechanical factors (e.g., loss of lung volume, retained secretions, pulmonary edema) usually does not resolve with bronchodilators. Restoration of lung volume with incentive spirometry or deep tidal ventilation increases radial traction on small airways. Reducing left ventricular filling pressures might relieve airway resistance caused by increased lung water, although interstitial fluid accumulation can persist. Also, extended contraction of airway smooth muscle obstructs venous and lymphatic flow, leading to airway wall edema that resolves slowly.

Decreased Compliance

Reduced pulmonary compliance increases the elastic work of breathing. In the extreme, low compliance causes progressive respiratory muscle fatigue, hypoventilation, and respiratory acidemia. Parenchymal changes also affect compliance. Reduction of FRC leads to small airway closure and distal lung collapse, requiring greater energy expenditure to re-expand the lung. Pulmonary edema increases the lung's weight and inertia and elevates surface tension by interfering with surfactant activity, making expansion more difficult. Pulmonary contusion or hemorrhage interferes with lung expansion, as do restrictive lung diseases, skeletal abnormalities, intrathoracic lesions, hemothorax, pneumothorax, or cardiomegaly. Obesity affects pulmonary compliance, especially when adipose tissue compresses the thoracic cage or increases intra-abdominal pressure in supine or lateral positions. Extrathoracic factors such as tight muscles of the chest or abdominal dressings and gas in the stomach or bowel reduce chest wall compliance. Most notably after intra-abdominal laparoscopic procedures, retained CO_2 may impair diaphragm movement. The CO_2 has the capability to dissecting into the thorax, creating either a pneumothorax or pneumomediastinum, which is usually a self-limited event as the CO_2 is relatively rapidly absorbed. There is usually no need for chest tube intervention. An intra-abdominal tumor, hemorrhage, ascites, bowel obstruction, or pregnancy impairs diaphragmatic excursion and reduces compliance.

Work of breathing is improved by resolving problems that reduce compliance. Allowing patients to recover in a semi-sitting (semi-Fowler) position reduces work of breathing. Incentive spirometry and chest physiotherapy help restore lung volume, as does positive end-expiratory pressure (PEEP) or continuous positive airway pressure (CPAP). In patients with COPD and highly compliant lungs, positive airway pressure might force the rib cage and diaphragms toward their excursion limits, accentuating inspiratory muscular effort.

Neuromuscular and Skeletal Problems

Postoperative airway obstruction and hypoventilation are accentuated by incomplete reversal of neuromuscular relaxation. Residual paralysis compromises airway patency, ability to overcome airway resistance, airway protection, and ability to clear secretions.[43] In the extreme, paralysis precludes effective spontaneous ventilation. Intraoperative use of shorter-acting relaxants might decrease the incidence of residual paralysis but does not eliminate the problem. Marginal reversal can be more dangerous than near-total paralysis because a weak, agitated patient exhibiting uncoordinated movements and airway obstruction is more easily identified. A somnolent patient exhibiting mild stridor and shallow ventilation from marginal neuromuscular function might be overlooked, allowing insidious hypoventilation and respiratory acidemia or regurgitation with aspiration to occur. PACU staff should be aware of patients who have received nondepolarizing muscle relaxants but no reversal agents because they often exhibit low levels of residual paralysis.[44] Safety of techniques designed to avoid reversal of short- and intermediate-duration relaxants has not been substantiated, and reversal of nondepolarizing relaxants is recommended.[6] The selective relaxant binding agent used widely in Europe and recently available in the United States, γ-cyclodextrins (i.e., Sugammadex), is a reversal drug that can avoid the side effects of other anticholinesterases and anticholinergics.[45] Patients with neuromuscular abnormalities such as myasthenia gravis, Eaton–Lambert syndrome, periodic paralysis, or muscular dystrophies exhibit exaggerated or prolonged responses to muscle relaxants. Even without relaxant administration, these patients can exhibit postoperative ventilatory insufficiency. Medications (e.g., antibiotics, furosemide, propranolol, phenytoin) potentiate neuromuscular relaxation, as does hypocalcemia or hypermagnesemia.

Diaphragmatic contraction is compromised in some postoperative patients, forcing more reliance on intercostal muscles and reducing the ability to overcome decreased compliance or increased ventilatory demands. Impairment of phrenic nerve function from interscalene block, trauma, or thoracic and neck operations can "paralyze" one or rarely both diaphragms.[25] Adequate ventilation will normally be maintained with only one diaphragm, and marginal ventilation by external intercostal muscles alone. However, with high work of breathing, muscle weakness, or increased ventilatory demands, a nonfunctional diaphragm impairs minute ventilation. Thoracic spinal or epidural blockade interferes with intercostal muscle function and reduces ventilatory reserve, especially in patients with COPD. Abnormal motor neuron function (e.g., Guillain–Barré syndrome, cervical spinal cord trauma), flail chest, or severe kyphosis or scoliosis can cause postoperative ventilatory insufficiency.

Simple tests help assess mechanical ability to ventilate. The ability to sustain head elevation in a supine position, a forced vital capacity of 10 to 12 mL/kg, an inspiratory pressure more negative than −25 cm H_2O, and tactile train-of-four assessment imply that strength of ventilatory muscles is adequate to sustain ventilation and to take a large enough breath to cough. However, none of these clinical end points reliably predicts recovery of airway protective reflexes,[44] and failure on these tests does not necessarily indicate the need for assisted ventilation.

The use of noninvasive mechanical ventilation techniques such as CPAP or bilevel ventilation can help safely extubate some patients earlier or prevent reintubation. By using these noninvasive techniques, patients can often overcome some of the above discussed issues interfering with normal respiration, thus reducing the risk of remaining intubated or reintubation. Units other than ICUs are able to manage these patients thereby offloading the burden of the ICU.

Occasionally, a clinical picture suggests ventilatory insufficiency when ventilation is adequate. Voluntary limitation of chest expansion to avoid pain (splinting) causes labored, rapid, shallow breathing characteristic of inadequate ventilation. Splinting seldom causes actual hypoventilation and usually improves with analgesia and repositioning. Ventilation with small tidal volumes due to thoracic restriction or reduced compliance seems to generate afferent input from pulmonary stretch receptors, leading to dyspnea, labored breathing, and accessory muscle recruitment in spite of appropriate minute ventilation. Occasional large, "satisfying" lung expansions often relieve these symptoms. Finally, spontaneous hyperventilation to compensate for a metabolic acidemia might generate tachypnea or labored breathing, which is mistaken for ventilatory insufficiency.

Increased Deadspace

Ventilation of unperfused deadspace or of poorly perfused alveoli with high ventilation/perfusion ($\dot{V}/\dot{Q}$) ratios is less effective in removing CO_2. Expansion of deadspace volume or reduction of tidal volume increases the fraction of each breath wasted in deadspace ($\dot{V}_D/\dot{V}_T$) and the amount of CO_2 from the previous exhalation that is rebreathed. A proportionally larger increase in total minute ventilation is required to meet any increase in CO_2 production. Patients with high $\dot{V}_D/\dot{V}_T$ are at greater risk for postoperative ventilatory failure.

Occasionally, an acute increase in deadspace contributes to respiratory acidemia in postoperative patients. Although upper airway deadspace is reduced after tracheal intubation and tracheostomy, excessive tubing volume or valve reversal in breathing circuits promotes rebreathing of CO_2. PEEP or CPAP elevates physiologic deadspace, especially in patients with high pulmonary compliance. Pulmonary embolization with air, thrombus, or cellular debris increases physiologic deadspace, although impact on CO_2 excretion is often compensated by accelerated minute ventilation from hypercarbic and hypoxic drives or reflex responses. Decreased cardiac output can transiently increase $\dot{V}_D/\dot{V}_T$ by decreasing perfusion to well-ventilated, nondependent lung and is the most common cause of acute increase in deadspace in the acute care setting. Irreversible increases in deadspace occur if adult respiratory distress syndrome (ARDS) related to sepsis, transfusion-related acute lung injury (TRALI), or hypoxia destroys pulmonary microvasculature. Deadspace may appear high if an inhalation interrupts the previous exhalation and spent alveolar gas is retained. This "gas trapping" occurs when high airway resistance lengthens the time required to exhale completely, or if improper inspiration/expiration ratios or high ventilatory rates are used during mechanical ventilation.

Increased Carbon Dioxide Production

Carbon dioxide production varies directly with metabolic rate, body temperature, and substrate availability. During anesthesia, CO_2 production falls to approximately 60% of the normal 2 to 3 mL/kg/min as hypothermia lowers metabolic activity and neuromuscular relaxation reduces tonic muscle contraction. Therefore, during recovery, metabolic rate and CO_2 production can increase by 40%. Shivering, high work of breathing, infection, sympathetic nervous system activity, or rapid carbohydrate metabolism during intravenous hyperalimentation accelerates CO_2 production. Malignant hyperthermia generates CO_2 production many times greater than normal, which rapidly exceeds ventilatory reserve and causes severe respiratory and metabolic acidemia. Even mild increases of CO_2 production can precipitate respiratory acidemia if low compliance, airway resistance, or neuromuscular paralysis interferes with ventilation. With the exception of adjusting hyperalimentation, improving work of breathing, reducing shivering, or treating hyperthermia, there is little yield from addressing CO_2 production in PACU patients.

Inadequate Postoperative Oxygenation

Systemic arterial partial pressure of oxygen (PaO_2) is the best indicator of pulmonary oxygen transfer from alveolar gas to pulmonary capillary blood. Arterial hemoglobin saturation monitored by pulse oximetry yields less information on alveolar-arterial gradients and is not helpful in assessing impact of hemoglobin dissociation curve shifts or carboxyhemoglobin.[46] Evaluation of metabolic acidemia or mixed venous oxygen content yields insight into peripheral oxygen delivery and utilization. Adequate arterial oxygenation does not mean that cardiac output, arterial perfusion pressure, or distribution of blood flow will maintain tissue oxygenation. Sepsis, hypotension, anemia, or hemoglobin dissociation abnormalities can generate tissue ischemia despite adequate oxygenation.

In postoperative patients, the acceptable lower limit for PaO_2 varies with individual patient characteristics. A PaO_2 below 65 to 70 mmHg causes significant hemoglobin desaturation, although tissue oxygen delivery might be maintained at lower levels. Maintaining PaO_2 between 80 and 100 mmHg (saturation 93% to 97%) ensures adequate oxygen availability. Little benefit is derived from elevating PaO_2 above 110 mmHg because hemoglobin is saturated and the amount of additional oxygen dissolved in plasma is negligible. During mechanical ventilation, a PaO_2 above 80 mmHg with 0.4 FiO_2 and 5-cm H_2O PEEP,[46] CPAP or spontaneous breathing trial usually predicts sustained adequate oxygenation after tracheal extubation.

Distribution of Ventilation

Loss of dependent lung volume commonly causes $\dot{V}/\dot{Q}$ mismatching and hypoxemia. A reduction in FRC decreases radial traction on small airways, leading to collapse and distal atelectasis that can worsen for 36 hours after surgery.[47] Reduced ventilation in dependent lung is particularly damaging because gravity directs pulmonary blood flow to dependent areas. Obese patients sustain large decreases in FRC during surgery. Older patients normally exhibit some airway closure at end expiration, and those with COPD have more severe closure that is exacerbated by small reductions in FRC. Retraction, packing, manipulation, or peritoneal insufflation during upper abdominal surgery reduces FRC, as does compression from leaning surgical assistants.[48] Prone, lithotomy, or Trendelenburg positions are disadvantageous, especially in obese patients. Right upper lobe collapse secondary to partial right main stem intubation is a frequently overlooked cause. During one-lung anesthesia, the weight of unsupported mediastinal contents, pressure from abdominal contents on the dependent diaphragm, and lung compression all reduce dependent lung volume. Gravity and lymphatic obstruction promote interstitial fluid accumulation and further $\dot{V}/\dot{Q}$ mismatching. This "down lung syndrome" may appear as unilateral pulmonary edema on the chest film.

Postoperatively, acute pulmonary edema from overhydration, ventricular dysfunction, airway obstruction, or increased capillary permeability (e.g., including TRALI, drug reactions) leads to hypoxemia by interfering with both $\dot{V}/\dot{Q}$ matching and diffusion of oxygen. Strong inspiratory efforts against an obstructed airway decrease FRC and promote negative-pressure pulmonary edema. Small airway occlusion from compression, retained secretions, or aspiration leads to distal hypoventilation and hypoxemia, as does main stem intubation. Pneumothorax or hemothorax also reduce lung volume.

Conservative measures that restore lung volume often improve oxygenation. If possible, patients should recover in a semisitting or reverse Trendelenburg position to reduce abdominal pressure on the diaphragms. Pain with ventilation encourages shallow breathing, so analgesia helps maintain FRC, especially with upper abdominal or chest wall incisions. Deep ventilation, cough, chest physiotherapy, and incentive spirometry seem to help expand FRC, mobilize secretions, and accustom a patient to incisional discomfort, but actual efficacy is debated.[49,50] For serious postoperative reduction of FRC, positive pressure is effective. CPAP (5 to 7 cm H_2O) or bilevel ventilation can be delivered by face mask for several hours until factors promoting loss of lung volume resolve. If hypoxemia is severe or patient acceptance of CPAP or the often more tolerable bilevel mask is poor, tracheal intubation is usually required. Intubation for delivery of noninvasive ventilation does not mandate positive-pressure ventilation. Ventilatory requirements should be assessed independently, considering Pa_{CO_2}, arterial pH, and work of breathing. Usually, 5 to 10 cm H_2O of CPAP or PEEP improves Pa_{O_2} without risking hypotension, increased intracranial pressure, or barotrauma. If Pa_{O_2} does not improve, one must re-evaluate the etiology. An occasional patient with ARDS or pulmonary contusion might require expiratory pressures in excess of 10 cm H_2O for improved oxygenation.

Tracheal intubation eliminates normal expiratory resistance and the "physiologic PEEP" (2 to 5 cm H_2O) that helps maintain lung volume during spontaneous ventilation. Exposing an intubated trachea to ambient pressure may cause a gradual reduction in FRC. Healthy, slender patients will often tolerate short periods of intubation without positive pressure, but generally it is prudent to use 5 cm H_2O CPAP for intubated postoperative patients.

Distribution of Perfusion

Poor distribution of pulmonary blood flow also interferes with $\dot{V}/\dot{Q}$ matching and oxygenation. Flow distribution is primarily determined by hydrodynamic factors (PA and venous pressures, vascular resistance), which are affected by gravity, airway pressure, lung volume, and cardiac dynamics. Flow distribution is modulated by hypoxic pulmonary vasoconstriction (HPV), which diverts flow from air spaces that exhibit low Pa_{O_2}. In postoperative patients, position affects oxygenation if gravity forces blood flow to areas with reduced ventilation. For example, placing a poorly ventilated lung in a dependent position can reduce Pa_{O_2}. Postoperative changes in PA pressure, airway pressure, and lung volume also have complex effects on blood flow distribution that can adversely affect $\dot{V}/\dot{Q}$ matching. Residual inhalation anesthetics, vasodilators, and sympathomimetics directly affect vascular tone and HPV, partially explaining larger alveolar-arterial oxygen gradients after general anesthesia. (Changes in distribution of ventilation also contribute.) Patients with liver cirrhosis exhibit poor $\dot{V}/\dot{Q}$ matching caused by small arteriovenous shunts that form throughout their lungs. Circulating endotoxin impairs HPV, contributing to hypoxemia in septic patients.

In the PACU, few interventions are useful to improve $\dot{V}/\dot{Q}$ matching by changing the distributions of pulmonary blood flow. It is best to maintain pulmonary arterial (PA) and airway pressures within an acceptable range. When possible, avoid placing an atelectatic or diseased lung in a dependent position. Placing poorly ventilated parenchyma in a nondependent position could improve $\dot{V}/\dot{Q}$ matching, but positioning a diseased lung in an "up" position may promote drainage of purulent material into the unaffected lung. Avoiding vasodilatory medications may improve Pa_{O_2} but benefits from the medication usually outweigh drawbacks of impaired HPV.

Inadequate Alveolar Pa_{O_2}

Postoperative hypoxemia is occasionally caused by a global reduction of Pa_{O_2}, usually from inadequate ventilation, and marked increase in Pa_{CO_2} (see the alveolar gas equation in Chapter 15). Hypoventilation must be severe to cause hypoxemia based on the alveolar gas equation, and can be completely masked by even small amounts of supplemental oxygen administration. Complete apnea or airway obstruction by a foreign body, soft-tissue edema, or laryngospasm as well as very high small airway resistance all lead to rapid depletion of alveolar oxygen, and preclude effective ventilation. If cessation of ventilation does occur, the rate of Pa_{O_2} decline varies with age, body habitus, degree of underlying illness, and initial Pa_{O_2} (Fig. 54-3).[41] Hypoxemia might also occur if opioids or residual anesthetic levels severely depress ventilatory drives. Partial airway obstruction does not usually reduce Pa_{O_2}, especially when patients are receiving supplemental oxygen. Increasing the oxygen content of the FRC with supplemental oxygen safeguards against hypoxemia from hypoventilation or airway obstruction, and eliminates the use of the pulse oximeter as a monitor of hypoventilation. Rarely, excessive concentrations of other gases reduce Pa_{O_2}. After general anesthesia, rapid outpouring of nitrous oxide displaces alveolar gas and can lower Pa_{O_2} if a patient is hypoventilating or breathing ambient air, but this "diffusion hypoxia" would usually occur before PACU admission. Volume displacement of oxygen could also occur during severe hypercarbia in a patient breathing ambient air, although acidemia is often a greater problem.

Reduced Mixed Venous $P\bar{v}_{O_2}$

Systemic venous partial pressure of oxygen $P\bar{v}_{O_2}$ is affected by >30 events/hour arterial oxygen content, cardiac output,

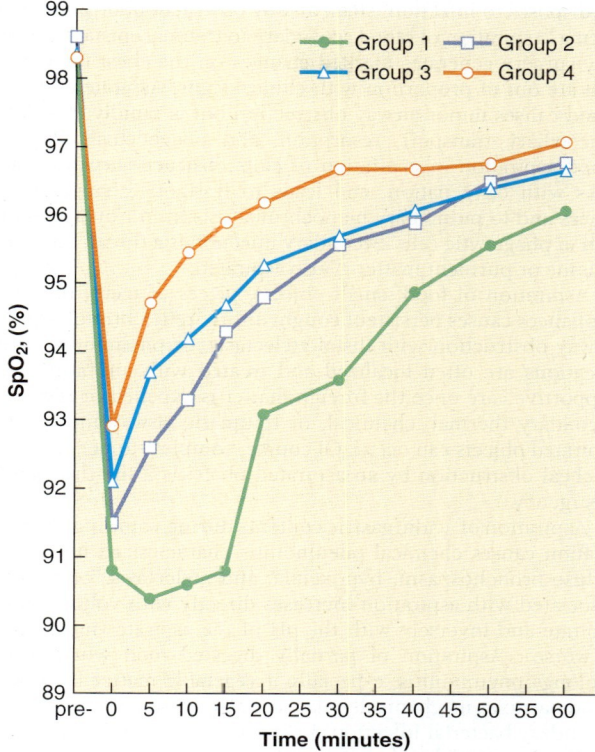

Figure 54-3 SpO₂ versus postanesthesia care unit time in patients spontaneously ventilating in room air after general anesthesia (Group 1, 0 to 1 year of age; group 2, 1 to 3 years; group 3, 3 to 14 years; group 4, 14 to 58 years). (Reprinted with permission from Xue FS, Huang YG, Tong SY, et al. A comparative study of early postoperative hypoxemia in infants, children, and adults undergoing elective plastic surgery. *Anesth Analg.* 1996;83:709.)

2% of women and 4% of men show overt symptoms of OSA.[51] These numbers are likely to increase as the population ages and become increasingly obese. In February 2014, the ASA Task Force on Perioperative Management of Patients with OSA issued guidelines based on the ASA scoring system for OSA and classifying patients as having mild, moderate, or severe OSA based on the apnea–hypopnea index (the number of apnea and hypopnea events per hour of sleep)[52]:

Mild OSA	apnea–hypopnea index	5–14 events/hour
Moderate OSA	apnea–hypopnea index	15–29 events/hour
Severe OSA	apnea–hypopnea index	>30 events/hour

The perioperative management of the OSA patient must start preoperatively with a well-planned anesthetic, taking into account the type, location, and recovery of surgery. Postoperative management concerns include analgesia, oxygenation, patient positioning, and monitoring. Regional anesthesia with minimal sedation is best for recovery versus increased use of opioids. Supplemental oxygen should be used immediately postoperatively. Patients who use CPAP or noninvasive positive-pressure ventilation should continue to use these therapies. Positioning should be used to minimize the patient's ability to obstruct the airway, which can be limited based on the type of surgery. Adult OSA patients show improvement in apnea–hypopnea index scores while in lateral, prone, and sitting positions compared with supine. With regard to monitoring, there is agreement among the consultants on the task force that pulse oximetry should be used until the patient's oxygen saturation remains above 90% on room air while sleeping. The use of telemetry for monitoring pulse oximetry, ECG, or ventilation can be beneficial in reducing adverse postoperative events and should be used on a patient need basis. With increasing studies in the area of OSA, the increased standardization of information regarding this patient population will lead to greater evidence-based treatment and supported clinical care.

Anemia

Preoperative hematocrit and intraoperative hemorrhage determine a patient's red cell mass and oxygen-carrying capacity after surgery. Reduction of hematocrit caused by dilution has less impact. The hematocrit at which oxygen delivery becomes insufficient to match tissue needs varies with cardiac reserve, oxygen consumption, hemoglobin dissociation, PaO₂, and blood flow distribution. The actual level at which shock, or lack of tissue oxygen delivery, occurs is known as the *critical DO₂ level*. For animals and humans who have normal myocardial function and are euvolemic, critical DO₂ requires at least 3 to 3.5 g/dL hemoglobin concentration. Of course, this level of hemoglobin may be too low to be an appropriate transfusion trigger. However, it does illustrate the large excess of hemoglobin available to meet metabolic O₂ demands. Each patient has a minimum hematocrit below which tissues use inefficient anaerobic metabolism, generating a lactic acidemia. Patients with vascular disease are at increased risk of vital organ ischemia as hematocrit falls. Work from the ASA and the cardiac anesthesia/surgery societies (Society of Thoracic surgeons and Society of Cardiovascular Anesthesiologists) published guidelines for transfusion and blood management. It is well accepted now that patients who are stable, not bleeding, and euvolemic can tolerate a hemoglobin of 6.0 g/dL. Transfusion may be of some benefit between 6 and 8 g/dL and it is rarely useful above 10 g/dL. Furthermore, transfusion of red cells to assist in weaning a patient from the ventilator has been shown to make the weaning process prolonged and/or make it far more difficult to discontinue mechanical ventilation.

distribution of peripheral blood flow, and tissue oxygen extraction. If arterial oxygen content decreases or tissue extraction increases, P$\bar{v}$O₂ falls. The lower the P$\bar{v}$O₂ in blood that is shunted or flows through low V̇/Q̇ units, the greater the reduction of PaO₂. Blood with a low P$\bar{v}$O₂ also extracts larger volumes of oxygen from alveolar gas, amplifying the effect of hypoventilation or airway obstruction on PaO₂. Very low P$\bar{v}$O₂ increases the risk of resorption atelectasis in poorly ventilated alveoli. In postoperative patients, shivering, infection, and hypermetabolism lower P$\bar{v}$O₂ by increasing peripheral oxygen extraction. Low cardiac output and hypotension also lower P$\bar{v}$O₂ by decreasing tissue oxygen delivery. Supplemental oxygen reduces the impact of low P$\bar{v}$O₂ on alveolar oxygen extraction and on arterial oxygenation.

Obstructive Sleep Apnea

Obstructive sleep apnea (OSA) is a syndrome in which patients exhibit a period of partial or complete obstruction of the upper airway. This obstruction in turn interrupts sleep patterns, resulting in daytime hypersomnolence, decreased ability to concentrate, increased irritability, as well as aggressive and distractible behavior in children. The airway obstruction may cause episodic oxygen desaturation, hypercarbia, and possibly lead to cardiac dysfunction. It is estimated that 9% of women and 24% of men in the United States show disordered breathing while asleep, and

Table 54-3 Common Oxygen Delivery Systems with Correlating O_2 Flow Rates to Delivered FiO_2 Ranges

System	O_2 Flow Rate (L/min)	FiO_2
Nasal cannula	1	0.21–0.24
	2	0.23–0.28
	3	0.27–0.32
	4	0.31–0.36
	5	0.35–0.40
	6	0.39–0.44
Simple mask	5	0.30–0.40
	8	0.40–0.60
Partial rebreathing mask	10	0.50–0.65
Nonrebreathing mask	10–15	0.60–near 1.00

Supplemental Oxygen

The incidence of hypoxemia in postoperative patients is high. In PACU patients placed on room air, 30% of patients younger than 1 year of age, 20% aged 1 to 3 years, 14% aged 3 to 14 years, and 7.8% of adults had hemoglobin saturations fall below 90%, with many falling below 85% (Fig. 54-3).[53] Clinical observation and assessment of cognitive function do not accurately screen for hypoxemia, so monitoring with pulse oximetry is essential throughout the PACU admission.[54] One cannot predict which patients will become hypoxemic or when hypoxemia will occur. Patients with lung disease or obesity, those recovering from thoracic or upper abdominal procedures, and those with preoperative hypoxemia are at increased risk.[55] Postoperative hypoxemia occurs in children, especially those with respiratory infections or chronic adenotonsillar hypertrophy. Hypoxemia occurs frequently after regional anesthesia.[21]

Supplemental oxygen should be administered only to patients at high risk of hypoxemia or with low SpO_2 readings (Table 54-3). However, some recommend supplemental oxygen be administered in the PACU during initial recovery and perhaps during transport to the PACU.[6] Supplemental oxygen does not address underlying causes of hypoxemia in postoperative patients, its use does not guarantee that hypoxemia will not occur, and it is likely to mask hypoventilation.[56] Although oxygen might cause minor mucosal drying, routine humidification is of little benefit unless intubation bypasses natural humidification. Oxygen apparatus can increase the risk of corneal abrasion during emergence.

2 Perioperative Aspiration

During anesthesia, depression of airway reflexes places patients at risk for intraoperative pulmonary aspiration that may manifest in the PACU, or for aspiration during recovery. Pulmonary morbidity from perioperative aspiration varies with the type and volume of the aspirate. Although aspiration of gastric contents is most widely feared, surgical patients also experience other aspiration syndromes.

Aspiration of clear oral secretions during induction, face mask ventilation, or emergence is common and usually insignificant. Cough, mild tracheal irritation, or transient laryngospasm are immediate sequelae, although large-volume aspiration predisposes to infection, small airway obstruction, or pulmonary edema. Aspiration of blood secondary to trauma, epistaxis, or airway surgery generates marked changes on the chest radiograph that are out of proportion with clinical signs. Aspirated "sterile" blood causes minor airway obstruction but is rapidly cleared by mucociliary transport, resorption, and phagocytosis. Massive blood aspiration or aspiration of clots obstructs airways, interferes with oxygenation, and leads to fibrinous changes in air spaces and to pulmonary hemochromatosis from iron accumulation in phagocytic cells. Secondary infection is a threat, especially if tissue or purulent matter is also aspirated.

Aspiration of food, small objects, pieces of teeth, or dental appliances causes persistent cough, diffuse reflex bronchospasm, airway obstruction with distal atelectasis, or pneumonia. Complications are often localized and treated with antibiotics and supportive care once the foreign matter is expelled or removed. Secondary thermal, chemical, or traumatic airway injury from aspirated objects can occur. Of course, complete upper airway or tracheal obstruction by an aspirated object is a life-threatening emergency.

Aspiration of acidic gastric contents during vomiting or regurgitation causes chemical pneumonitis characterized initially by diffuse bronchospasm, hypoxemia, and atelectasis.[57] Morbidity associated with aspiration increases directly with volume of the aspirate and inversely with the pH of the aspirate (more acidic is worse). Aspiration of partially digested food worsens and prolongs pneumonitis, especially if vegetable matter is present. Food particles mechanically obstruct airways and are a nidus for secondary bacterial infection. In serious cases, epithelial degeneration, interstitial and alveolar edema, and hemorrhage into air spaces rapidly progresses to ARDS with high-permeability pulmonary edema. Destruction of pneumocytes, decreased surfactant activity, hyaline membrane formation, and emphysematous changes can follow, leading to $\dot{V}/\dot{Q}$ mismatching and reduced compliance. Destruction of microvasculature increases pulmonary vascular resistance and deadspace ventilation.

The incidence of serious aspiration is relatively low in PACU patients, but the risk associated with aspiration is significant. Frequency of postoperative vomiting remains high, especially if gas has accumulated in the stomach. Protective airway reflexes such as cough, swallowing, and laryngospasm are suppressed by depressant medications such as inhalation anesthetics, sedatives, and opiates, so observe carefully patients with decreased levels of consciousness. Persisting effects of laryngeal nerve blocks or topical local anesthetics used to reduce airway irritability decrease postoperative airway protection, as does residual sedation. Reflexes are also impaired by residual neuromuscular paralysis.[44,58] Patients can sustain airway patency and spontaneous ventilation, pass a head lift test, have a tactile train-of-four T4/T1 ratio greater than 0.7, and still have impaired airway reflexes from residual paralysis. The T4/T1 ratio should exceed 0.9 before reflexes are completely competent.[58] Risk of aspiration also increases if reversal is omitted. Hypotension, hypoxemia, or acidemia cause both emesis and obtundation, increasing aspiration risk.

Preventing aspiration is critical because effective therapy is limited.[59] For patients at high risk, preoperative administration of nonparticulate antacids such as sodium citrate increases the pH of gastric fluid without excessively increasing volume. Avoid particulate antacids. Histamine type 2 receptor blockers such as famotidine or ranitidine reduce the volume and increase the pH of gastric secretions. Metoclopramide increases gastroesophageal sphincter tone and accelerates gastric emptying. Inserting a nasogastric tube is often ineffective to remove particulate matter and interferes with gastroesophageal sphincter integrity.

In the PACU, vigilance against aspiration is important. Trendelenburg position might promote regurgitation but aids in airway clearance if regurgitation or vomiting occurs. High-risk patients should not have the trachea extubated until airway reflexes are restored. Even though a patient is awake and able to follow commands he or she may still have depressed gag reflex for several hours after anesthesia. The introduction of opioids and other sedatives may turn a situation of relatively good airway protection into one of potential aspiration. Aspiration of acidic fluid can still occur around an inflated tracheal tube cuff, so nurses should frequently monitor the upper airway for secretions or vomitus. One should avoid cuff deflation until extubation because the rigid tube impairs laryngospasm, swallowing, and other protective reflexes. The pharynx should be suctioned and the trachea extubated at end inspiration with positive airway pressure to promote expulsion of material trapped below the cords but above the inflated cuff. Observation is essential after extubation because airway reflexes might be temporarily impaired. Anatomic distortion in the airway from soft tissue trauma or surgical intervention interferes with airway protection. Mandibular fixation makes expulsion of vomitus, blood, or secretions difficult, so have equipment for release of mandibular fixation available and ensure patients demonstrate cognitive and physical ability to clear the airway before the trachea is extubated.

Discovery of gastric secretions in the pharynx mandates immediate lateral head positioning (assuming cervical spine integrity) and suction of the airway. If airway reflexes are compromised, tracheal intubation is often appropriate. After intubation, the trachea is suctioned through the tracheal tube before positive-pressure ventilation, thus avoiding wide dissemination of aspirated material into distal airways. Instillation of saline or alkalotic solutions is not recommended. Assessing the pH of tracheal aspirate is useless because buffering is immediate. Checking pharyngeal aspirate pH is more accurate but of little practical value. Suspicion that aspiration has occurred mandates 24 to 48 hours of monitoring for development of aspiration pneumonitis. If the likelihood of aspiration is small in an ambulatory patient, outpatient follow-up can be done, assuming hypoxemia, cough, wheezing, or radiographic abnormalities do not appear within 4 to 6 hours. The patient should receive explicit instructions to contact a medical facility at the first appearance of malaise, fever, cough, chest pain, or other symptoms of pneumonitis. If likelihood of aspiration is high, the patient should be admitted to the hospital. Observation includes serial temperature checks, white blood cell counts with differential, chest radiograph, and blood gas determination. Chest physiotherapy, incentive spirometry, and restarting medications for pre-existing pulmonary conditions minimize the loss of lung volume, V̇/Q̇ mismatching, and infection. Fluffy infiltrates may appear on the chest radiograph any time within 24 hours. Hypoxemia might develop quickly or evolve insidiously as injury progresses, so frequent pulse oximetry monitoring is important.

If hypoxemia, increased airway resistance, consolidation, or pulmonary edema evolves, the patient should be supported with supplemental oxygen, PEEP, or CPAP. Mechanical ventilation may be necessary. Steroids yield no improvement and may increase the risk of bacterial superinfection. Bacterial infection does not always follow aspiration, so prophylactic antibiotics merely promote colonization by resistant organisms. If bacterial infection is apparent, institute antibiotic therapy based on culture results. If cultures are equivocal, use broad-spectrum antibiotics with coverage for Gram-negative rods and anaerobes, including *Bacteroides fragilis*. Overall therapy is similar to that for ARDS. Pulmonary edema from increased capillary permeability should not be treated with diuretics unless high filling pressures or hypervolemia exist.

Postoperative Renal Complications

Ability to Void

The ability to void should be assessed because opioids and autonomic side effects of regional anesthesia interfere with sphincter relaxation and promote urine retention. Urinary retention is common after urologic, inguinal, and genital surgery, and retention frequently delays discharge.[3] Observation after these operations is needed to determine if inability to urinate is a possible surgical complication. Neither the patient nor staff can accurately estimate bladder volume through sensation or palpation. An ultrasonic bladder scan helps assess bladder volume before discharge and avoid the archaic practice of routine "straight catheterization." It is reasonable to discharge selected ambulatory patients from the facility and inpatients to a floor before they void.[6,60,61] When inpatients are transferred prior to voiding, ensure urination can be monitored to avoid complications from urinary retention. Ambulatory patients who are discharged without voiding should receive a specific time interval in which to void (i.e., 10 to 12 hours after discharge). If retention persists, the patient must contact a health-care facility. High return rates after urologic procedures are related to urinary retention.[62]

Renal Tubular Function

Analysis of urine yields information about postoperative renal tubular function. Urine color is not useful for assessing concentrating ability, but it does assist recognition of hematuria, hemoglobinuria, or pyuria. Urine osmolarity (reflecting the number of particles in solution) is a more reliable index of tubular function than specific gravity, which is affected by molecular weight of solutes. An osmolarity above 450 mOsm/L indicates intact tubular concentrating ability. A urine sodium concentration far below or a potassium concentration above serum concentrations also indicates tubular viability, as does acidification or alkalinization of urine. Osmolarity, electrolyte, and pH values close to those in serum may indicate poor tubular function or acute tubular necrosis.

Inorganic fluoride released during metabolism of certain inhalation anesthetics (sevoflurane, enflurane, and methoxyflurane) can cause a transient reduction of tubular concentrating ability after long anesthetics. Higher fluoride levels cause renal tubular necrosis. Interaction of sevoflurane with dry carbon dioxide absorbents (often found in first cases or peripheral locations) generates compound A, a vinyl ether that degrades to release inorganic fluoride. Although transient impairment of protein retention and concentrating ability may occur, use of sevoflurane does not seriously affect renal function. This complication may be avoided entirely if lithium-based CO_2 absorbents are used.

Oliguria

Oliguria (≤0.5 mL/kg/hr) occurs frequently during recovery and usually reflects an appropriate renal response to hypovolemia. The stress response of surgery also increases antidiuretic hormone (ADH), which can lead to decreased urine output. However, decreased urine output might indicate abnormal renal function. The acceptable degree and duration of oliguria vary with baseline renal status, the surgical procedure, and the anticipated postoperative course. In patients without catheters, one should assess interval since last voiding, and bladder volume, to help differentiate oliguria from inability to void. One should check indwelling urinary catheters for kinking, for obstruction by blood clots or debris, and for the catheter tip being positioned above the urinary level in the bladder, and aggressively evaluate oliguria if intraoperative events could jeopardize renal function (e.g., aortic cross-clamping, severe hypotension, possible ureteral ligature, massive transfusion). Systemic blood pressure must be adequate for renal perfusion, based on preoperative pressures. Administration of desmopressin for hematologic purposes seldom affects postoperative urinary output. After urine is sent for electrolyte and osmolarity determinations, a 300- to 500-mL intravenous crystalloid bolus helps assess whether oliguria represents a renal response to hypovolemia. If output does not improve, consider a larger bolus or a diagnostic trial of furosemide, 5 mg intravenously. Furosemide increases urine output if oliguria reflects tubular resorption of fluid. Patients receiving chronic diuretic therapy might require a diuretic to maintain postoperative urine output.

Persistence of oliguria despite hydration, adequate perfusion pressure, and a furosemide challenge increases the likelihood of acute tubular necrosis, ureteral obstruction, renal artery or vein occlusion, or inappropriate ADH secretion. Cystoscopy, intravenous pyelography, angiography, or radionuclide scanning may help clarify renal status. Osmotic or loop diuretics may be useful to attenuate renal damage. The use of low-dose dopamine or dobutamine has not proven to improve renal function. Fenoldopam used perioperatively has been shown to reduce the risk of acute kidney injury for select high-risk cardiac surgical patients.[63] Consultation with a nephrologist is prudent.

Polyuria

Relying on high postoperative urinary output to gauge intravascular volume status or renal viability can be misleading. Profuse urine output often reflects generous intraoperative fluid administration, but osmotic diuresis caused by hyperglycemia and glycosuria is another common cause, particularly if glucose-containing crystalloid solutions are infusing. Polyuria might also reflect intraoperative diuretic administration. However, sustained polyuria (4 to 5 mL/kg/hr) can indicate abnormal regulation of water clearance or high-output renal failure, especially if urinary losses compromise intravascular volume and systemic blood pressure. Diabetes insipidus occurs secondary to intracranial surgery, pituitary ablation, head trauma, or increased intracranial pressure. A urine specific gravity of 1.005 or less and a urine osmolality 200 mOsm/kg or less are the hallmark of diabetes insipidus. A random plasma osmolality is generally above 285 mOsm/kg. Diagnostic or therapeutic administration of vasopressin is useful.

Metabolic Complications
Postoperative Acid–Base Disorders

Categorization of postoperative acid–base abnormalities into primary and compensatory disorders is difficult because rapidly changing pathophysiology can often generate multiple primary disorders.

Respiratory Acidemia

Respiratory acidemia is frequently encountered in PACU patients because anesthetics, opioids, and sedatives promote hypoventilation by depressing CNS sensitivity to pH and Pa_{CO_2}. In awake, spontaneously breathing patients with adequate analgesia, hypercarbia and acidemia are usually mild (Pa_{CO_2} 45 to 50 mmHg, pH 7.36 to 7.32). Deeply sedated patients exhibit more profound acidemia unless supplemental ventilation is administered. Patients with residual neuromuscular paralysis, increased airway resistance, or decreased pulmonary compliance might not sustain adequate ventilation despite an intact CNS drive, especially if CO_2 production is elevated by fever, shivering, or hyperalimentation. The kidneys require hours to generate a compensatory metabolic alkalosis, so compensation for acute postoperative respiratory acidemia is limited.

Symptoms of respiratory acidemia include agitation, confusion, ventilatory dissatisfaction, and tachypnea. Sympathetic nervous system response to low pH causes hypertension, tachycardia, and dysrhythmias. Respiratory acidemia caused by CNS depression often produces less intense signs of sympathetic nervous system activity. In patients with head injury, intracranial tumors, or cerebral edema, respiratory acidemia increases cerebral blood flow and intracranial pressure. At very low pH, catecholamines cannot interact with adrenergic receptors, so heart rate and blood pressure decrease precipitously. Treatment consists of correcting the imbalance between CO_2 production and alveolar ventilation. Raising the level of consciousness by the judicious reversal of opioids or benzodiazepines improves ventilatory drive. It is important to ensure that the patient does not have increased airway resistance or residual neuromuscular blockade. If spontaneous ventilation cannot maintain CO_2 excretion, tracheal intubation and mechanical ventilation are necessary. Reducing CO_2 production by controlling fever or shivering may be helpful.

Metabolic Acidemia

Evaluation of acute postoperative metabolic acidemia is relatively straightforward (Table 54-4). Occasionally, ketoacidosis occurs in diabetic patients. During ketoacidosis, serum glucose levels are elevated and ketones are detectable in blood or urine. Patients with renal failure or renal tubular acidosis usually exhibit a preoperative metabolic acidemia. Large volumes of saline infusions during surgery can generate a mild hyperchloremic, metabolic

Table 54-4 Causes of Acidemia
Normal anion gap acidosis
GI loss of bicarbonate
Diarrhea
Urinary diversion
GI fistulas or drains
Renal loss of bicarbonate
Renal tubular acidosis
Renal insufficiency
Recovery phase of ketoacidosis
Increased anion gap acidosis
Ketoacidosis (diabetic, alcoholic, severe cachexia)
Lactic acidosis (seizures, neuroleptic malignant syndrome, MH, severe asthma, pheochromocytoma, cardiogenic shock, hypovolemia, severe anemia, regional ischemia, sepsis, hypoglycemia)
Respiratory acidosis

GI, gastrointestinal; MH, malignant hyperthermia.

acidemia, but use of lactated Ringer solution avoids this problem.[64] Rarely, a patient manifests acidemia from toxic ingestion of aspirin or methanol. Once these unusual causes are excluded, postoperative metabolic acidemia almost always represents lactic acidemia secondary to insufficient delivery or utilization of oxygen in peripheral tissues. Peripheral hypoperfusion is often caused by low cardiac output (hypovolemia, cardiac failure, dysrhythmia) or peripheral vasodilation (sepsis, catecholamine depletion, sympathectomy). Arteriolar constriction from hypothermia or pressor administration reduces tissue perfusion and induces abnormal blood flow distribution. Hypoxemia, severe anemia, impaired hemoglobin dissociation, CO poisoning, and inability to use oxygen in the mitochondria (cyanide or arsenic poisoning) also generate lactic acidemia.

A spontaneously breathing patient will increase minute ventilation in response to metabolic acidemia and quickly generate a respiratory alkalosis to compensate for metabolic acidemia. However, general anesthetics and analgesics suppress this ventilatory response. The sympathetic response to acute postoperative metabolic acidemia is often milder than the response to respiratory acidemia because hydrogen and bicarbonate ions cross the blood–brain barrier with more difficulty than CO_2. Treatment consists of resolving the condition causing accumulation of metabolic acid. For example, ketoacidosis is treated with intravenous potassium, insulin, and glucose. Improving cardiac output or systemic blood pressure will reduce lactic acid production, as will rewarming. If conditions causing lactate accumulation are improved and acidemia is mild, renal excretion of hydrogen ions will restore normal pH. For severe or progressive acidemia, intravenous bicarbonate or calcium gluconate helps restore pH.

Respiratory Alkalemia

Pain or anxiety during emergence causes hyperventilation and acute respiratory alkalemia. Excessive mechanical ventilation also generates respiratory alkalemia, especially if hypothermia or paralysis has decreased CO_2 production. Pathologic causes of "central" hyperventilation include sepsis, cerebrovascular accident, or paradoxic CNS acidosis (an imbalance of bicarbonate concentration across the blood–brain barrier caused by prolonged hyperventilation). Acute respiratory alkalemia can generate confusion, dizziness, atrial dysrhythmias, and abnormal cardiac conduction. Alkalemia decreases cerebral blood flow, causing hypoperfusion and even stroke in patients with cerebrovascular disease. If the alkalemia is severe, reduced serum ionized calcium concentration precipitates muscle fasciculation or hypocalcemic tetany. Very high pH depresses cardiovascular, CNS, and catecholamine receptor functions. Metabolic compensation for acute respiratory alkalemia is limited because time constants for bicarbonate excretion are large. Treatment necessitates reducing alveolar ventilation, usually by administering analgesics and sedatives for pain and anxiety. Rebreathing of CO_2 has little application in the PACU.

Metabolic Alkalemia

Metabolic alkalemia is rare in PACU patients unless vomiting, gastric suctioning, dehydration, alkaline ingestion, or potassium-wasting diuretics caused an alkalemia that existed before surgery. Excessive intraoperative bicarbonate administration causes postoperative metabolic alkalemia, but alkalemia from metabolism of lactate or citrate usually does not appear within the first 24 hours. Respiratory compensation through retention of CO_2 is rapid but limited because hypoventilation eventually causes hypoxemia. Hydration and correction of hypochloremia and hypokalemia allow the kidney to excrete excess bicarbonate.

Glucose Disorders and Control

Adequate glucose control has been recommended to reduce morbidity in a variety of postsurgical patients. The control of glucose in diabetic and nondiabetic patients has been shown to reduce complications and hospital length of stay and improve patient outcomes. However, the potential for hypoglycemia and coma should not be discounted. Insulin therapy should be based on serum glucose levels and requires careful and timely monitoring of blood glucose levels to avoid hypoglycemia. This includes clear and concise hand off of information when patient care is transferred. Urine glucose measurements should be reserved to assess osmotic diuresis and estimate renal transport thresholds by comparison with serum levels.

Hyperglycemia

Glucose infusions and stress responses commonly elevate serum glucose levels after surgery. For most patients during anesthesia, glucose should not be included in maintenance intravenous solutions. Moderate postoperative hyperglycemia (150 to 250 mg/dL) resolves spontaneously and has little adverse effect in the nondiabetic patient. Higher glucose levels cause glycosuria with osmotic diuresis and interfere with serum electrolyte determinations. Severe hyperglycemia increases serum osmolality to a point that cerebral disequilibrium and hyperosmolar coma occur. Type 1 diabetic patients are at risk for ketoacidosis. Potassium replacement and serial blood glucose determinations are essential.

Hypoglycemia

Hypoglycemia in the PACU can be caused by endogenous insulin secretion or by excessive or inadvertent insulin administration. Serious postoperative hypoglycemia is rare and easily treated with intravenous 50% dextrose followed by glucose infusion. Either sedation or excessive sympathetic nervous system activity masks signs and symptoms of hypoglycemia after anesthesia. Diabetic patients and especially patients who have received insulin therapy intraoperatively must have serum glucose levels measured to avoid the serious problems related to hypoglycemia. Extreme care with documenting and reporting the use of insulin is paramount to provide safe and appropriate care.

Electrolyte Disorders

Hyponatremia

Postoperative hyponatremia occurs if free water is infused during surgery or if sodium-free irrigating solution is absorbed during transurethral prostatic resection or hysteroscopy. Accumulation of serum glycine or its metabolite, ammonia, might exacerbate symptoms. Free water retention is also caused by inappropriate ADH secretion, prolonged labor induction with oxytocin, or respiratory uptake of nebulized droplets. Theoretically, excessive infusion of isotonic saline leads to excretion of hypertonic urine, desalination, and iatrogenic hyponatremia. Symptoms of moderate hyponatremia include agitation, disorientation, visual disturbances, and nausea, whereas severe hyponatremia causes unconsciousness, impaired airway reflexes, and CNS irritability that progress to grand mal seizures. Therapy includes intravenous normal saline and intravenous furosemide to promote free water excretion. Infusion of hypertonic saline may be useful for severe hyponatremia, in which diligence not to increase serum sodium by 0.5 mEq/hr is needed to avoid CNS lesions or pulmonary edema. Monitor serum sodium concentration and osmolarity.

Hypokalemia

Postoperative hypokalemia is often inconsequential but might generate serious dysrhythmias, especially in patients taking digoxin. A potassium deficit caused by chronic diuretic therapy, nasogastric suctioning, or vomiting often underlies hypokalemia. Urinary and hemorrhagic losses, dilution, and insulin therapy generate acute hypokalemia that worsens during respiratory alkalemia. Excess sympathetic nervous system activity, infusion of calcium, or β-mimetic medications exacerbates effects of hypokalemia. Adding potassium to peripheral intravenous fluids often restores serum concentration, but concentrated solutions infused through a central catheter may be necessary. So often practitioners think 10 to 30 mEq of potassium will bring the patient back to normal. Potassium is an intracellular ion and a plasma potassium deficit is indicative of a far greater intracellular deficit. It is the intracellular-to-extracellular ratio that may well be important, and rapid changes can contribute to as many dysrhythmias as can mild hypokalemia alone.

Hyperkalemia

A high serum potassium level raises the suspicion of spurious hyperkalemia from a hemolyzed specimen or from sampling near an intravenous catheter containing potassium or banked blood. Postoperative hyperkalemia occurs after excessive potassium infusion or in patients with renal failure or malignant hyperthermia. Acute acidemia exacerbates hyperkalemia. Treatment with intravenous insulin and glucose acutely lowers potassium, whereas intravenous calcium counters myocardial effects. Hemodialysis may be necessary for high potassium levels or symptomatic patients.

Calcium and Magnesium

Although underlying parathyroid disease or massive fluid replacement reduces total body and ionized calcium, symptomatic hypocalcemia seldom occurs in the PACU. A rare patient might exhibit upper airway obstruction from hypocalcemia after parathyroid excision. Reduction of the ionized fraction by acute alkalemia may cause myocardial conduction and contractility abnormalities, decreased vascular tone, or tetany. Transfusion of blood containing chelating agents (e.g., citrate) rarely causes symptomatic hypocalcemia. Administration of calcium chloride or calcium gluconate to hypocalcemic patients improves cardiovascular dynamics.

Magnesium plays a key role in restoration of neuromuscular function after surgery and in maintenance of cardiac rhythm and conduction. Hypermagnesemia is rare because the kidneys are effective at excreting excessive magnesium. Obstetric patients who have been receiving magnesium for tocolysis or control of severe pregnancy-induced hypertension can present postoperatively hyporeflexivity, and at higher serum levels show prolonged atrioventricular conduction or complete heart block. Treatment entails intravenous calcium and diuretics.

Miscellaneous Complications

Incidental Trauma

Each patient admitted to the PACU should be carefully evaluated for traumatic complications. Discovery of a complication necessitates careful documentation, notification of physicians responsible for extended care, consultation with specialists, and follow-up.

Ocular Injuries and Visual Changes

Corneal abrasion caused by drying or by inadvertent eye contact during face mask ventilation or intubation is a common intraoperative eye injury. The incidence of this type of injury in a nonophthalmic patient is estimated to be between 0.034 and 0.17%, with the higher incidence related to prone or lateral positioning.[65] Corneal injury can occur during emergence in the PACU from patients rubbing their eyes, if a rigid oxygen face mask rides up on the eye, or if the eye is rubbed with a pulse oximeter probe and from eye make-up being rubbed in the eyes. Abrasions cause tearing, decreased visual acuity, pain, and photophobia. Fluorescein staining aids diagnosis. Abrasions usually heal spontaneously within 72 hours without scarring, but severe injury can cause cataract formation and impair vision. There is no standard treatment for corneal abrasions, but symptomatic treatment includes artificial tears, topical antibiotics, topical analgesics, and eye closure. Daily follow-up with patients with corneal abrasions should be done to verify healing and rule out other causes. If a patient has not had improvement in 48 hours, consultation with an ophthalmologist should be made.

Visual acuity is often impaired after anesthesia. Autonomic side effects of medications impair accommodation, and residual ocular lubricant clouds vision. Impairment of retinal perfusion by ocular compression generates postoperative visual disturbances ranging from loss of acuity to permanent blindness.[66,67] Ischemic optic atrophy can also occur in the absence of external compression.[68] Risk of blindness is higher after long procedures in the prone position, as well as in patients with vascular disease, pre-existing hypertension, diabetes, and sickle cell anemia. A significant percentage of postoperative patients suffer deficits in acuity unrelated to ocular trauma, some of whom require permanent refractive adjustment.[69] Anesthesiologists should be alert for visual impairment and check acuity when assessing patients at higher risk for ischemic optic atrophy.

Hearing Impairment

Hearing impairment after anesthesia and surgery is relatively common.[70] Although impairment is often subclinical, patients sometimes experience decreased auditory acuity, tinnitus, or roaring. Incidence of detectable hearing impairment is particularly high after dural puncture for spinal anesthesia (8% to 16%), and varies with needle size, needle type, and patient age. Impairment can be unilateral or bilateral and usually resolves spontaneously. Hearing loss also occurs after general anesthesia for both noncardiac and cardiac surgery, and is often related to disruption of the round window or tympanic membrane rupture. Eustachian tube inflammation and otitis secondary to endotracheal intubation can also impact hearing.

Oral, Pharyngeal, and Laryngeal Injuries

Laryngoscope blades, surgical instruments, rigid oral airways, and dentition can all cause trauma of oral soft tissues. Lip, tongue, or gum abrasions are treated with an ice pack and analgesia. Penetrating injuries caused by tissue entrapment between teeth and rigid devices may require topical antibiotics. After a traumatic tracheal intubation, hematoma or edema might cause partial upper airway obstruction. Nebulized racemic epinephrine often improves stridor more quickly than steroids. Dental damage can occur during airway manipulations or during emergence if a patient bites on a rigid oral airway or forcefully clenches his or her teeth. Document tooth or dental appliance damage, obtain a dental consultation, and observe for signs of foreign body aspiration.[71]

Sore throat and hoarseness after tracheal intubation occur in 20% to 50% of patients, depending on the degree of trauma during laryngoscopy and oropharyngeal suctioning, the duration of intubation, and the type of endotracheal tube. Mucosal irritation also presents as an unquenchable dryness in mouth and throat. The use of local anesthetic ointments to lubricate endotracheal tubes may cause additional mucosal irritation. Topical viscous lidocaine attenuates irritation from nasogastric tubes but may increase risk of aspiration during recovery. In children, the severity of postextubation laryngeal edema or tracheitis varies with age, intubation duration, and degree of trauma or tube movement. Most recover with cool mist therapy, but nebulized racemic epinephrine and dexamethasone may be needed in more severe cases. Laryngoscopy and intubation can also cause hypoglossal, lingual, or recurrent laryngeal nerve damage, vocal cord evulsion, desquamation of laryngeal or tracheal mucosa, edema or ulceration, and tracheal perforation. Postoperative sore throat and dysphagia also occurs without intubation, related to use of laryngeal mask airways,[72] oral airways, trauma from suctioning, or drying from unhumidified gases. Neck and jaw soreness is commonly seen after face mask anesthetics.

Nerve Injuries

Nerve injuries caused by improper positioning during anesthesia generate serious long-term complications.[73] Spinal cord injury can be caused by positioning for intubation or by hematoma accumulation after placement of neuraxial anesthetics. Peripheral nerve compression during general or regional anesthesia sometimes causes permanent sensory and motor deficits, as do stretch injuries from hyperextension of an extremity.[74] Any bruising or skin breakdown noted postoperatively should prompt evaluation for underlying nerve damage. Many postoperative neuropathies have no identifiable cause, particularly for ulnar neuropathy, which may be related to subtle positioning problems, pre-existing impairment, or sensitivity of the nerve to ischemia.[75] Every complaint of nonsurgical pain, numbness, or weakness from a postoperative patient should be carefully evaluated. In the event of neuropathic weakness, electromyographic studies may determine the location of the lesion and possible reversibility of the nerve deficit. Sensory neuropathies rarely last longer than 5 days and should be referred to a neurologist if the deficit exceeds this time or if it progresses.[76]

Postdural puncture headache may first occur in the PACU, although most appear within 24 to 48 hours. Headache is more frequent after difficult subarachnoid anesthesia with multiple attempts and after dural puncture during attempted epidural placement. Subarachnoid air bubbles from loss-of-resistance testing may contribute. In the PACU, treatment is supportive with hydration, analgesics, and positioning. In severe cases, early intervention with the definitive treatment of epidural blood patch might be considered. Nerve injury secondary to needle contact or intraneuronal injection during placement of regional anesthesia is rare but does occur.[74,77] In one study, 6.3% of 4,767 patients experienced paresthesia during placement of spinal anesthesia, but only 0.126% had persisting symptoms.[78] In the PACU, patients often complain of pain, focal numbness, residual paresthesia, or dysesthesia. Symptoms are usually transient. Administer analgesia, reassure the patient, document findings, and follow for the possibility of an evolving neurologic deficit.

During recovery from spinal anesthesia, some patients exhibit lower extremity discomfort, buttock pain, and other signs of sacral or lumbar neurologic irritation. This problem is more common in obese patients, after procedures in lithotomy position, and after spinal anesthesia with 5% lidocaine.[77] Symptoms are transient and treated supportively. Rarely, a patient exhibits headache and meningeal signs caused by chemical meningitis after injection of a spinal drug that is contaminated or outside the acceptable pH range.

Soft Tissue and Joint Injuries

If pressure points are improperly padded, soft tissue ischemia and necrosis occur, especially with lateral or prone positioning. Prolonged scalp pressure causes localized alopecia, whereas entrapment of ears, breasts, genitalia, or skin folds causes inflammation or necrosis. Regional ischemia from major arterial compression is rare. Thermal, electrical, or chemical burns from cautery equipment, preparatory solutions, or adhesives also occur. Extravasation of intravenous medications or fluids can cause sloughing, localized chemical neuropathy, or compartment syndromes. Excessive joint or muscle extension leads to postoperative backache, joint pain, stiffness, and even joint instability. After regional anesthesia, extremities must be properly secured and padded to prevent nerve injury.

Skeletal Muscle Pain

Postoperative muscle pain is caused by many intraoperative factors. Prolonged lack of motion or unusual muscle stretch during positioning often contributes to muscle stiffness and aching. Postoperative myalgia has been reported to range between 5% and 83% of patients after the use of succinylcholine,[79] whereas the pathogenesis of this myalgia remains unclear.[77,80] Acute myalgia also occurs after administration of other relaxants and in patients receiving no relaxant. Delayed-onset muscle fatigue can appear days after surgery and resolves spontaneously.

Hypothermia and Shivering

Although intraoperative temperature maintenance is a goal, patients still exhibit postoperative hypothermia. During anesthesia, heat is redistributed and also is lost by evaporation during skin preparation, by humidification of dry gases in the airway, and by radiation and convection from the skin and wound. Temperature reduction is accelerated by cold intravenous fluids and low ambient temperatures. The thermoregulatory threshold, below which humans actively regulate body temperature, is decreased during general anesthesia and is less effective under anesthesia. Ability to maintain body temperature is also compromised because paralysis and anesthesia impair shivering and thermoregulatory vasoconstriction, and because nonshivering thermogenesis is ineffective in adults. Rate of heat loss is similar during general or regional anesthesia, but rewarming is slower after regional anesthesia because residual vasodilation and paralysis impede heat generation and retention. Cachectic, traumatized, or burned patients experience greater temperature reduction, as do infants because of a low ratio of body mass-to-surface area.

Hypothermia complicates and prolongs care in the PACU.[81] Average PACU stay is increased by 40 to 90 minutes for hypothermic patients.[82] Postoperative hypothermia increases sympathetic nervous system activity with increased epinephrine and norepinephrine levels,[83] elevates peripheral vascular resistance, and decreases venous capacitance. Risk of myocardial ischemia[84] and dysrhythmia from mechanical myocardial stimulation is increased. Vasoconstriction interferes with the reliability of pulse oximetry and intra-arterial pressure monitoring. Hypoperfusion jeopardizes marginal tissue grafts and promotes tissue hypoxia and metabolic acidemia. The higher affinity of hemoglobin compromises oxygen unloading to hypothermic tissues. Platelet sequestration, decreased platelet function, and reduced clotting factor function contribute to coagulopathy. Moderate hyperglycemia occurs, cellular immune responses are compromised, and postoperative infection rates increase.[85] A decrease in the minimal alveolar concentration of inhalation anesthetics (5% to 7% per 1°C cooling) accentuates residual sedation. Low perfusion and impaired biotransformation might increase the duration of neuromuscular relaxants and sedatives. Moderate hypothermia (28° to 32°C) is associated with cardiac dysrhythmias. Severe hypothermia (≤28°C) interferes with cardiac rhythm generation and impulse conduction. On ECG, the PR, QRS, or QT intervals lengthen, and J waves appear. Spontaneous ventricular fibrillation occurs at temperatures less than 28°C.

During emergence, hypothalamic regulation generates shivering to increase endogenous heat production.[86] Shivering increases the risk of incidental trauma, disrupts medical devices, and interferes with ECG and pulse oximetry monitoring. Oxygen consumption and CO_2 production can increase 200%. Associated increases in minute ventilation and cardiac output might precipitate ventilatory failure in patients with limited reserve or myocardial ischemia in those with coronary artery disease.[84] Shivering is accentuated by tremors related to emergence from inhalation anesthesia. Tremors exhibit clonic and tonic components, and likely reflect decreased cortical influence on spinal cord reflexes.

Restoration of normothermia is an important goal during recovery. Forced-air warming devices are the most efficacious for treating hypothermia. Intravenous fluids and blood should be warmed. For most patients, shivering from mild-to-moderate hypothermia is uncomfortable but self-limited, and needs no treatment other than rewarming and reassurance. Many medications have been recommended to suppress shivering, but meperidine is most effective in conjunction rewarming.[6] Fentanyl has also been used with patients in whom meperidine is contraindicated. Withholding reversal of relaxants in ventilated, sedated patients attenuates shivering but increases rewarming time. If temperature is near normal (>36°C) and shivering is resolved, transfer from PACU to an inpatient floor or a discharge area is acceptable.

The Surgical Care Improvement Project sponsored by CMS, The Joint Commission (TJC), and other national partners is a program that uses several quality measures to help improve the safety and outcomes of surgical patients. One of those measures important to anesthesiologists is maintaining a patient's temperature above 36°C. Although this measure really begins with care in the operating room, the PACU has a 15-minute period from admission to observe a measured patient temperature of at least 36°C. Maintaining adequate temperature has been shown to reduce wound infections in surgical patients, producing better outcomes and reducing length of stay complications.

Hyperthermia

Hyperthermia is relatively uncommon in the PACU. Occasionally, a patient exhibits short-lived hyperthermia from close draping or aggressive intraoperative heat preservation. Postoperative fever sometimes reflects a pre-existing infection (e.g., sinusitis, upper respiratory or urinary tract infection) or an infection exacerbated by the surgical procedure (e.g., resection of infected tonsils or appendix, abscess drainage, urinary tract manipulation). Elevated temperature might indicate a drug or transfusion reaction. Muscarinic blocking agents such as atropine interfere with cooling and might contribute to fever, but they are seldom the cause in adults. Other hypermetabolic states such as thyroid storm must be considered. High fever occurs with malignant hyperthermia, but signs such as tachycardia, muscle rigidity, dysrhythmia, hyperventilation, and acidemia establish the diagnosis first.

Ambient cooling, chest physiotherapy, incentive spirometry, and antipyretics are usually sufficient to treat postoperative fever. One should withhold offending medications or blood products if a drug or transfusion reaction is suspected and notify the physician responsible for extended care to ensure postdischarge evaluation. Therapy for thyroid storm or malignant hyperthermia is well described elsewhere.

Persistent Sedation/Delayed Emergence

Approximately 90% of patients regain consciousness within 15 minutes of admission to the PACU; unconsciousness persisting for a greater period is considered prolonged. Even a highly susceptible patient should respond to a stimulus within 30 to 45 minutes after a reasonably conducted anesthetic. In a patient with prolonged sedation, one should research the level of preoperative responsiveness to uncover intoxication with drugs and alcohol or pre-existing mental dysfunction. One should note the time and amount of preoperative and intraoperative sedative medications, and review any unusual intraoperative events. The rate and character of spontaneous ventilation helps judge residual opioid effect; opioids are the *only* class of drugs that cause decreased respiratory rate. Physical assessment should include a tactile stimulus such as a light skin pinch, which elicits greater arousal than verbal stimulation, perhaps because sensory input is amplified through the reticular activating system. Diagnostic value of pupillary response is low.

Residual sedation from inhalation anesthetics might cause prolonged unconsciousness in obese patients, especially after long procedures, or when high concentrations are continued through the end of surgery. Prolonged sedation is less likely after anesthesia with low solubility agents such as sevoflurane or desflurane. Premedications that have sedative effects (e.g., diphenhydramine, hydroxyzine, promethazine, droperidol, lorazepam, midazolam, meclizine, and scopolamine) contribute to postoperative somnolence. Sedation from intraoperative opioid or sedative administration is dose-related. Opioids are the only drugs that cause bradypnea; thus, regardless of what other drug effects are present, if the respiratory rate is less than 14 to 16, then opioids are clearly affecting the patient's level of consciousness. To assess sedation from opioids, one can administer low-dose intravenous naloxone (0.04-mg increments every 2 minutes, up to 0.2 mg). With careful titration, respiratory depression and sedation can be reversed without dangerous reversal of analgesia. If unconsciousness is related to residual opioid effects, ventilatory rate and arousal will increase with 0.2 mg or less of intravenous naloxone, unless a patient has received a massive opioid overdose.

Flumazenil (0.2 mg/min intravenously to a total of 1.0 mg), a competitive benzodiazepine antagonist, differentiates sedation from midazolam and diazepam, although duration of action is short. Risk of inducing seizures must be considered in reversing chronic benzodiazepine users. Neither naloxone nor flumazenil should be used as a routine element of postoperative care.[6] Pharmaceutic reversal should be reserved for specific indications in individual patients. Administration of intravenous physostigmine (0.5 to 1 mg) counteracts but does not reverse sedation caused by inhalation anesthetics, other sedatives, and anticholinergics. If administration of naloxone, flumazenil, or physostigmine does not improve the level of consciousness, unconsciousness is most likely not related to reversible residual anesthetic medications. However, it is still possible that an unrecognized, preoperative overdose with depressant oral drugs (i.e., anticholinergic and antihistamines) is responsible.

The increasing use of dexmedetomidine for sedation cases can lead to persistent sedation in the PACU. These patients are usually easy to arouse and follow commands readily. They tend to have few respiratory issues unless other respiratory depressant medications have also been given. The minimal effect on respiratory drive by dexmedetomidine allows safe discharge from the PACU as long as the destination of the patient is sufficient to care for the level of sedation.

Profound residual neuromuscular paralysis could mimic unconsciousness by precluding any motor response to stimuli. This phenomenon could occur after gross overdosage, if reversal agents are omitted, in patients with unrecognized neuromuscular disease, with phase II blockade from succinylcholine, or its use in a patient with pseudocholinesterase deficiency. Observation of purposeful motion, spontaneous ventilation, or reflex muscular movement eliminates residual paralysis as an explanation. CNS depression secondary to intravenous local anesthetic toxicity or inadvertent subarachnoid injection can mimic postoperative coma. Children who were exhausted before surgery are often difficult to arouse after anesthesia, especially if sleep patterns are disrupted by emergency surgery at night. Hypothermia below 33°C impairs consciousness and increases the depressant effect of medications. Core temperatures below 30°C can cause fixed pupillary dilation, areflexia, and coma. A serum glucose level will eliminate severe hypoglycemia or hyperglycemic hyperosmolar coma as causes. Suspicion that unresponsiveness is caused by hypoglycemia indicates an immediate empiric trial of intravenous 50% dextrose. Hyposmolar states (<260 mOsm/L) such as acute hyponatremia (Na <125 mEq/L) are ruled out by checking serum electrolyte and osmolarity. Arterial blood gas analysis reveals CO_2 narcosis ($Paco_2$ >80 to 100 mmHg) as well as carboxyhemoglobin levels for carbon monoxide poisoning. A patient may also be feigning unresponsiveness or having a hysterical reaction that presents as unconsciousness, and is a diagnosis of exclusion.

If a diagnosis remains elusive, consult a neurologist for a thorough neurologic evaluation. Occasionally, unresponsiveness reflects subclinical grand mal seizures secondary to delirium tremens or an underlying seizure disorder. Cerebral anoxia from hypoperfusion or prolonged profound hypoxemia must be considered. In injured patients or those recovering from intracranial surgery, evaluate for unrecognized head trauma, intracerebral hemorrhage, or increased intracranial pressure. Patients sometimes awaken very slowly after long intracranial procedures.[88] Cerebral thromboembolism is another possibility in patients who have undergone internal jugular or subclavian cannulation. Patients with atrial fibrillation, carotid bruits, or hypercoagulable states are also at increased risk of thromboembolism. Paradoxical air or fat embolism through a right-to-left intracardiac shunt should be considered. After cardiac, proximal major vascular, or invasive neck surgery, risk of postoperative stroke ranges from 2.2% to 5.2%.[89] Postoperative cerebrovascular accidents in other patients are rare, showing a 0.03% to 0.08% incidence in the fourth decade but increasing to 3% to 4% by the eighth decade, and usually become evident after the PACU interval.[90]

Altered Mental Status

Recovering patients sometimes exhibit inappropriate mental reactions, ranging from lethargy and confusion to physical combativeness and extreme disorientation.

Emergence Reactions

Aside from the disturbance to staff and other patients, a stormy emergence reaction has significant medical consequences. The risk of incidental trauma increases, including contusion or fracture, corneal abrasion, and sprains from struggling. Thrashing jeopardizes suture lines, orthopedic fixations, vascular grafts, drains, tracheal tubes, and vascular catheters. Agitated patients manifest high levels of sympathetic nervous system tone, tachycardia, and hypertension. Less appreciated is the risk of injury to staff struggling to protect a combative patient.

For a short period after regaining consciousness, some patients appear unable to appropriately process sensory input. Most exhibit somnolence, slight disorientation, and sluggish mental reactions that rapidly clear. Others experience wide emotional swings such as weeping or escalating resistance to positioning and restraint. Predicting which patients will have adverse psychological reactions is difficult. Emergence delirium, which is prevalent in children and young adults, is difficult to predict preoperatively and does not appear to be related to specific types of anesthesia.[91] In young children, anxiety is heightened by parental separation. Heightened anxiety seems to be the one consistent factor in predicting emergence delirium.[92] Many therapies have been tried to prevent or stop emergence delirium in pediatric patients without much success; however, the use of dexmedetomidine has shown promise in reducing this phenomenon without increasing time to extubate or time to discharge.[93] Ketamine and propofol have also been used with some success.[94] Very young children may react inappropriately to sound when hearing acutely improves after myringotomies. Patients with reduced mental capacity, psychiatric disorders, organic brain dysfunction, or hostile preoperative interactions manifest those problems after surgery. Inability to speak due to oral fixation or tracheal intubation generates frustration or fear that exaggerates emergence reactions. Ethnic, cultural, and psychological characteristics play some role. A language barrier or a new postoperative hearing impairment accentuates an emergence reaction because input from PACU staff might not be understood. The incidence of stormy emergence is probably higher after procedures with high emotional significance. Recall of intraoperative events can generate severe panic and anxiety during emergence.[95] In patients who are physically dependent on alcohol, opioids, cocaine, or other illicit drugs, intoxication or withdrawal can elicit bizarre emergence behavior. Disorientation, paranoia, and combativeness occur after use of scopolamine as a premedication or antiemetic, which can be treated with intravenous physostigmine. Ketamine can cause dysphoria and hallucination, although acute reactions are rare. Etomidate can be a cause of restlessness.

Pain amplifies agitation, confusion, and aggressive behavior during emergence[96]; therefore, it is helpful to ensure adequate postoperative analgesia early in the PACU course. Urinary urgency or gastric distention from trapped gas generates discomfort and agitation, as do tight dressings, painful phlebotomy, and poor positioning. Endotracheal or nasogastric tubes and urinary catheters are also uncomfortable. Check for unusual pain sources such as corneal abrasion, entrapment of body parts, infiltrated vascular catheters, or small devices left beneath a patient. Nausea, dizziness, and pruritus are distressing during emergence. Some patients struggle to move from a supine into a more comfortable semisitting or lateral position, especially those with gastroesophageal reflux, pulmonary congestion, or obesity. Emerging patients often resist physical restraint. Residual paralysis elicits agitation or uncoordinated motions that make a patient appear disoriented and combative. Observation of weakness or a peculiar flapping nature of voluntary motion helps in the diagnosis. However, patients can appear fully recovered by head lift and train-of-four monitoring but still perceive impaired swallowing, visual acuity, and sense of strength.[97]

Combativeness, confusion, or disorientation might reflect respiratory dysfunction. Moderate hypoxemia often presents with clouded mentation, disorientation, and agitation resembling that caused by pain. Respiratory acidemia elicits profound agitation, although acidemia caused by ventilatory center depression generates less agitation because higher CNS functions are also depressed. Hypercarbia is more likely to cause lethargy or somnolence. Limitation of inspiratory volume by chest dressings, gastric distention, or splinting causes a vague dissatisfaction with lung inflation similar to air hunger. Inability to generate a forceful cough or clear secretions causes distress. Interstitial pulmonary edema elicits symptoms of air hunger before airway flooding occurs. Agitation can be profound, even with adequate ventilation and oxygenation.

Metabolic abnormalities interfere with lucidity. Lactic acidemia causes anxiety and mild disorientation; acute hyponatremia clouds the sensorium; and hypoglycemia causes first agitation and then diminished responsiveness. Seizure activity might mimic agitation and combativeness. Seizures should be higher in the differential diagnosis in patients with epilepsy, head trauma, and chronic alcohol or cocaine abuse. Cerebral hypoperfusion can produce disorientation, agitation, and combativeness, which can be seen after head trauma or space-occupying lesions. Action such as increasing the mean arterial pressure might be required to assure cerebral perfusion pressure.

There are few interventions that prevent combative emergence reactions.[92] Altered mental status is treated supportively because most emergence reactions often disappear within 10 to 15 minutes. Verbal reassurances that surgery is completed and that the patient is doing well are invaluable. One should use the patient's name frequently with reassurance of well-being, and stress the time and location. When practical, one should allow patients to choose their own position and provide adequate analgesia. In selected cases, parenteral sedation relieves fear or anxiety and smoothes emergence. Identifying whether a patient is reacting to pain or to anxiety is important. Benzodiazepines and barbiturates are ineffective analgesics, whereas opioids are poor anxiolytics. One should not administer sedative or analgesic medications if altered mental status might reflect a physiologic abnormality such as hypoxemia, hypoglycemia, hypotension, or acidemia, and use restraints only if a patient's or staff's safety is jeopardized.

Delirium and Cognitive Decline

A high percentage of elderly patients (5% to 50%) experience some degree of postoperative confusion, delirium, or cognitive decline.[98,99] Patients exhibit fluctuations in level of consciousness and orientation, or deterioration of memory, mental functions, and acquisition of new information. Delirium may be exhibited by two subtypes; hypoactive patients predominate, whereas a smaller percentage is hyperactive. The problem may be related to exacerbation of central cholinergic insufficiency by narcotics, sedatives, or anticholinergics. However, stress of surgery, fever, pain, emesis, sleep deprivation, and loss of routine undoubtedly contribute. Presence of pre-existing dementia, cognitive abnormalities,

organic brain syndrome, or hearing and visual impairment predicts postoperative delirium, as does evidence of physical infirmity such as high ASA physical status or lack of stress response to surgery. Cognitive dysfunction also occurs at lower incidence (15% greater than control) in younger patients, more frequently resolves within 3 months, and may be related to inactivity during recuperation.[100] Although signs often appear on the first to third postoperative day, onset is often evident in the PACU.

Overall, recovery of cognitive function is slower in the elderly.[101] Because older patients are often skilled at concealing declining capabilities, careful assessment of preoperative capabilities helps identify deficits that affect postoperative status. Postoperative lethargy, clouded sensorium, or delirium sometimes reflects an acute physiologic change. Hyperosmolarity from hyperglycemia or hypernatremia as well as hyponatremia can alter consciousness. Cerebral fluid shifts with decreased mentation occur in patients on dialysis and after rapid correction of severe dehydration. Patients receiving atropine premedication or chronic meperidine therapy might exhibit anticholinergic-induced delirium. Disorientation or clouded sensorium can reflect chronic use of psychogenic drugs, premedication with long-acting sedatives, or unrecognized intoxication. Life-threatening conditions such as seizures, hypoxemia, hypoglycemia, hypotension, acidemia, or cerebrovascular accident sometimes present with confusion, disorientation, inability to vocalize, or reduced level of consciousness, especially if earlier signs and symptoms are misinterpreted.

Although there is no anesthetic technique known to be better at avoiding postoperative delirium, there are things to avoid that might reduce its incidence.[102] Avoiding known factors such as benzodiazepines, anticholinergics, and meperidine will reduce a patient's risk.[103] Setting protocols to enhance a safe and efficient recovery begins with the initial planning of surgery. Recovery personnel in the PACU should be aware of and implement these protocols to remain consistent with the continuum of care. Pain management is a major factor for reducing the incidence of delirium. Ensure that patients are properly hydrated, remove catheters that are no longer needed, restore cognitive stimulation by returning eyeglasses and hearing aids, reorientate the patients, and provide frequent human interaction, all of which may aid in limiting or reducing delirium.

Postoperative Nausea and Vomiting

Postoperative nausea and vomiting (PONV) continues to be a significant challenge to be avoided after many types of anesthetics. Not only is PONV considered by many patients the most unpleasant aspect following an anesthetic, but many also describe it as their greatest fear of subsequent anesthetics.[104] Patients are often more concerned about PONV than pain or other risks associated with anesthesia and surgery. In addition to patients' dissatisfaction with nausea and vomiting, there exist medical risks (increased abdominal pressure, increased central venous pressure, aspiration of gastric contents, sympathetic nervous system response with increasing blood pressure and heart rate as well as parasympathetic responses producing bradycardia and hypotension). PONV represents a significant burden to be avoided due to patient satisfaction and safety as well as the economic impact of prolonged PACU stays and unanticipated admissions.

The incidence of PONV varies with many potential causes. Patients often experience nausea and emesis after discharge from the PACU, which may coincide with increased oral intake or waning effect of antiemetics. Surgeries associated with a higher risk of PONV are eye procedures, peritoneal or intestinal irritation, ear–nose–throat procedures, especially with middle ear manipulation, dental, and cosmetic procedures. Patient groups at increased risk are those with a previous history of PONV, a history of motion sickness, menstruating females, children over the age of two, obesity, and nonsmokers.[105] Perioperative factors that may increase the incidence include no PO intake (starvation, dehydration), autonomic imbalance, pain, and the effects of anesthetics on the chemotactic center.

Incidence of PONV is lower following regional rather than general anesthesia especially with decreased use of opioids.[106] The use of nonopioid analgesics may reduce the frequency of emesis while providing adequate pain control. Induction agents such as propofol and barbiturates are associated with reduced incidence compared to etomidate and ketamine. A total intravenous anesthetic (TIVA) technique with propofol greatly reduces PONV incidence compared to a pure inhalation anesthetic. There is little significant difference among inhalation agents, although sevoflurane and desflurane might generate slightly higher rates of nausea. The choice of anticholinergic reversal agents may be a contributing factor to PONV, but it remains unclear to what degree.

Several interventions have been evaluated and can be implemented to reduce the incidence of PONV. The use of meclizine 25 mg preoperatively for patients predisposed to motion sickness can be effective. Prophylaxis with 5-HT3 receptor antagonists (i.e., ondansetron) prior to emergence significantly reduces incidence and is cost effective. Dexamethasone also has antiemetic effects and can be used effectively with other prophylactic agents. Hydration is effective, easy, and cost effective. The use of droperidol prophylaxis decreased due to a 2001 FDA black box warning with prolonged QT on ECG as well as manufacturing issues beginning in 2013. The FDA letter regarding the use of droperidol did not address the usual prophylaxis dose of 0.625mg, but recommended ECG monitoring for 2 to 3 hours after administration. In September of 2011, the FDA came out with a similar safety announcement regarding prolonged QT with the use of ondansetron. There were no recommendations regarding routine ECG monitoring with the use of ondansetron but caution and monitoring should be used with those patients with known prolonged QT syndromes.[107] Rescue with nonselective antihistamines (i.e., promethazine) is effective, but caution is advised in patients where increased sedation can be problematic in children and patients with OSA. Acupuncture, acupressure, and TENS therapy can provide relief, but due to provider proficiency, patient acceptance, and proven efficacy compared to antiemetic medications, these methods are less frequently used.[108] More serious causes of nausea and vomiting such as hypotension, hypoxia, hypoglycemia, increased intracranial pressure, or gastric bleeding should be considered prior to treatment.

REFERENCES

1. Bothner U, Georgieff M, Schwilk B. The impact of minor perioperative anesthesia-related incidents, events, and complications on postanesthesia care unit utilization. *Anesth Analg.* 1999;89:506–513.
2. Cohen MM, O'Brien-Pallas LL, Copplestone C, et al. Nursing workload associated with adverse events in the postanesthesia care unit. *Anesthesiology.* 1999;91:1882–1890.
3. Pavlin DJ, Rapp SE, Polissar NL, et al. Factors affecting discharge time in adult outpatients. *Anesth Analg.* 1998;87:816–826.
4. Song D, Chung F, Ronayne M, et al. Fast-tracking (bypassing the PACU) does not reduce nursing workload after ambulatory surgery. *Br J Anaesth.* 2004;93:768–774.
5. Hines R, Barash PG, Watrous G, et al. Complications occurring in the postanesthesia care unit: A survey. *Anesth Analg.* 1992;74:503–509.
6. American Society of Anesthesiologists Task Force on Postanesthetic Care. Practice guidelines for postanesthetic care: a report by the American Society of Anesthesiologists Task Force on Postanesthetic Care. *Anesthesiology.* 2002;96:742–752.
7. Sullivan EE. Standards of perianesthesia nursing practice 2002. *J Perianesth Nurs.* 2002;17:275–276.
8. Swenson JD, Bay N, Loose E, et al. Outpatient management of continuous peripheral nerve catheters placed using ultrasound guidance: An experience in 620 patients. *Anesth Analg.* 2006;103:1436–1443.
9. Apfelbaum JL, Walawander CA, Grasela TH, et al. Eliminating intensive postoperative care in same-day surgery patients using short-acting anesthetics. *Anesthesiology.* 2002;97:66–74.
10. Pittet D, Stephan F, Hugonnet S, et al. Hand-cleansing during postanesthesia care. *Anesthesiology.* 2003;99:530–535.
11. Macario A, Weinger M, Carney S, et al. Which clinical anesthesia outcomes are important to avoid the perspective of patients? *Anesth Analg.* 1999;89:652–658.
12. Strassels SA, Chen C, Carr DB. Postoperative analgesia: economics, resource use, and patient satisfaction in an urban teaching hospital. *Anesth Analg.* 2002;94:130–137.
13. Apfelbaum JL, Chen C, Mehta SS, et al. Postoperative pain experience: Results from a national survey suggest postoperative pain continues to be undermanaged. *Anesth Analg.* 2003;97:534–540.
14. Rundshagen I, Schnabel K, Standl T, et al. Patients' vs nurses' assessments of postoperative pain and anxiety during patient- or nurse-controlled analgesia. *Br J Anaesth.* 1999;82:374–378.
15. American Society of Anesthesiologists Task Force on Acute Pain Management. Practice guidelines for acute pain management in the perioperative setting: An updated report by the American Society of Anesthesiologists Task Force on Acute Pain Management. *Anesthesiology.* 2004;100:1573–1581.
16. Chung F, Ritchie E, Su J. Postoperative pain in ambulatory surgery. *Anesth Analg.* 1997;85:808–816.
17. Wu CL, Berenholtz SM, Pronovost PJ, et al. Systematic review and analysis of postdischarge symptoms after outpatient surgery. *Anesthesiology.* 2002;96:994–1003.
18. Peng PW, Sandler AN. A review of the use of fentanyl analgesia in the management of acute pain in adults. *Anesthesiology.* 1999;90:576–599.
19. White PF. The role of non-opioid analgesic techniques in the management of pain after ambulatory surgery. *Anesth Analg.* 2002;94:577–585.
20. Gwirtz KH, Young JV, Byers RS, et al. The safety and efficacy of intrathecal opioid analgesia for acute postoperative pain: Seven years' experience with 5,969 surgical patients at Indiana university hospital. *Anesth Analg.* 1999;88:599–604.
21. de Leon-Casasola OA, Lema MJ. Postoperative epidural opioid analgesia: What are the choices? *Anesth Analg.* 1996;83:867–875.
22. Baig MK, Zmora O, Derdemezi J, et al. Use of the ON-Q pain management system is associated with decreased postoperative analgesic requirement: Double blind randomized placebo pilot study. *J Am Coll Surg.* 2006;202:297–305.
23. Capdevila X, Pirat P, Bringuier S, et al. Continuous peripheral nerve blocks in hospital wards after orthopedic surgery: A multicenter prospective analysis of the quality of postoperative analgesia and complications in 1,416 patients. *Anesthesiology.* 2005;103:1035–1045.
24. Ilfeld BM, Enneking FK. Continuous peripheral nerve blocks at home: A review. *Anesth Analg.* 2005;100:1822–1833.
25. Casati A, Fanelli G, Cedrati V, et al. Pulmonary function changes after interscalene brachial plexus anesthesia with 0.5% and 0.75% ropivacaine: A double-blinded comparison with 2% mepivacaine. *Anesth Analg.* 1999;88:587–592.
26. Aldrete JA. The post-anesthesia recovery score revisited. *J Clin Anesth.* 1995;7:89–91.
27. White PF, Song D. New criteria for fast-tracking after outpatient anesthesia: A comparison with the modified Aldrete's scoring system. *Anesth Analg.* 1999;88:1069–1072.
28. Standards for Postanesthesia Care (Approved by House of Delegates on October 12, 1988 and last amended on October 14, 2014). www.asahq.org Standards Guidelines Statements, Postanesthetic Care, 10.15.14 Standards for Post Anesthesia Care.
29. Noiseux N, Bracco D, Prieto I, et al. Do patients after off-pump coronary artery bypass grafting need the intensive care unit? A prospective audit of 85 patients. *Interact Cardiovasc Thorac Surg.* 2008;7:32–36.
30. Schweizer A, Khatchatourian G, Hohn L, et al. Opening of a new postanesthesia care unit: Impact on critical care utilization and complications following major vascular and thoracic surgery. *J Clin Anesth.* 2002;14:486–493.
31. Heland M, Retsas A. Establishing a cardiac surgery recovery unit within the post anaesthesia care unit. *Collegian.* 1999;6:10–13.
32. Baltimore JJ. Perianesthesia care of cardiac surgery patients: A CPAN review. *J Perianesth Nurs.* 2001;16:246–254.
33. Rose DK, Cohen MM, Wigglesworth DF, et al. Critical respiratory events in the postanesthesia care unit, patient, surgical, and anesthetic factors. *Anesthesiology.* 1994;81:410–418.
34. Schwilk B, Bothner U, Schraag S, et al. Perioperative respiratory events in smokers and nonsmokers undergoing general anaesthesia. *Acta Anaesthesiol Scand.* 1997;41:348–355.
35. Ballantyne JC, Carr DB, deFerranti S, et al. The comparative effects of postoperative analgesic therapies on pulmonary outcome: Cumulative meta-analyses of randomized, controlled trials. *Anesth Analg.* 1998;86:598–612.

36. Warner DO, Warner MA, Offord KP, et al. Airway obstruction and perioperative complications in smokers undergoing abdominal surgery. Anesthesiology. 1999;90:372–379.
37. Strauss SG, Lynn AM, Bratton SL, et al. Ventilatory response to CO_2 in children with obstructive sleep apnea from adenotonsillar hypertrophy. Anesth Analg. 1999;89:328–332.
38. Tait AR, Malviya S, Voepel-Lewis T, et al. Risk factors for perioperative adverse respiratory events in children with upper respiratory tract infections. Anesthesiology. 2001;95:299–306.
39. D'Honneur G, Lofaso F, Drummond GB, et al. Susceptibility to upper airway obstruction during partial neuromuscular block. Anesthesiology. 1998;88:371–378.
40. Asai T, Koga K, Vaughan RS. Respiratory complications associated with tracheal intubation and extubation. Br J Anaesth. 1998;80:767–775.
41. Benumof JL, Dagg R, Benumof R. Critical hemoglobin desaturation will occur before return to an unparalyzed state following 1 mg/kg intravenous succinylcholine. Anesthesiology. 1997;87:979–982.
42. Warner DO, Warner MA, Barnes RD, et al. Perioperative respiratory complications in patients with asthma. Anesthesiology. 1996;85:460–467.
43. Berg H, Roed J, Viby-Mogensen J, et al. Residual neuromuscular block is a risk factor for postoperative pulmonary complications: A prospective, randomised, and blinded study of postoperative pulmonary complications after atracurium, vecuronium and pancuronium. Acta Anaesthesiol Scand. 1997;41:1095–1103.
44. Debaene B, Plaud B, Dilly MP, et al. Residual paralysis in the PACU after a single intubating dose of nondepolarizing muscle relaxant with an intermediate duration of action. Anesthesiology. 2003;98:1042–1048.
45. de Boer HD, Driessen JJ, Marcus MA, et al. Reversal of rocuronium-induced (1.2 mg/kg) profound neuromuscular block by sugammadex: A multicenter, dose-finding and safety study. Anesthesiology. 2007;107:239–244.
46. Stoller JK, Kester L. Respiratory care protocols in postanesthesia care. J Perianesth Nurs. 1998;13:349–358.
47. Rothen HU, Sporre B, Engberg G, et al. Airway closure, atelectasis and gas exchange during general anaesthesia. Br J Anaesth. 1998;81:681–686.
48. Karayiannakis AJ, Makri GG, Mantzioka A, et al. Postoperative pulmonary function after laparoscopic and open cholecystectomy. Br J Anaesth. 1996;77:448–452.
49. Thomas JA, McIntosh JM. Are incentive spirometry, intermittent positive pressure breathing, and deep breathing exercises effective in the prevention of postoperative pulmonary complications after upper abdominal surgery? A systematic overview and meta-analysis. Phys Ther. 1994;74:3–10.
50. Overend TJ, Anderson CM, Lucy SD, et al. The effect of incentive spirometry on postoperative pulmonary complications: A systematic review. Chest. 2001;120:971–978.
51. Young T, Palta M, Dempsey J, et al. The occurrence of sleep-disordered breathing among middle-aged adults. N Engl J Med. 1993;328:1230–1235.
52. Xue FS, Huang YG, Tong SY, et al. A comparative study of early postoperative hypoxemia in infants, children, and adults undergoing elective plastic surgery. Anesth Analg. 1996;83:709–715.
53. Xue FS, Huang YG, Tong SY, et al. A comparative study of early post operative hypoxemia in infants, children and adults undergoing elective plastic surgery. Anesth Analg. 1996;83:709.
54. Moller JT, Johannessen NW, Espersen K, et al. Randomized evaluation of pulse oximetry in 20,802 Patients. II. Perioperative events and postoperative complications. Anesthesiology. 1993;78:445–453.
55. Xue FS, Li BW, Zhang GS, et al. The influence of surgical sites on early postoperative hypoxemia in adults undergoing elective surgery. Anesth Analg. 1999;88:213–219.
56. Moller JT, Wittrup M, Johansen SH. Hypoxemia in the postanesthesia care unit: An observer study. Anesthesiology. 1990;73:890–895.
57. Ng A, Smith G. Gastroesophageal reflux and aspiration of gastric contents in anesthetic practice. Anesth Analg. 2001;93:494–513.
58. Eriksson LI, Sundman E, Olsson R, et al. Functional assessment of the pharynx at rest and during swallowing in partially paralyzed humans: Aimultaneous videomanometry and mechanomyography of awake human volunteers. Anesthesiology. 1997;87:1035–1043.
59. Practice guidelines for preoperative fasting and the use of pharmacologic agents to reduce the risk of pulmonary aspiration: application to healthy patients undergoing elective procedures: a report by the American Society of Anesthesiologist Task Force on Preoperative Fasting. Anesthesiology. 1999;90:896–905.
60. Mulroy MF, Salinas FV, Larkin KL, et al. Ambulatory surgery patients may be discharged before voiding after short-acting spinal and epidural anesthesia. Anesthesiology. 2002;97:315–319.
61. Marshall SI, Chung F. Discharge criteria and complications after ambulatory surgery. Anesth Analg. 1999;88:508–517.
62. Twersky R, Fishman D, Homel P. What happens after discharge? Return hospital visits after ambulatory surgery. Anesth Analg. 1997;84:319–324.
63. Cogliati AA, Vellutini R, Nardini A, et al. Fenoldopam infusion for renal protection in high-risk cardiac surgery patients: A randomized clinical study. J Cardiothorac Vasc Anesth. 2007;21:847–850.
64. Waters JH, Gottlieb A, Schoenwald P, et al. Normal saline versus lactated Ringer's solution for intraoperative fluid management in patients undergoing abdominal aortic aneurysm repair: an outcome study. Anesth Analg. 2001;93:817–822.
65. Moos DD, Lind DM. Detection and treatment of perioperative corneal abrasions. J Perianesth Nurs. 2006;21:332–338.
66. Myers MA, Hamilton SR, Bogosian AJ, et al. Visual loss as a complication of spine surgery: A review of 37 cases. Spine. 1997;22:1325–1329.
67. Warner ME, Warner MA, Garrity JA, et al. The frequency of perioperative vision loss. Anesth Analg. 2001;93:1417–1421.
68. Williams EL, Hart WM Jr, Tempelhoff R. Postoperative ischemic optic neuropathy. Anesth Analg. 1995;80:1018–1029.
69. Warner ME, Fronapfel PJ, Hebl JR, et al. Perioperative visual changes. Anesthesiology. 2002;96:855–859.
70. Sprung J, Bourke DL, Contreras MG, et al. Perioperative hearing impairment. Anesthesiology. 2003;98:241–257.
71. Warner ME, Benenfeld SM, Warner MA, et al. Perianesthetic dental injuries: frequency, outcomes, and risk factors. Anesthesiology. 1999;90:1302–1305.
72. Brimacombe J, Holyoake L, Keller C, et al. Pharyngolaryngeal, neck, and jaw discomfort after anesthesia with the face mask and laryngeal mask airway at high and low cuff volumes in males and females. Anesthesiology. 2000;93:26–31.
73. Practice advisory for the prevention of perioperative peripheral neuropathies: A report by the American Society of Anesthesiologists Task Force on Prevention of Perioperative Peripheral Neuropathies. Anesthesiology. 2000;92:1168–1182.
74. Cheney FW, Domino KB, Caplan RA, et al. Nerve injury associated with anesthesia: A closed claims analysis. Anesthesiology. 1999;90:1062–1069.
75. Warner MA, Warner DO, Matsumoto JY, et al. Ulnar neuropathy in surgical patients. Anesthesiology. 1999;90:54–59.
76. Warner MA. Perioperative neuropathies. Mayo Clin Proc. 1998;73:567–574.
77. Auroy Y, Benhamou D, Bargues L, et al. Major complications of regional anesthesia in France: the SOS regional anesthesia hotline service. Anesthesiology. 2002;97:1274–1280.
78. Horlocker TT, McGregor DG, Matsushige DK, et al. A retrospective review of 4,767 consecutive spinal anesthetics: central nervous system complications: Perioperative outcomes group. Anesth Analg. 1997;84:578–584.
79. Schreiber JU, Mencke T, Biedler A, et al. Postoperative myalgia after succinylcholine: No evidence for an inflammatory origin. Anesth Analg. 2003;96:1640–1644.
80. Bettelli G. Which muscle relaxants should be used in day surgery and when. Curr Opin Anaesthesiol. 2006;19:600–605.
81. Sessler DI. Complications and treatment of mild hypothermia. Anesthesiology. 2001;95:531–543.
82. Lenhardt R, Marker E, Goll V, et al. Mild intraoperative hypothermia prolongs postanesthetic recovery. Anesthesiology. 1997;87:1318–1323.
83. Sun LS, Adams DC, Delphin E, et al. Sympathetic response during cardiopulmonary bypass: Mild versus moderate hypothermia. Crit Care Med. 1997;25:1990–1993.
84. Frank SM, Fleisher LA, Breslow MJ, et al. Perioperative maintenance of normothermia reduces the incidence of morbid cardiac events: A randomized clinical trial. JAMA. 1997;277:1127–1134.
85. Ammori JB, Sigakis M, Englesbe MJ, et al. Effect of intraoperative hyperglycemia during liver transplantation. J Surg Res. 2007;140:227–233.
86. De Witte J, Sessler DI. Perioperative shivering: physiology and pharmacology. Anesthesiology. 2002;96:467–484.
87. Zelcer J, Wells DG. Anaesthetic-related recovery room complications. Anaesth Intensive Care. 1987;15:168–174.
88. Schubert A, Mascha EJ, Bloomfield EL, et al. Effect of cranial surgery and brain tumor size on emergence from anesthesia. Anesthesiology. 1996;85:513–521.
89. Wong GY, Warner DO, Schroeder DR, et al. Risk of surgery and anesthesia for ischemic stroke. Anesthesiology. 2000;92:425–432.
90. Kim J, Gelb AW. Predicting perioperative stroke. J Neurosurg Anesthesiol. 1995;7:211–215.
91. Vlajkovic GP, Sindjelic RP. Emergence delirium in children: Many questions, few answers. Anesth Analg. 2007;104:84–91.
92. Voepel-Lewis T, Malviya S, Tait AR. A prospective cohort study of emergence agitation in the pediatric postanesthesia care unit. Anesth Analg. 2003;96:1625–1630.
93. Isik B, Arslan M, Tunga AD, et al. Dexmedetomidine decreases emergence agitation in pediatric patients after sevoflurane anesthesia without surgery. Paediatr Anaesth. 2006;16:748–753.
94. Abu-Shahwan I, Chowdary K. Ketamine is effective in decreasing the incidence of emergence agitation in children undergoing dental repair under sevoflurane general anesthesia. Paediatr Anaesth. 2007;17:846–850.
95. Schwender D, Kunze-Kronawitter H, Dietrich P, et al. Conscious awareness during general anaesthesia: patients' perceptions, emotions, cognition and reactions. Br J Anaesth. 1998;80:133–139.
96. Lynch EP, Lazor MA, Gellis JE, et al. The impact of postoperative pain on the development of postoperative delirium. Anesth Analg. 1998;86:781–785.

97. Kopman AF, Yee PS, Neuman GG. Relationship of the train-of-four fade ratio to clinical signs and symptoms of residual paralysis in awake volunteers. *Anesthesiology*. 1997;86:765–771.
98. Cook DJ, Rooke GA. Priorities in perioperative geriatrics. *Anesth Analg*. 2003;96:1823–1836.
99. Zakriya KJ, Christmas C, Wenz JFS, et al. Preoperative factors associated with postoperative change in confusion assessment method score in hip fracture patients. *Anesth Analg*. 2002;94:1628–1632.
100. Johnson T, Monk T, Rasmussen LS, et al. Postoperative cognitive dysfunction in middle-aged patients. *Anesthesiology*. 2002;96:1351–1357.
101. Dodds C, Allison J. Postoperative cognitive deficit in the elderly surgical patient. *Br J Anaesth*. 1998;81:449–462.
102. Card E, Pandharipande P, Tomes C, et al. Emergence from general anaesthesia and evolution of delirium signs in the post-anaesthesia car unit. *Br J Anaesth*. 2015;115:411–417.
103. Neufeld KJ, Leotsakos JM, Sieber FE, et al. Outcomes of early delirium diagnosis after general anesthesia in the elderly. *Anesth Analg*. 2013;117:471–478.
104. Kerger H, Turan A, Kredel M, et al. Patients' willingness to pay for anti-emetic treatment. *Acta Anaesthesiol Scand*. 2007;51:38–43.
105. Sinclair DR, Chung F, Mezei G. Can postoperative nausea and vomiting be predicted? *Anesthesiology*. 1999;91:109–118.
106. Williams BA, Kentor ML, Vogt MT, et al. Economics of nerve block pain management after anterior cruciate ligament reconstruction: Potential hospital cost savings via associated postanesthesia care unit bypass and same-day discharge. *Anesthesiology*. 2004;100:697–706.
107. Charbit B, Albaladejo P, Funck-Brentano C, et al. Prolongation of QTc interval after postoperative nausea and vomiting treatment by droperidol or ondansetron. *Anesthesiology*. 2005;102(6):1094–1100.
108. Lee A, Done ML. The use of nonpharmacologic techniques to prevent postoperative nausea and vomiting: a meta-analysis. *Anesth Analg*. 1999;88:1362–1369.

55 Acute Pain Management

STEPHEN M. MACRES • PETER G. MOORE • SCOTT M. FISHMAN

Acute Pain Defined
Anatomy of Acute Pain
   Pain Processing
Chemical Mediators of Transduction and Transmission
The Surgical Stress Response
Preventive Analgesia
Strategies for Acute Pain Management
Assessment of Acute Pain
Opioid Analgesics
Nonopioid Analgesic Adjuncts
Methods of Analgesia
   Patient-controlled Analgesia
   Neuraxial Analgesia
   Peripheral Nerve Blockade

Complications from Regional Anesthesia
Perioperative Pain Management of the Opioid-dependent Patient
Organization of Perioperative Pain Management Services
Special Considerations in the Perioperative Pain Management of Children
   Nonparenteral Analgesics
   Opioid Analgesics
   Patient-controlled Analgesia
   Epidural Neuraxial Analgesia
   Peripheral Nerve Blocks in Children
Conclusion

KEY POINTS

1. The inadequate relief of postoperative pain has adverse physiologic effects that can contribute to significant morbidity and mortality, resulting in the delay of patient recovery and return to daily activities.
2. The pain pathway is not "hardwired" and nociceptive input is not passively transmitted from the periphery to the brain. Tissue injury tends to fuel neuroplastic changes within the nervous system, which results in both peripheral and central sensitization.
3. In order for preventive analgesia to be successful, three critical principles must be adhered to: (1) The depth of analgesia must be adequate enough to block all nociceptive input during surgery, (2) the analgesic technique must be extensive enough to include the entire surgical field, and (3) the duration of analgesia must include both the surgical and postsurgical periods.
4. The various opioid analgesics available today have distinct pharmacologic differences that we can credit to their intricate interaction with the classical three main opioid receptors μ, δ, and κ. The opioid receptors are members of a G protein–coupled (guanosine triphosphate regulatory proteins) receptor family, which signals via a second messenger such as cyclic adenosine monophosphate or an ion channel.
5. Recommendations, which can decrease the risk of opioid-related respiratory depression, include the liberal use of opioid-sparing multimodal pharmacotherapy, regional anesthesia techniques and the continuous monitoring of patient ventilation with pulse oximetry and capnography, particularly in the high-risk individual.
6. The therapeutic benefit of nonsteroidal anti-inflammatory drugs is believed to be mediated through the inhibition of cyclooxygenase enzymes, types 1 and 2, which convert arachidonic acid to prostaglandins.
7. Short-term use of parecoxib and valdecoxib in patients following coronary artery bypass surgery is associated with an increased risk of thromboembolic events. The authors, therefore, do not recommend prescribing a cyclooxygenase-2 inhibitor for patients with a known history of coronary artery disease or cerebrovascular disease.
8. The five variables associated with all modes of patient-controlled analgesia include (1) bolus dose, (2) incremental (demand) dose, (3) lockout interval, (4) background infusion rate, and (5) 1- and 4-hour limits. A typical patient-controlled analgesia regimen in an otherwise healthy adult would be an incremental dose of 1 to 2 mg of morphine with an 8- to 10-minute lockout. The authors do not recommend a background infusion of opioid in the opioid-naive patient.
9. *Epidural analgesia* is a critical component of multimodal perioperative pain management and improved patient outcome. Meta-analyses investigating the efficacy of epidural analgesia found epidural analgesia to be superior to systemically administered opioids.
10. Continuous peripheral nerve block has proven to be an effective technique for postoperative pain management, which is superior to opioid analgesia with fewer opioid-related side effects and rare neurologic and infectious complications.
11. Should a perioperative nerve injury occur, it is incumbent on the physician to determine which combination of anesthetic, surgical, and patient risk factors are involved in any nerve injury and to not assume a priori that the regional anesthetic is the basis for the injury.
12. Ultrasound-guided regional anesthesia hastens the onset time of sensory and motor blockade and can decrease the performance time of a peripheral nerve block.
13. Although UGRA has not been shown to decrease the incidence of postoperative neurologic symptoms it is associated with a decreased risk for local anesthetic systemic toxicity and a lower incidence of pneumothorax following the performance of ultrasound-guided supraclavicular blockade.

> 14 The opioid-dependent patient is often identified just moments prior to surgery and the anesthesia team needs to be innovative. The anesthesiologist needs to be flexible enough to tailor an individual anesthetic that incorporates a multimodal approach, combining regional anesthesia with general anesthesia and nonopioid coanalgesics with opioid analgesics. Opioids remain the mainstay of perioperative pain management, and an adequate dose of opioid needs to be maintained to avoid precipitating withdrawal symptoms.
>
> 15 Perioperative management of the opioid-tolerant patient requires prudent use of both opioid and nonopioid analgesics as well as the application of site-specific regional anesthesia/analgesia.
>
> 16 The key components to establishing a successful perioperative pain management service begins with an institutional commitment to support the service. The team must be built around a physician leader with training and experience in pain medicine. There must be other anesthesiologists available to support the service.

Approximately 75 million surgical procedures are performed each year in the United States, and more than half are performed in the inpatient setting. Appropriate management of acute perioperative pain using multimodal or balanced analgesia is therefore crucial. In 1992 clinical practice guidelines were promulgated by the Agency for Health Care Policy and Research, which provided guidelines for physicians for the treatment of acute pain.[1] Soon thereafter the American Society of Anesthesiologists developed treatment guidelines for acute postoperative pain,[2] which has been recently updated and amended in a document promulgated by the American society of Pain Medicine, the American Society of Regional Anesthesia (ASRA), and the American Society of Anesthesiologists.[3] Despite significant advances in our knowledge and treatment of acute pain and dissemination of these guidelines, significant deficits continue to persist and the management **1** of acute postoperative pain is still less than optimal.

The inadequate relief of postoperative pain has adverse physiologic effects that can contribute to significant morbidity and mortality, resulting in the delay of patient recovery and return to daily activities.[4] In addition, poor postoperative pain control contributes to patient dissatisfaction with the surgical experience and may have adverse psychological consequences.[5] Poorly managed postoperative pain can also increase the incidence of persistent postoperative pain conditions. Because aggressive treatment of acute postoperative pain is considered to be so beneficial, the Joint Commission on Accreditation of Healthcare Organizations (JACHO) has declared that "pain is the fifth vital sign" and all institutions seeking accreditation from this group must develop pain management programs.

Acute Pain Defined

Acute pain has been defined as "the normal, predicted, physiologic response to an adverse chemical, thermal, or mechanical stimulus."[6] Generally, acute pain resolves within 1 month. However, poorly managed acute pain that might occur following surgery can produce pathophysiologic processes in both the peripheral and central nervous systems that have the potential to produce chronicity.[5] Acute pain–induced change in the central nervous system is known as *neuronal plasticity*. This can cause sensitization of the nervous system, resulting in allodynia and hyperalgesia. Surgical procedures that can be associated with chronic painful conditions include amputation of a limb, lateral thoracotomy, inguinal herniorrhaphy, abdominal hysterectomy, saphenous vein stripping, open cholecystectomy, nephrectomy, and mastectomy.[5]

Anatomy of Acute Pain

1 The nociceptive pathway is an afferent (Fig. 55-1) three-neuron dual ascending (e.g., anterolateral and dorsal column medial lemniscal pathways) system, with descending modulation (Fig. 55-2) from the cortex, thalamus, and brainstem.[7] Nociceptors are free nerve endings located in skin, muscle, bone, and connective tissue with cell bodies located in the dorsal root ganglia. The first-order neurons that make up the dual ascending system have their origins in the periphery as A-δ and polymodal C fibers (Table 55-1). A-δ fibers transmit "first pain," which is described as sharp or stinging in nature and is well localized. Polymodal C fibers transmit "second pain," which is more diffuse in nature and is associated with the affective and motivational aspects of pain. First-order neurons synapse on second-order neurons in the dorsal horn primarily within laminas I, II, and V, where they release excitatory amino acids and neuropeptides (Figs. 55-3 and 55-4). Some fibers can ascend or descend in Lissauer tract prior to terminating on neurons that project to higher centers. Second-order neurons consist of nociceptive-specific and wide dynamic-range (WDR) neurons. Nociceptive-specific neurons are located primarily in lamina I, respond only to noxious stimuli, and are thought to be involved in the sensory-discriminative aspects of pain. WDR neurons are predominantly located in laminae IV, V, and VI, respond to both nonnoxious and noxious input, and are involved with the affective–motivational component of pain. Axons of both nociceptive-specific and WDR neurons ascend the spinal cord via the dorsal column–medial lemniscus and the anterior lateral spinothalamic tract to synapse on third-order neurons in the contralateral thalamus, which then project to the somatosensory cortex, where nociceptive input is perceived as pain (Fig. 55-1).

Pain Processing

2 A key development in our understanding of pain processing is that the pain pathway is not "hardwired" and nociceptive input is not passively transmitted from the periphery to the brain.[8] Tissue injury tends to fuel neuroplastic changes within the nervous system, which results in both peripheral and central sensitization. Clinically this can manifest as *hyperalgesia,* which is **2** defined as an exaggerated pain response to a normally painful stimulus, and *allodynia,* which is defined as a painful response to a typically nonpainful stimulus (Fig. 55-5).[8]

The four elements of pain processing include (1) transduc- **3** tion, (2) transmission, (3) modulation, and (4) perception (Fig. 55-6). *Transduction* is the event whereby noxious thermal, chemical, or mechanical stimuli are converted into an action potential. *Transmission* occurs when the action potential is conducted through the nervous system via the first-, second-, and third-order neurons, which have cell bodies located in the dorsal root ganglion, dorsal horn, and thalamus, respectively. *Modulation* of pain transmission involves altering afferent neural transmission along the pain pathway. The dorsal horn of

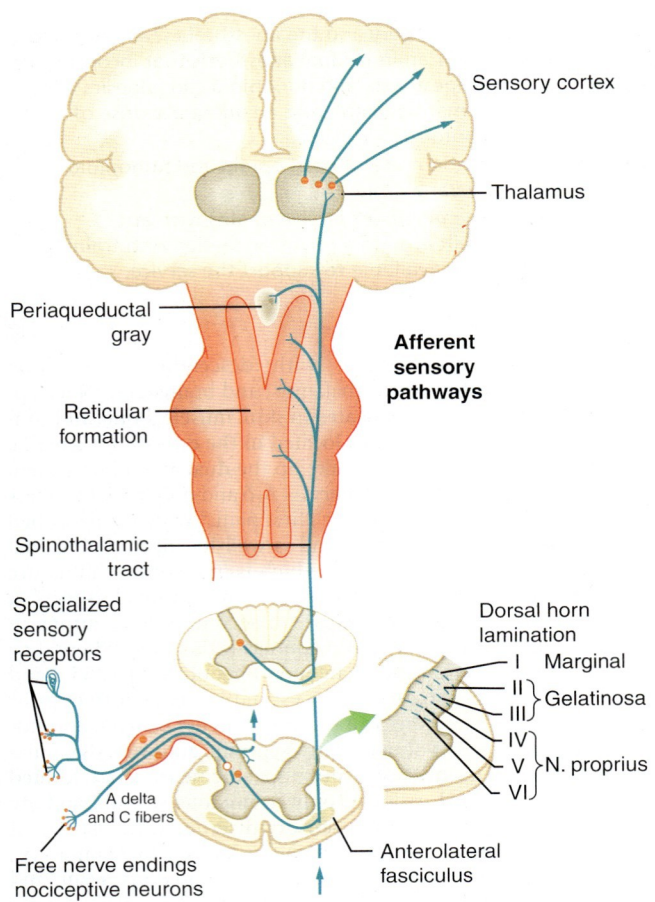

Figure 55-1 Afferent nociceptive pathway.

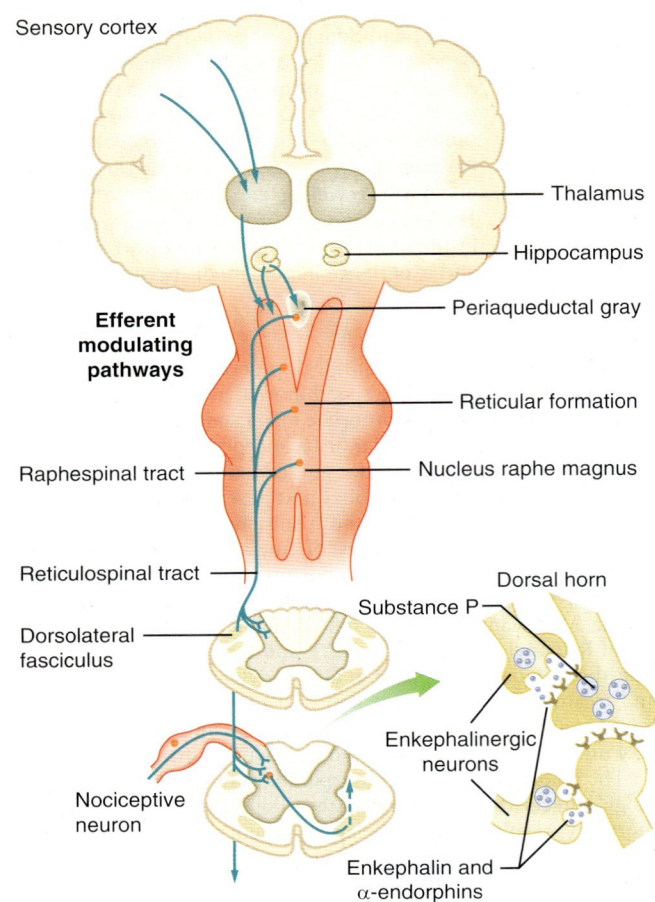

Figure 55-2 Efferent pathways involved in nociceptive regulation.

the spinal cord is the most common site for modulation of the pain pathway, and modulation can involve either *inhibition* or *augmentation* of the pain signals.[7] Examples of *inhibitory* spinal modulation include (1) release of inhibitory neurotransmitters such as γ-amino butyric acid (GABA) and glycine by intrinsic spinal neurons, and (2) activation of descending efferent neuronal pathways from the motor cortex, hypothalamus, periaqueductal gray matter, and the nucleus raphe magnus, which results in the release of norepinephrine, serotonin, and endorphins in

the dorsal horn. Spinal modulation, which results in *augmentation* of pain pathways, is manifested as central sensitization, which is a consequence of neuronal plasticity. The phenomenon of "wind-up" is a specific example of central plasticity that results from repetitive C-fiber stimulation of WDR neurons in the dorsal horn. *Perception* of pain is the final common pathway, which results from the integration of painful input into the somatosensory and limbic cortices. Generally speaking, traditional analgesic therapies have only targeted pain *perception*. A

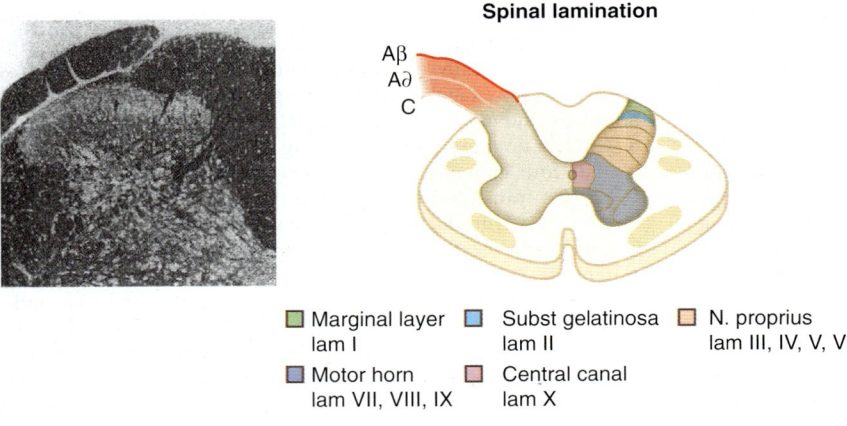

Figure 55-3 Schematic on the right showing the Rexed lamination and the approximate organization of the approach of the afferent to the spinal cord as they enter at the dorsal root entry zone and then penetrate into the dorsal horn to terminate in laminae I and II (A/C) or penetrate more deeply to loop upward to terminate as high as the dorsum of lamina III (Aβ). Inset on the left shows histologic appearance of the left dorsal quadrant, and large, myelinated axons. (Reprinted with permission from Warfield CA, Bajwa ZH, eds. *Principles and Practice of Pain Medicine*. 2nd ed. New York, NY: McGraw-Hill; 2004.)

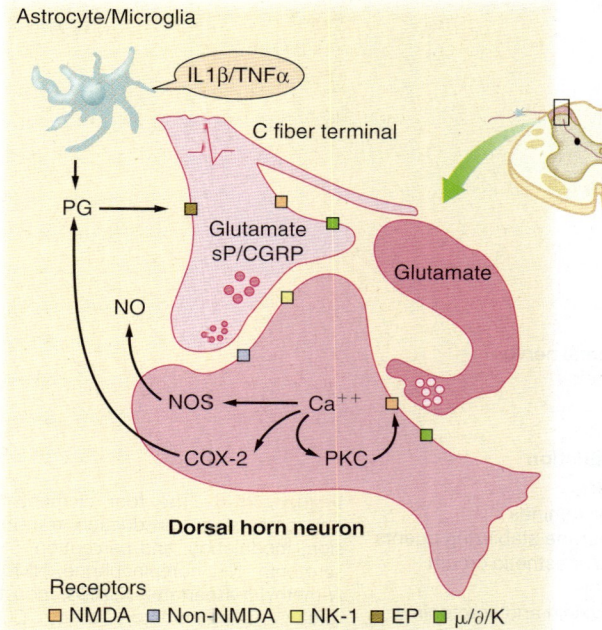

Figure 55-4 Schematic summarizing the organization of dorsal horn systems that contribute to the processing of nociceptive information. (1) Primary afferent C fibers release peptide (e.g., substance P [sP], calcitonin gene–related peptide [CGRP], and so on) and excitatory amino acid (glutamate) products. Small dorsal root ganglion (DRG) cells, as well as some postsynaptic elements contain nitric oxide synthase (NOS) and are able, upon depolarization, to release NO (nitric oxide). (2) Peptides and excitatory amino acids evoke excitation in second-order neurons. For glutamate, direct monosynaptic excitation is mediated by non–N-methyl-D-aspartate (NMDA) receptors (i.e., acute primary afferent excitation of WDR neurons is not mediated by the NMDA or neurokinin 1 [NK-1] receptor). (3) Interneurons excited by afferent barrage induce excitation in second-order neurons via an NMDA receptor. This leads to a marked increase in intracellular Ca^{2+} and the activation of kinases and phosphorylating enzymes. Prostaglandins (PGs) generated by cyclooxygenase-2 (COX-2) and NO by NOS are formed and released. These agents diffuse extracellularly and facilitate transmitter release (retrograde transmission) from primary and nonprimary afferent terminals, either by a direct cellular action (e.g., NO) or by an interaction with a specific class of receptors (e.g., EP receptors for prostanoids). (4) Nonneuronal sources of prostaglandins may include activated astrocytes and microglia that are stimulated by circulating cytokines, which are released secondary to peripheral nerve injury and inflammation. Terminal excitability can be altered by activation of a variety of receptors located on the sensory terminal, including those for, μ, δ, and κ opioids. (Adapted with permission from Warfield CA, Bajwa ZH, eds. *Principles and Practice of Pain Medicine*. 2nd ed. New York, NY: McGraw-Hill; 2004.)

Table 55-1 Primary Afferent Nerves

Fiber Class[a]	Velocity	Effective Stimuli
Aβ (myelinated) (12–20 μ dia)	Group II (>40–50 m/s)	Low-threshold mechanoreceptors Specialized nerve endings (Pacinian corpuscles)
Aδ (myelinated) (1–4 μ dia)	Group III (10 < x < 40 m/s)	Low-threshold mechanical or thermal High-threshold mechanical or thermal Specialized nerve endings
C (unmyelinated) (0.5–1.5 μ dia)	Group IV (<2 m/s)	High-threshold thermal, mechanical, and chemical Free nerve endings

[a]Aβ/Aδ/C is the Erlanger–Gasser classification and refers to axon size; II/III/IV is the Lloyd–Hunt classification and is defined on conduction velocity in muscle afferents. Because of the relationship between size and state of myelination with conduction velocity, these designations are often used interchangeably.
Reprinted with permission from Warfield CA, Bajwa ZH, eds. *Principles and Practice of Pain Medicine*. 2nd ed. New York, NY: McGraw-Hill; 2004:14.

multimodal approach to pain therapy should target all four elements of the pain processing pathway.

Chemical Mediators of Transduction and Transmission

Tissue damage following surgical procedures leads to the activation of small nociceptive nerve endings and local inflammatory cells (e.g., macrophages, mast cells, lymphocytes, and platelets) in the periphery. Antidromic release of substance P and glutamate from small nociceptive afferents results in vasodilation, extravasation of plasma proteins, and stimulation of inflammatory cells to release numerous algogenic substances (Table 55-2 and Fig. 55-7). This chemical milieu will both directly produce pain transduction via nociceptor stimulation as well as facilitate pain transduction by increasing the excitability of nociceptors. *Peripheral sensitization* of polymodal C fibers and high-threshold mechanoreceptors by these chemicals leads to *primary hyperalgesia*, which by definition is an exaggerated response to pain at the site of injury.

As is the case in the periphery, the dorsal horn of the spinal cord contains numerous transmitters and receptors involved in pain processing. Three classes of transmitter compounds integral to pain transmission include (1) the excitatory amino acids glutamate and aspartate, (2) the excitatory neuropeptides substance P and neurokinin A, and (3) the inhibitory amino acids

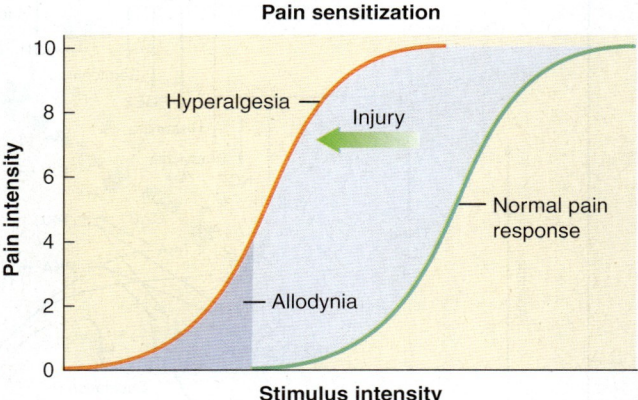

Figure 55-5 Pain sensitization. (From Dave Klemm, http:www.georgetown.edu/dml/facs/graphics/index.htm.)

Figure 55-6 The four elements of pain processing: transduction, transmission, modulation, and perception. 5HT, serotonin; NE, norepinephrine; NMDA, N-methyl-D-aspartate; NSAIDs, nonsteroidal anti-inflammatory drugs; CCK, cholecystokinin; NO, nitric oxide.

glycine and GABA. The various pain receptors include (1) the N-methyl-D-aspartate (NMDA), (2) the α-amino-3-hydroxy-5-methylisoxazole-4-proprionic acid (AMPA), (3) the kainate receptor, and (4) the metabotropic receptor (Fig. 55-8).

The AMPA and kainate receptors, which are sodium channel dependent, are essential for fast synaptic afferent input. On the other hand, the NMDA receptor, which is calcium channel dependent, is only activated following prolonged depolarization of the cell membrane. Release of substance P into the spinal cord will remove the magnesium block on the channel of the NMDA receptor, giving glutamate free access to the NMDA receptor. Repetitive C-fiber stimulation of WDR neurons in the dorsal horn at intervals of 0.5 to 1 Hz can precipitate the occurrence of windup and *central sensitization* (Fig. 55-9). This leads to *secondary hyperalgesia*, which, by definition, is an increased pain response evoked by stimuli outside the area of injury.

The Surgical Stress Response

Although similar, postoperative pain and the surgical stress response are not the same. Surgical stress causes release of cytokines (e.g., interleukin-1, interleukin-6, and tumor necrosis factor-α) and precipitates adverse neuroendocrine and sympathoadrenal responses, resulting in detrimental physiologic responses, particularly in high-risk patients.[5]

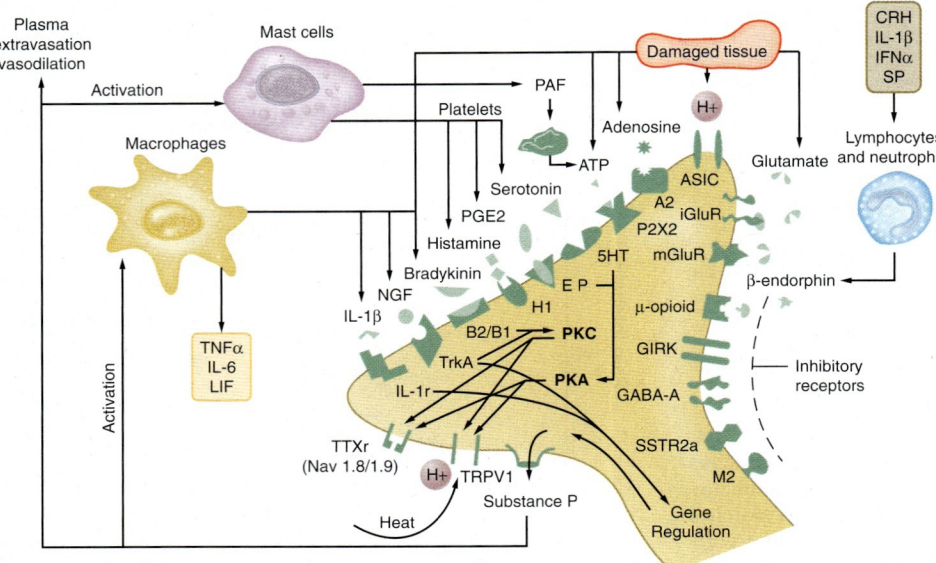

Figure 55-7 Schematic of the neurochemistry of somatosensory processing at peripheral sensory nerve endings. (Adapted with permission from Benzon HT, Raja SN, Molloy RE, et al., eds. *Essentials of Pain Medicine and Regional Anesthesia.* 2nd ed. Philadelphia, PA: Elsevier; 2005:8.)

Table 55-2 Algogenic Substances

Substance	Source	Effect
Bradykinin	Macrophages and plasma kininogen	Activates nociceptors
Serotonin	Platelets	Activates nociceptors
Histamine	Platelets and mast cells	Produces vasodilation, edema, and pruritus Potentiates the response of nociceptors to bradykinin
Prostaglandin	Tissue injury and cyclooxygenase pathway	Sensitizes nociceptors
Leukotriene	Tissue injury and lipooxygenase pathway	Sensitizes nociceptors
Excess H^+ ions	Tissue injury and ischemia	Increases pain and hyperalgesia associated with inflammation
Cytokines (e.g., interleukins and tissue necrosis factor)	Macrophages	Excites and sensitizes nociceptors
Adenosine	Tissue injury	Pain and hyperalgesia
Neurotransmitters (e.g., glutamate and substance P)	Antidromic release by peripheral nerve terminals following tissue injury	Substance P activates macrophages and mast cells Glutamate activates nociceptors
Nerve growth factor	Macrophages	Stimulates mast cells to release histamine and serotonin Induces heat hyperalgesia Sensitizes nociceptors

Data from Dougherty PM, Raja SN. Neurochemistry of somatosensory and pain processing. In: Benzon HT, Raja SN, Molloy RE, et al., eds. *Essentials of Pain Medicine and Regional Anesthesia*. Philadelphia, PA: Elsevier; 2005:7.

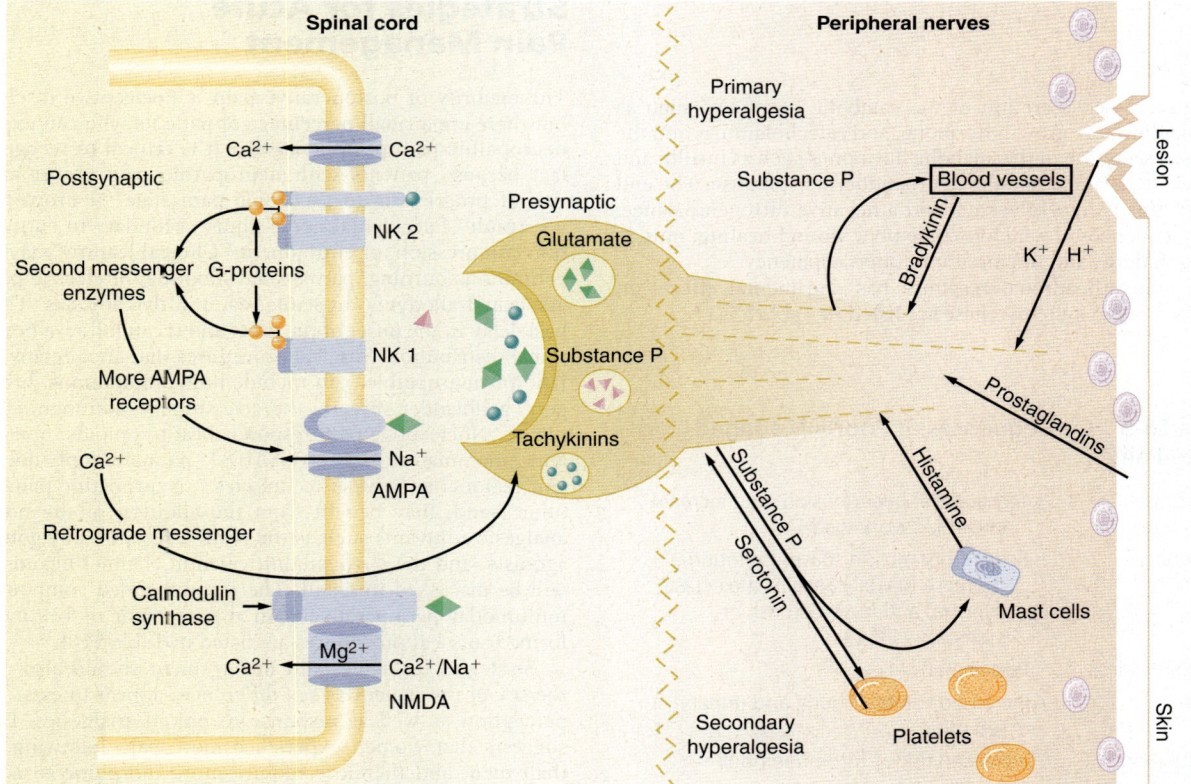

Figure 55-8 Schematic representation of peripheral and spinal mechanism involved in neuroplasticity. Primary hyperalgesia results from tissue release of toxic substances. These toxic substances spread to adjacent tissues, prolonging the hyperalgesic state (secondary hyperalgesia). As C fiber terminals increase in frequency of release of neurotransmitters, such as glutamate, substance P, tachykinins, brain-derived neurotrophic factor, and calcitonin gene–related peptide, the effects of these neurotransmitters are summated, resulting in prolonged depolarizations of second-order neurons (wind-up). Function changes at the second-order neuron occur as a result of neurotransmitter binding to postsynaptic receptors, which results in activity-dependent plasticity of the spinal cord. AMPA, α-amino-3-hydroxy-5-methyl-4-isoxazole propionic acid; NK, neurokinin; NMDA, *N*-methyl-D-aspartate.

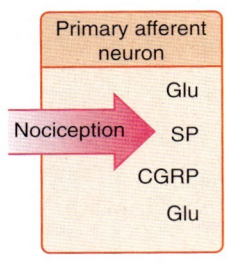
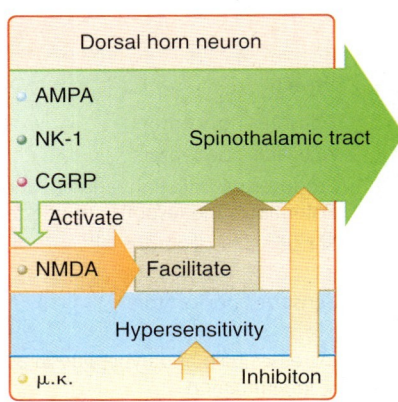

Figure 55-9 Primary nociceptive transmission in the spinal cord. Primary afferent nociceptive input is transmitted via α-amino-3-hydroxy-5-methyl-4-isoxazole propionic acid (AMPA), neurokinin-1 (NK1), and calcitonin gene–related peptide (CGRP) synapses, whose signals work their way to the thalamus. Glutaminergic (N-methyl-D-aspartate [NMDA]) synapses do not participate significantly in primary nociceptive transmission, but instead play a crucial role in spinal sensitization. Accordingly, even after complete NMDA blockade in the spinal cord, primary afferent nociceptive information is transmitted to the thalamus. NMDA antagonists thus have an antihyperalgesic rather than an analgesic effect in the spinal cord. Glu, glutamate; SP, substance P. (Adapted with permission from the International Association for the Study of Pain. Pain control updates. *IASP Newlett.* 2005;13[2]:3.)

Preventive Analgesia

Preventive analgesia includes any antinociceptive regimen delivered at any time during the perioperative period that will attenuate pain-induced sensitization. The term "preventive analgesia" replaces the older terminology "preemptive analgesia," which is defined as an analgesic regimen that is administered prior to surgical incision and is more effective at pain relief than the same regimen administered after surgery. Although use of the term preemptive analgesia has been popular in the past, evidence of its clinical benefit in humans has been mixed and the term should be considered obsolete.[10] The goal of preventive analgesia is to block the development of sustained pain. Theoretically, this occurs by preventing NMDA receptor activation in the dorsal horn that is associated with windup, facilitation, central sensitization expansion of receptive fields, and long-term potentiation, all of which can lead to a chronic pain state.[8] In order for preventive analgesia to be successful, three critical principles must be adhered to: (1) The depth of analgesia must be adequate enough to block all nociceptive input during surgery, (2) the analgesic technique must be extensive enough to include the entire surgical field, and (3) the duration of analgesia must include both the surgical and postsurgical periods. Patients with pre-existing chronic pain may not respond as well to these techniques because of pre-existing sensitization of the nervous system.[10]

Strategies for Acute Pain Management

The majority of postoperative pain is nociceptive in character, but there are a small percentage of patients who can experience neuropathic pain postoperatively. It is critical to recognize this fact because patients with neuropathic pain are at increased risk of progressing to a chronic pain state. Neuropathic pain is a result of accidental nerve injury secondary to cutting, traction compression, or entrapment.[5] Clinical features may include continuous burning, paroxysmal shooting, or electric pain with associated allodynia, hyperalgesia, and dysesthesias. There can be a delay in the onset of the pain, and it can follow a nondermatomal distribution. Surgical procedures that are a relatively high risk for neuropathic pain include limb amputations, breast surgery, gallbladder surgery, thoracic surgery, and inguinal hernia repair.[5] Nociceptive pain responds best to opioids, nonsteroidal anti-inflammatory drugs (NSAIDs), para-aminophenol agents, and regional anesthesia techniques.[11] Neuropathic pain, on the other hand, may benefit from the addition of the nonopioid analgesic adjuvants such as the NMDA receptor antagonists, α_2-agonists, and the $\alpha_2-\delta$ subunit calcium channel ligands, which will be discussed in detail. The recommended components for multimodal perioperative pain management of routinely performed surgical procedures are listed in Table 55-4.

Strategies for acute pain management should also consider the sex of the patient as sex differences appear to exist for pain perception as well as response to opioid analgesics. Evidence suggests that women experience more pain following surgery than men, and therefore require more morphine to achieve a similar level of pain relief.[12]

Finally, as knowledge of the human genome and understanding of the neurobiology of nociception evolve, we will be able to tailor pain management to the individual patient based on genetic variation. This strategy, known as pharmacogenetics, takes advantage of polymorphic genes, which can impact the pharmacokinetics of a drug by altering drug-metabolizing

The increased secretion of the catabolic hormones such as cortisol, glucagon, growth hormone, and catecholamines and the decreased secretion of the anabolic hormones such as insulin and testosterone characterize the neuroendocrine response. The end result of this is hyperglycemia and a negative nitrogen balance, the consequences of which include poor wound healing, muscle wasting, fatigue, and impaired immunocompetency.

The sympathoadrenal response has detrimental effects on numerous organ systems; these are listed in Table 55-3.[9]

Table 55-3 Consequences of Poorly Managed Acute Pain[5,9]

Cardiovascular	Tachycardia, hypertension, and increase in cardiac work load
Pulmonary	Respiratory muscle spasm (splinting), decrease in vital capacity, atelectasis, hypoxia, and increased risk of pulmonary infection
Gastrointestinal	Postoperative ileus
Renal	Increased risk of oliguria and urinary retention
Coagulation	Increased risk of thromboemboli
Immunologic	Impaired immune function
Muscular	Muscle weakness and fatigue. Limited mobility can increase the risk of thromboembolism
Psychological	Anxiety, fear, and frustration results in poor patient satisfaction

Table 55-4 Options for Components of Multimodal Therapy for Commonly Performed Surgeries

Type of Surgery	Systemic Pharmacologic Therapy	Local, Intra-articular, or Topical Techniques*	Regional Anesthetic Techniques*	Neuraxial Anesthetic Techniques*	Nonpharmacologic Therapies
Thoracotomy	Opioids[a] NSAIDs[b] and/or acetaminophen Gabapentin or pregabalin[b] IV ketamine[c]		Paravertebral block	Epidural with local anesthetic (with or without opioid), or intrathecal opioid	Cognitive modalities TENS
Open laparotomy	Opioids[a] NSAIDs[b] and/or acetaminophen Gabapentin or pregabalin[b] IV ketamine IV lidocaine	Local anesthetic at incision IV lidocaine infusion	Transversus abdominis plane block	Epidural with local anesthetic (with or without opioid), or intrathecal opioid	Cognitive modalities TENS
Total hip replacement	Opioids[a] NSAIDs[b] and/or acetaminophen Gabapentin or pregabalin[b] IV ketamine[c]	Intra-articular local anesthetic and/or opioid	Site-specific regional anesthetic technique with local anesthetic	Epidural with local anesthetic (with or without opioid), or intrathecal opioid	Cognitive modalities TENS
Total knee replacement	Opioids[a] NSAIDs[b] and/or acetaminophen Gabapentin or pregabalin[b] IV ketamine[c]	Intra-articular local anesthetic and/or opioid	Site-specific regional anesthetic technique with local anesthetic	Epidural with local anesthetic (with or without opioid), or intrathecal opioid	Cognitive modalities TENS
Spinal fusion	Opioids[a] Acetaminophen[d] Gabapentin or pregabalin[b] IV ketamine[c]	Local anesthetic at incision		Epidural with local anesthetic (with or without opioid), or intrathecal opioid	Cognitive modalities TENS
Cesarean section	Opioids[a] NSAIDs[b] and/or acetaminophen	Local anesthetic at incision	Transversus abdominal plane block	Epidural with local anesthetic (with or without opioid), or intrathecal opioid	Cognitive modalities TENS
Coronary artery bypass grafting	Opioids[a] Acetaminophen Gabapentin or pregabalin[b] IV ketamine[c]				Cognitive modalities TENS

Blank cells indicate techniques generally not used for the procedure in question.
*Intra-articular, peripheral regional, and neuraxial techniques typically not used together.
[a]Use IV PCA when parenteral route needed for more than a few hours and patients have adequate cognitive function to understand the device and safety limitations.
[b]May be administered preoperatively.
[c]On the basis of panel consensus, primarily consider for use in opioid-tolerant or otherwise complex patients.
[d]Use as adjunctive treatments.
NSAIDs, nonsteroidal anti-inflammatory drugs; TENS, transcutaneous electrical nerve stimulation. Reprinted with permission from Chou R, Gordon DB, de Leon-Casasola OA, et al. Management of postoperative pain: a clinical practice guideline from the American Pain Society, the American Society of Regional Anesthesia and Pain Medicine, and the American Society of Anesthesiologists' Committee on Regional Anesthesia, Executive Committee, and Administrative Council. J Pain. 2016;17(2):131–157.

enzymes, drug transport proteins, and drug receptors. The net effect will determine both the efficacy and side effects of individual drugs in each patient based on their personal genetic profile.

There are numerous examples of CYP (cytochrome P450) and UGT (Uridine 5′-diphospho-glucuronosyltransferase) genes that are polymorphic and will result in various responses to opioid analgesics. *Hydrocodone* is the most widely prescribed opioid analgesic in the United States. It has weak affinity for the μ receptor; however, demethylation by the CYP2D6 enzyme converts hydrocodone into hydromorphone, which has stronger μ receptor binding. Patients with the extensive metabolizer (EM) phenotype report better opioid effects and fewer adverse opioid effects than the patients with the poor metabolizer (PM) phenotype. Point-of-care phenotype-based dosing strategies would preclude

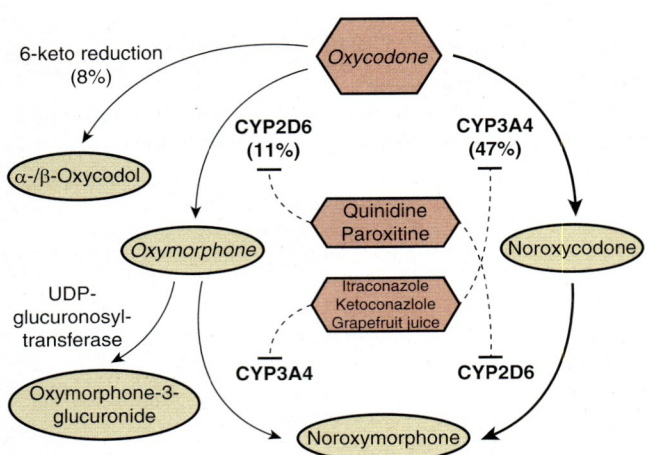

Figure 55-10 Oxycodone metabolism. (Adapted with permission from Landau R, Bollag LA, Kraft JC. Pharmacogenetics and anaesthesia: the value of genetic profiling. *Anaesthesia*. 2012;67(2):165–79.)

prescribing hydrocodone to patients with the poor metabolizer phenotype.

Oxycodone (Oxycontin, Percocet) is another commonly prescribed semisynthetic opioid analgesic that is used for the treatment of both acute and chronic pain. The drug is predominantly metabolized by CYP3A4 to inactive metabolites; however, approximately 11% of an oxycodone dose is cleared by CYP2D6 (Fig. 55-10) to produce the minor metabolite oxymorphone, which is reported to be eight times as potent as the parent drug. It is theoretically possible that toxicity or overdose could occur in CYP2D6 ultrarapid metabolizers or in patients who are concomitantly taking a CYP3A4 inhibitor (e.g., diltiazem, verapamil).

Both *codeine* and *tramadol* are examples of prodrugs that require metabolism by the CYP2D6 enzyme to an active intermediate that has analgesic effects. Whereas slow metabolizers of codeine display poor analgesia from the drug, rapid metabolizers can experience toxicity from the active metabolite, morphine (Fig. 55-11). Like codeine, tramadol is also a prodrug that requires CYP2D6 to be converted into the active metabolite O-desmethyltramadol. Poor metabolizers display incomplete analgesia. The frequency of poor metabolizers varies by ethnicity and is reported to be 8% in whites, 2% to 7% in African Americans and 0% to 0.5% in Asian populations. *Methadone* is also subject to genetic polymorphism secondary to modifications by genetic variations in CYP2D6, the OPRM1 μ opioid receptor, and the ABCB1 drug transport protein. Methadone fatalities are associated with the slow metabolizer phenotype.

Finally, genetic variants of the CYP2C9 enzyme and the melanocortin-1 receptor gene (*MC1R*) display poor metabolism of *celecoxib* and reduced effects of subcutaneous *lidocaine*, respectively. Future strategies will likely incorporate pharmacogenetic approaches to design individualized gene-based pain therapy for each patient, to optimize pain control and minimize adverse effects.[13,14]

Assessment of Acute Pain

The need for assessment of the patient in pain is illustrated by the postoperative patient who is said to be relatively pain-free, but who, on inspection, is lying almost completely still in bed. Too often, such a patient has had a recent cursory evaluation that included the traditional verbal analogue score (VAS) 0 to 10 scale ("on a scale of 0 to 10, with 0 being no pain and 10 being the worst pain you can imagine, how much pain are you in" from which the patient reported a low VAS score of 1/10) (Fig. 55-12). The treating team took that to be reassuring information and moved along. No one asked the patient about pain with movement, breathing, moving bowels, and so forth, all potentially important functional goals for the postoperative course that may be undermined by untreated pain.

A variety of well-studied pain measurement scales exist that can be helpful yet are not definitive. Unidimensional instruments such as the familiar numerical pain scale already mentioned, the visual analogue scale, and the "faces" (Fig. 55-12) pain rating scale can provide some degree of guidance about a patient's experience of pain, but all of these are completely subjective and are open to wide variation between subjects and within subjects at different times.

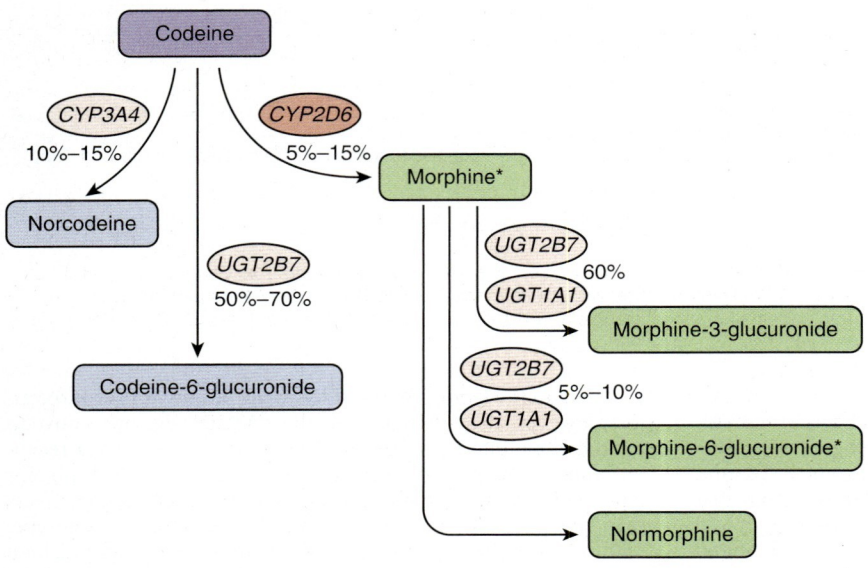

Figure 55-11 Codeine metabolism pathway in an individual with cytochrome P450 2D6 (CYP2D6) extensive metabolism. *Asterisks* denote active metabolites. (Adapted with permission from Crews KR, Gaedigk A, Dunnenberger HM, et al. Clinical Pharmacogenetics Implementation Consortium guidelines for cytochrome P450 2D6 genotype and codeine therapy: 2014 update. *Clin Pharmacol Ther*. 2014;95(4):376–382.)

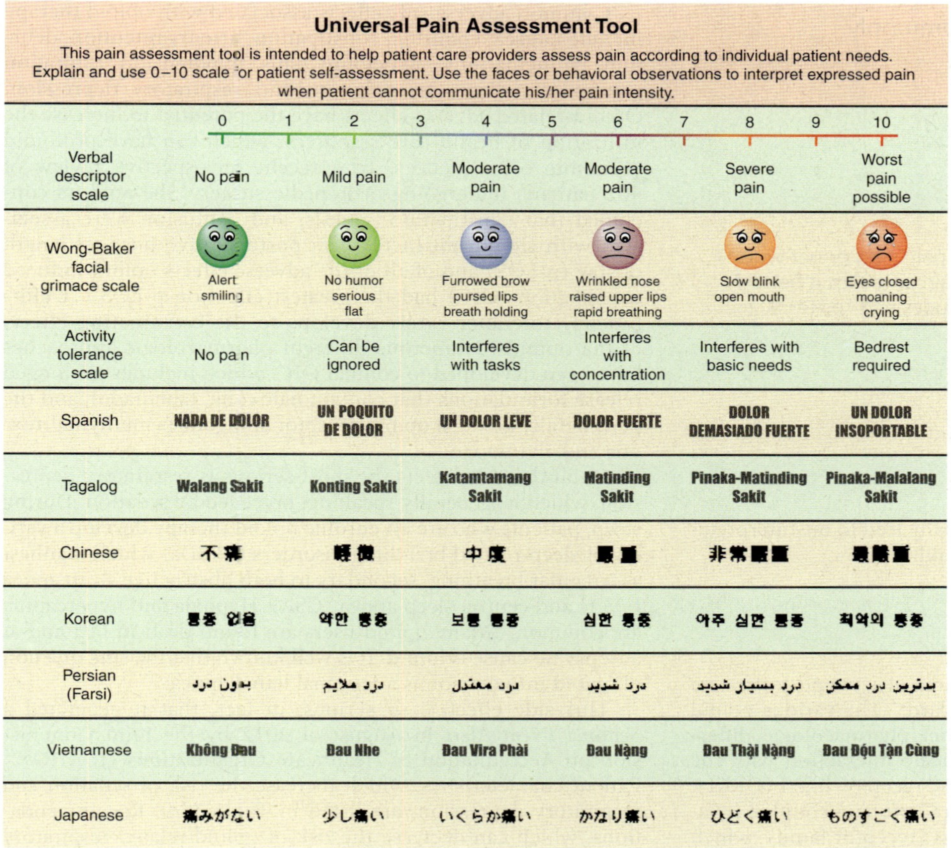

Universal Pain Assessment Tool

This pain assessment tool is intended to help patient care providers assess pain according to individual patient needs. Explain and use 0–10 scale for patient self-assessment. Use the faces or behavioral observations to interpret expressed pain when patient cannot communicate his/her pain intensity.

	0	1	2	3	4	5	6	7	8	9	10
Verbal descriptor scale	No pain		Mild pain		Moderate pain		Moderate pain		Severe pain		Worst pain possible
Wong-Baker facial grimace scale	Alert smiling		No humor serious flat		Furrowed brow pursed lips breath holding		Wrinkled nose raised upper lips rapid breathing		Slow blink open mouth		Eyes closed moaning crying
Activity tolerance scale	No pain		Can be ignored		Interferes with tasks		Interferes with concentration		Interferes with basic needs		Bedrest required
Spanish	NADA DE DOLOR		UN POQUITO DE DOLOR		UN DOLOR LEVE		DOLOR FUERTE		DOLOR DEMASIADO FUERTE		UN DOLOR INSOPORTABLE
Tagalog	Walang Sakit		Konting Sakit		Katamtamang Sakit		Matinding Sakit		Pinaka-Matinding Sakit		Pinaka-Malalang Sakit
Chinese	不痛		輕微		中度		嚴重		非常嚴重		最嚴重
Korean	통증 없음		약한 통증		보통 통증		심한 통증		아주 심한 통증		최악의 통증
Persian (Farsi)	بدون درد		درد ملایم		درد معتدل		درد شدید		درد بسیار شدید		بدترین درد ممکن
Vietnamese	Không Đau		Đau Nhẹ		Đau Vừa Phải		Đau Nặng		Đau Thật Nặng		Đau Đớn Tận Cùng
Japanese	痛みがない		少し痛い		いくらか痛い		かなり痛い		ひどく痛い		ものすごく痛い

Figure 55-12 Linear verbal analogue score and "faces" pain assessment tool.

Multidimensional instruments, such as the Mcgill Pain Questionnaire or the Brief Pain Inventory, provide a broader picture of a patient's experience, but are usually more cumbersome to administer and, in the end, suffer the same limitations as all other attempts to measure pain. A number of tools to assess cancer-related and noncancer chronic pain have been advanced and validated.[15] Most of these focus on persistent background pain and do not help identify intermittent or breakthrough pain. Several assessment scales specifically address breakthrough or episodic pain. The Breakthrough Pain Questionnaire was introduced by Portenoy and Hagen to assess breakthrough pain in cancer patients, and has also been studied in patients with acute noncancer pain, for which it can offer a picture of both breakthrough and background pain states.[16]

Ultimately, we are left with a maxim first attributed to Dr. John Bonica, the father of pain medicine: "Pain is what a patient says it is." The best way to begin assessing a patient's pain is to *ask* about it and *listen* to the answers. Attempts to reduce the experience to finite details may lead to failure to ask the right questions, distance us from our patients, focus us away from the whole person, and potentially miss golden diagnostic clues that could lead to effective interventions.

Effective treatment of acute pain requires assessment as well as vigilant reassessment to determine if the primary goals are met, adversity has occurred, or changes are necessary. Acute pain may be viewed as breakthrough, intermittent, or background in nature (Table 55-5). The assessment process for each of these is relatively similar and will help to resolve the related condition into broad pathophysiologic groups such as cancer versus noncancer, and nociceptive versus neuropathic, or mixed pain states. Such an approach supports a rational process for developing a useful differential diagnosis and approaches. Table 55-6 lists the common features of pain that are usually reviewed during the assessment for acute pain. A thorough physical examination must also be performed with particular attention to the neurologic examination, which may offer clues to aberrant neural processing. Such neurologic findings may indicate nerve injury, alerting the astute clinician to a neuropathic rather than a nociceptive pain state that requires a different analgesic approach.[17] A provocative physical examination may include examination of the affected areas with maneuvers that may provoke pain such as range of motion testing, walking, and cough. The benefits of provocative testing must outweigh the associated suffering incurred by the patient. Medical imaging is also a common part of the acute pain workup. Overemphasis on imaging data should,

Table 55-5 Three Classes of Acute Pain

Class	Description
Breakthrough	Pain that escalates above a persistent background pain
Transitory and intermittent	Pain that is episodic in the absence of background pain
Background	Pain that is persistent but may vary over time

Table 55-6 Features of Pain Commonly Addressed during Assessment

Onset of pain
Temporal pattern of pain
Site of pain
Radiation of pain
Quality (character) of pain
Intensity (severity) of pain
Exacerbating factors (what makes the pain start or get worse?)
Relieving factors (what prevents the pain or makes it better?)
Response to analgesics (including attitudes and concerns about opioids)
Response to other interventions
Associated physical symptoms
Associated psychological symptoms
Interference with activities of daily living

however, be avoided as this can potentially lead to misinterpretation of the patient's underlying pain syndrome.

Opioid Analgesics

Opioids are the mainstay for the treatment of acute postoperative pain, and morphine is the "gold standard." The various opioid analgesics available today have distinct pharmacologic differences that we can credit to their intricate interaction with the main opioid receptors: μ, δ, κ, and opioid receptor-like 1 (ORL1). The opioid receptors are members of a G protein–coupled (guanosine triphosphate regulatory proteins) receptor family, which signals via a second messenger such as cyclic adenosine monophosphate or an ion channel. In the ascending pain pathway, opioid receptors are located in three areas that include (1) the periphery, following inflammation; (2) the spinal cord dorsal horn; and (3) supraspinally in the brainstem, thalamus, and cortex. μ Opioid receptors are also found in the periaqueductal grey, the nucleus raphe magnus, and the rostral ventral medulla, which constitutes the descending inhibitory pain pathway. The three primary mechanisms of action for opioid analgesia at the level of the spinal cord include (1) inhibition of calcium influx presynaptically, resulting in inhibition of depolarization of the cell membrane and decreased release of neurotransmitters and neuropeptides into the synaptic cleft; (2) enhanced potassium efflux from the cell postsynaptically, resulting in hyperpolarization of the cell and a decrease in pain transmission, and (3) activation of a descending inhibitory pain circuit via inhibition of GABAergic transmission in the brainstem. Peripheral opioid receptors, which mediate analgesia, are located on primary afferent neurons. Activation of these receptors inhibits the release of pronociceptive and proinflammatory substances like substance P, which accounts for the analgesic and anti-inflammatory effects. The "broad-spectrum" opioid, methadone, has NMDA receptor antagonist properties and inhibits the reuptake of serotonin and norepinephrine, which may make it useful in the treatment of neuropathic pain.

There is great diversity in the available routes of administration of opioid analgesics. Table 55-7 is a list of relevant pharmacokinetic data. Table 55-8 offers equianalgesic dosing guidelines for the various opioids. The reader is referred to Perioperative Pain Management of the Opioid-Dependent Patient for a detailed discussion of incomplete cross-tolerance between the different opioids and dosing considerations.

Common adverse side effects associated with opioid therapy include nausea, vomiting, constipation, urinary retention, delirium, hallucinations, myoclonus, falls, hypotension, aspiration pneumonia, dizziness, sedation, and respiratory depression. Opioid-related adverse effects have the potential to increase the utilization of health-care resources, which can have profound economic consequences. In a recent retrospective review of 402 patients undergoing orthopedic surgery, the authors concluded that constipation, emesis, and confusion were associated with significant increase in postoperative hospital length of stay (p-LOS) and of all of the adverse effects opioid-induced constipation (OIC) had the greatest effect on p-LOS.[18] Unfortunately tolerance rarely develops to the constipating effects of the opioids. Numerous different pharmacologic approaches have been developed to combat OIC, which includes prolonged release formulations that contain naloxone, tapentadol, and the peripherally acting μ opioid receptor antagonists methylnaltrexone and alvimopan.[19]

Of all the side effects the most serious is respiratory depression, which is, generally speaking, preceded by sedation. During sleep, patients who are on chronic opioid therapy develop a variety of sleep-related breathing disorders (SRBDs) which manifest as irregular breathing, secondary to both obstructive sleep apnea (OSA) and central sleep apnea (CSA). Hypoxia and hypercapnia are common. "Many opioid users are found dead in bed and at autopsy no cause is found. It is well known that the sine qua non of opioid intoxication is a terminal lethal apnea."[20]

This side effect is so serious, in fact, that it generated a *Sentinel Event Alert* in August of 2012 by the Joint Commission on Accreditation of Healthcare Organizations (JCAHO).[21] Patient characteristics, which increase the risk of sedation and respiratory depression, are listed in Table 55-9. Recommendations, which can decrease the risk of opioid-related respiratory depression, include the liberal use of opioid-sparing multimodal pharmacotherapy, regional anesthesia techniques, and the continuous monitoring of patient ventilation with pulse oximetry and capnography, particularly in the high-risk individual. See Table 55-4 for recommendations for multimodal therapy for some commonly performed surgeries.

Respiratory assist devices can also be very helpful. Continuous positive airway pressure (CPAP) is recommended for the treatment of OSA in the opioid-dependent patient. However, patients can fail CPAP and CSA can emerge. These patients may be better candidates for either a bilevel device with backup rate or an adaptive servoventilation (ASV) device. A more comprehensive discussion of this topic is beyond the scope of this chapter and the reader is referred to the excellent review by Javaheri and Randerath.[20] Finally, Evzio is a take-home naloxone auto-injector that patients, family members, or caregivers can use in the event of an opioid overdose in the patient on chronic opioid therapy. The product received Food and Drug Administration (FDA) approval in April of 2014.

Other disconcerting side effects associated with the chronic use of opioids include opioid-induced hyperalgesia (OIH) and immune modulation. OIH is a relatively rare phenomenon whereby patients who are receiving opioids suddenly and paradoxically become more sensitive to pain despite continued treatment with opioids. Evidence suggests that OIH is more likely to develop following high doses of phenanthrene opioids such as morphine.[22,23] Changing the opioid to a phenyl piperidine derivative such as fentanyl may thwart OIH. There is also evidence that coadministration of an NMDA receptor antagonist can abolish opioid-induced tolerance and OIH.[22] Finally, opioid analgesics have profound immunomodulatory effects, which include inhibition of cellular and humoral immune functions, depressed natural killer cell activity, promotion of angiogenesis, and inhibition of

Table 55-7 Opioid Analgesic Pharmacokinetics[32]

Drug	Onset of Effect	Peak Effect	Duration of Effect	Elimination t½	VD (L/kg)	Protein Binding (%)	Metabolism Pathway	Active Metabolites	Major Excretion Pathway
Alfentanil	Immediate	1.5–2 min	<10 min	1.5–1.85 h	0.4–1	92%	Liver	—	Urine
Codeine	Oral: 10–30 min, IV: 15 min	0.5–1 h	Oral: 4–6 h, IV: 5 h	2.5–3 h	—	—	Liver	Morphine	Urine
Fentanyl injection	IV: immediate, IM: 7–8 min	—	IV: 0.5–1 h, IM: 1–2 h	3.65 h	4	Alters with increasing ionization	Liver	—	Urine
Fentanyl transdermal	—	24–72 h	72 h	≈17 h	6	Decreases with increasing ionization	Liver: CYP3A4	—	Urine
Fentanyl transmucosal	—	—	—	7 h	4	80–85%	Liver: CYP3A4	—	Urine
Hydromorphone	IM/SC: 15 min	0.5–1 h	IR: 4–5 h, ER: 24 h, IM/Subcutaneous: 4–5 h	IR: 2.3 h, ER: 18.6 h	≈4	8–20%	Liver: Glucuronidation	—	Urine
Levorphanol	Oral: 30 min	—	—	IM/Subcutaneous: 2.6 h	IV: 10–13	40%	—	—	—
Meperidine	IM: 15–30 min	Oral: 1 h	2–4 h	IV: 11–16 h	—	60–80%	Liver	Normeperidine	—
Methadone	Parenteral: 10–20 min Oral: 30–60 min	—	—	3–6 h (parent), <20 h (normeperidine)	—	—	—	—	—
Morphine sulfate	IM/SC: 10–30 min	Epidural: 10–15 min, Oral: 1 h	4 h	8–59 h	2–6	85–90%	Liver primarily CYP3A4 and to lesser extent CYP2D6	—	Urine and fecal
Oxycodone	Within 60 min	—	Subcutaneous/IM: 4–5 h	1.5–2 h	1–6	20–35%	Liver: glucuronidation	Morphine-6-glucuronide	Urine
Oxymorphone	Parenteral: 5–10 min	—	IR: 3–4 h CR: 12 h	IR: 3.2 h, CR: 4.5 h	2.6	45%	Liver: Somewhat involves CYP2D6	Noroxycodone and oxymorphone	Urine
Propoxyphene*	—	2–2.5 h	Parenteral: 3–6 h	1.3 h	≈3	—	Liver	—	Urine
Remifentanil	Rapid	—	—	6–12 h (parent), 30–36 h (norpropoxyphene)	—	80%	Liver	Norpropoxyphene	Urine
Sufentanil	IV: immediate, Epidural: 10 min	—	Epidural: 1.7 h	10–20 min	0.35	70%	Hydrolysis by esterases	—	Urine
Tramadol	—	—	2 h (tramadol), 3 h (M1, active metabolite)	2.7 h	—	91–93%, 79% in neonates	Liver and small intestine	—	—
	—	—	—	6.3 h (tramadol), 7.4 h (M1, active metabolite)	2.6–2.9	20%	Liver: CYP2D6 and CYP3A4	O-desmethyl-tramadol (M1) via CYP2D6	Urine

IV, intravenous; CT, cytochrome; IR, immediate release; ER, extended release; IM, intramuscular; SC, subcutaneous; CR, controlled release.

Table 55-8 Opioid Equianalgesic Dosing[158,189,190]

Drug	Dosage IV/IM/SQ	Oral (mg)
Morphine (MS Contin)	10 mg	30
Hydromorphone (Dilaudid)	1.5–2 mg	6–8
Hydrocodone (Vicodin)	NA	30–45
Oxymorphone (Opana IR and ER)	1 mg	10
Oxycodone (Percocet, Oxycontin)	10–15 mg	20
Levorphanol (Levo-Dromoran)	2 mg	4
Fentanyl	100 μg	NA
Meperidine (Demerol)	100 mg	300
Codeine	100 mg	200
Methadone	The conversion ratio for methadone is variable.	

IV, intravenous; IM, intramuscular; SQ, subcutaneous; IR, immediate release; ER, extended release.

apoptosis. Such effects can be beneficial or deleterious depending upon the clinical situation.[24,25]

Morphine is the prototype opioid and is the "gold standard" to which all other analgesics are compared. Although the plasma half-life of the drug is approximately 2 hours its analgesic duration of action is closer to 4 to 5 hours. Morphine undergoes hepatic glucuronidation to morphine-6-glucuronide and morphine-3-glucuronide, both of which are cleared by the kidney. Morphine-6-glucuronide is an active metabolite of morphine and is thought to be responsible for most of the analgesia associated with chronic dosing of the drug. Morphine-3-glucuronide, on the other hand, is considered to be devoid of analgesic activity. With chronic dosing these metabolites can accumulate and can be particularly problematic in patients with renal failure. Dosing adjustment is therefore necessary and monitoring of side effects is important. Morphine-6-glucuronide contributes to side effects such as drowsiness, nausea and vomiting, coma, and respiratory depression. Morphine-3-glucuronide, on the other hand, is thought to cause agitation, myoclonus, delirium, and hyperalgesia.

Hydromorphone is a semisynthetic opioid that has four to six times the potency of morphine. It is available for oral, rectal, parenteral, and neuraxial administration. Whereas the oral bioavailability of the drug is reported to be 20% to 50%, its bioavailability via the subcutaneous route is 78%, making it the ideal drug for long-term subcutaneous administration in the opioid-tolerant patient. Like morphine, hydromorphone is biotransformed in the liver. The active metabolites are dihydromorphine and dihydroisomorphine and the inactive metabolite is hydromorphone-3-glucuronide. Although hydromorphone has traditionally been the preferred opioid for patients with acute pain and impaired kidney function, evidence suggests that hydromorphone-3-glucuronide can accumulate in those with renal failure and may contribute to side effects such as neuroexcitation and cognitive impairment. Opioid-related side effects such as nausea, vomiting, sedation, cognitive impairment, and pruritus are reported to be less intense with hydromorphone vis-à-vis morphine. In fact, the incidence of pruritus following neuraxial administration of hydromorphone is reported to be approximately 5% versus the 11% to 77% range reported for neuraxial morphine.[26]

Codeine is an opioid agonist that has both analgesic and antitussive properties. In the United States, codeine is available for oral, subcutaneous, and intramuscular administration. As previously mentioned, codeine is a prodrug that is devoid of analgesic activity and requires metabolic conversion by the CYP2D6 enzyme into morphine, which has a 200-fold greater affinity for the μ-opioid receptor than the parent drug codeine. In *extensive metabolizers* O-demethylation of the drug by the CYP2D6 enzyme accounts for only 5% to 10% clearance of codeine; however, this conversion to morphine is critical for opioid activity (Fig. 55-11). In *poor metabolizers* and *ultrarapid* metabolizers codeine is contraindicated because of lack of efficacy in the former and the potential for toxicity in the latter (Table 55-10).[27]

Oxycodone (Oxycontin, Percocet) is used for the treatment of both acute and chronic pain and in the United States the drug is only available for oral administration. Please refer to the section Strategies for Acute Pain Management for further details. The drug is available only for oral administration. Oxycodone is predominantly metabolized by CYP3A4 to inactive metabolites; however, approximately 11% of an oxycodone dose is cleared by CYP2D6 to produce the minor metabolite oxymorphone, which is reported to be eight times as potent as the parent drug.[27] It is theoretically possible that toxicity or overdose could occur in CYP2D6 ultrarapid metabolizers or in patients who are concomitantly taking a CYP3A4 inhibitor (e.g., diltiazem, verapamil) (Fig. 55-10).

Fentanyl, a synthetic opioid chemically related to the phenylpiperidines, is a relatively selective μ receptor agonist, which is considered to have 80 times the potency of morphine following intravenous administration. It is extensively metabolized in the liver to norfentanyl and other inactive metabolites, which are excreted in the urine and bile. Fentanyl is therefore suitable for patients in renal failure. The drug is available for intravenous, subcutaneous, transdermal, transmucosal, and neuraxial administration. The transdermal administration of fentanyl using iontophoresis (Ionsys, The Medicine Company) is a novel on-demand drug delivery system that does not require venous access. Ionsys is designed to deliver a 40-μg dose of fentanyl over a 10-minute period of time following activation of the dose button and is strictly intended for inpatient use only.

Sufentanil, *alfentanil*, and *remifentanil* are analogues of fentanyl that have analgesic effects similar to those of morphine and the other μ receptor agonists. *Sufentanil* has approximately 1,000 times the potency of morphine and is primarily used in the operating room either intravenously or neuraxially.[28] Like fentanyl, sufentanil is very lipophilic, and although their pharmacokinetic and pharmacodynamic profiles are similar, sufentanil has a smaller

Table 55-9 Patients at Risk for Opioid-induced Sedation and Respiratory Depression

Sleep apnea
Morbid obesity
Snoring
Advancing age (>60 years)
Opioid naive
Following surgery of the upper abdomen or thorax
Patient with a history of opioid habituation
Increasing duration of general anesthesia
Additive or synergistic effects of other sedating drugs (e.g., antihistamines or benzodiazepines)
Cardiac and pulmonary comorbidities or major organ dysfunction
Thoracotomy
Smoker

© The Joint Commission. 2016; Reprinted with permission and adapted from the *Sentinel Event Alert*, Issue 49.

Table 55-10 Assignment of Likely Codeine Metabolism Phenotypes Based on Cytochrome P450 2D6 (*CYP2D6*) Diplotypes

Phenotype	Implications for Codeine Metabolism	Recommendations for Codeine Therapy	Classification of Recommendation for Codeine Therapy[a]	Considerations for Alternative Opioids
Ultrarapid metabolizer	Increased formation of morphine following codeine administration, leading to higher risk of toxicity	Avoid codeine use due to potential for toxicity.	Strong	Alternatives that are not affected by this CYP2D6 phenotype include morphine and nonopioid analgesics. Tramadol and, to a lesser extent, hydrocodone and oxycodone are not good alternatives because their metabolism is affected by CYP2D6 activity.[b,c]
Extensive metabolizer	Normal morphine formation	Use label-recommended age- or weight-specific dosing.	Strong	—
Intermediate metabolizer	Reduced morphine formation	Use label-recommended age- or weight-specific dosing. If no response, consider alternative analgesics such as morphine or a nonopioid.	Moderate	Monitor tramadol use for response.
Poor metabolizer	Greatly reduced morphine formation following codeine administration, leading to insufficient pain relief	Avoid codeine use due to lack of efficacy.	Strong	Alternatives that are not affected by this CYP2D6 phenotype include morphine and nonopioid analgesics. Tramadol and, to a lesser extent, hydrocodone and oxycodone are not good alternatives because their metabolism is affected by CYP2D6 activity; these agents should be avoided.[b,c]

[a] Rating scheme is described in Supplementary Data online.
[b,c] There is substantial evidence for decreased efficacy of tramadol in poor metabolizers and a single case report of toxicity in an ultrarapid metabolizer with renal impairment following tramadol use postsurgery. Use of other analgesics in CYP2D6 poor and ultrarapid metabolizers may therefore be preferable. Some other opioid analgesics, such as hydrocodone and oxycodone, are metabolized by CYP2D6. To avoid treatment complications, opioids that are not metabolized by CYP2D6 including morphine, oxymorphone, buprenorphine, fentanyl, methadone, and hydromorphone, along with nonopioid analgesics, may be considered as alternatives for use in CYP2D6 poor and ultrarapid metabolizers.
Reprinted with permission from Crews KR, Gaedigk A, Dunnenberger HM, et al. Clinical Pharmacogenetics Implementation Consortium guidelines for cytochrome P450 2D6 genotype and codeine therapy: 2014 update. *Clin Pharmacol Ther.* 2014;95(4):376–382.

volume of distribution and shorter elimination half-life.[28] The high intrinsic potency of sufentanil makes it an excellent choice for epidural analgesia in the opioid-dependent patient.[29] *Alfentanil* has approximately 10 times the potency of morphine and, like sufentanil, is used primarily in the operating room either intravenously or neuraxially. *Remifentanil* is an ultra–short-acting synthetic opioid. The potency of the drug is approximately equal to that of fentanyl. Remifentanil is rapidly degraded by tissue and plasma esterases, which accounts for its incredibly short terminal elimination half-life of 10 to 20 minutes.[28] Rapid clearance and lack of accumulation make this a very desirable opioid in the operative setting, particularly during neurosurgery when remifentanil is combined with propofol as part of a total intravenous anesthetic (TIVA). One disadvantage, however, is that discontinuation of a remifentanil infusion results in rapid loss of analgesia. There is also evidence to suggest that remifentanil infusions may be associated with the development of OIH. Further studies are clearly needed to better define this phenomenon.

Meperidine, a phenylpiperidine, is a synthetic μ opioid receptor agonist with a short half-life. The drug is recommended for the short-term management of acute pain only and has absolutely no role in the management of chronic pain. The drug is biotransformed by the liver to normeperidine, a potentially neurotoxic metabolite, which has a 12- to 16-hour half-life. Repetitive dosing of meperidine can cause accumulation of normeperidine, which may precipitate tremulousness, myoclonus, and seizures. It is therefore recommended that the total daily intravenous dose in an otherwise healthy adult without renal or central nervous system disease should not exceed 600 mg/day and should not be administered for longer than 48 hours.[30] We do not recommend administration of meperidine as an intravenous patient-controlled analgesia (PCA). The drug is contraindicated in patients receiving monoamine oxidase inhibitors, as this may precipitate a syndrome characterized by muscle rigidity, hyperpyrexia, and seizures.

Methadone is a relatively inexpensive synthetic opioid considered to be a broad-spectrum opioid because it is a (1) μ receptor

Table 55-11 Conversion Ratios from Morphine to Methadone[32,189,191]

Daily Chronic Oral Morphine Dose		Conversion Ratio (Oral Morphine: Oral Methadone)	
<100 mg	(e.g., 90 mg PO morphine)	3:1	(e.g., 30 mg PO methadone)
100–300 mg	(e.g., 300 mg PO morphine)	5:1	(e.g., 60 mg PO methadone)
300–600 mg	(e.g., 600 mg PO morphine)	10:1	(e.g., 60 mg PO methadone)
600–800 mg	(e.g., 720 mg PO morphine)	12:1	(e.g., 60 mg PO methadone)
800–1,000 mg	(e.g., 900 mg PO morphine)	15:1	(e.g., 60 mg PO methadone)
>1,000 mg	(e.g., 1,200 mg PO morphine)	20:1	(e.g., 60 mg PO methadone)

PO, by mouth.

agonist, (2) NMDA antagonist, and (3) inhibitor of monoamine transmitter reuptake, making it potentially useful for the treatment of neuropathic pain. The drug is well absorbed from the gastrointestinal tract with a reported bioavailability approximating 80%. The drug is extensively metabolized in the liver by the cytochrome P450 (CYP450) system to inactive metabolites, which are cleared in the bile and urine; unlike morphine, it is generally not necessary to adjust the dosage of methadone in patients with renal insufficiency. Methadone has an elimination half-life of 22 hours, and following a single dose the duration of analgesia is approximately 3 to 6 hours. With repetitive dosing, however, methadone can accumulate and slow tissue release into the blood stream can result in a long elimination half-life of up to 128 hours and duration of analgesia of 8 to 12 hours. This long half-life explains the potential risk for cumulative toxicity, and therefore the importance of monitoring for side effects such as excessive sedation and confusion following the initiation of an around-the-clock dosing regimen.

Finally, opioid rotation is a very useful technique to restore analgesic sensitivity in the highly tolerant patient, and methadone is a common choice for opioid rotation. Because cross-tolerance is incomplete, the calculated equianalgesic dose of any new opioid is always lower than expected. One must be particularly cautious, however, when converting from morphine to methadone as the morphine/methadone equianalgesic ratio appears to be curvilinear; whereas the morphine-to-methadone conversion ratio is 3:1 at morphine doses of less than 100 mg/day, the ratio is 20:1 at morphine doses of more than 1,000 mg/day (Table 55-11). Methadone is principally metabolized by the CYP3A4 subtype enzyme of the CYP450 system and, to a lesser extent, by the CYP1A2 and CYP2D6 subtypes. Consequently, there is the potential for numerous drug interactions with methadone, as shown in Table 55-12. Whereas inhibition of methadone metabolism will theoretically provoke toxicity, induction of methadone metabolism could potentially precipitate inadequate analgesia or even withdrawal symptoms. Frequent adjustments of the methadone dosage may therefore be required if medications are added to or eliminated from a patient's drug regimen. A rare side effect associated with methadone is a pause-dependent dysrhythmia associated with bradycardia, QT prolongation, and Torsades de pointe.

Buprenorphine is a highly lipophilic partial μ opioid receptor (MOR) agonist, κ receptor (KOR) antagonist, and ORL1 agonist. It is a lipophilic opioid with moderate intrinsic activity and a high affinity for the μ opioid receptor. The elimination half-life of the drug following intravenous administration is 1.2 to 7.2 hours (mean 2.2 hours). The terminal half-life of the drug following sublingual administration, however, is considerably longer secondary to sequestration of the drug in the oral mucosa and buccal fat. The drug is metabolized in the liver by the CYP3A4 enzyme to norbuprenorphine, a weak μ agonist responsible for respiratory depression. Buprenorphine and norbuprenorphine are rapidly conjugated via phase II reaction to buprenorphine-3-glucuronide and norbuprenorphine-3-glucuronide and neither metabolite decreases respiratory rate. In humans, buprenorphine is reported to have a ceiling effect for respiratory depression but not for analgesia. Buprenorphine is reported to be effective in a broader variety of pain phenotypes than fentanyl. In animal

Table 55-12 Methadone Drug Interactions

Clinical Significance	Increase Methadone Concentration/Effects	Decrease Methadone Concentration/Effects
Documented clinical effects	Ciprofloxacin (Cipro), diazepam (Valium), ethanol (acute use), fluconazole (Diflucan), urinary alkalinizers	Amprenavir (Agenerase), efavirenz (Sustiva), nelfinavir (Viracept), nevirapine (Viramune), phenobarbital, phenytoin (Dilantin), rifampin (Rifadin), ritonavir (Norvir), urinary acidifiers
Documented enzyme effects	Cimetidine (Tagamet), fluoxetine (Prozac)	Carbamazepine (Tegretol)
Clinical effects uncertain	Omeprazole (Prilosec), quinidine, paroxetine (Paxil)	
Predicted interaction	Delavirdine (Rescriptor), grapefruit juice, or fruit	Ethanol (chronic use)
No current clinical evidence	Ketoconazole (Nizoral), macrolide antibiotics (erythromycin, clarithromycin [Biaxin], troleandomycin [TAO]), tricyclic antidepressants, verapamil (Calan)	

models, it has proven to be efficacious in the treatment of neuropathic pain and in a human pain model it can block secondary hyperalgesia and central sensitization. Buprenorphine also produces less constipation and less cognitive dysfunction than other μ opioid receptor agonists and does not prolong the QTc interval like methadone.[31]

Buprenorphine is an excellent alternative for the treatment of acute pain in the patient who cannot tolerate morphine secondary to allergy or other sensitivity. In the adult patient the parenteral dose of buprenorphine is 300 μg, which is equivalent to 10 mg of morphine.[32] The recommended dosing interval is every 6 hours. Additional routes of administration include intramuscular, neuraxial, subcutaneous, sublingual, and transdermal.

A novel (off-label) route of administration of buprenorphine is the perineural application of the drug with local anesthetic. In an effort to prolong the duration of a single injection peripheral nerve block at the brachial and lumbar plexuses buprenorphine may be combined with a long-acting local anesthetic (bupivacaine or ropivacaine) with clonidine and dexamethasone and is referred to as *multimodal perineural analgesia*. This multimodal four-drug combination is reported to provide upwards of 40 hours of analgesia, which is vastly superior to less than 12 to 16 hours with a single long-acting local anesthetic! This single injection technique can be quite useful in austere environments or in situations which preclude placement of a continuous perineural catheter. The block can be performed quickly and offers an inexpensive alternative to a continuous perineural catheter. Please refer to the excellent review by Williams and colleagues for dosing guidelines.[33]

Tramadol (Ultram) and *Tapentadol (Nucynta)* are orally active, centrally acting synthetic analgesics possessing a novel mechanism of action which combines μ receptor agonist activity with monoamine reuptake inhibition. Whereas tramadol inhibits reuptake of both norepinephrine and serotonin, tapentadol only inhibits the reuptake of norepinephrine. Tramadol is a prodrug which is metabolized in the liver by the CYP450 CYP2D6 system to the active metabolite O-desmethyltramadol (M1), which has 200 times greater μ receptor affinity, greater potency, and longer half-life than the parent drug. This can be significant, because there can be an attenuated analgesic effect in the 5% to 15% of the population that has decreased CYP2D6 activity, as is the case with codeine. Tapentadol, on the other hand, is metabolized in the liver to an inactive metabolite via phase II glucuronidation and the drug does not require enzymatic conversion to an active drug. As such, tapentadol offers a distinct advantage over tramadol in terms of reduced variability in analgesia secondary to genetic polymorphism. Tapentadol metabolism will also not be subject to drug/drug interactions at the level of the CYP2D6 enzyme.[27,34]

Tramadol (Ultram) is indicated for mild to moderately severe acute pain. The drug is available as 50-mg tablets. Recommended dosing is 50 to 100 mg q 4 to 6 hours, not to exceed 400 mg in 24 hours. The drug is also available in extended release formulations and a combination product with acetaminophen. Tapentadol (Nucynta) is indicated for moderate to severe acute pain. It is available as 50-mg, 75-mg, and 100-mg tablets, which can be dosed q 4 to 6 hours not to exceed 700 mg on the first day of dosing and 600 mg every day thereafter. Tapentadol IR 50 and 75 mg provides postoperative analgesia similar to oxycodone IR 10 mg and with fewer gastrointestinal side effects. Advantages of tapentadol over tramadol include (1) lack of CYP450 drug interactions, (2) lower risk of seizures and serotonin syndrome, (3) superior analgesia, (4) fewer GI side effects, and (5) less variation in individual drug response secondary to genetic polymorphism.[35]

Both drugs should be administered with caution in patients at risk for respiratory depression. In addition, both drugs have the potential to produce serotonin syndrome (mental status changes, autonomic instability, and neuromuscular aberrations), particularly if administered with serotonergic drugs (selective serotonin reuptake inhibitors [SSRIs], selective norepinephrine uptake inhibitors, tricyclic antidepressants [TCAs], monamine oxidase inhibitors [MAOs] inhibitors, and triptans). Caution is advised when dosing these drugs in patients with a seizure disorder.

Nonopioid Analgesic Adjuncts

The *NSAIDs* are among the most commonly used drugs in the world because of their anti-inflammatory, analgesic, and antipyretic effects (Table 55-13). The therapeutic benefit of NSAIDs is believed to be mediated through the inhibition of cyclooxygenase (COX) enzymes (prostaglandin H_2 [PGH_2] synthetases), types 1 and 2, which convert arachidonic acid to PGH_2. The COX enzyme consists of two active sites: (1) the COX site and (2) the peroxidase site. NSAIDs mediate their effects by binding to the COX site (Fig. 55-13).

COX-1 is the constitutive enzyme that produces prostaglandins, which are important for general "house-keeping" functions such as gastric protection and hemostasis. COX-2, on the other hand, is the inducible form of the enzyme that produces prostaglandins that mediate pain, inflammation, fever, and carcinogenesis. Prostaglandin E_2 is the key mediator of both peripheral and central pain sensitization. Peripherally, prostaglandins do not directly mediate pain; rather, they contribute to hyperalgesia by sensitizing nociceptors to other mediators of pain sensation such as histamine and bradykinin.[36] Centrally, prostaglandins enhance pain transmission at the level of the dorsal horn by (1) increasing the release of substance P and glutamate from first-order pain neurons, (2) increasing the sensitivity of second-order pain neurons, and (3) inhibiting the release of neurotransmitters from the descending pain-modulating pathways.

NSAIDs have proved effective in the treatment of postoperative pain. In addition, they are opioid-sparing and can significantly decrease the incidence of opioid-related side effects such as postoperative nausea and vomiting and sedation.[37] Unlike the opioids, NSAIDs exhibit a "ceiling effect" with respect to maximum analgesic effects. Parenteral NSAIDs such as ketorolac are

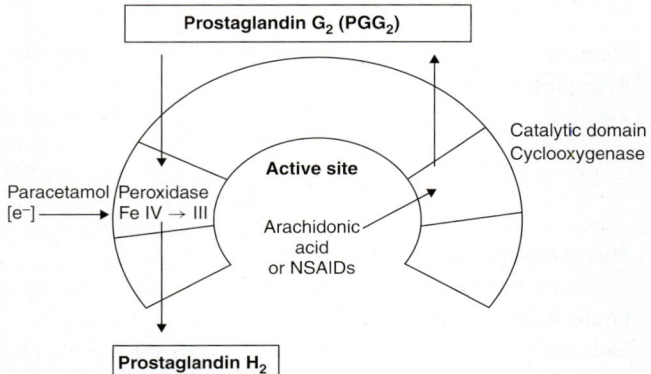

Figure 55-13 Paracetamol inhibits prostanoid synthesis. Arachidonic acid (AA) enters the active site of COX. The enzyme cyclizes AA and adds hydroperoxy group to form PGG2. This hydroperoxy group is reduced to the hydroxyl group of prostaglandin H2 (PGH2) by peroxidase. Paracetamol does not enter the active site COX but reduces Fe IV to Fe III and prevents activation of the peroxide catalytic moiety and therefore inhibits PGH$_2$ synthesis. NSAIDs, nonsteroidal anti-inflammatory drugs. (Adapted from Kam PCA, So A. COX-3: uncertainties and controversies. *Curr Anaesth Crit Care*. 2009;20:50.)

Table 55-13 Nonopioid Analgesics (Adult Dosing Guidelines)[30,32]

Drug	Route	Half-Life (h)	Dose (mg)	Comments
Para-aminophenols				
Acetaminophen	PO and IV	2	500–1,000 mg q4–6h Maximum daily dose (MDD) in the healthy adult is 4,000 mg. Intravenous dosing guidelines: Adult >50 kg: 1 g q4–6h not to exceed 4 g/day Adult <50 kg: 15mg/kg q4–6h not to exceed 3 g/day. Pedi >33 kg: 15 mg/kg q4–6h not to exceed 3 g/day. Pedi 10–33 kg: 15 mg/kg q4–6h not to exceed 2 g/day	Hepatotoxicity can occur in chronic alcoholics receiving therapeutic doses Administer intravenous formulation over 15 minutes
Salicylates				
Acetylsalicylic acid	PO	0.25	500–1,000 mg q4–6h MDD is 4,000 mg in the healthy adult	Salicylic acid has a $T_{1/2}$ 2–3 h at low doses and >20 h at higher doses. Because of the risk of Reyes syndrome avoid the use of aspirin in children <12 years old
Diflunisal	PO	8–12	500 mg q8–12h	Decrease the dose in the elderly to 500–1,000 mg/day
Choline magnesium trisalicylate	PO	9–17	Loading dose (LD) = 1,000 mg 1,000–1,500 mg q12h	Unlike aspirin does not increase bleeding time; MDD = 2,000–3,000 mg
NSAIDs Propionic Acids				
Ibuprofen Intravenous formulation (Caldolor) available in the United States in 2009.	PO and IV	2	400 mg q4–6h	Intravenous ibuprofen: Infuse over 30 minutes to avoid phlebitis Limit adult dose to 3,200 mg/day
Naproxen	PO	12–15	250 mg q6–8h	LD = 500 mg; MDD = 1,500 mg
Ketoprofen	PO	2.1	25–50 mg q6–8h	MDD = 300 mg
Oxaprozin	PO	42–50	600 mg q12–24h	MDD = 1,200 mg
Indolacetic Acids				
Indomethacin	PO	2	25 mg q8–12h	MDD = 200 mg
Sulindac	PO	7.8	150 mg q12h	MDD = 400 mg Active metabolite has a half-life of 16 h
Etodolac	PO	7.3	300–400 mg q8–12h	MDD = 1,000 mg
Pyrrolacetic Acids				
Ketorolac	IV	6	30 mg initially followed by 15–30 mg q6–8h not to exceed 5 days	MDD = 120 mg; hypovolemia should be corrected prior to administration Decrease the dose in the elderly (>65 years of age) and in renal failure
Phenylacetic Acids				
Diclofenac potassium	PO	2	50 mg q8h	MDD = 150 mg
Enolic Acids (Oxicams)				
Meloxicam	PO	15–20	7.5–15 mg q24h	COX-2 selectivity similar to celecoxib
Piroxicam	PO	50	20–40 mg q24h	
Naphthylalkanone				
Nabumetone	PO	22.5	500–750 mg q8–12h	LD = 1,000 mg MDD = 2,000 mg Active metabolite has half-life = 22.5 h
COX-2 Inhibitor				
Celecoxib	PO	11	100–200 mg q12h	LD = 400 mg; MDD = 400 mg Avoid this drug in patients with coronary heart disease, cerebrovascular disease or in patients allergic to sulfonamides

PO, by mouth; IV, intravenously; COX-2, cyclooxygenase; LD, loading dose; MDD, maximum daily dose.

commonly employed as part of a multimodal approach for acute perioperative pain management. The optimal dose of ketorolac for postoperative pain control is 15 to 30 mg intravenously every 6 to 8 hours, not to exceed 5 days. The dose should be decreased in patients with renal failure.

Despite the benefits of NSAIDs in the perioperative period they are not without some significant side effects. Platelet dysfunction, gastrointestinal ulceration, and an increased risk of nephrotoxicity are several reasons why the nonselective NSAIDs may be avoided in the perioperative period. The risk of nephrotoxicity is increased in patients with hypovolemia, congestive heart failure, and chronic renal insufficiency.[36] The COX-2–selective inhibitors were developed in an attempt to minimize their side effects. The COX-2–specific inhibitor celecoxib (Celebrex) is available in the United States. Rofecoxib (Vioxx) and valdecoxib (Bextra), also released in the same period, were recalled by the manufacturers because of concerns about adverse cardiovascular risks. Celecoxib is the only COX-2–specific inhibitor currently available in the United States for acute postoperative pain. The recommended oral loading dose is 400 mg followed by 200 mg orally every 12 hours for several days.

Unlike the nonselective NSAIDs, however, COX-2–specific inhibitors offer the potential advantages of a reduced incidence of gastrointestinal ulceration and they do not inhibit platelet function. Because prostaglandins play a crucial role in renal function through their effect on blood flow, natriuresis and glomerular filtration, traditional NSAIDs, and the COX-2 inhibitors can cause fluid retention and hypertension.

The authors, therefore, do not recommend prescribing a COX-2 inhibitor for patients with a known history of coronary artery disease or cerebrovascular disease. Both COX-1 and COX-2 play significant roles in bone fusion following fracture, and the use of the traditional NSAIDs has been found to inhibit the healing process, particularly following lumbar spinal fusion surgery. The effect of COX-2 inhibitors on bone fusion following orthopedic procedures continues to be controversial, and no recommendations can be made at this time. NSAIDs and COX-2–selective inhibitors should not be administered to patients with known hypersensitivity to the drugs or to patients with Samters triad (aka aspirin triad), which is a medical condition characterized by asthma, aspirin insensitivity, and nasal polyposis. Finally, avoid celecoxib and valdecoxib in patients with allergic-type reactions to sulfonamides.

The *para-aminophenol* derivative acetaminophen (paracetamol) has both analgesic and antipyretic properties, similar to aspirin, but is devoid of any anti-inflammatory effects. The drug is primarily a centrally acting inhibitor of the COX enzyme with minimal peripheral effects. Acetaminophen neither enters the active site of the COX enzyme nor binds to the COX site, but instead it prevents COX activation by reducing heme at the peroxidase site of the enzyme. In addition, there may be modulation of descending inhibitory serotoninergic pathways and the drug may act on the opioid, cannabinoid, transient potential receptor of vanilloid type 1 ($TRPV_1$), and NMDA receptors.[38] Acetaminophen is devoid of many of the side effects generally associated with the NSAIDs, such as gastrointestinal ulceration, impaired platelet function, adverse cardiorenal effects, and impairment of bone fusion following orthopedic procedures. Acetaminophen is opioid-sparing and can be used in conjunction with an NSAID as part of a multimodal analgesic program. The combination of acetaminophen with an NSAID is thought to provide analgesia that is superior to using either drug alone.[39] In adults, 2 g of oral acetaminophen is equivalent to 200 mg of celecoxib.

Intravenous acetaminophen (Ofirmev) was released in the United States in November of 2010. The drug is available as a 1 g (1,000 mg/100 mL) infusion that does not require reconstitution and can be infused through a peripheral intravenous (IV) line over 15 minutes. See Table 55-13 for dosing guidelines.

The *NMDA receptor antagonists* such as ketamine and dextromethorphan may be useful analgesic adjuncts. Excitatory neurotransmitter stimulation of the NMDA receptor is believed to be involved in the development and maintenance of several phenomena including (1) persistent postoperative pain, (2) hypersensitivity, windup, and allodynia, (3) opioid-induced tolerance, and (4) OIH. *Low-dose intravenous ketamine* has proven to be very effective in the management of perioperative pain. Numerous meta-analyses have described the opioid-sparing effect of the drug, and although the magnitude of the effect varies from one study to the next, it appears that the use of perioperative intravenous ketamine, for up to 48 hours postoperatively, can reduce opioid consumption by upwards of 40%.[40] Intravenous ketamine also reduces pain scores and no major complications have been reported following 48 hours of continuous infusion. Low-dose intravenous ketamine is defined as a bolus dose of ketamine that is 1 mg/kg or less or an infusion that is 1.2 mg/kg/hr or less (≤20 μg/kg/min).[40] The mechanism of action of ketamine is NMDA receptor blockade, but in addition the drug interacts with opioidergic, cholinergic, and monoaminergic receptors and blocks sodium channels.[41]

NMDA receptor antagonists may act synergistically when combined with an opioid. The ideal intravenous PCA morphine–ketamine combination ratio is 1:1 with an 8-minute lockout.[42] A double-blind study, however, demonstrates that the combination of ketamine (1 mg/mL) with morphine (1 mg/mL) administered as an intravenous PCA to patients following major abdominal surgery does not significantly improve pain relief.[43] In patients with morphine-resistant pain, however, the combination of 250 μg/kg of ketamine plus 15 μg/kg of morphine, as a bolus dose, has been reported to provide significant analgesia.[41] Results are promising, but more studies will certainly be required to clearly define the role of ketamine for postoperative analgesia.

Dextromethorphan, the d-isomer of the codeine analogue levorphanol, is a noncompetitive NMDA receptor antagonist that has been used for many years as an antitussive. Dextromethorphan does not have a direct analgesic effect; rather, analgesia is likely mediated by its NMDA receptor antagonism. The drug can be administered orally, intravenously, and intramuscularly. There is a sustained-release suspension available that contains dextromethorphan, 30 mg/5 mL, and is marketed as Delsym (Adams Respiratory Therapeutics). Following oral administration, the drug is metabolized to dextrorphan, which is the metabolite that accounts for most of the side effects, the most common of which are nausea and vomiting. Because the intravenous administration of large doses can lead to hypotension and tachycardia, the intramuscular route may be the preferred route of delivery. Dextromethorphan has been shown to both inhibit secondary hyperalgesia following peripheral burn injury and cause a reduction in temporal summation of pain. The preoperative administration of 150 mg of oral dextromethorphan can reduce the PCA morphine requirements of patients undergoing abdominal hysterectomy, and the preincisional administration of 120 mg of intramuscular dextromethorphan provides preemptive analgesia in patients undergoing elective upper abdominal surgery. Finally, a randomized double-blind placebo-controlled study has demonstrated that dextromethorphan dosed 200 mg orally every 8 hours (e.g., 2 hours prior to surgery, then 8 hours and 16 hours thereafter) can provide a modest reduction in morphine consumption following knee surgery.[44]

The α_2-*adrenergic agonists* clonidine (half-life, 9 to 12 hours) and dexmedetomidine (half-life, 2 hours) may be administered perioperatively to provide analgesia, sedation, and anxiolysis. The presynaptic activation of α_2-receptors that results in the decreased release of norepinephrine is believed to mediate analgesia. Whereas clonidine is a selective partial agonist for the α_2-adrenoreceptor, dexmedetomidine is superselective for the receptor. Their respective α_2/α_1 binding ratios are 220:1 for clonidine versus 1,620:1 for dexmedetomidine. Analgesia is mediated supraspinally (locus coeruleus), spinally (substantia gelatinosa), and peripherally. Dexmedetomidine is reported to have greater affinity for the 2A subtype of the receptor, which may account for the drug's superior analgesic properties vis-à-vis clonidine. Clonidine can be administered orally, transdermally, intravenously, perineurally, and neuraxially for perioperative pain management. Premedication with 5 µg/kg of oral clonidine in patients undergoing knee surgery can decrease the use of PCA morphine and decrease the incidence of postoperative nausea and vomiting. In addition, the combination of oral clonidine, 3 to 5 µg/kg with 0.2 mg/24 hours of transdermal clonidine can decrease postoperative PCA morphine requirement by 50% following prostatectomy surgery. In a double-blind, placebo-controlled study, investigators demonstrated that addition of 25 µg of intrathecal clonidine to a bupivacaine (15 mg) morphine (250 µg) spinal anesthetic cocktail, for total knee arthroplasty (TKA), could reduce postoperative morphine use and improve VAS pain scores at 24 hours.[45] In combination with a local anesthetic clonidine in doses of 0.5 to 1.0 µg/kg may enhance the efficacy and increase the duration of perineural blocks. A four-drug combination including bupivacaine (2.5 mg/mL), clonidine (3 µg/mL), buprenorphine (18 µg/mL), and dexamethasone (66 µg/mL) has been reported to provide greater than 24 hours of postoperative analgesia.[33] The authors of this study encourage further research in this area of motor-sparing perineural analgesia. Side effects from clonidine include sedation, hypotension, and bradycardia if the dose exceeds 150 µg.

Dexmedetomidine is a potent and highly selective α_2-adrenoreceptor agonist which demonstrates cardioprotective, neuroprotective, and renoprotective effects against hypoxic/ischemic injury.[46] The drug has been described as a useful and safe adjunct in numerous clinical situations, which include (1) premedication prior to intubation and extubation, (2) procedural sedation, (3) awake intubations, (4) as an adjuvant to regional anesthesia, (5) awake craniotomies, and (6) intraoperative and postoperative analgesia as part of a multimodal protocol. See Table 55-14 for dosing guidelines. The drug does not decrease gut motility and prevents postoperative nausea and vomiting and shivering. In the intensive care unit (ICU) dexmedetomidine has proven to be a very useful drug that decreases central nervous system sympathetic outflow in a dose-dependent manner. It provides adequate sedation without significant respiratory depression and analgesia that is opioid sparing. Unlike propofol and midazolam, dexmedetomidine is not a GABAergic drug, has no anticholinergic effects and promotes more physiological sleep pattern attributes, which attenuates neurocognitive impairment (delirium and agitation) and promotes early extubation and shorter length of stays (LOS) in the ICU.[47] The most frequently observed adverse effects associated with the use of dexmedetomidine are bradycardia and hypotension, which can be adequately treated with atropine, glycopyrrolate, and ephedrine.

The *gabapentinoids* (α_2-δ subunit calcium channel ligands), gabapentin (Neurontin) and pregabalin (Lyrica), are indicated for the treatment of partial onset seizures, neuropathic pain (e.g., postherpetic neuralgia), and other chronic pain states (e.g., fibromyalgia); however, there is now a growing body of evidence supporting the use of these drugs during the perioperative period to decrease postoperative pain and opioid use. Likewise, because the gabapentinoids can prevent the establishment of surgery-induced central sensitization, these drugs may play a role in preventing the transition from acute pain to chronic pain. As an added bonus, there is a decreased incidence of postoperative delirium, vomiting, pruritus, and urinary retention associated with the perioperative use of these drugs, probably secondary to their opioid-sparing effects. Common side effects associated with these drugs include sedation, headache, dizziness, and visual disturbances.[48,49]

Compared to traditional analgesics, which decrease afferent input from the site of tissue injury, the gabapentinoids decrease the hyperexcitability of dorsal horn neurons caused by tissue damage.[50] Although structurally similar to GABA these drugs are not GABAergic and do not bind $GABA_A$, $GABA_b$, $GABA_c$ radioligand sites or allosteric GABA receptor sites. The antinociceptive mechanism of action of the gabapentinoids has two aspects: modulation of the calcium-induced release of glutamate centrally in the dorsal horn, and activation of descending noradrenergic pathways in the spinal cord and brain (Fig. 55-14).[49]

When administered orally, both drugs are absorbed by amino acid carrier systems in the small intestines. The gastrointestinal absorption of *gabapentin* occurs only in the duodenum through a saturable transport system resulting in bioavailability that decreases with increasing doses. Consequently, increased doses of gabapentin result in incrementally smaller increases in plasma drug concentration (e.g., nonlinear pharmacokinetics).[51] *Pregabalin*, on the other hand, is absorbed throughout the small intestines through a nonsaturable transport system and has a linear pharmacokinetic profile (dose-independent absorption), and is more potent than gabapentin. Gabapentin oral absorption is significantly impaired by antacids, including bicitra. Both drugs are renally excreted and undergo insignificant liver metabolism.

Although the multimodal approach to perioperative pain management is to be applauded, we need to display caution when combining multiple pharmaceutical agents with different mechanisms of action ("poly-pharmacy") for fear of eliciting unacceptable side effects. The ideal multimodal drug combination should enhance analgesia while at the same time decrease drug-related adverse side effects. It is the general consensus that the gabapentinoids are opioid-sparing and effective in attenuating immediate postoperative pain; however, these drugs can also increase the risk of postoperative sedation, so great care should be taken when dosing these drugs, particularly in combination with opioid analgesics. Unfortunately, the optimal perioperative dosing

Table 55-14 Dexmedetomidine Dosing Guidelines

Route	Dose
Intravenous	Loading dose: 1 µg/kg over 10–20 minutes Maintenance dose: 0.2–0.7 µg/kg/hr
Intramuscular	2.5 µg/kg as premedication
Spinal	0.1–0.2 µg/kg
Epidural	1–2 µg/kg
Peripheral nerve block	1 µg/kg
Buccal	1–2 µg/kg
Intranasal	1–2 µg/kg

Reprinted with permission from Naaz S, Ozair E. Dexmedetomidine in current anaesthesia practice: a review. *J Clin Diagn Res.* 2014;8(10):GE01–GE04.

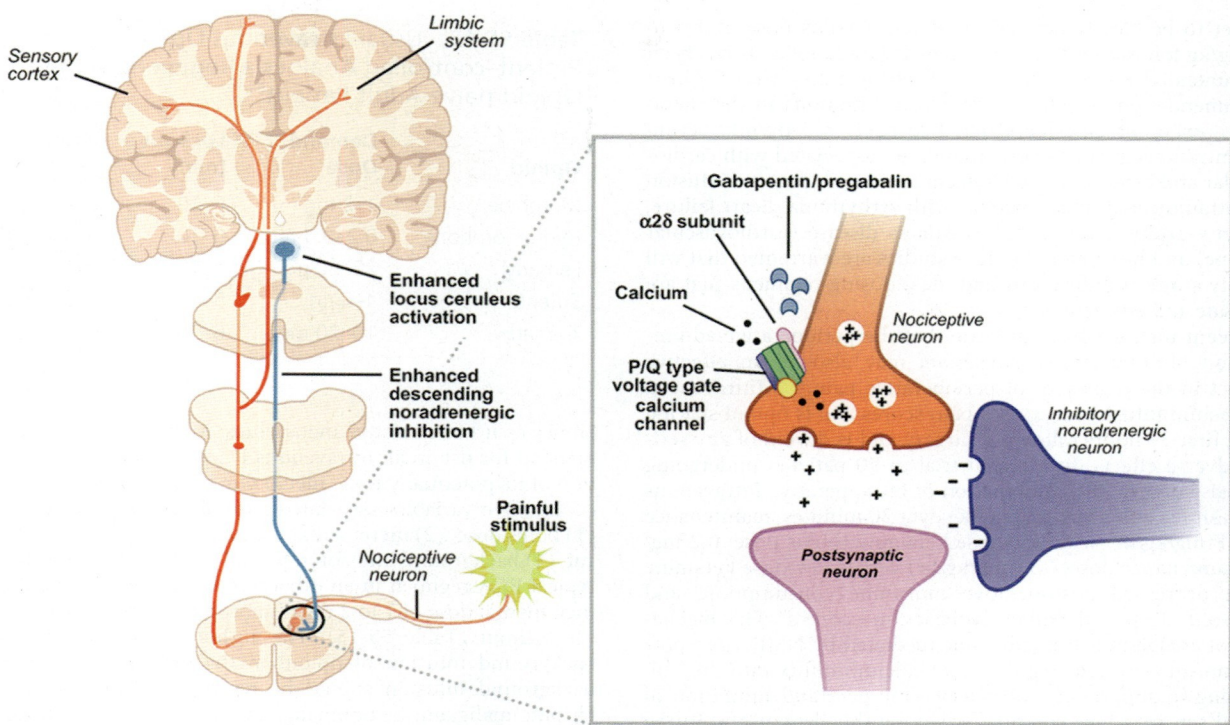

Figure 55-14 Hypothesized mechanisms of action of gabapentin. Gabapentin binds to the α-2δ subunit of voltage-gated P/Q type calcium channels. This binding appears to modulate the function and traffic of these channels, which appear on the synaptic bulb of presynaptic neurons. Calcium influx through these channels after a pain-evoked action potential is believed to trigger the fusion of synaptic vesicles with the neuronal membrane and consequent release of neurotransmitters in the dorsal horn of the spinal cord. Gabapentin may exert its analgesic effect by inhibiting or modulating this process. In addition, gabapentin may exert an analgesic effect by activating descending inhibitory noradrenergic pathways that regulate neurotransmission of pain signals in the dorsal horn of the spinal cord. (Reprinted with permission from Schmidt, PC, Ruchelli G, Mackey SC. Perioperative gabapentinoids: choice of agent, dose, timing, and effects on chronic postsurgical pain. *Anesthesiology*. 2013;119(5):1215–1221.)

regimen and treatment duration remain unclear. Preoperative dosing of gabapentin as high as 1,200 mg orally has been recommended; however, this may place the patient at an increased risk for postoperative respiratory depression. Patients at increased risk for postoperative respiratory depression include the elderly, the morbidly obese, and patients with OSA. In a recent retrospective study[52] involving patients undergoing total hip and knee arthroplasty, the authors suggest that premedication of patients with greater than 300 mg of gabapentin, as part of a multimodal analgesic regimen, is associated with an increased risk of postoperative respiratory depression. Unfortunately, these patients had also received a preoperative dose of sustained release oxycodone, which likewise put them at an increased risk for postoperative respiratory depression. In another placebo-controlled crossover study, the effects of pregabalin and remifentanil, alone and in combination, on analgesia, ventilation, and cognitive function were examined.[53] The authors concluded that the combination of the two drugs produced *additive* analgesia but *potentiated* respiratory depression and produced greater cognitive side effects. Prudence therefore dictates that great care should be taken when dosing gabapentinoids in combination with opioids. In the opioid-naive patient, the preoperative dose of gabapentin should rarely exceed 300 mg orally. In addition, gabapentinoids should not be combined with a preoperative dose of sustained release opioid. Only in rare circumstances, such as in the opioid-dependent patient or in the patient at increased risk for chronic postsurgical pain (e.g., thoracotomy), should higher doses of gabapentinoids be contemplated.[49]

Dosing of the gabapentinoids may be initiated preoperatively, intraoperatively, or postoperatively with equal efficacy. However, because it takes gabapentin and pregabalin 4 to 6 hours and 8 hours, respectively, to reach peak cerebrospinal fluid levels dosing of the drug the evening prior to surgery may ultimately prove to be the most beneficial method of administration.[49] Unfortunately, side effects such as dizziness, sedation, and confusion may preclude this approach. The postoperative dosing of the gabapentinoid may therefore be titrated based on side effects, with larger doses being prescribed during the evening. Dosing should be adjusted accordingly based on the patient's age, weight, and comorbidities (e.g., renal function). The ideal gabapentinoid dosing regimen that can optimize immediate postoperative pain and minimize the risk of postoperative respiratory depression, while reducing the development of chronic postsurgical pain, has yet to be elucidated and merits further investigation.

Following intravenous administration, the *local anesthetic* lidocaine has been shown to be analgesic, antihyperalgesic, and anti-inflammatory.[54,55] In vitro studies indicate that the beneficial effects of intravenous lidocaine are mediated by inhibitory actions on voltage-gated sodium channels, voltage-gated calcium channels, potassium channels, G protein–coupled receptors, NMDA receptors, and the glycinergic system.[56] The perioperative infusion of lidocaine has been shown to not only improve postoperative analgesia in patients recovering from laparoscopic colectomy but also decrease postoperative opioid requirements, attenuate postoperative ileus, and accelerate time to discharge from the hospital.[54,56] The ideal dose of systemic lidocaine has yet to be clearly defined; however, a bolus dose of 1.5 to 2.0 mg/kg followed by an infusion of 1.5 to 2 mg/kg/hr has been recommended for the treatment of perioperative pain.[56] These recommendations result in serum concentrations in the therapeutic range, which is considered to be 1 to 5 μg/mL. Serum concentrations greater than 5 μg/mL are associated with cardiovascular and central nervous system toxicity. Lidocaine infusion is contraindicated in any patient with arrhythmia, heart failure, coronary artery disease, Stokes–Adams disease (cardiovascular syncope) and heart block. Future studies are warranted that will identify surgical indications and ideal dosing regimens that are both safe and efficacious.

Recent meta-analyses indicate that the perioperative administration of intravenous *magnesium* may also be an effective adjunct in the treatment of perioperative pain.[57,58] Intravenous magnesium infusion decreases pain scores and is opioid sparing in the first 24 hours following surgery and is devoid of any serious adverse effects. In a recent trial of 50 patients undergoing scoliosis surgery, the combination of intraoperative intravenous magnesium (bolus dose: 50 mg/kg over 30 minutes, maintenance dose: 8 mg/kg/hr) with low-dose ketamine (bolus dose: 0.2 mg/kg, maintenance dose: 0.15 mg/kg/hr) versus low-dose ketamine alone, decreased postoperative morphine consumption, and improved sleep and patient satisfaction scores.[59] The mechanism of analgesia is thought to be mediated by NMDA receptor antagonism as well as regulation of calcium influx into the cell, resulting in suppression of neuropathic pain and inhibition of central sensitization, potentially making this drug useful in the opioid-tolerant patient.

The *glucocorticoids* are well known for their analgesic, anti-inflammatory, and antiemetic effects. Inhibition of cytosolic phospholipase A_2 upstream from the lipoxygenase and COX enzymes in the prostaglandin cascade most certainly accounts for both their anti-inflammatory and analgesic effects by inhibiting leukotriene and prostaglandin production. The mechanism of the antiemetic effect of the corticosteroids is less clearly understood but appears to be centrally mediated.[60] In combination with a gabapentinoid, acetaminophen, and an NSAID, dexamethasone is considered a useful component of a multimodal drug strategy to effectively attenuate postsurgical pain. The recommended preoperative intravenous dose is 0.11 to 0.2 mg/kg. Because the drug has been reported to cause perineal irritation in 50% to 70% of individuals following rapid administration, prudence dictates that the drug be diluted in 50 mL of normal saline and injected over 10 minutes prior to surgery.[61] In the opioid-tolerant patient, acute perioperative pain management can be challenging, and high dose intravenous dexamethasone, combined with a proton pump inhibitor, has been recommended as a useful therapeutic option.[62] Dexamethasone has also been administered via the perineural route as part of a four-drug cocktail. The perineural dose of dexamethasone should never exceed 1 mg per plexus![63]

Methods of Analgesia

Patient-controlled Analgesia

PCA is any technique of pain management that allows the patients to administer their own analgesia on demand. We will highlight some important aspects of PCA as a complete review of PCA is beyond the scope of this chapter; we refer the reader to the comprehensive review by Macintyre on this topic.[64] In the United States, the most commonly used drugs are morphine, hydromorphone, and fentanyl. Hydromorphone is recommended as an alternative in renal failure; however, fentanyl might be a better choice as it has no active metabolites. Meperidine is not recommended for use in an intravenous PCA secondary to accumulation of its potentially toxic metabolite normeperidine.

The five variables associated with all modes of PCA include (1) bolus dose, (2) incremental (demand) dose, (3) lockout interval, (4) background infusion rate, and (5) 1- and 4-hour limits. A typical PCA regimen in an otherwise healthy adult would be an incremental dose of 1 to 2 mg of morphine with an 8- to 10-minute lockout (Table 55-15). The authors do not recommend a background infusion of opioid in the opioid-naive patient. A background infusion should be reserved for the patient with chronic malignant or nonmalignant pain who is opioid-tolerant or in patients with persistent pain who have failed a trial of incremental PCA dosing. In the elderly, the dose of the PCA should be decreased. The relative risk factors for use of an opioid PCA are listed in Table 55-16. If more than two risk factors exist, you may want to avoid using a PCA in the standard dosing regimen and administer opioids only as needed.

Opioid-related side effects include nausea and vomiting, pruritus, sedation, and confusion. Consensus guidelines for the treatment of nausea and vomiting include prescribing various combinations of dopamine antagonists, serotonin antagonists, and glucocorticoids.[65] In addition, the perioperative systemic administration of an α_2-agonist (e.g., dexmedetomidine), which is both analgesic and opioid sparing, has been shown to reduce the incidence of postoperative nausea and vomiting.[66] Pruritus can be ameliorated with the use of diphenhydramine, hydroxyzine, or a low dose of an opioid antagonist (e.g., naloxone) or mixed agonist–antagonist (e.g., nalbuphine). Excessive sedation may respond to a change in the opioid; however, use of a multimodal analgesic technique, which incorporates the use of a regional anesthetic (e.g., epidural or peripheral nerve blockade), an NSAID, acetaminophen, or other nonopioid analgesics such as an NMDA receptor antagonist or an α_2-δ subunit calcium channel ligand, will have an opioid-sparing effect, which should attenuate opioid-induced sedation.

Table 55-15 Usual Intravenous Opioid Patient–controlled Analgesia Regimens in the Opioid-naive Adult Patient[64,192]

Opioid	Demand Dose	Lockout (min)	Basal Infusion
Morphine	1–2 mg	6–10	0–2 mg/hr
Hydromorphone	0.2–0.4 mg	6–10	0–0.4 mg/hr
Fentanyl	20–50 μg	5–10	0–60 μg/hr
Sufentanil	4–6 μg	5–10	0–8 μg/hr
Tramadol	10–20 mg	6–10	0–20 mg/hr

Table 55-16 Relative Risk Factors Associated with the Use of Patient-controlled Analgesia

Pulmonary disease
Obstructive sleep apnea
Renal or hepatic dysfunction
Congestive heart failure
Closed head injury
Altered mental status
Lactating mothers

Neuraxial Analgesia

Although opioid analgesics have been prescribed to patients for many centuries, the exact mechanism of action was not completely understood until 1971, when the opioid receptor was discovered. Within 5 years' time, Yaksh reported that morphine could produce spinally mediated analgesia in a rat model. Soon thereafter, in 1979 and 1981, respectively, Wang and then Onofrio reported significant pain relief following the neuraxial administration of morphine in patients with severe cancer-related pain. Since these discoveries, the intrathecal administration of opioids and the epidural administration of opioids plus a local anesthetic has produced significant comfort for our patients.

Epidural analgesia is a critical component of multimodal perioperative pain management and improved patient outcome. Meta-analysis investigating the efficacy of epidural analgesia found epidural analgesia to be superior to systemically administered opioids.[67] The efficacy of an epidural technique is determined by numerous factors that can include (1) catheter incision site congruency, (2) choice of analgesic drugs, (3) rates of infusion, (4) duration of epidural analgesia, and (5) type of pain assessment (rest versus dynamic). Ideally, the epidural catheter is positioned congruent with the surgical incision (Fig. 55-15). Thoracic epidural catheter placement is recommended for both thoracic and upper abdominal surgical procedures because of the observed improvement in coronary artery blood flow, attenuation of pulmonary complications, and the reduction in the duration of postoperative ileus. Combining a local anesthetic plus an opioid in the epidural space is believed to have a synergistic effect.[67] The optimal duration of epidural analgesia has not been determined, but recommendations are that the infusion be continued for at least 2 to 4 days. Other than analgesia, epidural infusions lasting less than 24 hours do not appear to offer any clear cardiovascular advantages.

Epidurally administered opioids have the distinct advantage of producing analgesia without causing significant sympatholytic effect or motor blockade. Analgesia occurs by way of a *spinal mechanism* and through a *supraspinal mechanism* following systemic adsorption. The spinal mechanism occurs following diffusion of the drug into the spinal fluid, and is determined by meningeal permeability. Opioids with intermediate lipophilicity (e.g., hydromorphone, alfentanil, and meperidine) have the ability to easily move between the aqueous and lipid regions of the arachnoid membrane and therefore have high meningeal permeability, which potentially confers higher bioavailability in the spinal cord. However, in a comprehensive review of the topic Bernards et al.[68] concluded that morphine has greater bioavailability in the spinal cord than alfentanil, fentanyl, and sufentanil.

In general, the epidural administration of hydrophilic opioids tends to have a slow onset, long duration, and a mechanism of action that is primarily spinal in nature. The epidural administration of lipophilic opioids, on the other hand, has a quick

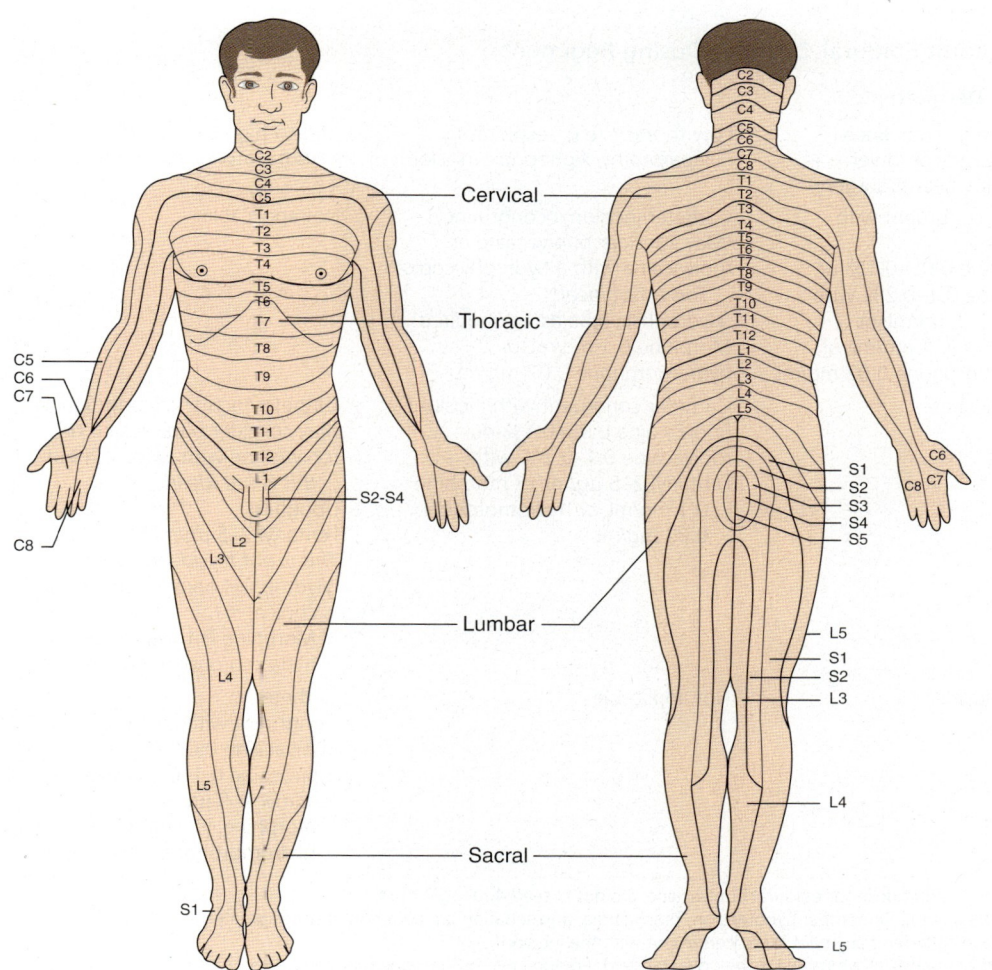

Figure 55-15 Dermatome guide for placement of epidural catheters.

onset, short duration, and a mechanism of action that is primarily supraspinal, secondary to rapid systemic uptake. However, the data are controversial and the site of action of lipophilic opioids such as fentanyl may primarily be determined by the mode of administration. Bolus administration of fentanyl appears to have a segmental analgesic effect whereas epidural infusion of fentanyl appears to have a nonsegmental (systemic) effect. There are some data, however, that suggest that there can be significant spinal mechanisms of action of the lipophilic opioids, particularly with the thoracic epidural infusion of fentanyl. In the opioid-tolerant patient taking more than 250 mg/day of oral morphine, sufentanil may be considered to be the epidural opioid of choice because of its high intrinsic activity.

As previously mentioned, local anesthetic–opioid combinations are the most common form of epidural infusion because the combination is considered to be synergistic. Local anesthetics have the unique ability to block the stress response by blocking afferent input to the spinal cord. Although bupivacaine plus fentanyl may be the most common combination, bupivacaine plus morphine makes more sense from a bioavailability point of view. Hydromorphone plus bupivacaine also makes very good sense as this combination has all the advantages of a hydrophilic opioid with excellent meningeal permeability but less risk of pruritus. Remember, epidural infusions may consist of just a hydrophilic opioid if the patient cannot tolerate side effects from the local anesthetic or if the epidural is incongruent with the surgical incision. Likewise, an epidural infusion may consist simply of a local anesthetic if the patient cannot tolerate opioid-related side effects, provided that the epidural is correctly placed and is congruent with the surgical incision. Table 55-17 contains epidural dosing guidelines.

Adjuvant medications, which may enhance analgesia, include clonidine and ketamine. Clonidine (2 µg/mL) can be combined with an opioid and a local anesthetic and is usually infused at a rate of 5 to 20 µg/hr. Side effects that limit its clinical usefulness include hypotension, bradycardia, and sedation. An epidural infusion consisting of ropivacaine 0.2%, fentanyl 5 µg/mL, and clonidine 2 µg/mL infused at a rate of 3 to 7 mL/hr following a TKA has been reported to cause no significant sedation in this dosage range.[69] The safety of epidurally administered ketamine has not been determined, and routine use cannot be recommended at this time.

A novel approach to postoperative pain control is extended-release epidural morphine (Depodur). The system consists of morphine encapsulated within a liposome delivery system, which provides controlled release of morphine for up to 48 hours. Double-blinded studies indicate that the epidural administration of liposomal morphine has proven to be efficacious in the treatment of postoperative pain associated with total hip arthroplasty (THA), TKA, and cesarean section. Depodur is approved only for lumbar epidural administration.

Intrathecal analgesia with a variety of drugs is a widely accepted practice for the treatment of both acute and chronic pain. Rathmell

Table 55-17 Guidelines for Adult Epidural Catheter Dosing Regimen[a,b]

Catheter Placement	Surgical Dermatome		
	Lumbar (e.g., total knee arthroplasty or lower extremity bypass surgery)	Low thoracic (e.g., exploratory laparotomy, xiphopubic incision)	Mid-to-high thoracic (e.g., thoracotomy, sternotomy)
Lumbar T_{12}–caudal	Catheter congruent with incision! Bupivacaine 0.05–0.1% or ropivacaine 0.1–0.2% with Fentanyl 2–5 µg/mL or morphine 0.1 mg/mL or hydromorphone 0.02 mg/mL	Catheter/incision incongruency! [c]May consider bupivacaine or ropivacaine with a hydrophilic opioid. This is not ideal! [d]Hydrophilic opioids are required! Morphine 0.1 mg/mL or hydromorphone 0.02 mg/mL	Not applicable
Low thoracic T_8 to T_{12}	Not applicable	Catheter congruent with incision! Bupivacaine 0.05–0.1% or ropivacaine 0.1–0.2% with Fentanyl 2–5 µg/mL or morphine 0.1 mg/mL or hydromorphone 0.02 mg/mL	Catheter/incision incongruency! May consider bupivacaine or ropivacaine with an opioid but this is not ideal! Lipophilic Fentanyl 2–5 µg/mL. This is not the ideal opioid! [d]Hydrophilic opioids are a better choice! 1. Morphine 0.1 mg/mL or 2. hydromorphone 0.02 mg/mL
Mid-to-high thoracic T_4 to T_8	Not applicable	Not applicable	Catheter Congruent with incision! Bupivacaine 0.05–0.1% or ropivacaine 0.1–0.2% with fentanyl 2–5 µg/mL or morphine 0.1 mg/mL or hydromorphone 0.02 mg/mL

[a]Rate of infusion, 2–10 mL/hr. Recommended adult dose for epidural bupivacaine. Do not exceed 400 mg/24 hr!
[b]May consider Clonidine 1–2 µg/mL in the epidural. Remember hypotension, bradycardia, and sedation are common at doses greater than 14 µg/hr.
[c]Local anesthetic efficacy is diminished if the catheter placement is not congruent with the incision!
[d]Hydrophilic opioids provide a broad band of analgesia! Morphine is the gold standard. Epidural hydromorphone may cause less pruritus.

et al.[70] have thoroughly reviewed the role of intrathecal analgesia for acute pain. Opioid analgesics, including morphine, hydromorphone, meperidine, methadone, fentanyl, and sufentanil, are the most commonly administered drugs for this purpose. Their distribution within the intrathecal space following administration is complex. Hydrophilic opioids (e.g., morphine) penetrate the spinal cord and bind to specific pre- and postsynaptic receptors within the dorsal horn. They traverse the dura slowly, bind to epidural fat poorly, and slowly enter the plasma. They tend to have a slow onset of action, long duration, and provide a broad band of analgesia. Delayed respiratory depression is more common with hydrophilic opioids secondary to rostral spread.[70] Lipophilic opioids (e.g., fentanyl), on the other hand, tend to bind to nonspecific receptors in the white matter. They rapidly cross the dura and are quickly sequestered into epidural fat and swiftly enter the systemic circulation. As a general rule lipophilic opioids tend to have a rapid onset of action, short duration, and a narrow band of analgesia. Delayed respiratory depression is less of a problem with the lipophilic opioids. Other side effects associated with intrathecal opioids include nausea and vomiting, urinary retention, and pruritus. The incidence of pruritus with intrathecal hydromorphone is reported to be significantly less than with morphine (refer to Table 55-18 for dosing guidelines).

Other useful analgesic additives include the α_2-agonists, NSAIDs, NMDA receptor antagonists, acetylcholinesterase inhibitors, adenosine, epinephrine, and benzodiazepines. The α_2-agonists alter pain transmission by binding to pre- and postsynaptic receptors within the dorsal horn of the spinal cord. Evidence suggests that intrathecal clonidine is synergistic with spinal local anesthetics, prolongs sensory and motor blockades, and causes less urinary retention than intrathecal morphine.[70] Intrathecal clonidine does not cause respiratory depression or pruritus. Intrathecal doses of 150 µg, however, are reported to increase the incidence of hypotension, bradycardia, and nausea[70] (refer to Table 55-19 for additional dosing recommendations). Anecdotal reports suggest that the neuraxial administration of an NSAID, either accidentally or intentionally, is both safe and effective. Further investigation for the treatment of postoperative pain is required to define the role of intrathecal NSAIDs as well as the acetylcholinesterase inhibitors, NMDA receptor antagonists, adenosine, and benzodiazepines.

Table 55-19 Intrathecal Analgesia: Other Dosing Guidelines[70,193]

Intrathecal Drug	Dosing	Comments
Clonidine	15–45 µg improves the quality of spinal blockade in outpatient surgery	Side effects increase significantly at intrathecal doses >150 µg
Epinephrine	0.1–0.6 mg Dose-related increase: 1. Return of motor function 2. Return of micturition	Not recommended for outpatient surgery
Neostigmine	6.25–50 µg Dose-related increase: 1. Motor blockade 2. Time for resolution of the block 3. Nausea and vomiting	Further studies of the appropriate intrathecal dose that optimizes analgesia while minimizing side effects are warranted

Table 55-18 Intrathecal Analgesia Dosing Guidelines[a,30,70]

Surgical Procedure	Intrathecal Drug Dose
Labor analgesia	Sufentanil 2.5–5 µg
Cesarean section (C-section)	Morphine 100 µg. The addition of clonidine 60 µg is synergistic and can increase the duration of spinal analgesia after C-section but also increases intraoperative sedation.
Outpatient knee arthroscopy	Fentanyl 10–25 µg will improve intraoperative analgesia without prolonging postoperative motor blockade.
Total knee arthroplasty	Morphine 100 µg
Total hip arthroplasty	Morphine 100 µg
Thoracotomy and major abdominal surgery	Morphine 500 µg. The incidence of side effects such as nausea and vomiting, urinary retention, pruritus and respiratory depression increase significantly with doses >300 µg.

[a]50–100 µg of intrathecal hydromorphone approximates 100–200 µg of intrathecal morphine.

Peripheral Nerve Blockade

Single-injection peripheral nerve blockade has been shown to provide pain control that is superior to opioids with fewer side effects.[71] Single-injection techniques are limited in duration but continuous peripheral nerve block (CPNB) techniques can extend the benefits of peripheral nerve blockade well into the postoperative period. CPNB has proven to be an effective technique for postoperative pain management; it is superior to opioid analgesia with fewer opioid-related side effects and rare neurologic and infectious complications.[72,73] The benefits of CPNB in the ambulatory setting include prolonged postoperative analgesia, facilitated discharge from the hospital, fewer opioid-related side effects, and greater patient satisfaction.[74] Since the previous iteration of this chapter, ultrasound-guided regional anesthesia (UGRA) has clearly become the primary peripheral nerve localization technique. Advantages of UGRA include not only decreased block performance time, block onset time, and local anesthetic requirements but also improved sensory block onset as well as improved block success. Likewise, UGRA has reduced the incidence of the dreaded complication of local anesthetic systemic toxicity (LAST).[75] Tables 55-20, 55-21, and 55-22 present indications and contraindications for specific peripheral nerve blocks. Table 55-23 has recommended dosing guidelines for CPNB.

The Brachial Plexus

Above the Clavicle

The *interscalene block* (ISB) is the ideal peripheral nerve block for painful orthopedic procedures on the shoulder and upper

Table 55-20 Brachial Plexus Blockade

Peripheral Nerve Block	Indications	Contraindications	Comments
Interscalene	Total shoulder arthroplasty and hemiarthroplasty Open rotator cuff repair Open anterior reconstruction Open reduction, internal fixation (ORIF) and joint fusion	Refusal by the patient, infection, or hematoma in the vicinity of the block, allergy to local anesthetics, and progressive neuropathy or lesion of unknown etiology In the anticoagulated patient follow the recommendations set forth for neuraxial blockade until practice guidelines for peripheral nerve blocks are promulgated	UGRA results in the following beneficial outcomes: • Faster block performance • Fewer needle passes • Decreased risk of vascular puncture • More rapid sensory block onset • Improved block success
Supraclavicular	Provides anesthesia to the entire upper extremity with a single injection of local anesthetic	See above	The incidence of pneumothorax with the use of US guidance is low.
Infraclavicular	This approach is ideally suited for surgery on the distal upper arm, the entire forearm, wrist, and hand Surgery distal to the elbow: Arteriovenous fistula, Colles' fracture, Dupuytren contracture release, wrist fusion, and ORIF Surgery on the forearm, wrist, and hand	See above Also chest deformities and healed but dislocated fractures of the clavicle	Ultrasound guidance can significantly improve the safety and effectiveness of this block. Catheter techniques can be useful.
Axillary	Hand surgery	See above	

Table 55-21 Lumbar and Sacral Plexus Blockade

Peripheral Nerve Block	Indications	Contraindications	Comments
Femoral nerve	Total knee arthroplasty (TKA) Anterior cruciate ligament repair, femoral neck fractures, and saphenous vein stripping Muscle biopsies involving the ventral, medial, or lateral thigh	See Table 55-20	Good choice for TKA May be combined with a sciatic nerve block for TKA Catheter techniques are useful. Ultrasound guidance confirms placement of the needle tip between the fascia iliaca and the iliopsoas muscle.
Adductor canal block	Total knee arthroplasty Any surgery on the medial aspect of the ankle		UGRA targets the saphenous nerve within the adductor canal.
Sciatic nerve	Above-the-knee amputation Combine with a lumbar plexus block Ankle joint replacement Ankle arthrodesis Calcaneal osteotomy Achilles tendon repair	See above	Numerous approaches have been described. The *parasacral approach* is the most cephalad. The *infragluteal parabiceps approach* is useful. Catheter techniques are useful for prolonged analgesia. Ultrasound guidance can confirm needle placement in the subgluteal space.
Popliteal fossa	Below-the-knee amputation Combine with a saphenous nerve block *Ankle surgery:* Triple arthrodesis, arthroscopy, and Achilles tendon repair *Foot surgery:* Bunion surgery and transmetatarsal amputation	See above	Lateral and posterior approaches have been described. Catheter insertion following ambulatory foot surgery can provide prolonged analgesia. Ultrasound guidance is very useful. Use the "seesaw" sign to confirm identification of the common peroneal and tibial nerves. May be combined with an adductor canal block to provide analgesia to the medial aspect of the ankle.

Table 55-22 Truncal Blocks

Peripheral Nerve Block	Indications	Contraindications	Comments
Paravertebral block	Breast surgery, thoracic and abdominal surgery, fractured ribs, postherpetic neuralgia	In the anticoagulated patient follow the recommendations set forth for neuraxial blockade	Numerous US guided approaches have been described.
Pectoralis block			
I	Breast expanders		
II	Mastectomies and sentinel node dissection		
Anterior serratus	Latissimus dorsi flap reconstruction and multiple rib fractures		
Transversus abdominis plane (TAP) block	Abdominal wall surgery		Unilateral TAP for surgery that does not cross the midline (e.g., renal transplant or appendectomy)
Subcostal TAP	Supra-umbilical incisions		Bilateral TAP for incisions that cross the midline (e.g., laparoscopic procedures)
Lateral TAP	Infra-umbilical incisions		
Posterior (QL) TAP	T5 to T10 spread		
Rectus sheath block	Midline abdominal surgical incision		
Transversalis fascia plane	Iliac crest bone graft		
Ilioinguinal/iliohypogastric nerve	Inguinal hernia repair		

arm such as repair of a rotator cuff or labral tear, acromioclavicular joint reconstruction, Bankart Procedure, proximal humerus fracture, and total shoulder arthroplasty. It is also indicated for vascular procedures performed on the shoulder and upper arm, but is a poor choice for forearm and hand surgery because the ulnar nerve is commonly spared. It is the most cephalad approach to the brachial plexus and was originally described by Winnie in 1970.[76]

Using ultrasound (US) guidance this is a relatively straight forward peripheral nerve block to perform. Although this block can be carried out using an in-plane or out-of-plane technique, the most common technique is a posterior in-plane approach with the transducer in an axial oblique plane. The needle tip is advanced under real time and is positioned adjacent to or within the brachial plexus sheath. The ideal position of the tip of the needle is unclear; however, Spence and colleagues[77] investigated this and suggest that conservative (periplexus) injection of local anesthetic adjacent to the brachial plexus sheath is as effective as aggressive (intraplexus) injection of local anesthetic within the brachial plexus sheath. Needle tip positioning within the brachial plexus sheath, however, does offer the advantage of using smaller volumes of local anesthetic while maintaining efficacy. When performing this block direct needle-to-nerve contact is not required for an effective interscalene block (ISB).[78] By avoiding direct needle-to-nerve contact you can maximize efficacy and minimize the risk of nerve injury. US-guided ISB has the advantage of minimizing vascular puncture and allows for multiple injections around the plexus, resulting in smaller volumes of local anesthetic and decreasing the risk of toxicity. Your end point for injection is real-time observation of hydrodissection of local anesthetic around the nerves.

Table 55-23 Recommended Dosing Regimen of Local Anesthetics for Continuous Peripheral Nerve Blockade[194,195]

Catheter	Agent	Rate of Infusion	PCA Bolus (mL)	Lockout (min)
Interscalene Infraclavicular	Ropivacaine 0.2% or bupivacaine 0.15–0.2%	5–8 mL/hr	2–4	15–20
Femoral	Ropivacaine 0.2% or bupivacaine 0.15–0.2%	5–10 mL/hr	5–10	30–60
Popliteal		5–8 mL/hr	2	15–20
Paravertebral	Ropivacaine 0.2%	0.1–0.2 mL/kg/hr	—	—
Bupivacaine 0.25% with 1:400,000 epinephrine		0.1 mL/kg/hr	—	—

PCA, patient-controlled analgesia.

Single-injection interscalene blockade for shoulder surgery reduces postoperative VAS pain scores, total opioid consumption, postoperative nausea and vomiting, time for request of first dose of analgesic, time to discharge, and unplanned hospital admissions.[79] Interscalene blockade provides postoperative analgesia, which is superior to subacromial bursae blockade, suprascapular nerve blockade, infusion of intra-articular local anesthetic, and parenteral opioids. To extend the period of postoperative analgesia, continuous catheter techniques have been successfully employed in both the inpatient and outpatient settings.

The *supraclavicular approach* to the brachial plexus provides anesthesia to the entire upper extremity with a single injection of local anesthetic. Indications for this block include arm, elbow, forearm (arteriovenous fistula creation), and hand (scaphoid fracture, trapeziectomy) surgeries. The supraclavicular approach is carried out at a point where the plexus is reduced to its fewest component parts, the superior, middle, and inferior trunks, as they pass under the clavicle and over the first rib.

In the now "classic" Kulenkampff description,[80] of this peripheral nerve block, needle insertion is 1 cm above the midpoint of the clavicle in a plane that is parallel to the patient's head and neck. This approach requires the elicitation of multiple paresthesias and multiple injections, and the incidence of pneumothorax has been reported to be as high as 0.5% to 5% with this technique. With the introduction of ultrasound guidance, however, the safety of this approach has improved dramatically. Real-time imaging of the needle tip in order to optimize its position not only decreases the risk of pneumothorax but also increases the quality and shortens the onset time of the block.[81,82] Single, double, and triple injection techniques have been described for this block.[83-85] It is unclear which technique is superior. The evidence to date, however, suggests that it is imperative that the advancing needle puncture the brachial plexus sheath, which can be appreciated as a palpable "fascial click." Local anesthetic can then be injected in divided doses within the perineural space, which can create a safe conduit for advancement of the needle into the space referred to as the "corner pocket," which is bordered by the subclavian artery medially, the first rib inferiorly, and the divisions of the brachial plexus superiorly and laterally. The ulnar nerve is commonly spared with the supraclavicular approach; however, the "corner pocket" technique (Fig. 55-16) is reported to block the ulnar nerve in at least 85% of cases when performed correctly.[83] Although ultrasound guidance has facilitated the performance of this block, unusual sonoanatomy (sonopathology), such as an aberrant transverse cervical artery, a dilated subclavian vein (secondary to elevated central venous pressure) and atypical locations of the brachial plexus can make this a challenging block to perform.[86,87] Although the supraclavicular approach is amenable to continuous catheter techniques, the literature on this subject is meager.

Below the Clavicle

The *infraclavicular block* is ideally suited for surgical procedures below the midhumerus such as the hand, wrist, forearm, or elbow.[88] The block targets the brachial plexus at the level of the cords where it is in close proximity to the axillary artery.[89] The popularity of this approach has been less than enthusiastic because of unreliable surface landmarks and the potential risks of pneumothorax and vascular puncture. Ultrasound guidance has, however, dramatically improved both the safety and efficacy of the infraclavicular approach and success rates are reported to be in the 90% to 100% range.[90]

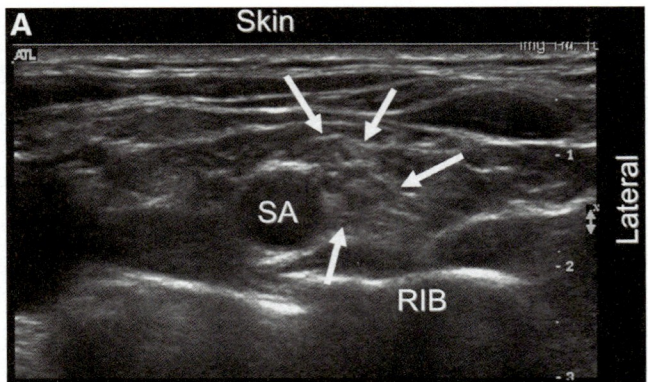
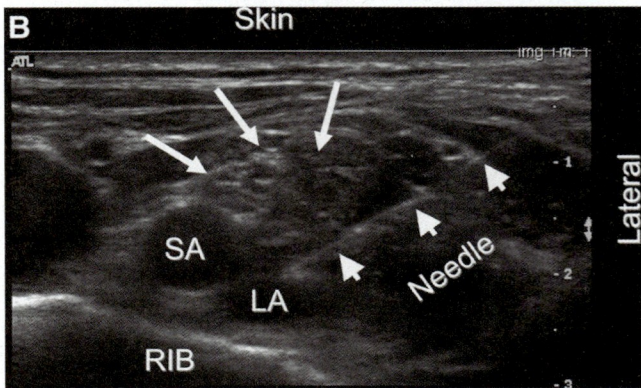

Figure 55-16 Ultrasound-guided supraclavicular nerve block. The long arrows highlight the brachial plexus at the level of the supraclavicular fossa. SA, subclavian artery; LA, local anesthetic. (Reprinted with permission from Soares LG, Brull R, Lai J, et al. Eight ball, corner pocket: the optimal needle position for ultrasound-guided supraclavicular block. *Reg Anesth Pain Med*. 2007;32:2.)

With the patient in the supine position the block is performed with the transducer placed below the clavicle in the delto-pectoral groove in a para-sagittal plane, which provides a short axis view of the axillary artery. Although this block may be performed with the arm adducted or abducted, the ideal position of the patient's arm is abducted to 90 degrees with the elbow flexed. This maneuver significantly displaces the clavicle in a cranial-posterior direction, and allows the needle to be inserted 2 to 4 cm cephalad to the transducer and anterior to the clavicle, resulting in a shallower approach with the needle, which optimizes the ultrasound image.[91] Use of an echogenic needle should facilitate performance of this peripheral nerve block, particularly if the angle of insertion becomes too steep. The optimal injection site is cranioposterior and adjacent to the axillary artery.[92] This area is closest to all three cords and potentially optimizes local anesthetic spread. A prospective randomized trial comparing ultrasound-guided infraclavicular blockade, with and without neurostimulation, has confirmed that the "U-shaped" distribution of local anesthetic around the posterior, medial, and lateral aspects of the axillary artery will reliably produce complete blockade of the brachial plexus (Fig. 55-17).[89]

A recent large-scale study documented the analgesic benefit and favorable safety profile of single-injection infraclavicular nerve blockade.[93] Placement of continuous infraclavicular nerve catheters has the advantage of providing prolonged analgesia for several days following surgery. Benefits include improved pain scores, decreased opioid requirements, less sedation, and less sleep disturbance with continuous infraclavicular nerve

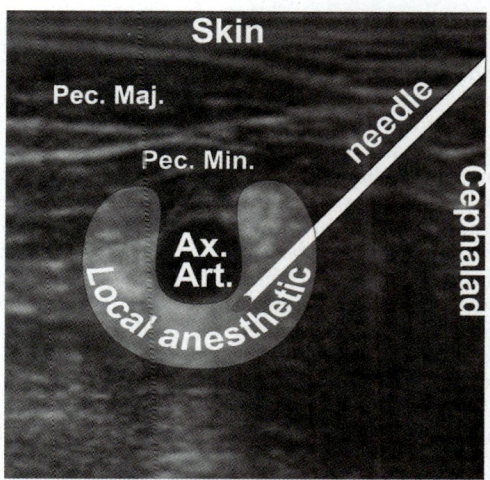

Figure 55-17 Ultrasound-guided infraclavicular nerve block. Ultrasonic anatomy, initial needle position, and desired U-shaped anesthetic distribution. Pec. Maj., pectoralis major muscle; Pec. Min., pectoralis minor muscle; Ax. Art., axillary artery. (Reprinted with permission from Dingemans E, Williams SR, Arcand G, et al. Neurostimulation in ultrasound-guided infraclavicular block. *Anestn Analg.* 2007;104:1274.)

blockade.[94] Although abduction of the arm is recommended the block can be performed with the arm *abducted* or *adducted*. This flexibility in positioning can be advantageous particularly in the trauma patient who has significant pain and limited mobility. Placement of continuous infraclavicular catheters provides the advantage of a secure point of insertion that will not dislodge easily with patient movement. It is also relatively easy to keep clean and sterile, particularly if the patient is to be discharged home with the catheter in situ to be removed at a later date.

The Lumbar Plexus

The lumbar plexus is formed from the ventral rami of the L1 to L4 spinal nerve roots, with a small contribution from T12 in some patients. The plexus lies within the substance of the psoas muscle in between the anterior and posterior masses and gives rise to the femoral (saphenous), obturator, lateral femoral cutaneous, ilioinguinal, iliohypogastric, and genitofemoral nerves. The nerves provide sensory innervation to the abdomen and groin, the anterior, lateral, and medial aspects of the thigh, the knee joint, and the medial part of the calf. Motor innervation is supplied to the abdominal muscles, the hip flexors, thigh adductors, and the quadriceps muscles. Numerous posterior and anterior approaches for lumbar plexus blockade (LPB) have been described[95] and the block is indicated for major surgeries of the hip and knee.

Posterior Approach (Psoas Compartment Block)

The posterior approach to the lumbar plexus reliably blocks the femoral, lateral femoral, and obturator nerves.[96] The block is performed with the patient in the lateral decubitus position, usually with the operative side in the uppermost (independent) position. The advantage of this position is that the block can be combined with a sciatic nerve block. The disadvantage, however, is the increased risk of epidural spread. When combined with sciatic nerve blockade, virtually any surgical procedure can be performed on the lower extremity. Although ultrasound-guided LPB has been described in the literature, it has not been studied extensively. Complications associated with the placement of a psoas compartment block includes epidural spread, spinal anesthesia, systemic toxicity, unilateral sympathectomy, renal subscapular hematoma, and neurologic injury.[97] Psoas compartment blockade should be avoided in the anticoagulated patient. The depth of the plexus in adults can make ultrasound guidance more challenging particularly in the obese patient, which will preclude its use, unless current ultrasound technology improves dramatically; however, in children ultrasound-guided LPB may prove to be efficacious.[98]

Anterior Approach (Femoral Nerve Block)

The femoral nerve is formed from the posterior divisions of the ventral rami of L2 to L4 and is the largest terminal branch of the lumbar plexus. The nerve emerges from the lower lateral border of the psoas muscle and passes beneath the inguinal ligament in the groove between the iliacus and psoas muscles. In the inguinal region the nerve is covered by two fascial layers, the fascia lata and fascia iliaca, and whereas the fascia lata separates the subcutaneous tissue from the muscle and vessels, the fascia iliaca completely envelopes both the iliopsoas muscle and the femoral nerve, physically separating the nerve from the femoral artery and vein.[99] Although the nerve can be visualized with ultrasound, both above and below the inguinal ligament, it is ideally visualized at the level of the inguinal crease, and at this level, the nerve is positioned approximately 0.5 cm lateral to the femoral artery. The nerve provides motor innervation to the quadriceps femoris, sartorius, and pectineus muscles as well as sensory innervation to the anterior thigh, knee, and the medial aspect of the lower extremity terminating as the saphenous nerve. Recent ultrasound-guided evidence indicates that the topographic relationship of the femoral nerve at the inguinal crease is *medial and lateral* to each other rather than *anterior and posterior* and both divisions are in close proximity to each other under the fascia iliaca.[100]

Femoral nerve block (FNB) is indicated for any surgery on the anterior aspect of the quadriceps muscle (biopsy or tendon repair), patella, TKA, anterior cruciate ligament repair or ankle surgery involving the medial aspect of the foot. Ultrasound-guided FNB is performed at the level of the femoral (inguinal) crease using a transverse cross-sectional (short-axis) view of the nerve as described by Ilfeld and colleagues.[101] Using an in-plane approach the needle is carefully advanced through the fascia iliaca and, while taking care to avoid direct needle-to-nerve contact, the needle is positioned either anterior or posterior to the nerve. Care must be taken to place the tip of the needle within the space between the fascia iliaca and the iliopsoas muscle lateral to the femoral artery (Fig. 55-18). Using incremental injection local anesthetic is administered into the perineural space and hydrodissection of local anesthetic around the nerve is confirmed.

Following TKA, ultrasound-guided FNB has been shown to provide analgesia that is superior to intravenous PCA alone and analgesia that is similar to epidural analgesia but without the hypotension associated with epidural analgesia.[102] Although both single shot and continuous catheter techniques have been described, a recent Cochrane Review indicates that continuous blockade may be superior to a single shot technique.[103] Evidence suggests, however, that continuous blockade of the femoral nerve can precipitate weakness of the quadriceps muscle, potentially increasing the risk of inpatient falls (IFs) following surgery.[104] Other independent risk factors for IF, completely unrelated to FNB, include advanced age, and increasing comorbidity burden such as sleep apnea, psychosis, obesity, and anemia.[105] The Centers for Medicare and Medicaid Services (CMS) have designated IF as a hospital-acquired condition that is a potentially avoidable event and they may not necessarily reimburse for related

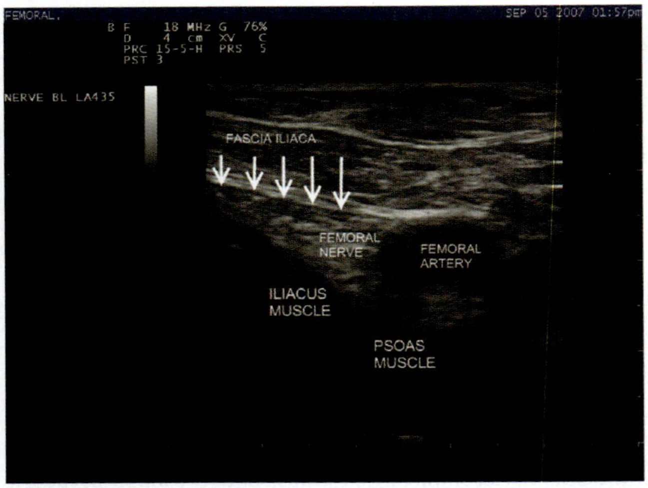

Figure 55-18 Ultrasound-guided femoral nerve blockade: Short axis ultrasound image of the infrainguinal structures. Femoral nerve blockade can be performed with a needle approach that is either in-plane or out-of-plane. The needle tip must be positioned within the space between the fascia iliaca and the iliopsoas muscle before local anesthetic is injected in order to achieve a successful block of the femoral nerve.

expenses. Comprehensive, multidisciplinary fall-prevention programs can eliminate the risk of IFs.

Saphenous nerve blockade is frequently combined with a lateral popliteal block or sciatic block for procedures involving the lower leg. The saphenous nerve is the only branch of the lumbar plexus below the knee and is the largest sensory terminal branch of the femoral nerve. The nerve provides sensory innervation to the medial, anteromedial, and posteromedial parts of the knee, leg, and medial malleolus and, in some people, the medial aspect of the large toe. Several approaches have been described at the level of the patella and medial malleolus; however, blockade of the nerve within the adductor canal (AC) has proven to be very popular. The AC is bounded by the sartorius, vastus medialis, and adductor muscles and contains the femoral vessels, saphenous nerve, the motor nerve to the vastus medialis, and occasionally the obturator nerve. The AC extends from the apex of the femoral triangle to the adductor hiatus.

Ultrasound-guided *adductor canal block* (ACB) is indicated for TKA, anterior cruciate ligament repair, medial menisectomy, and any surgery on the medial aspect of the ankle (total ankle arthroplasty and triple arthrodesis). The potential advantage of the ACB over the FNB is analgesia without significant motor blockade, theoretically decreasing the risk of IFs.[106] Although continuous AC catheters preserve quadriceps strength better than continuous femoral catheters there is evidence that femoral catheters may provide superior dynamic analgesia.[107] Generally speaking the ACB is performed at the mid-thigh level; however, the literature is confusing about what constitutes "mid-thigh"![108] Nevertheless, ultrasound-guided ACB is performed with the patient in the prone position with the operative leg externally rotated and the leg slightly flexed. In a transverse axial plane place a high-frequency linear transducer positioned on the medial aspect of the thigh to identify the femoral vessels coursing deep to the sartorius muscle. As the transducer is advanced caudally the femoral artery dives deep through the adductor hiatus. If the purpose of the ACB is to anesthetize both the saphenous nerve as well as the nerve to

the vastus medialis then the ideal needle entry point should be the distal thigh, within the AC, approximately 2 to 3 cm proximal to the adductor hiatus[109,110] or at the midpoint of the AC as defined by the ultrasound image of both the proximal and distal ends of the AC.[111] Injection at this point should provide analgesia to the anteromedial aspect of the knee joint, joint capsule, and retinaculum.[111] Needle insertion is in-plane using an anterior-lateral to posterior-medial direction.

Another very successful approach to femoral nerve blockade is the *fascia iliaca compartment block* (FICB). The injection site is distant from any neurovascular structures and therefore does not require neurostimulation to be successful.[97] The block has been described in both children and adults and is reported to be more successful than the 3-in-1 block. It is a large volume (30 to 60 mL) fascial plane block that targets both the femoral and lateral femoral cutaneous nerves, and is considered to be both a safer alternative to a lumbar plexus block and a critical component of a multimodal opioid-sparing technique for analgesia in the elderly patient with hip fracture. Advantages of this block, in the hip fracture patient, include (1) analgesia that allows positioning of the patient for neuraxial block, (2) opioid-sparing analgesia, (3) decreased length of hospital stay, and (4) less delirium.[112–114] The three techniques that have been described in the literature include the "landmark technique"[115] the supra-inguinal para-sagittal approach,[116] and the transverse approach in the inguinal crease.[117] When performing the supra-inguinal parasagittal approach it is recommended that you inject as proximally as possible to guarantee cephalad spread of local anesthetic into the pelvis (Figs. 55-19 and 55-20).[118]

Sacral Plexus

The sciatic nerve originates from the sacral plexus and is derived from the ventral rami of the fourth lumbar to the third sacral nerve roots. The three major components of the sciatic nerve include the tibial and common peroneal nerves and the posterior femoral cutaneous nerve to the thigh. The sciatic nerve provides sensory, motor, and some sympathetic innervation to the lower extremity, and its blockade, in combination with a femoral or saphenous nerve block, can provide complete anesthesia and

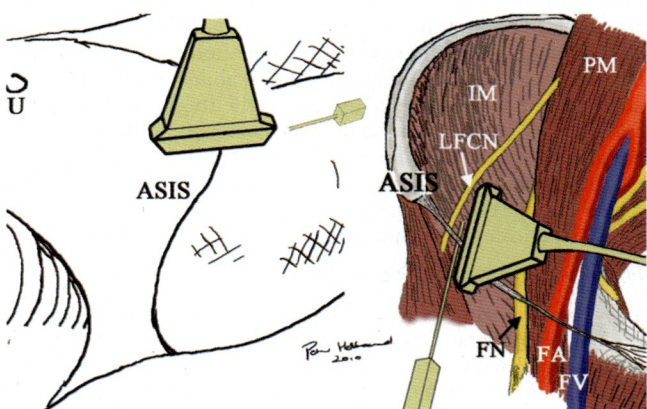

Figure 55-19 Probe and needle position and diagram of dissected iliac fossa showing anatomy for the suprainguinal fascia iliaca block. Iliacus muscle (IM), psoas muscle (PM), femoral nerve (FN), femoral artery (FA), femoral vein (FV), anterior superior iliac spine (ASIS), umbilicus (U), (LFCN) lateral femoral cutaneous nerve. (Reprinted with permission from Hebbard P, Ivanusic J, Sha S. Ultrasound-guided suprainguinal fascia iliaca block: a cadaveric evaluation of a novel approach. *Anaesthesia.* 2011;66:300–305.)

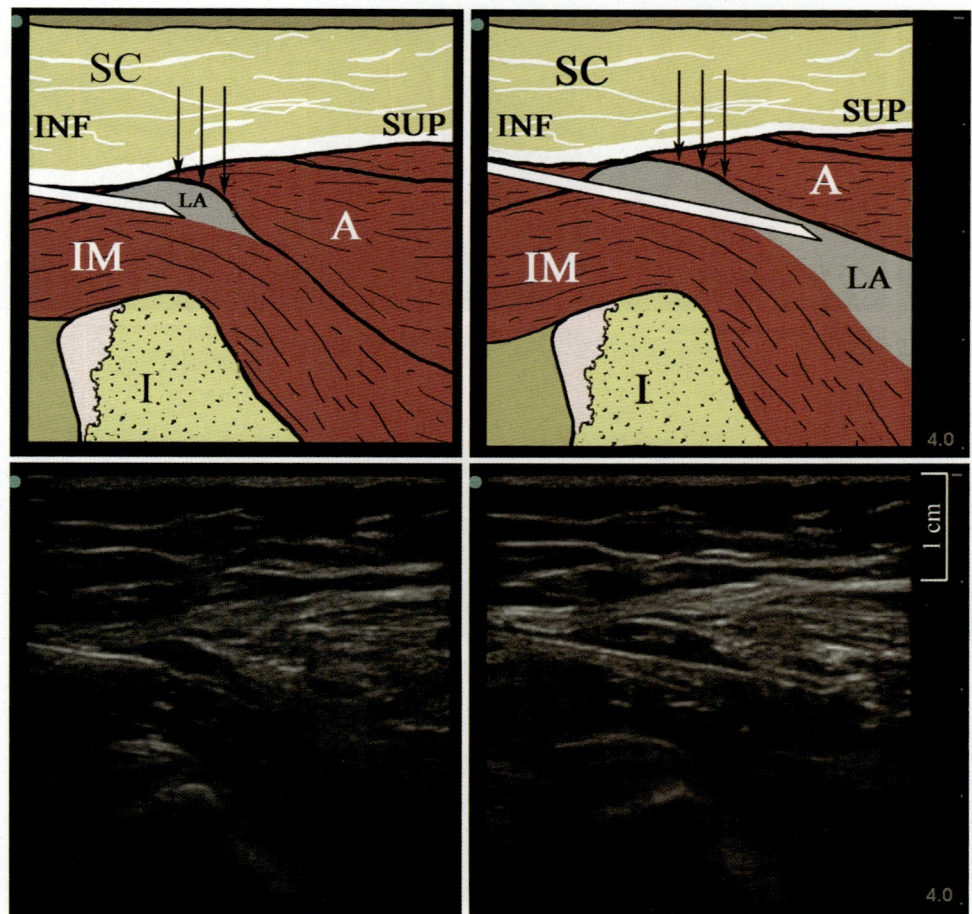

Figure 55-20 Sonograms during hydro-dissection (left image) and towards conclusion of block (right image) showing the collection of local anaesthetic (LA) beneath the fascia iliaca (*black arrows*) with the needle advanced through it. Iliacus muscle (IM), ilium (I) subcutaneous tissue (SC), abdominal muscles (A), inferior (INF), superior (SUP). (Reprinted with permission from Hebbard P, Ivanusic J, Sha S. Ultrasound-guided suprainguinal fascia iliaca block: a cadaveric evaluation of a novel approach. *Anaesthesia*. 2011;66:300–305.)

postoperative analgesia for lower extremity surgery. Sciatic nerve blockade has been proven useful in numerous surgical procedures, including THA and TKA, anterior cruciate ligament repair, complex outpatient knee surgeries, above- and below-the-knee amputations, as well as ankle and foot surgery. Although numerous proximal and distal techniques, using anterior, posterior, and lateral approaches to the sciatic nerve with the patient in the supine, prone lateral, and lithotomy positions, have been described, patient comfort is the key factor determining the optimal approach.

Sciatic nerve blockade within the popliteal fossa is probably one of the most common approaches. Sciatic nerve blockade at this level typically spares the posterior cutaneous nerve to the thigh, thus preserving hamstring function. This approach therefore has the added benefit of being less restrictive on ambulation, which is useful following ambulatory surgery. Compared with subcutaneous local anesthetic infiltration and ankle blockade, popliteal sciatic nerve blockade provides significantly longer postoperative analgesia and has a high degree of patient satisfaction.

Although single-shot sciatic nerve blockade can provide short-term analgesia, continuous popliteal sciatic nerve blockade with a peripheral nerve catheter can significantly extend the duration of postoperative analgesia and has been successfully implemented in both the inpatient and outpatient settings using an electronic infusion pump or a disposable elastomeric pump. Pain-related sleep disruption is less, and hospital LOS is shorter, which can potentially lead to a reduction in health-care costs.[119] Risks associated with at-home perineural infusions of local anesthetic include catheter site infection, nerve injury, and catheter migration with subsequent local anesthetic toxicity. Complications are relatively rare.[74,120]

Over the previous 5 years, ultrasound guidance has become the predominant technique for identifying the sciatic nerve within the popliteal space. It has significantly improved the accuracy of needle placement through real-time imaging of the nerve and has increased the rate of sensory block success through targeted circumferential spread of local anesthetic around the nerve.[121] The image of the sciatic nerve in the popliteal space varies depending on the type of transducer used, but the linear 5- to 12-MHz transducer provides the highest resolution image.[122] With the posterior approach and a short-axis (transverse cross-sectional) view, active or passive dorsiflexion of the foot can produce external rotation of the sciatic nerve around its central axis (seesaw sign) which facilitates its identification.[123]

In cadaveric models it has been demonstrated that a paraneural sheath envelopes the sciatic nerve.[124] Using high-definition ultrasound the paraneural sheath appears as a hyperechoic fascial layer between the epineurium of the nerve and the epimysium of the surrounding muscle (Fig. 55-21).[125] An injection deep to the paraneurium, within the paraneural space ("subparaneural" compartment), will, therefore, facilitate spread of local anesthetic along the length of the nerve and improve sensory blockade.[125] Likewise, subparaneural injection of local anesthetic at or above the bifurcation of the sciatic nerve in the popliteal

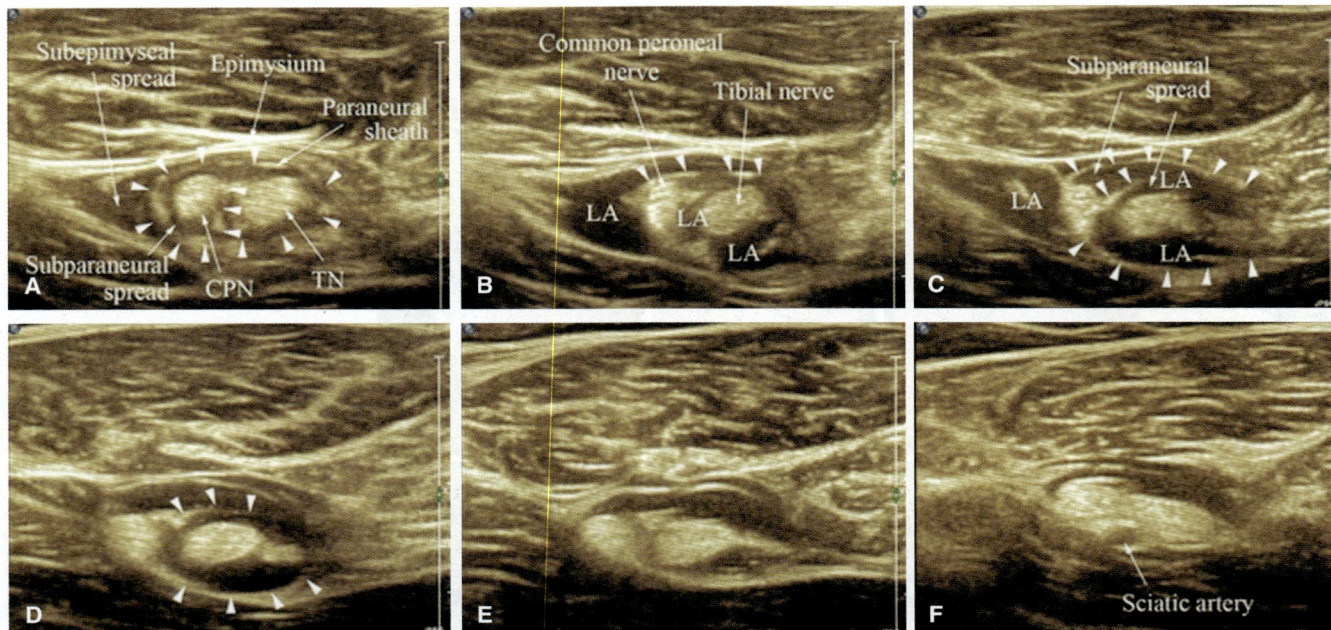

Figure 55-21 Sequence of transverse sonograms (distal to proximal) demonstrating the spread of the local anesthetic in both the subepimyseal and subparaneural compartments after an ultrasound-guided popliteal sciatic nerve block above its bifurcation. The paraneural sheath (*white arrow heads*) is interposed between the epimysium of the surrounding muscles and the outer surface (epineurium) of the sciatic nerve and its divisions. Note the extensive distal spread of the local anesthetic (LA), deep to the paraneural sheath, to encompass both the common peroneal (CPN) and tibial (TN) nerves. The individual paraneural sheath and subparaneural compartment of the CPN and TN are clearly delineated in **(C)**. Circumferential spread of the LA is also seen around the tibial nerve in **(D)**. (Reprinted with permission from Karmakar MK, Shariat AN, Pangthipampai P, et al. High-definition ultrasound imaging defines the paraneural sheath and the fascial compartment surrounding the sciatic nerve at the popliteal fossa. *Reg Anesth Pain Med*. 2013;38(5):447–451.

fossa has been shown to accelerate the onset time and increase the duration of sensory blockade.[126,127]

Truncal Blocks

Thoracic paravertebral block (TPB) can provide segmental analgesia for numerous surgical procedures including thoracotomy, mastectomy, nephrectomy, cholecystectomy and rib fractures, spinal surgery, and video-assisted thorascopic surgery, as well as inguinal and abdominal procedures. The paravertebral space (PVS) does not actually exist but is considered to be a potential space created by fluid distention of the tissues.[128] The PVS is defined anteriorly by the parietal pleura, posteriorly by the costotransverse ligament, superiorly by the occiput, inferiorly by the alar of the sacrum, and medially by the vertebral body, intervertebral disc, and the intervertebral foramen. Laterally, the PVS is contiguous with the intercostal space.[128] The PVS contains the anterior and posterior ramus of the spinal nerve root and the white and grey rami communicantes. Injection of local anesthetic into this potential space will therefore produce a dense sensory and sympathetic block resulting in unilateral segmental analgesia. Generally speaking, TBP is performed at the thoracic level. When performed in the lumbar region it is better known as a *psoas compartment block* and when performed at the cervical level it is referred to as a *deep cervical plexus block*.[128] TPB can be performed in the seated, prone, or lateral decubitus position. Although TPB has been performed using a blind percutaneous approach, the introduction of ultrasound guidance has improved the precision and decreased the complications associated with this procedure.

Different combinations of transducer positioning (transverse versus sagittal) and needle insertions (in-plane vs. out-of-plane) have resulted in the description of at least nine different ultrasound-guided approaches for TPB, the discussion of which is beyond the scope of this chapter.[129] Although the physician may have a preference for a specific transducer position it is recommended that a scout scan be performed utilizing both sagittal and transverse positioning prior to the performance of any block so important anatomic landmarks such as the pleura, superior costotransverse ligament (SCTL), and transverse process can be identified. The in-plane transverse technique (Fig. 55-22) is a tangential approach that inserts the needle in a lateral to medial direction that minimizes the risk of pleural puncture. However, there is a risk of epidural spread if the needle is advanced too close to the intervertebral foramen. The risk of epidural spread may be minimized by using an in-plane sagittal approach; however, this technique requires a steep insertion angle, which can make it difficult to image the tip of the needle.[129]

The advantages of TPB include lower postoperative VAS pain scores, a reduction in postoperative opioid consumption, and, therefore, less opioid-induced postoperative nausea and vomiting, less pain with movement, and shorter hospital stays. Continuous TPB compares favorably with thoracic epidurals for postthoracotomy analgesia. Continuous TPB provides analgesia that is equivalent to thoracic epidural blockade but without the side effects of hypotension, postoperative nausea and vomiting, and urinary retention[130] and may therefore be a reasonable alternative to a thoracic epidural catheter for postoperative analgesia.

Risks associated with the performance of TPB include pneumothorax, inadvertent entry of the block needle through the intervertebral foramen, epidural spread, and sympathetic blockade. Consequently, many practitioners may be uncomfortable performing this block and a reasonable alternative for chest

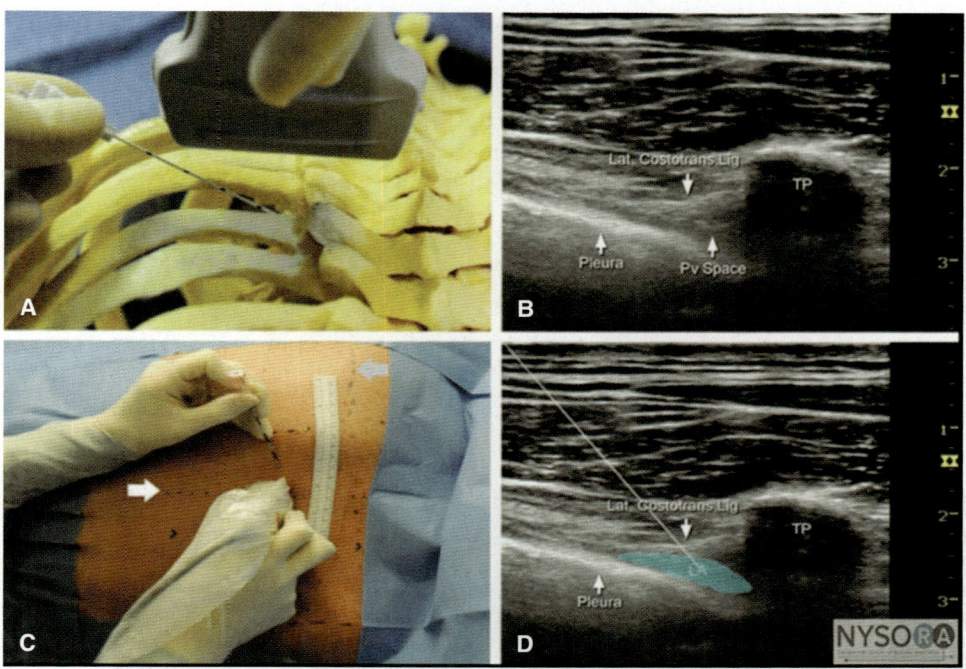

Figure 55-22 Ultrasound-guided thoracic paravertebral block. **A:** Transducer position and needle orientation. **B:** Corresponding ultrasound image. **C:** Patient is in oblique lateral position. >, spinous processes; gray arrow, left scapula; white arrow, paramedian line 3 cm (transverse processes). **D:** Needle insertion path and correct injection of local anesthetic. TP, transverse process. (Reprinted with permission from Vandepitte C, Pintaric TS, Gautier PE. Thoracic paravertebral block. NYSORA website. http://www.nysora.com/techniques/neuraxial-and-perineuraxial-techniques/ultrasound-guided/3277-thoracic-paravertebral-block.html. Published September 9, 2013.)

wall analgesia would be the less invasive *pectoral nerve block*. Pectoralis nerve blockade is an interfascial plane block, originally described by Blanco et al.[131] that deposits local anesthetic between the various muscle layers that consist of the pectoralis major, pectoralis minor, anterior serratus, and intercostal muscles. As part of a multimodal pain regimen pectoral nerve blockade has been demonstrated to significantly lower VAS pain scores and shorten the hospital stay for patients following modified radical mastectomy.[132] Ultrasound guidance has not only facilitated the performance of these blocks but also decreased the risk of inadvertent pneumothorax during execution of the block. All thoracic wall blocks are performed with the patient in the supine position with the arm abducted. The needle is inserted in-plane with the transducer in a medial-to-lateral direction.[131,133]

The *pectoralis I block* (PEC I) is indicated for any surgery on the pectoralis major muscle such as the insertion of breast expanders and subpectoral prosthesis. This block targets the lateral and median pectoral nerves within the fascial plane defined by the pectoralis major and pectoralis minor muscles at the level of the third rib. A total of 10 mL of local anesthetic is deposited at this level (Fig. 55-23).

The *pectoralis II block* (PEC II or modified PEC block) is indicated for more extensive chest wall surgery such as insertion of breast expanders and subpectoral prosthesis, tumorectomies, mastectomies, and sentinel node dissection. This block targets the lateral branches of the intercostal nerves that exit at the level of the mid-axillary line to innervate the breast and the skin from T2 to T6 as well as the long thoracic nerve. At the level of the third rib a total of 20 mL of local anesthetic is deposited between the serratus anterior muscle and either the pectoralis minor or the external intercostal muscle. This block is always combined with a PEC I block for extensive chest wall surgery such as mastectomy combined with placement of a tissue expander.

The *serratus plane block* is a relatively new block that is indicated for latissimus dorsi flap reconstruction and multiple rib fractures. The block is performed at the level of the fifth rib in the mid-axillary line and a total of 40 mL of local anesthetic is injected in the fascial plane defined by the latissimus dorsi and serratus anterior muscles.

The *transversus abdominis plane (TAP)* block is a volume-dependent compartmental field block that anesthetizes the anterior rami of the thoracolumbar spinal segmental nerves T7-L1 as they travel between the internal oblique (IO) and the transversus abdominis (TA) muscles. The TAP block provides both sensory and motor blockade of the abdominal wall and works best when postoperative pain is primarily of somatic and not visceral origin. This block can provide adequate postoperative analgesia in patients undergoing major abdominal surgery such as colorectal and renal transplant surgery, cesarean section, cholecystectomy, hysterectomy, inguinal herniorrhaphy, appendectomy, nephrectomy, bariatric surgery, gastrectomy, liver transplantation, and prostatectomy. Current evidence suggests that the TAP block is an essential component of multimodal analgesia, which can be opioid-sparing and is a reasonable alternative to epidural analgesia when placement of an epidural catheter is contraindicated.[134]

The TAP block was originally described in 2001 by Rafi[135] using a landmark method at the triangle of Petit (TOP), which is defined by the latissimus dorsi muscle posteriorly, the external oblique (EO) muscle anteriorly, and the iliac crest caudally. This is a blind approach that uses a "double-pop" technique to advance the needle into the appropriate fascial plane. Reliable identification of the TOP using the landmark approach can be difficult, particularly in the obese patient. Incorrect needle placement can result in positioning of the needle in the peritoneal cavity, which increases the risk of damage to visceral organs. The introduction of the ultrasound-guided TAP block has the advantage of real-time imaging of the EO, IO, and TA muscles with needle placement that can improve both the safety and efficacy of the TAP block when compared to the landmark technique. To date the three approaches that have been described in the literature include the lateral ("mid-axillary") approach, the "oblique subcostal" approach, and the posterior approach (aka the "quadratus lumborum" [QL] block) (Figs. 55-24 and 55-25).

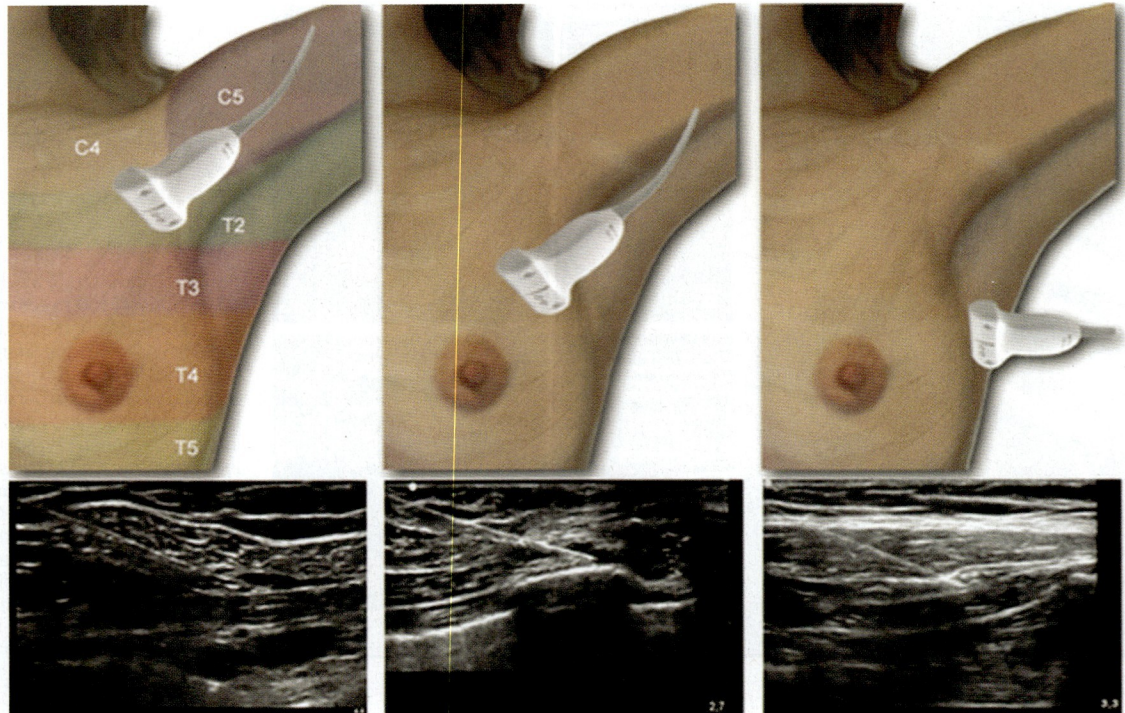

Figure 55-23. Graphic representing probe position and ultrasound image obtained during a Pecs I block (left), Pecs II block (middle) or a serratus plane block (right). (Reprinted with permission from Blanco R, Parras T, McDonnell JG, et al. Serratus plane block: a novel ultrasound-guided thoracic wall nerve block. *Anaesthesia.* 2013;68[11]:1107–1113.)

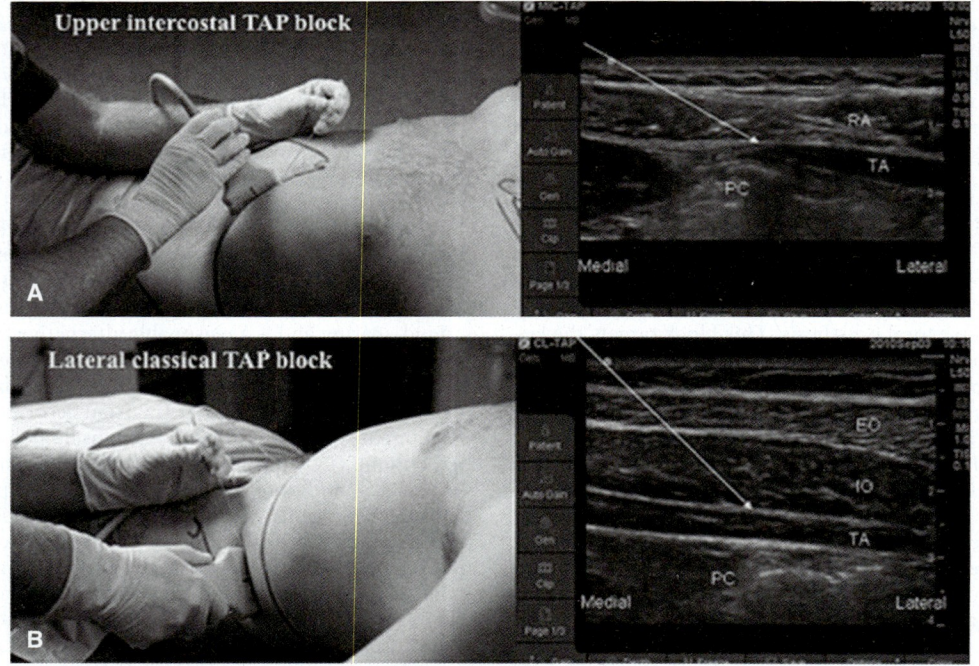

Figure 55-24 The bilateral dual (BD) TAP block. **A:** Upper intercostal TAP block. The needle is inserted above the rectus abdominis (RA) muscle and advanced in-plane to the transducer in a medial-to-lateral direction. The end point is beneath the RA and between the posterior rectus sheath and the transversus abdominis (TA) muscle. PC indicates peritoneal cavity; TAP, transversus abdominis plane. **B:** Lateral classic TAP block. The needle is inserted into the anterior axillary line beneath the thoracic cage and above the iliac crest. The needle is advanced in-plane to the transducer, and the end point is between the internal oblique (IO) and the transversus abdominis (TA) muscles. EO indicates external oblique muscle. (Reprinted with permission from Børglum J, Jensen K, Christensen AF, et al. Distribution patterns, dermatomal anesthesia, and ropivacaine serum concentration after bilateral dual TAP block. *Reg Anesth Pain Med.* 2012;37[3]: 294–301.)

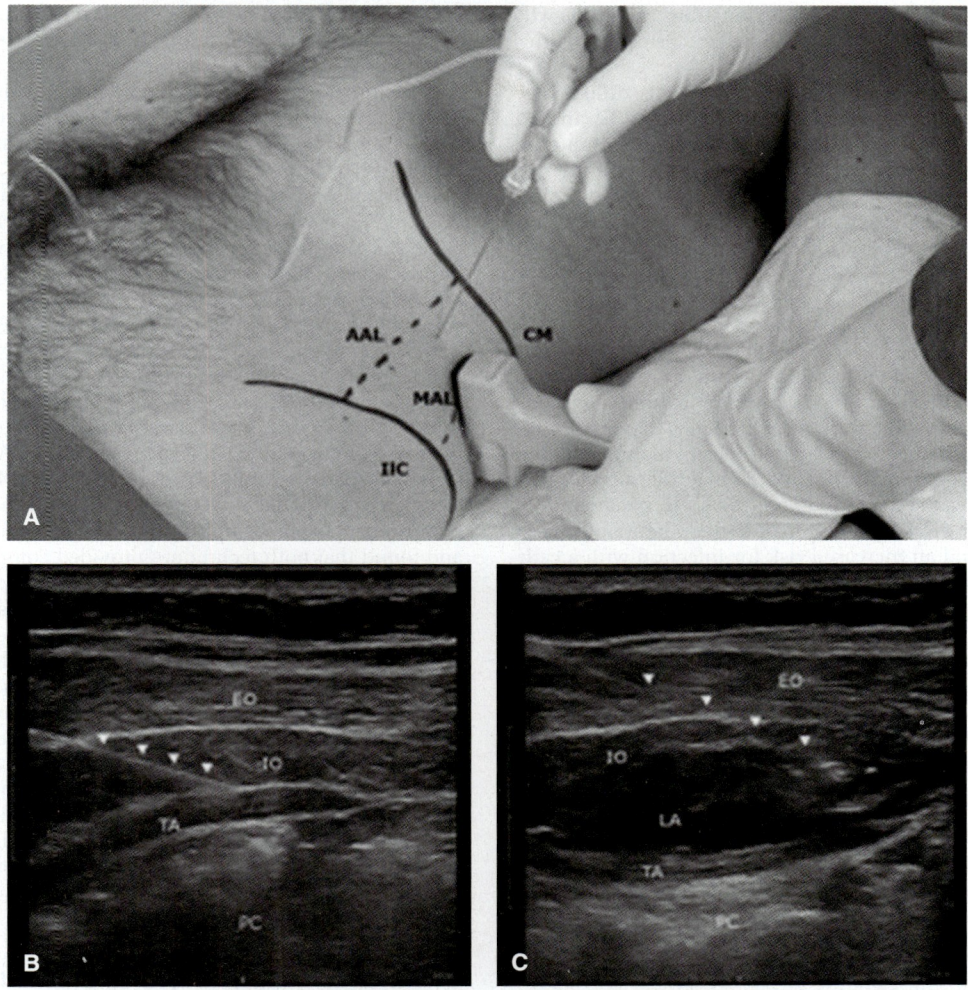

Figure 55-25 Photograph and ultrasonographic images demonstrating siting of the TAP block. **A:** Photograph of needle and transducer. **B:** Before injection of local anesthetic (LA). **C:** After injection of LA. The ultrasound transducer is placed in the transverse plane between the 12th rib or costal margin and the iliac crest. The end point of injection is 1 to 2 cm anterior to thoracolumbar fascia. The left side of the image is oriented medially, and the skin is at the top of the images. The needle is marked with *arrowheads*. PC indicates peritoneal cavity; CM, costal margin; IIC, iliac crest; AAL, anterior axillary line; MAL, medial axillary line; EO, external oblique; IO, internal oblique; TA, transversus abdominis. (Reprinted with permission from Støving K, Rothe C, Rosenstock CV, et al. Cutaneous sensory block area, muscle-relaxing effect, and block duration of the transversus abdominis plane block: a randomized, blinded, and placebo-controlled study in healthy volunteers. *Reg Anesth Pain Med*. 2015; 40[4]:355–362.)

Current recommendations suggest that the lateral TAP technique is well suited for infraumbilical (T10 to T12) incisions, and an oblique subcostal TAP for supraumbilical (T7 to T9) incisions. The role of the posterior TAP is unclear; however, it appears to provide better coverage of dermatomes[136] and more prolonged analgesia[137] compared to the lateral approach. Larger case series are recommended to better clarify the role of this novel block.

The *rectus sheath block* (RSB) is a regional anesthetic technique for use in adults to provide relaxation of the anterior abdominal wall during laparotomy. The RSB has been described in both adults and children and can provide effective postoperative analgesia for both umbilical and midline surgical incisions. The block is performed by depositing local anesthetic in the potential space between the rectus abdominis muscle and the posterior rectus sheath using an ultrasound-guided, in-plane, medial-to-lateral or lateral-to-medial approach. Complications associated with the block include intraperitoneal injection of local anesthetic, perforation of the bowel, and puncture of a mesenteric vessel.[134]

The *ilioinguinal/iliohypogastric* (II/IH) nerve block is indicated for analgesia following hernia repair in both adults and children and following orchidopexy and hydrocele repair in children. Both a landmark technique (two fascial "clicks") and a US-guided technique have been described; however, the US technique has been shown to be more reliable and potentially safer. Risks associated with this block include bowel puncture, bowel or pelvic hematoma, femoral nerve blockade, and elevated serum levels of local anesthetic. For the US-guided approach the patient is placed in the supine position and the anterior superior iliac spine (ASIS) is palpated. With a linear transducer positioned in the transverse plane with its lateral edge positioned at or above the ASIS the EO, IO, and TA muscles as well as the II and IH nerves and the deep circumflex iliac artery (DCIA) can be identified. Using an in-plane lateral-to-medial approach the block needle is carefully advanced into the neurovascular plane between the IO and TA muscles and with intermittent aspiration local anesthetic is carefully injected. Significant reduction of pain at rest and with mobilization has been demonstrated in adults who have received US-guided IL/IH nerve blockade prior to inguinal hernia repair.[138]

The *transversalis fascia plane* (TFP) block was designed to anesthetize the lateral cutaneous branches of the T12 and L1 nerves deep to the transversus abdominis muscle and anterior to the QL muscle. The block is indicated for patients undergoing iliac crest bone harvest, open appendectomy, and inguinal hernia repair. Complications, such as peritoneal puncture, are relatively rare because the peritoneum does not lie directly under the transversalis plane.[136]

Wound Infiltration

Recently, there has been an interest in continuous *intra-articular* and *periarticular* infiltration of local anesthetic with or without opioid for TKA. The advantage of the approach is that quadriceps strength can be maintained, thus facilitating ambulation and possibly earlier discharge from the hospital. A major disadvantage of this approach relates to reports of chondrolysis that may limit its usage. Other major disadvantages include the potential for large wound effusions and an increased risk for infection with a catheter in place. The *periarticular soft tissue injection* of local anesthetic combined with an NSAID (e.g., ropivacaine and ketorolac) combined with an intra-articular catheter for 24 hours has been described.[139] This technique appears to be safe and effective, and the risk of infection is minimized by removing the catheter on postoperative day 1.

Local infiltration analgesia (LIA) can be a useful technique for sustained reduction of perioperative pain following soft tissue and orthopedic surgeries. Multimodal analgesia that incorporates LIA is clearly superior to monotherapy-based regimens and has the advantage of being opioid sparing, and can reduce the number of opioid-related adverse events.[140] The efficacy of LIA has been compared to other popular modalities for perioperative analgesia following TKA with favorable results. A recent prospective, randomized, double-blind study compared LIA to intrathecal morphine in patients receiving a TKA and the authors concluded that LIA with ropivacaine provided better postoperative analgesia, earlier mobilization, and shorter hospital stay than intrathecal morphine.[141]

Both LIA and FNB demonstrate excellent perioperative analgesia following TKA; however, at the present time there is insufficient data supporting the superiority of one technique over the other.[103] Some orthopedic surgeons, however, prefer LIA because it is relatively easy and safe to perform intraoperatively and, unlike FNB, it has the advantage of preserving quadriceps strength, which can facilitate ambulation and potentially shorten the patients' hospital LOS. Direct infiltration of the wound with local anesthetic also has the potential advantage of decreasing inflammation and preventing central sensitization and ultimately neuropathic pain. The *periarticular* infiltration of a local anesthetic is technique dependent and requires careful administration of the drug into the posterior, inferior medial, superomedial, and superolateral capsules of the knee, as well as the periosteum, fascia, and subcuticular tissue.[142] Complications associated with LIA include systemic toxicity, infection, and wound dehiscence.

Although the perioperative administration of bupivacaine for acute perioperative pain control using LIA has proven to be quite efficacious, the duration of analgesia, unfortunately, is relatively short (<12 hours).[143] In an attempt to prolong the duration of analgesia a novel approach has been developed that encapsulates bupivacaine into microscopic lipid-based spherical particles (Depofoam). This *liposomal formulation of bupivacaine (Exparel)* is designed to release bupivacaine over a period of about 72 hours and in a recent efficacy analysis of 10 randomized, double-blind, single-dose wound infiltration studies, involving patients undergoing hernia repair, TKA, bunionectomy, breast augmentation, and hemorrhoidectomy, liposomal bupivacaine was shown to lower pain scores and reduce opioid consumption.[144]

Liposomal bupivacaine has been recommended as a superior alternative to bupivacaine HCl for LIA in TKA and in a recent phase II randomized dose-ranging study comparing various doses (133 mg, 266 mg, 399 mg, and 532 mg) of liposomal bupivacaine (Exparel) to bupivacaine HCl 150 mg, using LIA, liposomal bupivacaine (532 mg) was found to provide significantly greater analgesia for patients at rest.[140] Unfortunately, this dose of liposomal bupivacaine exceeds, by twofold, what is considered to be both safe and efficacious and is not FDA approved. Subsequently, a retrospective cohort study compared the periarticular injection of liposomal bupivacaine (266 mg) to the traditional periarticular injection of ropivacaine 400 mg (with morphine 5 mg and epinephrine 0.4 mg) for TKA and liposomal bupivacaine was found to provide pain control that was inferior to the less-expensive traditional periarticular injection.[142] Finally, a recent investigation compared liposomal bupivacaine (LIA) to single-injection FNB and found that both techniques provided comparable pain relief, and although the FNB group displayed greater postoperative knee flexion, the group that received LIA with liposomal bupivacaine demonstrated improved early ambulation and decreased LOS.[145]

Liposomal bupivacaine (Exparel) is intended for single-dose administration only and although the drug has been shown to be well tolerated at doses up to 532 mg, in five different surgical models, the maximum recommended dose, per the package insert, is 266 mg (20 mL). Combining liposomal bupivacaine with other drugs prior to administration is not recommended. The ideal multimodal, opioid-sparing, analgesic protocol following TKA has yet to be defined; however, it will more than likely consist of some combination of the aforementioned techniques. Further investigation is recommended to better define both the safety and efficacy of liposomal bupivacaine.

Continuous Peripheral Nerve Blockade Caveats

Interest in CPNB increased following the FDA warning in 1997 on the risk of spinal hematoma in patients who received epidural placement and low–molecular-weight heparin concurrently.[146] Although bleeding complications can be associated with the placement of CPNB catheters, the actual risks related to this technique are not well defined. Hemorrhagic complications, rather than neurologic deficits, appear to be the predominant risk associated with the performance of peripheral nerve blockade in the anticoagulated patient.[147] Major hemorrhage can occur following performance of psoas compartment blockade (e.g., LPB) and lumbar sympathetic blockade.[147] Special risk seems likely in any patient who may be anticoagulated perioperatively.[147]

Practice-based guidelines for the performance of *neuraxial techniques* in the anticoagulated patient are available online at the ASRA Web site at https://www.asra.com/advisory-guidelines. At the time of this publication, however, no consensus statement has been promulgated by the society outlining practice guidelines for the performance of *peripheral nerve blocks* in anticoagulated patients. Until guidelines are developed for the performance of peripheral nerve blockade in the anticoagulated patient, Horlocker et al.[147] recommend a conservative approach by adapting the guidelines set forth by ASRA (third edition) for the performance of neuraxial blockade, which they acknowledge may be overly restrictive. While work progresses on the Fourth Edition of the Practice Advisory, ASRA has developed a medical app that provides up to date, drug-specific guidelines, for antithrombotic and thrombolytic therapy use in the setting of regional anesthesia procedures. The app is available for your cell phone and can be downloaded from iTunes or Google Play.

Complications from Regional Anesthesia

The opinion of some that regional anesthesia is safer than general anesthesia may be based on the fact that regional anesthesia has been associated with reduced postoperative mortality secondary to thromboembolic phenomenon and myocardial infarction.[148,149] Nonetheless, data from the American Society of Anesthesiologists Closed Claims Project database suggests that the comparative safety of regional anesthesia in comparison to general anesthesia cannot be accurately determined. In a review of Closed Claims data, however, death is more common with claims involving general anesthesia and permanent-disabling and nondisabling temporary injuries are more often associated with regional anesthesia.[150] Serious complications associated with regional anesthesia include cardiac arrest, radiculopathy, cauda equina syndrome, and paraplegia. Fortunately, the incidence of severe anesthesia-related complications is rare (<0.1%); however, the incidence of cardiac arrest and neurologic complications is higher following spinal anesthesia than after all other types of regional procedures. The incidence of cardiac arrest following spinal anesthesia is 6.4 ± 1.2/10,000 versus 1.0 ± 0.4/10,000 for other forms of regional anesthesia. The incidence of neurologic injury after spinal anesthesia (6 ± 1/10,000 cases) is greater than all other regional techniques (e.g., epidural, peripheral nerve block, and intravenous regional anesthesia) combined (1.6 ± 0.5/10,000 cases).

Should a perioperative nerve injury occur, it is the responsibility of the physician to determine which combination of anesthetic, surgical, and patient risk factors are involved in any nerve injury and not assume a priori that the regional anesthetic is the reason. The risk factors for nerve injury are listed in Table 55-24. *Patient risk factors* for perioperative nerve injury may include any pre-existing systemic neuropathy (e.g., diabetes mellitus) or drug-induced neuropathy (e.g., vincristine or *cis*-platin).

Table 55-24 Risk Factors for Nerve Injury during the Performance of Regional Anesthesia

Variables	Risk Factors
Patient	Body habitus Pre-existing neurologic disorder (e.g., diabetes mellitus or patients who have received chemotherapy in the recent past) Male gender Advanced age
Surgical	Direct surgical trauma or stretch trauma Prolonged tourniquet time Hematoma Infection Tightly applied casts or surgical dressings Patient positioning
Regional anesthesia	Mechanical injury from the needle or catheter Chemical neurotoxicity from the local anesthetic Ischemic injury to the nerve

Table 55-25 Advantages of Ultrasound-guided Regional Anesthesia[152,196]

- Hastened block performance
- Fewer needle passes resulting in less patient discomfort and potentially a decreased risk of vascular puncture and hematoma formation in the anticoagulated patient
- Faster initial onset of the block
- Decreased dose of local anesthetic
- Preprocedural scanning can reveal anticipated as well as unanticipated structures such as hemodialysis catheters, ventriculoperitoneal shunts, vascular and neurologic anomalies

Risk factors for ulnar nerve injury include male sex, prolonged hospitalization, increasing age, extremes of body habitus, and diabetes. Diabetics, for example, has a decreased requirement for local anesthetic yet an increased risk for local anesthetic-induced nerve injury. This phenomenon has been described as the "double-crush" syndrome and proposes that axons injured at one site have an increased susceptibility to injury distally. Interestingly enough, in spite of this risk, regional anesthesia has been safely performed on patients with pre-existing ulnar neuropathy who underwent ulnar nerve transposition.[151]

Over the past quarter century ultrasound has become the preferred nerve localization technique that has truly transformed the practice of regional anesthesia. Direct visualization of the needle and the associated anatomic structures and real-time hydrodissection of local anesthetic around target nerves has been shown to hasten the onset of sensory and motor blockade, decrease performance time and the number of needle passes.[152] Although UGRA has not significantly reduced the incidence of postoperative neurologic symptoms, as compared to peripheral nerve stimulation technique, it has most definitely decreased the incidence of LAST and has had a meaningful impact on reducing the incidence of pneumothorax following supraclavicular nerve blockade.[152] Advantages associated with the use of UGRA are listed in Table 55-25. Relevant patient safety issues are listed in Table 55-26. See Chapters 22 (Local Anesthetics), 35 (Epidural and Spinal Anesthesia), and 36 (Peripheral Nerve Blockade)

Table 55-26 Ultrasound-guided Regional Anesthesia (UGRA) and Patient Safety[75,152]

1. Peripheral nerve injury
   1. The incidence of peripheral nerve injury with UGRA is similar to reports of nerve injury following the use of peripheral nerve stimulation (PNS).
2. Local anesthetic systemic toxicity
   1. Compared to PNS, UGRA decreases the risk of unintended vascular puncture but does not necessarily decrease the risk of local anesthetic toxicity.
3. Hemidiaphragmatic paresis (HDP)
   1. Low-volume UGRA of the brachial plexus can decrease the risk of HDP following an interscalene approach and almost eliminate it following a supraclavicular approach.
4. Pneumothorax (PTX)
   1. Because UGRA allows the anesthesiologist to directly visualize the pleura this should decrease the risk of PTX; however, PTX has been reported following the performance of UGRA.

for additional details on the reported complications of regional anesthesia.

Perioperative Pain Management of the Opioid-dependent Patient

Although this discussion focuses on the patient with chronic pain syndromes, these strategies for perioperative pain management are easily adaptable to other opioid-dependent populations. Chronic pain is defined as "pain without apparent biologic value that has persisted beyond the normal tissue healing time usually taken to be three months" (International Association for the Study of Pain) and "pain of a duration or intensity that adversely affects the function or well-being of the patient" (American Society of Anesthesiologists). Chronic pain is often associated with anxiety and depression, which may require treatment with various anxiolytics, antidepressants, anticonvulsants, antiarrhythmics, and skeletal muscle relaxants in addition to opioids. Symptoms unique to chronic pain include tight musculature, limited range of motion, and lack of energy, sleep disturbance, irritability, and social withdrawal. Associated psychiatric diagnoses may include hypochondriasis and psychosis.

Over the past decade, the percentage of patients with chronic pain for whom chronic opioids have been prescribed has increased dramatically. The United States has led the world in opioid prescribing for chronic pain. With only 4.6% of the world population the United States consumes 80% of the licit global supply of opioids.[153] The reason for this is twofold: (1) the more aggressive and compassionate treatment of chronic pain of malignant origin in cancer patients who are surviving longer and (2) to a much larger extent, the willingness of the medical community to treat pain of nonmalignant origin, such as osteoarthritis, with opioids.[154]

The goal of opioid therapy for chronic pain is improvement of pain, function, and quality of life. Unfortunately, recent evidence suggests that in spite of the increased use of opioids for chronic nonmalignant pain there have been no corresponding reductions in the rates of disability or improvements in health status.[155] Unacceptable opioid side effects and concerns about adverse hormonal effects and immune modulation from long-term exposure can cause patients to abandon therapy. Finally, long-term opioid use results in physical dependence, the potential for withdrawal symptoms on abrupt discontinuation of the opioid, and the development of OIH and tolerance. The U.S. FDA defines opioid tolerance as the use of the oral morphine equivalent of greater than or equal to 60 mg a day for 7 days or longer.[156] Recent evidence suggests that the opioid-tolerant patient can potentially have a complicated hospital course resulting in an increased LOS and high readmission rate.[156] A multimodal approach to pain management is highly recommended.

Physical dependence is a "physiologic state of adaptation to a specific psychoactive substance characterized by the emergence of a *withdrawal syndrome* during abstinence, which may be relieved in total or in part by re-administration of the substance." Opioid *withdrawal* is characterized by an increased sympathetic and parasympathetic response that results in hypertension, tachycardia, diaphoresis, abdominal cramping, and diarrhea. *Tolerance* is a rightward shift of the dose–response curve and by definition is "a state in which an increased dosage of a psychoactive substance is needed to produce a desired effect." Escalating doses of opioid may also be explained by an underlying progression of the disease state or by the development of OIH. Tolerance can be innate or acquired. Innate tolerance is a genetically predetermined sensitivity to a drug, whereas acquired tolerance can have a pharmacokinetic, learned, or pharmacodynamic basis. Pharmacokinetic tolerance involves a diminution in the effects of a drug because of changes in distribution and metabolism usually secondary to enzyme induction of the CYP450 system, which results in accelerated metabolism. Learned tolerance refers to compensatory behavior that masks intoxication. Pharmacodynamic tolerance refers to neuroadaptive changes that occur following chronic exposure to opioids, which may involve receptor desensitization secondary to receptor downregulation, internalization, and uncoupling of opioid receptors from G proteins. Opioids exhibit *cross-tolerance* to each other but the degree of cross-tolerance varies widely and is often incomplete.[157] Clinicians use incomplete cross-tolerance to their advantage to restore analgesic sensitivity in highly tolerant patients through opioid rotation.[157] Because cross-tolerance is incomplete, analgesia is restored with the new opioid at more than 50% below the predicted equianalgesic dose.[157] It must be stressed that the development of tolerance or physical dependence in no way implies that the patient is addicted to an opioid. *Addiction* is a biopsychosocial disease characterized by dysfunctional behavior that involves craving, compulsive use, loss of control, and the continued use of a drug in spite of adverse consequences. Finally, addiction should not be confused with *pseudoaddiction*, which, by definition, describes the patient who has behavioral features of addiction secondary to undertreatment of the pain syndrome. Pseudoaddiction is usually diagnosed retrospectively because once the dose of opioid is increased, pain resolves and aberrant behavior abates.

The onus for the identification of the opioid-dependent patient rests with the patient's surgical team, preoperative evaluation staff, and the anesthesia team.[158] Ideally the patient and the health-care teams will formulate a perioperative pain management plan prior to surgery, and the chronic pain service, if available, should be consulted. Often, however, the opioid-dependent patient is identified just moments prior to surgery and the anesthesia team needs to be innovative. The ideal perioperative pain management strategy, in the opioid-dependent patient, will involve a multimodal approach that employs regional analgesia techniques (neuraxial or peripheral nerve blockade) in conjunction with systemic nonopioid medications. Opioids, however, remain the mainstay of perioperative pain management, and an adequate dose of opioid needs to be maintained to avoid precipitating withdrawal symptoms (Table 55-27).

Preoperative management of the patient involves determining the patient's "baseline" opioid requirement, and on the day of surgery the patient should be instructed to take their normal opioid dose. If for some reason the patient neglects to take the opioid on the day of surgery, the anesthesiologist can administer an equivalent dose preoperatively. The opioid-dependent patient has increased opioid requirements, which are reported to be 30% to 100% greater than an opioid-naive patient[154]; therefore, during the preinduction period, the dose of fentanyl, morphine, or hydromorphone should be increased accordingly. Patients prescribed transdermal fentanyl patches are usually instructed to maintain their fentanyl patch into the operating room and this can serve as their baseline opioid requirement. Occasionally, however, in the case of major surgery, in which the risk of major blood loss or sepsis is significant, patients may be instructed to discontinue their transdermal patch, and an intravenous fentanyl infusion can be initiated to maintain adequate plasma concentrations. Patients maintained on methadone should continue their baseline dose throughout the perioperative period. In the United States, methadone is available for both oral and intravenous administration. The reader is reminded that patients receiving more than 200 mg of methadone per day can develop a prolonged QT interval, which places them at risk for

> **Table 55-27** Suggested Guidelines for Perioperative Pain Management in the Opioid-tolerant Patient
>
> **Preoperative**
> 1. Evaluation: Evaluation should include early recognition and high index of suspicion.
> 2. Identification: Identify factors such as total opioid dose requirement and previous surgery/trauma resulting in undermedication, inadequate analgesia, or relapse episodes.
> 3. Consultation: Meet with addiction specialists and pain specialists with regard to perioperative planning.
> 4. Reassurance: Discuss patient concerns related to pain control, anxiety, and risk of relapse.
> 5. Medication: Calculate opioid dose requirement and modes of administration; provide anxiolytics or other medications as clinically indicated.
>
> **Intraoperative**
> 1. Maintain baseline opioids (oral, transdermal, intravenous).
> 2. Increase intraoperative and postoperative opioid dose to compensate for tolerance.
> 3. Provide peripheral neural or plexus blockade; consider neuraxial analgesic techniques when clinically indicated.
> 4. Use nonopioids as analgesic adjuncts.
>
> **Postoperative**
> 1. Plan preoperatively for postoperative analgesia; formulate primary strategy as well as suitable alternatives.
> 2. Maintain baseline opioids.
> 3. Use multimodal analgesic techniques.
> 4. Patient-controlled analgesia: Use as primary therapy or as supplementation for epidural or regional techniques.
> 5. Continue neuraxial opioids: Intrathecal or epidural analgesia.
> 6. Maintain continuous neural blockade.
>
> **After Discharge**
> 1. If surgery provides complete pain relief, opioids should be slowly tapered, rather than abruptly discontinued.
> 2. Develop a pain management plan before hospital discharge. Provide adequate doses of opioid and nonopioid analgesics.
> 3. Arrange for a timely outpatient pain clinic follow-up or a visit with the patient's addictionologist.
>
> Data from Mitra S, Sinatra RS. Perioperative management of acute pain in the opioid-dependent patient. *Anesthesiology.* 2004;101:212.

Torsades de pointe. It is therefore recommended that a baseline electrocardiogram be obtained for comparison. Patients who are maintained on the partial opioid agonist buprenorphine may continue to receive the drug for postoperative pain control, and morphine, hydromorphone, or fentanyl may be administered to supplement analgesia if required.[159] Full antagonists (e.g., naloxone and naltrexone) and the partial agonists–antagonists (e.g., nalbuphine, pentazocine, and butorphanol) should be avoided because they will precipitate withdrawal symptoms in opioid-dependent patients.

Because it is well documented that the use of systemic non-opioid analgesics are opioid sparing in the opioid-naive patient it is reasonable to apply this experience to the opioid-tolerant patient. Drugs that should be part and parcel of any multimodal protocol for the perioperative care of the opioid-tolerant patient should include some combination of gabapentin or pregabalin, an NSAID or selective cyclooxygenase (COX-2) inhibitor, acetaminophen, dexamethasone, an NMDA receptor antagonist, α_2-receptor agonists, lidocaine, and magnesium.

Both *gabapentin* and *pregabalin* bind to the α-2δ subunit of voltage-gated P/Q-type calcium channels in the dorsal horn of the spinal cord and, by modulating the release of excitatory neurotransmitters from activated nociceptors, these drugs are believed to inhibit pain transmission and central sensitization.[49] They are both recommended for the treatment of perioperative pain in the opioid-tolerant patient.[62] Although gabapentin and pregabalin have similar mechanisms of action, pregabalin may be the preferred drug because of superior bioavailability and better diffusion into the central nervous system.[62]

The *NSAIDs* (e.g., ibuprofen and naproxen) have displayed proven efficacy for the treatment of postoperative pain and their opioid-sparing effect accounts for a significant reduction in opioid-related side effects, especially postoperative nausea and vomiting. Likewise, the analgesic effects of the *selective COX-2 inhibitors* are analogous to the NSAIDs. The recommended dose of celecoxib that reduces both postoperative pain and decreases opioid requirement is 400 mg orally 2 hours prior to surgery.[62,160]

Acetaminophen is an effective adjuvant in the treatment of postoperative pain, has an opioid-sparing effect, and decreases postoperative nausea and vomiting. The mechanism of action of the drug is elusive but is thought to involve inhibition of the COX enzyme via interaction at the peroxidase site, modulation of the descending inhibitory serotoninergic pathways, and opioid agonist effects. There is also evidence that the drug interacts with the endocannabinoid system, TRPV$_1$, and NMDA receptors,[161] which may make this drug particularly efficacious in the opioid-tolerant patient; however, more research into this intriguing area is warranted. The drug may be administered orally or intravenously; however, the intravenous route offers the advantage of earlier and higher peak plasma levels compared to oral acetaminophen, resulting in superior cerebrospinal fluid levels. The recommended adult dose in patients above 50 kg is 1,000 mg intravenously q 6 hours. The first dose may be administered just prior to surgery and continued postoperatively for as long as the patient is non per os (npo). In a single systematic qualitative review of 21 trials,[39] the authors conclude that the combination of an NSAID with acetaminophen demonstrates analgesia that is superior to either drug alone. Finally, dexamethasone may be beneficial, in the opioid-dependent patient, secondary to decreased neurotransmitter release and decreased production of the NMDA receptor antagonist kynurenic acid.[62] Although the recommended preoperative intravenous dose is 0.11 to 0.2 mg/kg[61] doses as high as 0.2 mg/kg have been administered as part of a multimodal analgesic strategy.[62] Future research strategies should focus on procedure-specific analgesic drug combinations, which can be specifically tailored to the patient that will provide optimal pain relief while minimizing side effects.

Intraoperative management of the opioid-dependent patient requires the prudent use of fentanyl, morphine, or hydromorphone in order to provide effective intraoperative anesthesia, postoperative analgesia, and to prevent opioid withdrawal. This requires the administration of the patients' baseline opioid requirement plus their intraoperative requirements secondary to surgical stimulation. Exact opioid dosing guidelines do not exist but because of receptor downregulation secondary to chronic opioid administration, opioid doses may need to be increased 30% to 100% vis-à-vis the opioid-naive patient. Because of receptor downregulation an alternative opioid may be useful in this setting. Opioid rotation takes advantage of the fact that the new opioid will bind a different opioid receptor subtype and be metabolized differently. Following the cancer pain model, the dose of the new opioid is less than 50% of the calculated equianalgesic dose because of incomplete cross-tolerance.[157] Although the alternative opioid may be administered for several days postoperatively, prudence dictates that a physician or pharmacist well versed in pain management convert the patient to the appropriate oral opioid regimen for discharge from the hospital.

The optimal intraoperative dose of opioid varies considerably from patient to patient; therefore, monitoring intraoperative vital signs such as heart rate, pupil size, and respiratory rate can be useful and allows the clinician to avoid the negative consequences of overdosing or underdosing the patient with opioid. Reversing neuromuscular blockade toward the end of a general anesthetic and allowing the patient to breathe spontaneously can be a prudent technique. Patients with a respiratory rate greater than 20 breaths per minute and significantly dilated pupils require additional opioid. Titrating fentanyl, morphine, or hydromorphone to a respiratory rate of 12 to 14 breaths per minute and a moderately miotic pupil is recommended. It is also recommended that patients who are receiving chronic methadone therapy may receive an additional intraoperative dose of 0.1 mg/kg intravenously, which can be titrated to hemodynamic effect and pupillary response.

Activation of the NMDA receptor by the second messenger protein kinase C (PKC) is reported to play a critical role in the development of opioid tolerance.[62] Inhibition of the NMDA receptor with the NMDA receptor antagonist ketamine can be a useful strategy in this patient population because it is reported to be effective at reversing morphine tolerance and restoring its effectiveness as an analgesic.[154] The recommended intraoperative dose of ketamine for the opioid-tolerant patient is 0.5 mg/kg as a bolus dose at the beginning of the case, followed by 10 µg/kg/min as an infusion for the duration of the case.[162] Low-dose ketamine may be continued into the postoperative period for up to 48 hours without any serious complications.

The α_2-adrenoreceptor agonists (e.g., dexmedetomidine and clonidine) have moderate analgesic effects and opioid-sparing effects in the opioid-naive patient. In the perioperative setting, they are sedating and anxiolytic and can decrease the stress response to surgery and postoperatively mitigate shivering, nausea and vomiting, and agitation. It is unclear at this time, however, what role, if any, this drug class would have specifically in the perioperative management of the opioid-tolerant patient, but they may be particularly valuable in the treatment of the opioid-tolerant patient because they attenuate opioid withdrawal symptoms and can reduce postoperative opioid requirements and pain.[158,163]

Intravenous lidocaine has been gaining acceptance as a drug that may be useful in a multimodal approach to perioperative pain management, particularly in the patient receiving abdominal surgery or in the patient in whom regional anesthesia is contraindicated. Systemic lidocaine displays analgesic, anti-inflammatory, and anti-hyperalgesic properties, which are mediated by inhibition of voltage-dependent sodium channels, NMDA receptors, and G protein–coupled receptors (GPCRs). Indirect blockade of the NMDA receptor through inhibition of PKC potentially makes this a useful drug in the opioid-tolerant patient.[164]

Like ketamine, intravenous magnesium is an NMDA receptor antagonist that can suppress neuropathic pain, potentiate morphine analgesia, attenuate morphine tolerance,[57] and has the ability to abolish the development of hyperalgesia and central sensitization,[165] which suggests that this drug would be particularly effective in the treatment of acute perioperative pain in the opioid-tolerant patient.[166] Because magnesium and ketamine bind to different sites on the NMDA receptor it has been posited that the combination of the two drugs may enhance analgesia through a "super-additive effect."[167] Future studies should focus on the ideal dosing regimen that maximizes analgesia while decreasing drug-related side effects.

Postoperative management of the opioid-dependent patient can be very challenging. Ideally, the optimal amount of opioid has been administered to the patient during the intraoperative period, allowing them to emerge from anesthesia comfortably sedated and pain-free. On arrival to the recovery room, intravenous opioids may be administered on an "as-needed" basis; however, initiation of an intravenous PCA opioid with both a basal and an incremental (bolus) dose will minimize the risk of breakthrough pain. The recommended basal infusion should equate to the patient's hourly preoperative oral opioid dose requirement as this will avoid precipitating withdrawal symptoms, and the bolus dose, as calculated from the background infusion, is the 1-hour dose of the background infusion. For example, a patient taking 90 mg of oral morphine per day equates to 30 mg of intravenous morphine per day, which can be administered as a basal morphine in fusion of 1.25 mg/hr. The bolus dose would be equivalent to 1.25 mg with a lockout interval of 6 to 10 minutes. Basal infusions are not required for patients who are maintained on their transdermal fentanyl patches as these provide adequate basal analgesia. Therefore, a fentanyl PCA with a bolus dose and an appropriate lockout interval is all that is required. Patients recovering from same-day surgery will be initially treated with intravenous doses of opioids in the recovery room; however, they can be quickly transitioned to an oral regimen consisting of their baseline opioid requirement plus an appropriate amount of short-acting opioid for breakthrough pain consistent with the invasiveness of the surgery.

Nonopioid coanalgesics are opioid-sparing and should be part and parcel of any multimodal perioperative pain management strategy in the opioid-dependent patient. Low-dose intravenous ketamine may be continued into the postoperative period; however, specific dosing recommendations are not available at this time. Please refer to the section on NMDA receptor antagonists for dosing guidelines. In a single case report, however, which involved an opioid-dependent trauma patient, ketamine was administered, postoperatively, at a starting dose of 10 µg/kg/min and then gradually tapered to 2.5 µg/kg/min over 45 minutes. This particular regimen provided significant pain control and was opioid sparing. The ketamine infusion was continued for 7 days without any adverse sequelae.[168]

The combination of both acetaminophen and a selective COX-2 inhibitor provides superior analgesia and is opioid-sparing. The administration of dexmedetomidine may also be particularly beneficial in the perioperative pain management of these patients. Likewise, the gabapentinoids, gabapentin, and pregabalin, display antihyperalgesic properties, have opioid-sparing effects in the opioid-naive patient, reduce OIH, and have been shown to reduce the incidence of postsurgical pain. The evidence suggests that it would be prudent to administer a gabapentinoid postoperatively for 10 to 14 days. Although both gabapentin and pregabalin are indicated, pregabalin is the preferred drug because of its superior pharmacokinetic profile. The recommended dosing regimen of pregabalin following TKA that reduces chronic pain is 300 mg 1 hour prior to surgery and for 14 days thereafter as a tapering regimen (150 to 50 mg twice daily).[169]

Regional anesthesia is highly recommended in this patient population. Peripheral nerve blockade as a single-injection technique or as a continuous catheter can be very useful. Likewise, if indicated, epidural analgesia should be part and parcel of the multimodal pain regimen for these patients. During the perioperative period, however, the epidural and systemic requirements for morphine have been reported to increase three to fourfold. Epidural infusions that have been recommended include a combination of fentanyl (2 to 5 µg/mL), morphine (0.1 to 0.2 mg/mL), or hydromorphone (0.02 to 0.04 mg/mL) combined with a local anesthetic such as bupivacaine (0.05% to 0.2%) or ropivacaine (0.1% to 0.2%). Switching to an opioid with high intrinsic efficacy may be useful. A combination of sufentanil (2 µg/mL) with 0.1% bupivacaine has been shown to be quite efficacious in an opioid-tolerant patient refractory to the analgesic effects of epidural morphine. The neuraxial administration of opioid is usually a very small fraction of the patient's baseline opioid requirement. Notwithstanding the fact that patients obtain excellent analgesia from the epidural, opioid serum levels and supraspinal receptor binding may not be totally adequate at preventing opioid withdrawal symptoms. It may therefore be necessary for the patient to receive at least part of their baseline opioid dose either orally or intravenously (PCA) to prevent opioid withdrawal symptoms. A physician well versed in chronic pain management and comfortable in the equianalgesic dosing of opioids via different routes of administration should ideally be involved in the care of the patient. Careful monitoring of the patient for excessive sedation or respiratory depression is mandatory, and caregivers in the recovery room and on the postsurgical units should be alerted to the potential risk for respiratory depression when parenteral and neuraxial opioids are combined.

Organization of Perioperative Pain Management Services

There is a growing recognition in the health-care industry that the undertreatment of pain is a widespread problem that cuts across all phases of patient care. The effective management of pain is a crucial component of good perioperative care and recovery from surgery. Unrelieved pain and inadequate pain relief have detrimental physiologic and psychological effects on patients by slowing recovery and creating burdens for patients and their families, and by increasing costs to the health-care system. Although the acute postoperative pain service plays an integral role in the pain management of the surgical patients, there are considerable barriers that challenge the establishment and/or effectiveness of acute pain teams in managing patients across the continuum of care. There is good evidence that the overall incidence of moderate-to-severe pain in surgical patients is about 25% to 40% despite the availability of pain treatment.[170] A major obstacle to the establishment of postoperative pain services is its cost in a privatized health system wherein limited reimbursement for postoperative care discourages the establishment of a service. The value of an acute pain service, apart from its benefit for patient care, also comes from the added value of reducing hospital costs by improving surgical outcome and by facilitating patient recovery and early discharge.[171] While providing direct patient care along previous lines such as the management of continuous epidural and regional catheter infusions and other modalities, the perioperative pain management service must also play a leading role in patient education and the education of other physicians, nurses, and caregivers to ensure their competence in effectively assessing, managing, and meeting a patient's needs. The success of a perioperative pain management team can be established not only in the context of the direct patient care that the team provides but also through its role in educating other health-care professionals and services as physician leaders responsible for setting clinical standards and practice guidelines in the health-care system.

The key components to establishing a successful perioperative pain management service begins with an institutional commitment to support the service. The team must be built around a physician leader with training and experience in pain medicine. There must be other anesthesiologists available to support the service. The institution must support the service, which may be manifest through support of a nurse coordinator or the availability of a pharmacist to consult on the many pharmaceutical issues that arise in patients on preoperative medications that may conflict with the perioperative pain management plan. The perioperative pain management chief is responsible for the development and implementation of clinical pathways and protocols that effectively enhance recovery following surgery. These protocols must include pain assessment tools that are adopted across the continuum of care by all caregivers.

Although it is convenient to regard postoperative pain primarily as acute pain caused by tissue injury associated with surgery, this may exclude other important factors that contribute to a patient's suffering following surgery. Acute postsurgical pain can also be caused by prolonged patient positioning or pressure effects from prolonged immobility. Many patients presenting for elective surgery may also suffer chronic pain from underlying illness or injury (e.g., degenerative diseases or malignancy) that may contribute significantly to the intensity of the postoperative pain experienced by the patient. Postoperative pain remains a substantial problem that is often masked by a patient's acceptance of pain as a natural consequence of surgery. Other common patient barriers include cultural and language barriers, stoicism and/or opiophobia, and personal experience or the experiences of friends and relatives. For these reasons, postoperative pain management begins preoperatively with patient education to alleviate the attendant anxiety, apprehension, and fear of surgery, to understand the patient's fears and concerns, and to come to an agreement with the patient that pain control is an expected goal of care. Education is also the key to changing attitudes of other caregivers to more effectively treat their patient's pain. In developing a perioperative pain service it is important to bear in mind that the importance of effective perioperative pain management extends well beyond the mere establishment of dedicated personnel; it must also encompass a leadership role in transforming the institutional culture to elevate the relief of pain and suffering to its place as a primary goal of patient care.[172]

Special Considerations in the Perioperative Pain Management of Children

Acute pain management in children undergoing surgery or invasive procedures offers several specific and unique challenges for the anesthesiologist. The challenges include the importance of support from the childs' parents and siblings, preoperative fear and anxiety in the child, developmental and communication issues, difficulties in evaluating pain and the effectiveness of treatment, and the child's reaction to pain, surgery, and the environment, including crying and resistance to care. These problems all summate to emphasize the importance of a holistic approach to pain management that focuses on family-centered care wherein significant efforts are made to reduce preoperative stress and anxiety and to engage the parents in gaining the cooperation of the child.[173] There is also good evidence that the level of preoperative anxiety and stress adversely impacts postoperative pain and recovery from surgery. A number of methods can be used to reduce preoperative anxiety in children. They include preoperative parental education and counseling about the operative experience,[174] distraction techniques including videos and music, handheld video games, game-playing with the support of the family and/or child life specialists, and parental presence coupled with oral midazolam (0.5 mg/kg) administration to ease anxiety associated with the transition to the induction of anesthesia. As parental behavior and attitudes can be major determinants of a child's behavior during the inhalational induction of anesthesia, the anesthesiologist is obliged to counsel and inform parents as to the importance of modulating their fear and anxiety should they want to be present during anesthetic induction.

Effective pain management in the postoperative period depends on effective assessment and the precision of the evaluation tools used to measure pain intensity.[175] A child's responses to pain may be variable and unpredictable because of their age and development, verbal communication skills, fear and anxiety, withdrawal, prior experiences, parental presence or absence, and the parent's reactions to the care.[176] A comprehensive approach to assessment that employs multiple assessment tools including behavioral responses offers the best option for success. The use of visual analogue "faces" pain scales referenced to the appropriate cultural identity of the patient can be useful in assessing postoperative pain severity. There is some question as to the value of parental or practitioner evaluation of a child's pain intensity relative to the visual analogue scale, but parents can play a key role in the assessment and management of their child's pain in the postoperative period, particularly when their child is reluctant to communicate or suffers from a cognitive disorder.[177]

Nonparenteral Analgesics

Nonopioid Analgesics

The use of nonopioid analgesics administered orally or by rectal suppository are important adjuvant analgesic therapies under a wide variety of circumstances. The release of intravenous acetaminophen (Ofirmev) in November 2011 has progressively replaced nonparenteral administration of acetaminophen in pediatric perioperative practice. See Table 55-13 for dosing guidelines in children. Intravenous acetaminophen can be used across a wide spectrum of surgical procedures and may be sufficient for outpatient procedures. Nonparenteral administration of acetaminophen either by oral administration (10 to 20 mg/kg) or by rectal suppository (20 to 40 mg/kg) after induction of anesthesia remains an acceptable alternative to parenteral administration. Although the short-term use of the NSAIDs (e.g., ibuprofen and ketorolac) are equipotent with acetaminophen and can be used with safety, the overall convenience and fewer side effects of acetaminophen have favored its use in children. Oral clonidine (4 µg/kg) given as a preoperative medication has also been used with good effect for sedation and postoperative pain management in children undergoing adenotonsillectomy. The greater degree of postoperative sedation with clonidine relative to other analgesics may limit its universal acceptance.

Opioid Analgesics

Codeine in combination with acetaminophen is commonly used with good effect for the management of moderate postoperative pain in the ambulatory patient.[178] Unfortunately, deaths have occurred post-operatively in children with obstructive sleep apnea who received codeine for pain control following tonsillectomy or adenoidectomy. Codeine is metabolized to morphine by the hepatic enzyme, CYP2D6, and ultra-rapid metabolizers of codeine appear to be at increased risk for unanticipated respiratory depression secondary to potentially fatal amounts of morphine in the body. Consequently, the FDA (Food and Drug Administration), has advised against the use of codeine in children and infants until additional clinical research can be performed to develop safer alternatives. The atypical opioid tramadol (3 mg/kg) has also been used as an oral preparation, usually in combination with midazolam (0.5 mg/kg) prior to the induction of anesthesia in children undergoing adenotonsillectomy. Oral tramadol can also be used for postoperative analgesia in children undergoing oral or dental procedures.[179] Intranasal sufentanil (0.2 µg/k) can also be used to manage preoperative anxiety and postoperative analgesia in children and may be more effective than oral tramadol.[179]

Patient-controlled Analgesia

PCA is established as an important postoperative pain management tool in adults and is increasingly used in older children to good effect.[180,181] There are safety concerns with the use of PCA in children that mandate a high level of surveillance with respect to the functioning of the equipment and careful patient monitoring that may be a limitation to its use in infants. PCA by proxy is a safety risk as there is no complete assurance that parents will be competent in assessing the intensity of their child's pain or be able to regulate the bolus dosages in order to avoid opioid overdosage.[182]

Epidural Neuraxial Analgesia

The use of epidural neuraxial analgesia either as a single-shot technique or as a continuous catheter technique has become a key component of the perioperative pain management plan for infants and young children undergoing abdominal, urologic, or orthopedic procedures.[183] The use of a single-shot "kiddy" caudal using a local anesthetic with morphine is effective in relieving pain associated with minor procedures in the outpatient setting. Although the overall morbidity is low, there is serious risk associated with epidural analgesia in children related to the systemic toxicity of the local anesthetic and the need to place the epidural under general anesthesia. The risk of irreversible cardiac toxicity, although primarily associated with the use of bupivacaine, can also occur with the ropivacaine and levobupivacaine at an incidence of about 30% to 50% relative to bupivacaine. The risks are increased in children with hepatic dysfunction or when large volumes of local anesthetic are injected into the epidural space through a small, sharp, immobile needle. In the rare event that cardiac toxicity occurs, the anesthesiologist must be prepared to initiate chest compressions and lung ventilation to minimize the risk of anoxic injury and immediately start an intravenous bolus infusion of 20% intralipid (1 to 2 mL/kg) followed by a continuous infusion (0.25 to 0.5 mL/kg/min) until normal cardiac rhythm and the circulation is restored.[184] Although the use of lipid emulsions can be successful in reversing cardiac arrest, their immediate availability does not excuse the anesthesiologist from taking all precautions to prevent systemic injection or absorption when performing the procedure.

Peripheral Nerve Blocks in Children

The introduction of small stimulating needles and ultrasound imaging along with long-acting local anesthetics and continuous catheter techniques in selected cases has resulted in an increase in the use of peripheral nerve blocks in children undergoing orthopedic extremity procedures.[185] The use of stimulating needles permits the anesthesiologist to place the injection after the child is anesthetized.[186] Because the child is unresponsive, it is important that the initial injection meets no resistance in order to avoid intraneural injection. Combined ilioinguinal and iliohypogastric nerve blocks performed under ultrasound guidance to reduce the volume of the injection have gained increasing interest for effective pain management in children undergoing inguinal herniorrhaphy.[187]

Conclusion

In October 2000, the U.S. Congress designated the decade beginning January 1, 2001, as the Decade of Pain Control and Research. The onus is on dedicated health-care professionals to provide our patients with the best care possible when it comes to pain and suffering, which applies directly to the perioperative state. Accomplishing this requires integration of information and systems from disparate disciplines within medicine. It challenges physicians to acquire a patient-focused perspective that provides the patient with a pleasant perioperative experience and enhanced recovery following surgery. In doing so, clinicians will be challenged to construct systems within hospitals to support such endeavors but will be able to show objective and meaningful outcomes with positive benefits to patients and to health-care organizations. The cost of ignoring pain and suffering has been widely cited to be in the billions of dollars each, but the cost in suffering is immeasurable. Anesthesiology has led the way in improving the overall pain care of the surgical patient and is positioned to lead medicine into a new era in which perioperative pain management is better, safer, more assured, and consistently available at the highest levels to all.

REFERENCES

1. United States Agency for Health Care Policy and Research. *Acute pain management operative or medical procedures and trauma.* Rockville, MD: U.S. Dept. of Health and Human Services Public Health Service Agency for Health Care Policy and Research; 1992.
2. American Society of Anesthesiologists Task Force on Acute Pain Management. Practice guidelines for acute pain management in the perioperative setting: an updated report by the American Society of Anesthesiologists Task Force on Acute Pain Management. *Anesthesiology.* 2012;116(2):248–273.
3. Chou R, Gordon DB, de Leon-Casasola OA, et al. Management of postoperative pain: a clinical practice guideline from the American Pain Society, the American Society of Regional Anesthesia and Pain Medicine, and the American Society of Anesthesiologists' Committee on Regional Anesthesia, Executive Committee, and Administrative Council. *J Pain.* 2016;17(2):131–157.
4. Wu CL, Naqibuddin M, Rowlingson AJ, et al. The effect of pain on health-related quality of life in the immediate postoperative period. *Anesth Analg.* 2003;97(4):1078–1085.
5. Joshi GP, Ogunnaike BO. Consequences of inadequate postoperative pain relief and chronic persistent postoperative pain. *Anesthesiol Clin North America.* 2005;23(1):21–36.
6. Carr DB, Goudas LC. Acute pain. *Lancet.* 1999;353(9169):2051–2058.
7. Raja SN, Dougherty PM. Anatomy and physiology of somatosensory and pain processing. In: Benzon HT, Raja SN, Molloy RE, et al., eds. *Essentials of Pain Medicine and Regional Anesthesia.* 2nd ed. Philadelphia, PA: Elsevier; 2005:1–6.
8. Wilder-Smith OH, Arendt-Nielsen L. Postoperative hyperalgesia: its clinical importance and relevance. *Anesthesiology.* 2006;104(3):601–607.
9. Rowlingson JC. Update on acute pain management. International Anesthesia Research Society Review Course Lectures, 2006:95–106.
10. Lavand'homme P. From preemptive to preventive analgesia: time to reconsider the role of perioperative peripheral nerve blocks? *Reg Anesth Pain Med.* 2011;36(1):4–6.
11. Taylor DR. Improving outcomes in acute pain management: optimizing patient selection. *Medscape Neurol Neurosurg.* 2004;6(2).
12. Cepeda MS, Carr DB. Women experience more pain and require more morphine than men to achieve a similar degree of analgesia. *Anesth Analg.* 2003;97(5):1464–1468.
13. Cohen M, Sadhasivam S, Vinks AA. Pharmacogenetics in perioperative medicine. *Curr Opin Anaesthesiol.* 2012;25(4):419–427.
14. Landau R, Bollag LA, Kraft JC. Pharmacogenetics and anaesthesia: the value of genetic profiling. *Anaesthesia.* 2012;67(2):165–179.
15. Caraceni A, Cherny N, Fainsinger R, et al. Pain measurement tools and methods in clinical research in palliative care: recommendations of an Expert Working Group of the European Association of Palliative Care. *J Pain Symptom Manage.* 2002;23(3):239–255.
16. Portenoy RK, Bennett DS, Rauck R, et al. Prevalence and characteristics of breakthrough pain in opioid-treated patients with chronic noncancer pain. *J Pain.* 2006;7(8):583–591.
17. Bennett M. The LANSS Pain Scale: the Leeds assessment of neuropathic symptoms and signs. *Pain.* 2001;92(1–2):147–157.
18. Pizzi LT, Toner R, Foley K, et al. Relationship between potential opioid-related adverse effects and hospital length of stay in patients receiving opioids after orthopedic surgery. *Pharmacotherapy.* 2012;32(6):502–514.
19. Camilleri M. Opioid-induced constipation: challenges and therapeutic opportunities. *Am J Gastroenterol.* 2011;106(5):835–842; quiz 843.
20. Javaheri S, Randerath WJ. Opioid-induced central sleep apnea: mechanisms and therapies. *Sleep Med Clin.* 2014;9:49–56.
21. Safe use of opioids in hospitals. *Sentinel Event Alert.* 2012;49:1–5.
22. Angst MS, Clark JD. Opioid-induced hyperalgesia: a qualitative systematic review. *Anesthesiology.* 2006;104(3):570–587.
23. Javaheri S, Randerath WJ. Opioid-induced central sleep apnea: mechanisms and therapies. *Sleep Medicine Clinics.* 2014;9(1):49–56.
24. Budd K. Pain management: is opioid immunosuppression a clinical problem? *Biomed Pharmacother.* 2006;60(7):310–317.
25. Gupta K, Kshirsagar S, Chang L, et al. Morphine stimulates angiogenesis by activating proangiogenic and survival-promoting signaling and promotes breast tumor growth. *Cancer Res.* 2002;62(15):4491–4498.
26. Sarhill N, Walsh D, Nelson KA. Hydromorphone: pharmacology and clinical applications in cancer patients. *Support Care Cancer.* 2001;9(2):84–96.
27. Crews KR, Gaedigk A, Dunnenberger HM, et al. Clinical Pharmacogenetics Implementation Consortium guidelines for cytochrome P450 2D6 genotype and codeine therapy: 2014 update. *Clin Pharmacol Ther.* 2014;95(4):376–382.
28. Mahajan G, Fishman SM. Major opioids in pain management. In: Benzon HT, Raja SN, Molloy RE, et al., eds. *Essentials of Pain Medicine and Regional Anesthesia.* 2nd ed. Philadelphia, PA: Elsevier; 2005:94–105.
29. Mitra S, Sinatra RS. Perioperative management of acute pain in the opioid-dependent patient. *Anesthesiology.* 2004;101(1):212–227.
30. American Pain Society. *Principles of Analgesic Use in the Treatment of Acute Pain and Cancer Pain.* 5th ed. American Pain Society; 2003.
31. Davis MP. Twelve reasons for considering buprenorphine as a frontline analgesic in the management of pain. *J Support Oncol.* 2012;10(6):209–219.
32. *Drug Facts and Comparisons,* ed. Wolters Kluwer Health, 2011.
33. Williams BA, Butt MT, Zeller JR, et al. Multimodal perineural analgesia with combined bupivacaine-clonidine-buprenorphine-dexamethasone: safe in vivo and chemically compatible in solution. *Pain Med.* 2015;16(1):186–198.
34. Frampton JE. Tapentadol immediate release: a review of its use in the treatment of moderate to severe acute pain. *Drugs.* 2010;70(13):1719–1743.
35. eMedExpert. Difference between Tramadol and Tapentadol. 2015, Jan; Available from: www.emedexpert.com/compare-meds/tramadol-vs-tapentadol Jan 2015.
36. Katz A. NSAIDs and COX-2 Selective Inhibitors. In: Benzon HT, Raja SN, Molloy RE, et al., eds. *Essentials of Pain Medicine and Regional Anesthesia.* 2nd ed. Philadelphia, PA: Elsevier; 2005:141–158.
37. Marret E, Kurdi O, Zufferey P, et al. Effects of nonsteroidal antiinflammatory drugs on patient-controlled analgesia morphine side effects: meta-analysis of randomized controlled trials. *Anesthesiology.* 2005;102(6):1249–1260.
38. Smith, H.S. Perioperative intravenous acetaminophen and NSAIDs. *Pain Med.* 2011;12(6):961–981.
39. Ong CK, Seymour RA, Lirk P, et al. Combining paracetamol (acetaminophen) with nonsteroidal antiinflammatory drugs: a qualitative systematic review of analgesic efficacy for acute postoperative pain. *Anesth Analg.* 2010;110(4):1170–1179.
40. Jouguelet-Lacoste J, La Colla L, Schilling D, et al. The use of intravenous infusion or single dose of low-dose ketamine for postoperative analgesia: a review of the current literature. *Pain Med.* 2015;16(2):383–403.
41. Weinbroum AA. A single small dose of postoperative ketamine provides rapid and sustained improvement in morphine analgesia in the presence of morphine-resistant pain. *Anesth Analg.* 2003;96(3):789–795.
42. Sveticic G, Gentilini A, Eichenberger U, et al. Combinations of morphine with ketamine for patient-controlled analgesia: a new optimization method. *Anesthesiology.* 2003;98(5):1195–1205.
43. Reeves M, Lindholm DE, Myles PS, et al. Adding ketamine to morphine for patient-controlled analgesia after major abdominal surgery: a double-blinded, randomized controlled trial. *Anesth Analg.* 2001;93(1):116–120.
44. Wadhwa A, Clarke D, Goodchild CS, et al. Large-dose oral dextromethorphan as an adjunct to patient-controlled analgesia with morphine after knee surgery. *Anesth Analg.* 2001;92(2):448–454.
45. Sites BD, Beach M, Biggs R, et al. Intrathecal clonidine added to a bupivacaine-morphine spinal anesthetic improves postoperative analgesia for total knee arthroplasty. *Anesth Analg.* 2003;96(4):1083–1088, table of contents.
46. Afonso J, Reis F. Dexmedetomidine: current role in anesthesia and intensive care. *Rev Bras Anestesiol.* 2012;62(1):118–133.
47. Pasin L, Landoni G, Nardelli P, et al. Dexmedetomidine reduces the risk of delirium, agitation and confusion in critically ill patients: a meta-analysis of randomized controlled trials. *J Cardiothorac Vasc Anesth.* 2014;28(6):1459–1466.

48. Clarke H, Bonin RP, Orser BA, et al. The prevention of chronic postsurgical pain using gabapentin and pregabalin: a combined systematic review and meta-analysis. *Anesth Analg*. 2012;115(2):428–442.
49. Schmidt PC, Ruchelli G, Mackey SC, et al. Perioperative gabapentinoids: choice of agent, dose, timing, and effects on chronic postsurgical pain. *Anesthesiology*. 2013;119(5):1215–1221.
50. Zhang J, Ho KY, Wang Y. Efficacy of pregabalin in acute postoperative pain: a meta-analysis. *Br J Anaesth*. 2011;106(4):454–462.
51. Gilron I. Gabapentin and pregabalin for chronic neuropathic and early post-surgical pain: current evidence and future directions. *Curr Opin Anaesthesiol*. 2007;20(5):456–472.
52. Weingarten TN, Jacob AK, Njathi CW, et al. Multimodal analgesic protocol and postanesthesia respiratory depression during phase I recovery after total joint arthroplasty. *Reg Anesth Pain Med*. 2015;40(4):330–336.
53. Myhre M, Diep LM, Stubhaug A. Pregabalin has analgesic, ventilatory, and cognitive effects in combination with remifentanil. *Anesthesiology*. 2016;124(1):141–149.
54. Kaba A, Laurent SR, Detroz BJ, et al. Intravenous lidocaine infusion facilitates acute rehabilitation after laparoscopic colectomy. *Anesthesiology*. 2007;106(1):11–18.
55. Ventham NT, Kennedy ED, Brady RR, et al. Efficacy of Intravenous Lidocaine for Postoperative Analgesia Following Laparoscopic Surgery: A Meta-Analysis. *World J Surg*. 2015;39(9):2220–2234.
56. van der Wal SE, van den Heuvel SA, Radema SA, et al. The in vitro mechanisms and in vivo efficacy of intravenous lidocaine on the neuroinflammatory response in acute and chronic pain. *Eur J Pain*. 2016;20(5):655–674.
57. Albrecht E, Kirkham KR, Liu SS, et al. Peri-operative intravenous administration of magnesium sulphate and postoperative pain: a meta-analysis. *Anaesthesia*. 2013;68(1):79–90.
58. De Oliveira GS Jr, Castro-Alves LJ, Khan JH, et al. Perioperative systemic magnesium to minimize postoperative pain: a meta-analysis of randomized controlled trials. *Anesthesiology*. 2013;119(1):178–190.
59. Jabbour HJ, Naccache NM, Jawish RJ, et al. Ketamine and magnesium association reduces morphine consumption after scoliosis surgery: prospective randomised double-blind study. *Acta Anaesthesiol Scand*. 2014;58(5):572–579.
60. Koç S, Memis D, Sut N. The preoperative use of gabapentin, dexamethasone, and their combination in varicocele surgery: A randomized controlled trial. *Anesth Analg*. 2007;105:1137–1142.
61. De Oliveira GS Jr, Almeida MD, Benzon HT, et al. Perioperative single dose systemic dexamethasone for postoperative pain: a meta-analysis of randomized controlled trials. *Anesthesiology*. 2011;115(3):575–588.
62. Mahathanaruk M, Hitt J, de LeonCasasola OA. Perioperative management of the opioid tolerant patient for orthopedic surgery. *Anesthesiol Clin*. 2014;32(4):923–932.
63. Williams BA, Ibinson JW, Mangione MP, et al. Research priorities regarding multimodal peripheral nerve blocks for postoperative analgesia and anesthesia based on hospital quality data extracted from over 1,300 cases (2011–2014). *Pain Med*. 2015;16(1):7–12.
64. Macintyre PE. Safety and efficacy of patient-controlled analgesia. *Br J Anaesth*. 2001;87(1):36–46.
65. Gan TJ, Diemunsch P, Habib AS, et al. Consensus guidelines for the management of postoperative nausea and vomiting. *Anesth Analg*. 2014;118(1):85–113.
66. Blaudszun G, Lysakowski C, Elia N, et al. Effect of perioperative systemic alpha2 agonists on postoperative morphine consumption and pain intensity: systematic review and meta-analysis of randomized controlled trials. *Anesthesiology*. 2012;116(6):1312–1322.
67. Block BM, Liu SS, Rowlingson AJ, et al. Efficacy of postoperative epidural analgesia: a meta-analysis. *JAMA*. 2003;290(18):2455–2463.
68. Bernards CM, Shen DD, Sterling ES, et al. Epidural, cerebrospinal fluid, and plasma pharmacokinetics of epidural opioids (part 1): differences among opioids. *Anesthesiology*. 2003;99(2):455–465.
69. Örster JG, Rosenberg PH. Small dose of clonidine mixed with low-dose ropivacaine and fentanyl for epidural analgesia after total knee arthroplasty. *Br J Anaesth*. 2004;93(5):670–677.
70. Rathmell JP, Lair TR, Nauman B. The role of intrathecal drugs in the treatment of acute pain. *Anesth Analg*. 2005;101(5 Suppl):S30–S43.
71. Sites BD, Beach M, Gallagher JD, et al. A single injection ultrasound-assisted femoral nerve block provides side effect-sparing analgesia when compared with intrathecal morphine in patients undergoing total knee arthroplasty. *Anesth Analg*. 2004;99(5):1539–1543.
72. Richman JM, Liu SS, Courpas G, et al. Does Continuous Peripheral Nerve Block Provide Superior Pain Control to Opioids? A Meta-Analysis. *Anesth Analg*. 2006;102:248–257.
73. Capdevila X, Pirat P, Bringuier S, et al. Continuous peripheral nerve blocks in hospital wards after orthopedic surgery: a multicenter prospective analysis of the quality of postoperative analgesia and complications in 1,416 patients. *Anesthesiology*. 2005;103(5):1035–1045.
74. Swenson JD, Bay N, Loose E, et al. Outpatient management of continuous peripheral nerve catheters placed using ultrasound guidance: an experience in 620 patients. *Anesth Analg*. 2006;103(6):1436–1443.
75. Neal JM, Brull R, Horn JL, et al. The Second American Society of Regional Anesthesia and Pain Medicine evidence-based medicine assessment of ultrasound guided regional anesthesia. *Reg Anesth Pain Med*. 2016;41(2):181–194.
76. Winnie AP. Interscalene brachial plexus block. *Anesth Analg*. 1970;49(3):455–466.
77. Spence BC, Beach ML, Gallagher JD, et al. Ultrasound-guided interscalene blocks: understanding where to inject the local anaesthetic. *Anaesthesia*. 2011;66(6):509–514.
78. Albrecht E, Kirkham KR, Taffé P, et al. The maximum effective needle-to-nerve distance for ultrasound-guided interscalene block: an exploratory study. *Reg Anesth Pain Med*. 2014;39(1):56–60.
79. Hadzic A, Williams BA, Karaca PE, et al. For outpatient rotator cuff surgery, nerve block anesthesia provides superior same-day recovery over general anesthesia. *Anesthesiology*. 2005;102(5):1001–1007.
80. Kulenkampf D. Anesthesia of the Brachial Plexus (German). *Zentralbl Chir*. 1911;38:1337–1350.
81. Perlas A, Chan VW, Simons M. Brachial plexus examination and localization using ultrasound and electrical stimulation: a volunteer study. *Anesthesiology*. 2003;99(2):429–435.
82. Perlas A, Lobo G, Lo N, et al. Ultrasound-guided supraclavicular block: outcome of 510 consecutive cases. *Reg Anesth Pain Med*. 2009;34(2):171–176.
83. Brull R, Chan VW. The corner pocket revisited. *Reg Anesth Pain Med*. 2011;36(3):308.
84. Roy, M, Nadeau MJ, Côté D, et al. Comparison of a single- or double-injection technique for ultrasound-guided supraclavicular block: a prospective, randomized, blinded controlled study. *Reg Anesth Pain Med*. 2012;37(1):55–59.
85. Arab SA, Alharbi MK, Nada EM, et al. Ultrasound-guided supraclavicular brachial plexus block: single versus triple injection technique for upper limb arteriovenous access surgery. *Anesth Analg*. 2014;118(5):1120–1125.
86. Sites BD, Macfarlane AJ, Sites VR, et al. Clinical sonopathology for the regional anesthesiologist: part 1: vascular and neural. *Reg Anesth Pain Med*. 2010;35(3):272–280.
87. Sites BD, Macfarlane AJ, Sites VR, et al. Clinical sonopathology for the regional anesthesiologist: part 2: bone, viscera, subcutaneous tissue, and foreign bodies. *Reg Anesth Pain Med*. 2010;35(3):281–289.
88. Bigeleisen P, Wilson M. A comparison of two techniques for ultrasound guided infraclavicular block. *Br J Anaesth*. 2006;96(4):502–507.
89. Dingemans E, Williams SR, Arcand G, et al. Neurostimulation in ultrasound-guided infraclavicular block: a prospective randomized trial. *Anesth Anlag*. 2007;104(5):1275–1280.
90. Sandhu NS, Capan LM. Ultrasound-guided infraclavicular brachial plexus block. *Br J Anaesth*. 2002;89(2):254–259.
91. Auyong DB, Gonzales J, Benonis JG. The Houdini clavicle: arm abduction and needle insertion site adjustment improves needle visibility for the infraclavicular nerve block. *Reg Anesth Pain Med*. 2010;35(4):403–404.
92. Sauter AR, Smith HJ, Stubhaug A, et al. Use of magnetic resonance imaging to define the anatomical location closest to all three cords of the infraclavicular brachial plexus. *Anesth Analg*. 2006;103(6):1574–1576.
93. Sandhu NS, Manne JS, Medabalmi PK, et al. Sonographically guided infraclavicular brachial plexus block in adults: a retrospective analysis of 1146 cases. *J Ultrasound Med*. 2006;25(12):1555–1561.
94. Ilfeld BM, Morey TE, Enneking FK. Infraclavicular perineural local anesthetic infusion: a comparison of three dosing regimens for postoperative analgesia. *Anesthesiology*. 2004;100(2):395–402.
95. Awad IT, Duggan EM. Posterior lumbar plexus block: anatomy, approaches, and techniques. *Reg Anesth Pain Med*. 2005;30(2):143–149.
96. Kaloul I, Guay J, Côté C, et al. The posterior lumbar plexus (psoas compartment) block and the three-in-one femoral nerve block provide similar postoperative analgesia after total knee replacement. *Can J Anaesth*. 2004;51(1):45–51.
97. Capdevila X, Coimbra C, Choquet O. Approaches to the lumbar plexus: success, risks, and results. *Reg Anesth Pain Med*. 2005;30(2):150–162.
98. Kirchmair L, Enna B, Mitterschiffthaler G, et al. Lumbar plexus in children. A sonographic study and its relevance to pediatric regional anesthesia. *Anesthesiology*. 2004;101(2):445–450.
99. Gray AT, Collins AB, Schafhalter-Zoppoth I. An introduction to femoral nerve and associated lumbar plexus nerve blocks under ultrasound guidance. *Techn Reg Anesth Pain Manag*. 2004;8(4):155–163.
100. Nader A, Malik K, Kendall MC, et al. Relationship between ultrasound imaging and eliciting motor response during femoral nerve stimulation. *J Ultrasound Med*. 2009;28(3):345–350.
101. Ilfeld BM, Loland VJ, Sandhu NS, et al. Continuous femoral nerve blocks: the impact of catheter tip location relative to the femoral nerve (anterior versus posterior) on quadriceps weakness and cutaneous sensory block. *Anesth Analg*. 2012;115(3):721–727.
102. Bauer MC, Pogatzki-Zahn EM, Zahn PK. Regional analgesia techniques for total knee replacement. *Curr Opin Anaesthesiol*. 2014;27(5):501–506.
103. Chan EY, Fransen M, Parker DA, et al. Femoral nerve blocks for acute postoperative pain after knee replacement surgery. *Cochrane Database Syst Rev*. 2014;5:CD009941.

104. Johnson RL, Kopp SL, Hebl JR, et al. Falls and major orthopaedic surgery with peripheral nerve blockade: a systematic review and meta-analysis. *Br J Anaesth*. 2013;110(4):518–528.
105. Memtsoudis SG, Danninger T, Rasul R, et al. Inpatient falls after total knee arthroplasty: the role of anesthesia type and peripheral nerve blocks. *Anesthesiology*. 2014;120(3):551–563.
106. Jæger P, Zaric D, Fomsgaard JS, et al. Adductor canal block versus femoral nerve block for analgesia after total knee arthroplasty: a randomized, double-blind study. *Reg Anesth Pain Med*. 2013;38(6):526–532.
107. Machi AT, Sztain JF, Kormylo NJ, et al. Discharge Readiness after Tricompartment Knee Arthroplasty: Adductor Canal versus Femoral Continuous Nerve Blocks—A Dual-center, Randomized Trial. *Anesthesiology*. 2015;123(2):444–456.
108. Bendtsen TF, Moriggl B, Chan V, et al. Redefining the adductor canal block. *Reg Anesth Pain Med*. 2014;39(5):442–443.
109. Bendtsen TF, Moriggl B, Chan V, et al. Defining adductor canal block. *Reg Anesth Pain Med*. 2014;39(3):253–254.
110. Manickam B, Perlas A, Duggan E, et al. Feasibility and efficacy of ultrasound-guided block of the saphenous nerve in the adductor canal. *Reg Anesth Pain Med*. 2009;34(6):578–580.
111. Burckett-St Laurant D, Peng P, Girón Arango L, et al. The Nerves of the Adductor Canal and the Innervation of the Knee: An Anatomic Study. *Reg Anesth Pain Med*. 2016 May-Jun 2016. 41(3):321–327.
112. Diakomi M, Papaioannou M, Mela A, et al. Preoperative fascia iliaca compartment block for positioning patients with hip fractures for central nervous blockade: a randomized trial. *Reg Anesth Pain Med*. 2014;39(5):394–398.
113. Dulaney-Cripe E, Hadaway S, Bauman R, et al. A continuous infusion fascia iliaca compartment block in hip fracture patients: a pilot study. *J Clin Med Res*. 2012;4(1):45–48.
114. Mouzopoulos G, Vasiliadis G, Lasanianos N, et al. Fascia iliaca block prophylaxis for hip fracture patients at risk for delirium: a randomized placebo-controlled study. *J Orthop Traumatol*. 2009;10(3):127–133.
115. Dalens B, Vanneuville G, Tanguy A. A Comparison of the fascia iliaca compartment block with the 3-in-1 block in children. *Anesth Analg*. 1989;69(6):705–713.
116. Hebbard P, Ivanusic J, Sha S. Ultrasound-guided supra-inguinal fascia iliaca block: a cadaveric evaluation of a novel approach. *Anaesthesia*. 2011;66(4):300–305.
117. Dolan J, Williams A, Murney E, et al. Ultrasound guided fascia iliaca block: a comparison with the loss of resistance technique. *Reg Anesth Pain Med*. 2008;33(6):526–531.
118. Vaughan B, Manley M, Stewart D, et al. Distal injection site may explain lack of analgesia from fascia iliaca block for total hip. *Reg Anesth Pain Med*. 2013;38(6):556–557.
119. Hunt KJ, Higgins TF, Carlston CV, et al. Continuous peripheral nerve blockade as postoperative analgesia for open treatment of calcaneal fractures. *J Orthop Trauma*. 2010;24(3):148–155.
120. Zaric D, Boysen K, Christiansen J, et al. Continuous popliteal sciatic nerve block for outpatient foot surgery–a randomized, controlled trial. *Acta Anaesthesiol Scand*. 2004;48(3):337–341.
121. Salinas FV. Evidence Basis for Ultrasound Guidance for Lower-Extremity Peripheral Nerve Block: Update 2016. *Reg Anesth Pain Med*. 2016;41(2):261–274.
122. Marhofer, P, Chan VW. Ultrasound-guided regional anesthesia: current concepts and future trends. *Anesthesia Analgesia*. 2007;104(5):1265–1269.
123. Schafhalter-Zoppoth I, Younger SJ, Collins AB, et al. The "seesaw" sign: improved sonographic identification of the sciatic nerve. *Anesthesiology*. 2004;101(3):808–809.
124. Andersen HL, Andersen SL, Tranum-Jensen J. Injection inside the paraneural sheath of the sciatic nerve: direct comparison among ultrasound imaging, macroscopic anatomy, and histologic analysis. *Reg Anesth Pain Med*. 2012;37(4):410–414.
125. Karmakar MK, Shariat AN, Pangthipampai P, et al. High-definition ultrasound imaging defines the paraneural sheath and the fascial compartments surrounding the sciatic nerve at the popliteal fossa. *Reg Anesth Pain Med*. 2013;38(5):447–451.
126. Tran DQ, González AP, Bernucci F, et al. A randomized comparison between bifurcation and prebifurcation subparaneural popliteal sciatic nerve blocks. *Anesth Analg*. 2013;116(5):1170–1175.
127. Choquet O, Noble GB, Abbal B, et al. Subparaneural versus circumferential extraneural injection at the bifurcation level in ultrasound-guided popliteal sciatic nerve blocks: a prospective, randomized, double-blind study. *Reg Anesth Pain Med*. 2014;39(4):306–311.
128. Richardson J. Paravertebral anesthesia and analgesia. *Can J Anaesth*. 2004;51(6):R1–R6.
129. Krediet AC, Moayeri N, van Geffen GJ, et al. Different Approaches to Ultrasound-guided Thoracic Paravertebral Block: An Illustrated Review. *Anesthesiology*. 2015;123(2):459–474.
130. Evans H, Steele SM, Nielsen KC, et al. Peripheral nerve blocks and continuous catheter techniques. *Anesthesiol Clin North America*. 2005;23(1):141–162.
131. Blanco R, Fajardo M, Parras Maldonado T. Ultrasound description of Pecs II (modified Pecs I): a novel approach to breast surgery. *Rev Esp Anestesiol Reanim*. 2012;59(9):470–475.
132. Bashandy GM, Abbas DN. Pectoral nerves I and II blocks in multimodal analgesia for breast cancer surgery: a randomized clinical trial. *Reg Anesth Pain Med*. 2015;40(1):68–74.
133. Blanco R, Parras T, McDonnell JG, et al. Serratus plane block: a novel ultrasound-guided thoracic wall nerve block. *Anaesthesia*. 2013;68(11):1107–1113.
134. Børglum J. Abdominal surgery: advances in the use of ultrasound guided truncal blocks for perioperative pain management. In: Derbel PF, ed. *Abdominal Surgery*. Rijeka, Croatia: InTech, 2012.
135. Rafi AN. Abdominal field block: a new approach via the lumbar triangle. *Anaesthesia*. 2001;56(10):1024–1026.
136. Abrahams M, Derby R, Horn JL. Update on Ultrasound for Truncal Blocks: A Review of the Evidence. *Reg Anesth Pain Med*. 2016;41(2):275–288.
137. Abdallah FW, Laffey JG, Halpern SH, et al. Duration of analgesic effectiveness after the posterior and lateral transversus abdominis plane block techniques for transverse lower abdominal incisions: a meta-analysis. *Br J Anaesth*. 2013;111(5):721–735.
138. Bærentzen F, Maschmann C, Jensen K, et al. Ultrasound-guided nerve block for inguinal hernia repair: a randomized, controlled, double-blind study. *Reg Anesth Pain Med*. 2012;37(5):502–507.
139. Vendittoli PA, Makinen P, Drolet P, et al. A multimodal analgesia protocol for total knee arthroplasty. A randomized, controlled study. *J Bone Joint Surg Am*. 2006;88(2):282–289.
140. Bramlett K, Onel E, Viscusi ER, et al. A randomized, double-blind, dose-ranging study comparing wound infiltration of DepoFoam bupivacaine, an extended-release liposomal bupivacaine, to bupivacaine HCl for postsurgical analgesia in total knee arthroplasty. *Knee*. 2012;19(5):530–536.
141. Essving P, Axelsson K, Åberg E, et al. Local infiltration analgesia versus intrathecal morphine for postoperative pain management after total knee arthroplasty: a randomized controlled trial. *Anesth Analg*. 2011;113(4):926–933.
142. Bagsby DT, Ireland PH, Meneghini RM. Liposomal bupivacaine versus traditional periarticular injection for pain control after total knee arthroplasty. *J Arthroplasty*. 2014;29(8):1687–1690.
143. Bergese SD, Ramamoorthy S, Patou G, et al. Efficacy profile of liposome bupivacaine, a novel formulation of bupivacaine for postsurgical analgesia. *J Pain Res*. 2012;5:107–116.
144. Viscusi ER, Sinatra R, Onel E, et al. The safety of liposome bupivacaine, a novel local analgesic formulation. *Clin J Pain*. 2014;30(2):102–110.
145. Surdam JW, Licini DJ, Baynes NT, et al. The use of exparel (liposomal bupivacaine) to manage postoperative pain in unilateral total knee arthroplasty patients. *J Arthroplasty*. 2015;30(2):325–329.
146. Horlocker TT, Wedel DJ. Neuraxial block and low-molecular-weight heparin: balancing perioperative analgesia and thromboprophylaxis. *Reg Anesth Pain Med*. 1998;23(6 Suppl 2):164–177.
147. Horlocker TT, Wedel DJ, Rowlingson JC, et al. Regional anesthesia in the patient receiving antithrombotic or thrombolytic therapy: American Society of Regional Anesthesia and Pain Medicine Evidence-Based Guidelines (Third Edition). *Reg Anesth Pain Med*. 2010;35(1):64–101.
148. Rodgers A, Walker N, Schug S, et al. Reduction of postoperative mortality and morbidity with epidural or spinal anaesthesia: results from overview of randomised trials. *BMJ*. 2000;321(7275):1493.
149. Tuman KJ, McCarthy RJ, March RJ, et al. Effects of epidural anesthesia and analgesia on coagulation and outcome after major vascular surgery. *Anesth Analg*. 1991;73(6):696–704.
150. Cheney, FW. High-severity injuries associated with regional anesthesia in the 1990's. *American Society of Anesthesiologists Newsletter*. 2001;65(6):6–8.
151. Hebl JR, Horlocker TT, Sorenson EJ, et al. Regional anesthesia does not increase the risk of postoperative neuropathy in patients undergoing ulnar nerve transposition. *Anesth Analg*. 2001;93(6):1606–1611.
152. Neal JM. Ultrasound-Guided Regional Anesthesia and Patient Safety: Update of an Evidence-Based Analysis. *Reg Anesth Pain Med*. 2016;41(2):195–204.
153. Manchikanti L, Singh A. Therapeutic opioids: a ten-year perspective on the complexities and complications of the escalating use, abuse, and nonmedical use of opioids. *Pain Physician*. 2008;11(2 Suppl):S63–S88.
154. Schug SA. Acute pain management in the opioid-tolerant patient. *Pain Manag*. 2012;2(6):581–591.
155. Sites BD, Beach ML, Davis MA. Increases in the use of prescription opioid analgesics and the lack of improvement in disability metrics among users. *Reg Anesth Pain Med*. 2014;39(1):6–12.
156. Gulur P, Williams L, Chaudhary S, et al. Opioid tolerance: a predictor of increased length of stay and higher readmission rates. *Pain Physician*. 2014;17(4):E503–E507.
157. Pasternak GW. Incomplete cross tolerance and multiple mu opioid peptide receptors. *Trends Pharmacol Sci*. 2001;22(2):67–70.
158. Carroll IR, Angst MS, Clark JD. Management of perioperative pain in patients chronically consuming opioids. *Reg Anesth Pain Med*. 2004;29(6):576–591.
159. Khanna IK, Pillarisetti S. Buprenorphine: an attractive opioid with underutilized potential in treatment of chronic pain. *J Pain Res*. 2015;8:859–870.
160. Derry S, Moore RA. Single dose oral celecoxib for acute postoperative pain in adults. *Cochrane Database Syst Rev*. 2013;10:CD004233.

161. Smith HS. Potential analgesic mechanisms of acetaminophen. *Pain Physician*. 2009;12(1):269–280.
162. Loftus RW, Yeager MP, Clark JA, et al. Intraoperative ketamine reduces perioperative opiate consumption in opiate-dependent patients with chronic back pain undergoing back surgery. *Anesthesiology*. 2010;113(3):639–646.
163. Ramaswamy S, Wilson JA, Colvin L. Non-opioid-based adjuvant analgesia in perioperative care. *Contin Educ Anaesth Crit Care Pain*. 2013;13(5):152–157.
164. de Menezes Couceiro TC, et al. Intravenous lidocaine to treat postoperative pain. *Rev Dor. São Paulo*. 2014;15(1):55–60.
165. Jabbour HJ, Naccache NM, Jawish RJ, et al. Ketamine and magnesium association reduces morphine consumption after scoliosis surgery: prospective randomised double-blind study. *Acta Anaesthesiol Scand*. 2014;58(5):572–579.
166. Naidu R, Flood P. Magnesium: Is There a Signal in the Noise? *Anesthesiology*. 2013;119(1):13–15.
167. Liu HT, Hollmann MW, Liu WH. Modulation of NMDA receptor function by ketamine and magnesium: Part I. *Anesth Analg*. 2001;92(5):1173–1181.
168. Haller G, Waeber JL, Infante NK. Ketamine combined with morphine for the management of pain in an opioid addict. *Anesthesiology*. 2002;96(5):1265–1266.
169. Buvanendran A, Kroin JS, Della Valle CJ. Perioperative oral pregabalin reduces chronic pain after total knee arthroplasty: a prospective, randomized, controlled trial. *Anesth Analg*. 2010;110(1):199–207.
170. Dolin SJ, Cashman JN, Bland JM. Effectiveness of acute postoperative pain management: I. Evidence from published data. *Br J Anaesth*. 2002;89(3):409–423.
171. Stadler M, Schlander M, Braeckman M, et al. A cost-utility and cost-effectiveness analysis of an acute pain service. *J Clin Anesth*. 2004;16(3):159–167.
172. Berry PH, Dahl JL. The new JCAHO pain standards: implications for pain management nurses. *Pain Manag Nurs*. 2000;1(1):3–12.
173. Kain ZN, Mayes LC, Caldwell-Andrews AA, et al. Preoperative anxiety, postoperative pain, and behavioral recovery in young children undergoing surgery. *Pediatrics*. 2006;118(2):651–658.
174. Wright KD, Stewart SH, Finley GA. Prevention and intervention strategies to alleviate preoperative anxiety in children: a critical review. *Behavior Modification*. 2007;31(1):52–79.
175. Voepel-Lewis T, Malviya S, Tait AR. A comparison of the clinical utility of pain assessment tools for children with cognitive impairment. *Anesth Analg*. 2008;106(1):72–78.
176. Taylor EM, Boyer K, Campbell FA. Pain in hospitalized children: a prospective cross-sectional survey of pain prevalence, intensity, assessment and management in a Canadian pediatric teaching hospital. *Pain Res Manag*. 2008;13(1):25–32.
177. Franck LS, Allen A, Oulton K. Making pain assessment more accessible to children and parents: can greater involvement improve the quality of care? *Clin J Pain*. 2007;23(4):331–338.
178. Moir MS, Bair E, Shinnick P, et al. Acetaminophen versus acetaminophen with codeine after pediatric tonsillectomy. *Laryngoscope*. 2000;110(11):1824–1827.
179. Bayrak F, Gunday I, Memis D, et al. A comparison of oral midazolam, oral tramadol, and intranasal sufentanil premedication in pediatric patients. *J Opioid Manag*. 2007;3(2):74–78.
180. Butkovic D, Kralik S, Matolic M, et al. Postoperative analgesia with intravenous fentanyl PCA vs epidural block after thoracoscopic pectus excavatum repair in children. *Br J Anaesth*. 2007;98(5):677–681.
181. Saudan S, Habre W, Ceroni D, et al. Safety and efficacy of patient controlled epidural analgesia following pediatric spinal surgery. *Paediatr Anaesth*. 2008;18(2):132–139.
182. Wuhrman E, Cooney MF, Dunwoody CJ, et al. Authorized and unauthorized ("PCA by proxy") dosing of analgesic infusion pumps: position statement with clinical practice recommendations. *Pain Manag Nurs*. 2007;8(1):4–11.
183. Ecoffey C. Pediatric regional anesthesia – update. Current Opinion in Anaesthesiology. *Paediatr Anaesth*. 2007;203(3):232–235.
184. Corman S.L, Skledar SL. Use of Lipid emulsion to reverse local anesthetic-induced toxicity. *Ann Pharmacother*. 2007;41(November):1873–1877.
185. Ganesh A, Rose JB, Wells L, et al. Continuous peripheral nerve blockade for inpatient and outpatient postoperative analgesia in children. *Anesth Analg*. 2007;105(5):1234–1242.
186. DeVera HV, Furukawa KT, Matson MD, et al. Regional techniques as an adjunct to general anesthesia for pediatric extremity and spine surgery. *J Pediatr Orthop*. 2006;26(6):801–804.
187. Weintraud M, Marhofer P, Bösenberg A, et al. Ilioinguinal/iliohypogastric blocks in children: where do we administer the local anesthetic without direct visualization? *Anesth Analg*. 2008;106(1):89–93.
188. Choi S, McCartney CJ. Evidence base for the use of ultrasound for upper extremity blocks: 2014 Update. *Reg Anesth Pain Med*. 2016;41(2):242–250.
189. Toombs JD, Kral LA. Methadone treatment for pain states. *Am Fam Phys*. 2005;71(17):1353–1358.
190. Hadi I, Morley-Forster PK, Dain S, et al. Perioperative management of the patient with chronic non-cancer pain. *Can J Anaesth*. 2006;53(12):1190–1199.
191. Ayonrinde OT, Bridge DT. The rediscovery of methadone for cancer pain management. *Med J Austr*. 2000;173(10):536–540.
192. Grass JA. Patient-controlled analgesia. *Anesth Analg*. 2005;101(Suppl):S44–S61.
193. Liu SS, McDonald SB. Current issues in spinal anesthesia. *Anesthesiology*. 2001;94(5):888–906.
194. Karmakar MK, Chui PT, Joynt GM, et al. Thoracic paravertebral block for management of pain associated with multiple fractured ribs in patients with concomitant lumbar spinal trauma. *Reg Anesth Pain Med*. 2001;26(2):169–173.
195. Liu S. Update in use of continuous perineural catheters for postoperative analgesia. IARS 2006 Review Course Lectures. *Anesth Analg*. 2006;(Suppl):64.
196. Liu SS, Ngeow JE, YaDeau JT. Ultrasound-guided regional anesthesia and analgesia: a qualitative review. *Reg Anesth Pain Med*. 2009;34(1):47–59.

56 Chronic Pain Management

HONORIO T. BENZON • ROBERT W. HURLEY • SALIM M. HAYEK

Anatomy, Physiology, and Neurochemistry of Somatosensory Pain Processing
  Primary Afferents and Peripheral Stimulation
  Neurochemistry of Peripheral Nerve and the Dorsal Root Ganglion
  Neurobiology of the Spinal Cord and Spinal Trigeminal Nucleus
  Neurobiology of Ascending Pathways
  Neurobiology of Descending Pathways
  Neurobiology of Supraspinal Structures Involved in Higher Cortical Processing
  Transition from Acute to Persistent or Chronic Nociception
Management of Common Pain Syndromes
  Low Back Pain: Radicular Pain Syndromes
  Low Back Pain: Facet Syndrome
  Buttock Pain: Sacroiliac Joint Syndrome and Piriformis Syndrome
  Myofascial Pain Syndrome and Fibromyalgia
Neuropathic Pain Syndromes
  Herpes Zoster and Postherpetic Neuralgia
  Diabetic Painful Neuropathy
  Complex Regional Pain Syndrome
  Human Immunodeficiency Virus Neuropathy
  Phantom Pain
Cancer Pain
  Neurolytic Blocks for Visceral Pain from Cancer
Pharmacologic Management of Pain
  Opioids
  Pharmacologic Treatments of Neuropathic Pain
Interventional Techniques
  Discography
  Thermal Annular Procedures
  Minimally Invasive Lumbar Decompression Procedure
  Vertebroplasty and Kyphoplasty
  Spinal Cord Stimulation
  Peripheral Nerve Stimulation
  Dorsal Root Ganglion Stimulation
  Occipital Nerve Stimulation
  Intrathecal Drug Delivery
Summary

KEY POINTS

1. A delta and C fibers, under normal conditions, transmit nociceptive (pain) information to the spinal cord from their free nerve endings in the periphery. In chronic pain conditions, the A beta fibers, which normally transmit nonnoxious information, also participate in nociceptive transmission.
2. Most randomized studies on the efficacy of epidural steroid injections show temporary relief of radicular pain. Studies on thermal rhizotomy of the medial branches, for relief of facet syndrome, show benefit that lasts 3 to 12 months. This relief avoids the usage of addicting opioids.
3. Injection of epidural local anesthetics and methylprednisolone, when performed three to four times during the acute stage of herpes zoster, may prevent the development of postherpetic neuralgia. Postherpetic neuralgia is mostly managed pharmacologically, although interventional techniques may be used in resistant cases.
4. Antidepressants and anticonvulsants are effective for treatment of neuropathic pain syndromes. Use of antidepressants is limited because of their side effects. Anticonvulsants have a more favorable side-effect profile and speed of therapeutic effect, which makes them the first line of treatment for these syndromes. Their efficacy is improved when combined with an opioid or an antidepressant.
5. Complex regional pain syndrome that does not respond to nerve blocks, physical therapy, and/or pharmacologic management may respond to spinal cord stimulation.
6. Opioids are the mainstay for cancer pain management and are effective in neuropathic pain, although at higher doses.
7. The majority of pain secondary to cancer is effectively managed pharmacologically with opioids, anticonvulsants, and antidepressants. Neurolysis of the visceral sympathetic system for pain secondary to abdominal or pelvic cancer relieves pain, decreases opioid consumption, and improves the patients' quality of life.
8. Vertebroplasty and kyphoplasty are indicated for vertebral compression fractures, although some studies question their efficacy.
9. Spinal cord stimulation is effective in patients with failed back syndrome and complex regional pain syndrome and may be effective in angina and critical limb ischemia.
10. Intrathecal drug delivery (IDD) systems are valuable options in cancer pain patients in whom opioids are ineffective at high doses or cause unacceptable side effects; however, noncancer pain patients seem to do best if they are on no- or low-doses of opioids prior to initiation of IDD.

Anatomy, Physiology, and Neurochemistry of Somatosensory Pain Processing

Primary Afferents and Peripheral Stimulation

A variety of mechanical, thermal, electrical, or chemical stimuli can result in the sensation and perception of pain. Information about these painful or noxious stimuli is transmitted to higher brain centers by receptors and neurons that are often distinct from those that carry innocuous somatic sensory information. The mammalian somatosensory system is subserved by four groups of afferent fibers differentiated by their anatomy, rate of transmission, and sensory modality transduced (Table 56-1).

The heavily myelinated large-diameter A beta (Aβ) fibers have specialized encapsulated nerve endings, which transduce innocuous or low-threshold mechanical stimulation. The activation of Aβ fibers has been invoked as a part of the mechanism for the production of pain relief by transcutaneous electrical nerve stimulators.[1] As well, it is becoming increasingly apparent that in chronic pain states, these fibers may indeed participate in pain signaling by adopting a "phenotype" similar to that of a C fiber (vide infra).[2]

The next groups of fibers represent the specialized sensory neurons that respond to actual or potential tissue damage, the nociceptors. The lightly myelinated medium-diameter A delta (Aδ) fibers and the unmyelinated small-diameter C fibers have free nerve endings that transduce noxious or high-threshold thermal, mechanical, and chemical stimulation. Patients with a mutation of the tyrosine kinase protein A, which is a component of the nerve growth factor receptor, fail to develop Aβ, Aδ, or C fibers and have no ability to sense pain.[3] Unlike receptors in the Aβ fibers, the Aδ and C fibers respond to stimulation of their receptive fields in a characteristic manner with slow adaptation and residual firing following the withdrawal of the stimulus. Although these two fiber groups respond similarly to stimulation, they mediate different aspects of pain sensation. The rapidly conducting Aδ fibers mediate the "first" pain or *epicritic pain*, which is well localized and is characterized as sharp or prickling. The slowly conducting C fibers mediate the "second" pain or *protopathic pain*, which temporally follows the epicritic pain and is poorly localized or diffuse and is characterized as burning or dull.[4]

The majority of Aδ and C nociceptors are polymodal and therefore are responsible for the transduction of noxious stimuli of different modalities. Nociceptive nerve endings are also located in muscle, the fascia, and adventitia of blood vessels, the knee joint, the dura, and the viscera. The primary afferent peripheral (distal) terminals express a variety of specific transducer channels that are sensitive over a range of stimulus intensities. When they are activated by the appropriate stimulus (thermal, chemical, or mechanical) these channels activate voltage-sensitive cation channels (NaV and CaV) and initiate an action potential. The sodium channel is of special interest following the discovery of its involvement in patients who are insensitive to pain. An epidemiologic study identified three Pakistani families with congenital insensitivity to pain. All were found to possess nonsense mutations of the *SCN9A* gene, resulting in truncation of the Nav1.7 isoform of the sodium channel.[5] Other mutations of this gene result in the impaired inactivation of this channel, which causes paroxysmal extreme pain disorder or hyperexcitability resulting in erythromelalgia.[6,7]

The understanding of the molecular underpinning of the sensory processing of pain has primarily come from studying the transient receptor potential (TRP) channels. The cloning and characterization of the "capsaicin" receptor of the TRP family of nonselective cation channels expanded the field immensely.[8] Members of this molecular family transduce thermal, mechanical, and chemical information in the periphery. The capsaicin receptor named *TRP vanilloid 1* (TRPV1), which responds to capsaicin and other vanilloid compounds and is also activated by acid and heat, provides an excellent example of the integration of multiple sensory modalities within a single neuron and is localized to nociceptors.[8] Furthermore, acidic environments can lower the activation threshold of the channel to heat stimuli. Therefore, the TRPV1 receptor may represent an important therapeutic target in inflammatory (acidic) pain conditions. Mice lacking the TRPV1 receptor are deficient in their response to thermal but not mechanical or other noxious stimuli.[9] These data suggest that this member of the family of TRP channels may play a role in the integration of noxious chemical and thermal stimuli while having relatively less to do with mechanical transduction.

Table 56-1 Primary Afferent Fibers and Their Function

Modality	Receptor	Fiber Type	Conduction Velocity and Diameter	Rate of Adaptation	Function
Proprioceptive	Golgi and Ruffini endings, muscle spindle afferents	Aα	70–120 m/s 15–20 µm	Slow and rapid	Muscle tension, length, and velocity
Mechanosensitive	Meissner, Ruffini, Pacinian corpuscles, and Merkel disc	Aβ	40–70 m/s 5–15 µm	Rapid (slow—Merkel)	Touch, flutter, motion, pressure, vibration
Thermoreceptive	Free nerve endings	Aδ	10–35 m/s 1–5 µm	Slow	Innocuous cold
	Free nerve endings	C	0.5–1 m/s <1 µm	Slow	Innocuous warmth
Nociceptive	Free nerve endings	Aδ	10–35 m/s 1–5 µm	Slow	Sharp pain
	Free nerve endings	C	0.5–1 m/s <1 µm	Slow	Burning pain

Neurochemistry of Peripheral Nerve and the Dorsal Root Ganglion

The nociceptive primary afferents, the Aδ and C fibers, represent the principal target of pharmacologic manipulation by the physician treating pain. Glutamate receptors, as well as opioid, substance P, somatostatin, and vanilloid receptors, have been identified on the peripheral endings of these nerve fibers. Although the transmission of acute nociceptive information is primarily by the Aδ and C fibers, a subset of the Aδ and C fibers are "thermoreceptors" that transduce innocuous cold and warm information, respectively. The cell bodies of primary afferents, regardless of the structure they innervate, make up the *dorsal root ganglia* (DRG) located just outside the spinal cord within the bony foramen.

Primary afferent activation results in a postsynaptic excitatory event in the spinal cord. Glutamate is the primary neurotransmitter serving this function. Acute activation events are mediated by the α-amino-3-hydroxy-5-methyl-4-isoxazole propionic acid (AMPA)-type glutamate receptor present on the dorsal horn neurons. This receptor produces a robust but short-lasting depolarization of the postsynaptic membrane by increasing sodium conductance and augmenting the activation of the N-methyl-D-aspartate (NMDA)-type glutamate receptor. In addition to glutamate, populations of primary afferents contain and release a variety of neuropeptides, including substance P, calcitonin gene–related peptide, adenosine triphosphate, adenosine, galanin, and somatostatin and growth factors, including brain-derived nerve growth factor.[10]

Neurobiology of the Spinal Cord and Spinal Trigeminal Nucleus

Primary afferent fibers enter the gray matter of the spinal cord through the *dorsal root entry zone* and innervate the spinal cord. The majority of heavily myelinated primary afferent fibers (Aα, Aβ) carrying sensory information, including tactile, pressure, and vibratory sense, enter in dorsal roots, traverse across the top of the dorsal horn of the spinal cord (Lissauer tract), and ascend ipsilaterally within the dorsal column and provide collateral branches into the gray matter of the dorsal horn. The small-diameter, lightly myelinated and unmyelinated fibers transmitting temperature and nociceptive information enter Lissauer tract and innervate the gray matter of the spinal cord. Unlike the heavily myelinated fibers, these fibers may also ascend rostrally or descend caudally through Lissauer tract before they innervate adjacent spinal levels.

The gray matter of the spinal cord is made up of synaptic terminations of primary afferents and the second-order neurons that form the first stage of processing and integration of sensory information. The gray matter of the spinal cord is divided into 10 laminae on the basis of histologic appearance. The dorsal horn includes laminae I to VI and represents the primary sensory complement of the spinal cord (Fig. 56-1). The ventral horn, including laminae VII to IX and lamina X, is involved in somatic motor and autonomic functions, respectively. *Somatic* C-fiber nociceptive afferent endings primarily terminate in the laminae I and II of the same and/or one to two adjacent spinal segments from which they entered from the periphery, whereas *visceral* C-fiber nociceptive afferents can terminate in the dorsal horn more than five segments rostrally or caudally. They terminate in the ipsilateral laminae I, II, V, X, and also in contralateral laminae V and X. Therefore, visceral afferents have a wider branching pattern and

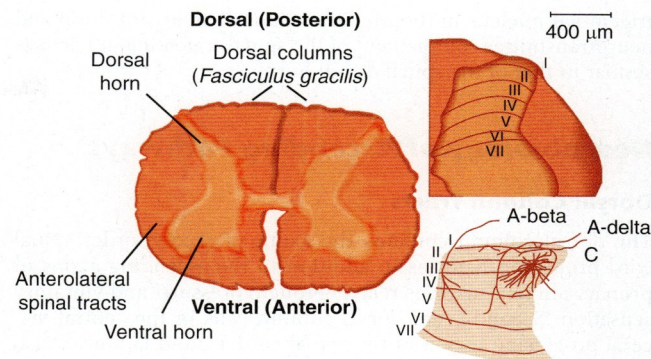

Figure 56-1 Histologic sections and schematic diagrams of the spinal dorsal horn. The histologic section at left is from the lumbar segment of the spinal cord. It is labeled to show the relationship between the major spinal somatosensory structures. The histologic section at right is from the rat lumbar spinal cord. The *outer heavy lines* show the boundary of the spinal gray matter and the *inner heavy lines* show the boundaries of Rexed laminae. These boundaries are established by the histologic characteristics of each zone, and the layers are identified by the Roman numerals. The drawing at the bottom illustrates the pattern of primary afferent innervation to the nonhuman primate spinal dorsal horn. The large myelinated (A-beta) fibers segregate to the dorsal aspect of an entering root and then track medially in the dorsal horn and terminate in layers III to V. The small myelinated (A-delta) fibers and C fibers that carry nociceptive information segregate ventrally in the entering roots, course laterally in the dorsal horn, and then largely terminate in the superficial layers (I and II) of the dorsal horn. (Adapted with permission from Raja SN, Dougherty PM. Anatomy and physiology of somatosensory and pain processing. In: Benzon HT, Raja SN, Molloy RE, et al., eds. *Essentials of Pain Medicine and Regional Anesthesia.* 2nd ed. Philadelphia, PA: Elsevier-Churchill Livingstone;2005:3.)

the nociceptive information they transmit is less localizable to a particular area of the body.

In addition to the primary afferent endings, neurons of the descending pathways and local interneurons also innervate the superficial dorsal horn (laminae I and II). The outer marginal layer or lamina I contain interneurons and cells that send axonal projections to the brainstem and midbrain structures. The substantia gelatinosa, or lamina II, also contains excitatory and inhibitory interneurons but fewer projection neurons. Laminae III and IV contain interneurons and the second-order neurons that make up the dorsal column pathways relaying nonnociceptive sensory and proprioceptive information. Laminae IV to VI contain interneurons and a modest portion of nociceptive projection neurons that distribute input to the brainstem and thalamus.

Nociceptive somatic input is primarily transmitted by second-order lamina I, IV, and V projection neurons as the contralateral spinothalamic tract (STT) pathway traveling to numerous brainstem regions and the thalamus.[11] There is a nociceptive visceral processing area in laminae III, IV, V, VII, and X. The visceral nociceptive input is relayed by second-order neurons whose axons travel within the dorsal column. Like the fibers transmitting nonnoxious sensory information, these fibers remain uncrossed until relayed with the crossed medial lemniscal fibers to the thalamus. The visceral pain information transmitted by the ventral STT is likely originating from cells also receiving somatic nociceptive input. Nociceptive and nonnociceptive sensory information from the head, neck, and dura transmitted via the trigeminal nerve innervates the dorsal horn of the spinal trigeminal nucleus in the caudal medulla. The organization and neurotransmitter complement of the spinal trigeminal nucleus is similar to that of the spinal dorsal horn.

Neurobiology of Ascending Pathways

Dorsal Column Tracts

The dorsal column contains the axons of second-order spinal cord projection neurons in addition to the ascending axons of primary afferent neurons relaying touch, pressure, and vibratory sensation. Second-order dorsal column cells in the central visceral processing region of the spinal cord around lamina X also respond to noxious visceral stimulation and converge on some of the thalamic cells receiving nociceptive information from the skin and other somatic structures.

Spinothalamic Tract

Spinothalamic tract (STT) neurons are the primary relay cells providing nociceptive input from the spinal cord to supraspinal levels. The axons of STT cells cross the midline of the spinal cord through the anterior white commissure and ascend primarily in the contralateral and anterolateral tracts. The axons of STT cells terminate primarily in the posterior complex of the thalamus, including the ventral posterior lateral and ventral posterior medial nuclei. Nonnoxious sensory input from the same body region converges on the same target thalamic neurons providing somatotopic encoding for localization of the input onto the cortical representation of the specific body region, allowing the ability to locate the source of the nociceptive input. The STT cells receiving noxious somatic input are predominantly situated in lamina I and the lateral aspect of the dorsal horn in laminae IV to V.[11] However, other STT neurons are scattered throughout the deep dorsal horn, intermediate region, including lamina X, and even in lamina VII of the ventral horn. These STT cells receive both somatic and visceral nociceptive information.

Spinohypothalamic, Limbic, and Cortical Connections

Pain is a sensory experience but also has an affective component to the perception of noxious stimuli. Pain can provoke fear, anxiety, and depression, resulting in autonomic responses, including increased heart rate and blood pressure as well as the endocrine stress response. These responses to noxious stimuli are mediated by the spinohypothalamic and spinoamygdalar pathways. In addition to their affective function, these regions are also thought to be involved in antinociception. Ascending axonal projections of these pathways arise predominantly from the spinal cord laminae I and X.

Neurobiology of Descending Pathways

The primary components of this descending pain inhibition system, but certainly not all-inclusive, is the "triad" of the periaqueductal gray (PAG), the rostral ventral medulla (RVM), and the dorsolateral pontine tegmentum (DLPT).[12] The PAG is an important site for the production of antinociception following electrical or chemical activation, or the injection of opioid receptor agonists. The endogenous opioid enkephalin is present within this nucleus, and opioid receptors of each subtype are present in this region. The PAG provides dense projections to the RVM, the locus coeruleus, and A7 nuclei.[13] Although the RVM can function as a relay nucleus in the production of antinociception by more cephalad midbrain structures, including the PAG, it also has a primary role in the suppression of nociceptive transmission at the level of the spinal cord. The suppression of nociceptive reflex behavior is mediated by the axons of RVM neurons that descend within the dorsolateral funiculus and terminate bilaterally in laminae I, II, V, VI, and VII of the spinal cord. Anatomic studies have shown that these axons terminate coincident with interneurons of the dorsal horn that are related to nociceptive transmission.[14] Consistent with the anatomic terminations of the RVM axons, physiologic studies have shown that stimulation of the RVM results in the inhibition of a population of nociceptive-specific neurons within the dorsal horn as well as selective inhibition of the nociceptive responses of wide-dynamic range neurons.[15] The DLPT is also an important component of spinal cord nociceptive modulation. It contains all of the noradrenergic neurons that project to the RVM and the spinal cord, and electrical stimulation of the DLPT sites produces spinal cord α_2-adrenergic receptor–mediated analgesia.[16]

Neurobiology of Supraspinal Structures Involved in Higher Cortical Processing

Higher cortical centers play a role in the perception of painful stimuli as well as the integration of the sensory-discriminative and affective components of the noxious stimulation. The localization of the neural structures involved in this perception and integration is still in its adolescence. The development of positron emission tomography and functional magnetic resonance imaging technologies has moved this research forward. These imaging technologies produce indirect evidence of neural activity related to pain stimulation. The primary and secondary somatosensory cortexes, the anterior cingulate gyrus, the insula, and the prefrontal cortex appear to be involved in the higher processing of somatic and visceral pain.[17] As the primary and secondary cortexes are known to be somatosensory processing regions, the imaging studies are consistent with a sensory-discriminative role of these structures. The insula and frontal cortex may contribute to memory and learning of events related to painful stimuli. The anterior cingulate cortex is thought to be involved in the analysis of the emotional significance of the painful input.

Transition from Acute to Persistent or Chronic Nociception

Pain sensation is unique among the somatosensory modalities in that it does not rapidly adapt to prolonged stimulation as do the other sensory modalities, such as fine touch. In fact, continued stimulation may produce greater noxious sensation or reduce the stimulus threshold or intensity that is necessary for the appreciation of the sensation as noxious. For instance, previously innocuous thermal or mechanical stimulation (e.g., warm water of a shower or the light touch of a towel) may be perceived as painful following a prior noxious stimulus (e.g., sunburn). This is termed *allodynia*. Another example of an altered pain state that may follow an acute injury is that of *hyperalgesia*, in which a previously noxious stimulus is perceived as more painful. The sensation of increased intensity of noxious stimulation at the site of the injury is the result of the sensitization of the peripheral nociceptors.

Persistent C fiber, but not Aβ fiber, the primary afferent activation of lamina I and lamina V (as occurs with tissue injury and inflammation), has been shown to enhance the response to subsequent stimulation and augment the size of the receptive field of the respective dorsal horn neuron. Therefore, afferent input from adjacent dermatomal areas now produces neuronal excitation. Furthermore, nonnoxious stimulation becomes increasingly able to activate these neurons. This general phenomenon has come to be termed *wind-up* or *central sensitization*.[18] This activation is thought to explain the allodynia and hyperalgesia observed surrounding the site of injury.

In addition to the alteration of the chemical milieu surrounding the primary afferent distal terminal that results from injury or persistent high-intensity stimulation, axonal sprouting and the formation of neuroma may occur. The neuroma may have an altered complement of ion channels, including an upregulation of sodium channels or a downregulation of potassium channels, which has the net result of increasing neuronal excitability and increasing nociceptive transmission. It has been shown that, following nerve damage, an increase in the expression of sodium channels occurs in the neuroma and the DRG. Numerous sodium channels exist on primary afferents; Nav1.8 and 1.9 subtypes are primarily found on C-fiber DRG cells. Genetic "knock-down" or removal of the Nav1.8 channel had no effect on baseline pain thresholds; however, it reversed nerve injury–evoked nociception.[19] Also following nerve damage, potassium currents have been shown to be reduced, suggesting a reduction in these channels contributing to spontaneous nociceptive activity. Consistent with this notion, it has been observed that potassium channel antagonists increase and potassium channel agonists decrease ectopic firing after peripheral nerve injury.[20]

Neuromas of injured primary afferents have altered sensitivity to a number of humoral factors, including cytokines, prostaglandins, and catecholamines. These factors are released from a variety of cell types, including inflammatory cells and neuronal support cells. Cytokines directly activate the nerve and neuroma through receptors that become expressed in the membrane after the nerve injury. A molecule that has been shown to have a prominent role following nerve damage is tumor necrosis factor subunit *alpha* (TNF-α).[21] Shortly after injury, TNF-α decreases potassium conductance, increasing neuronal excitability, whereas the long-term changes may be produced through the activation of second messenger systems, resulting in altered protein production. Application of TNF-α to the peripheral nerve results in hyperalgesia and systemic delivery of antibodies to TNF-α or TNF-α–binding protein reduces neuropathic pain.

Prostaglandins are also released from inflammatory cells following nerve and tissue damage. They can enhance the opening of Nav1.8 channels by acting though receptors on the afferent terminal.

Although acute noxious stimuli are transmitted to the spinal cord via Aδ and C fibers, the presence of allodynia is thought to be mediated by the activation of large-diameter Aβ fibers through what has been termed a *phenotypic* switch.[2] Prior to this peripheral injury, the Aβ fibers, unlike the C fibers, do not express substance P. However, following injury these fibers were able to express this neuropeptide.[22] These data therefore implicate Aβ fibers in the transmission of noxious peripheral stimulation and provide further support for the involvement of somatic Aβ fibers in at least some form of the allodynic pain states. Furthermore, the blockade of Aβ fibers results in a reduction in light-touch–evoked allodynia.[23] This phenotypic switch of Aβ fibers may represent another avenue for therapeutic intervention; however, the difficulty will be in differentiating between those Aβ fibers involved in noxious versus nonnoxious sensory information.

Management of Common Pain Syndromes

Low Back Pain: Radicular Pain Syndromes

The common causes of low back pain include radicular pain/radiculopathy from herniated disc or spinal/foraminal stenosis, facet syndrome, and internal disc disruption. Myofascial pain syndrome also causes back pain, whereas sacroiliac joint syndrome and piriformis syndrome cause mostly buttock pain but can present as low back pain or radicular pain. Radicular symptoms of pain, paresthesias, and numbness in a typical dermatomal distribution in the presence of objective signs of weakness, diminished reflexes, and positive straight-leg raise are secondary to pathology or dysfunction of the sensory spinal nerve roots. Low back pain, with or without radicular pain, is mostly due to lesions of the intervertebral discs and degenerative spinal disorders. Other causes include spinal metastasis, vertebral body fractures, infections, abdominal aortic aneurysm, and chronic pancreatic lesions.

Low back and radicular pain secondary to a herniated disc is due to mechanical nerve root compression and the subsequent inflammatory process. The presence of a herniated disc does not necessarily result in pain. Up to 36% of the general population[24] and up to 53% of pregnant women[25] can have an asymptomatic herniated disc. Follow-up studies on patients with a herniated disc show spontaneous regression without treatment, absence of symptoms in the presence of more abnormalities, and partial or complete resolution with treatment that includes medications, bed rest, physical therapy, traction, or epidural steroids.[26] If symptomatic, the patient usually presents with low back pain and radicular symptoms that include paresthesias as well as numbness and weakness in the distribution of the involved nerve root. Gait disturbances, loss of sensation, reduced muscle strength, and diminished reflexes involve the appropriate affected dermatomal distribution.

Inflammation in the spinal canal secondary to a herniated disc plays an important role in the causation of back and radicular pain. Herniated nucleus pulposus results in local release of cytokines and other inflammatory mediators that cause a chemical radiculitis. High levels of phospholipase A_2 activity were noted in human disc fragments removed at surgery from patients with symptomatic radiculopathy. Increased levels of the inflammatory cytokines interleukin-6 and interleukin-8 were noted from disc material taken from patients with known disc disease.[27] The application of disc material onto spinal nerve roots can induce functional and morphologic changes in the nerves. Disc cells express TNF-α, which, when applied to spinal nerve roots, causes changes similar to those seen after application of disc material; selective inhibition of TNF-α may reduce the intraneural edema.[28] A double-blind, placebo-controlled study showed that an intradiscal injection of 1.5 mg of etanercept, a TNF-α inhibitor, in a pain-generating disc did not reduce the pain scores or disability scores of patients with chronic discogenic pain or lumbosacral radiculopathy.[29] The use of the potent disease-modifying antirheumatic drugs, either intravenously or epidurally, in patients with low back pain is in its infancy. A review of the literature on the subject showed some studies to be of low quality, results that were inconclusive, or efficacies that were short-term.[30]

For patients with radicular symptoms who do not respond to conservative management, epidural steroid injections (ESIs) may be useful. Epidural steroids have an anti-inflammatory effect related to inhibition of phospholipase A_2 activity. In addition, steroids have an antinociceptive effect. The local application of methylprednisolone blocks transmission of C fibers but not the Aβ fibers. Several prospective randomized controlled studies have demonstrated short-term efficacy of ESIs for treatment of lumbar spine radiculopathy whereas others have not.[31,32] Another study demonstrated less leg pain and sensory deficit with ESI, but the incidence of surgery was the same between the steroid and the control groups.[33] For cervical ESIs, the few studies that have been done are mostly descriptive and their results were the same as in lumbar ESIs, that is, transient relief from the injections. The transient efficacy, that is, no more than 3 months, has to be viewed against the natural history of patients with herniated disc and spinal stenosis as these patients seem to do well over time with conservative management. The transient relief provided by ESIs may minimize the need for opioids and potent anti-inflammatory medications and their related side effects.[34] ESIs should be a component, but not the sole modality, of the conservative management of radicular pain.

A transforaminal approach can be employed to deposit steroid in the anterolateral epidural space, where the herniated disc is located, through the intervertebral foramina, and distally along the nerve root (Fig. 56-2). This approach is especially indicated in radicular pain specific to a single nerve root. Prospective randomized studies on transforaminal ESIs show the same results as with the interlaminar approach, that is, short-term efficacy of the injection.[35,36] The transforaminal approach has a better rationale than the midline interlaminar approach, and studies that compared the two approaches show better efficacy with the transforaminal approach.[37,38]

It is advisable that fluoroscopy be used in ESI, especially with the transforaminal approach, to assure insertion of the needle at the affected vertebral level and document the flow of the contrast medium (and the drug). Reassessment should be carried out 2 to 3 weeks after the initial injection. The use of multiple ESIs in a patient, with a short interval between injections, is not advised. If there is no response to an initial injection, it can be repeated once because some patients require a second injection before they respond. If there is partial response, up to three injections can be performed.

The complications of ESI may be due to the technique or from the injected drug, as well as the vehicle and additives. Complications related to the technique include needle trauma, vasospasm, and infection. Glucocorticoids reduce the hypoglycemic effect of insulin and interfere with blood glucose control in patients with diabetes mellitus. Insulin sensitivity may be impaired, there may be no change in the glycated hemoglobin (HbA_{1c}) levels, or the blood glucose can be increased for 1 week after ESIs. A single dose of 80 mg of methylprednisolone can suppress plasma cortisol levels and the ability to secrete cortisol in response to synthetic corticotropin for up to 3 weeks. Epidural triamcinolone, 80 mg, can suppress serum cortisol and corticotropin levels for up to 7 days after injection. The median recovery to normal levels occurs within 1 month after the last injection, and full recovery is at 3 months.[39]

Injury to the brain or spinal cord can occur with transforaminal ESIs.[40] The cerebral/cerebellar events can be ascribed to trauma to the vertebral artery, vasospasm from the injected steroid or dye, or embolism of the particulate steroid via the vertebral artery.[41,42] The spinal cord injuries can be ascribed to injury to the radicular artery accompanying the nerve root, spasm of the radicular artery from the injected dye or steroid, or embolism of the particulate steroid. The occurrence of adverse events at the lumbar level has been ascribed to intra-arterial injection into an abnormally low-lying artery of Adamkiewicz. These adverse events have also been described after injection of local anesthetic or dye, without steroid.[42] Huntoon[43] noted that the vertebral, ascending cervical, and deep cervical arteries supply segmental medullary vessels and that the ascending and deep cervical arteries are within 2 mm of the site of insertion of the needle for cervical transforaminal ESIs. The proximity of these arteries to the site of needle placement makes these blood vessels vulnerable to trauma or unintentional sites of injection of the steroid. Occlusion of the vessels occurs from the particulate steroids. Methylprednisolone acetate has the largest particle size, betamethasone the smallest particles, and triamcinolone acetonide is in between (Fig. 56-3).[42] Dexamethasone has no identifiable particles. Dexamethasone appears to be ideal for transforaminal ESIs; however, it is easily washed out from the epidural space, and preliminary studies showed its efficacy

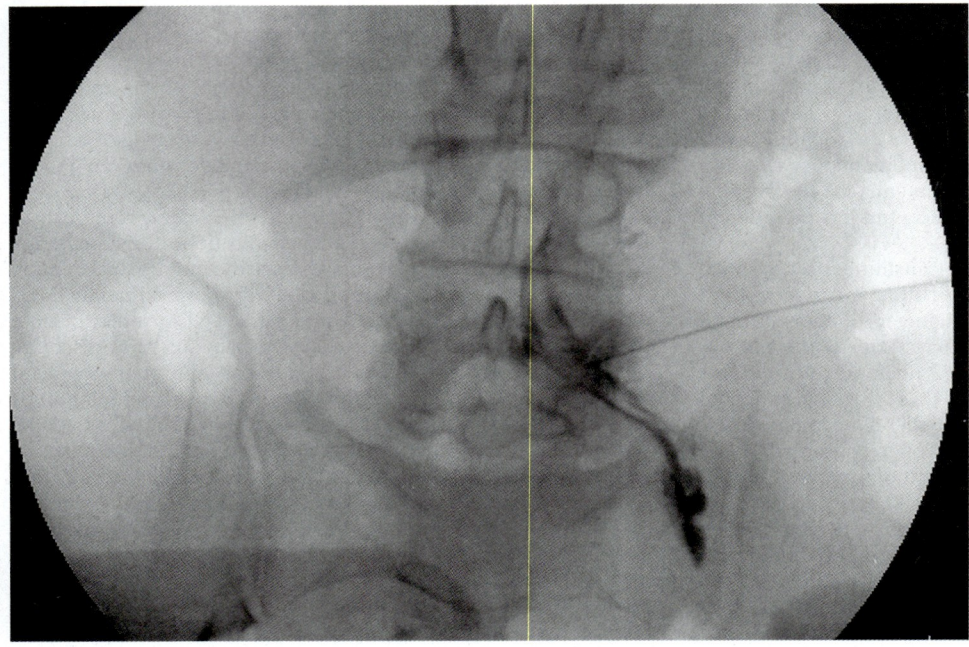

Figure 56-2 Right L5 transforaminal epidural injection. Note the spread of the contrast medium proximally into the lateral epidural space and distally along the nerve root.

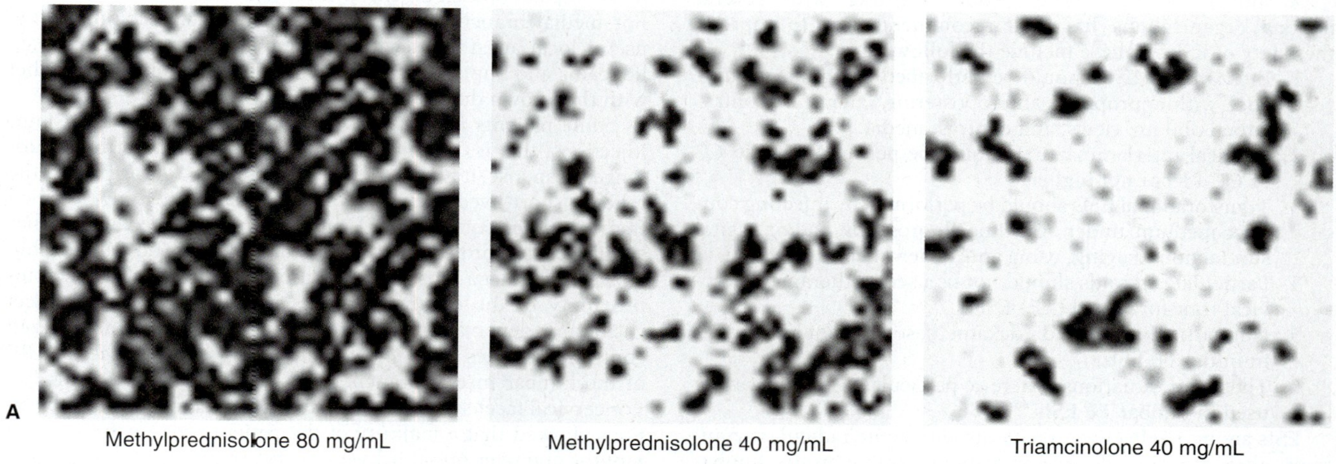

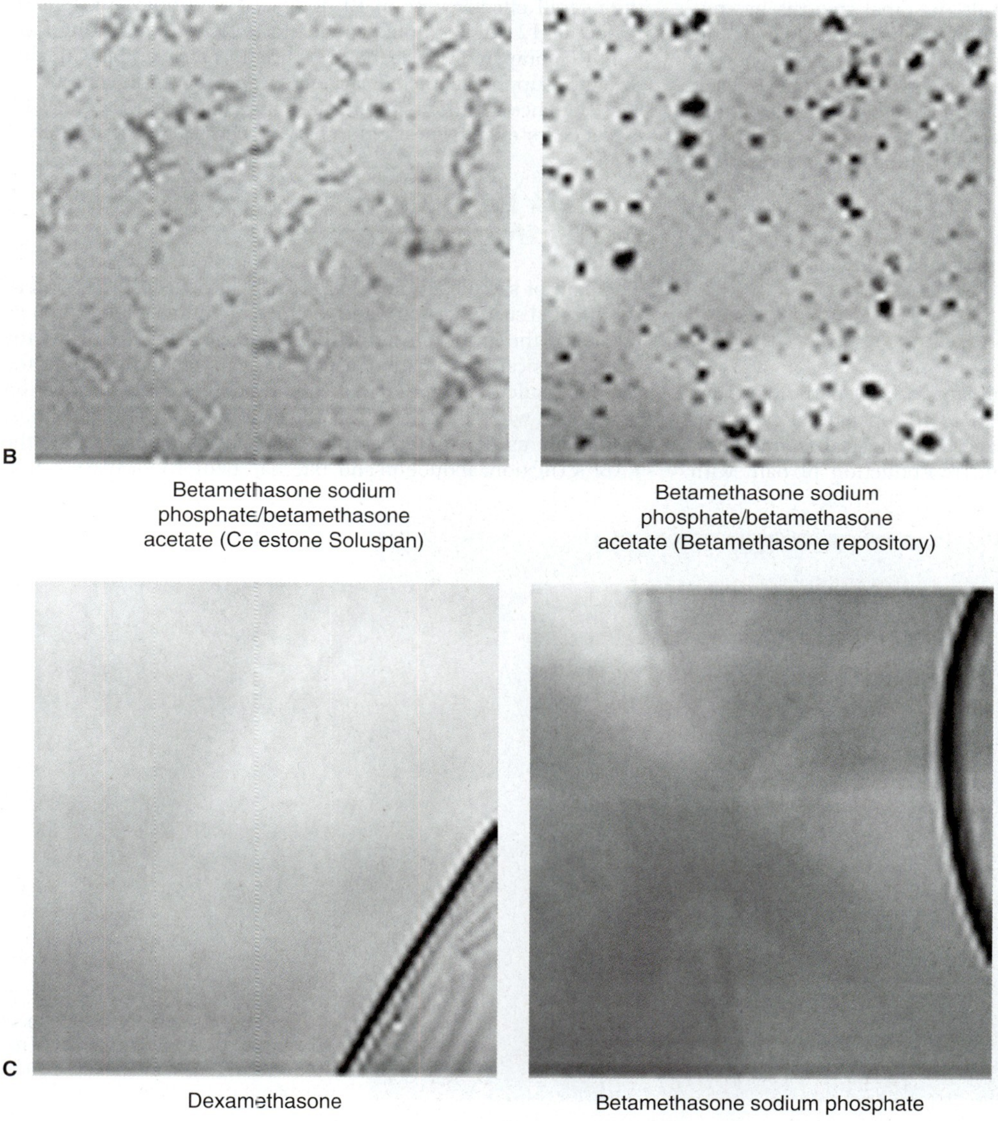

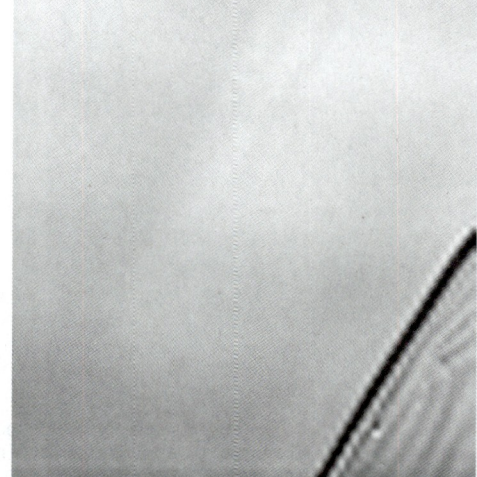
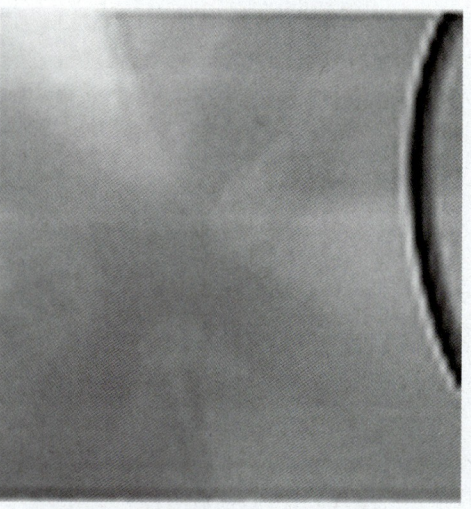

Figure 56-3 **A:** Typical microscopic appearances of methylprednisolone, 80 mg/mL and 40 mg/mL, and triamcinolone 40 mg/mL. The particles are amorphous in appearance. **B:** The particles of commercial betamethasone (Celestone Soluspan) are rodlike and lucent, whereas those of the compounded betamethasone (betamethasone repository) are amorphous. **C:** Note that dexamethasone is pure liquid. (Adapted with permission from Benzon HT, Chew TL, McCarthy R, et al. Comparison of the particle sizes of the different steroids and the effect of dilution: a review of the relative neurotoxicities of the steroids. *Anesthesiology*. 2007;106:331.)

to be of shorter duration than particulate steroids. Recent studies showed the efficacy of the nonparticulate dexamethasone to be the same as the particulate steroids.[44,45]

A multispecialty working group, together with several national organizations, has made recommendations to improve the safety of ESIs.[46] These include the following:

1. Interlaminar ESIs should be performed using image guidance with appropriate anteroposterior, lateral, or contralateral oblique views, and contrast media.
2. Cervical interlaminar ESI should be performed at C6-C7 or C7-T1 but not higher.
3. Transforaminal ESIs should be performed by injecting contrast medium under real-time fluoroscopy and/or digital subtraction imaging, using an AP view, before injection.
4. Particulate steroids should not be used in therapeutic cervical transforaminal (TF) ESIs.
5. Nonparticulate steroid (dexamethasone) should be used in initial TF ESIs.
6. There are situations where a particulate steroid can be used in lumbar TF ESIs.[46]

ESIs are more effective in patients with acute radicular symptoms; they are not effective in patients with chronic lumbar radiculopathy.[47] The efficacy of ESIs in spinal stenosis has not been established. It has been shown not to be better than an epidural local anesthetic.[48] However, local anesthetic may not be the appropriate control intervention because it also relieves back pain.[49] To have a long-term effect in spinal stenosis, ESIs should be part of a multidisciplinary approach.

Gabapentin appears to be effective in treating lumbosacral radicular pain.[50] However, ESIs resulted in greater reductions in worst leg pain and the patients experienced a positive outcome compared to gabapentin. Duloxetine was noted to be superior to placebo in treating the neuropathic component of chronic low back pain.[51]

Low Back Pain: Facet Syndrome

Patients with low back pain secondary to facet pathology have pain in the low back that radiates to the ipsilateral posterior thigh and usually ends at the knee. On physical examination there is paraspinal tenderness and reproduction of pain with extension–rotation maneuvers of the back. The diagnosis of facet syndrome is arrived at by a combination of the patient's history, physical examination findings, and a positive response to diagnostic medial branch blocks or facet joint injections (Fig. 56-4). For medial branch blocks, some investigators recommend the use of local anesthetics with different durations of effect (e.g., lidocaine and bupivacaine) and to correlate the duration of relief with the known duration of effect of the drug.

Some patients may have a prolonged response to facet joint injections, that is, up to 3 to 6 months. If the patient has a prolonged response, it is best to wait for recurrence of the pain. If the relief is short-lived, especially after medial branch blocks, then thermal radiofrequency (RF) rhizotomy of the medial branches should be performed. It appears that there is no relationship between the mean sensory stimulation threshold (which denotes proximity of the electrode to the nerve) during lumbar facet rhizotomy denervation and treatment outcome.[52] Randomized controlled studies have shown improvements after thermal RF of the lumbar medial branches that lasted 3 to 12 months.[53-55] For cervical facet syndrome, a systematic review of eight publications showed that a majority of the patients were pain free at 6 months and over one-third were pain-free at 1 year.[56] Regarding the overall effectiveness of RF for facet syndrome, a Cochrane review of 12 studies noted moderate evidence supporting facet joint RF compared to placebo over the short term and low quality evidence supporting the efficacy of RF over steroid injections.[57] A best evidence synthesis publication concluded there was level 2 evidence for effectiveness of lumbar and cervical RF neurotomy.[58]

Buttock Pain: Sacroiliac Joint Syndrome and Piriformis Syndrome

The pain of sacroiliac joint syndrome is located in the region of the affected sacroiliac joint and the medial buttock. The pain may radiate to the groin, posterior thigh, and occasionally below the knee. Physical examination usually reveals tenderness over the sacroiliac sulcus, reduction in the joint mobility, and reproduction of the pain when the affected sacroiliac joint is stressed. The most commonly used tests for sacroiliac joint dysfunction include the FABER (flexion, abduction and external rotation), or Patrick, test,

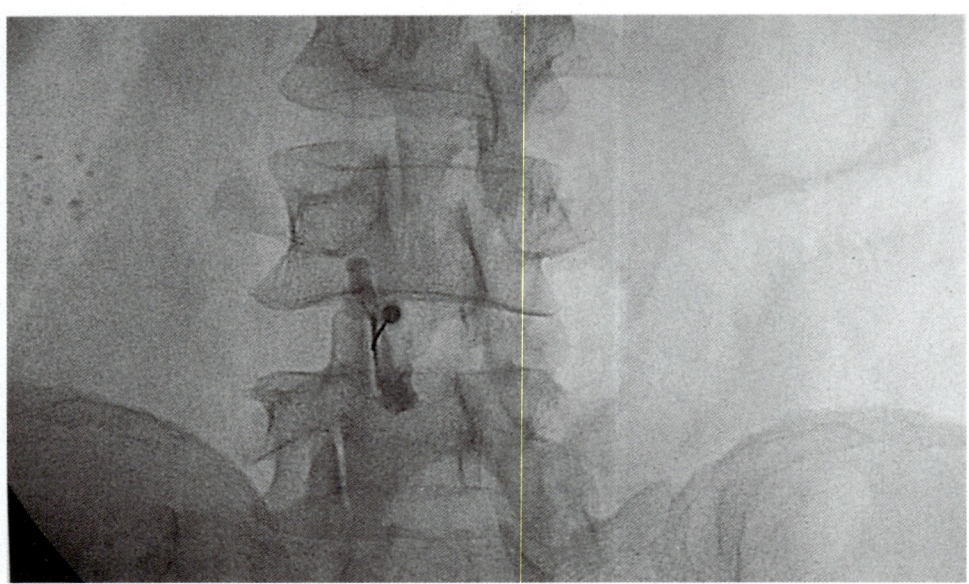

Figure 56-4 Left L4 to L5 facet joint injection. The injection of 5 mL of contrast medium demonstrates the extent of the joint capsule.

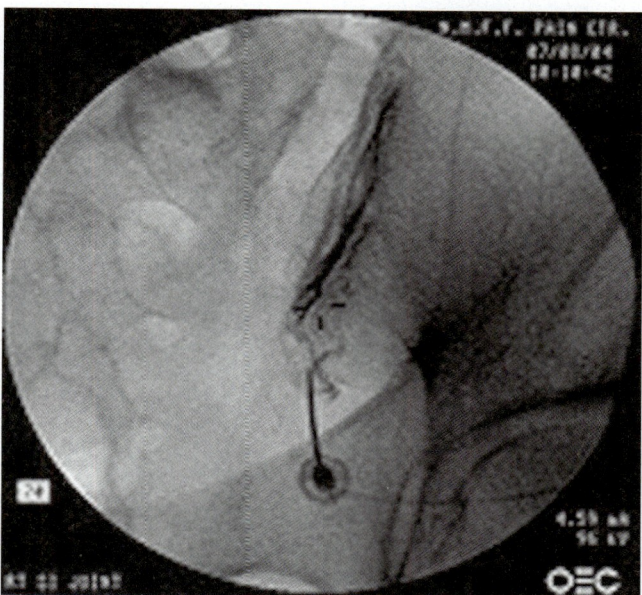

Figure 56-5 Sacroiliac joint injection. Note the spread of the contrast medium along the joint. (Adapted with permission from Benzon HT, Nader A. Hip, sacroiliac joint, and piriformis injections. In: Benzon HT, Rathmell J, Wu C, et al., eds. *Raj's Practical Management of Pain.* 4th ed. Philadelphia, PA: Mosby Elsevier;2008:1070.)

and the Gaenslen, Yeoman, sacroiliac shear, and Gillet tests. The FABER (Patrick) and the Yeoman test do not rule out hip pathology, whereas the Yeoman and the shear tests are more specific for sacroiliac joint syndrome. The presence of symptoms and physical examination findings suggestive of sacroiliac (SI) joint syndrome, pain on three of the provocative tests, and a positive response to SI joint injection are adequate to make the diagnosis of SI joint syndrome.

The treatments for SI joint syndrome include physical therapy, manipulation, intra-articular steroid injections (Fig. 56-5), RF denervation, and surgical fusion of the joint. Physical therapy and chiropractic manipulations are used extensively for the treatment of SI joint disease; however, there is no large outcome study validating their use. Intra-articular injections of steroid (40 to 80 mg of methylprednisolone or other depot steroid) and local anesthetic into the SI joint may result in a few months of pain relief, but again, no prospective controlled studies support their use.

Denervation of the lower portion of the SI joint may be achieved by the creation of bipolar RF strip lesions along the dorsal border of the SI joint in a leapfrog manner. It has been demonstrated that the use of a multilesion probe (Simplicity III, NeuroTherm) along the posterior sacral plate lateral to the foraminas can be effective for at least 6 months in approximately 50% of patients.[59] Local anesthetic blockade of the sensory innervation of the dorsal portion of the SI joint—the medial branch of the dorsal rami of L5 and the lateral branches of the dorsal rami of S1 to S3—can be performed when the relief from the SI joint injection is temporary. Relief from the local anesthetic block may last weeks to months when combined with physical therapy. Thermal RF lesioning of the lateral branches is performed for a more lasting relief. The bigger lesions created by the water-cooled RF technique (Fig. 56-6)[60] are inherently more effective because it accommodates for the variations in the location of the lateral branches along the lateral border of the sacral foraminas.

Piriformis Syndrome

Piriformis syndrome, another pain syndrome that originates in the buttocks, comprises 5% to 6% of patients referred for the treatment of back and leg pain. It occurs after trauma, surgery, and infection, or from compression of one of the components of the sciatic nerve as it runs between two divisions of the piriformis muscle.[61] Patients with piriformis syndrome complain of buttock pain with or without radiation to the ipsilateral leg. The buttock pain usually extends from the sacrum to the greater trochanter of the femur, whereas irritation of the sciatic nerve results in a buttock pain that radiates to the ipsilateral leg. Prolonged sitting, as in driving or biking, or getting up from a sitting position aggravates the pain.

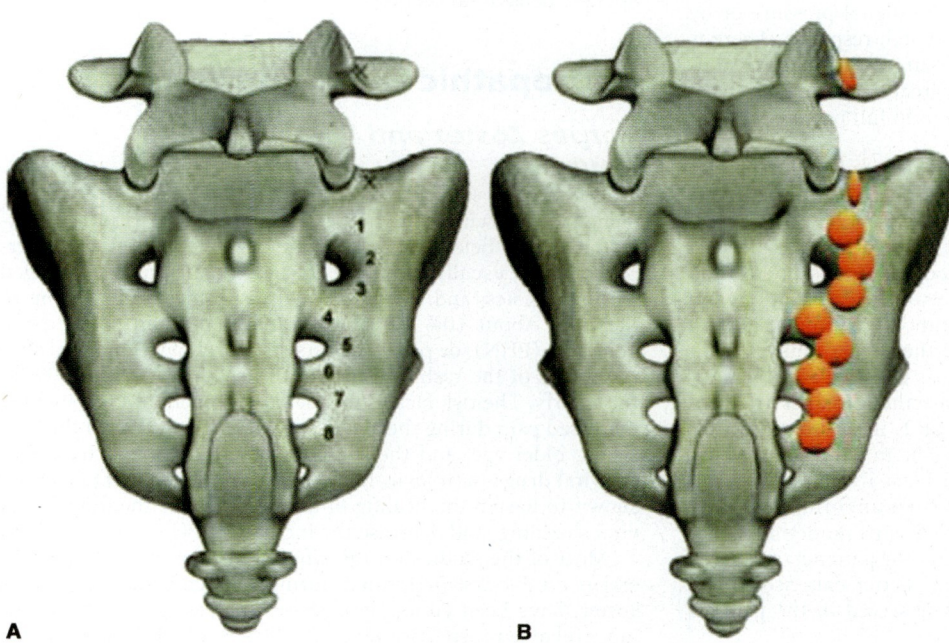

Figure 56-6 Target points (**A**) and expected lesions (**B**) from water-cooled radiofrequency denervation at the right L5 medial branch and the S1, S2, and S3 lateral branches. (Adapted with permission from Cohen SP, Hurley RW, Buckenmaier CC 3rd, et al. Randomized placebo-controlled study evaluating lateral branch radiofrequency denervation for sacroiliac joint pain. *Anesthesiology.* 2008;109:279–88.)

The pain is aggravated by hip flexion, adduction, and internal rotation. Neurologic examination is usually negative. There may be leg numbness when the sciatic nerve is irritated; the straight-leg test may be normal or limited. Three signs confirm the presence of piriformis syndrome[61]: (1) The *Pace sign*, wherein there is pain and weakness on resisted abduction of the hip in a patient who is seated with the hip flexed; (2) the *Lasègue sign*, wherein there is pain on flexion, adduction, and internal rotation of the hip in a patient who is supine (note that some clinicians also call pain on straight-leg raise the Lasègue sign); and (3) the *Freiberg sign*, wherein there is pain on forced internal rotation of the extended thigh. Note that the piriformis is an internal rotator of the flexed hip and an external rotator of the extended hip. The diagnosis of piriformis syndrome is made on clinical grounds. Electromyography may detect myopathic and neuropathic changes, including a delay in the H-reflex, with the affected leg in a flexed, adducted, and internally rotated (FAIR) position as compared with the same H-reflex in the normal anatomic position.

The treatments of piriformis syndrome include physical therapy combined with medications such as muscle relaxants, anti-inflammatory drugs, and analgesics to reduce the spasm, inflammation, and pain. Local anesthetic and steroid injections into the piriformis muscle may break the pain/muscle spasm cycle. Techniques involving identification of the piriformis muscle include the use of CT guidance, use of a nerve stimulator, or combined fluoroscopy–nerve stimulator guidance. A randomized study noted similar efficacy of the fluoroscopy- and ultrasound-guided piriformis injections.[62] There appears to be no difference between lidocaine and lidocaine with betamethasone.[63] If relief from the local anesthetic does not last, then the piriformis muscle is injected with 100 units of botulinum toxin A in 2 to 3 mL of local anesthetic.[64,65]

Myofascial Pain Syndrome and Fibromyalgia

Myofascial pain syndrome is a painful regional syndrome characterized by the presence of an active trigger point in a skeletal muscle. The trigger point can be felt as a palpable taut band and manipulation of the trigger point by digital pressure or by penetration by a needle may induce a twitch response. There is spot tenderness in the taut band; pressure on the tender nodule induces pain that the patient recognizes as an experienced pain pattern, and there may be limitation to full passive range of motion of the affected muscle.

The management of myofascial pain syndrome includes repeated applications of a cold spray over the trigger point in line with the involved muscle fibers, followed by gentle massage of the trigger point and stretching of the affected muscle. Physical therapy includes improving posture, body mechanics, relaxation techniques, trigger point massage, postisometric relaxation, and reciprocal inhibition. A part of a multimodal treatment is local anesthetic injection or dry needling of the trigger point. Recent studies show that dry needling may be as effective as local anesthetic injection; however, the local anesthetic makes the procedure less painful. Several injections at 2- to 3-week intervals, followed by physical therapy, may result in a long-term benefit. Botulinum toxin injections have been recommended but the results of clinical studies have not been uniform. In a study using an enriched protocol design (two groups randomized into botulinum toxin and placebo groups after the patients responded to an initial botulinum toxin injection), better pain scores and a reduced number of headaches were observed in the patients injected with botulinum toxin.[66]

Fibromyalgia

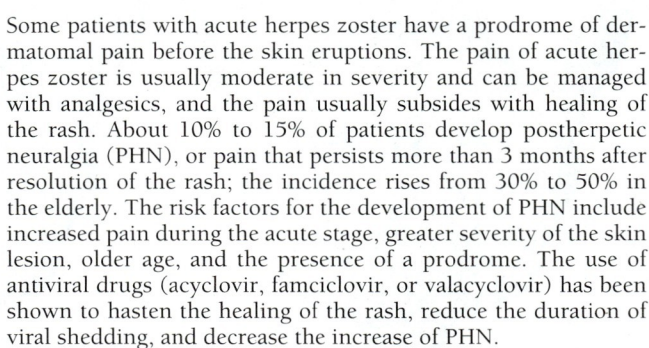

The American College of Rheumatology criteria for classification of fibromyalgia,[67] established in 1990, requires two components: a history of widespread pain for at least 3 months and allodynia to digital pressure at 11 or more of 18 anatomically defined tender points. The tender points are located in the occiput, the intertransverse spaces between C5 and C7, trapezii, supraspinatus, the second rib (just lateral to the costochondral junctions), lateral epicondyles, glutei, greater trochanters, and knees. In 2010, a new diagnostic paradigm was proposed that included a clinician-administered tool for widespread pain index (WPI) and the symptom severity (SS) scale of key characteristic signs and symptoms.[68]

There is a strong genetic and familial component to the development of fibromyalgia. Also, family members of fibromyalgia patients are more likely to have irritable bowel syndrome, temporomandibular disorders, headaches, and a host of other regional pain syndromes. They have higher concentrations of substance P and glutamate in cerebral spinal fluid (CSF) compared with normal controls.[69]

Opioidergic activity is normal or increased in fibromyalgia, and levels of cerebrospinal fluid enkephalins are roughly twice as high in these patients compared to healthy controls.[70] The increased activity of endogenous opioidergic systems explains clinicians' observations that opioids are ineffective in this syndrome. On the other hand, the principal metabolite of norepinephrine, 3-methoxy-4-hydroxyphenethylene glycol (MPHG) is lower in the CSF of patients with fibromyalgia. This may explain the efficacy of drugs that raise levels of both serotonin and norepinephrine (tricyclic antidepressants [TCAs], duloxetine, milnacipran, tramadol).

The optimal treatment of fibromyalgia supports a multifaceted program comprising pharmacologic and nonpharmacologic therapy.[71] Efficacious medications for treatment of fibromyalgia include two serotonin and norepinephrine receptor inhibitors (SNRIs) (duloxetine and milnacipran),[72,73] pregabalin, amitriptyline, gabapentin, and gamma-hydroxybutyrate (sodium oxybate).[74,75] Effective nondrug treatment includes patient education, supportive therapy, exercise programs (specifically low-intensity low-impact programs), and cognitive-behavioral and operant-behavioral therapy.

Neuropathic Pain Syndromes

Herpes Zoster and Postherpetic Neuralgia

Some patients with acute herpes zoster have a prodrome of dermatomal pain before the skin eruptions. The pain of acute herpes zoster is usually moderate in severity and can be managed with analgesics, and the pain usually subsides with healing of the rash. About 10% to 15% of patients develop postherpetic neuralgia (PHN), or pain that persists more than 3 months after resolution of the rash; the incidence rises from 30% to 50% in the elderly. The risk factors for the development of PHN include increased pain during the acute stage, greater severity of the skin lesion, older age, and the presence of a prodrome. The use of antiviral drugs (acyclovir, famciclovir, or valacyclovir) has been shown to hasten the healing of the rash, reduce the duration of viral shedding, and decrease the increase of PHN.

Most of the studies on the efficacy of neuraxial and peripheral nerve blocks, performed during the acute stage of herpes zoster, have been either retrospective or case series. However, more reliable prospective randomized controlled studies provide conflicting results. A study in which epidural methylprednisolone and bupivacaine was compared with acyclovir and prednisolone showed the epidural steroid group to have less pain (1.6% vs. 22%) and less allodynia (4% vs. 12%) at 1 year.[76] Another study in which standard therapy with oral antiviral medications and analgesics was compared with standard therapy and epidural methylprednisolone and bupivacaine noted less pain in the epidural group (48% vs. 58%) at 1 month but not at 3 months (21% vs. 28%).[77] The better results in this study may be related to the greater number of epidural injections (two to four vs. one). To be effective in preventing PHN, the blocks are preferably done within 2 weeks of the onset of rash.

The mainstay of treatment for PHN is pharmacologic management that includes anticonvulsants, opioids, and antidepressants. Although the antidepressants have been found to be effective, their use is precluded by the frequent occurrence of side effects. The side effects include anticholinergic effects such as tachycardia, dry mouth, constipation, and symptoms of prostatism in elderly males. Nortriptyline is preferred over amitriptyline because it is equally effective and better tolerated. Additional efficacious drugs include opioids and tramadol.[78,79] The anticonvulsants gabapentin and pregabalin are usually effective in the management of PHN.[80,81] The side effects of the drugs include somnolence, dizziness, and peripheral edema. Two studies showed that the combination of gabapentin and controlled-release morphine, and gabapentin and nortriptyline, were more effective and required lower daily dosages than when either drug was given alone.[82,83] Based on efficacy, antidepressants are the first choice for neuropathic pain syndromes, followed by opioids, tramadol, and gabapentin/pregabalin. When quality of life, side effects, prevention of addiction, and regulatory issues are considered important in addition to pain relief, then gabapentin/pregabalin may be the first drugs of choice. For the allodynia that accompanies PHN, a lidocaine patch is recommended. Capsaicin 8% topical patch can be used for localized pain.

Interventional techniques may be performed if medications do not control the pain of PHN. Intrathecal methylprednisolone, 60 mg in lidocaine, given once a week for four times, has been observed by some to be more effective in relieving PHN compared with intrathecal lidocaine or no treatment.[84] However, a study that tried to confirm the efficacy of intrathecal steroid had to be stopped because of lack of efficacy.[85] Based on possible risks and the lack of studies confirming its efficacy, a group of experts failed to arrive at a conclusive recommendation regarding the efficacy of intrathecal steroid for PHN.[86] Other interventional techniques for PHN are intrathecal alcohol and spinal cord stimulation (SCS).[87] When a spinal cord stimulator was placed in 28 patients with intractable PHN for 2 years, long-term pain relief was achieved in 23 patients and the median pain score decreased from 9 to 1.[88]

Diabetic Painful Neuropathy

Peripheral neuropathy may be present in approximately 65% of patients with insulin-dependent diabetes, most commonly distal symmetric polyneuropathy, followed by median nerve mononeuropathy at the wrist, and visceral autonomic neuropathy. The incidence of diabetic neuropathy increases with duration of diabetes, age, and degree of hyperglycemia; neuropathies generally develop after persistence of hyperglycemia for several years. The pathophysiology of diabetic neuropathy includes the polyol pathway, microvascular, and glycosylation end-product theories. All pathways result in chronic ischemia of the nerve.

The management of diabetic painful neuropathy (DPN) includes tight control of the patient's blood glucose and pharmacologic therapy. The anticonvulsants gabapentin and pregabalin appear to be effective in the management of DPN, with the efficacy of gabapentin enhanced by the addition of controlled-release morphine or nortriptyline.[82,83] The TCAs are also effective in DPN whereas the selective serotonin reuptake inhibitors are not as effective. The antidepressant duloxetine appears to be effective[89] and, together with its favorable side effect profile compared with the tricyclics, is now widely used in treatment of DPN. The European Federation of Neurological Sciences Task Force and the International Association for the Study of Pain (IASP) Neuropathic Pain Special Interest group (NeuPSIG) now recommend the serotonin–norepinephrine reuptake inhibitors (duloxetine, milnacipran) as the first-choice drugs for the treatment of DPN.[90,91] Finally, the opioids and tramadol are also effective in the treatment of DPN.

Complex Regional Pain Syndrome

Complex regional pain syndrome (CRPS) consists of two types. *CRPS type I* was originally termed *reflex sympathetic dystrophy*, whereas *CRPS type II* represents *causalgia*. The risk factors for the development of CRPS include previous trauma, nerve injury (for causalgia), previous surgery, work-related injuries, and female sex. The signs and symptoms of CRPS include spontaneous pain, hyperalgesia, allodynia, plus trophic, sudomotor, vasomotor abnormalities, and, finally, active and passive movement disorders. The clinical features of CRPS type II are the same as in CRPS type I except there is a preceding nerve injury in CRPS II. The IASP proposed diagnostic criteria for CRPS but because the criteria had a high diagnostic sensitivity with a low specificity, it resulted in overdiagnosis. The Budapest criteria, with high sensitivity and improved specificity, have supplanted the IASP criteria.[92]

Treatments for CRPS include sympathetic nerve blocks, physical therapy, and medications. Oral therapy includes gabapentin, memantine (an NMDA blocker), and alendronate.[93] Intravenous infusions include ketamine and bisphosphonates.[94] Ketamine can be given either as a 4- to 5-day infusion at 1 to 7 μg/kg/min (5 to 30 mg/hr in a 70-kg patient) or for 4 hours daily for 10 days at an infusion rate of 0.35 mg/kg/hr (24 mg/hr in a 70-kg person).[95,96] If ketamine infusion is employed, serial determinations of liver enzymes should be serially determined.[97] Intramuscular or subcutaneous calcitonin can also be used.[98] SCS should be considered if the patient does not respond to any of these treatments.[99,100]

Human Immunodeficiency Virus Neuropathy

Symptomatic neuropathy occurs in 10% to 35% of patients who are seropositive for human immunodeficiency virus (HIV), and pathologic abnormalities exist in almost all patients with end-stage AIDS. The sensory neuropathies associated with HIV include distal sensory polyneuropathy, the more common neuropathy related to the viral infection, and antiretroviral toxic neuropathy (ATN) secondary to the treatment. The clinical features of HIV sensory neuropathy typically include painful allodynia and hyperalgesia. The onset is gradual and most commonly involves the lower extremities. The neuropathy and dysesthesia progress from the distal to the more proximal structures. There is minimal subjective or objective motor involvement and this is generally limited to the intrinsic muscles of the foot.

The treatment of HIV sensory neuropathy is symptomatic and includes optimization of the patient's metabolic and nutritional status. Cessation or dose reduction of treatment with nucleoside reverse transcriptase inhibitors may improve the symptoms of ATN. The anticonvulsants, particularly lamotrigine (300 mg/day), can be effective therapy for HIV sensory neuropathy as well as ATN.[101] Gabapentin is also effective at doses of 1,200 to 3,600 mg/day.[102]

Phantom Pain

Nearly all patients with amputated extremities experience nonpainful sensations in the absent, phantom limb. As many as 60% of them experience pain. The onset of pain may be immediate but commonly occurs within the first few days following amputation. Approximately 50% of patients experience a decrease of their pain with time, whereas the other 50% report no change or an increase in pain over time. Phantom pain is caused by both peripheral and central factors. Peripheral mechanisms include neuromas, an increase in C-fiber activity, and sodium channel activation. Central mechanisms include abnormal firing of spinal internuncial neurons and supraspinal involvement secondary to the development of new synaptic connections in the cerebral cortex.

Numerous prophylactic measures have, with variable success, been undertaken in an attempt to reduce the incidence of phantom limb pain. These include perioperative epidural infusions of opioids and local anesthetics or clonidine, and continuous brachial plexus blockade with memantine. The treatment of phantom limb pain includes pharmacologic and nonpharmacologic measures. A systematic review noted level 2 evidence for the effectiveness of gabapentin, morphine, tramadol, intramuscular botulinum toxin, and epidural ketamine.[103] Nonpharmacologic measures include transcutaneous electrical nerve stimulation, spinal cord stimulators, and biofeedback. A combination of pharmacologic treatment with physical, psychological, or behavioral intervention is probably the most effective approach.

Cancer Pain

Significant pain is present in up to 25% of patients with cancer who are in active treatment and in up to 90% of patients with advanced cancer. The pain of cancer can be somatic, visceral, or neuropathic. Somatic pain tends to be responsive to opioids, nonsteroidal anti-inflammatory drugs (NSAIDs), or cyclooxygenase 2 inhibitors, and is also amenable to treatment with neural blockade. Visceral pain responds to sympathetic nerve blocks, and neuropathic pain is responsive to anticonvulsants, opioids, TCAs, serotonin–norepinephrine reuptake inhibitors, or combinations of these drugs.

Management of cancer pain should be multifaceted and include the following: (1) appropriate tumor-specific antineoplastic therapy, (2) pain medications, (3) interventional management, (4) behavioral and psychological management, and ultimately (5) hospice care. Pharmacologic therapies include opioids, antidepressants, anticonvulsants, NSAIDs, corticosteroids, oral local anesthetics, and topical analgesics. Opioids are the mainstay of treatment for cancer pain as approximately 75% to 95% of patients are responsive positively when appropriate guidelines are followed. Continuous intravenous opioid infusions can be performed during the later stages of the disease. Interventional treatments include neurolytic sympathetic nerve blocks and intrathecal opioids. Vertebroplasty or kyphoplasty may be required for vertebral compression syndromes.

Neurolytic Blocks for Visceral Pain from Cancer

Celiac Plexus Block

The celiac plexus innervates all of the abdominal viscera except the left side of the colon and the pelvic viscera. The plexus contains two large ganglia that receive sympathetic fibers from the greater, lesser, and least splanchnic nerves. It also receives parasympathetic fibers from the vagus nerve. The splanchnic nerves are located retroperitoneally at the level of the T12 and L1 vertebrae, and the celiac plexus is anterior to the crura of the diaphragm and surrounds the abdominal aorta and the celiac and superior mesenteric arteries.

Blockade of the celiac plexus can be achieved by the classic retrocrural approach, an anterocrural approach, or by neurolysis of the splanchnic nerves.[104] For the fluoroscopy-guided procedure, the tip of the needle is directed toward the body of L1 (Fig. 56-7). In the retrocrural approach, the tip of the needle is advanced approximately 1 cm anterior to the anterior and upper border of L1. In the anterocrural or transaortic approach, the tip of the needle is advanced through the lower portion of L1 and the aorta on the left side until blood can no longer be aspirated through the needle. For splanchnic nerve block, the tip of the needle is placed at the anterior portion of the T12 vertebral body. There appears to be no differences in efficacy between the three approaches.[104] Some clinicians perform an initial diagnostic block with a local anesthetic whereas others proceed immediately to a neurolytic block because the results of the diagnostic and neurolytic blocks may not be the same. Better results are usually seen with local anesthetics because of better spread (phenol is viscous and its vascular absorption may relieve pain). Fifty percent alcohol or 6% to 10% phenol is employed for the neurolytic block. The dosages

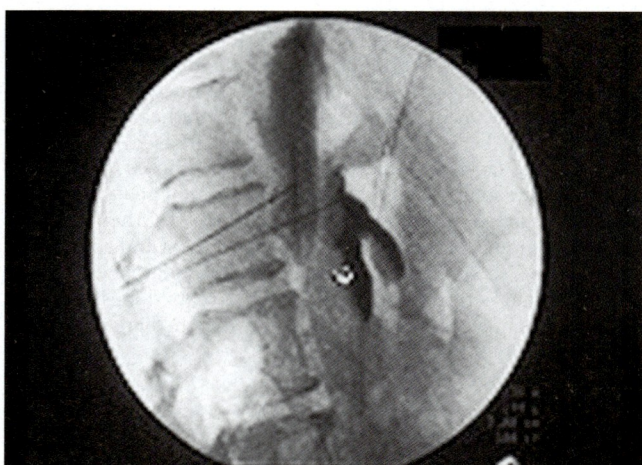

Figure 56-7 Retrocrural versus anterocrural approaches to neurolysis of the celiac plexus. Note that the tip of the needle is in the upper third of L1 and about 1 cm beyond the border of the vertebral body for the retrocrural technique; the spread of the contrast medium is cephalad. In contrast, the tip of the needle is the lower third of L1 and about 3 cm beyond the border of the vertebral body for the anterocrural technique; the spread of the contrast medium is caudad and in front of the aorta. (Adapted with permission from de Leon-Casasola OA. Neurolysis of the sympathetic axis for cancer pain management. In: Benzon HT, Rathmell J, Wu C, et al., eds. *Raj's Practical Management of Pain*. 4th ed. Philadelphia, PA: Mosby Elsevier;2008;918.)

of the neurolytic agents are 30 to 40 mL for the retrocrural and anterocrural approach, and 10 to 15 mL on each side for splanchnic nerve blockade. Complications from the celiac plexus block include orthostatic hypotension, back pain, retroperitoneal hematoma, reactive pleurisy, hiccups, hematuria, transient diarrhea, abdominal aortic dissection, transient motor paralysis, and paraplegia. The paraplegia and transient motor paralysis may be due to spasm of the lumbar segmental arteries that perfuse the spinal cord, direct vascular or neurologic injury, or retrograde spread to the nerve roots or spinal cord.

The efficacy of celiac plexus neurolysis in relieving pain from cancer of the upper abdomen has been substantiated in randomized controlled trials.[105,106] The end points of the studies were lower pain scores, less opioid consumption with a lower incidence of side effects, and equal or better quality of life. A meta-analysis of 21 retrospective studies in 1,145 patients concluded that adequate-to-excellent pain relief was achieved in 89% of the patients during the first 2 weeks following the block and partial-to-complete pain relief continued in 90% of the patients at the 3-month interval.[107] Using the GRADE (grading of recommendations assessment development, and evaluation) level of evidence, a European collaborative group gave a strong recommendation for the use of celiac plexus block for treatment of pancreatic cancer pain.[108]

Superior Hypogastric Plexus Block

Superior hypogastric plexus block is indicated for pelvic pain secondary to cancer and chronic nonmalignant conditions. The plexus is located in the retroperitoneum, bilaterally extending from the lower third of the fifth lumbar vertebra to the upper third of the first sacral vertebra. For blockade of the plexus, the patient is placed in the prone position and two 7-cm needles are inserted, under fluoroscopy, in medial and caudal directions until the tips lie anterior to the L5 to S1 intervertebral disc space. Alternatively, a single needle can be used through a transdiscal approach. After injection of contrast medium, 6 to 8 mL of local anesthetic is used for a diagnostic block while phenol or alcohol is employed for neurolysis. Anterior ultrasound-guided superior hypogastric plexus blocks appear to be effective for pelvic pain.[109] The factors associated with positive outcome include older age, and presence of bladder cancer.[110] The complications are minimal and include nerve root blockade secondary to retrograde spread of the injectate. Case reports support the efficacy of neurolytic superior hypogastric plexus block both in reducing pelvic pain secondary to cancer and in decreasing opioid consumption.

Ganglion Impar Block

Pain in the perineal area associated with malignancies can be treated with neurolysis of the ganglion impar (Walther ganglion), a solitary retroperitoneal structure located anteriorly to the sacrococcygeal junction. Visceral afferents innervating the perineum, distal rectum, anus, distal urethra, vulva, and distal third of vagina converge at the ganglion. For the procedure, the patient is usually prone. The transsacrococcygeal approach is easier to perform; a 20-gauge, 1.5-in needle is inserted through the sacrococcygeal ligament until the tip of the needle is just anterior to the anterior portion of the sacrum. Four to 8 mL of local anesthetic is used for diagnostic block and 8% to 10% phenol or 50% alcohol is used for neurolysis. Similar to superior hypogastric plexus blocks, there are no controlled studies on its efficacy, although case reports confirm its effectiveness in relieving perineal pain secondary to cancer.

Pharmacologic Management of Pain

Opioids

Morphine is the standard for opioid therapy for cancer pain (see Chapter 20, Opioids). It has a variable oral bioavailability between 10% and 45%. The metabolites of morphine include morphine-6-glucuronide, which causes additional analgesia, and morphine-3-glucuronide, which can cause adverse effects. Controlled-release preparations are available, reducing the need to take the drug frequently. The *numbers needed to treat* or NNT for 10 mg of morphine for postoperative pain is 2.9 and its *numbers needed to harm* or NNH is 9.1. Hydromorphone, a μ-receptor agonist, is three to five times more potent than morphine when given orally and five to seven times more potent when given parenterally. Its 3- to 4-hour duration of analgesic effect is similar to that of morphine. Pruritus, sedation, nausea, and vomiting occur less frequently compared with morphine. Its metabolite, hydromorphone-3-glucuronide, lacks analgesic property but possesses properties similar to that of morphine-3-glucuronide.

Methadone has a 60% to 95% bioavailability, high potency, and a long duration of action. It has ideal characteristics that include the lack of an active metabolite, additional salutary effects such as acting as an NMDA receptor antagonist and serotonin reuptake inhibitor, and it is inexpensive. Its potency compared with morphine ranges from 1:1 to 1:2 on acute dosing but can be 1:4 with chronic dosing. It has a long and unpredictable half-life of 8 to 80 hours that makes it difficult to achieve steady-state plasma concentrations, increasing the risk of accumulation and the need for careful and individualized dosing. There has been an "epidemic" of deaths due to unintentional overdose from methadone[111] because many physicians do not appreciate the consequences of the drug's long and unpredictable half-life. Methadone also causes cardiac rhythm abnormalities, including QT prolongation and Torsade de pointes. Most reports are based on high-dose maintenance (>120 mg) for the treatment of addiction; however, such occurrences have also been reported with lower dosages. Experts recommend disclosure of the dysrythmogenic property of the drug (especially for patients with cardiac disease), a screening electrocardiogram (ECG) before initiation of therapy, follow-up ECGs in patients who are taking over 100 mg daily, and risk stratification.[112] The risk should be discussed when the QTc interval is 450 to 500 ms and the methadone dose reduced or discontinued when the interval is greater than 500 ms.[112]

Oxycodone is mainly a prodrug, being active after conversion by the enzyme cytochrome P450 2D6 to oxymorphone (a μ-opioid agonist). Noroxycodone is its inactive metabolite. It has a high bioavailability (60%) and is associated with a low incidence of itching and hallucinations. It has an NNT of 2.5 in neuropathic pain; the oxycodone-to-morphine ratio is 1:1.5. The controlled-release preparation (OxyContin, Purdue Pharma) has good analgesic characteristics but became a popular drug for abuse prior to its reformulation to include abuse-deterrent technologies. Oxymorphone has greater affinity to the μ-receptor than morphine and has little or no affinity to the κ-opioid receptor. It is 10 times more potent than morphine when given intravenously. It has low histamine release, similar to fentanyl. Due to extensive first-pass hepatic metabolism, the bioavailability of oxymorphone is only 10%. However, its greater lipid solubility explains the rapid onset of analgesia. It should not be taken with alcohol because this increases its plasma concentration by as much as 300%. The efficacy of oxymorphone in chronic and cancer pain is similar to other opioids. Buprenorphine is a partial agonist at the μ-receptor, a κ-antagonist, and a weak δ-agonist. It has a rapid onset (30 minutes) when given orally and a long duration of action of 6 to 9 hours. Buprenorphine antagonizes the opioid effects of full agonists such as morphine or hydromorphone due to its partial opioid agonist pharmacodynamics.

The weak opioids include codeine, hydrocodone, tapentadol, and tramadol. Codeine is transformed to morphine via the enzyme cytochrome P450 2D6, and has an NNT of 16.7. Genetic factors can affect the effect of these drugs. Approximately 9% of Caucasians do not have the enzyme and do not experience analgesia from codeine.[113] Asians have a lower rate of codeine O-demethylation, resulting in less morphine formation. Children under 12 years of age lack maturity of the enzyme and cannot convert the drug to morphine, experiencing the drug's side effects with minimal analgesia.[114] Hydrocodone reaches peak serum concentrations within 1 to 2 hours and has a half-life of 2.5 to 4 hours. An additive effect is noted when ibuprofen is combined with hydrocodone.

Tramadol is a weak opioid agonist and a monoaminergic drug. It has bioavailability of 80% to 90%, low abuse potential, low incidence of constipation, and minimal risk of fatal respiratory depression, which is possibly limited to patients with severe renal failure. It has a dose-dependent efficacy, with NNTs of 8.5 for 50 mg, 5.3 for 75 mg, 4.8 for 100 mg, and 2.9 for 150 mg. The maximum dose of tramadol is 400 to 500 mg/day. Tapentadol is similar to tramadol and also has a dual mode of action as a μ-opioid agonist and a norepinephrine reuptake inhibitor. It is modestly stronger than tramadol. Tapentadol is FDA approved for moderate-to-severe acute pain, whereas its extended-release formulation is approved for moderate-to-severe chronic pain and diabetic neuropathy. Tapentadol has side effects and adverse reactions that are similar to those of tramadol, but has a higher risk of addiction and respiratory depression due to its opioid agonism. The oral equianalgesic doses of morphine 10 mg intravenously or 30 mg orally are (1) 200 mg of codeine, (2) 30 mg of hydrocodone, (3) 20 mg of oxycodone, (4) 150 mg of tramadol, and (5) 75 mg of tapentadol.

There is a public concern regarding the effect of opioids on driving performance. A 2013 study determined, contrary to older studies, that individuals receiving stable doses of 20 mg of morphine or equivalent are at increased risk for motor vehicle collisions and this risk increases substantially at doses above 120 mg.[115] Patients who have their opioid dose increased by greater than 30% over a period of 2 days show worsening of their cognitive performance.[116] Patients receiving stable low doses of opioids can probably drive, whereas those who are starting to take opioids, take moderate to high doses and those who had a recent increase in their dose should be warned about the hazards of driving.

Opioids are commonly used for cancer pain, with long-acting opioids supplemented by short-acting ones for breakthrough pain. Opioid monotherapy in cancer pain is rarely successful and adjuvants and procedural interventions are usually added for increased efficacy. The use of opioids for acute or short-term pain (<3 months) following surgery or traumatic injuries is well accepted and supported by the literature. The use of opioids for treatment of chronic (>3 months) noncancer pain is controversial. To date, there has been no randomized clinical trial establishing the efficacy of chronic opioid therapy for greater than 3 months.[117] Chronic opioid therapy is likely to be effective for long-term analgesia in a small subset of patients. Studies show them to be effective in the treatment of neuropathic pain, although at higher doses. Because of the undesirable issues associated with the use of opioids, such as addiction, aberrant behaviors, and regulatory issues, opioids are a third-line drug for neuropathic pain. The combination of a gabapentin and an opioid has been shown to result in better analgesia, fewer side effects, and lower doses of each drug. It should be noted that although individual studies show the efficacy of opioids in low back pain in the short term, a meta-analysis did not show reduced pain when compared with a placebo or a nonopioid control group.[118] Opioids, in addition to NSAIDs and muscle relaxants, may be efficacious for the short-term relief of acute low back pain, but the long-term efficacy of opioids (≥16 weeks) is unclear and cannot be recommended due to the established risks and harms of opioid therapy.[117,118] When treating fibromyalgia, tramadol, tapentadol, or a tramadol/acetaminophen combination are the only opioids that have been shown to be more effective than placebo. Other opioids, including pure opioid agonists, should not be used in the treatment of fibromyalgia and chronic widespread pain.

Opioids have significant risks and harm. The long-term use of opioids is associated with tolerance and physical dependence. The rates of substance-use disorders or opioid misuse reported in studies vary widely. A body of evidence suggests that among chronic pain patients receiving opioid therapy, 6% to 37% will exhibit aberrant drug-related behaviors, 8% to 16% will abuse their drugs, and approximately 2% to 14% may become addicted.[117] Factors predictive of increased risk for misuse included history of substance use disorder, history of sexual abuse, younger age, major depression, and use of psychotropic medications. Recent literature has supported the hypothesis that a subset of patients self-medicate with opioids to manage depression independent of pain.[119] This form of chemical coping is a factor to consider when opioid therapy is being considered.

Pharmacologic Treatments of Neuropathic Pain

NeuP-SIG of the IASP recently published a meta-analysis of 229 randomized double-blind studies, including nonpublished trials, of oral and topical medications used for neuropathic pain. The quality of each study was rated using GRADE. First-line medication recommendations included gabapentin, pregabalin, SNRIs, and TCAs. Second-line recommendations included capsaicin 8% patches, lidocaine patches, and tramadol. Third-line medications were botulinum toxin A and opioids.[120]

Antidepressants

TCAs have a serotonergic effect (interference with serotonin reuptake and alteration of serotonin binding to receptors in neural tissue), a noradrenergic effect (interaction with α-receptors), an opioidergic effect, blockade of the NMDA receptor complex, inhibition of the uptake of adenosine, and blockade of sodium and calcium channels. TCAs also have an anti-inflammatory effect in animal models of pain. The NNTs of antidepressants are comparable with those of opioids and anticonvulsants. Antidepressants also inhibit the histaminic, cholinergic, muscarinic, and nicotinic receptors, resulting in sedation, dry mouth, and urinary retention. TCAs, specifically amitriptyline and nortriptyline, have been shown to be effective in PHN.

Serotonin and norepinephrine receptor inhibitors (SNRIs) block the reuptake of serotonin and norepinephrine, with duloxetine having increased selectivity for serotonin. Venlafaxine has more serotonergic effects at lower doses but with greater noradrenergic activity at higher dosages. Duloxetine and milnacipran have preferential noradrenergic effect, have longer half-lives (12 and 8 hours respectively), and have no active metabolites. In addition to their antidepressant action, the SNRIs have an antinociceptive effect.[121,122] Duloxetine is effective in DPN and fibromyalgia and has a good safety profile for long-term use.[123,124] Patients with fibromyalgia have been shown to have improvements in fatigue, physical conditioning, and discomfort after milnacipran.[125,126] The efficacy of the SNRIs in DPN and fibromyalgia, coupled with the better side effect profile (free of cholinergic, histaminic, and α-adrenergic receptor effects, and less potential for drug interactions) in comparison to the TCAs, are probably the reasons for their increased preferential usage.[121] As stated previously, the European Federation of Neurological Sciences Task Force and the IASP NeuPSIG recommend the SNRIs as the first-choice drugs for the treatment of DPN.

TCAs have an NNT of 2.1 to 2.8 for treatment of PHN, 1.3 to 3.4 for DPN, and 1.7 for central pain. The side effects of antidepressants include cholinergic effects such as dry mouth, sedation, and urinary retention. Venlafaxine may cause hypertension and mania, and may exacerbate seizures. A gradual withdrawal is recommended for duloxetine to prevent agitation, anxiety, confusion, and hypomania. TCAs are more likely to cause weight gain compared with SNRIs. TCAs impair driving ability during the first week of treatment or during dose escalation, but driving performance returns to baseline shortly thereafter.[127] No impairment of driving ability apparently occurs with SNRIs. The recommended doses for the commonly used antidepressants are shown in Table 56-2. The serotonin specific reuptake inhibitors (SSRIs) (citalopram, paroxetine) show a limited effect on neuropathic pain.

Anticonvulsants

Neuropathic pain is associated with changes in sodium and calcium channel subunit expression, resulting in functional changes. In chronic nerve injury, there is redistribution and alteration of subunit compositions of sodium and calcium channels, resulting in spontaneous firing at ectopic sites along the sensory pathway. Sodium channel blockers inhibit spontaneous activities at neuromas, DRG, and at the dorsal horn of the spinal cord. Most anticonvulsants block sodium channels, explaining their efficacy in neuropathic pain syndromes. Other anticonvulsants act on ion channel systems, including $GABA_A$ receptor agonists (topiramate and felbamate), $GABA_A$ transaminase blockers (vigabatrin), $GABA_A$ transport blockers (tiagabine), and glutamate receptor antagonists (felbamate and topiramate). The other drugs directly block calcium channels (lamotrigine), T-type calcium channels (topiramate and zonisamide) and $α_2$-delta subunits (gabapentin and pregabalin). Randomized controlled studies demonstrate the efficacy of the anticonvulsants in several neuropathic pain syndromes including trigeminal neuralgia, PHN, DPN, HIV polyneuropathy, phantom limb pain, spinal cord injury (SCI) pain, and central poststroke pain.

Gabapentin is an effective drug in neuropathic pain (PHN, DPN, and SCI), multiple sclerosis pain, neuropathic cancer pain, and fibromyalgia. It has few side effects and lacks drug–drug interactions. Its median effective dose is 900 to 1,800 mg/day. Compared to gabapentin, pregabalin has an improved linear pharmacokinetic profile. It has been shown to be effective in PHN, DPN, and SCI pain. The maximum dose of pregabalin is 600 mg/day in patients with creatinine clearance more than 60 mL/min or 300 mg in patients with clearance of 30 to 60 mL/min. The popularity of gabapentin and pregabalin relates to the lack of drug interactions and their perceived speed of onset.[128]

Lamotrigine has been shown to be effective in HIV polyneuropathy, pain from SCI, trigeminal neuralgia, and central poststroke pain.[101] The most common side effect is rash, and use of lamotrigine is limited by the risk of Stevens–Johnson syndrome. Topiramate is effective in migraine prophylaxis, similar to divalproex. Oxcarbazepine is similar in chemical structure to carbamazepine and noted to be effective in trigeminal neuralgia with fewer side effects; its analgesic effect is fast and pain relief may be noted within 24 to 48 hours. The recommended doses of the commonly used anticonvulsants are in Table 56-2.

The side effects of anticonvulsants include dizziness, fatigue, somnolence, weight gain, peripheral edema (gabapentin and pregabalin); rash (lamotrigine); paresthesia, cognitive effects, weight loss (topiramate); hyponatremia; and low thyroid concentrations (oxcarbazepine).

Lidocaine Patch, Capsaicin Patch, Mexiletine, and Intravenous Lidocaine

The 5% lidocaine patch delivers lidocaine locally at the site of neuropathic pain generation, limiting its systemic effects and reducing its interactions with other concomitantly administered medications; analgesia is by local sodium channel blockade and not by its systemic effects. The patch contains 700 mg of lidocaine inside an adhesive. It is recommended that a maximum of three patches be applied for a maximum of 12 hr/day. Most patients experience pain relief within a few days of application. Others have a delayed response so it has been recommended that there should be a 2-week trial period. Some patients continue to experience relief between patch applications but others have pain when the patch is removed; clinicians recommend using the patch for 16 to 18 hours in these patients. The absorption of lidocaine is limited; only about 3% of the total dose applied is absorbed systemically.[129] The maximum plasma lidocaine concentration is usually achieved on the second day of a 12-hours-per-day patch application and is significantly lower than concentrations that are cardiotoxic. Clinical experience with the lidocaine patch has shown that it can be used effectively for patients with PHN.[130]

Capsaicin has been shown to defunctionalize TRPV1 nerve endings and reduce epidermal nerve fiber density.[131] The higher-concentration capsaicin 8% patch (Qutenza, Acorda Therapeutics) has been shown to be better than placebo and better than low-concentration (0.04%) capsaicin. It appears to be effective in PHN, DPN, and HIV neuropathy.[132,133] Its NNT, 30% relief, is 12 (6.4 to 70). Because of burning sensation during its placement, local

Table 56-2 Dosages (mg/day) of the Commonly Used Antidepressants and Anticonvulsants[a]

Antidepressants	Anticonvulsants
Amitriptyline: 10–300	Gabapentin: 900–3,600, tid
Doxepin: 30–300	Lamotrigine: 50–150
Nortriptyline: 50–150	Mexiletine: 300–1,350, tid
Desipramine: 25–300	Oxcarbazepine: 300–900, bid
Fluoxetine: 5–40	Pregabalin: 150–600, bid
Paroxetine: 20–40	Topiramate: 50–200, bid
Venlaflaxine: 37.5–300	
Duloxetine: 60–120, od or bid	
Milnacipran: 100–200 mg, 50–100 mg bid	

tid, three times a day; bid, twice a day; od, once daily.
[a]Unless indicated, dosing is once a day. Start with smallest possible dose and titrate to efficacy or side effects.

anesthetic cream applied 60 minutes before the patch is applied for 60 to 90 minutes. The 60-minute application is better tolerated and is similar in efficacy. There is an increase in pain 20 to 30 minutes after application, which disappears 2 to 3 hours after removal of the patch. Relief can be up to 12 weeks after one application. A maximum of four doses can be given at intervals of 12 weeks.[134]

Mexiletine is an oral analogue of lidocaine and has been used for diabetic neuropathy, thalamic stroke pain, spasticity, and myotonia but has been shown to only have modest efficacy. Its efficacy is similar to that of intravenous lidocaine, although a favorable response to intravenous lidocaine does not necessarily mean a similar response to mexiletine. The median recommended dose of mexiletine is 600 mg/per day.

Cannabinoids

Cannabis has been studied for treating neuropathic pain. Seven of the nine reviewed studies of nabiximols, a cannabinoid-based oral mucosal spray, were negative for the primary outcome of 50% pain reduction. Cannabinoids were therefore given a weak recommendation against use.[120] Another meta-analysis reviewed five randomized controlled trials that looked at inhaled (smoked) cannabis for treatment of chronic neuropathic pain and showed an NNT for short-term reduction in neuropathic pain similar to that of TCAs, SNRIs, and gabapentin. These studies are limited in the sample size, dose variability, lack of functional outcome variables, and short duration.[135] Nabiximols, but not delta-9-tetrahydrocannabinol (THC), were modestly effective in the treatment of cancer-related pain.[136] As of December 2015, the prescription and consumption of medical marijuana was legal in 23 states and the District of Columbia, although federally illegal. Dronabinol and nabilone, synthetic cannabinoids approved for nausea treatment, had no pain benefit in acute postsurgical pain clinical trials. Dronabinol did improve pain intensity in chronic pain patients who were opioid tolerant.[137]

Based on original studies, review articles, and meta-analysis publications, the recommended drugs for several different chronic pain syndromes are listed in Table 56-3.

Buprenorphine–Naloxone Therapy

Buprenorphine–naloxone (bup/nal in 4:1 ratio; Suboxone, Indivior Inc.) is a semisynthetic, sublingual tablet consisting of buprenorphine and naloxone in fixed 4:1 ratio. It has been noted to be effective in outpatient-based opioid addiction treatment and offers several advantages over methadone maintenance programs. As opioids are associated with adverse and social consequences, buprenorphine/naloxone has been prescribed as an alternative. A review of the literature showed it to be inadequate to provide pain relief in patients without opioid dependence or addiction.[138] In patients with chronic pain with opioid dependence or addiction, studies showed the drug to have some efficacy.[139,140]

Interventional Techniques

Discography

The symptoms of discogenic pain are nonspecific and include nonradicular back pain that is worse in the sitting position and with lifting maneuvers. The neurologic examination is usually normal; the MRI may show a high-intensity zone on the T2 sagittal images, indicating an annular tear. Treatments include stabilization, core strengthening, exercise training, back education, activity modification, and occasional ESIs for managing symptom exacerbation.

Diagnostic discography remains a useful tool in identifying painful intervertebral discs.[141] Some of the indications include (1) evaluation of abnormal discs to assess the extent of abnormality or correlation of the abnormality with clinical symptoms, (2) assessment of patients with persistent severe symptoms in whom diagnostic tests have failed to reveal which suspected disc is the source of pain, (3) assessment of discs before fusion to determine which discs within the proposed fusion segment are symptomatic, and (4) confirmation of a contained disc herniation or investigation of contrast distribution pattern before intradiscal procedures. Discography can be performed on an outpatient basis with fluoroscopic guidance, under light sedation. Antibiotic prophylaxis is recommended and may be administered either intradiscally or intravenously. The specifics of the technique are discussed by Derby et al.[142] Nonionic contrast is injected into the disc, preferably with a controlled injection system with pressure readout. The patient is asked to rate his or her pain on a 0 to 10 scale before and during injection, and whether the pain is *concordant*, that is, similar to the pain for which the patient is being evaluated.[143] The suggested end points for injection include (1) pain severity of 6 out of 10 or greater, (2) intradiscal pressure of less than 50 psi above opening pressure, or (3) a total of less than 3.5 mL of contrast medium has been injected. Anteroposterior and lateral images are taken to record the distribution of contrast medium and whether the contrast leaked outside the disc through a fissure in the annulus fibrosis. After recovery, the patient is sent for a postdiscography computed tomography (CT) scan, preferably within 4 hours of the discography.

Discitis is the most feared complication of discography; it is considerably decreased with prophylactic antibiotic use.[144] The diagnosis of discitis includes worsening back pain the week after discography, and elevated erythrocyte sedimentation rate and C-reactive protein that usually peaks 53 weeks after the procedure. The most common causative organism in discitis is

Table 56-3 Recommended Drugs for Chronic Pain Syndromes

Postherpetic Neuralgia	Diabetic Painful Neuropathy	Spinal Cord Injury	Fibromyalgia	Human Immunodeficiency Virus (HIV)
Pregabalin	Duloxetine	Pregabalin	Duloxetine	Lamotrigine
Gabapentin	Pregabalin	Gabapentin	Pregabalin	Gabapentin
Opioid	Gabapentin	Lamotrigine	Milnacipran	
Antidepressants	Antidepressants	IV lidocaine	Tramadol	
Tramadol		Mexilitine (±)		
Lidoderm patch (allodynia)				

Staphylococcus aureus. The possibility of disc injury after discography, resulting in disc degeneration and/or herniation from such procedures,[145] as well as the procedure's poor prognostic value for success of surgical fusion,[141] may have decreased the frequency with which the procedure is performed.

Thermal Annular Procedures

Intradiscal electrothermal therapy (IDET) is a procedure wherein a thermal resistance catheter is placed percutaneously in the posterolateral portion of the disc. Heat causes the collagen of the annulus fibrosis to contract. Two randomized sham-controlled studies examined IDET in discogenic pain patients, with one study showing significant improvements in pain scores and Oswestry Disability Index[146] and the other study demonstrating differences in pain or functional outcome between the IDET-treated and sham control groups.[147] The procedure was not approved by the Center for Medicare and Medicaid Services (CMS), leading to the near demise of its use in patients insured by commercial carriers and patients in the Veterans Administration system. Given the difficulty of navigating the IDET catheter in degenerated discs, a bilateral cooled RF approach—biacuplasty—was developed. A prospective sham-controlled study showed efficacy of biacuplasty compared to sham control at 6- and 12-months[148] and an open-label trial showed it to be superior to conventional medical management.[149] Similar to other thermal annular procedures, third-party insurance coverage remains extremely limited.

Minimally Invasive Lumbar Decompression Procedure

Spinal stenosis is narrowing of the spinal canal with compression of the nerve roots as demonstrated with a magnetic resonance imaging (MRI) or CT scan. Such canal narrowing can be secondary to hypertrophy of the ligamentum flavum or the facet joint. Low back pain from spinal stenosis is located in the low back area, buttocks, thighs, and/or legs in combination with neurogenic claudication, especially with erect posture (due to smaller spinal canal diameter in this position) or walking.[150] The minimally invasive lumbar decompression (MILD) procedure is a minimally invasive method of spinal decompression. It is indicated in patients with low back pain and neurogenic claudication associated with MRI or CT evidence of central canal stenosis secondary to ligamentum flavum hypertrophy in the lumbar segments.[151,152] The procedure involves limited percutaneous laminotomy and thinning of the ligamentum flavum to increase the critical diameter of the stenosed spinal canal. It can be performed under local anesthesia. A one- or, more usually, two-level decompression is performed. In contrast to surgical decompression with fusion wherein there is complete resection of the ligamentum flavum and bony posterior elements compressing the thecal sac and exiting nerve roots, the mild procedure only partially debulks the ligamentum flavum. Although initial reports were promising,[153,154] the procedure has not become commonplace because approval for payment by CMS (and subsequently commercial insurance carriers) was deferred pending a sham-controlled randomized trial.

Vertebroplasty and Kyphoplasty

Vertebroplasty and kyphoplasty are percutaneous interventional modalities to treat vertebral compression fractures (VCFs), a condition usually secondary to osteoporosis in elderly patients. Most healed VCFs are asymptomatic; pain may be experienced in acute or subacute VCF with bending, lifting, prolonged sitting or standing, or when the patient attempts to stand from a seated position. The pain is usually a deep back pain and there may be intercostal neuralgic symptoms or radiculitis and paravertebral muscle spasm. Pain is relieved by bed rest and the recumbent position. Radiography shows osteopenia or decreased bone mass; MRI is the imaging modality of choice as it detects bony edema associated with acute fracture with a very high sensitivity.

Vertebroplasty involves the injection of polymethylmethacrylate (PMMA) into the affected vertebral body; kyphoplasty involves the insertion of a balloon prior to the injection of the cement. These procedures lead to restoration of some of the decreased vertebral height, improved strength of the vertebral body, and decreased stress placed on the adjacent vertebrae. Both procedures are performed under fluoroscopic guidance. Vertebral body access is obtained through a uni- or bipedicular approach. The entire vertebral body does not have to be filled with cement to achieve pain relief; 2 mL is adequate for the procedure (Fig. 56-8). The patient remains supine for 3 to 5 hours after the procedure for assessment of neurologic status and observation for the occurrence of bleeding and hematomas. A CT scan is usually performed afterward for assessment of cement distribution and the occurrence of complications such as bleeding and leakage of the cement. Kyphoplasty involves the percutaneous introduction of a balloon into the vertebral body, inflation of the balloon, then filling of the balloon with PMMA that is more viscous than that used for vertebroplasty.

The complications of percutaneous vertebral augmentation include leakage of the cement and complications related to the procedure. The factors that contribute to cement leakage include the level of injection, severity of fracture, and the amount of cement injected. Neurologic complications include radiculopathy, spinal claudication, and paraplegia. Kyphoplasty may be associated with a lower rate of cement extravasation because of the higher viscosity of the PMMA that is used, the lower injection pressure employed, and the inflatable bone trap that seals

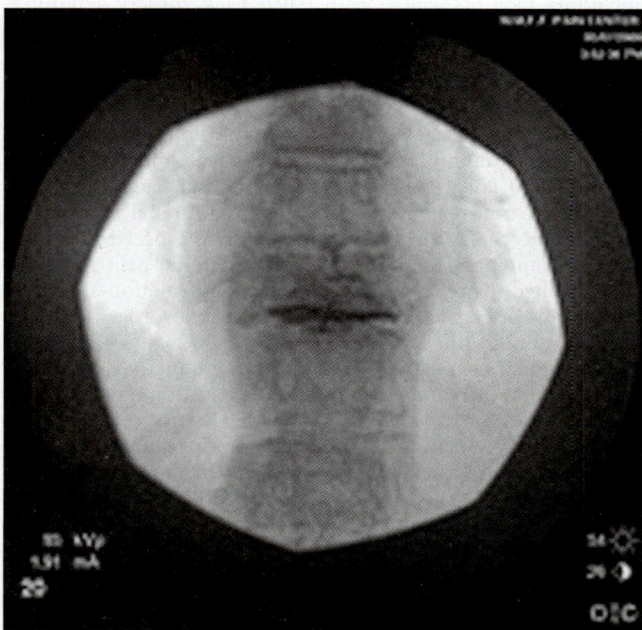

Figure 56-8 Vertebroplasty at T10 vertebral level. A total of 5 mL of cement was injected.

pathways for cement leakage.[155] Complications related to the procedure include infection, bleeding, and allergic reactions from the PMMA or contrast medium.

Initial results after vertebroplasty and kyphoplasty were good and complications were minimal.[156–160] More recent randomized controlled studies have not confirmed the beneficial effects of vertebroplasty in that improvements in pain and pain-related disability were similar to the improvements in the sham control group.[161,162] Although the conduct of the studies was criticized appropriately, questions about the mechanism and the effectiveness of this procedure remain unanswered.[163] Two randomized controlled studies showed the superiority of balloon kyphoplasty for VCFs in patients with osteoporosis or cancer when compared with a control nonsurgical care group.[164,165] These two randomized studies were partly criticized, in that funding of the study came from the maker of the device, and one of the authors was affiliated with the company. Final conclusions on the efficacy of these procedures await additional randomized controlled studies.

Spinal Cord Stimulation

The analgesic effect of spinal cord stimulation (SCS) may involve the *gate control theory,* neurotransmitter modulation in the spinal cord affecting pain pathways and suppression of sympathetic activity, with antidromic and activity supraspinal mechanisms also playing important roles. It is hypothesized that SCS increases the input of the large nerve fibers, thus closing the "gate" at the substantia gelatinosa of the dorsal horn of the spinal cord. SCS may alter the local neurochemistry at the dorsal horn, and there may be a decrease of the hyperexcitability of the wide dynamic neurons. It is correlated with increased levels of the inhibitory neurotransmitter GABA and a decrease of the excitatory neurotransmitters glutamate and aspartate.[166] In ischemic pain, the analgesia may be secondary to alteration of the sympathetic tone with restoration of a favorable oxygen supply-and-demand balance.

In the United States, SCS is approved "as an aid in the management of chronic intractable pain of the trunk and/or limbs, including pain associated with failed back surgery syndrome, low back pain and leg." Clinical indications for SCS implantation include patients with a diagnosis of post laminectomy syndrome, also known as failed back surgery syndrome (FBSS), CRPS, neuropathic pain syndromes, angina, and chronic critical limb ischemia and pain.[167–173] Many of these indications are considered off-label, including placement of all cervical spine stimulators. Patients who failed conservative therapy and had a temporary stimulation trial that has demonstrated pain relief after having passed a psychological evaluation generally proceed to permanent implantation. Many patients with chronic pain may have uncontrolled depressive symptoms and implantation should be avoided in patients with major psychological disorders. The general contraindications include systemic or local site of infection and abnormal coagulopathy. Complications include nerve and SCI, infection, hematoma, and lead breakage or migration.

Evidence supports the efficacy of SCS for treatment of persistent back and leg pain. In a randomized study, patients who were candidates for repeat laminectomy were randomized to either SCS or surgery.[167] At 6-month follow-up 67% of patients who had reoperation crossed over to SCS, but only 17% in the SCS group crossed over to repeat surgery. At the 3-year follow-up, the SCS group continued to have better outcomes compared with patients having repeat spine surgery. Overall, 47% of patients in the SCS group achieved 50% or more pain relief compared with 12% in the reoperation group ($p < 0.01$). The patients randomized to reoperation used significantly more opioids than those randomized to SCS. SCS is also superior to conservative medical management (CMM) in patients with FBSS. More recently, modifications to SCS parameters, in particular frequency rate and pattern, have shown improved efficacy in pain control. In particular, high frequency SCS at 10 kHz has shown superior pain relief in back and leg pain to conventional SCS (at low frequency 40 to 130 Hz) in long-term follow-up. Unlike conventional stimulation, SCS at 10 kHz is paresthesia free. In addition, sending packets of higher frequency stimulation at 500 Hz, in what has been referred to as burst SCS, has been shown to result in improved back and leg pain control compared to tonic stimulation, in a paresthesia-free fashion for the most part. Thus, there is sufficient evidence to support the efficacy of SCS for treating failed back syndrome in terms of sustained long-term pain relief with medication reduction, improvement in quality of life, increased patient satisfaction, increased ability to return to work, minimal side effects, and cost-effectiveness compared with alternative therapies; moreover the technique is reversible. Although the main indication for use of SCS in the United States is FBSS, it is a popular treatment for pain secondary to peripheral ischemia in Europe.

Studies examining the efficacy of SCS in CRPS have consisted of retrospective case series, prospective clinical studies, and a prospective randomized controlled study. In the randomized controlled study,[169] 54 patients with refractory CRPS who had failed previous therapies including surgical sympathectomy were randomized to either SCS with physiotherapy (SCS+PT) or PT alone. Using an intent-to-treat analysis at the 6-month follow-up, patients who were treated with SCS had a significantly greater reduction in pain, and a significantly higher percentage of patients graded their relief as much improved in terms of global perceived effect (a 7-scale outcome measure ranging from "worst ever" to "best ever"). These effects were maintained at 2 years but not at 5 years using an intent-to-treat analysis.[170] However, an as treated analysis of results at 5 years revealed significant improvement in the SCS+PT compared to the PT group. A meta-analysis[168] concluded that SCS is an effective tool in the management of CRPS and that a grade A level of evidence supports the efficacy of SCS in CRPS. A 12-year follow-up of a prospective cohort study showed SCS to provide an effective long-term pain treatment for 63% of the implanted patients.[171] For pain from peripheral ischemia and angina, most of the published literature consists of case series and case reports.

SCS electrodes are placed via a Touhy needle as shown in Figure 56-9.

Peripheral Nerve Stimulation

Electrical stimulation of a peripheral nerve can be used to treat neuropathic pain, ideally arising from a single nerve. When considering peripheral nerve stimulation (PNS) it is important to distinguish between open and percutaneous PNS approaches. In open PNS, nerve stimulation is made feasible with a circumferential (cuff) electrode that requires a surgical exposure of the target nerve. Application of high frequency (10 kHz) alternating current using a cuff electrode around a peripheral nerve has been shown to result in reversible complete neuronal conduction block. PNS of the sciatic or tibial nerve has shown promise in treating postamputation pain, and is now the subject of a large multicenter study. On the other hand, PNS involves the use of cylindrical percutaneous lead (originally designed for SCS) in close proximity to the target nerve or in the subcutaneous field area supplied by the target nerve. The former percutaneous approach requires target specificity and may be subject to lead migration and unwanted motor stimulation in mixed nerves. The

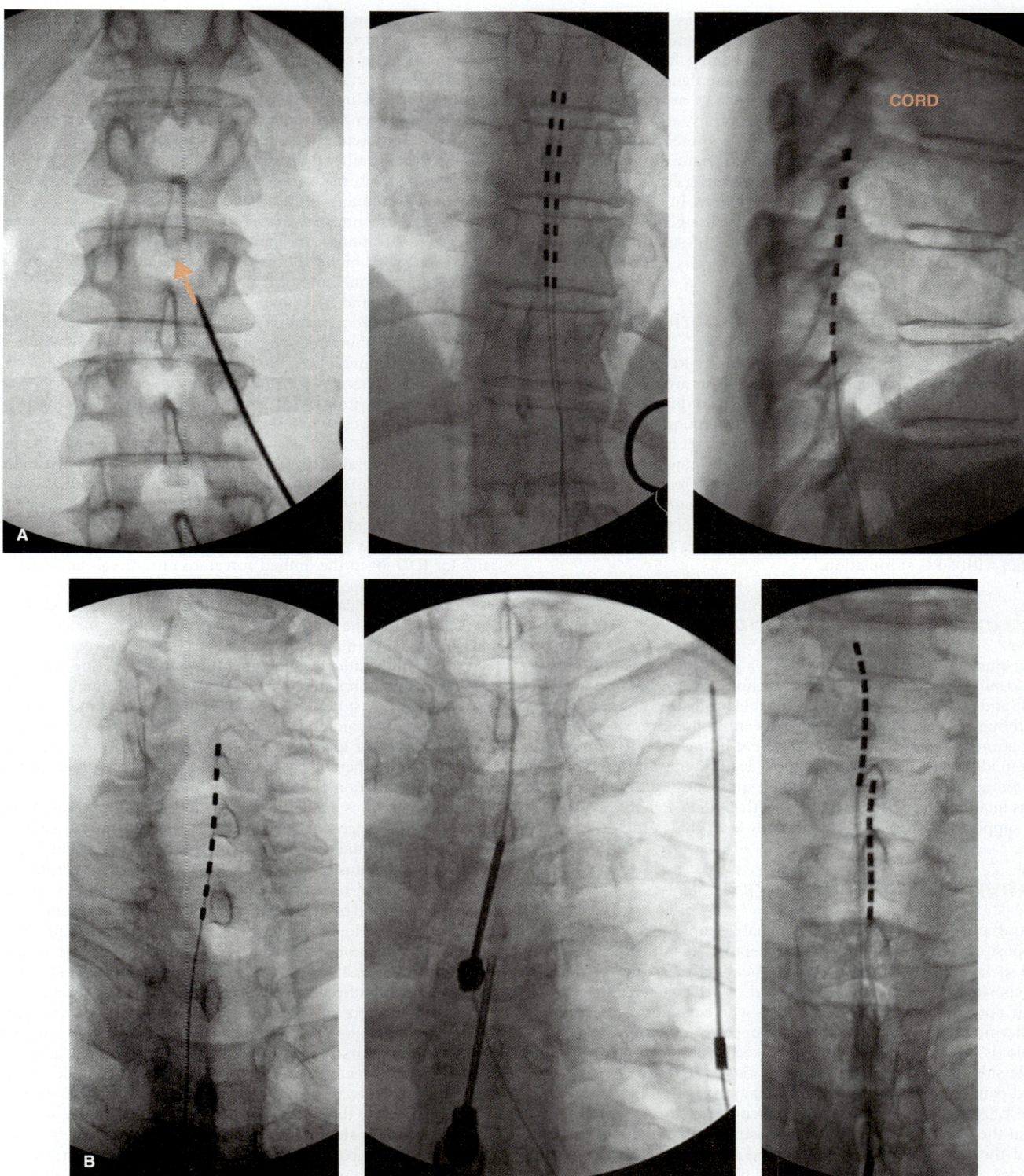

Figure 56-9 Placement of the epidural needle and the spinal cord electrodes at the thoracic (**A**) and cervical (**B**) levels.

latter percutaneous approach is referred to as peripheral nerve field stimulation and is less target specific and less technically challenging. It has been used for managing focal neuropathic pain such as occipital neuralgia, facial neuralgias, and PHN, and various other conditions such as refractory angina, abdominal pain, pelvic pain, knee pain after arthroplasty, and low back pain (in combination with SCS). It should be noted that most PNS studies are limited by their observational nature and absence of a control arm. As with patients who are being evaluated for SCS, neuropsychological testing may be valuable. In addition, before permanent implantation of the internal pulse generator, patients should have undergone a successful trial of stimulation with a predetermined therapeutic benefit.

Dorsal Root Ganglion Stimulation

A hybrid between SCS and PNS involves DRG stimulation. In DRG stimulation, special percutaneous leads are introduced, initially in the interlaminar epidural space, and directed toward the adjacent target DRG. Advantages of this technique involve targeting unique dermatomes and difficult-to-target areas, such as the foot, along with minimal-to-no positional changes in paresthesia intensity compared to conventional SCS. A recent comparative effectiveness study involving 152 CRPS patients randomized to DRG stimulation or paresthesia-based SCS showed a significantly greater proportion of patients achieving 50% or more pain relief with DRG stimulation.[174]

Occipital Nerve Stimulation

Occipital neurostimulation (ONS), a form of peripheral nerve field stimulation, is an innovative technique for providing reversible and effective therapy for intractable headache. The technique is thought to work via inhibition of central nociceptive impulses by stimulation of the superficial nerve branches of C2 and C3. As in all forms of neurostimulation, lead migration represents a potential technical failure that can require surgical replacement; this incidence is particularly high with ONS.[175] Reliable evidence to support the efficacy of this therapy is, at this point, lacking.

Intrathecal Drug Delivery

Intrathecal drug delivery (IDD) enables opioid to be directly deposited near the spinal cord receptors, resulting in analgesia at lower doses. An additional mechanism is the release of adenosine in the cerebrospinal fluid.[176] IDD systems are valuable options in chronic pain patients who have not responded to other modalities and in whom oral or transdermal medications/opioids are ineffective at reasonable doses, or cause unacceptable side effects. The main indications for IDD are cancer pain and pain of spinal origin, with the majority of pumps placed in the USA for FBSS. IDD allows the drug to be directly deposited near the spinal cord receptors, bypassing the blood–brain barrier and the first-pass effect encountered by systemic medications. Hence, medications that have limited blood–brain barrier permeability and medications whose target receptors are located in the spinal canal can be delivered more efficiently and at significantly lower doses. For pain applications, there are only two medications approved by the FDA for IDD: preservative-free morphine and the synthetic peptide ziconotide. Morphine, hydrocodone, or ziconotide are considered acceptable as first-line agents.[177]
A number of other medications are commonly used off-label, including hydromorphone, fentanyl, the local anesthetic bupivacaine, and the α_2 adrenergic agonist clonidine. Baclofen is FDA-approved for management of spasticity but otherwise has a limited role in pain applications.

Patients receiving intrathecal opioids develop tolerance not unlike what is seen with systemic opioids.[178] Side effects such as pruritus, urinary retention, and peripheral edema are more likely to occur with intrathecal than systemic administration of opioids. In addition, an 8% risk of developing an intrathecal catheter tip granuloma is unique to intrathecal opioid infusion. These are typically sterile inflammatory masses consisting of fibroblasts, macrophages, neutrophils, and monocytes.[179] Granuloma formation is increased with higher doses and concentrations of morphine and hydromorphone but not fentanyl. It is not mediated through opioid receptors and experiments suggest that granuloma formation may be related to dural mast cell degranulation occurring in response to morphine and hydromorphone but not fentanyl.

The overwhelming preponderance of IDD systems are placed for managing refractory chronic noncancer pain, primarily low back pain in the setting of previous lumbar spine surgery. In these cases, opioid dose escalation is concerning because it may predispose not only to intrathecal catheter tip granuloma but also to opioid-induced hyperalgesia. Several patient-related factors should be considered before instituting IDD systems for noncancer pain, including the patient's age, pain location, pain type and frequency, and baseline opioid consumption, as well as the patient's medical status. Patients with well-localized pain may be better candidates for IDD given the limited spread of intrathecal medications past the catheter tip; older patients are likely to have a slower rate of opioid dose escalation; a combination of bupivacaine with an opioid may slow the rate of opioid dose escalation; patients with neuropathic pain may escalate their opioid dose requirements more than other patients; and patients with neuropathic pain may respond to a combination of an opioid and bupivacaine.[180] Importantly, opioid consumption at baseline may be the most crucial determinant of opioid dose escalation and this has led to embracing the practice of low opioid dosing (sometimes referred to as "microdosing") whereby patients are weaned off systemic opioids prior to consideration of intrathecal administration.

A trial period is recommended before an intrathecal pump is permanently placed. A trial can be performed intrathecally or through the epidural space, by a single shot, intermittent bolus, or a continuous infusion. If a trial shows efficacy, then permanent implantation is performed. The placement of a permanent pump and catheter should be performed in the operating room under sterile conditions and intravenous antibiotics should be administered. Surgical considerations regarding IDD system implantation include choice of patient positioning (e.g., lateral decubitus vs. prone); type of anesthetic; intrathecal needle entry point (Fig. 56-10); eventual catheter tip location; site of pump placement; and a knowledge of the patient's lumbar spine anatomy, including prior spine surgery or pathology. A purse string suture should be placed in the fascia around the catheter to minimize cerebrospinal fluid leak. In the majority of patients, the only anatomical location that can reasonably accommodate the size of the pump is the abdominal wall on either side. The anatomic constraints are the bony borders of the iliac crest, and the costal margin. None of these should come in contact with the pump when the patient is seated because of discomfort and risk of damage to the pump or catheter. The pump pocket incision should be made to approximate the size of the pump. The incision can be carried down to the rectus fascia in thin patients. This is followed by tunneling through the subcutaneous tissues between the pump pocket and the posterior incision (Fig. 56-11). This must be done carefully to prevent accidental puncture of the peritoneum or even the pleura.

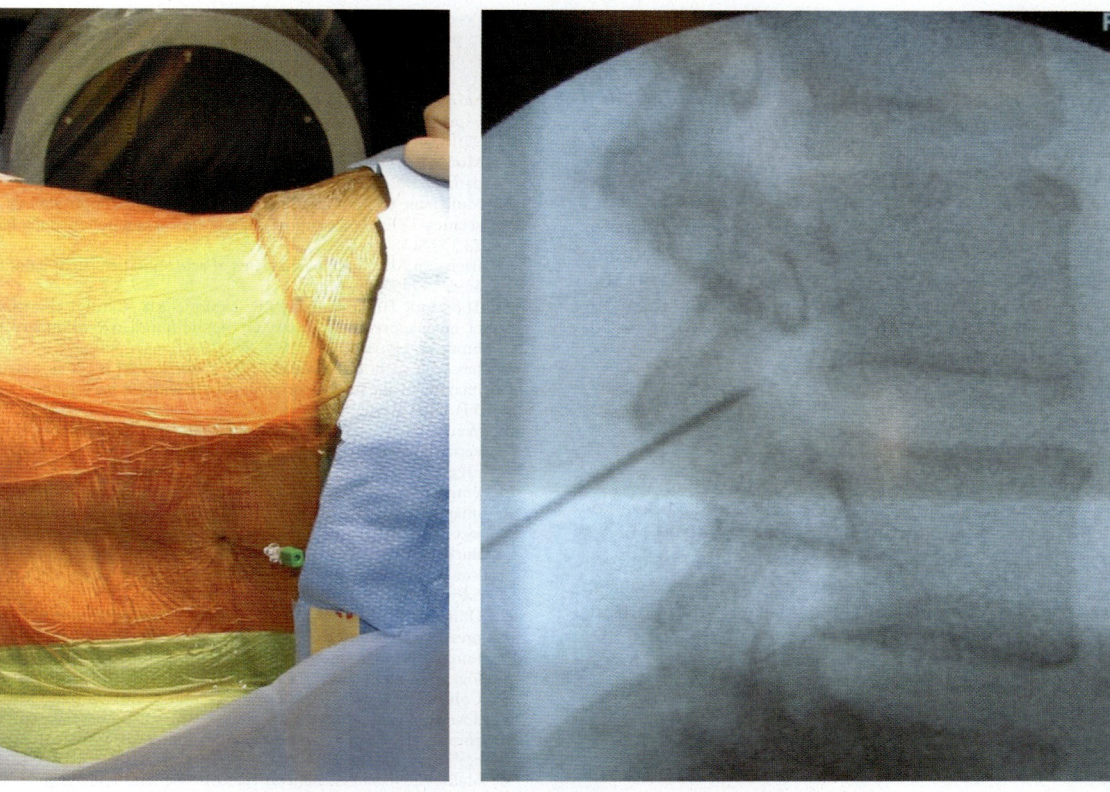

Figure 56-10 Placement of the intrathecal needle under fluoroscopy.

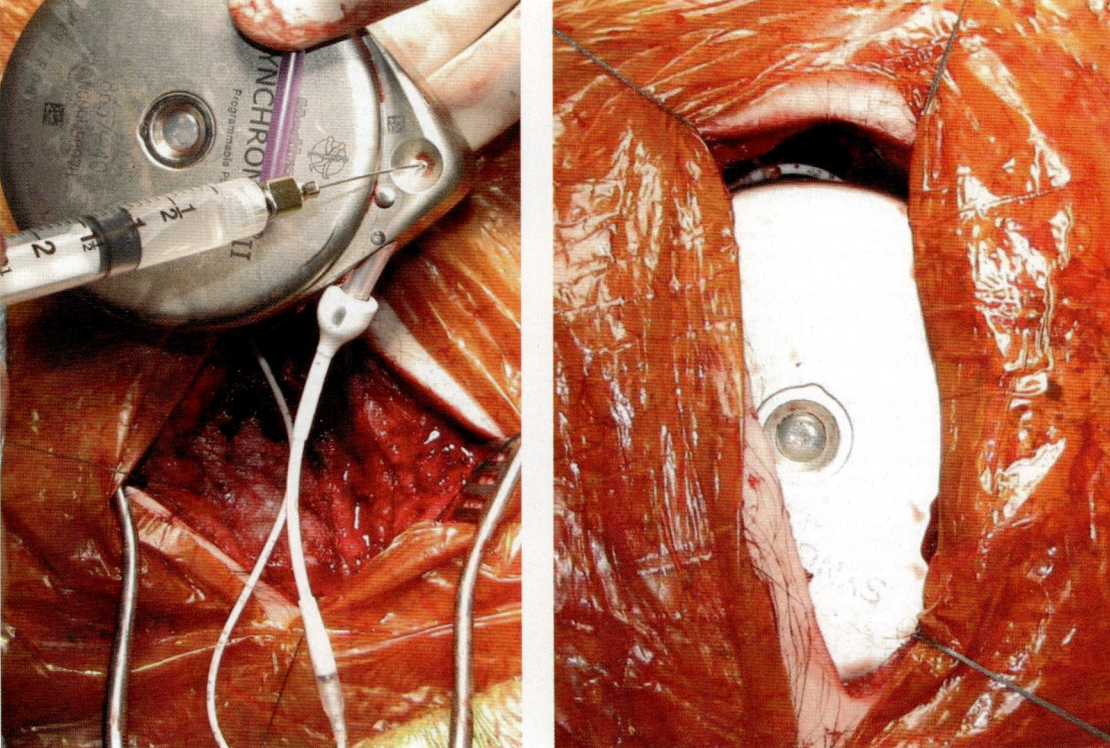

Figure 56-11 Connection of the intrathecal catheter to the programmable pump and confirmation of cerebrospinal fluid prior to placement in the pocket.

Complications of IDD systems can be divided into those related to the procedure/device and those related to the medications infused. Procedure/device-related complications include wound dehiscence, skin erosion over the device, infection, bleeding, CSF leak, seroma or hygroma collection, pump malfunction, and catheter kink or shear. Opioid-related complications include androgen deficiency, decreased testosterone levels and hypogonadism with increased risk of bone mineral deficiency, peripheral edema with morphine and hydromorphone, pruritus, urinary retention, and formation of an intrathecal granuloma. Bupivacaine may cause sensorimotor deficits and urinary retention and clonidine may cause hypotension. Details regarding management of intrathecal complications may be found in books on interventional pain management.

Summary

The proper treatment of pain, particularly chronic pain, is a unique field of medicine that is considered by some to be a specialty of its own, comparable to other major specialties such as medicine, surgery, and anesthesiology. The practice of chronic pain medicine involves a comprehensive knowledge of basic science, pharmacology, regional nerve blocks, and interventional procedures. The practice of chronic pain medicine is multidisciplinary and the anesthesiologist's role should complement that of physicians in other specialties, including physical medicine and rehabilitation, psychiatry, radiology, and surgery.

REFERENCES

1. Melzack R. Prolonged relief of pain by brief, intense transcutaneous somatic stimulation. *Pain.* 1975;1:357–373.
2. Neumann S, Doubell TP, Leslie T, et al. Inflammatory pain hypersensitivity mediated by phenotypic switch in myelinated primary sensory neurons. *Nature.* 1996;384:360–364.
3. Indo Y, Tsuruta M, Hayashida Y, et al. Mutations in the TRKA/NGF receptor gene in patients with congenital insensitivity to pain with anhidrosis. *Nat Genet.* 1996;13:485–488.
4. Fields HL. *Pain Syndromes in Neurology.* Boston, MA; London: Butterworths; 1990.
5. Cox JJ, Reimann F, Nicholas AK, et al. An SCN9A channelopathy causes congenital inability to experience pain. *Nature.* 2006;444:894–898.
6. Fertleman CR, Baker MD, Parker KA, et al. SCN9A mutations in paroxysmal extreme pain disorder: Allelic variants underlie distinct channel defects and phenotypes. *Neuron.* 2006;52:767–774.
7. Rush A, Dib-Hajj SD, Liu S, et al. A single sodium channel mutation produces hyper- or hypoexcitability in different types of neurons. *Proc Natl Acad Sci USA.* 2006;103:8245–8250.
8. Caterina MJ, Schumacher MA, Tominaga M, et al. The capsaicin receptor: A heat-activated ion channel in the pain pathway. *Nature.* 1997;389:816–824.
9. Caterina MJ, Leffler A, Malmberg AB, et al. Impaired nociception and pain sensation in mice lacking the capsaicin receptor. *Science.* 2000;288:306–313.
10. Honda CN, Lee CL. Immunohistochemistry of synaptic input and functional characterizations of neurons near the spinal central canal. *Brain Res.* 1985;343:120–128.
11. Willis WD, Kenshalo DR, Leonard RB. The cells of origin of the primate spinothalamic tract. *J Comp Neurol.* 1979;188:543–573.
12. Basbaum AI, Fields HL. The origin of descending pathways in the dorsolateral funiculus of the spinal cord of the cat and rat: further studies on the anatomy of pain modulation. *J Comp Neurol.* 1979;187:513–531.
13. Bajic D, Proudfit HL. Projections of neurons in the periaqueductal gray to pontine and medullary catecholamine cell groups involved in the modulation of nociception. *J Comp Neurol.* 1999;405:359–379.
14. Basbaum AI, Clanton C, Fields HL. Three bulbospinal pathways from the rostral medulla of the cat: An autoradiographic study of pain modulating systems. *J Comp Neurol.* 1978;178:209–224.
15. Duggan AW, Griersmith BT. Inhibition of the spinal transmission of nociceptive information by supraspinal stimulation in the cat. *Pain.* 1979;6:149–161.
16. Clark FM, Proudfit HK. The projection of noradrenergic neurons in the A7 catecholamine cell group to the spinal cord in the rat demonstrated by antero-grade tracing combined with immunocytochemistry. *Brain Res.* 1991;547:279–288.
17. Peyron R, Laurent B, Garcia-Larrea L. Functional imaging of brain responses to pain. A review and meta-analysis. *Neurophysiol Clin.* 2000;30:263–288.
18. Woolf CJ. Evidence for a central component of post-injury pain hypersensitivity. *Nature.* 1983;306:686–688.
19. Lai J, Gold M, Kim CS, et al. Inhibition of neuropathic pain by decreased expression of the tetrodotoxin-resistant sodium channel, NaV1.8. *Pain.* 2002;95:143–152.
20. Munro G, Dalby-Brown W. Kv7 (KCNQ) channel modulators and neuropathic pain. *J Med Chem.* 2007;50:2576–2582.
21. Mulleman D, Mammou S, Griffoul I, et al. Pathophysiology of disk-related sciatica. I.–Evidence supporting a chemical component. *Joint Bone Spine.* 2006;73:151–158.
22. Basbaum AI. Spinal mechanisms of acute and persistent pain. *Reg Anesth Pain Med.* 1999;24:59–67.
23. Torebjork HE, Lundberg LE, LaMotte RH. Central changes in processing of mechanoreceptive input in capsaicin-induced secondary hyperalgesia in humans. *J Physiol.* 1992;448:765–780.
24. Jensen MC, Brant-Zawadzki MN, Obuchowski N, et al. Magnetic resonance imaging of the lumbar spine in people without back pain. *N Eng J Med.* 1994;331:69–73.
25. Weinreb JC, Wolbarsht LB, Cohen JM, et al. Prevalence of lumbosacral intervertebral disc abnormalities in MR images of pregnant and asymptomatic non-pregnant women. *Radiology.* 1989;170:125–128.
26. Borenstein DG, O'Mara JW, Boden SD, et al. The value of magnetic resonance imaging of the lumbar spine to predict low back pain in asymptomatic subjects: A seven-year follow-up study. *J Bone Joint Surg Am.* 2001;83:1306–1311.
27. Burke JG, Watson RW, McCormack D, et al. Intervertebral discs which cause low back pain secrete high levels of proinflammatory mediators. *J Bone Joint Surg Br.* 2002;84:196–201.
28. Olmarker K, Rydevik B. Selective inhibition of tumor necrosis factor-alpha prevents nucleus induced thrombus formation, intraneural edema, and reduction of nerve conduction velocity: Possible implications for future pharmacologic treatment strategy of sciatica. *Spine.* 2001;26:863–869.
29. Cohen SP, Wenzell D, Hurley RW, et al. A double-blind placebo-controlled, dose-response pilot study evaluating intradiscal ethanercept in patients with chronic discogenic low back pain or lumbosacral radiculopathy. *Anesthesiology.* 2007;107:99–105.
30. Malik K, Nelson A, Benzon HT. Disease-modifying antirheumatic drugs for the treatment of low back pain: A systematic review of the literature. *Pain Pract.* 2016;16:629–641
31. Arden NK, Price C, Reading I, et al. WEST Study Group: A multicentre randomized controlled trial of epidural corticosteroid injections for sciatica: The WEST study. *Rheumatology.* 2005;44:1399–1406.
32. Wilson-MacDonald J, Burt G, Griffen D, et al. Epidural steroid injection for nerve root compression. A randomized, controlled trial. *J Bone Joint Surg Br.* 2005;87:352–355.
33. Carette S, Leclaire R, Marcoux S, et al. Epidural corticosteroid injections for sciatica due to herniated nucleus pulposus. *N Engl J Med.* 1997;336:1634–1640.
34. Benzon HT. The long journey of epidural steroid injections. *Reg Anesth Pain Med.* 2013;38:171–172
35. Karppinen J, Malmivaara A, Kurunlahti M, et al. Periradicular infiltration for sciatica: A randomized controlled trial. *Spine.* 2001;26:1059–1067.
36. Ng L, Chaudhary N, Sell P. The efficacy of corticosteroids in periradicular infiltration for chronic radicular pain: A randomized, double-blind, controlled trial. *Spine.* 2005;30:857–862.
37. Thomas E, Cyteval C, Abiad L, et al. Effect of transforaminal versus interspinous corticosteroid injection in discal radiculalgia—a prospective, randomized, double-blind study. *Clin Rheumatol.* 2003;22:299–304.
38. Ackerman WE 3rd, Ahmad M. The effect of lumbar epidural steroid injections in patients with lumbar disc herniations. *Anesth Analg.* 2007;104:1217–1222
39. Kay J, Findling JW, Raff H. Epidural triamcinolone suppresses the pituitary-adrenal axis in human subject. *Anesth Analg.* 1994;79:501–505
40. Rathmell JP, April C, Bogduk N. Cervical transforaminal injection of steroids. *Anesthesiology.* 2004;100:1595–1600.
41. Tiso RL, Cutler T, Catania JA, et al. Adverse central nervous system sequelae after selective transforaminal block: the role of corticosteroids. *Spine J.* 2004;4:468–474.
42. Benzon HT, Chew TL, McCarthy R, et al. Comparison of the particle sizes of the different steroids and the effect of dilution: A review of the relative neurotoxicities of the steroids. *Anesthesiology.* 2007;106:331–338.
43. Huntoon MA. Anatomy of the cervical intervertebral foramina: Vulnerable arteries and ischemic neurologic injuries after transforaminal epidural injections. *Pain.* 2005;117:104–111.
44. El-Yahchouchi C, Geske JR, Carter RE, et al. The noninferiority of the non-particulate steroid dexamethasone and triamcinolone in lumbar transforaminal epidural steroid injections. *Pain Med.* 2013;14:1650–1657.
45. Kennedy DJ, Plastaras C, Casey E, et al. Comparative effectiveness of lumbar transforaminal epidural steroid injections with particulate versus nonparticulate corticosteroids for lumbar radicular pain due to intervertebral disc herniation: A prospective, randomized, double-blind trial. *Pain Med.* 2014;15:548–555.

46. Rathmell JR, Benzon HT, Dreyfuss P, et al. Safeguards to prevent neurological complications after epidural steroid injections: Consensus opinions from a Multidisciplinary Working Group and national organizations. *Anesthesiology*. 2015;122:974–984
47. Iversen T, Solberg TK, Romner B, et al. Effect of caudal epidural steroid or saline injection in chronic lumbar radiculopathy: Muticentre, blinded, randomized controlled trial. *BMJ*. 2011;343:d5278.
48. Friedly JL, Comstock BA, Turner JA, et al. A randomized trial of epidural glucocorticoid injections for spinal stenosis. *N Eng J Med*. 2014; 371:11–21.
49. Bickett MC, Gupta A, Brown CH 4th, et al. Epidural injections for spinal pain: a systematic review and meta-analysis evaluating the "control" injections in randomized controlled trials. *Anesthesiology*. 2013;119:907–931.
50. Cohen SP, Hanling S, Bicket MC, et al. Epidural steroid injections compared with gabapentin for lumbosacral radicular pain: Multicenter randomized double blind comparative efficacy study. *BMJ*. 2015;350:h1748.
51. Schukro RP, Oehmke MJ, Geroldinger A, et al. Efficacy of duloxetine in chronic low back pain with neuropathic component: A randomized, double-blind, placebo-controlled crossover trial. *Anesthesiology*. 2016;124:150–158.
52. Cohen SP, Strassels SA, Kurihara C, et al. Does sensory stimulation threshold affect lumbar facet radiofrequency denervation outcomes: A prospective clinical correlation study. *Anesth Analg*. 2011;113:1233–1341.
53. van Wijk RM, Geurtz JW, Wynne HJ, et al. Radiofrequency denervation of lumbar facet joints in the treatment of chronic low back pain: A randomized, double-blind, sham lesion-trial. *Clin J Pain*. 2005;21:335–344.
54. Tekin I, Mirzai H, Ok G, et al. A comparison of conventional and pulsed radiofrequency in the treatment of chronic facet joint pain. *Clin J Pain*. 2007;23:524–529.
55. Nath S, Nath CA, Pettersson K. Percutaneous lumbar zygapophyseal (facet) joint neurotomy using radiofrequency current, in the management of chronic low back pain: a randomized double-blind trial. *Spine*. 2008;33:1291–1297.
56. Engel A, Rappard G, King W, et al; Standards Division of the International Spine Intervention Society. The effectiveness and risks of fluoroscopically-guided cervical medial branch thermal radiofrequency neurotomy: A systematic review with comprehensive analysis of the published data. *Pain Med*. 2016; 17:658–669.
57. Maas ET, Ostelo RW, Niemisto L, et al. Radiofrequency denervation for chronic low back pain. *Cochrane Database Syst Rev*. 2015;10:CD008572. doi: 10.1002/14651858.CD008572.pub2.
58. Manchikanti L, Kaye AD, Boswell MV, et al. A systematic review and best evidence synthesis of the effectiveness of therapeutic facet joint interventions in managing chronic spinal pain. *Pain Phsyician*. 2015;18:E535–E582
59. Schmidt PC, Pino CA, Vorenkamp KE. Sacroiliac joint radiofrequency ablation with probe: a case series of 60 patients. *Anesth Analg*. 2014;119:460–462.
60. Cohen SP, Hurley RW, Buckenmaier CC 3rd, et al. Randomized placebo-controlled study evaluating lateral branch radiofrequency denervation for sacroiliac joint pain. *Anesthesiology*. 2008;109:279–288.
61. Benzon HT, Katz JA, Benzon HA, et al. Piriformis syndrome: Anatomic considerations, a new injection technique, and a review of the literature. *Anesthesiology*. 2003;98:1442–1448.
62. Fowler IM, Tucker AA, Weimerskirch BP, et al. A randomized comparison of the efficacy of 2 techniques for piriformis injection: ultrasound-guided versus stimulator with fluoroscopic guidance. *Reg Anesth Pain Med*. 2014;39:126–132
63. Misirlioglu TO, Akgun P, Palamar D, et al. Piriformis syndrome: Comparison of the effectiveness of local anesthetic and corticosteroid injections: A double-blinded, randomized, controlled study. *Pain Physician*. 2015;18:163–171
64. Porta M. A comparative trial of botulinum toxin A and methylprednisolone for the treatment of myofascial pain syndrome and pain from chronic muscle spasm. *Pain*. 2000;85:101–105.
65. Jabbari B, Machado D. Treatment of refractory pain with botulinum toxins–an evidence-based review. *Pain Med*. 2011;12:1594–1606.
66. Nicol A, Wu II, Ferrante FM. Botulinum toxin type A injections for cervical and shoulder girdle myofascial pain using an enriched protocol design. *Anesth Analg*. 2014;118:1326–1335.
67. Wolfe F, Smythe HA, Yunus MB, et al. The American College of Rheumatology 1990 Criteria for the Classification of Fibromyalgia. *Arthritis Rheum*. 1990;33:160–172.
68. Wolfe F, Clauw DJ, Fitzcharles MA, et al. The American College of Rheumatology preliminary diagnostic criteria for fibromyalgia and measurement of symptom severity. *Arthritis Care Res*. 2010;62:600–610.
69. Sarchielli P, Di Filippo M, Nardi K, et al. Sensitization, glutamate, and the link between migraine and fibromyalgia. *Curr Pain Headache Rep*. 2007;11:343–351.
70. Baraniuk JN, Whalen G, Cunningham J, et al. Cerebrospinal fluid levels of opioid peptides in fibromyalgia and chronic low back pain. *BMC Musculoskelet Disord*. 2004;5:48.
71. Borchers AT, Gershwin ME. Fibromyalgia: A critical and comprehensive review. *Clin Rev Allergy Immunol*. 2015;49:100–151.
72. Arnold LM, Lu Y, Crofford LJ, et al. A double-blind, multicenter trial comparing duloxetine with placebo in the treatment of fibromyalgia patients with or without major depressive disorder. *Arthritis Rheum*. 2004;50:2974–2984.
73. Gendreau RM, Thorn MD, Gendreau JF, et al. The efficacy of milnacipran in fibromyalgia. *J Rheumatol*. 2005;32:1975–1985.
74. Crofford LJ, Mease PJ, Simpson SL, et al. Fibromyalgia relapse evaluation and efficacy for durability of meaningful relief (FREEDOM): A 6-month, double-blind, placebo-controlled trial with pregabalin. *Pain*. 2008;136:419–431.
75. Russell IJ, Perkins AT, Michalek JE. Oxybate SXB-26 Fibromyalgia Syndrome Study Group. Sodium oxybate relieves pain and improves function in fibromyalgia syndrome: A randomized, double-blind, placebo-controlled, multicenter clinical trial. *Arthritis Rheum*. 2009;60:299–309.
76. Pasqualucci A, Pasqualucci V, Galla F, et al. Prevention of postherpetic neuralgia: Acyclovir and prednisolone versus epidural local anesthetic and methylprednisolone. *Acta Anaesthesiol Scand*. 2000;44:910–918.
77. van Wijck AJ, Opstelten W, Moons KG, et al. The PINE study of epidural steroids local anaesthetics to prevent postherpetic neuralgia randomized controlled trial. *Lancet*. 2006;367:219–224.
78. Raja SN, Haythornthwaite JA, Papagallo M, et al. Opioids versus antidepressants in postherpetic neuralgia: A randomized placebo-controlled trial. *Neurology*. 2002;59:1015.
79. Boureau F, Legallicier P, Kabir-Ahmadi M. Tramadol in postherpetic neuralgia: A randomized, double-blind, placebo-controlled trial. *Pain*. 2003;104(1–2):323–331.
80. Dworkin RH, Corbin AE, Young JP, et al. Pregabalin for the treatment of postherpetic neuralgia: A randomized, placebo-controlled trial. *Neurology*. 2003;60:1274–1283.
81. Freynhagen R, Strojek K, Griesing T, et al. Efficacy of pregabalin in neuropathic pain evaluated in a 12-week, randomised, double-blind, multicentre, placebo-controlled trial of flexible- and fixed-dose regimens. *Pain*. 2005;115:254–263.
82. Gilron I, Bailey JM, Tu D, et al. Morphine, gabapentin, or their combination for neuropathic pain. *New Engl J Med*. 2005;352:1324–1334.
83. Gilron I, Bailey JM, Tu D, et al. Nortriptyline and gabapentin, alone and in combination for neuropathic pain: A double-blind, randomised controlled crossover trial. *Lancet*. 2009;374:1252–1261.
84. Kotani N, Kushikata T, Hashimoto H, et al. Intrathecal methylprednisolone for intractable postherpetic neuralgia. *N Engl J Med*. 2000;343:1514–1519.
85. Rijsdijk M, van Wijck AJ, Meulenhoff PC, et al. No beneficial effect of intrathecal methylprednisolone acetate in postherpetic neuralgia patients. *Eur J Pain*. 2013;17:714–723.
86. Dworkin RH, O'Connor AB, Kent J, et al; International Association for the Study of Pain Neuropathic Pain Special Interest Group. Interventional management of neuropathic pain: NeuPSIG recommendations. *Pain*. 2013;154:2249–2261.
87. Benzon HT, Chekka K, Darnule A, et al. Evidence-based case report: Intrathecal alcohol for postherpetic neuralgia. *Reg Anesth Pain Med*. 2009;34:514–521.
88. Harke H, Gretenkort P, Ladleif HU, et al. Spinal cord stimulation in postherpetic neuralgia and in acute herpes zoster. *Anesth Analg*. 2002;9:694–700.
89. Goldstein DJ, Lu Y, Detke MJ, et al. Duloxetine vs. placebo in patients with painful diabetic neuropathy. *Pain*. 2005;116:109–118.
90. Attal N, Cruccu G, Baron R, et al. European Federation of Neurological Sciences. EFNS guidelines on the pharmacological treatment of neuropathic pain: 2010 revision. *Eur J Neurol*. 2010;17:1113–1123.
91. Dworkin RH, O'Connor AB, Audette J, et al. Recommendations for the pharmacologic management of neuropathic pain: An overview and literature update. *Mayo Clin Proc*. 2010;85:S3–S14.
92. Harden RN, Bruehl S, Perez RS, et al. Validation of proposed diagnostic criteria (the "Budapest Criteria") for Complex Regional Pain Syndrome. *Pain*. 2010;150:268–274.
93. van de Vusse AC, Stomp-van den Berg SG, Kessels AH, et al. Randomised controlled trial of gabapentin in complex regional pain syndrome type 1. *BMC Neurol*. 2004;4;13.
94. Xu J, Yang J, Lin P, et al. Intravenous therapies for complex regional pain syndrome – a systematic review. *Anesth Analg*. 2016;122:843–856.
95. Sigtermans MJ, van Hilten JJ, Bauer MC, et al. Ketamine produces effective and long-term pain relief in patients with Complex Regional Pain Syndrome Type 1. *Pain*. 2009;145:304–311.
96. Schwartzman RJ, Alexander GM, Grothusen JR, et al. Outpatient intravenous ketamine for the treatment of complex regional pain syndrome: A double-blind placebo controlled study. *Pain*. 2009;147:107–115.
97. Noppers IM, Niesters M, Aarts LP, et al. Drug-induced liver injury following a repeated course of ketamine treatment for chronic pain in CRPS type 1 patients: A report of 3 cases. *Pain*. 2011;152(9):2173–2178.
98. Benzon HT, Liu SS, Buvanendran A. Evolving definitions and pharmacologic management of complex regional pain syndrome. *Anesth Analg*. 2016;122:601–604.
99. Kemler MA, De Vet HC, Barendse GA, et al. The effect of spinal cord stimulation in patients with chronic reflex sympathetic dystrophy: Two years' follow-up of the randomized controlled trial. *Ann Neurol*. 2004;55(1):13–18.
100. Kemler MA, de Vet HC, Barendse GA, et al. Effect of spinal cord stimulation for complex regional pain syndrome Type I: five year final follow-up of patients in a randomized controlled trial. *J Neurosurg*. 2008;108:292–298.

101. Simpson DM, McArthur JC, Olney R, et al. Lamotrigine Neuropathy Study HIV Team for HIV-associated painful sensory neuropathies: A placebo-controlled trial. *Neurology.* 2003;609:1508–1514.
102. Hahn K, Arendt G, Braun JS, et al. German Neuro-AIDS Working Group: A placebo-trial of gabapentin for painful HIV-associated sensory neuropathies. *J Neurol.* 2004;251:1260–1266.
103. McCormick C, Chang-Chien G, Marshall B, et al. Phantom limb pain: A systematic neuroanatomical-based review of pharmacologic management. *Pain Med.* 2014;15:292–305.
104. Ischia S, Ischia A, Polati E, et al. Three posterior percutaneous celiac plexus block: A prospective randomized study in 61 patients with pancreatic cancer pain. *Anesthesiology.* 1992;76:534–540.
105. Mercadante S. Celiac plexus block versus analgesics in pancreatic cancer pain. *Pain.* 1993;52:187–192.
106. Wong G, Schoeder DR, Carns PE, et al. Effect of neurolytic celiac plexus block on pain relief, quality of life, and survival in patients with unresectable pancreatic cancer. *JAMA.* 2004;291:1092–1099.
107. Eisenberg E, Carr DB, Chalmers TC. Neurolytic celiac plexus block for treatment of cancer pain: A meta-analysis. *Anesth Analg.* 1995;80:290–295.
108. Mercadante S, Klepstad P, Kurita GP, et al.; European Palliative Care Research Collaborative (EPCRC). Sympathetic blocks for visceral cancer pain management: A systematic review and EAPC recommendations. *Crit Rev Oncol Hematol.* 2015;96:577–583.
109. Mishra S, Bhatnagar S, Rana SP, et al. Efficacy of the anterior ultrasound-guided superior hypogastric plexus neurolysis in pelvic cancer pain in advanced gynecological cancer patients. *Pain Med.* 2013;14:837–842.
110. Kroll CE, Schartz B, Gonzalez-Fernandez M, et al. Factors associated with outcome after superior hypogastric plexus neurolysis in cancer patients. *Clin J Pain.* 2014;30:55–62.
111. Okie S. A flood of opioids: A rising tide of deaths. *New Engl J Med.* 2010;383:1981–1985.
112. Krantz MJ, Martin J, Stimmel B, et al. QTc interval screening in methadone treatment. *Ann Med.* 2009;150:387–395.
113. Somogyi AA, Barratt DT, Coller JK. Pharmacogenetics of opioids. *Clin Pharmacol Ther.* 2007;81:429–444.
114. Williams DG, Patel A, Howard RF. Pharmacogenetics of codeine metabolism in an urban population of children and its implications for analgesic reliability. *Br J Anaesth.* 2002;89:839–845.
115. Gomes T, Redelmeier DA, Juurlink DN, et al. Opioid dose and risk of road trauma in Canada: A population-based study. *JAMA Intern Med.* 2013;173:196–201.
116. Vainio A, Ollila J, Matikainen E, et al. Driving ability in cancer patients receiving long-morphine analgesia. *Lancet.* 1995;346:667.
117. Chou R, Turner JA, Devine EB, et al. The effectiveness and risks of long-term opioid therapy for chronic pain: A systematic review for a National Institute of Health Pathways to Prevention Workshop. *Ann Intern Med.* 2015;162:276–286.
118. Martell BA, O'Connor PG, Kerns RD, et al. Systematic review: Opioid treatment for chronic back pain: Prevalence, efficacy, and association with addiction. *Ann Int Med.* 2007;146:116–127.
119. Goesling J, Henry MJ, Moser SE, et al. Symptoms of depression are associated with opioid use regardless of pain severity and physical functioning among treatment seeking patients with chronic pain. *J Pain.* 2015;16:844–851.
120. Finnerup NB, Attal N, Harotounian S, et al. Pharmacotherapy for neuropathic pain in adults: a systematic review and meta-analysis. *Lancet Neurol.* 2015;14:162–173.
121. Watson CP, Gilron I, Sawynok J, et al. Nontricyclic analgesics and pain: Are serotonin norpeinephrine reuptake inhibitors (SNRIs) any better? *Pain.* 2011;152:2206–2210.
122. Bombolt SF, Mikkelsen JD, Blackburn-Munro G. Antinociceptive effects of the antidepressants amitriptyline, duloxetine, mirtazapine and citalopram in animal models of acute, persistent and neuropathic pain. *Neuropharmacology.* 2005;48:252–263.
123. Rashkin J, Pritchett YL, Wang F, et al. A double-blind, randomized multicenter trial comparing duloxetine with placebo in the management of diabetic peripheral neuropathic pain. *Pain Med.* 2005;6:346–356.
124. Arnold LM, Rosen A, Pritchett YL, et al. A randomized, double-blind, placebo-controlled trial of duloxetine in the treatment of women with fibromyalgia with or without major depressive disorder. *Pain.* 2005;119:5–15.
125. Clauw DJ, Mease P, Palmer RH, et al. Milnacipran for the treatment of fibromyalgia in adults: A 15-week, multicenter, randomized, double-blind, placebo-controlled, multiple-dose clinical trial. *Clin Ther.* 2008;30:1988–2004.
126. Mease PJ, Clauw DJ, Gendreau RM, et al. The efficacy and safety of milnacipran for treatment of fibromyalgia. A randomized, double-blind, placebo-controlled trial. *J Rheumatol.* 2009;36:398–409.
127. Ramaekers JG. Antidepressants and driver impairment: Empirical evidence from a standard on-the-road test. *J Clin Psychiatr.* 2003;64:20–29.
128. Sharma U, Griesing T, Emir B, et al. Time to onset of neuropathic pain reduction: A retrospective analysis of data from nine controlled trials of pregabalin for painful diabetic and postherpetic neuralgia. *Am J Ther.* 2010;17:577–585.
129. Campbell BJ, Rowbotham M, Davies PS, et al. Systemic absorption of topical lidocaine in normal volunteers, patients with post-herpetic neuralgia, and patients with acute herpes zoster. *J Pharm Sci.* 2002;91:1343–1350.
130. Rowbotham MC, Davies PS, Verkempinck C, et al. Lidocaine patch: Double-blind controlled study of new treatment method for postherpetic neuralgia. *Pain.* 1996;65:39–44.
131. Kennedy WR, Vanhove GF, Lu SP, et al. A randomized, controlled, open-label study of the long-term effects of NGX-4010, a high-concentration capsaicin patch, on epidermal nerve fiber density and sensory function in healthy volunteers. *J Pain.* 2010;11:579–587.
132. Backonja MM, Malan TP, Vanhove GF, et al. C102/106 Study Group:NGX-4010, a high-capsaicin patch, for the treatment of postherpetic neuralgia: A randomized, double-blind, controlled study with an open-label extension. *Pain Med.* 2010;11:600–608.
133. Simpson DM, Brown S, Tobias J. NGX-4010 C107 Study Group. Controlled trial of high-capsaicin patch for treatment of painful HIV neuropathy. *Neurology.* 2008;70:2305–2313.
134. Simpson DM, Gazda S, Brown S, et al. NGX-4010 C118 Study Group. Long-term safety of NGX-4010, a high-concentration capsaicin patch, in patients with peripheral neuropathic pain. *J Pain Symptom Manage.* 2010;39:1053–1064.
135. Deshpande A, Mailis-Gagnon A, Zoheiry N, et al. Efficacy and adverse effects of medical marijuana for chronic noncancer pain: Systematic review of randomized controlled trials. *Can Fam Physician.* 2015;61:e372–e381.
136. Johnson JR, Burnell-Nugent M, Lossignol D, et al. Multicenter, double-blind, randomized, placebo-controlled, parallel-group study of the efficacy, safety, and tolerability of THC:CBD extract and THC extract in patients with intractable cancer pain. *J Pain Symptom Manage.* 2010;39:167–179.
137. Narang S, Gibson D, Wasan AD, et al. Efficacy of dronabinol as an adjunct treatment for chronic pain patients on opioid therapy. *J Pain.* 2008;9:254–264.
138. Chen KY, Chen L, Mao J. Buprenorphine-naloxone therapy in pain management. *Anesthesiology.* 2014;120:1262–1274.
139. Neumann AM, Blondell RD, Jaanimägi U, et al. A preliminary study comparing methadone and buprenorphine in patients with chronic pain and coexistent opioid addiction. *J Addict Dis.* 2013;32:68–78.
140. Roux P, Sullivan MA, Cohen J, et al. Buprenorphine/naloxone as a promising therapeutic option for opioid abusing patients with chronic pain: Reduction of pain, opioid withdrawal symptoms, and abuse liability of oral oxycodone. *Pain.* 2013;154:1442–1448.
141. Pino CA, Ivie CS, Rathmell JP. Lumbar discography: Diagnostic role in discogenic pain. *Techn Reg Anesth Pain Manag.* 2009;13(2):85–92.
142. Derby R, Lee SH, Chen Y. Discograms: Cervical, thoracic, and lumbar. *Techn Reg Anesth Pain Manag.* 2005;9(2):97–105.
143. Derby R, Lee SH, Kim BJ, et al. Pressure-controlled lumbar discography in volunteers without low back symptoms. *Pain Med.* 2005;6:213–221.
144. Cohen SP, Larkin TM, Barna SA, et al. Lumbar discography: A comprehensive review of outcome studies, diagnostic accuracy, and principles. *Reg Anesth Pain Med.* 2005;30:163–183.
145. Carragee EJ, Don AS, Hurwitz EL, et al. 2009 ISSLS Prize Winner: Does discography cause accelerated progression of degeneration changes in the lumbar disc: A ten-year matched cohort study. *Spine.* 2009;34:2338–2345.
146. Pauza KJ, Howell S, Dreyfuss P, et al. A randomized, placebo-controlled trial of intradiscal electrothermal therapy for the treatment of discogenic low back pain. *Spine J.* 2004;4:27.
147. Freeman BJ, Fraser RD, Cain CM, et al. A randomized, double-blind, controlled trial: Intradiscal electrotheraml therapy versus placebo for the treatment of chronic discogenic low back pain. *Spine (Phila Pa 1976).* 2005;30:2369–2377.
148. Kapural L, Vrooman B, Srawar S, et al. A randomized, placebo-controlled trial of intradiscal radiofrequency, biacuplasty for treatment of discogenic lower back pain. *Pain Med.* 2013;14:362–373.
149. Desai MJ, Kapural L, Petersohn JD, et al. A prospective, randomized, multicenter, open-clinical trial comparing intradiscal biacupalsty to conventional medical management for discogenic lower back pain. *Spine (Phila Pa 1976).* 2016;41:1065–1074.
150. Kalichman L, Cole R, Kim DH, et al. Spinal stenosis prevalence and association with symptoms: The Framingham Study. *Spine J.* 2009;9:545–550.
151. Deer TR, Kapural L. New image-guided ultra-minimally invasive lumbar decompression method: The mild procedure. *Pain Physician.* 2010;13:35–41.
152. Costandi S, Chopko M, Mekhail M, et al. Lumbar spinal stenosis: Therapeutic options review. *Pain Pract.* 2015;15:68–81.
153. Lingreen R, Grider JS. Retrospective review of patient self-reported improvement and post-findings for mild (minimally invasive lumbar decompression). *Pain Physician.* 2010;13:555–560.
154. Chopko BW. A novel method for treatment of lumbar spinal stenosis in high-risk surgical candidates: Pilot study experience with percutaneous remodeling of ligamentum flavum and lamina. *J Neurosurg Spine.* 2011;14:46–50.
155. Philips FM, Wetzel FT, Leiberman I, et al. An in vivo comparison of the potential for extravertebral cement leak after vertebroplasty and kyphoplasty. *Spine.* 2002;27:2173–2178.
156. Diamond TH, Champion B, Clark WA. Management of acute osteoporotic vertebral fractures: A nonrandomized trial comparing percutaneous vertebroplasty with conservative therapy. *Am J Med.* 2003;114:257–265.

157. Perez-Higueras A, Alvarez L, Rossi RE, et al. Percutaneous vertebroplasty: Long-term clinical and radiological outcome. *Neuroradiology.* 2002;44:950–954.
158. Ledlie JT, Renfro MJ. Balloon kyphoplasty: One year outcomes in vertebral body height restoration, chronic pain, and activity levels. *J Neurosurg.* 2003;98:36–42.
159. Fourney DR, Schomer DF, Nader R, et al. Percutaneous vertebroplasty and kyphoplasty for painful vertebral body fractures in cancer patients. *J Neurosurg.* 2003;98:21–30.
160. Coumans JV, Reinhardt MK, Lieberman IH. Kyphoplasty for vertebral compression fractures: 1 year clinical outcomes from a prospective study. *J Neurosurg.* 2003;99:44–50.
161. Buchbinder R, Osborne RH, Ebeling PR, et al. A randomized trial of vertebroplasty for painful osteoporotic vertebral fractures. *N Engl J Med.* 2009;361:557–568.
162. Kallmes DF, Comstock BA, Heagerty PJ, et al. A randomized trial of vertebroplasty for osteoporotic spinal fractures. *N Engl J Med.* 2009;361:569–579.
163. Muijs SP, van Erkel AR, Dijkstra PD. Treatment of painful osteoporotic vertebral compression fractures: A brief review of the evidence for percutaneous vertebroplasty. *J Bone Joint Surg Br.* 2011;93:1149–1153.
164. Wardlaw D, Cummings SR, Van Meirhaeghe J, et al. Efficacy and safety of balloon kyphoplasty compared with non-surgical care for vertebral compression fracture (FREE): A randomised controlled trial. *Lancet.* 2009;373:1016–1024.
165. Berenson J, Pflugmacher R, Jarzem P, et al. Cancer Patient Fracture Evaluation (CAFE) Investigators. Balloon kyphoplasty versus non-surgical fracture management for treatment of painful vertebral body compression fractures in patients with cancer: A multicentre, randomised controlled trial. *Lancet Oncol.* 2011;12:225–235.
166. Linderoth B, Foreman R. Physiology of spinal cord stimulation: Review and update. *Neuromodulation.* 1999;3:150–164.
167. North RB, Kidd DH, Farrokhi F, et al. Spinal cord stimulation versus repeated lumbosacral spine surgery for chronic pain: A randomized controlled trial. *Neurosurgery.* 2005;51:106–107.
168. Taylor RS. Spinal cord stimulation in complex regional pain syndrome and refractory neuropathic back and leg pain/failed back surgery syndrome: Results of a systematic review and meta-analysis. *J Pain Sympt Manage.* 2006;31:S13–S19.
169. Kemler MA, Barendse GA, van Kleef M, et al. Spinal cord stimulation in patients with chronic reflex sympathetic dystrophy. *N Engl J Med.* 2000;343:618–624.
170. Kemler MA, de Vet HC, Barendse GA, et al. Spinal cord stimulation for chronic reflex sympathetic dystrophy – five year follow-up. *N Engl J Med.* 2006;354:2394–2396.
171. Geurts JW, Smits H, Kemler MA. Spinal cord stimulation for complex regional pain syndrome type I: a prospective cohort study with long-term follow-up. *Neuromodulation.* 2013;16:523–529.
172. Hautvast RW. Spinal cord stimulation in chronic intractable angina pectoris: A randomized, controlled efficacy study. *Am Heart J.* 1998;136:1114–1120.
173. Klomp HM. Spinal cord stimulation in critical limb ischemia: A randomized trial: ESES study group. *Lancet.* 1999;353:1040–1044.
174. Deer T. Prospective, randomized, multi-center, controlled clinical trial to assess the safety and efficacy of the spinal modulation Axium® Neurostimulator System in the treatment of chronic pain. Presented at the North American Neuromodulation Society Meeting, Las Vegas, Nevada. December 11, 2015.
175. Burns B, Watkins L, Goadsby PJ. Treatment of medically intractable cluster headache by occipital nerve stimulation: Long-term follow-up of eight patients. *Lancet.* 2007;369:1099–1106.
176. Eisenach JC, Hood DD, Curry R, et al. Intrathecal but not intravenous opioids release adenosine from the spinal cord. *Pain.* 2004;5:64.
177. Deer T, Krames ES, Hassenbusch SJ, et al. Polyanalgesic consensus conference 2007: Recommendations for the management of pain by intrathecal (intraspinal) drug delivery: Report of an interdisciplinary expert panel. *Neuromodulation.* 2007;10:300–328.
178. Hayek S, Joseph PN, Mekhail, NA. Pharmacology of intrathecally administered agents for treatment of spasticity and pain. *Seminars in Pain Medicine.* 2003;1:238–253.
179. Deer TR, Prager J, Levy R, et al. Polyanalgesic consensus conference-2012: Consensus on diagnosis, detection, and treatment of catheter-tip granulomas (inflammatory masses). *Neuromodulation.* 2012;15:483–495.
180. Hayek SM, Veizi E, Hanes M. Intrathecal hydromorphone and bupivacaine combination therapy for post-laminectomy syndrome optimized with patient-activated bolus device. *Pain Med.* 2016;17(3):561–571.

57 Critical Care Medicine

MATTHEW R. HALLMAN • CHRISTOPHER G. CHOUKALAS • STEVEN DEEM

Introduction
    Anesthesiologists and Critical Care Medicine
    Anesthesiology and Critical Care Medicine: The Future
    Critical Care Medicine: A Systems and Processes Approach
Processes of Care in the ICU
    Staffing
    Checklists
    Protocols and Care Bundles
    Resource Management
Neurologic and Neurosurgical Critical Care
    Neuromonitoring
    Diagnosis and Clinical Management of the Most Common Types of Neurologic Failure
Cardiovascular and Hemodynamic Aspects of Critical Care
    Types of Shock
    Monitoring and Resuscitation in Shock States
Acute Respiratory Failure
    Principles of Mechanical Ventilation
    Acute Respiratory Distress Syndrome

Acute Kidney Injury
Endocrine Aspects of Critical Care Medicine
    Glucose Management in Critical Illness
    Adrenal Function in Critical Illness
    Thyroid Function in Critical Illness
    Somatotropic Function in Critical Illness
Anemia and Transfusion Therapy in Critical Illness
Nutrition in the Critically Ill Patient
Sedation and Analgesia for the Critically Ill Patient
    Goals and Assessment
    Pharmacologic Management
    Delirium and Neurocognitive Complications
Complications in the ICU: Detection, Prevention, and Therapy
    Nosocomial Infections
    Stress Ulceration and Gastrointestinal Hemorrhage
    Venous Thromboembolism
    ICU-acquired Weakness
End of Life Care in the ICU

KEY POINTS

1. Simple and inexpensive interventions in the intensive care unit (ICU), such as the utilization of checklists, protocols, and care bundles can result in substantial improvements in patient outcomes.
2. The goal of resuscitation in brain injury is to prevent continuing cerebral insult after a primary injury has already occurred. This is accomplished by restoring cerebral blood flow, maintaining adequate cerebral perfusion pressure, reducing intracranial pressure, evacuating space occupying lesions, and avoiding fever, hyperglycemia, and hypoxia.
3. "Triple-H" therapy consisting of hypertension, hypervolemia, and hemodilution is no longer recommended for the treatment of cerebral vasospasm in subarachnoid hemorrhage. Instead, maintenance of euvolemia and a controlled stepwise trial of blood pressure augmentation in patients with suspected vasospasm is recommended.
4. Administration of thrombolytic therapy (rtPA) to patients presenting within 4.5 hours of onset of acute ischemic stroke results in improved neurologic outcome.
5. There are four general types of shock: hypovolemic, cardiogenic, distributive, and obstructive. The 28-day mortality for septic and cardiogenic shock, two of the most common types encountered in the ICU, are 20% to 40% and 70% to 80% respectively.
6. In patients with severe sepsis or septic shock, early and aggressive use of fluid resuscitation, appropriate antibiotics, infectious source control, and vasopressors/inotropes as needed improves survival.
7. Despite strong regional, local, and individual biases, there is little evidence to suggest that the mode of mechanical ventilation contributes significantly to any major outcome measure, and the choice of mode is largely one of clinician preference.
8. Separation from mechanical ventilation in patients who are recovering from respiratory failure is accelerated by respiratory therapy–driven protocols and daily trials of spontaneous breathing.
9. Ventilation with low tidal volume (6 mL/kg) in patients with acute lung injury and acute respiratory distress syndrome reduces mortality, compared to traditional tidal volumes (12 mL/kg).
10. Red blood cell transfusion in the ICU should be restricted (transfusion threshold hemoglobin <7 g/dL) with the possible exception of patients with active bleeding, early septic shock, acute myocardial infarction, unstable angina, or primary neurologic or neurosurgical problems.
11. Available evidence suggests that practices favoring light sedation, bolus administration versus continuous infusion of sedatives, and daily trials of awakening in ICU patients result in a variety of benefits, including a shortened duration of mechanical ventilation, decreased time in the ICU, and reduced mortality.
12. Delay in treatment of nosocomial infections is associated with increased mortality. Treatment should not be delayed pending diagnostic evaluation; rather treatment should be started after culture specimens are sent, and antibiotics then "de-escalated" after 48 to 72 hours to ensure adequate initial antibiotic treatment, but avoid long-term overuse of antibiotics.
13. End-of-life care is an important aspect of ICU care, and good communication between medical teams, patients, and their family members is required to ensure that delivered care is consistent with patient values and preferences. Patients at high risk of death or severely impaired functional recovery should be offered care focused on comfort and not just curative treatment. Palliative care can also be offered in conjunction with curative care.

Introduction

Anesthesiologists and Critical Care Medicine

Historically, Critical Care Medicine (CCM) evolved as a specialty nearly simultaneously in Europe and North America, but has followed different models in regards to the involvement of anesthesiologists. The first intensive care unit (ICU) in Europe may have been located in Denmark in the 1950s, and concurrently the first critical care physician, or "intensivist," may well have been an anesthesiologist.[1] Anesthesiologists continued to play a defining role in the development of CCM in most of Europe, Australia, New Zealand, Japan, and elsewhere, and comprise the majority of intensivists in many countries around the world today. In North America, anesthesiologists were also integral to the development of CCM as a specialty. However, in contrast to other countries, in the United States anesthesiologists have played a smaller role in the specialty, and today comprise a minority of the intensivist workforce.[2]

Although it has been suggested that the first ICU in North America was established at Johns Hopkins in 1923 to care for postoperative neurosurgical patients, it was not until the late 1950s and early 1960s that true multidisciplinary ICUs began to appear. Anesthesiologists played a natural role in the evolution of ICUs, given their familiarity with surgical resuscitation and mechanical ventilation. Early on, however, the concept of "intensivists" did not exist, and patients were often managed by their primary physician (be it a surgeon or an internist) and nurses, with formal or informal consultation given by specialists, including anesthesiologists.

In the early 1960s, the first CCM training program was established at the University of Pittsburgh under the direction of an anesthesiologist, Peter Safar, and the concept of "intensivist" was born. As defined by Dr. Safar, the qualities and qualifications of such an individual should include inquisitiveness, thoughtfulness, and a high level of motivation, action orientation, diplomacy, and scientific training. In the late 1960s, a group including Dr. Safar and another anesthesiologist, Ake Grenvik, were instrumental in inaugurating the Society of Critical Care Medicine (SCCM). Anesthesiologists working through SCCM were instrumental in developing the board certification process for CCM, and in 1986 the first CCM Certification examination was administered by the American Board of Anesthesiology.[3]

Anesthesiology and Critical Care Medicine: The Future

An increasing demand for intensivists is projected to continue through at least 2020,[2,4] driven largely by substantial evidence that intensivists increase the quality of ICU care and improve patient outcomes. In addition, the aging population is increasing the demand for critical care services. However, the supply of physician intensivists is not expected to keep pace, and instead is projected to decrease through 2025, leading to a worsening shortage of physician providers.[5] Anesthesiology as a specialty is ideally suited to help alleviate this shortage. Anesthesiologists are hospital-based, have sound fundamental training in physiology, pharmacology, invasive procedures, and monitoring, and have excellent historical and contemporary role models for the anesthesiologist as intensivist. In 2013 only 14% of new board certifications in CCM went to anesthesiologists, and less than 8% of graduating anesthesiology residents pursued critical care training.[6] Historically, economic and lifestyle considerations dissuaded many anesthesiology trainees from pursuing further training and careers in CCM. However, evolving reimbursement and staffing models are eliminating these disincentives in many practices. Furthermore, although the practice of CCM for anesthesiologists has historically been focused largely at academic centers, community practice opportunities are increasingly prevalent. While it seems certain that anesthesiologists will continue to play an important role in CCM worldwide, the current conditions in the United States are ideally suited for anesthesiologists wishing to pursue careers in CCM.

Critical Care Medicine: A Systems and Processes Approach

Critical care encompasses all disciplines of medicine. It is clearly beyond the scope of a single chapter to provide detailed coverage of all aspects of critical illness, including physiology, pathophysiology, and management of disease. In addition, many critical care issues are commonly encountered by anesthesiologists who practice solely in the operating room and are covered in detail elsewhere in this text. Thus, this chapter will focus on topics that are relatively unique to the ICU, but are widely applicable to the care of critically ill or injured patients. The entire chapter focuses on evidence-based practices that may improve both patient outcomes and health-care system performance in the perioperative setting.

Grading of levels of evidence and practice guidelines in an effort to improve clinical care has become standard practice. Several different grading systems exist, with no clear evidence that one is superior to another. Furthermore, given uncertainty about the methodology of grading systems and their effects on patient outcomes,[7] we have chosen not to include "grades" or levels of evidence in this chapter.

Processes of Care in the ICU

There is increasing pressure in medicine to deliver high quality care. With the passage of the Affordable Care Act (ACA) in 2010, the United States federal government provided a definition of high quality care and sought, among other things, to link quality care and reimbursement.[8] The six components of quality care according to the ACA are timely, effective, efficient, patient centered, equitable, and safe care. This legislation is rapidly changing many aspects of health-care delivery in the United States, and the ICU is no exception.[9]

A primary way to improve quality across a system is to reduce variability within the system. Processes of care are evidence-based organizational and individual practices that seek to improve the quality of care delivered by standardizing some aspects of health-care delivery. Although the number of potential process targets is nearly limitless, there are only a few that are widely agreed to improve the quality of care.

Staffing

As advances in medical and surgical therapeutics have increased the complexity of care for an aging and increasingly ill population of patients, it has become increasingly clear that the involvement of intensivists in the management of the critically ill patient is desirable.[10] However, the level of involvement is not clear. Numerous studies have suggested that mortality and other intermediate end points such as ICU length of stay, duration of mechanical ventilation, and cost can be reduced when "high-intensity" physician staffing models that mandate management or co-management by intensivists are used.[11–13] However, it does not appear that the addition of in-house nighttime attending physician intensivist staffing further improves outcomes compared to daytime only in-house attending physician staffing.[14,15] The best staffing model for a given ICU likely depends on many factors that are not yet fully understood.

Patient outcomes appear to be further improved by the addition of multidisciplinary providers to intensivist-led teams. Examples include pharmacist participation in daily rounds, as well as the inclusion of nurses, dieticians, and respiratory therapists. These practices significantly reduce costs and medication-related adverse events, and are also associated with decreased patient mortality.[16,17]

Checklists

[1] Despite the improvement in communication and information transfer that occurs with multidisciplinary teams, the high stress and massive volume of information in the ICU environment can lead to errors. Checklists have been widely implemented on ICU rounds as cognitive aides that serve as daily reminders to evaluate a limited number of interventions, preventative measures, bundles, and processes of care that can improve outcomes. Their implementation is associated with a decrease in mortality and ICU length of stay, and they cost virtually nothing.[18] It has been suggested that a checklist prompting consideration of potential interventions is more important than the specific interventions or protocols that are subsequently enacted, especially in ICUs with high-intensity staffing models.[19] Considering these potential benefits and the minimal economic investment required for checklist implementation, their use is strongly recommended. In fact, many of the care processes in this chapter commonly appear on checklists and should be considered with every patient, every day. Suggested content for consideration and inclusion in a daily ICU checklist is listed in Table 57-1. Content might be added or removed based on local ICU considerations.

Protocols and Care Bundles

The use of standardized protocols and care bundles has targeted improved timeliness and appropriateness of treatment for a variety of common ICU diagnoses, as well as prevention of common complications. For example, implementing a standardized order set for patients with septic shock may lower 28-day mortality.[20] Similarly, implementing a simple ventilator care bundle may reduce the incidence of ventilator-associated pneumonia (VAP) and antibiotic utilization.[21] Other studies have shown reduced rates of central line–associated bloodstream infections (CLABSIs) by implementing protocols and bundles.[22] An important additional benefit of utilizing standardized care processes is an improved ability to track outcomes and engage in quality assurance (QA) and quality improvement (QI) programs. As noted earlier, outcome tracking and reporting are now mandated and tied to reimbursement under the ACA.

Resource Management

In 2014 the Critical Care Societies Collaborative (CCSC) released a list of "Five Things Physicians and Patients Should Question" in critical care as part of the Choosing Wisely campaign. The campaign is designed to reduce unnecessary interventions that lack cost-effectiveness, and has been supported by many medical specialties. At the top of the CCM list is a recommendation to not order diagnostic studies (chest x-rays, blood gases, blood chemistries, cell counts, and electrocardiograms) at regular intervals (e.g., daily) without clear clinical indications. Compared with a practice of ordering tests only to answer clinical questions, or when doing so will affect management, the routine ordering of tests increases costs, does not benefit patients and may in fact harm them.[23] Additional recommendations including restrictive transfusion thresholds, avoiding oversedation and parenteral nutrition unless clearly indicated, and discussing end-of-life issues are addressed in other sections of this chapter. This type of effort to minimize unnecessary interventions recognizes both the financial impact such practice decisions have on individual patients and the health-care system overall, as well as the physician's role in providing not just effective, but efficient care.

Neurologic and Neurosurgical Critical Care

Neuromonitoring

There are many neuromonitoring techniques with both intraoperative and ICU applicability. Electroencephalogram (EEG), evoked potential monitors, near-infrared spectroscopy (NIRS), brain tissue oxygenation ($PbrO_2$), cerebral microdialysis, intracranial pressure (ICP) monitoring, transcranial Doppler (TCD) ultrasonography and jugular venous saturation (SjO_2) monitoring may all help in assessing pathophysiologic processes and adjusting therapy. These techniques are discussed in Chapters 26, 37, and 53, and will not be discussed in detail here.

Diagnosis and Clinical Management of the Most Common Types of Neurologic Failure

Traumatic Brain Injury

Traumatic brain injury (TBI) is the leading cause of death from blunt trauma, with an incidence of approximately 10 per 100,000 per year, and is the leading cause of death between 5 and 45 years of age. The most powerful predictors of poor outcome from injury through resuscitation are age greater than 55, poor pupillary reactivity, postresuscitation Glasgow Coma

Table 57-1 Suggested Daily Intensive Care Unit Checklist

- Spontaneous awakening trial
- Spontaneous breathing trial
- Nutrition/diet ordered
- Adequate sedation and analgesia
- Deep-venous thrombosis prophylaxis initiated
- Glucose control adequate
- Unnecessary labs and imaging discontinued
- Antibiotics discontinued
- Foley catheter removed
- Central venous catheter and arterial line removed
- Plan of the day reviewed

Scale (GCS), hypotension, hypoxia, and unfavorable intracranial diagnosis as established by radiological features (e.g., computed tomography [CT]). In addition, early hyperglycemia (>200 mg/dL) is a reliable independent predictor of poor outcome.

The GCS (see Chapter 53) is the most widely used clinical measure of injury severity in patients with TBI. The advantages of this scale are that it provides an objective method of measuring consciousness, it has high intra- and inter-rater reliability across observers with a wide variety of experience, and it has an excellent correlation with outcome. However, the GCS is not measurable in up to 25% to 45% of patients at admission, and is inaccurate when only the partial score is used, such as in patients with tracheal intubation whose verbal response cannot be assessed. TBI qualifies as severe when the GCS is 8 or less. The predictive value of the GCS at admission is about 69% for good neurologic outcome and 76% for unfavorable outcome. After 7 days these figures approximate 80% for both favorable and unfavorable outcome.[24]

Pupillary dilatation and light reactivity are also useful predictors of neurologic outcome after TBI. When both pupils are dilated and unreactive the likelihood of poor neurologic outcome or death is as high as 90% to 95%. When both pupils are reactive, the likelihood of poor neurologic outcome is approximately 30% to 40%, and the probability of good outcome is 50% to 70%.

In contrast, hypotension is a strong predictor of poor outcome in TBI. In one report, there was a 15-fold increased risk of mortality in patients with early hypotension and an 11-fold increase in mortality in patients with late hypotension.[25]

Radiological imaging is important in the diagnosis and prognosis of patients with TBI. A number of CT-based scoring systems have been developed and correlated with outcome, but the amount of midline shift appears to be the single most predictive feature of outcome. Subarachnoid blood, intraventricular blood, and diffuse axonal injury patterns portend worse outcomes, but epidural hematomas generally have better outcomes.[26] In addition, it should be noted that about one-third to one-half of TBI patients present with no imaging lesion at admission, but develop delayed lesions, which are associated with substantially worse neurologic outcome.

The goal of resuscitation in traumatic and other types of brain injury is to prevent continuing cerebral insult after a primary injury has already occurred. The extent of the primary cerebral injury is usually determined by the mechanism of the trauma, the cause, and duration of cerebral ischemia. A primary insult is often associated with intracranial hypertension and systemic hypotension, leading to decreased cerebral perfusion and brain ischemia. Concomitant hypoxemia aggravates brain hypoxia, especially in the presence of hyperthermia, which increases brain metabolic demand. The combined effect of these factors leads to secondary brain injury characterized by excitotoxicity, oxidative stress, and inflammation. The resulting cerebral ischemia may be the single most important secondary event to affect outcome following a cerebral insult. Prevention of secondary injury is the main goal of resuscitative efforts.

Traumatized areas of the brain manifest impaired autoregulation and disruption of the blood–brain barrier. If space-occupying lesions or edema are present, these will contribute to reduced brain compliance, leading to increased ICP and consequent reduction in cerebral blood flow. The rationale for attempting to optimize cerebral perfusion pressure (CPP) arises from the assumption that cerebral regions surrounding the primary lesion may be close to the ischemic threshold. Therefore, the goals of neuroresuscitation are to restore cerebral blood flow by maintenance of adequate CPP, reduction of ICP, evacuation of space-occupying lesions, initiation of therapies for cerebral protection, and avoidance of hypoxia.

Unfortunately, the ICU treatment of TBI is hindered by a lack of rigorous, randomized, controlled trials to prove benefit for many of the management strategies utilized today. The Brain Trauma Foundation has published Guidelines for the Management of Severe Traumatic Brain Injury, and revised them as recently as 2016.[27] However, only one recommendation in 28 subject areas is a Level 1 recommendation based on high quality evidence. Furthermore, even rigorous studies generate more debate than consensus, as exemplified by a recent randomized, controlled trial of ICP-guided therapy versus imaging and clinical examination-based treatment that found no benefit to ICP monitoring.[28] Thus, treatment remains largely based on pathophysiologic principles and uncontrolled trials. A general guideline for management of patients with severe TBI appears in Table 57-2. Basic principles of acute TBI management, including osmotherapy, are discussed further in Chapter 53; however, sedation, hyperventilation, hypothermia, corticosteroids, and anti-seizure prophylaxis are discussed in further detail later.

Sedation of neurologically impaired patients should typically be achieved with short-acting sedatives to allow for frequent assessment by neurologic examination.[29] Although no studies have investigated the effect of sedation on outcome in such patients, a common practice is to provide sedation with propofol, benzodiazepines, or dexmedetomidine in patients following TBI. These agents have favorable effects on cerebral oxygen balance, although propofol is more potent in this regard. Undesirable effects of sedatives can lead to a reduction in CPP due to hemodynamic depression, or to an increase in cerebral blood flow and a simultaneous increase in ICP.

Propofol rapidly penetrates the central nervous system and has rapid elimination kinetics. Despite the induction of systemic

Table 57-2 ICU Management of Patients with Severe Traumatic Brain Injury

Basic principles applied to all patients, assuming initial surgical management	• Head elevation 30–45 degrees[a] • CPP 60–70 Torr 　■ Euvolemia, vasopressors as needed 　■ ICP <20 Torr 　■ Mannitol, hypertonic saline 　■ CSF drainage • SaO_2 ≥95%; $PaCO_2$ 35–40 Torr • Temperature ≤37°C • Glucose 　■ <180 mg/dL • Sedation and analgesia • Early enteral nutrition • Seizure, stress ulcer, and DVT prophylaxis
Refractory intracranial hypertension Consider one or all of these interventions, depending on individual circumstances	• Optimized hyperventilation with SjO_2 and/or $PbrO_2$ monitoring • Barbiturate coma • Mild therapeutic hypothermia (33°–35°C) • Decompressive craniectomy

[a]Unless contraindicated by spine injury, hemodynamic instability, or otherwise.

ICU, intensive care unit; CPP, cerebral perfusion pressure; ICP, intracranial pressure; CSF, cerebrospinal fluid; SaO_2, arterial oxygen saturation; $PaCO_2$, arterial carbon dioxide tension; DVT, deep venous thrombosis; SjO_2, jugular venous oxygen saturation; $PbrO_2$, brain tissue oxygen tension.

hypotension, propofol decreases cerebral metabolism resulting in a coupled decline in cerebral blood flow, with a consequent decrease in ICP. Propofol's favorable pharmacologic and neurophysiologic profile has led to its widespread use in neurointensive care, and high-dose propofol has been advocated as a substitute for barbiturate therapy in patients with refractory intracranial hypertension. However, prolonged (>24 hours), high-dose (>80 μg/kg/min) propofol administration has been associated with lactic acidosis, cardiac failure, and death (propofol infusion syndrome) in children and adults with TBI.[30] Thus, the use of high-dose propofol to control refractory intracranial hypertension is not recommended, and barbiturates should be considered if ICP is not controlled by moderate doses of propofol.

The mechanisms by which barbiturates exert their cerebral protective effect appear to be mediated by a reduction in ICP via alteration in vascular tone, reduction of cerebral metabolic rate, and inhibition of free radical peroxidation. Although barbiturates are effective at reducing ICP, their routine use in TBI does not appear beneficial, and may in fact result in excess mortality in patients with diffuse brain injury.[31,32] This effect may in part relate to the profound cardiovascular depressant effects of barbiturates. Based on one small randomized trial, barbiturates do appear to reduce mortality in patients with refractory high ICP.[33] Thus, high-dose barbiturate therapy may be considered in hemodynamically stable, severe TBI patients with intracranial hypertension refractory to maximal medical and surgical ICP-lowering therapy. In some patients pentobarbital may induce cerebral hypoxia by reducing cerebral blood flow (CBF) in excess of metabolism, and therefore SjO_2 monitoring may be considered during barbiturate therapy.

The centrally acting α_2 agonist dexmedetomidine has both sedative and analgesic effects. Its most desirable property is that it can allow for a more interactive and awake patient than other sedatives. (See section on Sedation, later.) Although it has not been studied specifically in brain-injured patients, it has been shown that cerebral blood flow–cerebral metabolic rate of oxygen ($CMRO_2$) coupling remains intact in healthy volunteers during dexmedetomidine infusion.[34]

Although neuromuscular blockade may result in a fall in ICP, the routine use of neuromuscular blockade is discouraged because its use has been associated with longer ICU stays, a higher incidence of pneumonia, and a trend toward more frequent sepsis without any improvement in outcome.

Hyperventilation effectively reduces ICP by reducing cerebral blood flow. However, the role that hyperventilation should play in routine management of TBI is not clear. Primarily, there are concerns that hyperventilation may lead to critically low cerebral blood flow, resulting in worsening cerebral ischemia.[35] In small randomized trials, prophylactic hyperventilation has not proven to be beneficial in TBI.[36] Based on the available evidence, prolonged or prophylactic hyperventilation should be avoided after severe TBI, especially in the first 24 hours after the injury. Hyperventilation may be necessary for brief periods to reduce intracranial hypertension refractory to sedation, osmotic therapy, and cerebrospinal fluid (CSF) drainage, and should be guided by SjO_2 and/or $PbrO_2$.[37] A marked fall in either of these values suggests a harmful effect of hyperventilation, and that it should be reduced or discontinued.

Experimentally, hypothermia causes a reduction in cerebral metabolism by decreasing all cell functions related to neuronal electric activity and those responsible for cellular integrity. In addition, mild hypothermia has been shown to decrease the release of substrates associated with tissue injury such as glutamate and aspartate. However, numerous randomized trials of therapeutic mild hypothermia (33° to 35°C) in patients with TBI published over two decades and enrolling more than 1,000 total patients have failed to demonstrate a mortality benefit or improvement in neurologic outcome with hypothermia. In addition, a recent randomized, controlled trial of induced mild hypothermia for the treatment of refractory high ICP found worse outcomes at 6 months in the group treated with hypothermia.[38] Thus, induction of mild hypothermia in patients with TBI, either prophylactically or to treat high ICP, cannot be recommended.

An additional second-tier therapy to control refractory elevated ICP is decompressive craniectomy. While one large randomized trial of decompressive craniotomy for refractory high ICP in TBI (Decompressive Craniectomy [DECRA] trial) showed worse outcomes in the craniectomy group, a more recent large randomized trial of the same intervention with slightly different inclusion criteria (Randomized Evaluation of Surgery with Craniectomy for Uncontrollable Elevation of Intracranial Pressure [RESCUEicp] Trial) showed a survival benefit with craniectomy. The apparently contradictory results have not yet been incorporated into the guidelines.[40]

Corticosteroids to reduce posttraumatic inflammatory injury in TBI were advocated for 30 years or more, but without convincing evidence of benefit. The Corticosteroid Randomization after Significant Head Injury (CRASH) study, published in 2004, prospectively randomized over 10,000 patients presenting with acute TBI to receive high-dose methylprednisolone or placebo for 48 hours after hospital admission. Methylprednisolone administration was associated with an approximately 20% increase in the relative risk of death at 2 weeks in the entire cohort, and this detriment was evident across subgroups divided by severity and type of injury.[41] Thus, high-dose corticosteroids should not be administered as therapy for acute TBI.[37] Likewise, intravenous magnesium administration did not improve outcomes in patients with TBI, and might even have a negative effect in the treatment of significant brain injury.[42]

Anticonvulsants are effective at preventing early posttraumatic seizures within 7 days following TBI. However, the evidence does not indicate that prevention of early seizures improves outcome following TBI.[43] Seizures should therefore be treated on an as-needed basis.

Finally, it should be noted that use of albumin as fluid replacement therapy in patients with TBI has been associated with increased mortality in a subgroup analysis of a randomized controlled trial comparing saline and albumin.[44] Routine albumin administration to patients with TBI should be avoided.

Subarachnoid Hemorrhage

The incidence of subarachnoid hemorrhage (SAH) in the United States varies from 7.5 to 12.1 cases per 100,000 of population. The rupture of an intracranial aneurysm most commonly causes SAH. Other causes of SAH include trauma, vertebral and carotid artery dissection, dural and spinal arteriovenous malformations, mycotic aneurysms, sickle cell disease, cocaine abuse, coagulation disorders, and pituitary apoplexy. Aneurysmal SAH is associated with considerable morbidity and mortality, with one-third of SAH patients dead before receiving medical attention, and only one-third of patients being functional survivors.[45,46] The leading causes of death and disability are the direct effect of the initial bleed, cerebral vasospasm with resulting stroke, and rebleeding. Although the number of early deaths may not have changed substantially, the overall case fatality rate of aneurysmal SAH has fallen over time, and is reported in the 40% to 50% range in most studies.[47] Approximately 40% to 50% of survivors have good neurologic outcome after SAH, as measured by the modified Rankin scale.[47] Severity of the initial bleed is the most important determinant of SAH outcome.

At the time of aneurysm rupture, a large hemorrhage results in a critical reduction in cerebral blood flow due to an increase in ICP toward arterial diastolic values. The persistence of a no-flow pattern is associated with acute vasospasm and swelling of perivascular astrocytes, neuronal cells, and capillary endothelia. After SAH, injury to the posterior hypothalamus may stimulate release of norepinephrine from the adrenal medulla and sympathetic cardiac efferent nerves. The release of norepinephrine has been associated with ischemic changes in the subendocardium (neurogenic stunned myocardium or stress cardiomyopathy), cardiac dysrhythmias, and pulmonary edema.

In survivors of the initial bleed, management emphasizes early aneurysm control with either surgery or interventional neuroradiology (coiling). Approximately 10% to 23% of unsecured aneurysms will rebleed in the first 2 weeks, with approximately 6% occurring within the first 24 hours after the initial hemorrhage. Rebleeding is associated with a mortality rate of over 50%.[48] Early aneurysm occlusion substantially reduces the risk of this complication, and it is recommended that aneurysms be secured within 72 hours of rupture, and perhaps earlier in high-risk cases.

With the improvement of the operative management, delayed neurologic deterioration (DND)—due to cerebral vasospasm and delayed cerebral ischemia (DCI), cerebral edema, hydrocephalus, and the effects of fever and electrolyte abnormalities—has become an increasingly important cause of death and disability. In addition, patients can develop a number of medical problems related to either the SAH or associated critical illness.

Cerebral vasospasm after SAH is identified by angiography in up to 60% of patients, and is correlated with the amount and location of subarachnoid blood. A subsequent reduction in cerebral blood flow is ultimately responsible for the appearance of DCI, which occurs in approximately one-third of patients suffering from SAH. A systematic review of the literature found an overall death rate of 31% (vs. 17% in patients without vasospasm), permanent deficits in 35%, and good outcome in 34% of the patients who developed symptomatic vasospasm.[49] DCI typically presents as altered consciousness and/or transient focal neurologic deficits beyond the first 3 days after aneurysm rupture, typically peaks in 7 to 10 days, and resolves over 10 to 14 days. If severe, vasospasm can result in cerebral infarction and persistent neurologic deficits, which contribute to considerable long-term morbidity.

TCD has been used to identify and quantify cerebral vasospasm on the basis that blood flow velocity increases as the diameter of the vessel decreases. Changes in measured velocities over time may be more reliable than absolute values in predicting symptomatic vasospasm. Velocities greater than 200 cm/s have been associated with a high risk of infarction; however, there is poor correlation between TCD velocities and angiographic findings, especially for the posterior circulation.

Oral nimodipine (60 mg every 4 h for 21 days) is recognized as an effective treatment to improve neurologic outcome (reduction of cerebral infarction and poor functional outcome) and mortality in SAH patients with vasospasm.[50] Because angiographic studies do not demonstrate a difference in the frequency of vasospasm compared with a placebo-treated group, the benefits of nimodipine have been attributed to a cytoprotective effect related to the reduced availability of intracellular calcium and improved microvascular collateral flow. No other pharmacologic therapies to prevent or treat cerebral vasospasm have conclusively demonstrated effective results in clinical trials. Although earlier studies suggested that statins may have a protective effect in preventing cerebral vasospasm and DCI, subsequent randomized trials have not born this finding out.[51]

Hypervolemia, hypertension, and hemodilution (triple-H) therapy is historically one of the mainstays of prevention and treatment of cerebral ischemia associated with SAH-induced vasospasm, despite the lack of strong evidence for its effectiveness, especially for prophylactic use.[52] Triple-H therapy evolved from the observed association of hypovolemia with poor outcomes after SAH, cerebral blood flow dysregulation, and the beneficial rheologic effects of anemia on cerebral blood flow. However, current consensus guidelines recommend modification of this strategy to include maintenance of euvolemia, avoidance of intentional hemodilution, and a controlled trial of stepwise blood pressure augmentation in patients with suspected DCI.[53] In addition, discontinuation of nimodipine is recommended if its administration results in hypotension. Careful monitoring for cardiopulmonary complications of hemodynamic therapy is recommended.

Interventional neuroradiology with the use of balloon angioplasty can reverse or improve vasospasm-induced neurologic deficits if initiated early after the development of ischemic symptoms. Although observational data suggest a beneficial effect of angioplasty on long-term outcomes, these findings have not been confirmed in randomized, controlled trials, and the risks of angioplasty include intimal dissection, vessel rupture, ischemia, and infarction.

Hydrocephalus is another cause of neurologic dysfunction after SAH, occurring in 25% of patients surviving the hemorrhage. The presence of blood in the ventricular system obstructs ventricular drainage and CSF absorption sites (subarachnoid villi). Ventricular drainage is usually successful in improving neurologic symptoms due to hydrocephalus. A minority of patients will require a permanent ventriculoperitoneal shunt. Seizures also occur in 13% of patients with SAH, and are more common in patients with a neurologic deficit; thus, prophylactic anticonvulsant therapy may be considered.[53]

Hyponatremia occurs in 10% to 34% of patients after SAH. Hyponatremia usually develops several days after the hemorrhage and is attributed to two main causes: (1) a syndrome of inappropriate antidiuretic hormone (SIADH), which is associated with euvolemia or mild hypervolemia and an excess of free water, or (2) cerebral "salt wasting" with depletion of sodium and water. The differentiation of these two entities is difficult but important, because SIADH is treated by free-water restriction, whereas cerebral salt wasting is treated with volume repletion and sodium administration. Thus, assessment of intravascular volume status is a key component when deciding on the treatment regimen for hyponatremia associated with SAH. Urine electrolyte analysis is not discriminative, as urine sodium is high in both disorders, particularly in association with intravenous saline administration.

Other medical complications are relatively common after SAH and include pneumonia, neurogenic pulmonary edema and acute lung injury (ALI), stress (Takotsubo) cardiomyopathy, sepsis, and venous thromboembolism (VTE). Fever is highly prevalent after SAH and is associated with poor outcomes. Although fever is often due to noninfectious causes after SAH, a rigorous search for infection is necessary. Fever control is recommended during the risk period for DCI, particularly in high-risk patients.[53]

Acute Ischemic Stroke

Although the incidence of stroke has declined over the past few decades, stroke affects nearly 800,000 people annually, and was the fifth leading cause of death in the United States as of 2013.[54] Nearly 90% of strokes can be attributed to an ischemic mechanism such as atherosclerosis, thrombosis, cardio-embolism, or hypotension. Other major causes of stroke are intracerebral and subarachnoid hemorrhage. Unusual causes of stroke such as carotid artery dissection, hypercoagulation syndromes, or infective endocarditis should be considered in younger patients without apparent risk factors. Transient ischemic attacks may precede stroke and should be considered as a warning sign. The prognosis after stroke varies depending on the size and location of the lesion. In patients with acute ischemic stroke, the duration of coma appears to be the most important predictor of outcome and successful therapy.

Rapid clot lysis and restoration of circulation via systemic thrombolysis limits the extent of brain injury and improves outcome after thrombotic stroke. American Heart Association/American Stroke Association (AHA/ASA) guidelines recommend systemic thrombolysis using intravenous alteplase (rtPA) to patients presenting with acute ischemic stroke within 3 hours of symptom onset (barring contraindications), and up to 4.5 hours after symptom onset in select individuals.[55]

Accumulating evidence suggests that mechanical thrombectomy as an adjunct to systemic thrombolysis offers additional outcome benefits to select patients with ischemic stroke. Thus, the AHA/ASA guidelines recommend stent retrieval of clot in patients who have received intravenous alteplase within 4.5 hours of symptom onset, who have evidence of internal carotid or proximal middle cerebral artery (MCA) occlusion, and in whom treatment can be initiated within 6 hours of symptom onset.[56]

Neither unfractionated nor low-molecular-weight heparin have been shown to prevent progression or reduce the rate of stroke recurrence when administered within 48 hours of the acute event, and therefore are not recommended. In general, heparin is only recommended for early secondary prophylaxis in patients with suspected cardiac embolism. Aspirin 325 mg has been shown to reduce the risk of early recurrent ischemic stroke. It is recommended within 24 to 48 hours of stroke onset in most patients, but it does increase the risk of hemorrhagic stroke. The frequency of deep venous thrombosis in acute stroke is reduced by anticoagulants (e.g., low–molecular-weight heparin), but not by antiplatelet agents. However, it is unclear if the frequency of pulmonary embolism is also reduced.

The majority of patients with acute ischemic stroke present with severe arterial hypertension. In theory, permissive hypertension should be allowed after stroke because reduction of the CPP could compromise the viable brain surrounding the ischemic region (ischemic penumbra), although high-level evidence to support this recommendation is lacking. However, severe hypertension (blood pressure >220/120 mmHg) should be controlled because of increased risk of hemorrhagic transformation; a lower threshold is indicated after alteplase administration (blood pressure >185/110). If the stroke is accompanied by raised ICP due to cerebral edema, the principles of treatment of raised ICP discussed earlier for TBI similarly apply. Cytotoxic brain edema usually occurs 24 to 96 hours after acute ischemic stroke, and osmotherapy constitutes the basis of ICP reduction, and possibly hemicraniectomy in select patients (see later). Steroids are of no value in the treatment of ischemic stroke, and although some have advocated therapeutic hypothermia, there is insufficient evidence to recommend this approach in stroke outside of research settings. As with SAH, fever is associated with poor outcome after ischemic stroke, and close temperature monitoring and management are recommended. Hyperglycemia is also associated with poor outcome in ischemic stroke, and it is recommended to monitor and maintain blood glucose within the range of 140 to 180 mg/dL.[55]

Hemispheric MCA infarction with subsequent cerebral edema, increased ICP, and herniation (malignant MCA syndrome) is often fatal. Randomized trials demonstrate that hemicraniectomy improves survival in this setting.[57] However, this benefit may come at the expense of increased and often severe disability in survivors. This seems particularly true for patients greater than 60 years of age.[57,58] Cerebellar infarction can likewise result in fatal brainstem compression due to local edema. Case series suggest that suboccipital craniectomy can be life-saving in this situation, and that patients can recover with acceptable functional outcomes.[55,59]

Anoxic Brain Injury

Anoxic brain injury most commonly occurs as a result of cardiac arrest, either in- or out-of-hospital. Of patients who survive their initial cardiac arrest, in-hospital mortality ranges from approximately 50% to 90%, and a high percentage of survivors suffer brain injury with significant long-term disability. The pathophysiology of anoxic brain injury is multifactorial, and includes excitatory neurotransmitter release, accumulation of intracellular calcium, and oxygen free radical generation. Unfortunately, pharmacologic therapies aimed at several of these pathways, including barbiturates, benzodiazepines, corticosteroids, calcium channel antagonists, and free radical scavengers have failed to improve the outcome of anoxic brain injury.

Based largely on two small, single-center randomized trials published in 2002 that showed outcome benefits, mild therapeutic hypothermia (target temperature 33°C) has been widely applied to unconscious patients who survive initial resuscitation from cardiac arrest due to ventricular fibrillation or tachycardia.[60] However, a much larger, multicenter randomized trial published in 2013 found no benefit to targeting a temperature of 33°C compared to 36°C.[61] Based on this study, therapeutic hypothermia can no longer be recommended as routine therapy after cardiac arrest. Strict fever control with a target temperature of 36°C appears to result in similar outcomes.

Cardiovascular and Hemodynamic Aspects of Critical Care

Types of Shock

One of the most common and urgent requirements for critical care is the presence of shock. Shock is a state characterized by tissue oxygen delivery that is inadequate to meet demand. Often this is associated with circulatory instability and severe systemic hypotension. Shock states are commonly classified according to the primary cause of circulatory failure. Distributive (sometimes called vasodilatory) shock results from a reduction in systemic vascular resistance (SVR), often associated with an increased cardiac output (CO) as may happen in sepsis, anaphylaxis, or spinal cord injury. Cardiogenic shock results from left or right (or both) heart failure and is characterized by low CO and increased SVR. Hypovolemic shock is also associated with low CO and increased peripheral resistance, most commonly due to hemorrhage. Obstructive shock, as the name suggests, is characterized by an obstruction to forward flow such as may happen with a tension pneumothorax, pericardial tamponade, or pulmonary embolism. The most common form of shock encountered in the ICU depends on the type of ICU, but septic, cardiogenic, and hypovolemic shock are most common. Shock of all kinds is highly morbid and despite extensive research and aggressive management, the mortality from shock remains staggeringly high. Approximately 35% to 40% of patients die within 28 days of the onset of septic shock, and the mortality rate is 70% to 80% for patients with cardiogenic shock. The mortality from hypovolemic shock is highly variable and depends upon the etiology and the rapidity of recognition and treatment. Mortality from septic shock may be improving, as evidenced by the fact that control-group mortality in sepsis trials has decreased from 46% to approximately 20% between 2001[62] and 2014,[63-65] although this may reflect broader screening and inclusion of less sick patients than in past trials. Cardiogenic and septic shock are discussed in more detail in the following section, whereas the causes and treatment of hypovolemic and obstructive shock are discussed in Chapters 39 and 53.

Cardiogenic Shock

The hallmark of cardiogenic shock is primary pump failure, which itself may be caused by extensive myocardial infarction (MI), nonischemic cardiomyopathy, dysrhythmia, or mechanical complication (e.g., mitral regurgitation, ventricular septal defect). The pathophysiologic characteristics include a reduction in contractility, usually accompanied by dilatation of cardiac cavities and venous congestion. Determining the etiology of cardiogenic shock is of utmost importance because the treatment varies considerably based on the underlying mechanism. For example, the role of β-blockers in the management of nonischemic decompensated heart failure has evolved to be of increasing importance[66] and diuresis is frequently indicated, whereas in acute ischemic ST elevation MI (STEMI) β-blockers are critical and there is little role for acute diuresis. A 12-lead electrocardiogram (ECG), serum troponin measurements, B-type natriuretic peptide levels, and echocardiography should be obtained in all patients presenting with heart failure, and is helpful in differentiating between the various causes of heart failure.[67]

The onset of pump failure is associated with two compensatory mechanisms: a reflex vasoconstriction in systemic vessels causing an increase in left ventricle (LV) workload and myocardial oxygen demand, and a redistribution of blood volume toward the heart and the lungs.

Several studies have demonstrated that the incidence and severity of LV failure complicating acute MI are directly related to the extent of ventricular muscle necrosis. Consequently, therapy should minimize myocardial oxygen demand and raise oxygen delivery to the ischemic area. This goal is complicated by the fact that many resuscitative approaches to correct hypotension increase myocardial oxygen consumption (e.g., preload augmentation, inotropes, and vasopressors, as discussed later). In patients without hypotension, pharmacologic vasodilatation using nitroglycerin or sodium nitroprusside may reduce myocardial oxygen consumption and improve ventricular ejection by reducing LV afterload, and may also produce a shift of blood from the lungs to the periphery by reducing venous tone. Synthetic B-type natriuretic peptide (nesiritide) and dopamine agonists such as fenoldopam have similar effects, but have shown inconsistent benefit in large randomized trials and are not recommended for routine management.[68,69] When pharmacologic interventions are not sufficient to restore hemodynamic stability, the use of mechanical support with the insertion of intra-aortic balloon pump counterpulsation and ventricular assist devices can help unload the ventricles (see Chapter 39).

In patients with MI, coronary reperfusion can be achieved with systemic thrombolysis or, preferably, primary percutaneous coronary intervention (PCI). The American Heart Association/American College of Cardiology guidelines recommend treatment of STEMI by PCI within 90 minutes of presentation to PCI-capable centers, by thrombolytic therapy within 30 minutes of presentation to non–PCI-capable centers, or by rapid transfer under certain conditions of favorable timing.[70] Guidelines clearly favor PCI over fibrinolysis when both are feasible within the appropriate time frame. For patients with ischemia and cardiogenic shock, the addition of intra-aortic balloon counterpulsation to PCI in acute STEMI does not reduce infarct size[71] or mortality.[72] Data on the use of LV assist devices (LVADs) in the setting of acute ischemic cardiogenic shock are limited, but these may be effective devices to bridge patients in shock until recovery or transplant.[73]

Management of cardiac failure related to specific valvular abnormalities is discussed in Chapter 39.

Septic Shock

Septic shock is a form of distributive shock associated with infection and the activation of the systemic inflammatory response. It is usually characterized by a high CO, low SVR, hypotension, and regional blood flow redistribution that result in tissue hypoperfusion. Other noninfectious causes of distributive shock include acute spinal cord injury, pancreatitis, burns, fulminant hepatic failure, multiple traumatic injuries, toxic shock syndrome, anaphylatic and anaphylactoid reactions, and drug or toxin reactions, including insect bites, transfusion reactions, and heavy metal poisoning. Septic shock is the most common shock syndrome, accounting for roughly two-thirds of shock patients in broad critical care populations.[74] Severe sepsis and septic shock account for at least 10% of ICU admissions, and septic shock is more common in the very young and very old, in men than in women, and in black patients than in white patients.[75]

In patients with systemic infections, the physiologic response can be staged on a continuum from sepsis to severe sepsis and septic shock (Table 57-3).

The initiating event in septic shock appears to be the interaction between organism-specific ligands on pathogens and ligand-specific receptors (e.g., toll-like receptors, nucleotide-binding oligomerization domain–like receptors, and others) on cells of the innate immune system. The resulting release of immune mediators sets in motion a complex series of events that results in altered gene expression, T-cell differentiation, complement activation, elaboration of pro-coagulant processes, and the production and release of other immunomodulatory cytokines. Together, these events produce the septic phenotype (e.g., microthrombi, endothelial dysfunction, capillary leak, vasodilatation, effective hypovolemia, hypoperfusion, and organ failure).[75,76]

Although the calculated CO often increases, and echocardiography often shows hyperdynamic LV function in early sepsis, this may be secondary to the decrease in SVR that is a hallmark of septic shock. LV contractility itself is depressed in many patients. A global decrease in cardiac contractility, combined with relative hypovolemia, may reduce oxygen delivery to tissues. Even in the case of normal or seemingly adequate CO and oxygen delivery, metabolic needs are increased during sepsis, and the ability of the tissues to extract and utilize oxygen may be impaired. Thus, a metabolic acidosis may be present despite normal levels of oxygen transport.[77] A decrease in cellular oxygen extraction capacity may result from factors other than hypoperfusion, such as direct cellular damage by toxins and/or mediators or maldistribution of blood flow. The impact of impaired perfusion on organ function depends on individual susceptibility to hypoxia. Though hypoperfusion is the suspected cause of lactic acidosis in sepsis, various degrees of intermediary metabolic alterations may contribute to the increased

Table 57-3 Definitions of Sepsis and Organ Failure

Sepsis: Evidence of infection (either documented or suspected) and some of the following:

Core temperature <36°C or >38°C
Tachycardia >90 beats/min
Tachypnea >20 breaths/min while breathing spontaneously, or $PaCO_2$ <XX mmHg
White blood count >12,000 cells/mm^3, <4,000 cells/mm^3, or >10% immature forms
Altered mental status
Hypotension (SBP <90 mmHg, MAP <70 mmHg, XX >40 mmHg below normal or greater than 2 standard deviations below normal for age)
Hyperglycemia (serum glucose >140 mg/dL in the absence of diabetes)
Plasma C-reactive protein or procalcitonin elevation (>two standard deviations above normal)
Arterial hypoxemia (PaO_2:FiO_2 <300)
Coagulopathy (international normalized ratio >1.5)
Creatinine increase (rise in serum creatinine >0.5 mg/dL)

Severe Sepsis: Ongoing organ dysfunction attributed to infection that persists despite adequate fluid resuscitation:

Acute lung injury (PaO_2:FiO_2 <250 in absence of pneumonia as source of infection or PaO_2:FiO_2 <200 in presence of pneumonia as source of infection)
Lactic acid elevation (above the lab normal range)
Acute oliguria (urine output <0.5 mL/kg/hr for two or more hours despite adequate fluid resuscitation)
Coagulopathy (international normalized ratio >1.5)
Thrombocytopenia (<100,000/mL)
Bilirubin elevation (>2 mg/dL)

Septic Shock: Sepsis with hypotension, despite adequate fluid resuscitation

Multiple Organ Dysfunction Syndrome: Presence of several altered organ functions in an acutely ill patient such that homeostasis cannot be maintained without intervention

SBP, systolic blood pressure; MAP, mean arterial pressure.
Adapted with permission from: Dellinger RP, Levy MM, Rhodes A, et al. Surviving sepsis campaign: international guidelines for management of severe sepsis and septic shock. *Crit Care Med.* 2013;41:580–637.

Table 57-4 Management of Severe Sepsis and Septic Shock

- Initiation of early goal–directed resuscitation during the first 6 h after onset of sepsis
- Blood cultures to identify causative organisms before starting antibiotic therapy, and prompt imaging studies performed to identify potential source of infection
- Administration of empiric broad-spectrum antibiotics within 1 h of diagnosis, and reassessment of appropriate therapy upon availability of microbiology results
- Control of source of infection
- Administration of crystalloids as initial fluid resuscitation with consideration given to adding albumin when large volumes of crystalloid are required
- Avoidance of hetastarch formulations
- Initial fluid resuscitation volume of at least 30 mL/kg with additional fluid challenges continuing as long as there is hemodynamic improvement as assessed by either static or dynamic variables
- Use of norepinephrine as first-line vasopressor for a target MAP ≥65 mmHg
- Epinephrine may be added when an additional agent is needed
- Vasopressin may be added at a fixed rate as an adjunct to catecholamines, but should not be used alone
- Use of dopamine is recommended only in highly selected circumstances and should generally be avoided
- Consideration for dobutamine in low cardiac output states despite fluid resuscitation
- Targeting supranormal values of oxygen delivery is not recommended
- Stress-dose steroid therapy for septic shock only if blood pressure is poorly responsive to fluid and vasopressors
- Targeting a hemoglobin of 7–9 g/dL in the absence of tissue hypoperfusion, coronary artery disease, or acute hemorrhage
- Appropriate use of fresh frozen plasma and platelets
- Use of low tidal volume, limitation of inspiratory plateau pressure, and application of at least a minimal amount of positive end-expiratory pressure for ALI patients
- Elevation of the head of the bed to a semirecumbent position unless contraindicated
- Avoidance of routine use of pulmonary artery catheter in patients with ALI
- Use a conservative fluid strategy for patients with ALI who are not in shock
- Use of protocols for ventilation weaning and sedation/analgesia, with daily sedation interruption if using continuous infusion sedation
- Avoidance of neuromuscular blockade
- Use of bicarbonate to correct arterial pH above 7.15 is not recommended
- Consideration of limitation of life support when appropriate

ALI, acute lung injury.
Adapted with permission from: Dellinger RP, Levy MM, Rhodes A, et al. Surviving sepsis campaign: international guidelines for management of severe sepsis and septic shock. *Crit Care Med.* 2013;41:580–637.

lactate production independent of perfusion, or when tissue oxygen tension is normal.[77]

The hallmark of treatment of septic shock includes early antimicrobial therapy and source control, restoration of organ perfusion by augmenting circulating volume, stroke volume, and/or oxygen carrying capacity, and the management of the expected consequences of sepsis, organ failure, and critical care (e.g., infections, acute kidney injury [AKI], and VTE). These have been thoroughly investigated and discussed in the Surviving Sepsis Campaign Guidelines (summarized in Table 57-4), which provide an excellent review of the evidence for various components of therapy.[78]

Active screening protocols and resuscitation algorithms have enjoyed immense popularity and have been adopted widely, despite the lack of consistent benefit in organized trials[62–65] and poor adherence in evaluations of the implementation of care bundles.[79–81] Nevertheless, the practice of systematic, early, and aggressive attention, treatment, and monitoring has such tremendous face validity that these strategies are likely to remain the standard of care for some time.

Monitoring and Resuscitation in Shock States

The primary goal of monitoring patients in or at risk for shock is to identify and measure the presence of hemodynamic instability and inadequate tissue oxygen delivery, so that interventions can be undertaken to improve these perturbations. Invasive monitors used in shock states can be separated into those that assess hemodynamics and CO, and those that assess the degree to which the metabolic needs of the patient are being met.

Hemodynamic Monitoring

Adequate circulating volume is a necessary condition of adequate stroke volume and oxygen delivery, although assessing this volume is difficult. Intravascular pressure assessments such as the mean arterial pressure (MAP) and central venous pressure (CVP) have tremendous face validity, a historical track record, and are easy to measure and understand. However, these measures have their faults. Clinicians adhere poorly to MAP goals[82] and high-quality data linking active MAP management to improved outcomes remain elusive.[83,84] Moreover, given the typically poor correlation between various MAP measurement modalities,[84] its use as a proxy for hemodynamic information is suspect.[85] Similarly, the CVP is a poor predictor of whether a patient's stroke volume will respond to fluid.[86-88] Like monitoring CVP and MAP, the pulmonary artery catheter (PAC) has theoretical utility and is discussed at length in Chapter 26. However, despite the theoretical benefits, there are few data to support a positive effect of PAC utilization on mortality or other substantive outcome variables. Patient populations, including those with acute respiratory distress syndrome (ARDS), congestive heart failure, septic shock and high-risk surgical patients, have all been the subject of investigations targeting the effect of PAC use on outcome.[89,90] These trials have all failed to show benefit, and PAC use has greatly waned.

Echocardiography

Both transthoracic echocardiography (TTE), and transesophageal echocardiography (TEE) provide accurate diagnostic information with regard to dynamic ventricular function, valvular anatomy, pericardial anatomy, and intracardiac pressures. Although TEE has long been used in the operating room and is discussed in detail in Chapter 27 and Appendix 7, TTE use is becoming more widespread in the ICU as the size and cost of the equipment are decreasing. The major limitation of focused cardiac ultrasound is that it does not provide continuous monitoring and requires a high standard of training and experience. However, a number of studies have now shown that with limited training, critical care physicians can accurately and rapidly perform focused cardiac ultrasound examinations. In one study, intensivists were provided with 2 hours of formal didactic training followed by 4 hours of hands-on training in focused point-of-care cardiac ultrasound. Using formal TTEs obtained by professional sonographers and interpreted by attending cardiologists as a gold standard, the intensivists were able to correctly identify ventricular dysfunction over 80% of the time.[91] Moreover, the use of ultrasound in general, and cardiac ultrasound in particular, frequently identifies conditions that alter clinical management. The role of focused cardiac ultrasound in the management of the critically ill will likely expand in the future, because the availability of the equipment and the dearth of other noninvasive methods for answering the relevant clinical questions are simply too compelling. Both TTE and TEE applications are discussed in more detail in Appendix 7.

Dynamic Respiratory Indices

Positive pressure ventilation (PPV) has predictable effects on stroke volume in both normal subjects and critically ill patients, inasmuch as it reduces venous return and increases right ventricular afterload. During PPV there is an inspiratory reduction in right ventricular stroke volume due to decreased venous return and a subsequent reduction in LV end-diastolic volume appearing during the expiratory phase of the respiratory cycle. Therefore, the LV stroke volume varies cyclically with ventilation and is paralleled by a similar variation in systolic blood pressure and pulse pressure. These effects are more pronounced in patients on the steeper part of the Frank–Starling curve where, by definition, patients will enjoy a larger increase in stroke volume for a given increase in LV end-diastolic volume (i.e., a fluid bolus).

The relationship between these respirophasic changes in stroke volume and position on the Frank–Starling curve can be exploited to make inferences about a patient's likely response to fluid administration. A number of metrics to approximate these changes in stroke volume variation have been identified. These include systolic pressure variation (SPV) and pulse pressure variation, both of which utilize analysis of arterial waveforms. Thresholds indicating abnormal variation vary by device, but are generally in the range of 10% to 15%. The higher the degree of variation, the more stroke volume is changing with respiration, and, ultimately, the more likely the patient is to experience an increase in stroke volume with fluid administration. Compared to static measures such as CVP, systolic and pulse pressure variations are superior predictors of fluid responsiveness in patients with a variety of critical illnesses, including septic shock and ARDS, and following cardiac surgery.[86-88,92,93]

It should be noted that the use of these metrics has only been validated in patients who are tracheally intubated and receiving PPV. Spontaneous or noninvasive ventilation is associated with a different set of hemodynamic effects, and their relationship to volume responsiveness is being examined.[94] Furthermore, the majority of data were collected in patients receiving tidal volumes of at least 8 mL/kg, which is at the higher end of the acceptable range for patients with ARDS. Patients also need to be in a sinus rhythm; atrial fibrillation and frequent ectopy will alter the variation in arterial waveform amplitude independent of respirophasic changes, thereby exaggerating variation. Finally, because such analysis requires patients be synchronous with mechanical ventilation, study patients were generally deeply sedated, if not paralyzed. These pitfalls may limit generalizability of findings to patients in current ICUs, where a more restrictive approach to sedation and tidal volumes is frequently employed. Another important pitfall to dynamic respirophasic indices is that these measurements do not predict fluid responsiveness in patients with an open chest,[95] which may be becoming more frequent after complex cardiac surgery.[96]

Less-Invasive Cardiac Output Monitors

A host of less-invasive (relative to PAC) CO monitors have come to market in the last decade. Some exploit the analysis of the systemic arterial pulse contour, and a range of other modalities such as transesophageal Doppler and bio-reactance exist.

Pulse contour analysis (PCA) integrates the area under the curve of the arterial waveform to approximate stroke volume. Two commercially available devices utilize either lithium dilution (lithium injected through a peripheral IV—LiDCO [Lidco Ltd., London, UK]) or thermal dilution (saline injected through a central venous catheter—PiCCO [Pulsion, Feldkirchen, Germany]) for initial calibration. They then derive changes in CO using PCA. This approach correlates well with thermodilution CO derived from a PAC in a variety of conditions, and has the advantage of providing continuous measurement without necessitating the placement of a PAC.[97-100] The PiCCO device also allows for measurement of intrathoracic blood volume using transpulmonary thermodilution, and may be a more accurate reflection of preload than static CVP measurements. Although further validation of these techniques in critically ill patients is necessary, the use of PCA may obviate the need for PACs to measure CO, particularly if combined with the measurement of central venous oxygen saturation (ScvO$_2$) as an indicator of the balance between oxygen delivery and consumption.

A third PCA device, the FloTrac/Vigileo (Edwards Lifesciences, Irvine, CA), incorporates respirophasic changes into its calculation of stroke volume and, unlike the other two PCA devices, does not require a dilution calibration. Randomized trials of the device in high-risk surgical patients generally show a reduction in complications and improvement in surrogate markers (e.g., length of stay)[101,102]; however, controversy persists[103] and high-quality data in the ICU are lacking.

Transesophageal Doppler sonography utilizes a small esophageal probe to monitor descending aortic blood flow velocity continuously. When combined with the cross-sectional area of the aorta, the blood flow velocity allows for calculation of CO. Like the PCA devices discussed earlier, transesophageal Doppler shows good correlation with more traditional methods of CO measurement such as PAC, but its ability to alter meaningful outcomes in the ICU setting is not established.[104] The disadvantages of this technique are that it is inaccurate if not positioned correctly, is easily dislodged, and it does not measure the ascending aorta output or the aortic cross-sectional area directly, but instead uses nomograms to determine aortic cross-sectional area.[105]

Perhaps the least invasive of the CO monitors utilizes of the concept of bioreactance. These devices exploit the differential absorption of electrical current by pulsatile blood over time to estimate stroke volume. Using just four surface electrodes, the NICOM (Cheetah Medical, Newton Center, MA) is easy to place and has a low risk of complications. Although immediately appealing because of the simplicity, ease of use, and noninvasiveness, the CO derived from the NICOM does not seem to track well with other measures like the PAC[106,107] or transesophageal Doppler,[108] and as a part of a broader fluid resuscitation algorithm, the use of the device was not associated with improvements in relevant clinical outcomes.[109]

Metabolic Monitoring

Although an adequate circulation is necessary for resuscitation, occult hypoperfusion is possible in the setting of seemingly adequate hemodynamic conditions.[110] Once goals for an adequate circulation are met, metabolic goals can be addressed to detect and treat such cellular hypoperfusion, using lactate clearance and venous oximetry.

As the product of anaerobic metabolism, lactate is an indicator of insufficient oxygen delivery to cells. As elevated lactate level decreases, improved perfusion is assumed, and organ function should improve. Clearance of lactate as a goal of resuscitation has been studied recently in patients with septic[111] and undifferentiated shock.[112] Both studies randomized patients to resuscitation algorithms closely mimicking Rivers' early goal-directed therapy (EGDT) for severe sepsis, and showed that patients being treated according to lactate clearance did as well or better than those being treated according to traditional EGDT. Although the relationship between measured lactate and tissue hypoperfusion may not be as direct as it is physiologically intuitive,[77] these results suggest that lactate clearance is a reasonable monitoring strategy for the detection and resolution of hypoperfusion.

Venous oximetry, or assessment of mixed venous oxygen saturation (SvO$_2$), aims to measure postorgan bed oxygenation as a means to infer the oxygen extraction ratio and make further inference about adequacy of oxygen delivery. Measurement requires a PAC, which requires technical skill and carries risk of complications. SvO$_2$ and ScvO$_2$ reflect the relationship between oxygen delivery (DO$_2$) and oxygen consumption (VO$_2$). A somewhat less invasive and less costly alternative to placing a PAC for the measurement of SvO$_2$ is to measure ScvO$_2$ via a central venous catheter. ScvO$_2$ is approximately 5 mmHg higher than SvO$_2$ in critically ill patients, but appears to correlate well with SvO$_2$ during changes in hemodynamic status.[113] Because ScvO$_2$ approximates true SvO$_2$, trends in ScvO$_2$ closely mimic trends in SvO$_2$,[114] but this is somewhat controversial.[115,116] The use of venous oximetry gathered tremendous attention after the publication of EGDT using venous oximetry in patients with severe sepsis.[62]

The level of ScvO$_2$ has been associated with high mortality in sepsis. Supranormal levels, whether present at the outset of treatment or after treatment, may be a marker of altered oxygen utilization and are associated with a high mortality.[117,118] The impact of venous oximetry on outcome, however, is mixed. Achieving ScvO$_2$ more than 70% was independently associated with improved mortality in a retrospective analysis of sepsis care bundles (the only care factor positively associated with mortality),[79] although a much larger and similar analysis did not find the same favorable association between ScvO$_2$ and mortality.[80] Moreover, three recent, well-conducted attempts to replicate Rivers' initial trial have shown little benefit to EGDT, a central component of which is the assessment of ScvO$_2$.[63-65]

An important observation about monitoring technology must be recognized. Any individual technique is vulnerable to bias, contraindications, and error. Given the high stakes complexity of hemodynamic and metabolic assessment, the wisest approach is to understand the strengths and weaknesses of many possible strategies, apply the techniques most appropriate to a given patient with an eye toward possible bias, and interpret the information generated within the broader context of the patient's history, exam, and ever-changing clinical status.

Acute Respiratory Failure

Acute respiratory failure is characterized by a derangement in pulmonary gas exchange or an imbalance between the work of breathing and respiratory muscle capacity, and is usually accompanied by hypoxemia and/or hypercapnia. Indeed, in some cases respiratory failure may be caused by "nonrespiratory" issues (e.g., coma that results in the inability to protect the airway). Acute respiratory failure is a common phenomenon. Depending on the type of ICU, the majority of patients may be mechanically ventilated at any given time, and virtually all critically ill patients are mechanically ventilated for some portion of their ICU stay. Suffice it to say that the treatment of acute respiratory failure is primarily supportive, typically necessitates supplemental oxygen, and often requires mechanical ventilation with or without tracheal intubation. Acute respiratory failure typically resolves when the initiating condition is adequately treated. The following subsections will discuss basic principles of mechanical ventilation, some of the more challenging types of respiratory failure, and potential therapeutic approaches to respiratory failure.

Principles of Mechanical Ventilation

Mechanical ventilation in the ICU is provided through the application of positive pressure to the airway. At its simplest, a preset tidal volume (volume control) or inspiratory pressure (pressure control) and rate provide minimum minute ventilation. Any breathing that the patient does above this preset minute ventilation is either supported (continuous mandatory ventilation [CMV]) or not (intermittent mandatory ventilation [IMV]). However, ICU ventilators have become increasingly powerful and complex, capable of delivering high inspiratory flows, and utilizing microprocessors that simultaneously monitor and respond to multiple characteristics of the respiratory circuit. Thus, ventilatory modes used today include pressure support ventilation, pressure control ventilation, volume control ventilation, pressure-regulated volume control ventilation, high-frequency ventilation, proportional assist ventilation, airway pressure release ventilation, synchronous intermittent mandatory ventilation, and others. In reality, despite strong regional, local, and individual biases, there is little evidence to suggest that the mode of mechanical ventilation contributes significantly to any major outcome measure, and the choice of mode is at this point largely one of clinician preference. Thus, this discussion will not dwell on specific modes of ventilation.

Mechanical PPV has been traditionally considered supportive therapy that is applied until the initiating cause of respiratory failure improves sufficiently, such that the patient is able to breath without assistance. However, evidence suggests that mechanical ventilation may be injurious in certain settings. Traditionally, tidal volumes of 10 to 15 mL/kg were routinely used to ventilate patients in the ICU. The use of such "supraphysiologic" tidal volumes (normal resting tidal volumes are 5 to 7 mL/kg) evolved from the observation that the use of smaller-sized volumes was associated with the development of atelectasis and hypoxemia in anesthetized patients in the operating room. However, large tidal volumes can result in cardiovascular compromise, barotrauma, ventilator-induced or ventilator-associated lung injury (VILI or VALI), and excess mortality, as discussed later.

PPV results in increased intrathoracic pressure, which reduces venous return, and in turn results in reduced CO and blood pressure. In addition, PPV can result in alveolar overdistension and alveolar rupture, which manifests as pneumothorax, pneumomediastinum, and subcutaneous emphysema (barotrauma). Both of these effects are amplified in patients with obstructive lung disease (asthma and chronic obstructive lung disease [COPD]). In these patients, limitation of expiratory flow leads to air trapping and the development of intrinsic positive end-expiratory pressure, or "auto-PEEP." Air trapping results in alveolar overdistension and increases the risk of barotrauma, and auto-PEEP can contribute substantially to increased intrathoracic pressure and cardiovascular depression. Auto-PEEP cannot be measured without holding exhalation for a prolonged interval (expiratory pause) with both inspiratory and expiratory ventilator valves closed; thus, auto-PEEP may not be appreciated unless actively sought. Auto-PEEP can also be detected by observing a failure of expiratory flow to return to zero prior to initiation of the next breath.

The development of air trapping and auto-PEEP leads to significant morbidity and mortality in patients with obstructive lung disease. Thus, the ventilatory strategy in these patients should focus on prolongation of the expiratory time, limiting minute ventilation by using low tidal volumes (6 to 8 mL/kg or less) and a low rate (8 to 12 breaths per minute), and by reducing the inspiratory time of the respiratory cycle. Low minute ventilation is often associated with hypercapnia and respiratory acidosis (permissive hypercapnia); however, this does not appear to be harmful, and the benefits of reduced air trapping and auto-PEEP far outweigh any possible detriment. In order to decrease inspiratory time, the inspiratory flow rate must increase, and this results in increased peak airway pressure. However, most of the peak pressure is dissipated in the endotracheal tube and large airways, and more importantly, end-expiratory, static or plateau, and mean airway pressures will fall with increased expiratory time. In order to accomplish these goals, deep sedation is often required, and rarely neuromuscular blockade must be used. The adoption of this type of ventilatory strategy in the 1980s and 1990s was associated with a dramatic reduction in mortality due to acute, severe asthma and respiratory failure, from as high as 23% to less than 5%.[119]

In contrast to barotrauma, VILI or VALI refers to microscopic injury to the lung due to overdistension (volutrauma) and cyclic reopening of alveoli (atelectatrauma). VALI has been well-demonstrated in numerous experimental models, and is histologically similar to the features seen in ALI of other causes, with diffuse alveolar damage (DAD) and increased microvascular permeability.[120] In addition, VALI is associated with the systemic release of inflammatory mediators that may contribute to multiple organ failure. Clinically, patients felt to be at risk for VALI are those with abnormally low recruitable lung volumes, in particular those with ARDS. Thus, a "lung-protective" ventilatory strategy utilizing low tidal volume ventilation has been shown to reduce mortality when applied to patients with ARDS (see later). In addition, accumulating evidence suggests that the use of low tidal volume ventilation may reduce the risk of developing ARDS in critically ill patients.[121,122]

In summary, although tidal volumes of 10 to 12 mL/kg may still be indicated for some patients, in most cases an initial tidal volume of 8 mL/kg is probably appropriate, and volumes as low as 4 mL/kg may be appropriate in some cases. In addition, because lung volumes correlate with height rather than weight, tidal volume selection should be based on predicted or ideal body weight, rather than actual weight to avoid lung overdistension. Predicted body weight (PBW) can be calculated from the formula: PBW = 50 + 2.3 (height [inches] − 60) (males), or 45.5 + 2.3 (height [inches] − 60) (females).

Although mechanical ventilation generally implies tracheal intubation (translaryngeal or tracheotomy), noninvasive positive pressure ventilation (NPPV) or continuous positive airway pressure (CPAP) can be delivered via a tight-sealing nasal or full-face mask. NPPV is applied using either standard ICU ventilators (typically set to pressure support or pressure control modes, with or without PEEP) or specially designed ventilators that deliver CPAP or bi-level positive airway pressure (Bi-PAP). These dedicated noninvasive ventilators generate high gas flow, can cycle between a high inspiratory pressure and a lower expiratory pressure, and can sense and respond to patient inspiratory effort. Originally developed for home ventilation in patients with obstructive sleep apnea and chronic respiratory failure, newer models are targeted for use in the ICU and incorporate monitoring packages that allow assessment of delivered tidal volumes and respiratory patterns. However, there is no evidence that the type of ventilator used for NPPV affects patient outcome, and the choice of equipment is typically based on availability and familiarity.

NPPV compared to standard therapy has been associated with improved outcomes in a variety of causes of respiratory failure, including cardiogenic pulmonary edema, COPD, and ALI in immunosuppressed patients.[123,124] Improved outcomes include the avoidance of endotracheal intubation, a reduction in complications associated with intubation including VAP, and reduced mortality. However, NPPV is not without risk, and has been associated with increased complications, including a higher rate of MI in patients with cardiogenic pulmonary edema, and increased mortality in patients with respiratory failure after extubation.[125,126] Therefore, NPPV is best and most safely utilized when patient characteristics are ideal, including an awake, cooperative patient (with the exception of rapidly reversible obtundation due to hypercarbia), a low risk for regurgitation and aspiration of gastric contents, and a high likelihood that the process resulting in respiratory failure is rapidly reversible. Further research including larger, randomized trials of NPPV is necessary to better define the particular subgroups of patients who will benefit from this approach.

Another alternative to tracheal intubation and mechanical ventilation for patients with acute hypoxemic respiratory failure is the provision of oxygen through high flow nasal cannulae (HFNC), wherein a high concentration of heated and humidified oxygen is delivered at flow rates from 40 to 60 L/min. This technique not only delivers high inspired oxygen fraction (FiO_2) but also generates low levels of PEEP and may reduce the work of breathing. A number of studies, including two recent, moderately sized randomized controlled trials, have shown outcome benefits of HFNC for acute hypoxemic respiratory failure in comparison to NPPV and conventional therapy.[127,128] HFNC is thus a viable first-choice alternative to NPPV or tracheal intubation in select patients.

"Weaning" from mechanical ventilation is better termed "liberation" or "separation" from ventilation, because weaning implies that ventilation must be gradually withdrawn in order to allow respiratory muscle and patient adaptation to the process. In reality, separation from mechanical ventilation is more a function of the resolution of the cause of respiratory failure, rather than the technique used to withdraw ventilatory support. This is supported by a study showing that daily trials of unassisted ventilation (T-piece trials) resulted in more rapid separation from ventilation than other more gradual approaches, in particular IMV "weaning."[129] In addition, so-called "weaning parameters" are inadequate predictors of the success or failure of withdrawal of ventilatory support, and add little to routine management. Thus, the process of separation from mechanical ventilation is expedited when respiratory therapy–driven protocols are used that focus on daily assessment of the ability to breath without assistance, assuming improvement of the inciting process, adequate oxygenation, and hemodynamic stability.[130] Once the patient can breathe comfortably for 30 to 120 minutes without support, the trachea can be extubated, assuming that there are not other precluding factors such as airway abnormalities, coma, and so forth.

Acute Respiratory Distress Syndrome

ARDS is a syndrome of acute, hypoxemic respiratory failure marked pathologically by DAD, with resulting increased lung permeability and diffuse alveolar edema.[131] ARDS can occur as a result of direct injury to the lung (e.g., aspiration or pneumonia), or in association with extrapulmonary infection (sepsis) or injury (e.g., multiple trauma). ARDS and DAD are associated with an inflammatory cell infiltration of the lung, increased systemic markers of inflammation, and progression through exudative, fibroproliferative, and fibrotic phases of injury over days to weeks.

In order to better standardize the definition of ARDS for epidemiologic and research purposes, in 1994 a joint American-European Consensus Conference (AECC) proposed criteria for characterizing ARDS according to the severity of gas exchange abnormality, and distinguished ALI as a less severe version of ARDS, at least in terms of gas exchange.[132] Another multinational consensus conference convened in 2011 to refine the definition of ARDS; the resulting "Berlin Definition" eliminates the "ALI" term, adds more explicit criteria for the timing and presentation of the syndrome, and stratifies ARDS into three grades of severity according to gas exchange criteria.[133] Although the Berlin Definition performs better than the prior AECC definition in predicting mortality due to ARDS, its predictive value is still poor.

ARDS is highly prevalent in the ICU population and accounts for 10% to 15% of all ICU admissions.[134] Of predisposing factors, sepsis carries the highest risk (approximately 30%) and is the most common cause of ARDS. Mortality associated with ARDS appears to have fallen over the past 20 years, although this observation is mainly confined to randomized, controlled trials versus observational studies.[134,135] Moreover, ARDS mortality varies greatly with the population of patients studied; for example, ARDS mortality in trauma patients is 10% to 15%, whereas mortality in medical ICU patients is as high as 60%. Patients with ARDS continue to die primarily as a result of associated conditions (sepsis, multiple organ failure, etc.), and uncommonly die of hypoxemia per se.

Clinically, ARDS is characterized by reduced static thoracic (lung and chest wall) compliance and severe impairment of gas exchange, including high intrapulmonary shunt and dead space fraction. These mechanics and gas exchange abnormalities create a challenge in terms of optimizing mechanical ventilation, because maintenance of adequate oxygenation and carbon dioxide elimination are both problematic. In addition, although the ratio of PaO_2 to FiO_2 (P/F ratio) does not appear to predict mortality, high dead space fraction does, and may reflect the extent of pulmonary vascular injury.[136] Pulmonary hypertension often develops as the syndrome progresses, and can complicate hemodynamic management.

Although ARDS appears to be a diffuse process by chest x-ray, lung opacification is surprisingly heterogeneous when the lung is imaged by CT. Areas of dense opacification are frequently confined to the posterior, dependent portion of the lung, leaving a small, relatively normal, recruitable volume available for ventilation. This low recruitable lung volume has been termed the "baby lung," and has important implications for ventilatory management in ARDS, as discussed later.[120]

The treatment of ARDS is largely supportive, and includes aggressive treatment of inciting events, avoidance of complications, and mechanical ventilation. In regards to the latter, it is critical that tidal volumes and static ventilatory pressures are minimized in order to avoid further injury to the remaining relatively uninjured lung. A large, randomized, prospective trial found that a small tidal volume (6 mL/kg or less) and low static (plateau) airway pressure (≤30 cm H_2O) resulted in a relative mortality reduction of 22% when compared to a control group ventilated with tidal volumes of 12 mL/kg.[137] This approach was corroborated in a similar, smaller trial.[138] This is the only intervention that has been unequivocally proven to reduce mortality in patients with ARDS.

Because ARDS is marked by high intrapulmonary shunt, hypoxemia is relatively unresponsive to oxygen therapy. Thus, strategies to recruit collapsed lung are necessary. This is most commonly achieved by using PEEP. The optimal balance between PEEP and FiO_2 has been long debated, but at this point there is no strong evidence to favor either a "high PEEP, low FiO_2" or a "minimal PEEP, high FiO_2" strategy.[139] Other maneuvers to promote recruitment of lung include the use of esophageal manometry to titrate PEEP and tidal volume, recruitment maneuvers or sigh breaths, pressure controlled ventilation, airway pressure release ventilation, inverse ratio ventilation (prolonged inspiratory time), prone positioning, and high frequency ventilation. Of these techniques, prone positioning alone is associated with improved survival. A meta-analysis of seven randomized, controlled trials of patients with ARDS and ALI and a subsequent multicenter, randomized, controlled trial found a mortality benefit to prone positioning in patients with severe ARDS.[140,141] Unfortunately, the difficult logistics of prone positioning likely discourage early use of this potentially life-saving procedure. A number of studies have compared high frequency oscillatory ventilation to conventional ventilation for treatment of ARDS, including several multicenter, randomized controlled trials. However, this intervention is not associated with improved outcomes, as confirmed in a recent meta-analysis.[142]

Inhaled vasodilators such as nitric oxide (iNO) and prostaglandins also variably and transiently improve oxygenation in ARDS by improving blood flow to ventilated alveoli. However, several randomized, prospective trials have failed to show any relevant long-term outcome benefits associated with iNO administration to patients with ALI/ARDS.[143,144] Prostaglandins have not been as rigorously studied. Inhaled vasodilators may be useful as "rescue" therapy in selected patients with severe, refractory hypoxemia, although outcome benefits have not been established.

Given that ARDS is marked by high permeability pulmonary edema, it is intuitive that administration of excessive fluids be avoided. Results from a randomized, controlled trial found that a conservative fluid management strategy that emphasized diuresis resulted in improved oxygenation, more ventilator-free days, and more days not in the ICU, but no significant difference in mortality compared to liberal fluid management.[145] Another intervention to facilitate reduction of lung water in ARDS is co-administration of albumin with diuretics.[146] Similar improvements in fluid balance and oxygenation were again demonstrated, but this study was underpowered to detect a more meaningful mortality difference. Although a small study suggested that administration of inhaled β agonists might also enhance lung water clearance in patients with ARDS, a subsequent large randomized, controlled trial failed to show benefit to this therapy.[147]

Multiple therapies have been tested in an effort to halt the inflammatory and proliferative phases of injury, with mixed success. Corticosteroid administration to patients with ARDS has been associated with reduced mortality in two small, randomized trials and smaller case series and cohort studies.[148,149] A large randomized controlled trial sponsored by the ARDS Network randomized patients between days 7 and 28 of ARDS onset to methylprednisolone versus placebo.[150] Although there was no difference in 28-day mortality in the intention-to-treat analysis, patients receiving steroids between 7 and 14 days after ARDS onset appeared to benefit, but those starting treatment more than 14 days after ARDS onset appeared to suffer harm. Furthermore, the group receiving methylprednisolone had more ventilator-free days and shock-free days at day 28, in addition to improved oxygenation and respiratory system compliance. Thus, it appears that patients with ARDS may benefit from corticosteroid treatment within a narrow time window, but further study is necessary before strong conclusions can be drawn.

Additional areas of controversy in the management of patients with ARDS include the use of neuromuscular blockade and extracorporeal membrane oxygenation (ECMO). Although the use of neuromuscular blockade to facilitate mechanical ventilation of patients with ARDS has generally been on the decline due to fears of increased risk of critical illness myopathy, a French multicenter trial that randomized patients with severe ARDS (P/F ratio <150) to early treatment with cisatracurium versus placebo questions these fears.[151] The cisatracurium-treated group had a reduction in the adjusted hazard ratio for death, compared to the placebo group, and there was no increase in ICU-acquired paresis. Subsequent experimental data suggest that the benefits of neuromuscular blockade in ARDS may be due to anti-inflammatory effects of nicotinic receptor inhibition.[152] Reservations about this approach remain, however, and further research is necessary before routine neuromuscular blockade for severe ARDS can be recommended.

The use of ECMO to support patients with severe ARDS had resurgence during the influenza pandemic of 2009, with some observational data suggesting a survival benefit to ECMO.[153] In addition, a UK-based multicenter trial randomized patients with severe ARDS to consideration for ECMO at a specialized referral center versus conventional treatment at their originating hospital. Patients randomized to ECMO consideration had an increased likelihood of disability-free survival at 6 months.[154] Skepticism remains regarding the widespread use of ECMO for management of severe ARDS given the invasive nature of this approach, cost considerations, and need for transfer to specialized centers.

Acute Kidney Injury

AKI is reported to occur in up to 66% of critically ill patients.[155] In 2004, a consensus group proposed standard criteria for classifying the severity of renal injury and the associated outcomes.[156] The criteria, known as the RIFLE (risk of renal dysfunction, injury to the kidney, failure or loss of kidney function, and end-stage kidney disease) criteria, have been subsequently modified by the Acute Kidney Injury Network (AKIN) group, and most recently by the Kidney Disease: Improving Global Outcomes (KDIGO) group (Table 57-5).[157,158]

Table 57-5 Kidney Disease: Improving Global Outcomes (KDIGO) Classification of Acute Kidney Injury

Stage	Serum Creatinine	Urine Output	In-hospital Mortality Odds Ratio
1	↑ Serum Cr ≥1.5× baseline within 7 days OR ↑ Serum Cr ≥0.3 mg/dl within 48 h	<0.5 mL/kg/h for 6–12 h	2.5
2	↑ Serum Cr ≥2× baseline	<0.5 mL/kg/h for >12 h	5.4
3	↑ Serum Cr ≥3× baseline OR ↑ Serum Cr ≥4 mg/dL OR renal replacement therapy	<0.3 mL/kg/h for 24 h OR anuria × 12 h	10.1

OR, odds ratio.
Adapted from Kellum JA, Lameire N, Group KAGW. Diagnosis, evaluation, and management of acute kidney injury: a KDIGO summary (Part 1). *Crit Care.* 2013;17:204 and Mehta RL, Kellum JA, Shah SV, et al. Acute Kidney Injury Network: report of an initiative to improve outcomes in acute kidney injury. *Crit Care.* 2007;11(2):R31.

Despite the evolving definition of AKI, its incidence appears to be fairly stable over the past 20 years.[159] Moreover, the hospital mortality associated with AKI requiring dialysis has remained approximately 60% for nearly five decades.[159] This is discouraging when one considers reductions in mortality in association with other organ failures over the same time interval. The reasons for the lack of improvement in outcome are unclear, but likely include insensitive means for identifying patients with incipient renal failure and lack of effective preventive and therapeutic measures.

In the ICU, AKI occurs due to prerenal causes and tubular injury (acute tubular necrosis) in the vast majority of cases.[159] Other potential causes of AKI in the ICU include glomerulonephritis, vasculitis, interstitial nephritis, macro and microvascular disease (e.g., thrombotic thrombocytopenic purpura), toxins (nonsteroidal anti-inflammatory drugs, cisplatin, aminoglycosides, radiologic contrast, myoglobin, and hemoglobin), and urinary tract obstruction. The initial evaluation of AKI should focus on identifying easily correctable causes; thus, assessment of volume status utilizing functional hemodynamic monitoring, identification of nephrotoxic agents through careful history taking and medication review, urinalysis to identify possible glomerulonephritis or interstitial nephritis, and ultrasonography to rule out postrenal or obstructive sources of AKI are all important.

In incipient and established AKI, supportive care is the rule, with the focus on maintenance of euvolemia, avoidance of renal toxins, adjustment of medication doses, and monitoring of electrolytes and acid–base status. Pharmacologic approaches to the prevention and treatment of AKI have been uniformly disappointing. Current guidelines recommend against the use of low-dose dopamine, recombinant atrial natriuretic peptide, fenoldopam, colloid solutions, and diuretics for the prevention and treatment of AKI.[155] In the specific setting of contrast-induced nephropathy, the first intervention is avoidance of contrast exposure whenever possible. If contrast must be used, low- or iso-osmolar contrast agents, pre- and postcontrast exposure intravascular volume expansion with saline or sodium bicarbonate solutions, and possibly the use of oral (but not intravenous) N-acetyl cysteine may be useful.[155]

Although hemodialysis (i.e., renal replacement therapy [RRT]) is typically considered a supportive measure in AKI, recent interest has focused on the potential for RRT to improve renal recovery and reduce mortality. Research on RRT in the ICU has focused on the type, intensity, and dose of dialysis; the timing of initiation of RRT is also of interest, but has not been rigorously studied in this setting.

The intensity of RRT is determined by both the frequency of treatment and the degree of solute clearance per unit of time. Increased intensity of RRT has failed to improve outcomes in critically ill patients with AKI in two large, randomized clinical trials.[160,161] However, it should be noted that the prescribed intensity of RRT is seldom delivered in clinical practice owing to therapy interruptions for procedures or when filters require replacement. As such, efforts to ensure maximal delivery of the prescribed RRT dose are important.

Continuous renal replacement therapy (CRRT) (including continuous venovenous hemofiltration and hemodialysis) has long been known as a useful technique when hemodynamic instability is present. In contrast to intermittent hemodialysis, effective solute removal is possible with CRRT in the presence of arterial hypotension. Despite this theoretical advantage to CRRT, several studies, including a relatively large, multicenter randomized controlled trial, found no survival benefit to CRRT compared to intermittent hemodialysis.[162] The two techniques are considered equivalent.

Endocrine Aspects of Critical Care Medicine

Glucose Management in Critical Illness

Hyperglycemia is commonly encountered in critically ill patients and occurs in both diabetics and nondiabetics. Hyperglycemia results primarily because of increased glucose production and insulin resistance caused by inflammatory and hormonal mediators that are released in response to injury. Hyperglycemia may also be aggravated by various therapeutic and supportive interventions, including the use of corticosteroids and total parenteral nutrition. Although the risks of hyperglycemia for patients with diabetes who are ketosis-prone have long been appreciated, hyperglycemia is also detrimental to critically ill patients in a broader sense. Hyperglycemia is associated with increased risk of postoperative infection (wound and otherwise) and poor outcome in patients with stroke, TBI, and AKI.[155,163] In addition, the blood glucose level is a risk factor for mortality in diabetic patients admitted with acute MI.[164]

Given these considerations, strict glycemic control in critically ill patients has been advocated as leading to multiple outcome benefits. A single randomized controlled trial of surgical patients published in 2001 found that intensive insulin therapy (goal glucose <110 mg/dL) reduced ICU mortality by approximately 50% compared to more conventional therapy (goal glucose <215 mg/dL).[165] Based largely on the results of this one trial there was widespread adoption of protocols to target blood glucose between 80 and 110 mg/dL. Unfortunately, the benefits of the initial trial were not reproduced in multiple subsequent trials, and in fact an increased risk of hypoglycemia and associated harm have been observed.[166] After an additional large, multicenter, multinational randomized controlled trial of intensive insulin therapy (NICE-SUGAR [Normoglycemia in Intensive Care Evaluation–Survival Using Glucose Algorithm Regulation] study) showed increased mortality in the tight glucose control group, the practice of maintaining blood glucose between 80 and 110 mg/dL was widely abandoned.[167] Current serum glucose targets are somewhat variable, but most agree that 140 to 180 mg/dL is an acceptable goal in most patients.

Adrenal Function in Critical Illness

The stress response to injury includes an increase in serum cortisol levels in most critically ill patients.[168] However, adrenal insufficiency may also occur in critically ill patients for several reasons, including inhibition of adrenal stimulation or corticosteroid synthesis by drugs or cytokines and direct injury to or infection of the pituitary or adrenal glands.[169] Thus, adrenal insufficiency has been reported to occur with increased frequency in critically ill patients with trauma, burns, sepsis, and other conditions in comparison with the general population.

The diagnosis of adrenal insufficiency in critical illness is complicated by limitations of commonly used tests of adrenal function. Cortisol is highly protein bound, and serum proteins, including albumin, are commonly depressed in critically ill patients. Although total serum cortisol levels are low in critically ill patients with hypoproteinemia, free cortisol levels are elevated.[170] This suggests that older reports utilizing total serum cortisol levels in critically ill patients may overestimate the incidence of adrenal insufficiency. However, until free cortisol assays are more widely available, the diagnosis of adrenal insufficiency in critical illness must be based on clinical suspicion and total cortisol levels.

In addition to absolute adrenal insufficiency (low baseline cortisol and poor response to adrenocorticotropic hormone [ACTH] administration/stimulation), a condition of relative adrenal insufficiency (defined as an increase in serum cortisol of ≤9 μg/dL in response to ACTH administration, independent of the baseline cortisol level) has been described in patients in septic shock and with other illnesses. Low-normal baseline cortisol levels, high baseline cortisol levels, and a poor response to ACTH are all predictors of increased mortality in critical illness.[37]

Although high-dose corticosteroids for the treatment of septic shock are of no benefit, evidence suggests that lower doses (hydrocortisone 200 to 300 mg/day) can reduce dependency on vasopressors and shorten the duration of shock. Evidence for a mortality benefit is unclear, with some trials showing improved mortality and others showing lack of efficacy. A 2015 meta-analysis suggests that there is currently low quality evidence supporting a small mortality benefit with the use of low-dose hydrocortisone (200 to 300 mg/day or equivalent) in sepsis, but that the incidence of metabolic derangements is also increased.[171] Given the lack of clear benefit, current guidelines suggest a trial of low-dose hydrocortisone only in patients with vasopressor-dependent septic shock.[78] There does not appear to be an increased risk of gastric ulceration, superinfection, or neuromuscular weakness according to this analysis, but hypernatremia and hyperglycemia are more common in patients receiving steroids.

Thyroid Function in Critical Illness

Measures of thyroid function, including levels of thyrotropin (TSH), T_3, and T_4, are deranged in the majority of critically ill patients. Depression of T_3 occurs within hours of injury or illness and can persist for weeks. TSH levels may be normal initially, but fall to inappropriately low levels as illness progresses. T_4 levels are also often low, but can be normal or high. Low hormone levels may occur for a variety of reasons, including altered binding and metabolism early in the course of illness, and depressed neuroendocrine function with more prolonged courses. In addition, certain drugs (e.g., dopamine) can depress thyroid function through central mechanisms.[172] Low thyroid hormone levels, particularly T_3, correlate with the severity of illness and are associated with an increased risk of death.[168]

It is controversial whether the observed abnormalities in thyroid hormones represent an appropriate response to illness or true hypothyroidism; thus, the terms "euthyroid sick syndrome" and "nonthyroidal illness" have been coined to describe thyroid function abnormalities in critical illness. Furthermore, it is not clear whether replacement of thyroid hormones is indicated or beneficial in critical illness. T_3 administration to brain-dead organ donors appears to improve hemodynamic stability, although randomized trials have found minimal or no benefit to T_3 or T_4 administration in patients undergoing cardiopulmonary bypass and cardiac surgery.[173] In addition, several small studies have found no benefit to T_3 or T_4 administration to patients with a variety of critical illnesses. Larger, randomized prospective trials are necessary to define the role of routine thyroid hormone supplementation in nonthyroidal illness.

Importantly, true hypothyroidism may be present in the critically ill, particularly in the geriatric population, and should be considered in the face of refractory shock, adrenal insufficiency, unexplained coma, and prolonged, unexplained respiratory failure. True hypothyroidism is marked by an elevation of TSH (usually >25 mU/L) in the face of a low T_4 level.

Somatotropic Function in Critical Illness

Growth hormone (GH) levels are low in prolonged critical illness, and it has been conjectured that deficiencies of GH and insulin-like growth factor-1 (IGF-1) contribute to the muscle wasting seen in acute illness.[168] However, although small trials have found that GH administration can attenuate muscle catabolism in critical illness, a large, randomized trial found that administration of high-dose GH to critically ill patients resulted in increased mortality.[174] Thus, GH administration during critical illness cannot be advocated at this time, although further exploration of the benefits of smaller doses of GH may be warranted.

Anemia and Transfusion Therapy in Critical Illness

Anemia is a frequent if not obligate accompaniment of critical illness. The vast majority of patients admitted to the ICU are anemic at some point in their hospital stay, and approximately 40% of them will receive transfused blood.[175] Importantly, both anemia (hemoglobin [Hb] <9 g/dl) and the amount of transfused blood are independently associated with mortality.[176,177] However, this association does not denote cause and effect, particularly for anemia, which may just be a marker of the severity of illness.

The cause of anemia in critical illness is multifactorial, and related to blood loss from the primary injury or illness, iatrogenic blood loss due to daily blood sampling, nutritional deficiencies, and marrow suppression.[178] Given that approximately 13% of ICU patients may have iron, folate or vitamin B_{12} deficiencies, these parameters should be checked when consideration is given to blood transfusion.

Treatment of anemia in critical illness is the source of considerable debate. In unstressed subjects, severe anemia (Hb of 5 g/dL or less) is amazingly well tolerated due to physiologic compensations that maintain oxygen delivery and extraction. However, it has long been assumed that critically ill patients have less efficient compensatory mechanisms and reduced physiologic reserve, and thereby require a higher Hb concentration than unstressed individuals. Historically, this has translated to a red blood cell (RBC) transfusion threshold at an Hb concentration of approximately 10 g/dL. This is reflected in data from multiple studies supporting the prevalence of RBC transfusion in the ICU; approximately 40% of ICU patients receive an RBC transfusion at an average transfusion threshold of 8.5 g/dL.[175]

Transfusion of RBCs is not without risks including infection, transfusion-related acute lung injury (TRALI), transfusion-associated circulatory overload (TACO), transfusion-related immunomodulation (TRIM), microchimerism and more (see Chapter 17 for a more complete discussion of transfusion risks).[175] These negative effects of transfusion may help explain why a large, randomized, controlled trial of transfusion requirements in critical illness (the TRICC [transfusion requirements in critical care] study) found that 30-day mortality was not affected when a restrictive transfusion threshold (Hb <7 g/dL) was used, compared to a more conventional threshold of less than 10 g/dL.[179] Furthermore, a trend in mortality reduction favored the restrictive group, and various subgroups of patients (less than 55 years of age and less severely ill by APACHE [acute physiology and chronic health evaluation] scoring) had a significantly lower mortality when they were transfused using the restrictive strategy. A similar trial in pediatric patients found no mortality difference between restrictive and liberal transfusion strategies, suggesting that a restrictive strategy is safe in critically ill children.[180] More recent studies in patients with TBI[181] and acute upper gastrointestinal hemorrhage[182] confirm that restricting RBC transfusion to an Hb concentration of less than 7 g/dL reduces exposure to blood products, reduces complications, and in the case of upper gastrointestinal hemorrhage improves survival. Likewise, liberal RBC transfusion as part of goal-directed therapy that has been incorporated into the protocol for septic shock did not favorably affect outcomes.[183] These studies support clinical practice guidelines that recommend a restrictive transfusion practice in the ICU, with the possible exception of patients with active myocardial ischemia.[175]

Alternatives to the transfusion of RBCs for treatment of anemia are not currently available for widespread use. Several hemoglobin-based oxygen carriers (HBOCs) have been studied in clinical trials involving trauma and surgery, but results have been mixed, and none are currently FDA approved for use. Compassionate use of HBOCs in patients who have refused blood transfusion for religious reasons has been reported.

Prevention of anemia in critical illness is an appealing alternative to transfusion. One simple and potentially cost-saving approach is to reduce the volume and frequency of blood draws in the ICU. As noted earlier, iatrogenic blood loss is a major factor in the development of anemia of critical illness. Another potential approach is the administration of recombinant erythropoietin and iron. A large randomized controlled trial found that administration of recombinant erythropoietin to critically ill patients on day 3 of ICU stay and every week thereafter reduced transfusion requirements significantly, without affecting mortality or other outcome variables.[184] However, a subsequent randomized controlled trial with a lower recommended transfusion threshold found no reduction in blood transfusion in association with erythropoietin administration.[185] Although there was a reduction in mortality in trauma patients who received erythropoietin compared to placebo, a subsequent randomized, controlled trial in patients with TBI did not reveal an outcome benefit to the administration of erythropoietin.[181] Given the current high cost of erythropoietin, it is not a cost-effective alternative for general use in critical care at this time, but further investigation of its utility in trauma patients may be warranted.

Nutrition in the Critically Ill Patient

Critical illness can lead to hypermetabolic states, and if nutritional support is inadequate or delayed, patients are at immediate risk of malnutrition. Poor nutritional status is associated with increased mortality and morbidity among critically ill patients. Therefore, appropriate nutrition is an important aspect of critical care and adequate nutritional support should be considered a standard of care. What constitutes *adequate* nutritional support, however, remains less clear. Although current guidelines recommend providing 80% to 100% of predicted caloric needs as soon as possible during an ICU admission, a growing body of research suggests no harm to intentional underfeeding (providing 20% to 50% of predicted caloric needs).[186,187] Although over 200 formulas have been promoted for predicting daily calorie requirements of the critically ill patient, the American Society for Parenteral and Enteral Nutrition (ASPEN) and SCCM guidelines do not specify any specific formula.[188] It is acceptable to use a simple formula based on the patient's ideal body weight to calculate predicted caloric needs (25 to 30 kcal/kg/day), of which 15% to 20% should be represented by proteins (1.2 to 2 g/kg/day).

Feeding intolerance due to high gastric residual volume can be improved by the administration of gastric prokinetic agents and positioning an enteric tube postpyloric. However, a systematic review comparing gastric versus postpyloric feeding did not suggest a clinical benefit from postpyloric tube feeding with regard to pneumonia, ICU length of stay, and mortality.[189] There is some suggestion that intermittent enteral feeding, as opposed to a continuous feeding regimen, is more likely to allow earlier attainment of the enteral calorie goal.[190]

Most of the trials evaluating parenteral nutrition (PN) do not demonstrate any favorable impact on outcome. In fact, enteral nutrition (EN) is associated with lower infection risk and PN is associated with increased rates of complications and death. Therefore, EN is preferred over PN whenever possible because of its lower cost and less frequent complications.[191] Although not rigorously investigated, PN may be considered in patients unable to tolerate EN. There has been considerable debate regarding the timing of initiation of PN, with Canadian and American guidelines generally recommending delayed initiation, while European guidelines have recommended early initiation.[188,192] A prospective randomized trial comparing initiation of PN at or before ICU day 2 with PN initiation at ICU day 8 showed the delayed initiation group had a decrease in infections, shorter duration of mechanical ventilation, less need for RRT, and a cost savings.[193] However, it is unclear how long of a delay in initiating PN is acceptable, assuming that EN is contraindicated or not tolerated despite vigorous attempts. Overall, strategies to optimize delivery of EN (starting at the target rate, use of a feeding protocol with a higher threshold of gastric residuals volumes, use of motility agents, and use of small bowel feeding) and minimize the risks of EN (elevation of the head of the bed) should be considered. Studies that demonstrate a benefit from the use of supplemental PN in patients unable to tolerate adequate EN are lacking.[191]

Among special enteral formulations, immunonutrition has been hypothesized to influence infectious morbidity and mortality in critically ill patients via a beneficial effect on gastrointestinal immunologic function. This effect appears more likely in surgical patients, such as those with burns and those who are in trauma. Specific enteral formulations, particularly those with high concentrations of glutamine, have the strongest data to support their use.[194] The beneficial effects in medical ICU patients are less well established, and two recent randomized controlled trials found no benefit to nutritional supplementation with immunomodulatory agents in patients with ALI.[195,196] Trials supporting the administration of supplemental antioxidant micronutrients (selenium, zinc, and vitamins A, C, and E) are of overall low quality with high risk of bias and should be interpreted with caution.[197]

Sedation and Analgesia for the Critically Ill Patient

Goals and Assessment

Most patients in the ICU will experience some form of pain, agitation, or anxiety during their admission, and the indications for sedation and analgesia in the ICU are many. Although individual medications frequently provide multiple pharmacodynamic effects, including sedation, analgesia, and anxiolysis, it is helpful to think about these effects separately when selecting medications for an individual patient. For instance, painful procedures such as the insertion of indwelling catheters, endotracheal tubes, and thoracostomy tubes require analgesia, but often do not require anxiolysis or sedation. Conversely, agitated delirium or acute alcohol withdrawal do not require analgesia and are more appropriately treated with sedatives.

The goal of any sedation and analgesia strategy in the ICU is to provide enough medication to effectively treat patient symptoms, but to avoid adverse effects such as delirium, long-term cognitive deficits, and respiratory depression that are associated with overtreatment. The patient with an ideal level of sedation and analgesia is at reduced risk for dislodging catheters, removing monitoring devices, or falling out of bed. They are more likely to be synchronous with the mechanical ventilator, which improves oxygenation and reduces the risk of lung injury. They are also better able to participate with care, early mobilization, and physical and occupational therapy.

Assessing the adequacy of attempts to achieve these goals can be difficult. Several factors such as inter-individual variability, evolving severity of disease and organ dysfunction, variably intense pain stimuli and multiple drug interactions influence the analgesic and sedative needs of ICU patients. Therefore, it is important to titrate medications according to established therapeutic goals and reevaluate sedation requirements frequently. Several validated scales are available to assess sedation levels over time. The most commonly used are the Ramsay sedation scale, the Riker sedation–agitation scale (SAS), and the Richmond agitation–sedation scale (RASS). Features common to all of these scales are the ability to grade sedation over different depths and allow for indicators of agitation. There is no evidence that one scale is superior to another at this time, although the RASS has been more rigorously assessed for reliability and validity.[198,199] Similarly, there are a variety of validated pain scales. These scales are discussed in Chapter 55. The important point regarding assessment scales for pain, sedation, and delirium is that an assessment utilizing a validated scoring system should be made before and after every intervention to assess progress in achieving treatment goals.

Pharmacologic Management

Virtually any hypnotic-anxiolytic or opioid used in the operating room can be used in the ICU to provide sedation and analgesia, respectively. However, propofol, midazolam, and dexmedetomidine are the most commonly used hypnotic-anxiolytics. Each of these drugs has its own particular advantages and disadvantages, and detailed discussions of their properties can be found in Chapters 19 and 20. Some important considerations of their use in the ICU environment are discussed here.

Dexmedetomidine is unique in that its mechanism of action is profoundly different from that of propofol and benzodiazepines. It provides sedation without inducing unresponsiveness or coma, may have some analgesic effects,[200,201] and has little affect on respiratory drive. Generally speaking, however, dexmedetomidine is effective for patients who do not require deep sedation (e.g., patients with severe ARDS requiring aggressive mechanical ventilation). Because it does not reliably produce amnesia, it is not appropriate as a solo hypnotic-anxiolytic in patients requiring paralysis. Propofol is generally more effective in these settings, but can cause hypertriglyceridemia and lead to the potentially lethal "propofol infusion syndrome."

Benzodiazepines may be a good choice in patients who require deep sedation or amnesia (e.g., during the co-administration of neuromuscular blockers), but who have hypotension or shock. They are also effective in patients with alcohol withdrawal. Neither randomized nor retrospective data support dexmedetomidine use in patients with alcohol withdrawal, in terms of meaningful clinical outcome.[202,203] Although dexmedetomidine may reduce short-term benzodiazepine use in this situation, it does not reduce long-term use or improve symptom control.

Although the aforementioned physiologic rationale for the choice of a certain regimen exists, certain regimens may be superior in terms of patient outcomes of untoward neurocognitive effects, time on the ventilator, and length of stay. A large, well-conducted study[204] (two separate arms, no institutional cross-over) comparing dexmedetomidine with either propofol or midazolam demonstrated noninferiority for dexmedetomidine, although patients receiving propofol required less rescue sedation than those receiving dexmedetomidine. When compared to midazolam, dexmedetomidine may also be associated with a small reduction in the duration of mechanical ventilation, and it appears to provide significantly better patient responsiveness and cooperation compared to both drugs. Conversely, patients receiving dexmedetomidine were twice as likely as patients receiving propofol to have had cardiovascular instability. A trend toward higher mortality was observed in the dexmedetomidine group, but disappeared when all dexmedetomidine patients were compared to all propofol and midazolam patients. Interestingly, there was no difference between dexmedetomidine and midazolam on measures of agitation and delirium, whereas the difference between dexmedetomidine and propofol was statistically significant. A meta-analysis including 27 randomized trials comparing propofol versus midazolam suggested that tracheal extubation occurred earlier with the use of propofol for patients who were ventilated for a duration shorter than 36 hours.[205] However, no differences were found with regard to the ICU length of stay or mortality. Greater levels of hypotension and elevated triglyceride levels were observed with the use of propofol. Because the publication of this meta-analysis, an open label randomized trial demonstrated that a continuous infusion of propofol was associated with shorter length of mechanical ventilation and ICU stay compared to intermittent benzodiazepine administration.[206]

Opiates are a very common component of many ICU analgesia and sedation regimens, and are increasingly being used as single agents in certain types of patients[199] (e.g., patients with acute postoperative pain, with uncomplicated respiratory failure requiring modest degrees of mechanical ventilation, or who require sedation but do not tolerate hypnotic-anxiolytic drugs). Like dexmedetomidine, opiates do not reliably produce amnesia, and are not appropriate as single agents in patients who require paralysis. Morphine and fentanyl are the most commonly used opioids to provide analgesia in the ICU. Morphine should be avoided in patients with renal failure due to active metabolites that accumulate in the presence of impaired renal function.

Neuromuscular blockade may be occasionally indicated in ICU patients with severe ARDS with refractory hypoxemia. A single trial has demonstrated a benefit in mortality and ventilator-free days, but routine use is discouraged until these results are validated. Concerns remain that this practice may predispose to critical illness polyneuropathy and myopathy (see section on ICU-acquired Weakness), and an increased risk of nosocomial pneumonia.[207,208] Together, these studies underscore the fact that there is not likely to be a clearly, consistently superior regimen for all patients on all outcomes of interest, and careful consideration of the relative pros and cons must be undertaken for each individual patient.

Delirium and Neurocognitive Complications

Neurocognitive complications including delirium and prolonged cognitive dysfunction are associated with a number of sedative medications, and may be more common in patients treated with deeper levels of sedation. The distinguishing characteristics of delirium include an acute onset and fluctuating course, inattention, disorganized thinking, and altered level of consciousness. Structured screening instruments such as the Confusion Assessment Method for the ICU (CAM-ICU) are available, and their use in concert with proactive screening regimens are recommended for the diagnosis of delirium in the ICU.[209,210]

Critically ill patients are often deeply sedated, in part due to concerns for patient comfort, but also because of potential benefits afforded by a reduction in the sympathoadrenal response to injury. Although some literature supports the notion that benzodiazepine use may be associated with an increased frequency of delirium, two well-conducted trials failed to show a reduction in delirium in patients randomized to dexmedetomidine compared to benzodiazepine.[211,212] In addition, available evidence from observational and randomized trials suggests that practices favoring light sedation, bolus administration versus continuous infusion of sedatives, and promoting daily trials of awakening in ICU patients result in a variety of benefits, including a shortened duration of mechanical ventilation, decreased time in the ICU, and reduced mortality.[213-221]

Nonpharmacologic techniques including the use of both verbal and written communication, frequent reorientation, maintenance of a day–night cycle and noise reduction strategies can be used to improve comfort and safety and to reduce delirium and confusion. Antipsychotic medications like haloperidol and quetiapine are also being used more commonly in ICU sedation regimens, primarily to treat or prevent delirium or agitation, and to promote sleep or treat insomnia. The data for such use are limited and of poor quality. The only randomized, controlled trial of such use did show a reduction in periods of delirium with regular quetiapine administration, but the study was small.[222] SCCM guidelines specifically cite the lack of evidence for the use of haloperidol, atypical antipsychotics, or dexmedetomidine for the prevention of delirium.[199] Because those guidelines were issued in 2013, a retrospective study found an association between haloperidol use and an increase in next-day delirium, suggesting it is not effective for prevention.[223] A similar randomized trial[224] found no benefit. A systematic review of a number of pharmacologic prevention or treatment strategies (e.g., dexmedetomidine, various antipsychotics, cholinesterase inhibitors) resulted in a number of subtle findings and a high degree of heterogeneity for some comparisons, but trends generally favored pharmacologic intervention.[225] The relationship between delirium and antipsychotics as cause, prophylaxis, or treatment is not completely understood, and intervention decisions continue to require careful clinical assessment and follow-up.

The depth or use of sedation may also play a role in long-term outcomes after discharge from the ICU and hospital. Increasing evidence suggests that patients admitted to the ICU are at risk of developing symptoms of posttraumatic stress disorder,[226,227] delusional memories, and longer-term cognitive dysfunction. Approximately one-third will have signs and symptoms of cognitive dysfunction 12 months after discharge.[228] Interestingly, in this retrospective analysis, exposure to various sedative medications was not significantly associated with the development of longer-term cognitive dysfunction. Further, long-term follow-up of patients enrolled in sedation trials has not found sedation regimens promoting light sedation or daily awakening to be associated with increased long-term cognitive, psychological, or functional problems.[217,229,230]

Complications in the ICU: Detection, Prevention, and Therapy

Nosocomial Infections

Nosocomial infections are a major source of morbidity and mortality in the critically ill. At some level, nosocomial infections are unavoidable and occur because of the nature of intensive care—patients are critically ill with altered host defenses, they require invasive devices (endotracheal tubes, intravascular catheters, etc.) that provide portals of entry for infectious organisms, and they receive therapies that increase the risk of infection (e.g., glucocorticoids, PN). On the other hand, many nosocomial infections are preventable with relatively simple interventions.[231] This became more financially relevant in the United States in 2008, when the Center for Medicare and Medicaid Services (CMS) ceased reimbursing hospitals for treatment of preventable complications such as catheter-associated urinary tract infection (CAUTI) and catheter-related bloodstream infection (CRBSI).

Several types and sources of infections are relatively unique to ICU care and should be included in the differential diagnosis when signs suggestive of infection arise. These infections include sinusitis, VAP, CRBSI (also referred to as central line-associated bloodstream infection [CLABSI]), CAUTI, and invasive fungal infection.

Sinusitis

Radiographic sinusitis is common in critically ill patients with indwelling oral and nasal tubes. Nasotracheal intubation confers a greater risk than does orotracheal intubation of radiographic sinusitis, occurring in approximately 95% and 25% of patients with nasal and oral tubes after 1 week of intubation, respectively.[232] Several reports suggest that approximately 10% of radiographically diagnosed sinusitis is infected, as determined by quantitative cultures, although the incidence may be much higher. One study reported that bacterial sinusitis was responsible for 16% of fevers of unknown origin in a surgical ICU.[233] The organisms cultured from sinuses represent those that are responsible for other nosocomial infections, particularly VAP (staphylococcal species, enteric gram-negative bacteria, and non-lactose-fermenting gram-negative rods such as *Pseudomonas* and *Acinetobacter*). Bacterial sinusitis may predispose to the development of VAP, possibly because of microaspiration of infected secretions.

Prevention of sinusitis should focus on efforts to improve sinus drainage, including semirecumbent positioning and avoidance of nasal tubes. Bacterial sinusitis should be considered in patients with unexplained fever and leukocytosis in the ICU. If radiographic sinusitis is documented, any nasal tubes should be removed, and nasal irrigation and short-term administration of nasal decongestants should be considered. If the patient is severely ill, broad-spectrum antibiotic coverage should be considered. If these maneuvers do not result in resolution of signs and symptoms of sinusitis in 2 to 3 days, otolaryngologic consultation and consideration of sinus drainage procedures may be undertaken.

Ventilator-associated Pneumonia

Tracheal intubation and mechanical ventilation increase the risk of nosocomial pneumonia, thus the term VAP. The likelihood of developing VAP increases with the duration of mechanical ventilation, but the precise incidence is difficult to define due to substantial variability in how VAP is defined. Because VAP is widely associated with increased morbidity, it is an obvious target for QI interventions. In an effort to facilitate the study of such interventions the Centers for Disease Control and Prevention (CDC) implemented a standardized ventilator-associated event (VAE) surveillance program through the National Healthcare Safety Network (NHSN) in 2013.[234] Possible and probable VAP are specifically defined within the larger category of VAE. Importantly, in an effort to remove the subjective variability inherent to interpretation of radiographic studies, this definition of VAP does not make use of radiologic data, nor was it intended to be a clinical definition. Recent studies show inconsistent overlap in VAP detection when the NHSN and traditional definitions are simultaneously applied to the same population, with more cases of VAP detected using lower respiratory tract culture-based clinical criteria (that typically include a radiographic component) than with the NHSN criteria.[235] Given this caveat, recent studies utilizing the NHSN definition put the incidence at less than 4% per mechanical ventilation episode.[236,237] This contrasts with an incidence greater than 15% at 1 week of ICU and greater than 20% at 2 weeks described in older studies, and likely reflects increasing adherence to best practices for VAP prevention as well as changing definitions.[238]

Although the mortality in patients with VAP ranges between 30% and 70%, the attributable mortality (the number of patients who die because of VAP rather than with VAP) is more difficult to assess. This may be due to differences in the type of ICU, patient factors, diagnostic techniques across studies, or differences in the virulence of the causative pathogens. Although earlier work suggested an attributable mortality to VAP greater than 40%, more recent and rigorously conducted work suggests that the effect of VAP on mortality is minimal.[239]

VAP can be categorized as "early-onset," occurring within the first 48 to 72 hours of intubation/ventilation, or "late-onset," occurring thereafter (note that 4 days of mechanical ventilation is required in order for it to qualify as a VAE per the NHSN definition). Early-onset VAP is generally caused by organisms such as *Haemophilus influenzae, Streptococcus pneumoniae,* methicillin-sensitive *Staphylococcus aureus,* and other relatively antibiotic-sensitive oral flora that enter the trachea around the time of intubation. Late-onset VAP is associated with more virulent organisms such as methicillin-resistant *S. aureus, Pseudomonas aeruginosa,* and *Acinetobacter.* In general, early-onset organisms are associated with zero or low attributable mortality, whereas late-onset organisms, particularly *Pseudomonas* and *Acinetobacter* species, are associated with higher mortality.[240]

There are a number of interventions that can reduce the incidence of VAP, some of which are relatively simple and inexpensive, and others that are costlier and/or associated with some risk. The simplest and least expensive interventions are strict handwashing between patients, and semirecumbent positioning of the patient (head-of-bed angle at 30 degrees or greater from horizontal). Considering their negligible risks, these practices should be rigorously applied in all ICUs.

The use of acid suppression therapy to prevent gastrointestinal bleeding is more controversial. Acid-suppression therapies have been associated with increased VAP risk because they allow bacterial overgrowth in the stomach. Further, the risk of significant gastrointestinal bleeding is very low in the ICU, even in high-risk patients (those with coagulopathy or on mechanical ventilation). Thus, gastrointestinal acid suppression therapy may be reserved for high-risk patients, and sucralfate may be considered as an alternative agent to acid-suppressive regimens despite its potentially reduced effectiveness.

Somewhat more expensive interventions to reduce VAP that may be useful include specialized endotracheal tubes with subglottic suctioning ports and silver coatings. Although a meta-analysis supports the use of endotracheal tubes with subglottic suctioning ports to reduce the incidence of VAP and shorten both hospital and ICU length of stay, silver-coated tubes have not been proven beneficial in this regard.[241,242] Lending support to the use of subglottic suctioning tubes is a recent cost-benefit analysis that found the optimal strategy for VAP prevention includes their use.

Given that aspiration of gastric and oropharyngeal organisms appears to be a mechanism for the development of VAP, intervening to "decontaminate" these sites has been investigated. Although selective digestive decontamination (SDD) with non-absorbable antimicrobial agents remains controversial, a recent meta-analysis suggests that SDD may lower the incidence of VAP and bacteremia, as well as reduce mortality.[243] It is unclear if antibiotic resistance is increased with this practice. Limited oral decontamination with chlorhexidine has become more commonplace in many ICUs, but recent evidence also questions this practice.[244] Further clarification of the role of SDD and limited oral decontamination is expected following completion of two large multicenter randomized trials (ClinicalTrials.gov identifiers: NCT02389036 and NCT02208154).

An additional and important approach to reduce the overall mortality of VAP involves refinement of the diagnostic process and limitation of antibiotic therapy, to avoid the development and proliferation of antibiotic resistant organisms. As mentioned earlier, an invasive diagnostic strategy is likely more accurate than traditional clinical criteria to diagnose VAP. Invasive strategies typically involve collection of either tracheal aspirate specimens or bronchial–alveolar specimens using lavage or protected brushes, and then quantitating bacterial growth in the laboratory. Thus, VAP is diagnosed only when bacteria are seen within bronchoalveolar cells microscopically or when bacterial growth exceeds specific thresholds ($\geq 10^4$ colony-forming units/mL for bronchoalveolar lavage and $\geq 10^3$ colony-forming units/mL for protected brush specimens). Current Infectious Disease Society of America guidelines specify that tracheal aspirate specimens are equivalent to bronchial–alveolar specimens for VAP diagnosis, although the data supporting this recommendation are conflicting.[245–247] It therefore seems appropriate to favor collection of bronchial-alveolar specimens for VAP diagnosis when possible, while reserving tracheal aspirate specimens for instances when it is not feasible to obtain a bronchial-alveolar specimen.

It is clear that delay in treatment of nosocomial infections (including VAP) is associated with increased mortality. Treatment should not be delayed pending diagnostic evaluation; rather, treatment should be started after culture specimens are sent, if the clinical suspicion of VAP is high. Antibiotics can then be narrowed in spectrum or discontinued altogether depending on the results from quantitative cultures after 48 to 72 hours (Table 57-6). This approach is known as "de-escalating therapy" and is designed to ensure adequate antibiotic treatment up front, but avoid overuse of antibiotics in the long term.[240] Antibiotic selection should be predicated on hospital bacterial growth and resistance patterns. In general, for patients with early-onset VAP, antibiotics can be relatively narrow in spectrum and limited to a single agent. For late-onset VAP, broader spectrum antibiotics should be initiated and include agents from two different classes—resistant gram-negative organisms and methicillin-resistant *S. aureus.*

Table 57-6 Suggested Empiric Antibiotic Regimens for Common Intensive Care Unit Infections

Ventilator-associated pneumonia	
• Early (<72 hours of intubation and hospital admission)	Ceftriaxone PLUS azithromycin; consider adding vancomycin or linezolid if known history of MRSA
• Late (>72 hours of intubation or hospital admission)	Vancomycin OR linezolid AND cefepime; consider adding ciprofloxacin if high incidence of MDR GNRs
Bloodstream infections	Vancomycin OR linezolid AND cefepime
Urinary tract infections	
• Noncatheter-associated	Ceftriaxone
• Catheter-associated	Ceftazidime ADD vancomycin if GPCs on gram stain; CONSIDER meropenem instead of ceftazidime if concerned for MDR GNRs or ESBLs
C. difficile diarrhea	Vancomycin (oral dosing); IF shock, megacolon or ileus, then ADD IV metronidazole
Meningitis	
• Nonsurgical	Dexamethasone AND ceftriaxone AND vancomycin AND ampicillin AND acyclovir
• Postsurgical	Cefepime AND metronidazole AND vancomycin
Intra-abdominal infections	
• Community-acquired	Ceftriaxone AND metronidazole
• Hospital-acquired	Vancomycin AND either piperacillin-tazobactam OR meropenem
Sepsis, site unknown	Vancomycin AND meropenem Consider adding ciprofloxacin if concern for MDR GNRs or ESBLs

MDR, multi-drug resistant; MRSA, methicillin-resistant *Staphylococcus aureus*; GNR, gram-negative rods; GPC, gram-positive cocci; ESBL, extended spectrum β-lactamase. Initial antibiotic regimen should take into account local antibiograms. Antibiotic regimens should be narrowed once culture results are available.

The optimal duration of antibiotic therapy for VAP is not well defined. An often-cited meta-analysis found that 8 days of antibiotic therapy was effective for treatment of VAP in terms of mortality and recurrent infections, and resulted in more antibiotic-free days.[248] However, patients who had VAP caused by nonlactose–fermenting gram-negative rods (including *Pseudomonas*) had a higher infection recurrence rate if they received only an initial 8-day course of therapy. It is unclear whether intermediate courses of therapy would have avoided infection recurrence. Thus, it is reasonable to choose an 8-day course of therapy for many patients with VAP; however, if there is an inadequate early clinical response or infection with nonlactose–fermenting gram-negative rods a longer course should be considered.

Catheter-related Bloodstream Infections

As strictly defined by the CDC, CRBSI includes the following criteria: (1) clinical suspicion of catheter-related infection (including low likelihood of infection elsewhere), plus (2) positive culture of blood drawn from the catheter or a segment of catheter, plus (3) matching positive blood culture drawn from another site, preferably by direct venotomy or arterial puncture. Given this strict definition, the incidence of CRBSI is less than 5% in most studies. However, the incidence of bacteremia is affected by several factors, including the conditions and technique of insertion, type and location of catheter, and the duration of catheterization, and can vary widely from study to study. The attributable mortality of CRBSI is approximately 11%, which is much lower than that for primary bacteremia or bacteremia associated with another site of infection.[277] The cost associated with a CRBSI is quite high and estimated between $22,000 and $54,000.[22]

CRBSI is more likely when placement occurs under emergency conditions, and is reduced by the use of strict aseptic technique with full barrier precautions. This includes pre-insertion handwashing, full gown and gloves, and the use of a large barrier drape.[22] In addition, skin cleansing with chlorhexidine is more effective than other agents at reducing catheter-related infection. Attention to these practices can dramatically reduce catheter-related infection.[22,249,250] These simple interventions should be considered as standards of care and are recommended by the CDC.

CRBSI and bacteremia increase with the duration of catheterization, particularly for durations of greater than 2 days. However, routine catheter replacement at 3 or 7 days does not reduce the incidence of infection, and results in increased mechanical complications. Thus, routine guide-wire exchange of catheters is not recommended.

Catheters coated with either antiseptics (chlorhexidine and silver sulfadiazine) or antibiotics (rifampin and minocycline) reduce bacterial colonization of catheters as well as bacteremia. This effect becomes manifest only after days 5 to 6 of the catheter being in place; thus, the CDC recommends the use of antimicrobial-coated catheters in patients with an expected duration of catheterization of greater than 5 days, particularly if the local rate of CRBSI is high.[251] However, a large meta-analysis found that although coated catheters reduced the incidence of colonization and CRBSI, they did not reduce the incidence of clinically diagnosed sepsis or mortality.[252] Ultimately, key of strategies to reduce CRBSI are to limit the duration of insertion, and the need for continued central venous catheterization should be reviewed daily.[22,249] CRBSI may be insertion site-dependent, but adoption of these practices seem to be lessening the role that infectious concerns play when choosing a catheter insertion site.[253]

Catheter-related venous thrombosis occurs commonly, and is associated with an increased risk of infection. Routine flushing of catheter ports with heparin reduces both the incidence of thrombosis and infection. However, heparin solutions contain antimicrobial preservatives and it is unclear if the heparin or the preservative is responsible for the beneficial effect. In addition, heparin may induce thrombocytopenia. Therefore, the CDC does not recommend the routine use of heparin flushing.[251]

Organisms commonly responsible for catheter-related bacteremia include *S. epidermidis* and *S. aureus*, enteric gram-negative bacteria, *P. aeruginosa* and *Acinetobacter*, and occasionally *Enterococcal* species. Although coagulase-negative staphylococci are commonly isolated from blood cultures in the ICU, they are rarely responsible for true infection.[254] When catheter-related bacteremia is confirmed, the offending catheter should be removed and appropriate antibiotics continued for a minimum of 7 days. Longer courses should be considered for *S. aureus* bacteremia, given its predilection to cause endocarditis. Suspected CRBSI can be addressed by sending screening cultures drawn through the catheter and from a peripheral site. Guidewire exchange of the catheter with culture of the intracutaneous segment and tip can also be considered in this situation, but should a CRBSI be confirmed, the catheter should be removed, not exchanged. Depending on the patient's severity of illness, a strong suspicion of catheter-related bacteremia should trigger the institution of broad-spectrum antibiotic coverage, including coverage for methicillin-resistant staphylococcal species and nonlactose–fermenting gram-negative rods, until culture results return, with subsequent de-escalation of therapy. Similar to VAP, early appropriate antibiotic coverage of catheter-related bacteremia will likely reduce mortality, although this has not been systematically studied.

Urinary Tract Infection

The urinary tract is the second most common source of infection in the ICU, with infections occurring in up to one-third of patients. The incidence of CAUTI increases with the duration of bladder catheterization.[231,255] The responsible organisms are similar to those causing other nosocomial infections and include staphylococcal species, *Enterococcus,* enteric gram-negative bacteria, and nonlactose–fermenting gram-negative bacteria such as *Pseudomonas*. Bacteriuria is associated with bacteremia about 5% of the time. Similar to other ICU-acquired infections, CAUTIs are associated with increased mortality, although the attributable mortality is not clear.

Prevention of ICU-acquired CAUTI includes using careful handwashing and aseptic technique during catheter insertion and minimization of catheterization duration. The use of antimicrobial catheter coatings may also reduce the incidence of CAUTI, although the evidence is insufficient at this point to recommend general use of coated catheters.[255]

Invasive Fungal Infections

Invasive fungal infections in nonneutropenic patients are caused by *Candida* species in the vast majority of cases.[256] Risk factors for *Candida* infection include the presence of central venous catheters, recent abdominal surgery, anastomotic leakage and gastrointestinal perforation, dialysis-dependent renal failure, administration of PN, multiple broad-spectrum antibiotics, and steroids.[256] In addition to these factors, invasive *Aspergillus* and *Mucormycosis* are more typically associated with profound immunosuppression and diabetes, respectively.[257]

A significant clinical dilemma involves accurate and timely identification of invasive fungal infections. Positive cultures from sterile fluid remain the gold standard, but may take 72 to 96 hours to turn positive and may be positive in only 50% of autopsy-confirmed infections.[256] To improve accuracy and timeliness of the diagnosis, a number of molecular and serologic techniques have been developed. β-D-glucan is present in the cell wall of *Candida* and *Aspergillus* species, as well as *Pneumocystis jiroveci*, and an assay detecting its presence is approximately 80% sensitive and specific. A number of promising whole blood-based polymerase chain reaction (PCR) tests have also recently become available, with sensitivities above 90% in published trials and results available within hours of sample collection. However, they are expensive and have not yet been proven in clinical practice.[256] For diagnosis of *Aspergillus* and *Mucormycosis,* imaging with CT and magnetic resonance is invaluable, as biopsy and surgical debridement play an important role in management.[257]

Candida albicans is responsible for approximately 50% of invasive *Candida* infections in critically ill patients. *C. tropicalis, C. paraisopolis, C. glabrata,* and *C. krusei* account for the remainder.[256] In addition to simple bloodstream infection, *Candida* species are associated with CAUTI, postoperative peritonitis, and disseminated blood-borne infection. *Candida* is frequently cultured from the urine and sputum, but treatment is usually not necessary, as *Candida* pneumonia is unlikely and candiduria often clears without treatment, mostly with discontinuation of the bladder catheter. In addition, candiduria often recurs after initially successful antifungal therapy. True *Candida* peritonitis is also difficult to separate from contamination of culture specimens, but given that the mortality associated with *Candida* peritonitis is approximately 50%, treatment is warranted if clinical signs suggest infection. Similarly, candiduria and *Candida* in sputum cultures may be treated if there are systemic signs of infection, as colonization is a risk factor for invasive infection.

Disseminated blood-borne *Candida* infection can result in endophthalmitis, endocarditis, and hepatic and pulmonary abscesses. It is likely to occur when initial treatment of candidemia is delayed, and is associated with a high mortality. Prevention of invasive *Candida* infection involves avoidance of risk factors, including limitation of intravascular catheterization, PN, and antibiotic administration. Prophylactic therapy with fluconazole may be effective at reducing the risk of invasive *Candida* infection in high-risk patients, but this strategy has not been associated with improved mortality in the nonneutropenic population, and may increase the incidence of invasive infection with more resistant species, such as *C. glabrata* and *C. krusei*. Prophylactic therapy should be reserved for only the high-risk patient.[256] Empiric therapy should be considered in patients with a high likelihood of invasive *Candida* infection while awaiting culture results, as delay in treatment is associated with increased mortality. However, care should be taken to de-escalate therapy after several days in the absence of positive cultures or clinical response.

Documented *Candida* bloodstream infection should be treated aggressively, with therapy started promptly and continued for at least 2 weeks after the last positive blood culture. An ophthalmologic examination is warranted in patients with documented or suspected bloodstream infection, as patients with endophthalmitis may require longer courses of therapy. Intravascular catheters that are potential sources of bloodstream infection should be removed. Treatment of *Candida* infections has evolved over time, and current guidelines now recommend echinocandins such as caspofungin, micafungin, and anidulifungin as the first-line treatment in most settings.[258] Liposomal amphotericin B is generally reserved for refractory, life-threatening infections such as fungal endocarditis, invasive *Aspergillosis* and *Mucormycosis*. In addition, surgical debridement plays a key role in management of *Mucormycosis*.[257] Suggested empiric treatment of common ICU infections is outlined in Table 57-6.

Stress Ulceration and Gastrointestinal Hemorrhage

Gastric mucosal breakdown with resulting gastritis and ulceration (stress ulceration) can lead to gastrointestinal (GI) bleeding in the ICU. Clinically significant GI bleeding results in hemodynamic instability and/or a sudden fall in hematocrit that results in blood transfusion. The incidence of clinically

Table 57-7 Caprini Venous Thromboembolism Risk Assessment Model

1 Point	2 Points	3 Points	5 Points
Age 41–60 years	Age 61–74 years	Age >75 years	Stroke <1 month
Minor surgery	Arthroscopic surgery	Personal history of VTE	Elective lower extremity arthroplasty
Body mass index >25 kg/m^2	Major open surgery >45 min	Family history of VTE	Hip, pelvis, or leg fracture
Swollen legs	Laparoscopic surgery >45 min	Any thrombophilia	Acute spinal cord injury <1 month
Varicose veins	Bed rest >72 h	Elevated serum homocysteine	Multiple trauma <1 month
Pregnant or postpartum <1 month	Immobilizing plaster cast	Heparin-induced thrombocytopenia	
History of miscarriage	Central venous access		
Oral contraceptives or hormone replacement therapy			
Sepsis <1 month			
Serious lung disease <1 month			
Abnormal pulmonary function			
Acute myocardial infarction			
Congestive heart failure <1 month			
History of inflammatory bowel disease			
Medical patient on bed rest			

High risk: ≥5 points
Intermediate risk: 3–4 points
Low risk: 1–2 points
Very low risk: 0 points

VTE, venous thromboembolism.
Adapted with permission from Pollak AW, McBane RD 2nd. Succinct review of the new VTE prevention and management guidelines. *Mayo Clinic Proceedings.* 2014;89:394–408.

significant stress-related GI bleeding is relatively low—less than 5% in high-risk patients and less than 1% for low-risk patients.[259] The major risk factors for stress-related GI bleeding are mechanical ventilation and coagulopathy. Secondary risk factors among mechanically ventilated patients include renal failure, thermal injury, and possibly head injury, although the latter two factors have not been recently evaluated.[259] EN may protect against significant GI bleeding.[259]

Stress ulcer prophylaxis (SUP) strategies include acid suppression agents such as histamine type 2 receptor antagonists, proton pump inhibitors, and cytoprotective agents such as sucralfate. However, the agent of choice and related benefits are controversial for the following reasons: (1) recent meta-analyses suggest significant bias in published trials[261,262]; (2) methodological flaws in many of the studies, as well as significant practice changes that have occurred in other areas of care such as VAP prevention and the provision of nutrition because the original studies were published; (3) acid suppression may favor gastric colonization with enteric flora that may increase the risk of nosocomial pneumonia and *C. difficile* colitis.[261,263] Thus, although SUP is commonly used in critically ill patients, the utility of this intervention is unclear. Current evidence appears to support restricting their use to high-risk patients who are without EN for greater than 48 hours.

Venous Thromboembolism

VTE encompasses both deep venous thrombosis (DVT) and pulmonary embolism (PE), and occurs frequently in critically ill patients, with incidences of DVT of 10% to 30% and PE of 1.5% to 5%.[264] However, the reported incidence varies widely depending on the study design, DVT detection method, and patient population studied. Virtually all critically ill patients have one or more risk factors for VTE.[265] Determination of VTE risk is important in that it will help in choosing prophylactic therapy and in determining the level of suspicion for VTE in individual patients (Table 57-7).

In addition to classic lower extremity DVT, upper extremity DVT occurs with increased frequency in the ICU population. This is directly associated with the use of central venous catheters in the subclavian and internal jugular sites. Upper extremity DVT can result in PE in up to one-third of cases, with occasional fatalities. Catheter-related thrombosis is also associated with increased risk of CRBSI and bacteremia. Finally, upper extremity DVT is associated with considerable long-term morbidity, particularly related to postthrombotic syndrome.[266]

The literature supporting prophylactic measures to prevent VTE in the ICU population is relatively poor and generally shows differences only in intermediate end points (e.g., asymptomatic DVT), with no differences in the incidence of PE or death. In general, the risks of VTE prophylaxis, including heparin-induced thrombocytopenia and bleeding, must be weighed against the risk of VTE. It is generally agreed that high-risk patients without contraindications should receive pharmacologic prophylaxis, and low-risk patients with contraindications should receive mechanical prophylaxis with intermittent pneumatic compression devices. There are an ever-expanding number of medications that may be used for VTE chemoprophylaxis, but unfractionated heparin and low–molecular-weight heparin remain the most commonly used and most studied, with guidelines from professional societies updated regularly.[267] A number of validated scoring systems have been developed for both surgical and medical populations to assess VTE risk.[265] In patients at high risk for DVT with contraindications to anticoagulation, the preventative placement of a vena cava filter may be considered, although there are few data to support this practice. To reduce central venous catheter–associated thrombosis and infection, catheter tips should be positioned in the superior vena cava and catheters may be flushed with a dilute heparin solution. Heparin bonding of catheters may also reduce local thrombosis. Importantly, it should be recognized that the incidence of VTE in patients receiving pharmacologic prophylaxis remains substantial, ranging between 5% and 30% depending on the therapy and population studied.

Given the high incidence of asymptomatic DVT in critically ill patients, a high index of suspicion for VTE must be maintained. However, despite the high incidence of DVT, routine screening studies for DVT do not appear to improve clinical outcomes in the ICU. Thus, VTE should be considered in critically ill patients in the face of relatively nonspecific findings, such as unexplained tachycardia, tachypnea, fever, asymmetric extremity edema, and gas exchange abnormalities, including high dead space ventilation. Compression Doppler ultrasonography is the most commonly utilized test for diagnosis of DVT and has good positive and negative predictive value compared to contrast venography.[268] Helical chest CT has supplanted radionuclide ventilation–perfusion scanning as the primary test for the diagnosis of PE.[269] CT scanning can also be extended to include the extremities to diagnose DVT. However, ventilation–perfusion scanning and/or pulmonary angiography may have utility in specific circumstances, including in the presence of renal insufficiency (concerns about contrast-induced nephrotoxicity) or equivocal results on CT scan. In addition, pulmonary angiography may be the test of choice when the likelihood of PE is high and anticoagulation is contraindicated, necessitating immediate placement of a vena cava filter. D-dimer levels are not useful in the ICU population because they are frequently elevated and nonspecific in critically ill patients.

The mainstay of treatment for VTE is either unfractionated or low–molecular-weight heparin, which should be started prior to confirmatory studies if clinical suspicion is high. In situations of hemodynamic compromise, the use of systemic thrombolytic therapy may be life-saving. However, if bleeding risk is elevated, new catheter-directed thrombolysis and clot evacuation techniques, or open surgical thrombectomy, can be considered. The specific interventions are largely dependent on institutional capabilities and clinical circumstances.

For patients who have contraindications to anticoagulation or who have recurrent PE despite anticoagulation, vena cava filters can be placed in the superior or inferior vena cava, depending on DVT location. Ultimately, given the long-term thrombotic complications associated with these devices, patients with vena cava filters should be anticoagulated when no longer contraindicated, and the devices should be removed when they are no longer required.

ICU-acquired Weakness

The term ICU-acquired weakness (ICUAW) encompasses a wide variety of neuromuscular abnormalities developing as a consequence of critical illness. ICUAW is characterized by weakness that is symmetrical and bilateral, occurs during an ICU stay, and is not attributable to another specific etiology. The spectrum of illness ranges from subjective muscle fatigue to flaccid quadriplegia. Although various studies have attempted to distinguish neuropathic from myopathic syndromes, resulting in a bewildering list of associated acronyms, it is likely that there is considerable overlap between the two in terms of risk factors, presentation, and prognosis.[270]

ICUAW is associated with prolonged duration of mechanical ventilation, ICU stay, hospital stay, and mortality.[271] Prospective studies have shown that up to 11% of mechanically ventilated patients exhibit evidence of weakness at 24 hours. By 7 days the incidence may increase to 60%, and among those with ARDS and sepsis the number may be even higher.[271] In addition to sepsis, factors strongly associated with the development of ICUAW include duration of illness and hyperglycemia. Although corticosteroid and neuromuscular blocking drug administration have classically been associated with ICUAW, more recent evidence suggests that their use in modern ICUs is not associated with ICUAW. This is likely due to contemporary practice of using shorter-acting agents in lower doses and for much shorter courses than was historically the case.[272] Less specific contributors to the development of ICUAW include a catabolic nutritional state, systemic pro-inflammatory state, and generalized muscle unloading.[273]

Prevention of ICUAW centers on avoidance or minimization of contributory risk factors, including long courses of high-dose steroids, prolonged neuromuscular blockade, and hyperglycemia. High-quality evidence in support of specific interventions to prevent ICUAW exists only for avoidance of hyperglycemia. There is moderate-quality evidence that early mobilization may be beneficial.[274]

The diagnosis of ICUAW should be entertained in all critically ill patients with unexplained weakness. Electrodiagnostic studies can help confirm the diagnosis and rule out other, potentially treatable causes of weakness such as Guillain–Barré syndrome. Muscle biopsy is confirmatory in cases of myopathy, but given its invasive nature, biopsy is not warranted outside of research settings. Unfortunately, no specific, effective treatment for ICUAW has been identified; however, avoidance of potentially contributing agents and aggressive physical therapy is warranted. Discharge planning should include the potential need for long-term nursing and rehabilitative care.

End-of-Life Care in the ICU

Nearly 20% of patients in the United States die during a hospitalization with an ICU stay.[275] Consequently, the ICU is an important setting for delivering high-quality end-of-life care. Shared decision making and patient- and family-centered care require good communication between medical teams, patients, and their family members to ensure that delivered care is consistent with patient values and preferences. The Institute of Medicine Committee on Approaching Death released its report *Dying in America: Improving Quality and Honoring Individual Preferences Near the End of Life* in 2014. The report emphasizes the need for improved communication about end-of-life preferences between clinicians and patients in order to avoid unwanted treatment.[276] It is becoming more widely recognized that palliative care is one way to achieve this goal. Its implementation is associated with a higher quality of life, so much so that the CCSC Choosing Wisely campaign for critical care has recommended that patients at high risk of death or severely impaired functional recovery be offered care focused primarily on comfort, as an alternative to care focused primarily on a cure.[23] It is important to recognize that palliative care can also be offered in conjunction with curative care, and that intensivists play an important role in delivering palliative care in the ICU, in collaboration with palliative care specialists.

REFERENCES

1. Berthelsen PG, Cronqvist M. The first intensive care unit in the world: Copenhagen 1953. *Acta Anaesthesiol Scand.* 2003;47(10):1190–1195.
2. Angus DC, Kelley MA, Schmitz RJ, et al. Caring for the critically ill patient. Current and projected workforce requirements for care of the critically ill and

patients with pulmonary disease: can we meet the requirements of an aging population? *JAMA.* 2000;284(21):2762–2770.
3. Spielman FJ. Critical care medicine: anesthesiology steps forward. *Bull Anesth Hist.* 2003;21(1):12–13.
4. U.S. Health Resources and Services Administration. The critical care workforce: a study of the supply and demand for critical care physicians. Report to Congress. 2006. Available at: http://www.mc.vanderbilt.edu/documents/CAPNAH/files/criticalcare.pdf. Accessed January 3, 2017.
5. U.S. National Center for Health Workforce Analysis. Projecting the Supply of Non-Primary Care Specialty and Subspecialty Clinicians: 2010–2025. 2014. Available at: https://bhw.hrsa.gov/sites/default/files/bhw/nchwa/projections/clinicalspecialties.pdf. Accessed January 3, 2017.
6. American Board of Medical Specialties. *2013–2014 ABMS Board Certification Report.* Chicago, IL: Elsevier; 2014, 1–31.
7. Kavanagh BP. The GRADE system for rating clinical guidelines. *PLoS medicine.* 2009;6(9):e1000094.
8. States SaHoRotU. Patient protection and affordable care act. 2010.
9. Dogra AP, Dorman T. Critical care implications of the affordable care act. *Crit Care Med.* 2016;44:e168–e173.
10. Weled BJ, Adzhigirey LA, Hodgman TM, et al. Critical care delivery: the importance of process of care and ICU structure to improved outcomes: an update from the american college of critical care medicine task force on models of critical care. *Crit Care Med.* 2015;43(7):1520–1525.
11. Banerjee R, Naessens JM, Seferian EG, et al. Economic implications of nighttime attending intensivist coverage in a medical intensive care unit. *Crit Care Med.* 2011;39(6):1257–1262.
12. Nishisaki A, Pines JM, Lin R, et al. The impact of 24-hr, in-hospital pediatric critical care attending physician presence on process of care and patient outcomes. *Crit Care Med.* 2012;40(7):2190–2195.
13. Wilcox ME, Chong CA, Niven DJ, et al. Do intensivist staffing patterns influence hospital mortality following ICU admission? A systematic review and meta-analyses. *Crit Care Med.* 2013;41(10):2253–2274.
14. Kerlin MP, Small DS, Cooney E, et al. A randomized trial of nighttime physician staffing in an intensive care unit. *N Engl J Med.* 2013;368(23):2201–2209.
15. Wallace DJ, Angus DC, Barnato AE, et al. Nighttime intensivist staffing and mortality among critically ill patients. *N Engl J Med.* 2012;366(22):2093–2101.
16. Lane D, Ferri M, Lemaire J, et al. A systematic review of evidence-informed practices for patient care rounds in the ICU. *Crit Care Med.* 2013;41(8):2015–2029.
17. Kim MM, Barnato AE, Angus DC, et al. The effect of multidisciplinary care teams on intensive care unit mortality. *Arch Intern Med.* 2010;170(4):369–376.
18. Hales BM, Pronovost PJ. The checklist—a tool for error management and performance improvement. *J Crit Care.* 2006;21(3):231–235.
19. Vincent JL, Creteur J. Paradigm shifts in critical care medicine: the progress we have made. *Crit Care.* 2015;19 Suppl 3:S10.
20. Micek ST, Roubinian N, Heuring T, et al. Before-after study of a standardized hospital order set for the management of septic shock. *Crit Care Med.* 2006;34(11):2707–2713.
21. Morris AC, Hay AW, Swann DG, et al. Reducing ventilator-associated pneumonia in intensive care: impact of implementing a care bundle. *Crit Care Med.* 2011;39(10):2218–2224.
22. Pronovost P, Needham D, Berenholtz S, et al. An intervention to decrease catheter-related bloodstream infections in the ICU. *N Engl J Med.* 2006;355(26):2725–2732.
23. Critical Care Societies Collaborative Choosing wisely: five things physicians and patients should question. 2014. Available from: http://www.choosingwisely.org/clinician-lists - keyword = critical_care (accessed 22 Jan 2016).
24. Thatcher RW, Cantor DS, McAlaster R, et al. Comprehensive predictions of outcome in closed head-injured patients. The development of prognostic equations. *Ann N Y Acad Sci.* 1991;620:82–101.
25. Chesnut RM, Marshall SB, Piek J, et al. Early and late systemic hypotension as a frequent and fundamental source of cerebral ischemia following severe brain injury in the Traumatic Coma Data Bank. *Acta Neurochir Suppl (Wien).* 1993;59:121–125.
26. Nelson DW, Nystrom H, MacCallum RM, et al. Extended analysis of early computed tomography scans of traumatic brain injured patients and relations to outcome. *J Neurotrauma.* 2010;27(1):51–64.
27. Carney N, et al. Guidelines for the Management of Severe Traumatic Brain Injury, Fourth Edition. *Neurosurgery,* 2016.
28. Chesnut RM, Temkin N, Carney N, et al. A trial of intracranial-pressure monitoring in traumatic brain injury. *N Engl J Med.* 2012;367(26):2471–2481.
29. Mirski MA, Muffelman B, Ulatowski JA, et al. Sedation for the critically ill neurologic patient. *Crit Care Med.* 1995;23(12):2038–2053.
30. Cremer O, Moons, KG, Bouman, EA, et al. Long-term propofol infusion and cardiac failure in adult head-injured patients. *Lancet.* 2001;357:117–118.
31. Schwartz ML, Tator CH, Rowed DW, et al. The University of Toronto head injury treatment study: a prospective, randomized comparison of pentobarbital and mannitol. *Can J Neurol Sci.* 1984;11(4):434–440.
32. Ward JD, Becker DP, Miller JD, et al. Failure of prophylactic barbiturate coma in the treatment of severe head injury. *J Neurosurg.* 1985;62(3):383–388.

33. Eisenberg HM, Frankowski RF, Contant CF, et al. High-dose barbiturate control of elevated intracranial pressure in patients with severe head injury. *J Neurosurg.* 1988;69(1):15–23.
34. Drummond JC, Dao AV, Roth DM, et al. Effect of dexmedetomidine on cerebral blood flow velocity, cerebral metabolic rate, and carbon dioxide response in normal humans. *Anesthesiology.* 2008;108(2):225–232.
35. Robertson CS, Valadka AB, Hannay HJ, et al. Prevention of secondary ischemic insults after severe head injury. *Crit Care Med.* 1999;27(10):2086–2095.
36. Muizelaar JP, Marmarou A, Ward JD, et al. Adverse effects of prolonged hyperventilation in patients with severe head injury: a randomized clinical trial. *J Neurosurg.* 1991;75(5):731–739.
37. Lipiner-Friedman D, Sprung CL, Laterre PF, et al. Adrenal function in sepsis: the retrospective Corticus cohort study. *Crit Care Med.* 2007;35(4):1012–1018.
38. Andrews PJ, Sinclair HL, Rodriguez A, et al. Hypothermia for intracranial hypertension after traumatic brain injury. *N Engl J Med.* 2015;373(25):2403–2412.
39. Cooper DJ, Rosenfeld JV, Murray L, et al. Decompressive craniectomy in diffuse traumatic brain injury. *N Engl J Med.* 2011;364(16):1493–1502.
40. Hutchinson, PJ, et al. Trial of Decompressive Craniectomy for Traumatic Intracranial Hypertension. *N Engl J Med,* 2016;375(12):1119–1130.
41. Roberts I, Yates D, Sandercock P, et al. Effect of intravenous corticosteroids on death within 14 days in 10008 adults with clinically significant head injury (MRC CRASH trial): randomised placebo-controlled trial. *Lancet.* 2004;364 (9442):1321–1328.
42. Temkin NR, Anderson GD, Winn HR, et al. Magnesium sulfate for neuroprotection after traumatic brain injury: a randomised controlled trial. *Lancet Neurol.* 2007;6(1):29–38.
43. Temkin NR, Dikmen SS, Wilensky AJ, et al. A randomized, double-blind study of phenytoin for the prevention of post-traumatic seizures. *N Engl J Med.* 1990;323(8):497–502.
44. Myburgh J, Cooper J, Finfer S, et al. Saline or albumin for fluid resuscitation in patients with traumatic brain injury. *N Engl J Med.* 2007;357(9):874–884.
45. Kassell NF, Torner JC, Jane JA, et al. The International Cooperative Study on the Timing of Aneurysm Surgery. Part 2: Surgical results. *J Neurosurg.* 1990;73(1):37–47.
46. Kassell NF, Torner JC, Haley EC Jr, et al. The International Cooperative Study on the Timing of Aneurysm Surgery. Part 1: Overall management results. *J Neurosurg.* 1990;73(1):18–36.
47. Nieuwkamp DJ, Setz LE, Algra A, et al. Changes in case fatality of aneurysmal subarachnoid haemorrhage over time, according to age, sex, and region: a meta-analysis. *Lancet Neurol.* 2009;8(7):635–642.
48. van Donkelaar CE, Bakker NA, Veeger NJ, et al. Predictive factors for rebleeding after aneurysmal subarachnoid hemorrhage: rebleeding aneurysmal subarachnoid hemorrhage study. *Stroke.* 2015;46(8):2100–2106.
49. Dorsch NW. Cerebral arterial spasm—a clinical review. *Br J Neurosurg.* 1995;9(3):403–412.
50. Barker FG 2nd, Ogilvy CS. Efficacy of prophylactic nimodipine for delayed ischemic deficit after subarachnoid hemorrhage: a metaanalysis. *J Neurosurg.* 1996;84(3):405–414.
51. Liu J, Chen Q. Effect of statins treatment for patients with aneurysmal subarachnoid hemorrhage: a systematic review and meta-analysis of observational studies and randomized controlled trials. *Int J Clin Exp Med.* 2015;8(5):7198–7208.
52. Treggiari MM, Walder B, Suter PM, et al. Systematic review of the prevention of delayed ischemic neurological deficits with hypertension, hypervolemia, and hemodilution therapy following subarachnoid hemorrhage. *J Neurosurg.* 2003;98(5):978–984.
53. Diringer MN, Bleck TP, Claude Hemphill J 3rd, et al. Critical care management of patients following aneurysmal subarachnoid hemorrhage: recommendations from the Neurocritical Care Society's Multidisciplinary Consensus Conference. *Neurocrit Care.* 2011;15(2):211–240.
54. Mozaffarian D, Benjamin EJ, Go AS, et al. Heart disease and stroke statistics—2016 update: a report from the American Heart Association. *Circulation.* 2015. 133(4):e38–e360.
55. Jauch EC, Saver JL, Adams HP Jr, et al. Guidelines for the early management of patients with acute ischemic stroke: a guideline for healthcare professionals from the American Heart Association/American Stroke Association. *Stroke.* 2013;44(3):870–947.
56. Powers WJ, Derdeyn CP, Biller J, et al. 2015 American Heart Association/American Stroke Association focused update of the 2013 guidelines for the early management of patients with acute ischemic stroke regarding endovascular treatment: a guideline for healthcare professionals from the American Heart Association/American Stroke Association. *Stroke.* 2015;46(10):3020–3035.
57. Back L, Nagaraja V, Kapur A, et al. Role of decompressive hemicraniectomy in extensive middle cerebral artery strokes: a meta-analysis of randomised trials. *Intern Med J.* 2015;45(7):711–717.
58. Juttler E, Unterberg A, Woitzik J, et al. Hemicraniectomy in older patients with extensive middle-cerebral-artery stroke. *N Engl J Med.* 2014;370(12):1091–1100.
59. Chen HJ, Lee TC, Wei CP. Treatment of cerebellar infarction by decompressive suboccipital craniectomy. *Stroke.* 1992;23(7):957–961.

60. Hypothermia after Cardiac Arrest Study Group. Mild therapeutic hypothermia to improve the neurologic outcome after cardiac arrest. *N Engl J Med.* 2002;346(8):549–556.
61. Nielsen N, Wetterslev J, Cronberg T, et al. Targeted temperature management at 33 degrees C versus 36 degrees C after cardiac arrest. *N Engl J Med.* 2013;369(23):2197–2206.
62. Rivers E, Nguyen, B, Havstad, et al. Early goal-directed therapy in the treatment of severe sepsis and septic shock. *N Engl J Med.* 2001;345:1368–1377.
63. Group TAIatACT. Goal-directed resuscitation for patients with early septic shock. *N Engl J Med.* 2014;371:1496–1506.
64. Investigators TP. A randomized trial of protocol-based care for early septic shock. *N Engl J Med.* 2014;370:1683–1693.
65. Mouncey P, Osborn, TM, Power, GS, et al. Trial of early, goal-directed resuscitation for septic shock. *N Engl J Med.* 2015;372:1301–1311.
66. Prins K, Neill JM, Tyler JO, et al. Effects of beta-blockade withdrawal in acute decompensated heart failure. *JACC: Heart Failure.* 2015;3:647–653.
67. Jessup M, Abraham, WT, Casey, DE, et al. 2009 focused update: ACCF/AHA Guidelines for the Diagnosis and Management of Heart Failure in Adults: A report of the American College of Cardiology Foundation/American Heart Association Task Force on Practice Guidelines: Developed in collaboration with the International Society for Heart and Lung Transplantation. *Circulation.* 2009;119:1977–2016.
68. O'Connor C, Starling RC, Hernandez AF, et al. Effect of nesiritide in patients with acute decompensated heart failure. *New Engl J Med.* 2011;365:32–43.
69. Kelly J, Mentz RJ, Hasselbad V. Worsening heart failure during hospitalization for acute heart failure: insights from the Acute Study of Clinical Effectiveness of Nesiritide in Decompensated Heart Failure (ASCEND-HF). *Am Heart J.* 2015;170:298–305.
70. O'Gara P, Kushner FG. Aschiem DD, et al. 2013 ACCF/AHA guidelines for the management of ST-elevation myocardial infarction. *J Am Coll Cardiol.* 2013;61:78–140.
71. Patel M, Smalling RW, Thiele H, et al. Intra-aortic balloon counterpulsation and infarct size in patients with acute anterior myocardial infarction without shock: The CRISP AMI randomized trial. *JAMA.* 2011;306:1329–1337.
72. Thiele H, Zeymer U, Neumann F-J, et al. Intraaortic balloon support for myocardial infarction with cardiogenic shock. *N Engl J Med.* 2012;367:1287–1296.
73. Leshnower B, Gleason TG, O'Hara ML, et al. Safety and Efficacy of Left Ventricular Assist Device Support in Postmyocardial Infarction Cardiogenic Shock. *Ann Thorac Surg.* 2006;81:1365–1371.
74. DeBacker D, Biston P, Devriendt J, et al. Comparison of Dopamine and Norepinephrine in the Treatment of Shock. *N Engl J Med.* 2010;362:779–789.
75. Angus D, van der Pol. T. Severe sepsis and septic shock. *N Engl J Med.* 2013;369:840–851.
76. Russell J. Management of sepsis. *N Engl J Med.* 2006;355:1699–1713.
77. Marik P. The demise of early goal-directed therapy for severe sepsis and septic shock. *Acta Anaesth Scand.* 2015;59:561–567.
78. Dellinger RP, Levy MM, Rhodes A, et al. Surviving Sepsis Campaign guidelines for management of severe sepsis and septic shock. *Crit Care Med.* 2013;41:580–637.
79. Castellanos-Ortega A, Suberviola, B, Garcia-Astudillo, LA, et al. Impact of the Surviving Sepsis Campaign protocols on hospital length of stay and mortality in septic shock patients: Results of a three-year follow-up quasi-experimental study. *Crit Care Med.* 2010;38:1036–1043.
80. Levy M, Dellinger RP, Townsend SR, et al. The Surviving Sepsis Campaign: Results of an international guideline-based performance improvement program targeting severe sepsis. *Crit Care Med.* 2010;38:367–374.
81. Rhodes A, Phillips G, Beale R, et al. The Surviving Sepsis Campaign bundles and outcome: results from the International Multicentre Prevalence Study on Sepsis (the IMPreSS study). *Intensive Care Med.* 2015;41:1620–1628.
82. Takala J. Should we target blood pressure in sepsis? *Crit Care Med.* 2010;38(10):50–59.
83. Asfar P, Meziani F, Hamel JF, et al. High versus low blood-pressure target in patients with septic shock. *N Engl J Med.* 2014;370:1583–1593.
84. Wax D, Lin HM, Leibowitz AB. Invasive and concomitant noninvasive intraoperative blood pressure monitoring: observed differences in measurements and associated therapeutic interventions. *Anesthesiology.* 2011;115:973–978.
85. Magder S. The highs and lows of blood pressure: toward meaningful clinical targets in patients with shock. *Crit Care Med.* 2014;42:1241–1251.
86. Marik P, Cavallazzi R, Vasu T, et al. Dynamic changes in arterial waveform derived variables and fluid responsiveness in mechanically ventilated patients: a systematic review of the literature. *Crit Care Med.* 2009;37:2642–2647.
87. Marik P, Baram M, Vahid B. Does central venous pressure predict fluid responsiveness? A systematic review of the literature and the tale of the seven mares. *Chest.* 2008;134:172–178.
88. Marik P, Cavallazzi R. Does the central venous pressure predict fluid responsiveness? An updated meta-analysis and a plea for some common sense. *Crit Care Med.* 2013;41:177*–1781.
89. Richard C, Warszawski J, Anguel N, et al. Early use of the pulmonary artery catheter and outcomes in patients with shock and acute respiratory distress syndrome: A randomized controlled trial. *JAMA.* 2003;290:2713–2720.
90. Sandham J, Hull RD, Brant RF, et al. A randomized, controlled trial of the use of pulmonary-artery catheters in high-risk surgical patients. *N Engl J Med.* 2003;348:5–14.
91. Melamed R, Sprenkle MD, Ulstad VK, et al. Assessment of left ventricular function by intensivists using hand-held echocardiography. *Chest.* 2009;135:1416–1420.
92. Marik P, Corwin HL. Efficacy of red blood cell transfusion in the critically ill: A systematic review of the literature. *Crit Care Med.* 2008;36:2667–2674.
93. Yang X, Du B. Does pulse pressure variation predict fluid responsiveness in critically ill patients? A systematic review and meta-analysis. *Crit Care.* 2014;18:650–657.
94. Bronzwaer AS, Ouweneel DM, Stok WJ. Arterial pressure variation as a biomarker of preload dependency in spontaneously breathing subjects: a proof of principle. *PLoS One.* 2015;10:1–11.
95. De Wall E, Rex S, Kruitwagen CL, et al. Dynamic preload indicators fail to predict fluid responsiveness in open chest conditions. *Crit Care Med.* 2009;37:510–515.
96. Boeken U, Assmann A, Mehdiani A, et al. Open chest management after cardiac operations: outcome and timing of delayed sternal closure. *Europena J Cardiothorac Surg.* 2011;40:1146–1150.
97. Boyle M, Murgo M, Lawrence J, et al. Assessment of the accuracy of continuous cardiac output and pulse contour cardiac output in tracking cardiac index changes induced by volume load. *Aust Crit Care.* 2007;20:106–112.
98. Button D, Weibel, L, Reuthebuch, O, et al. Clinical evaluation of the FloTrac/Vigileo system and two established continuous cardiac output monitoring devices in patients undergoing cardiac surgery. *Br J Anaesth.* 2007;99:329–339.
99. Monnet X, Anguel N, Naudin B, et al. Arterial pressure-based cardiac output in septic patients: different accuracy of pulse contour and uncalibrated pressure waveform devices. *Crit Care.* 2010;14:109.
100. Sander M, von Heymann C, Foer A, et al. Pulse contour analysis after normothermic cardiopulmonary bypass in cardiac surgery patients. *Crit Care.* 2005;9:729–734.
101. Mayer J, Boldt, J, Mengistu, AM, et al. Goal-directed intraoperative therapy based on autocalibrated arterial pressure waveform analysis reduces hospital stay in high-risk surgical patients: a randomized, controlled trial. *Crit Care.* 2010;14:18–27.
102. Benes J, Chytra, I, Altmann, P, et al. Intraoperative fluid optimization using stroke volume variation in high risk surgical patients: results of prospective randomized study. *Crit Care.* 2010;14:118–133.
103. Giustiniano E, Morenghi E, Ruggieri N, et al. Cardiac output by Flotrac/Vigileo validation trials: are there reliable conclusions? *Rev Recent Clin Trials.* 2012;7:181–186.
104. Dark PM, Singer M. The validity of trans-esophageal Doppler ultrasonography as a measure of cardiac output in critically ill adults. *Intensive Care Med.* 2004;30(11):2060–2066.
105. Baillard C, Cohen, Y, Fosse, JP, et al. Haemodynamic measurements (continuous cardiac output and systemic vascular resistance) in critically ill patients: transoesophageal Doppler versus continuous thermodilution. *Anaesth Intensive Care.* 1999;27:33–37.
106. Fagnoul D, Vinvent JL, De Backer D. Cardiac output measurements using the bioreactance technique in critically ill patients. *Crit Care.* 2012;16:460–462.
107. Kupersztych-Hagege E, Teboul JL, Artigas A, et al. Bioreactance is not reliable for estimating cardiac output and the effects of passive leg raising in critically ill patients. *Br J Anaesth.* 2013;111:961–966.
108. Dubost C, Bougle, A, Hallynck, C, et al. Comparison of monitoring performance of bioreactance versus esophageal Doppler in pediatric patients. *Indian J Crit Care Med.* 2015;19:3–8.
109. Pestana D, Espinosa E, Eden A, et al. Perioperative goal-directed hemodynamic optimization using noninvasive cardiac output monitoring in major abdominal surgery: a prospective, randomized, multicenter, pragmatic trial: POEMAS study (PeriOperative goal-directed thErapy in Major Abdominal Surgery). *Anesth Analg.* 2014;119:579–587.
110. Abuleo G. Normotensive ischemic acute renal failure. *N Engl J Med.* 2007;357:797–805.
111. Jones A, Shapiro NI, Trzeciak S, et al. Lactate clearance vs central venous oxygen saturation as goals of early sepsis therapy: a randomized clinical trial. *JAMA.* 2010;303:739–746.
112. Jansen T, van Bommel J, Schoonderbeek FJ, et al. Early lactate-guided therapy in intensive care unit patients: a multicenter, open-label randomized controlled trial. *Am J Respir Crit Care Med.* 2010;182:752–761.
113. Reinhart K, Kuhn HJ, Hartog C, et al. Continuous central venous and pulmonary artery oxygen saturation monitoring in the critically ill. *Intensive Care Med.* 2004;30:1572–1578.
114. Reinhart K, Bloos F. The value of venous oximetry. *Curr Opin Crit Care.* 2005;11:259–263.
115. Chawla L, Zia H, Guttierrez G, et al. Lack of equivalence between central and mixed venous oxygen saturation. *Chest.* 2004;126:1891–1896.
116. Yazigi A, El-Khoury C, Jebara S, et al. Comparison of central venous to mixed venous oxygen saturation in patients with low cardiac index and filling pressures after coronary artery surgery. *J Cardiothorac Vasc Anesth.* 2008;22:77–83.

117. Pope J, Jones AE, Gaieski DF. Multicenter study of central venous oxygen saturation (ScvO2) as a predictor of mortality in patients with sepsis. *Ann Emerg Med.* 2010;55:40–46.
118. Murphy C, Schramm GE, Doherty JA. The importance of fluid management in acute lung injury secondary to septic shock. *Chest.* 2009;136:102–109.
119. Feihl F, Perret C. Permissive hypercapnia. How permissive should we be? *Am J Respir Crit Care Med.* 1994;150(6 Pt 1):1722–1737.
120. Moloney ED, Griffiths MJ. Protective ventilation of patients with acute respiratory distress syndrome. *Br J Anaesth.* 2004;92(2):261–270.
121. Determann RM, Royakkers A, Wolthuis EK, et al. Ventilation with lower tidal volumes as compared with conventional tidal volumes for patients without acute lung injury: a preventive randomized controlled trial. *Crit Care.* 2010;14(1):R1.
122. Gajic O, Frutos-Vivar F, Esteban A, et al. Ventilator settings as a risk factor for acute respiratory distress syndrome in mechanically ventilated patients. *Intensive Care Med.* 2005;31(7):922–926.
123. Nava S, Carbone G, DiBattista N, et al. Noninvasive ventilation in cardiogenic pulmonary edema: a multicenter randomized trial. *Am J Respir Crit Care Med.* 2003;168(12):1432–1437.
124. The American Thoracic Society, the European Respiratory Society, the European Society of Intensive Care Medicine, and the Société de Réanimation de Langue Française (approved by ATS Board of Directors, December 2000). International Consensus Conferences in Intensive Care Medicine: noninvasive positive pressure ventilation in acute Respiratory failure. *Am J Respir Crit Care Med.* 2001;163(1):283–291.
125. Esteban A, Frutos-Vivar F, Ferguson ND, et al. Noninvasive positive-pressure ventilation for respiratory failure after extubation. *N Engl J Med.* 2004;350(24):2452–2460.
126. Mehta S, Jay GD, Woolard RH, et al. Randomized, prospective trial of bilevel versus continuous positive airway pressure in acute pulmonary edema. *Crit Care Med.* 1997;25(4):620–628.
127. Frat JP, Thille AW, Mercat A, et al. High-flow oxygen through nasal cannula in acute hypoxemic respiratory failure. *N Engl J Med.* 2015;372(23):2185–2196.
128. Stephan F, Barrucand B, Petit P, et al. High-flow nasal oxygen vs noninvasive positive airway pressure in hypoxemic patients after cardiothoracic surgery: a randomized clinical trial. *JAMA.* 2015;313(23):2331–2339.
129. Esteban A, Frutos F, Tobin MJ, et al. A comparison of four methods of weaning patients from mechanical ventilation. Spanish Lung Failure Collaborative Group. *N Engl J Med.* 1995;332(6):345–350.
130. MacIntyre NR, Cook DJ, Ely EW Jr., et al. Evidence-based guidelines for weaning and discontinuing ventilatory support: a collective task force facilitated by the American College of Chest Physicians; the American Association for Respiratory Care; and the American College of Critical Care Medicine. *Chest.* 2001;120(6 Suppl):375S–395S.
131. Schuster DP. What is acute lung injury? What is ARDS? *Chest.* 1995;107 (6):1721–1726.
132. Bernard GR, Artigas A, Brigham KL, et al. Report of the American-European consensus conference on ARDS: definitions, mechanisms, relevant outcomes and clinical trial coordination. The Consensus Committee. *Intensive Care Med.* 1994;20(3):225–232.
133. Force ADT, Ranieri VM, Rubenfeld GD, et al. Acute respiratory distress syndrome: the Berlin Definition. *JAMA.* 2012;307(23):2526–2533.
134. Erickson SE, Martin GS, Davis JL, et al. Recent trends in acute lung injury mortality: 1996–2005. *Crit Care Med.* 2009;37(5):1574–1579.
135. Phua J, Badia JR, Adhikari NK, et al. Has mortality from acute respiratory distress syndrome decreased over time?: A systematic review. *Am J Respir Crit Care Med.* 2009;179(3):220–227.
136. Nuckton TJ, Alonso JA, Kallet RH, et al. Pulmonary dead-space fraction as a risk factor for death in the acute respiratory distress syndrome. *N Engl J Med.* 2002;346(17):1281–1286.
137. Ventilation with lower tidal volumes as compared with traditional tidal volumes for acute lung injury and the acute respiratory distress syndrome. The Acute Respiratory Distress Syndrome Network. *N Engl J Med.* 2000; 342(18):1301–1308.
138. Villar J, Kacmarek RM, Perez-Mendez L, et al. A high positive end-expiratory pressure, low tidal volume ventilatory strategy improves outcome in persistent acute respiratory distress syndrome: a randomized, controlled trial. *Crit Care Med.* 2006;34(5):1311–1318.
139. Santa Cruz R, Rojas JI, Nervi R, et al. High versus low positive end-expiratory pressure (PEEP) levels for mechanically ventilated adult patients with acute lung injury and acute respiratory distress syndrome. *Cochrane Database Syst Rev.* 2013;6:CD009098.
140. Sud S, Friedrich JO, Taccone P, et al. Prone ventilation reduces mortality in patients with acute respiratory failure and severe hypoxemia: systematic review and meta-analysis. *Intensive Care Med.* 2010;36(4):585–599.
141. Guerin C, Reignier J, Richard JC, et al. Prone positioning in severe acute respiratory distress syndrome. *N Engl J Med.* 2013;368(23):2159–2168.
142. Maitra S, Bhattacharjee S, Khanna P, et al. High-frequency ventilation does not provide mortality benefit in comparison with conventional lung-protective ventilation in acute respiratory distress syndrome: a meta-analysis of the randomized controlled trials. *Anesthesiology.* 2015;122(4):841–851.
143. Taylor RW, Zimmerman JL, Dellinger RP, et al. Low-dose inhaled nitric oxide in patients with acute lung injury: a randomized controlled trial. *JAMA.* 2004;291(13):1603–1609.
144. Sokol J, Jacobs SE, Bohn D. Inhaled nitric oxide for acute hypoxic respiratory failure in children and adults: a meta-analysis. *Anesth Analg.* 2003;97(4):989–998.
145. Wiedemann HP, Wheeler AP, Bernard GR, et al. Comparison of two fluid-management strategies in acute lung injury. *N Engl J Med.* 2006;354(24):2564–2575.
146. Martin GS, Moss M, Wheeler AP, et al. A randomized, controlled trial of furosemide with or without albumin in hypoproteinemic patients with acute lung injury. *Crit Care Med.* 2005;33(8):1681–1687.
147. Matthay MA, Brower RG, Carson S, et al. Randomized, placebo-controlled clinical trial of an aerosolized beta-agonist for treatment of acute lung injury. *Am J Respir Crit Care Med.* 2011;184(5):561–568.
148. Meduri GU, Headley AS, Golden E, et al. Effect of prolonged methylprednisolone therapy in unresolving acute respiratory distress syndrome: a randomized controlled trial. *JAMA.* 1998;280(2):159–165.
149. Meduri GU, Golden E, Freire AX, et al. Methylprednisolone infusion in early severe ARDS: results of a randomized controlled trial. *Chest.* 2007; 131(4):954–963.
150. Steinberg KP, Hudson LD, Goodman RB, et al. Efficacy and safety of corticosteroids for persistent acute respiratory distress syndrome. *N Engl J Med.* 2006;354(16):1671–1684.
151. Papazian L, Forel JM, Gacouin A, et al. Neuromuscular blockers in early acute respiratory distress syndrome. *N Engl J Med.* 2010;363:1107–1116.
152. Fanelli V, Morita Y, Cappello P, et al. neuromuscular blocking agent cisatracurium attenuates lung injury by inhibition of nicotinic acetylcholine receptor-alpha-1. *Anesthesiology.* 2016;124(1):132–140.
153. Noah MA, Peek GJ, Finney SJ, et al. Referral to an extracorporeal membrane oxygenation center and mortality among patients with severe 2009 influenza A(H1N1). *JAMA.* 2011;306(15):1659–1668.
154. Peek GJ, Elbourne D, Mugford M, et al. Randomised controlled trial and parallel economic evaluation of conventional ventilatory support versus extracorporeal membrane oxygenation for severe adult respiratory failure (CESAR). *Health Technol Assess.* 2010;14(35):1–46.
155. Hoste EA, De Corte W. Implementing the kidney disease: improving global outcomes/acute kidney injury guidelines in ICU patients. *Curr Opin Crit Care.* 2013;19(6):544–553.
156. Bellomo R, Ronco C, Kellum JA, et al. Acute renal failure: definition, outcome measures, animal models, fluid therapy and information technology needs: the Second International Consensus Conference of the Acute Dialysis Quality Initiative (ADQI) Group. *Crit Care.* 2004;8(4):R204–212.
157. Kellum JA, Lameire N, Group KAGW. Diagnosis, evaluation, and management of acute kidney injury: a KDIGO summary (Part 1). *Crit Care.* 2013;17(1):204.
158. Mehta RL, Kellum JA, Shah SV, et al. Acute Kidney Injury Network: report of an initiative to improve outcomes in acute kidney injury. *Crit Care.* 2007;11(2):R31.
159. Singri N, Ahya SN, Levin ML. Acute renal failure. *JAMA.* 2003;289(6):747–751.
160. The RENAL Replacement Therapy Study Investigators. Intensity of continuous renal-replacement therapy in critically ill patients. *N Engl J Med.* 2009;361(17):1627–1638.
161. Palevsky PM. Indications and timing of renal replacement therapy in acute kidney injury. *Crit Care Med.* 2008;36(4 Suppl):S224–228.
162. Vinsonneau C, Camus C, Combes A, et al. Continuous venovenous haemodiafiltration versus intermittent haemodialysis for acute renal failure in patients with multiple-organ dysfunction syndrome: a multicentre randomised trial. *Lancet.* 2006;368(9533):379–385.
163. McCowen KC, Malhotra A, Bistrian BR. Stress-induced hyperglycemia. *Crit Care Clin.* 2001;17(1):107–124.
164. Malmberg K, Norhammar A, Wedel H, et al. Glycometabolic state at admission: important risk marker of mortality in conventionally treated patients with diabetes mellitus and acute myocardial infarction: long-term results from the Diabetes and Insulin-Glucose Infusion in Acute Myocardial Infarction (DIGAMI) study. *Circulation.* 1999;99(20):2626–2632.
165. van den Berghe G, Wouters P, Weekers F, et al. Intensive insulin therapy in critically ill patients. *N Engl J Med.* 2001;345(19):1359–1367.
166. Wiener RS, Wiener DC, Larson RJ. Benefits and risks of tight glucose control in critically ill adults: a meta-analysis. *JAMA.* 2008;300(8):933–944.
167. Investigators N-SS, Finfer S, Chittock DR, Su SY, et al. Intensive versus conventional glucose control in critically ill patients. *N Engl J Med.* 2009;360(13):1283–1297.
168. Van den Berghe G, de Zegher F, Bouillon R. Clinical review 95: acute and prolonged critical illness as different neuroendocrine paradigms. *J Clin Endocrinol Metab.* 1998;83(6):1827–1834.
169. Cooper MS, Stewart PM. Corticosteroid insufficiency in acutely ill patients. *N Engl J Med.* 2003;348(8):727–734.
170. Hamrahian AH, Oseni TS, Arafah BM. Measurements of serum free cortisol in critically ill patients. *N Engl J Med.* 2004;350(16):1629–1638.
171. Annane D, Bellissant E, Bollaert PE, et al. Corticosteroids for treating sepsis. *Cochrane Database Syst Rev.* 2015;12:CD002243.

172. Van den Berghe G, de Zegher F, Lauwers P. Dopamine and the sick euthyroid syndrome in critical illness. *Clin Endocrinol (Oxf)*. 1994;41(6):731–737.
173. Bennett-Guerrero E, Jimenez JL, White WD, et al. Cardiovascular effects of intravenous triiodothyronine in patients undergoing coronary artery bypass graft surgery. A randomized, double-blind, placebo-controlled trial. Duke T3 study group. *JAMA*. 1996;275(9):687–692.
174. Takala J, Ruokonen E, Webster NR, et al. Increased mortality associated with growth hormone treatment in critically ill adults. *N Engl J Med*. 1999;341(11):785–792.
175. Napolitano LM, Kurek S, Luchette FA, et al. Clinical practice guideline: red blood cell transfusion in adult trauma and critical care. *Critical Care Medicine*. 2009;37(12):3124–3157.
176. Vincent JL, Baron JF, Reinhart K, et al. Anemia and blood transfusion in critically ill patients. *JAMA*. 2002;288(12):1499–1507.
177. Corwin HL, Gettinger A, Pearl RG, et al. The CRIT Study: Anemia and blood transfusion in the critically ill—current clinical practice in the United States. *Crit Care Med*. 2004;32(1):39–52.
178. Rodriguez RM, Corwin HL, Gettinger A, et al. Nutritional deficiencies and blunted erythropoietin response as causes of the anemia of critical illness. *J Crit Care*. 2001;16(1):36–41.
179. Hebert PC, Wells G, Blajchman MA, et al. A multicenter, randomized, controlled clinical trial of transfusion requirements in critical care. Transfusion Requirements in Critical Care Investigators, Canadian Critical Care Trials Group. *N Engl J Med*. 1999;340(6):409–417.
180. Lacroix J, Hebert PC, Hutchison JS, et al. Transfusion strategies for patients in pediatric intensive care units. *N Engl J Med*. 2007;356(16):1609–1619.
181. Robertson CS, Hannay HJ, Yamal JM, et al. Effect of erythropoietin and transfusion threshold on neurological recovery after traumatic brain injury: a randomized clinical trial. *JAMA*. 2014;312(1):36–47.
182. Villanueva C, Colomo A, Bosch A, et al. Transfusion strategies for acute upper gastrointestinal bleeding. *N Engl J Med*. 2013;368(1):11–21.
183. Pro CI, Yealy DM, Kellum JA, et al. A randomized trial of protocol-based care for early septic shock. *N Engl J Med*. 2014;370(18):1683–1693.
184. Corwin HL, Gettinger A, Pearl RG, et al. Efficacy of recombinant human erythropoietin in critically ill patients: a randomized controlled trial. *JAMA*. 2002;288(22):2827–2835.
185. Corwin HL, Gettinger A, Fabian TC, et al. Efficacy and safety of epoetin alfa in critically ill patients. *N Engl J Med*. 2007;357(10):965–976.
186. Arabi YM, Aldawood AS, Haddad SH, et al. Permissive underfeeding or standard enteral feeding in critically ill adults. *N Engl J Med*. 2015;372(25):2398–2408.
187. Marik PE, Hooper MH. Normocaloric versus hypocaloric feeding on the outcomes of ICU patients: a systematic review and meta-analysis. *Intensive Care Med*. 2016;42(3):316–323.
188. McClave SA, Martindale RG, Vanek VW, et al. Guidelines for the Provision and Assessment of Nutrition Support Therapy in the Adult Critically Ill Patient: Society of Critical Care Medicine (SCCM) and American Society for Parenteral and Enteral Nutrition (A.S.P.E.N.). *J Parenter Enteral Nutr*. 2009;33(3):277–316.
189. Marik PE, Zaloga GP. Gastric versus post-pyloric feeding: a systematic review. *Crit Care*. 2003;7(3):R46–51.
190. MacLeod JB, Lefton J, Houghton D, et al. Prospective randomized control trial of intermittent versus continuous gastric feeds for critically ill trauma patients. *J Trauma*. 2007;63(1):57–61.
191. Zaloga GP. Parenteral nutrition in adult inpatients with functioning gastrointestinal tracts: assessment of outcomes. *Lancet*. 2006;367(9516):1101–1111.
192. Singer P, Berger MM, Van den Berghe G, et al. ESPEN Guidelines on Parenteral Nutrition: intensive care. *Clin Nutr*. 2009;28(4):387–400.
193. Casaer MP, Mesotten D, Hermans G, et al. Early versus late parenteral nutrition in critically ill adults. *N Engl J Med*. 2011;365(6):506–517.
194. Chen QH, Yang Y, He HL, et al. The effect of glutamine therapy on outcomes in critically ill patients: a meta-analysis of randomized controlled trials. *Crit Care*. 2014;18(1):R8.
195. Rice TW, Wheeler AP, Thompson BT, et al. Enteral omega-3 fatty acid, gamma-linolenic acid, and antioxidant supplementation in acute lung injury. *JAMA*. 2011;306(14):1574–1581.
196. Stapleton RD, Martin TR, Weiss NS, et al. A phase II randomized placebo-controlled trial of omega-3 fatty acids for the treatment of acute lung injury. *Crit Care Med*. 2011;39(7):1655–1662.
197. Visser J, Labadarios D, Blaauw R. Micronutrient supplementation for critically ill adults: a systematic review and meta-analysis. *Nutrition*. 2011;27(7–8):745–758.
198. Ely E, Truman B, Shintani A, et al. Monitoring sedation status over time in ICU patients: reliability and validity of the Richmond Agitation-Sedation Scale (RASS). *JAMA*. 2003;289:2983–2991.
199. Barr J, Fraser GL, Puntillo K, et al. Clinical guidelines for the management of pain, agitation, and delirium in adult patients in the intensive care unit. *Crit Care Med*. 2013;41:263–306.
200. Tufangullari B, White PF, Peixoto MP, et al. Dexmedetomidine infusion during laparoscopic bariatric surgery: the effect on recovery outcome variables. *Anesth Analg*. 2008;106:1741–1748.
201. Feld JM, Hoffman WE, Stechert MM, et al. Fentanyl or dexmedetomidine combined with desflurane for bariatric surgery. *J Clin Anesth*. 2006;18:24–28.
202. VanderWeide L, Foster CJ, MacLaren R, et al. Evaluation of early dexmedetomidine addition to the standard of care for severe alcohol withdrawal in the ICU: a retrospective controlled cohort study. *J Intensive Care Med*. 2014:1–7.
203. Mueller S, Preslaski CR, Kiser TH, et al. A randomized, double-blind, placebo-controlled dose range study of dexmedetomidine as adjunctive therapy for alcohol withdrawal. *Crit Care Med*. 2014;42:1131–1139.
204. Jakob S, Ruokonen E, Grounds RM, et al. Dexmedetomidine vs midazolam or propofol for sedation during prolonged mechanical ventilation: two randomized controlled trials. *JAMA*. 2012;307:1151–1160.
205. Walder B, Elia N, Henzi I, et al. A lack of evidence of superiority of propofol versus midazolam for sedation in mechanically ventilated critically ill patients: a qualitative and quantitative systematic review. *Anesth Analg*. 2001;92:975–983.
206. Carson S, Kress JP, Rodgers JE, et al. A randomized trial of intermittent lorazepam versus propofol with daily interruption in mechanically ventilated patients. *Crit Care Med*. 2006;34:1326–1332.
207. Annane D. What is the evidence for harm of neuromuscular blockade and corticosteroid use in the intensive care unit? *Semin Respir Crit Care Med*. 2016;37:51–56.
208. Lipshutz A, Gropper MA. Intensive care unit-acquired muscle weakness: an ounce of prevention is worth a pound of cure. *Anesthesiology*. 2016;124:7–9.
209. Ely E, Inouye SK, Bernard GR, et al. Delirium in mechanically ventilated patients: Validity and reliability of the confusion assessment method for the intensive care unit (CAM-ICU). *JAMA*. 2001;286:2703–2710.
210. Bergeron N, Dubois MJ, Durmont M, et al. Intensive Care Delirium Screening Checklist: Evaluation of a new screening tool. *Intensive Care Med*. 2001;27:859–864.
211. Pandharipande P, Pun BT, Herr DL, et al. Effect of sedation with dexmedetomidine vs lorazepam on acute brain dysfunction in mechanically ventilated patients: The MENDS randomized controlled trial. *JAMA*. 2007;298:2644–2653.
212. Riker R, Shehabi Y, Bokesch PM, et al. Dexmedetomidine vs midazolam for sedation of critically ill patients: a randomized trial. *JAMA*. 2009;301:489–499.
213. Kollef M, Levy NT, Ahrens TS, et al. The use of continuous i.v. sedation is associated with prolongation of mechanical ventilation. *Chest*. 1998;114:541–548.
214. Brook A, Ahrens TS, Schaiff R, et al. Effect of a nursing-implemented sedation protocol on the duration of mechanical ventilation. *Crit Care Med*. 1999;27:2609–2615.
215. Kress J, Pohlman AS, O'Connor MF, et al. Daily interruption of sedative infusions in critically ill patients undergoing mechanical ventilation. *N Engl J Med*. 2000;342:1471–1477.
216. Girard TD, Kress JP, Fuchs BD, et al. Efficacy and safety of a paired sedation and ventilator weaning protocol for mechanically ventilated patients in intensive care (Awakening and Breathing Controlled trial): A randomised controlled trial. *Lancet*. 2008;371:126–134.
217. Treggiari M, Romand JA, Yanez ND, et al. Randomized trial of light versus deep sedation on mental health after critical illness. *Crit Care Med*. 2009;37:2527–2534.
218. Tanaka L, Azevedo LC, Park M, et al. Early sedation and clinical outcomes of mechanically ventilated patients: a prospective multicenter cohort study. *Crit Care*. 2014;18:R156.
219. Strom T, Martinussen T, Toft P. A protocol of no sedation for critically ill patients receiving mechanical ventilation: A randomised trial. *Lancet*. 2010;375:475–480.
220. Shehabi Y, Bellomo R, Reade MC, et al. Early intensive care sedation predicts long-term mortality in ventilated critically ill patients. *Am J Respir Crit Care Med*. 2012;186:724–731.
221. Laerkner E, Strom T, Toft P. No-sedation during mechanical ventilation: impact on patient's consciousness, nursing workload and costs. *Nurs Crit Care*. 2015;21:28–35.
222. Devlin J, Roberts RJ, Fong JJ, et al. Efficacy and safety of quetiapine in critically ill patients with delirium: A prospective, multicenter, randomized, double-blind, placebo-controlled pilot study. *Crit Care Med*. 2010;38:419–427.
223. Pisani M, Araujo KL, Murphy TE. Association of cumulative dose of haloperidol with next-day delirium in older medical ICU patients. *Crit Care Med*. 2015;43:996–1002.
224. Al-Qadheeb N, Skrobik Y, Schumaker G, et al. Preventing ICU subsyndromal delirium conversion to delirium with low-dose IV haloperidol: a double-blind, placebo-controlled pilot study. *Crit Care Med*. 2015:1–7.
225. Serafim R, Bozza FA, Soares M, et al. Pharmacologic prevention and treatment of delirium in intensive care patients: A systematic review. *J Crit Care*. 2015;30:799–807.
226. Samuelson K, Lundberg D, Fridlund B. Memory in relation to depth of sedation in adult mechanically ventilated intensive care patients. *Intensive Care Med*. 2004;32:660–667.
227. Girard T, Shintani, AK, Jackson, JC, et al. Risk factors for post-traumatic stress disorder symptoms following critical illness requiring mechanical ventilation: a prospective cohort study. *Crit Care*. 2007;11:28.

228. Pandharipande P, Girard TD, Jackson JC, et al. Long-term cognitive impairment after critical illness. *N Engl J Med.* 2013;369:1306–1316.
229. Jackson J, Girard TD, Gordon SM, et al. Long-term cognitive and psychological outcomes in the awakening and breathing controlled trial. *Am J Respir Crit Care Med.* 2010;182:183–191.
230. Kress J, Gehlbach B, Lacy M, et al. The long-term psychological effects of daily sedative interruption on critically ill patients. *Am J Respir Crit Care Med.* 2003;168:1457–1461.
231. Vincent JL. Nosocomial infections in adult intensive-care units. *Lancet.* 2003;361(9374):2068–2077.
232. Rouby JJ, Laurent P, Gosnach M, et al. Risk factors and clinical relevance of nosocomial maxillary sinusitis in the critically ill. *Am J Respir Crit Care Med.* 1994;150(3):776–783.
233. van Zanten AR, Dixon JM, Nipshagen MD, et al. Hospital-acquired sinusitis is a common cause of fever of unknown origin in orotracheally intubated critically ill patients. *Crit Care.* 2005;9(5):R583–R590.
234. Magill SS, Klompas M, Balk R, et al. Developing a new, national approach to surveillance for ventilator-associated events. *Crit Care Med.* 2013;41(11):2467–2475.
235. Klein Klouwenberg PM, van Mourik MS, Ong DS, et al. Electronic implementation of a novel surveillance paradigm for ventilator-associated events. Feasibility and validation. *Am J Respir Crit Care Med.* 2014;189(8):947–955.
236. Klompas M, Kleinman K, Murphy MV. Descriptive epidemiology and attributable morbidity of ventilator-associated events. *Infect Control Hosp Epidemiol.* 2014;35(5):502–510.
237. Klompas M, Anderson D, Trick W, et al. The preventability of ventilator-associated events. The CDC Prevention Epicenters Wake Up and Breathe Collaborative. *Am J Respir Crit Care Med.* 2015;191(3):292–301.
238. Cook DJ, Walter SD, Cook RJ, et al. Incidence of and risk factors for ventilator-associated pneumonia in critically ill patients. *Ann Intern Med.* 1998;129(6):433–440.
239. Bekaert M, Timsit JF, Vansteelandt S, et al. Attributable mortality of ventilator-associated pneumonia: a reappraisal using causal analysis. *Am J Respir Crit Care Med.* 2011;184(10):1133–1139.
240. Hoffken G, Niederman MS. Nosocomial pneumonia: the importance of a de-escalating strategy for antibiotic treatment of pneumonia in the ICU. *Chest.* 2002;122(6):2183–2196.
241. Muscedere J, Rewa O, McKechnie K, et al. Subglottic secretion drainage for the prevention of ventilator-associated pneumonia: a systematic review and meta-analysis. *Crit Care Med.* 2011;39(8):1985–1991.
242. Tokmaji G, Vermeulen H, Muller MC, et al. Silver-coated endotracheal tubes for prevention of ventilator-associated pneumonia in critically ill patients. *Cochrane Database Syst Rev.* 2015;8:CD009201.
243. Price R, MacLennan G, Glen J, et al. Selective digestive or oropharyngeal decontamination and topical oropharyngeal chlorhexidine for prevention of death in general intensive care: systematic review and network meta-analysis. *BMJ.* 2014;348:g2197.
244. Klompas M, Speck K, Howell MD, et al. Reappraisal of routine oral care with chlorhexidine gluconate for patients receiving mechanical ventilation: systematic review and meta-analysis. *JAMA Intern Med.* 2014;174(5):751–761.
245. American Thoracic Society and Infectious Diseases Society of America. Guidelines for the management of adults with hospital-acquired, ventilator-associated, and healthcare-associated pneumonia. *Am J Respir Crit Care Med.* 2005;171(4):388–416.
246. Scholte JB, van Dessel HA, Linssen CF, et al. Endotracheal aspirate and bronchoalveolar lavage fluid analysis: interchangeable diagnostic modalities in suspected ventilator-associated pneumonia? *J Clin Microbiol.* 2014;52(10):3597–3604.
247. Wood AY, Davit AJ 2nd, Ciraulo DL, et al. A prospective assessment of diagnostic efficacy of blind protective bronchial brushings compared to bronchoscope-assisted lavage, bronchoscope-directed brushings, and blind endotracheal aspirates in ventilator-associated pneumonia. *J Trauma.* 2003;55(5):825–834.
248. Pugh R, Grant C, Cooke RP, et al. Short-course versus prolonged-course antibiotic therapy for hospital-acquired pneumonia in critically ill adults. *Cochrane Database Syst Rev.* 2015;8:CD007577.
249. Berenholtz SM, Pronovost PJ, Lipsett PA, et al. Eliminating catheter-related bloodstream infections in the intensive care unit. *Crit Care Med.* 2004;32(10):2014–2020.
250. Kim JS, Holtom P, Vigen C. Reduction of catheter-related bloodstream infections through the use of a central venous line bundle: epidemiologic and economic consequences. *Am J Infect Control.* 2011;39(8):640–646.
251. O'Grady NP, Alexander M, Burns LA, et al. Guidelines for the prevention of intravascular catheter-related infections. *Clin Infect Dis.* 2011;52(9):e162–193.
252. Lai NM, Chaiyakunapruk N, Lai NA, et al. Catheter impregnation, coating or bonding for reducing central venous catheter-related infections in adults. *Cochrane Database Syst Rev.* 2013;6:CD007878.
253. Marik PE, Flemmer M, Harrison W. The risk of catheter-related bloodstream infection with femoral venous catheters as compared to subclavian and internal jugular venous catheters: a systematic review of the literature and meta-analysis. *Crit Care Med.* 2012;40(8):2479–2485.
254. Ringberg H, Thoren A, Bredberg A. Evaluation of coagulase-negative staphylococci in blood cultures. A prospective clinical and microbiological study. *Scand J Infect Dis.* 1991;23(3):315–323.
255. Tenke P, Koves B, Johansen TE. An update on prevention and treatment of catheter-associated urinary tract infections. *Curr Opin Infect Dis.* 2014;27(1):102–107.
256. McCarty TP, Pappas PG. Invasive candidiasis. *Infect Dis Clin North Am.* 2016;30(1):103–124.
257. Koehler P, Cornely OA. Contemporary strategies in the prevention and management of fungal infections. *Infect Dis Clin North Am.* 2016;30(1):265–275.
258. Pappas PG, Kauffman CA, Andes DR, et al. Clinical practice guideline for the management of candidiasis: 2016 update by the infectious diseases society of america. *Clin Infect Dis.* 2016;62(4):e1–e50.
259. Cook DJ, Fuller HD, Guyatt GH, et al. Risk factors for gastrointestinal bleeding in critically ill patients. Canadian Critical Care Trials Group. *N Engl J Med.* 1994;330(6):377–381.
260. Cook D, Heyland D, Griffith L, et al. Risk factors for clinically important upper gastrointestinal bleeding in patients requiring mechanical ventilation. Canadian Critical Care Trials Group. *Crit Care Med.* 1999;27(12):2812–2817.
261. Marik PE, Vasu T, Hirani A, et al. Stress ulcer prophylaxis in the new millennium: a systematic review and meta-analysis. *Crit Care Med.* 2010;38(11):2222–2228.
262. Krag M, Perner A, Wetterslev J, et al. Stress ulcer prophylaxis versus placebo or no prophylaxis in critically ill patients. A systematic review of randomised clinical trials with meta-analysis and trial sequential analysis. *Intensive Care Med.* 2014;40(1):11–22.
263. Buendgens L, Bruensing J, Matthes M, et al. Administration of proton pump inhibitors in critically ill medical patients is associated with increased risk of developing Clostridium difficile-associated diarrhea. *J Critical Care.* 2014;29(4):696e11–696e15.
264. Geerts W, Selby R. Prevention of venous thromboembolism in the ICU. *Chest.* 2003;124(6 Suppl):357S–363S.
265. Pollak AW, McBane RD 2nd. Succinct review of the new VTE prevention and management guidelines. *Mayo Clin Proc.* 2014;89(3):394–408.
266. Joffe HV, Goldhaber SZ. Upper-extremity deep vein thrombosis. *Circulation.* 2002;106(14):1874–1880.
267. Holbrook A, Schulman S, Witt DM, et al. Evidence-based management of anticoagulant therapy: Antithrombotic Therapy and Prevention of Thrombosis, 9th ed: American College of Chest Physicians Evidence-Based Clinical Practice Guidelines. *Chest.* 2012;141(2 Suppl):e152S–184S.
268. Kearon C, Ginsberg JS, Hirsh J. The role of venous ultrasonography in the diagnosis of suspected deep venous thrombosis and pulmonary embolism. *Ann Intern Med.* 1998;129(12):1044–1049.
269. Anderson DR, Kahn SR, Rodger MA, et al. Computed tomographic pulmonary angiography vs ventilation-perfusion lung scanning in patients with suspected pulmonary embolism: a randomized controlled trial. *JAMA.* 2007;298(23):2743–2753.
270. Deem S. Intensive-care-unit-acquired muscle weakness. *Respir Care.* 2006;51(9):1042–1052; discussion 1052–1043.
271. Hermans G, Van den Berghe G. Clinical review: intensive care unit acquired weakness. *Crit Care.* 2015;19:274.
272. Puthucheary Z, Rawal J, Ratnayake G, et al. Neuromuscular blockade and skeletal muscle weakness in critically ill patients: time to rethink the evidence? *Am J Respir Crit Care Med.* 2012;185(9):911–917.
273. Farhan H, Moreno-Duarte I, Latronico N, et al. Acquired muscle weakness in the surgical intensive care unit: nosology, epidemiology, diagnosis, and prevention. *Anesthesiology.* 2016;124(1):207–234.
274. Hermans G, De Jonghe B, Bruyninckx F, et al. Interventions for preventing critical illness polyneuropathy and critical illness myopathy. *Cochrane Database Syst Rev.* 2014;1:CD006832.
275. Angus DC, Barnato AE, Linde-Zwirble WT, et al. Use of intensive care at the end of life in the United States: an epidemiologic study. *Crit Care Med.* 2004;32(3):638–643.
276. Issues CoADAKE-o-L. Dying in America: Improving Quality and Honoring Individual Preferences Near the End of Life. 2014. Available from: http://www.nap.edu/read/18748/chapter/1.
277. Renaud B, Brun-Buisson C. Outcomes of primary and catheter-related bacteremia. A cohort and case-control study in critically ill patients. *Am J Respir Crit Care Med.* 2001;163:1584–1590.

58 Cardiopulmonary Resuscitation

CHARLES W. OTTO

History
Scope of the Problem
Ethical Issues: Do Not Resuscitate Orders in the Operating Room
Components of Resuscitation
Airway Management
  Foreign Body Airway Obstruction
Ventilation
  Physiology of Ventilation during Cardiopulmonary Resuscitation
  Techniques of Rescue Breathing
Circulation
  Physiology of Circulation during Closed-chest Compression
  Technique of Closed-chest Compression
  Alternative Methods of Circulatory Support
  Assessing the Adequacy of Circulation during Cardiopulmonary Resuscitation

Pharmacologic Therapy
  Routes of Administration
  Catecholamines and Vasopressors
  Amiodarone and Lidocaine
  Drugs Not Routinely Given during CPR
Electrical Therapy
  Electrical Pattern and Duration of Ventricular Fibrillation
  Defibrillators: Energy, Current, and Voltage
  Transthoracic Impedance
  Adverse Effects and Energy Requirements
Putting It All Together
  Time-sensitive Model of Ventricular Fibrillation
  Bystander CPR and Basic Life Support
  Advanced Life Support
  Rhythm Analysis and Defibrillation
Pediatric Cardiopulmonary Resuscitation
Postresuscitation Care
  Prognosis

KEY POINTS

1. Brain adenosine triphosphate is depleted after 4 to 6 minutes of no blood flow. It returns nearly to normal within 6 minutes of starting effective cardiopulmonary resuscitation (CPR).
2. Through living wills and other instruments, patients have begun placing limitations on medical treatment to include do not resuscitate orders, even while undergoing palliative surgical procedures.
3. The major components of resuscitation from cardiac arrest are airway, breathing, circulation, drugs, and electrical therapy (ABCDE).
4. Two theories for the mechanism of blood flow during closed-chest compression have been suggested: cardiac pump and thoracic pump.
5. During CPR, myocardial perfusion is 20% to 50% of normal, whereas cerebral perfusion is maintained at 50% to 90% of normal.
6. CPR has limited success, with only approximately 40% of victims being admitted to the hospital and 10% surviving to discharge.
7. End-tidal carbon dioxide has been found to be an excellent noninvasive guide to the adequacy of closed-chest compressions.
8. Effective uninterrupted chest compressions and defibrillation, if appropriate, should take precedence over medications.
9. Although there is some evidence of improved early restoration of spontaneous circulation in humans, there is no strong evidence that vasopressors improve long-term survival in human cardiac arrest.
10. After vasopressors, the drugs most likely to be of benefit during CPR are those that help suppress ectopic ventricular rhythms.
11. Ventricular fibrillation is the most common electrocardiogram pattern found during witnessed sudden cardiac arrest in adults.
12. Untreated ventricular fibrillation is a time-sensitive model with three phases: electrical, circulatory, and metabolic.
13. Arrest is less likely to be a sudden event and more likely related to progressive deterioration of respiratory and circulatory function in the pediatric age group.
14. For optimal outcome, successful restoration of spontaneous circulation must be followed by correction of reversible causes of arrest, including immediate coronary reperfusion and aggressive supportive care.

The current guidelines for cardiopulmonary resuscitation (2015 International Consensus on Cardiopulmonary Resuscitation and Emergency Cardiovascular Care Science with Treatment Recommendations) are an update to the 2010 guidelines (2010 American Heart Association [AHA] Guidelines for Cardiopulmonary Resuscitation and Emergency Cardiovascular Care) rather than a complete revision.[29,149] Thus, a number of figures remain the same between both editions. To assist the reader, the AHA has published web-based integrated guidelines, which are available at https://eccguidelines.heart.org/index.php/circulation/cpr-ecc-guidelines-2. In addition, the AHA limits the number of algorithms that can be reproduced outside their publications. Thus, we have included URLs to help you quickly locate algorithms online that were not able to be included within the chapter.

Treatment of cardiac and respiratory arrest is an integral part of anesthesia practice. The American Board of Anesthesiology states in its *Booklet of Information* that the "clinical management and teaching of cardiac, pulmonary, and neurologic resuscitation" are among the activities that define the specialty of anesthesiology. The cardiopulmonary physiology and pharmacology that form the basis of anesthesia practice are applicable to treating the victim of cardiac arrest. However, there is specialized knowledge relating to blood flow, ventilation, and pharmacology under the conditions of a cardiac arrest that must be understood to maintain leadership of the modern cardiopulmonary resuscitation (CPR) team. This chapter concentrates on those aspects of CPR that are different from the more common circumstances requiring cardiovascular support (e.g., shock, dysrhythmias).

History

Anesthesiologists have contributed many of the elements of modern CPR and continue to be active investigators and teachers in the field. Discoveries leading to current CPR practice have a long history recorded in many famous works.[1,2] The earliest reference may be the Bible story of Elisha breathing life back into the son of a Shunammite woman (2 Kings 4:34). In 1543, Andreas Vesalius[3] described tracheotomy and artificial ventilation. William Harvey's manual manipulation of the heart is well known. Early teaching of resuscitation was organized by the Society for the Recovery of Persons Apparently Drowned, founded in London in 1774. The combined techniques of modern CPR developed primarily from the fortuitous assemblage of innovative clinicians and researchers in Baltimore in the 1950s and early 1960s. Building on the long history of contributions from around the world, these investigators laid the framework for current CPR practice. In the late 1950s, mouth-to-mouth ventilation was established as the only effective means of artificial ventilation.[4-7] The internal defibrillator was developed in 1933,[8] but it was not applied successfully until 1947.[9] It was another decade before general use was made possible by the development of external cross-chest defibrillation.[10,11] Despite these advances, widespread resuscitation from cardiac arrest was not possible until Kouwenhoven et al.[12] described success with closed-chest cardiac massage in a series of patients. The final major component of modern CPR was added in 1963, when Redding and Pearson[13] described the improved success obtained by administering vasopressor drugs.

Scope of the Problem

Cardiovascular disease remains the most common cause of death in the industrialized world. Although cardiovascular mortality has been declining in the United States since the mid-1960s, more than 35% of all deaths are due to cardiovascular causes.[14] Of the 860,000 annual cardiovascular deaths, approximately half are related to coronary artery disease, the majority are sudden deaths, and 70% occur outside the hospital or in hospital emergency departments. Thus, CPR teaching and research tend to focus on myocardial ischemia as the primary cause of cardiac arrest. However, anesthesiologists are more likely than other practitioners to deal with causes other than myocardial infarction. CPR is symptomatic therapy, aimed at sustaining vital organ function until natural cardiac function is restored. The details of effective resuscitation technique are important. However, search for a remediable cause of the arrest must not be lost in excessive attention to mechanics. Brain adenosine triphosphate (ATP) is depleted after 4 to 6 minutes of no blood flow. It returns nearly to normal within 6 minutes of starting effective CPR. Studies in animals suggest that good neurologic outcome may be possible from 10- to 15-minute periods of normothermic cardiac arrest if good circulation is promptly restored.[15,16] In clinical practice, the severity of the underlying cardiac disease is the major determining factor in the success or failure of resuscitation attempts. Of those factors under control of the rescuers, poor outcomes are associated with long arrest times before CPR is begun, prolonged ventricular fibrillation (VF) without definitive therapy, and inadequate coronary and cerebral perfusion during cardiac massage. CPR begun by bystanders can more than double survival.[17] However, bystanders provide CPR only 25% to 30% of the time in sudden cardiac arrest. Optimal outcome from VF is obtained only if basic life support (BLS) is begun within 4 minutes of arrest and defibrillation applied within 8 minutes.[18] The importance of early defibrillation has been known for decades and is emphasized in CPR practice.[19,20] What is not as well recognized is the tendency to interrupt chest compressions frequently during a resuscitation attempt. Studies of emergency medical systems (EMSs) suggest that chest compressions are performed less than 50% of the time during a typical out-of-hospital resuscitation, being interrupted for pulse checks, intubations, starting intravenous catheters, defibrillation attempts, and moving the victim.[21] Because blood flow falls rapidly with cessation of compressions and resumes slowly with reinstitution of compressions, these interruptions are a major contributor to poor survival rates.

With an effective rapid-response EMS, initial resuscitation rates of 40% and survival to hospital discharge of 10% to 15% are possible after out-of-hospital arrests,[18,20] although the median reported survival to discharge with any first recorded rhythm is 6.4%.[22] Rates for survival to discharge from in-hospital arrest are about 18% in adults and 27% in children.[23] Within the hospital, the operating room is the location where CPR has the highest rate of success. Cardiac arrest occurs approximately seven times for every 10,000 anesthetics.[24] The cause for the arrest is anesthesia related approximately 4.5 times for every 10,000 anesthetics, but mortality from these arrests is only 0.4 per 10,000 anesthetics. Thus, resuscitation is successful approximately 90% of the time in anesthesia-related cardiac arrests.

Ethical Issues: Do Not Resuscitate Orders in the Operating Room

Although institution of CPR is standard medical care when an individual is found pulseless, terminally ill patients have become increasingly concerned about inappropriate application of life-sustaining procedures, including CPR. Through living wills and other instruments, patients have begun placing limitations on medical treatment to include do not resuscitate (DNR) orders, even while undergoing palliative surgical procedures. Such requests are generally accepted, even welcomed, by health-care workers. However, the operating room is one area of the hospital where DNR orders continue to cause ethical conflicts between medical personnel and patients.[25,26] There are ethically sound arguments on both sides of the issue as to whether DNR orders should be upheld in the operating room.

The patient's right to limit medical treatment, including refusing CPR, is firmly established in modern medical practice based on the ethical principle of respect for patient autonomy. A terminally ill patient can reject heroic measures such as resuscitation and still choose palliative therapy. If a surgical intervention will ameliorate symptoms or improve quality of life, there is no reason to withhold this treatment. Operative intervention increases the risk of cardiac arrest, and the patient may not want the burden of surviving in a worse condition than preoperatively. The possibility of death under anesthesia may be viewed as especially peaceful. Thus, the time that the DNR order provides the greatest protection against unwanted intervention is during surgery.

Despite these rather strong arguments for treating a DNR request in the operating room the same way it is treated elsewhere in the hospital, many operating room personnel are at least a little uneasy caring for these patients. Many surgeons require that DNR orders be suspended during the perioperative period or assume consent to surgery includes such suspension. There are multiple reasons for the reluctance to accept DNR status during surgery and anesthesia. Approximately 75% of cardiac arrests in the operating room are related to a surgical or anesthetic complication, and resuscitative attempts are highly successful.[24] Ethically, surgeons and anesthesiologists feel responsible for what happens to patients in the operating room: *primum non nocere* (first, do no harm). Although the physicians are highly diligent in monitoring and managing changes in the patient's status, complications and arrests do occur. Honoring a DNR order under these circumstances is frequently viewed as failure to treat a reversible process, and hence, tantamount to killing. This is an ethically sound view if the cause of arrest is readily identifiable and easily reversible and if treatment is likely to allow the patient to fulfill the objectives of coming to surgery.[25]

Institutionally, these ethical conflicts should be addressed by adoption of clear policies by hospitals.[27] For the individual patient, conflicts can be resolved by communication among the patient, family, and caregivers. A mutual decision can often be reached to suspend or severely limit a DNR order in the perioperative period if the patient understands the special circumstances of perioperative arrest, that interventions are brief and usually successful, and that the physicians support the patient's goals in coming to surgery and values in desiring not to prolong death. Many interventions commonly used in the operating room (mechanical ventilation, vasopressors, antidysrhythmics, blood products) may be considered forms of resuscitation in other situations. The only modalities that are not routine anesthetic care are cardiac massage and defibrillation. Therefore, the specific interventions included in a DNR status must be clarified with specific allowance made for methods necessary to perform anesthesia and surgery. A full discussion of this topic may be found in "Ethical Guidelines for the Anesthesia Care of Patients with Do-Not-Resuscitate Orders or Other Directives that Limit Treatment" by the American Society of Anesthesiologists (ASA), which is available on the ASA website (www.asahq.org).

Components of Resuscitation

[3] The major components of resuscitation from cardiac arrest are airway, breathing, circulation, drugs, and electrical therapy (ABCDE). Traditionally, these have been divided into two categories: basic life support (BLS), for those elements that can be performed without additional equipment—basic airway management, rescue breathing, and manual chest compressions (see AHA's basic cardiac arrest algorithm at http://bit.ly/2bYhiO8)—and advanced cardiac life support (ACLS), encompassing all the cognitive and technical skills necessary for resuscitation (see Fig. 58-1 and AHA's adult cardiac arrest algorithm at http://bit.ly/2c7wYJA). The lines between BLS and ACLS have tended to blur recently with the introduction of public-access automatic external defibrillators (AEDs) and the recognition that careful attention to uninterrupted, effective chest compressions improves outcome more than any advanced therapy. In the following sections, each of the components involved in resuscitation will be reviewed separately, followed by a discussion of combining the elements to achieve the best outcome.

Airway Management

The problem of airway obstruction caused by the tongue in the unconscious patient is familiar to the anesthesiologist. The techniques used for airway maintenance during anesthesia are applicable to the cardiac arrest victim. The primary method recommended to the public is the same head tilt–chin lift method commonly employed in the operating room.[28] The head is extended by pressure applied to the brow while the mandible is pulled forward by pressure on the front of the jaw, lifting the tongue away from the posterior pharynx. The jaw thrust maneuver (applying pressure behind the rami of the mandible) is an effective alternative. Properly inserted oropharyngeal or nasopharyngeal airways can be useful before intubation, recognizing the danger of inducing vomiting or laryngospasm in the semiconscious victim. Supraglottic airways (e.g., laryngeal mask airway, laryngeal tube, King airway, Combitube, etc.; see Chapter 28) have been used successfully in resuscitation attempts.[29] Tracheal intubation provides the best airway control, preventing aspiration and allowing the most effective ventilation. However, it should not be performed until adequate ventilation (preferably with supplemental oxygen) and chest compressions have been established. When other methods of establishing an airway are unsuccessful, translaryngeal ventilation or tracheotomy by cricothyroid puncture may be necessary.

Foreign Body Airway Obstruction

In 2004, unintentional choking or suffocation accounted for 5,891 deaths in the United States (approximately 0.2% of all deaths) and 725 of the victims were less than 1 year old.[14] Airway occlusion by a foreign object must be considered in any victim who suddenly stops breathing and becomes cyanotic and unconscious. It occurs most commonly during eating and is usually due to food, especially meat, impacting the laryngeal inlet, at the epiglottis or in the vallecula. Sudden death in restaurants from this cause is frequently mistaken for myocardial infarction, leading to the label "café coronary." Poorly chewed pieces of food, poor dentition or dentures, and elevated blood alcohol levels are the most common factors contributing to choking. The signs of total airway obstruction are the lack of air movement despite respiratory efforts and the inability of the victim to speak or cough. Cyanosis, unconsciousness, and cardiac arrest follow quickly. Partial airway obstruction will result in rasping or wheezing respirations accompanied by coughing. If the victim has good air movement and is able to cough forcefully, no intervention is indicated. However, if the cough weakens or cyanosis develops, the patient must be treated as if there were complete obstruction.

Mothers and friends have been pounding on the backs of choking victims for centuries. In 1974, Heimlich[30] proposed abdominal thrusts as a better method of relieving airway obstruction and, in 1976, Guildner et al.[31] reported that sternal thrusts were just as effective. Subsequently, there were multiple studies of these maneuvers. In clinical practice, Redding[32] observed that no maneuver was always successful and that each occasionally was successful when another had failed. To minimize confusion from teaching multiple techniques, the AHA has elected to emphasize the abdominal thrust maneuver (with chest thrusts as an alternative for the pregnant and massively obese).[29] This recommendation is made on the twofold premise that the abdominal

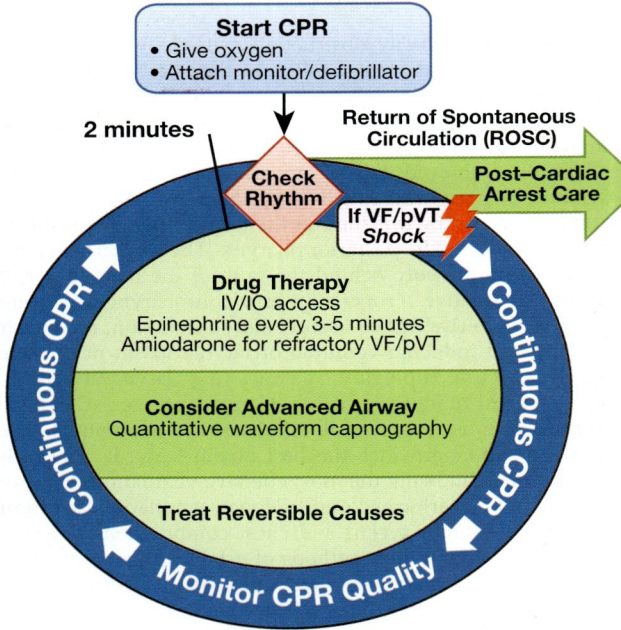

Figure 58-1 Advanced cardiac life support cardiac arrest circular algorithm. CPR, cardiopulmonary resuscitation; VF, ventricular fibrillation; VT, ventricular tachycardia; pVT, polymorphic ventricular tachycardia; IV, intravenous(ly); IO, intraosseous(ly); PetCO$_2$, partial pressure of end tidal carbon dioxide; J, joules. Reprinted with permission. 2015 American Heart Association Guidelines for CPR & ECC—Part 7: ACLS. ©2015 American Heart Association, Inc.

thrust is at least as effective as other techniques and that teaching one method simplifies education.

For the awake victim, abdominal thrusts are applied in the erect position (sitting or standing). The rescuer reaches around the victim from behind, placing the fist of one hand in the epigastrium between the xiphoid and umbilicus. The fist is grasped with the other hand and pressed into the epigastrium with a quick upward thrust. In the unconscious, thrusts are applied by kneeling astride the victim, placing the heel of one hand in the epigastrium and the other on top of the first hand. Care must be taken to ensure the xiphoid is not pushed into the abdominal contents and that the thrust is in the midline. Sternal thrusts are valuable in the massively obese or in women in advanced pregnancy. In the erect victim, the chest is encircled from behind, as in the abdominal maneuver, but the fist is placed in the midsternum. For the unconscious, thrusts are applied from the side of the supine victim with a hand position the same as for external cardiac compression. Back blows are applied directly over the thoracic spine between the scapulae. They must be delivered with force. Placing the victim in a head-down position (e.g., leaning over a chair) may help move the obstruction into the pharynx.

Whatever technique is used, each individual maneuver must be delivered as if it will relieve the obstruction. If the first attempt is unsuccessful, repeated attempts should be made because hypoxia-related muscular relaxation may eventually allow success. Complications of thrust maneuvers include laceration of the liver and spleen, gastric rupture, fractured ribs, and regurgitation.

In the unconscious victim, manual dislodgement of the obstruction should be tried only if solid material can be seen obstructing the airway. Grasping the object under direct visualization with a Magill forceps or ordinary instrument (e.g., ice tongs) may be used. Care must be taken not to push the foreign body deeper into the larynx. Blind finger sweeps and blind grasping with instruments are rarely successful and may cause damage to tonsils or other tissue. Finally, if the object cannot be dislodged, a cricothyroidotomy can be lifesaving.

Ventilation

The standard approach to the unresponsive victim is to follow opening of the airway with ventilation. When ventilation is provided in the rescue setting, mouth-to-mouth or mouth-to-nose ventilation is the most expeditious and effective method immediately available. Although inspired gas with this method will contain approximately 4% carbon dioxide and only approximately 17% oxygen (composition of exhaled air), it is sufficient to maintain viability.

Physiology of Ventilation during Cardiopulmonary Resuscitation

In the absence of an endotracheal tube, the distribution of gas between the lungs and stomach during positive-pressure ventilation will be determined by the relative impedance to flow into each (i.e., the opening pressure of the esophagus and the lung–thorax compliance). It is likely that esophageal opening pressure during cardiac arrest is no more than that found in anesthetized individuals (approximately 20 cm H_2O), and lung–thorax compliance is likely reduced. To avoid gastric insufflation, inspiratory airway pressures must be kept low.

Insufflation of air into the stomach during CPR leads to gastric distention, impeding ventilation and increasing the risk of regurgitation and gastric rupture. Avoiding gastric insufflation requires that peak inspiratory airway pressures stay below esophageal opening pressure. Partial airway obstruction by the tongue and pharyngeal tissues is a major cause of increased airway pressure contributing to gastric insufflation during CPR. Meticulous attention to airway management is necessary during rescue breathing. Recommended tidal volumes to cause a noticeable rise in the chest wall in most adults is 0.5 to 0.6 L. Each rescue breath should be given over 1 second during a pause in chest compressions.

Techniques of Rescue Breathing

While maintaining an open airway with the head tilt–jaw lift technique, the hand on the forehead pinches the nose, the rescuer takes a normal breath and seals the victim's mouth with the lips and exhales, watching for the chest to rise, indicating effective ventilation. For exhalation, the rescuer's mouth is removed from the victim, and the rescuer listens for escaping air while taking a breath. When both hands are being used in the jaw thrust maneuver of opening the airway, the cheek is used to seal the nose. For mouth-to-nose ventilation, the rescuer's lips surround the nose and the victim's lips are held closed. In some patients, the mouth must be allowed to open for exhalation with this technique. Give one breath over 1 second, take a normal breath, and give a second breath over 1 second. During CPR in adults and one-rescuer CPR in children, a pause for two breaths should be made after each 30 chest compressions. When there are two rescuers with a child victim, a pause for two breaths should be made after each 15 compressions.[29]

Several adjuncts to ventilation are available. Perhaps the most useful adjunct is a common mask, such as that used for anesthesia. The mask can be applied to the face and held in place with the thumbs and index fingers while the other fingers are used to apply jaw thrust. Breathing into the connector port of the mask provides ventilation. Mouth-to-mask ventilation may be more aesthetic than mouth-to-mouth ventilation and can be just as effective in trained hands. Masks are also available with one-way valves that direct the victim's exhaled gas away from the rescuer. Masks with integral nipple adapters are useful for providing supplemental oxygen. An oxygen flow of 10 L/min can raise the inspired concentration to 50%.

The self-inflating resuscitation bag and mask are the most common adjuncts used in rescue vehicles and hospitals. Although these devices have the advantages of noncontact and ability to use supplemental oxygen, they have been shown to be difficult for a single rescuer to apply properly to prevent substantial gas leak while maintaining a patent airway.[33] Tidal volumes with mouth-to-mouth and mouth-to-mask ventilation are often greater than those with the resuscitation bag. It is now recommended that if this device is to be used, two individuals manage the airway: one to hold the mask and maintain head position and one to squeeze the bag, using both hands.[34] The self-inflating resuscitation bag can also be used with supraglottic airways and endotracheal tubes.

Tracheal intubation provides the best control of ventilation without concern for gastric distention. With a supraglottic airway or an endotracheal tube in place, breathing can proceed without synchronizing ventilation with chest compressions. Blood flow during CPR slows rapidly when chest compressions are stopped and recovers slowly when they are resumed. Consequently, advanced airway placement should be accomplished without stopping chest compressions, if possible. Following placement, no pause should be made for ventilation, and one ventilation should be delivered every 6 seconds. Studies have not clearly demonstrated that any type of advanced airway management during resuscitation improves outcome over the self-inflating resuscitation bag and mask.[35]

Circulation

Physiology of Circulation during Closed-chest Compression

Two theories of the mechanism of blood flow during closed-chest compression have been suggested.[12,36] They are not mutually exclusive, and which mechanism predominates in humans continues to be debated.

Cardiac Pump Mechanism

The cardiac pump mechanism was originally proposed by Kouwenhoven et al.[12] and Jude et al.[37] According to this theory, pressure on the chest compresses the heart between the sternum and the spine. Compression raises the pressure in the ventricular chambers, closing the atrioventricular valves and ejecting blood into the lungs and aorta. During the relaxation phase of closed-chest compression, expansion of the thoracic cage causes a subatmospheric intrathoracic pressure, facilitating blood return. The mitral and tricuspid valves open, allowing blood to fill the ventricles. Pressure in the aorta causes aortic valve closure and coronary artery perfusion.

Thoracic Pump Mechanism

In 1976, Criley et al.[38] reported a patient undergoing cardiac catheterization who simultaneously developed VF and an episode of cough-hiccups. With every cough-hiccup, a significant arterial pressure was noted. This observation of self-administered "cough CPR" prompted further investigations on the mechanism of blood flow, and these studies produced the theory of a thoracic pump mechanism for blood flow during closed-chest compressions.[36] According to this theory, blood flows into the thorax during the relaxation phase of chest compressions in the same manner as that described for the cardiac pump mechanism.

During the compression phase, all intrathoracic structures are compressed equally by the rise in intrathoracic pressure caused by sternal depression, forcing blood out of the chest. Backward flow through the venous system is prevented by valves in the subclavian and internal jugular veins and by dynamic compression of the veins at the thoracic outlet by the increased intrathoracic pressure. Thicker, less compressible vessel walls prevent collapse on the arterial side, although arterial collapse will occur if intrathoracic pressure is raised enough.[39] The heart is a passive conduit with the atrioventricular valves remaining open during chest compression. Because there is a significant pressure difference between the carotid artery and jugular vein, blood flow to the head is favored. The lack of valves in the inferior vena cava results in less resistance to backward flow, and pressures in the arteries and veins below the diaphragm are nearly equal. This is consistent with the fact that there is little blood flow to organs below the diaphragm.[40,41]

It seems clear that fluctuations in intrathoracic pressure play a significant role in blood flow during CPR. It is also likely that compression of the heart occurs under some circumstances. Factors that influence the mechanism probably include the compliance and configuration of the chest wall, size of the heart, force of the sternal compressions, duration of cardiac arrest, and other undiscovered factors. It is likely that the predominant mechanism of blood flow varies from victim to victim and may even change from one mechanism to the the other during the resuscitation of the same victim.

Distribution of Blood Flow during Cardiopulmonary Resuscitation

Whatever the predominant mechanism, total body blood flow (cardiac output) is reduced from 10% to 33% of normal during experimental closed-chest cardiac massage. Similar severe reductions in flow are likely during clinical CPR in humans. Nearly all the blood flow is directed to organs above the diaphragm.[40,41] Myocardial perfusion is 20% to 50% of normal, whereas cerebral perfusion is maintained at 50% to 90% of normal. Abdominal visceral and lower extremity flow is reduced to 5% of normal. Total flow tends to decrease with time during CPR, but the relative distribution is not altered. Changes in CPR technique and the use of epinephrine may help sustain cardiac output over time.[41] Epinephrine improves flow to the brain and heart, whereas flow to organs below the diaphragm is unchanged or further reduced.

Gas Transport during Cardiopulmonary Resuscitation

During the low flow state of CPR, excretion of carbon dioxide (CO_2) (milliliters of CO_2 per minute in exhaled gas) is decreased from pre-arrest levels to approximately the same extent that cardiac output is reduced. This reduced CO_2 excretion is due primarily to shunting of blood flow away from the lower half of the body. The exhaled CO_2 reflects only the metabolism of the part of the body that is being perfused. In the nonperfused areas, CO_2 accumulates during CPR. When normal circulation is restored, the accumulated CO_2 is washed out, and a temporary increase in CO_2 excretion is seen.

Although CO_2 excretion is reduced during CPR, measurement of blood gases reveals an arterial respiratory alkalosis and a venous respiratory acidosis with a markedly elevated arteriovenous CO_2 difference.[42] The primary cause of these changes is the severely reduced cardiac output. Two factors account for the elevation of the venous partial pressure of CO_2 ($PvCO_2$). Buffering acid causes a reduction in serum bicarbonate, so the same blood CO_2 content results in a higher $PvCO_2$. In addition, the mixed venous CO_2 content is elevated. When flow to a tissue is reduced, all the CO_2 produced fails to be removed and CO_2 accumulates, raising the tissue partial pressure of CO_2. This allows more CO_2 to be carried in each aliquot of blood, and mixed venous CO_2 content increases. If flow remains constant, a new equilibrium is established in which all CO_2 produced in the tissue is removed but at a higher venous CO_2 content and partial pressure. In contrast to the venous blood, arterial CO_2 content and partial pressure ($PaCO_2$) are usually reduced during CPR. Although venous blood may have an increased CO_2, the marked reduction in cardiac output with maintained ventilation results in efficient CO_2 removal.

Decreased pulmonary blood flow during CPR causes a lack of perfusion to many nondependent alveoli. The alveolar gas of these lung units has no CO_2. Consequently, mixed alveolar CO_2 (i.e., end-tidal CO_2) will be low and correlate poorly with arterial CO_2. However, end-tidal CO_2 does correlate well with cardiac output during CPR. As flow increases, more alveoli become perfused, there is less alveolar dead space, and end-tidal CO_2 measurements rise.

Technique of Closed-chest Compression

Cardiac arrest should be assumed in an unresponsive individual with abnormal or absent breathing. The community or institution emergency response system should immediately be activated and chest compressions begun. In emergency circumstances, it is difficult to detect a pulse, even in a major artery (carotid, femoral, axillary). No more than 10 seconds should be taken to check for a pulse and, if a pulse is not definitely felt, chest compressions should be started. Witnessed sudden collapse with unresponsiveness in an adult in the absence of seizure activity is nearly always dysrhythmic cardiac arrest, and chest compressions should be started immediately.

Important considerations in performing closed-chest compressions are the position of the rescuer relative to the victim, the position of the rescuer's hands, and the rate and force of compression. The victim must be supine, the head level with the heart, for adequate brain perfusion. The victim must be on a firm surface. The rescuer should stand or kneel next to the victim's side. Compressions are performed most effectively if the rescuer's hips are on the same level, or slightly above the level of, the victim's chest.

Standard technique consists of the rhythmic application of pressure over the lower half of the sternum. The heel of one hand is placed on the lower sternum, and the other hand is placed on top of the first one. Great care must be taken to avoid pressing the xiphoid into the abdomen, which can lacerate the liver. Even with properly performed CPR, costochondral separation and rib fractures are common. Applying pressure on the ribs by improper hand placement increases these complications and risks puncturing the lung. Pressure on the sternum should be applied through the heel of the hand only, keeping the fingers free of the chest wall. The direction of force must be straight down on the sternum, with the arms straight and the elbows locked into position so the entire weight of the upper body is used to apply force. Inadequate chest recoil due to leaning on the chest during the relaxation phase has been demonstrated to be both common and deleterious to effective chest compressions. During relaxation, care must be taken to remove all pressure from the chest wall, but the hands should not lose contact with the chest wall.

The sternum must be depressed at least 2 to 2½ in (5 to 6 cm) in adults and teens. The duration of compression should be equal to that of relaxation, and the compression rate should be 100 to 120 times per minute. Push hard and push fast, minimizing interruptions in chest compressions. Allow a brief pause for two 1-second breaths after every 30 compressions. With an advanced airway in place, ventilations at a rate of 1 breath every 6 seconds should be interposed between compressions without a pause.

Alternative Methods of Circulatory Support

As currently practiced, CPR has limited success, with only approximately 40% of victims being admitted to the hospital and 10% surviving to discharge. Despite the occasional success of prolonged resuscitation, standard CPR will sustain most patients for only 15 to 30 minutes. If return of spontaneous circulation has not been achieved in that time, the outcome is dismal. Recognition of these limits and improved understanding of circulatory physiology during CPR have led to several proposals for alternatives to the standard techniques of closed-chest compression. The goals of the new methods are to provide better hemodynamics during CPR and thus improve survival and/or to extend the period of time during which CPR can successfully support viability. Unfortunately, none of the alternatives has proved reliably superior to the standard technique. According to the thoracic pump theory, elevation of intrathoracic pressure during chest compression should improve blood flow and pressure.[39] Studies of techniques that raise intrathoracic pressure (abdominal binding, simultaneous ventilation–compression) demonstrate that the elevated aortic pressure is offset by similar elevations in right atrial and intracranial pressures, so no improvement in myocardial or cerebral blood flow is found. These techniques are no longer recommended for use during CPR because survival is not improved when these techniques are compared with standard CPR.[43-45]

Interposed Abdominal Compression Cardiopulmonary Resuscitation

Interposed abdominal compression (IAC) is fundamentally different from abdominal binding. With this technique, an additional rescuer applies abdominal compressions manually during the relaxation phase of chest compression.[46] Abdominal pressure is released when chest compression begins. One large randomized trial of out-of-hospital cardiac arrest with IAC CPR found no improvement in survival compared with standard CPR,[47] but a subsequent in-hospital study demonstrated improved outcome.[48] The safety of IAC CPR has been established, and it may be considered for in-hospital CPR when there are sufficient personnel trained in its use. Further studies will be needed to establish out-of-hospital efficacy.

Mechanical Chest Compression Devices

Following the description of "cough CPR" and the development of the thoracic pump theory, a pneumatic vest device was developed that would simulate the events of vigorous coughing.[49] The most common modification is the *load-distributing band* (*LDB*) device, which uses a pneumatically or electronically actuated circumferential constricting band and backboard.[50] A high quality multicenter randomized controlled trial of the LDB versus manual CPR demonstrated equal survival to hospital discharge.[51] Case series also have used a number of piston-type devices to provide chest compressions with variable outcomes. The most commonly used is the *Lund University Cardiac Arrest System* (*LUCAS*) which is a gas (oxygen or air) or electric-powered piston that produces a consistent chest compression rate of 100/minute and a compression depth of 5 cm and which incorporates a suction cup attached to the sternum to return the sternum to the starting position.[52] These devices can be useful in circumstances where manual compressions are difficult or dangerous to perform (e.g., in a moving ambulance, in the angiography suite, or during prolonged resuscitation attempts). However, it can take considerable time to deploy and remove the device, prolonging the time chest compressions are not being performed and worsening outcome. Their use requires a well-trained team that can minimize hands-off time while applying and removing the device.

Active Compression–Decompression Cardiopulmonary Resuscitation

The active compression–decompression (ACD) technique developed from the anecdotal report of CPR performed with a plumber's helper applied to the anterior chest wall.[53] This suggested that active decompression of the chest wall might reduce intrathoracic pressure during the relaxation phase of chest compressions, leading to improved venous return, increased stroke volume with compression, and better blood flow. A suction device that can be applied to the chest wall to enable ACD was developed.[54] Hemodynamic studies of this technique in animals and humans have shown that coronary and cerebral perfusion may be somewhat improved with this method compared with standard CPR, although when epinephrine is used there is no difference between techniques.[54,55] Clinical trials of this technique have had mixed results, with four studies showing improved outcome and five showing no positive or negative effects. No survival benefit of ACD CPR over standard CPR was found in a meta-analysis of 10 trials involving 4,162 patients in the out-of-hospital setting and in a meta-analysis of two trials involving 826 patients in the in-hospital setting.[56]

Impedance Threshold Device

The impedance threshold device (ITD) is a valve that impedes air entry into the lungs during chest recoil of the relaxation phase of chest compressions, thus reducing intrathoracic pressure and increasing venous return to the thorax. Originally designed to be used with a cuffed endotracheal tube and ACD CPR (during which it would act to further increase the venous return of active decompression),[57] it can also be used with conventional CPR and a tight-fitting face mask or supraglottic airway.[58] Two randomized trials of out-of-hospital cardiac arrest comparing conventional CPR and the ITD with ACD CPR have shown improvement in short-term resuscitation.[57,59] One randomized trial of 8,718 out-of-hospital cardiac arrest victims undergoing standard CPR with an active versus sham ITD found no difference in short-term or long-term outcomes.[60] Although improved long-term survival has not been demonstrated, the ITD may be a useful adjunct for professionals trained in its use.

Invasive Techniques

In contrast to the closed-chest techniques, two invasive methods have been able to maintain cardiac and cerebral viability during long periods of cardiac arrest. In animal models, open-chest cardiac massage and extracorporeal CPR (ECPR) (cardiopulmonary bypass through the femoral artery and vein using a membrane oxygenator) can provide better hemodynamics, as well as better myocardial and cerebral perfusion, than closed-chest techniques.[61] Prompt restoration of blood flow and perfusion pressure with cardiopulmonary bypass can provide resuscitation with minimal neurologic deficit after 20 minutes of fibrillatory cardiac arrest in canines.[15] However, these techniques must be instituted relatively early (probably within 20 to 30 minutes of arrest) to be effective.[16,62] If open-chest massage is begun after 30 minutes of ineffective closed-chest compressions, survival is no better, although hemodynamics are improved.[63] The need to apply these maneuvers early in an arrest obviously limits the application. Early observational studies of ECPR have usually included a small number of subjects, younger patients with witnessed arrest, and potentially reversible conditions. Recent studies in Japan suggest ECPR applied rapidly after unsuccessful standard CPR combined with postresuscitation therapeutic hypothermia can significantly improve neurologically favorable survival. Before invasive procedures play a greater role in modern CPR, a method must be developed to predict, early in resuscitation, which patients will and will not respond to closed-chest compressions.

Assessing the Adequacy of Circulation during Cardiopulmonary Resuscitation

The adequacy of closed-chest compression is frequently judged by palpation of a pulse in the carotid or femoral vessels. The palpable pulse primarily reflects systolic pressure. Cardiac output correlates better with mean pressure and coronary perfusion with diastolic pressure. In the femoral area, the palpable pulse is as likely to be venous as arterial. Whenever possible, more accurate means of monitoring the efficacy of chest compressions should be used. The importance of monitoring CPR quality is stressed in the AHA ACLS circular algorithm (Fig. 58-1).

Return of spontaneous circulation with an arrested heart greatly depends on restoring oxygenated blood flow to the myocardium. In experimental models, a minimum blood flow of 15 to 20 mL/min/100 g of myocardium has been shown to be necessary for successful resuscitation.[64] Obtaining such flow depends on closed-chest compressions developing adequate cardiac output and coronary perfusion pressure. Similar to the beating heart, coronary perfusion during CPR occurs primarily in the relaxation phase (diastole) of chest compressions. In 1906, Crile and Dolley[65] suggested that a critical coronary perfusion pressure was necessary for successful resuscitation. This concept has been confirmed in numerous other reports.[41,64–74] During standard CPR, critical myocardial blood flow is associated with aortic diastolic pressure exceeding 40 mmHg. Because right atrial pressure can be elevated with some techniques, the aortic diastolic pressure minus the right atrial diastolic pressure is a more accurate reflection of coronary perfusion pressure. The critical coronary perfusion pressure is 15 to 25 mmHg. When invasive monitoring is available during CPR, adjustments in chest compression technique and epinephrine should be used to ensure critical perfusion pressures are exceeded. Damage to the myocardium from underlying disease may preclude survival no matter how effective the CPR efforts. However, vascular pressures below critical levels are associated with poor results even in patients who may be salvageable (Table 58-1).

Although invasive pressure monitoring may be ideal, it is rarely available during CPR. End-tidal CO_2 also has been found to be an excellent noninvasive guide to the adequacy of closed-chest compressions.[75] CO_2 excretion during CPR with an endotracheal tube in place is flow dependent rather than ventilation dependent. Because alveolar dead space is large in low-flow states, end-tidal CO_2 is very low (frequently <10 mmHg). If blood flow improves with better CPR technique, more alveoli are perfused

Table 58-1 Critical Variables Associated with Successful Resuscitation	
Variable	Amount
Myocardial blood flow (mL/min/100 g)	>15–20
Aortic diastolic pressure (mmHg)	>40
Coronary perfusion pressure (mmHg)	>15–25
End-tidal carbon dioxide (mmHg)	>10

and end-tidal CO_2 rises (usually to >20 mmHg with successful CPR). The earliest sign of return of spontaneous circulation is frequently a sudden increase in end-tidal CO_2 to over 40 mmHg. Within a wide range of cardiac outputs during CPR, end-tidal CO_2 correlates well with cardiac output,[76] coronary perfusion pressure,[77] and initial resuscitation.[78] End-tidal CO_2 correlates with survival in human CPR and can predict a poor outcome.[79,80] Patients with end-tidal CO_2 below 10 mmHg will not be resuscitated successfully. In the absence of invasive monitoring, end-tidal CO_2 using quantitative waveform capnography should be used to judge the effectiveness of chest compressions, whenever possible.[81] Attempts should be made to maximize the measured end-tidal CO_2 by alterations in technique or drug therapy. It should be remembered that sodium bicarbonate administration liberates CO_2 into the blood and causes a temporary increase in end-tidal CO_2. The elevation returns to baseline within 3 to 5 minutes of drug administration and end-tidal CO_2 monitoring can again be used for monitoring effectiveness of closed-chest compressions.

Pharmacologic Therapy

This discussion of drug therapy is confined to the use of drugs during CPR attempts to restore spontaneous circulation. The use of drugs to support the circulation when there is mechanical cardiac function is discussed elsewhere (see Chapters 13 and 14). During cardiac arrest, drug therapy is secondary to other interventions. Effective uninterrupted chest compressions and defibrillation, if appropriate, should take precedence over medications. Establishing intravenous access and pharmacologic therapy should come as soon as possible but after these critical interventions are established. Although vasopressors are firmly established as improving survival in animal models and there is some evidence of improved early restoration of spontaneous circulation in humans, there is no strong evidence that they improve long-term survival in human cardiac arrest.[82,83] The most common drugs and the appropriate adult doses are shown in Table 58-2. In addition, pharmacologic and other therapeutic approaches for the treatment of bradycardia and tachycardia are shown in Figures 58-2 and 58-3.

Routes of Administration

The preferred route of administration of all drugs during CPR is intravenous. The most rapid and highest drug levels occur with administration into a central vein. However, peripheral intravenous administration is also effective. The antecubital and external jugular veins are the sites of first choice for starting an infusion during resuscitation because inserting a central catheter usually necessitates stopping CPR. Because of poor blood flow below the diaphragm during CPR, drugs administered in the

Table 58-2 Adult Advanced Cardiac Life Support Drugs and Doses (Intravenous)

	Dose	Interval	Maximum
Epinephrine	1 mg	Every 3–5 min	None
If dose fails, consider new dose	3–7 mg	Every 3–5 min	None
Vasopressin	40 U	Alternative to epinephrine	—
Amiodarone	300 mg	Repeat 150 mg in 5 min	2 g
Lidocaine	1–1.5 mg/kg	Repeat 0.5–0.75 mg/kg in 5 min	3.0 mg/kg
Sodium bicarbonate	1 mEq/kg	As needed	Check pH

lower extremity may be extremely delayed or may not reach the sites of action. Even in the upper extremity, drugs may require 1 to 2 minutes to reach the central circulation. Onset of action may be accelerated if the drug bolus is followed by a 20- to 30-mL bolus of intravenous fluid. Intraosseous administration of fluids and medications is a good alternative to intravenous cannulation, allowing drug delivery similar to that of central venous administration. Commercial kits are available to facilitate intraosseous placement.

If intravenous or intraosseous access cannot be established, the endotracheal tube is an alternative route for administration of epinephrine, vasopressin, lidocaine, and atropine. Sodium

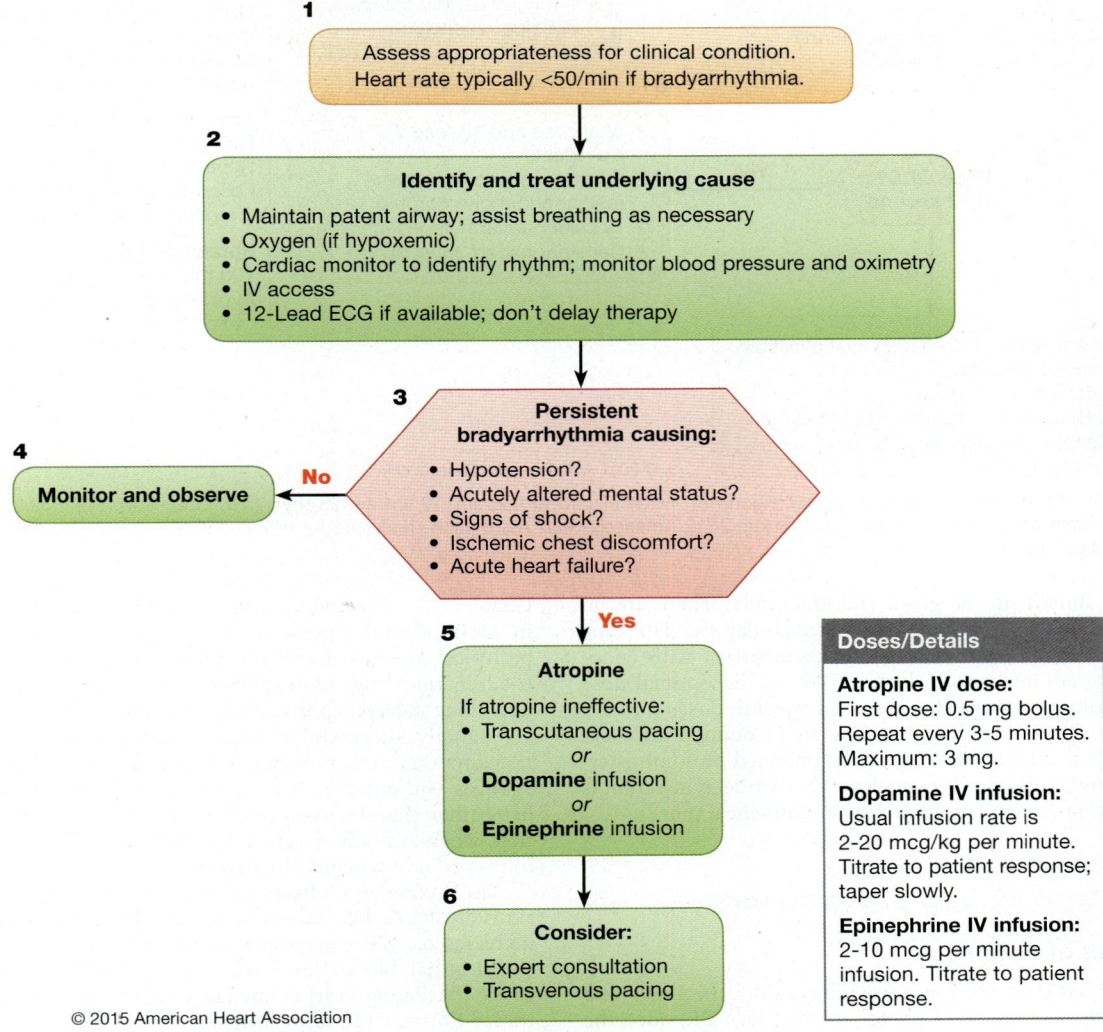

Figure 58-2 Adult bradycardia (with pulse) algorithm. ECG, electrocardiogram; IV, intravenous(ly). Reprinted with permission. 2015 American Heart Association Guidelines for CPR & ECC—Part 7: ACLS. ©2015 American Heart Association, Inc.

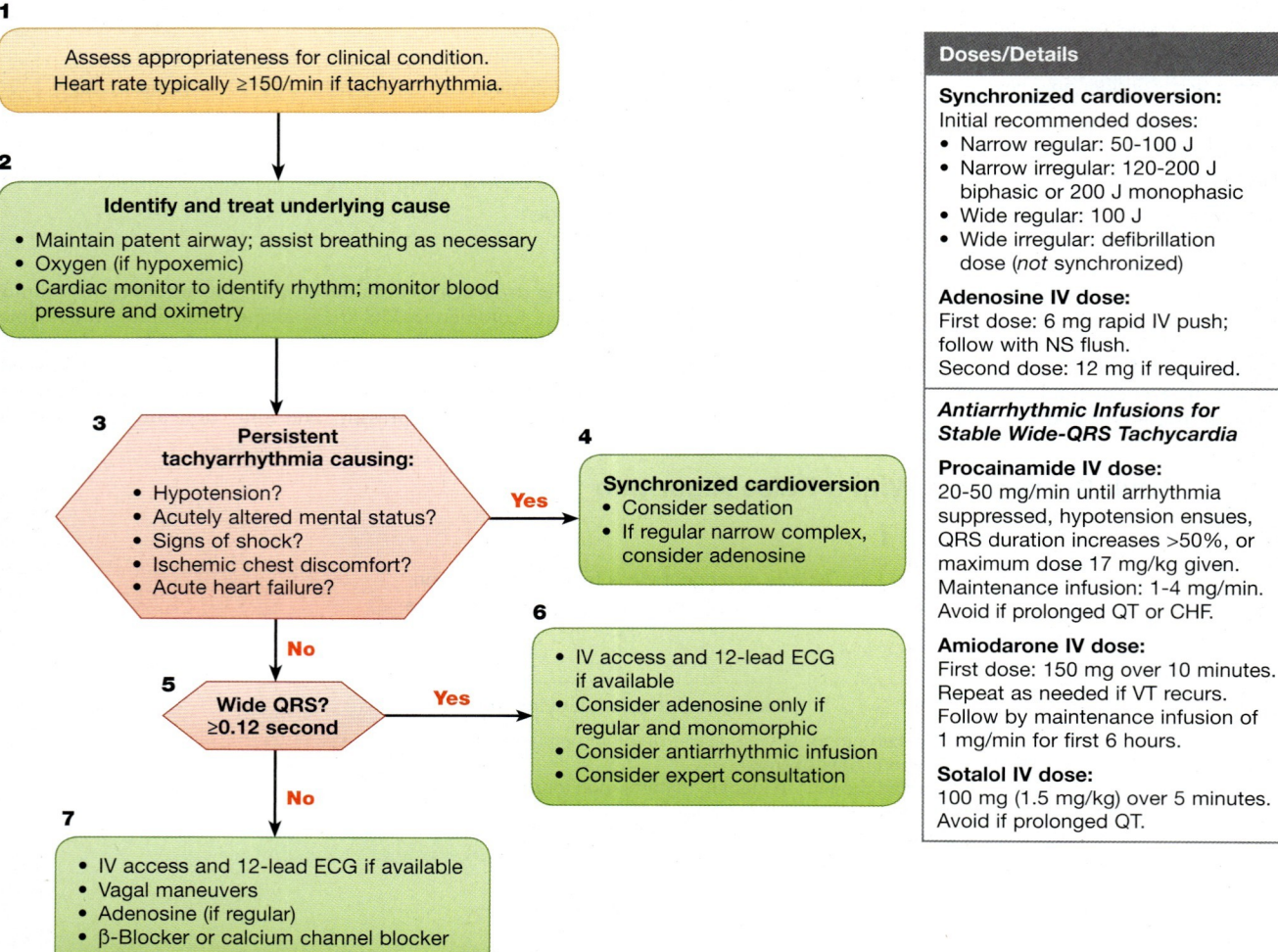

Figure 58-3 Adult tachycardia (with pulse) algorithm. ECG, electrocardiogram; IV, intravenous(ly); CHF, congestive heart failure; J, joules; VT, ventricular tachycardia. Reprinted with permission. 2015 American Heart Association Guidelines for CPR & ECC—Part 7: ACLS. ©2015 American Heart Association, Inc.

bicarbonate should not be given endotracheally. There are no data on endotracheal administration of amiodarone. The time to effect and drug levels achieved are inconsistent with endotracheal drug administration during CPR, so the optimal dose of drug is unknown using this route. In general, doses 2 to 2.5 times higher than the intravenous dose are recommended when this route is used. Better results may be obtained by administering 5- to 10-mL volumes. It is unclear whether deep injection is better than simple instillation into the endotracheal tube.

Catecholamines and Vasopressors

Mechanism of Action

Epinephrine has been used in resuscitation since the 1890s and has been the vasopressor of choice in modern CPR since the studies of Redding and Pearson[13,84] in the 1960s. The efficacy of epinephrine lies entirely in its α-adrenergic properties[71] (see Chapter 13). Peripheral vasoconstriction leads to an increase in aortic diastolic pressure, causing an increase in coronary perfusion pressure and myocardial blood flow.[41,85,86] All strong α-adrenergic drugs (epinephrine, phenylephrine, methoxamine, dopamine, norepinephrine), regardless of β-adrenergic potency, are equally successful in aiding resuscitation, as are strong nonadrenergic vasopressors (vasopressin).[13,84,87,88] β-Adrenergic agonists without α activity (isoproterenol, dobutamine) are no better than placebo. α-Adrenergic blockade precludes resuscitation, whereas β-adrenergic blockade has no effect on the ability to restore spontaneous circulation.[68,69]

The β-adrenergic effects of epinephrine are potentially deleterious during cardiac arrest. In the fibrillating heart, epinephrine increases oxygen consumption and decreases the endocardial-to-epicardial blood flow ratio. Myocardial lactate production in the fibrillating heart is unchanged after epinephrine administration during CPR, suggesting that the increased coronary blood flow does not improve the oxygen supply-to-demand ratio. Large doses of epinephrine increase deaths in swine early after resuscitation because of tachyarrhythmias and hypertension, an effect partially offset by metoprolol treatment. Despite these theoretical considerations, survival and neurologic outcome studies have shown no difference when epinephrine is compared with a pure α-agonist (methoxamine or phenylephrine) during CPR in animals[84,89] or humans.[83,90]

Epinephrine

When added to chest compressions, epinephrine helps develop the critical coronary perfusion pressure necessary to provide enough myocardial blood flow for restoration of spontaneous circulation. With invasive monitoring present during CPR, an arterial diastolic pressure of 40 mmHg or coronary perfusion pressure of 20 mmHg must be obtained with good chest-compression technique and/or epinephrine therapy (Table 58-1). In the absence of such monitoring, the dose of epinephrine must be chosen empirically. Since the studies of Redding and Pearson[13,84] in the 1960s, the standard intravenous dose used has been 0.5 to 1.0 mg. In the 1980s, animal studies suggested that higher doses of epinephrine in human CPR might improve myocardial and cerebral perfusion and improve success of resuscitation. Reports were published, including case reports and a series of children with historic controls, of return of spontaneous circulation when large doses (0.1 to 0.2 mg/kg) of epinephrine were given to patients who had failed resuscitation with standard doses.

Subsequent outcome studies did not demonstrate conclusively that higher doses of epinephrine improve survival. Eight adult prospective randomized clinical trials involving more than 9,000 cardiac arrest patients found no improvement in survival to hospital discharge or neurologic outcome, even in subgroups, when initial high-dose epinephrine (5 to 18 mg) is compared with standard doses (1 to 2 mg).[91-98] Some of the studies (and the cumulative data) suggest that there may be an improvement in immediate resuscitation with high-dose epinephrine. High doses apparently are not needed early in most cardiac arrests and could be deleterious under some circumstances. The use of high-dose epinephrine as rescue therapy when standard doses have failed has not been rigorously studied.

There is only one double-blind randomized control trial of epinephrine versus placebo reported from a single ambulance service in Australia.[99] Of the 534 patients, those receiving epinephrine had a 3.4 times greater chance of return of spontaneous circulation than those receiving placebo and a 2.3 times greater chance of hospital admission. Although more than twice as many patients receiving epinephrine survived to hospital discharge, this was not statistically significant because of the low numbers of survivors.

Current recommendations are to give 1 mg intravenously every 3 to 5 minutes in the adult. If this dose seems ineffective or to treat β-blocker or calcium channel blocker overdose, higher doses (3 to 7 mg) may be considered.

Vasopressin

Arginine vasopressin has been used as an alternative to epinephrine in a dose of 40 U intravenous/intraosseous (see Chapter 13). Vasopressin is a naturally occurring hormone (antidiuretic hormone) that, when administered in high doses, is a potent nonadrenergic vasoconstrictor, acting by stimulation of smooth muscle V_1 receptors. It is usually not recommended for conscious patients with coronary artery disease because the increased peripheral vascular resistance may provoke angina. The half-life in the intact circulation is 10 to 20 minutes and longer than epinephrine during CPR. Animal studies have demonstrated that vasopressin is as effective as or more effective than epinephrine in maintaining vital organ blood flow during CPR. Repeated doses during prolonged CPR in swine were associated with significantly improved rates of neurologically intact survival compared with epinephrine and placebo. Postresuscitation myocardial depression and splanchnic blood flow reduction are more marked with vasopressin than epinephrine, but they are transient and can be treated with low doses of dopamine.[100] Clinical studies indicate that vasopressin is as effective as epinephrine but have not definitively shown it to be superior. A small randomized, blinded study comparing vasopressin and standard-dose epinephrine in 40 patients with out-of-hospital VF found improved 24-hour survival with vasopressin but no difference in return of spontaneous circulation or survival to hospital discharge.[101] A larger, clinical trial of 200 inpatients found no difference between the drugs in survival for 1 hour or to hospital discharge.[102] In this study, response times were short, indicating that CPR outcome achieved with both vasopressin and epinephrine in short-term cardiac arrest may be comparable. The hemodynamic effects of vasopressin, compared with epinephrine, are especially impressive during long cardiac arrests. Thus, vasopressin may find most use in CPR during prolonged duration resuscitation. A multicenter, randomized study of 1,186 patients comparing vasopressin 40 U and epinephrine 1 mg for the first two doses of vasopressor during resuscitation from out-of-hospital cardiac arrest found no overall difference in survival to hospital admission (36% vs. 31%) or discharge (10% vs. 10%).[103] Overall, evidence currently suggests that, like other potent vasopressors, vasopressin is equivalent to but not better than epinephrine for use during CPR.

Amiodarone and Lidocaine

After vasopressors, the drugs most likely to be of benefit during CPR are those that help suppress ectopic ventricular rhythms. Amiodarone and lidocaine are used during cardiac arrest to aid defibrillation when VF is refractory to electrical countershock therapy or when fibrillation recurs following successful conversion. Lidocaine, primarily an antiectopic agent with few hemodynamic effects, tends to reverse the reduction in VF threshold caused by ischemia or infarction. It depresses automaticity by reducing the slope of phase 4 depolarization and reducing the heterogeneity of ventricular refractoriness.

Amiodarone is a pharmacologically complex drug with sodium, potassium, calcium, and α-adrenergic and β-adrenergic blocking properties that is useful for treatment of atrial and ventricular dysrhythmias. Amiodarone can cause hypotension and bradycardia when infused too rapidly in patients with an intact circulation.[104] This can usually be prevented by slowing the rate of drug infusion, or it can be treated with fluids, vasopressors, chronotropic agents, or temporary pacing. There are two randomized, blinded, placebo-controlled clinical trials in shock-resistant cardiac arrest victims demonstrating improved survival to hospital with amiodarone treatment, although there was no difference in survival to discharge.[105,106] Although weak, this is more evidence of efficacy than exists for lidocaine.

When VF or pulseless ventricular tachycardia is recognized, defibrillation should be attempted (see Fig. 58-1 and http://bit.ly/2c7wYJA). No antiarrhythmic agent has been shown to be superior to electrical defibrillation or more effective than placebo in the treatment of VF. Consequently, defibrillation should not be withheld or delayed to establish intravenous access or to administer drugs. When ventricular tachycardia or VF has not responded to or recurred following BLS, epinephrine, and defibrillation, amiodarone should be administered. In cardiac arrest, amiodarone is initially administered as a 300-mg rapid infusion. Supplemental infusions of 150 mg can be repeated as necessary for recurrent or resistant dysrhythmias to a maximum total daily dose of 2 g. (For dysrhythmias with an intact circulation, amiodarone is usually administered as 150 mg intravenously over 10 minutes, followed by 1 mg/min infusion for 6 hours and 0.5 mg/min thereafter.) Although lidocaine has no proven efficacy in cardiac arrest, it has few side effects. It is an alternative therapy in refractory fibrillation if amiodarone is not available. An initial bolus of 1 to 1.5 mg/kg should be given, and additional boluses of 0.5 to 0.75 mg/kg can be given every 5 to 10 minutes during CPR up to a total dose of 3 mg/kg.

Drugs Not Routinely Given during CPR

Atropine

Atropine sulfate enhances sinus node automaticity and atrioventricular conduction by its vagolytic effects. Although atropine has been given frequently during cardiac arrest associated with an electrocardiogram (ECG) pattern of asystole or slow pulseless electrical activity (PEA), neither animal nor human studies provide evidence that it actually improves outcome from asystolic or bradysystolic arrest.[107,108] The predominant cause of asystole and PEA is severe myocardial ischemia. Excessive parasympathetic tone probably contributes little to these rhythms during cardiac arrest in adults. Even in children, it is doubtful that parasympathetic tone plays a significant role during most arrests. Therefore, the most important treatment for asystole and PEA is effective chest compressions, ventilation, and epinephrine to improve coronary perfusion and myocardial oxygenation. There is no evidence that atropine is detrimental during cardiac arrest. However, *routine* use of atropine during cardiac arrest with these rhythms is unlikely to have benefit and is no longer recommended.

Sodium Bicarbonate

Although sodium bicarbonate was used commonly during CPR in the past, little evidence supports its efficacy. Use of sodium bicarbonate during resuscitation has been based on the theoretical considerations that acidosis lowers fibrillation threshold and impairs the physiologic response to catecholamines. But most studies have failed to demonstrate improved success of defibrillation or resuscitation with the use of bicarbonate.[109,110] The lack of effect of buffer therapy may be partially explained by the slow onset of metabolic acidosis during cardiac arrest. As measured by blood lactate or base deficit, acidosis does not become severe for 15 or 20 minutes of the cardiac arrest.[42,111]

In contrast to the lack of evidence that buffer therapy during CPR improves survival, the adverse effects of excessive sodium bicarbonate administration are well documented. In the past, metabolic alkalosis, hypernatremia, and hyperosmolarity were common after administration of bicarbonate during resuscitation attempts.[111,112] These abnormalities are associated with low resuscitation rates and poor outcomes.

Intravenous sodium bicarbonate combines with a hydrogen ion to produce carbonic acid that dissociates into CO_2 and water. The partial pressure of CO_2 in blood is temporarily elevated until the excess CO_2 is eliminated through the lungs. Tissue acidosis during CPR is caused primarily by the low blood flow and accumulation of CO_2 in the tissues.[42] Therefore, concern has been expressed that the liberation of CO_2 by bicarbonate administration would only worsen the existing problem. This is of particular concern within myocardial cells and the brain. CO_2 readily diffuses across cell membranes and the blood–brain barrier, whereas bicarbonate diffuses much more slowly. Thus, it is possible that sodium bicarbonate administration could result in a paradoxical worsening of intracellular and cerebral acidosis by further raising intracellular and cerebral CO_2 without a balancing increase in bicarbonate. Direct evidence for this effect has not been found. Use of clinically relevant doses causes no change in spinal fluid acid–base status or myocardial intracellular pH during bicarbonate administration.[113,114] Therefore, paradoxical acidosis from sodium bicarbonate therapy remains a concern primarily on theoretical grounds.

Routine use of sodium bicarbonate is not recommended for patients in cardiac arrest. Current practice restricts its use to arrests associated with hyperkalemia, severe pre-existing metabolic acidosis, and tricyclic or phenobarbital overdose. It may be considered for use in protracted resuscitation attempts after other modalities have been instituted and failed. When bicarbonate is used in these circumstances, the usual dose is 1 mEq/kg. However, dosing of sodium bicarbonate should be guided by blood–gas determination of acid–base status, whenever possible.

Calcium

With normal cardiovascular physiology, calcium increases myocardial contractility and enhances ventricular automaticity (see Chapter 12). Consequently, it has been advocated as a treatment for asystole and PEA. Early animal studies showed moderate success with calcium chloride in asphyxial arrest, although vasopressors were better.[13] In 1981, Dembo[115] reported dangerously high serum calcium levels (up to 18.2 mg/dL) during CPR and questioned the efficacy of calcium in cardiac arrest. Subsequently, several retrospective studies and prospective clinical trials during out-of-hospital cardiac arrest showed that calcium was no better than placebo in promoting resuscitation and survival from asystole or PEA.[116-119] Consequently, because of potentially deleterious effects, *routine* use of calcium is not recommended during CPR unless specific indications exist. Calcium may prove useful if hyperkalemia, hypocalcemia, or calcium channel blocker toxicity is present. There are no other indications for its use during CPR. When calcium is administered, the chloride salt is recommended because it produces higher and more consistent levels of ionized calcium than other salts. The usual dose is 2 to 4 mg/kg of the 10% solution administered slowly intravenously. Calcium gluconate contains one-third as much molecular calcium as does calcium chloride and requires metabolism of gluconate in the liver.

Electrical Therapy

Electrical Pattern and Duration of Ventricular Fibrillation

Ventricular fibrillation is the most common ECG pattern found during witnessed sudden cardiac arrest in adults. The only consistently effective treatment is electrical defibrillation. The most important controllable determinant of failure to resuscitate a patient with VF is the duration of fibrillation.[120] Other important factors, such as underlying disease and metabolic status, are largely beyond the control of rescuers. The fibrillating heart has high oxygen consumption, increasing myocardial ischemia and decreasing the time to irreversible cell damage. The longer VF continues, the more difficult it is to defibrillate and the less likely is successful resuscitation.[62,121] If defibrillation occurs within 1 minute of fibrillation, CPR is unnecessary for resuscitation. Initial resuscitation success following out-of-hospital fibrillation and survival to hospital discharge are improved the earlier that defibrillation is accomplished.[19,122]

The coarseness of the fibrillatory waves on the ECG may reflect the severity and duration of the myocardial insult and thus have prognostic significance.[123] However, the fibrillation amplitude seen on any one ECG lead varies with the orientation of that lead to the vector of the fibrillatory wave.[124] If the lead is oriented at right angles to the fibrillatory wave, a flat line can be seen. For this reason, the trace from a second lead or from a different position of paddle electrodes should always be inspected before a decision is made not to defibrillate. Low-*amplitude* fibrillatory waveforms are less likely to be associated with successful resuscitation and more likely to convert to asystole following defibrillation.[123] Similarly, low-*frequency* fibrillatory waveforms are associated with poor outcome, and the median frequency of the waveform correlates with myocardial perfusion during CPR and with success of defibrillation.[125,126] Multiple studies in animals and humans have shown that analysis of the VF waveform can predict, with varying reliability, the success of defibrillation attempts.[123,126–129] It is not yet clear whether such waveform analysis can predict success of resuscitation or direct modification of therapy prospectively. Catecholamines with β-adrenergic activity increase the vigor of fibrillation and the amplitude of the electrical activity, leading to the practice of administering epinephrine to make it "easier" to defibrillate. However, experimental work has shown that manipulation of the electrical pattern with epinephrine does not influence the success of defibrillation or reduce the energy needed for defibrillation.[121,130] Consequently, defibrillation should not be delayed for drug administration.

Defibrillators: Energy, Current, and Voltage

Defibrillators derive power from a line source of alternating current or an integral battery. The typical defibrillator consists of a variable transformer that stores direct current in a capacitor, a switch to charge the capacitor, and discharge switches to complete the circuit from capacitor to electrodes. Defibrillators are classified by the current waveform delivered: monophasic (current flows in one direction between electrodes) or biphasic (current reverses direction between electrodes during the shock). Older defibrillators used a monophasic damped half-sinusoid or a monophasic truncated exponential waveform. Many of these monophasic defibrillators may still be in use. All defibrillators currently on the market, including AEDs, deliver current in a truncated exponential (BTE), rectilinear (RLB), or pulsed biphasic waveform.

The AED is a device that monitors the ECG, recognizes VF, charges automatically, and gives a defibrillatory shock.[131] It has allowed the introduction of defibrillation into first-responder EMS networks and public access defibrillation because minimally trained individuals can incorporate defibrillation into BLS skills, improving survival in out-of-hospital arrest by reducing time to delivery of the first shock.[18–20,132] The algorithms these devices use to detect VF are accurate with nearly perfect specificity. They will not defibrillate a nonfibrillatory rhythm. Sensitivity rates are somewhat lower. They sometimes have trouble recognizing low-amplitude VF and can misinterpret pacemaker spikes as QRS complexes. Unfortunately, rhythm analysis can require up to 90 seconds, during which chest compressions are not being given. This may adversely influence the outcome in some circumstances.

Some defibrillators measure transthoracic impedance prior to the shock by passing a low-voltage current through the chest during the charge cycle.[133,134] This technology allows current-based defibrillation by adjusting the delivered energy for the measured resistance, permitting the use of low-energy shocks in appropriate patients and identification of victims needing higher energy.[135]

Defibrillation is accomplished by current passing through a critical mass of myocardium, causing simultaneous depolarization of the myofibrils. However, the output of defibrillators is indicated in energy units (joules or watt-seconds), not current (amperes). The relationships among energy, current, and impedance (resistance) are given by the following equations (standard units are indicated):

$$\text{Energy (joules)} = \text{Power (watts)} \times \text{Duration (seconds)} \quad (58\text{-}1)$$

$$\text{Power (watts)} = \text{Potential (volts)} \times \text{Current (amperes)} \quad (58\text{-}2)$$

$$\text{Current (amperes)} = \text{Potential (volts)}/\text{Resistance (ohms)} \quad (58\text{-}3)$$

$$\text{Current (amperes)} = \{\text{Energy (joules)}/[\text{Resistance (ohms)} \times \text{Duration (seconds)}]\}^{1/2} \quad (58\text{-}4)$$

From these equations, it can be determined that as the impedance between the paddle electrodes increases, the delivered energy will be reduced. Because internal resistance is low, the primary determinant of delivered energy will be transthoracic impedance. When transthoracic impedance is high, actual delivered energy will be lower. Even at a constant delivered energy, equation 58-4 indicates that the delivered current (the critical determinant of defibrillation) will be reduced as impedance increases. At high impedance and relatively low energy levels, current could be too low for defibrillation. Optimal results are obtained by keeping impedance as low as possible.

Transthoracic Impedance

Transthoracic impedance has been measured between 15 and 143 ohms in human defibrillation[136] (see Chapter 12). The average transthoracic impedance in human defibrillation is 70 to 80 ohms. Many of the important factors in minimizing transthoracic impedance are under the control of the rescuers. Resistance decreases with increasing electrode size, and studies suggest that optimal paddle size may be 13 cm in diameter.[137,138] For adults, handheld paddle electrodes and self-adhesive pad electrodes are most commonly 8 to 12 cm in diameter and work well in practice. Gel pads, electrode paste, or self-adhesive defibrillation or monitor pads specifically designed to conduct electricity in the defibrillation setting must be used.[137,138] When paste is used, it should be applied liberally to the paddle surface, especially the edges, to prevent burns and to obtain the maximum reduction in impedance. Transthoracic impedance is slightly, but significantly, higher during inspiration than during exhalation.[139] Air is a poor electrical conductor. Firm paddle pressure of at least 11 kg reduces resistance by improving paddle-to-skin contact and by expelling air from the lungs.[136] Resistance is probably of little clinical significance when reasonably proper technique and high-energy shocks are used. For lower energy shocks, great care should be taken to minimize resistance.

Adverse Effects and Energy Requirements

Repeated defibrillation with high energy in animals can be associated with dysrhythmias, ECG changes suggesting myocardial damage, and morphologic evidence of myocardial necrosis.[140,141] Whether similar injuries occur in humans is less certain. Slight elevations in creatine kinase–MB fractions have been measured in patients following cardioversion with high energies.[142] A higher incidence of atrioventricular block has been observed in patients receiving high-energy shocks than in patients receiving low-energy shock.[143] It seems likely that high-energy shocks, especially if repeated at close intervals, may result in myocardial damage. However, if energy is too low, the delivered current may be insufficient for defibrillation, especially when transthoracic impedance is high. There appears to be little risk of significant myocardial injury with currently recommended energy levels.

Older studies using monophasic waveform defibrillators found a general relationship between body size and energy requirements for defibrillation. Geddes et al.[144] observed that the current that is necessary for defibrillation in animals increased with increasing body mass. Children need less energy than adults, perhaps as low as 0.5 J/kg,[145] although the recommended dose is 2.0 to 4.0 J/kg, similar to that for adults.[29] Clinically, over the size range of adults, weight variability is not clinically significant and other factors are more important.[120] Studies of out-of-hospital and in-hospital arrests have demonstrated equal success when using monophasic shocks of 200 J or less initial energy compared with administering all shocks at energies 300 J or more.[143,146] Both monophasic and biphasic waveforms are successful in terminating VF. Neither waveform has been associated with better return of spontaneous circulation or survival.

Prior to 2005, the AHA recommendation for defibrillation with monophasic waveform devices was to use a stacked shock approach with an initial shock of 200 J followed immediately by a second shock at 200 to 300 J if the first was unsuccessful, followed, if both failed, by a third shock at 300 to 360 J.[147] However, the second and third shocks add limited incremental benefit and caused significant interruptions in chest compressions with reduced survival. With monophasic defibrillators, a single shock of 360 J should be given with immediate resumption of chest compressions (see Fig. 58-1 and http://bit.ly/2c7wYJA).

Biphasic shocks terminate VF at lower energies than any of the monophasic waveforms[148] and have an 85% to 98% first-shock success.[149] Selected energies from 150 to 200 J are generally effective with biphasic truncated exponential waveforms, and a selected energy of 120 J is effective with a rectilinear biphasic waveform. AEDs have the energy dose preselected. Most manual biphasic devices display the effective dose range and the user should select that dose. If the effective dose for a manual biphasic device is unknown, a dose of 200 J may be selected. This dose may not be optimal but falls within the effective dose range of nearly all biphasic devices. As with the monophasic devices, a single shock should be delivered with immediate resumption of chest compressions. If additional shocks are necessary, they may be given at the same or higher dose.

Putting It All Together

Since the mid-1970s, CPR has become widely practiced, facilitated by the efforts of the AHA, the International Red Cross, the European Resuscitation Council, and many other organizations around the world. The International Liaison Committee on Resuscitation, in conjunction with the AHA, periodically conducts an international review of the published science regarding CPR and emergency cardiac care. The resulting Consensus on Science and Treatment Recommendations[150] comprises the most complete evidence-based compilation of scientific data related to CPR practice. Individual organizations, including the AHA, use these data to develop guidelines for CPR practice. However, no common infrastructure exists that allows adoption of true international guidelines for CPR.

Following each consensus conference, the AHA refines and publishes specific guidelines for the teaching and practice of CPR in the United States.[29,147] These guidelines are developed because numerous individuals with varying levels of expertise (laypersons, emergency personnel, nurses, and physicians) need to be trained if CPR is to be effective in saving lives. For training to be effective, a standardized approach is needed. The AHA and other organizations also develop and sponsor courses at different levels of complexity for teaching CPR. The two levels of CPR care are referred to as *BLS* for ventilation and chest compressions without additional equipment, and *ACLS* for using all modalities available for resuscitation. Medical personnel need to be well versed in both levels of care. BLS is also appropriate for laypersons. The algorithms for approaching the patient with cardiac arrest published in the guidelines are familiar to all physicians and are reproduced in this chapter.

The AHA guidelines and algorithms are carefully researched using the best evidence and experts available. Until very recently, survival rates were dismal and remained stagnant for decades in spite of multiple updates to guidelines for CPR practice and many courses for lay public and health-care providers.[151] What has become clear in the past decade is that improvements in the standard clinical process of CPR may be more important to increase survival than any new intervention.[152] Standardized quality control of CPR practice is mandatory during any clinical trial if meaningful results are to be achieved. A continuous quality improvement model may be more relevant to improved outcomes than the randomized control trial. In addition, there is increasing awareness that the single approach to two pathophysiologically distinct entities (respiratory arrest and cardiac arrest) may not be optimal care for either. In the former, arrest occurs because of hypoxemia, and reoxygenating the blood by effective ventilation is mandatory for successful resuscitation. In the latter, arrest occurs because of cardiac dysrhythmia, usually with normal oxygenation, and attempts at ventilation during resuscitation, in fact, may be harmful. Recognizing these issues, the most recent refinement of the AHA guidelines emphasizes the importance of assessing the quality of CPR efforts and stresses the necessity of minimal interruptions in chest compressions throughout the resuscitation effort (see Fig. 58-1 and http://bit.ly/2c7wYJA).

Time-Sensitive Model of Ventricular Fibrillation

Weisfeldt and Becker[153] have described untreated VF as a time-sensitive model with three phases: electrical, circulatory, and metabolic. The *electrical phase* occurs during the first 4 to 5 minutes of the arrest, and early defibrillation is critical for success during this time. The *hemodynamic phase* follows for the next 10 to 15 minutes, when perfusing the myocardium and brain with oxygenated blood is critical. This is followed by what has been called the *metabolic phase*, when the ischemic injury to the heart is so great that it is not clear what interventions will be successful.

Prompt defibrillation during the electrical phase is when CPR has had the most dramatic effect and why public-access AED has proven beneficial. The longer VF continues, the more difficult it is to defibrillate and the less likely is successful resuscitation. AEDs have been employed successfully in many settings, including airplanes, airports, casinos, and in the community. The success of public access defibrillation was dramatically demonstrated by the results of installing AEDs in Chicago airports where, over the first 2 years, there was a 55% 1-year neurologically intact survival rate.[154] Similarly, when AEDs were installed in Las Vegas casinos and security personnel were instructed in their use, there was a 53% survival to discharge (74% in patients who received the shock within 3 minutes of collapse).[155] If an arrest is witnessed and a defibrillator or AED is immediately available, then defibrillation should be the first priority in resuscitation. However, in the usual out-of-hospital rescue with emergency medical technicians or paramedics doing the defibrillation, a rapid response is to apply the first shock in 6 to 7 minutes, and the time to first shock frequently is more than 10 minutes. Similar delays occur during in-hospital cardiac arrests.

With the onset of VF and cessation of coronary perfusion, the high oxygen consumption of the fibrillating heart causes the rapid depletion of myocardial high-energy phosphates, reducing the time to irreversible cell damage. Myocardial ATP levels during VF correlate with the success of defibrillation and postdefibrillation contractile function.[156] By about 4 minutes, the ATP levels in the heart have fallen to levels that make restoration of normal contractile function problematic. Effective chest compressions help replete or delay reductions in ATP by generating an adequate coronary perfusion pressure to restore myocardial blood flow. Therefore, the most important intervention during the hemodynamic phase of cardiac arrest is producing coronary perfusion with chest compressions before any attempt to defibrillate. In the absence of prompt defibrillation, the most important intervention for neurologically normal survival from cardiac arrest is restoration and maintenance of cerebral and myocardial blood flow. Because perfusion pressures generated by chest compressions are quite low compared with the intact circulation, any interruption of chest compressions markedly reduces the chances for neurologically normal survival. Therefore, any intervention that interrupts chest compressions is strongly discouraged.

Bystander CPR and Basic Life Support

Restoration of cerebral and myocardial blood flow must begin at the scene of the cardiac arrest. There are many studies documenting improved survival if bystanders provide CPR to the victim while awaiting arrival of EMS. Unfortunately, the incidence of bystander CPR has been falling for three decades. The reasons for a bystander's reluctance to intervene are multiple but seem to be primarily lack of training, the complexity of the task, and fear of harm. Many of these concerns focus on the mouth-to-mouth ventilation part of the CPR intervention.[157–159] One survey indicated that only 15% of laypersons would perform CPR with mouth-to-mouth ventilation on a stranger. When given the option of doing chest compressions only, 68% indicated they would perform CPR on a stranger.[159]

If the airway remains patent during CPR, chest compressions cause substantial air exchange. Early studies in anesthetized, paralyzed humans suggested that the airway would not remain open in the unconscious,[6,7] leading to the teaching that airway control and artificial ventilation must accompany chest compressions. However, there are considerable data to suggest that eliminating mouth-to-mouth ventilation early in the resuscitation of witnessed fibrillatory cardiac arrest is not detrimental to outcome and may improve survival. Data from the Belgian Cardiopulmonary Resuscitation (CPCR) Registry has demonstrated that 14-day survival and neurologic outcome are the same if bystanders initiate full BLS or perform chest compressions only. Both are significantly better than if the bystanders only do mouth-to-mouth ventilation or attempt no CPR.[160,161] A recent Japanese study found better survival in victims who received bystander chest compression–only CPR than in those who received both chest compressions and mouth-to-mouth ventilation from bystanders.[162]

The necessity for ventilation during BLS has been studied in animal models. Since 1993, there have been six studies containing data from 169 swine demonstrating that in prolonged fibrillatory cardiac arrest, neurologically intact survival is the same with chest compression–only resuscitation as with idealized standard CPR (as recommended by the 2000 AHA guidelines[147]), with a 15:2 compression-to-ventilation ratio when compressions are interrupted for only 4 seconds to provide ventilation.[163–166] However, it has been demonstrated that a single lay rescuer interrupts chest compressions for an average of 16 seconds to deliver the two recommended mouth-to-mouth ventilations.[167] When the 15:2 compression-to-ventilation ratio with 16-second pauses for ventilation was tested in the swine model of prolonged fibrillatory arrest, standard CPR resulted in just 13% 24-hour survival compared with 73% in animals receiving chest compressions only.[168]

Recognizing the deleterious effects of prolonged pauses in chest compressions for ventilation, the 2005 AHA guidelines changed the compression-to-ventilation ratio from 15:2 to 30:2, recommending that ventilation be done in 2 to 4 seconds. When the 30:2 ratio with a more realistic 16-second pause for ventilations is compared with continuous chest compressions without ventilation in the animal model, the 24-hour neurologically normal survival is only 42% in the 30:2 group compared with 70% in the continuous compressions group.[169]

Based on these studies, the Save Hearts in Arizona Registry and Education (SHARE) program began a public education program stressing immediate call to 911 and continuous chest compressions without ventilation in the case of witnessed unexpected sudden collapse in adults. The major advantage of this program is that lay individuals can be taught chest-compression-only CPR in a very short period with excellent retention. In Arizona between 2005 and 2009, the rate of bystander CPR increased from 28% to 40%, the rate of chest compression only CPR among bystanders increased from 20% to 76%, and rate of survival to hospital discharge during those years was 7.8% for those receiving standard CPR and 13.3% for those receiving chest compression–only CPR.[170] The importance of minimizing interruptions in chest compressions was emphasized in a science advisory by the AHA recommending "hands-only CPR" for the lay public.[171] For well-trained health-care providers operating within an organized EMS system, a randomized controlled trial of continuous chest compressions at 100/min with asynchronous ventilations at 10/min versus 30 compressions followed by a 5-second pause for two ventilations found no difference in survival or favorable neurologic function between the groups.[172]

Advanced Life Support

Recognizing that dysrhythmic arrest is most common in adults and the importance of establishing blood flow, the most recent AHA guidelines have recommended that CPR be initiated in the unresponsive individual with chest compressions before any attempt at ventilation when a single rescuer is present.[29] The principle of not interrupting chest compressions in order to maintain cerebral and myocardial perfusion applies to resuscitation attempts by health-care providers as well as lay bystanders. The adverse hemodynamic consequences of interrupting chest compressions have been well documented.[173] Blood flow stops almost immediately with cessation of chest compressions and returns slowly when they are resumed. Several compressions are necessary before perfusion pressures return to the levels obtained before compressions were stopped. This is particularly true for prolonged, repeated pauses for ventilation. But it is also relevant for the many other interruptions that occur during resuscitation: pulse checks, rhythm analysis, charging the defibrillator, stacked shocks, intubation, patient assessment, and intravenous line placement. Recent reports have documented that paramedics spend only about half the time during a resuscitation doing chest compressions, mostly because they are following the standard guidelines.[21,174]

Consequently it must be emphasized that chest compressions are to be paused only when absolutely necessary, and then for the shortest time possible. Intravenous line placement should not require cessation of chest compressions. Pulse checks occur only during pauses for rhythm analysis. Initial airway management may consist of insertion of an oropharyngeal airway and providing oxygen by mask with rescue breaths, assisted ventilation or intubation delayed until return of spontaneous circulation or until at least three cycles of compressions–rhythm analysis–shock are complete. A second rescuer's priorities should be obtaining intravenous access, delivering drugs, and relieving the individual giving chest compressions. If there are time and resources for airway management, ventilation and intubation are encouraged to take place while chest compressions continue.

Once ventilation begins, rescuers must be aware of the potentially deleterious effects of positive-pressure ventilation.[175,176] Positive-pressure ventilation increases intrathoracic pressure, reducing venous return, cardiac output, and coronary perfusion pressure and adversely affecting survival. These effects are amplified by the fact that physicians and paramedics often ventilate at rates that are many times the recommended 10 breaths per minute, even after extensive retraining.[174–177]

Rhythm Analysis and Defibrillation

As mentioned previously, after 4 to 5 minutes of VF, the myocardium is so depleted of high-energy phosphates that development of a normal contractile state is difficult, if not impossible. Therefore, immediate defibrillation during the circulatory phase is counterproductive, usually producing either asystole or PEA. In Seattle, it was noted that patients who had CPR prior to defibrillation had a better survival, and the improvement was accounted for by better results in the group of patients in whom the response time was greater than 4 minutes.[178] In a randomized trial of 200 out-of-hospital cardiac arrests in Oslo, there was a highly significant improvement in outcome if CPR was provided before defibrillation when the response time was greater than 5 minutes.[179] Consequently, resuscitation should be initiated with 200 continuous chest compressions at a rate of 100 per minute unless bystanders are already providing good chest compressions. Rhythm analysis and defibrillation, if indicated, follow. Pulse checks are done only during the period of rhythm analysis.

The interruption caused by stacked defibrillatory shocks was discussed previously. When combined with time for rhythm analysis and postshock pulse checks, this interruption may be unacceptably long or even fatal when an AED is in use instead of an experienced clinician interpreting the rhythm with a manual defibrillator.[180,181] The success rate of a single shock is between 70% and 85% with most monophasic waveform defibrillators and more than 90% with the newer biphasic waveform units. Despite this success, the postshock pulse check detects a pulse in only 2.5% of the victims. Recognizing these concerns, the current AHA guidelines recommend a single shock at 360 J for monophasic defibrillators and at the manufacturer's recommended power for biphasic units, with immediate resumption of 200 chest compressions before the next pulse/rhythm check.

In prolonged VF arrest, successful defibrillation almost always results in asystole or PEA, as indicated by the extremely small number of victims with a pulse following shocks. In fact, the standard laboratory model for PEA is prolonged VF followed by defibrillation, all without chest compressions. Immediately restarting chest compressions after defibrillation to provide coronary perfusion nearly always results in reversion to a perfusing rhythm. This certainly suggests that the best chance for restoration of spontaneous circulation following defibrillation will be by immediately resuming chest compressions without waiting to check a pulse or reanalyze the ECG rhythm.

Attention to the quality of CPR and minimizing interruptions in chest compressions has led to significant improvements in survival from cardiac arrest over the past decade. In rural Rock and Walworth counties in Wisconsin, in the 3 years preceding a change, there were 92 witnessed out-of-hospital adult cardiac arrests with an initially shockable rhythm; 18 of these victims survived and 14 (15%) were neurologically intact. In the first 3 years of applying a minimal-interruption approach in these counties, there were 89 witnessed out-of-hospital cardiac arrests; 42 (47%) of these patients survived and 35 (39%) were neurologically intact.[182] In two large metropolitan Arizona cities after institution of minimally interrupted cardiac resuscitation by the EMS, the rate of survival nearly tripled.[183] Among the 886 patients, survival to hospital discharge increased from 1.8% to 5.4%, and in the subgroup of 174 patients with witnessed cardiac arrest with VF, survival increased from 4.7% to 17.6%. These highly statistically significant results are encouraging in that they indicate a significant improvement in outcome from sudden cardiac death is possible.

Pediatric Cardiopulmonary Resuscitation

The principles of CPR discussed previously also apply to the child[13] in cardiac arrest. Arrest is less likely to be a sudden event and more likely related to progressive deterioration of respiratory and circulatory function in the pediatric age group. Airway and ventilation problems lead to asystole and PEA as the most common presenting rhythms. However, the consequences of myocardial and cerebral ischemia are the same as for the adult, and the basic approach to the unresponsive victim is similar. Although the higher incidence of respiratory arrest has led to emphasis on providing rescue breathing in children, the delay in providing ventilation is minimal when starting CPR with chest compressions and this approach is recommended in an unresponsive pulseless child (see AHA's Pediatric cardiac arrest algorithm for the single rescuer at http://bit.ly/2bYpScU and for two or more rescuers at http://bit.ly/2cMLpVH). The specific anatomic and physiologic considerations necessary for the child will be familiar to anesthesiologists. The special circumstance of neonatal resuscitation is discussed in Chapters 41 and 42.

The problem of airway management in the infant is well known to the anesthesiologist. Effective ventilation is especially critical because respiratory problems are frequently the cause for arrest. Mouth-to-mouth or mouth-to-nose and mouth (for infants) can be used as well as bag-valve-mask devices until intubation is possible. Cardiac compression in the infant is provided with two fingers on the midsternum or by encircling the chest with the hands and using the thumbs to provide compression. For the small child, compression can be provided with one hand on the midsternum. For both infants and children, compressions should be at least one-third the depth of the chest at a rate of 100 to 120/min. For a single rescuer, a 30:2 compression-to-ventilation ratio should be used and with two or more rescuers a 15:2 ratio is recommended.

The algorithm for pulseless arrest in the child is shown in Figure 58-4. Although defibrillation is less frequently necessary in

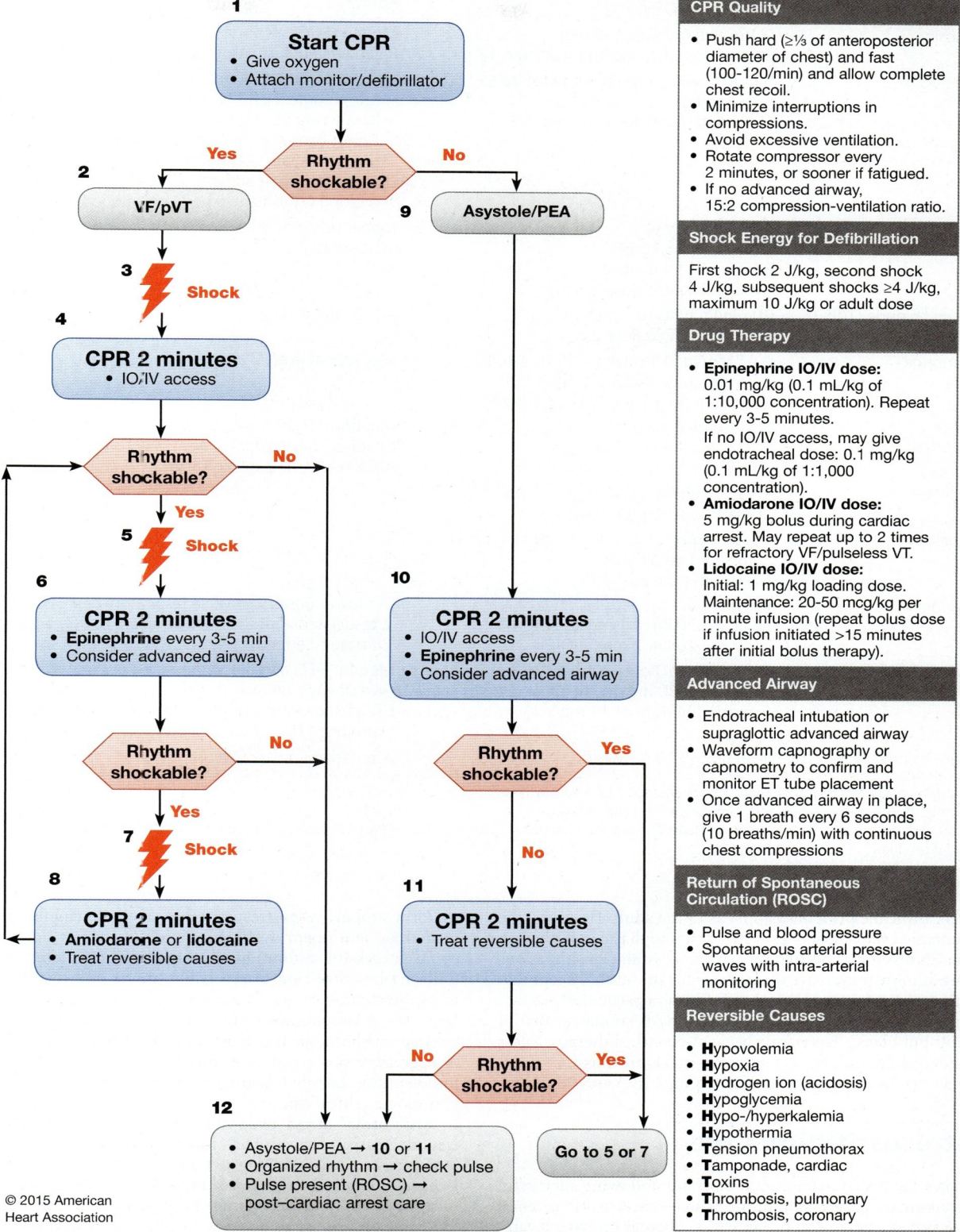

Figure 58-4 Pediatric advanced life support cardiac arrest algorithm. CPR, cardiopulmonary resuscitation; VF, ventricular fibrillation; VT, ventricular tachycardia; PEA, pulseless electrical activity; IV, intravenous(ly); IO, intraosseous(ly); J, joules. Reprinted with permission. 2015 American Heart Association Guidelines for CPR & ECC—Part 12: Pediatric Advanced Life Support. ©2015 American Heart Association, Inc.

Table 58-3 Medications for Pediatric Resuscitation

Drug	Dose	Remarks
Adenosine	0.1 mg/kg (maximum 6 mg) Second dose: 0.2 mg/kg (maximum 12 mg)	Monitor ECG Rapid IV/IO bolus with flush
Amiodarone	5 mg/kg IV/IO; may repeat twice up to 15 mg/kg Maximum single dose 300 mg	Monitor ECG and blood pressure; adjust administration rate to urgency (IV push during cardiac arrest, more slowly over 20–60 minutes with perfusing rhythm). Expert consultation strongly recommended prior to use when patient has a perfusing rhythm. Use caution when administering with other drugs that prolong QT (obtain expert consultation).
Atropine	0.02 mg/kg IV/IO 0.04–0.06 mg/kg ET[a] Repeat once if needed Maximum single dose 0.5 mg	Higher doses may be given with organophosphate poisoning
Calcium chloride (10%)	20 mg/kg IV/IO (0.2 mL/kg) Maximum single dose 2 g	Administer slowly
Epinephrine	0.01 mg/kg (0.1 mL/kg 1:10,000) IV/IO 0.01 mg/kg (0.1 mL/kg 1:1,000) ET[a] Maximum dose 1 mg IV/IO; 2.5 mg ET	May repeat every 3–5 min
Glucose	0.5–1.0 g/kg IV/IO	Newborn: 5–10 mL/kg $D_{10}W$ Children: 2–4 mL/kg $D_{25}W$ Adolescents: 1–2 mL/kg $D_{50}W$
Lidocaine	Bolus: 1 mg/kg IV/IO Infusion: 20–50 µg/kg/min	—
Magnesium sulfate	25–50 mg/kg IV/IO over 10–20 min; faster in torsades de pointes Maximum dose 2 g	—
Naloxone	Full reversal: ≤5 yr or ≤20 kg: 0.1 mg/kg IV/IO/ET[a] ≥5 yr or >20 kg: 2 mg IV/IO/ET[a]	Use lower doses to reverse respiratory depression associated with therapeutic opioid use (1–5 µg/kg titrate to effect)
Procainamide	15 mg/kg IV/IO over 30 to 60 min Adult dose: 20 mg/min IV infusion up to total maximum dose of 17 mg/kg	Monitor ECG and blood pressure Give slowly over 30–60 min Use caution when administering with other drugs that prolong QT
Sodium bicarbonate	1 mEq/kg IV/IO slowly	After adequate ventilation

ECG, electrocardiogram; IV, intravenous; IO, intraosseous; ET, endotracheal.
[a]Flush with 5 mL of normal saline and follow with five ventilations.
Reprinted with permission. 2015 American Heart Association Guidelines for CPR & ECC—Part 13: Neonatal Resuscitation ©2015 American Heart Association, Inc.

children, the same principles apply as in the adult. However, the recommended starting energy is 2 J/kg (monophasic or biphasic), which is doubled if defibrillation is unsuccessful. Considerations for drug administration are the same as for the adult, except that the interosseous route in the anterior tibia is a particularly attractive option in small children. Drug therapy is similar to that of the adult but plays a larger role because electrical therapy is less often needed (Table 58-3). The pediatric algorithms for bradycardia and tachycardia are shown in Figures 58-5 and 58-6.

Postresuscitation Care

The major factors contributing to mortality following successful resuscitation are progression of the primary disease and cerebral damage suffered as a result of the arrest. There is growing awareness that many potentially useful interventions during active CPR may not result in improved survival because of the lack of uniform supportive postresuscitation care, allowing progression to multisystem organ dysfunction and death. For optimal outcome, successful restoration of spontaneous circulation must be followed by correction of reversible causes of arrest, including immediate coronary reperfusion and aggressive supportive care (Fig. 58-7). Patients with successful restoration of spontaneous circulation should be transported to a facility with the capability of aggressive postarrest care, including percutaneous coronary intervention, targeted temperature management (TTM), and neurologic critical care.

Any cardiac arrest, even of brief duration, causes a generalized decrease in myocardial function similar to the regional hypokinesis seen following periods of regional ischemia. This is usually referred to as *global myocardial stunning* and can be mitigated with inotropic agents, if necessary. Active management following resuscitation appears to mitigate postischemic brain damage and improve neurologic outcomes. Although a significant number of patients have severe neurologic deficits following

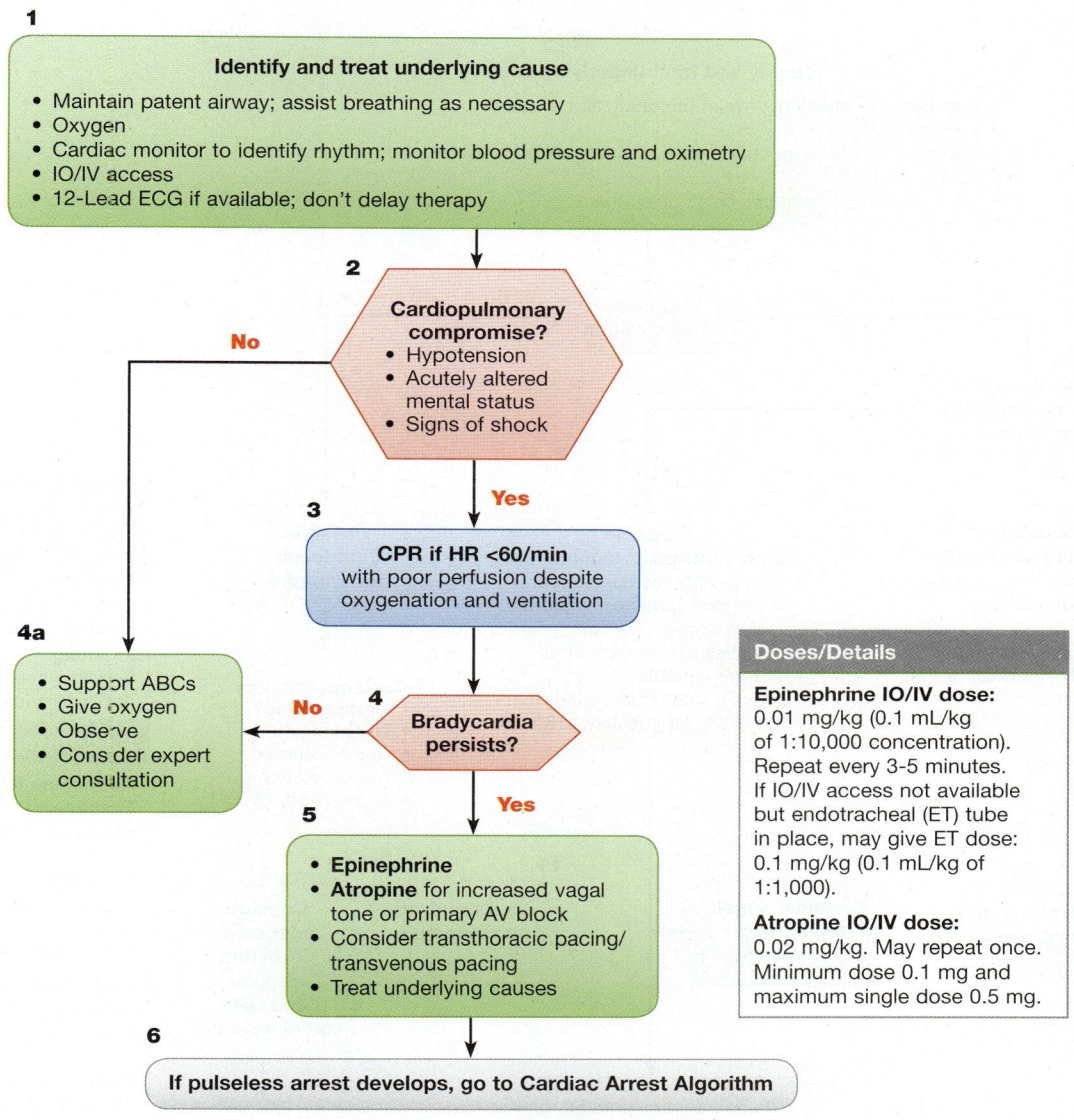

Figure 58-5 Pediatric advanced life support bradycardia (with pulse and poor perfusion) algorithm. ABCs, airway, breathing, and circulation; ECG, electrocardiogram; CPR, cardiopulmonary resuscitation; HR, heart rate; IV, intravenous(ly); IO, intraosseous(ly); AV, atrioventricular. Reprinted with permission. 2015 American Heart Association Guidelines for CPR & ECC—Part 12: Pediatric Advanced Life Support. ©2015 American Heart Association, Inc.

resuscitation, aggressive brain-oriented support does not seem to increase the proportion surviving in vegetative states.[184] Most severely damaged victims die of multisystem failure within 1 to 2 weeks.

When flow is restored following a period of global brain ischemia, three stages of cerebral reperfusion are seen in the ensuing 12 hours. Immediately following resuscitation, there are multifocal areas of the brain with no reflow. Within 1 hour, there is global hyperemia followed quickly by prolonged global hypoperfusion. Elevation of intracranial pressure is unusual following resuscitation from cardiac arrest. However, severe ischemic injury can lead to cerebral edema and increased intracranial pressure in the ensuing days. Nonconvulsive seizures are common postresuscitation with or without therapeutic hypothermia.[185] Continuous or frequent electroencephalography (EEG) for diagnosis of seizure should be performed on comatose patients and treatment instituted if indicated.

Postresuscitation support is focused on providing stable oxygenation and hemodynamics to minimize any further cerebral insult. A comatose patient should be maintained on mechanical ventilation for several hours to ensure adequate oxygenation and ventilation. Restlessness, coughing, or seizure activity should be aggressively treated with appropriate medications, including neuromuscular blockers, if necessary. Oxygen free radicals are a

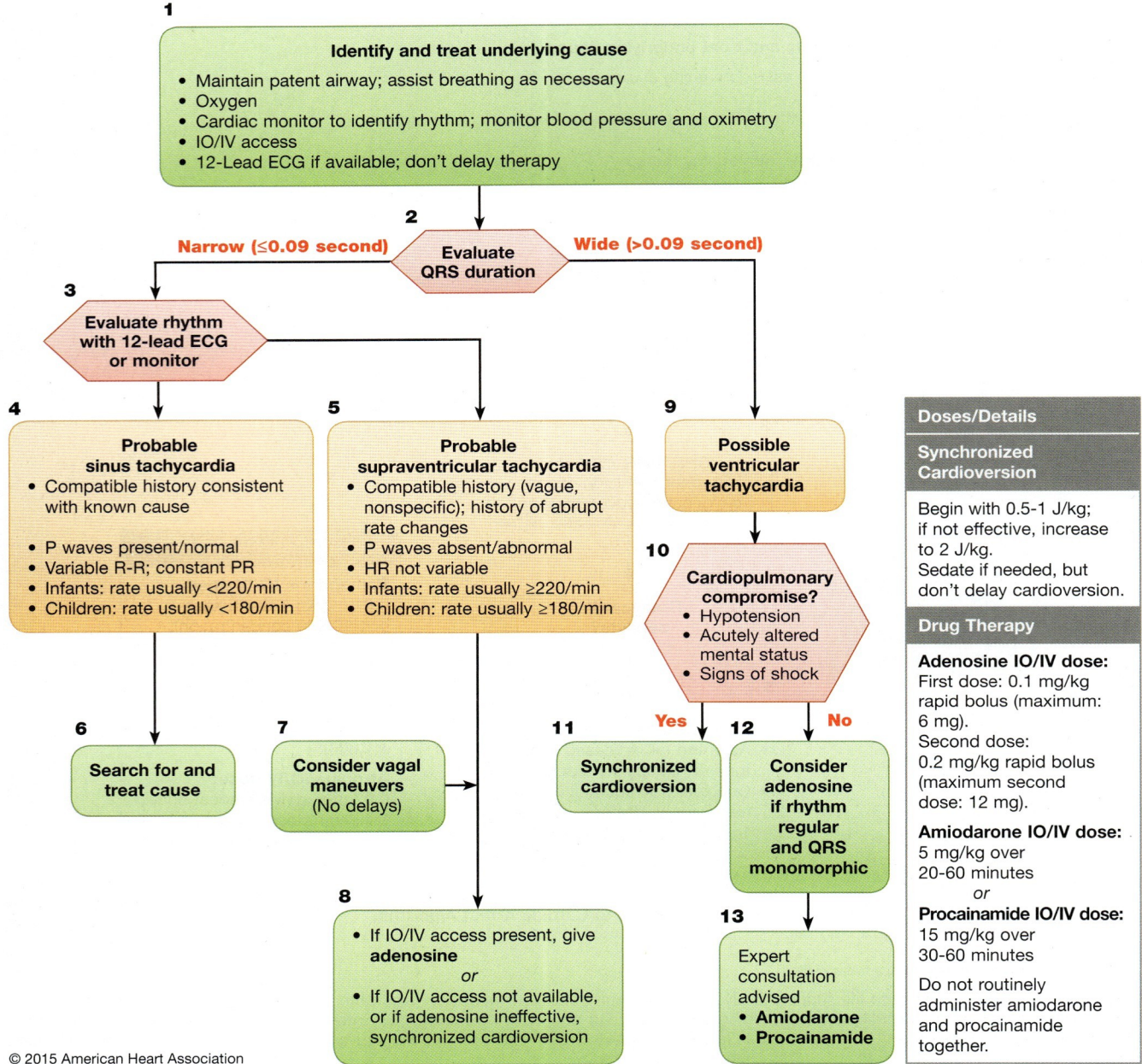

Figure 58-6 Pediatric advanced life support tachycardia (with pulse and poor perfusion) algorithm. ECG, electrocardiogram; HR, heart rate; IV, intravenous(ly); IO, intraosseous(ly); J, joules. Reprinted with permission. 2015 American Heart Association Guidelines for CPR & ECC—Part 12: Pediatric Advanced Life Support. ©2015 American Heart Association, Inc.

major cause of reperfusion injury and postresuscitation hyperoxia may contribute to poor neurologic outcome.[186–188] Following return of spontaneous circulation, inspired oxygen should be titrated to maintain oxygen saturation by pulse oximetry of at least 94% or an arterial PaO_2 above 100 mmHg as soon as possible. Hypocapnia ($PaCO_2$ <30 mmHg) should be avoided. Because cerebral autoregulation of blood flow is severely attenuated after cardiac arrest, both prolonged hypertension and hypotension are associated with a worsened outcome. Therefore, mean arterial pressure should be maintained at 90 to 110 mmHg. Hyperglycemia during cerebral ischemia is known to result in increased neurologic damage. Although it is unknown if high serum glucose in the postresuscitation period influences outcome, it seems prudent to control glucose in the 100 to 150 mg/dL range. Specific pharmacologic therapy directed at brain preservation has not been shown to have further benefit. Some animal trials of barbiturates were promising, but a large multicenter trial of thiopental found no improvement in neurologic status when this drug was

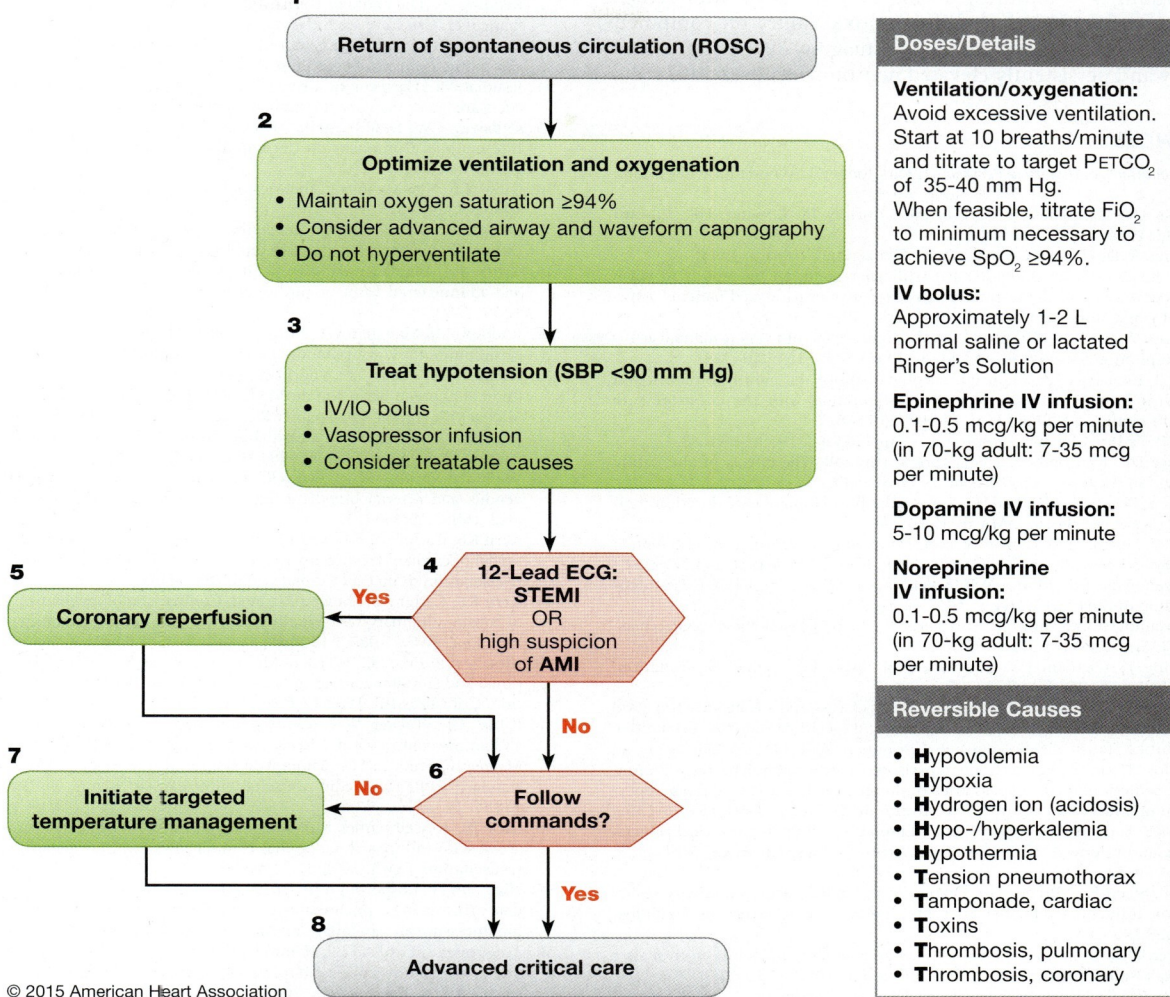

Figure 58-7 Postcardiac arrest care algorithm. SBP, systolic blood pressure; ECG, electrocardiogram; STEMI, ST elevation myocardial infarction; AMI, acute myocardial infarction; PetCO₂, partial pressure of end-tidal carbon dioxide; FiO₂, fraction of inspired oxygen; SpO₂, oxygen saturation by pulse oximetry; IV, intravenous(ly); IO, intraosseous(ly). Reprinted with permission. 2015 American Heart Association Guidelines for CPR & ECC—Part 8: Post-cardiac Arrest Care. ©2015 American Heart Association, Inc.

given following cardiac arrest.[184] Similar results were found with calcium channel blockers. Animal studies were encouraging, but a clinical trial found no improvement in outcome.[189]

In contrast to pharmacologic therapy, three more recent studies have demonstrated improved neurologic outcome with TTM (32° to 36°C) for 12 to 24 hours in cardiac arrest survivors who remained comatose after admission to the hospital.[190–192] The earlier trials used hypothermia and studied only patients whose initial rhythm was VF. A subsequent study found no difference in survival or neurologic outcome with TTM at 33° versus 36°C. These are the first studies to document improved neurologic outcome with a specific postarrest intervention. The International Liaison Committee on Resuscitation now recommends targeted temperature management for unconscious adult patients with return of spontaneous circulation after cardiac arrest at a constant temperature between 32° and 36°C for at least 24 hours.[193]

Prognosis

For the comatose survivor of CPR, the question of ultimate prognosis is important. Most patients who completely recover show rapid improvement in the first 48 hours. Predicting poor neurologic outcome (death or vegetative state) is difficult. It is generally agreed that poor outcome should not be predicted prior to 72 hours after return of spontaneous circulation in patients not undergoing hypothermia and that time should be extended for those receiving hypothermia.[194] At this time point, most comatose patients with a poor outcome have either no response or only extensor posturing to painful stimuli. But the false positive rate (a good outcome when a poor outcome is predicted) for this sign is high. So, decisions should not be made on this basis alone. Confirmatory signs that have nearly a 0% false positive rate are the absence of a pupillary light reflex at 72 hours and absence of the N20 wave on somatosensory evoked potentials at

24 to 72 hours. Less reliable confirmatory signs include unreactive burst suppression or status epilepticus on EEG, status myoclonus (lasting >30 minutes) during first 72 hours after return of spontaneous circulation, diffuse anoxic injury on computed tomography or magnetic resonance imaging of the brain, and markedly and persistently elevated neuron-specific endolase.[195]

REFERENCES

1. *Resuscitation: An Historical Perspective*. Park Ridge, IL: Wood Library Museum; 1976.
2. Brooks DK. *Resuscitation: Care of the Critically Ill*. London, UK: Edward Arnold; 1986.
3. Vesalius A. *De Humani Corporis*. Basel, Switzerland: Fabrica; 1543.
4. Elam JO, Brown ES, Elder JD Jr. Artificial respiration by mouth to mask method: A study of the respiratory gas exchange of paralyzed patients ventilated by operator's expired air. *N Engl J Med*. 1954;250:749–754.
5. Gordon AS, Frye CS, Gittelson L, et al. Mouth-to-mouth versus manual artificial respiration for children and adults. *JAMA*. 1958;167:320–328.
6. Safar P, Escarraga LA, Elam JO. A comparison of the mouth-to-mouth and mouth-to-airway methods of artificial respiration with the chest-pressure arm-lift methods. *N Engl J Med*. 1958;258:671–677.
7. Safar P. Failure of manual respiration. *J Appl Physiol*. 1959;14:84–88.
8. Hooker DR, Kouwenhoven WB, Langworthy OR. The effects of alternating current on the heart. *Am J Physiol*. 1933;103:444.
9. Beck CS, Pritchard WH, Feil HS. Ventricular fibrillation of long duration abolished by electric shock. *JAMA*. 1947;135:985.
10. Zoll PM, Linenthal AJ, Gibson W, et al. Termination of ventricular fibrillation in man by an externally applied electric shock. *N Engl J Med*. 1956;254:727–732.
11. Kouwenhoven WB, Milnor WR, Knickerbocker GG, et al. Closed-chest defibrillation of the heart. *Surgery*. 1957;42:550–561.
12. Kouwenhoven WB, Jude JR, Knickerbocker GG. Closed-chest cardiac massage. *JAMA*. 1960;173:1064–1067.
13. Redding JS, Pearson JW. Evaluation of drugs for cardiac resuscitation. *Anesthesiology*. 1963;24:203–207.
14. Rosamond W, Flegal K, Furie K, et al. Heart disease and stroke statistics 2008 update: a report from the American Heart Association Statistics Committee and Stroke Statistics Subcommittee. *Circulation*. 2008;117:e25–e146.
15. Angelos M, Safar P, Reich H. A comparison of cardiopulmonary resuscitation with cardiopulmonary bypass after prolonged cardiac arrest in dogs: reperfusion pressures and neurologic recovery. *Resuscitation*. 1991;21:121–135.
16. Kern KB, Sanders AB, Janas W, et al. Limitations of open-chest cardiac massage after prolonged, untreated cardiac arrest in dogs. *Ann Emerg Med*. 1991;20:761–767.
17. Wik L, Steen PA, Bircher HB. Quality of bystander cardiopulmonary resuscitation influences outcome after prehospital cardiac arrest. *Resuscitation*. 1994;28:195–203.
18. Weaver WD, Cobb LA, Hallstrom AP, et al. Factors influencing survival after out-of-hospital cardiac arrest. *J Am Coll Cardiol*. 1986;7:752–757.
19. Eisenberg MS, Copass MK, Halstrom AP, et al. Treatment of out-of-hospital cardiac arrest with rapid defibrillation by emergency medical technicians. *N Engl J Med*. 1980;302:1379–1383.
20. Weaver WD, Hill D, Fahrenbruch CE, et al. Use of the automatic external defibrillator in the management of out-of-hospital cardiac arrest. *N Engl J Med*. 1988;319:661–666.
21. Valenzuela TD, Kern KB, Clark LL, et al. Interruptions of chest compressions during emergency medical systems resuscitation. *Circulation*. 2005;112:1259–1265.
22. Nichol G, Stiell IG, Laupacis A, et al. A cumulative meta-analysis of the effectiveness of defibrillator-capable emergency medical services for victims of out-of-hospital cardiac arrest. *Ann Emerg Med*. 2005;46:512–525.
23. Nadkarni VM, Larkin GL, Peberdy MA, et al. First documented rhythm and clinical outcomes from in-hospital cardiac arrest among children and adults. *JAMA*. 2006;295:50–57.
24. Olsson GI, Hallen B. Cardiac arrest during anaesthesia: a computer-aided study of 250,543 anaesthetics. *Acta Anaesthesiol Scand*. 1988;32:653–664.
25. Cohen CB, Cohen PJ. Do-not-resuscitate orders in the operating room. *N Engl J Med*. 1991;325:1879–1882.
26. Walker RM. DNR in the OR. Resuscitation as an operative risk. *JAMA*. 1991;266:2407–2412.
27. Margolis JO, McGrath BJ, Kussin PS, et al. Do no resuscitate (DNR) orders during surgery: Ethical foundations for institutional policies in the United States. *Anesth Analg*. 1995;80:806–809.
28. Guildner CW. Resuscitation–opening the airway: A comparative study of techniques for opening an airway obstructed by the tongue. *JACEP*. 1976;5:588–590.
29. Emergency Cardiac Care Committee, Subcommittees and Task Forces, American Heart Association. 2010 American Heart Association guidelines for cardiopulmonary resuscitation and emergency cardiovascular care. *Circulation*. 2010;122:S640–S946.
30. Heimlich HJ. Pop goes the cafe coronary. *Emerg Med*. 1974;6:154.
31. Guildner CW, Williams D, Subtich T. Airway obstructed by foreign material: the Heimlich maneuver. *JACEP*. 1976;5:675–677.
32. Redding JS. The choking controversy: Critique of evidence on the Heimlich maneuver. *Crit Care Med*. 1979;7:475–479.
33. Harrison RR, Maull KI, Keenan RL, et al. Mouth-to-mask ventilation: a superior method of rescue breathing. *Ann Emerg Med*. 1982;11:74–76.
34. Jesudian MC, Harrison RR, Keenan RL, et al. Bag-valve-mask ventilation: two rescuers are better than one: Preliminary report. *Crit Care Med*. 1985;13:122–123.
35. Callaway CW, Soar J, Aibiki M, et al. Part 4: advanced life support: 2015 International Consensus on Cardiopulmonary Resuscitation and Emergency Cardiovascular.
36. Babbs CF. New versus old theories of blood flow during CPR. *Crit Care Med*. 1980;8:191–195.
37. Jude JR, Kouwenhoven WB, Knickerbocker GG. Cardiac arrest: report of application of external cardiac massage on 118 patients. *JAMA*. 1961;178:1063–1070.
38. Criley JM, Blaufuss AH, Kissel GL. Cough-induced cardiac compression: Self-administered form of cardiopulmonary resuscitation. *JAMA*. 1976;236:1246–1250.
39. Rudikoff MJ, Maughan WL, Effrom M, et al. Mechanisms of blood flow during cardiopulmonary resuscitation. *Circulation*. 1980;61:345–352.
40. Holmes HR, Babbs CF, Voorhees WD, et al. Influence of adrenergic drugs upon vital organ perfusion during CPR. *Crit Care Med*. 1980;8:137–140.
41. Michael JR, Guerci AD, Koehler RC, et al. Mechanisms by which epinephrine augments cerebral and myocardial perfusion during cardiopulmonary resuscitation in dogs. *Circulation*. 1984;69:822–835.
42. Weil MH, Rackow EC, Trevino R, et al. Difference in acid–base state between venous and arterial blood during cardiopulmonary resuscitation. *N Engl J Med*. 1986;315:153–156.
43. Kern KB, Carter AB, Showen RL, et al. Twenty-four-hour survival in a canine model of cardiac arrest comparing three methods of manual cardiopulmonary resuscitation. *J Am Coll Cardiol*. 1986;7:859–867.
44. Kern KB, Carter AB, Showen RL, et al. Comparison of mechanical techniques of cardiopulmonary resuscitation: survival and neurologic outcome in dogs. *Am J Emerg Med*. 1987;5:190–195.
45. Kirscher JP, Fine EG, Weisfeld ML, et al. Comparison of prehospital conventional and simultaneous compression–ventilation cardiopulmonary resuscitation. *Crit Care Med*. 1989;17:1263–1269.
46. Babbs CF, Tacker WA. Cardiopulmonary resuscitation with interposed abdominal compression. *Circulation*. 1986;74(Suppl 4):IV37–IV41.
47. Mateer JF, Stueven HA, Thompson BM, et al. Pre-hospital IAC-CPR versus standard CPR: Paramedic resuscitation of cardiac arrests. *Am J Emerg Med*. 1985;3:143–146.
48. Sack JB, Kesselbrenner MB, Bregman D. Survival from in-hospital cardiac arrest with interposed abdominal counterpulsation during cardiopulmonary resuscitation. *JAMA*. 1992;267:379–385.
49. Niemann JT, Rosborough JP, Criley JM, et al. Circulatory support during cardiac arrest using a pneumatic vest and abdominal binder with simultaneous high pressure airway inflation. *Ann Emerg Med*. 1984;13:767–770.
50. Timerman S, Cardoso LF, Ramires JA, et al. Improved hemodynamic performance with a novel chest compression device during treatment of in-hospital cardiac arrest. *Resuscitation*. 2004;61:273.
51. Wik L, Olsen JA, Persse D, et al. Manual vs. integrated automatic load-distributing band CPR with equal survival after out of hospital cardiac arrest: The randomized CIRC trial. *Resuscitation*. 2014;85:741–748.
52. Steen S, Liao Q, Pierre L, et al. Evaluation of LUCAS, a new device for automatic mechanical compression and active decompression resuscitation. *Resuscitation*. 2002;55:285–299.
53. Lurie KG, Lindo C, Chin J. CPR: The P stands for plumber's helper [letter]. *JAMA*. 1990;264:1661.
54. Cohen TJ, Tucker KJ, Lurie KG, et al. Active compression–decompression: a new method of cardiopulmonary resuscitation. *JAMA*. 1992;267:2916–2913.
55. Linder KH, Pfenniger EG, Lurie KG, et al. Effects of active compression–decompression resuscitation on myocardial and cerebral blood flow in pigs. *Circulation*. 1993;88:1254–1263.
56. Lafuente-Lafuente C, Melero-Bascones M. Active chest compression–decompression for cardiopulmonary resuscitation. *Cochrane Database Syst Rev*. 2004;(3):CD002751.
57. Plaisance P, Lurie KG, Payen D. Inspiratory impedance during active compression–decompression cardiopulmonary resuscitation: a randomized evaluation in patients in cardiac arrest. *Circulation*. 2000;101:989–994.
58. Aufderheide TP, Pirrallo RG, Provo TA, et al. Clinical evaluation of an inspiratory impedance threshold device during standard cardiopulmonary resuscitation in patients with out of hospital cardiac arrest. *Crit Care Med*. 2005;33:734–740.
59. Plaisance P, Lurie KG, Vicaut E, et al. Evaluation of an impedance threshold device in patients receiving active compression–decompression cardiopulmonary resuscitation for out of hospital cardiac arrest. *Resuscitation*. 2004;61:265–271.
60. Aufderheide TP, Nichol G, Rea TD, et al. A trial of an impedance threshold device in out-of-hospital cardiac arrest. *N Engl J Med*. 2011;365:798–806.

61. DeBehnke DJ, Angelos MG, Leasure JE. Comparison of standard external CPR, open-chest CPR, and cardiopulmonary bypass in a canine myocardial infarct model. *Ann Emerg Med.* 1991;20:754–760.
62. Sanders AB, Kern KB, Atlas M, et al. Importance of the duration of inadequate coronary perfusion pressure on resuscitation from cardiac arrest. *J Am Coll Cardiol.* 1985;6:113–118.
63. Kern KB, Sanders AB, Badylak SF, et al. Long term survival with open-chest cardiac massage after ineffective closed-chest compression in a canine preparation. *Circulation.* 1987;75:498–503.
64. Ralston SH, Voorhees WD, Babbs CF. Intrapulmonary epinephrine during prolonged CPR: improved regional blood flow and resuscitation in dogs. *Ann Emerg Med.* 1984;13:79–86.
65. Crile G, Dolley DH. Experimental research into resuscitation of dogs killed by anesthetics and asphyxia. *J Exp Med.* 1906;8:713–725.
66. Redding JS. Abdominal compression in cardiopulmonary resuscitation. *Anesth Analg.* 1971;50:658–675.
67. Pearson JW, Redding JS. Influence of peripheral vascular tone on cardiac resuscitation. *Anesth Analg.* 1965;44:746–752.
68. Yakaitis RW, Otto CW, Blitt CD. Relative importance of alpha and beta adrenergic receptors during resuscitation. *Crit Care Med.* 1979;7:293–296.
69. Otto CW, Yakaitis RW, Blitt CD. Mechanism of action of epinephrine in resuscitation from asphyxial arrest. *Crit Care Med.* 1981;9:321–324.
70. Ditchey RV, Winkler JV, Rhodes CA. Relative lack of coronary blood flow during closed-chest resuscitation in dogs. *Circulation.* 1982;66:297–302.
71. Otto CW, Yakaitis RW. The role of epinephrine in CPR: a reappraisal. *Ann Emerg Med.* 1984;13:840–843.
72. Sanders AB, Ewy GA, Taft TV. Prognostic and therapeutic importance of the aortic diastolic pressure in resuscitation from cardiac arrest. *Crit Care Med.* 1984;12:871–873.
73. Niemann JT, Criley JM, Rosborough JP, et al. Predictive indices of successful cardiac resuscitation after prolonged arrest and experimental cardiopulmonary resuscitation. *Ann Emerg Med.* 1985;14:521–528.
74. Paradis NA, Martin GB, Rivers EP, et al. Coronary perfusion pressure and the return of spontaneous circulation in human cardiopulmonary resuscitation. *JAMA.* 1990;263:1106–1113.
75. Kalenda Z. The capnogram as a guide to the efficacy of cardiac massage. *Resuscitation.* 1978;6:259–263.
76. Weil MH, Bisera J, Trevino RP. Cardiac output and end tidal carbon dioxide. *Crit Care Med.* 1985;13:907–909.
77. Sanders AB, Atlas M, Ewy GA, et al. Expired Pco_2 as an index of coronary perfusion pressure. *Am J Emerg Med.* 1985;3:147–149.
78. Sanders AB, Ewy GA, Fragg S, et al. Expired P_{CO_2} as a prognostic indicator of successful resuscitation from cardiac arrest. *Ann Emerg Med.* 1985;14:948–952.
79. Sanders AB, Kern KB, Otto CW, et al. End-tidal carbon dioxide monitoring during cardiopulmonary resuscitation: a prognostic indicator for survival. *JAMA.* 1989;262:1347–1351.
80. Levine RL, Wayne MA, Miller CC. End-tidal carbon dioxide and outcome of out-of-hospital cardiac arrest. *N Engl J Med.* 1997;337:301–306.
81. Kern KB, Sanders AB, Raife J, et al. A study of chest compression rates during cardiopulmonary resuscitation in humans: the importance of rate-directed compressions. *Arch Intern Med.* 1992;152:145–149.
82. Otto CW. Cardiovascular pharmacology II: The use of catecholamines, pressor agents, digitalis, and corticosteroids in CPR and emergency cardiac care. *Circulation.* 1986;74(Suppl 4):IV80–IV85.
83. Larabee TM. Vasopressors in cardiac arrest: a systematic review. *Resuscitation.* 2012;83:932–939.
84. Redding JS, Pearson JW. Resuscitation from ventricular fibrillation (drug therapy). *JAMA.* 1968;203:255–260.
85. Schleien CL, Dean JM, Koehler RC, et al. Effect of epinephrine on cerebral and myocardial perfusion in an infant animal preparation of cardiopulmonary resuscitation. *Circulation.* 1986;73:809–817.
86. Schleien CL, Koehler RC, Gervais H, et al. Organ blood flow and somatosensory-evoked potentials during and after cardiopulmonary resuscitation with epinephrine or phenylephrine. *Circulation.* 1989;79:1332–1342.
87. Otto CW, Yakaitis RW, Redding JS, et al. Comparison of dopamine, dobutamine, and epinephrine in CPR. *Crit Care Med.* 1981;9:640–643.
88. Lindner KH, Prengel AW, Pfenniger EG, et al. Vasopressin improves vital organ blood flow during closed-chest cardiopulmonary resuscitation in pigs. *Circulation.* 1995;91:215–221.
89. Brillman JC, Sanders AB, Otto CW, et al. A comparison of epinephrine and phenylephrine for resuscitation and neurologic outcome of cardiac arrest in dogs. *Ann Emerg Med.* 1987;16:11–17.
90. Silvast T, Saarnivaara L, Kinnunen A, et al. Comparison of adrenaline and phenylephrine in out-of-hospital CPR: a double-blind study. *Acta Anaesthesiol Scand.* 1985;29:610–613.
91. Linder KH, Ahnefeld FW, Prengel AW. Comparison of standard and high-dose adrenaline in the resuscitation of asystole and electromechanical dissociation. *Acta Anaesthesiol Scand.* 1991;35:253–256.
92. Stiell IB, Hebert PC, Weitzman BN, et al. High-dose epinephrine in adult cardiac arrest. *N Engl J Med.* 1992;327:1045–1050.
93. Brown CG, Martin DP, Pepe PE, et al. A comparison of standard-dose and high-dose epinephrine in cardiac arrest outside the hospital. *N Engl J Med.* 1992;327:1051–1055.
94. Callaham M, Madsen CD, Barton CW, et al. A randomized clinical trial of high-dose epinephrine and norepinephrine vs standard-dose epinephrine in prehospital cardiac arrest. *JAMA.* 1992;268:2667–2672.
95. Choux C, Gueugniaud P-Y, Barbieux A, et al. Standard doses versus repeated high doses of epinephrine in cardiac arrest outside the hospital. *Resuscitation.* 1995;29:3–9.
96. Gueugniaud P-Y, Mols P, Goldstein P, et al. A comparison of repeated high doses and repeated standard doses of epinephrine for cardiac arrest outside the hospital. *N Engl J Med.* 1998;339:1595–1601.
97. Lipman J, Wilson W, Kobilski S, et al. High-dose adrenaline in adult in-hospital asystolic cardiopulmonary resuscitation: a double-blind randomized trial. *Anaesth Intensive Care.* 1993;21:192–196.
98. Sherman BW, Munger MA, Foulke GE, et al. High-dose versus standard-dose epinephrine treatment of cardiac arrest after failure of standard therapy. *Pharmacotherapy.* 1997;17:242–247.
99. Jacobs IG, Finn JC, Jelinek GA, et al. Effect of adrenaline on survival in out-of-hospital cardiac arrest: a randomised double-blind placebo controlled trial. *Resuscitation.* 2011;82:1138–1143.
100. Prengel AW, Lindner KH, Keller A, et al. Cardiovascular function during the postresuscitation phase after cardiac arrest in pigs: a comparison of epinephrine versus vasopressin. *Crit Care Med.* 1996;24:2014–2019.
101. Lindner KH, Dirks B, Strohmenger HU, et al. Randomized comparison of epinephrine and vasopressin in patients with out-of-hospital ventricular fibrillation. *Lancet.* 1997;349:535–537.
102. Stiell IG, Hebert PC, Wells GA, et al. Vasopressin versus epinephrine for in hospital cardiac arrest: a randomized controlled trial. *Lancet.* 2001;358:105–109.
103. Wenzel V, Krismer AC, Arntz HR, et al. A comparison of vasopressin and epinephrine for out-of-hospital cardiopulmonary resuscitation. *N Engl J Med.* 2004;350:105–113.
104. Kowey PR, Levine JH, Herre JM, et al. Randomized, double-blind comparison of intravenous amiodarone and bretylium in the treatment of patients with recurrent hemodynamically destabilizing ventricular tachycardia or fibrillation. *Circulation.* 1995;92:3255–3263.
105. Kudenchuk PJ, Cobb LA, Copass MK, et al. Amiodarone for resuscitation after out of hospital cardiac arrest due to ventricular fibrillation. *N Engl J Med.* 1999;341:871–878.
106. Dorian P, Cass D, Schwartz B, et al. Amiodarone as compared with lidocaine for shock-resistant ventricular fibrillation. *N Engl J Med.* 2002;346:884–890.
107. Stueven HA, Tonsfeldt DJ, Thompson BM, et al. Atropine in asystole: human studies. *Ann Emerg Med.* 1984;13:815–817.
108. Coon GA, Clinton JE, Ruiz E. Use of atropine for brady-asystolic prehospital cardiac arrest. *Ann Emerg Med.* 1981;10:462–467.
109. Guerci AD, Chandra N, Johnson E, et al. Failure of sodium bicarbonate to improve resuscitation from ventricular fibrillation in dogs. *Circulation.* 1986;74(Suppl 4):IV75–IV79.
110. Federiuk CS, Sanders AB, Kern KB, et al. The effect of bicarbonate on resuscitation from cardiac arrest. *Ann Emerg Med.* 1991;20:1173–1177.
111. Bishop RL, Weisfeldt ML. Sodium bicarbonate administration during cardiac arrest: Effect on arterial pH, PCO_2, and osmolality. *JAMA.* 1976;235:506–509.
112. Mattar JA, Weil MH, Shubin H, et al. Cardiac arrest in the critically ill. II. Hyperosmolal states following cardiac arrest. *Am J Med.* 1974;56:162–168.
113. Sanders AB, Otto CW, Kern KB, et al. Acid–base balance in a canine model of cardiac arrest. *Ann Emerg Med.* 1988;17:667–671.
114. Kette F, Weil MH, von Planta MS, et al. Buffer agents do not reverse intra-myocardial acidosis during cardiac resuscitation. *Circulation.* 1990;81:1660–1666.
115. Dembo DH. Calcium in advanced life support. *Crit Care Med.* 1981;9:358–359.
116. Harrison EE, Amey BD. The use of calcium in cardiac resuscitation. *Am J Emerg Med.* 1983;1:267–273.
117. Stueven HA, Thompson BM, Aprahamian C, et al. Use of calcium in prehospital cardiac arrest. *Ann Emerg Med.* 1983;12:136–139.
118. Stueven HA, Thompson BM, Aprahamian C, et al. Calcium chloride: Reassessment of use in asystole. *Ann Emerg Med.* 1984;13:820–822.
119. Stueven HA, Thompson BM, Aprahamian C, et al. Lack of effectiveness of calcium chloride in refractory asystole. *Ann Emerg Med.* 1985;14:630–632.
120. Kerber RE, Sarnat W. Factors influencing the success of ventricular defibrillation in man. *Circulation.* 1979;60:226–230.
121. Yakaitis RW, Ewy GA, Otto CW, et al. Influence of time and therapy on ventricular defibrillation in dogs. *Crit Care Med.* 1980;8:157–163.
122. Weaver WD, Copass MD, Bufi D, et al. Improved neurologic recovery and survival after early defibrillation. *Circulation.* 1984;69:943–948.
123. Weaver WD, Cobb LA, Dennis D, et al. Amplitude of ventricular fibrillation waveform and outcome after cardiac arrest. *Ann Intern Med.* 1985;102:53–55.
124. Ewy GA, Dahl CF, Zimmermann M, et al. Ventricular fibrillation masquerading as ventricular standstill. *Crit Care Med.* 1981;9:841–844.
125. Stewart AJ, Allen JD, Adgey AAJ. Frequency analysis of ventricular fibrillation and resuscitation success. *Q J Med.* 1992;306:761–769.
126. Brown CG, Griffith RF, Ligten PV, et al. Median frequency: a new parameter for predicting defibrillation success rate. *Ann Emerg Med.* 1991;20:787–789.

127. Strohmenger HU, Lindner KH, Brown CG. Analysis of the ventricular fibrillation ECG signal amplitude and frequency parameters as predictors of countershock success in human. *Chest*. 1997;111:584–589.
128. Povoas HP, Weil MH, Tang W, et al. Predicting the success of defibrillation by electrocardiographic analysis. *Resuscitation*. 2002;53:77–82.
129. Stromenger HU, Eftestol T, Sunde K, et al. The predictive value of ventricular fibrillation electrocardiogram signal frequency and amplitude variables in patients with out-of-hospital cardiac arrest. *Anesth Analg*. 2001;93:1428–1433.
130. Otto CW, Yakaitis RW, Ewy GA. Effects of epinephrine on defibrillation in ischemic ventricular fibrillation. *Am J Emerg Med*. 1985;3:285–291.
131. Cummins RO, Eisenberg MS, Bergner L, et al. Sensitivity, accuracy and safety of an automatic external defibrillator: report of a field evaluation. *Lancet*. 1984;1:318–320.
132. Cummins RO, Eisenberg MS, Graves JR, et al. Automatic external defibrillators used by emergency medical technicians: a controlled clinical trial. *Circulation*. 1985;72(Suppl 3):8.
133. Kerber RE, Kouba C, Marines J, et al. Advance prediction of transthoracic impedance in human defibrillation and cardioversion: Importance of impedance in determining the success of low energy shocks. *Circulation*. 1984;70:303–308.
134. Kerber RE, McPherson D, Charbonnier R, et al. Automatic impedance-based energy adjustment for defibrillation: Experimental studies. *Circulation*. 1985; 71:136–140.
135. Lerman BB, DeMarco JP, Haines DE. Current-based versus energy-based ventricular defibrillation: a prospective study. *J Am Coll Cardiol*. 1988;12: 1259–1264.
136. Kerber RE, Grayzel J, Hoyt R, et al. Transthoracic resistance in human defibrillation: Influence of body weight, chest size, serial shocks, paddle size and paddle contact pressure. *Circulation*. 1981;63:676–682.
137. Connel PN, Ewy GA, Dahl CF, et al. Transthoracic impedance to defibrillation discharge: Effect of electrode size and electrode-chest wall interface. *J Electrocardiol*. 1973;6:313–91.
138. Ewy GA, Taren D. Comparison of paddle electrode pastes used for defibrillation. *Heart Lung*. 1977;6:847–850.
139. Ewy GA, Hellman DA, McClung S, et al. Influence of ventilation phase on transthoracic impedance and defibrillation effectiveness. *Crit Care Med*. 1980;8:164–166.
140. Dahl CF, Ewy GA, Warner ED, et al. Myocardial necrosis from direct current countershock. *Circulation*. 1974;50:956–961.
141. Warner ED, Dahl CF, Ewy GA. Myocardial injury from transthoracic defibrillator countershock. *Arch Pathol*. 1975;99:55–59.
142. Ehsani A, Ewy GA, Sobel BE. Effects of electrical countershock on serum creatine phosphokinase (CPK) isoenzyme activity. *Am J Cardiol*. 1976;37: 12–18.
143. Weaver WD, Cobb LA, Copass MK, et al. Ventricular defibrillation: a comparative trial using 175-J and 320-J shocks. *N Engl J Med*. 1982;307:1101–1106.
144. Geddes LA, Tacker WA, Rosborough JP, et al. Electrical dose for ventricular defibrillation of large and small animals using precordial electrodes. *J Clin Invest*. 1974;53:310–319.
145. Gutgesell HP, Tacker WA, Geddes LA, et al. Energy dose for defibrillation in children. *Pediatrics*. 1976;58:898–901.
146. Kerber RE, Jensen SR, Gascho JA, et al. Determinants of defibrillation: Prospective analysis of 183 patients. *Am J Cardiol*. 1983;52:739–745.
147. American Heart Association. Guidelines 2000 for cardiopulmonary resuscitation and emergency cardiovascular care: International Consensus on Science. *Circulation*. 2000;102(8):186–189.
148. Bardy GH, Marchlinski FE, Sharma AD, et al. Multicenter comparison of truncated biphasic shocks and standard damped sine wave monophasic shocks for transthoracic ventricular defibrillation. *Circulation*. 1996;94:2507–2514.
149. Morrison LJ, Henry RM, Ku V, et al. Single-shock defibrillation success in adult cardiac arrest: a systematic review. *Resuscitation*. 2013;84:1480–1486.
150. Hazinski MF, Nolan JP, Aickin R, et al. 2015 International consensus on cardiopulmonary resuscitation and emergency cardiovascular care science with treatment recommendations. *Circulation*. 2015;132(Suppl 1):S1.
151. Rea TD, Eisenberg MS, Becker LJ, et al. Temporal trends in sudden cardiac arrest: A 25-year emergency medical services perspective. *Circulation*. 2003;107:2780–2785.
152. Sanders AB. Cardiac arrest and the limitations of clinical trials. *N Engl J Med*. 2011;365:850–851.
153. Weisfeldt ML, Becker LB. Resuscitation after cardiac arrest: a 3-phase time-sensitive model. *JAMA*. 2002;288:3035–3038.
154. Caffrey SL, Willoughby PJ, Pepe PE, et al. Public use of automated external defibrillators. *N Engl J Med*. 2002;347:1242–1247.
155. Valenzulea TD, Roe DJ, Nichol G, et al. Outcomes of rapid defibrillation by security officers after cardiac arrest in casinos. *N Engl J Med*. 2000;343: 1206–1209.
156. Kern, KB, Garewal HS, Sanders AB, et al. Depletion of myocardial adenosine triphosphate during prolonged untreated ventricular fibrillation: Effect on defibrillation success. *Resuscitation*. 1990;20:221–229.
157. Ornato JP, Hallagan LF, McMahan SB, et al. Attitudes of BCLS instructors about mouth-to-mouth resuscitation during the AIDS epidemic. *Ann Emerg Med*. 1990; 19:151–156.
158. Brenner BE, Kauffman J. Reluctance of internists and medical nurses to perform mouth-to-mouth resuscitation. *Arch Intern Med*. 1993;153:1763–1769.
159. Locke CJ, Berg RA, Sanders AB, et al. Bystander cardiopulmonary resuscitation: concerns about mouth-to-mouth contact. *Arch Intern Med*. 1995;155: 938–943.
160. Bossaert L, Van Hoeyweghen R. The cerebral resuscitation study group: bystander cardiopulmonary resuscitation (CPR) in out-of-hospital cardiac arrest. *Resuscitation*. 1989;17(Suppl):S55–S69.
161. Van Hoeyweghen RJ, Bossaert LL, Mullie A, et al. Quality and efficiency of bystander CPR. *Resuscitation*. 1993;26:47–52.
162. SOS-KANTO study group. Cardiopulmonary resuscitation by bystanders with chest compression only (SOS-KANTO): an observational study. *Lancet*. 2007; 369:920–926.
163. Berg RA, Kern KB, Sanders AB, et al. Bystander cardiopulmonary resuscitation: Is ventilation necessary? *Circulation*. 1993;88:1907–1915.
164. Berg RA, Wilcoxson D, Hilwig RW, et al. The need for ventilatory support during bystander cardiopulmonary resuscitation. *Ann Emerg Med*. 1995;26:342–350.
165. Berg RA, Kern KB, Hilwig RW, et al. Assisted ventilation does not improve outcome in a porcine model of single-rescuer bystander cardiopulmonary resuscitation. *Circulation*. 1997;95:1635–1641.
166. Berg RA, Kern KB, Hilwig RW, et al. Assisted ventilation during 'bystander' CPR in a swine acute myocardial infarction model does not improve outcome. *Circulation*. 1997;96:4364–4371.
167. Assar D, Chamberlain D, Colquhoun M, et al. Randomized controlled trials of staged teaching for basic life support. 1. Skill acquisition at bronze stage. *Resuscitation*. 2000;45:7–15.
168. Kern KB, Hilwig R, Berg RA, et al. Importance of continuous chest compressions during cardiopulmonary resuscitation: improved outcome during a simulated single lay-rescuer scenario. *Circulation*. 2002;105:645–649.
169. Ewy GA, Zuercher M, Hilwig RW, et al. Improved neurological outcome with continuous chest compressions compared with 30:2 compressions-to-ventilations cardiopulmonary resuscitation in a realistic swine model of out-of-hospital cardiac arrest. *Circulation*. 2007;116:2525–2530.
170. Bobrow BJ, Spaite DW, Berg RA, et al. Chest compression-only CPR by lay rescuers and survival from out-of-hospital cardiac arrest. *JAMA*. 2010;304: 1447–1454.
171. Sayre MR, Berg RA, Cave DM, et al. Hands-only (compression-only) cardiopulmonary resuscitation: a call to action for bystander response to adults who experience out-of-hospital sudden cardiac arrest. A science advisory for the public from the American Heart Association Emergency Cardiovascular Care Committee. *Circulation*. 2008;117(16):2162–2167.
172. Nichol G, Leroux B, Wang H, et al. ROC Investigators. Trial of continuous or interrupted chest compressions during CPR. *N Engl J Med*. 2015;373(23): 2203–2214.
173. Berg RA, Sanders AB, Kern KB, et al. Adverse hemodynamic effects of interrupting chest compressions for rescue breathing during cardiopulmonary resuscitation for ventricular fibrillation cardiac arrest. *Circulation*. 2001;104: 2465–2470.
174. Wik L, Kramer-Johansen J, Myklebust H, et al. Quality of cardiopulmonary resuscitation during out-of-hospital cardiac arrest. *JAMA*. 2005;293:299–304.
175. Aufderheide TP, Sigudsson G, Pirrallo RG, et al. Hyperventilation-induced hypotension during cardiopulmonary resuscitation. *Circulation*. 2004;109: 1960–1965.
176. Aufderheide TP, Lurie K. Death by hyperventilation: a common and life-threatening problem during cardiopulmonary resuscitation. *Crit Care Med*. 2004;32(Suppl):S345–S351.
177. Milander MM, Hiscok PS, Sanders AB, et al. Chest compression and ventilation during cardiopulmonary resuscitation: The effects of audible tone guidance. *Acad Emerg Med*. 1995;2:708–713.
178. Cobb LA, Fahrenbruch CE, Walsh TR, et al. Influence of CPR prior to defibrillation in out-of-hospital ventricular fibrillation. *JAMA*. 1999;281:1182–1188.
179. Wik L, Hansen TB, Fylling F, et al. Delaying defibrillation to give basic cardiopulmonary resuscitation to patients with out-of-hospital ventricular fibrillation. *JAMA*. 2003;289:1389–1395.
180. Berg RA, Hilwig RE, Kern KB, et al. Automated external defibrillation versus manual defibrillation for prolonged ventricular fibrillation: lethal delays of chest compressions before and after countershocks. *Ann Emerg Med*. 2003;41:458–467.
181. Rea TD, Shah S, Kudenchuck PJ, et al. Automated external defibrillators: to what extent does the algorithm delay CPR? *Ann Emerg Med*. 2005;46:132–141.
182. Kellum MJ, Kennedy KW, Barney R, et al. Cardiocerebral resuscitation improves neurologically intact survival of patients with out-of-hospital cardiac arrest. *Ann Emerg Med*. 2008;52:253–255.
183. Bobrow BJ, Clark LL, Ewy GA, et al. Minimally interrupted cardiac resuscitation by emergency medical services for out-of-hospital cardiac arrest. *JAMA*. 2008; 299:1158–1165.
184. Abramson NS, Safar P, Detre KM, et al. Randomized clinical study of cardiopulmonary-cerebral resuscitation: Thiopental loading in comatose cardiac arrest survivors. *N Engl J Med*. 1986;314:397.
185. Rittenberger JC, Popescu A, Brenner RP, et al. Frequency and timing of nonconvulsive status epilepticus in comatose post-cardiac arrest subjects treated with hypothermia. *Neurocrit Care*. 2012;16:114–122.

186. Liu Y, Rosenthal RE, Haywood Y, et al. Normoxic ventilation after cardiac arrest reduces oxidation of brain lipids and improves neurological outcome. *Stroke*. 1998;29:1679–1686.
187. Zwemer CF, Whitesall SE, D'Alecy LG. Cardiopulmonary-cerebral resuscitation with 100% oxygen exacerbates neurological dysfunction following nine minutes of normothermic cardiac arrest in dogs. *Resuscitation*. 1994;27:159–170.
188. Lipinski CA, Hicks SD, Callaway CW. Normoxic ventilation during resuscitation and outcome from asphyxial cardiac arrest in rats. *Resuscitation*. 1999;42:221–229.
189. Brain Resuscitation Clinical Trial II study group. A randomized clinical study of a calcium-entry blocker (lidoflazine) in the treatment of comatose survivors of cardiac arrest. *N Engl J Med*. 1991;324:1225–1231.
190. Holzer M; The Hypothermia After Cardiac Arrest Study Group. Mild therapeutic hypothermia to improve the neurologic outcome after cardiac arrest. *N Engl J Med*. 2002;346:549–556.
191. Bernard SA, Gray TW, Buist MD, et al. Treatment of comatose survivors of out-of-hospital cardiac arrest with induced hypothermia. *N Engl J Med*. 2002;346:557–563.
192. Nielsen N, Wetterslev J, Cronberg T, et al. Targeted temperature management at 33°C versus 36°C after cardiac arrest. *N Engl J Med*. 2013;369:2197–2206.
193. Donnino M, Andersen LW, Berg KM, et al. Temperature management after cardiac arrest: An advisory statement by the Advanced Life Support Task Force of the International Liaison Committee on Resuscitation (ILCOR). *Circulation*. 2015;132:2448–2456.
194. Booth CM, Boone RH, Tomlinson G, et al. Is this patient dead, vegetative, or severely neurologically impaired? Assessing outcome for comatose survivors of cardiac arrest. *JAMA*. 2004;291:870–879.
195. Callaway CW, Donnino MW, Fink EL, et al. Part 8: post-cardiac arrest care: 2015 American Heart Association Guidelines Update for Cardiopulmonary Resuscitation and Emergency Cardiovascular Care. *Circulation*. 2015;132 (Suppl 2): S465–S482.

59 Disaster Preparedness

JOSEPH H. McISAAC III • CARIN A. HAGBERG • MICHAEL J. MURRAY

Introduction
Preparation
   Family Plan
   Government Plan
   Health-care Agency Plans
Role of Anesthesiologist in Managing Mass Casualties
   Triage
   Decontamination
   Emergency Department
   Operating Room Management
Chemical
   Nerve Agents
   Pulmonary Agents
   Blood Agents

Biologic
   History
   Smallpox
   Anthrax
   Plague
   Tularemia
   Botulism
   Hemorrhagic Fevers
Radiation—Nuclear
   Potential Sources of Ionizing Radiation Exposure
   Management
Explosives
Conclusion

KEY POINTS

1. There are certain principles that are common to all disaster events, independent of their etiology. As a group, anesthesiologists are well prepared to assist their communities in planning for and in caring for patients who sustain injury or harm from such events.

2. Often overlooked during emergency preparedness and disaster management training is the development of a family plan and a personal preparedness plan. The former is important whether one lives alone; has a pet, family, or friends living with him or her, or has legal responsibility for a loved one (elderly parents, disabled person). A plan should be in place that provides care for and information to loved ones.

3. Anesthesiologists' basic understanding of physiology and pharmacology, airway skills, fluid resuscitation expertise, ability to manage ventilators, and provide anesthesia both in and out of the operating rooms, is invaluable.

4. If assigned to triage patients, the anesthesiologist will be expected to classify patients into four groups: Those requiring immediate care, delayed care, minimal care (first aid), and expectant (no care).

5. If a patient presents with life-threatening injury, the patient is treated first and decontaminated afterward; otherwise all other patients are decontaminated in the triage area before they are evaluated and treated.

6. During a disaster, the anesthesiologist in charge of the schedule for the day should become the operating room medical director, co-locate with the operating room nurse in charge, and determine the status of ongoing cases. Surgeons in the midst of a procedure should be contacted and urged to finish as soon as possible. Elective cases should be postponed or cancelled.

7. In many disasters, infrastructure degradation plays a large part in reducing surgical capabilities at a time when demand is increased. Surgeons and anesthesiologists must consider what types of procedures can safely be undertaken and must prioritize care based on urgency and practicality.

8. There are three categories of biologic weapons. Category A are those weapons that are highly contagious, are associated with a high mortality rate, and have all the characteristics of a relatively ideal weapon of mass destruction.

9. The principle of disaster management following the release of ionizing radiation always involves containment (avoidance of bringing patients with material emitting ionizing radiation to the hospital). Therefore, as part of the containment process, to the extent possible, patients should be decontaminated at the site. Removal of clothing is critically important. β and γ rays and neutrons will no longer be present unless there is still material emitting this radiation on a person's clothing. Rather than guess whether radiation is still present it is best to disrobe patients and wash them with warm soapy water.

10. Orally administered potassium iodide can attenuate most radiation-induced thyroid effects, but must be given as quickly as possible because after 24 hours, there is little protective effect.

11. Because of the possibility of blast, thermal, and crush injuries that may occur along with radiation injury, the care of the injured may require the care of patients who have multiple combined injuries.

12. Patients who have sustained traumatic injury from an improvised explosive device but do not have third-degree burns should receive minimal amounts of intravenous crystalloid and should undergo "damage control resuscitation/surgery" as soon as possible.

13. Infrastructure degradation worsens the consequences of mass casualty events. Preparing to deliver care under austere circumstances, developing creative responses, and practicing (conducting simulations) regularly will mitigate the effects of a disaster and increase resilience for individuals, teams, and institutions.

Introduction

Hurricane Sandy, the Boston Marathon bombing, the Asiana plane crash, the pandemics caused by Ebola and Zika viruses are all events that entered our national consciousness, connoting vivid images of unfortunate circumstances. Although we cannot control, or even predict, the source of the next major disaster in the United States, it is far more likely to be Mother Nature and not an international terrorist who will be the force behind the destruction, but the latter scenario cannot be ignored. We can, however, control our preparedness and, therefore, our response to situations that result in mass casualties. As anesthesiologists, we have a responsibility not only to know our institution's disaster plan and our role therein but also to prepare our family members and ourselves so that we do not become unintended victims of the next disaster, which in turn would result in our unavailability to provide care during a disaster and in our becoming an additional burden to the health-care system.

The World Association for Disaster and Emergency Medicine (WADEM) provides a useful diagram for defining disaster nomenclature (Fig. 59-1).[1] A *mass casualty incident* (≤10 casualties arriving at a hospital simultaneously) typically refers to a situation that creates havoc within the hospital, but in these situations the hospital usually has the resources to manage the number of casualties arriving at its emergency department (ED). A *mass casualty event* (>10 casualties arriving at the ED) is one that has the potential to overwhelm a hospital's ability to respond

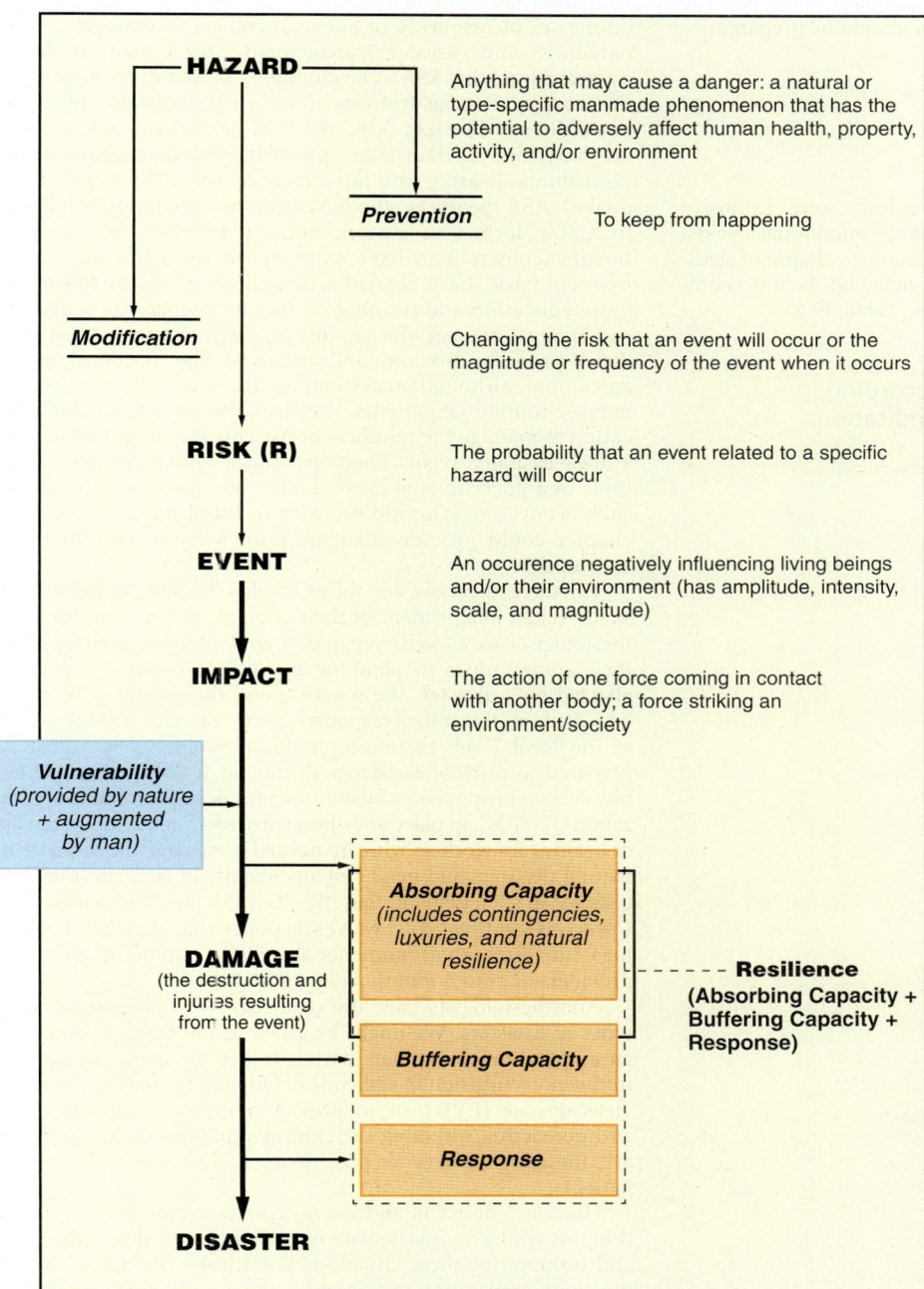

Figure 59-1 Diagrammatic descriptions of definitions. (Adapted from Task Force on Quality Control of Disaster Management, World Association for Disaster and Emergency Medicine, Nordic Society for Disaster Medicine. Health disaster management: guidelines for evaluation and research in the Utstein style. Volume I. Conceptual framework of disasters. *Prehosp Disaster Med*. 2003;17(Suppl). World Association for Disaster and Emergency Medicine website. https://wadem.org/wp-content/uploads/2016/03/intro.pdf.)

effectively. Certainly, the size of the hospital has bearing on how one defines a given situation, as larger hospitals have more resources to manage a larger number of casualties without being overwhelmed. Nonetheless, environmental factors also play a role in how effectively a hospital can respond to a situation. For example, a hospital's physical structure may be so damaged by an earthquake or a tornado that it is rendered inoperable, making it unsafe to provide care to its current patients, much less any new patients. As another example, flooding may result in the facility losing its external and its emergency back-up electrical power supply—making it, for all practical purposes, inoperable.

Mass-casualty incidents and events may result from any number of disasters, most commonly from naturally occurring events, but they may also result from human activity, both intentional and unintentional. The Joint Commission (TJC) lists the most likely disasters for which a hospital should be prepared:
- Air disaster
- Violence/security/active shooter
- Hurricane
- Tornado
- Water crisis
- Winter storm

Chemical, biologic, radiologic, nuclear, and explosive (CBRNE) attacks comprise the most likely intentional events, whereas industrial accidents, vehicle collisions, collapse of stadiums or other public structures, and fires make up the most commonly encountered unintentional events (Table 59-1).

Table 59-1 Types of Disasters According to the Joint Commission on Accreditation of Health-care Organizations

Natural
- **Meteorologic**
  - Hurricanes
  - Tornadoes
  - Floods
  - Mudslides
  - Extreme heat or cold
  - Forest fires
- **Geologic**
  - Earthquakes
  - Tsunamis
  - Volcanic eruptions
  - Lahars
- **Biologic**
  - Bacterial
  - Viral

Resulting from Human Activity
- **Unintentional**
  - Airplane/train/bus crash
  - Boat sinking
  - Fire
  - Nuclear accident
  - Industrial accident
  - Building collapses/sports stadium disaster
- **Intentional**
  - Chemical
  - Biologic
  - Radiologic
  - Nuclear
  - (High-yield) explosive

The first step in any disaster response plan is to mitigate or reduce the risk. The 2015 Sendai Framework lays out a path for international collaboration on disaster risk reduction.[2] The United States is also cognizant of the benefits to its foreign policy by assisting in humanitarian missions. The US Agency for International Development (USAID) spends a significant portion of its budget each year to provide humanitarian assistance in the wake of natural disasters such as floods, volcanic eruptions, and earthquakes. Of significance is that it spends just as much to mitigate the effects of future catastrophes.

The American Society of Anesthesiologists (ASA) recognized the importance of emergency preparedness and in the past decade established a Committee on Trauma and Emergency Preparedness (COTEP) and a Committee on Global Humanitarian Outreach (CGHO). The ASA has an extensive online set of resources to aid its members in emergency preparedness and disaster management.[3] As a member-driven organization, the ASA's development of these resources, for the most part, stems from members' requests to provide assistance during disasters (e.g., the 9-11 terrorist attack, numerous hurricanes and tornados, the 2010 Haitian earthquake, the Fukushima disaster, and most recently the 2015 Nepal earthquake). ASA members who have been involved in relief efforts, including former or current military members and international members who have experienced terrorism on a more frequent basis, have created a cacophony of voices calling for more education and training on how to prepare for a disaster and how to manage the victims of such disasters. Most residency program directors and anesthesiology residents would agree that although anesthesiologists are well prepared to manage individual patients, they lack the knowledge and education to manage the numbers of patients that might arise from a mass casualty event. There are entire books devoted to the topic and governments created large bureaucracies to address such events—so it would be naïve to think that a single book chapter could provide adequate knowledge to cope with all contingencies.

1 However, there are certain principles that are common to all such events, independent of their etiology, and as a group anesthesiologists are as well prepared, if not better prepared, to assist their communities in planning for and in caring for patients affected by a disaster. We must expend the energy to be better educated, as the initial response to any disaster always occurs at the local level; therefore, as anesthesiologists we must be prepared to provide assistance during such emergencies. Other physicians, hospital administrators, and nongovernment organizations (NGOs) all place anesthesia providers at the top of the list of health-care workers who are needed to manage the sequelae of natural disasters and mass casualty events. In fact, anesthesiologists are in such demand that the NGO Doctors Without Borders (*Medecins san Frontieres*) waives its policy that clinicians commit for 9- to 18-month assignments; there is an option for anesthesia providers of 1- to 3-month assignments.[4]

Anesthesiologists have the requisite skills to assist in many types of disasters. We might be asked to provide anesthesia for an amputation to facilitate extrication from rubble, to start an intravenous infusion in someone debilitated by diarrhea or Ebola virus disease (EVD), or to provide ventilatory support to an anthrax victim. Although the clinical situations are not customary, these are services we provide on a daily basis to individual patients.

However, disasters and mass casualty events are not something in which we participate on a daily basis; thus, education and training for these situations is critically important, beginning with preparation to respond to the most likely disasters that may occur in our respective geographic location. Even though natural and industrial disasters have occurred for millennia, the recent increasing use of CBRNE weapons by terrorists emphasizes the need for increased preparedness.

However, time and time again history demonstrates that enthusiasm for education is high after an event and then tapers off; maintaining that enthusiasm is difficult and therefore most, if not all, health-care facilities are not prepared to deal with mass casualty incidents, much less a mass casualty event, the exception being those facilities staffed by physicians with prior military training.[4-7] The majority of physicians most likely have not received adequate education to provide appropriate patient care in such situations. Rössler et al.[8] demonstrated that 24% of anesthesiologists who were deployed during humanitarian crises did not feel sufficiently prepared. Especially important for anesthesiologists who were deployed was the knowledge to repair and maintain anesthesia equipment, to perform peripheral nerve blocks using anatomic landmark techniques, to perform triage of mass casualties, and to treat patients with coexisting tropical disease.

In dealing with acts of terrorism, geography is not helpful in anticipating what might occur, but that is not to say that one cannot anticipate what to expect. One can learn from experience; terrorists have been successful, in their minds' eyes, with improvised explosive devices (IEDs), and even in those situations in which IEDs were not used, terrorists have chosen to use certain weapons of mass destruction (WMDs) more often than others. For example, a nerve agent, such as sarin, is most likely to be chosen as a chemical agent. Similarly, among biologic agents, anthrax, which was used in 2001, or smallpox would be the most likely choice because of the high lethality and infectivity associated with those two agents.[9,10] Twice in the past 20 years "dirty" bombs have either been planned or planted (and fortunately not used), so such devices would be the most likely source of radiation used by terrorists. However, to underscore what was stated here based on past experience, a natural or industrial event is more likely than a terrorist event.

One must also be cognizant that although he or she might never plan to participate in a humanitarian mission overseas and therefore thinks that there is no need to train to work in an austere environment, the environment may become very austere depending on the circumstances of the disaster in which one finds oneself. Any time a situation arises in which medical capability is significantly below standards to which we are accustomed in the United States (US), the anesthesiologist is practicing in an austere environment. This austerity might occur in a:

- Mass casualty event in which the number of cases overwhelms capacity
- Natural disaster in which the hospital is damaged or loses electricity or water
- Disaster (natural/industrial/terrorist) in which care is provided on site.

As described above, graduates of anesthesiology training programs in North America have the potential to cope well in such situations, provided that they understand the basic requisites of disaster management, the focus of this chapter.

Preparation

Family Plan

To manage the numbers of casualties that would be expected during a mass casualty, one must be prepared.[11,12] Often overlooked during emergency preparedness and disaster management training is the development of a family plan and a personal preparedness plan. A family plan is important whether one lives alone; has a pet, family, or friends living with him or her; or has legal responsibility for a loved one (elderly parents, disabled person). There are a number of websites that guide one through the creation of such a plan (Appendix A).[3] During hurricane Katrina, about 35% of policemen and firemen did not show up for work, which should not be surprising.[13] These individuals may have had to evacuate a parent in an assisted living facility or children in a day care center. Just as the military requires service members to have a family care plan (a Will and Last Testament as well!), as critically important health-care providers, we should also have family care plans. However, if you know that you will be unavailable during a disaster, then you have a responsibility to inform your employer or group of your personal situation. All family plans should include periodic family drills and updates. Plans might include situations such as what to do if there is a fire, what to do if parents do not make it home, the location of second copies of all-important documents, where to meet if the house or neighborhood is destroyed or not accessible. Many assume that they will be able to communicate with loved ones during a disaster but often cell phone towers are damaged or so many people are trying to use the system that the network is overwhelmed. Plan in advance so that you are prepared for these contingencies.

Just as service members have a duffel bag or sea bag packed with toiletries, bedding, change of clothes, money, flashlights, and battery-operated radio, those with such important roles as ours ideally should have a packed "bag" as well. In a hurricane, earthquake, flood, tornado, or huge solar flare, loss of electric power is very likely. ATMs, gas pumps, toll booths, and so on do not function without electricity—hence the need for some cash, flashlights, a battery-operated radio (to stay abreast of the news)—and a vehicle that has a fuel tank that is not empty!

Government Plan

In September 2011, the United States Department of Homeland Security published its first edition of a 111-page document, the National Preparedness Goal.[14] Table 59-2 lists the multiple issues for which the Federal Emergency Management Agency (FEMA) must prepare, and with which agencies it must coordinate: the US Departments of Justice, of Health and Human Services, of Agriculture, of Commerce, and of Defense. Of note is that within the "Response" section of the document, medical response is one of eleven types of responses for which the government has planned—a response which is under the auspices of the Department of Health and Human Services (DHHS). DHHS created and maintains a National Disaster Medical System (NDMS). Unfortunately, the system has not been adequately established and maintained. As highlighted by the US response to the earthquake in Haiti in 2010, the DHHS maintains only three International Medical Surgical Response Teams (IMSuRT), teams that were established with the idea that they would provide care to US citizens injured in areas of conflict. Unfortunately, only one is funded and equipped; and, prior to the earthquake in Haiti, it had been activated and used only once—namely, for the earthquake that occurred in 2003 in Bam, Iran. Other teams that DHHS maintains in its NDMS are:

- Disaster Medical Assistance Team (DMAT) is a team that can rapidly mobilize a staff of physicians, nurses, and other support personnel and set up emergency facilities and pharmaceutical dispensaries geographically as close as

Table 59-2 Issues for Which FEMA Must Prepare and Agencies with Which It Must Coordinate

Prevention	Protection	Mitigation	Response	Recovery
Forensics and attribution	Access control and identity verification	Community resilience	Critical transportation	Economic recovery
Intelligence and information sharing	Cybersecurity	Long-term vulnerability reduction	Environmental response/ health and safety	Health and social services
Interdiction and disruption	Intelligence and information sharing	Risk and disaster resilience assessment	Fatality management services	Housing
Screening, search, and detection	Interdiction and disruption	Threats and hazard identification	Infrastructure systems	Infrastructure systems
	Physical protective measures		Mass care services	Natural and cultural resources
	Risk management for protection programs and activities		Mass search and rescue operations	
	Screening, search, and detection		On-scene security and protection	
	Supply chain integrity and security		Operational communications	
			Public and private services and resources	
			Public health and medical services	
			Situational assessment	

possible to a disaster. The teams are self-sustaining for at least 72 hours before they require outside logistics. Just as the reserve military forces do, a DMAT is supposed to train one weekend per month. Not many surgeons and anesthesiologists have joined a DMAT, as the team does not have the capacity to perform surgical procedures!

- Disaster Mortuary Team (DMORT), as the name implies, is a team that manages large numbers of dead bodies following a mass casualty event and that has the capacity to conduct forensic examinations.
- National Veterinary Response Team (NVRT) is a team established to provide veterinary services, as well as zoonotic disease surveillance.

Most recently, the DHHS through its NDMS created an experimental Medical Specialty Enhancement Team (MSET). The MSET consists of a group of precredentialed anesthesiologists and surgeons (30 of each), along with a few pediatricians. The concept is that there would be a pool of specialists who would be activated during a crisis, whether domestic or international, and would have sufficient logistic support to ensure that the team could deploy to either a fixed facility or a field site. Once activated, MSET members would be federal employees during their deployments for a minimum of 2 weeks and would be protected by workers' compensation laws, the federal tort claims act, and the Uniformed Services Employment and Reemployment Rights Act (USERRA). DHHS knows that many anesthesia providers do not have time for monthly drills or frequent call ups that the DMATs have. Although MSET members would be encouraged to train with DMATs, participation in an MSET will require far less of an investment in time. However, if activated, members of the teams would be expected to deploy or risk being dropped from the team and program. The MSET is a work in progress and many of the details of logistics and training are unanswered, the hope being that once successfully established, the size and number of teams could be expanded and the teams better developed. The plan would be for any initial response to be local as such teams might take 2 or 3 days or longer to mobilize and deploy.

Health-care Agency Plans

In recent years, the US has endured several notable events: the anthrax attacks of 2000 and 2001, the destruction of the World Trade Center Towers on September 11, 2001, the SARS epidemic of 2004, and the continued devastation caused by nature (hurricanes, earthquakes, tornadoes, floods, and fires) and terrorists. Subsequently, TJC, the Centers for Medicare and Medicaid Services (CMS), and the American Hospital Association (AHA) have more closely monitored and evaluated hospitals' and communities' emergency preparedness. In 2003, TJC published "Health Care at the Crossroads: Strategies for Creating and Maintaining Community-Wide Emergency Preparedness Systems."[15] The white paper has not been updated, but emergency preparedness is one of the standards TJC uses to certify hospitals. Since 2003, TJC has hosted annual conferences and disseminates information to health-care systems to help them be better prepared. One of TJC's most recent publications, "Requirements for Emergency Management Oversight," attempts to provide a clear description of leadership-level oversight of emergency management in general and critical access hospitals.[16] To ensure that Medicare and Medicaid patients receive appropriate care during a disaster, the CMS has published a checklist that is meant to serve as a guide for health-care facilities to prepare for and to plan for disasters and emergencies.[17] Similarly, the AHA sends advisories to its member hospitals to provide them information on current scourges (e.g., management of patients with EVD or those infected with Zika virus).

Despite the best efforts of law enforcement, fire and rescue teams, and emergency medical agencies, hospitals will continue to play a vital role in helping communities respond to catastrophic events, whether natural, unintentional, or terrorist-initiated. TJC was proactive in recognizing that, "It is no longer sufficient to develop disaster plans and dust them off if a threat appears imminent. Rather a system of preparedness across communities must be in place every day."[15] Such a system is one that is best prepared to handle a surge in casualties or degradation of a facility's ability to handle any new patients following a disaster. The TJC acknowledged this need, despite decreasing health-care resources, for what it describes as "surge capacity" within healthcare systems to handle potentially hundreds, if not thousands or more, of patients who might be victims of catastrophic events. By planning and drilling, the TJC hopes to reduce the appeal to terrorists of using WMD as an effective means of terrorism, and to help communities better respond to natural disasters. The white paper TJC published focused on three major areas:

- Enlisting the community to develop the local response.
- Focusing on the key aspects of the system that prepare the community to mobilize to care for patients, protect its staff, and serve the public.
- Establishing the accountabilities, oversight, leadership, and sustainment of a community-preparedness system.[15]

Although the guidelines are not mandatory or required by law, all hospitals aspire to have TJC accreditation and from that perspective, the white paper was important in that hospitals do have biannual drills of their emergency preparedness and disaster management plans, sometimes coordinating with local law enforcement agencies and health departments and emergency medical response teams, to create as realistic scenarios as possible. Unfortunately, the participation of anesthesiology departments in these drills is often minimal. Drills are usually held on weekdays during working hours, times during which it is often difficult to spare anesthesia providers. Because anesthesiology departments are fully staffed and completely operational during those hours, hospital administrators certify that they can handle the number of casualties coming through their ED. Unfortunately, the drills are not very realistic—for financial reasons, surgical procedures are never delayed or canceled and the system is never tested at night or on weekends. At night, when there are minimal telecommunications personnel in place, how would a hospital mobilize its staff? Many have telephone "trees," but again, because they are not tested, many anesthesia providers have long since misplaced their contact information. Even if tested, how operational would the plan be during a major disaster when communication systems are overwhelmed? Short text messaging would be the best manner for departments to alert personnel to the disaster.

Other advantages to having anesthesiology departments actually participate in drills would be the establishment of trust with liaisons in the emergency response community and with local law enforcement agencies. How much better the outcome would have been if that had been the case in Moscow during the 2002 Nord-Ost siege when the Spetsnaz forces most likely used carfentanil against Chechen rebels without informing emergency response or hospital personnel, resulting in 170 deaths.[18]

Impediments to the establishment of effective response plans are not only financial but also based on a lack of awareness of what occurs during a disaster. As Israelis know from their years of dealing with suicide bombers, and as the Japanese found out during the release of sarin by an Aum Shinrikyo terrorist group in the Tokyo subway system in 1996, victims do NOT go to level I trauma centers, nor do they wait to be transported by emergency medical teams—they fan out in all directions to whatever health-care facility they can find, and they do so on foot, by private vehicles, or by whatever means available.[19]

St. Luke's Hospital in Tokyo found itself inundated with close to 900 patients within 90 minutes after the subway sarin attacks. The ED lobby entrance (almost the entire first floor of the hospital) was crammed with patients, none of whom had been decontaminated. The ensuing chaos was difficult to manage and delayed treatment for those who needed it most. The affected patients required treatment best understood by anesthesiologists who use cholinesterase inhibitors daily and best administered by intravenous lines inserted by these same providers.

Depending on available staff, including how many of the providers will actually respond to a mass casualty event or disaster, there may be insufficient personnel available to cover all rooms in the facility's operating suites. In addition, other areas of the hospital will continue to require coverage, such as the obstetric ward, intensive care, radiology, and endoscopy suites for both disaster-related care and routine emergencies. Creative staffing at higher ratios of coverage may be required to manage patient surges.

Other places anesthesia providers can assist in delivery of health care during a disaster include:

- Triage outside the hospital (who better to manage the pain or labored respiration of the expectant patient?)
- Decontamination (who better to evaluate for the presence of anticholinesterase [nerve] agents or cyanide toxicity?)
- Vascular access or airway management (made more difficult if wearing a hazard material, or HAZMAT, suit and even more difficult if one has never worn such a suit)
- Ventilator management in the intensive care unit (ICU) or in overflow areas of the hospital such as the post-anesthesia care unit (PACU) of patients with respiratory failure caused by a nerve agent or biologic agent

Role of Anesthesiologist in Managing Mass Casualties

It is difficult to anticipate every situation in which anesthesiologists could be requested to assist in managing mass casualty situations. For example, on October 26, 2002, terrorists held 750 hostages at the Nord-Ost Theater in Moscow. Many believe that the authorities instilled nebulized or volatile carfentanil into the air ducts of the opera house, thereby immobilizing the terrorists. Unfortunately, because of the incapacitating effect of the carfentanil, the hostages became victims too. Patients were transported from the theater to hospitals without any treatment prior to arrival. Ideally, anesthesiologists or other health-care providers with an opioid antagonist such as naloxone should have been readily available and present at the site to manage both casualties. Unfortunately, this was not the case.

Anesthesiologists' basic understanding of physiology and pharmacology, airway skills, fluid resuscitation expertise, and ability to manage ventilators and provide anesthesia, both in and out of the operating rooms, is invaluable. In these mass casualty situations, many patients suffer burns, fractures, lacerations, soft tissue trauma, and amputations that will require triage, stabilization in the emergency room or in another facility near the emergency room, and possibly more definitive treatment in the operating room or in the ICU.

During a mass casualty event, an anesthesiologist may well be requested to provide anesthetic services in an area other than the operating room or ICU. He or she will not know where they will be working until they report to the hospital and the command and control center has developed a plan to manage the event.[20] The site of the command and control center is pre-established and outlined in the hospital's emergency preparedness plan, but typically it is within the hospital's ED or in close proximity. Other entrances to the hospital are typically closed during a mass casualty event for the purposes of maintaining control of the numbers of patients that might present and to allow for decontamination of patients, if necessary, avoiding exposure of hospital personnel to contagious agents or transferrable substances, such as nerve agents. The lack of such control and decontamination of the Tokyo subway sarin attack victims in 1995 resulted in a number of health-care workers becoming ill by absorbing sarin from patients who had not been properly decontaminated.[19] Not only were they unable to work but they also became patients themselves, increasing the number of patients requiring care and consuming resources.

Triage

4 If assigned to triage patients, the anesthesiologist will be expected to classify patients into four groups—those requiring immediate care, delayed care, minimal care (first aid only), and expectant (no care, or comfort care only). The latter group includes those expected not to survive, or, because of the number of patients arriving, those for whom there are not adequate personnel or resources to adequately resuscitate without jeopardizing the lives of other patients who would not receive the care they require and for whom the prognosis is more favorable (Fig. 59-2). Experience has taught that initially triage officers are conservative; they try to save as many patients as possible, but over days, if not hours, they gain experience and become better at identifying patients for whom resources exist to improve outcome. In the future, biotechnology may play a role,[21] but at present hospitals must rely on physicians' experience and, again, because of their knowledge of the hospitals resources in both the operating room (OR) and the ICU, they may well be the ideal triage officer. He or she will have to assess and decide if patients fall into one of the four groups. "Expectant" patients are usually transported to an area separate from the ED, where they receive comfort care. Such a site must be situated so that newly arriving patients are not exposed to the sight of dying patients. Anesthesiologists may well be assigned to provide such care because of expertise in managing airways, in establishing intravenous access for the administration of medications, and our familiarity with the available anxiolytic and analgesic medications. As emotionally difficult as the process of identifying or managing patients not expected to survive is the assessment of patients who may have been injured or affected during a disaster but who do not appear to require treatment, yet might require delayed care. Various symptoms may be exhibited, depending on the type of agent, which will direct the appropriate therapy:

- Chemical (nerve) agents: If only headache, meiosis, rhinorrhea, and lacrimation after exposure, patients can be decontaminated (see later) and dismissed. Patients with dyspnea, bronchospasm, or arrhythmias will require treatment with atropine.
- Biologic agents: Fever, rash, dyspnea, cough. Antibiotics, antitoxins, antiviral agents, and supportive care.
- Radiation/nuclear: Nausea within 6 hours of exposure; because of the prevalence for those with this symptom, check leukocyte count, dismiss, and have the patient return in 48

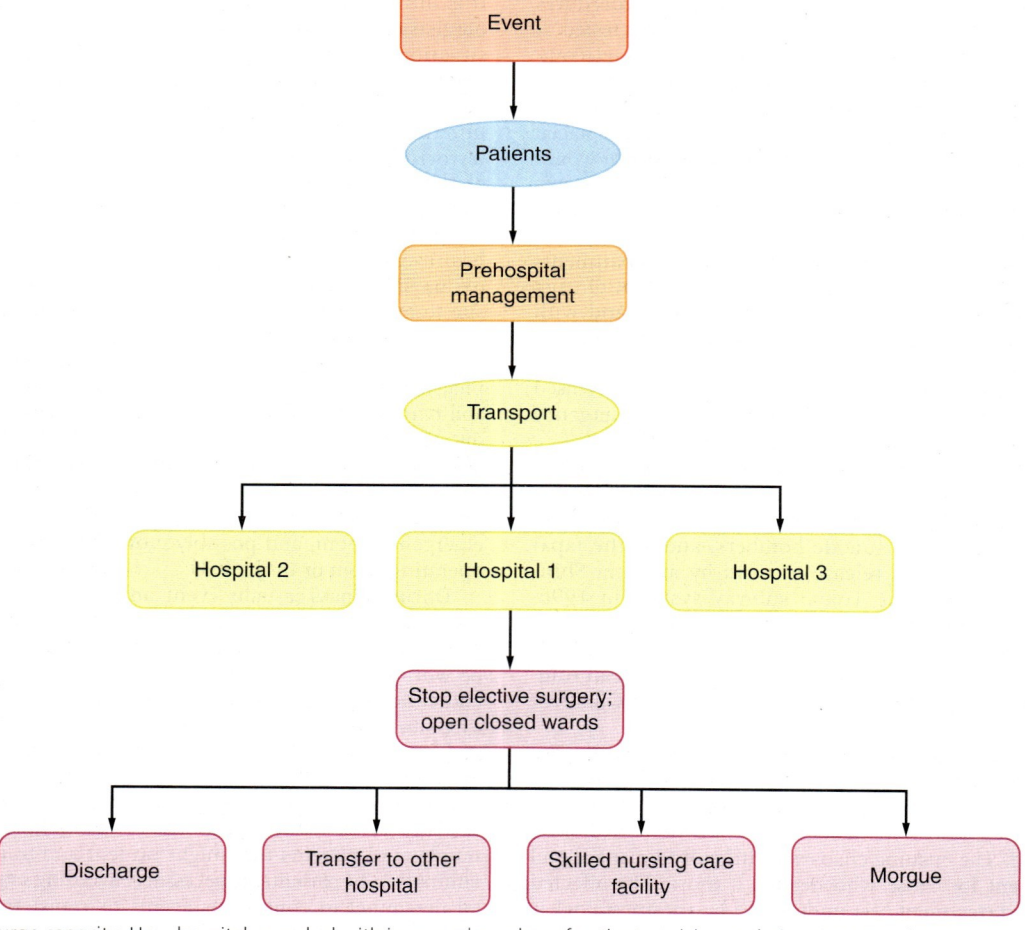

Figure 59-2 Surge capacity: How hospitals can deal with increased number of patients arriving at their emergency departments following a mass casualty event.

hours for repeat check—if no change in count, no therapy is indicated. There are several new therapies in development for mitigation of the effects of radiation exposure.
- Explosive: If tympanic membranes are intact and SpO_2 is within normal limits, other injuries are unlikely.

Decontamination

In most situations, those with proper training decontaminate people in contact with chemical agents or radioactive materials—the decontamination is normally performed first and then patients are evaluated and triaged. The principle is to limit the exposure of the patient to the agent and prevent contamination of caregivers. Off-gassing of some chemical agents can be problematic, especially with large numbers of exposed patients awaiting decontamination. Consideration should be given to providing lightweight "escape hoods" (available from multiple vendors) to reduce respiratory exposure before decontamination can be performed. The decontamination process is usually fairly straightforward; clothes are removed and individuals are washed with copious amounts of water (the contaminated water and apparel can present quite a challenge!); if individuals have been exposed to a chemical agent, a dilute solution of sodium hypochlorite 0.5% (household bleach) can be used.

However, if a patient presents with life-threatening injury, the patient is treated first and decontaminated afterward. Patients with severe chemical agent poisoning may present with acute respiratory failure requiring emergency tracheal intubation. In this scenario, an anesthesiologist would be assigned to the decontamination station. For obvious reasons, the intubation would have to be performed with the anesthesiologist wearing a HAZMAT or a biohazard suit with multiple-layered gloves and a gas mask. The suits are not insulated or cooled and if the decontamination is performed outside the hospital, the extremes of temperature can significantly hinder performance, as does the decreased manual dexterity, because of the gloves and the impairment in vision from the face hoods. Ideally, individuals with prior training would manage the airway intubation, but depending on circumstances, that may not happen. As many have learned from past experience, it is best to anticipate the unexpected, and to be flexible if the maximum numbers of patients are to be saved. Preparation of equipment and drugs before the arrival of contaminated patients decreases the difficulties with manual dexterity that are encountered while wearing the multiple-layered or rubber gloves. Consider securing the airway with a laryngeal mask airway, when indicated, rather than with a tracheal tube. Intraosseous cannulas are often easier to insert than intravenous cannulas when wearing HAZMAT personal protective equipment (PPE).

Emergency Department

Another place where an anesthesiologist might be assigned is the ED. While some level I trauma centers have an anesthesia team assigned to support the ED, many do not. Depending on the types of casualties, but especially for casualties from a violent explosion, anesthesiologists might be assigned to manage the airway and secure central venous access. Anesthesiologists should position themselves at the head of the bed and assume responsibility for the airway and venous access. For the former, it would be ideal to have two or three assistants (one providing in-line C-spine stabilization, another individual applying cricoid pressure, and a third individual administering medications.) Sometimes it is necessary to remind ED physicians and trauma surgeons that "A" (airway) and "B" (breathing) come before "C" (circulation); certainly, the primary and secondary surveys can be conducted during this critical time point but ventilation and oxygenation must be assured. Often, all three can be conducted simultaneously.

In previous industrial accidents and fires, appropriate management of the airway has been critical. Patients with large-area burns will require intravenous access for provision of intravascular volume resuscitation. Depending on the event (burn versus crush injury—protocols for fluid resuscitation vary), in patients with extensive soft tissue and skeletal muscle damage, alkalization of the urine with volume resuscitation and diuresis may be organ and life saving.

Operating Room Management

COTEP developed and published a checklist to assist the anesthesiologist in charge of the operative suite in prioritizing tasks for the management of a mass casualty event (Table 59-3).[3] The first task is to open the facility's operating manual (Environment of Care Manual in TDJ parlance) to the appropriate annex for the disaster, which hopefully will be hospital specific. Next, the disaster call-in tree is activated. Experience has shown that a branching tree of phone numbers is far better than a linear list. The anesthesiologist in charge should become the operating room medical director, co-locate with the operating room nurse in charge, and determine the status of on-going cases. Surgeons in the midst of procedures should be contacted and urged to finish as soon as possible. Elective cases should be postponed or cancelled. A list of available rooms and staff should be rapidly assembled and transmitted to the hospital emergency operations center (HEOC). Determine realistic staffing for the next 0 to 2, 2 to 12, and 12 to 24 hours. Free staff should be directed to set up open rooms to receive trauma patients. Support staff can be directed to resupply (oversupply) locations in anticipation of heavy use. Coordination with the PACU, blood bank, and ICUs will improve patient movement and space availability. It is advisable to send a senior anesthesiologist, especially one with critical care experience, to the ED to act as a liaison between the ED and the OR. This physician should have his or her own dedicated communications link with the operating rooms to transmit timely intelligence on the nature and number of surgical cases anticipated. The liaison can also act as an advisor to the ED. Some larger institutions can consider sending teams to the ED to help with triage and initial management of casualties. If HAZMATS are involved, consideration should be given to appropriate secondary decontamination, isolation techniques, PPE, and antidotes needed.

In many types of disasters, infrastructure degradation plays a large part in reducing surgical capabilities at a time when demand is increased. Surgeons and anesthesiologists must consider what types of procedures can safely be undertaken and must prioritize care based on urgency and practicality. Closed reduction of fractures or external fixation may be the most suitable options, other than amputation, for the orthopedic surgeon. General surgeons may lose the ability to do robotic or laparoscopic intra-abdominal surgery, and many intrathoracic and intracranial procedures will be impractical. Wong et al.[22] showed that burn dressing changes and extensive wound debridements were the most frequent planned surgical procedures after acute trauma. Although early in a mass casualty event, elective procedures are cancelled or delayed, there will be a backlog of patients requiring surgery. Falls, burns, motor vehicle accidents, and childbirth will continue to occur, possibly with increased frequency, depending on the disaster. As the community's infrastructure degrades over time, hygiene and

Table 59-3 Operating Room Procedures for Mass Casualty: Management Step by Step

Objective: To be able to manage the flow of patient care in operating rooms (ORs) during a mass casualty situation.

Steps: Indicate date and time for each item.

- Refer to facility's operations manual.
  Open up appropriate annex.
- Activate call-in tree.
  Assign an individual to activate. Use clerical personnel or automatic paging system, if available.
- Assess status of operating rooms.
  Determine staffing of ORs 0–2, 2–12, and 12–24 hours. Hold elective cases.
- Alert current ORs.
  Finish current surgical procedures as soon as possible and prepare to receive trauma.
- Assign staff.
  Set up for trauma/emergency cases.
- Anesthesia coordinator should become OR medical director.
  Work with OR nursing manager to facilitate communication and coordination of staff and facilities.
- Report OR status to hospital command center (HCC).
  Enter telephone, email address of HCC.
- Ensure adequate supplies.
  Coordinate with anesthesia techs/supply personnel to ensure adequate supplies of fluids, medications, disposables, etc.
- Contact the postanesthesia care unit.
  Accelerate transfer of patients to floors/ICUs in preparation for high volume of cases.
- Anesthesiologist should act as liaison in emergency department (ED).
  Send an experienced practitioner to the ED to act as a liaison (your eyes and ears) and keep communications open to anesthesia coordinator.
- Consider assembly of stat teams.
  Combination of anesthesia, surgical, nursing, respiratory personnel to triage, as needed.
- Hazardous material/weapons of mass destruction event.
  Review special personal protective procedures, such as decontamination and isolation techniques. Consider if part of the OR hallways should be considered "hot" or should have ventilation altered. Good resources include Chemical Hazards Emergency Medical Management and Radiation Emergency Medical Management websites.
- Coordinate with blood bank.
  Verify blood availability.
- Coordinate with other patient care areas.
  Intensive care units, obstetrics, pediatrics, etc. to ensure continuity of care for new and existing patients.

ICU, intensive care unit.
Developed by the Committee on Trauma and Emergency Preparedness.

sanitation becomes a problem. Increased respiratory infections, gastrointestinal (GI) disease, and wound infections are likely to increase. Loss of electrical power, which can result in loss of heating, air conditioning, and water may make it difficult to maintain normal operative and postoperative conditions. Patients may present dehydrated and some authors suggest liberalization of fasting guidelines to reduce intraoperative fluid needs and improve postoperative wound healing.[23]

Chemical

Nerve Agents

Prior to the last century, it was unthinkable that rogue states or terrorists would use chemical agents. During the First World War, more than one million soldiers and civilians were exposed to chemical gas injuries, with over 100,000 of them dying. In 1935, Italy invaded Abyssinia (Ethiopia) and during that invasion, sprayed mustard gas from aircrafts. When Japan invaded China in 1937, mustard, phosgene, and hydrogen cyanide were used. In that same year, German chemical laboratories produced the first nerve agent, tabun. During 1963 to 1967, Egypt used phosgene and mustard agents in support of South Yemen during the civil war in that country. When Iraq attacked Iran in the 1980s, mustard and nerve agents were used. In all these examples, chemical agents were used by the military during armed conflict. The governments mentioned have all signed the Chemical Weapons Convention. January 2012 marked the end of an era as, in compliance with the Chemical Weapons Convention ratified by the Senate in 1997, the US Army Chemical Materials Agency completed destruction of 27,000 tons of chemical weapons that it had manufactured and stored over the years.[24]

However, as one era ended another one had already begun. In 1994 and 1995, the use of the nerve agent sarin by the Japanese cult Aum Shinrikyo was a major turning point, because it was the first time that a terrorist group had used a nerve agent in a terrorist attack. More than 5,000 persons were evaluated at hospitals, approximately 1,000 of whom a had been exposed to the nerve agent, and 18 died. Both sides in the ongoing Syrian Civil War that started in 2013 have used chemical agents, including chlorine, mustard agent, and sarin. The nerve agents are so named because of their mechanism of action. The G series agents (GA, GB, GD, GF) were developed but never used by Germany during 1930s. They are considered nonpersistent, lasting in the environment a few minutes to a few days. The Novichok or V series agents (VE, VG, VM, VR, and VX) were manufactured by the USSR in 1980s. They persist in the environment and are 10 times more toxic that the G agents. VX is the only one ever fielded by the United States.

Similar to organophosphate insecticides and to the anticholinesterase (AChE) drugs that anesthesiologists use daily, nerve agents inhibit AChE. This inhibition results in excessive amounts of acetylcholine (the reason why a cholinergic agent such as atropine or glycopyrrolate is administered anytime we inject an AChE, such as neostigmine) at preganglionic muscarinic and postganglionic muscarinic and nicotinic receptors, leading to copious secretions, meiosis, arrhythmias, bronchospasm, tonic muscle contractions, respiratory paralysis, seizures, and death. A cholinergic agent and competitive muscarinic blocker (i.e., atropine or glycopyrrolate) is administered to attenuate and block the muscarinic side effects of the agents.

When anticipating a nerve agent attack, US military personnel pretreat themselves with low-dose pyridostigmine and don PPE; the latter prevents the agent from contacting and wetting skin from which it is readily absorbed, and low-dose pyridostigmine binds to AChE, preventing any nerve agent that is absorbed from binding to the enzyme. Pyridostigmine is a reversible drug that will be metabolized over time, whereas the nerve agents bind to AChE irreversibly.

US military personnel carry syringes of atropine and of pralidoxime chloride (2-PAM-CL), an oxime that reactivates AChE by removing the nerve agent from its binding site on the enzyme.

Spontaneous reactivation of enzyme complex is variable, which partly accounts for differences in acute toxicity between the nerve agents. 2-PAM-CL is administered to reactivate the dialkyl-phosphonyl AChE enzyme more quickly.[25] The most optimistic estimates are that after exposure 30 minutes will elapse before casualties are transported to EDs, the diagnosis of nerve agent attack is made, and the oxime can be administered. Thirty minutes is optimistic, given that there have been deaths at chemical weapons manufacturing facilities within 2 minutes of accidental exposure. Toxicity of the nerve agents is not just related to which agent, but also to the dose of agent to which one is exposed, and also the duration of exposure. However, if numbers of casualties arrive at a triage site outside a hospital ED, the sooner one administers an oxime, such as 2-PAM-CL, obidoxime, or HI-6, the better. Most of the nerve agents can be reversed with the exception of soman. With soman, aging of AChE occurs so fast that an oxime will have no effect. Even though aging occurs more slowly and reactivation occurs relatively rapidly in the case of nerve agents other than soman, early oxime administration is still clinically important in patients poisoned with these agents. Experimental studies on the treatment of nerve agent poisoning have to be interpreted with caution. Some studies have used prophylactic protocols, whereas the drugs concerned (atropine, oxime) would be given only to a civilian population after exposure. The experimental use of pyridostigmine before nerve agent exposure, although rational, is not of relevance in the civilian context. With the possible exception of the treatment of cyclosarin (GF) and soman poisoning, a review of available experimental evidence suggests that there are no clinically important differences between the different oximes in the treatment of nerve agent poisoning, if studies employing pretreatment with pyridostigmine are excluded.[25]

Diagnosis

Patients exposed to a nerve agent, either ingested, inhaled, or via the transdermal route. present with evidence of muscarinic site stimulation: airway, pupillary, and GI tract constriction; bradycardia; and activation of the glands within the eyes, nose, mouth, and sweat glands manifested by intense lacrimation, rhinorrhea, salivation, and sweating. The degree of exposure correlates with the amount of secretions produced. Nicotinic stimulation at preganglionic sites leads to tachycardia and hypertension, and at the nicotinic acetylcholine receptor on the neuromuscular junction, fasciculation, twitching, fatigue, and flaccid paralysis. The excessive parasympathetic activity leads to meiosis and loss of accommodation so that patients complain of blurred vision. Within the respiratory system, the increased parasympathetic activity leads to bronchorrhea and bronchoconstriction, which together with the respiratory muscle fatigue initially manifests as coughing, wheezing, and shortness of breath. The agent on the skin will produce localized sweating and fasciculation obvious to the naked eye. Within the cardiovascular system, activity within the muscarinic system leads to bradycardia, but depending on the degree of nicotinic activity in the preganglionic nodes, a patient's heart rate may be low, normal, or high. Within the GI tract, the increased parasympathetic activity leads to nausea, vomiting, diarrhea, and incontinence. This overall unopposed parasympathetic activity leads to a pneumonic of "DUMBBELS" (*d*iarrhea, *u*rination, *m*iosis, *b*ronchorrhea and *b*ronchoconstriction, *e*mesis, *l*acrimation, and *s*alivation).

Treatment

The toxicity of the nerve agents depends on the compound delivered, the dose that is delivered (LC), and the time (t) that an individual is exposed to that dose. For example, a patient exposed to 10 mg/m^3 of an agent for 10 minutes would have an LCt of 100 mg/min/m^3. The same could be achieved by being exposed to a concentration of 100 mg/m^3 for only 1 minute. The treatment for nerve agent poisoning is one with which every anesthesiologist is familiar. Atropine is a competitive muscarinic blocker. Pralidoxime chloride is the better long-term treatment as it reactivates AChE by removing the organophosphate compound. Atropine is administered at a dose of 2 to 6 mg or more and repeated every 5 to 10 minutes until secretions begin to decrease (i.e., until the patient is no longer salivating) and ventilation is improved. In severe casualties, 15 to 20 mg would not be unusual and some casualties have required gram amounts of atropine. The US military travels with automatic injectors containing 2 mg of atropine and 600 mg of 2-PAM-CL.

Depending on the extent of exposure, treatment differs. For minimal exposure, often seen with brief exposure to nerve agent vapor, patients may complain of headache and tightness in the chest and manifest meiosis, rhinorrhea, and salivation. Individuals must be removed from further exposure, clothing removed, topical atropine applied to the eye if pain is significant, and wet decontamination must be performed if there was any liquid exposure. With moderate exposure, the same signs are present, but the patient demonstrates more severe rhinorrhea, complains of dyspnea, and on examination, there is evidence of bronchospasm and muscle fasciculation. Patients with moderate (and severe) poisoning require treatment with atropine and 2-PAM-CL intramuscularly. Casualties again must have their clothing removed and if they were exposed to liquid nerve agent, they need to go through a wet decontamination process. With severe exposure, the same symptoms as mentioned above are present, but now the patient manifests severe respiratory compromise, flaccid paralysis, incontinence, arrhythmias, and convulsions. After decontamination the patient will require repetitive doses of intravenous atropine, along with intramuscular 2-PAM-CL, intravenous (IV) benzodiazepines to treat the seizures (caused by the muscarinic effects of the nerve agents within the central nervous system [CNS][26]), and intubation and mechanical ventilation, depending on the degree of respiratory compromise.

With nerve injury casualties, decontamination is critical. It needs to be done as quickly as possible, first by leaving the area of exposure. As commented at the beginning of this chapter, health care and emergency workers in Japan became victims themselves by standing unprotected in the subway cars in which there was sarin.[19] Patients are decontaminated by removing their clothing and washing with copious amounts of water and 0.5% hypochlorite (dilute household bleach). The bleach is not as critical as washing with copious amounts of water. Depending on the number of casualties, EDs may coordinate with the fire department. For example, they might arrange fire trucks side-by-side with a "chamber" established between the two trucks in which individuals can disrobe and be sprayed with water as they walk through the chamber. From there, depending upon the severity of the symptoms, they would receive atropine, 2-PAM-CL, and further treatment.

Pulmonary Agents

The so-called pulmonary agents are, by nature, gases at room temperature, and almost any gas could be considered a pulmonary agent if released in sufficient quantity in a closed environment to displace oxygen, thereby causing exposed subjects to die by asphyxiation. Chlorine and phosgene are considered the classic pulmonary agents and the two most likely to be used by terrorists. If quantities are released that are sufficient to displace oxygen, then death results from asphyxia. In addition, these two gases are extremely toxic to the lungs; individuals who survive the acute exposure if they have inhaled even small amounts often develop acute lung injury or acute respiratory distress syndrome (ARDS). However, the treatment is no different from what a critical care anesthesiologist would provide in managing a patient with Silo Filler's Disease or Farmer's Lung, which develops after exposure to nitrogen dioxide when a farm worker opens or enters a silo that has inadequate ventilation. The treatment of the resulting noncardiogenic pulmonary edema from NO_2 or the pulmonary agents is supportive: mechanical ventilation using small tidal volumes (6 to 8 mL/kg), peak airway pressures (<30 cm H_2O), positive end expiratory pressure, and inspired oxygen concentrations of 50% to 60% or less.

Blood Agents

The third and final class of chemical toxins includes the blood agents—hydrogen cyanide and cyanogen chloride. Because of the instability of the latter, hydrogen cyanide is more likely to be used by terrorists in a closed environment as an aerosol. Again, anesthesiologists are familiar with this class of substances because of our clinical use of sodium nitroprusside as an intravascular vasodilator, which has cyanide as a metabolite. Cyanide inhibits cellular respiration by interrupting the oxidative electron transfer process in mitochondria. The treatment for cyanide toxicity is similar to what anesthesiologists would do for a patient who had an accidental overdose of sodium nitroprusside: Intravenous thiosulfate and supportive care, including tracheal intubation, ventilation with 100% oxygen, and inotropes and vasopressors to stabilize the cardiovascular system.

Biologic

History

This section includes a discussion that considers the naturally occurring infectious agents, as well as those agents most likely to be used by terrorists. Many of the latter caused plagues in the past or were used as weapons. Infectious organisms have been used as biologic weapons since the dawn of history. Ghengis Khan is reported to have used cats infected with fleas bearing the plague to destroy towns in his conquest of Asia. In the 1770s, British forces distributed blankets that harbored smallpox virus to American Indians, killing more than 50% of the infected tribes. In World War II, Unit 731, a Japanese military unit, is reported to have dropped plague-infected fleas over populated areas of China, causing outbreaks of plague and killing several hundred thousand people.[27]

The ideal biologic agent is one that has the greatest potential for adverse public health consequences, generating mass casualties, and with potential for easy large-scale dissemination that could cause mass hysteria and civil disruption. Such a weapon should be relatively easy to produce, inexpensive, highly infectious, and contagious, resulting in widespread morbidity and mortality. To be effective, there should be little or no natural immunity, which is currently the case with diseases such as smallpox for which we no longer routinely vaccinate individuals, except in the military and in high-risk public health areas. There are three categories of biologic weapons (Table 59-4). Category A includes weapons that are highly contagious, that

Table 59-4 Biologic Agents Used for Warfare

Category A: Highly contagious and fit all the characteristics of a relatively ideal biologic agent
Bacillus anthracis (anthrax)
Variola major (smallpox)
Yersinia pestis (plague)
Clostridium botulinum (botulism)
Francisella tularensis (tularemia)
Viral hemorrhagic fever (Ebola, Lassa, Marburg, Argentine)
Category B: Relatively easy to disseminate but have low mortality rates
Coxiella burnetii (Q fever)
Vibrio cholerae (cholera)
Burkholderia mallei (glanders)
Enteric pathogens (*E. coli* 0157:H7, *Salmonella, Shigella*)
Cholera, cryptosporidium
Various encephalitic viruses
Various biologic toxins
Category C: Emerging pathogens that might be engineered for biologic warfare
Various equine encephalitic viruses

are associated with a high mortality rate, and that have all the characteristics of a relatively ideal weapon of mass destruction.

Smallpox

The last case of naturally occurring smallpox in the world was reported in 1977 in Somalia.[28] In 1978, two laboratory workers were infected with the disease in the United Kingdom.[28] In 1980, the World Health Organization (WHO) announced that the world was free of this scourge. Terrorists might consider using smallpox as a weapon because an increasing number of people no longer carry immunity. Routine vaccination for smallpox is no longer performed, except in the military and for some public health-care workers considered at high risk of contracting the disease (individuals whom the government would rely on to staff vaccination stations if there were a breakout).[28] Forty to eighty percent of patients exposed to the smallpox virus will become infected with the disease. Smallpox is highly infective, requiring only 10 to 100 organisms to infect an individual. The mortality rate is approximately 30% in unvaccinated patients and as high as 50% if smallpox occurs in communities that have no native immunity against smallpox. The protective effect of the smallpox vaccine decreases with time, but even at 20 years, the vaccine would provide some protection.

When an unvaccinated person is initially infected, she or he develops a prodrome of malaise, headache, and backache, with the onset of fever to as high as 40°C. The fever decreases over the next 3 or 4 days, at which time a rash develops. This progression is in contradistinction to chickenpox, in which the rash develops at the same time as the fever. Unlike chickenpox, smallpox has a predilection for the distal extremities and face, though no part of the body is spared. Also, all lesions in a patient with smallpox are at the same stage, whereas with chickenpox, lesions are at multiple different stages: papules, vesicles, pustules, and scabs. Most cases of smallpox are transmitted through aerosolized droplets that are inhaled, but clothes and blankets that have come in contact with pustules, until the scab falls off, are infectious; the organism can be transmitted in these linens.

Smallpox has probably been present in humans since 10,000 BC. It is transmitted human to human, and if used as a bioterrorism agent, would likely be dispersed by aerosols in the environment with the hope that multiple humans would be infected and would transmit the virus to other humans. There is evidence that the former Soviet Union developed transgenic smallpox viruses that are very infectious and for which the US vaccine may not be completely protective. The time of onset after exposure to such a virus might be very short. Currently there are only two WHO-approved depositories of smallpox, at the Centers for Disease Control and Prevention (CDC) in Atlanta, Georgia, and at the Institute of Virus Preparations in Russia. With the collapse of the Soviet Union, there was a concern that some stores of smallpox made it into rogue countries that may have developed their own biologic weapons.

A look at how the WHO eradicated smallpox might be helpful in understanding how the United States has prepared to respond to smallpox as a biologic weapon. In the eighteenth century, 400,000 Europeans a year were dying from smallpox. Though only 1% of patients who survive smallpox become blind, it accounted for one-third of all cases of blindness in Europe. The WHO eradicated smallpox by identifying patients with smallpox and placing them in strict quarantine. Such patients are readily identified because of the presence of smallpox lesions on the face. Patients were quarantined and all their contacts were vaccinated, because there was a 3- to 7-day window with the naturally occurring virus before the patient developed symptoms and signs of smallpox.[29]

Vaccination against smallpox is controversial. The vaccine is made from a live vaccinia virus developed in calf lymph, but is not an attenuated smallpox virus itself. Smallpox is a member of the Orthodox genus of the poxviridae family of double-stranded deoxyribonucleic acid (DNA) viruses that also contain cowpox, monkey pox, and vaccinia. In the event of a documented case of smallpox, the CDC plans to quarantine the patient and immediate patient contacts within a certain geographic area would be vaccinated. There are stockpiles of vaccines placed strategically throughout the United States just for such an event. A bifurcated needle is dipped into the reconstituted vaccine and then 10 to 15 points of entry are made into the dermis of the upper deltoid. Because of the side effects of smallpox vaccinations, people with immunologic disorders, eczema (active or with a history of severe eczema), and pregnant or nursing women should not receive the vaccine. The CDC monitors for adverse side effects of vaccination; most are not serious, such as fever, rash, and malaise, although two cases of cardiomyopathy have been reported.[30] There is no plan to vaccinate the entire US population following an isolated case.

Many obstacles have been overcome to develop second- and third-generation smallpox vaccines. Before 2001, the vaccine that was used, Dryvax (similar to what Jenner used in the 18th century), contained live attenuated virus and was the reason that immunocompromised individuals developed adverse events when vaccinated. From 2001 to the present, Acambis Modified Vaccinia Ankara (ACAM) has been used to vaccinate against smallpox. Dryvax and ACAM are fairly similar, though the latter may be a little safer to use than Dryvax, but not so much safer than when immunocompromised individuals are offered the vaccine. To avoid the dangers of a live vaccine, an inactive vaccine (modified vaccinia Ankara [MVA; Imvamune]) was developed[31]; the United States has a contract to purchase 20 million doses. The available evidence is that even immunocompromised individuals, such as those with HIV infection, might tolerate immunization. The CDC and the states' departments of health will implement their quarantine and vaccination plans should an index case or cluster cases occur.

Anthrax

Bacillus anthracis (anthrax) was probably used as a biologic weapon in the Middle Ages, when troops laying siege to a town would catapult infected animal carcasses over the ramparts into the inhabited areas. For reasons discussed later, this method was not a particularly effective method of infecting the native population. During the twentieth century, several countries, including the United States, Great Britain, Russia, and Iraq, studied ways to "weaponize" anthrax. Normally, if anthrax spores are inhaled, they clump in the nasal pharynx. To be weaponized, *B. anthracis* must be finely ground so that it readily aerosolizes and can get to and deposit in the terminal bronchioles and alveoli.[32] Inhalation anthrax, which was relatively uncommon in the past, has an 80% fatality rate. One of the letters that was mailed in the anthrax attacks of 2001 contained 2 g of weapons-grade anthrax. With a median lethal dose (LD_{50}) of 1,000 spores, under optimal conditions, this was enough material to infect 50 million individuals. In a terrorist attack, for maximum effect, anthrax could be aerosolized and sprayed from airplanes or delivered through a dispersion device mounted on top of a missile. The attacks on North America in 2001 and the accidental release of spores at a biologic facility in the city of Sverdlovsk in the former Soviet Union in 1979 are illustrative of the potential of anthrax as a weapon. In the United States, 5 of 11 cases resulted in death (45% mortality rate); in the former Soviet Union, 66 of 77 died (86% mortality rate).[33] The Aum Shinrikyo also released anthrax spores in Tokyo in 1993. Fortunately, they used a nonpathogenic strain of anthrax and so there were no casualties.[32] As demonstrated in 2001 in the United States, terrorists are sophisticated enough that they might be successful in obtaining and releasing weapons-grade anthrax. Such attacks, even if detected early,[34] would create mass hysteria and greatly affect the entire country and world.[35]

Anthrax is a gram-positive, spore-forming bacillus that is transmitted to humans from contaminated animals, their byproducts, or carcasses. Spores may persist in soil for years. The disease is all but gone from North America, but is still prevalent in many developing countries, and herbivores, especially cattle, usually die within 24 to 48 hours of contracting the disease. The carcass has such a large number of organisms, that humans, who are relatively resistant to infection, can be exposed and contract the disease.[36]

There are three primary types of anthrax infection: Cutaneous, inhalation, and GI. Ninety-five percent of cases are cutaneous. From a public health perspective, inhalation anthrax is most concerning, as it usually affects 2,000 to 20,000 people worldwide per annum. People can be exposed through contact with animals in an agricultural or industrial setting (i.e., a rendering plant or tanning facility, or, as mentioned previously, in the production of biologic weapons).[37]

Anthrax has additional appeal to bioterrorists because inhalation anthrax is difficult to detect. It manifests as an influenza-like disease with fever, myalgias, malaise, and a nonproductive cough with or without chest pain.[38] After a few days, the patient appears to get better, but then a couple of days later the patient becomes much more ill with dyspnea, cyanosis, hemoptysis, stridor, and chest pain. The most notable finding on physical examination and laboratory testing is a widened mediastinum. Usually when a patient develops profound dyspnea, death ensues within 1 to 2 days. In the past, penicillin G was the treatment of choice, but since weaponized anthrax has been engineered to be resistant to penicillin G, ciprofloxacin or doxycycline is more commonly used. In the outbreaks in Florida, Washington DC, and New Jersey, contacts of infected patients or people exposed to the spores were treated with ciprofloxacin or doxycycline. A more recent study concluded that this drug regimen is the best strategy for managing a small-scale attack, as occurred in 2001.[39]

Plague

The oldest cases of *Yersinia pestis* (bubonic plague) were documented in China in the third century. *Y. pestis* has been thought to be the etiologic agent in multiple epidemics and three pandemics, the first of which was during the Roman emperor Justinian's reign; the second pandemic was during the 14th century—the Black Death—and killed one-third of the population of Europe; and the last was at the end of the 19th century and killed millions in China and India.[40] The first documented use of plague as a biologic weapon was in 1346 when the Tartars in their siege of the fortress at Kaffa catapulted infected corpses into the city.[27] The plague was used by Unit 731 to infect large areas of China, and as many as 200,000 Chinese may have died. More recently, the United States and Russia have studied *Y. pestis* as a bioagent, examining ways to aerosolize and ways to distribute the bacillus. Surprisingly, the organism is only viable for approximately 60 minutes after being distributed; if dispersed by an airplane, its viability would limit its infectivity for only 10 km from the dispersion site.

Y. pestis is a nonmotile, gram-positive bacillus. Rodents and fleas are its natural hosts, and they re-infect each other by fleas biting infected rodents. Soil can be contaminated and therefore rodents can acquire the disease simply by digging in an infected area. Humans are an accidental host and they usually acquire the disease from a fleabite, though rarely there can be direct inoculation of infected material into a person. Direct person-to-person transmission occurs with pneumonic plague.

There are two types of plague: Bubonic and pneumonic. With bubonic plague, after a fleabite, there is a 2- to 6-day incubation period, at which time there is the sudden onset of fever, chills, weakness, and headache. Intense painful swelling occurs in the lymph nodes, usually in the groin, axilla, or neck. These swellings or buboes are typically oval in nature, 1 to 10 cm in diameter, and extremely tender. Up to 25% of patients will have pustules, papules, or skin lesions near these buboes. Without treatment, patients become septic, develop septic shock with cyanosis and gangrene in peripheral tissues, leading to the "black death" descriptor that was used during the pandemics in Europe. As mentioned, material from these buboes is infective only if inoculated into human tissue. However, patients who have bubonic plague can seed their lungs, in which case they develop pneumonic plague. During coughing, they aerosolize *Y. pestis*, which is highly contagious. Mortality for either form of the disease is above 50%. Diagnosis is made with a Gram stain or culture of organisms from blood, sputum, or buboes. The treatment of choice is streptomycin, but chloramphenicol and tetracycline are acceptable alternatives. Patients with pneumonic plague should be managed as one would manage a patient with drug resistance to tuberculosis, because the respiratory secretions are highly infectious. There is currently no vaccine against *Y. pestis*.

Tularemia

Francisella tularensis (tularemia) has some similarities to anthrax and plague, but is not nearly as dangerous. It was studied as a biologic weapon in the twentieth century because it is highly infectious, requiring an inoculum of perhaps as small as only ten organisms.[41] During World War II, tularemia developed in soldiers along the German-Russian front and was thought secondary to the use of *F. tularensis* as a biologic weapon. The fact that both armies were infected underscores one of the dangers of using infectious agents as biologic weapons. Often these are dispersed with aerosols, and despite the best predictions of air currents, they are notoriously unpredictable; with the shifting air currents, one's own troops could become infected. Unit 731 of the Japanese army also studied the use of *F. tularensis* as a biologic weapon, and the United States and Russia were known to have grown large quantities of *F. tularensis*.

F. tularensis is a gram-negative, pleomorphic rod. There are several animal hosts, with the cotton-tailed rabbit being one of the most susceptible. Normally, humans acquire *tularensis* through direct contact of an infected animal or from the bite of an infected tick or deerfly.[41] Occasionally, the ingestion of infected food or inhalation of a small amount of aerosol will initiate the disease. There are two strains of *F. tularensis*, Jellison A and B, with the B strain being relatively innocuous; in North America the A strain is quite virulent. Normally, a patient will develop a cutaneous ulcer at the site of entry after contact with an animal. As few as 10 or 50 organisms can invade the body through either hair follicles or mini abrasions. The incubation period is 2 to 6 days, at which time there is swelling and ulceration at the site of entry. As the swelling continues, the skin eventually breaks, creating an ulcer, which develops a necrotic base that becomes black as it scars. It is likely that *F. tularensis* would be delivered as an aerosol from an airplane, in which case, following inhalation, there is a 3- to 5-day incubation period, and then the onset of disease is marked with fever, pharyngitis, bronchitis, pneumonia, pleuritis, and hilar lymphadenopathy. Mortality rate for pneumonic tularemia is 5% to 15%.

The treatment of choice for tularemia is streptomycin, though gentamicin, tetracycline, and chloramphenicol have been used. There is concern that the former Soviet Union, perhaps the United States, and perhaps terrorists have engineered *F. tularensis* to be resistant to a number of agents. Prophylaxis with streptomycin, ciprofloxacin, or doxycycline has been recommended in the past for individuals exposed to the organism. There was a vaccine comprised of an attenuated whole organism strain, but it is no longer available.

Botulism

The first known work with *Clostridium botulinum* (botulism) as a biologic weapon was in World War II. Both the Germans and Japanese military and scientific communities experimented with *C. botulinum*. Unit 731 fed pure cultures of *C. botulinum* to Chinese captives with devastating effects. Both the United States and former Soviet Union are known to have produced large quantities of *C. botulinum* toxin, as have Iraq, Iran, Syria, and North Korea. In fact, after the first Gulf War, Iraq admitted to having over 19,000 L of concentrated botulism toxin, of which almost half was loaded on military weapons.[42] Nineteen thousand liters of botulinum toxin is enough to kill the world's population three times over! More recently, Aum Shinrikyo, the cult in Japan, dispersed aerosols of botulinum toxin on three different occasions in Japan. Fortunately, their dispersal methods were associated with multiple problems and no one was injured. Of concern is that a terrorist organization working with a rogue state could acquire and use botulinum as a bioterrorist weapon.

Botulism manifests as neuroparalysis caused by the toxin from *C. botulinum*. Unlike all the other biologic weapons mentioned previously, it is not caused by a live organism and, therefore, is not contagious. The organism from which botulinum toxin is derived is a gram-positive spore, which is an obligatory anaerobe, widely distributed in soil and in marine and agricultural products. Humans ingest C. botulinum without apparent effects until the organism begins to release toxins, of which there are several. Toxins are distributed from the GI tract, or from the lungs if inhaled, in the bloodstream to cholinergic nerve endings, where they block the release of acetylcholine at muscarinic and nicotinic receptors by inhibiting the intracellular fusion of the vesicles containing acetylcholine to nerve terminal membrane for release into the synaptic cleft. This mechanism is the exact opposite of the chemical nerve agents such as sarin, which result in an increase in the amount of acetylcholine at the cholinergic receptors, but the end result is the same. Patients develop a progressive weakness and a flaccid paralysis that begins in the extremities and progress until the respiratory muscles cease to contract. Of note, C. botulinum toxin is the most potent poison known to humans; the LD_{100} dose is only 1 pg.[43]

Shortly after ingestion or inhalation of the toxin, the incubation period is between 2 hours and 8 days, but most commonly between 12 and 36 hours.[44] As muscles become weak, patients develop diplopia, dysphonia, dysarthria, dysphagia, and eventually dyspnea and finally paralysis. Along with the effects noted within the skeletal muscle system caused by the lack of acetylcholine at the nicotinic receptor, muscarinic blockade results in decreased salivation, ileus, and urinary retention, again the opposite of what is seen with nerve agent poisoning.

Toxins can be removed through gastric lavage, use of cathartics, and with enemas. The treatment of patients includes the use of a trivalent antitoxin. Patients with profound respiratory embarrassment should have their airways protected and mechanical ventilation initiated. Without the use of antitoxin, it takes the patient 2 to 8 weeks to recover. The mortality rate is quoted as 5% to 10%.

Hemorrhagic Fevers

There are a number of viral hemorrhagic fevers that are listed as category A agents, including the arena viruses (Lassa fever and others), bunya viruses (hanta), flaviviruses (Dengue), and filoviruses (Ebola and Marburg). There are at least 18 viruses that cause human hemorrhagic fevers, which form a special group of viruses characterized by viral replication in lymphoid cells, after which patients develop fever and myalgia with an incubation of anywhere from 2 to 18 days, depending on the agent itself and the amount that is inhaled or inoculated across the dermis. They encompass syndromes that vary from febrile hemorrhagic fever with edema to septic shock, which rapidly leads to death. Both the United States and the former Soviet Union have experimented and have weaponized several of these viruses. Studies in nonhuman primates suggest that the agents are highly infectious, requiring only a few virions to produce illness.[44] The Aum Shinrikyo cult in Japan went to Africa in the 1990s to try to obtain an Ebola virus, which they planned to weaponize but fortunately, they were unsuccessful. There is no known incident where these agents have been used as a biologic weapon, but the natural outbreak of EVD during 2014–2015 spurred considerable investment in research and development into diagnostic tests and treatment with antivirals of the filoviruses (Ebola viruses and Marburg viruses).[45]

The viruses are single-stranded, ribonucleic acid (RNA) viruses that have a rodent or insect reservoir (bats are the natural reservoirs of Ebola virus)[46] and are communicated to humans by inhalation of an aerosol, through contact with an infected animal, or the bite of an infected insect. Humans are not a reservoir for the virus. The hemorrhagic fevers are contagious, and significant person-to-person transmission has occurred. The incubation period is within several days of contact or inhalation of the agent, at which time patients present with fever, myalgia, and evidence of a capillary leak (systemic leak or pulmonary edema), thrombocytopenia, and disseminated intravascular coagulation (DIC). The fatality rate, depending on the specific virus used, is anywhere from 2% to 60%. However, in the 2014–2015 EVD pandemic, as of March 3, 2016, the CDC and WHO reported that there had been 15,250 confirmed cases and that there were 11,316 deaths, for a fatality rate of about 75%.[47] There are no specific antiviral therapies for this class of viruses. Ribavirin, interferon-α, and hyperimmune globulin are often administered, with ribavirin being more protective against some of the viruses than others, but unfortunately one does not initially know what the etiologic agent is when the patient first presents.

Administration of convalescent serum and ZMapp (Mapp Biopharmaceutical, San Diego, CA, USA), a mixture of monoclonal antibodies, has been shown to be effective if treatment is begun early enough. An experimental vaccine is being tested. The 2014–2015 outbreak demonstrated that Ebola presents a significant risk to health-care workers, especially during the late stages of the disease. High-level PPE is required to be worn by health-care workers whenever aerosols are generated, such as during suctioning, intubation, and bronchoscopy. Even flushing a toilet to dispose of bodily secretions has been shown to aerosolize viral particles. PPE is donned under observation prior to entering a patient's negative pressure isolation room. Proper doffing after patient contact is equally critical to avoid infection. The ASA website has an extensive protocol along with videos.[48] PPE can take as long as 30 minutes to put on and remove. Emergency intubation thus becomes impractical. All airway management should therefore be anticipatory. Elective surgery should be avoided. Every effort should be made to perform emergency procedures in the patient's isolation room. Equipment can be brought to the bedside and left afterward. If it is necessary to transport patients, staff must wear appropriate PPE and the patient, ideally, should be transported in an isopod. Intraoperative procedures should be established and practiced to avoid staff exposure.

Dengue fever, Chikungunya, and Zika virus disease have become increasingly prevalent across the tropics and subtropics. Dengue, Chikungunya, and Zika are viruses transmitted through *Aedes aegypti* and *Aedes albopictus* mosquitoes. In 2016, there was an outbreak of Zika in the Americas. Most infected patients were asymptomatic or had minor disease consisting of fever and rash. However, Zika virus infection has been associated with an increased incidence of microcephaly in babies born to infected mothers and an increase in Guillain–Barré disease. All three diseases can be transmitted through blood contamination and Zika virus has also been transmitted sexually. Current guidance suggests higher levels of PPE when participating in aerosol-generating procedures. Pregnant caregivers should consider higher levels of protection due to the apparent increased risk to the fetus from Zika infection.[49] At present, there is no vaccine for Zika virus infection and care of infected patients is supportive.

Radiation—Nuclear

The greatest likelihood for dealing with patients who are exposed to ionizing radiation would come from a nuclear power plant or reactor accident, then from a terrorist action, and lastly from a detonation of a nuclear bomb. With respect to nuclear power plants, the US Nuclear Regulatory Commission has not found that people living adjacent to the plants have increased rates of cancer; however, the commision continues to study the issue.[50] Unfortunately, that was not the case when there was release of radioactive material as has occurred in the past at Chernobyl, and most recently at the Fukushima Daiichi nuclear power plant in Japan following the earthquake and tsunami on March 11, 2011. Because the details of the disaster in Japan are still not completely clear, this discussion will focus on Chernobyl; it is claimed that the meltdown that occurred in Japan released only 10% as much radiation as occurred at Chernobyl.[51]

On April 26, 1986, workers at the Chernobyl nuclear power plant did not recognize or respond to evidence that one of the reactors was malfunctioning, with loss of cooling capacity and an explosion of the nuclear reactor.[52] Two workers died as a direct effect of the explosion, while those who remained in shielded areas survived unless they went to fight the fire, in which case they eventually died of radiation injury. Short-term γ and β emissions from the explosion and subsequent γ and β radiation from the reactor core debris killed many more, with long-term health effects to the entire community. Because of a lack of protective clothing and respirators, the radioactive material that exploded into the atmosphere rained down for several days, affecting many more workers and thousands of civilians. Primary sources of radiation were iodine-131, strontium-90, and cesium-137. During the subsequent 24 hours, 140,000 people were evacuated and potassium iodide tablets were distributed to as many people in the area as possible. Two hundred and thirty patients were subsequently hospitalized, with many patients succumbing to infections because of bone marrow suppression, and in those patients in whom bone marrow transplantation was attempted, 17 of 19 died because of associated radiation burns. All told, radiation burns caused 21 deaths. Oropharyngeal burns occurred in 28 patients. Over the next several years, the average radiation exposure around Chernobyl was four times normal due to residual ground contamination. Almost two decades later, the effects of Chernobyl continue to be felt in the immediate vicinity and in the area down-wind from the reactor site.[52] The experience from Chernobyl reveals the kind of injuries that anesthesiologists can anticipate from nuclear accidents, including radiation burns, bone marrow suppression, the destruction of the lining of the GI tract, GI bleeding with translocation of bacteria, infection, sepsis, septic shock, and death. As evidenced by the experiences in Chernobyl, potassium iodide is indicated to protect the thyroid gland from taking up iodine-131, and other drugs are being considered, such as 5-androstenediol.

There have been other situations from which we can learn during which people have been exposed to ionizing radiation. On March 28, 1979, at the Three Mile Island nuclear power plant, the number 2 nuclear reactor overheated, and because the pressure relief valve failed to close, radioactive coolant was released into the containment facility.[53] As is often the case, there were numerous communication missteps, which resulted in the release of inconsistent information, generating genuine fear among individuals living nearby the nuclear power plant. There were no biologic effects of the event, but severe psychological sequelae did result.

On September 13, 1987, in Goiania, Brazil, a lead canister containing between 1,400 and 1,600 curies of cesium-137 contaminated 250 people; four of them died, and many others had short- and long-term health sequelae.[54] Mitigation efforts required the removal of 6,000 tons of clothing, furniture, dirt, trees, and other materials. The cesium had been left in a building in a lead canister when it was abandoned by its occupants; the canister was taken, opened by looters, and children played with the material.

Potential Sources of Ionizing Radiation Exposure

We are exposed to radiation on an annual basis from cosmic radiation, radon, medical devices, and in multiple stores and factories. In essence, half of our exposure comes from natural sources, with most of the remaining exposure originating from medical imaging and devices.[50] A chest radiograph leads to 5 to 10 millirem (mrem) of exposure, whereas a computed tomographic scan can result in 5,000 mrem of exposure.

Obviously, the greatest concern is the exposure to ionizing radiation that is unintentional—as occurred at the Chernobyl nuclear power plants. Intentional exposure threats are the result of military conflict or terrorism. With respect to the former, the two situations in which this occurred were in Hiroshima and Nagasaki in 1945. In Hiroshima, the bomb ("Little Boy") was only a 12.5-kiloton bomb, which killed an estimated 66,000 people and injured 69,000 more. The bomb that fell at Nagasaki ("Fat Boy") was a 22-kiloton plutonium implosion bomb, which killed between 39,000 and 74,000 people, with 75,000 people sustaining severe injuries. We learned from that experience that the majority of casualties are from the initial blast, fire, and the collapse of buildings. Radiation exposure subsequently killed many more. With any nuclear explosion, many individuals will be injured or die from the primary effect of the blast. Patients could have burn, crush, or radiation injury, or any combination thereof.

More recently, we have come to recognize that exposure to ionizing radiation may be as a result of terrorism. The most likely event will be the use of a dispersion device such as a conventional weapon or bomb surrounded with radionuclides such as cesium or strontium. In fact, in 1987, Iraq tested a 1-ton "dirty" bomb, and in 1996, Islamic terrorists in Chechnya placed a bomb packed with cesium-137 in a Moscow park that did not explode. While a radiation dispersion device remains the most likely event, terrorists could also target a nuclear power plant using a commercial jet, munitions, or internal sabotage.

While a blast, crush, or thermal injury is readily apparent, the effects of ionizing radiation are usually not apparent. Anesthesiologists should be familiar with types of ionizing radiation, which include α particles, β particles, γ rays, x-rays, and neutrons. One also needs to understand how radiation is measured (Table 59-5). There are several methods, which take into account not only the decay rate of a radioactive isotope (becquerel [Bq] or a curie [Ci]) but also the dose absorbed, usually quantified as the amount absorbed by any type of tissue or material. The radiation-absorbed dose (rad or Gray [Gy]) is the international system of units (SI) method for denoting the amount of energy deposited in joules per kilogram. One Gy equals 100 rad. A sievert is the SI unit for measurement of *human* exposure to radiation in joules per kilogram, with 1 Sv = 100 rem (roentgen equivalent for man).

In a nuclear accident or catastrophe, patients could have several types of radiation exposure. They may receive external radiation from an x-ray–emitting device or from γ rays or β particles, they may be contaminated with debris emitting ionized radiation, or they might inhale gaseous radioactive material.[55] Some of this material can become incorporated into tissue as radioactive iodine isotopes would. In order to protect individuals, the distance from the source or explosion is important, as are the amount of shielding, the time one is exposed, and the amount of radioactive material to which one is exposed. Human tissue will

Table 59-5 Radiation Exposure Terms

Term	Definition	Equivalence
Becquerel (Bq)	SI unit for measurement of radioactivity, defined as decay events per second 1 Bq = 1 disintegration per second	
Curie (Ci)	Traditional measure of radioactivity, as measured by radioactivity decay	1 Ci = 0.7×10^{10} disintegrations per second
Radiation-absorbed dose (rad)	Dose deposited by any type of radiation, in any type of tissue or material	1 rad = 0.01 Gy
Gray (Gy)	SI unit for the energy deposited by any type of radiation, in joules per kilogram	1 Gy = 100 rad
Roentgen equivalent man (rem)	Unit of human exposure to radiation	1 rem = 0.01 Sv
Sievert (Sv)	SI unit for measurement of human exposure to radiation, in joules per kilogram	1 Sv = 100 rem

SI, International System of units.

block α particles (though if inhaled, α particles can penetrate up to 50 μm into the pulmonary epithelium material, leading to the development of lung cancer), but will not stop β particles or γ rays. Aluminum shields stop β particles, but γ rays can penetrate even concrete walls and lead is required to shield for both γ and x-rays.

The most likely injury from ionizing radiation is to those tissues that have the greatest turnover rate, that is, the sensitivity of tissues to radiation (from greatest to least) is for lymphoid, GI, reproductive, dermal, bone marrow, and nervous system tissue. In reality, the response of lymphoid and bone marrow to ionizing radiation cause the greatest problems. The thrombocytopenia, granulocytopenia, and the GI injury lead to bleeding and bacterial translocation across the GI epithelium, the net result of which is sepsis and bleeding—the hallmarks of acute radiation syndrome, which lead to death.

Because ionizing radiation is invisible, affected individuals may appear normal. Patients who present with nausea, vomiting, diarrhea, and fever are likely to have severe acute radiation syndrome. Hypotension, erythema, and CNS dysfunction will manifest later. "Short-term" effects such as these, however, may not appear until days to weeks after the exposure, depending on the amount of exposure (as little as 0.75 to 1 Gy), whereas hematopoietic syndrome (severe lymphoid and bone marrow suppression) results from exposure to 3 to 6 Gy and may lead to death within 8 to 50 days. Long-term effects include thyroid cancer and psychological injury, as has been documented many times in the past.

Management

Should a radiation disaster occur, it would be followed by a huge coordinated local, state, and federal response, which at the federal level would include the US Department of Homeland Security, the Department of Energy, the Department of Justice, FEMA, the Environmental Protection Agency, and the Nuclear Regulatory Commission. Of most importance, depending on the type of catastrophe, would be the immediate evacuation of the area. If evacuation is impossible, a safe place should be sought within the home or building. The principles of disaster management always involve containment (avoid bringing patients with material emitting ionizing radiation to the hospital). Therefore, as part of the containment process, to the extent possible, patients should be decontaminated at the site. Removal of clothing is critically important. β and γ rays and neutrons will no longer be present on the patient unless there is still material emitting this radiation on a person's clothing. Rather than guess whether radiation is still present, it is best to disrobe patients. In previous mass casualty situations, maintenance of casualties' privacy has been a concern, but not one with an easy solution. Afterward, patients' skin should be washed with warm soapy water. Depending on the number of casualties, decontamination areas may have to be set up outside of hospitals, especially because individuals will arrive by private vehicles or on foot. Take care to isolate patients' personal belongings, giving the same consideration to biologic fluids—including saliva, blood, urine, and stool (all of which may be contaminated with radioisotopes and may therefore require special precautions when being handled)—as for clothing.

Potassium iodide can attenuate most of the radiation-induced thyroid effects, but must be given as quickly as possible because there is little protective effect if it is given more than 24 hours after exposure. Treatment is largely supportive, as these patients will develop acute radiation syndrome manifested by bleeding and sepsis. Treatment guidelines for management of postirradiation sepsis have been developed and advocated by the military.[56] The use of granulocyte colony–stimulating factor may be of benefit. Other treatments would include oral and GI decontamination using nasopharyngeal lavage, oral lavage and brushing, early stomach lavage, or administration of emetic and osmotic laxatives. Blocking agents include potassium iodide and strontium lactate. Mobilizing agents include ammonium chloride, calcium gluconate, and diuretics, which may enhance renal excretion. Chelation therapy that has been recommended includes calcium diethylenetriamine pentaacetic acid (DTPA) as an initial dose and then zinc DTPA.[57] Granulocyte macrophage colony–stimulating factor and thrombopoietin or interleukin-11, though postulated, have not been proven to be of benefit. For individuals with a contaminated GI tract, selective decontamination may be helpful, though this again has not been demonstrated to be of benefit in this situation.[58]

Unfortunately, because of the possibility of blast, thermal, and crush injuries, along with the radiation injury, the care of the injured may require the care of patients who have multiple combined injuries. The initial response should be as per the advanced trauma life support (ATLS) guidelines, which include an assessment of the airway, breathing, and circulation, and extent of trauma and then decontamination of the patient, after which the patient is stabilized and further evaluated. Wounds must be considered contaminated. "Dirty wounds" should not be closed but cleaned and debrided, excised, and observed. Unfortunately, in this situation, there is also the possibility that there may be the combined effects of a radiation-releasing event and the use of either chemical or biologic agents.[58] Because of the variety of types of terrorism, some of it reportedly government sponsored, communities and the US government have had to plan for the detonation of a nuclear device on US soil.[59,60]

Explosives

Management of traumatic injury is covered in Chapter 53, but a chapter on disaster management would not be complete without mentioning the use of explosive devices by terrorists. As the media reports daily, particularly in Afghanistan, the use of IEDs is the terrorist's favorite weapon. Patients have burns, fractures, lacerations, multiple shrapnel injuries, soft tissue trauma, and traumatic amputations. As the weapons have become more sophisticated and powerful, the extent of injuries has increased significantly. In 2012, US military personnel experienced more multiple-than single-traumatic extremity amputations.[61]

Patients with any evidence of burns to the face or airway will require appropriate airway management. Patients should be intubated, awake if possible, because a significant number of these patients will have mild-to-moderate glottic edema at the time of intubation. Those patients with burns must be managed aggressively with respect to fluid resuscitation. With isolated total body surface injury, fluid resuscitation is aggressive. With polytrauma and no third-degree burns, "damage control resuscitation/surgery" is the norm.[62] The patient's body temperature is maintained and surgery is performed as soon as possible to stop the bleeding, thereby decreasing the need for blood products and the chances of developing a dilutional coagulopathy. Patients who do develop a coagulopathy appear to benefit from a ratio of packed red blood cells to fresh frozen plasma to platelets of 1:1:1.[63,64] One study has demonstrated that tranexamic acid decreases the need for additional blood products. In patients with crush injury and markedly elevated creatine phosphokinase, alkalinization of the urine-forced diuresis may attenuate renal failure from myoglobinuria.

Conclusion

Although it is unlikely that an anesthesiologist will be at the initial site of a natural or intentional disaster, it could happen. Most likely, anesthesiologists will become involved if the hospital at which they work provides care for a number of these patients. Anesthesiologists could find themselves involved in triage, in the ED, OR, or ICU.[65] As suggested for several of these situations, airway management and ventilator management may be critical, as would the establishment of intravascular access and volume resuscitation.

Obviously, it is critical to have a high index of suspicion if you are managing the index case, or two or more patients, with presenting signs and symptoms that are suggestive of the use of a biologic weapon. The individual who is the point of contact for the index case should notify the hospital infectious disease specialist and the local and state health departments. Factors that might indicate the intentional release of a biologic agent would include unusual temporal or geographic clustering of cases, an uncommon age distribution, or a significant number of cases (more than one) of acute flaccid paralysis that might suggest use of botulinum toxin.

If called to the hospital to be involved in managing such a catastrophe, the anesthesiologist must review basic decontamination and isolation techniques and, as mentioned previously, must follow those guidelines scrupulously. It is clear that anesthesiologists have the requisite training and experience to be of vital importance in managing such casualties. However, based on their training, they may not be emotionally prepared to manage these patients. They must remember that unlike their normal practice, they may have to triage patients, accept the fact that the standard of care may be different, and focus their efforts on interventions that will carry the greatest benefit for the greatest number of casualties.

This process begins when the anesthesiologist gets the call at home or in the hospital regarding an impending mass casualty event. She or he must first report to the command and control center and, though most likely they may work in the operating room, they could also be used in the triage area in the ED or in the ICU. Of utmost importance is familiarity with the hospital's disaster plan. One must also develop one's own family care plan in anticipation of absence from the home for extended periods of time. Ensuring one's own safety through the appropriate use of protective devices to serve as barriers against radiologic, biologic, and chemical weapons is also of vital importance. Infrastructure degradation worsens the consequences of mass casualty events. Preparing to deliver care under austere circumstances, developing creative responses, and practicing (simulations) regularly will mitigate the effects of a disaster and increase resilience for individuals, teams, and institutions.

Appendix A. Disaster Preparedness Planning Guide for Families (from FEMA)

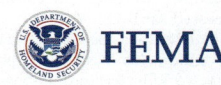

Family Emergency Plan

Make sure your family has a plan in case of an emergency. Before an emergency happens, sit down together and decide how you will get in contact with each other, where you will go, and what you will do in an emergency. Keep a copy of this plan in your emergency supply kit or another safe place where you can access it in the event of a disaster.

Out-of-Town Contact Name: _____ Telephone Number: _____
Email: _____
Neighborhood Meeting Place: _____ Telephone Number: _____
Regional Meeting Place: _____ Telephone Number: _____
Evacuation Location: _____ Telephone Number: _____

Fill out the following information for each family member and keep it up to date.

Name: _____ Social Security Number: _____
Date of Birth: _____ Important Medical Information: _____

Name: _____ Social Security Number: _____
Date of Birth: _____ Important Medical Information: _____

Name: _____ Social Security Number: _____
Date of Birth: _____ Important Medical Information: _____

Name: _____ Social Security Number: _____
Date of Birth: _____ Important Medical Information: _____

Name: _____ Social Security Number: _____
Date of Birth: _____ Important Medical Information: _____

Name: _____ Social Security Number: _____
Date of Birth: _____ Important Medical Information: _____

Write down where your family spends the most time: work, school, and other places you frequent. Schools, daycare providers, workplaces, and apartment buildings should all have site-specific emergency plans that you and your family need to know about.

Work Location One
Address: _____
Phone Number: _____
Evacuation Location: _____

Work Location Two
Address: _____
Phone Number: _____
Evacuation Location: _____

Work Location Three
Address: _____
Phone Number: _____
Evacuation Location: _____

Other places you frequent
Address: _____
Phone Number: _____
Evacuation Location: _____

School Location One
Address: _____
Phone Number: _____
Evacuation Location: _____

School Location Two
Address: _____
Phone Number: _____
Evacuation Location: _____

School Location Three
Address: _____
Phone Number: _____
Evacuation Location: _____

Other place you frequent
Address: _____
Phone Number: _____
Evacuation Location: _____

Important Information	Name	Telephone Number	Policy Number
Doctor(s):			
Other:			
Pharmacist:			
Medical Insurance:			
Homeowner's/Rental Insurance:			
Veterinarian/Kennel (for pets):			

Dial 911 for Emergencies

REFERENCES

1. World Association for Disaster and Emergency Management (WADEM) Health Disaster Management. Guidelines for evaluation and research. WADEM website. http://wadem.org/guidelines.html. Published 2003. Accessed April 11, 2016.
2. United Nations. Sendai framework for disaster risk reduction 2015–2030. PreventionWeb website. http://www.preventionweb.net/files/43291_sendaiframeworkfordrren.pdf. Published 2015. Accessed August 15, 2016.
3. American Society of Anesthesiologists (ASA). Committee on Trauma and Emergency Preparedness (COTEP). ASA website. https://www.asahq.org/resources/resources-from-asa-committees/committee-on-trauma-and-emergency-preparedness. Published 2015. Accessed April 11, 2016.
4. Doctors Without Borders/Médecins Sans Frontières (MSF). Who we need. Doctors Without Borders website. http://www.doctorswithoutborders.org/work-us/work-field/who-we-need/anesthesiologists-nurse-anesthetists. Published 2013. Accessed April 11, 2016.
5. Dara SI, Ashton RW, Farmer JC. Engendering enthusiasm for sustainable disaster critical care response: why this is of consequence to critical care professionals? *Crit Care*. 2005;9(2):125–127.
6. Gomez D, Haas B, Ahmed N, et al. Disaster preparedness of Canadian trauma centres: the perspective of medical directors of trauma. *Can J Surg*. 2011;54(1):9–16.
7. Ciraulo DL, Frykberg ER, Feliciano DV, et al. A survey assessment of the level of preparedness for domestic terrorism and mass casualty incidents among eastern association for the surgery of trauma members. *J Trauma*. 2004;56(5):1033–1039.
8. Rössler B, Marhofer P, Hüpfl M, et al. Preparedness of anesthesiologists working in humanitarian disasters. *Disaster Med Public Health Prep*. 2013;7(4):408–412.
9. Moore ZS, Seward JF, Lane JM. Smallpox. *Lancet*. 2006;367(9508):425–435.
10. Tepper M, Whitehead J. Clinical predictors of bioterrorism-related inhalational anthrax. *Lancet*. 2005;365(9455):214.
11. Lynch DK. Plan ahead. *Anesth Analg*. 2010;110(3):653–654.
12. Merchant RM, Leigh JE, Lurie N. Health care volunteers and disaster response—first, be prepared. *N Engl J Med*. 2010;362(10):872–873.
13. Masterson L, Steffen C, Brin M, et al. Willingness to respond: Of emergency department personnel and their predicted participation in mass casualty terrorist events. *J Emerg Med*. 2009;36(1):43–49.
14. US Department of Homeland Security (USDHS) Federal Emergency Management Agency (FEMA). National preparedness goal. FEMA website. http://www.fema.gov. Accessed April 11, 2016.
15. The Joint Commission on Accreditation of Healthcare Organizations (TJC). Health care at the crossroads: strategies for creating and sustaining community-wide emergency preparedness systems. TJC website. http://www.jointcommission.org/assets/1/18/health_care_at_the_crossroads.pdf. Published 2003. Accessed April 11, 2016.
16. Joint Commission on Accreditation of Healthcare Organizations (TJC). Emergency management oversight requirements. TJC website. http://www.jointcommission.org/assets/1/18/JCP0713_Emergency_Mgmt_Oversight.pdf. Published 2013. Accessed March 21, 2016.
17. US Department of Health and Human Services. Emergency preparedness checklist. Centers for Medicaid and Medicare Services website. http//cms.gov/medicare/provider-enrollment-and-certification/surveycertemergprep/downloads/sandc_epchecklist_provider.pdf. Published 2013. Accessed April 11, 2016.
18. Enserink M, Stone R. Questions swirl over knockout gas used in hostage crisis. *Science*. 2002;298:1150–1151.
19. Okumura T, Takasu N, Ishimatsu S, et al. Report on 640 victims of the Tokyo subway sarin attack. *Ann Emerg Med*. 1996;28(2):129–135.
20. Zane RD, Prestipino AL. Implementing the hospital emergency incident command system: an integrated delivery system's experience. *Prehosp Disaster Med*. 2004;19(4):311–317.
21. Goransson Nyberg A, Stricklin D, Sellstrom A. Mass casualties and healthcare following the release of toxic chemicals or radioactive material: contribution of modern biotechnology. *Int J Environ Res Public Health*. 2011;8(12):4521–4549.
22. Wong EG, Dominguez L, Trelles M, et al. Operative trauma in low-resource settings: the experience of Medicins Sans Frontieres in environments of conflict, post conflict, and disaster. *J Surg*. 2015;157(5):850–856.
23. Jawa RS, Zakrison TL, Richards AT, et al. Facilitating safer surgery and anesthesia in a disaster zone. *Am J Surg*. 2012;204(3):406–409.
24. Chemical, Biological, Radiological, and Nuclear Defense Information Analysis Center (CBRNIAC). U.S. Army Chemical Materials agency creates a safer tomorrow. *CBRNIAC Newsletter*. 2012;13(2):4–7.
25. Kassa J, Karasova JZ, Musilek K, et al. A comparison of the neuroprotective efficacy of newly developed oximes (K117, K127) and currently available oxime (obidoxime) in tabun-poisoned rats. *Toxicol Mech Methods*. 2009;19(3):232–238.
26. Aroniadou-Anderjaska V, Figueiredo TH, Apland JP, et al. Primary brain targets of nerve agents: the role of the amygdala in comparison to the hippocampus. *Neurotoxicol*. 2009;30(5):772–776.
27. Beeching NJ, Dance DA, Miller AR, et al. Biological warfare and bioterrorism. *BMJ*. 2002;324(7333):336–339.
28. Breman JG, Henderson DA. Diagnosis and management of smallpox. *N Engl J Med*. 2002;346(17):1300–1308.
29. Choo CW. The World Health Organization smallpox eradication programme. http://choo.fis.utoronto.ca/fis/courses/lis2102/KO.WHO.case.html. Published 2012. Accessed April 11, 2016.
30. Centers for Disease Control and Prevention (CDC). Smallpox vaccine adverse events among civilians—United States, March 4–10, 2003. *JAMA*. 2003;289(15):1921–1922.
31. Frey SE, Newman FK, Kennedy JS, et al. Clinical and immunologic responses to multiple doses of IMVAMUNE (modified vaccinia Ankara) followed by Dryvax challenge. *Vaccine*. 2007;25(51):8562–8573.
32. Inglesby TV, Henderson DA, Bartlett JG, et al. Anthrax as a biological weapon: medical and public health management. Working Group on Civilian Biodefense. *JAMA*. 1999;281(18):1735–1745.
33. Kalamas AG. Anthrax. *Anesthesiol Clin North Am*. 2004;22(3):533–540.
34. Janse I, Hamidjaja RA, Bok JM, et al. Reliable detection of Bacillus anthracis, Francisella tularensis and Yersinia pestis by using multiplex qPCR including internal controls for nucleic acid extraction and amplification. *BMC Microbiol*. 2010;10:314.
35. Martin G. Anthrax: lessons learned from the U.S. Capitol experience. *Mil Med*. 2003;168(9):9–14.
36. Swartz MN. Recognition and management of anthrax: an update. *N Engl J Med*. 2001;345(22):1621–1626.
37. Dixon TC, Meselson M, Guillemin J, et al. Anthrax. *N Engl J Med*. 1999;341(11):815–826.
38. Shafazand S, Doyle R, Ruoss S, et al. Inhalational anthrax: epidemiology, diagnosis, and management. *Chest*. 1999;116(5):1369–1376.
39. Schmitt B, Dobrez D, Parada JP, et al. Responding to a small-scale bioterrorist anthrax attack: cost-effectiveness analysis comparing pre-attack vaccination with postattack antibiotic treatment and vaccination. *Arch Intern Med*. 2007;167(7):655–662.
40. Prentice MB, Rahalison L. Plague. *Lancet*. 2007;369(9568):1196–1207.
41. Zietz BP, Dunkelberg H. The history of the plague and the research on the causative agent Yersinia pestis. *Int J Hyg Environ Health*. 2004;207(2):165–178.
42. Josko D. Botulin toxin: a weapon in terrorism. *Clin Lab Sci*. 2004;17(1):30–34.
43. Franz DR, Jahrling PB, McClain DJ, et al. Clinical recognition and management of patients exposed to biological warfare agents. *Clin Lab Med*. 2001;21(3):435–473.
44. Bhalla DK, Warheit DB. Biological agents with potential for misuse: a historical perspective and defensive measures. *Toxicol Appl Pharmacol*. 2004;199(1):71–84.
45. Kuhn JH, Dodd LE, Wahl-Jensen V, et al. Evaluation of perceived threat differences posed by filovirus variants. *Biosecur Bioterror*. 2011;9(4):361–371.
46. Murray MJ. Ebola virus disease: a review of its past and present. *Anesth Analg*. 2015;121:798–809.
47. Centers for Disease Control and Prevention (CDC). 2014 Ebola outbreak in West Africa. CDC website. http://www.cdc.gov/vhf/ebola/outbreaks/2014-west-africa/index.html. Published 2014. Accessed April 11, 2016.
48. American Society of Anesthesiologists (ASA) Committee on Trauma and Emergency Preparedness (COTEP). Ebola information. ASA website. https://www.asahq.org/resources/clinical-information/ebola-information#4. Published 2016. Accessed April 11, 2016.
49. Centers for Disease Control and Prevention (CDC). Zika virus. CDC website. http://www.cdc.gov/zika/index.html. Published 2016. Accessed March 4, 2016.
50. US Nuclear Regulatory Commission, Office of Public Affairs. Fact Sheet on Biological Effects of Radiation. http://www.nrc.gov/ Published 2011. Accessed April 10, 2016.
51. Masamichi CN, Haruyasu N, Hiroaki T, et al. Preliminary estimation of release amounts of ^{131}I and ^{137}Cs accidentally discharged from the Fukushima Daiichi nuclear power plant into the atmosphere. *J Nucl Sci Tech*. 2011;(7):1129–1134.
52. Shibata Y, Yamashita S, Masyakin VB, et al. 15 years after Chernobyl: new evidence of thyroid cancer. *Lancet*. 2001;358(9297):1965–1966.
53. Collins DL. Human responses to the threat of or exposure to ionizing radiation at Three Mile Island, Pennsylvania, and Goiania, Brazil. *Mil Med*. 2002;167(2):137–138.
54. Collins DL, de Carvalho AB. Chronic stress from the Goiania 137Cs radiation accident. *Behav Med*. 1993;18(4):149–157.
55. Ibrahim SA, Simon SL, Bouville A, et al. Alimentary tract absorption (f1 values) for radionuclides in local and regional fallout from nuclear tests. *Health Phys*. 2010;99(2):233–251.
56. Brook I, Elliott TB, Ledney GD, et al. Management of postirradiation sepsis. *Mil Med*. 2002;167(2):105–106.
57. Knudson GB, Elliott TB, Brook I, et al. Nuclear, biological, and chemical combined injuries and countermeasures on the battlefield. *Mil Med*. 2002;167(2):95–97.
58. Shi C, Lu S. Radiation injuries. *Int J Low Extrem Wounds*. 2011;10(3):120–121.

59. Sternberg S. Experts plan for how to deal with nuclear terror strike. USA Today website. http://www.usatoday.com/news/nation/2011-03-15-nuke-med14_ST_N.htm. Published March 15, 2011. Accessed April 10, 2016.
60. National Security Staff Interagency Policy Coordination Subcommittee for Preparedness and Response to Radiological and Nuclear Threats. *Planning Guidance for Response to a Nuclear Detonation*. 2nd Ed. Washington DC, US Environmental Protection Agency; 2010.
61. Zoroya G. IEDs contribute to increase in multiple amputations. USA Today website. http://www.usatoday.com/news/military/story/2012-06-04/IEDamputations-military-Afghanistan/55385376/1. Published June 4, 2012. Accessed. April 4, 2016.
62. Holcomb JB, Jenkins D, Rhee P, et al. Damage control resuscitation: directly addressing the early coagulopathy of trauma. *J Trauma*. 2007;62(2):307–310.
63. CRASH-2 Collaborators, Roberts I, Shakur H, Afolabi A, et al. The importance of early treatment with tranexamic acid in bleeding trauma patients: an exploratory analysis of the CRASH-2 randomised controlled trial. *Lancet*. 2011;377(9771):1101.e1–e2.
64. Borgman MA, Spinella PC, Perkins JG, et al. The ratio of blood products transfused affects mortality in patients receiving massive transfusions at a combat support hospital. *J Trauma*. 2007;63(4):805–813.
65. Baker DJ. Management of casualties from terrorist chemical and biological attack: a key role for the anaesthetist. *Br J Anaesth*. 2002;89(2):211–214.

Section 10
APPENDICES

1. Formulas
2. Atlas of Electrocardiography
3. Pacemaker and Implantable Cardiac Defibrillator Protocols
4. American Society of Anesthesiologists Standards, Guidelines, and Statements
5. The Airway Approach Algorithm and Difficult Airway Algorithm
6. Malignant Hyperthermia Protocol
7. Herbal Medications
8. Atlas of Ultrasound and Echocardiography (eBook only)

APPENDIX 1
Formulas

Hemodynamic Formulas

Hemodynamic Variables: Calculations and Normal Values

Variable	Calculation	Normal Values
Cardiac index (CI)	CO/BSA	2.5–4.0 L/min/m^2
Stroke volume (SV)	CO × 1000/HR	60–90 mL/beat
Stroke index (SI)	SV/BSA	40–60 mL/beat/m^2
Mean arterial pressure (MAP)	Diastolic pressure + 1/3 pulse pressure	80–120 mmHg
Systemic vascular resistance (SVR)	$\frac{MAP - \overline{CVP}}{CO} \times 79.9$	1,200–1,500 dyne-cm-sec^{-5}
Pulmonary vascular resistance (PVR)	$\frac{\overline{PAP} - \overline{PCWP}}{CO} \times 79.9$	100–300 dyne-cm-sec^{-5}
Right ventricular stroke work index (RVSWI)	0.0136 (PAP − CVP) × SI	5–9 g-m/beat/m^2
Left ventricular stroke work index (LWSWI)	0.0136 (MAP − PCWP) × SI	45–60 g-m/beat/m^2

HR, heart rate; CVP, mean central venous pressure; PAP, mean pulmonary artery pressure; BSA, body surface area; CO, cardiac output; PCWP, pulmonary capillary wedge pressure; MAP, mean arterial blood pressure.

Respiratory Formulas

	Normal Values (70 kg)
Alveolar oxygen tension $P_AO_2 = (P_B - 47) F_{IO_2} - P_ACO_2$	110 mmHg ($F_{IO_2} = 0.21$)
Alveolar-arterial oxygen gradient $AaO_2 = P_AO_2 - P_aO_2$	<10 mmHg ($F_{IO_2} = 0.21$)
Arterial-to-alveolar oxygen ratio, a/A ratio	>0.75
Arterial oxygen content $CaO_2 = (SaO_2)(Hb \times 1.34) + P_aO_2 (0.0031)$	21 mL/100 mL
Mixed venous oxygen content $C\bar{V}O_2 = (S\bar{V}O_2)(Hb \times 1.34) + P\bar{V}O_2 (0.0031)$	15 mL/100 mL
Arterial-venous oxygen content difference $aVO_2 = CaO_2 - C\bar{V}O_2$	4–6 mL/100 mL
Intrapulmonary shunt $\dot{Q}s/\dot{Q}T = (CCO_2 - CaO_2)/(CCO_2 - C\bar{V}O_2)$ $CCO_2 = (Hb \times 1.34) + (P_AO_2 \times 0.0031)$	<5%
Physiologic dead space $\dot{V}D/\dot{V}T = (P_aCO_2 - P_ECO_2)/P_aCO_2$	0.33
Oxygen consumption $\dot{V}O_2 = CO(CaO_2 - C\dot{V}O_2)$	240 mL/min
Oxygen transport $O_2T = CO(CaO_2)$	1,000 mL/min

CaO_2, arterial oxygen content; $C\dot{V}O_2$, mixed venous oxygen content; CCO_2, pulmonary capillary oxygen content; CO, cardiac output; F_{IO_2}, fraction inspired oxygen; O_2T, oxygen transport; P_B, barometric pressure; $\dot{Q}s/\dot{Q}T$, intrapulmonary shunt; P_ACO_2, alveolar carbon dioxide tension; P_aCO_2, arterial carbon dioxide tension; P_AO_2, alveolar oxygen tension; P_aO_2, arterial oxygen tension; P_ECO_2, expired carbon dioxide tension; V_D, dead space gas volume; V_T, tidal volume; VO_2, oxygen consumption (minute).

Lung Volumes and Capacities

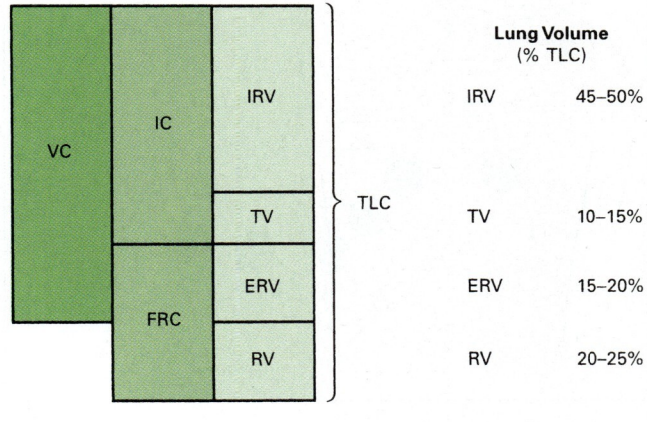

Lung Volume	(% TLC)
IRV	45–50%
TV	10–15%
ERV	15–20%
RV	20–25%

		Normal Values (70 kg)
Vital capacity	VC	4,800 mL
Inspiratory capacity	IC	3,800 mL
Functional residual capacity	FRC	2,400 mL
Inspiratory reserve volume	IRV	3,500 mL
Tidal volume	TV	1,500 mL
Expiratory reserve volume	ERV	1,200 mL
Residual volume	RV	1,200 mL
Total lung capacity	TLC	6,000 mL

APPENDIX 2
Atlas of Electrocardiography

GINA C. BADESCU • BENJAMIN M. SHERMAN • JAMES R. ZAIDAN • PAUL G. BARASH

Lead Placement		
	Electrode	
	Positive	*Negative*
Bipolar Leads		
I	LA	RA
II	LL	RA
III	LL	LA
Augmented Unipolar		
aVR	RA	LA, LL
aVL	LA	RA, LL
aVF	LL	RA, LA
Precordial		
V_1	4 ICS–RSB	
V_2	4 ICS–LSB	
V_3	Midway between V_2 and V_4	
V_4	5 ICS–MCL	
V_5	5 ICS–AAL	
V_6	5 ICS–MAL	

Abbrev.	Meaning
LA	Left arm
RA	Right arm
LL	Left leg
ICS	Intercostal space
RSB	Right sternal border
LSB	Left sternal border
MCL	Midclavicular line
AAL	Anterior axillary line
MAL	Midaxillary line

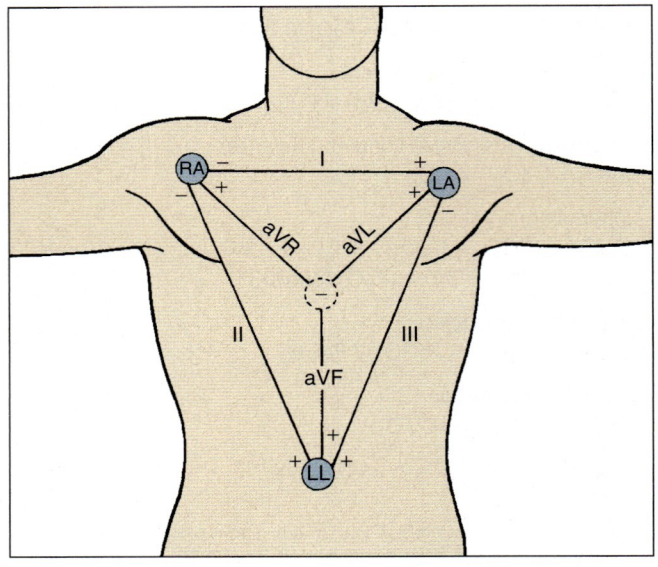

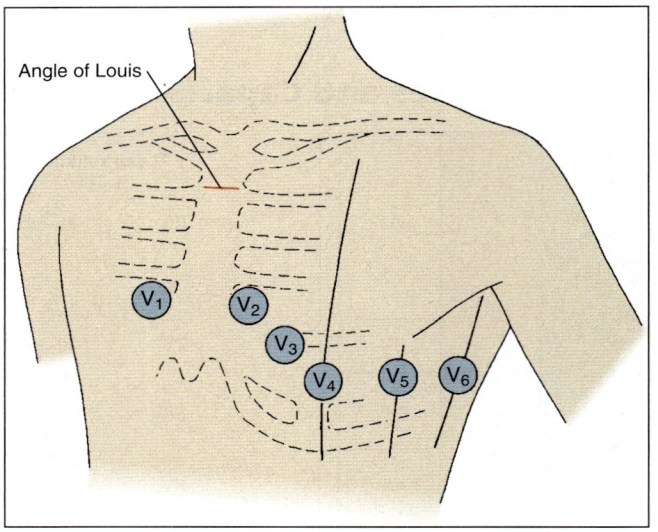

Sections and images of this appendix were developed, in part, for both Barash PG, Cullen BF, Cahalan MK, et al, eds. *Clinical Anesthesia*. 8th ed. Philadelphia, PA: Wolters Kluwer Health; 2016 and Kaplan JA, Reich DL, Savino JS, eds. *Kaplan's Cardiac Anesthesia: The Echo Era*. Philadelphia, PA: Elsevier; 2011, with permission of the editors and publishers.

The Normal Electrocardiogram—Cardiac Cycle

The normal electrocardiogram is composed of waves (P, QRS, T, and U) and intervals (PR, QRS, ST, and QT).

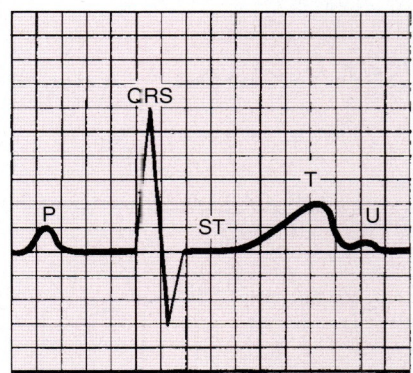

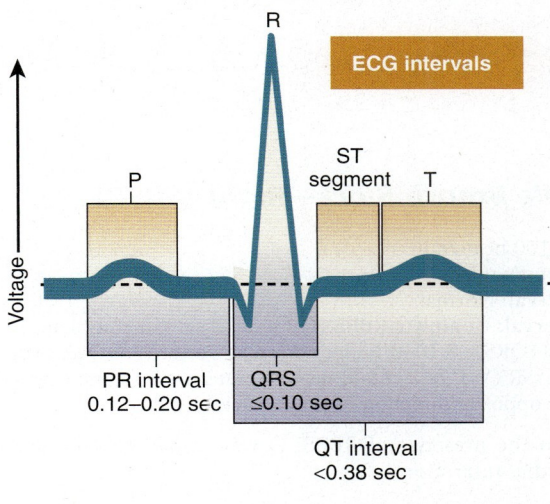

ECG intervals

Atrial Fibrillation

Rate: Variable (~150–200 beats/min)
Rhythm: Irregular
PR interval: No P wave; PR interval not discernible
QT interval: QRS normal

Note: Must be differentiated from atrial flutter: (1) absence of flutter waves and presence of fibrillatory line; (2) flutter usually associated with higher ventricular rates (>150 beats/min). Loss of atrial contraction reduces cardiac output (10%–20%). Mural atrial thrombi may develop. Considered controlled if ventricular rate is <100 beats/min.

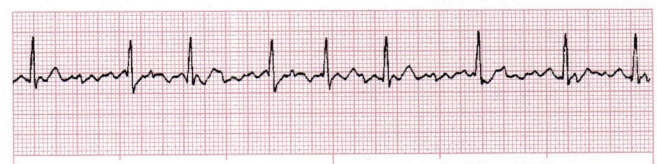

Atrial Flutter

Rate: Rapid, atrial usually regular (250–350 beats/min); ventricular usually regular (<100 beats/min)
Rhythm: Atrial and ventricular regular
PR interval: Flutter (F) waves are saw-toothed. PR interval cannot be measured.
QT interval: QRS usually normal; ST segment and T waves are not identifiable.

Note: Vagal maneuvers will slow ventricular response, simplifying recognition of the F waves.

II

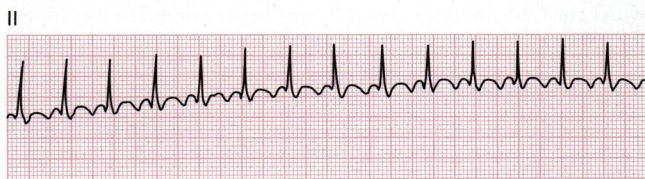

Atrioventricular Block (First Degree)

Rate: 60–100 beats/min
Rhythm: Regular
PR interval: Prolonged (>0.20 sec) and constant
QT interval: Normal

Note: Usually clinically insignificant; may be early harbinger of drug toxicity.

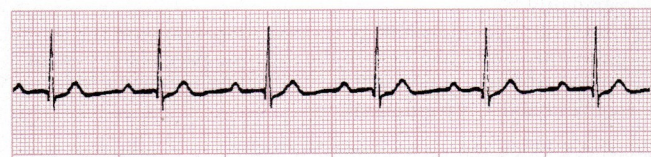

Atrioventricular Block (Second Degree), Mobitz Type I/Wenckebach Block

Rate: 60–100 beats/min
Rhythm: Atrial regular; ventricular irregular
PR interval: P wave normal; PR interval progressively lengthens with each cycle until QRS complex is dropped (dropped beat). PR interval following dropped beat is shorter than normal.
QT interval: QRS complex normal but dropped periodically.

Note: Commonly seen in trained athletes and with drug toxicity.

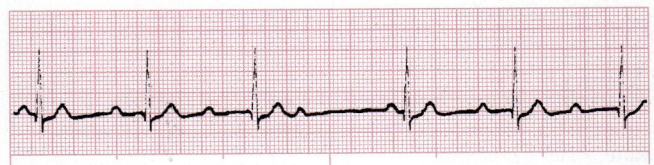

5 Atrioventricular Block (Second Degree), Mobitz Type II

Rate: <100 beats/min
Rhythm: Atrial regular; ventricular regular or irregular
PR interval: P waves normal, but some are not followed by QRS complex.
QT interval: Normal but may have widened QRS complex if block is at level of bundle branch. ST segment and T wave may be abnormal, depending on location of block.

Note: In contrast to Mobitz type I block, the PR and RR intervals are constant and the dropped QRS occurs without warning. The wider the QRS complex (block lower in the conduction system), the greater the amount of myocardial damage.

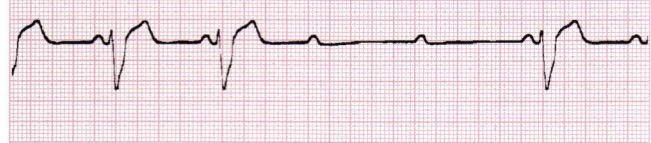

6 Atrioventricular Block (Third Degree), Complete Heart Block

Rate: <45 beats/min
Rhythm: Atrial regular; ventricular regular; no relationship between P wave and QRS complex.
PR interval: Variable because atria and ventricles beat independently.
QT interval: QRS morphology variable, depending on the origin of the ventricular beat in the intrinsic pacemaker system (atrioventricular junctional vs. ventricular pacemaker). ST segment and T wave normal.

Note: AV block represents complete failure of conduction from atria to ventricles (no P wave is conducted to the ventricle). The atrial rate is faster than ventricular rate. P waves have no relationship to QRS complexes (e.g., they are electrically disconnected). In contrast, with AV dissociation, the P wave is conducted through the AV node and the atrial and ventricular rate are similar. Immediate treatment with atropine or isoproterenol is required if cardiac output is reduced. Consideration should be given to insertion of a pacemaker. Seen as a complication of mitral valve replacement.

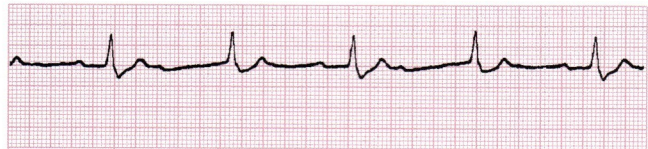

7 Bundle-Branch Block—Left (LBBB)

Rate: <100 beats/min
Rhythm: Regular
PR interval: Normal
QT interval: Complete LBBB (QRS >0.12 sec); incomplete LBBB (QRS = 0.10–0.12 sec); lead V_1 negative RS complex; I, aVL, V_6 wide R wave without Q or S component. ST segment and T-wave direction opposite direction of the R wave.

Note: LBBB does not occur in healthy patients and usually indicates serious heart disease with a poor prognosis. In patients with LBBB, insertion of a pulmonary artery catheter may lead to complete heart block.

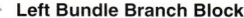
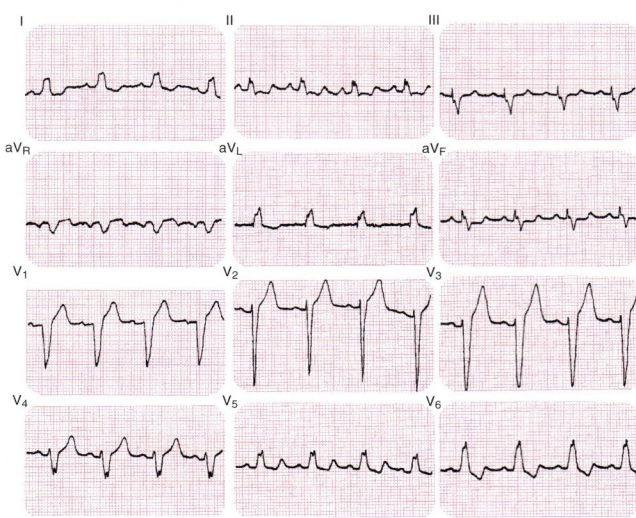

8 Bundle Branch Block—Right (RBBB)

Rate: <100 beats/min
Rhythm: Regular
PR interval: Normal
QT interval: Complete RBBB (QRS >0.12 sec); incomplete RBBB (QRS = 0.10–0.12 sec). Varying patterns of QRS complex; rSR (V_1); RS, wide R with M pattern. ST segment and T wave opposite direction of the R wave.

Note: In the presence of RBBB, Q waves may be seen with a myocardial infarction.

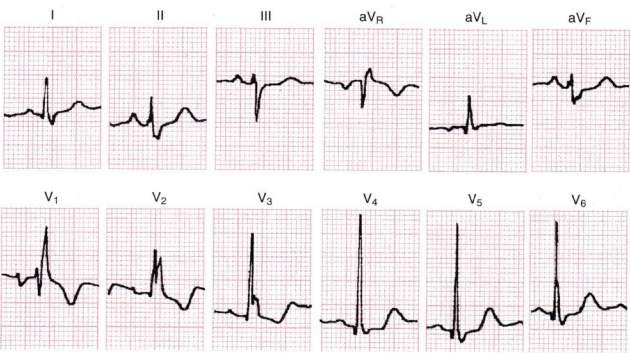

Coronary Artery Disease

9 ◂ *Transmural Myocardial Infarction (TMI)*

Q waves seen on ECG, useful in confirming diagnosis, are associated with poorer prognosis and more significant hemodynamic impairment. Arrhythmias frequently complicate course. Small Q waves may be normal variant. For myocardial infarction (MI), Q waves >0.04 seconds or depth exceeds one-third of R wave. For inferior wall MI, differentiate from RVH by axis deviation.

Myocardial Infarction			
Anatomic Site	**Leads**	**ECG Changes**	**Coronary Artery**
Inferior	II, III, AVF	Q, ↑ST, ↑T	Right

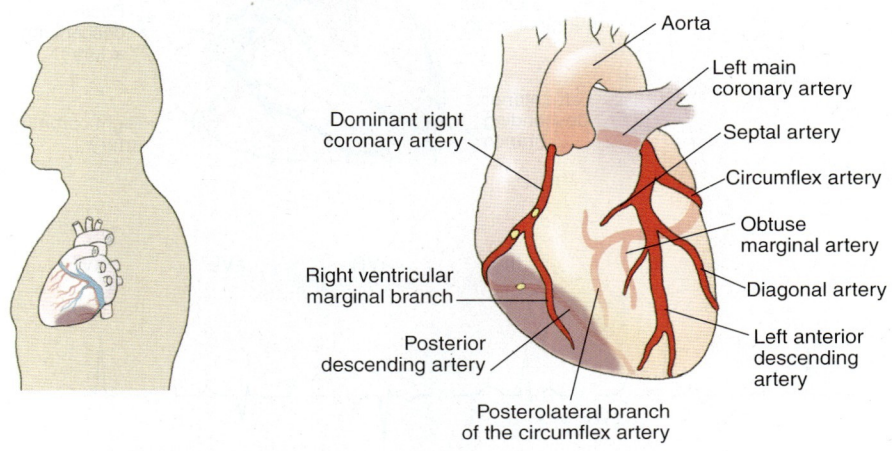

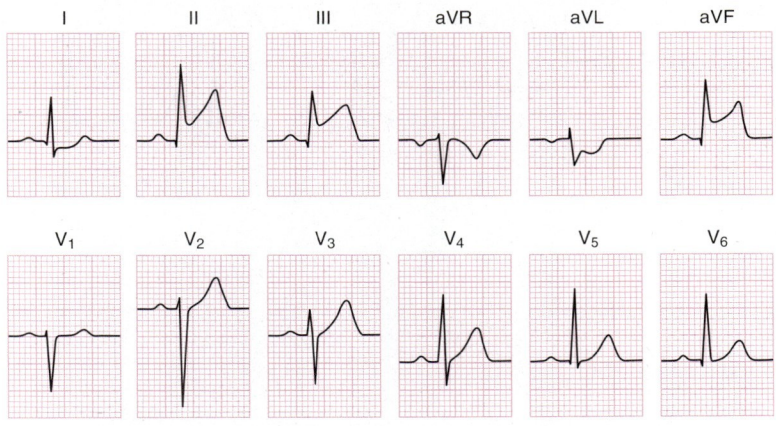

Myocardial Infarction

Anatomic Site	Leads	ECG Changes	Coronary Artery
Posterior	V_1–V_2	↑R, ↓ST, ↓T	Posterior descending

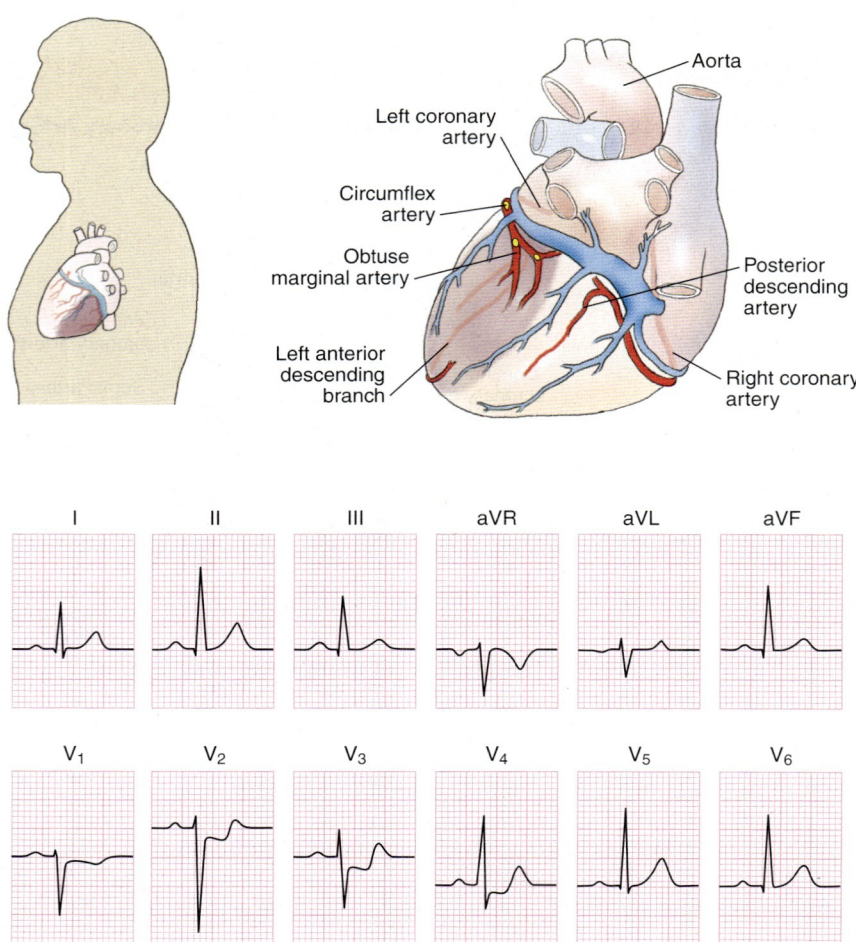

Myocardial Infarction

Anatomic Site	Leads	ECG Changes	Coronary Artery
Lateral	I, aVL, V_5–V_6	Q, ↑ST, ↑T	Left circumflex

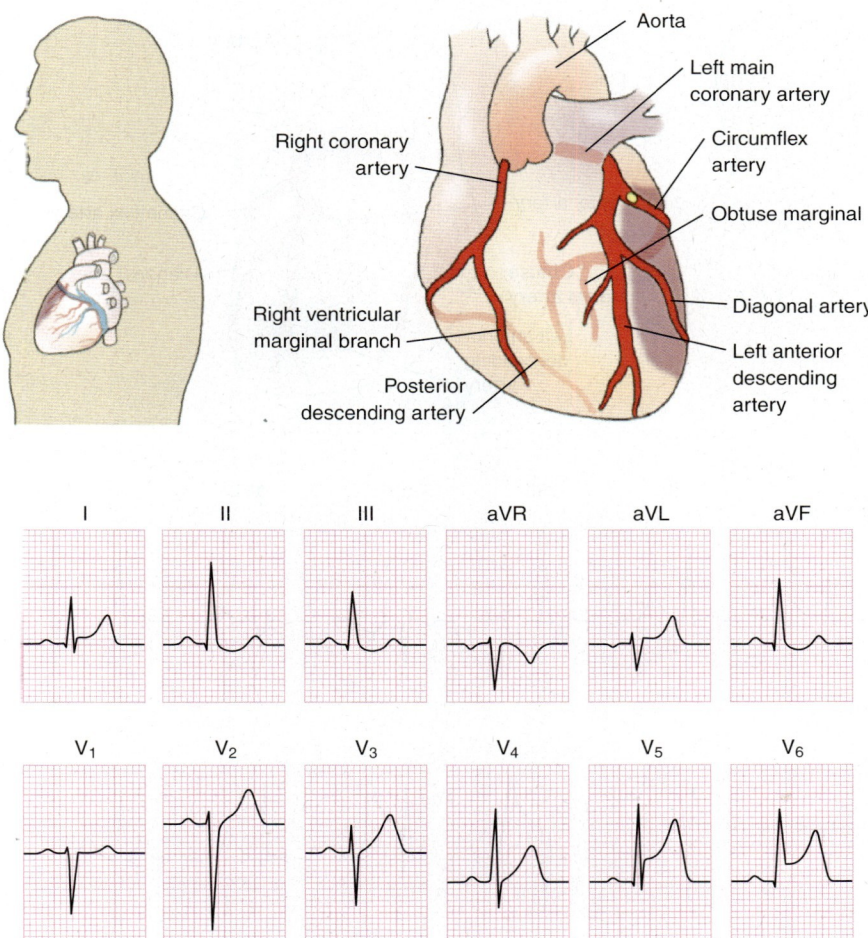

Myocardial Infarction

Anatomic Site	Leads	ECG Changes	Coronary Artery
Anterior	I, aVL, V$_1$–V$_4$	Q, ↑ST, ↑T	Left anterior descending

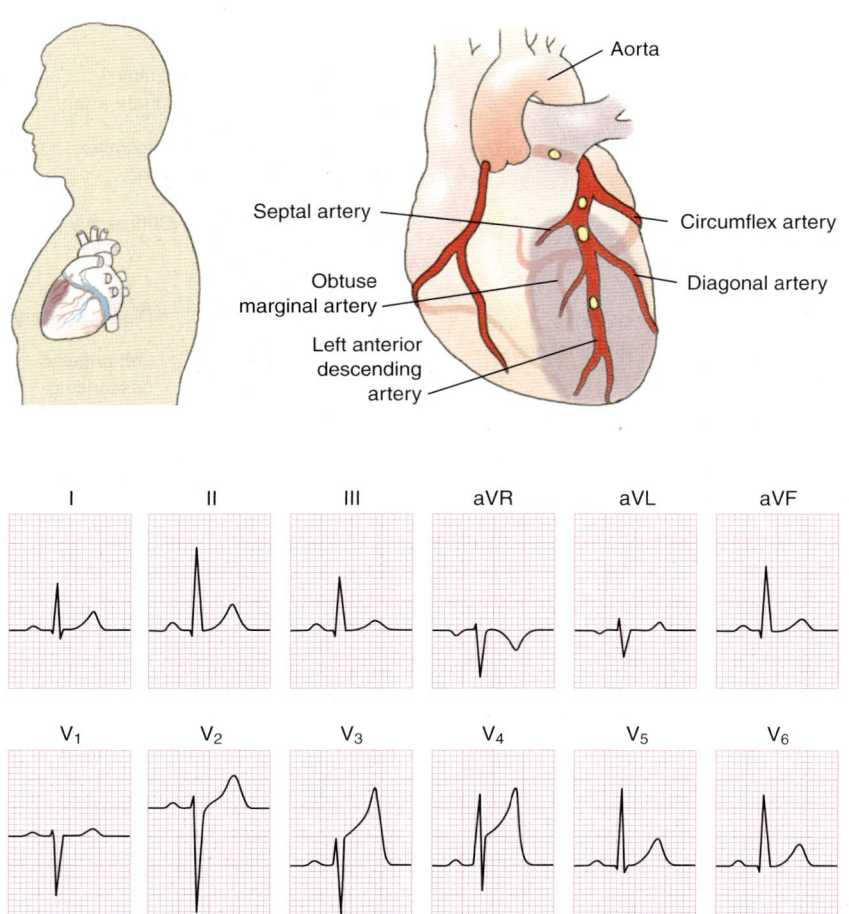

Myocardial Infarction

Anatomic Site	Leads	ECG Changes	Coronary Artery
Anteroseptal	V_1–V_4	Q, ↑ST, ↑T	Left anterior descending

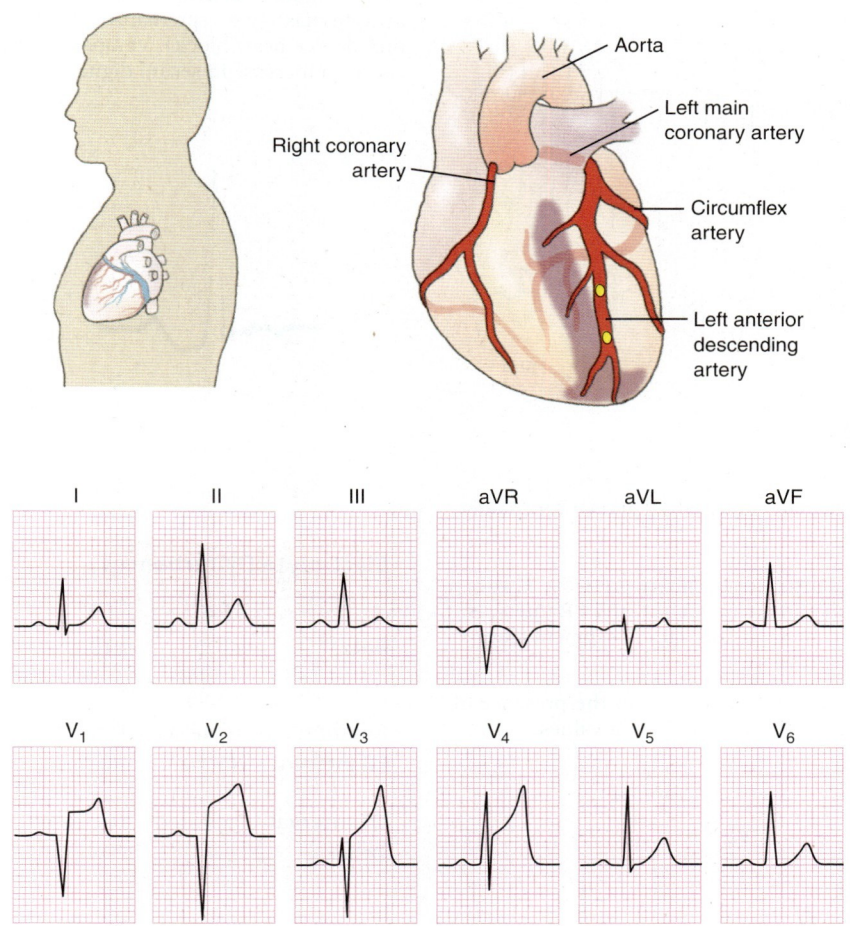

Subendocardial Myocardial Infarction (SEMI)

Persistent ST-segment depression and/or T-wave inversion in the absence of Q wave. Usually requires additional laboratory data (e.g., isoenzymes) to confirm diagnosis. Anatomic site of coronary lesion is similar to that of TMI electrocardiographically.

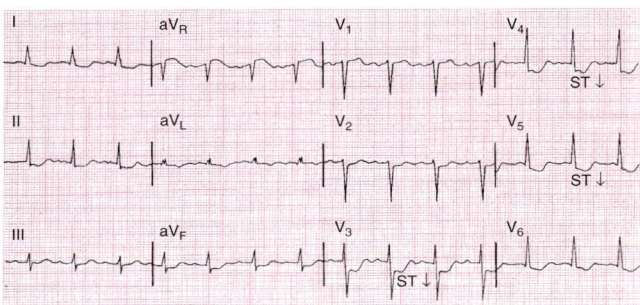

Myocardial Ischemia

Rate: Variable
Rhythm: Usually regular but may show atrial and/or ventricular arrhythmias.
PR interval: Normal
QT interval: ST segment depressed; J-point depression; T-wave inversion; conduction disturbances. (**A**) TP and PR intervals are baseline for ST-segment deviation. (**B**) ST-segment elevation. (**C**) ST-segment depression.

Note: Intraoperative ischemia usually is seen in the presence of "normal" vital signs (e.g., ± 20% of preinduction values).

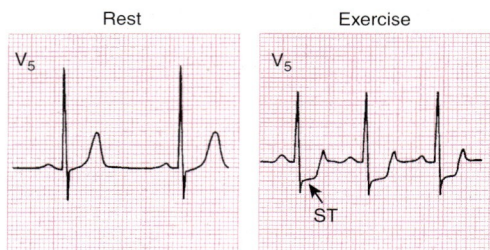

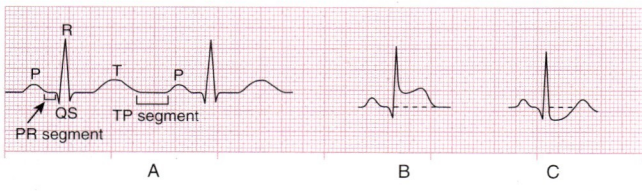

Digitalis Effect

Rate: <100 beats/min
Rhythm: Regular
PR interval: Normal or prolonged
QT interval: ST-segment sloping ("digitalis effect")

Note: Digitalis toxicity can be the cause of many common arrhythmias (e.g., premature ventricular contractions, second-degree heart block). Verapamil, quinidine, and amiodarone cause an increase in serum digitalis concentration.

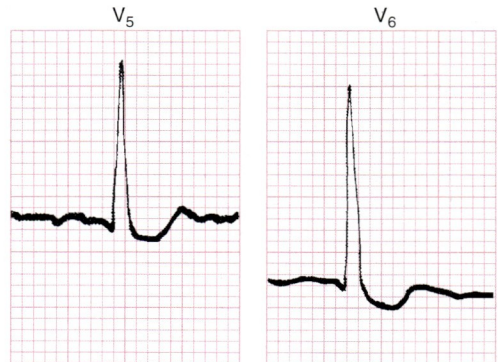

Electrolyte Disturbances

	$\downarrow Ca^{2+}$	$\uparrow Ca^{2+}$	$\downarrow K^+$	$\uparrow K^+$
Rate	<100 beats/min	<100 beats/min	<100 beats/min	<100 beats/min
Rhythm	Regular	Regular	Regular	Regular
PR interval	Normal	Normal/increased	Normal	Normal
QT interval	Increased	Decreased	Normal	Increased
Other			T wave flat, U wave	T wave peaked

Note: ECG changes usually do not correlate with serum calcium. Hypocalcemia rarely causes arrhythmias in the absence of hypokalemia. In contrast, abnormalities in serum potassium concentration can be diagnosed by ECG. Similarly, in the clinical range, magnesium concentrations are rarely associated with unique ECG patterns. The presence of a U wave (>1.5 mm in height) can also be seen in left main coronary artery disease, with certain medications and long QT syndrome.

Calcium

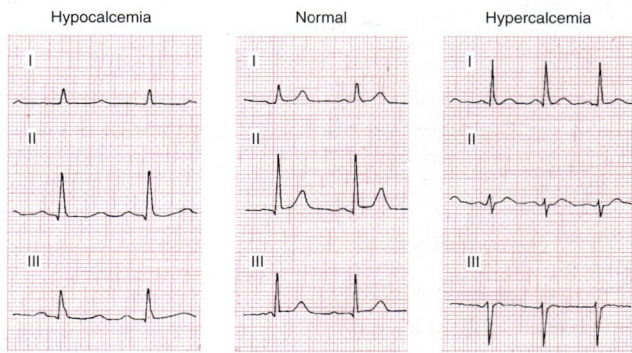

Potassium

Hypokalemia (K⁺ = 1.9 mEq/L)

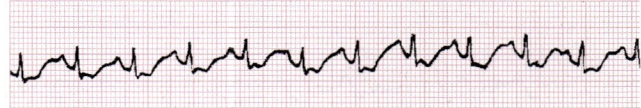

Hyperkalemia (K⁺ = 7.9 mEq/L)

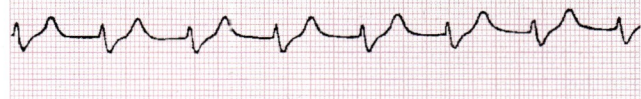

Hypothermia

Rate: <60 beats/min
Rhythm: Sinus
PR interval: Prolonged
QT interval: Prolonged

Note: Seen at temperatures below 33°C with ST-segment elevation (J point or Osborn wave). Tremor due to shivering or Parkinson disease may interfere with ECG interpretation and may be confused with atrial flutter. May represent normal variant of early ventricular repolarization. (*Arrow* indicates J point or Osborn waves.)

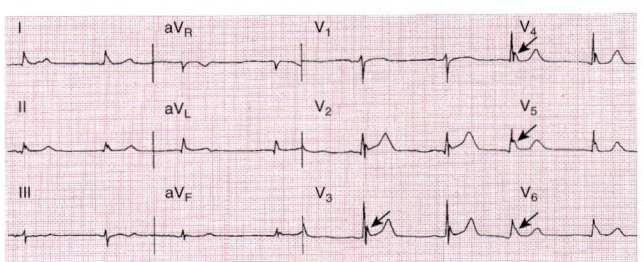

Multifocal Atrial Tachycardia

Rate: 100–200 beats/min
Rhythm: Irregular
PR interval: Consecutive P waves are of varying shape.
QT interval: Normal

Note: Seen in patients with severe lung disease. Vagal maneuvers have no effect. At heart rates <100 beats/min, it may appear as wandering atrial pacemaker. May be mistaken for atrial fibrillation. Treatment is of the causative disease process.

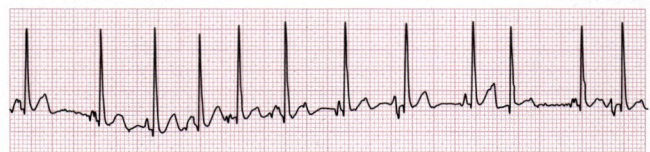

Paroxysmal Atrial Tachycardia (PAT)

Rate: 150–250 beats/min
Rhythm: Regular
PR interval: Difficult to distinguish because of tachycardia obscuring P wave. P wave may precede, be included in, or follow QRS complex.
QT interval: Normal, but ST segment and T wave may be difficult to distinguish.

Note: Therapy depends on the degree of hemodynamic compromise. Carotid sinus massage, or other vagal maneuvers, may terminate rhythm or decrease heart rate. In contrast to management of PAT in awake patients, synchronized cardioversion, rather than pharmacologic treatment, is preferred in hemodynamically unstable anesthetized patients.

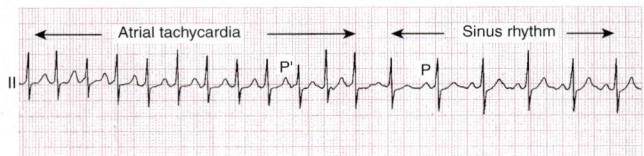

Pericarditis

Rate: Variable
Rhythm: Variable
PR interval: Normal
QT interval: Diffuse ST and T-wave changes with no Q wave and seen in more leads than a myocardial infarction.

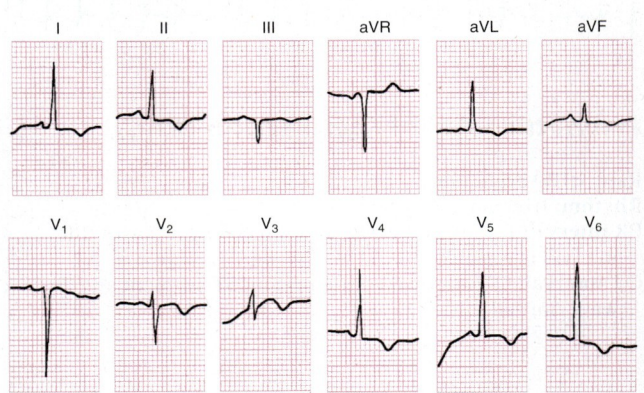

Pericardial Tamponade

Rate: Variable
Rhythm: Variable
PR interval: Low-voltage P wave
QT interval: Seen as electrical alternans with low-voltage complexes and varying amplitude of P, QRS, and T waves with each heart beat.

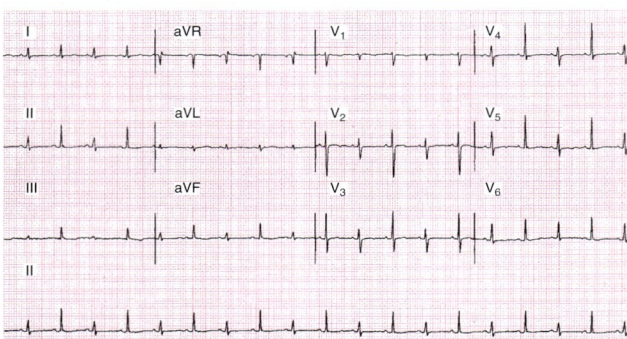

Pneumothorax

Rate: Variable
Rhythm: Variable
PR interval: Normal
QT interval: Normal

Note: Common ECG abnormalities include right-axis deviation, decreased QRS amplitude, and inverted T waves V_1–V_6. Differentiate from pulmonary embolus. May present as electrical alternans; thus, pericardial effusion should be ruled out.

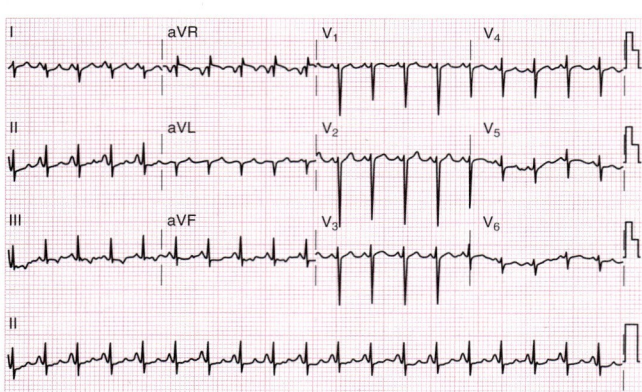

Premature Atrial Contraction (PAC)

Rate: <100 beats/min
Rhythm: Irregular
PR interval: P waves may be lost in preceding T waves. PR interval is variable.
QT interval: QRS normal configuration; ST segment and T wave normal.

Note: Nonconducted PAC appearance similar to that of sinus arrest; T waves with PAC may be distorted by inclusion of P wave in the T wave.

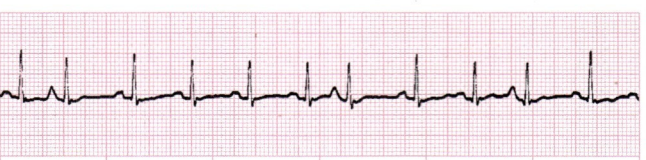

Premature Ventricular Contraction (PVC)

Rate: Usually <100 beats/min
Rhythm: Irregular
PR interval: P wave and PR interval absent; retrograde conduction of P wave can be seen.
QT interval: Wide QRS (>0.12 sec); ST segment cannot be evaluated (e.g., ischemia); T wave opposite direction of QRS with compensatory pause. Fourth and eighth beats are PVCs.

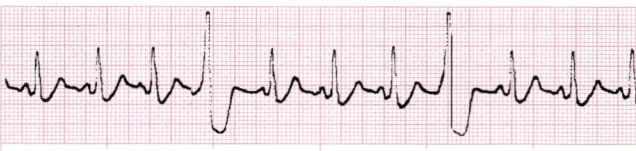

Pulmonary Embolus

Rate: >100 beats/min
Rhythm: Sinus
PR interval: P-pulmonale waveform
QT interval: Q waves in leads III and aVF

Note: Classic ECG signs S1Q3T3 with T-wave inversion also seen in V_1–V_4 and RV strain (ST depression V_1–V_4). May present with atrial fibrillation or flutter.

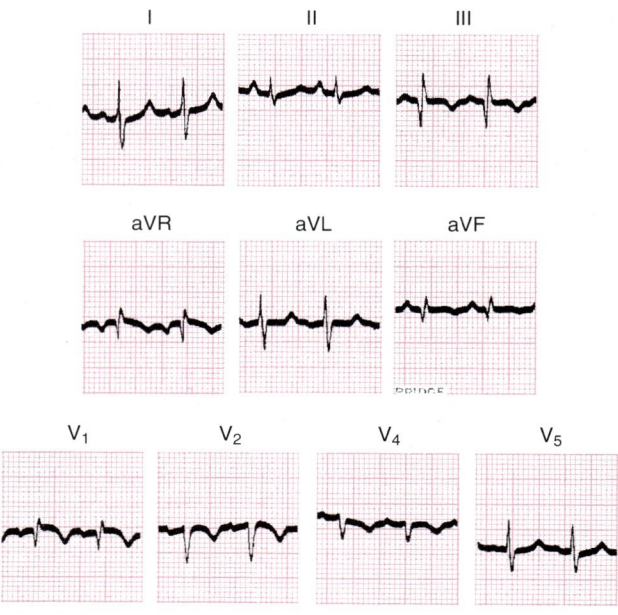

Sinus Bradycardia

Rate: <60 beats/min
Rhythm: Sinus
PR interval: Normal
QT interval: Normal

Note: Seen in trained athletes as normal variant.

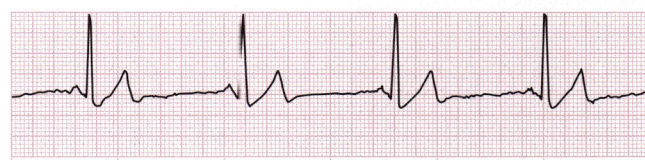

Sinus Arrhythmia

Rate: 60–100 beats/min
Rhythm: Sinus
PR interval: Normal
QT interval: R-R interval variable

Note: Heart rate increases with inhalation and decreases with exhalation + 10%–20% (respiratory). Nonrespiratory sinus arrhythmia seen in elderly with heart disease. Also seen with increased intracranial pressure.

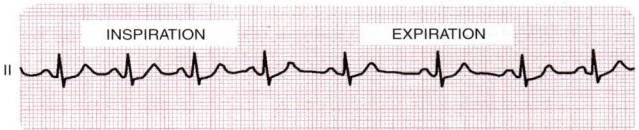

Sinus Arrest

Rate: <60 beats/min
Rhythm: Varies
PR interval: Variable
QT interval: Variable

Note: Rhythm depends on the cardiac pacemaker firing in the absence of sinoatrial stimulus (atrial pacemaker 60–75 beats/min; junctional 40–60 beats/min; ventricular 30–45 beats/min). Junctional rhythm most common. Occasional P waves may be seen (retrograde P wave).

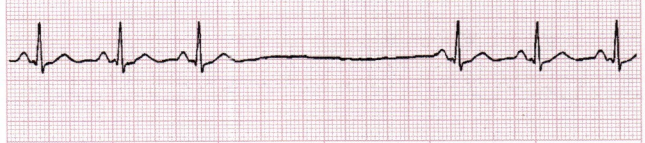

Sinus Tachycardia

Rate: 100–160 beats/min
Rhythm: Regular
PR interval: Normal; P wave may be difficult to see.
QT interval: Normal

Note: Should be differentiated from paroxysmal atrial tachycardia (PAT). With PAT, carotid massage terminates arrhythmia. Sinus tachycardia may respond to vagal maneuvers but reappears as soon as vagal stimulus is removed.

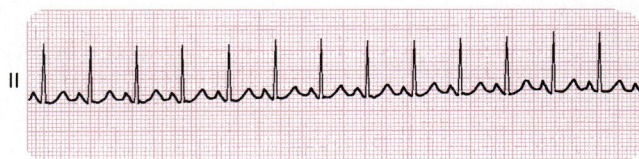

Subarachnoid Hemorrhage

Rate: <60 beats/min
Rhythm: Sinus
PR interval: Normal
QT interval: T-wave inversion is deep and wide. Prominent U waves are seen. Sinus arrythmias are observed. Q waves may be seen and may mimick acute coronary syndrome.

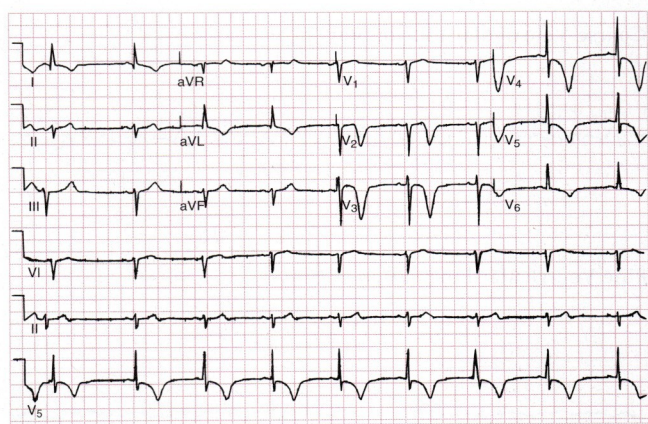

Torsades de Pointes

Rate: 150–250 beats/min
Rhythm: No atrial component seen; ventricular rhythm regular or irregular.
PR interval: P wave buried in QRS complex.
QT interval: QRS complexes usually wide and with phasic variation twisting around a central axis (a few complexes point upward, then a few point downward). ST segments and T waves difficult to discern.

Note: Type of ventricular tachycardia associated with prolonged QT interval. Seen with electrolyte disturbances (e.g., hypokalemia, hypocalcemia, and hypomagnesemia) and bradycardia. Administering standard antiarrhythmics (lidocaine, procainamide, etc.) may worsen torsades de pointes. Prevention includes treatment of the electrolyte disturbance. Treatment includes shortening of the QT interval, pharmacologically or by pacing; unstable polymorphic VT is treated with immediate defibrillation.

Torsades de Pointes: Sustained

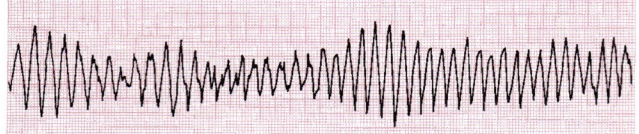

29 ▸ Ventricular Fibrillation

Rate: Absent
Rhythm: None
PR interval: Absent
QT interval: Absent

Note: "Pseudoventricular fibrillation" may be the result of a monitor malfunction (e.g., ECG lead disconnect). Always check for carotid pulse before instituting therapy.

Coarse Ventricular Fibrillation

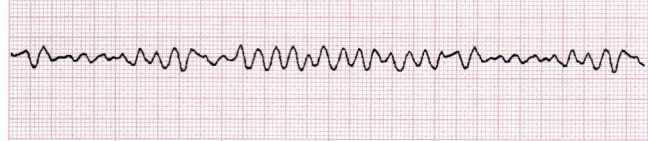

Fine Ventricular Fibrillation

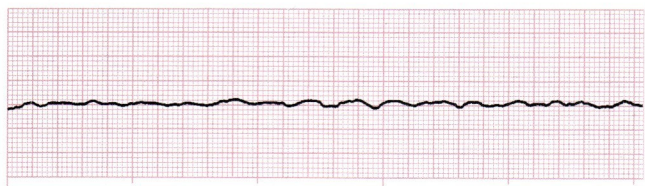

30 ▸ Ventricular Tachycardia

Rate: 100–250 beats/min
Rhythm: No atrial component seen; ventricular rhythm irregular or regular.
PR interval: Absent; retrograde P wave may be seen in QRS complex.
QT interval: Wide, bizarre QRS complex. ST segment and T wave difficult to determine.

Note: In the presence of hemodynamic compromise, VT with a pulse is treated with immediate synchronized cardioversion, whereas VT without a pulse is treated with immediate defibrillation. If the patient is stable, with short bursts of ventricular tachycardia, pharmacologic management is preferred. Should be differentiated from supraventricular tachycardia with aberrancy (SVT-A). Compensatory pause and atrioventricular dissociation suggest a PVC. P waves and SR′ (V_1) and slowing to vagal stimulus also suggest SVT-A.

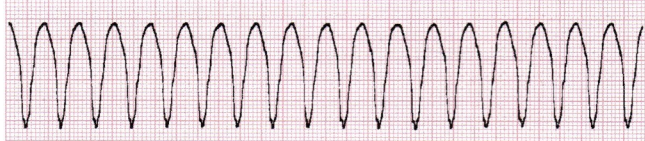

Wolff-Parkinson-White Syndrome (WPW) ▸ 31

Rate: <100 beats/min
Rhythm: Regular
PR interval: P wave normal; PR interval short (<0.12 sec)
QT interval: Duration (>0.10 sec) with slurred QRS complex (delta wave). Type A has delta wave, RBBB, with upright QRS complex V_1. Type B has delta wave and downward QRS-V_1. ST segment and T wave usually normal.

Note: Digoxin should be avoided in the presence of WPW because it increases conduction through the accessory bypass tract (bundle of Kent) and decreases AV node conduction; consequently, ventricular fibrillation can occur.

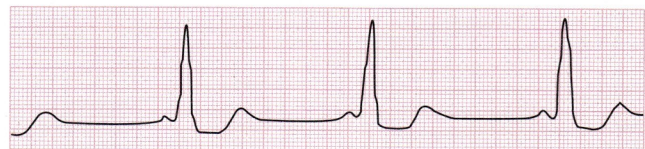

Atrial Pacing ▸ 32

Pacemaker Tracings

Atrial pacing as demonstrated in this figure is used when the atrial impulse can proceed through the AV node. Examples are sinus bradycardia and junctional rhythms associated with clinically significant decreases in blood pressure. (*Arrows* are pacemaker spikes.)

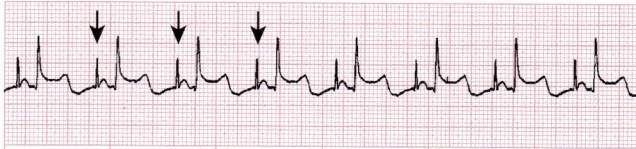

33 ◀ Ventricular Pacing

In this tracing, ventricular pacing is evident by absence of atrial wave (P wave) and pacemaker spike preceding QRS complex. Ventricular pacing is employed in the presence of bradycardia secondary to AV block or atrial fibrillation. (*Arrows* are pacemaker spikes.)

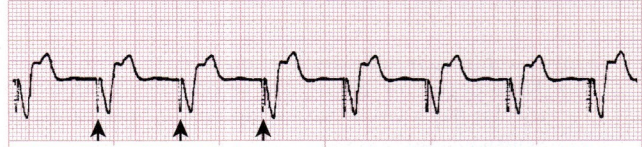

34 ◀ DDD Pacing

DDD pacing, one of the most commonly used pacing modes, paces and senses both the right atrium and right ventricle (A-V sequential pacing). Each atrial and the right ventricular complex are preceded by a pacemaker spike.

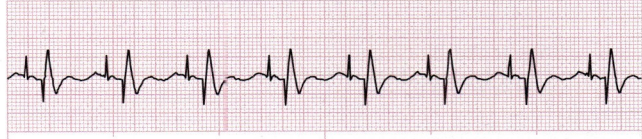

Acknowledgments

Illustrations in this appendix are reprinted from Aehlert B. *ECGs Made Easy*. 4th ed. St. Louis: Mosby/Elsevier; 2011; Goldberger AL. *Clinical Electrocardiography: A Simplified Approach*. 7th ed. Philadelphia: Mosby/Elsevier; 2006; Groh WJ, Zipes DP. Neurological disorders and cardiovascular disease. In: Bonow RO, Mann DL, Zipes DP, et al, eds. *Braunwald's Heart Disease: A Textbook of Cardiovascular Medicine*. 9th ed. Philadelphia: Saunders/Elsevier; 2012; Huszar RJ. *Basic Dysrhythmias: Interpretation and Management*. 2nd ed. St Louis: Mosby Lifeline; 1994; and Soltani P, Malozzi CM, Saleh BA, et al. Electrocardiogram manifestation of spontaneous pneumothorax. *Am J Emerg Med* 2009;27:750.e1–e5.

APPENDIX 3
Pacemaker and Implantable Cardiac Defibrillator Protocols

GINA C. BADESCU • BENJAMIN M. SHERMAN • JAMES R. ZAIDAN • PAUL G. BARASH

Pacemakers

Pacemakers are devices that deliver electrical energy and control the patient's cardiac conduction system when necessary (Table 3-2).

Indications for Permanent Pacemaker Implantation

1. Sinus node dysfunction[1]
   - Patients with documented symptomatic bradycardia or chronotropic incompetence
   - Patients with bradycardia induced by essential medical regimen
   - Patients with syncopal episodes and induced sinus bradycardia or pauses on electrophysiologic studies
   - Patients with symptoms and heart rate less than 40 bpm
2. Atrioventricular node dysfunction
   - Third-degree or high-grade second-degree atrioventricular block (AVB) with symptomatic bradycardia or ventricular arrhythmias
   - Third-degree AVB or high-grade second-degree AVB with medication-induced bradycardia
   - Asymptomatic third-degree AVB with documented asystole longer than 3 seconds or longer than 5 seconds if atrial fibrillation is present
   - Third-degree AVB s/p AV node ablation, or postoperative third-degree AVB that is not expected to recover
   - Neuromuscular disorders with third-degree AVB: Erb dystrophy, Kearns–Sayre syndrome, myotonic muscular dystrophy
   - Second-degree AVB with symptomatic bradycardia, or exercise-induced AVB
3. Bifascicular block and:
   - Type II second- or third-degree AVB

Table 3-1 Abbreviation Table

Abbrev	Meaning	Abbrev	Meaning
3D	three dimensional	ICD	implantable cardiac defibrillators
ASA	American Society of Anesthesiologists	ILR	implantable loop recorder
ATP	antitachycardia pacing	LV	left ventricle
AV	atrioventricular	LVOT	left ventricular outflow tract
AVB	atrioventricular block	MRI	magnetic resonance imaging
BPEG	British Pacing and Electrophysiology Group	NASPE	North American Society of Pacing and Electrophysiology
bpm	beats per minute		
CAD	coronary artery disease	NBG	N (NASPE), B (BPEG), G (GENERIC)
CIED	cardiac implantable electronic devices	PG	pulse generator
CPB	cardiopulmonary bypass	PP	external cardioversion–defibrillation pads or paddles
CRP	current return pad	RA	right atrium
CRT-D	cardiac resynchronization therapy—defibrillation	R&R	rate and rhythm
CT	cautery tool	RF	radio frequency
DCM	dilated cardiomyopathy	RT	radiation therapy
ECG	electrocardiogram	RV	right ventricle
ECT	electroconvulsive therapy	SCD	sudden cardiac death
EF	ejection fraction	SND	sinus node dysfunction
EMI	electromagnetic interference	STEMI	ST-segment elevation myocardial infarction
HCM	hypertrophic cardiomyopathy	TUNA	transurethral needle ablation
HR	heart rate	TURP	transurethral resection of prostate
HRS	Heart Rhythm Society	VT	ventricular tachycardia
HV	HV interval	VF	ventricular fibrillation

- Alternating bundle branch block
- Syncope
4. Second- or third-degree AVB after an ST elevation myocardial infarction (STEMI)
5. Hypersensitive carotid sinus syndrome and neurocardiogenic syncope
6. Cardiac transplantation patients who develop persistent inappropriate bradycardia
7. Other conditions:
   - Neuromuscular disease
   - Cardiac sarcoidosis with development of AVB
   - Central obstructive sleep apnea
8. Prevention and termination of certain arrhythmias (e.g., supraventricular tachycardia)
9. Hemodynamic indications:
   - Cardiac resynchronization therapy (CRT) in patients with ejection fraction (EF) below 35% and QRS greater than 120 msec
   - Hypertrophic cardiomyopathy and sinus node dysfunction (SND) or AV node dysfunction
10. Congenital heart diseases

Implantable Cardiac Defibrillators

Implantable cardiac defibrillators (ICDs) are rhythm management devices, which consist of a generator and a lead system.[2] One lead is usually placed in the right atrium and the second lead in the right ventricular apex (Table 3-3). A specific type of ICD is the biventricular pacemaker, used for CRT. This device will have a third lead placed in the coronary sinus to pace the left ventricular (LV) lateral wall in synchrony with the right ventricle (RV), in the patient with EF below 35% and a QRS duration longer than 120 msec.[1]

Indications for ICD Implantation

1. Secondary prevention of sudden cardiac death (SCD) patients with a previous ventricular tachycardia/fibrillation (VT/VF) cardiac arrest
   - Patients with coronary artery disease (CAD) who survived one cardiac arrest (if >48 h after an acute MI)
   - Patients with nonischemic dilated cardiomyopathy and
   - Hypertrophic cardiomyopathy
   - Arrhythmogenic right ventricular (RV) dysplasia
   - Genetic proarrhythmic syndromes with one prior episode of VT/VF; include long and short QT syndrome, Brugada syndrome, catecholaminergic polymorphic VT, idiopathic VF
   - Syncope with inducible sustained VT: when the arrhythmia is assumed to be the reason the syncope
2. Primary prevention of SCD
   - Includes all the subgroups from the secondary prevention that are considered high risk but did not yet have an episode of VT/VF.

Potential Intraoperative Problems with CIEDs

Electromagnetic interference (EMI) with the device is more likely when electrocautery is used above the umbilicus in a patient with a CIED implanted in subclavicular region. For generators placed elsewhere (e.g., abdominal site), expert opinion also points to the 15-cm rule, which is a distance of 15 cm around the generator or cardiac leads with the highest risk of interference.[3]

EMI leads to:
1. Inhibition of pacemaker by EMI
2. Inappropriate delivery of antitachycardia therapy by ICD
3. Changes in lead parameters:
   - Atrial mode switching
   - Inappropriate ventricular sensing
   - Electrical reset
   - Increase in ventricular thresholds
4. "Runaway" pacemaker[4]
5. Pacemaker failure after direct contact with electrocautery and cardioversion
6. Conversion from VOO (Table 3-2) back to backup mode (reprogramming)
7. Transient of permanent loss of capture
8. Dislodgement of leads during atrial fibrillation ablation procedures[5]
9. Rate adaptive pacing (interaction of minute ventilation sensor with ECG/plethysmography)
10. Oversensing and inhibition with use of lithotripsy
11. Noise reversal mode
12. Myocardial burns
13. Radiofrequency ablation and therapeutic radiation are associated with a high risk of interference similar to EMI, due to long exposure to current. Grant et al. reported in a recent study that the most notable risk factor for malfunction of CIED in patients undergoing radiation therapy was neutron producing radiotherapy (RT). The incident CIED dose up to 5.4 Gy did not correlate with CIED malfunction,

Table 3-2   Generic Pacemaker Code: NASPE/BPEG Revised (2002)

Position I, Pacing Chamber(s)	Position II, Sensing Chamber(s)	Position III, Response(s) to Sensing	Position IV, Programmability	Position V, Multisite Pacing
O = none	O = none	O = none	O = none	O = none
A = atrium	A = atrium	I = inhibited	R = rate modulation	A = atrium
V = ventricle	V = ventricle	T = triggered		V = ventricle
D = dual (A + V)	D = dual (A + V)	D = dual (T + I)		D = dual (A + V)

NBG: N refers to North American Society of Pacing and Electrophysiology (NASPE), now called the Heart Rhythm Society (HRS); B refers to British Pacing and Electrophysiology Group (BPEG); and G refers to generic.

Reproduced with permission from Practice advisory for perioperative management of patients with cardiac rhythm management devices: pacemakers and implantable cardioverter-defibrillators. A report by the American Society of Anesthesiologists Task Force on Perioperative Management of Patients with Cardiac Rhythm Management Devices. Anesthesiology. 2011;114:247–261.

Table 3-3 Generic Defibrillator Code (NBG): NASPE/BPEG

Position I, Shock Chamber(s)	Position II, Antitachycardia Pacing Chamber(s)	Position III, Tachycardia Detection	Position IV,[a] Antibradycardia Pacing Chamber(s)
O = none	O = none	E = electrogram	O = none
A = atrium	A = atrium	H = hemodynamic	A = atrium
V = ventricle	V = ventricle		V = ventricle
D = dual (A + V)	D = dual (A + V)		D = dual (A + V)

[a]For robust identification, position IV is expanded into its complete NBG code. For example, a biventricular pacing defibrillator with ventricular shock and antitachycardia pacing functionality would be identified as VVE-DDDRV, assuming that the pacing section was programmed DDDRV. Currently, no hemodynamic sensors have been approved for tachycardia detection (position III).

Reproduced with permission from Practice advisory for perioperative management of patients with cardiac rhythm management devices: pacemakers and implantable cardioverter-defibrillators. A report by the American Society of Anesthesiologists Task Force on Perioperative Management of Patients with Cardiac Rhythm Management Devices. *Anesthesiology.* 2011;114:247–261.

leading to the conclusion that it is possible that surgical relocation of the CIED may be minimized if nonneutron-producing RT is to be delivered.[6]

14. Scanning wand. A case report recently published by Plakke et al. documented a case of asystole induced by interference of the scanning wand with the temporary pacemaker with epicardial pacing wires placed routinely at separation from cardiopulmonary bypass.[7] Publication of this case report gave rise to a controversy, the manufacturer stating that the scanning wand was used off-label, without properly following the instruction manual and placing most of the blame for the incident on the anesthesiologist.[8] This resulted in the provider's response of how responsibility is assigned with the use of this device.[9] This clearly begs the more important question of how do we get the health-care providers appropriately educated on use of such devices.

General Principles of Perioperative Management of Patients with CIEDs

- The perioperative management of the patient with a CIED is via an individualized recommendation, made by the CIED team (electrophysiologist, cardiologist), in collaboration with members of the surgical/anesthesia team (perioperative team).[3] The recommendations should not be made by the industry representative without supervision by a physician who is qualified to manage these devices.
- The perioperative team should provide information to the CIED team regarding the upcoming procedure (Table 3-4).
- The CIED team should, in turn, provide information about the device and a recommendation for perioperative management of the device (Table 3-5).
- The patient with a pacemaker should have had an interrogation of the device in the 12 months prior to the surgical procedure, whereas the patient with an ICD should have had the device interrogated within 6 months prior to the scheduled procedure.
- The inactivation of the ICD or programming of a pacemaker to asynchronous mode is recommended when EMI is likely to occur.
- In patients in whom the ICD antiarrhythmia detection is turned off, the external defibrillator, with the pads positioned on the patient, is immediately available and ready to deliver therapy.
- In cases in which EMI is likely, the function of the CIED can be altered either by ferrous magnet or by reprogramming. See below for magnet response for ICD.
- Magnet response: Placing a magnet over a pacemaker generator will turn the pacemaker to asynchronous mode in most models. Placing a magnet over an

Table 3-4 Essential Elements of the Information Given to the CIED Physician

- Type of procedure
- Anatomic location of surgical procedure
- Patient position during the procedure
- Will monopolar electrosurgery be used? (If so, anatomic location of EMI delivery.)
- Will other sources of EMI likely be present?
- Will cardioversion or defibrillation be used?
- Surgical venue (operating room, procedure suite, etc.)
- Anticipated postprocedural arrangements (anticipated discharge to home <23 hours, inpatient admission to critical care bed, telemetry bed)
- Unusual circumstances: Cardiothoracic or chest wall surgical procedure that could impair/damage or encroach upon the CIED leads, anticipated large blood loss, operation in close proximity to CIED

Reprinted with permission from Crossley GH, Poole JE, Rozner MA, et al. The Heart Rhythm Society (HRS)/American Society of Anesthesiologists (ASA) Expert Consensus Statement on the Perioperative Management of Patients with Implantable Defibrillators, Pacemakers, and Arrhythmia Monitors: Facilities and Patient Management. This document was developed as a joint project with the American Society of Anesthesiologists (ASA), and in collaboration with the American Heart Association (AHA), and the Society of Thoracic Surgeons (STS). *Heart Rhythm.* 2011;8(7):1114–1154.

Table 3-5 Essential Elements of the Preoperative CIED Evaluation to Be Provided to the Operative Team

- Date of last device interrogation
- Type of device: Pacemaker ICD, CRT-D, CRT-P, ILR, implantable hemodynamic monitor
- Manufacturer and model
- Indication for device
  - Pacemaker: Sick sinus syndrome, AV block, syncope
  - ICD: Primary or secondary prevention
  - Cardiac resynchronization therapy
- Battery longevity documented as >3 months
- Are any of the leads <3 months old?
- Programming
  - Pacing mode and programmed lower rate
  - ICD therapy
    - Lowest heart rate for shock delivery
    - Lowest heart rate for ATP delivery
  - Rate-responsive sensor type, if programmed on
- Is the patient pacemaker dependent, and what is the underlying rhythm and heart rate if it can be determined?
- What is the response of this device to magnet placement
  - Magnet pacing rate for a pacemaker
  - Pacing amplitude response to magnet function
  - Will ICD detections resume automatically with removal of the magnet? Does this device allow for magnet application function to be disabled? If so, document programming of patient's device for this feature.
- Any alert status on CIED generator or lead
- Last pacing threshold: Document adequate safety margin with the date of that threshold

Reprinted with permission from Crossley GH, Poole JE, Rozner MA, et al. The Heart Rhythm Society (HRS)/American Society of Anesthesiologists (ASA) Expert Consensus Statement on the Perioperative Management of Patients with Implantable Defibrillators, Pacemakers, and Arrhythmia Monitors: Facilities and Patient Management. This document was developed as a joint project with the American Society of Anesthesiologists (ASA), and in collaboration with the American Heart Association (AHA), and the Society of Thoracic Surgeons (STS). Heart Rhythm. 2011;8(7):1114–1154.

ICD will suspend the arrhythmia detection. It will *not* switch the pacemaker function to asynchronous mode; therefore, in patients who are pacemaker dependent, the team must be aware of the risk of inhibition of the pacemaker by the EMI. If EMI is likely to occur, the recommendation is to reprogram the CIED prior to the case, by turning the arrhythmia detection function to off and program the pacemaker to asynchronous mode. Because a minority of models do not respond to magnet application in the fashion described above, it is always recommended to contact the manufacturer and confirm the response to magnet for the specific model one is dealing with.

- Complications related to application of magnet are rare. However, recent publication of a case report of three patients with intraoperative complications related to inadequate preoperative evaluation of the CIED and knowledge about response to magnet application underline the importance of following the ASA and HRS guidelines and gain knowledge about these issues preoperatively, as the complications are most of the time acute and severe.[10]

Risk Mitigation Strategies

- Use bipolar cautery where possible.[3]
- Use short bursts of monopolar cautery, 5 seconds or less.
- Place the return current pad in such a way to avoid crossing the generator.
- Have rescue equipment, including external pacemaker/defibrillator, immediately available for all patients with CIED.
- Activating the electrocautery in the area of the generator, even if the active electrode is not touching the patient, will cause interference.

Anesthesia Device Services

In the last few years, perioperative management of rhythm devices has become a more active focus of the Surgery and Anesthesia Departments in different institutions across the country. This is due to the increasing number of patients that present for surgery with one of these devices in place, posing real scheduling and management challenges, with the most concerning issue being scheduling delay. The Anesthesiology Department at the University of Washington evaluated management of CIED in the perioperative period by an Anesthesia Device Service (ADS) versus the Electrophysiology/Cardiology Service (EPCS) over a period of 4 years (2009–2013).[11]

The ADS was developed with help and training from the EPCS and managed 548 patients during this time, with no major complications or safety concerns and at the end of the 4 years obtained a slight reduction in the scheduling delays. Most errors made by the ADS were with restoration of the demand features postoperatively in the patients where the asynchronous mode was used during surgery, whereas the EPCS failed mostly at following the recommendations of the perioperative management of CIEDs by the HRS, published in 2011.[12]

The creation of such a service is a serious undertaking, necessitating training of anesthesiologists and a very close collaboration between the Anesthesiology and Cardiology Departments. However, it is conceivable that in the future this type of service will become an integral part of the perioperative surgical home, particularly in high volume centers where the scheduling delays have a serious impact.

Table 3-6 and Figure 3-1 are examples of approaches to perioperative management of patients with CIEDs.[13]

Recommendations for Postoperative Follow-Up of Patients with CIEDs (Tables 3-7, 3-8 and 3-9)

Optimization of Pacing after Cardiopulmonary Bypass

Separation from CPB is usually associated with a conduction abnormality, from first-degree AV block, sinus bradycardia, to third-degree AV block, or interventricular delays.[14]

1. **Lead placement:** Right atrial (RA) lead: place at the cephalic atrial wall, between the atrial appendages. Right ventricular lead: place at the level of the right ventricle outflow tract (RVOT). For the patient with obstructive cardiomyopathy, the RV lead is better placed in the RV

Table 3-6 Example of a Stepwise Approach to the Perioperative Management of the Patient with a CIED

Perioperative Period	Patient/CIED Condition	Intervention
Preoperative evaluation	Patient has CIED Determine CIED type (PM, ICD, CRT)	Focused history Focused physical examination Manufacturer's CIED identification card Chest x-ray (no data available) Supplemental resources[a]
	Determine if patient is CIED-dependent for pacing function	Verbal history Bradyarrhythmia symptoms Atrioventricular node ablation No spontaneous ventricular activity[b]
	Determine CIED function	Comprehensive CIED evaluation[c] Determine if pacing pulses are present and create paced beats
Preoperative preparation	EMI unlikely during procedure	If EMI is unlikely, then special precautions are not needed
	EMI likely; CIED is PM	Reprogram to asynchronous mode when indicated Suspend rate adaptive functions[d]
	EMI likely; CIED is ICD	Suspend antitachyarrhythmia functions. If patient is dependent on pacing function, then alter pacing function as above
	EMI likely; All CIED	Use bipolar cautery; ultrasonic scalpel
	Intraoperative physiologic changes likely (e.g., bradycardia, ischemia)	Temporary pacing and cardioversion–defibrillation available Plan for possible adverse CIED-patient interaction
Intraoperative management	Monitoring	Electrocardiographic monitoring per ASA standard Peripheral pulse monitoring
	Electrocautery interference	CT/CRP no current through PG/leads Avoid proximity of CT to PG/leads Short bursts at lowest possible energy Use bipolar cautery; ultrasonic scalpel
	RF catheter ablation	Avoid contact of RF catheter with PG/leads RF current path far away from PG/leads Discuss these concerns with operator
	Lithotripsy	Do not focus lithotripsy beam near PG R-wave triggers lithotripsy? Disable atrial pacing
	MRI	Generally contraindicated If required, consult ordering physician, cardiologist, radiologist, and manufacturer
	Radiation therapy	PG/leads must be outside of RT field Possible surgical relocation of PG Verify PG function during/after RT course
	ECT	Consult with ordering physician, patient's cardiologist, a CIED service, or CIED manufacturer
Emergency defibrillation-cardioversion	ICD: magnet-disabled	Terminate all EMI sources Remove magnet to re-enable therapies Observe for appropriate therapies
	ICD: programming disabled	Programming to re-enable therapies or proceed directly with external cardioversion/defibrillation
	ICD: either of above	Minimize current flow through PG/leads PP as far as possible from PG PP perpendicular to major axis PG/leads To extent possible, PP in anterior–posterior location
	Regardless of CIED type	Use clinically appropriate cardioversion/defibrillation energy
Postoperative management	Immediate postoperative period	Monitor cardiac R&R continuously Back-up pacing and cardioversion/defibrillation capability
	Postoperative interrogation and restoration of CIED function	Interrogation to assess function Settings appropriate?[e] Is CIED an ICD?[f] Use cardiology/PM-ICD service if needed

[a]Manufacturer's databases, pacemaker clinic records, cardiology consultation
[b]With cardiac rhythm management device (CRMD) programmed VVI at lowest programmable rate.
[c]Ideally, CIED function assessed by interrogation, with function altered by reprogramming if required.
[d]Most times this will be necessary; when in doubt, assume so.
[e]If necessary, reprogram appropriate setting.
[f]Restore all antitachycardia therapies.
Reprinted with permission from Practice advisory for perioperative management of patients with cardiac rhythm management devices: pacemakers and implantable cardioverter-defibrillators. A report by the American Society of Anesthesiologists Task Force on Perioperative Management of Patients with Cardiac Rhythm Management Devices. Anesthesiology. 2011;114:247–261.

Table 3-7 Specific Procedures and Writing Committee Recommendations on Postoperative CIED Evaluation

Procedure	Recommendation
Monopolar electrosurgery	CIED evaluated[a] within 1 month from procedure unless Table 3-8 criteria are fulfilled
External cardioversion	CIED evaluated[a] prior to discharge or transfer from cardiac telemetry
Radiofrequency ablation	CIED evaluated[a] prior to discharge or transfer from cardiac telemetry
Electroconvulsive therapy	CIED evaluated[a] within 1 month from procedure unless fulfilling Table 3-8 criteria
Nerve conduction studies (ENG)	No additional CIED evaluation beyond routine
Ocular procedures	No additional CIED evaluation beyond routine
Therapeutic radiation	CIED evaluated prior to discharge or transfer from cardiac telemetry; remote monitoring optimal; some instances may indicate interrogation after each treatment (see text)
TUNA/TURP	No additional CIED evaluation beyond routine
Hysteroscopic ablation	No additional CIED evaluation beyond routine
Lithotripsy	CIED evaluated[a] within 1 month from procedure unless fulfilling Table 3-8 criteria
Endoscopy	No additional CIED evaluation beyond routine
Iontophoresis	No additional CIED evaluation beyond routine
Photodynamic therapy	No additional CIED evaluation beyond routine
X-ray/CT scans/mammography	No additional CIED evaluation beyond routine

[a]This evaluation is intended to reveal electrical reset. Therefore, an interrogation alone is needed. This can be accomplished in person or by remote telemetry.

CIED, cardiac implantable electronic device; CT, computed tomography; TUNA, transurethral needle ablation; TURP, transurethral resection of prostate.

Reprinted with permission from Crossley GH, Poole JE, Rozner MA, et al. The Heart Rhythm Society (HRS)/American Society of Anesthesiologists (ASA) Expert Consensus Statement on the Perioperative Management of Patients with Implantable Defibrillators, Pacemakers, and Arrhythmia Monitors: Facilities and Patient Management. This document was developed as a joint project with the American Society of Anesthesiologists (ASA), and in collaboration with the American Heart Association (AHA), and the Society of Thoracic Surgeons (STS). *Heart Rhythm.* 2011;8(7):1114–1154.

Table 3-8 Indications for the Interrogation of CIEDs prior to Patient Discharge or Transfer from a Cardiac Telemetry Environment

- Patients with CIEDs reprogrammed prior to the procedure that left the device nonfunctional such as disabling tachycardia detection in an ICD.
- Patients with CIEDs who underwent hemodynamically challenging surgeries such as cardiac surgery or significant vascular surgery (e.g., abdominal aortic aneurysmal repair).[a]
- Patients with CIEDs who experienced significant intraoperative events including cardiac arrest requiring temporary pacing or cardiopulmonary resuscitation and those who required external electrical cardioversion.
- Emergent surgery where the site of EMI exposure was above the umbilicus
- Cardiothoracic surgery
- Patients with CIEDs who underwent certain types of procedures (Table 3-7) that emit EMI with a greater probability of affecting device function.
- Patients with CIEDs who have logistical limitations that would prevent reliable device evaluation within 1 month from their procedure

[a]The general purpose of this interrogation is to assure that reset did not occur. In these cases, a full evaluation including threshold evaluations is suggested.

CIED, cardiac implantable electrical device; EMI, electromagnetic interference; ICD, implantable cardiac defibrillator.

Reprinted with permission from Crossley GH, Poole JE, Rozner MA, et al. The Heart Rhythm Society (HRS)/American Society of Anesthesiologists (ASA) Expert Consensus Statement on the Perioperative Management of Patients with Implantable Defibrillators, Pacemakers, and Arrhythmia Monitors: Facilities and Patient Management. This document was developed as a joint project with the American Society of Anesthesiologists (ASA), and in collaboration with the American Heart Association (AHA), and the Society of Thoracic Surgeons (STS). *Heart Rhythm.* 2011;8(7):1114–1154.

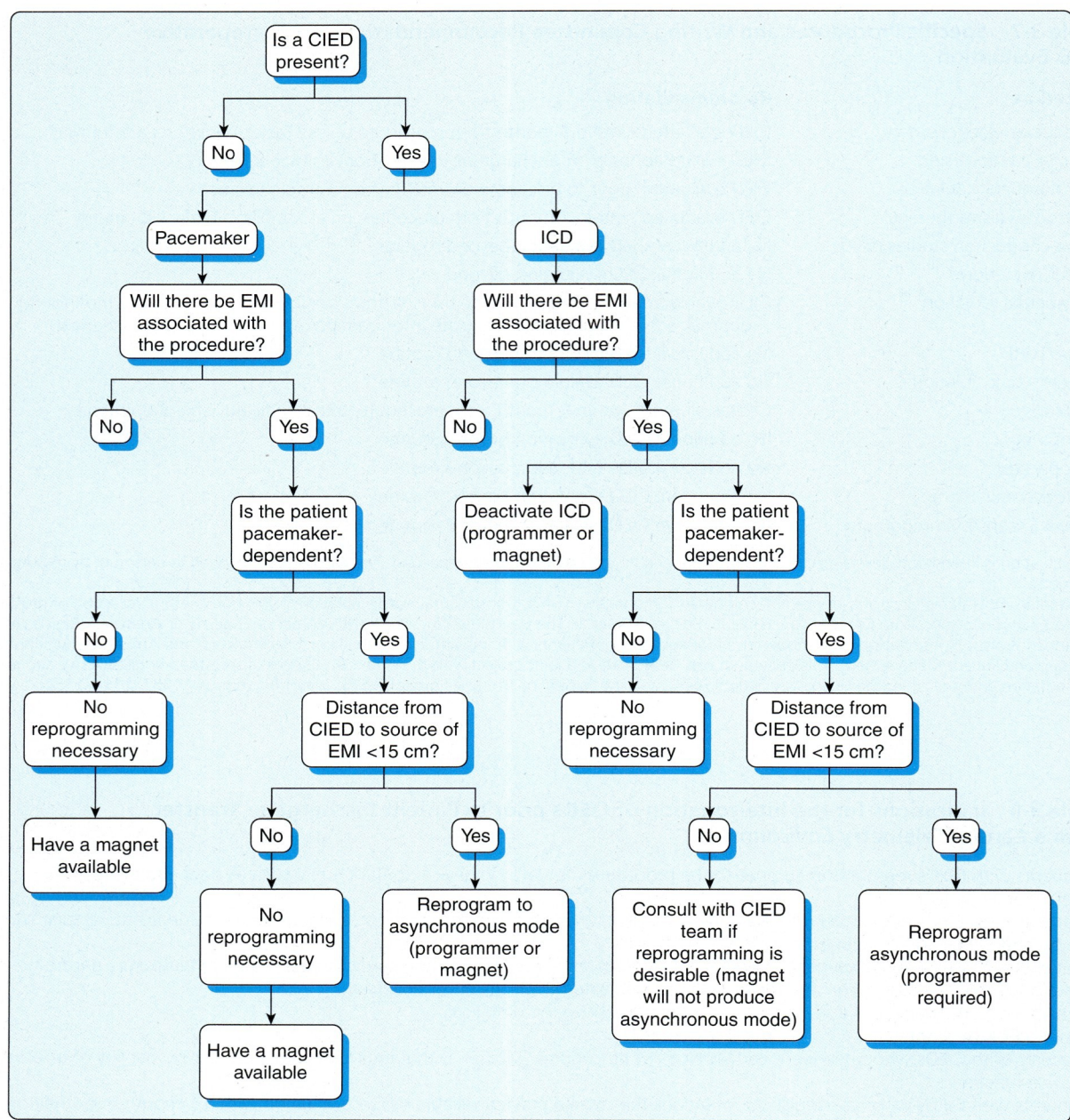

Figure 3-1 Example of an algorithm for perioperative management of patients with CIEDs. (Reprinted with permission from Stone ME, Salter B, Fischer A. Perioperative management of patients with cardiac implantable electronic devices. *Br J Anaesth*. 2011;107(Suppl 1):i16–i26.)

Table 3-9 Treatment of Pacemaker Failure

Rate	Possible Response
Adequate to maintain blood pressure	1. Oxygen, airway control 2. Place magnet over pacemaker 3. Atropine if sinus bradycardia
Severe bradycardia and hypotension	1. Oxygen, airway control 2. Place magnet over pacemaker 3. Other types of pacing if magnet does not activate the pacemaker (transcutaneous, esophageal, or transvenous) 4. Atropine if sinus bradycardia 5. Isoproterenol to increase ventricular rate
No escape rhythm	1. Cardiopulmonary resuscitation 2. Place magnet over pacemaker 3. Other types of pacing if magnet does not activate the pacemaker (transcutaneous, esophageal, or transvenous) 4. Isoproterenol to increase ventricular rate

Reprinted with permission from Zaidan JR, Youngberg JA, Lake CL, et al., eds., *Cardiac, Vascular and Thoracic Anesthesia*. New York. NY: Churchill Livingstone; 2000.

apex, for less dynamic obstruction of the LVOT. Biventricular pacing is initiated for patients with intraventricular conduction lesions and dyssynchrony of contraction. Place the LV lead at the basal posterolateral wall, and hook the two ventricular leads through a y piece to the ventricular output of the temporary pacemaker box.

2. **Rate:** program to obtain the best improvement in cardiac output and improvement in mixed venous saturation and arterial blood pressure.
3. **AV delay:** In patients with LV dysfunction, we can maximize the contribution of the atria to the preload. Use pulse wave Doppler through the mitral valve inflow, and modify the AV delay to obtain a clear E and A waveforms, and to ensure that the A wave finishes before the onset of the QRS; the closure of the mitral valve should happen at the end of the A wave, but before any diastolic mitral regurgitation.
4. **Pacing mode:** Three modes are explained here. In the patient with normal AV conduction, AAI mode allows for increase in HR and a physiologic depolarization of the ventricles. If inhibition by electrocautery is a concern, use asynchronous pacing in AOO mode (Table 3-2). For the patient with AV conduction delay, DOO or DDI should be used. DDI mode also avoids tracking of rapid atrial rates in case of post bypass atrial fibrillation.
5. **Biventricular pacing**[14,15] in patients with EF below 35% and QRS longer than 120 msec acute biventricular pacing improves torsion and mechanics of contraction, particularly in patients with mitral regurgitation due to papillary muscle dyssynchrony. Speckle-tracking, 3D echocardiography, M-mode definition of septal to wall motion delay, color Doppler tissue imaging, and analysis of segmental velocity are used to characterize ventricular dyssynchrony. Currently, available temporary pacemakers only allow biventricular pacing through a Y connection of the two ventricular epicardial wires to the ventricular output of the box. Acute CRT leads to an increase in myocardial performance with a slight decrease in myocardial oxygen consumption.

REFERENCES

1. Epstein AE, Dimarco JP, Ellenbogen KA, et al. ACC/AHA/HRS 2008 guidelines for device-based therapy of cardiac rhythm abnormalities: executive summary. *Heart Rhythm*. 2008;5:934–955.
2. Stone KR, McPherson CA. Assessment and management of patients with pacemakers and implantable cardioverter defibrillators. *Crit Care Med*. 2004;32:S155–165.
3. Crossley GH, Poole JE, Rozner MA, et al. The Heart Rhythm Society (HRS)/American Society of Anesthesiologists (ASA) Expert Consensus Statement on the perioperative management of patients with implantable defibrillators, pacemakers and arrhythmia monitors: facilities and patient management this document was developed as a joint project with the American Society of Anesthesiologists (ASA), and in collaboration with the American Heart Association (AHA), and the Society of Thoracic Surgeons (STS). *Heart Rhythm*. 2011;8:1114–1154.
4. Heller LI. Surgical electrocautery and the runaway pacemaker syndrome. *Pacing Clin Electrophysiol*. 1990;13:1084–1085.
5. Lakkireddy D, Patel D, Ryschon K, et al. Safety and efficacy of radiofrequency energy catheter ablation of atrial fibrillation in patients with pacemakers and implantable cardiac defibrillators. *Heart Rhythm*. 2005;2:1309–1316.
6. Grant JD, Jensen GL, Tang C, et al. Radiotherapy-induced malfunction in contemporary cardiovascular implantable electronic devices: clinical incidence and predictors. *JAMA Oncol*. 2015;1:624–632.
7. Plakke MJ, Maisonave Y, Daley SM, et al. Radiofrequency scanning for retained surgical items can cause electromagnetic interference and pacing inhibition if an asynchronous pacing mode is not applied. *A A Case Rep*. 2016;6:143–145.
8. Kane T. Editorial comment: manufacturer's response. *A A Case Rep*. 2016;6:142.
9. Rozner MA, Schultheis L, Schulman PM. The unstated Murphy's Law of the operating room: if something goes wrong, blame anesthesia. *A A Case Rep*. 2016;6:139–141.
10. Schulman PM, Rozner MA. Case report: use caution when applying magnets to pacemakers or defibrillators for surgery. *Anesth Analg*. 2013; 117:422–427.
11. Rooke GA, Lombaard SA, Van Norman GA, et al. Initial experience of an anesthesiology-based service for perioperative management of pacemakers and implantable cardioverter defibrillators. *Anesthesiology*. 2015;123:1024–1032.
12. Rozner MA, Schulman PM. Creating an anesthesiologist-run pacemaker and defibrillator service: closing the perioperative care gap for these patients. *Anesthesiology*. 2015;123:990–992.
13. Stone ME, Salter A, Fischer G. Perioperative management of patients with cardiac implantable electronic devices. *Br J Anaesth*. 2011;107(Suppl 1):i16–i26.
14. Chua J, Schwarzenberger JA, Mahajan A. Optimization of pacing after cardiopulmonary bypass. *J Cardiothorac Vasc Anest*. 2012;26:291–301.
15. Wang DY, Richmond ME, Quinn TA, et al. Optimized temporary biventricular pacing acutely improves intraoperative cardiac output after weaning from cardiopulmonary bypass: a substudy of a randomized clinical trial. *J Thorac Cardiovasc Surg*. 2011;141:1002–1008.

APPENDIX 4
American Society of Anesthesiologists Standards, Guidelines, and Statements

Committee of Origin: Standards and Practice Parameters

(Approved by the ASA House of Delegates on October 21, 1986, and last amended on October 20, 2010, with an effective date of July 1, 2011)

These standards apply to all anesthesia care although, in emergency circumstances, appropriate life support measures take precedence. These standards may be exceeded at any time based on the judgment of the responsible anesthesiologist. They are intended to encourage quality patient care, but observing them cannot guarantee any specific patient outcome. They are subject to revision from time to time, as warranted by the evolution of technology and practice. They apply to all general anesthetics, regional anesthetics, and monitored anesthesia care. This set of standards addresses only the issue of basic anesthetic monitoring, which is one component of anesthesia care. In certain rare or unusual circumstances, (1) some of these methods of monitoring may be clinically impractical, and (2) appropriate use of the described monitoring methods may fail to detect untoward clinical developments. Brief interruptions of continual* monitoring may be unavoidable. These standards are not intended for application to the care of the obstetrical patient in labor or in the conduct of pain management.

Standard I

Qualified anesthesia personnel shall be present in the room throughout the conduct of all general anesthetics, regional anesthetics, and monitored anesthesia care.

Objective

Because of the rapid changes in patient status during anesthesia, qualified anesthesia personnel shall be continuously present to monitor the patient and provide anesthesia care. In the event there is a direct known hazard, for example, radiation, to the anesthesia personnel which might require intermittent remote observation of the patient, some provision for monitoring the patient must be made. In the event that an emergency requires the temporary absence of the person primarily responsible for the anesthetic, the best judgment of the anesthesiologist will be exercised in comparing the emergency with the anesthetized patient's condition and in the selection of the person left responsible for the anesthetic during the temporary absence.

---

*Note that "continual" is defined as "repeated regularly and frequently in steady rapid succession" whereas "continuous" means "prolonged without any interruption at any time."

Standard II

During all anesthetics, the patient's oxygenation, ventilation, circulation, and temperature shall be continually evaluated.

Oxygenation

Objective

To ensure adequate oxygen concentration in the inspired gas and the blood during all anesthetics.

Methods

1. Inspired gas: During every administration of general anesthesia using an anesthesia machine, the concentration of oxygen in the patient breathing system shall be measured by an oxygen analyzer with a low oxygen concentration limit alarm in use.†
2. Blood oxygenation: During all anesthetics, a quantitative method of assessing oxygenation such as pulse oximetry shall be employed.† When the pulse oximeter is utilized, the variable pitch pulse tone and the low threshold alarm shall be audible to the anesthesiologist or the anesthesia care team personnel.† Adequate illumination and exposure of the patient are necessary to assess color.†

Ventilation

Objective

To ensure adequate ventilation of the patient during all anesthetics.

Methods

1. Every patient receiving general anesthesia shall have the adequacy of ventilation continually evaluated. Qualitative clinical signs such as chest excursion, observation of the reservoir breathing bag, and auscultation of breath sounds are useful. Continual monitoring for the presence of expired carbon dioxide shall be performed unless invalidated by the nature of the patient, procedure, or equipment. Quantitative monitoring of the volume of expired gas is strongly encouraged.†
2. When an endotracheal tube or laryngeal mask is inserted, its correct positioning must be verified by clinical assessment and by identification of carbon dioxide in the expired gas. Continual end-tidal carbon dioxide analysis, in use from the time of endotracheal tube/laryngeal mask

---

†Under extenuating circumstances, the responsible anesthesiologist may waive the requirements marked with a dagger (†); it is recommended that when this is done, it should be so stated (including the reasons) in a note in the patient's medical record.

placement, until extubation/removal or initiating transfer to a postoperative care location, shall be performed using a quantitative method such as capnography, capnometry, or mass spectroscopy.[†] When capnography or capnometry is utilized, the end-tidal CO_2 alarm shall be audible to the anesthesiologist or the anesthesia care team personnel.[†]
3. When ventilation is controlled by a mechanical ventilator, there shall be in continuous use a device that is capable of detecting disconnection of components of the breathing system. The device must give an audible signal when its alarm threshold is exceeded.
4. During regional anesthesia (with no sedation) or local anesthesia (with no sedation), the adequacy of ventilation shall be evaluated by continual observation of qualitative clinical signs. During moderate or deep sedation the adequacy of ventilation shall be evaluated by continual observation of qualitative clinical signs and monitoring for the presence of exhaled carbon dioxide unless precluded or invalidated by the nature of the patient, procedure, or equipment.

Circulation

Objective

To ensure the adequacy of the patient's circulatory function during all anesthetics.

Methods

1. Every patient receiving anesthesia shall have the electrocardiogram continuously displayed from the beginning of anesthesia until preparing to leave the anesthetizing location.[†]
2. Every patient receiving anesthesia shall have arterial blood pressure and heart rate determined and evaluated at least every 5 minutes.[†]
3. Every patient receiving general anesthesia shall have, in addition to the above, circulatory function continually evaluated by at least one of the following: palpation of a pulse, auscultation of heart sounds, monitoring of a tracing of intra-arterial pressure, ultrasound peripheral pulse monitoring, or pulse plethysmography or oximetry.

Body Temperature

Objective

To aid in the maintenance of appropriate body temperature during all anesthetics.

Methods

Every patient receiving anesthesia shall have temperature monitored when clinically significant changes in body temperature are intended, anticipated, or suspected.

Continuum of Depth of Sedation: Definition of General Anesthesia and Levels of Sedation/Analgesia*

Committee of Origin: Quality Management and Departmental Administration

(Approved by the ASA House of Delegates on October 13, 1999, and last amended on October 15, 2014)

	Minimal Sedation (Anxiolysis)	Moderate Sedation/ Analgesia (Conscious Sedation)	Deep Sedation/ Analgesia	General Anesthesia
Responsiveness	Normal response to verbal stimulation	Purposeful[†] response to verbal or tactile stimulation	Purposeful[†] response following repeated or painful stimulation	Unarousable even with painful stimulus
Airway	Unaffected	No intervention required	Intervention may be required	Intervention often required
Spontaneous Ventilation	Unaffected	Adequate	May be inadequate	Frequently inadequate
Cardiovascular Function	Unaffected	Usually maintained	Usually maintained	May be impaired

Minimal Sedation (Anxiolysis) is a drug-induced state during which patients respond normally to verbal commands. Although cognitive function and physical coordination may be impaired, airway reflexes, and ventilatory and cardiovascular functions are unaffected.

Moderate Sedation/Analgesia (Conscious Sedation) is a drug-induced depression of consciousness during which patients respond purposefully[†] to verbal commands, either alone or accompanied by light tactile stimulation. No interventions are required to maintain a patent airway, and spontaneous ventilation is adequate. Cardiovascular function is usually maintained.

Deep Sedation/Analgesia is a drug-induced depression of consciousness during which patients cannot be easily aroused but respond purposefully[†] following repeated or painful stimulation.

---

*Monitored Anesthesia Care ("MAC") does not describe the continuum of depth of sedation, rather it describes "a specific anesthesia service in which an anesthesiologist has been requested to participate in the care of a patient undergoing a diagnostic or therapeutic procedure."
[†]Reflex withdrawal from a painful stimulus is NOT considered a purposeful response.

The ability to independently maintain ventilatory function may be impaired. Patients may require assistance in maintaining a patent airway, and spontaneous ventilation may be inadequate. Cardiovascular function is usually maintained.

General Anesthesia is a drug-induced loss of consciousness during which patients are not arousable, even by painful stimulation. The ability to independently maintain ventilatory function is often impaired. Patients often require assistance in maintaining a patent airway, and positive pressure ventilation may be required because of depressed spontaneous ventilation or drug-induced depression of neuromuscular function. Cardiovascular function may be impaired.

Because sedation is a continuum, it is not always possible to predict how an individual patient will respond. Hence, practitioners intending to produce a given level of sedation should be able to rescue† patients whose level of sedation becomes deeper than initially intended. Individuals administering Moderate Sedation/Analgesia (Conscious Sedation) should be able to rescue† patients who enter a state of Deep Sedation/Analgesia, while those administering Deep Sedation/Analgesia should be able to rescue† patients who enter a state of General Anesthesia.

Basic Standards for Preanesthesia Care

Committee of Origin: Standards and Practice Parameters

(Approved by the ASA House of Delegates on October 14, 1987, and last affirmed on October 28, 2015)

These standards apply to all patients who receive anesthesia care. Under exceptional circumstances, these standards may be modified. When this is the case, the circumstances shall be documented in the patient's record.

An anesthesiologist shall be responsible for determining the medical status of the patient and developing a plan of anesthesia care.

The anesthesiologist, before the delivery of anesthesia care, is responsible for:
1. Reviewing the available medical record.
2. Interviewing and performing a focused examination of the patient to:
   a. Discuss the medical history, including previous anesthetic experiences and medical therapy.
   b. Assess those aspects of the patient's physical condition that might affect decisions regarding perioperative risk and management.
3. Ordering and reviewing pertinent available tests and consultations as necessary for the delivery of anesthesia care.
4. Ordering appropriate preoperative medications.
5. Ensuring that consent has been obtained for the anesthesia care.
6. Documenting in the chart that the above has been performed.

---

†Rescue of a patient from a deeper level of sedation than intended is an intervention by a practitioner proficient in airway management and advanced life support. The qualified practitioner corrects adverse physiologic consequences of the deeper-than-intended level of sedation (such as hypoventilation, hypoxia and hypotension) and returns the patient to the originally intended level of sedation. It is not appropriate to continue the procedure at an unintended level of sedation.

Standards for Postanesthesia Care

Committee of Origin: Standards and Practice Parameters

(Approved by the ASA House of Delegates on October 27, 2004, and last amended on October 15, 2014)

These standards apply to postanesthesia care in all locations. These standards may be exceeded based on the judgment of the responsible anesthesiologist. They are intended to encourage quality patient care, but cannot guarantee any specific patient outcome. They are subject to revision from time to time as warranted by the evolution of technology and practice.

Standard I

All patients who have received general anesthesia, regional anesthesia or monitored anesthesia care shall receive appropriate postanesthesia management.**
1. A Postanesthesia Care Unit (PACU) or an area which provides equivalent postanesthesia care (for example, a Surgical Intensive Care Unit) shall be available to receive patients after anesthesia care. All patients who receive anesthesia care shall be admitted to the PACU or its equivalent **except** by specific order of the anesthesiologist responsible for the patient's care.
2. The medical aspects of care in the PACU (or equivalent area) shall be governed by policies and procedures which have been reviewed and approved by the Department of Anesthesiology.
3. The design, equipment, and staffing of the PACU shall meet requirements of the facility's accrediting and licensing bodies.

Standard II

A patient transported to the PACU shall be accompanied by a member of the anesthesia care team who is knowledgeable about the patient's condition. The patient shall be continually evaluated and treated during transport with monitoring and support appropriate to the patient's condition.

Standard III

Upon arrival in the PACU, the patient shall be re-evaluated and a verbal report provided to the responsible PACU nurse by the member of the anesthesia care team who accompanies the patient.
1. The patient's status on arrival in the PACU shall be documented.
2. Information concerning the preoperative condition and the surgical/anesthetic course shall be transmitted to the PACU nurse.
3. The member of the Anesthesia Care Team shall remain in the PACU until the PACU nurse accepts responsibility for the nursing care of the patient.

Standard IV

The patient's condition shall be evaluated continually in the PACU.
1. The patient shall be observed and monitored by methods appropriate to the patient's medical condition. Particular attention should be given to monitoring oxygenation,

---

**Refer to *Perianesthesia Nursing Standards, Practice Recommendations and Interpretive Statements*, published by ASPAN, for issues of nursing care.

ventilation, circulation, level of consciousness, and temperature. During recovery from all anesthetics, a quantitative method of assessing oxygenation such as pulse oximetry shall be employed in the initial phase of recovery.[§] This is not intended for application during the recovery of the obstetrical patient in whom regional anesthesia was used for labor and vaginal delivery.
2. An accurate written report of the PACU period shall be maintained. Use of an appropriate PACU scoring system is encouraged for each patient on admission, at appropriate intervals prior to discharge and at the time of discharge.
3. General medical supervision and coordination of patient care in the PACU should be the responsibility of an anesthesiologist.
4. There shall be a policy to assure the availability in the facility of a physician capable of managing complications and providing cardiopulmonary resuscitation for patients in the PACU.

Standard V

A physician is responsible for the discharge of the patient from the postanesthesia care unit.
1. When discharge criteria are used, they must be approved by the Department of Anesthesiology and the medical staff. They may vary depending upon whether the patient is discharged to a hospital room, to the Intensive Care Unit, to a short stay unit or home.
2. In the absence of the physician responsible for the discharge, the PACU nurse shall determine that the patient meets the discharge criteria. The name of the physician accepting responsibility for discharge shall be noted on the record.

[§]Under extenuating circumstances, the responsible anesthesiologist may waive the requirements marked with an asterisk (*); it is recommended that when this is done, it should be so stated (including the reasons) in a note in the patient's medical record.

Practice Advisory for the Prevention and Management of Operating Room Fires

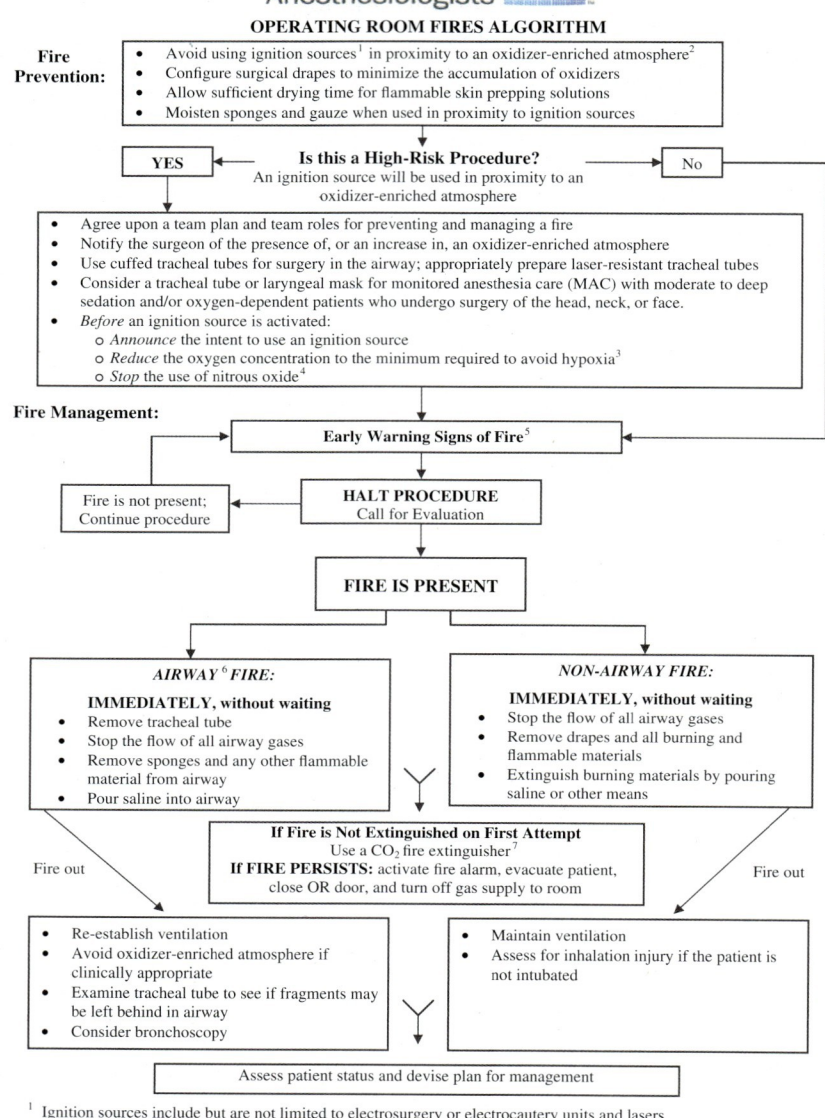

Figure 1 Operating room fires algorithm. CO_2, carbon dioxide; OR, operating room. (From Caplan RA, Barker SJ, Connis RT, et al; American Society of Anesthesiologists Task Force on Operating Room Fires. Practice advisory for the Prevention and Management of Operating Room Fires: a report by the American Society of Anesthesiologists Task Force on Operating Room Fires. *Anesthesiology*. 2008;108:786–801, with permission.)

OR Fire Prevention Algorithm*

Start Here

Is patient at risk for surgical fire?
Procedures involving the head, neck and upper chest (above T5) *and* use of an ignition source in proximity to an oxidizer.

→ **NO** → Proceed, but frequently reassess for changes in fire risk.

↓ **YES**

Nurses and surgeons avoid pooling of alcohol-based skin preparations and allow adequate drying time. Prior to initial use of electrocautery, communication occurs between surgeon and anesthesia professional.

↓

Does patient require oxygen supplementation?

→ **NO** → Use room air sedation.

↓ **YES**

Is >30% oxygen concentration required to maintain oxygen saturation?

→ **NO** → Use delivery device such as a blender or common gas outlet to maintain oxygen below 30%.

↓ **YES**

Secure airway with endotracheal tube or supraglottic device.

Although securing the airway is preferred, for cases where using an airway device is undesirable or not feasible, oxygen accumulation may be minimized by air insufflation over the face and open draping to provide wide exposure of the surgical site to the atmosphere.

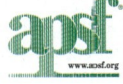

Provided as an educational resource by the **Anesthesia Patient Safety Foundation**
Copyright ©2014 Anesthesia Patient Safety Foundation   www.apsf.org

The following organizations have indicated their support for APSF's efforts to increase awareness of the potential for surgical fires in at-risk patients: American Society of Anesthesiologists, American Association of Nurse Anesthetists, American Academy of Anesthesiologist Assistants, American College of Surgeons, American Society of Anesthesia Technologists and Technicians, American Society of PeriAnesthesia Nurses, Association of periOperative Registered Nurses, ECRI Institute, Food and Drug Administration Safe Use Initiative, National Patient Safety Foundation, The Joint Commission

---

*This is not an ASA document but is included because of its relevance to fire safety. (http://www.apsf.org/newsletters/html/Handouts/ORFireAlgorithmPoster8.5×11.pdf)

Position on Monitored Anesthesia Care

Committee of Origin: Economics

(Approved by the House of Delegates on October 25, 2005, and last amended on October 16, 2013)

Monitored anesthesia care is a specific anesthesia service for a diagnostic or therapeutic procedure. Indications for monitored anesthesia care include the nature of the procedure, the patient's clinical condition and/or the potential need to convert to a general or regional anesthetic.

Monitored anesthesia care includes all aspects of anesthesia care—a preprocedure visit, intraprocedure care, and postprocedure anesthesia management. During monitored anesthesia care, the anesthesiologist provides or medically directs a number of specific services, including but not limited to:
- Diagnosis and treatment of clinical problems that occur during the procedure
- Support of vital functions
- Administration of sedatives, analgesics, hypnotics, anesthetic agents, or other medications as necessary for patient safety
- Psychological support and physical comfort
- Provision of other medical services as needed to complete the procedure safely.

Monitored anesthesia care may include varying levels of sedation, analgesia, and anxiolysis as necessary. The provider of monitored anesthesia care must be prepared and qualified to convert to general anesthesia when necessary. If the patient loses consciousness and the ability to respond purposefully, the anesthesia care is a general anesthetic, irrespective of whether airway instrumentation is required.

Monitored anesthesia care is a physician service provided to an individual patient. It should be subject to the same level of payment as general or regional anesthesia. Accordingly, the ASA Relative Value Guide provides for the use of proper base units, time and any appropriate modifier units as the basis for determining payment.

Distinguishing Monitored Anesthesia Care ("MAC") from Moderate Sedation/Analgesia (Conscious Sedation)

Committee of Origin: Economics

(Approved by the ASA House of Delegates on October 27, 2004, last amended on October 21, 2009, and reaffirmed on October 16, 2013)

Moderate Sedation/Analgesia (Conscious Sedation; hereinafter known as Moderate Sedation) is a physician service recognized in the CPT procedural coding system. During Moderate Sedation, a physician supervises or personally administers sedative and/or analgesic medications that can allay patient anxiety and control pain during a diagnostic or therapeutic procedure. Such drug-induced depression of a patient's level of consciousness to a "moderate" level of sedation, as defined in The Joint Commission (TJC) standards, is intended to facilitate the successful performance of the diagnostic or therapeutic procedure while providing patient comfort and cooperation. Physicians providing moderate sedation must be qualified to recognize "deep" sedation, manage its consequences and adjust the level of sedation to a "moderate" or lesser level. The continual assessment of the effects of sedative or analgesic medications on the level of consciousness and on cardiac and respiratory function is an integral element of this service.

The American Society of Anesthesiologists has defined Monitored Anesthesia Care (*see Position on Monitored Anesthesia Care, updated on October 16, 2013*). This physician service can be distinguished from Moderate Sedation in several ways. An essential component of MAC is the anesthesia assessment and management of a patient's actual or anticipated physiological derangements or medical problems that may occur during a diagnostic or therapeutic procedure. While Monitored Anesthesia Care may include the administration of sedatives and/or analgesics often used for Moderate Sedation, the provider of MAC must be prepared and qualified to convert to general anesthesia when necessary. Additionally, a provider's ability to intervene to rescue a patient's airway from any sedation-induced compromise is a prerequisite to the qualifications to provide Monitored Anesthesia Care. By contrast, Moderate Sedation is not expected to induce depths of sedation that would impair the patient's own ability to maintain the integrity of his or her airway. These components of Monitored Anesthesia Care are unique aspects of an anesthesia service that are not part of Moderate Sedation.

The administration of sedatives, hypnotics, analgesics, as well as anesthetic drugs commonly used for the induction and maintenance of general anesthesia is often, but not always, a part of Monitored Anesthesia Care. In some patients who may require only minimal sedation, MAC is often indicated because even small doses of these medications could precipitate adverse physiologic responses that would necessitate acute clinical interventions and resuscitation. If a patient's condition and/or a procedural requirement is likely to require sedation to a "deep" level or even to a transient period of general anesthesia, only a practitioner privileged to provide anesthesia services should be allowed to manage the sedation. Due to the strong likelihood that "deep" sedation may, with or without intention, transition to general anesthesia, the skills of an anesthesia provider are necessary to manage the effects of general anesthesia on the patient as well as to return the patient quickly to a state of "deep" or lesser sedation.

Like all anesthesia services, Monitored Anesthesia Care includes an array of postprocedure responsibilities beyond the expectations of practitioners providing Moderate Sedation, including assuring a return to full consciousness, relief of pain, management of adverse physiological responses or side effects from medications administered during the procedure, as well as the diagnosis and treatment of co-existing medical problems.

Monitored Anesthesia Care allows for the safe administration of a maximal depth of sedation in excess of that provided during Moderate Sedation. The ability to adjust the sedation level from full consciousness to general anesthesia during the course of a procedure provides maximal flexibility in matching sedation level to patient needs and procedural requirements. In situations where the procedure is more invasive or when the patient is especially fragile, optimizing sedation level is necessary to achieve ideal procedural conditions.

In summary, Monitored Anesthesia Care is a physician service that is clearly distinct from Moderate Sedation due to the expectations and qualifications of the provider who must be able to utilize all anesthesia resources to support life and to provide patient comfort and safety during a diagnostic or therapeutic procedure.

Ethical Guidelines for the Anesthesia Care of Patients with Do-Not-Resuscitate Orders or Other Directives That Limit Treatment

Committee of Origin: Ethics

(Approved by the ASA House of Delegates on October 17, 2001, and last amended on October 16, 2013)

These guidelines apply both to patients with decision-making capacity and also to patients without decision-making capacity who have previously expressed their preferences.

I. Given the diversity of published opinions and cultures within our society, an essential element of preoperative preparation and perioperative care for patients with Do-Not-Resuscitate (DNR) orders or other directives that limit treatment is communication among involved parties. It is necessary to document relevant aspects of this communication.

II. Policies automatically suspending DNR orders or other directives that limit treatment prior to procedures involving anesthetic care may not sufficiently address a patient's rights to self-determination in a responsible and ethical manner. Such policies, if they exist, should be reviewed and revised, as necessary, to reflect the content of these guidelines.

III. The administration of anesthesia necessarily involves some practices and procedures that might be viewed as "resuscitation" in other settings. Prior to procedures requiring anesthetic care, any existing directives to limit the use of resuscitation procedures (that is, do-not-resuscitate orders and/or advance directives) should, when possible, be reviewed with the patient or designated surrogate. As a result of this review, the status of these directives should be clarified or modified based on the preferences of the patient. One of the three following alternatives may provide for a satisfactory outcome in many cases.

   A. Full Attempt at Resuscitation: The patient or designated surrogate may request the full suspension of existing directives during the anesthetic and immediate postoperative period, thereby consenting to the use of any resuscitation procedures that may be appropriate to treat clinical events that occur during this time.

   B. Limited Attempt at Resuscitation Defined With Regard to Specific Procedures: The patient or designated surrogate may elect to continue to refuse certain specific resuscitation procedures (e.g., chest compressions, defibrillation, or tracheal intubation). The anesthesiologist should inform the patient or designated surrogate about which procedures are (1) essential to the success of the anesthesia and the proposed procedure, and (2) which procedures are not essential and may be refused.

   C. Limited Attempt at Resuscitation Defined With Regard to the Patient's Goals and Values: The patient or designated surrogate may allow the anesthesiologist and surgical/procedural team to use clinical judgment in determining which resuscitation procedures are appropriate in the context of the situation and the patient's stated goals and values. For example, some patients may want full resuscitation procedures to be used to manage adverse clinical events that are believed to be quickly and easily reversible, but to refrain from treatment for conditions that are likely to result in permanent sequelae, such as neurologic impairment or unwanted dependence upon life-sustaining technology.

IV. Any clarifications or modifications made to the patient's directive should be documented in the medical record. In cases where the patient or designated surrogate requests that the anesthesiologist use clinical judgment in determining which resuscitation procedures are appropriate, the anesthesiologist should document the discussion with particular attention to the stated goals and values of the patient.

V. Plans for postoperative/postprocedural care should indicate if or when the original, pre-existent directive to limit the use of resuscitation procedures will be reinstated. This occurs when the patient leaves the postanesthesia care unit or when the patient has recovered from the acute effects of anesthesia and surgery/procedure. Consideration should be given to whether continuing to provide the patient with a time-limited or event-limited postoperative/postprocedure trial of therapy would help the patient or surrogate better evaluate whether continued therapy would be consistent with the patient's goals.

VI. It is important to discuss and document whether there are to be any exceptions to the injunction(s) against intervention should there occur a specific recognized complication of the surgery/procedure or anesthesia.

VII. Concurrence on these issues by the primary physician (if not the surgeon/proceduralist of record), the surgeon/proceduralist and the anesthesiologist is desirable. If possible, these physicians should meet together with the patient (or the patient's legal representative) when these issues are discussed. This duty of the patient's physicians is deemed to be of such importance that it should not be delegated. Other members of the health-care team who are (or will be) directly involved with the patient's care during the planned procedure should, if feasible, be included in this process.

VIII. Should conflicts arise, the following resolution processes are recommended:

   A. When an anesthesiologist finds the patient's or surgeon's/proceduralist's limitations of intervention decisions to be irreconcilable with one's own moral views, then the anesthesiologist should withdraw in a nonjudgmental fashion, providing an alternative for care in a timely fashion.

   B. When an anesthesiologist finds the patient's or surgeon's/proceduralist's limitation of intervention decisions to be in conflict with generally accepted standards of care, ethical practice or institutional policies, then the anesthesiologist should voice such concerns and present the situation to the appropriate institutional body.

   C. If these alternatives are not feasible within the time frame necessary to prevent further morbidity or suffering, then in accordance with the American Medical Association's Principles of Medical Ethics, care should proceed with reasonable adherence to the patient's directives, being mindful of the patient's goals and values.

IX. A representative from the hospital's anesthesiology service should establish a liaison with surgical, procedural, and nursing services for presentation, discussion and procedural application of these guidelines. Hospital staff should be made aware of the proceedings of these discussions and the motivations for them.

X. Modification of these guidelines may be appropriate when they conflict with local standards or policies, and in those emergency situations involving patients lacking decision-making capacity whose intentions have not been previously expressed.

Practice Guidelines for Preoperative Fasting and Use of Pharmacologic Agents to Reduce Risk of Pulmonary Aspiration: Application to Healthy Patients Undergoing Elective Procedures

Committee of Origin: Standards and Practice Parameters

(Approved by the ASA House of Delegates on October 17, 2001, and last amended on October 26, 2016)

Summary of Fasting Recommendations

A. Fasting Recommendations*

Ingested Material	Minimum Fasting Period[†]
• Clear liquids[‡]	2h
• Breast milk	4h
• Infant formula	6h
• Nonhuman milk[§]	6h
• Light meal**	6h
• Fried foods, fatty foods, or meat	Additional fasting time (e.g., 8 or more hours) may be needed

*These recommendations apply to healthy patients who are undergoing elective procedures. They are not intended for women in labor. Following the guidelines does not guarantee complete gastric emptying.
[†]The fasting periods noted above apply to all ages.
[‡]Examples of clear liquids include water, fruit juices without pulp, carbonated beverages, clear tea, and black coffee.
[§]Since nonhuman milk is similar to solids in gastric emptying time, the amount ingested must be considered when determining an appropriate fasting period.
**A light meal typically consists of toast and clear liquids. Meals that include fried or fatty foods or meat may prolong gastric emptying time. Additional fasting time (e.g., 8 or more hours) may be needed in these cases. Both the amount and type of foods ingested must be considered when determining an appropriate fasting period.

These recommendations apply to healthy patients who are undergoing elective procedures. They are not intended for women in labor. Following the Guidelines does not guarantee complete gastric emptying. The fasting periods noted above apply to patients of all ages.

Examples of clear liquids include water, fruit juices without pulp, carbonated beverages, clear tea, and black coffee. Because nonhuman milk is similar to solids in gastric emptying time, the amount ingested must be considered when determining an appropriate fasting period.

A light meal typically consists of toast and clear liquids. Meals that include fried or fatty foods or meat may prolong gastric emptying time. Additional fasting time (e.g., 8 h or more) may be needed in these cases. Both the amount and type of food ingested must be considered when determining an appropriate fasting period.

Summary of Pharmacologic Recommendations

B. Pharmacologic Recommendations

Medication Type and Common Examples	Recommendation
Gastrointestinal stimulants:	
• Metoclopramide	May be used/no routine use
Gastric acid secretion blockers:	
• Cimetidine	May be used/no routine use
• Famotidine	May be used/no routine use
• Ranitidine	May be used/no routine use
• Omeprazole	May be used/no routine use
• Lansoprazole	May be used/no routine use
Antacids:	
• Sodium citrate	May be used/no routine use
• Sodium bicarbonate	May be used/no routine use
• Magnesium trisilicate	May be used/no routine use
Antiemetics:	
• Ondansetron	May be used/no routine use
Anticholinergics:	
• Atropine	No use
• Scopolamine	No use
• Glycopyrrolate	No use
Combinations of the medications above:	No routine use

APPENDIX 5
The Airway Approach Algorithm and Difficult Airway Algorithm

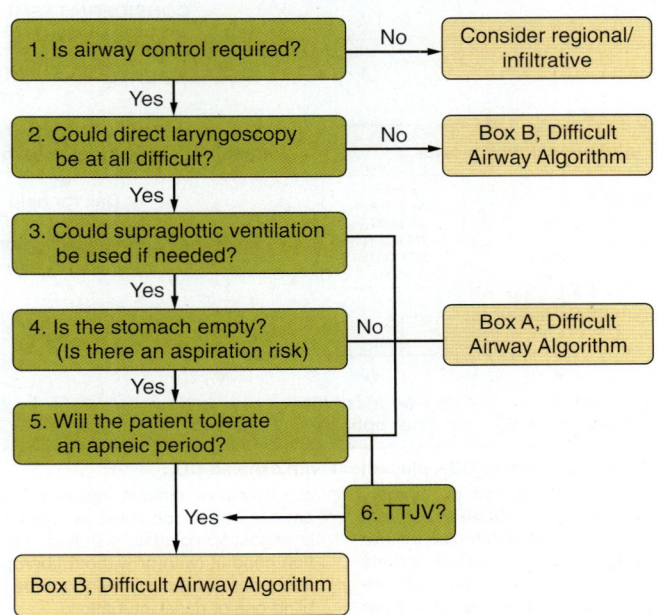

Figure 1 The airway approach algorithm: A decision tree approach to entry into the American Society of Anesthesiologists difficult airway algorithm. TTJV, transtracheal jet ventilation. (From Rosenblatt WH, Sukhupragarn W. Airway management. In: Barash PG, Cullen BF, Stoelting RK, et al., eds. Clinical Anesthesia. 7th ed. Philadelphia: Lippincott Williams & Wilkins; 2013:788, with permission.)

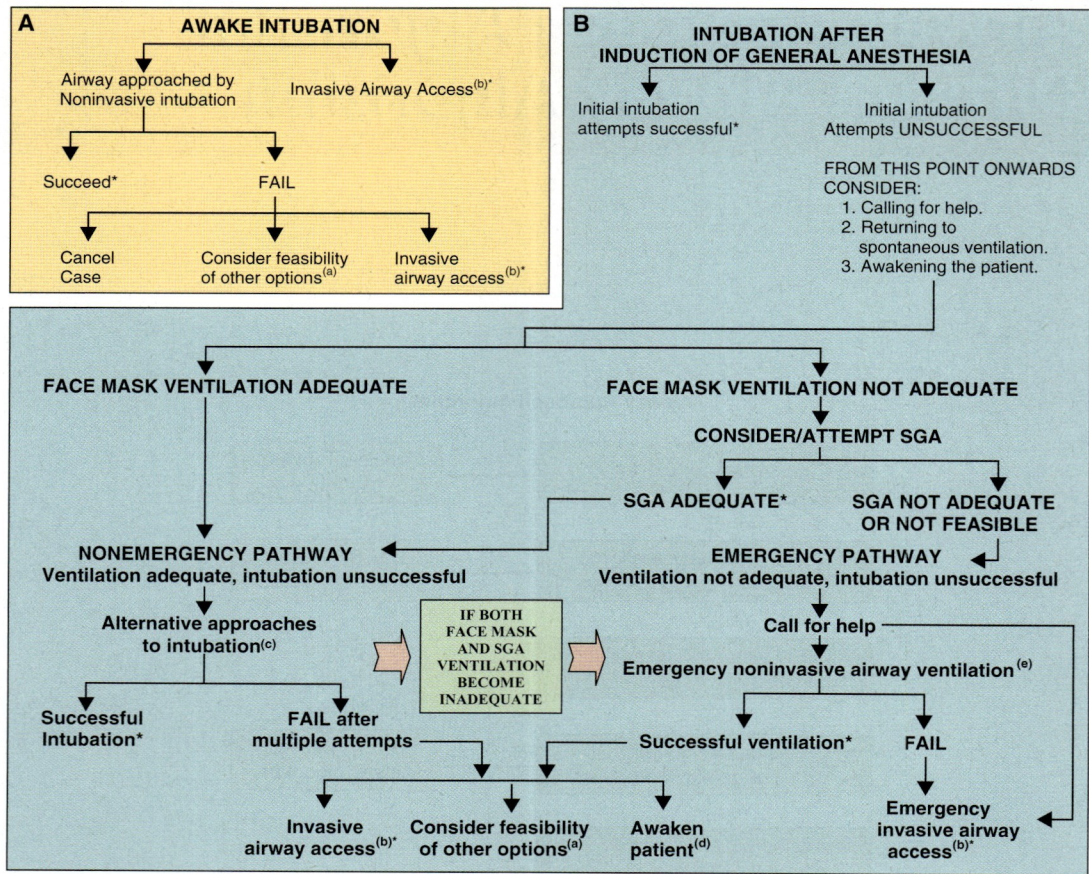

*Confirm ventilation, tracheal intubation, or SGA placement with exhaled CO_2.

a. Other options include (but are not limited to): surgery utilizing face mask or supraglottic airway (SGA) anesthesia (e.g., LMA, ILMA, laryngeal tube), local anesthesia infiltration or regional nerve blockade. Pursuit of these options usually implies that mask ventilation will not be problematic. Therefore, these options may be of limited value if this step in the algorithm has been reached via the Emergency Pathway.

b. Invasive airway access includes surgical or percutaneous airway, jet ventilation, and retrograde intubation.

c. Alternative difficult intubation approaches include (but are not limited to): video-assisted laryngoscopy, alternative laryngoscope blades, SGA (e.g., LMA or ILMA) as an intubation conduit (with or without fiberoptic guidance), fiberoptic intubation, intubating stylet or tube changer, light wand, and blind oral or nasal intubation.

d. Consider re-preparation of the patient for awake intubation or canceling surgery.

e. Emergency non-invasive airway ventilation consists of a SGA.

Figure 2 The American Society of Anesthesiologists difficult airway algorithm. **A:** Awake intubation. **B:** Intubation after induction of general anesthesia. (Reprinted with permission from Apfelbaum JL, Hagberg CA, Caplan RA, et al; American Society of Anesthesiologists Task Force on Management of the Difficult Airway. Practice guidelines for management of the difficult airway: an updated report by the American Society of Anesthesiologists Task Force on Management of the Difficult Airway. *Anesthesiology.* 2013;118(2):251–270.)

APPENDIX 6
Malignant Hyperthermia Protocol

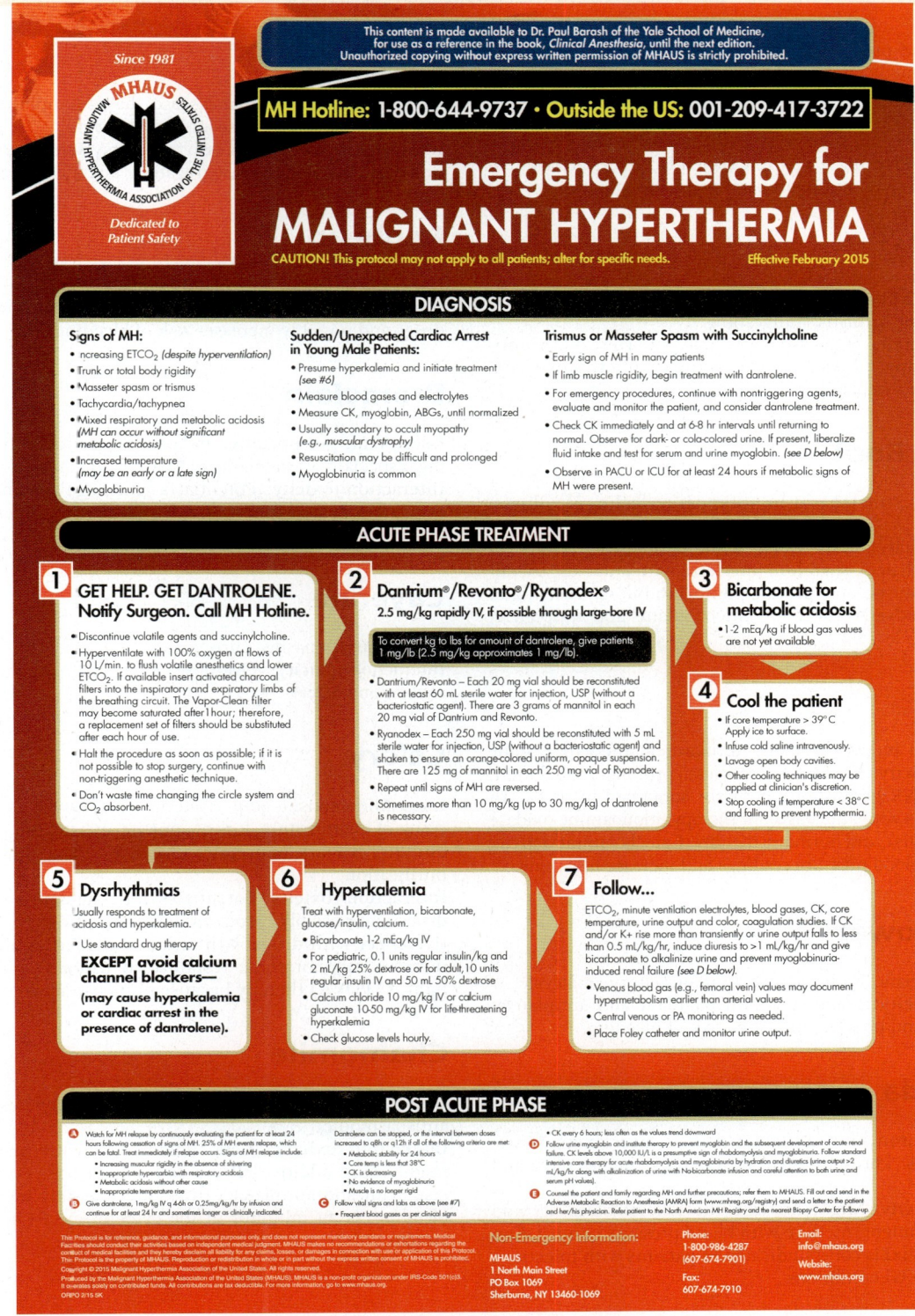

Reproduced with permission of the Malignant Hyperthermia Association of the United States (http://www.mhaus.org/).

APPENDIX 7
Herbal Medications

The authors and publisher have exerted every effort to ensure that the herbal medication selection in this appendix is in accord with current recommendations and practice at the time of publication.

The editors wish to acknowledge the contribution of Stella A. Haddadin, BSc, PharmD, Yale–New Haven Hospital, Department of Pharmacy Services, in the preparation of this appendix.

Alfalfa

Uses: Diuretic, kidney, bladder and prostate conditions, hyperglycemia, asthma, arthritis, indigestion
Interaction/toxicity: Excessive use may interfere with anticoagulant therapy, potentiate drug-induced photosensitivity, and interfere with hormone therapy.

Angelica Root

Uses: Gastrointestinal spasm, loss of appetite, feeling of fullness, and flatulence
Interaction/toxicity: Can cause photodermatitis, claims to increase stomach acid, therefore interferes with antacids, sucralfate, H2 antagonists, and proton pump inhibitors. Potentiates the effects and adverse effects of anticoagulants and antiplatelet drugs.

Anise

Uses: Dyspepsia and as a pediatric antiflatulent and expectorant
Interaction/toxicity: Excessive doses can prolong coagulation, increasing PT/INR because of coumarin contained in anise. An interaction exists with anticoagulant therapy, monoamine oxidase inhibitors (MAOIs), and hormone therapy. Catecholamine activity might increase blood pressure readings and increase heart rate.

Arnica Flower

Uses: Antiphlogistic, antiseptic, anti-inflammatory, analgesic
Interaction/toxicity: Potentiates anticoagulant and antiplatelet effect of drugs and possibly increases risk of bleeding.

Asafoetida

Uses: Chronic bronchitis, asthma, pertussis, hoarseness, hysteria, flatulent colic, chronic gastric, dyspepsia, irritable colon, and convulsions
Interaction/toxicity: Might increase the risk of bleeding, and excessive doses might interfere with blood pressure control. Can irritate GI tract and is contraindicated in patients with infectious or inflammatory GI conditions.

Bilberry

Uses: Peripheral vascular disease, diabetes, ophthalmologic diseases, peptic ulcer disease and scleroderma
Interaction/toxicity: Excessive use may interfere with coagulation and inhibit platelet aggregation; alters glucose regulation.

Bogbean

Uses: Rheumatism, loss of appetite, dyspepsia
Interaction/toxicity: Potentiates anticoagulant and antiplatelet drugs and possibly increases risk of bleeding.

Bromelain

Uses: Acute postoperative and posttraumatic conditions of swelling, especially of the nasal and paranasal sinuses, osteoarthritis
Interaction/toxicity: Potentiates anticoagulant and antiplatelet drugs and possibly increases risk of bleeding. Increases plasma and urine tetracycline level.

Cayenne

Uses: Muscle spasms, chronic pain
Interaction/toxicity: Overdose may cause hypothermia. May cause skin blisters.

Celery

Uses: Rheumatism, gout, hysteria, nervousness, weight loss as a result of malnutrition, loss of appetite, exhaustion, sedative, mild diuretic, urinary antiseptic, digestive aid, antiflatulent, blood purification
Interaction/toxicity: Potentiates anticoagulant and antiplatelet drugs and possibly increases risk of bleeding. There is an additive effect with drugs with sedative properties and may cause increase in phototoxic response to psoralen plus ultraviolet light A (PUVA) therapy because of its psoralen content.

Chamomile

Uses: Flatulence, nervous diarrhea, restlessness, insomnia, antispasmodic
Interaction/toxicity: Concomitant use with benzodiazepines might cause additive effects and side effects. Potentiates anticoagulant and antiplatelet drugs and possibly increases risk of bleeding. Is an inhibitor of the cytochrome P450 3A4 enzyme system.

Clove

Uses: Flatulence, nausea, and vomiting
Interaction/toxicity: Potentiates anticoagulant and antiplatelet drugs and possibly increases risk of bleeding.

Dandelion

Uses: Diuretic, GI disorders and anti-inflammatory effect
Interaction/toxicity: Excessive use may interfere with coagulation and inhibit platelet aggregation; alters glucose regulation. Do not use in the presence of biliary obstruction. Interactions with digoxin, lithium, insulin, oral hypoglycemics, cytochrome P450, ciprofloxacin, disulfram and metronidazole.

Danshen

Uses: Circulation problems, cardiovascular diseases, chronic hepatitis, abdominal masses, insomnia because of palpitations and tight chest, acne, psoriasis, eczema, aids in wound healing
Interaction/toxicity: Potentiates anticoagulant and antiplatelet drugs and possibly increases risk of bleeding. Increases the cardiovascular effects and side effects of digoxin.

Devil's Claw

Uses: Osteoarthritis, rheumatoid arthritis, gout, myalgia, fibrositis
Interaction/toxicity: Can affect heart rate, contractility of heart, and blood pressure. Might decrease blood glucose levels and have additive effects with medications used for diabetes. May cause an increase in gastric acid secretions.

Dong Quai

Uses: Gynecologic ailments, menopausal symptoms
Interaction/toxicity: Potentiates anticoagulant and antiplatelet drugs and possibly increases risk of bleeding.

Echinacea

Uses: Common colds, urinary tract infections
Interaction/toxicity: May cause hepatotoxicity especially with other concomitant hepatotoxins. Antagonizes steroids and immunosuppressants. May possess immunosuppressive activity after long-term use.

Ephedra

Uses: Diet aid, bacteriostatic, antitussive
Interaction/toxicity: May cause arrhythmias with inhalation anesthetics and cardiac glycosides. Life-threatening reaction with MAOIs. May cause depletion of catecholamines and lead to perioperative hemodynamic instability. Can cause death.

Fenugreek

Uses: Lower blood sugar in diabetics
Interaction/toxicity: Potentiates anticoagulant and antiplatelet drugs and possibly increases risk of bleeding. Inhibits corticosteroid drug activity, interferes with hormone therapy, can alter blood glucose control, and potentiate effect of MAOIs.

Feverfew

Uses: Migraine prophylaxis, antipyretic
Interaction/toxicity: Inhibit platelet activity. Potentiates anticoagulants. Abrupt withdrawal may cause rebound headaches. Uterine stimulant. Associated with serotonin syndrome.

Fish Oil

Uses: Cardiovascular disease, colon cancer, psychiatric disorders, diabetes, inflammatory disease, inflammatory bowel diseases, premenstrual syndrome and scleroderma
Interaction/toxicity: Excessive use may interfere with coagulation and inhibit platelet aggregation; alters glucose regulation; potentiates anti-hypertensive drugs.

Flaxseed Oil

Uses: Cardiovascular disease, colon cancer, psychiatric disorders, diabetes, inflammatory disease, inflammatory bowel diseases, breast cancer and depression
Interaction/toxicity: Excessive use may interfere with coagulation and inhibit platelet aggregation; alters glucose regulation.

Garlic (Pertains to Supplement Product)

Uses: Lower lipids, antihypertensive, antiplatelet, antioxidant, antithrombolytic
Interaction/toxicity: Potentiates anticoagulants, especially in the presence of drugs that inhibit platelet function. Potentiates vasodilator drugs and antihypertensives. May decrease blood glucose levels as a result of increased serum insulin levels.

Ginger (Pertains to Supplement Product)

Uses: Antinauseant, antispasmodic
Interaction/toxicity: Inhibits thromboxane synthetase. Potentiates anticoagulants. May alter effects of calcium channel blockers.

Ginkgo

Uses: Circulatory stimulant, inhibit platelets
Interaction/toxicity: Potentiates anticoagulants, especially in the presence of aspirin, NSAIDs, heparin, and warfarin.

Ginseng

Uses: Antioxidant
Interaction/toxicity: Antagonize anticoagulants. Avoid use of sympathetic stimulants, which may result in tachycardia or hypertension. Possesses hypoglycemic effects. Potentiates digoxin and MAOIs.

Goldenseal

Uses: Diuretic, anti-inflammatory, hemostatic
Interaction/toxicity: May worsen edema and hypertension. Oxytocic possesses activity.

Grape Seed

Uses: Anti-oxidant, cardiovascular disorders, peripheral circulatory disorders, multiple sclerosis, Parkinson disease
Interaction/toxicity: Excessive use may interfere with coagulation and inhibit platelet aggregation; may inhibit xanthine oxidase.

Green Tea

Uses: Improves cognitive performance, lowers cholesterol and triglycerides, aids in the prevention of breast, bladder, esophageal, and pancreatic cancers. Decreased risk of Parkinson disease, gingivitis, obesity
Interaction/toxicity: Concomitant use might inhibit effect of adenosine and antagonize effect of warfarin. Because of the caffeine content, there is an increase in cardiac inotropic effects of beta-adrenergic agonist drugs, an increase in the effects and toxicity of clozapine, and an increased risk of agitation, tremors, and insomnia in combination with ephedrine. It might precipitate hypertensive crisis with MAOIs as well. Might reduce sedative effects of benzodiazepines.

Horse Chestnut

Uses: Scleroderma, peripheral vascular disorders, varicose veins and relieving pain, tiredness, tension, swelling in legs, itching, and edema
Interaction/toxicity: Excessive use may interfere with coagulation and inhibit platelet aggregation; phosphodiesterase inhibitor and alters glucose regulation. Potentiates anticoagulant and antiplatelet drugs and possibly increases risk of bleeding, hypoglycemic effects, might interfere with binding of protein binding drugs.

Kava-Kava

Uses: Anxiolytic, analgesic
Interaction/toxicity: Potentiates barbiturates, opioids, and benzodiazepines.

Licorice

Uses: Heal gastric and duodenal ulcers
Interaction/toxicity: May cause hypertension, hypokalemia, and edema.

Lovage Root

Uses: Used for inflammation of the lower urinary tract and prevention of kidney gravel; in "irrigation therapy," it is used as a mild diuretic
Interaction/toxicity: Might increase sodium retention and interfere with diuretic therapy.

Meadowsweet

Uses: Supportive therapy for colds
Interaction/toxicity: Can potentiate narcotic effects. Contains a salicylate constituent.

Onions

Uses: Loss of appetite, preventing atherosclerosis, dyspepsia, fever, colds, cough, tendency toward infection, and inflammation of the mouth and pharynx
Interaction/toxicity: May enhance antidiabetic drug effects and alter blood sugar control. Might enhance antiplatelet drug activity and increase bleeding risk.

Papain

Uses: Inflammation and swelling in patient with pharyngitis
Interaction/toxicity: Concomitant use with anticoagulant and antiplatelet drugs may increase risk of bleeding.

Parsley

Uses: Breath freshener, urinary tract infections, and kidney or bladder stones
Interaction/toxicity: Might interfere with oral anticoagulant therapy because of the vitamin K contained in parsley. May interfere with diuretic therapy by enhancing sodium retention. Might potentiate MAOI drug therapy.

Passion Flower

Uses: Generalized anxiety disorder
Interaction/toxicity: Concomitant use with barbiturates can increase drug-induced sleep time; can potentiate the effects of sedatives and tranquilizers, including sedative effects of antihistamines.

Quassia

Uses: Anorexia, indigestion, fever, mouthwash, as an anthelmintic for thread worms, nematodes, and ascaris
Interaction/toxicity: Stimulates gastric acid and might oppose effect of antacids and H2 antagonists. Excessive doses might have additive effects with anticoagulant therapy with Coumadin. Concomitant use of potassium-depleting diuretics or stimulant laxative abuse might increase risk of cardiac glycoside toxicity as a result of potassium loss.

Red Clover

Uses: Hot flashes
Interaction/toxicity: Can increase the anticoagulant effects and bleeding risk because of its Coumarin content. May interfere with hormone replacement therapy or oral contraceptives, and may interfere with tamoxifen because of its potential estrogenic effects. Can inhibit cytochrome P450 (cyp450) 3A4.

Saw Palmetto

Uses: Benign prostatic hypertrophy, antiandrogenic
Interaction/toxicity: Potentiates birth control pills and estrogens. May cause hypertension.

St. John's Wort

Uses: Depression, anxiety
Interaction/toxicity: Possible interaction/toxicity with MAOIs and meperidine. May prolong anesthetic effects. Potentiates digoxin. May decrease effects of warfarin, steroids, and possibly benzodiazepines and calcium channel blockers.

Sweet Clover

Uses: Chronic venous insufficiency, including leg pain and heaviness, night-time leg cramps, itching and swelling, for supportive treatment of thrombophlebitis, lymphatic congestion, postthrombotic syndromes, and hemorrhoids
Interaction/toxicity: Use with hepatotoxic drugs might increase risk of hepatotoxicity. Concomitant use with anticoagulant and antiplatelet drugs may increase risk of bleeding.

Turmeric

Uses: Dyspepsia, jaundice, hepatitis, flatulence, abdominal bloating
Interaction/toxicity: Concomitant use with anticoagulant and antiplatelet drugs may increase risk of bleeding.

Valerian

Uses: Sedative, anxiolytic
Interaction/toxicity: Potentiates barbiturates and anesthetics. May blunt symptoms of benzodiazepine withdrawal.

Vitamin E

Uses: Vitamin E deficiency, heart disease
Interaction/toxicity: Concomitant use with anticoagulant and antiplatelet drugs may increase risk of bleeding. Might prevent tolerance to nitrates.

Willow Bark

Uses: Lower back pain, fever, rheumatic ailments, headache
Interaction/toxicity: Enough salicylate is present in willow bark to cause drug interactions common to salicylates or aspirin. Can impair effectiveness of beta-adrenergic blockers, probenecid, and sulfinpyrazone. Can increase effects, side effects, or toxicity of alcohol, anticoagulants, carbonic anhydrase inhibitors, heparin, methotrexate, NSAIDs, sulfonylureas, and valproic acid.

Index

Note: Page number followed by f and t indicates figure and table respectively.

A

A alpha (Aα) fibers, 1608t, 1609
AANA. *See* American Association of Nurse Anesthetists (AANA)
ABA. *See* American Board of Anesthesiology (ABA)
Abciximab, 206, 450
Abdominal aortic aneurysms, 1127
Abdominal compartment syndrome, 1529–1530, 1529f
Abdominal compression, prone position and, 821–822
Abdominal superficial surgery, 1250
Abdominal thrust maneuver, 1663–1664
Abdominal trauma, 1509–1511, 1510t
Abdominal wall lift, 1263
A beta (Aβ) fibers
    blockade of, 1611
    characteristics, 1608, 1608t
    phenotypic switch, 1611
Abiomed Impella (Abiomed), 1103
ABMS. *See* American Board of Medical Specialties (ABMS)
Abruptio placentae, 1160
Absolute shunt, 373, 375
ACA. *See* Affordable Care Act (ACA)
Academic anesthesiologists, 44–45
    advancement issues, 45
    compensation issues, 45
    department characteristics, 44–45
    faculty roles, 45
Acambis Modified Vaccinia Ankara (ACAM), 1697
Accelerated intravascular coagulation and fibrinolysis (AICF), 1308
Acceleromyography (AMG), 547–548
Accessory lumen, flexible scope, 798
Accessory obturator nerve, 962
Accountable care organizations (ACO), 27, 53–54
Accreditation Council for Graduate Medical Education (ACGME), 27, 70
Acetaminophen, 515, 517, 1232
    for acute perioperative pain, 1599
    characteristics, 1579
    dosing guidelines, 1578t
    for pediatric patients, 1221
Acetazolamide, 1378, 1381
Acetylcholine (ACh), 302, 302f, 342, 352–353, 528, 528f
    mobilization of, 529
    release of, 529
Acetylcholinesterase inhibitors. *See* Anticholinesterase agents
N-acetylcysteine, 324
Acetylsalicylic acid, dosing guidelines, 1578t
ACGME. *See* Accreditation Council for Graduate Medical Education (ACGME)
ACh. *See* Acetylcholine (ACh)
Acid–base disorders
    metabolic acidosis, 1407
    metabolic alkalosis, 1407
    mixed, 1408, 1408f
    postoperative, 1552
        metabolic acidemia, 1552–1553, 1552t
        metabolic alkalemia, 1553
        respiratory acidemia, 1552
        respiratory alkalemia, 1553
    respiratory acidosis, 1408
    respiratory alkalosis, 1408

Acid–base equilibrium, 385
Acid–base interpretation
    equilibrium, 385
    metabolic acidosis, 386–387, 386t, 387t
    metabolic alkalosis, 385–386, 385t, 386t
    practical approach to, 388–390, 388t
    respiratory acidosis, 388, 388t
    respiratory alkalosis, 387
    Stewart approach to, 385
    and treatment, 384–388
Acid-fast bacilli (AFB), 80
ACO. *See* Accountable care organizations (ACO)
Acquired hemophilia, 446
Acquired Immune Deficiency Syndrome (AIDS), 79
Acromegaly, 1353
Actin, 284
Activated clotting time (ACT), 425–426, 1092
Activated partial thromboplastin time (APTT), 425, 1443
Activated protein C (APC), 423
Active compression-decompression (ACD) technique, 1667
Active transport, 242
Activity of daily living (ADL), 905–906
Acute chest syndrome (ACS), 635
Acute compartment syndrome (ACS), 1453
Acute fatty liver of pregnancy (AFLP), 1306, 1306t, 1307
Acute glaucoma, 1396. *See also* Glaucoma
Acute hemolytic transfusion reactions (AHTRs), 438–439
Acute hepatitis, 1304–1305
    diagnosis of, 1304
    HAV, 1304
    HBV, 1304
    HCV, 1304–1305
    HDV, 1304
    HEV, 1304
Acute intermittent porphyria (AIP), 623, 624t
Acute kidney injury (AKI), 1401, 1405, 1408–1409, 1529, 1529t
    cardiac surgery and, 1415, 1416f
    in ICU, 1645–1646, 1645t
    intrinsic, 1408
    nephrotoxins and perioperative, 1409–1410, 1409t
    noncardiac surgical procedures and, 1415–1417
    postrenal, 1408–1409
    prerenal azotemia, 1408
    prerenal factors causing, 1408
    prevention, during emergency surgery, 1416
Acute kidney injury network (AKIN), 1529
Acute liver failure (ALF), 1302–1304, 1471
    antibiotics for, 1303
    cerebral hyperemia associated with, 1303
    coagulopathy in, 1304
    corticosteroids for, 1303
    due to drug-related toxicity, 1302
    encephalopathy, grades of, 1302, 1302t
    etiologies of, 1302
    hypotension in, 1304
    laboratory analysis, 1302t
    natural history, 1302
Acute lung injury (ALI)
    risk factors for, 1031
    thoracic surgery and, 1031
Acute normovolemic hemodilution (ANH), 442–443

Acute opioid tolerance, 510
Acute postgastric reduction surgery (APGARS) neuropathy, 1286
Acute postoperative pulmonary edema, 1361
Acute respiratory distress syndrome (ARDS), 1644–1645
Acute respiratory failure, 1642–1644
Acute traumatic coagulopathy (ATC), 1499
Acute tubular necrosis (ATN), 1288
Addiction, 1598
    in anesthesiologists, 82–83
    characteristics of, 82
    untreated, 83
Addison's disease
    anesthetic considerations, 1337–1338
    clinical presentation, 1337
    diagnosis of, 1337
    steroid replacement during perioperative period, 1338, 1339f
    treatment of, 1337–1338
Additives to local anesthetics
    $β_2$-adrenergic agonists, 571
    epinephrine, 570, 570t
    liposomes, 571–572
    opioids, 571
    solutions, alkalinization of, 570–571
    steroids, 571, 571f
Adductor canal block (ACB), 1590
Adductor pollicis muscle (APM), 530, 537, 548f
A delta (Aδ) fibers, 508, 1608
    function, 1608t, 1609
Adenoidectomy, 1358
    recommendation of American Academy of Otolaryngology, 1363t
Adenosine, 855t
Adenosine diphosphate (ADP), 421
Adenosine receptors, 348
Adenosine triphosphatase (ATPase) pump, 404
Adenosine triphosphate (ATP), 1014, 1662
Adjuncts drugs, ocular surgery, 1378–1379, 1379t
Adjuncts, ocular surgery, 1387–1388
Adjustable pressure-limiting (APL), 645
Adrenal cortex
    adrenal insufficiency, 1337–1338, 1338t
    Cushing syndrome, 1336
    function, 1335
    glucocorticoid
        physiology, 1335
        therapy, 1338, 1339t
    mineralocorticoid
        excess, 1337
        insufficiency, 1339
        physiology, 1335, 1336f
Adrenal–cortical suppression, 599
Adrenal disorders, 599–600
Adrenalectomy, 1336, 1435
Adrenal insufficiency, in critical illness, 1646–1647
Adrenal medulla, 1339–1343, 1340f
Adrenergic receptors, 254
    numbers and sensitivity of, 348–349
Adrenocorticotropic hormone (ACTH), 517, 1018
Adriani, John, 18
Adult bradycardia (with pulse) algorithm, 1669f
Adult tachycardia (with pulse) algorithm, 1670f
Advanced cardiac life support cardiac arrest circular algorithm, 1664f
Advanced maternal age (AMA), 1156, 1164

1749

Advanced practice registered nurses (APRN), 32
Adverse event, response to, 43–44
AEDs. *See* Automatic external defibrillators (AEDs)
AFB. *See* Acid-fast bacilli (AFB)
Afferent fibers, 1608, 1608t
Affordable Care Act (ACA), 27, 28, 1633
Age/aging
   age-related macular degeneration and, 1392
   body composition, changes in, 900, 900f
   cardiovascular, 902, 904
   central nervous system, 901
   demographics of, 897–898
   drug pharmacology and, 901–902, 901f, 902f, 903t
   economics of, 897–898, 898f
   frailty, concept of, 899
   functional reserve and, 899
   kidney, 900
   liver, 900
   on perioperative complications and associated mortality, 909t
   physiologic, 899–900
   physiology of organ, 900–905
   postdural puncture headache and, 938
   process of, 898–900, 899f
   pulmonary, 904–905, 905f
   respiratory function and, 366
   thermoregulation and, 905
Age Discrimination Act, 84
Age-related macular degeneration
   blindness, 1392
   treatment for, 1392
Agonists, 254, 255, 255f
AIDS. *See* Acquired Immune Deficiency Syndrome (AIDS)
Airborne precautions (Check), 77
Air embolization, 823
Air-Q, 777f, 778, 787
Airtraq AVANT, 786
Airtraq optical laryngoscope, 786, 786f
Airway, 768
   anatomy, 768–769
      bronchi, 769
      cricoid cartilage, 769
      cricothyroid membrane, 768–769, 769f
      infants and adults, larynx of, 768t
      laryngeal skeleton, 768
      trachea, 769
   difficult, 791
   epiglottitis, 1366
   evaluation and intervention, in trauma patient, 1489
      airway obstruction, 1489
      cervical spine injury, 1490–1492
      direct airway damage, 1492–1493
      full stomach, 1489–1490
      head, eye and vascular injuries, 1490
   examination, components of, 589t
   foreign body aspiration, 1366–1367, 1367f
   infants
      anatomy, 1220–1221
         alveolar ventilation, 1220–1221
         comparison with adults, 1220t
         cricoid ring, 1220
         pseudostratified, columnar epithelium, 1220
         trachea, 1220
      physiology, 1220–1221
   laryngotracheobronchitis, 1366
   laser surgery of, 1367–1368, 1368t
   management, 767–768
      airway anatomy and, 768–769
      anesthesia induction and, 773–791
      during cardiopulmonary resuscitation, 1663–1664
      difficult and failed, 791–797
      flexible intubation scopes in, 797–800
      history and physical examination and, 770–773, 770t, 771t
      history of, 769–770
      preoxygenation and, 773
   maxillofacial trauma, 1370–1371
   nasal surgery of, 1368–1369, 1369f
   neonate, anatomy of, 1186–1187, 1186f
   obstruction, in trauma patient, 1489
   resistance, 1545–1546
   skull base surgery, 1369–1370
   surgery, 1364–1365
      bronchoscopy, 1365, 1365t
      stridor, 1364–1365, 1364t
   upper infections, 1370
Airway Approach Algorithm (AAA), 792, 1741f
Airway bougies, 801–802
Airway distress, 1220
Airway exchange catheters (AECs), 790, 791f
Airway obstruction, foreign body, 1663
Airway reflexes, protective, sedation and, 837–838
Airway resistance, 1225
Airway Scope, 786, 786f
AKI. *See* Acute kidney injury (AKI)
ALA-dehydratase-deficient porphyria (ADP), 623, 624t
Alanine aminotransferase (ALT), 1300
Alarm fatigue, 69
Albumin, 395, 429, 1222
Albuminuria, 1346
Alcoholic hepatitis, 1305
   therapy for, 1305
Alcoholics Anonymous (AA), 83
Alcohol, in pregnancy, 1165
Alcohol septal ablation, 890
Aldosterone, 391, 1404
Alemtuzumab (Campath), 1464
Alfentanil, 14, 512, 830, 855t, 1412, 1575
   context-sensitive plasma half-time for, 264f
   dose ranges
      effect of age on, 903t
   pharmacokinetics, 1573t
Algogenic substances, 1567t
Ali, H. H., 16
Alkaloids, 302f, 303
Alleles, 144
Allen, Freeman, 82
Allen test, 715
Allergic reactions, 67–68, 68t, 204, 438. *See also* Hypersensitivity reactions
   in anesthesiologists, 68
   drugs and agents implicated in, 214, 215–217, 215t
   evaluation of patients with, 214–215
   intraoperative, 208–209, 209t
   life-threatening, 214
   perioperative management, 214–215
   testing for, 215
Allodynia, 510, 1563, 1610, 1616, 1617
Alloimmune hemolytic anemia, 634
Alloimmunization, 439–440
Allometric scaling, 257
α_1-Acid glycoprotein concentration, in children, 1222
α_2-Adrenergic agonists, 571, 1579–1580
α-Adrenergic receptors, 343, 345–347
   in central nervous system, 346
   in coronary arteries, 346
   in myocardium, 346
   in peripheral vessels, 346
α_1-Adrenoceptor antagonists, 314–315
α_2-Adrenoceptor antagonists, 315–316
   clonidine, 315–316
   dexmedetomidine, 316
α_2-Agonists, 933
α-Amino-3-hydroxy-5-methylisoxazole-4-proprionic acid (AMPA), 1566, 1568f
α-Fetoprotein (AFP), 1207
α-Glucosidase inhibitors, 1345
α-Melanocyte-stimulating hormone (αMSH), 517
Alprazolam, in patients with renal failure, 1412
Alternating current (AC)
   capacitance in, 120f
   description of, 110
   electrical shock hazards, 111, 111f
   leakage currents and, 120f
Alternative circuits, 8
Alternative hypothesis, 170
Altitude, ventilatory response to, 369
Alveolar-capillary membrane, 363–364
Alveolar dead space ventilation, 372, 373
Alveolar pressure, 372
Alveolar transmural pressure gradient, 364. *See also* Lung
Alveolar ventilation, 1220–1221
   FRC ratio in infants, 1224
Alvimopan, 1572
Alzheimer disease (AD), 620
AMA. *See* American Medical Association (AMA)
Ambu aScope 3 flexible intubation scope, 798, 799f
Ambulatory anesthesia
   airway adjuncts, 858
   fasting guidelines, 851t
   intraoperative management
      caudal anesthesia, 855
      regional techniques, 854
      sedation and analgesia, 857
      spinal anesthesia, 854
   postanesthesia care
      nausea and vomiting, 860
      reversal of muscle relaxants, 859
   postsurgical pain, 860
   preoperative screening, 851
   procedures, 848–851
Ambulatory laparoscopic surgery, 1263
American Academy of Chest Physicians (AACP), 1454
American Association of Nurse Anesthetists (AANA), 32, 33, 36, 702
American Association of Oral and Maxillofacial Surgeons, 872
American Board of Anesthesiology (ABA), 22, 32
American Board of Medical Specialties (ABMS), 35
American Cancer Society, on lung cancer, 1030
American Conference of Governmental Industrial Hygienists, 66
American Council for Graduate Medical Education, 35
American Geriatrics Society, 897
American Heart Association (AHA), 590
   SBE prophylaxis recommendations, 1237t
American Heart Association Advanced Cardiac Life Support (ACLS) protocol, 869
American Medical Association (AMA), 22
American National Emergency X-Radiography Utilization Study (NEXUS), 1490
American National Standards Institute (ANSI), 11, 648
American Nurses Credentialing Center, 32
American Osteopathic Association, 33–34
American Society for Regional Anesthesia, 19
American Society of Anesthesiologists (ASA), 11, 28, 66, 430, 586, 648, 702, 897, 953, 1688
   Basic Standards for Preanesthesia Care, 37, 1734
   Continuum of Depth of Sedation, 1733-1734
   Difficult Airway Algorithm, 37

Difficult Airway Algorithm (ASA-DAA), 791–796, 791f, 1742f
fasting guidelines, 1233 1233t, 1740
Guidelines for Determining Anesthesia Machine Obsolescence, 41
Guidelines for the Ethical Practice of Anesthesiology, 33
Newsletter, 33
physical status classification, 590t
Practice Advisories, 38
Practice Advisory for Preanesthesia Evaluation, 37
Practice Guideline, 37
Practice Guidelines for Obstetrical Anesthesia, 37
Practice Management Conference, 33
Relative Value Guide, 48
resource materials through, 33
standards for basic anesthetic monitoring, 1732–1740
standards for Postanesthesia Care, 37, 1539, 1734-1735
standards of practice, 37
Visual Loss Registry, 821
website, 33
American Society of Post Anesthesia Nurses, 37
American Society of Regional Anesthesia (ASRA), 19, 22, 953, 1454
American Spinal Cord Association (ASIA) Impairment Scale, 1023t
Americans with Disabilities Act, 83
Ames test, 480
Ametop, 1244
Aminoamides, 569
Amino esters, 13, 569
Aminophylline, 1035
Aminosteroid nondepolarizing neuromuscular blocking agents, 534t, 535–536
Amiodarone, during CPR, 1671–1672
Amitriptyline, 1617
   dosage range, 1621t
   for fibromyalgia, 1616
Ammonia, 1302–1303
Amnesia, 234
AMPA-type glutamate receptor, 1609
Amphetamines, in pregnancy, 1166, 1166t
Amsorb, 135
Amylin analogs, 1345
Amyotrophic lateral sclerosis (ALS), 621–622
Anaesthetists' Travel Club, 22
Analgesia, 935
   epidural, 1199
   intrathecal, 1584–1585, 1585t
   for knee, surgery to, 1451–1452, 1451t
   methods of, 1582–1597
   neuraxial, 1583–1585, 1584t, 1585t
   nonopioid adjuncts, 1577–1582, 1578t
   for opioids, 508–510
   for orthopedic surgery, 1446t
   patient-controlled, 1582, 1582t
   spinal mechanism, 1583
   supraspinal mechanism, 1583
   topical, 1387
Analysis of variance, 173
Anaphylatoxins, 210
   biologic effects of, 210t
Anaphylaxis, 204, 208
   arachidonic acid metabolites, 210
   chemical mediators of, 209
   IgE-mediated pathophysiology, 209–210, 209f
   management of, 211–212
      airway evaluation, 213
      anesthetic drugs, discontinuation of, 212
      antihistamines, 213
      bicarbonate, 213
      bronchodilators, 213
      catecholamines, 213
      corticosteroids, 213
      epinephrine administration, 213
      during general anesthesia, 212t
      oxygen administration, 212
      refractory hypotension, 213
      volume expansion, 212–213
   non–IgE-mediated reactions, 210–211
   peptide mediators of, 209–210
   recognition of, 210
Andersen disease, 629
Andersen–Tawil syndrome (ATS), 616
Andrews, Edmund, 7
Android (central) obesity, 1278
Anemia, 636, 1549
   of chronic kidney disease, 1411
   in critical illness, 1647–1648
   hemolytic, 633–634
   nutritional deficiency, 633
   oxygen delivery with, 633t
   physiologic compensation for, 431–433, 432t
   types of, 633t
Anesthesia, 220–221. *See also* Postanesthesia recovery
   academic, 22
   apparatus checkout recommendations, 698–699
   for complex spine surgery, 1023–1024
   conduct of
      intraoperative management, 906–907, 907f
      perioperative complications, 908–911, 908f
      postoperative care, 907–908
      preoperative visit, 905–906
   delivery, ASA guidelines, 701–704
   delivery systems, early, 7–8, 7f
   equipment maintenance and service, 41
   before ether, 2–5
   history of, 1–23
   management of, 614, 615, 618, 619, 620, 622, 624–625, 632, 636, 637–638, 639, 640–641
   measurement of anesthetic potency, 221
   multisite model for, 236f
   for neurosurgery, 1003–1024
      cerebral perfusion, 1011–1013
      cerebral protection, 1013–1014
      management, 1014–1016
      monitoring, 1009–1011
      neuroanatomy, 1004–1006, 1004f, 1005f, 1006f, 1007f, 1007t
      neurophysiology, 1007–1008, 1008f
      pathophysiology, 1008–1009, 1009f
      procedures, 1016–1022
   non-OR, scheduling of, 58
   and obstructive pulmonary disease, 379
   physical and psychological, 2
   principles, equipment, and standards, 5–11
   and professionalism, 21–23
   and restrictive pulmonary disease, 379–380
   safety standards, 11
   for spine trauma, 1023–1024
   subspecialties
      cardiovascular anesthesia, 19–20
      neuroanesthesia, 20
      obstetric anesthesia, 20–21
      regional anesthesia, 17–19
      transfusion medicine, 21
   transplant, 1458–1481. *See also* Transplantation
   and traumatic brain injury, 1022–1023
   ventilators, 684–687
      bellows, 685–686, 685f
      classification of, 684 hazards, 686–687
      problems, 686–687, 686f
Anesthesia and Analgesia, 21
Anesthesia drug, cost of, 62
Anesthesia face mask, 773–775, 774f
Anesthesia Information Management Systems (AIMS), 727
Anesthesia machine, 646f–647f
   function of, 645
   generic two-gas, 652f
Anesthesia Machine Workbook (AMW), 668
Anesthesia maintenance
   in elective surgery, 1248
   fluid maintenance requirements, 1248–1249
   for preventing blood loss, 1248–1249
   techniques, 1247–1248
Anesthesia Patient Safety Foundation (APSF), 33, 41, 668, 702
   information resources through, 32–33
   on technology training, 41
   website, 33
Anesthesia preoperative evaluation clinic (APEC), 59
Anesthesia Quality Institute (AQI), 32, 103, 843
Anesthesia risk
   mortality/morbidity, 91, 92t–97t
   National Practitioner Data Bank (NPDB), 100
   risk management after adverse outcome, 99–100
   checklists, 98, 98t
   concept, 97–98
   "Do Not Resuscitate" (DNR) and, 100
   informed consent, 98–99
   record keeping, 99
Anesthesia workstations (AWS), 1224
   alarm devices, 660
   anatomy of, 656
      high-pressure circuit, 656
      intermediate-pressure circuit, 656
      low-pressure circuit, 656
   anesthetic breathing circuit, 679–681
      Bain circuit, 679–680, 680f
      circle breathing system, 680–681
      Mapleson breathing systems, 679–680, 679f
   carbon dioxide absorbents, 681–683
      absorptive capacity, 682
      canisters, 681
      chemistry of, 681–682
      comparisons, 683t
      indicators, 682
      interactions of inhaled anesthetics with, 682–683, 683t
   checkout of, 652, 652f
      ASA 2008 guidelines for developing institution-specific, 701–704
      circle system evaluation, 654–655, 655f
      gas supply lines, 653–654
      guidelines for preanesthesia procedures, 700–701
      low-pressure circuit leak test, 653–654, 654f
      negative-pressure leak test, 654, 654f
      oxygen analyzer calibration, 652–653
      oxygen flush positive-pressure leak test, 653, 654f
      recommendations, 698–699
      self-tests, 655, 655f
   cylinder supply source, 657–658, 658f
   definition, 645
   electronic alarm devices and pneumatic, 660
   electronic flowmeter, 664–665, 664f, 665f
   equipment failure, 648
   flowmeter assembly, 661–664, 661f
      annular space, 662f
      components of, 662–663, 662f
      conventional flowmeters, operating principles of, 662, 662f
      flow control valve assembly, 661f, 662
      oxygen, 661f
      problems with, 663–664, 663f
      subassembly, 661f, 662–663
   functions, comparison of, 649t–651t

Anesthesia workstations (*continued*)
  GE-Datex-Ohmeda Link-25 Proportion-Limiting Control System, 665–667, 666f
  machine intermediate-pressure system, 659
  machine outlet check valve, 653
  nitrous oxide, 658–659
  oxygen failure cutoff valves, 660, 660f
  oxygen flush valve, 667–668
  oxygen pressure regulators, 660–661
  oxygen ratio monitor controller, 666–667, 666f
  oxygen supply pressure failure safety devices, 659–661
  pipeline supply source, 656–657
  pneumatic and electronic alarm devices, 660
  pneumatics, 656
  pre-use procedures, 646, 648
  proportioning systems, 665–667, 666f
  safety features of, 648
  sensitive oxygen ratio controller, 666–667, 666f
  software simulation, 668–679
  standards, 646, 648
  two-gas machine, 652f
  vaporizers, 668
    D-Vapor for desflurane, 673–676, 674f, 675t, 676f
    GE-Datex-Ohmeda Aladin Cassette, 676–678, 677f, 678f
    Maquet FLOW-i electronic injector, 647f, 669t, 679
    models and characteristics, 678t
    physics of, 668–669, 669t
    Tec 6 for desflurane, 673–676, 674f, 675t, 676f, 677f
    variable bypass, 669–673
  variations, 688–691
    Apollo workstation, 689–690
    Datex-Ohmeda S/5 ADU, 688–689, 688f
    Dräger Medical Narkomed 6000 Series, 689–690, 690f
    Fabius GS, 690
    GE Healthcare Aisys Carestation, 688–689, 688f
    Maquet Flow-i workstation, 690-691, 690f, 691f
  ventilators, 684–687
    bellows, 685–686, 685f
    classification of, 684 hazards, 686–687
    problems, 686–687, 686f
  waste gas scavenging systems, 691–695
Anesthesiologists, 2
  as Clinical Director of OR, 56
  job market for, 44
  participation in facility activities, 35–36
  in preoperative screening clinics, 55
  relationship with facility staff, 36
  types of practice, 44–47
    academic practice, 44–45
    private practice, 45–47
Anesthesiology, 242
Anesthesiology practice
  administrative components
    adverse event, response to, 43–44
    anesthesia equipment and equipment maintenance, 40–42
    certification maintenance, 35
    credentialing process and clinical privileges, 33–35
    malpractice insurance, 42–43
    meetings and case discussion, 39–40
    MOCA process, 35
    operational and information resources, 32–33
    policy and procedure, 39
    professional staff participation and relationships, 35–36
  standards of practice, 36–39
  support staff, 40
  bundled payment model, 27–28
  cost and quality issues, 61–62
  essentials, 44–56
    accountable care organizations, 53–54
    antitrust considerations, 49–50
    billing and collecting, 47–49, 49t
    electronic medical records, 54–55
    evolving practice arrangements, 51–53
    exclusive service contracts, 50–51
    HIPAA, 54
    hospital subsidies, 51
    job market, 44
    management intricacies, 54
    perioperative medicine and hospital care, 55–56
    types of practice, 44–47
  multispecialty, 31–32
  operating room management, 56–61
    organization, 56–57
    personnel issues, 60–61
    scheduling cases, 57–60
  PSH, 28–30
  service line, 30–31
Anesthesiology Residency Review Committee, 27
Anesthetic agents
  antibiotics, 538
  anticonvulsants, 538
  β-receptor antagonists, 538
  calcium channel antagonists, 538
  corticosteroids, 538
  depolarizing and nondepolarizing, 537
  genetic variability in response to, 157–158
  history of use of, 11–17
  with inhalational agents, 537–538
  local anesthetics, 538
  nondepolarizing, 537
Anesthetic breathing circuit, 679–681
  Bain circuit, 679–680, 680f
  circle breathing system, 680–681
  Mapleson breathing systems, 679–680, 679f
Anesthetic effects in vitro and whole-animal anesthesia, link between, 230–233
  genetic approaches, 230–232
  pharmacologic approaches, 230
Anesthetic gases, 66–67, 66t
  behavioral effects, 66
  cancer, 66
  NIOSH recommendations, 66
  nitrous oxide exposure, 66
  OSHA and, 68
  reproductive outcomes, 66
  trace levels, 67
  waste, exposure to, 66–67
Anesthetic potency, 157
Anesthetic target sites, chemical nature of
  anesthetic binding to proteins, 222–223
  lipid theories of anesthesia, 222
  lipid *versus* protein targets, 222
  Meyer–Overton rule, 221, 221f, 222
  protein theories of anesthesia, 222
Angiogenesis, in wound healing, 193
Angiography, 885
Angiotensin converting enzyme inhibitors, 328–329, 328f, 1409
Angiotensin I, 350
Angiotensin II, 1404
Angiotensin receptor blockers (ARBs), 329, 1409
Anion gap (AG), 1407
Ankle, surgery to, 1452
Anoci-association, 19
Anoxic brain injury, 1638
Anrep effect, 286
ANS. *See* Autonomic nervous system (ANS)
ANSI. *See* American National Standards Institute (ANSI)
Antacids, 604–605
Antagonists, 254
Antepartum hemorrhage, 1159–1160
Anterior cerebral artery (ACA), 1005
Anterior cruciate ligament (ACL), 1452
Anterior ischemic optic neuropathy, postsurgical, 1395
Anterior mediastinal mass (AMM), 1236–1237
  tracheal intubation for, 1237
Anterior motor root, 919
Anthrax, 1697–1698
Anti-$β_2$-glycoprotein-1 (A$β$GP), 426–427
Antibiotics, 189–191
  anaphylactic reactions to, 215
  prophylactic, 53
  recommendations for, 190t
  before thoracic surgery, 1035
Antibodies, 205–206, 205f
  classes and properties of, 206t
Anticardiolipin antibodies (ACLA), 426–427
Anticholinergics, 608, 608t, 1186, 1225
Anticholinesterase agents, 550–553
Anticonvulsants, in TBI, 1636
Antidiuretic hormone (ADH), 335, 391, 1018, 1353–1354, 1403–1404, 1551–1552
  secretion of, 1353–1354
Antiemetics, history of use of, 16–17
Antiepileptic drugs (AEDs), 619–620, 620t
Antifactor Xa activity (aFXa), 427
Antifibrinolytic therapy, 453, 1526
Antigens, 205, 205t
Antihistamines, for anaphylactic reactions, 213
Antihypertensive therapy, in preeclampsia, 1158
Antiphospholipid antibodies (APLA), 425
Antiretroviral therapy, prophylactic, 80
Antisepsis, 187, 189
Antisialagogue, awake intubation and, 794
Antithrombin-III (AT-III), 423
Antithrombotics, ASRA guidelines for, 1449t
Antithymocyte globulin (ATG), in immunosuppressive therapy, 1464
Antitrust laws, 49
Anxiety Reduction, 851–852
Anxiolysis, 1242, 1733
  distraction techniques, 1242
  parental presence at induction of anesthesia, 1242
  pharmacologic sedation, 1242–1243
Aortic aneurysms, 1090, 1127
  formation of, 1127–1128
  rupture, 1128
Aortic dissection, 1089, 1128
  anesthetic considerations, 1089, 1089t
  hemodynamic goals, 1089t
  type A, 1089
  type B, 1089
Aortic input impedance, 290
Aortic reconstruction, 1127–1133
  anesthetic management, 1132–1133
  aortic cross-clamp placement, 1128, 1128f
  aortic occlusion and reperfusion pathophysiology, 1128–1130, 1129t
  renal hemodynamics and renal protection, 1130–1131
  spinal cord ischemia and protection, 1131–1132
Aortic stenosis
  anesthetic considerations, 1083–1084
  clinical factors with, 1082
  hemodynamic goals, 1083t
  pathophysiology, 1082–1083, 1083f
Aortic valve insufficiency (AI), 1085–1086
  anesthetic considerations, 1085–1086

hemodynamic goals, 1086t
pathophysiology, 1084f, 1085
Aortocaval syndrome, 811
Aortoiliac occlusive disease (AIOD), 1133
Aoyagi, Takuo, 10
APEC. *See* Anesthesia preoperative evaluation clinic (APEC)
Apert's disease, 1220
Apixaban, 427, 451
Aplysia, 226
Apnea, 367t
   in neonates, 1202
Apneic oxygenation, 773
Apneusis, 367t
Apneustic ventilation, 367t
Apollo workstation, 689–690
Apoptosis, 1221
Apraclonidine, 358
APRN. *See* Advanced practice registered nurses (APRN)
Arachidonic acid metabolites, 210
Arachnoid mater, 917–918, 918f
ARDS. *See* Acute respiratory distress syndrome (ARDS)
Arecoline, 302f
Arginine vasopressin (AVP), 400, 1304
   during CPR, 1671
Arm, surgery to, 1447
   anesthetic management, 1448
   approach, 1447–1448
   positioning, 1447–1448, 1447f
Arndt blocker, 1048–1049, 1048f
Arousal, 234
Arrestins, 254
Arrhythmias, 474–475, 474f
Arterial blood gas analysis, preoperative, 1032
Arterial oxygenation
   assessment of, 375
   monitoring of
      contraindications, 710
      indications, 710
      principles of operation, 709, 709f
      problems and limitations, 710
      use and interpretation, 709
Arterial waveform analysis, in cardiac output monitoring
   contraindications, 723
   indications, 723
   principles of operation, 721–723, 722f
   problems and limitations, 723–724
   use and interpretation, 723
Arteriovenous malformations (AVM), 1019–1020
Artery of Adamkiewicz, 1131
Arthritis, 600
Articular processes, vertebral, 916
ASA. *See* American Society of Anesthesiologists (ASA)
Ascending pathways, neurobiology of, 1610
Ascites, 1313–1314
ASCVD. *See* Atherosclerotic cardiovascular disease (ASCVD)
Aspartate aminotransferase (AST), 1300
Aspiration, perioperative, 1550–1551
Aspirin, 53, 449
Assessment of Blood Consumption (ABC) score, 1495
Asthma, 597, 1234–1235
   preoperative bronchodilator therapy for, 1234–1235
   steroids for, 1234
ASTM F1850–00 standard, 659
Atherosclerotic cardiovascular disease (ASCVD), 1112
   coronary artery disease and, 1114
   and disease in other areas of body, 1113–1114, 1114f

medical optimization prior to surgery, 1114–1119
myocardial infarction and, 1114
pathophysiology of, 1113
preoperative anesthesia evaluation, 1119–1120
risk factors for, 1113
vulnerable plaque model, 1113
Atomic mass units (AMU), 658
Atracurium, 211, 535t, 537, 1230, 1412, 1413
Atrial natriuretic peptide (ANP), 1404
Atropine, 304–306, 305t, 342, 350, 355, 355f, 355t, 608, 1186, 1247, 1694
   for awake intubation, 794
   during cardiac arrest, 1672
   toxicity, 306, 306t
Augmented gas inflow, 465
Aura-I, 787
Autologous blood conservation (ABC), 441–444
Automatic external defibrillators (AEDs), 1663, 1673
Automatic implantable cardioverter defibrillator (AICD), 126
Autonomic control, 233–234
Autonomic dysfunction, 1309
Autonomic dysreflexia (AD), 1024
Autonomic nervous system (ANS), 333–334, 476, 476f
   adrenergic receptors, 343–349, 343f, 344t, 345t
      α-adrenergic receptors, 343, 345–347
      β-adrenergic receptors, 347
      location of, 343f
   agonists, 342
   ANS ganglion, 336
   antagonists, 342
   central, 334–335
   cholinergic receptors, 342–343
   dopaminergic receptors, 347–348
   efferent ANS, 336f
   functional anatomy, 334–342
   heart and, 338
   lung and, 338–339
   nerve fibers, 336, 336t
   parasympathetic nervous system, 334, 337–338
      transmission, 339–340
   peripheral, 335–342, 335f
   peripheral circulation, 338
   pharmacology, 351
      antimuscarinic drugs, 355–356, 355f, 355t
      direct cholinomimetics, 352–353, 352f
      ganglionic drugs, 351–352
      indirect cholinomimetics, 353–354, 354f
      mode of action, 351
      muscarinic agonists, 352
      muscarinic antagonists, 354–355
   reflexes and interactions, 349–350
   sympathetic nervous system, 334, 336–337
      transmission, 340–342
   syndromes and regulation, 356–359
      diabetic neuropathy, 358
      Horner syndrome, 357–358, 357f
      orthostatic hypotension, 358
   transmission, 339, 339f
Avian influenza A, 74
AVPU system, for assessment of consciousness, 1500–1501, 1500t
Awake craniotomy, 1021–1022
Awake fiberoptic intubation, 1513
Awake intubation, 792, 794–796
Axillary blocks, 972–974, 973f
Axillary roll, 817
Ayre, Phillip, 8
Azathioprine, 1465

B

Babesia species, 437
Bacillus anthracis (anthrax), 1697–1698
Backache, 937
Background/leak channels, 226
Backward–upward–rightward pressure (BURP) maneuver, 781
Baclofen, 855t
Bainbridge reflex, 349
Bain circuit, 679–680, 680f
Bain–Spoerel apparatus, 8
Banting, Frederick, 11
Barbiturates, 371, 499–501, 500t, 1014, 1284
   clinical uses, 501
   pharmacodynamics, 500
      cardiovascular effects, 501
      central nervous system effects, 500–501
      respiratory system effects, 501
   pharmacokinetics, 500
   side effects, 501
   in TBI, 1636
Bardeen, Charles, 22
Bariatric surgery, 1279
Barker, Arthur, 18
Barnard, Christian, 1476
Barometric pressure, 375, 464
Baroreceptors, 349–350
Basal ganglia, 1004
Basic cardiac life support (BLS) certification, 869
Basiliximab, in immunosuppressive therapy, 1464
Basophils, 206
Bayesian inference, 172
B cells, 205
Bean bag, 817
Becker muscular dystrophy (BMD), 613, 1236
Beckwith–Wiedemann syndrome, 1206–1207
Beer–Lambert law, 710
Belatacept, in immunosuppressive therapy, 1464
Belladonna alkaloids, 355–356
Bellows classification, 684, 685f. *See also* Anesthesia workstations
Benchmarks, performance-based pay and, 53
Bennett, Abram E., 15
Bennett and Bird valve, 8
   usage of, 9
Benzocaine, 13
   for awake intubation, 795
Benzodiazepines, 498, 498t, 606–607, 606t, 852, 1233, 1284, 1319, 1412, 1649
   for awake intubation, 794
   clinical uses, 499, 499t
   diazepam, 606–607
   lorazepam, 606–607, 607f
   metabolism and clearance, 498t
   midazolam, 606, 607f
   for monitored anesthetic care, 832–833
   pharmacodynamics, 499, 499t
   pharmacokinetics, 498–499, 499t
   pharmacologic variables of, 606t
   side effects, 499
Benzylisoquinolinium nondepolarizing neuromuscular blocking agents, 535t
Berci, George, 770
Berman intubating oral airways, 800, 800f
$β_2$-Adrenergic agonists, 571
β-Adrenergic blocking drug, 1381
β-Adrenergic receptors, 347
$β_2$-Adrenoceptor agonist, 313
β-Adrenoceptor antagonists. *See* β-Blockers
β-Blockers, 316, 602–603
   adverse effects, 319
   atenolol, 317t, 320
   cardiovascular effects of, 316–321, 317t, 318f
   carvedilol, 317t, 320–321
   esmolol, 317t, 320

β-Blockers (continued)
  for ischemia, 1081
  labetalol, 317t, 320
  metoprolol, 317t, 320
  prophylactic, 53
  propranolol, 316, 317t, 319–320
  topical, 319
  vascular surgery and, 1115–1116
Betamethasone (Celestone Soluspan), 1612, 1613f
Betaxolol, 1381
Bethanechol, 302f, 303, 353
Bezold–Jarisch reflex, 935
Bias, management of, 168–169
Bier, August, 17, 19
Bier block, 19
Big Data, 179
Bile salts, 1307
Bilevel positive airway pressure (BiPAP), 1292
Billing process
  for anesthesiology services, 48
  HIPAA Privacy Rule and, 54
  prospective payments, 52
  tracking data on computer, 48, 49t
Billroth, Theodore, 19
Binomial probability distribution function, 174
Bioavailability, 243
Biologic disaster, 1696–1699
Biologic hypothesis, 169
Biomarkers, in perioperative medicine, 151–155
Biopsy, liver, 1301
Biotransformation reactions, 244
  phase I reactions, 244–245
Bird and Bennett valves, 8
Bird, Forrest, 9
Birt–Hogg–Dubé syndrome, 1418
BIS. See Bispectral index (BIS)
Bispectral index (BIS), 494, 550, 840–841, 907, 1224
Bispectrum, 725
Bisphosphonates, 412
Bixby, E. May, 12
Bladder exstrophy, 1435
Blalock, Alfred, 19
Blalock–Taussig shunt, 19
Blinding, 169
Blind nasal intubation, 769
Blindness, prone position and, 820–821
Block adjuvants, ocular surgery, 1387–1388
Blocks
  adductor canal, 1586t, 1590
  ankle, 996–998
  Bier, 19
  brachial plexus, 967–974, 1200, 1585, 1586t, 1588–1589, 1588f, 1589f
    axillary block, 972–974, 973f
    infraclavicular block, 970–972, 971f
    interscalene block, 967–969, 968f
    median nerve, 975–977, 976f
    radial nerve, 974–975, 974f
    supraclavicular block, 969–970, 969f
    ulnar nerve, 976f, 977
  caudal, 1199, 1199f, 1249–1250
  cervical plexus, 954–955, 955f, 965–967, 966f
  deep cervical plexus, 1592
  deep peroneal nerve, 997–998, 997f
  epidural, 1250
  fascia iliaca compartment, 1590, 1590f, 1591f
  femoral nerve/fascia iliaca, 988–989, 989f, 1586t, 1589–1590, 1590f
  iliohypogastric nerve, 978, 984–985, 985f, 1595–1596
  ilioinguinal nerve, 978, 984–985, 985f, 1199-1200, 1200f, 1595–1596
  infraorbital nerve, 964
  intercostal nerves, 978–980, 979f
  intravenous regional anesthesia (Bier block), 977–978
  lateral femoral cutaneous nerve, 989, 1200
  local anesthetics, 1587t
  lower extremity, 986
  lumbar plexus, 986–988, 986f, 987f, 1586t, 1589–1590, 1590f, 1591f
    terminal nerves of, 988–991
  mandibular nerve, 965, 965f
  maxillary nerve, 964–965, 965f
  mental nerve, 964
  neurosurgical, 1200
  obturator nerve, 989–990, 990f
  occipital nerve, 967
  paravertebral, 980–982, 980f, 982f
  pectoralis nerve, 1593
  penile, 985–986, 1199
  peribulbar (extraconal), 1383–1386, 1384f
  peripheral nerve, 945–998, 1291–1292, 1585. See also Peripheral nerve blocks (PNBs)
  popliteal fossa, 1586t
  posterior tibial nerve, 996, 997f
  psoas compartment, 1589
  rectus sheath, 978, 983–984, 984f, 1595
  retrobulbar (intraconal), 1383–1386, 1384f
  sacral plexus, 1586t, 1590–1592, 1592f
  saphenous nerve, 990–991, 991f, 998, 1590
  scheduling, 58
  sciatic nerve, 1586t
    anterior, 995–996, 995f
    posterior, 991–995, 992f, 993f, 994f
  semilunar (gasserian) ganglion, 954f, 963
  serratus plane, 1593
  spinal, 1250
  superficial trigeminal nerve, 963–964, 964f
  supraorbital nerve, 963–964, 964f
  supratrochlear nerve, 964
  sural nerve, 996–997
  TAP, 1200, 1200f
  thoracic paravertebral, 1592–1593
  transversalis fascia plane, 1596
  transversus abdominis plane, 978, 982–983, 983f, 984f, 1593, 1594f, 1595, 1595f
  trigeminal nerve, 954, 954f, 963–965
  truncal, 1587t, 1592–1596, 1593f–1595f
  trunk nerve, 978–985
  upper extremity, 967–978
  Winnie, 19
Blood
  collection, 428
  compatibility testing, 430
  component processing and storage, 428–429
  component production, 428–430, 428t
  conservation strategies, 441–444, 442t
  cryoprecipitate, 434, 435t
  fibrinogen concentrates, 435
  new, 1525
  pathogen inactivation, 429–430
  perioperative salvage, 443–444
  plasma derivatives, 429
  plasma products, 433–434, 434t
  platelets, 433, 433t
  product administration, risks of, 435–441
    infectious, 435–437, 436t
    noninfectious, 437–441, 438t
  products and transfusion thresholds, 430–435
  RBC and platelet substitutes, 430
  red blood cells, 430–433
Blood-borne pathogens, 71
Blood Conservation Clinical Practice Guidelines, 431
Blood flow
  distribution of, 372, 372f
  velocity calculations, 743f
Blood pressure
  in children, 1221t
  intermittent noninvasive monitoring of
    contraindications, 716
    indications, 716
    principles of operation, 715–716
    problems and limitations, 716–717
    use and interpretation, 716, 716f
  invasive monitoring of
    arterial cannulation, 713–714, 713t
    contraindications, 714
    indications, 714
    principles of operation, 713
    problems and limitations, 714–715, 715f
    use and interpretation, 713–714, 713t
Blood transfusion therapy, 21, 1248–1249
Blood urea nitrogen (BUN), 395, 596, 1405
Blue baby, 19
Blue bloaters, 1032
Blunt cardiac injury (BCI), 1506–1507, 1507f, 1509t
B-mode echocardiography, 733–734
Bodok seal, 657
Body fluid compartments, 390
Body mass index (BMI), 1278
Body temperature, monitoring of
  contraindications, 724
  indications, 724
  principles of operation, 724
  problems and limitations, 724
  use and interpretation, 724
Bohr equation, 374
Boiling point of liquid, 668
Bolus, 947
Bolus–Elimination–Infusion (BET) scheme, 263, 263t
Bone Cement Implantation Syndrome (BCIS), 1454
Bonfils Intubation Fiberscope (BIF), 783
Bonica, John J., 19
Boothby, Walter, 8
Booth, Harold, 12
Botulinum toxin A, 1616
Botulism, 1698–1699
Bovet, Daniel, 16
Bovine spongiform encephalopathy, 80
Bowditch effect, 289–290
Boyle-Davis gag, 6
Boyle, Henry E. G. "Cockie," 8
Boyle machines, 8
Boyle's law, 657, 951, 952f
BPCI. See Bundled Payments for Care Improvement (BPCI)
BPF. See Bronchopleural fistula (BPF)
Brachial plexopathy, 824–825, 824f
Brachial plexus, 956–959, 957f
  axillary, 1586t
  blocks, 967–974, 1200
    axillary, 972–974, 973f
    infraclavicular, 970–972, 971f
    interscalene, 967–969, 968f
    median nerve, 975–977, 976f
    radial nerve, 974–975, 974f
    supraclavicular, 969–970, 969f
    ulnar nerve, 976f, 977
  infraclavicular, 1586t
  injuries, 821, 821f
  interscalene, 1586t
  neuropathy, 813
  for pain management, 1585, 1586t, 1588–1589, 1588f, 1589f
  supraclavicular, 1586t
  terminal nerves of, 957, 958f
Bradycardia, 935
  causes of, 1247, 1247t
  hypoxia and, 1247
  incidence of, 1247
  treatment of, 1247

Brain, 1004–1006
  anatomy of, 1004–1006, 1004f
  arteries, 1005
  blood supply in, 1005
  cerebral blood flow in, 1007–1008
  compartments
    infratentorium, 1005
    supratentorium, 1004–1005, 1004f
  CSF flows, 1005–1006, 1006f
  edema in, 1009
  extrapyramidal system of, 1004
  homeostasis of, 1012–1013
  intracranial hypertension and, 1009
  limbic system of, 1005
  neurophysiology, 1007–1008, 1008f
  structures, functionality of, 107t
  venous system of, 1005, 1005f
Brain damage, causes of, 104
Brain-dead donors, 1459–1460
  anesthesiology setup for, 1459t
  anesthetic management during organ harvest, 1460
  cardiac organs evaluation, 1459, 1460
  central venous pressure monitoring, 1460
  hemodynamic instability in, 1459
  lung removal, 1460
Brainstem, 1005
Brainstem auditory evoked potentials (BAEPs), 1009, 1010–1011, 1010f
Brain surgery, 20
Braun, Heinrich, 18, 19
Breach of duty, 103
Breast tissue ischemia, 821
Breath-holding, ventilatory response to, 369–370
Breathing, 366
  chemical control of, 370–371, 370f
Breath sounds, preoperative evaluation, 1031
Bredenfeld, Elisabeth, 13
British Committee for Standards in Haemotology (BCSH), 431
British Medical Journal, 20
Broca's index, 1278
Bronchial blockers, in lung separation, 1047, 1047t
Bronchiolar smooth muscle tone, 478, 479f.
  See also Inhaled anesthetics
Bronchodilators, anaphylactic reactions and, 213
Bronchopleural fistula (BPF), 1062
  anesthesia for, 1062–1063
Bronchopulmonary lavage, 1064–1065
Bronchoscopy, 1056–1058, 1365, 1365t
  complications of, 1058
  fiberoptic, 1058
  general anesthesia for, 1057
  indications for, 1056t
  instruments for, 1057t
  local anesthesia for, 1057
  rigid, 1057–1058
Brooke formulas, for fluid resuscitation, 1515–1516, 1515t
Brown, W. Easson, 11
B-type natriuretic peptide (BNP), 153
Bubble flowmeters, 9
Budd–Chiari syndrome, 1304
Bullae, 1063–1064
Bullard laryngoscope, 7
Bullard, Roger, 7
Bullet oscilloscope, 10
Bundled Payments for Care Improvement (BPCI), 28
Buphthalmos, 1377
Bupivacaine, 14, 1189–1190, 1250
  dosage, 1190
  metabolism, 1190
  neonatal jaundice and, 1148
  toxicity, 1190

Buprenorphine, 520, 855t
  for acute postoperative pain, 1576–1577
Buprenorphine–naloxone therapy, 1622
Buretrol, 1248
Burkhardt, Ludwig, 13
Burkitt lymphoma, 75
Burn injuries, 1511–1516
  airway complications, 1512–1514
  carbon monoxide toxicity and, 1514, 1514t
  cyanide toxicity, 1514–1515
  fluid replacement, 1515–1516, 1515t
  mechanism of, 1511–1512, 1512t, 1513t
  ventilation and intensive care, 1514
Burnout, 81–82
Bursa-derived (B-cell) lymphocytes, 205
Burst suppression ratio (BSR), 725
Butorphanol, for obstetric analgesia, 1149
Buttock pain, management of, 1614–1616
Butyrylcholinesterase. *See* Pseudocholinesterase
Bypass *versus* Angioplasty in Severe Ischaemia of the Leg (BASIL) trial, 1138

C

CABG. *See* Coronary artery bypass graft (CABG)
Caenorhabditis elegans, 224, 230–231
Caglieri, Guido, 18
Calcific aortic stenosis, 890
Calcineurin inhibitors (CNIs), 1464
Calcitonin, 412
Calcitriol, 409
Calcium, 1554
  during CPR, 1672
  hypercalcemia, 411–412
  hypocalcemia, 409–411
  physiologic role, 409
Calcium channel blockers, 325–328, 326t
  clevidipine, 326t, 327
  diltiazem, 326t, 327–328
  for ischemia, 1081–1082
  nicardipine, 326t, 327
  nifedipine, 325, 326t, 327
  nimodipine, 326t, 327
  verapamil, 326t, 328
Calcium hydroxide lime (Amsorb), 681
Calverley, Roderick, 11
Canadian cervical spine rule, 1491–1492, 1492f
Cancer, 65
Candida albicans, 1653
Candida infection, 1653
Candidate gene approach, 147
Cannabinoids, 1622
Cannizzaro reaction, 1227
Capacitance, 110–111, 110f
Capacitors, 110
Capillary glycocalyx, 395
Capitation, prospective payments and, 52
Capnography, 10–11, 711. *See also* Anesthesia
Capnometry, 711, 1241
Capnothorax, 1271
Capsaicin patch, 1621–1622
Capsaicin receptor, 1608
Carbamylcholine, 302f, 303
Carbon dioxide (CO_2)
  absorbents, anesthesia workstations, 681–683
    absorptive capacity, 682
    canisters, 681
    chemistry of, 681–682
    comparisons, 683t
    indicators, 682
    interactions of inhaled anesthetics with, 682–683, 683t
  absorption, 9, 9f. *See also* Anesthesia
  extravasation, 1270–1272
  insufflation, 1262
  transport, 371–376

Carbon monoxide
  diffusing capacity (D_{LCO}), 378
  toxicity
    burns victims and, 1514
    symptoms of, 1514t
Carboprost, 1160t
Carboxyhemoglobin (COHb), 709, 1514, 1514t
Cardiac anatomy, 278
  architecture, 278–279, 278f
  coronary blood supply, 280–281, 280f
  valve structure, 279
Cardiac cycle, 286–287
Cardiac implantable electronic devices (CIEDs)
  anesthesia device services, 1727
  intraoperative problems with, 1725–1726
  perioperative management, 1726–1727, 1726t–1728t
  postoperative evaluation and management, 1727, 1729t, 1730f, 1731, 1731f
  risk mitigation strategies, 1727
Cardiac index (CI), 1265, 1708
Cardiac murmurs, classification of, 1107t
Cardiac myocyte
  calcium–myofilament interaction, 285
  contractile apparatus, 283–285
  myosin–actin interaction, 285–286
  ultrastructure, 283
Cardiac output (CO) monitoring
  arterial waveform analysis in
    contraindications, 723
    indications, 723
    principles of operation, 721–723, 722f
    problems and limitations, 723–724
    use and interpretation, 723
  pulmonary arterial catheter in
    contraindications, 721
    indications, 720–721
    principles of operation, 720
    problems and limitations, 721
    use and interpretation, 720
Cardiac resynchronization therapy (CRT), 1477–1478
Cardiac surgery. *See also* Cardiopulmonary bypass (CPB)
  acute kidney injury and, 1415, 1416f
  anesthetics, choice of, 1095–1096
    induction drugs, 1096
    neuromuscular blocking drugs, 1096
    opioids, 1096
  antifibrinolytic use in, 1092
  aortic diseases, 1089–1090
  blood conservation in, 1092
  and cardiac tamponade, 1105–1106
  cardiopulmonary bypass, 1090–1093
  children with congenital heart disease and, 1106–1108
  coronary artery disease, 1078–1082
  drug therapy and, preoperative, 1093
  history and growth of, 19–20
  intraoperative management, 1096–1104
    cardiopulmonary bypass, 1097–1099, 1098t
    discontinuation of CPB, 1099–1101, 1099f–1101f, 1099t, 1100t
    incision to bypass, 1097
    induction and intubation, 1097
    intra-aortic balloon pump, 1101–1102, 1102f
    postbypass bleeding, 1104
    preincision period, 1097
    preinduction period, 1097
    preparation, 1096, 1096t
    rewarming, 1099
    ventricular assist device, 1102–1104
  minimally invasive, 1104–1105
  monitoring techniques, 1094–1095
    arterial blood pressure, 1094

Cardiac surgery (continued)
  central nervous system function and complications, 1095
  central venous pressure, 1094
  echocardiography, 1095
  electrocardiogram, 1094
  pulmonary artery catheter, 1094–1095
  pulse oximeter, 1094
  temperature, 1094
  pain management, postoperative, 1106
  physical examination, preoperative, 1093–1094, 1094t
  premedication, 1094
  preoperative visit, 1093
  valvular heart disease, 1082–1089
  ventricular dysfunction and, 1093, 1093t
Cardiac tamponade, 1105–1106
Cardiogenic shock, 1638, 1639
CardioMed endotracheal ventilation catheter, 790
Cardiomyopathy of pregnancy, 1162–1163
Cardioplegia
  anterograde, 1093
  retrograde, 1093
Cardiopulmonary bypass (CPB), 1090–1093
  anticoagulation, 1091–1092
  brain monitoring during, 1095
  checklist before initiating, 1098t
  checklist before separation from, 1099t
  checklist during, 1098t
  circuits, 1090–1091, 1090f
  discontinuation of, 1099–1101, 1100f, 1100t
  heat exchanger, 1091
  intraoperative autologous hemodilution, 1092
  intraoperative management, 1097–1099, 1098t, 1099t
  monitoring and management during, 1097–1099
  myocardial protection, 1092–1093
  oxygenators, 1091
  postcardiopulmonary bypass, 1104
  prime, 1091
  pump, 1091
Cardiopulmonary pressures, calculation of, 747t
Cardiopulmonary resuscitation (CPR), 1662
  adult bradycardia (with pulse) algorithm, 1669f
  adult tachycardia (with pulse) algorithm, 1670f
  advanced life support, 1675–1676
  AHA ACLS circular algorithm, 1664f
  airway management, 1663–1664
  blood flow during, 1665, 1666
  bystander CPR and basic life support (BLS), 1675
  cardiac arrest and, 1662
  circulation, 1665–1668
  components of, 1663
  drug therapy, 1668–1672, 1669t
    amiodarone and lidocaine, 1671–1672
    catecholamines and vasopressors, 1670–1671
    routes of administration, 1668–1670
  electrical therapy, 1672–1674
  historical perspective, 1662
  pediatric, 1676–1678
  postcardiac arrest care algorithm, 1681f
  postresuscitation care, 1678–1681
  prognosis, 1681–1682
  rhythm analysis and defibrillation, 1676
  ventilation, 1664–1665
Cardiovascular aging, 902, 904
Cardiovascular anesthesia, 19–20
Cardiovascular disease, 590–596, 591f, 591t, 593t, 594f, 595f, 1662
  atherosclerotic, risk for, 592

cardiac testing, indications for, 592–593
cardiovascular implantable electronic devices, patients with, 596
coronary angiography in, 594-595
electrocardiogram for, 593
exercise tolerance, importance of, 592, 593t
noninvasive testing for, 593–594
patients with coronary artery stents, 595–596, 595f
perioperative coronary interventions, 595
surgical procedure, importance of, 592
ventricular and valvular function, assessment of, 594
Cardiovascular effects, inhalational anesthetics, 1225-1226
Cardiovascular implantable electronic devices (CIEDs), 596
Cardiovascular system
  during laparoscopy, 1264–1265, 1265t
    cardiac filling pressures and volumes, 1265
    changes in cardiac index, 1265
    disruption of esophageal hiatus during, 1265
    increased IAP, 1265
    mean arterial pressure, 1264, 1265
    systemic vascular resistance, 1264, 1265
  pediatric, 1221
  preoperative evaluation, 1031–1032
  prevention and treatment
    vasopressors, 935–936, 937f
    volume, 935
  subarachnoid, 935, 936f
Carlens tube, 1041, 1042f
Carotid artery stenting, 1134–1135
Carotid endarterectomy (CEA), 1122
  anesthetic considerations, 1124–1127
  neurophysiologic monitoring during, 1122–1124, 1123f
    carotid stump pressure, 1124
    electroencephalography, 1123–1124, 1123f
    motor evoked potentials, 1124
    nearinfrared spectroscopy, 1124
    somatosensory evoked potentials, 1124
    transcranial Doppler (TCD), 1124
  postoperative considerations, 1127
  preoperative evaluation and preparation, 1122
Carotid intima-media thickness (CIMT), 1114
Carotid surgery, 1020–1021
Carpal tunnel syndrome, 1287
Case discussion, 39–40
Cataract surgery, 1373–1374, 1374t
Catecholamines, 340, 340f
  during CPR, 1670–1671
  inactivation, 341–342, 341f
  peripheral SNS activity, 340–342
  pharmacology, 306–309, 307f, 308–309t
  regulation, 341
  synthesis of, 341, 341f
Catechol-O-methyltransferase (COMT), 342
Categorical binary data, 174
Categorical variables, 166
Cathelin, Fernand, 18
Catheter-related blood stream infections (CRBSI), 53
  in ICU, 1652–1653
Catheters
  for peripheral nerve blocks, 951–952
  pulmonary artery, 707, 717–718, 720, 721
    in cardiac output monitoring, 720–721
    oximetric, 720–721
Cathode ray oscilloscopes, 10
Cauda equina, 919
Caudal anesthesia, 1199
Caudal blocks, 855
  anesthesia for, 1249–1250
Caudal epidural block, 1199, 1199f

CCM. See Critical care medicine (CCM)
CDC. See Centers for Disease Control and Prevention (CDC)
CEA. See Carotid endarterectomy (CEA)
Cebranopadol, 507
Celecoxib (Celebrex), 1579
  dosing guidelines, 1578t
Celiac plexus block, 1618–1619, 1618f
Cell-mediated immunity, 205
Cell salvage, intraoperative, 1092
Center for Medicare and Medicaid Innovation, 28
Center for Medicare and Medicaid Services (CMS), 27–28, 48, 53, 842, 1543
Centers for Disease Control and Prevention (CDC), 71
Central anticholinergic syndrome, 356, 356t
Central chemoreceptors, 369
Central dogma of molecular biology, complexity of, 144, 144f
Central limit theorem, 172
Central line-associated blood stream infections (CLABSIs), 1634
Central nervous system (CNS), 74, 368
  aging, 901
  anesthetics and
    amnesia, 234
    autonomic control, 233–234
    immobility, 233
    unconsciousness, 234–235
  depressants, 1377
  diseases
    Alzheimer disease, 620
    amyotrophic lateral sclerosis, 621–622
    Creutzfeldt–Jakob disease, 622
    epilepsy, 619–620, 620t
    Huntington disease, 621
    multiple sclerosis, 619
    Parkinson disease, 620–621
  function, monitoring of, 1009–1011, 1010f
  infants
    cerebral blood flow, 1221
    neuroapoptosis, 1221
    NMDA and $GABA_A$ receptors antagonists, 1221
    oxygen consumption of brain, 1221
    physiology, 1221
  mechanisms of local anesthetics, 564–565
  structures, functionality of, 107t
  subarachnoid and epidural anesthesia
    differential nerve block, 935
    site of action, 934–935
  toxicity of, 575–576
  transfer of drugs across, 242
Central opioid analgesia, 508–509, 509f
Central/plasma compartment, 249
Central sensitization, 1611
Central venous cannulas, monitoring of
  contraindications, 719, 719t
  indications, 718–719
  principles of operation, 717–718, 717f
  problems and limitations, 719–720
  use and interpretation, 718, 718f
Central venous pressure (CVP), 717, 1641
  monitoring, thoracic surgery and, 1036
Centrifugal pumps (CPs), 1091
Cephalosporins, 609, 1238
Cerebellar infarction, 1638
Cerebral aneurysms, 886
  surgery, 1018–1019, 1018t, 1019t
Cerebral blood flow (CBF), 471, 471f
  in brain, 1007–1008
  and hypercapnia, 472
  and hypocapnia, 472
Cerebral cortex, 235, 334
Cerebral edema, 1303

Cerebral hyperperfusion syndrome (CHS), 1127
Cerebral ischemia, 1120
Cerebral metabolic rate, 471
   of oxygen consumption, 1007
Cerebral metabolism, 1012–1013
Cerebral microdialysis, 1013
Cerebral oximetry, 1013
Cerebral oxygenation, 1012–1013
Cerebral protection
   glucose and cerebral ischemia, 1014
   hypothermia, 1013–1014
   ischemic and reperfusion, 1013
   pharmacologic therapy for, 1014
   practical approach, 1014
Cerebral salt wasting, 1637
Cerebrospinal fluid (CSF), 17, 369, 918, 1005–1006, 1006f
Cerebrovascular resistance (CVR), 1007, 1008
Certified Registered Nurse Anesthetists (CRNA), 28
Cervical airway injuries, 1492–1493, 1493t
Cervical plexus, 954–955, 955f
   blocks, 966–967
      deep, 966
      superficial, 966–967, 966f
Cervical spine injuries, 1490
   airway management in, 1491–1492, 1491f
   causes of, 1490
   initial evaluation, 1490–1491
Cervical strap muscles, 362
Cesarean delivery
   advanced maternal age and, 1164
   anesthesia for, 1152
      general anesthesia, 1153–1154
      neuraxial anesthesia, 1152–1153
   indications for, 1152
C1 esterase inhibitor (C1-INH), 211
C fibers, 508, 569, 1608, 1608t
Chagas, 437
Chandy maneuver, 788
Channeled scopes, 786
CHD. See Congenital heart disease (CHD)
Cheater plug, 117, 117f
Checklists, ICU, 1634
Chelation therapy, 1701
Chemical, biologic, radiologic, nuclear, and explosive (CBRNE), 1688
Chemical dependence, 85
Chemical disaster, 1694–1696
Chemical injury, 942
Chemicals, occupational exposure from, 66
Chemokines, 205
Chemoreceptor trigger zone (CTZ), 523
Chen, MeiYu, 11
Chest injuries, 1505–1509
   blunt cardiac injury, 1506–1507, 1507f, 1509t
   chest wall injury, 1505
   diaphragmatic injury, 1509
   penetrating cardiac injury, 1506
   pericardial tamponade, 1506
   pleural injury, 1505–1506
   pulmonary contusion, 1506
   thoracic aortic injury, 1507–1509, 1508f, 1508t
Chest radiography, preoperative, 1031
Chest wall injury, 1505
Chickenpox, 74
Child–Pugh score, modified, 1316t
Children
   heart rates in, 1221t
   ideal body weight in, 1237
   obesity in, 1237–1238, 1238t
Chimney graft, 1136
Chi-square test, 174–175
Chlorhexidine, 185–186, 923
   in hand washing, 185–186

Chloroform à la reine, 5
Chloroform, and obstetrics, 4–5. See also Anesthesia
Chloroprocaine, 855t, 932–933, 934, 942, 1148, 1153, 1190–1191
Chlorpromazine, 17
Chlorpropamide, 404
Cholestatic diseases, 1307, 1314–1315
Choline, 302f, 303
Choline magnesium trisalicylate, 1578t
Cholinergic agonists, 302–303, 302f, 303t
Cholinergic drugs, 302. See also specific types
Cholinesterase disorders, 625, 625t
Cholinesterase inhibitors (anticholinesterases), 304, 304f
Choriocapillaris, 1374
Chronic hepatocellular disease, 1315
Chronic immune suppression, complications of, 1463t
Chronic kidney disease (CKD), 1410–1415
Chronic obstructive pulmonary disease (COPD), 362
Chronic opioid tolerance, 510–511
Chronic pain, 1598
Chronic pain management, lawsuits and, 105
Chronic regional pain syndrome (CRPS), 495
Churchill-Davidson, H., 16
Chvostek sign, 411, 1407
CIEDs. See Cardiac implantable electronic devices (CIEDs)
Cigarette smoking, 602
   effects on pulmonary function, 380, 597
   thoracic surgery and, 1030, 1034–1035
Cimetidine, 604
Cincinnati Individual Transfusion Trigger (CITT), 1496
Circle breathing system, 680–681
Circle of Willis, 714, 1005, 1005f, 1122, 1122f
Circulation, during cardiopulmonary resuscitation
   adequacy of, assessment of, 1668
   circulatory support, alternative methods of, 1667
      active compression-decompression CPR, 1667
      impedance threshold device, 1667
      interposed abdominal compression, 1667
      invasive techniques, 1667–1668
      mechanical chest compression devices, 1667
   closed-chest compression and, 1665
      blood flow during CPR, 1666
      cardiac pump mechanism, 1665
      gas transport during CPR, 1666
      technique of, 1666–1667
      thoracic pump mechanism, 1665–1666
Circumcision of newborns, 1435
Cirrhosis and portal hypertension, 1307–1314
   ascites, 1313–1314
   cardiac manifestations, 1308–1309
   hemostasis, 1307–1308
   hepatic encephalopathy, 1312–1313
   pulmonary complications, 1310–1311
   renal dysfunction in, 1309–1310
   varices, 1314
Cis-atracurium, 480, 535t, 537, 1230–1231
   dose ranges, effect of aging on, 903t
   in neonates, 1188
Citrate, 441
CJD. See Creutzfeldt-Jakob disease (CJD)
Clamp and sew technique, 1509
Clarke, William E., 3
Clarus Video System, 783, 783f
Classic laryngeal mask airway (cLMA), 1239
Clevidipine, 326f, 327
Clinical actionability, 149
Clinical Director of OR, 56

Clinical Genome Resource (ClinGen), 149
Clinical privileges, 33–35
   anticompetitive contracts and, 50
   blanket privileges, 35
   privilege renewals, 34
Clinical utility, 149
Clinical validity, 149
Clonidine, 315–316, 855t, 874, 1243, 1579–1580
Cloquet, Jules, 2
Closed-chest compression
   circulation during, 1665–1666
   technique of, 1666–1667
Closed-circuit anesthesia, 712
Clostridium botulinum (botulism), 1698–1699
Clostridium difficile, 74
   hand washing in prevention of, 184
Clot lysis index, 1308
Clover bag, 7
Clover, Joseph, 5, 7, 10, 769
Clubbing, preoperative evaluation, 1031
C-MAC system, 785, 785f
CME. See Continuing medical education (CME)
CMS. See Center for Medicare and Medicaid Services (CMS)
CMV. See Cytomegalovirus (CMV)
CNS. See Central nervous system (CNS)
Coagulation
   inhibitors, 425
   laboratory evaluation of, 425
Coagulopathy, in trauma patient, 1524–1525
Cocaine, 13, 17
   for awake intubation, 795
   history of use of, 13
   as local anesthetic, 17
   ophthalmic use, 1380
   during pregnancy, 1201
   in pregnancy, 1165–1166
Coccyx, description, 916
Cochrane Library, 179
Codeine, 14, 1232, 1412, 1570, 1570f, 1574
   pharmacokinetics, 1573t
Codesmith, Albert, 10
Coding, billing and, 47
Codman, Charles, 10
Coefficient of determination, 175
Cognitive dysfunction, 97
Cohen blocker, 1048f, 1049
Cold cardioplegia, 1093
Collagen deposition, wound healing, 194
Collins, Vincent, 11
Colloid osmotic pressure, 395
Colloids, 395–397
   versus crystalloid intravenous fluids, 396t
   infusions on intracranial pressure, 396
   and traumatic brain injury, 396
Color-flow Doppler (CFD), 743–744, 744f, 745f
Combined pharmacokinetic–pharmacodynamic model, 256
Combined spinal/epidural (CSE) analgesia
   for cesarean delivery, 1153
   drug dosing, 929, 929f
   for labor and vaginal delivery, 1151
   technique, 928–929, 929f
   trouble shooting, 929, 929f
Committee on Emergency Preparedness and Trauma (COTEP), 1688
Committee on Global Humanitarian Outreach (CGHO), 1688
Commotio cordis, 1507
Communication, in operating room management, 57
Comorbid injuries, 1023–1024
Compartmental models, pharmacokinetics
   one-compartment model, 250–251
   three-compartment model, 252–253, 252f
   two-compartment model, 251–252, 251f

Compartment syndrome, 816, 1511
  causes of, 816
  perioperative, 816
Competition
  antitrust considerations, 49–50
  exclusive service contracts and, 50–51
Competitive antagonists, 254
Complement, 207, 207f
  activation, 207, 210–211
  release of, 195
Complex regional pain syndrome (CRPS), 1617
Complex sleep apnea (CSA), 1572
Composite tissue transplantation, 1472–1473
Compound A, 481, 482f
  induced nephrotoxicity, 1227
Compound muscle action potentials (CMAPs), 1010
Compressed air injection technique (CAIT), 951, 952f
Compulsory random drug testing, 83
Computed tomography (CT), 887, 1301
  in abdominal trauma, 1509–1510, 1510t
Computer-assisted personalized sedation (CAPS) devices, 843
Computerized Provider Order Entry (CPOE) systems, 727
Conditioning pain modulation (CPM), 505, 509
Conduction anesthesia, 18
Conductive airways, 363
Conductors, 110
Condylar process, 1251
Confidence factor, 172
Confidence intervals (CIs), 172
Conflict, 69–70
Confusion Assessment Method for the ICU (CAM-ICU), 1650
Congenital diaphragmatic hernia (CDH), 1204
  anesthetic technique in, 1205
  clinical presentation, 1204, 1205, 1205f
  diagnosis of, 1204–1205
  embryology, 1204, 1204f
  incidence of, 1204
  perioperative care, 1205
  postoperative care, 1205–1206
  preoperative care, 1205, 1206f
Congenital erythropoietic porphyria (CEP), 624, 624t
Congenital heart disease (CHD)
  children with, anesthesia for, 1106–1108, 1106t
    anesthetic and intraoperative management, 1107
    cardiac evaluations, 1107
    laboratory evaluations, 1106–1107
    monitoring, 1107
    physical examination, 1106
    premedication, 1107
    tracheal extubation and postoperative ventilation, 1107–1108
Congenital muscular dystrophy (CMD), 614
Congenital myopathies, 612–614, 613t
Congenital rubella syndrome (CRS), 75
Congestive heart failure (CHF), 1476
Conivaptan, 402
Conjugation reactions, 245
Conjunctiva, 1375
Conjunctival edema, 820
Connective tissues diseases, 636
  adverse effects of drugs used to treat, 637t
  inflammatory myopathies (dermatomyositis/polymyositis), 639
  rheumatoid arthritis, 636–638
  systemic lupus erythematosus, 637t, 638
  systemic sclerosis (scleroderma), 639
Constant pressure variable orifice flowmeters, 662

Context-sensitive decrement times, 264–265, 265f
Context-sensitive half-time, 264, 264f, 511, 511f, 829–831, 829f, 830f
Continuing medical education (CME), 31
Continuous interval data, 166
Continuous peripheral nerve block (CPNB), 1585
Continuous positive airway pressure (CPAP), 365, 1572, 1643
  to nondependent lung, 1052–1053
Continuous quality improvement, 91
Continuous renal replacement therapy (CRRT), 1646
Continuous-wave (CW) Doppler echocardiography, 743
Contoured supine posture, 811, 811f
Contract law, 103
Control groups, 168–169
Conus elasticus, 768
Convection, 371
Convenience sampling, 168
Cook Airway Exchange Catheters, 790
Cook TTJV catheter, 803
Coping mechanisms, 81
Copper Kettle, 9, 10
Copy number variants (CNVs), 144, 144f
Cormack–Lehane laryngeal view scoring system, 781, 782f
Corneal abrasion, 97, 1393, 1554
Cornea transplantation, 1465
Corning, Leonard, 18
Coronary artery bypass grafting (CABG), 475, 592, 1078
Coronary artery disease (CAD), 587
  CABG surgery and, 1078–1082
    anesthetic, choice of, 1080
    coronary blood flow, 1078–1079
    hemodynamic goals, 1079, 1079t
    intravenous sedative hypnotics for, 1080
    ischemia, monitoring for, 1079–1080
    ischemia, treatment of, 1080–1082, 1081t
    myocardial oxygen demand, 1078
    myocardial oxygen supply, 1078, 1078f
    opioids for, 1080
    volatile anesthetics for, 1080
Coronary Artery Revascularization Prophylaxis (CARP) trial, 1118
Coronary blood supply, 280–281, 280f, 281f
Coronary physiology, 282–283
Coronary sinus sampling, 147
Coronary vascular reserve, 1078
Coronary vascular resistance, 282
Cor pulmonale, 1358, 1358f
Corssen, Guenter, 13
Cortical blindness, 1396
Corticosteroids, 1464
  anaphylactic reactions and, 213
  antiemetic effects of, 17
  in ARDS, 1645
  in TBI, 1636
Costotransverse joint, 959
Costovertebral articulations, 959
Costovertebral joint, 959
Cotton, Frederick, 8
Cough
  thoracic surgery and, 1030
  ventilation and, 368
Couvelaire uterus, 1160
COX-2 inhibitors, 875
CPAP. See Continuous positive airway pressure (CPAP)
CPB. See Cardiopulmonary bypass (CPB)
CPR. See Cardiopulmonary resuscitation (CPR)
CPT. See Current procedural terminology (CPT)
Cranium, 1004

Crawford needle, 923f
CRBSI. See Catheter-related blood stream infections (CRBSI)
C-reactive protein (CRP), 153
  high sensitivity CRP (hs-CRP), 153
Credentialing process, 33–35
  central, 33
  documentation for, 34–35
  economic provisions, 49
  need of, 33–34
  references, 34
Cremophor EL, 13
Creutzfeldt–Jakob disease (CJD), 80, 622
Cricoid cartilage, 769
Cricothyroid membrane (CTM), 768–769, 802
Cricothyroidotomy, 1664
Cricothyrotomy, 802
Cricotracheal ligament, 769
Crile, George W., 10
Critical care medicine (CCM), 1633. See also Intensive care unit (ICU)
  anesthesiologists and, 1633
  cardiovascular aspects, 1638–1642
  endocrine aspects, 1646–1647
  hemodynamic aspects, 1638–1642
  neurological and neurosurgical care, 1634–1638
Critical Care Societies Collaborative (CCSC), 1634
Critical incidents, 101
Critical temperature (CT), 658
CRNA. See Certified Registered Nurse Anesthetists (CRNA)
Cromolyn sodium, before thoracic surgery, 1035
Cross-sectional study, 167
Crouzon's disease, 1220
CRRT. See Continuous renal replacement therapy (CRRT)
CRS. See Congenital rubella syndrome (CRS)
Cryoprecipitate, 434, 435t, 1526
Cryptorchidism, 1435
Crystalloids, 395–397
  versus colloids, 396t
  infusions on intracranial pressure, 396
  for resuscitation, 1496, 1516
CSF. See Cerebrospinal fluid (CSF)
Curare, 14, 15
Curbelo, Martinez, 18
Current
  density, 112
  effect on cells, 110–111
  effect on humans, 112t
  electrical shock and, 111–112
  of light bulbs, 113f
  wattage and, 110
Current procedural terminology (CPT), 48
Current Researches in Anesthesia and Analgesia, 21
Cushing, Harvey, 10
Cushing's disease, 1237, 1336
Cutoff effects, 222
Cyanide toxicity, 1696
  in burned patients, 1514–1515
Cyanosis, preoperative evaluation, 1031
Cyclic adenosine monophosphate (cAMP), 213, 409
Cyclodextrins, 789
Cyclooxygenase (COX) enzymes, 1577, 1579
Cyclopentolate, ophthalmic use, 1380
Cyclopropane, 11, 15, 769
Cyclopropyl-methoxycarbonyl metomidate (CPMM), 502, 502f
Cyclosporine, in immunosuppressive therapy, 1464
Cylinder pressure regulator, 657
CYP2B6, 513
CYP2D6, 517

CYP450 enzyme systems, 1222, 1222f
    CYP450 2D6 enzyme, 1232
    CYP450 2E1 enzyme, 1226
Cystectomy surgery, 1422–1423
    diversion procedures, 1424
    ileal conduit, 1424
    intraoperative considerations, 1423
    partial, 1423
    postoperative considerations, 1423
    preoperative considerations, 1423
    radical, 1424
    simple, 1423
Cystoscopy, 1428
Cytochrome oxidase systems, 1375, 1375f
Cytochrome P450C9 (CYP2C9), 158
Cytochrome P450D6 (CYP2D6), 158
Cytochromes P450 (CYP), 245, 245t
Cytokines, 205, 206
Cytomegalovirus (CMV), 75, 428, 437
    congenital, 75
    primary, 75
Cytotoxic edema, brain, 1009
Cytotoxic reactions, 207–208, 208f

D

Dabigatran, 451
Daclizumab, in immunosuppressive therapy, 1464
Dacryocystorhinostomy, 1375
Dalton's law, 375, 462
Damage control resuscitation, 1496
Dantrolene, 1230, 1235
DAPT. See Dual antiplatelet therapy (DAPT)
Data
    structure, 166
    types, 166t
Datex-Ohmeda anesthesia
    machines, 656
    workstations, 653
Datex-Ohmeda S/5 ADU, 688–689, 688f
Datex-Ohmeda Tec 6 desflurane vaporizer, 668
Datex S5/ADU, 664f
Da Vinci Surgical System, 1264
Davis, Hamilton, 11
Davis, S. Griffith, 10
Davy, Humphry, 3
D-dimers, 425
Decamethonium, 16
Decastrello, A., 21
Decompressive craniectomy, in TBI, 1636
Decontamination, 1693
Deep-brain stimulators (DBS), 621
Deep cervical plexus block, 1592
Deep hypothermic circulatory arrest (DHCA), 1019
Deep peroneal nerve, 962
    blocks, 997–998, 997f
Defibrillation, 1672–1673
Deglutition, 368
Degrees of freedom, 171
Delayed hemolytic transfusion reactions (DHTRs), 439
Deliberate intervention, 167
Delirium, 13
Delta hepatitis, 75
De Motu Cordis, 12
Denervated heart, 350
Denis, Jean Baptiste, 21
Dental injury complaints, 97
Department of Health and Human Services (DHHS), 1689
Dependent variables, 166
Depositions, in malpractice lawsuits, 105
Depression, 84
    preoperative, 197

Dermatome, 919, 920f
Dermatomyositis (DM), 639
Descending pathways, neurobiology of, 1610
Descriptive statistics, 166–167
Desensitization, 254
Desflurane, 12, 460, 468, 471, 472, 481, 1222, 1288, 1306
    airway reflex, 1225
    airway resistance, 1225
    carbon dioxide production, rate of, 1227
    changes in blood pressure, 1226
    heart rate, effect on, 1226
    hepatic dysfunction, 1226-1227
    minimum alveolar concentration of, 1225
    in neonates, 1189
    oxygen consumption, 1226
    respiratory rate, 1225
    risk of nephrotoxicity, 1226
    washin of, 1224
Desipramine, 1621t
Desmopressin (DDAVP), 453, 1353
Dexamethasone, 855t, 875, 1009, 1016, 1249, 1253, 1254
Dexmedetomidine, 316, 496, 496f, 496t, 1233, 1243, 1286, 1287, 1412, 1580, 1580t, 1649
    for awake intubation, 794
    clinical uses, 497
    dose ranges, effect of aging on, 903t
    for monitored anesthetic care, 836
    in neonates, 1186–1187
    pharmacodynamics, 496, 497f
    pharmacokinetics, 496
    side effects, 497–498
    in TBI, 1636
Dextromethorphan, 1579
Dextrose, 392–393
Diabetes insipidus, 1353
Diabetes mellitus (DM), 592, 598–599, 1234, 1343
    anesthetic management
        intraoperative, 1347–1348
        preoperative, 1345–1347
    classification, 1343–1344
    diabetic ketoacidosis, 1351–1352, 1352t
    diagnosis of, 1344, 1345t
    end-organ complications of, 1346–1347
    glucose-lowering drugs, properties of, 1346t
    glucose-lowering regimen and preoperative counseling, 1347
    glycemic control
        in critically ill patients, 1350t
        perioperative, 1349, 1349f
        preoperative, 1347
    glycemic goals, 1349–1350
    hyperglycemia and, 1348, 1348f
        perioperative, management of, 1350–1351
    hyperosmolar nonketotic coma and, 1351
    hypoglycemia, 1352
    perioperative outcomes, 1348, 1348f
    physiology, 1344
    in pregnancy, 1163
    treatment of, 1344–1345
    type 1, 1351
    type 2, 1351
Diabetic ketoacidosis (DKA), 1163, 1347, 1351–1352, 1352t
Diabetic neuropathy, 358
Diabetic painful neuropathy, 1617
Diagnosis codes, and billing, 48
Diameter indexing, 11
Diameter Index Safety System (DISS), 657, 659f
Diaphragmatic injury, 1509
Diarrheal disease, 74
Diastolic dysfunction, 1308

Diastolic function, determinants of, 293–298, 293t
    atrial function, 297–298
    LV filling and compliance, invasive assessment of, 294–295
    LV relaxation, invasive assessment of, 294
    noninvasive analysis, 295–296, 296f
    pericardium, 296–297
Diastolic heart failure, 293–294
Diazepam, 606–607, 855t
Dichotomous data, 166
Diclofenac, 1232
    dosing guidelines, 1578t
Diencephalon, 1004
Die perorale Intubation, 5
Diethyl ether, 3
Differential block, 935
    nerves, 568
Difficult airway algorithm, 791–797
    Airway Approach Algorithm, 792–793
    ASA Difficult Airway Algorithm (ASA-DAA), 791–796, 791f, 1742f
    awake airway management, 794–796
    clinical scenarios and, 796–797
    invasive airway, 793–794
    regional anesthesia in, 792, 793t
    Vortex approach, 793, 793f, 793t
Diffusing capacity for carbon monoxide, 1033–1034
Diffusion, 371
    hypoxia, 459, 468
Diflunisal, dosing guidelines, 1578t
Digitalis glycosides, 323
Digitalis purpurea, 323
Diisopropylphenol, 1227–1228
2,6-diisopropylphenol. See Propofol
Dilaudid. See Hydromorphone
Diltiazem, 326t, 327–328
Dilute Russell viper venom time (DRVVT), 427
Dimer, 1392
Dimethyl fumarate, 619
Dinoprostone, 1160t
Dioscorides, 2
Dipeptidyl-peptidase-4 inhibitors, 1345
Diphenhydramine, 607
Dipivefrin, 1380
Diprivan, 1245
Direct current (DC)
    description of, 110
    electrical shock hazards, 111, 111f
Direct gating, 228
Direct laryngoscopy, 778–780
Direct thrombin inhibitors (DTIs), 425, 426
Disability, in anesthesiologists, 84
Disaster Medical Assistance Team (DMAT), 1689
Disaster Mortuary Team (DMORT), 1690
Disasters and mass casualty events, 1687–1689
    anesthesiologist in, role of, 1691–1694
        decontamination, 1693
        emergency department, 1693
        operating room management, 1693–1694, 1694t
        triage, 1692–1693
    biologic, 1696–1699
        anthrax, 1697–1698
        botulism, 1698–1699
        hemorrhagic fevers, 1699
        plague, 1698
        smallpox, 1696–1697
        tularemia, 1698
    chemical
        blood agents, 1696
        nerve agents, 1694–1695
        pulmonary agents, 1695–1696
    definitions related to, 1687
    explosives, 1702

Disasters and mass casualty events (*continued*)
  preparation for
    family plan, 1689, 1703
    government plan, 1689–1690
    health-care agency plans, 1690–1691
  radiation, 1699–1702
  types of disasters, 1688
Disciplinary action, 83
Discounted fee-for-service arrangements, 51
Discovery phase, in malpractice lawsuits, 106
Discrete interval data, 166
Disseminated intravascular coagulation (DIC), 425, 447–449, 1300, 1308
  common disorders associated with, 448t
  scoring algorithm for diagnosis of, 449t
Distal (collecting duct) acting diuretics, 1415
Distal convoluted tubule diuretics, 1415
Distraction techniques, 1242
  preschool-age children, 1242
  younger children, 1242
Diuretics
  distal (collecting duct) acting, 1415
  distal convoluted tubule, 1415
  loop, 1415
  mechanisms of action, 1413–1415, 1414f
  osmotic, 1414
  proximal tubule, 1414
DNA viruses, 74–75
Dobutamine, 308–309t, 312–313
Dobutamine stress echocardiogram (DSE), 593–594
Documentation
  anesthesia equipment, 41
  for credentialing process, 33
  meetings and case discussion, 39
  pay for performance and, 53
  policy and procedure, 39
Dogliotti, Achille M., 19
Domino, Edward, 13
Donation after cardiac death (DCD), 1459, 1460–1461, 1461t
Donor nephrectomy, 1419–1420
DonorNet, 1458
Do not resuscitate (DNR) orders, 1662–1663, 1739-1740
Dopamine, 308–309t, 312, 340, 343, 1415
Dopaminergic agonists, 1415
Dopaminergic (DA) receptor, 343, 347
  in central nervous system, 348
  in kidney and mesentery, 348
  in myocardium, 347
  in peripheral vessels, 347–348
δ-Opioid receptor (DOR), 507–508
Doppler echocardiography, 742–744, 743f
  color-flow, 743–744
  continuous-wave, 743, 744f–745f
  mitral regurgitation, 745f
  pulsed-wave, 743, 744f
  spectral, 743
Doppler effect, 742
Doppler equation, 742–743
Doppler flow detection device, 714
Doppler shift, 1011
Dorrance, George, 6
Dorsal column tracts, 1610
Dorsal respiratory group (DRG), 367
Dorsal root ganglion (DRG), 1609
  stimulation, 1626
Dorsolateral pontine tegmentum (DLPT), 1610
Double burst stimulation (DBS), 542f, 543t, 544
Double insulation, 122
Double-lumen endobronchial tubes, 1041–1045
  checking for proper position of, 1043, 1044f
  malposition of, 1043–1045, 1045f
  placement of, 1043
  Robertshaw-design, 1041–1042, 1042f
  rubber–silicone left-sided, 1042–1043

Double-lung transplantation, 1475
Doughty technique, epidural anesthesia, 927, 928f
Downregulation of receptors, 254
Down syndrome, 589, 1220, 1253
Doxacurium, 535t, 537, 1412
Doxepin, 1621t
Draeger, Heinrich, 8
Dräger Apollo workstation, 665f
Dräger Fabius GS ventilator, 684f
Dräger Medical Narkomed 6000 Series, 689–690, 690f
Dräger Oxygen Ratio Monitor Controller/ Sensitive Oxygen Ratio Controller, 666–667, 666f
Droperidol, 14, 17, 855t
Drosophila, 231
Drug abuse, 82, 85
Drug Enforcement Administration (DEA) certificate, 868
Drug-induced hyperkalemia, 407
Drug-induced liver injury (DILI), 1305–1306
  clinical chemistry criteria for, 1305t
Drug-induced sleep endoscopy (DISE), 1360
Drug interactions, 258
  absorption of drug and, 259
  drug distribution and, 259
  drug metabolism and, 259–260, 260t
  pharmaceutical, 258–259
  pharmacodynamic, 260
  pharmacokinetic, 259–260
  response surface models of, 270–271, 270f, 271f, 272t
  in vitro interactions, 258
  in vivo interactions, 258–259
Drug patches, 243
Drugs, anesthetic, 242. *See also* Pharmacodynamics; Pharmacokinetics
  bioavailability, 243
  biotransformation reactions, 244
  closed-loop infusions, 269–270
  cytochromes P450 enzymes, 245, 245t
  distribution, 244
  drug metabolism, variations in, 245–246
  elimination clearance, 244
  first-pass metabolism, 243
  hepatic drug clearance, 246–248, 247f, 248t
  hydrophilic, 242
  inhalational administration, 244
  intramuscular and subcutaneous administration, 243
  intrathecal, epidural, and perineural injection, 243–244
  intravenous administration, 243
  lipophilic, 243
  oral administration, 243
  phase I reactions, 244–245
  phase II reactions, 245
  redistribution, 244
  renal drug clearance, 246, 246t
  soft, 266
  therapeutic index, 243
  transcutaneous administration, 243
  transfer across membranes, 242–243
Dry sounds (wheezes), 1031
Dryvax, 1697
D-tubocurarine, 16
Dual antiplatelet therapy (DAPT), 1116, 1117
Duchenne muscular dystrophy (DMD), 613, 1236, 1445
Duloxetine, 359, 1616, 1621t
  for chronic pain, 1622t
Dupotet, Charles, 2
Dura mater, 917, 917f, 918f
Duty
  breach of, 103
  owed to patients, 103

D-vapor for desflurane vaporizers, 673–676, 674f, 675t, 676f
  dial setting *versus* flow through restrictor R2, 675t
  fresh gas flow rate *versus* working pressure, 675t
  operating principles of, 674–675, 674f
  output, 675–676, 675t
  safety features, 676
  variable bypass vaporizers and, 673–674
Dynamic Gas Scavenging System (DGSS), 694f, 695
Dynamic genomics, 145–146
Dynorphin A, 508
Dysfibrinogenemia, 1307
Dysphoria, preoperative assessments, 197
Dyspnea, thoracic surgery and, 1030
Dysrhythmias, 719
  thoracic surgery and, 1036
Dystrophin protein complex, 1236

E

ε-Aminocaproic acid (EACA), 1470, 1526
Ears
  mastoid, 1363–1364
  middle ear, 1363–1364
  myringotomy, 1363
  surgery, 1363–1364, 1364f
  tube insertion, 1363
Eastern Association for the Surgery of Trauma (EAST), 1530f, 1531
Eaton–Lambert syndrome. *See* Myasthenic syndrome
Ebola
  precautions, 73t
  viruses, 1699
EBV. *See* Epstein-Barr virus (EBV)
Ecallantide, 211
Ecarin, 427
Ecarin clotting time (ECT), 425, 426
Echocardiography, 731–764
  and aorta, diseases of, 757–759
  beam shape in, 733, 733f
  B-mode, 733–734
  and cardiac masses, 759–760
  and congenital heart disease, 760, 760f
  Doppler, 742–744, 743f
    color-flow, 743–744
    continuous-wave, 743, 744f–745f
    pulsed-wave, 743, 744f
    spectral, 743
  epiaortic, 761
  epicardial, 761
  focused transthoracic cardiac ultrasound, 762–764
  hemodynamic assessments and, 744–746
    pressure assessment, 745–746, 746f
    valve area, 745, 746f
    volumetric flow assessments, 744–745, 745f
  left ventricular diastolic function, evaluation of, 750–753
  M-mode, 734, 734f
  outside operating room, 761-762
  principles and technology of
    image display, 733–734, 734f
    instrumentation, 733, 733f
    physics of sound, 732, 732f
    signal processing, 733
    sound transmission in tissue, properties of, 732–733
    spatial *versus* dynamic image quality, 734–735
  procedures, 760–761
  resolution of, 733
  systolic function, evaluation of, 746–750

Index 1761

three-dimensional, 741–742, 742f
transducers in, 733
transesophageal examination, 735–742
   contraindication to probe placement, 735
   orientation, 735–736, 736f
   probe insertion, 735
   probe manipulation, 735
   safety, 735
   three-dimensional, 741–742
   two-dimensional, 736–741
   two-dimensional, 734, 734f, 736–741, 737f–741f
ultrasound-guided central vein cannulation in, 760–761, 761f
valvular heart disease, evaluation of, 753–757, 757t
Echothiophate, 304, 354, 1380
Eclampsia, 1156–1159. See also Hypertensive disorders of pregnancy
Economic credentialing, 50
ECT. See Electroconvulsive therapy (ECT)
E-cylinders, 657–658, 658f, 659f
Edema, from fluid replacement therapy, 1515
Edoxaban, 451
Edrophonium, 304f, 550–551, 554
  dose ranges, effect of aging on, 903t
  in neonates, 1188
Edwards, Waldo, 18
Effector cells, 206
Efficacy, drug, 255
Egg allergy, 1238
Egg lecithin, 1245
EHR. See Electronic health records (EHR)
Eihorn, Alfred, 13
Einthoven, Willem, 10
Eisenmenger syndrome, 1162
Eisleb, Otto, 14
Ejection fraction, 293
E & J Resuscitator, 8
Ekenstam, B., 14
ELA-Max, 1244
Elam, James, 9
Elastic work (W_{el}), 365, 365f
  lung, 364–365
Elbow surgery, 1448–1449
Elective surgery, 1248
Electrical cables, 114f
Electrical outlets
  grounded, 115f, 117f
  hospital-grade, 124, 124f
  ungrounded, 118f–119f
Electrical power
  grounded, 113–117
  ungrounded, 117–120
Electrical shocks
  alternating current and, 111
  direct current and, 111
  sources of, 111–112, 112f, 112t
Electrical therapy, during CPR, 1672–1674
  adverse effects and energy requirements, 1673–1674
  defibrillators, 1673
  electrical pattern and ventricular fibrillation duration, 1672–1673
  transthoracic impedance, 1673
Electricity, principles of, 109–110
Electrocardiograms (ECGs)
  atrial fibrillation, 1711
  atrial flutter, 1711
  atrial pacing, 1722
  atrioventricular block (complete heart block), 1712
  atrioventricular block (first degree), 1711
  atrioventricular block (Mobitz type I/ Wenckebach block), 1711
  atrioventricular block (Mobitz type II), 1712

atrioventricular block (second degree), 1711
bundle-branch block, left (LBBB), 1712
bundle-branch block, right (RBBB), 1712
DDD pacing, 1723
digitalis effect, 1718
hypercalcemia, 1719
hyperkalemia, 1719
hypocalcemia, 1719
hypokalemia, 1719
hypothermia, 1719
multifocal atrial tachycardia, 1719
myocardial ischemia, 1718
normal, 1711
paroxysmal atrial tachycardia, 1719
pericardial tamponade, 1720
pericarditis, 1719
pneumothorax, 1720
premature atrial contraction, 1720
premature ventricular contraction, 1720
preoperative, 1031
pulmonary embolus, 1720
sinus arrest, 1721
sinus arrhythmia, 1721
sinus bradycardia, 1721
sinus tachycardia, 1721
subarachnoid hemorrhage, 1721
subendocardial myocardial infarction, 1718
torsades de pointes, 1721–1722
transmural myocardial infarction, 1713–1717
ventricular fibrillation, 1722
ventricular pacing, 1723
ventricular tachycardia, 1722
Wolff-Parkinson-White syndrome, 1722
Electrocardiography, 10–11, 1709. See also Anesthesia; Electrocardiograms (ECGs)
Electrocautery, 125, 709
Electroconvulsive therapy (ECT), 15, 893
Electroencephalography (EEG), 471
  for carotid surgery, 1123
  signals, monitoring of
    contraindications, 726–727
    indications, 725–726
    principles of operation, 724–725
    problems and limitations, 727
    use and interpretation, 725, 726f
Electrolyte disorders
  of calcium balance, 1406–1407
  of magnesium balance, 1406–1407
  of phosphorus balance, 1406–1407
  of potassium balance, 1406
  of sodium balance, 1406
Electrolytes
  calcium, 409–412
  magnesium, 414–415
  phosphate, 412–414
  potassium, 404–409
  regulation of total body, 398t
  sodium, 398–404
Electromagnetic interference (EMI), 128–129
Electromyography (EMG), 547, 1009, 1010, 1011
Electronic fetal monitor, 1166
Electronic flowmeter, 664–665, 664f, 665f
Electronic health records (EHR), 31, 99
Electronic medical records (EMR), 54–55
Electrosurgery, 125–127, 125f, 126f
Electrosurgical unit (ESU), 126–128, 126f, 134–135
  bipolar, 126
  unipolar, 126
Elimination clearance, 244, 249, 252
Elimination half-life, 249–250
Elliotson, John, 2
Elliptocytosis, 633–634
Emergence agitation, 1253
Emergency medical systems (EMSs), 1662
Emery-Dreifuss muscular dystrophy, 613, 1236

Employee Retirement Income Security Act, 84
Empyema, 1062
  anesthesia for, 1062–1063
EMR. See Electronic medical records (EMR)
Encyclopedia of DNA Elements (ENCODE), 148
End-diastolic pressure–volume relationship (EDPVR), 288
Endocarditis prophylaxis, 1237
  antibiotic regimen for, 1237
  SBE prophylaxis, 1237t
Endocrine disease, 598–600, 599t
  adrenal disorders, 599–600
  diabetes mellitus, 598–599
  thyroid and parathyroid diseases, 599, 599t
End-of-life care, in ICU, 1655
Endogenous calcium antagonist, 414
Endogenous opioid system, 507–508
Endoleak, 1137
  types of, 1137, 1138f
Endoneurium, 564
Endoplasmic reticulum protein (ERp58), 67
Endorphins, 1354
Endoscopic retrograde cholangiopancreatography (ERCP), 889–890, 1301
Endothelin, 283
Endotracheal tube (ETT), 20, 1125
Endovascular aortic repair, 1135–1138
  anesthetic management, 1136–1137
  complications, 1137–1138
  EVAR risk assessment model, 1135–1136
  evolution of, 1136
Endovascular surgery, 1134
  carotid artery stenting, 1134–1135
  endovascular aortic repair, 1135–1138
  peripheral artery disease and, 1138–1139
End-plate potential (EPP), 529
End-stage liver disease (ESLD), 1467
  multisystem complications of, 1467t
End-stage renal disease (ESRD), 1410
  prevalence of, 1465
End-systolic pressure–volume relation (ESPVR), 288
End-tidal CO_2 ($ETCO_2$), 711–712, 711f, 712t
End-tidal $PaCO_2$ ($PETCO_2$) determination, 374
Enflurane, 12, 460f, 1223, 1306
  carbon dioxide, rate of production of, 1227
Enhanced recovery after surgery (ERAS), 30, 398, 1539
Enk flow modulator, 803, 803f
Enteral nutrition (EN), 1648
Enteric infections, 74
Enterobacter cloacae, 437
Enterococcus spp., vancomycin-resistant, 187
Enumeration data. See Categorical binary data
Enzyme immunoassays (EIAs), 427
Enzyme-linked immunosorbent assay (ELISA), 215
Enzyme systems, maturity in children, 1222
Eosinophilic chemotactic factor of anaphylaxis (ECF-A), 209–210
Eosinophils, 206
Ephedrine, 314, 855t, 935
Epiaortic echocardiography, 761
Epicardial echocardiography, 761
Epicritic pain, 1608
Epidemiology, 175–176
Epidermal growth factor (EGF) release, 192
Epidermolysis bullosa, 639–641, 640f
Epidural abscesses, prevention of, 189
Epidural analgesia, in labor and vaginal delivery, 1150–1151
Epidural anesthesia, 854, 914–942, 1250. See also specific anesthetic agents
  anatomy, 915
    cerebrospinal fluid, 918
    epidural space, 916–917, 917f

Epidural anesthesia (continued)
  ligaments, 916, 916f
  meninges, 917–918, 917f, 918f, 919f
  spinal cord, 919, 920f
  spine, ultrasound of, 919, 920f, 921f
  vertebrae, 915–916, 916f
 approach, 923–924, 924f
 cardiovascular physiology, 935–936, 937f
 central nervous system physiology, 934–935
 combined, 928–929
 complications, 937–942
  backache, 937
  chemical injury, 942
  headache, 938–939
  hearing loss, 939
  high block/total subarachnoid spinal block, 939
  hypoperfusion, 941
  mass lesions, 940–941, 940f, 941f
  needle trauma, 939–940, 939f, 940f
  neurologic injury, 939–942, 940f, 941f
  spinal stenosis, 941–942
  systemic toxicity, 939
 continuous, 926–928
 contraindications, 915
 efficiency and, 930
 gastrointestinal system physiology, 936
 indications, 915
 needles, 923, 923f, 924f
 neuraxial anesthesia and outcome, 915
 patient preparation
  equipment, 922, 922t
  positioning, 922–923, 922f, 923f
  skin preparation, 923
 pharmacology
  adjuvants, 933
  onset and duration, 932–933, 933t
  recommendations, 932t
  spread of block, 932, 932f
  test doses, 933–934, 934f
 physiology, 934–937
 respiratory system physiology, 936
 subarachnoid anesthesia and, 919–920, 919f, 920f
 technique, 922–930, 924f, 925f, 926f
  air versus saline, 926–927
  choice of, 929–930
  Doughty, 927, 928f
  epidural catheter, 927–928
  intermittent versus continuous, 927, 927f
 temperature homeostasis, 937
Epidural blood patch, 938–939
Epidural neuraxial analgesia, 1602
Epidural space
 compartments of, 917f
 description, 916–917
Epidural steroid injections (ESIs)
 complications, 1612
 efficacy of, 1612
 for low back pain, 1611–1612
 safety of, 1614
 steroids for, 1612
 transforaminal, 1612, 1612f
Epigenetics, 147
Epigenome-wide association studies (EWAS), 147
Epiglottitis, 1366
Epilepsy surgery, 1021
Epinephrine, 308–309t, 309–311, 314, 421, 570, 570t, 855t, 931, 933, 1247, 1250, 1253
 during anaphylactic shock, 213
 during CPR, 1670–1671
 ophthalmic use, 1380
 test dose, in obstetrics, 1152
Epineurium, 564, 565f
Episcleral membrane. See Tenon capsule
Epithelialization, wound healing, 194

Epsilon-aminocaproic acid (EACA), 424
Epstein–Barr virus (EBV), 71
Eptifibatide, 450
Equipment
 classic laryngeal mask airway, 1239
 failure, 40
 of independent anesthesiologists, 61
 for infants and children, 1239–1240
 maintenance of, 40–42
 Microcuff tube, 1240
 service, 41
ERAS. See Enhanced recovery after surgery (ERAS)
Ergonomics, 69–70
Ergot alkaloids (Methergine), 1160t
ERp58. See Endoplasmic reticulum protein (ERp58)
Errors, in hypothesis testing, 170, 170t
Erythromycin, 1347
Erythropoietic protoporphyria (EPP), 624, 624t
Erythropoietin, 428, 443
Escherichia coli, 437
Eschmann introducer, 801–802
Esmolol, for ischemia, 1081
Esophageal tracheal Combitube, 801, 802f
Esophageal tubes with laryngeal openings, 801
Esophagogastroduodenoscopy, 1314
Ethanol, in hand washing, 184. See also Alcohol
Ether anesthesia, 3–4, 4f
The ether controversy, 4
Ethyl chloride, 11
Ethylene, 11
Ethylenediaminetetraacetic acid (EDTA), 489, 1245
Ethyl vinyl ether, 12
Ethyl violet, 682
Etidocaine, 14
Etodolac, dosing guidelines, 1578t
Etomidate, 13, 14, 492–493, 492f, 492t, 906, 1245, 1412
 clearance and volume of distribution, 1228
 clinical uses, 493
 dose of, 1228
 dose ranges, effect of aging on, 903t
 half-life of, 1228
 pharmacodynamics, 493
 pharmacokinetics, 492, 493t
 side effects, 493
Eucapnic ventilation, 369
Euglobulin clot lysis time (ECLT), 1308
Eupnea, 367t
European Carotid Surgery Trial (ECST), 1122
European Economic Union, 41
European Society of Anaesthesiology (ESA), 431
European Society of Cardiology (ESC), 603
Eutectic mixture of local anesthetics (EMLA), 1191, 1244
Excimer laser, 1392
Exclusive service contracts, 50–51
Exercise oximetry, 1033
Exercise tolerance, thoracic surgery and, 1031
Exogenous opioids, classification of, 511
Experimental constraints, 168
Expert witnesses, 104
Expiratory chin drop, 774
Expiratory reserve volume, 376
Expiratory ventilatory assistance, 803
Expired gases, monitoring of
 contraindications, 712
 indications, 712
 principles of operation, 710–711, 710f
 problems and limitations, 712–713
 use and interpretation, 711–712, 711f, 711t, 712f
Explanatory variables, 166
Explosive devices, use of, by terrorists, 1702
Extended criteria donors (ECDs), 1458
External ventricular drains (EVDs), 1012
Extracellular fluid (ECF), 1183–1184

Extracellular matrix deposition, wound healing, 194
Extracellular volume (ECV), 386, 390
 regulation of, 390–391, 392f
Extracorporeal CPR (ECPR), 1667–1668
Extracorporeal membrane oxygenation (ECMO), 1103, 1476, 1480
 in ARDS, 1645
Extremity injuries, 1511
Eye injuries, 97
Eyelids, 1375
 akinesia of, 1385
EZ blocker, 1048f, 1049

F

FABER Patrick test, 1615
Fabius GS workstations, 689–690, 690f
Facemask ventilation, 773–775, 774f
Face rests, 820
Facet syndrome, 1614, 1614f
Facilitated diffusion, 242
Facioscapulohumeral muscular dystrophy, 614
Factor V Leiden (FVL), 153, 426
Failed back surgery syndrome (FBSS), 1624
Fail-safe valve, 656
Fair Labor Standards Act, 84
Family plan, for disaster management, 1689, 1703
Famotidine, 604, 787
Fanconi–Bickel syndrome, 629
Farmer's Lung, 1696
Fascia iliaca block, 988–989, 989f, 1590, 1590f, 1591f
Fast-twitch muscle fibers, 362
Fat embolus syndrome (FES), 1453–1454, 1454t
Fatigue, 70–71
Faulconer, Albert, 11
FDA. See Food and Drug Administration (FDA)
Febrile nonhemolytic transfusion reactions (FNHTRs), 429, 437–438
Federal Emergency Management Agency (FEMA), 1689, 1690t
Federal laws, 83
Federal Tax Relief and Healthcare Act, 53
Federal Trade Commission, 50
Federation Credentials Verification Service, 34
Federation of State Medical Boards, 34
Fell, George, 5
Fell–O'Dwyer apparatus, 5
Femoral arterial thermodilution (FATD), 721
Femoral nerve, 961–962, 962f
 block, 988–989, 989f, 1450, 1452, 1589–1590, 1590f
 catheters, 856
Fenoldopam, 313–314, 1415
Fentanyl, 14, 511–512, 511f, 512, 607–608, 855t, 874, 931, 1231, 1248, 1250, 1288, 1412, 1574
 context-sensitive plasma half-time for, 264f
 dose ranges, effect of aging on, 903t
 in neonates, 1187
 for pain relief, 515–516, 515f, 1574
 patient–controlled regimens, 1582t
 pharmacokinetics, 1573t
Fetal asphyxia, 1169
Fetal heart rate (FHR)
 acceleration of, 1166
 baseline, 1166
 decelerations, 1166–1167, 1167f
 monitoring, 1166–1167, 1167f
 three-tiered system for evaluation of, 1167, 1168f
 variable decelerations, 1167
Fetal monitoring, 1166–1168
 electronic, 1166–1167, 1167f
 pulse oximetry, 1168
 scalp pH testing, 1168

Fetus, drug transfer to, 1147–1148
Fiberoptic laryngoscopy, 1196
Fibrinogen, 1526
   concentrates, 435
   replacement, indications for, 435t
Fibrinolysis, 423–424, 424f
   inhibition of, 423–424
Fibroblasts
   differentiation of, 194
   in wound healing, 194
Fibromyalgia, 1616
   definition, 1616
   management of, 1616
Fick equation, 464
Fick principle, 1147
Filum terminale, 917
Fingernails, hand hygiene and, 187
Fire, in operating room
   drills, 135
   ignition sources, 131–132, 132t
   prevention and management of, 130t
   safety, 130–137, 135f–137f
   triangle, 131f
   types of, 131
Fisher Grade System, 1018, 1019t
Fisher's exact test, 174
Flail chest, 1493–1494
Flasher, 8
Flexible fiberoptic bronchoscope, 7
Flexible scope-aided intubation, 797–800, 798f
   contraindications to, 797, 798t
   elements of, 798–799
   failure of, reasons for, 798t
   hang-up, 799
   indication for, 797
   intubating oral airways, 799–800, 800f
   use of, 799–800, 799f, 800t
FloTrac, 721, 723, 1642
Flow control valve assemblies, 661f, 662
Flow cytometry, 146
Flowmeters, 9
   bubble, 9
   electronic, 664–665, 664f, 665f
   problems with
      ambiguous scale, 663–664
      inaccuracy, 663
      leaks, 663, 663f
   scale, 663
   sequence, 663f
   subassembly, 661f, 662–663
      flow tubes, 662
      indicator floats and float stops, 662–663
      safety features of, 663
      scale, 663
Flow-over, vaporization, 670
Flow tubes, 662
Flow–volume loops, 378, 378f, 1032, 1033f
Fluid creep, 1515
Fluid dehydration, 1248
Fluid management, 1288
   assessment, 397–398
   blood transfusion therapy, 1248–1249
   colloids, crystalloids, and hypertonic solutions, 395–397
   elective surgery, 1248
   fluid replacement therapy, 391–393
   general principles, 1248
   monitoring, 397–398
   for pain management, 1249–1250
      caudal blockade, 1249–1250
      epidural block, 1250
      spinal block, 1250
   physiology, 390–391
   prophylaxis for postoperative vomiting, 1249
   for regional anesthesia, 1249–1250
   surgical fluid requirements, 393–395

Fluid replacement therapy
   dextrose, 392–393
   water, sodium, and potassium: maintenance requirements for, 391–392, 393t
Fluid resuscitation
   in burned patient, 1515–1516, 1515t
   in hemorrhagic shock, 1496–1497, 1496t
Flumazenil, 860, 1556
Fluorine, 12
Fluoromethyl-2,2-difluoro-1-(trifluoromethyl) vinyl ether, 1227
Fluotec, 10
Fluoxetine, 1621t
Fluroxene, 12
Focused abdominal sonography for trauma (FAST), 1510
Focused transthoracic cardiac ultrasound (FoCUS), 762–764, 762f
   exam views, 762, 763f–764f
   transthoracic echo, 763, 763t
FOCUS trial, 1117
Food and Drug Administration (FDA), 37, 648
   Medical Device Problem Reporting system, 41
Foot drop, 824
Foot, surgery to, 1452
Forbes/Cori disease, 626, 629
Forced duction test (FDT), 1378–1379
Forced expiratory flow, 377
Forced expiratory volume (FEV), 377
   in one second (FEV_1), 366, 936
Forced expired volume in 1 second (FEV_1), 1032
Forced vital capacity (FVC), 377, 602, 936, 1032
Foregger, Richard von, 8
Foreign body
   airway obstruction, 1663–1664
   aspiration, 1366–1367, 1367f
Forest plot, 179, 180f
Fortuitous, 11
Fospropofol, 502
   for monitored anesthetic care, 832
Fournier gangrene, 1436
Fractional area change (FAC), 293, 748f, 750
Frailty, concept of, 899
Frame rate, 734–735
Francisella tularensis (tularemia), 1698
Frank–Starling effect, 286
F ratios, 173
Frazier, Charles, 20
Freiberg sign, piriformis syndrome, 1616
Freon, 12
Fresh frozen plasma (FFP), 428, 1526
Fresh gas flow (FGF), 462, 656
Freud, Sigmund, 13, 17, 82
Frova Intubating Introducer, 802
Full prone position, 819–820, 820f
Full stomach
   induction, 1241–1242
   trauma, 1489–1490
Functional Airway Assessment (FAA), 779
Functional airway divisions, 363t
Functional endoscopic sinus surgery (FESS), 1368
Functional residual capacity (FRC), 362, 365, 376, 464, 1181, 1266
   measurement, 376–377
   on obesity, 1279, 1280f
Fungal infections, in ICU, 1653
FVL. See Factor V Leiden (FVL)

G

GABA-activated ion channels, 228–229
Gabapentin (Neurontin), 1580–1582, 1581f, 1599, 1616
   in chronic pain, 1622t
   dosage range, 1621t

   in neuropathic pain, 1621
   side effects, 1621
Gabapentinoids, 1580–1582
Gaenslen test, 1615
Gallamine, 16
Galvanic cell analyzers, 708
Gamma-hydroxybutyrate, 1616
Ganglion impar block, 1619
Gantry-style lifting device, 1289
Gas diffusion, 371. See also Oxygen
Gases
   in mixtures, 462
   in solution, 462
GASnet, 33
Gas trapping, 376
Gastric acidity, reduction of, 787
Gastric contents, control of, 786, 787t
Gastrointestinal endoscopy, 872
Gastrointestinal system, 936
Gastroschisis, 1206–1207, 1207f
   antenatal diagnosis of, 1207
   perioperative care, 1207–1208, 1208f
   postoperative care, 1208
   preoperative care, 1207
Gauge pressure, 656
Gauss, Carl, 20
GE Aisys Carestation, 664–665
GE-Datex-Ohmeda, 665
   Aladin cassette vaporizers, 668, 676–678, 677f, 678f
   Excel machines, 667
   Link-25 Proportion-Limiting Control System, 665–667, 666f
General anesthesia, 220, 1734
   for carotid endarterectomy, 1125
   for cesarean delivery, 1153–1154
   for preeclamptic patients, 1159
   for vaginal delivery, 1152
General Anesthesia *versus* Local Anesthesia for carotid surgery (GALA) trial, 1125
General damages, defined, 104
Genetic association studies, 147–149
Genetic variants
   and neurologic outcomes, 155–156
   perioperative kidney outcomes and, 156
   and postoperative event-free survival, 155
   postoperative lung injury, risk for, 156–157
Genitofemoral nerve, 961
1,000 Genomes Project, 148
Genome-wide association studies (GWAS), 147, 148, 154
Genome-wide scan, 147
Genomics
   dynamic, 145–146
   and perioperative risk profiling, 149–157, 149t–152t
   static, 145, 146
Gestational diabetes mellitus, 1163
Giardia lamblia, 74
Gibbon, John, 19
Gillet test, 1615
Gillies, Harold, 6
Gingivostomatitis, 74
Glasgow Coma Scale (GCS), 1635
   for assessment of consciousness, 1500–1501, 1501t
Glaucoma, 1376–1377
   closed-angle/acute, 1376–1377
   open-angle/chronic, 1376–1377
GLIC, 223
Gliderite Rigid Stylet, 784
Glidescope, 770
   blade, 784, 784f
Glidescope Titanium, 785
Glinides, 1345
Global myocardial stunning, 1678

Glomerular filtration rate (GFR), 391, 1183, 1403–1405
  estimates of, 1404–1405
Glossopharyngeal nerve, 795–796
Gloves, 187
Glucagon, 1344
Glucagon-like peptide-1 (GLP-1), 1345
Glucocorticoids, 412, 1582
Glucosedependent insulinotropic polypeptide (GIP), 1345
Glucose-lowering drugs, properties of, 1346t
Glucose management, in critical illness, 1646
Glucose-6-phosphate dehydrogenase (G6PD) deficiency, 634, 634t
Glutamate-activated ion channels, 227–228
Glutamine, 1303
Glycemic lability index (GLI), 1348
Glycerol, 1381
Glycine, 229
Glycocalyx, 935
Glycogen branching enzyme (GBE), 629
Glycogen storage diseases (GSD), 625–626, 626f, 627t–628t, 629
Glycopyrrolate, 304–306, 305t, 355, 355f, 355t, 608, 1186
  for awake intubation, 794
Goldan, Ormond, 18
Goldman nasal mask, 7
Golgi tendon organs, 368, 1608t
Gordh, Torsten, 22
Government plan, for disaster management, 1689–1690
GP IIb/IIIa receptor antagonists, 450
G-protein–coupled receptors (GPCRs), 421, 508
G-proteins, 254
Graft-*versus*-host disease (GVHD), 428
Granulation tissue, in wound healing, 193, 194
Great Influenza, 73
Greene needle, 923f
Griffith, Harold, 15
Ground fault circuit interrupter (GFCI), 122, 122f, 129
Grounding, shock hazards and, 112–113
Ground plates, 125
Ground wires, 122
Growth factors, in epithelialization, 194
Growth hormone (GH), 1018, 1647
Guarded-receptor theory, 568
Guedel, Arthur, 6, 22, 769
Guillain–Barré syndrome (GBS), 618–619
Gum elastic bougie, 802
GWAS. *See* Genome-wide association studies (GWAS)
Gwathmey, James Tayloe, 8
Gynecoid (peripheral) obesity, 1278

H

HAE. *See* Hereditary angioedema (HAE)
Haemophilus influenzae type B, 1366
Hall, Richard, 17
Halothane, 10, 12, 66, 460f, 1223, 1223f, 1247, 1305
  airway reflex, 1225
  carbon dioxide production, rate of, 1227
  changes in blood pressure, 1226
  heart rate, effect on, 1225, 1226
  hepatic dysfunction, 1226-1227
  hepatitis, 1227, 1305–1306
  minimum alveolar concentration of, 1225
  myocardial contractility, 1226
  in neonates, 1189
  oxygen consumption, 1226
  versus sevoflurane, 1226
  speed of washout, 1224
Halsted, William, 17, 18, 82

Hand hygiene
  barriers to, 186
  indications for, 186t
  infection control and, 184–187
  for nurses in ICU, 187
  technique, 186t
  WHO's "5 Moments" for, 186-187, 188f
Hand, surgery to, 1448–1449
Haplotype analysis, 144
Haplotypes, 144
Haptens, 205, 205t
Harmel, Merel, 19
Harvey, William, 12
HBeAg. *See* Hepatitis B e antigen (HBeAg)
HBsAg. *See* Hepatitis B surface antigen (HBsAg)
HBV. *See* Hepatitis B virus (HBV)
HCV. *See* Hepatitis C virus (HCV)
HCW. *See* Health-care workers (HCW)
Headache, 938–939
Head and neck surgery, fire risks, 131
Head coverings, in infection control, 187
Head-down positions, 824
  complications of, 824–825
    brachial plexopathy, 824–825, 824f
    head and neck injury, 824
    robotic procedures and, 824
Head-elevated positions
  complications of, 823–824
    air embolus, 823
    edema of face, tongue, and neck, 823
    midcervical tetraplegia, 823
    postural hypotension, 823
    sciatic nerve injury, 824
  lateral position with elevated head, 822–823, 823f
  sitting, 822, 822f
  supine recumbent position, 822
Head injury, 1499–1500, 1500t
  anesthetic management, 1502
  complications, 1500
  diagnosis of, 1500–1501, 1500t
    consciousness, assessment of, 1500–1501, 1500t
    CT scanning, 1501
    neurologic examination, 1500
    pupillary reaction, 1501
  management of, 1501–1502, 1503t
Head tilt-chin lift method, 1663
Health-care agency plans, for disaster management, 1690–1691
Healthcare Facilities Accreditation Program (HFAP), 847
Health-care workers (HCW), 73
Health Insurance Portability and Accountability Act (HIPAA), 54
Hearing impairment, 1554
Hearing loss, 939
Heart, 278. *See also* Cardiac anatomy
  coronary blood supply, 280–281, 280f, 281f
  denervated, 350
  impulse conduction, 281–282
Heart disease, during pregnancy, 1161–1163
Heart failure with normal ejection fraction (HFNEF), 293–294
Heart–lung transplantation, 1476
HeartMate, 1477, 1477f
Heart rate, 282
  in children, 1221t
Heart transplantation, 1476
  intraoperative management, 1479–1480, 1479f, 1480t
  left ventricular assist devices, 1476–1478, 1477f
  pediatric, 1480
  preanesthetic considerations, 1478–1479
  recipient selection, 1478
Heat exchanger, 1091

Heat, in electrical circuits, 110
Heidbrink, Jay, 8
Heliox, 1253
HELLP syndrome, 1157, 1158, 1306–1307
Heme, 623
Hemisacralization, 916
Hemodialysis, 1646
Hemodynamics, 473, 473f
  formulas, 1708
  monitoring, of trauma patients, 1516–1518, 1517t, 1518f
Hemoglobin, 431
Hemoglobin-based oxygen carriers (HBOCs), 1648
Hemoglobinopathies, 634–636, 634t
Hemoglobin oxygen desaturation, 1245
Hemolytic anemias, 633–634
Hemophilias, 446
Hemorrhage, obstetric. *See* Obstetric hemorrhage
Hemorrhagic fever, 1699
Hemorrhagic retinopathy, postsurgical, 1394
Hemostasis, 1307–1308
  acquired disorders of
    disseminated intravascular coagulopathy, 447–449, 448t
    liver disease, 447
    vitamin K deficiency, 447
  anticoagulation and pharmacologic therapy
    ADP receptor antagonists, 449
    cyclooxygenase inhibitors, 449
    GP IIb/IIIa receptor antagonists, 450
    heparin-induced thrombocytopenia, 451-452
    heparin therapy, 451
    monitoring of, 427
    oral anticoagulants, 450-451, 451t
    parenteral direct thrombin inhibitors, 452
    phosphodiesterase inhibitors, 449
    vitamin K antagonists, 450
    Xa antagonists, 451
  antifibrinolytic therapy, 453
  desmopressin, 453
  diagnosis, 444–449
  disorders of, 444–449
  hereditary hypercoagulability, 446–447
  laboratory evaluation of, 422–427
  primary, 420, 421f
    activation, 421–422
    adherence, 420–421
    antiplatelet medications, mechanisms of, 422
    diagnosis, 444disorders of, 444–446
    inhibition, 422
    laboratory evaluation of, 424–425
    stabilization, 422
    treatment, 444
  prothrombin complex concentrates and, 452–453
  recombinant activated factor VIIs, 452
  secondary, 422–423, 422f
    clotting factors, inhibition of, 423, 423f
    disorders of, 446–447
    hemophilias, 446–447
    laboratory evaluation of, 425–426
  treatment, 444–449
  viscoelastic testing, 426
Hemostatic biomarkers, 153
Hemostatic resuscitation protocols, 1161, 1498, 1498t
Henderson–Hasselbalch equation, 385, 1147
Henderson, Velyien, 11
Henry's law, 462
HEPA. *See* High-efficiency particulate air (HEPA)
Heparin anticoagulation testing, 427
Heparin-induced thrombocytopenia (HIT), 451-452, 1092
Hepatic and hepatobiliary diseases, 1301–1307
  acute liver failure, 1302–1304
  acute viral hepatitis, 1304–1305

alcoholic hepatitis, 1305
drug-induced liver injury, 1305–1306
pregnancy-related liver diseases, 1306–1307
Hepatic artery thrombosis (HAT), 1471
Hepatic drug clearance, 246–248, 247f
Hepatic dysfunction
blood tests in, 1301t
differential diagnosis of, 1301t
Hepatic encephalopathy (HE), 1312–1313
nomenclature of, 1313t
precipitating factors in, 1313t
West Haven criteria, 1312t
Hepatic function, assessment of
aspartate aminotransferase/alanine aminotransferase ratio, 1300
blood tests and differential diagnosis, 1301t
grades of encephalopathy, 1302t
laboratory tests, 1300
monoethylglycinexylidide (MEGX) test, 1300
serum albumin and coagulation testing, 1300
tests for synthetic function, 1300
Hepatitis, 428. *See also* Acute hepatitis
Hepatitis A, 78
Hepatitis B e antigen (HBeAg), 78
Hepatitis B surface antigen (HBsAg), 78
Hepatitis B virus (HBV), 71, 78, 78f, 436
acute, 78
vaccine, 78
Hepatitis C virus (HCV), 71, 78–79, 436
Hepatobiliary imaging, 1300–1301
abdominal x-rays, 1301
CT scanning, 1301
ERCP, 1301
MRI, 1301
THC, 1301
ultrasonography, 1301
Hepatocellular carcinoma (HCC), 1315
Hepatopulmonary syndrome (HPS), 1310–1311, 1469
staging of, 1310t
Hepatorenal syndrome (HRS), 1305, 1470
Herbal medications, 1744-1747
Herb, Isabella, 11
Hereditary angioedema (HAE), 207, 211
Hereditary coproporphyria (HCP), 623, 624t
Hereditary disorders of platelets, 444-445
Hereditary elliptocytosis, 633–634
Hereditary hypercoagulability, 446-447
Hereditary spherocytosis 633–634
Hering–Breuer reflex, 368
Hernia repair in neonate, 1212
anesthetic techniques for, 1212–1213
discharge after, 1213
regional anesthesia for, 1213
Hernia surgery, 1235
Heroin, 507
Herpes simplex viruses (HSV), 74
Herpes zoster, 1616–1617
Herrick, James, 10
Hers disease, 629
Hexobarbital (Evipal), 13
Hibernating myocardium, 1079
Hibiclens, chemical injury, 1393
Hickman, Henry Hill, 3
High block/total subarachnoid spinal block, 939
High-efficiency particulate air (HEPA), 80
High-frequency jet ventilation (HFJV), 887
High-frequency ventilation, 1062
Hill, Bradford, 175
Hingson, Robert, 18
HIPAA. *See* Health Insurance Portability and Accountability Act (HIPAA)
Hip, surgery to, 1449
ambulatory, 1451
anesthesia technique, 1450
approach, 1449–1450

blood loss and transfusion, 1451
positioning, 1449–1450, 1450f
Hirudin, 1092
Histamine, 348
Histamine, nonimmunologic release of, 211, 211f
Histamine-2 receptor antagonists, 604
Histamine receptors, release of, 192
HIV. *See* Human immunodeficiency virus (HIV)
Holladay, H. A., 16
Holmes, Mackinnon, 19
Hoover sign, 1031
Horner syndrome, 357–358, 357f
Horsely, Sir Victor, 20
Hospital risk management program, 97
Hospitals
anesthesiologists in, 44, 53
subsidies by, 51
House
with modern style wiring, 116f
with older style wiring, 115f
HPS. *See* Hepatopulmonary syndrome (HPS)
HPV. *See* Hypoxic pulmonary vasoconstriction (HPV)
HRSV. *See* Human respiratory syncytial virus (HRSV)
HSV. *See* Herpes simplex viruses (HSV)
5-HT$_3$ receptors, 229
Human factor analysis, 69
Human Genome Project, 148, 159–160
Human genomic variation, 144, 144f
Human immunodeficiency virus (HIV), 71, 428, 436
infection, occupational, 79
neuropathy, 1617–1618
risk of, 79–80
in United States, 79
Humanized antibodies, 1464
Human leukocyte antigen (HLA), 428
Human neutrophil antigen (HNA), 1527
Human respiratory syncytial virus (HRSV), 73, 74
Human stem cell transplantation (HSCT), 629
Human T-cell lymphotropic virus-1 (HTLV-1), 436–437
Human T-cell lymphotropic virus-2 (HTLV-2), 436–437
Humoral immunity, 205
Hunt and Hess Grading Scale, 1018, 1018t
Hunter syndrome, 629
Huntington disease (HD), 621
Hunt, Reid, 16
Hurler syndrome, 629, 632
Hustead needle, 923f
Hybrid pediatric cardiac surgery, 1108
Hybrid rate constants, 251
Hyde v Jefferson Parish, 51
Hydralazine, 325
in preeclampsia, 1158
Hydrocephalus, 1211–1212, 1637
Hydrocodone, 1570–1571
Hydrocortisone, 412
Hydrolysis, 244
Hydromorphone, 855t, 1232, 1254
for acute postoperative pain, 1574
dose ranges, effect of aging on, 903t
patient–controlled regimens, 1582t
pharmacokinetics, 1573t
Hydrophilic drugs, 242
Hydrotherapy, 1149
Hydroxyethyl starch (HES), 395–396
Hyperalgesia, 510, 1563, 1565, 1566, 1610
Hyperbilirubinemia, 1314
Hypercalcemia, 411–412, 1407
bone resorption and, 412
malignancy and, 412

total serum calcium and, 411
treatment of, 412
Hypercapnia, 472
Hypercarbia, 538, 1266t
Hypercoagulability, hereditary, 446-447
Hyperemesis gravidarum, 1306
Hyperglycemia, 1014, 1553
in critically ill patients, 1646
critically ill patients and, 1117
diabetes mellitus and, 1348, 1348f
modulators of perioperative, 1349f
perioperative, management of, 1350–1351
Hyperglycemic hyperosmolar state (HHS), 1351–1352
Hyperhomocysteinemia, 427
Hyperkalemia, 1187–1188, 1406, 1554
cause of, 407
in chronic renal failure, 1410t
diagnosis of, 407
drug-induced, 407
electrocardiographic (ECG) manifestations of, 407f
manifestations of, 407
symptoms and signs of, 407
treatment of, 408–409, 408f, 409t
Hyperkalemic periodic paralysis (hyperPP), 615–616, 616t
Hypermagnesemia, 415, 1407, 1554
Hypernatremia, 1406
clinical consequences of, 403
diabetes insipidus and, 403
management of, 404
neurologic symptoms of, 403
treatment of, 403–404, 403t, 404f
Hyperosmolar nonketotic coma, 1351
Hyperparathyroidism, 1332–1334
anesthetic considerations, 1334
treatment, 1334
Hyperphosphatemia, 413–414, 1407
Hyperpolarization-activated cyclic nucleotide-gated channels (HCN channels), 227
Hypersensitivity reactions, 207
type I, 207, 207f
type II, 207–208, 208f
type III, 208, 208f
type IV, 208, 208f
Hypertension, 592
Hypertensive disorders of pregnancy, 1156–1159
anesthetic management, 1159
chronic hypertension, 1156
with superimposed preeclampsia, 1156
gestational hypertension, 1156
preeclampsia/eclampsia, 1156
treatment of, 1158–1159
Hyperthermia, 608, 1556
malignant, pediatrics, 1235–1236
Hyperthyroidism, 1329–1331
anesthetic considerations, 1330–1331
causes of, 1329t
manifestations of, 1329
treatment, 1330–1331, 1330t
Hypertonicity, 395
Hypertonic solutions, 395–397, 1378
advantages and disadvantages, 397t
clinical implications of, 396–397
Hypertrophic cardiomyopathy, 1084–1085
anesthetic considerations, 1084–1085
hemodynamic goals, 1084t
pathophysiology, 1084, 1084f
Hypertrophic obstructive cardiomyopathy (HOCM), 1468
Hyperventilation, 370
Hypervolemia, hypertension, and hemodilution (triple-H) therapy, 1637
Hypnomidate, 13

Index

Hypocalcemia, 1226, 1407
  causes of, 409
  clinical manifestations, 410, 410t
  diagnostic evaluation, 411
  symptoms, 410
  treatment of, 411, 411t
Hypocapnia, 472
Hypoglycemia, 1248, 1251, 1348, 1352, 1553
Hypokalemia, 538, 1226, 1406, 1554
  causes of, 405
  diagnostic flow chart for, 406f
  evaluation of, 405–406
  symptoms and signs of, 405
  treatment of, 406–407, 406t
Hypokalemic periodic paralysis (hypoPP), 616
Hypomagnesemia, 414–415, 415t, 1226, 1407
Hyponatremia, 623, 1248, 1251, 1406, 1553–1554
  defined, 399
  euvolemic, 400
  evaluation algorithm, 399f
  hemodialysis in, 403
  neurologic symptoms, 402
  serum osmolality, 399–400
  signs and symptoms, 399, 400, 1429
  sodium, 399–403
  treatment of, 401–403, 401f
Hypoparathyroidism, 1334–1335
  clinical features of, 1334–1335
  treatment of, 1335
Hypoperfusion, 941
Hypophosphatemia, 413, 413t, 1407, 1463
Hypospadias, 1435
Hypotension, 935
  after trauma, 1523–1524
Hypotensive bradycardic events (HBE), 1447
Hypothalamus, 334-335, 1004, 1005
Hypothermia, 937, 1013–1014, 1555–1556
  diagnosis of, 1525
  perioperative, 840
  systemic, 1092–1093
  in trauma patient, 1524, 1525
  treatment of
    antifibrinolytic agents, 1526
    cryoprecipitate, 1526
    factor VIIa, 1526–1527
    fibrinogen, 1526
    fresh frozen plasma, 1526
    hemostasis, 1525–1526
    platelets, 1526
    prothrombin complex concentrate (factor IX complex), 1527
    red blood cell transfusion, 1525–1526
    transfusion-related lung injury, 1527
Hypothesis formulation, 169–170, 170t
Hypothesis testing, 171, 174–175
Hypothyroidism, 1226, 1331–1332
  anesthetic considerations, 1331–1332
  causes of, 1331t
Hypovolemia, 1520–1522, 1521f
  correction of, 1248
Hypoxemia, 1289
Hypoxia, 496, 1247, 1266t
Hypoxic pulmonary vasoconstriction (HPV), 373, 479, 1054–1055
  anesthetics on, effects of, 1055–1056
  determinants of, 1056
  potentiators of, 1056

I

IARS. *See* International Anesthesia Research Society (IARS)
Ibuprofen, 1232
  dosing guidelines, 1578t
  for postoperative pain, 1599
ICDs. *See* Implantable cardiac defibrillators (ICDs)
ICU. *See* Intensive care unit (ICU)
ICU-acquired weakness (ICUAW), 1655
Idarucizumab, 206, 427
Ideal body weight (IBW), 1278
I-Gel, 777f, 778
Ikeda, Shigeto, 7
Ileal conduit surgery, 1424
Iliohypogastric nerve block, 978, 984–985, 985f
Ilioinguinal/iliohypogastric (II/IH) nerve block, 1595–1596
Ilioinguinal nerve block, 978, 984–985, 985f, 1199–1200, 1200f
IL-2 receptor (CD25) antagonists, 1464
Image-guided laryngoscopy, 783
Immobility, 233
Immune function, effects of anesthesia on, 207
Immune hemolytic anemias, 634
Immune suppression, complications of, 1463t
Immune system, 204–205
Immunity, 71
Immunoglobulins (Igs), 429. *See also* Antibodies
Immunonutrition, 1648
Immunosuppressive agents, 1463–1465
  antibodies
    monoclonal, 1464
    polyclonal, 1464
  calcineurin inhibitors, 1464
  corticosteroids, 1464
  mesenchymal stem cells (MSCs) infusion, 1465
  mTOR inhibitors, 1464–1465
  mycophenolate mofetil, 1465
  purine antagonists, 1465
Impairment, 84
Impedance, 110
Impedance threshold device (ITD), 1667
Implantable cardiac defibrillators (ICDs), 1382, 1725
  indications for, 1725
Implantable gastric stimulator, 1279
Impotence surgery and medication, 1434, 1434f
Improvised explosive devices (IEDs), 1689
Impulse conduction, 281–282
Inamrinone, 321–322
Inclusion-body myositis (IBM), 639
Independent practice associations, 52
Index of autoregulation, 1011
Indocyanine green (ICG) elimination, 1300
Indomethacin, dosing guidelines, 1578t
Inductance, 111
Induction techniques, pediatric
  emergency drugs, availability of, 1241
  equipment, 1239–1240
  full stomach and rapid sequence induction, 1241–1242
  laryngospasm, management of, 1246–1247, 1246f
  patient monitoring system, 1240
    anesthetic depth, 1241
    capnography, 1240
    temperature, 1240–1241
  preoperative preparation
    inhalational, 1243–1244
    intramuscular, 1245
    intravenous, 1244–1245
    mask phobia, challenges with, 1244, 1244f
    parental presence, 1242
    rectal, 1245
  problems
    bradycardia, 1247, 1247t
    hemoglobin oxygen desaturation, 1245
    hypoxia, 1247
    laryngospasm, 1245–1247, 1246f, 1246t
Infant
  versus adult
    lung volumes, 1181f
    respiratory values, 1181t
  blood component therapy in, 1184
  cardiovascular system of, 1179–1180, 1179f, 1180f
  changes at birth, 1179–1180, 1180f
  fetal circulation in, 1179–1180, 1179f, 1180f
  fluid and electrolyte therapy in, 1183–1184
  hepatic system in, 1184–1185
  physiology of, 1178–1191
  pulmonary system of, 1181–1183, 1181f, 1182f, 1183f
  renal system of, 1183
  transition period of, 1178–1191
Infection, thoracic surgery and, 1035
Infectious diseases
  airborne precautions, 72t
  contact precautions, 72t
  droplet precautions, 72t
  standard precautions, 71t
  transmission-based precautions, 71–72
Infectious hazards. *See under* Occupational health
Inferential statistics, 171
Inflammation biomarkers, 152–153
Inflammatory myopathies, 639
Inflammatory neuropathies, 618
Influenza pandemics. *See under* Respiratory viruses
Influenza viruses. *See under* Respiratory viruses
Informed consent, 98–99
Infraclavicular blocks, 970–972, 971f, 1588–1589
Infrared absorption spectrophotometry (IRAS), 710
Infused fluids, distribution of, 390, 391f
Inguinal nerves, 960
Inhalational anesthetics, 1222–1227, 1223t
  pharmacodynamics, 1225–1227, 1225f
    BIS readings, 1226
    cardiovascular effects, 1225–1226
    central nervous system, 1226
    cerebral blood flow changes, 1226
    cerebral metabolic rate for oxygen, 1226
    cerebral vascular resistance, 1226
    cerebrovasodilatation, 1226
    EEG activity, 1226
    hepatic changes, 1226-1227
    renal effects, 1226
    respiration, effects on, 1225
    in vitro metabolism, 1227
  pharmacokinetics, 1223–1225, 1223t, 1223f
    mode of ventilation, 1224
    shunts, effect of, 1224
    speed of washout, 1224-1225
  physicochemical properties, 1222, 1223t
  washin ratio for, 1223
  washout times for, 1235t
Inhalation labor analgesia, 1151–1152
Inhaled anesthetics, 3, 11–12, 459–482. *See also* Anesthesia
  alterations in neurophysiology, 471–473
  alveolar concentration of, 462
  anesthetic metabolism, 482
  autonomic nervous system, 476, 476f
  autoregulation, 471
  bronchiolar smooth muscle tone, 478, 479f
  carbon dioxide
    absorbers, anesthetic degradation by, 481–482
    response to, 477–478, 478f
  cerebral blood flow, 471, 471f
  cerebral metabolic rate, 471
  cerebral protection, 472
  chemical structure of, 460f
  circulatory system, 473–476
  clinical overview, 468–469
  clinical utility, 482

for induction of anesthesia, 482
for maintenance of anesthesia, 482
coronary steal, 475
distribution (tissue uptake), 464–465
electroencephalogram, 471
elimination, 467–468, 467f
features of, 461
fetal development, effects on, 480–481
flow–metabolism coupling, 471
fluoride-induced nephrotoxicity, 482
genetic effects, 480–481
hemodynamics, 473, 473f
hepatic effects, 479
hypercapnia, 472
hypocapnia, 472
hypoxemia, response to 477–478, 478f
intracerebral pressure, 471–472
malignant hyperthermia, 479–480
metabolism, 465
minimum alveolar concentration, 469–471, 469t, 470f, 470t
mucociliary function, 478
myocardial contractility, 474, 474f
myocardial ischemia, 475
neuromuscular system, 479–480
neuropharmacology of, 469–473
nitrous oxide, 472–473, 474
obstetric use, 480–481
overpressurization and concentration effect, 465
perfusion effects, 466
pharmacokinetic principles, 460–468
pharmacology of, 1223t
physical characteristics of, 461–462, 461t
postoperative cognitive dysfunction, 472
processed electroencephalograms and neuromonitoring, 472
pulmonary system, 476–479
pulmonary vascular resistance, 478–479
second gas effect, 465, 465f, 466f
spontaneous ventilation, 474–475
uptake and distribution, 463–464
usage of, 460
ventilation
 effects, 465–466, 466f, 476–477, 477f
 mechanics, 477
 perfusion mismatching, 466, 467f
volatile anesthetics, 482
 cardioprotection from, 475
Inhaled nitric oxide (iNO), 1476
Inhaled volatile anesthetic agents, physical properties of, 669t
Inherited disorders
 cholinesterase disorders, 625
 glycogen storage diseases, 625–629
 hemoglobinopathies, 634–636
 hemolytic anemias, 633–634
 malignant hyperthermia, 622–623
 mucopolysaccharidoses, 629, 630t–631t, 632
 nutritional deficiency anemias, 633
 osteogenesis imperfecta, 632–633
 porphyrias, 623–625
Inhibition of $GABA_A$ channels, 229
Innovar, 14
Insertions–deletions, 144 144f
Inspiratory capacity, 376
Inspiratory paradox, 1031
Insulators, 110
Insulin, 1344
Insulin resistance syndrome, 1283
Insurance, malpractice, 42–43
Integrating, artificial skin substitute, 1523
Intensive care unit (ICU), 36, 1633
 acute kidney injury in, 1645–1646
 acute respiratory failure in, 1642–1645
 anemia and transfusion therapy in, 1647–1648

end-of-life care in, 1655
nosocomial infections in, 1650–1652
 catheter-related blood stream infections, 1652–1653
 invasive fungal infections, 1653
 sinusitis, 1650
 urinary tract infection, 1653
 ventilator-associated pneumonia, 1650–1652
nutrition in, 1648
processes of care in, 1633–1634
 checklists, 1634, 1634t
 protocols and care bundles, 1634
 resource management, 1634
 staffing, 1633–1634
sedation and analgesia in, 1648–1650
stress ulceration and gastrointestinal hemorrhage in, 1653–1654
venous thromboembolism in, 1654–1655
weakness in, 1655
Intensive insulin therapy (IIT), 1349–1350
Intercompartmental clearance, 252
Intercostal nerves, 959
 blocks, 978–980, 979f
Interleukins, 207
Intermediate response variables, 166
Intermittent claudication (IC), 1133
International Anesthesia Research Society (IARS), 21
International collection of diseases (ICD), 48
International College of Anesthetists, 21
International Electrotechnical Commission (IEC), 648
International Guidelines for the Selection of Lung Transplant Candidates, 1473, 1473t
International HapMap Project, 148
International Medical Surgical Response Teams (IMSuRT), 1689
International normalized ratio (INR), 427, 600, 1454
International Organization for Standards (ISO), 648
International Society for Heart and Lung Transplantation registry, 1473, 1475
International society transfusion guidelines, 431t
Interpersonal relationships, stress and, 56
Interposed abdominal compression (IAC), 1667
Interscalene blocks (ISB), 967–969, 968f, 1585, 1587–1588, 1588f, 1589f
Interspinous ligament, 916
Interstitial edema, brain, 1009
Interstitial fluid volume (IFV), 390
Interval-strength effect, 290
Interval variables, 166
Intestinal transplantation, 1472
Intocostrin, 16
Intra-abdominal injuries, 1270
Intra-abdominal pressure (IAP), 1265
Intra-aortic balloon pump, 1101–1102
 complications with, 1102
 indications and contraindications for, 1102t
Intrabdominal fluid extravasation (IAFE), 1451
Intracellular fluid (ICF), 1183
Intracellular volume (ICV), 390
Intracranial hypertension, 1009
Intracranial pressure (ICP), 1008–1009, 1009f
 effect of volatile anesthetics on, 471–472
 in head injury, 1501–1502
 hyperventilation and, 1471
 management protocol, 1303, 1303t
 monitoring, 1012, 1012f, 1471
Intradermal testing, 215
Intradermal water injection, 1149
Intradiscal electrothermal therapy (IDET), 1623

Intrahepatic cholestasis of pregnancy (ICP), 1306, 1306t
Intralipid, 947, 953, 1248, 1602
Intramuscular induction of anesthesia, 1245
Intraocular pressure (IOP), 608
 during anesthesia, 1375–1376
 influencing factors, 1376
 maintenance of, 1375–1376
 neuromuscular blocking drugs on, 1378–1379, 1378f
 succinylcholine on, 1378–1379, 1379t
Intraocular surgery, 1390
Intraoperative blood salvage (IOBS), 443
Intraoperative bronchodilator therapy, 1235
Intrapleural pressure, 364. See also Lung
Intrathecal drug delivery (IDD), 1626, 1627f, 1628
Intravenous anesthetics, 12–13, 486–502
 barbiturates, 499–501, 500f, 500t
 benzodiazepines, 498–499, 498t, 499t
 cyclopropyl-methoxycarbonyl metomidate, 502
 dexmedetomidine, 496–498, 496f, 496t, 497f
 etomidate, 492–493, 492f, 492t, 493t, 1228
 fospropofol, 502
 ketamine, 493–496, 493f, 493t, 495f, 1228
 neuromuscular blocking agents, 1228–1231
 opioids, 1231–1233
 pharmacokinetics, 486–489, 487f, 488f, 489f
 properties of, 487t
 propofol, 489–492, 490t, 491f, 502, 1227–1228
 remimazolam, 501-502, 501f
 Sedasys, 502
 sedatives, 1233
 THRX-918661/AZD-3043, 502
Intravenous drugs, 1227–1233
 etomidate, 1228
 ketamine, 1228
 neuromuscular blocking agents, 1228–1231
  atracurium, 1230
  cis-atracurium, 1230–1231
  neostigmine, 1231
  rocuronium, 1230
  succinylcholine, 1228–1230
  sugammadex, 1231
 opioids, 1231–1233
  acetaminophen, 1232
  codeine, 1232
  diclofenac, 1232
  fentanyl, 1231
  hydromorphone, 1232
  ibuprofen, 1232
  ketorolac, 1232
  meperidine, 1231
  morphine, 1231
  remifentanil, 1231–1232
 propofol, 1227–1228
 sedatives, 1233
  dexmedetomidine, 1233
  midazolam, 1233
Intravenous induction of anesthesia, 1244–1245
Intravenous regional anesthesia (Bier block), 977–978
Intrinsic acute kidney injury, 1408
Intubating oral airways, 799–800, 800f
Intubation skills, 70
Ion channels, anesthetic actions on, 225
 ligand-gated, 227–230
 voltage-dependent, 225–227
Ionizing radiation, exposure to, 1699–1702
Ionophores, 254
Ipratropium, 306, 306f
Iron deficiency anemia, 633
Iron overload, 441
Ischemia, 1013
 reversible, 1078–1079

Ischemic optic neuropathy, 820, 1394–1396
  anterior, 1395
  posterior, 1395–1396
Ischemic stroke, 1637–1638
Islet transplants, 1472
Isobologram, 270–271, 270f, 271f
Isoconcentration nomogram, 263–264, 263f
Isoflurane, 12, 20, 460, 460f, 468, 475, 1080, 1223, 1251, 1288, 1306
  airway reflex, 1225
  autoregulation, effect on, 1226
  carbon dioxide production, rate of, 1227
  changes in blood pressure, 1226
  heart rate, effect on, 1226
  hepatic dysfunction, 1226-1227
  in neonates, 1189
  oxygen consumption, 1226
  risk of nephrotoxicity, 1226
  speed of washout, 1224, 1225
Iso-Gard LIM, 120, 122
Isolated power system (IPS), 117, 119–120
  faulty equipment on, 119f
  leakage current, 120, 120f
  safety feature of, 119f
  in wet locations, 129
Isolation transformers, 117, 118f, 119, 119f
Isoproterenol, 308–309t, 313, 350, 1247, 1479, 1481
Isovolumic relaxation time (IVRT), 295

J
Jackson blade, 6
Jackson, Dennis, 9
Janeway, Henry, 6
Janssen, Paul, 13, 14
Jarman, Ronald, 13
Jaw thrust maneuver, 774, 1663
JCAHO. *See* Joint Commission for the Accreditation of Healthcare Organizations (JCAHO)
John Snow's inhaler, 7f
Johnson, Enid, 15
Johnstone, Michael, 12
Joint Commission, 35, 1688, 1690–1691
  standards, 38
Joint Commission on Accreditation of Healthcare Organizations (JCAHO), 35, 702, 1563
Joint injuries, 1555
Joules, definition, 110
J-tip injector, 1244
Jugular bulb venous oximetry, 1012

K
Kabat-Zinn, Jon, 85
Kalenda, Zden, 11
Kaplan, Joel, 19
Kaye, Geoffry, 21
Keats, Arthur, 20
Keown, Kenneth, 19
Kessel v Monongahela County General Hospital, 51
Ketamine, 13, 228, 493, 493f, 493t, 855t, 874, 1243, 1245, 1247–1248, 1412, 1557, 1579
  bolus dose of, 1579
  clinical uses
    analgesia, 494-495
    anesthesia, 494
    chronic pain, 495
    depression, 495
    sedation, 494
  effective blood concentration of, 1228
  half-life for, 1228
  intramuscular use, 1228
  intranasal dose of, 1228
  with midazolam, 1228
  for monitored anesthetic care, 835–836
  in neonates, 1186
  for obstetric analgesia, 1150
  as perioperative analgesia, 1228
  pharmacodynamics, 494, 495f
  pharmacokinetics, 493–494
  as premedication, 1228
  as racemic mixture, 1228
  rectal dose of, 1228
  side effects, 1228
    cardiovascular, 496
    central nervous system, 496
    intracranial pressure/seizure issues, 496
    respiratory, 496
Ketoprofen, dosing guidelines, 1578t
Ketorolac, 14, 855t, 1232
  dosing guidelines, 1578t
Kettle, Copper, 9
Khoka, 13
Kidney, 1401
  α receptors in, 346–347
  β receptors in, 347
  clinical assessment of, 1404–1406
Kidney Donor Profile Index (KCPI), 1465
Kidney Donor Risk Index (KDRI), 1465
Kidney donors, living, 1461
Kidney rest, 817
Kinemyography (KMG), 548
King Laryngeal Tube, 777–778, 777f
KingVision Video Laryngoscope, 786
Kinins, 210
Knee surgery
  ambulatory, 1452
  analgesia for, 1451–1452, 1451t
  anesthesia technique, 1451
  ankle, 1452
  foot, 1452
  positioning, 1451
  total knee arthroplasty, 1451
Knowledge-based alarms, 69
Koller, Carl, 13, 17
κ-Opioid receptor (KOR), 507–508
Korotkoff sounds, 716
Krantz, John C., 12
Krönig, Bernhardt, 20
Kruskal–Wallis one-way analysis of variance, 174
Kuhn, Franz, 9, 769
Kupffer cells, 1299
Kyphoplasty, 1623–1624

L
LA appendage, 297–298
Labat, Gaston, 19
Labetalol, 1380
  for ischemia, 1081
Labor analgesia, 1148–1149
  general anesthesia, 1152
  inhalation, 1151–1152
  medications, 1149
    ketamine, 1150
    opioids, 1149–1150
  nonpharmacologic methods, 1149
  regional analgesia, 1150
    combined spinal/epidural analgesia, 1151
    epidural analgesia, 1150–1151
    paracervical block, 1151
    paravertebral lumbar sympathetic block, 1151
    pudendal nerve block, 1151
    spinal analgesia, 1151
Labor pain, remifentanil for, 524
Labor support, continuous, 1149
Lacrimal drainage system, 1375
Lambert–Eaton syndrome (LEMS), 618
  versus myasthenia gravis, 618t

Laminar flow, lung, 365–366
Lamont, Austin, 19
Lamotrigine
  for chronic pain, 1622t
  dosage range, 1621t
  side effects, 1621
The Lancet, 4
Landsteiner, Karl, 21
Lansoprazole, 787
Laparoscopic adjustable gastric banding (LAGB), 1279
Laparoscopy, 1288
  in abdominal trauma, 1510, 1510t
  airway edema and, 1272
  anesthetic technique
    body temperature, 1269
    fluid management, 1269
    inhaled anesthetics, 1268
    intraoperative monitoring, 1268
    maintenance, 1268
    mechanical ventilation, 1268–1269
    neuromuscular blockade, 1268
    nitrous oxide, 1268
    pharmacologic adjuncts, 1268
    propofol, 1268
  brachial plexus injuries and, 1272
  intraoperative complications
    capnothorax, 1271
    cardiopulmonary complications, 1266t, 1270
    hypercarbia, 1266t
    hypoxia, 1266t
    intra-abdominal injuries, 1270
    subcutaneous emphysema, 1270–1271
    venous gas embolism, 1271–1272, 1272f
  ocular injuries and, 1272
  patient shifting and falls injury and, 1272
  peripheral nerve injuries and, 1272
  physiological impact of
    cardiovascular system, 1264–1265, 1265t
    end-tidal CO_2 ($ETCO_2$) levels, 1266
    functional residual capacity, 1266
    pulmonary changes, 1265t
    regional perfusion effects, 1267, 1267t
    respiratory system, 1265–1267, 1265t, 1266t
    splanchnic, renal, and cerebral blood flow, changes in, 1267
  postoperative complications
    respiratory dysfunction, 1272
    venous thrombosis, 1273
  postoperative management
    acute pain management, 1273
    PONV, 1273
  surgery
    ambulatory, 1263
    approach for, 1262–1263
    benefits of, 1262t
    disadvantages of, 1263t
    patient positioning during, 1263
    robotic, 1263–1264, 1264f, 1264t
LA pressure (LAP), 1086–1087
Laryngeal injuries, 1493, 1493t
Laryngeal mask airway (LMA), 7, 770, 775, 775f, 1225, 1287, 1360
  insertion of, 775–776, 776f
  LMA Classic, 775
  LMA Flexible, 775f, 776–777
  LMA ProSeal, 775, 778
  size, 775
Laryngeal Tube Suction (LTS-D), 777–778
Laryngeal view scoring system, 781, 782f
Laryngology, 1363
Laryngoscope, 6
Laryngospasm, 774, 1245–1247, 1253
  clinical findings in, 1246

factors associated with, 1246t
  management of, 1246–1247, 1246f
Laryngotracheobronchitis (LTB), 1366
Larynx, 768
Lasègue sign, piriformis syndrome, 1616
Laser Doppler flowmetry (LDF), 1011–1012
LaserFlex tube, 133, 133f
Laser goggles, 134
Lasers, fires and, 131, 133
Laser surgery
  of airway, 1367–1368, 1368t
  corrective, 1392
  principles of, 1392
Lasertubus laser resistant ET tube, 133, 133f
Lasing medium, 132
LAST. *See* Local anesthetic systemic toxicity (LAST)
Latent heat of vaporization, 669
Lateral cutaneous nerve of thigh, 961, 962f
Lateral femoral cutaneous nerve block, 1200
Lateral positions, 816–817
  complications of, 817, 819
    eyes and ears, 817, 819
    neck, 819
    suprascapular nerve, 819
  flexed, 817
    kidney position, 817 819f
    lateral jackknife position, 817, 818f
  semisupine and semiprone, 817, 818f
  standard, 817, 817f
Latex allergy, 215–216, 1238
Latex gloves, 68t
Laudanum, 2
Laughing gas, 3
Laurence–Moon–Biedl syndrome, 1237
Lawen, Arthur, 15
Lawn chair position. *See* Contoured supine posture
Law of Laplace, 282, 286 290
Lawsuits, anesthesia-related, 104–105, 104f
Leakage currents, 120, 120f, 123, 123f
Leake, Chauncey, 11
Leak test, 654, 654f
Lean body weight (LBW), 1278
Lee, E. W., 18
LeFort I-III fractures, 1370–1371
Left anterior descending artery (LDA), 280–281
Left circumflex artery (LCCA), 280–281
Left ventricular assist devices (LVADs), 1102, 1476–1478, 1477f
Left ventricular diastolic dysfunction, 293–294, 294t
Left ventricular end-diastolic pressure (LVEDP), 717
Left ventricular end-diastolic volume (LVEDV), 717
Left ventricular mass index (LVMI), 626
Left ventricular stroke work index (LWSWI), 1708
Legal issues
  credentialing process, 33–35
  equipment failures, 40
Lemmon, William, 18
Lessinger airway, 769
Leukoagglutinins, 210
Leukocyte histamine, 215
Leukoreduction (LR), 428
Leukotrienes, 210
Level of significance, 170
Levitan First Pass Success Scope, 783
Levobupivacaine, 1190, 1250
Levodopa, 621
Levorphanol, pharmacokinetics, 1573t
Levosimendan, 322–323, 322t
Lewis, Thomas, 10
Liability

insurance, 42, 43
  malpractice insurance and, 40–41
  vicarious, 32
Libby Zion case, 70
LiDCOrapid, 721, 723
Lidocaine, 13, 19, 567, 568, 569, 571, 573f, 575, 575t, 855t, 872, 1153, 1190, 1222
  for awake intubation, 795
  for chronic pain, 1622t
  during CPR, 1671–1672
  patch, 1621–1622
Lidoderm patch (allodynia), for chronic pain, 1622t
Ligaments, 916, 916f
Ligamentum flavum, 916
Ligamentum nuchae, 916
Ligand-gated ion channels, anesthetic effects on, 227–230
  GABA-activated ion channels, 228–229
  glutamate-activated ion channels, 227–228
  5-HT$_3$ receptors, 229
Ligand-gated receptors, 229
Light bulbs
  circuits, 116f
  resistance of, 113f
  wiring of sockets, 116f
Limb-girdle muscular dystrophy (LGMD), 613–614
Limbic system, brain, 1005
Linear regression analysis, 175
Line isolation monitors (LIMs), 120, 121f, 122
  function of, 120, 122
  meter for, 120, 121f
  in operating rooms, 130
Lingual tonsil hyperplasia, 779, 780f
Lipophilic drugs, 243
Liposomal bupivacaine (Exparel), 1596
Liposomal morphine, 855t
Liposomes, 571–572
Liposuction, 871
Lister, Baron, 10
Liston, Robert, 2
Litholyme, 683
Litigation, 99
Liver. *See also* Hepatic function, assessment of; Hepatobiliary imaging
  abdominal x-rays for disease of, 1301
  apoferritin system, 1299
  biopsy, 1301
  Clichy criteria for transplantation, 1303
  CT scanning for disease of, 1301
  and drug toxicity, 1305
  ERCP for disease of, 1301
  hepatobiliary imaging for disease of, 1300–1301
  intraoperative management
    anesthetic techniques, 1317–1318
    hepatic resection, 1320–1321, 1320f
    monitoring and vascular access, 1317
    pharmacokinetic and pharmacodynamic alterations, 1318–1319
    transjugular intrahepatic portosystemic shunt procedure, 1319–1320, 1319f
    vasopressors, 1319
    volume resuscitation, 1319
  King's college selection criteria for transplantation, 1303, 1304t
  microcirculation of, 1299
  MRI for disease of, 1301
  postoperative dysfunction of, 1321–1322
    causes, 1321t
    hyperbilirubinemia, 1321–1322, 1322t
  preoperative management
    hepatic evaluation, 1316
    risks, 1316–1317
  as reservoir for blood, 1299

role in health, 1298–1300
  acetyl-CoA generation, 1299
  deamination of amino acids, 1300
  hepatic blood flow, 1299
  in protein metabolism, 1299
  THC for disease of, 1301
  ultrasonography for disease of, 1301
Liver disease, 600
Liver donors, living, 1462–1463, 1462f, 1463f
Liver function tests (LFTs), 1300
Liver transplantation
  acute liver failure, 1471
  coagulation management, 1469–1471
  diagnoses leading to, 1468t
  intraoperative procedures, 1469–1471
    anhepatic phase, 1470
    dissection phase, 1469–1470
    neohepatic phase, 1471
    reperfusion phase, 1470–1471
  pediatric, 1471
  phases, 1469–1471
  preoperative considerations, 1467–1469
    cardiac disease, 1468
    hepatopulmonary syndrome, 1469
    hypertrophic obstructive cardiomyopathy, 1468
    MELD Score, 1467–1468
    PELD Score, 1467–1468
    portopulmonary hypertension, 1468
    screening for infectious diseases, 1468
  pulmonary embolism and, 1470
  renal dysfunction in, 1468
LMA. *See* Laryngeal mask airway (LMA)
LMA Fastrach, 787–788
Load (current), definition, 111
Load-distributing band (LDB) device, 1667
Local anesthetics (LAs), 13–14, 538, 564–580
  activity and potency of, 569–570, 570t
  additives to
    β_2-adrenergic agonists, 571
    epinephrine, 570, 570t
    liposomes, 571–572
    opioids, 571
    solutions, alkalinization of, 570–571
    steroids, 571, 571f
  allergy to, 217, 580
  application of, 567
  for awake airway management, 794–796
  binding site, 568f
  cardiovascular toxicity of, 576–577, 576f–577f
  central nervous system toxicity of, 575–576
  clinical pharmacokinetics of, 572t, 573–575, 573t, 574t, 575f, 575t
  clinical use of, 574t, 575
  distribution of, 572–573, 573t
  dosing regimen of, for continuous peripheral nerve blockade, 1587t
  elimination of, 573
  future therapeutics and modalities of, 580, 580f
  mechanisms of
    central nervous system, 564–565
    molecular, 567–568, 567f, 568f
    nerve blockade, 568–569, 568f
    nerves, anatomy of, 564–565, 565f, 566t
    neural conduction, electrophysiology of, 565–567
    voltage-gated sodium channels, electrophysiology of, 565–567, 566f, 567t
  myotoxicity of, 579, 579f
  neural toxicity of, 578–579
  pharmacodynamics of, 569–572
  pharmacokinetics of, 572–575
  pharmacology of, 569–572
  physiochemical properties of, 569–570, 569t

Local anesthetics (continued)
  skin testing for, 217
  solutions, alkalinization of, 570–571
  systemic absorption of, 572, 572t, 573f
  systemic toxicity of, 575–578, 575t, 578t
  transient neurologic symptoms, 579, 579t
Local anesthetic systemic toxicity (LAST), 1153, 1155, 1585, 1586t, 1587t
Local infiltration analgesia (LIA), 1596
Loevenhart, Arthur, 22
Löfgren, Nils, 13
Logistic regression, 176
  multivariable, 176–177
Long, Crawford Williamson, 3
Long Island Society of Anesthetists, 21
Longitudinal studies, 167–168
Loop diuretics, 1415
Loperamide, 243
Lorazepam, 606–607, 607f
Lossen, Wilhelm, 13
Low back pain, 1611–1614
Low-density lipoproteins (LDLs), 1113
Lower esophageal sphincter (LES), 1146
Lower extremity compartment syndrome, 812, 813
Lower extremity, orthopedic surgery to, 1449–1452
Lower gastrointestinal tract obstruction, 1210, 1210f
Lower limit of autoregulation (LLA), 1007–1008
Lower, Richard, 12
Low-flow scavenging systems, 695
Low flow wizard (LFW), 665, 665f
Low lymph flow paradox, 395
Low-molecular-weight heparin (LMWH), 427
Low-pressure circuit (LPC), 644
  leak test, 653–654, 654f
Lucas, George, 11
Luckhardt, Arno, 11
Ludwig angina, 1370
Luft, K., 11
Lumbar backache, 816
Lumbar epidural anesthesia, for cesarean delivery, 1152–1153
Lumbar plexus, 959–960
  block, 986–988, 986f, 987f, 1450
  for pain management, 1586t, 1589–1590, 1590f, 1591f
  terminal nerves of, 961–962, 988–991
Lumbar puncture, 18
Lundquist, Bengt, 13
Lund University Cardiac Arrest System (LUCAS), 1667
Lundy, John, 13, 22
Lung
  divisions of, 363t
  elastic work, 364–365
  functional anatomy of, 362–364
  increased airway resistance, 366
  mechanics, 364–366, 365f
  physiologic dead space, 373–374
  physiologic shunt, 374–376
  resistance to gas flow, 365–366
  structures, 362–364
  volumes and capacities, 376–377, 376f
Lung cancer, 1030, 1030f
  cigarette smoking and, 1030
  incidence of, 1030
  thoracic surgery for. See Thoracic surgery
Lung cysts, 1063–1064
Lung isolation, 1041
  and lung separation, 1041
Lung separation, 1041
  double-lumen endobronchial tubes for, 1041–1045
  in patient with difficult airway, 1046–1150
  tracheostomy patient and, 1045–1046

Lung transplantation, 1473
  indications for, 1473
  inhaled nitric oxide and, 1476
  intraoperative management
    double-lung transplantation, 1475
    pediatric lung transplantation, 1475
    single-lung transplantation, 1474–1475
  pediatric, 1475
  primary graft dysfunction, 1475–1476
  recipient selection, 1473–1474, 1473t
  surgical options for, 1473
Lung volumes
  and capacities, 1709
  effects of anesthesia and surgery on, 1032
Lung water, reduction of, 1645
Lupus anticoagulants (LAs), 425
LV coronary perfusion pressure, 1078
LV diastolic pressure (LVDP), 1078
Lymnea stagnalis, 226
Lymphoblastic T cell lymphoma, 1237
Lymphomas, 1237
Lysine analogs, 453

M

MAC. See Monitored anesthesia care (MAC)
Macewan, William, 5
Machine intermediate-pressure system, 659
Macintosh blade, 6, 780–781
Macintosh, Robert, 6
MACRA. See Medicare Access and CHIP Reauthorization Act of 2015 (MACRA)
Macrophages, 206
Macroshocks, 111
  effects of, 112t
Mad cow disease, 80
Magill angulated forceps, 6
Magill, Ivan, 769
Magill tube, 6, 769
Magnesium, 855t, 1554
  hypermagnesemia, 415, 1407
  hypomagnesemia, 414–415, 415t, 1407
  physiologic role, 414
Magnesium sulfate, for preeclampsia, 1158
Magnetic resonance imaging (MRI), 68
  for C-spine injury, 1491
Mainstream capnography, 1240
Maintenance of Certification in Anesthesiology (MOCA), 35
Major adverse cardiac events (MACE), 590–591, 1114, 1116
Malignant hyperthermia (MH), 469, 479–480, 532, 539t, 587, 622, 623f, 1235–1236
  clinical grading scale, 624t
  management of
    acute MH, 622–623, 624t
    susceptible patient, 623, 624t
  protocol, 1743
  safe versus unsafe drugs in, 624t
  treatment of acute episode of, 624t
Malignant Hyperthermia Association of the United States (MHAUS), 623
Mallampati airway classification, 589, 589t
Mallampati score, 779
Malnourishment, albumin concentration and, 1222
Maloetine, 16
Malpractice insurance, 42–43
Mammalian target of rapamycin (mTOR), 898
  inhibitors, 1464–1465
Managed care organizations (MCO), 36
  pay for performance issues, 53
  prospective payments and, 52
Management companies, practice for, 47
The Management of Pain (Bonica), 19
Mandibular nerve blocks, 965, 965f

Mandragora, analgesics of, 2
Mannitol, 1381, 1414
Mann–Whitney rank sum test, 174
Manual bolus, 262–263
Manual for Anesthesia Department Organization and Management, 33
Manual inline stabilization (MILS), of neck, 1491
Mapleson breathing systems, 679–680, 679f
Maquet FLOW-i electronic injector vaporizers, 647f, 669t, 679
Maquet Flow-i workstation, 690-691, 690f, 691f
Marburg viruses, 1699
Marey law, 349
Marijuana, in pregnancy, 1165
Masimo Rad-5, 1514
Mask phobia, 1244, 1244f
Maslach Burnout Inventory (MBI), 82
Mass casualty event, 1687
Mass casualty incident, 1687
Massive Transfusion Score (MTS), 1496
Mass lesions, 940–941, 940f, 941f
Mast cells, 206
Matas, Rudolph, 18
Maternal age, advanced, 1156
Matrix (M) protein, 73
Maxillary nerve blocks, 964–965, 965f
Maxillofacial surgery, 872
Maxillofacial trauma, 1370–1371, 1492
Maximal oxygen consumption, 1033–1034
Maximum voluntary ventilation (MVV), 377, 1032
MBI. See Maslach Burnout Inventory (MBI)
MBSR. See Mindfulness-based stress reduction (MBSR)
MCA. See Middle cerebral artery (MCA)
McArdle disease, 629
Mcgill Pain Questionnaire, 1571
McGrath Mac, 785
McGrath Mac X blade, 786
McGrath Series 5 videolaryngoscope, 784f, 785
McIntyre, A. R., 15
McKesson, E. I., 22
McMechan, Francis Hoffer, 21
MCO. See Managed care organizations (MCO)
McQuiston, William, 19
Mean, 167
Mean amplitude of glycemic excursions (MAGE), 1348
Mean arterial pressure (MAP), 716, 1007–1008, 1641, 1708
Mean Residence Time (MRT), 252
Measles (rubeola), 75, 76t–77t
Measles, mumps, rubella (MMR), 75
Mechanical chest compression devices, 1667
Mechanical circulatory support (MCS), 1100, 1103
Mechanical sling lifting devices, 1289
Mechanical ventilation, 1288–1289
  in ICU, 1642–1644
Mechanomyography (MMG), 547
Meconium aspiration, 1182–1183, 1183f
Medecins san Frontieres, 1688
Median, 167
Median nerve, 958
  blocks, 975–977, 976f
  injuries to, 814
Median power frequency (MPF), 725
Mediastinal mass, diagnostic procedures for, 1059–1061
  mediastinoscopy, 1060–1061
  thoracoscopy, 1061
  video-assisted thoracoscopic surgery, 1061
Mediastinal shift, 1038, 1039f
Medical and Family Leave Act, 84
Medic Alert bracelets, 217
Medical Specialty Enhancement Team (MSET), 1690

Medicare Access and CHIP Reauthorization Act of 2015 (MACRA), 32
Medicare payments, 103
Medulla oblongata, 335
Medullary centers, 367
Meetings, 39–40
Megaloblastic anemia, 632
Meissner corpuscles, 1608t
MELD Score, 1316–1317, 1467–1468
Melker emergency cricothyrotomy catheter set, 804
Meloxicam,
   dosing guidelines, 1578t
Membrane oxygenators, 1091
Meninges
   anatomy, 917–918, 917f
   arachnoid mater, 917–918, 918f
   dura mater, 917, 917f, 918f
   pia mater, 918, 919f
Meperidine, 14, 507, 607–608, 855t, 1231, 1412, 1575
   dose ranges, effect of aging on, 903t
   for labor pain, 1149
   pharmacokinetics, 1573t
Mepivacaine, 14
Mercapturic acid, 245
Merit Based Incentive Payment System, 32
Merkel disc, 1608t
Mesenchymal stem cells (MSCs) infusion, 1465
Mesmerism, 2
Meta-analyses, 179
Metabolic acidemia, 1552–1553, 1552t
Metabolic acidosis, 386–387, 1407
   anesthetic risk associated with, 387
   differential diagnosis of, 386t
   preoperative assessment for, 387
   during prolonged surgery, 389t
   respiratory compensation in, 386t
   in trauma patients, 1527
   treatment of, 387
   ventilatory compensation for, 387t
Metabolic alkalemia, 1553
Metabolic alkalosis, 385–386, 1407
   factors to maintain, 386t
   generation of, 385t
   to nausea and vomiting, 389t
   respiratory compensation in, 386t
   treatment of, 386
Metabolic derangements, 441
Metabolic syndrome, 592, 1283–1284
   conditions with, 1283
   National Cholesterol Education Program (NCEP) Adult Treatment Panel III (ATP III), 1283
Metabolomic tools, 147
Methacholine, 302f, 303
Methadone, 513
   for acute postoperative pain, 1575–1576, 1576t
   aging and dosage of, 903t
   conversion of morphine to, 1576t
   drug interactions with, 1576t
   in neonates, 1187
   pharmacokinetics, 1573t
Methemoglobin (MetHb), 709
Methicillin-resistant *Staphylococcus aureus* (MRSA), 187
Methionine synthetase (MS), 480
Method-mode (M-mode) echocardiography, 734, 734f
Methoxyflurane, 12, 1226
Methyl methacrylate, 67
Methylprednisolone acetate, 1612, 1613f
Metoclopramide, 17, 348, 605, 1347
Metoprolol, for ischemia, 1081
Metubine, 16

Mexiletine, 1622
   dosage range, 1621t
   side effects, 1621
Mexilitine
   for chronic pain, 1622t
Meyer–Overton rule, 221, 221f
   exceptions to, 222
MG. *See* Myasthenia gravis (MG)
Michenfelder, John D. "Jack," 20
Microangiopathic hemolytic anemia (MAHA), 1306–1307
Microaspiration, 787
Micrognathia, 1220
Microsatellites, 144, 144f
Microshocks, 111–112, 123–124, 123f, 124f
   current density in, 123
   effects of, 112t
   to electrically susceptible patients, 124f
Midazolam, 498, 498f, 499t, 606, 607f, 855t, 860, 1221, 1233, 1243
   for acute perioperative pain in pediatric patients, 1602
   and diazepam, 833t
   dose, 852, 852f
   dose ranges, effect of aging on, 903t
   for monitored anesthetic care, 832–833, 833f
   in neonates, 1186
   properties of, 498–499
   versus remimazolam, 501f
Midcervical tetraplegia, 823
Middle cerebral artery (MCA), 1005
   occlusion, 1638
Miller blade, 780–781, 781f
Miller, Robert, 6
Millikan, Glen, 10
Milnacipran, 1616, 1621t
   for chronic pain, 1622t
Milrinone, 321, 322t
Mindfulness-based stress reduction (MBSR), 85
Miniature end-plate potentials (MEPPs), 529
Minimally invasive direct coronary artery bypass (MIDCAB), 1104
Minimally invasive lumbar decompression (MILD), 1623
Minimally invasive procedures, 1262
   advantages, 1262t
   hemodynamic effects of, 1264
   patient position during, 1263
Minimum alveolar concentration (MAC), 157, 221, 370, 469–471, 469f, 470t, 516, 831, 1198, 1198f, 1223, 1225
   effect of age on, 470–471, 470f
   factors decreasing, 470t
   factors increasing, 469t
Misoprostol, 1160t
Mitochondrial myopathies, 1236
Mitral regurgitation (MR), 1087–1089
   acute-onset, 1088
   anesthetic considerations, 1088–1089
   Doppler echocardiography, 745f
   etiology, 1087
   hemodynamic goals, 1088t
   mechanisms of, 1088t
   pathophysiology, 1087–1088
Mitral stenosis, 1086–1087
   anesthetic considerations, 1087
   cause of, 1086
   hemodynamic goals, 1087t
   pathophysiology, 1086–1087
Mitral valve, 279
Mivacurium, 535t, 537, 1412
   dose ranges, effect of aging on, 903t
Mixed acid–base disorders, 1408, 1408f
MMR. *See* Measles, mumps, rubella (MMR)
MOCA. *See* Maintenance of Certification in Anesthesiology (MOCA)

Modafinil, 70
Mode, 167
Model for End-Stage Liver Disease (MELD) score, 600
Moderate sedation/analgesia, 826–827, 1733
Modified Child–Pugh score, 1316t
Modified vaccinia Ankara (MVA), 1697
Modulated-receptor theory, 568
Modulation, pain processing, 1563–1564
Monitored anesthesia care (MAC), 826, 1289, 1382
   ASA on, 827, 827t, 1738
   context-sensitive half-time, 829–831, 829f, 830f
   distribution of drug, 828–829
   drug interactions, 831
   drugs for
      benzodiazepines, 832–833
      dexmedetomidine, 836
      fospropofol, 832
      ketamine, 835–836
      opioids, 833–834
      patient-controlled sedation and analgesia, 836–837
      propofol, 831–832, 832t
      remifentanil, 834–835
      sedative–hypnotics, 836
   elimination half-time, 829
   and moderate sedation/analgesia, 826–827, 1738
   monitoring during, 839–843
      ASA standards, 839
      auscultation, 839
      bispectral index, 840–841
      capnography, 839–840
      cardiovascular system, 840
      communication and observation, 839
      Continuum of Depth of Sedation, 841t
      local anesthetic toxicity, 841–842
      pulse oximetry, 839
      SEDASYS, 843
      sedation and analgesia, by nonanesthesiologists, 842–843
      temperature monitoring, 840
   pharmacologic basis of, 828
   by Physician Anesthesiologist, 826
   preoperative evaluation, 827–828
   respiratory function and, 837–838
   supplemental oxygen administration, 838–839
   techniques of, 828
   terminology related to, 826–827
Monitoring techniques, 707–728
   of arterial oxygenation by pulse oximetry, 709–710
   of body temperature, 724
   of cardiac output by arterial waveform analysis, 721–724
   of cardiac output by pulmonary arterial catheter, 720–721
   of central venous and right-heart pressures, 717–720
   of expired gases, 710–713
   future trends in, 727–728
   of inspired oxygen concentration, 708
   of processed EEG signals, 724–727
   systemic blood pressure, intermittent, noninvasive monitoring of, 713–715, 715–717
Monoamine oxidase (MAO), 342
Monoamine oxidase inhibitors (MAOIs), 358–359
Monochlorodifluoromethane, 12
Morbid obesity, 1278
Morch "Respirator," 8
Morch, Trier, 8

Morphine, 2, 12, 507, 512, 513f, 607–608, 855t, 1231, 1248, 1254, 1412
   for acute pain, 1574
   cardiovascular effects, 523
   conversion of methadone to, 1576t
   dose ranges, effect of aging on, 903t
   in neonates, 1187
   in neuroanesthesia, 20
   for pain relief, 515, 515f
   patient–controlled regimens, 1582t
   and scopolamine, 20
Morphine-3-glucuronide (M3G), 512, 1574
Morphine-6-glucuronide (M6G), 512, 1574
Morphine sulfate, pharmacokinetics, 1573t
Morquio syndrome, 629
Morris, Lucien, 9
Mortality, and morbidity, anesthesia-related, 91, 92t–97t
Morton, William Thomas Green, 3
Motor-evoked potentials (MEPs), 472, 1009, 1010, 1010f, 1011, 1444
Mouth-to-mask ventilation, 1665
Mouth-to-nose ventilation, 1665
MRI. See Magnetic resonance imaging (MRI)
Mucociliary function, 478. See also Inhaled anesthetics
Mucolytic drugs, before thoracic surgery, 1035
Mucopolysaccharidoses (MPS), 629, 630t–631t, 632
Multicenter Perioperative Outcomes Group (MPOG), 179
Multiorgan failure (MOF), 1499
Multiple sclerosis (MS), 619
Multivariable linear regression, 176
Multivariate index scores, 772
μ-Opioid receptor (MOR), 507
Muromonab-CD3, in immunosuppression, 1464
Muscarine, 302f
Muscarinic antagonists, 304–306, 305t
   toxicity, 306, 306t
Muscarinic receptors, 342
Muscle paralysis, 858
Muscle relaxants, 1412–1413, 1413t. See also Neuromuscular blocking agents (NMBAs)
   development of, 15t
   and direct laryngoscopy, 801
   history of, 14–16, 15t, 16f
Muscular dystrophy, 612–614, 613f, 614f
   types of, 613t
Musculocutaneous nerve, 958–959
Musculoskeletal diseases, 613f
   congenital myopathies, 612–614, 613t
   muscular dystrophy, 612–614, 613f, 613t, 614f
   myotonic dystrophy, 614–615, 615t
Myasthenia gravis (MG), 616–617, 1065–1068
   anesthesia, management of, 617
   clinical classification, 1065t
   clinical presentations of, 617t
   diagnosis, 1065
   disorders associated with, 1066t
   general anesthesia for, 1066–1068
   versus Lambert–Eaton syndrome, 618t
   medical therapy, 1065–1066, 1066t
   Osserman staging system for, 617t
   postoperative care, 1068
   postoperative respiratory failure, 1068
   vecuronium in, 617f
Myasthenic syndrome, 1068
Mycobacterium tuberculosis, 80
Mycophenolate mofetil, in immunosuppression, 1465
Myelomeningocele
   clinical presentation, 1210–1211
   perioperative care, 1211
   postoperative care, 1211
   preoperative care, 1211
Myocardial contractility, 292–293, 474, 474f
Myocardial infarction (MI), 589
   during pregnancy, 1163
Myocardial Infarction and Cardiac Arrest (MICA), 590
Myocardial protection, 1092–1093
Myocardium, 278, 278f
Myofascial pain syndrome, 1616
Myogenic reflex theory, 1403
Myopathies, 1236
Myosin, 283–284, 284f
Myotonic dystrophy, 614–615
   classification of, 615t
   management of anesthesia, 615
   type 1, 615, 615t
   type 2, 615, 615t
Myxedema, 1331–1332, 1332t

N

NA. See Narcotics Anonymous (NA)
Nabiximols, 1622
Nabumetone, dosing guidelines, 1578t
NACOR. See National Anesthesia Clinical Outcomes Registry (NACOR)
Nalbuphine, for obstetric analgesia, 1149
Naloxone, 506, 509, 510, 511, 513, 520, 1149
Naltrexone, 511
Naproxen
   for acute perioperative pain, 1599
   dosing guidelines, 1578t
Narcotics Anonymous (NA), 83
Nasal surgery of airway, 1368–1369, 1369f
National Anesthesia Clinical Outcomes Registry (NACOR), 33, 55
National Center for Immunization and Respiratory Diseases (NCIRD), 75, 103
National Clinical Outcomes Registry (NACOR), 179
National Council of State Boards of Nursing, 32
National Healthcare Safety Network (NHSN), 1651
National Institute for Occupational Safety and Health (NIOSH), 66, 480, 691
National Practitioner Data Bank (NPDB), 34, 100
National Safety Council, 1487
National Surgery Quality Program (NSQIP), 179
National Veterinary Response Team (NVRT), 1690
Natriuretic peptides, 153–154
Nausea, 858
NCIRD. See National Center for Immunization and Respiratory Diseases (NCIRD)
Neck injury, 1504–1505
Necrotizing autoimmune myositis (NAM), 639
Necrotizing enterocolitis (NEC), 1212
Needles
   for epidural anesthesia, 923, 923f, 924f
   ophthalmic anesthesia, complications of, 1385t
   for peripheral nerve blocks, 950–951
   Quincke, 923f
   for regional anesthesia, 950–951
   spinal anesthesia, 923, 923f, 924f
   trauma, 939–940, 939f, 940f
Negative pressure pulmonary edema, 1253
Neodymium:yttrium-aluminum-garnet (Nd:YAG) laser, 1392
Neomycin, 1303
Neonatal anesthesia
   anesthetic agents, neurodevelopmental effects of, 1203
   anesthetic management of neonate, 1191–1201
   infant, physiology and transition period of, 1178–1191
   postoperative apnea and, 1202
   pregnancy, maternal drug use during, 1201
   respiratory distress syndrome and, 1202
   retinopathy of prematurity and, 1202–1203
   surgical procedures in neonates, 1203–1214
   temperature control and, 1201–1202
   thermogenesis and, 1201–1202
Neonatal period, 1178
Neonatal resuscitation algorithm, 1170f
Neonates
   airway, anatomy of, 1185–1186, 1186f
   anesthetic drugs in, 1186–1191
      anticholinergics, 1186
      cis-atracurium, 1188
      desflurane, 1189
      dexmedetomidine, 1186–1187
      edrophonium, 1188
      fentanyl, 1187
      halothane, 1189
      isoflurane, 1189
      ketamine, 1186
      local, 1189–1191
      methadone, 1187
      midazolam, 1186
      morphine, 1187
      neostigmine, 1188
      neuromuscular blocking agents, 1187–1188
      nondepolarizing agents, 1188
      opioids, 1187
      pancuronium, 1188
      propofol, 1186
      remifentanil, 1187
      rocuronium, 1188
      sedative/hypnotics, 1186
      sevoflurane, 1189
      succinylcholine, 1187–1188
      vecuronium, 1188
      volatile agents, 1188–1189
   anesthetic management of, 1191
   baroreceptors, 1180
   blood component therapy in, 1184
   blood gas values in, 1181t
   cardiac output in, 1180
   fluid and electrolyte therapy in, 1183–1184
   heart, 1180
   intraoperative considerations for
      airway management, 1195–1196, 1196f, 1197f
      anesthetic dose requirements, 1198, 1198f
      anesthetic systems, 1195–1196, 1197t
      induction of anesthesia, 1195
      monitoring, 1193–1195
      surgical requirements, impact of, 1197
      uptake and distribution of anesthetics, 1197–1198
   local anesthetic solutions in, 1189–1191
      amides, 1189
      bupivacaine, 1189–1190
      2-chloroprocaine, 1190–1191
      ester, 1190
      levobupivacaine, 1190
      lidocaine, 1190
      management of, 1191
      ropivacaine, 1190
   myocardial function in, 1180
   oxygen for, 1180
   postoperative pain management in, 1200–1201, 1201t
      intravenous analgesia, 1201
      oral routes of medications, 1200
      rectal routes of medications, 1201
   postoperative ventilation in, 1201
   preoperative considerations for
      history, 1191–1192, 1192t
      laboratory investigations, 1193
      physical examination, 1192–1193
      preanesthetic plan, 1193
      premedication, 1193

regional anesthesia techniques in, 1198–1200, 1198t
  brachial plexus block, 1200
  caudal epidural block, 1199, 1199f
  epidural analgesia, 1199
  ilioinguinal nerve block, 1199-1200, 1200f
  lateral femoral cutaneous nerve block, 1200
  neurosurgical blocks, 1200
  penile block, 1199
  spinal anesthesia, 1198–1199
  TAP block, 1200, 1200f
special considerations in
  maternal drug use during pregnancy, 1201
  neurodevelopmental effects of anesthetic agents, 1203
  postoperative apnea, 1202
  respiratory distress syndrome, 1202
  retinopathy of prematurity, 1202–1203
  temperature control, 1201–1202
  thermogenesis, 1201–1202
surgical procedures in, 1203–1214
  central venous catheter, placement of, 1214
  congenital diaphragmatic hernia, 1204–1206
  gastroschisis, 1206–1208
  hydrocephalus, 1211–1212
  inguinal hernia repair, 1212–1213
  lower gastrointestinal tract obstruction, 1210
  myelomeningocele, 1210–1211
  necrotizing enterocolitis, 1212
  omphalocele, 1206–1208
  patent ductus arteriosus, ligation of, 1213–1214
  pyloric stenosis, 1213
  tracheoesophageal fistula, 1208–1209
  upper gastrointestinal tract obstruction, 1209–1210
topical anesthesia in, 1191
ventilator strategies in, 1197t
Neostigmine, 304f, 550–554, 553f, 789, 855t, 1231
  dose ranges, effect of aging on, 903t
  in neonates, 1188
Neosynephrine, 1234
Neovascularization, wound healing, 193–194
Nephrectomy, 1417, 1418f, 1435
  donor, 1419–1420
  incision for, 1417
  intraoperative considerations, 1419
  laparoscopic and robotic, 1420–1422
  nephron-sparing partial, 1417, 1420
  pneumoperitoneum, physiology of, 1422, 1422t
  postoperative considerations, 1419
  preoperative considerations, 1417–1419
  radical, 1420
  simple, 1419–1420
Nephrolithiasis, emergency treatment of, 1436
Nephrology, perioperative
  acid–base disorders, 1407–1408, 1408f
  acute kidney conditions, 1408–1410
  chronic kidney disease, 1410–1415
  electrolyte disorders, 1406–1407
  high renal-risk surgical procedures, 1415–1417
  pathophysiology, 1405
Nephron-sparing partial nephrectomy, 1417, 1420
Nerve damage, 104
Nephrotoxins, 1408
  and perioperative acute kidney injury, 1409–1410, 1409t
Nerves
  agents, 1694–1695
  anatomy of, 564–565

blockade, mechanisms of, 568–569, 568f
fibers, classification of, 566t
injuries, 1555
Neu, M., 9
Neural inertia, 220
Neuraxial anesthesia, 914–942, 1290–1291. See also specific anesthetic agents
  ASRA guidelines for, 1449t
  and hypotension, 1154
  for prostatectomy, 1425
Neuroanatomy, 1004–1006, 1004f, 1005f, 1006f, 1007f, 1007t
Neuroanesthesia, 20
Neuroapoptosis, 1221
Neurogenic shock, 1503
Neuroleptic malignant syndrome (NMS), 621
Neurologic and Adaptive Capacities Score (NACS), 480
Neurologic injury, 939–942, 940f, 941f
Neuromonitoring, in ICU, 1634
Neuromuscular blocking agents (NMBAs), 216, 527–560, 528f, 529f, 1228-1231, 1378–1379, 1378f. See also specific agents
  altered responses to, 538, 539t
  anaphylactic reactions to, 217
  classification, 530
  definition, 528
  depolarizing, 530–533
    characteristics of, 530, 531f
    clinical uses, 533
    contraindications, 533
    neuromuscular effects, 530
    pharmacodynamic properties of, 531t
    pharmacokinetic properties of, 531t
    pharmacology of, 530–531
    side effects of, 531–533, 532f
      anaphylaxis, 533
      fasciculations, 532
      hyperkalemia, 532
      intracranial pressure, 532
      intragastric pressure, 532
      intraocular pressure, 532
      malignant hyperthermia, 532
      masseter muscle spasm, 532–533
      myalgias, 532
  drug interactions
    antibiotics, 538
    anticonvulsants, 538
    β-receptor antagonists, 538
    calcium channel antagonists, 538
    corticosteroids, 538
    depolarizing and nondepolarizing, 537
    with inhalational agents, 537–538
    with local anesthetics, 538
    nondepolarizing, 537
  duration of action for, 530
  management of, 549t
  monitoring
    and clinical applications, 548, 549t, 550, 550f, 550t
    differential muscle sensitivity, 548, 548f
    electrode placement, 548
    modalities, 539, 541–544, 541f–542f, 543t
    and risk-benefit ratio, 538–539
    stimulator characteristics, 539, 540f
    testing and recording response, 544–548, 545t–547t
  morphology of neuromuscular junction, 528, 528f, 529f
  nerve stimulation, 528–529
  nondepolarizing, 530, 533–537
    aminosteroid compounds, 534t, 535–536
    characteristics, 533
    classification of depth of, 550t
    onset and duration of action, 535, 536f
    pharmacology, 533–534, 534t, 535t

    tetrahydroisoquinoline (benzylisoquinolinium) derivatives, 537
  onset of action (onset time) for, 530
  pharmacologic characteristics, 530, 530f
  pharmacology of, 528–530
  physiology of, 528–530
  postsynaptic events, 529
  presynaptic events, 529
  receptor up- and downregulation, 530
  recovery index of, 530
  reversal agents
    anticholinesterase agents, 550–553
    drug shortages and clinical impact, 553–554
    edrophonium, 554
    neostigmine, 551–554
    neuromuscular block, 556, 557t–559t
    in patients with neuromuscular disorders, 556
    sugammadex, 554–557, 557f, 560
  usage of, 528
Neuromuscular junction (NMJ), 528
  morphology of, 528, 528f, 529f
Neuronal excitability, 224
Neuronal plasticity, 1563
Neurosurgery, anesthesia for, 1003–1024
  airway management, 1015
  arteriovenous malformations, 1019–1020
  carotid surgery, 1020–1021
  for cerebral aneurysm, 1018–1019
  cerebral perfusion, 1011–1013
  cerebral protection, 1013–1014
  craniotomy, 1021–1022
  emergence, 1016
  endovascular treatment, 1018–1019
  for epilepsy, 1021
  fluids and electrolytes maintenance, 1015–1016
  glucose management, 1016
  induction of anesthesia, 1015
  maintenance of anesthesia, 1015
  management, 1014–1016
  monitoring, 1009–1011
  neuroanatomy, 1004–1006, 1004f, 1005f, 1006f, 1007f, 1007t
  neurophysiology, 1007–1008, 1008f
  pathophysiology, 1008–1009, 1009f
  for pituitary, 1018
  preoperative evaluation, 1014–1015
  procedures, 1016–1022
  transfusion therapy, 1016
  for tumors, 1016–1018
  ventilatory management, 1015
Neurosurgical blocks, 1200
Neutral grounded power system, 113, 113f
Neutrophils, 206
Newborn resuscitation, in delivery room, 1168–1172
  APGAR score, 1171, 1172t
  diagnostic procedures, 1172
  EXIT procedure, 1172
  fetal asphyxia, 1169
  neonatal adaptations at birth, 1169
  resuscitation, 1169–1171, 1170f
    chest compressions, 1171
    initial appraisal of newborn, 1169, 1171
    initial stabilization, 1171
    medications and volume expansion, 1171
    respirations and heart rate assessment, 1171
    therapeutic guidelines, 1171t
    ventilation, 1171
Newborns. See also Infant; Neonates
  circumcision of, 1435
  period, 1178
Newsletter (ASA), 33
New York Society of Anesthetists, 21, 22

Next-generation sequencing (NGS) technology, 147
Ngai, Shuh-Hsun, 10
Nicardipine, 326t, 327
NICOM, 1642
Nicotine, 351
Nicotinic acetylcholine receptors (nAChRs), 528, 529, 529f
Nicotinic effect, 342
Niemann, Albert, 13
Nifedipine, 325, 326t, 327
Night call, 70–71
Nimodipine, 326t, 327, 1637
NIOSH. See National Institute for Occupational Safety and Health (NIOSH)
Nirvaquine, 13
Nitroglycerin, 324, 1639
  for myocardial ischemia, 1080–1081
Nitroprusside, in preeclampsia, 1158–1159
Nitrous oxide (N_2O), 3, 469, 472–473, 474, 1243, 1288
  for analgesia during labor, 1151
  and anesthesia machine, 658–659
  production of, 3
  solubilities of, 1381t
Nitrovasodilators, 324–325
  nitroglycerin, 324
  sodium nitroprusside, 324–325
N-methyl-D-aspartate (NMDA) receptors, 494, 508, 1566, 1568f, 1579, 1600, 1609
Nociception/orphanin FQ (NOP) receptor, 507, 508
Nociceptors, 508, 1608
Nodes of Ranvier, 564, 565f
Noise pollution, 68–69, 69t
Nominal variables, 166
Nonalcoholic fatty liver disease (NAFLD), 1315–1316
Nonalcoholic steatohepatitis (NASH), 1309, 1468
Non-A, non-B hepatitis (NANBH), 75
Noncardiac surgical procedures, 1415–1417
Noncompartmental pharmacokinetic methods, 252
Noncompetitive antagonists, 254
Non-Hodgkin's lymphoma, 1237
Nonimmobilizers, 222
Noninvasive positive pressure ventilation (NPPV), 1287, 1643–1644
Nonoperating room anesthesia (NORA)
  Arrhythmia classification, 892t
  ASA standards for, 882t
  computed tomography, 887
  continuum of anesthesia, 883, 883t
  electroconvulsive therapy, 893
  environmental considerations for, 863–885
  equipment required for, 868t
  gastroenterology, 872, 889, 890
  hypersensitivity reactions, 885, 886t
  interventional cardiology, 890–893
  interventional neuroradiology, 886–887
  intravenous contrast agents, 885
  magnetic resonance imaging, 888
  nonoperating room procedures, 885–893
  orthopedics and podiatry, 872
  patient safety in, 882–883
  patient transfer, 883
  pediatric sedation, 888
  positron emission tomography, 889
  preprocedural checklists, 882–883
  procedures, 881t
  radiation therapy, 888–889
  radiofrequency ablation, 887
  sedation and anesthesia, 883
  standards of care for, 883
  three-step paradigm for, 881t
  X-rays and fluoroscopy, 883–885

Nonopioid receptors, 508
Nonparametric tests, 174
Nonsteroidal anti-inflammatory drugs (NSAIDs), 14, 449, 853, 1232–1233, 1409, 1577, 1578t, 1579, 1599
Norepinephrine (NE), 308–309t, 311–312, 339, 340–342, 935
Norketamine, 1228
Normal equation, 166
Normal saline, 1248
North American Symptomatic Carotid Endarterectomy (NASCET) trial, 1121–1122
Nortriptyline, 1621t
Nosocomial infections, in ICU, 1650–1653
Nosworthy, Michael, 22
NP. See Nucleoprotein (NP)
NSAIDs. See Nonsteroidal anti-inflammatory drugs (NSAIDs)
Nucleoprotein (NP), 73
Nucleus basalis of Meynert (NBM), 235
Null hypothesis, 170, 171
Numerous Cases of Surgical Operations Without Pain in the Mesmeric State, 2
Nu-trake, 804
Nutritional deficiency anemias, 633
Nutrition, in critically ill patient, 1648
Nyquist limit, 743

O

Obesity
  abnormalities of liver, 1278, 1283, 1284
  ambulatory anesthesia in, 1292–1293
  android, 1278
  anesthetic implications of, 1280t
  cardiovascular effects of, 1237–1238
  in children, 1237–1238
  classification on waist circumference, 1278, 1278t
  conditions, 1278
  critical care, 1293
  definitions, 1278
    children, 1237–1238
    World Health Organization (WHO), 1277
  drug dosing, 1238t
  epidemiology, 1277–1279
  expiratory reserve volume (ERV), effect on, 1279
  functional residual capacity (FRC), effect on, 1279, 1280f
  glomerular hyperfiltration of, 1283
  gynecoid (peripheral), 1278
  incidence of severe pneumonitis, 1288
  insulin resistance, 1238
  intraoperative considerations
    airway management, 1287–1288, 1287f
    anesthesia care and sedation, monitored, 1289–1290
    emergence, 1289, 1289f
    equipment and monitoring, 1287
    fluid management, 1288
    induction and maintenance, 1288
    mechanical ventilation, 1288–1289
    neuraxial anesthesia, 1290–1291
    peripheral nerve blocks, 1291–1292
    regional anesthesia, 1290–1292
  intravenous drug dosing in, 1285t
  management of
    antiobesity medications, 1278
    bariatric surgery, 1279
    combined procedures, 1279
    lifestyle counseling, 1278
    malabsorptive procedures, 1279
    medical therapy, 1278–1279
    restrictive procedures, 1279
  medical consequences of, 1280t
  morbid, 1278
  morbidity and mortality, postoperative, 1293
  pathophysiology
    cardiovascular system, 1281–1283, 1281f, 1282f
    gastrointestinal system, 1283
    hematologic system, 1281–1283
    renal and endocrine systems, 1283–1284
    respiratory system, 1279–1281, 1280f
  perioperative respiratory events, 1238
  pharmacology
    perioperative agents, 1284, 1286
    principles, 1284, 1284f
  postoperative considerations
    analgesia, 1292, 1292t
    monitoring, 1292
    ventilatory evaluation and management, 1292
  in pregnancy, 1163–1164
  preoperative evaluation, 1286–1287
    airway assessment, 1286
    cardiopulmonary systems, 1286
    hematologic issues, 1286–1287
    metabolic and nutritional abnormalities, 1286
  and resuscitation, 1293
  volume of drug distribution in, 1284
Obesity hypoventilation (Pickwickian) syndrome (OHS), 1281
Observational study, 167
Observer's Assessment of Alertness/Sedation Scale, 841t
Obstetrical anesthesia, 20–21, 1144–1174
  cesarean delivery and, 1152–1154
  complications, 1154–1155
    hypotension, 1154–1155
    local anesthetic systemic toxicity, 1155
    maternal mortality, 1154
    nerve injury, 1155
    postdural puncture headache, 1155
    pulmonary aspiration, 1154
    total spinal anesthesia, 1155
  fetal monitoring, 1166–1168
  high-risk parturients, management of, 1155–1164
  labor and vaginal delivery and, 1148–1152
  nonobstetric surgery in pregnant woman, 1172–1174
  physiologic changes of pregnancy and, 1145–1146
  placental transfer and fetal exposure to anesthetic drugs, 1147–1148
  preterm delivery and, 1164–1165
  substance abuse and, 1165–116
Obstetric hemorrhage, 1159–1161
Obstructive pulmonary disease, anesthesia and, 379
Obstructive sleep apnea (OSA), 506, 518, 589, 597–598, 1228, 1280–1281, 1358–1360, 1549
  overnight polysomnography for, 1281
  pediatrics, preoperative assessments, 1235
Obturator nerve, 962
  block, 989–990, 990f
Occipital nerve, 955–956, 956f
  blocks, 967
Occipital neurostimulation (ONS), 1626
Occupational health
  emotional considerations
    addiction, 82–83
    aging anesthesiologist, 84
    burnout, 81–82
    disability, 84
    impairment, 84
    mortality rates, 84

stress, 81
substance use, 82–83
suicide, 84–85
infectious hazards
Creutzfeldt–Jakob disease, 80
DNA viruses, 74–75
measles (rubeola), 75
OSHA standards, 71–72
pathogenic human retroviruses, 79–80
prion diseases, 80
respiratory viruses, 73–74
rubella, 75
standard precautions, 71–72, 71t–72t
transmission-based precautions, 71–72
tuberculosis, 80–81
viral hepatitis, 75, 77t, 78–79
viruses in smoke plumes, 81
physical hazards
allergic reactions, 67–68
anesthetic gases, 66–67
chemicals, 67
ergonomics/human factors, 69–70
fatigue, 70–71
night call, 70–71
noise pollution, 68–69, 69t
radiation, 68
work hours, 70–71
wellness
fitness, 85
lifestyle-related diseases, 85
mindfullness, 85–86
nutrition/diet, 85, 86f
Occupational HIV infection, 79–80
Occupational Safety and Health Administration (OSHA), 68, 868
standards, 71–72
Ocular anatomy, 1374–1375, 1374f
Ocular injuries, 1272
Ocular physiology, 1375–1377
aqueous humor, formation and drainage of, 1375, 1375f
glaucoma, 1376–1377
intraocular pressure, maintenance of, 1375–1376
Oculocardiac reflex, 1379
Oculopharyngeal muscular dystrophy, 614
Oculosympathetic paresis. See Horner syndrome
O'Dwyer, Joseph, 5, 769
Office-based anesthesia (OBA)
accreditation, 870–871
advantages, 864–865
anesthetic agents for, 873–875
anesthetic techniques, 873–875
business aspects, 876
causes of injury, 866t
disadvantages, 864–865
equipment required for, 868t
historical perspective of, 864–865
legal aspects, 876
office selection, 868–871
otolaryngology procedures, 873
patient selection, 866–867, 867t
postanesthesia care unit, 875
procedure selection, 871–873
regulations, 875–876
safety issues, 865–866
state regulation of, 864t
surgeon selection, 867–868
Off-pump coronary artery bypass (OPCAB), 1104–1105
Ohmeda Excel 210 machines, 667
Ohmeda Modulus II plus machines, 667
Ohm's law, 109
OKT3 monoclonal antibody, 1464
Oleum vitrioli dulce, 3
Oliguria, 1551–1552

Omeprazole, 787
Omphalocele, 1206–1207, 1206f
antenatal diagnosis of, 1207
perioperative care, 1207–1208
postoperative care, 1208
preoperative care, 1207
On Chloroform and Other Anaesthetics, 5
Oncotic pressure, 395
Ondansetron, 17, 1249, 1254
One-lung ventilation (OLV), 479
indications for
absolute, 1040–1041, 1041t
relative, 1041, 1041t
lung separation
double-lumen endobronchial tubes, 1041–1045
in patient with difficult airway, 1046–1050
in patient with permanent tracheostomy, 1045–1046
management of, 1050–1054
clinical approach, 1053–1054, 1053t
confirmation of position of DLT, 1051
dependent lung, PEEP to, 1052
inspired oxygen fraction, 1051
nondependent lung, CPAP to, 1052–1053
tidal volume and respiratory rate, 1051–1052
nitric oxide and, 1056
physiology of, 1038–1040, 1038f–1040f
On the Inhalation of the Vapour of Ether, 5
Operating room (OR), 586
conductive flooring, 127
construction of, 129–130
contamination, sources of, 66t
electrical power to, 117, 118f
electrical safety in, 126–127
electromagnetic interference, 128–129
environmental hazards, 127–128, 127f
fire
algorithm, 1736f, 1737
drills, 135
ignition sources, 131–132, 132t
prevention and management of, 130t, 1736f
safety, 130–137, 135f–137f
triangle, 131f
types of, 131
ground fault circuit interrupters in, 122, 122f
grounding of equipment, 113t
management, anesthesiologists in, 56–61
organization, 56–57
personnel issues, 60–61
scheduling cases, 57–60
Ophthalmic drugs, anesthetic ramifications of
anticholinesterase agents, 1380
betaxolol, 1381
cocaine, 1380
cyclopentolate, 1380
epinephrine, 1380
intraocular perfluorocarbons, 1381, 1381t
phenylephrine, 1380–1381
systemic, 1381
timolol, 1381
Ophthalmologic procedures, 872
Ophthalmologic surgery
adjuncts and, 1387–1388
anesthesia, effects of
adjuncts drugs, 1378–1379, 1379t
central nervous system depressants, 1377
hyperventilation, 1377
hypothermia, 1377
hypoventilation, 1377
temperature, 1377
ventilation, 1377
anesthesia techniques, 1383–1389
choice of, 1387–1388
anesthetic management in

intraocular surgery, 1390, 1390t
laser therapy, 1392
"open-eye, full-stomach" encounters, 1389–1390
retinal detachment surgery, 1390–1391
strabismus surgery, 1391–1392
block adjuvants and, 1387–1388
cannula-based anesthesia, 1386–1387, 1387f
"open-eye, full-stomach" encounters, 1389–1390
postoperative complications, 1392–1396
acute glaucoma, 1396
chemical injury, 1393
corneal abrasion, 1393
cortical blindness, 1396
hemorrhagic retinopathy, 1394
ischemic optic neuropathy, 1394–1396
mild visual symptoms, 1393
photic injury, 1393
postcataract ptosis, 1396
retinal ischemia, 1394
preoperative evaluation
anesthesia options, 1383
establishing rapport and assessing medical condition, 1381–1383
safety protocols, 1383
side of anesthesia, 1383
techniques of anesthesia, 1383–1389
principles of monitored anesthesia care, 1388–1389
requirements of, 1374t
topical analgesia, 1387
Opiate pain relievers (OPR), 82
Opioid-induced hyperalgesia (OIH), 505, 508, 510–511, 1572
and tolerance, 510–511
Opioid-induced respiratory depression
incidence and risk factors of, 518–520, 519f
mechanisms, 518, 518f
monitoring, 521–522, 522f, 523f
versus opioid analgesia, 520, 521f
reversal of, 520–521
Opioids, 14, 505–524, 571, 607–608, 853, 933, 1231–1233, 1289, 1290, 1412. *See also specific drug*
acetaminophen, 1232
agonists, 511
analgesics for acute pain, 1572, 1573t, 1574–1577
antagonists, 511
for cardiac surgery, 1080
central analgesia, 508–509, 509f
chemical structures of, 507f
for chronic pain, 1622t
codeine, 1232
diclofenac, 1232
endogenous system, 507–508
equianalgesic dosing, 1574t
exogenous, classification of, 511
fentanyl, 1231
gender differences, 524
history, 506–507
hydromorphone, 1232
ibuprofen, 1232
induced respiratory depression, 518–522, 518f–519f, 521f–523f
ketorolac, 1232
for labor analgesia, 1149–1150
mechanisms, 508–511
meperidine, 1231
metabolism, 512–513
for monitored anesthetic care, 833–834
morphine, 1231
multiple, targeting of, 508
natural, 511
in neonates, 1187

Opioids (continued)
  nonopioid receptors and, 508
  OIH and, 510–511
  for pain management, 1619–1620
  pain relief and, 514–516, 514f
  peripheral analgesia, 509–510, 510f
  pharmacodynamics, 514–517, 514f
  pharmacogenetics, 517–518, 517f
  pharmacokinetic–pharmacodynamic models of, 513–514, 514f
  pharmacokinetics, 511–512, 511f
  potency, 511
  in pregnancy, 1165
  remifentanil, 524, 1231–1232
  respiratory depression and, 1574t
  sedation and, 1574t
  semisynthetic, 511
  side effects, 522
    cardiovascular effects, 523–524
    postoperative nausea and vomiting, 522–523
    smooth muscle effects, 523
  synthetic, 511
  tolerance, 510–511, 1598
  withdrawal, 1598
Opium, 506
OPR. See Opiate pain relievers (OPR)
Opsonization, 206
Optical stylets, 783
Optimal external laryngeal manipulation, 781
OR. See Operating room (OR)
Oral premedications for children, 1243
Orbital cone, 1384
Orchiopexy, 1435
Order statistics, 174
Ordinal data, 166
Oré, Pierre, 12
Organ aging, physiology of, 900
  body composition, changes in, 900, 900f
  cardiovascular, 902, 904
  central nervous system, 901
  drug pharmacology and, 901–902, 901f, 902f, 903t
  kidney, 900
  liver, 900
  pulmonary, 904–905, 905f
  thermoregulation and, 905
Organ donors, anesthetic management of, 1459–1463
  brain-dead donors, 1459–1460
  donation after cardiac death, 1460–1461, 1461t
  living kidney donors, 1461
  living liver donors, 1462–1463
Organ dysfunction, 538
Organic anion polypeptide transporters (OATPs), 243
Organophosphate poisoning, 354
Organophosphates, 304
Orlistat, 1279
Oropharyngeal airway, obstruction of, 1358
Orotracheal intubation, 20
Orthomyxoviridae, 73
Orthopedic surgery
  analgesia for, 1446t
  anesthesia for, 1441–1454
  anesthetic technique, selection of, 1442
  to lower extremity, 1449–1452
    anesthetic techniques for, 1451t
    hip, 1449–1451, 1450f
    knee, 1451–1452
    nerve blocks for, 1451t
    pelvis, 1449–1451
  pediatric, 1452–1453
  preoperative assessment, 1442
  special considerations
    acute compartment syndrome, 1453
    amputation, 1453
    fat embolus syndrome, 1453–1454, 1454t
    microvascular surgery, 1453
    thromboprophylaxis, 1454
    tourniquets, 1453
    venous thromboembolism, 1454
  spine surgery, anesthesia for
    blood conservation in, 1443
    complications of, 1445–1446
    injury, 1444
    muscular disorders, 1445
    positioning for, 1443, 1443f
    postoperative care, 1445
    preoperative evaluation for, 1442–1443
    scoliosis, 1444–1445
    spinal cord monitoring, 1444
    vertebral column disease, 1445
  to upper extremity, 1446–1449
    elbow, wrist, and hand, 1448–1449
    shoulder, 1447–1448
    upper arm, 1447–1448
Orthostatic hypotension, 358
OSHA. See Occupational Safety and Health Administration (OSHA)
Osmolality, 395
Osmolarity, 395
Osmotic demyelination syndrome, 402
Osmotic diuretics, 1414
Osserman staging system for myasthenia gravis, 617t
Osteogenesis imperfecta (OI), 632–633, 632t
Otolaryngologic surgery, anesthesia for
  adult surgery, 1367–1371
  airway evaluation, 1357
  pediatric
    airway emergencies, 1366–1367
    ear, nose, and throat surgery, 1357–1365
    surgery, 1367–1371
Ottenberg, Reuben, 21
Outcome of care, 101
Out-of-plane (OOP) needling, 949, 950f
Ovassapian intubating oral airway, 800, 800f
Overnight polysomnography (OPS), 1281
Overwhelming postsplenectomy infection (OPSI), 634
Oxaprozin, dosing guidelines, 1578t
Oxcarbazepine
  dosage range, 1621t
  side effects, 1621
Oxidations, 244–245
Oxybarbiturate, 13
Oxycodone, 1570, 1570f, 1574
  pharmacokinetics, 1573t
Oxygen
  analyzer calibration, 652–653. See also Anesthesia workstations
  concentration, monitoring of
    contraindications, 708
    galvanic cell analyzers, 708
    indications, 708
    paramagnetic oxygen analyzers, 708
    polarographic oxygen analyzers, 708
    principles of operation, 708
    problems and limitations, 708
    use and interpretation, 708
  delivery as a goal of management, 398
  desaturation, 1245, 1253
  flowmeter assembly, 661f
  flush positive-pressure leak test, 653, 654f
  flush valve, 667–668
  thoracic surgery and, 1037–1038
  transport of
    bulk flow of gas, 371
    gas diffusion, 371
    physiologic dead space, 373–374
    physiologic shunt, 374–376
    ventilation and perfusion, distribution of, 372–373, 372f, 373f
Oxygen consumption index (VO_2I), 1519
Oxygen delivery index (DO_2I), 1519
Oxygen delivery meters, high-pressure, 803
Oxygen failure cutoff valves, 656, 660, 660f
Oxygen Failure Protection Device (OFPD), 660, 661f
Oxygen Ratio Monitor Controller (ORMC), 666–667, 666f
Oxymetazoline, 1234
Oxymorphone, pharmacokinetics, 1573t
Oxytocin, 1160t

P

PA. See Pulmonary artery (PA)
PAC. See Pulmonary artery catheter (PAC)
Pacemakers, 1724
  permanent, indications for, 1724–1725
Pace sign, piriformis syndrome, 1616
Pacinian corpuscles, 1608t
$PaCO_2$, 1008
  determination of, 374
  ventilatory responses to, 374
PACU. See Postanesthesia care unit (PACU)
PAD. See Peripheral artery disease; Peripheral artery disease (PAD)
Padding materials, 811
Pagés–Dogliotti single-injection technique, 18
Pagés, Fidel, 19
Pain. See also Pain management
  acute, 1563
    anatomy of, 1563–1565, 1564f, 1565f, 1565t, 1566f
    assessment of, 1570–1572, 1571f, 1572t
    in children, management of, 1601–1603
    classes of, 1571t
    definition, 1563
    management, strategies for, 1568–1570, 1569t, 1570f
    and methods of analgesia, 1582–1597
    nonopioid analgesic adjuncts for, 1577–1582, 1578t, 1602
    opioid analgesics for, 1572, 1573t, 1574–1577
    opioid-dependent patient, management of, 1598–1601, 1599t
    pain processing, 1563–1565, 1565f, 1566f
    perioperative pain management services for, 1601
    poor management, consequences of, 1568t
    preventive analgesia for, 1568
    and regional anesthesia, 1597–1598, 1597t
    surgical stress response to, 1566, 1568
  allogenic substances, 1567t
  cancer, 1618–1619
    celiac plexus block, 1618–1619, 1618f
    cortical connections, 1610
    ganglion impar block, 1619
    higher cortical processing, 1610
    limbic connections, 1610
  neuropathic, 1568
  perception, 1564–1565
  postoperative, 1254
  processing
    acute to persistent/chronic nociception, transition from, 1610–1611
    anatomy of, 1608–1611
    ascending pathways, 1610
    cortical, neurobiology of supraspinal structures, 1610
    descending pathways, 1610
    neurochemistry of, 1608–1611
    peripheral nerve and dorsal root ganglion, 1609

peripheral stimulation, 1608, 1608t
physiology of, 1608–1611
primary afferents, 1608, 1608t
spinal cord and spinal trigeminal nucleus, 1609–1610, 1609f
receptors, 1566
sensation, 1610
sensitization, 1565f
spinohypothalamic connections, 1610
superior hypogastric plexus block, 1619
syndromes, management of
buttock pain, 1614–1616
complex regional pain, 1617
diabetic painful neuropathy, 1617
facet, 1614, 1614f
fibromyalgia, 1616
herpes zoster, 1616–1617
HIV sensory neuropathy, 1617–1618
low back pain, 1611–1614
myofascial pain, 1616
neuropathic pain, 1616–1618
phantom limb, 1613
piriformis, 1615–1616
postherpetic neuralgia, 1616–1617
radicular pain, 1611–1614, 1612f, 1613f
sacroiliac joint, 1614–1615, 1615f
transduction, chemical mediators of, 1565–1566, 1566f, 1567f, 1567t
transmission, chemical mediators of, 1565–1566, 1566f, 1567f, 1567t

Pain management
drugs for chronic, 1622t
fluid for, 1249–1250
caudal blockade, 1249–1250
epidural block, 1250
spinal block, 1250
interventional techniques
discography, 1622–1623
dorsal root ganglion stimulation, 1626
intradiscal electrothermal therapy, 1623
intrathecal drug delivery, 1626, 1627f, 1628
kyphoplasty, 1623–1624
minimally invasive lumbar decompression procedure, 1623
occipital neurostimulation, 1626
peripheral nerve stimulation, 1624, 1626
spinal cord stimulation, 1624, 1625f
vertebroplasty, 1623–1624, 1623f
pharmacologic, 1619–1622
anticonvulsants, 1621, 1621t
antidepressants, 1620–1621, 1621t
buprenorphine–naloxone therapy, 1622
cannabinoids, 1622
capsaicin patch, 1621–1622
intravenous lidocaine, 1621–1622
lidocaine patch, 1621–1622
mexiletine, 1622
of neuropathic pain, 1620–1622
opioids, 1619–1620

Pain response, genetic variability in, 158
Pal, Jacob, 14
Pancreas transplantation, 1472
Pancuronium, 534t, 535–536, 1412
dose ranges, effect of aging on, 903t
in neonates, 1188
Papillary muscle, 279
Papillomatosis of vocal cords, 1363
Paracervical block, for labor and vaginal delivery, 1151
Paracetamol, 1577f, 1579
Paradoxical breathing, 1038, 1039f
Paraglossal approach, 782
Paramagnetic oxygen analyzers, 708
Parametric test statistics, 172
Paraplegia, 816

Parasympatholytics, before thoracic surgery, 1035
Parathyroid diseases, 599, 599t
Parathyroidectomy, 1334
Parathyroid glands, 1332–1335
anesthesia for parathyroid surgery, 1334
calcium physiology, 1332, 1333f
hyperparathyroidism, 1332–1334
hypoparathyroidism, 1334–1335
Parathyroid hormone (PTH), 409
Paravertebral block, 980–982, 980f, 982f
Paravertebral lumbar sympathetic block
for labor and vaginal delivery, 1151
Paravertebral spaces (PVS), 956, 1592
Pardee, Harold, 10
Parecoxib, 855t
Parental presence at induction of anesthesia (PPIA), 1242
Parenteral direct thrombin inhibitors, 452
Parenteral nutrition (PN), 1648
Park bench position, 822–823, 823f
Parkinson disease (PD), 620–621
Parkland formulas, for fluid resuscitation, 1515–1516, 1515f
Paroxetine, 1621t
Partial agonists, 254
Partial pressure of gas, 462
Partial thromboplastin time (PTT), 1092, 1307
Passive transport, 242
Patent ductus arteriosus (PDA), ligation of, 1213–1214
Pathogenic human retroviruses, 79–80
occupational risk of HIV transmission, 79
postexposure treatment, 80
prophylactic antiretroviral therapy, 80
Pathogen inactivation, 429–430. See also Blood
Patient-controlled analgesia (PCA), 1554
for adult patient, 1582, 1582t
for children, 1602
during monitored anesthesia care, 836–837
risk factors with, 1582t
Patient-controlled epidural analgesia (PCEA), 1150
Patient monitoring, pediatric anesthesia, 1240
anesthetic depth, 1241
capnography, 1240
temperature, 1240–1241
Patient positioning, 809. See also specific position
and complications, 809–825
general principles, 809–811
head-down positions, 824
complications of, 824–825
head-elevated positions
complications of, 823–824
lateral position with elevated head, 822–823, 823f
sitting, 822, 822f
supine recumbent position, 822
ischemia and, 811
lateral positions, 816–817
complications of, 817, 819
flexed, 817, 818f
semisupine and semiprone, 817, 818f
standard, 817, 817f
prone position
complications of, 820–822
full prone, 819–820, 820f
supine position
complications of, 813–816
contoured, 811, 811f
horizontal, 810f, 811
lateral uterine/abdominal mass displacement, 811
lithotomy, 811–813, 812f, 813f
and tissue damage, 810–811
Patient Protection and Affordable Care Act, 27, 28

Patient transfer device (PTD), lifting device, 1289, 1289f
Pay for performance (P4P program), 53
PCA. See Pulse contour analysis (PCA)
PEAA. See Percutaneous emergency airway access
Pectoralis nerve blockade, 1593
Pediatric advanced life support cardiac arrest algorithm, 1677f
Pediatric anesthesia emergence delirium (PAED), 1253
Pediatric cardiopulmonary resuscitation, 1676–1678
advanced life support cardiac arrest algorithm, 1677f
bradycardia, algorithm for, 1679f
medications for resuscitation, 1678t
tachycardia, algorithm for, 1680f
Pediatric heart transplantation, 1480
Pediatric liver transplantation, 1471
Pediatric lung transplantation, 1475
Pediatric orthopedic anesthesia, 1452–1453
Pediatric patients
anesthesia in
emergence and recovery from, 1250–1251, 1252t
induction of, 1239–1242. See also Induction techniques, pediatric
perioperative pain in
management of, 1602
nonopioid analgesics, 1602
opioid analgesics, 1602
Pediatric Regional Anesthesia Network (PRAN), 1453
Pediatric renal transplantation, 1467
Pediatric surgical urologic disorders, 1435
Pediatric tracheal tube sizes, 782, 782t
PEEP. See Positive end-expiratory pressure (PEEP)
Peer review organizations, 38
PELD Score, 1467–1468
Pelvic fractures, 1511
Pelvis, surgery to, 1449
ambulatory, 1451
anesthesia technique, 1450
approach, 1449–1450
blood loss and transfusion, 1451
positioning, 1449–1450, 1450f
Pemphigus, 641
Penetrating cardiac injury, 1506
Penicillin allergy, 1238
Penicillin skin testing, 215
Penile block, 985–986, 1199
Pentax Airway Scope, 786f
PEP. See Postexposure prophylaxis (PEP)
PEPline. See Post-Exposure Prophylaxis Hotline
Percent fractional area change, 748f, 750
Percent Fractional Shortening (%FS), 748, 749–750
Percent of glottic opening (POGO) score, 781
Percutaneous coronary intervention (PCI), 1639
Percutaneous cricothyrotomy systems, 804
Percutaneous emergency airway access (PEAA), 792, 802–804, 803f
Percutaneous nephrolithotomy (PNL), 1433
Percutaneous Transtracheal Jet Ventilation (PTJV), 803
Percutaneous Ventricular Assist Devices, 890
Periaqueductal gray (PAG), 508, 1610
Pericardial tamponade, 1506
Pericardium, 296–297, 297f
Perifornical area (PF), 235
Perineural Human Research Drugs, 855t
Perineurium, 564
Perioperative aspiration, 1550–1551
Perioperative atrial fibrillation (PoAF), 154–155

Perioperative Beta Blockade (POBBLE) trial, 1115
Perioperative blood cell salvage, 441
Perioperative genomics, 142
PeriOperative ISchemic Evaluation (POISE-1) trial, 1115
Perioperative medicine, anesthesiologists in, 55–56
Perioperative pain management, anesthetic administration for
  caudal blockade, 1249–1250
  epidural block, 1250
  spinal block, 1250
Perioperative precision medicine, 141–142, 143f
Perioperative surgical home (PSH), 28–30, 29f, 897
Peripheral arterial catheterization, thoracic surgery and, 1036
Peripheral artery disease (PAD)
  endovascular management of, 1138–1139
  endovascular repair of, 1138–1139
  surgery for, 1133–1134
Peripheral chemoreceptors, 368–369
Peripheral nerve blocks (PNBs), 945–998, 1291–1292, 1585
  assessment and monitoring, 952
  benefits of, 945–946
  bolus for, 947
  brachial plexus, 1585, 1586t, 1588–1589, 1588f, 1589f
  caveats, 1596–1597
  in children, 1602–1603
  clinical anatomy, 953–963
    head and neck, 954–956, 954f, 955f, 956f
    lower extremity, 960–963, 960f–962f
    spine, 955f, 956
    trunk, 959–960, 960f
    upper extremity, 956–959, 957f–958f
  complications, prevention of, 952–953
  continuous, 1585, 1587t
  continuous-infusion catheter kits for, 951–952
  and discharge criteria, 952
  documentation for, 947
  drug selection and toxicity, 953
  general principles and equipment, 946–953
  head and neck techniques, 963–967
    cervical plexus blocks, 965–967
    occipital nerve blocks, 967
    trigeminal nerve blocks, 963–965
  lower extremity techniques, 986–998
    ankle block, 996–998, 997f
    psoas compartment block, 986–988, 986f, 987f
    sciatic nerve block, 991–996, 992f, 993f, 994f, 995f
    separate blocks of terminal nerves, 988–991, 989f, 990f, 991f
  lumbar plexus, 1586t, 1589–1590, 1590f, 1591f
  monitoring for, 947
  nerve damage and other complications, 953
  for pain management, 1585–1597
  patient selection for, 952–953
  penile block, 985–986
  premedication for, 947
  sacral plexus, 1586t, 1590–1592, 1592f
  sedation for, 947
  setup for, 946–947, 946f
    block room supplies, 946–947
    catheters, 951–952
    needles, 950–951
  techniques for
    nerve stimulation, 948, 948f
    ultrasound imaging, 948–950, 950f, 951t
  trunk nerve blocks, 978–985
    ilioinguinal and iliohypogastric nerve blocks, 984–985, 985f
    intercostal nerve block, 978–980, 979f
    paravertebral block, 980–982, 980f, 982f
    rectus sheath block, 983–984, 984f
    transversus abdominis plane block, 982–983, 983f
  upper extremity techniques, 967–978
    brachial plexus block, 967–974
    intravenous regional anesthesia (Bier block), 977–978
    terminal block, 974–977
  US-guided, 949
  wound infiltration, 1596
Peripheral nerves, neurochemistry of, 1609
Peripheral nerve stimulation (PNS), 888, 1624, 1626
Peripheral opioid analgesia, 509–510, 510f
Periportal necrosis, 1157
Periscope stent, 1136, 1136f
Peritonsillar abscess, 1361
Permanent gases, 461
Peroneal nerves, 961
Per se rule, Sherman Antitrust Act, 50
Persistent pulmonary hypertension of newborn (PPHN), 1182
Personality, 81
Personal protective equipment (PPE), 72
P-glycoprotein (P-gp), 243, 517–518
Phantom limb pain, 1618
Pharmacodynamics, 252, 460
  concentration–response relationships, 255–258
  definition, 460
  dose–response relationships, 255
  drug–receptor interactions, 253–255
  effect of hypovolemia on, 1521, 1521f
  intravenous anesthetics and, 261–272
  renal system, 1226–1227
  respiration, 1225–1226
  in vitro metabolism, 1227
Pharmacodynamic variability, 157
  perioperative drugs and, 158, 159t
Pharmacogenomics, 157
  and anesthesia, 157–159
Pharmacokinetic–pharmacodynamic (PKPD) model
  combined, 256
  of opioids, 513–514, 514t
Pharmacokinetics, 242. *See also specific drugs*
  compartmental models, 248
    one-compartment model, 250–251
    three-compartment model, 252–253, 252f
    two-compartment model, 251–252, 251f
  definition, 460
  drug absorption and administration routes
    inhalational administration, 244
    intramuscular and subcutaneous administration, 243
    intrathecal, epidural, and perineural injection, 243–244
    intravenous administration, 243
    oral administration, 243
    transcutaneous administration, 243
    transfer across membranes, 242–243
  drug distribution, 244
  drug elimination, 244
    biotransformation reactions, 244
    cytochromes P450 enzymes, 245, 245t
    elimination clearance, 244
    hepatic drug clearance, 246–248, 247f, 248t
    phase I reactions, 244–245
    phase II reactions, 245
    renal drug clearance, 246, 246t
  drug metabolism
    chronologic variations in, 246
    genetic variations in, 245–246
  effect of hepatic or renal disease on, 250
  effect of hypovolemia on, 1521, 1521f
  elimination half-life, 249–250
  first-order kinetic process, 248
  half-life of, 248–249, 249t
  front-end, 268–269
  high-risk, 158–159
  intravenous anesthetics, 261–272, 486–489, 487f, 488f, 489f
  noncompartmental (stochastic) models, 253
  nonlinear, 250
  opioid analgesic, 1573t
  physiologic models, 248
  total drug clearance, 249
  volume of distribution, 249
Pharmacokinetic variability, 157
  perioperative drugs and, 158, 159t
Pharmacology
  age/aging and, 901–902
  age and absorption of drugs, 1221–1222
  bioavailability, factors influencing, 1221–1222
  developmental, 1221–1223
  free fraction of medications, 1222
  inhalational anesthetics
    pharmacodynamics, 1225–1227
    pharmacokinetics, 1223–1225
    pharmacology of, 1223t
    washin and washout of, 1223t
  intravenous
    etomidate, 1228
    ketamine, 1228
    neuromuscular blocking agents, 1228–1231
    opioids, 1231–1233
    propofol, 1227–1228
    sedatives, 1233
  metabolism in liver, 1222
  midazolam, 1221
  in obesity
    perioperative agents, 1284, 1286
    principles, 1284, 1284f
  phase 1 reactions, 1222, 1222f
  phase 2 reactions, 1222
  proteins binding medications, 1222
  rectal venous administration, effect of, 1222
  route of administration, 1222
Pharyngeal bulb gasway, 769
Pharyngitis, 74
Phencyclidine (PCP), 13, 493, 494
Phenobarbital, 13
Phenotypes, perioperative, 142t
Phenotypic switch, A beta (Aβ) fibers, 1611
Phenoxybenzamine, 315
Phentermine (Adipex-P), 1278–1279
Phentolamine, 315
Phenylephrine, 308–309t, 314, 346, 855t, 931, 935
  for maternal hypotension, 1154
  ophthalmic use, 1380–1381
Pheochromocytoma
  anesthetic considerations, 1341–1343
  clinical presentation, 1340
  description, 1340
  diagnosis of, 1340–1341, 1341f
  drugs in management of, 1342t
Phlebotomy, 428
Pholcodine, 1228
Phosphate
  hyperphosphatemia, 413–414, 1407
  hypophosphatemia, 413, 1407
  physiologic role, 412–413
Phosphodiesterase inhibitors, 321–322, 322t, 1035
Phosphodiesterase isoenzyme (PDE III), type III, 321
Phosphoinositides, 409
Phospholamban, 285
Pholine iodide. *See* Echothiophate

Phospholipase C (PLC), 421
Photic injury, 1393
Photoaffinity-labeling reagents, 223
Photoplethysmographic pulse wave, 716
Physical dependence, 1593
Physical hazards. See under Occupational health
Physician–hospital organizations, 52
Physician Quality Reporting System (PQRS), 33
Physiologic dead space, 373–374
    assessment of, 374
Physiologic shunt, 374–375
    assessment of, 375
    calculation of, 375–376
Physostigmine, 304f, 306, 354, 354t, 550
Pia mater, 918, 919f
PiCCO device, 721, 1641–1642
Pickwickian syndrome, 1281
Pierre-Robin syndrome, 7, 1220
Pilocarpine, 302f, 303
Pin indexing, 11
Pin Index Safety System (PISS), 657
Pink puffers, 1032
Pioglitazone (Actos), 1345
Pipecuronium, 16, 534t, 536, 1412
    dose ranges, effect of aging on, 903t
Piperidines, 512–513
Piriformis syndromes, management of, 1615–1616
Piroxicam, dosing guidelines, 1578t
Pi's Pillow, 779
Pitkin, G. P., 18
Pituitary gland, 1352–1354
    anatomy, 1352
    anterior pituitary, 1352–1353
    posterior pituitary, 1353–1354
Pituitary surgery, 1018
Placebo-induced analgesia, 508–509
Placenta accreta, 1160
Placenta, drug transfer through, 1147–1148
Placental ischemia, 1156, 1156f
Placenta previa, 1160
Plague, 1698
Plasma cholinesterase. See Pseudocholinesterase
Plasma derivatives, 429. See also Blood
Plasma-Lyte, for kidney transplantation, 1466
Plasma products, 433–434, 434t
Plasmin activator inhibitor-1 (PAI-1), 1308
Plasminogen, 423
Plasminogen activation inhibitor-1 (PAI-1), 153, 423, 424f, 1283
Plasmodium species, 437
Platelet-activating factor (PAF), 210
Platelet function tests (PFTs), 424
Platelets, 420, 433, 1526
    activation, 421–422
    dysfunction, causes of, 433t
    hereditary disorders of, 445
    pathways, 421f
    storage, 429
    transfusion, indications for, 433t
Pleural injury, 1505–1506
Pneumonia, 74
Pneumoperitoneum, 1262, 1263, 1264, 1265, 1288
    physiology of, 1422, 1422t
Poiseuille's law, 365
Polarographic oxygen analyzers, 708
Policy and procedure manual, 39
Polycythemia, 1106
Polymethylmethacrylate (PMMA), 1623–1624
Polymorphism, 144, 245
Polymorphonuclear leukocytes, 206
Polymyositis (PM), 639
Polyuria, 403, 1552
Pompe disease, 626
Pons, 335

Pontine centers, 368
PONV. See Postoperative nausea and vomiting (PONV)
Poppy (*Papaver somniferum*), 14
Population parameters, 166
Population pharmacokinetic modeling, 252
Population pharmacokinetic–pharmacodynamic (PKPD) model, 256–257
Population variance, 167
Porphyria cutanea tarda (PCT), 624, 624t
Porphyrias, 623–625
    acute, 623–624
    anesthesia, management of, 624–625
    drugs to precipitate, 625t
    types of, 624t
Portal hypertension, 1314
Portopulmonary hypertension (PPHTN), 1310–1311, 1468
Positive end-expiratory pressure (PEEP), 907, 1015, 1289, 1644
    to dependent lung, 1052, 1052f
Positive pressure ventilation (PPV), 1015, 1641, 1643
Postanesthesia care, standards for, 1538
Postanesthesia care units (PACUs), 36, 66
    admission to, 1540, 1541t
    altered mental status in
        delirium and cognitive decline, 1558
        emergence reactions, 1557–1558
    ASA standards of, 1539
    cardiovascular complications in, 1543–1544
    complications in, 1251–1254
        emergence agitation, 1253
        laryngospasm, 1253
        negative pressure pulmonary edema, 1253
        oxygen desaturation, 1253
        postoperative pain, 1254
        postoperative stridor, 1253
        vomiting, 1253–1254
    discharge criteria from, 1542–1543, 1543t
    hypercarbia in, 1544
    hyperthermia in, 1556
    hypothermia in, 1555–1556
    hypoventilation in, 1544
    levels of care, 1539
    metabolic complications in
        electrolyte disorders, 1553–1554
        glucose disorders and control, 1553
        postoperative acid–base abnormalities, 1552–1553
    muscle pain in, 1555
    nursing skills for, 1251
    pain management in, 1540–1542, 1542f
    persistent sedation/delayed emergence in, 1556–1557
    postoperative evaluation in, 1543
    postoperative nausea and vomiting in, 1558–1559
    postoperative pulmonary dysfunction in, 1544
        airway resistance, 1545–1546, 1545f
        alveolar PAO_2, inadequate, 1548, 1549f
        anemia, 1549
        carbon dioxide production, 1547
        deadspace, increase in, 1547
        distribution of ventilation, 1547–1548
        mixed venous Po_2, reduced, 1548–1549
        neuromuscular and skeletal problems, 1546–1547
        obstructive sleep apnea, 1549
        perfusion, distribution of, 1548
        perioperative aspiration, 1550–1551
        postoperative oxygenation, inadequate, 1547
        reduced compliance, 1546
        respiratory drive, inadequate, 1544–1545
        supplemental oxygen, 1550
        ventilation, inadequate, 1544

    postoperative renal complications in
        ability to void, 1551
        oliguria, 1551–1552
        polyuria, 1552
        renal tubular function, 1551
    safety in, 1540
    shivering in, 1555–1556
    transportation of children to, 1251–1252, 1252f
    traumatic complications in, 1554
        hearing impairment, 1554
        nerve injuries, 1555
        ocular injuries and visual changes, 1554
        oral, pharyngeal, and laryngeal injuries, 1554–1555
        soft tissue and joint injuries, 1555
    value and economics of, 1538–1539
Postanesthesia recovery, 1538
    cardiovascular complications in, 1543–1544
    levels of care, 1539
    postanesthesia care unit and, 1538–1539. See also Postanesthesia care units (PACUs)
    postoperative evaluation, 1543
    safety in, 1540
    standards for care, 1538
    triage, 1539–1540
Postanesthetic triage, 1539–1540
Postcataract ptosis, 1396
Postdischarge nausea and vomiting (PDNV), 858
Postdural puncture headaches (PDPHs), 923, 938–939, 1151, 1155
Posterior cerebral arteries (PCAs), 1005
Posterior communicating artery (PCOM), 1005
Posterior descending coronary artery (PDA), 280
Posterior ischemic optic neuropathy, postsurgical, 1395–1396
Posterior sensory root, 919
Posterior tibial nerve block, 996, 997f
Posterior urethral valves (PUVs), 1435
Postexposure prophylaxis (PEP), 78
Post-Exposure Prophylaxis Hotline (PEPline), 72
Postextubation stridor, 1253
Postherpetic neuralgia (PHN), 1616–1617
Postoperative blood salvage (POBS), 443–444
Postoperative cognitive dysfunction (POCD), 472, 620, 909–911
Postoperative nausea and vomiting (PONV), 13, 469, 522–523, 587–588
    in adults, 588t
    and laparoscopic surgery, 1273
    in PACU, 1558–1559
    treatment for, 16–17
Postoperative pulmonary complications (PPCs), 362, 381
Postoperative stridor, 1253
Postoperative vomiting (POV) management, 1243
    prophylaxis for, 1249
Postpartum hemorrhage, 1160, 1160t
Postrenal acute kidney injury, 1408–1409
Postresuscitation care, 1678–1681
Posttetanic count (PTC), 541f, 543t, 544
Posttransfusion purpura (PTP), 440–441
Postural hypotension, 823
Potassium
    hyperkalemia, 407–409
    hypokalemia, 405–407
    physiologic role, 404–405
    renal loss, causes of, 405t
Potassium channels, 226
Potassium iodide, 1701
Potassium titanyl phosphate (KTP) laser, 132
Potency, drug, 255
Potent agents, 461
Potent anesthetics, 461
Potentiation, 228, 228f

Power, 109, 110
Power failures, contingency plans, 128
PPD. See Purified protein derivative (PPD)
PPE. See Personal protective equipment (PPE)
P4P program. See Pay for performance
P pulmonale, 1031
PQRS. See Physician Quality Reporting System (PQRS)
Practice Advisories, 37
Practice guidelines, 37–38
Practice Guidelines for Obstetrical Anesthesia, 37
Practice Guidelines for Perioperative Blood Management, 430
Practice Guidelines for Sedation and Analgesia by Non-Anesthesiologists, 826
Practice management
  antitrust considerations, 49–50
  case discussions, 39–40
  cost issues, 38
  exclusive service contracts, 50–51
  malpractice insurance, 42–43
  meetings, 39–40
  policy and procedures, 39
  support staff, 40
Prader–Willi syndrome, 1237
Pralidoxime (2-PAM), 304
Pralidoxime chloride (2-PAM-CL), 1694
Pravaz, Charles Gabriel, 12
Prazosin, 314, 315, 343
Preanesthesia checkout (PAC) procedures
  background, 700
  general considerations, 700
  objectives, 700
  personnel performing, 700
  principles, 700–701
Precision factor, 172
Precision medicine, 142
Precision Medicine Initiative, 142
Predicted body weight (PBW), 1278
Preeclampsia, 1156–1159, 1306. See also Hypertensive disorders of pregnancy
Pre-exposure prophylaxis (PrEP), 80
Preferred provider organizations, 52
Pregabalin (Lyrica), 1580, 1599
  for chronic pain, 1622t
  dosage range, 1621t
  for fibromyalgia, 1616
  side effects, 1621
Preganglionic sympathetic fibers, 935
Preganglionic sympathetic neurons, 919
Pregestational diabetes, 1163
Pregnancy
  heart disease during, 1161–1163
    cardiomyopathy of pregnancy, 1162–1163
    congenital heart disease, 1161–1162
    coronary artery disease and myocardial infarction, 1163
    primary pulmonary hypertension, 1162
    sudden arrhythmic death syndrome, 1163
    valvular heart disease, 1162, 1162t
  hyperparathyroidism in, 1332–1333
  liver diseases, 1306–1307
  nonobstetric surgery in, 1172–1174
  obesity in, 1163–1164
  pheochromocytomas in, 1342
  physiologic changes of, 1145–1146, 1145t
    cardiovascular, 1145
    drug responses, 1146
    gastrointestinal, 1146
    hematologic, 1145
    metabolism, 1146
    respiratory, 1145–1146
  substance abuse in, 1165–1166
Preoperative assessments, 586–609
  antibiotic prophylaxis, 608–609
  changing concepts in, 586

clinical effects, 588t
healthy patient, approach to, 586–590, 587t
laboratory testing
  chest x-ray, 602
  coagulation, 601
  complete blood count, 601
  defining normal values, 600
  hemoglobin concentration, 601
  pregnancy testing, 601–602
  pulmonary function tests, 602
  risks and costs versus benefits, 600–602
medications/allergies, 588–589, 588t
pediatrics
  allergies, 1238
  anesthetic risks, consent/assent for, 1239
  anterior mediastinal mass, 1236–1237
  asthma, 1234–1235
  endocarditis prophylaxis, 1237, 1237t
  of ex-premature infants, 1235
  fasting guidelines, 1233–1234, 1233t
  gastric emptying times, 1233–1234
  laboratory testing, 1234
  malignant hyperthermia, 1235–1236
  medical, surgical, and family histories, 1238
  obesity, 1237–1238, 1238t
  obstructive sleep apnea, 1235
  physical examination, 1238–1239
  risk of regurgitation and aspiration, 1233–1234
  sickle cell disease, 1236
  upper respiratory tract infections, 1234, 1234t
PONV, 587–588, 588t
premedication, 605–608, 606t, 607f, 608t
preparation
  current medications/treatment of coexisting diseases, 602–603
  patient, 609
  smoking cessation, 602
psychological preparation, 605, 605t
pulmonary aspiration, prevention of, 603–605, 603t, 604t, 1740
response to previous anesthetics, 587–588
summary of, 602
surgical procedures, classification of, 587t
systemic disease, evaluation of
  arthritis, 600
  cardiovascular disease, 590–596, 591f, 591t, 593f, 594f, 595f
  endocrine disease, 598–600, 599t
  liver disease, 600
  pulmonary disease, 596–598, 596t
  renal disease, 600
systems approach for
  airway, 589, 589t
  cardiovascular system, 589–590
  endocrine system, 590
  neurologic system, 590
  pulmonary system, 589
Preoperative autologous blood donation (PAD), 441, 442
Preoperative Endoscopic Airway Evaluation (PEAE), 797
Preoperative physical examination, pediatric
  airway examination, 1238–1239
  cardiovascular examination, 1239
  respiratory examination, 1239
Preoperative pregnancy test, 1234
Preoperative preparation, pediatric
  anxiolysis, 1242–1243
    distraction techniques, 1242
  induction techniques
    inhalational, 1243–1244
    intramuscular, 1245
    intravenous, 1244–1245
    parental presence, 1242
    rectal, 1245

mask phobia, challenges with, 1244, 1244f
postoperative vomiting (POV) management, 1243
Preoperative pulmonary function testing, 378–379
Preoxygenation, 773
PrEP. See Pre-exposure prophylaxis (PrEP)
Prerenal azotemia, 1408
Pressure-controlled ventilation (PCV), 684, 1052, 1240, 1475
Pressure recording analytical method (PRAM), 724
Pressure-sensor shutoff valve, 660, 660f
Pressure support–assisted ventilation, 684
Pressure–volume diagram, 288, 288f, 289f
Presynaptic effects, 224–225
Preterm delivery, 1164–1165
Preterm labor, 1164–1165
Primary graft dysfunction (PGD), 1475–1476
Primary hemostasis, 420, 421f
  activation, 421–422
  adherence, 420–421
  antiplatelet medications, mechanisms of, 422
  disorders of, 444–446
  inhibition, 422
  laboratory evaluation of, 424–425
  stabilization, 422
Primary hyperalgesia, 1565
Primary pulmonary hypertension (PPH), 1162
Primary survey, of trauma patient, 1488
Prime, 1091
Primrose cuffed oropharyngeal tube, 769
Prion diseases, 80
Privacy officer, 54
Private practice, 45–46
  billing issues, 47–49
  as employee, 46–47
  with group, 45–46
  as hospital employee, 46–47
  independent, 45
  for management company, 47
  in office-based setting, 47
Probability, 170
Probability distribution, 166
Procaine (Novocaine), 13, 18, 19
Production pressure, 70
Professional liability
  anesthesia–related lawsuits, 104–105, 104f
  response to lawsuits, 105
  tort system
    breach of duty, 103
    causation, 103–104
    damages, 104
    duty, 103
    standard of care, 104
Prolactin, secretion, 1353
Promethazine (Phenergan), 17
Prone position
  complications of, 820–822
    abdominal compression, 821–822
    brachial plexus injuries, 821, 821f
    breast injuries, 821
    eyes and ears, 820–821
    neck problems, 821
    stoma and genitals, 822
  full prone, 819–820, 820f
Propensity score matching, 177–178
Prophylactic antiretroviral therapy, 80
Prophylaxis, for postoperative vomiting, 1249
Propofol, 13, 489, 489f, 490t, 725, 860, 1241, 1245, 1247–1248, 1557
  BET scheme for, 263t
  clinical uses, 491–492
  dose ranges, effect of aging on, 903t
  effect of obesity, 1285t, 1288
  formulations, 502

for monitored anesthetic care, 831–832, 832t
in neonates, 1186
pharmacodynamics, 490–491
pharmacokinetics, 489–490
pharmacokinetics of, 262
side effects, 492
in TBI, 1635-1636
Propofol infusion syndrome (PRIS), 487, 492, 1228, 1248
Proportional-integral-derivative (PID) controllers, 269
Propoxyphene, pharmacokinetics, 1573t
Propranolol, for ischemia, 1081
Proprioception, ventilation and, 368
Prospective (cohort) study, 167
Prostaglandin D_2, 210
Prostaglandin E, 1157
Prostaglandin E2, 348
Prostaglandins, 210, 1404
Prostatectomy, 1424
   intraoperative considerations, 1425
   laparoscopic and robotic, 1425–1427, 1426f
   neuraxial anesthesia for, 1425
   postoperative considerations, 1425
   preoperative considerations, 1424, 1424f
   radical, 1425
   simple, 1425
Protamine, 1104
Protected health information, 54
Protein C, 427
Protein C-ase, 423
Proteinuria, placental ischemia and, 1157
Proteome, 146
Proteomics, 146
Prothrombin complex concentrates (PCCs), 429, 453, 1527
Prothrombin time (PT), 425
Proton pump inhibitors (PPIs), 604
Protopathic pain, 1608
Proximal tubule diuretics, 1414
Proximate cause, tort and, 103
Prozac (fluoxetine), 359
Pseudoaddiction, 1598
Pseudocholinesterase, 531, 1229–1230
   variants, 1229t
Pseudococaine solutions, 1380
Pseudohyperkalemia, 408
Pseudotolerance, 324, 511
PSH. See Perioperative Surgical Home (PSH)
Psoas compartment block
   anatomy, 986–988
   landmarks for, 986f
   for perioperative acute pain, 1589, 1592
   ultrasound-guided, 987f
Ptosis, 1396
Pudendal nerve block, for labor and vaginal delivery, 1151
Pulmonary aging, 904–905, 905f
Pulmonary artery (PA), 37
Pulmonary artery catheters (PACs), 19, 707, 717–718, 720, 721, 1079, 1094–1095
   in cardiac output monitoring
      contraindications, 721
      indications, 720–721
      principles of operation, 720
      problems and limitations, 721
      use and interpretation, 720
      oximetric, 720–721
   thoracic surgery and, 1036–1037
Pulmonary aspiration, 801, 1740
Pulmonary capillary wedge pressure (PCWP), 718, 1037
Pulmonary contusion, 1506
Pulmonary disease, 596–598, 596t
   asthma, 597

obstructive sleep apnea, 597–598
tobacco use and, 597
Pulmonary dysfunction, postoperative, 1544
   airway resistance, 1545–1546, 1545f
   alveolar PAO_2, inadequate, 1548, 1549f
   anemia, 1549
   carbon dioxide production, 1547
   deadspace, increase in, 1547
   distribution of ventilation, 1547–1548
   mixed venous Po_2, reduced, 1548–1549
   neuromuscular and skeletal problems, 1546–1547
   obstructive sleep apnea, 1549
   perfusion, distribution of, 1548
   perioperative aspiration, 1550–1551
   postoperative oxygenation, inadequate, 1547
   reduced compliance, 1546
   respiratory drive, inadequate, 1544–1545
   supplemental oxygen, 1550
   ventilation, inadequate, 1544
Pulmonary embolism, after liver transplantation, 1470
Pulmonary function
   cigarette smoking, effects on, 380
   postoperative, 380–381
   practical application of, 378–379
   preoperative assessment, 378–379
   testing, 376–378, 379t, 602, 1466
      bronchodilator therapy and, 1032–1033
      preoperative, 1032
Pulmonary hypertension, 1162
Pulmonary rehabilitation, before thoracic surgery, 1035
Pulmonary vascular resistance (PVR), 478–479, 1308, 1708
Pulmonary vascular system, 364
Pulmonic valve, 279
Pulmotor, 8
Pulsatility index, 1011
Pulse contour analysis (PCA), 1641–1642
Pulsed-wave (PW) Doppler echocardiography, 743, 744f
Pulse oximeter, 1243
Pulse oximetry, 10–11. See also Anesthesia
   for arterial oxygenation monitoring
      contraindications, 710
      indications, 710
      principles of operation, 709, 709f
      problems and limitations, 710
      use and interpretation, 709
   fetal, 1168
   thoracic surgery and, 1037–1038
Pulse pressure variation (PPV), 1036
Pulse repetition frequency, 734
   in pulsed-wave Doppler, 743
   of sound pulses, 734
Pulsiocath thermistor-tipped catheter, 1516
Pumping effect, 671
Punitive damages, defined, 104
Purified protein derivative (PPD), 72
Purine antagonists, 1465
Purtscher retinopathy, 1394
Pyloric stenosis, 1213
   anesthetic management, 1213
   laparoscopic repair of, 1213f
Pyridostigmine, 304f, 551, 1694
Pyruvate kinase deficiency, 634

Q

QA. See Quality assurance (QA)
QCDR. See Qualified Clinical Data Registry (QCDR)
QMDA. See Quality Management and Departmental Administrative (QMDA)
Qualified Clinical Data Registry (QCDR), 32, 55

Quality assurance (QA), 35
   credentialing and, 33–35
   meetings, 39–40
Quality improvement
   in anesthesia, 100–101
   Joint Commission requirements for, 102
   outcome measurement, 101–102
Quality Management and Departmental Administrative (QMDA), 33
Quality of care, 101
Quarterly Anesthesia Supplement, 21
Quetelet's index, 1278
Quicktrach transtracheal catheter, 804
Quincke, Heinrich, 18
Quincke needle, 923f

R

Rabeprazole, 787
RAC. See Recovery Audit Contractor (RAC)
Radial artery catheter, thoracic surgery and, 1036
Radial nerve
   anatomy, 957–958
   blocks, 974–975, 974f
   compression, 814
Radiation disaster, 1699–1702
Radical nephrectomy, 1420
   with inferior vena cava tumor thrombus, 1420, 1421f
Radicular pain syndromes, 1611–1614, 1612f, 1613f
Radioallergoscrbent test (RAST), 215
Radiofrequency ablation, 887
Radio frequency identification (RFID), 727
Raman scattering devices, 710
Ramsay sedation scale, 1649
Random allocation
   concealment of, 169
   of treatment groups, 169
Randomized controlled trial (RCT), 168
Random sampling, 168
Ranitidine, 604
Rapacuronium, 16, 211
Rapid infuser systems, 1524
Rapid response teams, 55
Rapid sequence induction (RSI), 786, 787, 1241–1242, 1288
RASS. See Richmond Agitation Sedation Scale (RASS)
Rasvussin translaryngeal catheters, 803
Rate of restoration of flow velocity, 1011
Raventos, James, 12
Recombinant activated factor VIIs, 452
Recommended exposure limits, for waste anesthetic gases, 66
Record keeping, 99
Recovery Audit Contractor (RAC), 33
Recovery index of NMBAs, 530
Rectal induction of anesthesia, 1245
Rectus sheath block (RSB), 978, 983–984, 984f, 1595
Recurrent laryngeal nerve, 768, 796
Red blood cells (RBC), 430–433
   perioperative salvage, 443–444
   and platelet substitutes, 430
   preservation, 429
Redistribution, 460
Reductive reactions, 245
References
   dates/position only, 34
   telephone verification, 34
Reflection, of sound, 732
Refraction, of sound, 732
Refractory ascites, 1313
Refrigeration anesthesia, 2

Regional anesthesia, 17–19, 945. *See also* Peripheral nerve blocks (PNBs)
   complications from, 1597–1598, 1597t
   definition of, 17
   for hernia repair in neonate, 1213
   in infants and children, 1249–1250
   needles for, 950–951
   in neonates, 1198–1200, 1198t
   for orthopedic surgical procedures, 1441–1442
   for pain management, 1585–1597
      complications from, 1597–1598, 1597t
   for upper extremity surgery, 1446–1449, 1448t
Regular insulin sliding scale (RISS), 1351
Rehn, Ludwig, 19
Relative rate (RR), 83
Remifentanil, 14, 266, 512–513, 725, 855t, 1231–1232, 1248, 1288, 1412
   context-sensitive plasma half-time for, 264f
   dose ranges, effect of aging on, 903t
   for labor pain, 524
   for monitored anesthetic care, 834–835
   in neonates, 1187
   for pain relief, 516, 516f, 517f, 1575
   pharmacokinetics, 1573t
Remimazolam, 266, 501-502
   versus midazolam, 501f
Renal anatomy and physiology
   glomerular filtration, 1403–1404
   gross anatomy, 1401–1402, 1402f
   kidney, clinical assessment of, 1404–1406
   structure and function, correlation of, 1402–1403
   ultrastructure, 1401–1402, 1402f
Renal blood flow (RBF) autoregulation, 1403, 1403f
Renal disease, 600
Renal drug clearance, 246, 246t
Renal dysfunction, liver transplantation and, 1468
Renal failure
   anesthetic agents in, 1411
   in crush syndrome, 1529
   drug prescribing in, 1411
   factors contributing to chronic, 1410t
Renal function tests, 1404–1406
Renal transplantation
   intraoperative procedures, 1466–1467
      anesthesia, 1466
      glucose control, 1466–1467
      hemodynamic management, 1466
      incision, 1466
      renal blood flow, maintenance of, 1466
      transfusion, 1467
   pain management after, 1467
   pediatric, 1467
   preoperative considerations, 1465–1466, 1465t
      cardiovascular function, 1465–1466
      diabetic control, 1466
      hypercoagulable states, 1466
      kidney allocation, 1465, 1466
      preoperative dialysis, 1466
      pulmonary function tests, 1466
   surgical complications of, 1467
Renal vasodilator mechanisms, 1404
Rendell-Baker, Leslie, 11
Renin, 350
Renin–angiotensin–aldosterone system, 1404
Renin–angiotensin system (RAS) blockers, 1116
Repeated measurement experiments, 173
Reperfusion, 1013
Rescue breathing, 1665
Research design, 167–168, 167t
Residual volume, 376
Res ipsa loquitur, 104
Respirators, 366
Respiratory acidemia, 1552

Respiratory acidosis, 388, 388t, 1408
Respiratory airways, 363–364
Respiratory alkalemia, 1553
Respiratory alkalosis, 387, 1408
Respiratory centers, 367, 367f
Respiratory distress syndrome (RDS), 1202
   in neonates, 1202
Respiratory dysfunction, 1272
Respiratory formulas, 1709
Respiratory pattern, preoperative evaluation, 1031
Respiratory system
   function in anesthesia, 361–381
   pattern terminology, 367t
   subarachnoid and epidural anesthesia, 936
Respiratory viruses, 73–74
   avian influenza A, 74
   HRSV, 74
   influenza pandemics, 73–74
   influenza viruses, 73
Response variables, 166
Restrictive pulmonary disease, anesthesia and, 379
Resuscitation associated coagulopathy (RAC), 1499
Reticular activating system (RAS), 234
Reticular formation (RF), 234
Retina, 1374–1375
Retinal detachment surgery, 1390–1391
Retinal ischemia, postsurgical, 1394
Retinopathy of prematurity (ROP), 1202–1203
Retrograde autologous priming (RAP), 1092
Retrograde wire intubation (RWI), 802, 802t
Retrospective (case-control) study, 167–168
Reverse loading technique, 785
Revised Cardiac Risk Index (RCRI), 590, 591, 591t
Rheumatic disease, 1082
Rheumatoid arthritis (RA), 589, 636–638
   management of anesthesia, 637–638
   manifestations of, 637t
   MRI of cervical spine in, 638f
Richmond Agitation Sedation Scale (RASS), 726, 1649
Rifaximin, 1303
Right coronary artery (RCA), 280–281
Right heart pressures, monitoring of
   contraindications, 719, 719t
   indications, 718–719
   principles of operation, 717–718, 717f
   problems and limitations, 719–720
   use and interpretation, 718, 718f
Right ventricular outflow tract (RVOT), 720
Right ventricular stroke work index (RVSWI), 1708
Rigid bronchoscopes, 9
Riker sedation-agitation scale (SAS), 1649
Riluzole, 622
Risk corridors, 52
Risk management
   adverse event responses and, 99–100
   in anesthesia, 98
   case discussions, 39–40
   concept, 97–98
   "Do Not Resuscitate," 100
   informed consent and, 98–99
   Jehovah's Witnesses and, 100
   meetings, 39–40
   record keeping and, 99
Rituximab, 1464
Riva Rocci cuff, 10
Rivaroxaban, 427, 451
Robertshaw, Frank, 7
Robotic laparoscopic surgery, 1263–1264, 1264f, 1264t
Robust statistics, 174

Rocuronium, 16, 211, 534t, 536, 1230, 1413
   dose ranges, effect of aging on, 903t
   in neonates, 1188
Rofecoxib (Vioxx), 1579
Roller pumps, 1091
Ropivacaine, 14, 1190, 1250
   safety of, 14
Rosiglitazone (Avandia), 1345
Rostroventral medulla (RVM), 508, 1610
Rotameters, 9
Rotavirus, 74
ROTEM, 1519, 1520
Roux-en-Y gastric bypass (RYGB), 1279
Rovenstine, Emery A., 6, 19
Rowbotham, Stanley, 6, 769
RR. *See* Relative rate (RR)
Rubella, 75
Ruffini corpuscles, 1608t
RugLoop, 267
Rule of reason, Sherman Antitrust Act, 49–50
Ryanodex, 1235
Rynd, Francis, 12

S

Sacral hiatus, 916
Sacral plexus, 960–961, 960f–961f
   blockade, 1586t, 1590–1592, 1592f
Sacroiliac joint syndromes, 1614–1615, 1615f
Sacroiliac shear test, 1615
Sacrum, description, 916
Sadove, Max Samuel, 19
Safe harbor networks, 50
Safety/utility functions, respiratory depression, 520, 521f
SAH. *See* Subarachnoid hemorrhage (SAH)
Salt-wasting syndrome, 400
Sample test statistic, 170
Sampling, 168
Saphenous nerve, 961, 961f, 963
   block, 990–991, 991f, 998, 1590
Sarcolemma, 283
Sarcoplasmic reticulum (SR), 622
Sargeant, Percy, 20
SARS. *See* Severe acute respiratory syndrome (SARS)
SARS-associated coronavirus (SARS-CoV), 74
Saturated vapor pressure (SVP), 658, 668–669, 669f
Save Hearts in Arizona Registry and Education (SHARE) program, 1675
Sayres, Louis Albert, 14
Scanlon Early Neonatal Neurobehavioral Scale, 480
Scapular winging, 813–814, 814f
Scavenging equipment, 66
Scavenging systems, waste gas, 691–695
   components, 691–694, 692f
      gas-collecting assembly, 692
      gas-disposal assembly, 692f, 694
      gas-disposal assembly conduit, 692f, 694
      interfaces, 692–693, 693f
      positive- and negative-pressure relief, 693f, 694
      positive-pressure relief only, 693, 693f
      transfer means, 692
   hazards, 694–695
   low-flow, 695
Schaumann, O., 14
Scheduling, 57–60
   after–hours coverage, 61
   block scheduling, 58
   computerized scheduling, 59
   offsite procedures, 58–59
   open scheduling, 58
   preoperative clinic and, 59–60
   type of schedules, 58–59

Scherzer, Carl von, 13
Schleich, Carl Ludwig, 18
Schmidt, Erwin, 22
Schwann cells, 564, 565f
Sciatic nerve, 961
  blocks
    anterior, 995–996, 995f
    posterior, 991–995, 992f, 993f, 994f
  injury to, 824
Scientific Registry of Transplant Recipients, 459
Sclera, coat of eye, 1374
Scoliosis, 1444–1445
  surgery for, 1442–1443
Scopolamine, 2, 13, 20, 304–306, 305t, 355, 355f, 355t, 608
  and morphine, 20
  in obstetric anesthesia, 20
Secondary hemostasis, 422–423, 422f
  clotting factors, inhibition of, 423, 423f
  disorders of, 446–447
  laboratory evaluation of, 425
Secondary hyperalgesia, 1566
Secondary survey, of trauma patient, 1488–1489
Second gas effect, 465, 465f, 466f
Second messengers, 254
Sedasys, 502
SEDASYS (computer-assisted personalized sedation), 843
Sedation–agitation scale, 726
Sedation and analgesia, for critically ill patient, 1648–1650
  goals and assessment, 1648–1649
  neurocognitive complications, 1649–1650
  pharmacological management, 1649
Sedation, levels of, 1733-1734
Sedative/hypnotics, in neonates, 1186
Seifert, M. J., 22
Seldinger technique, 713–714
Selective digestive decontamination (SDD), 1651
Selective serotonin reuptake inhibitors (SSRI), 359
Self-inflating resuscitation bag (SIRB), 652, 652f, 1665
Self-tests, 655, 655f
Self-tolerance, 205
Sellick maneuver, 787
2015 Sendai Framework, 1688
Sensitive Oxygen Ratio Controller (S-ORC), 666–667, 666f
Sensory-evoked potentials (SEPs), 472
Sentinel events, 101
Sepsis, 1312
Septic shock, 1639–1640, 1640t
Sequential compression devices (SCDs), 1293
Serotonin, 348, 421
Serotonin syndrome, 260, 261t
Serratus plane block, 1593
Sertürner, Freidrich A. W., 14
Serum–ascites albumin gradient (SAAG), 1313
Service contract, exclusive, 50–51
Severe acute respiratory syndrome (SARS), 71, 74
Severinghaus, John, 10
Severino, 2
Sevoflurane, 12, 460, 468, 471–472, 481–482, 682, 1223, 1224, 1225, 1288
  airway reflex, 1225
  autoregulation, effect on, 1226
  carbon dioxide production, rate of, 1227
  on cardiac conduction system, 1225-1226
  changes in blood pressure, 1226
  degradation via Canrizzaro reaction, 1227
  electroencephalogram during, 1226
  versus halothane, 1226
  hepatic dysfunction, 1226-1227
  minimum alveolar concentration of, 1225
  myoclonic movement, 1226
  in neonates, 1189
  oxygen consumption, 1226
  QT interval, 1226
  respiratory rate, 1225
  seizures in hyperventilation, 1226
  speed of washout, 1224
  washin of, 1224
SGR. See Sustainable growth rate (SGR)
Shared decision–making, 99
Shattock, Samuel, 21
SHEA. See Society for Healthcare Epidemiology of America (SHEA)
Sheridan, David, 7
Sherman Antitrust Act, 49
Shikani Seeing Optical Stylet (SOS), 783, 783f
Shipway airway, 769
Shivering in PACU, 1555–1556
Shock
  absorber, 15
  cardiogenic, 1638, 1639
  causes, 1494–1495, 1496t
  distributive, 1638
  hemorrhagic, 1494–1495
    bleeding sources, control of, 1495
    hemoglobin measurement in, 1498
    hemostatic resuscitation protocols in, 1498, 1498t
    initial fluid resuscitation in, response to, 1496–1497, 1496t
    severity of, evaluation of, 1495
    trauma life support classification of, 1496t
    in trauma patient, 1495–1499, 1496t
    vicious cycle/lethal triad in, 1499, 1499f
  hypovolemic, 1638
  in ICU, 1638
  management of, 1494–1499
  monitoring and resuscitation in, 1640–1641
    dynamic respiratory indices, 1641
    echocardiography, 1641
    hemodynamic monitoring, 1641
    less-invasive cardiac output monitors, 1641–1642
    metabolic monitoring, 1642
  obstructive, 1638
  septic, 1639–1640, 1640t
  types of, 1638–1642
Shock index (SI), 1495
Shock wave lithotripsy (SWL), 1432–1433, 1433t
Short circuit, 111
Shoulder, surgery to, 1447
  anesthetic management, 1448
  approach, 1447–1448
  positioning, 1447–1448, 1447f
Shukys, Julius, 12
Shunt effect, 375
Sicard, Jean Athanase, 18
Sickle cell disease (SCD), 634–636, 1236
  anesthesia, management of, 635–636
  cellular and tissue injury in, 635t
  complications of, 635t
  hemoglobin concentrations, 1236
  perioperative preparation, 1236
  sickle trait, 1236
Silo Filler's Disease, 1696
Simpson, James Young, 4
Single-donor platelets, 428
Single-lung transplantation, 1474–1475
Single nucleotide polymorphisms (SNPs), 144, 144f
Single twitch (ST) stimulation, 539, 541–542, 541f, 543t
Sinusitis, in ICU, 1650
Sirolimus (Rapamycin), in immunosuppression, 1464
Sise, Lincoln, 18
Sister chromatid exchanges (SCE), 480
Skeletal muscle channelopathies, 615, 615t
  Andersen–Tawil syndrome, 616
  Guillain–Barré syndrome, 618–619
  hyperkalemic periodic paralysis, 615–616, 616t
  hypokalemic periodic paralysis, 616
  Lambert–Eaton syndrome, 618
  myasthenia gravis, 616–617, 617f, 617t
S–ketamine, 1223
Skin care, 187t
Skin disorders, 639
  epidermolysis bullosa, 639–641, 640f
  pemphigus, 641
Skin testing, 215
Skull base surgery, 1369–1370
Sleep
  apnea, 1358–1360
  deprivation, 70
  loss, 70
Sleep disordered breathing (SDB), 1358–1360
Slogoff, Stephen, 20
Smalhout, Bob, 11
Smallpox, 1696–1697
Smith, Robert, 10
Smoke plumes, viruses in, 81
Smoking, 602
  in pregnancy, 1165
Smooth muscle effects, 523. See also Opioids
Sniffing position, 5
Sniff Position Pillow, 779
Snorkel stent, 1136, 1136f
Snow, John, 5
Soak time, definition, 946
Society for Advancement of Geriatric Anesthesia, 897
Society for Healthcare Epidemiology of America (SHEA), 73
Society for Vascular Surgery Vascular Quality Initiative (SVS-VQI), 1115
Society of Cardiovascular Anesthesiologists, 431
Society of Critical Care Medicine (SCCM), 1633
Society of Thoracic Surgeons, 431
Society of Thoracic Surgeons National Database, 179
Soda lime, 681
Sodium
  hypernatremia, 403–404
  hyponatremia, 399–403
  physiologic role, 398–399, 398t
  tubular reabsorption of, 1403–1404
Sodium bicarbonate, 933
  during CPR, 1672
Sodium-glucose cotransporter 2 (SGLT2) inhibitors, 1345
Sodium nitroprusside (SNP), 324–325, 1639
  for myocardial ischemia, 1081
Sodium thiopental, 1245
Soft tissue injuries, 1555
Solubility, gas molecules, 462
Somatosensory-evoked potentials (SSEPs), 493, 935, 1009, 1010, 1010f, 1011, 1444
Somatotropic function, in critical illness, 1647
Soporifics, 2
Sound
  amplitude of wave, 732
  attenuation, 732–733
  intensity of, 732
  physics of, 732
  signal processing, 733
  transmission in tissues, 732–733
  velocity of, 732
  wave, 732, 732f
Special damage, defined, 104
Specific heat, definition of, 669

Spectral edge frequency (SEF), 725
Speers, Louise, 12
Spetzler–Martin Grading System, 1020t
Spherocytosis, 633–634
Spinal analgesia, for labor and vaginal delivery, 1151
Spinal anesthesia, 17, 914–942, 1198–1199. *See also specific anesthetic agents*
   anatomy, 915
      cerebrospinal fluid, 918
      epidural space, 916–917, 917f
      ligaments, 916, 916f
      meninges, 917–918, 917f, 918f, 919f
      spinal cord, 919, 920f
      spine, ultrasound of, 919, 920f, 921f
      vertebrae, 915–916, 916f
   approach, 923–924, 924f
   cardiovascular physiology, 935–936, 937f
   central nervous system physiology, 934–935
   for cesarean delivery, 1152
   combined, 928–929
   complications, 937–942
      backache, 937
      chemical injury, 942
      headache, 938–939
      hearing loss, 939
      high block/total subarachnoid spinal block, 939
      hypoperfusion, 941
      mass lesions, 940–941, 940f, 941f
      needle trauma, 939–940, 939f, 940f
      neurologic injury, 939–942, 940f, 941f
      spinal stenosis, 941–942
      systemic toxicity, 939
   continuous, 926–928
   contraindications, 915
   efficiency and, 930
   gastrointestinal system physiology, 936
   indications, 915
   needles, 923, 923f, 924f
   neuraxial anesthesia and outcome, 915
   patient preparation
      equipment, 922, 922t
      positioning, 922–923, 922f, 923f
      skin preparation, 923
   pharmacology
      adjuvants, 931
      local anesthetic dose, 930
      patient variables, 930
      spread and duration, 930, 930f, 931f, 931t
   respiratory system physiology, 936
   temperature homeostasis, 937
Spinal cord, 1006f
   anatomy, 919, 920f
   blood supply, 1006, 1007f
   injury, 1023–1024, 1444
      complications, 1024
      initial management, 1023–1024
      intraoperative management, 1024
   intraoperative monitoring of, 1444
   monitoring, 1444
   neurobiology of, 1609–1610
   neurophysiology, 1007–1008, 1008f
   stimulation, 1624, 1625f
   structures, functionality of, 107t
   tracts, 1006f
Spinal cord injured children without radiologic abnormalities (SCIWORA), 1491
Spinal cord injury
   anesthetic considerations in, 1504
   evaluation of, 1502–1503
   hemodynamic management of, 1504
   initial management in, 1503
      immobilization, 1503–1504
      intubation, 1503–1504
   respiratory complications in, 1504, 1504f

Spinal cord ischemia, 1131–1132
Spinal cord perfusion pressure (SCPP), 1008
Spinal nerves, 919
   anatomy, 955f, 956
   lamination, 1564f
   lumbar, 959–960
   origin of, 919
Spinal shock, 1503
Spinal stenosis, 941–942
Spinal trigeminal nucleus, neurobiology of, 1609–1610
Spine surgery
   blood conservation in, 1443
   complications of, 1445–1446
   injury, 1444
   muscular disorders, 1445
   positioning for, 1443, 1443f
   postoperative care, 1445
   preoperative evaluation for, 1442–1443
   scoliosis, 1444–1445
   spinal cord monitoring, 1444
   vertebral column disease, 1445
Spinohypothalamic connections, 1610
Spinothalamic tract (STT), 1610
Spinous process, 915–916
SpiraLith, 683
Spirometry, thoracic surgery and, 1032
Spiropulsator, 8
Split-lung function tests, 1033
Sprotte needle, 923f
Sputum culture, 1030
Stacking, 1287–1288
Staffing, in ICU, 1633–1634
Standard error of the mean, 172
Standard of care, 36–39
   defined, 36
   sources of information on, 36
Standard precautions, 71–72, 71t–72t
Standards for Basic Anesthetic Monitoring, 43, 1732-1740
Stanpump, 267
Staphylococcus, 437
Staphyloma, 1385
Starling law of capillary filtration, 395
Static genomics, 145, 146
Statins, 603
Statistical analysis
   Bayesian methods, 172
   hypothesis formulation, 169–170, 170t
   inferential statistics, 171
   logic of proof, 170
   P value, 171–172
   sample size calculations, 170
Statistical hypothesis, 169
Statistical resources, 181
Statistics, 165–166
Steady-state concentration, 262
Steinbüchel, Richard von, 20
Sternal thrusts, 1664
Steroids, 571, 571f
   before thoracic surgery, 1035
Stewart approach, to acid–base interpretation, 385
Stovaine, 18
Strabismus surgery, 1390t, 1391–1392
Strata, 168
Stray capacitance, 110–111
Stress, 81
Stress-induced analgesia, 508
Stress-induced hyperglycemia, 1348
Stressors, 85
Stress ulcer prophylaxis (SUP) strategies, 1654
Stridor, 1253, 1364–1365, 1364t
Stroke. *See also* Carotid endarterectomy (CEA)
   ischemic, 1120–1121, 1637–1638
Stroke index (SI), 1708

Stroke volume (SV), 723, 1708
Stroke volume variation (SVV), 723
Structure, in quality of care, 100
Student's t test, 172–173
Study designs
   blinding, 169
   control groups, 168–169
   elements of, 168
   experimental constraints, 168
   sampling methods, 168
   types of, 167–168
Study of the Effect of Nosocomial Infection Control (SENIC), 196
Stunning, 1079
Sturli, A., 21
Subarachnoid anesthesia, 914–942. *See also specific anesthetic agents*
   anatomy, 915
      cerebrospinal fluid, 918
      epidural space, 916–917, 917f
      ligaments, 916, 916f
      meninges, 917–918, 917f, 918f, 919f
      spinal cord, 919, 920f
      spine, ultrasound of, 919, 920f, 921f
      vertebrae, 915–916, 916f
   approach, 923–924, 924f
   combined, 928–929
   complications, 937–942
      backache, 937
      chemical injury, 942
      headache, 938–939
      hearing loss, 939
      high block/total subarachnoid spinal block, 939
      hypoperfusion, 941
      mass lesions, 940–941, 940f, 941f
      needle trauma, 939–940, 939f, 940f
      neurologic injury, 939–942, 940f, 941f
      spinal stenosis, 941–942
      systemic toxicity, 939
   continuous, 926–928
   contraindications, 915
   efficiency and, 930
   epidural anesthesia and, 919–920, 919f, 920f
   indications, 915
   needles, 923, 923f, 924f
   neuraxial anesthesia and outcome, 915
   patient preparation
      equipment, 922, 922t
      positioning, 922–923, 922f, 923f
      skin preparation, 923
   pharmacology
      adjuvants, 931
      local anesthetic dose, 930
      patient variables, 930
      spread and duration, 930, 930f, 931f, 931t
Subarachnoid hemorrhage (SAH), 1009, 1018, 1636–1637
Subarachnoid space, 917
Subcutaneous emphysema, 1270–1271
Subdural space, 917, 917f
Subsidies, by hospitals, 51
Substance abuse, 82–83
   in pregnancy, 1165–1166
Substantial factor test, 103
Succinylcholine (SCh), 16, 530–533, 1228–1230, 1243, 1245, 1288, 1378, 1412
   characteristics of, 530, 531f
   clinical uses, 533
   contraindications, 533
   dose of, 1229
   dose ranges, effect of aging on, 903t
   in neonates, 1187–1188
   neuromuscular effects, 530
   pharmacodynamic properties of, 531t
   pharmacokinetic properties of, 531t

pharmacology of, 530–531
side effects of, 531–533, 532f, 1229-1230
   anaphylaxis, 533
   fasciculations, 532
   hyperkalemia, 532
   intracranial pressure, 532
   intragastric pressure, 532
   intraocular pressure, 532
   malignant hyperthermia, 532
   masseter muscle spasm, 532–533
   myalgias, 532
Suckling, Charles, 12
Sudden arrhythmic death syndrome (SADS), 1163
Sufentanil, 14, 512, 855t, 931, 1243, 1245, 1574–1575, 1602
  context-sensitive plasma half-time for, 264f
  dose ranges, effect of aging on, 903t
  for pain relief, 516
  patient–controlled regimens, 1582t
  pharmacokinetics, 1573
Sugammadex, 258, 527, 536, 554, 1231, 1413
  calabadion, 557, 560
  clinical use, 555–556
  neuromuscular block, reversal of, 556, 560
  pharmacokinetics, 554
  pharmacology, 554, 555f
  re-establishment of block after reversal, 557, 560
  side effects and safety, 554–555
Suicide, 84–85
Sulfonylureas, 1345
Sulindac, dosing guidelines, 1578t
Summary statistics, 166
Superficial peroneal nerve, 963
Superficial trigeminal nerve blocks, 963–964, 964f
Superior hypogastric plexus block, 1619
Superior laryngeal nerve, 796
Superselective anesthesia functional examination (SAFE), 887
Superselective ophthalmic artery chemotherapy (SOAC), 1379
Supine hypotensive syndrome, 811
Supine position
  complications of, 813–816
    arm complications, 816, 816f
    axillary trauma from humeral head, 814
    backache and paraplegia, 816
    brachial plexus neuropathy, 813
    compartment syndrome, 816
    long thoracic nerve dysfunction, 813–814
    median nerve dysfunction, 814
    radial nerve compression, 814
    root injuries, 813
    sternal retraction, 813
    ulnar neuropathy, 814–816, 815f
  contoured, 811, 811f
  horizontal, 810f, 811
  lateral uterine/abdominal mass displacement, 811
  lithotomy, 811–813, 812f, 813f
    exaggerated, 812–813, 813f
    high, 812, 813f
    low, 812, 812f
    standard, 811–812, 812f
Supplemental oxygen, administration of, 838–839
Support staff, need for, 49
Suprachoroidal space, 1374
Supraclavicular blocks, 969–970, 969f
  contraindications, 1585t
  indications, 1586t
  ultrasound-guided, 1538f
Supraglottic airway (SGA), 769–770, 775–778, 1196, 1383. *See also* Laryngeal mask airway (LMA)

Air-Q, 777f, 778
and bronchospasm, 777
cardiopulmonary resuscitation and, 801
complications of, 777f
contraindications to, 777
in failed airway, 800–804
I-Gel, 777f, 778
intubating, 787–788
King Laryngeal Tube, 777–778, 777f
removal, 777
second-generation, 778, 778t
Supraglottitis, 1366
Supraorbital nerve, route of, 954
Suprascapular nerve, 819
Supraspinous ligament, 916
Sural nerve, 963
  block, 996–997
Surge capacity, 1691, 1692f
Surgical fluid requirements
  fluid losses, water and electrolyte composition of, 393
  perioperative fluid infusion rates on clinical outcomes, 393–395, 393f, 394f
Surgical home model, of care, 29f
Surgical safety checklist elements, 98, 98t
Surgical site infections (SSIs)
  antibiotic prophylaxis, 189–191, 189f
  definition of, 185t
  frequency of, 184f
Surgical stress response, 1354, 1566, 1568
Surviving Sepsis Campaign Guidelines, 1640t
Sustainable growth rate (SGR), 32
Swish and swallow (local anesthetic), 795
Sword, Brian, 9
Sympathomimetics
  ephedrine, 314
  phenylephrine, 314
  before thoracic surgery, 1035
Synaptic cleft, 528, 528f
Synaptic transmission, 224–225
Synchronized intermittent mandatory ventilation (S-IMV), 684
Syndrome of inappropriate antidiuretic hormone (SIADH), 400, 400t, 1018–1019, 1637
  criteria for diagnosis of, 401t
Syndrome X, 1283–1284
Synera, 1244
Systematic reviews, 178–179
Systemic hypothermia, 1092–1093
Systemic lupus erythematosus (SLE), 637t, 638
Systemic sclerosis (Scleroderma), 639
Systemic toxicity, 939
Systemic vascular resistance (SVR), 723, 1708
Systolic blood pressure (SBP), 1495
  normal, 1495
  in trauma patient, 1495, 1495f
Systolic function
  determinants of, 288–293, 289f
    afterload, 290–292, 291f
    heart rate, 289–290
    myocardial contractility, 292–293
    preload, 290
  evaluation of, 746–750
    left ventricular cavity, 749–750, 749f
    left ventricular walls, 747–749, 747f–748f, 749t
Systolic pressure variation (SPV), 1036
Systolic pulse variation, 723

T

Tabern, Donalee, 13
Tacrolimus, 1464
Tait, Dudley, 18
Tandem Heart, 1477
Tapentadol, 507, 1577

Target-controlled infusion (TCI), 266–268, 266f, 267f
Tarui disease, 629
Taveaux, R., 16
TB. *See* Tuberculosis (TB)
TBI. *See* Traumatic brain injury (TBI)
T cells
  helper, 205
  suppressor, 205
Teamwork, anesthesia professionals and, 56
Tec 6 for desflurane vaporizers, 673–676, 674f, 675t, 676f, 677f
  dial setting *versus* flow through restrictor R2, 675t
  fresh gas flow rate *versus* working pressure, 675t
  operating principles of, 674–675, 674f
  output, 675–676, 675t
  safety features, 676
  variable bypass vaporizers and, 673–674
TECOTA. *See* Temperature Compensated Trichloroethylene Air (TECOTA)
TEE. *See* Transesophageal echocardiography (TEE)
Temperature
  axillary, 1241
  core, 1240–1241
  modalities for maintaining warmth, 1241
  monitoring, 1240–1241
    during monitored anesthesia care, 840
  of operating room, 1241
  thermoregulatory homeostasis, for infants and children, 1241
Temperature Compensated Trichloroethylene Air (TECOTA), 10
Tenon capsule, 1387
Tension pneumothorax, 1494, 1505
Teratomas, 1237
Teriflunomide, 619
Terminal effector plexuses, 339
Terminal nerves
  of brachial plexus, 957, 958f
  of lumbar plexus, 961–962
Terrell, Ross, 12
Tertiary survey, of trauma patient, 1489
Testicular torsion, 1435–1436
Tetanic stimulation (TET), 541f, 543, 543t
Teter, Charles, 8
Tetracaine, 13, 18
  for awake intubation, 795
Thalamic reticular nuclei (TRN), 235
Thalamus, 235, 1004
Thalassemia, 636
Therapeutic index, 243
Therapeutic threshold, of drug, 257–258
Therapeutic window, 258
Thermal conductivity, 669
Thermal radiofrequency lesioning, 1614
Thermodilution Cardiac Output (TCO), 720–721
Thermogenesis, 1201–1202
Thermoreceptors, 1609
Thermoregulation aging, 905
Thermosensory fibers, afferent, 1608t
Thiamylal (Surital®), 13
Thiobarbiturates, 13
Thiopental (Pentothal®), 13, 242, 499–500, 500f, 1245
  clinical uses, 501
  dose ranges, effect of aging on, 903t
  pharmacodynamics, 500–501
  pharmacokinetics, 500
  side effects, 501
Thoracic airway injuries, 1493
Thoracic aortic aneurysms, 1127
Thoracic aortic injury, 1507–1509, 1508f, 1508t

Thoracic outlet obstruction, 821
Thoracic paravertebral block (TPB), 1592–1593
Thoracic pump mechanism, 1665–1666
Thoracic surgery
  anesthesia for, 1029–1072
    bronchoscopy, 1056–1058
    choice of, 1054
  cardiovascular system, evaluation of, 1031–1032
  complications
    atelectasis, 1070
    bleeding and respiratory, 1071
    cardiovascular, 1070–1071
    neurologic, 1071–1072
  history examination, 1031
  hypoxic pulmonary vasoconstriction, 1054–1056
  intraoperative monitoring, 1035–1040
  lung resectability, evaluation for, 1032–1034
  mediastinal mass, diagnostic procedures for, 1059–1061
  one-lung ventilation, 1040–1050
    management of, 1050–1954
  physical examination, 1030–1031
  postoperative pain management, 1068–1070
  preoperative evaluation, 1030–1034
  preoperative preparation, 1034–1035
  pulmonary function testing, 1032–1034
  pulmonary rehabilitation and, 1035
  risk with, 1030
Thoratec CentriMag, 1103
Thoratec Heartmate II, 1103
Thorax, anatomy, 362
Three-dimensional echocardiography, 741–742, 742f
Thrombin, 422
Thrombin-activated fibrinolysis inhibitor (TAFI), 423–424, 1308
Thromboelastography (TEG), 1308, 1470, 1519–1520, 1519f, 1520f
Thromboembolic disorders
  acquired risk factors for, 426–427
  congenital risk factors for, 426
  diagnosis of, 426–427
Thromboembolism, 1530–1531, 1531f
Thrombomodulin, 423
Thromboprophylaxis, 1454
Thromboxane A_2 (TxA$_2$), 283, 421
Thrust maneuver, 1663–1664
THRX-918661/AZD-3043, 502
Thymomas, 1237
Thymus-derived cells (T cells), 205
Thyroid diseases, 599, 599t, 1237
Thyroid function, in critical illness, 1647
Thyroid function tests, 1328–1329, 1329t
  for assessing thyroid hormone binding, 1328–1329
  radioactive iodine uptake, 1329
  serum thyroxine, 1328
  serum triiodothyronine, 1328
  thyroid-stimulating hormone, 1329
Thyroid-stimulating hormone (TSH), 1018
  function of, 1327–1328
  release of, 1327–1328
  tests for, 1328
Thyroid storm
  description of, 1330
  management of, 1330t
Thyrotoxicosis, management of, 1330
Thyrotropin. See Thyroid–stimulating hormone (TSH)
Thyrotropin-releasing hormone, 1327
Thyroxine (T4)
  secretion of, 1327–1328, 1328f
  serum level testing, 1328
Thyroxine-binding globulin (TBG), 1328

Tibial nerve, 961, 962–963
Ticagrelor, 449
Tidal volume, 376
Time gating, pulsed wave Doppler in, 743
Time to maximum effect compartment concentration, 268
Time Weighted Average (TWA), 66
Timolol, ophthalmic use, 1381
Tiotropium, 306, 306f
Tipping of vaporizer, 672–673
Tirofiban, 450
Tissue factor pathway inhibitor (TFPI), 423
Tissue hypoxia, clinical indications of, 432t
Tissue oxygenation, equations for, 432t
Tissue plasminogen activator (tPA), 423, 1308
Tissue solubility, 1224
Title VII of the Civil Rights Act, 84
Tobacco, 592, 597
  abuse, in pregnancy, 1165
Tolerance, definition, 1598
Tolvaptan, 402
Tonic blockade, 567
Tonicity, 395
Tonsillectomy, 6, 1358
  anesthetic management for, 1360–1361
  complications, 1361–1363, 1361f, 1362f
  recommendation of American Academy of Otolaryngology, 1363t
Tonsillotomy, 1360
Topiramate (Topamax), 1279
  dosage range, 1621t
  in migraine prophylaxis, 1279
  side effects, 1621
Total body sodium, 398
Total body surface area (TBSA), 1511–1512, 1513t
Total body water (TBW), 390, 1183, 1278
Total drug clearance, 249
Total hip arthroplasty (THA), 1449
Total intravenous anesthesia (TIVA), 515, 725, 868, 1011, 1247–1248
Total knee arthroplasty (TKA), 1449, 1451–1452
Total shoulder arthroplasty (TSA), 1447
Tourniquets, 1453
Tovell, Ralph, 11
Toxicants, 131
  operating room fires and, 131
  risks of, 131
Tracheal extubation, 788–791
  complications of, 789t
  deep, 789
  difficult, 790–791
  failure, 789
  patients at risk for complications after, 790, 790t
  postsurgical, 789t
Tracheal intubation, 5–7, 6f, 769, 772, 1665. See also Anesthesia
  blind, 788
  direct laryngoscope blades, 780–783
  direct laryngoscopy, 778–780
  fiberoptic-assisted, 7
  optical stylets, 783
Tracheal resection and reconstruction, 1064
Tracheal tubes, for infants and children, 1240
Tracheoesophageal fistula (TEF), 1208, 1208f
  anesthetic considerations, 1209
  clinical presentation, 1208–1209
  closure, 1209
  postoperative care, 1209
  repair, endoscopic methods for, 1209
Tracheostomy, fire safety, 133–134
Traffic patterns, operating room, 189
Train-of-four (TOF), 527, 533, 541f, 542, 543t, 544t, 551–553, 552f
Tramadol, 508, 855t, 1570, 1570f, 1577

for chronic pain, 1622t
  patient–controlled regimens, 1582t
  for perioperative pain in pediatric patients, 1602
  pharmacokinetics, 1573t
Tranexamic acid (TXA), 424, 1161, 1443, 1526
Transcranial Doppler ultrasonography (TCD), 1011
Transcription, 144–145
Transcriptome, 146
Transcutaneous electrical nerve stimulation (TENS), 1149
Transdermal scopolamine, 305
Transducers, 732
  sound production, 732, 732f
  ultrasound
    beam shape, 733
    resolution, 733
Transduction, pain processing, 1563
Transesophageal echocardiography (TEE), 290, 735, 1317, 1463, 1494
  CABG surgery and, 1079–1080
  contraindications, 735
  intraoperative, 1037
  orientation, 735–736, 736f
  probe insertion, 735
  probe manipulation, 735
  safety, 735
  thoracic surgery and, 1037
  three-dimensional, 741–742
  two-dimensional, 734–741
    descending aortic short- and long-axis views, 741, 741f
    goals of, 736–741
    midesophageal aortic valve short-axis view, 739, 739f
    midesophageal ascending aorta (AA) long-axis view, 737, 738f
    midesophageal ascending aorta short-axis view, 737, 738f, 739
    midesophageal bicaval view, 740, 740f
    midesophageal four-chamber view, 736, 737f
    midesophageal long-axis view, 737, 738f
    midesophageal right ventricular inflow–outflow view, 739–740, 739f
    midesophageal two-chamber view, 737, 737f
    transgastric midpapillary short-axis view, 740–741, 740f
Transforming growth factor β (TGF–β), 192
Transfusion-associated cardiovascular overload (TACO), 441
Transfusion-associated graft-versus-host disease (TA-GVHD), 440
Transfusion medicine, 21
Transfusion-related acute lung injury (TRALI), 429, 440, 1527
Transfusion-related immunomodulation (TRIM), 429, 439
Transfusion therapy, in critical illness, 1647–1648
Transfusion-transmitted infections, 436t
Transhepatic cholangiography (THC), 1301
Transient ischemic attack (TIA), 1121
Transient neurological symptoms (TNS), 579, 579t, 942, 1452
Transient receptor potential (TRP) channels, 1608
Transitional airways, 363
Transjugular intrahepatic portosystemic shunt (TIPS), 887, 1319–1320, 1319f
Transmission
  pain processing, 1563
  precautions, 71–72
Transnasal Humidified Rapid-Insufflation Ventilatory Exchange (THRIVE), 773

Transplantation, 1458–1459
  composite tissue, 1472–1473
  corneal, 1465
  heart, 1476–1480
  heart–lung, 1476
  immunosuppressive agents, 1463–1465
  liver, 1467–1471
  lung, 1473–1476
  management of patient for nontransplant surgery, 1480–1481
  organ donors, anesthetic management of, 1459–1463
  pancreas and islet, 1472
  renal, 1465–1467
  small bowel and multivisceral, 1472
Transplant recipients, and nontransplant surgery, 1480–1481
Transpulmonary pressure, 364, 372. *See also* Lung
Transthoracic echocardiography (TTE)
  hemodynamic monitoring, 1517–1518, 1517t, 1518f
  in ICU, 1641
Transthoracic impedance, 1673
Transurethral endoscopy, 1427–1430
Transurethral resection of bladder tumor (TURBT), 1422, 1427–1430
Transurethral resection of prostate (TURP), 1427, 1428
Transurethral resection (TUR) syndrome, 1428–1430, 1429t
  clinical manifestations of, 1430
  irrigating solutions for, 1429t
  treatment of, 1430t
Transurethral surveillance and resection procedures, 1427
  cystoscopy, 1428
  intraoperative considerations, 1428
  irrigating solutions for, 1428–1430, 1429t
  postoperative considerations, 1428
  preoperative considerations, 1427
  prostate resection, 1428
  transurethral bladder tumor resection, 1428
  transurethral resection syndrome, 1428–1430
  ureteroscopy, 1428
Transversalis fascial plane (TFP) block, 983, 1596
Transverse process, description, 915
Transversus abdominis plane (TAP), 1542
  block, 978, 982–983, 983f, 984f, 1200, 1200f, 1593, 1594f, 1595, 1595f
Trauma, 1487–1488
  anesthetic and adjunct drugs in, 1520–1523
    airway compromise and, 1520
    burns and, 1522–1523
    cardiac injury and, 1522
    head and open eye injuries and, 1522
    hypovolemia and, 1520–1522, 1521f
  initial evaluation and resuscitation, 1488–1489, 1488f
    airway evaluation and intervention, 1489–1493
    breathing abnormalities, management of, 1493–1494
    primary survey, 1488
    rapid overview, 1488
    secondary survey, 1488–1489
    shock, management of, 1494–1499
    tertiary survey, 1489
  intraoperative complications, management of
    coagulation abnormalities, 1524–1525
    electrolyte and acid–base disturbances, 1527
    hypothermia, 1524
    intraoperative death, 1527–1528, 1528t
    persistent hypotension, 1523–1524
  monitoring in
    coagulation, 1519–1520, 1519f
    hemodynamic, 1516–1518, 1517t, 1518f
    organ perfusion and oxygen utilization, 1519
    oxygenation, 1518–1519
    urine output, 1518
  morbidity and mortality rate, 1487–1488
  operative management, 1516-1528
    abdominal and pelvic injuries, 1509–1511
    anesthetic and adjunct drugs, 1520–1523
    burns, 1511–1516
    chest injury, 1505–1509
    extremity injuries, 1511
    head injury, 1499–1502
    intraoperative complications, 1523–1528
    monitoring , 1516–1520
    neck injury, 1504–1505
  spine and spinal cord injury, 1502–1504
  postoperative considerations, early, 1528
    abdominal compartment syndrome, 1529–1530, 1529f
    acute kidney injury, 1529, 1529t
    thromboembolism, 1530–1531, 1531f
    ventilatory support, 1529
Traumatic brain injury (TBI), 1634–1636
  and anesthesia, 1022–1023
  and colloids, 396
  ICU treatment of, 1635–1636, 1635t
  predictors of poor outcome from, 1634–1635
  radiological imaging in, 1635
  resuscitation in, 1635
Traveler's diarrhea, 74
Treacher Collins syndrome, 1220
TREK-1 channels, 227
Trendelenburg (head-up) position, 1265
Trepanation, 20
Treppe effect, 289, 323
Triage, 1692–1693
Triamcinolone, 855t
Triamcinolone acetonide, 1612, 1613f
Tricuspid regurgitation, 1286
Tricuspid valve, 279
Tricyclic antidepressants, 359
Trifluoroacetyl (TFA), 1306
Trifluoroethyl vinyl ether, 12
Trigeminal nerve
  anatomy, 954
  blocks, 954, 954f, 963–965
  branches of, 954f
Trigeminocardiac reflex (TCR), 1379
3,3′,5-triiodothyronine (T3), 1327–1328, 1328f
Trimethaphan, 352
tris-Hydroxymethyl aminomethane (THAM), 387
Trocars, 1262
Tropomyosin, 284, 284f
Troponin proteins, 284–285
Troponin T, 285
Troposmia, 1243
Trousseau, Emile, 769
Trousseau sign, 411, 1335, 1407
TRP vanilloid 1 (TRPV1), 1608
Trunk nerve blocks, 978–985
Trypanosoma cruzi (Chagas disease), 428
t test, 172–173
Tube exchangers, 1046–1147
Tuberculosis (TB), 80–81
Tuberomammillary nucleus (TMN), 234, 234f
D-Tubocurare (dTC), 351
Tubuloglomerular feedback, 1403
Tuffier, Theodor, 17, 18
Tularemia, 1698
Tumor necrosis factor, 206
Tumor necrosis factor alpha (TNF-α), 1611
Tuohy, Edward, 18
Tuohy needle, 923f
Turbulent flow, lung, 366
TWA. *See* Time Weighted Average (TWA)

Twilight Sleep, 20
Two-dimensional echocardiography, 734, 734f, 736–741, 737f–741f
Two-tail alternative hypothesis, 170
Type 1 diabetes, 1351
Type 2 diabetes, 1351
Type 0 GSD, 629
Type I error, 170
Type II error, 170
Tyrosine kinase protein A, 1608

U

Ulnar nerve
  anatomy, 959
  blocks, 976f, 977
  injury, 1597
Ulnar neuropathy, 814–816, 815f
Ultimum moriens, 369
Ultrafiltration, 1092
Ultrasound
  in abdominal trauma, 1510, 1510t
  for airway evaluation, 772–773
  in anterior sciatic nerve block, 995–996, 995f
  in axillary block, 972–973, 973f
  in deep peroneal nerve, 997–998, 997f
  in femoral nerve/fascia iliaca block, 988–989, 989f
  in iliohypogastric nerve block, 985, 985f
  in ilioinguinal nerve block, 985, 985f
  in infraclavicular block, 971–972, 971f
  in intercostal nerve block, 979–980, 979f
  in interscalene block, 968, 968f
  in lumbar plexus block, 987, 987f
  in median nerve block, 976, 976f
  in obturator nerve block, 989–990, 990f
  in paravertebral block, 981, 982f
  in peripheral nerve blocks, 948–950, 950f, 951t
  in posterior sciatic nerve block, 992, 992f, 993f, 994f
  in posterior tibial nerve, 996, 997f
  in radial nerve block, 974–975, 974f
  in rectus sheath block, 983–984, 984f
  in saphenous nerve block, 991, 991f
  in supraclavicular block, 969f, 970
  transducers
    beam shape, 733
    resolution, 733
  in transversus abdominis plane block, 982–983, 983f
  in ulnar nerve block, 976f, 977
Ultrasound-guided regional anesthesia (UGRA), 1585
Umbrella coverage, 42
Unconsciousness, anesthetic-induced, 234–235
Uncoupling, 471
Uniblocker, 1048f, 1049
Uniformed Services Employment and Reemployment Rights Act (USERRA), 1690
Unitary theory of anesthesia, 221
United Network of Organ Sharing (UNOS), 458
Univent tube, 1047–1048, 1047f
Upper airway infections, 1370
Upper extremities
  cutaneous innervation, 958f
  nerve blocks, 956–959
  orthopedic surgery to, 1446–1449
  terminal nerves, 958f
Upper Gastrointestinal Endoscopy, 889
Upper gastrointestinal tract obstruction, 1209–1210
Upper respiratory tract infections (URTIs), 851, 1234
  criteria to cancel anesthesia, 1234t
  perioperative respiratory complications, 1234

UR. *See* Utilization reviews (UR)
Uremic syndrome, 1410, 1410t, 1411t
  cardiovascular complications of, 1410
Ureteropelvic junction obstruction (UPJO), 1435
Ureteroscopy, 1428
  for removal of stones, 1433
Urethral catheters, 10
Urinalysis and urine characteristics, 1405–1406
Urinary tract infection (UTI), in ICU, 1653
Urine
  output monitoring, 1518
  renal function and, 1405–1406
  specific gravity, 1405–1406
Urogynecology, 1433–1434
  adrenalectomy for, 1435
  impotence surgery and medication, 1434, 1434f
  nephrectomy, 1435
  pediatric surgical urologic disorders, 1435
  reconstructive procedures, 1435
Urokinase, 423
Urolithiasis, therapies for, 1430, 1431f
  intraoperative considerations, 1432
  kidney stone types, 1431t
  laparoscopic pyelolithotomy/nephrectomy, 1433
  open pyelolithotomy/nephrectomy, 1433
  percutaneous nephrolithotomy, 1433
  postoperative considerations, 1432
  preoperative considerations, 1432
  shock wave lithotripsy, 1432–1433, 1433t
  ureteroscopy for removal of stones, 1433
Urologic emergencies, 1435
  Fournier gangrene, 1436
  nephrolithiasis, emergency treatment of, 1436
  testicular torsion, 1435–1436
Urologic surgery, 1401–1436
  anesthetic considerations for, 1417
US Agency for International Development (USAID), 1688
U.S. Bureau of Labor, 65
Use-dependent blockade, 567–568
U.S. Environmental Protection Agency, 67
U.S. National Library of Medicine (USNLM), 847
Uterotonic therapy, 1160, 1160t
UTI. *See* Urinary tract infection (UTI)
Utilization reviews (UR), 38
Uveal tract, coat of eye, 1374

V

Vacuum-supported retention devices, 817
Vagus nerve, 337
Valdecoxib (Bextra), 1579
Valine, 635
Valsalva maneuver, 349
Valvular heart disease, 1082–1089
  aortic insufficiency, 1085–1086
  aortic stenosis, 1082–1084
  hypertrophic cardiomyopathy, 1084–1085
  mitral regurgitation, 1087–1089
  mitral stenosis, 1086–1087
  in pregnancy, 1162
Vancomycin, 191
Vanilloid receptors, 1609
Vanillylmandelic acid, 342
  structure of, 1341f
VAP. *See* Ventilator-associated pneumonia (VAP)
Vaporizers, 9–10. *See also* Anesthesia
  anesthesia workstations, 668
    D-Vapor for desflurane, 673–676, 674f, 675t, 676f
    GE-Datex-Ohmeda Aladin Cassette, 676–678, 677f, 678f
    misfilling of, 672
    models and characteristics, 678t
  in MRI suite, 673
  overfilling of, 673
  physics of, 668–669, 669t
  Tec 6 for desflurane, 673–676, 674f, 675t, 676f, 677f
  tipping of, 672–673
  variable bypass, 669–673
  calibrated, 9
  leaks, 673
  Maquet FLOW-i electronic injector, 647f, 669t, 679
  models and characteristics, 678t
Vapor pressure, 668–669, 669f
Vaptans, 402
Variability, data, 167
Variable bypass vaporizers, 669–673
  hazards
    improper filling, 673
    leaks, 673
    misfilling, 672
    in MRI suite, 673
    simultaneous inhaled anesthetic administration, 673
    tipping, 672–673
  operating principles of, 670, 670f
  output, influencing factors, 671
    fresh gas composition, 672, 672f
    fresh gas flow rate, 671
    intermittent back pressure, 671
    temperature, 671, 671f
  safety features, 672
Variance, 167
Variant Creutzfeldt–Jakob disease (vCJD), 428, 437
Varicella-zoster immune globulin (VariZIG), 75
Varicella-zoster virus (VZV), 74
Varices, 1314
Variegate porphyria (VP), 623, 624t
VariZIG. *See* Varicella-zoster immune globulin (VariZIG)
Vascular surgery
  atherosclerotic disease and, 1113–1120
  endovascular procedures (*see* Endovascular surgery)
  open
    aortic reconstruction, 1127–1133
    cerebrovascular disease, 1120–1127
    peripheral artery disease, 1133–1134
Vasculogenesis, wound healing, 194
Vasoconstrictors, 931
  for ischemia, 1081
Vasogenic edema, brain, 1009
Vaso-occlusive crisis (VOC), 635
Vasopressin, 323–324, 391, 421, 1353
  anaphylactic reactions and, 213
  during CPR, 1671
Vasopressors, during CPR, 1670–1671
Vecuronium, 16, 534t, 536
  dose ranges, effect of aging on, 903t
  in neonates, 1188
Venlafaxine, 1621t
Venous admixture, 375
Venous air embolism (VAE), 823, 1015, 1445–1446
Venous baroreceptors, 349
Venous gas embolism, 1271–1272
Venous oximetry, 1642
Venous thromboembolism (VTE), 1273, 1307, 1454
  in critically ill patients, 1654–1655, 1654t
  in trauma patients, 1530–1531, 1530f
Venovenous bypass (VVB), 1469
Ventilation, 366
  apneustic, 367t
  during cardiopulmonary resuscitation, 1664–1665
  chemical control of, 368–371
  control of, 366–371, 367f
  distribution of, 372
  muscles of, 362
  perfusion relationships, 372–373, 373f
  reflex control of, 368
  thoracic surgery and, 1038
Ventilation–perfusion ratio (VQI), 376
Ventilator-associated event (VAE) surveillance program, 1651
Ventilator-associated lung injury (VALI), 1643
Ventilator-associated pneumonia (VAP), 1634, 1650–1652, 1652t
Ventilators, 8–9
  anesthesia workstations, 684–688
  strategies in neonates, 1197t
Ventilators, anesthesia workstations, 684–688
  bellows, 685–686, 685f
  classification, 684
    bellows, 684
    circuit designation, 684
    cycling mechanism, 684
    drive mechanism, 684
    power source, 684
  hazards, 686–687
  problems, 686
    bellows assembly, 687 circle system, 686–687, 686f
    control assembly, 687
    power supply, 687
Venting systems, 81
Ventrain, 803–804, 803f
Ventral respiratory group (VRG), 367
Ventral tegmental area (VTA), 235
Ventricular assist devices (VAD), 1102–1104
Ventricular fibrillation. *See also* Cardiopulmonary resuscitation (CPR)
  sudden cardiac arrest and, 1672
  time-sensitive model of, 1674–1675
Ventricular interdependence, 297
Ventrolateral posterior optic nucleus (VLPO), 234–235, 234f
Verapamil, 326t, 328
  for ischemia, 1081–1082
Verbal analog score (VAS), 1570
Veress needle, 1262
Vernitrol, 10
Vertebral body processes, 956
Vertebral canal, 915, 916
Vertebral column disease, 1445
Vertebral compression fractures (VCFs), 1623–1624
Vertebral notches, 916
Vertebroplasty, 1623–1624, 1623f
Vessel-rich group (VRG), 462–463
Veterans Affairs Cooperative Studies (VACS) Program, 1122
Vicarious liability, 33
Video-assisted thoracoscopic surgery (VATS), 1209, 1214, 1506
Videolaryngoscopy (VL), 767, 783–786
Vigilance, 69
Vigileo, 1642
Vinethene (divinyl ether), 11
Viral hepatitis, 75, 77t, 78–79
Viral infections, 71
Virtual Anesthesia Machine (VAM), 668, 668f
Viruses, in smoke plumes, 81
Viscoelastic testing, 426
Viscoelastic whole-blood clotting, 425, 426
Vision loss, 1446
  ischemic optic neuropathy and, 820
  prone position and, 820–821
Visual disturbances, after anesthesia, 1393
Visual evoked potentials (VEPs), 1009, 1011
Vital capacity, 370, 376–377

Vitamin D
  function of, 1333f
  hyperparathyroidism and, 1332–1333
Vitamin K, 1307
  deficiency, 447
Vitreoretinal surgery, 1387
Vitreous humor, 1374–1375
VivaSight-DL disposable DLT, 1042
Vocal cord dysfunction, 758
Vocal cord topicalization, 796
Vocal folds, 768
Volatile anesthetics, physiochemical properties of, 461t
Voltage-dependent calcium channels (VDCCs), 226, 227
Voltage-dependent ion channels, anesthetic effects on, 225–227
Voltage-gated sodium channels, 565–567, 566f, 567t
Voltage–sensitive cation channels, 1608
Volume of distribution at peak effect, 268
Volwiler, Ernest H., 13
Vomiting, 1253–1254
Von Gierke disease, 625–626
von Hippel–Lindau syndrome, 1340, 1418
von Willebrand disease (vWD), 425, 445
  classification of inherited, 445
  diagnosis of, 445
  treatment, 445-446
Vorapaxar, 450
VZV. See Varicella-zoster virus (VZV)

W

WAG. See Waste anesthetic gases (WAG)
Wakefulness, 234
Wake-up test, spinal cord, 1444
Warfarin, 450, 1300
  anticoagulation, 427
Washin
  curve for inhalational anesthetics, 1223–1224, 1223f
  of desflurane, 1224
  of halothane in children, 1223, 1223f
  of less soluble anesthetics, 1224
  order in anesthetics, 1223
  ratio, 1223
  of sevoflurane, 1224

Washout times, for inhalational anesthetics, 1235t
Waste anesthetic gases (WAG), 65, 66–67
Waste gas scavenging systems, 691–695
  components, 691–694, 692f
    gas-collecting assembly, 692
    gas-disposal assembly, 692f, 694
    gas-disposal assembly conduit, 692f, 694
    interfaces, 692–693, 693f
    positive- and negative-pressure relief, 693f, 694
    positive-pressure relief only, 693, 693f
    transfer means, 692
  hazards, 694–695
  low-flow, 695
Water
  body composition and, 900
  tubular reabsorption of, 1403–1404
Water–bubble flowmeters, 8
Waters, Ralph, 6, 9, 11, 22, 769
Wynands, J. Earl, 19
Weaning, from mechanical ventilation, 1644
Weapons of mass destruction (WMD), 1689
Wedged hepatic venous pressure (WHVP), 1314
Wellbutrin, 359
Wellness. See under Occupational health
West Haven criteria for semiquantitative grading of mental state, 1312t
West Nile virus (WNV), 437
Wet sounds (crackles), 1031
Wheezing, thoracic surgery and, 1035
Whitacre needle, 923f
White, Samuel S., 8
Whole-blood–derived platelets, 428
Whole-genome expression analysis, 146
Wiliams intubating oral airways, 800, 800f
Wilson frame, 820, 821
Wind-up, 1611
Winnie block, 19
Wiring
  modern style, 116f
  older style, 115f
  of sockets, 116f
Wolff–Parkinson–White syndrome, 282
Wood, Alexander, 12
Wood, Paul, 22
Woodworth phenomenon, 286
Work hours, 70–71
Workload, hand washing statistics and, 186

World Association for Disaster and Emergency Management (WADEM), 1687
World Federation of Neurological Surgeons Grading Scale, 1018, 1019t
World Health Organization, Surgery Safety Checklist, 57
Wound healing
  dysregulation of, 197
  granulation tissue in, 194
  initial responses, 192
  maturation phase, 194–195
  mechanisms of, 191–195
  patient management
    intraoperative, 197–199, 197t
    intravascular volume management, 197–199, 199t
    postoperative, 199–200, 199t
    preoperative preparation, 196–197
  processes of, 191f
  proliferation phase, 193–194
  remodeling phase, 194–195
  resistance to infection, 192–193
  stress and, 197
Wound perfusion, 195–196
Wren, Christopher, 12
Wrist, surgery to, 1448–1449
Wu-scope, 7
Wu, Tzu-Lang, 7

X

Xenon, 12, 468–469, 1221, 1222-1223
X-linked erythropoietic protoporphyria (XLP), 624, 624t

Y

Yeoman test, 1615
Yersinia pestis, 1698
Yttrium-aluminum-garnet (YAG) laser, 132, 1392

Z

Zero crossing frequency (ZXF), 725
Zika virus, 1699
ZMapp, 1699
Z score, 172
Zyban, 359